KEEP YOUR ENTIRE DRUG REFERENCE LIBRARY COMPLETELY UP-TO-DATE WITH THESE KEY VOLUMES

1997 PHYSICIANS' DESK REFERENCE®

Physicians have turned to PDR® for the latest word on prescription drugs for over 50 years! Today, PDR is still considered the standard prescription drug reference and can be found in virtually every physician's office, hospital, and pharmacy in the United States. In fact, nine out of ten doctors consider PDR their most important reference source. Now the 51st Edition will soon be available and your old edition will be obsolete.

You'll find the most complete data on over 4,000 drugs by product and generic name (both in the same convenient index), manufacturer, and category. PDR provides complete medical information, usage and warnings, and product overviews that summarize listings, plus more than 2,000 full-size, full-color photos cross-referenced to the drug. $71.95

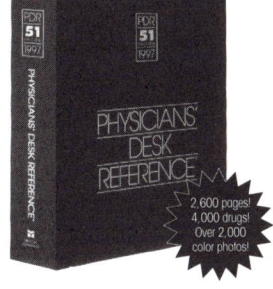

1997 PDR GUIDE TO DRUG INTERACTIONS, SIDE EFFECTS, INDICATIONS, CONTRAINDICATIONS™

The most up-to-date listings in four vital areas: **Interactions:** identify potential problems with drug combinations by brand and generic name. **Side Effects:** look up specific sign, symptom, or abnormality to see if any drugs the patient is taking might be the problem. **Indications:** a complete list of all drugs indicated—all cross-referenced to your 1997 PDR! The new *Contraindications Index* lists all drugs that must not be prescribed in the presence of a given medical condition. $49.95

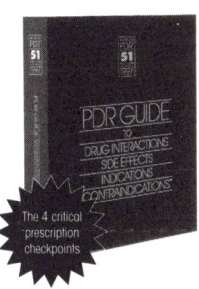

PDR® MEDICAL DICTIONARY

More than 100,000 entries! 1,900+ pages include a complete Medical Etymology section to help the reader understand medical/scientific word formation. Includes a comprehensive cross-reference table of generic and brand-name pharmaceuticals and manufacturers, plus a 31-page appendix containing useful charts on scales, temperatures, temperature equivalents, metric and SI units, weights and measures, laboratory and reference values, blood groups and much more. $44.95

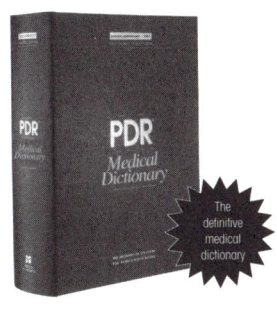

PDR® GENERICS™

Here is the most comprehensive reference of its kind, providing complete prescribing and pricing information on nearly 40,000 medications, both brand and generic.

Compiled, edited, and reviewed by a team of 400 pharmacists and physicians, it includes complete pricing data–including average package prices—the average unit cost of each dosage form and strength, each alternative's therapeutic equivalency, and identification of companies approved to manufacture the drug. $79.95

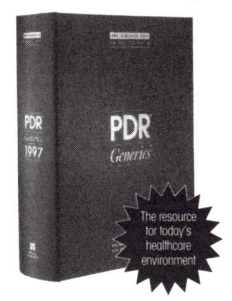

1997 PDR FOR NONPRESCRIPTION DRUGS®

The acknowledged authority offers full FDA-approved descriptions of the most commonly used OTC medicines, four separate indices and in-depth data on ingredients, indications, and drug interactions. Includes a valuable new *Companion Drug Index* that lists common diseases and frequently encountered side effects, along with the prescription drugs associated with them, plus OTC products recommended for symptomatic relief. $44.95

1997 PDR FOR OPHTHALMOLOGY®

The definitive reference filled with accurate, up-to-date information specifically for the eye-care professional. It provides detailed reference data on drugs and equipment used in the fields of ophthalmology and optometry. Its comprehensive coverage includes lens types and their uses… specialized instrumentation… color product photographs… a detailed encyclopedia of pharmaceuticals in ophthalmology… five full indices… an extensive bibliography… and much more. $46.95

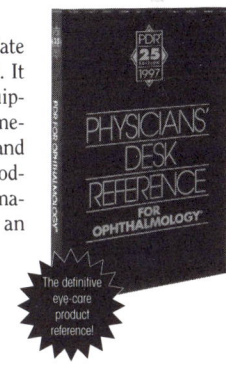

Complete your 1997 PDR® Library NOW! Enclose payment and save shipping costs.

(P7) _____ copies 1997 Physicians' Desk Reference $71.95 ea. ....$_____

(T7) _____ copies 1997 PDR Supplements A&B (payment must be enclosed) $21.95 set ....$_____

(N7) _____ copies 1997 PDR for Nonprescription Drugs $44.95 ea. ....$_____

(G7) _____ copies 1997 PDR Guide to Drug Interactions, Side Effects, Indications, Contraindications $49.95 ea. ....$_____

(O7) _____ copies 1997 PDR for Ophthalmology $46.95 ea. ....$_____

(J7) _____ copies PDR Medical Dictionary $44.95 ea. ....$_____

(X7) _____ copies 1997 PDR Generics $79.95 ea. ....$_____

Shipping & handling ....$_____

Sales Tax (FL, GA, IA, & NJ) ....$_____

TOTAL AMOUNT OF ORDER ....$_____

Prices slightly higher outside U.S. and all customs, duty and other taxes are the customer's responsibility. We cannot ship to P.O. box numbers.

PLEASE INDICATE METHOD OF PAYMENT:

☐ **PAYMENT ENCLOSED** (shipping & handling FREE)

☐ Check payable to PDR   ☐ VISA   ☐ MasterCard   ☐ Discover   ☐ American Express

Account No.   Exp. Date

Telephone No.   Signature

☐ **BILL ME LATER** (Add $6.25 per book for shipping and handling)

☐ **SAVE TIME AND MONEY EVERY YEAR AS A SUBSCRIBER.** Check here to enter a standing order for future editions of publications ordered. They will be shipped to you automatically, after advance notice, and you are guaranteed earliest delivery and free shipping and handling.

577858

Name

Address

City/State/Zip

Mail this order form to: Physicians' Desk Reference, P.O. Box 10689, Des Moines, IA 50336

ELECTRONIC PDR® ORDER FORM

Please send me the following:
___ 1997 POCKET PDR® unit with 1997 PDR® DataCard, which provides six essential topics on every Rx product in PDR. ....$199.95 each
___ 1997 POCKET PDR® DESKTOP SYSTEM with 1997 PDR® DataCard. ....$249.95 each

Please send me the following DataCards checked below.
- ☐ 1997 PDR (DataCard only)..$99.95 $_____
- ☐ The Merck Manual, 16th Edition ....$99.95 $_____
- ☐ The Medical Letter® Handbook of Adverse Drug Interactions ....$99.95 $_____
- ☐ Washington University Manual of Medical Therapeutics ....$69.95 $_____
- ☐ Harrison's Principles of Internal Medicine Companion Handbook, 13th Edition. ....$79.95 $_____
- ☐ Organiz-It (Personal Organizer) ....$69.95 $_____
- ☐ DSM-IV™: Diagnostic and Statistical Manual of Mental Disorders ....$79.95 $_____
- ☐ Principles of Surgery Companion Handbook, Sixth Edition ....$79.95 $_____

Please send me the 1997 PDR® Electronic library™ as indicated below. I understand each annual subscription includes 2 updates.
___ PDR® ELECTRONIC LIBRARY...................................$595.00 each $_____
Check diskette format for software: ☐ 5¼" ☐ 3½"
___ The Merck Manual..$99.95 each $_____
___ Stedman's Medical Dictionary..............................$79.95 each $_____
___ PDR Family Guides (Windows only) ....$29.95 each $_____
___ PDR Drug ID (Windows only) ....$39.95 each $_____
___ Stedman's PLUS Spell Checker 3.0 (Windows only) compatible with Word Perfect 5.1 and higher, Microsoft Word for Windows 2.0 ....$99.95 each $_____
___ Griffith's 5-Minute Clinical Consult (Windows only) ..$59.95 each $_____

Sales Tax (FL, GA, IA, NJ) $_____
Total Amount of Order $_____

PLEASE INDICATE METHOD OF PAYMENT
☐ Check payable to PDR.
☐ VISA ☐ MasterCard ☐ Discover ☐ Amex

ACCT. NO. _____

EXP. DATE _____ TELEPHONE _____

SIGNATURE _____

Prices slightly higher outside U.S. and all customs, duty and other taxes are the customer's responsibility.

For Faster Service: CALL TOLL-FREE 1-800-232-7379 or FAX to (201) 573-4956. Do not mail confirmation order in addition to this fax.

NAME _____

ADDRESS _____

CITY _____ STATE _____ ZIP _____

PDR electronic products are sold under annual license agreements.

3700EG

Detach along dotted line and mail in an envelope to: Physicians' Desk Reference®, Five Paragon Drive, Montvale, NJ 07645

Access the Latest Drug Data with Electronic Speed!

Put instant PDR power in the palm of your hand!
Portable...Practical...Powerful...Compact...Versatile...Economical!

1997 POCKET PDR®

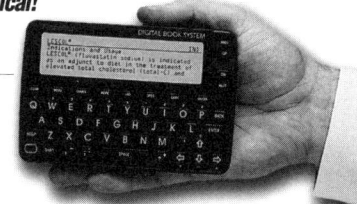

Here's the PDR you can use anywhere — on rounds and calls, at the office or clinic, at home. At the touch of a button, you can easily call up the full text of 6 key topics for every prescription drug fully described in PDR:
- ◆ Indications ◆ Adverse Reactions ◆ Warnings
- ◆ Contraindications ◆ How Supplied
- ◆ Dosage and Administration

This tiny electronic marvel gives you instant access to thousands of pages of data on more than 3,000 prescription drugs. Access the same FDA-approved information contained in the 1997 PDR and PDR for Ophthalmology, including coverage of the latest drugs.

Fast and convenient — Combining powerful search capabilities with key facts on every Rx drug in PDR and PDR for Ophthalmology®, POCKET PDR instantly delivers the essential guidance you need.

Simple and easy to use — Just key in the first few letters of a drug's brand or generic name, choose from the list of drugs that match, and you have the information you want. You can also access the information you need through a new comprehensive therapeutic class index.

Truly portable —The POCKET PDR measures just 5 1/4" x 3 1/4" x 1/2", weighs less than five ounces, and fits easily in any shirt or coat pocket. Just pull out your POCKET PDR, press a few buttons and get accurate drug data instantly.

State of the art — POCKET PDR uses the popular Franklin DBS-2 Digital Book System Unit with interchangeable 45 MB DataCards. No other hand-held electronic data storage and retrieval system can beat its performance.

In addition to the 1997 PDR DataCard, POCKET PDR can be used with the large number of available medical reference DataCards. Snap a second DataCard into your POCKET PDR, and instantly switch from PDR to another medical reference. $199.95

A 12-month limited warranty against manufacturing defects and 4 lithium batteries are included.

- ◆ **1997 PDR.** The same FDA-approved prescription drug data found in the 1997 PDR on indications, contraindications, warnings, adverse reactions, dosage and administration, and how supplied. Available 2/97. $129.95
- ◆ **The Merck Manual,** 16th edition (Merck Research Labs). Reference in seconds, the causes, symptoms, evaluation, and treatment of virtually every known disorder in medicine. $99.95
- ◆ **The Medical Letter® Handbook of Adverse Drug Interactions** (The Medical Letter®). Check adverse interactions for up to 20 drugs at a time. Search by brand or generic drug name. $99.95
- ◆ **The Washington University Manual of Medical Therapeutics,** 28th edition (Little, Brown & Co.). Reference therapeutic and diagnostic information in seconds for a broad spectrum of illnesses. 69.95
- ◆ **Harrison's Principles of Internal Medicine Companion Handbook,** 13th Edition (McGraw-Hill). Summarizes the diagnosis and treatment of all disorders commonly seen in clinical settings. $79.95
- ◆ **Organiz-It!** Personal organizer stores thousands of addresses, phone numbers, appointments and expense records. Contains calculator, world time clock and more. $69.95.
- ◆ **DSM-IV™: Diagnostic and Statistical manual of Mental Disorders** (American Psychiatric Press). The standard for information on psychiatric disorders. $79.95
- ◆ **Principles of Surgery, Companion Handbook,** Sixth Edition (McGraw-Hill). Summarizes the standard reference on surgery with instant search and retrieval capabilities, allowing storage of notes directly in the text. $79.95

Speed diagnosis and prescribing with fast, flexible access to all the medical references you need in one fully integrated system.

PDR® ELECTRONIC LIBRARY™

- ◆ **PDR ELECTRONIC LIBRARY**, now available on CD-ROM, is a single integrated system that instantly gives you all the information you need on the most current editions of:
  ◆ Physicians' Desk Reference® ◆ PDR® Supplements ◆ PDR for Ophthalmology® ◆ PDR for Nonprescription Drugs® ◆ PDR Guide to Drug Interactions, Side Effects, Indications, and Contraindications™ $595.00

Choose from the large and growing selection of optional modules for the PDR Electronic Library:

- ◆ **The Merck Manual** (available for DOS or Windows) $99.95
- ◆ **Stedman's Medical Dictionary** (DOS or Windows) $79.95
- ◆ **PDR® Family Guides Patient Leaflets** (Windows only) — Based on the official labeling in PDR, this easy-to-use electronic guide gives the authoritative, accurate facts patients need in plain, no-nonsense language. $29.95
- ◆ **PDR Drug ID** (Windows only)— A pharmaceutical imprint database that provides fast and accurate identification of virtually any prescription drug. $39.95
- ◆ **Stedman's PLUS Spell Checker 3.0** (Windows only)— 300,000+ medical and pharmaceutical terms add to the power of your word processor. Compatible with Wordperfect 5.1 and higher, Microsoft Word for Windows 2.0 and 6.0, Lotus AmiPro 3.0 and 3.1. $99.95
- ◆ **Griffith's 5-Minute Clinical Consult** (Windows only) — Provides clinical information for over 1,000 disorders including diagnosis, treatment, medication, follow-up. $59.95

Equipment required: IBM PC-compatible computer, DOS 3.1 or later, MS-DOS CD-ROM Extensions, 640K main memory, CD-ROM drive, 10 MB free on hard drive.

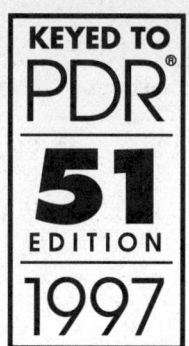

PDR GUIDE
TO
DRUG INTERACTIONS
SIDE EFFECTS
INDICATIONS
CONTRAINDICATIONS™

Interactions Index (White Pages)	1
Food Interactions Cross-Reference (Blue Pages)	1233
Side Effects Index (Pink Pages)	1241
Indications Index (Yellow Pages)	1493
Contraindications Index (Green Pages)	1589

Editor • Mukesh Mehta, RPh

Index Editors: Ann Ben Larbi; Thomas L. Fleming, RPh; Marion Gray, RPh; Lila A. Noueihed, RPh; Sarah G. Terzides

Physicians' Desk Reference Staff — *Medical Consultant:* Ronald Arky, MD, Charles S. Davidson Professor of Medicine and Master, Francis Weld Peabody Society, Harvard Medical School; *Executive Vice President, Directory Services:* Paul A. Konowitch; *Vice President of Product Management:* Stephen B. Greenberg; *Product Managers:* Cy S. Caine, Mark A. Friedman; *National Sales Manager:* Dikran N. Barsamian; *Senior Account Manager:* Anthony Sorce; *Account Managers:* Donald V. Bruccoleri, Lawrence C. Keary, Jeffrey M. Keller, Jeffrey F. Pfohl, P. Anthony Pinsonault; *Trade Sales Manager:* Robin B. Bartlett; *Trade Sales Account Executive:* Bill Gaffney; *Direct Marketing Manager:* Robert W. Chapman; *Marketing Communications Manager:* Maryann Malorgio; *Director, Professional Support Services:* Mukesh Mehta, RPh; *Senior Drug Information Specialist:* Thomas Fleming, RPh; *Drug Information Specialist:* Marion Gray, RPh; *Vice President of Production:* David A. Pitler; *Vice President, Contract Services/Fulfillment:* Steven R. Andreazza; *Contracts and Support Services Director:* Marjorie A. Duffy; *Fulfillment Manager:* Stephen Schweikhart; *Manager, Database Administration:* Lynne Handler; *Director of Production, Annuals:* Carrie Williams; *Manager of Production, Annuals:* Kimberly Hiller-Vivas; *Senior Production Coordinators:* Amy B. Brooks, Dawn B. McCall; *Production Coordinator:* Mary Ellen R. Breun; *Index/Format Manager:* Jeffrey D. Schaefer; *Senior Format Editor:* Gregory J. Westley; *Assistant Index Editor:* Eileen C. Idzik; *Art Associate:* Joan K. Akerlind; *Electronic Publishing Coordinator:* Joanne M. Pearson; *Senior Digital Imaging Coordinator:* Shawn W. Cahill; *Digital Imaging Coordinator:* Frank J. McElroy, III; *Editor, Special Projects:* David W. Sifton

Copyright © 1997 and published by Medical Economics Company, Inc. at Montvale, NJ 07645-1742. All rights reserved. None of the content of this publication may be reproduced, stored in a retrieval system, resold, redistributed, or transmitted in any form or by any means (electronic, mechanical, photocopying, recording, or otherwise) without the prior written permission of the publisher. PHYSICIANS' DESK REFERENCE®, PDR®, PDR For Nonprescription Drugs®, PDR For Ophthalmology®, Pocket PDR®, and The PDR® Family Guide to Prescription Drugs® are registered trademarks used herein under license. PDR Guide to Drug Interactions, Side Effects, Indications, Contraindications™, PDR® Generics™, PDR® Medical Dictionary™, PDR® Nurse's Handbook™, PDR® Nurse's Dictionary™, The PDR® Family Guide to Women's Health and Prescription Drugs™, The PDR® Family Guide to Nutrition and Health™, PDR® Electronic Library™, and PDR® Drug Interactions, Side Effects, Indications, Contraindications Diskettes™ are trademarks used herein under license.

Officers of Medical Economics: *President and Chief Executive Officer:* Curtis B. Allen; *Vice President, Human Resources:* Pamela M. Bilash; *Vice President, Finance, and Chief Financial Officer:* Thomas W. Ehardt; *Executive Vice President:* Richard F. Kiernan; *Executive Vice President, Directory Services:* Paul A. Konowitch; *Executive Vice President, Magazine Publishing:* Thomas F. Rice; *Senior Vice President, Operations:* John R. Ware; *Vice President, Information Services, and Chief Information Officer:* Edward J. Zecchini

ISBN: 1-56363-206-3

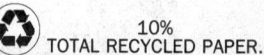

FOREWORD

For fully 10 years now, the *PDR Guide* has been providing clinicians with fast solutions to complex prescribing dilemmas. This year, we're pleased to add yet another important decision-making tool: *PDR's* new Contraindications Index. This convenient cross-reference permits you to instantly identify and eliminate from consideration all drugs that must NOT be used in the presence of a given medical condition.

The Contraindications Index joins the *PDR Guide's* three other indices to provide you with the nation's most exhaustive database of official prescribing information. Extracted from the FDA-approved labeling in *Physicians' Desk Reference®*, *PDR For Nonprescription Drugs®*, and *PDR For Ophthalmology®*, the entries in the *PDR Guide* cover more than 2,900 drug products. With every listing cross-referenced to the underlying text, the book presents you with a quick, reliable means for screening any patient regimen for potential conflicts and problems.

There are many ways to use the Guide:

- To check for potential interactions, turn to the white pages. In this section you'll find an entry for each product described in *PDR* and its companion volumes. Listed are compounds and dietary items that may interact with the product, as well as the specific brands containing each compound. A brief description of the interaction also appears. (Because product labeling varies in the scope of its interaction reporting, be sure to check the listing for each product in the patient's regimen.)

- If you suspect an interaction with a specific dietary item, turn to the blue pages. There you will find potential drug/food and drug/alcohol interactions cross-referenced alphabetically by the name or type of food. Each entry includes a list of implicated drugs and a brief description of each interaction.

- To single out the most likely source of a side effect, check the pink pages. They contain an alphabetical list of the more than 3,600 distinct reactions cited throughout *PDR* and its companion volumes. Each entry includes an alphabetical list of the brands that have been associated with the problem. To help target the most likely offenders, incidence data are included whenever found in the official labeling.

- If you need to locate an alternative to a problem medication—or simply want to review the full range of options for a particular diagnosis—turn to the yellow pages. Here each indication found in *PDR* and its companions is listed alphabetically, with a cross-reference to all brands approved for that purpose. For easy comparison, the listings include the generic name and manufacturer of each product. (Only FDA-approved indications are referenced.)

- When therapy is complicated by other medical conditions, turn to the green pages to quickly eliminate contraindicated drugs from consideration. Here each contraindication cited in *PDR* is listed alphabetically, together with the drugs to avoid in its presence.

Please note that all entries in the Guide are derived directly from the FDA-sanctioned prescribing information published by *PDR*. Therefore the only products listed are those described in *Physicians' Desk Reference* and its companion volumes; and the only facts presented are those that appear in these books.

Although all three *PDR* volumes have been carefully sifted for pertinent facts during compilation of the Guide, please remember that the publisher does not guarantee that the entries are totally accurate or complete. Also remember that important qualifications and extenuations of these facts may reside in the underlying text. Use this guide as a convenient cross-reference; but consult the *PDR* text, as well as the medical literature, when more detailed information is needed.

For your additional convenience, *PDR* now supplements the Guide and its other printed references with a variety of electronic prescribing aids:

- *Pocket PDR®* — A handheld personal electronic database of key sections from the prescription-drug listings in *PDR*.

- *PDR® Electronic Library™* — A Windows-compatible CD-ROM with a complete database of *PDR* prescribing information, electronically searchable for instant retrieval. A standard subscription includes *PDR's* sophisticated prescription-screening program and an exhaustive file of chemical structures, illus-

trations, and full-color product photographs. Optional enhancements include the complete contents of *The Merck Manual* and *Stedman's Medical Dictionary*, as well as a handy file of patient handouts drawn from *PDR's* consumer handbook, *The PDR® Family Guide to Prescription Drugs®*. The disc is available for use on individual PCs and PC networks.

- *PDR® Drug Interactions, Side Effects, Indications, Contraindications Diskettes™* — An electronic version of the *PDR Guide* capable of automatically screening a 20-drug regimen for conflicts, then proposing alternatives for any problematic medication.

- *PDR Database Services* — A preformatted text file suitable for integration in large mainframe-based information systems.

In the current cost-conscious healthcare environment, you should also be aware of the newest volume in the *PDR* family of references. Entitled *PDR® Generics™*, this exhaustive pharmaceutical reference includes generic monographs covering virtually all prescription drugs. For all therapeutically equivalent products, it provides brand/generic unit cost comparisons and average generic prices by package size. Also included are the average wholesale prices of all available supplies. Drugs in this volume are indexed by brand and generic name, therapeutic category, and indication. Off-label indications are included.

Also noteworthy are the *PDR® Nurse's Handbook™*, a specially designed drug reference with complete coverage of nursing implications, and the *PDR® Nurse's Dictionary™*, a pocket-sized guide to essential clinical terminology. For desk use, there's also the *PDR® Medical Dictionary*, an authoritative reference that combines a complete medical lexicon with *PDR's* unparalleled database of brand and generic drug names.

For more information on any of these important references, please call, toll-free, 1-800-232-7379 or fax 201-573-4956.

SECTION 1

INTERACTIONS INDEX

Cataloged in this section are all interactions found during a review of the labeling published in *PDR, PDR For Nonprescription Drugs,* and *PDR For Ophthalmology.* The list is arranged alphabetically by brand or, when applicable, generic name.

Whenever appropriate, each brand-name heading is followed by a summary of the major pharmaceutical categories with which the product is said to interact. Beneath this summary is an alphabetical list of the compounds in these categories, each followed by a brief notation regarding the results of concurrent administration with the brand in question. After each notation is an alphabetical list of the brands of the compound found in *PDR* and its companion volumes. Page numbers refer to the 1997 editions of *PDR* and *PDR*

For Ophthalmology and the 1996 edition of *PDR For Nonprescription Drugs,* which is published later each year. A key to the symbols denoting the companion volumes appears in the bottom margin of every other page.

Following the list of interactive drugs is a similar list of foods. Note that interactions with alcohol are listed here as well.

This index lists only interactions cited in official prescribing information as published by *PDR.* Because product labeling varies in the scope of its interaction reporting, the most prudent course is to check each product in the patient's regimen. Note also that cross-sensitivity reactions and effects on laboratory results are not included in the listings.

ACES ANTIOXIDANT SOFT GELS
(Beta Carotene, Vitamin C, Vitamin E, Selenium) 647
None cited in PDR database.

A AND D MEDICATED DIAPER RASH OINTMENT
(Petrolatum, White, Zinc Oxide) 757
None cited in PDR database.

A AND D OINTMENT
(Petrolatum, Lanolin) 757
None cited in PDR database.

AMO ENDOSOL (BALANCED SALT SOLUTION)
(Balanced Salt Solution) 229
None cited in PDR database.

AMO VITRAX VISCOELASTIC SOLUTION
(Sodium Hyaluronate) 229
None cited in PDR database.

AMVISC PLUS
(Sodium Hyaluronate) 327
None cited in PDR database.

A-200 LICE CONTROL SPRAY
(Permethrin) 672
None cited in PDR database.

A-200 LICE KILLING GEL
(Piperonyl Butoxide, Pyrethrum Extract) 672
None cited in PDR database.

A-200 LICE KILLING SHAMPOO
(Piperonyl Butoxide, Pyrethrum Extract) 672
None cited in PDR database.

AVC CREAM
(Sulfanilamide) 1245
None cited in PDR database.

AVC SUPPOSITORIES
(Sulfanilamide) 1245
None cited in PDR database.

ABBOKINASE
(Urokinase) 403
May interact with anticoagulants and certain other agents. Compounds in these categories include:

Aspirin (Altered platelet function; aspirin is not recommended for treatment of fever). Products include:
  Alka-Seltzer Cherry Effervescent Antacid and Pain Reliever 609
  Alka-Seltzer Extra Strength Effervescent Antacid and Pain Reliever 609
  Alka-Seltzer Lemon Lime Effervescent Antacid and Pain Reliever 609
  Alka-Seltzer Original Effervescent Antacid and Pain Reliever 609
  Alka-Seltzer Plus 611
  Alka-Seltzer Plus Sinus Medicine .. 611
  Ascriptin 650
  Arthritis Strength BC Powder 631
  BC Cold Powder Multi-Symptom Formula (Cold-Sinus-Allergy) 631
  BC Cold Powder Non-Drowsy Formula (Cold-Sinus) 631
  BC Powder 631
  Genuine Bayer Aspirin Tablets & Caplets 618
  Extra Strength Bayer Arthritis Pain Regimen Formula 615
  Extra Strength Bayer Aspirin Caplets & Tablets 617
  Extended-Release Bayer 8-Hour Aspirin 616
  Extra Strength Bayer Plus Aspirin Caplets 617
  Extra Strength Bayer PM Aspirin Plus Sleep Aid 617
  Aspirin Regimen Bayer 81 mg Tablets with Calcium 615
  Aspirin Regimen Bayer Adult Low Strength 81 mg Tablets 613
  Aspirin Regimen Bayer Children's Chewable Aspirin 616
  Aspirin Regimen Bayer Regular Strength 325 mg Caplets 613
  Bufferin Analgesic Tablets 636
  Arthritis Strength Bufferin Analgesic Caplets 637
  Extra Strength Bufferin Analgesic Tablets 637
  Cama Arthritis Pain Reliever 748
  Darvon Compound-65 Pulvules ... 1475
  Easprin 1971
  Ecotrin 2625
  Ecotrin Enteric Coated Aspirin Maximum Strength Tablets and Caplets 775
  Ecotrin Enteric Coated Aspirin Regular Strength Tablets 2625
  Empirin Aspirin Tablets 818
  Excedrin Extra-Strength Analgesic Tablets, Caplets, and Geltabs 734
  Fiorinal Capsules 2388
  Fiorinal with Codeine Capsules .. 2390
  Fiorinal Tablets 2388
  Goody's Extra Strength Headache Powders 632
  Goody's Extra Strength Pain Relief Tablets 632
  Halfprin Tablets 1413
  Norgesic 1554
  Percodan Tablets 955
  Percodan-Demi Tablets 956
  Robaxisal Tablets 2246
  Soma Compound w/Codeine Tablets 2784
  Soma Compound Tablets 2783
  St. Joseph Adult Chewable Aspirin (81 mg.) 768
  Talwin Compound 2466
  Vanquish Analgesic Caplets 627

Dalteparin Sodium (Increased risk of hemorrhage). Products include:
  Fragmin Injection 2088

Dicumarol (Increased risk of hemorrhage).
  No products indexed under this heading.

Enoxaparin (Increased risk of hemorrhage). Products include:
  Lovenox Injection 2187

Heparin Calcium (Increased risk of hemorrhage).
  No products indexed under this heading.

Heparin Sodium (Increased risk of hemorrhage). Products include:
  Heparin Lock Flush Solution 2831
  Heparin Sodium Injection 2832
  Heparin Sodium Vials 1486

Indomethacin (Altered platelet function). Products include:
  Indocin 1723

IMPORTANT NOTE: Always consult each drug listing in the patient's regimen for possible interactions.

Abbokinase | Interactions Index | 2

Indomethacin Sodium Trihydrate (Altered platelet function). Products include:
Indocin I.V. ... 1727
Phenylbutazone (Altered platelet function).
No products indexed under this heading.
Warfarin Sodium (Increased risk of hemorrhage). Products include:
Coumadin ... 941

ABBOKINASE OPEN-CATH
(Urokinase) ... 405
May interact with:

Aspirin (Concomitant use with aspirin for treatment of fever should be avoided). Products include:
Alka-Seltzer Cherry Effervescent Antacid and Pain Reliever ... ▣ 609
Alka-Seltzer Extra Strength Effervescent Antacid and Pain Reliever ... ▣ 609
Alka-Seltzer Lemon Lime Effervescent Antacid and Pain Reliever ... ▣ 609
Alka-Seltzer Original Effervescent Antacid and Pain Reliever ... ▣ 609
Alka-Seltzer Plus ... ▣ 611
Alka-Seltzer Plus Sinus Medicine ... ▣ 611
Ascriptin ... ▣ 650
Arthritis Strength BC Powder ... ▣ 631
BC Cold Powder Multi-Symptom Formula (Cold-Sinus-Allergy) ... ▣ 631
BC Cold Powder Non-Drowsy Formula (Cold-Sinus) ... ▣ 631
BC Powder ... ▣ 631
Genuine Bayer Aspirin Tablets & Caplets ... ▣ 618
Extra Strength Bayer Arthritis Pain Regimen Formula ... ▣ 615
Extra Strength Bayer Aspirin Caplets & Tablets ... ▣ 617
Extended-Release Bayer 8-Hour Aspirin ... ▣ 616
Extra Strength Bayer Plus Aspirin Caplets ... ▣ 617
Extra Strength Bayer PM Aspirin Plus Sleep Aid ... ▣ 617
Aspirin Regimen Bayer 81 mg Tablets with Calcium ... ▣ 615
Aspirin Regimen Bayer Adult Low Strength 81 mg Tablets ... ▣ 613
Aspirin Regimen Bayer Children's Chewable Aspirin ... ▣ 616
Aspirin Regimen Bayer Regular Strength 325 mg Caplets ... ▣ 613
Bufferin Analgesic Tablets ... ▣ 636
Arthritis Strength Bufferin Analgesic Caplets ... ▣ 637
Extra Strength Bufferin Analgesic Tablets ... ▣ 637
Cama Arthritis Pain Reliever ... ▣ 748
Darvon Compound-65 Pulvules ... 1475
Easprin ... 1971
Ecotrin ... 2625
Ecotrin Enteric Coated Aspirin Maximum Strength Tablets and Caplets ... ▣ 775
Ecotrin Enteric Coated Aspirin Regular Strength Tablets ... 2625
Empirin Aspirin Tablets ... ▣ 818
Excedrin Extra-Strength Analgesic Tablets, Caplets, and Geltabs ... 734
Fiorinal Capsules ... 2388
Fiorinal with Codeine Capsules ... 2390
Fiorinal Tablets ... 2388
Goody's Extra Strength Headache Powders ... ▣ 632
Goody's Extra Strength Pain Relief Tablets ... ▣ 632
Halfprin Tablets ... 1413
Norgesic ... 1554
Percodan Tablets ... 955
Percodan-Demi Tablets ... 956
Robaxisal Tablets ... 2246
Soma Compound w/Codeine Tablets ... 2784
Soma Compound Tablets ... 2783
St. Joseph Adult Chewable Aspirin (81 mg.) ... ▣ 768
Talwin Compound ... 2466
Vanquish Analgesic Caplets ... ▣ 627

ABELCET INJECTION
(Amphotericin B) ... 1540
May interact with antineoplastics, corticosteroids, cardiac glycosides, imidazoles, aminoglycosides, muscle relaxants, and certain other agents. Compounds in these categories include:

ACTH (Concurrent use may potentiate hypokalemia which could predispose the patient to cardiac dysfunction).
No products indexed under this heading.
Altretamine (Concurrent use may enhance the potential for renal toxicity, bronchospasm, and hypotension). Products include:
Hexalen Capsules ... 2760
Amikacin Sulfate (Concurrent use may enhance the potential for drug-induced renal toxicity). Products include:
Amikacin Sulfate Injection, USP ... 523
Amikacin Sulfate Injection, USP ... 981
Amikin Injectable ... 502
Anastrozole (Concurrent use may enhance the potential for renal toxicity, bronchospasm, and hypotension). Products include:
Arimidex Tablets ... 2932
Asparaginase (Concurrent use may enhance the potential for renal toxicity, bronchospasm, and hypotension). Products include:
Elspar ... 1700
Atracurium Besylate (Amphotericin B-induced hypokalemia may enhance the curariform effect of skeletal muscle relaxants). Products include:
Tracrium Injection ... 1155
Baclofen (Amphotericin B-induced hypokalemia may enhance the curariform effect of skeletal muscle relaxants). Products include:
Lioresal Intrathecal ... 1634
Lioresal Tablets ... 847
Betamethasone Acetate (Concurrent use may potentiate hypokalemia which could predispose the patient to cardiac dysfunction). Products include:
Celestone Soluspan Suspension ... 2484
Betamethasone Sodium Phosphate (Concurrent use may potentiate hypokalemia which could predispose the patient to cardiac dysfunction). Products include:
Celestone Soluspan Suspension ... 2484
Bicalutamide (Concurrent use may enhance the potential for renal toxicity, bronchospasm, and hypotension). Products include:
Casodex Tablets ... 2934
Bleomycin Sulfate (Concurrent use may enhance the potential for renal toxicity, bronchospasm, and hypotension). Products include:
Blenoxane ... 697
Busulfan (Concurrent use may enhance the potential for renal toxicity, bronchospasm, and hypotension). Products include:
Myleran Tablets ... 1209
Carboplatin (Concurrent use may enhance the potential for renal toxicity, bronchospasm, and hypotension). Products include:
Paraplatin for Injection ... 713
Carisoprodol (Amphotericin B-induced hypokalemia may enhance the curariform effect of skeletal muscle relaxants). Products include:
Soma Compound w/Codeine Tablets ... 2784
Soma Compound Tablets ... 2783
Soma Tablets ... 2782
Carmustine (BCNU) (Concurrent use may enhance the potential for renal toxicity, bronchospasm, and hypotension). Products include:
BiCNU ... 696
Chlorambucil (Concurrent use may enhance the potential for renal toxicity, bronchospasm, and hypotension). Products include:
Leukeran Tablets ... 1205
Chlorzoxazone (Amphotericin B-induced hypokalemia may enhance the curariform effect of skeletal muscle relaxants). Products include:
Parafon Forte DSC Caplets ... 1590
Cisatracurium Besylate (Amphotericin B-induced hypokalemia may enhance the curariform effect of skeletal muscle relaxants). Products include:
Nimbex Injection ... 1131
Cisplatin (Concurrent use may enhance the potential for renal toxicity, bronchospasm, and hypotension). Products include:
Platinol for Injection ... 717
Platinol-AQ Injection ... 719
Clotrimazole (Antagonism between amphotericin B and imidazole derivatives, which inhibit ergosterol synthesis, has been reported; clinical significance of this finding has not been determined). Products include:
Prescription Strength Desenex AF Cream ... ▣ 653
Lotrimin ... 2514
Lotrimin AF Antifungal Cream, Lotion and Solution ... ▣ 766
Lotrisone Cream ... 2515
Mycelex OTC Cream Antifungal ... ▣ 622
Mycelex Troches ... 601
Mycelex-7 Vaginal Cream Antifungal ... ▣ 622
Mycelex-7 Vaginal Antifungal Cream with 7 Disposable Applicators ... ▣ 623
Mycelex-7 Vaginal Inserts Antifungal ... ▣ 623
Mycelex-7 Combination-Pack Vaginal Inserts & External Vulvar Cream ... ▣ 623
Mycelex-G 500 mg Vaginal Tablets 602
Cortisone Acetate (Concurrent use may potentiate hypokalemia which could predispose the patient to cardiac dysfunction). Products include:
Cortone Acetate Sterile Suspension ... 1663
Cortone Acetate Tablets ... 1664
Cyclobenzaprine Hydrochloride (Amphotericin B-induced hypokalemia may enhance the curariform effect of skeletal muscle relaxants). Products include:
Flexeril Tablets ... 1701
Cyclophosphamide (Concurrent use may enhance the potential for renal toxicity, bronchospasm, and hypotension). Products include:
Cytoxan ... 700
Cyclosporine (Concurrent initiation of cyclosporine and Abelcet within several days of bone marrow ablation may be associated with increased nephrotoxicity). Products include:
Neoral ... 2405
Sandimmune ... 2416
Dacarbazine (Concurrent use may enhance the potential for renal toxicity, bronchospasm, and hypotension). Products include:
DTIC-Dome ... 593
Dantrolene Sodium (Amphotericin B-induced hypokalemia may enhance the curariform effect of skeletal muscle relaxants). Products include:
Dantrium Capsules ... 2131
Dantrium Intravenous ... 2132
Daunorubicin Citrate (Concurrent use may enhance the potential for renal toxicity, bronchospasm, and hypotension). Products include:
DaunoXome ... 1842
Daunorubicin Hydrochloride (Concurrent use may enhance the potential for renal toxicity, bronchospasm, and hypotension). Products include:
Cerubidine for Injection ... 634
Deslanoside (Concurrent use may induce hypokalemia and may potentiate digitalis toxicity).
No products indexed under this heading.
Dexamethasone (Concurrent use may potentiate hypokalemia which could predispose the patient to cardiac dysfunction). Products include:
AK-Trol Ointment & Suspension ... ◉ 205
Decadron Elixir ... 1676
Decadron Tablets ... 1678
Decaspray Topical Aerosol ... 1689
Maxitrol Ophthalmic Ointment and Suspension ... ◉ 222
TobraDex Ophthalmic Suspension and Ointment ... 469
Dexamethasone Acetate (Concurrent use may potentiate hypokalemia which could predispose the patient to cardiac dysfunction). Products include:
Dalalone D.P. Injectable ... 1009
Decadron-LA Sterile Suspension ... 1687
Dexamethasone Sodium Phosphate (Concurrent use may potentiate hypokalemia which could predispose the patient to cardiac dysfunction). Products include:
Decadron Phosphate Injection ... 1680
Decadron Phosphate Sterile Ophthalmic Ointment ... 1684
Decadron Phosphate Sterile Ophthalmic Solution ... 1685
Decadron Phosphate Topical Cream ... 1686
Decadron Phosphate with Xylocaine Injection, Sterile ... 1683
Dexacort Phosphate in Respihaler .. 1606
Dexacort Phosphate in Turbinaire .. 1607
NeoDecadron Sterile Ophthalmic Ointment ... 1755
NeoDecadron Sterile Ophthalmic Solution ... 1756
NeoDecadron Topical Cream ... 1757
Digitoxin (Concurrent use may induce hypokalemia and may potentiate digitalis toxicity). Products include:
Crystodigin Tablets ... 1472
Digoxin (Concurrent use may induce hypokalemia and may potentiate digitalis toxicity). Products include:
Lanoxicaps ... 1110
Lanoxin Elixir Pediatric ... 1113
Lanoxin Injection ... 1116
Lanoxin Injection Pediatric ... 1119
Lanoxin Tablets ... 1121
Docetaxel (Concurrent use may enhance the potential for renal toxicity, bronchospasm, and hypotension). Products include:
Taxotere for Injection Concentrate 2204
Doxacurium Chloride (Amphotericin B-induced hypokalemia may enhance the curariform effect of skeletal muscle relaxants). Products include:
Nuromax Injection ... 1136
Doxorubicin Hydrochloride (Concurrent use may enhance the potential for renal toxicity, bronchospasm, and hypotension). Products include:
Adriamycin PFS ... 2056
Adriamycin RDF ... 2056
Doxil ... 2613
Doxorubicin Astra ... 531
Rubex for Injection ... 721

(▣ Described in PDR For Nonprescription Drugs) (◉ Described in PDR For Ophthalmology)

3 **Interactions Index** **Abelcet**

Estramustine Phosphate Sodium (Concurrent use may enhance the potential for renal toxicity, bronchospasm, and hypotension). Products include:
- Emcyt Capsules ... 2085

Etoposide (Concurrent use may enhance the potential for renal toxicity, bronchospasm, and hypotension). Products include:
- Etoposide Injection ... 539
- VePesid Capsules and Injection ... 727

Floxuridine (Concurrent use may enhance the potential for renal toxicity, bronchospasm, and hypotension). Products include:
- Sterile FUDR ... 2284

Fluconazole (Antagonism between amphotericin B and imidazole derivatives, which inhibit ergosterol synthesis, has been reported; clinical significance of this finding has not been determined). Products include:
- Diflucan Tablets, Injection, and Oral Suspension ... 2003

Flucytosine (Concurrent use may increase the toxicity of flucytosine by possibly increasing its cellular uptake and/or impairing its renal excretion). Products include:
- Ancobon Capsules ... 2254

Fludrocortisone Acetate (Concurrent use may potentiate hypokalemia which could predispose the patient to cardiac dysfunction). Products include:
- Florinef Acetate Tablets ... 506

Fluorouracil (Concurrent use may enhance the potential for renal toxicity, bronchospasm, and hypotension). Products include:
- Efudex ... 2280
- Fluoroplex Topical Solution & Cream 1% ... 475
- Fluorouracil Injection ... 2282

Flutamide (Concurrent use may enhance the potential for renal toxicity, bronchospasm, and hypotension). Products include:
- Eulexin Capsules ... 2498

Gemcitabine Hydrochloride (Concurrent use may enhance the potential for renal toxicity, bronchospasm, and hypotension). Products include:
- Gemzar for Injection ... 1482

Gentamicin Sulfate (Concurrent use may enhance the potential for drug-induced renal toxicity). Products include:
- Garamycin Cream 0.1% ... 2501
- Garamycin Injectable ... 2502
- Garamycin Ointment 0.1% ... 2501
- Garamycin Ophthalmic ... 2501
- Genoptic Sterile Ophthalmic Solution ... ⊙ 241
- Genoptic Sterile Ophthalmic Ointment ... ⊙ 241
- Gentak ... ⊙ 209
- Pred-G Liquifilm Sterile Ophthalmic Suspension ... ⊙ 248
- Pred-G S.O.P. Sterile Ophthalmic Ointment ... ⊙ 249

Hydrocortisone (Concurrent use may potentiate hypokalemia which could predispose the patient to cardiac dysfunction). Products include:
- Anusol-HC Cream 2.5% ... 1953
- Aquanil HC Lotion ... 1989
- Maximum Strength Cortaid Spray ▣ 800
- CORTENEMA ... 2713
- Cortisporin Ointment ... 1074
- Cortisporin Ophthalmic Ointment Sterile ... 1074
- Cortisporin Ophthalmic Suspension Sterile ... 1075
- Cortisporin Otic Solution Sterile ... 1076
- Cortisporin Otic Suspension Sterile 1077
- Cortizone-5 ... ▣ 795
- Cortizone-10 ... ▣ 795
- Hydrocortone Tablets ... 1715
- Hytone ... 922
- Hytone Ointment 2 ½% ... 923
- Massengill Medicated Soft Cloth Towelettes ... 2628
- Pediotic Suspension Sterile ... 1140
- Preparation H Hydrocortisone 1% Cream ... ▣ 843
- ProctoCream-HC 2.5% ... 2552
- VōSoL HC Otic Solution ... 2786

Hydrocortisone Acetate (Concurrent use may potentiate hypokalemia which could predispose the patient to cardiac dysfunction). Products include:
- Analpram-HC Rectal Cream 1% and 2.5% ... 993
- Anusol HC-1 Hydrocortisone Anti-Itch Ointment ... ▣ 810
- Anusol-HC Suppositories ... 1954
- Caldecort Anti-Itch Hydrocortisone Cream ... ▣ 651
- Coly-Mycin S Otic w/Neomycin & Hydrocortisone ... 1965
- Cortaid ... ▣ 800
- Cortifoam ... 2540
- Cortisporin Cream ... 1073
- Epifoam ... 2543
- Hydrocortone Acetate Sterile Suspension ... 1712
- Mantadil Cream ... 1124
- Nupercainal Hydrocortisone 1% Cream ... ▣ 661
- Pramosone Cream, Lotion & Ointment ... 995
- ProctoFoam-HC ... 2552
- Terra-Cortril Ophthalmic Suspension ... 2033

Hydrocortisone Sodium Phosphate (Concurrent use may potentiate hypokalemia which could predispose the patient to cardiac dysfunction). Products include:
- Hydrocortone Phosphate Injection, Sterile ... 1713

Hydrocortisone Sodium Succinate (Concurrent use may potentiate hypokalemia which could predispose the patient to cardiac dysfunction).
- No products indexed under this heading.

Hydroxyurea (Concurrent use may enhance the potential for renal toxicity, bronchospasm, and hypotension). Products include:
- Hydrea Capsules ... 705

Idarubicin Hydrochloride (Concurrent use may enhance the potential for renal toxicity, bronchospasm, and hypotension). Products include:
- Idamycin Injection ... 2096

Ifosfamide (Concurrent use may enhance the potential for renal toxicity, bronchospasm, and hypotension). Products include:
- IFEX ... 706

Interferon alfa-2A, Recombinant (Concurrent use may enhance the potential for renal toxicity, bronchospasm, and hypotension). Products include:
- Roferon-A Injection ... 2308

Interferon alfa-2B, Recombinant (Concurrent use may enhance the potential for renal toxicity, bronchospasm, and hypotension). Products include:
- Intron A for Injection ... 2506

Irinotecan Hydrochloride (Concurrent use may enhance the potential for renal toxicity, bronchospasm, and hypotension).
- No products indexed under this heading.

Kanamycin Sulfate (Concurrent use may enhance the potential for drug-induced renal toxicity).
- No products indexed under this heading.

Ketoconazole (Antagonism between amphotericin B and imidazole derivatives, which inhibit ergosterol synthesis, has been reported; clinical significance of this finding has not been determined). Products include:
- Nizoral 2% Cream ... 1344
- Nizoral 2% Shampoo ... 1344
- Nizoral Tablets ... 1345

Leukocyte transfusions (Acute pulmonary toxicity has been reported in patients receiving intravenous amphotericin B and leukocyte transfusions).

Levamisole Hydrochloride (Concurrent use may enhance the potential for renal toxicity, bronchospasm, and hypotension). Products include:
- Ergamisol Tablets ... 1340

Lomustine (CCNU) (Concurrent use may enhance the potential for renal toxicity, bronchospasm, and hypotension). Products include:
- CeeNU Capsules ... 699

Mechlorethamine Hydrochloride (Concurrent use may enhance the potential for renal toxicity, bronchospasm, and hypotension). Products include:
- Mustargen ... 1752

Megestrol Acetate (Concurrent use may enhance the potential for renal toxicity, bronchospasm, and hypotension). Products include:
- Megace Oral Suspension ... 708
- Megace Tablets ... 710

Melphalan (Concurrent use may enhance the potential for renal toxicity, bronchospasm, and hypotension). Products include:
- Alkeran Tablets ... 1198

Mercaptopurine (Concurrent use may enhance the potential for renal toxicity, bronchospasm, and hypotension). Products include:
- Purinethol Tablets ... 1214

Metaxalone (Amphotericin B-induced hypokalemia may enhance the curariform effect of skeletal muscle relaxants). Products include:
- Skelaxin Tablets ... 793

Methocarbamol (Amphotericin B-induced hypokalemia may enhance the curariform effect of skeletal muscle relaxants). Products include:
- Robaxin Injectable ... 2245
- Robaxin Tablets ... 2246
- Robaxisal Tablets ... 2246

Methotrexate Sodium (Concurrent use may enhance the potential for renal toxicity, bronchospasm, and hypotension). Products include:
- Methotrexate Sodium Tablets, Injection, for Injection and LPF Injection ... 1322

Methylprednisolone Acetate (Concurrent use may potentiate hypokalemia which could predispose the patient to cardiac dysfunction).
- No products indexed under this heading.

Methylprednisolone Sodium Succinate (Concurrent use may potentiate hypokalemia which could predispose the patient to cardiac dysfunction).
- No products indexed under this heading.

Metocurine Iodide (Amphotericin B-induced hypokalemia may enhance the curariform effect of skeletal muscle relaxants). Products include:
- Metubine Iodide Vials ... 932

Miconazole (Antagonism between amphotericin B and imidazole derivatives, which inhibit ergosterol synthesis, has been reported; clinical significance of this finding has not been determined).
- No products indexed under this heading.

Miconazole Nitrate (Antagonism between amphotericin B and imidazole derivatives, which inhibit ergosterol synthesis, has been reported; clinical significance of this finding has not been determined). Products include:
- Prescription Strength Desenex Spray Powder and Spray Liquid ▣ 653
- Lotrimin AF Antifungal Spray Liquid, Spray Powder, Spray Deodorant Powder, Powder and Jock Itch Spray Powder ... ▣ 766
- Monistat Dual-Pak ... 1906
- Monistat 3 Vaginal Suppositories ... 1905
- Monistat-Derm (miconazole nitrate 2%) Cream ... 1944
- Ting Antifungal Spray Powder ... ▣ 666

Mitomycin (Mitomycin-C) (Concurrent use may enhance the potential for renal toxicity, bronchospasm, and hypotension). Products include:
- Mutamycin for Injection ... 712

Mitotane (Concurrent use may enhance the potential for renal toxicity, bronchospasm, and hypotension). Products include:
- Lysodren Tablets ... 707

Mitoxantrone Hydrochloride (Concurrent use may enhance the potential for renal toxicity, bronchospasm, and hypotension). Products include:
- Novantrone for Injection ... 1327

Mivacurium Chloride (Amphotericin B-induced hypokalemia may enhance the curariform effect of skeletal muscle relaxants). Products include:
- Mivacron ... 1125

Orphenadrine Citrate (Amphotericin B-induced hypokalemia may enhance the curariform effect of skeletal muscle relaxants). Products include:
- Norflex ... 1554
- Norgesic ... 1554

Paclitaxel (Concurrent use may enhance the potential for renal toxicity, bronchospasm, and hypotension). Products include:
- Taxol Injection ... 723

Pancuronium Bromide (Amphotericin B-induced hypokalemia may enhance the curariform effect of skeletal muscle relaxants).
- No products indexed under this heading.

Pentamidine Isethionate (Concurrent use may enhance the potential for drug-induced renal toxicity).
- No products indexed under this heading.

Prednisolone Acetate (Concurrent use may potentiate hypokalemia which could predispose the patient to cardiac dysfunction). Products include:
- AK-CIDE ... ⊙ 203
- AK-CIDE Ointment ... ⊙ 203
- Blephamide Liquifilm Sterile Ophthalmic Suspension ... 472
- Blephamide Ointment ... ⊙ 234
- Econopred & Econopred Plus Ophthalmic Suspensions ... ⊙ 216
- Poly-Pred Liquifilm ... ⊙ 246
- Pred Forte ... ⊙ 247
- Pred Mild ... ⊙ 250
- Pred-G Liquifilm Sterile Ophthalmic Suspension ... ⊙ 248
- Pred-G S.O.P. Sterile Ophthalmic Ointment ... ⊙ 249

IMPORTANT NOTE: Always consult each drug listing in the patient's regimen for possible interactions.

Prednisolone Sodium Phosphate (Concurrent use may potentiate hypokalemia which could predispose the patient to cardiac dysfunction). Products include:
AK-PRED .... ⊚ 204
Hydeltrasol Injection, Sterile 1708
Pediapred Oral Solution 1618

Prednisolone Tebutate (Concurrent use may potentiate hypokalemia which could predispose the patient to cardiac dysfunction). Products include:
Hydeltra-T.B.A. Sterile Suspension 1710

Prednisone (Concurrent use may potentiate hypokalemia which could predispose the patient to cardiac dysfunction).
No products indexed under this heading.

Procarbazine Hydrochloride (Concurrent use may enhance the potential for renal toxicity, bronchospasm, and hypotension). Products include:
Matulane Capsules 2300

Rocuronium Bromide (Amphotericin B-induced hypokalemia may enhance the curariform effect of skeletal muscle relaxants). Products include:
Zemuron Injection 1885

Streptomycin Sulfate (Concurrent use may enhance the potential for drug-induced renal toxicity). Products include:
Streptomycin Sulfate Injection 2031

Streptozocin (Concurrent use may enhance the potential for renal toxicity, bronchospasm, and hypotension). Products include:
Zanosar Sterile Powder 2119

Succinylcholine Chloride (Amphotericin B-induced hypokalemia may enhance the curariform effect of skeletal muscle relaxants). Products include:
Anectine 1062

Tamoxifen Citrate (Concurrent use may enhance the potential for renal toxicity, bronchospasm, and hypotension). Products include:
Nolvadex Tablets 2957

Teniposide (Concurrent use may enhance the potential for renal toxicity, bronchospasm, and hypotension). Products include:
Vumon for Injection 729

Thioguanine (Concurrent use may enhance the potential for renal toxicity, bronchospasm, and hypotension). Products include:
Thioguanine Tablets, Tabloid Brand 1225

Thiotepa (Concurrent use may enhance the potential for renal toxicity, bronchospasm, and hypotension). Products include:
Thioplex (Thiotepa For Injection) 1329

Tobramycin (Concurrent use may enhance the potential for drug-induced renal toxicity). Products include:
AKTOB .... ⊚ 207
TobraDex Ophthalmic Suspension and Ointment 469
Tobrex Ophthalmic Ointment and Solution .... ⊚ 226

Tobramycin Sulfate (Concurrent use may enhance the potential for drug-induced renal toxicity). Products include:
Nebcin Vials, Hyporets & ADD-Vantage 1518

Topotecan Hydrochloride (Concurrent use may enhance the potential for renal toxicity, bronchospasm, and hypotension). Products include:
Hycamtin for Injection 2665

Triamcinolone (Concurrent use may potentiate hypokalemia which could predispose the patient to cardiac dysfunction).
No products indexed under this heading.

Triamcinolone Acetonide (Concurrent use may potentiate hypokalemia which could predispose the patient to cardiac dysfunction). Products include:
Azmacort Oral Inhaler 2175
Nasacort AQ Nasal Spray 2191
Nasacort Nasal Inhaler 2189

Triamcinolone Diacetate (Concurrent use may potentiate hypokalemia which could predispose the patient to cardiac dysfunction).
No products indexed under this heading.

Triamcinolone Hexacetonide (Concurrent use may potentiate hypokalemia which could predispose the patient to cardiac dysfunction).
No products indexed under this heading.

Tubocurarine Chloride (Amphotericin B-induced hypokalemia may enhance the curariform effect of skeletal muscle relaxants).
No products indexed under this heading.

Vecuronium Bromide (Amphotericin B-induced hypokalemia may enhance the curariform effect of skeletal muscle relaxants). Products include:
Norcuron for Injection 1875

Vincristine Sulfate (Concurrent use may enhance the potential for renal toxicity, bronchospasm, and hypotension). Products include:
Oncovin Solution Vials & Hyporets 1521

Vinorelbine Tartrate (Concurrent use may enhance the potential for renal toxicity, bronchospasm, and hypotension). Products include:
Navelbine Injection 1212

Zidovudine (Potential for increased myelotoxicity and nephrotoxicity). Products include:
Retrovir Capsules 1216
Retrovir I.V. Infusion 1221
Retrovir Syrup 1216

AC SLIM CAP
(Nutritional Supplement) 461
May interact with monoamine oxidase inhibitors. Compounds in this category include:

Furazolidone (Concurrent use requires advice from a health care practitioner). Products include:
Furoxone 2221

Isocarboxazid (Concurrent use requires advice from a health care practitioner).
No products indexed under this heading.

Phenelzine Sulfate (Concurrent use requires advice from a health care practitioner). Products include:
Nardil 1977

Selegiline Hydrochloride (Concurrent use requires advice from a health care practitioner). Products include:
Eldepryl Capsules 2729

Tranylcypromine Sulfate (Concurrent use requires advice from a health care practitioner). Products include:
Parnate Tablets 2679

ACCUPRIL TABLETS
(Quinapril Hydrochloride) 1950
May interact with diuretics, potassium sparing diuretics, potassium preparations, tetracyclines, lithium preparations, and certain other agents. Compounds in these categories include:

Amiloride Hydrochloride (Occasional excessive reduction of blood pressure; potential for hyperkalemia). Products include:
Midamor Tablets 1746
Moduretic Tablets 1748

Bendroflumethiazide (Occasional excessive reduction of blood pressure).
No products indexed under this heading.

Bumetanide (Occasional excessive reduction of blood pressure). Products include:
Bumex 2260

Chlorothiazide (Occasional excessive reduction of blood pressure). Products include:
Aldoclor Tablets 1638
Diupres Tablets 1691
Diuril Oral 1694

Chlorothiazide Sodium (Occasional excessive reduction of blood pressure). Products include:
Diuril Sodium Intravenous 1693

Chlorthalidone (Occasional excessive reduction of blood pressure). Products include:
Combipres Tablets 682
Tenoretic Tablets 2963
Thalitone 1293

Demeclocycline Hydrochloride (Reduced absorption of tetracycline by approximately 28% to 37%). Products include:
Declomycin Tablets 1421

Doxycycline Calcium (Reduced absorption of tetracycline by approximately 28% to 37%). Products include:
Vibramycin Calcium Oral Suspension Syrup 2038

Doxycycline Hyclate (Reduced absorption of tetracycline by approximately 28% to 37%). Products include:
Doryx Capsules 1970
Vibramycin Hyclate Capsules 2038
Vibramycin Hyclate Intravenous ... 2040
Vibra-Tabs Film Coated Tablets ... 2038

Doxycycline Monohydrate (Reduced absorption of tetracycline by approximately 28% to 37%). Products include:
Monodox Capsules 1858
Vibramycin Monohydrate for Oral Suspension 2038

Ethacrynic Acid (Occasional excessive reduction of blood pressure). Products include:
Edecrin Tablets 1698

Furosemide (Occasional excessive reduction of blood pressure). Products include:
Lasix Injection, Oral Solution and Tablets 1267

Hydrochlorothiazide (Occasional excessive reduction of blood pressure). Products include:
Aldactazide Tablets 2556
Aldoril Tablets 1644
Apresazide Capsules 824
Capozide Tablets 744
Dyazide Capsules 2653
Esidrix Tablets 839
Esimil Tablets 840
HydroDIURIL Tablets 1716
Hydropres Tablets 1718
Hyzaar Tablets 1720
Inderide Tablets 2838
Inderide LA Long Acting Capsules 2840
Lopressor HCT Tablets 850
Lotensin HCT Tablets 855
Moduretic Tablets 1748
Oretic Tablets 450
Prinzide Tablets 1780
Ser-Ap-Es Tablets 867
Timolide Tablets 1791
Vaseretic Tablets 1810
Zestoretic Tablets 2968
Ziac 1459

Hydroflumethiazide (Occasional excessive reduction of blood pressure). Products include:
Diucardin Tablets 2824

Indapamide (Occasional excessive reduction of blood pressure).
No products indexed under this heading.

Lithium Carbonate (Increased serum lithium levels and symptoms of lithium toxicity). Products include:
Eskalith 2658
Lithium Carbonate Capsules & Tablets 2352
Lithonate/Lithotabs/Lithobid 2721

Lithium Citrate (Increased serum lithium levels and symptoms of lithium toxicity).
No products indexed under this heading.

Methacycline Hydrochloride (Reduced absorption of tetracycline by approximately 28% to 37%).
No products indexed under this heading.

Methyclothiazide (Occasional excessive reduction of blood pressure). Products include:
Enduron Tablets 424

Metolazone (Occasional excessive reduction of blood pressure). Products include:
Mykrox Tablets 1617
Zaroxolyn Tablets 1625

Minocycline Hydrochloride (Reduced absorption of tetracycline by approximately 28% to 37%). Products include:
DYNACIN Capsules 1627
Minocin Intravenous 1428
Minocin Oral Suspension 1431
Minocin Pellet-Filled Capsules 1429

Oxytetracycline Hydrochloride (Reduced absorption of tetracycline by approximately 28% to 37%). Products include:
TERAK Ointment .... ⊚ 210
Terra-Cortril Ophthalmic Suspension 2033
Terramycin with Polymyxin B Sulfate Ophthalmic Ointment 2035
Urobiotic-250 Capsules 2038

Polythiazide (Occasional excessive reduction of blood pressure). Products include:
Minizide Capsules 2016

Potassium Acid Phosphate (Potential for hyperkalemia). Products include:
K-Phos Original Formula 'Sodium Free' Tablets 633

Potassium Bicarbonate (Potential for hyperkalemia). Products include:
Alka-Seltzer Gold Effervescent Antacid .... ⊞ 611

Potassium Chloride (Potential for hyperkalemia). Products include:
Chlor-3 Condiment 1003
Colyte and Colyte-flavored 2540
GoLYTELY 694
K-Dur Microburst Release System (potassium chloride, USP) E.R. Tablets 1364
K-Lor Powder Packets 438
K-Norm Capsules 1615
K-Tab Filmtab 439
Micro-K 2237
Micro-K LS Packets 2238
NuLYTELY 694
Cherry Flavor NuLYTELY 694
Rum-K Syrup 1004
Slow-K Extended-Release Tablets 869

(⊞ Described in PDR For Nonprescription Drugs)   (⊚ Described in PDR For Ophthalmology)

Interactions Index

Potassium Citrate (Potential for hyperkalemia). Products include:
- Polycitra Syrup ... 574
- Polycitra-K Crystals ... 574
- Polycitra-K Oral Solution ... 575
- Polycitra-LC ... 574
- Urocit-K Tablets ... 1828

Potassium Gluconate (Potential for hyperkalemia).
No products indexed under this heading.

Potassium Phosphate, Dibasic (Potential for hyperkalemia).
No products indexed under this heading.

Potassium Phosphate, Monobasic (Potential for hyperkalemia). Products include:
- K-Phos Neutral Tablets ... 633
- K-Phos Original Formula 'Sodium Free' Tablets ... 633

Spironolactone (Occasional excessive reduction of blood pressure; potential for hyperkalemia). Products include:
- Aldactazide Tablets ... 2556
- Aldactone Tablets ... 2558

Tetracycline Hydrochloride (Reduced absorption of tetracycline by approximately 28% to 37%). Products include:
- Achromycin V Capsules ... 1417
- Helidac Therapy ... 2135

Torsemide (Occasional excessive reduction of blood pressure). Products include:
- Demadex Tablets and Injection ... 691

Triamterene (Occasional excessive reduction of blood pressure; potential for hyperkalemia). Products include:
- Dyazide Capsules ... 2653
- Dyrenium Capsules ... 2655

Food Interactions

Diet, high-lipid (Rate and extent of Quinapril absorption are diminished moderately).

ACCUTANE CAPSULES
(Isotretinoin) ... 2252
May interact with:

Vitamin A (Additive Vitamin A toxicity). Products include:
- Aquasol A Vitamin A Capsules, USP ... 525
- Aquasol A Parenteral ... 526
- Breath + Plus ... 603
- Materna Tablets ... 1427
- Megadose ... 513
- One-A-Day Antioxidant Plus ... 625

Food Interactions

Dairy products (Increases oral absorption of isotretinoin).

Food, unspecified (Increases oral absorption of isotretinoin).

ACCUZYME OINTMENT
(Papain, Urea) ... 1236
None cited in PDR database.

ACEL-IMUNE DIPHTHERIA AND TETANUS TOXOIDS AND ACELLULAR PERTUSSIS VACCINE ADSORBED
(Diphtheria & Tetanus Toxoids and Acellular Pertussis Vaccine) ... 1415
May interact with immunosuppressive agents, corticosteroids, cytotoxic drugs, alkylating agents, anticoagulants, and certain other agents. Compounds in these categories include:

Azathioprine (Reduces response to active immunization procedures). Products include:
- Azathioprine Tablets ... 2349
- Imuran ... 1103

Betamethasone Acetate (Reduces response to active immunization procedures). Products include:
- Celestone Soluspan Suspension ... 2484

Betamethasone Sodium Phosphate (Reduces response to active immunization procedures). Products include:
- Celestone Soluspan Suspension ... 2484

Bleomycin Sulfate (Reduces response to active immunization procedures). Products include:
- Blenoxane ... 697

Busulfan (Reduces response to active immunization procedures). Products include:
- Myleran Tablets ... 1209

Carmustine (BCNU) (Reduces response to active immunization procedures). Products include:
- BiCNU ... 696

Chlorambucil (Reduces response to active immunization procedures). Products include:
- Leukeran Tablets ... 1205

Cortisone Acetate (Reduces response to active immunization procedures). Products include:
- Cortone Acetate Sterile Suspension ... 1663
- Cortone Acetate Tablets ... 1664

Cyclophosphamide (Reduces response to active immunization procedures). Products include:
- Cytoxan ... 700

Cyclosporine (Reduces response to active immunization procedures). Products include:
- Neoral ... 2405
- Sandimmune ... 2416

Dacarbazine (Reduces response to active immunization procedures). Products include:
- DTIC-Dome ... 593

Dalteparin Sodium (Caution should be exercised). Products include:
- Fragmin Injection ... 2088

Daunorubicin Hydrochloride (Reduces response to active immunization procedures). Products include:
- Cerubidine for Injection ... 634

Dexamethasone (Reduces response to active immunization procedures). Products include:
- AK-Trol Ointment & Suspension ... 205
- Decadron Elixir ... 1676
- Decadron Tablets ... 1678
- Decaspray Topical Aerosol ... 1689
- Maxitrol Ophthalmic Ointment and Suspension ... 222
- TobraDex Ophthalmic Suspension and Ointment ... 469

Dexamethasone Acetate (Reduces response to active immunization procedures). Products include:
- Dalalone D.P. Injectable ... 1009
- Decadron-LA Sterile Suspension ... 1687

Dexamethasone Sodium Phosphate (Reduces response to active immunization procedures). Products include:
- Decadron Phosphate Injection ... 1680
- Decadron Phosphate Sterile Ophthalmic Ointment ... 1684
- Decadron Phosphate Sterile Ophthalmic Solution ... 1685
- Decadron Phosphate Topical Cream ... 1686
- Decadron Phosphate with Xylocaine Injection, Sterile ... 1683
- Dexacort Phosphate in Respihaler ... 1606
- Dexacort Phosphate in Turbinaire ... 1607
- NeoDecadron Sterile Ophthalmic Ointment ... 1755
- NeoDecadron Sterile Ophthalmic Solution ... 1756
- NeoDecadron Topical Cream ... 1757

Dicumarol (Caution should be exercised).
No products indexed under this heading.

Doxorubicin Hydrochloride (Reduces response to active immunization procedures). Products include:
- Adriamycin PFS ... 2056
- Adriamycin RDF ... 2056
- Doxil ... 2613
- Doxorubicin Astra ... 531
- Rubex for Injection ... 721

Enoxaparin (Caution should be exercised). Products include:
- Lovenox Injection ... 2187

Fludrocortisone Acetate (Reduces response to active immunization procedures). Products include:
- Florinef Acetate Tablets ... 506

Fluorouracil (Reduces response to active immunization procedures). Products include:
- Efudex ... 2280
- Fluoroplex Topical Solution & Cream 1% ... 475
- Fluorouracil Injection ... 2282

Heparin Calcium (Caution should be exercised).
No products indexed under this heading.

Heparin Sodium (Caution should be exercised). Products include:
- Heparin Lock Flush Solution ... 2831
- Heparin Sodium Injection ... 2832
- Heparin Sodium Vials ... 1486

Hydrocortisone (Reduces response to active immunization procedures). Products include:
- Anusol-HC Cream 2.5% ... 1953
- Aquanil HC Lotion ... 1989
- Maximum Strength Cortaid Spray ... 800
- CORTENEMA ... 2713
- Cortisporin Ointment ... 1074
- Cortisporin Ophthalmic Ointment Sterile ... 1074
- Cortisporin Ophthalmic Suspension Sterile ... 1075
- Cortisporin Otic Solution Sterile ... 1076
- Cortisporin Otic Suspension Sterile ... 1077
- Cortizone-5 ... 795
- Cortizone-10 ... 795
- Hydrocortone Tablets ... 1715
- Hytone ... 922
- Hytone Ointment 2 ½% ... 923
- Massengill Medicated Soft Cloth Towelettes ... 2628
- Pediotic Suspension Sterile ... 1140
- Preparation H Hydrocortisone 1% Cream ... 843
- ProctoCream-HC 2.5% ... 2552
- VōSoL HC Otic Solution ... 2786

Hydrocortisone Acetate (Reduces response to active immunization procedures). Products include:
- Analpram-HC Rectal Cream 1% and 2.5% ... 993
- Anusol HC-1 Hydrocortisone Anti-Itch Ointment ... 810
- Anusol-HC Suppositories ... 1954
- Caldecort Anti-Itch Hydrocortisone Cream ... 651
- Coly-Mycin S Otic w/Neomycin & Hydrocortisone ... 1965
- Cortaid ... 800
- Cortifoam ... 2540
- Cortisporin Cream ... 1073
- Epifoam ... 2543
- Hydrocortone Acetate Sterile Suspension ... 1712
- Mantadil Cream ... 1124
- Nupercainal Hydrocortisone 1% Cream ... 661
- Pramosone Cream, Lotion & Ointment ... 995
- ProctoFoam-HC ... 2552
- Terra-Cortril Ophthalmic Suspension ... 2033

Hydrocortisone Sodium Phosphate (Reduces response to active immunization procedures). Products include:
- Hydrocortone Phosphate Injection, Sterile ... 1713

Hydrocortisone Sodium Succinate (Reduces response to active immunization procedures).
No products indexed under this heading.

Hydroxyurea (Reduces response to active immunization procedures). Products include:
- Hydrea Capsules ... 705

Immune Globulin (Human) (Reduces response to active immunization procedures).
No products indexed under this heading.

Immune Globulin Intravenous (Human) (Reduces response to active immunization procedures).
No products indexed under this heading.

Lomustine (CCNU) (Reduces response to active immunization procedures). Products include:
- CeeNU Capsules ... 699

Mechlorethamine Hydrochloride (Reduces response to active immunization procedures). Products include:
- Mustargen ... 1752

Melphalan (Reduces response to active immunization procedures). Products include:
- Alkeran Tablets ... 1198

Methotrexate Sodium (Reduces response to active immunization procedures). Products include:
- Methotrexate Sodium Tablets, Injection, for Injection and LPF Injection ... 1322

Methylprednisolone Acetate (Reduces response to active immunization procedures).
No products indexed under this heading.

Methylprednisolone Sodium Succinate (Reduces response to active immunization procedures).
No products indexed under this heading.

Mitotane (Reduces response to active immunization procedures). Products include:
- Lysodren Tablets ... 707

Mitoxantrone Hydrochloride (Reduces response to active immunization procedures). Products include:
- Novantrone for Injection ... 1327

Muromonab-CD3 (Reduces response to active immunization procedures). Products include:
- Orthoclone OKT3 Sterile Solution ... 1892

Mycophenolate Mofetil (Reduces response to active immunization procedures). Products include:
- CellCept Capsules ... 2265

Prednisolone Acetate (Reduces response to active immunization procedures). Products include:
- AK-CIDE ... 203
- AK-CIDE Ointment ... 203
- Blephamide Liquifilm Sterile Ophthalmic Suspension ... 472
- Blephamide Ointment ... 234
- Econopred & Econopred Plus Ophthalmic Suspensions ... 216
- Poly-Pred Liquifilm ... 246
- Pred Forte ... 247
- Pred Mild ... 250
- Pred-G Liquifilm Sterile Ophthalmic Suspension ... 248
- Pred-G S.O.P. Sterile Ophthalmic Ointment ... 249

Prednisolone Sodium Phosphate (Reduces response to active immunization procedures). Products include:
- AK-PRED ... 204
- Hydeltrasol Injection, Sterile ... 1708
- Pediapred Oral Solution ... 1618

IMPORTANT NOTE: Always consult each drug listing in the patient's regimen for possible interactions.

Acel-Imune

Prednisolone Tebutate (Reduces response to active immunization procedures). Products include:
Hydeltra-T.B.A. Sterile Suspension 1710

Prednisone (Reduces response to active immunization procedures).
No products indexed under this heading.

Procarbazine Hydrochloride (Reduces response to active immunization procedures). Products include:
Matulane Capsules 2300

Tacrolimus (Reduces response to active immunization procedures). Products include:
Prograf 1028

Tamoxifen Citrate (Reduces response to active immunization procedures). Products include:
Nolvadex Tablets 2957

Thiotepa (Reduces response to active immunization procedures). Products include:
Thioplex (Thiotepa For Injection) 1329

Triamcinolone (Reduces response to active immunization procedures).
No products indexed under this heading.

Triamcinolone Acetonide (Reduces response to active immunization procedures). Products include:
Azmacort Oral Inhaler 2175
Nasacort AQ Nasal Spray 2191
Nasacort Nasal Inhaler 2189

Triamcinolone Diacetate (Reduces response to active immunization procedures).
No products indexed under this heading.

Triamcinolone Hexacetonide (Reduces response to active immunization procedures).
No products indexed under this heading.

Vincristine Sulfate (Reduces response to active immunization procedures). Products include:
Oncovin Solution Vials & Hyporets 1521

Warfarin Sodium (Caution should be exercised). Products include:
Coumadin 941

ACHROMYCIN V CAPSULES
(Tetracycline Hydrochloride) 1417
May interact with oral anticoagulants, penicillins, antacids, oral contraceptives, and certain other agents. Compounds in these categories include:

Aluminum Carbonate (Impaired absorption of tetracycline). Products include:
Basaljel Capsules 2810
Basaljel Suspension 2810
Basaljel Tablets 2810

Aluminum Hydroxide (Impaired absorption of tetracycline). Products include:
ALternaGEL Liquid 1358
Maximum Strength Ascriptin 650
Cama Arthritis Pain Reliever 748
Gaviscon Extra Strength Relief Formula Antacid Tablets 778
Gaviscon Extra Strength Relief Formula Liquid Antacid 779
Gaviscon Liquid Antacid 779
Gelusil Antacid-Anti-gas Liquid 819
Gelusil Antacid-Anti-gas Tablets 819
Maalox Antacid/Anti-Gas Tablets 889
Maalox Heartburn Relief Suspension 658
Maalox Antacid Liquid 888
Extra Strength Maalox Antacid/Anti-Gas Liquid and Tablets 888
Mylanta 1359
Tempo Soft Antacid 799

Aluminum Hydroxide Gel (Impaired absorption of tetracycline). Products include:
ALternaGEL Liquid 675
Aludrox Oral Suspension 850
Amphojel Suspension 2802
Amphojel Suspension without Flavor 2802
Amphojel Tablets 2802
Ascriptin 650
Gaviscon Antacid Tablets 778
Gaviscon-2 Antacid Tablets 779
Mylanta Liquid 676
Mylanta Double Strength Liquid 676
Nephrox Suspension 671

Amoxicillin Trihydrate (Interference with bactericidal action of penicillin). Products include:
Amoxil 2631
Augmentin 2637
Augmentin Tablets 2640

Ampicillin (Interference with bactericidal action of penicillin). Products include:
Omnipen Capsules 2872
Omnipen for Oral Suspension 2873

Ampicillin Sodium (Interference with bactericidal action of penicillin). Products include:
Unasyn 2035

Ampicillin Trihydrate (Interference with bactericidal action of penicillin).
No products indexed under this heading.

Azlocillin Sodium (Interference with bactericidal action of penicillin).
No products indexed under this heading.

Bacampicillin Hydrochloride (Interference with bactericidal action of penicillin). Products include:
Spectrobid Tablets 2030

Carbenicillin Disodium (Interference with bactericidal action of penicillin).
No products indexed under this heading.

Carbenicillin Indanyl Sodium (Interference with bactericidal action of penicillin). Products include:
Geocillin Tablets 2009

Desogestrel (Reduced efficacy and increased incidence of breakthrough bleeding). Products include:
Desogen Tablets 1867
Ortho-Cept 1907

Dicloxacillin Sodium (Interference with bactericidal action of penicillin).
No products indexed under this heading.

Dicumarol (Depressed plasma prothombin activity; downward adjustment of anticoagulant dosage may be necessary).
No products indexed under this heading.

Ethinyl Estradiol (Reduced efficacy and increased incidence of breakthrough bleeding). Products include:
Brevicon 2563
Demulen 2580
Desogen Tablets 1867
Levlen/Tri-Levlen 646
Lo/Ovral Tablets 2852
Lo/Ovral-28 Tablets 2857
Modicon 1928
Nordette-21 Tablets 2863
Nordette-28 Tablets 2866
Norinyl 2563
Ortho-Cept 1907
Ortho-Cyclen/Ortho Tri-Cyclen 1914
Ortho-Novum 1928
Ortho-Cyclen/Ortho Tri-Cyclen 1914
Ovcon 765
Ovral Tablets 2877
Ovral-28 Tablets 2878
Levlen/Tri-Levlen 646
Tri-Norinyl 2607
Triphasil-21 Tablets 2919
Triphasil-28 Tablets 2924

Ethynodiol Diacetate (Reduced efficacy and increased incidence of breakthrough bleeding). Products include:
Demulen 2580

Levonorgestrel (Reduced efficacy and increased incidence of breakthrough bleeding). Products include:
Levlen/Tri-Levlen 646
Nordette-21 Tablets 2863
Nordette-28 Tablets 2866
Norplant System 2868
Levlen/Tri-Levlen 646
Triphasil-21 Tablets 2919
Triphasil-28 Tablets 2924

Magaldrate (Impaired absorption of tetracycline).
No products indexed under this heading.

Magnesium Hydroxide (Impaired absorption of tetracycline). Products include:
Aludrox Oral Suspension 850
Ascriptin 650
Di-Gel Antacid/Anti-Gas 762
Gelusil Antacid-Anti-gas Liquid 819
Gelusil Antacid-Anti-gas Tablets 819
Maalox Antacid/Anti-Gas Tablets 889
Maalox Antacid Liquid 888
Extra Strength Maalox Antacid/Anti-Gas Liquid and Tablets 888
Mylanta Fast-Acting 1359
Mylanta Gelcaps Antacid 678
Fast-Acting Mylanta Liquid Antacid 1359
Mylanta Tablets 677
Maximum-Strength Fast-Acting Mylanta Liquid Antacid 1359
Mylanta Double Strength Tablets 677
Phillips' Milk of Magnesia Liquid 627
Rolaids Antacid Tablets 807
Tempo Soft Antacid 799

Magnesium Oxide (Impaired absorption of tetracycline). Products include:
Beelith Tablets 632
Bufferin Analgesic Tablets 636
Arthritis Strength Bufferin Analgesic Caplets 637
Extra Strength Bufferin Analgesic Tablets 637
Caltrate PLUS 681
Cama Arthritis Pain Reliever 748
Mag-Ox 400 666
Uro-Mag 666

Mestranol (Reduced efficacy and increased incidence of breakthrough bleeding). Products include:
Norinyl 2563
Ortho-Novum 1928

Mezlocillin Sodium (Interference with bactericidal action of penicillin). Products include:
Mezlin 594
Mezlin Pharmacy Bulk Package 597

Nafcillin Sodium (Interference with bactericidal action of penicillin).
No products indexed under this heading.

Norethindrone (Reduced efficacy and increased incidence of breakthrough bleeding). Products include:
Brevicon 2563
Micronor Tablets 1903
Modicon 1928
Norinyl 2563
Nor-Q D Tablets 2598
Ortho-Novum 1928
Ovcon 765
Tri-Norinyl 2607

Norethynodrel (Reduced efficacy and increased incidence of breakthrough bleeding).
No products indexed under this heading.

Norgestimate (Reduced efficacy and increased incidence of breakthrough bleeding). Products include:
Ortho-Cyclen/Ortho Tri-Cyclen 1914
Ortho-Cyclen/Ortho Tri-Cyclen 1914

Norgestrel (Reduced efficacy and increased incidence of breakthrough bleeding). Products include:
Lo/Ovral Tablets 2852
Lo/Ovral-28 Tablets 2857
Ovral Tablets 2877
Ovral-28 Tablets 2878
Ovrette Tablets 2878

Penicillin G Benzathine (Interference with bactericidal action of penicillin). Products include:
Bicillin C-R Injection 2810
Bicillin C-R 900/300 Injection 2812
Bicillin L-A Injection 2813

Penicillin G Potassium (Interference with bactericidal action of penicillin). Products include:
Pfizerpen for Injection 2022

Penicillin G Procaine (Interference with bactericidal action of penicillin). Products include:
Bicillin C-R Injection 2810
Bicillin C-R 900/300 Injection 2812

Penicillin G Sodium (Interference with bactericidal action of penicillin).
No products indexed under this heading.

Penicillin V Potassium (Interference with bactericidal action of penicillin). Products include:
Pen•Vee K 2879

Sodium Bicarbonate (Impaired absorption of tetracycline). Products include:
Alka-Seltzer Cherry Effervescent Antacid and Pain Reliever 609
Alka-Seltzer Extra Strength Effervescent Antacid and Pain Reliever 609
Alka-Seltzer Gold Effervescent Antacid 611
Alka-Seltzer Lemon Lime Effervescent Antacid and Pain Reliever 609
Alka-Seltzer Original Effervescent Antacid and Pain Reliever 609
Arm & Hammer Pure Baking Soda 648
Colyte and Colyte-flavored 2540
GoLYTELY 694
Massengill Disposable Douches 780
Massengill Liquid Concentrate 780
NuLYTELY 694
Cherry Flavor NuLYTELY 694

Ticarcillin Disodium (Interference with bactericidal action of penicillin). Products include:
Ticar for Injection 2704
Timentin for Injection 2706

Warfarin Sodium (Depressed plasma prothombin activity; downward adjustment of anticoagulant dosage may be necessary). Products include:
Coumadin 941

Food Interactions
Dairy products (Interfers with absorption of oral forms of tetracycline).

Food, unspecified (Interfers with absorption of oral forms of tetracycline).

ACID MANTLE CREME
(Petrolatum, White) 747
None cited in PDR database.

ACI-JEL THERAPEUTIC VAGINAL JELLY
(Acetic Acid, Oxyquinoline Sulfate) 1903
None cited in PDR database.

ACLOVATE CREAM
(Alclometasone Dipropionate) 1061
None cited in PDR database.

ACLOVATE OINTMENT
(Alclometasone Dipropionate) 1061
None cited in PDR database.

(◨ Described in PDR For Nonprescription Drugs)   (◉ Described in PDR For Ophthalmology)

ACTHIB
(Haemophilus B Conjugate Vaccine) .. 893

May interact with immunosuppressive agents, alkylating agents, cytotoxic drugs, corticosteroids, and anticoagulants. Compounds in these categories include:

Azathioprine (May reduce the immune response to vaccine). Products include:
- Azathioprine Tablets 2349
- Imuran 1103

Betamethasone Acetate (Corticosteroids, when used in greater than physiologic doses, may reduce the immune response to vaccine). Products include:
- Celestone Soluspan Suspension 2484

Betamethasone Sodium Phosphate (Corticosteroids, when used in greater than physiologic doses, may reduce the immune response to vaccine). Products include:
- Celestone Soluspan Suspension 2484

Bleomycin Sulfate (May reduce the immune response to vaccine). Products include:
- Blenoxane 697

Busulfan (May reduce the immune response to vaccine). Products include:
- Myleran Tablets 1209

Carmustine (BCNU) (May reduce the immune response to vaccine). Products include:
- BiCNU 696

Chlorambucil (May reduce the immune response to vaccine). Products include:
- Leukeran Tablets 1205

Cortisone Acetate (Corticosteroids, when used in greater than physiologic doses, may reduce the immune response to vaccine). Products include:
- Cortone Acetate Sterile Suspension 1663
- Cortone Acetate Tablets 1664

Cyclophosphamide (May reduce the immune response to vaccine). Products include:
- Cytoxan 700

Cyclosporine (May reduce the immune response to vaccine). Products include:
- Neoral 2405
- Sandimmune 2416

Dacarbazine (May reduce the immune response to vaccine). Products include:
- DTIC-Dome 593

Dalteparin Sodium (Use with caution). Products include:
- Fragmin Injection 2088

Daunorubicin Hydrochloride (May reduce the immune response to vaccine). Products include:
- Cerubidine for Injection 634

Dexamethasone (Corticosteroids, when used in greater than physiologic doses, may reduce the immune response to vaccine). Products include:
- AK-Trol Ointment & Suspension .... ⊚ 205
- Decadron Elixir 1676
- Decadron Tablets 1678
- Decaspray Topical Aerosol 1689
- Maxitrol Ophthalmic Ointment and Suspension .... ⊚ 222
- TobraDex Ophthalmic Suspension and Ointment 469

Dexamethasone Acetate (Corticosteroids, when used in greater than physiologic doses, may reduce the immune response to vaccine). Products include:
- Dalalone D.P. Injectable 1009
- Decadron-LA Sterile Suspension...... 1687

Dexamethasone Sodium Phosphate (Corticosteroids, when used in greater than physiologic doses, may reduce the immune response to vaccine). Products include:
- Decadron Phosphate Injection 1680
- Decadron Phosphate Sterile Ophthalmic Ointment 1684
- Decadron Phosphate Sterile Ophthalmic Solution 1685
- Decadron Phosphate Topical Cream 1686
- Decadron Phosphate with Xylocaine Injection, Sterile 1683
- Dexacort Phosphate in Respihaler .. 1606
- Dexacort Phosphate in Turbinaire ... 1607
- NeoDecadron Sterile Ophthalmic Ointment 1755
- NeoDecadron Sterile Ophthalmic Solution 1756
- NeoDecadron Topical Cream 1757

Dicumarol (Use with caution).
No products indexed under this heading.

Doxorubicin Hydrochloride (May reduce the immune response to vaccine). Products include:
- Adriamycin PFS 2056
- Adriamycin RDF 2056
- Doxil 2613
- Doxorubicin Astra 531
- Rubex for Injection 721

Enoxaparin (Use with caution). Products include:
- Lovenox Injection 2187

Fludrocortisone Acetate (Corticosteroids, when used in greater than physiologic doses, may reduce the immune response to vaccine). Products include:
- Florinef Acetate Tablets 506

Fluorouracil (May reduce the immune response to vaccine). Products include:
- Efudex 2280
- Fluoroplex Topical Solution & Cream 1% 475
- Fluorouracil Injection 2282

Heparin Calcium (Use with caution).
No products indexed under this heading.

Heparin Sodium (Use with caution). Products include:
- Heparin Lock Flush Solution 2831
- Heparin Sodium Injection 2832
- Heparin Sodium Vials 1486

Hydrocortisone (Corticosteroids, when used in greater than physiologic doses, may reduce the immune response to vaccine). Products include:
- Anusol-HC Cream 2.5% 1953
- Aquanil HC Lotion 1989
- Maximum Strength Cortaid Spray ⊞ 800
- CORTENEMA 2713
- Cortisporin Ointment 1074
- Cortisporin Ophthalmic Ointment Sterile 1074
- Cortisporin Ophthalmic Suspension Sterile 1075
- Cortisporin Otic Solution Sterile 1076
- Cortisporin Otic Suspension Sterile 1077
- Cortizone-5 .... ⊞ 795
- Cortizone-10 .... ⊞ 795
- Hydrocortone Tablets 1715
- Hytone 922
- Hytone Ointment 2½% 923
- Massengill Medicated Soft Cloth Towelettes 2628
- Pediotic Suspension Sterile ... 1140
- Preparation H Hydrocortisone 1% Cream .... ⊞ 843
- ProctoCream-HC 2.5% 2552
- VōSoL HC Otic Solution 2786

Hydrocortisone Acetate (Corticosteroids, when used in greater than physiologic doses, may reduce the immune response to vaccine). Products include:
- Analpram-HC Rectal Cream 1% and 2.5% 993
- Anusol HC-1 Hydrocortisone Anti-Itch Ointment .... ⊞ 810
- Anusol-HC Suppositories 1954
- Caldecort Anti-Itch Hydrocortisone Cream .... ⊞ 651
- Coly-Mycin S Otic w/Neomycin & Hydrocortisone 1965
- Cortaid .... ⊞ 800
- Cortifoam 2540
- Cortisporin Cream 1073
- Epifoam 2543
- Hydrocortone Acetate Sterile Suspension 1712
- Mantadil Cream 1124
- Nupercainal Hydrocortisone 1% Cream .... ⊞ 661
- Pramosone Cream, Lotion & Ointment 995
- ProctoFoam-HC 2552
- Terra-Cortril Ophthalmic Suspension 2033

Hydrocortisone Sodium Phosphate (Corticosteroids, when used in greater than physiologic doses, may reduce the immune response to vaccine). Products include:
- Hydrocortone Phosphate Injection, Sterile 1713

Hydrocortisone Sodium Succinate (Corticosteroids, when used in greater than physiologic doses, may reduce the immune response to vaccine).
No products indexed under this heading.

Hydroxyurea (May reduce the immune response to vaccine). Products include:
- Hydrea Capsules 705

Immune Globulin (Human) (May reduce the immune response to vaccine).
No products indexed under this heading.

Lomustine (CCNU) (May reduce the immune response to vaccine). Products include:
- CeeNU Capsules 699

Mechlorethamine Hydrochloride (May reduce the immune response to vaccine). Products include:
- Mustargen 1752

Melphalan (May reduce the immune response to vaccine). Products include:
- Alkeran Tablets 1198

Methotrexate Sodium (May reduce the immune response to vaccine). Products include:
- Methotrexate Sodium Tablets, Injection, for Injection and LPF Injection 1322

Methylprednisolone Acetate (Corticosteroids, when used in greater than physiologic doses, may reduce the immune response to vaccine).
No products indexed under this heading.

Methylprednisolone Sodium Succinate (Corticosteroids, when used in greater than physiologic doses, may reduce the immune response to vaccine).
No products indexed under this heading.

Mitotane (May reduce the immune response to vaccine). Products include:
- Lysodren Tablets 707

Mitoxantrone Hydrochloride (May reduce the immune response to vaccine). Products include:
- Novantrone for Injection 1327

Muromonab-CD3 (May reduce the immune response to vaccine). Products include:
- Orthoclone OKT3 Sterile Solution .. 1892

Mycophenolate Mofetil (May reduce the immune response to vaccine). Products include:
- CellCept Capsules 2265

Prednisolone Acetate (Corticosteroids, when used in greater than physiologic doses, may reduce the immune response to vaccine). Products include:
- AK-CIDE .... ⊚ 203
- AK-CIDE Ointment .... ⊚ 203
- Blephamide Liquifilm Sterile Ophthalmic Suspension 472
- Blephamide Ointment .... ⊚ 234
- Econopred & Econopred Plus Ophthalmic Suspensions .. ⊚ 216
- Poly-Pred Liquifilm .... ⊚ 246
- Pred Forte .... ⊚ 247
- Pred Mild .... ⊚ 250
- Pred-G Liquifilm Sterile Ophthalmic Suspension .... ⊚ 248
- Pred-G S.O.P. Sterile Ophthalmic Ointment .... ⊚ 249

Prednisolone Sodium Phosphate (Corticosteroids, when used in greater than physiologic doses, may reduce the immune response to vaccine). Products include:
- AK-PRED .... ⊚ 204
- Hydeltrasol Injection, Sterile 1708
- Pediapred Oral Solution 1618

Prednisolone Tebutate (Corticosteroids, when used in greater than physiologic doses, may reduce the immune response to vaccine). Products include:
- Hydeltra-T.B.A. Sterile Suspension 1710

Prednisone (Corticosteroids, when used in greater than physiologic doses, may reduce the immune response to vaccine).
No products indexed under this heading.

Procarbazine Hydrochloride (May reduce the immune response to vaccine). Products include:
- Matulane Capsules 2300

Tacrolimus (May reduce the immune response to vaccine). Products include:
- Prograf 1028

Tamoxifen Citrate (May reduce the immune response to vaccine). Products include:
- Nolvadex Tablets 2957

Thiotepa (May reduce the immune response to vaccine). Products include:
- Thioplex (Thiotepa For Injection) 1329

Triamcinolone (Corticosteroids, when used in greater than physiologic doses, may reduce the immune response to vaccine).
No products indexed under this heading.

Triamcinolone Acetonide (Corticosteroids, when used in greater than physiologic doses, may reduce the immune response to vaccine). Products include:
- Azmacort Oral Inhaler 2175
- Nasacort AQ Nasal Spray ... 2191
- Nasacort Nasal Inhaler 2189

Triamcinolone Diacetate (Corticosteroids, when used in greater than physiologic doses, may reduce the immune response to vaccine).
No products indexed under this heading.

Triamcinolone Hexacetonide (Corticosteroids, when used in greater than physiologic doses, may reduce the immune response to vaccine).
No products indexed under this heading.

Vincristine Sulfate (May reduce the immune response to vaccine). Products include:
- Oncovin Solution Vials & Hyporets 1521

Warfarin Sodium (Use with caution). Products include:
- Coumadin 941

IMPORTANT NOTE: Always consult each drug listing in the patient's regimen for possible interactions.

ACTHREL FOR INJECTION
(Corticorelin Ovine Triflutate) 2990
May interact with:

Dexamethasone (The plasma ACTH response to corticorelin injection is inhibited or blunted in normal subjects pretreated with dexamethasone). Products include:
- AK-Trol Ointment & Suspension .... ⊚ 205
- Decadron Elixir 1676
- Decadron Tablets 1678
- Decaspray Topical Aerosol 1689
- Maxitrol Ophthalmic Ointment and Suspension .... ⊚ 222
- TobraDex Ophthalmic Suspension and Ointment 469

Dexamethasone Acetate (The plasma ACTH response to corticorelin injection is inhibited or blunted in normal subjects pretreated with dexamethasone). Products include:
- Dalalone D.P. Injectable 1009
- Decadron-LA Sterile Suspension 1687

Dexamethasone Sodium Phosphate (The plasma ACTH response to corticorelin injection is inhibited or blunted in normal subjects pretreated with dexamethasone). Products include:
- Decadron Phosphate Injection 1680
- Decadron Phosphate Sterile Ophthalmic Ointment 1684
- Decadron Phosphate Sterile Ophthalmic Solution 1685
- Decadron Phosphate Topical Cream 1686
- Decadron Phosphate with Xylocaine Injection, Sterile 1683
- Dexacort Phosphate in Respihaler .. 1606
- Dexacort Phosphate in Turbinaire .. 1607
- NeoDecadron Sterile Ophthalmic Ointment 1755
- NeoDecadron Sterile Ophthalmic Solution 1756
- NeoDecadron Topical Cream 1757

Heparin Sodium (A possible interaction between corticorelin and heparin may be associated with a major hypotensive reaction; use of heparin to maintain i.v. canula patency during corticorelin test is not recommended). Products include:
- Heparin Lock Flush Solution 2831
- Heparin Sodium Injection 2832
- Heparin Sodium Vials 1486

ACTIFED ALLERGY DAYTIME/NIGHTTIME CAPLETS
(Diphenhydramine Hydrochloride, Pseudoephedrine Hydrochloride) .... ■□ 808
May interact with monoamine oxidase inhibitors, hypnotics and sedatives, tranquilizers, and certain other agents. Compounds in these categories include:

Alprazolam (May increase drowsiness effect). Products include:
- Xanax Tablets 2115

Buspirone Hydrochloride (May increase drowsiness effect). Products include:
- BuSpar Tablets 738

Chlordiazepoxide (May increase drowsiness effect). Products include:
- Limbitrol 2333

Chlordiazepoxide Hydrochloride (May increase drowsiness effect). Products include:
- Librax Capsules 2330
- Librium Capsules 2331
- Librium Injectable 2332

Chlorpromazine (May increase drowsiness effect). Products include:
- Thorazine Suppositories 2701

Chlorpromazine Hydrochloride (May increase drowsiness effect). Products include:
- Thorazine 2701

Chlorprothixene (May increase drowsiness effect).
No products indexed under this heading.

Chlorprothixene Hydrochloride (May increase drowsiness effect).
No products indexed under this heading.

Clorazepate Dipotassium (May increase drowsiness effect). Products include:
- Tranxene 459

Diazepam (May increase drowsiness effect). Products include:
- Dizac (diazepam injectable emulsion) CIV 1862
- Valium Injectable 2336
- Valium Tablets 2335

Droperidol (May increase drowsiness effect). Products include:
- Inapsine Injection 462

Estazolam (May increase drowsiness effect). Products include:
- ProSom Tablets 457

Ethchlorvynol (May increase drowsiness effect). Products include:
- Placidyl Capsules 456

Ethinamate (May increase drowsiness effect).
No products indexed under this heading.

Fluphenazine Decanoate (May increase drowsiness effect). Products include:
- Prolixin Decanoate 510

Fluphenazine Enanthate (May increase drowsiness effect). Products include:
- Prolixin Enanthate 510

Fluphenazine Hydrochloride (May increase drowsiness effect). Products include:
- Prolixin 510

Flurazepam Hydrochloride (May increase drowsiness effect). Products include:
- Dalmane Capsules 2329

Furazolidone (Concurrent and/or sequential use is not recommended). Products include:
- Furoxone 2221

Glutethimide (May increase drowsiness effect).
No products indexed under this heading.

Haloperidol (May increase drowsiness effect). Products include:
- Haldol Injection, Tablets and Concentrate 1585

Haloperidol Decanoate (May increase drowsiness effect). Products include:
- Haldol Decanoate 1587

Hydroxyzine Hydrochloride (May increase drowsiness effect). Products include:
- Atarax Tablets & Syrup 1992
- Marax Tablets & DF Syrup 2015
- Vistaril Intramuscular Solution 2042

Isocarboxazid (Concurrent and/or sequential use is not recommended).
No products indexed under this heading.

Lorazepam (May increase drowsiness effect). Products include:
- Ativan Injection 2805
- Ativan Tablets 2807

Loxapine Hydrochloride (May increase drowsiness effect). Products include:
- Loxitane 1426

Loxapine Succinate (May increase drowsiness effect). Products include:
- Loxitane Capsules 1426

Meprobamate (May increase drowsiness effect). Products include:
- Miltown Tablets 2780
- PMB 200 and PMB 400 2890

Mesoridazine Besylate (May increase drowsiness effect). Products include:
- Serentil 689

Midazolam Hydrochloride (May increase drowsiness effect). Products include:
- Versed Injection 2324

Molindone Hydrochloride (May increase drowsiness effect). Products include:
- Moban Tablets and Concentrate 1036

Oxazepam (May increase drowsiness effect). Products include:
- Serax Capsules 2916
- Serax Tablets 2916

Perphenazine (May increase drowsiness effect). Products include:
- Etrafon 2495
- Triavil Tablets 1800
- Trilafon 2532

Phenelzine Sulfate (Concurrent and/or sequential use is not recommended). Products include:
- Nardil 1977

Prazepam (May increase drowsiness effect).
No products indexed under this heading.

Prochlorperazine (May increase drowsiness effect). Products include:
- Compazine 2644

Promethazine Hydrochloride (May increase drowsiness effect). Products include:
- Mepergan Injection 2859
- Phenergan with Codeine 2883
- Phenergan with Dextromethorphan 2885
- Phenergan Injection 2880
- Phenergan Suppositories 2882
- Phenergan Syrup 2881
- Phenergan Tablets 2882
- Phenergan VC 2886
- Phenergan VC with Codeine 2888

Propofol (May increase drowsiness effect). Products include:
- Diprivan Injectable Emulsion 2939

Quazepam (May increase drowsiness effect). Products include:
- Doral Tablets 2773

Secobarbital Sodium (May increase drowsiness effect). Products include:
- Seconal Sodium Pulvules 1529

Selegiline Hydrochloride (Concurrent and/or sequential use is not recommended). Products include:
- Eldepryl Capsules 2729

Temazepam (May increase drowsiness effect). Products include:
- Restoril Capsules 2413

Thioridazine Hydrochloride (May increase drowsiness effect). Products include:
- Mellaril 2398

Thiothixene (May increase drowsiness effect). Products include:
- Navane Capsules and Concentrate 2018
- Navane Intramuscular 2019

Tranylcypromine Sulfate (Concurrent and/or sequential use is not recommended). Products include:
- Parnate Tablets 2679

Triazolam (May increase drowsiness effect). Products include:
- Halcion Tablets 2093

Trifluoperazine Hydrochloride (May increase drowsiness effect). Products include:
- Stelazine 2692

Zolpidem Tartrate (May increase drowsiness effect). Products include:
- Ambien Tablets 2559

Food Interactions

Alcohol (May increase drowsiness effect).

ACTIFED COLD & ALLERGY TABLETS
(Pseudoephedrine Hydrochloride, Triprolidine Hydrochloride) .... ■□ 807
May interact with monoamine oxidase inhibitors, hypnotics and sedatives, tranquilizers, and certain other agents. Compounds in these categories include:

Alprazolam (May increase drowsiness effect). Products include:
- Xanax Tablets 2115

Buspirone Hydrochloride (May increase drowsiness effect). Products include:
- BuSpar Tablets 738

Chlordiazepoxide (May increase drowsiness effect). Products include:
- Limbitrol 2333

Chlordiazepoxide Hydrochloride (May increase drowsiness effect). Products include:
- Librax Capsules 2330
- Librium Capsules 2331
- Librium Injectable 2332

Chlorpromazine (May increase drowsiness effect). Products include:
- Thorazine Suppositories 2701

Chlorpromazine Hydrochloride (May increase drowsiness effect). Products include:
- Thorazine 2701

Chlorprothixene (May increase drowsiness effect).
No products indexed under this heading.

Chlorprothixene Hydrochloride (May increase drowsiness effect).
No products indexed under this heading.

Clorazepate Dipotassium (May increase drowsiness effect). Products include:
- Tranxene 459

Diazepam (May increase drowsiness effect). Products include:
- Dizac (diazepam injectable emulsion) CIV 1862
- Valium Injectable 2336
- Valium Tablets 2335

Droperidol (May increase drowsiness effect). Products include:
- Inapsine Injection 462

Estazolam (May increase drowsiness effect). Products include:
- ProSom Tablets 457

Ethchlorvynol (May increase drowsiness effect). Products include:
- Placidyl Capsules 456

Ethinamate (May increase drowsiness effect).
No products indexed under this heading.

Fluphenazine Decanoate (May increase drowsiness effect). Products include:
- Prolixin Decanoate 510

Fluphenazine Enanthate (May increase drowsiness effect). Products include:
- Prolixin Enanthate 510

Fluphenazine Hydrochloride (May increase drowsiness effect). Products include:
- Prolixin 510

Flurazepam Hydrochloride (May increase drowsiness effect). Products include:
- Dalmane Capsules 2329

Furazolidone (Concurrent and/or sequential use is not recommended). Products include:
- Furoxone 2221

Glutethimide (May increase drowsiness effect).
No products indexed under this heading.

(■□ Described in PDR For Nonprescription Drugs)   (⊚ Described in PDR For Ophthalmology)

Haloperidol (May increase drowsiness effect). Products include:
Haldol Injection, Tablets and Concentrate 1585
Haloperidol Decanoate (May increase drowsiness effect). Products include:
Haldol Decanoate 1587
Hydroxyzine Hydrochloride (May increase drowsiness effect). Products include:
Atarax Tablets & Syrup 1992
Marax Tablets & DF Syrup 2015
Vistaril Intramuscular Solution 2042
Isocarboxazid (Concurrent and/or sequential use is not recommended).
No products indexed under this heading.
Lorazepam (May increase drowsiness effect). Products include:
Ativan Injection 2805
Ativan Tablets 2807
Loxapine Hydrochloride (May increase drowsiness effect). Products include:
Loxitane 1426
Loxapine Succinate (May increase drowsiness effect). Products include:
Loxitane Capsules 1426
Meprobamate (May increase drowsiness effect). Products include:
Miltown Tablets 2780
PMB 200 and PMB 400 2890
Mesoridazine Besylate (May increase drowsiness effect). Products include:
Serentil 689
Midazolam Hydrochloride (May increase drowsiness effect). Products include:
Versed Injection 2324
Molindone Hydrochloride (May increase drowsiness effect). Products include:
Moban Tablets and Concentrate 1036
Oxazepam (May increase drowsiness effect). Products include:
Serax Capsules 2916
Serax Tablets 2916
Perphenazine (May increase drowsiness effect). Products include:
Etrafon 2495
Triavil Tablets 1800
Trilafon 2532
Phenelzine Sulfate (Concurrent and/or sequential use is not recommended). Products include:
Nardil 1977
Prazepam (May increase drowsiness effect).
No products indexed under this heading.
Prochlorperazine (May increase drowsiness effect). Products include:
Compazine 2644
Promethazine Hydrochloride (May increase drowsiness effect). Products include:
Mepergan Injection 2859
Phenergan with Codeine 2883
Phenergan with Dextromethorphan 2885
Phenergan Injection 2880
Phenergan Suppositories 2882
Phenergan Syrup 2881
Phenergan Tablets 2882
Phenergan VC 2886
Phenergan VC with Codeine 2888
Propofol (May increase drowsiness effect). Products include:
Diprivan Injectable Emulsion 2939
Quazepam (May increase drowsiness effect). Products include:
Doral Tablets 2773
Secobarbital Sodium (May increase drowsiness effect). Products include:
Seconal Sodium Pulvules 1529

Selegiline Hydrochloride (Concurrent and/or sequential use is not recommended). Products include:
Eldepryl Capsules 2729
Temazepam (May increase drowsiness effect). Products include:
Restoril Capsules 2413
Thioridazine Hydrochloride (May increase drowsiness effect). Products include:
Mellaril 2398
Thiothixene (May increase drowsiness effect). Products include:
Navane Capsules and Concentrate 2018
Navane Intramuscular 2019
Tranylcypromine Sulfate (Concurrent and/or sequential use is not recommended). Products include:
Parnate Tablets 2679
Triazolam (May increase drowsiness effect). Products include:
Halcion Tablets 2093
Trifluoperazine Hydrochloride (May increase drowsiness effect). Products include:
Stelazine 2692
Zolpidem Tartrate (May increase drowsiness effect). Products include:
Ambien Tablets 2559

Food Interactions
Alcohol (May increase drowsiness effect).

ACTIFED COLD & SINUS CAPLETS AND TABLETS
(Acetaminophen, Pseudoephedrine Hydrochloride, Triprolidine Hydrochloride) 808
May interact with monoamine oxidase inhibitors, hypnotics and sedatives, tranquilizers, and certain other agents. Compounds in these categories include:

Alprazolam (May increase drowsiness effect). Products include:
Xanax Tablets 2115
Buspirone Hydrochloride (May increase drowsiness effect). Products include:
BuSpar Tablets 738
Chlordiazepoxide (May increase drowsiness effect). Products include:
Limbitrol 2333
Chlordiazepoxide Hydrochloride (May increase drowsiness effect). Products include:
Librax Capsules 2330
Librium Capsules 2331
Librium Injectable 2332
Chlorpromazine (May increase drowsiness effect). Products include:
Thorazine Suppositories 2701
Chlorpromazine Hydrochloride (May increase drowsiness effect). Products include:
Thorazine 2701
Chlorprothixene (May increase drowsiness effect).
No products indexed under this heading.
Chlorprothixene Hydrochloride (May increase drowsiness effect).
No products indexed under this heading.
Clorazepate Dipotassium (May increase drowsiness effect). Products include:
Tranxene 459
Diazepam (May increase drowsiness effect). Products include:
Dizac (diazepam injectable emulsion) CIV 1862
Valium Injectable 2336
Valium Tablets 2335
Droperidol (May increase drowsiness effect). Products include:
Inapsine Injection 462

Estazolam (May increase drowsiness effect). Products include:
ProSom Tablets 457
Ethchlorvynol (May increase drowsiness effect). Products include:
Placidyl Capsules 456
Ethinamate (May increase drowsiness effect).
No products indexed under this heading.
Fluphenazine Decanoate (May increase drowsiness effect). Products include:
Prolixin Decanoate 510
Fluphenazine Enanthate (May increase drowsiness effect). Products include:
Prolixin Enanthate 510
Fluphenazine Hydrochloride (May increase drowsiness effect). Products include:
Prolixin 510
Flurazepam Hydrochloride (May increase drowsiness effect). Products include:
Dalmane Capsules 2329
Furazolidone (Concurrent and/or sequential use is not recommended). Products include:
Furoxone 2221
Glutethimide (May increase drowsiness effect).
No products indexed under this heading.
Haloperidol (May increase drowsiness effect). Products include:
Haldol Injection, Tablets and Concentrate 1585
Haloperidol Decanoate (May increase drowsiness effect). Products include:
Haldol Decanoate 1587
Hydroxyzine Hydrochloride (May increase drowsiness effect). Products include:
Atarax Tablets & Syrup 1992
Marax Tablets & DF Syrup 2015
Vistaril Intramuscular Solution 2042
Isocarboxazid (Concurrent and/or sequential use is not recommended).
No products indexed under this heading.
Lorazepam (May increase drowsiness effect). Products include:
Ativan Injection 2805
Ativan Tablets 2807
Loxapine Hydrochloride (May increase drowsiness effect). Products include:
Loxitane 1426
Loxapine Succinate (May increase drowsiness effect). Products include:
Loxitane Capsules 1426
Meprobamate (May increase drowsiness effect). Products include:
Miltown Tablets 2780
PMB 200 and PMB 400 2890
Mesoridazine Besylate (May increase drowsiness effect). Products include:
Serentil 689
Midazolam Hydrochloride (May increase drowsiness effect). Products include:
Versed Injection 2324
Molindone Hydrochloride (May increase drowsiness effect). Products include:
Moban Tablets and Concentrate 1036
Oxazepam (May increase drowsiness effect). Products include:
Serax Capsules 2916
Serax Tablets 2916
Perphenazine (May increase drowsiness effect). Products include:
Etrafon 2495

Triavil Tablets 1800
Trilafon 2532
Phenelzine Sulfate (Concurrent and/or sequential use is not recommended). Products include:
Nardil 1977
Prazepam (May increase drowsiness effect).
No products indexed under this heading.
Prochlorperazine (May increase drowsiness effect). Products include:
Compazine 2644
Promethazine Hydrochloride (May increase drowsiness effect). Products include:
Mepergan Injection 2859
Phenergan with Codeine 2883
Phenergan with Dextromethorphan 2885
Phenergan Injection 2880
Phenergan Suppositories 2882
Phenergan Syrup 2881
Phenergan Tablets 2882
Phenergan VC 2886
Phenergan VC with Codeine 2888
Propofol (May increase drowsiness effect). Products include:
Diprivan Injectable Emulsion 2939
Quazepam (May increase drowsiness effect). Products include:
Doral Tablets 2773
Secobarbital Sodium (May increase drowsiness effect). Products include:
Seconal Sodium Pulvules 1529
Selegiline Hydrochloride (Concurrent and/or sequential use is not recommended). Products include:
Eldepryl Capsules 2729
Temazepam (May increase drowsiness effect). Products include:
Restoril Capsules 2413
Thioridazine Hydrochloride (May increase drowsiness effect). Products include:
Mellaril 2398
Thiothixene (May increase drowsiness effect). Products include:
Navane Capsules and Concentrate 2018
Navane Intramuscular 2019
Tranylcypromine Sulfate (Concurrent and/or sequential use is not recommended). Products include:
Parnate Tablets 2679
Triazolam (May increase drowsiness effect). Products include:
Halcion Tablets 2093
Trifluoperazine Hydrochloride (May increase drowsiness effect). Products include:
Stelazine 2692
Zolpidem Tartrate (May increase drowsiness effect). Products include:
Ambien Tablets 2559

Food Interactions
Alcohol (May increase drowsiness effect).

ACTIFED SINUS DAYTIME/NIGHTTIME TABLETS AND CAPLETS
(Acetaminophen, Diphenhydramine Hydrochloride, Pseudoephedrine Hydrochloride) 809
May interact with hypnotics and sedatives, monoamine oxidase inhibitors, tranquilizers, and certain other agents. Compounds in these categories include:

Alprazolam (May increase drowsiness effect). Products include:
Xanax Tablets 2115
Buspirone Hydrochloride (May increase drowsiness effect). Products include:
BuSpar Tablets 738

IMPORTANT NOTE: Always consult each drug listing in the patient's regimen for possible interactions.

Actifed Sinus Interactions Index 10

Chlordiazepoxide (May increase drowsiness effect). Products include:
Limbitrol 2333

Chlordiazepoxide Hydrochloride (May increase drowsiness effect). Products include:
Librax Capsules 2330
Librium Capsules 2331
Librium Injectable 2332

Chlorpromazine (May increase drowsiness effect). Products include:
Thorazine Suppositories 2701

Chlorpromazine Hydrochloride (May increase drowsiness effect). Products include:
Thorazine 2701

Chlorprothixene (May increase drowsiness effect).
No products indexed under this heading.

Chlorprothixene Hydrochloride (May increase drowsiness effect).
No products indexed under this heading.

Clorazepate Dipotassium (May increase drowsiness effect). Products include:
Tranxene 459

Diazepam (May increase drowsiness effect). Products include:
Dizac (diazepam injectable emulsion) CIV 1862
Valium Injectable 2336
Valium Tablets 2335

Droperidol (May increase drowsiness effect). Products include:
Inapsine Injection 462

Estazolam (May increase drowsiness effect). Products include:
ProSom Tablets 457

Ethchlorvynol (May increase drowsiness effect). Products include:
Placidyl Capsules 456

Ethinamate (May increase drowsiness effect).
No products indexed under this heading.

Fluphenazine Decanoate (May increase drowsiness effect). Products include:
Prolixin Decanoate 510

Fluphenazine Enanthate (May increase drowsiness effect). Products include:
Prolixin Enanthate 510

Fluphenazine Hydrochloride (May increase drowsiness effect). Products include:
Prolixin 510

Flurazepam Hydrochloride (May increase drowsiness effect). Products include:
Dalmane Capsules 2329

Furazolidone (Concurrent and/or sequential use is not recommended). Products include:
Furoxone 2221

Glutethimide (May increase drowsiness effect).
No products indexed under this heading.

Haloperidol (May increase drowsiness effect). Products include:
Haldol Injection, Tablets and Concentrate 1585

Haloperidol Decanoate (May increase drowsiness effect). Products include:
Haldol Decanoate 1587

Hydroxyzine Hydrochloride (May increase drowsiness effect). Products include:
Atarax Tablets & Syrup 1992
Marax Tablets & DF Syrup 2015
Vistaril Intramuscular Solution 2042

Isocarboxazid (Concurrent and/or sequential use is not recommended).
No products indexed under this heading.

Lorazepam (May increase drowsiness effect). Products include:
Ativan Injection 2805
Ativan Tablets 2807

Loxapine Hydrochloride (May increase drowsiness effect). Products include:
Loxitane 1426

Loxapine Succinate (May increase drowsiness effect). Products include:
Loxitane Capsules 1426

Meprobamate (May increase drowsiness effect). Products include:
Miltown Tablets 2780
PMB 200 and PMB 400 2890

Mesoridazine Besylate (May increase drowsiness effect). Products include:
Serentil 689

Midazolam Hydrochloride (May increase drowsiness effect). Products include:
Versed Injection 2324

Molindone Hydrochloride (May increase drowsiness effect). Products include:
Moban Tablets and Concentrate 1036

Oxazepam (May increase drowsiness effect). Products include:
Serax Capsules 2916
Serax Tablets 2916

Perphenazine (May increase drowsiness effect). Products include:
Etrafon 2495
Triavil Tablets 1800
Trilafon 2532

Phenelzine Sulfate (Concurrent and/or sequential use is not recommended). Products include:
Nardil 1977

Prazepam (May increase drowsiness effect).
No products indexed under this heading.

Prochlorperazine (May increase drowsiness effect). Products include:
Compazine 2644

Promethazine Hydrochloride (May increase drowsiness effect). Products include:
Mepergan Injection 2859
Phenergan with Codeine 2883
Phenergan with Dextromethorphan 2885
Phenergan Injection 2880
Phenergan Suppositories 2882
Phenergan Syrup 2881
Phenergan Tablets 2882
Phenergan VC 2886
Phenergan VC with Codeine 2888

Propofol (May increase drowsiness effect). Products include:
Diprivan Injectable Emulsion 2939

Quazepam (May increase drowsiness effect). Products include:
Doral Tablets 2773

Secobarbital Sodium (May increase drowsiness effect). Products include:
Seconal Sodium Pulvules 1529

Selegiline Hydrochloride (Concurrent and/or sequential use is not recommended). Products include:
Eldepryl Capsules 2729

Temazepam (May increase drowsiness effect). Products include:
Restoril Capsules 2413

Thioridazine Hydrochloride (May increase drowsiness effect). Products include:
Mellaril 2398

Thiothixene (May increase drowsiness effect). Products include:
Navane Capsules and Concentrate 2018
Navane Intramuscular 2019

Tranylcypromine Sulfate (Concurrent and/or sequential use is not recommended). Products include:
Parnate Tablets 2679

Triazolam (May increase drowsiness effect). Products include:
Halcion Tablets 2093

Trifluoperazine Hydrochloride (May increase drowsiness effect). Products include:
Stelazine 2692

Zolpidem Tartrate (May increase drowsiness effect). Products include:
Ambien Tablets 2559

Food Interactions

Alcohol (May increase drowsiness effect).

ACTIGALL CAPSULES

(Ursodiol) 818

May interact with oral contraceptives, bile acid sequestering agents, lipid-lowering drugs, estrogens, and certain other agents. Compounds in these categories include:

Aluminum Carbonate (Aluminum-based antacids have been shown to absorb bile acids in vitro and may be expected to interfere with the action of ursodiol). Products include:
Basaljel Capsules 2810
Basaljel Suspension 2810
Basaljel Tablets 2810

Aluminum Hydroxide (Aluminum-based antacids have been shown to absorb bile acids in vitro and may be expected to interfere with the action of ursodiol). Products include:
ALternaGEL Liquid 1358
Maximum Strength Ascriptin ▣ 650
Cama Arthritis Pain Reliever ▣ 748
Gaviscon Extra Strength Relief Formula Antacid Tablets ▣ 778
Gaviscon Extra Strength Relief Formula Liquid Antacid ▣ 779
Gaviscon Liquid Antacid ▣ 779
Gelusil Antacid-Anti-gas Liquid ▣ 819
Gelusil Antacid-Anti-gas Tablets ▣ 819
Maalox Antacid/Anti-Gas Tablets 889
Maalox Heartburn Relief Suspension ▣ 658
Maalox Antacid Liquid 888
Extra Strength Maalox Antacid/Anti-Gas Liquid and Tablets 888
Mylanta 1359
Tempo Soft Antacid ▣ 799

Aluminum Hydroxide Gel (Aluminum-based antacids have been shown to absorb bile acids in vitro and may be expected to interfere with the action of ursodiol). Products include:
ALternaGEL Liquid ▣ 675
Aludrox Oral Suspension ▣ 850
Amphojel Suspension 2802
Amphojel Suspension without Flavor 2802
Amphojel Tablets 2802
Ascriptin ▣ 650
Gaviscon Antacid Tablets ▣ 778
Gaviscon-2 Antacid Tablets ▣ 779
Mylanta Liquid ▣ 676
Mylanta Double Strength Liquid ▣ 676
Nephrox Suspension ▣ 671

Chlorotrianisene (Estrogens increase hepatic cholesterol secretion and encourage cholesterol gallstone formation and hence may counteract the effectiveness of ursodiol).
No products indexed under this heading.

Cholestyramine (Reduces absorption of ursodiol and may interfere with its action). Products include:
Questran 774

Clofibrate (Clofibrate increases hepatic cholesterol secretion and encourages cholesterol gallstone formation and hence counteracts the effectiveness of ursodiol). Products include:
Atromid-S Capsules 2808

Colestipol Hydrochloride (Reduces absorption of ursodiol and may interfere with its action). Products include:
Colestid 2073

Desogestrel (Oral contraceptives increase hepatic cholesterol secretion and encourage cholesterol gallstone formation and hence may counteract the effectiveness of ursodiol). Products include:
Desogen Tablets 1867
Ortho-Cept 1907

Dienestrol (Estrogens increase hepatic cholesterol secretion and encourage cholesterol gallstone formation and hence may counteract the effectiveness of ursodiol). Products include:
Ortho Dienestrol Cream 1922

Diethylstilbestrol (Estrogens increase hepatic cholesterol secretion and encourage cholesterol gallstone formation and hence may counteract the effectiveness of ursodiol). Products include:
Diethylstilbestrol Tablets 1477

Estradiol (Estrogens increase hepatic cholesterol secretion and encourage cholesterol gallstone formation and hence may counteract the effectiveness of ursodiol). Products include:
Climara Transdermal System 640
Estrace Cream and Tablets 751
Estraderm Transdermal System 842
Estring Vaginal Ring 2086
Vivelle Transdermal System 880

Estrogens, Conjugated (Estrogens increase hepatic cholesterol secretion and encourage cholesterol gallstone formation and hence may counteract the effectiveness of ursodiol). Products include:
PMB 200 and PMB 400 2890
Premarin Intravenous 2893
Premarin Tablets 2896
Premarin Vaginal Cream 2898
Premphase 2900
Prempro 2905

Estrogens, Esterified (Estrogens increase hepatic cholesterol secretion and encourage cholesterol gallstone formation and hence may counteract the effectiveness of ursodiol). Products include:
ESTRATAB Tablets (0.3, 0.625, 1.25, 2.5 mg) 2715
Estratest 2718
Menest Tablets 2671

Estropipate (Estrogens increase hepatic cholesterol secretion and encourage cholesterol gallstone formation and hence may counteract the effectiveness of ursodiol). Products include:
Ogen Tablets 2103
Ogen Vaginal Cream 2106
Ortho-Est 1925

Ethinyl Estradiol (Estrogens increase hepatic cholesterol secretion and encourage cholesterol gallstone formation and hence may counteract the effectiveness of ursodiol). Products include:
Brevicon 2563
Demulen 2580
Desogen Tablets 1867
Levlen/Tri-Levlen 646
Lo/Ovral Tablets 2852
Lo/Ovral-28 Tablets 2857
Modicon 1928
Nordette-21 Tablets 2863

11 **Interactions Index** **Activase**

Nordette-28 Tablets 2866
Norinyl 2563
Ortho-Cept 1907
Ortho-Cyclen/Ortho-Tri-Cyclen 1914
Ortho-Novum 1928
Ortho-Cyclen/Ortho Tri-Cyclen 1914
Ovcon 765
Ovral Tablets 2877
Ovral-28 Tablets 2878
Levlen/Tri-Levlen 646
Tri-Norinyl 2607
Triphasil-21 Tablets 2919
Triphasil-28 Tablets 2924

Ethynodiol Diacetate (Oral contraceptives increase hepatic cholesterol secretion and encourage cholesterol gallstone formation and hence may counteract the effectiveness of ursodiol). Products include:
Demulen 2580

Fluvastatin Sodium (Lipid-lowering drugs may increase hepatic cholesterol secretion and may encourage cholesterol gallstone formation and hence may counteract the effectiveness of ursodiol). Products include:
Lescol Capsules 2395

Gemfibrozil (Lipid-lowering drugs may increase hepatic cholesterol secretion and may encourage cholesterol gallstone formation and hence may counteract the effectiveness of ursodiol). Products include:
Lopid Tablets 1974

Levonorgestrel (Oral contraceptives increase hepatic cholesterol secretion and encourage cholesterol gallstone formation and hence may counteract the effectiveness of ursodiol). Products include:
Levlen/Tri-Levlen 646
Nordette-21 Tablets 2863
Nordette-28 Tablets 2866
Norplant System 2868
Levlen/Tri-Levlen 646
Triphasil-21 Tablets 2919
Triphasil-28 Tablets 2924

Lovastatin (Lipid-lowering drugs may increase hepatic cholesterol secretion and may encourage cholesterol gallstone formation and hence may counteract the effectiveness of ursodiol). Products include:
Mevacor Tablets 1742

Mestranol (Oral contraceptives increase hepatic cholesterol secretion and encourage cholesterol gallstone formation and hence may counteract the effectiveness of ursodiol). Products include:
Norinyl 2563
Ortho-Novum 1928

Norethindrone (Oral contraceptives increase hepatic cholesterol secretion and encourage cholesterol gallstone formation and hence may counteract the effectiveness of ursodiol). Products include:
Brevicon 2563
Micronor Tablets 1903
Modicon 1928
Norinyl 2563
Nor-Q D Tablets 2598
Ortho-Novum 1928
Ovcon 765
Tri-Norinyl 2607

Norethynodrel (Oral contraceptives increase hepatic cholesterol secretion and encourage cholesterol gallstone formation and hence may counteract the effectiveness of ursodiol).
No products indexed under this heading.

Norgestimate (Oral contraceptives increase hepatic cholesterol secretion and encourage cholesterol gallstone formation and hence may counteract the effectiveness of ursodiol). Products include:
Ortho-Cyclen/Ortho-Tri-Cyclen 1914
Ortho-Cyclen/Ortho Tri-Cyclen 1914

Norgestrel (Oral contraceptives increase hepatic cholesterol secretion and encourage cholesterol gallstone formation and hence may counteract the effectiveness of ursodiol). Products include:
Lo/Ovral Tablets 2852
Lo/Ovral-28 Tablets 2857
Ovral Tablets 2877
Ovral-28 Tablets 2878
Ovrette Tablets 2878

Polyestradiol Phosphate (Estrogens increase hepatic cholesterol secretion and encourage cholesterol gallstone formation and hence may counteract the effectiveness of ursodiol).
No products indexed under this heading.

Pravastatin Sodium (Lipid-lowering drugs may increase hepatic cholesterol secretion and may encourage cholesterol gallstone formation and hence may counteract the effectiveness of ursodiol). Products include:
Pravachol Tablets 770

Probucol (Lipid-lowering drugs may increase hepatic cholesterol secretion and may encourage cholesterol gallstone formation and hence may counteract the effectiveness of ursodiol).
No products indexed under this heading.

Quinestrol (Estrogens increase hepatic cholesterol secretion and encourage cholesterol gallstone formation and hence may counteract the effectiveness of ursodiol).
No products indexed under this heading.

Simvastatin (Lipid-lowering drugs may increase hepatic cholesterol secretion and may encourage cholesterol gallstone formation and hence may counteract the effectiveness of ursodiol). Products include:
Zocor Tablets 1821

ACTIMMUNE

(Interferon Gamma-1B) 1043
May interact with:

Bone Marrow Depressants, unspecified (Caution should be exercised when administering with other potentially myelosuppressive agents).

ACTIVASE

(Alteplase, Recombinant) 1045
May interact with oral anticoagulants, platelet inhibitors, and certain other agents. Compounds in these categories include:

Aspirin (Increased risk of bleeding). Products include:
Alka-Seltzer Cherry Effervescent Antacid and Pain Reliever ND 609
Alka-Seltzer Extra Strength Effervescent Antacid and Pain Reliever ND 609
Alka-Seltzer Lemon Lime Effervescent Antacid and Pain Reliever ND 609
Alka-Seltzer Original Effervescent Antacid and Pain Reliever ND 609
Alka-Seltzer Plus ND 611
Alka-Seltzer Plus Sinus Medicine ND 611
Ascriptin ND 650
Arthritis Strength BC Powder ND 631
BC Cold Powder Multi-Symptom Formula (Cold-Sinus-Allergy) ND 631
BC Cold Powder Non-Drowsy Formula (Cold-Sinus) ND 631
BC Powder ND 631
Genuine Bayer Aspirin Tablets & Caplets ND 618
Extra Strength Bayer Arthritis Pain Regimen Formula ND 615
Extra Strength Bayer Aspirin Caplets & Tablets ND 617
Extended-Release Bayer 8-Hour Aspirin ND 616
Extra Strength Bayer Plus Aspirin Caplets ND 617
Extra Strength Bayer PM Aspirin Plus Sleep Aid ND 617
Aspirin Regimen Bayer 81 mg Tablets with Calcium ND 615
Aspirin Regimen Bayer Adult Low Strength 81 mg Tablets ND 613
Aspirin Regimen Bayer Children's Chewable Aspirin ND 616
Aspirin Regimen Bayer Regular Strength 325 mg Caplets ND 613
Bufferin Analgesic Tablets ND 636
Arthritis Strength Bufferin Analgesic Caplets ND 637
Extra Strength Bufferin Analgesic Tablets ND 637
Cama Arthritis Pain Reliever ND 748
Darvon Compound-65 Pulvules 1475
Easprin 1971
Ecotrin 2625
Ecotrin Enteric Coated Aspirin Maximum Strength Tablets and Caplets ND 775
Ecotrin Enteric Coated Aspirin Regular Strength Tablets 2625
Empirin Aspirin Tablets ND 818
Excedrin Extra-Strength Analgesic Tablets, Caplets, and Geltabs 734
Fiorinal Capsules 2388
Fiorinal with Codeine Capsules 2390
Fiorinal Tablets 2388
Goody's Extra Strength Headache Powders ND 632
Goody's Extra Strength Pain Relief Tablets ND 632
Halfprin Tablets 1413
Norgesic 1554
Percodan Tablets 955
Percodan-Demi Tablets 956
Robaxisal Tablets 2246
Soma Compound w/Codeine Tablets 2784
Soma Compound Tablets 2783
St. Joseph Adult Chewable Aspirin (81 mg.) ND 768
Talwin Compound 2466
Vanquish Analgesic Caplets ND 627

Azlocillin Sodium (Increased risk of bleeding).
No products indexed under this heading.

Carbenicillin Indanyl Sodium (Increased risk of bleeding). Products include:
Geocillin Tablets 2009

Choline Magnesium Trisalicylate (Increased risk of bleeding). Products include:
Trilisate 2155

Diclofenac Potassium (Increased risk of bleeding). Products include:
Cataflam Tablets 833

Diclofenac Sodium (Increased risk of bleeding). Products include:
Voltaren Ophthalmic Sterile Ophthalmic Solution ◎ 264
Cataflam/Voltaren/Voltaren-XR 833

Dicumarol (Increased risk of bleeding).
No products indexed under this heading.

Diflunisal (Increased risk of bleeding). Products include:
Dolobid Tablets 1695

Dipyridamole (Increased risk of bleeding). Products include:
Persantine Tablets 686

Fenoprofen Calcium (Increased risk of bleeding). Products include:
Nalfon 200 Pulvules & Nalfon Tablets 933

Flurbiprofen (Increased risk of bleeding).
No products indexed under this heading.

Heparin Calcium (Increased risk of bleeding).
No products indexed under this heading.

Heparin Sodium (Increased risk of bleeding). Products include:
Heparin Lock Flush Solution 2831
Heparin Sodium Injection 2832
Heparin Sodium Vials 1486

Ibuprofen (Increased risk of bleeding). Products include:
Advil Cold and Sinus Caplets and Tablets ND 837
Advil Ibuprofen Tablets, Caplets and Gel Caplets ND 836
Children's Motrin Ibuprofen Oral Suspension 1558
IBU Tablets 1389
Ibuprohm ND 713
Motrin IB Caplets, Tablets, and Gelcaps ND 802
Motrin Ibuprofen Suspension, Oral Drops, Chewable Tablets, Caplets 1563
Nuprin Ibuprofen/Analgesic Tablets & Caplets ND 645
Vicks DayQuil SINUS Pressure & PAIN Relief with IBUPROFEN ND 735

Indomethacin (Increased risk of bleeding). Products include:
Indocin 1723

Indomethacin Sodium Trihydrate (Increased risk of bleeding). Products include:
Indocin I.V. 1727

Ketoprofen (Increased risk of bleeding). Products include:
Actron Caplets and Tablets ND 608
Orudis Capsules 2874
Orudis KT ND 842
Oruvail Capsules 2874

Magnesium Salicylate (Increased risk of bleeding). Products include:
Backache Caplets ND 635
Doan's Extra-Strength Analgesic ND 653
Extra Strength Doan's P.M. ND 653
Doan's Regular Strength Analgesic ND 654
Mobigesic Tablets ND 607

Meclofenamate Sodium (Increased risk of bleeding).
No products indexed under this heading.

Mefenamic Acid (Increased risk of bleeding). Products include:
Ponstel 1982

Mezlocillin Sodium (Increased risk of bleeding). Products include:
Mezlin 594
Mezlin Pharmacy Bulk Package 597

Nafcillin Sodium (Increased risk of bleeding).
No products indexed under this heading.

Naproxen (Increased risk of bleeding). Products include:
Anaprox/Naprosyn 2277

Naproxen Sodium (Increased risk of bleeding). Products include:
Aleve 2124
Anaprox/Naprosyn 2277
Naprelan Tablets 2861

Penicillin G Benzathine (Increased risk of bleeding). Products include:
Bicillin C-R Injection 2810
Bicillin C-R 900/300 Injection 2812
Bicillin L-A Injection 2813

Penicillin G Procaine (Increased risk of bleeding). Products include:
Bicillin C-R Injection 2810
Bicillin C-R 900/300 Injection 2812

Phenylbutazone (Increased risk of bleeding).
No products indexed under this heading.

IMPORTANT NOTE: Always consult each drug listing in the patient's regimen for possible interactions.

Activase — Interactions Index — 12

Piroxicam (Increased risk of bleeding). Products include:
   Feldene Capsules 2008

Salsalate (Increased risk of bleeding). Products include:
   Disalcid 1549
   Mono-Gesic Tablets 810
   Salflex Tablets 791

Sulindac (Increased risk of bleeding). Products include:
   Clinoril Tablets 1658

Ticarcillin Disodium (Increased risk of bleeding). Products include:
   Ticar for Injection 2704
   Timentin for Injection 2706

Ticlopidine Hydrochloride (Increased risk of bleeding). Products include:
   Ticlid Tablets 2317

Tolmetin Sodium (Increased risk of bleeding). Products include:
   Tolectin (200, 400 and 600 mg) .. 1591

Warfarin Sodium (Increased risk of bleeding). Products include:
   Coumadin 941

ACTRON CAPLETS AND TABLETS
(Ketoprofen) 608

Food Interactions
Alcohol (Patients consuming 3 or more alcohol-containing drinks per day should consult their physician for advice on when and how they should take Actron).

ACULAR STERILE OPHTHALMIC SOLUTION
(Ketorolac Tromethamine) 470
None cited in PDR database.

ACUTRIM 16 HOUR STEADY CONTROL APPETITE SUPPRESSANT
(Phenylpropanolamine Hydrochloride) 648
See Acutrim Late Day Strength Appetite Suppressant

ACUTRIM LATE DAY STRENGTH APPETITE SUPPRESSANT
(Phenylpropanolamine Hydrochloride) 648
May interact with monoamine oxidase inhibitors and certain other agents. Compounds in these categories include:

Furazolidone (Do not use concomitantly). Products include:
   Furoxone 2221

Isocarboxazid (Do not use concomitantly).
   No products indexed under this heading.

Nasal decongestants, unspecified (Concurrent use is not recommended).

Phenelzine Sulfate (Do not use concomitantly). Products include:
   Nardil 1977

Phenylpropanolamine Containing Anorectics (Concurrent use not recommended).

Prescription Drugs, unspecified (Concurrent use not recommended).

Selegiline Hydrochloride (Do not use concomitantly). Products include:
   Eldepryl Capsules 2729

Tranylcypromine Sulfate (Do not use concomitantly). Products include:
   Parnate Tablets 2679

ACUTRIM MAXIMUM STRENGTH APPETITE SUPPRESSANT
(Phenylpropanolamine Hydrochloride) 648
See Acutrim Late Day Strength Appetite Suppressant

ADAGEN (PEGADEMASE BOVINE) INJECTION
(Pegademase Bovine) 988
May interact with:

Vidarabine Monohydrate (Concomitant use can substantially alter activities of Adagen).
   No products indexed under this heading.

ADALAT CAPSULES (10 MG AND 20 MG)
(Nifedipine) 580
May interact with beta blockers, cardiac glycosides, oral anticoagulants, and certain other agents. Compounds in these categories include:

Acebutolol Hydrochloride (Increased likelihood of congestive heart failure, severe hypotension, or exacerbation of angina). Products include:
   Sectral Capsules 2914

Atenolol (Increased likelihood of congestive heart failure, severe hypotension, or exacerbation of angina). Products include:
   Tenoretic Tablets 2963
   Tenormin Tablets and I.V. Injection 2965

Betaxolol Hydrochloride (Increased likelihood of congestive heart failure, severe hypotension, or exacerbation of angina). Products include:
   Betoptic Ophthalmic Solution ... 465
   Betoptic S Ophthalmic Suspension 467
   Kerlone Tablets 2588

Bisoprolol Fumarate (Increased likelihood of congestive heart failure, severe hypotension, or exacerbation of angina). Products include:
   Zebeta Tablets 1457
   Ziac 1459

Carteolol Hydrochloride (Increased likelihood of congestive heart failure, severe hypotension, or exacerbation of angina). Products include:
   Cartrol Tablets 413
   Ocupress Ophthalmic Solution, 1% Sterile 297

Cimetidine (Increased peak nifedipine plasma levels). Products include:
   Tagamet HB Tablets 786
   Tagamet Tablets 2694

Cimetidine Hydrochloride (Increased peak nifedipine plasma levels). Products include:
   Tagamet 2694

Deslanoside (Isolated reports of elevated digoxin levels).
   No products indexed under this heading.

Dicumarol (Increased prothrombin time).
   No products indexed under this heading.

Digitoxin (Isolated reports of elevated digoxin levels). Products include:
   Crystodigin Tablets 1472

Digoxin (Isolated reports of elevated digoxin levels). Products include:
   Lanoxicaps 1110
   Lanoxin Elixir Pediatric 1113
   Lanoxin Injection 1116
   Lanoxin Injection Pediatric 1119
   Lanoxin Tablets 1121

Esmolol Hydrochloride (Increased likelihood of congestive heart failure, severe hypotension, or exacerbation of angina). Products include:
   Brevibloc (esmolol HCl) Injection 1860

Labetalol Hydrochloride (Increased likelihood of congestive heart failure, severe hypotension, or exacerbation of angina). Products include:
   Normodyne Injection 2519
   Normodyne Tablets 2522
   Trandate 1158

Levobunolol Hydrochloride (Increased likelihood of congestive heart failure, severe hypotension, or exacerbation of angina). Products include:
   Betagan 230

Metipranolol Hydrochloride (Increased likelihood of congestive heart failure, severe hypotension, or exacerbation of angina). Products include:
   OptiPranolol (Metipranolol 0.3%) Sterile Ophthalmic Solution 256

Metoprolol Succinate (Increased likelihood of congestive heart failure, severe hypotension, or exacerbation of angina). Products include:
   Toprol-XL Tablets 560

Metoprolol Tartrate (Increased likelihood of congestive heart failure, severe hypotension, or exacerbation of angina). Products include:
   Lopressor 848
   Lopressor HCT Tablets 850

Nadolol (Increased likelihood of congestive heart failure, severe hypotension, or exacerbation of angina).
   No products indexed under this heading.

Penbutolol Sulfate (Increased likelihood of congestive heart failure, severe hypotension, or exacerbation of angina). Products include:
   Levatol Tablets 2547

Pindolol (Increased likelihood of congestive heart failure, severe hypotension, or exacerbation of angina). Products include:
   Visken Tablets 2428

Propranolol Hydrochloride (Increased likelihood of congestive heart failure, severe hypotension, or exacerbation of angina). Products include:
   Inderal 2834
   Inderal LA Long Acting Capsules 2836
   Inderide Tablets 2838
   Inderide LA Long Acting Capsules .. 2840

Quinidine Gluconate (Decreased plasma level of quinidine). Products include:
   Quinaglute Dura-Tabs Tablets ... 644

Quinidine Polygalacturonate (Decreased plasma level of quinidine). Products include:
   Cardioquin Tablets 2146

Quinidine Sulfate (Decreased plasma level of quinidine). Products include:
   Quinidex Extentabs 2240

Ranitidine Hydrochloride (Produces smaller, non-significant increases in peak nifedipine plasma levels and AUC). Products include:
   Zantac 1182
   Zantac Injection 1180
   Zantac Syrup 1182

Sotalol Hydrochloride (Increased likelihood of congestive heart failure, severe hypotension, or exacerbation of angina). Products include:
   Betapace Tablets 637

Timolol Hemihydrate (Increased likelihood of congestive heart failure, severe hypotension, or exacerbation of angina). Products include:
   Betimol 0.25%, 0.5% 259

Timolol Maleate (Increased likelihood of congestive heart failure, severe hypotension, or exacerbation of angina). Products include:
   Blocadren Tablets 1654
   Timolide Tablets 1791
   Timoptic in Ocudose 1796
   Timoptic Sterile Ophthalmic Solution 1794
   Timoptic-XE 1798

Warfarin Sodium (Increased prothrombin time). Products include:
   Coumadin 941

ADALAT CC
(Nifedipine) 582
May interact with beta blockers, cardiac glycosides, oral anticoagulants, narcotic analgesics, and certain other agents. Compounds in these categories include:

Acebutolol Hydrochloride (Combination of nifedipine and beta blocker may increase the likelihood of congestive heart failure, severe hypotension, or exacerbation of angina). Products include:
   Sectral Capsules 2914

Alfentanil Hydrochloride (Potential for severe hypotension and/or increased fluid volume requirements cannot be ruled out when nifedipine is co-administered with beta blocker and narcotic analgesic). Products include:
   Alfenta Injection 1334

Atenolol (Combination of nifedipine and beta blocker may increase the likelihood of congestive heart failure, severe hypotension, or exacerbation of angina). Products include:
   Tenoretic Tablets 2963
   Tenormin Tablets and I.V. Injection 2965

Betaxolol Hydrochloride (Combination of nifedipine and beta blocker may increase the likelihood of congestive heart failure, severe hypotension, or exacerbation of angina). Products include:
   Betoptic Ophthalmic Solution ... 465
   Betoptic S Ophthalmic Suspension 467
   Kerlone Tablets 2588

Bisoprolol Fumarate (Combination of nifedipine and beta blocker may increase the likelihood of congestive heart failure, severe hypotension, or exacerbation of angina). Products include:
   Zebeta Tablets 1457
   Ziac 1459

Buprenorphine (Potential for severe hypotension and/or increased fluid volume requirements cannot be ruled out when nifedipine is co-administered with beta blocker and narcotic analgesic). Products include:
   Buprenex Injectable 2170

Carteolol Hydrochloride (Combination of nifedipine and beta blocker may increase the likelihood of congestive heart failure, severe hypotension, or exacerbation of angina). Products include:
   Cartrol Tablets 413
   Ocupress Ophthalmic Solution, 1% Sterile 297

Cimetidine (Both the peak plasma level of nifedipine and AUC may increase in the presence of cimetidine). Products include:
   Tagamet HB Tablets 786
   Tagamet Tablets 2694

(Described in PDR For Nonprescription Drugs)   (Described in PDR For Ophthalmology)

Cimetidine Hydrochloride (Both the peak plasma level of nifedipine and AUC may increase in the presence of cimetidine). Products include:
- Tagamet ... 2694

Codeine Phosphate (Potential for severe hypotension and/or increased fluid volume requirements cannot be ruled out when nifedipine is co-administered with beta blocker and narcotic analgesic). Products include:
- Brontex ... 2130
- Dimetane-DC Cough Syrup ... 2232
- Fioricet with Codeine Capsules ... 2387
- Fiorinal with Codeine Capsules ... 2390
- Nucofed ... 2225
- Phenergan with Codeine ... 2883
- Phenergan VC with Codeine ... 2888
- Robitussin A-C Syrup ... 2248
- Robitussin-DAC Syrup ... 2249
- Ryna ... ⊞ 804
- Soma Compound w/Codeine Tablets ... 2784
- Tylenol with Codeine ... 1592

Deslanoside (Potential of elevated digoxin levels).
- No products indexed under this heading.

Dezocine (Potential for severe hypotension and/or increased fluid volume requirements cannot be ruled out when nifedipine is co-administered with beta blocker and narcotic analgesic). Products include:
- Dalgan Injection ... 529

Dicumarol (Rare reports of increased prothrombin time).
- No products indexed under this heading.

Digitoxin (Potential of elevated digoxin levels). Products include:
- Crystodigin Tablets ... 1472

Digoxin (Potential of elevated digoxin levels). Products include:
- Lanoxicaps ... 1110
- Lanoxin Elixir Pediatric ... 1113
- Lanoxin Injection ... 1116
- Lanoxin Injection Pediatric ... 1119
- Lanoxin Tablets ... 1121

Esmolol Hydrochloride (Combination of nifedipine and beta blocker may increase the likelihood of congestive heart failure, severe hypotension, or exacerbation of angina). Products include:
- Brevibloc (esmolol HCl) Injection ... 1860

Fentanyl (Potential for severe hypotension and/or increased fluid volume requirements cannot be ruled out when nifedipine is co-administered with beta blocker, narcotic analgesic and high dose fentanyl anesthesia). Products include:
- Duragesic Transdermal System ... 1336

Fentanyl Citrate (Potential for severe hypotension and/or increased fluid volume requirements cannot be ruled out when nifedipine is co-administered with beta blocker, narcotic analgesic and high-dose fentanyl anesthesia). Products include:
- Sublimaze Injection ... 463

Hydrocodone Bitartrate (Potential for severe hypotension and/or increased fluid volume requirements cannot be ruled out when nifedipine is co-administered with beta blocker and narcotic analgesic). Products include:
- Codiclear DH Syrup ... 808
- Duratuss HD Elixir ... 2750
- Histussin D Liquid ... 670
- Hycodan Tablets and Syrup ... 946
- Hycomine Compound Tablets ... 948
- Hycomine ... 947
- Hycotuss Expectorant Syrup ... 950
- Hydrocet Capsules ... 787
- Lorcet 10/650 Tablets ... 1016
- Lortab ... 2751
- Tussend ... 1830
- Tussend Expectorant ... 1831
- Vicodin Tablets ... 1404
- Vicodin ES Tablets ... 1405
- Vicodin HP Tablets ... 1403
- Vicodin Tuss Expectorant ... 1406
- Zydone Capsules ... 967

Hydrocodone Polistirex (Potential for severe hypotension and/or increased fluid volume requirements cannot be ruled out when nifedipine is co-administered with beta blocker and narcotic analgesic). Products include:
- Tussionex Pennkinetic Extended-Release Suspension ... 1624

Hydromorphone Hydrochloride (Potential for severe hypotension and/or increased fluid volume requirements cannot be ruled out when nifedipine is co-administered with beta blocker and narcotic analgesic). Products include:
- Dilaudid Ampules ... 1382
- Dilaudid Cough Syrup ... 1383
- Dilaudid-HP Injection ... 1384
- Dilaudid-HP Lyophilized Powder 250 mg ... 1384
- Dilaudid ... 1382
- Dilaudid Oral Liquid ... 1386
- Dilaudid ... 1382
- Dilaudid Tablets - 8 mg ... 1386

Labetalol Hydrochloride (Combination of nifedipine and beta blocker may increase the likelihood of congestive heart failure, severe hypotension, or exacerbation of angina). Products include:
- Normodyne Injection ... 2519
- Normodyne Tablets ... 2522
- Trandate ... 1158

Levobunolol Hydrochloride (Combination of nifedipine and beta blocker may increase the likelihood of congestive heart failure, severe hypotension, or exacerbation of angina). Products include:
- Betagan ... ◉ 230

Levorphanol Tartrate (Potential for severe hypotension and/or increased fluid volume requirements cannot be ruled out when nifedipine is co-administered with beta blocker and narcotic analgesic). Products include:
- Levo-Dromoran ... 2297

Meperidine Hydrochloride (Potential for severe hypotension and/or increased fluid volume requirements cannot be ruled out when nifedipine is co-administered with beta blocker and narcotic analgesic). Products include:
- Demerol ... 2438
- Mepergan Injection ... 2859

Methadone Hydrochloride (Potential for severe hypotension and/or increased fluid volume requirements cannot be ruled out when nifedipine is co-administered with beta blocker and narcotic analgesic). Products include:
- Methadone Hydrochloride Oral Concentrate ... 2356
- Methadone Hydrochloride Oral Solution & Tablets ... 2357

Metipranolol Hydrochloride (Combination of nifedipine and beta blocker may increase the likelihood of congestive heart failure, severe hypotension, or exacerbation of angina). Products include:
- OptiPranolol (Metipranolol 0.3%) Sterile Ophthalmic Solution ... ◉ 256

Metoprolol Succinate (Combination of nifedipine and beta blocker may increase the likelihood of congestive heart failure, severe hypotension, or exacerbation of angina). Products include:
- Toprol-XL Tablets ... 560

Metoprolol Tartrate (Combination of nifedipine and beta blocker may increase the likelihood of congestive heart failure, severe hypotension, or exacerbation of angina). Products include:
- Lopressor ... 848
- Lopressor HCT Tablets ... 850

Morphine Sulfate (Potential for severe hypotension and/or increased fluid volume requirements cannot be ruled out when nifedipine is co-administered with beta blocker and narcotic analgesic). Products include:
- Astramorph/PF Injection, USP (Preservative-Free) ... 526
- Duramorph Injection ... 983
- Infumorph 200 and Infumorph 500 Sterile Solutions ... 985
- Kadian Capsules ... 2948
- MS Contin Tablets ... 2149
- MSIR ... 2152
- Oramorph SR (Morphine Sulfate Sustained Release Tablets) ... 2359
- RMS Suppositories CII ... 2766
- Roxanol ... 2365

Nadolol (Combination of nifedipine and beta blocker may increase the likelihood of congestive heart failure, severe hypotension, or exacerbation of angina).
- No products indexed under this heading.

Opium Alkaloids (Potential for severe hypotension and/or increased fluid volume requirements cannot be ruled out when nifedipine is co-administered with beta blocker and narcotic analgesic).
- No products indexed under this heading.

Oxycodone Hydrochloride (Potential for severe hypotension and/or increased fluid volume requirements cannot be ruled out when nifedipine is co-administered with beta blocker and narcotic analgesic). Products include:
- OxyContin Tablets ... 2163
- OxyIR Capsules ... 2167
- Percocet Tablets ... 955
- Percodan Tablets ... 955
- Percodan-Demi Tablets ... 956
- Roxicodone Tablets, Oral Solution & Intensol (Oxycodone) ... 2366
- Tylox Capsules ... 1593

Penbutolol Sulfate (Combination of nifedipine and beta blocker may increase the likelihood of congestive heart failure, severe hypotension, or exacerbation of angina). Products include:
- Levatol Tablets ... 2547

Pindolol (Combination of nifedipine and beta blocker may increase the likelihood of congestive heart failure, severe hypotension, or exacerbation of angina). Products include:
- Visken Tablets ... 2428

Propoxyphene Hydrochloride (Potential for severe hypotension and/or increased fluid volume requirements cannot be ruled out when nifedipine is co-administered with beta blocker and narcotic analgesic). Products include:
- Darvon ... 1475
- Wygesic Tablets ... 2930

Propoxyphene Napsylate (Potential for severe hypotension and/or increased fluid volume requirements cannot be ruled out when nifedipine is co-administered with beta blocker and narcotic analgesic). Products include:
- Darvon-N/Darvocet-N ... 1473

Propranolol Hydrochloride (Combination of nifedipine and beta blocker may increase the likelihood of congestive heart failure, severe hypotension, or exacerbation of angina). Products include:
- Inderal ... 2834
- Inderal LA Long Acting Capsules ... 2836
- Inderide Tablets ... 2838
- Inderide LA Long Acting Capsules ... 2840

Quinidine Gluconate (Rare reports of decreased plasma level of quinidine). Products include:
- Quinaglute Dura-Tabs Tablets ... 644

Quinidine Polygalacturonate (Rare reports of decreased plasma level of quinidine). Products include:
- Cardioquin Tablets ... 2146

Quinidine Sulfate (Rare reports of decreased plasma level of quinidine). Products include:
- Quinidex Extentabs ... 2240

Ranitidine Hydrochloride (Produces smaller, non-significant increases in peak nifedipine plasma levels and AUC). Products include:
- Zantac ... 1182
- Zantac Injection ... 1180
- Zantac Syrup ... 1182

Sotalol Hydrochloride (Combination of nifedipine and beta blocker may increase the likelihood of congestive heart failure, severe hypotension, or exacerbation of angina). Products include:
- Betapace Tablets ... 637

Sufentanil Citrate (Potential for severe hypotension and/or increased fluid volume requirements cannot be ruled out when nifedipine is co-administered with beta blocker and narcotic analgesic). Products include:
- Sufenta Injection ... 1355

Timolol Hemihydrate (Combination of nifedipine and beta blocker may increase the likelihood of congestive heart failure, severe hypotension, or exacerbation of angina). Products include:
- Betimol 0.25%, 0.5% ... ◉ 259

Timolol Maleate (Combination of nifedipine and beta blocker may increase the likelihood of congestive heart failure, severe hypotension, or exacerbation of angina). Products include:
- Blocadren Tablets ... 1654
- Timolide Tablets ... 1791
- Timoptic in Ocudose ... 1796
- Timoptic Sterile Ophthalmic Solution ... 1794
- Timoptic-XE ... 1798

Warfarin Sodium (Rare reports of increased prothrombin time). Products include:
- Coumadin ... 941

Food Interactions

Diet, high-lipid (High fat meal increases peak plasma nifedipine concentrations by 60%, a prolongation in the time to peak concentration, but no significant change in the AUC; administer on an empty stomach).

ADAPIN CAPSULES
(Doxepin Hydrochloride) ... 1542
May interact with antidepressant drugs, phenothiazines, monoamine oxidase inhibitors, quinidine, and

IMPORTANT NOTE: Always consult each drug listing in the patient's regimen for possible interactions.

Adapin Interactions Index 14

certain other agents. Compounds in these categories include:

Amitriptyline Hydrochloride (Certain antidepressants are metabolized by cytochrome P450 2D6 isoenzyme and may make normal metabolizers resemble poor metabolizers resulting in higher than expected plasma levels of tricyclic antidepressants). Products include:

Elavil ... 2945
Etrafon ... 2495
Limbitrol ... 2333
Triavil Tablets ... 1800

Amoxapine (Certain antidepressants are metabolized by cytochrome P450 2D6 isoenzyme and may make normal metabolizers resemble poor metabolizers resulting in higher than expected plasma levels of tricyclic antidepressants). Products include:

Asendin Tablets ... 1419

Bupropion Hydrochloride (Certain antidepressants are metabolized by cytochrome P450 2D6 isoenzyme and may make normal metabolizers resemble poor metabolizers resulting in higher than expected plasma levels of tricyclic antidepressants). Products include:

Wellbutrin Tablets ... 1177

Chlorpromazine (Phenothiazines are metabolized by cytochrome P450 2D6 isoenzyme and may make normal metabolizers resemble poor metabolizers resulting in higher than expected plasma levels of tricyclic antidepressants). Products include:

Thorazine Suppositories ... 2701

Chlorpromazine Hydrochloride (Phenothiazines are metabolized by cytochrome P450 2D6 isoenzyme and may make normal metabolizers resemble poor metabolizers resulting in higher than expected plasma levels of tricyclic antidepressants). Products include:

Thorazine ... 2701

Cimetidine (Co-administration has been reported to produce clinically significant fluctuations in steady-state serum concentrations of various tricyclic antidepressants; serious anticholinergic symptoms, such as severe dry mouth, urinary retention and blurred vision have been reported). Products include:

Tagamet HB Tablets ... ▣ 786
Tagamet Tablets ... 2694

Cimetidine Hydrochloride (Co-administration has been reported to produce clinically significant fluctuations in steady-state serum concentrations of various tricyclic antidepressants; serious anticholinergic symptoms, such as severe dry mouth, urinary retention and blurred vision have been reported). Products include:

Tagamet ... 2694

Desipramine Hydrochloride (Certain antidepressants are metabolized by cytochrome P450 2D6 isoenzyme and may make normal metabolizers resemble poor metabolizers resulting in higher than expected plasma levels of tricyclic antidepressants). Products include:

Norpramin Tablets ... 1273

Flecainide Acetate (Certain antiarrhythmics, such as flecainide, are metabolized by cytochrome P450 2D6 isoenzyme and may make normal metabolizers resemble poor metabolizers resulting in higher than expected plasma levels of tricyclic antidepressants). Products include:

Tambocor Tablets ... 1555

Fluoxetine Hydrochloride (May inhibit the activity of cytochrome P450 2D6 isoenzyme and may make normal metabolizers resemble poor metabolizers resulting in higher than expected plasma levels of tricyclic antidepressants; due to long half-life of fluoxetine, at least 5 weeks should elapse before initiating TCA treatment in a patient being withdrawn from fluoxetine). Products include:

Prozac Pulvules & Liquid, Oral Solution ... 935

Fluphenazine Decanoate (Phenothiazines are metabolized by cytochrome P450 2D6 isoenzyme and may make normal metabolizers resemble poor metabolizers resulting in higher than expected plasma levels of tricyclic antidepressants). Products include:

Prolixin Decanoate ... 510

Fluphenazine Enanthate (Phenothiazines are metabolized by cytochrome P450 2D6 isoenzyme and may make normal metabolizers resemble poor metabolizers resulting in higher than expected plasma levels of tricyclic antidepressants). Products include:

Prolixin Enanthate ... 510

Fluphenazine Hydrochloride (Phenothiazines are metabolized by cytochrome P450 2D6 isoenzyme and may make normal metabolizers resemble poor metabolizers resulting in higher than expected plasma levels of tricyclic antidepressants). Products include:

Prolixin ... 510

Furazolidone (Co-administration of tricyclic antidepressants and MAO inhibitor has produced serious side effects and even death; concurrent and/or sequential use is contraindicated). Products include:

Furoxone ... 2221

Imipramine Hydrochloride (Certain antidepressants are metabolized by cytochrome P450 2D6 isoenzyme and may make normal metabolizers resemble poor metabolizers resulting in higher than expected plasma levels of tricyclic antidepressants). Products include:

Tofranil Ampuls ... 873
Tofranil Tablets ... 875

Imipramine Pamoate (Certain antidepressants are metabolized by cytochrome P450 2D6 isoenzyme and may make normal metabolizers resemble poor metabolizers resulting in higher than expected plasma levels of tricyclic antidepressants). Products include:

Tofranil-PM Capsules ... 876

Isocarboxazid (Co-administration of tricyclic antidepressants and MAO inhibitor has produced serious side effects and even death; concurrent and/or sequential use is contraindicated).

No products indexed under this heading.

Maprotiline Hydrochloride (Certain antidepressants are metabolized by cytochrome P450 2D6 isoenzyme and may make normal metabolizers resemble poor metabolizers resulting in higher than expected plasma levels of tricyclic antidepressants). Products include:

Ludiomil Tablets ... 861

Mesoridazine Besylate (Phenothiazines are metabolized by cytochrome P450 2D6 isoenzyme and may make normal metabolizers resemble poor metabolizers resulting in higher than expected plasma levels of tricyclic antidepressants). Products include:

Serentil ... 689

Methotrimeprazine (Phenothiazines are metabolized by cytochrome P450 2D6 isoenzyme and may make normal metabolizers resemble poor metabolizers resulting in higher than expected plasma levels of tricyclic antidepressants). Products include:

Levoprome ... 1321

Mirtazapine (Certain antidepressants are metabolized by cytochrome P450 2D6 isoenzyme and may make normal metabolizers resemble poor metabolizers resulting in higher than expected plasma levels of tricyclic antidepressants). Products include:

Remeron Tablets ... 1878

Nefazodone Hydrochloride (Certain antidepressants are metabolized by cytochrome P450 2D6 isoenzyme and may make normal metabolizers resemble poor metabolizers resulting in higher than expected plasma levels of tricyclic antidepressants). Products include:

Serzone Tablets ... 776

Nortriptyline Hydrochloride (Certain antidepressants are metabolized by cytochrome P450 2D6 isoenzyme and may make normal metabolizers resemble poor metabolizers resulting in higher than expected plasma levels of tricyclic antidepressants). Products include:

Pamelor ... 2409

Paroxetine Hydrochloride (Selective serotonin reuptake inhibitors, such as paroxetine may have variable extent of inhibition of P450 2D6; potential for higher than expected plasma levels of tricyclic antidepressants). Products include:

Paxil Tablets ... 2681

Perphenazine (Phenothiazines are metabolized by cytochrome P450 2D6 isoenzyme and may make normal metabolizers resemble poor metabolizers resulting in higher than expected plasma levels of tricyclic antidepressants). Products include:

Etrafon ... 2495
Triavil Tablets ... 1800
Trilafon ... 2532

Phenelzine Sulfate (Co-administration of tricyclic antidepressants and MAO inhibitor has produced serious side effects and even death; concurrent and/or sequential use is contraindicated). Products include:

Nardil ... 1977

Prochlorperazine (Phenothiazines are metabolized by cytochrome P450 2D6 isoenzyme and may make normal metabolizers resemble poor metabolizers resulting in higher than expected plasma levels of tricyclic antidepressants). Products include:

Compazine ... 2644

Promethazine Hydrochloride (Phenothiazines are metabolized by cytochrome P450 2D6 isoenzyme and may make normal metabolizers resemble poor metabolizers resulting in higher than expected plasma levels of tricyclic antidepressants). Products include:

Mepergan Injection ... 2859
Phenergan with Codeine ... 2883
Phenergan with Dextromethorphan 2885
Phenergan Injection ... 2880
Phenergan Suppositories ... 2882
Phenergan Syrup ... 2881
Phenergan Tablets ... 2882
Phenergan VC ... 2886
Phenergan VC with Codeine ... 2888

Propafenone Hydrochloride (Certain antiarrhythmics, such as propafenone, are metabolized by cytochrome P450 2D6 isoenzyme and may make normal metabolizers resemble poor metabolizers resulting in higher than expected plasma levels of tricyclic antidepressants). Products include:

Rythmol Tablets–150mg, 225mg, 300mg ... 1399

Protriptyline Hydrochloride (Certain antidepressants are metabolized by cytochrome P450 2D6 isoenzyme and may make normal metabolizers resemble poor metabolizers resulting in higher than expected plasma levels of tricyclic antidepressants). Products include:

Vivactil Tablets ... 1820

Quinidine Gluconate (May inhibit the activity of cytochrome P450 2D6 isoenzyme and may make normal metabolizers resemble poor metabolizers resulting in higher than expected plasma levels of tricyclic antidepressants). Products include:

Quinaglute Dura-Tabs Tablets ... 644

Quinidine Polygalacturonate (May inhibit the activity of cytochrome P450 2D6 isoenzyme and may make normal metabolizers resemble poor metabolizers resulting in higher than expected plasma levels of tricyclic antidepressants). Products include:

Cardioquin Tablets ... 2146

Quinidine Sulfate (May inhibit the activity of cytochrome P450 2D6 isoenzyme and may make normal metabolizers resemble poor metabolizers resulting in higher than expected plasma levels of tricyclic antidepressants). Products include:

Quinidex Extentabs ... 2240

Selegiline Hydrochloride (Co-administration of tricyclic antidepressants and MAO inhibitor has produced serious side effects and even death; concurrent and/or sequential use is contraindicated). Products include:

Eldepryl Capsules ... 2729

Sertraline Hydrochloride (Selective serotonin reuptake inhibitors, such as sertraline, may have variable extent of inhibition of P450 2D6; potential for higher than expected plasma levels of tricyclic antidepressants). Products include:

Zoloft Tablets ... 2051

Thioridazine Hydrochloride (Phenothiazines are metabolized by cytochrome P450 2D6 isoenzyme and may make normal metabolizers resemble poor metabolizers resulting in higher than expected plasma levels of tricyclic antidepressants). Products include:

Mellaril ... 2398

(▣ Described in PDR For Nonprescription Drugs) (◉ Described in PDR For Ophthalmology)

Tranylcypromine Sulfate (Co-administration of tricyclic antidepressants and MAO inhibitor has produced serious side effects and even death; concurrent and/or sequential use is contraindicated). Products include:

Parnate Tablets ... 2679

Trazodone Hydrochloride (Certain antidepressants are metabolized by cytochrome P450 2D6 isoenzyme and may make normal metabolizers resemble poor metabolizers resulting in higher than expected plasma levels of tricyclic antidepressants). Products include:

Desyrel and Desyrel Dividose ... 504

Trifluoperazine Hydrochloride (Phenothiazines are metabolized by cytochrome P450 2D6 isoenzyme and may make normal metabolizers resemble poor metabolizers resulting in higher than expected plasma levels of tricyclic antidepressants). Products include:

Stelazine ... 2692

Trimipramine Maleate (Certain antidepressants are metabolized by cytochrome P450 2D6 isoenzyme and may make normal metabolizers resemble poor metabolizers resulting in higher than expected plasma levels of tricyclic antidepressants). Products include:

Surmontil Capsules ... 2917

Venlafaxine Hydrochloride (Certain antidepressants are metabolized by cytochrome P450 2D6 isoenzyme and may make normal metabolizers resemble poor metabolizers resulting in higher than expected plasma levels of tricyclic antidepressants). Products include:

Effexor ... 2825

Food Interactions

Alcohol (Doxepin may potentiate the CNS depressant effects of alcohol).

ADATOSIL 5000

(Silicone Oil) ... ◎ 265

None cited in PDR database.

ADDERALL TABLETS

(Amphetamine Aspartate, Amphetamine Sulfate, Dextroamphetamine Saccharate, Dextroamphetamine Sulfate) ... 2209

May interact with monoamine oxidase inhibitors, urinary alkalizing agents, tricyclic antidepressants, antihistamines, antihypertensives, thiazides, veratrum alkaloids, and certain other agents. Compounds in these categories include:

Acebutolol Hydrochloride (Amphetamines may antagonize the hypotensive effects of antihypertensives). Products include:

Sectral Capsules ... 2914

Acetazolamide (Acetazolamide produces alkaline urine and thereby decreasing urinary excretion; increases blood levels resulting in potentiation of the action of amphetamines). Products include:

Diamox Sequels (Sustained Release) ... ◎ 318
Diamox Tablets ... ◎ 317

Acetazolamide Sodium (Acetazolamide produces alkaline urine and thereby decreasing urinary excretion; increases blood levels resulting in potentiation of the action of amphetamines). Products include:

Diamox Intravenous ... ◎ 317

Acrivastine (Amphetamines may counteract the sedative effect of antihistamines). Products include:

Semprex-D Capsules ... 1620

Amitriptyline Hydrochloride (Enhanced activity of tricyclic antidepressants or sympathomimetics; possible increases in the brain concentration of *d*-amphetamine resulting in potentiated cardiovascular effects). Products include:

Elavil ... 2945
Etrafon ... 2495
Limbitrol ... 2333
Triavil Tablets ... 1800

Amlodipine Besylate (Amphetamines may antagonize the hypotensive effects of antihypertensives). Products include:

Lotrel Capsules ... 858
Norvasc Tablets ... 2020

Ammonium Chloride (Increases the concentration of the ionized species of the amphetamine molecule, thereby increasing urinary excretion; lowers blood levels and efficacy of amphetamines).

No products indexed under this heading.

Amoxapine (Enhanced activity of tricyclic antidepressants or sympathomimetics; possible increases in the brain concentration of *d*-amphetamine resulting in potentiated cardiovascular effects). Products include:

Asendin Tablets ... 1419

Astemizole (Amphetamines may counteract the sedative effect of antihistamines). Products include:

Hismanal Tablets ... 1341

Atenolol (Amphetamines may antagonize the hypotensive effects of antihypertensives). Products include:

Tenoretic Tablets ... 2963
Tenormin Tablets and I.V. Injection 2965

Azatadine Maleate (Amphetamines may counteract the sedative effect of antihistamines). Products include:

Trinalin Repetabs Tablets ... 1373

Benazepril Hydrochloride (Amphetamines may antagonize the hypotensive effects of antihypertensives). Products include:

Lotensin Tablets ... 852
Lotensin HCT Tablets ... 855
Lotrel Capsules ... 858

Bendroflumethiazide (Some thiazides produce alkaline urine, thereby decreasing urinary excretion of amphetamines; potential for increase in blood levels resulting in potentiation of the action of amphetamines).

No products indexed under this heading.

Betaxolol Hydrochloride (Amphetamines may antagonize the hypotensive effects of antihypertensives). Products include:

Betoptic Ophthalmic Solution ... 465
Betoptic S Ophthalmic Suspension 467
Kerlone Tablets ... 2588

Bisoprolol Fumarate (Amphetamines may antagonize the hypotensive effects of antihypertensives). Products include:

Zebeta Tablets ... 1457
Ziac ... 1459

Bromodiphenhydramine Hydrochloride (Amphetamines may counteract the sedative effect of antihistamines).

No products indexed under this heading.

Brompheniramine Maleate (Amphetamines may counteract the sedative effect of antihistamines). Products include:

Alka-Seltzer Plus Sinus Medicine ... 611
Bromfed Capsules (Extended-Release) ... 1832
Bromfed Syrup ... 712
Bromfed Tablets ... 1832
Bromfed-DM Cough Syrup ... 1832
Bromfed-PD Capsules (Extended-Release) ... 1832
Dimetane-DC Cough Syrup ... 2232
Dimetane-DX Cough Syrup ... 2233
Dimetapp Allergy Dye-Free Elixir ... 838
Dimetapp Allergy Sinus Caplets ... 838
Dimetapp Cold & Allergy Chewable Tablets ... 838
Dimetapp Cold & Cough Liqui-Gels ... 839
Dimetapp Cold & Fever Suspension ... 839
Dimetapp DM Elixir ... 840
Dimetapp Elixir ... 840
Dimetapp Extentabs ... 841
Dimetapp Tablets/Liqui-Gels ... 841
Rondec Chewable Tablets ... 974
Vicks DayQuil Allergy Relief 12-Hour Extended Release Tablets ... 733
Vicks DayQuil Allergy Relief 4-Hour Tablets ... 733

Captopril (Amphetamines may antagonize the hypotensive effects of antihypertensives). Products include:

Capoten Tablets ... 740
Capozide Tablets ... 744

Carteolol Hydrochloride (Amphetamines may antagonize the hypotensive effects of antihypertensives). Products include:

Cartrol Tablets ... 413
Ocupress Ophthalmic Solution, 1% Sterile ... ◎ 297

Cetirizine Hydrochloride (Amphetamines may counteract the sedative effect of antihistamines). Products include:

Zyrtec Tablets ... 2053

Chlorothiazide (Some thiazides produce alkaline urine, thereby decreasing urinary excretion of amphetamines; potential for increase in blood levels resulting in potentiation of the action of amphetamines). Products include:

Aldoclor Tablets ... 1638
Diupres Tablets ... 1691
Diuril Oral ... 1694

Chlorothiazide Sodium (Some thiazides produce alkaline urine, thereby decreasing urinary excretion of amphetamines; potential for increase in blood levels resulting in potentiation of the action of amphetamines). Products include:

Diuril Sodium Intravenous ... 1693

Chlorpheniramine Maleate (Amphetamines may counteract the sedative effect of antihistamines). Products include:

Alka-Seltzer Plus Cold Medicine ... 611
Alka-Seltzer Plus Cold Medicine Liqui-Gels ... 612
Alka-Seltzer Plus Cold & Cough Medicine ... 611
Alka-Seltzer Plus Cold & Cough Medicine Liqui-Gels ... 612
Alka-Seltzer Plus Flu & Body Aches Effervescent Tablets ... 612
Allerest Maximum Strength ... 649
Allerest Sinus Pain Formula ... 649
Ana-Kit Anaphylaxis Emergency Treatment Kit ... 611
Atrohist Pediatric Capsules ... 1603
Atrohist Plus Tablets ... 1605
BC Cold Powder Multi-Symptom Formula (Cold-Sinus-Allergy) ... 631
Cerose DM ... 853
Cheracol Plus Head Cold/Cough Formula ... 741
Children's TYLENOL Cold Multi-Symptom Chewable Tablets and Liquid ... 1559
Children's TYLENOL Cold Plus Cough Multi Symptom Chewable Tablets and Liquid ... 1560
Children's TYLENOL Flu Suspension Liquid ... 1560
Children's Vicks DayQuil Allergy Relief ... 730
Children's Vicks NyQuil Cold/Cough Relief ... 731
Chlor-Trimeton Allergy Decongestant Tablets ... 759
Chlor-Trimeton Allergy Tablets ... 758
Allergy-Sinus Comtrex Multi-Symptom Allergy-Sinus Formula Tablets and Caplets ... 639
Comtrex Multi-Symptom ... 638
Contac Continuous Action Nasal Decongestant/Antihistamine 12 Hour Capsules ... 773
Contac Maximum Strength Continuous Action Decongestant/Antihistamine 12 Hour Caplets ... 772
Contac Severe Cold and Flu Formula Caplets ... 773
Coricidin Cold + Flu Tablets ... 760
Coricidin Cough + Cold Tablets ... 760
Coricidin 'D' Decongestant Tablets ... 760
D.A. II Tablets ... 972
D.A. Chewable Tablets ... 970
Dura-Tap/PD Capsules ... 970
Dura-Vent/DA Tablets ... 972
Efidac 24 Chlorpheniramine ... 655
Extendryl ... 1003
Fedahist Gyrocaps ... 2545
Hycomine Compound Tablets ... 948
Kronofed-A ... 994
Nolamine Timed-Release Tablets ... 790
Novahistine Elixir ... 782
Ornade Spansule Capsules ... 2678
PediaCare Cough-Cold Chewable Tablets and Liquid ... 1569
PediaCare NightRest Cough-Cold Liquid ... 1569
Pediatric Vicks 44m Cough & Cold Relief ... 737
Pyrroxate Caplets ... 742
Ryna ... 804
Sinarest ... 663
Sine-Off Sinus Medicine ... 784
Singlet Tablets ... 785
Sinulin Tablets ... 792
Sinutab Sinus Allergy Medication, Maximum Strength Tablets and Caplets ... 823
Sudafed Cold & Allergy Tablets ... 826
Teldrin 12 Hour Antihistamine/Nasal Decongestant Allergy Relief Capsules ... 786
TheraFlu Flu and Cold Medicine ... 750
Theraflu Maximum Strength Flu and Cold Medicine For Sore Throat ... 751
TheraFlu Flu, Cold and Cough Medicine ... 750
TheraFlu Maximum Strength Nighttime Flu, Cold & Cough Medicine ... 751
Triaminic Night Time ... 754
Triaminic Syrup ... 755
Triaminic Triaminicol Cold & Cough ... 756
Triaminicin Tablets ... 756
Tussend ... 1830
TYLENOL Allergy Sinus, Maximum Strength Caplets and Gelcaps ... 1571
TYLENOL Cold Medication, Multi-Symptom Formula Tablets and Caplets ... 1572
TYLENOL Cold Medication, Multi-Symptom Hot Liquid Packets ... 1572
Vicks 44 LiquiCaps Cough, Cold & Flu Relief ... 728
Vicks 44M Cough, Cold & Flu Relief ... 729

Chlorpheniramine Polistirex (Amphetamines may counteract the sedative effect of antihistamines). Products include:

Tussionex Pennkinetic Extended-Release Suspension ... 1624

Chlorpheniramine Tannate (Amphetamines may counteract the sedative effect of antihistamines). Products include:

Atrohist Pediatric Suspension ... 1604
Atrohist Pediatric Suspension Dye-Free ... 1604
Rynatan ... 2781
Rynatuss ... 2782

IMPORTANT NOTE: Always consult each drug listing in the patient's regimen for possible interactions.

Adderall / Interactions Index

Chlorpromazine (Blocks dopamine and norepinephrine reuptake resulting in inhibition of central stimulating effects). Products include:
- Thorazine Suppositories ... 2701

Chlorpromazine Hydrochloride (Blocks dopamine and norepinephrine reuptake resulting in inhibition of central stimulating effects). Products include:
- Thorazine ... 2701

Chlorthalidone (Amphetamines may antagonize the hypotensive effects of antihypertensives). Products include:
- Combipres Tablets ... 682
- Tenoretic Tablets ... 2963
- Thalitone ... 1293

Clemastine Fumarate (Amphetamines may counteract the sedative effect of antihistamines). Products include:
- Tavist Syrup ... 2426
- Tavist Tablets ... 2427
- Tavist-1 12 Hour Relief Tablets ... 749
- Tavist-D 12 Hour Relief Tablets ... 750

Clomipramine Hydrochloride (Enhanced activity of tricyclic antidepressants or sympathomimetics; possible increases in the brain concentration of d-amphetamine resulting in potentiated cardiovascular effects). Products include:
- Anafranil Capsules ... 819

Clonidine (Amphetamines may antagonize the hypotensive effects of antihypertensives). Products include:
- Catapres-TTS ... 680

Clonidine Hydrochloride (Amphetamines may antagonize the hypotensive effects of antihypertensives). Products include:
- Catapres Tablets ... 679
- Combipres Tablets ... 682

Cryptenamine Preparations (Amphetamines inhibit the hypotensive effect of veratrum alkaloids).
No products indexed under this heading.

Cyproheptadine Hydrochloride (Amphetamines may counteract the sedative effect of antihistamines). Products include:
- Periactin ... 1767

Deserpidine (Amphetamines may antagonize the hypotensive effects of antihypertensives).
No products indexed under this heading.

Desipramine Hydrochloride (Enhanced activity of tricyclic antidepressants or sympathomimetics; possible increases in the brain concentration of d-amphetamine resulting in potentiated cardiovascular effects). Products include:
- Norpramin Tablets ... 1273

Dexchlorpheniramine Maleate (Amphetamines may counteract the sedative effect of antihistamines).
No products indexed under this heading.

Diazoxide (Amphetamines may antagonize the hypotensive effects of antihypertensives). Products include:
- Hyperstat I.V. Injection ... 2504
- Proglycem ... 575

Diltiazem Hydrochloride (Amphetamines may antagonize the hypotensive effects of antihypertensives). Products include:
- Cardizem CD Capsules ... 1251
- Cardizem SR Capsules ... 1255
- Cardizem Injectable ... 1253
- Cardizem Tablets ... 1257
- Dilacor XR Extended-release Capsules ... 2183
- Tiazac Capsules ... 1019

Diphenhydramine Citrate (Amphetamines may counteract the sedative effect of antihistamines). Products include:
- Excedrin P.M. Analgesic/Sleeping Aid Tablets, Caplets, Liquigels ... 735

Diphenhydramine Hydrochloride (Amphetamines may counteract the sedative effect of antihistamines). Products include:
- Actifed Allergy Daytime/Nighttime Caplets ... 808
- Actifed Sinus Daytime/Nighttime Tablets and Caplets ... 809
- Extra Strength Bayer PM Aspirin Plus Sleep Aid ... 617
- Benadryl Allergy Chewables ... 811
- Benadryl Allergy/Cold Tablets ... 811
- Benadryl Allergy Decongestant Liquid Medication ... 812
- Benadryl Allergy Decongestant Tablets ... 812
- Benadryl Allergy Liquid Medication ... 813
- Benadryl Allergy ... 811
- Benadryl Allergy Sinus Headache Caplets ... 813
- Benadryl Dye-Free Allergy Liquigel Softgels ... 813
- Benadryl Dye-Free Allergy Liquid Medication ... 814
- Benadryl Itch Relief Stick Extra Strength ... 814
- Benadryl Cream ... 814
- Benadryl Gel ... 815
- Benadryl Spray ... 815
- Benadryl Injection ... 1955
- Contac Day & Night Cold/Flu Night Caplets ... 772
- Contac Night Allergy/Sinus Caplets ... 771
- Extra Strength Doan's P.M. ... 653
- Excedrin P.M. Analgesic/Sleeping Aid Tablets, Caplets, Liquigels ... 643
- Nytol QuickCaps Caplets ... 632
- Sleepinal Night-time Sleep Aid Capsules and Softgels ... 798
- TYLENOL Allergy Sinus NightTime, Maximum Strength Caplets ... 1571
- TYLENOL Flu NightTime, Maximum Strength Gelcaps ... 1575
- TYLENOL Flu NightTime, Maximum Strength Hot Medication Packets ... 1575
- TYLENOL PM Pain Reliever/Sleep Aid, Extra Strength Gelcaps, Caplets, Geltabs ... 1576
- TYLENOL Severe Allergy Medication Caplets ... 1571
- Maximum Strength Unisom Sleepgels ... 1990
- Unisom With Pain Relief-Nighttime Sleep Aid and Pain Reliever ... 1991

Diphenylpyraline Hydrochloride (Amphetamines may counteract the sedative effect of antihistamines).
No products indexed under this heading.

Doxazosin Mesylate (Amphetamines may antagonize the hypotensive effects of antihypertensives). Products include:
- Cardura Tablets ... 1993

Doxepin Hydrochloride (Enhanced activity of tricyclic antidepressants or sympathomimetics; possible increases in the brain concentration of d-amphetamine resulting in potentiated cardiovascular effects). Products include:
- Adapin Capsules ... 1542
- Sinequan ... 2028
- Zonalon Cream ... 1042

Enalapril Maleate (Amphetamines may antagonize the hypotensive effects of antihypertensives). Products include:
- Vaseretic Tablets ... 1810
- Vasotec Tablets ... 1816

Enalaprilat (Amphetamines may antagonize the hypotensive effects of antihypertensives). Products include:
- Vasotec I.V. ... 1814

Esmolol Hydrochloride (Amphetamines may antagonize the hypotensive effects of antihypertensives). Products include:
- Brevibloc (esmolol HCl) Injection ... 1860

Ethosuximide (Amphetamines may delay intestinal absorption of ethosuximide). Products include:
- Zarontin Capsules ... 1986
- Zarontin Syrup ... 1986

Felodipine (Amphetamines may antagonize the hypotensive effects of antihypertensives). Products include:
- Plendil Extended-Release Tablets ... 514

Fosinopril Sodium (Amphetamines may antagonize the hypotensive effects of antihypertensives). Products include:
- Monopril Tablets ... 762

Fosphenytoin Sodium (Co-administration may produce a synergistic anticonvulsant action). Products include:
- Cerebyx Injection ... 1956

Furazolidone (MAO inhibitors slow amphetamine metabolism thereby potentiating and increasing their effects resulting in hypertensive crises; concurrent and/or sequential use is contraindicated). Products include:
- Furoxone ... 2221

Furosemide (Amphetamines may antagonize the hypotensive effects of antihypertensives). Products include:
- Lasix Injection, Oral Solution and Tablets ... 1267

Glutamic Acid Hydrochloride (Gastrointestinal acidifying agents lower absorption of amphetamines, blood levels and efficacy).
No products indexed under this heading.

Guanabenz Acetate (Amphetamines may antagonize the hypotensive effects of antihypertensives).
No products indexed under this heading.

Guanethidine Monosulfate (Gastrointestinal acidifying agents lower absorption of amphetamines, blood levels and efficacy; amphetamines may antagonize the hypotensive effects of antihypertensives). Products include:
- Esimil Tablets ... 840
- Ismelin Tablets ... 845

Haloperidol (Blocks dopamine and norepinephrine reuptake resulting in inhibition of central stimulating effects). Products include:
- Haldol Injection, Tablets and Concentrate ... 1585

Haloperidol Decanoate (Blocks dopamine and norepinephrine reuptake resulting in inhibition of central stimulating effects). Products include:
- Haldol Decanoate ... 1587

Hydralazine Hydrochloride (Amphetamines may antagonize the hypotensive effects of antihypertensives). Products include:
- Apresazide Capsules ... 824
- Apresoline Hydrochloride Tablets ... 826
- Hydralazine Hydrochloride Injection USP ... 2712
- Ser-Ap-Es Tablets ... 867

Hydrochlorothiazide (Some thiazides produce alkaline urine, thereby decreasing urinary excretion of amphetamines; potential for increase in blood levels resulting in potentiation of the action of amphetamines). Products include:
- Aldactazide Tablets ... 2556
- Aldoril Tablets ... 1644
- Apresazide Capsules ... 824
- Capozide Tablets ... 744
- Dyazide Capsules ... 2653
- Esidrix Tablets ... 839
- Esimil Tablets ... 840
- HydroDIURIL Tablets ... 1716
- Hydropres Tablets ... 1718
- Hyzaar Tablets ... 1720
- Inderide Tablets ... 2838
- Inderide LA Long Acting Capsules ... 2840
- Lopressor HCT Tablets ... 850
- Lotensin HCT Tablets ... 855
- Moduretic Tablets ... 1748
- Oretic Tablets ... 450
- Prinzide Tablets ... 1780
- Ser-Ap-Es Tablets ... 867
- Timolide Tablets ... 1791
- Vaseretic Tablets ... 1810
- Zestoretic Tablets ... 2968
- Ziac ... 1459

Hydroflumethiazide (Some thiazides produce alkaline urine, thereby decreasing urinary excretion of amphetamines; potential for increase in blood levels resulting in potentiation of the action of amphetamines). Products include:
- Diucardin Tablets ... 2824

Imipramine Hydrochloride (Enhanced activity of tricyclic antidepressants or sympathomimetics; possible increases in the brain concentration of d-amphetamine resulting in potentiated cardiovascular effects). Products include:
- Tofranil Ampuls ... 873
- Tofranil Tablets ... 875

Imipramine Pamoate (Enhanced activity of tricyclic antidepressants or sympathomimetics; possible increases in the brain concentration of d-amphetamine resulting in potentiated cardiovascular effects). Products include:
- Tofranil-PM Capsules ... 876

Indapamide (Amphetamines may antagonize the hypotensive effects of antihypertensives).
No products indexed under this heading.

Isocarboxazid (MAO inhibitors slow amphetamine metabolism, thereby potentiating and increasing their effects resulting in hypertensive crises; concurrent and/or sequential use is contraindicated).
No products indexed under this heading.

Isradipine (Amphetamines may antagonize the hypotensive effects of antihypertensives). Products include:
- DynaCirc Capsules ... 2381
- DynaCirc CR Tablets ... 2383

Labetalol Hydrochloride (Amphetamines may antagonize the hypotensive effects of antihypertensives). Products include:
- Normodyne Injection ... 2519
- Normodyne Tablets ... 2522
- Trandate ... 1158

Lisinopril (Amphetamines may antagonize the hypotensive effects of antihypertensives). Products include:
- Prinivil Tablets ... 1776
- Prinzide Tablets ... 1780
- Zestoretic Tablets ... 2968
- Zestril Tablets ... 2972

Lithium Carbonate (Inhibits anti-obesity and stimulating effects of amphetamines). Products include:
- Eskalith ... 2658
- Lithium Carbonate Capsules & Tablets ... 2352
- Lithonate/Lithotabs/Lithobid ... 2721

Loratadine (Amphetamines may counteract the sedative effect of antihistamines). Products include:
- Claritin Tablets ... 2485
- Claritin-D Tablets ... 2487

(▣ Described in PDR For Nonprescription Drugs)   (◉ Described in PDR For Ophthalmology)

Losartan Potassium (Amphetamines may antagonize the hypotensive effects of antihypertensives). Products include:
   Cozaar Tablets 1668
   Hyzaar Tablets 1720

Maprotiline Hydrochloride (Enhanced activity of tricyclic antidepressants or sympathomimetics; possible increases in the brain concentration of d-amphetamine resulting in potentiated cardiovascular effects). Products include:
   Ludiomil Tablets.......................... 861

Mecamylamine Hydrochloride (Amphetamines may antagonize the hypotensive effects of antihypertensives). Products include:
   Inversine Tablets 1729

Meperidine Hydrochloride (Amphetamine potentiates the analgesic effect of meperidine). Products include:
   Demerol 2438
   Mepergan Injection 2859

Methdilazine Hydrochloride (Amphetamines may counteract the sedative effect of antihistamines).
   No products indexed under this heading.

Methenamine (Acidifying agents used in methenamine therapy increase the urinary excretion and reduce the efficacy of amphetamines). Products include:
   Urised Tablets 2123

Methenamine Hippurate (Acidifying agents used in methenamine therapy increase the urinary excretion and reduce the efficacy of amphetamines).
   No products indexed under this heading.

Methenamine Mandelate (Acidifying agents used in methenamine therapy increase the urinary excretion and reduce the efficacy of amphetamines). Products include:
   Uroqid-Acid No. 2 Tablets 633

Methyclothiazide (Some thiazides produce alkaline urine, thereby decreasing urinary excretion of amphetamines; potential for increase in blood levels resulting in potentiation of the action of amphetamines). Products include:
   Enduron Tablets.......................... 424

Methyldopa (Amphetamines may antagonize the hypotensive effects of antihypertensives). Products include:
   Aldoclor Tablets 1638
   Aldomet Oral 1640
   Aldoril Tablets 1644

Methyldopate Hydrochloride (Amphetamines may antagonize the hypotensive effects of antihypertensives). Products include:
   Aldomet Ester HCl Injection 1642

Metolazone (Amphetamines may antagonize the hypotensive effects of antihypertensives). Products include:
   Mykrox Tablets 1617
   Zaroxolyn Tablets 1625

Metoprolol Succinate (Amphetamines may antagonize the hypotensive effects of antihypertensives). Products include:
   Toprol-XL Tablets 560

Metoprolol Tartrate (Amphetamines may antagonize the hypotensive effects of antihypertensives). Products include:
   Lopressor 848
   Lopressor HCT Tablets 850

Metyrosine (Amphetamines may antagonize the hypotensive effects of antihypertensives). Products include:
   Demser Capsules....................... 1690

Minoxidil (Amphetamines may antagonize the hypotensive effects of antihypertensives).
   No products indexed under this heading.

Moexipril Hydrochloride (Amphetamines may antagonize the hypotensive effects of antihypertensives). Products include:
   Univasc Tablets 2553

Nadolol (Amphetamines may antagonize the hypotensive effects of antihypertensives).
   No products indexed under this heading.

Nicardipine Hydrochloride (Amphetamines may antagonize the hypotensive effects of antihypertensives). Products include:
   Cardene Capsules 2261
   Cardene I.V. 2815
   Cardene SR Capsules................ 2264

Nifedipine (Amphetamines may antagonize the hypotensive effects of antihypertensives). Products include:
   Adalat Capsules (10 mg and 20 mg) 580
   Adalat CC 582
   Procardia Capsules 2024
   Procardia XL Extended Release Tablets 2026

Nisoldipine (Amphetamines may antagonize the hypotensive effects of antihypertensives). Products include:
   Sular Tablets 2961

Nitroglycerin (Amphetamines may antagonize the hypotensive effects of antihypertensives). Products include:
   Deponit NTG Transdermal Delivery System 2541
   Nitro-Bid IV 1270
   Nitro-Bid Ointment 1272
   Nitro-Dur (nitroglycerin) Transdermal Infusion System 1365
   Nitrolingual Spray 2193
   Nitrostat Tablets 1981
   Transderm-Nitro Transdermal Therapeutic System 878

Norepinephrine Hydrochloride (Amphetamines enhance the adrenergic effect of norepinephrine).

Nortriptyline Hydrochloride (Enhanced activity of tricyclic antidepressants or sympathomimetics; possible increases in the brain concentration of d-amphetamine resulting in potentiated cardiovascular effects). Products include:
   Pamelor 2409

Penbutolol Sulfate (Amphetamines may antagonize the hypotensive effects of antihypertensives). Products include:
   Levatol Tablets 2547

Phenelzine Sulfate (MAO inhibitors slow amphetamine metabolism, thereby potentiating and increasing their effects resulting in hypertensive crises; concurrent and/or sequential use is contraindicated). Products include:
   Nardil 1977

Phenobarbital (Amphetamines may delay intestinal absorption of phenobarbital; co-administration may produce a synergistic anticonvulsant action). Products include:
   Arco-Lase Plus Tablets 513
   Bellergal-S Tablets 2375
   Donnatal 2234
   Donnatal Extentabs 2234
   Donnatal Tablets 2234
   Phenobarbital Elixir and Tablets 1523
   Quadrinal Tablets 1398

Phenoxybenzamine Hydrochloride (Amphetamines may antagonize the hypotensive effects of antihypertensives). Products include:
   Dibenzyline Capsules 2650

Phentolamine Mesylate (Amphetamines may antagonize the hypotensive effects of antihypertensives). Products include:
   Regitine Vials 864

Phenytoin (Amphetamines may delay intestinal absorption of phenytoin; co-administration may produce a synergistic anticonvulsant action). Products include:
   Dilantin Infatabs 1967
   Dilantin-125 Suspension 1969

Phenytoin Sodium (Amphetamines may delay intestinal absorption of phenytoin; co-administration may produce a synergistic anticonvulsant action). Products include:
   Dilantin Kapseals 1965

Pindolol (Amphetamines may antagonize the hypotensive effects of antihypertensives). Products include:
   Visken Tablets 2428

Polythiazide (Some thiazides produce alkaline urine, thereby decreasing urinary excretion of amphetamines; potential for increase in blood levels resulting in potentiation of the action of amphetamines). Products include:
   Minizide Capsules 2016

Potassium Citrate (Increases the concentration of the non-ionized species of the amphetamine molecule, thereby decreasing urinary excretion; potential for higher blood levels and efficacy of amphetamines). Products include:
   Polycitra Syrup 574
   Polycitra-K Crystals 574
   Polycitra-K Oral Solution 575
   Polycitra-LC 574
   Urocit-K Tablets 1828

Prazosin Hydrochloride (Amphetamines may antagonize the hypotensive effects of antihypertensives). Products include:
   Minipress Capsules 2015
   Minizide Capsules 2016

Promethazine Hydrochloride (Amphetamines may counteract the sedative effect of antihistamines). Products include:
   Mepergan Injection 2859
   Phenergan with Codeine 2883
   Phenergan with Dextromethorphan 2885
   Phenergan Injection 2880
   Phenergan Suppositories 2882
   Phenergan Syrup 2881
   Phenergan Tablets 2882
   Phenergan VC 2886
   Phenergan VC with Codeine 2888

Propoxyphene Hydrochloride (In cases of propoxyphene overdosage, amphetamine CNS stimulation is potentiated and fatal convulsions can occur). Products include:
   Darvon 1475
   Wygesic Tablets 2930

Propoxyphene Napsylate (In cases of propoxyphene overdosage, amphetamine CNS stimulation is potentiated and fatal convulsions can occur). Products include:
   Darvon-N/Darvocet-N 1473

Propranolol Hydrochloride (Amphetamines may antagonize the hypotensive effects of antihypertensives). Products include:
   Inderal 2834
   Inderal LA Long Acting Capsules 2836
   Inderide Tablets 2838
   Inderide LA Long Acting Capsules .. 2840

Protriptyline Hydrochloride (Enhanced activity of tricyclic antidepressants or sympathomimetics; possible increases in the brain concentration of d-amphetamine resulting in potentiated cardiovascular effects). Products include:
   Vivactil Tablets 1820

Pyrilamine Maleate (Amphetamines may counteract the sedative effect of antihistamines). Products include:
   4-Way Fast Acting Nasal Spray (regular & mentholated) 644
   Maximum Strength Multi-Symptom Formula Midol 621
   PMS Multi-Symptom Formula Midol 622

Pyrilamine Tannate (Amphetamines may counteract the sedative effect of antihistamines). Products include:
   Atrohist Pediatric Suspension 1604
   Atrohist Pediatric Suspension Dye-Free 1604
   Rynatan 2781

Quinapril Hydrochloride (Amphetamines may antagonize the hypotensive effects of antihypertensives). Products include:
   Accupril Tablets 1950

Ramipril (Amphetamines may antagonize the hypotensive effects of antihypertensives). Products include:
   Altace Capsules 1238

Rauwolfia Serpentina (Amphetamines may antagonize the hypotensive effects of antihypertensives).
   No products indexed under this heading.

Rescinnamine (Amphetamines may antagonize the hypotensive effects of antihypertensives).
   No products indexed under this heading.

Reserpine (Gastrointestinal acidifying agents lower absorption of amphetamines, blood levels and efficacy; amphetamines may antagonize the hypotensive effects of antihypertensives). Products include:
   Diupres Tablets 1691
   Hydropres Tablets 1718
   Ser-Ap-Es Tablets 867

Selegiline Hydrochloride (MAO inhibitors slow amphetamine metabolism thereby potentiating and increasing their effects resulting in hypertensive crises; concurrent and/or sequential use is contraindicated). Products include:
   Eldepryl Capsules 2729

Sodium Acid Phosphate (Increases the concentration of the ionized species of the amphetamine molecule, thereby increasing urinary excretion; lowers blood levels and efficacy of amphetamines). Products include:
   Uroqid-Acid No. 2 Tablets 633

Sodium Bicarbonate (Systemic sodium bicarbonate, a gastrointestinal alkalinizing agent, increases absorption of amphetamines). Products include:
   Alka-Seltzer Cherry Effervescent Antacid and Pain Reliever 609
   Alka-Seltzer Extra Strength Effervescent Antacid and Pain Reliever 609
   Alka-Seltzer Gold Effervescent Antacid 611
   Alka-Seltzer Lemon Lime Effervescent Antacid and Pain Reliever 609
   Alka-Seltzer Original Effervescent Antacid and Pain Reliever 609
   Arm & Hammer Pure Baking Soda 648
   Colyte and Colyte-flavored........ 2540
   GoLYTELY 694

IMPORTANT NOTE: Always consult each drug listing in the patient's regimen for possible interactions.

Massengill Disposable Douches ▣ 780
Massengill Liquid Concentrate ▣ 780
NuLYTELY 694
Cherry Flavor NuLYTELY 694

Sodium Citrate (Increases the concentration of the non-ionized species of the amphetamine molecule, thereby decreasing urinary excretion; potential for higher blood levels and efficacy of amphetamines). Products include:

Bicitra 573
Polycitra 574
Salix SST Lozenges Saliva Stimulant ▣ 757

Sodium Nitroprusside (Amphetamines may antagonize the hypotensive effects of antihypertensives).

No products indexed under this heading.

Sotalol Hydrochloride (Amphetamines may antagonize the hypotensive effects of antihypertensives). Products include:

Betapace Tablets 637

Spirapril Hydrochloride (Amphetamines may antagonize the hypotensive effects of antihypertensives).

No products indexed under this heading.

Terazosin Hydrochloride (Amphetamines may antagonize the hypotensive effects of antihypertensives). Products include:

Hytrin Capsules 434

Terfenadine (Amphetamines may counteract the sedative effect of antihistamines). Products include:

Seldane Tablets 1284
Seldane-D Extended-Release Tablets 1286

Timolol Maleate (Amphetamines may antagonize the hypotensive effects of antihypertensives). Products include:

Blocadren Tablets 1654
Timolide Tablets 1791
Timoptic in Ocudose 1796
Timoptic Sterile Ophthalmic Solution 1794
Timoptic-XE 1798

Torsemide (Amphetamines may antagonize the hypotensive effects of antihypertensives). Products include:

Demadex Tablets and Injection 691

Trandolapril (Amphetamines may antagonize the hypotensive effects of antihypertensives). Products include:

Mavik Tablets 1407

Tranylcypromine Sulfate (MAO inhibitors slow amphetamine metabolism, thereby potentiating and increasing their effects resulting in hypertensive crises; concurrent and/or sequential use is contraindicated). Products include:

Parnate Tablets 2679

Trimeprazine Tartrate (Amphetamines may counteract the sedative effect of antihistamines).

No products indexed under this heading.

Trimethaphan Camsylate (Amphetamines may antagonize the hypotensive effects of antihypertensives).

No products indexed under this heading.

Trimipramine Maleate (Enhanced activity of tricyclic antidepressants or sympathomimetics; possible increases in the brain concentration of *d*-amphetamine resulting in potentiated cardiovascular effects). Products include:

Surmontil Capsules 2917

Tripelennamine Hydrochloride (Amphetamines may counteract the sedative effect of antihistamines). Products include:

PBZ Tablets 863
PBZ-SR Tablets 862

Triprolidine Hydrochloride (Amphetamines may counteract the sedative effect of antihistamines). Products include:

Actifed Cold & Allergy Tablets ▣ 807
Actifed Cold & Sinus Caplets and Tablets ▣ 808

Verapamil Hydrochloride (Amphetamines may antagonize the hypotensive effects of antihypertensives). Products include:

Calan SR Caplets 2571
Calan Tablets 2568
Covera-HS Tablets 2573
Isoptin Injectable 1391
Isoptin Oral Tablets 1393
Isoptin SR Tablets 1395
Verelan Capsules 1455

Vitamin C (Ascorbic acid lowers absorption of amphetamines, blood levels and efficacy). Products include:

ACES Antioxidant Soft Gels ▣ 647
Chromagen Capsules 2470
Chromagen FA 2471
Chromagen Forte 2471
Dexatrim Maximum Strength Plus Vitamin C/Caffeine-Free Caplets ▣ 795
Ester-C Mineral Ascorbates Powder ▣ 673
Fero-Folic-500 Filmtab 433
Fero-Grad-500 Filmtab 434
Halls Vitamin C Drops ▣ 807
Irospan 1000
Materna Tablets 1427
Niferex w/Vitamin C Tablets 811
One-A-Day Antioxidant Plus ▣ 625
Protegra Antioxidant Vitamin & Mineral Supplement ▣ 685
Sunkist Children's Chewable Multivitamins - Plus Extra C ▣ 665
Sunkist Vitamin C ▣ 666
Trinsicon Capsules 2759
Venolax ▣ 686
Vitron-C Tablets ▣ 667

Food Interactions

Fruit juices, unspecified (Lowers absorption of amphetamines, blood levels and efficacy).

ADENOCARD INJECTION

(Adenosine) 1021

May interact with xanthine bronchodilators, cardiac glycosides, and certain other agents. Compounds in these categories include:

Aminophylline (The effects of adenosine are antagonized by co-administration with methylxanthines, such as theophylline; larger doses of adenosine may be required or adenosine may not be effective).

No products indexed under this heading.

Caffeine (The effects of adenosine are antagonized by co-administration with methylxanthines, such as caffeine; larger doses of adenosine may be required or adenosine may not be effective). Products include:

Arthritis Strength BC Powder ▣ 631
BC Powder ▣ 631
Cafergot 2376
DHCplus Capsules 2148
Darvon Compound-65 Pulvules 1475
Esgic-plus Capsules 1012
Esgic-plus Tablets 1012
Aspirin Free Excedrin Analgesic Caplets and Geltabs 734
Excedrin Extra-Strength Analgesic Tablets, Caplets, and Geltabs 734
Fioricet Tablets 2386
Fioricet with Codeine Capsules 2387
Fiorinal Capsules 2388
Fiorinal with Codeine Capsules 2390
Fiorinal Tablets 2388
Goody's Extra Strength Headache Powders ▣ 632
Goody's Extra Strength Pain Relief Tablets ▣ 632
Maximum Strength Multi-Symptom Formula Midol ▣ 621
No Doz Maximum Strength Caplets ▣ 644
Norgesic 1554
Vanquish Analgesic Caplets ▣ 627
Wigraine Tablets 1884

Carbamazepine (Adenosine decreases the conduction through AV node, higher degrees of heart block may be produced in the presence of carbamazepine). Products include:

Atretol Tablets 569
Tegretol/Tegretol-XR 870

Deslanoside (The use of adenosine in patients receiving digitalis may be rarely associated with ventricular fibrillation).

No products indexed under this heading.

Digitoxin (The use of adenosine in patients receiving digitalis may be rarely associated with ventricular fibrillation). Products include:

Crystodigin Tablets 1472

Digoxin (The use of adenosine in patients receiving digitalis may be rarely associated with ventricular fibrillation). Products include:

Lanoxicaps 1110
Lanoxin Elixir Pediatric 1113
Lanoxin Injection 1116
Lanoxin Injection Pediatric 1119
Lanoxin Tablets 1121

Dipyridamole (Adenosine effects are potentiated by dipyridamole; smaller doses of adenosine may be effective with concurrent use). Products include:

Persantine Tablets 686

Dyphylline (The effects of adenosine are antagonized by co-administration with methylxanthines, such as theophylline; larger doses of adenosine may be required or adenosine may not be effective). Products include:

Lufyllin & Lufyllin-400 Tablets 2778
Lufyllin-GG Elixir & Tablets 2779

Theophylline (The effects of adenosine are antagonized by co-administration with methylxanthines, such as theophylline; larger doses of adenosine may be required or adenosine may not be effective). Products include:

Marax Tablets & DF Syrup 2015
Quibron 2227

Theophylline Anhydrous (The effects of adenosine are antagonized by co-administration with methylxanthines, such as theophylline; larger doses of adenosine may be required or adenosine may not be effective). Products include:

Aerolate 1003
Primatene Tablets ▣ 844
Respbid Tablets 687
Slo-bid Gyrocaps 2201
Theo-24 Extended Release Capsules 2753
Theo-Dur Extended-Release Tablets 1367
Theo-X Extended-Release Tablets 793
Uni-Dur Extended-Release Tablets 1374
Uniphyl 400 mg and 600 mg Tablets 2157

Theophylline Calcium Salicylate (The effects of adenosine are antagonized by co-administration with methylxanthines, such as theophylline; larger doses of adenosine may be required or adenosine may not be effective). Products include:

Quadrinal Tablets 1398

Theophylline Sodium Glycinate (The effects of adenosine are antagonized by co-administration with methylxanthines, such as theophylline; larger doses of adenosine may be required or adenosine may not be effective).

No products indexed under this heading.

ADENOSCAN

(Adenosine) 1022

May interact with beta blockers, cardiac glycosides, calcium channel blockers, adenosine receptor antagonists, and nucleoside transport inhibitors. Compounds in these categories include:

Acebutolol Hydrochloride (Potential for additive or synergistic depressant effects on the SA or AV nodes; adenosine should be used with caution in the presence of these agents; no adverse interactions have been reported when co-administered). Products include:

Sectral Capsules 2914

Aminophylline (The vasoactive effects of adenosine are inhibited by adenosine receptor antagonists such as alkylxanthines).

No products indexed under this heading.

Amlodipine Besylate (Potential for additive or synergistic depressant effects on the SA or AV nodes; adenosine should be used with caution in the presence of these agents; no adverse interactions have been reported when co-administered). Products include:

Lotrel Capsules 858
Norvasc Tablets 2020

Atenolol (Potential for additive or synergistic depressant effects on the SA or AV nodes; adenosine should be used with caution in the presence of these agents; no adverse interactions have been reported when co-administered). Products include:

Tenoretic Tablets 2963
Tenormin Tablets and I.V. Injection 2965

Bepridil Hydrochloride (Potential for additive or synergistic depressant effects on the SA or AV nodes; adenosine should be used with caution in the presence of these agents; no adverse interactions have been reported when co-administered). Products include:

Vascor Tablets (200 and 300 mg) 1597

Betaxolol Hydrochloride (Potential for additive or synergistic depressant effects on the SA or AV nodes; adenosine should be used with caution in the presence of these agents; no adverse interactions have been reported when co-administered). Products include:

Betoptic Ophthalmic Solution 465
Betoptic S Ophthalmic Suspension 467
Kerlone Tablets 2588

Bisoprolol Fumarate (Potential for additive or synergistic depressant effects on the SA or AV nodes; adenosine should be used with caution in the presence of these agents; no adverse interactions have been reported when co-administered). Products include:

Zebeta Tablets 1457
Ziac 1459

Caffeine (The vasoactive effects of adenosine are inhibited by adenosine receptor antagonists such as alkylxanthines). Products include:

Arthritis Strength BC Powder ▣ 631
BC Powder ▣ 631
Cafergot 2376

(▣ Described in PDR For Nonprescription Drugs) (◉ Described in PDR For Ophthalmology)

19 **Interactions Index** **Adipex-P**

DHCplus Capsules 2148
Darvon Compound-65 Pulvules 1475
Esgic-plus Capsules 1012
Esgic-plus Tablets 1012
Aspirin Free Excedrin Analgesic Caplets and Geltabs 734
Excedrin Extra-Strength Analgesic Tablets, Caplets, and Geltabs 734
Fioricet Tablets 2386
Fioricet with Codeine Capsules 2387
Fiorinal Capsules 2388
Fiorinal with Codeine Capsules 2390
Fiorinal Tablets 2388
Goody's Extra Strength Headache Powders .... BD 632
Goody's Extra Strength Pain Relief Tablets .... BD 632
Maximum Strength Multi-Symptom Formula Midol .... BD 621
No Doz Maximum Strength Caplets .... BD 644
Norgesic 1554
Vanquish Analgesic Caplets .... BD 627
Wigraine Tablets 1884

Carteolol Hydrochloride (Potential for additive or synergistic depressant effects on the SA or AV nodes; adenosine should be used with caution in the presence of these agents; no adverse interactions have been reported when co-administered). Products include:
Cartrol Tablets 413
Ocupress Ophthalmic Solution, 1% Sterile .... ◉ 297

Deslanoside (Potential for additive or synergistic depressant effects on the SA or AV nodes; adenosine should be used with caution in the presence of these agents; no adverse interactions have been reported when co-administered).
No products indexed under this heading.

Digitoxin (Potential for additive or synergistic depressant effects on the SA or AV nodes; adenosine should be used with caution in the presence of these agents; no adverse interactions have been reported when co-administered). Products include:
Crystodigin Tablets 1472

Digoxin (Potential for additive or synergistic depressant effects on the SA or AV nodes; adenosine should be used with caution in the presence of these agents; no adverse interactions have been reported when co-administered). Products include:
Lanoxicaps 1110
Lanoxin Elixir Pediatric 1113
Lanoxin Injection 1116
Lanoxin Injection Pediatric 1119
Lanoxin Tablets 1121

Diltiazem Hydrochloride (Potential for additive or synergistic depressant effects on the SA or AV nodes; adenosine should be used with caution in the presence of these agents; no adverse interactions have been reported when co-administered). Products include:
Cardizem CD Capsules 1251
Cardizem SR Capsules 1255
Cardizem Injectable 1253
Cardizem Tablets 1257
Dilacor XR Extended-release Capsules 2183
Tiazac Capsules 1019

Dipyridamole (Vasoactive effects of adenosine are potentiated by nucleoside transport inhibited). Products include:
Persantine Tablets 686

Dyphylline (The vasoactive effects of adenosine are inhibited by adenosine receptor antagonists such as alkylxanthines). Products include:
Lufyllin & Lufyllin-400 Tablets 2778
Lufyllin-GG Elixir & Tablets 2779

Esmolol Hydrochloride (Potential for additive or synergistic depressant effects on the SA or AV nodes; adenosine should be used with caution in the presence of these agents; no adverse interactions have been reported when co-administered). Products include:
Brevibloc (esmolol HCl) Injection 1860

Felodipine (Potential for additive or synergistic depressant effects on the SA or AV nodes; adenosine should be used with caution in the presence of these agents; no adverse interactions have been reported when co-administered). Products include:
Plendil Extended-Release Tablets 514

Isradipine (Potential for additive or synergistic depressant effects on the SA or AV nodes; adenosine should be used with caution in the presence of these agents; no adverse interactions have been reported when co-administered). Products include:
DynaCirc Capsules 2381
DynaCirc CR Tablets 2383

Labetalol Hydrochloride (Potential for additive or synergistic depressant effects on the SA or AV nodes; adenosine should be used with caution in the presence of these agents; no adverse interactions have been reported when co-administered). Products include:
Normodyne Injection 2519
Normodyne Tablets 2522
Trandate 1158

Levobunolol Hydrochloride (Potential for additive or synergistic depressant effects on the SA or AV nodes; adenosine should be used with caution in the presence of these agents; no adverse interactions have been reported when co-administered). Products include:
Betagan .... ◉ 230

Metipranolol Hydrochloride (Potential for additive or synergistic depressant effects on the SA or AV nodes; adenosine should be used with caution in the presence of these agents; no adverse interactions have been reported when co-administered). Products include:
OptiPranolol (Metipranolol 0.3%) Sterile Ophthalmic Solution .... ◉ 256

Metoprolol Succinate (Potential for additive or synergistic depressant effects on the SA or AV nodes; adenosine should be used with caution in the presence of these agents; no adverse interactions have been reported when co-administered). Products include:
Toprol-XL Tablets 560

Metoprolol Tartrate (Potential for additive or synergistic depressant effects on the SA or AV nodes; adenosine should be used with caution in the presence of these agents; no adverse interactions have been reported when co-administered). Products include:
Lopressor 848
Lopressor HCT Tablets 850

Nadolol (Potential for additive or synergistic depressant effects on the SA or AV nodes; adenosine should be used with caution in the presence of these agents; no adverse interactions have been reported when co-administered).
No products indexed under this heading.

Nicardipine Hydrochloride (Potential for additive or synergistic depressant effects on the SA or AV nodes; adenosine should be used with caution in the presence of these agents; no adverse interactions have been reported when co-administered). Products include:
Cardene Capsules 2261
Cardene I.V. 2815
Cardene SR Capsules 2264

Nifedipine (Potential for additive or synergistic depressant effects on the SA or AV nodes; adenosine should be used with caution in the presence of these agents; no adverse interactions have been reported when co-administered). Products include:
Adalat Capsules (10 mg and 20 mg) 580
Adalat CC 582
Procardia Capsules 2024
Procardia XL Extended Release Tablets 2026

Nimodipine (Potential for additive or synergistic depressant effects on the SA or AV nodes; adenosine should be used with caution in the presence of these agents; no adverse interactions have been reported when co-administered). Products include:
Nimotop Capsules 603

Nisoldipine (Potential for additive or synergistic depressant effects on the SA or AV nodes; adenosine should be used with caution in the presence of these agents; no adverse interactions have been reported when co-administered). Products include:
Sular Tablets 2961

Penbutolol Sulfate (Potential for additive or synergistic depressant effects on the SA or AV nodes; adenosine should be used with caution in the presence of these agents; no adverse interactions have been reported when co-administered). Products include:
Levatol Tablets 2547

Pindolol (Potential for additive or synergistic depressant effects on the SA or AV nodes; adenosine should be used with caution in the presence of these agents; no adverse interactions have been reported when co-administered). Products include:
Visken Tablets 2428

Propranolol Hydrochloride (Potential for additive or synergistic depressant effects on the SA or AV nodes; adenosine should be used with caution in the presence of these agents; no adverse interactions have been reported when co-administered). Products include:
Inderal 2834
Inderal LA Long Acting Capsules 2836
Inderide Tablets 2838
Inderide LA Long Acting Capsules 2840

Sotalol Hydrochloride (Potential for additive or synergistic depressant effects on the SA or AV nodes; adenosine should be used with caution in the presence of these agents; no adverse interactions have been reported when co-administered). Products include:
Betapace Tablets 637

Theophylline (The vasoactive effects of adenosine are inhibited by adenosine receptor antagonists such as alkylxanthines). Products include:
Marax Tablets & DF Syrup 2015
Quibron 2227

Theophylline Anhydrous (The vasoactive effects of adenosine are inhibited by adenosine receptor antagonists such as alkylxanthines). Products include:
Aerolate 1003
Primatene Tablets .... BD 844
Respbid Tablets 687
Slo-bid Gyrocaps 2201
Theo-24 Extended Release Capsules 2753
Theo-Dur Extended-Release Tablets 1367
Theo-X Extended-Release Tablets 793
Uni-Dur Extended-Release Tablets 1374
Uniphyl 400 mg and 600 mg Tablets 2157

Theophylline Calcium Salicylate (The vasoactive effects of adenosine are inhibited by adenosine receptor antagonists such as alkylxanthines). Products include:
Quadrinal Tablets 1398

Theophylline Sodium Glycinate (The vasoactive effects of adenosine are inhibited by adenosine receptor antagonists such as alkylxanthines).
No products indexed under this heading.

Timolol Hemihydrate (Potential for additive or synergistic depressant effects on the SA or AV nodes; adenosine should be used with caution in the presence of these agents; no adverse interactions have been reported when co-administered). Products include:
Betimol 0.25%, 0.5% .... ◉ 259

Timolol Maleate (Potential for additive or synergistic depressant effects on the SA or AV nodes; adenosine should be used with caution in the presence of these agents; no adverse interactions have been reported when co-administered). Products include:
Blocadren Tablets 1654
Timolide Tablets 1791
Timoptic in Ocudose 1796
Timoptic Sterile Ophthalmic Solution 1794
Timoptic-XE 1798

Verapamil Hydrochloride (Potential for additive or synergistic depressant effects on the SA or AV nodes; adenosine should be used with caution in the presence of these agents; no adverse interactions have been reported when co-administered). Products include:
Calan SR Caplets 2571
Calan Tablets 2568
Covera-HS Tablets 2573
Isoptin Injectable 1391
Isoptin Oral Tablets 1393
Isoptin SR Tablets 1395
Verelan Capsules 1455

ADIPEX-P TABLETS AND CAPSULES
(Phentermine Hydrochloride) 1035
May interact with monoamine oxidase inhibitors, insulin, and certain other agents. Compounds in these categories include:

Furazolidone (Contraindication; hypertensive crisis may result). Products include:
Furoxone 2221

Guanethidine Monosulfate (Decreased hypotensive effect of guanethidine). Products include:
Esimil Tablets 840
Ismelin Tablets 845

Insulin, Human (Insulin requirement may be altered).
No products indexed under this heading.

IMPORTANT NOTE: Always consult each drug listing in the patient's regimen for possible interactions.

Adipex-P — Interactions Index

Insulin, Human Isophane Suspension (Insulin requirement may be altered). Products include:
   Novolin N Human Insulin 10 ml Vials 1846

Insulin, Human NPH (Insulin requirement may be altered). Products include:
   Humulin N, 100 Units 1495
   Novolin N PenFill 1.5 ml Cartridges Durable Insulin Delivery System 1849
   Novolin N Prefilled Syringe Disposable Insulin Delivery System 1850

Insulin, Human Regular (Insulin requirement may be altered). Products include:
   Humulin R, 100 Units 1497
   Novolin R Human Insulin 10 ml Vials 1846
   Novolin R PenFill 1.5 ml Cartridges Durable Insulin Delivery System 1849
   Novolin R Prefilled Syringe Disposable Insulin Delivery System 1850
   Velosulin BR Human Insulin 10 ml Vials 1847

Insulin, Human, Zinc Suspension (Insulin requirement may be altered). Products include:
   Humulin L, 100 Units 1494
   Humulin U, 100 Units 1498
   Novolin L Human Insulin 10 ml Vials 1846

Insulin Lispro, Human (Insulin requirement may be altered). Products include:
   Humalog Injection 1488

Insulin, NPH (Insulin requirement may be altered). Products include:
   NPH, 100 Units 1502
   Pork NPH, 100 Units 1506
   Purified Pork NPH Isophane Insulin 1852

Insulin, Regular (Insulin requirement may be altered). Products include:
   Regular, 100 Units 1503
   Pork Regular, 100 Units 1507
   Pork Regular (Concentrated), 500 Units 1508
   Purified Pork Regular Insulin ... 1852

Insulin, Zinc Crystals (Insulin requirement may be altered). Products include:
   NPH, 100 Units 1502

Insulin, Zinc Suspension (Insulin requirement may be altered). Products include:
   Iletin I 1501
   Lente, 100 Units 1501
   Iletin II 1504
   Pork Lente, 100 Units 1504
   Purified Pork Lente Insulin 1852

Isocarboxazid (Contraindication; hypertensive crisis may result).
   No products indexed under this heading.

Phenelzine Sulfate (Contraindication; hypertensive crisis may result). Products include:
   Nardil 1977

Selegiline Hydrochloride (Contraindication; hypertensive crisis may result). Products include:
   Eldepryl Capsules 2729

Tranylcypromine Sulfate (Contraindication; hypertensive crisis may result). Products include:
   Parnate Tablets 2679

Food Interactions

Alcohol (May result in adverse drug interaction).

ADRIAMYCIN PFS

(Doxorubicin Hydrochloride) 2056
May interact with antineoplastics and certain other agents. Compounds in these categories include:

Altretamine (Doxorubicin may potentiate the toxicity of other anticancer therapies). Products include:
   Hexalen Capsules 2760

Anastrozole (Doxorubicin may potentiate the toxicity of other anticancer therapies). Products include:
   Arimidex Tablets 2932

Asparaginase (Doxorubicin may potentiate the toxicity of other anticancer therapies). Products include:
   Elspar 1700

Bicalutamide (Doxorubicin may potentiate the toxicity of other anticancer therapies). Products include:
   Casodex Tablets 2934

Bleomycin Sulfate (Doxorubicin may potentiate the toxicity of other anticancer therapies). Products include:
   Blenoxane 697

Busulfan (Doxorubicin may potentiate the toxicity of other anticancer therapies). Products include:
   Myleran Tablets 1209

Carboplatin (Doxorubicin may potentiate the toxicity of other anticancer therapies). Products include:
   Paraplatin for Injection 713

Carmustine (BCNU) (Doxorubicin may potentiate the toxicity of other anticancer therapies). Products include:
   BiCNU 696

Chlorambucil (Doxorubicin may potentiate the toxicity of other anticancer therapies). Products include:
   Leukeran Tablets 1205

Cisplatin (Doxorubicin may potentiate the toxicity of other anticancer therapies). Products include:
   Platinol for Injection 717
   Platinol-AQ Injection 719

Cyclophosphamide (Doxorubicin may potentiate the toxicity of other anticancer therapies; serious irreversible myocardial toxicity; exacerbation of cyclophosphamide-induced hemorrhagic cystitis). Products include:
   Cytoxan 700

Cyclosporine (Concurrent use may induce coma and/or seizures). Products include:
   Neoral 2405
   Sandimmune 2416

Cytarabine (Combination therapy results in necrotizing colitis, typhilitis, bloody stools and severe infections). Products include:
   Cytosar-U Sterile Powder 2077

Dacarbazine (Doxorubicin may potentiate the toxicity of other anticancer therapies). Products include:
   DTIC-Dome 593

Daunorubicin Citrate (Doxorubicin may potentiate the toxicity of other anticancer therapies). Products include:
   DaunoXome 1842

Daunorubicin Hydrochloride (Doxorubicin may potentiate the toxicity of other anticancer therapies). Products include:
   Cerubidine for Injection 634

Docetaxel (Doxorubicin may potentiate the toxicity of other anticancer therapies). Products include:
   Taxotere for Injection Concentrate 2204

Estramustine Phosphate Sodium (Doxorubicin may potentiate the toxicity of other anticancer therapies). Products include:
   Emcyt Capsules 2085

Etoposide (Doxorubicin may potentiate the toxicity of other anticancer therapies). Products include:
   Etoposide Injection 539
   VePesid Capsules and Injection 727

Floxuridine (Doxorubicin may potentiate the toxicity of other anticancer therapies). Products include:
   Sterile FUDR 2284

Fluorouracil (Doxorubicin may potentiate the toxicity of other anticancer therapies). Products include:
   Efudex 2280
   Fluoroplex Topical Solution & Cream 1% 475
   Fluorouracil Injection 2282

Flutamide (Doxorubicin may potentiate the toxicity of other anticancer therapies). Products include:
   Eulexin Capsules 2498

Fosphenytoin Sodium (Potential for decreased phenytoin levels with concurrent use). Products include:
   Cerebyx Injection 1956

Gemcitabine Hydrochloride (Doxorubicin may potentiate the toxicity of other anticancer therapies). Products include:
   Gemzar for Injection 1482

Hydroxyurea (Doxorubicin may potentiate the toxicity of other anticancer therapies). Products include:
   Hydrea Capsules 705

Idarubicin Hydrochloride (Doxorubicin may potentiate the toxicity of other anticancer therapies; concurrent use is contraindicated in patients who have received previous treatment with complete cumulative doses of idarubicin). Products include:
   Idamycin Injection 2096

Ifosfamide (Doxorubicin may potentiate the toxicity of other anticancer therapies). Products include:
   IFEX 706

Interferon alfa-2A, Recombinant (Doxorubicin may potentiate the toxicity of other anticancer therapies). Products include:
   Roferon-A Injection 2308

Interferon alfa-2B, Recombinant (Doxorubicin may potentiate the toxicity of other anticancer therapies). Products include:
   Intron A for Injection 2506

Irinotecan Hydrochloride (Doxorubicin may potentiate the toxicity of other anticancer therapies).
   No products indexed under this heading.

Levamisole Hydrochloride (Doxorubicin may potentiate the toxicity of other anticancer therapies). Products include:
   Ergamisol Tablets 1340

Live Virus Vaccines (Administration of live vaccine to immunocompromised patients, including those undergoing cytotoxic chemotherapy, may be hazardous).

Lomustine (CCNU) (Doxorubicin may potentiate the toxicity of other anticancer therapies). Products include:
   CeeNU Capsules 699

Mechlorethamine Hydrochloride (Doxorubicin may potentiate the toxicity of other anticancer therapies). Products include:
   Mustargen 1752

Megestrol Acetate (Doxorubicin may potentiate the toxicity of other anticancer therapies). Products include:
   Megace Oral Suspension 708
   Megace Tablets 710

Melphalan (Doxorubicin may potentiate the toxicity of other anticancer therapies). Products include:
   Alkeran Tablets 1198

Mercaptopurine (Enhanced hepatotoxicity of 6-mercaptopurine). Products include:
   Purinethol Tablets 1214

Methotrexate Sodium (Doxorubicin may potentiate the toxicity of other anticancer therapies). Products include:
   Methotrexate Sodium Tablets, Injection, for Injection and LPF Injection 1322

Mitomycin (Mitomycin-C) (Doxorubicin may potentiate the toxicity of other anticancer therapies). Products include:
   Mutamycin for Injection 712

Mitotane (Doxorubicin may potentiate the toxicity of other anticancer therapies). Products include:
   Lysodren Tablets 707

Mitoxantrone Hydrochloride (Doxorubicin may potentiate the toxicity of other anticancer therapies). Products include:
   Novantrone for Injection 1327

Paclitaxel (Doxorubicin may potentiate the toxicity of other anticancer therapies). Products include:
   Taxol Injection 723

Phenobarbital (Increases the elimination of doxorubicin). Products include:
   Arco-Lase Plus Tablets 513
   Bellergal-S Tablets 2375
   Donnatal 2234
   Donnatal Extentabs 2234
   Donnatal Tablets 2234
   Phenobarbital Elixir and Tablets 1523
   Quadrinal Tablets 1398

Phenytoin (Potential for decreased phenytoin levels with concurrent use). Products include:
   Dilantin Infatabs 1967
   Dilantin-125 Suspension 1969

Phenytoin Sodium (Potential for decreased phenytoin levels with concurrent use). Products include:
   Dilantin Kapseals 1965

Procarbazine Hydrochloride (Doxorubicin may potentiate the toxicity of other anticancer therapies). Products include:
   Matulane Capsules 2300

Streptozocin (May inhibit the hepatic metabolism; doxorubicin may potentiate the toxicity of other anticancer therapies). Products include:
   Zanosar Sterile Powder 2119

Tamoxifen Citrate (Doxorubicin may potentiate the toxicity of other anticancer therapies). Products include:
   Nolvadex Tablets 2957

Teniposide (Doxorubicin may potentiate the toxicity of other anticancer therapies). Products include:
   Vumon for Injection 729

Thioguanine (Doxorubicin may potentiate the toxicity of other anticancer therapies). Products include:
   Thioguanine Tablets, Tabloid Brand 1225

Thiotepa (Doxorubicin may potentiate the toxicity of other anticancer therapies). Products include:
   Thioplex (Thiotepa For Injection) 1329

Topotecan Hydrochloride (Doxorubicin may potentiate the toxicity of other anticancer therapies). Products include:
   Hycamtin for Injection 2665

Vincristine Sulfate (Doxorubicin may potentiate the toxicity of other anticancer therapies). Products include:

Oncovin Solution Vials & Hyporets 1521

ADRIAMYCIN RDF

(Doxorubicin Hydrochloride) 2056

See **Adriamycin PFS**

ADVERA SPECIALIZED COMPLETE NUTRITION

(Nutritional Beverage)..........................2337

None cited in PDR database.

ADVIL COLD AND SINUS CAPLETS AND TABLETS

(Ibuprofen, Pseudoephedrine Hydrochloride).................................... 837

May interact with monoamine oxidase inhibitors. Compounds in this category include:

Furazolidone (Concurrent and/or sequential use is not recommended). Products include:

Furoxone 2221

Isocarboxazid (Concurrent and/or sequential use is not recommended).

No products indexed under this heading.

Phenelzine Sulfate (Concurrent and/or sequential use is not recommended). Products include:

Nardil 1977

Selegiline Hydrochloride (Concurrent and/or sequential use is not recommended). Products include:

Eldepryl Capsules 2729

Tranylcypromine Sulfate (Concurrent and/or sequential use is not recommended). Products include:

Parnate Tablets 2679

ADVIL IBUPROFEN TABLETS, CAPLETS AND GEL CAPLETS

(Ibuprofen)... 836

May interact with:

Acetaminophen (Concurrent administration should not be undertaken without physician's direction). Products include:

Actifed Cold & Sinus Caplets and Tablets 808
Actifed Sinus Daytime/Nighttime Tablets and Caplets 809
Alka-Seltzer Fast Relief Caplets...... 610
Alka-Seltzer Plus Liqui-Gels............ 612
Alka-Seltzer Plus Flu & Body Aches Effervescent Tablets............ 612
Alka-Seltzer Plus Flu & Body Aches Liqui-Gels Non-Drowsy Formula 613
Alka-Seltzer Plus Night-Time Cold Medicine Liqui-Gels.................... 612
Allerest No Drowsiness 649
Allerest Sinus Pain Formula 649
Axocet Capsules............................. 2469
Benadryl Allergy/Cold Tablets.......... 811
Benadryl Allergy Sinus Headache Caplets 813
Children's TYLENOL acetaminophen Chewable Tablets, Elixir, Suspension Liquid, and Suspension Drops................................. 1559
Children's TYLENOL Cold Multi-Symptom Chewable Tablets and Liquid 1559
Children's TYLENOL Cold Plus Cough Multi Symptom Chewable Tablets and Liquid.................... 1560
Children's TYLENOL Flu Suspension Liquid 1560
Allergy-Sinus Comtrex Multi-Symptom Allergy-Sinus Formula Tablets and Caplets 639
Comtrex Multi-Symptom.................. 638
Comtrex Non-Drowsy...................... 640
Contac Day Allergy/Sinus Caplets ... 771
Contac Day & Night 772
Contac Night Allergy/Sinus Caplets 771
Contac Severe Cold and Flu Formula Caplets 773
Contac Severe Cold & Flu Non-Drowsy 774
Coricidin Cold + Flu Tablets............ 760
Coricidin 'D' Decongestant Tablets 760
DHCplus Capsules......................... 2148
Darvon-N/Darvocet-N 1473
Dimetapp Allergy Sinus Caplets 838
Dimetapp Cold & Fever Suspension 839
Drixoral Cold and Flu Extended-Release Tablets........................... 764
Drixoral Cough + Sore Throat Liquid Caps 763
Drixoral Allergy/Sinus Extended Release Tablets.......................... 765
Esgic-plus Capsules 1012
Esgic-plus Tablets 1012
Aspirin Free Excedrin Analgesic Caplets and Geltabs 734
Excedrin Extra-Strength Analgesic Tablets, Caplets, and Geltabs........ 734
Excedrin P.M. Analgesic/Sleeping Aid Tablets, Caplets, Liquigels...... 735
Fioricet Tablets 2386
Fioricet with Codeine Capsules 2387
Goody's Extra Strength Headache Powders 632
Goody's Extra Strength Pain Relief Tablets 632
Hycomine Compound Tablets 948
Hydrocet Capsules 787
Infants' TYLENOL acetaminophen Suspension Drops 1559
Infants' TYLENOL Cold Decongestant & Fever-Reducer Drops 1561
Junior Strength TYLENOL acetaminophen Coated Caplets and Chewable Tablets......................... 1562
Lorcet 10/650 Tablets 1016
Lortab 2751
Lurline PMS Tablets 1000
Maximum Strength Multi-Symptom Formula Midol 621
PMS Multi-Symptom Formula Midol 622
Maximum Strength Midol Teen Multi-Symptom Formula 621
Midrin Capsules 788
Panodol Tablets and Caplets 783
Children's Panadol Chewable Tablets, Liquid, Infant's Drops 783
Percocet Tablets 955
Percogesic Analgesic Tablets........... 727
Phrenilin 790
Pyrroxate Caplets 742
Robitussin Cold, Cough & Flu Liqui-Gels 844
Robitussin Night-Time Cold Formula 847
Sedapap Tablets 50 mg/650 mg .. 1826
Sinarest 663
Sine-Aid Maximum Strength Sinus Headache Gelcaps, Caplets and Tablets 1570
Sine-Off No Drowsiness Formula Caplets 784
Sine-Off Sinus Medicine 784
Singlet Tablets 785
Sinulin Tablets 792
Sinutab Sinus Allergy Medication, Maximum Strength Tablets and Caplets 823
Sinutab Sinus Medication, Maximum Strength Without Drowsiness Formula, Tablets & Caplets 824
Sudafed Cold and Cough Liquid Caps 826
Sudafed Severe Cold Formula Caplets 828
Sudafed Severe Cold Formula Tablets 828
Sudafed Sinus Caplets...................... 829
Sudafed Sinus Tablets...................... 829
Talacen Caplets 2464
TheraFlu Flu and Cold Medicine 750
Theraflu Maximum Strength Flu and Cold Medicine For Sore Throat 751
TheraFlu Flu, Cold and Cough Medicine 750
TheraFlu Maximum Strength Nighttime Flu, Cold & Cough Medicine 751
TheraFlu Maximum Strength Non-Drowsy Formula Flu, Cold & Cough Medicine 751
TheraFlu Maximum Strength, Non-Drowsy Formula Flu, Cold and Cough Caplets 752
Theraflu Maximum Strength Sinus Non-Drowsy Formula Caplets 752
Triaminic Sore Throat Formula 755
Triaminicin Tablets 756
TYLENOL acetaminophen Extended Relief Caplets 1570
TYLENOL acetaminophen, Extra Strength Adult Liquid Pain Reliever 1570
TYLENOL acetaminophen, Extra Strength Gelcaps, Geltabs, Caplets, Tablets 1570
TYLENOL acetaminophen, Regular Strength Caplets and Tablets....... 1570
TYLENOL Allergy Sinus, Maximum Strength Caplets and Gelcaps 1571
TYLENOL Allergy Sinus NightTime, Maximum Strength Caplets........... 1571
TYLENOL Cold Medication, Multi-Symptom Formula Tablets and Caplets 1572
TYLENOL Cold Medication, Multi-Symptom Hot Liquid Packets........ 1572
TYLENOL Cold Medication, No Drowsiness Formula Caplets and Gelcaps 1572
TYLENOL Cold Severe Congestion Caplets 1573
TYLENOL Cough Medication, Multi Symptom 1574
TYLENOL Cough Medication with Decongestant, Multi Symptom...... 1574
TYLENOL Flu No Drowsiness Formula, Maximum Strength Gelcaps 1575
TYLENOL Flu NightTime, Maximum Strength Gelcaps 1575
TYLENOL Flu NightTime, Maximum Strength Hot Medication Packets 1575
TYLENOL Headache Plus Pain Reliever with Antacid, Extra Strength Caplets 705
TYLENOL PM Pain Reliever/Sleep Aid, Extra Strength Gelcaps, Caplets, Geltabs 1576
TYLENOL Severe Allergy Medication Caplets 1571
TYLENOL Sinus, Maximum Strength Geltabs, Gelcaps, Caplets and Tablets 1576
Tylenol with Codeine 1592
Tylox Capsules 1593
Unisom With Pain Relief-Nighttime Sleep Aid and Pain Reliever........... 1991
Vanquish Analgesic Caplets 627
Vicks 44 LiquiCaps Cough, Cold & Flu Relief.................................. 728
Vicks 44M Cough, Cold & Flu Relief... 729
Vicks DayQuil LiquiCaps/Liquid Multi-Symptom Cold/Flu Relief .. 734
Vicks Nyquil Hot Therapy................. 735
Vicks NyQuil LiquiCaps/Liquid Multi-Symptom Cold/Flu Relief, Original and Cherry Flavors........... 736
Vicodin Tablets 1404
Vicodin ES Tablets 1405
Vicodin HP Tablets 1403
Wygesic Tablets 2930
Zydone Capsules 967

Aspirin (Concurrent administration should not be undertaken without physician's direction). Products include:

Alka-Seltzer Cherry Effervescent Antacid and Pain Reliever 609
Alka-Seltzer Extra Strength Effervescent Antacid and Pain Reliever 609
Alka-Seltzer Lemon Lime Effervescent Antacid and Pain Reliever 609
Alka-Seltzer Original Effervescent Antacid and Pain Reliever 609
Alka-Seltzer Plus 611
Alka-Seltzer Plus Sinus Medicine .. 611
Ascriptin 650
Arthritis Strength BC Powder........... 631
BC Cold Powder Multi-Symptom Formula (Cold-Sinus-Allergy) 631
BC Cold Powder Non-Drowsy Formula (Cold-Sinus)..................... 631
BC Powder 631
Genuine Bayer Aspirin Tablets & Caplets 618
Extra Strength Bayer Arthritis Pain Regimen Formula 615
Extra Strength Bayer Aspirin Caplets & Tablets 617
Extended-Release Bayer 8-Hour Aspirin 616
Extra Strength Bayer Plus Aspirin Caplets 617
Extra Strength Bayer PM Aspirin Plus Sleep Aid 617
Aspirin Regimen Bayer 81 mg Tablets with Calcium 615
Aspirin Regimen Bayer Adult Low Strength 81 mg Tablets 613
Aspirin Regimen Bayer Children's Chewable Aspirin......................... 616
Aspirin Regimen Bayer Regular Strength 325 mg Caplets 613
Bufferin Analgesic Tablets................ 636
Arthritis Strength Bufferin Analgesic Caplets 637
Extra Strength Bufferin Analgesic Tablets 637
Cama Arthritis Pain Reliever............. 748
Darvon Compound-65 Pulvules 1475
Easprin 1971
Ecotrin 2625
Ecotrin Enteric Coated Aspirin Maximum Strength Tablets and Caplets 775
Ecotrin Enteric Coated Aspirin Regular Strength Tablets 2625
Empirin Aspirin Tablets 818
Excedrin Extra-Strength Analgesic Tablets, Caplets, and Geltabs........ 734
Fiorinal Capsules 2388
Fiorinal with Codeine Capsules 2390
Fiorinal Tablets 2388
Goody's Extra Strength Headache Powders 632
Goody's Extra Strength Pain Relief Tablets 632
Halfprin Tablets 1413
Norgesic... 1554
Percodan Tablets 955
Percodan-Demi Tablets 956
Robaxisal Tablets........................... 2246
Soma Compound w/Codeine Tablets 2784
Soma Compound Tablets................. 2783
St. Joseph Adult Chewable Aspirin (81 mg.) 768
Talwin Compound 2466
Vanquish Analgesic Caplets 627

AEROBID INHALER SYSTEM

(Flunisolide) 1004

None cited in PDR database.

AEROBID-M INHALER SYSTEM

(Flunisolide) 1004

None cited in PDR database.

AEROLATE JR. T.D. CAPSULES

(Theophylline Anhydrous)....................1003

None cited in PDR database.

AEROLATE LIQUID

(Theophylline Anhydrous)....................1003

None cited in PDR database.

AEROLATE SR. T.D. CAPSULES

(Theophylline Anhydrous)....................1003

None cited in PDR database.

AEROLATE III T.D. CAPSULES

(Theophylline Anhydrous)....................1003

None cited in PDR database.

AFRIN CHERRY SCENTED NASAL SPRAY 0.05%

(Oxymetazoline Hydrochloride) 757

None cited in PDR database.

AFRIN EXTRA MOISTURIZING NASAL SPRAY

(Oxymetazoline Hydrochloride) 757

None cited in PDR database.

IMPORTANT NOTE: Always consult each drug listing in the patient's regimen for possible interactions.

Afrin　　　　　　　Interactions Index

AFRIN MENTHOL NASAL SPRAY, 0.05%
(Oxymetazoline Hydrochloride) 757
None cited in PDR database.

AFRIN NASAL SPRAY 0.05% AND NASAL SPRAY PUMP
(Oxymetazoline Hydrochloride) 757
None cited in PDR database.

AFRIN NOSE DROPS 0.05%
(Oxymetazoline Hydrochloride) 757
None cited in PDR database.

AFRIN SALINE MIST
(Sodium Chloride) 758
None cited in PDR database.

AFRIN SINUS
(Oxymetazoline Hydrochloride) 757
None cited in PDR database.

AIRET ALBUTEROL SULFATE INHALATION SOLUTION
(Albuterol Sulfate) 1602
May interact with sympathomimetic aerosol bronchodilators, monoamine oxidase inhibitors, tricyclic antidepressants, beta blockers, and certain other agents. Compounds in these categories include:

Acebutolol Hydrochloride (Effect of each other inhibited). Products include:
　Sectral Capsules 2914

Albuterol (Concurrent use should be avoided). Products include:
　Proventil Inhalation Aerosol 2524
　Ventolin Inhalation Aerosol and Refill 1170

Amitriptyline Hydrochloride (Action of albuterol on the vascular system may be potentiated). Products include:
　Elavil 2945
　Etrafon 2495
　Limbitrol 2333
　Triavil Tablets 1800

Amoxapine (Action of albuterol on the vascular system may be potentiated). Products include:
　Asendin Tablets 1419

Atenolol (Effect of each other inhibited). Products include:
　Tenoretic Tablets 2963
　Tenormin Tablets and I.V. Injection 2965

Betaxolol Hydrochloride (Effect of each other inhibited). Products include:
　Betoptic Ophthalmic Solution 465
　Betoptic S Ophthalmic Suspension 467
　Kerlone Tablets 2588

Bisoprolol Fumarate (Effect of each other inhibited). Products include:
　Zebeta Tablets 1457
　Ziac 1459

Bitolterol Mesylate (Concurrent use should be avoided). Products include:
　Tornalate Solution for Inhalation, 0.2% 976
　Tornalate Metered Dose Inhaler 978

Carteolol Hydrochloride (Effect of each other inhibited). Products include:
　Cartrol Tablets 413
　Ocupress Ophthalmic Solution, 1% Sterile ...... ⊚ 297

Clomipramine Hydrochloride (Action of albuterol on the vascular system may be potentiated). Products include:
　Anafranil Capsules 819

Desipramine Hydrochloride (Action of albuterol on the vascular system may be potentiated). Products include:
　Norpramin Tablets 1273

Doxepin Hydrochloride (Action of albuterol on the vascular system may be potentiated). Products include:
　Adapin Capsules 1542
　Sinequan 2028
　Zonalon Cream 1042

Epinephrine (Do not use concomitantly). Products include:
　EPIFRIN ...... ⊚ 237
　EpiPen 808
　Marcaine with Epinephrine 2446
　Primatene Mist 843
　Sensorcaine with Epinephrine Injection 554
　Sus-Phrine Injection 1017
　Xylocaine with Epinephrine Injections 562

Epinephrine Bitartrate (Do not use concomitantly). Products include:
　Sensorcaine-MPF with Epinephrine Injection 554

Epinephrine Hydrochloride (Do not use concomitantly). Products include:
　Ana-Kit Anaphylaxis Emergency Treatment Kit 611

Esmolol Hydrochloride (Effect of each other inhibited). Products include:
　Brevibloc (esmolol HCl) Injection 1860

Furazolidone (Action of albuterol on the vascular system may be potentiated). Products include:
　Furoxone 2221

Imipramine Hydrochloride (Action of albuterol on the vascular system may be potentiated). Products include:
　Tofranil Ampuls 873
　Tofranil Tablets 875

Imipramine Pamoate (Action of albuterol on the vascular system may be potentiated). Products include:
　Tofranil-PM Capsules 876

Isocarboxazid (Action of albuterol on the vascular system may be potentiated).
No products indexed under this heading.

Isoetharine (Concurrent use should be avoided). Products include:
　Bronkometer Aerosol 2432
　Bronkosol Solution 2432
　Isoetharine Inhalation Solution, USP, Arm-a-Med 545

Isoproterenol Hydrochloride (Concurrent use should be avoided). Products include:
　Isuprel Hydrochloride Solution 2443
　Isuprel Injection 2441
　Isuprel Mistometer 2442

Labetalol Hydrochloride (Effect of each other inhibited). Products include:
　Normodyne Injection 2519
　Normodyne Tablets 2522
　Trandate 1158

Levobunolol Hydrochloride (Effect of each other inhibited). Products include:
　Betagan ...... ⊚ 230

Maprotiline Hydrochloride (Action of albuterol on the vascular system may be potentiated). Products include:
　Ludiomil Tablets 861

Metaproterenol Sulfate (Concurrent use should be avoided). Products include:
　Alupent 672
　Metaproterenol Sulfate Inhalation Solution, USP, Arm-a-Med 547

Metipranolol Hydrochloride (Effect of each other inhibited). Products include:
　OptiPranolol (Metipranolol 0.3%) Sterile Ophthalmic Solution ...... ⊚ 256

Metoprolol Succinate (Effect of each other inhibited). Products include:
　Toprol-XL Tablets 560

Metoprolol Tartrate (Effect of each other inhibited). Products include:
　Lopressor 848
　Lopressor HCT Tablets 850

Nadolol (Effect of each other inhibited).
No products indexed under this heading.

Nortriptyline Hydrochloride (Action of albuterol on the vascular system may be potentiated). Products include:
　Pamelor 2409

Penbutolol Sulfate (Effect of each other inhibited). Products include:
　Levatol Tablets 2547

Phenelzine Sulfate (Action of albuterol on the vascular system may be potentiated). Products include:
　Nardil 1977

Pindolol (Effect of each other inhibited). Products include:
　Visken Tablets 2428

Pirbuterol Acetate (Concurrent use should be avoided). Products include:
　Maxair Autohaler 1550
　Maxair Inhaler 1552

Propranolol Hydrochloride (Effect of each other inhibited). Products include:
　Inderal 2834
　Inderal LA Long Acting Capsules 2836
　Inderide Tablets 2838
　Inderide LA Long Acting Capsules 2840

Protriptyline Hydrochloride (Action of albuterol on the vascular system may be potentiated). Products include:
　Vivactil Tablets 1820

Salmeterol Xinafoate (Concurrent use should be avoided). Products include:
　Serevent Inhalation Aerosol 1149

Selegiline Hydrochloride (Action of albuterol on the vascular system may be potentiated). Products include:
　Eldepryl Capsules 2729

Sotalol Hydrochloride (Effect of each other inhibited). Products include:
　Betapace Tablets 637

Terbutaline Sulfate (Concurrent use should be avoided). Products include:
　Brethaire Inhaler 830
　Brethine Ampuls 832
　Brethine Tablets 831
　Bricanyl Subcutaneous Injection 1247
　Bricanyl Tablets 1248

Timolol Hemihydrate (Effect of each other inhibited). Products include:
　Betimol 0.25%, 0.5% ...... ⊚ 259

Timolol Maleate (Effect of each other inhibited). Products include:
　Blocadren Tablets 1654
　Timolide Tablets 1791
　Timoptic in Ocudose 1796
　Timoptic Sterile Ophthalmic Solution 1794
　Timoptic-XE 1798

Tranylcypromine Sulfate (Action of albuterol on the vascular system may be potentiated). Products include:
　Parnate Tablets 2679

Trimipramine Maleate (Action of albuterol on the vascular system may be potentiated). Products include:
　Surmontil Capsules 2917

AK-CIDE
(Prednisolone Acetate, Sulfacetamide Sodium) ...... ⊚ 203
None cited in PDR database.

AK-CIDE OINTMENT
(Prednisolone Acetate, Sulfacetamide Sodium) ...... ⊚ 203
None cited in PDR database.

AK-FLUOR INJECTION 10% AND 25%
(Fluorescein Sodium) ...... ⊚ 204
None cited in PDR database.

AKINETON INJECTION
(Biperiden Hydrochloride) 1380
May interact with tricyclic antidepressants, phenothiazines, antihistamines, antipsychotic agents, and certain other agents. Compounds in these categories include:

Acrivastine (Central anticholinergic syndrome). Products include:
　Semprex-D Capsules 1620

Amitriptyline Hydrochloride (Central anticholinergic syndrome). Products include:
　Elavil 2945
　Etrafon 2495
　Limbitrol 2333
　Triavil Tablets 1800

Amoxapine (Central anticholinergic syndrome). Products include:
　Asendin Tablets 1419

Astemizole (Central anticholinergic syndrome). Products include:
　Hismanal Tablets 1341

Azatadine Maleate (Central anticholinergic syndrome). Products include:
　Trinalin Repetabs Tablets 1373

Bromodiphenhydramine Hydrochloride (Central anticholinergic syndrome).
No products indexed under this heading.

Brompheniramine Maleate (Central anticholinergic syndrome). Products include:
　Alka-Seltzer Plus Sinus Medicine 611
　Bromfed Capsules (Extended-Release) 1832
　Bromfed Syrup 712
　Bromfed Tablets 1832
　Bromfed-DM Cough Syrup 1832
　Bromfed-PD Capsules (Extended-Release) 1832
　Dimetane-DC Cough Syrup 2232
　Dimetane-DX Cough Syrup 2233
　Dimetapp Allergy Dye-Free Elixir 838
　Dimetapp Allergy Sinus Caplets 838
　Dimetapp Cold & Allergy Chewable Tablets 838
　Dimetapp Cold & Cough Liqui-Gels 839
　Dimetapp Cold & Fever Suspension 839
　Dimetapp DM Elixir 840
　Dimetapp Elixir 840
　Dimetapp Extentabs 841
　Dimetapp Tablets/Liqui-Gels 841
　Rondec Chewable Tablets 974
　Vicks DayQuil Allergy Relief 12-Hour Extended Release Tablets 733
　Vicks DayQuil Allergy Relief 4-Hour Tablets 733

(Described in PDR For Nonprescription Drugs)　　　　　　(⊚ Described in PDR For Ophthalmology)

Cetirizine Hydrochloride (Central anticholinergic syndrome). Products include:
Zyrtec Tablets 2053

Chlorpheniramine Maleate (Central anticholinergic syndrome). Products include:
Alka-Seltzer Plus Cold Medicine .... ⊞ 611
Alka-Seltzer Plus Cold Medicine Liqui-Gels .... ⊞ 612
Alka-Seltzer Plus Cold & Cough Medicine .... ⊞ 611
Alka-Seltzer Plus Cold & Cough Medicine Liqui-Gels .... ⊞ 612
Alka-Seltzer Plus Flu & Body Aches Effervescent Tablets ...... ⊞ 612
Allerest Maximum Strength .... ⊞ 649
Allerest Sinus Pain Formula .... ⊞ 649
Ana-Kit Anaphylaxis Emergency Treatment Kit 611
Atrohist Pediatric Capsules 1603
Atrohist Plus Tablets 1605
BC Cold Powder Multi-Symptom Formula (Cold-Sinus-Allergy) 631
Cerose DM .... ⊞ 853
Cheracol Plus Head Cold/Cough Formula .... ⊞ 741
Children's TYLENOL Cold Multi-Symptom Chewable Tablets and Liquid 1559
Children's TYLENOL Cold Plus Cough Multi Symptom Chewable Tablets and Liquid 1560
Children's TYLENOL Flu Suspension Liquid 1560
Children's Vicks DayQuil Allergy Relief .... ⊞ 730
Children's Vicks NyQuil Cold/Cough Relief .... ⊞ 731
Chlor-Trimeton Allergy Decongestant Tablets .... ⊞ 759
Chlor-Trimeton Allergy Tablets ...... ⊞ 758
Allergy-Sinus Comtrex Multi-Symptom Allergy-Sinus Formula Tablets and Caplets .... ⊞ 639
Comtrex Multi-Symptom .... ⊞ 638
Contac Continuous Action Nasal Decongestant/Antihistamine 12 Hour Capsules .... ⊞ 773
Contac Maximum Strength Continuous Action Decongestant/Antihistamine 12 Hour Caplets .. 772
Contac Severe Cold and Flu Formula Caplets 773
Coricidin Cold + Flu Tablets .... ⊞ 760
Coricidin Cough + Cold Tablets ... ⊞ 760
Coricidin 'D' Decongestant Tablets .... ⊞ 760
D.A. II Tablets 972
D.A. Chewable Tablets 970
Dura-Tap/PD Capsules 970
Dura-Vent/DA Tablets 972
Efidac 24 Chlorpheniramine .... ⊞ 655
Extendryl 1003
Fedahist Gyrocaps 2545
Hycomine Compound Tablets 948
Kronofed-A 994
Nolamine Timed-Release Tablets 790
Novahistine Elixir .... ⊞ 782
Ornade Spansule Capsules 2678
PediaCare Cough-Cold Chewable Tablets and Liquid 1569
PediaCare NightRest Cough-Cold Liquid 1569
Pediatric Vicks 44m Cough & Cold Relief .... ⊞ 737
Pyrroxate Caplets .... ⊞ 742
Ryna .... ⊞ 804
Sinarest .... ⊞ 663
Sine-Off Sinus Medicine .... ⊞ 784
Singlet Tablets .... ⊞ 785
Sinulin Tablets 792
Sinutab Sinus Allergy Medication, Maximum Strength Tablets and Caplets .... ⊞ 823
Sudafed Cold & Allergy Tablets ..... ⊞ 826
Teldrin 12 Hour Antihistamine/Nasal Decongestant Allergy Relief Capsules .... ⊞ 786
TheraFlu Flu and Cold Medicine .... ⊞ 750
Theraflu Maximum Strength Flu and Cold Medicine For Sore Throat .... ⊞ 751
TheraFlu Flu, Cold and Cough Medicine .... ⊞ 750
TheraFlu Maximum Strength Nighttime Flu, Cold & Cough Medicine .... ⊞ 751
Triaminic Night Time .... ⊞ 754
Triaminic Syrup .... ⊞ 755

Triaminic Triaminicol Cold & Cough .... ⊞ 756
Triaminicin Tablets .... ⊞ 756
Tussend 1830
TYLENOL Allergy Sinus, Maximum Strength Caplets and Gelcaps ... 1571
TYLENOL Cold Medication, Multi-Symptom Formula Tablets and Caplets 1572
TYLENOL Cold Medication, Multi-Symptom Hot Liquid Packets ... 1572
Vicks 44 LiquiCaps Cough, Cold & Flu Relief .... ⊞ 728
Vicks 44M Cough, Cold & Flu Relief .... ⊞ 729

Chlorpheniramine Polistirex (Central anticholinergic syndrome). Products include:
Tussionex Pennkinetic Extended-Release Suspension 1624

Chlorpheniramine Tannate (Central anticholinergic syndrome). Products include:
Atrohist Pediatric Suspension 1604
Atrohist Pediatric Suspension Dye-Free 1604
Rynatan 2781
Rynatuss 2782

Chlorpromazine (Central anticholinergic syndrome). Products include:
Thorazine Suppositories 2701

Chlorprothixene (Central anticholinergic syndrome).
No products indexed under this heading.

Chlorprothixene Hydrochloride (Central anticholinergic syndrome).
No products indexed under this heading.

Clemastine Fumarate (Central anticholinergic syndrome). Products include:
Tavist Syrup 2426
Tavist Tablets 2427
Tavist-1 12 Hour Relief Tablets ... ⊞ 749
Tavist-D 12 Hour Relief Tablets ... ⊞ 750

Clomipramine Hydrochloride (Central anticholinergic syndrome). Products include:
Anafranil Capsules 819

Clorazepate Dipotassium (Central anticholinergic syndrome). Products include:
Tranxene 459

Clozapine (Central anticholinergic syndrome). Products include:
Clozaril Tablets 2377

Cyproheptadine Hydrochloride (Central anticholinergic syndrome). Products include:
Periactin 1767

Desipramine Hydrochloride (Central anticholinergic syndrome). Products include:
Norpramin Tablets 1273

Dexchlorpheniramine Maleate (Central anticholinergic syndrome).
No products indexed under this heading.

Diphenhydramine Citrate (Central anticholinergic syndrome). Products include:
Excedrin P.M. Analgesic/Sleeping Aid Tablets, Caplets, Liquigels 735

Diphenhydramine Hydrochloride (Central anticholinergic syndrome). Products include:
Actifed Allergy Daytime/Nighttime Caplets .... ⊞ 808
Actifed Sinus Daytime/Nighttime Tablets and Caplets .... ⊞ 809
Extra Strength Bayer PM Aspirin Plus Sleep Aid .... ⊞ 617
Benadryl Allergy Chewables .... ⊞ 811
Benadryl Allergy/Cold Tablets ..... ⊞ 811
Benadryl Allergy Decongestant Liquid Medication .... ⊞ 812
Benadryl Allergy Decongestant Tablets .... ⊞ 812
Benadryl Allergy Liquid Medication .... ⊞ 813

Benadryl Allergy .... ⊞ 811
Benadryl Allergy Sinus Headache Caplets .... ⊞ 813
Benadryl Dye-Free Allergy Liquigel Softgels .... ⊞ 813
Benadryl Dye-Free Allergy Liquid Medication .... ⊞ 814
Benadryl Itch Relief Stick Extra Strength .... ⊞ 814
Benadryl Cream .... ⊞ 814
Benadryl Gel .... ⊞ 815
Benadryl Spray .... ⊞ 815
Benadryl Injection 1955
Contac Day & Night Cold/Flu Night Caplets .... ⊞ 772
Contac Night Allergy/Sinus Caplets .... ⊞ 771
Extra Strength Doan's P.M. .... ⊞ 653
Excedrin P.M. Analgesic/Sleeping Aid Tablets, Caplets, Liquigels ... ⊞ 643
Nytol QuickCaps Caplets .... ⊞ 632
Sleepinal Night-time Sleep Aid Capsules and Softgels .... ⊞ 798
TYLENOL Allergy Sinus NightTime, Maximum Strength Caplets 1571
TYLENOL Flu NightTime, Maximum Strength Gelcaps 1575
TYLENOL Flu NightTime, Maximum Strength Hot Medication Packets 1575
TYLENOL PM Pain Reliever/Sleep Aid, Extra Strength Gelcaps, Caplets, Geltabs 1576
TYLENOL Severe Allergy Medication Caplets 1571
Maximum Strength Unisom Sleepgels 1990
Unisom With Pain Relief-Nighttime Sleep Aid and Pain Reliever 1991

Diphenylpyraline Hydrochloride (Central anticholinergic syndrome).
No products indexed under this heading.

Doxepin Hydrochloride (Central anticholinergic syndrome). Products include:
Adapin Capsules 1542
Sinequan 2028
Zonalon Cream 1042

Fluphenazine Decanoate (Central anticholinergic syndrome). Products include:
Prolixin Decanoate 510

Fluphenazine Enanthate (Central anticholinergic syndrome). Products include:
Prolixin Enanthate 510

Fluphenazine Hydrochloride (Central anticholinergic syndrome). Products include:
Prolixin 510

Haloperidol (Central anticholinergic syndrome). Products include:
Haldol Injection, Tablets and Concentrate 1585

Haloperidol Decanoate (Central anticholinergic syndrome). Products include:
Haldol Decanoate 1587

Imipramine Hydrochloride (Central anticholinergic syndrome). Products include:
Tofranil Ampuls 873
Tofranil Tablets 875

Imipramine Pamoate (Central anticholinergic syndrome). Products include:
Tofranil-PM Capsules 876

Loratadine (Central anticholinergic syndrome). Products include:
Claritin Tablets 2485
Claritin-D Tablets 2487

Loxapine Hydrochloride (Central anticholinergic syndrome). Products include:
Loxitane 1426

Loxapine Succinate (Central anticholinergic syndrome). Products include:
Loxitane Capsules 1426

Maprotiline Hydrochloride (Central anticholinergic syndrome). Products include:
Ludiomil Tablets 861

Meperidine Hydrochloride (Central anticholinergic syndrome). Products include:
Demerol 2438
Mepergan Injection 2859

Mesoridazine Besylate (Central anticholinergic syndrome). Products include:
Serentil 689

Methdilazine Hydrochloride (Central anticholinergic syndrome).
No products indexed under this heading.

Methotrimeprazine (Central anticholinergic syndrome). Products include:
Levoprome 1321

Molindone Hydrochloride (Central anticholinergic syndrome). Products include:
Moban Tablets and Concentrate 1036

Nortriptyline Hydrochloride (Central anticholinergic syndrome). Products include:
Pamelor 2409

Perphenazine (Central anticholinergic syndrome). Products include:
Etrafon 2495
Triavil Tablets 1800
Trilafon 2532

Prochlorperazine (Central anticholinergic syndrome). Products include:
Compazine 2644

Promethazine Hydrochloride (Central anticholinergic syndrome). Products include:
Mepergan Injection 2859
Phenergan with Codeine 2883
Phenergan with Dextromethorphan .. 2885
Phenergan Injection 2880
Phenergan Suppositories 2882
Phenergan Syrup 2881
Phenergan Tablets 2882
Phenergan VC 2886
Phenergan VC with Codeine 2888

Protriptyline Hydrochloride (Central anticholinergic syndrome). Products include:
Vivactil Tablets 1820

Pyrilamine Maleate (Central anticholinergic syndrome syndrome). Products include:
4-Way Fast Acting Nasal Spray (regular & mentholated) .... ⊞ 644
Maximum Strength Multi-Symptom Formula Midol .... ⊞ 621
PMS Multi-Symptom Formula Midol .... ⊞ 622

Pyrilamine Tannate (Central anticholinergic syndrome). Products include:
Atrohist Pediatric Suspension 1604
Atrohist Pediatric Suspension Dye-Free 1604
Rynatan 2781

Quinidine Gluconate (Central anticholinergic syndrome). Products include:
Quinaglute Dura-Tabs Tablets 644

Quinidine Polygalacturonate (Central anticholinergic syndrome). Products include:
Cardioquin Tablets 2146

Quinidine Sulfate (Central anticholinergic syndrome). Products include:
Quinidex Extentabs 2240

Risperidone (Central anticholinergic syndrome). Products include:
Risperdal Tablets 1348

Terfenadine (Central anticholinergic syndrome). Products include:
Seldane Tablets 1284
Seldane-D Extended-Release Tablets 1286

IMPORTANT NOTE: Always consult each drug listing in the patient's regimen for possible interactions.

Thioridazine Hydrochloride (Central anticholinergic syndrome). Products include:
  Mellaril 2398
Thiothixene (Central anticholinergic syndrome). Products include:
  Navane Capsules and Concentrate 2018
  Navane Intramuscular 2019
Trifluoperazine Hydrochloride (Central anticholinergic syndrome). Products include:
  Stelazine 2692
Trimeprazine Tartrate (Central anticholinergic syndrome).
  No products indexed under this heading.
Trimipramine Maleate (Central anticholinergic syndrome). Products include:
  Surmontil Capsules................................ 2917
Tripelennamine Hydrochloride (Central anticholinergic syndrome). Products include:
  PBZ Tablets 863
  PBZ-SR Tablets.................................. 862
Triprolidine Hydrochloride (Central anticholinergic syndrome). Products include:
  Actifed Cold & Allergy Tablets........ 807
  Actifed Cold & Sinus Caplets and Tablets 808

AKINETON TABLETS
(Biperiden Hydrochloride) 1380
  See Akineton Injection

AK-PRED
(Prednisolone Sodium Phosphate) .. 204
None cited in PDR database.

AK-SPORE OINTMENT
(Bacitracin Zinc, Neomycin Sulfate, Polymyxin B Sulfate) 205
None cited in PDR database.

AK-SPORE SOLUTION
(Gramicidin, Neomycin Sulfate, Polymyxin B Sulfate) 205
None cited in PDR database.

AKTOB
(Tobramycin) 207
None cited in PDR database.

AK-TROL OINTMENT & SUSPENSION
(Dexamethasone, Neomycin Sulfate, Polymyxin B Sulfate) 205
None cited in PDR database.

AKORN ANTIOXIDANTS
(Vitamins with Minerals) 206
None cited in PDR database.

AKPRO
(Dipivefrin Hydrochloride) 206
None cited in PDR database.

ALBALON SOLUTION WITH LIQUIFILM
(Naphazoline Hydrochloride)............. 229
May interact with monoamine oxidase inhibitors, tricyclic antidepressants, and certain other agents. Compounds in these categories include:

Amitriptyline Hydrochloride (May potentiate the pressor effect of naphazoline). Products include:
  Elavil 2945
  Etrafon 2495
  Limbitrol 2333
  Triavil Tablets 1800
Amoxapine (May potentiate the pressor effect of naphazoline). Products include:
  Asendin Tablets 1419

Clomipramine Hydrochloride (May potentiate the pressor effect of naphazoline). Products include:
  Anafranil Capsules 819
Desipramine Hydrochloride (May potentiate the pressor effect of naphazoline). Products include:
  Norpramin Tablets 1273
Doxepin Hydrochloride (May potentiate the pressor effect of naphazoline). Products include:
  Adapin Capsules 1542
  Sinequan 2028
  Zonalon Cream 1042
Furazolidone (Severe hypertensive crisis). Products include:
  Furoxone 2221
Imipramine Hydrochloride (May potentiate the pressor effect of naphazoline). Products include:
  Tofranil Ampuls 873
  Tofranil Tablets 875
Imipramine Pamoate (May potentiate the pressor effect of naphazoline). Products include:
  Tofranil-PM Capsules 876
Isocarboxazid (Severe hypertensive crisis).
  No products indexed under this heading.
Maprotiline Hydrochloride (May potentiate the pressor effect of naphazoline). Products include:
  Ludiomil Tablets.......................... 861
Nortriptyline Hydrochloride (May potentiate the pressor effect of naphazoline). Products include:
  Pamelor 2409
Phenelzine Sulfate (Severe hypertensive crisis). Products include:
  Nardil 1977
Protriptyline Hydrochloride (May potentiate the pressor effect of naphazoline). Products include:
  Vivactil Tablets 1820
Selegiline Hydrochloride (Severe hypertensive crisis). Products include:
  Eldepryl Capsules 2729
Tranylcypromine Sulfate (Severe hypertensive crisis). Products include:
  Parnate Tablets 2679
Trimipramine Maleate (May potentiate the pressor effect of naphazoline). Products include:
  Surmontil Capsules 2917

ALBENZA TABLETS
(Albendazole) 2629
May interact with:

Cimetidine (Co-administration has resulted in increased albendazole sulfoxide concentrations in bile and cystic fluid in hydatid cyst). Products include:
  Tagamet HB Tablets................... 786
  Tagamet Tablets 2694
Cimetidine Hydrochloride (Co-administration has resulted in increased albendazole sulfoxide concentrations in bile and cystic fluid in hydatid cyst). Products include:
  Tagamet....................................... 2694
Dexamethasone (Co-administration has resulted in higher steady-state trough concentrations of albendazole sulfoxide). Products include:
  AK-Trol Ointment & Suspension 205
  Decadron Elixir 1676
  Decadron Tablets 1678
  Decaspray Topical Aerosol 1689
  Maxitrol Ophthalmic Ointment and Suspension 222
  TobraDex Ophthalmic Suspension and Ointment 469

Dexamethasone Acetate (Co-administration has resulted in higher steady-state trough concentrations of albendazole sulfoxide). Products include:
  Dalalone D.P. Injectable 1009
  Decadron-LA Sterile Suspension ... 1687
Dexamethasone Sodium Phosphate (Co-administration has resulted in higher steady-state trough concentrations of albendazole sulfoxide). Products include:
  Decadron Phosphate Injection 1680
  Decadron Phosphate Sterile Ophthalmic Ointment.......................... 1684
  Decadron Phosphate Sterile Ophthalmic Solution 1685
  Decadron Phosphate Topical Cream 1686
  Decadron Phosphate with Xylocaine Injection, Sterile 1683
  Dexacort Phosphate in Respihaler .. 1606
  Dexacort Phosphate in Turbinaire .. 1607
  NeoDecadron Sterile Ophthalmic Ointment 1755
  NeoDecadron Sterile Ophthalmic Solution 1756
  NeoDecadron Topical Cream 1757
Praziquantel (Co-administration has resulted in increased maximum plasma concentration and area under the curve of albendazole sulfoxide). Products include:
  Biltricide Tablets 584

Food Interactions
Diet, high-lipid (Oral bioavailability appears to be enhanced when albendazole is co-administered with a fatty meal).

ALBUMINAR-5, ALBUMIN (HUMAN) U.S.P. 5%
(Albumin (Human)) 795
None cited in PDR database.

ALBUMINAR-25, ALBUMIN (HUMAN) U.S.P. 25%
(Albumin (Human)) 796
None cited in PDR database.

NATURAL MD BASIC RX
(Vitamins, Multiple)........................... 602
None cited in PDR database.

ALBUTEROL SULFATE, USP SOLUTION FOR INHALATION, ARM-A-MED
(Albuterol Sulfate) 522
May interact with sympathomimetic aerosol bronchodilators, monoamine oxidase inhibitors, tricyclic antidepressants, beta blockers, and drugs which lower serum potassium (selected). Compounds in these categories include:

Acebutolol Hydrochloride (Beta-receptor blocking agents and albuterol inhibit effect of each other). Products include:
  Sectral Capsules 2914
Albuterol (Concurrent use with other sympathomimetic aerosol bronchodilators should be avoided). Products include:
  Proventil Inhalation Aerosol 2524
  Ventolin Inhalation Aerosol and Refill 1170
Amitriptyline Hydrochloride (Action of albuterol on the vascular system may be potentiated). Products include:
  Elavil 2945
  Etrafon 2495
  Limbitrol 2333
  Triavil Tablets 1800
Amoxapine (Action of albuterol on the vascular system may be potentiated). Products include:
  Asendin Tablets 1419

Atenolol (Beta-receptor blocking agents and albuterol inhibit effect of each other). Products include:
  Tenoretic Tablets 2963
  Tenormin Tablets and I.V. Injection 2965
Bendroflumethiazide (Potential for hypokalemic effect with concurrent use).
  No products indexed under this heading.
Betamethasone Acetate (Potential for hypokalemic effect with concurrent use). Products include:
  Celestone Soluspan Suspension 2484
Betamethasone Sodium Phosphate (Potential for hypokalemic effect with concurrent use). Products include:
  Celestone Soluspan Suspension 2484
Betaxolol Hydrochloride (Beta-receptor blocking agents and albuterol inhibit effect of each other). Products include:
  Betoptic Ophthalmic Solution............ 465
  Betoptic S Ophthalmic Suspension 467
  Kerlone Tablets 2588
Bisoprolol Fumarate (Beta-receptor blocking agents and albuterol inhibit effect of each other). Products include:
  Zebeta Tablets 1457
  Ziac 1459
Bitolterol Mesylate (Concurrent use with other sympathomimetic aerosol bronchodilators should be avoided). Products include:
  Tornalate Solution for Inhalation, 0.2%.. 976
  Tornalate Metered Dose Inhaler .. 978
Carteolol Hydrochloride (Beta-receptor blocking agents and albuterol inhibit effect of each other). Products include:
  Cartrol Tablets 413
  Ocupress Ophthalmic Solution, 1% Sterile 297
Chlorothiazide (Potential for hypokalemic effect with concurrent use). Products include:
  Aldoclor Tablets 1638
  Diupres Tablets 1691
  Diuril Oral 1694
Chlorothiazide Sodium (Potential for hypokalemic effect with concurrent use). Products include:
  Diuril Sodium Intravenous 1693
Clomipramine Hydrochloride (Action of albuterol on the vascular system may be potentiated). Products include:
  Anafranil Capsules 819
Cortisone Acetate (Potential for hypokalemic effect with concurrent use). Products include:
  Cortone Acetate Sterile Suspension 1663
  Cortone Acetate Tablets 1664
Desipramine Hydrochloride (Action of albuterol on the vascular system may be potentiated). Products include:
  Norpramin Tablets 1273
Dexamethasone (Potential for hypokalemic effect with concurrent use). Products include:
  AK-Trol Ointment & Suspension 205
  Decadron Elixir 1676
  Decadron Tablets 1678
  Decaspray Topical Aerosol 1689
  Maxitrol Ophthalmic Ointment and Suspension 222
  TobraDex Ophthalmic Suspension and Ointment 469
Dexamethasone Acetate (Potential for hypokalemic effect with concurrent use). Products include:
  Dalalone D.P. Injectable 1009
  Decadron-LA Sterile Suspension 1687

Interactions Index — Albuterol Sulfate, USP

Dexamethasone Sodium Phosphate (Potential for hypokalemic effect with concurrent use). Products include:
- Decadron Phosphate Injection ... 1680
- Decadron Phosphate Sterile Ophthalmic Ointment ... 1684
- Decadron Phosphate Sterile Ophthalmic Solution ... 1685
- Decadron Phosphate Topical Cream ... 1686
- Decadron Phosphate with Xylocaine Injection, Sterile ... 1683
- Dexacort Phosphate in Respihaler .. 1606
- Dexacort Phosphate in Turbinaire .. 1607
- NeoDecadron Sterile Ophthalmic Ointment ... 1755
- NeoDecadron Sterile Ophthalmic Solution ... 1756
- NeoDecadron Topical Cream ... 1757

Doxepin Hydrochloride (Action of albuterol on the vascular system may be potentiated). Products include:
- Adapin Capsules ... 1542
- Sinequan ... 2028
- Zonalon Cream ... 1042

Esmolol Hydrochloride (Beta-receptor blocking agents and albuterol inhibit effect of each other). Products include:
- Brevibloc (esmolol HCl) Injection ... 1860

Furazolidone (Action of albuterol on the vascular system may be potentiated). Products include:
- Furoxone ... 2221

Hydrochlorothiazide (Potential for hypokalemic effect with concurrent use). Products include:
- Aldactazide Tablets ... 2556
- Aldoril Tablets ... 1644
- Apresazide Capsules ... 824
- Capozide Tablets ... 744
- Dyazide Capsules ... 2653
- Esidrix Tablets ... 839
- Esimil Tablets ... 840
- HydroDIURIL Tablets ... 1716
- Hydropres Tablets ... 1718
- Hyzaar Tablets ... 1720
- Inderide Tablets ... 2838
- Inderide LA Long Acting Capsules .. 2840
- Lopressor HCT Tablets ... 850
- Lotensin HCT Tablets ... 855
- Moduretic Tablets ... 1748
- Oretic Tablets ... 450
- Prinzide Tablets ... 1780
- Ser-Ap-Es Tablets ... 867
- Timolide Tablets ... 1791
- Vaseretic Tablets ... 1810
- Zestoretic Tablets ... 2968
- Ziac ... 1459

Hydrocortisone (Potential for hypokalemic effect with concurrent use). Products include:
- Anusol-HC Cream 2.5% ... 1953
- Aquanil HC Lotion ... 1989
- Maximum Strength Cortaid Spray ... 800
- CORTENEMA ... 2713
- Cortisporin Ointment ... 1074
- Cortisporin Ophthalmic Ointment Sterile ... 1074
- Cortisporin Ophthalmic Suspension Sterile ... 1075
- Cortisporin Otic Solution Sterile ... 1076
- Cortisporin Otic Suspension Sterile ... 1077
- Cortizone-5 ... 795
- Cortizone-10 ... 795
- Hydrocortone Tablets ... 1715
- Hytone ... 922
- Hytone Ointment 2 ½% ... 923
- Massengill Medicated Soft Cloth Towelettes ... 2628
- Pediotic Suspension Sterile ... 1140
- Preparation H Hydrocortisone 1% Cream ... 843
- ProctoCream-HC 2.5% ... 2552
- VōSoL HC Otic Solution ... 2786

Hydrocortisone Acetate (Potential for hypokalemic effect with concurrent use). Products include:
- Analpram-HC Rectal Cream 1% and 2.5% ... 993
- Anusol HC-1 Hydrocortisone Anti-Itch Ointment ... 810
- Anusol-HC Suppositories ... 1954
- Caldecort Anti-Itch Hydrocortisone Cream ... 651
- Coly-Mycin S Otic w/Neomycin & Hydrocortisone ... 1965
- Cortaid ... 800
- Cortifoam ... 2540
- Cortisporin Cream ... 1073
- Epifoam ... 2543
- Hydrocortone Acetate Sterile Suspension ... 1712
- Mantadil Cream ... 1124
- Nupercainal Hydrocortisone 1% Cream ... 661
- Pramosone Cream, Lotion & Ointment ... 995
- ProctoFoam-HC ... 2552
- Terra-Cortril Ophthalmic Suspension ... 2033

Hydrocortisone Sodium Phosphate (Potential for hypokalemic effect with concurrent use). Products include:
- Hydrocortone Phosphate Injection, Sterile ... 1713

Hydrocortisone Sodium Succinate (Potential for hypokalemic effect with concurrent use).
- No products indexed under this heading.

Hydroflumethiazide (Potential for hypokalemic effect with concurrent use). Products include:
- Diucardin Tablets ... 2824

Imipramine Hydrochloride (Action of albuterol on the vascular system may be potentiated). Products include:
- Tofranil Ampuls ... 873
- Tofranil Tablets ... 875

Imipramine Pamoate (Action of albuterol on the vascular system may be potentiated). Products include:
- Tofranil-PM Capsules ... 876

Isocarboxazid (Action of albuterol on the vascular system may be potentiated).
- No products indexed under this heading.

Isoetharine (Concurrent use with other sympathomimetic aerosol bronchodilators should be avoided). Products include:
- Bronkometer Aerosol ... 2432
- Bronkosol Solution ... 2432
- Isoetharine Inhalation Solution, USP, Arm-a-Med ... 545

Isoproterenol Hydrochloride (Concurrent use with other sympathomimetic aerosol bronchodilators should be avoided). Products include:
- Isuprel Hydrochloride Solution ... 2443
- Isuprel Injection ... 2441
- Isuprel Mistometer ... 2442

Labetalol Hydrochloride (Beta-receptor blocking agents and albuterol inhibit effect of each other). Products include:
- Normodyne Injection ... 2519
- Normodyne Tablets ... 2522
- Trandate ... 1158

Levobunolol Hydrochloride (Beta-receptor blocking agents and albuterol inhibit effect of each other). Products include:
- Betagan ... 230

Maprotiline Hydrochloride (Action of albuterol on the vascular system may be potentiated). Products include:
- Ludiomil Tablets ... 861

Metaproterenol Sulfate (Concurrent use with other sympathomimetic aerosol bronchodilators should be avoided). Products include:
- Alupent ... 672
- Metaproterenol Sulfate Inhalation Solution, USP, Arm-a-Med ... 547

Methyclothiazide (Potential for hypokalemic effect with concurrent use). Products include:
- Enduron Tablets ... 424

Methylprednisolone Acetate (Potential for hypokalemic effect with concurrent use).
- No products indexed under this heading.

Methylprednisolone Sodium Succinate (Potential for hypokalemic effect with concurrent use).
- No products indexed under this heading.

Metipranolol Hydrochloride (Beta-receptor blocking agents and albuterol inhibit effect of each other). Products include:
- OptiPranolol (Metipranolol 0.3%) Sterile Ophthalmic Solution ... 256

Metoprolol Succinate (Beta-receptor blocking agents and albuterol inhibit effect of each other). Products include:
- Toprol-XL Tablets ... 560

Metoprolol Tartrate (Beta-receptor blocking agents and albuterol inhibit effect of each other). Products include:
- Lopressor ... 848
- Lopressor HCT Tablets ... 850

Nadolol (Beta-receptor blocking agents and albuterol inhibit effect of each other).
- No products indexed under this heading.

Nortriptyline Hydrochloride (Action of albuterol on the vascular system may be potentiated). Products include:
- Pamelor ... 2409

Penbutolol Sulfate (Beta-receptor blocking agents and albuterol inhibit effect of each other). Products include:
- Levatol Tablets ... 2547

Phenelzine Sulfate (Action of albuterol on the vascular system may be potentiated). Products include:
- Nardil ... 1977

Pindolol (Beta-receptor blocking agents and albuterol inhibit effect of each other). Products include:
- Visken Tablets ... 2428

Pirbuterol Acetate (Concurrent use with other sympathomimetic aerosol bronchodilators should be avoided). Products include:
- Maxair Autohaler ... 1550
- Maxair Inhaler ... 1552

Polythiazide (Potential for hypokalemic effect with concurrent use). Products include:
- Minizide Capsules ... 2016

Prednisolone Acetate (Potential for hypokalemic effect with concurrent use). Products include:
- AK-CIDE ... 203
- AK-CIDE Ointment ... 203
- Blephamide Liquifilm Sterile Ophthalmic Suspension ... 472
- Blephamide Ointment ... 234
- Econopred & Econopred Plus Ophthalmic Suspensions ... 216
- Poly-Pred Liquifilm ... 246
- Pred Forte ... 247
- Pred Mild ... 250
- Pred-G Liquifilm Sterile Ophthalmic Suspension ... 248
- Pred-G S.O.P. Sterile Ophthalmic Ointment ... 249

Prednisolone Sodium Phosphate (Potential for hypokalemic effect with concurrent use). Products include:
- AK-PRED ... 204
- Hydeltrasol Injection, Sterile ... 1708
- Pediapred Oral Solution ... 1618

Prednisolone Tebutate (Potential for hypokalemic effect with concurrent use). Products include:
- Hydeltra-T.B.A. Sterile Suspension ... 1710

Prednisone (Potential for hypokalemic effect with concurrent use).
- No products indexed under this heading.

Propranolol Hydrochloride (Beta-receptor blocking agents and albuterol inhibit effect of each other). Products include:
- Inderal ... 2834
- Inderal LA Long Acting Capsules ... 2836
- Inderide Tablets ... 2838
- Inderide LA Long Acting Capsules .. 2840

Protriptyline Hydrochloride (Action of albuterol on the vascular system may be potentiated). Products include:
- Vivactil Tablets ... 1820

Salmeterol Xinafoate (Concurrent use with other sympathomimetic aerosol bronchodilators should be avoided). Products include:
- Serevent Inhalation Aerosol ... 1149

Selegiline Hydrochloride (Action of albuterol on the vascular system may be potentiated). Products include:
- Eldepryl Capsules ... 2729

Sotalol Hydrochloride (Beta-receptor blocking agents and albuterol inhibit effect of each other). Products include:
- Betapace Tablets ... 637

Terbutaline Sulfate (Concurrent use with other sympathomimetic aerosol bronchodilators should be avoided). Products include:
- Brethaire Inhaler ... 830
- Brethine Ampuls ... 832
- Brethine Tablets ... 831
- Bricanyl Subcutaneous Injection ... 1247
- Bricanyl Tablets ... 1248

Timolol Hemihydrate (Beta-receptor blocking agents and albuterol inhibit effect of each other). Products include:
- Betimol 0.25%, 0.5% ... 259

Timolol Maleate (Beta-receptor blocking agents and albuterol inhibit effect of each other). Products include:
- Blocadren Tablets ... 1654
- Timolide Tablets ... 1791
- Timoptic in Ocudose ... 1796
- Timoptic Sterile Ophthalmic Solution ... 1794
- Timoptic-XE ... 1798

Tranylcypromine Sulfate (Action of albuterol on the vascular system may be potentiated). Products include:
- Parnate Tablets ... 2679

Triamcinolone (Potential for hypokalemic effect with concurrent use).
- No products indexed under this heading.

Triamcinolone Acetonide (Potential for hypokalemic effect with concurrent use). Products include:
- Azmacort Oral Inhaler ... 2175
- Nasacort AQ Nasal Spray ... 2191
- Nasacort Nasal Inhaler ... 2189

Triamcinolone Diacetate (Potential for hypokalemic effect with concurrent use).
- No products indexed under this heading.

Triamcinolone Hexacetonide (Potential for hypokalemic effect with concurrent use).
- No products indexed under this heading.

IMPORTANT NOTE: Always consult each drug listing in the patient's regimen for possible interactions.

Albuterol Sulfate, USP — Interactions Index

Trimipramine Maleate (Action of albuterol on the vascular system may be potentiated). Products include:
- Surmontil Capsules 2917

ALDACTAZIDE TABLETS
(Spironolactone, Hydrochlorothiazide) 2556
May interact with potassium preparations, diuretics, potassium sparing diuretics, loop diuretics, lithium preparations, oral hypoglycemic agents, insulin, cardiac glycosides, glucocorticoids, ACE inhibitors, and certain other agents. Compounds in these categories include:

Acarbose (Hydrochlorothiazide may raise blood glucose levels; dose adjustment of hypoglycemic agents may be necessary). Products include:
- Precose 604

ACTH (Hypokalemia may develop as a result of profound diuresis, particularly when co-administered).
- No products indexed under this heading.

Amiloride Hydrochloride (Concomitant use has been associated with severe hyperkalemia; concurrent use should be avoided). Products include:
- Midamor Tablets 1746
- Moduretic Tablets 1748

Benazepril Hydrochloride (Concomitant use has been associated with severe hyperkalemia; concurrent use should be avoided). Products include:
- Lotensin Tablets 852
- Lotensin HCT Tablets 855
- Lotrel Capsules 858

Bendroflumethiazide (Co-administration may result in dilutional hyponatremia, manifested by dry mouth, thirst, drowsiness, and lethargy).
- No products indexed under this heading.

Betamethasone Acetate (Hypokalemia may develop as a result of profound diuresis, particularly when co-administered with glucocorticoids). Products include:
- Celestone Soluspan Suspension 2484

Betamethasone Sodium Phosphate (Hypokalemia may develop as a result of profound diuresis, particularly when co-administered with glucocorticoids). Products include:
- Celestone Soluspan Suspension 2484

Bumetanide (Hypokalemia may develop as a result of profound diuresis, particularly when co-administered with loop diuretics). Products include:
- Bumex 2260

Captopril (Concomitant use has been associated with severe hyperkalemia; concurrent use should be avoided). Products include:
- Capoten Tablets 740
- Capozide Tablets 744

Chlorothiazide (Co-administration may result in dilutional hyponatremia, manifested by dry mouth, thirst, drowsiness, and lethargy). Products include:
- Aldoclor Tablets 1638
- Diupres Tablets 1691
- Diuril Oral 1694

Chlorothiazide Sodium (Co-administration may result in dilutional hyponatremia, manifested by dry mouth, thirst, drowsiness, and lethargy). Products include:
- Diuril Sodium Intravenous 1693

Chlorpropamide (Hydrochlorothiazide may raise blood glucose levels; dose adjustment of hypoglycemic agents may be necessary). Products include:
- Diabinese Tablets 2002

Chlorthalidone (Co-administration may result in dilutional hyponatremia, manifested by dry mouth, thirst, drowsiness, and lethargy). Products include:
- Combipres Tablets 682
- Tenoretic Tablets 2963
- Thalitone 1293

Cortisone Acetate (Hypokalemia may develop as a result of profound diuresis, particularly when co-administered with glucocorticoids). Products include:
- Cortone Acetate Sterile Suspension 1663
- Cortone Acetate Tablets 1664

Deslanoside (Hypokalemia induced by thiazides may exaggerate the effects of digitalis therapy).
- No products indexed under this heading.

Dexamethasone (Hypokalemia may develop as a result of profound diuresis, particularly when co-administered with glucocorticoids). Products include:
- AK-Trol Ointment & Suspension .... ⊙ 205
- Decadron Elixir 1676
- Decadron Tablets 1678
- Decaspray Topical Aerosol 1689
- Maxitrol Ophthalmic Ointment and Suspension .... ⊙ 222
- TobraDex Ophthalmic Suspension and Ointment 469

Dexamethasone Acetate (Hypokalemia may develop as a result of profound diuresis, particularly when co-administered with glucocorticoids). Products include:
- Dalalone D.P. Injectable 1009
- Decadron-LA Sterile Suspension 1687

Dexamethasone Sodium Phosphate (Hypokalemia may develop as a result of profound diuresis, particularly when co-administered with glucocorticoids). Products include:
- Decadron Phosphate Injection 1680
- Decadron Phosphate Sterile Ophthalmic Ointment 1684
- Decadron Phosphate Sterile Ophthalmic Solution 1685
- Decadron Phosphate Topical Cream 1686
- Decadron Phosphate with Xylocaine Injection, Sterile 1683
- Dexacort Phosphate in Respihaler 1606
- Dexacort Phosphate in Turbinaire 1607
- NeoDecadron Sterile Ophthalmic Ointment 1755
- NeoDecadron Sterile Ophthalmic Solution 1756
- NeoDecadron Topical Cream 1757

Digitoxin (Hypokalemia induced by thiazides may exaggerate the effects of digitalis therapy). Products include:
- Crystodigin Tablets 1472

Digoxin (Spironolactone may increase the half-life of digoxin resulting in increased serum digoxin levels and subsequent digitalis toxicity; hypokalemia induced by thiazides may exaggerate the effects of digitalis therapy). Products include:
- Lanoxicaps 1110
- Lanoxin Elixir Pediatric 1113
- Lanoxin Injection 1116
- Lanoxin Injection Pediatric 1119
- Lanoxin Tablets 1121

Enalapril Maleate (Concomitant use has been associated with severe hyperkalemia; concurrent use should be avoided). Products include:
- Vaseretic Tablets 1810

- Vasotec Tablets 1816

Enalaprilat (Concomitant use has been associated with severe hyperkalemia; concurrent use should be avoided). Products include:
- Vasotec I.V. 1814

Ethacrynic Acid (Hypokalemia may develop as a result of profound diuresis, particularly when co-administered with loop diuretics). Products include:
- Edecrin Tablets 1698

Fludrocortisone Acetate (Hypokalemia may develop as a result of profound diuresis, particularly when co-administered with glucocorticoids). Products include:
- Florinef Acetate Tablets 506

Fosinopril Sodium (Concomitant use has been associated with severe hyperkalemia; concurrent use should be avoided). Products include:
- Monopril Tablets 762

Furosemide (Hypokalemia may develop as a result of profound diuresis, particularly when co-administered with loop diuretics). Products include:
- Lasix Injection, Oral Solution and Tablets 1267

Glimepiride (Hydrochlorothiazide may raise blood glucose levels; dose adjustment of hypoglycemic agents may be necessary). Products include:
- Amaryl Tablets 1241

Glipizide (Hydrochlorothiazide may raise blood glucose levels; dose adjustment of hypoglycemic agents may be necessary). Products include:
- Glucotrol Tablets 2011
- Glucotrol XL Extended Release Tablets 2012

Glyburide (Hydrochlorothiazide may raise blood glucose levels; dose adjustment of hypoglycemic agents may be necessary). Products include:
- DiaBeta Tablets 1265
- Glynase PresTab Tablets 2091
- Micronase Tablets 2099

Hydrocortisone (Hypokalemia may develop as a result of profound diuresis, particularly when co-administered with glucocorticoids). Products include:
- Anusol-HC Cream 2.5% 1953
- Aquanil HC Lotion 1989
- Maximum Strength Cortaid Spray .... ⊞ 800
- CORTENEMA 2713
- Cortisporin Ointment 1074
- Cortisporin Ophthalmic Ointment Sterile 1074
- Cortisporin Ophthalmic Suspension Sterile 1075
- Cortisporin Otic Solution Sterile 1076
- Cortisporin Otic Suspension Sterile 1077
- Cortizone-5 .... ⊞ 795
- Cortizone-10 .... ⊞ 795
- Hydrocortone Tablets 1715
- Hytone 922
- Hytone Ointment 2 ½% 923
- Massengill Medicated Soft Cloth Towelettes 2628
- Pediotic Suspension Sterile 1140
- Preparation H Hydrocortisone 1% Cream .... ⊞ 843
- ProctoCream-HC 2.5% 2552
- VōSoL HC Otic Solution 2786

Hydrocortisone Acetate (Hypokalemia may develop as a result of profound diuresis, particularly when co-administered with glucocorticoids). Products include:
- Analpram-HC Rectal Cream 1% and 2.5% 993
- Anusol HC-1 Hydrocortisone Anti-Itch Ointment .... ⊞ 810
- Anusol-HC Suppositories 1954
- Caldecort Anti-Itch Hydrocortisone Cream .... ⊞ 651

- Coly-Mycin S Otic w/Neomycin & Hydrocortisone 1965
- Cortaid .... ⊞ 800
- Cortifoam 2540
- Cortisporin Cream 1073
- Epifoam 2543
- Hydrocortone Acetate Sterile Suspension 1712
- Mantadil Cream 1124
- Nupercainal Hydrocortisone 1% Cream .... ⊞ 661
- Pramosone Cream, Lotion & Ointment 995
- ProctoFoam-HC 2552
- Terra-Cortril Ophthalmic Suspension 2033

Hydrocortisone Sodium Phosphate (Hypokalemia may develop as a result of profound diuresis, particularly when co-administered with glucocorticoids). Products include:
- Hydrocortone Phosphate Injection, Sterile 1713

Hydrocortisone Sodium Succinate (Hypokalemia may develop as a result of profound diuresis, particularly when co-administered with glucocorticoids).
- No products indexed under this heading.

Hydroflumethiazide (Co-administration may result in dilutional hyponatremia, manifested by dry mouth, thirst, drowsiness, and lethargy). Products include:
- Diucardin Tablets 2824

Indapamide (Co-administration may result in dilutional hyponatremia, manifested by dry mouth, thirst, drowsiness, and lethargy).
- No products indexed under this heading.

Indomethacin (Concomitant use has been associated with severe hyperkalemia). Products include:
- Indocin 1723

Indomethacin Sodium Trihydrate (Concomitant use has been associated with severe hyperkalemia). Products include:
- Indocin I.V. 1727

Insulin, Human (Hydrochlorothiazide may raise blood glucose levels; dose adjustment of insulin may be necessary).
- No products indexed under this heading.

Insulin, Human Isophane Suspension (Hydrochlorothiazide may raise blood glucose levels; dose adjustment of insulin may be necessary). Products include:
- Novolin N Human Insulin 10 ml Vials 1846

Insulin, Human NPH (Hydrochlorothiazide may raise blood glucose levels; dose adjustment of insulin may be necessary). Products include:
- Humulin N, 100 Units 1495
- Novolin N PenFill 1.5 ml Cartridges Durable Insulin Delivery System 1849
- Novolin N Prefilled Syringe Disposable Insulin Delivery System 1850

Insulin, Human Regular (Hydrochlorothiazide may raise blood glucose levels; dose adjustment of insulin may be necessary). Products include:
- Humulin R, 100 Units 1497
- Novolin R Human Insulin 10 ml Vials 1846
- Novolin R PenFill 1.5 ml Cartridges Durable Insulin Delivery System 1849
- Novolin R Prefilled Syringe Disposable Insulin Delivery System 1850
- Velosulin BR Human Insulin 10 ml Vials 1847

(⊞ Described in PDR For Nonprescription Drugs) (⊙ Described in PDR For Ophthalmology)

Interactions Index

Insulin, Human, Zinc Suspension (Hydrochlorothiazide may raise blood glucose levels; dose adjustment of insulin may be necessary). Products include:
- Humulin L, 100 Units 1494
- Humulin U, 100 Units 1498
- Novolin L Human Insulin 10 ml Vials 1846

Insulin Lispro, Human (Hydrochlorothiazide may raise blood glucose levels; dose adjustment of insulin may be necessary). Products include:
- Humalog Injection 1488

Insulin, NPH (Hydrochlorothiazide may raise blood glucose levels; dose adjustment of insulin may be necessary). Products include:
- NPH, 100 Units 1502
- Pork NPH, 100 Units 1506
- Purified Pork NPH Isophane Insulin 1852

Insulin, Regular (Hydrochlorothiazide may raise blood glucose levels; dose adjustment of insulin may be necessary). Products include:
- Regular, 100 Units 1503
- Pork Regular, 100 Units 1507
- Pork Regular (Concentrated), 500 Units 1508
- Purified Pork Regular Insulin 1852

Insulin, Zinc Crystals (Hydrochlorothiazide may raise blood glucose levels; dose adjustment of insulin may be necessary). Products include:
- NPH, 100 Units 1502

Insulin, Zinc Suspension (Hydrochlorothiazide may raise blood glucose levels; dose adjustment of insulin may be necessary). Products include:
- Iletin I 1501
- Lente, 100 Units 1501
- Iletin II 1504
- Pork Lente, 100 Units 1504
- Purified Pork Lente Insulin 1852

Lisinopril (Concomitant use has been associated with severe hyperkalemia; concurrent use should be avoided). Products include:
- Prinivil Tablets 1776
- Prinzide Tablets 1780
- Zestoretic Tablets 2968
- Zestril Tablets 2972

Lithium Carbonate (Concurrent use of diuretic with lithium is not recommended as it may produce lithium toxicity). Products include:
- Eskalith 2658
- Lithium Carbonate Capsules & Tablets 2352
- Lithonate/Lithotabs/Lithobid 2721

Lithium Citrate (Concurrent use of diuretic with lithium is not recommended as it may produce lithium toxicity).
- No products indexed under this heading.

Metformin Hydrochloride (Hydrochlorothiazide may raise blood glucose levels; dose adjustment of hypoglycemic agents may be necessary). Products include:
- Glucophage Tablets 754

Methyclothiazide (Co-administration may result in dilutional hyponatremia, manifested by dry mouth, thirst, drowsiness, and lethargy). Products include:
- Enduron Tablets 424

Methylprednisolone Acetate (Hypokalemia may develop as a result of profound diuresis, particularly when co-administered with glucocorticoids).
- No products indexed under this heading.

Methylprednisolone Sodium Succinate (Hypokalemia may develop as a result of profound diuresis, particularly when co-administered with glucocorticoids).
- No products indexed under this heading.

Metolazone (Co-administration may result in dilutional hyponatremia, manifested by dry mouth, thirst, drowsiness, and lethargy). Products include:
- Mykrox Tablets 1617
- Zaroxolyn Tablets 1625

Moexipril Hydrochloride (Concomitant use has been associated with severe hyperkalemia; concurrent use should be avoided). Products include:
- Univasc Tablets 2553

Norepinephrine Bitartrate (Reduced vascular responsiveness to norepinephrine). Products include:
- Levophed Bitartrate Injection 2445

Polythiazide (Co-administration may result in dilutional hyponatremia, manifested by dry mouth, thirst, drowsiness, and lethargy). Products include:
- Minizide Capsules 2016

Potassium Acid Phosphate (Concurrent use with excessive potassium intake may cause hyperkalemia leading to cardiac irregularities). Products include:
- K-Phos Original Formula 'Sodium Free' Tablets 633

Potassium Bicarbonate (Concurrent use with excessive potassium intake may cause hyperkalemia leading to cardiac irregularities). Products include:
- Alka-Seltzer Gold Effervescent Antacid .... ⊛ 611

Potassium Chloride (Concurrent use with excessive potassium intake may cause hyperkalemia leading to cardiac irregularities). Products include:
- Chlor-3 Condiment 1003
- Colyte and Colyte-flavored 2540
- GoLYTELY 694
- K-Dur Microburst Release System (potassium chloride, USP) E.R. Tablets 1364
- K-Lor Powder Packets 438
- K-Norm Capsules 1615
- K-Tab Filmtab 439
- Micro-K 2237
- Micro-K LS Packets 2238
- NuLYTELY 694
- Cherry Flavor NuLYTELY 694
- Rum-K Syrup 1004
- Slow-K Extended-Release Tablets 869

Potassium Citrate (Concurrent use with excessive potassium intake may cause hyperkalemia leading to cardiac irregularities). Products include:
- Polycitra Syrup 574
- Polycitra-K Crystals 574
- Polycitra-K Oral Solution 575
- Polycitra-LC 574
- Urocit-K Tablets 1828

Potassium Gluconate (Concurrent use with excessive potassium intake may cause hyperkalemia leading to cardiac irregularities).
- No products indexed under this heading.

Potassium Phosphate, Dibasic (Concurrent use with excessive potassium intake may cause hyperkalemia leading to cardiac irregularities).
- No products indexed under this heading.

Potassium Phosphate, Monobasic (Concurrent use with excessive potassium intake may cause hyperkalemia leading to cardiac irregularities). Products include:
- K-Phos Neutral Tablets 633
- K-Phos Original Formula 'Sodium Free' Tablets 633

Prednisolone Acetate (Hypokalemia may develop as a result of profound diuresis, particularly when co-administered with glucocorticoids). Products include:
- AK-CIDE .... ⊛ 203
- AK-CIDE Ointment .... ⊛ 203
- Blephamide Liquifilm Sterile Ophthalmic Suspension 472
- Blephamide Ointment .... ⊛ 234
- Econopred & Econopred Plus Ophthalmic Suspensions .... ⊛ 216
- Poly-Pred Liquifilm .... ⊛ 246
- Pred Forte .... ⊛ 247
- Pred Mild .... ⊛ 250
- Pred-G Liquifilm Sterile Ophthalmic Suspension .... ⊛ 248
- Pred-G S.O.P. Sterile Ophthalmic Ointment .... ⊛ 249

Prednisolone Sodium Phosphate (Hypokalemia may develop as a result of profound diuresis, particularly when co-administered with glucocorticoids). Products include:
- AK-PRED .... ⊛ 204
- Hydeltrasol Injection, Sterile 1708
- Pediapred Oral Solution 1618

Prednisolone Tebutate (Hypokalemia may develop as a result of profound diuresis, particularly when co-administered with glucocorticoids). Products include:
- Hydeltra-T.B.A. Sterile Suspension 1710

Prednisone (Hypokalemia may develop as a result of profound diuresis, particularly when co-administered with glucocorticoids).
- No products indexed under this heading.

Quinapril Hydrochloride (Concomitant use has been associated with severe hyperkalemia; concurrent use should be avoided). Products include:
- Accupril Tablets 1950

Ramipril (Concomitant use has been associated with severe hyperkalemia; concurrent use should be avoided). Products include:
- Altace Capsules 1238

Spirapril Hydrochloride (Concomitant use has been associated with severe hyperkalemia; concurrent use should be avoided).
- No products indexed under this heading.

Tolazamide (Hydrochlorothiazide may raise blood glucose levels; dose adjustment of hypoglycemic agents may be necessary).
- No products indexed under this heading.

Tolbutamide (Hydrochlorothiazide may raise blood glucose levels; dose adjustment of hypoglycemic agents may be necessary).
- No products indexed under this heading.

Torsemide (Hypokalemia may develop as a result of profound diuresis, particularly when co-administered with loop diuretics). Products include:
- Demadex Tablets and Injection 691

Trandolapril (Concomitant use has been associated with severe hyperkalemia; concurrent use should be avoided). Products include:
- Mavik Tablets 1407

Triamcinolone (Hypokalemia may develop as a result of profound diuresis, particularly when co-administered with glucocorticoids).
- No products indexed under this heading.

Triamcinolone Acetonide (Hypokalemia may develop as a result of profound diuresis, particularly when co-administered with glucocorticoids). Products include:
- Azmacort Oral Inhaler 2175
- Nasacort AQ Nasal Spray 2191
- Nasacort Nasal Inhaler 2189

Triamcinolone Diacetate (Hypokalemia may develop as a result of profound diuresis, particularly when co-administered with glucocorticoids).
- No products indexed under this heading.

Triamcinolone Hexacetonide (Hypokalemia may develop as a result of profound diuresis, particularly when co-administered with glucocorticoids).
- No products indexed under this heading.

Triamterene (Concomitant use has been associated with severe hyperkalemia; concurrent use should be avoided). Products include:
- Dyazide Capsules 2653
- Dyrenium Capsules 2655

Tubocurarine Chloride (Thiazides may increase the responsiveness to tubocurarine).
- No products indexed under this heading.

ALDACTONE TABLETS

(Spironolactone) 2558
May interact with potassium preparations, antihypertensives, diuretics, potassium sparing diuretics, ganglionic blocking agents, ACE inhibitors, and certain other agents. Compounds in these categories include:

Acebutolol Hydrochloride (Aldactone potentiates effects of other antihypertensives). Products include:
- Sectral Capsules 2914

Amiloride Hydrochloride (Concomitant use has been associated with severe hyperkalemia; concurrent use should be avoided). Products include:
- Midamor Tablets 1746
- Moduretic Tablets 1748

Amlodipine Besylate (Aldactone potentiates effects of other antihypertensives). Products include:
- Lotrel Capsules 858
- Norvasc Tablets 2020

Atenolol (Aldactone potentiates effects of other antihypertensives). Products include:
- Tenoretic Tablets 2963
- Tenormin Tablets and I.V. Injection 2965

Benazepril Hydrochloride (Concomitant use has been associated with severe hyperkalemia; concurrent use should be avoided). Products include:
- Lotensin Tablets 852
- Lotensin HCT Tablets 855
- Lotrel Capsules 858

Bendroflumethiazide (Co-administration may result in hyponatremia, manifested by dry mouth, thirst, drowsiness, and lethargy; Aldactone potentiates effects of the diuretics).
- No products indexed under this heading.

Betaxolol Hydrochloride (Aldactone potentiates effects of other antihypertensives). Products include:
- Betoptic Ophthalmic Solution 465
- Betoptic S Ophthalmic Suspension 467

IMPORTANT NOTE: Always consult each drug listing in the patient's regimen for possible interactions.

Aldactone **Interactions Index** 28

Kerlone Tablets ... 2588

Bisoprolol Fumarate (Aldactone potentiates effects of other antihypertensives). Products include:

Zebeta Tablets ... 1457
Ziac ... 1459

Bumetanide (Co-administration may result in hyponatremia, manifested by dry mouth, thirst, drowsiness, and lethargy; Aldactone potentiates effects of the diuretics). Products include:

Bumex ... 2260

Captopril (Concomitant use has been associated with severe hyperkalemia; concurrent use should be avoided). Products include:

Capoten Tablets ... 740
Capozide Tablets ... 744

Carteolol Hydrochloride (Aldactone potentiates effects of other antihypertensives). Products include:

Cartrol Tablets ... 413
Ocupress Ophthalmic Solution, 1% Sterile ... ◉ 297

Chlorothiazide (Co-administration may result in hyponatremia, manifested by dry mouth, thirst, drowsiness, and lethargy; Aldactone potentiates effects of the diuretics). Products include:

Aldoclor Tablets ... 1638
Diupres Tablets ... 1691
Diuril Oral ... 1694

Chlorothiazide Sodium (Co-administration may result in hyponatremia, manifested by dry mouth, thirst, drowsiness, and lethargy; Aldactone potentiates effects of the diuretics). Products include:

Diuril Sodium Intravenous ... 1693

Chlorthalidone (Co-administration may result in hyponatremia, manifested by dry mouth, thirst, drowsiness, and lethargy; Aldactone potentiates effects of the diuretics). Products include:

Combipres Tablets ... 682
Tenoretic Tablets ... 2963
Thalitone ... 1293

Clonidine (Aldactone potentiates effects of other antihypertensives). Products include:

Catapres-TTS ... 680

Clonidine Hydrochloride (Aldactone potentiates effects of other antihypertensives). Products include:

Catapres Tablets ... 679
Combipres Tablets ... 682

Deserpidine (Aldactone potentiates effects of other antihypertensives).

No products indexed under this heading.

Diazoxide (Aldactone potentiates effects of other antihypertensives). Products include:

Hyperstat I.V. Injection ... 2504
Proglycem ... 575

Digoxin (Spironolactone may increase the half-life of digoxin resulting in increased serum digoxin levels and subsequent digitalis toxicity). Products include:

Lanoxicaps ... 1110
Lanoxin Elixir Pediatric ... 1113
Lanoxin Injection ... 1116
Lanoxin Injection Pediatric ... 1119
Lanoxin Tablets ... 1121

Diltiazem Hydrochloride (Aldactone potentiates effects of other antihypertensives). Products include:

Cardizem CD Capsules ... 1251
Cardizem SR Capsules ... 1255
Cardizem Injectable ... 1253
Cardizem Tablets ... 1257
Dilacor XR Extended-release Capsules ... 2183
Tiazac Capsules ... 1019

Doxazosin Mesylate (Aldactone potentiates effects of other antihypertensives). Products include:

Cardura Tablets ... 1993

Enalapril Maleate (Concomitant use has been associated with severe hyperkalemia; concurrent use should be avoided). Products include:

Vaseretic Tablets ... 1810
Vasotec Tablets ... 1816

Enalaprilat (Concomitant use has been associated with severe hyperkalemia; concurrent use should be avoided). Products include:

Vasotec I.V. ... 1814

Esmolol Hydrochloride (Aldactone potentiates effects of other antihypertensives). Products include:

Brevibloc (esmolol HCl) Injection ... 1860

Ethacrynic Acid (Co-administration may result in hyponatremia, manifested by dry mouth, thirst, drowsiness, and lethargy; Aldactone potentiates effects of the diuretics). Products include:

Edecrin Tablets ... 1698

Felodipine (Aldactone potentiates effects of other antihypertensives). Products include:

Plendil Extended-Release Tablets ... 514

Fosinopril Sodium (Concomitant use has been associated with severe hyperkalemia; concurrent use should be avoided). Products include:

Monopril Tablets ... 762

Furosemide (Co-administration may result in hyponatremia, manifested by dry mouth, thirst, drowsiness, and lethargy; Aldactone potentiates effects of the diuretics). Products include:

Lasix Injection, Oral Solution and Tablets ... 1267

Guanabenz Acetate (Aldactone potentiates effects of other antihypertensives).

No products indexed under this heading.

Guanethidine Monosulfate (Aldactone potentiates effects of other antihypertensives). Products include:

Esimil Tablets ... 840
Ismelin Tablets ... 845

Hydralazine Hydrochloride (Aldactone potentiates effects of other antihypertensives). Products include:

Apresazide Capsules ... 824
Apresoline Hydrochloride Tablets ... 826
Hydralazine Hydrochloride Injection USP ... 2712
Ser-Ap-Es Tablets ... 867

Hydrochlorothiazide (Co-administration may result in hyponatremia, manifested by dry mouth, thirst, drowsiness, and lethargy; Aldactone potentiates effects of the diuretics). Products include:

Aldactazide Tablets ... 2556
Aldoril Tablets ... 1644
Apresazide Capsules ... 824
Capozide Tablets ... 744
Dyazide Capsules ... 2653
Esidrix Tablets ... 839
Esimil Tablets ... 840
HydroDIURIL Tablets ... 1716
Hydropres Tablets ... 1718
Hyzaar Tablets ... 1720
Inderide Tablets ... 2838
Inderide LA Long Acting Capsules ... 2840
Lopressor HCT Tablets ... 850
Lotensin HCT Tablets ... 855
Moduretic Tablets ... 1748
Oretic Tablets ... 450
Prinzide Tablets ... 1780
Ser-Ap-Es Tablets ... 867
Timolide Tablets ... 1791
Vaseretic Tablets ... 1810
Zestoretic Tablets ... 2968
Ziac ... 1459

Hydroflumethiazide (Co-administration may result in hyponatremia, manifested by dry mouth, thirst, drowsiness, and lethargy; Aldactone potentiates effects of the diuretics). Products include:

Diucardin Tablets ... 2824

Indapamide (Co-administration may result in hyponatremia, manifested by dry mouth, thirst, drowsiness, and lethargy; Aldactone potentiates effects of the diuretics).

No products indexed under this heading.

Indomethacin (Concomitant use has been associated with severe hyperkalemia). Products include:

Indocin ... 1723

Indomethacin Sodium Trihydrate (Concomitant use has been associated with severe hyperkalemia). Products include:

Indocin I.V. ... 1727

Isradipine (Aldactone potentiates effects of other antihypertensives). Products include:

DynaCirc Capsules ... 2381
DynaCirc CR Tablets ... 2383

Labetalol Hydrochloride (Aldactone potentiates effects of other antihypertensives). Products include:

Normodyne Injection ... 2519
Normodyne Tablets ... 2522
Trandate ... 1158

Lisinopril (Concomitant use has been associated with severe hyperkalemia; concurrent use should be avoided). Products include:

Prinivil Tablets ... 1776
Prinzide Tablets ... 1780
Zestoretic Tablets ... 2968
Zestril Tablets ... 2972

Losartan Potassium (Aldactone potentiates effects of other antihypertensives). Products include:

Cozaar Tablets ... 1668
Hyzaar Tablets ... 1720

Mecamylamine Hydrochloride (Aldactone potentiates effects of other antihypertensives; the dosage of ganglionic blocking agents should be reduced by at least 50%). Products include:

Inversine Tablets ... 1729

Methyclothiazide (Co-administration may result in hyponatremia, manifested by dry mouth, thirst, drowsiness, and lethargy; Aldactone potentiates effects of the diuretics). Products include:

Enduron Tablets ... 424

Methyldopa (Aldactone potentiates effects of other antihypertensives). Products include:

Aldoclor Tablets ... 1638
Aldomet Oral ... 1640
Aldoril Tablets ... 1644

Methyldopate Hydrochloride (Aldactone potentiates effects of other antihypertensives). Products include:

Aldomet Ester HCl Injection ... 1642

Metolazone (Co-administration may result in hyponatremia, manifested by dry mouth, thirst, drowsiness, and lethargy; Aldactone potentiates effects of the diuretics). Products include:

Mykrox Tablets ... 1617
Zaroxolyn Tablets ... 1625

Metoprolol Succinate (Aldactone potentiates effects of other antihypertensives). Products include:

Toprol-XL Tablets ... 560

Metoprolol Tartrate (Aldactone potentiates effects of other antihypertensives). Products include:

Lopressor ... 848
Lopressor HCT Tablets ... 850

Metyrosine (Aldactone potentiates effects of other antihypertensives). Products include:

Demser Capsules ... 1690

Minoxidil (Aldactone potentiates effects of other antihypertensives).

No products indexed under this heading.

Moexipril Hydrochloride (Concomitant use has been associated with severe hyperkalemia; concurrent use should be avoided). Products include:

Univasc Tablets ... 2553

Nadolol (Aldactone potentiates effects of other antihypertensives).

No products indexed under this heading.

Nicardipine Hydrochloride (Aldactone potentiates effects of other antihypertensives). Products include:

Cardene Capsules ... 2261
Cardene I.V. ... 2815
Cardene SR Capsules ... 2264

Nifedipine (Aldactone potentiates effects of other antihypertensives). Products include:

Adalat Capsules (10 mg and 20 mg) ... 580
Adalat CC ... 582
Procardia Capsules ... 2024
Procardia XL Extended Release Tablets ... 2026

Nisoldipine (Aldactone potentiates effects of other antihypertensives). Products include:

Sular Tablets ... 2961

Nitroglycerin (Aldactone potentiates effects of other antihypertensives). Products include:

Deponit NTG Transdermal Delivery System ... 2541
Nitro-Bid IV ... 1270
Nitro-Bid Ointment ... 1272
Nitro-Dur (nitroglycerin) Transdermal Infusion System ... 1365
Nitrolingual Spray ... 2193
Nitrostat Tablets ... 1981
Transderm-Nitro Transdermal Therapeutic System ... 878

Norepinephrine Bitartrate (Reduced vascular responsiveness to norepinephrine). Products include:

Levophed Bitartrate Injection ... 2445

Penbutolol Sulfate (Aldactone potentiates effects of other antihypertensives). Products include:

Levatol Tablets ... 2547

Phenoxybenzamine Hydrochloride (Aldactone potentiates effects of other antihypertensives). Products include:

Dibenzyline Capsules ... 2650

Phentolamine Mesylate (Aldactone potentiates effects of other antihypertensives). Products include:

Regitine Vials ... 864

Pindolol (Aldactone potentiates effects of other antihypertensives). Products include:

Visken Tablets ... 2428

Polythiazide (Co-administration may result in hyponatremia, manifested by dry mouth, thirst, drowsiness, and lethargy; Aldactone potentiates effects of the diuretics). Products include:

Minizide Capsules ... 2016

Potassium Acid Phosphate (Concurrent use with excessive potassium intake may cause hyperkalemia; concurrent use should be avoided). Products include:

K-Phos Original Formula 'Sodium Free' Tablets ... 633

(▣ Described in PDR For Nonprescription Drugs) (◉ Described in PDR For Ophthalmology)

Potassium Bicarbonate (Concurrent use with excessive potassium intake may cause hyperkalemia; concurrent use should be avoided). Products include:

Alka-Seltzer Gold Effervescent Antacid .... ⊂⊃ 611

Potassium Chloride (Concurrent use with excessive potassium intake may cause hyperkalemia; concurrent use should be avoided). Products include:

Chlor-3 Condiment 1003
Colyte and Colyte-flavored 2540
GoLYTELY 694
K-Dur Microburst Release System (potassium chloride, USP) E.R. Tablets 1364
K-Lor Powder Packets 438
K-Norm Capsules 1615
K-Tab Filmtab 439
Micro-K 2237
Micro-K LS Packets 2238
NuLYTELY 694
Cherry Flavor NuLYTELY 694
Rum-K Syrup 1004
Slow-K Extended-Release Tablets ... 869

Potassium Citrate (Concurrent use with excessive potassium intake may cause hyperkalemia; concurrent use should be avoided). Products include:

Polycitra Syrup 574
Polycitra-K Crystals 574
Polycitra-K Oral Solution 575
Polycitra-LC 574
Urocit-K Tablets 1828

Potassium Gluconate (Concurrent use with excessive potassium intake may cause hyperkalemia; concurrent use should be avoided).

No products indexed under this heading.

Potassium Phosphate, Dibasic (Concurrent use with excessive potassium intake may cause hyperkalemia; concurrent use should be avoided).

No products indexed under this heading.

Potassium Phosphate, Monobasic (Concurrent use with excessive potassium intake may cause hyperkalemia; concurrent use should be avoided). Products include:

K-Phos Neutral Tablets 633
K-Phos Original Formula 'Sodium Free' Tablets 633

Prazosin Hydrochloride (Aldactone potentiates effects of other antihypertensives). Products include:

Minipress Capsules 2015
Minizide Capsules 2016

Propranolol Hydrochloride (Aldactone potentiates effects of other antihypertensives). Products include:

Inderal 2834
Inderal LA Long Acting Capsules ... 2836
Inderide Tablets 2838
Inderide LA Long Acting Capsules .. 2840

Quinapril Hydrochloride (Concomitant use has been associated with severe hyperkalemia; concurrent use should be avoided). Products include:

Accupril Tablets 1950

Ramipril (Concomitant use has been associated with severe hyperkalemia; concurrent use should be avoided). Products include:

Altace Capsules 1238

Rauwolfia Serpentina (Aldactone potentiates effects of other antihypertensives).

No products indexed under this heading.

Rescinnamine (Aldactone potentiates effects of other antihypertensives).

No products indexed under this heading.

Reserpine (Aldactone potentiates effects of other antihypertensives). Products include:

Diupres Tablets 1691
Hydropres Tablets 1718
Ser-Ap-Es Tablets 867

Sodium Nitroprusside (Aldactone potentiates effects of other antihypertensives).

No products indexed under this heading.

Sotalol Hydrochloride (Aldactone potentiates effects of other antihypertensives). Products include:

Betapace Tablets 637

Spirapril Hydrochloride (Concomitant use has been associated with severe hyperkalemia; concurrent use should be avoided).

No products indexed under this heading.

Terazosin Hydrochloride (Aldactone potentiates effects of other antihypertensives). Products include:

Hytrin Capsules 434

Timolol Maleate (Aldactone potentiates effects of other antihypertensives). Products include:

Blocadren Tablets 1654
Timolide Tablets 1791
Timoptic in Ocudose 1796
Timoptic Sterile Ophthalmic Solution 1794
Timoptic-XE 1798

Torsemide (Co-administration may result in hyponatremia, manifested by dry mouth, thirst, drowsiness, and lethargy; Aldactone potentiates effects of the diuretics). Products include:

Demadex Tablets and Injection 691

Trandolapril (Concomitant use has been associated with severe hyperkalemia; concurrent use should be avoided). Products include:

Mavik Tablets 1407

Triamterene (Concomitant use has been associated with severe hyperkalemia; concurrent use should be avoided). Products include:

Dyazide Capsules 2653
Dyrenium Capsules 2655

Trimethaphan Camsylate (Aldactone potentiates effects of other antihypertensives; the dosage of ganglionic blocking agents should be reduced by at least 50%).

No products indexed under this heading.

Verapamil Hydrochloride (Aldactone potentiates effects of other antihypertensives). Products include:

Calan SR Caplets 2571
Calan Tablets 2568
Covera-HS Tablets 2573
Isoptin Injectable 1391
Isoptin Oral Tablets 1393
Isoptin SR Tablets 1395
Verelan Capsules 1455

Food Interactions

Diet, potassium-rich (Concurrent use with diet rich in potassium should not ordinarily be given with spironolactone since this may result in hyperkalemia).

ALDOCLOR TABLETS
(Methyldopa, Chlorothiazide) 1638
May interact with antihypertensives, general anesthetics, corticosteroids, insulin, lithium preparations, oral hypoglycemic agents, non-steroidal anti-inflammatory agents, monoamine oxidase inhibitors, barbiturates, narcotic analgesics, cardiac glycosides, and certain other agents. Compounds in these categories include:

Acarbose (Dosage adjustment of the antidiabetic drug may be required). Products include:

Precose 604

Acebutolol Hydrochloride (Potentiation of antihypertensive effect). Products include:

Sectral Capsules 2914

ACTH (Hypokalemia may result).

No products indexed under this heading.

Alfentanil Hydrochloride (Aggravates orthostatic hypotension). Products include:

Alfenta Injection 1334

Amlodipine Besylate (Potentiation of antihypertensive effect). Products include:

Lotrel Capsules 858
Norvasc Tablets 2020

Aprobarbital (Aggravates orthostatic hypotension).

No products indexed under this heading.

Atenolol (Potentiation of antihypertensive effect). Products include:

Tenoretic Tablets 2963
Tenormin Tablets and I.V. Injection 2965

Benazepril Hydrochloride (Potentiation of antihypertensive effect). Products include:

Lotensin Tablets 852
Lotensin HCT Tablets 855
Lotrel Capsules 858

Bendroflumethiazide (Potentiation of antihypertensive effect).

No products indexed under this heading.

Betamethasone Acetate (Hypokalemia may result). Products include:

Celestone Soluspan Suspension 2484

Betamethasone Sodium Phosphate (Hypokalemia may result). Products include:

Celestone Soluspan Suspension 2484

Betaxolol Hydrochloride (Potentiation of antihypertensive effect). Products include:

Betoptic Ophthalmic Solution 465
Betoptic S Ophthalmic Suspension .. 467
Kerlone Tablets 2588

Bisoprolol Fumarate (Potentiation of antihypertensive effect). Products include:

Zebeta Tablets 1457
Ziac 1459

Buprenorphine (Aggravates orthostatic hypotension). Products include:

Buprenex Injectable 2170

Butabarbital (Aggravates orthostatic hypotension).

No products indexed under this heading.

Butalbital (Aggravates orthostatic hypotension). Products include:

Axocet Capsules 2469
Esgic-plus Capsules 1012
Esgic-plus Tablets 1012
Fioricet Tablets 2386
Fioricet with Codeine Capsules 2387
Fiorinal Capsules 2388
Fiorinal with Codeine Capsules 2390
Fiorinal Tablets 2388
Phrenilin 790
Sedapap Tablets 50 mg/650 mg 1826

Captopril (Potentiation of antihypertensive effect). Products include:

Capoten Tablets 740
Capozide Tablets 744

Carteolol Hydrochloride (Potentiation of antihypertensive effects). Products include:

Cartrol Tablets 413

Ocupress Ophthalmic Solution, 1% Sterile .... ⊂⊃ 297

Chlorothiazide Sodium (Potentiation of antihypertensive effect). Products include:

Diuril Sodium Intravenous 1693

Chlorpropamide (Dosage adjustment of the antidiabetic drug may be required). Products include:

Diabinese Tablets 2002

Chlorthalidone (Potentiation of antihypertensive effect). Products include:

Combipres Tablets 682
Tenoretic Tablets 2963
Thalitone 1293

Cholestyramine (Cholestyramine resin has the potential of binding thiazide diuretics and reducing absorption from the gastrointestinal tract). Products include:

Questran 774

Clonidine (Potentiation of antihypertensive effect). Products include:

Catapres-TTS 680

Clonidine Hydrochloride (Potentiation of antihypertensive effect). Products include:

Catapres Tablets 679
Combipres Tablets 682

Codeine Phosphate (Aggravates orthostatic hypotension). Products include:

Brontex 2130
Dimetane-DC Cough Syrup 2232
Fioricet with Codeine Capsules 2387
Fiorinal with Codeine Capsules 2390
Nucofed 2225
Phenergan with Codeine 2883
Phenergan VC with Codeine 2888
Robitussin A-C Syrup 2248
Robitussin-DAC Syrup 2249
Ryna .... ⊂⊃ 804
Soma Compound w/Codeine Tablets 2784
Tylenol with Codeine 1592

Colestipol Hydrochloride (Colestipole resin has the potential of binding thiazide diuretics and reducing absorption from the gastrointestinal tract). Products include:

Colestid 2073

Cortisone Acetate (Hypokalemia may result). Products include:

Cortone Acetate Sterile Suspension 1663
Cortone Acetate Tablets 1664

Deserpidine (Potentiation of antihypertensive effect).

No products indexed under this heading.

Deslanoside (Thiazide-induced hypokalemia may cause cardiac arrhythmia and may also sensitize or exaggerate the response of the heart to the toxic effects of digitalis).

No products indexed under this heading.

Dexamethasone (Hypokalemia may result). Products include:

AK-Trol Ointment & Suspension .... ⊂⊃ 205
Decadron Elixir 1676
Decadron Tablets 1678
Decaspray Topical Aerosol 1689
Maxitrol Ophthalmic Ointment and Suspension .... ⊂⊃ 222
TobraDex Ophthalmic Suspension and Ointment 469

Dexamethasone Acetate (Hypokalemia may result). Products include:

Dalalone D.P. Injectable 1009
Decadron-LA Sterile Suspension 1687

Dexamethasone Sodium Phosphate (Hypokalemia may result). Products include:

Decadron Phosphate Injection 1680
Decadron Phosphate Sterile Ophthalmic Ointment 1684
Decadron Phosphate Sterile Ophthalmic Solution 1685

IMPORTANT NOTE: Always consult each drug listing in the patient's regimen for possible interactions.

Aldoclor Interactions Index 30

Decadron Phosphate Topical Cream ... 1686
Decadron Phosphate with Xylocaine Injection, Sterile ... 1683
Dexacort Phosphate in Respihaler .. 1606
Dexacort Phosphate in Turbinaire .. 1607
NeoDecadron Sterile Ophthalmic Ointment ... 1755
NeoDecadron Sterile Ophthalmic Solution ... 1756
NeoDecadron Topical Cream ... 1757

Dezocine (Aggravates orthostatic hypotension). Products include:
Dalgan Injection ... 529

Diazoxide (Potentiation of antihypertensive effects). Products include:
Hyperstat I.V. Injection ... 2504
Proglycem ... 575

Diclofenac Potassium (May result in reduced diuretic effect). Products include:
Cataflam Tablets ... 833

Diclofenac Sodium (May result in reduced diuretic effect). Products include:
Voltaren Ophthalmic Sterile Ophthalmic Solution ... ⊙ 264
Cataflam/Voltaren/Voltaren-XR ... 833

Digitoxin (Thiazide-induced hypokalemia may cause cardiac arrhythmia and may also sensitize or exaggerate the response of the heart to the toxic effects of digitalis). Products include:
Crystodigin Tablets ... 1472

Digoxin (Thiazide-induced hypokalemia may cause cardiac arrhythmia and may also sensitize or exaggerate the response of the heart to the toxic effects of digitalis). Products include:
Lanoxicaps ... 1110
Lanoxin Elixir Pediatric ... 1113
Lanoxin Injection ... 1116
Lanoxin Injection Pediatric ... 1119
Lanoxin Tablets ... 1121

Diltiazem Hydrochloride (Potentiation of antihypertensive effect). Products include:
Cardizem CD Capsules ... 1251
Cardizem SR Capsules ... 1255
Cardizem Injectable ... 1253
Cardizem Tablets ... 1257
Dilacor XR Extended-release Capsules ... 2183
Tiazac Capsules ... 1019

Doxazosin Mesylate (Potentiation of antihypertensive effect). Products include:
Cardura Tablets ... 1993

Enalapril Maleate (Potentiation of antihypertensive effect). Products include:
Vaseretic Tablets ... 1810
Vasotec Tablets ... 1816

Enalaprilat (Potentiation of antihypertensive effect). Products include:
Vasotec I.V. ... 1814

Enflurane (May require reduced dose of anesthetics).
No products indexed under this heading.

Esmolol Hydrochloride (Potentiation of antihypertensive effect). Products include:
Brevibloc (esmolol HCl) Injection ... 1860

Etodolac (May result in reduced diuretic effect). Products include:
Lodine Capsules and Tablets ... 2849

Felodipine (Potentiation of antihypertensive effect). Products include:
Plendil Extended-Release Tablets ... 514

Fenoprofen Calcium (May result in reduced diuretic effects). Products include:
Nalfon 200 Pulvules & Nalfon Tablets ... 933

Fentanyl (Aggravates orthostatic hypotension). Products include:
Duragesic Transdermal System ... 1336

Fentanyl Citrate (Aggravates orthostatic hypotension). Products include:
Sublimaze Injection ... 463

Fludrocortisone Acetate (Hypokalemia may result). Products include:
Florinef Acetate Tablets ... 506

Flurbiprofen (May result in reduced diuretic effect).
No products indexed under this heading.

Fosinopril Sodium (Potentiation of antihypertensive effect). Products include:
Monopril Tablets ... 762

Furazolidone (Concurrent use is contraindicated). Products include:
Furoxone ... 2221

Furosemide (Potentiation of antihypertensive effect). Products include:
Lasix Injection, Oral Solution and Tablets ... 1267

Glimepiride (Dosage adjustment of the antidiabetic drug may be required). Products include:
Amaryl Tablets ... 1241

Glipizide (Dosage adjustment of the antidiabetic drug may be required). Products include:
Glucotrol Tablets ... 2011
Glucotrol XL Extended Release Tablets ... 2012

Glyburide (Dosage adjustment of the antidiabetic drug may be required). Products include:
DiaBeta Tablets ... 1265
Glynase PresTab Tablets ... 2091
Micronase Tablets ... 2099

Guanabenz Acetate (Potentiation of antihypertensive effect).
No products indexed under this heading.

Guanethidine Monosulfate (Potentiation of antihypertensive effect). Products include:
Esimil Tablets ... 840
Ismelin Tablets ... 845

Hydralazine Hydrochloride (Potentiation of antihypertensive effect). Products include:
Apresazide Capsules ... 824
Apresoline Hydrochloride Tablets .. 826
Hydralazine Hydrochloride Injection USP ... 2712
Ser-Ap-Es Tablets ... 867

Hydrochlorothiazide (Potentiation of antihypertensive effect). Products include:
Aldactazide Tablets ... 2556
Aldoril Tablets ... 1644
Apresazide Capsules ... 824
Capozide Tablets ... 744
Dyazide Capsules ... 2653
Esidrix Tablets ... 839
Esimil Tablets ... 840
HydroDIURIL Tablets ... 1716
Hydropres Tablets ... 1718
Hyzaar Tablets ... 1720
Inderide Tablets ... 2838
Inderide LA Long Acting Capsules .. 2840
Lopressor HCT Tablets ... 850
Lotensin HCT Tablets ... 855
Moduretic Tablets ... 1748
Oretic Tablets ... 450
Prinzide Tablets ... 1780
Ser-Ap-Es Tablets ... 867
Timolide Tablets ... 1791
Vaseretic Tablets ... 1810
Zestoretic Tablets ... 2968
Ziac ... 1459

Hydrocodone Bitartrate (Aggravates orthostatic hypotension). Products include:
Codiclear DH Syrup ... 808
Duratuss HD Elixir ... 2750
Histussin D Liquid ... 670
Hycodan Tablets and Syrup ... 946
Hycomine Compound Tablets ... 948
Hycomine ... 947
Hycotuss Expectorant Syrup ... 950
Hydrocet Capsules ... 787
Lorcet 10/650 Tablets ... 1016
Lortab ... 2751
Tussend ... 1830
Tussend Expectorant ... 1831
Vicodin Tablets ... 1404
Vicodin ES Tablets ... 1405
Vicodin HP Tablets ... 1403
Vicodin Tuss Expectorant ... 1406
Zydone Capsules ... 967

Hydrocodone Polistirex (Aggravates orthostatic hypotension). Products include:
Tussionex Pennkinetic Extended-Release Suspension ... 1624

Hydrocortisone (Hypokalemia may result). Products include:
Anusol-HC Cream 2.5% ... 1953
Aquanil HC Lotion ... 1989
Maximum Strength Cortaid Spray ▣ 800
CORTENEMA ... 2713
Cortisporin Ointment ... 1074
Cortisporin Ophthalmic Ointment Sterile ... 1074
Cortisporin Ophthalmic Suspension Sterile ... 1075
Cortisporin Otic Solution Sterile ... 1076
Cortisporin Otic Suspension Sterile 1077
Cortizone-5 ... ▣ 795
Cortizone-10 ... ▣ 795
Hydrocortone Tablets ... 1715
Hytone ... 922
Hytone Ointment 2 ½% ... 923
Massengill Medicated Soft Cloth Towelettes ... 2628
Pediotic Suspension Sterile ... 1140
Preparation H Hydrocortisone 1% Cream ... ▣ 843
ProctoCream-HC 2.5% ... 2552
VōSoL HC Otic Solution ... 2786

Hydrocortisone Acetate (Hypokalemia may result). Products include:
Analpram-HC Rectal Cream 1% and 2.5% ... 993
Anusol HC-1 Hydrocortisone Anti-Itch Ointment ... ▣ 810
Anusol-HC Suppositories ... 1954
Caldecort Anti-Itch Hydrocortisone Cream ... ▣ 651
Coly-Mycin S Otic w/Neomycin & Hydrocortisone ... 1965
Cortaid ... ▣ 800
Cortifoam ... 2540
Cortisporin Cream ... 1073
Epifoam ... 2543
Hydrocortone Acetate Sterile Suspension ... 1712
Mantadil Cream ... 1124
Nupercainal Hydrocortisone 1% Cream ... ▣ 661
Pramosone Cream, Lotion & Ointment ... 995
ProctoFoam-HC ... 2552
Terra-Cortril Ophthalmic Suspension ... 2033

Hydrocortisone Sodium Phosphate (Hypokalemia may result). Products include:
Hydrocortone Phosphate Injection, Sterile ... 1713

Hydrocortisone Sodium Succinate (Hypokalemia may result).
No products indexed under this heading.

Hydroflumethiazide (Potentiation of antihypertensive effect). Products include:
Diucardin Tablets ... 2824

Hydromorphone Hydrochloride (Aggravates orthostatic hypotension). Products include:
Dilaudid Ampules ... 1382
Dilaudid Cough Syrup ... 1383
Dilaudid-HP Injection ... 1384
Dilaudid-HP Lyophilized Powder 250 mg ... 1384
Dilaudid ... 1382
Dilaudid Oral Liquid ... 1386
Dilaudid ... 1382
Dilaudid Tablets - 8 mg ... 1386

Ibuprofen (May result in reduced diuretic effects). Products include:
Advil Cold and Sinus Caplets and Tablets ... ▣ 837
Advil Ibuprofen Tablets, Caplets and Gel Caplets ... ▣ 836
Children's Motrin Ibuprofen Oral Suspension ... 1558
IBU Tablets ... 1389
Ibuprohm ... ▣ 713
Motrin IB Caplets, Tablets, and Gelcaps ... ▣ 802
Motrin Ibuprofen Suspension, Oral Drops, Chewable Tablets, Caplets ... 1563
Nuprin Ibuprofen/Analgesic Tablets & Caplets ... ▣ 645
Vicks DayQuil SINUS Pressure & PAIN Relief with IBUPROFEN ... ▣ 735

Indapamide (Potentiation of antihypertensive effect).
No products indexed under this heading.

Indomethacin (May result in reduced diuretic effects). Products include:
Indocin ... 1723

Indomethacin Sodium Trihydrate (May result in reduced diuretic effects). Products include:
Indocin I.V. ... 1727

Insulin, Human (May alter insulin requirements).
No products indexed under this heading.

Insulin, Human Isophane Suspension (May alter insulin requirements). Products include:
Novolin N Human Insulin 10 ml Vials ... 1846

Insulin, Human NPH (May alter insulin requirements). Products include:
Humulin N, 100 Units ... 1495
Novolin N PenFill 1.5 ml Cartridges Durable Insulin Delivery System ... 1849
Novolin N Prefilled Syringe Disposable Insulin Delivery System ... 1850

Insulin, Human Regular (May alter insulin requirements). Products include:
Humulin R, 100 Units ... 1497
Novolin R Human Insulin 10 ml Vials ... 1846
Novolin R PenFill 1.5 ml Cartridges Durable Insulin Delivery System ... 1849
Novolin R Prefilled Syringe Disposable Insulin Delivery System ... 1850
Velosulin BR Human Insulin 10 ml Vials ... 1847

Insulin, Human, Zinc Suspension (May alter insulin requirements). Products include:
Humulin L, 100 Units ... 1494
Humulin U, 100 Units ... 1498
Novolin L Human Insulin 10 ml Vials ... 1846

Insulin Lispro, Human (May alter insulin requirements). Products include:
Humalog Injection ... 1488

Insulin, NPH (May alter insulin requirements). Products include:
NPH, 100 Units ... 1502
Pork NPH, 100 Units ... 1506
Purified Pork NPH Isophane Insulin ... 1852

Insulin, Regular (May alter insulin requirements). Products include:
Regular, 100 Units ... 1503
Pork Regular, 100 Units ... 1507
Pork Regular (Concentrated), 500 Units ... 1508
Purified Pork Regular Insulin ... 1852

Insulin, Zinc Crystals (May alter insulin requirements). Products include:
NPH, 100 Units ... 1502

(▣ Described in PDR For Nonprescription Drugs) (⊙ Described in PDR For Ophthalmology)

Insulin, Zinc Suspension (May alter insulin requirements). Products include:
- Iletin I 1501
- Lente, 100 Units 1501
- Iletin II 1504
- Pork Lente, 100 Units 1504
- Purified Pork Lente Insulin 1852

Isocarboxazid (Concurrent use is contraindicated).
No products indexed under this heading.

Isoflurane (May require reduced dose of anesthetics).
No products indexed under this heading.

Isradipine (Potentiation of antihypertensive effect). Products include:
- DynaCirc Capsules 2381
- DynaCirc CR Tablets 2383

Ketamine Hydrochloride (May require reduced dose of anesthetics).
No products indexed under this heading.

Ketoprofen (May result in reduced diuretic effects). Products include:
- Actron Caplets and Tablets 608
- Orudis Capsules 2874
- Orudis KT 842
- Oruvail Capsules 2874

Ketorolac Tromethamine (May result in reduced diuretic effect). Products include:
- Acular Sterile Ophthalmic Solution 470
- Toradol 2319

Labetalol Hydrochloride (Potentiation of antihypertensive effect). Products include:
- Normodyne Injection 2519
- Normodyne Tablets 2522
- Trandate 1158

Levorphanol Tartrate (Aggravates orthostatic hypotension). Products include:
- Levo-Dromoran 2297

Lisinopril (Potentiation of antihypertensive effect). Products include:
- Prinivil Tablets 1776
- Prinzide Tablets 1780
- Zestoretic Tablets 2968
- Zestril Tablets 2972

Lithium Carbonate (High risk of lithium toxicity). Products include:
- Eskalith 2658
- Lithium Carbonate Capsules & Tablets 2352
- Lithonate/Lithotabs/Lithobid 2721

Lithium Citrate (High risk of lithium toxicity).
No products indexed under this heading.

Losartan Potassium (Potentiation of antihypertensive effect). Products include:
- Cozaar Tablets 1668
- Hyzaar Tablets 1720

Mecamylamine Hydrochloride (Potentiation of antihypertensive effect). Products include:
- Inversine Tablets 1729

Meclofenamate Sodium (May result in reduced diuretic effects).
No products indexed under this heading.

Mefenamic Acid (May result in reduced diuretic effects). Products include:
- Ponstel 1982

Meperidine Hydrochloride (Aggravates orthostatic hypotension). Products include:
- Demerol 2438
- Mepergan Injection 2859

Mephobarbital (Aggravates orthostatic hypotension). Products include:
- Mebaral Tablets 2452

Metformin Hydrochloride (Dosage adjustment of the antidiabetic drug may be required). Products include:
- Glucophage Tablets 754

Methadone Hydrochloride (Aggravates orthostatic hypotension). Products include:
- Methadone Hydrochloride Oral Concentrate 2356
- Methadone Hydrochloride Oral Solution & Tablets 2357

Methohexital Sodium (May require reduced dose of anesthetics).
No products indexed under this heading.

Methoxyflurane (May require reduced dose of anesthetics).
No products indexed under this heading.

Methyclothiazide (Potentiation of antihypertensive effect). Products include:
- Enduron Tablets 424

Methyldopate Hydrochloride (Potentiation of antihypertensive effect). Products include:
- Aldomet Ester HCl Injection 1642

Methylprednisolone Acetate (Hypokalemia may result).
No products indexed under this heading.

Methylprednisolone Sodium Succinate (Hypokalemia may result).
No products indexed under this heading.

Metolazone (Potentiation of antihypertensive effect). Products include:
- Mykrox Tablets 1617
- Zaroxolyn Tablets 1625

Metoprolol Succinate (Potentiation of antihypertensive effect). Products include:
- Toprol-XL Tablets 560

Metoprolol Tartrate (Potentiation of antihypertensive effect). Products include:
- Lopressor 848
- Lopressor HCT Tablets 850

Metyrosine (Potentiation of antihypertensive effect). Products include:
- Demser Capsules 1690

Minoxidil (Potentiation of antihypertensive effect).
No products indexed under this heading.

Moexipril Hydrochloride (Potentiation of antihypertensive effect). Products include:
- Univasc Tablets 2553

Morphine Sulfate (Aggravates orthostatic hypotension). Products include:
- Astramorph/PF Injection, USP (Preservative-Free) 526
- Duramorph Injection 983
- Infumorph 200 and Infumorph 500 Sterile Solutions 985
- Kadian Capsules 2948
- MS Contin Tablets 2149
- MSIR 2152
- Oramorph SR (Morphine Sulfate Sustained Release Tablets) 2359
- RMS Suppositories CII 2766
- Roxanol 2365

Nabumetone (May result in reduced diuretic effect). Products include:
- Relafen Tablets 2688

Nadolol (Potentiation of antihypertensive effect).
No products indexed under this heading.

Naproxen (May result in reduced diuretic effects). Products include:
- Anaprox/Naprosyn 2277

Naproxen Sodium (May result in reduced diuretic effects). Products include:
- Aleve 2124
- Anaprox/Naprosyn 2277
- Naprelan Tablets 2861

Nicardipine Hydrochloride (Potentiation of antihypertensive effects). Products include:
- Cardene Capsules 2261
- Cardene I.V. 2815
- Cardene SR Capsules 2264

Nifedipine (Potentiation of antihypertensive effect). Products include:
- Adalat Capsules (10 mg and 20 mg) 580
- Adalat CC 582
- Procardia Capsules 2024
- Procardia XL Extended Release Tablets 2026

Nisoldipine (Potentiation of antihypertensive effect). Products include:
- Sular Tablets 2961

Nitroglycerin (Potentiation of antihypertensive effect). Products include:
- Deponit NTG Transdermal Delivery System 2541
- Nitro-Bid IV 1270
- Nitro-Bid Ointment 1272
- Nitro-Dur (nitroglycerin) Transdermal Infusion System 1365
- Nitrolingual Spray 2193
- Nitrostat Tablets 1981
- Transderm-Nitro Transdermal Therapeutic System 878

Norepinephrine Bitartrate (May decrease arterial responsiveness to norepinephrine). Products include:
- Levophed Bitartrate Injection 2445

Opium Alkaloids (Aggravates orthostatic hypotension).
No products indexed under this heading.

Oxaprozin (May result in reduced diuretic effect). Products include:
- Daypro Caplets 2578

Oxycodone Hydrochloride (Aggravates orthostatic hypotension). Products include:
- OxyContin Tablets 2163
- OxyIR Capsules 2167
- Percocet Tablets 955
- Percodan Tablets 955
- Percodan-Demi Tablets 956
- Roxicodone Tablets, Oral Solution & Intensol (Oxycodone) 2366
- Tylox Capsules 1593

Penbutolol Sulfate (Potentiation of antihypertensive effects). Products include:
- Levatol Tablets 2547

Pentobarbital Sodium (Aggravates orthostatic hypotension). Products include:
- Nembutal Sodium Capsules 440
- Nembutal Sodium Solution 442
- Nembutal Sodium Suppositories 444

Phenelzine Sulfate (Concurrent use is contraindicated). Products include:
- Nardil 1977

Phenobarbital (Aggravates orthostatic hypotension). Products include:
- Arco-Lase Plus Tablets 513
- Bellergal-S Tablets 2375
- Donnatal 2234
- Donnatal Extentabs 2234
- Donnatal Tablets 2234
- Phenobarbital Elixir and Tablets 1523
- Quadrinal Tablets 1398

Phenoxybenzamine Hydrochloride (Potentiation of antihypertensive effect). Products include:
- Dibenzyline Capsules 2650

Phentolamine Mesylate (Potentiation of antihypertensive effect). Products include:
- Regitine Vials 864

Phenylbutazone (May result in reduced diuretic effects).
No products indexed under this heading.

Pindolol (Potentiation of antihypertensive effect). Products include:
- Visken Tablets 2428

Piroxicam (May result in reduced diuretic effects). Products include:
- Feldene Capsules 2008

Polythiazide (Potentiation of antihypertensive effect). Products include:
- Minizide Capsules 2016

Prazosin Hydrochloride (Potentiation of antihypertensive effect). Products include:
- Minipress Capsules 2015
- Minizide Capsules 2016

Prednisolone Acetate (Hypokalemia may result). Products include:
- AK-CIDE .... ◉ 203
- AK-CIDE Ointment .... ◉ 203
- Blephamide Liquifilm Sterile Ophthalmic Suspension 472
- Blephamide Ointment .... ◉ 234
- Econopred & Econopred Plus Ophthalmic Suspensions .... ◉ 216
- Poly-Pred Liquifilm .... ◉ 246
- Pred Forte .... ◉ 247
- Pred Mild .... ◉ 250
- Pred-G Liquifilm Sterile Ophthalmic Suspension .... ◉ 248
- Pred-G S.O.P. Sterile Ophthalmic Ointment .... ◉ 249

Prednisolone Sodium Phosphate (Hypokalemia may result). Products include:
- AK-PRED .... ◉ 204
- Hydeltrasol Injection, Sterile 1708
- Pediapred Oral Solution 1618

Prednisolone Tebutate (Hypokalemia may result). Products include:
- Hydeltra-T.B.A. Sterile Suspension 1710

Prednisone (Hypokalemia may result).
No products indexed under this heading.

Propofol (May require reduced dose of anesthetics). Products include:
- Diprivan Injectable Emulsion 2939

Propoxyphene Hydrochloride (Aggravates orthostatic hypotension). Products include:
- Darvon 1475
- Wygesic Tablets 2930

Propoxyphene Napsylate (Aggravates orthostatic hypotension). Products include:
- Darvon-N/Darvocet-N 1473

Propranolol Hydrochloride (Potentiation of antihypertensive effect). Products include:
- Inderal 2834
- Inderal LA Long Acting Capsules 2836
- Inderide Tablets 2838
- Inderide LA Long Acting Capsules 2840

Quinapril Hydrochloride (Potentiation of antihypertensive effect). Products include:
- Accupril Tablets 1950

Ramipril (Potentiation of antihypertensive effect). Products include:
- Altace Capsules 1238

Rauwolfia Serpentina (Potentiation of antihypertensive effect).
No products indexed under this heading.

Rescinnamine (Potentiation of antihypertensive effect).
No products indexed under this heading.

Reserpine (Potentiation of antihypertensive effect). Products include:
- Diupres Tablets 1691
- Hydropres Tablets 1718
- Ser-Ap-Es Tablets 867

IMPORTANT NOTE: Always consult each drug listing in the patient's regimen for possible interactions.

Interactions Index

Aldoclor

Secobarbital Sodium (Aggravates orthostatic hypotension). Products include:
- Seconal Sodium Pulvules ... 1529

Selegiline Hydrochloride (Concurrent use is contraindicated). Products include:
- Eldepryl Capsules ... 2729

Sevoflurane (May require reduced dose of anesthetics).
- No products indexed under this heading.

Sodium Nitroprusside (Potentiation of antihypertensive effect).
- No products indexed under this heading.

Sotalol Hydrochloride (Potentiation of antihypertensive effect). Products include:
- Betapace Tablets ... 637

Spirapril Hydrochloride (Potentiation of antihypertensive effect).
- No products indexed under this heading.

Sufentanil Citrate (Aggravates orthostatic hypotension). Products include:
- Sufenta Injection ... 1355

Sulindac (May result in reduced diuretic effects). Products include:
- Clinoril Tablets ... 1658

Terazosin Hydrochloride (Potentiation of antihypertensive effect). Products include:
- Hytrin Capsules ... 434

Thiamylal Sodium (Aggravates orthostatic hypotension).
- No products indexed under this heading.

Timolol Maleate (Potentiation of antihypertensive effect). Products include:
- Blocadren Tablets ... 1654
- Timolide Tablets ... 1791
- Timoptic in Ocudose ... 1796
- Timoptic Sterile Ophthalmic Solution ... 1794
- Timoptic-XE ... 1798

Tolazamide (Dosage adjustment of the antidiabetic drug may be required).
- No products indexed under this heading.

Tolbutamide (Dosage adjustment of the antidiabetic drug may be required).
- No products indexed under this heading.

Tolmetin Sodium (May result in reduced diuretic effects). Products include:
- Tolectin (200, 400 and 600 mg) ... 1591

Torsemide (Potentiation of antihypertensive effect). Products include:
- Demadex Tablets and Injection ... 691

Tranylcypromine Sulfate (Concurrent use is contraindicated). Products include:
- Parnate Tablets ... 2679

Triamcinolone (Hypokalemia may result).
- No products indexed under this heading.

Triamcinolone Acetonide (Hypokalemia may result). Products include:
- Azmacort Oral Inhaler ... 2175
- Nasacort AQ Nasal Spray ... 2191
- Nasacort Nasal Inhaler ... 2189

Triamcinolone Diacetate (Hypokalemia may result).
- No products indexed under this heading.

Triamcinolone Hexacetonide (Hypokalemia may result).
- No products indexed under this heading.

Trimethaphan Camsylate (Potentiation of antihypertensive effect).
- No products indexed under this heading.

Tubocurarine Chloride (Increased responsiveness to tubocurarine).
- No products indexed under this heading.

Verapamil Hydrochloride (Potentiation of antihypertensive effect). Products include:
- Calan SR Caplets ... 2571
- Calan Tablets ... 2568
- Covera-HS Tablets ... 2573
- Isoptin Injectable ... 1391
- Isoptin Oral Tablets ... 1393
- Isoptin SR Tablets ... 1395
- Verelan Capsules ... 1455

Food Interactions

Alcohol (Aggravates orthostatic hypotension).

ALDOMET ESTER HCL INJECTION
(Methyldopate Hydrochloride) ... 1642
May interact with general anesthetics, antihypertensives, lithium preparations, monoamine oxidase inhibitors, and certain other agents. Compounds in these categories include:

Acebutolol Hydrochloride (Potentiation of antihypertensive effect). Products include:
- Sectral Capsules ... 2914

Amlodipine Besylate (Potentiation of antihypertensive effect). Products include:
- Lotrel Capsules ... 858
- Norvasc Tablets ... 2020

Atenolol (Potentiation of antihypertensive effect). Products include:
- Tenoretic Tablets ... 2963
- Tenormin Tablets and I.V. Injection ... 2965

Benazepril Hydrochloride (Potentiation of antihypertensive effect). Products include:
- Lotensin Tablets ... 852
- Lotensin HCT Tablets ... 855
- Lotrel Capsules ... 858

Bendroflumethiazide (Potentiation of antihypertensive effect).
- No products indexed under this heading.

Betaxolol Hydrochloride (Potentiation of antihypertensive effect). Products include:
- Betoptic Ophthalmic Solution ... 465
- Betoptic S Ophthalmic Suspension ... 467
- Kerlone Tablets ... 2588

Bisoprolol Fumarate (Potentiation of antihypertensive effect). Products include:
- Zebeta Tablets ... 1457
- Ziac ... 1459

Captopril (Potentiation of antihypertensive effect). Products include:
- Capoten Tablets ... 740
- Capozide Tablets ... 744

Carteolol Hydrochloride (Potentiation of antihypertensive effect). Products include:
- Cartrol Tablets ... 413
- Ocupress Ophthalmic Solution, 1% Sterile ... ⊙ 297

Chlorothiazide (Potentiation of antihypertensive effect). Products include:
- Aldoclor Tablets ... 1638
- Diupres Tablets ... 1691
- Diuril Oral ... 1694

Chlorothiazide Sodium (Potentiation of antihypertensive effect). Products include:
- Diuril Sodium Intravenous ... 1693

Chlorthalidone (Potentiation of antihypertensive effect). Products include:
- Combipres Tablets ... 682
- Tenoretic Tablets ... 2963
- Thalitone ... 1293

Clonidine (Potentiation of antihypertensive effect). Products include:
- Catapres-TTS ... 680

Clonidine Hydrochloride (Potentiation of antihypertensive effect). Products include:
- Catapres Tablets ... 679
- Combipres Tablets ... 682

Deserpidine (Potentiation of antihypertensive effect).
- No products indexed under this heading.

Diazoxide (Potentiation of antihypertensive effect). Products include:
- Hyperstat I.V. Injection ... 2504
- Proglycem ... 575

Diltiazem Hydrochloride (Potentiation of antihypertensive effect). Products include:
- Cardizem CD Capsules ... 1251
- Cardizem SR Capsules ... 1255
- Cardizem Injectable ... 1253
- Cardizem Tablets ... 1257
- Dilacor XR Extended-release Capsules ... 2183
- Tiazac Capsules ... 1019

Doxazosin Mesylate (Potentiation of antihypertensive effect). Products include:
- Cardura Tablets ... 1993

Enalapril Maleate (Potentiation of antihypertensive effect). Products include:
- Vaseretic Tablets ... 1810
- Vasotec Tablets ... 1816

Enalaprilat (Potentiation of antihypertensive effect). Products include:
- Vasotec I.V. ... 1814

Enflurane (May require reduced dose of anesthetics).
- No products indexed under this heading.

Esmolol Hydrochloride (Potentiation of antihypertensive effect). Products include:
- Brevibloc (esmolol HCl) Injection ... 1860

Felodipine (Potentiation of antihypertensive effect). Products include:
- Plendil Extended-Release Tablets ... 514

Fosinopril Sodium (Potentiation of antihypertensive effect). Products include:
- Monopril Tablets ... 762

Furazolidone (Concurrent use is contraindicated). Products include:
- Furoxone ... 2221

Furosemide (Potentiation of antihypertensive effect). Products include:
- Lasix Injection, Oral Solution and Tablets ... 1267

Guanabenz Acetate (Potentiation of antihypertensive effect).
- No products indexed under this heading.

Guanethidine Monosulfate (Potentiation of antihypertensive effect). Products include:
- Esimil Tablets ... 840
- Ismelin Tablets ... 845

Hydralazine Hydrochloride (Potentiation of antihypertensive effect). Products include:
- Apresazide Capsules ... 824
- Apresoline Hydrochloride Tablets ... 826
- Hydralazine Hydrochloride Injection USP ... 2712
- Ser-Ap-Es Tablets ... 867

Hydrochlorothiazide (Potentiation of antihypertensive effect). Products include:
- Aldactazide Tablets ... 2556
- Aldoril Tablets ... 1644
- Apresazide Capsules ... 824
- Capozide Tablets ... 744
- Dyazide Capsules ... 2653
- Esidrix Tablets ... 839
- Esimil Tablets ... 840
- HydroDIURIL Tablets ... 1716
- Hydropres Tablets ... 1718
- Hyzaar Tablets ... 1720
- Inderide Tablets ... 2838
- Inderide LA Long Acting Capsules ... 2840
- Lopressor HCT Tablets ... 850
- Lotensin HCT Tablets ... 855
- Moduretic Tablets ... 1748
- Oretic Tablets ... 450
- Prinzide Tablets ... 1780
- Ser-Ap-Es Tablets ... 867
- Timolide Tablets ... 1791
- Vaseretic Tablets ... 1810
- Zestoretic Tablets ... 2968
- Ziac ... 1459

Hydroflumethiazide (Potentiation of antihypertensive effect). Products include:
- Diucardin Tablets ... 2824

Indapamide (Potentiation of antihypertensive effect).
- No products indexed under this heading.

Isocarboxazid (Concurrent use is contraindicated).
- No products indexed under this heading.

Isoflurane (May require reduced dose of anesthetics).
- No products indexed under this heading.

Isradipine (Potentiation of antihypertensive effect). Products include:
- DynaCirc Capsules ... 2381
- DynaCirc CR Tablets ... 2383

Ketamine Hydrochloride (May require reduced dose of anesthetics).
- No products indexed under this heading.

Labetalol Hydrochloride (Potentiation of antihypertensive effect). Products include:
- Normodyne Injection ... 2519
- Normodyne Tablets ... 2522
- Trandate ... 1158

Lisinopril (Potentiation of antihypertensive effects). Products include:
- Prinivil Tablets ... 1776
- Prinzide Tablets ... 1780
- Zestoretic Tablets ... 2968
- Zestril Tablets ... 2972

Lithium Carbonate (Potential for lithium toxicity). Products include:
- Eskalith ... 2658
- Lithium Carbonate Capsules & Tablets ... 2352
- Lithonate/Lithotabs/Lithobid ... 2721

Lithium Citrate (Potential for lithium toxicity).
- No products indexed under this heading.

Losartan Potassium (Potentiation of antihypertensive effect). Products include:
- Cozaar Tablets ... 1668
- Hyzaar Tablets ... 1720

Mecamylamine Hydrochloride (Potentiation of antihypertensive effect). Products include:
- Inversine Tablets ... 1729

Methohexital Sodium (May require reduced dose of anesthetics).
- No products indexed under this heading.

Methoxyflurane (May require reduced dose of anesthetics).
- No products indexed under this heading.

Methyclothiazide (Potentiation of antihypertensive effect). Products include:
- Enduron Tablets ... 424

(▣ Described in PDR For Nonprescription Drugs) (⊙ Described in PDR For Ophthalmology)

Methyldopa (Potentiation of antihypertensive effect). Products include:
- Aldoclor Tablets 1638
- Aldomet Oral 1640
- Aldoril Tablets 1644

Metolazone (Potentiation of antihypertensive effect). Products include:
- Mykrox Tablets 1617
- Zaroxolyn Tablets 1625

Metoprolol Succinate (Potentiation of antihypertensive effect). Products include:
- Toprol-XL Tablets 560

Metoprolol Tartrate (Potentiation of antihypertensive effect). Products include:
- Lopressor 848
- Lopressor HCT Tablets 850

Metyrosine (Potentiation of antihypertensive effect). Products include:
- Demser Capsules 1690

Minoxidil (Potentiation of antihypertensive effect).
- No products indexed under this heading.

Moexipril Hydrochloride (Potentiation of antihypertensive effect). Products include:
- Univasc Tablets 2553

Nadolol (Potentiation of antihypertensive effect).
- No products indexed under this heading.

Nicardipine Hydrochloride (Potentiation of antihypertensive effect). Products include:
- Cardene Capsules 2261
- Cardene I.V. 2815
- Cardene SR Capsules 2264

Nifedipine (Potentiation of antihypertensive effect). Products include:
- Adalat Capsules (10 mg and 20 mg) 580
- Adalat CC 582
- Procardia Capsules 2024
- Procardia XL Extended Release Tablets 2026

Nisoldipine (Potentiation of antihypertensive effect). Products include:
- Sular Tablets 2961

Nitroglycerin (Potentiation of antihypertensive effect). Products include:
- Deponit NTG Transdermal Delivery System 2541
- Nitro-Bid IV 1270
- Nitro-Bid Ointment 1272
- Nitro-Dur (nitroglycerin) Transdermal Infusion System 1365
- Nitrolingual Spray 2193
- Nitrostat Tablets 1981
- Transderm-Nitro Transdermal Therapeutic System 878

Penbutolol Sulfate (Potentiation of antihypertensive effect). Products include:
- Levatol Tablets 2547

Phenelzine Sulfate (Concurrent use is contraindicated). Products include:
- Nardil 1977

Phenoxybenzamine Hydrochloride (Potentiation of antihypertensive effect). Products include:
- Dibenzyline Capsules 2650

Phentolamine Mesylate (Potentiation of antihypertensive effect). Products include:
- Regitine Vials 864

Pindolol (Potentiation of antihypertensive effect). Products include:
- Visken Tablets 2428

Polythiazide (Potentiation of antihypertensive effect). Products include:
- Minizide Capsules 2016

Prazosin Hydrochloride (Potentiation of antihypertensive effect). Products include:
- Minipress Capsules 2015
- Minizide Capsules 2016

Propofol (May require reduced dose of anesthetics). Products include:
- Diprivan Injectable Emulsion 2939

Propranolol Hydrochloride (Potentiation of antihypertensive effect). Products include:
- Inderal 2834
- Inderal LA Long Acting Capsules 2836
- Inderide Tablets 2838
- Inderide LA Long Acting Capsules 2840

Quinapril Hydrochloride (Potentiation of antihypertensive effect). Products include:
- Accupril Tablets 1950

Ramipril (Potentiation of antihypertensive effect). Products include:
- Altace Capsules 1238

Rauwolfia Serpentina (Potentiation of antihypertensive effect).
- No products indexed under this heading.

Rescinnamine (Potentiation of antihypertensive effect).
- No products indexed under this heading.

Reserpine (Potentiation of antihypertensive effect). Products include:
- Diupres Tablets 1691
- Hydropres Tablets 1718
- Ser-Ap-Es Tablets 867

Selegiline Hydrochloride (Concurrent use is contraindicated). Products include:
- Eldepryl Capsules 2729

Sevoflurane (May require reduced dose of anesthetics).
- No products indexed under this heading.

Sodium Nitroprusside (Potentiation of antihypertensive effect).
- No products indexed under this heading.

Sotalol Hydrochloride (Potentiation of antihypertensive effect). Products include:
- Betapace Tablets 637

Spirapril Hydrochloride (Potentiation of antihypertensive effect).
- No products indexed under this heading.

Terazosin Hydrochloride (Potentiation of antihypertensive effect). Products include:
- Hytrin Capsules 434

Timolol Maleate (Potentiation of antihypertensive effect). Products include:
- Blocadren Tablets 1654
- Timolide Tablets 1791
- Timoptic in Ocudose 1796
- Timoptic Sterile Ophthalmic Solution 1794
- Timoptic-XE 1798

Torsemide (Potentiation of antihypertensive effect). Products include:
- Demadex Tablets and Injection 691

Tranylcypromine Sulfate (Concurrent use is contraindicated). Products include:
- Parnate Tablets 2679

Trimethaphan Camsylate (Potentiation of antihypertensive effect).
- No products indexed under this heading.

Verapamil Hydrochloride (Potentiation of antihypertensive effect). Products include:
- Calan SR Caplets 2571
- Calan Tablets 2568
- Covera-HS Tablets 2573
- Isoptin Injectable 1391
- Isoptin Oral Tablets 1393
- Isoptin SR Tablets 1395
- Verelan Capsules 1455

ALDOMET ORAL SUSPENSION
(Methyldopa) 1640

May interact with antihypertensives, general anesthetics, lithium preparations, monoamine oxidase inhibitors, and certain other agents. Compounds in these categories include:

Acebutolol Hydrochloride (Potentiation of antihypertensive effect). Products include:
- Sectral Capsules 2914

Amlodipine Besylate (Potentiation of antihypertensive effect). Products include:
- Lotrel Capsules 858
- Norvasc Tablets 2020

Atenolol (Potentiation of antihypertensive effect). Products include:
- Tenoretic Tablets 2963
- Tenormin Tablets and I.V. Injection 2965

Benazepril Hydrochloride (Potentiation of antihypertensive effect). Products include:
- Lotensin Tablets 852
- Lotensin HCT Tablets 855
- Lotrel Capsules 858

Bendroflumethiazide (Potentiation of antihypertensive effect).
- No products indexed under this heading.

Betaxolol Hydrochloride (Potentiation of antihypertensive effect). Products include:
- Betoptic Ophthalmic Solution 465
- Betoptic S Ophthalmic Suspension 467
- Kerlone Tablets 2588

Bisoprolol Fumarate (Potentiation of antihypertensive effect). Products include:
- Zebeta Tablets 1457
- Ziac 1459

Captopril (Potentiation of antihypertensive effect). Products include:
- Capoten Tablets 740
- Capozide Tablets 744

Carteolol Hydrochloride (Potentiation of antihypertensive effect). Products include:
- Cartrol Tablets 413
- Ocupress Ophthalmic Solution, 1% Sterile 297

Chlorothiazide (Potentiation of antihypertensive effect). Products include:
- Aldoclor Tablets 1638
- Diupres Tablets 1691
- Diuril Oral 1694

Chlorothiazide Sodium (Potentiation of antihypertensive effect). Products include:
- Diuril Sodium Intravenous 1693

Chlorthalidone (Potentiation of antihypertensive effect). Products include:
- Combipres Tablets 682
- Tenoretic Tablets 2963
- Thalitone 1293

Clonidine (Potentiation of antihypertensive effect). Products include:
- Catapres-TTS 680

Clonidine Hydrochloride (Potentiation of antihypertensive effect). Products include:
- Catapres Tablets 679
- Combipres Tablets 682

Deserpidine (Potentiation of antihypertensive effect).
- No products indexed under this heading.

Diazoxide (Potentiation of antihypertensive effect). Products include:
- Hyperstat I.V. Injection 2504
- Proglycem 575

Diltiazem Hydrochloride (Potentiation of antihypertensive effect). Products include:
- Cardizem CD Capsules 1251
- Cardizem SR Capsules 1255
- Cardizem Injectable 1253
- Cardizem Tablets 1257
- Dilacor XR Extended-release Capsules 2183
- Tiazac Capsules 1019

Doxazosin Mesylate (Potentiation of antihypertensive effect). Products include:
- Cardura Tablets 1993

Enalapril Maleate (Potentiation of antihypertensive effect). Products include:
- Vaseretic Tablets 1810
- Vasotec Tablets 1816

Enalaprilat (Potentiation of antihypertensive effect). Products include:
- Vasotec I.V. 1814

Enflurane (May require reduced dose of anesthetics).
- No products indexed under this heading.

Esmolol Hydrochloride (Potentiation of antihypertensive effect). Products include:
- Brevibloc (esmolol HCl) Injection 1860

Felodipine (Potentiation of antihypertensive effect). Products include:
- Plendil Extended-Release Tablets 514

Fosinopril Sodium (Potentiation of antihypertensive effect). Products include:
- Monopril Tablets 762

Furazolidone (Concurrent use is contraindicated). Products include:
- Furoxone 2221

Furosemide (Potentiation of antihypertensive effect). Products include:
- Lasix Injection, Oral Solution and Tablets 1267

Guanabenz Acetate (Potentiation of antihypertensive effect).
- No products indexed under this heading.

Guanethidine Monosulfate (Potentiation of antihypertensive effect). Products include:
- Esimil Tablets 840
- Ismelin Tablets 845

Hydralazine Hydrochloride (Potentiation of antihypertensive effect). Products include:
- Apresazide Capsules 824
- Apresoline Hydrochloride Tablets 826
- Hydralazine Hydrochloride Injection USP 2712
- Ser-Ap-Es Tablets 867

Hydrochlorothiazide (Potentiation of antihypertensive effect). Products include:
- Aldactazide Tablets 2556
- Aldoril Tablets 1644
- Apresazide Capsules 824
- Capozide Tablets 744
- Dyazide Capsules 2653
- Esidrix Tablets 839
- Esimil Tablets 840
- HydroDIURIL Tablets 1716
- Hydropres Tablets 1718
- Hyzaar Tablets 1720
- Inderide Tablets 2838
- Inderide LA Long Acting Capsules 2840
- Lopressor HCT Tablets 850
- Lotensin HCT Tablets 855
- Moduretic Tablets 1748
- Oretic Tablets 450
- Prinzide Tablets 1780
- Ser-Ap-Es Tablets 867
- Timolide Tablets 1791
- Vaseretic Tablets 1810
- Zestoretic Tablets 2968
- Ziac 1459

Hydroflumethiazide (Potentiation of antihypertensive effect). Products include:
- Diucardin Tablets 2824

IMPORTANT NOTE: Always consult each drug listing in the patient's regimen for possible interactions.

Indapamide (Potentiation of antihypertensive effect).
No products indexed under this heading.

Isocarboxazid (Concurrent use is contraindicated).
No products indexed under this heading.

Isoflurane (May require reduced dose of anesthetics).
No products indexed under this heading.

Isradipine (Potentiation of antihypertensive effect). Products include:
DynaCirc Capsules 2381
DynaCirc CR Tablets 2383

Ketamine Hydrochloride (May require reduced dose of anesthetics).
No products indexed under this heading.

Labetalol Hydrochloride (Potentiation of antihypertensive effect). Products include:
Normodyne Injection 2519
Normodyne Tablets 2522
Trandate 1158

Lisinopril (Potentiation of antihypertensive effect). Products include:
Prinivil Tablets 1776
Prinzide Tablets 1780
Zestoretic Tablets 2968
Zestril Tablets 2972

Lithium Carbonate (Potential for lithium toxicity). Products include:
Eskalith 2658
Lithium Carbonate Capsules & Tablets 2352
Lithonate/Lithotabs/Lithobid 2721

Lithium Citrate (Potential for lithium toxicity).
No products indexed under this heading.

Losartan Potassium (Potentiation of antihypertensive effect). Products include:
Cozaar Tablets 1668
Hyzaar Tablets 1720

Mecamylamine Hydrochloride (Potentiation of antihypertensive effect). Products include:
Inversine Tablets 1729

Methohexital Sodium (May require reduced dose of anesthetics).
No products indexed under this heading.

Methoxyflurane (May require reduced dose of anesthetics).
No products indexed under this heading.

Methyclothiazide (Potentiation of antihypertensive effect). Products include:
Enduron Tablets 424

Methyldopate Hydrochloride (Potentiation of antihypertensive effect). Products include:
Aldomet Ester HCl Injection 1642

Metolazone (Potentiation of antihypertensive effect). Products include:
Mykrox Tablets 1617
Zaroxolyn Tablets 1625

Metoprolol Succinate (Potentiation of antihypertensive effect). Products include:
Toprol-XL Tablets 560

Metoprolol Tartrate (Potentiation of antihypertensive effect). Products include:
Lopressor 848
Lopressor HCT Tablets 850

Metyrosine (Potentiation of antihypertensive effect). Products include:
Demser Capsules 1690

Minoxidil (Potentiation of antihypertensive effect).
No products indexed under this heading.

Moexipril Hydrochloride (Potentiation of antihypertensive effect). Products include:
Univasc Tablets 2553

Nadolol (Potentiation of antihypertensive effect).
No products indexed under this heading.

Nicardipine Hydrochloride (Potentiation of antihypertensive effect). Products include:
Cardene Capsules 2261
Cardene I.V. 2815
Cardene SR Capsules 2264

Nifedipine (Potentiation of antihypertensive effect). Products include:
Adalat Capsules (10 mg and 20 mg) 580
Adalat CC 582
Procardia Capsules 2024
Procardia XL Extended Release Tablets 2026

Nisoldipine (Potentiation of antihypertensive effect). Products include:
Sular Tablets 2961

Nitroglycerin (Potentiation of antihypertensive effect). Products include:
Deponit NTG Transdermal Delivery System 2541
Nitro-Bid IV 1270
Nitro-Bid Ointment 1272
Nitro-Dur (nitroglycerin) Transdermal Infusion System 1365
Nitrolingual Spray 2193
Nitrostat Tablets 1981
Transderm-Nitro Transdermal Therapeutic System 878

Penbutolol Sulfate (Potentiation of antihypertensive effect). Products include:
Levatol Tablets 2547

Phenelzine Sulfate (Concurrent use is contraindicated). Products include:
Nardil 1977

Phenoxybenzamine Hydrochloride (Potentiation of antihypertensive effect). Products include:
Dibenzyline Capsules 2650

Phentolamine Mesylate (Potentiation of antihypertensive effect). Products include:
Regitine Vials 864

Pindolol (Potentiation of antihypertensive effect). Products include:
Visken Tablets 2428

Polythiazide (Potentiation of antihypertensive effect). Products include:
Minizide Capsules 2016

Prazosin Hydrochloride (Potentiation of antihypertensive effect). Products include:
Minipress Capsules 2015
Minizide Capsules 2016

Propofol (May require reduced dose of anesthetics). Products include:
Diprivan Injectable Emulsion 2939

Propranolol Hydrochloride (Potentiation of antihypertensive effect). Products include:
Inderal 2834
Inderal LA Long Acting Capsules 2836
Inderide Tablets 2838
Inderide LA Long Acting Capsules .. 2840

Quinapril Hydrochloride (Potentiation of antihypertensive effect). Products include:
Accupril Tablets 1950

Ramipril (Potentiation of antihypertensive effect). Products include:
Altace Capsules 1238

Rauwolfia Serpentina (Potentiation of antihypertensive effect).
No products indexed under this heading.

Rescinnamine (Potentiation of antihypertensive effect).
No products indexed under this heading.

Reserpine (Potentiation of antihypertensive effect). Products include:
Diupres Tablets 1691
Hydropres Tablets 1718
Ser-Ap-Es Tablets 867

Selegiline Hydrochloride (Concurrent use is contraindicated). Products include:
Eldepryl Capsules 2729

Sevoflurane (May require reduced dose of anesthetics).
No products indexed under this heading.

Sodium Nitroprusside (Potentiation of antihypertensive effect).
No products indexed under this heading.

Sotalol Hydrochloride (Potentiation of antihypertensive effect). Products include:
Betapace Tablets 637

Spirapril Hydrochloride (Potentiation of antihypertensive effect).
No products indexed under this heading.

Terazosin Hydrochloride (Potentiation of antihypertensive effect). Products include:
Hytrin Capsules 434

Timolol Maleate (Potentiation of antihypertensive effect). Products include:
Blocadren Tablets 1654
Timolide Tablets 1791
Timoptic in Ocudose 1796
Timoptic Sterile Ophthalmic Solution 1794
Timoptic-XE 1798

Torsemide (Potentiation of antihypertensive effect). Products include:
Demadex Tablets and Injection 691

Tranylcypromine Sulfate (Concurrent use is contraindicated). Products include:
Parnate Tablets 2679

Trimethaphan Camsylate (Potentiation of antihypertensive effect).
No products indexed under this heading.

Verapamil Hydrochloride (Potentiation of antihypertensive effect). Products include:
Calan SR Caplets 2571
Calan Tablets 2568
Covera-HS Tablets 2573
Isoptin Injectable 1391
Isoptin Oral Tablets 1393
Isoptin SR Tablets 1395
Verelan Capsules 1455

ALDOMET TABLETS
(Methyldopa) 1640
See Aldomet Oral Suspension

ALDORIL TABLETS
(Methyldopa, Hydrochlorothiazide) 1644
May interact with corticosteroids, antihypertensives, general anesthetics, insulin, non-steroidal anti-inflammatory agents, barbiturates, narcotic analgesics, monoamine oxidase inhibitors, oral hypoglycemic agents, lithium preparations, cardiac glycosides, and certain other agents. Compounds in these categories include:

Acarbose (Dosage adjustment of the antidiabetic drug may be required). Products include:
Precose 604

Acebutolol Hydrochloride (Potentiation of antihypertensive effect). Products include:
Sectral Capsules 2914

ACTH (Hypokalemia may result).
No products indexed under this heading.

Alfentanil Hydrochloride (Aggravates orthostatic hypotension). Products include:
Alfenta Injection 1334

Amlodipine Besylate (Potentiation of antihypertensive effect). Products include:
Lotrel Capsules 858
Norvasc Tablets 2020

Aprobarbital (Aggravates orthostatic hypotension).
No products indexed under this heading.

Atenolol (Potentiation of antihypertensive effect). Products include:
Tenoretic Tablets 2963
Tenormin Tablets and I.V. Injection 2965

Benazepril Hydrochloride (Potentiation of antihypertensive effect). Products include:
Lotensin Tablets 852
Lotensin HCT Tablets 855
Lotrel Capsules 858

Bendroflumethiazide (Potentiation of antihypertensive effect).
No products indexed under this heading.

Betamethasone Acetate (Hypokalemia may result). Products include:
Celestone Soluspan Suspension 2484

Betamethasone Sodium Phosphate (Hypokalemia may result). Products include:
Celestone Soluspan Suspension 2484

Betaxolol Hydrochloride (Potentiation of antihypertensive effect). Products include:
Betoptic Ophthalmic Solution. 465
Betoptic S Ophthalmic Suspension 467
Kerlone Tablets 2588

Bisoprolol Fumarate (Potentiation of antihypertensive effect). Products include:
Zebeta Tablets 1457
Ziac 1459

Buprenorphine (Aggravates orthostatic hypotension). Products include:
Buprenex Injectable 2170

Butabarbital (Aggravates orthostatic hypotension).
No products indexed under this heading.

Butalbital (Aggravates orthostatic hypotension). Products include:
Axocet Capsules 2469
Esgic-plus Capsules 1012
Esgic-plus Tablets 1012
Fioricet Tablets 2386
Fioricet with Codeine Capsules .. 2387
Fiorinal Capsules 2388
Fiorinal with Codeine Capsules .. 2390
Fiorinal Tablets 2388
Phrenilin 790
Sedapap Tablets 50 mg/650 mg .. 1826

Captopril (Potentiation of antihypertensive effect). Products include:
Capoten Tablets 740
Capozide Tablets 744

Carteolol Hydrochloride (Potentiation of antihypertensive effect). Products include:
Cartrol Tablets 413
Ocupress Ophthalmic Solution, 1% Sterile .... ⊚ 297

Chlorothiazide (Potentiation of antihypertensive effect). Products include:
Aldoclor Tablets 1638
Diupres Tablets 1691
Diuril Oral 1694

Chlorothiazide Sodium (Potentiation of antihypertensive effect). Products include:
Diuril Sodium Intravenous 1693

(▧ Described in PDR For Nonprescription Drugs)   (⊚ Described in PDR For Ophthalmology)

Chlorpropamide (Dosage adjustment of the antidiabetic drug may be required). Products include:
- Diabinese Tablets ... 2002

Chlorthalidone (Potentiation of antihypertensive effect). Products include:
- Combipres Tablets ... 682
- Tenoretic Tablets ... 2963
- Thalitone ... 1293

Cholestyramine (Binds the hydrochlorothiazide and reduces its absorption from gastrointestinal tract by up to 85%). Products include:
- Questran ... 774

Clonidine (Potentiation of antihypertensive effect). Products include:
- Catapres-TTS ... 680

Clonidine Hydrochloride (Potentiation of antihypertensive effect). Products include:
- Catapres Tablets ... 679
- Combipres Tablets ... 682

Codeine Phosphate (Aggravates orthostatic hypotension). Products include:
- Brontex ... 2130
- Dimetane-DC Cough Syrup ... 2232
- Fioricet with Codeine Capsules ... 2387
- Fiorinal with Codeine Capsules ... 2390
- Nucofed ... 2225
- Phenergan with Codeine ... 2883
- Phenergan VC with Codeine ... 2888
- Robitussin A-C Syrup ... 2248
- Robitussin-DAC Syrup ... 2249
- Ryna ... ⊞ 804
- Soma Compound w/Codeine Tablets ... 2784
- Tylenol with Codeine ... 1592

Colestipol Hydrochloride (Binds the hydrochlorothiazide and reduces its absorption from gastrointestinal tract by up to 43%). Products include:
- Colestid ... 2073

Cortisone Acetate (Hypokalemia may result). Products include:
- Cortone Acetate Sterile Suspension ... 1663
- Cortone Acetate Tablets ... 1664

Deserpidine (Potentiation of antihypertensive effect).
- No products indexed under this heading.

Deslanoside (Hypokalemia may exaggerate cardiac toxicity of digitalis).
- No products indexed under this heading.

Dexamethasone (Hypokalemia may result). Products include:
- AK-Trol Ointment & Suspension ... ◉ 205
- Decadron Elixir ... 1676
- Decadron Tablets ... 1678
- Decaspray Topical Aerosol ... 1689
- Maxitrol Ophthalmic Ointment and Suspension ... ◉ 222
- TobraDex Ophthalmic Suspension and Ointment ... 469

Dexamethasone Acetate (Hypokalemia may result). Products include:
- Dalalone D.P. Injectable ... 1009
- Decadron-LA Sterile Suspension ... 1687

Dexamethasone Sodium Phosphate (Hypokalemia may result). Products include:
- Decadron Phosphate Injection ... 1680
- Decadron Phosphate Sterile Ophthalmic Ointment ... 1684
- Decadron Phosphate Sterile Ophthalmic Solution ... 1685
- Decadron Phosphate Topical Cream ... 1686
- Decadron Phosphate with Xylocaine Injection, Sterile ... 1683
- Dexacort Phosphate in Respihaler ... 1606
- Dexacort Phosphate in Turbinaire ... 1607
- NeoDecadron Sterile Ophthalmic Ointment ... 1755
- NeoDecadron Sterile Ophthalmic Solution ... 1756
- NeoDecadron Topical Cream ... 1757

Dezocine (Aggravates orthostatic hypotension). Products include:
- Dalgan Injection ... 529

Diazoxide (Potentiation of antihypertensive effect). Products include:
- Hyperstat I.V. Injection ... 2504
- Proglycem ... 575

Diclofenac Potassium (May result in reduced diuretic effect). Products include:
- Cataflam Tablets ... 833

Diclofenac Sodium (May result in reduced diuretic effect). Products include:
- Voltaren Ophthalmic Sterile Ophthalmic Solution ... ◉ 264
- Cataflam/Voltaren/Voltaren-XR ... 833

Digitoxin (Hypokalemia may exaggerate cardiac toxicity of digitalis). Products include:
- Crystodigin Tablets ... 1472

Digoxin (Hypokalemia may exaggerate cardiac toxicity of digitalis). Products include:
- Lanoxicaps ... 1110
- Lanoxin Elixir Pediatric ... 1113
- Lanoxin Injection ... 1116
- Lanoxin Injection Pediatric ... 1119
- Lanoxin Tablets ... 1121

Diltiazem Hydrochloride (Potentiation of antihypertensive effect). Products include:
- Cardizem CD Capsules ... 1251
- Cardizem SR Capsules ... 1255
- Cardizem Injectable ... 1253
- Cardizem Tablets ... 1257
- Dilacor XR Extended-release Capsules ... 2183
- Tiazac Capsules ... 1019

Doxazosin Mesylate (Potentiation of antihypertensive effect). Products include:
- Cardura Tablets ... 1993

Enalapril Maleate (Potentiation of antihypertensive effect). Products include:
- Vaseretic Tablets ... 1810
- Vasotec Tablets ... 1816

Enalaprilat (Potentiation of antihypertensive effect). Products include:
- Vasotec I.V. ... 1814

Enflurane (May require reduced dose of anesthetics).
- No products indexed under this heading.

Esmolol Hydrochloride (Potentiation of antihypertenisive effect). Products include:
- Brevibloc (esmolol HCl) Injection ... 1860

Etodolac (May result in reduced diuretic effect). Products include:
- Lodine Capsules and Tablets ... 2849

Felodipine (Potentiation of antihypertensive effect). Products include:
- Plendil Extended-Release Tablets ... 514

Fenoprofen Calcium (May result in reduced diuretic effects). Products include:
- Nalfon 200 Pulvules & Nalfon Tablets ... 933

Fentanyl (Aggravates orthostatic hypotension). Products include:
- Duragesic Transdermal System ... 1336

Fentanyl Citrate (Aggravates orthostatic hypotension). Products include:
- Sublimaze Injection ... 463

Fludrocortisone Acetate (Hypokalemia may result). Products include:
- Florinef Acetate Tablets ... 506

Flurbiprofen (May result in reduced diuretic effect).
- No products indexed under this heading.

Fosinopril Sodium (Potentiation of antihypertensive effect). Products include:
- Monopril Tablets ... 762

Furazolidone (Concurrent use is contraindicated). Products include:
- Furoxone ... 2221

Furosemide (Potentiation of antihypertensive effect). Products include:
- Lasix Injection, Oral Solution and Tablets ... 1267

Glimepiride (Dosage adjustment of the antidiabetic drug may be required). Products include:
- Amaryl Tablets ... 1241

Glipizide (Dosage adjustment of the antidiabetic drug may be required). Products include:
- Glucotrol Tablets ... 2011
- Glucotrol XL Extended Release Tablets ... 2012

Glyburide (Dosage adjustment of the antidiabetic drug may be required). Products include:
- DiaBeta Tablets ... 1265
- Glynase PresTab Tablets ... 2091
- Micronase Tablets ... 2099

Guanabenz Acetate (Potentiation of antihypertensive effect).
- No products indexed under this heading.

Guanethidine Monosulfate (Potentiation of antihypertensive effect). Products include:
- Esimil Tablets ... 840
- Ismelin Tablets ... 845

Hydralazine Hydrochloride (Potentiation of antihypertensive effect). Products include:
- Apresazide Capsules ... 824
- Apresoline Hydrochloride Tablets ... 826
- Hydralazine Hydrochloride Injection USP ... 2712
- Ser-Ap-Es Tablets ... 867

Hydrocodone Bitartrate (Aggravates orthostatic hypotension). Products include:
- Codiclear DH Syrup ... 808
- Duratuss HD Elixir ... 2750
- Histussin D Liquid ... 670
- Hycodan Tablets and Syrup ... 946
- Hycomine Compound Tablets ... 948
- Hycomine ... 947
- Hycotuss Expectorant Syrup ... 950
- Hydrocet Capsules ... 787
- Lorcet 10/650 Tablets ... 1016
- Lortab ... 2751
- Tussend ... 1830
- Tussend Expectorant ... 1831
- Vicodin Tablets ... 1404
- Vicodin ES Tablets ... 1405
- Vicodin HP Tablets ... 1403
- Vicodin Tuss Expectorant ... 1406
- Zydone Capsules ... 967

Hydrocodone Polistirex (Aggravates orthostatic hypotension). Products include:
- Tussionex Pennkinetic Extended-Release Suspension ... 1624

Hydrocortisone (Hypokalemia may result). Products include:
- Anusol-HC Cream 2.5% ... 1953
- Aquanil HC Lotion ... 1989
- Maximum Strength Cortaid Spray ... ⊞ 800
- CORTENEMA ... 2713
- Cortisporin Ointment ... 1074
- Cortisporin Ophthalmic Ointment Sterile ... 1074
- Cortisporin Ophthalmic Suspension Sterile ... 1075
- Cortisporin Otic Solution Sterile ... 1076
- Cortisporin Otic Suspension Sterile ... 1077
- Cortizone-5 ... ⊞ 795
- Cortizone-10 ... ⊞ 795
- Hydrocortone Tablets ... 1715
- Hytone ... 922
- Hytone Ointment 2 ½% ... 923
- Massengill Medicated Soft Cloth Towelettes ... 2628
- Pediotic Suspension Sterile ... 1140
- Preparation H Hydrocortisone 1% Cream ... ⊞ 843
- ProctoCream-HC 2.5% ... 2552
- VōSoL HC Otic Solution ... 2786

Hydrocortisone Acetate (Hypokalemia may result). Products include:
- Analpram-HC Rectal Cream 1% and 2.5% ... 993
- Anusol HC-1 Hydrocortisone Anti-Itch Ointment ... ⊞ 810
- Anusol-HC Suppositories ... 1954
- Caldecort Anti-Itch Hydrocortisone Cream ... ⊞ 651
- Coly-Mycin S Otic w/Neomycin & Hydrocortisone ... 1965
- Cortaid ... ⊞ 800
- Cortifoam ... 2540
- Cortisporin Cream ... 1073
- Epifoam ... 2543
- Hydrocortone Acetate Sterile Suspension ... 1712
- Mantadil Cream ... 1124
- Nupercainal Hydrocortisone 1% Cream ... ⊞ 661
- Pramosone Cream, Lotion & Ointment ... 995
- ProctoFoam-HC ... 2552
- Terra-Cortril Ophthalmic Suspension ... 2033

Hydrocortisone Sodium Phosphate (Hypokalemia may result). Products include:
- Hydrocortone Phosphate Injection, Sterile ... 1713

Hydrocortisone Sodium Succinate (Hypokalemia may result).
- No products indexed under this heading.

Hydroflumethiazide (Potentiation of antihypertensive effect). Products include:
- Diucardin Tablets ... 2824

Hydromorphone Hydrochloride (Aggravates orthostatic hypotension). Products include:
- Dilaudid Ampules ... 1382
- Dilaudid Cough Syrup ... 1383
- Dilaudid-HP Injection ... 1384
- Dilaudid-HP Lyophilized Powder 250 mg ... 1384
- Dilaudid ... 1382
- Dilaudid Oral Liquid ... 1386
- Dilaudid ... 1382
- Dilaudid Tablets - 8 mg ... 1386

Ibuprofen (May result in reduced diuretic effects). Products include:
- Advil Cold and Sinus Caplets and Tablets ... ⊞ 837
- Advil Ibuprofen Tablets, Caplets and Gel Caplets ... ⊞ 836
- Children's Motrin Ibuprofen Oral Suspension ... 1558
- IBU Tablets ... 1389
- Ibuprohm ... ⊞ 713
- Motrin IB Caplets, Tablets, and Gelcaps ... ⊞ 802
- Motrin Ibuprofen Suspension, Oral Drops, Chewable Tablets, Caplets ... 1563
- Nuprin Ibuprofen/Analgesic Tablets & Caplets ... ⊞ 645
- Vicks DayQuil SINUS Pressure & PAIN Relief with IBUPROFEN ... ⊞ 735

Indapamide (Potentiation of antihypertensive effect).
- No products indexed under this heading.

Indomethacin (May result in reduced diuretic effects). Products include:
- Indocin ... 1723

Indomethacin Sodium Trihydrate (May result in reduced diuretic effects). Products include:
- Indocin I.V. ... 1727

Insulin, Human (Insulin requirement may be altered).
- No products indexed under this heading.

Insulin, Human Isophane Suspension (Insulin requirement may be altered). Products include:
- Novolin N Human Insulin 10 ml Vials ... 1846

IMPORTANT NOTE: Always consult each drug listing in the patient's regimen for possible interactions.

Aldoril — Interactions Index

Insulin, Human NPH (Insulin requirement may be altered). Products include:
- Humulin N, 100 Units ... 1495
- Novolin N PenFill 1.5 ml Cartridges Durable Insulin Delivery System ... 1849
- Novolin N Prefilled Syringe Disposable Insulin Delivery System ... 1850

Insulin, Human Regular (Insulin requirement may be altered). Products include:
- Humulin R, 100 Units ... 1497
- Novolin R Human Insulin 10 ml Vials ... 1846
- Novolin R PenFill 1.5 ml Cartridges Durable Insulin Delivery System ... 1849
- Novolin R Prefilled Syringe Disposable Insulin Delivery System ... 1850
- Velosulin BR Human Insulin 10 ml Vials ... 1847

Insulin, Human, Zinc Suspension (Insulin requirement may be altered). Products include:
- Humulin L, 100 Units ... 1494
- Humulin U, 100 Units ... 1498
- Novolin L Human Insulin 10 ml Vials ... 1846

Insulin Lispro, Human (Insulin requirement may be altered). Products include:
- Humalog Injection ... 1488

Insulin, NPH (Insulin requirement may be altered). Products include:
- NPH, 100 Units ... 1502
- Pork NPH, 100 Units ... 1506
- Purified Pork NPH Isophane Insulin ... 1852

Insulin, Regular (Insulin requirement may be altered). Products include:
- Regular, 100 Units ... 1503
- Pork Regular, 100 Units ... 1507
- Pork Regular (Concentrated), 500 Units ... 1508
- Purified Pork Regular Insulin ... 1852

Insulin, Zinc Crystals (Insulin requirement may be altered). Products include:
- NPH, 100 Units ... 1502

Insulin, Zinc Suspension (Insulin requirement may be altered). Products include:
- Iletin I ... 1501
- Lente, 100 Units ... 1501
- Iletin II ... 1504
- Pork Lente, 100 Units ... 1504
- Purified Pork Lente Insulin ... 1852

Isocarboxazid (Concurrent use is contraindicated).
No products indexed under this heading.

Isoflurane (May require reduced dose of anesthetics).
No products indexed under this heading.

Isradipine (Potentiation of antihypertensive effect). Products include:
- DynaCirc Capsules ... 2381
- DynaCirc CR Tablets ... 2383

Ketamine Hydrochloride (May require reduced dose of anesthetics).
No products indexed under this heading.

Ketoprofen (May result in reduced diuretic effects). Products include:
- Actron Caplets and Tablets ... ⊞ 608
- Orudis Capsules ... 2874
- Orudis KT ... ⊞ 842
- Oruvail Capsules ... 2874

Ketorolac Tromethamine (May result in reduced diuretic effect). Products include:
- Acular Sterile Ophthalmic Solution ... 470
- Toradol ... 2319

Labetalol Hydrochloride (Potentiation of antihypertensive effect). Products include:
- Normodyne Injection ... 2519
- Normodyne Tablets ... 2522
- Trandate ... 1158

Levorphanol Tartrate (Aggravates orthostatic hypotension). Products include:
- Levo-Dromoran ... 2297

Lisinopril (Potentiation of antihypertensive effect). Products include:
- Prinivil Tablets ... 1776
- Prinzide Tablets ... 1780
- Zestoretic Tablets ... 2968
- Zestril Tablets ... 2972

Lithium Carbonate (High risk of lithium toxicity). Products include:
- Eskalith ... 2658
- Lithium Carbonate Capsules & Tablets ... 2352
- Lithonate/Lithotabs/Lithobid ... 2721

Lithium Citrate (High risk of lithium toxicity).
No products indexed under this heading.

Losartan Potassium (Potentiation of antihypertensive effect). Products include:
- Cozaar Tablets ... 1668
- Hyzaar Tablets ... 1720

Mecamylamine Hydrochloride (Potentiation of antihypertensive effect). Products include:
- Inversine Tablets ... 1729

Meclofenamate Sodium (May result in reduced diuretic effects).
No products indexed under this heading.

Mefenamic Acid (May result in reduced diuretic effects). Products include:
- Ponstel ... 1982

Meperidine Hydrochloride (Aggravates orthostatic hypotension). Products include:
- Demerol ... 2438
- Mepergan Injection ... 2859

Mephobarbital (Aggravates orthostatic hypotension). Products include:
- Mebaral Tablets ... 2452

Metformin Hydrochloride (Dosage adjustment of the antidiabetic drug may be required). Products include:
- Glucophage Tablets ... 754

Methadone Hydrochloride (Aggravates orthostatic hypotension). Products include:
- Methadone Hydrochloride Oral Concentrate ... 2356
- Methadone Hydrochloride Oral Solution & Tablets ... 2357

Methohexital Sodium (May require reduced dose of anesthetics).
No products indexed under this heading.

Methoxyflurane (May require reduced dose of anesthetics).
No products indexed under this heading.

Methyclothiazide (Potentiation of antihypertensive effect). Products include:
- Enduron Tablets ... 424

Methyldopate Hydrochloride (Potentiation of antihypertensive effect). Products include:
- Aldomet Ester HCl Injection ... 1642

Methylprednisolone Acetate (Hypokalemia may result).
No products indexed under this heading.

Methylprednisolone Sodium Succinate (Hypokalemia may result).
No products indexed under this heading.

Metolazone (Potentiation of antihypertensive effect). Products include:
- Mykrox Tablets ... 1617
- Zaroxolyn Tablets ... 1625

Metoprolol Succinate (Potentiation of antihypertensive effect). Products include:
- Toprol-XL Tablets ... 560

Metoprolol Tartrate (Potentiation of antihypertensive effect). Products include:
- Lopressor ... 848
- Lopressor HCT Tablets ... 850

Metyrosine (Potentiation of antihypertensive effect). Products include:
- Demser Capsules ... 1690

Minoxidil (Potentiation of antihypertensive effect).
No products indexed under this heading.

Moexipril Hydrochloride (Potentiation of antihypertensive effect). Products include:
- Univasc Tablets ... 2553

Morphine Sulfate (Aggravates orthostatic hypotension). Products include:
- Astramorph/PF Injection, USP (Preservative-Free) ... 526
- Duramorph Injection ... 983
- Infumorph 200 and Infumorph 500 Sterile Solutions ... 985
- Kadian Capsules ... 2948
- MS Contin Tablets ... 2149
- MSIR ... 2152
- Oramorph SR (Morphine Sulfate Sustained Release Tablets) ... 2359
- RMS Suppositories CII ... 2766
- Roxanol ... 2365

Nabumetone (May result in reduced diuretic effect). Products include:
- Relafen Tablets ... 2688

Nadolol (Potentiation of antihypertensive effect).
No products indexed under this heading.

Naproxen (May result in reduced diuretic effects). Products include:
- Anaprox/Naprosyn ... 2277

Naproxen Sodium (May result in reduced diuretic effects). Products include:
- Aleve ... 2124
- Anaprox/Naprosyn ... 2277
- Naprelan Tablets ... 2861

Nicardipine Hydrochloride (Potentiation of antihypertensive effect). Products include:
- Cardene Capsules ... 2261
- Cardene I.V. ... 2815
- Cardene SR Capsules ... 2264

Nifedipine (Potentiation of antihypertensive effect). Products include:
- Adalat Capsules (10 mg and 20 mg) ... 580
- Adalat CC ... 582
- Procardia Capsules ... 2024
- Procardia XL Extended Release Tablets ... 2026

Nisoldipine (Potentiation of antihypertensive effect). Products include:
- Sular Tablets ... 2961

Nitroglycerin (Potentiation of antihypertensive effect). Products include:
- Deponit NTG Transdermal Delivery System ... 2541
- Nitro-Bid IV ... 1270
- Nitro-Bid Ointment ... 1272
- Nitro-Dur (nitroglycerin) Transdermal Infusion System ... 1365
- Nitrolingual Spray ... 2193
- Nitrostat Tablets ... 1981
- Transderm-Nitro Transdermal Therapeutic System ... 878

Norepinephrine Bitartrate (Decreased arterial responsiveness to norepinephrine). Products include:
- Levophed Bitartrate Injection ... 2445

Opium Alkaloids (Aggravates orthostatic hypotension).
No products indexed under this heading.

Oxaprozin (May result in reduced diuretic effect). Products include:
- Daypro Caplets ... 2578

Oxycodone Hydrochloride (Aggravates orthostatic hypotension). Products include:
- OxyContin Tablets ... 2163
- OxyIR Capsules ... 2167
- Percocet Tablets ... 955
- Percodan Tablets ... 955
- Percodan-Demi Tablets ... 956
- Roxicodone Tablets, Oral Solution & Intensol (Oxycodone) ... 2366
- Tylox Capsules ... 1593

Penbutolol Sulfate (Potentiation of antihypertensive effect). Products include:
- Levatol Tablets ... 2547

Pentobarbital Sodium (Aggravates orthostatic hypotension). Products include:
- Nembutal Sodium Capsules ... 440
- Nembutal Sodium Solution ... 442
- Nembutal Sodium Suppositories ... 444

Phenelzine Sulfate (Concurrent use is contraindicated). Products include:
- Nardil ... 1977

Phenobarbital (Aggravates orthostatic hypotension). Products include:
- Arco-Lase Plus Tablets ... 513
- Bellergal-S Tablets ... 2375
- Donnatal ... 2234
- Donnatal Extentabs ... 2234
- Donnatal Tablets ... 2234
- Phenobarbital Elixir and Tablets ... 1523
- Quadrinal Tablets ... 1398

Phenoxybenzamine Hydrochloride (Potentiation of antihypertensive effect). Products include:
- Dibenzyline Capsules ... 2650

Phentolamine Mesylate (Potentiation of antihypertensive effect). Products include:
- Regitine Vials ... 864

Phenylbutazone (May result in reduced diuretic effects).
No products indexed under this heading.

Pindolol (Potentiation of antihypertensive effect). Products include:
- Visken Tablets ... 2428

Piroxicam (May result in reduced diuretic effects). Products include:
- Feldene Capsules ... 2008

Polythiazide (Potentiation of antihypertensive effect). Products include:
- Minizide Capsules ... 2016

Prazosin Hydrochloride (Potentiation of antihypertensive effect). Products include:
- Minipress Capsules ... 2015
- Minizide Capsules ... 2016

Prednisolone Acetate (Hypokalemia may result). Products include:
- AK-CIDE ... ⊚ 203
- AK-CIDE Ointment ... ⊚ 203
- Blephamide Liquifilm Sterile Ophthalmic Suspension ... ⊚ 472
- Blephamide Ointment ... ⊚ 234
- Econopred & Econopred Plus Ophthalmic Suspensions ... ⊚ 216
- Poly-Pred Liquifilm ... ⊚ 246
- Pred Forte ... ⊚ 247
- Pred Mild ... ⊚ 250
- Pred-G Liquifilm Sterile Ophthalmic Suspension ... ⊚ 248
- Pred-G S.O.P. Sterile Ophthalmic Ointment ... ⊚ 249

Prednisolone Sodium Phosphate (Hypokalemia may result). Products include:
- AK-PRED ... ⊚ 204
- Hydeltrasol Injection, Sterile ... 1708
- Pediapred Oral Solution ... 1618

Prednisolone Tebutate (Hypokalemia may result). Products include:
- Hydeltra-T.B.A. Sterile Suspension ... 1710

(⊞ Described in PDR For Nonprescription Drugs)   (⊚ Described in PDR For Ophthalmology)

Prednisone (Hypokalemia may result).
- No products indexed under this heading.

Propofol (May require reduced dose of anesthetics). Products include:
- Diprivan Injectable Emulsion 2939

Propoxyphene Hydrochloride (Aggravates orthostatic hypotension). Products include:
- Darvon 1475
- Wygesic Tablets 2930

Propoxyphene Napsylate (Aggravates orthostatic hypotension). Products include:
- Darvon-N/Darvocet-N 1473

Propranolol Hydrochloride (Potentiation of antihypertensive effect). Products include:
- Inderal 2834
- Inderal LA Long Acting Capsules 2836
- Inderide Tablets 2838
- Inderide LA Long Acting Capsules .. 2840

Quinapril Hydrochloride (Potentiation of antihypertensive effect). Products include:
- Accupril Tablets 1950

Ramipril (Potentiation of antihypertensive effect). Products include:
- Altace Capsules 1238

Rauwolfia Serpentina (Potentiation of antihypertensive effect).
- No products indexed under this heading.

Rescinnamine (Potentiation of antihypertensive effect).
- No products indexed under this heading.

Reserpine (Potentiation of antihypertensive effect). Products include:
- Diupres Tablets 1691
- Hydropres Tablets 1718
- Ser-Ap-Es Tablets 867

Secobarbital Sodium (Aggravates orthostatic hypotension). Products include:
- Seconal Sodium Pulvules 1529

Selegiline Hydrochloride (Concurrent use is contraindicated). Products include:
- Eldepryl Capsules 2729

Sevoflurane (May require reduced dose of anesthetics).
- No products indexed under this heading.

Sodium Nitroprusside (Potentiation of antihypertensive effect).
- No products indexed under this heading.

Sotalol Hydrochloride (Potentiation of antihypertensive effect). Products include:
- Betapace Tablets 637

Spirapril Hydrochloride (Potentiation of antihypertensive effect).
- No products indexed under this heading.

Sufentanil Citrate (Aggravates orthostatic hypotension). Products include:
- Sufenta Injection 1355

Sulindac (May result in reduced diuretic effects). Products include:
- Clinoril Tablets 1658

Terazosin Hydrochloride (Potentiation of antihypertensive effect). Products include:
- Hytrin Capsules 434

Thiamylal Sodium (Aggravates orthostatic hypotension).
- No products indexed under this heading.

Timolol Maleate (Potentiation of antihypertensive effect). Products include:
- Blocadren Tablets 1654
- Timolide Tablets 1791
- Timoptic in Ocudose 1796
- Timoptic Sterile Ophthalmic Solution 1794
- Timoptic-XE 1798

Tolazamide (Dosage adjustment of the antidiabetic drug may be required).
- No products indexed under this heading.

Tolbutamide (Dosage adjustment of the antidiabetic drug may be required).
- No products indexed under this heading.

Tolmetin Sodium (May result in reduced diuretic effects). Products include:
- Tolectin (200, 400 and 600 mg) .. 1591

Torsemide (Potentiation of antihypertensive effect). Products include:
- Demadex Tablets and Injection 691

Tranylcypromine Sulfate (Concurrent use is contraindicated). Products include:
- Parnate Tablets 2679

Triamcinolone (Hypokalemia may result).
- No products indexed under this heading.

Triamcinolone Acetonide (Hypokalemia may result). Products include:
- Azmacort Oral Inhaler 2175
- Nasacort AQ Nasal Spray 2191
- Nasacort Nasal Inhaler 2189

Triamcinolone Diacetate (Hypokalemia may result).
- No products indexed under this heading.

Triamcinolone Hexacetonide (Hypokalemia may result).
- No products indexed under this heading.

Trimethaphan Camsylate (Potentiation of antihypertensive effect).
- No products indexed under this heading.

Tubocurarine Chloride (Increased responsiveness to tubocurarine).
- No products indexed under this heading.

Verapamil Hydrochloride (Potentiation of antihypertensive effect). Products include:
- Calan SR Caplets 2571
- Calan Tablets 2568
- Covera-HS Tablets 2573
- Isoptin Injectable 1391
- Isoptin Oral Tablets 1393
- Isoptin SR Tablets 1395
- Verelan Capsules 1455

Food Interactions

Alcohol (Aggravates orthostatic hypotension).

ALEVE

(Naproxen Sodium) 2124
May interact with:

Acetaminophen (Concurrent administration is not recommended unless advised by a physician). Products include:
- Actifed Cold & Sinus Caplets and Tablets 808
- Actifed Sinus Daytime/Nighttime Tablets and Caplets 809
- Alka-Seltzer Fast Relief Caplets 610
- Alka-Seltzer Plus Liqui-Gels 612
- Alka-Seltzer Plus Flu & Body Aches Effervescent Tablets 612
- Alka-Seltzer Plus Flu & Body Aches Liqui-Gels Non-Drowsy Formula 613
- Alka-Seltzer Plus Night-Time Cold Medicine Liqui-Gels 612
- Allerest No Drowsiness 649
- Allerest Sinus Pain Formula 649
- Axocet Capsules 2469
- Benadryl Allergy/Cold Tablets 811
- Benadryl Allergy Sinus Headache Caplets 813
- Children's TYLENOL acetaminophen Chewable Tablets, Elixir, Suspension Liquid, and Suspension Drops 1559
- Children's TYLENOL Cold Multi-Symptom Chewable Tablets and Liquid 1559
- Children's TYLENOL Cold Plus Cough Multi Symptom Chewable Tablets and Liquid 1560
- Children's TYLENOL Flu Suspension Liquid 1560
- Allergy-Sinus Comtrex Multi-Symptom Allergy-Sinus Formula Tablets and Caplets 639
- Comtrex Multi-Symptom 638
- Comtrex Non-Drowsy 640
- Contac Day Allergy/Sinus Caplets 771
- Contac Day & Night 772
- Contac Night Allergy/Sinus Caplets 771
- Contac Severe Cold and Flu Formula Caplets 773
- Contac Severe Cold & Flu Non-Drowsy 774
- Coricidin Cold + Flu Tablets 760
- Coricidin 'D' Decongestant Tablets 760
- DHCplus Capsules 2148
- Darvon-N/Darvocet-N 1473
- Dimetapp Allergy Sinus Caplets 838
- Dimetapp Cold & Fever Suspension 839
- Drixoral Cold and Flu Extended-Release Tablets 764
- Drixoral Cough + Sore Throat Liquid Caps 763
- Drixoral Allergy/Sinus Extended Release Tablets 765
- Esgic-plus Capsules 1012
- Esgic-plus Tablets 1012
- Aspirin Free Excedrin Analgesic Caplets and Geltabs 734
- Excedrin Extra-Strength Analgesic Tablets, Caplets, and Geltabs 734
- Excedrin P.M. Analgesic/Sleeping Aid Tablets, Caplets, Liquigels 735
- Fioricet Tablets 2386
- Fioricet with Codeine Capsules 2387
- Goody's Extra Strength Headache Powders 632
- Goody's Extra Strength Pain Relief Tablets 632
- Hycomine Compound Tablets 948
- Hydrocet Capsules 787
- Infants' TYLENOL acetaminophen Suspension Drops 1559
- Infants' TYLENOL Cold Decongestant & Fever-Reducer Drops 1561
- Junior Strength TYLENOL acetaminophen Coated Caplets and Chewable Tablets 1562
- Lorcet 10/650 Tablets 1016
- Lortab 2751
- Lurline PMS Tablets 1000
- Maximum Strength Multi-Symptom Formula Midol 621
- PMS Multi-Symptom Formula Midol 622
- Maximum Strength Midol Teen Multi-Symptom Formula 621
- Midrin Capsules 788
- Panodol Tablets and Caplets 783
- Children's Panadol Chewable Tablets, Liquid, Infant's Drops 783
- Percocet Tablets 955
- Percogesic Analgesic Tablets 727
- Phrenilin 790
- Pyrroxate Caplets 742
- Robitussin Cold, Cough & Flu Liqui-Gels 844
- Robitussin Night-Time Cold Formula 847
- Sedapap Tablets 50 mg/650 mg .. 1826
- Sinarest 663
- Sine-Aid Maximum Strength Sinus Headache Gelcaps, Caplets and Tablets 1570
- Sine-Off No Drowsiness Formula Caplets 784
- Sine-Off Sinus Medicine 784
- Singlet Tablets 785
- Sinulin Tablets 792
- Sinutab Sinus Allergy Medication, Maximum Strength Tablets and Caplets 823
- Sinutab Sinus Medication, Maximum Strength Without Drowsiness Formula, Tablets & Caplets 824
- Sudafed Cold and Cough Liquid Caps 826
- Sudafed Severe Cold Formula Caplets 828
- Sudafed Severe Cold Formula Tablets 828
- Sudafed Sinus Caplets 829
- Sudafed Sinus Tablets 829
- Talacen Caplets 2464
- TheraFlu Flu and Cold Medicine 750
- Theraflu Maximum Strength Flu and Cold Medicine For Sore Throat 751
- TheraFlu Flu, Cold and Cough Medicine 750
- TheraFlu Maximum Strength Nighttime Flu, Cold & Cough Medicine 751
- TheraFlu Maximum Strength Non-Drowsy Formula Flu, Cold & Cough Medicine 751
- TheraFlu Maximum Strength, Non-Drowsy Formula Flu, Cold and Cough Caplets 752
- Theraflu Maximum Strength Sinus Non-Drowsy Formula Caplets 752
- Triaminic Sore Throat Formula 755
- Triaminicin Tablets 756
- TYLENOL acetaminophen Extended Relief Caplets 1570
- TYLENOL acetaminophen, Extra Strength Adult Liquid Pain Reliever 1570
- TYLENOL acetaminophen, Extra Strength Gelcaps, Geltabs, Caplets, Tablets 1570
- TYLENOL acetaminophen, Regular Strength Caplets and Tablets 1570
- TYLENOL Allergy Sinus, Maximum Strength Caplets and Gelcaps 1571
- TYLENOL Allergy Sinus NightTime, Maximum Strength Caplets 1571
- TYLENOL Cold Medication, Multi-Symptom Formula Tablets and Caplets 1572
- TYLENOL Cold Medication, Multi-Symptom Hot Liquid Packets 1572
- TYLENOL Cold Medication, No Drowsiness Formula Caplets and Gelcaps 1572
- TYLENOL Cold Severe Congestion Caplets 1573
- TYLENOL Cough Medication, Multi Symptom 1574
- TYLENOL Cough Medication with Decongestant, Multi Symptom 1574
- TYLENOL Flu No Drowsiness Formula, Maximum Strength Gelcaps 1575
- TYLENOL Flu NightTime, Maximum Strength Gelcaps 1575
- TYLENOL Flu NightTime, Maximum Strength Hot Medication Packets 1575
- TYLENOL Headache Plus Pain Reliever with Antacid, Extra Strength Caplets 705
- TYLENOL PM Pain Reliever/Sleep Aid, Extra Strength Gelcaps, Caplets, Geltabs 1576
- TYLENOL Severe Allergy Medication Caplets 1571
- TYLENOL Sinus, Maximum Strength Geltabs, Gelcaps, Caplets and Tablets 1576
- Tylenol with Codeine 1592
- Tylox Capsules 1593
- Unisom With Pain Relief-Nighttime Sleep Aid and Pain Reliever 1991
- Vanquish Analgesic Caplets 627
- Vicks 44 LiquiCaps Cough, Cold & Flu Relief 728
- Vicks 44M Cough, Cold & Flu Relief 729
- Vicks DayQuil LiquiCaps/Liquid Multi-Symptom Cold/Flu Relief .. 734
- Vicks Nyquil Hot Therapy 735
- Vicks NyQuil LiquiCaps/Liquid Multi-Symptom Cold/Flu Relief, Original and Cherry Flavors 736
- Vicodin Tablets 1404
- Vicodin ES Tablets 1405
- Vicodin HP Tablets 1403
- Wygesic Tablets 2930
- Zydone Capsules 967

IMPORTANT NOTE: Always consult each drug listing in the patient's regimen for possible interactions.

Interactions Index

Aleve

Aspirin (Concurrent administration is not recommended unless advised by a physician). Products include:
- Alka-Seltzer Cherry Effervescent Antacid and Pain Reliever 609
- Alka-Seltzer Extra Strength Effervescent Antacid and Pain Reliever 609
- Alka-Seltzer Lemon Lime Effervescent Antacid and Pain Reliever 609
- Alka-Seltzer Original Effervescent Antacid and Pain Reliever 609
- Alka-Seltzer Plus 611
- Alka-Seltzer Plus Sinus Medicine 611
- Ascriptin 650
- Arthritis Strength BC Powder 631
- BC Cold Powder Multi-Symptom Formula (Cold-Sinus-Allergy) 631
- BC Cold Powder Non-Drowsy Formula (Cold-Sinus) 631
- BC Powder 631
- Genuine Bayer Aspirin Tablets & Caplets 618
- Extra Strength Bayer Arthritis Pain Regimen Formula 615
- Extra Strength Bayer Aspirin Caplets & Tablets 617
- Extended-Release Bayer 8-Hour Aspirin 616
- Extra Strength Bayer Plus Aspirin Caplets 617
- Extra Strength Bayer PM Aspirin Plus Sleep Aid 617
- Aspirin Regimen Bayer 81 mg Tablets with Calcium 615
- Aspirin Regimen Bayer Adult Low Strength 81 mg Tablets 613
- Aspirin Regimen Bayer Children's Chewable Aspirin 616
- Aspirin Regimen Bayer Regular Strength 325 mg Caplets 613
- Bufferin Analgesic Tablets 636
- Arthritis Strength Bufferin Analgesic Caplets 637
- Extra Strength Bufferin Analgesic Tablets 637
- Cama Arthritis Pain Reliever 748
- Darvon Compound-65 Pulvules 1475
- Easprin 1971
- Ecotrin 2625
- Ecotrin Enteric Coated Aspirin Maximum Strength Tablets and Caplets 775
- Ecotrin Enteric Coated Aspirin Regular Strength Tablets 2625
- Empirin Aspirin Tablets 818
- Excedrin Extra-Strength Analgesic Tablets, Caplets, and Geltabs 734
- Fiorinal Capsules 2388
- Fiorinal with Codeine Capsules 2390
- Fiorinal Tablets 2388
- Goody's Extra Strength Headache Powders 632
- Goody's Extra Strength Pain Relief Tablets 632
- Halfprin Tablets 1413
- Norgesic 1554
- Percodan Tablets 955
- Percodan-Demi Tablets 956
- Robaxisal Tablets 2246
- Soma Compound w/Codeine Tablets 2784
- Soma Compound Tablets 2783
- St. Joseph Adult Chewable Aspirin (81 mg.) 768
- Talwin Compound 2466
- Vanquish Analgesic Caplets 627

Ibuprofen (Concurrent administration is not recommended unless advised by a physician). Products include:
- Advil Cold and Sinus Caplets and Tablets 837
- Advil Ibuprofen Tablets, Caplets and Gel Caplets 836
- Children's Motrin Ibuprofen Oral Suspension 1558
- IBU Tablets 1389
- Ibuprohm 713
- Motrin IB Caplets, Tablets, and Gelcaps 802
- Motrin Ibuprofen Suspension, Oral Drops, Chewable Tablets, Caplets 1563
- Nuprin Ibuprofen/Analgesic Tablets & Caplets 645
- Vicks DayQuil SINUS Pressure & PAIN Relief with IBUPROFEN 735

Naproxen (Concurrent administration is not recommended unless advised by a physician). Products include:
- Anaprox/Naprosyn 2277

Food Interactions

Alcohol (Concurrent use should be undertaken with the physician's consultation).

ALFENTA INJECTION
(Alfentanil Hydrochloride) 1334
May interact with central nervous system depressants, certain other agents, and monoamine oxidase inhibitors. Compounds in these categories include:

Alprazolam (Enhances CNS and cardiovascular effects). Products include:
- Xanax Tablets 2115

Aprobarbital (Enhances CNS and cardiovascular effects).
No products indexed under this heading.

Buprenorphine (Enhances CNS and cardiovascular effects). Products include:
- Buprenex Injectable 2170

Buspirone Hydrochloride (Enhances CNS and cardiovascular effects). Products include:
- BuSpar Tablets 738

Butabarbital (Enhances CNS and cardiovascular effects).
No products indexed under this heading.

Butalbital (Enhances CNS and cardiovascular effects). Products include:
- Axocet Capsules 2469
- Esgic-plus Capsules 1012
- Esgic-plus Tablets 1012
- Fioricet Tablets 2386
- Fioricet with Codeine Capsules 2387
- Fiorinal Capsules 2388
- Fiorinal with Codeine Capsules 2390
- Fiorinal Tablets 2388
- Phrenilin 790
- Sedapap Tablets 50 mg/650 mg .. 1826

Chlordiazepoxide (Enhances CNS and cardiovascular effects). Products include:
- Limbitrol 2333

Chlordiazepoxide Hydrochloride (Enhances CNS and cardiovascular effects). Products include:
- Librax Capsules 2330
- Librium Capsules 2331
- Librium Injectable 2332

Chlorpromazine (Enhances CNS and cardiovascular effects). Products include:
- Thorazine Suppositories 2701

Chlorpromazine Hydrochloride (Enhances CNS and cardiovascular effects). Products include:
- Thorazine 2701

Chlorprothixene (Enhances CNS and cardiovascular effects).
No products indexed under this heading.

Chlorprothixene Hydrochloride (Enhances CNS and cardiovascular effects).
No products indexed under this heading.

Chlorprothixene Lactate (Enhances CNS and cardiovascular effects).
No products indexed under this heading.

Cimetidine (Reduces the clearance of alfentanil). Products include:
- Tagamet HB Tablets 786
- Tagamet Tablets 2694

Cimetidine Hydrochloride (Reduces the clearance of alfentanil). Products include:
- Tagamet 2694

Clorazepate Dipotassium (Enhances CNS and cardiovascular effects). Products include:
- Tranxene 459

Clozapine (Enhances CNS and cardiovascular effects). Products include:
- Clozaril Tablets 2377

Codeine Phosphate (Enhances CNS and cardiovascular effects). Products include:
- Brontex 2130
- Dimetane-DC Cough Syrup 2232
- Fioricet with Codeine Capsules 2387
- Fiorinal with Codeine Capsules 2390
- Nucofed 2225
- Phenergan with Codeine 2883
- Phenergan VC with Codeine 2888
- Robitussin A-C Syrup 2248
- Robitussin-DAC Syrup 2249
- Ryna 804
- Soma Compound w/Codeine Tablets 2784
- Tylenol with Codeine 1592

Desflurane (Enhances CNS and cardiovascular effects). Products include:
- Suprane (desflurane, USP) 1865

Dezocine (Enhances CNS and cardiovascular effects). Products include:
- Dalgan Injection 529

Diazepam (Enhances CNS and cardiovascular effects; vasodilation, hypotension, delayed recovery). Products include:
- Dizac (diazepam injectable emulsion) CIV 1862
- Valium Injectable 2336
- Valium Tablets 2335

Droperidol (Enhances CNS and cardiovascular effects). Products include:
- Inapsine Injection 462

Enflurane (Enhances CNS and cardiovascular effects).
No products indexed under this heading.

Erythromycin (Inhibits Alfenta clearance and may increase or prolong respiratory depression). Products include:
- A/T/S 2% Acne Topical Gel 1244
- A/T/S 2% Acne Topical Solution 1244
- Benzamycin Topical Gel 919
- E-Mycin Tablets 1388
- Emgel 2% Topical Gel 1081
- ERYC 1972
- Erycette (erythromycin 2%) Topical Solution 1943
- Ery-Tab Tablets 426
- Erythromycin Base Filmtab 430
- Erythromycin Delayed-Release Capsules, USP 431
- Ilotycin Ophthalmic Ointment 928
- PCE Dispertab Tablets 453
- T-Stat 2.0% Topical Solution and Pads 2797
- THERAMYCIN Z 2% Solution 1629

Erythromycin Estolate (Inhibits Alfenta clearance and may increase or prolong respiratory depression). Products include:
- Ilosone 927

Erythromycin Ethylsuccinate (Inhibits Alfenta clearance and may increase or prolong respiratory depression). Products include:
- E.E.S. 427
- EryPed 425
- Pediazole Suspension 2340

Erythromycin Glucoptate (Inhibits Alfenta clearance and may increase or prolong respiratory depression). Products include:
- Ilotycin Gluceptate, IV, Vials 929

Erythromycin Lactobionate (Inhibits Alfenta clearance and may increase or prolong respiratory depression).
No products indexed under this heading.

Erythromycin Stearate (Inhibits Alfenta clearance and may increase or prolong respiratory depression). Products include:
- Erythrocin Stearate Filmtab 429

Estazolam (Enhances CNS and cardiovascular effects). Products include:
- ProSom Tablets 457

Ethchlorvynol (Enhances CNS and cardiovascular effects). Products include:
- Placidyl Capsules 456

Ethinamate (Enhances CNS and cardiovascular effects).
No products indexed under this heading.

Fentanyl (Enhances CNS and cardiovascular effects). Products include:
- Duragesic Transdermal System 1336

Fentanyl Citrate (Enhances CNS and cardiovascular effects). Products include:
- Sublimaze Injection 463

Fluphenazine Decanoate (Enhances CNS and cardiovascular effects). Products include:
- Prolixin Decanoate 510

Fluphenazine Enanthate (Enhances CNS and cardiovascular effects). Products include:
- Prolixin Enanthate 510

Fluphenazine Hydrochloride (Enhances CNS and cardiovascular effects). Products include:
- Prolixin 510

Flurazepam Hydrochloride (Enhances CNS and cardiovascular effects). Products include:
- Dalmane Capsules 2329

Furazolidone (Severe and unpredictable potentiation of MAO inhibitors has been reported for other opioid analgesics, and rarely with alfentanil; concurrent use should be undertaken very carefully). Products include:
- Furoxone 2221

Glutethimide (Enhances CNS and cardiovascular effects).
No products indexed under this heading.

Haloperidol (Enhances CNS and cardiovascular effects). Products include:
- Haldol Injection, Tablets and Concentrate 1585

Haloperidol Decanoate (Enhances CNS and cardiovascular effects). Products include:
- Haldol Decanoate 1587

Hydrocodone Bitartrate (Enhances CNS and cardiovascular effects). Products include:
- Codiclear DH Syrup 808
- Duratuss HD Elixir 2750
- Histussin D Liquid 670
- Hycodan Tablets and Syrup 946
- Hycomine Compound Tablets 948
- Hycomine 947
- Hycotuss Expectorant Syrup 950
- Hydrocet Capsules 787
- Lorcet 10/650 Tablets 1016
- Lortab 2751
- Tussend 1830
- Tussend Expectorant 1831
- Vicodin Tablets 1404
- Vicodin ES Tablets 1405
- Vicodin HP Tablets 1403
- Vicodin Tuss Expectorant 1406
- Zydone Capsules 967

(◨ Described in PDR For Nonprescription Drugs)   (◉ Described in PDR For Ophthalmology)

Hydrocodone Polistirex (Enhances CNS and cardiovascular effects). Products include:
Tussionex Pennkinetic Extended-Release Suspension ... 1624

Hydroxyzine Hydrochloride (Enhances CNS and cardiovascular effects). Products include:
Atarax Tablets & Syrup ... 1992
Marax Tablets & DF Syrup ... 2015
Vistaril Intramuscular Solution ... 2042

Isocarboxazid (Severe and unpredictable potentiation of MAO inhibitors has been reported for other opioid analgesics, and rarely with alfentanil; concurrent use should be undertaken very carefully).
No products indexed under this heading.

Isoflurane (Enhances CNS and cardiovascular effects).
No products indexed under this heading.

Ketamine Hydrochloride (Enhances CNS and cardiovascular effects).
No products indexed under this heading.

Levomethadyl Acetate Hydrochloride (Enhances CNS and cardiovascular effects). Products include:
Orlaam Oral Solution ... 2361

Levorphanol Tartrate (Enhances CNS and cardiovascular effects). Products include:
Levo-Dromoran ... 2297

Lorazepam (Enhances CNS and cardiovascular effects). Products include:
Ativan Injection ... 2805
Ativan Tablets ... 2807

Loxapine Hydrochloride (Enhances CNS and cardiovascular effects). Products include:
Loxitane ... 1426

Loxapine Succinate (Enhances CNS and cardiovascular effects). Products include:
Loxitane Capsules ... 1426

Meperidine Hydrochloride (Enhances CNS and cardiovascular effects). Products include:
Demerol ... 2438
Mepergan Injection ... 2859

Mephobarbital (Enhances CNS and cardiovascular effects). Products include:
Mebaral Tablets ... 2452

Meprobamate (Enhances CNS and cardiovascular effects). Products include:
Miltown Tablets ... 2780
PMB 200 and PMB 400 ... 2890

Mesoridazine Besylate (Enhances CNS and cardiovascular effects). Products include:
Serentil ... 689

Methadone Hydrochloride (Enhances CNS and cardiovascular effects). Products include:
Methadone Hydrochloride Oral Concentrate ... 2356
Methadone Hydrochloride Oral Solution & Tablets ... 2357

Methohexital Sodium (Enhances CNS and cardiovascular effects).
No products indexed under this heading.

Methotrimeprazine (Enhances CNS and cardiovascular effects). Products include:
Levoprome ... 1321

Methoxyflurane (Enhances CNS and cardiovascular effects).
No products indexed under this heading.

Midazolam Hydrochloride (Enhances CNS and cardiovascular effects). Products include:
Versed Injection ... 2324

Molindone Hydrochloride (Enhances CNS and cardiovascular effects). Products include:
Moban Tablets and Concentrate ... 1036

Morphine Sulfate (Enhances CNS and cardiovascular effects). Products include:
Astramorph/PF Injection, USP (Preservative-Free) ... 526
Duramorph Injection ... 983
Infumorph 200 and Infumorph 500 Sterile Solutions ... 985
Kadian Capsules ... 2948
MS Contin Tablets ... 2149
MSIR ... 2152
Oramorph SR (Morphine Sulfate Sustained Release Tablets) ... 2359
RMS Suppositories CII ... 2766
Roxanol ... 2365

Opium Alkaloids (Enhances CNS and cardiovascular effects).
No products indexed under this heading.

Oxazepam (Enhances CNS and cardiovascular effects). Products include:
Serax Capsules ... 2916
Serax Tablets ... 2916

Oxycodone Hydrochloride (Enhances CNS and cardiovascular effects). Products include:
OxyContin Tablets ... 2163
OxyIR Capsules ... 2167
Percocet Tablets ... 955
Percodan Tablets ... 955
Percodan-Demi Tablets ... 956
Roxicodone Tablets, Oral Solution & Intensol (Oxycodone) ... 2366
Tylox Capsules ... 1593

Pentobarbital Sodium (Enhances CNS and depressant effects). Products include:
Nembutal Sodium Capsules ... 440
Nembutal Sodium Solution ... 442
Nembutal Sodium Suppositories ... 444

Perphenazine (Enhances CNS and cardiovascular effects). Products include:
Etrafon ... 2495
Triavil Tablets ... 1800
Trilafon ... 2532

Phenelzine Sulfate (Severe and unpredictable potentiation of MAO inhibitors has been reported for other opioid analgesics, and rarely with alfentanil; concurrent use should be undertaken very carefully). Products include:
Nardil ... 1977

Phenobarbital (Enhances CNS and cardiovascular effects). Products include:
Arco-Lase Plus Tablets ... 513
Bellergal-S Tablets ... 2375
Donnatal ... 2234
Donnatal Extentabs ... 2234
Donnatal Tablets ... 2234
Phenobarbital Elixir and Tablets ... 1523
Quadrinal Tablets ... 1398

Prazepam (Enhances CNS and cardiovascular effects).
No products indexed under this heading.

Prochlorperazine (Enhances CNS and cardiovascular effects). Products include:
Compazine ... 2644

Promethazine Hydrochloride (Enhances CNS and cardiovascular effects). Products include:
Mepergan Injection ... 2859
Phenergan with Codeine ... 2883
Phenergan with Dextromethorphan ... 2885
Phenergan Injection ... 2880
Phenergan Suppositories ... 2882
Phenergan Syrup ... 2881
Phenergan Tablets ... 2882
Phenergan VC ... 2886
Phenergan VC with Codeine ... 2888

Propofol (Enhances CNS and cardiovascular effects). Products include:
Diprivan Injectable Emulsion ... 2939

Propoxyphene Hydrochloride (Enhances CNS and cardiovascular effects). Products include:
Darvon ... 1475
Wygesic Tablets ... 2930

Propoxyphene Napsylate (Enhances CNS and cardiovascular effects). Products include:
Darvon-N/Darvocet-N ... 1473

Quazepam (Enhances CNS and cardiovascular effects). Products include:
Doral Tablets ... 2773

Risperidone (Enhances CNS and cardiovascular effects). Products include:
Risperdal Tablets ... 1348

Secobarbital Sodium (Enhances CNS and cardiovascular effects). Products include:
Seconal Sodium Pulvules ... 1529

Selegiline Hydrochloride (Severe and unpredictable potentiation of MAO inhibitors has been reported for other opioid analgesics, and rarely with alfentanil; concurrent use should be undertaken very carefully). Products include:
Eldepryl Capsules ... 2729

Sevoflurane (Enhances CNS and cardiovascular effects).
No products indexed under this heading.

Sufentanil Citrate (Enhances CNS and cardiovascular effects). Products include:
Sufenta Injection ... 1355

Temazepam (Enhances CNS and cardiovascular effects). Products include:
Restoril Capsules ... 2413

Thiamylal Sodium (Enhances CNS and cardiovascular effects).
No products indexed under this heading.

Thioridazine Hydrochloride (Enhances CNS and cardiovascular effects). Products include:
Mellaril ... 2398

Thiothixene (Enhances CNS and cardiovascular effects). Products include:
Navane Capsules and Concentrate ... 2018
Navane Intramuscular ... 2019

Tranylcypromine Sulfate (Severe and unpredictable potentiation of MAO inhibitors has been reported for other opioid analgesics, and rarely with alfentanil; concurrent use should be undertaken very carefully). Products include:
Parnate Tablets ... 2679

Triazolam (Enhances CNS and cardiovascular effects). Products include:
Halcion Tablets ... 2093

Trifluoperazine Hydrochloride (Enhances CNS and cardiovascular effects). Products include:
Stelazine ... 2692

Zolpidem Tartrate (Enhances CNS and cardiovascular effects). Products include:
Ambien Tablets ... 2559

ALFERON N INJECTION
(Interferon Alfa-N3 (Human Leukocyte Derived)) ... 2142
None cited in PDR database.

ALITRAQ SPECIALIZED ELEMENTAL NUTRITION WITH GLUTAMINE
(L-Glutamine, Nutritional Supplement) ... 2337
None cited in PDR database.

ALKA-MINTS CHEWABLE ANTACID
(Calcium Carbonate) ... 609
May interact with:

Prescription Drugs, unspecified (Antacids may interact with certain unspecified prescription drugs; concurrent use is not recommended).

ALKA-SELTZER CHERRY EFFERVESCENT ANTACID AND PAIN RELIEVER
(Aspirin, Sodium Bicarbonate, Citric Acid) ... 609
See Alka-Seltzer Original Effervescent Antacid and Pain Reliever

ALKA-SELTZER EXTRA STRENGTH EFFERVESCENT ANTACID AND PAIN RELIEVER
(Aspirin, Sodium Bicarbonate, Citric Acid) ... 609
See Alka-Seltzer Original Effervescent Antacid and Pain Reliever

ALKA-SELTZER FAST RELIEF CAPLETS
(Acetaminophen, Calcium Carbonate) ... 610
May interact with:

Prescription Drugs, unspecified (Effects not specified).

ALKA-SELTZER GOLD EFFERVESCENT ANTACID
(Citric Acid, Potassium Bicarbonate, Sodium Bicarbonate) ... 611
May interact with:

Prescription Drugs, unspecified (Antacids may interact with certain unspecified prescription drugs; check with your doctor).

ALKA-SELTZER LEMON LIME EFFERVESCENT ANTACID AND PAIN RELIEVER
(Aspirin, Sodium Citrate) ... 609
See Alka-Seltzer Original Effervescent Antacid and Pain Reliever

ALKA-SELTZER ORIGINAL EFFERVESCENT ANTACID AND PAIN RELIEVER
(Aspirin, Citric Acid, Sodium Bicarbonate) ... 609
May interact with oral anticoagulants, oral hypoglycemic agents, antigout agents, and certain other agents. Compounds in these categories include:

Acarbose (Concurrent use is not recommended unless directed by a doctor). Products include:
Precose ... 604

Allopurinol (Concurrent use is not recommended unless directed by a doctor). Products include:
Zyloprim Tablets ... 1194

Antiarthritic Drugs, unspecified (Concurrent use is not recommended unless directed by a doctor).

Chlorpropamide (Concurrent use is not recommended unless directed by a doctor). Products include:
Diabinese Tablets ... 2002

IMPORTANT NOTE: Always consult each drug listing in the patient's regimen for possible interactions.

Dicumarol (Concurrent use is not recommended unless directed by a doctor).
No products indexed under this heading.

Glimepiride (Concurrent use is not recommended unless directed by a doctor). Products include:
Amaryl Tablets 1241

Glipizide (Concurrent use is not recommended unless directed by a doctor). Products include:
Glucotrol Tablets 2011
Glucotrol XL Extended Release Tablets 2012

Glyburide (Concurrent use is not recommended unless directed by a doctor). Products include:
DiaBeta Tablets 1265
Glynase PresTab Tablets 2091
Micronase Tablets 2099

Metformin Hydrochloride (Concurrent use is not recommended unless directed by a doctor). Products include:
Glucophage Tablets 754

Prescription Drugs, unspecified (Antacids may interact with certain unspecified prescription drugs; concurrent use is not recommended unless directed by a doctor).

Probenecid (Concurrent use is not recommended unless directed by a doctor). Products include:
Benemid Tablets 1651
ColBENEMID Tablets 1662

Sulfinpyrazone (Concurrent use is not recommended unless directed by a doctor). Products include:
Anturane 823

Tolazamide (Concurrent use is not recommended unless directed by a doctor).
No products indexed under this heading.

Tolbutamide (Concurrent use is not recommended unless directed by a doctor).
No products indexed under this heading.

Warfarin Sodium (Concurrent use is not recommended unless directed by a doctor). Products include:
Coumadin 941

ALKA-SELTZER PLUS COLD MEDICINE

(Chlorpheniramine Maleate, Aspirin, Phenylpropanolamine Bitartrate) ▣ 611
See **Alka-Seltzer Plus Cold & Cough Medicine**

ALKA-SELTZER PLUS COLD MEDICINE LIQUI-GELS

(Chlorpheniramine Maleate, Pseudoephedrine Hydrochloride, Acetaminophen) .... ▣ 612
See **Alka-Seltzer Plus Night-Time Cold Medicine Liqui-Gels**

ALKA-SELTZER PLUS COLD & COUGH MEDICINE

(Aspirin, Chlorpheniramine Maleate, Dextromethorphan Hydrobromide, Phenylpropanolamine Bitartrate) .... ▣ 611
May interact with hypnotics and sedatives, tranquilizers, oral anticoagulants, antihypertensives, monoamine oxidase inhibitors, oral hypoglycemic agents, insulin, antigout agents, and certain other agents. Compounds in these categories include:

Acarbose (Concurrent use with drugs for diabetes is not recommended). Products include:
Precose 604

Acebutolol Hydrochloride (Concurrent use with drugs for blood pressure is not recommended). Products include:
Sectral Capsules 2914

Allopurinol (Concurrent use with drugs for gout is not recommended). Products include:
Zyloprim Tablets 1194

Alprazolam (May increase drowsiness effect). Products include:
Xanax Tablets 2115

Amlodipine Besylate (Concurrent use with drugs for blood pressure is not recommended). Products include:
Lotrel Capsules 858
Norvasc Tablets 2020

Antiarthritic Drugs, unspecified (Concurrent use with unspecified arthritis drugs is not recommended).

Atenolol (Concurrent use with drugs for blood pressure is not recommended). Products include:
Tenoretic Tablets 2963
Tenormin Tablets and I.V. Injection 2965

Benazepril Hydrochloride (Concurrent use with drugs for blood pressure is not recommended). Products include:
Lotensin Tablets 852
Lotensin HCT Tablets 855
Lotrel Capsules 858

Bendroflumethiazide (Concurrent use with drugs for blood pressure is not recommended).
No products indexed under this heading.

Betaxolol Hydrochloride (Concurrent use with drugs for blood pressure is not recommended). Products include:
Betoptic Ophthalmic Solution 465
Betoptic S Ophthalmic Suspension 467
Kerlone Tablets 2588

Bisoprolol Fumarate (Concurrent use with drugs for blood pressure is not recommended). Products include:
Zebeta Tablets 1457
Ziac 1459

Buspirone Hydrochloride (May increase drowsiness effect). Products include:
BuSpar Tablets 738

Captopril (Concurrent use with drugs for blood pressure is not recommended). Products include:
Capoten Tablets 740
Capozide Tablets 744

Carteolol Hydrochloride (Concurrent use with drugs for blood pressure is not recommended). Products include:
Cartrol Tablets 413
Ocupress Ophthalmic Solution, 1% Sterile .... ◎ 297

Chlordiazepoxide (May increase drowsiness effect). Products include:
Limbitrol 2333

Chlordiazepoxide Hydrochloride (May increase drowsiness effect). Products include:
Librax Capsules 2330
Librium Capsules 2331
Librium Injectable 2332

Chlorothiazide (Concurrent use with drugs for blood pressure is not recommended). Products include:
Aldoclor Tablets 1638
Diupres Tablets 1691
Diuril Oral 1694

Chlorothiazide Sodium (Concurrent use with drugs for blood pressure is not recommended). Products include:
Diuril Sodium Intravenous 1693

Chlorpromazine (May increase drowsiness effect). Products include:
Thorazine Suppositories 2701

Chlorpromazine Hydrochloride (May increase drowsiness effect). Products include:
Thorazine 2701

Chlorpropamide (Concurrent use with drugs for diabetes is not recommended). Products include:
Diabinese Tablets 2002

Chlorprothixene (May increase drowsiness effect).
No products indexed under this heading.

Chlorprothixene Hydrochloride (May increase drowsiness effect).
No products indexed under this heading.

Chlorthalidone (Concurrent use with drugs for blood pressure is not recommended). Products include:
Combipres Tablets 682
Tenoretic Tablets 2963
Thalitone 1293

Clonidine (Concurrent use with drugs for blood pressure is not recommended). Products include:
Catapres-TTS 680

Clonidine Hydrochloride (Concurrent use with drugs for blood pressure is not recommended). Products include:
Catapres Tablets 679
Combipres Tablets 682

Clorazepate Dipotassium (May increase drowsiness effect). Products include:
Tranxene 459

Deserpidine (Concurrent use with drugs for blood pressure is not recommended).
No products indexed under this heading.

Diazepam (May increase drowsiness effect). Products include:
Dizac (diazepam injectable emulsion) CIV 1862
Valium Injectable 2336
Valium Tablets 2335

Diazoxide (Concurrent use with drugs for blood pressure is not recommended). Products include:
Hyperstat I.V. Injection 2504
Proglycem 575

Dicumarol (Concurrent use with anticoagulant is not recommended).
No products indexed under this heading.

Diltiazem Hydrochloride (Concurrent use with drugs for blood pressure is not recommended). Products include:
Cardizem CD Capsules 1251
Cardizem SR Capsules 1255
Cardizem Injectable 1253
Cardizem Tablets 1257
Dilacor XR Extended-release Capsules 2183
Tiazac Capsules 1019

Doxazosin Mesylate (Concurrent use with drugs for blood pressure is not recommended). Products include:
Cardura Tablets 1993

Droperidol (May increase drowsiness effect). Products include:
Inapsine Injection 462

Enalapril Maleate (Concurrent use with drugs for blood pressure is not recommended). Products include:
Vaseretic Tablets 1810
Vasotec Tablets 1816

Enalaprilat (Concurrent use with drugs for blood pressure is not recommended). Products include:
Vasotec I.V. 1814

Esmolol Hydrochloride (Concurrent use with drugs for blood pressure is not recommended). Products include:
Brevibloc (esmolol HCl) Injection ... 1860

Estazolam (May increase drowsiness effect). Products include:
ProSom Tablets 457

Ethchlorvynol (May increase drowsiness effect). Products include:
Placidyl Capsules 456

Ethinamate (May increase drowsiness effect).
No products indexed under this heading.

Felodipine (Concurrent use with drugs for blood pressure is not recommended). Products include:
Plendil Extended-Release Tablets 514

Fluphenazine Decanoate (May increase drowsiness effect). Products include:
Prolixin Decanoate 510

Fluphenazine Enanthate (May increase drowsiness effect). Products include:
Prolixin Enanthate 510

Fluphenazine Hydrochloride (May increase drowsiness effect). Products include:
Prolixin 510

Flurazepam Hydrochloride (May increase drowsiness effect). Products include:
Dalmane Capsules 2329

Fosinopril Sodium (Concurrent use with drugs for blood pressure is not recommended). Products include:
Monopril Tablets 762

Furazolidone (Concurrent and/or sequential use is not recommended). Products include:
Furoxone 2221

Furosemide (Concurrent use with drugs for blood pressure is not recommended). Products include:
Lasix Injection, Oral Solution and Tablets 1267

Glimepiride (Concurrent use with drugs for diabetes is not recommended). Products include:
Amaryl Tablets 1241

Glipizide (Concurrent use with drugs for diabetes is not recommended). Products include:
Glucotrol Tablets 2011
Glucotrol XL Extended Release Tablets 2012

Glutethimide (May increase drowsiness effect).
No products indexed under this heading.

Glyburide (Concurrent use with drugs for diabetes is not recommended). Products include:
DiaBeta Tablets 1265
Glynase PresTab Tablets 2091
Micronase Tablets 2099

Guanabenz Acetate (Concurrent use with drugs for blood pressure is not recommended).
No products indexed under this heading.

Guanethidine Monosulfate (Concurrent use with drugs for blood pressure is not recommended). Products include:
Esimil Tablets 840
Ismelin Tablets 845

(▣ Described in PDR For Nonprescription Drugs) (◎ Described in PDR For Ophthalmology)

Interactions Index

Haloperidol (May increase drowsiness effect). Products include:
- Haldol Injection, Tablets and Concentrate 1585

Haloperidol Decanoate (May increase drowsiness effect). Products include:
- Haldol Decanoate 1587

Hydralazine Hydrochloride (Concurrent use with drugs for blood pressure is not recommended). Products include:
- Apresazide Capsules 824
- Apresoline Hydrochloride Tablets .. 826
- Hydralazine Hydrochloride Injection USP 2712
- Ser-Ap-Es Tablets 867

Hydrochlorothiazide (Concurrent use with drugs for blood pressure is not recommended). Products include:
- Aldactazide Tablets 2556
- Aldoril Tablets 1644
- Apresazide Capsules 824
- Capozide Tablets 744
- Dyazide Capsules 2653
- Esidrix Tablets 839
- Esimil Tablets 840
- HydroDIURIL Tablets 1716
- Hydropres Tablets 1718
- Hyzaar Tablets 1720
- Inderide Tablets 2838
- Inderide LA Long Acting Capsules .. 2840
- Lopressor HCT Tablets 850
- Lotensin HCT Tablets 855
- Moduretic Tablets 1748
- Oretic Tablets 450
- Prinzide Tablets 1780
- Ser-Ap-Es Tablets 867
- Timolide Tablets 1791
- Vaseretic Tablets 1810
- Zestoretic Tablets 2968
- Ziac 1459

Hydroflumethiazide (Concurrent use with drugs for blood pressure is not recommended). Products include:
- Diucardin Tablets 2824

Hydroxyzine Hydrochloride (May increase drowsiness effect). Products include:
- Atarax Tablets & Syrup 1992
- Marax Tablets & DF Syrup 2015
- Vistaril Intramuscular Solution 2042

Indapamide (Concurrent use with drugs for blood pressure is not recommended).
- No products indexed under this heading.

Insulin, Human (Concurrent use with drugs for diabetes is not recommended).
- No products indexed under this heading.

Insulin, Human Isophane Suspension (Concurrent use with drugs for diabetes is not recommended). Products include:
- Novolin N Human Insulin 10 ml Vials 1846

Insulin, Human NPH (Concurrent use with drugs for diabetes is not recommended). Products include:
- Humulin N, 100 Units 1495
- Novolin N PenFill 1.5 ml Cartridges Durable Insulin Delivery System 1849
- Novolin N Prefilled Syringe Disposable Insulin Delivery System 1850

Insulin, Human Regular (Concurrent use with drugs for diabetes is not recommended). Products include:
- Humulin R, 100 Units 1497
- Novolin R Human Insulin 10 ml Vials 1846
- Novolin R PenFill 1.5 ml Cartridges Durable Insulin Delivery System 1849
- Novolin R Prefilled Syringe Disposable Insulin Delivery System 1850
- Velosulin BR Human Insulin 10 ml Vials 1847

Insulin, Human, Zinc Suspension (Concurrent use with drugs for diabetes is not recommended). Products include:
- Humulin L, 100 Units 1494
- Humulin U, 100 Units 1498
- Novolin L Human Insulin 10 ml Vials 1846

Insulin Lispro, Human (Concurrent use with drugs for diabetes is not recommended). Products include:
- Humalog Injection 1488

Insulin, NPH (Concurrent use with drugs for diabetes is not recommended). Products include:
- NPH, 100 Units 1502
- Pork NPH, 100 Units 1506
- Purified Pork NPH Isophane Insulin 1852

Insulin, Regular (Concurrent use with drugs for diabetes is not recommended). Products include:
- Regular, 100 Units 1503
- Pork Regular, 100 Units 1507
- Pork Regular (Concentrated), 500 Units 1508
- Purified Pork Regular Insulin 1852

Insulin, Zinc Crystals (Concurrent use with drugs for diabetes is not recommended). Products include:
- NPH, 100 Units 1502

Insulin, Zinc Suspension (Concurrent use with drugs for diabetes is not recommended). Products include:
- Iletin I 1501
- Lente, 100 Units 1501
- Iletin II 1504
- Pork Lente, 100 Units 1504
- Purified Pork Lente Insulin 1852

Isocarboxazid (Concurrent and/or sequential use is not recommended).
- No products indexed under this heading.

Isradipine (Concurrent use with drugs for blood pressure is not recommended). Products include:
- DynaCirc Capsules 2381
- DynaCirc CR Tablets 2383

Labetalol Hydrochloride (Concurrent use with drugs for blood pressure is not recommended). Products include:
- Normodyne Injection 2519
- Normodyne Tablets 2522
- Trandate 1158

Lisinopril (Concurrent use with drugs for blood pressure is not recommended). Products include:
- Prinivil Tablets 1776
- Prinzide Tablets 1780
- Zestoretic Tablets 2968
- Zestril Tablets 2972

Lorazepam (May increase drowsiness effect). Products include:
- Ativan Injection 2805
- Ativan Tablets 2807

Losartan Potassium (Concurrent use with drugs for blood pressure is not recommended). Products include:
- Cozaar Tablets 1668
- Hyzaar Tablets 1720

Loxapine Hydrochloride (May increase drowsiness effect). Products include:
- Loxitane 1426

Loxapine Succinate (May increase drowsiness effect). Products include:
- Loxitane Capsules 1426

Mecamylamine Hydrochloride (Concurrent use with drugs for blood pressure is not recommended). Products include:
- Inversine Tablets 1729

Meprobamate (May increase drowsiness effect). Products include:
- Miltown Tablets 2780
- PMB 200 and PMB 400 2890

Mesoridazine Besylate (May increase drowsiness effect). Products include:
- Serentil 689

Metformin Hydrochloride (Concurrent use with drugs for diabetes is not recommended). Products include:
- Glucophage Tablets 754

Methyclothiazide (Concurrent use with drugs for blood pressure is not recommended). Products include:
- Enduron Tablets 424

Methyldopa (Concurrent use with drugs for blood pressure is not recommended). Products include:
- Aldoclor Tablets 1638
- Aldomet Oral 1640
- Aldoril Tablets 1644

Methyldopate Hydrochloride (Concurrent use with drugs for blood pressure is not recommended). Products include:
- Aldomet Ester HCl Injection 1642

Metolazone (Concurrent use with drugs for blood pressure is not recommended). Products include:
- Mykrox Tablets 1617
- Zaroxolyn Tablets 1625

Metoprolol Succinate (Concurrent use with drugs for blood pressure is not recommended). Products include:
- Toprol-XL Tablets 560

Metoprolol Tartrate (Concurrent use with drugs for blood pressure is not recommended). Products include:
- Lopressor 848
- Lopressor HCT Tablets 850

Metyrosine (Concurrent use with drugs for blood pressure is not recommended). Products include:
- Demser Capsules 1690

Midazolam Hydrochloride (May increase drowsiness effect). Products include:
- Versed Injection 2324

Minoxidil (Concurrent use with drugs for blood pressure is not recommended).
- No products indexed under this heading.

Moexipril Hydrochloride (Concurrent use with drugs for blood pressure is not recommended). Products include:
- Univasc Tablets 2553

Molindone Hydrochloride (May increase drowsiness effect). Products include:
- Moban Tablets and Concentrate 1036

Nadolol (Concurrent use with drugs for blood pressure is not recommended).
- No products indexed under this heading.

Nicardipine Hydrochloride (Concurrent use with drugs for blood pressure is not recommended). Products include:
- Cardene Capsules 2261
- Cardene I.V. 2815
- Cardene SR Capsules 2264

Nifedipine (Concurrent use with drugs for blood pressure is not recommended). Products include:
- Adalat Capsules (10 mg and 20 mg) 580
- Adalat CC 582
- Procardia Capsules 2024
- Procardia XL Extended Release Tablets 2026

Nisoldipine (Concurrent use with drugs for blood pressure is not recommended). Products include:
- Sular Tablets 2961

Nitroglycerin (Concurrent use with drugs for blood pressure is not recommended). Products include:
- Deponit NTG Transdermal Delivery System 2541
- Nitro-Bid IV 1270
- Nitro-Bid Ointment 1272
- Nitro-Dur (nitroglycerin) Transdermal Infusion System 1365
- Nitrolingual Spray 2193
- Nitrostat Tablets 1981
- Transderm-Nitro Transdermal Therapeutic System 878

Oxazepam (May increase drowsiness effect). Products include:
- Serax Capsules 2916
- Serax Tablets 2916

Penbutolol Sulfate (Concurrent use with drugs for blood pressure is not recommended). Products include:
- Levatol Tablets 2547

Perphenazine (May increase drowsiness effect). Products include:
- Etrafon 2495
- Triavil Tablets 1800
- Trilafon 2532

Phenelzine Sulfate (Concurrent and/or sequential use is not recommended). Products include:
- Nardil 1977

Phenoxybenzamine Hydrochloride (Concurrent use with drugs for blood pressure is not recommended). Products include:
- Dibenzyline Capsules 2650

Phentolamine Mesylate (Concurrent use with drugs for blood pressure is not recommended). Products include:
- Regitine Vials 864

Pindolol (Concurrent use with drugs for blood pressure is not recommended). Products include:
- Visken Tablets 2428

Polythiazide (Concurrent use with drugs for blood pressure is not recommended). Products include:
- Minizide Capsules 2016

Prazepam (May increase drowsiness effect).
- No products indexed under this heading.

Prazosin Hydrochloride (Concurrent use with drugs for blood pressure is not recommended). Products include:
- Minipress Capsules 2015
- Minizide Capsules 2016

Probenecid (Concurrent use with drugs for gout is not recommended). Products include:
- Benemid Tablets 1651
- ColBENEMID Tablets 1662

Prochlorperazine (May increase drowsiness effect). Products include:
- Compazine 2644

Promethazine Hydrochloride (May increase drowsiness effect). Products include:
- Mepergan Injection 2859
- Phenergan with Codeine 2883
- Phenergan with Dextromethorphan 2885
- Phenergan Injection 2880
- Phenergan Suppositories 2882
- Phenergan Syrup 2881
- Phenergan Tablets 2882
- Phenergan VC 2888
- Phenergan VC with Codeine 2888

Propofol (May increase drowsiness effect). Products include:
- Diprivan Injectable Emulsion 2939

IMPORTANT NOTE: Always consult each drug listing in the patient's regimen for possible interactions.

Propranolol Hydrochloride (Concurrent use with drugs for blood pressure is not recommended). Products include:
- Inderal 2834
- Inderal LA Long Acting Capsules 2836
- Inderide Tablets 2838
- Inderide LA Long Acting Capsules 2840

Quazepam (May increase drowsiness effect). Products include:
- Doral Tablets 2773

Quinapril Hydrochloride (Concurrent use with drugs for blood pressure is not recommended). Products include:
- Accupril Tablets 1950

Ramipril (Concurrent use with drugs for blood pressure is not recommended). Products include:
- Altace Capsules 1238

Rauwolfia Serpentina (Concurrent use with drugs for blood pressure is not recommended).
- No products indexed under this heading.

Rescinnamine (Concurrent use with drugs for blood pressure is not recommended).
- No products indexed under this heading.

Reserpine (Concurrent use with drugs for blood pressure is not recommended). Products include:
- Diupres Tablets 1691
- Hydropres Tablets 1718
- Ser-Ap-Es Tablets 867

Secobarbital Sodium (May increase drowsiness effect). Products include:
- Seconal Sodium Pulvules 1529

Selegiline Hydrochloride (Concurrent and/or sequential use is not recommended). Products include:
- Eldepryl Capsules 2729

Sodium Nitroprusside (Concurrent use with drugs for blood pressure is not recommended).
- No products indexed under this heading.

Sotalol Hydrochloride (Concurrent use with drugs for blood pressure is not recommended). Products include:
- Betapace Tablets 637

Spirapril Hydrochloride (Concurrent use with drugs for blood pressure is not recommended).
- No products indexed under this heading.

Sulfinpyrazone (Concurrent use with drugs for gout is not recommended). Products include:
- Anturane 823

Temazepam (May increase drowsiness effect). Products include:
- Restoril Capsules 2413

Terazosin Hydrochloride (Concurrent use with drugs for blood pressure is not recommended). Products include:
- Hytrin Capsules 434

Thioridazine Hydrochloride (May increase drowsiness effect). Products include:
- Mellaril 2398

Thiothixene (May increase drowsiness effect). Products include:
- Navane Capsules and Concentrate 2018
- Navane Intramuscular 2019

Timolol Maleate (Concurrent use with drugs for blood pressure is not recommended). Products include:
- Blocadren Tablets 1654
- Timolide Tablets 1791
- Timoptic in Ocudose 1796
- Timoptic Sterile Ophthalmic Solution 1794
- Timoptic-XE 1798

Tolazamide (Concurrent use with drugs for diabetes is not recommended).
- No products indexed under this heading.

Tolbutamide (Concurrent use with drugs for diabetes is not recommended).
- No products indexed under this heading.

Torsemide (Concurrent use with drugs for blood pressure is not recommended). Products include:
- Demadex Tablets and Injection 691

Tranylcypromine Sulfate (Concurrent and/or sequential use is not recommended). Products include:
- Parnate Tablets 2679

Triazolam (May increase drowsiness effect). Products include:
- Halcion Tablets 2093

Trifluoperazine Hydrochloride (May increase drowsiness effect). Products include:
- Stelazine 2692

Trimethaphan Camsylate (Concurrent use with drugs for blood pressure is not recommended).
- No products indexed under this heading.

Verapamil Hydrochloride (Concurrent use with drugs for blood pressure is not recommended). Products include:
- Calan SR Caplets 2571
- Calan Tablets 2568
- Covera-HS Tablets 2573
- Isoptin Injectable 1391
- Isoptin Oral Tablets 1393
- Isoptin SR Tablets 1395
- Verelan Capsules 1455

Warfarin Sodium (Concurrent use with anticoagulant is not recommended). Products include:
- Coumadin 941

Zolpidem Tartrate (May increase drowsiness effect). Products include:
- Ambien Tablets 2559

Food Interactions

Alcohol (May increase drowsiness effect).

ALKA-SELTZER PLUS COLD & COUGH MEDICINE LIQUI-GELS

(Dextromethorphan Hydrobromide, Chlorpheniramine Maleate, Pseudoephedrine Hydrochloride, Acetaminophen) ◙ 612

See **Alka-Seltzer Plus Night-Time Cold Medicine Liqui-Gels**

ALKA-SELTZER PLUS FLU & BODY ACHES EFFERVESCENT TABLETS

(Acetaminophen, Chlorpheniramine Maleate, Dextromethorphan Hydrobromide, Phenylpropanolamine Hydrochloride) ◙ 612

May interact with monoamine oxidase inhibitors, tranquilizers, hypnotics and sedatives, and certain other agents. Compounds in these categories include:

Alprazolam (May increase drowsiness effect). Products include:
- Xanax Tablets 2115

Buspirone Hydrochloride (May increase drowsiness effect). Products include:
- BuSpar Tablets 738

Chlordiazepoxide (May increase drowsiness effect). Products include:
- Limbitrol 2333

Chlordiazepoxide Hydrochloride (May increase drowsiness effect). Products include:
- Librax Capsules 2330
- Librium Capsules 2331
- Librium Injectable 2332

Chlorpromazine (May increase drowsiness effect). Products include:
- Thorazine Suppositories 2701

Chlorpromazine Hydrochloride (May increase drowsiness effect). Products include:
- Thorazine 2701

Chlorprothixene (May increase drowsiness effect).
- No products indexed under this heading.

Chlorprothixene Hydrochloride (May increase drowsiness effect).
- No products indexed under this heading.

Clorazepate Dipotassium (May increase drowsiness effect). Products include:
- Tranxene 459

Diazepam (May increase drowsiness effect). Products include:
- Dizac (diazepam injectable emulsion) CIV 1862
- Valium Injectable 2336
- Valium Tablets 2335

Droperidol (May increase drowsiness effect). Products include:
- Inapsine Injection 462

Estazolam (May increase drowsiness effect). Products include:
- ProSom Tablets 457

Ethchlorvynol (May increase drowsiness effect). Products include:
- Placidyl Capsules 456

Ethinamate (May increase drowsiness effect).
- No products indexed under this heading.

Fluphenazine Decanoate (May increase drowsiness effect). Products include:
- Prolixin Decanoate 510

Fluphenazine Enanthate (May increase drowsiness effect). Products include:
- Prolixin Enanthate 510

Fluphenazine Hydrochloride (May increase drowsiness effect). Products include:
- Prolixin 510

Flurazepam Hydrochloride (May increase drowsiness effect). Products include:
- Dalmane Capsules 2329

Furazolidone (Concurrent and/or sequential use is not recommended). Products include:
- Furoxone 2221

Glutethimide (May increase drowsiness effect).
- No products indexed under this heading.

Haloperidol (May increase drowsiness effect). Products include:
- Haldol Injection, Tablets and Concentrate 1585

Haloperidol Decanoate (May increase drowsiness effect). Products include:
- Haldol Decanoate 1587

Hydroxyzine Hydrochloride (May increase drowsiness effect). Products include:
- Atarax Tablets & Syrup 1992
- Marax Tablets & DF Syrup 2015
- Vistaril Intramuscular Solution 2042

Isocarboxazid (Concurrent and/or sequential use is not recommended).
- No products indexed under this heading.

Lorazepam (May increase drowsiness effect). Products include:
- Ativan Injection 2805
- Ativan Tablets 2807

Loxapine Hydrochloride (May increase drowsiness effect). Products include:
- Loxitane 1426

Loxapine Succinate (May increase drowsiness effect). Products include:
- Loxitane Capsules 1426

Meprobamate (May increase drowsiness effect). Products include:
- Miltown Tablets 2780
- PMB 200 and PMB 400 2890

Mesoridazine Besylate (May increase drowsiness effect). Products include:
- Serentil 689

Midazolam Hydrochloride (May increase drowsiness effect). Products include:
- Versed Injection 2324

Molindone Hydrochloride (May increase drowsiness effect). Products include:
- Moban Tablets and Concentrate 1036

Oxazepam (May increase drowsiness effect). Products include:
- Serax Capsules 2916
- Serax Tablets 2916

Perphenazine (May increase drowsiness effect). Products include:
- Etrafon 2495
- Triavil Tablets 1800
- Trilafon 2532

Phenelzine Sulfate (Concurrent and/or sequential use is not recommended). Products include:
- Nardil 1977

Prazepam (May increase drowsiness effect).
- No products indexed under this heading.

Prochlorperazine (May increase drowsiness effect). Products include:
- Compazine 2644

Promethazine Hydrochloride (May increase drowsiness effect). Products include:
- Mepergan Injection 2859
- Phenergan with Codeine 2883
- Phenergan with Dextromethorphan 2885
- Phenergan Injection 2880
- Phenergan Suppositories 2882
- Phenergan Syrup 2881
- Phenergan Tablets 2882
- Phenergan VC 2886
- Phenergan VC with Codeine 2888

Propofol (May increase drowsiness effect). Products include:
- Diprivan Injectable Emulsion 2939

Quazepam (May increase drowsiness effect). Products include:
- Doral Tablets 2773

Secobarbital Sodium (May increase drowsiness effect). Products include:
- Seconal Sodium Pulvules 1529

Selegiline Hydrochloride (Concurrent and/or sequential use is not recommended). Products include:
- Eldepryl Capsules 2729

Temazepam (May increase drowsiness effect). Products include:
- Restoril Capsules 2413

Thioridazine Hydrochloride (May increase drowsiness effect). Products include:
- Mellaril 2398

Thiothixene (May increase drowsiness effect). Products include:
- Navane Capsules and Concentrate 2018
- Navane Intramuscular 2019

(◙ Described in PDR For Nonprescription Drugs) (◉ Described in PDR For Ophthalmology)

Tranylcypromine Sulfate (Concurrent and/or sequential use is not recommended). Products include:
Parnate Tablets 2679
Triazolam (May increase drowsiness effect). Products include:
Halcion Tablets 2093
Trifluoperazine Hydrochloride (May increase drowsiness effect). Products include:
Stelazine 2692
Zolpidem Tartrate (May increase drowsiness effect). Products include:
Ambien Tablets 2559

Food Interactions
Alcohol (May increase drowsiness effect).

ALKA-SELTZER PLUS FLU & BODY ACHES LIQUI-GELS NON-DROWSY FORMULA
(Acetaminophen, Dextromethorphan Hydrobromide, Pseudoephedrine Hydrochloride) 613
May interact with monoamine oxidase inhibitors. Compounds in this category include:

Furazolidone (Concurrent and/or sequential use is not recommended). Products include:
Furoxone 2221
Isocarboxazid (Concurrent and/or sequential use is not recommended).
No products indexed under this heading.
Phenelzine Sulfate (Concurrent and/or sequential use is not recommended). Products include:
Nardil 1977
Selegiline Hydrochloride (Concurrent use with drugs is not recommended). Products include:
Eldepryl Capsules 2729
Tranylcypromine Sulfate (Concurrent and/or sequential use is not recommended). Products include:
Parnate Tablets 2679

ALKA-SELTZER PLUS NIGHT-TIME COLD MEDICINE
(Aspirin, Phenylpropanolamine Bitartrate, Doxylamine Succinate, Dextromethorphan Hydrobromide) 611
See Alka-Seltzer Plus Cold & Cough Medicine

ALKA-SELTZER PLUS NIGHT-TIME COLD MEDICINE LIQUI-GELS
(Dextromethorphan Hydrobromide, Doxylamine Succinate, Pseudoephedrine Hydrochloride, Acetaminophen) 612
May interact with hypnotics and sedatives, tranquilizers, monoamine oxidase inhibitors, antihypertensives, and certain other agents. Compounds in these categories include:

Acebutolol Hydrochloride (Concurrent use with drugs for blood pressure is not recommended). Products include:
Sectral Capsules 2914
Alprazolam (May increase drowsiness effect). Products include:
Xanax Tablets 2115
Amlodipine Besylate (Concurrent use with drugs for blood pressure is not recommended). Products include:
Lotrel Capsules 858
Norvasc Tablets 2020

Atenolol (Concurrent use with drugs for blood pressure is not recommended). Products include:
Tenoretic Tablets 2963
Tenormin Tablets and I.V. Injection 2965
Benazepril Hydrochloride (Concurrent use with drugs for blood pressure is not recommended). Products include:
Lotensin Tablets 852
Lotensin HCT Tablets 855
Lotrel Capsules 858
Bendroflumethiazide (Concurrent use with drugs for blood pressure is not recommended).
No products indexed under this heading.
Betaxolol Hydrochloride (Concurrent use with drugs for blood pressure is not recommended). Products include:
Betoptic Ophthalmic Solution 465
Betoptic S Ophthalmic Suspension 467
Kerlone Tablets 2588
Bisoprolol Fumarate (Concurrent use with drugs for blood pressure is not recommended). Products include:
Zebeta Tablets 1457
Ziac 1459
Buspirone Hydrochloride (May increase drowsiness effect). Products include:
BuSpar Tablets 738
Captopril (Concurrent use with drugs for blood pressure is not recommended). Products include:
Capoten Tablets 740
Capozide Tablets 744
Carteolol Hydrochloride (Concurrent use with drugs for blood pressure is not recommended). Products include:
Cartrol Tablets 413
Ocupress Ophthalmic Solution, 1% Sterile 297
Chlordiazepoxide (May increase drowsiness effect). Products include:
Limbitrol 2333
Chlordiazepoxide Hydrochloride (May increase drowsiness effect). Products include:
Librax Capsules 2330
Librium Capsules 2331
Librium Injectable 2332
Chlorothiazide (Concurrent use with drugs for blood pressure is not recommended). Products include:
Aldoclor Tablets 1638
Diupres Tablets 1691
Diuril Oral 1694
Chlorothiazide Sodium (Concurrent use with drugs for blood pressure is not recommended). Products include:
Diuril Sodium Intravenous 1693
Chlorpromazine (May increase drowsiness effect). Products include:
Thorazine Suppositories 2701
Chlorpromazine Hydrochloride (May increase drowsiness effect). Products include:
Thorazine 2701
Chlorprothixene (May increase drowsiness effect).
No products indexed under this heading.
Chlorprothixene Hydrochloride (May increase drowsiness effect).
No products indexed under this heading.
Chlorthalidone (Concurrent use with drugs for blood pressure is not recommended). Products include:
Combipres Tablets 682
Tenoretic Tablets 2963
Thalitone 1293

Clonidine (Concurrent use with drugs for blood pressure is not recommended). Products include:
Catapres-TTS 680
Clonidine Hydrochloride (Concurrent use with drugs for blood pressure is not recommended). Products include:
Catapres Tablets 679
Combipres Tablets 682
Clorazepate Dipotassium (May increase drowsiness effect). Products include:
Tranxene 459
Deserpidine (Concurrent use with drugs for blood pressure is not recommended).
No products indexed under this heading.
Diazepam (May increase drowsiness effect). Products include:
Dizac (diazepam injectable emulsion) CIV 1862
Valium Injectable 2336
Valium Tablets 2335
Diazoxide (Concurrent use with drugs for blood pressure is not recommended). Products include:
Hyperstat I.V. Injection 2504
Proglycem 575
Diltiazem Hydrochloride (Concurrent use with drugs for blood pressure is not recommended). Products include:
Cardizem CD Capsules 1251
Cardizem SR Capsules 1255
Cardizem Injectable 1253
Cardizem Tablets 1257
Dilacor XR Extended-release Capsules 2183
Tiazac Capsules 1019
Doxazosin Mesylate (Concurrent use with drugs for blood pressure is not recommended). Products include:
Cardura Tablets 1993
Droperidol (May increase drowsiness effect). Products include:
Inapsine Injection 462
Enalapril Maleate (Concurrent use with drugs for blood pressure is not recommended). Products include:
Vaseretic Tablets 1810
Vasotec Tablets 1816
Enalaprilat (Concurrent use with drugs for blood pressure is not recommended). Products include:
Vasotec I.V. 1814
Esmolol Hydrochloride (Concurrent use with drugs for blood pressure is not recommended). Products include:
Brevibloc (esmolol HCl) Injection 1860
Estazolam (May increase drowsiness effect). Products include:
ProSom Tablets 457
Ethchlorvynol (May increase drowsiness effect). Products include:
Placidyl Capsules 456
Ethinamate (May increase drowsiness effect).
No products indexed under this heading.
Felodipine (Concurrent use with drugs for blood pressure is not recommended). Products include:
Plendil Extended-Release Tablets 514
Fluphenazine Decanoate (May increase drowsiness effect). Products include:
Prolixin Decanoate 510
Fluphenazine Enanthate (May increase drowsiness effect). Products include:
Prolixin Enanthate 510

Fluphenazine Hydrochloride (May increase drowsiness effect). Products include:
Prolixin 510
Flurazepam Hydrochloride (May increase drowsiness effect). Products include:
Dalmane Capsules 2329
Fosinopril Sodium (Concurrent use with drugs for blood pressure is not recommended). Products include:
Monopril Tablets 762
Furazolidone (Concurrent and/or sequential use is not recommended). Products include:
Furoxone 2221
Furosemide (Concurrent use with drugs for blood pressure is not recommended). Products include:
Lasix Injection, Oral Solution and Tablets 1267
Glutethimide (May increase drowsiness effect).
No products indexed under this heading.
Guanabenz Acetate (Concurrent use with drugs for blood pressure is not recommended).
No products indexed under this heading.
Guanethidine Monosulfate (Concurrent use with drugs for blood pressure is not recommended). Products include:
Esimil Tablets 840
Ismelin Tablets 845
Haloperidol (May increase drowsiness effect). Products include:
Haldol Injection, Tablets and Concentrate 1585
Haloperidol Decanoate (May increase drowsiness effect). Products include:
Haldol Decanoate 1587
Hydralazine Hydrochloride (Concurrent use with drugs for blood pressure is not recommended). Products include:
Apresazide Capsules 824
Apresoline Hydrochloride Tablets .. 826
Hydralazine Hydrochloride Injection USP 2712
Ser-Ap-Es Tablets 867
Hydrochlorothiazide (Concurrent use with drugs for blood pressure is not recommended). Products include:
Aldactazide Tablets 2556
Aldoril Tablets 1644
Apresazide Capsules 824
Capozide Tablets 744
Dyazide Capsules 2653
Esidrix Tablets 839
Esimil Tablets 840
HydroDIURIL Tablets 1716
Hydropres Tablets 1718
Hyzaar Tablets 1720
Inderide Tablets 2838
Inderide LA Long Acting Capsules .. 2840
Lopressor HCT Tablets 850
Lotensin HCT Tablets 855
Moduretic Tablets 1748
Oretic Tablets 450
Prinzide Tablets 1780
Ser-Ap-Es Tablets 867
Timolide Tablets 1791
Vaseretic Tablets 1810
Zestoretic Tablets 2968
Ziac 1459
Hydroflumethiazide (Concurrent use with drugs for blood pressure is not recommended). Products include:
Diucardin Tablets 2824
Hydroxyzine Hydrochloride (May increase drowsiness effect). Products include:
Atarax Tablets & Syrup 1992
Marax Tablets & DF Syrup 2015
Vistaril Intramuscular Solution 2042

IMPORTANT NOTE: Always consult each drug listing in the patient's regimen for possible interactions.

Alka-Seltzer Plus Liqui-Gels Interactions Index 44

Indapamide (Concurrent use with drugs for blood pressure is not recommended).
No products indexed under this heading.

Isocarboxazid (Concurrent and/or sequential use is not recommended).
No products indexed under this heading.

Isradipine (Concurrent use with drugs for blood pressure is not recommended). Products include:
DynaCirc Capsules ... 2381
DynaCirc CR Tablets ... 2383

Labetalol Hydrochloride (Concurrent use with drugs for blood pressure is not recommended). Products include:
Normodyne Injection ... 2519
Normodyne Tablets ... 2522
Trandate ... 1158

Lisinopril (Concurrent use with drugs for blood pressure is not recommended). Products include:
Prinivil Tablets ... 1776
Prinzide Tablets ... 1780
Zestoretic Tablets ... 2968
Zestril Tablets ... 2972

Lorazepam (May increase drowsiness effect). Products include:
Ativan Injection ... 2805
Ativan Tablets ... 2807

Losartan Potassium (Concurrent use with drugs for blood pressure is not recommended). Products include:
Cozaar Tablets ... 1668
Hyzaar Tablets ... 1720

Loxapine Hydrochloride (May increase drowsiness effect). Products include:
Loxitane ... 1426

Loxapine Succinate (May increase drowsiness effect). Products include:
Loxitane Capsules ... 1426

Mecamylamine Hydrochloride (Concurrent use with drugs for blood pressure is not recommended). Products include:
Inversine Tablets ... 1729

Meprobamate (May increase drowsiness effect). Products include:
Miltown Tablets ... 2780
PMB 200 and PMB 400 ... 2890

Mesoridazine Besylate (May increase drowsiness effect). Products include:
Serentil ... 689

Methyclothiazide (Concurrent use with drugs for blood pressure is not recommended). Products include:
Enduron Tablets ... 424

Methyldopa (Concurrent use with drugs for blood pressure is not recommended). Products include:
Aldoclor Tablets ... 1638
Aldomet Oral ... 1640
Aldoril Tablets ... 1644

Methyldopate Hydrochloride (Concurrent use with drugs for blood pressure is not recommended). Products include:
Aldomet Ester HCl Injection ... 1642

Metolazone (Concurrent use with drugs for blood pressure is not recommended). Products include:
Mykrox Tablets ... 1617
Zaroxolyn Tablets ... 1625

Metoprolol Succinate (Concurrent use with drugs for blood pressure is not recommended). Products include:
Toprol-XL Tablets ... 560

Metoprolol Tartrate (Concurrent use with drugs for blood pressure is not recommended). Products include:
Lopressor ... 848
Lopressor HCT Tablets ... 850

Metyrosine (Concurrent use with drugs for blood pressure is not recommended). Products include:
Demser Capsules ... 1690

Midazolam Hydrochloride (May increase drowsiness effect). Products include:
Versed Injection ... 2324

Minoxidil (Concurrent use with drugs for blood pressure is not recommended).
No products indexed under this heading.

Moexipril Hydrochloride (Concurrent use with drugs for blood pressure is not recommended). Products include:
Univasc Tablets ... 2553

Molindone Hydrochloride (May increase drowsiness effect). Products include:
Moban Tablets and Concentrate ... 1036

Nadolol (Concurrent use with drugs for blood pressure is not recommended).
No products indexed under this heading.

Nicardipine Hydrochloride (Concurrent use with drugs for blood pressure is not recommended). Products include:
Cardene Capsules ... 2261
Cardene I.V. ... 2815
Cardene SR Capsules ... 2264

Nifedipine (Concurrent use with drugs for blood pressure is not recommended). Products include:
Adalat Capsules (10 mg and 20 mg) ... 580
Adalat CC ... 582
Procardia Capsules ... 2024
Procardia XL Extended Release Tablets ... 2026

Nisoldipine (Concurrent use with drugs for blood pressure is not recommended). Products include:
Sular Tablets ... 2961

Nitroglycerin (Concurrent use with drugs for blood pressure is not recommended). Products include:
Deponit NTG Transdermal Delivery System ... 2541
Nitro-Bid IV ... 1270
Nitro-Bid Ointment ... 1272
Nitro-Dur (nitroglycerin) Transdermal Infusion System ... 1365
Nitrolingual Spray ... 2193
Nitrostat Tablets ... 1981
Transderm-Nitro Transdermal Therapeutic System ... 878

Oxazepam (May increase drowsiness effect). Products include:
Serax Capsules ... 2916
Serax Tablets ... 2916

Penbutolol Sulfate (Concurrent use with drugs for blood pressure is not recommended). Products include:
Levatol Tablets ... 2547

Perphenazine (May increase drowsiness effect). Products include:
Etrafon ... 2495
Triavil Tablets ... 1800
Trilafon ... 2532

Phenelzine Sulfate (Concurrent and/or sequential use is not recommended). Products include:
Nardil ... 1977

Phenoxybenzamine Hydrochloride (Concurrent use with drugs for blood pressure is not recommended). Products include:
Dibenzyline Capsules ... 2650

Phentolamine Mesylate (Concurrent use with drugs for blood pressure is not recommended). Products include:
Regitine Vials ... 864

Pindolol (Concurrent use with drugs for blood pressure is not recommended). Products include:
Visken Tablets ... 2428

Polythiazide (Concurrent use with drugs for blood pressure is not recommended). Products include:
Minizide Capsules ... 2016

Prazepam (May increase drowsiness effect).
No products indexed under this heading.

Prazosin Hydrochloride (Concurrent use with drugs for blood pressure is not recommended). Products include:
Minipress Capsules ... 2015
Minizide Capsules ... 2016

Prochlorperazine (May increase drowsiness effect). Products include:
Compazine ... 2644

Promethazine Hydrochloride (May increase drowsiness effect). Products include:
Mepergan Injection ... 2859
Phenergan with Codeine ... 2883
Phenergan with Dextromethorphan 2885
Phenergan Injection ... 2880
Phenergan Suppositories ... 2882
Phenergan Syrup ... 2881
Phenergan Tablets ... 2882
Phenergan VC ... 2886
Phenergan VC with Codeine ... 2888

Propofol (May increase drowsiness effect). Products include:
Diprivan Injectable Emulsion ... 2939

Propranolol Hydrochloride (Concurrent use with drugs for blood pressure is not recommended). Products include:
Inderal ... 2834
Inderal LA Long Acting Capsules ... 2836
Inderide Tablets ... 2838
Inderide LA Long Acting Capsules .. 2840

Quazepam (May increase drowsiness effect). Products include:
Doral Tablets ... 2773

Quinapril Hydrochloride (Concurrent use with drugs for blood pressure is not recommended). Products include:
Accupril Tablets ... 1950

Ramipril (Concurrent use with drugs for blood pressure is not recommended). Products include:
Altace Capsules ... 1238

Rauwolfia Serpentina (Concurrent use with drugs for blood pressure is not recommended).
No products indexed under this heading.

Rescinnamine (Concurrent use with drugs for blood pressure is not recommended).
No products indexed under this heading.

Reserpine (Concurrent use with drugs for blood pressure is not recommended). Products include:
Diupres Tablets ... 1691
Hydropres Tablets ... 1718
Ser-Ap-Es Tablets ... 867

Secobarbital Sodium (May increase drowsiness effect). Products include:
Seconal Sodium Pulvules ... 1529

Selegiline Hydrochloride (Concurrent and/or sequential use is not recommended). Products include:
Eldepryl Capsules ... 2729

Sodium Nitroprusside (Concurrent use with drugs for blood pressure is not recommended).
No products indexed under this heading.

Sotalol Hydrochloride (Concurrent use with drugs for blood pressure is not recommended). Products include:
Betapace Tablets ... 637

Spirapril Hydrochloride (Concurrent use with drugs for blood pressure is not recommended).
No products indexed under this heading.

Temazepam (May increase drowsiness effect). Products include:
Restoril Capsules ... 2413

Terazosin Hydrochloride (Concurrent use with drugs for blood pressure is not recommended). Products include:
Hytrin Capsules ... 434

Thioridazine Hydrochloride (May increase drowsiness effect). Products include:
Mellaril ... 2398

Thiothixene (May increase drowsiness effect). Products include:
Navane Capsules and Concentrate 2018
Navane Intramuscular ... 2019

Timolol Maleate (Concurrent use with drugs for blood pressure is not recommended). Products include:
Blocadren Tablets ... 1654
Timolide Tablets ... 1791
Timoptic in Ocudose ... 1796
Timoptic Sterile Ophthalmic Solution ... 1794
Timoptic-XE ... 1798

Torsemide (Concurrent use with drugs for blood pressure is not recommended). Products include:
Demadex Tablets and Injection ... 691

Tranylcypromine Sulfate (Concurrent and/or sequential use is not recommended). Products include:
Parnate Tablets ... 2679

Triazolam (May increase drowsiness effect). Products include:
Halcion Tablets ... 2093

Trifluoperazine Hydrochloride (May increase drowsiness effect). Products include:
Stelazine ... 2692

Trimethaphan Camsylate (Concurrent use with drugs for blood pressure is not recommended).
No products indexed under this heading.

Verapamil Hydrochloride (Concurrent use with drugs for blood pressure is not recommended). Products include:
Calan SR Caplets ... 2571
Calan Tablets ... 2568
Covera-HS Tablets ... 2573
Isoptin Injectable ... 1391
Isoptin Oral Tablets ... 1393
Isoptin SR Tablets ... 1395
Verelan Capsules ... 1455

Zolpidem Tartrate (May increase drowsiness effect). Products include:
Ambien Tablets ... 2559

Food Interactions

Alcohol (May increase drowsiness effect).

ALKA-SELTZER PLUS SINUS MEDICINE
(Phenylpropanolamine Bitartrate, Aspirin, Brompheniramine Maleate) ▣ 611
See **Alka-Seltzer Plus Cold & Cough Medicine**

(▣ Described in PDR For Nonprescription Drugs) (◉ Described in PDR For Ophthalmology)

ALKERAN FOR INJECTION
(Melphalan Hydrochloride)..................1196
May interact with:

Carmustine (BCNU) (Reduced threshold for BCNU lung toxicity). Products include:
BiCNU 696

Cisplatin (Affects melphalan kinetics by inducing renal dysfunction and subsequently altering melphalan clearance). Products include:
Platinol for Injection 717
Platinol-AQ Injection 719

Cyclosporine (Potential for severe renal failure). Products include:
Neoral 2405
Sandimmune 2416

Nalidixic Acid (Increased incidence of severe hemorrhagic necrotic enterocolitis). Products include:
NegGram 2453

ALKERAN TABLETS
(Melphalan).................................1198
None cited in PDR database.

ALLEREST MAXIMUM STRENGTH
(Chlorpheniramine Maleate, Pseudoephedrine Hydrochloride)..... 649
May interact with monoamine oxidase inhibitors, hypnotics and sedatives, tranquilizers, and certain other agents. Compounds in these categories include:

Alfentanil Hydrochloride (Concurrent use produces additive effects). Products include:
Alfenta Injection 1334

Alprazolam (Concurrent use produces additive effects). Products include:
Xanax Tablets 2115

Aprobarbital (Concurrent use produces additive effects).
No products indexed under this heading.

Buprenorphine (Concurrent use produces additive effects). Products include:
Buprenex Injectable 2170

Buspirone Hydrochloride (Concurrent use produces additive effects). Products include:
BuSpar Tablets 738

Butabarbital (Concurrent use produces additive effects).
No products indexed under this heading.

Butalbital (Concurrent use produces additive effects). Products include:
Axocet Capsules 2469
Esgic-plus Capsules 1012
Esgic-plus Tablets 1012
Fioricet Tablets 2386
Fioricet with Codeine Capsules 2387
Fiorinal Capsules 2388
Fiorinal with Codeine Capsules 2390
Fiorinal Tablets 2388
Phrenilin 790
Sedapap Tablets 50 mg/650 mg .. 1826

Chlordiazepoxide (Concurrent use produces additive effects). Products include:
Limbitrol 2333

Chlordiazepoxide Hydrochloride (Concurrent use produces additive effects). Products include:
Librax Capsules 2330
Librium Capsules 2331
Librium Injectable 2332

Chlorpromazine (Concurrent use produces additive effects). Products include:
Thorazine Suppositories 2701

Chlorpromazine Hydrochloride (Concurrent use produces additive effects). Products include:
Thorazine 2701

Chlorprothixene (Concurrent use produces additive effects).
No products indexed under this heading.

Chlorprothixene Hydrochloride (Concurrent use produces additive effects).
No products indexed under this heading.

Clorazepate Dipotassium (Concurrent use produces additive effects). Products include:
Tranxene 459

Clozapine (Concurrent use produces additive effects). Products include:
Clozaril Tablets 2377

Codeine Phosphate (Concurrent use produces additive effects). Products include:
Brontex 2130
Dimetane-DC Cough Syrup 2232
Fioricet with Codeine Capsules 2387
Fiorinal with Codeine Capsules 2390
Nucofed 2225
Phenergan with Codeine 2883
Phenergan VC with Codeine 2888
Robitussin A-C Syrup 2248
Robitussin-DAC Syrup 2249
Ryna 804
Soma Compound w/Codeine Tablets 2784
Tylenol with Codeine 1592

Desflurane (Concurrent use produces additive effects). Products include:
Suprane (desflurane, USP) 1865

Dezocine (Concurrent use produces additive effects). Products include:
Dalgan Injection 529

Diazepam (Concurrent use produces additive effects). Products include:
Dizac (diazepam injectable emulsion) CIV 1862
Valium Injectable 2336
Valium Tablets 2335

Droperidol (Concurrent use produces additive effects). Products include:
Inapsine Injection 462

Enflurane (Concurrent use produces additive effects).
No products indexed under this heading.

Estazolam (Concurrent use produces additive effects). Products include:
ProSom Tablets 457

Ethchlorvynol (Concurrent use produces additive effects). Products include:
Placidyl Capsules 456

Ethinamate (Concurrent use produces additive effects).
No products indexed under this heading.

Fentanyl (Concurrent use produces additive effects). Products include:
Duragesic Transdermal System 1336

Fentanyl Citrate (Concurrent use produces additive effects). Products include:
Sublimaze Injection 463

Fluphenazine Decanoate (Concurrent use produces additive effects). Products include:
Prolixin Decanoate 510

Fluphenazine Enanthate (Concurrent use produces additive effects). Products include:
Prolixin Enanthate 510

Fluphenazine Hydrochloride (Concurrent use produces additive effects). Products include:
Prolixin 510

Flurazepam Hydrochloride (Concurrent use produces additive effects). Products include:
Dalmane Capsules 2329

Furazolidone (Concurrent and/or sequential use is not recommended). Products include:
Furoxone 2221

Glutethimide (Concurrent use produces additive effects).
No products indexed under this heading.

Haloperidol (Concurrent use produces additive effects). Products include:
Haldol Injection, Tablets and Concentrate 1585

Haloperidol Decanoate (Concurrent use produces additive effects). Products include:
Haldol Decanoate 1587

Hydrocodone Bitartrate (Concurrent use produces additive effects). Products include:
Codiclear DH Syrup 808
Duratuss HD Elixir 2750
Histussin D Liquid 670
Hycodan Tablets and Syrup 946
Hycomine Compound Tablets 948
Hycomine 947
Hycotuss Expectorant Syrup 950
Hydrocet Capsules 787
Lorcet 10/650 Tablets 1016
Lortab 2751
Tussend 1830
Tussend Expectorant 1831
Vicodin Tablets 1404
Vicodin ES Tablets 1405
Vicodin HP Tablets 1403
Vicodin Tuss Expectorant 1406
Zydone Capsules 967

Hydrocodone Polistirex (Concurrent use produces additive effects). Products include:
Tussionex Pennkinetic Extended-Release Suspension 1624

Hydroxyzine Hydrochloride (Concurrent use produces additive effects). Products include:
Atarax Tablets & Syrup 1992
Marax Tablets & DF Syrup 2015
Vistaril Intramuscular Solution 2042

Isocarboxazid (Concurrent and/or sequential use is not recommended).
No products indexed under this heading.

Isoflurane (Concurrent use produces additive effects).
No products indexed under this heading.

Ketamine Hydrochloride (Concurrent use produces additive effects).
No products indexed under this heading.

Levomethadyl Acetate Hydrochloride (Concurrent use produces additive effects). Products include:
Orlaam Oral Solution 2361

Levorphanol Tartrate (Concurrent use produces additive effects). Products include:
Levo-Dromoran 2297

Lorazepam (Concurrent use produces additive effects). Products include:
Ativan Injection 2805
Ativan Tablets 2807

Loxapine Hydrochloride (Concurrent use produces additive effects). Products include:
Loxitane 1426

Loxapine Succinate (Concurrent use produces additive effects). Products include:
Loxitane Capsules 1426

Meperidine Hydrochloride (Concurrent use produces additive effects). Products include:
Demerol 2438
Mepergan Injection 2859

Mephobarbital (Concurrent use produces additive effects). Products include:
Mebaral Tablets 2452

Meprobamate (Concurrent use produces additive effects). Products include:
Miltown Tablets 2780
PMB 200 and PMB 400 2890

Mesoridazine Besylate (Concurrent use produces additive effects). Products include:
Serentil 689

Methadone Hydrochloride (Concurrent use produces additive effects). Products include:
Methadone Hydrochloride Oral Concentrate 2356
Methadone Hydrochloride Oral Solution & Tablets 2357

Methohexital Sodium (Concurrent use produces additive effects).
No products indexed under this heading.

Methotrimeprazine (Concurrent use produces additive effects). Products include:
Levoprome 1321

Methoxyflurane (Concurrent use produces additive effects).
No products indexed under this heading.

Midazolam Hydrochloride (Concurrent use produces additive effects). Products include:
Versed Injection 2324

Molindone Hydrochloride (Concurrent use produces additive effects). Products include:
Moban Tablets and Concentrate 1036

Morphine Sulfate (Concurrent use produces additive effects). Products include:
Astramorph/PF Injection, USP (Preservative-Free) 526
Duramorph Injection 983
Infumorph 200 and Infumorph 500 Sterile Solutions 985
Kadian Capsules 2948
MS Contin Tablets 2149
MSIR 2152
Oramorph SR (Morphine Sulfate Sustained Release Tablets) 2359
RMS Suppositories CII 2766
Roxanol 2365

Opium Alkaloids (Concurrent use produces additive effects).
No products indexed under this heading.

Oxazepam (Concurrent use produces additive effects). Products include:
Serax Capsules 2916
Serax Tablets 2916

Oxycodone Hydrochloride (Concurrent use produces additive effects). Products include:
OxyContin Tablets 2163
OxyIR Capsules 2167
Percocet Tablets 955
Percodan Tablets 955
Percodan-Demi Tablets 956
Roxicodone Tablets, Oral Solution & Intensol (Oxycodone) 2366
Tylox Capsules 1593

Pentobarbital Sodium (Concurrent use produces additive effects). Products include:
Nembutal Sodium Capsules 440
Nembutal Sodium Solution 442
Nembutal Sodium Suppositories ... 444

Perphenazine (Concurrent use produces additive effects). Products include:
Etrafon 2495
Triavil Tablets 1800

IMPORTANT NOTE: Always consult each drug listing in the patient's regimen for possible interactions.

Allerest Maximum — Interactions Index — 46

Trilafon.................................... 2532
Phenelzine Sulfate (Concurrent and/or sequential use is not recommended). Products include:
Nardil 1977
Phenobarbital (Concurrent use produces additive effects). Products include:
Arco-Lase Plus Tablets 513
Bellergal-S Tablets 2375
Donnatal 2234
Donnatal Extentabs 2234
Donnatal Tablets 2234
Phenobarbital Elixir and Tablets ... 1523
Quadrinal Tablets 1398
Prazepam (Concurrent use produces additive effects).
No products indexed under this heading.
Prochlorperazine (Concurrent use produces additive effects). Products include:
Compazine 2644
Promethazine Hydrochloride (Concurrent use produces additive effects). Products include:
Mepergan Injection 2859
Phenergan with Codeine 2883
Phenergan with Dextromethorphan 2885
Phenergan Injection 2880
Phenergan Suppositories 2882
Phenergan Syrup 2881
Phenergan Tablets 2882
Phenergan VC 2886
Phenergan VC with Codeine 2888
Propofol (Concurrent use produces additive effects). Products include:
Diprivan Injectable Emulsion 2939
Propoxyphene Hydrochloride (Concurrent use produces additive effects). Products include:
Darvon 1475
Wygesic Tablets 2930
Propoxyphene Napsylate (Concurrent use produces additive effects). Products include:
Darvon-N/Darvocet-N 1473
Quazepam (Concurrent use produces additive effects). Products include:
Doral Tablets 2773
Risperidone (Concurrent use produces additive effects). Products include:
Risperdal Tablets 1348
Secobarbital Sodium (Concurrent use produces additive effects). Products include:
Seconal Sodium Pulvules 1529
Selegiline Hydrochloride (Concurrent and/or sequential use is not recommended). Products include:
Eldepryl Capsules 2729
Sufentanil Citrate (Concurrent use produces additive effects). Products include:
Sufenta Injection 1355
Temazepam (Concurrent use produces additive effects). Products include:
Restoril Capsules 2413
Thiamylal Sodium (Concurrent use produces additive effects).
No products indexed under this heading.
Thioridazine Hydrochloride (Concurrent use produces additive effects). Products include:
Mellaril 2398
Thiothixene (Concurrent use produces additive effects). Products include:
Navane Capsules and Concentrate 2018
Navane Intramuscular 2019
Tranylcypromine Sulfate (Concurrent use and/or sequential use is not recommended). Products include:
Parnate Tablets 2679

Triazolam (Concurrent use produces additive effects). Products include:
Halcion Tablets 2093
Trifluoperazine Hydrochloride (Concurrent use produces additive effects). Products include:
Stelazine 2692
Zolpidem Tartrate (Concurrent use produces additive effects). Products include:
Ambien Tablets 2559

Food Interactions
Alcohol (May increase drowsiness).

ALLEREST NO DROWSINESS
(Acetaminophen, Pseudoephedrine Hydrochloride)................ 649
See Allerest Maximum Strength

ALLEREST SINUS PAIN FORMULA
(Acetaminophen, Chlorpheniramine Maleate, Pseudoephedrine Hydrochloride)................ 649
See Allerest Maximum Strength

ALL-FLEX ARCING SPRING DIAPHRAGM (SEE ALSO ORTHO DIAPHRAGM KITS)
(Diaphragm).............................. 1921
None cited in PDR database.

ALOMIDE OPHTHALMIC SOLUTION
(Lodoxamide Tromethamine)............. 465
None cited in PDR database.

ALPHA KERI MOISTURE RICH BODY OIL
(Lanolin Oil)............................ 635
None cited in PDR database.

ALTACE CAPSULES
(Ramipril)................................. 1238
May interact with potassium sparing diuretics, diuretics, potassium preparations, lithium preparations, and certain other agents. Compounds in these categories include:

Amiloride Hydrochloride (May result in excessive reduction of blood pressure after initiation of therapy; increased risk of hyperkalemia). Products include:
Midamor Tablets 1746
Moduretic Tablets 1748
Bendroflumethiazide (May result in excessive reduction of blood pressure after initiation of therapy).
No products indexed under this heading.
Bumetanide (May result in excessive reduction of blood pressure after initiation of therapy). Products include:
Bumex 2260
Chlorothiazide (May result in excessive reduction of blood pressure after initiation of therapy). Products include:
Aldoclor Tablets 1638
Diupres Tablets 1691
Diuril Oral 1694
Chlorothiazide Sodium (May result in excessive reduction of blood pressure after initiation of therapy). Products include:
Diuril Sodium Intravenous 1693
Chlorthalidone (May result in excessive reduction of blood pressure after initiation of therapy). Products include:
Combipres Tablets 682
Tenoretic Tablets 2963
Thalitone 1293

Ethacrynic Acid (May result in excessive reduction of blood pressure after initiation of therapy). Products include:
Edecrin Tablets 1698
Furosemide (May result in excessive reduction of blood pressure after initiation of therapy). Products include:
Lasix Injection, Oral Solution and Tablets 1267
Hydrochlorothiazide (May result in excessive reduction of blood pressure after initiation of therapy). Products include:
Aldactazide Tablets 2556
Aldoril Tablets 1644
Apresazide Capsules 824
Capozide Tablets 744
Dyazide Capsules 2653
Esidrix Tablets 839
Esimil Tablets 840
HydroDIURIL Tablets 1716
Hydropres Tablets 1718
Hyzaar Tablets 1720
Inderide Tablets 2838
Inderide LA Long Acting Capsules .. 2840
Lopressor HCT Tablets 850
Lotensin HCT Tablets 855
Moduretic Tablets 1748
Oretic Tablets 450
Prinzide Tablets 1780
Ser-Ap-Es Tablets 867
Timolide Tablets 1791
Vaseretic Tablets 1810
Zestoretic Tablets 2968
Ziac 1459
Hydroflumethiazide (May result in excessive reduction of blood pressure after initiation of therapy). Products include:
Diucardin Tablets 2824
Indapamide (May result in excessive reduction of blood pressure after initiation of therapy).
No products indexed under this heading.
Lithium Carbonate (Increased serum lithium levels and symptoms of lithium toxicity). Products include:
Eskalith 2658
Lithium Carbonate Capsules & Tablets 2352
Lithonate/Lithotabs/Lithobid 2721
Lithium Citrate (Increased serum lithium levels and symptoms of lithium toxicity).
No products indexed under this heading.
Methyclothiazide (May result in excessive reduction of blood pressure after initiation of therapy). Products include:
Enduron Tablets 424
Metolazone (May result in excessive reduction of blood pressure after initiation of therapy). Products include:
Mykrox Tablets 1617
Zaroxolyn Tablets 1625
Polythiazide (May result in excessive reduction of blood pressure after initiation of therapy). Products include:
Minizide Capsules 2016
Potassium Acid Phosphate (Increased risk of hyperkalemia). Products include:
K-Phos Original Formula 'Sodium Free' Tablets 633
Potassium Bicarbonate (Increased risk of hyperkalemia). Products include:
Alka-Seltzer Gold Effervescent Antacid 611
Potassium Chloride (Increased risk of hyperkalemia). Products include:
Chlor-3 Condiment 1003
Colyte and Colyte-flavored 2540
GoLYTELY 694

K-Dur Microburst Release System (potassium chloride, USP) E.R. Tablets 1364
K-Lor Powder Packets 438
K-Norm Capsules 1615
K-Tab Filmtab 439
Micro-K 2237
Micro-K LS Packets 2238
NuLYTELY 694
Cherry Flavor NuLYTELY 694
Rum-K Syrup 1004
Slow-K Extended-Release Tablets 869
Potassium Citrate (Increased risk of hyperkalemia). Products include:
Polycitra Syrup 574
Polycitra-K Crystals 574
Polycitra-K Oral Solution 575
Polycitra-LC 574
Urocit-K Tablets 1828
Potassium Gluconate (Increased risk of hyperkalemia).
No products indexed under this heading.
Potassium Phosphate, Dibasic (Increased risk of hyperkalemia).
No products indexed under this heading.
Potassium Phosphate, Monobasic (Increased risk of hyperkalemia). Products include:
K-Phos Neutral Tablets 633
K-Phos Original Formula 'Sodium Free' Tablets 633
Spironolactone (May result in excessive reduction of blood pressure after initiation of therapy; increased risk of hyperkalemia). Products include:
Aldactazide Tablets 2556
Aldactone Tablets 2558
Torsemide (May result in excessive reduction of blood pressure after initiation of therapy). Products include:
Demadex Tablets and Injection .. 691
Triamterene (May result in excessive reduction of blood pressure after initiation of therapy; increased risk of hyperkalemia). Products include:
Dyazide Capsules 2653
Dyrenium Capsules 2655

Food Interactions
Food, unspecified (The rate of absorption is reduced, not the extent of absorption).
Salt substitutes, potassium-containing (Increases risk of hyperkalemia).

ALTERNAGEL LIQUID
(Aluminum Hydroxide)............. 1358
May interact with tetracyclines. Compounds in this category include:

Demeclocycline Hydrochloride (Should not be taken concurrently). Products include:
Declomycin Tablets 1421
Doxycycline Calcium (Should not be taken concurrently). Products include:
Vibramycin Calcium Oral Suspension Syrup 2038
Doxycycline Hyclate (Should not be taken concurrently). Products include:
Doryx Capsules 1970
Vibramycin Hyclate Capsules 2038
Vibramycin Hyclate Intravenous 2040
Vibra-Tabs Film Coated Tablets . 2038
Doxycycline Monohydrate (Should not be taken concurrently). Products include:
Monodox Capsules 1858
Vibramycin Monohydrate for Oral Suspension 2038
Methacycline Hydrochloride (Should not be taken concurrently).
No products indexed under this heading.

(◨ Described in PDR For Nonprescription Drugs) (⊙ Described in PDR For Ophthalmology)

Minocycline Hydrochloride (Should not be taken concurrently). Products include:

- DYNACIN Capsules 1627
- Minocin Intravenous 1428
- Minocin Oral Suspension 1431
- Minocin Pellet-Filled Capsules 1429

Oxytetracycline (Should not be taken concurrently). Products include:

- Terramycin Intramuscular Solution 2034

Oxytetracycline Hydrochloride (Should not be taken concurrently). Products include:

- TERAK Ointment ..... ◉ 210
- Terra-Cortril Ophthalmic Suspension 2033
- Terramycin with Polymyxin B Sulfate Ophthalmic Ointment 2035
- Urobiotic-250 Capsules 2038

Tetracycline Hydrochloride (Should not be taken concurrently). Products include:

- Achromycin V Capsules 1417
- Helidac Therapy 2135

ALUPENT INHALATION AEROSOL

(Metaproterenol Sulfate) 672
See **Alupent Inhalation Solution**

ALUPENT INHALATION SOLUTION

(Metaproterenol Sulfate) 672

May interact with monoamine oxidase inhibitors, tricyclic antidepressants, and sympathomimetic aerosol bronchodilators. Compounds in these categories include:

Albuterol (Possible potentiation of adrenergic effects with beta adrenergic aerosol bronchodilators). Products include:

- Proventil Inhalation Aerosol 2524
- Ventolin Inhalation Aerosol and Refill 1170

Amitriptyline Hydrochloride (The action of beta adrenergic agonists on the vascular system may be potentiated). Products include:

- Elavil 2945
- Etrafon 2495
- Limbitrol 2333
- Triavil Tablets 1800

Amoxapine (The action of beta adrenergic agonists on the vascular system may be potentiated). Products include:

- Asendin Tablets 1419

Bitolterol Mesylate (Possible potentiation of adrenergic effects with beta adrenergic aerosol bronchodilators). Products include:

- Tornalate Solution for Inhalation, 0.2% 976
- Tornalate Metered Dose Inhaler 978

Clomipramine Hydrochloride (The action of beta adrenergic agonists on the vascular system may be potentiated). Products include:

- Anafranil Capsules 819

Desipramine Hydrochloride (The action of beta adrenergic agonists on the vascular system may be potentiated). Products include:

- Norpramin Tablets 1273

Doxepin Hydrochloride (The action of beta adrenergic agonists on the vascular system may be potentiated). Products include:

- Adapin Capsules 1542
- Sinequan 2028
- Zonalon Cream 1042

Furazolidone (The action of beta adrenergic agonists on the vascular system may be potentiated). Products include:

- Furoxone 2221

Imipramine Hydrochloride (The action of beta adrenergic agonists on the vascular system may be potentiated). Products include:

- Tofranil Ampuls 873
- Tofranil Tablets 875

Imipramine Pamoate (The action of beta adrenergic agonists on the vascular system may be potentiated). Products include:

- Tofranil-PM Capsules 876

Isocarboxazid (The action of beta adrenergic agonists on the vascular system may be potentiated).

No products indexed under this heading.

Isoetharine (Possible potentiation of adrenergic effects with beta adrenergic aerosol bronchodilators). Products include:

- Bronkometer Aerosol 2432
- Bronkosol Solution 2432
- Isoetharine Inhalation Solution, USP, Arm-a-Med 545

Isoproterenol Hydrochloride (Possible potentiation of adrenergic effects with beta adrenergic aerosol bronchodilators). Products include:

- Isuprel Hydrochloride Solution 2443
- Isuprel Injection 2441
- Isuprel Mistometer 2442

Maprotiline Hydrochloride (The action of beta adrenergic agonists on the vascular system may be potentiated). Products include:

- Ludiomil Tablets 861

Nortriptyline Hydrochloride (The action of beta adrenergic agonists on the vascular system may be potentiated). Products include:

- Pamelor 2409

Phenelzine Sulfate (The action of beta adrenergic agonists on the vascular system may be potentiated). Products include:

- Nardil 1977

Pirbuterol Acetate (Possible potentiation of adrenergic effects with beta adrenergic aerosol bronchodilators). Products include:

- Maxair Autohaler 1550
- Maxair Inhaler 1552

Protriptyline Hydrochloride (The action of beta adrenergic agonists on the vascular system may be potentiated). Products include:

- Vivactil Tablets 1820

Salmeterol Xinafoate (Possible potentiation of adrenergic effects with beta adrenergic aerosol bronchodilators). Products include:

- Serevent Inhalation Aerosol 1149

Selegiline Hydrochloride (The action of beta adrenergic agonists on the vascular system may be potentiated). Products include:

- Eldepryl Capsules 2729

Terbutaline Sulfate (Possible potentiation of adrenergic effects with beta adrenergic aerosol bronchodilators). Products include:

- Brethaire Inhaler 830
- Brethine Ampuls 832
- Brethine Tablets 831
- Bricanyl Subcutaneous Injection 1247
- Bricanyl Tablets 1248

Tranylcypromine Sulfate (The action of beta adrenergic agonists on the vascular system may be potentiated). Products include:

- Parnate Tablets 2679

Trimipramine Maleate (The action of beta adrenergic agonists on the vascular system may be potentiated). Products include:

- Surmontil Capsules 2917

ALUPENT SYRUP

(Metaproterenol Sulfate) 672
See **Alupent Inhalation Solution**

ALUPENT TABLETS

(Metaproterenol Sulfate) 672
See **Alupent Inhalation Solution**

AMARYL TABLETS

(Glimepiride) 1241

May interact with non-steroidal anti-inflammatory agents, salicylates, sulfonamides, monoamine oxidase inhibitors, beta blockers, oral anticoagulants, diuretics, thiazides, corticosteroids, phenothiazines, thyroid preparations, estrogens, oral contraceptives, sympathomimetics, and certain other agents. Compounds in these categories include:

Acebutolol Hydrochloride (May potentiate hypoglycemic action). Products include:

- Sectral Capsules 2914

Albuterol (Sympathomimetics tend to produce hyperglycemia and concurrent use may lead to loss of control). Products include:

- Proventil Inhalation Aerosol 2524
- Ventolin Inhalation Aerosol and Refill 1170

Albuterol Sulfate (Sympathomimetics tend to produce hyperglycemia and concurrent use may lead to loss of control). Products include:

- Airet Albuterol Sulfate Inhalation Solution 1602
- Albuterol Sulfate, USP Solution for Inhalation, Arm-a-Med 522
- Proventil Inhalation Solution 0.083% 2527
- Proventil Repetabs Tablets 2529
- Proventil Solution for Inhalation 0.5% 2525
- Proventil Syrup 2528
- Proventil Tablets 2529
- Ventolin Inhalation Solution 1171
- Ventolin Nebules Inhalation Solution 1172
- Ventolin Rotacaps for Inhalation 1173
- Ventolin Syrup 1175
- Ventolin Tablets 1176
- Volmax Extended-Release Tablets 1835

Amiloride Hydrochloride (Diuretics tend to produce hyperglycemia and concurrent use may lead to loss of control). Products include:

- Midamor Tablets 1746
- Moduretic Tablets 1748

Aspirin (Co-administration of aspirin (1 g tid) led to a 34% decrease in the mean glimepiride AUC and, therefore, a 34% increase in the mean CL/f; no hypoglycemic symptoms were reported). Products include:

- Alka-Seltzer Cherry Effervescent Antacid and Pain Reliever 609
- Alka-Seltzer Extra Strength Effervescent Antacid and Pain Reliever 609
- Alka-Seltzer Lemon Lime Effervescent Antacid and Pain Reliever 609
- Alka-Seltzer Original Effervescent Antacid and Pain Reliever 609
- Alka-Seltzer Plus 611
- Alka-Seltzer Plus Sinus Medicine 611
- Ascriptin 650
- Arthritis Strength BC Powder 631
- BC Cold Powder Multi-Symptom Formula (Cold-Sinus-Allergy) 631
- BC Cold Powder Non-Drowsy Formula (Cold-Sinus) 631
- BC Powder 631
- Genuine Bayer Aspirin Tablets & Caplets 618
- Extra Strength Bayer Arthritis Pain Regimen Formula 615
- Extra Strength Bayer Aspirin Caplets & Tablets 617
- Extended-Release Bayer 8-Hour Aspirin 616
- Extra Strength Bayer Plus Aspirin Caplets 617
- Extra Strength Bayer PM Aspirin Plus Sleep Aid 617
- Aspirin Regimen Bayer 81 mg Tablets with Calcium 615
- Aspirin Regimen Bayer Adult Low Strength 81 mg Tablets 613
- Aspirin Regimen Bayer Children's Chewable Aspirin 616
- Aspirin Regimen Bayer Regular Strength 325 mg Caplets 613
- Bufferin Analgesic Tablets 636
- Arthritis Strength Bufferin Analgesic Caplets 637
- Extra Strength Bufferin Analgesic Tablets 637
- Cama Arthritis Pain Reliever 748
- Darvon Compound-65 Pulvules 1475
- Easprin 1971
- Ecotrin 2625
- Ecotrin Enteric Coated Aspirin Maximum Strength Tablets and Caplets 775
- Ecotrin Enteric Coated Aspirin Regular Strength Tablets 2625
- Empirin Aspirin Tablets 818
- Excedrin Extra-Strength Analgesic Tablets, Caplets, and Geltabs 734
- Fiorinal Capsules 2388
- Fiorinal with Codeine Capsules 2390
- Fiorinal Tablets 2388
- Goody's Extra Strength Headache Powders 632
- Goody's Extra Strength Pain Relief Tablets 632
- Halfprin Tablets 1413
- Norgesic 1554
- Percodan Tablets 955
- Percodan-Demi Tablets 956
- Robaxisal Tablets 2246
- Soma Compound w/Codeine Tablets 2784
- Soma Compound Tablets 2783
- St. Joseph Adult Chewable Aspirin (81 mg.) 768
- Talwin Compound 2466
- Vanquish Analgesic Caplets 627

Atenolol (May potentiate hypoglycemic action). Products include:

- Tenoretic Tablets 2963
- Tenormin Tablets and I.V. Injection 2965

Bendroflumethiazide (Thiazides tend to produce hyperglycemia and concurrent use may lead to loss of control).

No products indexed under this heading.

Betamethasone Acetate (Corticosteroids tend to produce hyperglycemia and concurrent use may lead to loss of control). Products include:

- Celestone Soluspan Suspension 2484

Betamethasone Sodium Phosphate (Corticosteroids tend to produce hyperglycemia and concurrent use may lead to loss of control). Products include:

- Celestone Soluspan Suspension 2484

Betaxolol Hydrochloride (May potentiate hypoglycemic action). Products include:

- Betoptic Ophthalmic Solution 465
- Betoptic S Ophthalmic Suspension 467
- Kerlone Tablets 2588

Bisoprolol Fumarate (May potentiate hypoglycemic action). Products include:

- Zebeta Tablets 1457
- Ziac 1459

Bumetanide (Diuretics tend to produce hyperglycemia and concurrent use may lead to loss of control). Products include:

- Bumex 2260

Carteolol Hydrochloride (May potentiate hypoglycemic action). Products include:

- Cartrol Tablets 413
- Ocupress Ophthalmic Solution, 1% Sterile ..... ◉ 297

Chloramphenicol (May potentiate hypoglycemic action). Products include:

- Chloromycetin Ophthalmic Ointment, 1% ..... ◉ 298

IMPORTANT NOTE: Always consult each drug listing in the patient's regimen for possible interactions.

Amaryl Tablets — Interactions Index

Chloromycetin Ophthalmic Solution 299
Chloroptic S.O.P. 236
Chloroptic Sterile Ophthalmic Solution 236

Chloramphenicol Palmitate (May potentiate hypoglycemic action).
  No products indexed under this heading.

Chloramphenicol Sodium Succinate (May potentiate hypoglycemic action). Products include:
  Chloromycetin Sodium Succinate 1960

Chlorothiazide (Thiazides tend to produce hyperglycemia and concurrent use may lead to loss of control). Products include:
  Aldoclor Tablets 1638
  Diupres Tablets 1691
  Diuril Oral 1694

Chlorothiazide Sodium (Thiazides tend to produce hyperglycemia and concurrent use may lead to loss of control). Products include:
  Diuril Sodium Intravenous 1693

Chlorotrianisene (Estrogens tend to produce hyperglycemia and concurrent use may lead to loss of control).
  No products indexed under this heading.

Chlorpromazine (Phenothiazines tend to produce hyperglycemia and concurrent use may lead to loss of control). Products include:
  Thorazine Suppositories 2701

Chlorpromazine Hydrochloride (Phenothiazines tend to produce hyperglycemia and concurrent use may lead to loss of control). Products include:
  Thorazine 2701

Chlorpropamide (May potentiate hypoglycemic action). Products include:
  Diabinese Tablets 2002

Chlorthalidone (Diuretics tend to produce hyperglycemia and concurrent use may lead to loss of control). Products include:
  Combipres Tablets 682
  Tenoretic Tablets 2963
  Thalitone 1293

Choline Magnesium Trisalicylate (May potentiate hypoglycemic action; clinical trials data indicate no evidence of significant adverse interaction with concurrent use). Products include:
  Trilisate 2155

Cortisone Acetate (Corticosteroids tend to produce hyperglycemia and concurrent use may lead to loss of control). Products include:
  Cortone Acetate Sterile Suspension 1663
  Cortone Acetate Tablets 1664

Desogestrel (Oral contraceptives tend to produce hyperglycemia and concurrent use may lead to loss of control). Products include:
  Desogen Tablets 1867
  Ortho-Cept 1907

Dexamethasone (Corticosteroids tend to produce hyperglycemia and concurrent use may lead to loss of control). Products include:
  AK-Trol Ointment & Suspension .... ⊙ 205
  Decadron Elixir 1676
  Decadron Tablets 1678
  Decaspray Topical Aerosol 1689
  Maxitrol Ophthalmic Ointment and Suspension .... ⊙ 222
  TobraDex Ophthalmic Suspension and Ointment 469

Dexamethasone Acetate (Corticosteroids tend to produce hyperglycemia and concurrent use may lead to loss of control). Products include:
  Dalalone D.P. Injectable 1009
  Decadron-LA Sterile Suspension 1687

Dexamethasone Sodium Phosphate (Corticosteroids tend to produce hyperglycemia and concurrent use may lead to loss of control). Products include:
  Decadron Phosphate Injection 1680
  Decadron Phosphate Sterile Ophthalmic Ointment 1684
  Decadron Phosphate Sterile Ophthalmic Solution 1685
  Decadron Phosphate Topical Cream 1686
  Decadron Phosphate with Xylocaine Injection, Sterile 1683
  Dexacort Phosphate in Respihaler .. 1606
  Dexacort Phosphate in Turbinaire .. 1607
  NeoDecadron Sterile Ophthalmic Ointment 1755
  NeoDecadron Sterile Ophthalmic Solution 1756
  NeoDecadron Topical Cream 1757

Diclofenac Potassium (May potentiate hypoglycemic action). Products include:
  Cataflam Tablets 833

Diclofenac Sodium (May potentiate hypoglycemic action). Products include:
  Voltaren Ophthalmic Sterile Ophthalmic Solution .... ⊙ 264
  Cataflam/Voltaren/Voltaren-XR 833

Dicumarol (May potentiate hypoglycemic action).
  No products indexed under this heading.

Dienestrol (Estrogens tend to produce hyperglycemia and concurrent use may lead to loss of control). Products include:
  Ortho Dienestrol Cream 1922

Diethylstilbestrol (Estrogens tend to produce hyperglycemia and concurrent use may lead to loss of control). Products include:
  Diethylstilbestrol Tablets 1477

Diflunisal (May potentiate hypoglycemic action; clinical trials data indicate no evidence of significant adverse interaction with concurrent use). Products include:
  Dolobid Tablets 1695

Dobutamine Hydrochloride (Sympathomimetics tend to produce hyperglycemia and concurrent use may lead to loss of control). Products include:
  Dobutrex Solution Vials 1480

Dopamine Hydrochloride (Sympathomimetics tend to produce hyperglycemia and concurrent use may lead to loss of control).
  No products indexed under this heading.

Ephedrine Hydrochloride (Sympathomimetics tend to produce hyperglycemia and concurrent use may lead to loss of control). Products include:
  Primatene Tablets .... ▣ 844
  Quadrinal Tablets 1398

Ephedrine Sulfate (Sympathomimetics tend to produce hyperglycemia and concurrent use may lead to loss of control). Products include:
  Marax Tablets & DF Syrup 2015

Ephedrine Tannate (Sympathomimetics tend to produce hyperglycemia and concurrent use may lead to loss of control). Products include:
  Rynatuss 2782

Epinephrine (Sympathomimetics tend to produce hyperglycemia and concurrent use may lead to loss of control). Products include:
  EPIFRIN .... ⊙ 237
  EpiPen 808
  Marcaine with Epinephrine 2446
  Primatene Mist .... ▣ 843
  Sensorcaine with Epinephrine Injection 554
  Sus-Phrine Injection 1017
  Xylocaine with Epinephrine Injections 562

Epinephrine Bitartrate (Sympathomimetics tend to produce hyperglycemia and concurrent use may lead to loss of control). Products include:
  Sensorcaine-MPF with Epinephrine Injection 554

Epinephrine Hydrochloride (Sympathomimetics tend to produce hyperglycemia and concurrent use may lead to loss of control). Products include:
  Ana-Kit Anaphylaxis Emergency Treatment Kit 611

Esmolol Hydrochloride (May potentiate hypoglycemic action). Products include:
  Brevibloc (esmolol HCl) Injection 1860

Estradiol (Estrogens tend to produce hyperglycemia and concurrent use may lead to loss of control). Products include:
  Climara Transdermal System 640
  Estrace Cream and Tablets 751
  Estraderm Transdermal System 842
  Estring Vaginal Ring 2086
  Vivelle Transdermal System 880

Estrogens, Conjugated (Estrogens tend to produce hyperglycemia and concurrent use may lead to loss of control). Products include:
  PMB 200 and PMB 400 2890
  Premarin Intravenous 2893
  Premarin Tablets 2896
  Premarin Vaginal Cream 2898
  Premphase 2900
  Prempro 2905

Estrogens, Esterified (Estrogens tend to produce hyperglycemia and concurrent use may lead to loss of control). Products include:
  ESTRATAB Tablets (0.3, 0.625, 1.25, 2.5 mg) 2715
  Estratest 2718
  Menest Tablets 2671

Estropipate (Estrogens tend to produce hyperglycemia and concurrent use may lead to loss of control). Products include:
  Ogen Tablets 2103
  Ogen Vaginal Cream 2106
  Ortho-Est 1925

Ethacrynic Acid (Diuretics tend to produce hyperglycemia and concurrent use may lead to loss of control). Products include:
  Edecrin Tablets 1698

Ethinyl Estradiol (Oral contraceptives tend to produce hyperglycemia and concurrent use may lead to loss of control). Products include:
  Brevicon 2563
  Demulen 2580
  Desogen Tablets 1867
  Levlen/Tri-Levlen 646
  Lo/Ovral Tablets 2852
  Lo/Ovral-28 Tablets 2857
  Modicon 1928
  Nordette-21 Tablets 2863
  Nordette-28 Tablets 2866
  Norinyl 2563
  Ortho-Cept 1907
  Ortho-Cyclen/Ortho-Tri-Cyclen 1914
  Ortho-Novum 1928
  Ortho-Cyclen/Ortho Tri-Cyclen 1914
  Ovcon 765
  Ovral Tablets 2877
  Ovral-28 Tablets 2878
  Levlen/Tri-Levlen 646
  Tri-Norinyl 2607
  Triphasil-21 Tablets 2919
  Triphasil-28 Tablets 2924

Ethynodiol Diacetate (Oral contraceptives tend to produce hyperglycemia and concurrent use may lead to loss of control). Products include:
  Demulen 2580

Etodolac (May potentiate hypoglycemic action). Products include:
  Lodine Capsules and Tablets 2849

Fenoprofen Calcium (May potentiate hypoglycemic action). Products include:
  Nalfon 200 Pulvules & Nalfon Tablets 933

Fludrocortisone Acetate (Corticosteroids tend to produce hyperglycemia and concurrent use may lead to loss of control). Products include:
  Florinef Acetate Tablets 506

Fluphenazine Decanoate (Phenothiazines tend to produce hyperglycemia and concurrent use may lead to loss of control). Products include:
  Prolixin Decanoate 510

Fluphenazine Enanthate (Phenothiazines tend to produce hyperglycemia and concurrent use may lead to loss of control). Products include:
  Prolixin Enanthate 510

Fluphenazine Hydrochloride (Phenothiazines tend to produce hyperglycemia and concurrent use may lead to loss of control). Products include:
  Prolixin 510

Flurbiprofen (May potentiate hypoglycemic action).
  No products indexed under this heading.

Furazolidone (May potentiate hypoglycemic action). Products include:
  Furoxone 2221

Furosemide (Diuretics tend to produce hyperglycemia and concurrent use may lead to loss of control). Products include:
  Lasix Injection, Oral Solution and Tablets 1267

Glipizide (May potentiate hypoglycemic action). Products include:
  Glucotrol Tablets 2011
  Glucotrol XL Extended Release Tablets 2012

Glyburide (May potentiate hypoglycemic action). Products include:
  DiaBeta Tablets 1265
  Glynase PresTab Tablets 2091
  Micronase Tablets 2099

Hydrochlorothiazide (Thiazides tend to produce hyperglycemia and concurrent use may lead to loss of control). Products include:
  Aldactazide Tablets 2556
  Aldoril Tablets 1644
  Apresazide Capsules 824
  Capozide Tablets 744
  Dyazide Capsules 2653
  Esidrix Tablets 839
  Esimil Tablets 840
  HydroDIURIL Tablets 1716
  Hydropres Tablets 1718
  Hyzaar Tablets 1720
  Inderide Tablets 2838
  Inderide LA Long Acting Capsules .. 2840
  Lopressor HCT Tablets 850
  Lotensin HCT Tablets 855
  Moduretic Tablets 1748
  Oretic Tablets 450
  Prinzide Tablets 1780
  Ser-Ap-Es Tablets 867
  Timolide Tablets 1791
  Vaseretic Tablets 1810
  Zestoretic Tablets 2968
  Ziac 1459

(▣ Described in PDR For Nonprescription Drugs)   (⊙ Described in PDR For Ophthalmology)

Hydrocortisone (Corticosteroids tend to produce hyperglycemia and concurrent use may lead to loss of control). Products include:
- Anusol-HC Cream 2.5% 1953
- Aquanil HC Lotion 1989
- Maximum Strength Cortaid Spray ▣ 800
- CORTENEMA 2713
- Cortisporin Ointment 1074
- Cortisporin Ophthalmic Ointment Sterile 1074
- Cortisporin Ophthalmic Suspension Sterile 1075
- Cortisporin Otic Solution Sterile .. 1076
- Cortisporin Otic Suspension Sterile 1077
- Cortizone-5 .... ▣ 795
- Cortizone-10 .... ▣ 795
- Hydrocortone Tablets 1715
- Hytone 922
- Hytone Ointment 2 ½% 923
- Massengill Medicated Soft Cloth Towelettes 2628
- Pediotic Suspension Sterile 1140
- Preparation H Hydrocortisone 1% Cream .... ▣ 843
- ProctoCream-HC 2.5% 2552
- VōSoL HC Otic Solution 2786

Hydrocortisone Acetate (Corticosteroids tend to produce hyperglycemia and concurrent use may lead to loss of control). Products include:
- Analpram-HC Rectal Cream 1% and 2.5% 993
- Anusol HC-1 Hydrocortisone Anti-Itch Ointment .... ▣ 810
- Anusol-HC Suppositories 1954
- Caldecort Anti-Itch Hydrocortisone Cream .... ▣ 651
- Coly-Mycin S Otic w/Neomycin & Hydrocortisone 1965
- Cortaid .... ▣ 800
- Cortifoam 2540
- Cortisporin Cream 1073
- Epifoam 2543
- Hydrocortone Acetate Sterile Suspension 1712
- Mantadil Cream 1124
- Nupercainal Hydrocortisone 1% Cream .... ▣ 661
- Pramosone Cream, Lotion & Ointment 995
- ProctoFoam-HC 2552
- Terra-Cortril Ophthalmic Suspension 2033

Hydrocortisone Sodium Phosphate (Corticosteroids tend to produce hyperglycemia and concurrent use may lead to loss of control). Products include:
- Hydrocortone Phosphate Injection, Sterile 1713

Hydrocortisone Sodium Succinate (Corticosteroids tend to produce hyperglycemia and concurrent use may lead to loss of control).
No products indexed under this heading.

Hydroflumethiazide (Thiazides tend to produce hyperglycemia and concurrent use may lead to loss of control). Products include:
- Diucardin Tablets 2824

Ibuprofen (May potentiate hypoglycemic action). Products include:
- Advil Cold and Sinus Caplets and Tablets .... ▣ 837
- Advil Ibuprofen Tablets, Caplets and Gel Caplets .... ▣ 836
- Children's Motrin Ibuprofen Oral Suspension 1558
- IBU Tablets 1389
- Ibuprohm 713
- Motrin IB Caplets, Tablets, and Gelcaps .... ▣ 802
- Motrin Ibuprofen Suspension, Oral Drops, Chewable Tablets, Caplets 1563
- Nuprin Ibuprofen/Analgesic Tablets & Caplets .... ▣ 645
- Vicks DayQuil SINUS Pressure & PAIN Relief with IBUPROFEN .... ▣ 735

Indapamide (Diuretics tend to produce hyperglycemia and concurrent use may lead to loss of control).
No products indexed under this heading.

Indomethacin (May potentiate hypoglycemic action). Products include:
- Indocin 1723

Indomethacin Sodium Trihydrate (May potentiate hypoglycemic action). Products include:
- Indocin I.V. 1727

Isocarboxazid (May potentiate hypoglycemic action).
No products indexed under this heading.

Isoniazid (Isoniazid tends to produce hyperglycemia and concurrent use may lead to loss of control). Products include:
- Nydrazid Injection 509
- Rifamate Capsules 1278
- Rifater 1280

Isoproterenol Hydrochloride (Sympathomimetics tend to produce hyperglycemia and concurrent use may lead to loss of control). Products include:
- Isuprel Hydrochloride Solution .. 2443
- Isuprel Injection 2441
- Isuprel Mistometer 2442

Isoproterenol Sulfate (Sympathomimetics tend to produce hyperglycemia and concurrent use may lead to loss of control). Products include:
- Norisodrine with Calcium Iodide Syrup 446

Ketoprofen (May potentiate hypoglycemic action). Products include:
- Actron Caplets and Tablets .... ▣ 608
- Orudis Capsules 2874
- Orudis KT .... ▣ 842
- Oruvail Capsules 2874

Ketorolac Tromethamine (May potentiate hypoglycemic action). Products include:
- Acular Sterile Ophthalmic Solution 470
- Toradol 2319

Labetalol Hydrochloride (May potentiate hypoglycemic action). Products include:
- Normodyne Injection 2519
- Normodyne Tablets 2522
- Trandate 1158

Levobunolol Hydrochloride (May potentiate hypoglycemic action). Products include:
- Betagan .... ⓒ 230

Levonorgestrel (Oral contraceptives tend to produce hyperglycemia and concurrent use may lead to loss of control). Products include:
- Levlen/Tri-Levlen 646
- Nordette-21 Tablets 2863
- Nordette-28 Tablets 2866
- Norplant System 2868
- Levlen/Tri-Levlen 646
- Triphasil-21 Tablets 2919
- Triphasil-28 Tablets 2924

Levothyroxine Sodium (Thyroid products tend to produce hyperglycemia and concurrent use may lead to loss of control). Products include:
- Eltroxin Tablets 2214
- Levothroid Tablets 1015
- Levothyroxine Sodium, USP for Injection 546
- Levoxyl Tablets 918
- Synthroid 1410

Liothyronine Sodium (Thyroid products tend to produce hyperglycemia and concurrent use may lead to loss of control). Products include:
- Cytomel Tablets 2647
- Triostat Injection 2708

Liotrix (Thyroid products tend to produce hyperglycemia and concurrent use may lead to loss of control).
No products indexed under this heading.

Magnesium Salicylate (May potentiate hypoglycemic action; clinical trials data indicate no evidence of significant adverse interaction with concurrent use). Products include:
- Backache Caplets .... ▣ 635
- Doan's Extra-Strength Analgesic ▣ 653
- Extra Strength Doan's P.M. ...... ▣ 653
- Doan's Regular Strength Analgesic .... ▣ 654
- Mobigesic Tablets .... ▣ 607

Meclofenamate Sodium (May potentiate hypoglycemic action).
No products indexed under this heading.

Mefenamic Acid (May potentiate hypoglycemic action). Products include:
- Ponstel 1982

Mesoridazine Besylate (Phenothiazines tend to produce hyperglycemia and concurrent use may lead to loss of control). Products include:
- Serentil 689

Mestranol (Oral contraceptives tend to produce hyperglycemia and concurrent use may lead to loss of control). Products include:
- Norinyl 2563
- Ortho-Novum 1928

Metaproterenol Sulfate (Sympathomimetics tend to produce hyperglycemia and concurrent use may lead to loss of control). Products include:
- Alupent 672
- Metaproterenol Sulfate Inhalation Solution, USP, Arm-a-Med 547

Metaraminol Bitartrate (Sympathomimetics tend to produce hyperglycemia and concurrent use may lead to loss of control). Products include:
- Aramine Injection 1649

Methotrimeprazine (Phenothiazines tend to produce hyperglycemia and concurrent use may lead to loss of control). Products include:
- Levoprome 1321

Methoxamine Hydrochloride (Sympathomimetics tend to produce hyperglycemia and concurrent use may lead to loss of control). Products include:
- Vasoxyl Injection 1169

Methyclothiazide (Thiazides tend to produce hyperglycemia and concurrent use may lead to loss of control). Products include:
- Enduron Tablets 424

Methylprednisolone Acetate (Corticosteroids tend to produce hyperglycemia and concurrent use may lead to loss of control).
No products indexed under this heading.

Methylprednisolone Sodium Succinate (Corticosteroids tend to produce hyperglycemia and concurrent use may lead to loss of control).
No products indexed under this heading.

Metipranolol Hydrochloride (May potentiate hypoglycemic action). Products include:
- OptiPranolol (Metipranolol 0.3%) Sterile Ophthalmic Solution ...... ⓒ 256

Metolazone (Diuretics tend to produce hyperglycemia and concurrent use may lead to loss of control). Products include:
- Mykrox Tablets 1617
- Zaroxolyn Tablets 1625

Metoprolol Succinate (May potentiate hypoglycemic action). Products include:
- Toprol-XL Tablets 560

Metoprolol Tartrate (May potentiate hypoglycemic action). Products include:
- Lopressor 848
- Lopressor HCT Tablets 850

Miconazole (A potential interaction between oral miconazole and oral hypoglycemic agents leading to severe hypoglycemia has been reported).
No products indexed under this heading.

Nabumetone (May potentiate hypoglycemic action). Products include:
- Relafen Tablets 2688

Nadolol (May potentiate hypoglycemic action).
No products indexed under this heading.

Naproxen (May potentiate hypoglycemic action). Products include:
- Anaprox/Naprosyn 2277

Naproxen Sodium (May potentiate hypoglycemic action). Products include:
- Aleve 2124
- Anaprox/Naprosyn 2277
- Naprelan Tablets 2861

Nicotinic Acid (Nicotinic acid tends to produce hyperglycemia and concurrent use may lead to loss of control).
No products indexed under this heading.

Norepinephrine Bitartrate (Sympathomimetics tend to produce hyperglycemia and concurrent use may lead to loss of control). Products include:
- Levophed Bitartrate Injection 2445

Norethindrone (Oral contraceptives tend to produce hyperglycemia and concurrent use may lead to loss of control). Products include:
- Brevicon 2563
- Micronor Tablets 1903
- Modicon 1928
- Norinyl 2563
- Nor-Q D Tablets 2598
- Ortho-Novum 1928
- Ovcon 765
- Tri-Norinyl 2607

Norethynodrel (Oral contraceptives tend to produce hyperglycemia and concurrent use may lead to loss of control).
No products indexed under this heading.

Norgestimate (Oral contraceptives tend to produce hyperglycemia and concurrent use may lead to loss of control). Products include:
- Ortho-Cyclen/Ortho-Tri-Cyclen .. 1914
- Ortho-Cyclen/Ortho Tri-Cyclen .. 1914

Norgestrel (Oral contraceptives tend to produce hyperglycemia and concurrent use may lead to loss of control). Products include:
- Lo/Ovral Tablets 2852
- Lo/Ovral-28 Tablets 2857
- Ovral Tablets 2877
- Ovral-28 Tablets 2878
- Ovrette Tablets 2878

Oxaprozin (May potentiate hypoglycemic action). Products include:
- Daypro Caplets 2578

Penbutolol Sulfate (May potentiate hypoglycemic action). Products include:
- Levatol Tablets 2547

Perphenazine (Phenothiazines tend to produce hyperglycemia and concurrent use may lead to loss of control). Products include:
- Etrafon 2495
- Triavil Tablets 1800
- Trilafon 2532

IMPORTANT NOTE: Always consult each drug listing in the patient's regimen for possible interactions.

Amaryl Tablets Interactions Index 50

Phenelzine Sulfate (May potentiate hypoglycemic action). Products include:
- Nardil 1977

Phenylbutazone (May potentiate hypoglycemic action).
- No products indexed under this heading.

Phenylephrine Bitartrate (Sympathomimetics tend to produce hyperglycemia and concurrent use may lead to loss of control).
- No products indexed under this heading.

Phenylephrine Hydrochloride (Sympathomimetics tend to produce hyperglycemia and concurrent use may lead to loss of control). Products include:
- Atrohist Plus Tablets 1605
- Cerose DM .... ⊞ 853
- D.A. II Tablets 972
- D.A. Chewable Tablets 970
- Dura-Vent/DA Tablets 972
- Extendryl 1003
- 4-Way Fast Acting Nasal Spray (regular & mentholated) .... ⊞ 644
- Hemorid .... ⊞ 797
- Hycomine Compound Tablets 948
- Neo-Synephrine Hydrochloride 1% Carpuject 2455
- Neo-Synephrine Hydrochloride 1% Injection 2455
- Neo-Synephrine Hydrochloride (Ophthalmic) 2456
- Neo-Synephrine .... ⊞ 624
- Novahistine Elixir .... ⊞ 782
- Phenergan VC 2886
- Phenergan VC with Codeine 2888
- Preparation H .... ⊞ 842
- Tympagesic Ear Drops 2476
- Vicks Sinex Nasal Spray and Ultra Fine Mist .... ⊞ 738

Phenylephrine Tannate (Sympathomimetics tend to produce hyperglycemia and concurrent use may lead to loss of control). Products include:
- Atrohist Pediatric Suspension 1604
- Atrohist Pediatric Suspension Dye-Free 1604
- Rynatan 2781
- Rynatuss 2782

Phenylpropanolamine Hydrochloride (Sympathomimetics tend to produce hyperglycemia and concurrent use may lead to loss of control). Products include:
- Acutrim .... ⊞ 648
- Atrohist Plus Tablets 1605
- BC Cold Powder Multi-Symptom Formula (Cold-Sinus-Allergy) .... ⊞ 631
- BC Cold Powder Non-Drowsy Formula (Cold-Sinus) .... ⊞ 631
- Cheracol Plus Head Cold/Cough Formula .... ⊞ 741
- Comtrex Multi-Symptom Cold Reliever Liqui-Gels .... ⊞ 638
- Comtrex Multi-Symptom Non-Drowsy Liqui-gels .... ⊞ 640
- Contac Continuous Action Nasal Decongestant/Antihistamine 12 Hour Capsules .... ⊞ 773
- Contac Maximum Strength Continuous Action Decongestant/Antihistamine 12 Hour Caplets .... ⊞ 772
- Contac Severe Cold and Flu Formula Caplets .... ⊞ 773
- Coricidin 'D' Decongestant Tablets .... ⊞ 760
- Dexatrim .... ⊞ 795
- Dexatrim Plus Vitamins Caplets .... ⊞ 796
- Dimetane-DC Cough Syrup 2232
- Dimetapp Allergy Sinus Caplets .... ⊞ 838
- Dimetapp Cold & Allergy Chewable Tablets .... ⊞ 838
- Dimetapp Cold & Cough Liqui-Gels .... ⊞ 839
- Dimetapp DM Elixir .... ⊞ 840
- Dimetapp Elixir .... ⊞ 840
- Dimetapp Extentabs .... ⊞ 841
- Dimetapp Tablets/Liqui-Gels .... ⊞ 841
- Dura-Vent Tablets 971
- Entex LA Tablets 972
- Exgest LA Tablets 787
- Hycomine 947
- Nolamine Timed-Release Tablets 790
- Ornade Spansule Capsules 2678
- Propagest Tablets 791
- Pyrroxate Caplets .... ⊞ 742
- Robitussin-CF .... ⊞ 846
- Sinulin Tablets 792
- Tavist-D 12 Hour Relief Tablets .... ⊞ 750
- Teldrin 12 Hour Antihistamine/Nasal Decongestant Allergy Relief Capsules .... ⊞ 786
- Triaminic Expectorant .... ⊞ 753
- Triaminic Syrup .... ⊞ 755
- Triaminic Triaminicol Cold & Cough .... ⊞ 756
- Triaminic DM Syrup .... ⊞ 756
- Triaminicin Tablets .... ⊞ 756
- Vicks DayQuil Allergy Relief 12-Hour Extended Release Tablets .... ⊞ 733
- Vicks DayQuil Allergy Relief 4-Hour Tablets .... ⊞ 733
- Vicks DayQuil SINUS Pressure & CONGESTION Relief .... ⊞ 734

Phenytoin (Phenytoin tends to produce hyperglycemia and concurrent use may lead to loss of control). Products include:
- Dilantin Infatabs 1967
- Dilantin-125 Suspension 1969

Phenytoin Sodium (Phenytoin tends to produce hyperglycemia and concurrent use may lead to loss of control). Products include:
- Dilantin Kapseals 1965

Pindolol (May potentiate hypoglycemic action). Products include:
- Visken Tablets 2428

Pirbuterol Acetate (Sympathomimetics tend to produce hyperglycemia and concurrent use may lead to loss of control). Products include:
- Maxair Autohaler 1550
- Maxair Inhaler 1552

Piroxicam (May potentiate hypoglycemic action). Products include:
- Feldene Capsules 2008

Polyestradiol Phosphate (Estrogens tend to produce hyperglycemia and concurrent use may lead to loss of control).
- No products indexed under this heading.

Polythiazide (Thiazides tend to produce hyperglycemia and concurrent use may lead to loss of control). Products include:
- Minizide Capsules 2016

Prednisolone Acetate (Corticosteroids tend to produce hyperglycemia and concurrent use may lead to loss of control). Products include:
- AK-CIDE .... ◉ 203
- AK-CIDE Ointment .... ◉ 203
- Blephamide Liquifilm Sterile Ophthalmic Suspension 472
- Blephamide Ointment .... ◉ 234
- Econopred & Econopred Plus Ophthalmic Suspensions .... ◉ 216
- Poly-Pred Liquifilm .... ◉ 246
- Pred Forte .... ◉ 247
- Pred Mild .... ◉ 250
- Pred-G Liquifilm Sterile Ophthalmic Suspension .... ◉ 248
- Pred-G S.O.P. Sterile Ophthalmic Ointment .... ◉ 249

Prednisolone Sodium Phosphate (Corticosteroids tend to produce hyperglycemia and concurrent use may lead to loss of control). Products include:
- AK-PRED .... ◉ 204
- Hydeltrasol Injection, Sterile 1708
- Pediapred Oral Solution 1618

Prednisolone Tebutate (Corticosteroids tend to produce hyperglycemia and concurrent use may lead to loss of control). Products include:
- Hydeltra-T.B.A. Sterile Suspension 1710

Prednisone (Corticosteroids tend to produce hyperglycemia and concurrent use may lead to loss of control).
- No products indexed under this heading.

Probenecid (May potentiate hypoglycemic action). Products include:
- Benemid Tablets 1651
- ColBENEMID Tablets 1662

Prochlorperazine (Phenothiazines tend to produce hyperglycemia and concurrent use may lead to loss of control). Products include:
- Compazine 2644

Promethazine Hydrochloride (Phenothiazines tend to produce hyperglycemia and concurrent use may lead to loss of control). Products include:
- Mepergan Injection 2859
- Phenergan with Codeine 2883
- Phenergan with Dextromethorphan 2885
- Phenergan Injection 2880
- Phenergan Suppositories 2882
- Phenergan Syrup 2881
- Phenergan Tablets 2882
- Phenergan VC 2886
- Phenergan VC with Codeine 2888

Propranolol Hydrochloride (Co-administration increases C_{max}, AUC, and T½ of glimepiride by 23%, 22%, and 15% respectively and it decreases CL/f by 18%; no evidence of clinically significant adverse interactions). Products include:
- Inderal 2834
- Inderal LA Long Acting Capsules 2836
- Inderide Tablets 2838
- Inderide LA Long Acting Capsules 2840

Pseudoephedrine Hydrochloride (Sympathomimetics tend to produce hyperglycemia and concurrent use may lead to loss of control). Products include:
- Actifed Allergy Daytime/Nighttime Caplets .... ⊞ 808
- Actifed Cold & Allergy Tablets .... ⊞ 807
- Actifed Cold & Sinus Caplets and Tablets .... ⊞ 808
- Actifed Sinus Daytime/Nighttime Tablets and Caplets .... ⊞ 809
- Advil Cold and Sinus Caplets and Tablets .... ⊞ 837
- Alka-Seltzer Plus Liqui-Gels .... ⊞ 612
- Alka-Seltzer Plus Flu & Body Aches Liqui-Gels Non-Drowsy Formula .... ⊞ 613
- Alka-Seltzer Plus Night-Time Cold Medicine Liqui-Gels .... ⊞ 612
- Allerest Maximum Strength .... ⊞ 649
- Allerest No Drowsiness .... ⊞ 649
- Allerest Sinus Pain Formula .... ⊞ 649
- Atrohist Pediatric Capsules 1603
- Benadryl Allergy/Cold Tablets .... ⊞ 811
- Benadryl Allergy Decongestant Liquid Medication .... ⊞ 812
- Benadryl Allergy Decongestant Tablets .... ⊞ 812
- Benadryl Allergy Sinus Headache Caplets .... ⊞ 813
- Benylin Multisymptom .... ⊞ 816
- Bromfed Capsules (Extended-Release) 1832
- Bromfed Syrup .... ⊞ 712
- Bromfed Tablets 1832
- Bromfed-DM Cough Syrup 1832
- Bromfed-PD Capsules (Extended-Release) 1832
- Children's TYLENOL Cold Multi-Symptom Chewable Tablets and Liquid 1559
- Children's TYLENOL Cold Plus Cough Multi Symptom Chewable Tablets and Liquid 1560
- Children's TYLENOL Flu Suspension Liquid 1560
- Children's Vicks DayQuil Allergy Relief .... ⊞ 730
- Children's Vicks NyQuil Cold/Cough Relief .... ⊞ 731
- Allergy-Sinus Comtrex Multi-Symptom Allergy-Sinus Formula Tablets and Caplets .... ⊞ 639
- Comtrex Multi-Symptom .... ⊞ 638
- Comtrex Multi-Symptom Non-Drowsy Caplets .... ⊞ 640
- Congess 1003
- Contac Day Allergy/Sinus Caplets ⊞ 771
- Contac Day & Night .... ⊞ 772
- Contac Night Allergy/Sinus Caplets .... ⊞ 771
- Contac Severe Cold & Flu Non-Drowsy .... ⊞ 774
- Deconsal II Tablets 1605
- Dimetane-DX Cough Syrup 2233
- Dimetapp Cold & Fever Suspension .... ⊞ 839
- Dimetapp Decongestant Pediatric Drops .... ⊞ 840
- Dorcol Children's Cough Syrup .... ⊞ 748
- Drixoral Cough + Congestion Liquid Caps .... ⊞ 763
- Dura-Tap/PD Capsules 970
- Duratuss Tablets 2750
- Duratuss HD Elixir 2750
- Efidac/24 .... ⊞ 655
- Entex PSE Tablets 973
- Fedahist Gyrocaps 2545
- Guaifed 1833
- Guaifed Syrup .... ⊞ 712
- Guaimax-D Tablets 809
- Histussin D Liquid 670
- Infants' TYLENOL Cold Decongestant & Fever-Reducer Drops 1561
- Kronofed-A 994
- Novahistine DMX .... ⊞ 782
- Nucofed 2225
- PediaCare Cough-Cold Chewable Tablets and Liquid 1569
- PediaCare Infants' Decongestant Drops 1569
- PediaCare Infants' Drops Decongestant Plus Cough 1569
- PediaCare NightRest Cough-Cold Liquid 1569
- Pediatric Vicks 44d Cough & Head Congestion Relief .... ⊞ 736
- Pediatric Vicks 44m Cough & Cold Relief .... ⊞ 737
- Robitussin Cold & Cough Liqui-Gels .... ⊞ 844
- Robitussin Cold, Cough & Flu Liqui-Gels .... ⊞ 844
- Robitussin Maximum Strength Cough & Cold .... ⊞ 847
- Robitussin Night-Time Cold Formula .... ⊞ 847
- Robitussin Pediatric Cough & Cold Formula .... ⊞ 848
- Robitussin Pediatric Drops .... ⊞ 849
- Robitussin Severe Congestion Liqui-Gels .... ⊞ 845
- Robitussin-DAC Syrup 2249
- Robitussin-PE .... ⊞ 846
- Rondec Oral Drops 974
- Rondec Syrup 974
- Rondec Tablet 974
- Rondec Chewable Tablets 974
- Rondec-TR Tablet 974
- Ryna .... ⊞ 804
- Seldane-D Extended-Release Tablets 1286
- Semprex-D Capsules 1620
- Sinarest .... ⊞ 663
- Sine-Aid Maximum Strength Sinus Headache Gelcaps, Caplets and Tablets 1570
- Sine-Off No Drowsiness Formula Caplets .... ⊞ 784
- Sine-Off Sinus Medicine .... ⊞ 784
- Singlet Tablets .... ⊞ 785
- Sinutab Non-Drying Liquid Caps .... ⊞ 823
- Sinutab Sinus Allergy Medication, Maximum Strength Tablets and Caplets .... ⊞ 823
- Sinutab Sinus Medication, Maximum Strength Without Drowsiness Formula, Tablets & Caplets .... ⊞ 824
- Sudafed Children's Cold & Cough Liquid Medication .... ⊞ 825
- Sudafed Children's Nasal Decongestant Liquid Medication .... ⊞ 826
- Sudafed Cold & Allergy Tablets .... ⊞ 826
- Sudafed Cold and Cough Liquid Caps .... ⊞ 826
- Sudafed Nasal Decongestant Tablets, 30 mg .... ⊞ 825
- Sudafed Nasal Decongestant Tablets, 60 mg .... ⊞ 825
- Sudafed Non-Drying Sinus Liquid Caps .... ⊞ 827
- Sudafed Pediatric Nasal Decongestant Liquid Oral Drops .... ⊞ 827

Interactions Index

Sudafed Severe Cold Formula Caplets 828
Sudafed Severe Cold Formula Tablets 828
Sudafed Sinus Caplets 829
Sudafed Sinus Tablets 829
Sudafed 12 Hour Caplets 824
Syn-Rx Tablets 1622
Syn-Rx DM Tablets 1623
TheraFlu Flu and Cold Medicine 750
TheraFlu Maximum Strength Flu and Cold Medicine For Sore Throat 751
TheraFlu Flu, Cold and Cough Medicine 750
TheraFlu Maximum Strength Nighttime Flu, Cold & Cough Medicine 751
TheraFlu Maximum Strength Non-Drowsy Formula Flu, Cold & Cough Medicine 751
TheraFlu Maximum Strength, Non-Drowsy Formula Flu, Cold and Cough Caplets 752
Theraflu Maximum Strength Sinus Non-Drowsy Formula Caplets 752
Triaminic AM Cough and Decongestant Formula 753
Triaminic AM Decongestant Formula 753
Triaminic Infant Oral Decongestant Drops 754
Triaminic Night Time 754
Triaminic Sore Throat Formula 755
Tussend 1830
Tussend Expectorant 1831
TYLENOL Allergy Sinus, Maximum Strength Caplets and Gelcaps 1571
TYLENOL Allergy Sinus NightTime, Maximum Strength Caplets 1571
TYLENOL Cold Medication, Multi-Symptom Formula Tablets and Caplets 1572
TYLENOL Cold Medication, Multi-Symptom Hot Liquid Packets 1572
TYLENOL Cold Medication, No Drowsiness Formula Caplets and Gelcaps 1572
TYLENOL Cold Severe Congestion Caplets 1573
TYLENOL Cough Medication with Decongestant, Multi Symptom 1574
TYLENOL Flu No Drowsiness Formula, Maximum Strength Gelcaps 1575
TYLENOL Flu NightTime, Maximum Strength Gelcaps 1575
TYLENOL Flu NightTime, Maximum Strength Hot Medication Packets 1575
TYLENOL Sinus, Maximum Strength Geltabs, Gelcaps, Caplets and Tablets 1576
Vicks 44 LiquiCaps Cough, Cold & Flu Relief 728
Vicks 44 LiquiCaps Non-Drowsy Cough & Cold Relief 729
Vicks 44D Cough & Head Congestion Relief 728
Vicks 44M Cough, Cold & Flu Relief 729
Vicks DayQuil LiquiCaps/Liquid Multi-Symptom Cold/Flu Relief 734
Vicks DayQuil SINUS Pressure & PAIN Relief with IBUPROFEN 735
Vicks Nyquil Hot Therapy 735
Vicks NyQuil LiquiCaps/Liquid Multi-Symptom Cold/Flu Relief, Original and Cherry Flavors 736

Pseudoephedrine Sulfate (Sympathomimetics tend to produce hyperglycemia and concurrent use may lead to loss of control). Products include:
Chlor-Trimeton Allergy Decongestant Tablets 759
Claritin-D Tablets 2487
Drixoral Cold and Allergy Sustained-Action Tablets 763
Drixoral Cold and Flu Extended-Release Tablets 764
Drixoral Non-Drowsy Formula Extended-Release Tablets 764
Drixoral Allergy/Sinus Extended Release Tablets 765
Trinalin Repetabs Tablets 1373

Quinestrol (Estrogens tend to produce hyperglycemia and concurrent use may lead to loss of control).
No products indexed under this heading.

Salmeterol Xinafoate (Sympathomimetics tend to produce hyperglycemia and concurrent use may lead to loss of control). Products include:
Serevent Inhalation Aerosol 1149

Salsalate (May potentiate hypoglycemic action; clinical trials data indicate no evidence of significant adverse interaction with concurrent use). Products include:
Disalcid 1549
Mono-Gesic Tablets 810
Salflex Tablets 791

Selegiline Hydrochloride (May potentiate hypoglycemic action). Products include:
Eldepryl Capsules 2729

Sotalol Hydrochloride (May potentiate hypoglycemic action). Products include:
Betapace Tablets 637

Spironolactone (Diuretics tend to produce hyperglycemia and concurrent use may lead to loss of control). Products include:
Aldactazide Tablets 2556
Aldactone Tablets 2558

Sulfacytine (May potentiate hypoglycemic action).

Sulfamethizole (May potentiate hypoglycemic action). Products include:
Urobiotic-250 Capsules 2038

Sulfamethoxazole (May potentiate hypoglycemic action). Products include:
Bactrim DS Tablets 2257
Bactrim I.V. Infusion 2255
Bactrim 2257
Gantanol Tablets 2285
Septra 1146
Septra I.V. Infusion 1142
Septra I.V. Infusion ADD-Vantage Vials 1144
Septra 1146

Sulfasalazine (May potentiate hypoglycemic action). Products include:
Azulfidine 2059

Sulfinpyrazone (May potentiate hypoglycemic action). Products include:
Anturane 823

Sulfisoxazole (May potentiate hypoglycemic action). Products include:
Gantrisin Tablets 2286

Sulfisoxazole Diolamine (May potentiate hypoglycemic action).
No products indexed under this heading.

Sulindac (May potentiate hypoglycemic action). Products include:
Clinoril Tablets 1658

Terbutaline Sulfate (Sympathomimetics tend to produce hyperglycemia and concurrent use may lead to loss of control). Products include:
Brethaire Inhaler 830
Brethine Ampuls 832
Brethine Tablets 831
Bricanyl Subcutaneous Injection 1247
Bricanyl Tablets 1248

Thioridazine Hydrochloride (Phenothiazines tend to produce hyperglycemia and concurrent use may lead to loss of control). Products include:
Mellaril 2398

Thyroglobulin (Thyroid products tend to produce hyperglycemia and concurrent use may lead to loss of control).
No products indexed under this heading.

Thyroid (Thyroid products tend to produce hyperglycemia and concurrent use may lead to loss of control).
No products indexed under this heading.

Thyroxine (Thyroid products tend to produce hyperglycemia and concurrent use may lead to loss of control).
No products indexed under this heading.

Thyroxine Sodium (Thyroid products tend to produce hyperglycemia and concurrent use may lead to loss of control).
No products indexed under this heading.

Timolol Hemihydrate (May potentiate hypoglycemic action). Products include:
Betimol 0.25%, 0.5% 259

Timolol Maleate (May potentiate hypoglycemic action). Products include:
Blocadren Tablets 1654
Timolide Tablets 1791
Timoptic in Ocudose 1796
Timoptic Sterile Ophthalmic Solution 1794
Timoptic-XE 1798

Tolazamide (May potentiate hypoglycemic action).
No products indexed under this heading.

Tolbutamide (May potentiate hypoglycemic action).
No products indexed under this heading.

Tolmetin Sodium (May potentiate hypoglycemic action). Products include:
Tolectin (200, 400 and 600 mg) .. 1591

Torsemide (Diuretics tend to produce hyperglycemia and concurrent use may lead to loss of control). Products include:
Demadex Tablets and Injection 691

Tranylcypromine Sulfate (May potentiate hypoglycemic action). Products include:
Parnate Tablets 2679

Triamcinolone (Corticosteroids tend to produce hyperglycemia and concurrent use may lead to loss of control).
No products indexed under this heading.

Triamcinolone Acetonide (Corticosteroids tend to produce hyperglycemia and concurrent use may lead to loss of control). Products include:
Azmacort Oral Inhaler 2175
Nasacort AQ Nasal Spray 2191
Nasacort Nasal Inhaler 2189

Triamcinolone Diacetate (Corticosteroids tend to produce hyperglycemia and concurrent use may lead to loss of control).
No products indexed under this heading.

Triamcinolone Hexacetonide (Corticosteroids tend to produce hyperglycemia and concurrent use may lead to loss of control).
No products indexed under this heading.

Triamterene (Diuretics tend to produce hyperglycemia and concurrent use may lead to loss of control). Products include:
Dyazide Capsules 2653
Dyrenium Capsules 2655

Trifluoperazine Hydrochloride (Phenothiazines tend to produce hyperglycemia and concurrent use may lead to loss of control). Products include:
Stelazine 2692

Warfarin Sodium (May potentiate hypoglycemic action). Products include:
Coumadin 941

Food Interactions

Meal, unspecified (When glimepiride is given with meals the mean T_{max} is slightly increased (12%) and mean C_{max} and AUC are slightly decreased).

AMBIEN TABLETS

(Zolpidem Tartrate) 2559
May interact with central nervous system depressants and certain other agents. Compounds in these categories include:

Alfentanil Hydrochloride (Potential for enhanced CNS depressant effects of zolpidem). Products include:
Alfenta Injection 1334

Alprazolam (Potential for enhanced CNS depressant effects of zolpidem). Products include:
Xanax Tablets 2115

Aprobarbital (Potential for enhanced CNS depressant effects of zolpidem).
No products indexed under this heading.

Buprenorphine (Potential for enhanced CNS depressant effects of zolpidem). Products include:
Buprenex Injectable 2170

Buspirone Hydrochloride (Potential for enhanced CNS depressant effects of zolpidem). Products include:
BuSpar Tablets 738

Butabarbital (Potential for enhanced CNS depressant effects of zolpidem).
No products indexed under this heading.

Butalbital (Potential for enhanced CNS depressant effects of zolpidem). Products include:
Axocet Capsules 2469
Esgic-plus Capsules 1012
Esgic-plus Tablets 1012
Fioricet Tablets 2386
Fioricet with Codeine Capsules 2387
Fiorinal Capsules 2388
Fiorinal with Codeine Capsules 2390
Fiorinal Tablets 2388
Phrenilin 790
Sedapap Tablets 50 mg/650 mg .. 1826

Chlordiazepoxide (Potential for enhanced CNS depressant effects of zolpidem). Products include:
Limbitrol 2333

Chlordiazepoxide Hydrochloride (Potential for enhanced CNS depressant effects of zolpidem). Products include:
Librax Capsules 2330
Librium Capsules 2331
Librium Injectable 2332

Chlorpromazine (Additive effect of decreased alertness and psychomotor performance; potential for enhanced CNS depressant effects of zolpidem). Products include:
Thorazine Suppositories 2701

Chlorpromazine Hydrochloride (Additive effect of decreased alertness and psychomotor performance; potential for enhanced CNS depressant effects of zolpidem). Products include:
Thorazine 2701

IMPORTANT NOTE: Always consult each drug listing in the patient's regimen for possible interactions.

Ambien | Interactions Index | 52

Chlorprothixene (Potential for enhanced CNS depressant effects of zolpidem).
No products indexed under this heading.

Chlorprothixene Hydrochloride (Potential for enhanced CNS depressant effects of zolpidem).
No products indexed under this heading.

Chlorprothixene Lactate (Potential for enhanced CNS depressant effects of zolpidem).
No products indexed under this heading.

Clorazepate Dipotassium (Potential for enhanced CNS depressant effects of zolpidem). Products include:
Tranxene 459

Clozapine (Potential for enhanced CNS depressant effects of zolpidem). Products include:
Clozaril Tablets 2377

Codeine Phosphate (Potential for enhanced CNS depressant effects of zolpidem). Products include:
Brontex 2130
Dimetane-DC Cough Syrup 2232
Fioricet with Codeine Capsules 2387
Fiorinal with Codeine Capsules 2390
Nucofed 2225
Phenergan with Codeine 2883
Phenergan VC with Codeine 2888
Robitussin A-C Syrup 2248
Robitussin-DAC Syrup 2249
Ryna .... ▣ 804
Soma Compound w/Codeine Tablets 2784
Tylenol with Codeine 1592

Desflurane (Potential for enhanced CNS depressant effects of zolpidem). Products include:
Suprane (desflurane, USP) 1865

Dezocine (Potential for enhanced CNS depressant effects of zolpidem). Products include:
Dalgan Injection 529

Diazepam (Potential for enhanced CNS depressant effects of zolpidem). Products include:
Dizac (diazepam injectable emulsion) CIV 1862
Valium Injectable 2336
Valium Tablets 2335

Droperidol (Potential for enhanced CNS depressant effects of zolpidem). Products include:
Inapsine Injection 462

Enflurane (Potential for enhanced CNS depressant effects of zolpidem).
No products indexed under this heading.

Estazolam (Potential for enhanced CNS depressant effects of zolpidem). Products include:
ProSom Tablets 457

Ethchlorvynol (Potential for enhanced CNS depressant effects of zolpidem). Products include:
Placidyl Capsules 456

Ethinamate (Potential for enhanced CNS depressant effects of zolpidem).
No products indexed under this heading.

Fentanyl (Potential for enhanced CNS depressant effects of zolpidem). Products include:
Duragesic Transdermal System 1336

Fentanyl Citrate (Potential for enhanced CNS depressant effects of zolpidem). Products include:
Sublimaze Injection 463

Flumazenil (Flumazenil reverses sedative/hypnotic effects of Zolpidem). Products include:
Romazicon 2311

Fluphenazine Decanoate (Potential for enhanced CNS depressant effects of zolpidem). Products include:
Prolixin Decanoate 510

Fluphenazine Enanthate (Potential for enhanced CNS depressant effects of zolpidem). Products include:
Prolixin Enanthate 510

Fluphenazine Hydrochloride (Potential for enhanced CNS depressant effects of zolpidem). Products include:
Prolixin 510

Flurazepam Hydrochloride (Potential for enhanced CNS depressant effects of zolpidem). Products include:
Dalmane Capsules 2329

Glutethimide (Potential for enhanced CNS depressant effects of zolpidem).
No products indexed under this heading.

Haloperidol (Potential for enhanced CNS depressant effects of zolpidem). Products include:
Haldol Injection, Tablets and Concentrate 1585

Haloperidol Decanoate (Potential for enhanced CNS depressant effects of zolpidem). Products include:
Haldol Decanoate 1587

Hydrocodone Bitartrate (Potential for enhanced CNS depressant effects of zolpidem). Products include:
Codiclear DH Syrup 808
Duratuss HD Elixir 2750
Histussin D Liquid 670
Hycodan Tablets and Syrup 946
Hycomine Compound Tablets 948
Hycomine 947
Hycotuss Expectorant Syrup 950
Hydrocet Capsules 787
Lorcet 10/650 Tablets 1016
Lortab 2751
Tussend 1830
Tussend Expectorant 1831
Vicodin Tablets 1404
Vicodin ES Tablets 1405
Vicodin HP Tablets 1403
Vicodin Tuss Expectorant 1406
Zydone Capsules 967

Hydrocodone Polistirex (Potential for enhanced CNS depressant effects of zolpidem). Products include:
Tussionex Pennkinetic Extended-Release Suspension 1624

Hydroxyzine Hydrochloride (Potential for enhanced CNS depressant effects of zolpidem). Products include:
Atarax Tablets & Syrup 1992
Marax Tablets & DF Syrup 2015
Vistaril Intramuscular Solution 2042

Imipramine Hydrochloride (Co-administration produces 20% decrease in peak levels of imipramine with an additive effect of decreased alertness). Products include:
Tofranil Ampuls 873
Tofranil Tablets 875

Imipramine Pamoate (Co-administration produces 20% decrease in peak levels of imipramine with an additive effect of decreased alertness). Products include:
Tofranil-PM Capsules 876

Isoflurane (Potential for enhanced CNS depressant effects of zolpidem).
No products indexed under this heading.

Ketamine Hydrochloride (Potential for enhanced CNS depressant effects of zolpidem).
No products indexed under this heading.

Levomethadyl Acetate Hydrochloride (Potential for enhanced CNS depressant effects of zolpidem). Products include:
Orlaam Oral Solution 2361

Levorphanol Tartrate (Potential for enhanced CNS depressant effects of zolpidem). Products include:
Levo-Dromoran 2297

Lorazepam (Potential for enhanced CNS depressant effects of zolpidem). Products include:
Ativan Injection 2805
Ativan Tablets 2807

Loxapine Hydrochloride (Potential for enhanced CNS depressant effects of zolpidem). Products include:
Loxitane 1426

Loxapine Succinate (Potential for enhanced CNS depressant effects of zolpidem). Products include:
Loxitane Capsules 1426

Meperidine Hydrochloride (Potential for enhanced CNS depressant effects of zolpidem). Products include:
Demerol 2438
Mepergan Injection 2859

Mephobarbital (Potential for enhanced CNS depressant effects of zolpidem). Products include:
Mebaral Tablets 2452

Meprobamate (Potential for enhanced CNS depressant effects of zolpidem). Products include:
Miltown Tablets 2780
PMB 200 and PMB 400 2890

Mesoridazine Besylate (Potential for enhanced CNS depressant effects of zolpidem). Products include:
Serentil 689

Methadone Hydrochloride (Potential for enhanced CNS depressant effects of zolpidem). Products include:
Methadone Hydrochloride Oral Concentrate 2356
Methadone Hydrochloride Oral Solution & Tablets 2357

Methohexital Sodium (Potential for enhanced CNS depressant effects of zolpidem).
No products indexed under this heading.

Methotrimeprazine (Potential for enhanced CNS depressant effects of zolpidem). Products include:
Levoprome 1321

Methoxyflurane (Potential for enhanced CNS depressant effects of zolpidem).
No products indexed under this heading.

Midazolam Hydrochloride (Potential for enhanced CNS depressant effects of zolpidem). Products include:
Versed Injection 2324

Molindone Hydrochloride (Potential for enhanced CNS depressant effects of zolpidem). Products include:
Moban Tablets and Concentrate 1036

Morphine Sulfate (Potential for enhanced CNS depressant effects of zolpidem). Products include:
Astramorph/PF Injection, USP (Preservative-Free) 526
Duramorph Injection 983
Infumorph 200 and Infumorph 500 Sterile Solutions 985
Kadian Capsules 2948
MS Contin Tablets 2149
MSIR 2152
Oramorph SR (Morphine Sulfate Sustained Release Tablets) 2359
RMS Suppositories CII 2766
Roxanol 2365

Opium Alkaloids (Potential for enhanced CNS depressant effects of zolpidem).
No products indexed under this heading.

Oxazepam (Potential for enhanced CNS depressant effects of zolpidem). Products include:
Serax Capsules 2916
Serax Tablets 2916

Oxycodone Hydrochloride (Potential for enhanced CNS depressant effects of zolpidem). Products include:
OxyContin Tablets 2163
OxyIR Capsules 2167
Percocet Tablets 955
Percodan Tablets 955
Percodan-Demi Tablets 956
Roxicodone Tablets, Oral Solution & Intensol (Oxycodone) 2366
Tylox Capsules 1593

Pentobarbital Sodium (Potential for enhanced CNS depressant effects of zolpidem). Products include:
Nembutal Sodium Capsules 440
Nembutal Sodium Solution 442
Nembutal Sodium Suppositories 444

Perphenazine (Potential for enhanced CNS depressant effects of zolpidem). Products include:
Etrafon 2495
Triavil Tablets 1800
Trilafon 2532

Phenobarbital (Potential for enhanced CNS depressant effects of zolpidem). Products include:
Arco-Lase Plus Tablets 513
Bellergal-S Tablets 2375
Donnatal 2234
Donnatal Extentabs 2234
Donnatal Tablets 2234
Phenobarbital Elixir and Tablets 1523
Quadrinal Tablets 1398

Prazepam (Potential for enhanced CNS depressant effects of zolpidem).
No products indexed under this heading.

Prochlorperazine (Potential for enhanced CNS depressant effects of zolpidem). Products include:
Compazine 2644

Promethazine Hydrochloride (Potential for enhanced CNS depressant effects of zolpidem). Products include:
Mepergan Injection 2859
Phenergan with Codeine 2883
Phenergan with Dextromethorphan 2885
Phenergan Injection 2880
Phenergan Suppositories 2882
Phenergan Syrup 2881
Phenergan Tablets 2882
Phenergan VC 2886
Phenergan VC with Codeine 2888

Propofol (Potential for enhanced CNS depressant effects of zolpidem). Products include:
Diprivan Injectable Emulsion 2939

Propoxyphene Hydrochloride (Potential for enhanced CNS depressant effects of zolpidem). Products include:
Darvon 1475
Wygesic Tablets 2930

Propoxyphene Napsylate (Potential for enhanced CNS depressant effects of zolpidem). Products include:
Darvon-N/Darvocet-N 1473

Quazepam (Potential for enhanced CNS depressant effects of zolpidem). Products include:
Doral Tablets 2773

(▣ Described in PDR For Nonprescription Drugs) (◉ Described in PDR For Ophthalmology)

Risperidone (Potential for enhanced CNS depressant effects of zolpidem). Products include:
Risperdal Tablets 1348

Secobarbital Sodium (Potential for enhanced CNS depressant effects of zolpidem). Products include:
Seconal Sodium Pulvules 1529

Sevoflurane (Potential for enhanced CNS depressant effects of zolpidem).
No products indexed under this heading.

Sufentanil Citrate (Potential for enhanced CNS depressant effects of zolpidem). Products include:
Sufenta Injection 1355

Temazepam (Potential for enhanced CNS depressant effects of zolpidem). Products include:
Restoril Capsules 2413

Thiamylal Sodium (Potential for enhanced CNS depressant effects of zolpidem).
No products indexed under this heading.

Thioridazine Hydrochloride (Potential for enhanced CNS depressant effects of zolpidem). Products include:
Mellaril 2398

Thiothixene (Potential for enhanced CNS depressant effects of zolpidem). Products include:
Navane Capsules and Concentrate ... 2018
Navane Intramuscular 2019

Triazolam (Potential for enhanced CNS depressant effects of zolpidem). Products include:
Halcion Tablets 2093

Trifluoperazine Hydrochloride (Potential for enhanced CNS depressant effects of zolpidem). Products include:
Stelazine 2692

Food Interactions

Alcohol (Co-administration produces additive effects on psychomotor performance).

Meal, unspecified (Mean AUC and C_{max} decreased by 15% and 25% respectively, while T_{max} was prolonged by 60%; for faster sleep onset, Ambien should not be administered with or immediately after meal).

AMEN TABLETS
(Medroxyprogesterone Acetate) 785
May interact with estrogens and certain other agents. Compounds in these categories include:

Aminoglutethimide (Concomitant administration may depress the bioavailability of Amen). Products include:
Cytadren Tablets 837

Chlorotrianisene (Potential for adverse effects on carbohydrate and lipid metabolism).
No products indexed under this heading.

Dienestrol (Potential for adverse effects on carbohydrate and lipid metabolism). Products include:
Ortho Dienestrol Cream 1922

Diethylstilbestrol (Potential for adverse effects on carbohydrate and lipid metabolism). Products include:
Diethylstilbestrol Tablets 1477

Estradiol (Potential for adverse effects on carbohydrate and lipid metabolism). Products include:
Climara Transdermal System 640
Estrace Cream and Tablets 751
Estraderm Transdermal System 842
Estring Vaginal Ring 2086
Vivelle Transdermal System 880

Estrogens, Conjugated (Potential for adverse effects on carbohydrate and lipid metabolism). Products include:
PMB 200 and PMB 400 2890
Premarin Intravenous 2893
Premarin Tablets 2896
Premarin Vaginal Cream 2898
Premphase 2900
Prempro 2905

Estrogens, Esterified (Potential for adverse effects on carbohydrate and lipid metabolism). Products include:
ESTRATAB Tablets (0.3, 0.625, 1.25, 2.5 mg) 2715
Estratest 2718
Menest Tablets 2671

Estropipate (Potential for adverse effects on carbohydrate and lipid metabolism). Products include:
Ogen Tablets 2103
Ogen Vaginal Cream 2106
Ortho-Est 1925

Ethinyl Estradiol (Potential for adverse effects on carbohydrate and lipid metabolism). Products include:
Brevicon 2563
Demulen 2580
Desogen Tablets 1867
Levlen/Tri-Levlen 646
Lo/Ovral Tablets 2852
Lo/Ovral-28 Tablets 2857
Modicon 1928
Nordette-21 Tablets 2863
Nordette-28 Tablets 2866
Norinyl 2563
Ortho-Cept 1907
Ortho-Cyclen/Ortho-Tri-Cyclen 1914
Ortho-Novum 1928
Ortho-Cyclen/Ortho Tri-Cyclen 1914
Ovcon 765
Ovral Tablets 2877
Ovral-28 Tablets 2878
Levlen/Tri-Levlen 646
Tri-Norinyl 2607
Triphasil-21 Tablets 2919
Triphasil-28 Tablets 2924

Polyestradiol Phosphate (Potential for adverse effects on carbohydrate and lipid metabolism).
No products indexed under this heading.

Quinestrol (Potential for adverse effects on carbohydrate and lipid metabolism).
No products indexed under this heading.

AMERICAINE ANESTHETIC LUBRICANT
(Benzocaine) 1603
None cited in PDR database.

AMERICAINE HEMORRHOIDAL OINTMENT
(Benzocaine) 649
None cited in PDR database.

AMERICAINE OTIC TOPICAL ANESTHETIC EAR DROPS
(Benzocaine) 1603
None cited in PDR database.

AMERICAINE TOPICAL ANESTHETIC FIRST AID OINTMENT
(Benzocaine) 649
None cited in PDR database.

AMERICAINE TOPICAL ANESTHETIC SPRAY
(Benzocaine) 649
None cited in PDR database.

AMICAR SYRUP, TABLETS, AND INJECTION
(Aminocaproic Acid) 1312
None cited in PDR database.

AMIKACIN SULFATE INJECTION, USP
(Amikacin Sulfate) 523
May interact with aminoglycosides, beta-lactams antibiotics, cephalosporins, neuromuscular blocking agents, anesthetics, and certain other agents. Compounds in these categories include:

Alfentanil Hydrochloride (Increased potential for neuromuscular blockade and respiratory paralysis). Products include:
Alfenta Injection 1334

Amphotericin B (Concurrent and/or sequential use may increase the potential for increased toxicity, especially nephrotoxicity or neurotoxicity). Products include:
Abelcet Injection 1540
Fungizone Intravenous 507
Fungizone Oral Suspension 704

Atracurium Besylate (Increased potential for neuromuscular blockade and respiratory paralysis). Products include:
Tracrium Injection 1155

Aztreonam (In vitro mixing may result in a significant mutual inactivation; a reduction in serum half-life or serum levels may occur when administered separately, especially in patients with severely impaired renal function). Products include:
Azactam for Injection 736

Bacitracin Zinc (Concurrent and/or sequential use may increase the potential for increased toxicity, especially nephrotoxicity or neurotoxicity). Products include:
AK-Spore Ointment 205
Betadine Brand First Aid Antibiotics & Moisturizer Ointment 2144
Cortisporin Ointment 1074
Cortisporin Ophthalmic Ointment Sterile 1074
Mycitracin 803
Neosporin Ointment 821
Neosporin Plus Maximum Strength Ointment 822
Neosporin Ophthalmic Ointment Sterile 1130
Polysporin Ointment 822
Polysporin Ophthalmic Ointment Sterile 1140
Polysporin Powder 823

Cefaclor (Co-administration of parenteral aminoglycosides with cephalosporins has resulted in increased nephrotoxicity; concomitant cephalosporins may spuriously elevate creatinine determinations). Products include:
Ceclor Pulvules & Suspension 1470

Cefadroxil (Co-administration of parenteral aminoglycosides with cephalosporins has resulted in increased nephrotoxicity; concomitant cephalosporins may spuriously elevate creatinine determinations). Products include:
Duricef Capsules, Tablets, and Oral Suspension 750

Cefamandole Nafate (Co-administration of parenteral aminoglycosides with cephalosporins has resulted in increased nephrotoxicity; concomitant cephalosporins may spuriously elevate creatinine determinations). Products include:
Mandol Vials, Faspak & ADD-Vantage 1516

Cefazolin Sodium (Co-administration of parenteral aminoglycosides with cephalosporins has resulted in increased nephrotoxicity; concomitant cephalosporins may spuriously elevate creatinine determinations). Products include:
Ancef Injection 2632
Kefzol Vials, Faspak & ADD-Vantage 1511

Cefixime (Co-administration of parenteral aminoglycosides with cephalosporins has resulted in increased nephrotoxicity; concomitant cephalosporins may spuriously elevate creatinine determinations). Products include:
Suprax 1443

Cefmetazole Sodium (Co-administration of parenteral aminoglycosides with cephalosporins has resulted in increased nephrotoxicity; concomitant cephalosporins may spuriously elevate creatinine determinations).
No products indexed under this heading.

Cefonicid Sodium (Co-administration of parenteral aminoglycosides with cephalosporins has resulted in increased nephrotoxicity; concomitant cephalosporins may spuriously elevate creatinine determinations). Products include:
Monocid Injection 2674

Cefoperazone Sodium (Co-administration of parenteral aminoglycosides with cephalosporins has resulted in increased nephrotoxicity; concomitant cephalosporins may spuriously elevate creatinine determinations). Products include:
Cefobid Intravenous/Intramuscular 1996
Cefobid Pharmacy Bulk Package - Not for Direct Infusion 1999

Ceforanide (Co-administration of parenteral aminoglycosides with cephalosporins has resulted in increased nephrotoxicity; concomitant cephalosporins may spuriously elevate creatinine determinations).
No products indexed under this heading.

Cefotaxime Sodium (Co-administration of parenteral aminoglycosides with cephalosporins has resulted in increased nephrotoxicity; concomitant cephalosporins may spuriously elevate creatinine determinations). Products include:
Claforan Sterile and Injection 1259

Cefotetan (Co-administration of parenteral aminoglycosides with cephalosporins has resulted in increased nephrotoxicity; concomitant cephalosporins may spuriously elevate creatinine determinations). Products include:
Cefotan 2936

Cefoxitin Sodium (Co-administration of parenteral aminoglycosides with cephalosporins has resulted in increased nephrotoxicity; concomitant cephalosporins may spuriously elevate creatinine determinations). Products include:
Mefoxin 1734
Mefoxin Premixed Intravenous Solution 1737

Cefpodoxime Proxetil (Co-administration of parenteral aminoglycosides with cephalosporins has resulted in increased nephrotoxicity; concomitant cephalosporins may spuriously elevate creatinine determinations). Products include:
Vantin for Oral Suspension and Vantin Tablets 2112

Cefprozil (Co-administration of parenteral aminoglycosides with cephalosporins has resulted in increased nephrotoxicity; concomitant cephalosporins may spuriously elevate creatinine determinations). Products include:
Cefzil Tablets and Oral Suspension 747

IMPORTANT NOTE: Always consult each drug listing in the patient's regimen for possible interactions.

Ceftazidime (Co-administration of parenteral aminoglycosides with cephalosporins has resulted in increased nephrotoxicity; concomitant cephalosporins may spuriously elevate creatinine determinations). Products include:

- Ceptaz 1070
- Fortaz 1092
- Tazicef for Injection 2697
- Tazidime Vials, Faspak & ADD-Vantage 1531

Ceftizoxime Sodium (Co-administration of parenteral aminoglycosides with cephalosporins has resulted in increased nephrotoxicity; concomitant cephalosporins may spuriously elevate creatinine determinations). Products include:

- Cefizox for Intramuscular or Intravenous Use 1025

Ceftriaxone Sodium (Co-administration of parenteral aminoglycosides with cephalosporins has resulted in increased nephrotoxicity; concomitant cephalosporins may spuriously elevate creatinine determinations). Products include:

- Rocephin Injectable Vials, ADD-Vantage, Galaxy Container 2305

Cefuroxime Axetil (Co-administration of parenteral aminoglycosides with cephalosporins has resulted in increased nephrotoxicity; concomitant cephalosporins may spuriously elevate creatinine determinations). Products include:

- Ceftin 1067

Cefuroxime Sodium (Co-administration of parenteral aminoglycosides with cephalosporins has resulted in increased nephrotoxicity; concomitant cephalosporins may spuriously elevate creatinine determinations). Products include:

- Kefurox Vials, Faspak & ADD-Vantage 1509
- Zinacef 1184

Cephalexin (Co-administration of parenteral aminoglycosides with cephalosporins has resulted in increased nephrotoxicity; concomitant cephalosporins may spuriously elevate creatinine determinations). Products include:

- Keflex Pulvules & Oral Suspension 930

Cephaloridine (Concurrent and/or sequential use may increase the potential for increased toxicity, especially nephrotoxicity or neurotoxicity).

Cephalothin Sodium (Co-administration of parenteral aminoglycosides with cephalosporins has resulted in increased nephrotoxicity; concomitant cephalosporins may spuriously elevate creatinine determinations).

Cephapirin Sodium (Co-administration of parenteral aminoglycosides with cephalosporins has resulted in increased nephrotoxicity; concomitant cephalosporins may spuriously elevate creatinine determinations).

No products indexed under this heading.

Cephradine (Co-administration of parenteral aminoglycosides with cephalosporins has resulted in increased nephrotoxicity; concomitant cephalosporins may spuriously elevate creatinine determinations).

No products indexed under this heading.

Chlorothiazide Sodium (When administered intravenously, diuretics may enhance aminoglycoside toxicity by altering antibiotic concentrations in serum and tissue). Products include:

- Diuril Sodium Intravenous 1693

Cilastatin Sodium (*In vitro* mixing may result in a significant mutual inactivation; a reduction in serum half-life or serum levels may occur when administered separately, especially in patients with severely impaired renal function). Products include:

- Primaxin I.M. 1770
- Primaxin I.V. 1772

Cisatracurium Besylate (Increased potential for neuromuscular blockade and respiratory paralysis). Products include:

- Nimbex Injection 1131

Cisplatin (Concurrent and/or sequential use may increase the potential for increased toxicity, especially nephrotoxicity or neurotoxicity). Products include:

- Platinol for Injection 717
- Platinol-AQ Injection 719

Colistin Sulfate (Concurrent and/or sequential use may increase the potential for increased toxicity, especially nephrotoxicity or neurotoxicity). Products include:

- Coly-Mycin S Otic w/Neomycin & Hydrocortisone 1965

Doxacurium Chloride (Increased potential for neuromuscular blockade and respiratory paralysis). Products include:

- Nuromax Injection 1136

Enflurane (Increased potential for neuromuscular blockade and respiratory paralysis).

No products indexed under this heading.

Ethacrynic Acid (Potential for increased ototoxicity; concurrent use should be avoided). Products include:

- Edecrin Tablets 1698

Fentanyl Citrate (Increased potential for neuromuscular blockade and respiratory paralysis). Products include:

- Sublimaze Injection 463

Furosemide (Potential for increased ototoxicity; concurrent use should be avoided). Products include:

- Lasix Injection, Oral Solution and Tablets 1267

Gentamicin Sulfate (Concurrent and/or sequential use may increase the potential for increased toxicity, especially nephrotoxicity or neurotoxicity). Products include:

- Garamycin Cream 0.1% 2501
- Garamycin Injectable 2502
- Garamycin Ointment 0.1% 2501
- Garamycin Ophthalmic 2501
- Genoptic Sterile Ophthalmic Solution .... ◉ 241
- Genoptic Sterile Ophthalmic Ointment .... ◉ 241
- Gentak .... ◉ 209
- Pred-G Liquifilm Sterile Ophthalmic Suspension .... ◉ 248
- Pred-G S.O.P. Sterile Ophthalmic Ointment .... ◉ 249

Halothane (Increased potential for neuromuscular blockade and respiratory paralysis). Products include:

- Fluothane 2830

Imipenem (*In vitro* mixing may result in a significant mutual inactivation; a reduction in serum half-life or serum levels may occur when administered separately, especially in patients with severely impaired renal function). Products include:

- Primaxin I.M. 1770
- Primaxin I.V. 1772

Isoflurane (Increased potential for neuromuscular blockade and respiratory paralysis).

No products indexed under this heading.

Kanamycin Sulfate (Concurrent and/or sequential use may increase the potential for increased toxicity, especially nephrotoxicity or neurotoxicity).

No products indexed under this heading.

Ketamine Hydrochloride (Increased potential for neuromuscular blockade and respiratory paralysis).

No products indexed under this heading.

Loracarbef (Co-administration of parenteral aminoglycosides with cephalosporins has resulted in increased nephrotoxicity; concomitant cephalosporins may spuriously elevate creatinine determinations). Products include:

- Lorabid Suspension and Pulvules 1513

Methohexital Sodium (Increased potential for neuromuscular blockade and respiratory paralysis).

No products indexed under this heading.

Metocurine Iodide (Increased potential for neuromuscular blockade and respiratory paralysis). Products include:

- Metubine Iodide Vials 932

Midazolam Hydrochloride (Increased potential for neuromuscular blockade and respiratory paralysis). Products include:

- Versed Injection 2324

Mivacurium Chloride (Increased potential for neuromuscular blockade and respiratory paralysis). Products include:

- Mivacron 1125

Pancuronium Bromide (Increased potential for neuromuscular blockade and respiratory paralysis).

No products indexed under this heading.

Paromomycin Sulfate (Concurrent and/or sequential use may increase the potential for increased toxicity, especially nephrotoxicity or neurotoxicity).

No products indexed under this heading.

Polymyxin B Sulfate (Concurrent and/or sequential use may increase the potential for increased toxicity, especially nephrotoxicity or neurotoxicity). Products include:

- AK-Spore .... ◉ 205
- AK-Trol Ointment & Suspension .... ◉ 205
- Betadine Brand First Aid Antibiotics & Moisturizer Ointment 2144
- Cortisporin Cream 1073
- Cortisporin Ointment 1074
- Cortisporin Ophthalmic Ointment Sterile 1074
- Cortisporin Ophthalmic Suspension Sterile 1075
- Cortisporin Otic Solution Sterile 1076
- Cortisporin Otic Suspension Sterile 1077
- Maxitrol Ophthalmic Ointment and Suspension .... ◉ 222
- Mycitracin .... ▣ 803
- Neosporin G.U. Irrigant Sterile 1130
- Neosporin Ointment .... ▣ 821
- Neosporin Plus Maximum Strength Cream .... ▣ 821
- Neosporin Plus Maximum Strength Ointment .... ▣ 822
- Neosporin Ophthalmic Ointment Sterile 1130
- Neosporin Ophthalmic Solution Sterile 1131
- Pediotic Suspension Sterile 1140
- Poly-Pred Liquifilm .... ◉ 246
- Polysporin Ointment .... ▣ 822
- Polysporin Ophthalmic Ointment Sterile 1140
- Polysporin Powder .... ▣ 823
- Polytrim Ophthalmic Solution Sterile 479
- TERAK Ointment .... ◉ 210
- Terramycin with Polymyxin B Sulfate Ophthalmic Ointment 2035

Propofol (Increased potential for neuromuscular blockade and respiratory paralysis). Products include:

- Diprivan Injectable Emulsion 2939

Rocuronium Bromide (Increased potential for neuromuscular blockade and respiratory paralysis). Products include:

- Zemuron Injection 1885

Streptomycin Sulfate (Concurrent and/or sequential use may increase the potential for increased toxicity, especially nephrotoxicity or neurotoxicity). Products include:

- Streptomycin Sulfate Injection 2031

Succinylcholine Chloride (Increased potential for neuromuscular blockade and respiratory paralysis). Products include:

- Anectine 1062

Sufentanil Citrate (Increased potential for neuromuscular blockade and respiratory paralysis). Products include:

- Sufenta Injection 1355

Thiamylal Sodium (Increased potential for neuromuscular blockade and respiratory paralysis).

No products indexed under this heading.

Tobramycin (Concurrent and/or sequential use may increase the potential for increased toxicity, especially nephrotoxicity or neurotoxicity). Products include:

- AKTOB .... ◉ 207
- TobraDex Ophthalmic Suspension and Ointment 469
- Tobrex Ophthalmic Ointment and Solution .... ◉ 226

Tobramycin Sulfate (Concurrent and/or sequential use may increase the potential for increased toxicity, especially nephrotoxicity or neurotoxicity). Products include:

- Nebcin Vials, Hyporets & ADD-Vantage 1518

Torsemide (When administered intravenously, diuretics may enhance aminoglycoside toxicity by altering antibiotic concentrations in serum and tissue). Products include:

- Demadex Tablets and Injection 691

Tubocurarine Chloride (Increased potential for neuromuscular blockade and respiratory paralysis).

No products indexed under this heading.

Vancomycin Hydrochloride (Concurrent and/or sequential use may increase the potential for increased toxicity, especially nephrotoxicity or neurotoxicity). Products include:

- Vancocin HCl, Oral Solution & Pulvules 1536
- Vancocin HCl, Vials & ADD-Vantage 1534

Vecuronium Bromide (Increased potential for neuromuscular blockade and respiratory paralysis). Products include:

- Norcuron for Injection 1875

(▣ Described in PDR For Nonprescription Drugs) (◉ Described in PDR For Ophthalmology)

Viomycin (Concurrent and/or sequential use may increase the potential for increased toxicity, especially nephrotoxicity or neurotoxicity).

AMIKACIN SULFATE INJECTION, USP
(Amikacin Sulfate) 981
May interact with aminoglycosides, anesthetics, cephalosporins, neuromuscular blocking agents, penicillins, and certain other agents. Compounds in these categories include:

Alfentanil Hydrochloride (Increased potential for neuromuscular blockade and respiratory paralysis). Products include:
Alfenta Injection 1334

Amoxicillin Trihydrate (Potential for mutual inactivation and a reduction in serum half-life may occur). Products include:
Amoxil 2631
Augmentin 2637
Augmentin Tablets 2640

Amphotericin B (Concurrent and/or sequential use may increase the potential for increased toxicity). Products include:
Abelcet Injection 1540
Fungizone Intravenous 507
Fungizone Oral Suspension 704

Ampicillin Sodium (Potential for mutual inactivation and a reduction in serum half-life may occur). Products include:
Unasyn 2035

Atracurium Besylate (Increased potential for neuromuscular blockade and respiratory paralysis). Products include:
Tracrium Injection 1155

Azlocillin Sodium (Potential for mutual inactivation and a reduction in serum half-life may occur).
No products indexed under this heading.

Bacampicillin Hydrochloride (Potential for mutual inactivation and a reduction in serum half-life may occur). Products include:
Spectrobid Tablets 2030

Bacitracin Zinc (Concurrent and/or sequential use may increase the potential for increased toxicity). Products include:
AK-Spore Ointment .... ◎ 205
Betadine Brand First Aid Antibiotics & Moisturizer Ointment ... 2144
Cortisporin Ointment 1074
Cortisporin Ophthalmic Ointment Sterile 1074
Mycitracin .... ◎■ 803
Neosporin Ointment .... ◎■ 821
Neosporin Plus Maximum Strength Ointment .... ◎■ 822
Neosporin Ophthalmic Ointment Sterile 1130
Polysporin Ointment .... ◎■ 822
Polysporin Ophthalmic Ointment Sterile 1140
Polysporin Powder .... ◎■ 823

Carbenicillin Indanyl Sodium (Potential for mutual inactivation and a reduction in serum half-life may occur). Products include:
Geocillin Tablets 2009

Cefaclor (Potential for increased nephrotoxicity and concomitant cephalosporins may spuriously elevate creatinine determinations). Products include:
Ceclor Pulvules & Suspension ... 1470

Cefadroxil (Potential for increased nephrotoxicity and concomitant cephalosporins may spuriously elevate creatinine determinations). Products include:
Duricef Capsules, Tablets, and Oral Suspension 750

Cefamandole Nafate (Potential for increased nephrotoxicity and concomitant cephalosporins may spuriously elevate creatinine determinations). Products include:
Mandol Vials, Faspak & ADD-Vantage 1516

Cefazolin Sodium (Potential for increased nephrotoxicity and concomitant cephalosporins may spuriously elevate creatinine determinations). Products include:
Ancef Injection 2632
Kefzol Vials, Faspak & ADD-Vantage 1511

Cefixime (Potential for increased nephrotoxicity and concomitant cephalosporins may spuriously elevate creatinine determinations). Products include:
Suprax 1443

Cefmetazole Sodium (Potential for increased nephrotoxicity and concomitant cephalosporins may spuriously elevate creatinine determinations).
No products indexed under this heading.

Cefonicid Sodium (Potential for increased nephrotoxicity and concomitant cephalosporins may spuriously elevate creatinine determinations). Products include:
Monocid Injection 2674

Cefoperazone Sodium (Potential for increased nephrotoxicity and concomitant cephalosporins may spuriously elevate creatinine determinations). Products include:
Cefobid Intravenous/Intramuscular 1996
Cefobid Pharmacy Bulk Package - Not for Direct Infusion 1999

Ceforanide (Potential for increased nephrotoxicity and concomitant cephalosporins may spuriously elevate creatinine determinations).
No products indexed under this heading.

Cefotaxime Sodium (Potential for increased nephrotoxicity and concomitant cephalosporins may spuriously elevate creatinine determinations). Products include:
Claforan Sterile and Injection ... 1259

Cefotetan (Potential for increased nephrotoxicity and concomitant cephalosporins may spuriously elevate creatinine determinations). Products include:
Cefotan 2936

Cefoxitin Sodium (Potential for increased nephrotoxicity and concomitant cephalosporins may spuriously elevate creatinine determinations). Products include:
Mefoxin 1734
Mefoxin Premixed Intravenous Solution 1737

Cefpodoxime Proxetil (Potential for increased nephrotoxicity and concomitant cephalosporins may spuriously elevate creatinine determinations). Products include:
Vantin for Oral Suspension and Vantin Tablets 2112

Cefprozil (Potential for increased nephrotoxicity and concomitant cephalosporins may spuriously elevate creatinine determinations). Products include:
Cefzil Tablets and Oral Suspension 747

Ceftazidime (Potential for increased nephrotoxicity and concomitant cephalosporins may spuriously elevate creatinine determinations). Products include:
Ceptaz 1070
Fortaz 1092
Tazicef for Injection 2697
Tazidime Vials, Faspak & ADD-Vantage 1531

Ceftizoxime Sodium (Potential for increased nephrotoxicity and concomitant cephalosporins may spuriously elevate creatinine determinations). Products include:
Cefizox for Intramuscular or Intravenous Use 1025

Ceftriaxone Sodium (Potential for increased nephrotoxicity and concomitant cephalosporins may spuriously elevate creatinine determinations). Products include:
Rocephin Injectable Vials, ADD-Vantage, Galaxy Container ... 2305

Cefuroxime Axetil (Potential for increased nephrotoxicity and concomitant cephalosporins may spuriously elevate creatinine determinations). Products include:
Ceftin 1067

Cefuroxime Sodium (Potential for increased nephrotoxicity and concomitant cephalosporins may spuriously elevate creatinine determinations). Products include:
Kefurox Vials, Faspak & ADD-Vantage 1509
Zinacef 1184

Cephalexin (Potential for increased nephrotoxicity and concomitant cephalosporins may spuriously elevate creatinine determinations). Products include:
Keflex Pulvules & Oral Suspension 930

Cephaloridine (Concurrent and/or sequential use may increase the potential for increased toxicity).

Cephalothin Sodium (Potential for increased nephrotoxicity and concomitant cephalosporins may spuriously elevate creatinine determinations).

Cephapirin Sodium (Potential for increased nephrotoxicity and concomitant cephalosporins may spuriously elevate creatinine determinations).
No products indexed under this heading.

Cephradine (Potential for increased nephrotoxicity and concomitant cephalosporins may spuriously elevate creatinine determinations).
No products indexed under this heading.

Cisatracurium Besylate (Increased potential for neuromuscular blockade and respiratory paralysis). Products include:
Nimbex Injection 1131

Cisplatin (Concurrent and/or sequential use may increase the potential for increased toxicity). Products include:
Platinol for Injection 717
Platinol-AQ Injection 719

Colistin Sulfate (Concurrent and/or sequential use may increase the potential for increased toxicity). Products include:
Coly-Mycin S Otic w/Neomycin & Hydrocortisone 1965

Dicloxacillin Sodium (Potential for mutual inactivation and a reduction in serum half-life may occur).
No products indexed under this heading.

Doxacurium Chloride (Increased potential for neuromuscular blockade and respiratory paralysis). Products include:
Nuromax Injection 1136

Enflurane (Increased potential for neuromuscular blockade and respiratory paralysis).
No products indexed under this heading.

Ethacrynic Acid (Potential for increased ototoxicity; concurrent use should be avoided). Products include:
Edecrin Tablets 1698

Fentanyl Citrate (Increased potential for neuromuscular blockade and respiratory paralysis). Products include:
Sublimaze Injection 463

Furosemide (Potential for increased ototoxicity; concurrent use should be avoided). Products include:
Lasix Injection, Oral Solution and Tablets 1267

Gentamicin Sulfate (Concurrent and/or sequential use may increase the potential for increased toxicity). Products include:
Garamycin Cream 0.1% 2501
Garamycin Injectable 2502
Garamycin Ointment 0.1% 2501
Garamycin Ophthalmic 2501
Genoptic Sterile Ophthalmic Solution .... ◎ 241
Genoptic Sterile Ophthalmic Ointment .... ◎ 241
Gentak .... ◎ 209
Pred-G Liquifilm Sterile Ophthalmic Suspension .... ◎ 248
Pred-G S.O.P. Sterile Ophthalmic Ointment .... ◎ 249

Halothane (Increased potential for neuromuscular blockade and respiratory paralysis). Products include:
Fluothane 2830

Isoflurane (Increased potential for neuromuscular blockade and respiratory paralysis).
No products indexed under this heading.

Kanamycin Sulfate (Concurrent and/or sequential use may increase the potential for increased toxicity).
No products indexed under this heading.

Ketamine Hydrochloride (Increased potential for neuromuscular blockade and respiratory paralysis).
No products indexed under this heading.

Lithium Carbonate (Increased potential for neuromuscular blockade and respiratory paralysis). Products include:
Eskalith 2658
Lithium Carbonate Capsules & Tablets 2352
Lithonate/Lithotabs/Lithobid ... 2721

Lithium Citrate (Increased potential for neuromuscular blockade and respiratory paralysis).
No products indexed under this heading.

Loracarbef (Potential for increased nephrotoxicity and concomitant cephalosporins may spuriously elevate creatinine determinations). Products include:
Lorabid Suspension and Pulvules 1513

Methohexital Sodium (Increased potential for neuromuscular blockade and respiratory paralysis).
No products indexed under this heading.

Metocurine Iodide (Increased potential for neuromuscular blockade and respiratory paralysis). Products include:
Metubine Iodide Vials 932

IMPORTANT NOTE: Always consult each drug listing in the patient's regimen for possible interactions.

Mezlocillin Sodium (Potential for mutual inactivation and a reduction in serum half-life may occur). Products include:

Mezlin ... 594
Mezlin Pharmacy Bulk Package ... 597

Midazolam Hydrochloride (Increased potential for neuromuscular blockade and respiratory paralysis). Products include:

Versed Injection ... 2324

Mivacurium Chloride (Increased potential for neuromuscular blockade and respiratory paralysis). Products include:

Mivacron ... 1125

Nafcillin Sodium (Potential for mutual inactivation and a reduction in serum half-life may occur).

No products indexed under this heading.

Pancuronium Bromide (Increased potential for neuromuscular blockade and respiratory paralysis).

No products indexed under this heading.

Paromomycin Sulfate (Concurrent and/or sequential use may increase the potential for increased toxicity).

No products indexed under this heading.

Penicillin G Benzathine (Potential for mutual inactivation and a reduction in serum half-life may occur). Products include:

Bicillin C-R Injection ... 2810
Bicillin C-R 900/300 Injection ... 2812
Bicillin L-A Injection ... 2813

Penicillin G Potassium (Potential for mutual inactivation and a reduction in serum half-life may occur). Products include:

Pfizerpen for Injection ... 2022

Penicillin G Procaine (Potential for mutual inactivation and a reduction in serum half-life may occur). Products include:

Bicillin C-R Injection ... 2810
Bicillin C-R 900/300 Injection ... 2812

Penicillin G Sodium (Potential for mutual inactivation and a reduction in serum half-life may occur).

No products indexed under this heading.

Penicillin V Potassium (Potential for mutual inactivation and a reduction in serum half-life may occur). Products include:

Pen•Vee K ... 2879

Polymyxin B Sulfate (Concurrent and/or sequential use may increase the potential for increased toxicity). Products include:

AK-Spore ... ⊙ 205
AK-Trol Ointment & Suspension ... ⊙ 205
Betadine Brand First Aid Antibiotics & Moisturizer Ointment ... 2144
Cortisporin Cream ... 1073
Cortisporin Ointment ... 1074
Cortisporin Ophthalmic Ointment Sterile ... 1074
Cortisporin Ophthalmic Suspension Sterile ... 1075
Cortisporin Otic Solution Sterile ... 1076
Cortisporin Otic Suspension Sterile 1077
Maxitrol Ophthalmic Ointment and Suspension ... ⊙ 222
Mycitracin ... ▣ 803
Neosporin G.U. Irrigant Sterile ... 1130
Neosporin Ointment ... ▣ 821
Neosporin Plus Maximum Strength Cream ... ▣ 821
Neosporin Plus Maximum Strength Ointment ... ▣ 822
Neosporin Ophthalmic Ointment Sterile ... 1130
Neosporin Ophthalmic Solution Sterile ... 1131
Pediotic Suspension Sterile ... 1140
Poly-Pred Liquifilm ... ⊙ 246
Polysporin Ointment ... ▣ 822
Polysporin Ophthalmic Ointment Sterile ... 1140
Polysporin Powder ... ▣ 823
Polytrim Ophthalmic Solution Sterile ... 479
TERAK Ointment ... ⊙ 210
Terramycin with Polymyxin B Sulfate Ophthalmic Ointment ... 2035

Propofol (Increased potential for neuromuscular blockade and respiratory paralysis). Products include:

Diprivan Injectable Emulsion ... 2939

Rocuronium Bromide (Increased potential for neuromuscular blockade and respiratory paralysis). Products include:

Zemuron Injection ... 1885

Streptomycin Sulfate (Concurrent and/or sequential use may increase the potential for increased toxicity). Products include:

Streptomycin Sulfate Injection ... 2031

Succinylcholine Chloride (Increased potential for neuromuscular blockade and respiratory paralysis). Products include:

Anectine ... 1062

Sufentanil Citrate (Increased potential for neuromuscular blockade and respiratory paralysis). Products include:

Sufenta Injection ... 1355

Thiamylal Sodium (Increased potential for neuromuscular blockade and respiratory paralysis).

No products indexed under this heading.

Ticarcillin Disodium (Potential for mutual inactivation and a reduction in serum half-life may occur). Products include:

Ticar for Injection ... 2704
Timentin for Injection ... 2706

Tobramycin (Concurrent and/or sequential use may increase the potential for increased toxicity). Products include:

AKTOB ... ⊙ 207
TobraDex Ophthalmic Suspension and Ointment ... 469
Tobrex Ophthalmic Ointment and Solution ... ⊙ 226

Tobramycin Sulfate (Concurrent and/or sequential use may increase the potential for increased toxicity). Products include:

Nebcin Vials, Hyporets & ADD-Vantage ... 1518

Tubocurarine Chloride (Increased potential for neuromuscular blockade and respiratory paralysis).

No products indexed under this heading.

Vancomycin Hydrochloride (Concurrent and/or sequential use may increase the potential for increased toxicity). Products include:

Vancocin HCl, Oral Solution & Pulvules ... 1536
Vancocin HCl, Vials & ADD-Vantage ... 1534

Vecuronium Bromide (Increased potential for neuromuscular blockade and respiratory paralysis). Products include:

Norcuron for Injection ... 1875

Viomycin (Concurrent and/or sequential use may increase the potential for increased toxicity).

AMIKIN INJECTABLE

(Amikacin Sulfate) ... 502

May interact with aminoglycosides, cephalosporins, penicillins, neuromuscular blocking agents, anesthetics, and certain other agents. Compounds in these categories include:

Alfentanil Hydrochloride (Increased potential for neuromuscular blockade and respiratory paralysis). Products include:

Alfenta Injection ... 1334

Amoxicillin Trihydrate (Potential for mutual inactivation and a reduction in serum half-life may occur). Products include:

Amoxil ... 2631
Augmentin ... 2637
Augmentin Tablets ... 2640

Amphotericin B (Concurrent and/or sequential use may increase the potential for increased toxicity). Products include:

Abelcet Injection ... 1540
Fungizone Intravenous ... 507
Fungizone Oral Suspension ... 704

Ampicillin Sodium (Potential for mutual inactivation and a reduction in serum half-life may occur). Products include:

Unasyn ... 2035

Atracurium Besylate (Increased potential for neuromuscular blockade and respiratory paralysis). Products include:

Tracrium Injection ... 1155

Azlocillin Sodium (Potential for mutual inactivation and a reduction in serum half-life may occur).

No products indexed under this heading.

Bacampicillin Hydrochloride (Potential for mutual inactivation and a reduction in serum half-life may occur). Products include:

Spectrobid Tablets ... 2030

Bacitracin Zinc (Concurrent and/or sequential use may increase the potential for increased toxicity). Products include:

AK-Spore Ointment ... ⊙ 205
Betadine Brand First Aid Antibiotics & Moisturizer Ointment ... 2144
Cortisporin Ointment ... 1074
Cortisporin Ophthalmic Ointment Sterile ... 1074
Mycitracin ... ▣ 803
Neosporin Ointment ... ▣ 821
Neosporin Plus Maximum Strength Ointment ... ▣ 822
Neosporin Ophthalmic Ointment Sterile ... 1130
Polysporin Ointment ... ▣ 822
Polysporin Ophthalmic Ointment Sterile ... 1140
Polysporin Powder ... ▣ 823

Carbenicillin Indanyl Sodium (Potential for mutual inactivation and a reduction in serum half-life may occur). Products include:

Geocillin Tablets ... 2009

Cefaclor (Potential for increased nephrotoxicity and concomitant cephalosporins may spuriously elevate creatinine determinations). Products include:

Ceclor Pulvules & Suspension ... 1470

Cefadroxil (Potential for increased nephrotoxicity and concomitant cephalosporins may spuriously elevate creatinine determinations). Products include:

Duricef Capsules, Tablets, and Oral Suspension ... 750

Cefamandole Nafate (Potential for increased nephrotoxicity and concomitant cephalosporins may spuriously elevate creatinine determinations). Products include:

Mandol Vials, Faspak & ADD-Vantage ... 1516

Cefazolin Sodium (Potential for increased nephrotoxicity and concomitant cephalosporins may spuriously elevate creatinine determinations). Products include:

Ancef Injection ... 2632
Kefzol Vials, Faspak & ADD-Vantage ... 1511

Cefixime (Potential for increased nephrotoxicity and concomitant cephalosporins may spuriously elevate creatinine determinations). Products include:

Suprax ... 1443

Cefmetazole Sodium (Potential for increased nephrotoxicity and concomitant cephalosporins may spuriously elevate creatinine determinations).

No products indexed under this heading.

Cefonicid Sodium (Potential for increased nephrotoxicity and concomitant cephalosporins may spuriously elevate creatinine determinations). Products include:

Monocid Injection ... 2674

Cefoperazone Sodium (Potential for increased nephrotoxicity and concomitant cephalosporins may spuriously elevate creatinine determinations). Products include:

Cefobid Intravenous/Intramuscular 1996
Cefobid Pharmacy Bulk Package - Not for Direct Infusion ... 1999

Ceforanide (Potential for increased nephrotoxicity and concomitant cephalosporins may spuriously elevate creatinine determinations).

No products indexed under this heading.

Cefotaxime Sodium (Potential for increased nephrotoxicity and concomitant cephalosporins may spuriously elevate creatinine determinations). Products include:

Claforan Sterile and Injection ... 1259

Cefotetan (Potential for increased nephrotoxicity and concomitant cephalosporins may spuriously elevate creatinine determinations). Products include:

Cefotan ... 2936

Cefoxitin Sodium (Potential for increased nephrotoxicity and concomitant cephalosporins may spuriously elevate creatinine determinations). Products include:

Mefoxin ... 1734
Mefoxin Premixed Intravenous Solution ... 1737

Cefpodoxime Proxetil (Potential for increased nephrotoxicity and concomitant cephalosporins may spuriously elevate creatinine determinations). Products include:

Vantin for Oral Suspension and Vantin Tablets ... 2112

Cefprozil (Potential for increased nephrotoxicity and concomitant cephalosporins may spuriously elevate creatinine determinations). Products include:

Cefzil Tablets and Oral Suspension 747

Ceftazidime (Potential for increased nephrotoxicity and concomitant cephalosporins may spuriously elevate creatinine determinations). Products include:

Ceptaz ... 1070
Fortaz ... 1092
Tazicef for Injection ... 2697
Tazidime Vials, Faspak & ADD-Vantage ... 1531

(▣ Described in PDR For Nonprescription Drugs) (⊙ Described in PDR For Ophthalmology)

Interactions Index — Aminohippurate Sodium

Ceftizoxime Sodium (Potential for increased nephrotoxicity and concomitant cephalosporins may spuriously elevate creatinine determinations). Products include:
Cefizox for Intramuscular or Intravenous Use 1025

Ceftriaxone Sodium (Potential for increased nephrotoxicity and concomitant cephalosporins may spuriously elevate creatinine determinations). Products include:
Rocephin Injectable Vials, ADD-Vantage, Galaxy Container 2305

Cefuroxime Axetil (Potential for increased nephrotoxicity and concomitant cephalosporins may spuriously elevate creatinine determinations). Products include:
Ceftin 1067

Cefuroxime Sodium (Potential for increased nephrotoxicity and concomitant cephalosporins may spuriously elevate creatinine determinations). Products include:
Kefurox Vials, Faspak & ADD-Vantage 1509
Zinacef 1184

Cephalexin (Potential for increased nephrotoxicity and concomitant cephalosporins may spuriously elevate creatinine determinations). Products include:
Keflex Pulvules & Oral Suspension 930

Cephaloridine (Concurrent and/or sequential use may increase the potential for increased toxicity).

Cephalothin Sodium (Potential for increased nephrotoxicity and concomitant cephalosporins may spuriously elevate creatinine determinations).

Cephapirin Sodium (Potential for increased nephrotoxicity and concomitant cephalosporins may spuriously elevate creatinine determinations).
No products indexed under this heading.

Cephradine (Potential for increased nephrotoxicity and concomitant cephalosporins may spuriously elevate creatinine determinations).
No products indexed under this heading.

Cisatracurium Besylate (Increased potential for neuromuscular blockade and respiratory paralysis). Products include:
Nimbex Injection 1131

Cisplatin (Concurrent and/or sequential use may increase the potential for increased toxicity). Products include:
Platinol for Injection 717
Platinol-AQ Injection 719

Colistin Sulfate (Concurrent and/or sequential use may increase the potential for increased toxicity). Products include:
Coly-Mycin S Otic w/Neomycin & Hydrocortisone 1965

Dicloxacillin Sodium (Potential for mutual inactivation and a reduction in serum half-life may occur).
No products indexed under this heading.

Doxacurium Chloride (Increased potential for neuromuscular blockade and respiratory paralysis). Products include:
Nuromax Injection 1136

Enflurane (Increased potential for neuromuscular blockade and respiratory paralysis).
No products indexed under this heading.

Ethacrynic Acid (Potential for increased ototoxicity; concurrent use should be avoided). Products include:
Edecrin Tablets 1698

Fentanyl Citrate (Increased potential for neuromuscular blockade and respiratory paralysis). Products include:
Sublimaze Injection 463

Furosemide (Potential for increased ototoxicity; concurrent use should be avoided). Products include:
Lasix Injection, Oral Solution and Tablets 1267

Gentamicin Sulfate (Concurrent and/or sequential use may increase the potential for increased toxicity). Products include:
Garamycin Cream 0.1% 2501
Garamycin Injectable 2502
Garamycin Ointment 0.1% 2501
Garamycin Ophthalmic 2501
Genoptic Sterile Ophthalmic Solution .... ⊙ 241
Genoptic Sterile Ophthalmic Ointment .... ⊙ 241
Gentak .... ⊙ 209
Pred-G Liquifilm Sterile Ophthalmic Suspension .... ⊙ 248
Pred-G S.O.P. Sterile Ophthalmic Ointment .... ⊙ 249

Halothane (Increased potential for neuromuscular blockade and respiratory paralysis). Products include:
Fluothane 2830

Isoflurane (Increased potential for neuromuscular blockade and respiratory paralysis).
No products indexed under this heading.

Kanamycin Sulfate (Concurrent and/or sequential use may increase the potential for increased toxicity).
No products indexed under this heading.

Ketamine Hydrochloride (Increased potential for neuromuscular blockade and respiratory paralysis).
No products indexed under this heading.

Lithium Carbonate (Increased potential for neuromuscular blockade and respiratory paralysis). Products include:
Eskalith 2658
Lithium Carbonate Capsules & Tablets 2352
Lithonate/Lithotabs/Lithobid 2721

Lithium Citrate (Increased potential for neuromuscular blockade and respiratory paralysis).
No products indexed under this heading.

Loracarbef (Potential for increased nephrotoxicity and concomitant cephalosporins may spuriously elevate creatinine determinations). Products include:
Lorabid Suspension and Pulvules 1513

Methohexital Sodium (Increased potential for neuromuscular blockade and respiratory paralysis).
No products indexed under this heading.

Metocurine Iodide (Increased potential for neuromuscular blockade and respiratory paralysis). Products include:
Metubine Iodide Vials 932

Mezlocillin Sodium (Potential for mutual inactivation and a reduction in serum half-life may occur). Products include:
Mezlin 594
Mezlin Pharmacy Bulk Package 597

Midazolam Hydrochloride (Increased potential for neuromuscular blockade and respiratory paralysis). Products include:
Versed Injection 2324

Mivacurium Chloride (Increased potential for neuromuscular blockade and respiratory paralysis). Products include:
Mivacron 1125

Nafcillin Sodium (Potential for mutual inactivation and a reduction in serum half-life may occur).
No products indexed under this heading.

Pancuronium Bromide (Increased potential for neuromuscular blockade and respiratory paralysis).
No products indexed under this heading.

Paromomycin Sulfate (Concurrent and/or sequential use may increase the potential for increased toxicity).
No products indexed under this heading.

Penicillin G Benzathine (Potential for mutual inactivation and a reduction in serum half-life may occur). Products include:
Bicillin C-R Injection 2810
Bicillin C-R 900/300 Injection 2812
Bicillin L-A Injection 2813

Penicillin G Potassium (Potential for mutual inactivation and a reduction in serum half-life may occur). Products include:
Pfizerpen for Injection 2022

Penicillin G Procaine (Potential for mutual inactivation and a reduction in serum half-life may occur). Products include:
Bicillin C-R Injection 2810
Bicillin C-R 900/300 Injection 2812

Penicillin G Sodium (Potential for mutual inactivation and a reduction in serum half-life may occur).
No products indexed under this heading.

Penicillin V Potassium (Potential for mutual inactivation and a reduction in serum half-life may occur). Products include:
Pen•Vee K 2879

Polymyxin B Sulfate (Concurrent and/or sequential use may increase the potential for increased toxicity). Products include:
AK-Spore .... ⊙ 205
AK-Trol Ointment & Suspension .... ⊙ 205
Betadine Brand First Aid Antibiotics & Moisturizer Ointment ... 2144
Cortisporin Cream 1073
Cortisporin Ointment 1074
Cortisporin Ophthalmic Ointment Sterile 1074
Cortisporin Ophthalmic Suspension Sterile 1075
Cortisporin Otic Solution Sterile 1076
Cortisporin Otic Suspension Sterile 1077
Maxitrol Ophthalmic Ointment and Suspension .... ⊙ 222
Mycitracin .... ⊙ 803
Neosporin G.U. Irrigant Sterile 1130
Neosporin Ointment .... ⊙ 821
Neosporin Plus Maximum Strength Cream .... ⊙ 821
Neosporin Plus Maximum Strength Ointment .... ⊙ 822
Neosporin Ophthalmic Ointment Sterile 1130
Neosporin Ophthalmic Solution Sterile 1131
Pediotic Suspension Sterile 1140
Poly-Pred Liquifilm .... ⊙ 246
Polysporin Ointment .... ⊙ 822
Polysporin Ophthalmic Ointment Sterile 1140
Polysporin Powder .... ⊙ 823
Polytrim Ophthalmic Solution Sterile 479
TERAK Ointment .... ⊙ 210

Terramycin with Polymyxin B Sulfate Ophthalmic Ointment 2035

Propofol (Increased potential for neuromuscular blockade and respiratory paralysis). Products include:
Diprivan Injectable Emulsion ... 2939

Rocuronium Bromide (Increased potential for neuromuscular blockade and respiratory paralysis). Products include:
Zemuron Injection 1885

Streptomycin Sulfate (Concurrent and/or sequential use may increase the potential for increased toxicity). Products include:
Streptomycin Sulfate Injection 2031

Succinylcholine Chloride (Increased potential for neuromuscular blockade and respiratory paralysis). Products include:
Anectine 1062

Sufentanil Citrate (Increased potential for neuromuscular blockade and respiratory paralysis). Products include:
Sufenta Injection 1355

Thiamylal Sodium (Increased potential for neuromuscular blockade and respiratory paralysis).
No products indexed under this heading.

Ticarcillin Disodium (Potential for mutual inactivation and a reduction in serum half-life may occur). Products include:
Ticar for Injection 2704
Timentin for Injection 2706

Tobramycin (Concurrent and/or sequential use may increase the potential for increased toxicity). Products include:
AKTOB .... ⊙ 207
TobraDex Ophthalmic Suspension and Ointment 469
Tobrex Ophthalmic Ointment and Solution .... ⊙ 226

Tobramycin Sulfate (Concurrent and/or sequential use may increase the potential for increased toxicity). Products include:
Nebcin Vials, Hyporets & ADD-Vantage 1518

Tubocurarine Chloride (Increased potential for neuromuscular blockade and respiratory paralysis).
No products indexed under this heading.

Vancomycin Hydrochloride (Concurrent and/or sequential use may increase the potential for increased toxicity). Products include:
Vancocin HCl, Oral Solution & Pulvules 1536
Vancocin HCl, Vials & ADD-Vantage 1534

Vecuronium Bromide (Increased potential for neuromuscular blockade and respiratory paralysis). Products include:
Norcuron for Injection 1875

Viomycin (Concurrent and/or sequential use may increase the potential for increased toxicity).

AMINO-CERV
(Urea, Benzalkonium Chloride, L-Cystine, Sodium Propionate, Methionine, Inositol) 1827
None cited in PDR database.

AMINOHIPPURATE SODIUM INJECTION
(Aminohippurate Sodium) 1646
May interact with sulfonamides and certain other agents. Compounds in these categories include:

Bendroflumethiazide (Renal clearance measurements impaired).

IMPORTANT NOTE: Always consult each drug listing in the patient's regimen for possible interactions.

Aminohippurate Sodium — Interactions Index

No products indexed under this heading.

Chlorothiazide (Renal clearance measurements impaired). Products include:
- Aldoclor Tablets 1638
- Diupres Tablets 1691
- Diuril Oral 1694

Chlorothiazide Sodium (Renal clearance measurements impaired). Products include:
- Diuril Sodium Intravenous 1693

Chlorpropamide (Renal clearance measurements impaired). Products include:
- Diabinese Tablets 2002

Glipizide (Renal clearance measurements impaired). Products include:
- Glucotrol Tablets 2011
- Glucotrol XL Extended Release Tablets 2012

Glyburide (Renal clearance measurements impaired). Products include:
- DiaBeta Tablets 1265
- Glynase PresTab Tablets 2091
- Micronase Tablets 2099

Hydrochlorothiazide (Renal clearance measurements impaired). Products include:
- Aldactazide Tablets 2556
- Aldoril Tablets 1644
- Apresazide Capsules 824
- Capozide Tablets 744
- Dyazide Capsules 2653
- Esidrix Tablets 839
- Esimil Tablets 840
- HydroDIURIL Tablets 1716
- Hydropres Tablets 1718
- Hyzaar Tablets 1720
- Inderide Tablets 2838
- Inderide LA Long Acting Capsules .. 2840
- Lopressor HCT Tablets 850
- Lotensin HCT Tablets 855
- Moduretic Tablets 1748
- Oretic Tablets 450
- Prinzide Tablets 1780
- Ser-Ap-Es Tablets 867
- Timolide Tablets 1791
- Vaseretic Tablets 1810
- Zestoretic Tablets 2968
- Ziac 1459

Hydroflumethiazide (Renal clearance measurements impaired). Products include:
- Diucardin Tablets 2824

Methyclothiazide (Renal clearance measurements impaired). Products include:
- Enduron Tablets 424

Polythiazide (Renal clearance measurements impaired). Products include:
- Minizide Capsules 2016

Probenecid (Tubular secretion of PAH depressed). Products include:
- Benemid Tablets 1651
- ColBENEMID Tablets 1662

Procaine Hydrochloride (Renal clearance measurements impaired). Products include:
- Novocain Hydrochloride for Spinal Anesthesia 2457

Sulfamethizole (Renal clearance measurements impaired). Products include:
- Urobiotic-250 Capsules 2038

Sulfamethoxazole (Renal clearance measurements impaired). Products include:
- Bactrim DS Tablets 2257
- Bactrim I.V. Infusion 2255
- Bactrim 2257
- Gantanol Tablets 2285
- Septra 1146
- Septra I.V. Infusion 1142
- Septra I.V. Infusion ADD-Vantage Vials 1144
- Septra 1146

Sulfasalazine (Renal clearance measurements impaired). Products include:
- Azulfidine 2059

Sulfinpyrazone (Renal clearance measurements impaired). Products include:
- Anturane 823

Sulfisoxazole (Renal clearance measurements impaired). Products include:
- Gantrisin Tablets 2286

Sulfisoxazole Diolamine (Renal clearance measurements impaired). No products indexed under this heading.

Tolazamide (Renal clearance measurements impaired). No products indexed under this heading.

Tolbutamide (Renal clearance measurements impaired). No products indexed under this heading.

AMINOPLEX CAPSULES (Amino Acid Preparations) ... 2749
None cited in PDR database.

AMINOTATE CAPSULES (Amino Acid Preparations) ... 2749
None cited in PDR database.

AMOXIL CAPSULES AND CHEWABLE TABLETS (Amoxicillin Trihydrate) 2631
May interact with:

Probenecid (Concurrent administration delays excretion of amoxicillin). Products include:
- Benemid Tablets 1651
- ColBENEMID Tablets 1662

AMOXIL PEDIATRIC DROPS, POWDER FOR ORAL SUSPENSION (Amoxicillin Trihydrate) 2631
See Amoxil Capsules and Chewable Tablets

AMPHOJEL SUSPENSION (Aluminum Hydroxide Gel) 2802
May interact with tetracyclines. Compounds in this category include:

Demeclocycline Hydrochloride (Concurrent administration should be avoided). Products include:
- Declomycin Tablets 1421

Doxycycline Calcium (Concurrent administration should be avoided). Products include:
- Vibramycin Calcium Oral Suspension Syrup 2038

Doxycycline Hyclate (Concurrent administration should be avoided). Products include:
- Doryx Capsules 1970
- Vibramycin Hyclate Capsules 2038
- Vibramycin Hyclate Intravenous .. 2040
- Vibra-Tabs Film Coated Tablets .. 2038

Doxycycline Monohydrate (Concurrent administration should be avoided). Products include:
- Monodox Capsules 1858
- Vibramycin Monohydrate for Oral Suspension 2038

Methacycline Hydrochloride (Concurrent administration should be avoided). No products indexed under this heading.

Minocycline Hydrochloride (Concurrent administration should be avoided). Products include:
- DYNACIN Capsules 1627
- Minocin Intravenous 1428
- Minocin Oral Suspension 1431
- Minocin Pellet-Filled Capsules .. 1429

Oxytetracycline (Concurrent administration should be avoided). Products include:
- Terramycin Intramuscular Solution 2034

Oxytetracycline Hydrochloride (Concurrent administration should be avoided). Products include:
- TERAK Ointment .... ⊙ 210
- Terra-Cortril Ophthalmic Suspension 2033
- Terramycin with Polymyxin B Sulfate Ophthalmic Ointment 2035
- Urobiotic-250 Capsules 2038

Prescription Drugs, unspecified (Effect resulting from coadministration not specified).

Tetracycline Hydrochloride (Concurrent administration should be avoided). Products include:
- Achromycin V Capsules 1417
- Helidac Therapy 2135

AMPHOJEL SUSPENSION WITHOUT FLAVOR (Aluminum Hydroxide Gel) 2802
See Amphojel Suspension

AMPHOJEL TABLETS (Aluminum Hydroxide Gel) 2802
See Amphojel Suspension

ANAFRANIL CAPSULES (Clomipramine Hydrochloride) 819
May interact with sympathomimetics, anticholinergics, central nervous system depressants, monoamine oxidase inhibitors, barbiturates, thyroid preparations, quinidine, phenothiazines, antidepressant drugs, and certain other agents. Compounds in these categories include:

Albuterol (Due to structural similarity to other tricyclic antidepressants, concurrent use requires close supervision). Products include:
- Proventil Inhalation Aerosol 2524
- Ventolin Inhalation Aerosol and Refill 1170

Albuterol Sulfate (Due to structural similarity to other tricyclic antidepressants, concurrent use requires close supervision). Products include:
- Airet Albuterol Sulfate Inhalation Solution 1602
- Albuterol Sulfate, USP Solution for Inhalation, Arm-a-Med 522
- Proventil Inhalation Solution 0.083% 2527
- Proventil Repetabs Tablets 2529
- Proventil Solution for Inhalation 0.5% 2525
- Proventil Syrup 2528
- Proventil Tablets 2529
- Ventolin Inhalation Solution 1171
- Ventolin Nebules Inhalation Solution 1172
- Ventolin Rotacaps for Inhalation 1173
- Ventolin Syrup 1175
- Ventolin Tablets 1176
- Volmax Extended-Release Tablets .. 1835

Alfentanil Hydrochloride (Co-administration may exaggerate patient's response to CNS depressants). Products include:
- Alfenta Injection 1334

Alprazolam (Co-administration may exaggerate patient's response to CNS depressants). Products include:
- Xanax Tablets 2115

Amitriptyline Hydrochloride (Many antidepressants are substrates for P450 2D6 and may make normal metabolizers resemble poor metabolizers resulting in higher than expected plasma levels of tricyclic antidepressants). Products include:
- Elavil 2945
- Etrafon 2495
- Limbitrol 2333

- Triavil Tablets 1800

Amoxapine (Many antidepressants are substrates for P450 2D6 and may make normal metabolizers resemble poor metabolizers resulting in higher than expected plasma levels of tricyclic antidepressants). Products include:
- Asendin Tablets 1419

Aprobarbital (Co-administration may exaggerate patient's response to CNS depressants; plasma levels of several closely related tricyclic antidepressants have been decreased by the concomitant hepatic enzyme inducers, such as barbiturates).
No products indexed under this heading.

Atropine Sulfate (Clomipramine has anticholinergic properties; concurrent use requires close supervision). Products include:
- Arco-Lase Plus Tablets 513
- Atrohist Plus Tablets 1605
- Donnatal 2234
- Donnatal Extentabs 2234
- Donnatal Tablets 2234
- Lomotil 2591
- Motofen Tablets 789
- Urised Tablets 2123

Belladonna Alkaloids (Clomipramine has anticholinergic properties; concurrent use requires close supervision). Products include:
- Bellergal-S Tablets 2375
- Hyland's Bedwetting Tablets ... ⊡ 788
- Hyland's EnurAid Tablets ...... ⊡ 789
- Hyland's Headache Tablets ..... ⊡ 790
- Hyland's Teething Tablets ..... ⊡ 790
- Similasan Eye Drops #1 .... ⊡ 769

Benztropine Mesylate (Clomipramine has anticholinergic properties; concurrent use requires close supervision). Products include:
- Cogentin 1661

Biperiden Hydrochloride (Clomipramine has anticholinergic properties; concurrent use requires close supervision). Products include:
- Akineton 1380

Buprenorphine (Co-administration may exaggerate patient's response to CNS depressants). Products include:
- Buprenex Injectable 2170

Bupropion Hydrochloride (Many antidepressants are substrates for P450 2D6 and may make normal metabolizers resemble poor metabolizers resulting in higher than expected plasma levels of tricyclic antidepressants). Products include:
- Wellbutrin Tablets 1177

Buspirone Hydrochloride (Co-administration may exaggerate patient's response to CNS depressants). Products include:
- BuSpar Tablets 738

Butabarbital (Co-administration may exaggerate patient's response to CNS depressants; plasma levels of several closely related tricyclic antidepressants have been decreased by the concomitant hepatic enzyme inducers, such as barbiturates).
No products indexed under this heading.

Butalbital (Co-administration may exaggerate patient's response to CNS depressants; plasma levels of several closely related tricyclic antidepressants have been decreased by the concomitant hepatic enzyme inducers, such as barbiturates). Products include:
- Axocet Capsules 2469
- Esgic-plus Capsules 1012
- Esgic-plus Tablets 1012
- Fioricet Tablets 2386
- Fioricet with Codeine Capsules .. 2387

(⊡ Described in PDR For Nonprescription Drugs)   (⊙ Described in PDR For Ophthalmology)

Fiorinal Capsules 2388
Fiorinal with Codeine Capsules 2390
Fiorinal Tablets 2388
Phrenilin 790
Sedapap Tablets 50 mg/650 mg .. 1826

Chlordiazepoxide (Co-administration may exaggerate patient's response to CNS depressants). Products include:
Limbitrol 2333

Chlordiazepoxide Hydrochloride (Co-administration may exaggerate patient's response to CNS depressants). Products include:
Librax Capsules 2330
Librium Capsules 2331
Librium Injectable 2332

Chlorpromazine (Phenothiazines are substrates for P450 2D6 and may make normal metabolizers resemble poor metabolizers resulting in higher than expected plasma levels of tricyclic antidepressants; co-administration may exaggerate patient's response to CNS depressants). Products include:
Thorazine Suppositories 2701

Chlorpromazine Hydrochloride (Phenothiazines are substrates for P450 2D6 and may make normal metabolizers resemble poor metabolizers resulting in higher than expected plasma levels of tricyclic antidepressants; co-administration may exaggerate patient's response to CNS depressants). Products include:
Thorazine 2701

Chlorprothixene (Co-administration may exaggerate patient's response to CNS depressants).
No products indexed under this heading.

Chlorprothixene Hydrochloride (Co-administration may exaggerate patient's response to CNS depressants).
No products indexed under this heading.

Chlorprothixene Lactate (Co-administration may exaggerate patient's response to CNS depressants).
No products indexed under this heading.

Cimetidine (Plasma levels of several closely related tricyclic antidepressants have been reported to be increased by co-administration of hepatic enzyme inhibitors, such as cimetidine). Products include:
Tagamet HB Tablets 786
Tagamet Tablets 2694

Cimetidine Hydrochloride (Plasma levels of several closely related tricyclic antidepressants have been reported to be increased by co-administration of hepatic enzyme inhibitors, such as cimetidine). Products include:
Tagamet 2694

Clidinium Bromide (Clomipramine has anticholinergic properties; concurrent use requires close supervision). Products include:
Librax Capsules 2330

Clonidine (Due to structural similarity to other tricyclic antidepressants, pharmacological effects of clonidine may be blocked). Products include:
Catapres-TTS 680

Clonidine Hydrochloride (Due to structural similarity to other tricyclic antidepressants, pharmacological effects of clonidine may be blocked). Products include:
Catapres Tablets 679

Combipres Tablets 682

Clorazepate Dipotassium (Co-administration may exaggerate patient's response to CNS depressants). Products include:
Tranxene 459

Clozapine (Co-administration may exaggerate patient's response to CNS depressants). Products include:
Clozaril Tablets 2377

Codeine Phosphate (Co-administration may exaggerate patient's response to CNS depressants). Products include:
Brontex 2130
Dimetane-DC Cough Syrup 2232
Fioricet with Codeine Capsules 2387
Fiorinal with Codeine Capsules 2390
Nucofed 2225
Phenergan with Codeine 2883
Phenergan VC with Codeine 2888
Robitussin A-C Syrup 2248
Robitussin-DAC Syrup 2249
Ryna 804
Soma Compound w/Codeine Tablets 2784
Tylenol with Codeine 1592

Desflurane (Co-administration may exaggerate patient's response to CNS depressants). Products include:
Suprane (desflurane, USP) 1865

Desipramine Hydrochloride (Many antidepressants are substrates for P450 2D6 and may make normal metabolizers resemble poor metabolizers resulting in higher than expected plasma levels of tricyclic antidepressants). Products include:
Norpramin Tablets 1273

Dezocine (Co-administration may exaggerate patient's response to CNS depressants). Products include:
Dalgan Injection 529

Diazepam (Co-administration may exaggerate patient's response to CNS depressants). Products include:
Dizac (diazepam injectable emulsion) CIV 1862
Valium Injectable 2336
Valium Tablets 2335

Dicyclomine Hydrochloride (Clomipramine has anticholinergic properties; concurrent use requires close supervision). Products include:
Bentyl 1246

Digoxin (Clomipramine is highly protein bound, and co-administration with digoxin, another highly protein bound drug, may cause an increase in plasma concentrations of either drug, potentially resulting in adverse effects). Products include:
Lanoxicaps 1110
Lanoxin Elixir Pediatric 1113
Lanoxin Injection 1116
Lanoxin Injection Pediatric 1119
Lanoxin Tablets 1121

Dobutamine Hydrochloride (Due to structural similarity to other tricyclic antidepressants, concurrent use requires close supervision). Products include:
Dobutrex Solution Vials 1480

Dopamine Hydrochloride (Due to structural similarity to other tricyclic antidepressants, concurrent use requires close supervision).
No products indexed under this heading.

Doxepin Hydrochloride (Many antidepressants are substrates for P450 2D6 and may make normal metabolizers resemble poor metabolizers resulting in higher than expected plasma levels of tricyclic antidepressants). Products include:
Adapin Capsules 1542

Sinequan 2028
Zonalon Cream 1042

Droperidol (Co-administration may exaggerate patient's response to CNS depressants). Products include:
Inapsine Injection 462

Enflurane (Co-administration may exaggerate patient's response to CNS depressants).
No products indexed under this heading.

Ephedrine Hydrochloride ().
Products include:
Primatene Tablets 844
Quadrinal Tablets 1398

Ephedrine Sulfate (Due to structural similarity to other tricyclic antidepressants, concurrent use requires close supervision). Products include:
Marax Tablets & DF Syrup 2015

Ephedrine Tannate (Due to structural similarity to other tricyclic antidepressants, concurrent use requires close supervision). Products include:
Rynatuss 2782

Epinephrine (Due to structural similarity to other tricyclic antidepressants, concurrent use requires close supervision). Products include:
EPIFRIN 237
EpiPen 808
Marcaine with Epinephrine 2446
Primatene Mist 843
Sensorcaine with Epinephrine Injection 554
Sus-Phrine Injection 1017
Xylocaine with Epinephrine Injections 562

Epinephrine Bitartrate (Due to structural similarity to other tricyclic antidepressants, concurrent use requires close supervision). Products include:
Sensorcaine-MPF with Epinephrine Injection 554

Epinephrine Hydrochloride (Due to structural similarity to other tricyclic antidepressants, concurrent use requires close supervision). Products include:
Ana-Kit Anaphylaxis Emergency Treatment Kit 611

Estazolam (Co-administration may exaggerate patient's response to CNS depressants). Products include:
ProSom Tablets 457

Ethchlorvynol (Co-administration may exaggerate patient's response to CNS depressants). Products include:
Placidyl Capsules 456

Ethinamate (Co-administration may exaggerate patient's response to CNS depressants).
No products indexed under this heading.

Fentanyl (Co-administration may exaggerate patient's response to CNS depressants). Products include:
Duragesic Transdermal System 1336

Fentanyl Citrate (Co-administration may exaggerate patient's response to CNS depressants). Products include:
Sublimaze Injection 463

Flecainide Acetate (Type 1C antiarrhythmics, such as flecainide, are substrates for P450 2D6 and may make normal metabolizers resemble poor metabolizers resulting in higher than expected plasma levels of tricyclic antidepressants). Products include:
Tambocor Tablets 1555

Fluoxetine Hydrochloride (Plasma levels of several closely related tricyclic antidepressants have been reported to be increased by co-administration of hepatic enzyme inhibitors, such as fluoxetine; due to long half-life of fluoxetine, at least 5 weeks should elapse before initiating TCA treatment in a patient being withdrawn from fluoxetine). Products include:
Prozac Pulvules & Liquid, Oral Solution 935

Fluphenazine Decanoate (Phenothiazines are substrates for P450 2D6 and may make normal metabolizers resemble poor metabolizers resulting in higher than expected plasma levels of tricyclic antidepressants; co-administration may exaggerate patient's response to CNS depressants). Products include:
Prolixin Decanoate 510

Fluphenazine Enanthate (Phenothiazines are substrates for P450 2D6 and may make normal metabolizers resemble poor metabolizers resulting in higher than expected plasma levels of tricyclic antidepressants; co-administration may exaggerate patient's response to CNS depressants). Products include:
Prolixin Enanthate 510

Fluphenazine Hydrochloride (Phenothiazines are substrates for P450 2D6 and may make normal metabolizers resemble poor metabolizers resulting in higher than expected plasma levels of tricyclic antidepressants; co-administration may exaggerate patient's response to CNS depressants). Products include:
Prolixin 510

Flurazepam Hydrochloride (Co-administration may exaggerate patient's response to CNS depressants). Products include:
Dalmane Capsules 2329

Fosphenytoin Sodium (Plasma levels of several closely related tricyclic antidepressants have been decreased by the concomitant hepatic enzyme inducers, such as phenytoin). Products include:
Cerebyx Injection 1956

Furazolidone (Clomipramine should not be given in combination, or within 14 days before or after treatment with an MAO inhibitor; hyperpyretic crisis, seizures, coma, and death have been reported in patients receiving such combinations). Products include:
Furoxone 2221

Glutethimide (Co-administration may exaggerate patient's response to CNS depressants).
No products indexed under this heading.

Glycopyrrolate (Clomipramine has anticholinergic properties; concurrent use requires close supervision). Products include:
Robinul Forte Tablets 2247
Robinul Injectable 2247
Robinul Tablets 2247

Guanadrel Sulfate (Due to structural similarity to other tricyclic antidepressants, pharmacological effects of guanadrel may be blocked). Products include:
Hylorel Tablets 1613

IMPORTANT NOTE: Always consult each drug listing in the patient's regimen for possible interactions.

Anafranil / Interactions Index

Guanethidine Monosulfate (Due to structural similarity to other tricyclic antidepressants, pharmacological effects of guanethidine may be blocked). Products include:
- Esimil Tablets 840
- Ismelin Tablets 845

Haloperidol (Concurrent use increases plasma concentrations of clomipramine; co-administration may exaggerate patient's response to CNS depressants). Products include:
- Haldol Injection, Tablets and Concentrate 1585

Haloperidol Decanoate (Concurrent use increases plasma concentrations of clomipramine; co-administration may exaggerate patient's response to CNS depressants). Products include:
- Haldol Decanoate 1587

Hydrocodone Bitartrate (Co-administration may exaggerate patient's response to CNS depressants). Products include:
- Codiclear DH Syrup 808
- Duratuss HD Elixir 2750
- Histussin D Liquid 670
- Hycodan Tablets and Syrup 946
- Hycomine Compound Tablets 948
- Hycomine 947
- Hycotuss Expectorant Syrup 950
- Hydrocet Capsules 787
- Lorcet 10/650 Tablets 1016
- Lortab 2751
- Tussend 1830
- Tussend Expectorant 1831
- Vicodin Tablets 1404
- Vicodin ES Tablets 1405
- Vicodin HP Tablets 1403
- Vicodin Tuss Expectorant 1406
- Zydone Capsules 967

Hydrocodone Polistirex (Co-administration may exaggerate patient's response to CNS depressants). Products include:
- Tussionex Pennkinetic Extended-Release Suspension 1624

Hydromorphone Hydrochloride (Co-administration may exaggerate patient's response to CNS depressants). Products include:
- Dilaudid Ampuls 1382
- Dilaudid Cough Syrup 1383
- Dilaudid-HP Injection 1384
- Dilaudid-HP Lyophilized Powder 250 mg 1384
- Dilaudid 1382
- Dilaudid Oral Liquid 1386
- Dilaudid 1382
- Dilaudid Tablets - 8 mg 1386

Hydroxyzine Hydrochloride (Co-administration may exaggerate patient's response to CNS depressants). Products include:
- Atarax Tablets & Syrup 1992
- Marax Tablets & DF Syrup 2015
- Vistaril Intramuscular Solution 2042

Hyoscyamine (Clomipramine has anticholinergic properties; concurrent use requires close supervision). Products include:
- Cystospaz Tablets 2123
- Urised Tablets 2123

Hyoscyamine Sulfate (Clomipramine has anticholinergic properties; concurrent use requires close supervision). Products include:
- Arco-Lase Plus Tablets 513
- Atrohist Plus Tablets 1605
- Cystospaz-M Capsules 2123
- Donnatal 2234
- Donnatal Extentabs 2234
- Donnatal Tablets 2234
- Kutrase Capsules 2546
- Levsin/Levsinex/Levbid 2549

Imipramine Hydrochloride (Many antidepressants are substrates for P450 2D6 and may make normal metabolizers resemble poor metabolizers resulting in higher than expected plasma levels of tricyclic antidepressants). Products include:
- Tofranil Ampuls 873
- Tofranil Tablets 875

Imipramine Pamoate (Many antidepressants are substrates for P450 2D6 and may make normal metabolizers resemble poor metabolizers resulting in higher than expected plasma levels of tricyclic antidepressants). Products include:
- Tofranil-PM Capsules 876

Ipratropium Bromide (Clomipramine has anticholinergic properties; concurrent use requires close supervision). Products include:
- Atrovent Inhalation Aerosol 674
- Atrovent Inhalation Solution 675
- Atrovent Nasal Spray 0.03% 676
- Atrovent Nasal Spray 0.06% 678

Isocarboxazid (Clomipramine should not be given in combination, or within 14 days before or after treatment with an MAO inhibitor; hyperpyretic crisis, seizures, coma, and death have been reported in patients receiving such combinations).
- No products indexed under this heading.

Isoflurane (Co-administration may exaggerate patient's response to CNS depressants).
- No products indexed under this heading.

Isoproterenol Hydrochloride (Due to structural similarity to other tricyclic antidepressants, concurrent use requires close supervision). Products include:
- Isuprel Hydrochloride Solution 2443
- Isuprel Injection 2441
- Isuprel Mistometer 2442

Isoproterenol Sulfate (Due to structural similarity to other tricyclic antidepressants, concurrent use requires close supervision). Products include:
- Norisodrine with Calcium Iodide Syrup 446

Ketamine Hydrochloride (Co-administration may exaggerate patient's response to CNS depressants).
- No products indexed under this heading.

Levomethadyl Acetate Hydrochloride (Co-administration may exaggerate patient's response to CNS depressants). Products include:
- Orlaam Oral Solution 2361

Levorphanol Tartrate (Co-administration may exaggerate patient's response to CNS depressants). Products include:
- Levo-Dromoran 2297

Levothyroxine Sodium (Co-administration increases the possibility of cardiac toxicity). Products include:
- Eltroxin Tablets 2214
- Levothroid Tablets 1015
- Levothyroxine Sodium, USP for Injection 546
- Levoxyl Tablets 918
- Synthroid 1410

Liothyronine Sodium (Co-administration increases the possibility of cardiac toxicity). Products include:
- Cytomel Tablets 2647
- Triostat Injection 2708

Liotrix (Co-administration increases the possibility of cardiac toxicity).
- No products indexed under this heading.

Lorazepam (Co-administration may exaggerate patient's response to CNS depressants). Products include:
- Ativan Injection 2805
- Ativan Tablets 2807

Loxapine Hydrochloride (Co-administration may exaggerate patient's response to CNS depressants). Products include:
- Loxitane 1426

Loxapine Succinate (Co-administration may exaggerate patient's response to CNS depressants). Products include:
- Loxitane Capsules 1426

Maprotiline Hydrochloride (Many antidepressants are substrates for P450 2D6 and may make normal metabolizers resemble poor metabolizers resulting in higher than expected plasma levels of tricyclic antidepressants). Products include:
- Ludiomil Tablets 861

Mepenzolate Bromide (Clomipramine has anticholinergic properties; concurrent use requires close supervision).
- No products indexed under this heading.

Meperidine Hydrochloride (Co-administration may exaggerate patient's response to CNS depressants). Products include:
- Demerol 2438
- Mepergan Injection 2859

Mephobarbital (Co-administration may exaggerate patient's response to CNS depressants; plasma levels of several closely related tricyclic antidepressants have been decreased by the concomitant hepatic enzyme inducers, such as barbiturates). Products include:
- Mebaral Tablets 2452

Meprobamate (Co-administration may exaggerate patient's response to CNS depressants). Products include:
- Miltown Tablets 2780
- PMB 200 and PMB 400 2890

Mesoridazine Besylate (Phenothiazines are substrates for P450 2D6 and may make normal metabolizers resemble poor metabolizers resulting in higher than expected plasma levels of tricyclic antidepressants; co-administration may exaggerate patient's response to CNS depressants). Products include:
- Serentil 689

Metaproterenol Sulfate (Due to structural similarity to other tricyclic antidepressants, concurrent use requires close supervision). Products include:
- Alupent 672
- Metaproterenol Sulfate Inhalation Solution, USP, Arm-a-Med 547

Metaraminol Bitartrate (Due to structural similarity to other tricyclic antidepressants, concurrent use requires close supervision). Products include:
- Aramine Injection 1649

Methadone Hydrochloride (Co-administration may exaggerate patient's response to CNS depressants). Products include:
- Methadone Hydrochloride Oral Concentrate 2356
- Methadone Hydrochloride Oral Solution & Tablets 2357

Methohexital Sodium (Co-administration may exaggerate patient's response to CNS depressants).
- No products indexed under this heading.

Methotrimeprazine (Phenothiazines are substrates for P450 2D6 and may make normal metabolizers resemble poor metabolizers resulting in higher than expected plasma levels of tricyclic antidepressants; co-administration may exaggerate patient's response to CNS depressants). Products include:
- Levoprome 1321

Methoxamine Hydrochloride (Due to structural similarity to other tricyclic antidepressants, concurrent use requires close supervision). Products include:
- Vasoxyl Injection 1169

Methoxyflurane (Co-administration may exaggerate patient's response to CNS depressants).
- No products indexed under this heading.

Methylphenidate Hydrochloride (Plasma levels of several closely related tricyclic antidepressants have been increased by the co-administration). Products include:
- Ritalin 866

Midazolam Hydrochloride (Co-administration may exaggerate patient's response to CNS depressants). Products include:
- Versed Injection 2324

Mirtazapine (Many antidepressants are substrates for P450 2D6 and may make normal metabolizers resemble poor metabolizers resulting in higher than expected plasma levels of tricyclic antidepressants). Products include:
- Remeron Tablets 1878

Molindone Hydrochloride (Co-administration may exaggerate patient's response to CNS depressants). Products include:
- Moban Tablets and Concentrate 1036

Morphine Sulfate (Co-administration may exaggerate patient's response to CNS depressants). Products include:
- Astramorph/PF Injection, USP (Preservative-Free) 526
- Duramorph Injection 983
- Infumorph 200 and Infumorph 500 Sterile Solutions 985
- Kadian Capsules 2948
- MS Contin Tablets 2149
- MSIR 2152
- Oramorph SR (Morphine Sulfate Sustained Release Tablets) 2359
- RMS Suppositories CII 2766
- Roxanol 2365

Nefazodone Hydrochloride (Many antidepressants are substrates for P450 2D6 and may make normal metabolizers resemble poor metabolizers resulting in higher than expected plasma levels of tricyclic antidepressants). Products include:
- Serzone Tablets 776

Norepinephrine Bitartrate (Due to structural similarity to other tricyclic antidepressants, concurrent use requires close supervision). Products include:
- Levophed Bitartrate Injection 2445

(■ Described in PDR For Nonprescription Drugs) (◆ Described in PDR For Ophthalmology)

Nortriptyline Hydrochloride (Many antidepressants are substrates for P450 2D6 and may make normal metabolizers resemble poor metabolizers resulting in higher than expected plasma levels of tricyclic antidepressants). Products include:

Pamelor 2409

Opium Alkaloids (Co-administration may exaggerate patient's response to CNS depressants).

No products indexed under this heading.

Oxazepam (Co-administration may exaggerate patient's response to CNS depressants). Products include:

Serax Capsules 2916
Serax Tablets 2916

Oxybutynin Chloride (Clomipramine has anticholinergic properties; concurrent use requires close supervision). Products include:

Ditropan 1267

Oxycodone Hydrochloride (Co-administration may exaggerate patient's response to CNS depressants). Products include:

OxyContin Tablets 2163
OxyIR Capsules 2167
Percocet Tablets 955
Percodan Tablets 955
Percodan-Demi Tablets 956
Roxicodone Tablets, Oral Solution & Intensol (Oxycodone) 2366
Tylox Capsules 1593

Paroxetine Hydrochloride (Selective serotonin reuptake inhibitors, such as sertraline, may have variable extent of inhibition of P450 2D6; potential for higher than expected plasma levels of tricyclic antidepressants). Products include:

Paxil Tablets 2681

Pentobarbital Sodium (Co-administration may exaggerate patient's response to CNS depressants; plasma levels of several closely related tricyclic antidepressants have been decreased by the concomitant hepatic enzyme inducers, such as barbiturates). Products include:

Nembutal Sodium Capsules 440
Nembutal Sodium Solution 442
Nembutal Sodium Suppositories 444

Perphenazine (Phenothiazines are substrates for P450 2D6 and may make normal metabolizers resemble poor metabolizers resulting in higher than expected plasma levels of tricyclic antidepressants; co-administration may exaggerate patient's response to CNS depressants). Products include:

Etrafon 2495
Triavil Tablets 1800
Trilafon 2532

Phenelzine Sulfate (Clomipramine should not be given in combination, or within 14 days before or after treatment with an MAO inhibitor; hyperpyretic crisis, seizures, coma, and death have been reported in patients receiving such combinations). Products include:

Nardil 1977

Phenobarbital (Concurrent use increases plasma concentrations of phenobarbital; co-administration may exaggerate patient's response to CNS depressants; plasma levels of several closely related tricyclic antidepressants have been decreased by the concomitant hepatic enzyme inducers, such as barbiturates). Products include:

Arco-Lase Plus Tablets 513
Bellergal-S Tablets 2375
Donnatal 2234
Donnatal Extentabs 2234
Donnatal Tablets 2234
Phenobarbital Elixir and Tablets 1523
Quadrinal Tablets 1398

Phenylephrine Bitartrate (Due to structural similarity to other tricyclic antidepressants, concurrent use requires close supervision).

No products indexed under this heading.

Phenylephrine Hydrochloride (Due to structural similarity to other tricyclic antidepressants, concurrent use requires close supervision). Products include:

Atrohist Plus Tablets 1605
Cerose DM 853
D.A. II Tablets 972
D.A. Chewable Tablets 970
Dura-Vent/DA Tablets 972
Extendryl 1003
4-Way Fast Acting Nasal Spray (regular & mentholated) 644
Hemorid 797
Hycomine Compound Tablets 948
Neo-Synephrine Hydrochloride 1% Carpuject 2455
Neo-Synephrine Hydrochloride 1% Injection 2455
Neo-Synephrine Hydrochloride (Ophthalmic) 2456
Neo-Synephrine 624
Novahistine Elixir 782
Phenergan VC 2886
Phenergan VC with Codeine 2888
Preparation H 842
Tympagesic Ear Drops 2476
Vicks Sinex Nasal Spray and Ultra Fine Mist 738

Phenylephrine Tannate (Due to structural similarity to other tricyclic antidepressants, concurrent use requires close supervision). Products include:

Atrohist Pediatric Suspension 1604
Atrohist Pediatric Suspension Dye-Free 1604
Rynatan 2781
Rynatuss 2782

Phenylpropanolamine Hydrochloride (Due to structural similarity to other tricyclic antidepressants, concurrent use requires close supervision). Products include:

Acutrim 648
Atrohist Plus Tablets 1605
BC Cold Powder Multi-Symptom Formula (Cold-Sinus-Allergy) 631
BC Cold Powder Non-Drowsy Formula (Cold-Sinus) 631
Cheracol Plus Head Cold/Cough Formula 741
Comtrex Multi-Symptom Cold Reliever Liqui-Gels 638
Comtrex Multi-Symptom Non-Drowsy Liqui-gels 640
Contac Continuous Action Nasal Decongestant/Antihistamine 12 Hour Capsules 773
Contac Maximum Strength Continuous Action Decongestant/Antihistamine 12 Hour Caplets 772
Contac Severe Cold and Flu Formula Caplets 773
Coricidin 'D' Decongestant Tablets 760
Dexatrim 795
Dexatrim Plus Vitamins Caplets 796
Dimetane-DC Cough Syrup 2232
Dimetapp Allergy Sinus Caplets 838
Dimetapp Cold & Allergy Chewable Tablets 838
Dimetapp Cold & Cough Liqui-Gels 839
Dimetapp DM Elixir 840
Dimetapp Elixir 840
Dimetapp Extentabs 841
Dimetapp Tablets/Liqui-Gels 841
Dura-Vent Tablets 971
Entex LA Tablets 972
Exgest LA Tablets 787
Hycomine 947
Nolamine Timed-Release Tablets 790
Ornade Spansule Capsules 2678
Propagest Tablets 791
Pyrroxate Caplets 742
Robitussin-CF 846
Sinulin Tablets 792
Tavist-D 12 Hour Relief Tablets 750
Teldrin 12 Hour Antihistamine/Nasal Decongestant Allergy Relief Capsules 786
Triaminic Expectorant 753
Triaminic Syrup 755
Triaminic Triaminicol Cold & Cough 756
Triaminic DM Syrup 756
Triaminicin Tablets 756
Vicks DayQuil Allergy Relief 12-Hour Extended Release Tablets 733
Vicks DayQuil Allergy Relief 4-Hour Tablets 733
Vicks DayQuil SINUS Pressure & CONGESTION Relief 734

Phenytoin (Plasma levels of several closely related tricyclic antidepressants have been decreased by the concomitant hepatic enzyme inducers, such as phenytoin). Products include:

Dilantin Infatabs 1967
Dilantin-125 Suspension 1969

Phenytoin Sodium (Plasma levels of several closely related tricyclic antidepressants have been decreased by the concomitant hepatic enzyme inducers, such as phenytoin). Products include:

Dilantin Kapseals 1965

Pirbuterol Acetate (Due to structural similarity to other tricyclic antidepressants, concurrent use requires close supervision). Products include:

Maxair Autohaler 1550
Maxair Inhaler 1552

Prazepam (Co-administration may exaggerate patient's response to CNS depressants).

No products indexed under this heading.

Prochlorperazine (Phenothiazines are substrates for P450 2D6 and may make normal metabolizers resemble poor metabolizers resulting in higher than expected plasma levels of tricyclic antidepressants; co-administration may exaggerate patient's response to CNS depressants). Products include:

Compazine 2644

Procyclidine Hydrochloride (Clomipramine has anticholinergic properties; concurrent use requires close supervision). Products include:

Kemadrin Tablets 1105

Promethazine Hydrochloride (Phenothiazines are substrates for P450 2D6 and may make normal metabolizers resemble poor metabolizers resulting in higher than expected plasma levels of tricyclic antidepressants; co-administration may exaggerate patient's response to CNS depressants). Products include:

Mepergan Injection 2859
Phenergan with Codeine 2883
Phenergan with Dextromethorphan 2885
Phenergan Injection 2880
Phenergan Suppositories 2882
Phenergan Syrup 2881
Phenergan Tablets 2882
Phenergan VC 2886
Phenergan VC with Codeine 2888

Propafenone Hydrochloride (Type 1C antiarrhythmics, such as propafenone, are substrates for P450 2D6 and may make normal metabolizers resemble poor metabolizers resulting in higher than expected plasma levels of tricyclic antidepressants). Products include:

Rythmol Tablets–150mg, 225mg, 300mg 1399

Propantheline Bromide (Clomipramine has anticholinergic properties; concurrent use requires close supervision). Products include:

Pro-Banthine Tablets 2226

Propofol (Co-administration may exaggerate patient's response to CNS depressants). Products include:

Diprivan Injectable Emulsion 2939

Propoxyphene Hydrochloride (Co-administration may exaggerate patient's response to CNS depressants). Products include:

Darvon 1475
Wygesic Tablets 2930

Propoxyphene Napsylate (Co-administration may exaggerate patient's response to CNS depressants). Products include:

Darvon-N/Darvocet-N 1473

Protriptyline Hydrochloride (Many antidepressants are substrates for P450 2D6 and may make normal metabolizers resemble poor metabolizers resulting in higher than expected plasma levels of tricyclic antidepressants). Products include:

Vivactil Tablets 1820

Pseudoephedrine Hydrochloride (Due to structural similarity to other tricyclic antidepressants, concurrent use requires close supervision). Products include:

Actifed Allergy Daytime/Nighttime Caplets 808
Actifed Cold & Allergy Tablets 807
Actifed Cold & Sinus Caplets and Tablets 808
Actifed Sinus Daytime/Nighttime Tablets and Caplets 809
Advil Cold and Sinus Caplets and Tablets 837
Alka-Seltzer Plus Liqui-Gels 612
Alka-Seltzer Plus Flu & Body Aches Liqui-Gels Non-Drowsy Formula 613
Alka-Seltzer Plus Night-Time Cold Medicine Liqui-Gels 612
Allerest Maximum Strength 649
Allerest No Drowsiness 649
Allerest Sinus Pain Formula 649
Atrohist Pediatric Capsules 1603
Benadryl Allergy/Cold Tablets 811
Benadryl Allergy Decongestant Liquid Medication 812
Benadryl Allergy Decongestant Tablets 812
Benadryl Allergy Sinus Headache Caplets 813
Benylin Multisymptom 816
Bromfed Capsules (Extended-Release) 1832
Bromfed Syrup 712
Bromfed Tablets 1832
Bromfed-DM Cough Syrup 1832
Bromfed-PD Capsules (Extended-Release) 1832
Children's TYLENOL Cold Multi-Symptom Chewable Tablets and Liquid 1559
Children's TYLENOL Cold Plus Cough Multi Symptom Chewable Tablets and Liquid 1560
Children's TYLENOL Flu Suspension Liquid 1560
Children's Vicks DayQuil Allergy Relief 730
Children's Vicks NyQuil Cold/Cough Relief 731
Allergy-Sinus Comtrex Multi-Symptom Allergy-Sinus Formula Tablets and Caplets 639
Comtrex Multi-Symptom 638
Comtrex Multi-Symptom Non-Drowsy Caplets 640
Congess 1003
Contac Day Allergy/Sinus Caplets 771
Contac Day & Night 772
Contac Night Allergy/Sinus Caplets 771
Contac Severe Cold & Flu Non-Drowsy 774
Deconsal II Tablets 1605
Dimetane-DX Cough Syrup 2233
Dimetapp Cold & Fever Suspension 839
Dimetapp Decongestant Pediatric Drops 840
Dorcol Children's Cough Syrup 748
Drixoral Cough + Congestion Liquid Caps 763

IMPORTANT NOTE: Always consult each drug listing in the patient's regimen for possible interactions.

Anafranil — Interactions Index

Dura-Tap/PD Capsules ... 970
Duratuss Tablets ... 2750
Duratuss HD Elixir ... 2750
Efidac/24 ... 655
Entex PSE Tablets ... 973
Fedahist Gyrocaps ... 2545
Guaifed ... 1833
Guaifed Syrup ... 712
Guaimax-D Tablets ... 809
Histussin D Liquid ... 670
Infants' TYLENOL Cold Decongestant & Fever-Reducer Drops ... 1561
Kronofed-A ... 994
Novahistine DMX ... 782
Nucofed ... 2225
PediaCare Cough-Cold Chewable Tablets and Liquid ... 1569
PediaCare Infants' Decongestant Drops ... 1569
PediaCare Infants' Drops Decongestant Plus Cough ... 1569
PediaCare NightRest Cough-Cold Liquid ... 1569
Pediatric Vicks 44d Cough & Head Congestion Relief ... 736
Pediatric Vicks 44m Cough & Cold Relief ... 737
Robitussin Cold & Cough Liqui-Gels ... 844
Robitussin Cold, Cough & Flu Liqui-Gels ... 844
Robitussin Maximum Strength Cough & Cold ... 847
Robitussin Night-Time Cold Formula ... 847
Robitussin Pediatric Cough & Cold Formula ... 848
Robitussin Pediatric Drops ... 849
Robitussin Severe Congestion Liqui-Gels ... 845
Robitussin-DAC Syrup ... 2249
Robitussin-PE ... 846
Rondec Oral Drops ... 974
Rondec Syrup ... 974
Rondec Tablet ... 974
Rondec Chewable Tablets ... 974
Rondec-TR Tablet ... 974
Ryna ... 804
Seldane-D Extended-Release Tablets ... 1286
Semprex-D Capsules ... 1620
Sinarest ... 663
Sine-Aid Maximum Strength Sinus Headache Gelcaps, Caplets and Tablets ... 1570
Sine-Off No Drowsiness Formula Caplets ... 784
Sine-Off Sinus Medicine ... 784
Singlet Tablets ... 785
Sinutab Non-Drying Liquid Caps ... 823
Sinutab Sinus Allergy Medication, Maximum Strength Tablets and Caplets ... 823
Sinutab Sinus Medication, Maximum Strength Without Drowsiness Formula, Tablets & Caplets ... 824
Sudafed Children's Cold & Cough Liquid Medication ... 825
Sudafed Children's Nasal Decongestant Liquid Medication ... 826
Sudafed Cold & Allergy Tablets ... 826
Sudafed Cold and Cough Liquid Caps ... 826
Sudafed Nasal Decongestant Tablets, 30 mg ... 825
Sudafed Nasal Decongestant Tablets, 60 mg ... 825
Sudafed Non-Drying Sinus Liquid Caps ... 827
Sudafed Pediatric Nasal Decongestant Liquid Oral Drops ... 827
Sudafed Severe Cold Formula Caplets ... 828
Sudafed Severe Cold Formula Tablets ... 828
Sudafed Sinus Caplets ... 829
Sudafed Sinus Tablets ... 829
Sudafed 12 Hour Caplets ... 824
Syn-Rx Tablets ... 1622
Syn-Rx DM Tablets ... 1623
TheraFlu Flu and Cold Medicine ... 750
Theraflu Maximum Strength Flu and Cold Medicine For Sore Throat ... 751
TheraFlu Flu, Cold and Cough Medicine ... 750
TheraFlu Maximum Strength Nighttime Flu, Cold & Cough Medicine ... 751
TheraFlu Maximum Strength Non-Drowsy Formula Flu, Cold & Cough Medicine ... 751
TheraFlu Maximum Strength, Non-Drowsy Formula Flu, Cold and Cough Caplets ... 752
Theraflu Maximum Strength Sinus Non-Drowsy Formula Caplets ... 752
Triaminic AM Cough and Decongestant Formula ... 753
Triaminic AM Decongestant Formula ... 753
Triaminic Infant Oral Decongestant Drops ... 754
Triaminic Night Time ... 754
Triaminic Sore Throat Formula ... 755
Tussend ... 1830
Tussend Expectorant ... 1831
TYLENOL Allergy Sinus, Maximum Strength Caplets and Gelcaps ... 1571
TYLENOL Allergy Sinus NightTime, Maximum Strength Caplets ... 1571
TYLENOL Cold Medication, Multi-Symptom Formula Tablets and Caplets ... 1572
TYLENOL Cold Medication, Multi-Symptom Hot Liquid Packets ... 1572
TYLENOL Cold Medication, No Drowsiness Formula Caplets and Gelcaps ... 1572
TYLENOL Cold Severe Congestion Caplets ... 1573
TYLENOL Cough Medication with Decongestant, Multi Symptom ... 1574
TYLENOL Flu No Drowsiness Formula, Maximum Strength Gelcaps ... 1575
TYLENOL Flu NightTime, Maximum Strength Gelcaps ... 1575
TYLENOL Flu NightTime, Maximum Strength Hot Medication Packets ... 1575
TYLENOL Sinus, Maximum Strength Geltabs, Gelcaps, Caplets and Tablets ... 1576
Vicks 44 LiquiCaps Cough, Cold & Flu Relief ... 728
Vicks 44 LiquiCaps Non-Drowsy Cough & Cold Relief ... 729
Vicks 44D Cough & Head Congestion Relief ... 728
Vicks 44M Cough, Cold & Flu Relief ... 729
Vicks DayQuil LiquiCaps/Liquid Multi-Symptom Cold/Flu Relief ... 734
Vicks DayQuil SINUS Pressure & PAIN Relief with IBUPROFEN ... 735
Vicks Nyquil Hot Therapy ... 735
Vicks NyQuil LiquiCaps/Liquid Multi-Symptom Cold/Flu Relief, Original and Cherry Flavors ... 736

Pseudoephedrine Sulfate (Due to structural similarity to other tricyclic antidepressants, concurrent use requires close supervision). Products include:
Chlor-Trimeton Allergy Decongestant Tablets ... 759
Claritin-D Tablets ... 2487
Drixoral Cold and Allergy Sustained-Action Tablets ... 763
Drixoral Cold and Flu Extended-Release Tablets ... 764
Drixoral Non-Drowsy Formula Extended-Release Tablets ... 764
Drixoral Allergy/Sinus Extended Release Tablets ... 765
Trinalin Repetabs Tablets ... 1373

Quazepam (Co-administration may exaggerate patient's response to CNS depressants). Products include:
Doral Tablets ... 2773

Quinidine Gluconate (May inhibit the activity of cytochrome P450 2D6 isoenzyme and may make normal metabolizers resemble poor metabolizers resulting in higher than expected plasma levels of tricyclic antidepressants). Products include:
Quinaglute Dura-Tabs Tablets ... 644

Quinidine Polygalacturonate (May inhibit the activity of cytochrome P450 2D6 isoenzyme and may make normal metabolizers resemble poor metabolizers resulting in higher than expected plasma levels of tricyclic antidepressants). Products include:
Cardioquin Tablets ... 2146

Quinidine Sulfate (May inhibit the activity of cytochrome P450 2D6 isoenzyme and may make normal metabolizers resemble poor metabolizers resulting in higher than expected plasma levels of tricyclic antidepressants). Products include:
Quinidex Extentabs ... 2240

Risperidone (Co-administration may exaggerate patient's response to CNS depressants). Products include:
Risperdal Tablets ... 1348

Salmeterol Xinafoate (Due to structural similarity to other tricyclic antidepressants, concurrent use requires close supervision). Products include:
Serevent Inhalation Aerosol ... 1149

Scopolamine (Clomipramine has anticholinergic properties; concurrent use requires close supervision). Products include:
Transderm Scōp Transdermal Therapeutic System ... 890

Scopolamine Hydrobromide (Clomipramine has anticholinergic properties; concurrent use requires close supervision). Products include:
Atrohist Plus Tablets ... 1605
Donnatal ... 2234
Donnatal Extentabs ... 2234
Donnatal Tablets ... 2234

Secobarbital Sodium (Co-administration may exaggerate patient's response to CNS depressants; plasma levels of several closely related tricyclic antidepressants have been decreased by the concomitant hepatic enzyme inducers, such as barbiturates). Products include:
Seconal Sodium Pulvules ... 1529

Selegiline Hydrochloride (Clomipramine should not be given in combination, or within 14 days before or after treatment with an MAO inhibitor; hyperpyretic crisis, seizures, coma, and death have been reported in patients receiving such combinations). Products include:
Eldepryl Capsules ... 2729

Sertraline Hydrochloride (Selective serotonin reuptake inhibitors, such as sertraline, may have variable extent of inhibition of P450 2D6; potential for higher than expected plasma levels of tricyclic antidepressants). Products include:
Zoloft Tablets ... 2051

Sevoflurane (Co-administration may exaggerate patient's response to CNS depressants).
No products indexed under this heading.

Sufentanil Citrate (Co-administration may exaggerate patient's response to CNS depressants). Products include:
Sufenta Injection ... 1355

Temazepam (Co-administration may exaggerate patient's response to CNS depressants). Products include:
Restoril Capsules ... 2413

Terbutaline Sulfate (Due to structural similarity to other tricyclic antidepressants, concurrent use requires close supervision). Products include:
Brethaire Inhaler ... 830
Brethine Ampuls ... 832
Brethine Tablets ... 831
Bricanyl Subcutaneous Injection ... 1247
Bricanyl Tablets ... 1248

Thiamylal Sodium (Co-administration may exaggerate patient's response to CNS depressants; plasma levels of several closely related tricyclic antidepressants have been decreased by the concomitant hepatic enzyme inducers, such as barbiturates).
No products indexed under this heading.

Thioridazine Hydrochloride (Phenothiazines are substrates for P450 2D6 and may make normal metabolizers resemble poor metabolizers resulting in higher than expected plasma levels of tricyclic antidepressants; co-administration may exaggerate patient's response to CNS depressants). Products include:
Mellaril ... 2398

Thiothixene (Co-administration may exaggerate patient's response to CNS depressants). Products include:
Navane Capsules and Concentrate ... 2018
Navane Intramuscular ... 2019

Thyroglobulin (Co-administration increases the possibility of cardiac toxicity).
No products indexed under this heading.

Thyroid (Co-administration increases the possibility of cardiac toxicity).
No products indexed under this heading.

Thyroxine (Co-administration increases the possibility of cardiac toxicity).
No products indexed under this heading.

Thyroxine Sodium (Co-administration increases the possibility of cardiac toxicity).
No products indexed under this heading.

Tranylcypromine Sulfate (Clomipramine should not be given in combination, or within 14 days before or after treatment with an MAO inhibitor; hyperpyretic crisis, seizures, coma, and death have been reported in patients receiving such combinations). Products include:
Parnate Tablets ... 2679

Trazodone Hydrochloride (Many antidepressants are substrates for P450 2D6 and may make normal metabolizers resemble poor metabolizers resulting in higher than expected plasma levels of tricyclic antidepressants). Products include:
Desyrel and Desyrel Dividose ... 504

Triazolam (Co-administration may exaggerate patient's response to CNS depressants). Products include:
Halcion Tablets ... 2093

Tridihexethyl Chloride (Clomipramine has anticholinergic properties; concurrent use requires close supervision).
No products indexed under this heading.

(▣ Described in PDR For Nonprescription Drugs) (◉ Described in PDR For Ophthalmology)

Trifluoperazine Hydrochloride (Phenothiazines are substrates for P450 2D6 and may make normal metabolizers resemble poor metabolizers resulting in higher than expected plasma levels of tricyclic antidepressants; co-administration may exaggerate patient's response to CNS depressants). Products include:
- Stelazine ... 2692

Trihexyphenidyl Hydrochloride (Clomipramine has anticholinergic properties; concurrent use requires close supervision). Products include:
- Artane ... 1418

Trimipramine Maleate (Many antidepressants are substrates for P450 2D6 and may make normal metabolizers resemble poor metabolizers resulting in higher than expected plasma levels of tricyclic antidepressants). Products include:
- Surmontil Capsules ... 2917

Venlafaxine Hydrochloride (Many antidepressants are substrates for P450 2D6 and may make normal metabolizers resemble poor metabolizers resulting in higher than expected plasma levels of tricyclic antidepressants). Products include:
- Effexor ... 2825

Warfarin Sodium (Clomipramine is highly protein bound, and co-administration with warfarin, another highly protein bound drug, may cause an increase in plasma concentrations of either drug, potentially resulting in adverse effects). Products include:
- Coumadin ... 941

Zolpidem Tartrate (Co-administration may exaggerate patient's response to CNS depressants). Products include:
- Ambien Tablets ... 2559

Food Interactions

Alcohol (Co-administration may exaggerate patient's response to alcohol).

ANA-KIT ANAPHYLAXIS EMERGENCY TREATMENT KIT

(Epinephrine Hydrochloride, Chlorpheniramine Maleate) ... 611

May interact with tricyclic antidepressants, sympathomimetics, cardiac glycosides, beta blockers, ergot-containing drugs, phenothiazines, insulin, oral hypoglycemic agents, and certain other agents. Compounds in these categories include:

Acarbose (Diabetics may require an increased dose of oral hypoglycemic drugs). Products include:
- Precose ... 604

Acebutolol Hydrochloride (Antagonizes the cardiostimulating and bronchodilating effects of epinephrine). Products include:
- Sectral Capsules ... 2914

Albuterol (Additive effects may be detrimental to the patient). Products include:
- Proventil Inhalation Aerosol ... 2524
- Ventolin Inhalation Aerosol and Refill ... 1170

Albuterol Sulfate (Additive effects may be detrimental to the patient). Products include:
- Airet Albuterol Sulfate Inhalation Solution ... 1602
- Albuterol Sulfate, USP Solution for Inhalation, Arm-a-Med ... 522
- Proventil Inhalation Solution 0.083% ... 2527
- Proventil Repetabs Tablets ... 2529
- Proventil Solution for Inhalation 0.5% ... 2525
- Proventil Syrup ... 2528
- Proventil Tablets ... 2529
- Ventolin Inhalation Solution ... 1171
- Ventolin Nebules Inhalation Solution ... 1172
- Ventolin Rotacaps for Inhalation ... 1173
- Ventolin Syrup ... 1175
- Ventolin Tablets ... 1176
- Volmax Extended-Release Tablets .. 1835

Amitriptyline Hydrochloride (Potentiation of epinephrine). Products include:
- Elavil ... 2945
- Etrafon ... 2495
- Limbitrol ... 2333
- Triavil Tablets ... 1800

Amoxapine (Potentiation of epinephrine). Products include:
- Asendin Tablets ... 1419

Atenolol (Antagonizes the cardiostimulating and bronchodilating effects of epinephrine). Products include:
- Tenoretic Tablets ... 2963
- Tenormin Tablets and I.V. Injection 2965

Betaxolol Hydrochloride (Antagonizes the cardiostimulating and bronchodilating effects of epinephrine). Products include:
- Betoptic Ophthalmic Solution ... 465
- Betoptic S Ophthalmic Suspension 467
- Kerlone Tablets ... 2588

Bisoprolol Fumarate (Antagonizes the cardiostimulating and bronchodilating effects of epinephrine). Products include:
- Zebeta Tablets ... 1457
- Ziac ... 1459

Carteolol Hydrochloride (Antagonizes the cardiostimulating and bronchodilating effects of epinephrine). Products include:
- Cartrol Tablets ... 413
- Ocupress Ophthalmic Solution, 1% Sterile ... ◉ 297

Chlorpheniramine Polistirex (Potentiation of epinephrine). Products include:
- Tussionex Pennkinetic Extended-Release Suspension ... 1624

Chlorpheniramine Tannate (Potentiation of epinephrine). Products include:
- Atrohist Pediatric Suspension ... 1604
- Atrohist Pediatric Suspension Dye-Free ... 1604
- Rynatan ... 2781
- Rynatuss ... 2782

Chlorpromazine (May reverse the pressor effects of epinephrine). Products include:
- Thorazine Suppositories ... 2701

Chlorpromazine Hydrochloride (May reverse the pressor effects of epinephrine). Products include:
- Thorazine ... 2701

Chlorpropamide (Diabetics may require an increased dose of oral hypoglycemic drugs). Products include:
- Diabinese Tablets ... 2002

Clomipramine Hydrochloride (Potentiation of epinephrine). Products include:
- Anafranil Capsules ... 819

Desipramine Hydrochloride (Potentiation of epinephrine). Products include:
- Norpramin Tablets ... 1273

Deslanoside (Cardiac glycosides may sensitize the myocardium to beta-adrenergic stimulation and cardiac arrhythmias more likely).
- No products indexed under this heading.

Dexchlorpheniramine Maleate (Potentiation of epinephrine).
- No products indexed under this heading.

Digitoxin (Cardiac glycosides may sensitize the myocardium to beta-adrenergic stimulation and cardiac arrhythmias more likely). Products include:
- Crystodigin Tablets ... 1472

Digoxin (Cardiac glycosides may sensitize the myocardium to beta-adrenergic stimulation and cardiac arrhythmias more likely). Products include:
- Lanoxicaps ... 1110
- Lanoxin Elixir Pediatric ... 1113
- Lanoxin Injection ... 1116
- Lanoxin Injection Pediatric ... 1119
- Lanoxin Tablets ... 1121

Dihydroergotamine Mesylate (May reverse the pressor effects of epinephrine). Products include:
- D.H.E. 45 Injection ... 2381

Diphenhydramine Citrate (Potentiation of epinephrine). Products include:
- Excedrin P.M. Analgesic/Sleeping Aid Tablets, Caplets, Liquigels ... 735

Diphenhydramine Hydrochloride (Potentiation of epinephrine). Products include:
- Actifed Allergy Daytime/Nighttime Caplets ... 808
- Actifed Sinus Daytime/Nighttime Tablets and Caplets ... 809
- Extra Strength Bayer PM Aspirin Plus Sleep Aid ... 617
- Benadryl Allergy Chewables ... 811
- Benadryl Allergy/Cold Tablets ... 811
- Benadryl Allergy Decongestant Liquid Medication ... 812
- Benadryl Allergy Decongestant Tablets ... 812
- Benadryl Allergy Liquid Medication ... 813
- Benadryl Allergy ... 811
- Benadryl Allergy Sinus Headache Caplets ... 813
- Benadryl Dye-Free Allergy Liqui-gel Softgels ... 813
- Benadryl Dye-Free Allergy Liquid Medication ... 814
- Benadryl Itch Relief Stick Extra Strength ... 814
- Benadryl Cream ... 814
- Benadryl Gel ... 815
- Benadryl Spray ... 815
- Benadryl Injection ... 1955
- Contac Day & Night Cold/Flu Night Caplets ... 772
- Contac Night Allergy/Sinus Caplets ... 771
- Extra Strength Doan's P.M. ... 653
- Excedrin P.M. Analgesic/Sleeping Aid Tablets, Caplets, Liquigels ... 643
- Nytol QuickCaps Caplets ... 632
- Sleepinal Night-time Sleep Aid Capsules and Softgels ... 798
- TYLENOL Allergy Sinus NightTime, Maximum Strength Caplets ... 1571
- TYLENOL Flu NightTime, Maximum Strength Gelcaps ... 1575
- TYLENOL Flu NightTime, Maximum Strength Hot Medication Packets ... 1575
- TYLENOL PM Pain Reliever/Sleep Aid, Extra Strength Gelcaps, Caplets, Geltabs ... 1576
- TYLENOL Severe Allergy Medication Caplets ... 1571
- Maximum Strength Unisom Sleepgels ... 1990
- Unisom With Pain Relief-Nighttime Sleep Aid and Pain Reliever ... 1991

Dobutamine Hydrochloride (Additive effects may be detrimental to the patient). Products include:
- Dobutrex Solution Vials ... 1480

Dopamine Hydrochloride (Additive effects may be detrimental to the patient).
- No products indexed under this heading.

Doxepin Hydrochloride (Potentiation of epinephrine). Products include:
- Adapin Capsules ... 1542
- Sinequan ... 2028
- Zonalon Cream ... 1042

Ephedrine Hydrochloride (Additive effects may be detrimental to the patient). Products include:
- Primatene Tablets ... 844
- Quadrinal Tablets ... 1398

Ephedrine Sulfate (Additive effects may be detrimental to the patient). Products include:
- Marax Tablets & DF Syrup ... 2015

Ephedrine Tannate (Additive effects may be detrimental to the patient). Products include:
- Rynatuss ... 2782

Epinephrine (Additive effects may be detrimental to the patient). Products include:
- EPIFRIN ... ◉ 237
- EpiPen ... 808
- Marcaine with Epinephrine ... 2446
- Primatene Mist ... 843
- Sensorcaine with Epinephrine Injection ... 554
- Sus-Phrine Injection ... 1017
- Xylocaine with Epinephrine Injections ... 562

Epinephrine Bitartrate (Additive effects may be detrimental to the patient). Products include:
- Sensorcaine-MPF with Epinephrine Injection ... 554

Ergotamine Tartrate (May reverse the pressor effects of epinephrine). Products include:
- Bellergal-S Tablets ... 2375
- Cafergot ... 2376
- Ergomar Tablets ... 1543
- Wigraine Tablets ... 1884

Esmolol Hydrochloride (Antagonizes the cardiostimulating and bronchodilating effects of epinephrine). Products include:
- Brevibloc (esmolol HCl) Injection 1860

Fluphenazine Decanoate (May reverse the pressor effects of epinephrine). Products include:
- Prolixin Decanoate ... 510

Fluphenazine Enanthate (May reverse the pressor effects of epinephrine). Products include:
- Prolixin Enanthate ... 510

Fluphenazine Hydrochloride (May reverse the pressor effects of epinephrine). Products include:
- Prolixin ... 510

Glimepiride (Diabetics may require an increased dose of oral hypoglycemic drugs). Products include:
- Amaryl Tablets ... 1241

Glipizide (Diabetics may require an increased dose of oral hypoglycemic drugs). Products include:
- Glucotrol Tablets ... 2011
- Glucotrol XL Extended Release Tablets ... 2012

Glyburide (Diabetics may require an increased dose of oral hypoglycemic drugs). Products include:
- DiaBeta Tablets ... 1265
- Glynase PresTab Tablets ... 2091
- Micronase Tablets ... 2099

Imipramine Hydrochloride (Potentiation of epinephrine). Products include:
- Tofranil Ampuls ... 873
- Tofranil Tablets ... 875

Imipramine Pamoate (Potentiation of epinephrine). Products include:
- Tofranil-PM Capsules ... 876

Insulin, Human (Diabetics may require an increased dose of insulin).
- No products indexed under this heading.

IMPORTANT NOTE: Always consult each drug listing in the patient's regimen for possible interactions.

Insulin, Human Isophane Suspension (Diabetics may require an increased dose of insulin). Products include:
- Novolin N Human Insulin 10 ml Vials ... 1846

Insulin, Human NPH (Diabetics may require an increased dose of insulin). Products include:
- Humulin N, 100 Units ... 1495
- Novolin N PenFill 1.5 ml Cartridges Durable Insulin Delivery System ... 1849
- Novolin N Prefilled Syringe Disposable Insulin Delivery System ... 1850

Insulin, Human Regular (Diabetics may require an increased dose of insulin). Products include:
- Humulin R, 100 Units ... 1497
- Novolin R Human Insulin 10 ml Vials ... 1846
- Novolin R PenFill 1.5 ml Cartridges Durable Insulin Delivery System ... 1849
- Novolin R Prefilled Syringe Disposable Insulin Delivery System ... 1850
- Velosulin BR Human Insulin 10 ml Vials ... 1847

Insulin, Human, Zinc Suspension (Diabetics may require an increased dose of insulin). Products include:
- Humulin L, 100 Units ... 1494
- Humulin U, 100 Units ... 1498
- Novolin L Human Insulin 10 ml Vials ... 1846

Insulin Lispro, Human (Diabetics may require an increased dose of insulin). Products include:
- Humalog Injection ... 1488

Insulin, NPH (Diabetics may require an increased dose of insulin). Products include:
- NPH, 100 Units ... 1502
- Pork NPH, 100 Units ... 1506
- Purified Pork NPH Isophane Insulin ... 1852

Insulin, Regular (Diabetics may require an increased dose of insulin). Products include:
- Regular, 100 Units ... 1503
- Pork Regular, 100 Units ... 1507
- Pork Regular (Concentrated), 500 Units ... 1508
- Purified Pork Regular Insulin ... 1852

Insulin, Zinc Crystals (Diabetics may require an increased dose of insulin). Products include:
- NPH, 100 Units ... 1502

Insulin, Zinc Suspension (Diabetics may require an increased dose of insulin). Products include:
- Iletin I ... 1501
- Lente, 100 Units ... 1501
- Iletin II ... 1504
- Pork Lente, 100 Units ... 1504
- Purified Pork Lente Insulin ... 1852

Isoproterenol Hydrochloride (Additive effects may be detrimental to the patient). Products include:
- Isuprel Hydrochloride Solution ... 2443
- Isuprel Injection ... 2441
- Isuprel Mistometer ... 2442

Isoproterenol Sulfate (Additive effects may be detrimental to the patient). Products include:
- Norisodrine with Calcium Iodide Syrup ... 446

Labetalol Hydrochloride (Antagonizes the cardiostimulating and bronchodilating effects of epinephrine). Products include:
- Normodyne Injection ... 2519
- Normodyne Tablets ... 2522
- Trandate ... 1158

Levobunolol Hydrochloride (Antagonizes the cardiostimulating and bronchodilating effects of epinephrine). Products include:
- Betagan ... ⊚ 230

Levothyroxine Sodium (Potentiation of epinephrine). Products include:
- Eltroxin Tablets ... 2214
- Levothroid Tablets ... 1015
- Levothyroxine Sodium, USP for Injection ... 546
- Levoxyl Tablets ... 918
- Synthroid ... 1410

Maprotiline Hydrochloride (Potentiation of epinephrine). Products include:
- Ludiomil Tablets ... 861

Mercurial Diuretics (Mercurial diuretics may sensitize the myocardium to beta-adrenergic stimulation and cardiac arrhythmias more likely).

Mesoridazine Besylate (May reverse the pressor effects of epinephrine). Products include:
- Serentil ... 689

Metaproterenol Sulfate (Additive effects may be detrimental to the patient). Products include:
- Alupent ... 672
- Metaproterenol Sulfate Inhalation Solution, USP, Arm-a-Med ... 547

Metaraminol Bitartrate (Additive effects may be detrimental to the patient). Products include:
- Aramine Injection ... 1649

Metformin Hydrochloride (Diabetics may require an increased dose of oral hypoglycemic drugs). Products include:
- Glucophage Tablets ... 754

Methotrimeprazine (May reverse the pressor effects of epinephrine). Products include:
- Levoprome ... 1321

Methoxamine Hydrochloride (Additive effects may be detrimental to the patient). Products include:
- Vasoxyl Injection ... 1169

Methylergonovine Maleate (May reverse the pressor effects of epinephrine). Products include:
- Methergine ... 2401

Methysergide Maleate (May reverse the pressor effects of epinephrine). Products include:
- Sansert Tablets ... 2424

Metipranolol Hydrochloride (Antagonizes the cardiostimulating and bronchodilating effects of epinephrine). Products include:
- OptiPranolol (Metipranolol 0.3%) Sterile Ophthalmic Solution ... ⊚ 256

Metoprolol Succinate (Antagonizes the cardiostimulating and bronchodilating effects of epinephrine). Products include:
- Toprol-XL Tablets ... 560

Metoprolol Tartrate (Antagonizes the cardiostimulating and bronchodilating effects of epinephrine). Products include:
- Lopressor ... 848
- Lopressor HCT Tablets ... 850

Nadolol (Antagonizes the cardiostimulating and bronchodilating effects of epinephrine).
No products indexed under this heading.

Norepinephrine Bitartrate (Additive effects may be detrimental to the patient). Products include:
- Levophed Bitartrate Injection ... 2445

Nortriptyline Hydrochloride (Potentiation of epinephrine). Products include:
- Pamelor ... 2409

Penbutolol Sulfate (Antagonizes the cardiostimulating and bronchodilating effects of epinephrine). Products include:
- Levatol Tablets ... 2547

Perphenazine (May reverse the pressor effects of epinephrine). Products include:
- Etrafon ... 2495
- Triavil Tablets ... 1800
- Trilafon ... 2532

Phentolamine Mesylate (Antagonizes the vasoconstrictive and hypertensive effects of epinephrine). Products include:
- Regitine Vials ... 864

Phenylephrine Bitartrate (Additive effects may be detrimental to the patient).
No products indexed under this heading.

Phenylephrine Hydrochloride (Additive effects may be detrimental to the patient). Products include:
- Atrohist Plus Tablets ... 1605
- Cerose DM ... •◻ 853
- D.A. II Tablets ... 972
- D.A. Chewable Tablets ... 970
- Dura-Vent/DA Tablets ... 972
- Extendryl ... 1003
- 4-Way Fast Acting Nasal Spray (regular & mentholated) ... •◻ 644
- Hemorid ... •◻ 797
- Hycomine Compound Tablets ... 948
- Neo-Synephrine Hydrochloride 1% Carpuject ... 2455
- Neo-Synephrine Hydrochloride 1% Injection ... 2455
- Neo-Synephrine Hydrochloride (Ophthalmic) ... 2456
- Neo-Synephrine ... •◻ 624
- Novahistine Elixir ... •◻ 782
- Phenergan VC ... 2886
- Phenergan VC with Codeine ... 2888
- Preparation H ... •◻ 842
- Tympagesic Ear Drops ... 2476
- Vicks Sinex Nasal Spray and Ultra Fine Mist ... •◻ 738

Phenylephrine Tannate (Additive effects may be detrimental to the patient). Products include:
- Atrohist Pediatric Suspension ... 1604
- Atrohist Pediatric Suspension Dye-Free ... 1604
- Rynatan ... 2781
- Rynatuss ... 2782

Phenylpropanolamine Hydrochloride (Additive effects may be detrimental to the patient). Products include:
- Acutrim ... •◻ 648
- Atrohist Plus Tablets ... 1605
- BC Cold Powder Multi-Symptom Formula (Cold-Sinus-Allergy) ... •◻ 631
- BC Cold Powder Non-Drowsy Formula (Cold-Sinus) ... •◻ 631
- Cheracol Plus Head Cold/Cough Formula ... •◻ 741
- Comtrex Multi-Symptom Cold Reliever Liqui-Gels ... •◻ 638
- Comtrex Multi-Symptom Non-Drowsy Liqui-gels ... •◻ 640
- Contac Continuous Action Nasal Decongestant/Antihistamine 12 Hour Capsules ... •◻ 773
- Contac Maximum Strength Continuous Action Decongestant/Antihistamine 12 Hour Caplets ... •◻ 772
- Contac Severe Cold and Flu Formula Caplets ... •◻ 773
- Coricidin 'D' Decongestant Tablets ... •◻ 760
- Dexatrim ... •◻ 795
- Dexatrim Plus Vitamins Caplets ... •◻ 796
- Dimetane-DC Cough Syrup ... 2232
- Dimetapp Allergy Sinus Caplets ... •◻ 838
- Dimetapp Cold & Allergy Chewable Tablets ... •◻ 838
- Dimetapp Cold & Cough Liqui-Gels ... •◻ 839
- Dimetapp DM Elixir ... •◻ 840
- Dimetapp Elixir ... •◻ 840
- Dimetapp Extentabs ... •◻ 841
- Dimetapp Tablets/Liqui-Gels ... •◻ 841
- Dura-Vent Tablets ... 971
- Entex LA Tablets ... 972
- Exgest LA Tablets ... 787
- Hycomine ... 947
- Nolamine Timed-Release Tablets ... 790
- Ornade Spansule Capsules ... 2678
- Propagest Tablets ... 791

Pyrroxate Caplets ... •◻ 742
Robitussin-CF ... •◻ 846
Sinulin Tablets ... 792
Tavist-D 12 Hour Relief Tablets ... •◻ 750
Teldrin 12 Hour Antihistamine/Nasal Decongestant Allergy Relief Capsules ... •◻ 786
Triaminic Expectorant ... •◻ 753
Triaminic Syrup ... •◻ 755
Triaminic Triaminicol Cold & Cough ... •◻ 756
Triaminic DM Syrup ... •◻ 755
Triaminicin Tablets ... •◻ 756
Vicks DayQuil Allergy Relief 12-Hour Extended Release Tablets ... •◻ 733
Vicks DayQuil Allergy Relief 4-Hour Tablets ... •◻ 733
Vicks DayQuil SINUS Pressure & CONGESTION Relief ... •◻ 734

Pindolol (Antagonizes the cardiostimulating and bronchodilating effects of epinephrine). Products include:
- Visken Tablets ... 2428

Pirbuterol Acetate (Additive effects may be detrimental to the patient). Products include:
- Maxair Autohaler ... 1550
- Maxair Inhaler ... 1552

Prochlorperazine (May reverse the pressor effects of epinephrine). Products include:
- Compazine ... 2644

Promethazine Hydrochloride (May reverse the pressor effects of epinephrine). Products include:
- Mepergan Injection ... 2859
- Phenergan with Codeine ... 2883
- Phenergan with Dextromethorphan ... 2885
- Phenergan Injection ... 2880
- Phenergan Suppositories ... 2882
- Phenergan Syrup ... 2881
- Phenergan Tablets ... 2882
- Phenergan VC ... 2886
- Phenergan VC with Codeine ... 2888

Propranolol Hydrochloride (Antagonizes the cardiostimulating and bronchodilating effects of epinephrine). Products include:
- Inderal ... 2834
- Inderal LA Long Acting Capsules ... 2836
- Inderide Tablets ... 2838
- Inderide LA Long Acting Capsules ... 2840

Protriptyline Hydrochloride (Potentiation of epinephrine). Products include:
- Vivactil Tablets ... 1820

Pseudoephedrine Hydrochloride (Additive effects may be detrimental to the patient). Products include:
- Actifed Allergy Daytime/Nighttime Caplets ... •◻ 808
- Actifed Cold & Allergy Caplets ... •◻ 807
- Actifed Cold & Sinus Caplets and Tablets ... •◻ 808
- Actifed Sinus Daytime/Nighttime Tablets and Caplets ... •◻ 809
- Advil Cold and Sinus Caplets and Tablets ... •◻ 837
- Alka-Seltzer Plus Liqui-Gels ... •◻ 612
- Alka-Seltzer Plus Flu & Body Aches Liqui-Gels Non-Drowsy Formula ... •◻ 613
- Alka-Seltzer Plus Night-Time Cold Medicine Liqui-Gels ... •◻ 612
- Allerest Maximum Strength ... •◻ 649
- Allerest No Drowsiness ... •◻ 649
- Allerest Sinus Pain Formula ... •◻ 649
- Atrohist Pediatric Capsules ... 1603
- Benadryl Allergy/Cold Tablets ... •◻ 811
- Benadryl Allergy Decongestant Liquid Medication ... •◻ 812
- Benadryl Allergy Decongestant Tablets ... •◻ 812
- Benadryl Allergy Sinus Headache Caplets ... •◻ 813
- Benylin Multisymptom ... •◻ 816
- Bromfed Capsules (Extended-Release) ... 1832
- Bromfed Syrup ... •◻ 712
- Bromfed Tablets ... 1832
- Bromfed-DM Cough Syrup ... 1832
- Bromfed-PD Capsules (Extended-Release) ... 1832

(•◻ Described in PDR For Nonprescription Drugs)   (⊚ Described in PDR For Ophthalmology)

65 **Interactions Index** **Androderm**

Children's TYLENOL Cold Multi-Symptom Chewable Tablets and Liquid ... 1559
Children's TYLENOL Cold Plus Cough Multi Symptom Chewable Tablets and Liquid ... 1560
Children's TYLENOL Flu Suspension Liquid ... 1560
Children's Vicks DayQuil Allergy Relief ... 730
Children's Vicks NyQuil Cold/Cough Relief ... 731
Allergy-Sinus Comtrex Multi-Symptom Allergy-Sinus Formula Tablets and Caplets ... 639
Comtrex Multi-Symptom ... 638
Comtrex Multi-Symptom Non-Drowsy Caplets ... 640
Congess ... 1003
Contac Day Allergy/Sinus Caplets ... 771
Contac Day & Night ... 772
Contac Night Allergy/Sinus Caplets ... 771
Contac Severe Cold & Flu Non-Drowsy ... 774
Deconsal II Tablets ... 1605
Dimetane-DX Cough Syrup ... 2233
Dimetapp Cold & Fever Suspension ... 839
Dimetapp Decongestant Pediatric Drops ... 840
Dorcol Children's Cough Syrup ... 748
Drixoral Cough + Congestion Liquid Caps ... 763
Dura-Tap/PD Capsules ... 970
Duratuss Tablets ... 2750
Duratuss HD Elixir ... 2750
Efidac/24 ... 655
Entex PSE Tablets ... 973
Fedahist Gyrocaps ... 2545
Guaifed ... 1833
Guaifed Syrup ... 712
Guaimax-D Tablets ... 809
Histussin D Liquid ... 670
Infants' TYLENOL Cold Decongestant & Fever-Reducer Drops ... 1561
Kronofed-A ... 994
Novahistine DMX ... 782
Nucofed ... 2225
PediaCare Cough-Cold Chewable Tablets and Liquid ... 1569
PediaCare Infants' Decongestant Drops ... 1569
PediaCare Infants' Drops Decongestant Plus Cough ... 1569
PediaCare NightRest Cough-Cold Liquid ... 1569
Pediatric Vicks 44d Cough & Head Congestion Relief ... 736
Pediatric Vicks 44m Cough & Cold Relief ... 737
Robitussin Cold & Cough Liqui-Gels ... 844
Robitussin Cold, Cough & Flu Liqui-Gels ... 844
Robitussin Maximum Strength Cough & Cold ... 847
Robitussin Night-Time Cold Formula ... 847
Robitussin Pediatric Cough & Cold Formula ... 848
Robitussin Pediatric Drops ... 849
Robitussin Severe Congestion Liqui-Gels ... 845
Robitussin-DAC Syrup ... 2249
Robitussin-PE ... 846
Rondec Oral Drops ... 974
Rondec Syrup ... 974
Rondec Tablet ... 974
Rondec Chewable Tablets ... 974
Rondec-TR Tablet ... 974
Ryna ... 804
Seldane-D Extended-Release Tablets ... 1286
Semprex-D Capsules ... 1620
Sinarest ... 663
Sine-Aid Maximum Strength Sinus Headache Gelcaps, Caplets and Tablets ... 1570
Sine-Off No Drowsiness Formula Caplets ... 784
Sine-Off Sinus Medicine ... 784
Singlet Tablets ... 785
Sinutab Non-Drying Liquid Caps ... 823
Sinutab Sinus Allergy Medication, Maximum Strength Tablets and Caplets ... 823
Sinutab Sinus Medication, Maximum Strength Without Drowsiness Formula, Tablets & Caplets ... 824
Sudafed Children's Cold & Cough Liquid Medication ... 825
Sudafed Children's Nasal Decongestant Liquid Medication ... 826
Sudafed Cold & Allergy Tablets ... 826
Sudafed Cold and Cough Liquid Caps ... 826
Sudafed Nasal Decongestant Tablets, 30 mg ... 825
Sudafed Nasal Decongestant Tablets, 60 mg ... 825
Sudafed Non-Drying Sinus Liquid Caps ... 827
Sudafed Pediatric Nasal Decongestant Liquid Oral Drops ... 827
Sudafed Severe Cold Formula Caplets ... 828
Sudafed Severe Cold Formula Tablets ... 828
Sudafed Sinus Caplets ... 829
Sudafed Sinus Tablets ... 829
Sudafed 12 Hour Caplets ... 824
Syn-Rx Tablets ... 1622
Syn-Rx DM Tablets ... 1623
TheraFlu Flu and Cold Medicine ... 750
Theraflu Maximum Strength Flu and Cold Medicine For Sore Throat ... 751
TheraFlu Flu, Cold and Cough Medicine ... 750
TheraFlu Maximum Strength Nighttime Flu, Cold & Cough Medicine ... 751
TheraFlu Maximum Strength Non-Drowsy Formula Flu, Cold & Cough Medicine ... 751
TheraFlu Maximum Strength, Non-Drowsy Formula Flu, Cold and Cough Caplets ... 752
Theraflu Maximum Strength Sinus Non-Drowsy Formula Caplets ... 752
Triaminic AM Cough and Decongestant Formula ... 753
Triaminic AM Decongestant Formula ... 753
Triaminic Infant Oral Decongestant Drops ... 754
Triaminic Night Time ... 754
Triaminic Sore Throat Formula ... 755
Tussend ... 1830
Tussend Expectorant ... 1831
TYLENOL Allergy Sinus, Maximum Strength Caplets and Gelcaps ... 1571
TYLENOL Allergy Sinus NightTime, Maximum Strength Caplets ... 1571
TYLENOL Cold Medication, Multi-Symptom Formula Tablets and Caplets ... 1572
TYLENOL Cold Medication, Multi-Symptom Hot Liquid Packets ... 1572
TYLENOL Cold Medication, No Drowsiness Formula Caplets and Gelcaps ... 1572
TYLENOL Cold Severe Congestion Caplets ... 1573
TYLENOL Cough Medication with Decongestant, Multi Symptom ... 1574
TYLENOL Flu No Drowsiness Formula, Maximum Strength Gelcaps ... 1575
TYLENOL Flu NightTime, Maximum Strength Gelcaps ... 1575
TYLENOL Flu NightTime, Maximum Strength Hot Medication Packets ... 1575
TYLENOL Sinus, Maximum Strength Geltabs, Gelcaps, Caplets and Tablets ... 1576
Vicks 44 LiquiCaps Cough, Cold & Flu Relief ... 728
Vicks 44 LiquiCaps Non-Drowsy Cough & Cold Relief ... 729
Vicks 44D Cough & Head Congestion Relief ... 728
Vicks 44M Cough, Cold & Flu Relief ... 729
Vicks DayQuil LiquiCaps/Liquid Multi-Symptom Cold/Flu Relief ... 734
Vicks DayQuil SINUS Pressure & PAIN Relief with IBUPROFEN ... 735
Vicks Nyquil Hot Therapy ... 735
Vicks NyQuil LiquiCaps/Liquid Multi-Symptom Cold/Flu Relief, Original and Cherry Flavors ... 736

Pseudoephedrine Sulfate (Additive effects may be detrimental to the patient). Products include:
Chlor-Trimeton Allergy Decongestant Tablets ... 759
Claritin-D Tablets ... 2487
Drixoral Cold and Allergy Sustained-Action Tablets ... 763
Drixoral Cold and Flu Extended-Release Tablets ... 764
Drixoral Non-Drowsy Formula Extended-Release Tablets ... 764
Drixoral Allergy/Sinus Extended Release Tablets ... 765
Trinalin Repetabs Tablets ... 1373

Salmeterol Xinafoate (Additive effects may be detrimental to the patient). Products include:
Serevent Inhalation Aerosol ... 1149

Sotalol Hydrochloride (Antagonizes the cardiostimulating and bronchodilating effects of epinephrine). Products include:
Betapace Tablets ... 637

Terbutaline Sulfate (Additive effects may be detrimental to the patient). Products include:
Brethaire Inhaler ... 830
Brethine Ampuls ... 832
Brethine Tablets ... 831
Bricanyl Subcutaneous Injection ... 1247
Bricanyl Tablets ... 1248

Thioridazine Hydrochloride (May reverse the pressor effects of epinephrine). Products include:
Mellaril ... 2398

Timolol Hemihydrate (Antagonizes the cardiostimulating and bronchodilating effects of epinephrine). Products include:
Betimol 0.25%, 0.5% ... ◉ 259

Timolol Maleate (Antagonizes the cardiostimulating and bronchodilating effects of epinephrine). Products include:
Blocadren Tablets ... 1654
Timolide Tablets ... 1791
Timoptic in Ocudose ... 1796
Timoptic Sterile Ophthalmic Solution ... 1794
Timoptic-XE ... 1798

Tolazamide (Diabetics may require an increased dose of oral hypoglycemic drugs).
No products indexed under this heading.

Tolbutamide (Diabetics may require an increased dose of oral hypoglycemic drugs).
No products indexed under this heading.

Trifluoperazine Hydrochloride (May reverse the pressor effects of epinephrine). Products include:
Stelazine ... 2692

Trimeprazine Tartrate (Potentiation of epinephrine).
No products indexed under this heading.

Trimipramine Maleate (Potentiation of epinephrine). Products include:
Surmontil Capsules ... 2917

Tripelennamine Hydrochloride (Potentiation of epinephrine). Products include:
PBZ Tablets ... 863
PBZ-SR Tablets ... 862

ANALPRAM-HC RECTAL CREAM 1% AND 2.5%
(Hydrocortisone Acetate, Pramoxine Hydrochloride) ... 993
None cited in PDR database.

ANAPROX TABLETS
(Naproxen Sodium) ... 2277
See **EC-Naprosyn Delayed-Release Tablets**

ANAPROX DS TABLETS
(Naproxen Sodium) ... 2277
See **EC-Naprosyn Delayed-Release Tablets**

ANCEF INJECTION
(Cefazolin Sodium) ... 2632
May interact with:

Probenecid (Increased and prolonged cephalosporin blood levels). Products include:
Benemid Tablets ... 1651
ColBENEMID Tablets ... 1662

ANCOBON CAPSULES
(Flucytosine) ... 2254
May interact with:

Amphotericin B (Antifungal synergism). Products include:
Abelcet Injection ... 1540
Fungizone Intravenous ... 507
Fungizone Oral Suspension ... 704

Cytosine Arabinoside (Inactivation of Ancobon's antifungal activity).

Drugs That Impair Glomerular Filtration (Biological half-life of Ancobon may be prolonged).

ANDRODERM TESTOSTERONE TRANSDERMAL SYSTEM
(Testosterone) ... 2634
May interact with oral anticoagulants, insulin, and certain other agents. Compounds in these categories include:

Dicumarol (Potential for decreased requirements of oral anticoagulants).
No products indexed under this heading.

Insulin, Human (In diabetic patients androgens may decrease blood glucose and, therefore, insulin requirements).
No products indexed under this heading.

Insulin, Human Isophane Suspension (In diabetic patients androgens may decrease blood glucose and, therefore, insulin requirements). Products include:
Novolin N Human Insulin 10 ml Vials ... 1846

Insulin, Human NPH (In diabetic patients androgens may decrease blood glucose and, therefore, insulin requirements). Products include:
Humulin N, 100 Units ... 1495
Novolin N PenFill 1.5 ml Cartridges Durable Insulin Delivery System ... 1849
Novolin N Prefilled Syringe Disposable Insulin Delivery System ... 1850

Insulin, Human Regular (In diabetic patients androgens may decrease blood glucose and, therefore, insulin requirements). Products include:
Humulin R, 100 Units ... 1497
Novolin R Human Insulin 10 ml Vials ... 1846
Novolin R PenFill 1.5 ml Cartridges Durable Insulin Delivery System ... 1849
Novolin R Prefilled Syringe Disposable Insulin Delivery System ... 1850
Velosulin BR Human Insulin 10 ml Vials ... 1847

Insulin, Human, Zinc Suspension (In diabetic patients androgens may decrease blood glucose and, therefore, insulin requirements). Products include:
Humulin L, 100 Units ... 1494
Humulin U, 100 Units ... 1498
Novolin L Human Insulin 10 ml Vials ... 1846

IMPORTANT NOTE: Always consult each drug listing in the patient's regimen for possible interactions.

Androderm / Interactions Index

Insulin Lispro, Human (In diabetic patients androgens may decrease blood glucose and, therefore, insulin requirements). Products include:
- Humalog Injection 1488

Insulin, NPH (In diabetic patients androgens may decrease blood glucose and, therefore, insulin requirements). Products include:
- NPH, 100 Units 1502
- Pork NPH, 100 Units 1506
- Purified Pork NPH Isophane Insulin 1852

Insulin, Regular (In diabetic patients androgens may decrease blood glucose and, therefore, insulin requirements). Products include:
- Regular, 100 Units 1503
- Pork Regular, 100 Units 1507
- Pork Regular (Concentrated), 500 Units 1508
- Purified Pork Regular Insulin 1852

Insulin, Zinc Crystals (In diabetic patients androgens may decrease blood glucose and, therefore, insulin requirements). Products include:
- NPH, 100 Units 1502

Insulin, Zinc Suspension (In diabetic patients androgens may decrease blood glucose and, therefore, insulin requirements). Products include:
- Iletin I 1501
- Lente, 100 Units 1501
- Iletin II 1504
- Pork Lente, 100 Units 1504
- Purified Pork Lente Insulin 1852

Oxyphenbutazone (Concurrent administration may result in elevated serum levels of oxyphenbutazone).

Warfarin Sodium (Potential for decreased requirements of oral anticoagulants). Products include:
- Coumadin 941

ANDROID CAPSULES, 10 MG
(Methyltestosterone) 1297
May interact with oral anticoagulants, insulin, and certain other agents. Compounds in these categories include:

Dicumarol (Decreased anticoagulant requirements).
No products indexed under this heading.

Insulin, Human (In diabetic patients the metabolic effects of androgens may decrease blood glucose and insulin requirements).
No products indexed under this heading.

Insulin, Human Isophane Suspension (In diabetic patients the metabolic effects of androgens may decrease blood glucose and insulin requirements). Products include:
- Novolin N Human Insulin 10 ml Vials 1846

Insulin, Human NPH (In diabetic patients the metabolic effects of androgens may decrease blood glucose and insulin requirements). Products include:
- Humulin N, 100 Units 1495
- Novolin N PenFill 1.5 ml Cartridges Durable Insulin Delivery System 1849
- Novolin N Prefilled Syringe Disposable Insulin Delivery System 1850

Insulin, Human Regular (In diabetic patients the metabolic effects of androgens may decrease blood glucose and insulin requirements). Products include:
- Humulin R, 100 Units 1497
- Novolin R Human Insulin 10 ml Vials 1846
- Novolin R PenFill 1.5 ml Cartridges Durable Insulin Delivery System 1849
- Novolin R Prefilled Syringe Disposable Insulin Delivery System 1850
- Velosulin BR Human Insulin 10 ml Vials 1847

Insulin, Human, Zinc Suspension (In diabetic patients the metabolic effects of androgens may decrease blood glucose and insulin requirements). Products include:
- Humulin L, 100 Units 1494
- Humulin U, 100 Units 1498
- Novolin L Human Insulin 10 ml Vials 1846

Insulin Lispro, Human (In diabetic patients the metabolic effects of androgens may decrease blood glucose and insulin requirements). Products include:
- Humalog Injection 1488

Insulin, NPH (In diabetic patients the metabolic effects of androgens may decrease blood glucose and insulin requirements). Products include:
- NPH, 100 Units 1502
- Pork NPH, 100 Units 1506
- Purified Pork NPH Isophane Insulin 1852

Insulin, Regular (In diabetic patients the metabolic effects of androgens may decrease blood glucose and insulin requirements). Products include:
- Regular, 100 Units 1503
- Pork Regular, 100 Units 1507
- Pork Regular (Concentrated), 500 Units 1508
- Purified Pork Regular Insulin 1852

Insulin, Zinc Crystals (In diabetic patients the metabolic effects of androgens may decrease blood glucose and insulin requirements). Products include:
- NPH, 100 Units 1502

Insulin, Zinc Suspension (In diabetic patients the metabolic effects of androgens may decrease blood glucose and insulin requirements). Products include:
- Iletin I 1501
- Lente, 100 Units 1501
- Iletin II 1504
- Pork Lente, 100 Units 1504
- Purified Pork Lente Insulin 1852

Oxyphenbutazone (Concurrent use may result in elevated serum levels of oxyphenbutazone).

Warfarin Sodium (Decreased anticoagulant requirements). Products include:
- Coumadin 941

ANECTINE INJECTION
(Succinylcholine Chloride) 1062
See **Anectine Sterile Powder Flo-Pack**

ANECTINE STERILE POWDER FLO-PACK
(Succinylcholine Chloride) 1062
May interact with beta blockers, monoamine oxidase inhibitors, oral contraceptives, glucocorticoids, neuromuscular blocking agents, and certain other agents. Compounds in these categories include:

Acebutolol Hydrochloride (Enhances neuromuscular blocking action). Products include:
- Sectral Capsules 2914

Antibiotics, non-penicillin, unspecified (Enhances neuromuscular blocking action).

Anticancer Drugs, unspecified (Prolong respiratory depression).

Aprotinin (Enhances neuromuscular blocking action). Products include:
- Trasylol 607

Atenolol (Enhances neuromuscular blocking action). Products include:
- Tenoretic Tablets 2963
- Tenormin Tablets and I.V. Injection 2965

Atracurium Besylate (Possible synergistic or antagonistic effect if co-administered during the same procedure). Products include:
- Tracrium Injection 1155

Betamethasone Acetate (Chronic use of glucocorticoids enhances neuromuscular blocking effect by reducing plasma cholinesterase activity). Products include:
- Celestone Soluspan Suspension 2484

Betamethasone Sodium Phosphate (Chronic use of glucocorticoids enhances neuromuscular blocking effect by reducing plasma cholinesterase activity). Products include:
- Celestone Soluspan Suspension 2484

Betaxolol Hydrochloride (Enhances neuromuscular blocking action). Products include:
- Betoptic Ophthalmic Solution 465
- Betoptic S Ophthalmic Suspension 467
- Kerlone Tablets 2588

Bisoprolol Fumarate (Enhances neuromuscular blocking action). Products include:
- Zebeta Tablets 1457
- Ziac 1459

Carteolol Hydrochloride (Enhances neuromuscular blocking action). Products include:
- Cartrol Tablets 413
- Ocupress Ophthalmic Solution, 1% Solution .... ⊙ 297

Chloroquine Hydrochloride (Enhances neuromuscular blocking action). Products include:
- Aralen Hydrochloride Injection 2430

Chloroquine Phosphate (Enhances neuromuscular blocking action). Products include:
- Aralen Phosphate Tablets 2431

Cisatracurium Besylate (Possible synergistic or antagonistic effect if co-administered during the same procedure). Products include:
- Nimbex Injection 1131

Cortisone Acetate (Chronic use of glucocorticoids enhances neuromuscular blocking effect by reducing plasma cholinesterase activity). Products include:
- Cortone Acetate Sterile Suspension 1663
- Cortone Acetate Tablets 1664

Desflurane (Enhances neuromuscular blocking action). Products include:
- Suprane (desflurane, USP) 1865

Desogestrel (Chronic use of oral contraceptives enhances neuromuscular blocking effect by reducing plasma cholinesterase activity). Products include:
- Desogen Tablets 1867
- Ortho-Cept 1907

Dexamethasone (Chronic use of glucocorticoids enhances neuromuscular blocking effect by reducing plasma cholinesterase activity). Products include:
- AK-Trol Ointment & Suspension .... ⊙ 205
- Decadron Elixir 1676
- Decadron Tablets 1678
- Decaspray Topical Aerosol 1689
- Maxitrol Ophthalmic Ointment and Suspension .... ⊙ 222
- TobraDex Ophthalmic Suspension and Ointment 469

Dexamethasone Acetate (Chronic use of glucocorticoids enhances neuromuscular blocking effect by reducing plasma cholinesterase activity). Products include:
- Dalalone D.P. Injectable 1009
- Decadron-LA Sterile Suspension 1687

Dexamethasone Sodium Phosphate (Chronic use of glucocorticoids enhances neuromuscular blocking effect by reducing plasma cholinesterase activity). Products include:
- Decadron Phosphate Injection 1680
- Decadron Phosphate Sterile Ophthalmic Ointment 1684
- Decadron Phosphate Sterile Ophthalmic Solution 1685
- Decadron Phosphate Topical Cream 1686
- Decadron Phosphate with Xylocaine Injection, Sterile 1683
- Dexacort Phosphate in Respihaler 1606
- Dexacort Phosphate in Turbinaire 1607
- NeoDecadron Sterile Ophthalmic Ointment 1755
- NeoDecadron Sterile Ophthalmic Solution 1756
- NeoDecadron Topical Cream 1757

Diethyl Ether (Enhances neuromuscular blocking action).

Doxacurium Chloride (Possible synergistic or antagonistic effect if co-administered during the same procedure). Products include:
- Nuromax Injection 1136

Echothiophate Iodide (Prolongs respiratory depression). Products include:
- Phospholine Iodide .... ⊙ 323

Esmolol Hydrochloride (Enhances neuromuscular blocking action). Products include:
- Brevibloc (esmolol HCl) Injection 1860

Ethinyl Estradiol (Chronic use of oral contraceptives enhances neuromuscular blocking effect by reducing plasma cholinesterase activity). Products include:
- Brevicon 2563
- Demulen 2580
- Desogen Tablets 1867
- Levlen/Tri-Levlen 646
- Lo/Ovral Tablets 2852
- Lo/Ovral-28 Tablets 2857
- Modicon 1928
- Nordette-21 Tablets 2863
- Nordette-28 Tablets 2866
- Norinyl 2563
- Ortho-Cept 1907
- Ortho-Cyclen/Ortho-Tri-Cyclen 1914
- Ortho-Novum 1928
- Ortho-Cyclen/Ortho Tri-Cyclen 1914
- Ovcon 765
- Ovral Tablets 2877
- Ovral-28 Tablets 2878
- Levlen/Tri-Levlen 646
- Tri-Norinyl 2607
- Triphasil-21 Tablets 2919
- Triphasil-28 Tablets 2924

Ethynodiol Diacetate (Chronic use of oral contraceptives enhances neuromuscular blocking effect by reducing plasma cholinesterase activity). Products include:
- Demulen 2580

Fludrocortisone Acetate (Chronic use of glucocorticoids enhances neuromuscular blocking effect by reducing plasma cholinesterase activity). Products include:
- Florinef Acetate Tablets 506

Furazolidone (Chronic use of certain unspecified MAO inhibitors enhances neuromuscular blocking effect by reducing plasma cholinesterase activity). Products include:
- Furoxone 2221

(▩ Described in PDR For Nonprescription Drugs)   (⊙ Described in PDR For Ophthalmology)

Hydrocortisone (Chronic use of glucocorticoids enhances neuromuscular blocking effect by reducing plasma cholinesterase activity). Products include:

Anusol-HC Cream 2.5%	1953
Aquanil HC Lotion	1989
Maximum Strength Cortaid Spray	800
CORTENEMA	2713
Cortisporin Ointment	1074
Cortisporin Ophthalmic Ointment Sterile	1074
Cortisporin Ophthalmic Suspension Sterile	1075
Cortisporin Otic Solution Sterile	1076
Cortisporin Otic Suspension Sterile	1077
Cortizone-5	795
Cortizone-10	795
Hydrocortone Tablets	1715
Hytone	922
Hytone Ointment 2 ½%	923
Massengill Medicated Soft Cloth Towelettes	2628
Pediotic Suspension Sterile	1140
Preparation H Hydrocortisone 1% Cream	843
ProctoCream-HC 2.5%	2552
VōSoL HC Otic Solution	2786

Hydrocortisone Acetate (Chronic use of glucocorticoids enhances neuromuscular blocking effect by reducing plasma cholinesterase activity). Products include:

Analpram-HC Rectal Cream 1% and 2.5%	993
Anusol HC-1 Hydrocortisone Anti-Itch Ointment	810
Anusol-HC Suppositories	1954
Caldecort Anti-Itch Hydrocortisone Cream	651
Coly-Mycin S Otic w/Neomycin & Hydrocortisone	1965
Cortaid	800
Cortifoam	2540
Cortisporin Cream	1073
Epifoam	2543
Hydrocortone Acetate Sterile Suspension	1712
Mantadil Cream	1124
Nupercainal Hydrocortisone 1% Cream	661
Pramosone Cream, Lotion & Ointment	995
ProctoFoam-HC	2552
Terra-Cortril Ophthalmic Suspension	2033

Hydrocortisone Sodium Phosphate (Chronic use of glucocorticoids enhances neuromuscular blocking effect by reducing plasma cholinesterase activity). Products include:

Hydrocortone Phosphate Injection, Sterile	1713

Hydrocortisone Sodium Succinate (Chronic use of glucocorticoids enhances neuromuscular blocking effect by reducing plasma cholinesterase activity).

No products indexed under this heading.

Isocarboxazid (Chronic use of certain unspecified MAO inhibitors enhances neuromuscular blocking effect by reducing plasma cholinesterase activity).

No products indexed under this heading.

Isoflurane (Enhances neuromuscular blocking action).

No products indexed under this heading.

Labetalol Hydrochloride (Enhances neuromuscular blocking action). Products include:

Normodyne Injection	2519
Normodyne Tablets	2522
Trandate	1158

Levobunolol Hydrochloride (Enhances neuromuscular blocking action). Products include:

Betagan	230

Levonorgestrel (Chronic use of oral contraceptives enhances neuromuscular blocking effect by reducing plasma cholinesterase activity). Products include:

Levlen/Tri-Levlen	646
Nordette-21 Tablets	2863
Nordette-28 Tablets	2866
Norplant System	2868
Levlen/Tri-Levlen	646
Triphasil-21 Tablets	2919
Triphasil-28 Tablets	2924

Lidocaine Hydrochloride (Enhances neuromuscular blocking action). Products include:

Decadron Phosphate with Xylocaine Injection, Sterile	1683
Unguentine Plus	712
Xylocaine Injections	562

Lithium Carbonate (Enhances neuromuscular blocking action). Products include:

Eskalith	2658
Lithium Carbonate Capsules & Tablets	2352
Lithonate/Lithotabs/Lithobid	2721

Magnesium Sulfate Injection (Enhances neuromuscular blocking action).

Mestranol (Chronic use of oral contraceptives enhances neuromuscular blocking effect by reducing plasma cholinesterase activity). Products include:

Norinyl	2563
Ortho-Novum	1928

Methylprednisolone Acetate (Chronic use of glucocorticoids enhances neuromuscular blocking effect by reducing plasma cholinesterase activity).

No products indexed under this heading.

Methylprednisolone Sodium Succinate (Chronic use of glucocorticoids enhances neuromuscular blocking effect by reducing plasma cholinesterase activity).

No products indexed under this heading.

Metipranolol Hydrochloride (Enhances neuromuscular blocking action). Products include:

OptiPranolol (Metipranolol 0.3%) Sterile Ophthalmic Solution	256

Metoclopramide Hydrochloride (Enhances neuromuscular blocking action). Products include:

Reglan	2243

Metocurine Iodide (Possible synergistic or antagonistic effect if co-administered during the same procedure). Products include:

Metubine Iodide Vials	932

Metoprolol Succinate (Enhances neuromuscular blocking action). Products include:

Toprol-XL Tablets	560

Metoprolol Tartrate (Enhances neuromuscular blocking action). Products include:

Lopressor	848
Lopressor HCT Tablets	850

Mivacurium Chloride (Possible synergistic or antagonistic effect if co-administered during the same procedure). Products include:

Mivacron	1125

Nadolol (Enhances neuromuscular blocking action).

No products indexed under this heading.

Norethindrone (Chronic use of oral contraceptives enhances neuromuscular blocking effect by reducing plasma cholinesterase activity). Products include:

Brevicon	2563
Micronor Tablets	1903
Modicon	1928
Norinyl	2563
Nor-Q D Tablets	2598
Ortho-Novum	1928
Ovcon	765
Tri-Norinyl	2607

Norethynodrel (Chronic use of oral contraceptives enhances neuromuscular blocking effect by reducing plasma cholinesterase activity).

No products indexed under this heading.

Norgestimate (Chronic use of oral contraceptives enhances neuromuscular blocking effect by reducing plasma cholinesterase activity). Products include:

Ortho-Cyclen/Ortho-Tri-Cyclen	1914
Ortho-Cyclen/Ortho-Tri-Cyclen	1914

Norgestrel (Chronic use of oral contraceptives enhances neuromuscular blocking effect by reducing plasma cholinesterase activity). Products include:

Lo/Ovral Tablets	2852
Lo/Ovral-28 Tablets	2857
Ovral Tablets	2877
Ovral-28 Tablets	2878
Ovrette Tablets	2878

Oxytocin (Enhances neuromuscular blocking action). Products include:

Syntocinon Injection	2425

Oxytocin (Nasal Spray) (Enhances neuromuscular blocking action).

Pancuronium Bromide (Possible synergistic or antagonistic effect if co-administered during the same procedure).

No products indexed under this heading.

Penbutolol Sulfate (Enhances neuromuscular blocking action). Products include:

Levatol Tablets	2547

Phenelzine Sulfate (Chronic use of certain unspecified MAO inhibitors enhances neuromuscular blocking effect by reducing plasma cholinesterase activity). Products include:

Nardil	1977

Pindolol (Enhances neuromuscular blocking action). Products include:

Visken Tablets	2428

Prednisolone Acetate (Chronic use of glucocorticoids enhances neuromuscular blocking effect by reducing plasma cholinesterase activity). Products include:

AK-CIDE	203
AK-CIDE Ointment	203
Blephamide Liquifilm Sterile Ophthalmic Suspension	472
Blephamide Ointment	234
Econopred & Econopred Plus Ophthalmic Suspensions	216
Poly-Pred Liquifilm	246
Pred Forte	247
Pred Mild	250
Pred-G Liquifilm Sterile Ophthalmic Suspension	248
Pred-G S.O.P. Sterile Ophthalmic Ointment	249

Prednisolone Sodium Phosphate (Chronic use of glucocorticoids enhances neuromuscular blocking effect by reducing plasma cholinesterase activity). Products include:

AK-PRED	204
Hydeltrasol Injection, Sterile	1708
Pediapred Oral Solution	1618

Prednisolone Tebutate (Chronic use of glucocorticoids enhances neuromuscular blocking effect by reducing plasma cholinesterase activity). Products include:

Hydeltra-T.B.A. Sterile Suspension	1710

Prednisone (Chronic use of glucocorticoids enhances neuromuscular blocking effect by reducing plasma cholinesterase activity).

No products indexed under this heading.

Procainamide Hydrochloride (Enhances neuromuscular blocking action). Products include:

Procanbid Extended-Release Tablets	1983

Promazine Hydrochloride (Enhances neuromuscular blocking action).

No products indexed under this heading.

Propranolol Hydrochloride (Enhances neuromuscular blocking action). Products include:

Inderal	2834
Inderal LA Long Acting Capsules	2836
Inderide Tablets	2838
Inderide LA Long Acting Capsules	2840

Quinidine Gluconate (Enhances neuromuscular blocking action). Products include:

Quinaglute Dura-Tabs Tablets	644

Quinidine Polygalacturonate (Enhances neuromuscular blocking action). Products include:

Cardioquin Tablets	2146

Quinidine Sulfate (Enhances neuromuscular blocking action). Products include:

Quinidex Extentabs	2240

Quinine (Enhances neuromuscular blocking action).

Rocuronium Bromide (Possible synergistic or antagonistic effect if co-administered during the same procedure). Products include:

Zemuron Injection	1885

Selegiline Hydrochloride (Chronic use of certain unspecified MAO inhibitors enhances neuromuscular blocking effect by reducing plasma cholinesterase activity). Products include:

Eldepryl Capsules	2729

Sotalol Hydrochloride (Enhances neuromuscular blocking action). Products include:

Betapace Tablets	637

Terbutaline Sulfate (Enhances neuromuscular blocking action). Products include:

Brethaire Inhaler	830
Brethine Ampuls	832
Brethine Tablets	831
Bricanyl Subcutaneous Injection	1247
Bricanyl Tablets	1248

Timolol Hemihydrate (Enhances neuromuscular blocking action). Products include:

Betimol 0.25%, 0.5%	259

Timolol Maleate (Enhances neuromuscular blocking action). Products include:

Blocadren Tablets	1654
Timolide Tablets	1791
Timoptic in Ocudose	1796
Timoptic Sterile Ophthalmic Solution	1794
Timoptic-XE	1798

Tranylcypromine Sulfate (Chronic use of certain unspecified MAO inhibitors enhances neuromuscular blocking effect by reducing plasma cholinesterase activity). Products include:

Parnate Tablets	2679

Triamcinolone (Chronic use of glucocorticoids enhances neuromuscular blocking effect by reducing plasma cholinesterase activity).

No products indexed under this heading.

IMPORTANT NOTE: Always consult each drug listing in the patient's regimen for possible interactions.

Anectine — Interactions Index

Triamcinolone Acetonide (Chronic use of glucocorticoids enhances neuromuscular blocking effect by reducing plasma cholinesterase activity). Products include:

- Azmacort Oral Inhaler ... 2175
- Nasacort AQ Nasal Spray ... 2191
- Nasacort Nasal Inhaler ... 2189

Triamcinolone Diacetate (Chronic use of glucocorticoids enhances neuromuscular blocking effect by reducing plasma cholinesterase activity).
No products indexed under this heading.

Triamcinolone Hexacetonide (Chronic use of glucocorticoids enhances neuromuscular blocking effect by reducing plasma cholinesterase activity).
No products indexed under this heading.

Trimethaphan Camsylate (Enhances neuromuscular blocking action).
No products indexed under this heading.

Vecuronium Bromide (Possible synergistic or antagonistic effect if co-administered during the same procedure). Products include:

- Norcuron for Injection ... 1875

ANTABUSE TABLETS
(Disulfiram) ... 2802
May interact with oral anticoagulants and certain other agents. Compounds in these categories include:

Dicumarol (Prolonged prothrombin time).
No products indexed under this heading.

Isoniazid (Potential for the appearance of unsteady gait or marked changes in mental status). Products include:

- Nydrazid Injection ... 509
- Rifamate Capsules ... 1278
- Rifater ... 1280

Metronidazole (Psychotic reactions due to combined toxicity). Products include:

- Flagyl 375 Capsules ... 2587
- Flagyl I.V. RTU ... 2373
- Helidac Therapy ... 2135
- MetroCream ... 1034
- MetroGel ... 1034
- MetroGel-Vaginal ... 917
- Protostat Tablets ... 1939

Metronidazole Hydrochloride (Psychotic reactions due to combined toxicity). Products include:

- Flagyl I.V. ... 2373

Paraldehyde (Contraindicated).

Phenytoin (Phenytoin intoxication). Products include:

- Dilantin Infatabs ... 1967
- Dilantin-125 Suspension ... 1969

Phenytoin Sodium (Phenytoin intoxication). Products include:

- Dilantin Kapseals ... 1965

Warfarin Sodium (Prolonged prothrombin time). Products include:

- Coumadin ... 941

Food Interactions
Alcohol (Antabuse plus alcohol, even small amounts, produces flushing, throbbing in head and neck, respiratory difficulty, headache and other serious reactions including convulsions and death; concurrent use is contraindicated).

ANTILIRIUM INJECTABLE
(Physostigmine Salicylate) ... 1007
May interact with:

Atropine Sulfate (Atropine antagonizes the action of Physostigmine). Products include:

- Arco-Lase Plus Tablets ... 513
- Atrohist Plus Tablets ... 1605
- Donnatal ... 2234
- Donnatal Extentabs ... 2234
- Donnatal Tablets ... 2234
- Lomotil ... 2591
- Motofen Tablets ... 789
- Urised Tablets ... 2123

Decamethonium (Concurrent administration contraindicated).

Succinylcholine Chloride (Concurrent administration contraindicated). Products include:

- Anectine ... 1062

ANTIVENIN (BLACK WIDOW SPIDER)
(Black Widow Spider Antivenin (Equine)) ... 1647
None cited in PDR database.

ANTIVENIN (CROTALIDAE) POLYVALENT
(Antivenin (Crotalidae) Polyvalent) ... 2803
May interact with beta blockers. Compounds in this category include:

Acebutolol Hydrochloride (Potential for increased severity of acute and prolonged anaphylaxis). Products include:

- Sectral Capsules ... 2914

Atenolol (Potential for increased severity of acute and prolonged anaphylaxis). Products include:

- Tenoretic Tablets ... 2963
- Tenormin Tablets and I.V. Injection ... 2965

Betaxolol Hydrochloride (Potential for increased severity of acute and prolonged anaphylaxis). Products include:

- Betoptic Ophthalmic Solution ... 465
- Betoptic S Ophthalmic Suspension ... 467
- Kerlone Tablets ... 2588

Bisoprolol Fumarate (Potential for increased severity of acute and prolonged anaphylaxis). Products include:

- Zebeta Tablets ... 1457
- Ziac ... 1459

Carteolol Hydrochloride (Potential for increased severity of acute and prolonged anaphylaxis). Products include:

- Cartrol Tablets ... 413
- Ocupress Ophthalmic Solution, 1% Sterile ... ⊚ 297

Esmolol Hydrochloride (Potential for increased severity of acute and prolonged anaphylaxis). Products include:

- Brevibloc (esmolol HCl) Injection ... 1860

Labetalol Hydrochloride (Potential for increased severity of acute and prolonged anaphylaxis). Products include:

- Normodyne Injection ... 2519
- Normodyne Tablets ... 2522
- Trandate ... 1158

Levobunolol Hydrochloride (Potential for increased severity of acute and prolonged anaphylaxis). Products include:

- Betagan ... ⊚ 230

Metipranolol Hydrochloride (Potential for increased severity of acute and prolonged anaphylaxis). Products include:

- OptiPranolol (Metipranolol 0.3%) Sterile Ophthalmic Solution ... ⊚ 256

Metoprolol Succinate (Potential for increased severity of acute and prolonged anaphylaxis). Products include:

- Toprol-XL Tablets ... 560

Metoprolol Tartrate (Potential for increased severity of acute and prolonged anaphylaxis). Products include:

- Lopressor ... 848
- Lopressor HCT Tablets ... 850

Nadolol (Potential for increased severity of acute and prolonged anaphylaxis).
No products indexed under this heading.

Penbutolol Sulfate (Potential for increased severity of acute and prolonged anaphylaxis). Products include:

- Levatol Tablets ... 2547

Pindolol (Potential for increased severity of acute and prolonged anaphylaxis). Products include:

- Visken Tablets ... 2428

Propranolol Hydrochloride (Potential for increased severity of acute and prolonged anaphylaxis). Products include:

- Inderal ... 2834
- Inderal LA Long Acting Capsules ... 2836
- Inderide Tablets ... 2838
- Inderide LA Long Acting Capsules ... 2840

Sotalol Hydrochloride (Potential for increased severity of acute and prolonged anaphylaxis). Products include:

- Betapace Tablets ... 637

Timolol Hemihydrate (Potential for increased severity of acute and prolonged anaphylaxis). Products include:

- Betimol 0.25%, 0.5% ... ⊚ 259

Timolol Maleate (Potential for increased severity of acute and prolonged anaphylaxis). Products include:

- Blocadren Tablets ... 1654
- Timolide Tablets ... 1791
- Timoptic in Ocudose ... 1796
- Timoptic Sterile Ophthalmic Solution ... 1794
- Timoptic-XE ... 1798

ANTIVERT, ANTIVERT/25 TABLETS, & ANTIVERT/50 TABLETS
(Meclizine Hydrochloride) ... 1992

Food Interactions
Alcohol (Concurrent use should be avoided).

ANTURANE CAPSULES
(Sulfinpyrazone) ... 823
May interact with oral anticoagulants, salicylates, sulfonylureas, insulin, and certain other agents. Compounds in these categories include:

Aspirin (Uricosuric action antagonized). Products include:

- Alka-Seltzer Cherry Effervescent Antacid and Pain Reliever ... ▣ 609
- Alka-Seltzer Extra Strength Effervescent Antacid and Pain Reliever ... ▣ 609
- Alka-Seltzer Lemon Lime Effervescent Antacid and Pain Reliever ... ▣ 609
- Alka-Seltzer Original Effervescent Antacid and Pain Reliever ... ▣ 609
- Alka-Seltzer Plus ... ▣ 611
- Alka-Seltzer Plus Sinus Medicine ... ▣ 611
- Ascriptin ... ▣ 650
- Arthritis Strength BC Powder ... ▣ 631
- BC Cold Powder Multi-Symptom Formula (Cold-Sinus-Allergy) ... ▣ 631
- BC Cold Powder Non-Drowsy Formula (Cold-Sinus) ... ▣ 631
- BC Powder ... ▣ 631
- Genuine Bayer Aspirin Tablets & Caplets ... ▣ 618
- Extra Strength Bayer Arthritis Pain Regimen Formula ... ▣ 615
- Extra Strength Bayer Aspirin Caplets & Tablets ... ▣ 617
- Extended-Release Bayer 8-Hour Aspirin ... ▣ 616
- Extra Strength Bayer Plus Aspirin Caplets ... ▣ 617
- Extra Strength Bayer PM Aspirin Plus Sleep Aid ... ▣ 617
- Aspirin Regimen Bayer 81 mg Tablets with Calcium ... ▣ 615
- Aspirin Regimen Bayer Adult Low Strength 81 mg Tablets ... ▣ 613
- Aspirin Regimen Bayer Children's Chewable Aspirin ... ▣ 616
- Aspirin Regimen Bayer Regular Strength 325 mg Caplets ... ▣ 613
- Bufferin Analgesic Tablets ... ▣ 636
- Arthritis Strength Bufferin Analgesic Caplets ... ▣ 637
- Extra Strength Bufferin Analgesic Tablets ... ▣ 637
- Cama Arthritis Pain Reliever ... ▣ 748
- Darvon Compound-65 Pulvules ... 1475
- Easprin ... 1971
- Ecotrin ... 2625
- Ecotrin Enteric Coated Aspirin Maximum Strength Tablets and Caplets ... ▣ 775
- Ecotrin Enteric Coated Aspirin Regular Strength Tablets ... 2625
- Empirin Aspirin Tablets ... ▣ 818
- Excedrin Extra-Strength Analgesic Tablets, Caplets, and Geltabs ... 734
- Fiorinal Capsules ... 2388
- Fiorinal with Codeine Capsules ... 2390
- Fiorinal Tablets ... 2388
- Goody's Extra Strength Headache Powders ... ▣ 632
- Goody's Extra Strength Pain Relief Tablets ... ▣ 632
- Halfprin Tablets ... 1413
- Norgesic ... 1554
- Percodan Tablets ... 955
- Percodan-Demi Tablets ... 956
- Robaxisal Tablets ... 2246
- Soma Compound w/Codeine Tablets ... 2784
- Soma Compound Tablets ... 2783
- St. Joseph Adult Chewable Aspirin (81 mg.) ... ▣ 768
- Talwin Compound ... 2466
- Vanquish Analgesic Caplets ... ▣ 627

Chlorpropamide (Potentiated). Products include:

- Diabinese Tablets ... 2002

Choline Magnesium Trisalicylate (Uricosuric action antagonized). Products include:

- Trilisate ... 2155

Dicumarol (Action of coumarin-type anticoagulants may be accentuated).
No products indexed under this heading.

Diflunisal (Uricosuric action antagonized). Products include:

- Dolobid Tablets ... 1695

Glimepiride (Potentiated). Products include:

- Amaryl Tablets ... 1241

Glipizide (Potentiated). Products include:

- Glucotrol Tablets ... 2011
- Glucotrol XL Extended Release Tablets ... 2012

Glyburide (Potentiated). Products include:

- DiaBeta Tablets ... 1265
- Glynase PresTab Tablets ... 2091
- Micronase Tablets ... 2099

Insulin, Human (Potentiated).
No products indexed under this heading.

Insulin, Human Isophane Suspension (Potentiated). Products include:

- Novolin N Human Insulin 10 ml Vials ... 1846

Insulin, Human NPH (Potentiated). Products include:

- Humulin N, 100 Units ... 1495

(▣ Described in PDR For Nonprescription Drugs)   (⊚ Described in PDR For Ophthalmology)

Novolin N PenFill 1.5 ml Cartridges Durable Insulin Delivery System 1849
Novolin N Prefilled Syringe Disposable Insulin Delivery System 1850

Insulin, Human Regular (Potentiated). Products include:
Humulin R, 100 Units 1497
Novolin R Human Insulin 10 ml Vials 1846
Novolin R PenFill 1.5 ml Cartridges Durable Insulin Delivery System 1849
Novolin R Prefilled Syringe Disposable Insulin Delivery System 1850
Velosulin BR Human Insulin 10 ml Vials 1847

Insulin, Human, Zinc Suspension (Potentiated). Products include:
Humulin L, 100 Units 1494
Humulin U, 100 Units 1498
Novolin L Human Insulin 10 ml Vials 1846

Insulin Lispro, Human (Potentiated). Products include:
Humalog Injection 1488

Insulin, NPH (Potentiated). Products include:
NPH, 100 Units 1502
Pork NPH, 100 Units.................... 1506
Purified Pork NPH Isophane Insulin 1852

Insulin, Regular (Potentiated). Products include:
Regular, 100 Units 1503
Pork Regular, 100 Units 1507
Pork Regular (Concentrated), 500 Units 1508
Purified Pork Regular Insulin 1852

Insulin, Zinc Crystals (Potentiated). Products include:
NPH, 100 Units 1502

Insulin, Zinc Suspension (Potentiated). Products include:
Iletin I 1501
Lente, 100 Units 1501
Iletin II 1504
Pork Lente, 100 Units.................. 1504
Purified Pork Lente Insulin 1852

Magnesium Salicylate (Uricosuric action antagonized). Products include:
Backache Caplets ....⊞ 635
Doan's Extra-Strength Analgesic ....⊞ 653
Extra Strength Doan's P.M. ....⊞ 653
Doan's Regular Strength Analgesic ....⊞ 654
Mobigesic Tablets ....⊞ 607

Salsalate (Uricosuric action antagonized). Products include:
Disalcid 1549
Mono-Gesic Tablets 810
Salflex Tablets 791

Sulfisoxazole (Potentiated). Products include:
Gantrisin Tablets 2286

Tolazamide (Potentiated).
No products indexed under this heading.

Tolbutamide (Potentiated).
No products indexed under this heading.

Warfarin Sodium (Action of coumarin-type anticoagulants may be accentuated). Products include:
Coumadin 941

ANTURANE TABLETS
(Sulfinpyrazone) 823
See **Anturane Capsules**

ANUSOL HEMORRHOIDAL OINTMENT
(Pramoxine Hydrochloride, Zinc Oxide, Mineral Oil) ....⊞ 810
None cited in PDR database.

ANUSOL HEMORRHOIDAL SUPPOSITORIES
(Starch) ....⊞ 810
None cited in PDR database.

ANUSOL HC-1 HYDROCORTISONE ANTI-ITCH OINTMENT
(Hydrocortisone Acetate) ....⊞ 810
None cited in PDR database.

ANUSOL-HC CREAM 2.5%
(Hydrocortisone) 1953
None cited in PDR database.

ANUSOL-HC SUPPOSITORIES
(Hydrocortisone Acetate) 1954
None cited in PDR database.

APRESAZIDE CAPSULES
(Hydralazine Hydrochloride, Hydrochlorothiazide) 824
May interact with monoamine oxidase inhibitors, corticosteroids, antihypertensives, insulin, narcotic analgesics, barbiturates, cardiac glycosides, non-steroidal anti-inflammatory agents, lithium preparations, and certain other agents. Compounds in these categories include:

Acebutolol Hydrochloride (Additive or potentiated action). Products include:
Sectral Capsules 2914

ACTH (Concomitant use may result in hypokalemia).
No products indexed under this heading.

Alfentanil Hydrochloride (May potentiate orthostatic hypotension). Products include:
Alfenta Injection 1334

Amlodipine Besylate (Additive or potentiated action). Products include:
Lotrel Capsules 858
Norvasc Tablets 2020

Aprobarbital (May potentiate orthostatic hypotension).
No products indexed under this heading.

Atenolol (Additive or potentiated action). Products include:
Tenoretic Tablets 2963
Tenormin Tablets and I.V. Injection ... 2965

Benazepril Hydrochloride (Additive or potentiated action). Products include:
Lotensin Tablets 852
Lotensin HCT Tablets 855
Lotrel Capsules 858

Bendroflumethiazide (Additive or potentiated action).
No products indexed under this heading.

Betamethasone Acetate (Concomitant use may result in hypokalemia). Products include:
Celestone Soluspan Suspension 2484

Betamethasone Sodium Phosphate (Concomitant use may result in hypokalemia). Products include:
Celestone Soluspan Suspension 2484

Betaxolol Hydrochloride (Additive or potentiated action). Products include:
Betoptic Ophthalmic Solution 465
Betoptic S Ophthalmic Suspension ... 467
Kerlone Tablets 2588

Bisoprolol Fumarate (Additive or potentiated action). Products include:
Zebeta Tablets 1457
Ziac 1459

Buprenorphine (May potentiate orthostatic hypotension). Products include:
Buprenex Injectable 2170

Butabarbital (May potentiate orthostatic hypotension).
No products indexed under this heading.

Butalbital (May potentiate orthostatic hypotension). Products include:
Axocet Capsules 2469
Esgic-plus Capsules 1012
Esgic-plus Tablets 1012
Fioricet Tablets 2386
Fioricet with Codeine Capsules 2387
Fiorinal Capsules 2388
Fiorinal with Codeine Capsules 2390
Fiorinal Tablets 2388
Phrenilin 790
Sedapap Tablets 50 mg/650 mg .. 1826

Captopril (Additive or potentiated action). Products include:
Capoten Tablets 740
Capozide Tablets 744

Carteolol Hydrochloride (Additive or potentiated action). Products include:
Cartrol Tablets 413
Ocupress Ophthalmic Solution, 1% Sterile ....ⓒ 297

Chlorothiazide (Additive or potentiated action). Products include:
Aldoclor Tablets 1638
Diupres Tablets 1691
Diuril Oral 1694

Chlorothiazide Sodium (Additive or potentiated action). Products include:
Diuril Sodium Intravenous 1693

Chlorthalidone (Additive or potentiated action). Products include:
Combipres Tablets 682
Tenoretic Tablets 2963
Thalitone 1293

Cholestyramine (Impairs the oral absorption of hydrochlorothiazide from gastrointestinal tract by up to 85%). Products include:
Questran 774

Clonidine (Additive or potentiated action). Products include:
Catapres-TTS................................ 680

Clonidine Hydrochloride (Additive or potentiated action). Products include:
Catapres Tablets 679
Combipres Tablets 682

Codeine Phosphate (May potentiate orthostatic hypotension). Products include:
Brontex 2130
Dimetane-DC Cough Syrup 2232
Fioricet with Codeine Capsules 2387
Fiorinal with Codeine Capsules 2390
Nucofed 2225
Phenergan with Codeine 2883
Phenergan VC with Codeine 2888
Robitussin A-C Syrup 2248
Robitussin-DAC Syrup 2249
Ryna ....⊞ 804
Soma Compound w/Codeine Tablets 2784
Tylenol with Codeine 1592

Colestipol Hydrochloride (Impairs the oral absorption of hydrochlorothiazide from gastrointestinal tract by up to 43%). Products include:
Colestid 2073

Cortisone Acetate (Concomitant use may result in hypokalemia). Products include:
Cortone Acetate Sterile Suspension 1663
Cortone Acetate Tablets 1664

Deserpidine (Additive or potentiated action).
No products indexed under this heading.

Deslanoside (Hypokalemia can exaggerate cardiotoxicity of digitalis).
No products indexed under this heading.

Dexamethasone (Concomitant use may result in hypokalemia). Products include:
AK-Trol Ointment & Suspension .... ⓒ 205
Decadron Elixir 1676
Decadron Tablets 1678
Decaspray Topical Aerosol 1689
Maxitrol Ophthalmic Ointment and Suspension .... ⓒ 222
TobraDex Ophthalmic Suspension and Ointment............................ 469

Dexamethasone Acetate (Concomitant use may result in hypokalemia). Products include:
Dalalone D.P. Injectable 1009
Decadron-LA Sterile Suspension ... 1687

Dexamethasone Sodium Phosphate (Concomitant use may result in hypokalemia). Products include:
Decadron Phosphate Injection 1680
Decadron Phosphate Sterile Ophthalmic Ointment 1684
Decadron Phosphate Sterile Ophthalmic Solution 1685
Decadron Phosphate Topical Cream 1686
Decadron Phosphate with Xylocaine Injection, Sterile 1683
Dexacort Phosphate in Respihaler .. 1606
Dexacort Phosphate in Turbinaire .. 1607
NeoDecadron Sterile Ophthalmic Ointment 1755
NeoDecadron Sterile Ophthalmic Solution 1756
NeoDecadron Topical Cream 1757

Dezocine (May potentiate orthostatic hypotension). Products include:
Dalgan Injection 529

Diazoxide (Profound hypotensive episodes may occur when diazoxide injection and hydralazine are used concomitantly). Products include:
Hyperstat I.V. Injection 2504
Proglycem 575

Diclofenac Potassium (Concurrent administration may reduce the diuretic, natriuretic and antihypertensive effects of thiazide diuretics). Products include:
Cataflam Tablets 833

Diclofenac Sodium (Concurrent administration may reduce the diuretic, natriuretic and antihypertensive effects of thiazide diuretics). Products include:
Voltaren Ophthalmic Sterile Ophthalmic Solution .... ⓒ 264
Cataflam/Voltaren/Voltaren-XR 833

Digitoxin (Hypokalemia can exaggerate cardiotoxicity of digitalis). Products include:
Crystodigin Tablets 1472

Digoxin (Hypokalemia can exaggerate cardiotoxicity of digitalis). Products include:
Lanoxicaps 1110
Lanoxin Elixir Pediatric 1113
Lanoxin Injection 1116
Lanoxin Injection Pediatric 1119
Lanoxin Tablets 1121

Diltiazem Hydrochloride (Additive or potentiated action). Products include:
Cardizem CD Capsules 1251
Cardizem SR Capsules 1255
Cardizem Injectable 1253
Cardizem Tablets 1257
Dilacor XR Extended-release Capsules 2183
Tiazac Capsules 1019

Doxazosin Mesylate (Additive or potentiated action). Products include:
Cardura Tablets 1993

Enalapril Maleate (Additive or potentiated action). Products include:
Vaseretic Tablets 1810
Vasotec Tablets 1816

Enalaprilat (Additive or potentiated action). Products include:
Vasotec I.V. 1814

Epinephrine (Pressor responses may be reduced). Products include:
EPIFRIN .... ⓒ 237

IMPORTANT NOTE: Always consult each drug listing in the patient's regimen for possible interactions.

Apresazide | Interactions Index | 70

EpiPen 808
Marcaine with Epinephrine 2446
Primatene Mist ◘ 843
Sensorcaine with Epinephrine Injection 554
Sus-Phrine Injection 1017
Xylocaine with Epinephrine Injections 562

Epinephrine Bitartrate (Pressor responses may be reduced). Products include:
Sensorcaine-MPF with Epinephrine Injection 554

Esmolol Hydrochloride (Additive or potentiated action). Products include:
Brevibloc (esmolol HCl) Injection 1860

Etodolac (Concurrent administration may reduce the diuretic, natriuretic and antihypertensive effects of thiazide diuretics). Products include:
Lodine Capsules and Tablets 2849

Felodipine (Additive or potentiated action). Products include:
Plendil Extended-Release Tablets 514

Fenoprofen Calcium (Concurrent administration may reduce the diuretic, natriuretic and antihypertensive effects of thiazide diuretics). Products include:
Nalfon 200 Pulvules & Nalfon Tablets 933

Fentanyl (May potentiate orthostatic hypotension). Products include:
Duragesic Transdermal System 1336

Fentanyl Citrate (May potentiate orthostatic hypotension). Products include:
Sublimaze Injection 463

Fludrocortisone Acetate (Concomitant use may result in hypokalemia). Products include:
Florinef Acetate Tablets 506

Flurbiprofen (Concurrent administration may reduce the diuretic, natriuretic and antihypertensive effects of thiazide diuretics).
No products indexed under this heading.

Fosinopril Sodium (Additive or potentiated action). Products include:
Monopril Tablets 762

Furazolidone (MAO inhibitors should be used with caution in patients receiving hydralazine). Products include:
Furoxone 2221

Furosemide (Additive or potentiated action). Products include:
Lasix Injection, Oral Solution and Tablets 1267

Guanabenz Acetate (Additive or potentiated action).
No products indexed under this heading.

Guanethidine Monosulfate (Additive or potentiated action). Products include:
Esimil Tablets 840
Ismelin Tablets 845

Hydrocodone Bitartrate (May potentiate orthostatic hypotension). Products include:
Codiclear DH Syrup 808
Duratuss HD Elixir 2750
Histussin D Liquid 670
Hycodan Tablets and Syrup 946
Hycomine Compound Tablets 948
Hycomine 947
Hycotuss Expectorant Syrup 950
Hydrocet Capsules 787
Lorcet 10/650 Tablets 1016
Lortab 2751
Tussend 1830
Tussend Expectorant 1831
Vicodin Tablets 1404
Vicodin ES Tablets 1405
Vicodin HP Tablets 1403
Vicodin Tuss Expectorant 1406
Zydone Capsules 967

Hydrocodone Polistirex (May potentiate orthostatic hypotension). Products include:
Tussionex Pennkinetic Extended-Release Suspension 1624

Hydrocortisone (Concomitant use may result in hypokalemia). Products include:
Anusol-HC Cream 2.5% 1953
Aquanil HC Lotion 1989
Maximum Strength Cortaid Spray ◘ 800
CORTENEMA 2713
Cortisporin Ointment 1074
Cortisporin Ophthalmic Ointment Sterile 1074
Cortisporin Ophthalmic Suspension Sterile 1075
Cortisporin Otic Solution Sterile 1076
Cortisporin Otic Suspension Sterile 1077
Cortizone-5 ◘ 795
Cortizone-10 ◘ 795
Hydrocortone Tablets 1715
Hytone 922
Hytone Ointment 2 ½% 923
Massengill Medicated Soft Cloth Towelettes 2628
Pediotic Suspension Sterile 1140
Preparation H Hydrocortisone 1% Cream ◘ 843
ProctoCream-HC 2.5% 2552
VōSoL HC Otic Solution 2786

Hydrocortisone Acetate (Concomitant use may result in hypokalemia). Products include:
Analpram-HC Rectal Cream 1% and 2.5% 993
Anusol HC-1 Hydrocortisone Anti-Itch Ointment ◘ 810
Anusol-HC Suppositories 1954
Caldecort Anti-Itch Hydrocortisone Cream ◘ 651
Coly-Mycin S Otic w/Neomycin & Hydrocortisone 1965
Cortaid ◘ 800
Cortifoam 2540
Cortisporin Cream 1073
Epifoam 2543
Hydrocortone Acetate Sterile Suspension 1712
Mantadil Cream 1124
Nupercainal Hydrocortisone 1% Cream ◘ 661
Pramosone Cream, Lotion & Ointment 995
ProctoFoam-HC 2552
Terra-Cortril Ophthalmic Suspension 2033

Hydrocortisone Sodium Phosphate (Concomitant use may result in hypokalemia). Products include:
Hydrocortone Phosphate Injection, Sterile 1713

Hydrocortisone Sodium Succinate (Concomitant use may result in hypokalemia).
No products indexed under this heading.

Hydroflumethiazide (Additive or potentiated action). Products include:
Diucardin Tablets 2824

Hydromorphone Hydrochloride (May potentiate orthostatic hypotension). Products include:
Dilaudid Ampules 1382
Dilaudid Cough Syrup 1383
Dilaudid-HP Injection 1384
Dilaudid-HP Lyophilized Powder 250 mg 1384
Dilaudid 1382
Dilaudid Oral Liquid 1386
Dilaudid 1382
Dilaudid Tablets - 8 mg 1386

Ibuprofen (Concurrent administration may reduce the diuretic, natriuretic and antihypertensive effects of thiazide diuretics). Products include:
Advil Cold and Sinus Caplets and Tablets ◘ 837
Advil Ibuprofen Tablets, Caplets and Gel Caplets ◘ 836
Children's Motrin Ibuprofen Oral Suspension 1558
IBU Tablets 1389
Ibuprohm ◘ 713
Motrin IB Caplets, Tablets, and Gelcaps ◘ 802
Motrin Ibuprofen Suspension, Oral Drops, Chewable Tablets, Caplets 1563
Nuprin Ibuprofen/Analgesic Tablets & Caplets ◘ 645
Vicks DayQuil SINUS Pressure & PAIN Relief with IBUPROFEN ◘ 735

Indapamide (Additive or potentiated action).
No products indexed under this heading.

Indomethacin (Concurrent administration may reduce the diuretic, natriuretic and antihypertensive effects of thiazide diuretics). Products include:
Indocin 1723

Indomethacin Sodium Trihydrate (Concurrent administration may reduce the diuretic, natriuretic and antihypertensive effects of thiazide diuretics). Products include:
Indocin I.V. 1727

Insulin, Human (Insulin requirements may be altered).
No products indexed under this heading.

Insulin, Human Isophane Suspension (Insulin requirements may be altered). Products include:
Novolin N Human Insulin 10 ml Vials 1846

Insulin, Human NPH (Insulin requirements may be altered). Products include:
Humulin N, 100 Units 1495
Novolin N PenFill 1.5 ml Cartridges Durable Insulin Delivery System 1849
Novolin N Prefilled Syringe Disposable Insulin Delivery System 1850

Insulin, Human Regular (Insulin requirements may be altered). Products include:
Humulin R, 100 Units 1497
Novolin R Human Insulin 10 ml Vials 1846
Novolin R PenFill 1.5 ml Cartridges Durable Insulin Delivery System 1849
Novolin R Prefilled Syringe Disposable Insulin Delivery System 1850
Velosulin BR Human Insulin 10 ml Vials 1847

Insulin, Human, Zinc Suspension (Insulin requirements may be altered). Products include:
Humulin L, 100 Units 1494
Humulin U, 100 Units 1498
Novolin L Human Insulin 10 ml Vials 1846

Insulin Lispro, Human (Insulin requirements may be altered). Products include:
Humalog Injection 1488

Insulin, NPH (Insulin requirements may be altered). Products include:
NPH, 100 Units 1502
Pork NPH, 100 Units 1506
Purified Pork NPH Isophane Insulin 1852

Insulin, Regular (Insulin requirements may be altered). Products include:
Regular, 100 Units 1503
Pork Regular, 100 Units 1507
Pork Regular (Concentrated), 500 Units 1508
Purified Pork Regular Insulin 1852

Insulin, Zinc Crystals (Insulin requirements may be altered). Products include:
NPH, 100 Units 1502

Insulin, Zinc Suspension (Insulin requirements may be altered). Products include:
Iletin I 1501
Lente, 100 Units 1501
Iletin II 1504
Pork Lente, 100 Units 1504
Purified Pork Lente Insulin 1852

Isocarboxazid (MAO inhibitors should be used with caution in patients receiving hydralazine).
No products indexed under this heading.

Isradipine (Additive or potentiated action). Products include:
DynaCirc Capsules 2381
DynaCirc CR Tablets 2383

Ketoprofen (Concurrent administration may reduce the diuretic, natriuretic and antihypertensive effects of thiazide diuretics). Products include:
Actron Caplets and Tablets ◘ 608
Orudis Capsules 2874
Orudis KT ◘ 842
Oruvail Capsules 2874

Ketorolac Tromethamine (Concurrent administration may reduce the diuretic, natriuretic and antihypertensive effects of thiazide diuretics). Products include:
Acular Sterile Ophthalmic Solution 470
Toradol 2319

Labetalol Hydrochloride (Additive or potentiated action). Products include:
Normodyne Injection 2519
Normodyne Tablets 2522
Trandate 1158

Levorphanol Tartrate (May potentiate orthostatic hypotension). Products include:
Levo-Dromoran 2297

Lisinopril (Additive or potentiated action). Products include:
Prinivil Tablets 1776
Prinzide Tablets 1780
Zestoretic Tablets 2968
Zestril Tablets 2972

Lithium Carbonate (Lithium renal clearance is reduced by thiazides, increasing the risk of lithium toxicity). Products include:
Eskalith 2658
Lithium Carbonate Capsules & Tablets 2352
Lithonate/Lithotabs/Lithobid 2721

Lithium Citrate (Lithium renal clearance is reduced by thiazides, increasing the risk of lithium toxicity).
No products indexed under this heading.

Losartan Potassium (Additive or potentiated action). Products include:
Cozaar Tablets 1668
Hyzaar Tablets 1720

Mecamylamine Hydrochloride (Additive or potentiated action). Products include:
Inversine Tablets 1729

Meclofenamate Sodium (Concurrent administration may reduce the diuretic, natriuretic and antihypertensive effects of thiazide diuretics).
No products indexed under this heading.

Mefenamic Acid (Concurrent administration may reduce the diuretic, natriuretic and antihypertensive effects of thiazide diuretics). Products include:
Ponstel 1982

Meperidine Hydrochloride (May potentiate orthostatic hypotension). Products include:
Demerol 2438
Mepergan Injection 2859

(◘ Described in PDR For Nonprescription Drugs) (◉ Described in PDR For Ophthalmology)

71 **Interactions Index** **Apresazide**

Mephobarbital (May potentiate orthostatic hypotension). Products include:
Mebaral Tablets 2452

Methadone Hydrochloride (May potentiate orthostatic hypotension). Products include:
Methadone Hydrochloride Oral Concentrate 2356
Methadone Hydrochloride Oral Solution & Tablets 2357

Methyclothiazide (Additive or potentiated action). Products include:
Enduron Tablets 424

Methyldopa (Co-administration has resulted in rare reports of hemolytic anemia). Products include:
Aldoclor Tablets 1638
Aldomet Oral 1640
Aldoril Tablets 1644

Methyldopate Hydrochloride (Co-administration has resulted in rare reports of hemolytic anemia). Products include:
Aldomet Ester HCl Injection 1642

Methylprednisolone (Concomitant use may result in hypokalemia).
No products indexed under this heading.

Methylprednisolone Acetate (Concomitant use may result in hypokalemia).
No products indexed under this heading.

Methylprednisolone Sodium Succinate (Concomitant use may result in hypokalemia).
No products indexed under this heading.

Metolazone (Additive or potentiated action). Products include:
Mykrox Tablets 1617
Zaroxolyn Tablets 1625

Metoprolol Succinate (Additive or potentiated action). Products include:
Toprol-XL Tablets 560

Metoprolol Tartrate (Additive or potentiated action). Products include:
Lopressor 848
Lopressor HCT Tablets 850

Metyrosine (Additive or potentiated action). Products include:
Demser Capsules 1690

Minoxidil (Additive or potentiated action).
No products indexed under this heading.

Moexipril Hydrochloride (Additive or potentiated action). Products include:
Univasc Tablets 2553

Morphine Sulfate (May potentiate orthostatic hypotension). Products include:
Astramorph/PF Injection, USP (Preservative-Free) 526
Duramorph Injection 983
Infumorph 200 and Infumorph 500 Sterile Solutions 985
Kadian Capsules 2948
MS Contin Tablets 2149
MSIR 2152
Oramorph SR (Morphine Sulfate Sustained Release Tablets) 2359
RMS Suppositories CII 2766
Roxanol 2365

Nabumetone (Concurrent administration may reduce the diuretic, natriuretic and antihypertensive effects of thiazide diuretics). Products include:
Relafen Tablets 2688

Nadolol (Additive or potentiated action).
No products indexed under this heading.

Naproxen (Concurrent administration may reduce the diuretic, natriuretic and antihypertensive effects of thiazide diuretics). Products include:
Anaprox/Naprosyn 2277

Naproxen Sodium (Concurrent administration may reduce the diuretic, natriuretic and antihypertensive effects of thiazide diuretics). Products include:
Aleve 2124
Anaprox/Naprosyn 2277
Naprelan Tablets 2861

Nicardipine Hydrochloride (Additive or potentiated action). Products include:
Cardene Capsules 2261
Cardene I.V. 2815
Cardene SR Capsules 2264

Nifedipine (Additive or potentiated action). Products include:
Adalat Capsules (10 mg and 20 mg) 580
Adalat CC 582
Procardia Capsules 2024
Procardia XL Extended Release Tablets 2026

Nisoldipine (Additive or potentiated action). Products include:
Sular Tablets 2961

Nitroglycerin (Additive or potentiated action). Products include:
Deponit NTG Transdermal Delivery System 2541
Nitro-Bid IV 1270
Nitro-Bid Ointment 1272
Nitro-Dur (nitroglycerin) Transdermal Infusion System 1365
Nitrolingual Spray 2193
Nitrostat Tablets 1981
Transderm-Nitro Transdermal Therapeutic System 878

Norepinephrine Bitartrate (Decreased arterial response to norepinephrine). Products include:
Levophed Bitartrate Injection 2445

Opium Alkaloids (May potentiate orthostatic hypotension).
No products indexed under this heading.

Oxaprozin (Concurrent administration may reduce the diuretic, natriuretic and antihypertensive effects of thiazide diuretics). Products include:
Daypro Caplets 2578

Oxycodone Hydrochloride (May potentiate orthostatic hypotension). Products include:
OxyContin Tablets 2163
OxyIR Capsules 2167
Percocet Tablets 955
Percodan Tablets 955
Percodan-Demi Tablets 956
Roxicodone Tablets, Oral Solution & Intensol (Oxycodone) 2366
Tylox Capsules 1593

Penbutolol Sulfate (Additive or potentiated action). Products include:
Levatol Tablets 2547

Pentobarbital Sodium (May potentiate orthostatic hypotension). Products include:
Nembutal Sodium Capsules 440
Nembutal Sodium Solution 442
Nembutal Sodium Suppositories 444

Phenelzine Sulfate (MAO inhibitors should be used with caution in patients receiving hydralazine). Products include:
Nardil 1977

Phenobarbital (May potentiate orthostatic hypotension). Products include:
Arco-Lase Plus Tablets 513
Bellergal-S Tablets 2375
Donnatal 2234
Donnatal Extentabs 2234
Donnatal Tablets 2234
Phenobarbital Elixir and Tablets 1523
Quadrinal Tablets 1398

Phenoxybenzamine Hydrochloride (Additive or potentiated action). Products include:
Dibenzyline Capsules 2650

Phentolamine Mesylate (Additive or potentiated action). Products include:
Regitine Vials 864

Phenylbutazone (Concurrent administration may reduce the diuretic, natriuretic and antihypertensive effects of thiazide diuretics).
No products indexed under this heading.

Pindolol (Additive or potentiated action). Products include:
Visken Tablets 2428

Piroxicam (Concurrent administration may reduce the diuretic, natriuretic and antihypertensive effects of thiazide diuretics). Products include:
Feldene Capsules 2008

Polythiazide (Additive or potentiated action). Products include:
Minizide Capsules 2016

Prazosin Hydrochloride (Additive or potentiated action). Products include:
Minipress Capsules 2015
Minizide Capsules 2016

Prednisolone Acetate (Concomitant use may result in hypokalemia). Products include:
AK-CIDE .... ⊙ 203
AK-CIDE Ointment .... ⊙ 203
Blephamide Liquifilm Sterile Ophthalmic Suspension 472
Blephamide Ointment .... ⊙ 234
Econopred & Econopred Plus Ophthalmic Suspensions .... ⊙ 216
Poly-Pred Liquifilm .... ⊙ 246
Pred Forte .... ⊙ 247
Pred Mild .... ⊙ 250
Pred-G Liquifilm Sterile Ophthalmic Suspension .... ⊙ 248
Pred-G S.O.P. Sterile Ophthalmic Ointment .... ⊙ 249

Prednisolone Sodium Phosphate (Concomitant use may result in hypokalemia). Products include:
AK-PRED .... ⊙ 204
Hydeltrasol Injection, Sterile 1708
Pediapred Oral Solution 1618

Prednisolone Tebutate (Concomitant use may result in hypokalemia). Products include:
Hydeltra-T.B.A. Sterile Suspension 1710

Prednisone (Concomitant use may result in hypokalemia).
No products indexed under this heading.

Propoxyphene Hydrochloride (May potentiate orthostatic hypotension). Products include:
Darvon 1475
Wygesic Tablets 2930

Propoxyphene Napsylate (May potentiate orthostatic hypotension). Products include:
Darvon-N/Darvocet-N 1473

Propranolol Hydrochloride (Additive or potentiated action). Products include:
Inderal 2834
Inderal LA Long Acting Capsules 2836
Inderide Tablets 2838
Inderide LA Long Acting Capsules 2840

Quinapril Hydrochloride (Additive or potentiated action). Products include:
Accupril Tablets 1950

Ramipril (Additive or potentiated action). Products include:
Altace Capsules 1238

Rauwolfia Serpentina (Additive or potentiated action).
No products indexed under this heading.

Rescinnamine (Additive or potentiated action).
No products indexed under this heading.

Reserpine (Additive or potentiated action). Products include:
Diupres Tablets 1691
Hydropres Tablets 1718
Ser-Ap-Es Tablets 867

Secobarbital Sodium (May potentiate orthostatic hypotension). Products include:
Seconal Sodium Pulvules 1529

Selegiline Hydrochloride (MAO inhibitors should be used with caution in patients receiving hydralazine). Products include:
Eldepryl Capsules 2729

Sodium Nitroprusside (Additive or potentiated action).
No products indexed under this heading.

Sotalol Hydrochloride (Additive or potentiated action). Products include:
Betapace Tablets 637

Spirapril Hydrochloride (Additive or potentiated action).
No products indexed under this heading.

Sufentanil Citrate (May potentiate orthostatic hypotension). Products include:
Sufenta Injection 1355

Sulindac (Concurrent administration may reduce the diuretic, natriuretic and antihypertensive effects of thiazide diuretics). Products include:
Clinoril Tablets 1658

Terazosin Hydrochloride (Additive or potentiated action). Products include:
Hytrin Capsules 434

Thiamylal Sodium (May potentiate orthostatic hypotension).
No products indexed under this heading.

Timolol Maleate (Additive or potentiated action). Products include:
Blocadren Tablets 1654
Timolide Tablets 1791
Timoptic in Ocudose 1796
Timoptic Sterile Ophthalmic Solution 1794
Timoptic-XE 1798

Tolmetin Sodium (Concurrent administration may reduce the diuretic, natriuretic and antihypertensive effects of thiazide diuretics). Products include:
Tolectin (200, 400 and 600 mg) .. 1591

Torsemide (Additive or potentiated action). Products include:
Demadex Tablets and Injection 691

Trandolapril (Additive or potentiated action). Products include:
Mavik Tablets 1407

Tranylcypromine Sulfate (MAO inhibitors should be used with caution in patients receiving hydralazine). Products include:
Parnate Tablets 2679

Triamcinolone (Concomitant use may result in hypokalemia).
No products indexed under this heading.

Triamcinolone Acetonide (Concomitant use may result in hypokalemia). Products include:
Azmacort Oral Inhaler 2175
Nasacort AQ Nasal Spray 2191
Nasacort Nasal Inhaler 2189

IMPORTANT NOTE: Always consult each drug listing in the patient's regimen for possible interactions.

Triamcinolone Diacetate (Concomitant use may result in hypokalemia).
No products indexed under this heading.
Triamcinolone Hexacetonide (Concomitant use may result in hypokalemia).
No products indexed under this heading.
Trimethaphan Camsylate (Additive or potentiated action).
No products indexed under this heading.
Tubocurarine Chloride (Increased responsiveness to tubocurarine).
No products indexed under this heading.
Verapamil Hydrochloride (Additive or potentiated action). Products include:

- Calan SR Caplets 2571
- Calan Tablets 2568
- Covera-HS Tablets 2573
- Isoptin Injectable 1391
- Isoptin Oral Tablets 1393
- Isoptin SR Tablets 1395
- Verelan Capsules 1455

Food Interactions

Alcohol (May potentiate orthostatic hypotension).
Food, unspecified (Enhances gastrointestinal absorption of hydrochlorothiazide).

APRESOLINE HYDROCHLORIDE TABLETS

(Hydralazine Hydrochloride) 826
May interact with monoamine oxidase inhibitors and certain other agents. Compounds in these categories include:

Diazoxide (Profound hypotensive episodes may occur when diazoxide injection and hydralazine are used concomitantly). Products include:

- Hyperstat I.V. Injection 2504
- Proglycem 575

Furazolidone (MAO inhibitors should be used with caution in patients receiving hydralazine). Products include:

- Furoxone 2221

Isocarboxazid (MAO inhibitors should be used with caution in patients receiving hydralazine).
No products indexed under this heading.
Phenelzine Sulfate (MAO inhibitors should be used with caution in patients receiving hydralazine). Products include:

- Nardil 1977

Selegiline Hydrochloride (MAO inhibitors should be used with caution in patients receiving hydralazine). Products include:

- Eldepryl Capsules 2729

Tranylcypromine Sulfate (MAO inhibitors should be used with caution in patients receiving hydralazine). Products include:

- Parnate Tablets 2679

Food Interactions

Food, unspecified (Administration of hydralazine with food results in higher plasma levels).

AQUAMEPHYTON INJECTION

(Phytonadione) 1648
May interact with oral anticoagulants. Compounds in this category include:

Dicumarol (Temporary resistance to anticoagulants).
No products indexed under this heading.
Warfarin Sodium (Temporary resistance to anticoagulants). Products include:

- Coumadin 941

AQUANIL HC LOTION

(Hydrocortisone) 1989
None cited in PDR database.

AQUAPHOR HEALING OINTMENT

(Petrolatum, Mineral Oil) 636
None cited in PDR database.

AQUAPHOR HEALING OINTMENT, ORIGINAL FORMULA

(Mineral Oil, Petrolatum) 636
None cited in PDR database.

AQUASOL A VITAMIN A CAPSULES, USP

(Vitamin A) 525
May interact with oral contraceptives. Compounds in this category include:

Desogestrel (Potential for a significant increase in plasma vitamin A levels). Products include:

- Desogen Tablets 1867
- Ortho-Cept 1907

Ethinyl Estradiol (Potential for a significant increase in plasma vitamin A levels). Products include:

- Brevicon 2563
- Demulen 2580
- Desogen Tablets 1867
- Levlen/Tri-Levlen 646
- Lo/Ovral Tablets 2852
- Lo/Ovral-28 Tablets 2857
- Modicon 1928
- Nordette-21 Tablets 2863
- Nordette-28 Tablets 2866
- Norinyl 2563
- Ortho-Cept 1907
- Ortho-Cyclen/Ortho-Tri-Cyclen 1914
- Ortho-Novum 1928
- Ortho-Cyclen/Ortho Tri-Cyclen 1914
- Ovcon 765
- Ovral Tablets 2877
- Ovral-28 Tablets 2878
- Levlen/Tri-Levlen 646
- Tri-Norinyl 2607
- Triphasil-21 Tablets 2919
- Triphasil-28 Tablets 2924

Ethynodiol Diacetate (Potential for a significant increase in plasma vitamin A levels). Products include:

- Demulen 2580

Levonorgestrel (Potential for a significant increase in plasma vitamin A levels). Products include:

- Levlen/Tri-Levlen 646
- Nordette-21 Tablets 2863
- Nordette-28 Tablets 2866
- Norplant System 2868
- Levlen/Tri-Levlen 646
- Triphasil-21 Tablets 2919
- Triphasil-28 Tablets 2924

Mestranol (Potential for a significant increase in plasma vitamin A levels). Products include:

- Norinyl 2563
- Ortho-Novum 1928

Norethindrone (Potential for a significant increase in plasma vitamin A levels). Products include:

- Brevicon 2563
- Micronor Tablets 1903
- Modicon 1928
- Norinyl 2563
- Nor-Q D Tablets 2598
- Ortho-Novum 1928
- Ovcon 765
- Tri-Norinyl 2607

Norethynodrel (Potential for a significant increase in plasma vitamin A levels).
No products indexed under this heading.
Norgestimate (Potential for a significant increase in plasma vitamin A levels). Products include:

- Ortho-Cyclen/Ortho-Tri-Cyclen 1914
- Ortho-Cyclen/Ortho Tri-Cyclen 1914

Norgestrel (Potential for a significant increase in plasma vitamin A levels). Products include:

- Lo/Ovral Tablets 2852
- Lo/Ovral-28 Tablets 2857
- Ovral Tablets 2877
- Ovral-28 Tablets 2878
- Ovrette Tablets 2878

AQUASOL A PARENTERAL

(Vitamin A) 526
May interact with oral contraceptives. Compounds in this category include:

Desogestrel (Potential for a significant increase in plasma vitamin A levels). Products include:

- Desogen Tablets 1867
- Ortho-Cept 1907

Ethinyl Estradiol (Potential for a significant increase in plasma vitamin A levels). Products include:

- Brevicon 2563
- Demulen 2580
- Desogen Tablets 1867
- Levlen/Tri-Levlen 646
- Lo/Ovral Tablets 2852
- Lo/Ovral-28 Tablets 2857
- Modicon 1928
- Nordette-21 Tablets 2863
- Nordette-28 Tablets 2866
- Norinyl 2563
- Ortho-Cept 1907
- Ortho-Cyclen/Ortho-Tri-Cyclen 1914
- Ortho-Novum 1928
- Ortho-Cyclen/Ortho Tri-Cyclen 1914
- Ovcon 765
- Ovral Tablets 2877
- Ovral-28 Tablets 2878
- Levlen/Tri-Levlen 646
- Tri-Norinyl 2607
- Triphasil-21 Tablets 2919
- Triphasil-28 Tablets 2924

Ethynodiol Diacetate (Potential for a significant increase in plasma vitamin A levels). Products include:

- Demulen 2580

Levonorgestrel (Potential for a significant increase in plasma vitamin A levels). Products include:

- Levlen/Tri-Levlen 646
- Nordette-21 Tablets 2863
- Nordette-28 Tablets 2866
- Norplant System 2868
- Levlen/Tri-Levlen 646
- Triphasil-21 Tablets 2919
- Triphasil-28 Tablets 2924

Mestranol (Potential for a significant increase in plasma vitamin A levels). Products include:

- Norinyl 2563
- Ortho-Novum 1928

Norethindrone (Potential for a significant increase in plasma vitamin A levels). Products include:

- Brevicon 2563
- Micronor Tablets 1903
- Modicon 1928
- Norinyl 2563
- Nor-Q D Tablets 2598
- Ortho-Novum 1928
- Ovcon 765
- Tri-Norinyl 2607

Norethynodrel (Potential for a significant increase in plasma vitamin A levels).
No products indexed under this heading.
Norgestimate (Potential for a significant increase in plasma vitamin A levels). Products include:

- Ortho-Cyclen/Ortho-Tri-Cyclen 1914
- Ortho-Cyclen/Ortho Tri-Cyclen 1914

Norgestrel (Potential for a significant increase in plasma vitamin A levels). Products include:

- Lo/Ovral Tablets 2852
- Lo/Ovral-28 Tablets 2857
- Ovral Tablets 2877
- Ovral-28 Tablets 2878
- Ovrette Tablets 2878

ARALEN HYDROCHLORIDE INJECTION

(Chloroquine Hydrochloride) 2430
May interact with:

Hepatotoxic Drugs, unspecified (Concurrent use requires caution).

ARALEN PHOSPHATE TABLETS

(Chloroquine Phosphate) 2431
May interact with:

Hepatotoxic Drugs, unspecified (Caution should be exercised when used in conjunction with known hepatotoxic drugs).

ARAMINE INJECTION

(Metaraminol Bitartrate) 1649
May interact with cardiac glycosides, monoamine oxidase inhibitors, tricyclic antidepressants, and certain other agents. Compounds in these categories include:

Amitriptyline Hydrochloride (Potentiates pressor effect). Products include:

- Elavil 2945
- Etrafon 2495
- Limbitrol 2333
- Triavil Tablets 1800

Amoxapine (Potentiates pressor effect). Products include:

- Asendin Tablets 1419

Clomipramine Hydrochloride (Potentiates pressor effect). Products include:

- Anafranil Capsules 819

Desipramine Hydrochloride (Potentiates pressor effect). Products include:

- Norpramin Tablets 1273

Deslanoside (May cause ectopic arrhythmic reaction).
No products indexed under this heading.
Digitoxin (May cause ectopic arrhythmic reaction). Products include:

- Crystodigin Tablets 1472

Digoxin (May cause ectopic arrhythmic reaction). Products include:

- Lanoxicaps 1110
- Lanoxin Elixir Pediatric 1113
- Lanoxin Injection 1116
- Lanoxin Injection Pediatric 1119
- Lanoxin Tablets 1121

Doxepin Hydrochloride (Potentiates pressor effect). Products include:

- Adapin Capsules 1542
- Sinequan 2028
- Zonalon Cream 1042

Furazolidone (Potentiates pressor effect). Products include:

- Furoxone 2221

Halothane (Concurrent use should be avoided). Products include:

- Fluothane 2830

Imipramine Hydrochloride (Potentiates pressor effect). Products include:

- Tofranil Ampuls 873
- Tofranil Tablets 875

Imipramine Pamoate (Potentiates pressor effect). Products include:

- Tofranil-PM Capsules 876

Isocarboxazid (Potentiates pressor effect).
No products indexed under this heading.
Maprotiline Hydrochloride (Potentiates pressor effect). Products include:
Ludiomil Tablets 861
Nortriptyline Hydrochloride (Potentiates pressor effect). Products include:
Pamelor 2409
Phenelzine Sulfate (Potentiates pressor effect). Products include:
Nardil 1977
Protriptyline Hydrochloride (Potentiates pressor effect). Products include:
Vivactil Tablets 1820
Selegiline Hydrochloride (Potentiates pressor effect). Products include:
Eldepryl Capsules 2729
Tranylcypromine Sulfate (Potentiates pressor effect). Products include:
Parnate Tablets 2679
Trimipramine Maleate (Potentiates pressor effect). Products include:
Surmontil Capsules 2917

ARCO-LASE PLUS TABLETS
(Amylase, Cellulase, Lipase, Protease, Hyoscyamine Sulfate, Phenobarbital) 513
None cited in PDR database.

ARCO-LASE TABLETS
(Amylase, Lipase, Cellulase, Protease) 513
None cited in PDR database.

AREDIA FOR INJECTION
(Pamidronate Disodium) 827
None cited in PDR database.

ARIMIDEX TABLETS
(Anastrozole) 2932
None cited in PDR database.

ARM & HAMMER PURE BAKING SODA
(Sodium Bicarbonate) 648
May interact with:

Prescription Drugs, unspecified (Antacids may interact with certain unspecified prescription drugs; consult your physician).

ARTANE ELIXIR
(Trihexyphenidyl Hydrochloride) ...1418
May interact with:

Levodopa (The usual dose of each may need to be reduced when used concomitantly). Products include:
Atamet Tablets 567
Larodopa Tablets 2296
Sinemet Tablets 959
Sinemet CR Tablets 961

ARTANE TABLETS
(Trihexyphenidyl Hydrochloride) ...1418
See **Artane Elixir**

ARTHRICARE ODOR FREE RUB
(Capsaicin, Menthol, Methyl Nicotinate) 667
None cited in PDR database.

ARTHRICARE TRIPLE MEDICATED RUB
(Menthol, Methyl Nicotinate, Methyl Salicylate) 667

None cited in PDR database.

ASACOL DELAYED-RELEASE TABLETS
(Mesalamine) 2129
None cited in PDR database.

ARTHRITIS PAIN ASCRIPTIN
(Aspirin Buffered, Calcium Carbonate) 650
See **Regular Strength Ascriptin Tablets**

MAXIMUM STRENGTH ASCRIPTIN
(Aspirin Buffered, Calcium Carbonate) 650
See **Regular Strength Ascriptin Tablets**

REGULAR STRENGTH ASCRIPTIN TABLETS
(Aspirin Buffered, Calcium Carbonate) 650
May interact with oral anticoagulants, oral hypoglycemic agents, antigout agents, and certain other agents. Compounds in these categories include:

Acarbose (Concurrent use is not recommended unless directed by a doctor). Products include:
Precose 604
Allopurinol (Concurrent use is not recommended unless directed by a doctor). Products include:
Zyloprim Tablets 1194
Antiarthritic Drugs, unspecified (Concurrent use is not recommended unless directed by a doctor).
Chlorpropamide (Concurrent use is not recommended unless directed by a doctor). Products include:
Diabinese Tablets 2002
Dicumarol (Concurrent use is not recommended unless directed by a doctor).
No products indexed under this heading.
Glimepiride (Concurrent use is not recommended unless directed by a doctor). Products include:
Amaryl Tablets 1241
Glipizide (Concurrent use is not recommended unless directed by a doctor). Products include:
Glucotrol Tablets 2011
Glucotrol XL Extended Release Tablets 2012
Glyburide (Concurrent use is not recommended unless directed by a doctor). Products include:
DiaBeta Tablets 1265
Glynase PresTab Tablets 2091
Micronase Tablets 2099
Metformin Hydrochloride (Concurrent use is not recommended unless directed by a doctor). Products include:
Glucophage Tablets 754
Prescription Drugs, unspecified (Antacids may interact with certain unspecified prescription drugs).
Probenecid (Concurrent use is not recommended unless directed by a doctor). Products include:
Benemid Tablets 1651
ColBENEMID Tablets 1662
Sulfinpyrazone (Concurrent use is not recommended unless directed by a doctor). Products include:
Anturane 823

Tolazamide (Concurrent use is not recommended unless directed by a doctor).
No products indexed under this heading.
Tolbutamide (Concurrent use is not recommended unless directed by a doctor).
No products indexed under this heading.
Warfarin Sodium (Concurrent use is not recommended unless directed by a doctor). Products include:
Coumadin 941

ASENDIN TABLETS
(Amoxapine) 1419
May interact with monoamine oxidase inhibitors, anticholinergics, barbiturates, central nervous system depressants, selective serotonin reuptake inhibitors, antidepressant drugs, phenothiazines, and certain other agents. Compounds in these categories include:

Alfentanil Hydrochloride (Enhanced response to central nervous system depressants). Products include:
Alfenta Injection 1334
Alprazolam (Enhanced response to central nervous system depressants). Products include:
Xanax Tablets 2115
Amitriptyline Hydrochloride (Concomitant use of amoxapine with other drugs that inhibit cytochrome $P_{450}IID_6$ may require lower than usual doses prescribed for either drug). Products include:
Elavil 2945
Etrafon 2495
Limbitrol 2333
Triavil Tablets 1800
Aprobarbital (Enhanced response to barbiturates).
No products indexed under this heading.
Atropine Sulfate (Paralytic ileus may occur). Products include:
Arco-Lase Plus Tablets 513
Atrohist Plus Tablets 1605
Donnatal 2234
Donnatal Extentabs 2234
Donnatal Tablets 2234
Lomotil 2591
Motofen Tablets 789
Urised Tablets 2123
Belladonna Alkaloids (Paralytic ileus may occur). Products include:
Bellergal-S Tablets 2375
Hyland's Bedwetting Tablets 788
Hyland's EnurAid Tablets 789
Hyland's Headache Tablets 790
Hyland's Teething Tablets 790
Similasan Eye Drops #1 769
Benztropine Mesylate (Paralytic ileus may occur). Products include:
Cogentin 1661
Biperiden Hydrochloride (Paralytic ileus may occur). Products include:
Akineton 1380
Buprenorphine (Enhanced response to central nervous system depressants). Products include:
Buprenex Injectable 2170
Bupropion Hydrochloride (Concomitant use of amoxapine with other drugs that inhibit cytochrome $P_{450}IID_6$ may require lower than usual doses prescribed for either drug). Products include:
Wellbutrin Tablets 1177
Buspirone Hydrochloride (Enhanced response to central nervous system depressants). Products include:
BuSpar Tablets 738

Butabarbital (Enhanced response to barbiturates).
No products indexed under this heading.
Butalbital (Enhanced response to barbiturates). Products include:
Axocet Capsules 2469
Esgic-plus Capsules 1012
Esgic-plus Tablets 1012
Fioricet Tablets 2386
Fioricet with Codeine Capsules ... 2387
Fiorinal Capsules 2388
Fiorinal with Codeine Capsules .. 2390
Fiorinal Tablets 2388
Phrenilin 790
Sedapap Tablets 50 mg/650 mg .. 1826
Chlordiazepoxide (Enhanced response to central nervous system depressants). Products include:
Limbitrol 2333
Chlordiazepoxide Hydrochloride (Enhanced response to central nervous system depressants). Products include:
Librax Capsules 2330
Librium Capsules 2331
Librium Injectable 2332
Chlorpromazine (Concomitant use of amoxapine with other drugs that inhibit cytochrome $P_{450}IID_6$ may require lower than usual doses prescribed for either drug; enhanced response to central nervous system depressants). Products include:
Thorazine Suppositories 2701
Chlorpromazine Hydrochloride (Concomitant use of amoxapine with other drugs that inhibit cytochrome $P_{450}IID_6$ may require lower than usual doses prescribed for either drug). Products include:
Thorazine 2701
Chlorprothixene (Enhanced response to central nervous system depressants).
No products indexed under this heading.
Chlorprothixene Hydrochloride (Enhanced response to central nervous system depressants).
No products indexed under this heading.
Chlorprothixene Lactate (Enhanced response to central nervous system depressants).
No products indexed under this heading.
Cimetidine (Significant increase in serum levels of several tricyclic antidepressants; not documented with Asendin; concomitant use of amoxapine with other drugs that inhibit cytochrome $P_{450}11D_6$ may require lower than usual doses prescribed for either drug). Products include:
Tagamet HB Tablets 786
Tagamet Tablets 2694
Cimetidine Hydrochloride (Significant increase in serum levels of several tricyclic antidepressants; not documented with Asendin; concomitant use of amoxapine with other drugs that inhibit cytochrome $P_{450}11D_6$ may require lower than usual doses prescribed for either drug). Products include:
Tagamet 2694
Clidinium Bromide (Paralytic ileus may occur; enhanced response to central nervous system depressants). Products include:
Librax Capsules 2330
Clorazepate Dipotassium (Enhanced response to central nervous system depressants). Products include:
Tranxene 459

IMPORTANT NOTE: Always consult each drug listing in the patient's regimen for possible interactions.

Asendin Tablets | Interactions Index | 74

Clozapine (Enhanced response to central nervous system depressants). Products include:
Clozaril Tablets ... 2377

Codeine Phosphate (Enhanced response to central nervous system depressants). Products include:
Brontex ... 2130
Dimetane-DC Cough Syrup ... 2232
Fioricet with Codeine Capsules ... 2387
Fiorinal with Codeine Capsules ... 2390
Nucofed ... 2225
Phenergan with Codeine ... 2883
Phenergan VC with Codeine ... 2888
Robitussin A-C Syrup ... 2248
Robitussin-DAC Syrup ... 2249
Ryna ... ▣ 804
Soma Compound w/Codeine Tablets ... 2784
Tylenol with Codeine ... 1592

Desflurane (Enhanced response to central nervous system depressants). Products include:
Suprane (desflurane, USP) ... 1865

Desipramine Hydrochloride (Concomitant use of amoxapine with other drugs that inhibit cytochrome $P_{450}IID_6$ may require lower than usual doses prescribed for either drug). Products include:
Norpramin Tablets ... 1273

Dezocine (Enhanced response to central nervous system depressants). Products include:
Dalgan Injection ... 529

Diazepam (Enhanced response to central nervous system depressants). Products include:
Dizac (diazepam injectable emulsion) CIV ... 1862
Valium Injectable ... 2336
Valium Tablets ... 2335

Dicyclomine Hydrochloride (Paralytic ileus may occur). Products include:
Bentyl ... 1246

Doxepin Hydrochloride (Concomitant use of amoxapine with other drugs that inhibit cytochrome $P_{450}IID_6$ may require lower than usual doses prescribed for either drug). Products include:
Adapin Capsules ... 1542
Sinequan ... 2028
Zonalon Cream ... 1042

Droperidol (Enhanced response to central nervous system depressants). Products include:
Inapsine Injection ... 462

Enflurane (Enhanced response to central nervous system depressants).
No products indexed under this heading.

Estazolam (Enhanced response to central nervous system depressants). Products include:
ProSom Tablets ... 457

Ethchlorvynol (Enhanced response to central nervous system depressants). Products include:
Placidyl Capsules ... 456

Ethinamate (Enhanced response to central nervous system depressants).
No products indexed under this heading.

Ethopropazine Hydrochloride (Paralytic ileus may occur).

Fentanyl (Enhanced response to central nervous system depressants). Products include:
Duragesic Transdermal System ... 1336

Fentanyl Citrate (Enhanced response to central nervous system depressants). Products include:
Sublimaze Injection ... 463

Flecainide Acetate (Concomitant use of amoxapine with other drugs that inhibit cytochrome $P_{450}IID_6$ may require lower than usual doses prescribed for either drug). Products include:
Tambocor Tablets ... 1555

Fluoxetine Hydrochloride (Concomitant use of amoxapine with other drugs that inhibit cytochrome $P_{450}IID_6$ may require lower than usual doses prescribed for either drug; sufficient time must elapse before initiating Asendin treatment in a patient being withdrawn from fluoxetine due to its long half-life). Products include:
Prozac Pulvules & Liquid, Oral Solution ... 935

Fluphenazine Decanoate (Concomitant use of amoxapine with other drugs that inhibit cytochrome $P_{450}IID_6$ may require lower than usual doses prescribed for either drug; enhanced response to central nervous system depressants). Products include:
Prolixin Decanoate ... 510

Fluphenazine Enanthate (Concomitant use of amoxapine with other drugs that inhibit cytochrome $P_{450}IID_6$ may require lower than usual doses prescribed for either drug; enhanced response to central nervous system depressants). Products include:
Prolixin Enanthate ... 510

Fluphenazine Hydrochloride (Concomitant use of amoxapine with other drugs that inhibit cytochrome $P_{450}IID_6$ may require lower than usual doses prescribed for either drug; enhanced response to central nervous system depressants). Products include:
Prolixin ... 510

Flurazepam Hydrochloride (Enhanced response to central nervous system depressants). Products include:
Dalmane Capsules ... 2329

Fluvoxamine Maleate (Concomitant use of amoxapine with other drugs that inhibit cytochrome $P_{450}IID_6$ may require lower than usual doses prescribed for either drug Enhanced response to barbiturates). Products include:
LUVOX Tablets ... 2723

Furazolidone (Concurrent and/or sequential use may result in hyperpyretic crises, severe convulsions, and fatalities; coadministration is contraindicated). Products include:
Furoxone ... 2221

Glutethimide (Enhanced response to central nervous system depressants).
No products indexed under this heading.

Glycopyrrolate (Paralytic ileus may occur). Products include:
Robinul Forte Tablets ... 2247
Robinul Injectable ... 2247
Robinul Tablets ... 2247

Haloperidol (Enhanced response to central nervous system depressants). Products include:
Haldol Injection, Tablets and Concentrate ... 1585

Haloperidol Decanoate (Enhanced response to central nervous system depressants). Products include:
Haldol Decanoate ... 1587

Hydrocodone Bitartrate (Enhanced response to central nervous system depressants). Products include:
Codiclear DH Syrup ... 808
Duratuss HD Elixir ... 2750
Histussin D Liquid ... 670
Hycodan Tablets and Syrup ... 946
Hycomine Compound Tablets ... 948
Hycomine ... 947
Hycotuss Expectorant Syrup ... 950
Hydrocet Capsules ... 787
Lorcet 10/650 Tablets ... 1016
Lortab ... 2751
Tussend ... 1830
Tussend Expectorant ... 1831
Vicodin Tablets ... 1404
Vicodin ES Tablets ... 1405
Vicodin HP Tablets ... 1403
Vicodin Tuss Expectorant ... 1406
Zydone Capsules ... 967

Hydrocodone Polistirex (Enhanced response to central nervous system depressants). Products include:
Tussionex Pennkinetic Extended-Release Suspension ... 1624

Hydroxyzine Hydrochloride (Enhanced response to central nervous system depressants). Products include:
Atarax Tablets & Syrup ... 1992
Marax Tablets & DF Syrup ... 2015
Vistaril Intramuscular Solution ... 2042

Hyoscyamine (Paralytic ileus may occur). Products include:
Cystospaz Tablets ... 2123
Urised Tablets ... 2123

Hyoscyamine Sulfate (Paralytic ileus may occur). Products include:
Arco-Lase Plus Tablets ... 513
Atrohist Plus Tablets ... 1605
Cystospaz-M Capsules ... 2123
Donnatal ... 2234
Donnatal Extentabs ... 2234
Donnatal Tablets ... 2234
Kutrase Capsules ... 2546
Levsin/Levsinex/Levbid ... 2549

Imipramine Hydrochloride (Concomitant use of amoxapine with other drugs that inhibit cytochrome $P_{450}IID_6$ may require lower than usual doses prescribed for either drug). Products include:
Tofranil Ampuls ... 873
Tofranil Tablets ... 875

Imipramine Pamoate (Concomitant use of amoxapine with other drugs that inhibit cytochrome $P_{450}IID_6$ may require lower than usual doses prescribed for either drug). Products include:
Tofranil-PM Capsules ... 876

Ipratropium Bromide (Paralytic ileus may occur). Products include:
Atrovent Inhalation Aerosol ... 674
Atrovent Inhalation Solution ... 675
Atrovent Nasal Spray 0.03% ... 676
Atrovent Nasal Spray 0.06% ... 678

Isocarboxazid (Concurrent and/or sequential use may result in hyperpyretic crises, severe convulsions, and fatalities; coadministration is contraindicated).
No products indexed under this heading.

Isoflurane (Enhanced response to central nervous system depressants).
No products indexed under this heading.

Ketamine Hydrochloride (Enhanced response to central nervous system depressants).
No products indexed under this heading.

Levomethadyl Acetate Hydrochloride (Enhanced response to central nervous system depressants). Products include:
Orlaam Oral Solution ... 2361

Levorphanol Tartrate (Enhanced response to central nervous system depressants). Products include:
Levo-Dromoran ... 2297

Lorazepam (Enhanced response to central nervous system depressants). Products include:
Ativan Injection ... 2805
Ativan Tablets ... 2807

Loxapine Hydrochloride (Enhanced response to central nervous system depressants). Products include:
Loxitane ... 1426

Loxapine Succinate (Enhanced response to central nervous system depressants). Products include:
Loxitane Capsules ... 1426

Maprotiline Hydrochloride (Concomitant use of amoxapine with other drugs that inhibit cytochrome $P_{450}IID_6$ may require lower than usual doses prescribed for either drug). Products include:
Ludiomil Tablets ... 861

Mepenzolate Bromide (Paralytic ileus may occur).
No products indexed under this heading.

Meperidine Hydrochloride (Enhanced response to central nervous system depressants). Products include:
Demerol ... 2438
Mepergan Injection ... 2859

Mephobarbital (Enhanced response to barbiturates). Products include:
Mebaral Tablets ... 2452

Meprobamate (Enhanced response to central nervous system depressants). Products include:
Miltown Tablets ... 2780
PMB 200 and PMB 400 ... 2890

Mesoridazine Besylate (Concomitant use of amoxapine with other drugs that inhibit cytochrome $P_{450}IID_6$ may require lower than usual doses prescribed for either drug; enhanced response to central nervous system depressants). Products include:
Serentil ... 689

Methadone Hydrochloride (Enhanced response to central nervous system depressants). Products include:
Methadone Hydrochloride Oral Concentrate ... 2356
Methadone Hydrochloride Oral Solution & Tablets ... 2357

Methohexital Sodium (Enhanced response to central nervous system depressants).
No products indexed under this heading.

Methotrimeprazine (Concomitant use of amoxapine with other drugs that inhibit cytochrome $P_{450}IID_6$ may require lower than usual doses prescribed for either drug; enhanced response to central nervous system depressants). Products include:
Levoprome ... 1321

Methoxyflurane (Enhanced response to central nervous system depressants).
No products indexed under this heading.

Midazolam Hydrochloride (Enhanced response to central nervous system depressants). Products include:
Versed Injection ... 2324

(▣ Described in PDR For Nonprescription Drugs) (◉ Described in PDR For Ophthalmology)

Interactions Index

Molindone Hydrochloride (Enhanced response to central nervous system depressants). Products include:
- Moban Tablets and Concentrate 1036

Morphine Sulfate (Enhanced response to central nervous system depressants). Products include:
- Astramorph/PF Injection, USP (Preservative-Free) 526
- Duramorph Injection 983
- Infumorph 200 and Infumorph 500 Sterile Solutions 985
- Kadian Capsules 2948
- MS Contin Tablets 2149
- MSIR 2152
- Oramorph SR (Morphine Sulfate Sustained Release Tablets) 2359
- RMS Suppositories CII 2766
- Roxanol 2365

Nefazodone Hydrochloride (Concomitant use of amoxapine with other drugs that inhibit cytochrome $P_{450}IID_6$ may require lower than usual doses prescribed for either drug). Products include:
- Serzone Tablets 776

Nortriptyline Hydrochloride (Concomitant use of amoxapine with other drugs that inhibit cytochrome $P_{450}IID_6$ may require lower than usual doses prescribed for either drug). Products include:
- Pamelor 2409

Opium Alkaloids (Enhanced response to central nervous system depressants).
- No products indexed under this heading.

Oxazepam (Enhanced response to central nervous system depressants). Products include:
- Serax Capsules 2916
- Serax Tablets 2916

Oxybutynin Chloride (Paralytic ileus may occur). Products include:
- Ditropan 1267

Oxycodone Hydrochloride (Enhanced response to central nervous system depressants). Products include:
- OxyContin Tablets 2163
- OxyIR Capsules 2167
- Percocet Tablets 955
- Percodan Tablets 955
- Percodan-Demi Tablets 956
- Roxicodone Tablets, Oral Solution & Intensol (Oxycodone) 2366
- Tylox Capsules 1593

Oxyphenonium Bromide (Paralytic ileus may occur).

Paroxetine Hydrochloride (Concomitant use of amoxapine with other drugs that inhibit cytochrome $P_{450}IID_6$ may require lower than usual doses prescribed for either drug). Products include:
- Paxil Tablets 2681

Pentobarbital Sodium (Enhanced response to barbiturates). Products include:
- Nembutal Sodium Capsules 440
- Nembutal Sodium Solution 442
- Nembutal Sodium Suppositories 444

Perphenazine (Concomitant use of amoxapine with other drugs that inhibit cytochrome $P_{450}IID_6$ may require lower than usual doses prescribed for either drug; enhanced response to central nervous system depressants). Products include:
- Etrafon 2495
- Triavil Tablets 1800
- Trilafon 2532

Phenelzine Sulfate (Concurrent and/or sequential use may result in hyperpyretic crises, severe convulsions, and fatalities; coadministration is contraindicated). Products include:
- Nardil 1977

Phenobarbital (Enhanced response to barbiturates). Products include:
- Arco-Lase Plus Tablets 513
- Bellergal-S Tablets 2375
- Donnatal 2234
- Donnatal Extentabs 2234
- Donnatal Tablets 2234
- Phenobarbital Elixir and Tablets 1523
- Quadrinal Tablets 1398

Prazepam (Enhanced response to central nervous system depressants).
- No products indexed under this heading.

Prochlorperazine (Concomitant use of amoxapine with other drugs that inhibit cytochrome $P_{450}IID_6$ may require lower than usual doses prescribed for either drug; enhanced response to central nervous system depressants). Products include:
- Compazine 2644

Procyclidine Hydrochloride (Paralytic ileus may occur). Products include:
- Kemadrin Tablets 1105

Promethazine Hydrochloride (Concomitant use of amoxapine with other drugs that inhibit cytochrome $P_{450}IID_6$ may require lower than usual doses prescribed for either drug; enhanced response to central nervous system depressants). Products include:
- Mepergan Injection 2859
- Phenergan with Codeine 2883
- Phenergan with Dextromethorphan 2885
- Phenergan Injection 2880
- Phenergan Suppositories 2882
- Phenergan Syrup 2881
- Phenergan Tablets 2882
- Phenergan VC 2886
- Phenergan VC with Codeine 2888

Propafenone Hydrochloride (Concomitant use of amoxapine with other drugs that inhibit cytochrome $P_{450}IID_6$ may require lower than usual doses prescribed for either drug). Products include:
- Rythmol Tablets–150mg, 225mg, 300mg 1399

Propantheline Bromide (Paralytic ileus may occur). Products include:
- Pro-Banthine Tablets 2226

Propofol (Enhanced response to central nervous system depressants). Products include:
- Diprivan Injectable Emulsion 2939

Propoxyphene Hydrochloride (Enhanced response to central nervous system depressants). Products include:
- Darvon 1475
- Wygesic Tablets 2930

Propoxyphene Napsylate (Enhanced response to central nervous system depressants). Products include:
- Darvon-N/Darvocet-N 1473

Protriptyline Hydrochloride (Concomitant use of amoxapine with other drugs that inhibit cytochrome $P_{450}IID_6$ may require lower than usual doses prescribed for either drug). Products include:
- Vivactil Tablets 1820

Quazepam (Enhanced response to central nervous system depressants). Products include:
- Doral Tablets 2773

Quinidine Gluconate (Concomitant use of amoxapine with other drugs that inhibit cytochrome $P_{450}IID_6$ may require lower than usual doses prescribed for either drug). Products include:
- Quinaglute Dura-Tabs Tablets 644

Quinidine Polygalacturonate (Concomitant use of amoxapine with other drugs that inhibit cytochrome $P_{450}IID_6$ may require lower than usual doses prescribed for either drug). Products include:
- Cardioquin Tablets 2146

Quinidine Sulfate (Concomitant use of amoxapine with other drugs that inhibit cytochrome $P_{450}IID_6$ may require lower than usual doses prescribed for either drug). Products include:
- Quinidex Extentabs 2240

Risperidone (Enhanced response to central nervous system depressants). Products include:
- Risperdal Tablets 1348

Scopolamine (Paralytic ileus may occur). Products include:
- Transderm Scōp Transdermal Therapeutic System 890

Scopolamine Hydrobromide (Paralytic ileus may occur). Products include:
- Atrohist Plus Tablets 1605
- Donnatal 2234
- Donnatal Extentabs 2234
- Donnatal Tablets 2234

Secobarbital Sodium (Enhanced response to barbiturates). Products include:
- Seconal Sodium Pulvules 1529

Selegiline Hydrochloride (Concurrent and/or sequential use may result in hyperpyretic crises, severe convulsions, and fatalities; coadministration is contraindicated). Products include:
- Eldepryl Capsules 2729

Sertraline Hydrochloride (Concomitant use of amoxapine with other drugs that inhibit cytochrome $P_{450}IID_6$ may require lower than usual doses prescribed for either drug). Products include:
- Zoloft Tablets 2051

Sevoflurane (Enhanced response to central nervous system depressants).
- No products indexed under this heading.

Sufentanil Citrate (Enhanced response to central nervous system depressants). Products include:
- Sufenta Injection 1355

Temazepam (Enhanced response to central nervous system depressants). Products include:
- Restoril Capsules 2413

Thiamylal Sodium (Enhanced response to barbiturates).
- No products indexed under this heading.

Thioridazine Hydrochloride (Concomitant use of amoxapine with other drugs that inhibit cytochrome $P_{450}IID_6$ may require lower than usual doses prescribed for either drug; enhanced response to central nervous system depressants). Products include:
- Mellaril 2398

Thiothixene (Enhanced response to central nervous system depressants). Products include:
- Navane Capsules and Concentrate 2018
- Navane Intramuscular 2019

Tranylcypromine Sulfate (Concurrent and/or sequential use may result in hyperpyretic crises, severe convulsions, and fatalities; coadministration is contraindicated). Products include:
- Parnate Tablets 2679

Trazodone Hydrochloride (Concomitant use of amoxapine with other drugs that inhibit cytochrome $P_{450}IID_6$ may require lower than usual doses prescribed for either drug). Products include:
- Desyrel and Desyrel Dividose 504

Triazolam (Enhanced response to central nervous system depressants). Products include:
- Halcion Tablets 2093

Tridihexethyl Chloride (Paralytic ileus may occur).
- No products indexed under this heading.

Trifluoperazine Hydrochloride (Concomitant use of amoxapine with other drugs that inhibit cytochrome $P_{450}IID_6$ may require lower than usual doses prescribed for either drug; enhanced response to central nervous system depressants). Products include:
- Stelazine 2692

Trihexyphenidyl Hydrochloride (Paralytic ileus may occur). Products include:
- Artane 1418

Trimipramine Maleate (Concomitant use of amoxapine with other drugs that inhibit cytochrome $P_{450}IID_6$ may require lower than usual doses prescribed for either drug). Products include:
- Surmontil Capsules 2917

Venlafaxine Hydrochloride (Concomitant use of amoxapine with other drugs that inhibit cytochrome $P_{450}IID_6$ may require lower than usual doses prescribed for either drug). Products include:
- Effexor 2825

Zolpidem Tartrate (Enhanced response to central nervous system depressants). Products include:
- Ambien Tablets 2559

Food Interactions
Alcohol (Enhanced response to alcohol).

ASPERCREME CREME, LOTION ANALGESIC RUB
(Trolamine Salicylate) 794
None cited in PDR database.

ASTRAMORPH/PF INJECTION, USP (PRESERVATIVE-FREE)
(Morphine Sulfate) 526
May interact with central nervous system depressants, psychotropics, antihistamines, antipsychotic agents, tricyclic antidepressants, monoamine oxidase inhibitors, hypnotics and sedatives, phenothiazines, butyrophenones, anticoagulants, parenterally administered corticosteroids, and certain other agents. Compounds in these categories include:

Acrivastine (Potentiation of depressant effects of morphine). Products include:
- Semprex-D Capsules 1620

Alfentanil Hydrochloride (Potentiation of depressant effects of morphine). Products include:
- Alfenta Injection 1334

IMPORTANT NOTE: Always consult each drug listing in the patient's regimen for possible interactions.

Astramorph/PF Interactions Index 76

Alprazolam (Potentiation of depressant effects of morphine). Products include:
Xanax Tablets ... 2115

Amitriptyline Hydrochloride (Potentiation of depressant effects of morphine). Products include:
Elavil ... 2945
Etrafon ... 2495
Limbitrol ... 2333
Triavil Tablets ... 1800

Amoxapine (Potentiation of depressant effects of morphine). Products include:
Asendin Tablets ... 1419

Aprobarbital (Potentiation of depressant effects of morphine).
No products indexed under this heading.

Astemizole (Potentiation of depressant effects of morphine). Products include:
Hismanal Tablets ... 1341

Azatadine Maleate (Potentiation of depressant effects of morphine). Products include:
Trinalin Repetabs Tablets ... 1373

Bromodiphenhydramine Hydrochloride (Potentiation of depressant effects of morphine).
No products indexed under this heading.

Brompheniramine Maleate (Potentiation of depressant effects of morphine). Products include:
Alka-Seltzer Plus Sinus Medicine .. ▣ 611
Bromfed Capsules (Extended-Release) ... 1832
Bromfed Syrup ... ▣ 712
Bromfed Tablets ... 1832
Bromfed-DM Cough Syrup ... 1832
Bromfed-PD Capsules (Extended-Release) ... 1832
Dimetane-DC Cough Syrup ... 2232
Dimetane-DX Cough Syrup ... 2233
Dimetapp Allergy Dye-Free Elixir ... ▣ 838
Dimetapp Allergy Sinus Caplets ... ▣ 838
Dimetapp Cold & Allergy Chewable Tablets ... ▣ 838
Dimetapp Cold & Cough Liqui-Gels ... ▣ 839
Dimetapp Cold & Fever Suspension ... ▣ 839
Dimetapp DM Elixir ... ▣ 840
Dimetapp Elixir ... ▣ 840
Dimetapp Extentabs ... ▣ 841
Dimetapp Tablets/Liqui-Gels ... ▣ 841
Rondec Chewable Tablets ... 974
Vicks DayQuil Allergy Relief 12-Hour Extended Release Tablets ... ▣ 733
Vicks DayQuil Allergy Relief 4-Hour Tablets ... ▣ 733

Buprenorphine (Potentiation of depressant effects of morphine). Products include:
Buprenex Injectable ... 2170

Buspirone Hydrochloride (Potentiation of depressant effects of morphine). Products include:
BuSpar Tablets ... 738

Butabarbital (Potentiation of depressant effects of morphine).
No products indexed under this heading.

Butalbital (Potentiation of depressant effects of morphine). Products include:
Axocet Capsules ... 2469
Esgic-plus Capsules ... 1012
Esgic-plus Tablets ... 1012
Fioricet Tablets ... 2386
Fioricet with Codeine Capsules ... 2387
Fiorinal Capsules ... 2388
Fiorinal with Codeine Capsules ... 2390
Fiorinal Tablets ... 2388
Phrenilin ... 790
Sedapap Tablets 50 mg/650 mg .. 1826

Cetirizine Hydrochloride (Potentiation of depressant effects of morphine). Products include:
Zyrtec Tablets ... 2053

Chlordiazepoxide (Potentiation of depressant effects of morphine). Products include:
Limbitrol ... 2333

Chlordiazepoxide Hydrochloride (Potentiation of depressant effects of morphine). Products include:
Librax Capsules ... 2330
Librium Capsules ... 2331
Librium Injectable ... 2332

Chlorpheniramine Maleate (Potentiation of depressant effects of morphine). Products include:
Alka-Seltzer Plus Cold Medicine ... ▣ 611
Alka-Seltzer Plus Cold Medicine Liqui-Gels ... ▣ 612
Alka-Seltzer Plus Cold & Cough Medicine ... ▣ 611
Alka-Seltzer Plus Cold & Cough Medicine Liqui-Gels ... ▣ 612
Alka-Seltzer Plus Flu & Body Aches Effervescent Tablets ... ▣ 612
Allerest Maximum Strength ... ▣ 649
Allerest Sinus Pain Formula ... ▣ 649
Ana-Kit Anaphylaxis Emergency Treatment Kit ... 611
Atrohist Pediatric Capsules ... 1603
Atrohist Plus Tablets ... 1605
BC Cold Powder Multi-Symptom Formula (Cold-Sinus-Allergy) ... ▣ 631
Cerose DM ... ▣ 853
Cheracol Plus Head Cold/Cough Formula ... ▣ 741
Children's TYLENOL Cold Multi-Symptom Chewable Tablets and Liquid ... 1559
Children's TYLENOL Cold Plus Cough Multi Symptom Chewable Tablets and Liquid ... 1560
Children's TYLENOL Flu Suspension Liquid ... 1560
Children's Vicks DayQuil Allergy Relief ... ▣ 730
Children's Vicks NyQuil Cold/Cough Relief ... ▣ 731
Chlor-Trimeton Allergy Decongestant Tablets ... ▣ 759
Chlor-Trimeton Allergy Tablets ... ▣ 758
Allergy-Sinus Comtrex Multi-Symptom Allergy-Sinus Formula Tablets and Caplets ... ▣ 639
Comtrex Multi-Symptom ... ▣ 638
Contac Continuous Action Nasal Decongestant/Antihistamine 12 Hour Capsules ... ▣ 773
Contac Maximum Strength Continuous Action Decongestant/Antihistamine 12 Hour Caplets .. ▣ 772
Contac Severe Cold and Flu Formula Caplets ... ▣ 773
Coricidin Cold + Flu Tablets ... ▣ 760
Coricidin Cough + Cold Tablets ... ▣ 760
Coricidin 'D' Decongestant Tablets ... ▣ 760
D.A. II Tablets ... 972
D.A. Chewable Tablets ... 970
Dura-Tap/PD Capsules ... 970
Dura-Vent/DA Tablets ... 972
Efidac 24 Chlorpheniramine ... ▣ 655
Extendryl ... 1003
Fedahist Gyrocaps ... 2545
Hycomine Compound Tablets ... 948
Kronofed-A ... 994
Nolamine Timed-Release Tablets ... 790
Novahistine Elixir ... ▣ 782
Ornade Spansule Capsules ... 2678
PediaCare Cough-Cold Chewable Tablets and Liquid ... 1569
PediaCare NightRest Cough-Cold Liquid ... 1569
Pediatric Vicks 44m Cough & Cold Relief ... ▣ 737
Pyrroxate Caplets ... ▣ 742
Ryna ... ▣ 804
Sinarest ... ▣ 663
Sine-Off Sinus Medicine ... ▣ 784
Singlet Tablets ... ▣ 785
Sinulin Tablets ... 792
Sinutab Sinus Allergy Medication, Maximum Strength Tablets and Caplets ... ▣ 823
Sudafed Cold & Allergy Tablets ... ▣ 826
Teldrin 12 Hour Antihistamine/Nasal Decongestant Allergy Relief Capsules ... ▣ 786
TheraFlu Flu and Cold Medicine ... ▣ 750
Theraflu Maximum Strength Flu and Cold Medicine For Sore Throat ... ▣ 751
TheraFlu Flu, Cold and Cough Medicine ... ▣ 750
TheraFlu Maximum Strength Nighttime Flu, Cold & Cough Medicine ... ▣ 751
Triaminic Night Time ... ▣ 754
Triaminic Syrup ... ▣ 755
Triaminic Triaminicol Cold & Cough ... ▣ 756
Triaminicin Tablets ... ▣ 756
Tussend ... 1830
TYLENOL Allergy Sinus, Maximum Strength Caplets and Gelcaps ... 1571
TYLENOL Cold Medication, Multi-Symptom Formula Tablets and Caplets ... 1572
TYLENOL Cold Medication, Multi-Symptom Hot Liquid Packets ... 1572
Vicks 44 LiquiCaps Cough, Cold & Flu Relief ... ▣ 728
Vicks 44M Cough, Cold & Flu Relief ... ▣ 729

Chlorpheniramine Polistirex (Potentiation of depressant effects of morphine). Products include:
Tussionex Pennkinetic Extended-Release Suspension ... 1624

Chlorpheniramine Tannate (Potentiation of depressant effects of morphine). Products include:
Atrohist Pediatric Suspension ... 1604
Atrohist Pediatric Suspension Dye-Free ... 1604
Rynatan ... 2781
Rynatuss ... 2782

Chlorpromazine (Potentiation of depressant effects of morphine; increased risk of respiratory depression). Products include:
Thorazine Suppositories ... 2701

Chlorpromazine Hydrochloride (Potentiation of depressant effects of morphine). Products include:
Thorazine ... 2701

Chlorprothixene (Potentiation of depressant effects of morphine; increased risk of respiratory depression).
No products indexed under this heading.

Chlorprothixene Hydrochloride (Potentiation of depressant effects of morphine; increased risk of respiratory depression).
No products indexed under this heading.

Chlorprothixene Lactate (Potentiation of depressant effects of morphine).
No products indexed under this heading.

Clemastine Fumarate (Potentiation of depressant effects of morphine). Products include:
Tavist Syrup ... 2426
Tavist Tablets ... 2427
Tavist-1 12 Hour Relief Tablets ... ▣ 749
Tavist-D 12 Hour Relief Tablets ... ▣ 750

Clomipramine Hydrochloride (Potentiation of depressant effects of morphine). Products include:
Anafranil Capsules ... 819

Clorazepate Dipotassium (Potentiation of depressant effects of morphine). Products include:
Tranxene ... 459

Clozapine (Potentiation of depressant effects of morphine; increased risk of respiratory depression). Products include:
Clozaril Tablets ... 2377

Codeine Phosphate (Potentiation of depressant effects of morphine). Products include:
Brontex ... 2130
Dimetane-DC Cough Syrup ... 2232
Fioricet with Codeine Capsules ... 2387
Fiorinal with Codeine Capsules ... 2390
Nucofed ... 2225
Phenergan with Codeine ... 2883
Phenergan VC with Codeine ... 2888
Robitussin A-C Syrup ... 2248
Robitussin-DAC Syrup ... 2249
Ryna ... ▣ 804
Soma Compound w/Codeine Tablets ... 2784
Tylenol with Codeine ... 1592

Cyproheptadine Hydrochloride (Potentiation of depressant effects of morphine). Products include:
Periactin ... 1767

Dalteparin Sodium (Administration of morphine by epidural or intrathecal route is contraindicated in presence of concomitant anticoagulant therapy). Products include:
Fragmin Injection ... 2088

Desflurane (Potentiation of depressant effects of morphine). Products include:
Suprane (desflurane, USP) ... 1865

Desipramine Hydrochloride (Potentiation of depressant effects of morphine). Products include:
Norpramin Tablets ... 1273

Dexamethasone Acetate (Administration of morphine by epidural or intrathecal route is contraindicated in presence of concomitantly administered parenteral corticosteroids within 2 weeks). Products include:
Dalalone D.P. Injectable ... 1009
Decadron-LA Sterile Suspension ... 1687

Dexamethasone Sodium Phosphate (Administration of morphine by epidural or intrathecal route is contraindicated in presence of concomitantly administered parenteral corticosteroids within 2 weeks). Products include:
Decadron Phosphate Injection ... 1680
Decadron Phosphate Sterile Ophthalmic Ointment ... 1684
Decadron Phosphate Sterile Ophthalmic Solution ... 1685
Decadron Phosphate Topical Cream ... 1686
Decadron Phosphate with Xylocaine Injection, Sterile ... 1683
Dexacort Phosphate in Respihaler .. 1606
Dexacort Phosphate in Turbinaire .. 1607
NeoDecadron Sterile Ophthalmic Ointment ... 1755
NeoDecadron Sterile Ophthalmic Solution ... 1756
NeoDecadron Topical Cream ... 1757

Dexchlorpheniramine Maleate (Potentiation of depressant effects of morphine).
No products indexed under this heading.

Dezocine (Potentiation of depressant effects of morphine). Products include:
Dalgan Injection ... 529

Diazepam (Potentiation of depressant effects of morphine). Products include:
Dizac (diazepam injectable emulsion) CIV ... 1862
Valium Injectable ... 2336
Valium Tablets ... 2335

Dicumarol (Administration of morphine by epidural or intrathecal route is contraindicated in presence of concomitant anticoagulant therapy).
No products indexed under this heading.

Diphenhydramine Citrate (Potentiation of depressant effects of morphine). Products include:
Excedrin P.M. Analgesic/Sleeping Aid Tablets, Caplets, Liquigels ... 735

Diphenhydramine Hydrochloride (Potentiation of depressant effects of morphine). Products include:
Actifed Allergy Daytime/Nighttime Caplets ... ▣ 808

(▣ Described in PDR For Nonprescription Drugs) (◉ Described in PDR For Ophthalmology)

Interactions Index

Actifed Sinus Daytime/Nighttime Tablets and Caplets ... 809
Extra Strength Bayer PM Aspirin Plus Sleep Aid ... 617
Benadryl Allergy Chewables ... 811
Benadryl Allergy/Cold Tablets ... 811
Benadryl Allergy Decongestant Liquid Medication ... 812
Benadryl Allergy Decongestant Tablets ... 812
Benadryl Allergy Liquid Medication ... 813
Benadryl Allergy ... 811
Benadryl Allergy Sinus Headache Caplets ... 813
Benadryl Dye-Free Allergy Liquigel Softgels ... 813
Benadryl Dye-Free Allergy Liquid Medication ... 814
Benadryl Itch Relief Stick Extra Strength ... 814
Benadryl Cream ... 814
Benadryl Gel ... 815
Benadryl Spray ... 815
Benadryl Injection ... 1955
Contac Day & Night Cold/Flu Night Caplets ... 772
Contac Night Allergy/Sinus Caplets ... 771
Extra Strength Doan's P.M. ... 653
Excedrin P.M. Analgesic/Sleeping Aid Tablets, Caplets, Liquigels ... 643
Nytol QuickCaps Caplets ... 632
Sleepinal Night-time Sleep Aid Capsules and Softgels ... 798
TYLENOL Allergy Sinus NightTime, Maximum Strength Caplets ... 1571
TYLENOL Flu NightTime, Maximum Strength Gelcaps ... 1575
TYLENOL Flu NightTime, Maximum Strength Hot Medication Packets ... 1575
TYLENOL PM Pain Reliever/Sleep Aid, Extra Strength Gelcaps, Caplets, Geltabs ... 1576
TYLENOL Severe Allergy Medication Caplets ... 1571
Maximum Strength Unisom Sleepgels ... 1990
Unisom With Pain Relief-Nighttime Sleep Aid and Pain Reliever ... 1991

Diphenylpyraline Hydrochloride (Potentiation of depressant effects of morphine).
No products indexed under this heading.

Doxepin Hydrochloride (Potentiation of depressant effects of morphine). Products include:
Adapin Capsules ... 1542
Sinequan ... 2028
Zonalon Cream ... 1042

Droperidol (Potentiation of depressant effects of morphine). Products include:
Inapsine Injection ... 462

Enflurane (Potentiation of depressant effects of morphine).
No products indexed under this heading.

Enoxaparin (Administration of morphine by epidural or intrathecal route is contraindicated in presence of concomitant anticoagulant therapy). Products include:
Lovenox Injection ... 2187

Estazolam (Potentiation of depressant effects of morphine). Products include:
ProSom Tablets ... 457

Ethchlorvynol (Potentiation of depressant effects of morphine). Products include:
Placidyl Capsules ... 456

Ethinamate (Potentiation of depressant effects of morphine).
No products indexed under this heading.

Fentanyl (Potentiation of depressant effects of morphine). Products include:
Duragesic Transdermal System ... 1336

Fentanyl Citrate (Potentiation of depressant effects of morphine). Products include:
Sublimaze Injection ... 463

Fluphenazine Decanoate (Potentiation of depressant effects of morphine; increased risk of respiratory depression). Products include:
Prolixin Decanoate ... 510

Fluphenazine Enanthate (Potentiation of depressant effects of morphine; increased risk of respiratory depression). Products include:
Prolixin Enanthate ... 510

Fluphenazine Hydrochloride (Potentiation of depressant effects of morphine; increased risk of respiratory depression). Products include:
Prolixin ... 510

Flurazepam Hydrochloride (Potentiation of depressant effects of morphine). Products include:
Dalmane Capsules ... 2329

Furazolidone (Concomitant use potentiates depressant effects of morphine). Products include:
Furoxone ... 2221

Glutethimide (Potentiation of depressant effects of morphine).
No products indexed under this heading.

Haloperidol (Potentiation of depressant effects of morphine). Products include:
Haldol Injection, Tablets and Concentrate ... 1585

Haloperidol Decanoate (Potentiation of depressant effects of morphine; increased risk of respiratory depression). Products include:
Haldol Decanoate ... 1587

Heparin Calcium (Administration of morphine by epidural or intrathecal route is contraindicated in presence of concomitant anticoagulant therapy).
No products indexed under this heading.

Heparin Sodium (Administration of morphine by epidural or intrathecal route is contraindicated in presence of concomitant anticoagulant therapy). Products include:
Heparin Lock Flush Solution ... 2831
Heparin Sodium Injection ... 2832
Heparin Sodium Vials ... 1486

Hydrocodone Bitartrate (Potentiation of depressant effects of morphine). Products include:
Codiclear DH Syrup ... 808
Duratuss HD Elixir ... 2750
Histussin D Liquid ... 670
Hycodan Tablets and Syrup ... 946
Hycomine Compound Tablets ... 948
Hycomine ... 947
Hycotuss Expectorant Syrup ... 950
Hydrocet Capsules ... 787
Lorcet 10/650 Tablets ... 1016
Lortab ... 2751
Tussend ... 1830
Tussend Expectorant ... 1831
Vicodin Tablets ... 1404
Vicodin ES Tablets ... 1405
Vicodin HP Tablets ... 1403
Vicodin Tuss Expectorant ... 1406
Zydone Capsules ... 967

Hydrocodone Polistirex (Potentiation of depressant effects of morphine). Products include:
Tussionex Pennkinetic Extended-Release Suspension ... 1624

Hydrocortisone Acetate (Administration of morphine by epidural or intrathecal route is contraindicated in presence of concomitantly administered parenteral corticosteroids within 2 weeks). Products include:
Analpram-HC Rectal Cream 1% and 2.5% ... 993
Anusol HC-1 Hydrocortisone Anti-Itch Ointment ... 810
Anusol-HC Suppositories ... 1954
Caldecort Anti-Itch Hydrocortisone Cream ... 651
Coly-Mycin S Otic w/Neomycin & Hydrocortisone ... 1965
Cortaid ... 800
Cortifoam ... 2540
Cortisporin Cream ... 1073
Epifoam ... 2543
Hydrocortone Acetate Sterile Suspension ... 1712
Mantadil Cream ... 1124
Nupercainal Hydrocortisone 1% Cream ... 661
Pramosone Cream, Lotion & Ointment ... 995
ProctoFoam-HC ... 2552
Terra-Cortril Ophthalmic Suspension ... 2033

Hydrocortisone Sodium Phosphate (Administration of morphine by epidural or intrathecal route is contraindicated in presence of concomitantly administered parenteral corticosteroids within 2 weeks). Products include:
Hydrocortone Phosphate Injection, Sterile ... 1713

Hydrocortisone Sodium Succinate (Administration of morphine by epidural or intrathecal route is contraindicated in presence of concomitantly administered parenteral corticosteroids within 2 weeks).
No products indexed under this heading.

Hydroxyzine Hydrochloride (Potentiation of depressant effects of morphine). Products include:
Atarax Tablets & Syrup ... 1992
Marax Tablets & DF Syrup ... 2015
Vistaril Intramuscular Solution ... 2042

Imipramine Hydrochloride (Potentiation of depressant effects of morphine). Products include:
Tofranil Ampuls ... 873
Tofranil Tablets ... 875

Imipramine Pamoate (Potentiation of depressant effects of morphine). Products include:
Tofranil-PM Capsules ... 876

Isocarboxazid (Concomitant use potentiates depressant effects of morphine).
No products indexed under this heading.

Isoflurane (Potentiation of depressant effects of morphine).
No products indexed under this heading.

Ketamine Hydrochloride (Potentiation of depressant effects of morphine).
No products indexed under this heading.

Levomethadyl Acetate Hydrochloride (Potentiation of depressant effects of morphine). Products include:
Orlaam Oral Solution ... 2361

Levorphanol Tartrate (Potentiation of depressant effects of morphine). Products include:
Levo-Dromoran ... 2297

Lithium Carbonate (Potentiation of depressant effects of morphine; increased risk of respiratory depression). Products include:
Eskalith ... 2658
Lithium Carbonate Capsules & Tablets ... 2352
Lithonate/Lithotabs/Lithobid ... 2721

Lithium Citrate (Potentiation of depressant effects of morphine; increased risk of respiratory depression).
No products indexed under this heading.

Loratadine (Potentiation of depressant effects of morphine). Products include:
Claritin Tablets ... 2485
Claritin-D Tablets ... 2487

Lorazepam (Potentiation of depressant effects of morphine). Products include:
Ativan Injection ... 2805
Ativan Tablets ... 2807

Loxapine Hydrochloride (Potentiation of depressant effects of morphine; increased risk of respiratory depression). Products include:
Loxitane ... 1426

Loxapine Succinate (Potentiation of depressant effects of morphine). Products include:
Loxitane Capsules ... 1426

Maprotiline Hydrochloride (Potentiation of depressant effects of morphine). Products include:
Ludiomil Tablets ... 861

Meperidine Hydrochloride (Potentiation of depressant effects of morphine). Products include:
Demerol ... 2438
Mepergan Injection ... 2859

Mephobarbital (Potentiation of depressant effects of morphine). Products include:
Mebaral Tablets ... 2452

Meprobamate (Potentiation of depressant effects of morphine). Products include:
Miltown Tablets ... 2780
PMB 200 and PMB 400 ... 2890

Mesoridazine Besylate (Potentiation of depressant effects of morphine; increased risk of respiratory depression). Products include:
Serentil ... 689

Methadone Hydrochloride (Potentiation of depressant effects of morphine). Products include:
Methadone Hydrochloride Oral Concentrate ... 2356
Methadone Hydrochloride Oral Solution & Tablets ... 2357

Methdilazine Hydrochloride (Potentiation of depressant effects of morphine).
No products indexed under this heading.

Methohexital Sodium (Potentiation of depressant effects of morphine).
No products indexed under this heading.

Methotrimeprazine (Potentiation of depressant effects of morphine). Products include:
Levoprome ... 1321

Methoxyflurane (Potentiation of depressant effects of morphine).
No products indexed under this heading.

Methylprednisolone Acetate (Administration of morphine by epidural or intrathecal route is contraindicated in presence of concomitantly administered parenteral corticosteroids within 2 weeks).
No products indexed under this heading.

Methylprednisolone Sodium Succinate (Administration of morphine by epidural or intrathecal route is contraindicated in presence of concomitantly administered parenteral corticosteroids within 2 weeks).
No products indexed under this heading.

Midazolam Hydrochloride (Potentiation of depressant effects of morphine). Products include:
Versed Injection ... 2324

IMPORTANT NOTE: Always consult each drug listing in the patient's regimen for possible interactions.

Astramorph/PF — Interactions Index

Molindone Hydrochloride (Potentiation of depressant effects of morphine; increased risk of respiratory depression with neuroleptics). Products include:
- Moban Tablets and Concentrate 1036

Nortriptyline Hydrochloride (Potentiation of depressant effects of morphine). Products include:
- Pamelor 2409

Opium Alkaloids (Potentiation of depressant effects of morphine).
- No products indexed under this heading.

Oxazepam (Potentiation of depressant effects of morphine). Products include:
- Serax Capsules 2916
- Serax Tablets 2916

Oxycodone Hydrochloride (Potentiation of depressant effects of morphine). Products include:
- OxyContin Tablets 2163
- OxyIR Capsules 2167
- Percocet Tablets 955
- Percodan Tablets 955
- Percodan-Demi Tablets 956
- Roxicodone Tablets, Oral Solution & Intensol (Oxycodone) 2366
- Tylox Capsules 1593

Pentobarbital Sodium (Potentiation of depressant effects of morphine). Products include:
- Nembutal Sodium Capsules 440
- Nembutal Sodium Solution 442
- Nembutal Sodium Suppositories 444

Perphenazine (Potentiation of depressant effects of morphine). Products include:
- Etrafon 2495
- Triavil Tablets 1800
- Trilafon 2532

Phenelzine Sulfate (Concomitant use potentiates depressant effects of morphine). Products include:
- Nardil 1977

Phenobarbital (Potentiation of depressant effects of morphine). Products include:
- Arco-Lase Plus Tablets 513
- Bellergal-S Tablets 2375
- Donnatal 2234
- Donnatal Extentabs 2234
- Donnatal Tablets 2234
- Phenobarbital Elixir and Tablets 1523
- Quadrinal Tablets 1398

Pimozide (Potentiation of depressant effects of morphine; increased risk of respiratory depression). Products include:
- Orap Tablets 1037

Prazepam (Potentiation of depressant effects of morphine).
- No products indexed under this heading.

Prednisolone Acetate (Administration of morphine by epidural or intrathecal route is contraindicated in presence of concomitantly administered parenteral corticosteroids within 2 weeks). Products include:
- AK-CIDE ...... ⊙ 203
- AK-CIDE Ointment ...... ⊙ 203
- Blephamide Liquifilm Sterile Ophthalmic Suspension 472
- Blephamide Ointment ...... ⊙ 234
- Econopred & Econopred Plus Ophthalmic Suspensions ...... ⊙ 216
- Poly-Pred Liquifilm ...... ⊙ 246
- Pred Forte ...... ⊙ 247
- Pred Mild ...... ⊙ 250
- Pred-G Liquifilm Sterile Ophthalmic Suspension ...... ⊙ 248
- Pred-G S.O.P. Sterile Ophthalmic Ointment ...... ⊙ 249

Prednisolone Sodium Phosphate (Administration of morphine by epidural or intrathecal route is contraindicated in presence of concomitantly administered parenteral corticosteroids within 2 weeks). Products include:
- AK-PRED ...... ⊙ 204
- Hydeltrasol Injection, Sterile 1708
- Pediapred Oral Solution 1618

Prednisolone Tebutate (Administration of morphine by epidural or intrathecal route is contraindicated in presence of concomitantly administered parenteral corticosteroids within 2 weeks). Products include:
- Hydeltra-T.B.A. Sterile Suspension 1710

Prochlorperazine (Potentiation of depressant effects of morphine; increased risk of respiratory depression). Products include:
- Compazine 2644

Promethazine Hydrochloride (Potentiation of depressant effects of morphine; increased risk of respiratory depression). Products include:
- Mepergan Injection 2859
- Phenergan with Codeine 2883
- Phenergan with Dextromethorphan 2885
- Phenergan Injection 2880
- Phenergan Suppositories 2882
- Phenergan Syrup 2881
- Phenergan Tablets 2882
- Phenergan VC 2886
- Phenergan VC with Codeine 2888

Propofol (Potentiation of depressant effects of morphine). Products include:
- Diprivan Injectable Emulsion 2939

Propoxyphene Hydrochloride (Potentiation of depressant effects of morphine). Products include:
- Darvon 1475
- Wygesic Tablets 2930

Propoxyphene Napsylate (Potentiation of depressant effects of morphine). Products include:
- Darvon-N/Darvocet-N 1473

Protriptyline Hydrochloride (Potentiation of depressant effects of morphine). Products include:
- Vivactil Tablets 1820

Pyrilamine Maleate (Potentiation of depressant effects of morphine). Products include:
- 4-Way Fast Acting Nasal Spray (regular & mentholated) ...... ■□ 644
- Maximum Strength Multi-Symptom Formula Midol ...... ■□ 621
- PMS Multi-Symptom Formula Midol ...... ■□ 622

Pyrilamine Tannate (Potentiation of depressant effects of morphine). Products include:
- Atrohist Pediatric Suspension 1604
- Atrohist Pediatric Suspension Dye-Free 1604
- Rynatan 2781

Quazepam (Potentiation of depressant effects of morphine). Products include:
- Doral Tablets 2773

Risperidone (Potentiation of depressant effects of morphine). Products include:
- Risperdal Tablets 1348

Secobarbital Sodium (Potentiation of depressant effects of morphine). Products include:
- Seconal Sodium Pulvules 1529

Selegiline Hydrochloride (Concomitant use potentiates depressant effects of morphine). Products include:
- Eldepryl Capsules 2729

Sevoflurane (Potentiation of depressant effects of morphine).
- No products indexed under this heading.

Sufentanil Citrate (Potentiation of depressant effects of morphine). Products include:
- Sufenta Injection 1355

Temazepam (Potentiation of depressant effects of morphine). Products include:
- Restoril Capsules 2413

Terfenadine (Potentiation of depressant effects of morphine). Products include:
- Seldane Tablets 1284
- Seldane-D Extended-Release Tablets 1286

Thiamylal Sodium (Potentiation of depressant effects of morphine).
- No products indexed under this heading.

Thioridazine Hydrochloride (Potentiation of depressant effects of morphine; increased risk of respiratory depression). Products include:
- Mellaril 2398

Thiothixene (Potentiation of depressant effects of morphine; increased risk of respiratory depression). Products include:
- Navane Capsules and Concentrate 2018
- Navane Intramuscular 2019

Tranylcypromine Sulfate (Concomitant use potentiates depressant effects of morphine). Products include:
- Parnate Tablets 2679

Triamcinolone Acetonide (Administration of morphine by epidural or intrathecal route is contraindicated in presence of concomitantly administered parenteral corticosteroids within 2 weeks). Products include:
- Azmacort Oral Inhaler 2175
- Nasacort AQ Nasal Spray 2191
- Nasacort Nasal Inhaler 2189

Triamcinolone Diacetate (Administration of morphine by epidural or intrathecal route is contraindicated in presence of concomitantly administered parenteral corticosteroids within 2 weeks).
- No products indexed under this heading.

Triamcinolone Hexacetonide (Administration of morphine by epidural or intrathecal route is contraindicated in presence of concomitantly administered parenteral corticosteroids within 2 weeks).
- No products indexed under this heading.

Triazolam (Potentiation of depressant effects of morphine). Products include:
- Halcion Tablets 2093

Trifluoperazine Hydrochloride (Potentiation of depressant effects of morphine; increased risk of respiratory depression). Products include:
- Stelazine 2692

Trimeprazine Tartrate (Potentiation of depressant effects of morphine).
- No products indexed under this heading.

Trimipramine Maleate (Potentiation of depressant effects of morphine). Products include:
- Surmontil Capsules 2917

Tripelennamine Hydrochloride (Potentiation of depressant effects of morphine). Products include:
- PBZ 863
- PBZ-SR Tablets 862

Triprolidine Hydrochloride (Potentiation of depressant effects of morphine). Products include:
- Actifed Cold & Allergy Tablets ...... ■□ 807
- Actifed Cold & Sinus Caplets and Tablets ...... ■□ 808

Warfarin Sodium (Administration of morphine by epidural or intrathecal route is contraindicated in presence of concomitant anticoagulant therapy). Products include:
- Coumadin 941

Zolpidem Tartrate (Potentiation of depressant effects of morphine). Products include:
- Ambien Tablets 2559

Food Interactions

Alcohol (Potentiation of depressant effects of morphine).

ATAMET TABLETS
(Carbidopa, Levodopa) 567
May interact with monoamine oxidase inhibitors, antihypertensives, tricyclic antidepressants, phenothiazines, and butyrophenones. Compounds in these categories include:

Acebutolol Hydrochloride (Potential for symptomatic postural hypotension). Products include:
- Sectral Capsules 2914

Amitriptyline Hydrochloride (Potential for rare adverse reactions, including hypertension and dyskinesia). Products include:
- Elavil 2945
- Etrafon 2495
- Limbitrol 2333
- Triavil Tablets 1800

Amlodipine Besylate (Potential for symptomatic postural hypotension). Products include:
- Lotrel Capsules 858
- Norvasc Tablets 2020

Amoxapine (Potential for rare adverse reactions, including hypertension and dyskinesia). Products include:
- Asendin Tablets 1419

Atenolol (Potential for symptomatic postural hypotension). Products include:
- Tenoretic Tablets 2963
- Tenormin Tablets and I.V. Injection 2965

Benazepril Hydrochloride (Potential for symptomatic postural hypotension). Products include:
- Lotensin Tablets 852
- Lotensin HCT Tablets 855
- Lotrel Capsules 858

Bendroflumethiazide (Potential for symptomatic postural hypotension).
- No products indexed under this heading.

Betaxolol Hydrochloride (Potential for symptomatic postural hypotension). Products include:
- Betoptic Ophthalmic Solution 465
- Betoptic S Ophthalmic Suspension 467
- Kerlone Tablets 2588

Bisoprolol Fumarate (Potential for symptomatic postural hypotension). Products include:
- Zebeta Tablets 1457
- Ziac 1459

Captopril (Potential for symptomatic postural hypotension). Products include:
- Capoten Tablets 740
- Capozide Tablets 744

Carteolol Hydrochloride (Potential for symptomatic postural hypotension). Products include:
- Cartrol Tablets 413
- Ocupress Ophthalmic Solution, 1% Sterile ...... ⊙ 297

Chlorothiazide (Potential for symptomatic postural hypotension). Products include:
- Aldoclor Tablets 1638
- Diupres Tablets 1691
- Diuril Oral 1694

(■□ Described in PDR For Nonprescription Drugs)   (⊙ Described in PDR For Ophthalmology)

79 Interactions Index Atamet

Chlorothiazide Sodium (Potential for symptomatic postural hypotension). Products include:
Diuril Sodium Intravenous ... 1693

Chlorpromazine (Reduces therapeutic effect of levodopa). Products include:
Thorazine Suppositories ... 2701

Chlorpromazine Hydrochloride (Reduces therapeutic effect of levodopa). Products include:
Thorazine ... 2701

Chlorthalidone (Potential for symptomatic postural hypotension). Products include:
Combipres Tablets ... 682
Tenoretic Tablets ... 2963
Thalitone ... 1293

Clomipramine Hydrochloride (Potential for rare adverse reactions, including hypertension and dyskinesia). Products include:
Anafranil Capsules ... 819

Clonidine (Potential for symptomatic postural hypotension). Products include:
Catapres-TTS ... 680

Clonidine Hydrochloride (Potential for symptomatic postural hypotension). Products include:
Catapres Tablets ... 679
Combipres Tablets ... 682

Deserpidine (Potential for symptomatic postural hypotension).
No products indexed under this heading.

Desipramine Hydrochloride (Potential for rare adverse reactions, including hypertension and dyskinesia). Products include:
Norpramin Tablets ... 1273

Diazoxide (Potential for symptomatic postural hypotension). Products include:
Hyperstat I.V. Injection ... 2504
Proglycem ... 575

Diltiazem Hydrochloride (Potential for symptomatic postural hypotension). Products include:
Cardizem CD Capsules ... 1251
Cardizem SR Capsules ... 1255
Cardizem Injectable ... 1253
Cardizem Tablets ... 1257
Dilacor XR Extended-release Capsules ... 2183
Tiazac Capsules ... 1019

Doxazosin Mesylate (Potential for symptomatic postural hypotension). Products include:
Cardura Tablets ... 1993

Doxepin Hydrochloride (Potential for rare adverse reactions, including hypertension and dyskinesia). Products include:
Adapin Capsules ... 1542
Sinequan ... 2028
Zonalon Cream ... 1042

Enalapril Maleate (Potential for symptomatic postural hypotension). Products include:
Vaseretic Tablets ... 1810
Vasotec Tablets ... 1816

Enalaprilat (Potential for symptomatic postural hypotension). Products include:
Vasotec I.V. ... 1814

Esmolol Hydrochloride (Potential for symptomatic postural hypotension). Products include:
Brevibloc (esmolol HCl) Injection ... 1860

Felodipine (Potential for symptomatic postural hypotension). Products include:
Plendil Extended-Release Tablets ... 514

Fluphenazine Decanoate (Reduces therapeutic effect of levodopa). Products include:
Prolixin Decanoate ... 510

Fluphenazine Enanthate (Reduces therapeutic effect of levodopa). Products include:
Prolixin Enanthate ... 510

Fluphenazine Hydrochloride (Reduces therapeutic effect of levodopa). Products include:
Prolixin ... 510

Fosinopril Sodium (Potential for symptomatic postural hypotension). Products include:
Monopril Tablets ... 762

Furazolidone (Concurrent use is contraindicated). Products include:
Furoxone ... 2221

Furosemide (Potential for symptomatic postural hypotension). Products include:
Lasix Injection, Oral Solution and Tablets ... 1267

Guanabenz Acetate (Potential for symptomatic postural hypotension).
No products indexed under this heading.

Guanethidine Monosulfate (Potential for symptomatic postural hypotension). Products include:
Esimil Tablets ... 840
Ismelin Tablets ... 845

Haloperidol (Reduces therapeutic effect of levodopa). Products include:
Haldol Injection, Tablets and Concentrate ... 1585

Haloperidol Decanoate (Reduces therapeutic effect of levodopa). Products include:
Haldol Decanoate ... 1587

Hydralazine Hydrochloride (Potential for symptomatic postural hypotension). Products include:
Apresazide Capsules ... 824
Apresoline Hydrochloride Tablets ... 826
Hydralazine Hydrochloride Injection USP ... 2712
Ser-Ap-Es Tablets ... 867

Hydrochlorothiazide (Potential for symptomatic postural hypotension). Products include:
Aldactazide Tablets ... 2556
Aldoril Tablets ... 1644
Apresazide Capsules ... 824
Capozide Tablets ... 744
Dyazide Capsules ... 2653
Esidrix Tablets ... 839
Esimil Tablets ... 840
HydroDIURIL Tablets ... 1716
Hydropres Tablets ... 1718
Hyzaar Tablets ... 1720
Inderide Tablets ... 2838
Inderide LA Long Acting Capsules ... 2840
Lopressor HCT Tablets ... 850
Lotensin HCT Tablets ... 855
Moduretic Tablets ... 1748
Oretic Tablets ... 450
Prinzide Tablets ... 1780
Ser-Ap-Es Tablets ... 867
Timolide Tablets ... 1791
Vaseretic Tablets ... 1810
Zestoretic Tablets ... 2968
Ziac ... 1459

Hydroflumethiazide (Potential for symptomatic postural hypotension). Products include:
Diucardin Tablets ... 2824

Imipramine Hydrochloride (Potential for rare adverse reactions, including hypertension and dyskinesia). Products include:
Tofranil Ampuls ... 873
Tofranil Tablets ... 875

Imipramine Pamoate (Potential for rare adverse reactions, including hypertension and dyskinesia). Products include:
Tofranil-PM Capsules ... 876

Indapamide (Potential for symptomatic postural hypotension).
No products indexed under this heading.

Isocarboxazid (Concurrent use is contraindicated).
No products indexed under this heading.

Isradipine (Potential for symptomatic postural hypotension). Products include:
DynaCirc Capsules ... 2381
DynaCirc CR Tablets ... 2383

Labetalol Hydrochloride (Potential for symptomatic postural hypotension). Products include:
Normodyne Injection ... 2519
Normodyne Tablets ... 2522
Trandate ... 1158

Lisinopril (Potential for symptomatic postural hypotension). Products include:
Prinivil Tablets ... 1776
Prinzide Tablets ... 1780
Zestoretic Tablets ... 2968
Zestril Tablets ... 2972

Losartan Potassium (Potential for symptomatic postural hypotension). Products include:
Cozaar Tablets ... 1668
Hyzaar Tablets ... 1720

Maprotiline Hydrochloride (Potential for rare adverse reactions, including hypertension and dyskinesia). Products include:
Ludiomil Tablets ... 861

Mecamylamine Hydrochloride (Potential for symptomatic postural hypotension). Products include:
Inversine Tablets ... 1729

Mesoridazine Besylate (Reduces therapeutic effect of levodopa). Products include:
Serentil ... 689

Methotrimeprazine (Reduces therapeutic effect of levodopa). Products include:
Levoprome ... 1321

Methyclothiazide (Potential for symptomatic postural hypotension). Products include:
Enduron Tablets ... 424

Methyldopa (Potential for symptomatic postural hypotension). Products include:
Aldoclor Tablets ... 1638
Aldomet Oral ... 1640
Aldoril Tablets ... 1644

Methyldopate Hydrochloride (Potential for symptomatic postural hypotension). Products include:
Aldomet Ester HCl Injection ... 1642

Metolazone (Potential for symptomatic postural hypotension). Products include:
Mykrox Tablets ... 1617
Zaroxolyn Tablets ... 1625

Metoprolol Succinate (Potential for symptomatic postural hypotension). Products include:
Toprol-XL Tablets ... 560

Metoprolol Tartrate (Potential for symptomatic postural hypotension). Products include:
Lopressor ... 848
Lopressor HCT Tablets ... 850

Metyrosine (Potential for symptomatic postural hypotension). Products include:
Demser Capsules ... 1690

Minoxidil (Potential for symptomatic postural hypotension).
No products indexed under this heading.

Moexipril Hydrochloride (Potential for symptomatic postural hypotension). Products include:
Univasc Tablets ... 2553

Nadolol (Potential for symptomatic postural hypotension).
No products indexed under this heading.

Nicardipine Hydrochloride (Potential for symptomatic postural hypotension). Products include:
Cardene Capsules ... 2261
Cardene I.V. ... 2815
Cardene SR Capsules ... 2264

Nifedipine (Potential for symptomatic postural hypotension). Products include:
Adalat Capsules (10 mg and 20 mg) ... 580
Adalat CC ... 582
Procardia Capsules ... 2024
Procardia XL Extended Release Tablets ... 2026

Nisoldipine (Potential for symptomatic postural hypotension). Products include:
Sular Tablets ... 2961

Nitroglycerin (Potential for symptomatic postural hypotension). Products include:
Deponit NTG Transdermal Delivery System ... 2541
Nitro-Bid IV ... 1270
Nitro-Bid Ointment ... 1272
Nitro-Dur (nitroglycerin) Transdermal Infusion System ... 1365
Nitrolingual Spray ... 2193
Nitrostat Tablets ... 1981
Transderm-Nitro Transdermal Therapeutic System ... 878

Nortriptyline Hydrochloride (Potential for rare adverse reactions, including hypertension and dyskinesia). Products include:
Pamelor ... 2409

Papaverine Hydrochloride (Beneficial effects of levodopa reversed in Parkinson's disease). Products include:
Papaverine Hydrochloride Vials and Ampoules ... 1523

Penbutolol Sulfate (Potential for symptomatic postural hypotension). Products include:
Levatol Tablets ... 2547

Perphenazine (Reduces therapeutic effect of levodopa). Products include:
Etrafon ... 2495
Triavil Tablets ... 1800
Trilafon ... 2532

Phenelzine Sulfate (Concurrent use is contraindicated). Products include:
Nardil ... 1977

Phenoxybenzamine Hydrochloride (Potential for symptomatic postural hypotension). Products include:
Dibenzyline Capsules ... 2650

Phentolamine Mesylate (Potential for symptomatic postural hypotension). Products include:
Regitine Vials ... 864

Phenytoin (Beneficial effects of levodopa reversed in Parkinson's disease). Products include:
Dilantin Infatabs ... 1967
Dilantin-125 Suspension ... 1969

Phenytoin Sodium (Beneficial effects of levodopa reversed in Parkinson's disease). Products include:
Dilantin Kapseals ... 1965

Pindolol (Potential for symptomatic postural hypotension). Products include:
Visken Tablets ... 2428

Polythiazide (Potential for symptomatic postural hypotension). Products include:
Minizide Capsules ... 2016

Prazosin Hydrochloride (Potential for symptomatic postural hypotension). Products include:
Minipress Capsules ... 2015
Minizide Capsules ... 2016

IMPORTANT NOTE: Always consult each drug listing in the patient's regimen for possible interactions.

Atamet

Prochlorperazine (Reduces therapeutic effect of levodopa). Products include:
- Compazine 2644

Promethazine Hydrochloride (Reduces therapeutic effect of levodopa). Products include:
- Mepergan Injection 2859
- Phenergan with Codeine 2883
- Phenergan with Dextromethorphan 2885
- Phenergan Injection 2880
- Phenergan Suppositories 2882
- Phenergan Syrup 2881
- Phenergan Tablets 2882
- Phenergan VC 2886
- Phenergan VC with Codeine ... 2888

Propranolol Hydrochloride (Potential for symptomatic postural hypotension). Products include:
- Inderal 2834
- Inderal LA Long Acting Capsules ... 2836
- Inderide Tablets 2838
- Inderide LA Long Acting Capsules .. 2840

Protriptyline Hydrochloride (Potential for rare adverse reactions, including hypertension and dyskinesia). Products include:
- Vivactil Tablets 1820

Quinapril Hydrochloride (Potential for symptomatic postural hypotension). Products include:
- Accupril Tablets 1950

Ramipril (Potential for symptomatic postural hypotension). Products include:
- Altace Capsules 1238

Rauwolfia Serpentina (Potential for symptomatic postural hypotension).
- No products indexed under this heading.

Rescinnamine (Potential for symptomatic postural hypotension).
- No products indexed under this heading.

Reserpine (Potential for symptomatic postural hypotension). Products include:
- Diupres Tablets 1691
- Hydropres Tablets 1718
- Ser-Ap-Es Tablets 867

Sodium Nitroprusside (Potential for symptomatic postural hypotension).
- No products indexed under this heading.

Sotalol Hydrochloride (Potential for symptomatic postural hypotension). Products include:
- Betapace Tablets 637

Spirapril Hydrochloride (Potential for symptomatic postural hypotension).
- No products indexed under this heading.

Terazosin Hydrochloride (Potential for symptomatic postural hypotension). Products include:
- Hytrin Capsules 434

Thioridazine Hydrochloride (Reduces therapeutic effect of levodopa). Products include:
- Mellaril 2398

Timolol Maleate (Potential for symptomatic postural hypotension). Products include:
- Blocadren Tablets 1654
- Timolide Tablets 1791
- Timoptic in Ocudose 1796
- Timoptic Sterile Ophthalmic Solution 1794
- Timoptic-XE 1798

Torsemide (Potential for symptomatic postural hypotension). Products include:
- Demadex Tablets and Injection ... 691

Tranylcypromine Sulfate (Concurrent use is contraindicated). Products include:
- Parnate Tablets 2679

Trifluoperazine Hydrochloride (Reduces therapeutic effect of levodopa). Products include:
- Stelazine 2692

Trimethaphan Camsylate (Potential for symptomatic postural hypotension).
- No products indexed under this heading.

Trimipramine Maleate (Potential for rare adverse reactions, including hypertension and dyskinesia). Products include:
- Surmontil Capsules 2917

Verapamil Hydrochloride (Potential for symptomatic postural hypotension). Products include:
- Calan SR Caplets 2571
- Calan Tablets 2568
- Covera-HS Tablets 2573
- Isoptin Injectable 1391
- Isoptin Oral Tablets 1393
- Isoptin SR Tablets 1395
- Verelan Capsules 1455

Food Interactions

Diet high in protein (Levodopa competes with certain amino acids, the absorption of levodopa may be impaired in some patients on a high protein diet).

ATARAX TABLETS & SYRUP

(Hydroxyzine Hydrochloride) 1992
May interact with narcotic analgesics, barbiturates, central nervous system depressants, and certain other agents. Compounds in these categories include:

Alfentanil Hydrochloride (The potentiating action of hydroxyzine must be considered when it is used concurrently). Products include:
- Alfenta Injection 1334

Alprazolam (The potentiating action of hydroxyzine must be considered when it is used concurrently). Products include:
- Xanax Tablets 2115

Aprobarbital (The potentiating action of hydroxyzine must be considered when it is used concurrently).
- No products indexed under this heading.

Buprenorphine (The potentiating action of hydroxyzine must be considered when it is used concurrently). Products include:
- Buprenex Injectable 2170

Buspirone Hydrochloride (The potentiating action of hydroxyzine must be considered when it is used concurrently). Products include:
- BuSpar Tablets 738

Butabarbital (The potentiating action of hydroxyzine must be considered when it is used concurrently).
- No products indexed under this heading.

Butalbital (The potentiating action of hydroxyzine must be considered when it is used concurrently). Products include:
- Axocet Capsules 2469
- Esgic-plus Capsules 1012
- Esgic-plus Tablets 1012
- Fioricet Tablets 2386
- Fioricet with Codeine Capsules ... 2387
- Fiorinal Capsules 2388
- Fiorinal with Codeine Capsules ... 2390
- Fiorinal Tablets 2388
- Phrenilin 790
- Sedapap Tablets 50 mg/650 mg .. 1826

Chlordiazepoxide (The potentiating action of hydroxyzine must be considered when it is used concurrently). Products include:
- Limbitrol 2333

Chlordiazepoxide Hydrochloride (The potentiating action of hydroxyzine must be considered when it is used concurrently). Products include:
- Librax Capsules 2330
- Librium Capsules 2331
- Librium Injectable 2332

Chlorpromazine (The potentiating action of hydroxyzine must be considered when it is used concurrently). Products include:
- Thorazine Suppositories 2701

Chlorpromazine Hydrochloride (The potentiating action of hydroxyzine must be considered when it is used concurrently). Products include:
- Thorazine 2701

Chlorprothixene (The potentiating action of hydroxyzine must be considered when it is used concurrently).
- No products indexed under this heading.

Chlorprothixene Hydrochloride (The potentiating action of hydroxyzine must be considered when it is used concurrently).
- No products indexed under this heading.

Chlorprothixene Lactate (The potentiating action of hydroxyzine must be considered when it is used concurrently).
- No products indexed under this heading.

Clorazepate Dipotassium (The potentiating action of hydroxyzine must be considered when it is used concurrently). Products include:
- Tranxene 459

Clozapine (The potentiating action of hydroxyzine must be considered when it is used concurrently). Products include:
- Clozaril Tablets 2377

Codeine Phosphate (The potentiating action of hydroxyzine must be considered when it is used concurrently). Products include:
- Brontex 2130
- Dimetane-DC Cough Syrup 2232
- Fioricet with Codeine Capsules ... 2387
- Fiorinal with Codeine Capsules ... 2390
- Nucofed 2225
- Phenergan with Codeine 2883
- Phenergan VC with Codeine ... 2888
- Robitussin A-C Syrup 2248
- Robitussin-DAC Syrup 2249
- Ryna .... ◆□ 804
- Soma Compound w/Codeine Tablets 2784
- Tylenol with Codeine 1592

Desflurane (The potentiating action of hydroxyzine must be considered when it is used concurrently). Products include:
- Suprane (desflurane, USP) 1865

Dezocine (The potentiating action of hydroxyzine must be considered when it is used concurrently). Products include:
- Dalgan Injection 529

Diazepam (The potentiating action of hydroxyzine must be considered when it is used concurrently). Products include:
- Dizac (diazepam injectable emulsion) CIV 1862
- Valium Injectable 2336
- Valium Tablets 2335

Droperidol (The potentiating action of hydroxyzine must be considered when it is used concurrently). Products include:
- Inapsine Injection 462

Enflurane (The potentiating action of hydroxyzine must be considered when it is used concurrently).
- No products indexed under this heading.

Estazolam (The potentiating action of hydroxyzine must be considered when it is used concurrently). Products include:
- ProSom Tablets 457

Ethchlorvynol (The potentiating action of hydroxyzine must be considered when it is used concurrently). Products include:
- Placidyl Capsules 456

Ethinamate (The potentiating action of hydroxyzine must be considered when it is used concurrently).
- No products indexed under this heading.

Fentanyl (The potentiating action of hydroxyzine must be considered when it is used concurrently). Products include:
- Duragesic Transdermal System 1336

Fentanyl Citrate (The potentiating action of hydroxyzine must be considered when it is used concurrently). Products include:
- Sublimaze Injection 463

Fluphenazine Decanoate (The potentiating action of hydroxyzine must be considered when it is used concurrently). Products include:
- Prolixin Decanoate 510

Fluphenazine Enanthate (The potentiating action of hydroxyzine must be considered when it is used concurrently). Products include:
- Prolixin Enanthate 510

Fluphenazine Hydrochloride (The potentiating action of hydroxyzine must be considered when it is used concurrently). Products include:
- Prolixin 510

Flurazepam Hydrochloride (The potentiating action of hydroxyzine must be considered when it is used concurrently). Products include:
- Dalmane Capsules 2329

Glutethimide (The potentiating action of hydroxyzine must be considered when it is used concurrently).
- No products indexed under this heading.

Haloperidol (The potentiating action of hydroxyzine must be considered when it is used concurrently). Products include:
- Haldol Injection, Tablets and Concentrate 1585

Haloperidol Decanoate (The potentiating action of hydroxyzine must be considered when it is used concurrently). Products include:
- Haldol Decanoate 1587

Hydrocodone Bitartrate (The potentiating action of hydroxyzine must be considered when it is used concurrently). Products include:
- Codiclear DH Syrup 808
- Duratuss HD Elixir 2750
- Histussin D Liquid 670
- Hycodan Tablets and Syrup ... 946
- Hycomine Compound Tablets ... 948
- Hycomine 947
- Hycotuss Expectorant Syrup .. 950
- Hydrocet Capsules 787
- Lorcet 10/650 Tablets 1016
- Lortab 2751
- Tussend 1830
- Tussend Expectorant 1831

(◆□ Described in PDR For Nonprescription Drugs) (◉ Described in PDR For Ophthalmology)

Vicodin Tablets 1404
Vicodin ES Tablets 1405
Vicodin HP Tablets 1403
Vicodin Tuss Expectorant 1406
Zydone Capsules 967

Hydrocodone Polistirex (The potentiating action of hydroxyzine must be considered when it is used concurrently). Products include:
Tussionex Pennkinetic Extended-Release Suspension 1624

Hydromorphone Hydrochloride (The potentiating action of hydroxyzine must be considered when it is used concurrently). Products include:
Dilaudid Ampules 1382
Dilaudid Cough Syrup 1383
Dilaudid-HP Injection 1384
Dilaudid-HP Lyophilized Powder 250 mg 1384
Dilaudid 1382
Dilaudid Oral Liquid 1386
Dilaudid 1382
Dilaudid Tablets - 8 mg 1386

Isoflurane (The potentiating action of hydroxyzine must be considered when it is used concurrently).
No products indexed under this heading.

Ketamine Hydrochloride (The potentiating action of hydroxyzine must be considered when it is used concurrently).
No products indexed under this heading.

Levomethadyl Acetate Hydrochloride (The potentiating action of hydroxyzine must be considered when it is used concurrently). Products include:
Orlaam Oral Solution 2361

Levorphanol Tartrate (The potentiating action of hydroxyzine must be considered when it is used concurrently). Products include:
Levo-Dromoran 2297

Lorazepam (The potentiating action of hydroxyzine must be considered when it is used concurrently). Products include:
Ativan Injection 2805
Ativan Tablets 2807

Loxapine Hydrochloride (The potentiating action of hydroxyzine must be considered when it is used concurrently). Products include:
Loxitane 1426

Loxapine Succinate (The potentiating action of hydroxyzine must be considered when it is used concurrently). Products include:
Loxitane Capsules 1426

Meperidine Hydrochloride (The potentiating action of hydroxyzine must be considered when it is used concurrently). Products include:
Demerol 2438
Mepergan Injection 2859

Mephobarbital (The potentiating action of hydroxyzine must be considered when it is used concurrently). Products include:
Mebaral Tablets 2452

Meprobamate (The potentiating action of hydroxyzine must be considered when it is used concurrently). Products include:
Miltown Tablets 2780
PMB 200 and PMB 400 2890

Mesoridazine Besylate (The potentiating action of hydroxyzine must be considered when it is used concurrently). Products include:
Serentil 689

Methadone Hydrochloride (The potentiating action of hydroxyzine must be considered when it is used concurrently). Products include:
Methadone Hydrochloride Oral Concentrate 2356
Methadone Hydrochloride Oral Solution & Tablets 2357

Methohexital Sodium (The potentiating action of hydroxyzine must be considered when it is used concurrently).
No products indexed under this heading.

Methotrimeprazine (The potentiating action of hydroxyzine must be considered when it is used concurrently). Products include:
Levoprome 1321

Methoxyflurane (The potentiating action of hydroxyzine must be considered when it is used concurrently).
No products indexed under this heading.

Midazolam Hydrochloride (The potentiating action of hydroxyzine must be considered when it is used concurrently). Products include:
Versed Injection 2324

Molindone Hydrochloride (The potentiating action of hydroxyzine must be considered when it is used concurrently). Products include:
Moban Tablets and Concentrate 1036

Morphine Sulfate (The potentiating action of hydroxyzine must be considered when it is used concurrently). Products include:
Astramorph/PF Injection, USP (Preservative-Free) 526
Duramorph Injection 983
Infumorph 200 and Infumorph 500 Sterile Solutions 985
Kadian Capsules 2948
MS Contin Tablets 2149
MSIR 2152
Oramorph SR (Morphine Sulfate Sustained Release Tablets) 2359
RMS Suppositories CII 2766
Roxanol 2365

Non-narcotic Analgesics, unspecified (Potentiated action of non-narcotic analgesics).

Opium Alkaloids (The potentiating action of hydroxyzine must be considered when it is used concurrently).
No products indexed under this heading.

Oxazepam (The potentiating action of hydroxyzine must be considered when it is used concurrently). Products include:
Serax Capsules 2916
Serax Tablets 2916

Oxycodone Hydrochloride (The potentiating action of hydroxyzine must be considered when it is used concurrently). Products include:
OxyContin Tablets 2163
OxyIR Capsules 2167
Percocet Tablets 955
Percodan Tablets 955
Percodan-Demi Tablets 956
Roxicodone Tablets, Oral Solution & Intensol (Oxycodone) 2366
Tylox Capsules 1593

Pentobarbital Sodium (The potentiating action of hydroxyzine must be considered when it is used concurrently). Products include:
Nembutal Sodium Capsules 440
Nembutal Sodium Solution 442
Nembutal Sodium Suppositories 444

Perphenazine (The potentiating action of hydroxyzine must be considered when it is used concurrently). Products include:
Etrafon 2495

Triavil Tablets 1800
Trilafon 2532

Phenobarbital (The potentiating action of hydroxyzine must be considered when it is used concurrently). Products include:
Arco-Lase Plus Tablets 513
Bellergal-S Tablets 2375
Donnatal 2234
Donnatal Extentabs 2234
Donnatal Tablets 2234
Phenobarbital Elixir and Tablets 1523
Quadrinal Tablets 1398

Prazepam (The potentiating action of hydroxyzine must be considered when it is used concurrently).
No products indexed under this heading.

Prochlorperazine (The potentiating action of hydroxyzine must be considered when it is used concurrently). Products include:
Compazine 2644

Promethazine Hydrochloride (The potentiating action of hydroxyzine must be considered when it is used concurrently). Products include:
Mepergan Injection 2859
Phenergan with Codeine 2883
Phenergan with Dextromethorphan 2885
Phenergan Injection 2880
Phenergan Suppositories 2882
Phenergan Syrup 2881
Phenergan Tablets 2882
Phenergan VC 2886
Phenergan VC with Codeine 2888

Propofol (The potentiating action of hydroxyzine must be considered when it is used concurrently). Products include:
Diprivan Injectable Emulsion 2939

Propoxyphene Hydrochloride (The potentiating action of hydroxyzine must be considered when it is used concurrently). Products include:
Darvon 1475
Wygesic Tablets 2930

Propoxyphene Napsylate (The potentiating action of hydroxyzine must be considered when it is used concurrently). Products include:
Darvon-N/Darvocet-N 1473

Quazepam (The potentiating action of hydroxyzine must be considered when it is used concurrently). Products include:
Doral Tablets 2773

Risperidone (The potentiating action of hydroxyzine must be considered when it is used concurrently). Products include:
Risperdal Tablets 1348

Secobarbital Sodium (The potentiating action of hydroxyzine must be considered when it is used concurrently). Products include:
Seconal Sodium Pulvules 1529

Sevoflurane (The potentiating action of hydroxyzine must be considered when it is used concurrently).
No products indexed under this heading.

Sufentanil Citrate (The potentiating action of hydroxyzine must be considered when it is used concurrently). Products include:
Sufenta Injection 1355

Temazepam (The potentiating action of hydroxyzine must be considered when it is used concurrently). Products include:
Restoril Capsules 2413

Thiamylal Sodium (The potentiating action of hydroxyzine must be considered when it is used concurrently).
No products indexed under this heading.

Thioridazine Hydrochloride (The potentiating action of hydroxyzine must be considered when it is used concurrently). Products include:
Mellaril 2398

Thiothixene (The potentiating action of hydroxyzine must be considered when it is used concurrently). Products include:
Navane Capsules and Concentrate 2018
Navane Intramuscular 2019

Triazolam (The potentiating action of hydroxyzine must be considered when it is used concurrently). Products include:
Halcion Tablets 2093

Trifluoperazine Hydrochloride (The potentiating action of hydroxyzine must be considered when it is used concurrently). Products include:
Stelazine 2692

Zolpidem Tartrate (The potentiating action of hydroxyzine must be considered when it is used concurrently). Products include:
Ambien Tablets 2559

Food Interactions
Alcohol (Increased effect of alcohol).

ATIVAN INJECTION
(Lorazepam) 2805
May interact with phenothiazines, barbiturates, monoamine oxidase inhibitors, narcotic analgesics, central nervous system depressants, and certain other agents. Compounds in these categories include:

Alfentanil Hydrochloride (Additive CNS depressant effects). Products include:
Alfenta Injection 1334

Alprazolam (Additive CNS depressant effects). Products include:
Xanax Tablets 2115

Aprobarbital (Additive CNS depressant effects).
No products indexed under this heading.

Buprenorphine (Additive CNS depressant effects). Products include:
Buprenex Injectable 2170

Buspirone Hydrochloride (Additive CNS depressant effects). Products include:
BuSpar Tablets 738

Butabarbital (Additive CNS depressant effects).
No products indexed under this heading.

Butalbital (Additive CNS depressant effects). Products include:
Axocet Capsules 2469
Esgic-plus Capsules 1012
Esgic-plus Tablets 1012
Fioricet Tablets 2386
Fioricet with Codeine Capsules 2387
Fiorinal Capsules 2388
Fiorinal with Codeine Capsules 2390
Fiorinal Tablets 2388
Phrenilin 790
Sedapap Tablets 50 mg/650 mg .. 1826

Chlordiazepoxide (Additive CNS depressant effects). Products include:
Limbitrol 2333

Chlordiazepoxide Hydrochloride (Additive CNS depressant effects). Products include:
Librax Capsules 2330

IMPORTANT NOTE: Always consult each drug listing in the patient's regimen for possible interactions.

Ativan Injection **Interactions Index** **82**

Librium Capsules 2331
Librium Injectable 2332

Chlorpromazine (Additive CNS depressant effects). Products include:
Thorazine Suppositories 2701

Chlorprothixene (Additive CNS depressant effects).
No products indexed under this heading.

Chlorprothixene Hydrochloride (Additive CNS depressant effects).
No products indexed under this heading.

Chlorprothixene Lactate (Additive CNS depressant effects).
No products indexed under this heading.

Clorazepate Dipotassium (Additive CNS depressant effects). Products include:
Tranxene 459

Clozapine (Additive CNS depressant effects). Products include:
Clozaril Tablets 2377

Codeine Phosphate (Additive CNS depressant effects). Products include:
Brontex 2130
Dimetane-DC Cough Syrup 2232
Fioricet with Codeine Capsules 2387
Fiorinal with Codeine Capsules 2390
Nucofed 2225
Phenergan with Codeine 2883
Phenergan VC with Codeine 2888
Robitussin A-C Syrup 2248
Robitussin-DAC Syrup 2249
Ryna ▣ 804
Soma Compound w/Codeine Tablets 2784
Tylenol with Codeine 1592

Desflurane (Additive CNS depressant effects). Products include:
Suprane (desflurane, USP) 1865

Dezocine (Additive CNS depressant effects). Products include:
Dalgan Injection 529

Diazepam (Additive CNS depressant effects). Products include:
Dizac (diazepam injectable emulsion) CIV 1862
Valium Injectable 2336
Valium Tablets 2335

Droperidol (Additive CNS depressant effects). Products include:
Inapsine Injection 462

Enflurane (Additive CNS depressant effects).
No products indexed under this heading.

Estazolam (Additive CNS depressant effects). Products include:
ProSom Tablets 457

Ethchlorvynol (Additive CNS depressant effects). Products include:
Placidyl Capsules 456

Ethinamate (Additive CNS depressant effects).
No products indexed under this heading.

Fentanyl (Additive CNS depressant effects). Products include:
Duragesic Transdermal System 1336

Fentanyl Citrate (Additive CNS depressant effects). Products include:
Sublimaze Injection 463

Fluphenazine Decanoate (Additive CNS depressant effects). Products include:
Prolixin Decanoate 510

Fluphenazine Enanthate (Additive CNS depressant effects). Products include:
Prolixin Enanthate 510

Fluphenazine Hydrochloride (Additive CNS depressant effects). Products include:
Prolixin 510

Flurazepam Hydrochloride (Additive CNS depressant effects). Products include:
Dalmane Capsules 2329

Furazolidone (Additive CNS depressant effects). Products include:
Furoxone 2221

Glutethimide (Additive CNS depressant effects).
No products indexed under this heading.

Haloperidol (Additive CNS depressant effects). Products include:
Haldol Injection, Tablets and Concentrate 1585

Haloperidol Decanoate (Additive CNS depressant effects). Products include:
Haldol Decanoate 1587

Hydrocodone Bitartrate (Additive CNS depressant effects). Products include:
Codiclear DH Syrup 808
Duratuss HD Elixir 2750
Histussin D Liquid 670
Hycodan Tablets and Syrup 946
Hycomine Compound Tablets 948
Hycomine 947
Hycotuss Expectorant Syrup 950
Hydrocet Capsules 787
Lorcet 10/650 Tablets 1016
Lortab 2751
Tussend 1830
Tussend Expectorant 1831
Vicodin Tablets 1404
Vicodin ES Tablets 1405
Vicodin HP Tablets 1403
Vicodin Tuss Expectorant 1406
Zydone Capsules 967

Hydrocodone Polistirex (Additive CNS depressant effects). Products include:
Tussionex Pennkinetic Extended-Release Suspension 1624

Hydromorphone Hydrochloride (Additive CNS depressant effects). Products include:
Dilaudid Ampules 1382
Dilaudid Cough Syrup 1383
Dilaudid-HP Injection 1384
Dilaudid-HP Lyophilized Powder 250 mg 1384
Dilaudid 1382
Dilaudid Oral Liquid 1386
Dilaudid 1382
Dilaudid Tablets - 8 mg 1386

Hydroxyzine Hydrochloride (Additive CNS depressant effects). Products include:
Atarax Tablets & Syrup 1992
Marax Tablets & DF Syrup 2015
Vistaril Intramuscular Solution 2042

Isocarboxazid (Additive CNS depressant effects).
No products indexed under this heading.

Isoflurane (Additive CNS depressant effects).
No products indexed under this heading.

Ketamine Hydrochloride (Additive CNS depressant effects).
No products indexed under this heading.

Levomethadyl Acetate Hydrochloride (Additive CNS depressant effects). Products include:
Orlaam Oral Solution 2361

Levorphanol Tartrate (Additive CNS depressant effects). Products include:
Levo-Dromoran 2297

Loxapine Hydrochloride (Additive CNS depressant effects). Products include:
Loxitane 1426

Loxapine Succinate (Additive CNS depressant effects). Products include:
Loxitane Capsules 1426

Meperidine Hydrochloride (Additive CNS depressant effects). Products include:
Demerol 2438
Mepergan Injection 2859

Mephobarbital (Additive CNS depressant effects). Products include:
Mebaral Tablets 2452

Meprobamate (Additive CNS depressant effects). Products include:
Miltown Tablets 2780
PMB 200 and PMB 400 2890

Mesoridazine Besylate (Additive CNS depressant effects). Products include:
Serentil 689

Methadone Hydrochloride (Additive CNS depressant effects). Products include:
Methadone Hydrochloride Oral Concentrate 2356
Methadone Hydrochloride Oral Solution & Tablets 2357

Methohexital Sodium (Additive CNS depressant effects).
No products indexed under this heading.

Methotrimeprazine (Additive CNS depressant effects). Products include:
Levoprome 1321

Methoxyflurane (Additive CNS depressant effects).
No products indexed under this heading.

Midazolam Hydrochloride (Additive CNS depressant effects). Products include:
Versed Injection 2324

Molindone Hydrochloride (Additive CNS depressant effects). Products include:
Moban Tablets and Concentrate 1036

Morphine Sulfate (Additive CNS depressant effects). Products include:
Astramorph/PF Injection, USP (Preservative-Free) 526
Duramorph Injection 983
Infumorph 200 and Infumorph 500 Sterile Solutions 985
Kadian Capsules 2948
MS Contin Tablets 2149
MSIR 2152
Oramorph SR (Morphine Sulfate Sustained Release Tablets) 2359
RMS Suppositories CII 2766
Roxanol 2365

Opium Alkaloids (Additive CNS depressant effects).
No products indexed under this heading.

Oxazepam (Additive CNS depressant effects). Products include:
Serax Capsules 2916
Serax Tablets 2916

Oxycodone Hydrochloride (Additive CNS depressant effects). Products include:
OxyContin Tablets 2163
OxyIR Capsules 2167
Percocet Tablets 955
Percodan Tablets 955
Percodan-Demi Tablets 956
Roxicodone Tablets, Oral Solution & Intensol (Oxycodone) 2366
Tylox Capsules 1593

Pentobarbital Sodium (Additive CNS depressant effects). Products include:
Nembutal Sodium Capsules 440
Nembutal Sodium Solution 442
Nembutal Sodium Suppositories 444

Perphenazine (Additive CNS depressant effects). Products include:
Etrafon 2495
Triavil Tablets 1800
Trilafon 2532

Phenelzine Sulfate (Additive CNS depressant effects). Products include:
Nardil 1977

Phenobarbital (Additive CNS depressant effects). Products include:
Arco-Lase Plus Tablets 513
Bellergal-S Tablets 2375
Donnatal 2234
Donnatal Extentabs 2234
Donnatal Tablets 2234
Phenobarbital Elixir and Tablets 1523
Quadrinal Tablets 1398

Prazepam (Additive CNS depressant effects).
No products indexed under this heading.

Prochlorperazine (Additive CNS depressant effects). Products include:
Compazine 2644

Promethazine Hydrochloride (Additive CNS depressant effects). Products include:
Mepergan Injection 2859
Phenergan with Codeine 2883
Phenergan with Dextromethorphan 2885
Phenergan Injection 2880
Phenergan Suppositories 2882
Phenergan Syrup 2881
Phenergan Tablets 2882
Phenergan VC 2886
Phenergan VC with Codeine 2888

Propofol (Additive CNS depressant effects). Products include:
Diprivan Injectable Emulsion 2939

Propoxyphene Hydrochloride (Additive CNS depressant effects). Products include:
Darvon 1475
Wygesic Tablets 2930

Propoxyphene Napsylate (Additive CNS depressant effects). Products include:
Darvon-N/Darvocet-N 1473

Quazepam (Additive CNS depressant effects). Products include:
Doral Tablets 2773

Risperidone (Additive CNS depressant effects). Products include:
Risperdal Tablets 1348

Scopolamine (Increased incidence of sedation, hallucinations, and irrational behavior). Products include:
Transderm Scōp Transdermal Therapeutic System 890

Scopolamine Hydrobromide (Increased incidence of sedation, hallucinations, and irrational behavior). Products include:
Atrohist Plus Tablets 1605
Donnatal 2234
Donnatal Extentabs 2234
Donnatal Tablets 2234

Secobarbital Sodium (Additive CNS depressant effects). Products include:
Seconal Sodium Pulvules 1529

Selegiline Hydrochloride (Additive CNS depressant effects). Products include:
Eldepryl Capsules 2729

Sevoflurane (Additive CNS depressant effects).
No products indexed under this heading.

Sufentanil Citrate (Additive CNS depressant effects). Products include:
Sufenta Injection 1355

Temazepam (Additive CNS depressant effects). Products include:
Restoril Capsules 2413

Thiamylal Sodium (Additive CNS depressant effects).
No products indexed under this heading.

(▣ Described in PDR For Nonprescription Drugs) (◉ Described in PDR For Ophthalmology)

Thioridazine Hydrochloride (Additive CNS depressant effects). Products include:
Mellaril 2398
Thiothixene (Additive CNS depressant effects). Products include:
Navane Capsules and Concentrate 2018
Navane Intramuscular 2019
Tranylcypromine Sulfate (Additive CNS depressant effects). Products include:
Parnate Tablets 2679
Triazolam (Additive CNS depressant effects). Products include:
Halcion Tablets 2093
Trifluoperazine Hydrochloride (Additive CNS depressant effects). Products include:
Stelazine 2692
Zolpidem Tartrate (Additive CNS depressant effects). Products include:
Ambien Tablets 2559

Food Interactions
Alcohol (Additive CNS depressant effects).

ATIVAN TABLETS
(Lorazepam) 2807
May interact with barbiturates, central nervous system depressants, and certain other agents. Compounds in these categories include:

Alfentanil Hydrochloride (Diminished tolerance for other CNSD when used concurrently). Products include:
Alfenta Injection 1334
Alprazolam (Diminished tolerance for other CNSD when used concurrently). Products include:
Xanax Tablets 2115
Aprobarbital (Diminished tolerance for other CNSD when used concurrently; potential for increased CNS-depressant effects).
No products indexed under this heading.
Buprenorphine (Diminished tolerance for other CNSD when used concurrently). Products include:
Buprenex Injectable 2170
Buspirone Hydrochloride (Diminished tolerance for other CNSD when used concurrently). Products include:
BuSpar Tablets 738
Butabarbital (Diminished tolerance for other CNSD when used concurrently; potential for increased CNS-depressant effects).
No products indexed under this heading.
Butalbital (Diminished tolerance for other CNSD when used concurrently; potential for increased CNS-depressant effects). Products include:
Axocet Capsules 2469
Esgic-plus Capsules 1012
Esgic-plus Tablets 1012
Fioricet Tablets 2386
Fioricet with Codeine Capsules ... 2387
Fiorinal Capsules 2388
Fiorinal with Codeine Capsules ... 2390
Fiorinal Tablets 2388
Phrenilin 790
Sedapap Tablets 50 mg/650 mg .. 1826
Chlordiazepoxide (Diminished tolerance for other CNSD when used concurrently). Products include:
Limbitrol 2333
Chlordiazepoxide Hydrochloride (Diminished tolerance for other CNSD when used concurrently). Products include:
Librax Capsules 2330
Librium Capsules 2331
Librium Injectable 2332
Chlorpromazine (Diminished tolerance for other CNSD when used concurrently). Products include:
Thorazine Suppositories 2701
Chlorpromazine Hydrochloride (Diminished tolerance for other CNSD when used concurrently). Products include:
Thorazine 2701
Chlorprothixene (Diminished tolerance for other CNSD when used concurrently).
No products indexed under this heading.
Chlorprothixene Hydrochloride (Diminished tolerance for other CNSD when used concurrently).
No products indexed under this heading.
Chlorprothixene Lactate (Diminished tolerance for other CNSD when used concurrently).
No products indexed under this heading.
Clorazepate Dipotassium (Diminished tolerance for other CNSD when used concurrently). Products include:
Tranxene 459
Clozapine (Diminished tolerance for other CNSD when used concurrently). Products include:
Clozaril Tablets 2377
Codeine Phosphate (Diminished tolerance for other CNSD when used concurrently). Products include:
Brontex 2130
Dimetane-DC Cough Syrup 2232
Fioricet with Codeine Capsules ... 2387
Fiorinal with Codeine Capsules ... 2390
Nucofed 2225
Phenergan with Codeine 2883
Phenergan VC with Codeine 2888
Robitussin A-C Syrup 2248
Robitussin-DAC Syrup 2249
Ryna 804
Soma Compound w/Codeine Tablets 2784
Tylenol with Codeine 1592
Desflurane (Diminished tolerance for other CNSD when used concurrently). Products include:
Suprane (desflurane, USP) 1865
Dezocine (Diminished tolerance for other CNSD when used concurrently). Products include:
Dalgan Injection 529
Diazepam (Diminished tolerance for other CNSD when used concurrently). Products include:
Dizac (diazepam injectable emulsion) CIV 1862
Valium Injectable 2336
Valium Tablets 2335
Droperidol (Diminished tolerance for other CNSD when used concurrently). Products include:
Inapsine Injection 462
Enflurane (Diminished tolerance for other CNSD when used concurrently).
No products indexed under this heading.
Estazolam (Diminished tolerance for other CNSD when used concurrently). Products include:
ProSom Tablets 457
Ethchlorvynol (Diminished tolerance for other CNSD when used concurrently). Products include:
Placidyl Capsules 456
Ethinamate (Diminished tolerance for other CNSD when used concurrently).
No products indexed under this heading.
Fentanyl (Diminished tolerance for other CNSD when used concurrently). Products include:
Duragesic Transdermal System 1336
Fentanyl Citrate (Diminished tolerance for other CNSD when used concurrently). Products include:
Sublimaze Injection 463
Fluphenazine Decanoate (Diminished tolerance for other CNSD when used concurrently). Products include:
Prolixin Decanoate 510
Fluphenazine Enanthate (Diminished tolerance for other CNSD when used concurrently). Products include:
Prolixin Enanthate 510
Fluphenazine Hydrochloride (Diminished tolerance for other CNSD when used concurrently). Products include:
Prolixin 510
Flurazepam Hydrochloride (Diminished tolerance for other CNSD when used concurrently). Products include:
Dalmane Capsules 2329
Glutethimide (Diminished tolerance for other CNSD when used concurrently).
No products indexed under this heading.
Haloperidol (Diminished tolerance for other CNSD when used concurrently). Products include:
Haldol Injection, Tablets and Concentrate 1585
Haloperidol Decanoate (Diminished tolerance for other CNSD when used concurrently). Products include:
Haldol Decanoate 1587
Hydrocodone Bitartrate (Diminished tolerance for other CNSD when used concurrently). Products include:
Codiclear DH Syrup 808
Duratuss HD Elixir 2750
Histussin D Liquid 670
Hycodan Tablets and Syrup 946
Hycomine Compound Tablets 948
Hycomine 947
Hycotuss Expectorant Syrup 950
Hydrocet Capsules 787
Lorcet 10/650 Tablets 1016
Lortab 2751
Tussend 1830
Tussend Expectorant 1831
Vicodin Tablets 1404
Vicodin ES Tablets 1405
Vicodin HP Tablets 1403
Vicodin Tuss Expectorant 1406
Zydone Capsules 967
Hydrocodone Polistirex (Diminished tolerance for other CNSD when used concurrently). Products include:
Tussionex Pennkinetic Extended-Release Suspension 1624
Hydroxyzine Hydrochloride (Diminished tolerance for other CNSD when used concurrently). Products include:
Atarax Tablets & Syrup 1992
Marax Tablets & DF Syrup 2015
Vistaril Intramuscular Solution 2042
Isoflurane (Diminished tolerance for other CNSD when used concurrently).
No products indexed under this heading.
Ketamine Hydrochloride (Diminished tolerance for other CNSD when used concurrently).
No products indexed under this heading.
Levomethadyl Acetate Hydrochloride (Diminished tolerance for other CNSD when used concurrently). Products include:
Orlaam Oral Solution 2361
Levorphanol Tartrate (Diminished tolerance for other CNSD when used concurrently). Products include:
Levo-Dromoran 2297
Loxapine Hydrochloride (Diminished tolerance for other CNSD when used concurrently). Products include:
Loxitane 1426
Loxapine Succinate (Diminished tolerance for other CNSD when used concurrently). Products include:
Loxitane Capsules 1426
Meperidine Hydrochloride (Diminished tolerance for other CNSD when used concurrently). Products include:
Demerol 2438
Mepergan Injection 2859
Mephobarbital (Diminished tolerance for other CNSD when used concurrently; potential for increased CNS-depressant effects). Products include:
Mebaral Tablets 2452
Meprobamate (Diminished tolerance for other CNSD when used concurrently). Products include:
Miltown Tablets 2780
PMB 200 and PMB 400 2890
Mesoridazine Besylate (Diminished tolerance for other CNSD when used concurrently). Products include:
Serentil 689
Methadone Hydrochloride (Diminished tolerance for other CNSD when used concurrently). Products include:
Methadone Hydrochloride Oral Concentrate 2356
Methadone Hydrochloride Oral Solution & Tablets 2357
Methohexital Sodium (Diminished tolerance for other CNSD when used concurrently).
No products indexed under this heading.
Methotrimeprazine (Diminished tolerance for other CNSD when used concurrently). Products include:
Levoprome 1321
Methoxyflurane (Diminished tolerance for other CNSD when used concurrently).
No products indexed under this heading.
Midazolam Hydrochloride (Diminished tolerance for other CNSD when used concurrently). Products include:
Versed Injection 2324
Molindone Hydrochloride (Diminished tolerance for other CNSD when used concurrently). Products include:
Moban Tablets and Concentrate .. 1036
Morphine Sulfate (Diminished tolerance for other CNSD when used concurrently). Products include:
Astramorph/PF Injection, USP (Preservative-Free) 526
Duramorph Injection 983
Infumorph 200 and Infumorph 500 Sterile Solutions 985
Kadian Capsules 2948
MS Contin Tablets 2149
MSIR 2152
Oramorph SR (Morphine Sulfate Sustained Release Tablets) 2359
RMS Suppositories CII 2766
Roxanol 2365

IMPORTANT NOTE: Always consult each drug listing in the patient's regimen for possible interactions.

Opium Alkaloids (Diminished tolerance for other CNSD when used concurrently).
No products indexed under this heading.

Oxazepam (Diminished tolerance for other CNSD when used concurrently). Products include:
Serax Capsules 2916
Serax Tablets 2916

Oxycodone Hydrochloride (Diminished tolerance for other CNSD when used concurrently). Products include:
OxyContin Tablets 2163
OxyIR Capsules 2167
Percocet Tablets 955
Percodan Tablets 955
Percodan-Demi Tablets 956
Roxicodone Tablets, Oral Solution & Intensol (Oxycodone) 2366
Tylox Capsules 1593

Pentobarbital Sodium (Diminished tolerance for other CNSD when used concurrently; potential for increased CNS-depressant effects). Products include:
Nembutal Sodium Capsules 440
Nembutal Sodium Solution 442
Nembutal Sodium Suppositories 444

Perphenazine (Diminished tolerance for other CNSD when used concurrently). Products include:
Etrafon 2495
Triavil Tablets 1800
Trilafon 2532

Phenobarbital (Diminished tolerance for other CNSD when used concurrently; potential for increased CNS-depressant effects). Products include:
Arco-Lase Plus Tablets 513
Bellergal-S Tablets 2375
Donnatal 2234
Donnatal Extentabs 2234
Donnatal Tablets 2234
Phenobarbital Elixir and Tablets 1523
Quadrinal Tablets 1398

Prazepam (Diminished tolerance for other CNSD when used concurrently).
No products indexed under this heading.

Prochlorperazine (Diminished tolerance for other CNSD when used concurrently). Products include:
Compazine 2644

Promethazine Hydrochloride (Diminished tolerance for other CNSD when used concurrently). Products include:
Mepergan Injection 2859
Phenergan with Codeine 2883
Phenergan with Dextromethorphan 2885
Phenergan Injection 2880
Phenergan Suppositories 2882
Phenergan Syrup 2881
Phenergan Tablets 2882
Phenergan VC 2886
Phenergan VC with Codeine 2888

Propofol (Diminished tolerance for other CNSD when used concurrently). Products include:
Diprivan Injectable Emulsion 2939

Propoxyphene Hydrochloride (Diminished tolerance for other CNSD when used concurrently). Products include:
Darvon 1475
Wygesic Tablets 2930

Propoxyphene Napsylate (Diminished tolerance for other CNSD when used concurrently). Products include:
Darvon-N/Darvocet-N 1473

Quazepam (Diminished tolerance for other CNSD when used concurrently). Products include:
Doral Tablets 2773

Risperidone (Diminished tolerance for other CNSD when used concurrently). Products include:
Risperdal Tablets 1348

Secobarbital Sodium (Diminished tolerance for other CNSD when used concurrently; potential for increased CNS-depressant effects). Products include:
Seconal Sodium Pulvules 1529

Sevoflurane (Diminished tolerance for other CNSD when used concurrently).
No products indexed under this heading.

Sufentanil Citrate (Diminished tolerance for other CNSD when used concurrently). Products include:
Sufenta Injection 1355

Temazepam (Diminished tolerance for other CNSD when used concurrently). Products include:
Restoril Capsules 2413

Thiamylal Sodium (Diminished tolerance for other CNSD when used concurrently; potential for increased CNS-depressant effects).
No products indexed under this heading.

Thioridazine Hydrochloride (Diminished tolerance for other CNSD when used concurrently). Products include:
Mellaril 2398

Thiothixene (Diminished tolerance for other CNSD when used concurrently). Products include:
Navane Capsules and Concentrate 2018
Navane Intramuscular 2019

Triazolam (Diminished tolerance for other CNSD when used concurrently). Products include:
Halcion Tablets 2093

Trifluoperazine Hydrochloride (Diminished tolerance for other CNSD when used concurrently). Products include:
Stelazine 2692

Zolpidem Tartrate (Diminished tolerance for other CNSD when used concurrently). Products include:
Ambien Tablets 2559

Food Interactions

Alcohol (Diminished tolerance for alcohol when used concurrently; potential for increased CNS-depressant effects).

ATRETOL TABLETS
(Carbamazepine) 569
May interact with calcium channel blockers, monoamine oxidase inhibitors, lithium preparations, anticonvulsants, oral contraceptives, xanthine bronchodilators, and certain other agents. Compounds in these categories include:

Aminophylline (Half-life of theophyllin is shortened when concurrently administered).
No products indexed under this heading.

Amlodipine Besylate (Concomitant administration has been reported to result in elevated plasma levels of carbamazepine resulting in toxicity is some cases). Products include:
Lotrel Capsules 858
Norvasc Tablets 2020

Bepridil Hydrochloride (Concomitant administration has been reported to result in elevated plasma levels of carbamazepine resulting in toxicity is some cases). Products include:
Vascor Tablets (200 and 300 mg) 1597

Cimetidine (Concomitant administration has been reported to result in elevated plasma levels of carbamazepine resulting in toxicity is some cases). Products include:
Tagamet HB Tablets .... ▣ 786
Tagamet Tablets 2694

Cimetidine Hydrochloride (Concomitant administration has been reported to result in elevated plasma levels of carbamazepine resulting in toxicity is some cases). Products include:
Tagamet 2694

Desogestrel (Potential for breakthrough bleeding in patients receiving concomitant oral contraceptives; reliability may be adversely affected). Products include:
Desogen Tablets 1867
Ortho-Cept 1907

Diltiazem Hydrochloride (Concomitant administration has been reported to result in elevated plasma levels of carbamazepine resulting in toxicity is some cases). Products include:
Cardizem CD Capsules 1251
Cardizem SR Capsules 1255
Cardizem Injectable 1253
Cardizem Tablets 1257
Dilacor XR Extended-release Capsules 2183
Tiazac Capsules 1019

Divalproex Sodium (Potential for an increase in the ratio of active 10,11-epoxide metabolite to parent compound; valproic acid serum levels may be reduced when divalproex is administered with carbamazepine; combination therapy with other anticonvulsant has resulted in alteration of thyroid function). Products include:
Depakote Tablets 418

Doxycycline Calcium (Half-life of doxycyclline is shortened when concurrently administered). Products include:
Vibramycin Calcium Oral Suspension Syrup 2038

Doxycycline Hyclate (Half-life of doxycyclline is shortened when concurrently administered). Products include:
Doryx Capsules 1970
Vibramycin Hyclate Capsules 2038
Vibramycin Hyclate Intravenous 2040
Vibra-Tabs Film Coated Tablets 2038

Doxycycline Monohydrate (Half-life of doxycyclline is shortened when concurrently administered). Products include:
Monodox Capsules 1858
Vibramycin Monohydrate for Oral Suspension 2038

Dyphylline (Half-life of theophyllin is shortened when concurrently administered). Products include:
Lufyllin & Lufyllin-400 Tablets 2778
Lufyllin-GG Elixir & Tablets 2779

Erythromycin (Concomitant administration has been reported to result in elevated plasma levels of carbamazepine resulting in toxicity is some cases). Products include:
A/T/S 2% Acne Topical Gel 1244
A/T/S 2% Acne Topical Solution 1244
Benzamycin Topical Gel 919
E-Mycin Tablets 1388
Emgel 2% Topical Gel 1081
ERYC 1972
Erycette (erythromycin 2%) Topical Solution 1943
Ery-Tab Tablets 426
Erythromycin Base Filmtab 430
Erythromycin Delayed-Release Capsules, USP 431
Ilotycin Ophthalmic Ointment 928
PCE Dispertab Tablets 453
T-Stat 2.0% Topical Solution and Pads 2797
THERAMYCIN Z 2% Solution 1629

Erythromycin Estolate (Concomitant administration has been reported to result in elevated plasma levels of carbamazepine resulting in toxicity is some cases). Products include:
Ilosone 927

Erythromycin Ethylsuccinate (Concomitant administration has been reported to result in elevated plasma levels of carbamazepine resulting in toxicity is some cases). Products include:
E.E.S. 427
EryPed 425
Pediazole Suspension 2340

Erythromycin Gluceptate (Concomitant administration has been reported to result in elevated plasma levels of carbamazepine resulting in toxicity is some cases). Products include:
Ilotycin Gluceptate, IV, Vials 929

Erythromycin Stearate (Concomitant administration has been reported to result in elevated plasma levels of carbamazepine resulting in toxicity is some cases). Products include:
Erythrocin Stearate Filmtab 429

Ethinyl Estradiol (Potential for breakthrough bleeding in patients receiving concomitant oral contraceptives; reliability may be adversely affected). Products include:
Brevicon 2563
Demulen 2580
Desogen Tablets 1867
Levlen/Tri-Levlen 646
Lo/Ovral Tablets 2852
Lo/Ovral-28 Tablets 2857
Modicon 1928
Nordette-21 Tablets 2863
Nordette-28 Tablets 2866
Norinyl 2563
Ortho-Cept 1907
Ortho-Cyclen/Ortho-Tri-Cyclen 1914
Ortho-Novum 1928
Ortho-Cyclen/Ortho Tri-Cyclen 1914
Ovcon 765
Ovral Tablets 2877
Ovral-28 Tablets 2878
Levlen/Tri-Levlen 646
Tri-Norinyl 2607
Triphasil-21 Tablets 2919
Triphasil-28 Tablets 2924

Ethosuximide (Combination therapy with other anticonvulsant has resulted in alteration of thyroid function). Products include:
Zarontin Capsules 1986
Zarontin Syrup 1986

Ethotoin (Combination therapy with other anticonvulsant has resulted in alteration of thyroid function). Products include:
Peganone Tablets 455

Ethynodiol Diacetate (Potential for breakthrough bleeding in patients receiving concomitant oral contraceptives; reliability may be adversely affected). Products include:
Demulen 2580

Felbamate (Combination therapy with other anticonvulsant has resulted in alteration of thyroid function). Products include:
Felbatol 2774

Felodipine (Concomitant administration has been reported to result in elevated plasma levels of carbamazepine resulting in toxicity is some cases). Products include:
Plendil Extended-Release Tablets 514

Furazolidone (On theoretical grounds concurrent and/or sequential use is contraindicated). Products include:
  Furoxone 2221

Haloperidol (Haloperidol serum levels may be reduced when it is administered with carbamazepine). Products include:
  Haldol Injection, Tablets and Concentrate 1585

Haloperidol Decanoate (Haloperidol serum levels may be reduced when it is administered with carbamazepine). Products include:
  Haldol Decanoate.................... 1587

Isocarboxazid (On theoretical grounds concurrent and/or sequential use is contraindicated).
  No products indexed under this heading.

Isoniazid (Concomitant administration has been reported to result in elevated plasma levels of carbamazepine resulting in toxicity in some cases). Products include:
  Nydrazid Injection 509
  Rifamate Capsules 1278
  Rifater 1280

Isradipine (Concomitant administration has been reported to result in elevated plasma levels of carbamazepine resulting in toxicity is some cases). Products include:
  DynaCirc Capsules 2381
  DynaCirc CR Tablets 2383

Lamotrigine (Combination therapy with other anticonvulsant has resulted in alteration of thyroid function). Products include:
  Lamictal Tablets 1105

Levonorgestrel (Potential for breakthrough bleeding in patients receiving concomitant oral contraceptives; reliability may be adversely affected). Products include:
  Levlen/Tri-Levlen 646
  Nordette-21 Tablets 2863
  Nordette-28 Tablets 2866
  Norplant System 2868
  Levlen/Tri-Levlen 646
  Triphasil-21 Tablets 2919
  Triphasil-28 Tablets 2924

Lithium Carbonate (Concomitant administration may increase the risk of neurotoxic side effects). Products include:
  Eskalith 2658
  Lithium Carbonate Capsules & Tablets 2352
  Lithonate/Lithotabs/Lithobid 2721

Lithium Citrate (Concomitant administration may increase the risk of neurotoxic side effects).
  No products indexed under this heading.

Mephenytoin (Combination therapy with other anticonvulsant has resulted in alteration of thyroid function). Products include:
  Mesantoin Tablets 2400

Mestranol (Potential for breakthrough bleeding in patients receiving concomitant oral contraceptives; reliability may be adversely affected). Products include:
  Norinyl 2563
  Ortho-Novum............................ 1928

Methsuximide (Combination therapy with other anticonvulsant has resulted in alteration of thyroid function). Products include:
  Celontin Kapseals 1955

Nicardipine Hydrochloride (Concomitant administration has been reported to result in elevated plasma levels of carbamazepine resulting in toxicity is some cases). Products include:
  Cardene Capsules 2261
  Cardene I.V. 2815
  Cardene SR Capsules.............. 2264

Nifedipine (Concomitant administration has been reported to result in elevated plasma levels of carbamazepine resulting in toxicity is some cases). Products include:
  Adalat Capsules (10 mg and 20 mg) 580
  Adalat CC 582
  Procardia Capsules 2024
  Procardia XL Extended Release Tablets 2026

Nimodipine (Concomitant administration has been reported to result in elevated plasma levels of carbamazepine resulting in toxicity is some cases). Products include:
  Nimotop Capsules 603

Nisoldipine (Concomitant administration has been reported to result in elevated plasma levels of carbamazepine resulting in toxicity is some cases). Products include:
  Sular Tablets 2961

Norethindrone (Potential for breakthrough bleeding in patients receiving concomitant oral contraceptives; reliability may be adversely affected). Products include:
  Brevicon 2563
  Micronor Tablets 1903
  Modicon 1928
  Norinyl 2563
  Nor-Q D Tablets 2598
  Ortho-Novum............................ 1928
  Ovcon 765
  Tri-Norinyl 2607

Norethynodrel (Potential for breakthrough bleeding in patients receiving concomitant oral contraceptives; reliability may be adversely affected).
  No products indexed under this heading.

Norgestimate (Potential for breakthrough bleeding in patients receiving concomitant oral contraceptives; reliability may be adversely affected). Products include:
  Ortho-Cyclen/Ortho-Tri-Cyclen 1914
  Ortho-Cyclen/Ortho Tri-Cyclen 1914

Norgestrel (Potential for breakthrough bleeding in patients receiving concomitant oral contraceptives; reliability may be adversely affected). Products include:
  Lo/Ovral Tablets 2852
  Lo/Ovral-28 Tablets.................. 2857
  Ovral Tablets 2877
  Ovral-28 Tablets 2878
  Ovrette Tablets 2878

Paramethadione (Combination therapy with other anticonvulsant has resulted in alteration of thyroid function).
  No products indexed under this heading.

Phenacemide (Combination therapy with other anticonvulsant has resulted in alteration of thyroid function). Products include:
  Phenurone Tablets 455

Phenelzine Sulfate (On theoretical grounds concurrent and/or sequential use is contraindicated). Products include:
  Nardil 1977

Phenobarbital (Simultaneous administration produces a marked lowering of serum levels of carbamazepine; combination therapy with other anticonvulsant has resulted in alteration of thyroid function). Products include:
  Arco-Lase Plus Tablets 513
  Bellergal-S Tablets 2375
  Donnatal 2234
  Donnatal Extentabs................... 2234
  Donnatal Tablets 2234
  Phenobarbital Elixir and Tablets 1523
  Quadrinal Tablets 1398

Phensuximide (Combination therapy with other anticonvulsant has resulted in alteration of thyroid function).
  No products indexed under this heading.

Phenytoin (Simultaneous administration produces a marked lowering of serum levels of carbamazepine; half-life of phenytoin is shortened when concurrently administered; combination therapy with other anticonvulsant has resulted in alteration of thyroid function). Products include:
  Dilantin Infatabs....................... 1967
  Dilantin-125 Suspension 1969

Phenytoin Sodium (Simultaneous administration produces a marked lowering of serum levels of carbamazepine; half-life of phenytoin is shortened when concurrently administered; combination therapy with other anticonvulsant has resulted in alteration of thyroid function). Products include:
  Dilantin Kapseals 1965

Primidone (Simultaneous administration produces a marked lowering of serum levels of carbamazepine; combination therapy with other anticonvulsant has resulted in alteration of thyroid function). Products include:
  Mysoline.................................... 2860

Propoxyphene Hydrochloride (Concomitant administration has been reported to result in elevated plasma levels of carbamazepine resulting in toxicity is some cases). Products include:
  Darvon 1475
  Wygesic Tablets 2930

Propoxyphene Napsylate (Concomitant administration has been reported to result in elevated plasma levels of carbamazepine resulting in toxicity is some cases). Products include:
  Darvon-N/Darvocet-N 1473

Selegiline Hydrochloride (On theoretical grounds concurrent and/or sequential use is contraindicated). Products include:
  Eldepryl Capsules 2729

Theophylline (Half-life of theophyllin is shortened when concurrently administered). Products include:
  Marax Tablets & DF Syrup...... 2015
  Quibron 2227

Theophylline Anhydrous (Half-life of theophyllin is shortened when concurrently administered). Products include:
  Aerolate 1003
  Primatene Tablets 844
  Respbid Tablets 687
  Slo-bid Gyrocaps 2201
  Theo-24 Extended Release Capsules 2753
  Theo-Dur Extended-Release Tablets 1367
  Theo-X Extended-Release Tablets 793
  Uni-Dur Extended-Release Tablets.. 1374
  Uniphyl 400 mg and 600 mg Tablets 2157

Theophylline Calcium Salicylate (Half-life of theophyllin is shortened when concurrently administered). Products include:
  Quadrinal Tablets 1398

Theophylline Sodium Glycinate (Half-life of theophyllin is shortened when concurrently administered).
  No products indexed under this heading.

Tranylcypromine Sulfate (On theoretical grounds concurrent and/or sequential use is contraindicated). Products include:
  Parnate Tablets 2679

Trimethadione (Combination therapy with other anticonvulsant has resulted in alteration of thyroid function).
  No products indexed under this heading.

Valproic Acid (Potential for an increase in the ratio of active 10,11-epoxide metabolite to parent compound; valproic acid serum levels may be reduced when valproic acid is administered with carbamazepine; combination therapy with other anticonvulsant has resulted in alteration of thyroid function). Products include:
  Depakene 416

Verapamil Hydrochloride (Concomitant administration has been reported to result in elevated plasma levels of carbamazepine resulting in toxicity is some cases). Products include:
  Calan SR Caplets 2571
  Calan Tablets 2568
  Covera-HS Tablets 2573
  Isoptin Injectable 1391
  Isoptin Oral Tablets 1393
  Isoptin SR Tablets 1395
  Verelan Capsules 1455

Warfarin Sodium (Half-life of warfarin is shortened when concurrently administered). Products include:
  Coumadin 941

ATROHIST PEDIATRIC CAPSULES

(Chlorpheniramine Maleate, Pseudoephedrine Hydrochloride) 1603
May interact with monoamine oxidase inhibitors, beta blockers, veratrum alkaloids, central nervous system depressants, and certain other agents. Compounds in these categories include:

Acebutolol Hydrochloride (Increases the effects of sympathomimetics). Products include:
  Sectral Capsules 2914

Alfentanil Hydrochloride (Potential for additive effects). Products include:
  Alfenta Injection 1334

Alprazolam (Potential for additive effects). Products include:
  Xanax Tablets 2115

Aprobarbital (Potential for additive effects).
  No products indexed under this heading.

Atenolol (Increases the effects of sympathomimetics). Products include:
  Tenoretic Tablets 2963
  Tenormin Tablets and I.V. Injection ... 2965

Betaxolol Hydrochloride (Increases the effects of sympathomimetics). Products include:
  Betoptic Ophthalmic Solution... 465
  Betoptic S Ophthalmic Suspension ... 467
  Kerlone Tablets 2588

IMPORTANT NOTE: Always consult each drug listing in the patient's regimen for possible interactions.

Atrohist — Interactions Index

Bisoprolol Fumarate (Increases the effects of sympathomimetics). Products include:
- Zebeta Tablets 1457
- Ziac 1459

Buprenorphine (Potential for additive effects). Products include:
- Buprenex Injectable 2170

Buspirone Hydrochloride (Potential for additive effects). Products include:
- BuSpar Tablets 738

Butabarbital (Potential for additive effects).
No products indexed under this heading.

Butalbital (Potential for additive effects). Products include:
- Axocet Capsules 2469
- Esgic-plus Capsules 1012
- Esgic-plus Tablets 1012
- Fioricet Tablets 2386
- Fioricet with Codeine Capsules 2387
- Fiorinal Capsules 2388
- Fiorinal with Codeine Capsules 2390
- Fiorinal Tablets 2388
- Phrenilin 790
- Sedapap Tablets 50 mg/650 mg .. 1826

Carteolol Hydrochloride (Increases the effects of sympathomimetics). Products include:
- Cartrol Tablets 413
- Ocupress Ophthalmic Solution, 1% Sterile .... ⊚ 297

Chlordiazepoxide (Potential for additive effects). Products include:
- Limbitrol 2333

Chlordiazepoxide Hydrochloride (Potential for additive effects). Products include:
- Librax Capsules 2330
- Librium Capsules 2331
- Librium Injectable 2332

Chlorpromazine (Potential for additive effects). Products include:
- Thorazine Suppositories 2701

Chlorpromazine Hydrochloride (Potential for additive effects). Products include:
- Thorazine 2701

Chlorprothixene (Potential for additive effects).
No products indexed under this heading.

Chlorprothixene Hydrochloride (Potential for additive effects).
No products indexed under this heading.

Chlorprothixene Lactate (Potential for additive effects).
No products indexed under this heading.

Clorazepate Dipotassium (Potential for additive effects). Products include:
- Tranxene 459

Clozapine (Potential for additive effects). Products include:
- Clozaril Tablets 2377

Codeine Phosphate (Potential for additive effects). Products include:
- Brontex 2130
- Dimetane-DC Cough Syrup 2232
- Fioricet with Codeine Capsules 2387
- Fiorinal with Codeine Capsules 2390
- Nucofed 2225
- Phenergan with Codeine 2883
- Phenergan VC with Codeine 2888
- Robitussin A-C Syrup 2248
- Robitussin-DAC Syrup 2249
- Ryna .... ▣ 804
- Soma Compound w/Codeine Tablets 2784
- Tylenol with Codeine 1592

Cryptenamine Preparations (Reduced antihypertensive effects).

Desflurane (Potential for additive effects). Products include:
- Suprane (desflurane, USP) 1865

Dezocine (Potential for additive effects). Products include:
- Dalgan Injection 529

Diazepam (Potential for additive effects). Products include:
- Dizac (diazepam injectable emulsion) CIV 1862
- Valium Injectable 2336
- Valium Tablets 2335

Droperidol (Potential for additive effects). Products include:
- Inapsine Injection 462

Enflurane (Potential for additive effects).
No products indexed under this heading.

Esmolol Hydrochloride (Increases the effects of sympathomimetics). Products include:
- Brevibloc (esmolol HCl) Injection 1860

Estazolam (Potential for additive effects). Products include:
- ProSom Tablets 457

Ethchlorvynol (Potential for additive effects). Products include:
- Placidyl Capsules 456

Ethinamate (Potential for additive effects).
No products indexed under this heading.

Fentanyl (Potential for additive effects). Products include:
- Duragesic Transdermal System 1336

Fentanyl Citrate (Potential for additive effects). Products include:
- Sublimaze Injection 463

Fluphenazine Decanoate (Potential for additive effects). Products include:
- Prolixin Decanoate 510

Fluphenazine Enanthate (Potential for additive effects). Products include:
- Prolixin Enanthate 510

Fluphenazine Hydrochloride (Potential for additive effects). Products include:
- Prolixin 510

Flurazepam Hydrochloride (Potential for additive effects). Products include:
- Dalmane Capsules 2329

Furazolidone (Increases the effects of sympathomimetics; concurrent and/or sequential use is contraindicated). Products include:
- Furoxone 2221

Glutethimide (Potential for additive effects).
No products indexed under this heading.

Haloperidol (Potential for additive effects). Products include:
- Haldol Injection, Tablets and Concentrate 1585

Haloperidol Decanoate (Potential for additive effects). Products include:
- Haldol Decanoate 1587

Hydrocodone Bitartrate (Potential for additive effects). Products include:
- Codiclear DH Syrup 808
- Duratuss HD Elixir 2750
- Histussin D Liquid 670
- Hycodan Tablets and Syrup 946
- Hycomine Compound Tablets 948
- Hycomine 947
- Hycotuss Expectorant Syrup 950
- Hydrocet Capsules 787
- Lorcet 10/650 Tablets 1016
- Lortab 2751
- Tussend 1830
- Tussend Expectorant 1831
- Vicodin Tablets 1404
- Vicodin ES Tablets 1405
- Vicodin HP Tablets 1403
- Vicodin Tuss Expectorant 1406
- Zydone Capsules 967

Hydrocodone Polistirex (Potential for additive effects). Products include:
- Tussionex Pennkinetic Extended-Release Suspension 1624

Hydroxyzine Hydrochloride (Potential for additive effects). Products include:
- Atarax Tablets & Syrup 1992
- Marax Tablets & DF Syrup 2015
- Vistaril Intramuscular Solution 2042

Isocarboxazid (Increases the effects of sympathomimetics; concurrent and/or sequential use is contraindicated).
No products indexed under this heading.

Isoflurane (Potential for additive effects).
No products indexed under this heading.

Ketamine Hydrochloride (Potential for additive effects).
No products indexed under this heading.

Labetalol Hydrochloride (Increases the effects of sympathomimetics). Products include:
- Normodyne Injection 2519
- Normodyne Tablets 2522
- Trandate 1158

Levobunolol Hydrochloride (Increases the effects of sympathomimetics). Products include:
- Betagan .... ⊚ 230

Levomethadyl Acetate Hydrochloride (Potential for additive effects). Products include:
- Orlaam Oral Solution 2361

Levorphanol Tartrate (Potential for additive effects). Products include:
- Levo-Dromoran 2297

Lorazepam (Potential for additive effects). Products include:
- Ativan Injection 2805
- Ativan Tablets 2807

Loxapine Hydrochloride (Potential for additive effects). Products include:
- Loxitane 1426

Loxapine Succinate (Potential for additive effects). Products include:
- Loxitane Capsules 1426

Mecamylamine Hydrochloride (Reduced antihypertensive effects). Products include:
- Inversine Tablets 1729

Meperidine Hydrochloride (Potential for additive effects). Products include:
- Demerol 2438
- Mepergan Injection 2859

Mephobarbital (Potential for additive effects). Products include:
- Mebaral Tablets 2452

Meprobamate (Potential for additive effects). Products include:
- Miltown Tablets 2780
- PMB 200 and PMB 400 2890

Mesoridazine Besylate (Potential for additive effects). Products include:
- Serentil 689

Methadone Hydrochloride (Potential for additive effects). Products include:
- Methadone Hydrochloride Oral Concentrate 2356
- Methadone Hydrochloride Oral Solution & Tablets 2357

Methohexital Sodium (Potential for additive effects).
No products indexed under this heading.

Methotrimeprazine (Potential for additive effects). Products include:
- Levoprome 1321

Methoxyflurane (Potential for additive effects).
No products indexed under this heading.

Methyldopa (Reduced antihypertensive effects). Products include:
- Aldoclor Tablets 1638
- Aldomet Oral 1640
- Aldoril Tablets 1644

Methyldopate Hydrochloride (Reduced antihypertensive effects). Products include:
- Aldomet Ester HCl Injection 1642

Metipranolol Hydrochloride (Increases the effects of sympathomimetics). Products include:
- OptiPranolol (Metipranolol 0.3%) Sterile Ophthalmic Solution .... ⊚ 256

Metoprolol Succinate (Increases the effects of sympathomimetics). Products include:
- Toprol-XL Tablets 560

Metoprolol Tartrate (Increases the effects of sympathomimetics). Products include:
- Lopressor 848
- Lopressor HCT Tablets 850

Midazolam Hydrochloride (Potential for additive effects). Products include:
- Versed Injection 2324

Molindone Hydrochloride (Potential for additive effects). Products include:
- Moban Tablets and Concentrate 1036

Morphine Sulfate (Potential for additive effects). Products include:
- Astramorph/PF Injection, USP (Preservative-Free) 526
- Duramorph Injection 983
- Infumorph 200 and Infumorph 500 Sterile Solutions 985
- Kadian Capsules 2948
- MS Contin Tablets 2149
- MSIR 2152
- Oramorph SR (Morphine Sulfate Sustained Release Tablets) 2359
- RMS Suppositories CII 2766
- Roxanol 2365

Nadolol (Increases the effects of sympathomimetics).
No products indexed under this heading.

Opium Alkaloids (Potential for additive effects).
No products indexed under this heading.

Oxazepam (Potential for additive effects). Products include:
- Serax Capsules 2916
- Serax Tablets 2916

Oxycodone Hydrochloride (Potential for additive effects). Products include:
- OxyContin Tablets 2163
- OxyIR Capsules 2167
- Percocet Tablets 955
- Percodan Tablets 955
- Percodan-Demi Tablets 956
- Roxicodone Tablets, Oral Solution & Intensol (Oxycodone) 2366
- Tylox Capsules 1593

Penbutolol Sulfate (Increases the effects of sympathomimetics). Products include:
- Levatol Tablets 2547

Pentobarbital Sodium (Potential for additive effects). Products include:
- Nembutal Sodium Capsules 440
- Nembutal Sodium Solution 442
- Nembutal Sodium Suppositories 444

Perphenazine (Potential for additive effects). Products include:
- Etrafon 2495
- Triavil Tablets 1800
- Trilafon 2532

(▣ Described in PDR For Nonprescription Drugs) (⊚ Described in PDR For Ophthalmology)

87 **Interactions Index** **Atrohist Pediatric**

Phenelzine Sulfate (Increases the effects of sympathomimetics; concurrent and/or sequential use is contraindicated). Products include:
Nardil ... 1977

Phenobarbital (Potential for additive effects). Products include:
Arco-Lase Plus Tablets ... 513
Bellergal-S Tablets ... 2375
Donnatal ... 2234
Donnatal Extentabs ... 2234
Donnatal Tablets ... 2234
Phenobarbital Elixir and Tablets ... 1523
Quadrinal Tablets ... 1398

Pindolol (Increases the effects of sympathomimetics). Products include:
Visken Tablets ... 2428

Prazepam (Potential for additive effects).
No products indexed under this heading.

Prochlorperazine (Potential for additive effects). Products include:
Compazine ... 2644

Promethazine Hydrochloride (Potential for additive effects). Products include:
Mepergan Injection ... 2859
Phenergan with Codeine ... 2883
Phenergan with Dextromethorphan 2885
Phenergan Injection ... 2880
Phenergan Suppositories ... 2882
Phenergan Syrup ... 2881
Phenergan Tablets ... 2882
Phenergan VC ... 2886
Phenergan VC with Codeine ... 2888

Propofol (Potential for additive effects). Products include:
Diprivan Injectable Emulsion ... 2939

Propoxyphene Hydrochloride (Potential for additive effects). Products include:
Darvon ... 1475
Wygesic Tablets ... 2930

Propoxyphene Napsylate (Potential for additive effects). Products include:
Darvon-N/Darvocet-N ... 1473

Propranolol Hydrochloride (Increases the effects of sympathomimetics). Products include:
Inderal ... 2834
Inderal LA Long Acting Capsules ... 2836
Inderide Tablets ... 2838
Inderide LA Long Acting Capsules .. 2840

Quazepam (Potential for additive effects). Products include:
Doral Tablets ... 2773

Reserpine (Reduced antihypertensive effects). Products include:
Diupres Tablets ... 1691
Hydropres Tablets ... 1718
Ser-Ap-Es Tablets ... 867

Risperidone (Potential for additive effects). Products include:
Risperdal Tablets ... 1348

Secobarbital Sodium (Potential for additive effects). Products include:
Seconal Sodium Pulvules ... 1529

Selegiline Hydrochloride (Increases the effects of sympathomimetics; concurrent and/or sequential use is contraindicated). Products include:
Eldepryl Capsules ... 2729

Sevoflurane (Potential for additive effects).
No products indexed under this heading.

Sotalol Hydrochloride (Increases the effects of sympathomimetics). Products include:
Betapace Tablets ... 637

Sufentanil Citrate (Potential for additive effects). Products include:
Sufenta Injection ... 1355

Temazepam (Potential for additive effects). Products include:
Restoril Capsules ... 2413

Thiamylal Sodium (Potential for additive effects).
No products indexed under this heading.

Thioridazine Hydrochloride (Potential for additive effects). Products include:
Mellaril ... 2398

Thiothixene (Potential for additive effects). Products include:
Navane Capsules and Concentrate 2018
Navane Intramuscular ... 2019

Timolol Hemihydrate (Increases the effects of sympathomimetics). Products include:
Betimol 0.25%, 0.5% ... ◉ 259

Timolol Maleate (Increases the effects of sympathomimetics). Products include:
Blocadren Tablets ... 1654
Timolide Tablets ... 1791
Timoptic in Ocudose ... 1796
Timoptic Sterile Ophthalmic Solution ... 1794
Timoptic-XE ... 1798

Tranylcypromine Sulfate (Increases the effects of sympathomimetics; concurrent and/or sequential use is contraindicated). Products include:
Parnate Tablets ... 2679

Triazolam (Potential for additive effects). Products include:
Halcion Tablets ... 2093

Trifluoperazine Hydrochloride (Potential for additive effects). Products include:
Stelazine ... 2692

Zolpidem Tartrate (Potential for additive effects). Products include:
Ambien Tablets ... 2559

Food Interactions

Alcohol (Potential for additive effects).

ATROHIST PEDIATRIC SUSPENSION

(Chlorpheniramine Tannate, Phenylephrine Tannate, Pyrilamine Tannate) ... 1604

May interact with monoamine oxidase inhibitors, central nervous system depressants, tranquilizers, hypnotics and sedatives, and certain other agents. Compounds in these categories include:

Alfentanil Hydrochloride (Potential for additive central nervous system effects). Products include:
Alfenta Injection ... 1334

Alprazolam (Potential for additive central nervous system effects). Products include:
Xanax Tablets ... 2115

Aprobarbital (Potential for additive central nervous system effects).
No products indexed under this heading.

Buprenorphine (Potential for additive central nervous system effects). Products include:
Buprenex Injectable ... 2170

Buspirone Hydrochloride (Potential for additive central nervous system effects). Products include:
BuSpar Tablets ... 738

Butabarbital (Potential for additive central nervous system effects).
No products indexed under this heading.

Butalbital (Potential for additive central nervous system effects). Products include:
Axocet Capsules ... 2469
Esgic-plus Capsules ... 1012
Esgic-plus Tablets ... 1012
Fioricet Tablets ... 2386
Fioricet with Codeine Capsules ... 2387
Fiorinal Capsules ... 2388
Fiorinal with Codeine Capsules ... 2390
Fiorinal Tablets ... 2388
Phrenilin ... 790
Sedapap Tablets 50 mg/650 mg .. 1826

Chlordiazepoxide (Potential for additive central nervous system effects). Products include:
Limbitrol ... 2333

Chlordiazepoxide Hydrochloride (Potential for additive central nervous system effects). Products include:
Librax Capsules ... 2330
Librium Capsules ... 2331
Librium Injectable ... 2332

Chlorpromazine (Potential for additive central nervous system effects). Products include:
Thorazine Suppositories ... 2701

Chlorpromazine Hydrochloride (Potential for additive central nervous system effects). Products include:
Thorazine ... 2701

Chlorprothixene (Potential for additive central nervous system effects).
No products indexed under this heading.

Chlorprothixene Hydrochloride (Potential for additive central nervous system effects).
No products indexed under this heading.

Chlorprothixene Lactate (Potential for additive central nervous system effects).
No products indexed under this heading.

Clorazepate Dipotassium (Potential for additive central nervous system effects). Products include:
Tranxene ... 459

Clozapine (Potential for additive central nervous system effects). Products include:
Clozaril Tablets ... 2377

Codeine Phosphate (Potential for additive central nervous system effects). Products include:
Brontex ... 2130
Dimetane-DC Cough Syrup ... 2232
Fioricet with Codeine Capsules ... 2387
Fiorinal with Codeine Capsules ... 2390
Nucofed ... 2225
Phenergan with Codeine ... 2883
Phenergan VC with Codeine ... 2888
Robitussin A-C Syrup ... 2248
Robitussin-DAC Syrup ... 2249
Ryna ... 804
Soma Compound w/Codeine Tablets ... 2784
Tylenol with Codeine ... 1592

Desflurane (Potential for additive central nervous system effects). Products include:
Suprane (desflurane, USP) ... 1865

Dezocine (Potential for additive central nervous system effects). Products include:
Dalgan Injection ... 529

Diazepam (Potential for additive central nervous system effects). Products include:
Dizac (diazepam injectable emulsion) CIV ... 1862
Valium Injectable ... 2336
Valium Tablets ... 2335

Droperidol (Potential for additive central nervous system effects). Products include:
Inapsine Injection ... 462

Enflurane (Potential for additive central nervous system effects).
No products indexed under this heading.

Estazolam (Potential for additive central nervous system effects). Products include:
ProSom Tablets ... 457

Ethchlorvynol (Potential for additive central nervous system effects). Products include:
Placidyl Capsules ... 456

Ethinamate (Potential for additive central nervous system effects).
No products indexed under this heading.

Fentanyl (Potential for additive central nervous system effects). Products include:
Duragesic Transdermal System ... 1336

Fentanyl Citrate (Potential for additive central nervous system effects). Products include:
Sublimaze Injection ... 463

Fluphenazine Decanoate (Potential for additive central nervous system effects). Products include:
Prolixin Decanoate ... 510

Fluphenazine Enanthate (Potential for additive central nervous system effects). Products include:
Prolixin Enanthate ... 510

Fluphenazine Hydrochloride (Potential for additive central nervous system effects). Products include:
Prolixin ... 510

Flurazepam Hydrochloride (Potential for additive central nervous system effects). Products include:
Dalmane Capsules ... 2329

Furazolidone (Prolongs and intensifies the anticholingeric effects of antihistamines and the overall effects of sympathomimetics; concurrent and/or sequential treatment should not be undertaken). Products include:
Furoxone ... 2221

Glutethimide (Potential for additive central nervous system effects).
No products indexed under this heading.

Haloperidol (Potential for additive central nervous system effects). Products include:
Haldol Injection, Tablets and Concentrate ... 1585

Haloperidol Decanoate (Potential for additive central nervous system effects). Products include:
Haldol Decanoate ... 1587

Hydrocodone Bitartrate (Potential for additive central nervous system effects). Products include:
Codiclear DH Syrup ... 808
Duratuss HD Elixir ... 2750
Histussin D Liquid ... 670
Hycodan Tablets and Syrup ... 946
Hycomine Compound Tablets ... 948
Hycomine ... 947
Hycotuss Expectorant Syrup ... 950
Hydrocet Capsules ... 787
Lorcet 10/650 Tablets ... 1016
Lortab ... 2751
Tussend ... 1830
Tussend Expectorant ... 1831
Vicodin Tablets ... 1404
Vicodin ES Tablets ... 1405
Vicodin HP Tablets ... 1403
Vicodin Tuss Expectorant ... 1406
Zydone Capsules ... 967

Hydrocodone Polistirex (Potential for additive central nervous system effects). Products include:
Tussionex Pennkinetic Extended-Release Suspension ... 1624

Hydroxyzine Hydrochloride (Potential for additive central nervous system effects). Products include:
Atarax Tablets & Syrup ... 1992
Marax Tablets & DF Syrup ... 2015
Vistaril Intramuscular Solution ... 2042

IMPORTANT NOTE: Always consult each drug listing in the patient's regimen for possible interactions.

Isocarboxazid (Prolongs and intensifies the anticholingeric effects of antihistamines and the overall effects of sympathomimetics; concurrent and/or sequential treatment should not be undertaken).
No products indexed under this heading.
Isoflurane (Potential for additive central nervous system effects).
No products indexed under this heading.
Ketamine Hydrochloride (Potential for additive central nervous system effects).
No products indexed under this heading.
Levomethadyl Acetate Hydrochloride (Potential for additive central nervous system effects). Products include:
Orlaam Oral Solution ... 2361
Levorphanol Tartrate (Potential for additive central nervous system effects). Products include:
Levo-Dromoran ... 2297
Lorazepam (Potential for additive central nervous system effects). Products include:
Ativan Injection ... 2805
Ativan Tablets ... 2807
Loxapine Hydrochloride (Potential for additive central nervous system effects). Products include:
Loxitane ... 1426
Loxapine Succinate (Potential for additive central nervous system effects). Products include:
Loxitane Capsules ... 1426
Meperidine Hydrochloride (Potential for additive central nervous system effects). Products include:
Demerol ... 2438
Mepergan Injection ... 2859
Mephobarbital (Potential for additive central nervous system effects). Products include:
Mebaral Tablets ... 2452
Meprobamate (Potential for additive central nervous system effects). Products include:
Miltown Tablets ... 2780
PMB 200 and PMB 400 ... 2890
Mesoridazine Besylate (Potential for additive central nervous system effects). Products include:
Serentil ... 689
Methadone Hydrochloride (Potential for additive central nervous system effects). Products include:
Methadone Hydrochloride Oral Concentrate ... 2356
Methadone Hydrochloride Oral Solution & Tablets ... 2357
Methohexital Sodium (Potential for additive central nervous system effects).
No products indexed under this heading.
Methotrimeprazine (Potential for additive central nervous system effects). Products include:
Levoprome ... 1321
Methoxyflurane (Potential for additive central nervous system effects).
No products indexed under this heading.
Midazolam Hydrochloride (Potential for additive central nervous system effects). Products include:
Versed Injection ... 2324
Molindone Hydrochloride (Potential for additive central nervous system effects). Products include:
Moban Tablets and Concentrate ... 1036
Morphine Sulfate (Potential for additive central nervous system effects). Products include:
Astramorph/PF Injection, USP (Preservative-Free) ... 526
Duramorph Injection ... 983
Infumorph 200 and Infumorph 500 Sterile Solutions ... 985
Kadian Capsules ... 2948
MS Contin Tablets ... 2149
MSIR ... 2152
Oramorph SR (Morphine Sulfate Sustained Release Tablets) ... 2359
RMS Suppositories CII ... 2766
Roxanol ... 2365
Opium Alkaloids (Potential for additive central nervous system effects).
No products indexed under this heading.
Oxazepam (Potential for additive central nervous system effects). Products include:
Serax Capsules ... 2916
Serax Tablets ... 2916
Oxycodone Hydrochloride (Potential for additive central nervous system effects). Products include:
OxyContin Tablets ... 2163
OxyIR Capsules ... 2167
Percocet Tablets ... 955
Percodan Tablets ... 955
Percodan-Demi Tablets ... 956
Roxicodone Tablets, Oral Solution & Intensol (Oxycodone) ... 2366
Tylox Capsules ... 1593
Pentobarbital Sodium (Potential for additive central nervous system effects). Products include:
Nembutal Sodium Capsules ... 440
Nembutal Sodium Solution ... 442
Nembutal Sodium Suppositories ... 444
Perphenazine (Potential for additive central nervous system effects). Products include:
Etrafon ... 2495
Triavil Tablets ... 1800
Trilafon ... 2532
Phenelzine Sulfate (Prolongs and intensifies the anticholingeric effects of antihistamines and the overall effects of sympathomimetics; concurrent and/or sequential treatment should not be undertaken). Products include:
Nardil ... 1977
Phenobarbital (Potential for additive central nervous system effects). Products include:
Arco-Lase Plus Tablets ... 513
Bellergal-S Tablets ... 2375
Donnatal ... 2234
Donnatal Extentabs ... 2234
Donnatal Tablets ... 2234
Phenobarbital Elixir and Tablets ... 1523
Quadrinal Tablets ... 1398
Prazepam (Potential for additive central nervous system effects).
No products indexed under this heading.
Prochlorperazine (Potential for additive central nervous system effects). Products include:
Compazine ... 2644
Promethazine Hydrochloride (Potential for additive central nervous system effects). Products include:
Mepergan Injection ... 2859
Phenergan with Codeine ... 2883
Phenergan with Dextromethorphan 2885
Phenergan Injection ... 2880
Phenergan Suppositories ... 2882
Phenergan Syrup ... 2881
Phenergan Tablets ... 2882
Phenergan VC ... 2886
Phenergan VC with Codeine ... 2888
Propofol (Potential for additive central nervous system effects). Products include:
Diprivan Injectable Emulsion ... 2939
Propoxyphene Hydrochloride (Potential for additive central nervous system effects). Products include:
Darvon ... 1475
Wygesic Tablets ... 2930
Propoxyphene Napsylate (Potential for additive central nervous system effects). Products include:
Darvon-N/Darvocet-N ... 1473
Quazepam (Potential for additive central nervous system effects). Products include:
Doral Tablets ... 2773
Risperidone (Potential for additive central nervous system effects). Products include:
Risperdal Tablets ... 1348
Secobarbital Sodium (Potential for additive central nervous system effects). Products include:
Seconal Sodium Pulvules ... 1529
Selegiline Hydrochloride (Prolongs and intensifies the anticholingeric effects of antihistamines and the overall effects of sympathomimetics; concurrent and/or sequential treatment should not be undertaken). Products include:
Eldepryl Capsules ... 2729
Sevoflurane (Potential for additive central nervous system effects).
No products indexed under this heading.
Sufentanil Citrate (Potential for additive central nervous system effects). Products include:
Sufenta Injection ... 1355
Temazepam (Potential for additive central nervous system effects). Products include:
Restoril Capsules ... 2413
Thiamylal Sodium (Potential for additive central nervous system effects).
No products indexed under this heading.
Thioridazine Hydrochloride (Potential for additive central nervous system effects). Products include:
Mellaril ... 2398
Thiothixene (Potential for additive central nervous system effects). Products include:
Navane Capsules and Concentrate 2018
Navane Intramuscular ... 2019
Tranylcypromine Sulfate (Prolongs and intensifies the anticholingeric effects of antihistamines and the overall effects of sympathomimetics; concurrent and/or sequential treatment should not be undertaken). Products include:
Parnate Tablets ... 2679
Triazolam (Potential for additive central nervous system effects). Products include:
Halcion Tablets ... 2093
Trifluoperazine Hydrochloride (Potential for additive central nervous system effects). Products include:
Stelazine ... 2692
Zolpidem Tartrate (Potential for additive central nervous system effects). Products include:
Ambien Tablets ... 2559

Food Interactions

Alcohol (Potential for additive central nervous system effects).

ATROHIST PEDIATRIC SUSPENSION DYE-FREE

(Chlorpheniramine Tannate, Phenylephrine Tannate, Pyrilamine Tannate) ... 1604
May interact with central nervous system depressants, hypnotics and sedatives, tranquilizers, monoamine oxidase inhibitors, and certain other agents. Compounds in these categories include:
Alfentanil Hydrochloride (Potential for additive central nervous system effects). Products include:
Alfenta Injection ... 1334
Alprazolam (Potential for additive central nervous system effects). Products include:
Xanax Tablets ... 2115
Aprobarbital (Potential for additive central nervous system effects).
No products indexed under this heading.
Buprenorphine (Potential for additive central nervous system effects). Products include:
Buprenex Injectable ... 2170
Buspirone Hydrochloride (Potential for additive central nervous system effects). Products include:
BuSpar Tablets ... 738
Butabarbital (Potential for additive central nervous system effects).
No products indexed under this heading.
Butalbital (Potential for additive central nervous system effects). Products include:
Axocet Capsules ... 2469
Esgic-plus Capsules ... 1012
Esgic-plus Tablets ... 1012
Fioricet Tablets ... 2386
Fioricet with Codeine Capsules ... 2387
Fiorinal Capsules ... 2388
Fiorinal with Codeine Capsules ... 2390
Fiorinal Tablets ... 2388
Phrenilin ... 790
Sedapap Tablets 50 mg/650 mg .. 1826
Chlordiazepoxide (Potential for additive central nervous system effects). Products include:
Limbitrol ... 2333
Chlordiazepoxide Hydrochloride (Potential for additive central nervous system effects). Products include:
Librax Capsules ... 2330
Librium Capsules ... 2331
Librium Injectable ... 2332
Chlorpromazine (Potential for additive central nervous system effects). Products include:
Thorazine Suppositories ... 2701
Chlorpromazine Hydrochloride (Potential for additive central nervous system effects). Products include:
Thorazine ... 2701
Chlorprothixene (Potential for additive central nervous system effects).
No products indexed under this heading.
Chlorprothixene Hydrochloride (Potential for additive central nervous system effects).
No products indexed under this heading.
Chlorprothixene Lactate (Potential for additive central nervous system effects).
No products indexed under this heading.
Clorazepate Dipotassium (Potential for additive central nervous system effects). Products include:
Tranxene ... 459

(▭ Described in PDR For Nonprescription Drugs) (◉ Described in PDR For Ophthalmology)

89 Interactions Index Atrohist Pediatric Dye-Free

Clozapine (Potential for additive central nervous system effects). Products include:
Clozaril Tablets ... 2377

Codeine Phosphate (Potential for additive central nervous system effects). Products include:
Brontex ... 2130
Dimetane-DC Cough Syrup ... 2232
Fioricet with Codeine Capsules ... 2387
Fiorinal with Codeine Capsules ... 2390
Nucofed ... 2225
Phenergan with Codeine ... 2883
Phenergan VC with Codeine ... 2888
Robitussin A-C Syrup ... 2248
Robitussin-DAC Syrup ... 2249
Ryna ... 804
Soma Compound w/Codeine Tablets ... 2784
Tylenol with Codeine ... 1592

Desflurane (Potential for additive central nervous system effects). Products include:
Suprane (desflurane, USP) ... 1865

Dezocine (Potential for additive central nervous system effects). Products include:
Dalgan Injection ... 529

Diazepam (Potential for additive central nervous system effects). Products include:
Dizac (diazepam injectable emulsion) CIV ... 1862
Valium Injectable ... 2336
Valium Tablets ... 2335

Droperidol (Potential for additive central nervous system effects). Products include:
Inapsine Injection ... 462

Enflurane (Potential for additive central nervous system effects).
No products indexed under this heading.

Estazolam (Potential for additive central nervous system effects). Products include:
ProSom Tablets ... 457

Ethchlorvynol (Potential for additive central nervous system effects). Products include:
Placidyl Capsules ... 456

Ethinamate (Potential for additive central nervous system effects).
No products indexed under this heading.

Fentanyl (Potential for additive central nervous system effects). Products include:
Duragesic Transdermal System ... 1336

Fentanyl Citrate (Potential for additive central nervous system effects). Products include:
Sublimaze Injection ... 463

Fluphenazine Decanoate (Potential for additive central nervous system effects). Products include:
Prolixin Decanoate ... 510

Fluphenazine Enanthate (Potential for additive central nervous system effects). Products include:
Prolixin Enanthate ... 510

Fluphenazine Hydrochloride (Potential for additive central nervous system effects). Products include:
Prolixin ... 510

Flurazepam Hydrochloride (Potential for additive central nervous system effects). Products include:
Dalmane Capsules ... 2329

Furazolidone (Prolongs and intensifies the anticholinergic effects of antihistamines and the overall effects of sympathomimetics; concurrent and/or sequential use is not recommended). Products include:
Furoxone ... 2221

Glutethimide (Potential for additive central nervous system effects).
No products indexed under this heading.

Haloperidol (Potential for additive central nervous system effects). Products include:
Haldol Injection, Tablets and Concentrate ... 1585

Haloperidol Decanoate (Potential for additive central nervous system effects). Products include:
Haldol Decanoate ... 1587

Hydrocodone Bitartrate (Potential for additive central nervous system effects). Products include:
Codiclear DH Syrup ... 808
Duratuss HD Elixir ... 2750
Histussin D Liquid ... 670
Hycodan Tablets and Syrup ... 946
Hycomine Compound Tablets ... 948
Hycomine ... 947
Hycotuss Expectorant Syrup ... 950
Hydrocet Capsules ... 787
Lorcet 10/650 Tablets ... 1016
Lortab ... 2751
Tussend ... 1830
Tussend Expectorant ... 1831
Vicodin Tablets ... 1404
Vicodin ES Tablets ... 1405
Vicodin HP Tablets ... 1403
Vicodin Tuss Expectorant ... 1406
Zydone Capsules ... 967

Hydrocodone Polistirex (Potential for additive central nervous system effects). Products include:
Tussionex Pennkinetic Extended-Release Suspension ... 1624

Hydroxyzine Hydrochloride (Potential for additive central nervous system effects). Products include:
Atarax Tablets & Syrup ... 1992
Marax Tablets & DF Syrup ... 2015
Vistaril Intramuscular Solution ... 2042

Isocarboxazid (Prolongs and intensifies the anticholinergic effects of antihistamines and the overall effects of sympathomimetics; concurrent and/or sequential use is not recommended).
No products indexed under this heading.

Isoflurane (Potential for additive central nervous system effects).
No products indexed under this heading.

Ketamine Hydrochloride (Potential for additive central nervous system effects).
No products indexed under this heading.

Levomethadyl Acetate Hydrochloride (Potential for additive central nervous system effects). Products include:
Orlaam Oral Solution ... 2361

Levorphanol Tartrate (Potential for additive central nervous system effects). Products include:
Levo-Dromoran ... 2297

Lorazepam (Potential for additive central nervous system effects). Products include:
Ativan Injection ... 2805
Ativan Tablets ... 2807

Loxapine Hydrochloride (Potential for additive central nervous system effects). Products include:
Loxitane ... 1426

Loxapine Succinate (Potential for additive central nervous system effects). Products include:
Loxitane Capsules ... 1426

Meperidine Hydrochloride (Potential for additive central nervous system effects). Products include:
Demerol ... 2438
Mepergan Injection ... 2859

Mephobarbital (Potential for additive central nervous system effects). Products include:
Mebaral Tablets ... 2452

Meprobamate (Potential for additive central nervous system effects). Products include:
Miltown Tablets ... 2780
PMB 200 and PMB 400 ... 2890

Mesoridazine Besylate (Potential for additive central nervous system effects). Products include:
Serentil ... 689

Methadone Hydrochloride (Potential for additive central nervous system effects). Products include:
Methadone Hydrochloride Oral Concentrate ... 2356
Methadone Hydrochloride Oral Solution & Tablets ... 2357

Methohexital Sodium (Potential for additive central nervous system effects).
No products indexed under this heading.

Methotrimeprazine (Potential for additive central nervous system effects). Products include:
Levoprome ... 1321

Methoxyflurane (Potential for additive central nervous system effects).
No products indexed under this heading.

Midazolam Hydrochloride (Potential for additive central nervous system effects). Products include:
Versed Injection ... 2324

Molindone Hydrochloride (Potential for additive central nervous system effects). Products include:
Moban Tablets and Concentrate ... 1036

Morphine Sulfate (Potential for additive central nervous system effects). Products include:
Astramorph/PF Injection, USP (Preservative-Free) ... 526
Duramorph Injection ... 983
Infumorph 200 and Infumorph 500 Sterile Solutions ... 985
Kadian Capsules ... 2948
MS Contin Tablets ... 2149
MSIR ... 2152
Oramorph SR (Morphine Sulfate Sustained Release Tablets) ... 2359
RMS Suppositories CII ... 2766
Roxanol ... 2365

Opium Alkaloids (Potential for additive central nervous system effects).
No products indexed under this heading.

Oxazepam (Potential for additive central nervous system effects). Products include:
Serax Capsules ... 2916
Serax Tablets ... 2916

Oxycodone Hydrochloride (Potential for additive central nervous system effects). Products include:
OxyContin Tablets ... 2163
OxyIR Capsules ... 2167
Percocet Tablets ... 955
Percodan Tablets ... 955
Percodan-Demi Tablets ... 956
Roxicodone Tablets, Oral Solution & Intensol (Oxycodone) ... 2366
Tylox Capsules ... 1593

Pentobarbital Sodium (Potential for additive central nervous system effects). Products include:
Nembutal Sodium Capsules ... 440
Nembutal Sodium Solution ... 442
Nembutal Sodium Suppositories ... 444

Perphenazine (Potential for additive central nervous system effects). Products include:
Etrafon ... 2495
Triavil Tablets ... 1800
Trilafon ... 2532

Phenelzine Sulfate (Prolongs and intensifies the anticholinergic effects of antihistamines and the overall effects of sympathomimetics; concurrent and/or sequential use is not recommended). Products include:
Nardil ... 1977

Phenobarbital (Potential for additive central nervous system effects). Products include:
Arco-Lase Plus Tablets ... 513
Bellergal-S Tablets ... 2375
Donnatal ... 2234
Donnatal Extentabs ... 2234
Donnatal Tablets ... 2234
Phenobarbital Elixir and Tablets ... 1523
Quadrinal Tablets ... 1398

Prazepam (Potential for additive central nervous system effects).
No products indexed under this heading.

Prochlorperazine (Potential for additive central nervous system effects). Products include:
Compazine ... 2644

Promethazine Hydrochloride (Potential for additive central nervous system effects). Products include:
Mepergan Injection ... 2859
Phenergan with Codeine ... 2883
Phenergan with Dextromethorphan 2885
Phenergan Injection ... 2880
Phenergan Suppositories ... 2882
Phenergan Syrup ... 2881
Phenergan Tablets ... 2882
Phenergan VC ... 2886
Phenergan VC with Codeine ... 2888

Propofol (Potential for additive central nervous system effects). Products include:
Diprivan Injectable Emulsion ... 2939

Propoxyphene Hydrochloride (Potential for additive central nervous system effects). Products include:
Darvon ... 1475
Wygesic Tablets ... 2930

Propoxyphene Napsylate (Potential for additive central nervous system effects). Products include:
Darvon-N/Darvocet-N ... 1473

Quazepam (Potential for additive central nervous system effects). Products include:
Doral Tablets ... 2773

Risperidone (Potential for additive central nervous system effects). Products include:
Risperdal Tablets ... 1348

Secobarbital Sodium (Potential for additive central nervous system effects). Products include:
Seconal Sodium Pulvules ... 1529

Selegiline Hydrochloride (Prolongs and intensifies the anticholinergic effects of antihistamines and the overall effects of sympathomimetics; concurrent and/or sequential use is not recommended). Products include:
Eldepryl Capsules ... 2729

Sevoflurane (Potential for additive central nervous system effects).
No products indexed under this heading.

Sufentanil Citrate (Potential for additive central nervous system effects). Products include:
Sufenta Injection ... 1355

Temazepam (Potential for additive central nervous system effects). Products include:
Restoril Capsules ... 2413

Thiamylal Sodium (Potential for additive central nervous system effects).
No products indexed under this heading.

IMPORTANT NOTE: Always consult each drug listing in the patient's regimen for possible interactions.

Atrohist Pediatric Dye-Free — Interactions Index

Thioridazine Hydrochloride (Potential for additive central nervous system effects). Products include:
- Mellaril 2398

Thiothixene (Potential for additive central nervous system effects). Products include:
- Navane Capsules and Concentrate .. 2018
- Navane Intramuscular 2019

Tranylcypromine Sulfate (Prolongs and intensifies the anticholinergic effects of antihistamines and the overall effects of sympathomimetics; concurrent and/or sequential use is not recommended). Products include:
- Parnate Tablets 2679

Triazolam (Potential for additive central nervous system effects). Products include:
- Halcion Tablets 2093

Trifluoperazine Hydrochloride (Potential for additive central nervous system effects). Products include:
- Stelazine 2692

Zolpidem Tartrate (Potential for additive central nervous system effects). Products include:
- Ambien Tablets 2559

Food Interactions

Alcohol (Potential for additive central nervous system effects).

ATROHIST PLUS TABLETS

(Chlorpheniramine Maleate, Phenylpropanolamine Hydrochloride, Phenylephrine Hydrochloride, Hyoscyamine Sulfate, Atropine Sulfate, Scopolamine Hydrobromide) 1605
May interact with monoamine oxidase inhibitors, hypnotics and sedatives, tranquilizers, and certain other agents. Compounds in these categories include:

Alprazolam (Possible additive drowsiness effects). Products include:
- Xanax Tablets 2115

Buspirone Hydrochloride (Possible additive drowsiness effects). Products include:
- BuSpar Tablets 738

Chlordiazepoxide (Possible additive drowsiness effects). Products include:
- Limbitrol 2333

Chlordiazepoxide Hydrochloride (Possible additive drowsiness effects). Products include:
- Librax Capsules 2330
- Librium Capsules 2331
- Librium Injectable 2332

Chlorpromazine (Possible additive drowsiness effects). Products include:
- Thorazine Suppositories 2701

Chlorpromazine Hydrochloride (Possible additive drowsiness effects). Products include:
- Thorazine 2701

Chlorprothixene (Possible additive drowsiness effects).
No products indexed under this heading.

Chlorprothixene Hydrochloride (Possible additive drowsiness effects).
No products indexed under this heading.

Clorazepate Dipotassium (Possible additive drowsiness effects). Products include:
- Tranxene 459

Diazepam (Possible additive drowsiness effects). Products include:
- Dizac (diazepam injectable emulsion) CIV 1862
- Valium Injectable 2336
- Valium Tablets 2335

Droperidol (Possible additive drowsiness effects). Products include:
- Inapsine Injection 462

Estazolam (Possible additive drowsiness effects). Products include:
- ProSom Tablets 457

Ethchlorvynol (Possible additive drowsiness effects). Products include:
- Placidyl Capsules 456

Ethinamate (Possible additive drowsiness effects).
No products indexed under this heading.

Fluphenazine Decanoate (Possible additive drowsiness effects). Products include:
- Prolixin Decanoate 510

Fluphenazine Enanthate (Possible additive drowsiness effects). Products include:
- Prolixin Enanthate 510

Fluphenazine Hydrochloride (Possible additive drowsiness effects). Products include:
- Prolixin 510

Flurazepam Hydrochloride (Possible additive drowsiness effects). Products include:
- Dalmane Capsules 2329

Furazolidone (Concomitant and/or sequential use with monoamine oxidase inhibitors is contraindicated). Products include:
- Furoxone 2221

Glutethimide (Possible additive drowsiness effects).
No products indexed under this heading.

Haloperidol (Possible additive drowsiness effects). Products include:
- Haldol Injection, Tablets and Concentrate 1585

Haloperidol Decanoate (Possible additive drowsiness effects). Products include:
- Haldol Decanoate 1587

Hydroxyzine Hydrochloride (Possible additive drowsiness effects). Products include:
- Atarax Tablets & Syrup 1992
- Marax Tablets & DF Syrup ... 2015
- Vistaril Intramuscular Solution ... 2042

Isocarboxazid (Concomitant and/or sequential use with monoamine oxidase inhibitors is contraindicated).
No products indexed under this heading.

Lorazepam (Possible additive drowsiness effects). Products include:
- Ativan Injection 2805
- Ativan Tablets 2807

Loxapine Hydrochloride (Possible additive drowsiness effects). Products include:
- Loxitane 1426

Loxapine Succinate (Possible additive drowsiness effects). Products include:
- Loxitane Capsules 1426

Meprobamate (Possible additive drowsiness effects). Products include:
- Miltown Tablets 2780
- PMB 200 and PMB 400 2890

Mesoridazine Besylate (Possible additive drowsiness effects). Products include:
- Serentil 689

Midazolam Hydrochloride (Possible additive drowsiness effects). Products include:
- Versed Injection 2324

Molindone Hydrochloride (Possible additive drowsiness effects). Products include:
- Moban Tablets and Concentrate 1036

Oxazepam (Possible additive drowsiness effects). Products include:
- Serax Capsules 2916
- Serax Tablets 2916

Perphenazine (Possible additive drowsiness effects). Products include:
- Etrafon 2495
- Triavil Tablets 1800
- Trilafon 2532

Phenelzine Sulfate (Concomitant and/or sequential use with monoamine oxidase inhibitors is contraindicated). Products include:
- Nardil 1977

Prazepam (Possible additive drowsiness effects).
No products indexed under this heading.

Prochlorperazine (Possible additive drowsiness effects). Products include:
- Compazine 2644

Promethazine Hydrochloride (Possible additive drowsiness effects). Products include:
- Mepergan Injection 2859
- Phenergan with Codeine 2883
- Phenergan with Dextromethorphan ... 2885
- Phenergan Injection 2880
- Phenergan Suppositories 2882
- Phenergan Syrup 2881
- Phenergan Tablets 2882
- Phenergan VC 2886
- Phenergan VC with Codeine .. 2888

Propofol (Possible additive drowsiness effects). Products include:
- Diprivan Injectable Emulsion ... 2939

Quazepam (Possible additive drowsiness effects). Products include:
- Doral Tablets 2773

Secobarbital Sodium (Possible additive drowsiness effects). Products include:
- Seconal Sodium Pulvules 1529

Selegiline Hydrochloride (Concomitant and/or sequential use with monoamine oxidase inhibitors is contraindicated). Products include:
- Eldepryl Capsules 2729

Temazepam (Possible additive drowsiness effects). Products include:
- Restoril Capsules 2413

Thioridazine Hydrochloride (Possible additive drowsiness effects). Products include:
- Mellaril 2398

Thiothixene (Possible additive drowsiness effects). Products include:
- Navane Capsules and Concentrate .. 2018
- Navane Intramuscular 2019

Tranylcypromine Sulfate (Concomitant and/or sequential use with monoamine oxidase inhibitors is contraindicated). Products include:
- Parnate Tablets 2679

Triazolam (Possible additive drowsiness effects). Products include:
- Halcion Tablets 2093

Trifluoperazine Hydrochloride (Possible additive drowsiness effects). Products include:
- Stelazine 2692

Zolpidem Tartrate (Possible additive drowsiness effects). Products include:
- Ambien Tablets 2559

Food Interactions

Alcohol (Possible additive drowsiness effects).

ATROMID-S CAPSULES

(Clofibrate) 2808
May interact with anticoagulants and certain other agents. Compounds in these categories include:

Dalteparin Sodium (To prevent bleeding complications, anticoagulant dosage should be reduced generally by one-half). Products include:
- Fragmin Injection 2088

Dicumarol (To prevent bleeding complications, anticoagulant dosage should be reduced generally by one-half).
No products indexed under this heading.

Enoxaparin (To prevent bleeding complications, anticoagulant dosage should be reduced generally by one-half). Products include:
- Lovenox Injection 2187

Heparin Calcium (To prevent bleeding complications, anticoagulant dosage should be reduced generally by one-half).
No products indexed under this heading.

Heparin Sodium (To prevent bleeding complications, anticoagulant dosage should be reduced generally by one-half). Products include:
- Heparin Lock Flush Solution ... 2831
- Heparin Sodium Injection ... 2832
- Heparin Sodium Vials 1486

Lovastatin (Potential for fulminant rhabdomyolysis, myopathy, and acute renal failure). Products include:
- Mevacor Tablets 1742

Phenytoin (Atromid-S may displace phenytoin from its binding site). Products include:
- Dilantin Infatabs 1967
- Dilantin-125 Suspension 1969

Phenytoin Sodium (Atromid-S may displace phenytoin from its binding site). Products include:
- Dilantin Kapseals 1965

Tolbutamide (Increased hypoglycemic effect; Atromid-S may displace tolbutamide from its binding site).
No products indexed under this heading.

Warfarin Sodium (To prevent bleeding complications, anticoagulant dosage should be reduced generally by one-half). Products include:
- Coumadin 941

ATROVENT INHALATION AEROSOL

(Ipratropium Bromide) 674
None cited in PDR database.

ATROVENT INHALATION SOLUTION

(Ipratropium Bromide) 675
None cited in PDR database.

ATROVENT NASAL SPRAY 0.03%

(Ipratropium Bromide) 676
May interact with anticholinergics. Compounds in this category include:

Interactions Index / Augmentin

Atropine Sulfate (Some potential for an additive interaction with other concomitantly administered anticholinergic drugs). Products include:
- Arco-Lase Plus Tablets 513
- Atrohist Plus Tablets 1605
- Donnatal 2234
- Donnatal Extentabs 2234
- Donnatal Tablets 2234
- Lomotil 2591
- Motofen Tablets 789
- Urised Tablets 2123

Belladonna Alkaloids (Some potential for an additive interaction with other concomitantly administered anticholinergic drugs). Products include:
- Bellergal-S Tablets 2375
- Hyland's Bedwetting Tablets 788
- Hyland's EnurAid Tablets 789
- Hyland's Headache Tablets 790
- Hyland's Teething Tablets 790
- Similasan Eye Drops #1 769

Benztropine Mesylate (Some potential for an additive interaction with other concomitantly administered anticholinergic drugs). Products include:
- Cogentin 1661

Biperiden Hydrochloride (Some potential for an additive interaction with other concomitantly administered anticholinergic drugs). Products include:
- Akineton 1380

Clidinium Bromide (Some potential for an additive interaction with other concomitantly administered anticholinergic drugs). Products include:
- Librax Capsules 2330

Dicyclomine Hydrochloride (Some potential for an additive interaction with other concomitantly administered anticholinergic drugs). Products include:
- Bentyl 1246

Glycopyrrolate (Some potential for an additive interaction with other concomitantly administered anticholinergic drugs). Products include:
- Robinul Forte Tablets 2247
- Robinul Injectable 2247
- Robinul Tablets 2247

Hyoscyamine (Some potential for an additive interaction with other concomitantly administered anticholinergic drugs). Products include:
- Cystospaz Tablets 2123
- Urised Tablets 2123

Hyoscyamine Sulfate (Some potential for an additive interaction with other concomitantly administered anticholinergic drugs). Products include:
- Arco-Lase Plus Tablets 513
- Atrohist Plus Tablets 1605
- Cystospaz-M Capsules 2123
- Donnatal 2234
- Donnatal Extentabs 2234
- Donnatal Tablets 2234
- Kutrase Capsules 2546
- Levsin/Levsinex/Levbid 2549

Mepenzolate Bromide (Some potential for an additive interaction with other concomitantly administered anticholinergic drugs).
- No products indexed under this heading.

Oxybutynin Chloride (Some potential for an additive interaction with other concomitantly administered anticholinergic drugs). Products include:
- Ditropan 1267

Procyclidine Hydrochloride (Some potential for an additive interaction with other concomitantly administered anticholinergic drugs). Products include:
- Kemadrin Tablets 1105

Propantheline Bromide (Some potential for an additive interaction with other concomitantly administered anticholinergic drugs). Products include:
- Pro-Banthine Tablets 2226

Scopolamine (Some potential for an additive interaction with other concomitantly administered anticholinergic drugs). Products include:
- Transderm Scop Transdermal Therapeutic System 890

Scopolamine Hydrobromide (Some potential for an additive interaction with other concomitantly administered anticholinergic drugs). Products include:
- Atrohist Plus Tablets 1605
- Donnatal 2234
- Donnatal Extentabs 2234
- Donnatal Tablets 2234

Tridihexethyl Chloride (Some potential for an additive interaction with other concomitantly administered anticholinergic drugs).
- No products indexed under this heading.

Trihexyphenidyl Hydrochloride (Some potential for an additive interaction with other concomitantly administered anticholinergic drugs). Products include:
- Artane 1418

ATROVENT NASAL SPRAY 0.06%
(Ipratropium Bromide) 678
May interact with anticholinergics. Compounds in this category include:

Atropine Sulfate (Some potential for an additive interaction with other concomitantly administered anticholinergic drugs). Products include:
- Arco-Lase Plus Tablets 513
- Atrohist Plus Tablets 1605
- Donnatal 2234
- Donnatal Extentabs 2234
- Donnatal Tablets 2234
- Lomotil 2591
- Motofen Tablets 789
- Urised Tablets 2123

Belladonna Alkaloids (Some potential for an additive interaction with other concomitantly administered anticholinergic drugs). Products include:
- Bellergal-S Tablets 2375
- Hyland's Bedwetting Tablets 788
- Hyland's EnurAid Tablets 789
- Hyland's Headache Tablets 790
- Hyland's Teething Tablets 790
- Similasan Eye Drops #1 769

Benztropine Mesylate (Some potential for an additive interaction with other concomitantly administered anticholinergic drugs). Products include:
- Cogentin 1661

Biperiden Hydrochloride (Some potential for an additive interaction with other concomitantly administered anticholinergic drugs). Products include:
- Akineton 1380

Clidinium Bromide (Some potential for an additive interaction with other concomitantly administered anticholinergic drugs). Products include:
- Librax Capsules 2330

Dicyclomine Hydrochloride (Some potential for an additive interaction with other concomitantly administered anticholinergic drugs). Products include:
- Bentyl 1246

Glycopyrrolate (Some potential for an additive interaction with other concomitantly administered anticholinergic drugs). Products include:
- Robinul Forte Tablets 2247
- Robinul Injectable 2247
- Robinul Tablets 2247

Hyoscyamine (Some potential for an additive interaction with other concomitantly administered anticholinergic drugs). Products include:
- Cystospaz Tablets 2123
- Urised Tablets 2123

Hyoscyamine Sulfate (Some potential for an additive interaction with other concomitantly administered anticholinergic drugs). Products include:
- Arco-Lase Plus Tablets 513
- Atrohist Plus Tablets 1605
- Cystospaz-M Capsules 2123
- Donnatal 2234
- Donnatal Extentabs 2234
- Donnatal Tablets 2234
- Kutrase Capsules 2546
- Levsin/Levsinex/Levbid 2549

Mepenzolate Bromide (Some potential for an additive interaction with other concomitantly administered anticholinergic drugs).
- No products indexed under this heading.

Oxybutynin Chloride (Some potential for an additive interaction with other concomitantly administered anticholinergic drugs). Products include:
- Ditropan 1267

Procyclidine Hydrochloride (Some potential for an additive interaction with other concomitantly administered anticholinergic drugs). Products include:
- Kemadrin Tablets 1105

Propantheline Bromide (Some potential for an additive interaction with other concomitantly administered anticholinergic drugs). Products include:
- Pro-Banthine Tablets 2226

Scopolamine (Some potential for an additive interaction with other concomitantly administered anticholinergic drugs). Products include:
- Transderm Scop Transdermal Therapeutic System 890

Scopolamine Hydrobromide (Some potential for an additive interaction with other concomitantly administered anticholinergic drugs). Products include:
- Atrohist Plus Tablets 1605
- Donnatal 2234
- Donnatal Extentabs 2234
- Donnatal Tablets 2234

Tridihexethyl Chloride (Some potential for an additive interaction with other concomitantly administered anticholinergic drugs).
- No products indexed under this heading.

Trihexyphenidyl Hydrochloride (Some potential for an additive interaction with other concomitantly administered anticholinergic drugs). Products include:
- Artane 1418

A/T/S 2% ACNE TOPICAL GEL
(Erythromycin) 1244
May interact with:

Concomitant Topical Acne Therapy (Potential for cumulative irritant effect).

A/T/S 2% ACNE TOPICAL SOLUTION
(Erythromycin) 1244
May interact with:

Concomitant Topical Acne Therapy (Potential for cumulative irritant effect).

ATTENUVAX
(Measles Virus Vaccine Live) 1650
May interact with immunosuppressive agents. Compounds in this category include:

Azathioprine (Concurrent use in individuals on immunosuppressive therapy is contraindicated). Products include:
- Azathioprine Tablets 2349
- Imuran 1103

Cyclosporine (Concurrent use in individuals on immunosuppressive therapy is contraindicated). Products include:
- Neoral 2405
- Sandimmune 2416

Immune Globulin (Human) (Concurrent use in individuals on immunosuppressive therapy is contraindicated).
- No products indexed under this heading.

Muromonab-CD3 (Concurrent use in individuals on immunosuppressive therapy is contraindicated). Products include:
- Orthoclone OKT3 Sterile Solution .. 1892

Mycophenolate Mofetil (Concurrent use in individuals on immunosuppressive therapy is contraindicated). Products include:
- CellCept Capsules 2265

Tacrolimus (Concurrent use in individuals on immunosuppressive therapy is contraindicated). Products include:
- Prograf 1028

AUGMENTIN CHEWABLE TABLETS
(Amoxicillin Trihydrate, Clavulanate Potassium) 2637
See **Augmentin Tablets**

AUGMENTIN POWDER FOR ORAL SUSPENSION
(Amoxicillin Trihydrate, Clavulanate Potassium) 2637
See **Augmentin Tablets**

AUGMENTIN TABLETS
(Amoxicillin Trihydrate, Clavulanate Potassium) 2640
May interact with:

Allopurinol (Substantially increased incidence of rashes has been reported with ampicillin; no data with Augmentin and allopurinol administered concurrently). Products include:
- Zyloprim Tablets 1194

Probenecid (Decreases the renal tubular secretion of amoxicillin; concurrent use may result in increased and prolonged blood levels of amoxicillin; co-administration is not recommended). Products include:
- Benemid Tablets 1651
- ColBENEMID Tablets 1662

IMPORTANT NOTE: Always consult each drug listing in the patient's regimen for possible interactions.

Augmentin **Interactions Index** 92

AURALGAN OTIC SOLUTION
(Antipyrine, Benzocaine, Glycerin) 2810
None cited in PDR database.

AVONEX
(Interferon Beta-1a) 662
May interact with:

Bone Marrow Depressants, unspecified (Co-administration with myelosuppressive agents requires careful patient monitoring).

AXID PULVULES
(Nizatidine) 1468
May interact with:

Aspirin (Increased serum salicylate levels when nizatidine is given concurrently with very high doses (3,900 mg) of aspirin). Products include:
- Alka-Seltzer Cherry Effervescent Antacid and Pain Reliever .... ▣ 609
- Alka-Seltzer Extra Strength Effervescent Antacid and Pain Reliever .... ▣ 609
- Alka-Seltzer Lemon Lime Effervescent Antacid and Pain Reliever .... ▣ 609
- Alka-Seltzer Original Effervescent Antacid and Pain Reliever .... ▣ 609
- Alka-Seltzer Plus .... ▣ 611
- Alka-Seltzer Plus Sinus Medicine .. ▣ 611
- Ascriptin .... ▣ 650
- Arthritis Strength BC Powder......... ▣ 631
- BC Cold Powder Multi-Symptom Formula (Cold-Sinus-Allergy) ...... ▣ 631
- BC Cold Powder Non-Drowsy Formula (Cold-Sinus) .... ▣ 631
- BC Powder .... ▣ 631
- Genuine Bayer Aspirin Tablets & Caplets .... ▣ 618
- Extra Strength Bayer Arthritis Pain Regimen Formula .... ▣ 615
- Extra Strength Bayer Aspirin Caplets & Tablets .... ▣ 617
- Extended-Release Bayer 8-Hour Aspirin .... ▣ 616
- Extra Strength Bayer Plus Aspirin Caplets .... ▣ 617
- Extra Strength Bayer PM Aspirin Plus Sleep Aid .... ▣ 617
- Aspirin Regimen Bayer 81 mg Tablets with Calcium .... ▣ 615
- Aspirin Regimen Bayer Adult Low Strength 81 mg Tablets .... ▣ 613
- Aspirin Regimen Bayer Children's Chewable Aspirin .... ▣ 616
- Aspirin Regimen Bayer Regular Strength 325 mg Caplets .... ▣ 613
- Bufferin Analgesic Tablets........ ▣ 636
- Arthritis Strength Bufferin Analgesic Caplets .... ▣ 637
- Extra Strength Bufferin Analgesic Tablets .... ▣ 637
- Cama Arthritis Pain Reliever........ ▣ 748
- Darvon Compound-65 Pulvules 1475
- Easprin 1971
- Ecotrin 2625
- Ecotrin Enteric Coated Aspirin Maximum Strength Tablets and Caplets .... ▣ 775
- Ecotrin Enteric Coated Aspirin Regular Strength Tablets 2625
- Empirin Aspirin Tablets .... ▣ 818
- Excedrin Extra-Strength Analgesic Tablets, Caplets, and Geltabs........ 734
- Fiorinal Capsules 2388
- Fiorinal with Codeine Capsules 2390
- Fiorinal Tablets 2388
- Goody's Extra Strength Headache Powders .... ▣ 632
- Goody's Extra Strength Pain Relief Tablets .... ▣ 632
- Halfprin Tablets 1413
- Norgesic 1554
- Percodan Tablets 955
- Percodan-Demi Tablets 956
- Robaxisal Tablets 2246
- Soma Compound w/Codeine Tablets 2784
- Soma Compound Tablets 2783
- St. Joseph Adult Chewable Aspirin (81 mg.) .... ▣ 768
- Talwin Compound 2466
- Vanquish Analgesic Caplets .... ▣ 627

AXOCET CAPSULES
(Acetaminophen, Butalbital)................2469
May interact with monoamine oxidase inhibitors, narcotic analgesics, general anesthetics, hypnotics and sedatives, tranquilizers, central nervous system depressants, and certain other agents. Compounds in these categories include:

Alfentanil Hydrochloride (Co-administration may cause increased CNS depression). Products include:
- Alfenta Injection 1334

Alprazolam (Co-administration may cause increased CNS depression). Products include:
- Xanax Tablets 2115

Aprobarbital (Co-administration may cause increased CNS depression).
- No products indexed under this heading.

Buprenorphine (Co-administration may cause increased CNS depression). Products include:
- Buprenex Injectable 2170

Buspirone Hydrochloride (Co-administration may cause increased CNS depression). Products include:
- BuSpar Tablets 738

Butabarbital (Co-administration may cause increased CNS depression).
- No products indexed under this heading.

Chlordiazepoxide (Co-administration may cause increased CNS depression). Products include:
- Limbitrol 2333

Chlordiazepoxide Hydrochloride (Co-administration may cause increased CNS depression). Products include:
- Librax Capsules 2330
- Librium Capsules 2331
- Librium Injectable 2332

Chlorpromazine (Co-administration may cause increased CNS depression). Products include:
- Thorazine Suppositories 2701

Chlorpromazine Hydrochloride (Co-administration may cause increased CNS depression). Products include:
- Thorazine 2701

Chlorprothixene (Co-administration may cause increased CNS depression).
- No products indexed under this heading.

Chlorprothixene Hydrochloride (Co-administration may cause increased CNS depression).
- No products indexed under this heading.

Chlorprothixene Lactate (Co-administration may cause increased CNS depression).
- No products indexed under this heading.

Clorazepate Dipotassium (Co-administration may cause increased CNS depression). Products include:
- Tranxene 459

Clozapine (Co-administration may cause increased CNS depression). Products include:
- Clozaril Tablets 2377

Codeine Phosphate (Co-administration may cause increased CNS depression). Products include:
- Brontex 2130
- Dimetane-DC Cough Syrup 2232
- Fioricet with Codeine Capsules 2387
- Fiorinal with Codeine Capsules 2390
- Nucofed 2225
- Phenergan with Codeine 2883
- Phenergan VC with Codeine 2888
- Robitussin A-C Syrup 2248
- Robitussin-DAC Syrup 2249
- Ryna .... ▣ 804
- Soma Compound w/Codeine Tablets 2784
- Tylenol with Codeine 1592

Desflurane (Co-administration may cause increased CNS depression). Products include:
- Suprane (desflurane, USP) 1865

Dezocine (Co-administration may cause increased CNS depression). Products include:
- Dalgan Injection 529

Diazepam (Co-administration may cause increased CNS depression). Products include:
- Dizac (diazepam injectable emulsion) CIV 1862
- Valium Injectable 2336
- Valium Tablets 2335

Droperidol (Co-administration may cause increased CNS depression). Products include:
- Inapsine Injection 462

Enflurane (Co-administration may cause increased CNS depression).
- No products indexed under this heading.

Estazolam (Co-administration may cause increased CNS depression). Products include:
- ProSom Tablets 457

Ethchlorvynol (Co-administration may cause increased CNS depression). Products include:
- Placidyl Capsules 456

Ethinamate (Co-administration may cause increased CNS depression).
- No products indexed under this heading.

Fentanyl (Co-administration may cause increased CNS depression). Products include:
- Duragesic Transdermal System........ 1336

Fentanyl Citrate (Co-administration may cause increased CNS depression). Products include:
- Sublimaze Injection 463

Fluphenazine Decanoate (Co-administration may cause increased CNS depression). Products include:
- Prolixin Decanoate 510

Fluphenazine Enanthate (Co-administration may cause increased CNS depression). Products include:
- Prolixin Enanthate 510

Fluphenazine Hydrochloride (Co-administration may cause increased CNS depression). Products include:
- Prolixin 510

Flurazepam Hydrochloride (Co-administration may cause increased CNS depression). Products include:
- Dalmane Capsules 2329

Furazolidone (The CNS effects of butalbital may be potentiated by monoamine oxidase inhibitors). Products include:
- Furoxone 2221

Glutethimide (Co-administration may cause increased CNS depression).
- No products indexed under this heading.

Haloperidol (Co-administration may cause increased CNS depression). Products include:
- Haldol Injection, Tablets and Concentrate 1585

Haloperidol Decanoate (Co-administration may cause increased CNS depression). Products include:
- Haldol Decanoate 1587

Hydrocodone Bitartrate (Co-administration may cause increased CNS depression). Products include:
- Codiclear DH Syrup 808
- Duratuss HD Elixir 2750
- Histussin D Liquid 670
- Hycodan Tablets and Syrup 946
- Hycomine Compound Tablets 948
- Hycomine 947
- Hycotuss Expectorant Syrup 950
- Hydrocet Capsules 787
- Lorcet 10/650 Tablets 1016
- Lortab 2751
- Tussend 1830
- Tussend Expectorant 1831
- Vicodin Tablets 1404
- Vicodin ES Tablets 1405
- Vicodin HP Tablets 1403
- Vicodin Tuss Expectorant 1406
- Zydone Capsules 967

Hydrocodone Polistirex (Co-administration may cause increased CNS depression). Products include:
- Tussionex Pennkinetic Extended-Release Suspension 1624

Hydromorphone Hydrochloride (Co-administration may cause increased CNS depression). Products include:
- Dilaudid Ampules 1382
- Dilaudid Cough Syrup 1383
- Dilaudid-HP Injection 1384
- Dilaudid-HP Lyophilized Powder 250 mg 1384
- Dilaudid 1382
- Dilaudid Oral Liquid 1386
- Dilaudid 1382
- Dilaudid Tablets - 8 mg 1386

Hydroxyzine Hydrochloride (Co-administration may cause increased CNS depression). Products include:
- Atarax Tablets & Syrup 1992
- Marax Tablets & DF Syrup 2015
- Vistaril Intramuscular Solution 2042

Isocarboxazid (The CNS effects of butalbital may be potentiated by monoamine oxidase inhibitors).
- No products indexed under this heading.

Isoflurane (Co-administration may cause increased CNS depression).
- No products indexed under this heading.

Ketamine Hydrochloride (Co-administration may cause increased CNS depression).
- No products indexed under this heading.

Levomethadyl Acetate Hydrochloride (Co-administration may cause increased CNS depression). Products include:
- Orlaam Oral Solution 2361

Levorphanol Tartrate (Co-administration may cause increased CNS depression). Products include:
- Levo-Dromoran 2297

Lorazepam (Co-administration may cause increased CNS depression). Products include:
- Ativan Injection 2805
- Ativan Tablets 2807

Loxapine Hydrochloride (Co-administration may cause increased CNS depression). Products include:
- Loxitane 1426

Loxapine Succinate (Co-administration may cause increased CNS depression). Products include:
- Loxitane Capsules 1426

Meperidine Hydrochloride (Co-administration may cause increased CNS depression). Products include:
- Demerol 2438
- Mepergan Injection 2859

Mephobarbital (Co-administration may cause increased CNS depression). Products include:
- Mebaral Tablets 2452

(▣ Described in PDR For Nonprescription Drugs) (◉ Described in PDR For Ophthalmology)

Meprobamate (Co-administration may cause increased CNS depression). Products include:
Miltown Tablets 2780
PMB 200 and PMB 400 2890

Mesoridazine Besylate (Co-administration may cause increased CNS depression). Products include:
Serentil 689

Methadone Hydrochloride (Co-administration may cause increased CNS depression). Products include:
Methadone Hydrochloride Oral Concentrate 2356
Methadone Hydrochloride Oral Solution & Tablets 2357

Methohexital Sodium (Co-administration may cause increased CNS depression).
No products indexed under this heading.

Methoxyflurane (Co-administration may cause increased CNS depression).
No products indexed under this heading.

Midazolam Hydrochloride (Co-administration may cause increased CNS depression). Products include:
Versed Injection 2324

Molindone Hydrochloride (Co-administration may cause increased CNS depression). Products include:
Moban Tablets and Concentrate 1036

Morphine Sulfate (Co-administration may cause increased CNS depression). Products include:
Astramorph/PF Injection, USP (Preservative-Free) 526
Duramorph Injection 983
Infumorph 200 and Infumorph 500 Sterile Solutions 985
Kadian Capsules 2948
MS Contin Tablets 2149
MSIR 2152
Oramorph SR (Morphine Sulfate Sustained Release Tablets) 2359
RMS Suppositories CII 2766
Roxanol 2365

Opium Alkaloids (Co-administration may cause increased CNS depression).
No products indexed under this heading.

Oxazepam (Co-administration may cause increased CNS depression). Products include:
Serax Capsules 2916
Serax Tablets 2916

Oxycodone Hydrochloride (Co-administration may cause increased CNS depression). Products include:
OxyContin Tablets 2163
OxyIR Capsules 2167
Percocet Tablets 955
Percodan Tablets 955
Percodan-Demi Tablets 956
Roxicodone Tablets, Oral Solution & Intensol (Oxycodone) 2366
Tylox Capsules 1593

Pentobarbital Sodium (Co-administration may cause increased CNS depression). Products include:
Nembutal Sodium Capsules 440
Nembutal Sodium Solution 442
Nembutal Sodium Suppositories 444

Perphenazine (Co-administration may cause increased CNS depression). Products include:
Etrafon 2495
Triavil Tablets 1800
Trilafon 2532

Phenelzine Sulfate (The CNS effects of butalbital may be potentiated by monoamine oxidase inhibitors). Products include:
Nardil 1977

Phenobarbital (Co-administration may cause increased CNS depression). Products include:
Arco-Lase Plus Tablets 513

Bellergal-S Tablets 2375
Donnatal 2234
Donnatal Extentabs 2234
Donnatal Tablets 2234
Phenobarbital Elixir and Tablets 1523
Quadrinal Tablets 1398

Prazepam (Co-administration may cause increased CNS depression).
No products indexed under this heading.

Prochlorperazine (Co-administration may cause increased CNS depression). Products include:
Compazine 2644

Promethazine Hydrochloride (Co-administration may cause increased CNS depression). Products include:
Mepergan Injection 2859
Phenergan with Codeine 2883
Phenergan with Dextromethorphan ... 2885
Phenergan Injection 2880
Phenergan Suppositories 2882
Phenergan Syrup 2881
Phenergan Tablets 2882
Phenergan VC 2886
Phenergan VC with Codeine 2888

Propofol (Co-administration may cause increased CNS depression). Products include:
Diprivan Injectable Emulsion 2939

Propoxyphene Hydrochloride (Co-administration may cause increased CNS depression). Products include:
Darvon 1475
Wygesic Tablets 2930

Propoxyphene Napsylate (Co-administration may cause increased CNS depression). Products include:
Darvon-N/Darvocet-N 1473

Quazepam (Co-administration may cause increased CNS depression). Products include:
Doral Tablets 2773

Risperidone (Co-administration may cause increased CNS depression). Products include:
Risperdal Tablets 1348

Secobarbital Sodium (Co-administration may cause increased CNS depression). Products include:
Seconal Sodium Pulvules 1529

Selegiline Hydrochloride (The CNS effects of butalbital may be potentiated by monoamine oxidase inhibitors). Products include:
Eldepryl Capsules 2729

Sevoflurane (Co-administration may cause increased CNS depression).
No products indexed under this heading.

Sufentanil Citrate (Co-administration may cause increased CNS depression). Products include:
Sufenta Injection 1355

Temazepam (Co-administration may cause increased CNS depression). Products include:
Restoril Capsules 2413

Thiamylal Sodium (Co-administration may cause increased CNS depression).
No products indexed under this heading.

Thioridazine Hydrochloride (Co-administration may cause increased CNS depression). Products include:
Mellaril 2398

Thiothixene (Co-administration may cause increased CNS depression). Products include:
Navane Capsules and Concentrate .. 2018
Navane Intramuscular 2019

Tranylcypromine Sulfate (The CNS effects of butalbital may be potentiated by monoamine oxidase inhibitors). Products include:
Parnate Tablets 2679

Triazolam (Co-administration may cause increased CNS depression). Products include:
Halcion Tablets 2093

Trifluoperazine Hydrochloride (Co-administration may cause increased CNS depression). Products include:
Stelazine 2692

Zolpidem Tartrate (Co-administration may cause increased CNS depression). Products include:
Ambien Tablets 2559

Food Interactions
Alcohol (Concurrent use may cause increased CNS depression).

AYGESTIN TABLETS
(Norethindrone Acetate) 990
None cited in PDR database.

AYR SALINE NASAL DROPS
(Sodium Chloride) 606
None cited in PDR database.

AYR SALINE NASAL GEL
(Sodium Chloride) 606
None cited in PDR database.

AYR SALINE NASAL MIST
(Sodium Chloride) 606
None cited in PDR database.

AZACTAM FOR INJECTION
(Aztreonam) 736
May interact with aminoglycosides and certain other agents. Compounds in these categories include:

Amikacin Sulfate (Renal function should be monitored if used concurrently or if higher dosages of aminoglycosides are used). Products include:
Amikacin Sulfate Injection, USP 523
Amikacin Sulfate Injection, USP 981
Amikin Injectable 502

Cefoxitin Sodium (Beta-lactamase inducing antibiotics may antagonize aztreonam). Products include:
Mefoxin 1734
Mefoxin Premixed Intravenous Solution 1737

Gentamicin Sulfate (Renal function should be monitored if used concurrently or if higher dosages of aminoglycosides are used). Products include:
Garamycin Cream 0.1% 2501
Garamycin Injectable 2502
Garamycin Ointment 0.1% 2501
Garamycin Ophthalmic 2501
Genoptic Sterile Ophthalmic Solution 241
Genoptic Sterile Ophthalmic Ointment 241
Gentak 209
Pred-G Liquifilm Sterile Ophthalmic Suspension 248
Pred-G S.O.P. Sterile Ophthalmic Ointment 249

Kanamycin Sulfate (Renal function should be monitored if used concurrently or if higher dosages of aminoglycosides are used).
No products indexed under this heading.

Streptomycin Sulfate (Renal function should be monitored if used concurrently or if higher dosages of aminoglycosides are used). Products include:
Streptomycin Sulfate Injection 2031

Tobramycin (Renal function should be monitored if used concurrently or if higher dosages of aminoglycosides are used). Products include:
AKTOB 207
TobraDex Ophthalmic Suspension and Ointment 469
Tobrex Ophthalmic Ointment and Solution 226

Tobramycin Sulfate (Renal function should be monitored if used concurrently or if higher dosages of aminoglycosides are used). Products include:
Nebcin Vials, Hyporets & ADD-Vantage 1518

AZATHIOPRINE TABLETS
(Azathioprine) 2349
May interact with ACE inhibitors and certain other agents. Compounds in these categories include:

Allopurinol (Inhibits the principal pathway for detoxification of azathioprine; reduce azathioprine dosage by $1/3$ to $1/4$ the usual dose). Products include:
Zyloprim Tablets 1194

Benazepril Hydrochloride (Co-administration has been reported to induce severe leukopenia). Products include:
Lotensin Tablets 852
Lotensin HCT Tablets 855
Lotrel Capsules 858

Captopril (Co-administration has been reported to induce severe leukopenia). Products include:
Capoten Tablets 740
Capozide Tablets 744

Enalapril Maleate (Co-administration has been reported to induce severe leukopenia). Products include:
Vaseretic Tablets 1810
Vasotec Tablets 1816

Enalaprilat (Co-administration has been reported to induce severe leukopenia). Products include:
Vasotec I.V. 1814

Fosinopril Sodium (Co-administration has been reported to induce severe leukopenia). Products include:
Monopril Tablets 762

Lisinopril (Co-administration has been reported to induce severe leukopenia). Products include:
Prinivil Tablets 1776
Prinzide Tablets 1780
Zestoretic Tablets 2968
Zestril Tablets 2972

Moexipril Hydrochloride (Co-administration has been reported to induce severe leukopenia). Products include:
Univasc Tablets 2553

Quinapril Hydrochloride (Co-administration has been reported to induce severe leukopenia). Products include:
Accupril Tablets 1950

Ramipril (Co-administration has been reported to induce severe leukopenia). Products include:
Altace Capsules 1238

Spirapril Hydrochloride (Co-administration has been reported to induce severe leukopenia).
No products indexed under this heading.

Sulfamethoxazole (Co-administration with sulfamethoxazole/trimethoprim may lead to exaggerated leukopenia, especially in renal transplant recipients). Products include:
Bactrim DS Tablets 2257

IMPORTANT NOTE: Always consult each drug listing in the patient's regimen for possible interactions.

Azathioprine — Interactions Index

Bactrim I.V. Infusion 2255
Bactrim 2257
Gantanol Tablets 2285
Septra 1146
Septra I.V. Infusion 1142
Septra I.V. Infusion ADD-Vantage Vials 1144
Septra 1146

Trandolapril (Co-administration has been reported to induce severe leukopenia). Products include:
Mavik Tablets 1407

Trimethoprim (Co-administration with sulfamethoxazole/trimethoprim may lead to exaggerated leukopenia, especially in renal transplant recipients). Products include:
Bactrim DS Tablets 2257
Bactrim I.V. Infusion 2255
Bactrim 2257
Proloprim Tablets 1141
Septra 1146
Septra I.V. Infusion 1142
Septra I.V. Infusion ADD-Vantage Vials 1144
Septra 1146
Trimpex Tablets 2323

AZELEX
(Azelaic Acid) 471
None cited in PDR database.

AZMACORT ORAL INHALER
(Triamcinolone Acetonide) 2175
May interact with:

Prednisone (Potential for increased likelihood of HPA suppression).
No products indexed under this heading.

AZULFIDINE EN-TABS
(Sulfasalazine) 2059
See Azulfidine Tablets

AZULFIDINE TABLETS
(Sulfasalazine) 2059
May interact with:

Digoxin (Reduced absorption of digoxin). Products include:
Lanoxicaps 1110
Lanoxin Elixir Pediatric 1113
Lanoxin Injection 1116
Lanoxin Injection Pediatric 1119
Lanoxin Tablets 1121

Folic Acid (Reduced absorption of folic acid). Products include:
Cefol Filmtab 415
Chromagen FA 2471
Chromagen Forte 2471
Fero-Folic-500 Filmtab 433
Iberet-Folic-500 Filmtab 433
Materna Tablets 1427
Mega-B 513
Megadose 513
Nephro-Fer Rx Tablets 2168
Nephro-Vite + Fe Tablets 2170
Nephro-Vite Rx Tablets 2170
Niferex-150 Forte Capsules 811
Slow Fe with Folic Acid 890
Trinsicon Capsules 2759

ARTHRITIS STRENGTH BC POWDER
(Aspirin, Salicylamide, Caffeine) 631
See BC Cold Powder Multi-Symptom Formula (Cold-Sinus-Allergy)

BC COLD POWDER MULTI-SYMPTOM FORMULA (COLD-SINUS-ALLERGY)
(Aspirin, Phenylpropanolamine Hydrochloride, Chlorpheniramine Maleate) 631
May interact with monoamine oxidase inhibitors and certain other agents. Compounds in these categories include:

Furazolidone (Concurrent use not recommended; consult your doctor). Products include:
Furoxone 2221

Isocarboxazid (Concurrent use not recommended; consult your doctor).
No products indexed under this heading.

Phenelzine Sulfate (Concurrent use not recommended; consult your doctor). Products include:
Nardil 1977

Selegiline Hydrochloride (Concurrent use not recommended; consult your doctor). Products include:
Eldepryl Capsules 2729

Tranylcypromine Sulfate (Concurrent use not recommended; consult your doctor). Products include:
Parnate Tablets 2679

Food Interactions
Alcohol (Concurrent use not recommended; consult your doctor).

BC COLD POWDER NON-DROWSY FORMULA (COLD-SINUS)
(Aspirin, Phenylpropanolamine Hydrochloride) 631
See BC Cold Powder Multi-Symptom Formula (Cold-Sinus-Allergy)

BC POWDER
(Aspirin, Salicylamide, Caffeine) 631
See BC Cold Powder Multi-Symptom Formula (Cold-Sinus-Allergy)

BACKACHE CAPLETS
(Magnesium Salicylate) 635
May interact with oral anticoagulants and certain other agents. Compounds in these categories include:

Antiarthritic Drugs, unspecified (Concurrent use is not recommended).

Antidiabetic Drugs, unspecified (Concurrent use is not recommended).

Antigout Drugs, unspecified (Concurrent use is not recommended).

Dicumarol (Concurrent use is not recommended).
No products indexed under this heading.

Warfarin Sodium (Concurrent use is not recommended). Products include:
Coumadin 941

BACTRIM DS TABLETS
(Trimethoprim, Sulfamethoxazole) 2257
May interact with thiazides, oral anticoagulants, and certain other agents. Compounds in these categories include:

Bendroflumethiazide (Increased incidence of thrombocytopenia with purpura in elderly).
No products indexed under this heading.

Chlorothiazide (Increased incidence of thrombocytopenia with purpura in elderly). Products include:
Aldoclor Tablets 1638
Diupres Tablets 1691
Diuril Oral 1694

Chlorothiazide Sodium (Increased incidence of thrombocytopenia with purpura in elderly). Products include:
Diuril Sodium Intravenous 1693

Dicumarol (Prolonged prothrombin time).
No products indexed under this heading.

Hydrochlorothiazide (Increased incidence of thrombocytopenia with purpura in elderly). Products include:
Aldactazide Tablets 2556
Aldoril Tablets 1644
Apresazide Capsules 824
Capozide Tablets 744
Dyazide Capsules 2653
Esidrix Tablets 839
Esimil Tablets 840
HydroDIURIL Tablets 1716
Hydropres Tablets 1718
Hyzaar Tablets 1720
Inderide Tablets 2838
Inderide LA Long Acting Capsules .. 2840
Lopressor HCT Tablets 850
Lotensin HCT Tablets 855
Moduretic Tablets 1748
Oretic Tablets 450
Prinzide Tablets 1780
Ser-Ap-Es Tablets 867
Timolide Tablets 1791
Vaseretic Tablets 1810
Zestoretic Tablets 2968
Ziac 1459

Hydroflumethiazide (Increased incidence of thrombocytopenia with purpura in elderly). Products include:
Diucardin Tablets 2824

Methotrexate Sodium (Increased free methotrexate concentrations). Products include:
Methotrexate Sodium Tablets, Injection, for Injection and LPF Injection 1322

Methyclothiazide (Increased incidence of thrombocytopenia with purpura in elderly). Products include:
Enduron Tablets 424

Phenytoin (Decreased hepatic metabolism of phenytoin). Products include:
Dilantin Infatabs 1967
Dilantin-125 Suspension 1969

Phenytoin Sodium (Decreased hepatic metabolism of phenytoin). Products include:
Dilantin Kapseals 1965

Polythiazide (Increased incidence of thrombocytopenia with purpura in elderly). Products include:
Minizide Capsules 2016

Warfarin Sodium (Prolonged prothrombin time). Products include:
Coumadin 941

BACTRIM I.V. INFUSION
(Trimethoprim, Sulfamethoxazole) 2255
May interact with thiazides, oral anticoagulants, and certain other agents. Compounds in these categories include:

Bendroflumethiazide (Increased incidence of thrombocytopenia with purpura in elderly).
No products indexed under this heading.

Chlorothiazide (Increased incidence of thrombocytopenia with purpura in elderly). Products include:
Aldoclor Tablets 1638
Diupres Tablets 1691
Diuril Oral 1694

Chlorothiazide Sodium (Increased incidence of thrombocytopenia with purpura in elderly). Products include:
Diuril Sodium Intravenous 1693

Dicumarol (Prolonged prothrombin time).
No products indexed under this heading.

Hydrochlorothiazide (Increased incidence of thrombocytopenia with purpura in elderly). Products include:
Aldactazide Tablets 2556
Aldoril Tablets 1644
Apresazide Capsules 824
Capozide Tablets 744
Dyazide Capsules 2653
Esidrix Tablets 839
Esimil Tablets 840
HydroDIURIL Tablets 1716
Hydropres Tablets 1718
Hyzaar Tablets 1720
Inderide Tablets 2838
Inderide LA Long Acting Capsules .. 2840
Lopressor HCT Tablets 850
Lotensin HCT Tablets 855
Moduretic Tablets 1748
Oretic Tablets 450
Prinzide Tablets 1780
Ser-Ap-Es Tablets 867
Timolide Tablets 1791
Vaseretic Tablets 1810
Zestoretic Tablets 2968
Ziac 1459

Hydroflumethiazide (Increased incidence of thrombocytopenia with purpura in elderly). Products include:
Diucardin Tablets 2824

Methotrexate Sodium (Increased free methotrexate concentrations). Products include:
Methotrexate Sodium Tablets, Injection, for Injection and LPF Injection 1322

Methyclothiazide (Increased incidence of thrombocytopenia with purpura in elderly). Products include:
Enduron Tablets 424

Phenytoin (Decreased hepatic metabolism of phenytoin). Products include:
Dilantin Infatabs 1967
Dilantin-125 Suspension 1969

Phenytoin Sodium (Decreased hepatic metabolism of phenytoin). Products include:
Dilantin Kapseals 1965

Polythiazide (Increased incidence of thrombocytopenia with purpura in elderly). Products include:
Minizide Capsules 2016

Warfarin Sodium (Prolonged prothrombin time). Products include:
Coumadin 941

BACTRIM PEDIATRIC SUSPENSION
(Trimethoprim, Sulfamethoxazole) ... 2257
See Bactrim DS Tablets

BACTRIM TABLETS
(Trimethoprim, Sulfamethoxazole) ... 2257
See Bactrim DS Tablets

BACTROBAN NASAL
(Mupirocin Calcium) 2643
None cited in PDR database.

BACTROBAN OINTMENT
(Mupirocin) 2642
None cited in PDR database.

BALMEX OINTMENT
(Zinc Oxide) 631
None cited in PDR database.

(⊞ Described in PDR For Nonprescription Drugs)   (⊙ Described in PDR For Ophthalmology)

BARRI-CARE ANTIMICROBIAL BARRIER OINTMENT
(Chloroxylenol) 646
None cited in PDR database.

BASALJEL CAPSULES
(Aluminum Carbonate) 2810
May interact with tetracyclines. Compounds in this category include:

Demeclocycline Hydrochloride (Concurrent oral administration should be avoided). Products include:
- Declomycin Tablets 1421

Doxycycline Calcium (Concurrent oral administration should be avoided). Products include:
- Vibramycin Calcium Oral Suspension Syrup 2038

Doxycycline Hyclate (Concurrent oral administration should be avoided). Products include:
- Doryx Capsules 1970
- Vibramycin Hyclate Capsules 2038
- Vibramycin Hyclate Intravenous 2040
- Vibra-Tabs Film Coated Tablets 2038

Doxycycline Monohydrate (Concurrent oral administration should be avoided). Products include:
- Monodox Capsules 1858
- Vibramycin Monohydrate for Oral Suspension 2038

Methacycline Hydrochloride (Concurrent oral administration should be avoided).
- No products indexed under this heading.

Minocycline Hydrochloride (Concurrent oral administration should be avoided). Products include:
- DYNACIN Capsules 1627
- Minocin Intravenous 1428
- Minocin Oral Suspension 1431
- Minocin Pellet-Filled Capsules 1429

Oxytetracycline (Concurrent oral administration should be avoided). Products include:
- Terramycin Intramuscular Solution 2034

Oxytetracycline Hydrochloride (Concurrent oral administration should be avoided). Products include:
- TERAK Ointment .... ◎ 210
- Terra-Cortril Ophthalmic Suspension 2033
- Terramycin with Polymyxin B Sulfate Ophthalmic Ointment 2035
- Urobiotic-250 Capsules 2038

Tetracycline Hydrochloride (Concurrent oral administration should be avoided). Products include:
- Achromycin V Capsules 1417
- Helidac Therapy 2135

BASALJEL SUSPENSION
(Aluminum Carbonate) 2810
See **Basaljel Capsules**

BASALJEL TABLETS
(Aluminum Carbonate) 2810
See **Basaljel Capsules**

GENUINE BAYER ASPIRIN TABLETS & CAPLETS
(Aspirin) 618
May interact with oral anticoagulants and certain other agents. Compounds in these categories include:

Aluminum Carbonate (Concurrent administration of nonabsorbable antacids may alter the rate of absorption of aspirin, thereby resulting in a decreased acetylsalicylic acid/salicylate ratio in plasma). Products include:
- Basaljel Capsules 2810
- Basaljel Suspension 2810
- Basaljel Tablets 2810

Aluminum Hydroxide (Concurrent administration of nonabsorbable antacids may alter the rate of absorption of aspirin, thereby resulting in a decreased acetylsalicylic acid/salicylate ratio in plasma). Products include:
- ALternaGEL Liquid 1358
- Maximum Strength Ascriptin 650
- Cama Arthritis Pain Reliever 748
- Gaviscon Extra Strength Relief Formula Antacid Tablets 778
- Gaviscon Extra Strength Relief Formula Liquid Antacid 779
- Gaviscon Liquid Antacid 779
- Gelusil Antacid-Anti-gas Liquid 819
- Gelusil Antacid-Anti-gas Tablets 819
- Maalox Antacid/Anti-Gas Tablets 889
- Maalox Heartburn Relief Suspension 658
- Maalox Antacid Liquid 888
- Extra Strength Maalox Antacid/Anti-Gas Liquid and Tablets 888
- Mylanta 1359
- Tempo Soft Antacid 799

Aluminum Hydroxide Gel (Concurrent administration of nonabsorbable antacids may alter the rate of absorption of aspirin, thereby resulting in a decreased acetylsalicylic acid/salicylate ratio in plasma). Products include:
- ALternaGEL Liquid 675
- Aludrox Oral Suspension 850
- Amphojel Suspension 2802
- Amphojel Suspension without Flavor 2802
- Amphojel Tablets 2802
- Ascriptin 650
- Gaviscon Antacid Tablets 778
- Gaviscon-2 Antacid Tablets 779
- Mylanta Liquid 676
- Mylanta Double Strength Liquid 676
- Nephrox Suspension 671

Antiarthritic Drugs, unspecified (Effect not specified).

Antidiabetic Drugs, unspecified (Effect not specified).

Antigout Drugs, unspecified (Effect not specified).

Dicumarol (Effect not specified).
- No products indexed under this heading.

Magnesium Hydroxide (Concurrent administration of nonabsorbable antacids may alter the rate of absorption of aspirin, thereby resulting in a decreased acetylsalicylic acid/salicylate ratio in plasma). Products include:
- Aludrox Oral Suspension 850
- Ascriptin 650
- Di-Gel Antacid/Anti-Gas 762
- Gelusil Antacid-Anti-gas Liquid 819
- Gelusil Antacid-Anti-gas Tablets 819
- Maalox Antacid/Anti-Gas Tablets 889
- Maalox Antacid Liquid 888
- Extra Strength Maalox Antacid/Anti-Gas Liquid and Tablets 888
- Mylanta Fast-Acting 1359
- Mylanta Gelcaps Antacid 678
- Fast-Acting Mylanta Liquid Antacid 1359
- Mylanta Tablets 677
- Maximum-Strength Fast-Acting Mylanta Liquid Antacid 1359
- Mylanta Double Strength Tablets 677
- Phillips' Milk of Magnesia Liquid 627
- Rolaids Antacid Tablets 807
- Tempo Soft Antacid 799

Magnesium Oxide (Concurrent administration of nonabsorbable antacids may alter the rate of absorption of aspirin, thereby resulting in a decreased acetylsalicylic acid/salicylate ratio in plasma). Products include:
- Beelith Tablets 632
- Bufferin Analgesic Tablets 636
- Arthritis Strength Bufferin Analgesic Caplets 637
- Extra Strength Bufferin Analgesic Tablets 637
- Caltrate PLUS 681
- Cama Arthritis Pain Reliever 748
- Mag-Ox 400 666
- Uro-Mag 666

Sodium Bicarbonate (Concurrent administration of absorbable antacids at therapeutic doses may increase the clearance of salicylates in some individuals). Products include:
- Alka-Seltzer Cherry Effervescent Antacid and Pain Reliever 609
- Alka-Seltzer Extra Strength Effervescent Antacid and Pain Reliever 609
- Alka-Seltzer Gold Effervescent Antacid 611
- Alka-Seltzer Lemon Lime Effervescent Antacid and Pain Reliever 609
- Alka-Seltzer Original Effervescent Antacid and Pain Reliever 609
- Arm & Hammer Pure Baking Soda 648
- Colyte and Colyte-flavored 2540
- GoLYTELY 694
- Massengill Disposable Douches 780
- Massengill Liquid Concentrate 780
- NuLYTELY 694
- Cherry Flavor NuLYTELY 694

Warfarin Sodium (Effect not specified). Products include:
- Coumadin 941

EXTRA STRENGTH BAYER ARTHRITIS PAIN REGIMEN FORMULA
(Aspirin, Enteric Coated) 615
May interact with oral anticoagulants and certain other agents. Compounds in these categories include:

Antiarthritic Drugs, unspecified (Concurrent use not recommended; consult your doctor).

Antidiabetic Drugs, unspecified (Concurrent use not recommended; consult your doctor).

Antigout Drugs, unspecified (Concurrent use not recommended; consult your doctor).

Dicumarol (Concurrent use not recommended; consult your doctor).
- No products indexed under this heading.

Warfarin Sodium (Concurrent use not recommended; consult your doctor). Products include:
- Coumadin 941

EXTRA STRENGTH BAYER ASPIRIN CAPLETS & TABLETS
(Aspirin) 617
May interact with oral anticoagulants and certain other agents. Compounds in these categories include:

Antiarthritic Drugs, unspecified (Effect not specified).

Antidiabetic Drugs, unspecified (Effect not specified).

Antigout Drugs, unspecified (Effect not specified).

Dicumarol (Effect not specified).
- No products indexed under this heading.

Warfarin Sodium (Effect not specified). Products include:
- Coumadin 941

EXTENDED-RELEASE BAYER 8-HOUR ASPIRIN
(Aspirin) 616
May interact with oral anticoagulants and certain other agents. Compounds in these categories include:

Antiarthritic Drugs, unspecified (Effect not specified).

Antidiabetic Drugs, unspecified (Effect not specified).

Antigout Drugs, unspecified (Effect not specified).

Dicumarol (Effect not specified).
- No products indexed under this heading.

Warfarin Sodium (Effect not specified). Products include:
- Coumadin 941

EXTRA STRENGTH BAYER PLUS ASPIRIN CAPLETS
(Aspirin, Calcium Carbonate) 617
May interact with oral anticoagulants and certain other agents. Compounds in these categories include:

Antiarthritic Drugs, unspecified (Concurrent use is not recommended unless directed by a doctor).

Antidiabetic Drugs, unspecified (Concurrent use is not recommended unless directed by a doctor).

Antigout Drugs, unspecified (Concurrent use is not recommended unless directed by a doctor).

Dicumarol (Concurrent use is not recommended unless directed by a doctor).
- No products indexed under this heading.

Warfarin Sodium (Concurrent use is not recommended unless directed by a doctor). Products include:
- Coumadin 941

EXTRA STRENGTH BAYER PM ASPIRIN PLUS SLEEP AID
(Aspirin, Diphenhydramine Hydrochloride) 617
May interact with oral anticoagulants, hypnotics and sedatives, tranquilizers, and certain other agents. Compounds in these categories include:

Alprazolam (Concurrent use not recommended). Products include:
- Xanax Tablets 2115

Antiarthritic Drugs, unspecified (Concurrent use not recommended; consult your doctor).

Antidiabetic Drugs, unspecified (Concurrent use not recommended; consult your doctor).

Antigout Drugs, unspecified (Concurrent use not recommended; consult your doctor).

Buspirone Hydrochloride (Concurrent use not recommended). Products include:
- BuSpar Tablets 738

Chlordiazepoxide (Concurrent use not recommended). Products include:
- Limbitrol 2333

Chlordiazepoxide Hydrochloride (Concurrent use not recommended). Products include:
- Librax Capsules 2330
- Librium Capsules 2331
- Librium Injectable 2332

Chlorpromazine (Concurrent use not recommended). Products include:
- Thorazine Suppositories 2701

Chlorpromazine Hydrochloride (Concurrent use not recommended). Products include:
- Thorazine 2701

Chlorprothixene (Concurrent use not recommended).
- No products indexed under this heading.

IMPORTANT NOTE: Always consult each drug listing in the patient's regimen for possible interactions.

Interactions Index

Bayer PM Extra

Chlorprothixene Hydrochloride (Concurrent use not recommended).
No products indexed under this heading.

Clorazepate Dipotassium (Concurrent use not recommended). Products include:
Tranxene 459

Diazepam (Concurrent use not recommended). Products include:
Dizac (diazepam injectable emulsion) CIV 1862
Valium Injectable 2336
Valium Tablets 2335

Dicumarol (Concurrent use not recommended; consult your doctor).
No products indexed under this heading.

Droperidol (Concurrent use not recommended). Products include:
Inapsine Injection 462

Estazolam (Concurrent use not recommended). Products include:
ProSom Tablets 457

Ethchlorvynol (Concurrent use not recommended). Products include:
Placidyl Capsules 456

Ethinamate (Concurrent use not recommended).
No products indexed under this heading.

Fluphenazine Decanoate (Concurrent use not recommended). Products include:
Prolixin Decanoate 510

Fluphenazine Enanthate (Concurrent use not recommended). Products include:
Prolixin Enanthate 510

Fluphenazine Hydrochloride (Concurrent use not recommended). Products include:
Prolixin 510

Flurazepam Hydrochloride (Concurrent use not recommended). Products include:
Dalmane Capsules 2329

Glutethimide (Concurrent use not recommended).
No products indexed under this heading.

Haloperidol (Concurrent use not recommended). Products include:
Haldol Injection, Tablets and Concentrate 1585

Haloperidol Decanoate (Concurrent use not recommended). Products include:
Haldol Decanoate 1587

Hydroxyzine Hydrochloride (Concurrent use not recommended). Products include:
Atarax Tablets & Syrup 1992
Marax Tablets & DF Syrup 2015
Vistaril Intramuscular Solution 2042

Lorazepam (Concurrent use not recommended). Products include:
Ativan Injection 2805
Ativan Tablets 2807

Loxapine Hydrochloride (Concurrent use not recommended). Products include:
Loxitane 1426

Loxapine Succinate (Concurrent use not recommended). Products include:
Loxitane Capsules 1426

Meprobamate (Concurrent use not recommended). Products include:
Miltown Tablets 2780
PMB 200 and PMB 400 2890

Mesoridazine Besylate (Concurrent use not recommended). Products include:
Serentil 689

Midazolam Hydrochloride (Concurrent use not recommended). Products include:
Versed Injection 2324

Molindone Hydrochloride (Concurrent use not recommended). Products include:
Moban Tablets and Concentrate 1036

Oxazepam (Concurrent use not recommended). Products include:
Serax Capsules 2916
Serax Tablets 2916

Perphenazine (Concurrent use not recommended). Products include:
Etrafon 2495
Triavil Tablets 1800
Trilafon 2532

Prazepam (Concurrent use not recommended).
No products indexed under this heading.

Prochlorperazine (Concurrent use not recommended). Products include:
Compazine 2644

Promethazine Hydrochloride (Concurrent use not recommended). Products include:
Mepergan Injection 2859
Phenergan with Codeine 2883
Phenergan with Dextromethorphan 2885
Phenergan Injection 2880
Phenergan Suppositories 2882
Phenergan Syrup 2881
Phenergan Tablets 2882
Phenergan VC 2886
Phenergan VC with Codeine 2888

Propofol (Concurrent use not recommended). Products include:
Diprivan Injectable Emulsion 2939

Quazepam (Concurrent use not recommended). Products include:
Doral Tablets 2773

Secobarbital Sodium (Concurrent use not recommended). Products include:
Seconal Sodium Pulvules 1529

Temazepam (Concurrent use not recommended). Products include:
Restoril Capsules 2413

Thioridazine Hydrochloride (Concurrent use not recommended). Products include:
Mellaril 2398

Thiothixene (Concurrent use not recommended). Products include:
Navane Capsules and Concentrate 2018
Navane Intramuscular 2019

Triazolam (Concurrent use not recommended). Products include:
Halcion Tablets 2093

Trifluoperazine Hydrochloride (Concurrent use not recommended). Products include:
Stelazine 2692

Warfarin Sodium (Concurrent use not recommended; consult your doctor). Products include:
Coumadin 941

Zolpidem Tartrate (Concurrent use not recommended). Products include:
Ambien Tablets 2559

Food Interactions
Alcohol (Avoid concurrent use).

ASPIRIN REGIMEN BAYER 81 MG TABLETS WITH CALCIUM
(Aspirin, Calcium Carbonate) .... ▣ 615
May interact with oral anticoagulants, oral hypoglycemic agents, antigout agents, and certain other agents. Compounds in these categories include:

Acarbose (Concurrent use should be avoided unless directed by a doctor). Products include:
Precose 604

Allopurinol (Concurrent use should be avoided unless directed by a doctor). Products include:
Zyloprim Tablets 1194

Antiarthritic Drugs, unspecified (Concurrent use should be avoided unless directed by a doctor).

Chlorpropamide (Concurrent use should be avoided unless directed by a doctor). Products include:
Diabinese Tablets 2002

Dicumarol (Concurrent use should be avoided unless directed by a doctor).
No products indexed under this heading.

Glimepiride (Concurrent use should be avoided unless directed by a doctor). Products include:
Amaryl Tablets 1241

Glipizide (Concurrent use should be avoided unless directed by a doctor). Products include:
Glucotrol Tablets 2011
Glucotrol XL Extended Release Tablets 2012

Glyburide (Concurrent use should be avoided unless directed by a doctor). Products include:
DiaBeta Tablets 1265
Glynase PresTab Tablets 2091
Micronase Tablets 2099

Metformin Hydrochloride (Concurrent use should be avoided unless directed by a doctor). Products include:
Glucophage Tablets 754

Probenecid (Concurrent use should be avoided unless directed by a doctor). Products include:
Benemid Tablets 1651
ColBENEMID Tablets 1662

Sulfinpyrazone (Concurrent use should be avoided unless directed by a doctor). Products include:
Anturane 823

Tolazamide (Concurrent use should be avoided unless directed by a doctor).
No products indexed under this heading.

Tolbutamide (Concurrent use should be avoided unless directed by a doctor).
No products indexed under this heading.

Warfarin Sodium (Concurrent use should be avoided unless directed by a doctor). Products include:
Coumadin 941

ASPIRIN REGIMEN BAYER ADULT LOW STRENGTH 81 MG TABLETS
(Aspirin, Enteric Coated) .... ▣ 613
See Aspirin Regimen Bayer Regular Strength 325 mg Caplets

ASPIRIN REGIMEN BAYER CHILDREN'S CHEWABLE ASPIRIN
(Aspirin) .... ▣ 616
May interact with oral anticoagulants and certain other agents. Compounds in these categories include:

Antiarthritic Drugs, unspecified (Effect not specified).

Antidiabetic Drugs, unspecified (Effect not specified).

Antigout Drugs, unspecified (Effect not specified).

Dicumarol (Effect not specified).
No products indexed under this heading.

Warfarin Sodium (Effect not specified). Products include:
Coumadin 941

ASPIRIN REGIMEN BAYER REGULAR STRENGTH 325 MG CAPLETS
(Aspirin, Enteric Coated) .... ▣ 613
May interact with oral anticoagulants, antigout agents, antacids containing aluminium, calcium and magnesium, and certain other agents. Compounds in these categories include:

Allopurinol (Effect not specified). Products include:
Zyloprim Tablets 1194

Aluminum Carbonate (Concurrent use of absorbable antacids at therapeutic doses may increase the clearance of salicylates in some individuals). Products include:
Basaljel Capsules 2810
Basaljel Suspension 2810
Basaljel Tablets 2810

Aluminum Hydroxide (Concurrent use of absorbable antacids at therapeutic doses may increase the clearance of salicylates in some individuals). Products include:
ALternaGEL Liquid 1358
Maximum Strength Ascriptin ... ▣ 650
Cama Arthritis Pain Reliever ... ▣ 748
Gaviscon Extra Strength Relief Formula Antacid Tablets ...... ▣ 778
Gaviscon Extra Strength Relief Formula Liquid Antacid .... ▣ 779
Gaviscon Liquid Antacid .... ▣ 779
Gelusil Antacid-Anti-gas Liquid ▣ 819
Gelusil Antacid-Anti-gas Tablets ▣ 819
Maalox Antacid/Anti-Gas Tablets 889
Maalox Heartburn Relief Suspension .... ▣ 658
Maalox Antacid Liquid 888
Extra Strength Maalox Antacid/Anti-Gas Liquid and Tablets 888
Mylanta 1359
Tempo Soft Antacid .... ▣ 799

Aluminum Hydroxide Gel (Concurrent use of absorbable antacids at therapeutic doses may increase the clearance of salicylates in some individuals). Products include:
ALternaGEL Liquid .... ▣ 675
Aludrox Oral Suspension .... ▣ 850
Amphojel Suspension 2802
Amphojel Suspension without Flavor 2802
Amphojel Tablets 2802
Ascriptin .... ▣ 650
Gaviscon Antacid Tablets .... ▣ 778
Gaviscon-2 Antacid Tablets ..... ▣ 779
Mylanta Liquid .... ▣ 676
Mylanta Double Strength Liquid ▣ 676
Nephrox Suspension .... ▣ 671

Antiarthritic Drugs, unspecified (Effect not specified).

Antidiabetic Drugs, unspecified (Effect not specified).

Dicumarol (Effect not specified).
No products indexed under this heading.

Magaldrate (Concurrent use of absorbable antacids at therapeutic doses may increase the clearance of salicylates in some individuals).
No products indexed under this heading.

Magnesium Hydroxide (Concurrent use of absorbable antacids at therapeutic doses may increase the clearance of salicylates in some individuals). Products include:
Aludrox Oral Suspension .... ▣ 850
Ascriptin .... ▣ 650
Di-Gel Antacid/Anti-Gas .... ▣ 762

(▣ Described in PDR For Nonprescription Drugs)　　　　　　　　　　　　　　　　　　　(⊙ Described in PDR For Ophthalmology)

Interactions Index

Gelusil Antacid-Anti-gas Liquid 819
Gelusil Antacid-Anti-gas Tablets 819
Maalox Antacid/Anti-Gas Tablets 889
Maalox Antacid Liquid 888
Extra Strength Maalox Antacid/
    Anti-Gas Liquid and Tablets 888
Mylanta Fast-Acting 1359
Mylanta Gelcaps Antacid 678
Fast-Acting Mylanta Liquid Antacid 1359
Mylanta Tablets 677
Maximum-Strength Fast-Acting
    Mylanta Liquid Antacid 1359
Mylanta Double Strength Tablets .. 677
Phillips' Milk of Magnesia Liquid..... 627
Rolaids Antacid Tablets 807
Tempo Soft Antacid 799

Magnesium Oxide (Concurrent use of absorbable antacids at therapeutic doses may increase the clearance of salicylates in some individuals). Products include:
Beelith Tablets 632
Bufferin Analgesic Tablets 636
Arthritis Strength Bufferin Analgesic Caplets 637
Extra Strength Bufferin Analgesic Tablets 637
Caltrate PLUS 681
Cama Arthritis Pain Reliever 748
Mag-Ox 400 666
Uro-Mag 666

Probenecid (Effect not specified). Products include:
Benemid Tablets 1651
ColBENEMID Tablets 1662

Sodium Bicarbonate (Concurrent use of nonabsorbable antacids may alter the rate of absorption of aspirin resulting in a decreased acetylsalicylic acid/salicylate ratio in plasma). Products include:
Alka-Seltzer Cherry Effervescent Antacid and Pain Reliever 609
Alka-Seltzer Extra Strength Effervescent Antacid and Pain Reliever 609
Alka-Seltzer Gold Effervescent Antacid 611
Alka-Seltzer Lemon Lime Effervescent Antacid and Pain Reliever 609
Alka-Seltzer Original Effervescent Antacid and Pain Reliever 609
Arm & Hammer Pure Baking Soda 648
Colyte and Colyte-flavored 2540
GoLYTELY 694
Massengill Disposable Douches 780
Massengill Liquid Concentrate 780
NuLYTELY 694
Cherry Flavor NuLYTELY 694

Sulfinpyrazone (Effect not specified). Products include:
Anturane 823

Warfarin Sodium (Effect not specified). Products include:
Coumadin 941

BEANO
(Alpha Galactosidase Enzyme) 602
May interact with monoamine oxidase inhibitors. Compounds in this category include:

Furazolidone (Concurrent use should be avoided). Products include:
Furoxone 2221

Isocarboxazid (Concurrent use should be avoided).
No products indexed under this heading.

Phenelzine Sulfate (Concurrent use should be avoided). Products include:
Nardil 1977

Selegiline Hydrochloride (Concurrent use should be avoided). Products include:
Eldepryl Capsules 2729

Tranylcypromine Sulfate (Concurrent use should be avoided). Products include:
Parnate Tablets 2679

BECLOVENT INHALATION AEROSOL AND REFILL
(Beclomethasone Dipropionate) 1063
May interact with:

Prednisone (Combined administration of alternate-day prednisone systemic treatment and orally inhaled beclomethasone increases likelihood of HPA suppression compared to therapeutic dose of either one alone).
No products indexed under this heading.

BECONASE AQ NASAL SPRAY
(Beclomethasone Dipropionate) 1065
None cited in PDR database.

BECONASE INHALATION AEROSOL
(Beclomethasone Dipropionate) 1065
None cited in PDR database.

BEELITH TABLETS
(Magnesium Oxide, Vitamin B_6) 632
May interact with:

Prescription Drugs, unspecified (Concurrent use should be avoided).

BELLERGAL-S TABLETS
(Phenobarbital, Ergotamine Tartrate, Belladonna Alkaloids) 2375
May interact with oral anticoagulants, tricyclic antidepressants, phenothiazines, narcotic analgesics, beta blockers, estrogens, central nervous system depressants, doxycycline, quinidine, and certain other agents. Compounds in these categories include:

Acebutolol Hydrochloride (A possible interaction may result in excessive vasoconstriction). Products include:
Sectral Capsules 2914

Alfentanil Hydrochloride (Combined use may result in a potentiation of the depressant action). Products include:
Alfenta Injection 1334

Alprazolam (Combined use may result in a potentiation of the depressant action). Products include:
Xanax Tablets 2115

Amitriptyline Hydrochloride (Combined use may result in a potentiation of the depressant action; additive anticholinergic effect). Products include:
Elavil 2945
Etrafon 2495
Limbitrol 2333
Triavil Tablets 1800

Amoxapine (Combined use may result in a potentiation of the depressant action; additive anticholinergic effect). Products include:
Asendin Tablets 1419

Aprobarbital (Combined use may result in a potentiation of the depressant action).
No products indexed under this heading.

Atenolol (A possible interaction may result in excessive vasoconstriction). Products include:
Tenoretic Tablets 2963
Tenormin Tablets and I.V. Injection 2965

Betaxolol Hydrochloride (A possible interaction may result in excessive vasoconstriction). Products include:
Betoptic Ophthalmic Solution 465
Betoptic S Ophthalmic Suspension 467

Kerlone Tablets 2588

Bisoprolol Fumarate (A possible interaction may result in excessive vasoconstriction). Products include:
Zebeta Tablets 1457
Ziac 1459

Buprenorphine (Combined use may result in a potentiation of the depressant action). Products include:
Buprenex Injectable 2170

Buspirone Hydrochloride (Combined use may result in a potentiation of the depressant action). Products include:
BuSpar Tablets 738

Butabarbital (Combined use may result in a potentiation of the depressant action).
No products indexed under this heading.

Butalbital (Combined use may result in a potentiation of the depressant action). Products include:
Axocet Capsules 2469
Esgic-plus Capsules 1012
Esgic-plus Tablets 1012
Fioricet Tablets 2386
Fioricet with Codeine Capsules 2387
Fiorinal Capsules 2388
Fiorinal with Codeine Capsules 2390
Fiorinal Tablets 2388
Phrenilin 790
Sedapap Tablets 50 mg/650 mg .. 1826

Carteolol Hydrochloride (A possible interaction may result in excessive vasoconstriction). Products include:
Cartrol Tablets 413
Ocupress Ophthalmic Solution, 1% Sterile 297

Chlordiazepoxide (Combined use may result in a potentiation of the depressant action). Products include:
Limbitrol 2333

Chlordiazepoxide Hydrochloride (Combined use may result in a potentiation of the depressant action). Products include:
Librax Capsules 2330
Librium Capsules 2331
Librium Injectable 2332

Chlorotrianisene (Phenobarbital, through enzyme induction, is shown to metabolize estrogen at an increased rate; consideration should be given to alternate methods of contraception, if avoidance of pregnancy is critical).
No products indexed under this heading.

Chlorpromazine (Combined use may result in a potentiation of the depressant action). Products include:
Thorazine Suppositories 2701

Chlorpromazine Hydrochloride (Combined use may result in a potentiation of the depressant action). Products include:
Thorazine 2701

Chlorprothixene (Combined use may result in a potentiation of the depressant action).
No products indexed under this heading.

Chlorprothixene Hydrochloride (Combined use may result in a potentiation of the depressant action).
No products indexed under this heading.

Chlorprothixene Lactate (Combined use may result in a potentiation of the depressant action).
No products indexed under this heading.

Bellergal-S

Clomipramine Hydrochloride (Combined use may result in a potentiation of the depressant action; additive anticholinergic effect). Products include:
Anafranil Capsules 819

Clorazepate Dipotassium (Combined use may result in a potentiation of the depressant action). Products include:
Tranxene 459

Clozapine (Combined use may result in a potentiation of the depressant action). Products include:
Clozaril Tablets 2377

Codeine Phosphate (Combined use may result in a potentiation of the depressant action). Products include:
Brontex 2130
Dimetane-DC Cough Syrup 2232
Fioricet with Codeine Capsules 2387
Fiorinal with Codeine Capsules 2390
Nucofed 2225
Phenergan with Codeine 2883
Phenergan VC with Codeine 2888
Robitussin A-C Syrup 2248
Robitussin-DAC Syrup 2249
Ryna 804
Soma Compound w/Codeine Tablets 2784
Tylenol with Codeine 1592

Desflurane (Combined use may result in a potentiation of the depressant action). Products include:
Suprane (desflurane, USP) 1865

Desipramine Hydrochloride (Combined use may result in a potentiation of the depressant action; additive anticholinergic effect). Products include:
Norpramin Tablets 1273

Dezocine (Combined use may result in a potentiation of the depressant action). Products include:
Dalgan Injection 529

Diazepam (Combined use may result in a potentiation of the depressant action). Products include:
Dizac (diazepam injectable emulsion) CIV 1862
Valium Injectable 2336
Valium Tablets 2335

Dicumarol (Phenobarbital may lower the plasma levels of oral anticoagulant and may cause a decrease in anticoagulant activity).
No products indexed under this heading.

Dienestrol (Phenobarbital, through enzyme induction, is shown to metabolize estrogen at an increased rate; consideration should be given to alternate methods of contraception, if avoidance of pregnancy is critical). Products include:
Ortho Dienestrol Cream 1922

Diethylstilbestrol (Phenobarbital, through enzyme induction, is shown to metabolize estrogen at an increased rate; consideration should be given to alternate methods of contraception, if avoidance of pregnancy is critical). Products include:
Diethylstilbestrol Tablets 1477

Divalproex Sodium (Valproate appears to decrease barbiturate metabolism, therefore barbiturate blood levels should be monitored). Products include:
Depakote Tablets 418

Doxepin Hydrochloride (Combined use may result in a potentiation of the depressant action; additive anticholinergic effect). Products include:
Adapin Capsules 1542
Sinequan 2028
Zonalon Cream 1042

IMPORTANT NOTE: Always consult each drug listing in the patient's regimen for possible interactions.

Bellergal-S **Interactions Index** **98**

Doxycycline Calcium (Phenobarbital, through enzyme induction, is shown to metabolize doxycycline at an increased rate). Products include:
Vibramycin Calcium Oral Suspension Syrup 2038

Doxycycline Hyclate (Phenobarbital, through enzyme induction, is shown to metabolize doxycycline at an increased rate). Products include:
Doryx Capsules 1970
Vibramycin Hyclate Capsules 2038
Vibramycin Hyclate Intravenous 2040
Vibra-Tabs Film Coated Tablets 2038

Doxycycline Monohydrate (Phenobarbital, through enzyme induction, is shown to metabolize doxycycline at an increased rate). Products include:
Monodox Capsules 1858
Vibramycin Monohydrate for Oral Suspension 2038

Droperidol (Combined use may result in a potentiation of the depressant action). Products include:
Inapsine Injection 462

Enflurane (Combined use may result in a potentiation of the depressant action).
No products indexed under this heading.

Esmolol Hydrochloride (A possible interaction may result in excessive vasoconstriction). Products include:
Brevibloc (esmolol HCl) Injection 1860

Estazolam (Combined use may result in a potentiation of the depressant action). Products include:
ProSom Tablets 457

Estradiol (Phenobarbital, through enzyme induction, is shown to metabolize estrogen at an increased rate; consideration should be given to alternate methods of contraception, if avoidance of pregnancy is critical). Products include:
Climara Transdermal System 640
Estrace Cream and Tablets 751
Estraderm Transdermal System 842
Estring Vaginal Ring 2086
Vivelle Transdermal System 880

Estrogens, Conjugated (Phenobarbital, through enzyme induction, is shown to metabolize estrogen at an increased rate; consideration should be given to alternate methods of contraception, if avoidance of pregnancy is critical). Products include:
PMB 200 and PMB 400 2890
Premarin Intravenous 2893
Premarin Tablets 2896
Premarin Vaginal Cream 2898
Premphase 2900
Prempro 2905

Estrogens, Esterified (Phenobarbital, through enzyme induction, is shown to metabolize estrogen at an increased rate; consideration should be given to alternate methods of contraception, if avoidance of pregnancy is critical). Products include:
ESTRATAB Tablets (0.3, 0.625, 1.25, 2.5 mg) 2715
Estratest 2718
Menest Tablets 2671

Estropipate (Phenobarbital, through enzyme induction, is shown to metabolize estrogen at an increased rate; consideration should be given to alternate methods of contraception, if avoidance of pregnancy is critical). Products include:
Ogen Tablets 2103
Ogen Vaginal Cream 2106
Ortho-Est 1925

Ethchlorvynol (Combined use may result in a potentiation of the depressant action). Products include:
Placidyl Capsules 456

Ethinamate (Combined use may result in a potentiation of the depressant action).
No products indexed under this heading.

Ethinyl Estradiol (Phenobarbital, through enzyme induction, is shown to metabolize estrogen at an increased rate; consideration should be given to alternate methods of contraception, if avoidance of pregnancy is critical). Products include:
Brevicon 2563
Demulen 2580
Desogen Tablets 1867
Levlen/Tri-Levlen 646
Lo/Ovral Tablets 2852
Lo/Ovral-28 Tablets 2857
Modicon 1928
Nordette-21 Tablets 2863
Nordette-28 Tablets 2866
Norinyl 2563
Ortho-Cept 1907
Ortho-Cyclen/Ortho-Tri-Cyclen 1914
Ortho-Novum 1928
Ortho-Cyclen/Ortho Tri-Cyclen 1914
Ovcon 765
Ovral Tablets 2877
Ovral-28 Tablets 2878
Levlen/Tri-Levlen 646
Tri-Norinyl 2607
Triphasil-21 Tablets 2919
Triphasil-28 Tablets 2924

Fentanyl (Combined use may result in a potentiation of the depressant action). Products include:
Duragesic Transdermal System 1336

Fentanyl Citrate (Combined use may result in a potentiation of the depressant action). Products include:
Sublimaze Injection 463

Fluphenazine Decanoate (Combined use may result in a potentiation of the depressant action). Products include:
Prolixin Decanoate 510

Fluphenazine Enanthate (Combined use may result in a potentiation of the depressant action). Products include:
Prolixin Enanthate 510

Fluphenazine Hydrochloride (Combined use may result in a potentiation of the depressant action). Products include:
Prolixin 510

Flurazepam Hydrochloride (Combined use may result in a potentiation of the depressant action). Products include:
Dalmane Capsules 2329

Glutethimide (Combined use may result in a potentiation of the depressant action).
No products indexed under this heading.

Griseofulvin (Phenobarbital, through enzyme induction, is shown to metabolize griseofulvin at an increased rate). Products include:
Fulvicin P/G Tablets 2499
Fulvicin P/G 165 & 330 Tablets 2500
Grifulvin V (griseofulvin tablets) Microsize (griseofulvin oral suspension) Microsize 1944
Gris-PEG Tablets, 125 mg & 250 mg 476

Haloperidol (Combined use may result in a potentiation of the depressant action). Products include:
Haldol Injection, Tablets and Concentrate 1585

Haloperidol Decanoate (Combined use may result in a potentiation of the depressant action). Products include:
Haldol Decanoate 1587

Hydrocodone Bitartrate (Combined use may result in a potentiation of the depressant action). Products include:
Codiclear DH Syrup 808
Duratuss HD Elixir 2750
Histussin D Liquid 670
Hycodan Tablets and Syrup 946
Hycomine Compound Tablets 948
Hycomine 947
Hycotuss Expectorant Syrup 950
Hydrocet Capsules 787
Lorcet 10/650 Tablets 1016
Lortab 2751
Tussend 1830
Tussend Expectorant 1831
Vicodin Tablets 1404
Vicodin ES Tablets 1405
Vicodin HP Tablets 1403
Vicodin Tuss Expectorant 1406
Zydone Capsules 967

Hydrocodone Polistirex (Combined use may result in a potentiation of the depressant action). Products include:
Tussionex Pennkinetic Extended-Release Suspension 1624

Hydromorphone Hydrochloride (Combined use may result in a potentiation of the depressant action). Products include:
Dilaudid Ampules 1382
Dilaudid Cough Syrup 1383
Dilaudid-HP Injection 1384
Dilaudid-HP Lyophilized Powder 250 mg 1384
Dilaudid 1382
Dilaudid Oral Liquid 1386
Dilaudid 1382
Dilaudid Tablets - 8 mg 1386

Hydroxyzine Hydrochloride (Combined use may result in a potentiation of the depressant action). Products include:
Atarax Tablets & Syrup 1992
Marax Tablets & DF Syrup 2015
Vistaril Intramuscular Solution 2042

Imipramine Hydrochloride (Combined use may result in a potentiation of the depressant action; additive anticholinergic effect). Products include:
Tofranil Ampuls 873
Tofranil Tablets 875

Imipramine Pamoate (Combined use may result in a potentiation of the depressant action; additive anticholinergic effect). Products include:
Tofranil-PM Capsules 876

Isoflurane (Combined use may result in a potentiation of the depressant action).
No products indexed under this heading.

Ketamine Hydrochloride (Combined use may result in a potentiation of the depressant action).
No products indexed under this heading.

Labetalol Hydrochloride (A possible interaction may result in excessive vasoconstriction). Products include:
Normodyne Injection 2519
Normodyne Tablets 2522
Trandate 1158

Levobunolol Hydrochloride (A possible interaction may result in excessive vasoconstriction). Products include:
Betagan ..... ◉ 230

Levomethadyl Acetate Hydrochloride (Combined use may result in a potentiation of the depressant action). Products include:
Orlaam Oral Solution 2361

Levorphanol Tartrate (Combined use may result in a potentiation of the depressant action). Products include:
Levo-Dromoran 2297

Lorazepam (Combined use may result in a potentiation of the depressant action). Products include:
Ativan Injection 2805
Ativan Tablets 2807

Loxapine Hydrochloride (Combined use may result in a potentiation of the depressant action). Products include:
Loxitane 1426

Loxapine Succinate (Combined use may result in a potentiation of the depressant action). Products include:
Loxitane Capsules 1426

Maprotiline Hydrochloride (Combined use may result in a potentiation of the depressant action; additive anticholinergic effect). Products include:
Ludiomil Tablets 861

Meperidine Hydrochloride (Combined use may result in a potentiation of the depressant action). Products include:
Demerol 2438
Mepergan Injection 2859

Mephobarbital (Combined use may result in a potentiation of the depressant action). Products include:
Mebaral Tablets 2452

Meprobamate (Combined use may result in a potentiation of the depressant action). Products include:
Miltown Tablets 2780
PMB 200 and PMB 400 2890

Mesoridazine Besylate (Combined use may result in a potentiation of the depressant action). Products include:
Serentil 689

Methadone Hydrochloride (Combined use may result in a potentiation of the depressant action). Products include:
Methadone Hydrochloride Oral Concentrate 2356
Methadone Hydrochloride Oral Solution & Tablets 2357

Methohexital Sodium (Combined use may result in a potentiation of the depressant action).
No products indexed under this heading.

Methotrimeprazine (Combined use may result in a potentiation of the depressant action). Products include:
Levoprome 1321

Methoxyflurane (Combined use may result in a potentiation of the depressant action).
No products indexed under this heading.

Metipranolol Hydrochloride (A possible interaction may result in excessive vasoconstriction). Products include:
OptiPranolol (Metipranolol 0.3%) Sterile Ophthalmic Solution ..... ◉ 256

Metoprolol Succinate (A possible interaction may result in excessive vasoconstriction). Products include:
Toprol-XL Tablets 560

Metoprolol Tartrate (A possible interaction may result in excessive vasoconstriction). Products include:
Lopressor 848
Lopressor HCT Tablets 850

(▭ Described in PDR For Nonprescription Drugs) (◉ Described in PDR For Ophthalmology)

Interactions Index

Midazolam Hydrochloride (Combined use may result in a potentiation of the depressant action). Products include:
- Versed Injection 2324

Molindone Hydrochloride (Combined use may result in a potentiation of the depressant action). Products include:
- Moban Tablets and Concentrate ... 1036

Morphine Sulfate (Combined use may result in a potentiation of the depressant action). Products include:
- Astramorph/PF Injection, USP (Preservative-Free) 526
- Duramorph Injection 983
- Infumorph 200 and Infumorph 500 Sterile Solutions 985
- Kadian Capsules 2948
- MS Contin Tablets 2149
- MSIR 2152
- Oramorph SR (Morphine Sulfate Sustained Release Tablets) 2359
- RMS Suppositories CII 2766
- Roxanol 2365

Nadolol (A possible interaction may result in excessive vasoconstriction).
- No products indexed under this heading.

Nortriptyline Hydrochloride (Combined use may result in a potentiation of the depressant action; additive anticholinergic effect). Products include:
- Pamelor 2409

Opium Alkaloids (Combined use may result in a potentiation of the depressant action).
- No products indexed under this heading.

Oxazepam (Combined use may result in a potentiation of the depressant action). Products include:
- Serax Capsules 2916
- Serax Tablets 2916

Oxycodone Hydrochloride (Combined use may result in a potentiation of the depressant action). Products include:
- OxyContin Tablets 2163
- OxyIR Capsules 2167
- Percocet Tablets 955
- Percodan Tablets 955
- Percodan-Demi Tablets 956
- Roxicodone Tablets, Oral Solution & Intensol (Oxycodone) 2366
- Tylox Capsules 1593

Penbutolol Sulfate (A possible interaction may result in excessive vasoconstriction). Products include:
- Levatol Tablets 2547

Pentobarbital Sodium (Combined use may result in a potentiation of the depressant action). Products include:
- Nembutal Sodium Capsules 440
- Nembutal Sodium Solution 442
- Nembutal Sodium Suppositories 444

Perphenazine (Combined use may result in a potentiation of the depressant action). Products include:
- Etrafon 2495
- Triavil Tablets 1800
- Trilafon 2532

Phenytoin (Variable effect on phenytoin metabolism with possible accelerating effect). Products include:
- Dilantin Infatabs 1967
- Dilantin-125 Suspension 1969

Phenytoin Sodium (Variable effect on phenytoin metabolism with possible accelerating effect). Products include:
- Dilantin Kapseals 1965

Pindolol (A possible interaction may result in excessive vasoconstriction). Products include:
- Visken Tablets 2428

Polyestradiol Phosphate (Phenobarbital, through enzyme induction, is shown to metabolize estrogen at an increased rate; consideration should be given to alternate methods of contraception, if avoidance of pregnancy is critical).
- No products indexed under this heading.

Prazepam (Combined use may result in a potentiation of the depressant action).
- No products indexed under this heading.

Prochlorperazine (Combined use may result in a potentiation of the depressant action). Products include:
- Compazine 2644

Promethazine Hydrochloride (Combined use may result in a potentiation of the depressant action). Products include:
- Mepergan Injection 2859
- Phenergan with Codeine 2883
- Phenergan with Dextromethorphan 2885
- Phenergan Injection 2880
- Phenergan Suppositories 2882
- Phenergan Syrup 2881
- Phenergan Tablets 2882
- Phenergan VC 2886
- Phenergan VC with Codeine 2888

Propofol (Combined use may result in a potentiation of the depressant action). Products include:
- Diprivan Injectable Emulsion 2939

Propoxyphene Hydrochloride (Combined use may result in a potentiation of the depressant action). Products include:
- Darvon 1475
- Wygesic Tablets 2930

Propoxyphene Napsylate (Combined use may result in a potentiation of the depressant action). Products include:
- Darvon-N/Darvocet-N 1473

Propranolol Hydrochloride (A possible interaction may result in excessive vasoconstriction). Products include:
- Inderal 2834
- Inderal LA Long Acting Capsules 2836
- Inderide Tablets 2838
- Inderide LA Long Acting Capsules .. 2840

Protriptyline Hydrochloride (Combined use may result in a potentiation of the depressant action; additive anticholinergic effect). Products include:
- Vivactil Tablets 1820

Quazepam (Combined use may result in a potentiation of the depressant action). Products include:
- Doral Tablets 2773

Quinestrol (Phenobarbital, through enzyme induction, is shown to metabolize estrogen at an increased rate; consideration should be given to alternate methods of contraception, if avoidance of pregnancy is critical).
- No products indexed under this heading.

Quinidine Gluconate (Phenobarbital, through enzyme induction, is shown to metabolize quinidine at an increased rate). Products include:
- Quinaglute Dura-Tabs Tablets 644

Quinidine Polygalacturonate (Phenobarbital, through enzyme induction, is shown to metabolize quinidine at an increased rate). Products include:
- Cardioquin Tablets 2146

Quinidine Sulfate (Phenobarbital, through enzyme induction, is shown to metabolize quinidine at an increased rate). Products include:
- Quinidex Extentabs 2240

Risperidone (Combined use may result in a potentiation of the depressant action). Products include:
- Risperdal Tablets 1348

Secobarbital Sodium (Combined use may result in a potentiation of the depressant action). Products include:
- Seconal Sodium Pulvules 1529

Sevoflurane (Combined use may result in a potentiation of the depressant action).
- No products indexed under this heading.

Sotalol Hydrochloride (A possible interaction may result in excessive vasoconstriction). Products include:
- Betapace Tablets 637

Sufentanil Citrate (Combined use may result in a potentiation of the depressant action). Products include:
- Sufenta Injection 1355

Temazepam (Combined use may result in a potentiation of the depressant action). Products include:
- Restoril Capsules 2413

Thiamylal Sodium (Combined use may result in a potentiation of the depressant action).
- No products indexed under this heading.

Thioridazine Hydrochloride (Combined use may result in a potentiation of the depressant action). Products include:
- Mellaril 2398

Thiothixene (Combined use may result in a potentiation of the depressant action). Products include:
- Navane Capsules and Concentrate .. 2018
- Navane Intramuscular 2019

Timolol Hemihydrate (A possible interaction may result in excessive vasoconstriction). Products include:
- Betimol 0.25%, 0.5% 259

Timolol Maleate (A possible interaction may result in excessive vasoconstriction). Products include:
- Blocadren Tablets 1654
- Timolide Tablets 1791
- Timoptic in Ocudose 1796
- Timoptic Sterile Ophthalmic Solution 1794
- Timoptic-XE 1798

Triazolam (Combined use may result in a potentiation of the depressant action). Products include:
- Halcion Tablets 2093

Trifluoperazine Hydrochloride (Combined use may result in a potentiation of the depressant action). Products include:
- Stelazine 2692

Trimipramine Maleate (Combined use may result in a potentiation of the depressant action; additive anticholinergic effect). Products include:
- Surmontil Capsules 2917

Valproic Acid (Valproate appears to decrease barbiturate metabolism, therefore barbiturate blood levels should be monitored). Products include:
- Depakene 416

Warfarin Sodium (Phenobarbital may lower the plasma levels of oral anticoagulant and may cause a decrease in anticoagulant activity). Products include:
- Coumadin 941

Zolpidem Tartrate (Combined use may result in a potentiation of the depressant action). Products include:
- Ambien Tablets 2559

Food Interactions

Alcohol (Combined use may result in a potentiation of the depressant action).

BENADRYL ALLERGY CHEWABLES
(Diphenhydramine Hydrochloride) .. 811
May interact with monoamine oxidase inhibitors, hypnotics and sedatives, tranquilizers, and certain other agents. Compounds in these categories include:

Alprazolam (May increase drowsiness effect). Products include:
- Xanax Tablets 2115

Buspirone Hydrochloride (May increase drowsiness effect). Products include:
- BuSpar Tablets 738

Chlordiazepoxide (May increase drowsiness effect). Products include:
- Limbitrol 2333

Chlordiazepoxide Hydrochloride (May increase drowsiness effect). Products include:
- Librax Capsules 2330
- Librium Capsules 2331
- Librium Injectable 2332

Chlorpromazine (May increase drowsiness effect). Products include:
- Thorazine Suppositories 2701

Chlorpromazine Hydrochloride (May increase drowsiness effect). Products include:
- Thorazine 2701

Chlorprothixene (May increase drowsiness effect).
- No products indexed under this heading.

Chlorprothixene Hydrochloride (May increase drowsiness effect).
- No products indexed under this heading.

Clorazepate Dipotassium (May increase drowsiness effect). Products include:
- Tranxene 459

Diazepam (May increase drowsiness effect). Products include:
- Dizac (diazepam injectable emulsion) CIV 1862
- Valium Injectable 2336
- Valium Tablets 2335

Droperidol (May increase drowsiness effect). Products include:
- Inapsine Injection 462

Estazolam (May increase drowsiness effect). Products include:
- ProSom Tablets 457

Ethchlorvynol (May increase drowsiness effect). Products include:
- Placidyl Capsules 456

Ethinamate (May increase drowsiness effect).
- No products indexed under this heading.

Fluphenazine Decanoate (May increase drowsiness effect). Products include:
- Prolixin Decanoate 510

Fluphenazine Enanthate (May increase drowsiness effect). Products include:
- Prolixin Enanthate 510

Fluphenazine Hydrochloride (May increase drowsiness effect). Products include:
- Prolixin 510

Flurazepam Hydrochloride (May increase drowsiness effect). Products include:
- Dalmane Capsules 2329

IMPORTANT NOTE: Always consult each drug listing in the patient's regimen for possible interactions.

Furazolidone (Concurrent and/or sequential use is not recommended). Products include:
Furoxone ... 2221
Glutethimide (May increase drowsiness effect).
No products indexed under this heading.
Haloperidol (May increase drowsiness effect). Products include:
Haldol Injection, Tablets and Concentrate ... 1585
Haloperidol Decanoate (May increase drowsiness effect). Products include:
Haldol Decanoate ... 1587
Hydroxyzine Hydrochloride (May increase drowsiness effect). Products include:
Atarax Tablets & Syrup ... 1992
Marax Tablets & DF Syrup ... 2015
Vistaril Intramuscular Solution ... 2042
Isocarboxazid (Concurrent and/or sequential use is not recommended).
No products indexed under this heading.
Lorazepam (May increase drowsiness effect). Products include:
Ativan Injection ... 2805
Ativan Tablets ... 2807
Loxapine Hydrochloride (May increase drowsiness effect). Products include:
Loxitane ... 1426
Loxapine Succinate (May increase drowsiness effect). Products include:
Loxitane Capsules ... 1426
Meprobamate (May increase drowsiness effect). Products include:
Miltown Tablets ... 2780
PMB 200 and PMB 400 ... 2890
Mesoridazine Besylate (May increase drowsiness effect). Products include:
Serentil ... 689
Midazolam Hydrochloride (May increase drowsiness effect). Products include:
Versed Injection ... 2324
Molindone Hydrochloride (May increase drowsiness effect). Products include:
Moban Tablets and Concentrate ... 1036
Oxazepam (May increase drowsiness effect). Products include:
Serax Capsules ... 2916
Serax Tablets ... 2916
Perphenazine (May increase drowsiness effect). Products include:
Etrafon ... 2495
Triavil Tablets ... 1800
Trilafon ... 2532
Phenelzine Sulfate (Concurrent and/or sequential use is not recommended). Products include:
Nardil ... 1977
Prazepam (May increase drowsiness effect).
No products indexed under this heading.
Prochlorperazine (May increase drowsiness effect). Products include:
Compazine ... 2644
Promethazine Hydrochloride (May increase drowsiness effect). Products include:
Mepergan Injection ... 2859
Phenergan with Codeine ... 2883
Phenergan with Dextromethorphan 2885
Phenergan Injection ... 2880
Phenergan Suppositories ... 2882
Phenergan Syrup ... 2881
Phenergan Tablets ... 2882
Phenergan VC ... 2886
Phenergan VC with Codeine ... 2888
Propofol (May increase drowsiness effect). Products include:
Diprivan Injectable Emulsion ... 2939
Quazepam (May increase drowsiness effect). Products include:
Doral Tablets ... 2773
Secobarbital Sodium (May increase drowsiness effect). Products include:
Seconal Sodium Pulvules ... 1529
Selegiline Hydrochloride (Concurrent and/or sequential use is not recommended). Products include:
Eldepryl Capsules ... 2729
Temazepam (May increase drowsiness effect). Products include:
Restoril Capsules ... 2413
Thioridazine Hydrochloride (May increase drowsiness effect). Products include:
Mellaril ... 2398
Thiothixene (May increase drowsiness effect). Products include:
Navane Capsules and Concentrate 2018
Navane Intramuscular ... 2019
Tranylcypromine Sulfate (Concurrent and/or sequential use is not recommended). Products include:
Parnate Tablets ... 2679
Triazolam (May increase drowsiness effect). Products include:
Halcion Tablets ... 2093
Trifluoperazine Hydrochloride (May increase drowsiness effect). Products include:
Stelazine ... 2692
Zolpidem Tartrate (May increase drowsiness effect). Products include:
Ambien Tablets ... 2559

Food Interactions

Alcohol (May increase drowsiness effect).

BENADRYL ALLERGY/COLD TABLETS
(Acetaminophen, Diphenhydramine Hydrochloride, Pseudoephedrine Hydrochloride) ... ▣ 811
May interact with monoamine oxidase inhibitors, hypnotics and sedatives, tranquilizers, and certain other agents. Compounds in these categories include:

Alprazolam (May increase drowsiness effect). Products include:
Xanax Tablets ... 2115
Buspirone Hydrochloride (May increase drowsiness effect). Products include:
BuSpar Tablets ... 738
Chlordiazepoxide (May increase drowsiness effect). Products include:
Limbitrol ... 2333
Chlordiazepoxide Hydrochloride (May increase drowsiness effect). Products include:
Librax Capsules ... 2330
Librium Capsules ... 2331
Librium Injectable ... 2332
Chlorpromazine (May increase drowsiness effect). Products include:
Thorazine Suppositories ... 2701
Chlorpromazine Hydrochloride (May increase drowsiness effect). Products include:
Thorazine ... 2701
Chlorprothixene (May increase drowsiness effect).
No products indexed under this heading.
Chlorprothixene Hydrochloride (May increase drowsiness effect).
No products indexed under this heading.
Clorazepate Dipotassium (May increase drowsiness effect). Products include:
Tranxene ... 459
Diazepam (May increase drowsiness effect). Products include:
Dizac (diazepam injectable emulsion) CIV ... 1862
Valium Injectable ... 2336
Valium Tablets ... 2335
Droperidol (May increase drowsiness effect). Products include:
Inapsine Injection ... 462
Estazolam (May increase drowsiness effect). Products include:
ProSom Tablets ... 457
Ethchlorvynol (May increase drowsiness effect). Products include:
Placidyl Capsules ... 456
Ethinamate (May increase drowsiness effect).
No products indexed under this heading.
Fluphenazine Decanoate (May increase drowsiness effect). Products include:
Prolixin Decanoate ... 510
Fluphenazine Enanthate (May increase drowsiness effect). Products include:
Prolixin Enanthate ... 510
Fluphenazine Hydrochloride (May increase drowsiness effect). Products include:
Prolixin ... 510
Flurazepam Hydrochloride (May increase drowsiness effect). Products include:
Dalmane Capsules ... 2329
Furazolidone (Concurrent and/or sequential use is not recommended). Products include:
Furoxone ... 2221
Glutethimide (May increase drowsiness effect).
No products indexed under this heading.
Haloperidol (May increase drowsiness effect). Products include:
Haldol Injection, Tablets and Concentrate ... 1585
Haloperidol Decanoate (May increase drowsiness effect). Products include:
Haldol Decanoate ... 1587
Hydroxyzine Hydrochloride (May increase drowsiness effect). Products include:
Atarax Tablets & Syrup ... 1992
Marax Tablets & DF Syrup ... 2015
Vistaril Intramuscular Solution ... 2042
Isocarboxazid (Concurrent and/or sequential use is not recommended).
No products indexed under this heading.
Lorazepam (May increase drowsiness effect). Products include:
Ativan Injection ... 2805
Ativan Tablets ... 2807
Loxapine Hydrochloride (May increase drowsiness effect). Products include:
Loxitane ... 1426
Loxapine Succinate (May increase drowsiness effect). Products include:
Loxitane Capsules ... 1426
Meprobamate (May increase drowsiness effect). Products include:
Miltown Tablets ... 2780
PMB 200 and PMB 400 ... 2890
Mesoridazine Besylate (May increase drowsiness effect). Products include:
Serentil ... 689
Midazolam Hydrochloride (May increase drowsiness effect). Products include:
Versed Injection ... 2324
Molindone Hydrochloride (May increase drowsiness effect). Products include:
Moban Tablets and Concentrate ... 1036
Oxazepam (May increase drowsiness effect). Products include:
Serax Capsules ... 2916
Serax Tablets ... 2916
Perphenazine (May increase drowsiness effect). Products include:
Etrafon ... 2495
Triavil Tablets ... 1800
Trilafon ... 2532
Phenelzine Sulfate (Concurrent and/or sequential use is not recommended). Products include:
Nardil ... 1977
Prazepam (May increase drowsiness effect).
No products indexed under this heading.
Prochlorperazine (May increase drowsiness effect). Products include:
Compazine ... 2644
Promethazine Hydrochloride (May increase drowsiness effect). Products include:
Mepergan Injection ... 2859
Phenergan with Codeine ... 2883
Phenergan with Dextromethorphan 2885
Phenergan Injection ... 2880
Phenergan Suppositories ... 2882
Phenergan Syrup ... 2881
Phenergan Tablets ... 2882
Phenergan VC ... 2886
Phenergan VC with Codeine ... 2888
Propofol (May increase drowsiness effect). Products include:
Diprivan Injectable Emulsion ... 2939
Quazepam (May increase drowsiness effect). Products include:
Doral Tablets ... 2773
Secobarbital Sodium (May increase drowsiness effect). Products include:
Seconal Sodium Pulvules ... 1529
Selegiline Hydrochloride (Concurrent and/or sequential use is not recommended). Products include:
Eldepryl Capsules ... 2729
Temazepam (May increase drowsiness effect). Products include:
Restoril Capsules ... 2413
Thioridazine Hydrochloride (May increase drowsiness effect). Products include:
Mellaril ... 2398
Thiothixene (May increase drowsiness effect). Products include:
Navane Capsules and Concentrate 2018
Navane Intramuscular ... 2019
Tranylcypromine Sulfate (Concurrent and/or sequential use is not recommended). Products include:
Parnate Tablets ... 2679
Triazolam (May increase drowsiness effect). Products include:
Halcion Tablets ... 2093
Trifluoperazine Hydrochloride (May increase drowsiness effect). Products include:
Stelazine ... 2692
Zolpidem Tartrate (May increase drowsiness effect). Products include:
Ambien Tablets ... 2559

Food Interactions

Alcohol (May increase drowsiness effect).

BENADRYL ALLERGY DECONGESTANT LIQUID MEDICATION
(Diphenhydramine Hydrochloride, Pseudoephedrine Hydrochloride) ... ▣ 812
May interact with hypnotics and sedatives, tranquilizers, monoamine oxidase inhibitors, and certain other

(▣ Described in PDR For Nonprescription Drugs) (◎ Described in PDR For Ophthalmology)

agents. Compounds in these categories include:

Alprazolam (May increase drowsiness effect; consult your physician). Products include:
- Xanax Tablets 2115

Buspirone Hydrochloride (May increase drowsiness effect; consult your physician). Products include:
- BuSpar Tablets 738

Chlordiazepoxide (May increase drowsiness effect; consult your physician). Products include:
- Limbitrol 2333

Chlordiazepoxide Hydrochloride (May increase drowsiness effect; consult your physician). Products include:
- Librax Capsules 2330
- Librium Capsules 2331
- Librium Injectable 2332

Chlorpromazine (May increase drowsiness effect; consult your physician). Products include:
- Thorazine Suppositories 2701

Chlorpromazine Hydrochloride (May increase drowsiness effect; consult your physician). Products include:
- Thorazine 2701

Chlorprothixene (May increase drowsiness effect; consult your physician).
- No products indexed under this heading.

Chlorprothixene Hydrochloride (May increase drowsiness effect; consult your physician).
- No products indexed under this heading.

Clorazepate Dipotassium (May increase drowsiness effect; consult your physician). Products include:
- Tranxene 459

Diazepam (May increase drowsiness effect; consult your physician). Products include:
- Dizac (diazepam injectable emulsion) CIV 1862
- Valium Injectable 2336
- Valium Tablets 2335

Droperidol (May increase drowsiness effect; consult your physician). Products include:
- Inapsine Injection 462

Estazolam (May increase drowsiness effect; consult your physician). Products include:
- ProSom Tablets 457

Ethchlorvynol (May increase drowsiness effect; consult your physician). Products include:
- Placidyl Capsules 456

Ethinamate (May increase drowsiness effect; consult your physician).
- No products indexed under this heading.

Fluphenazine Decanoate (May increase drowsiness effect; consult your physician). Products include:
- Prolixin Decanoate 510

Fluphenazine Enanthate (May increase drowsiness effect; consult your physician). Products include:
- Prolixin Enanthate 510

Fluphenazine Hydrochloride (May increase drowsiness effect; consult your physician). Products include:
- Prolixin 510

Flurazepam Hydrochloride (May increase drowsiness effect; consult your physician). Products include:
- Dalmane Capsules 2329

Furazolidone (Concurrent and/or sequential use is not recommended). Products include:
- Furoxone 2221

Glutethimide (May increase drowsiness effect; consult your physician).
- No products indexed under this heading.

Haloperidol (May increase drowsiness effect; consult your physician). Products include:
- Haldol Injection, Tablets and Concentrate 1585

Haloperidol Decanoate (May increase drowsiness effect; consult your physician). Products include:
- Haldol Decanoate 1587

Hydroxyzine Hydrochloride (May increase drowsiness effect; consult your physician). Products include:
- Atarax Tablets & Syrup 1992
- Marax Tablets & DF Syrup 2015
- Vistaril Intramuscular Solution 2042

Isocarboxazid (Concurrent and/or sequential use is not recommended).
- No products indexed under this heading.

Lorazepam (May increase drowsiness effect; consult your physician). Products include:
- Ativan Injection 2805
- Ativan Tablets 2807

Loxapine Hydrochloride (May increase drowsiness effect; consult your physician). Products include:
- Loxitane 1426

Loxapine Succinate (May increase drowsiness effect; consult your physician). Products include:
- Loxitane Capsules 1426

Meprobamate (May increase drowsiness effect; consult your physician). Products include:
- Miltown Tablets 2780
- PMB 200 and PMB 400 2890

Mesoridazine Besylate (May increase drowsiness effect; consult your physician). Products include:
- Serentil 689

Midazolam Hydrochloride (May increase drowsiness effect; consult your physician). Products include:
- Versed Injection 2324

Molindone Hydrochloride (May increase drowsiness effect; consult your physician). Products include:
- Moban Tablets and Concentrate 1036

Oxazepam (May increase drowsiness effect; consult your physician). Products include:
- Serax Capsules 2916
- Serax Tablets 2916

Perphenazine (May increase drowsiness effect; consult your physician). Products include:
- Etrafon 2495
- Triavil Tablets 1800
- Trilafon 2532

Phenelzine Sulfate (Concurrent and/or sequential use is not recommended). Products include:
- Nardil 1977

Prazepam (May increase drowsiness effect; consult your physician).
- No products indexed under this heading.

Prochlorperazine (May increase drowsiness effect; consult your physician). Products include:
- Compazine 2644

Promethazine Hydrochloride (May increase drowsiness effect; consult your physician). Products include:
- Mepergan Injection 2859
- Phenergan with Codeine 2883
- Phenergan with Dextromethorphan 2885
- Phenergan Injection 2880
- Phenergan Suppositories 2882
- Phenergan Syrup 2881
- Phenergan Tablets 2882
- Phenergan VC 2886
- Phenergan VC with Codeine 2888

Propofol (May increase drowsiness effect; consult your physician). Products include:
- Diprivan Injectable Emulsion 2939

Quazepam (May increase drowsiness effect; consult your physician). Products include:
- Doral Tablets 2773

Secobarbital Sodium (May increase drowsiness effect; consult your physician). Products include:
- Seconal Sodium Pulvules 1529

Selegiline Hydrochloride (Concurrent and/or sequential use is not recommended). Products include:
- Eldepryl Capsules 2729

Temazepam (May increase drowsiness effect; consult your physician). Products include:
- Restoril Capsules 2413

Thioridazine Hydrochloride (May increase drowsiness effect; consult your physician). Products include:
- Mellaril 2398

Thiothixene (May increase drowsiness effect; consult your physician). Products include:
- Navane Capsules and Concentrate 2018
- Navane Intramuscular 2019

Tranylcypromine Sulfate (Concurrent and/or sequential use is not recommended). Products include:
- Parnate Tablets 2679

Triazolam (May increase drowsiness effect; consult your physician). Products include:
- Halcion Tablets 2093

Trifluoperazine Hydrochloride (May increase drowsiness effect; consult your physician). Products include:
- Stelazine 2692

Zolpidem Tartrate (May increase drowsiness effect; consult your physician). Products include:
- Ambien Tablets 2559

Food Interactions

Alcohol (May increase drowsiness effect; avoid concurrent use).

BENADRYL ALLERGY DECONGESTANT TABLETS
(Diphenhydramine Hydrochloride, Pseudoephedrine Hydrochloride) 812

May interact with hypnotics and sedatives, tranquilizers, monoamine oxidase inhibitors, and certain other agents. Compounds in these categories include:

Alprazolam (May increase the drowsiness effect). Products include:
- Xanax Tablets 2115

Buspirone Hydrochloride (May increase the drowsiness effect). Products include:
- BuSpar Tablets 738

Chlordiazepoxide (May increase the drowsiness effect). Products include:
- Limbitrol 2333

Chlordiazepoxide Hydrochloride (May increase the drowsiness effect). Products include:
- Librax Capsules 2330
- Librium Capsules 2331
- Librium Injectable 2332

Chlorpromazine (May increase the drowsiness effect). Products include:
- Thorazine Suppositories 2701

Chlorpromazine Hydrochloride (May increase the drowsiness effect). Products include:
- Thorazine 2701

Chlorprothixene (May increase the drowsiness effect).
- No products indexed under this heading.

Chlorprothixene Hydrochloride (May increase the drowsiness effect).
- No products indexed under this heading.

Clorazepate Dipotassium (May increase the drowsiness effect). Products include:
- Tranxene 459

Diazepam (May increase the drowsiness effect). Products include:
- Dizac (diazepam injectable emulsion) CIV 1862
- Valium Injectable 2336
- Valium Tablets 2335

Droperidol (May increase the drowsiness effect). Products include:
- Inapsine Injection 462

Estazolam (May increase the drowsiness effect). Products include:
- ProSom Tablets 457

Ethchlorvynol (May increase the drowsiness effect). Products include:
- Placidyl Capsules 456

Ethinamate (May increase the drowsiness effect).
- No products indexed under this heading.

Fluphenazine Decanoate (May increase the drowsiness effect). Products include:
- Prolixin Decanoate 510

Fluphenazine Enanthate (May increase the drowsiness effect). Products include:
- Prolixin Enanthate 510

Fluphenazine Hydrochloride (May increase the drowsiness effect). Products include:
- Prolixin 510

Flurazepam Hydrochloride (May increase the drowsiness effect). Products include:
- Dalmane Capsules 2329

Furazolidone (Concurrent and/or sequential use is not recommended). Products include:
- Furoxone 2221

Glutethimide (May increase the drowsiness effect).
- No products indexed under this heading.

Haloperidol (May increase the drowsiness effect). Products include:
- Haldol Injection, Tablets and Concentrate 1585

Haloperidol Decanoate (May increase the drowsiness effect). Products include:
- Haldol Decanoate 1587

Hydroxyzine Hydrochloride (May increase the drowsiness effect). Products include:
- Atarax Tablets & Syrup 1992
- Marax Tablets & DF Syrup 2015
- Vistaril Intramuscular Solution 2042

Isocarboxazid (Concurrent and/or sequential use is not recommended).
- No products indexed under this heading.

Lorazepam (May increase the drowsiness effect). Products include:
- Ativan Injection 2805
- Ativan Tablets 2807

IMPORTANT NOTE: Always consult each drug listing in the patient's regimen for possible interactions.

Benadryl Decongestant / **Interactions Index** 102

Loxapine Hydrochloride (May increase the drowsiness effect). Products include:
Loxitane 1426

Loxapine Succinate (May increase the drowsiness effect). Products include:
Loxitane Capsules 1426

Meprobamate (May increase the drowsiness effect). Products include:
Miltown Tablets 2780
PMB 200 and PMB 400 2890

Mesoridazine Besylate (May increase the drowsiness effect). Products include:
Serentil 689

Midazolam Hydrochloride (May increase the drowsiness effect). Products include:
Versed Injection 2324

Molindone Hydrochloride (May increase the drowsiness effect). Products include:
Moban Tablets and Concentrate 1036

Oxazepam (May increase the drowsiness effect). Products include:
Serax Capsules 2916
Serax Tablets 2916

Perphenazine (May increase the drowsiness effect). Products include:
Etrafon 2495
Triavil Tablets 1800
Trilafon 2532

Phenelzine Sulfate (Concurrent and/or sequential use is not recommended). Products include:
Nardil 1977

Prazepam (May increase the drowsiness effect).
No products indexed under this heading.

Prochlorperazine (May increase the drowsiness effect). Products include:
Compazine 2644

Promethazine Hydrochloride (May increase the drowsiness effect). Products include:
Mepergan Injection 2859
Phenergan with Codeine 2883
Phenergan with Dextromethorphan 2885
Phenergan Injection 2880
Phenergan Suppositories 2882
Phenergan Syrup 2881
Phenergan Tablets 2882
Phenergan VC 2886
Phenergan VC with Codeine .. 2888

Propofol (May increase the drowsiness effect). Products include:
Diprivan Injectable Emulsion .. 2939

Quazepam (May increase the drowsiness effect). Products include:
Doral Tablets 2773

Secobarbital Sodium (May increase the drowsiness effect). Products include:
Seconal Sodium Pulvules 1529

Selegiline Hydrochloride (Concurrent and/or sequential use is not recommended). Products include:
Eldepryl Capsules 2729

Temazepam (May increase the drowsiness effect). Products include:
Restoril Capsules 2413

Thioridazine Hydrochloride (May increase the drowsiness effect). Products include:
Mellaril 2398

Thiothixene (May increase the drowsiness effect). Products include:
Navane Capsules and Concentrate ... 2018
Navane Intramuscular 2019

Tranylcypromine Sulfate (Concurrent and/or sequential use is not recommended). Products include:
Parnate Tablets 2679

Triazolam (May increase the drowsiness effect). Products include:
Halcion Tablets 2093

Trifluoperazine Hydrochloride (May increase the drowsiness effect). Products include:
Stelazine 2692

Zolpidem Tartrate (May increase the drowsiness effect). Products include:
Ambien Tablets 2559

Food Interactions
Alcohol (Increases the drowsiness effect; avoid concomitant use).

BENADRYL ALLERGY LIQUID MEDICATION
(Diphenhydramine Hydrochloride) .. ▩ 813
May interact with hypnotics and sedatives, tranquilizers, and certain other agents. Compounds in these categories include:

Alprazolam (May increase drowsiness effect; consult your physician). Products include:
Xanax Tablets 2115

Buspirone Hydrochloride (May increase drowsiness effect; consult your physician). Products include:
BuSpar Tablets 738

Chlordiazepoxide (May increase drowsiness effect; consult your physician). Products include:
Limbitrol 2333

Chlordiazepoxide Hydrochloride (May increase drowsiness effect; consult your physician). Products include:
Librax Capsules 2330
Librium Capsules 2331
Librium Injectable 2332

Chlorpromazine (May increase drowsiness effect; consult your physician). Products include:
Thorazine Suppositories 2701

Chlorpromazine Hydrochloride (May increase drowsiness effect; consult your physician). Products include:
Thorazine 2701

Chlorprothixene (May increase drowsiness effect; consult your physician).
No products indexed under this heading.

Chlorprothixene Hydrochloride (May increase drowsiness effect; consult your physician).
No products indexed under this heading.

Clorazepate Dipotassium (May increase drowsiness effect; consult your physician). Products include:
Tranxene 459

Diazepam (May increase drowsiness effect; consult your physician). Products include:
Dizac (diazepam injectable emulsion) CIV 1862
Valium Injectable 2336
Valium Tablets 2335

Droperidol (May increase drowsiness effect; consult your physician). Products include:
Inapsine Injection 462

Estazolam (May increase drowsiness effect; consult your physician). Products include:
ProSom Tablets 457

Ethchlorvynol (May increase drowsiness effect; consult your physician). Products include:
Placidyl Capsules 456

Ethinamate (May increase drowsiness effect; consult your physician).
No products indexed under this heading.

Fluphenazine Decanoate (May increase drowsiness effect; consult your physician). Products include:
Prolixin Decanoate 510

Fluphenazine Enanthate (May increase drowsiness effect; consult your physician). Products include:
Prolixin Enanthate 510

Fluphenazine Hydrochloride (May increase drowsiness effect; consult your physician). Products include:
Prolixin 510

Flurazepam Hydrochloride (May increase drowsiness effect; consult your physician). Products include:
Dalmane Capsules 2329

Glutethimide (May increase drowsiness effect; consult your physician).
No products indexed under this heading.

Haloperidol (May increase drowsiness effect; consult your physician). Products include:
Haldol Injection, Tablets and Concentrate 1585

Haloperidol Decanoate (May increase drowsiness effect; consult your physician). Products include:
Haldol Decanoate 1587

Hydroxyzine Hydrochloride (May increase drowsiness effect; consult your physician). Products include:
Atarax Tablets & Syrup 1992
Marax Tablets & DF Syrup 2015
Vistaril Intramuscular Solution 2042

Lorazepam (May increase drowsiness effect; consult your physician). Products include:
Ativan Injection 2805
Ativan Tablets 2807

Loxapine Hydrochloride (May increase drowsiness effect; consult your physician). Products include:
Loxitane 1426

Loxapine Succinate (May increase drowsiness effect; consult your physician). Products include:
Loxitane Capsules 1426

Meprobamate (May increase drowsiness effect; consult your physician). Products include:
Miltown Tablets 2780
PMB 200 and PMB 400 2890

Mesoridazine Besylate (May increase drowsiness effect; consult your physician). Products include:
Serentil 689

Midazolam Hydrochloride (May increase drowsiness effect; consult your physician). Products include:
Versed Injection 2324

Molindone Hydrochloride (May increase drowsiness effect; consult your physician). Products include:
Moban Tablets and Concentrate 1036

Oxazepam (May increase drowsiness effect; consult your physician). Products include:
Serax Capsules 2916
Serax Tablets 2916

Perphenazine (May increase drowsiness effect; consult your physician). Products include:
Etrafon 2495
Triavil Tablets 1800
Trilafon 2532

Prazepam (May increase drowsiness effect; consult your physician).
No products indexed under this heading.

Prochlorperazine (May increase drowsiness effect; consult your physician). Products include:
Compazine 2644

Promethazine Hydrochloride (May increase drowsiness effect; consult your physician). Products include:
Mepergan Injection 2859
Phenergan with Codeine 2883
Phenergan with Dextromethorphan 2885
Phenergan Injection 2880
Phenergan Suppositories 2882
Phenergan Syrup 2881
Phenergan Tablets 2882
Phenergan VC 2886
Phenergan VC with Codeine . 2888

Propofol (May increase drowsiness effect; consult your physician). Products include:
Diprivan Injectable Emulsion . 2939

Quazepam (May increase drowsiness effect; consult your physician). Products include:
Doral Tablets 2773

Secobarbital Sodium (May increase drowsiness effect; consult your physician). Products include:
Seconal Sodium Pulvules 1529

Temazepam (May increase drowsiness effect; consult your physician). Products include:
Restoril Capsules 2413

Thioridazine Hydrochloride (May increase drowsiness effect; consult your physician). Products include:
Mellaril 2398

Thiothixene (May increase drowsiness effect; consult your physician). Products include:
Navane Capsules and Concentrate ... 2018
Navane Intramuscular 2019

Triazolam (May increase drowsiness effect; consult your physician). Products include:
Halcion Tablets 2093

Trifluoperazine Hydrochloride (May increase drowsiness effect; consult your physician). Products include:
Stelazine 2692

Zolpidem Tartrate (May increase drowsiness effect; consult your physician). Products include:
Ambien Tablets 2559

Food Interactions
Alcohol (Increases drowsiness effect).

BENADRYL ALLERGY KAPSEALS
(Diphenhydramine Hydrochloride) .. ▩ 811
May interact with hypnotics and sedatives, tranquilizers, and certain other agents. Compounds in these categories include:

Alprazolam (May increase drowsiness effect). Products include:
Xanax Tablets 2115

Buspirone Hydrochloride (May increase drowsiness effect). Products include:
BuSpar Tablets 738

Chlordiazepoxide (May increase drowsiness effect). Products include:
Limbitrol 2333

Chlordiazepoxide Hydrochloride (May increase drowsiness effect). Products include:
Librax Capsules 2330
Librium Capsules 2331
Librium Injectable 2332

Chlorpromazine (May increase drowsiness effect). Products include:
Thorazine Suppositories 2701

Chlorpromazine Hydrochloride (May increase drowsiness effect). Products include:
Thorazine 2701

(▩ Described in PDR For Nonprescription Drugs)   (⊙ Described in PDR For Ophthalmology)

Chlorprothixene (May increase drowsiness effect).
No products indexed under this heading.

Chlorprothixene Hydrochloride (May increase drowsiness effect).
No products indexed under this heading.

Clorazepate Dipotassium (May increase drowsiness effect). Products include:
Tranxene 459

Diazepam (May increase drowsiness effect). Products include:
Dizac (diazepam injectable emulsion) CIV 1862
Valium Injectable 2336
Valium Tablets 2335

Droperidol (May increase drowsiness effect). Products include:
Inapsine Injection 462

Estazolam (May increase drowsiness effect). Products include:
ProSom Tablets 457

Ethchlorvynol (May increase drowsiness effect). Products include:
Placidyl Capsules 456

Ethinamate (May increase drowsiness effect).
No products indexed under this heading.

Fluphenazine Decanoate (May increase drowsiness effect). Products include:
Prolixin Decanoate 510

Fluphenazine Enanthate (May increase drowsiness effect). Products include:
Prolixin Enanthate 510

Fluphenazine Hydrochloride (May increase drowsiness effect). Products include:
Prolixin 510

Flurazepam Hydrochloride (May increase drowsiness effect). Products include:
Dalmane Capsules 2329

Glutethimide (May increase drowsiness effect).
No products indexed under this heading.

Haloperidol (May increase drowsiness effect). Products include:
Haldol Injection, Tablets and Concentrate 1585

Haloperidol Decanoate (May increase drowsiness effect). Products include:
Haldol Decanoate 1587

Hydroxyzine Hydrochloride (May increase drowsiness effect). Products include:
Atarax Tablets & Syrup 1992
Marax Tablets & DF Syrup 2015
Vistaril Intramuscular Solution 2042

Lorazepam (May increase drowsiness effect). Products include:
Ativan Injection 2805
Ativan Tablets 2807

Loxapine Hydrochloride (May increase drowsiness effect). Products include:
Loxitane 1426

Loxapine Succinate (May increase drowsiness effect). Products include:
Loxitane Capsules 1426

Meprobamate (May increase drowsiness effect). Products include:
Miltown Tablets 2780
PMB 200 and PMB 400 2890

Mesoridazine Besylate (May increase drowsiness effect). Products include:
Serentil 689

Midazolam Hydrochloride (May increase drowsiness effect). Products include:
Versed Injection 2324

Molindone Hydrochloride (May increase drowsiness effect). Products include:
Moban Tablets and Concentrate 1036

Oxazepam (May increase drowsiness effect). Products include:
Serax Capsules 2916
Serax Tablets 2916

Perphenazine (May increase drowsiness effect). Products include:
Etrafon 2495
Triavil Tablets 1800
Trilafon 2532

Prazepam (May increase drowsiness effect).
No products indexed under this heading.

Prochlorperazine (May increase drowsiness effect). Products include:
Compazine 2644

Promethazine Hydrochloride (May increase drowsiness effect). Products include:
Mepergan Injection 2859
Phenergan with Codeine 2883
Phenergan with Dextromethorphan 2885
Phenergan Injection 2880
Phenergan Suppositories 2882
Phenergan Syrup 2881
Phenergan Tablets 2882
Phenergan VC 2886
Phenergan VC with Codeine 2888

Propofol (May increase drowsiness effect). Products include:
Diprivan Injectable Emulsion 2939

Quazepam (May increase drowsiness effect). Products include:
Doral Tablets 2773

Secobarbital Sodium (May increase drowsiness effect). Products include:
Seconal Sodium Pulvules 1529

Temazepam (May increase drowsiness effect). Products include:
Restoril Capsules 2413

Thioridazine Hydrochloride (May increase drowsiness effect). Products include:
Mellaril 2398

Thiothixene (May increase drowsiness effect). Products include:
Navane Capsules and Concentrate 2018
Navane Intramuscular 2019

Triazolam (May increase drowsiness effect). Products include:
Halcion Tablets 2093

Trifluoperazine Hydrochloride (May increase drowsiness effect). Products include:
Stelazine 2692

Zolpidem Tartrate (May increase drowsiness effect). Products include:
Ambien Tablets 2559

Food Interactions

Alcohol (May increase drowsiness effect).

BENADRYL ALLERGY TABLETS

(Diphenhydramine Hydrochloride) .. ▣ 811
See **Benadryl Allergy Kapseals**

BENADRYL ALLERGY SINUS HEADACHE CAPLETS

(Diphenhydramine Hydrochloride, Pseudoephedrine Hydrochloride, Acetaminophen) .... ▣ 813
May interact with hypnotics and sedatives, tranquilizers, monoamine oxidase inhibitors, and certain other agents. Compounds in these categories include:

Alprazolam (May increase drowsiness effect). Products include:
Xanax Tablets 2115

Buspirone Hydrochloride (May increase drowsiness effect). Products include:
BuSpar Tablets 738

Chlordiazepoxide (May increase drowsiness effect). Products include:
Limbitrol 2333

Chlordiazepoxide Hydrochloride (May increase drowsiness effect). Products include:
Librax Capsules 2330
Librium Capsules 2331
Librium Injectable 2332

Chlorpromazine (May increase drowsiness effect). Products include:
Thorazine Suppositories 2701

Chlorpromazine Hydrochloride (May increase drowsiness effect). Products include:
Thorazine 2701

Chlorprothixene (May increase drowsiness effect).
No products indexed under this heading.

Chlorprothixene Hydrochloride (May increase drowsiness effect).
No products indexed under this heading.

Clorazepate Dipotassium (May increase drowsiness effect). Products include:
Tranxene 459

Diazepam (May increase drowsiness effect). Products include:
Dizac (diazepam injectable emulsion) CIV 1862
Valium Injectable 2336
Valium Tablets 2335

Droperidol (May increase drowsiness effect). Products include:
Inapsine Injection 462

Estazolam (May increase drowsiness effect). Products include:
ProSom Tablets 457

Ethchlorvynol (May increase drowsiness effect). Products include:
Placidyl Capsules 456

Ethinamate (May increase drowsiness effect).
No products indexed under this heading.

Fluphenazine Decanoate (May increase drowsiness effect). Products include:
Prolixin Decanoate 510

Fluphenazine Enanthate (May increase drowsiness effect). Products include:
Prolixin Enanthate 510

Fluphenazine Hydrochloride (May increase drowsiness effect). Products include:
Prolixin 510

Flurazepam Hydrochloride (May increase drowsiness effect). Products include:
Dalmane Capsules 2329

Furazolidone (Concurrent and/or sequential use is not recommended). Products include:
Furoxone 2221

Glutethimide (May increase drowsiness effect).
No products indexed under this heading.

Haloperidol (May increase drowsiness effect). Products include:
Haldol Injection, Tablets and Concentrate 1585

Haloperidol Decanoate (May increase drowsiness effect). Products include:
Haldol Decanoate 1587

Hydroxyzine Hydrochloride (May increase drowsiness effect). Products include:
Atarax Tablets & Syrup 1992
Marax Tablets & DF Syrup 2015
Vistaril Intramuscular Solution 2042

Isocarboxazid (Concurrent and/or sequential use is not recommended).
No products indexed under this heading.

Lorazepam (May increase drowsiness effect). Products include:
Ativan Injection 2805
Ativan Tablets 2807

Loxapine Hydrochloride (May increase drowsiness effect). Products include:
Loxitane 1426

Loxapine Succinate (May increase drowsiness effect). Products include:
Loxitane Capsules 1426

Meprobamate (May increase drowsiness effect). Products include:
Miltown Tablets 2780
PMB 200 and PMB 400 2890

Mesoridazine Besylate (May increase drowsiness effect). Products include:
Serentil 689

Midazolam Hydrochloride (May increase drowsiness effect). Products include:
Versed Injection 2324

Molindone Hydrochloride (May increase drowsiness effect). Products include:
Moban Tablets and Concentrate 1036

Oxazepam (May increase drowsiness effect). Products include:
Serax Capsules 2916
Serax Tablets 2916

Perphenazine (May increase drowsiness effect). Products include:
Etrafon 2495
Triavil Tablets 1800
Trilafon 2532

Phenelzine Sulfate (Concurrent and/or sequential use is not recommended). Products include:
Nardil 1977

Prazepam (May increase drowsiness effect).
No products indexed under this heading.

Prochlorperazine (May increase drowsiness effect). Products include:
Compazine 2644

Promethazine Hydrochloride (May increase drowsiness effect). Products include:
Mepergan Injection 2859
Phenergan with Codeine 2883
Phenergan with Dextromethorphan 2885
Phenergan Injection 2880
Phenergan Suppositories 2882
Phenergan Syrup 2881
Phenergan Tablets 2882
Phenergan VC 2886
Phenergan VC with Codeine 2888

Propofol (May increase drowsiness effect). Products include:
Diprivan Injectable Emulsion 2939

Quazepam (May increase drowsiness effect). Products include:
Doral Tablets 2773

Secobarbital Sodium (May increase drowsiness effect). Products include:
Seconal Sodium Pulvules 1529

Selegiline Hydrochloride (Concurrent and/or sequential use is not recommended). Products include:
Eldepryl Capsules 2729

IMPORTANT NOTE: Always consult each drug listing in the patient's regimen for possible interactions.

Benadryl Allergy Sinus — Interactions Index

Temazepam (May increase drowsiness effect). Products include:
- Restoril Capsules 2413

Thioridazine Hydrochloride (May increase drowsiness effect). Products include:
- Mellaril 2398

Thiothixene (May increase drowsiness effect). Products include:
- Navane Capsules and Concentrate 2018
- Navane Intramuscular 2019

Tranylcypromine Sulfate (Concurrent and/or sequential use is not recommended). Products include:
- Parnate Tablets 2679

Triazolam (May increase drowsiness effect). Products include:
- Halcion Tablets 2093

Trifluoperazine Hydrochloride (May increase drowsiness effect). Products include:
- Stelazine 2692

Zolpidem Tartrate (May increase drowsiness effect). Products include:
- Ambien Tablets 2559

Food Interactions
Alcohol (May increase drowsiness effect).

BENADRYL DYE-FREE ALLERGY LIQUI-GEL SOFTGELS
(Diphenhydramine Hydrochloride) .. 📖 813
May interact with hypnotics and sedatives, tranquilizers, and certain other agents. Compounds in these categories include:

Alprazolam (May increase the drowsiness effect). Products include:
- Xanax Tablets 2115

Buspirone Hydrochloride (May increase the drowsiness effect). Products include:
- BuSpar Tablets 738

Chlordiazepoxide (May increase the drowsiness effect). Products include:
- Limbitrol 2333

Chlordiazepoxide Hydrochloride (May increase the drowsiness effect). Products include:
- Librax Capsules 2330
- Librium Capsules 2331
- Librium Injectable 2332

Chlorpromazine (May increase the drowsiness effect). Products include:
- Thorazine Suppositories 2701

Chlorpromazine Hydrochloride (May increase the drowsiness effect). Products include:
- Thorazine 2701

Chlorprothixene (May increase the drowsiness effect).
- No products indexed under this heading.

Chlorprothixene Hydrochloride (May increase the drowsiness effect).
- No products indexed under this heading.

Clorazepate Dipotassium (May increase the drowsiness effect). Products include:
- Tranxene 459

Diazepam (May increase the drowsiness effect). Products include:
- Dizac (diazepam injectable emulsion) CIV 1862
- Valium Injectable 2336
- Valium Tablets 2335

Droperidol (May increase the drowsiness effect). Products include:
- Inapsine Injection 462

Estazolam (May increase the drowsiness effect). Products include:
- ProSom Tablets 457

Ethchlorvynol (May increase the drowsiness effect). Products include:
- Placidyl Capsules 456

Ethinamate (May increase the drowsiness effect).
- No products indexed under this heading.

Fluphenazine Decanoate (May increase the drowsiness effect). Products include:
- Prolixin Decanoate 510

Fluphenazine Enanthate (May increase the drowsiness effect). Products include:
- Prolixin Enanthate 510

Fluphenazine Hydrochloride (May increase the drowsiness effect). Products include:
- Prolixin 510

Flurazepam Hydrochloride (May increase the drowsiness effect). Products include:
- Dalmane Capsules 2329

Glutethimide (May increase the drowsiness effect).
- No products indexed under this heading.

Haloperidol (May increase the drowsiness effect). Products include:
- Haldol Injection, Tablets and Concentrate 1585

Haloperidol Decanoate (May increase the drowsiness effect). Products include:
- Haldol Decanoate 1587

Hydroxyzine Hydrochloride (May increase the drowsiness effect). Products include:
- Atarax Tablets & Syrup 1992
- Marax Tablets & DF Syrup . 2015
- Vistaril Intramuscular Solution 2042

Lorazepam (May increase the drowsiness effect). Products include:
- Ativan Injection 2805
- Ativan Tablets 2807

Loxapine Hydrochloride (May increase the drowsiness effect). Products include:
- Loxitane 1426

Loxapine Succinate (May increase the drowsiness effect). Products include:
- Loxitane Capsules 1426

Meprobamate (May increase the drowsiness effect). Products include:
- Miltown Tablets 2780
- PMB 200 and PMB 400 2890

Mesoridazine Besylate (May increase the drowsiness effect). Products include:
- Serentil 689

Midazolam Hydrochloride (May increase the drowsiness effect). Products include:
- Versed Injection 2324

Molindone Hydrochloride (May increase the drowsiness effect). Products include:
- Moban Tablets and Concentrate 1036

Oxazepam (May increase the drowsiness effect). Products include:
- Serax Capsules 2916
- Serax Tablets 2916

Perphenazine (May increase the drowsiness effect). Products include:
- Etrafon 2495
- Triavil Tablets 1800
- Trilafon 2532

Prazepam (May increase the drowsiness effect). Products include:
- No products indexed under this heading.

Prochlorperazine (May increase the drowsiness effect). Products include:
- Compazine 2644

Promethazine Hydrochloride (May increase the drowsiness effect). Products include:
- Mepergan Injection 2859
- Phenergan with Codeine 2883
- Phenergan with Dextromethorphan 2885
- Phenergan Injection 2880
- Phenergan Suppositories ... 2882
- Phenergan Syrup 2881
- Phenergan Tablets 2882
- Phenergan VC 2886
- Phenergan VC with Codeine 2888

Propofol (May increase the drowsiness effect). Products include:
- Diprivan Injectable Emulsion 2939

Quazepam (May increase the drowsiness effect). Products include:
- Doral Tablets 2773

Secobarbital Sodium (May increase the drowsiness effect). Products include:
- Seconal Sodium Pulvules ... 1529

Temazepam (May increase the drowsiness effect). Products include:
- Restoril Capsules 2413

Thioridazine Hydrochloride (May increase the drowsiness effect). Products include:
- Mellaril 2398

Thiothixene (May increase the drowsiness effect). Products include:
- Navane Capsules and Concentrate 2018
- Navane Intramuscular 2019

Triazolam (May increase the drowsiness effect). Products include:
- Halcion Tablets 2093

Trifluoperazine Hydrochloride (May increase the drowsiness effect). Products include:
- Stelazine 2692

Zolpidem Tartrate (May increase the drowsiness effect). Products include:
- Ambien Tablets 2559

Food Interactions
Alcohol (May increase the drowsiness effect).

BENADRYL DYE-FREE ALLERGY LIQUID MEDICATION
(Diphenhydramine Hydrochloride) .. 📖 814
May interact with hypnotics and sedatives, tranquilizers, and certain other agents. Compounds in these categories include:

Alprazolam (May increase the drowsiness effect). Products include:
- Xanax Tablets 2115

Buspirone Hydrochloride (May increase the drowsiness effect). Products include:
- BuSpar Tablets 738

Chlordiazepoxide (May increase the drowsiness effect). Products include:
- Limbitrol 2333

Chlordiazepoxide Hydrochloride (May increase the drowsiness effect). Products include:
- Librax Capsules 2330
- Librium Capsules 2331
- Librium Injectable 2332

Chlorpromazine (May increase the drowsiness effect). Products include:
- Thorazine Suppositories 2701

Chlorpromazine Hydrochloride (May increase the drowsiness effect). Products include:
- Thorazine 2701

Chlorprothixene (May increase the drowsiness effect).
- No products indexed under this heading.

Chlorprothixene Hydrochloride (May increase the drowsiness effect).
- No products indexed under this heading.

Clorazepate Dipotassium (May increase the drowsiness effect). Products include:
- Tranxene 459

Diazepam (May increase the drowsiness effect). Products include:
- Dizac (diazepam injectable emulsion) CIV 1862
- Valium Injectable 2336
- Valium Tablets 2335

Droperidol (May increase the drowsiness effect). Products include:
- Inapsine Injection 462

Estazolam (May increase the drowsiness effect). Products include:
- ProSom Tablets 457

Ethchlorvynol (May increase the drowsiness effect). Products include:
- Placidyl Capsules 456

Ethinamate (May increase the drowsiness effect).
- No products indexed under this heading.

Fluphenazine Decanoate (May increase the drowsiness effect). Products include:
- Prolixin Decanoate 510

Fluphenazine Enanthate (May increase the drowsiness effect). Products include:
- Prolixin Enanthate 510

Fluphenazine Hydrochloride (May increase the drowsiness effect). Products include:
- Prolixin 510

Flurazepam Hydrochloride (May increase the drowsiness effect). Products include:
- Dalmane Capsules 2329

Glutethimide (May increase the drowsiness effect).
- No products indexed under this heading.

Haloperidol (May increase the drowsiness effect). Products include:
- Haldol Injection, Tablets and Concentrate 1585

Haloperidol Decanoate (May increase the drowsiness effect). Products include:
- Haldol Decanoate 1587

Hydroxyzine Hydrochloride (May increase the drowsiness effect). Products include:
- Atarax Tablets & Syrup 1992
- Marax Tablets & DF Syrup . 2015
- Vistaril Intramuscular Solution 2042

Lorazepam (May increase the drowsiness effect). Products include:
- Ativan Injection 2805
- Ativan Tablets 2807

Loxapine Hydrochloride (May increase the drowsiness effect). Products include:
- Loxitane 1426

Loxapine Succinate (May increase the drowsiness effect). Products include:
- Loxitane Capsules 1426

Meprobamate (May increase the drowsiness effect). Products include:
- Miltown Tablets 2780
- PMB 200 and PMB 400 2890

Mesoridazine Besylate (May increase the drowsiness effect). Products include:
- Serentil 689

(📖 Described in PDR For Nonprescription Drugs) (⊚ Described in PDR For Ophthalmology)

Interactions Index — Benadryl Injection

Midazolam Hydrochloride (May increase the drowsiness effect). Products include:
- Versed Injection 2324

Molindone Hydrochloride (May increase the drowsiness effect). Products include:
- Moban Tablets and Concentrate 1036

Oxazepam (May increase the drowsiness effect). Products include:
- Serax Capsules 2916
- Serax Tablets 2916

Perphenazine (May increase the drowsiness effect). Products include:
- Etrafon 2495
- Triavil Tablets 1800
- Trilafon 2532

Prazepam (May increase the drowsiness effect).
No products indexed under this heading.

Prochlorperazine (May increase the drowsiness effect). Products include:
- Compazine 2644

Promethazine Hydrochloride (May increase the drowsiness effect). Products include:
- Mepergan Injection 2859
- Phenergan with Codeine 2883
- Phenergan with Dextromethorphan 2885
- Phenergan Injection 2880
- Phenergan Suppositories 2882
- Phenergan Syrup 2881
- Phenergan Tablets 2882
- Phenergan VC 2886
- Phenergan VC with Codeine 2888

Propofol (May increase the drowsiness effect). Products include:
- Diprivan Injectable Emulsion 2939

Quazepam (May increase the drowsiness effect). Products include:
- Doral Tablets 2773

Secobarbital Sodium (May increase the drowsiness effect). Products include:
- Seconal Sodium Pulvules 1529

Temazepam (May increase the drowsiness effect). Products include:
- Restoril Capsules 2413

Thioridazine Hydrochloride (May increase the drowsiness effect). Products include:
- Mellaril 2398

Thiothixene (May increase the drowsiness effect). Products include:
- Navane Capsules and Concentrate 2018
- Navane Intramuscular 2019

Triazolam (May increase the drowsiness effect). Products include:
- Halcion Tablets 2093

Trifluoperazine Hydrochloride (May increase the drowsiness effect). Products include:
- Stelazine 2692

Zolpidem Tartrate (May increase the drowsiness effect). Products include:
- Ambien Tablets 2559

Food Interactions
Alcohol (May increase the drowsiness effect).

BENADRYL ITCH RELIEF STICK EXTRA STRENGTH
(Diphenhydramine Hydrochloride, Zinc Acetate) 814
None cited in PDR database.

BENADRYL ITCH STOPPING CREAM EXTRA STRENGTH
(Diphenhydramine Hydrochloride, Zinc Acetate) 814
See Benadryl Itch Stopping Cream Original Strength

BENADRYL ITCH STOPPING CREAM ORIGINAL STRENGTH
(Diphenhydramine Hydrochloride, Zinc Acetate) 814
May interact with:

Diphenhydramine (Concurrent use with other diphenhydramine-containing product is not recommended).
No products indexed under this heading.

BENADRYL ITCH STOPPING GEL EXTRA STRENGTH
(Diphenhydramine Hydrochloride, Zinc Acetate) 815
See Benadryl Itch Stopping Gel Original Strength

BENADRYL ITCH STOPPING GEL ORIGINAL STRENGTH
(Diphenhydramine Hydrochloride, Zinc Acetate) 815
May interact with:

Diphenhydramine (Concurrent use with other diphenhydramine-containing product is not recommended).
No products indexed under this heading.

BENADRYL ITCH STOPPING SPRAY EXTRA STRENGTH
(Diphenhydramine Hydrochloride, Zinc Acetate) 815
See Benadryl Itch Stopping Spray Original Strength

BENADRYL ITCH STOPPING SPRAY ORIGINAL STRENGTH
(Diphenhydramine Hydrochloride, Zinc Acetate) 815
None cited in PDR database.

BENADRYL PARENTERAL
(Diphenhydramine Hydrochloride) 1955
May interact with central nervous system depressants, monoamine oxidase inhibitors, and certain other agents. Compounds in these categories include:

Alfentanil Hydrochloride (Additive effects). Products include:
- Alfenta Injection 1334

Alprazolam (Additive effects). Products include:
- Xanax Tablets 2115

Aprobarbital (Additive effects).
No products indexed under this heading.

Buprenorphine (Additive effects). Products include:
- Buprenex Injectable 2170

Buspirone Hydrochloride (Additive effects). Products include:
- BuSpar Tablets 738

Butabarbital (Additive effects).
No products indexed under this heading.

Butalbital (Additive effects). Products include:
- Axocet Capsules 2469
- Esgic-plus Capsules 1012
- Esgic-plus Tablets 1012
- Fioricet Tablets 2386
- Fioricet with Codeine Capsules 2387
- Fiorinal Capsules 2388
- Fiorinal with Codeine Capsules 2390
- Fiorinal Tablets 2388
- Phrenilin 790
- Sedapap Tablets 50 mg/650 mg 1826

Chlordiazepoxide (Additive effects). Products include:
- Limbitrol 2333

Chlordiazepoxide Hydrochloride (Additive effects). Products include:
- Librax Capsules 2330
- Librium Capsules 2331
- Librium Injectable 2332

Chlorpromazine (Additive effects). Products include:
- Thorazine Suppositories 2701

Chlorprothixene (Additive effects).
No products indexed under this heading.

Chlorprothixene Hydrochloride (Additive effects). Products include:
No products indexed under this heading.

Chlorprothixene Lactate (Additive effects).
No products indexed under this heading.

Clorazepate Dipotassium (Additive effects). Products include:
- Tranxene 459

Clozapine (Additive effects). Products include:
- Clozaril Tablets 2377

Codeine Phosphate (Additive effects). Products include:
- Brontex 2130
- Dimetane-DC Cough Syrup 2232
- Fioricet with Codeine Capsules 2387
- Fiorinal with Codeine Capsules 2390
- Nucofed 2225
- Phenergan with Codeine 2883
- Phenergan VC with Codeine 2888
- Robitussin A-C Syrup 2248
- Robitussin-DAC Syrup 2249
- Ryna 804
- Soma Compound w/Codeine Tablets 2784
- Tylenol with Codeine 1592

Desflurane (Additive effects). Products include:
- Suprane (desflurane, USP) 1865

Dezocine (Additive effects). Products include:
- Dalgan Injection 529

Diazepam (Additive effects). Products include:
- Dizac (diazepam injectable emulsion) CIV 1862
- Valium Injectable 2336
- Valium Tablets 2335

Droperidol (Additive effects). Products include:
- Inapsine Injection 462

Enflurane (Additive effects).
No products indexed under this heading.

Estazolam (Additive effects). Products include:
- ProSom Tablets 457

Ethchlorvynol (Additive effects). Products include:
- Placidyl Capsules 456

Ethinamate (Additive effects).
No products indexed under this heading.

Fentanyl (Additive effects). Products include:
- Duragesic Transdermal System 1336

Fentanyl Citrate (Additive effects). Products include:
- Sublimaze Injection 463

Fluphenazine Decanoate (Additive effects). Products include:
- Prolixin Decanoate 510

Fluphenazine Enanthate (Additive effects). Products include:
- Prolixin Enanthate 510

Fluphenazine Hydrochloride (Additive effects). Products include:
- Prolixin 510

Flurazepam Hydrochloride (Additive effects). Products include:
- Dalmane Capsules 2329

Furazolidone (Anticholinergic effects of antihistamines prolonged and intensified). Products include:
- Furoxone 2221

Glutethimide (Additive effects).
No products indexed under this heading.

Haloperidol (Additive effects). Products include:
- Haldol Injection, Tablets and Concentrate 1585

Haloperidol Decanoate (Additive effects). Products include:
- Haldol Decanoate 1587

Hydrocodone Bitartrate (Additive effects). Products include:
- Codiclear DH Syrup 808
- Duratuss HD Elixir 2750
- Histussin D Liquid 670
- Hycodan Tablets and Syrup 946
- Hycomine Compound Tablets 948
- Hycomine 947
- Hycotuss Expectorant Syrup 950
- Hydrocet Capsules 787
- Lorcet 10/650 Tablets 1016
- Lortab 2751
- Tussend 1830
- Tussend Expectorant 1831
- Vicodin Tablets 1404
- Vicodin ES Tablets 1405
- Vicodin HP Tablets 1403
- Vicodin Tuss Expectorant 1406
- Zydone Capsules 967

Hydrocodone Polistirex (Additive effects). Products include:
- Tussionex Pennkinetic Extended-Release Suspension 1624

Hydroxyzine Hydrochloride (Additive effects). Products include:
- Atarax Tablets & Syrup 1992
- Marax Tablets & DF Syrup 2015
- Vistaril Intramuscular Solution 2042

Isocarboxazid (Anticholinergic effects of antihistamines prolonged and intensified).
No products indexed under this heading.

Isoflurane (Additive effects).
No products indexed under this heading.

Ketamine Hydrochloride (Additive effects).
No products indexed under this heading.

Levomethadyl Acetate Hydrochloride (Additive effects). Products include:
- Orlaam Oral Solution 2361

Levorphanol Tartrate (Additive effects). Products include:
- Levo-Dromoran 2297

Lorazepam (Additive effects). Products include:
- Ativan Injection 2805
- Ativan Tablets 2807

Loxapine Hydrochloride (Additive effects). Products include:
- Loxitane 1426

Loxapine Succinate (Additive effects). Products include:
- Loxitane Capsules 1426

Meperidine Hydrochloride (Additive effects). Products include:
- Demerol 2438
- Mepergan Injection 2859

Mephobarbital (Additive effects). Products include:
- Mebaral Tablets 2452

Meprobamate (Additive effects). Products include:
- Miltown Tablets 2780
- PMB 200 and PMB 400 2890

Mesoridazine Besylate (Additive effects). Products include:
- Serentil 689

IMPORTANT NOTE: Always consult each drug listing in the patient's regimen for possible interactions.

Benadryl Injection

Methadone Hydrochloride (Additive effects). Products include:
- Methadone Hydrochloride Oral Concentrate ... 2356
- Methadone Hydrochloride Oral Solution & Tablets ... 2357

Methohexital Sodium (Additive effects).
No products indexed under this heading.

Methotrimeprazine (Additive effects). Products include:
- Levoprome ... 1321

Methoxyflurane (Additive effects).
No products indexed under this heading.

Midazolam Hydrochloride (Additive effects). Products include:
- Versed Injection ... 2324

Molindone Hydrochloride (Additive effects). Products include:
- Moban Tablets and Concentrate ... 1036

Morphine Sulfate (Additive effects). Products include:
- Astramorph/PF Injection, USP (Preservative-Free) ... 526
- Duramorph Injection ... 983
- Infumorph 200 and Infumorph 500 Sterile Solutions ... 985
- Kadian Capsules ... 2948
- MS Contin Tablets ... 2149
- MSIR ... 2152
- Oramorph SR (Morphine Sulfate Sustained Release Tablets) ... 2359
- RMS Suppositories CII ... 2766
- Roxanol ... 2365

Opium Alkaloids (Additive effects).
No products indexed under this heading.

Oxazepam (Additive effects). Products include:
- Serax Capsules ... 2916
- Serax Tablets ... 2916

Oxycodone Hydrochloride (Additive effects). Products include:
- OxyContin Tablets ... 2163
- OxyIR Capsules ... 2167
- Percocet Tablets ... 955
- Percodan Tablets ... 955
- Percodan-Demi Tablets ... 956
- Roxicodone Tablets, Oral Solution & Intensol (Oxycodone) ... 2366
- Tylox Capsules ... 1593

Pentobarbital Sodium (Additive effects). Products include:
- Nembutal Sodium Capsules ... 440
- Nembutal Sodium Solution ... 442
- Nembutal Sodium Suppositories ... 444

Perphenazine (Additive effects). Products include:
- Etrafon ... 2495
- Triavil Tablets ... 1800
- Trilafon ... 2532

Phenelzine Sulfate (Anticholinergic effects of antihistamines prolonged and intensified). Products include:
- Nardil ... 1977

Phenobarbital (Additive effects). Products include:
- Arco-Lase Plus Tablets ... 513
- Bellergal-S Tablets ... 2375
- Donnatal ... 2234
- Donnatal Extentabs ... 2234
- Donnatal Tablets ... 2234
- Phenobarbital Elixir and Tablets ... 1523
- Quadrinal Tablets ... 1398

Prazepam (Additive effects).
No products indexed under this heading.

Prochlorperazine (Additive effects). Products include:
- Compazine ... 2644

Promethazine Hydrochloride (Additive effects). Products include:
- Mepergan Injection ... 2859
- Phenergan with Codeine ... 2883
- Phenergan with Dextromethorphan ... 2885
- Phenergan Injection ... 2880
- Phenergan Suppositories ... 2882
- Phenergan Syrup ... 2881
- Phenergan Tablets ... 2882
- Phenergan VC ... 2886
- Phenergan VC with Codeine ... 2888

Propofol (Additive effects). Products include:
- Diprivan Injectable Emulsion ... 2939

Propoxyphene Hydrochloride (Additive effects). Products include:
- Darvon ... 1475
- Wygesic Tablets ... 2930

Propoxyphene Napsylate (Additive effects). Products include:
- Darvon-N/Darvocet-N ... 1473

Quazepam (Additive effects). Products include:
- Doral Tablets ... 2773

Risperidone (Additive effects). Products include:
- Risperdal Tablets ... 1348

Secobarbital Sodium (Additive effects). Products include:
- Seconal Sodium Pulvules ... 1529

Selegiline Hydrochloride (Anticholinergic effects of antihistamines prolonged and intensified). Products include:
- Eldepryl Capsules ... 2729

Sevoflurane (Additive effects).
No products indexed under this heading.

Sufentanil Citrate (Additive effects). Products include:
- Sufenta Injection ... 1355

Temazepam (Additive effects). Products include:
- Restoril Capsules ... 2413

Thiamylal Sodium (Additive effects).
No products indexed under this heading.

Thioridazine Hydrochloride (Additive effects). Products include:
- Mellaril ... 2398

Thiothixene (Additive effects). Products include:
- Navane Capsules and Concentrate ... 2018
- Navane Intramuscular ... 2019

Tranylcypromine Sulfate (Anticholinergic effects of antihistamines prolonged and intensified). Products include:
- Parnate Tablets ... 2679

Triazolam (Additive effects). Products include:
- Halcion Tablets ... 2093

Trifluoperazine Hydrochloride (Additive effects). Products include:
- Stelazine ... 2692

Zolpidem Tartrate (Additive effects). Products include:
- Ambien Tablets ... 2559

Food Interactions

Alcohol (Additive effects).

BENADRYL STERI-VIALS, AMPOULES, AND STERI-DOSE SYRINGE
(Diphenhydramine Hydrochloride) ... 1955
See **Benadryl Parenteral**

BENEMID TABLETS
(Probenecid) ... 1651
May interact with salicylates, penicillins, beta-lactams antibiotics, sulfonamides, sulfonylureas, and certain other agents. Compounds in these categories include:

Acetaminophen (Co-administration increases the mean plasma elimination half-life of acetaminophen which can lead to increased plasma concentrations). Products include:
- Actifed Cold & Sinus Caplets and Tablets ... 808
- Actifed Sinus Daytime/Nighttime Tablets and Caplets ... 809
- Alka-Seltzer Fast Relief Caplets ... 610
- Alka-Seltzer Plus Liqui-Gels ... 612
- Alka-Seltzer Plus Flu & Body Aches Effervescent Tablets ... 612
- Alka-Seltzer Plus Flu & Body Aches Liqui-Gels Non-Drowsy Formula ... 613
- Alka-Seltzer Plus Night-Time Cold Medicine Liqui-Gels ... 612
- Allerest No Drowsiness ... 649
- Allerest Sinus Pain Formula ... 649
- Axocet Capsules ... 2469
- Benadryl Allergy/Cold Tablets ... 811
- Benadryl Allergy Sinus Headache Caplets ... 813
- Children's TYLENOL acetaminophen Chewable Tablets, Elixir, Suspension Liquid, and Suspension Drops ... 1559
- Children's TYLENOL Cold Multi-Symptom Chewable Tablets and Liquid ... 1559
- Children's TYLENOL Cold Plus Cough Multi Symptom Chewable Tablets and Liquid ... 1560
- Children's TYLENOL Flu Suspension Liquid ... 1560
- Comtrex Multi-Symptom Allergy-Sinus Formula Tablets and Caplets ... 639
- Comtrex Multi-Symptom ... 638
- Comtrex Non-Drowsy ... 640
- Contac Day Allergy/Sinus Caplets ... 771
- Contac Day & Night ... 772
- Contac Night Allergy/Sinus Caplets ... 771
- Contac Severe Cold and Flu Formula Caplets ... 773
- Contac Severe Cold & Flu Non-Drowsy ... 774
- Coricidin Cold + Flu Tablets ... 760
- Coricidin 'D' Decongestant Tablets ... 760
- DHCplus Capsules ... 2148
- Darvon-N/Darvocet-N ... 1473
- Dimetapp Allergy Sinus Caplets ... 838
- Dimetapp Cold & Fever Suspension ... 839
- Drixoral Cold and Flu Extended-Release Tablets ... 764
- Drixoral Cough + Sore Throat Liquid Caps ... 763
- Drixoral Allergy/Sinus Extended Release Tablets ... 765
- Esgic-plus Capsules ... 1012
- Esgic-plus Tablets ... 1012
- Aspirin Free Excedrin Analgesic Caplets and Geltabs ... 734
- Excedrin Extra-Strength Analgesic Tablets, Caplets, and Geltabs ... 734
- Excedrin P.M. Analgesic/Sleeping Aid Tablets, Caplets, Liquigels ... 735
- Fioricet Tablets ... 2386
- Fioricet with Codeine Capsules ... 2387
- Goody's Extra Strength Headache Powders ... 632
- Goody's Extra Strength Pain Relief Tablets ... 632
- Hycomine Compound Tablets ... 948
- Hydrocet Capsules ... 787
- Infants' TYLENOL acetaminophen Suspension Drops ... 1559
- Infants' TYLENOL Cold Decongestant & Fever-Reducer Drops ... 1561
- Junior Strength TYLENOL acetaminophen Coated Caplets and Chewable Tablets ... 1562
- Lorcet 10/650 Tablets ... 1016
- Lortab ... 2751
- Lurline PMS Tablets ... 1000
- Maximum Strength Multi-Symptom Formula Midol ... 621
- PMS Multi-Symptom Formula Midol ... 622
- Maximum Strength Midol Teen Multi-Symptom Formula ... 621
- Midrin Capsules ... 788
- Panodol Tablets and Caplets ... 783
- Children's Panadol Chewable Tablets, Liquid, Infant's Drops ... 783
- Percocet Tablets ... 955
- Percogesic Analgesic Tablets ... 727
- Phrenilin ... 790
- Pyrroxate Caplets ... 742
- Robitussin Cold, Cough & Flu Liqui-Gels ... 844
- Robitussin Night-Time Cold Formula ... 847
- Sedapap Tablets 50 mg/650 mg ... 1826
- Sinarest ... 663
- Sine-Aid Maximum Strength Sinus Headache Gelcaps, Caplets and Tablets ... 1570
- Sine-Off No Drowsiness Formula Caplets ... 784
- Sine-Off Sinus Medicine ... 784
- Singlet Tablets ... 785
- Sinulin Tablets ... 792
- Sinutab Sinus Allergy Medication, Maximum Strength Tablets and Caplets ... 823
- Sinutab Sinus Medication, Maximum Strength Without Drowsiness Formula, Tablets & Caplets ... 824
- Sudafed Cold and Cough Liquid Caps ... 826
- Sudafed Severe Cold Formula Caplets ... 828
- Sudafed Severe Cold Formula Tablets ... 828
- Sudafed Sinus Caplets ... 829
- Sudafed Sinus Tablets ... 829
- Talacen Caplets ... 2464
- TheraFlu Flu and Cold Medicine ... 750
- Theraflu Maximum Strength Flu and Cold Medicine For Sore Throat ... 751
- TheraFlu Flu, Cold and Cough Medicine ... 750
- TheraFlu Maximum Strength Nighttime Flu, Cold & Cough Medicine ... 751
- TheraFlu Maximum Strength Non-Drowsy Formula Flu, Cold & Cough Medicine ... 751
- TheraFlu Maximum Strength, Non-Drowsy Formula Flu, Cold and Cough Caplets ... 752
- Theraflu Maximum Strength Sinus Non-Drowsy Formula Caplets ... 752
- Triaminic Sore Throat Formula ... 755
- Triaminicin Tablets ... 756
- TYLENOL acetaminophen Extended Relief Caplets ... 1570
- TYLENOL acetaminophen, Extra Strength Adult Liquid Pain Reliever ... 1570
- TYLENOL acetaminophen, Extra Strength Gelcaps, Geltabs, Caplets, Tablets ... 1570
- TYLENOL acetaminophen, Regular Strength Caplets and Tablets ... 1570
- TYLENOL Allergy Sinus, Maximum Strength Caplets and Gelcaps ... 1571
- TYLENOL Allergy Sinus NightTime, Maximum Strength Caplets ... 1571
- TYLENOL Cold Medication, Multi-Symptom Formula Tablets and Caplets ... 1572
- TYLENOL Cold Medication, Multi-Symptom Hot Liquid Packets ... 1572
- TYLENOL Cold Medication, No Drowsiness Formula Caplets and Gelcaps ... 1572
- TYLENOL Cold Severe Congestion Caplets ... 1573
- TYLENOL Cough Medication, Multi Symptom ... 1574
- TYLENOL Cough Medication with Decongestant, Multi Symptom ... 1574
- TYLENOL Flu No Drowsiness Formula, Maximum Strength Gelcaps ... 1575
- TYLENOL Flu NightTime, Maximum Strength Gelcaps ... 1575
- TYLENOL Flu NightTime, Maximum Strength Hot Medication Packets ... 1575
- TYLENOL Headache Plus Pain Reliever with Antacid, Extra Strength Caplets ... 705
- TYLENOL PM Pain Reliever/Sleep Aid, Extra Strength Gelcaps, Caplets, Geltabs ... 1576
- TYLENOL Severe Allergy Medication Caplets ... 1571
- TYLENOL Sinus, Maximum Strength Geltabs, Gelcaps, Caplets and Tablets ... 1576
- Tylenol with Codeine ... 1592
- Tylox Capsules ... 1593
- Unisom With Pain Relief-Nighttime Sleep Aid and Pain Reliever ... 1991
- Vanquish Analgesic Caplets ... 627
- Vicks 44 LiquiCaps Cough, Cold & Flu Relief ... 728
- Vicks 44M Cough, Cold & Flu Relief ... 729
- Vicks DayQuil LiquiCaps/Liquid Multi-Symptom Cold/Flu Relief ... 734

- Vicks Nyquil Hot Therapy 735
- Vicks NyQuil LiquiCaps/Liquid Multi-Symptom Cold/Flu Relief, Original and Cherry Flavors 736
- Vicodin Tablets 1404
- Vicodin ES Tablets 1405
- Vicodin HP Tablets 1403
- Wygesic Tablets 2930
- Zydone Capsules 967

Aminosalicylic Acid (Probenecid inhibits renal transport of aminosalicylic acid). Products include:

- PASER Granules 1333

Aminohippurate Sodium (Probenecid inhibits renal transport of amino hippuric acid). Products include:

- Aminohippurate Sodium Injection .. 1646

Amoxicillin Trihydrate (Concurrent use of therapeutic dose of probenecid and penicillin or other beta-lactams results in higher plasma concentrations of penicillin or beta-lactam antibiotics resulting in increased side effects such as psychic disturbances). Products include:

- Amoxil 2631
- Augmentin 2637
- Augmentin Tablets 2640

Ampicillin (Concurrent use of therapeutic dose of probenecid and penicillin or other beta-lactams results in higher plasma concentrations of penicillin or beta-lactam antibiotics resulting in increased side effects such as psychic disturbances). Products include:

- Omnipen Capsules 2872
- Omnipen for Oral Suspension 2873

Ampicillin Sodium (Concurrent use of therapeutic dose of probenecid and penicillin or other beta-lactams results in higher plasma concentrations of penicillin or beta-lactam antibiotics resulting in increased side effects such as psychic disturbances). Products include:

- Unasyn 2035

Ampicillin Trihydrate (Concurrent use of therapeutic dose of probenecid and penicillin or other beta-lactams results in higher plasma concentrations of penicillin or beta-lactam antibiotics resulting in increased side effects such as psychic disturbances).

No products indexed under this heading.

Aspirin (Concurrent use with salicylates is contraindicated because salicylates antagonize the uricosuric action of probenecid). Products include:

- Alka-Seltzer Cherry Effervescent Antacid and Pain Reliever 609
- Alka-Seltzer Extra Strength Effervescent Antacid and Pain Reliever 609
- Alka-Seltzer Lemon Lime Effervescent Antacid and Pain Reliever 609
- Alka-Seltzer Original Effervescent Antacid and Pain Reliever 609
- Alka-Seltzer Plus 611
- Alka-Seltzer Plus Sinus Medicine .. 611
- Ascriptin 650
- Arthritis Strength BC Powder 631
- BC Cold Powder Multi-Symptom Formula (Cold-Sinus-Allergy) 631
- BC Cold Powder Non-Drowsy Formula (Cold-Sinus) 631
- BC Powder 631
- Genuine Bayer Aspirin Tablets & Caplets 618
- Extra Strength Bayer Arthritis Pain Regimen Formula 615
- Extra Strength Bayer Aspirin Caplets & Tablets 617
- Extended-Release Bayer 8-Hour Aspirin 616
- Extra Strength Bayer Plus Aspirin Caplets 617
- Extra Strength Bayer PM Aspirin Plus Sleep Aid 617
- Aspirin Regimen Bayer 81 mg Tablets with Calcium 615
- Aspirin Regimen Bayer Adult Low Strength 81 mg Tablets 613
- Aspirin Regimen Bayer Children's Chewable Aspirin 616
- Aspirin Regimen Bayer Regular Strength 325 mg Caplets 613
- Bufferin Analgesic Tablets 636
- Arthritis Strength Bufferin Analgesic Caplets 637
- Extra Strength Bufferin Analgesic Tablets 637
- Cama Arthritis Pain Reliever 748
- Darvon Compound-65 Pulvules 1475
- Easprin 1971
- Ecotrin 2625
- Ecotrin Enteric Coated Aspirin Maximum Strength Tablets and Caplets 775
- Ecotrin Enteric Coated Aspirin Regular Strength Tablets 2625
- Empirin Aspirin Tablets 818
- Excedrin Extra-Strength Analgesic Tablets, Caplets, and Geltabs 734
- Fiorinal Capsules 2388
- Fiorinal with Codeine Capsules 2390
- Fiorinal Tablets 2388
- Goody's Extra Strength Headache Powders 632
- Goody's Extra Strength Pain Relief Tablets 632
- Halfprin Tablets 1413
- Norgesic 1554
- Percodan Tablets 955
- Percodan-Demi Tablets 956
- Robaxisal Tablets 2246
- Soma Compound w/Codeine Tablets 2784
- Soma Compound Tablets 2783
- St. Joseph Adult Chewable Aspirin (81 mg.) 768
- Talwin Compound 2466
- Vanquish Analgesic Caplets 627

Azlocillin Sodium (Concurrent use of therapeutic dose of probenecid and penicillin or other beta-lactams results in higher plasma concentrations of penicillin or beta-lactam antibiotics resulting in increased side effects such as psychic disturbances).

No products indexed under this heading.

Aztreonam (Concurrent use of therapeutic dose of probenecid and penicillin or other beta-lactams results in higher plasma concentrations of penicillin or beta-lactam antibiotics resulting in increased side effects such as psychic disturbances). Products include:

- Azactam for Injection 736

Bacampicillin Hydrochloride (Concurrent use of therapeutic dose of probenecid and penicillin or other beta-lactams results in higher plasma concentrations of penicillin or beta-lactam antibiotics resulting in increased side effects such as psychic disturbances). Products include:

- Spectrobid Tablets 2030

Bendroflumethiazide (Probenecid produces insignificant increase in free sulfonamide plasma concentrations but a significant increase in total sulfonamide plasma levels).

No products indexed under this heading.

Carbenicillin Disodium (Concurrent use of therapeutic dose of probenecid and penicillin or other beta-lactams results in higher plasma concentrations of penicillin or beta-lactam antibiotics resulting in increased side effects such as psychic disturbances).

No products indexed under this heading.

Carbenicillin Indanyl Sodium (Concurrent use of therapeutic dose of probenecid and penicillin or other beta-lactams results in higher plasma concentrations of penicillin or beta-lactam antibiotics resulting in increased side effects such as psychic disturbances). Products include:

- Geocillin Tablets 2009

Cefaclor (Concurrent use of therapeutic dose of probenecid and penicillin or other beta-lactams results in higher plasma concentrations of penicillin or beta-lactam antibiotics resulting in increased side effects such as psychic disturbances). Products include:

- Ceclor Pulvules & Suspension 1470

Cefadroxil (Concurrent use of therapeutic dose of probenecid and penicillin or other beta-lactams results in higher plasma concentrations of penicillin or beta-lactam antibiotics resulting in increased side effects such as psychic disturbances). Products include:

- Duricef Capsules, Tablets, and Oral Suspension 750

Cefamandole Nafate (Concurrent use of therapeutic dose of probenecid and penicillin or other beta-lactams results in higher plasma concentrations of penicillin or beta-lactam antibiotics resulting in increased side effects such as psychic disturbances). Products include:

- Mandol Vials, Faspak & ADD-Vantage 1516

Cefazolin Sodium (Concurrent use of therapeutic dose of probenecid and penicillin or other beta-lactams results in higher plasma concentrations of penicillin or beta-lactam antibiotics resulting in increased side effects such as psychic disturbances). Products include:

- Ancef Injection 2632
- Kefzol Vials, Faspak & ADD-Vantage 1511

Cefixime (Concurrent use of therapeutic dose of probenecid and penicillin or other beta-lactams results in higher plasma concentrations of penicillin or beta-lactam antibiotics resulting in increased side effects such as psychic disturbances). Products include:

- Suprax 1443

Cefmetazole Sodium (Concurrent use of therapeutic dose of probenecid and penicillin or other beta-lactams results in higher plasma concentrations of penicillin or beta-lactam antibiotics resulting in increased side effects such as psychic disturbances).

No products indexed under this heading.

Cefonicid Sodium (Concurrent use of therapeutic dose of probenecid and penicillin or other beta-lactams results in higher plasma concentrations of penicillin or beta-lactam antibiotics resulting in increased side effects such as psychic disturbances). Products include:

- Monocid Injection 2674

Cefoperazone Sodium (Concurrent use of therapeutic dose of probenecid and penicillin or other beta-lactams results in higher plasma concentrations of penicillin or beta-lactam antibiotics resulting in increased side effects such as psychic disturbances). Products include:

- Cefobid Intravenous/Intramuscular 1996
- Cefobid Pharmacy Bulk Package-Not for Direct Infusion 1999

Ceforanide (Concurrent use of therapeutic dose of probenecid and penicillin or other beta-lactams results in higher plasma concentrations of penicillin or beta-lactam antibiotics resulting in increased side effects such as psychic disturbances).

No products indexed under this heading.

Cefotaxime Sodium (Concurrent use of therapeutic dose of probenecid and penicillin or other beta-lactams results in higher plasma concentrations of penicillin or beta-lactam antibiotics resulting in increased side effects such as psychic disturbances). Products include:

- Claforan Sterile and Injection 1259

Cefotetan (Concurrent use of therapeutic dose of probenecid and penicillin or other beta-lactams results in higher plasma concentrations of penicillin or beta-lactam antibiotics resulting in increased side effects such as psychic disturbances). Products include:

- Cefotan 2936

Cefoxitin Sodium (Concurrent use of therapeutic dose of probenecid and penicillin or other beta-lactams results in higher plasma concentrations of penicillin or beta-lactam antibiotics resulting in increased side effects such as psychic disturbances). Products include:

- Mefoxin 1734
- Mefoxin Premixed Intravenous Solution 1737

Cefpodoxime Proxetil (Concurrent use of therapeutic dose of probenecid and penicillin or other beta-lactams results in higher plasma concentrations of penicillin or beta-lactam antibiotics resulting in increased side effects such as psychic disturbances). Products include:

- Vantin for Oral Suspension and Vantin Tablets 2112

Cefprozil (Concurrent use of therapeutic dose of probenecid and penicillin or other beta-lactams results in higher plasma concentrations of penicillin or beta-lactam antibiotics resulting in increased side effects such as psychic disturbances). Products include:

- Cefzil Tablets and Oral Suspension 747

Ceftazidime (Concurrent use of therapeutic dose of probenecid and penicillin or other beta-lactams results in higher plasma concentrations of penicillin or beta-lactam antibiotics resulting in increased side effects such as psychic disturbances). Products include:

- Ceptaz 1070
- Fortaz 1092
- Tazicef for Injection 2697
- Tazidime Vials, Faspak & ADD-Vantage 1531

Ceftizoxime Sodium (Concurrent use of therapeutic dose of probenecid and penicillin or other beta-lactams results in higher plasma concentrations of penicillin or beta-lactam antibiotics resulting in increased side effects such as psychic disturbances). Products include:

- Cefizox for Intramuscular or Intravenous Use 1025

IMPORTANT NOTE: Always consult each drug listing in the patient's regimen for possible interactions.

Ceftriaxone Sodium (Concurrent use of therapeutic dose of probenecid and penicillin or other beta-lactams results in higher plasma concentrations of penicillin or beta-lactam antibiotics resulting in increased side effects such as psychic disturbances). Products include:
- Rocephin Injectable Vials, ADD-Vantage, Galaxy Container 2305

Cefuroxime Axetil (Concurrent use of therapeutic dose of probenecid and penicillin or other beta-lactams results in higher plasma concentrations of penicillin or beta-lactam antibiotics resulting in increased side effects such as psychic disturbances). Products include:
- Ceftin 1067

Cefuroxime Sodium (Concurrent use of therapeutic dose of probenecid and penicillin or other beta-lactams results in higher plasma concentrations of penicillin or beta-lactam antibiotics resulting in increased side effects such as psychic disturbances). Products include:
- Kefurox Vials, Faspak & ADD-Vantage 1509
- Zinacef 1184

Cephalexin (Concurrent use of therapeutic dose of probenecid and penicillin or other beta-lactams results in higher plasma concentrations of penicillin or beta-lactam antibiotics resulting in increased side effects such as psychic disturbances). Products include:
- Keflex Pulvules & Oral Suspension 930

Cephalothin Sodium (Concurrent use of therapeutic dose of probenecid and penicillin or other beta-lactams results in higher plasma concentrations of penicillin or beta-lactam antibiotics resulting in increased side effects such as psychic disturbances).

Cephapirin Sodium (Concurrent use of therapeutic dose of probenecid and penicillin or other beta-lactams results in higher plasma concentrations of penicillin or beta-lactam antibiotics resulting in increased side effects such as psychic disturbances).
- No products indexed under this heading.

Cephradine (Concurrent use of therapeutic dose of probenecid and penicillin or other beta-lactams results in higher plasma concentrations of penicillin or beta-lactam antibiotics resulting in increased side effects such as psychic disturbances).
- No products indexed under this heading.

Chlorothiazide (Probenecid produces insignificant increase in free sulfonamide plasma concentrations but a significant increase in total sulfonamide plasma levels). Products include:
- Aldoclor Tablets 1638
- Diupres Tablets 1691
- Diuril Oral 1694

Chlorothiazide Sodium (Probenecid produces insignificant increase in free sulfonamide plasma concentrations but a significant increase in total sulfonamide plasma levels). Products include:
- Diuril Sodium Intravenous 1693

Chlorpropamide (Probenecid may prolong or enhance the action of oral sulfonylureas and thereby increase the risk of hypoglycemia). Products include:
- Diabinese Tablets 2002

Choline Magnesium Trisalicylate (Concurrent use with salicylates is contraindicated because salicylates antagonize the uricosuric action of probenecid). Products include:
- Trilisate 2155

Cilastatin Sodium (Concurrent use of therapeutic dose of probenecid and penicillin or other beta-lactams results in higher plasma concentrations of penicillin or beta-lactam antibiotics resulting in increased side effects such as psychic disturbances). Products include:
- Primaxin I.M. 1770
- Primaxin I.V. 1772

Dicloxacillin Sodium (Concurrent use of therapeutic dose of probenecid and penicillin or other beta-lactams results in higher plasma concentrations of penicillin or beta-lactam antibiotics resulting in increased side effects such as psychic disturbances).
- No products indexed under this heading.

Diflunisal (Concurrent use with salicylates is contraindicated because salicylates antagonize the uricosuric action of probenecid). Products include:
- Dolobid Tablets 1695

Glimepiride (Probenecid may prolong or enhance the action of oral sulfonylureas and thereby increase the risk of hypoglycemia). Products include:
- Amaryl Tablets 1241

Glipizide (Probenecid may prolong or enhance the action of oral sulfonylureas and thereby increase the risk of hypoglycemia). Products include:
- Glucotrol Tablets 2011
- Glucotrol XL Extended Release Tablets 2012

Glyburide (Probenecid may prolong or enhance the action of oral sulfonylureas and thereby increase the risk of hypoglycemia). Products include:
- DiaBeta Tablets 1265
- Glynase PresTab Tablets 2091
- Micronase Tablets 2099

Hydrochlorothiazide (Probenecid produces insignificant increase in free sulfonamide plasma concentrations but a significant increase in total sulfonamide plasma levels). Products include:
- Aldactazide Tablets 2556
- Aldoril Tablets 1644
- Apresazide Capsules 824
- Capozide Tablets 744
- Dyazide Capsules 2653
- Esidrix Tablets 839
- Esimil Tablets 840
- HydroDIURIL Tablets 1716
- Hydropres Tablets 1718
- Hyzaar Tablets 1720
- Inderide Tablets 2838
- Inderide LA Long Acting Capsules .. 2840
- Lopressor HCT Tablets 850
- Lotensin HCT Tablets 855
- Moduretic Tablets 1748
- Oretic Tablets 450
- Prinzide Tablets 1780
- Ser-Ap-Es Tablets 867
- Timolide Tablets 1791
- Vaseretic Tablets 1810
- Zestoretic Tablets 2968
- Ziac 1459

Hydroflumethiazide (Probenecid produces insignificant increase in free sulfonamide plasma concentrations but a significant increase in total sulfonamide plasma levels). Products include:
- Diucardin Tablets 2824

Imipenem (Concurrent use of therapeutic dose of probenecid and penicillin or other beta-lactams results in higher plasma concentrations of penicillin or beta-lactam antibiotics resulting in increased side effects such as psychic disturbances). Products include:
- Primaxin I.M. 1770
- Primaxin I.V. 1772

Indomethacin (Co-administration increases the mean plasma elimination half-life of indomethacin which can lead to increased plasma concentrations). Products include:
- Indocin 1723

Indomethacin Sodium Trihydrate (Co-administration increases the mean plasma elimination half-life of indomethacin which can lead to increased plasma concentrations). Products include:
- Indocin I.V. 1727

Ketamine Hydrochloride (Potential for prolonged anesthesia based on animal data).
- No products indexed under this heading.

Ketoprofen (Co-administration increases the mean plasma elimination half-life of ketoprofen which can lead to increased plasma concentrations). Products include:
- Actron Caplets and Tablets .... ▣ 608
- Orudis Capsules 2874
- Orudis KT .... ▣ 842
- Oruvail Capsules 2874

Loracarbef (Concurrent use of therapeutic dose of probenecid and penicillin or other beta-lactams results in higher plasma concentrations of penicillin or beta-lactam antibiotics resulting in increased side effects such as psychic disturbances). Products include:
- Lorabid Suspension and Pulvules.... 1513

Lorazepam (Co-administration increases the mean plasma elimination half-life of lorazepam which can lead to increased plasma concentrations). Products include:
- Ativan Injection 2805
- Ativan Tablets 2807

Magnesium Salicylate (Concurrent use with salicylates is contraindicated because salicylates antagonize the uricosuric action of probenecid). Products include:
- Backache Caplets .... ▣ 635
- Doan's Extra-Strength Analgesic.... ▣ 653
- Extra Strength Doan's P.M. .... ▣ 653
- Doan's Regular Strength Analgesic .... ▣ 654
- Mobigesic Tablets .... ▣ 607

Meclofenamate Sodium (Co-administration increases the mean plasma elimination half-life of meclofenamate which can lead to increased plasma concentrations).
- No products indexed under this heading.

Methotrexate Sodium (Increased plasma concentrations of methotrexate which may result in methotrexate toxicity; dosage of methotrexate may need to be reduced and serum levels may need to be monitored if given concurrently). Products include:
- Methotrexate Sodium Tablets, Injection, for Injection and LPF Injection 1322

Methyclothiazide (Probenecid produces insignificant increase in free sulfonamide plasma concentrations but a significant increase in total sulfonamide plasma levels). Products include:
- Enduron Tablets 424

Mezlocillin Sodium (Concurrent use of therapeutic dose of probenecid and penicillin or other beta-lactams results in higher plasma concentrations of penicillin or beta-lactam antibiotics resulting in increased side effects such as psychic disturbances). Products include:
- Mezlin 594
- Mezlin Pharmacy Bulk Package 597

Nafcillin Sodium (Concurrent use of therapeutic dose of probenecid and penicillin or other beta-lactams results in higher plasma concentrations of penicillin or beta-lactam antibiotics resulting in increased side effects such as psychic disturbances).
- No products indexed under this heading.

Naproxen (Co-administration increases the mean plasma elimination half-life of naproxen which can lead to increased plasma concentrations). Products include:
- Anaprox/Naprosyn 2277

Naproxen Sodium (Co-administration increases the mean plasma elimination half-life of naproxen which can lead to increased plasma concentrations). Products include:
- Aleve 2124
- Anaprox/Naprosyn 2277
- Naprelan Tablets 2861

Penicillin G Benzathine (Concurrent use of therapeutic dose of probenecid and penicillin or other beta-lactams results in higher plasma concentrations of penicillin or beta-lactam antibiotics resulting in increased side effects such as psychic disturbances). Products include:
- Bicillin C-R Injection 2810
- Bicillin C-R 900/300 Injection 2812
- Bicillin L-A Injection 2813

Penicillin G Potassium (Concurrent use of therapeutic dose of probenecid and penicillin or other beta-lactams results in higher plasma concentrations of penicillin or beta-lactam antibiotics resulting in increased side effects such as psychic disturbances). Products include:
- Pfizerpen for Injection 2022

Penicillin G Procaine (Concurrent use of therapeutic dose of probenecid and penicillin or other beta-lactams results in higher plasma concentrations of penicillin or beta-lactam antibiotics resulting in increased side effects such as psychic disturbances). Products include:
- Bicillin C-R Injection 2810
- Bicillin C-R 900/300 Injection 2812

Penicillin G Sodium (Concurrent use of therapeutic dose of probenecid and penicillin or other beta-lactams results in higher plasma concentrations of penicillin or beta-lactam antibiotics resulting in increased side effects such as psychic disturbances).
- No products indexed under this heading.

109 **Interactions Index** **Bentyl**

Penicillin V Potassium (Concurrent use of therapeutic dose of probenecid and penicillin or other beta-lactams results in higher plasma concentrations of penicillin or beta-lactam antibiotics resulting in increased side effects such as psychic disturbances). Products include:
- Pen•Vee K 2879

Polythiazide (Probenecid produces insignificant increase in free sulfonamide plasma concentrations but a significant increase in total sulfonamide plasma levels). Products include:
- Minizide Capsules 2016

Pyrazinamide (Pyrazinamide antagonizes the uricosuric action of probenecid). Products include:
- Pyrazinamide Tablets 1442
- Rifater 1280

Rifampin (Co-administration increases the mean plasma elimination half-life of rifampin which can lead to increased plasma concentrations). Products include:
- Rifadin 1276
- Rifamate Capsules 1278
- Rifater 1280
- Rimactane Capsules 865

Salsalate (Concurrent use with salicylates is contraindicated because salicylates antagonize the uricosuric action of probenecid). Products include:
- Disalcid 1549
- Mono-Gesic Tablets 810
- Salflex Tablets 791

Sodium Thiopental (Patients receiving probenecid require less thiopental for induction of anesthesia).
- No products indexed under this heading.

Sulfacytine (Probenecid produces insignificant increase in free sulfonamide plasma concentrations but a significant increase in total sulfonamide plasma levels).

Sulfamethizole (Probenecid produces insignificant increase in free sulfonamide plasma concentrations but a significant increase in total sulfonamide plasma levels). Products include:
- Urobiotic-250 Capsules 2038

Sulfamethoxazole (Probenecid produces insignificant increase in free sulfonamide plasma concentrations but a significant increase in total sulfonamide plasma levels). Products include:
- Bactrim DS Tablets 2257
- Bactrim I.V. Infusion 2255
- Bactrim 2257
- Gantanol Tablets 2285
- Septra 1146
- Septra I.V. Infusion 1142
- Septra I.V. Infusion ADD-Vantage Vials 1144
- Septra 1146

Sulfasalazine (Probenecid produces insignificant increase in free sulfonamide plasma concentrations but a significant increase in total sulfonamide plasma levels). Products include:
- Azulfidine 2059

Sulfinpyrazone (Probenecid produces insignificant increase in free sulfonamide plasma concentrations but a significant increase in total sulfonamide plasma levels). Products include:
- Anturane 823

Sulfisoxazole (Probenecid produces insignificant increase in free sulfonamide plasma concentrations but a significant increase in total sulfonamide plasma levels). Products include:
- Gantrisin Tablets 2286

Sulfisoxazole Diolamine (Probenecid produces insignificant increase in free sulfonamide plasma concentrations but a significant increase in total sulfonamide plasma levels).
- No products indexed under this heading.

Sulindac (Co-administration has slight effect on plasma sulfide levels but plasma levels of sulindac and sulfone are increased; modest reduction in uricosuric action of probenecid). Products include:
- Clinoril Tablets 1658

Ticarcillin Disodium (Concurrent use of therapeutic dose of probenecid and penicillin or other beta-lactams results in higher plasma concentrations of penicillin or beta-lactam antibiotics resulting in increased side effects such as psychic disturbances). Products include:
- Ticar for Injection 2704
- Timentin for Injection 2706

Tolazamide (Probenecid may prolong or enhance the action of oral sulfonylureas and thereby increase the risk of hypoglycemia).
- No products indexed under this heading.

Tolbutamide (Probenecid may prolong or enhance the action of oral sulfonylureas and thereby increase the risk of hypoglycemia).
- No products indexed under this heading.

BENGAY EXTERNAL ANALGESIC PRODUCTS
(Menthol, Methyl Salicylate) ..... ⊡ 714
None cited in PDR database.

BENOQUIN CREAM 20%
(Monobenzone) 1298
None cited in PDR database.

BENTYL 10 MG CAPSULES
(Dicyclomine Hydrochloride) 1246
May interact with antacids, agents used to treat achlorhydria and/or to test gastric secretion, nitrates and nitrites, monoamine oxidase inhibitors, phenothiazines, antihistamines, narcotic analgesics, tricyclic antidepressants, benzodiazepines, corticosteroids, sympathomimetics, antiglaucoma agents, anticholinergics, quinidine, and certain other agents. Compounds in these categories include:

Acetazolamide (Effects of antiglaucoma agents antagonized). Products include:
- Diamox Sequels (Sustained Release) ..... ⊙ 318
- Diamox Tablets ..... ⊙ 317

Acetylcholine Chloride (Effects of antiglaucoma agents antagonized). Products include:
- Miochol-E with Iocare Steri-Tags and Miochol-E System Pak ..... ⊙ 263

Acrivastine (Increases certain actions or side effects). Products include:
- Semprex-D Capsules 1620

Albuterol (Increases certain actions or side effects). Products include:
- Proventil Inhalation Aerosol 2524
- Ventolin Inhalation Aerosol and Refill 1170

Albuterol Sulfate (Increases certain actions or side effects). Products include:
- Airet Albuterol Sulfate Inhalation Solution 1602
- Albuterol Sulfate, USP Solution for Inhalation, Arm-a-Med 522
- Proventil Inhalation Solution 0.083% 2527
- Proventil Repetabs Tablets 2529
- Proventil Solution for Inhalation 0.5% 2525
- Proventil Syrup 2528
- Proventil Tablets 2529
- Ventolin Inhalation Solution 1171
- Ventolin Nebules Inhalation Solution 1172
- Ventolin Rotacaps for Inhalation 1173
- Ventolin Syrup 1175
- Ventolin Tablets 1176
- Volmax Extended-Release Tablets 1835

Alfentanil Hydrochloride (Increases certain actions or side effects). Products include:
- Alfenta Injection 1334

Alprazolam (Increases certain actions or side effects). Products include:
- Xanax Tablets 2115

Aluminum Carbonate (Antacids may interfere with the absorption of anticholinergic agents, simultaneous use of these drugs should be avoided). Products include:
- Basaljel Capsules 2810
- Basaljel Suspension 2810
- Basaljel Tablets 2810

Aluminum Hydroxide (Antacids may interfere with the absorption of anticholinergic agents, simultaneous use of these drugs should be avoided). Products include:
- ALternaGEL Liquid 1358
- Maximum Strength Ascriptin ..... ⊡ 650
- Cama Arthritis Pain Reliever ..... ⊡ 748
- Gaviscon Extra Strength Relief Formula Antacid Tablets ..... ⊡ 778
- Gaviscon Extra Strength Relief Formula Liquid Antacid ..... ⊡ 779
- Gaviscon Liquid Antacid ..... ⊡ 779
- Gelusil Antacid-Anti-gas Liquid ..... ⊡ 819
- Gelusil Antacid-Anti-gas Tablets ..... ⊡ 819
- Maalox Antacid/Anti-Gas Tablets 889
- Maalox Heartburn Relief Suspension ..... ⊡ 658
- Maalox Antacid Liquid 888
- Extra Strength Maalox Antacid/Anti-Gas Liquid and Tablets 888
- Mylanta 1359
- Tempo Soft Antacid ..... ⊡ 799

Aluminum Hydroxide Gel (Antacids may interfere with the absorption of anticholinergic agents, simultaneous use of these drugs should be avoided). Products include:
- ALternaGEL Liquid ..... ⊡ 675
- Aludrox Oral Suspension ..... ⊡ 850
- Amphojel Suspension 2802
- Amphojel Suspension without Flavor 2802
- Amphojel Tablets 2802
- Ascriptin ..... ⊡ 650
- Gaviscon Antacid Tablets ..... ⊡ 778
- Gaviscon-2 Antacid Tablets ..... ⊡ 779
- Mylanta Liquid ..... ⊡ 676
- Mylanta Double Strength Liquid ..... ⊡ 676
- Nephrox Suspension ..... ⊡ 671

Amantadine Hydrochloride (Increases certain actions or side effects). Products include:
- Symmetrel Capsules 965
- Symmetrel Syrup 963

Amitriptyline Hydrochloride (Increases certain actions or side effects). Products include:
- Elavil 2945
- Etrafon 2495
- Limbitrol 2333
- Triavil Tablets 1800

Amoxapine (Increases certain actions or side effects). Products include:
- Asendin Tablets 1419

Amyl Nitrite (Increases certain actions and side effects).
- No products indexed under this heading.

Astemizole (Increases certain actions or side effects). Products include:
- Hismanal Tablets 1341

Atropine Sulfate (Increases certain actions or side effects). Products include:
- Arco-Lase Plus Tablets 513
- Atrohist Plus Tablets 1605
- Donnatal 2234
- Donnatal Extentabs 2234
- Donnatal Tablets 2234
- Lomotil 2591
- Motofen Tablets 789
- Urised Tablets 2123

Azatadine Maleate (Increases certain actions or side effects). Products include:
- Trinalin Repetabs Tablets 1373

Belladonna Alkaloids (Increases certain actions or side effects). Products include:
- Bellergal-S Tablets 2375
- Hyland's Bedwetting Tablets ..... ⊡ 788
- Hyland's EnurAid Tablets ..... ⊡ 789
- Hyland's Headache Tablets ..... ⊡ 790
- Hyland's Teething Tablets ..... ⊡ 790
- Similasan Eye Drops #1 ..... ⊡ 769

Benztropine Mesylate (Increases certain actions or side effects). Products include:
- Cogentin 1661

Betamethasone Acetate (Concurrent use in the presence of increased intraocular pressure may be hazardous). Products include:
- Celestone Soluspan Suspension 2484

Betamethasone Sodium Phosphate (Concurrent use in the presence of increased intraocular pressure may be hazardous). Products include:
- Celestone Soluspan Suspension 2484

Betaxolol Hydrochloride (Effects of antiglaucoma agents antagonized). Products include:
- Betoptic Ophthalmic Solution 465
- Betoptic S Ophthalmic Suspension 467
- Kerlone Tablets 2588

Biperiden Hydrochloride (Increases certain actions or side effects). Products include:
- Akineton 1380

Bromodiphenhydramine Hydrochloride (Increases certain actions or side effects).
- No products indexed under this heading.

Brompheniramine Maleate (Increases certain actions or side effects). Products include:
- Alka-Seltzer Plus Sinus Medicine ..... ⊡ 611
- Bromfed Capsules (Extended-Release) 1832
- Bromfed Syrup ..... ⊡ 712
- Bromfed Tablets 1832
- Bromfed-DM Cough Syrup 1832
- Bromfed-PD Capsules (Extended-Release) 1832
- Dimetane-DC Cough Syrup 2232
- Dimetane-DX Cough Syrup 2233
- Dimetapp Allergy Dye-Free Elixir ..... ⊡ 838
- Dimetapp Allergy Sinus Caplets ..... ⊡ 838
- Dimetapp Cold & Allergy Chewable Tablets ..... ⊡ 838
- Dimetapp Cold & Cough Liqui-Gels ..... ⊡ 839
- Dimetapp Cold & Fever Suspension ..... ⊡ 839
- Dimetapp DM Elixir ..... ⊡ 840
- Dimetapp Elixir ..... ⊡ 840
- Dimetapp Extentabs ..... ⊡ 841
- Dimetapp Tablets/Liqui-Gels ..... ⊡ 841
- Rondec Chewable Tablets 974
- Vicks DayQuil Allergy Relief 12-Hour Extended Release Tablets ..... ⊡ 733
- Vicks DayQuil Allergy Relief 4-Hour Tablets ..... ⊡ 733

IMPORTANT NOTE: Always consult each drug listing in the patient's regimen for possible interactions.

Bentyl Interactions Index 110

Buprenorphine (Increases certain actions or side effects). Products include:
- Buprenex Injectable ... 2170

Carbachol (Effects of antiglaucoma agents antagonized). Products include:
- Carbastat Intraocular Solution ... ⊙ 260
- Isopto Carbachol Ophthalmic Solution ... ⊙ 221
- MIOSTAT Intraocular Solution ... ⊙ 222

Cetirizine Hydrochloride (Increases certain actions or side effects). Products include:
- Zyrtec Tablets ... 2053

Chlordiazepoxide (Increases certain actions or side effects). Products include:
- Limbitrol ... 2333

Chlordiazepoxide Hydrochloride (Increases certain actions or side effects). Products include:
- Librax Capsules ... 2330
- Librium Capsules ... 2331
- Librium Injectable ... 2332

Chlorpheniramine Maleate (Increases certain actions or side effects). Products include:
- Alka-Seltzer Plus Cold Medicine ... ▣ 611
- Alka-Seltzer Plus Cold Medicine Liqui-Gels ... ▣ 612
- Alka-Seltzer Plus Cold & Cough Medicine ... ▣ 611
- Alka-Seltzer Plus Cold & Cough Medicine Liqui-Gels ... ▣ 612
- Alka-Seltzer Plus Flu & Body Aches Effervescent Tablets ... ▣ 612
- Allerest Maximum Strength ... ▣ 649
- Allerest Sinus Pain Formula ... ▣ 649
- Ana-Kit Anaphylaxis Emergency Treatment Kit ... 611
- Atrohist Pediatric Capsules ... 1603
- Atrohist Plus Tablets ... 1605
- BC Cold Powder Multi-Symptom Formula (Cold-Sinus-Allergy) ... ▣ 631
- Cerose DM ... ▣ 853
- Cheracol Plus Head Cold/Cough Formula ... ▣ 741
- Children's TYLENOL Cold Multi-Symptom Chewable Tablets and Liquid ... 1559
- Children's TYLENOL Cold Plus Cough Multi Symptom Chewable Tablets and Liquid ... 1560
- Children's TYLENOL Flu Suspension Liquid ... 1560
- Children's Vicks DayQuil Allergy Relief ... ▣ 730
- Children's Vicks NyQuil Cold/Cough Relief ... ▣ 731
- Chlor-Trimeton Allergy Decongestant Tablets ... ▣ 759
- Chlor-Trimeton Allergy Tablets ... ▣ 758
- Allergy-Sinus Comtrex Multi-Symptom Allergy-Sinus Formula Tablets and Caplets ... ▣ 639
- Comtrex Multi-Symptom ... ▣ 638
- Contac Continuous Action Nasal Decongestant/Antihistamine 12 Hour Capsules ... ▣ 773
- Contac Maximum Strength Continuous Action Decongestant/Antihistamine 12 Hour Caplets ... ▣ 772
- Contac Severe Cold and Flu Formula Caplets ... ▣ 773
- Coricidin Cold + Flu Tablets ... ▣ 760
- Coricidin Cough + Cold Tablets ... ▣ 760
- Coricidin 'D' Decongestant Tablets ... ▣ 760
- D.A. II Tablets ... 972
- D.A. Chewable Tablets ... 970
- Dura-Tap/PD Capsules ... 970
- Dura-Vent/DA Tablets ... 972
- Efidac 24 Chlorpheniramine ... ▣ 655
- Extendryl ... 1003
- Fedahist Gyrocaps ... 2545
- Hycomine Compound Tablets ... 948
- Kronofed-A ... 994
- Nolamine Timed-Release Tablets ... 790
- Novahistine Elixir ... ▣ 782
- Ornade Spansule Capsules ... 2678
- PediaCare Cough-Cold Chewable Tablets and Liquid ... 1569
- PediaCare NightRest Cough-Cold Liquid ... 1569
- Pediatric Vicks 44m Cough & Cold Relief ... ▣ 737
- Pyrroxate Caplets ... ▣ 742
- Ryna ... ▣ 804
- Sinarest ... ▣ 663
- Sine-Off Sinus Medicine ... ▣ 784
- Singlet Tablets ... ▣ 785
- Sinulin Tablets ... 792
- Sinutab Sinus Allergy Medication, Maximum Strength Tablets and Caplets ... ▣ 823
- Sudafed Cold & Allergy Tablets ... ▣ 826
- Teldrin 12 Hour Antihistamine/Nasal Decongestant Allergy Relief Capsules ... ▣ 786
- TheraFlu Flu and Cold Medicine ... ▣ 750
- Theraflu Maximum Strength Flu and Cold Medicine For Sore Throat ... ▣ 751
- TheraFlu Flu, Cold and Cough Medicine ... ▣ 750
- TheraFlu Maximum Strength Nighttime Flu, Cold & Cough Medicine ... ▣ 751
- Triaminic Night Time ... ▣ 754
- Triaminic Syrup ... ▣ 755
- Triaminic Triaminicol Cold & Cough ... ▣ 756
- Triaminicin Tablets ... ▣ 756
- Tussend ... 1830
- TYLENOL Allergy Sinus, Maximum Strength Caplets and Gelcaps ... 1571
- TYLENOL Cold Medication, Multi-Symptom Formula Tablets and Caplets ... 1572
- TYLENOL Cold Medication, Multi-Symptom Hot Liquid Packets ... 1572
- Vicks 44 LiquiCaps Cough, Cold & Flu Relief ... ▣ 728
- Vicks 44M Cough, Cold & Flu Relief ... ▣ 729

Chlorpheniramine Polistirex (Increases certain actions or side effects). Products include:
- Tussionex Pennkinetic Extended-Release Suspension ... 1624

Chlorpheniramine Tannate (Increases certain actions or side effects). Products include:
- Atrohist Pediatric Suspension ... 1604
- Atrohist Pediatric Suspension Dye-Free ... 1604
- Rynatan ... 2781
- Rynatuss ... 2782

Chlorpromazine (Increases certain actions or side effects). Products include:
- Thorazine Suppositories ... 2701

Chlorpromazine Hydrochloride (Increases certain actions or side effects). Products include:
- Thorazine ... 2701

Clemastine Fumarate (Increases certain actions or side effects). Products include:
- Tavist Syrup ... 2426
- Tavist Tablets ... 2427
- Tavist-1 12 Hour Relief Tablets ... ▣ 749
- Tavist-D 12 Hour Relief Tablets ... ▣ 750

Clidinium Bromide (Increases certain actions or side effects). Products include:
- Librax Capsules ... 2330

Clomipramine Hydrochloride (Increases certain actions or side effects). Products include:
- Anafranil Capsules ... 819

Clonazepam (Increases certain actions or side effects). Products include:
- Klonopin Tablets ... 2294

Clorazepate Dipotassium (Increases certain actions or side effects). Products include:
- Tranxene ... 459

Codeine Phosphate (Increases certain actions or side effects). Products include:
- Brontex ... 2130
- Dimetane-DC Cough Syrup ... 2232
- Fioricet with Codeine Capsules ... 2387
- Fiorinal with Codeine Capsules ... 2390
- Nucofed ... 2225
- Phenergan with Codeine ... 2883
- Phenergan VC with Codeine ... 2888
- Robitussin A-C Syrup ... 2248
- Robitussin-DAC Syrup ... 2249
- Ryna ... ▣ 804
- Soma Compound w/Codeine Tablets ... 2784
- Tylenol with Codeine ... 1592

Cortisone Acetate (Concurrent use in the presence of increased intraocular pressure may be hazardous). Products include:
- Cortone Acetate Sterile Suspension ... 1663
- Cortone Acetate Tablets ... 1664

Cyproheptadine Hydrochloride (Increases certain actions or side effects). Products include:
- Periactin ... 1767

Demecarium Bromide (Effects of antiglaucoma agents antagonized). Products include:
- Humorsol Sterile Ophthalmic Solution ... 1707

Desipramine Hydrochloride (Increases certain actions or side effects). Products include:
- Norpramin Tablets ... 1273

Dexamethasone (Concurrent use in the presence of increased intraocular pressure may be hazardous). Products include:
- AK-Trol Ointment & Suspension ... ⊙ 205
- Decadron Elixir ... 1676
- Decadron Tablets ... 1678
- Decaspray Topical Aerosol ... 1689
- Maxitrol Ophthalmic Ointment and Suspension ... ⊙ 222
- TobraDex Ophthalmic Suspension and Ointment ... 469

Dexamethasone Acetate (Concurrent use in the presence of increased intraocular pressure may be hazardous). Products include:
- Dalalone D.P. Injectable ... 1009
- Decadron-LA Sterile Suspension ... 1687

Dexamethasone Sodium Phosphate (Concurrent use in the presence of increased intraocular pressure may be hazardous). Products include:
- Decadron Phosphate Injection ... 1680
- Decadron Phosphate Sterile Ophthalmic Ointment ... 1684
- Decadron Phosphate Sterile Ophthalmic Solution ... 1685
- Decadron Phosphate Topical Cream ... 1686
- Decadron Phosphate with Xylocaine Injection, Sterile ... 1683
- Dexacort Phosphate in Respihaler ... 1606
- Dexacort Phosphate in Turbinaire ... 1607
- NeoDecadron Sterile Ophthalmic Ointment ... 1755
- NeoDecadron Sterile Ophthalmic Solution ... 1756
- NeoDecadron Topical Cream ... 1757

Dexchlorpheniramine Maleate (Increases certain actions or side effects).
- No products indexed under this heading.

Dezocine (Increases certain actions or side effects). Products include:
- Dalgan Injection ... 529

Diazepam (Increases certain actions or side effects). Products include:
- Dizac (diazepam injectable emulsion) CIV ... 1862
- Valium Injectable ... 2336
- Valium Tablets ... 2335

Dichlorphenamide (Effects of antiglaucoma agents antagonized). Products include:
- Daranide Tablets ... 1676

Digoxin (Co-administration with anticholinergic agents may affect gastrointestinal absorption of slowly dissolving dosage forms of digoxin; increased serum digoxin concentrations may result). Products include:
- Lanoxicaps ... 1110
- Lanoxin Elixir Pediatric ... 1113
- Lanoxin Injection ... 1116
- Lanoxin Injection Pediatric ... 1119
- Lanoxin Tablets ... 1121

Diphenhydramine Citrate (Increases certain actions or side effects). Products include:
- Excedrin P.M. Analgesic/Sleeping Aid Tablets, Caplets, Liquigels ... 735

Diphenhydramine Hydrochloride (Increases certain actions or side effects). Products include:
- Actifed Allergy Daytime/Nighttime Caplets ... ▣ 808
- Actifed Sinus Daytime/Nighttime Tablets and Caplets ... ▣ 809
- Extra Strength Bayer PM Aspirin Plus Sleep Aid ... ▣ 617
- Benadryl Allergy Chewables ... ▣ 811
- Benadryl Allergy/Cold Tablets ... ▣ 811
- Benadryl Allergy Decongestant Liquid Medication ... ▣ 812
- Benadryl Allergy Decongestant Tablets ... ▣ 812
- Benadryl Allergy Liquid Medication ... ▣ 813
- Benadryl Allergy ... ▣ 811
- Benadryl Allergy Sinus Headache Caplets ... ▣ 813
- Benadryl Dye-Free Allergy Liquigel Softgels ... ▣ 813
- Benadryl Dye-Free Allergy Liquid Medication ... ▣ 814
- Benadryl Itch Relief Stick Extra Strength ... ▣ 814
- Benadryl Cream ... ▣ 814
- Benadryl Gel ... ▣ 815
- Benadryl Spray ... ▣ 815
- Benadryl Injection ... 1955
- Contac Day & Night Cold/Flu Night Caplets ... ▣ 772
- Contac Night Allergy/Sinus Caplets ... ▣ 771
- Extra Strength Doan's P.M. ... ▣ 653
- Excedrin P.M. Analgesic/Sleeping Aid Tablets, Caplets, Liquigels ... ▣ 643
- Nytol QuickCaps Caplets ... ▣ 632
- Sleepinal Night-time Sleep Aid Capsules and Softgels ... ▣ 798
- TYLENOL Allergy Sinus NightTime, Maximum Strength Caplets ... 1571
- TYLENOL Flu NightTime, Maximum Strength Gelcaps ... 1575
- TYLENOL Flu NightTime, Maximum Strength Hot Medication Packets ... 1575
- TYLENOL PM Pain Reliever/Sleep Aid, Extra Strength Gelcaps, Caplets, Geltabs ... 1576
- TYLENOL Severe Allergy Medication Caplets ... 1571
- Maximum Strength Unisom Sleepgels ... 1990
- Unisom With Pain Relief-Nighttime Sleep Aid and Pain Reliever ... 1991

Dipivefrin Hydrochloride (Effects of antiglaucoma agents antagonized). Products include:
- AKPRO ... ⊙ 206
- PROPINE with C CAP Compliance Cap ... ⊙ 251

Dobutamine Hydrochloride (Increases certain actions or side effects). Products include:
- Dobutrex Solution Vials ... 1480

Dopamine Hydrochloride (Increases certain actions or side effects).
- No products indexed under this heading.

Doxepin Hydrochloride (Increases certain actions or side effects). Products include:
- Adapin Capsules ... 1542
- Sinequan ... 2028
- Zonalon Cream ... 1042

Echothiophate Iodide (Effects of antiglaucoma agents antagonized). Products include:
- Phospholine Iodide ... ⊙ 323

Ephedrine Hydrochloride (Increases certain actions or side effects). Products include:
- Primatene Tablets ... ▣ 844
- Quadrinal Tablets ... 1398

(▣ Described in PDR For Nonprescription Drugs) (⊙ Described in PDR For Ophthalmology)

Ephedrine Sulfate (Increases certain actions or side effects). Products include:
- Marax Tablets & DF Syrup ... 2015

Ephedrine Tannate (Increases certain actions or side effects). Products include:
- Rynatuss ... 2782

Epinephrine (Increases certain actions or side effects). Products include:
- EPIFRIN ... ⊙ 237
- EpiPen ... 808
- Marcaine with Epinephrine ... 2446
- Primatene Mist ... ▣ 843
- Sensorcaine with Epinephrine Injection ... 554
- Sus-Phrine Injection ... 1017
- Xylocaine with Epinephrine Injections ... 562

Epinephrine Bitartrate (Increases certain actions or side effects). Products include:
- Sensorcaine-MPF with Epinephrine Injection ... 554

Epinephrine Hydrochloride (Increases certain actions or side effects). Products include:
- Ana-Kit Anaphylaxis Emergency Treatment Kit ... 611

Epinephryl Borate (Increases certain actions or side effects).
- No products indexed under this heading.

Erythrityl Tetranitrate (Increases certain actions and side effects).
- No products indexed under this heading.

Estazolam (Increases certain actions or side effects). Products include:
- ProSom Tablets ... 457

Fentanyl (Increases certain actions or side effects). Products include:
- Duragesic Transdermal System ... 1336

Fentanyl Citrate (Increases certain actions or side effects). Products include:
- Sublimaze Injection ... 463

Fludrocortisone Acetate (Concurrent use in the presence of increased intraocular pressure may be hazardous). Products include:
- Florinef Acetate Tablets ... 506

Fluphenazine Decanoate (Increases certain actions or side effects). Products include:
- Prolixin Decanoate ... 510

Fluphenazine Enanthate (Increases certain actions or side effects). Products include:
- Prolixin Enanthate ... 510

Fluphenazine Hydrochloride (Increases certain actions or side effects). Products include:
- Prolixin ... 510

Flurazepam Hydrochloride (Increases certain actions or side effects). Products include:
- Dalmane Capsules ... 2329

Furazolidone (Co-administration with MAO inhibitors may increase certain actions or side effects of anticholinergic drugs). Products include:
- Furoxone ... 2221

Glutamic Acid Hydrochloride (Antagonizes the inhibiting effects on gastric hydrochloric acid).
- No products indexed under this heading.

Glycopyrrolate (Increases certain actions or side effects). Products include:
- Robinul Forte Tablets ... 2247
- Robinul Injectable ... 2247
- Robinul Tablets ... 2247

Halazepam (Increases certain actions or side effects).
- No products indexed under this heading.

Hydrocodone Bitartrate (Increases certain actions or side effects). Products include:
- Codiclear DH Syrup ... 808
- Duratuss HD Elixir ... 2750
- Histussin D Liquid ... 670
- Hycodan Tablets and Syrup ... 946
- Hycomine Compound Tablets ... 948
- Hycomine ... 947
- Hycotuss Expectorant Syrup ... 950
- Hydrocet Capsules ... 787
- Lorcet 10/650 Tablets ... 1016
- Lortab ... 2751
- Tussend ... 1830
- Tussend Expectorant ... 1831
- Vicodin Tablets ... 1404
- Vicodin ES Tablets ... 1405
- Vicodin HP Tablets ... 1403
- Vicodin Tuss Expectorant ... 1406
- Zydone Capsules ... 967

Hydrocodone Polistirex (Increases certain actions or side effects). Products include:
- Tussionex Pennkinetic Extended-Release Suspension ... 1624

Hydrocortisone (Concurrent use in the presence of increased intraocular pressure may be hazardous). Products include:
- Anusol-HC Cream 2.5% ... 1953
- Aquanil HC Lotion ... 1989
- Maximum Strength Cortaid Spray ▣ 800
- CORTENEMA ... 2713
- Cortisporin Ointment ... 1074
- Cortisporin Ophthalmic Ointment Sterile ... 1074
- Cortisporin Ophthalmic Suspension Sterile ... 1075
- Cortisporin Otic Solution Sterile ... 1076
- Cortisporin Otic Suspension Sterile 1077
- Cortizone-5 ... ▣ 795
- Cortizone-10 ... ▣ 795
- Hydrocortone Tablets ... 1715
- Hytone ... 922
- Hytone Ointment 2 ½% ... 923
- Massengill Medicated Soft Cloth Towelettes ... 2628
- Pediotic Suspension Sterile ... 1140
- Preparation H Hydrocortisone 1% Cream ... ▣ 843
- ProctoCream-HC 2.5% ... 2552
- VōSoL HC Otic Solution ... 2786

Hydrocortisone Acetate (Concurrent use in the presence of increased intraocular pressure may be hazardous). Products include:
- Analpram-HC Rectal Cream 1% and 2.5% ... 993
- Anusol HC-1 Hydrocortisone Anti-Itch Ointment ... ▣ 810
- Anusol-HC Suppositories ... 1954
- Caldecort Anti-Itch Hydrocortisone Cream ... ▣ 651
- Coly-Mycin S Otic w/Neomycin & Hydrocortisone ... 1965
- Cortaid ... ▣ 800
- Cortifoam ... 2540
- Cortisporin Cream ... 1073
- Epifoam ... 2543
- Hydrocortone Acetate Sterile Suspension ... 1712
- Mantadil Cream ... 1124
- Nupercainal Hydrocortisone 1% Cream ... ▣ 661
- Pramosone Cream, Lotion & Ointment ... 995
- ProctoFoam-HC ... 2552
- Terra-Cortril Ophthalmic Suspension ... 2033

Hydrocortisone Sodium Phosphate (Concurrent use in the presence of increased intraocular pressure may be hazardous). Products include:
- Hydrocortone Phosphate Injection, Sterile ... 1713

Hydrocortisone Sodium Succinate (Concurrent use in the presence of increased intraocular pressure may be hazardous).
- No products indexed under this heading.

Hydromorphone Hydrochloride (Increases certain actions or side effects). Products include:
- Dilaudid Ampules ... 1382
- Dilaudid Cough Syrup ... 1383
- Dilaudid-HP Injection ... 1384
- Dilaudid-HP Lyophilized Powder 250 mg ... 1384
- Dilaudid ... 1382
- Dilaudid Oral Liquid ... 1386
- Dilaudid ... 1382
- Dilaudid Tablets - 8 mg ... 1386

Hyoscyamine (Increases certain actions or side effects). Products include:
- Cystospaz Tablets ... 2123
- Urised Tablets ... 2123

Hyoscyamine Sulfate (Increases certain actions or side effects). Products include:
- Arco-Lase Plus Tablets ... 513
- Atrohist Plus Tablets ... 1605
- Cystospaz-M Capsules ... 2123
- Donnatal ... 2234
- Donnatal Extentabs ... 2234
- Donnatal Tablets ... 2234
- Kutrase Capsules ... 2546
- Levsin/Levsinex/Levbid ... 2549

Imipramine Hydrochloride (Increases certain actions or side effects). Products include:
- Tofranil Ampuls ... 873
- Tofranil Tablets ... 875

Imipramine Pamoate (Increases certain actions or side effects). Products include:
- Tofranil-PM Capsules ... 876

Ipratropium Bromide (Increases certain actions or side effects). Products include:
- Atrovent Inhalation Aerosol ... 674
- Atrovent Inhalation Solution ... 675
- Atrovent Nasal Spray 0.03% ... 676
- Atrovent Nasal Spray 0.06% ... 678

Isocarboxazid (Co-administration with MAO inhibitors may increase certain actions or side effects of anticholinergic drugs).
- No products indexed under this heading.

Isoflurophate (Effects of antiglaucoma agents antagonized).
- No products indexed under this heading.

Isoproterenol Hydrochloride (Increases certain actions or side effects). Products include:
- Isuprel Hydrochloride Solution ... 2443
- Isuprel Injection ... 2441
- Isuprel Mistometer ... 2442

Isoproterenol Sulfate (Increases certain actions or side effects). Products include:
- Norisodrine with Calcium Iodide Syrup ... 446

Isosorbide Dinitrate (Increases certain actions and side effects). Products include:
- Dilatrate-SR Capsules ... 2542
- Isordil Sublingual Tablets ... 2845
- Isordil Tembids ... 2847
- Isordil Titradose Tablets ... 2848
- Sorbitrate ... 2959

Isosorbide Mononitrate (Increases certain actions and side effects). Products include:
- Imdur ... 1362
- Ismo Tablets ... 2844
- Monoket Tablets ... 2550

Levobunolol Hydrochloride (Effects of antiglaucoma agents antagonized). Products include:
- Betagan ... ⊙ 230

Levorphanol Tartrate (Increases certain actions or side effects). Products include:
- Levo-Dromoran ... 2297

Loratadine (Increases certain actions or side effects). Products include:
- Claritin Tablets ... 2485
- Claritin-D Tablets ... 2487

Lorazepam (Increases certain actions or side effects). Products include:
- Ativan Injection ... 2805
- Ativan Tablets ... 2807

Magaldrate (Antacids may interfere with the absorption of anticholinergic agents, simultaneous use of these drugs should be avoided).
- No products indexed under this heading.

Magnesium Hydroxide (Antacids may interfere with the absorption of anticholinergic agents, simultaneous use of these drugs should be avoided). Products include:
- Aludrox Oral Suspension ... ▣ 850
- Ascriptin ... ▣ 650
- Di-Gel Antacid/Anti-Gas ... ▣ 762
- Gelusil Antacid-Anti-gas Liquid ... ▣ 819
- Gelusil Antacid-Anti-gas Tablets ... ▣ 819
- Maalox Antacid/Anti-Gas Tablets ... 889
- Maalox Antacid Liquid ... 888
- Extra Strength Maalox Antacid/Anti-Gas Liquid and Tablets ... 888
- Mylanta Fast-Acting ... 1359
- Mylanta Gelcaps Antacid ... ▣ 678
- Fast-Acting Mylanta Liquid Antacid 1359
- Mylanta Tablets ... ▣ 677
- Maximum-Strength Fast-Acting Mylanta Liquid Antacid ... 1359
- Mylanta Double Strength Tablets .. ▣ 677
- Phillips' Milk of Magnesia Liquid ... ▣ 627
- Rolaids Antacid Tablets ... ▣ 807
- Tempo Soft Antacid ... ▣ 799

Magnesium Oxide (Antacids may interfere with the absorption of anticholinergic agents, simultaneous use of these drugs should be avoided). Products include:
- Beelith Tablets ... 632
- Bufferin Analgesic Tablets ... ▣ 636
- Arthritis Strength Bufferin Analgesic Caplets ... ▣ 637
- Extra Strength Bufferin Analgesic Tablets ... ▣ 637
- Caltrate PLUS ... ▣ 681
- Cama Arthritis Pain Reliever ... ▣ 748
- Mag-Ox 400 ... 666
- Uro-Mag ... 666

Maprotiline Hydrochloride (Increases certain actions or side effects). Products include:
- Ludiomil Tablets ... 861

Mepenzolate Bromide (Increases certain actions or side effects).
- No products indexed under this heading.

Meperidine Hydrochloride (Increases certain actions or side effects). Products include:
- Demerol ... 2438
- Mepergan Injection ... 2859

Mesoridazine Besylate (Increases certain actions or side effects). Products include:
- Serentil ... 689

Metaproterenol Sulfate (Increases certain actions or side effects). Products include:
- Alupent ... 672
- Metaproterenol Sulfate Inhalation Solution, USP, Arm-a-Med ... 547

Metaraminol Bitartrate (Increases certain actions or side effects). Products include:
- Aramine Injection ... 1649

Methadone Hydrochloride (Increases certain actions or side effects). Products include:
- Methadone Hydrochloride Oral Concentrate ... 2356
- Methadone Hydrochloride Oral Solution & Tablets ... 2357

Methazolamide (Effects of antiglaucoma agents antagonized). Products include:
- GlaucTabs ... ⊙ 209
- Neptazane Tablets ... ⊙ 320

IMPORTANT NOTE: Always consult each drug listing in the patient's regimen for possible interactions.

Bentyl | Interactions Index | 112

Methdilazine Hydrochloride (Increases certain actions or side effects).
No products indexed under this heading.

Methotrimeprazine (Increases certain actions or side effects). Products include:
Levoprome 1321

Methoxamine Hydrochloride (Increases certain actions or side effects). Products include:
Vasoxyl Injection 1169

Methylprednisolone Acetate (Concurrent use in the presence of increased intraocular pressure may be hazardous).
No products indexed under this heading.

Methylprednisolone Sodium Succinate (Concurrent use in the presence of increased intraocular pressure may be hazardous).
No products indexed under this heading.

Metoclopramide Hydrochloride (Gastrointestinal motility effects of metoclopramide may be antagonized). Products include:
Reglan 2243

Midazolam Hydrochloride (Increases certain actions or side effects). Products include:
Versed Injection 2324

Morphine Sulfate (Increases certain actions or side effects). Products include:
Astramorph/PF Injection, USP (Preservative-Free) 526
Duramorph Injection 983
Infumorph 200 and Infumorph 500 Sterile Solutions 985
Kadian Capsules 2948
MS Contin Tablets 2149
MSIR 2152
Oramorph SR (Morphine Sulfate Sustained Release Tablets) 2359
RMS Suppositories CII 2766
Roxanol 2365

Nitroglycerin (Increases certain actions and side effects). Products include:
Deponit NTG Transdermal Delivery System 2541
Nitro-Bid IV 1270
Nitro-Bid Ointment 1272
Nitro-Dur (nitroglycerin) Transdermal Infusion System 1365
Nitrolingual Spray 2193
Nitrostat Tablets 1981
Transderm-Nitro Transdermal Therapeutic System 878

Norepinephrine Bitartrate (Increases certain actions or side effects). Products include:
Levophed Bitartrate Injection 2445

Nortriptyline Hydrochloride (Increases certain actions or side effects). Products include:
Pamelor 2409

Opium Alkaloids (Increases certain actions or side effects).
No products indexed under this heading.

Oxazepam (Increases certain actions or side effects). Products include:
Serax Capsules 2916
Serax Tablets 2916

Oxybutynin Chloride (Increases certain actions or side effects). Products include:
Ditropan 1267

Oxycodone Hydrochloride (Increases certain actions or side effects). Products include:
OxyContin Tablets 2163
OxyIR Capsules 2167
Percocet Tablets 955
Percodan Tablets 955
Percodan-Demi Tablets 956
Roxicodone Tablets, Oral Solution & Intensol (Oxycodone) 2366
Tylox Capsules 1593

Pentaerythritol Tetranitrate (Increases certain actions and side effects).
No products indexed under this heading.

Pentagastrin (Antagonizes the inhibiting effects on gastric hydrochloric acid). Products include:
Peptavlon 2997

Perphenazine (Increases certain actions or side effects). Products include:
Etrafon 2495
Triavil Tablets 1800
Trilafon 2532

Phenelzine Sulfate (Co-administration with MAO inhibitors may increase certain actions or side effects of anticholinergic drugs). Products include:
Nardil 1977

Phenylephrine Bitartrate (Increases certain actions or side effects).
No products indexed under this heading.

Phenylephrine Hydrochloride (Increases certain actions or side effects). Products include:
Atrohist Plus Tablets 1605
Cerose DM .... ▣ 853
D.A. II Tablets 972
D.A. Chewable Tablets 970
Dura-Vent/DA Tablets 972
Extendryl 1003
4-Way Fast Acting Nasal Spray (regular & mentholated) .... ▣ 644
Hemorid .... ▣ 797
Hycomine Compound Tablets 948
Neo-Synephrine Hydrochloride 1% Carpuject 2455
Neo-Synephrine Hydrochloride 1% Injection 2455
Neo-Synephrine Hydrochloride (Ophthalmic) 2456
Neo-Synephrine .... ▣ 624
Novahistine Elixir .... ▣ 782
Phenergan VC 2886
Phenergan VC with Codeine 2888
Preparation H .... ▣ 842
Tympagesic Ear Drops 2476
Vicks Sinex Nasal Spray and Ultra Fine Mist .... ▣ 738

Phenylephrine Tannate (Increases certain actions or side effects). Products include:
Atrohist Pediatric Suspension 1604
Atrohist Pediatric Suspension Dye-Free 1604
Rynatan 2781
Rynatuss 2782

Phenylpropanolamine Hydrochloride (Increases certain actions or side effects). Products include:
Acutrim .... ▣ 648
Atrohist Plus Tablets 1605
BC Cold Powder Multi-Symptom Formula (Cold-Sinus-Allergy) .... ▣ 631
BC Cold Powder Non-Drowsy Formula (Cold-Sinus) .... ▣ 631
Cheracol Plus Head Cold/Cough Formula .... ▣ 741
Comtrex Multi-Symptom Cold Reliever Liqui-Gels .... ▣ 638
Comtrex Multi-Symptom Non-Drowsy Liqui-gels .... ▣ 640
Contac Continuous Action Nasal Decongestant/Antihistamine 12 Hour Capsules .... ▣ 773
Contac Maximum Strength Continuous Action Decongestant/Antihistamine 12 Hour Caplets .... ▣ 772
Contac Severe Cold and Flu Formula Caplets .... ▣ 773
Coricidin 'D' Decongestant Tablets .... ▣ 760
Dexatrim .... ▣ 795
Dexatrim Plus Vitamins Caplets .... ▣ 796
Dimetane-DC Cough Syrup 2232
Dimetapp Allergy Sinus Caplets .... ▣ 838
Dimetapp Cold & Allergy Chewable Tablets .... ▣ 838
Dimetapp Cold & Cough Liqui-Gels .... ▣ 839
Dimetapp DM Elixir .... ▣ 840
Dimetapp Elixir .... ▣ 840
Dimetapp Extentabs .... ▣ 841
Dimetapp Tablets/Liqui-Gels .... ▣ 841
Dura-Vent Tablets 971
Entex LA Tablets 972
Exgest LA Tablets 787
Hycomine 947
Nolamine Timed-Release Tablets 790
Ornade Spansule Capsules 2678
Propagest Tablets 791
Pyrroxate Caplets .... ▣ 742
Robitussin-CF .... ▣ 846
Sinulin Tablets 792
Tavist-D 12 Hour Relief Tablets .... ▣ 750
Teldrin 12 Hour Antihistamine/Nasal Decongestant Allergy Relief Capsules .... ▣ 786
Triaminic Expectorant .... ▣ 753
Triaminic Syrup .... ▣ 755
Triaminic Triaminicol Cold & Cough .... ▣ 756
Triaminic DM Syrup .... ▣ 756
Triaminicin Tablets .... ▣ 756
Vicks DayQuil Allergy Relief 12-Hour Extended Release Tablets .... ▣ 733
Vicks DayQuil Allergy Relief 4-Hour Tablets .... ▣ 733
Vicks DayQuil SINUS Pressure & CONGESTION Relief .... ▣ 734

Pilocarpine (Effects of antiglaucoma agents antagonized). Products include:
Ocusert Pilo-20 and Pilo-40 Ocular Therapeutic Systems .... ⊙ 252

Pilocarpine Hydrochloride (Effects of antiglaucoma agents antagonized). Products include:
Isopto Carpine Ophthalmic Solution .... ⊙ 221
Pilopine HS Ophthalmic Gel .... ⊙ 224
Salagen Tablets 1546

Pirbuterol Acetate (Increases certain actions or side effects). Products include:
Maxair Autohaler 1550
Maxair Inhaler 1552

Prazepam (Increases certain actions or side effects).
No products indexed under this heading.

Prednisolone Acetate (Concurrent use in the presence of increased intraocular pressure may be hazardous). Products include:
AK-CIDE .... ⊙ 203
AK-CIDE Ointment .... ⊙ 203
Blephamide Liquifilm Sterile Ophthalmic Suspension 472
Blephamide Ointment .... ⊙ 234
Econopred & Econopred Plus Ophthalmic Suspensions .... ⊙ 216
Poly-Pred Liquifilm .... ⊙ 246
Pred Forte .... ⊙ 247
Pred Mild .... ⊙ 250
Pred-G Liquifilm Sterile Ophthalmic Suspension .... ⊙ 248
Pred-G S.O.P. Sterile Ophthalmic Ointment .... ⊙ 249

Prednisolone Sodium Phosphate (Concurrent use in the presence of increased intraocular pressure may be hazardous). Products include:
AK-PRED .... ⊙ 204
Hydeltrasol Injection, Sterile 1708
Pediapred Oral Solution 1618

Prednisolone Tebutate (Concurrent use in the presence of increased intraocular pressure may be hazardous). Products include:
Hydeltra-T.B.A. Sterile Suspension 1710

Prednisone (Concurrent use in the presence of increased intraocular pressure may be hazardous).
No products indexed under this heading.

Prochlorperazine (Increases certain actions or side effects). Products include:
Compazine 2644

Procyclidine Hydrochloride (Increases certain actions or side effects). Products include:
Kemadrin Tablets 1105

Promethazine Hydrochloride (Increases certain actions or side effects). Products include:
Mepergan Injection 2859
Phenergan with Codeine 2883
Phenergan with Dextromethorphan 2885
Phenergan Injection 2880
Phenergan Suppositories 2882
Phenergan Syrup 2881
Phenergan Tablets 2882
Phenergan VC 2886
Phenergan VC with Codeine 2888

Propantheline Bromide (Increases certain actions or side effects). Products include:
Pro-Banthine Tablets 2226

Propoxyphene Hydrochloride (Increases certain actions or side effects). Products include:
Darvon 1475
Wygesic Tablets 2930

Propoxyphene Napsylate (Increases certain actions or side effects). Products include:
Darvon-N/Darvocet-N 1473

Protriptyline Hydrochloride (Increases certain actions or side effects). Products include:
Vivactil Tablets 1820

Pseudoephedrine Hydrochloride (Increases certain actions or side effects). Products include:
Actifed Allergy Daytime/Nighttime Caplets .... ▣ 808
Actifed Cold & Allergy Tablets .... ▣ 807
Actifed Cold & Sinus Caplets and Tablets .... ▣ 808
Actifed Sinus Daytime/Nighttime Tablets and Caplets .... ▣ 809
Advil Cold and Sinus Caplets and Tablets .... ▣ 837
Alka-Seltzer Plus Liqui-Gels .... ▣ 612
Alka-Seltzer Plus Flu & Body Aches Liqui-Gels Non-Drowsy Formula .... ▣ 613
Alka-Seltzer Plus Night-Time Cold Medicine Liqui-Gels .... ▣ 612
Allerest Maximum Strength .... ▣ 649
Allerest No Drowsiness .... ▣ 649
Allerest Sinus Pain Formula .... ▣ 649
Atrohist Pediatric Capsules 1603
Benadryl Allergy/Cold Tablets .... ▣ 811
Benadryl Allergy Decongestant Liquid Medication .... ▣ 812
Benadryl Allergy Decongestant Tablets .... ▣ 812
Benadryl Allergy Sinus Headache Caplets .... ▣ 813
Benylin Multisymptom .... ▣ 816
Bromfed Capsules (Extended-Release) 1832
Bromfed Syrup .... ▣ 712
Bromfed Tablets 1832
Bromfed-DM Cough Syrup 1832
Bromfed-PD Capsules (Extended-Release) 1832
Children's TYLENOL Cold Multi-Symptom Chewable Tablets and Liquid 1559
Children's TYLENOL Cold Plus Cough Multi Symptom Chewable Tablets and Liquid 1560
Children's TYLENOL Flu Suspension Liquid 1560
Children's Vicks DayQuil Allergy Relief .... ▣ 730
Children's Vicks NyQuil Cold/Cough Relief .... ▣ 731
Allergy-Sinus Comtrex Multi-Symptom Allergy-Sinus Formula Tablets and Caplets .... ▣ 639
Comtrex Multi-Symptom .... ▣ 638
Comtrex Multi-Symptom Non-Drowsy Caplets .... ▣ 640
Congess 1003
Contac Day Allergy/Sinus Caplets ▣ 771
Contac Day & Night .... ▣ 772
Contac Night Allergy/Sinus Caplets .... ▣ 771
Contac Severe Cold & Flu Non-Drowsy .... ▣ 774
Deconsal II Tablets 1605
Dimetane-DX Cough Syrup 2233

(▣ Described in PDR For Nonprescription Drugs) (⊙ Described in PDR For Ophthalmology)

113 Interactions Index Bentyl

Dimetapp Cold & Fever Suspension ... 839
Dimetapp Decongestant Pediatric Drops ... 840
Dorcol Children's Cough Syrup ... 748
Drixoral Cough + Congestion Liquid Caps ... 763
Dura-Tap/PD Capsules ... 970
Duratuss Tablets ... 2750
Duratuss HD Elixir ... 2750
Efidac/24 ... 655
Entex PSE Tablets ... 973
Fedahist Gyrocaps ... 2545
Guaifed ... 1833
Guaifed Syrup ... 712
Guaimax-D Tablets ... 809
Histussin D Liquid ... 670
Infants' TYLENOL Cold Decongestant & Fever-Reducer Drops ... 1561
Kronofed-A ... 994
Novahistine DMX ... 782
Nucofed ... 2225
PediaCare Cough-Cold Chewable Tablets and Liquid ... 1569
PediaCare Infants' Decongestant Drops ... 1569
PediaCare Infants' Drops Decongestant Plus Cough ... 1569
PediaCare NightRest Cough-Cold Liquid ... 1569
Pediatric Vicks 44d Cough & Head Congestion Relief ... 736
Pediatric Vicks 44m Cough & Cold Relief ... 737
Robitussin Cold & Cough Liqui-Gels ... 844
Robitussin Cold, Cough & Flu Liqui-Gels ... 844
Robitussin Maximum Strength Cough & Cold ... 847
Robitussin Night-Time Cold Formula ... 847
Robitussin Pediatric Cough & Cold Formula ... 848
Robitussin Pediatric Drops ... 849
Robitussin Severe Congestion Liqui-Gels ... 845
Robitussin-DAC Syrup ... 2249
Robitussin-PE ... 846
Rondec Oral Drops ... 974
Rondec Syrup ... 974
Rondec Tablet ... 974
Rondec Chewable Tablets ... 974
Rondec-TR Tablet ... 974
Ryna ... 804
Seldane-D Extended-Release Tablets ... 1286
Semprex-D Capsules ... 1620
Sinarest ... 663
Sine-Aid Maximum Strength Sinus Headache Gelcaps, Caplets and Tablets ... 1570
Sine-Off No Drowsiness Formula Caplets ... 784
Sine-Off Sinus Medicine ... 784
Singlet Tablets ... 785
Sinutab Non-Drying Liquid Caps ... 823
Sinutab Sinus Allergy Medication, Maximum Strength Tablets and Caplets ... 823
Sinutab Sinus Medication, Maximum Strength Without Drowsiness Formula, Tablets & Caplets ... 824
Sudafed Children's Cold & Cough Liquid Medication ... 825
Sudafed Children's Nasal Decongestant Liquid Medication ... 826
Sudafed Cold & Allergy Tablets ... 826
Sudafed Cold and Cough Liquid Caps ... 826
Sudafed Nasal Decongestant Tablets, 30 mg ... 825
Sudafed Nasal Decongestant Tablets, 60 mg ... 825
Sudafed Non-Drying Sinus Liquid Caps ... 827
Sudafed Pediatric Nasal Decongestant Liquid Oral Drops ... 827
Sudafed Severe Cold Formula Caplets ... 828
Sudafed Severe Cold Formula Tablets ... 828
Sudafed Sinus Caplets ... 829
Sudafed Sinus Tablets ... 829
Sudafed 12 Hour Caplets ... 824
Syn-Rx Tablets ... 1622
Syn-Rx DM Tablets ... 1623
TheraFlu Flu and Cold Medicine ... 750
Theraflu Maximum Strength Flu and Cold Medicine For Sore Throat ... 751
TheraFlu Flu, Cold and Cough Medicine ... 750
TheraFlu Maximum Strength Nighttime Flu, Cold & Cough Medicine ... 751
TheraFlu Maximum Strength Non-Drowsy Formula Flu, Cold & Cough Medicine ... 751
TheraFlu Maximum Strength, Non-Drowsy Formula Flu, Cold and Cough Caplets ... 752
Theraflu Maximum Strength Sinus Non-Drowsy Formula Caplets ... 752
Triaminic AM Cough and Decongestant Formula ... 753
Triaminic AM Decongestant Formula ... 753
Triaminic Infant Oral Decongestant Drops ... 754
Triaminic Night Time ... 754
Triaminic Sore Throat Formula ... 755
Tussend ... 1830
Tussend Expectorant ... 1831
TYLENOL Allergy Sinus, Maximum Strength Caplets and Gelcaps ... 1571
TYLENOL Allergy Sinus NightTime, Maximum Strength Caplets ... 1571
TYLENOL Cold Medication, Multi-Symptom Formula Tablets and Caplets ... 1572
TYLENOL Cold Medication, Multi-Symptom Hot Liquid Packets ... 1572
TYLENOL Cold Medication, No Drowsiness Formula Caplets and Gelcaps ... 1572
TYLENOL Cold Severe Congestion Caplets ... 1573
TYLENOL Cough Medication with Decongestant, Multi Symptom ... 1574
TYLENOL Flu No Drowsiness Formula, Maximum Strength Gelcaps ... 1575
TYLENOL Flu NightTime, Maximum Strength Gelcaps ... 1575
TYLENOL Flu NightTime, Maximum Strength Hot Medication Packets ... 1575
TYLENOL Sinus, Maximum Strength Geltabs, Gelcaps, Caplets and Tablets ... 1576
Vicks 44 LiquiCaps Cough, Cold & Flu Relief ... 728
Vicks 44 LiquiCaps Non-Drowsy Cough & Cold Relief ... 729
Vicks 44D Cough & Head Congestion Relief ... 728
Vicks 44M Cough, Cold & Flu Relief ... 729
Vicks DayQuil LiquiCaps/Liquid Multi-Symptom Cold/Flu Relief ... 734
Vicks DayQuil SINUS Pressure & PAIN Relief with IBUPROFEN ... 735
Vicks Nyquil Hot Therapy ... 735
Vicks NyQuil LiquiCaps/Liquid Multi-Symptom Cold/Flu Relief, Original and Cherry Flavors ... 736

Pseudoephedrine Sulfate (Increases certain actions or side effects). Products include:
Chlor-Trimeton Allergy Decongestant Tablets ... 759
Claritin-D Tablets ... 2487
Drixoral Cold and Allergy Sustained-Action Tablets ... 763
Drixoral Cold and Flu Extended-Release Tablets ... 764
Drixoral Non-Drowsy Formula Extended-Release Tablets ... 764
Drixoral Allergy/Sinus Extended Release Tablets ... 765
Trinalin Repetabs Tablets ... 1373

Pyrilamine Maleate (Increases certain actions or side effects). Products include:
4-Way Fast Acting Nasal Spray (regular & mentholated) ... 644
Maximum Strength Multi-Symptom Formula Midol ... 621
PMS Multi-Symptom Formula Midol ... 622

Pyrilamine Tannate (Increases certain actions or side effects). Products include:
Atrohist Pediatric Suspension ... 1604
Atrohist Pediatric Suspension Dye-Free ... 1604
Rynatan ... 2781

Quazepam (Increases certain actions or side effects). Products include:
Doral Tablets ... 2773

Quinidine Gluconate (Co-administration with antiarrhythmic agents of class 1, such as quinidine, may increase certain actions or side effects of anticholinergic drugs). Products include:
Quinaglute Dura-Tabs Tablets ... 644

Quinidine Polygalacturonate (Co-administration with antiarrhythmic agents of class 1, such as quinidine, may increase certain actions or side effects of anticholinergic drugs). Products include:
Cardioquin Tablets ... 2146

Quinidine Sulfate (Co-administration with antiarrhythmic agents of class 1, such as quinidine, may increase certain actions or side effects of anticholinergic drugs). Products include:
Quinidex Extentabs ... 2240

Salmeterol Xinafoate (Increases certain actions or side effects). Products include:
Serevent Inhalation Aerosol ... 1149

Scopolamine (Increases certain actions or side effects). Products include:
Transderm Scōp Transdermal Therapeutic System ... 890

Scopolamine Hydrobromide (Increases certain actions or side effects). Products include:
Atrohist Plus Tablets ... 1605
Donnatal ... 2234
Donnatal Extentabs ... 2234
Donnatal Tablets ... 2234

Selegiline Hydrochloride (Co-administration with MAO inhibitors may increase certain actions or side effects of anticholinergic drugs). Products include:
Eldepryl Capsules ... 2729

Sodium Bicarbonate (Antacids may interfere with the absorption of anticholinergic agents, simultaneous use of these drugs should be avoided). Products include:
Alka-Seltzer Cherry Effervescent Antacid and Pain Reliever ... 609
Alka-Seltzer Extra Strength Effervescent Antacid and Pain Reliever ... 609
Alka-Seltzer Gold Effervescent Antacid ... 611
Alka-Seltzer Lemon Lime Effervescent Antacid and Pain Reliever ... 609
Alka-Seltzer Original Effervescent Antacid and Pain Reliever ... 609
Arm & Hammer Pure Baking Soda ... 648
Colyte and Colyte-flavored ... 2540
GoLYTELY ... 694
Massengill Disposable Douches ... 780
Massengill Liquid Concentrate ... 780
NuLYTELY ... 694
Cherry Flavor NuLYTELY ... 694

Sufentanil Citrate (Increases certain actions or side effects). Products include:
Sufenta Injection ... 1355

Temazepam (Increases certain actions or side effects). Products include:
Restoril Capsules ... 2413

Terbutaline Sulfate (Increases certain actions or side effects). Products include:
Brethaire Inhaler ... 830
Brethine Ampuls ... 832
Brethine Tablets ... 831
Bricanyl Subcutaneous Injection ... 1247
Bricanyl Tablets ... 1248

Terfenadine (Increases certain actions or side effects). Products include:
Seldane Tablets ... 1284
Seldane-D Extended-Release Tablets ... 1286

Thioridazine Hydrochloride (Increases certain actions or side effects). Products include:
Mellaril ... 2398

Timolol Maleate (Effects of antiglaucoma agents antagonized). Products include:
Blocadren Tablets ... 1654
Timolide Tablets ... 1791
Timoptic in Ocudose ... 1796
Timoptic Sterile Ophthalmic Solution ... 1794
Timoptic-XE ... 1798

Tranylcypromine Sulfate (Co-administration with MAO inhibitors may increase certain actions or side effects of anticholinergic drugs). Products include:
Parnate Tablets ... 2679

Triamcinolone (Concurrent use in the presence of increased intraocular pressure may be hazardous).
No products indexed under this heading.

Triamcinolone Acetonide (Concurrent use in the presence of increased intraocular pressure may be hazardous). Products include:
Azmacort Oral Inhaler ... 2175
Nasacort AQ Nasal Spray ... 2191
Nasacort Nasal Inhaler ... 2189

Triamcinolone Diacetate (Concurrent use in the presence of increased intraocular pressure may be hazardous).
No products indexed under this heading.

Triamcinolone Hexacetonide (Concurrent use in the presence of increased intraocular pressure may be hazardous).
No products indexed under this heading.

Triazolam (Increases certain actions or side effects). Products include:
Halcion Tablets ... 2093

Tridihexethyl Chloride (Increases certain actions or side effects).
No products indexed under this heading.

Trifluoperazine Hydrochloride (Increases certain actions or side effects). Products include:
Stelazine ... 2692

Trihexyphenidyl Hydrochloride (Increases certain actions or side effects). Products include:
Artane ... 1418

Trimeprazine Tartrate (Increases certain actions or side effects).
No products indexed under this heading.

Trimipramine Maleate (Increases certain actions or side effects). Products include:
Surmontil Capsules ... 2917

Tripelennamine Hydrochloride (Increases certain actions or side effects). Products include:
PBZ Tablets ... 863
PBZ-SR Tablets ... 862

Triprolidine Hydrochloride (Increases certain actions or side effects). Products include:
Actifed Cold & Allergy Tablets ... 807
Actifed Cold & Sinus Caplets and Tablets ... 808

BENTYL INJECTION
(Dicyclomine Hydrochloride) ... 1246
See **Bentyl 10 mg Capsules**

IMPORTANT NOTE: Always consult each drug listing in the patient's regimen for possible interactions.

BENTYL SYRUP
(Dicyclomine Hydrochloride) 1246
See **Bentyl 10 mg Capsules**

BENTYL 20 MG TABLETS
(Dicyclomine Hydrochloride) 1246
See **Bentyl 10 mg Capsules**

BENYLIN ADULT FORMULA COUGH SUPPRESSANT
(Dextromethorphan Hydrobromide) .... ▣ 817
May interact with monoamine oxidase inhibitors. Compounds in this category include:

Furazolidone (Concurrent and/or sequential use should be avoided). Products include:
  Furoxone 2221

Isocarboxazid (Concurrent and/or sequential use should be avoided).
  No products indexed under this heading.

Phenelzine Sulfate (Concurrent and/or sequential use should be avoided). Products include:
  Nardil 1977

Selegiline Hydrochloride (Concurrent and/or sequential use should be avoided). Products include:
  Eldepryl Capsules 2729

Tranylcypromine Sulfate (Concurrent and/or sequential use should be avoided). Products include:
  Parnate Tablets 2679

BENYLIN EXPECTORANT
(Dextromethorphan Hydrobromide, Guaifenesin) .... ▣ 816
May interact with monoamine oxidase inhibitors. Compounds in this category include:

Furazolidone (Concurrent and/or sequential use is not recommended). Products include:
  Furoxone 2221

Isocarboxazid (Concurrent and/or sequential use is not recommended).
  No products indexed under this heading.

Phenelzine Sulfate (Concurrent and/or sequential use is not recommended). Products include:
  Nardil 1977

Selegiline Hydrochloride (Concurrent and/or sequential use is not recommended). Products include:
  Eldepryl Capsules 2729

Tranylcypromine Sulfate (Concurrent and/or sequential use is not recommended.). Products include:
  Parnate Tablets 2679

BENYLIN MULTISYMPTOM
(Dextromethorphan Hydrobromide, Pseudoephedrine Hydrochloride, Guaifenesin) .... ▣ 816
May interact with monoamine oxidase inhibitors. Compounds in this category include:

Furazolidone (Concurrent and/or sequential use is not recommended). Products include:
  Furoxone 2221

Isocarboxazid (Concurrent and/or sequential use is not recommended).
  No products indexed under this heading.

Phenelzine Sulfate (Concurrent and/or sequential use is not recommended). Products include:
  Nardil 1977

Selegiline Hydrochloride (Concurrent and/or sequential use is not recommended). Products include:
  Eldepryl Capsules 2729

Tranylcypromine Sulfate (Concurrent and/or sequential use is not recommended). Products include:
  Parnate Tablets 2679

BENYLIN PEDIATRIC COUGH SUPPRESSANT
(Dextromethorphan Hydrobromide) .... ▣ 817
May interact with monoamine oxidase inhibitors. Compounds in this category include:

Furazolidone (Concurrent and/or sequential use should be avoided). Products include:
  Furoxone 2221

Isocarboxazid (Concurrent and/or sequential use should be avoided).
  No products indexed under this heading.

Phenelzine Sulfate (Concurrent and/or sequential use should be avoided). Products include:
  Nardil 1977

Selegiline Hydrochloride (Concurrent and/or sequential use should be avoided). Products include:
  Eldepryl Capsules 2729

Tranylcypromine Sulfate (Concurrent and/or sequential use should be avoided). Products include:
  Parnate Tablets 2679

BENZAC 5 & 10 GEL
(Benzoyl Peroxide) 1031
None cited in PDR database.

BENZAC AC 2½%, 5%, AND 10% WATER-BASE GEL
(Benzoyl Peroxide) 1031
None cited in PDR database.

BENZAC AC WASH 2½%, 5%, 10% WATER-BASE CLEANSER
(Benzoyl Peroxide) 1031
None cited in PDR database.

BENZAC W WASH 5 & 10 WATER-BASE CLEANSER
(Benzoyl Peroxide) 1031
None cited in PDR database.

BENZAC W 2½, 5 & 10 WATER-BASE GEL
(Benzoyl Peroxide) 1031
None cited in PDR database.

BENZAMYCIN TOPICAL GEL
(Erythromycin, Benzoyl Peroxide) 919
May interact with:

Concomitant Topical Acne Therapy (Possible cumulative irritancy effect may occur).

BENZASHAVE MEDICATED SHAVE CREAM 5% AND 10%
(Benzoyl Peroxide) 1627
None cited in PDR database.

BEROCCA PLUS TABLETS
(Vitamins with Minerals) 2259
May interact with:

Levodopa (Decreased efficacy). Products include:
  Atamet Tablets 567
  Larodopa Tablets 2296
  Sinemet Tablets 959
  Sinemet CR Tablets 961

BEROCCA TABLETS
(Vitamin B Complex With Vitamin C) 2259
May interact with:

Levodopa (Decreased efficacy). Products include:
  Atamet Tablets 567
  Larodopa Tablets 2296
  Sinemet Tablets 959
  Sinemet CR Tablets 961

BETADINE BRAND FIRST AID ANTIBIOTICS & MOISTURIZER OINTMENT
(Polymyxin B Sulfate, Bacitracin Zinc) 2144
None cited in PDR database.

BETADINE DISPOSABLE MEDICATED DOUCHE
(Povidone Iodine) 2144
None cited in PDR database.

BETADINE FIRST AID CREAM
(Povidone Iodine) 2144
None cited in PDR database.

BETADINE MEDICATED DOUCHE
(Povidone Iodine) 2144
None cited in PDR database.

BETADINE MEDICATED GEL
(Povidone Iodine) 2144
None cited in PDR database.

BETADINE MEDICATED VAGINAL SUPPOSITORIES
(Povidone Iodine) 2145
None cited in PDR database.

BETADINE OINTMENT
(Povidone Iodine) 2145
None cited in PDR database.

BETADINE PRE-MIXED MEDICATED DISPOSABLE DOUCHE
(Povidone Iodine) 2144
None cited in PDR database.

BETADINE SKIN CLEANSER
(Povidone Iodine) 2145
None cited in PDR database.

BETADINE SOLUTION
(Povidone Iodine) 2145
None cited in PDR database.

BETADINE 5% STERILE OPHTHALMIC PREP SOLUTION
(Povidone Iodine) .... ⊚ 266
None cited in PDR database.

BETADINE SURGICAL SCRUB
(Povidone Iodine) 2145
None cited in PDR database.

BETAGAN LIQUIFILM
(Levobunolol Hydrochloride) .... ⊚ 230
See **BETAGAN Liquifilm with C CAP Compliance Cap**

BETAGAN LIQUIFILM WITH C CAP COMPLIANCE CAP
(Levobunolol Hydrochloride) .... ⊚ 230
May interact with beta blockers, phenothiazines, cardiac glycosides, and certain other agents. Compounds in these categories include:

Acebutolol Hydrochloride (Co-administration with oral beta blockers may result in additive effect either on intraocular pressure or on the known systemic effects of beta blockade). Products include:
  Sectral Capsules 2914

Atenolol (Co-administration with oral beta blockers may result in additive effect either on intraocular pressure or on the known systemic effects of beta blockade). Products include:
  Tenoretic Tablets 2963
  Tenormin Tablets and I.V. Injection 2965

Betaxolol Hydrochloride (Co-administration with oral beta blockers may result in additive effect either on intraocular pressure or on the known systemic effects of beta blockade). Products include:
  Betoptic Ophthalmic Solution............ 465
  Betoptic S Ophthalmic Suspension ... 467
  Kerlone Tablets 2588

Bisoprolol Fumarate (Co-administration with oral beta blockers may result in additive effect either on intraocular pressure or on the known systemic effects of beta blockade). Products include:
  Zebeta Tablets 1457
  Ziac 1459

Carteolol Hydrochloride (Co-administration with oral beta blockers may result in additive effect either on intraocular pressure or on the known systemic effects of beta blockade). Products include:
  Cartrol Tablets 413
  Ocupress Ophthalmic Solution, 1% Sterile .... ⊚ 297

Chlorpromazine (Co-administration with phenothiazine-related compounds may have an additive hypotensive effect due to inhibition of each other's metabolism). Products include:
  Thorazine Suppositories 2701

Chlorpromazine Hydrochloride (Co-administration with phenothiazine-related compounds may have an additive hypotensive effect due to inhibition of each other's metabolism). Products include:
  Thorazine 2701

Deserpidine (Possible additive effects and production of hypotension and/or bradycardia when beta blocker is concurrently used with catecholamine-depleting drugs).
  No products indexed under this heading.

Deslanoside (Co-administration with digitalis and calcium channel blockers may have an additive effect on prolonging atrioventricular conduction time).
  No products indexed under this heading.

Digitoxin (Co-administration with digitalis and calcium channel blockers may have an additive effect on prolonging atrioventricular conduction time). Products include:
  Crystodigin Tablets 1472

Digoxin (Co-administration with digitalis and calcium channel blockers may have an additive effect on prolonging atrioventricular conduction time). Products include:
  Lanoxicaps 1110
  Lanoxin Elixir Pediatric 1113
  Lanoxin Injection 1116
  Lanoxin Injection Pediatric................. 1119
  Lanoxin Tablets 1121

(▣ Described in PDR For Nonprescription Drugs) (⊚ Described in PDR For Ophthalmology)

Epinephrine (Concurrent use in patients with history of atopy or severe anaphylactic reaction to allergens may be unresponsive to the usual doses of epinephrine used to treat anaphylactic reaction; mydriasis may result with concomitant epinephrine). Products include:
EPIFRIN .... ⊙ 237
EpiPen 808
Marcaine with Epinephrine 2446
Primatene Mist .... ▣ 843
Sensorcaine with Epinephrine Injection 554
Sus-Phrine Injection 1017
Xylocaine with Epinephrine Injections 562

Epinephrine Hydrochloride (Concurrent use in patients with history of atopy or severe anaphylactic reaction to allergens may be unresponsive to the usual doses of epinephrine used to treat anaphylactic reaction; mydriasis may result with concomitant epinephrine). Products include:
Ana-Kit Anaphylaxis Emergency Treatment Kit 611

Esmolol Hydrochloride (Co-administration with oral beta blockers may result in additive effect either on intraocular pressure or on the known systemic effects of beta blockade). Products include:
Brevibloc (esmolol HCl) Injection 1860

Fluphenazine Decanoate (Co-administration with phenothiazine-related compounds may have an additive hypotensive effect due to inhibition of each other's metabolism). Products include:
Prolixin Decanoate 510

Fluphenazine Enanthate (Co-administration with phenothiazine-related compounds may have an additive hypotensive effect due to inhibition of each other's metabolism). Products include:
Prolixin Enanthate 510

Fluphenazine Hydrochloride (Co-administration with phenothiazine-related compounds may have an additive hypotensive effect due to inhibition of each other's metabolism). Products include:
Prolixin 510

Labetalol Hydrochloride (Co-administration with oral beta blockers may result in additive effect either on intraocular pressure or on the known systemic effects of beta blockade). Products include:
Normodyne Injection 2519
Normodyne Tablets 2522
Trandate 1158

Mesoridazine Besylate (Co-administration with phenothiazine-related compounds may have an additive hypotensive effect due to inhibition of each other's metabolism). Products include:
Serentil 689

Methotrimeprazine (Co-administration with phenothiazine-related compounds may have an additive hypotensive effect due to inhibition of each other's metabolism). Products include:
Levoprome 1321

Metipranolol Hydrochloride (Co-administration with oral beta blockers may result in additive effect either on intraocular pressure or on the known systemic effects of beta blockade). Products include:
OptiPranolol (Metipranolol 0.3%) Sterile Ophthalmic Solution .... ⊙ 256

Metoprolol Succinate (Co-administration with oral beta blockers may result in additive effect either on intraocular pressure or on the known systemic effects of beta blockade). Products include:
Toprol-XL Tablets 560

Metoprolol Tartrate (Co-administration with oral beta blockers may result in additive effect either on intraocular pressure or on the known systemic effects of beta blockade). Products include:
Lopressor 848
Lopressor HCT Tablets 850

Nadolol (Co-administration with oral beta blockers may result in additive effect either on intraocular pressure or on the known systemic effects of beta blockade).
No products indexed under this heading.

Penbutolol Sulfate (Co-administration with oral beta blockers may result in additive effect either on intraocular pressure or on the known systemic effects of beta blockade). Products include:
Levatol Tablets 2547

Perphenazine (Co-administration with phenothiazine-related compounds may have an additive hypotensive effect due to inhibition of each other's metabolism). Products include:
Etrafon 2495
Triavil Tablets 1800
Trilafon 2532

Pindolol (Co-administration with oral beta blockers may result in additive effect either on intraocular pressure or on the known systemic effects of beta blockade). Products include:
Visken Tablets 2428

Prochlorperazine (Co-administration with phenothiazine-related compounds may have an additive hypotensive effect due to inhibition of each other's metabolism). Products include:
Compazine 2644

Promethazine Hydrochloride (Co-administration with phenothiazine-related compounds may have an additive hypotensive effect due to inhibition of each other's metabolism). Products include:
Mepergan Injection 2859
Phenergan with Codeine 2883
Phenergan with Dextromethorphan 2885
Phenergan Injection 2880
Phenergan Suppositories 2882
Phenergan Syrup 2881
Phenergan Tablets 2882
Phenergan VC 2886
Phenergan VC with Codeine 2888

Propranolol Hydrochloride (Co-administration with oral beta blockers may result in additive effect either on intraocular pressure or on the known systemic effects of beta blockade). Products include:
Inderal 2834
Inderal LA Long Acting Capsules ... 2836
Inderide Tablets 2838
Inderide LA Long Acting Capsules .. 2840

Rauwolfia Serpentina (Possible additive effects and production of hypotension and/or bradycardia when beta blocker is concurrently used with catecholamine-depleting drugs).
No products indexed under this heading.

Rescinnamine (Possible additive effects and production of hypotension and/or bradycardia when beta blocker is concurrently used with catecholamine-depleting drugs).
No products indexed under this heading.

Reserpine (Possible additive effects and production of hypotension and/or bradycardia when beta blocker is concurrently used with catecholamine-depleting drugs). Products include:
Diupres Tablets 1691
Hydropres Tablets 1718
Ser-Ap-Es Tablets 867

Sotalol Hydrochloride (Co-administration with oral beta blockers may result in additive effect either on intraocular pressure or on the known systemic effects of beta blockade). Products include:
Betapace Tablets 637

Thioridazine Hydrochloride (Co-administration with phenothiazine-related compounds may have an additive hypotensive effect due to inhibition of each other's metabolism). Products include:
Mellaril 2398

Timolol Maleate (Co-administration with oral beta blockers may result in additive effect either on intraocular pressure or on the known systemic effects of beta blockade). Products include:
Blocadren Tablets 1654
Timolide Tablets 1791
Timoptic in Ocudose 1796
Timoptic Sterile Ophthalmic Solution 1794
Timoptic-XE 1798

Trifluoperazine Hydrochloride (Co-administration with phenothiazine-related compounds may have an additive hypotensive effect due to inhibition of each other's metabolism). Products include:
Stelazine 2692

BETAPACE TABLETS
(Sotalol Hydrochloride) 637
May interact with drugs that prolong the qt interval, cardiac glycosides, calcium channel blockers, catecholamine depleting drugs, insulin, oral hypoglycemic agents, beta$_2$ agonists, antiarrhythmics, and certain other agents. Compounds in these categories include:

Acarbose (Potential for hyperglycemia; symptoms of hypoglycemia may be masked; dosage of antidiabetic drugs may require adjustment). Products include:
Precose 604

Acebutolol Hydrochloride (Potential for prolonged refractoriness; concomitant therapy is not recommended). Products include:
Sectral Capsules 2914

Adenosine (Potential for prolonged refractoriness; concomitant therapy is not recommended). Products include:
Adenocard Injection 1021
Adenoscan 1022

Albuterol (Beta-agonist may have to be administered in increased dosage when used concomitantly). Products include:
Proventil Inhalation Aerosol 2524

Ventolin Inhalation Aerosol and Refill 1170

Albuterol Sulfate (Beta-agonist may have to be administered in increased dosage when used concomitantly). Products include:
Airet Albuterol Sulfate Inhalation Solution 1602
Albuterol Sulfate, USP Solution for Inhalation, Arm-a-Med 522
Proventil Inhalation Solution 0.083% 2527
Proventil Repetabs Tablets 2529
Proventil Solution for Inhalation 0.5% 2525
Proventil Syrup 2528
Proventil Tablets 2529
Ventolin Inhalation Solution 1171
Ventolin Nebules Inhalation Solution 1172
Ventolin Rotacaps for Inhalation ... 1173
Ventolin Syrup 1175
Ventolin Tablets 1176
Volmax Extended-Release Tablets .. 1835

Amiodarone Hydrochloride (Potential for prolonged refractoriness; concomitant therapy is not recommended; caution is advised if used concurrently due to sotalol's effect on cardiac repolarization (QTc prolongation) torsade de pointes, a polymorphic ventricular tachycardia with prolonged QT interval). Products include:
Cordarone Intravenous 2821
Cordarone Tablets 2818

Amitriptyline Hydrochloride (Caution is advised if used concurrently due to sotalol's effect on cardiac repolarization (QTc prolongation) torsade de pointes, a polymorphic ventricular tachycardia with prolonged QT interval). Products include:
Elavil 2945
Etrafon 2495
Limbitrol 2333
Triavil Tablets 1800

Amlodipine Besylate (Possible additive effects on AV conduction or ventricular conduction; co-administration may result in hypotension). Products include:
Lotrel Capsules 858
Norvasc Tablets 2020

Amoxapine (Caution is advised if used concurrently due to sotalol's effect on cardiac repolarization (QTc prolongation) torsade de pointes, a polymorphic ventricular tachycardia with prolonged QT interval). Products include:
Asendin Tablets 1419

Astemizole (Caution is advised if used concurrently due to sotalol's effect on cardiac repolarization (QTc prolongation) torsade de pointes, a polymorphic ventricular tachycardia with prolonged QT interval). Products include:
Hismanal Tablets 1341

Bepridil Hydrochloride (Possible additive effects on AV conduction or ventricular conduction; co-administration may result in hypotension). Products include:
Vascor Tablets (200 and 300 mg) 1597

Bitolterol Mesylate (Beta-agonist may have to be administered in increased dosage when used concomitantly). Products include:
Tornalate Solution for Inhalation, 0.2% 976
Tornalate Metered Dose Inhaler ... 978

IMPORTANT NOTE: Always consult each drug listing in the patient's regimen for possible interactions.

Betapace — Interactions Index

Bretylium Tosylate (Potential for prolonged refractoriness; concomitant therapy is not recommended; caution is advised if used concurrently due to sotalol's effect on cardiac repolarization (QTc prolongation) torsade de pointes, a polymorphic ventricular tachycardia with prolonged QT interval).
    No products indexed under this heading.

Chlorpromazine (Caution is advised if used concurrently due to sotalol's effect on cardiac repolarization (QTc prolongation) torsade de pointes, a polymorphic ventricular tachycardia with prolonged QT interval). Products include:
    Thorazine Suppositories 2701

Chlorpromazine Hydrochloride (Caution is advised if used concurrently due to sotalol's effect on cardiac repolarization (QTc prolongation) torsade de pointes, a polymorphic ventricular tachycardia with prolonged QT interval). Products include:
    Thorazine 2701

Chlorpropamide (Potential for hyperglycemia; symptoms of hypoglycemia may be masked; dosage of antidiabetic drugs may require adjustment). Products include:
    Diabinese Tablets 2002

Clomipramine Hydrochloride (Caution is advised if used concurrently due to sotalol's effect on cardiac repolarization (QTc prolongation) torsade de pointes, a polymorphic ventricular tachycardia with prolonged QT interval). Products include:
    Anafranil Capsules 819

Clonidine (Beta-blocking drugs may potentiate the rebound hypertension sometimes observed after discontinuation of clonidine). Products include:
    Catapres-TTS 680

Clonidine Hydrochloride (Beta-blocking drugs may potentiate the rebound hypertension sometimes observed after discontinuation of clonidine). Products include:
    Catapres Tablets 679
    Combipres Tablets 682

Deserpidine (Produces an excessive reduction of resting sympathetic nervous tone).
    No products indexed under this heading.

Desipramine Hydrochloride (Caution is advised if used concurrently due to sotalol's effect on cardiac repolarization (QTc prolongation) torsade de pointes, a polymorphic ventricular tachycardia with prolonged QT interval). Products include:
    Norpramin Tablets 1273

Deslanoside (Potential for proarrhythmic events when co-administered).
    No products indexed under this heading.

Digitoxin (Potential for proarrhythmic events when co-administered). Products include:
    Crystodigin Tablets 1472

Digoxin (Potential for proarrhythmic events when co-administered). Products include:
    Lanoxicaps 1110
    Lanoxin Elixir Pediatric 1113
    Lanoxin Injection 1116
    Lanoxin Injection Pediatric 1119
    Lanoxin Tablets 1121

Diltiazem Hydrochloride (Possible additive effects on AV conduction or ventricular conduction; co-administration may result in hypotension). Products include:
    Cardizem CD Capsules 1251
    Cardizem SR Capsules 1255
    Cardizem Injectable 1253
    Cardizem Tablets 1257
    Dilacor XR Extended-release Capsules 2183
    Tiazac Capsules 1019

Disopyramide Phosphate (Potential for prolonged refractoriness; concomitant therapy is not recommended; caution is advised if used concurrently due to sotalol's effect on cardiac repolarization (QTc prolongation) torsade de pointes, a polymorphic ventricular tachycardia with prolonged QT interval). Products include:
    Norpace 2596

Doxepin Hydrochloride (Caution is advised if used concurrently due to sotalol's effect on cardiac repolarization (QTc prolongation) torsade de pointes, a polymorphic ventricular tachycardia with prolonged QT interval). Products include:
    Adapin Capsules 1542
    Sinequan 2028
    Zonalon Cream 1042

Ephedrine Hydrochloride (Beta-agonist may have to be administered in increased dosage when used concomitantly). Products include:
    Primatene Tablets 844
    Quadrinal Tablets 1398

Ephedrine Sulfate (Beta-agonist may have to be administered in increased dosage when used concomitantly). Products include:
    Marax Tablets & DF Syrup 2015

Ephedrine Tannate (Beta-agonist may have to be administered in increased dosage when used concomitantly). Products include:
    Rynatuss 2782

Epinephrine (Beta-agonist may have to be administered in increased dosage when used concomitantly). Products include:
    EPIFRIN 237
    EpiPen 808
    Marcaine with Epinephrine 2446
    Primatene Mist 843
    Sensorcaine with Epinephrine Injection 554
    Sus-Phrine Injection 1017
    Xylocaine with Epinephrine Injections 562

Epinephrine Hydrochloride (Beta-agonist may have to be administered in increased dosage when used concomitantly; potential for unresponsiveness to the usual dose of epinephrine to treat allergic reaction). Products include:
    Ana-Kit Anaphylaxis Emergency Treatment Kit 611

Ethylnorepinephrine Hydrochloride (Beta-agonist may have to be administered in increased dosage when used concomitantly).
    No products indexed under this heading.

Felodipine (Possible additive effects on AV conduction or ventricular conduction; co-administration may result in hypotension). Products include:
    Plendil Extended-Release Tablets 514

Flecainide Acetate (Potential for prolonged refractoriness; concomitant therapy is not recommended; caution is advised if used concurrently due to sotalol's effect on cardiac repolarization (QTc prolongation) torsade de pointes, a polymorphic ventricular tachycardia with prolonged QT interval). Products include:
    Tambocor Tablets 1555

Fluphenazine Decanoate (Caution is advised if used concurrently due to sotalol's effect on cardiac repolarization (QTc prolongation) torsade de pointes, a polymorphic ventricular tachycardia with prolonged QT interval). Products include:
    Prolixin Decanoate 510

Fluphenazine Enanthate (Caution is advised if used concurrently due to sotalol's effect on cardiac repolarization (QTc prolongation) torsade de pointes, a polymorphic ventricular tachycardia with prolonged QT interval). Products include:
    Prolixin Enanthate 510

Fluphenazine Hydrochloride (Caution is advised if used concurrently due to sotalol's effect on cardiac repolarization (QTc prolongation) torsade de pointes, a polymorphic ventricular tachycardia with prolonged QT interval). Products include:
    Prolixin 510

Glimepiride (Potential for hyperglycemia; symptoms of hypoglycemia may be masked; dosage of antidiabetic drugs may require adjustment). Products include:
    Amaryl Tablets 1241

Glipizide (Potential for hyperglycemia; symptoms of hypoglycemia may be masked; dosage of antidiabetic drugs may require adjustment). Products include:
    Glucotrol Tablets 2011
    Glucotrol XL Extended Release Tablets 2012

Glyburide (Potential for hyperglycemia; symptoms of hypoglycemia may be masked; dosage of antidiabetic drugs may require adjustment). Products include:
    DiaBeta Tablets 1265
    Glynase PresTab Tablets 2091
    Micronase Tablets 2099

Guanethidine Monosulfate (Produces an excessive reduction of resting sympathetic nervous tone). Products include:
    Esimil Tablets 840
    Ismelin Tablets 845

Imipramine Hydrochloride (Caution is advised if used concurrently due to sotalol's effect on cardiac repolarization (QTc prolongation) torsade de pointes, a polymorphic ventricular tachycardia with prolonged QT interval). Products include:
    Tofranil Ampuls 873
    Tofranil Tablets 875

Imipramine Pamoate (Caution is advised if used concurrently due to sotalol's effect on cardiac repolarization (QTc prolongation) torsade de pointes, a polymorphic ventricular tachycardia with prolonged QT interval). Products include:
    Tofranil-PM Capsules 876

Insulin, Human (Potential for hyperglycemia; symptoms of hypoglycemia may be masked; dosage of insulin may require adjustment).
    No products indexed under this heading.

Insulin, Human Isophane Suspension (Potential for hyperglycemia; symptoms of hypoglycemia may be masked; dosage of insulin may require adjustment). Products include:
    Novolin N Human Insulin 10 ml Vials 1846

Insulin, Human NPH (Potential for hyperglycemia; symptoms of hypoglycemia may be masked; dosage of insulin may require adjustment). Products include:
    Humulin N, 100 Units 1495
    Novolin N PenFill 1.5 ml Cartridges Durable Insulin Delivery System 1849
    Novolin N Prefilled Syringe Disposable Insulin Delivery System 1850

Insulin, Human Regular (Potential for hyperglycemia; symptoms of hypoglycemia may be masked; dosage of insulin may require adjustment). Products include:
    Humulin R, 100 Units 1497
    Novolin R Human Insulin 10 ml Vials 1846
    Novolin R PenFill 1.5 ml Cartridges Durable Insulin Delivery System 1849
    Novolin R Prefilled Syringe Disposable Insulin Delivery System 1850
    Velosulin BR Human Insulin 10 ml Vials 1847

Insulin, Human, Zinc Suspension (Potential for hyperglycemia; symptoms of hypoglycemia may be masked; dosage of insulin may require adjustment). Products include:
    Humulin L, 100 Units 1494
    Humulin U, 100 Units 1498
    Novolin L Human Insulin 10 ml Vials 1846

Insulin Lispro, Human (Potential for hyperglycemia; symptoms of hypoglycemia may be masked; dosage of insulin may require adjustment). Products include:
    Humalog Injection 1488

Insulin, NPH (Potential for hyperglycemia; symptoms of hypoglycemia may be masked; dosage of insulin may require adjustment). Products include:
    NPH, 100 Units 1502
    Pork NPH, 100 Units 1506
    Purified Pork NPH Isophane Insulin 1852

Insulin, Regular (Potential for hyperglycemia; symptoms of hypoglycemia may be masked; dosage of insulin may require adjustment). Products include:
    Regular, 100 Units 1503
    Pork Regular, 100 Units 1507
    Pork Regular (Concentrated), 500 Units 1508
    Purified Pork Regular Insulin 1852

Insulin, Zinc Crystals (Potential for hyperglycemia; symptoms of hypoglycemia may be masked; dosage of insulin may require adjustment). Products include:
    NPH, 100 Units 1502

Insulin, Zinc Suspension (Potential for hyperglycemia; symptoms of hypoglycemia may be masked; dosage of insulin may require adjustment). Products include:
    Iletin I 1501
    Lente, 100 Units 1501
    Iletin II 1504
    Pork Lente, 100 Units 1504
    Purified Pork Lente Insulin 1852

(■□ Described in PDR For Nonprescription Drugs)   (◉ Described in PDR For Ophthalmology)

Isoetharine (Beta-agonist may have to be administered in increased dosage when used concomitantly). Products include:
Bronkometer Aerosol 2432
Bronkosol Solution 2432
Isoetharine Inhalation Solution, USP, Arm-a-Med 545

Isoproterenol Hydrochloride (Beta-agonist may have to be administered in increased dosage when used concomitantly). Products include:
Isuprel Hydrochloride Solution 2443
Isuprel Injection 2441
Isuprel Mistometer 2442

Isoproterenol Sulfate (Beta-agonist may have to be administered in increased dosage when used concomitantly). Products include:
Norisodrine with Calcium Iodide Syrup 446

Isradipine (Possible additive effects on AV conduction or ventricular conduction; co-administration may result in hypotension). Products include:
DynaCirc Capsules 2381
DynaCirc CR Tablets 2383

Lidocaine Hydrochloride (Potential for prolonged refractoriness; concomitant therapy is not recommended; caution is advised if used concurrently due to sotalol's effect on cardiac repolarization (QTc prolongation) torsade de pointes, a polymorphic ventricular tachycardia with prolonged QT interval). Products include:
Decadron Phosphate with Xylocaine Injection, Sterile 1683
Unguentine Plus 712
Xylocaine Injections 562

Maprotiline Hydrochloride (Caution is advised if used concurrently due to sotalol's effect on cardiac repolarization (QTc prolongation) torsade de pointes, a polymorphic ventricular tachycardia with prolonged QT interval). Products include:
Ludiomil Tablets 861

Mesoridazine (Caution is advised if used concurrently due to sotalol's effect on cardiac repolarization (QTc prolongation) torsade de pointes, a polymorphic ventricular tachycardia with prolonged QT interval).

Metaproterenol Sulfate (Beta-agonist may have to be administered in increased dosage when used concomitantly). Products include:
Alupent 672
Metaproterenol Sulfate Inhalation Solution, USP, Arm-a-Med 547

Metformin Hydrochloride (Potential for hyperglycemia; symptoms of hypoglycemia may be masked; dosage of antidiabetic drugs may require adjustment). Products include:
Glucophage Tablets 754

Mexiletine Hydrochloride (Potential for prolonged refractoriness; concomitant therapy is not recommended; caution is advised if used concurrently due to sotalol's effect on cardiac repolarization (QTc prolongation) torsade de pointes, a polymorphic ventricular tachycardia with prolonged QT interval). Products include:
Mexitil Capsules 684

Moricizine Hydrochloride (Potential for prolonged refractoriness; concomitant therapy is not recommended). Products include:
Ethmozine Tablets 2217

Nicardipine Hydrochloride (Possible additive effects on AV conduction or ventricular conduction; co-administration may result in hypotension). Products include:
Cardene Capsules 2261
Cardene I.V. 2815
Cardene SR Capsules 2264

Nifedipine (Possible additive effects on AV conduction or ventricular conduction; co-administration may result in hypotension). Products include:
Adalat Capsules (10 mg and 20 mg) 580
Adalat CC 582
Procardia Capsules 2024
Procardia XL Extended Release Tablets 2026

Nimodipine (Possible additive effects on AV conduction or ventricular conduction; co-administration may result in hypotension). Products include:
Nimotop Capsules 603

Nisoldipine (Possible additive effects on AV conduction or ventricular conduction; co-administration may result in hypotension). Products include:
Sular Tablets 2961

Nortriptyline Hydrochloride (Caution is advised if used concurrently due to sotalol's effect on cardiac repolarization (QTc prolongation) torsade de pointes, a polymorphic ventricular tachycardia with prolonged QT interval). Products include:
Pamelor 2409

Perphenazine (Caution is advised if used concurrently due to sotalol's effect on cardiac repolarization (QTc prolongation) torsade de pointes, a polymorphic ventricular tachycardia with prolonged QT interval). Products include:
Etrafon 2495
Triavil Tablets 1800
Trilafon 2532

Pirbuterol Acetate (Beta-agonist may have to be administered in increased dosage when used concomitantly). Products include:
Maxair Autohaler 1550
Maxair Inhaler 1552

Procainamide Hydrochloride (Potential for prolonged refractoriness; concomitant therapy is not recommended; caution is advised if used concurrently due to sotalol's effect on cardiac repolarization (QTc prolongation) torsade de pointes, a polymorphic ventricular tachycardia with prolonged QT interval). Products include:
Procanbid Extended-Release Tablets 1983

Prochlorperazine (Caution is advised if used concurrently due to sotalol's effect on cardiac repolarization (QTc prolongation) torsade de pointes, a polymorphic ventricular tachycardia with prolonged QT interval). Products include:
Compazine 2644

Promethazine Hydrochloride (Caution is advised if used concurrently due to sotalol's effect on cardiac repolarization (QTc prolongation) torsade de pointes, a polymorphic ventricular tachycardia with prolonged QT interval). Products include:
Mepergan Injection 2859
Phenergan with Codeine 2883
Phenergan with Dextromethorphan ... 2885
Phenergan Injection 2880
Phenergan Suppositories 2882
Phenergan Syrup 2881
Phenergan Tablets 2882
Phenergan VC 2886
Phenergan VC with Codeine 2888

Propafenone Hydrochloride (Potential for prolonged refractoriness; concomitant therapy is not recommended; caution is advised if used concurrently due to sotalol's effect on cardiac repolarization (QTc prolongation) torsade de pointes, a polymorphic ventricular tachycardia with prolonged QT interval). Products include:
Rythmol Tablets–150mg, 225mg, 300mg 1399

Propranolol Hydrochloride (Potential for prolonged refractoriness; concomitant therapy is not recommended). Products include:
Inderal 2834
Inderal LA Long Acting Capsules 2836
Inderide Tablets 2838
Inderide LA Long Acting Capsules ... 2840

Protriptyline Hydrochloride (Caution is advised if used concurrently due to sotalol's effect on cardiac repolarization (QTc prolongation) torsade de pointes, a polymorphic ventricular tachycardia with prolonged QT interval). Products include:
Vivactil Tablets 1820

Quinidine Gluconate (Potential for prolonged refractoriness; concomitant therapy is not recommended; caution is advised if used concurrently due to sotalol's effect on cardiac repolarization (QTc prolongation) torsade de pointes, a polymorphic ventricular tachycardia with prolonged QT interval). Products include:
Quinaglute Dura-Tabs Tablets 644

Quinidine Polygalacturonate (Potential for prolonged refractoriness; concomitant therapy is not recommended; caution is advised if used concurrently due to sotalol's effect on cardiac repolarization (QTc prolongation) torsade de pointes, a polymorphic ventricular tachycardia with prolonged QT interval). Products include:
Cardioquin Tablets 2146

Quinidine Sulfate (Potential for prolonged refractoriness; concomitant therapy is not recommended; caution is advised if used concurrently due to sotalol's effect on cardiac repolarization (QTc prolongation) torsade de pointes, a polymorphic ventricular tachycardia with prolonged QT interval). Products include:
Quinidex Extentabs 2240

Rauwolfia Serpentina (Produces an excessive reduction of resting sympathetic nervous tone).
No products indexed under this heading.

Rescinnamine (Produces an excessive reduction of resting sympathetic nervous tone).
No products indexed under this heading.

Reserpine (Produces an excessive reduction of resting sympathetic nervous tone). Products include:
Diupres Tablets 1691
Hydropres Tablets 1718
Ser-Ap-Es Tablets 867

Salmeterol Xinafoate (Beta-agonist may have to be administered in increased dosage when used concomitantly). Products include:
Serevent Inhalation Aerosol 1149

Terbutaline Sulfate (Beta-agonist may have to be administered in increased dosage when used concomitantly). Products include:
Brethaire Inhaler 830
Brethine Ampuls 832
Brethine Tablets 831
Bricanyl Subcutaneous Injection 1247
Bricanyl Tablets 1248

Terfenadine (Caution is advised if used concurrently due to sotalol's effect on cardiac repolarization (QTc prolongation) torsade de pointes, a polymorphic ventricular tachycardia with prolonged QT interval). Products include:
Seldane Tablets 1284
Seldane-D Extended-Release Tablets 1286

Thioridazine Hydrochloride (Caution is advised if used concurrently due to sotalol's effect on cardiac repolarization (QTc prolongation) torsade de pointes, a polymorphic ventricular tachycardia with prolonged QT interval). Products include:
Mellaril 2398

Tocainide Hydrochloride (Potential for prolonged refractoriness; concomitant therapy is not recommended; caution is advised if used concurrently due to sotalol's effect on cardiac repolarization (QTc prolongation) torsade de pointes, a polymorphic ventricular tachycardia with prolonged QT interval). Products include:
Tonocard Tablets 519

Tolazamide (Potential for hyperglycemia; symptoms of hypoglycemia may be masked; dosage of antidiabetic drugs may require adjustment).
No products indexed under this heading.

Tolbutamide (Potential for hyperglycemia; symptoms of hypoglycemia may be masked; dosage of antidiabetic drugs may require adjustment).
No products indexed under this heading.

Trifluoperazine Hydrochloride (Caution is advised if used concurrently due to sotalol's effect on cardiac repolarization (QTc prolongation) torsade de pointes, a polymorphic ventricular tachycardia with prolonged QT interval). Products include:
Stelazine 2692

Trimipramine Maleate (Caution is advised if used concurrently due to sotalol's effect on cardiac repolarization (QTc prolongation) torsade de pointes, a polymorphic ventricular tachycardia with prolonged QT interval). Products include:
Surmontil Capsules 2917

Verapamil Hydrochloride (Potential for prolonged refractoriness; concomitant therapy is not recommended; possible additive effects on AV conduction or ventricular conduction; co-administration may result in hypotension). Products include:
Calan SR Caplets 2571
Calan Tablets 2568
Covera-HS Tablets 2573
Isoptin Injectable 1391
Isoptin Oral Tablets 1393
Isoptin SR Tablets 1395
Verelan Capsules 1455

Food Interactions
Meal, unspecified (Reduces oral absorption by 20%).

IMPORTANT NOTE: Always consult each drug listing in the patient's regimen for possible interactions.

BETASEPT SURGICAL SCRUB
(Chlorhexidine Gluconate) 2145
None cited in PDR database.

BETASERON FOR SC INJECTION
(Interferon Beta-1b) 653
None cited in PDR database.

BETIMOL 0.25%, 0.5%
(Timolol Hemihydrate) .... ◉ 259
May interact with beta blockers, calcium channel blockers, cardiac glycosides, and certain other agents. Compounds in these categories include:

Acebutolol Hydrochloride (Concurrent use with systemic beta blockers may result in additive effect either on the intraocular pressure or the known systemic effect of beta blockade). Products include:
- Sectral Capsules 2914

Amlodipine Besylate (Possible atrioventricular conduction disturbances, left ventricular failure, and hypotension). Products include:
- Lotrel Capsules 858
- Norvasc Tablets 2020

Atenolol (Concurrent use with systemic beta blockers may result in additive effect either on the intraocular pressure or the known systemic effect of beta blockade). Products include:
- Tenoretic Tablets 2963
- Tenormin Tablets and I.V. Injection 2965

Bepridil Hydrochloride (Possible atrioventricular conduction disturbances, left ventricular failure, and hypotension). Products include:
- Vascor Tablets (200 and 300 mg) 1597

Betaxolol Hydrochloride (Concurrent use with systemic beta blockers may result in additive effect either on the intraocular pressure or the known systemic effect of beta blockade). Products include:
- Betoptic Ophthalmic Solution 465
- Betoptic S Ophthalmic Suspension 467
- Kerlone Tablets 2588

Bisoprolol Fumarate (Concurrent use with systemic beta blockers may result in additive effect either on the intraocular pressure or the known systemic effect of beta blockade). Products include:
- Zebeta Tablets 1457
- Ziac 1459

Carteolol Hydrochloride (Concurrent use with systemic beta blockers may result in additive effect either on the intraocular pressure or the known systemic effect of beta blockade). Products include:
- Cartrol Tablets 413
- Ocupress Ophthalmic Solution, 1% Sterile .... ◉ 297

Deslanoside (Concomitant use of beta blockers with digitalis and calcium antagonists may have additive effects in prolonging atrioventricular conduction time).
- No products indexed under this heading.

Digitoxin (Concomitant use of beta blockers with digitalis and calcium antagonists may have additive effects in prolonging atrioventricular conduction time). Products include:
- Crystodigin Tablets 1472

Digoxin (Concomitant use of beta blockers with digitalis and calcium antagonists may have additive effects in prolonging atrioventricular conduction time). Products include:
- Lanoxicaps 1110
- Lanoxin Elixir Pediatric 1113
- Lanoxin Injection 1116
- Lanoxin Injection Pediatric 1119
- Lanoxin Tablets 1121

Diltiazem Hydrochloride (Possible atrioventricular conduction disturbances, left ventricular failure, and hypotension). Products include:
- Cardizem CD Capsules 1251
- Cardizem SR Capsules 1255
- Cardizem Injectable 1253
- Cardizem Tablets 1257
- Dilacor XR Extended-release Capsules 2183
- Tiazac Capsules 1019

Epinephrine (Patients with a history of atopy or anaphylactic reactions to a variety of allergens may be unresponsive to the usual dose of injectable epinephrine used to treat allergic reactions). Products include:
- EPIFRIN .... ◉ 237
- EpiPen 808
- Marcaine with Epinephrine 2446
- Primatene Mist .... ▣ 843
- Sensorcaine with Epinephrine Injection 554
- Sus-Phrine Injection 1017
- Xylocaine with Epinephrine Injections 562

Epinephrine Bitartrate (Patients with a history of atopy or anaphylactic reactions to a variety of allergens may be unresponsive to the usual dose of injectable epinephrine used to treat allergic reactions). Products include:
- Sensorcaine-MPF with Epinephrine Injection 554

Esmolol Hydrochloride (Concurrent use with systemic beta blockers may result in additive effect either on the intraocular pressure or the known systemic effect of beta blockade). Products include:
- Brevibloc (esmolol HCl) Injection 1860

Felodipine (Possible atrioventricular conduction disturbances, left ventricular failure, and hypotension). Products include:
- Plendil Extended-Release Tablets 514

Isradipine (Possible atrioventricular conduction disturbances, left ventricular failure, and hypotension). Products include:
- DynaCirc Capsules 2381
- DynaCirc CR Tablets 2383

Labetalol Hydrochloride (Concurrent use with systemic beta blockers may result in additive effect either on the intraocular pressure or the known systemic effect of beta blockade). Products include:
- Normodyne Injection 2519
- Normodyne Tablets 2522
- Trandate 1158

Levobunolol Hydrochloride (Concurrent use with systemic beta blockers may result in additive effect either on the intraocular pressure or the known systemic effect of beta blockade). Products include:
- Betagan .... ◉ 230

Metipranolol Hydrochloride (Concurrent use with systemic beta blockers may result in additive effect either on the intraocular pressure or the known systemic effect of beta blockade). Products include:
- OptiPranolol (Metipranolol 0.3%) Sterile Ophthalmic Solution .... ◉ 256

Metoprolol Succinate (Concurrent use with systemic beta blockers may result in additive effect either on the intraocular pressure or the known systemic effect of beta blockade). Products include:
- Toprol-XL Tablets 560

Metoprolol Tartrate (Concurrent use with systemic beta blockers may result in additive effect either on the intraocular pressure or the known systemic effect of beta blockade). Products include:
- Lopressor 848
- Lopressor HCT Tablets 850

Nadolol (Concurrent use with systemic beta blockers may result in additive effect either on the intraocular pressure or the known systemic effect of beta blockade).
- No products indexed under this heading.

Nicardipine Hydrochloride (Possible atrioventricular conduction disturbances, left ventricular failure, and hypotension). Products include:
- Cardene Capsules 2261
- Cardene I.V. 2815
- Cardene SR Capsules 2264

Nifedipine (Possible atrioventricular conduction disturbances, left ventricular failure, and hypotension). Products include:
- Adalat Capsules (10 mg and 20 mg) 580
- Adalat CC 582
- Procardia Capsules 2024
- Procardia XL Extended Release Tablets 2026

Nimodipine (Possible atrioventricular conduction disturbances, left ventricular failure, and hypotension). Products include:
- Nimotop Capsules 603

Nisoldipine (Possible atrioventricular conduction disturbances, left ventricular failure, and hypotension). Products include:
- Sular Tablets 2961

Penbutolol Sulfate (Concurrent use with systemic beta blockers may result in additive effect either on the intraocular pressure or the known systemic effect of beta blockade). Products include:
- Levatol Tablets 2547

Pindolol (Concurrent use with systemic beta blockers may result in additive effect either on the intraocular pressure or the known systemic effect of beta blockade). Products include:
- Visken Tablets 2428

Propranolol Hydrochloride (Concurrent use with systemic beta blockers may result in additive effect either on the intraocular pressure or the known systemic effect of beta blockade). Products include:
- Inderal 2834
- Inderal LA Long Acting Capsules 2836
- Inderide Tablets 2838
- Inderide LA Long Acting Capsules .. 2840

Reserpine (Possible additive effects and the production of hypotension and/or marked bradycardia). Products include:
- Diupres Tablets 1691
- Hydropres Tablets 1718
- Ser-Ap-Es Tablets 867

Sotalol Hydrochloride (Concurrent use with systemic beta blockers may result in additive effect either on the intraocular pressure or the known systemic effect of beta blockade). Products include:
- Betapace Tablets 637

Timolol Maleate (Concurrent use with systemic beta blockers may result in additive effect either on the intraocular pressure or the known systemic effect of beta blockade). Products include:
- Blocadren Tablets 1654
- Timolide Tablets 1791
- Timoptic in Ocudose 1796
- Timoptic Sterile Ophthalmic Solution 1794
- Timoptic-XE 1798

Verapamil Hydrochloride (Possible atrioventricular conduction disturbances, left ventricular failure, and hypotension). Products include:
- Calan SR Caplets 2571
- Calan Tablets 2568
- Covera-HS Tablets 2573
- Isoptin Injectable 1391
- Isoptin Oral Tablets 1393
- Isoptin SR Tablets 1395
- Verelan Capsules 1455

BETOPTIC OPHTHALMIC SOLUTION
(Betaxolol Hydrochloride) 465
May interact with beta blockers, general anesthetics, catecholamine depleting drugs, adrenergic augmenting psychotropics, and certain other agents. Compounds in these categories include:

Acebutolol Hydrochloride (Potential additive effects either on the intraocular pressure or on the known systemic effects of beta blockade). Products include:
- Sectral Capsules 2914

Atenolol (Potential additive effects either on the intraocular pressure or on the known systemic effects of beta blockade). Products include:
- Tenoretic Tablets 2963
- Tenormin Tablets and I.V. Injection 2965

Bisoprolol Fumarate (Potential additive effects either on the intraocular pressure or on the known systemic effects of beta blockade). Products include:
- Zebeta Tablets 1457
- Ziac 1459

Carteolol Hydrochloride (Potential additive effects either on the intraocular pressure or on the known systemic effects of beta blockade). Products include:
- Cartrol Tablets 413
- Ocupress Ophthalmic Solution, 1% Sterile .... ◉ 297

Deserpidine (Possible additive effects and the production of hypotension and/or bradycardia).
- No products indexed under this heading.

Enflurane (Impairment of heart's ability to respond to beta-adrenergically mediated sympathetic reflex stimuli).
- No products indexed under this heading.

Esmolol Hydrochloride (Potential additive effects either on the intraocular pressure or on the known systemic effects of beta blockade). Products include:
- Brevibloc (esmolol HCl) Injection 1860

Guanethidine Monosulfate (Possible additive effects and the production of hypotension and/or bradycardia). Products include:
- Esimil Tablets 840
- Ismelin Tablets 845

Isocarboxazid (Exercise caution when used concomitantly).
- No products indexed under this heading.

Isoflurane (Impairment of heart's ability to respond to beta-adrenergically mediated sympathetic reflex stimuli).
- No products indexed under this heading.

Ketamine Hydrochloride (Impairment of heart's ability to respond to beta-adrenergically mediated sympathetic reflex stimuli).
- No products indexed under this heading.

(▣ Described in PDR For Nonprescription Drugs) (◉ Described in PDR For Ophthalmology)

Labetalol Hydrochloride (Potential additive effects either on the intraocular pressure or on the known systemic effects of beta blockade). Products include:
- Normodyne Injection 2519
- Normodyne Tablets 2522
- Trandate 1158

Levobunolol Hydrochloride (Potential additive effects either on the intraocular pressure or on the known systemic effects of beta blockade). Products include:
- Betagan .... ⓒ 230

Methohexital Sodium (Impairment of heart's ability to respond to beta-adrenergically mediated sympathetic reflex stimuli).
No products indexed under this heading.

Methoxyflurane (Impairment of heart's ability to respond to beta-adrenergically mediated sympathetic reflex stimuli).
No products indexed under this heading.

Metipranolol Hydrochloride (Potential additive effects either on the intraocular pressure or on the known systemic effects of beta blockade). Products include:
- OptiPranolol (Metipranolol 0.3%) Sterile Ophthalmic Solution .... ⓒ 256

Metoprolol Succinate (Potential additive effects either on the intraocular pressure or on the known systemic effects of beta blockade). Products include:
- Toprol-XL Tablets 560

Metoprolol Tartrate (Potential additive effects either on the intraocular pressure or on the known systemic effects of beta blockade). Products include:
- Lopressor 848
- Lopressor HCT Tablets 850

Nadolol (Potential additive effects either on the intraocular pressure or on the known systemic effects of beta blockade).
No products indexed under this heading.

Pargyline Hydrochloride (Exercise caution when used concomitantly).
No products indexed under this heading.

Penbutolol Sulfate (Potential additive effects either on the intraocular pressure or on the known systemic effects of beta blockade). Products include:
- Levatol Tablets 2547

Phenelzine Sulfate (Exercise caution when used concomitantly). Products include:
- Nardil 1977

Pindolol (Potential additive effects either on the intraocular pressure or on the known systemic effects of beta blockade). Products include:
- Visken Tablets 2428

Propofol (Impairment of heart's ability to respond to beta-adrenergically mediated sympathetic reflex stimuli). Products include:
- Diprivan Injectable Emulsion 2939

Propranolol Hydrochloride (Potential additive effects either on the intraocular pressure or on the known systemic effects of beta blockade). Products include:
- Inderal 2834
- Inderal LA Long Acting Capsules 2836
- Inderide Tablets 2838
- Inderide LA Long Acting Capsules .. 2840

Rauwolfia Serpentina (Possible additive effects and the production of hypotension and/or bradycardia).
No products indexed under this heading.

Rescinnamine (Possible additive effects and the production of hypotension and/or bradycardia).
No products indexed under this heading.

Reserpine (Possible additive effects and the production of hypotension and/or bradycardia). Products include:
- Diupres Tablets 1691
- Hydropres Tablets 1718
- Ser-Ap-Es Tablets 867

Sevoflurane (Impairment of heart's ability to respond to beta-adrenergically mediated sympathetic reflex stimuli).
No products indexed under this heading.

Sotalol Hydrochloride (Potential additive effects either on the intraocular pressure or on the known systemic effects of beta blockade). Products include:
- Betapace Tablets 637

Timolol Hemihydrate (Potential additive effects either on the intraocular pressure or on the known systemic effects of beta blockade). Products include:
- Betimol 0.25%, 0.5% .... ⓒ 259

Timolol Maleate (Potential additive effects either on the intraocular pressure or on the known systemic effects of beta blockade). Products include:
- Blocadren Tablets 1654
- Timolide Tablets 1791
- Timoptic in Ocudose 1796
- Timoptic Sterile Ophthalmic Solution 1794
- Timoptic-XE 1798

Tranylcypromine Sulfate (Exercise caution when used concomitantly). Products include:
- Parnate Tablets 2679

BETOPTIC S OPHTHALMIC SUSPENSION
(Betaxolol Hydrochloride) 467
May interact with beta blockers, adrenergic augmenting psychotropics, and certain other agents. Compounds in these categories include:

Acebutolol Hydrochloride (Co-administration with oral beta blockers may result in additive effect either on intraocular pressure or on the known systemic effect of beta blockade). Products include:
- Sectral Capsules 2914

Atenolol (Co-administration with oral beta blockers may result in additive effect either on intraocular pressure or on the known systemic effect of beta blockade). Products include:
- Tenoretic Tablets 2963
- Tenormin Tablets and I.V. Injection 2965

Bisoprolol Fumarate (Co-administration with oral beta blockers may result in additive effect either on intraocular pressure or on the known systemic effect of beta blockade). Products include:
- Zebeta Tablets 1457
- Ziac 1459

Carteolol Hydrochloride (Co-administration with oral beta blockers may result in additive effect either on intraocular pressure or on the known systemic effect of beta blockade). Products include:
- Cartrol Tablets 413
- Ocupress Ophthalmic Solution, 1% Sterile .... ⓒ 297

Deserpidine (Possible additive effects and production of hypotension and/or bradycardia when beta blocker is concurrently used with catecholamine depleting drugs).
No products indexed under this heading.

Epinephrine (Concurrent use in patients with history of atopy or severe anaphylactic reaction to allergens may be unresponsive to the usual doses of epinephrine used to treat anaphylactic reaction). Products include:
- EPIFRIN .... ⓒ 237
- EpiPen 808
- Marcaine with Epinephrine 2446
- Primatene Mist .... ⓒ 843
- Sensorcaine with Epinephrine Injection 554
- Sus-Phrine Injection 1017
- Xylocaine with Epinephrine Injections 562

Epinephrine Hydrochloride (Concurrent use in patients with history of atopy or severe anaphylactic reaction to allergens may be unresponsive to the usual doses of epinephrine used to treat anaphylactic reaction). Products include:
- Ana-Kit Anaphylaxis Emergency Treatment Kit 611

Esmolol Hydrochloride (Co-administration with oral beta blockers may result in additive effect either on intraocular pressure or on the known systemic effect of beta blockade). Products include:
- Brevibloc (esmolol HCl) Injection 1860

Isocarboxazid (Exercise caution when used concurrently with adrenergic psychotropic drugs).
No products indexed under this heading.

Labetalol Hydrochloride (Co-administration with oral beta blockers may result in additive effect either on intraocular pressure or on the known systemic effect of beta blockade). Products include:
- Normodyne Injection 2519
- Normodyne Tablets 2522
- Trandate 1158

Levobunolol Hydrochloride (Co-administration with oral beta blockers may result in additive effect either on intraocular pressure or on the known systemic effect of beta blockade). Products include:
- Betagan .... ⓒ 230

Metipranolol Hydrochloride (Co-administration with oral beta blockers may result in additive effect either on intraocular pressure or on the known systemic effect of beta blockade). Products include:
- OptiPranolol (Metipranolol 0.3%) Sterile Ophthalmic Solution .... ⓒ 256

Metoprolol Succinate (Co-administration with oral beta blockers may result in additive effect either on intraocular pressure or on the known systemic effect of beta blockade). Products include:
- Toprol-XL Tablets 560

Metoprolol Tartrate (Co-administration with oral beta blockers may result in additive effect either on intraocular pressure or on the known systemic effect of beta blockade). Products include:
- Lopressor 848
- Lopressor HCT Tablets 850

Nadolol (Co-administration with oral beta blockers may result in additive effect either on intraocular pressure or on the known systemic effect of beta blockade).
No products indexed under this heading.

Pargyline Hydrochloride (Exercise caution when used concurrently with adrenergic psychotropic drugs).
No products indexed under this heading.

Penbutolol Sulfate (Co-administration with oral beta blockers may result in additive effect either on intraocular pressure or on the known systemic effect of beta blockade). Products include:
- Levatol Tablets 2547

Phenelzine Sulfate (Exercise caution when used concurrently with adrenergic psychotropic drugs). Products include:
- Nardil 1977

Pindolol (Co-administration with oral beta blockers may result in additive effect either on intraocular pressure or on the known systemic effect of beta blockade). Products include:
- Visken Tablets 2428

Propranolol Hydrochloride (Co-administration with oral beta blockers may result in additive effect either on intraocular pressure or on the known systemic effect of beta blockade). Products include:
- Inderal 2834
- Inderal LA Long Acting Capsules 2836
- Inderide Tablets 2838
- Inderide LA Long Acting Capsules .. 2840

Rauwolfia Serpentina (Possible additive effects and production of hypotension and/or bradycardia when beta blocker is concurrently used with catecholamine depleting drugs).
No products indexed under this heading.

Rescinnamine (Possible additive effects and production of hypotension and/or bradycardia when beta blocker is concurrently used with catecholamine depleting drugs).
No products indexed under this heading.

Reserpine (Possible additive effects and production of hypotension and/or bradycardia when beta blocker is concurrently used with catecholamine depleting drugs). Products include:
- Diupres Tablets 1691
- Hydropres Tablets 1718
- Ser-Ap-Es Tablets 867

Sotalol Hydrochloride (Co-administration with oral beta blockers may result in additive effect either on intraocular pressure or on the known systemic effect of beta blockade). Products include:
- Betapace Tablets 637

Timolol Hemihydrate (Co-administration with oral beta blockers may result in additive effect either on the known systemic effect of beta blockade). Products include:
- Betimol 0.25%, 0.5% .... ⓒ 259

Timolol Maleate (Co-administration with oral beta blockers may result in additive effect either on the intraocular pressure or on the known systemic effect of beta blockade). Products include:
- Blocadren Tablets 1654
- Timolide Tablets 1791
- Timoptic in Ocudose 1796
- Timoptic Sterile Ophthalmic Solution 1794
- Timoptic-XE 1798

Tranylcypromine Sulfate (Exercise caution when used concurrently with adrenergic psychotropic drugs). Products include:
- Parnate Tablets 2679

IMPORTANT NOTE: Always consult each drug listing in the patient's regimen for possible interactions.

BIAVAX II
(Rubella & Mumps Virus Vaccine Live) 1653
May interact with:

Azathioprine (Contraindication). Products include:
Azathioprine Tablets 2349
Imuran 1103

Cyclosporine (Contraindication). Products include:
Neoral 2405
Sandimmune 2416

Immune Globulin (Human) (Contraindication).
No products indexed under this heading.

Immune Globulin Intravenous (Human) (Contraindication).

Muromonab-CD3 (Contraindication). Products include:
Orthoclone OKT3 Sterile Solution .. 1892

BIAXIN FILMTAB
(Clarithromycin) 406
May interact with xanthine bronchodilators, oral anticoagulants, and certain other agents. Compounds in these categories include:

Alfentanil Hydrochloride (Co-administration can be associated with elevation in alfentanil serum levels). Products include:
Alfenta Injection 1334

Aminophylline (Potential for increased serum theophylline concentration).
No products indexed under this heading.

Astemizole (Co-administration can be associated with elevation in astemizole serum levels). Products include:
Hismanal Tablets 1341

Bromocriptine Mesylate (Co-administration can be associated with elevation in bromocriptine serum levels). Products include:
Parlodel 2411

Carbamazepine (Potential for increased serum concentration of carbamazepine). Products include:
Atretol Tablets 569
Tegretol/Tegretol-XR 870

Cisapride (Co-administration can be associated with elevation in cisapride serum levels). Products include:
Propulsid 1346

Cyclosporine (Co-administration can be associated with elevation in cyclosporine serum levels). Products include:
Neoral 2405
Sandimmune 2416

Dicumarol (Co-administration may result in the potentiation of oral anticoagulant effects).
No products indexed under this heading.

Digoxin (Concomitant use has resulted in elevated digoxin serum concentrations and some patients have shown signs of digoxin toxicity, including arrhythmias). Products include:
Lanoxicaps 1110
Lanoxin Elixir Pediatric 1113
Lanoxin Injection 1116
Lanoxin Injection Pediatric 1119
Lanoxin Tablets 1121

Dihydroergotamine Mesylate (Concurrent use is associated with acute ergot toxicity characterized by severe peripheral vasospasm and dysesthesia). Products include:
D.H.E. 45 Injection 2381

Disopyramide Phosphate (Co-administration can be associated with elevation in disopyramide serum levels). Products include:
Norpace 2596

Divalproex Sodium (Co-administration can be associated with elevation in valproate serum levels). Products include:
Depakote Tablets 418

Dyphylline (Potential for increased serum theophylline concentration). Products include:
Lufyllin & Lufyllin-400 Tablets 2778
Lufyllin-GG Elixir & Tablets 2779

Ergotamine Tartrate (Concurrent use is associated with acute ergot toxicity characterized by severe peripheral vasospasm and dysesthesia). Products include:
Bellergal-S Tablets 2375
Cafergot 2376
Ergomar Tablets 1543
Wigraine Tablets 1884

Fluconazole (Co-administration has resulted in increases in the mean steady-state clarithromycin C_{min} and AUC). Products include:
Diflucan Tablets, Injection, and Oral Suspension 2003

Fosphenytoin Sodium (Co-administration can be associated with elevation in phenytoin serum levels). Products include:
Cerebyx Injection 1956

Hexobarbital (Co-administration can be associated with elevation in hexobarbital serum levels).

Lovastatin (Co-administration can be associated with elevation in lovastatin serum levels). Products include:
Mevacor Tablets 1742

Omeprazole (Co-administration increases the steady-state plasma concentrations, $C_{max}AUC_{0-24}$, and $T^{1}/_{2}$ of omeprazole). Products include:
Prilosec Delayed-Release Capsules 516

Phenytoin (Co-administration can be associated with elevation in phenytoin serum levels). Products include:
Dilantin Infatabs 1967
Dilantin-125 Suspension 1969

Phenytoin Sodium (Co-administration can be associated with elevation in phenytoin serum levels). Products include:
Dilantin Kapseals 1965

Pimozide (Co-administration can be associated with elevation in pimozide serum levels). Products include:
Orap Tablets 1037

Terfenadine (Co-administration may increase plasma concentration of terfenadine active metabolite by 3-fold; concurrent use in patients with preexisting cardiac abnormalities or electrolyte disturbances is contraindicated). Products include:
Seldane Tablets 1284
Seldane-D Extended-Release Tablets 1286

Theophylline (Potential for increased serum theophylline concentration). Products include:
Marax Tablets & DF Syrup 2015
Quibron 2227

Theophylline Anhydrous (Potential for increased serum theophylline concentration). Products include:
Aerolate 1003
Primatene Tablets .... ▣ 844
Respbid Tablets 687
Slo-bid Gyrocaps 2201
Theo-24 Extended Release Capsules 2753
Theo-Dur Extended-Release Tablets 1367
Theo-X Extended-Release Tablets .. 793
Uni-Dur Extended-Release Tablets .. 1374
Uniphyl 400 mg and 600 mg Tablets 2157

Theophylline Calcium Salicylate (Potential for increased serum theophylline concentration). Products include:
Quadrinal Tablets 1398

Theophylline Sodium Glycinate (Potential for increased serum theophylline concentration).
No products indexed under this heading.

Triazolam (Concomitant use has resulted in CNS effects, including somnolence and confusion potentially due to decrease in clearance of triazolam resulting in increased pharmacological effects). Products include:
Halcion Tablets 2093

Valproic Acid (Co-administration can be associated with elevation in valproate serum levels). Products include:
Depakene 416

Warfarin Sodium (Co-administration may result in the potentiation of oral anticoagulant effects). Products include:
Coumadin 941

Zidovudine (Potential for decreased steady-state zidovudine concentration). Products include:
Retrovir Capsules 1216
Retrovir I.V. Infusion 1221
Retrovir Syrup 1216

Food Interactions

Food, unspecified (Food slightly delays both the onset of absorption and the formation of the active metabolite, but does not affect the extent of bioavailability; Biaxin may be administered without regard to food).

BIAXIN GRANULES
(Clarithromycin) 406
See **Biaxin Filmtab**

BICHLORACETIC ACID KAHLENBERG
(Dichloroacetic Acid) 1233
None cited in PDR database.

BICILLIN C-R INJECTION
(Penicillin G Procaine, Penicillin G Benzathine) 2810
May interact with tetracyclines and certain other agents. Compounds in these categories include:

Demeclocycline Hydrochloride (May antagonize the bactericidal effect of penicillin). Products include:
Declomycin Tablets 1421

Doxycycline Calcium (May antagonize the bactericidal effect of penicillin). Products include:
Vibramycin Calcium Oral Suspension Syrup 2038

Doxycycline Hyclate (May antagonize the bactericidal effect of penicillin). Products include:
Doryx Capsules 1970
Vibramycin Hyclate Capsules 2038
Vibramycin Hyclate Intravenous 2040
Vibra-Tabs Film Coated Tablets 2038

Doxycycline Monohydrate (May antagonize the bactericidal effect of penicillin). Products include:
Monodox Capsules 1858
Vibramycin Monohydrate for Oral Suspension 2038

Methacycline Hydrochloride (May antagonize the bactericidal effect of penicillin).
No products indexed under this heading.

Minocycline Hydrochloride (May antagonize the bactericidal effect of penicillin). Products include:
DYNACIN Capsules 1627
Minocin Intravenous 1428
Minocin Oral Suspension 1431
Minocin Pellet-Filled Capsules 1429

Oxytetracycline Hydrochloride (May antagonize the bactericidal effect of penicillin). Products include:
TERAK Ointment .... ◉ 210
Terra-Cortril Ophthalmic Suspension 2033
Terramycin with Polymyxin B Sulfate Ophthalmic Ointment 2035
Urobiotic-250 Capsules 2038

Probenecid (Increases serum penicillin levels). Products include:
Benemid Tablets 1651
ColBENEMID Tablets 1662

Tetracycline Hydrochloride (May antagonize the bactericidal effect of penicillin). Products include:
Achromycin V Capsules 1417
Helidac Therapy 2135

BICILLIN C-R 900/300 INJECTION
(Penicillin G Procaine, Penicillin G Benzathine) 2812
May interact with tetracyclines and certain other agents. Compounds in these categories include:

Demeclocycline Hydrochloride (May antagonize the bactericidal effect of penicillin). Products include:
Declomycin Tablets 1421

Doxycycline Calcium (May antagonize the bactericidal effect of penicillin). Products include:
Vibramycin Calcium Oral Suspension Syrup 2038

Doxycycline Hyclate (May antagonize the bactericidal effect of penicillin). Products include:
Doryx Capsules 1970
Vibramycin Hyclate Capsules 2038
Vibramycin Hyclate Intravenous 2040
Vibra-Tabs Film Coated Tablets 2038

Doxycycline Monohydrate (May antagonize the bactericidal effect of penicillin). Products include:
Monodox Capsules 1858
Vibramycin Monohydrate for Oral Suspension 2038

Methacycline Hydrochloride (May antagonize the bactericidal effect of penicillin).
No products indexed under this heading.

Minocycline Hydrochloride (May antagonize the bactericidal effect of penicillin). Products include:
DYNACIN Capsules 1627
Minocin Intravenous 1428
Minocin Oral Suspension 1431
Minocin Pellet-Filled Capsules 1429

Oxytetracycline Hydrochloride (May antagonize the bactericidal effect of penicillin). Products include:
TERAK Ointment .... ◉ 210
Terra-Cortril Ophthalmic Suspension 2033
Terramycin with Polymyxin B Sulfate Ophthalmic Ointment 2035
Urobiotic-250 Capsules 2038

(▣ Described in PDR For Nonprescription Drugs) (◉ Described in PDR For Ophthalmology)

Probenecid (Concurrent administration increases and prolongs serum penicillin levels). Products include:
- Benemid Tablets ... 1651
- ColBENEMID Tablets ... 1662

Tetracycline Hydrochloride (May antagonize the bactericidal effect of penicillin). Products include:
- Achromycin V Capsules ... 1417
- Helidac Therapy ... 2135

BICILLIN L-A INJECTION
(Penicillin G Benzathine) ... 2813
May interact with tetracyclines and certain other agents. Compounds in these categories include:

Demeclocycline Hydrochloride (May antagonize the bactericidal effect of penicillin). Products include:
- Declomycin Tablets ... 1421

Doxycycline Calcium (May antagonize the bactericidal effect of penicillin). Products include:
- Vibramycin Calcium Oral Suspension Syrup ... 2038

Doxycycline Hyclate (May antagonize the bactericidal effect of penicillin). Products include:
- Doryx Capsules ... 1970
- Vibramycin Hyclate Capsules ... 2038
- Vibramycin Hyclate Intravenous ... 2040
- Vibra-Tabs Film Coated Tablets ... 2038

Doxycycline Monohydrate (May antagonize the bactericidal effect of penicillin). Products include:
- Monodox Capsules ... 1858
- Vibramycin Monohydrate for Oral Suspension ... 2038

Methacycline Hydrochloride (May antagonize the bactericidal effect of penicillin).
- No products indexed under this heading.

Minocycline Hydrochloride (May antagonize the bactericidal effect of penicillin). Products include:
- DYNACIN Capsules ... 1627
- Minocin Intravenous ... 1428
- Minocin Oral Suspension ... 1431
- Minocin Pellet-Filled Capsules ... 1429

Oxytetracycline Hydrochloride (May antagonize the bactericidal effect of penicillin). Products include:
- TERAK Ointment ... 210
- Terra-Cortril Ophthalmic Suspension ... 2033
- Terramycin with Polymyxin B Sulfate Ophthalmic Ointment ... 2035
- Urobiotic-250 Capsules ... 2038

Probenecid (Increases serum penicillin levels). Products include:
- Benemid Tablets ... 1651
- ColBENEMID Tablets ... 1662

Tetracycline Hydrochloride (May antagonize the bactericidal effect of penicillin). Products include:
- Achromycin V Capsules ... 1417
- Helidac Therapy ... 2135

BICITRA
(Sodium Citrate, Citric Acid) ... 573
May interact with:

Aluminum Carbonate (Avoid concomitant use of aluminum-based antacids). Products include:
- Basaljel Capsules ... 2810
- Basaljel Suspension ... 2810
- Basaljel Tablets ... 2810

Aluminum Hydroxide (Avoid concomitant use of aluminum-based antacids). Products include:
- ALternaGEL Liquid ... 1358
- Maximum Strength Ascriptin ... 650
- Cama Arthritis Pain Reliever ... 748
- Gaviscon Extra Strength Relief Formula Antacid Tablets ... 778
- Gaviscon Extra Strength Relief Formula Liquid Antacid ... 779
- Gaviscon Liquid Antacid ... 779
- Gelusil Antacid-Anti-gas Liquid ... 819
- Gelusil Antacid-Anti-gas Tablets ... 819
- Maalox Antacid/Anti-Gas Tablets ... 889
- Maalox Heartburn Relief Suspension ... 658
- Maalox Antacid Liquid ... 888
- Extra Strength Maalox Antacid/Anti-Gas Liquid and Tablets ... 888
- Mylanta ... 1359
- Tempo Soft Antacid ... 799

Aluminum Hydroxide Gel (Avoid concomitant use of aluminum-based antacids). Products include:
- ALternaGEL Liquid ... 675
- Aludrox Oral Suspension ... 850
- Amphojel Suspension ... 2802
- Amphojel Suspension without Flavor ... 2802
- Amphojel Tablets ... 2802
- Ascriptin ... 650
- Gaviscon Antacid Tablets ... 778
- Gaviscon-2 Antacid Tablets ... 779
- Mylanta Liquid ... 676
- Mylanta Double Strength Liquid ... 676
- Nephrox Suspension ... 671

BICNU
(Carmustine (BCNU)) ... 696
None cited in PDR database.

BICOZENE CREME
(Benzocaine, Resorcinol) ... 747
None cited in PDR database.

BILTRICIDE TABLETS
(Praziquantel) ... 584
None cited in PDR database.

BIOCLATE, ANTIHEMOPHILIC FACTOR (RECOMBINANT)
(Antihemophilic Factor (Recombinant)) ... 797
None cited in PDR database.

BIO-COMPLEX 5000 GENTLE FOAMING CLEANSER
(Aloe Vera) ... 830
None cited in PDR database.

BIO-COMPLEX 5000 REVITALIZING CONDITIONER
(Cleanser) ... 830
None cited in PDR database.

BIO-COMPLEX 5000 REVITALIZING SHAMPOO
(Cleanser) ... 830
None cited in PDR database.

BIO-GINKGO 24/6 TABLETS
(Ginkgo Biloba) ... 2984
None cited in PDR database.

BIO-GINKGO 27/7 TABLETS
(Ginkgo Biloba) ... 2984
None cited in PDR database.

BIOLEAN
(Nutritional Supplement) ... 830
May interact with anorexiants and antidepressant drugs. Compounds in these categories include:

Amitriptyline Hydrochloride (Concurrent use is not recommended). Products include:
- Elavil ... 2945
- Etrafon ... 2495
- Limbitrol ... 2333
- Triavil Tablets ... 1800

Amoxapine (Concurrent use is not recommended). Products include:
- Asendin Tablets ... 1419

Amphetamine Resins (Concurrent use is not recommended).
- No products indexed under this heading.

Benzphetamine Hydrochloride (Concurrent use is not recommended).
- No products indexed under this heading.

Bupropion Hydrochloride (Concurrent use is not recommended). Products include:
- Wellbutrin Tablets ... 1177

Desipramine Hydrochloride (Concurrent use is not recommended). Products include:
- Norpramin Tablets ... 1273

Dextroamphetamine Sulfate (Concurrent use is not recommended). Products include:
- Adderall Tablets ... 2209
- Dexedrine ... 2648
- DextroStat-Dextroamphetamine Sulfate Tablets ... 2211

Diethylpropion Hydrochloride (Concurrent use is not recommended).
- No products indexed under this heading.

Doxepin Hydrochloride (Concurrent use is not recommended). Products include:
- Adapin Capsules ... 1542
- Sinequan ... 2028
- Zonalon Cream ... 1042

Fenfluramine Hydrochloride (Concurrent use is not recommended). Products include:
- Pondimin Tablets ... 2239

Fluoxetine Hydrochloride (Concurrent use is not recommended). Products include:
- Prozac Pulvules & Liquid, Oral Solution ... 935

Imipramine Hydrochloride (Concurrent use is not recommended). Products include:
- Tofranil Ampuls ... 873
- Tofranil Tablets ... 875

Imipramine Pamoate (Concurrent use is not recommended). Products include:
- Tofranil-PM Capsules ... 876

Isocarboxazid (Concurrent use is not recommended).
- No products indexed under this heading.

Maprotiline Hydrochloride (Concurrent use is not recommended). Products include:
- Ludiomil Tablets ... 861

Mazindol (Concurrent use is not recommended). Products include:
- Sanorex Tablets ... 2423

Methamphetamine Hydrochloride (Concurrent use is not recommended). Products include:
- Desoxyn Gradumet Tablets ... 422

Nefazodone Hydrochloride (Concurrent use is not recommended). Products include:
- Serzone Tablets ... 776

Nortriptyline Hydrochloride (Concurrent use is not recommended). Products include:
- Pamelor ... 2409

Paroxetine Hydrochloride (Concurrent use is not recommended). Products include:
- Paxil Tablets ... 2681

Phendimetrazine Tartrate (Concurrent use is not recommended). Products include:
- Bontril Slow-Release Capsules ... 786
- Prelu-2 Timed Release Capsules ... 687

Phenelzine Sulfate (Concurrent use is not recommended). Products include:
- Nardil ... 1977

Phenmetrazine Hydrochloride (Concurrent use is not recommended).
- No products indexed under this heading.

Protriptyline Hydrochloride (Concurrent use is not recommended). Products include:
- Vivactil Tablets ... 1820

Sertraline Hydrochloride (Concurrent use is not recommended). Products include:
- Zoloft Tablets ... 2051

Tranylcypromine Sulfate (Concurrent use is not recommended). Products include:
- Parnate Tablets ... 2679

Trazodone Hydrochloride (Concurrent use is not recommended). Products include:
- Desyrel and Desyrel Dividose ... 504

Trimipramine Maleate (Concurrent use is not recommended). Products include:
- Surmontil Capsules ... 2917

Venlafaxine Hydrochloride (Concurrent use is not recommended). Products include:
- Effexor ... 2825

BIOLEAN ACCELERATOR
(Nutritional Supplement) ... 831
May interact with antidepressant drugs and anorexiants. Compounds in these categories include:

Amitriptyline Hydrochloride (Effect of concurrent use is not specified). Products include:
- Elavil ... 2945
- Etrafon ... 2495
- Limbitrol ... 2333
- Triavil Tablets ... 1800

Amoxapine (Effect of concurrent use is not specified). Products include:
- Asendin Tablets ... 1419

Amphetamine Resins (Effect of concurrent use is not specified).
- No products indexed under this heading.

Benzphetamine Hydrochloride (Effect of concurrent use is not specified).
- No products indexed under this heading.

Bupropion Hydrochloride (Effect of concurrent use is not specified). Products include:
- Wellbutrin Tablets ... 1177

Desipramine Hydrochloride (Effect of concurrent use is not specified). Products include:
- Norpramin Tablets ... 1273

Dextroamphetamine Sulfate (Effect of concurrent use is not specified). Products include:
- Adderall Tablets ... 2209
- Dexedrine ... 2648
- DextroStat-Dextroamphetamine Sulfate Tablets ... 2211

Diethylpropion Hydrochloride (Effect of concurrent use is not specified).
- No products indexed under this heading.

Doxepin Hydrochloride (Effect of concurrent use is not specified). Products include:
- Adapin Capsules ... 1542
- Sinequan ... 2028
- Zonalon Cream ... 1042

Fenfluramine Hydrochloride (Effect of concurrent use is not specified). Products include:
- Pondimin Tablets ... 2239

IMPORTANT NOTE: Always consult each drug listing in the patient's regimen for possible interactions.

BioLean Accelerator / Interactions Index

Fluoxetine Hydrochloride (Effect of concurrent use is not specified). Products include:
- Prozac Pulvules & Liquid, Oral Solution 935

Imipramine Hydrochloride (Effect of concurrent use is not specified). Products include:
- Tofranil Ampuls 873
- Tofranil Tablets 875

Imipramine Pamoate (Effect of concurrent use is not specified). Products include:
- Tofranil-PM Capsules 876

Isocarboxazid (Effect of concurrent use is not specified).
- No products indexed under this heading.

Maprotiline Hydrochloride (Effect of concurrent use is not specified). Products include:
- Ludiomil Tablets 861

Mazindol (Effect of concurrent use is not specified). Products include:
- Sanorex Tablets 2423

Methamphetamine Hydrochloride (Effect of concurrent use is not specified). Products include:
- Desoxyn Gradumet Tablets 422

Nefazodone Hydrochloride (Effect of concurrent use is not specified). Products include:
- Serzone Tablets 776

Nortriptyline Hydrochloride (Effect of concurrent use is not specified). Products include:
- Pamelor 2409

Paroxetine Hydrochloride (Effect of concurrent use is not specified). Products include:
- Paxil Tablets 2681

Phendimetrazine Tartrate (Effect of concurrent use is not specified). Products include:
- Bontril Slow-Release Capsules 786
- Prelu-2 Timed Release Capsules 687

Phenelzine Sulfate (Effect of concurrent use is not specified). Products include:
- Nardil 1977

Phenmetrazine Hydrochloride (Effect of concurrent use is not specified).
- No products indexed under this heading.

Protriptyline Hydrochloride (Effect of concurrent use is not specified). Products include:
- Vivactil Tablets 1820

Sertraline Hydrochloride (Effect of concurrent use is not specified). Products include:
- Zoloft Tablets 2051

Tranylcypromine Sulfate (Effect of concurrent use is not specified). Products include:
- Parnate Tablets 2679

Trazodone Hydrochloride (Effect of concurrent use is not specified). Products include:
- Desyrel and Desyrel Dividose 504

Trimipramine Maleate (Effect of concurrent use is not specified). Products include:
- Surmontil Capsules 2917

Venlafaxine Hydrochloride (Effect of concurrent use is not specified). Products include:
- Effexor 2825

BIOLEAN FREE
(Amino Acid Preparations, Nutritional Supplement) 831
May interact with monoamine oxidase inhibitors, anorexiants, and certain other agents. Compounds in these categories include:

Amphetamine Resins (Concurrent use is not recommended).
- No products indexed under this heading.

Benzphetamine Hydrochloride (Concurrent use is not recommended).
- No products indexed under this heading.

Caffeine-containing medications (Concurrent caffeine intake should be minimized.)

Dextroamphetamine Sulfate (Concurrent use is not recommended). Products include:
- Adderall Tablets 2209
- Dexedrine 2648
- DextroStat-Dextroamphetamine Sulfate Tablets 2211

Diethylpropion Hydrochloride (Concurrent use is not recommended).
- No products indexed under this heading.

Fenfluramine Hydrochloride (Concurrent use is not recommended). Products include:
- Pondimin Tablets 2239

Furazolidone (Concurrent use is not recommended). Products include:
- Furoxone 2221

Isocarboxazid (Concurrent use is not recommended).
- No products indexed under this heading.

Mazindol (Concurrent use is not recommended). Products include:
- Sanorex Tablets 2423

Methamphetamine Hydrochloride (Concurrent use is not recommended). Products include:
- Desoxyn Gradumet Tablets 422

Phendimetrazine Tartrate (Concurrent use is not recommended). Products include:
- Bontril Slow-Release Capsules 786
- Prelu-2 Timed Release Capsules 687

Phenelzine Sulfate (Concurrent use is not recommended). Products include:
- Nardil 1977

Phenmetrazine Hydrochloride (Concurrent use is not recommended).
- No products indexed under this heading.

Selegiline Hydrochloride (Concurrent use is not recommended). Products include:
- Eldepryl Capsules 2729

Tranylcypromine Sulfate (Concurrent use is not recommended). Products include:
- Parnate Tablets 2679

Food Interactions
Beverages, caffeine-containing (Concurrent caffeine intake should be minimized.)

BIOLEAN LIPOTRIM
(Nutritional Supplement) 832
None cited in PDR database.

BIOLEAN MEAL
(Nutritional Beverage) 832
None cited in PDR database.

BION TEARS
(Lubricant) 214
None cited in PDR database.

BLENOXANE
(Bleomycin Sulfate) 697
May interact with:

Filgrastim (Some published reports indicate that the risk of pulmonary toxicity may be increased with concurrent use). Products include:
- Neupogen for Injection 495

BLEPH-10 OPHTHALMIC OINTMENT 10%
(Sulfacetamide Sodium) 472
May interact with silver preparations. Compounds in this category include:

Silver Nitrate (Incompatible).
- No products indexed under this heading.

BLEPH-10 OPHTHALMIC SOLUTION 10%
(Sulfacetamide Sodium) 472
May interact with silver preparations. Compounds in this category include:

Silver Nitrate (Incompatible).
- No products indexed under this heading.

BLEPHAMIDE LIQUIFILM STERILE OPHTHALMIC SUSPENSION
(Prednisolone Acetate, Sulfacetamide Sodium) 472
May interact with para-aminobenzoic acid based local anesthetics and certain other agents. Compounds in these categories include:

Procaine Hydrochloride (Local anesthetics related to p-amino benzoic acid may antagonize the action of the sulfonamides). Products include:
- Novocain Hydrochloride for Spinal Anesthesia 2457

Silver Nitrate (Blephamide ophthalmic suspension is incompatible with silver preparations).
- No products indexed under this heading.

Tetracaine Hydrochloride (Local anesthetics related to p-amino benzoic acid may antagonize the action of the sulfonamides). Products include:
- Cetacaine Topical Anesthetic 812
- Pontocaine Hydrochloride for Spinal Anesthesia 2460

BLEPHAMIDE OINTMENT
(Sulfacetamide Sodium, Prednisolone Acetate) 234
May interact with silver preparations and para-aminobenzoic acid based local anesthetics. Compounds in these categories include:

Procaine Hydrochloride (May antagonize the action of sulfonamide). Products include:
- Novocain Hydrochloride for Spinal Anesthesia 2457

Silver Nitrate (Blephamide ointment is incompatible with silver preparations).
- No products indexed under this heading.

Tetracaine Hydrochloride (May antagonize the action of sulfonamide). Products include:
- Cetacaine Topical Anesthetic 812
- Pontocaine Hydrochloride for Spinal Anesthesia 2460

BLOCADREN TABLETS
(Timolol Maleate) 1654
May interact with cardiac glycosides, insulin, oral hypoglycemic agents, catecholamine depleting drugs, calcium channel blockers, non-steroidal anti-inflammatory agents, and certain other agents. Compounds in these categories include:

Acarbose (Beta blockers may mask the signs and symptoms of acute hypoglycemia). Products include:
- Precose 604

Amlodipine Besylate (AV conduction disturbances; left ventricular failure). Products include:
- Lotrel Capsules 858
- Norvasc Tablets 2020

Bepridil Hydrochloride (AV conduction disturbances; left ventricular failure). Products include:
- Vascor Tablets (200 and 300 mg) 1597

Chlorpropamide (Beta blockers may mask the signs and symptoms of acute hypoglycemia). Products include:
- Diabinese Tablets 2002

Diclofenac Potassium (Blunting of the antihypertensive effect). Products include:
- Cataflam Tablets 833

Diclofenac Sodium (Blunting of the antihypertensive effect). Products include:
- Voltaren Ophthalmic Sterile Ophthalmic Solution 264
- Cataflam/Voltaren/Voltaren-XR 833

Digitoxin (Additive effects in prolonging AV conduction time). Products include:
- Crystodigin Tablets 1472

Digoxin (Additive effects in prolonging AV conduction time). Products include:
- Lanoxicaps 1110
- Lanoxin Elixir Pediatric 1113
- Lanoxin Injection 1116
- Lanoxin Injection Pediatric 1119
- Lanoxin Tablets 1121

Diltiazem Hydrochloride (AV conduction disturbances; left ventricular failure). Products include:
- Cardizem CD Capsules 1251
- Cardizem SR Capsules 1255
- Cardizem Injectable 1253
- Cardizem Tablets 1257
- Dilacor XR Extended-release Capsules 2183
- Tiazac Capsules 1019

Epinephrine (Patients with a history of atopy or severe anaphylactic reaction to variety of allergens may be unresponsive to the usual dose of epinephrine to treat anaphylactic reactions). Products include:
- EPIFRIN 237
- EpiPen 808
- Marcaine with Epinephrine 2446
- Primatene Mist 843
- Sensorcaine with Epinephrine Injection 554
- Sus-Phrine Injection 1017
- Xylocaine with Epinephrine Injections 562

Epinephrine Hydrochloride (Patients with a history of atopy or severe anaphylactic reaction to variety of allergens may be unresponsive to the usual dose of epinephrine to treat anaphylactic reactions). Products include:
- Ana-Kit Anaphylaxis Emergency Treatment Kit 611

Etodolac (Blunting of the antihypertensive effect). Products include:
- Lodine Capsules and Tablets 2849

Felodipine (AV conduction disturbances; left ventricular failure). Products include:
- Plendil Extended-Release Tablets 514

Fenoprofen Calcium (Blunting of the antihypertensive effect). Products include:
- Nalfon 200 Pulvules & Nalfon Tablets 933

(▣ Described in PDR For Nonprescription Drugs)   (⊙ Described in PDR For Ophthalmology)

123 **Interactions Index** **Bonine Tablets**

Flurbiprofen (Blunting of the antihypertensive effect).
No products indexed under this heading.

Glimepiride (Beta blockers may mask the signs and symptoms of acute hypoglycemia). Products include:
Amaryl Tablets 1241

Glipizide (Beta blockers may mask the signs and symptoms of acute hypoglycemia). Products include:
Glucotrol Tablets 2011
Glucotrol XL Extended Release Tablets 2012

Glyburide (Beta blockers may mask the signs and symptoms of acute hypoglycemia). Products include:
DiaBeta Tablets 1265
Glynase PresTab Tablets 2091
Micronase Tablets 2099

Guanethidine Monosulfate (Additive effects; hypotension and/or bradycardia). Products include:
Esimil Tablets 840
Ismelin Tablets 845

Ibuprofen (Blunting of the antihypertensive effect). Products include:
Advil Cold and Sinus Caplets and Tablets 837
Advil Ibuprofen Tablets, Caplets and Gel Caplets 836
Children's Motrin Ibuprofen Oral Suspension 1558
IBU Tablets 1389
Ibuprohm 713
Motrin IB Caplets, Tablets, and Gelcaps 802
Motrin Ibuprofen Suspension, Oral Drops, Chewable Tablets, Caplets 1563
Nuprin Ibuprofen/Analgesic Tablets & Caplets 645
Vicks DayQuil SINUS Pressure & PAIN Relief with IBUPROFEN 735

Indomethacin (Blunting of the antihypertensive effect). Products include:
Indocin 1723

Indomethacin Sodium Trihydrate (Blunting of the antihypertensive effect). Products include:
Indocin I.V. 1727

Insulin, Human Isophane Suspension (Beta blockers may mask the signs and symptoms of acute hypoglycemia). Products include:
Novolin N Human Insulin 10 ml Vials 1846

Insulin, Human NPH (Beta blockers may mask the signs and symptoms of acute hypoglycemia). Products include:
Humulin N, 100 Units 1495
Novolin N PenFill 1.5 ml Cartridges Durable Insulin Delivery System 1849
Novolin N Prefilled Syringe Disposable Insulin Delivery System 1850

Insulin, Human Regular (Beta blockers may mask the signs and symptoms of acute hypoglycemia). Products include:
Humulin R, 100 Units 1497
Novolin R Human Insulin 10 ml Vials 1846
Novolin R PenFill 1.5 ml Cartridges Durable Insulin Delivery System 1849
Novolin R Prefilled Syringe Disposable Insulin Delivery System 1850
Velosulin BR Human Insulin 10 ml Vials 1847

Insulin, Human, Zinc Suspension (Beta blockers may mask the signs and symptoms of acute hypoglycemia). Products include:
Humulin L, 100 Units 1494
Humulin U, 100 Units 1498
Novolin L Human Insulin 10 ml Vials 1846

Insulin Lispro, Human (Beta blockers may mask the signs and symptoms of acute hypoglycemia). Products include:
Humalog Injection 1488

Insulin, NPH (Beta blockers may mask the signs and symptoms of acute hypoglycemia). Products include:
NPH, 100 Units 1502
Pork NPH, 100 Units 1506
Purified Pork NPH Isophane Insulin 1852

Insulin, Regular (Beta blockers may mask the signs and symptoms of acute hypoglycemia). Products include:
Regular, 100 Units 1503
Pork Regular, 100 Units 1507
Pork Regular (Concentrated), 500 Units 1508
Purified Pork Regular Insulin 1852

Insulin, Zinc Crystals (Beta blockers may mask the signs and symptoms of acute hypoglycemia). Products include:
NPH, 100 Units 1502

Insulin, Zinc Suspension (Beta blockers may mask the signs and symptoms of acute hypoglycemia). Products include:
Iletin I 1501
Lente, 100 Units 1501
Iletin II 1504
Pork Lente, 100 Units 1504
Purified Pork Lente Insulin 1852

Isradipine (AV conduction disturbances; left ventricular failure). Products include:
DynaCirc Capsules 2381
DynaCirc CR Tablets 2383

Ketoprofen (Blunting of the antihypertensive effect). Products include:
Actron Caplets and Tablets 608
Orudis Capsules 2874
Orudis KT 842
Oruvail Capsules 2874

Ketorolac Tromethamine (Blunting of the antihypertensive effect). Products include:
Acular Sterile Ophthalmic Solution 470
Toradol 2319

Meclofenamate Sodium (Blunting of the antihypertensive effect).
No products indexed under this heading.

Mefenamic Acid (Blunting of the antihypertensive effect). Products include:
Ponstel 1982

Metformin Hydrochloride (Beta blockers may mask the signs and symptoms of acute hypoglycemia). Products include:
Glucophage Tablets 754

Nabumetone (Blunting of the antihypertensive effect). Products include:
Relafen Tablets 2688

Naproxen (Blunting of the antihypertensive effect). Products include:
Anaprox/Naprosyn 2277

Naproxen Sodium (Blunting of the antihypertensive effect). Products include:
Aleve 2124
Anaprox/Naprosyn 2277
Naprelan Tablets 2861

Nicardipine Hydrochloride (AV conduction disturbances; left ventricular failure). Products include:
Cardene Capsules 2261
Cardene I.V. 2815
Cardene SR Capsules 2264

Nifedipine (Hypotension). Products include:
Adalat Capsules (10 mg and 20 mg) 580
Adalat CC 582
Procardia Capsules 2024
Procardia XL Extended Release Tablets 2026

Nimodipine (AV conduction disturbances; left ventricular failure). Products include:
Nimotop Capsules 603

Nisoldipine (AV conduction disturbances; left ventricular failure). Products include:
Sular Tablets 2961

Oxaprozin (Blunting of the antihypertensive effect). Products include:
Daypro Caplets 2578

Phenylbutazone (Blunting of the antihypertensive effect).
No products indexed under this heading.

Piroxicam (Blunting of the antihypertensive effect). Products include:
Feldene Capsules 2008

Reserpine (Additive effects; hypotension and/or bradycardia). Products include:
Diupres Tablets 1691
Hydropres Tablets 1718
Ser-Ap-Es Tablets 867

Sulindac (Blunting of the antihypertensive effect). Products include:
Clinoril Tablets 1658

Tolazamide (Beta blockers may mask the signs and symptoms of acute hypoglycemia).
No products indexed under this heading.

Tolbutamide (Beta blockers may mask the signs and symptoms of acute hypoglycemia).
No products indexed under this heading.

Tolmetin Sodium (Blunting of the antihypertensive effect). Products include:
Tolectin (200, 400 and 600 mg) .. 1591

Verapamil Hydrochloride (AV conduction disturbances; left ventricular failure). Products include:
Calan SR Caplets 2571
Calan Tablets 2568
Covera-HS Tablets 2573
Isoptin Injectable 1391
Isoptin Oral Tablets 1393
Isoptin SR Tablets 1395
Verelan Capsules 1455

BONINE TABLETS
(Meclizine Hydrochloride) 1990
May interact with hypnotics and sedatives, tranquilizers, and certain other agents. Compounds in these categories include:

Alprazolam (May increase drowsiness effect). Products include:
Xanax Tablets 2115

Buspirone Hydrochloride (May increase drowsiness effect). Products include:
BuSpar Tablets 738

Chlordiazepoxide (May increase drowsiness effect). Products include:
Limbitrol 2333

Chlordiazepoxide Hydrochloride (May increase drowsiness effect). Products include:
Librax Capsules 2330
Librium Capsules 2331
Librium Injectable 2332

Chlorpromazine (May increase drowsiness effect). Products include:
Thorazine Suppositories 2701

Chlorprothixene (May increase drowsiness effect).
No products indexed under this heading.

Chlorprothixene Hydrochloride (May increase drowsiness effect).
No products indexed under this heading.

Clorazepate Dipotassium (May increase drowsiness effect). Products include:
Tranxene 459

Diazepam (May increase drowsiness effect). Products include:
Dizac (diazepam injectable emulsion) CIV 1862
Valium Injectable 2336
Valium Tablets 2335

Droperidol (May increase drowsiness effect). Products include:
Inapsine Injection 462

Estazolam (May increase drowsiness effect). Products include:
ProSom Tablets 457

Ethchlorvynol (May increase drowsiness effect). Products include:
Placidyl Capsules 456

Ethinamate (May increase drowsiness effect).
No products indexed under this heading.

Fluphenazine Decanoate (May increase drowsiness effect). Products include:
Prolixin Decanoate 510

Fluphenazine Enanthate (May increase drowsiness effect). Products include:
Prolixin Enanthate 510

Fluphenazine Hydrochloride (May increase drowsiness effect). Products include:
Prolixin 510

Flurazepam Hydrochloride (May increase drowsiness effect). Products include:
Dalmane Capsules 2329

Glutethimide (May increase drowsiness effect).
No products indexed under this heading.

Haloperidol (May increase drowsiness effect). Products include:
Haldol Injection, Tablets and Concentrate 1585

Haloperidol Decanoate (May increase drowsiness effect). Products include:
Haldol Decanoate 1587

Hydroxyzine Hydrochloride (May increase drowsiness effect). Products include:
Atarax Tablets & Syrup 1992
Marax Tablets & DF Syrup 2015
Vistaril Intramuscular Solution 2042

Lorazepam (May increase drowsiness effect). Products include:
Ativan Injection 2805
Ativan Tablets 2807

Loxapine Hydrochloride (May increase drowsiness effect). Products include:
Loxitane 1426

Loxapine Succinate (May increase drowsiness effect). Products include:
Loxitane Capsules 1426

Meprobamate (May increase drowsiness effect). Products include:
Miltown Tablets 2780
PMB 200 and PMB 400 2890

Mesoridazine Besylate (May increas drowsiness effect). Products include:
Serentil 689

Midazolam Hydrochloride (May increase drowsiness effect). Products include:
Versed Injection 2324

Molindone Hydrochloride (May increase drowsiness effect). Products include:
Moban Tablets and Concentrate 1036

IMPORTANT NOTE: Always consult each drug listing in the patient's regimen for possible interactions.

Bonine Tablets / Interactions Index

Oxazepam (May increase drowsiness effect). Products include:
- Serax Capsules 2916
- Serax Tablets 2916

Perphenazine (May increase drowsiness effect). Products include:
- Etrafon 2495
- Triavil Tablets 1800
- Trilafon 2532

Prazepam (May increase drowsiness effect).
- No products indexed under this heading.

Prochlorperazine (May increase drowsiness effect). Products include:
- Compazine 2644

Promethazine Hydrochloride (May increase drowsiness effect). Products include:
- Mepergan Injection 2859
- Phenergan with Codeine ... 2883
- Phenergan with Dextromethorphan ... 2885
- Phenergan Injection 2880
- Phenergan Suppositories ... 2882
- Phenergan Syrup 2881
- Phenergan Tablets 2882
- Phenergan VC 2886
- Phenergan VC with Codeine ... 2888

Propofol (May increase drowsiness effect). Products include:
- Diprivan Injectable Emulsion ... 2939

Quazepam (May increase drowsiness effect). Products include:
- Doral Tablets 2773

Secobarbital Sodium (May increase drowsiness effect). Products include:
- Seconal Sodium Pulvules ... 1529

Temazepam (May increase drowsiness effect). Products include:
- Restoril Capsules 2413

Thioridazine Hydrochloride (May increase drowsiness effect). Products include:
- Mellaril 2398

Thiothixene (May increase drowsiness effect). Products include:
- Navane Capsules and Concentrate ... 2018
- Navane Intramuscular 2019

Triazolam (May increase drowsiness effect). Products include:
- Halcion Tablets 2093

Trifluoperazine Hydrochloride (May increase drowsiness effect). Products include:
- Stelazine 2692

Zolpidem Tartrate (May increase drowsiness effect). Products include:
- Ambien Tablets 2559

Food Interactions

Alcohol (May increase drowsiness effect).

BONTRIL SLOW-RELEASE CAPSULES
(Phendimetrazine Tartrate) 786
May interact with monoamine oxidase inhibitors, insulin, and certain other agents. Compounds in these categories include:

Furazolidone (Potential for hypertensive crisis). Products include:
- Furoxone 2221

Guanethidine Monosulfate (Hypotensive effect of guanethidine may be decreased). Products include:
- Esimil Tablets 840
- Ismelin Tablets 845

Insulin, Human (Insulin requirement may be altered).
- No products indexed under this heading.

Insulin, Human Isophane Suspension (Insulin requirement may be altered). Products include:
- Novolin N Human Insulin 10 ml Vials 1846

Insulin, Human NPH (Insulin requirement may be altered). Products include:
- Humulin N, 100 Units 1495
- Novolin N PenFill 1.5 ml Cartridges Durable Insulin Delivery System 1849
- Novolin N Prefilled Syringe Disposable Insulin Delivery System ... 1850

Insulin, Human Regular (Insulin requirement may be altered). Products include:
- Humulin R, 100 Units 1497
- Novolin R Human Insulin 10 ml Vials 1846
- Novolin R PenFill 1.5 ml Cartridges Durable Insulin Delivery System 1849
- Novolin R Prefilled Syringe Disposable Insulin Delivery System ... 1850
- Velosulin BR Human Insulin 10 ml Vials 1847

Insulin, Human, Zinc Suspension (Insulin requirement may be altered). Products include:
- Humulin L, 100 Units 1494
- Humulin U, 100 Units 1498
- Novolin L Human Insulin 10 ml Vials 1846

Insulin Lispro, Human (Insulin requirement may be altered). Products include:
- Humalog Injection 1488

Insulin, NPH (Insulin requirement may be altered). Products include:
- NPH, 100 Units 1502
- Pork NPH, 100 Units 1506
- Purified Pork NPH Isophane Insulin 1852

Insulin, Regular (Insulin requirement may be altered). Products include:
- Regular, 100 Units 1503
- Pork Regular, 100 Units ... 1507
- Pork Regular (Concentrated), 500 Units 1508
- Purified Pork Regular Insulin ... 1852

Insulin, Zinc Crystals (Insulin requirement may be altered). Products include:
- NPH, 100 Units 1502

Insulin, Zinc Suspension (Insulin requirement may be altered). Products include:
- Iletin I 1501
- Lente, 100 Units 1501
- Iletin II 1504
- Pork Lente, 100 Units 1504
- Purified Pork Lente Insulin ... 1852

Isocarboxazid (Potential for hypertensive crisis).
- No products indexed under this heading.

Phenelzine Sulfate (Potential for hypertensive crisis). Products include:
- Nardil 1977

Selegiline Hydrochloride (Potential for hypertensive crisis). Products include:
- Eldepryl Capsules 2729

Tranylcypromine Sulfate (Potential for hypertensive crisis). Products include:
- Parnate Tablets 2679

BOROFAX SKIN PROTECTANT OINTMENT
(Zinc Oxide, Petrolatum, White) ...... ▣ 817
None cited in PDR database.

BOTOX (BOTULINUM TOXIN TYPE A) PURIFIED NEUROTOXIN COMPLEX
(Botulinum Toxin Type A) 473
None cited in PDR database.

BREATH + PLUS
(Vitamin A, Vitamin E) .... ▣ 603
None cited in PDR database.

BRETHAIRE INHALER
(Terbutaline Sulfate) 830
May interact with monoamine oxidase inhibitors, tricyclic antidepressants, beta blockers, sympathomimetic aerosol bronchodilators, and certain other agents. Compounds in these categories include:

Acebutolol Hydrochloride (Beta receptor blocking agents and terbutaline sulfate inhibit each other). Products include:
- Sectral Capsules 2914

Albuterol (Concomitant therapy with other sympathomimetic aerosol bronchodilators should be avoided). Products include:
- Proventil Inhalation Aerosol ... 2524
- Ventolin Inhalation Aerosol and Refill 1170

Amitriptyline Hydrochloride (May potentiate action of terbutaline sulfate on vascular system). Products include:
- Elavil 2945
- Etrafon 2495
- Limbitrol 2333
- Triavil Tablets 1800

Amoxapine (May potentiate action of terbutaline sulfate on vascular system). Products include:
- Asendin Tablets 1419

Atenolol (Beta receptor blocking agents and terbutaline sulfate inhibit each other). Products include:
- Tenoretic Tablets 2963
- Tenormin Tablets and I.V. Injection ... 2965

Betaxolol Hydrochloride (Beta receptor blocking agents and terbutaline sulfate inhibit each other). Products include:
- Betoptic Ophthalmic Solution ... 465
- Betoptic S Ophthalmic Suspension ... 467
- Kerlone Tablets 2588

Bisoprolol Fumarate (Beta receptor blocking agents and terbutaline sulfate inhibit each other). Products include:
- Zebeta Tablets 1457
- Ziac 1459

Bitolterol Mesylate (Concomitant therapy with other sympathomimetic aerosol bronchodilators should be avoided). Products include:
- Tornalate Solution for Inhalation, 0.2% 976
- Tornalate Metered Dose Inhaler ... 978

Carteolol Hydrochloride (Beta receptor blocking agents and terbutaline sulfate inhibit each other). Products include:
- Cartrol Tablets 413
- Ocupress Ophthalmic Solution, 1% Sterile .... ◉ 297

Clomipramine Hydrochloride (May potentiate action of terbutaline sulfate on vascular system). Products include:
- Anafranil Capsules 819

Desipramine Hydrochloride (May potentiate action of terbutaline sulfate on vascular system). Products include:
- Norpramin Tablets 1273

Doxepin Hydrochloride (May potentiate action of terbutaline sulfate on vascular system). Products include:
- Adapin Capsules 1542
- Sinequan 2028
- Zonalon Cream 1042

Epinephrine (Concomitant administration is not advised). Products include:
- EPIFRIN .... ◉ 237
- EpiPen 808
- Marcaine with Epinephrine ... 2446
- Primatene Mist .... ▣ 843
- Sensorcaine with Epinephrine Injection 554

- Sus-Phrine Injection 1017
- Xylocaine with Epinephrine Injections 562

Epinephrine Bitartrate (Concomitant administration is not advised). Products include:
- Sensorcaine-MPF with Epinephrine Injection 554

Epinephrine Hydrochloride (Concomitant administration is not advised). Products include:
- Ana-Kit Anaphylaxis Emergency Treatment Kit 611

Esmolol Hydrochloride (Beta receptors blocking agents and terbutaline sulfate inhibit each other). Products include:
- Brevibloc (esmolol HCl) Injection ... 1860

Furazolidone (May potentiate action of terbutaline sulfate on vascular system). Products include:
- Furoxone 2221

Imipramine Hydrochloride (May potentiate action of terbutaline sulfate on vascular system). Products include:
- Tofranil Ampuls 873
- Tofranil Tablets 875

Imipramine Pamoate (May potentiate action of terbutaline sulfate on vascular system). Products include:
- Tofranil-PM Capsules 876

Isocarboxazid (May potentiate action of terbutaline sulfate on vascular system).
- No products indexed under this heading.

Isoetharine (Concomitant therapy with other sympathomimetic aerosol bronchodilators should be avoided). Products include:
- Bronkometer Aerosol 2432
- Bronkosol Solution 2432
- Isoetharine Inhalation Solution, USP, Arm-a-Med 545

Isoproterenol Hydrochloride (Concomitant therapy with other sympathomimetic aerosol bronchodilators should be avoided). Products include:
- Isuprel Hydrochloride Solution ... 2443
- Isuprel Injection 2441
- Isuprel Mistometer 2442

Isoproterenol Sulfate (Concomitant administration is not advised). Products include:
- Norisodrine with Calcium Iodide Syrup 446

Labetalol Hydrochloride (Beta receptor blocking agents and terbutaline sulfate inhibit each other). Products include:
- Normodyne Injection 2519
- Normodyne Tablets 2522
- Trandate 1158

Levobunolol Hydrochloride (Beta receptor blocking agents and terbutaline sulfate inhibit each other). Products include:
- Betagan .... ◉ 230

Maprotiline Hydrochloride (May potentiate action of terbutaline sulfate on vascular system). Products include:
- Ludiomil Tablets 861

Metaproterenol Sulfate (Concomitant therapy with other sympathomimetic aerosol bronchodilators should be avoided). Products include:
- Alupent 672
- Metaproterenol Sulfate Inhalation Solution, USP, Arm-a-Med ... 547

Metipranolol Hydrochloride (Beta receptor blocking agents and terbutaline sulfate inhibit each other). Products include:
- OptiPranolol (Metipranolol 0.3%) Sterile Ophthalmic Solution ... ◉ 256

(▣ Described in PDR For Nonprescription Drugs)   (◉ Described in PDR For Ophthalmology)

Metoprolol Succinate (Beta receptor blocking agents and terbutaline sulfate inhibit each other). Products include:
- Toprol-XL Tablets 560

Metoprolol Tartrate (Beta receptor blocking agents and terbutaline sulfate inhibit each other). Products include:
- Lopressor 848
- Lopressor HCT Tablets 850

Nadolol (Beta receptor blocking agents and terbutaline sulfate inhibit each other).
- No products indexed under this heading.

Nortriptyline Hydrochloride (May potentiate action of terbutaline sulfate on vascular system). Products include:
- Pamelor 2409

Penbutolol Sulfate (Beta receptor blocking agents and terbutaline sulfate inhibit each other). Products include:
- Levatol Tablets 2547

Phenelzine Sulfate (May potentiate action of terbutaline sulfate on vascular system). Products include:
- Nardil 1977

Pindolol (Beta receptor blocking agents and terbutaline sulfate inhibit each other). Products include:
- Visken Tablets 2428

Pirbuterol Acetate (Concomitant therapy with other sympathomimetic aerosol bronchodilators should be avoided). Products include:
- Maxair Autohaler 1550
- Maxair Inhaler 1552

Propranolol Hydrochloride (Beta receptor blocking agents and terbutaline sulfate inhibit each other). Products include:
- Inderal 2834
- Inderal LA Long Acting Capsules 2836
- Inderide Tablets 2838
- Inderide LA Long Acting Capsules .. 2840

Protriptyline Hydrochloride (May potentiate action of terbutaline sulfate on vascular system). Products include:
- Vivactil Tablets 1820

Salmeterol Xinafoate (Concomitant therapy with other sympathomimetic aerosol bronchodilators should be avoided). Products include:
- Serevent Inhalation Aerosol 1149

Selegiline Hydrochloride (May potentiate action of terbutaline sulfate on vascular system). Products include:
- Eldepryl Capsules 2729

Sotalol Hydrochloride (Beta receptor blocking agents and terbutaline sulfate inhibit each other). Products include:
- Betapace Tablets 637

Timolol Hemihydrate (Beta receptor blocking agents and terbutaline sulfate inhibit each other). Products include:
- Betimol 0.25%, 0.5% .... ◉ 259

Timolol Maleate (Beta receptor blocking agents and terbutaline sulfate inhibit each other). Products include:
- Blocadren Tablets 1654
- Timolide Tablets 1791
- Timoptic in Ocudose 1796
- Timoptic Sterile Ophthalmic Solution 1794
- Timoptic-XE 1798

Tranylcypromine Sulfate (May potentiate action of terbutaline sulfate on vascular system). Products include:
- Parnate Tablets 2679

Trimipramine Maleate (May potentiate action of terbutaline sulfate on vascular system). Products include:
- Surmontil Capsules 2917

BRETHINE AMPULS

(Terbutaline Sulfate) 832

May interact with sympathomimetics, monoamine oxidase inhibitors, and tricyclic antidepressants. Compounds in these categories include:

Albuterol (Combined effect on cardiovascular system may be deleterious). Products include:
- Proventil Inhalation Aerosol 2524
- Ventolin Inhalation Aerosol and Refill 1170

Albuterol Sulfate (Combined effect on cardiovascular system may be deleterious). Products include:
- Airet Albuterol Sulfate Inhalation Solution 1602
- Albuterol Sulfate, USP Solution for Inhalation, Arm-a-Med 522
- Proventil Inhalation Solution 0.083% 2527
- Proventil Repetabs Tablets 2529
- Proventil Solution for Inhalation 0.5% 2525
- Proventil Syrup 2528
- Proventil Tablets 2529
- Ventolin Inhalation Solution 1171
- Ventolin Nebules Inhalation Solution 1172
- Ventolin Rotacaps for Inhalation 1173
- Ventolin Syrup 1175
- Ventolin Tablets 1176
- Volmax Extended-Release Tablets .. 1835

Amitriptyline Hydrochloride (The action of beta-adrenergic agonists on the vascular system may be potentiated). Products include:
- Elavil 2945
- Etrafon 2495
- Limbitrol 2333
- Triavil Tablets 1800

Amoxapine (The action of beta-adrenergic agonists on the vascular system may be potentiated). Products include:
- Asendin Tablets 1419

Clomipramine Hydrochloride (The action of beta-adrenergic agonists on the vascular system may be potentiated). Products include:
- Anafranil Capsules 819

Desipramine Hydrochloride (The action of beta-adrenergic agonists on the vascular system may be potentiated). Products include:
- Norpramin Tablets 1273

Dobutamine Hydrochloride (Combined effect on cardiovascular system may be deleterious). Products include:
- Dobutrex Solution Vials 1480

Dopamine Hydrochloride (Combined effect on cardiovascular system may be deleterious).
- No products indexed under this heading.

Doxepin Hydrochloride (The action of beta-adrenergic agonists on the vascular system may be potentiated). Products include:
- Adapin Capsules 1542
- Sinequan 2028
- Zonalon Cream 1042

Ephedrine Hydrochloride (Combined effect on cardiovascular system may be deleterious). Products include:
- Primatene Tablets .... ▣ 844
- Quadrinal Tablets 1398

Ephedrine Sulfate (Combined effect on cardiovascular system may be deleterious). Products include:
- Marax Tablets & DF Syrup 2015

Ephedrine Tannate (Combined effect on cardiovascular system may be deleterious). Products include:
- Rynatuss 2782

Epinephrine (Combined effect on cardiovascular system may be deleterious). Products include:
- EPIFRIN .... ◉ 237
- EpiPen 808
- Marcaine with Epinephrine 2446
- Primatene Mist .... ▣ 843
- Sensorcaine with Epinephrine Injection 554
- Sus-Phrine Injection 1017
- Xylocaine with Epinephrine Injections 562

Epinephrine Bitartrate (Combined effect on cardiovascular system may be deleterious). Products include:
- Sensorcaine-MPF with Epinephrine Injection 554

Epinephrine Hydrochloride (Combined effect on cardiovascular system may be deleterious). Products include:
- Ana-Kit Anaphylaxis Emergency Treatment Kit 611

Furazolidone (The action of beta-adrenergic agonists on the vascular system may be potentiated). Products include:
- Furoxone 2221

Imipramine Hydrochloride (The action of beta-adrenergic agonists on the vascular system may be potentiated). Products include:
- Tofranil Ampuls 873
- Tofranil Tablets 875

Imipramine Pamoate (The action of beta-adrenergic agonists on the vascular system may be potentiated). Products include:
- Tofranil-PM Capsules 876

Isocarboxazid (The action of beta-adrenergic agonists on the vascular system may be potentiated).
- No products indexed under this heading.

Isoproterenol Hydrochloride (Combined effect on cardiovascular system may be deleterious). Products include:
- Isuprel Hydrochloride Solution 2443
- Isuprel Injection 2441
- Isuprel Mistometer 2442

Isoproterenol Sulfate (Combined effect on cardiovascular system may be deleterious). Products include:
- Norisodrine with Calcium Iodide Syrup 446

Maprotiline Hydrochloride (The action of beta-adrenergic agonists on the vascular system may be potentiated). Products include:
- Ludiomil Tablets 861

Metaproterenol Sulfate (Combined effect on cardiovascular system may be deleterious). Products include:
- Alupent 672
- Metaproterenol Sulfate Inhalation Solution, USP, Arm-a-Med 547

Metaraminol Bitartrate (Combined effect on cardiovascular system may be deleterious). Products include:
- Aramine Injection 1649

Norepinephrine Bitartrate (Combined effect on cardiovascular system may be deleterious). Products include:
- Levophed Bitartrate Injection 2445

Nortriptyline Hydrochloride (The action of beta-adrenergic agonists on the vascular system may be potentiated). Products include:
- Pamelor 2409

Phenelzine Sulfate (The action of beta-adrenergic agonists on the vascular system may be potentiated). Products include:
- Nardil 1977

Phenylephrine Bitartrate (Combined effect on cardiovascular system may be deleterious).
- No products indexed under this heading.

Phenylephrine Hydrochloride (Combined effect on cardiovascular system may be deleterious). Products include:
- Atrohist Plus Tablets 1605
- Cerose DM .... ▣ 853
- D.A. II Tablets 972
- D.A. Chewable Tablets 970
- Dura-Vent/DA Tablets 972
- Extendryl 1003
- 4-Way Fast Acting Nasal Spray (regular & mentholated) .... ▣ 644
- Hemorid .... ▣ 797
- Hycomine Compound Tablets 948
- Neo-Synephrine Hydrochloride 1% Carpuject 2455
- Neo-Synephrine Hydrochloride 1% Injection 2455
- Neo-Synephrine Hydrochloride (Ophthalmic) 2456
- Neo-Synephrine .... ▣ 624
- Novahistine Elixir .... ▣ 782
- Phenergan VC 2886
- Phenergan VC with Codeine 2888
- Preparation H .... ▣ 842
- Tympagesic Ear Drops 2476
- Vicks Sinex Nasal Spray and Ultra Fine Mist .... ▣ 738

Phenylephrine Tannate (Combined effect on cardiovascular system may be deleterious). Products include:
- Atrohist Pediatric Suspension 1604
- Atrohist Pediatric Suspension Dye-Free 1604
- Rynatan 2781
- Rynatuss 2782

Phenylpropanolamine Hydrochloride (Combined effect on cardiovascular system may be deleterious). Products include:
- Acutrim .... ▣ 648
- Atrohist Plus Tablets 1605
- BC Cold Powder Multi-Symptom Formula (Cold-Sinus-Allergy) .... ▣ 631
- BC Cold Powder Non-Drowsy Formula (Cold-Sinus) .... ▣ 631
- Cheracol Plus Head Cold/Cough Formula .... ▣ 741
- Comtrex Multi-Symptom Cold Reliever Liqui-Gels .... ▣ 638
- Comtrex Multi-Symptom Non-Drowsy Liqui-gels .... ▣ 640
- Contac Continuous Action Nasal Decongestant/Antihistamine 12 Hour Capsules .... ▣ 773
- Contac Maximum Strength Continuous Action Decongestant/Antihistamine 12 Hour Caplets .... ▣ 772
- Contac Severe Cold and Flu Formula Caplets .... ▣ 773
- Coricidin 'D' Decongestant Tablets .... ▣ 760
- Dexatrim .... ▣ 795
- Dexatrim Plus Vitamins Caplets .... ▣ 796
- Dimetane-DC Cough Syrup 2232
- Dimetapp Allergy Sinus Caplets .... ▣ 838
- Dimetapp Cold & Allergy Chewable Tablets .... ▣ 838
- Dimetapp Cold & Cough Liqui-Gels .... ▣ 839
- Dimetapp DM Elixir .... ▣ 840
- Dimetapp Elixir .... ▣ 840
- Dimetapp Extentabs .... ▣ 841
- Dimetapp Tablets/Liqui-Gels .... ▣ 841
- Dura-Vent Tablets 971
- Entex LA Tablets 972
- Exgest LA Tablets 787
- Hycomine 947
- Nolamine Timed-Release Tablets 790
- Ornade Spansule Capsules 2678
- Propagest Tablets 791
- Pyrroxate Caplets .... ▣ 742
- Robitussin-CF .... ▣ 846
- Sinulin Tablets 792
- Tavist-D 12 Hour Relief Tablets .... ▣ 750

IMPORTANT NOTE: Always consult each drug listing in the patient's regimen for possible interactions.

Brethine — Interactions Index

Teldrin 12 Hour Antihistamine/Nasal Decongestant Allergy Relief Capsules	⊡ 786
Triaminic Expectorant	⊡ 753
Triaminic Syrup	⊡ 755
Triaminic Triaminicol Cold & Cough	⊡ 756
Triaminic DM Syrup	⊡ 756
Triaminicin Tablets	⊡ 756
Vicks DayQuil Allergy Relief 12-Hour Extended Release Tablets	⊡ 733
Vicks DayQuil Allergy Relief 4-Hour Tablets	⊡ 733
Vicks DayQuil SINUS Pressure & CONGESTION Relief	⊡ 734

Pirbuterol Acetate (Combined effect on cardiovascular system may be deleterious). Products include:

Maxair Autohaler	1550
Maxair Inhaler	1552

Protriptyline Hydrochloride (The action of beta-adrenergic agonists on the vascular system may be potentiated). Products include:

Vivactil Tablets	1820

Pseudoephedrine Hydrochloride (Combined effect on cardiovascular system may be deleterious). Products include:

Actifed Allergy Daytime/Nighttime Caplets	⊡ 808
Actifed Cold & Allergy Tablets	⊡ 807
Actifed Cold & Sinus Caplets and Tablets	⊡ 808
Actifed Sinus Daytime/Nighttime Tablets and Caplets	⊡ 809
Advil Cold and Sinus Caplets and Tablets	⊡ 837
Alka-Seltzer Plus Liqui-Gels	⊡ 612
Alka-Seltzer Plus Flu & Body Aches Liqui-Gels Non-Drowsy Formula	⊡ 613
Alka-Seltzer Plus Night-Time Cold Medicine Liqui-Gels	⊡ 612
Allerest Maximum Strength	⊡ 649
Allerest No Drowsiness	⊡ 649
Allerest Sinus Pain Formula	⊡ 649
Atrohist Pediatric Capsules	1603
Benadryl Allergy/Cold Tablets	⊡ 811
Benadryl Allergy Decongestant Liquid Medication	⊡ 812
Benadryl Allergy Decongestant Tablets	⊡ 812
Benadryl Allergy Sinus Headache Caplets	⊡ 813
Benylin Multisymptom	⊡ 816
Bromfed Capsules (Extended-Release)	1832
Bromfed Syrup	⊡ 712
Bromfed Tablets	1832
Bromfed-DM Cough Syrup	1832
Bromfed-PD Capsules (Extended-Release)	1832
Children's TYLENOL Cold Multi-Symptom Chewable Tablets and Liquid	1559
Children's TYLENOL Cold Plus Cough Multi Symptom Chewable Tablets and Liquid	1560
Children's TYLENOL Flu Suspension Liquid	1560
Children's Vicks DayQuil Allergy Relief	⊡ 730
Children's Vicks NyQuil Cold/Cough Relief	⊡ 731
Allergy-Sinus Comtrex Multi-Symptom Allergy-Sinus Formula Tablets and Caplets	⊡ 639
Comtrex Multi-Symptom	⊡ 638
Comtrex Multi-Symptom Non-Drowsy Caplets	⊡ 640
Congess	1003
Contac Day Allergy/Sinus Caplets	⊡ 771
Contac Day & Night	⊡ 772
Contac Night Allergy/Sinus Caplets	⊡ 771
Contac Severe Cold & Flu Non-Drowsy	⊡ 774
Deconsal II Tablets	1605
Dimetane-DX Cough Syrup	2233
Dimetapp Cold & Fever Suspension	⊡ 839
Dimetapp Decongestant Pediatric Drops	⊡ 840
Dorcol Children's Cough Syrup	⊡ 748
Drixoral Cough + Congestion Liquid Caps	763
Dura-Tap/PD Capsules	970
Duratuss Tablets	2750
Duratuss HD Elixir	2750
Efidac/24	⊡ 655
Entex PSE Tablets	973
Fedahist Gyrocaps	2545
Guaifed	1833
Guaifed Syrup	⊡ 712
Guaimax-D Tablets	809
Histussin D Liquid	670
Infants' TYLENOL Cold Decongestant & Fever-Reducer Drops	1561
Kronofed-A	994
Novahistine DMX	⊡ 782
Nucofed	2225
PediaCare Cough-Cold Chewable Tablets and Liquid	1569
PediaCare Infants' Decongestant Drops	1569
PediaCare Infants' Drops Decongestant Plus Cough	1569
PediaCare NightRest Cough-Cold Liquid	1569
Pediatric Vicks 44d Cough & Head Congestion Relief	⊡ 736
Pediatric Vicks 44m Cough & Cold Relief	⊡ 737
Robitussin Cold & Cough Liqui-Gels	⊡ 844
Robitussin Cold, Cough & Flu Liqui-Gels	⊡ 844
Robitussin Maximum Strength Cough & Cold	⊡ 847
Robitussin Night-Time Cold Formula	⊡ 847
Robitussin Pediatric Cough & Cold Formula	⊡ 848
Robitussin Pediatric Drops	⊡ 849
Robitussin Severe Congestion Liqui-Gels	⊡ 845
Robitussin-DAC Syrup	2249
Robitussin-PE	⊡ 846
Rondec Oral Drops	974
Rondec Syrup	974
Rondec Tablet	974
Rondec Chewable Tablets	974
Rondec-TR Tablet	974
Ryna	⊡ 804
Seldane-D Extended-Release Tablets	1286
Semprex-D Capsules	1620
Sinarest	⊡ 663
Sine-Aid Maximum Strength Sinus Headache Gelcaps, Caplets and Tablets	1570
Sine-Off No Drowsiness Formula Caplets	⊡ 784
Sine-Off Sinus Medicine	⊡ 784
Singlet Tablets	⊡ 785
Sinutab Non-Drying Liquid Caps	⊡ 823
Sinutab Sinus Allergy Medication, Maximum Strength Tablets and Caplets	⊡ 823
Sinutab Sinus Medication, Maximum Strength Without Drowsiness Formula, Tablets & Caplets	⊡ 824
Sudafed Children's Cold & Cough Liquid Medication	⊡ 825
Sudafed Children's Nasal Decongestant Liquid Medication	⊡ 826
Sudafed Cold & Allergy Tablets	⊡ 826
Sudafed Cold and Cough Liquid Caps	⊡ 826
Sudafed Nasal Decongestant Tablets, 30 mg	⊡ 825
Sudafed Nasal Decongestant Tablets, 60 mg	⊡ 825
Sudafed Non-Drying Sinus Liquid Caps	⊡ 827
Sudafed Pediatric Nasal Decongestant Liquid Oral Drops	⊡ 827
Sudafed Severe Cold Formula Caplets	⊡ 828
Sudafed Severe Cold Formula Tablets	⊡ 828
Sudafed Sinus Caplets	⊡ 829
Sudafed Sinus Tablets	⊡ 829
Sudafed 12 Hour Caplets	⊡ 824
Syn-Rx Tablets	1622
Syn-Rx DM Tablets	1623
TheraFlu Flu and Cold Medicine	⊡ 750
Theraflu Maximum Strength Flu and Cold Medicine For Sore Throat	⊡ 751
TheraFlu Flu, Cold and Cough Medicine	⊡ 750
TheraFlu Maximum Strength Nighttime Flu, Cold & Cough Medicine	⊡ 751
TheraFlu Maximum Strength Non-Drowsy Formula Flu, Cold & Cough Medicine	⊡ 751
TheraFlu Maximum Strength, Non-Drowsy Formula Flu, Cold and Cough Caplets	⊡ 752
Theraflu Maximum Strength Sinus Non-Drowsy Formula Caplets	⊡ 752
Triaminic AM Cough and Decongestant Formula	⊡ 753
Triaminic AM Decongestant Formula	⊡ 753
Triaminic Infant Oral Decongestant Drops	⊡ 754
Triaminic Night Time	⊡ 754
Triaminic Sore Throat Formula	⊡ 755
Tussend	1830
Tussend Expectorant	1831
TYLENOL Allergy Sinus, Maximum Strength Caplets and Gelcaps	1571
TYLENOL Allergy Sinus NightTime, Maximum Strength Caplets	1571
TYLENOL Cold Medication, Multi-Symptom Formula Tablets and Caplets	1572
TYLENOL Cold Medication, Multi-Symptom Hot Liquid Packets	1572
TYLENOL Cold Medication, No Drowsiness Formula Caplets and Gelcaps	1572
TYLENOL Cold Severe Congestion Caplets	1573
TYLENOL Cough Medication with Decongestant, Multi Symptom	1574
TYLENOL Flu No Drowsiness Formula, Maximum Strength Gelcaps	1575
TYLENOL Flu NightTime, Maximum Strength Gelcaps	1575
TYLENOL Flu NightTime, Maximum Strength Hot Medication Packets	1575
TYLENOL Sinus, Maximum Strength Geltabs, Gelcaps, Caplets and Tablets	1576
Vicks 44 LiquiCaps Cough, Cold & Flu Relief	⊡ 728
Vicks 44 LiquiCaps Non-Drowsy Cough & Cold Relief	⊡ 729
Vicks 44D Cough & Head Congestion Relief	⊡ 728
Vicks 44M Cough, Cold & Flu Relief	⊡ 729
Vicks DayQuil LiquiCaps/Liquid Multi-Symptom Cold/Flu Relief	⊡ 734
Vicks DayQuil SINUS Pressure & PAIN Relief with IBUPROFEN	⊡ 735
Vicks Nyquil Hot Therapy	⊡ 735
Vicks NyQuil LiquiCaps/Liquid Multi-Symptom Cold/Flu Relief, Original and Cherry Flavors	⊡ 736

Pseudoephedrine Sulfate (Combined effect on cardiovascular system may be deleterious). Products include:

Chlor-Trimeton Allergy Decongestant Tablets	⊡ 759
Claritin-D Tablets	2487
Drixoral Cold and Allergy Sustained-Action Tablets	⊡ 763
Drixoral Cold and Flu Extended-Release Tablets	⊡ 764
Drixoral Non-Drowsy Formula Extended-Release Tablets	⊡ 764
Drixoral Allergy/Sinus Extended Release Tablets	⊡ 765
Trinalin Repetabs Tablets	1373

Salmeterol Xinafoate (Combined effect on cardiovascular system may be deleterious). Products include:

Serevent Inhalation Aerosol	1149

Selegiline Hydrochloride (The action of beta-adrenergic agonists on the vascular system may be potentiated). Products include:

Eldepryl Capsules	2729

Tranylcypromine Sulfate (The action of beta-adrenergic agonists on the vascular system may be potentiated). Products include:

Parnate Tablets	2679

Trimipramine Maleate (The action of beta-adrenergic agonists on the vascular system may be potentiated). Products include:

Surmontil Capsules	2917

BRETHINE TABLETS
(Terbutaline Sulfate) 831

May interact with sympathomimetics. Compounds in this category include:

Albuterol (Concomitant use not recommended; combined effect on the cardiovascular system may be deleterious). Products include:

Proventil Inhalation Aerosol	2524
Ventolin Inhalation Aerosol and Refill	1170

Albuterol Sulfate (Concomitant use not recommended; combined effect on the cardiovascular system may be deleterious). Products include:

Airet Albuterol Sulfate Inhalation Solution	1602
Albuterol Sulfate, USP Solution for Inhalation, Arm-a-Med	522
Proventil Inhalation Solution 0.083%	2527
Proventil Repetabs Tablets	2529
Proventil Solution for Inhalation 0.5%	2525
Proventil Syrup	2528
Proventil Tablets	2529
Ventolin Inhalation Solution	1171
Ventolin Nebules Inhalation Solution	1172
Ventolin Rotacaps for Inhalation	1173
Ventolin Syrup	1175
Ventolin Tablets	1176
Volmax Extended-Release Tablets	1835

Dobutamine Hydrochloride (Concomitant use not recommended; combined effect on the cardiovascular system may be deleterious). Products include:

Dobutrex Solution Vials	1480

Dopamine Hydrochloride (Concomitant use not recommended; combined effect on the cardiovascular system may be deleterious).

No products indexed under this heading.

Ephedrine Hydrochloride (Concomitant use not recommended; combined effect on the cardiovascular system may be deleterious). Products include:

Primatene Tablets	⊡ 844
Quadrinal Tablets	1398

Ephedrine Sulfate (Concomitant use not recommended; combined effect on the cardiovascular system may be deleterious). Products include:

Marax Tablets & DF Syrup	2015

Ephedrine Tannate (Concomitant use not recommended; combined effect on the cardiovascular system may be deleterious). Products include:

Rynatuss	2782

Epinephrine (Concomitant use not recommended; combined effect on the cardiovascular system may be deleterious). Products include:

EPIFRIN	⊙ 237
EpiPen	808
Marcaine with Epinephrine	2446
Primatene Mist	⊡ 843
Sensorcaine with Epinephrine Injection	554
Sus-Phrine Injection	1017
Xylocaine with Epinephrine Injections	562

Epinephrine Bitartrate (Concomitant use not recommended; combined effect on the cardiovascular system may be deleterious). Products include:

Sensorcaine-MPF with Epinephrine Injection	554

Epinephrine Hydrochloride (Concomitant use not recommended; combined effect on the cardiovascular system may be deleterious). Products include:

Ana-Kit Anaphylaxis Emergency Treatment Kit	611

(⊡ Described in PDR For Nonprescription Drugs)   (⊙ Described in PDR For Ophthalmology)

Isoproterenol Hydrochloride
(Concomitant use not recommended; combined effect on the cardiovascular system may be deleterious). Products include:

Isuprel Hydrochloride Solution	2443
Isuprel Injection	2441
Isuprel Mistometer	2442

Isoproterenol Sulfate
(Concomitant use not recommended; combined effect on the cardiovascular system may be deleterious). Products include:

Norisodrine with Calcium Iodide Syrup	446

Metaproterenol Sulfate
(Concomitant use not recommended; combined effect on the cardiovascular system may be deleterious). Products include:

Alupent	672
Metaproterenol Sulfate Inhalation Solution, USP, Arm-a-Med	547

Metaraminol Bitartrate
(Concomitant use not recommended; combined effect on the cardiovascular system may be deleterious). Products include:

Aramine Injection	1649

Methoxamine Hydrochloride
(Concomitant use not recommended; combined effect on the cardiovascular system may be deleterious). Products include:

Vasoxyl Injection	1169

Norepinephrine Bitartrate
(Concomitant use not recommended; combined effect on the cardiovascular system may be deleterious). Products include:

Levophed Bitartrate Injection	2445

Phenylephrine Bitartrate
(Concomitant use not recommended; combined effect on the cardiovascular system may be deleterious).

No products indexed under this heading.

Phenylephrine Hydrochloride
(Concomitant use not recommended; combined effect on the cardiovascular system may be deleterious). Products include:

Atrohist Plus Tablets	1605
Cerose DM	853
D.A. II Tablets	972
D.A. Chewable Tablets	970
Dura-Vent/DA Tablets	972
Extendryl	1003
4-Way Fast Acting Nasal Spray (regular & mentholated)	644
Hemorid	797
Hycomine Compound Tablets	948
Neo-Synephrine Hydrochloride 1% Carpuject	2455
Neo-Synephrine Hydrochloride 1% Injection	2455
Neo-Synephrine Hydrochloride (Ophthalmic)	2456
Neo-Synephrine	624
Novahistine Elixir	782
Phenergan VC	2886
Phenergan VC with Codeine	2888
Preparation H	842
Tympagesic Ear Drops	2476
Vicks Sinex Nasal Spray and Ultra Fine Mist	738

Phenylephrine Tannate
(Concomitant use not recommended; combined effect on the cardiovascular system may be deleterious). Products include:

Atrohist Pediatric Suspension	1604
Atrohist Pediatric Suspension Dye-Free	1604
Rynatan	2781
Rynatuss	2782

Phenylpropanolamine Hydrochloride
(Concomitant use not recommended; combined effect on the cardiovascular system may be deleterious). Products include:

Acutrim	648
Atrohist Plus Tablets	1605
BC Cold Powder Multi-Symptom Formula (Cold-Sinus-Allergy)	631
BC Cold Powder Non-Drowsy Formula (Cold-Sinus)	631
Cheracol Plus Head Cold/Cough Formula	741
Comtrex Multi-Symptom Cold Reliever Liqui-Gels	638
Comtrex Multi-Symptom Non-Drowsy Liqui-gels	640
Contac Continuous Action Nasal Decongestant/Antihistamine 12 Hour Capsules	773
Contac Maximum Strength Continuous Action Decongestant/Antihistamine 12 Hour Caplets	772
Contac Severe Cold and Flu Formula Caplets	773
Coricidin 'D' Decongestant Tablets	760
Dexatrim	795
Dexatrim Plus Vitamins Caplets	796
Dimetane-DC Cough Syrup	2232
Dimetapp Allergy Sinus Caplets	838
Dimetapp Cold & Allergy Chewable Tablets	838
Dimetapp Cold & Cough Liqui-Gels	839
Dimetapp DM Elixir	840
Dimetapp Elixir	840
Dimetapp Extentabs	841
Dimetapp Tablets/Liqui-Gels	841
Dura-Vent Tablets	971
Entex LA Tablets	972
Exgest LA Tablets	787
Hycomine	947
Nolamine Timed-Release Tablets	790
Ornade Spansule Capsules	2678
Propagest Tablets	791
Pyrroxate Caplets	742
Robitussin-CF	846
Sinulin Tablets	792
Tavist-D 12 Hour Relief Tablets	750
Teldrin 12 Hour Antihistamine/Nasal Decongestant Allergy Relief Capsules	786
Triaminic Expectorant	753
Triaminic Syrup	755
Triaminic Triaminicol Cold & Cough	756
Triaminic DM Syrup	756
Triaminicin Tablets	756
Vicks DayQuil Allergy Relief 12-Hour Extended Release Tablets	733
Vicks DayQuil Allergy Relief 4-Hour Tablets	733
Vicks DayQuil SINUS Pressure & CONGESTION Relief	734

Pirbuterol Acetate
(Concomitant use not recommended; combined effect on the cardiovascular system may be deleterious). Products include:

Maxair Autohaler	1550
Maxair Inhaler	1552

Pseudoephedrine Hydrochloride
(Concomitant use not recommended; combined effect on the cardiovascular system may be deleterious). Products include:

Actifed Allergy Daytime/Nighttime Caplets	808
Actifed Cold & Allergy Tablets	807
Actifed Cold & Sinus Caplets and Tablets	808
Actifed Sinus Daytime/Nighttime Tablets and Caplets	809
Advil Cold and Sinus Caplets and Tablets	837
Alka-Seltzer Plus Liqui-Gels	612
Alka-Seltzer Plus Flu & Body Aches Liqui-Gels Non-Drowsy Formula	613
Alka-Seltzer Plus Night-Time Cold Medicine Liqui-Gels	612
Allerest Maximum Strength	649
Allerest No Drowsiness	649
Allerest Sinus Pain Formula	649
Atrohist Pediatric Capsules	1603
Benadryl Allergy/Cold Tablets	811
Benadryl Allergy Decongestant Liquid Medication	812
Benadryl Allergy Decongestant Tablets	812
Benadryl Allergy Sinus Headache Caplets	813
Benylin Multisymptom	816
Bromfed Capsules (Extended-Release)	1832
Bromfed Syrup	712
Bromfed Tablets	1832
Bromfed-DM Cough Syrup	1832
Bromfed-PD Capsules (Extended-Release)	1832
Children's TYLENOL Cold Multi-Symptom Chewable Tablets and Liquid	1559
Children's TYLENOL Cold Plus Cough Multi Symptom Chewable Tablets and Liquid	1560
Children's TYLENOL Flu Suspension Liquid	1560
Children's Vicks DayQuil Allergy Relief	730
Children's Vicks NyQuil Cold/Cough Relief	731
Allergy-Sinus Comtrex Multi-Symptom Allergy-Sinus Formula Tablets and Caplets	639
Comtrex Multi-Symptom	638
Comtrex Multi-Symptom Non-Drowsy Caplets	640
Congess	1003
Contac Day Allergy/Sinus Caplets	771
Contac Day & Night	772
Contac Night Allergy/Sinus Caplets	771
Contac Severe Cold & Flu Non-Drowsy	774
Deconsal II Tablets	1605
Dimetane-DX Cough Syrup	2233
Dimetapp Cold & Fever Suspension	839
Dimetapp Decongestant Pediatric Drops	840
Dorcol Children's Cough Syrup	748
Drixoral Cough + Congestion Liquid Caps	763
Dura-Tap/PD Capsules	970
Duratuss Tablets	2750
Duratuss HD Elixir	2750
Efidac/24	655
Entex PSE Tablets	973
Fedahist Gyrocaps	2545
Guaifed	1833
Guaifed Syrup	712
Guaimax-D Tablets	809
Histussin D Liquid	670
Infants' TYLENOL Cold Decongestant & Fever-Reducer Drops	1561
Kronofed-A	994
Novahistine DMX	782
Nucofed	2225
PediaCare Cough-Cold Chewable Tablets and Liquid	1569
PediaCare Infants' Decongestant Drops	1569
PediaCare Infants' Drops Decongestant Plus Cough	1569
PediaCare NightRest Cough-Cold Liquid	1569
Pediatric Vicks 44d Cough & Head Congestion Relief	736
Pediatric Vicks 44m Cough & Cold Relief	737
Robitussin Cold & Cough Liqui-Gels	844
Robitussin Cold, Cough & Flu Liqui-Gels	844
Robitussin Maximum Strength Cough & Cold	847
Robitussin Night-Time Cold Formula	847
Robitussin Pediatric Cough & Cold Formula	848
Robitussin Pediatric Drops	849
Robitussin Severe Congestion Liqui-Gels	845
Robitussin-DAC Syrup	2249
Robitussin-PE	846
Rondec Oral Drops	974
Rondec Syrup	974
Rondec Tablet	974
Rondec Chewable Tablets	974
Rondec-TR Tablet	804
Ryna	804
Seldane-D Extended-Release Tablets	1286
Semprex-D Capsules	1620
Sinarest	663
Sine-Aid Maximum Strength Sinus Headache Gelcaps, Caplets and Tablets	1570
Sine-Off No Drowsiness Formula Caplets	784
Sine-Off Sinus Medicine	784
Singlet Tablets	785
Sinutab Non-Drying Liquid Caps	823
Sinutab Sinus Allergy Medication, Maximum Strength Tablets and Caplets	823
Sinutab Sinus Medication, Maximum Strength Without Drowsiness Formula, Tablets & Caplets	824
Sudafed Children's Cold & Cough Liquid Medication	825
Sudafed Children's Nasal Decongestant Liquid Medication	826
Sudafed Cold & Allergy Tablets	826
Sudafed Cold and Cough Liquid Caps	826
Sudafed Nasal Decongestant Tablets, 30 mg	825
Sudafed Nasal Decongestant Tablets, 60 mg	825
Sudafed Non-Drying Nasal Liquid Caps	827
Sudafed Pediatric Nasal Decongestant Liquid Oral Drops	827
Sudafed Severe Cold Formula Caplets	828
Sudafed Severe Cold Formula Tablets	828
Sudafed Sinus Caplets	829
Sudafed Sinus Tablets	829
Sudafed 12 Hour Caplets	824
Syn-Rx Tablets	1622
Syn-Rx DM Tablets	1623
TheraFlu Flu and Cold Medicine	750
Theraflu Maximum Strength Flu and Cold Medicine For Sore Throat	751
TheraFlu Flu, Cold and Cough Medicine	750
TheraFlu Maximum Strength Nighttime Flu, Cold & Cough Medicine	751
TheraFlu Maximum Strength Non-Drowsy Formula Flu, Cold & Cough Medicine	751
TheraFlu Maximum Strength, Non-Drowsy Formula Flu, Cold and Cough Caplets	752
Theraflu Maximum Strength Sinus Non-Drowsy Formula Caplets	752
Triaminic AM Cough and Decongestant Formula	753
Triaminic AM Decongestant Formula	753
Triaminic Infant Oral Decongestant Drops	754
Triaminic Night Time	754
Triaminic Sore Throat Formula	755
Tussend	1830
Tussend Expectorant	1831
TYLENOL Allergy Sinus, Maximum Strength Caplets and Gelcaps	1571
TYLENOL Allergy Sinus NightTime, Maximum Strength Caplets	1571
TYLENOL Cold Medication, Multi-Symptom Formula Tablets and Caplets	1572
TYLENOL Cold Medication, Multi-Symptom Hot Liquid Packets	1572
TYLENOL Cold Medication, No Drowsiness Formula Caplets and Gelcaps	1572
TYLENOL Cold Severe Congestion Caplets	1573
TYLENOL Cough Medication with Decongestant, Multi Symptom	1574
TYLENOL Flu No Drowsiness Formula, Maximum Strength Gelcaps	1575
TYLENOL Flu NightTime, Maximum Strength Gelcaps	1575
TYLENOL Flu NightTime, Maximum Strength Hot Medication Packets	1575
TYLENOL Sinus, Maximum Strength Geltabs, Gelcaps, Caplets and Tablets	1576
Vicks 44 LiquiCaps Cough, Cold & Flu Relief	728
Vicks 44 LiquiCaps Non-Drowsy Cough & Cold Relief	729
Vicks 44D Cough & Head Congestion Relief	728
Vicks 44M Cough, Cold & Flu Relief	729
Vicks DayQuil LiquiCaps/Liquid Multi-Symptom Cold/Flu Relief	734
Vicks DayQuil SINUS Pressure & PAIN Relief with IBUPROFEN	735
Vicks Nyquil Hot Therapy	735
Vicks NyQuil LiquiCaps/Liquid Multi-Symptom Cold/Flu Relief, Original and Cherry Flavors	736

IMPORTANT NOTE: Always consult each drug listing in the patient's regimen for possible interactions.

Brethine Tablets — Interactions Index

Pseudoephedrine Sulfate (Concomitant use not recommended; combined effect on the cardiovascular system may be deleterious). Products include:
- Chlor-Trimeton Allergy Decongestant Tablets 759
- Claritin-D Tablets 2487
- Drixoral Cold and Allergy Sustained-Action Tablets 763
- Drixoral Cold and Flu Extended-Release Tablets 764
- Drixoral Non-Drowsy Formula Extended-Release Tablets 764
- Drixoral Allergy/Sinus Extended Release Tablets 765
- Trinalin Repetabs Tablets 1373

Salmeterol Xinafoate (Concomitant use not recommended; combined effect on the cardiovascular system may be deleterious). Products include:
- Serevent Inhalation Aerosol 1149

BREVIBLOC (ESMOLOL HCL) INJECTION
(Esmolol Hydrochloride) 1860
May interact with:

Deserpidine (Potential for additive effect; hypotension or marked bradycardia which may result in vertigo, syncope, or postural hypotension).
No products indexed under this heading.

Digoxin (Increased digoxin levels by 10-20% when concomitantly administered by intravenous route). Products include:
- Lanoxicaps 1110
- Lanoxin Elixir Pediatric 1113
- Lanoxin Injection 1116
- Lanoxin Injection Pediatric 1119
- Lanoxin Tablets 1121

Dopamine Hydrochloride (Concurrent use is not recommended to control supraventricular tachycardia because of the danger of blocking cardiac contractility when systemic vascular resistance is high).
No products indexed under this heading.

Epinephrine Hydrochloride (Concurrent use is not recommended to control supraventricular tachycardia because of the danger of blocking cardiac contractility when systemic vascular resistance is high; potential for unresponsiveness to the usual dose of epinephrine to treat allergic reaction). Products include:
- Ana-Kit Anaphylaxis Emergency Treatment Kit 611

Morphine Sulfate (Intravenous morphine increases Brevibloc steady-state blood levels by 46%). Products include:
- Astramorph/PF Injection, USP (Preservative-Free) 526
- Duramorph Injection 983
- Infumorph 200 and Infumorph 500 Sterile Solutions 985
- Kadian Capsules 2948
- MS Contin Tablets 2149
- MSIR 2152
- Oramorph SR (Morphine Sulfate Sustained Release Tablets) 2359
- RMS Suppositories CII 2766
- Roxanol 2365

Norepinephrine Hydrochloride (Concurrent use is not recommended to control supraventricular tachycardia because of the danger of blocking cardiac contractility when systemic vascular resistance is high).

Reserpine (Potential for additive effect; hypotension or marked bradycardia which may result in vertigo, syncope, or postural hypotension). Products include:
- Diupres Tablets 1691
- Hydropres Tablets 1718
- Ser-Ap-Es Tablets 867

Succinylcholine Chloride (Prolonged neuromuscular blockade from 5 minutes to eight minutes). Products include:
- Anectine 1062

Verapamil Hydrochloride (Potential for fatal cardiac arrests in patients with depressed myocardial function). Products include:
- Calan SR Caplets 2571
- Calan Tablets 2568
- Covera-HS Tablets 2573
- Isoptin Injectable 1391
- Isoptin Oral Tablets 1393
- Isoptin SR Tablets 1395
- Verelan Capsules 1455

Warfarin Sodium (Brevibloc concentrations were equivocally higher when given with Warfarin). Products include:
- Coumadin 941

BREVICON 21-DAY TABLETS
(Norethindrone, Ethinyl Estradiol) 2563
May interact with barbiturates, tetracyclines, and certain other agents. Compounds in these categories include:

Ampicillin (Potential for reduced efficacy and increased incidence of breakthrough bleeding and menstrual irregularities with concomitant use). Products include:
- Omnipen Capsules 2872
- Omnipen for Oral Suspension 2873

Ampicillin Sodium (Potential for reduced efficacy and increased incidence of breakthrough bleeding and menstrual irregularities with concomitant use). Products include:
- Unasyn 2035

Aprobarbital (Potential for reduced efficacy and increased incidence of breakthrough bleeding and menstrual irregularities with concomitant use).
No products indexed under this heading.

Butabarbital (Potential for reduced efficacy and increased incidence of breakthrough bleeding and menstrual irregularities with concomitant use).
No products indexed under this heading.

Butalbital (Potential for reduced efficacy and increased incidence of breakthrough bleeding and menstrual irregularities with concomitant use). Products include:
- Axocet Capsules 2469
- Esgic-plus Capsules 1012
- Esgic-plus Tablets 1012
- Fioricet Tablets 2386
- Fioricet with Codeine Capsules 2387
- Fiorinal Capsules 2388
- Fiorinal with Codeine Capsules 2390
- Fiorinal Tablets 2388
- Phrenilin 790
- Sedapap Tablets 50 mg/650 mg 1826

Demeclocycline Hydrochloride (Potential for reduced efficacy and increased incidence of breakthrough bleeding and menstrual irregularities with concomitant use). Products include:
- Declomycin Tablets 1421

Doxycycline Calcium (Potential for reduced efficacy and increased incidence of breakthrough bleeding and menstrual irregularities with concomitant use). Products include:
- Vibramycin Calcium Oral Suspension Syrup 2038

Doxycycline Hyclate (Potential for reduced efficacy and increased incidence of breakthrough bleeding and menstrual irregularities with concomitant use). Products include:
- Doryx Capsules 1970
- Vibramycin Hyclate Capsules 2038
- Vibramycin Hyclate Intravenous 2040
- Vibra-Tabs Film Coated Tablets 2038

Doxycycline Monohydrate (Potential for reduced efficacy and increased incidence of breakthrough bleeding and menstrual irregularities with concomitant use). Products include:
- Monodox Capsules 1858
- Vibramycin Monohydrate for Oral Suspension 2038

Fosphenytoin Sodium (Potential for reduced efficacy and increased incidence of breakthrough bleeding and menstrual irregularities with concomitant use). Products include:
- Cerebyx Injection 1956

Griseofulvin (Potential for reduced efficacy and increased incidence of breakthrough bleeding and menstrual irregularities with concomitant use). Products include:
- Fulvicin P/G Tablets 2499
- Fulvicin P/G 165 & 330 Tablets 2500
- Grifulvin V (griseofulvin tablets) Microsize (griseofulvin oral suspension) Microsize 1944
- Gris-PEG Tablets, 125 mg & 250 mg 476

Mephobarbital (Potential for reduced efficacy and increased incidence of breakthrough bleeding and menstrual irregularities with concomitant use). Products include:
- Mebaral Tablets 2452

Methacycline Hydrochloride (Potential for reduced efficacy and increased incidence of breakthrough bleeding and menstrual irregularities with concomitant use).
No products indexed under this heading.

Minocycline Hydrochloride (Potential for reduced efficacy and increased incidence of breakthrough bleeding and menstrual irregularities with concomitant use). Products include:
- DYNACIN Capsules 1627
- Minocin Intravenous 1428
- Minocin Oral Suspension 1431
- Minocin Pellet-Filled Capsules 1429

Oxytetracycline Hydrochloride (Potential for reduced efficacy and increased incidence of breakthrough bleeding and menstrual irregularities with concomitant use). Products include:
- TERAK Ointment 210
- Terra-Cortril Ophthalmic Suspension 2033
- Terramycin with Polymyxin B Sulfate Ophthalmic Ointment 2035
- Urobiotic-250 Capsules 2038

Pentobarbital Sodium (Potential for reduced efficacy and increased incidence of breakthrough bleeding and menstrual irregularities with concomitant use). Products include:
- Nembutal Sodium Capsules 440
- Nembutal Sodium Solution 442
- Nembutal Sodium Suppositories 444

Phenobarbital (Potential for reduced efficacy and increased incidence of breakthrough bleeding and menstrual irregularities with concomitant use). Products include:
- Arco-Lase Plus Tablets 513
- Bellergal-S Tablets 2375
- Donnatal 2234
- Donnatal Extentabs 2234
- Donnatal Tablets 2234
- Phenobarbital Elixir and Tablets 1523
- Quadrinal Tablets 1398

Phenylbutazone (Potential for reduced efficacy and increased incidence of breakthrough bleeding and menstrual irregularities with concomitant use).
No products indexed under this heading.

Phenytoin (Potential for reduced efficacy and increased incidence of breakthrough bleeding and menstrual irregularities with concomitant use). Products include:
- Dilantin Infatabs 1967
- Dilantin-125 Suspension 1969

Phenytoin Sodium (Potential for reduced efficacy and increased incidence of breakthrough bleeding and menstrual irregularities with concomitant use). Products include:
- Dilantin Kapseals 1965

Rifampin (Co-administration has been associated with reduced efficacy and increased incidence of breakthrough bleeding and menstrual irregularities). Products include:
- Rifadin 1276
- Rifamate Capsules 1278
- Rifater 1280
- Rimactane Capsules 865

Secobarbital Sodium (Potential for reduced efficacy and increased incidence of breakthrough bleeding and menstrual irregularities with concomitant use). Products include:
- Seconal Sodium Pulvules 1529

Tetracycline Hydrochloride (Potential for reduced efficacy and increased incidence of breakthrough bleeding and menstrual irregularities with concomitant use). Products include:
- Achromycin V Capsules 1417
- Helidac Therapy 2135

Thiamylal Sodium (Potential for reduced efficacy and increased incidence of breakthrough bleeding and menstrual irregularities with concomitant use).
No products indexed under this heading.

BREVICON 28-DAY TABLETS
(Norethindrone, Ethinyl Estradiol) 2563
See Brevicon 21-Day Tablets

BREVOXYL-4 GEL
(Benzoyl Peroxide) 2732
None cited in PDR database.

BREVOXYL-8 GEL
(Benzoyl Peroxide) 2732
None cited in PDR database.

BREVOXYL CLEANSING LOTION
(Benzoyl Peroxide) 2732
None cited in PDR database.

BRICANYL SUBCUTANEOUS INJECTION
(Terbutaline Sulfate) 1247
May interact with sympathomimetic bronchodilators, monoamine oxidase inhibitors, tricyclic antidepressants, and beta blockers. Compounds in these categories include:

Acebutolol Hydrochloride (Blocked pulmonary effects; may produce severe asthma attacks in asthmatic patients). Products include:
- Sectral Capsules 2914

Albuterol (Deleterious cardiovascular effects). Products include:
- Proventil Inhalation Aerosol 2524

(■ Described in PDR For Nonprescription Drugs)   (⊙ Described in PDR For Ophthalmology)

129 **Interactions Index** **Bricanyl Tablets**

Ventolin Inhalation Aerosol and Refill ... 1170

Albuterol Sulfate (Deleterious cardiovascular effects). Products include:

Airet Albuterol Sulfate Inhalation Solution ... 1602
Albuterol Sulfate, USP Solution for Inhalation, Arm-a-Med ... 522
Proventil Inhalation Solution 0.083% ... 2527
Proventil Repetabs Tablets ... 2529
Proventil Solution for Inhalation 0.5% ... 2525
Proventil Syrup ... 2528
Proventil Tablets ... 2529
Ventolin Inhalation Solution ... 1171
Ventolin Nebules Inhalation Solution ... 1172
Ventolin Rotacaps for Inhalation ... 1173
Ventolin Syrup ... 1175
Ventolin Tablets ... 1176
Volmax Extended-Release Tablets .. 1835

Amitriptyline Hydrochloride (Potentiates terbutaline's vascular effects). Products include:

Elavil ... 2945
Etrafon ... 2495
Limbitrol ... 2333
Triavil Tablets ... 1800

Amoxapine (Potentiates terbutaline's vascular effects). Products include:

Asendin Tablets ... 1419

Atenolol (Blocked pulmonary effects; may produce severe asthma attacks in asthmatic patients). Products include:

Tenoretic Tablets ... 2963
Tenormin Tablets and I.V. Injection 2965

Betaxolol Hydrochloride (Blocked pulmonary effects; may produce severe asthma attacks in asthmatic patients). Products include:

Betoptic Ophthalmic Solution ... 465
Betoptic S Ophthalmic Suspension 467
Kerlone Tablets ... 2588

Bisoprolol Fumarate (Blocked pulmonary effects; may produce severe asthma attacks in asthmatic patients). Products include:

Zebeta Tablets ... 1457
Ziac ... 1459

Bitolterol Mesylate (Deleterious cardiovascular effects). Products include:

Tornalate Solution for Inhalation, 0.2% ... 976
Tornalate Metered Dose Inhaler ... 978

Carteolol Hydrochloride (Blocked pulmonary effects; may produce severe asthma attacks in asthmatic patients). Products include:

Cartrol Tablets ... 413
Ocupress Ophthalmic Solution, 1% Sterile ... ◉ 297

Clomipramine Hydrochloride (Potentiates terbutaline's vascular effects). Products include:

Anafranil Capsules ... 819

Desipramine Hydrochloride (Potentiates terbutaline's vascular effects). Products include:

Norpramin Tablets ... 1273

Doxepin Hydrochloride (Potentiates terbutaline's vascular effects). Products include:

Adapin Capsules ... 1542
Sinequan ... 2028
Zonalon Cream ... 1042

Ephedrine Hydrochloride (Deleterious cardiovascular effects). Products include:

Primatene Tablets ... ▣ 844
Quadrinal Tablets ... 1398

Ephedrine Sulfate (Deleterious cardiovascular effects). Products include:

Marax Tablets & DF Syrup ... 2015

Ephedrine Tannate (Deleterious cardiovascular effects). Products include:

Rynatuss ... 2782

Epinephrine (Deleterious cardiovascular effects). Products include:

EPIFRIN ... ◉ 237
EpiPen ... 808
Marcaine with Epinephrine ... 2446
Primatene Mist ... ▣ 843
Sensorcaine with Epinephrine Injection ... 554
Sus-Phrine Injection ... 1017
Xylocaine with Epinephrine Injections ... 562

Epinephrine Hydrochloride (Deleterious cardiovascular effects). Products include:

Ana-Kit Anaphylaxis Emergency Treatment Kit ... 611

Esmolol Hydrochloride (Blocked pulmonary effects; may produce severe asthma attacks in asthmatic patients). Products include:

Brevibloc (esmolol HCl) Injection 1860

Ethylnorepinephrine Hydrochloride (Deleterious cardiovascular effects).

No products indexed under this heading.

Furazolidone (Potentiates terbutaline's vascular effects). Products include:

Furoxone ... 2221

Imipramine Hydrochloride (Potentiates terbutaline's vascular effects). Products include:

Tofranil Ampuls ... 873
Tofranil Tablets ... 875

Imipramine Pamoate (Potentiates terbutaline's vascular effects). Products include:

Tofranil-PM Capsules ... 876

Isocarboxazid (Potentiates terbutaline's vascular effects).

No products indexed under this heading.

Isoetharine (Deleterious cardiovascular effects). Products include:

Bronkometer Aerosol ... 2432
Bronkosol Solution ... 2432
Isoetharine Inhalation Solution, USP, Arm-a-Med ... 545

Isoproterenol Hydrochloride (Deleterious cardiovascular effects). Products include:

Isuprel Hydrochloride Solution ... 2443
Isuprel Injection ... 2441
Isuprel Mistometer ... 2442

Isoproterenol Sulfate (Deleterious cardiovascular effects). Products include:

Norisodrine with Calcium Iodide Syrup ... 446

Labetalol Hydrochloride (Blocked pulmonary effects; may produce severe asthma attacks in asthmatic patients). Products include:

Normodyne Injection ... 2519
Normodyne Tablets ... 2522
Trandate ... 1158

Levobunolol Hydrochloride (Blocked pulmonary effects; may produce severe asthma attacks in asthmatic patients). Products include:

Betagan ... ◉ 230

Maprotiline Hydrochloride (Potentiates terbutaline's vascular effects). Products include:

Ludiomil Tablets ... 861

Metaproterenol Sulfate (Deleterious cardiovascular effects). Products include:

Alupent ... 672
Metaproterenol Sulfate Inhalation Solution, USP, Arm-a-Med ... 547

Metipranolol Hydrochloride (Blocked pulmonary effects; may produce severe asthma attacks in asthmatic patients). Products include:

OptiPranolol (Metipranolol 0.3%) Sterile Ophthalmic Solution ... ◉ 256

Metoprolol Succinate (Blocked pulmonary effects; may produce severe asthma attacks in asthmatic patients). Products include:

Toprol-XL Tablets ... 560

Metoprolol Tartrate (Blocked pulmonary effects; may produce severe asthma attacks in asthmatic patients). Products include:

Lopressor ... 848
Lopressor HCT Tablets ... 850

Nadolol (Blocked pulmonary effects; may produce severe asthma attacks in asthmatic patients).

No products indexed under this heading.

Nortriptyline Hydrochloride (Potentiates terbutaline's vascular effects). Products include:

Pamelor ... 2409

Penbutolol Sulfate (Blocked pulmonary effects; may produce severe asthma attacks in asthmatic patients). Products include:

Levatol Tablets ... 2547

Phenelzine Sulfate (Potentiates terbutaline's vascular effects). Products include:

Nardil ... 1977

Pindolol (Blocked pulmonary effects; may produce severe asthma attacks in asthmatic patients). Products include:

Visken Tablets ... 2428

Pirbuterol Acetate (Deleterious cardiovascular effects). Products include:

Maxair Autohaler ... 1550
Maxair Inhaler ... 1552

Propranolol Hydrochloride (Blocked pulmonary effects; may produce severe asthma attacks in asthmatic patients). Products include:

Inderal ... 2834
Inderal LA Long Acting Capsules ... 2836
Inderide Tablets ... 2838
Inderide LA Long Acting Capsules .. 2840

Protriptyline Hydrochloride (Potentiates terbutaline's vascular effects). Products include:

Vivactil Tablets ... 1820

Salmeterol Xinafoate (Deleterious cardiovascular effects). Products include:

Serevent Inhalation Aerosol ... 1149

Selegiline Hydrochloride (Potentiates terbutaline's vascular effects). Products include:

Eldepryl Capsules ... 2729

Sotalol Hydrochloride (Blocked pulmonary effects; may produce severe asthma attacks in asthmatic patients). Products include:

Betapace Tablets ... 637

Timolol Hemihydrate (Blocked pulmonary effects; may produce severe asthma attacks in asthmatic patients). Products include:

Betimol 0.25%, 0.5% ... ◉ 259

Timolol Maleate (Blocked pulmonary effects; may produce severe asthma attacks in asthmatic patients). Products include:

Blocadren Tablets ... 1654
Timolide Tablets ... 1791
Timoptic in Ocudose ... 1796
Timoptic Sterile Ophthalmic Solution ... 1794
Timoptic-XE ... 1798

Tranylcypromine Sulfate (Potentiates terbutaline's vascular effects). Products include:

Parnate Tablets ... 2679

Trimipramine Maleate (Potentiates terbutaline's vascular effects). Products include:

Surmontil Capsules ... 2917

BRICANYL TABLETS

(Terbutaline Sulfate) ... 1248

May interact with sympathomimetic bronchodilators, monoamine oxidase inhibitors, tricyclic antidepressants, and beta blockers. Compounds in these categories include:

Acebutolol Hydrochloride (Blocked pulmonary effects; may produce severe asthma attacks in asthmatic patients). Products include:

Sectral Capsules ... 2914

Albuterol (Deleterious cardiovascular effects). Products include:

Proventil Inhalation Aerosol ... 2524
Ventolin Inhalation Aerosol and Refill ... 1170

Albuterol Sulfate (Deleterious cardiovascular effects). Products include:

Airet Albuterol Sulfate Inhalation Solution ... 1602
Albuterol Sulfate, USP Solution for Inhalation, Arm-a-Med ... 522
Proventil Inhalation Solution 0.083% ... 2527
Proventil Repetabs Tablets ... 2529
Proventil Solution for Inhalation 0.5% ... 2525
Proventil Syrup ... 2528
Proventil Tablets ... 2529
Ventolin Inhalation Solution ... 1171
Ventolin Nebules Inhalation Solution ... 1172
Ventolin Rotacaps for Inhalation ... 1173
Ventolin Syrup ... 1175
Ventolin Tablets ... 1176
Volmax Extended-Release Tablets .. 1835

Amitriptyline Hydrochloride (Potentiates terbutaline's vascular effects). Products include:

Elavil ... 2945
Etrafon ... 2495
Limbitrol ... 2333
Triavil Tablets ... 1800

Amoxapine (Potentiates terbutaline's vascular effects). Products include:

Asendin Tablets ... 1419

Atenolol (Blocked pulmonary effects; may produce severe asthma attacks in asthmatic patients). Products include:

Tenoretic Tablets ... 2963
Tenormin Tablets and I.V. Injection 2965

Betaxolol Hydrochloride (Blocked pulmonary effects; may produce severe asthma attacks in asthmatic patients). Products include:

Betoptic Ophthalmic Solution ... 465
Betoptic S Ophthalmic Suspension 467
Kerlone Tablets ... 2588

Bisoprolol Fumarate (Blocked pulmonary effects; may produce severe asthma attacks in asthmatic patients). Products include:

Zebeta Tablets ... 1457
Ziac ... 1459

Bitolterol Mesylate (Deleterious cardiovascular effects). Products include:

Tornalate Solution for Inhalation, 0.2% ... 976
Tornalate Metered Dose Inhaler ... 978

Carteolol Hydrochloride (Blocked pulmonary effects; may produce severe asthma attacks in asthmatic patients). Products include:

Cartrol Tablets ... 413

IMPORTANT NOTE: Always consult each drug listing in the patient's regimen for possible interactions.

Bricanyl Tablets · Interactions Index · 130

Ocupress Ophthalmic Solution, 1% Sterile .... ⊙ 297

Clomipramine Hydrochloride (Potentiates terbutaline's vascular effects). Products include:
Anafranil Capsules 819

Desipramine Hydrochloride (Potentiates terbutaline's vascular effects). Products include:
Norpramin Tablets 1273

Doxepin Hydrochloride (Potentiates terbutaline's vascular effects). Products include:
Adapin Capsules 1542
Sinequan 2028
Zonalon Cream 1042

Ephedrine Hydrochloride (Deleterious cardiovascular effects). Products include:
Primatene Tablets .... ◘ 844
Quadrinal Tablets 1398

Ephedrine Sulfate (Deleterious cardiovascular effects). Products include:
Marax Tablets & DF Syrup 2015

Ephedrine Tannate (Deleterious cardiovascular effects). Products include:
Rynatuss 2782

Epinephrine (Deleterious cardiovascular effects). Products include:
EPIFRIN .... ⊙ 237
EpiPen 808
Marcaine with Epinephrine 2446
Primatene Mist .... ◘ 843
Sensorcaine with Epinephrine Injection 554
Sus-Phrine Injection 1017
Xylocaine with Epinephrine Injections 562

Epinephrine Hydrochloride (Deleterious cardiovascular effects). Products include:
Ana-Kit Anaphylaxis Emergency Treatment Kit 611

Esmolol Hydrochloride (Blocked pulmonary effects; may produce severe asthma attacks in asthmatic patients). Products include:
Brevibloc (esmolol HCl) Injection 1860

Ethylnorepinephrine Hydrochloride (Deleterious cardiovascular effects).
No products indexed under this heading.

Furazolidone (Potentiates terbutaline's vascular effects). Products include:
Furoxone 2221

Imipramine Hydrochloride (Potentiates terbutaline's vascular effects). Products include:
Tofranil Ampuls 873
Tofranil Tablets 875

Imipramine Pamoate (Potentiates terbutaline's vascular effects). Products include:
Tofranil-PM Capsules 876

Isocarboxazid (Potentiates terbutaline's vascular effects).
No products indexed under this heading.

Isoetharine (Deleterious cardiovascular effects). Products include:
Bronkometer Aerosol 2432
Bronkosol Solution 2432
Isoetharine Inhalation Solution, USP, Arm-a-Med 545

Isoproterenol Hydrochloride (Deleterious cardiovascular effects). Products include:
Isuprel Hydrochloride Solution 2443
Isuprel Injection 2441
Isuprel Mistometer 2442

Isoproterenol Sulfate (Deleterious cardiovascular effects). Products include:
Norisodrine with Calcium Iodide Syrup 446

Labetalol Hydrochloride (Blocked pulmonary effects; may produce severe asthma attacks in asthmatic patients). Products include:
Normodyne Injection 2519
Normodyne Tablets 2522
Trandate 1158

Levobunolol Hydrochloride (Blocked pulmonary effects; may produce severe asthma attacks in asthmatic patients). Products include:
Betagan .... ⊙ 230

Maprotiline Hydrochloride (Potentiates terbutaline's vascular effects). Products include:
Ludiomil Tablets 861

Metaproterenol Sulfate (Deleterious cardiovascular effects). Products include:
Alupent 672
Metaproterenol Sulfate Inhalation Solution, USP, Arm-a-Med 547

Metipranolol Hydrochloride (Blocked pulmonary effects; may produce severe asthma attacks in asthmatic patients). Products include:
OptiPranolol (Metipranolol 0.3%) Sterile Ophthalmic Solution .... ⊙ 256

Metoprolol Succinate (Blocked pulmonary effects; may produce severe asthma attacks in asthmatic patients). Products include:
Toprol-XL Tablets 560

Metoprolol Tartrate (Blocked pulmonary effects; may produce severe asthma attacks in asthmatic patients). Products include:
Lopressor 848
Lopressor HCT Tablets 850

Nadolol (Blocked pulmonary effects; may produce severe asthma attacks in asthmatic patients).
No products indexed under this heading.

Nortriptyline Hydrochloride (Potentiates terbutaline's vascular effects). Products include:
Pamelor 2409

Penbutolol Sulfate (Blocked pulmonary effects; may produce severe asthma attacks in asthmatic patients). Products include:
Levatol Tablets 2547

Phenelzine Sulfate (Potentiates terbutaline's vascular effects). Products include:
Nardil 1977

Pindolol (Blocked pulmonary effects; may produce severe asthma attacks in asthmatic patients). Products include:
Visken Tablets 2428

Pirbuterol Acetate (Deleterious cardiovascular effects). Products include:
Maxair Autohaler 1550
Maxair Inhaler 1552

Propranolol Hydrochloride (Blocked pulmonary effects; may produce severe asthma attacks in asthmatic patients). Products include:
Inderal 2834
Inderal LA Long Acting Capsules 2836
Inderide Tablets 2838
Inderide LA Long Acting Capsules 2840

Protriptyline Hydrochloride (Potentiates terbutaline's vascular effects). Products include:
Vivactil Tablets 1820

Salmeterol Xinafoate (Deleterious cardiovascular effects). Products include:
Serevent Inhalation Aerosol 1149

Selegiline Hydrochloride (Potentiates terbutaline's vascular effects). Products include:
Eldepryl Capsules 2729

Sotalol Hydrochloride (Blocked pulmonary effects; may produce severe asthma attacks in asthmatic patients). Products include:
Betapace Tablets 637

Timolol Hemihydrate (Blocked pulmonary effects; may produce severe asthma attacks in asthmatic patients). Products include:
Betimol 0.25%, 0.5% .... ⊙ 259

Timolol Maleate (Blocked pulmonary effects; may produce severe asthma attacks in asthmatic patients). Products include:
Blocadren Tablets 1654
Timolide Tablets 1791
Timoptic in Ocudose 1796
Timoptic Sterile Ophthalmic Solution 1794
Timoptic-XE 1798

Tranylcypromine Sulfate (Potentiates terbutaline's vascular effects). Products include:
Parnate Tablets 2679

Trimipramine Maleate (Potentiates terbutaline's vascular effects). Products include:
Surmontil Capsules 2917

BROMFED CAPSULES (EXTENDED-RELEASE)

(Brompheniramine Maleate, Pseudoephedrine Hydrochloride) 1832
May interact with central nervous system depressants, monoamine oxidase inhibitors, beta blockers, veratrum alkaloids, and certain other agents. Compounds in these categories include:

Acebutolol Hydrochloride (Increased sympathomimetic effect). Products include:
Sectral Capsules 2914

Alfentanil Hydrochloride (Additive effects). Products include:
Alfenta Injection 1334

Alprazolam (Additive effects). Products include:
Xanax Tablets 2115

Aprobarbital (Additive effects).
No products indexed under this heading.

Atenolol (Increased sympathomimetic effect). Products include:
Tenoretic Tablets 2963
Tenormin Tablets and I.V. Injection 2965

Betaxolol Hydrochloride (Increased sympathomimetic effect). Products include:
Betoptic Ophthalmic Solution 465
Betoptic S Ophthalmic Suspension 467
Kerlone Tablets 2588

Bisoprolol Fumarate (Increased sympathomimetic effect). Products include:
Zebeta Tablets 1457
Ziac 1459

Buprenorphine (Additive effects). Products include:
Buprenex Injectable 2170

Buspirone Hydrochloride (Additive effects). Products include:
BuSpar Tablets 738

Butabarbital (Additive effects).
No products indexed under this heading.

Butalbital (Additive effects). Products include:
Axocet Capsules 2469
Esgic-plus Capsules 1012
Esgic-plus Tablets 1012
Fioricet Tablets 2386
Fioricet with Codeine Capsules 2387
Fiorinal Capsules 2388
Fiorinal with Codeine Capsules 2390
Fiorinal Tablets 2388
Phrenilin 790
Sedapap Tablets 50 mg/650 mg .. 1826

Carteolol Hydrochloride (Increased sympathomimetic effect). Products include:
Cartrol Tablets 413
Ocupress Ophthalmic Solution, 1% Sterile .... ⊙ 297

Chlordiazepoxide (Additive effects). Products include:
Limbitrol 2333

Chlordiazepoxide Hydrochloride (Additive effects). Products include:
Librax Capsules 2330
Librium Capsules 2331
Librium Injectable 2332

Chlorpromazine (Additive effects). Products include:
Thorazine Suppositories 2701

Chlorprothixene (Additive effects).
No products indexed under this heading.

Chlorprothixene Hydrochloride (Additive effects).
No products indexed under this heading.

Chlorprothixene Lactate (Additive effects).
No products indexed under this heading.

Clorazepate Dipotassium (Additive effects). Products include:
Tranxene 459

Clozapine (Additive effects). Products include:
Clozaril Tablets 2377

Codeine Phosphate (Additive effects). Products include:
Brontex 2130
Dimetane-DC Cough Syrup 2232
Fioricet with Codeine Capsules 2387
Fiorinal with Codeine Capsules 2390
Nucofed 2225
Phenergan with Codeine 2883
Phenergan VC with Codeine 2888
Robitussin A-C Syrup 2248
Robitussin-DAC Syrup 2249
Ryna .... ◘ 804
Soma Compound w/Codeine Tablets 2784
Tylenol with Codeine 1592

Cryptenamine Preparations (Reduced antihypertensive effects).

Desflurane (Additive effects). Products include:
Suprane (desflurane, USP) 1865

Dezocine (Additive effects). Products include:
Dalgan Injection 529

Diazepam (Additive effects). Products include:
Dizac (diazepam injectable emulsion) CIV 1862
Valium Injectable 2336
Valium Tablets 2335

Droperidol (Additive effects). Products include:
Inapsine Injection 462

Enflurane (Additive effects).
No products indexed under this heading.

Esmolol Hydrochloride (Increased sympathomimetic effect). Products include:
Brevibloc (esmolol HCl) Injection ... 1860

Estazolam (Additive effects). Products include:
ProSom Tablets 457

Ethchlorvynol (Additive effects). Products include:
Placidyl Capsules 456

Ethinamate (Additive effects).
No products indexed under this heading.

Fentanyl (Additive effects). Products include:
Duragesic Transdermal System 1336

(◘ Described in PDR For Nonprescription Drugs) (⊙ Described in PDR For Ophthalmology)

Fentanyl Citrate (Additive effects). Products include:
- Sublimaze Injection 463

Fluphenazine Decanoate (Additive effects). Products include:
- Prolixin Decanoate 510

Fluphenazine Enanthate (Additive effects). Products include:
- Prolixin Enanthate 510

Fluphenazine Hydrochloride (Additive effects). Products include:
- Prolixin 510

Flurazepam Hydrochloride (Additive effects). Products include:
- Dalmane Capsules 2329

Furazolidone (Increased sympathomimetic effect; concurrent therapy is contraindicated). Products include:
- Furoxone 2221

Glutethimide (Additive effects). No products indexed under this heading.

Haloperidol (Additive effects). Products include:
- Haldol Injection, Tablets and Concentrate 1585

Haloperidol Decanoate (Additive effects). Products include:
- Haldol Decanoate 1587

Hydrocodone Bitartrate (Additive effects). Products include:
- Codiclear DH Syrup 808
- Duratuss HD Elixir 2750
- Histussin D Liquid 670
- Hycodan Tablets and Syrup 946
- Hycomine Compound Tablets 948
- Hycomine 947
- Hycotuss Expectorant Syrup 950
- Hydrocet Capsules 787
- Lorcet 10/650 Tablets 1016
- Lortab 2751
- Tussend 1830
- Tussend Expectorant 1831
- Vicodin Tablets 1404
- Vicodin ES Tablets 1405
- Vicodin HP Tablets 1403
- Vicodin Tuss Expectorant 1406
- Zydone Capsules 967

Hydrocodone Polistirex (Additive effects). Products include:
- Tussionex Pennkinetic Extended-Release Suspension 1624

Hydroxyzine Hydrochloride (Additive effects). Products include:
- Atarax Tablets & Syrup 1992
- Marax Tablets & DF Syrup 2015
- Vistaril Intramuscular Solution 2042

Isocarboxazid (Increased sympathomimetic effect; concurrent therapy is contraindicated). No products indexed under this heading.

Isoflurane (Additive effects). No products indexed under this heading.

Ketamine Hydrochloride (Additive effects). No products indexed under this heading.

Labetalol Hydrochloride (Increased sympathomimetic effect). Products include:
- Normodyne Injection 2519
- Normodyne Tablets 2522
- Trandate 1158

Levobunolol Hydrochloride (Increased sympathomimetic effect). Products include:
- Betagan 230

Levomethadyl Acetate Hydrochloride (Additive effects). Products include:
- Orlaam Oral Solution 2361

Levorphanol Tartrate (Additive effects). Products include:
- Levo-Dromoran 2297

Lorazepam (Additive effects). Products include:
- Ativan Injection 2805

- Ativan Tablets 2807

Loxapine Hydrochloride (Additive effects). Products include:
- Loxitane 1426

Loxapine Succinate (Additive effects). Products include:
- Loxitane Capsules 1426

Mecamylamine Hydrochloride (Reduced antihypertensive effects). Products include:
- Inversine Tablets 1729

Meperidine Hydrochloride (Additive effects). Products include:
- Demerol 2438
- Mepergan Injection 2859

Mephobarbital (Additive effects). Products include:
- Mebaral Tablets 2452

Meprobamate (Additive effects). Products include:
- Miltown Tablets 2780
- PMB 200 and PMB 400 2890

Mesoridazine Besylate (Additive effects). Products include:
- Serentil 689

Methadone Hydrochloride (Additive effects). Products include:
- Methadone Hydrochloride Oral Concentrate 2356
- Methadone Hydrochloride Oral Solution & Tablets 2357

Methohexital Sodium (Additive effects). No products indexed under this heading.

Methotrimeprazine (Additive effects). Products include:
- Levoprome 1321

Methoxyflurane (Additive effects). No products indexed under this heading.

Methyldopa (Reduced antihypertensive effects). Products include:
- Aldoclor Tablets 1638
- Aldomet Oral 1640
- Aldoril Tablets 1644

Methyldopate Hydrochloride (Reduced antihypertensive effects). Products include:
- Aldomet Ester HCl Injection 1642

Metipranolol Hydrochloride (Increased sympathomimetic effect). Products include:
- OptiPranolol (Metipranolol 0.3%) Sterile Ophthalmic Solution 256

Metoprolol Succinate (Increased sympathomimetic effect). Products include:
- Toprol-XL Tablets 560

Metoprolol Tartrate (Increased sympathomimetic effect). Products include:
- Lopressor 848
- Lopressor HCT Tablets 850

Midazolam Hydrochloride (Additive effects). Products include:
- Versed Injection 2324

Molindone Hydrochloride (Additive effects). Products include:
- Moban Tablets and Concentrate 1036

Morphine Sulfate (Additive effects). Products include:
- Astramorph/PF Injection, USP (Preservative-Free) 526
- Duramorph Injection 983
- Infumorph 200 and Infumorph 500 Sterile Solutions 985
- Kadian Capsules 2948
- MS Contin Tablets 2149
- MSIR 2152
- Oramorph SR (Morphine Sulfate Sustained Release Tablets) 2359
- RMS Suppositories CII 2766
- Roxanol 2365

Nadolol (Increased sympathomimetic effect). No products indexed under this heading.

Opium Alkaloids (Additive effects). No products indexed under this heading.

Oxazepam (Additive effects). Products include:
- Serax Capsules 2916
- Serax Tablets 2916

Oxycodone Hydrochloride (Additive effects). Products include:
- OxyContin Tablets 2163
- OxyIR Capsules 2167
- Percocet Tablets 955
- Percodan Tablets 955
- Percodan-Demi Tablets 956
- Roxicodone Tablets, Oral Solution & Intensol (Oxycodone) 2366
- Tylox Capsules 1593

Penbutolol Sulfate (Increased sympathomimetic effect). Products include:
- Levatol Tablets 2547

Pentobarbital Sodium (Additive effects). Products include:
- Nembutal Sodium Capsules 440
- Nembutal Sodium Solution 442
- Nembutal Sodium Suppositories 444

Perphenazine (Additive effects). Products include:
- Etrafon 2495
- Triavil Tablets 1800
- Trilafon 2532

Phenelzine Sulfate (Increased sympathomimetic effect; concurrent therapy is contraindicated). Products include:
- Nardil 1977

Phenobarbital (Additive effects). Products include:
- Arco-Lase Plus Tablets 513
- Bellergal-S Tablets 2375
- Donnatal 2234
- Donnatal Extentabs 2234
- Donnatal Tablets 2234
- Phenobarbital Elixir and Tablets 1523
- Quadrinal Tablets 1398

Pindolol (Increased sympathomimetic effect). Products include:
- Visken Tablets 2428

Prazepam (Additive effects). No products indexed under this heading.

Prochlorperazine (Additive effects). Products include:
- Compazine 2644

Promethazine Hydrochloride (Additive effects). Products include:
- Mepergan Injection 2859
- Phenergan with Codeine 2883
- Phenergan with Dextromethorphan 2885
- Phenergan Injection 2880
- Phenergan Suppositories 2882
- Phenergan Syrup 2881
- Phenergan Tablets 2882
- Phenergan VC 2886
- Phenergan VC with Codeine 2888

Propofol (Additive effects). Products include:
- Diprivan Injectable Emulsion 2939

Propoxyphene Hydrochloride (Additive effects). Products include:
- Darvon 1475
- Wygesic Tablets 2930

Propoxyphene Napsylate (Additive effects). Products include:
- Darvon-N/Darvocet-N 1473

Propranolol Hydrochloride (Increased sympathomimetic effect). Products include:
- Inderal 2834
- Inderal LA Long Acting Capsules 2836
- Inderide Tablets 2838
- Inderide LA Long Acting Capsules 2840

Quazepam (Additive effects). Products include:
- Doral Tablets 2773

Reserpine (Reduced antihypertensive effects). Products include:
- Diupres Tablets 1691
- Hydropres Tablets 1718
- Ser-Ap-Es Tablets 867

Risperidone (Additive effects). Products include:
- Risperdal Tablets 1348

Secobarbital Sodium (Additive effects). Products include:
- Seconal Sodium Pulvules 1529

Selegiline Hydrochloride (Increased sympathomimetic effect; concurrent therapy is contraindicated). Products include:
- Eldepryl Capsules 2729

Sevoflurane (Additive effects). No products indexed under this heading.

Sotalol Hydrochloride (Increased sympathomimetic effect). Products include:
- Betapace Tablets 637

Sufentanil Citrate (Additive effects). Products include:
- Sufenta Injection 1355

Temazepam (Additive effects). Products include:
- Restoril Capsules 2413

Thiamylal Sodium (Additive effects). No products indexed under this heading.

Thioridazine Hydrochloride (Additive effects). Products include:
- Mellaril 2398

Thiothixene (Additive effects). Products include:
- Navane Capsules and Concentrate 2018
- Navane Intramuscular 2019

Timolol Hemihydrate (Increased sympathomimetic effect). Products include:
- Betimol 0.25%, 0.5% 259

Timolol Maleate (Increased sympathomimetic effect). Products include:
- Blocadren Tablets 1654
- Timolide Tablets 1791
- Timoptic in Ocudose 1796
- Timoptic Sterile Ophthalmic Solution 1794
- Timoptic-XE 1798

Tranylcypromine Sulfate (Increased sympathomimetic effect; concurrent therapy is contraindicated). Products include:
- Parnate Tablets 2679

Triazolam (Additive effects). Products include:
- Halcion Tablets 2093

Trifluoperazine Hydrochloride (Additive effects). Products include:
- Stelazine 2692

Zolpidem Tartrate (Additive effects). Products include:
- Ambien Tablets 2559

Food Interactions
Alcohol (Additive effects).

BROMFED SYRUP
(Brompheniramine Maleate, Pseudoephedrine Hydrochloride) 712
May interact with monoamine oxidase inhibitors, hypnotics and sedatives, tranquilizers, and certain other agents. Compounds in these categories include:

Alprazolam (May increase drowsiness effect). Products include:
- Xanax Tablets 2115

Buspirone Hydrochloride (May increase drowsiness effect). Products include:
- BuSpar Tablets 738

Chlordiazepoxide (May increase drowsiness effect). Products include:
- Limbitrol 2333

Chlordiazepoxide Hydrochloride (May increase drowsiness effect). Products include:
- Librax Capsules 2330

IMPORTANT NOTE: Always consult each drug listing in the patient's regimen for possible interactions.

Interactions Index

Bromfed Syrup

Librium Capsules 2331
Librium Injectable 2332

Chlorpromazine (May increase drowsiness effect). Products include:
Thorazine Suppositories 2701

Chlorpromazine Hydrochloride (May increase drowsiness effect). Products include:
Thorazine 2701

Chlorprothixene (May increase drowsiness effect).
No products indexed under this heading.

Chlorprothixene Hydrochloride (May increase drowsiness effect).
No products indexed under this heading.

Clorazepate Dipotassium (May increase drowsiness effect). Products include:
Tranxene 459

Diazepam (May increase drowsiness effect). Products include:
Dizac (diazepam injectable emulsion) CIV 1862
Valium Injectable 2336
Valium Tablets 2335

Droperidol (May increase drowsiness effect). Products include:
Inapsine Injection 462

Estazolam (May increase drowsiness effect). Products include:
ProSom Tablets 457

Ethchlorvynol (May increase drowsiness effect). Products include:
Placidyl Capsules 456

Ethinamate (May increase drowsiness effect).
No products indexed under this heading.

Fluphenazine Decanoate (May increase drowsiness effect). Products include:
Prolixin Decanoate 510

Fluphenazine Enanthate (May increase drowsiness effect). Products include:
Prolixin Enanthate 510

Fluphenazine Hydrochloride (May increase drowsiness effect). Products include:
Prolixin 510

Flurazepam Hydrochloride (May increase drowsiness effect). Products include:
Dalmane Capsules 2329

Furazolidone (Concurrent and/or sequential use is not recommended). Products include:
Furoxone 2221

Glutethimide (May increase drowsiness effect).
No products indexed under this heading.

Haloperidol (May increase drowsiness effect). Products include:
Haldol Injection, Tablets and Concentrate 1585

Haloperidol Decanoate (May increase drowsiness effect). Products include:
Haldol Decanoate 1587

Hydroxyzine Hydrochloride (May increase drowsiness effect). Products include:
Atarax Tablets & Syrup 1992
Marax Tablets & DF Syrup 2015
Vistaril Intramuscular Solution 2042

Isocarboxazid (Concurrent and/or sequential use is not recommended).
No products indexed under this heading.

Lorazepam (May increase drowsiness effect). Products include:
Ativan Injection 2805
Ativan Tablets 2807

Loxapine Hydrochloride (May increase drowsiness effect). Products include:
Loxitane 1426

Loxapine Succinate (May increase drowsiness effect). Products include:
Loxitane Capsules 1426

Meprobamate (May increase drowsiness effect). Products include:
Miltown Tablets 2780
PMB 200 and PMB 400 2890

Mesoridazine Besylate (May increase drowsiness effect). Products include:
Serentil 689

Midazolam Hydrochloride (May increase drowsiness effect). Products include:
Versed Injection 2324

Molindone Hydrochloride (May increase drowsiness effect). Products include:
Moban Tablets and Concentrate ... 1036

Oxazepam (May increase drowsiness effect). Products include:
Serax Capsules 2916
Serax Tablets 2916

Perphenazine (May increase drowsiness effect). Products include:
Etrafon 2495
Triavil Tablets 1800
Trilafon 2532

Phenelzine Sulfate (Concurrent and/or sequential use is not recommended). Products include:
Nardil 1977

Prazepam (May increase drowsiness effect).
No products indexed under this heading.

Prochlorperazine (May increase drowsiness effect). Products include:
Compazine 2644

Promethazine Hydrochloride (May increase drowsiness effect). Products include:
Mepergan Injection 2859
Phenergan with Codeine 2883
Phenergan with Dextromethorphan 2885
Phenergan Injection 2880
Phenergan Suppositories 2882
Phenergan Syrup 2881
Phenergan Tablets 2882
Phenergan VC 2886
Phenergan VC with Codeine 2888

Propofol (May increase drowsiness effect). Products include:
Diprivan Injectable Emulsion 2939

Quazepam (May increase drowsiness effect). Products include:
Doral Tablets 2773

Secobarbital Sodium (May increase drowsiness effect). Products include:
Seconal Sodium Pulvules 1529

Selegiline Hydrochloride (Concurrent and/or sequential use is not recommended). Products include:
Eldepryl Capsules 2729

Temazepam (May increase drowsiness effect). Products include:
Restoril Capsules 2413

Thioridazine Hydrochloride (May increase drowsiness effect). Products include:
Mellaril 2398

Thiothixene (May increase drowsiness effect). Products include:
Navane Capsules and Concentrate 2018
Navane Intramuscular 2019

Tranylcypromine Sulfate (Concurrent and/or sequential use is not recommended). Products include:
Parnate Tablets 2679

Triazolam (May increase drowsiness effect). Products include:
Halcion Tablets 2093

Trifluoperazine Hydrochloride (May increase drowsiness effect). Products include:
Stelazine 2692

Zolpidem Tartrate (May increase drowsiness effect). Products include:
Ambien Tablets 2559

Food Interactions

Alcohol (May increase drowsiness effect).

BROMFED TABLETS
(Brompheniramine Maleate, Pseudoephedrine Hydrochloride) 1832
See **Bromfed Capsules (Extended-Release)**

BROMFED-DM COUGH SYRUP
(Brompheniramine Maleate, Pseudoephedrine Hydrochloride, Dextromethorphan Hydrobromide) 1832
May interact with central nervous system depressants, tranquilizers, hypnotics and sedatives, monoamine oxidase inhibitors, antihypertensives, and certain other agents. Compounds in these categories include:

Acebutolol Hydrochloride (Sympathomimetic, pseudoephedrine, may reduce the effects of antihypertensives). Products include:
Sectral Capsules 2914

Alfentanil Hydrochloride (Potential for additive effects). Products include:
Alfenta Injection 1334

Alprazolam (Potential for additive effects). Products include:
Xanax Tablets 2115

Amlodipine Besylate (Sympathomimetic, pseudoephedrine, may reduce the effects of antihypertensives). Products include:
Lotrel Capsules 858
Norvasc Tablets 2020

Aprobarbital (Potential for additive effects).
No products indexed under this heading.

Atenolol (Sympathomimetic, pseudoephedrine, may reduce the effects of antihypertensives). Products include:
Tenoretic Tablets 2963
Tenormin Tablets and I.V. Injection 2965

Benazepril Hydrochloride (Sympathomimetic, pseudoephedrine, may reduce the effects of antihypertensives). Products include:
Lotensin Tablets 852
Lotensin HCT Tablets 855
Lotrel Capsules 858

Bendroflumethiazide (Sympathomimetic, pseudoephedrine, may reduce the effects of antihypertensives).
No products indexed under this heading.

Betaxolol Hydrochloride (Sympathomimetic, pseudoephedrine, may reduce the effects of antihypertensives). Products include:
Betoptic Ophthalmic Solution 465
Betoptic S Ophthalmic Suspension 467
Kerlone Tablets 2588

Bisoprolol Fumarate (Sympathomimetic, pseudoephedrine, may reduce the effects of antihypertensives). Products include:
Zebeta Tablets 1457
Ziac 1459

Buprenorphine (Potential for additive effects). Products include:
Buprenex Injectable 2170

Buspirone Hydrochloride (Potential for additive effects). Products include:
BuSpar Tablets 738

Butabarbital (Potential for additive effects).
No products indexed under this heading.

Butalbital (Potential for additive effects). Products include:
Axocet Capsules 2469
Esgic-plus Capsules 1012
Esgic-plus Tablets 1012
Fioricet Tablets 2386
Fioricet with Codeine Capsules ... 2387
Fiorinal Capsules 2388
Fiorinal with Codeine Capsules ... 2390
Fiorinal Tablets 2388
Phrenilin 790
Sedapap Tablets 50 mg/650 mg .. 1826

Captopril (Sympathomimetic, pseudoephedrine, may reduce the effects of antihypertensives). Products include:
Capoten Tablets 740
Capozide Tablets 744

Carteolol Hydrochloride (Sympathomimetic, pseudoephedrine, may reduce the effects of antihypertensives). Products include:
Cartrol Tablets 413
Ocupress Ophthalmic Solution, 1% Sterile .... ⊙ 297

Chlordiazepoxide (Potential for additive effects). Products include:
Limbitrol 2333

Chlordiazepoxide Hydrochloride (Potential for additive effects). Products include:
Librax Capsules 2330
Librium Capsules 2331
Librium Injectable 2332

Chlorothiazide (Sympathomimetic, pseudoephedrine, may reduce the effects of antihypertensives). Products include:
Aldoclor Tablets 1638
Diupres Tablets 1691
Diuril Oral 1694

Chlorothiazide Sodium (Sympathomimetic, pseudoephedrine, may reduce the effects of antihypertensives). Products include:
Diuril Sodium Intravenous 1693

Chlorpromazine (Potential for additive effects). Products include:
Thorazine Suppositories 2701

Chlorpromazine Hydrochloride (Potential for additive effects). Products include:
Thorazine 2701

Chlorprothixene (Potential for additive effects).
No products indexed under this heading.

Chlorprothixene Hydrochloride (Potential for additive effects).
No products indexed under this heading.

Chlorprothixene Lactate (Potential for additive effects).
No products indexed under this heading.

Chlorthalidone (Sympathomimetic, pseudoephedrine, may reduce the effects of antihypertensives). Products include:
Combipres Tablets 682
Tenoretic Tablets 2963
Thalitone 1293

Clonidine (Sympathomimetic, pseudoephedrine, may reduce the effects of antihypertensives). Products include:
Catapres-TTS 680

Clonidine Hydrochloride (Sympathomimetic, pseudoephedrine, may reduce the effects of antihypertensives). Products include:
Catapres Tablets 679

(▣ Described in PDR For Nonprescription Drugs)   (⊙ Described in PDR For Ophthalmology)

Combipres Tablets ... 682

Clorazepate Dipotassium (Potential for additive effects). Products include:
Tranxene ... 459

Clozapine (Potential for additive effects). Products include:
Clozaril Tablets ... 2377

Codeine Phosphate (Potential for additive effects). Products include:
Brontex ... 2130
Dimetane-DC Cough Syrup ... 2232
Fioricet with Codeine Capsules ... 2387
Fiorinal with Codeine Capsules ... 2390
Nucofed ... 2225
Phenergan with Codeine ... 2883
Phenergan VC with Codeine ... 2888
Robitussin A-C Syrup ... 2248
Robitussin-DAC Syrup ... 2249
Ryna ... 804
Soma Compound w/Codeine Tablets ... 2784
Tylenol with Codeine ... 1592

Deserpidine (Sympathomimetic, pseudoephedrine, may reduce the effects of antihypertensives).
No products indexed under this heading.

Desflurane (Potential for additive effects). Products include:
Suprane (desflurane, USP) ... 1865

Dezocine (Potential for additive effects). Products include:
Dalgan Injection ... 529

Diazepam (Potential for additive effects). Products include:
Dizac (diazepam injectable emulsion) CIV ... 1862
Valium Injectable ... 2336
Valium Tablets ... 2335

Diazoxide (Sympathomimetic, pseudoephedrine, may reduce the effects of antihypertensives). Products include:
Hyperstat I.V. Injection ... 2504
Proglycem ... 575

Diltiazem Hydrochloride (Sympathomimetic, pseudoephedrine, may reduce the effects of antihypertensives). Products include:
Cardizem CD Capsules ... 1251
Cardizem SR Capsules ... 1255
Cardizem Injectable ... 1253
Cardizem Tablets ... 1257
Dilacor XR Extended-release Capsules ... 2183
Tiazac Capsules ... 1019

Doxazosin Mesylate (Sympathomimetic, pseudoephedrine, may reduce the effects of antihypertensives). Products include:
Cardura Tablets ... 1993

Droperidol (Potential for additive effects). Products include:
Inapsine Injection ... 462

Enalapril Maleate (Sympathomimetic, pseudoephedrine, may reduce the effects of antihypertensives). Products include:
Vaseretic Tablets ... 1810
Vasotec Tablets ... 1816

Enalaprilat (Sympathomimetic, pseudoephedrine, may reduce the effects of antihypertensives). Products include:
Vasotec I.V. ... 1814

Enflurane (Potential for additive effects).
No products indexed under this heading.

Esmolol Hydrochloride (Sympathomimetic, pseudoephedrine, may reduce the effects of antihypertensives). Products include:
Brevibloc (esmolol HCl) Injection ... 1860

Estazolam (Potential for additive effects). Products include:
ProSom Tablets ... 457

Ethchlorvynol (Potential for additive effects). Products include:
Placidyl Capsules ... 456

Ethinamate (Potential for additive effects).
No products indexed under this heading.

Felodipine (Sympathomimetic, pseudoephedrine, may reduce the effects of antihypertensives). Products include:
Plendil Extended-Release Tablets ... 514

Fentanyl (Potential for additive effects). Products include:
Duragesic Transdermal System ... 1336

Fentanyl Citrate (Potential for additive effects). Products include:
Sublimaze Injection ... 463

Fluphenazine Decanoate (Potential for additive effects). Products include:
Prolixin Decanoate ... 510

Fluphenazine Enanthate (Potential for additive effects). Products include:
Prolixin Enanthate ... 510

Fluphenazine Hydrochloride (Potential for additive effects). Products include:
Prolixin ... 510

Flurazepam Hydrochloride (Potential for additive effects). Products include:
Dalmane Capsules ... 2329

Fosinopril Sodium (Sympathomimetic, pseudoephedrine, may reduce the effects of antihypertensives). Products include:
Monopril Tablets ... 762

Furazolidone (Prolongs and intensifies the anticholinergic effects; enhances pseudoephedrine effects; concurrent use is contraindicated). Products include:
Furoxone ... 2221

Furosemide (Sympathomimetic, pseudoephedrine, may reduce the effects of antihypertensives). Products include:
Lasix Injection, Oral Solution and Tablets ... 1267

Glutethimide (Potential for additive effects).
No products indexed under this heading.

Guanabenz Acetate (Sympathomimetic, pseudoephedrine, may reduce the effects of antihypertensives).
No products indexed under this heading.

Guanethidine Monosulfate (Sympathomimetic, pseudoephedrine, may reduce the effects of antihypertensives). Products include:
Esimil Tablets ... 840
Ismelin Tablets ... 845

Haloperidol (Potential for additive effects). Products include:
Haldol Injection, Tablets and Concentrate ... 1585

Haloperidol Decanoate (Potential for additive effects). Products include:
Haldol Decanoate ... 1587

Hydralazine Hydrochloride (Sympathomimetic, pseudoephedrine, may reduce the effects of antihypertensives). Products include:
Apresazide Capsules ... 824
Apresoline Hydrochloride Tablets ... 826
Hydralazine Hydrochloride Injection USP ... 2712
Ser-Ap-Es Tablets ... 867

Hydrochlorothiazide (Sympathomimetic, pseudoephedrine, may reduce the effects of antihypertensives). Products include:
Aldactazide Tablets ... 2556
Aldoril Tablets ... 1644
Apresazide Capsules ... 824
Capozide Tablets ... 744
Dyazide Capsules ... 2653
Esidrix Tablets ... 839
Esimil Tablets ... 840
HydroDIURIL Tablets ... 1716
Hydropres Tablets ... 1718
Hyzaar Tablets ... 1720
Inderide Tablets ... 2838
Inderide LA Long Acting Capsules ... 2840
Lopressor HCT Tablets ... 850
Lotensin HCT Tablets ... 855
Moduretic Tablets ... 1748
Oretic Tablets ... 450
Prinzide Tablets ... 1780
Ser-Ap-Es Tablets ... 867
Timolide Tablets ... 1791
Vaseretic Tablets ... 1810
Zestoretic Tablets ... 2968
Ziac ... 1459

Hydrocodone Bitartrate (Potential for additive effects). Products include:
Codiclear DH Syrup ... 808
Duratuss HD Elixir ... 2750
Histussin D Liquid ... 670
Hycodan Tablets and Syrup ... 946
Hycomine Compound Tablets ... 948
Hycomine ... 947
Hycotuss Expectorant Syrup ... 950
Hydrocet Capsules ... 787
Lorcet 10/650 Tablets ... 1016
Lortab ... 2751
Tussend ... 1830
Tussend Expectorant ... 1831
Vicodin Tablets ... 1404
Vicodin ES Tablets ... 1405
Vicodin HP Tablets ... 1403
Vicodin Tuss Expectorant ... 1406
Zydone Capsules ... 967

Hydrocodone Polistirex (Potential for additive effects). Products include:
Tussionex Pennkinetic Extended-Release Suspension ... 1624

Hydroflumethiazide (Sympathomimetic, pseudoephedrine, may reduce the effects of antihypertensives). Products include:
Diucardin Tablets ... 2824

Hydroxyzine Hydrochloride (Potential for additive effects). Products include:
Atarax Tablets & Syrup ... 1992
Marax Tablets & DF Syrup ... 2015
Vistaril Intramuscular Solution ... 2042

Indapamide (Sympathomimetic, pseudoephedrine, may reduce the effects of antihypertensives).
No products indexed under this heading.

Isocarboxazid (Prolongs and intensifies the anticholinergic effects; enhances pseudoephedrine effects; concurrent use is contraindicated).
No products indexed under this heading.

Isoflurane (Potential for additive effects).
No products indexed under this heading.

Isradipine (Sympathomimetic, pseudoephedrine, may reduce the effects of antihypertensives). Products include:
DynaCirc Capsules ... 2381
DynaCirc CR Tablets ... 2383

Ketamine Hydrochloride (Potential for additive effects).
No products indexed under this heading.

Labetalol Hydrochloride (Sympathomimetic, pseudoephedrine, may reduce the effects of antihypertensives). Products include:
Normodyne Injection ... 2519
Normodyne Tablets ... 2522
Trandate ... 1158

Levomethadyl Acetate Hydrochloride (Potential for additive effects). Products include:
Orlaam Oral Solution ... 2361

Levorphanol Tartrate (Potential for additive effects). Products include:
Levo-Dromoran ... 2297

Lisinopril (Sympathomimetic, pseudoephedrine, may reduce the effects of antihypertensives). Products include:
Prinivil Tablets ... 1776
Prinzide Tablets ... 1780
Zestoretic Tablets ... 2968
Zestril Tablets ... 2972

Lorazepam (Potential for additive effects). Products include:
Ativan Injection ... 2805
Ativan Tablets ... 2807

Losartan Potassium (Sympathomimetic, pseudoephedrine, may reduce the effects of antihypertensives). Products include:
Cozaar Tablets ... 1668
Hyzaar Tablets ... 1720

Loxapine Hydrochloride (Potential for additive effects). Products include:
Loxitane ... 1426

Loxapine Succinate (Potential for additive effects). Products include:
Loxitane Capsules ... 1426

Mecamylamine Hydrochloride (Sympathomimetic, pseudoephedrine, may reduce the effects of antihypertensives). Products include:
Inversine Tablets ... 1729

Meperidine Hydrochloride (Potential for additive effects). Products include:
Demerol ... 2438
Mepergan Injection ... 2859

Mephobarbital (Potential for additive effects). Products include:
Mebaral Tablets ... 2452

Meprobamate (Potential for additive effects). Products include:
Miltown Tablets ... 2780
PMB 200 and PMB 400 ... 2890

Mesoridazine Besylate (Potential for additive effects). Products include:
Serentil ... 689

Methadone Hydrochloride (Potential for additive effects). Products include:
Methadone Hydrochloride Oral Concentrate ... 2356
Methadone Hydrochloride Oral Solution & Tablets ... 2357

Methohexital Sodium (Potential for additive effects).
No products indexed under this heading.

Methotrimeprazine (Potential for additive effects). Products include:
Levoprome ... 1321

Methoxyflurane (Potential for additive effects).
No products indexed under this heading.

Methyclothiazide (Sympathomimetic, pseudoephedrine, may reduce the effects of antihypertensives). Products include:
Enduron Tablets ... 424

Methyldopa (Sympathomimetic, pseudoephedrine, may reduce the effects of antihypertensives). Products include:
Aldoclor Tablets ... 1638
Aldomet Oral ... 1640
Aldoril Tablets ... 1644

IMPORTANT NOTE: Always consult each drug listing in the patient's regimen for possible interactions.

Methyldopate Hydrochloride (Sympathomimetic, pseudoephedrine, may reduce the effects of antihypertensives). Products include:
- Aldomet Ester HCl Injection 1642

Metolazone (Sympathomimetic, pseudoephedrine, may reduce the effects of antihypertensives). Products include:
- Mykrox Tablets 1617
- Zaroxolyn Tablets 1625

Metoprolol Succinate (Sympathomimetic, pseudoephedrine, may reduce the effects of antihypertensives). Products include:
- Toprol-XL Tablets 560

Metoprolol Tartrate (Sympathomimetic, pseudoephedrine, may reduce the effects of antihypertensives). Products include:
- Lopressor 848
- Lopressor HCT Tablets 850

Metyrosine (Sympathomimetic, pseudoephedrine, may reduce the effects of antihypertensives). Products include:
- Demser Capsules 1690

Midazolam Hydrochloride (Potential for additive effects). Products include:
- Versed Injection 2324

Minoxidil (Sympathomimetic, pseudoephedrine, may reduce the effects of antihypertensives).
- No products indexed under this heading.

Moexipril Hydrochloride (Sympathomimetic, pseudoephedrine, may reduce the effects of antihypertensives). Products include:
- Univasc Tablets 2553

Molindone Hydrochloride (Potential for additive effects). Products include:
- Moban Tablets and Concentrate 1036

Morphine Sulfate (Potential for additive effects). Products include:
- Astramorph/PF Injection, USP (Preservative-Free) 526
- Duramorph Injection 983
- Infumorph 200 and Infumorph 500 Sterile Solutions 985
- Kadian Capsules 2948
- MS Contin Tablets 2149
- MSIR 2152
- Oramorph SR (Morphine Sulfate Sustained Release Tablets) 2359
- RMS Suppositories CII 2766
- Roxanol 2365

Nadolol (Sympathomimetic, pseudoephedrine, may reduce the effects of antihypertensives).
- No products indexed under this heading.

Nicardipine Hydrochloride (Sympathomimetic, pseudoephedrine, may reduce the effects of antihypertensives). Products include:
- Cardene Capsules 2261
- Cardene I.V. 2815
- Cardene SR Capsules 2264

Nifedipine (Sympathomimetic, pseudoephedrine, may reduce the effects of antihypertensives). Products include:
- Adalat Capsules (10 mg and 20 mg) 580
- Adalat CC 582
- Procardia Capsules 2024
- Procardia XL Extended Release Tablets 2026

Nisoldipine (Sympathomimetic, pseudoephedrine, may reduce the effects of antihypertensives). Products include:
- Sular Tablets 2961

Nitroglycerin (Sympathomimetic, pseudoephedrine, may reduce the effects of antihypertensives). Products include:
- Deponit NTG Transdermal Delivery System 2541
- Nitro-Bid IV 1270
- Nitro-Bid Ointment 1272
- Nitro-Dur (nitroglycerin) Transdermal Infusion System 1365
- Nitrolingual Spray 2193
- Nitrostat Tablets 1981
- Transderm-Nitro Transdermal Therapeutic System 878

Opium Alkaloids (Potential for additive effects).
- No products indexed under this heading.

Oxazepam (Potential for additive effects). Products include:
- Serax Capsules 2916
- Serax Tablets 2916

Oxycodone Hydrochloride (Potential for additive effects). Products include:
- OxyContin Tablets 2163
- OxyIR Capsules 2167
- Percocet Tablets 955
- Percodan Tablets 955
- Percodan-Demi Tablets 956
- Roxicodone Tablets, Oral Solution & Intensol (Oxycodone) 2366
- Tylox Capsules 1593

Penbutolol Sulfate (Sympathomimetic, pseudoephedrine, may reduce the effects of antihypertensives). Products include:
- Levatol Tablets 2547

Pentobarbital Sodium (Potential for additive effects). Products include:
- Nembutal Sodium Capsules 440
- Nembutal Sodium Solution 442
- Nembutal Sodium Suppositories 444

Perphenazine (Potential for additive effects). Products include:
- Etrafon 2495
- Triavil Tablets 1800
- Trilafon 2532

Phenelzine Sulfate (Prolongs and intensifies the anticholinergic effects; enhances pseudoephedrine effects; concurrent use is contraindicated). Products include:
- Nardil 1977

Phenobarbital (Potential for additive effects). Products include:
- Arco-Lase Plus Tablets 513
- Bellergal-S Tablets 2375
- Donnatal 2234
- Donnatal Extentabs 2234
- Donnatal Tablets 2234
- Phenobarbital Elixir and Tablets 1523
- Quadrinal Tablets 1398

Phenoxybenzamine Hydrochloride (Sympathomimetic, pseudoephedrine, may reduce the effects of antihypertensives). Products include:
- Dibenzyline Capsules 2650

Phentolamine Mesylate (Sympathomimetic, pseudoephedrine, may reduce the effects of antihypertensives). Products include:
- Regitine Vials 864

Pindolol (Sympathomimetic, pseudoephedrine, may reduce the effects of antihypertensives). Products include:
- Visken Tablets 2428

Polythiazide (Sympathomimetic, pseudoephedrine, may reduce the effects of antihypertensives). Products include:
- Minizide Capsules 2016

Prazepam (Potential for additive effects).
- No products indexed under this heading.

Prazosin Hydrochloride (Sympathomimetic, pseudoephedrine, may reduce the effects of antihypertensives). Products include:
- Minipress Capsules 2015
- Minizide Capsules 2016

Prochlorperazine (Potential for additive effects). Products include:
- Compazine 2644

Promethazine Hydrochloride (Potential for additive effects). Products include:
- Mepergan Injection 2859
- Phenergan with Codeine 2883
- Phenergan with Dextromethorphan ... 2885
- Phenergan Injection 2880
- Phenergan Suppositories 2882
- Phenergan Syrup 2881
- Phenergan Tablets 2882
- Phenergan VC 2886
- Phenergan VC with Codeine 2888

Propofol (Potential for additive effects). Products include:
- Diprivan Injectable Emulsion 2939

Propoxyphene Hydrochloride (Potential for additive effects). Products include:
- Darvon 1475
- Wygesic Tablets 2930

Propoxyphene Napsylate (Potential for additive effects). Products include:
- Darvon-N/Darvocet-N 1473

Propranolol Hydrochloride (Sympathomimetic, pseudoephedrine, may reduce the effects of antihypertensives). Products include:
- Inderal 2834
- Inderal LA Long Acting Capsules 2836
- Inderide Tablets 2838
- Inderide LA Long Acting Capsules ... 2840

Quazepam (Potential for additive effects). Products include:
- Doral Tablets 2773

Quinapril Hydrochloride (Sympathomimetic, pseudoephedrine, may reduce the effects of antihypertensives). Products include:
- Accupril Tablets 1950

Ramipril (Sympathomimetic, pseudoephedrine, may reduce the effects of antihypertensives). Products include:
- Altace Capsules 1238

Rauwolfia Serpentina (Sympathomimetic, pseudoephedrine, may reduce the effects of antihypertensives).
- No products indexed under this heading.

Rescinnamine (Sympathomimetic, pseudoephedrine, may reduce the effects of antihypertensives).
- No products indexed under this heading.

Reserpine (Sympathomimetic, pseudoephedrine, may reduce the effects of antihypertensives). Products include:
- Diupres Tablets 1691
- Hydropres Tablets 1718
- Ser-Ap-Es Tablets 867

Risperidone (Potential for additive effects). Products include:
- Risperdal Tablets 1348

Secobarbital Sodium (Potential for additive effects). Products include:
- Seconal Sodium Pulvules 1529

Selegiline Hydrochloride (Prolongs and intensifies the anticholinergic effects; enhances pseudoephedrine effects; concurrent use is contraindicated). Products include:
- Eldepryl Capsules 2729

Sevoflurane (Potential for additive effects).
- No products indexed under this heading.

Sodium Nitroprusside (Sympathomimetic, pseudoephedrine, may reduce the effects of antihypertensives).
- No products indexed under this heading.

Sotalol Hydrochloride (Sympathomimetic, pseudoephedrine, may reduce the effects of antihypertensives). Products include:
- Betapace Tablets 637

Spirapril Hydrochloride (Sympathomimetic, pseudoephedrine, may reduce the effects of antihypertensives).
- No products indexed under this heading.

Sufentanil Citrate (Potential for additive effects). Products include:
- Sufenta Injection 1355

Temazepam (Potential for additive effects). Products include:
- Restoril Capsules 2413

Terazosin Hydrochloride (Sympathomimetic, pseudoephedrine, may reduce the effects of antihypertensives). Products include:
- Hytrin Capsules 434

Thiamylal Sodium (Potential for additive effects).
- No products indexed under this heading.

Thioridazine Hydrochloride (Potential for additive effects). Products include:
- Mellaril 2398

Thiothixene (Potential for additive effects). Products include:
- Navane Capsules and Concentrate 2018
- Navane Intramuscular 2019

Timolol Maleate (Sympathomimetic, pseudoephedrine, may reduce the effects of antihypertensives). Products include:
- Blocadren Tablets 1654
- Timolide Tablets 1791
- Timoptic in Ocudose 1796
- Timoptic Sterile Ophthalmic Solution 1794
- Timoptic-XE 1798

Torsemide (Sympathomimetic, pseudoephedrine, may reduce the effects of antihypertensives). Products include:
- Demadex Tablets and Injection 691

Tranylcypromine Sulfate (Prolongs and intensifies the anticholinergic effects; enhances pseudoephedrine effects; concurrent use is contraindicated). Products include:
- Parnate Tablets 2679

Triazolam (Potential for additive effects). Products include:
- Halcion Tablets 2093

Trifluoperazine Hydrochloride (Potential for additive effects). Products include:
- Stelazine 2692

Trimethaphan Camsylate (Sympathomimetic, pseudoephedrine, may reduce the effects of antihypertensives).
- No products indexed under this heading.

Verapamil Hydrochloride (Sympathomimetic, pseudoephedrine, may reduce the effects of antihypertensives). Products include:
- Calan SR Caplets 2571
- Calan Tablets 2568
- Covera-HS Tablets 2573
- Isoptin Injectable 1391
- Isoptin Oral Tablets 1393
- Isoptin SR Tablets 1395
- Verelan Capsules 1455

Zolpidem Tartrate (Potential for additive effects). Products include:
- Ambien Tablets 2559

Food Interactions
Alcohol (Potential for additive effects).

BROMFED-PD CAPSULES (EXTENDED-RELEASE)
(Brompheniramine Maleate, Pseudoephedrine Hydrochloride) 1832
See Bromfed Capsules (Extended-Release)

BRONKOMETER AEROSOL
(Isoetharine) 2432
See Bronkosol Solution

BRONKOSOL SOLUTION
(Isoetharine) 2432
May interact with sympathomimetics. Compounds in this category include:

Albuterol (May cause excessive tachycardia due to direct cardiac stimulation). Products include:
- Proventil Inhalation Aerosol 2524
- Ventolin Inhalation Aerosol and Refill 1170

Albuterol Sulfate (May cause excessive tachycardia due to direct cardiac stimulation). Products include:
- Airet Albuterol Sulfate Inhalation Solution 1602
- Albuterol Sulfate, USP Solution for Inhalation, Arm-a-Med 522
- Proventil Inhalation Solution 0.083% 2527
- Proventil Repetabs Tablets 2529
- Proventil Solution for Inhalation 0.5% 2525
- Proventil Syrup 2528
- Proventil Tablets 2529
- Ventolin Inhalation Solution 1171
- Ventolin Nebules Inhalation Solution 1172
- Ventolin Rotacaps for Inhalation 1173
- Ventolin Syrup 1175
- Ventolin Tablets 1176
- Volmax Extended-Release Tablets .. 1835

Dobutamine Hydrochloride (May cause excessive tachycardia due to direct cardiac stimulation). Products include:
- Dobutrex Solution Vials 1480

Dopamine Hydrochloride (May cause excessive tachycardia due to direct cardiac stimulation).
No products indexed under this heading.

Ephedrine Hydrochloride (May cause excessive tachycardia due to direct cardiac stimulation). Products include:
- Primatene Tablets .... ▣ 844
- Quadrinal Tablets 1398

Ephedrine Sulfate (May cause excessive tachycardia due to direct cardiac stimulation). Products include:
- Marax Tablets & DF Syrup 2015

Ephedrine Tannate (May cause excessive tachycardia due to direct cardiac stimulation). Products include:
- Rynatuss 2782

Epinephrine (May cause excessive tachycardia due to direct cardiac stimulation). Products include:
- EPIFRIN .... ⊙ 237
- EpiPen 808
- Marcaine with Epinephrine 2446
- Primatene Mist .... ▣ 843
- Sensorcaine with Epinephrine Injection 554
- Sus-Phrine Injection 1017
- Xylocaine with Epinephrine Injections 562

Epinephrine Bitartrate (May cause excessive tachycardia due to direct cardiac stimulation). Products include:
- Sensorcaine-MPF with Epinephrine Injection 554

Epinephrine Hydrochloride (May cause excessive tachycardia due to direct cardiac stimulation). Products include:
- Ana-Kit Anaphylaxis Emergency Treatment Kit 611

Isoproterenol Hydrochloride (May cause excessive tachycardia due to direct cardiac stimulation). Products include:
- Isuprel Hydrochloride Solution 2443
- Isuprel Injection 2441
- Isuprel Mistometer 2442

Isoproterenol Sulfate (May cause excessive tachycardia due to direct cardiac stimulation). Products include:
- Norisodrine with Calcium Iodide Syrup 446

Metaproterenol Sulfate (May cause excessive tachycardia due to direct cardiac stimulation). Products include:
- Alupent 672
- Metaproterenol Sulfate Inhalation Solution, USP, Arm-a-Med 547

Metaraminol Bitartrate (May cause excessive tachycardia due to direct cardiac stimulation). Products include:
- Aramine Injection 1649

Methoxamine Hydrochloride (May cause excessive tachycardia due to direct cardiac stimulation). Products include:
- Vasoxyl Injection 1169

Norepinephrine Bitartrate (May cause excessive tachycardia due to direct cardiac stimulation). Products include:
- Levophed Bitartrate Injection 2445

Phenylephrine Bitartrate (May cause excessive tachycardia due to direct cardiac stimulation).
No products indexed under this heading.

Phenylephrine Hydrochloride (May cause excessive tachycardia due to direct cardiac stimulation). Products include:
- Atrohist Plus Tablets 1605
- Cerose DM .... ▣ 853
- D.A. II Tablets 972
- D.A. Chewable Tablets 970
- Dura-Vent/DA Tablets 972
- Extendryl 1003
- 4-Way Fast Acting Nasal Spray (regular & mentholated) .... ▣ 644
- Hemoril .... ▣ 797
- Hycomine Compound Tablets 948
- Neo-Synephrine Hydrochloride 1% Carpuject 2455
- Neo-Synephrine Hydrochloride 1% Injection 2455
- Neo-Synephrine Hydrochloride (Ophthalmic) 2456
- Neo-Synephrine 624
- Novahistine Elixir .... ▣ 782
- Phenergan VC 2886
- Phenergan VC with Codeine 2888
- Preparation H .... ▣ 842
- Tympagesic Ear Drops 2476
- Vicks Sinex Nasal Spray and Ultra Fine Mist .... ▣ 738

Phenylephrine Tannate (May cause excessive tachycardia due to direct cardiac stimulation). Products include:
- Atrohist Pediatric Suspension 1604
- Atrohist Pediatric Suspension Dye-Free 1604
- Rynatan 2781
- Rynatuss 2782

Phenylpropanolamine Hydrochloride (May cause excessive tachycardia due to direct cardiac stimulation). Products include:
- Acutrim 648
- Atrohist Plus Tablets 1605
- BC Cold Powder Multi-Symptom Formula (Cold-Sinus-Allergy) ... ▣ 631
- BC Cold Powder Non-Drowsy Formula (Cold-Sinus) .... ▣ 631
- Cheracol Plus Head Cold/Cough Formula .... ▣ 741
- Comtrex Multi-Symptom Cold Reliever Liqui-Gels .... ▣ 638
- Comtrex Multi-Symptom Non-Drowsy Liqui-gels .... ▣ 640
- Contac Continuous Action Nasal Decongestant/Antihistamine 12 Hour Capsules .... ▣ 773
- Contac Maximum Strength Continuous Action Decongestant/Antihistamine 12 Hour Caplets .. ▣ 772
- Contac Severe Cold and Flu Formula Caplets .... ▣ 773
- Coricidin 'D' Decongestant Tablets .... ▣ 760
- Dexatrim .... ▣ 795
- Dexatrim Plus Vitamins Caplets .. ▣ 796
- Dimetane-DC Cough Syrup 2232
- Dimetapp Allergy Sinus Caplets ... ▣ 838
- Dimetapp Cold & Allergy Chewable Tablets .... ▣ 838
- Dimetapp Cold & Cough Liqui-Gels .... ▣ 839
- Dimetapp DM Elixir .... ▣ 840
- Dimetapp Elixir .... ▣ 840
- Dimetapp Extentabs .... ▣ 841
- Dimetapp Tablets/Liqui-Gels .... ▣ 841
- Dura-Vent Tablets 971
- Entex LA Tablets 972
- Exgest LA Tablets 787
- Hycomine 947
- Nolamine Timed-Release Tablets 790
- Ornade Spansule Capsules 2678
- Propagest Tablets 791
- Pyrroxate Caplets .... ▣ 742
- Robitussin-CF .... ▣ 846
- Sinulin Tablets 792
- Tavist-D 12 Hour Relief Tablets .. ▣ 750
- Teldrin 12 Hour Antihistamine/Nasal Decongestant Allergy Relief Capsules .... ▣ 786
- Triaminic Expectorant .... ▣ 753
- Triaminic Syrup .... ▣ 755
- Triaminic Triaminicol Cold & Cough .... ▣ 756
- Triaminic DM Syrup .... ▣ 756
- Triaminicin Tablets .... ▣ 756
- Vicks DayQuil Allergy Relief 12-Hour Extended Release Tablets .. ▣ 733
- Vicks DayQuil Allergy Relief 4-Hour Tablets .... ▣ 733
- Vicks DayQuil SINUS Pressure & CONGESTION Relief................ ▣ 734

Pirbuterol Acetate (May cause excessive tachycardia due to direct cardiac stimulation). Products include:
- Maxair Autohaler 1550
- Maxair Inhaler 1552

Pseudoephedrine Hydrochloride (May cause excessive tachycardia due to direct cardiac stimulation). Products include:
- Actifed Allergy Daytime/Nighttime Caplets .... ▣ 808
- Actifed Cold & Allergy Tablets .. ▣ 807
- Actifed Cold & Sinus Caplets and Tablets .... ▣ 808
- Actifed Sinus Daytime/Nighttime Tablets and Caplets .... ▣ 809
- Advil Cold and Sinus Caplets and Tablets .... ▣ 837
- Alka-Seltzer Plus Liqui-Gels..... ▣ 612
- Alka-Seltzer Plus Flu & Body Aches Liqui-Gels Non-Drowsy Formula .... ▣ 613
- Alka-Seltzer Plus Night-Time Cold Medicine Liqui-Gels .... ▣ 612
- Allerest Maximum Strength .... ▣ 649
- Allerest No Drowsiness .... ▣ 649
- Allerest Sinus Pain Formula ..... ▣ 649
- Atrohist Pediatric Capsules 1603
- Benadryl Allergy/Cold Tablets.. ▣ 811
- Benadryl Allergy Decongestant Liquid Medication .... ▣ 812
- Benadryl Allergy Decongestant Tablets .... ▣ 812
- Benadryl Allergy Sinus Headache Caplets .... ▣ 813
- Benylin Multisymptom .... ▣ 816
- Bromfed Capsules (Extended-Release) 1832
- Bromfed Syrup .... ▣ 712
- Bromfed Tablets 1832
- Bromfed-DM Cough Syrup 1832
- Bromfed-PD Capsules (Extended-Release) 1832
- Children's TYLENOL Cold Multi-Symptom Chewable Tablets and Liquid 1559
- Children's TYLENOL Cold Plus Cough Multi Symptom Chewable Tablets and Liquid 1560
- Children's TYLENOL Flu Suspension Liquid 1560
- Children's Vicks DayQuil Allergy Relief .... ▣ 730
- Children's Vicks NyQuil Cold/Cough Relief .... ▣ 731
- Allergy-Sinus Comtrex Multi-Symptom Allergy-Sinus Formula Tablets and Caplets .... ▣ 639
- Comtrex Multi-Symptom.......... ▣ 638
- Comtrex Multi-Symptom Non-Drowsy Caplets .... ▣ 640
- Congess 1003
- Contac Day Allergy/Sinus Caplets . ▣ 771
- Contac Day & Night .... ▣ 772
- Contac Night Allergy/Sinus Caplets .... ▣ 771
- Contac Severe Cold & Flu Non-Drowsy .... ▣ 774
- Deconsal II Tablets 1605
- Dimetane-DX Cough Syrup 2233
- Dimetapp Cold & Fever Suspension .... ▣ 839
- Dimetapp Decongestant Pediatric Drops .... ▣ 840
- Dorcol Children's Cough Syrup.. ▣ 748
- Drixoral Cough + Congestion Liqui Caps .... ▣ 763
- Dura-Tap/PD Capsules 970
- Duratuss Tablets 2750
- Duratuss HD Elixir 2750
- Efidac/24 .... ▣ 655
- Entex PSE Tablets 973
- Fedahist Gyrocaps 2545
- Guaifed 1833
- Guaifed Syrup .... ▣ 712
- Guaimax-D Tablets 809
- Histussin D Liquid 670
- Infants' TYLENOL Cold Decongestant & Fever-Reducer Drops 1561
- Kronofed-A 994
- Novahistine DMX .... ▣ 782
- Nucofed 2225
- PediaCare Cough-Cold Chewable Tablets and Liquid 1569
- PediaCare Infants' Decongestant Drops 1569
- PediaCare Infants' Drops Decongestant Plus Cough 1569
- PediaCare NightRest Cough-Cold Liquid 1569
- Pediatric Vicks 44d Cough & Head Congestion Relief .... ▣ 736
- Pediatric Vicks 44m Cough & Cold Relief .... ▣ 737
- Robitussin Cold & Cough Liqui-Gels .... ▣ 844
- Robitussin Cold, Cough & Flu Liqui-Gels .... ▣ 844
- Robitussin Maximum Strength Cough & Cold .... ▣ 847
- Robitussin Night-Time Cold Formula .... ▣ 847
- Robitussin Pediatric Cough & Cold Formula .... ▣ 848
- Robitussin Pediatric Drops ...... ▣ 849
- Robitussin Severe Congestion Liqui-Gels .... ▣ 845
- Robitussin-DAC Syrup 2249
- Robitussin-PE .... ▣ 846
- Rondec Oral Drops 974
- Rondec Syrup 974
- Rondec Tablet 974
- Rondec Chewable Tablets 974
- Rondec-TR Tablet 974
- Ryna 804
- Seldane-D Extended-Release Tablets 1286
- Semprex-D Capsules 1620
- Sinarest .... ▣ 663
- Sine-Aid Maximum Strength Sinus Headache Gelcaps, Caplets and Tablets 1570
- Sine-Off No Drowsiness Formula Caplets .... ▣ 784
- Sine-Off Sinus Medicine .... ▣ 784
- Singlet Tablets .... ▣ 785
- Sinutab Non-Drying Liquid Caps .. ▣ 823
- Sinutab Sinus Allergy Medication, Maximum Strength Tablets and Caplets .... ▣ 823
- Sinutab Sinus Medication, Maximum Strength Without Drowsiness Formula, Tablets & Caplets .... ▣ 824

IMPORTANT NOTE: Always consult each drug listing in the patient's regimen for possible interactions.

Bronkosol — Interactions Index

Sudafed Children's Cold & Cough Liquid Medication ... 825
Sudafed Children's Nasal Decongestant Liquid Medication ... 826
Sudafed Cold & Allergy Tablets ... 826
Sudafed Cold and Cough Liquid Caps ... 826
Sudafed Nasal Decongestant Tablets, 30 mg. ... 825
Sudafed Nasal Decongestant Tablets, 60 mg ... 825
Sudafed Non-Drying Sinus Liquid Caps ... 827
Sudafed Pediatric Nasal Decongestant Liquid Oral Drops ... 827
Sudafed Severe Cold Formula Caplets ... 828
Sudafed Severe Cold Formula Tablets ... 828
Sudafed Sinus Caplets ... 829
Sudafed Sinus Tablets ... 829
Sudafed 12 Hour Caplets ... 824
Syn-Rx Tablets ... 1622
Syn-Rx DM Tablets ... 1623
TheraFlu Flu and Cold Medicine ... 750
Theraflu Maximum Strength Flu and Cold Medicine For Sore Throat ... 751
TheraFlu Flu, Cold and Cough Medicine ... 750
TheraFlu Maximum Strength Nighttime Flu, Cold & Cough Medicine ... 751
TheraFlu Maximum Strength Non-Drowsy Formula Flu, Cold & Cough Medicine ... 751
TheraFlu Maximum Strength, Non-Drowsy Formula Flu, Cold and Cough Caplets ... 752
Theraflu Maximum Strength Sinus Non-Drowsy Formula Caplets ... 752
Triaminic AM Cough and Decongestant Formula ... 753
Triaminic AM Decongestant Formula ... 753
Triaminic Infant Oral Decongestant Drops ... 754
Triaminic Night Time ... 754
Triaminic Sore Throat Formula ... 755
Tussend ... 1830
Tussend Expectorant ... 1831
TYLENOL Allergy Sinus, Maximum Strength Caplets and Gelcaps ... 1571
TYLENOL Allergy Sinus NightTime, Maximum Strength Caplets ... 1571
TYLENOL Cold Medication, Multi-Symptom Formula Tablets and Caplets ... 1572
TYLENOL Cold Medication, Multi-Symptom Hot Liquid Packets ... 1572
TYLENOL Cold Medication, No Drowsiness Formula Caplets and Gelcaps ... 1572
TYLENOL Cold Severe Congestion Caplets ... 1573
TYLENOL Cough Medication with Decongestant, Multi Symptom ... 1574
TYLENOL Flu No Drowsiness Formula, Maximum Strength Gelcaps ... 1575
TYLENOL Flu NightTime, Maximum Strength Gelcaps ... 1575
TYLENOL Flu NightTime, Maximum Strength Hot Medication Packets ... 1575
TYLENOL Sinus, Maximum Strength Geltabs, Gelcaps, Caplets and Tablets ... 1576
Vicks 44 LiquiCaps Cough, Cold & Flu Relief ... 728
Vicks 44 LiquiCaps Non-Drowsy Cough & Cold Relief ... 729
Vicks 44D Cough & Head Congestion Relief ... 728
Vicks 44M Cough, Cold & Flu Relief ... 729
Vicks DayQuil LiquiCaps/Liquid Multi-Symptom Cold/Flu Relief ... 734
Vicks DayQuil SINUS Pressure & PAIN Relief with IBUPROFEN ... 735
Vicks Nyquil Hot Therapy ... 735
Vicks NyQuil LiquiCaps/Liquid Multi-Symptom Cold/Flu Relief, Original and Cherry Flavors ... 736

Pseudoephedrine Sulfate (May cause excessive tachycardia due to direct cardiac stimulation). Products include:
Chlor-Trimeton Allergy Decongestant Tablets ... 759
Claritin-D Tablets ... 2487

Drixoral Cold and Allergy Sustained-Action Tablets ... 763
Drixoral Cold and Flu Extended-Release Tablets ... 764
Drixoral Non-Drowsy Formula Extended-Release Tablets ... 764
Drixoral Allergy/Sinus Extended Release Tablets ... 765
Trinalin Repetabs Tablets ... 1373

Salmeterol Xinafoate (May cause excessive tachycardia due to direct cardiac stimulation). Products include:
Serevent Inhalation Aerosol ... 1149

Terbutaline Sulfate (May cause excessive tachycardia due to direct cardiac stimulation). Products include:
Brethaire Inhaler ... 830
Brethine Ampuls ... 832
Brethine Tablets ... 831
Bricanyl Subcutaneous Injection ... 1247
Bricanyl Tablets ... 1248

BRONTEX LIQUID
(Codeine Phosphate, Guaifenesin) ... 2130
See **Brontex Tablets**

BRONTEX TABLETS
(Codeine Phosphate, Guaifenesin) ... 2130
May interact with central nervous system depressants, hypnotics and sedatives, tranquilizers, antidepressant drugs, narcotic analgesics, and certain other agents. Compounds in these categories include:

Alfentanil Hydrochloride (Potential for greater sedation). Products include:
Alfenta Injection ... 1334

Alprazolam (Potential for greater sedation). Products include:
Xanax Tablets ... 2115

Amitriptyline Hydrochloride (Potential for greater sedation). Products include:
Elavil ... 2945
Etrafon ... 2495
Limbitrol ... 2333
Triavil Tablets ... 1800

Amoxapine (Potential for greater sedation). Products include:
Asendin Tablets ... 1419

Aprobarbital (Potential for greater sedation).
No products indexed under this heading.

Buprenorphine (Potential for greater sedation). Products include:
Buprenex Injectable ... 2170

Bupropion Hydrochloride (Potential for greater sedation). Products include:
Wellbutrin Tablets ... 1177

Buspirone Hydrochloride (Potential for greater sedation). Products include:
BuSpar Tablets ... 738

Butabarbital (Potential for greater sedation).
No products indexed under this heading.

Butalbital (Potential for greater sedation). Products include:
Axocet Capsules ... 2469
Esgic-plus Capsules ... 1012
Esgic-plus Tablets ... 1012
Fioricet Tablets ... 2386
Fioricet with Codeine Capsules ... 2387
Fiorinal Capsules ... 2388
Fiorinal with Codeine Capsules ... 2390
Fiorinal Tablets ... 2388
Phrenilin ... 790
Sedapap Tablets 50 mg/650 mg ... 1826

Chlordiazepoxide (Potential for greater sedation). Products include:
Limbitrol ... 2333

Chlordiazepoxide Hydrochloride (Potential for greater sedation). Products include:
Librax Capsules ... 2330

Librium Capsules ... 2331
Librium Injectable ... 2332

Chlorpromazine (Potential for greater sedation). Products include:
Thorazine Suppositories ... 2701

Chlorpromazine Hydrochloride (Potential for greater sedation). Products include:
Thorazine ... 2701

Chlorprothixene (Potential for greater sedation).
No products indexed under this heading.

Chlorprothixene Hydrochloride (Potential for greater sedation).
No products indexed under this heading.

Chlorprothixene Lactate (Potential for greater sedation).
No products indexed under this heading.

Clorazepate Dipotassium (Potential for greater sedation). Products include:
Tranxene ... 459

Clozapine (Potential for greater sedation). Products include:
Clozaril Tablets ... 2377

Desflurane (Potential for greater sedation). Products include:
Suprane (desflurane, USP) ... 1865

Desipramine Hydrochloride (Potential for greater sedation). Products include:
Norpramin Tablets ... 1273

Dezocine (Potential for greater sedation). Products include:
Dalgan Injection ... 529

Diazepam (Potential for greater sedation). Products include:
Dizac (diazepam injectable emulsion) CIV ... 1862
Valium Injectable ... 2336
Valium Tablets ... 2335

Doxepin Hydrochloride (Potential for greater sedation). Products include:
Adapin Capsules ... 1542
Sinequan ... 2028
Zonalon Cream ... 1042

Droperidol (Potential for greater sedation). Products include:
Inapsine Injection ... 462

Enflurane (Potential for greater sedation).
No products indexed under this heading.

Estazolam (Potential for greater sedation). Products include:
ProSom Tablets ... 457

Ethchlorvynol (Potential for greater sedation). Products include:
Placidyl Capsules ... 456

Ethinamate (Potential for greater sedation).
No products indexed under this heading.

Fentanyl (Potential for greater sedation). Products include:
Duragesic Transdermal System ... 1336

Fentanyl Citrate (Potential for greater sedation). Products include:
Sublimaze Injection ... 463

Fluoxetine Hydrochloride (Potential for greater sedation). Products include:
Prozac Pulvules & Liquid, Oral Solution ... 935

Fluphenazine Decanoate (Potential for greater sedation). Products include:
Prolixin Decanoate ... 510

Fluphenazine Enanthate (Potential for greater sedation). Products include:
Prolixin Enanthate ... 510

Fluphenazine Hydrochloride (Potential for greater sedation). Products include:
Prolixin ... 510

Flurazepam Hydrochloride (Potential for greater sedation). Products include:
Dalmane Capsules ... 2329

Glutethimide (Potential for greater sedation).
No products indexed under this heading.

Haloperidol (Potential for greater sedation). Products include:
Haldol Injection, Tablets and Concentrate ... 1585

Haloperidol Decanoate (Potential for greater sedation). Products include:
Haldol Decanoate ... 1587

Hydrocodone Bitartrate (Potential for greater sedation). Products include:
Codiclear DH Syrup ... 808
Duratuss HD Elixir ... 2750
Histussin D Liquid ... 670
Hycodan Tablets and Syrup ... 946
Hycomine Compound Tablets ... 948
Hycomine ... 947
Hycotuss Expectorant Syrup ... 950
Hydrocet Capsules ... 787
Lorcet 10/650 Tablets ... 1016
Lortab ... 2751
Tussend ... 1830
Tussend Expectorant ... 1831
Vicodin Tablets ... 1404
Vicodin ES Tablets ... 1405
Vicodin HP Tablets ... 1403
Vicodin Tuss Expectorant ... 1406
Zydone Capsules ... 967

Hydrocodone Polistirex (Potential for greater sedation). Products include:
Tussionex Pennkinetic Extended-Release Suspension ... 1624

Hydromorphone Hydrochloride (Potential for greater sedation). Products include:
Dilaudid Ampules ... 1382
Dilaudid Cough Syrup ... 1383
Dilaudid-HP Injection ... 1384
Dilaudid-HP Lyophilized Powder 250 mg ... 1384
Dilaudid ... 1382
Dilaudid Oral Liquid ... 1386
Dilaudid ... 1382
Dilaudid Tablets - 8 mg. ... 1386

Hydroxyzine Hydrochloride (Potential for greater sedation). Products include:
Atarax Tablets & Syrup ... 1992
Marax Tablets & DF Syrup ... 2015
Vistaril Intramuscular Solution ... 2042

Imipramine Hydrochloride (Potential for greater sedation). Products include:
Tofranil Ampuls ... 873
Tofranil Tablets ... 875

Imipramine Pamoate (Potential for greater sedation). Products include:
Tofranil-PM Capsules ... 876

Isocarboxazid (Potential for greater sedation).
No products indexed under this heading.

Isoflurane (Potential for greater sedation).
No products indexed under this heading.

Ketamine Hydrochloride (Potential for greater sedation).
No products indexed under this heading.

Levomethadyl Acetate Hydrochloride (Potential for greater sedation). Products include:
Orlaam Oral Solution ... 2361

(■ Described in PDR For Nonprescription Drugs)   (◉ Described in PDR For Ophthalmology)

Levorphanol Tartrate (Potential for greater sedation). Products include:
Levo-Dromoran 2297
Lorazepam (Potential for greater sedation). Products include:
Ativan Injection 2805
Ativan Tablets 2807
Loxapine Hydrochloride (Potential for greater sedation). Products include:
Loxitane 1426
Loxapine Succinate (Potential for greater sedation). Products include:
Loxitane Capsules 1426
Maprotiline Hydrochloride (Potential for greater sedation). Products include:
Ludiomil Tablets 861
Meperidine Hydrochloride (Potential for greater sedation). Products include:
Demerol 2438
Mepergan Injection 2859
Mephobarbital (Potential for greater sedation). Products include:
Mebaral Tablets 2452
Meprobamate (Potential for greater sedation). Products include:
Miltown Tablets 2780
PMB 200 and PMB 400 2890
Mesoridazine Besylate (Potential for greater sedation). Products include:
Serentil 689
Methadone Hydrochloride (Potential for greater sedation). Products include:
Methadone Hydrochloride Oral Concentrate 2356
Methadone Hydrochloride Oral Solution & Tablets............. 2357
Methohexital Sodium (Potential for greater sedation).
No products indexed under this heading.
Methotrimeprazine (Potential for greater sedation). Products include:
Levoprome 1321
Methoxyflurane (Potential for greater sedation).
No products indexed under this heading.
Midazolam Hydrochloride (Potential for greater sedation). Products include:
Versed Injection 2324
Molindone Hydrochloride (Potential for greater sedation). Products include:
Moban Tablets and Concentrate 1036
Morphine Sulfate (Potential for greater sedation). Products include:
Astramorph/PF Injection, USP (Preservative-Free) 526
Duramorph Injection 983
Infumorph 200 and Infumorph 500 Sterile Solutions 985
Kadian Capsules 2948
MS Contin Tablets 2149
MSIR 2152
Oramorph SR (Morphine Sulfate Sustained Release Tablets) 2359
RMS Suppositories CII 2766
Roxanol 2365
Nefazodone Hydrochloride (Potential for greater sedation). Products include:
Serzone Tablets 776
Nortriptyline Hydrochloride (Potential for greater sedation). Products include:
Pamelor 2409
Opium Alkaloids (Potential for greater sedation).
No products indexed under this heading.

Oxazepam (Potential for greater sedation). Products include:
Serax Capsules 2916
Serax Tablets 2916
Oxycodone Hydrochloride (Potential for greater sedation). Products include:
OxyContin Tablets................ 2163
OxyIR Capsules 2167
Percocet Tablets 955
Percodan Tablets 955
Percodan-Demi Tablets 956
Roxicodone Tablets, Oral Solution & Intensol (Oxycodone) 2366
Tylox Capsules 1593
Paroxetine Hydrochloride (Potential for greater sedation). Products include:
Paxil Tablets 2681
Pentobarbital Sodium (Potential for greater sedation). Products include:
Nembutal Sodium Capsules 440
Nembutal Sodium Solution 442
Nembutal Sodium Suppositories 444
Perphenazine (Potential for greater sedation). Products include:
Etrafon 2495
Triavil Tablets 1800
Trilafon 2532
Phenelzine Sulfate (Potential for greater sedation). Products include:
Nardil 1977
Phenobarbital (Potential for greater sedation). Products include:
Arco-Lase Plus Tablets 513
Bellergal-S Tablets 2375
Donnatal 2234
Donnatal Extentabs 2234
Donnatal Tablets 2234
Phenobarbital Elixir and Tablets 1523
Quadrinal Tablets 1398
Prazepam (Potential for greater sedation).
No products indexed under this heading.
Prochlorperazine (Potential for greater sedation). Products include:
Compazine 2644
Promethazine Hydrochloride (Potential for greater sedation). Products include:
Mepergan Injection 2859
Phenergan with Codeine 2883
Phenergan with Dextromethorphan 2885
Phenergan Injection 2880
Phenergan Suppositories 2882
Phenergan Syrup 2881
Phenergan Tablets 2882
Phenergan VC 2886
Phenergan VC with Codeine 2888
Propofol (Potential for greater sedation). Products include:
Diprivan Injectable Emulsion 2939
Propoxyphene Hydrochloride (Potential for greater sedation). Products include:
Darvon 1475
Wygesic Tablets 2930
Propoxyphene Napsylate (Potential for greater sedation). Products include:
Darvon-N/Darvocet-N 1473
Protriptyline Hydrochloride (Potential for greater sedation). Products include:
Vivactil Tablets 1820
Quazepam (Potential for greater sedation). Products include:
Doral Tablets 2773
Risperidone (Potential for greater sedation). Products include:
Risperdal Tablets 1348
Secobarbital Sodium (Potential for greater sedation). Products include:
Seconal Sodium Pulvules 1529

Sertraline Hydrochloride (Potential for greater sedation). Products include:
Zoloft Tablets 2051
Sevoflurane (Potential for greater sedation).
No products indexed under this heading.
Sufentanil Citrate (Potential for greater sedation). Products include:
Sufenta Injection 1355
Temazepam (Potential for greater sedation). Products include:
Restoril Capsules 2413
Thiamylal Sodium (Potential for greater sedation).
No products indexed under this heading.
Thioridazine Hydrochloride (Potential for greater sedation). Products include:
Mellaril 2398
Thiothixene (Potential for greater sedation). Products include:
Navane Capsules and Concentrate 2018
Navane Intramuscular 2019
Tranylcypromine Sulfate (Potential for greater sedation). Products include:
Parnate Tablets 2679
Trazodone Hydrochloride (Potential for greater sedation). Products include:
Desyrel and Desyrel Dividose 504
Triazolam (Potential for greater sedation). Products include:
Halcion Tablets 2093
Trifluoperazine Hydrochloride (Potential for greater sedation). Products include:
Stelazine 2692
Trimipramine Maleate (Potential for greater sedation). Products include:
Surmontil Capsules 2917
Venlafaxine Hydrochloride (Potential for greater sedation). Products include:
Effexor 2825
Zolpidem Tartrate (Potential for greater sedation). Products include:
Ambien Tablets 2559

Food Interactions
Alcohol (Potential for greater sedation).

BUFFERIN ANALGESIC TABLETS
(Aspirin) .... ▣ 636
May interact with:

Aluminum Carbonate (Concurrent administration of nonabsorbable antacids may alter the rate of absorption of aspirin). Products include:
Basaljel Capsules 2810
Basaljel Suspension 2810
Basaljel Tablets 2810
Aluminum Hydroxide (Concurrent administration of nonabsorbable antacids may alter the rate of absorption of aspirin). Products include:
ALternaGEL Liquid 1358
Maximum Strength Ascriptin ...... ▣ 650
Cama Arthritis Pain Reliever ...... ▣ 748
Gaviscon Extra Strength Relief Formula Antacid Tablets..... ▣ 778
Gaviscon Extra Strength Relief Formula Liquid Antacid ..... ▣ 779
Gaviscon Liquid Antacid ...... ▣ 779
Gelusil Antacid-Anti-gas Liquid ...... ▣ 819
Gelusil Antacid-Anti-gas Tablets ...... ▣ 819
Maalox Antacid/Anti-Gas Tablets.... 889
Maalox Heartburn Relief Suspension ...... ▣ 658
Maalox Antacid Liquid 888
Extra Strength Maalox Antacid/Anti-Gas Liquid and Tablets 888
Mylanta 1359
Tempo Soft Antacid .... ▣ 799
Aluminum Hydroxide Gel (Concurrent administration of nonabsorbable antacids may alter the rate of absorption of aspirin). Products include:
ALternaGEL Liquid .... ▣ 675
Aludrox Oral Suspension .... ▣ 850
Amphojel Suspension 2802
Amphojel Suspension without Flavor 2802
Amphojel Tablets 2802
Ascriptin .... ▣ 650
Gaviscon Antacid Tablets ... ▣ 778
Gaviscon-2 Antacid Tablets ▣ 779
Mylanta Liquid .... ▣ 676
Mylanta Double Strength Liquid ... ▣ 676
Nephrox Suspension .... ▣ 671
Antiarthritic Drugs, unspecified (Effect not specified).
Anticoagulant Drugs, unspecified (Effect not specified).
Antidiabetic Drugs, unspecified (Effect not specified).
Antigout Drugs, unspecified (Effect not specified).
Magnesium Hydroxide (Concurrent administration of nonabsorbable antacids may alter the rate of absorption of aspirin). Products include:
Aludrox Oral Suspension .... ▣ 850
Ascriptin .... ▣ 650
Di-Gel Antacid/Anti-Gas ..... ▣ 762
Gelusil Antacid-Anti-gas Liquid ▣ 819
Gelusil Antacid-Anti-gas Tablets .... ▣ 819
Maalox Antacid/Anti-Gas Tablets.... 889
Maalox Antacid Liquid 888
Extra Strength Maalox Antacid/Anti-Gas Liquid and Tablets 888
Mylanta Fast-Acting 1359
Mylanta Gelcaps Antacid .... ▣ 678
Fast-Acting Mylanta Liquid Antacid 1359
Mylanta Tablets .... ▣ 677
Maximum-Strength Fast-Acting Mylanta Liquid Antacid 1359
Mylanta Double Strength Tablets ▣ 677
Phillips' Milk of Magnesia Liquid.... ▣ 627
Rolaids Antacid Tablets ...... ▣ 807
Tempo Soft Antacid .... ▣ 799
Magnesium Oxide (Concurrent administration of nonabsorbable antacids may alter the rate of absorption of aspirin). Products include:
Beelith Tablets 632
Bufferin Analgesic Tablets... ▣ 636
Arthritis Strength Bufferin Analgesic Caplets .... ▣ 637
Extra Strength Bufferin Analgesic Tablets .... ▣ 637
Caltrate PLUS .... ▣ 681
Cama Arthritis Pain Reliever ▣ 748
Mag-Ox 400 666
Uro-Mag 666
Sodium Bicarbonate (Concurrent administration with absorbable antacids may increase the clearance of salicylates). Products include:
Alka-Seltzer Cherry Effervescent Antacid and Pain Reliever ...... ▣ 609
Alka-Seltzer Extra Strength Effervescent Antacid and Pain Reliever .... ▣ 609
Alka-Seltzer Gold Effervescent Antacid .... ▣ 611
Alka-Seltzer Lemon Lime Effervescent Antacid and Pain Reliever .... ▣ 609
Alka-Seltzer Original Effervescent Antacid and Pain Reliever ...... ▣ 609
Arm & Hammer Pure Baking Soda .... ▣ 648
Colyte and Colyte-flavored ... 2540
GoLYTELY 694
Massengill Disposable Douches ... ▣ 780
Massengill Liquid Concentrate ▣ 780
NuLYTELY 694
Cherry Flavor NuLYTELY ... 694

IMPORTANT NOTE: Always consult each drug listing in the patient's regimen for possible interactions.

Bufferin / Interactions Index

ARTHRITIS STRENGTH BUFFERIN ANALGESIC CAPLETS
(Aspirin) .... ▣ 637
May interact with:

Antiarthritic Drugs, unspecified (Effect not specified).
Anticoagulant Drugs, unspecified (Effect not specified).
Antidiabetic Drugs, unspecified (Effect not specified).
Antigout Drugs, unspecified (Effect not specified).

EXTRA STRENGTH BUFFERIN ANALGESIC TABLETS
(Aspirin) .... ▣ 637
May interact with:

Antiarthritic Drugs, unspecified (Effect not specified).
Anticoagulant Drugs, unspecified (Effect not specified).
Antidiabetic Drugs, unspecified (Effect not specified).
Antigout Drugs, unspecified (Effect not specified).

BUGS BUNNY COMPLETE CHILDREN'S CHEWABLE VITAMINS + MINERALS WITH IRON AND CALCIUM (SUGAR FREE)
(Vitamins with Minerals) .... ▣ 620
None cited in PDR database.

BUGS BUNNY WITH EXTRA C CHILDREN'S CHEWABLE VITAMINS (SUGAR FREE)
(Vitamins with Minerals) .... ▣ 621
None cited in PDR database.

BUGS BUNNY PLUS IRON CHILDREN'S CHEWABLE VITAMINS (SUGAR FREE)
(Vitamins with Iron) .... ▣ 619
None cited in PDR database.

BUMEX INJECTION
(Bumetanide) 2260
May interact with aminoglycosides, lithium preparations, antihypertensives, and certain other agents. Compounds in these categories include:

Acebutolol Hydrochloride (Antihypertensive effect potentiated). Products include:
Sectral Capsules 2914

Amikacin Sulfate (Potential for ototoxicity and/or nephrotoxicity). Products include:
Amikacin Sulfate Injection, USP 523
Amikacin Sulfate Injection, USP 981
Amikin Injectable 502

Amlodipine Besylate (Antihypertensive effect potentiated). Products include:
Lotrel Capsules 858
Norvasc Tablets 2020

Atenolol (Antihypertensive effect potentiated). Products include:
Tenoretic Tablets 2963
Tenormin Tablets and I.V. Injection 2965

Benazepril Hydrochloride (Antihypertensive effect potentiated). Products include:
Lotensin Tablets 852
Lotensin HCT Tablets 855
Lotrel Capsules 858

Bendroflumethiazide (Antihypertensive effect potentiated).
No products indexed under this heading.

Betaxolol Hydrochloride (Antihypertensive effect potentiated). Products include:
Betoptic Ophthalmic Solution 465
Betoptic S Ophthalmic Suspension .. 467
Kerlone Tablets 2588

Bisoprolol Fumarate (Antihypertensive effect potentiated). Products include:
Zebeta Tablets 1457
Ziac 1459

Captopril (Antihypertensive effect potentiated). Products include:
Capoten Tablets 740
Capozide Tablets 744

Carteolol Hydrochloride (Antihypertensive effect potentiated). Products include:
Cartrol Tablets 413
Ocupress Ophthalmic Solution, 1% Sterile .... ⊙ 297

Chlorothiazide (Antihypertensive effect potentiated). Products include:
Aldoclor Tablets 1638
Diupres Tablets 1691
Diuril Oral 1694

Chlorothiazide Sodium (Antihypertensive effect potentiated). Products include:
Diuril Sodium Intravenous 1693

Chlorthalidone (Antihypertensive effect potentiated). Products include:
Combipres Tablets 682
Tenoretic Tablets 2963
Thalitone 1293

Clonidine (Antihypertensive effect potentiated). Products include:
Catapres-TTS......................... 680

Clonidine Hydrochloride (Antihypertensive effect potentiated). Products include:
Catapres Tablets 679
Combipres Tablets 682

Deserpidine (Antihypertensive effect potentiated).
No products indexed under this heading.

Diazoxide (Antihypertensive effect potentiated). Products include:
Hyperstat I.V. Injection 2504
Proglycem 575

Diltiazem Hydrochloride (Antihypertensive effect potentiated). Products include:
Cardizem CD Capsules 1251
Cardizem SR Capsules 1255
Cardizem Injectable 1253
Cardizem Tablets 1257
Dilacor XR Extended-release Capsules 2183
Tiazac Capsules 1019

Doxazosin Mesylate (Antihypertensive effect potentiated). Products include:
Cardura Tablets 1993

Enalapril Maleate (Antihypertensive effect potentiated). Products include:
Vaseretic Tablets 1810
Vasotec Tablets 1816

Enalaprilat (Antihypertensive effect potentiated). Products include:
Vasotec I.V. 1814

Esmolol Hydrochloride (Antihypertensive effect potentiated). Products include:
Brevibloc (esmolol HCl) Injection ... 1860

Felodipine (Antihypertensive effect potentiated). Products include:
Plendil Extended-Release Tablets ... 514

Fosinopril Sodium (Antihypertensive effect potentiated). Products include:
Monopril Tablets 762

Furosemide (Antihypertensive effect potentiated). Products include:
Lasix Injection, Oral Solution and Tablets 1267

Gentamicin Sulfate (Potential for ototoxicity and/or nephrotoxicity). Products include:
Garamycin Cream 0.1% 2501
Garamycin Injectable 2502
Garamycin Ointment 0.1% 2501
Garamycin Ophthalmic 2501
Genoptic Sterile Ophthalmic Solution .... ⊙ 241
Genoptic Sterile Ophthalmic Ointment .... ⊙ 241
Gentak .... ⊙ 209
Pred-G Liquifilm Sterile Ophthalmic Suspension .... ⊙ 248
Pred-G S.O.P. Sterile Ophthalmic Ointment .... ⊙ 249

Guanabenz Acetate (Antihypertensive effect potentiated).
No products indexed under this heading.

Guanethidine Monosulfate (Antihypertensive effect potentiated). Products include:
Esimil Tablets 840
Ismelin Tablets 845

Hydralazine Hydrochloride (Antihypertensive effect potentiated). Products include:
Apresazide Capsules 824
Apresoline Hydrochloride Tablets .. 826
Hydralazine Hydrochloride Injection USP 2712
Ser-Ap-Es Tablets 867

Hydrochlorothiazide (Antihypertensive effect potentiated). Products include:
Aldactazide Tablets 2556
Aldoril Tablets 1644
Apresazide Capsules 824
Capozide Tablets 744
Dyazide Capsules 2653
Esidrix Tablets 839
Esimil Tablets 840
HydroDIURIL Tablets 1716
Hydropres Tablets 1718
Hyzaar Tablets 1720
Inderide Tablets 2838
Inderide LA Long Acting Capsules .. 2840
Lopressor HCT Tablets 850
Lotensin HCT Tablets 855
Moduretic Tablets 1748
Oretic Tablets 450
Prinzide Tablets 1780
Ser-Ap-Es Tablets 867
Timolide Tablets 1791
Vaseretic Tablets 1810
Zestoretic Tablets 2968
Ziac 1459

Hydroflumethiazide (Antihypertensive effect potentiated). Products include:
Diucardin Tablets 2824

Indapamide (Antihypertensive effect potentiated).
No products indexed under this heading.

Indomethacin (Decreased plasma renin activity). Products include:
Indocin 1723

Indomethacin Sodium Trihydrate (Decreased plasma renin activity). Products include:
Indocin I.V. 1727

Isradipine (Antihypertensive effect potentiated). Products include:
DynaCirc Capsules 2381
DynaCirc CR Tablets 2383

Kanamycin Sulfate (Potential for ototoxicity and/or nephrotoxicity).
No products indexed under this heading.

Labetalol Hydrochloride (Antihypertensive effect potentiated). Products include:
Normodyne Injection 2519
Normodyne Tablets 2522
Trandate 1158

Lisinopril (Antihypertensive effect potentiated). Products include:
Prinivil Tablets 1776
Prinzide Tablets 1780
Zestoretic Tablets 2968
Zestril Tablets 2972

Lithium Carbonate (Reduced renal clearance and added high risk of lithium toxicity). Products include:
Eskalith 2658
Lithium Carbonate Capsules & Tablets 2352
Lithonate/Lithotabs/Lithobid 2721

Lithium Citrate (Reduced renal clearance and added high risk of lithium toxicity).
No products indexed under this heading.

Losartan Potassium (Antihypertensive effect potentiated). Products include:
Cozaar Tablets 1668
Hyzaar Tablets 1720

Mecamylamine Hydrochloride (Antihypertensive effect potentiated). Products include:
Inversine Tablets 1729

Methyclothiazide (Antihypertensive effect potentiated). Products include:
Enduron Tablets 424

Methyldopa (Antihypertensive effect potentiated). Products include:
Aldoclor Tablets 1638
Aldomet Oral 1640
Aldoril Tablets 1644

Methyldopate Hydrochloride (Antihypertensive effect potentiated). Products include:
Aldomet Ester HCl Injection 1642

Metolazone (Antihypertensive effect potentiated). Products include:
Mykrox Tablets 1617
Zaroxolyn Tablets 1625

Metoprolol Succinate (Antihypertensive effect potentiated). Products include:
Toprol-XL Tablets 560

Metoprolol Tartrate (Antihypertensive effect potentiated). Products include:
Lopressor 848
Lopressor HCT Tablets 850

Metyrosine (Antihypertensive effect potentiated). Products include:
Demser Capsules 1690

Minoxidil (Antihypertensive effect potentiated).
No products indexed under this heading.

Moexipril Hydrochloride (Antihypertensive effect potentiated). Products include:
Univasc Tablets 2553

Nadolol (Antihypertensive effect potentiated).
No products indexed under this heading.

Nicardipine Hydrochloride (Antihypertensive effect potentiated). Products include:
Cardene Capsules 2261
Cardene I.V. 2815
Cardene SR Capsules 2264

Nifedipine (Antihypertensive effect potentiated). Products include:
Adalat Capsules (10 mg and 20 mg) 580
Adalat CC 582
Procardia Capsules 2024
Procardia XL Extended Release Tablets 2026

Nisoldipine (Antihypertensive effect potentiated). Products include:
Sular Tablets 2961

(▣ Described in PDR For Nonprescription Drugs)   (⊙ Described in PDR For Ophthalmology)

Nitroglycerin (Antihypertensive effect potentiated). Products include:
 Deponit NTG Transdermal Delivery System ... 2541
 Nitro-Bid IV ... 1270
 Nitro-Bid Ointment ... 1272
 Nitro-Dur (nitroglycerin) Transdermal Infusion System ... 1365
 Nitrolingual Spray ... 2193
 Nitrostat Tablets ... 1981
 Transderm-Nitro Transdermal Therapeutic System ... 878

Penbutolol Sulfate (Antihypertensive effect potentiated). Products include:
 Levatol Tablets ... 2547

Phenoxybenzamine Hydrochloride (Antihypertensive effect potentiated). Products include:
 Dibenzyline Capsules ... 2650

Phentolamine Mesylate (Antihypertensive effect potentiated). Products include:
 Regitine Vials ... 864

Pindolol (Antihypertensive effect potentiated). Products include:
 Visken Tablets ... 2428

Polythiazide (Antihypertensive effect potentiated). Products include:
 Minizide Capsules ... 2016

Prazosin Hydrochloride (Antihypertensive effect potentiated). Products include:
 Minipress Capsules ... 2015
 Minizide Capsules ... 2016

Probenecid (Decreases natriuresis and hyperreninemia; concurrent use should be avoided). Products include:
 Benemid Tablets ... 1651
 ColBENEMID Tablets ... 1662

Propranolol Hydrochloride (Antihypertensive effect potentiated). Products include:
 Inderal ... 2834
 Inderal LA Long Acting Capsules ... 2836
 Inderide Tablets ... 2838
 Inderide LA Long Acting Capsules .. 2840

Quinapril Hydrochloride (Antihypertensive effect potentiated). Products include:
 Accupril Tablets ... 1950

Ramipril (Antihypertensive effect potentiated). Products include:
 Altace Capsules ... 1238

Rauwolfia Serpentina (Antihypertensive effect potentiated).
 No products indexed under this heading.

Rescinnamine (Antihypertensive effect potentiated).
 No products indexed under this heading.

Reserpine (Antihypertensive effect potentiated). Products include:
 Diupres Tablets ... 1691
 Hydropres Tablets ... 1718
 Ser-Ap-Es Tablets ... 867

Sodium Nitroprusside (Antihypertensive effect potentiated).
 No products indexed under this heading.

Sotalol Hydrochloride (Antihypertensive effect potentiated). Products include:
 Betapace Tablets ... 637

Spirapril Hydrochloride (Antihypertensive effect potentiated).
 No products indexed under this heading.

Streptomycin Sulfate (Potential for ototoxicity and/or nephrotoxicity). Products include:
 Streptomycin Sulfate Injection ... 2031

Terazosin Hydrochloride (Antihypertensive effect potentiated). Products include:
 Hytrin Capsules ... 434

Timolol Maleate (Antihypertensive effect potentiated). Products include:
 Blocadren Tablets ... 1654
 Timolide Tablets ... 1791
 Timoptic in Ocudose ... 1796
 Timoptic Sterile Ophthalmic Solution ... 1794
 Timoptic-XE ... 1798

Tobramycin (Potential for ototoxicity and/or nephrotoxicity). Products include:
 AKTOB ... 207
 TobraDex Ophthalmic Suspension and Ointment ... 469
 Tobrex Ophthalmic Ointment and Solution ... 226

Tobramycin Sulfate (Potential for ototoxicity and/or nephrotoxicity). Products include:
 Nebcin Vials, Hyporets & ADD-Vantage ... 1518

Torsemide (Antihypertensive effect potentiated). Products include:
 Demadex Tablets and Injection ... 691

Trimethaphan Camsylate (Antihypertensive effect potentiated).
 No products indexed under this heading.

Verapamil Hydrochloride (Antihypertensive effect potentiated). Products include:
 Calan SR Caplets ... 2571
 Calan Tablets ... 2568
 Covera-HS Tablets ... 2573
 Isoptin Injectable ... 1391
 Isoptin Oral Tablets ... 1393
 Isoptin SR Tablets ... 1395
 Verelan Capsules ... 1455

BUMEX TABLETS
(Bumetanide) ... 2260
See **Bumex Injection**

BUPRENEX INJECTABLE
(Buprenorphine) ... 2170
May interact with central nervous system depressants, narcotic analgesics, general anesthetics, antihistamines, benzodiazepines, monoamine oxidase inhibitors, phenothiazines, hypnotics and sedatives, tranquilizers, and certain other agents. Compounds in these categories include:

Acrivastine (Increased CNS depression). Products include:
 Semprex-D Capsules ... 1620

Alfentanil Hydrochloride (Increased CNS depression). Products include:
 Alfenta Injection ... 1334

Alprazolam (Increased CNS depression). Products include:
 Xanax Tablets ... 2115

Aprobarbital (Increased CNS depression).
 No products indexed under this heading.

Astemizole (Increased CNS depression). Products include:
 Hismanal Tablets ... 1341

Azatadine Maleate (Increased CNS depression). Products include:
 Trinalin Repetabs Tablets ... 1373

Bromodiphenhydramine Hydrochloride (Increased CNS depression).
 No products indexed under this heading.

Brompheniramine Maleate (Increased CNS depression). Products include:
 Alka-Seltzer Plus Sinus Medicine .. 611
 Bromfed Capsules (Extended-Release) ... 1832
 Bromfed Syrup ... 712
 Bromfed Tablets ... 1832
 Bromfed-DM Cough Syrup ... 1832
 Bromfed-PD Capsules (Extended-Release) ... 1832
 Dimetane-DC Cough Syrup ... 2232
 Dimetane-DX Cough Syrup ... 2233
 Dimetapp Allergy Dye-Free Elixir .. 838
 Dimetapp Allergy Sinus Caplets ... 838
 Dimetapp Cold & Allergy Chewable Tablets ... 838
 Dimetapp Cold & Cough Liqui-Gels ... 839
 Dimetapp Cold & Fever Suspension ... 839
 Dimetapp DM Elixir ... 840
 Dimetapp Elixir ... 840
 Dimetapp Extentabs ... 841
 Dimetapp Tablets/Liqui-Gels ... 841
 Rondec Chewable Tablets ... 974
 Vicks DayQuil Allergy Relief 12-Hour Extended Release Tablets .. 733
 Vicks DayQuil Allergy Relief 4-Hour Tablets ... 733

Buspirone Hydrochloride (Increased CNS depression). Products include:
 BuSpar Tablets ... 738

Butabarbital (Increased CNS depression).
 No products indexed under this heading.

Butalbital (Increased CNS depression). Products include:
 Axocet Capsules ... 2469
 Esgic-plus Capsules ... 1012
 Esgic-plus Tablets ... 1012
 Fioricet ... 2386
 Fioricet with Codeine Capsules ... 2387
 Fiorinal ... 2388
 Fiorinal with Codeine Capsules ... 2390
 Fiorinal Tablets ... 2388
 Phrenilin ... 790
 Sedapap Tablets 50 mg/650 mg .. 1826

Cetirizine Hydrochloride (Increased CNS depression). Products include:
 Zyrtec Tablets ... 2053

Chlordiazepoxide (Increased CNS depression). Products include:
 Limbitrol ... 2333

Chlordiazepoxide Hydrochloride (Increased CNS depression). Products include:
 Librax Capsules ... 2330
 Librium Capsules ... 2331
 Librium Injectable ... 2332

Chlorpheniramine Maleate (Increased CNS depression). Products include:
 Alka-Seltzer Plus Cold Medicine 611
 Alka-Seltzer Plus Cold Medicine Liqui-Gels ... 612
 Alka-Seltzer Plus Cold & Cough Medicine ... 611
 Alka-Seltzer Plus Cold & Cough Medicine Liqui-Gels ... 612
 Alka-Seltzer Plus Flu & Body Aches Effervescent Tablets ... 612
 Allerest Maximum Strength ... 649
 Allerest Sinus Pain Formula ... 649
 Ana-Kit Anaphylaxis Emergency Treatment Kit ... 611
 Atrohist Pediatric Capsules ... 1603
 Atrohist Plus Tablets ... 1605
 BC Cold Powder Multi-Symptom Formula (Cold-Sinus-Allergy) ... 631
 Cerose DM ... 853
 Cheracol Plus Head Cold/Cough Formula ... 741
 Children's TYLENOL Cold Multi-Symptom Chewable Tablets and Liquid ... 1559
 Children's TYLENOL Cold Plus Cough Multi Symptom Chewable Tablets and Liquid ... 1560
 Children's TYLENOL Flu Suspension Liquid ... 1560
 Children's Vicks DayQuil Allergy Relief ... 730
 Children's Vicks NyQuil Cold/Cough Relief ... 731
 Chlor-Trimeton Allergy Decongestant Tablets ... 759
 Chlor-Trimeton Allergy Tablets ... 758
 Allergy-Sinus Comtrex Multi-Symptom Allergy-Sinus Formula Tablets and Caplets ... 639
 Comtrex Multi-Symptom ... 638
 Contac Continuous Action Nasal Decongestant/Antihistamine 12 Hour Capsules ... 773
 Contac Maximum Strength Continuous Action Decongestant/Antihistamine 12 Hour Caplets .. 772
 Contac Severe Cold and Flu Formula Caplets ... 773
 Coricidin Cold + Flu Tablets ... 760
 Coricidin Cough + Cold Tablets ... 760
 Coricidin 'D' Decongestant Tablets ... 760
 D.A. II Tablets ... 972
 D.A. Chewable Tablets ... 970
 Dura-Tap/PD Capsules ... 970
 Dura-Vent/DA Tablets ... 972
 Efidac 24 Chlorpheniramine ... 655
 Extendryl ... 1003
 Fedahist Gyrocaps ... 2545
 Hycomine Compound Tablets ... 948
 Kronofed-A ... 994
 Nolamine Timed-Release Tablets ... 790
 Novahistine Elixir ... 782
 Ornade Spansule Capsules ... 2678
 PediaCare Cough-Cold Chewable Tablets and Liquid ... 1569
 PediaCare NightRest Cough-Cold Liquid ... 1569
 Pediatric Vicks 44m Cough & Cold Relief ... 737
 Pyrroxate Caplets ... 742
 Ryna ... 804
 Sinarest ... 663
 Sine-Off Sinus Medicine ... 784
 Singlet Tablets ... 785
 Sinulin Tablets ... 792
 Sinutab Sinus Allergy Medication, Maximum Strength Tablets and Caplets ... 823
 Sudafed Cold & Allergy Tablets ... 826
 Teldrin 12 Hour Antihistamine/Nasal Decongestant Allergy Relief Capsules ... 786
 TheraFlu Flu and Cold Medicine ... 750
 Theraflu Maximum Strength Flu and Cold Medicine For Sore Throat ... 751
 TheraFlu Flu, Cold and Cough Medicine ... 750
 TheraFlu Maximum Strength Nighttime Flu, Cold & Cough Medicine ... 751
 Triaminic Night Time ... 754
 Triaminic Syrup ... 755
 Triaminic Triaminicol Cold & Cough ... 756
 Triaminicin Tablets ... 756
 Tussend ... 1830
 TYLENOL Allergy Sinus, Maximum Strength Caplets and Gelcaps ... 1571
 TYLENOL Cold Medication, Multi-Symptom Formula Tablets and Caplets ... 1572
 TYLENOL Cold Medication, Multi-Symptom Hot Liquid Packets ... 1572
 Vicks 44 LiquiCaps Cough, Cold & Flu Relief ... 728
 Vicks 44M Cough, Cold & Flu Relief ... 729

Chlorpheniramine Polistirex (Increased CNS depression). Products include:
 Tussionex Pennkinetic Extended-Release Suspension ... 1624

Chlorpheniramine Tannate (Increased CNS depression). Products include:
 Atrohist Pediatric Suspension ... 1604
 Atrohist Pediatric Suspension Dye-Free ... 1604
 Rynatan ... 2781
 Rynatuss ... 2782

Chlorpromazine (Increased CNS depression). Products include:
 Thorazine Suppositories ... 2701

Chlorprothixene (Increased CNS depression).
 No products indexed under this heading.

Chlorprothixene Hydrochloride (Increased CNS depression).
 No products indexed under this heading.

Chlorprothixene Lactate (Increased CNS depression).
 No products indexed under this heading.

IMPORTANT NOTE: Always consult each drug listing in the patient's regimen for possible interactions.

Buprenex Interactions Index 140

Clemastine Fumarate (Increased CNS depression). Products include:
Tavist Syrup ... 2426
Tavist Tablets ... 2427
Tavist-1 12 Hour Relief Tablets ... ▣ 749
Tavist-D 12 Hour Relief Tablets ... ▣ 750

Clorazepate Dipotassium (Increased CNS depression). Products include:
Tranxene ... 459

Clozapine (Increased CNS depression). Products include:
Clozaril Tablets ... 2377

Codeine Phosphate (Increased CNS depression). Products include:
Brontex ... 2130
Dimetane-DC Cough Syrup ... 2232
Fioricet with Codeine Capsules ... 2387
Fiorinal with Codeine Capsules ... 2390
Nucofed ... 2225
Phenergan with Codeine ... 2883
Phenergan VC with Codeine ... 2888
Robitussin A-C Syrup ... 2248
Robitussin-DAC Syrup ... 2249
Ryna ... ▣ 804
Soma Compound w/Codeine Tablets ... 2784
Tylenol with Codeine ... 1592

Cyproheptadine Hydrochloride (Increased CNS depression). Products include:
Periactin ... 1767

Desflurane (Increased CNS depression). Products include:
Suprane (desflurane, USP) ... 1865

Dexchlorpheniramine Maleate (Increased CNS depression).
No products indexed under this heading.

Dezocine (Increased CNS depression). Products include:
Dalgan Injection ... 529

Diazepam (Concurrent use has resulted in respiratory and cardiovascular collapse; increased CNS depression). Products include:
Dizac (diazepam injectable emulsion) CIV ... 1862
Valium Injectable ... 2336
Valium Tablets ... 2335

Diphenhydramine Citrate (Increased CNS depression). Products include:
Excedrin P.M. Analgesic/Sleeping Aid Tablets, Caplets, Liquigels ... 735

Diphenhydramine Hydrochloride (Increased CNS depression). Products include:
Actifed Allergy Daytime/Nighttime Caplets ... ▣ 808
Actifed Sinus Daytime/Nighttime Tablets and Caplets ... ▣ 809
Extra Strength Bayer PM Aspirin Plus Sleep Aid ... ▣ 617
Benadryl Allergy Chewables ... ▣ 811
Benadryl Allergy/Cold Tablets ... ▣ 811
Benadryl Allergy Decongestant Liquid Medication ... ▣ 812
Benadryl Allergy Decongestant Tablets ... ▣ 812
Benadryl Allergy Liquid Medication ... ▣ 813
Benadryl Allergy ... ▣ 811
Benadryl Allergy Sinus Headache Caplets ... ▣ 813
Benadryl Dye-Free Allergy Liqui-gel Softgels ... ▣ 813
Benadryl Dye-Free Allergy Liquid Medication ... ▣ 814
Benadryl Itch Relief Stick Extra Strength ... ▣ 814
Benadryl Cream ... ▣ 814
Benadryl Gel ... ▣ 815
Benadryl Spray ... ▣ 815
Benadryl Injection ... 1955
Contac Day & Night Cold/Flu Night Caplets ... ▣ 772
Contac Night Allergy/Sinus Caplets ... ▣ 771
Extra Strength Doan's P.M. ... ▣ 653
Excedrin P.M. Analgesic/Sleeping Aid Tablets, Caplets, Liquigels ... ▣ 643
Nytol QuickCaps Caplets ... ▣ 632
Sleepinal Night-time Sleep Aid Capsules and Softgels ... ▣ 798
TYLENOL Allergy Sinus NightTime, Maximum Strength Caplets ... 1571
TYLENOL Flu NightTime, Maximum Strength Gelcaps ... 1575
TYLENOL Flu NightTime, Maximum Strength Hot Medication Packets ... 1575
TYLENOL PM Pain Reliever/Sleep Aid, Extra Strength Gelcaps, Caplets, Geltabs ... 1576
TYLENOL Severe Allergy Medication Caplets ... 1571
Maximum Strength Unisom Sleepgels ... 1990
Unisom With Pain Relief-Nighttime Sleep Aid and Pain Reliever ... 1991

Diphenylpyraline Hydrochloride (Increased CNS depression).
No products indexed under this heading.

Droperidol (Increased CNS depression). Products include:
Inapsine Injection ... 462

Enflurane (Increased CNS depression).
No products indexed under this heading.

Estazolam (Increased CNS depression). Products include:
ProSom Tablets ... 457

Ethchlorvynol (Increased CNS depression). Products include:
Placidyl Capsules ... 456

Ethinamate (Increased CNS depression).
No products indexed under this heading.

Fentanyl (Increased CNS depression). Products include:
Duragesic Transdermal System ... 1336

Fentanyl Citrate (Increased CNS depression). Products include:
Sublimaze Injection ... 463

Fluphenazine Decanoate (Increased CNS depression). Products include:
Prolixin Decanoate ... 510

Fluphenazine Enanthate (Increased CNS depression). Products include:
Prolixin Enanthate ... 510

Fluphenazine Hydrochloride (Increased CNS depression). Products include:
Prolixin ... 510

Flurazepam Hydrochloride (Increased CNS depression). Products include:
Dalmane Capsules ... 2329

Furazolidone (Effect unspecified; caution should be exercised). Products include:
Furoxone ... 2221

Glutethimide (Increased CNS depression).
No products indexed under this heading.

Halazepam (Increased CNS depression).
No products indexed under this heading.

Haloperidol (Increased CNS depression). Products include:
Haldol Injection, Tablets and Concentrate ... 1585

Haloperidol Decanoate (Increased CNS depression). Products include:
Haldol Decanoate ... 1587

Hydrocodone Bitartrate (Increased CNS depression). Products include:
Codiclear DH Syrup ... 808
Duratuss HD Elixir ... 2750
Histussin D Liquid ... 670
Hycodan Tablets and Syrup ... 946
Hycomine Compound Tablets ... 948
Hycomine ... 947
Hycotuss Expectorant Syrup ... 950
Hydrocet Capsules ... 787
Lorcet 10/650 Tablets ... 1016
Lortab ... 2751
Tussend ... 1830
Tussend Expectorant ... 1831
Vicodin Tablets ... 1404
Vicodin ES Tablets ... 1405
Vicodin HP Tablets ... 1403
Vicodin Tuss Expectorant ... 1406
Zydone Capsules ... 967

Hydrocodone Polistirex (Increased CNS depression). Products include:
Tussionex Pennkinetic Extended-Release Suspension ... 1624

Hydromorphone Hydrochloride (Increased CNS depression). Products include:
Dilaudid Ampules ... 1382
Dilaudid Cough Syrup ... 1383
Dilaudid-HP Injection ... 1384
Dilaudid-HP Lyophilized Powder 250 mg ... 1384
Dilaudid ... 1382
Dilaudid Oral Liquid ... 1386
Dilaudid ... 1382
Dilaudid Tablets - 8 mg ... 1386

Hydroxyzine Hydrochloride (Increased CNS depression). Products include:
Atarax Tablets & Syrup ... 1992
Marax Tablets & DF Syrup ... 2015
Vistaril Intramuscular Solution ... 2042

Isocarboxazid (Effect unspecified; caution should be exercised).
No products indexed under this heading.

Isoflurane (Increased CNS depression).
No products indexed under this heading.

Ketamine Hydrochloride (Increased CNS depression).
No products indexed under this heading.

Levomethadyl Acetate Hydrochloride (Increased CNS depression). Products include:
Orlaam Oral Solution ... 2361

Levorphanol Tartrate (Increased CNS depression). Products include:
Levo-Dromoran ... 2297

Loratadine (Increased CNS depression). Products include:
Claritin Tablets ... 2485
Claritin-D Tablets ... 2487

Lorazepam (Increased CNS depression). Products include:
Ativan Injection ... 2805
Ativan Tablets ... 2807

Loxapine Hydrochloride (Increased CNS depression). Products include:
Loxitane ... 1426

Loxapine Succinate (Increased CNS depression). Products include:
Loxitane Capsules ... 1426

Meperidine Hydrochloride (Increased CNS depression). Products include:
Demerol ... 2438
Mepergan Injection ... 2859

Mephobarbital (Increased CNS depression). Products include:
Mebaral Tablets ... 2452

Meprobamate (Increased CNS depression). Products include:
Miltown Tablets ... 2780
PMB 200 and PMB 400 ... 2890

Mesoridazine Besylate (Increased CNS depression). Products include:
Serentil ... 689

Methadone Hydrochloride (Increased CNS depression). Products include:
Methadone Hydrochloride Oral Concentrate ... 2356
Methadone Hydrochloride Oral Solution & Tablets ... 2357

Methdilazine Hydrochloride (Increased CNS depression).
No products indexed under this heading.

Methohexital Sodium (Increased CNS depression).
No products indexed under this heading.

Methotrimeprazine (Increased CNS depression). Products include:
Levoprome ... 1321

Methoxyflurane (Increased CNS depression).
No products indexed under this heading.

Midazolam Hydrochloride (Increased CNS depression). Products include:
Versed Injection ... 2324

Molindone Hydrochloride (Increased CNS depression). Products include:
Moban Tablets and Concentrate ... 1036

Morphine Sulfate (Increased CNS depression). Products include:
Astramorph/PF Injection, USP (Preservative-Free) ... 526
Duramorph Injection ... 983
Infumorph 200 and Infumorph 500 Sterile Solutions ... 985
Kadian Capsules ... 2948
MS Contin Tablets ... 2149
MSIR ... 2152
Oramorph SR (Morphine Sulfate Sustained Release Tablets) ... 2359
RMS Suppositories CII ... 2766
Roxanol ... 2365

Opium Alkaloids (Increased CNS depression).
No products indexed under this heading.

Oxazepam (Increased CNS depression). Products include:
Serax Capsules ... 2916
Serax Tablets ... 2916

Oxycodone Hydrochloride (Increased CNS depression). Products include:
OxyContin Tablets ... 2163
OxyIR Capsules ... 2167
Percocet Tablets ... 955
Percodan Tablets ... 955
Percodan-Demi Tablets ... 956
Roxicodone Tablets, Oral Solution & Intensol (Oxycodone) ... 2366
Tylox Capsules ... 1593

Pentobarbital Sodium (Increased CNS depression). Products include:
Nembutal Sodium Capsules ... 440
Nembutal Sodium Solution ... 442
Nembutal Sodium Suppositories ... 444

Perphenazine (Increased CNS depression). Products include:
Etrafon ... 2495
Triavil Tablets ... 1800
Trilafon ... 2532

Phenelzine Sulfate (Effect unspecified; caution should be exercised). Products include:
Nardil ... 1977

Phenobarbital (Increased CNS depression). Products include:
Arco-Lase Plus Tablets ... 513
Bellergal-S Tablets ... 2375
Donnatal ... 2234
Donnatal Extentabs ... 2234
Donnatal Tablets ... 2234
Phenobarbital Elixir and Tablets ... 1523
Quadrinal Tablets ... 1398

Phenprocoumon (Potential for purpura).

Prazepam (Increased CNS depression).
No products indexed under this heading.

Prochlorperazine (Increased CNS depression). Products include:
Compazine ... 2644

(▣ Described in PDR For Nonprescription Drugs) (◉ Described in PDR For Ophthalmology)

Promethazine Hydrochloride (Increased CNS depression). Products include:
- Mepergan Injection ... 2859
- Phenergan with Codeine ... 2883
- Phenergan with Dextromethorphan ... 2885
- Phenergan Injection ... 2880
- Phenergan Suppositories ... 2882
- Phenergan Syrup ... 2881
- Phenergan Tablets ... 2882
- Phenergan VC ... 2886
- Phenergan VC with Codeine ... 2888

Propofol (Increased CNS depression). Products include:
- Diprivan Injectable Emulsion ... 2939

Propoxyphene Hydrochloride (Increased CNS depression). Products include:
- Darvon ... 1475
- Wygesic Tablets ... 2930

Propoxyphene Napsylate (Increased CNS depression). Products include:
- Darvon-N/Darvocet-N ... 1473

Pyrilamine Maleate (Increased CNS depression). Products include:
- 4-Way Fast Acting Nasal Spray (regular & mentholated) ... 644
- Maximum Strength Multi-Symptom Formula Midol ... 621
- PMS Multi-Symptom Formula Midol ... 622

Pyrilamine Tannate (Increased CNS depression). Products include:
- Atrohist Pediatric Suspension ... 1604
- Atrohist Pediatric Suspension Dye-Free ... 1604
- Rynatan ... 2781

Quazepam (Increased CNS depression). Products include:
- Doral Tablets ... 2773

Risperidone (Increased CNS depression). Products include:
- Risperdal Tablets ... 1348

Secobarbital Sodium (Increased CNS depression). Products include:
- Seconal Sodium Pulvules ... 1529

Selegiline Hydrochloride (Effect unspecified; caution should be exercised). Products include:
- Eldepryl Capsules ... 2729

Sevoflurane (Increased CNS depression).
- No products indexed under this heading.

Sufentanil Citrate (Increased CNS depression). Products include:
- Sufenta Injection ... 1355

Temazepam (Increased CNS depression). Products include:
- Restoril Capsules ... 2413

Terfenadine (Increased CNS depression). Products include:
- Seldane Tablets ... 1284
- Seldane-D Extended-Release Tablets ... 1286

Thiamylal Sodium (Increased CNS depression).
- No products indexed under this heading.

Thioridazine Hydrochloride (Increased CNS depression). Products include:
- Mellaril ... 2398

Thiothixene (Increased CNS depression). Products include:
- Navane Capsules and Concentrate ... 2018
- Navane Intramuscular ... 2019

Tranylcypromine Sulfate (Effect unspecified; caution should be exercised). Products include:
- Parnate Tablets ... 2679

Triazolam (Increased CNS depression). Products include:
- Halcion Tablets ... 2093

Trifluoperazine Hydrochloride (Increased CNS depression). Products include:
- Stelazine ... 2692

Trimeprazine Tartrate (Increased CNS depression).
- No products indexed under this heading.

Tripelennamine Hydrochloride (Increased CNS depression). Products include:
- PBZ Tablets ... 863
- PBZ-SR Tablets ... 862

Triprolidine Hydrochloride (Increased CNS depression). Products include:
- Actifed Cold & Allergy Tablets ... 807
- Actifed Cold & Sinus Caplets and Tablets ... 808

Zolpidem Tartrate (Increased CNS depression). Products include:
- Ambien Tablets ... 2559

Food Interactions
Alcohol (Increased CNS depression).

BUSPAR TABLETS
(Buspirone Hydrochloride) ... 738
May interact with monoamine oxidase inhibitors and certain other agents. Compounds in these categories include:

Digoxin (In vitro buspirone may displace less firmly bound drugs like digoxin; the clinical significance is unknown). Products include:
- Lanoxicaps ... 1110
- Lanoxin Elixir Pediatric ... 1113
- Lanoxin Injection ... 1116
- Lanoxin Injection Pediatric ... 1119
- Lanoxin Tablets ... 1121

Furazolidone (Co-administration may pose a hazard due to potential for elevated blood pressure; concomitant administration is not recommended). Products include:
- Furoxone ... 2221

Haloperidol (Increased serum haloperidol concentrations). Products include:
- Haldol Injection, Tablets and Concentrate ... 1585

Haloperidol Decanoate (Increased serum haloperidol concentrations). Products include:
- Haldol Decanoate ... 1587

Isocarboxazid (Co-administration may pose a hazard due to potential for elevated blood pressure; concomitant administration is not recommended).
- No products indexed under this heading.

Phenelzine Sulfate (Co-administration may pose a hazard due to potential for elevated blood pressure; concomitant administration is not recommended). Products include:
- Nardil ... 1977

Psychotropic drugs, unspecified (Concomitant use of BuSpar with other CNS-active drugs should be approached with caution).

Selegiline Hydrochloride (Co-administration may pose a hazard due to potential for elevated blood pressure; concomitant administration is not recommended). Products include:
- Eldepryl Capsules ... 2729

Tranylcypromine Sulfate (Co-administration may pose a hazard due to potential for elevated blood pressure; concomitant administration is not recommended). Products include:
- Parnate Tablets ... 2679

Trazodone Hydrochloride (Possible SGPT elevation). Products include:
- Desyrel and Desyrel Dividose ... 504

Warfarin Sodium (Single report of prolonged prothrombin time in a patient on other tightly protein bound drugs). Products include:
- Coumadin ... 941

Food Interactions
Alcohol (Concomitant use should be avoided).

Food, unspecified (Food may decrease presystemic clearance of buspirone).

BUTISOL SODIUM ELIXIR & TABLETS
(Butabarbital Sodium) ... 2768
May interact with oral anticoagulants, corticosteroids, central nervous system depressants, monoamine oxidase inhibitors, hypnotics and sedatives, tranquilizers, doxycycline, antihistamines, and certain other agents. Compounds in these categories include:

Acrivastine (Co-administration may produce additive CNS depressant effects). Products include:
- Semprex-D Capsules ... 1620

Alfentanil Hydrochloride (Co-administration may produce additive CNS depressant effects). Products include:
- Alfenta Injection ... 1334

Alprazolam (Co-administration may produce additive CNS depressant effects). Products include:
- Xanax Tablets ... 2115

Aprobarbital (Co-administration may produce additive CNS depressant effects).
- No products indexed under this heading.

Astemizole (Co-administration may produce additive CNS depressant effects). Products include:
- Hismanal Tablets ... 1341

Azatadine Maleate (Co-administration may produce additive CNS depressant effects). Products include:
- Trinalin Repetabs Tablets ... 1373

Betamethasone Acetate (Barbiturates appear to enhance the metabolism of exogenous corticosteroids through the induction of hepatic microsomal enzymes). Products include:
- Celestone Soluspan Suspension ... 2484

Betamethasone Sodium Phosphate (Barbiturates appear to enhance the metabolism of exogenous corticosteroids through the induction of hepatic microsomal enzymes). Products include:
- Celestone Soluspan Suspension ... 2484

Bromodiphenhydramine Hydrochloride (Co-administration may produce additive CNS depressant effects).
- No products indexed under this heading.

Brompheniramine Maleate (Co-administration may produce additive CNS depressant effects). Products include:
- Alka-Seltzer Plus Sinus Medicine ... 611
- Bromfed Capsules (Extended-Release) ... 1832
- Bromfed Syrup ... 712
- Bromfed Tablets ... 1832
- Bromfed-DM Cough Syrup ... 1832
- Bromfed-PD Capsules (Extended-Release) ... 1832
- Dimetane-DC Cough Syrup ... 2232
- Dimetane-DX Cough Syrup ... 2233
- Dimetapp Allergy Dye-Free Elixir ... 838
- Dimetapp Allergy Sinus Caplets ... 838
- Dimetapp Cold & Allergy Chewable Tablets ... 838
- Dimetapp Cold & Cough Liqui-Gels ... 839
- Dimetapp Cold & Fever Suspension ... 839
- Dimetapp DM Elixir ... 840
- Dimetapp Elixir ... 840
- Dimetapp Extentabs ... 841
- Dimetapp Tablets/Liqui-Gels ... 841
- Rondec Chewable Tablets ... 974
- Vicks DayQuil Allergy Relief 12-Hour Extended Release Tablets ... 733
- Vicks DayQuil Allergy Relief 4-Hour Tablets ... 733

Buprenorphine (Co-administration may produce additive CNS depressant effects). Products include:
- Buprenex Injectable ... 2170

Buspirone Hydrochloride (Co-administration may produce additive CNS depressant effects). Products include:
- BuSpar Tablets ... 738

Butabarbital (Co-administration may produce additive CNS depressant effects).
- No products indexed under this heading.

Butalbital (Co-administration may produce additive CNS depressant effects). Products include:
- Axocet Capsules ... 2469
- Esgic-plus Capsules ... 1012
- Esgic-plus Tablets ... 1012
- Fioricet Tablets ... 2386
- Fioricet with Codeine Capsules ... 2387
- Fiorinal Capsules ... 2388
- Fiorinal with Codeine Capsules ... 2390
- Fiorinal Tablets ... 2388
- Phrenilin ... 790
- Sedapap Tablets 50 mg/650 mg ... 1826

Cetirizine Hydrochloride (Co-administration may produce additive CNS depressant effects). Products include:
- Zyrtec Tablets ... 2053

Chlordiazepoxide (Co-administration may produce additive CNS depressant effects). Products include:
- Limbitrol ... 2333

Chlordiazepoxide Hydrochloride (Co-administration may produce additive CNS depressant effects). Products include:
- Librax Capsules ... 2330
- Librium Capsules ... 2331
- Librium Injectable ... 2332

Chlorpheniramine Maleate (Co-administration may produce additive CNS depressant effects). Products include:
- Alka-Seltzer Plus Cold Medicine ... 611
- Alka-Seltzer Plus Cold Medicine Liqui-Gels ... 612
- Alka-Seltzer Plus Cold & Cough Medicine ... 611
- Alka-Seltzer Plus Cold & Cough Medicine Liqui-Gels ... 612
- Alka-Seltzer Plus Flu & Body Aches Effervescent Tablets ... 612
- Allerest Maximum Strength ... 649
- Allerest Sinus Pain Formula ... 649
- Ana-Kit Anaphylaxis Emergency Treatment Kit ... 611
- Atrohist Pediatric Capsules ... 1603
- Atrohist Plus Tablets ... 1605
- BC Cold Powder Multi-Symptom Formula (Cold-Sinus-Allergy) ... 631
- Cerose DM ... 853
- Cheracol Plus Head Cold/Cough Formula ... 741
- Children's TYLENOL Cold Multi-Symptom Chewable Tablets and Liquid ... 1559
- Children's TYLENOL Cold Plus Cough Multi Symptom Chewable Tablets and Liquid ... 1560
- Children's TYLENOL Flu Suspension Liquid ... 1560
- Children's Vicks DayQuil Allergy Relief ... 730
- Children's Vicks NyQuil Cold/Cough Relief ... 731
- Chlor-Trimeton Allergy Decongestant Tablets ... 759
- Chlor-Trimeton Allergy Tablets ... 758

IMPORTANT NOTE: Always consult each drug listing in the patient's regimen for possible interactions.

Butisol Sodium / Interactions Index

Allergy-Sinus Comtrex Multi-Symptom Allergy-Sinus Formula Tablets and Caplets ... 639
Comtrex Multi-Symptom ... 638
Contac Continuous Action Nasal Decongestant/Antihistamine 12 Hour Capsules ... 773
Contac Maximum Strength Continuous Action Decongestant/Antihistamine 12 Hour Caplets .. 772
Contac Severe Cold and Flu Formula Capsules ... 773
Coricidin Cold + Flu Tablets ... 760
Coricidin Cough + Cold Tablets ... 760
Coricidin 'D' Decongestant Tablets ... 760
D.A. II Tablets ... 972
D.A. Chewable Tablets ... 970
Dura-Tap/PD Capsules ... 970
Dura-Vent/DA Tablets ... 972
Efidac 24 Chlorpheniramine ... 655
Extendryl ... 1003
Fedahist Gyrocaps ... 2545
Hycomine Compound Tablets ... 948
Kronofed-A ... 994
Nolamine Timed-Release Tablets ... 790
Novahistine Elixir ... 782
Ornade Spansule Capsules ... 2678
PediaCare Cough-Cold Chewable Tablets and Liquid ... 1569
PediaCare NightRest Cough-Cold Liquid ... 1569
Pediatric Vicks 44m Cough & Cold Relief ... 737
Pyrroxate Caplets ... 742
Ryna ... 804
Sinarest ... 663
Sine-Off Sinus Medicine ... 784
Singlet Tablets ... 785
Sinulin Tablets ... 792
Sinutab Sinus Allergy Medication, Maximum Strength Tablets and Caplets ... 823
Sudafed Cold & Allergy Tablets ... 826
Teldrin 12 Hour Antihistamine/Nasal Decongestant Allergy Relief Capsules ... 786
TheraFlu Flu and Cold Medicine ... 750
Theraflu Maximum Strength Flu and Cold Medicine For Sore Throat ... 751
TheraFlu Flu, Cold and Cough Medicine ... 750
TheraFlu Maximum Strength Nighttime Flu, Cold & Cough Medicine ... 751
Triaminic Night Time ... 754
Triaminic Syrup ... 755
Triaminic Triaminicol Cold & Cough ... 756
Triaminicin Tablets ... 756
Tussend ... 1830
TYLENOL Allergy Sinus, Maximum Strength Caplets and Gelcaps ... 1571
TYLENOL Cold Medication, Multi-Symptom Formula Tablets and Caplets ... 1572
TYLENOL Cold Medication, Multi-Symptom Hot Liquid Packets ... 1572
Vicks 44 LiquiCaps Cough, Cold & Flu Relief ... 728
Vicks 44M Cough, Cold & Flu Relief ... 729

Chlorpheniramine Polistirex
(Co-administration may produce additive CNS depressant effects). Products include:
Tussionex Pennkinetic Extended-Release Suspension ... 1624

Chlorpheniramine Tannate
(Co-administration may produce additive CNS depressant effects). Products include:
Atrohist Pediatric Suspension ... 1604
Atrohist Pediatric Suspension Dye-Free ... 1604
Rynatan ... 2781
Rynatuss ... 2782

Chlorpromazine
(Co-administration may produce additive CNS depressant effects). Products include:
Thorazine Suppositories ... 2701

Chlorpromazine Hydrochloride
(Co-administration may produce additive CNS depressant effects). Products include:
Thorazine ... 2701

Chlorprothixene
(Co-administration may produce additive CNS depressant effects).
No products indexed under this heading.

Chlorprothixene Hydrochloride
(Co-administration may produce additive CNS depressant effects).
No products indexed under this heading.

Chlorprothixene Lactate
(Co-administration may produce additive CNS depressant effects).
No products indexed under this heading.

Clemastine Fumarate
(Co-administration may produce additive CNS depressant effects). Products include:
Tavist Syrup ... 2426
Tavist Tablets ... 2427
Tavist-1 12 Hour Relief Tablets ... 749
Tavist-D 12 Hour Relief Tablets ... 750

Clorazepate Dipotassium
(Co-administration may produce additive CNS depressant effects). Products include:
Tranxene ... 459

Clozapine
(Co-administration may produce additive CNS depressant effects). Products include:
Clozaril Tablets ... 2377

Codeine Phosphate
(Co-administration may produce additive CNS depressant effects). Products include:
Brontex ... 2130
Dimetane-DC Cough Syrup ... 2232
Fioricet with Codeine Capsules ... 2387
Fiorinal with Codeine Capsules ... 2390
Nucofed ... 2225
Phenergan with Codeine ... 2883
Phenergan VC with Codeine ... 2888
Robitussin A-C Syrup ... 2248
Robitussin-DAC Syrup ... 2249
Ryna ... 804
Soma Compound w/Codeine Tablets ... 2784
Tylenol with Codeine ... 1592

Cortisone Acetate
(Barbiturates appear to enhance the metabolism of exogenous corticosteroids through the induction of hepatic microsomal enzymes). Products include:
Cortone Acetate Sterile Suspension ... 1663
Cortone Acetate Tablets ... 1664

Cyproheptadine Hydrochloride
(Co-administration may produce additive CNS depressant effects). Products include:
Periactin ... 1767

Desflurane
(Co-administration may produce additive CNS depressant effects). Products include:
Suprane (desflurane, USP) ... 1865

Dexamethasone
(Barbiturates appear to enhance the metabolism of exogenous corticosteroids through the induction of hepatic microsomal enzymes). Products include:
AK-Trol Ointment & Suspension ... 205
Decadron Elixir ... 1676
Decadron Tablets ... 1678
Decaspray Topical Aerosol ... 1689
Maxitrol Ophthalmic Ointment and Suspension ... 222
TobraDex Ophthalmic Suspension and Ointment ... 469

Dexamethasone Acetate
(Barbiturates appear to enhance the metabolism of exogenous corticosteroids through the induction of hepatic microsomal enzymes). Products include:
Dalalone D.P. Injectable ... 1009
Decadron-LA Sterile Suspension ... 1687

Dexamethasone Sodium Phosphate
(Barbiturates appear to enhance the metabolism of exogenous corticosteroids through the induction of hepatic microsomal enzymes). Products include:
Decadron Phosphate Injection ... 1680
Decadron Phosphate Sterile Ophthalmic Ointment ... 1684
Decadron Phosphate Sterile Ophthalmic Solution ... 1685
Decadron Phosphate Topical Cream ... 1686
Decadron Phosphate with Xylocaine Injection, Sterile ... 1683
Dexacort Phosphate in Respihaler ... 1755
Dexacort Phosphate in Turbinaire .. 1607
NeoDecadron Sterile Ophthalmic Ointment ... 1755
NeoDecadron Sterile Ophthalmic Solution ... 1756
NeoDecadron Topical Cream ... 1757

Dexchlorpheniramine Maleate
(Co-administration may produce additive CNS depressant effects).
No products indexed under this heading.

Dezocine
(Co-administration may produce additive CNS depressant effects). Products include:
Dalgan Injection ... 529

Diazepam
(Co-administration may produce additive CNS depressant effects). Products include:
Dizac (diazepam injectable emulsion) CIV ... 1862
Valium Injectable ... 2336
Valium Tablets ... 2335

Dicumarol
(Barbiturates can induce hepatic microsomal enzymes resulting in increased metabolism and decreased anticoagulant response of oral anticoagulants).
No products indexed under this heading.

Diphenhydramine Citrate
(Co-administration may produce additive CNS depressant effects). Products include:
Excedrin P.M. Analgesic/Sleeping Aid Tablets, Caplets, Liquigels ... 735

Diphenhydramine Hydrochloride
(Co-administration may produce additive CNS depressant effects). Products include:
Actifed Allergy Daytime/Nighttime Caplets ... 808
Actifed Sinus Daytime/Nighttime Tablets and Caplets ... 809
Extra Strength Bayer PM Aspirin Plus Sleep Aid ... 617
Benadryl Allergy Chewables ... 811
Benadryl Allergy/Cold Tablets ... 811
Benadryl Allergy Decongestant Liquid Medication ... 812
Benadryl Allergy Decongestant Tablets ... 812
Benadryl Allergy Liquid Medication ... 813
Benadryl Allergy ... 811
Benadryl Allergy Sinus Headache Caplets ... 813
Benadryl Dye-Free Allergy Liquigel Softgels ... 813
Benadryl Dye-Free Allergy Liquid Medication ... 814
Benadryl Itch Relief Stick Extra Strength ... 814
Benadryl Cream ... 814
Benadryl Gel ... 815
Benadryl Spray ... 815
Benadryl Injection ... 1955
Contac Day & Night Cold/Flu Night Caplets ... 772
Contac Night Allergy/Sinus Caplets ... 771
Extra Strength Doan's P.M. ... 653
Excedrin P.M. Analgesic/Sleeping Aid Tablets, Caplets, Liquigels ... 643
Nytol QuickCaps Caplets ... 632
Sleepinal Night-time Sleep Aid Capsules and Softgels ... 798
TYLENOL Allergy Sinus NightTime, Maximum Strength Caplets ... 1571
TYLENOL Flu NightTime, Maximum Strength Gelcaps ... 1575
TYLENOL Flu NightTime, Maximum Strength Hot Medication Packets ... 1575
TYLENOL PM Pain Reliever/Sleep Aid, Extra Strength Gelcaps, Caplets, Geltabs ... 1576
TYLENOL Severe Allergy Medication Caplets ... 1571
Maximum Strength Unisom Sleepgels ... 1990
Unisom With Pain Relief-Nighttime Sleep Aid and Pain Reliever ... 1991

Diphenylpyraline Hydrochloride
(Co-administration may produce additive CNS depressant effects).
No products indexed under this heading.

Divalproex Sodium
(Valproic acid appears to decrease the barbiturate metabolism). Products include:
Depakote Tablets ... 418

Doxycycline Calcium
(Barbiturates, such as phenobarbital, have been shown to shorten the half-life of doxycycline through the induction of hepatic microsomal enzymes that metabolize the antibiotic). Products include:
Vibramycin Calcium Oral Suspension Syrup ... 2038

Doxycycline Hyclate
(Barbiturates, such as phenobarbital, have been shown to shorten the half-life of doxycycline through the induction of hepatic microsomal enzymes that metabolize the antibiotic). Products include:
Doryx Capsules ... 1970
Vibramycin Hyclate Capsules ... 2038
Vibramycin Hyclate Intravenous ... 2040
Vibra-Tabs Film Coated Tablets ... 2038

Doxycycline Monohydrate
(Barbiturates, such as phenobarbital, have been shown to shorten the half-life of doxycycline through the induction of hepatic microsomal enzymes that metabolize the antibiotic). Products include:
Monodox Capsules ... 1858
Vibramycin Monohydrate for Oral Suspension ... 2038

Droperidol
(Co-administration may produce additive CNS depressant effects). Products include:
Inapsine Injection ... 462

Enflurane
(Co-administration may produce additive CNS depressant effects).
No products indexed under this heading.

Estazolam
(Co-administration may produce additive CNS depressant effects). Products include:
ProSom Tablets ... 457

Ethchlorvynol
(Co-administration may produce additive CNS depressant effects). Products include:
Placidyl Capsules ... 456

Ethinamate
(Co-administration may produce additive CNS depressant effects).
No products indexed under this heading.

Ethinyl Estradiol
(Barbiturates, such as phenobarbital, may decrease the effect of estradiol by increasing its metabolism; an alternate form of contraceptive method might be suggested). Products include:
Brevicon ... 2563
Demulen ... 2580
Desogen Tablets ... 1867
Levlen/Tri-Levlen ... 646
Lo/Ovral ... 2852
Lo/Ovral-28 Tablets ... 2857
Modicon ... 1928
Nordette-21 Tablets ... 2863
Nordette-28 Tablets ... 2866
Norinyl ... 2563
Ortho-Cept ... 1907

(▣ Described in PDR For Nonprescription Drugs)   (⊙ Described in PDR For Ophthalmology)

143 **Interactions Index** **Butisol Sodium**

Ortho-Cyclen/Ortho-Tri-Cyclen 1914
Ortho-Novum 1928
Ortho-Cyclen/Ortho Tri-Cyclen 1914
Ovcon 765
Ovral Tablets 2877
Ovral-28 Tablets 2878
Levlen/Tri-Levlen 646
Tri-Norinyl 2607
Triphasil-21 Tablets 2919
Triphasil-28 Tablets 2924

Fentanyl (Co-administration may produce additive CNS depressant effects). Products include:
Duragesic Transdermal System 1336

Fentanyl Citrate (Co-administration may produce additive CNS depressant effects). Products include:
Sublimaze Injection 463

Fludrocortisone Acetate (Barbiturates appear to enhance the metabolism of exogenous corticosteroids through the induction of hepatic microsomal enzymes). Products include:
Florinef Acetate Tablets 506

Fluphenazine Decanoate (Co-administration may produce additive CNS depressant effects). Products include:
Prolixin Decanoate 510

Fluphenazine Enanthate (Co-administration may produce additive CNS depressant effects). Products include:
Prolixin Enanthate 510

Fluphenazine Hydrochloride (Co-administration may produce additive CNS depressant effects). Products include:
Prolixin 510

Flurazepam Hydrochloride (Co-administration may produce additive CNS depressant effects). Products include:
Dalmane Capsules 2329

Fosphenytoin Sodium (The effect of barbiturates on the metabolism of phenytoin appears to be variable). Products include:
Cerebyx Injection 1956

Furazolidone (MAO inhibitors prolong the effects of barbiturates probably by inhibiting barbiturate metabolism). Products include:
Furoxone 2221

Glutethimide (Co-administration may produce additive CNS depressant effects).
No products indexed under this heading.

Griseofulvin (Barbiturates, such as phenobarbital, appear to interfere with the absorption of orally administered griseofulvin, thus decreasing its blood levels). Products include:
Fulvicin P/G Tablets 2499
Fulvicin P/G 165 & 330 Tablets 2500
Grifulvin V (griseofulvin tablets) Microsize (griseofulvin oral suspension) Microsize 1944
Gris-PEG Tablets, 125 mg & 250 mg 476

Haloperidol (Co-administration may produce additive CNS depressant effects). Products include:
Haldol Injection, Tablets and Concentrate 1585

Haloperidol Decanoate (Co-administration may produce additive CNS depressant effects). Products include:
Haldol Decanoate 1587

Hydrocodone Bitartrate (Co-administration may produce additive CNS depressant effects). Products include:
Codiclear DH Syrup 808
Duratuss HD Elixir 2750
Histussin D Liquid 670
Hycodan Tablets and Syrup 946
Hycomine Compound Tablets 948
Hycomine 947
Hycotuss Expectorant Syrup 950
Hydrocet Capsules 787
Lorcet 10/650 Tablets 1016
Lortab 2751
Tussend 1830
Tussend Expectorant 1831
Vicodin Tablets 1404
Vicodin ES Tablets 1405
Vicodin HP Tablets 1403
Vicodin Tuss Expectorant 1406
Zydone Capsules 967

Hydrocodone Polistirex (Co-administration may produce additive CNS depressant effects). Products include:
Tussionex Pennkinetic Extended-Release Suspension 1624

Hydrocortisone (Barbiturates appear to enhance the metabolism of exogenous corticosteroids through the induction of hepatic microsomal enzymes). Products include:
Anusol-HC Cream 2.5% 1953
Aquanil HC Lotion 1989
Maximum Strength Cortaid Spray 800
CORTENEMA 2713
Cortisporin Ointment 1074
Cortisporin Ophthalmic Ointment Sterile 1074
Cortisporin Ophthalmic Suspension Sterile 1075
Cortisporin Otic Solution Sterile 1076
Cortisporin Otic Suspension Sterile 1077
Cortizone-5 795
Cortizone-10 795
Hydrocortone Tablets 1715
Hytone 922
Hytone Ointment 2 ½% 923
Massengill Medicated Soft Cloth Towelettes 2628
Pediotic Suspension Sterile 1140
Preparation H Hydrocortisone 1% Cream 843
ProctoCream-HC 2.5% 2552
VōSoL HC Otic Solution 2786

Hydrocortisone Acetate (Barbiturates appear to enhance the metabolism of exogenous corticosteroids through the induction of hepatic microsomal enzymes). Products include:
Analpram-HC Rectal Cream 1% and 2.5% 993
Anusol HC-1 Hydrocortisone Anti-Itch Ointment 810
Anusol-HC Suppositories 1954
Caldecort Anti-Itch Hydrocortisone Cream 651
Coly-Mycin S Otic w/Neomycin & Hydrocortisone 1965
Cortaid 800
Cortifoam 2540
Cortisporin Cream 1073
Epifoam 2543
Hydrocortone Acetate Sterile Suspension 1712
Mantadil Cream 1124
Nupercainal Hydrocortisone 1% Cream 661
Pramosone Cream, Lotion & Ointment 995
ProctoFoam-HC 2552
Terra-Cortril Ophthalmic Suspension 2033

Hydrocortisone Sodium Phosphate (Barbiturates appear to enhance the metabolism of exogenous corticosteroids through the induction of hepatic microsomal enzymes). Products include:
Hydrocortone Phosphate Injection, Sterile 1713

Hydrocortisone Sodium Succinate (Barbiturates appear to enhance the metabolism of exogenous corticosteroids through the induction of hepatic microsomal enzymes).
No products indexed under this heading.

Hydromorphone Hydrochloride (Co-administration may produce additive CNS depressant effects). Products include:
Dilaudid Ampules 1382
Dilaudid Cough Syrup 1383
Dilaudid-HP Injection 1384
Dilaudid-HP Lyophilized Powder 250 mg 1384
Dilaudid 1382
Dilaudid Oral Liquid 1386
Dilaudid 1382
Dilaudid Tablets - 8 mg 1386

Hydroxyzine Hydrochloride (Co-administration may produce additive CNS depressant effects). Products include:
Atarax Tablets & Syrup 1992
Marax Tablets & DF Syrup 2015
Vistaril Intramuscular Solution 2042

Isocarboxazid (MAO inhibitors prolong the effects of barbiturates probably by inhibiting barbiturate metabolism).
No products indexed under this heading.

Isoflurane (Co-administration may produce additive CNS depressant effects).
No products indexed under this heading.

Ketamine Hydrochloride (Co-administration may produce additive CNS depressant effects).
No products indexed under this heading.

Levomethadyl Acetate Hydrochloride (Co-administration may produce additive CNS depressant effects). Products include:
Orlaam Oral Solution 2361

Levorphanol Tartrate (Co-administration may produce additive CNS depressant effects). Products include:
Levo-Dromoran 2297

Loratadine (Co-administration may produce additive CNS depressant effects). Products include:
Claritin Tablets 2485
Claritin-D Tablets 2487

Lorazepam (Co-administration may produce additive CNS depressant effects). Products include:
Ativan Injection 2805
Ativan Tablets 2807

Loxapine Hydrochloride (Co-administration may produce additive CNS depressant effects). Products include:
Loxitane 1426

Loxapine Succinate (Co-administration may produce additive CNS depressant effects). Products include:
Loxitane Capsules 1426

Meperidine Hydrochloride (Co-administration may produce additive CNS depressant effects). Products include:
Demerol 2438
Mepergan Injection 2859

Mephobarbital (Co-administration may produce additive CNS depressant effects). Products include:
Mebaral Tablets 2452

Meprobamate (Co-administration may produce additive CNS depressant effects). Products include:
Miltown Tablets 2780
PMB 200 and PMB 400 2890

Mesoridazine Besylate (Co-administration may produce additive CNS depressant effects). Products include:
Serentil 689

Methadone Hydrochloride (Co-administration may produce additive CNS depressant effects). Products include:
Methadone Hydrochloride Oral Concentrate 2356
Methadone Hydrochloride Oral Solution & Tablets 2357

Methdilazine Hydrochloride (Co-administration may produce additive CNS depressant effects).
No products indexed under this heading.

Methohexital Sodium (Co-administration may produce additive CNS depressant effects).
No products indexed under this heading.

Methotrimeprazine (Co-administration may produce additive CNS depressant effects). Products include:
Levoprome 1321

Methoxyflurane (Co-administration may produce additive CNS depressant effects).
No products indexed under this heading.

Methylprednisolone Acetate (Barbiturates appear to enhance the metabolism of exogenous corticosteroids through the induction of hepatic microsomal enzymes).
No products indexed under this heading.

Methylprednisolone Sodium Succinate (Barbiturates appear to enhance the metabolism of exogenous corticosteroids through the induction of hepatic microsomal enzymes).
No products indexed under this heading.

Midazolam Hydrochloride (Co-administration may produce additive CNS depressant effects). Products include:
Versed Injection 2324

Molindone Hydrochloride (Co-administration may produce additive CNS depressant effects). Products include:
Moban Tablets and Concentrate 1036

Morphine Sulfate (Co-administration may produce additive CNS depressant effects). Products include:
Astramorph/PF Injection, USP (Preservative-Free) 526
Duramorph Injection 983
Infumorph 200 and Infumorph 500 Sterile Solutions 985
Kadian Capsules 2948
MS Contin Tablets 2149
MSIR 2152
Oramorph SR (Morphine Sulfate Sustained Release Tablets) 2359
RMS Suppositories CII 2766
Roxanol 2365

Opium Alkaloids (Co-administration may produce additive CNS depressant effects).
No products indexed under this heading.

Oxazepam (Co-administration may produce additive CNS depressant effects). Products include:
Serax Capsules 2916
Serax Tablets 2916

Oxycodone Hydrochloride (Co-administration may produce additive CNS depressant effects). Products include:
OxyContin Tablets 2163
OxyIR Capsules 2167
Percocet Tablets 955
Percodan Tablets 955
Percodan-Demi Tablets 956
Roxicodone Tablets, Oral Solution & Intensol (Oxycodone) 2366
Tylox Capsules 1593

IMPORTANT NOTE: Always consult each drug listing in the patient's regimen for possible interactions.

Pentobarbital Sodium (Co-administration may produce additive CNS depressant effects). Products include:
Nembutal Sodium Capsules 440
Nembutal Sodium Solution 442
Nembutal Sodium Suppositories...... 444

Perphenazine (Co-administration may produce additive CNS depressant effects). Products include:
Etrafon 2495
Triavil Tablets 1800
Trilafon.. 2532

Phenelzine Sulfate (MAO inhibitors prolong the effects of barbiturates probably by inhibiting barbiturate metabolism). Products include:
Nardil 1977

Phenobarbital (Co-administration may produce additive CNS depressant effects). Products include:
Arco-Lase Plus Tablets 513
Bellergal-S Tablets 2375
Donnatal 2234
Donnatal Extentabs............................ 2234
Donnatal Tablets 2234
Phenobarbital Elixir and Tablets...... 1523
Quadrinal Tablets 1398

Phenytoin (The effect of barbiturates on the metabolism of phenytoin appears to be variable). Products include:
Dilantin Infatabs................................ 1967
Dilantin-125 Suspension 1969

Phenytoin Sodium (The effect of barbiturates on the metabolism of phenytoin appears to be variable). Products include:
Dilantin Kapseals 1965

Prazepam (Co-administration may produce additive CNS depressant effects).
No products indexed under this heading.

Prednisolone Acetate (Barbiturates appear to enhance the metabolism of exogenous corticosteroids through the induction of hepatic microsomal enzymes). Products include:
AK-CIDE .... ⊙ 203
AK-CIDE Ointment.............................. ⊙ 203
Blephamide Liquifilm Sterile Ophthalmic Suspension........................... 472
Blephamide Ointment .... ⊙ 234
Econopred & Econopred Plus Ophthalmic Suspensions .... ⊙ 216
Poly-Pred Liquifilm .... ⊙ 246
Pred Forte.. ⊙ 247
Pred Mild... ⊙ 250
Pred-G Liquifilm Sterile Ophthalmic Suspension .... ⊙ 248
Pred-G S.O.P. Sterile Ophthalmic Ointment .... ⊙ 249

Prednisolone Sodium Phosphate (Barbiturates appear to enhance the metabolism of exogenous corticosteroids through the induction of hepatic microsomal enzymes). Products include:
AK-PRED .... ⊙ 204
Hydeltrasol Injection, Sterile............ 1708
Pediapred Oral Solution 1618

Prednisolone Tebutate (Barbiturates appear to enhance the metabolism of exogenous corticosteroids through the induction of hepatic microsomal enzymes). Products include:
Hydeltra-T.B.A. Sterile Suspension 1710

Prednisone (Barbiturates appear to enhance the metabolism of exogenous corticosteroids through the induction of hepatic microsomal enzymes).
No products indexed under this heading.

Prochlorperazine (Co-administration may produce additive CNS depressant effects). Products include:
Compazine 2644

Promethazine Hydrochloride (Co-administration may produce additive CNS depressant effects). Products include:
Mepergan Injection 2859
Phenergan with Codeine................... 2883
Phenergan with Dextromethorphan 2885
Phenergan Injection 2880
Phenergan Suppositories 2882
Phenergan Syrup 2881
Phenergan Tablets 2882
Phenergan VC 2886
Phenergan VC with Codeine 2888

Propofol (Co-administration may produce additive CNS depressant effects). Products include:
Diprivan Injectable Emulsion 2939

Propoxyphene Hydrochloride (Co-administration may produce additive CNS depressant effects). Products include:
Darvon 1475
Wygesic Tablets 2930

Propoxyphene Napsylate (Co-administration may produce additive CNS depressant effects). Products include:
Darvon-N/Darvocet-N 1473

Pyrilamine Maleate (Co-administration may produce additive CNS depressant effects). Products include:
4-Way Fast Acting Nasal Spray (regular & mentholated)............... ▣ 644
Maximum Strength Multi-Symptom Formula Midol .... ▣ 621
PMS Multi-Symptom Formula Midol .... ▣ 622

Pyrilamine Tannate (Co-administration may produce additive CNS depressant effects). Products include:
Atrohist Pediatric Suspension 1604
Atrohist Pediatric Suspension Dye-Free 1604
Rynatan 2781

Quazepam (Co-administration may produce additive CNS depressant effects). Products include:
Doral Tablets 2773

Risperidone (Co-administration may produce additive CNS depressant effects). Products include:
Risperdal Tablets............................... 1348

Secobarbital Sodium (Co-administration may produce additive CNS depressant effects). Products include:
Seconal Sodium Pulvules 1529

Selegiline Hydrochloride (MAO inhibitors prolong the effects of barbiturates probably by inhibiting barbiturate metabolism). Products include:
Eldepryl Capsules 2729

Sevoflurane (Co-administration may produce additive CNS depressant effects).
No products indexed under this heading.

Sufentanil Citrate (Co-administration may produce additive CNS depressant effects). Products include:
Sufenta Injection 1355

Temazepam (Co-administration may produce additive CNS depressant effects). Products include:
Restoril Capsules.............................. 2413

Terfenadine (Co-administration may produce additive CNS depressant effects). Products include:
Seldane Tablets 1284
Seldane-D Extended-Release Tablets 1286

Thiamylal Sodium (Co-administration may produce additive CNS depressant effects).
No products indexed under this heading.

Thioridazine Hydrochloride (Co-administration may produce additive CNS depressant effects). Products include:
Mellaril 2398

Thiothixene (Co-administration may produce additive CNS depressant effects). Products include:
Navane Capsules and Concentrate 2018
Navane Intramuscular 2019

Tranylcypromine Sulfate (MAO inhibitors prolong the effects of barbiturates probably by inhibiting barbiturate metabolism). Products include:
Parnate Tablets 2679

Triamcinolone (Barbiturates appear to enhance the metabolism of exogenous corticosteroids through the induction of hepatic microsomal enzymes).
No products indexed under this heading.

Triamcinolone Acetonide (Barbiturates appear to enhance the metabolism of exogenous corticosteroids through the induction of hepatic microsomal enzymes). Products include:
Azmacort Oral Inhaler 2175
Nasacort AQ Nasal Spray.................. 2191
Nasacort Nasal Inhaler 2189

Triamcinolone Diacetate (Barbiturates appear to enhance the metabolism of exogenous corticosteroids through the induction of hepatic microsomal enzymes).
No products indexed under this heading.

Triamcinolone Hexacetonide (Barbiturates appear to enhance the metabolism of exogenous corticosteroids through the induction of hepatic microsomal enzymes).
No products indexed under this heading.

Triazolam (Co-administration may produce additive CNS depressant effects). Products include:
Halcion Tablets.................................. 2093

Trifluoperazine Hydrochloride (Co-administration may produce additive CNS depressant effects). Products include:
Stelazine 2692

Trimeprazine Tartrate (Co-administration may produce additive CNS depressant effects).
No products indexed under this heading.

Tripelennamine Hydrochloride (Co-administration may produce additive CNS depressant effects). Products include:
PBZ Tablets 863
PBZ-SR Tablets.................................. 862

Triprolidine Hydrochloride (Co-administration may produce additive CNS depressant effects). Products include:
Actifed Cold & Allergy Tablets......... ▣ 807
Actifed Cold & Sinus Caplets and Tablets .... ▣ 808

Valproic Acid (Valproic acid appears to decrease the bartiturate metabolism). Products include:
Depakene 416

Warfarin Sodium (Barbiturates can induce hepatic microsomal enzymes resulting in increased metabolism and decreased anticoagulant response of oral anticoagulants). Products include:
Coumadin 941

Zolpidem Tartrate (Co-administration may produce additive CNS depressant effects). Products include:
Ambien Tablets.................................. 2559

Food Interactions

Alcohol (Concurrent use may produce additive CNS depressant effects).

CAFERGOT SUPPOSITORIES

(Ergotamine Tartrate, Caffeine)..........2376
See **Cafergot Tablets**

CAFERGOT TABLETS

(Ergotamine Tartrate, Caffeine)..........2376
May interact with vasopressors, macrolide antibiotics, and certain other agents. Compounds in these categories include:

Azithromycin (Elevates blood levels; potential for vasospastic reactions). Products include:
Zithromax 2043
Zithromax Tablets 2046

Clarithromycin (Elevates blood levels; potential for vasospastic reactions). Products include:
Biaxin 406

Dirithromycin (Elevates blood levels; potential for vasospastic reactions). Products include:
Dynabac... 668

Dopamine Hydrochloride (Potential for extreme hypertension; concurrent administration should be avoided).
No products indexed under this heading.

Epinephrine Bitartrate (Potential for extreme hypertension; concurrent administration should be avoided). Products include:
Sensorcaine-MPF with Epinephrine Injection 554

Epinephrine Hydrochloride (Potential for extreme hypertension; concurrent administration should be avoided). Products include:
Ana-Kit Anaphylaxis Emergency Treatment Kit 611

Erythromycin (Elevates blood levels; potential for vasospastic reactions). Products include:
A/T/S 2% Acne Topical Gel............. 1244
A/T/S 2% Acne Topical Solution..... 1244
Benzamycin Topical Gel 919
E-Mycin Tablets 1388
Emgel 2% Topical Gel...................... 1081
ERYC... 1972
Erycette (erythromycin 2%) Topical Solution....................................... 1943
Ery-Tab Tablets 426
Erythromycin Base Filmtab 430
Erythromycin Delayed-Release Capsules, USP................................ 431
Ilotycin Ophthalmic Ointment........... 928
PCE Dispertab Tablets 453
T-Stat 2.0% Topical Solution and Pads 2797
THERAMYCIN Z 2% Solution........... 1629

Erythromycin Estolate (Elevates blood levels; potential for vasospastic reactions). Products include:
Ilosone 927

Erythromycin Ethylsuccinate (Elevates blood levels; potential for vasospastic reactions). Products include:
E.E.S. 427
EryPed 425
Pediazole Suspension 2340

Erythromycin Gluceptate (Elevates blood levels; potential for vasospastic reactions). Products include:
Ilotycin Gluceptate, IV, Vials 929

Erythromycin Stearate (Elevates blood levels; potential for vasospastic reactions). Products include:
Erythrocin Stearate Filmtab 429

Metaraminol Bitartrate (Potential for extreme hypertension; concurrent administration should be avoided). Products include:
Aramine Injection.............................. 1649

(▣ Described in PDR For Nonprescription Drugs) (⊙ Described in PDR For Ophthalmology)

Interactions Index — Calan SR Caplets

Methoxamine Hydrochloride (Potential for extreme hypertension; concurrent administration should be avoided). Products include:
- Vasoxyl Injection ... 1169

Nicotine (Provokes vasoconstriction in some patients; predisposing to a greater ischemic response). Products include:
- Habitrol Nicotine Transdermal System ... 884
- Nicotrol NS Nicotine Nasal Spray ... 1565
- Nicotrol Nicotine Transdermal System ... 1568
- Prostep (nicotine transdermal system) ... 1439

Nicotine Polacrilex (Provokes vasoconstriction in some patients; predisposing to a greater ischemic response).
- No products indexed under this heading.

Norepinephrine Bitartrate (Potential for extreme hypertension; concurrent administration should be avoided). Products include:
- Levophed Bitartrate Injection ... 2445

Phenylephrine Hydrochloride (Potential for extreme hypertension; concurrent administration should be avoided). Products include:
- Atrohist Plus Tablets ... 1605
- Cerose DM ... 853
- D.A. II Tablets ... 972
- D.A. Chewable Tablets ... 970
- Dura-Vent/DA Tablets ... 972
- Extendryl ... 1003
- 4-Way Fast Acting Nasal Spray (regular & mentholated) ... 644
- Hemoril ... 797
- Hycomine Compound Tablets ... 948
- Neo-Synephrine Hydrochloride 1% Carpuject ... 2455
- Neo-Synephrine Hydrochloride 1% Injection ... 2455
- Neo-Synephrine Hydrochloride (Ophthalmic) ... 2456
- Neo-Synephrine ... 624
- Novahistine Elixir ... 782
- Phenergan VC ... 2886
- Phenergan VC with Codeine ... 2888
- Preparation H ... 842
- Tympagesic Ear Drops ... 2476
- Vicks Sinex Nasal Spray and Ultra Fine Mist ... 738

Propranolol Hydrochloride (Potentiates vasoconstrictive action). Products include:
- Inderal ... 2834
- Inderal LA Long Acting Capsules ... 2836
- Inderide Tablets ... 2838
- Inderide LA Long Acting Capsules ... 2840

Troleandomycin (Elevates blood levels; potential for vasospastic reactions). Products include:
- Tao Capsules ... 2033

CALADRYL CLEAR LOTION
(Pramoxine Hydrochloride, Zinc Acetate) ... 817
None cited in PDR database.

CALADRYL CREAM FOR KIDS
(Calamine, Pramoxine Hydrochloride) ... 817
None cited in PDR database.

CALADRYL LOTION
(Calamine, Pramoxine Hydrochloride) ... 817
None cited in PDR database.

CALAN SR CAPLETS
(Verapamil Hydrochloride) ... 2571
May interact with beta blockers, lithium preparations, nondepolarizing neuromuscular blocking agents, inhalant anesthetics, alpha adrenergic blockers, cardiac glycosides, diuretics, ACE inhibitors, vasodilators, and certain other agents. Compounds in these categories include:

Acebutolol Hydrochloride (Additive effect on lowering blood pressure; additive negative effects on heart rate, atrioventricular conduction, and/or cardiac contractility). Products include:
- Sectral Capsules ... 2914

Amiloride Hydrochloride (Additive effect on lowering blood pressure). Products include:
- Midamor Tablets ... 1746
- Moduretic Tablets ... 1748

Aminophylline (Verapamil may inhibit the clearance and increase the plasma levels of theophylline).
- No products indexed under this heading.

Atenolol (Additive effect on lowering blood pressure; additive negative effects on heart rate, atrioventricular conduction, and/or cardiac contractility; variable effect in atenolol clearance). Products include:
- Tenoretic Tablets ... 2963
- Tenormin Tablets and I.V. Injection ... 2965

Atracurium Besylate (Activity of neuromuscular blocking agents potentiated). Products include:
- Tracrium Injection ... 1155

Benazepril Hydrochloride (Additive effect on lowering blood pressure). Products include:
- Lotensin Tablets ... 852
- Lotensin HCT Tablets ... 855
- Lotrel Capsules ... 858

Bendroflumethiazide (Additive effect on lowering blood pressure).
- No products indexed under this heading.

Betaxolol Hydrochloride (Additive effect on lowering blood pressure; additive negative effects on heart rate, atrioventricular conduction, and/or cardiac contractility). Products include:
- Betoptic Ophthalmic Solution ... 465
- Betoptic S Ophthalmic Suspension ... 467
- Kerlone Tablets ... 2588

Bisoprolol Fumarate (Additive effect on lowering blood pressure; additive negative effects on heart rate, atrioventricular conduction, and/or cardiac contractility). Products include:
- Zebeta Tablets ... 1457
- Ziac ... 1459

Bumetanide (Additive effect on lowering blood pressure). Products include:
- Bumex ... 2260

Captopril (Additive effect on lowering blood pressure). Products include:
- Capoten Tablets ... 740
- Capozide Tablets ... 744

Carbamazepine (Increased concentrations of carbamazepine). Products include:
- Atretol Tablets ... 569
- Tegretol/Tegretol-XR ... 870

Carteolol Hydrochloride (Additive effect on lowering blood pressure; additive negative effects on heart rate, atrioventricular conduction, and/or cardiac contractility). Products include:
- Cartrol Tablets ... 413
- Ocupress Ophthalmic Solution, 1% Sterile ... 297

Chlorothiazide (Additive effect on lowering blood pressure). Products include:
- Aldoclor Tablets ... 1638
- Diupres Tablets ... 1691
- Diuril Oral ... 1694

Chlorothiazide Sodium (Additive effect on lowering blood pressure). Products include:
- Diuril Sodium Intravenous ... 1693

Chlorthalidone (Additive effect on lowering blood pressure). Products include:
- Combipres Tablets ... 682
- Tenoretic Tablets ... 2963
- Thalitone ... 1293

Cimetidine (Possible reduction in verapamil clearance). Products include:
- Tagamet HB Tablets ... 786
- Tagamet Tablets ... 2694

Cimetidine Hydrochloride (Possible reduction in verapamil clearance). Products include:
- Tagamet ... 2694

Cisatracurium Besylate (Activity of neuromuscular blocking agents potentiated). Products include:
- Nimbex Injection ... 1131

Clonidine (Additive effect on lowering blood pressure). Products include:
- Catapres-TTS ... 680

Clonidine Hydrochloride (Additive effect on lowering blood pressure). Products include:
- Catapres Tablets ... 679
- Combipres Tablets ... 682

Cyclosporine (Possible increase in serum levels of cyclosporine). Products include:
- Neoral ... 2405
- Sandimmune ... 2416

Desflurane (Excessive cardiovascular depression). Products include:
- Suprane (desflurane, USP) ... 1865

Deslanoside (Chronic verapamil treatment can increase serum digoxin levels and this can result in digitalis toxicity).
- No products indexed under this heading.

Diazoxide (Additive effect on lowering blood pressure). Products include:
- Hyperstat I.V. Injection ... 2504
- Proglycem ... 575

Digitoxin (Chronic verapamil treatment can increase serum digoxin levels and this can result in digitalis toxicity). Products include:
- Crystodigin Tablets ... 1472

Digoxin (Chronic verapamil treatment can increase serum digoxin levels and this can result in digitalis toxicity). Products include:
- Lanoxicaps ... 1110
- Lanoxin Elixir Pediatric ... 1113
- Lanoxin Injection ... 1116
- Lanoxin Injection Pediatric ... 1119
- Lanoxin Tablets ... 1121

Disopyramide Phosphate (Do not administer concomitantly). Products include:
- Norpace ... 2596

Doxazosin Mesylate (May result in a reduction in blood pressure that is excessive in some patients). Products include:
- Cardura Tablets ... 1993

Dyphylline (Verapamil may inhibit the clearance and increase the plasma levels of theophylline). Products include:
- Lufyllin & Lufyllin-400 Tablets ... 2778
- Lufyllin-GG Elixir & Tablets ... 2779

Enalapril Maleate (Additive effect on lowering blood pressure). Products include:
- Vaseretic Tablets ... 1810
- Vasotec Tablets ... 1816

Enalaprilat (Additive effect on lowering blood pressure). Products include:
- Vasotec I.V. ... 1814

Enflurane (Excessive cardiovascular depression).
- No products indexed under this heading.

Epoprostenol Sodium (Additive effect on lowering blood pressure). Products include:
- Flolan for Injection ... 1085

Esmolol Hydrochloride (Additive effect on lowering blood pressure; additive negative effects on heart rate, atrioventricular conduction, and/or cardiac contractility). Products include:
- Brevibloc (esmolol HCl) Injection ... 1860

Ethacrynic Acid (Additive effect on lowering blood pressure). Products include:
- Edecrin Tablets ... 1698

Flecainide Acetate (Possible additive effects on myocardial contractility, AV conduction, and repolarization). Products include:
- Tambocor Tablets ... 1555

Fosinopril Sodium (Additive effect on lowering blood pressure). Products include:
- Monopril Tablets ... 762

Furosemide (Additive effect on lowering blood pressure). Products include:
- Lasix Injection, Oral Solution and Tablets ... 1267

Guanabenz Acetate (Additive effect on lowering blood pressure).
- No products indexed under this heading.

Guanadrel Sulfate (Additive effect on lowering blood pressure). Products include:
- Hylorel Tablets ... 1613

Guanethidine Monosulfate (Additive effect on lowering blood pressure). Products include:
- Esimil Tablets ... 840
- Ismelin Tablets ... 845

Halothane (Excessive cardiovascular depression). Products include:
- Fluothane ... 2830

Hydralazine Hydrochloride (Additive effect on lowering blood pressure). Products include:
- Apresazide Capsules ... 824
- Apresoline Hydrochloride Tablets ... 826
- Hydralazine Hydrochloride Injection USP ... 2712
- Ser-Ap-Es Tablets ... 867

Hydrochlorothiazide (Additive effect on lowering blood pressure). Products include:
- Aldactazide Tablets ... 2556
- Aldoril Tablets ... 1644
- Apresazide Capsules ... 824
- Capozide Tablets ... 744
- Dyazide Capsules ... 2653
- Esidrix Tablets ... 839
- Esimil Tablets ... 840
- HydroDIURIL Tablets ... 1716
- Hydropres Tablets ... 1718
- Hyzaar Tablets ... 1720
- Inderide Tablets ... 2838
- Inderide LA Long Acting Capsules ... 2840
- Lopressor HCT Tablets ... 850
- Lotensin HCT Tablets ... 855
- Moduretic Tablets ... 1748
- Oretic Tablets ... 450
- Prinzide Tablets ... 1780
- Ser-Ap-Es Tablets ... 867
- Timolide Tablets ... 1791
- Vaseretic Tablets ... 1810
- Zestoretic Tablets ... 2968
- Ziac ... 1459

Hydroflumethiazide (Additive effect on lowering blood pressure). Products include:
- Diucardin Tablets ... 2824

IMPORTANT NOTE: Always consult each drug listing in the patient's regimen for possible interactions.

Calan SR Caplets Interactions Index 146

Indapamide (Additive effect on lowering blood pressure).
No products indexed under this heading.

Isoflurane (Excessive cardiovascular depression).
No products indexed under this heading.

Labetalol Hydrochloride (Additive effect on lowering blood pressure; additive negative effects on heart rate, atrioventricular conduction, and/or cardiac contractility). Products include:
Normodyne Injection ... 2519
Normodyne Tablets ... 2522
Trandate ... 1158

Levobunolol Hydrochloride (Additive effect on lowering blood pressure; additive negative effects on heart rate, atrioventricular conduction, and/or cardiac contractility). Products include:
Betagan ... ⊙ 230

Lisinopril (Additive effect on lowering blood pressure). Products include:
Prinivil Tablets ... 1776
Prinzide Tablets ... 1780
Zestoretic Tablets ... 2968
Zestril Tablets ... 2972

Lithium Carbonate (Possible lowering of serum lithium levels; possible increased sensitivity to effects of lithium). Products include:
Eskalith ... 2658
Lithium Carbonate Capsules & Tablets ... 2352
Lithonate/Lithotabs/Lithobid ... 2721

Lithium Citrate (Possible lowering of serum lithium levels; possible increased sensitivity to effects of lithium).
No products indexed under this heading.

Mecamylamine Hydrochloride (Additive effect on lowering blood pressure). Products include:
Inversine Tablets ... 1729

Methoxyflurane (Excessive cardiovascular depression).
No products indexed under this heading.

Methyclothiazide (Additive effect on lowering blood pressure). Products include:
Enduron Tablets ... 424

Methyldopa (Additive effect on lowering blood pressure). Products include:
Aldoclor Tablets ... 1638
Aldomet Oral ... 1640
Aldoril Tablets ... 1644

Methyldopate Hydrochloride (Additive effect on lowering blood pressure). Products include:
Aldomet Ester HCl Injection ... 1642

Metipranolol Hydrochloride (Additive effect on lowering blood pressure; additive negative effects on heart rate, atrioventricular conduction, and/or cardiac contractility). Products include:
OptiPranolol (Metipranolol 0.3%) Sterile Ophthalmic Solution ... ⊙ 256

Metocurine Iodide (Activity of neuromuscular blocking agents potentiated). Products include:
Metubine Iodide Vials ... 932

Metolazone (Additive effect on lowering blood pressure). Products include:
Mykrox Tablets ... 1617
Zaroxolyn Tablets ... 1625

Metoprolol Succinate (Additive effect on lowering blood pressure; additive negative effects on heart rate, atrioventricular conduction, and/or cardiac contractility). Products include:
Toprol-XL Tablets ... 560

Metoprolol Tartrate (Additive effect on lowering blood pressure; additive negative effects on heart rate, atrioventricular conduction, and/or cardiac contractility; decrease in metoprolol clearance). Products include:
Lopressor ... 848
Lopressor HCT Tablets ... 850

Metyrosine (Additive effect on lowering blood pressure). Products include:
Demser Capsules ... 1690

Minoxidil (Additive effect on lowering blood pressure).
No products indexed under this heading.

Mivacurium Chloride (Activity of neuromuscular blocking agents potentiated). Products include:
Mivacron ... 1125

Moexipril Hydrochloride (Additive effect on lowering blood pressure). Products include:
Univasc Tablets ... 2553

Nadolol (Additive effect on lowering blood pressure; additive negative effects on heart rate, atrioventricular conduction, and/or cardiac contractility).
No products indexed under this heading.

Pancuronium Bromide (Activity of neuromuscular blocking agents potentiated).
No products indexed under this heading.

Penbutolol Sulfate (Additive effect on lowering blood pressure; additive negative effects on heart rate, atrioventricular conduction, and/or cardiac contractility). Products include:
Levatol Tablets ... 2547

Phenobarbital (Verapamil clearance may be increased). Products include:
Arco-Lase Plus Tablets ... 513
Bellergal-S Tablets ... 2375
Donnatal ... 2234
Donnatal Extentabs ... 2234
Donnatal Tablets ... 2234
Phenobarbital Elixir and Tablets ... 1523
Quadrinal Tablets ... 1398

Phenoxybenzamine Hydrochloride (Additive effect on lowering blood pressure). Products include:
Dibenzyline Capsules ... 2650

Phentolamine Mesylate (Additive effect on lowering blood pressure). Products include:
Regitine Vials ... 864

Pindolol (Additive effect on lowering blood pressure; additive negative effects on heart rate, atrioventricular conduction, and/or cardiac contractility). Products include:
Visken Tablets ... 2428

Polythiazide (Additive effect on lowering blood pressure). Products include:
Minizide Capsules ... 2016

Prazosin Hydrochloride (May result in a reduction in blood pressure that is excessive in some patients). Products include:
Minipress Capsules ... 2015
Minizide Capsules ... 2016

Propranolol Hydrochloride (Additive effect on lowering blood pressure; additive negative effects on heart rate, atrioventricular conduction, and/or cardiac contractility; decrease in propranolol clearance). Products include:
Inderal ... 2834
Inderal LA Long Acting Capsules ... 2836
Inderide Tablets ... 2838
Inderide LA Long Acting Capsules ... 2840

Quinapril Hydrochloride (Additive effect on lowering blood pressure). Products include:
Accupril Tablets ... 1950

Quinidine Gluconate (Hypotension in patients with hypertrophic cardiomyopathy). Products include:
Quinaglute Dura-Tabs Tablets ... 644

Quinidine Polygalacturonate (Hypotension in patients with hypertrophic cardiomyopathy). Products include:
Cardioquin Tablets ... 2146

Quinidine Sulfate (Hypotension in patients with hypertrophic cardiomyopathy). Products include:
Quinidex Extentabs ... 2240

Ramipril (Additive effect on lowering blood pressure). Products include:
Altace Capsules ... 1238

Rifampin (Reduced oral verapamil bioavailability). Products include:
Rifadin ... 1276
Rifamate Capsules ... 1278
Rifater ... 1280
Rimactane Capsules ... 865

Rocuronium Bromide (Activity of neuromuscular blocking agents potentiated). Products include:
Zemuron Injection ... 1885

Sotalol Hydrochloride (Additive effect on lowering blood pressure; additive negative effects on heart rate, atrioventricular conduction, and/or cardiac contractility). Products include:
Betapace Tablets ... 637

Spirapril Hydrochloride (Additive effect on lowering blood pressure).
No products indexed under this heading.

Spironolactone (Additive effect on lowering blood pressure). Products include:
Aldactazide Tablets ... 2556
Aldactone Tablets ... 2558

Succinylcholine Chloride (Potentiation of neuromuscular blockers). Products include:
Anectine ... 1062

Terazosin Hydrochloride (May result in a reduction in blood pressure that is excessive in some patients). Products include:
Hytrin Capsules ... 434

Theophylline (Verapamil may inhibit the clearance and increase the plasma levels of theophylline). Products include:
Marax Tablets & DF Syrup ... 2015
Quibron ... 2227

Theophylline Anhydrous (Verapamil may inhibit the clearance and increase the plasma levels of theophylline). Products include:
Aerolate ... 1003
Primatene Tablets ... ▣ 844
Respbid Tablets ... 687
Slo-bid Gyrocaps ... 2201
Theo-24 Extended Release Capsules ... 2753
Theo-Dur Extended-Release Tablets ... 1367
Theo-X Extended-Release Tablets ... 793
Uni-Dur Extended-Release Tablets ... 1374
Uniphyl 400 mg and 600 mg Tablets ... 2157

Theophylline Calcium Salicylate (Verapamil may inhibit the clearance and increase the plasma levels of theophylline). Products include:
Quadrinal Tablets ... 1398

Theophylline Sodium Glycinate (Verapamil may inhibit the clearance and increase the plasma levels of theophylline).
No products indexed under this heading.

Timolol Hemihydrate (Additive effect on lowering blood pressure; additive negative effects on heart rate, atrioventricular conduction, and/or cardiac contractility). Products include:
Betimol 0.25%, 0.5% ... ⊙ 259

Timolol Maleate (Additive effect on lowering blood pressure; additive negative effects on heart rate, atrioventricular conduction, and/or cardiac contractility). Products include:
Blocadren Tablets ... 1654
Timolide Tablets ... 1791
Timoptic in Ocudose ... 1796
Timoptic Sterile Ophthalmic Solution ... 1794
Timoptic-XE ... 1798

Torsemide (Additive effect on lowering blood pressure). Products include:
Demadex Tablets and Injection ... 691

Trandolapril (Additive effect on lowering blood pressure). Products include:
Mavik Tablets ... 1407

Triamterene (Additive effect on lowering blood pressure). Products include:
Dyazide Capsules ... 2653
Dyrenium Capsules ... 2655

Vecuronium Bromide (Activity of neuromuscular blocking agents potentiated). Products include:
Norcuron for Injection ... 1875

Food Interactions

Food, unspecified (Produces decreased bioavailability (AUC) but a narrower peak-to-trough ratio).

CALAN TABLETS
(Verapamil Hydrochloride) ... 2568
May interact with beta blockers, cardiac glycosides, lithium preparations, diuretics, ACE inhibitors, vasodilators, nondepolarizing neuromuscular blocking agents, inhalant anesthetics, and certain other agents. Compounds in these categories include:

Acebutolol Hydrochloride (Additive negative effects on heart rate, AV conduction and/or cardiac contractility; additive hypotensive effect). Products include:
Sectral Capsules ... 2914

Amiloride Hydrochloride (Additive effect on lowering blood pressure). Products include:
Midamor Tablets ... 1746
Moduretic Tablets ... 1748

Aminophylline (Verapamil may inhibit the clearance and increase the plasma levels of theophylline).
No products indexed under this heading.

Atenolol (Additive negative effects on heart rate, AV conduction and/or cardiac contractility; additive hypotensive effect; variable effect in atenolol clearance). Products include:
Tenoretic Tablets ... 2963
Tenormin Tablets and I.V. Injection 2965

(▣ Described in PDR For Nonprescription Drugs) (⊙ Described in PDR For Ophthalmology)

Interactions Index — Calan Tablets

Atracurium Besylate (Activity of neuromuscular blocking agents potentiated). Products include:
Tracrium Injection ... 1155

Benazepril Hydrochloride (Additive effect on lowering blood pressure). Products include:
Lotensin Tablets ... 852
Lotensin HCT Tablets ... 855
Lotrel Capsules ... 858

Bendroflumethiazide (Additive effect on lowering blood pressure).
No products indexed under this heading.

Betaxolol Hydrochloride (Additive negative effects on heart rate, AV conduction and/or cardiac contractility; additive hypotensive effect). Products include:
Betoptic Ophthalmic Solution ... 465
Betoptic S Ophthalmic Suspension ... 467
Kerlone Tablets ... 2588

Bisoprolol Fumarate (Additive negative effects on heart rate, AV conduction and/or cardiac contractility; additive hypotensive effect). Products include:
Zebeta Tablets ... 1457
Ziac ... 1459

Bumetanide (Additive effect on lowering blood pressure). Products include:
Bumex ... 2260

Captopril (Additive effect on lowering blood pressure). Products include:
Capoten Tablets ... 740
Capozide Tablets ... 744

Carbamazepine (Increased carbamazepine concentrations). Products include:
Atretol Tablets ... 569
Tegretol/Tegretol-XR ... 870

Carteolol Hydrochloride (Additive negative effects on heart rate, AV conduction and/or cardiac contractility; additive hypotensive effect). Products include:
Cartrol Tablets ... 413
Ocupress Ophthalmic Solution, 1% Sterile ... 297

Chlorothiazide (Additive effect on lowering blood pressure). Products include:
Aldoclor Tablets ... 1638
Diupres Tablets ... 1691
Diuril Oral ... 1694

Chlorothiazide Sodium (Additive effect on lowering blood pressure). Products include:
Diuril Sodium Intravenous ... 1693

Chlorthalidone (Additive effect on lowering blood pressure). Products include:
Combipres Tablets ... 682
Tenoretic Tablets ... 2963
Thalitone ... 1293

Cimetidine (Possible reduction in verapamil clearance). Products include:
Tagamet HB Tablets ... 786
Tagamet Tablets ... 2694

Cimetidine Hydrochloride (Possible reduction in verapamil clearance). Products include:
Tagamet ... 2694

Cisatracurium Besylate (Activity of neuromuscular blocking agents potentiated). Products include:
Nimbex Injection ... 1131

Clonidine (Additive effect on lowering blood pressure). Products include:
Catapres-TTS ... 680

Clonidine Hydrochloride (Additive effect on lowering blood pressure). Products include:
Catapres Tablets ... 679
Combipres Tablets ... 682

Cyclosporine (Possible increase in serum levels of cyclosporine). Products include:
Neoral ... 2405
Sandimmune ... 2416

Desflurane (Excessive cardiovascular depression). Products include:
Suprane (desflurane, USP) ... 1865

Deslanoside (Chronic verapamil treatment can increase serum digoxin levels and this can result in digitalis toxicity).
No products indexed under this heading.

Diazoxide (Additive effect on lowering blood pressure). Products include:
Hyperstat I.V. Injection ... 2504
Proglycem ... 575

Digitoxin (Chronic verapamil treatment can increase serum digoxin levels and this can result in digitalis toxicity). Products include:
Crystodigin Tablets ... 1472

Digoxin (Chronic verapamil treatment can increase serum digoxin levels and this can result in digitalis toxicity). Products include:
Lanoxicaps ... 1110
Lanoxin Elixir Pediatric ... 1113
Lanoxin Injection ... 1116
Lanoxin Injection Pediatric ... 1119
Lanoxin Tablets ... 1121

Disopyramide Phosphate (Do not administer concomitantly). Products include:
Norpace ... 2596

Dyphylline (Verapamil may inhibit the clearance and increase the plasma levels of theophylline). Products include:
Lufyllin & Lufyllin-400 Tablets ... 2778
Lufyllin-GG Elixir & Tablets ... 2779

Enalapril Maleate (Additive effect on lowering blood pressure). Products include:
Vaseretic Tablets ... 1810
Vasotec Tablets ... 1816

Enalaprilat (Additive effect on lowering blood pressure). Products include:
Vasotec I.V. ... 1814

Enflurane (Excessive cardiovascular depression).
No products indexed under this heading.

Epoprostenol Sodium (Additive effect on lowering blood pressure). Products include:
Flolan for Injection ... 1085

Esmolol Hydrochloride (Additive negative effects on heart rate, AV conduction and/or cardiac contractility; additive hypotensive effect). Products include:
Brevibloc (esmolol HCl) Injection ... 1860

Ethacrynic Acid (Additive effect on lowering blood pressure). Products include:
Edecrin Tablets ... 1698

Flecainide Acetate (Possible additive negative inotropic effect and prolongation of AV conduction). Products include:
Tambocor Tablets ... 1555

Fosinopril Sodium (Additive effect on lowering blood pressure). Products include:
Monopril Tablets ... 762

Furosemide (Additive effect on lowering blood pressure). Products include:
Lasix Injection, Oral Solution and Tablets ... 1267

Guanabenz Acetate (Additive effect on lowering blood pressure).
No products indexed under this heading.

Guanadrel Sulfate (Additive effect on lowering blood pressure). Products include:
Hylorel Tablets ... 1613

Guanethidine Monosulfate (Additive effect on lowering blood pressure). Products include:
Esimil Tablets ... 840
Ismelin Tablets ... 845

Halothane (Excessive cardiovascular depression). Products include:
Fluothane ... 2830

Hydralazine Hydrochloride (Additive effect on lowering blood pressure). Products include:
Apresazide Capsules ... 824
Apresoline Hydrochloride Tablets ... 826
Hydralazine Hydrochloride Injection USP ... 2712
Ser-Ap-Es Tablets ... 867

Hydrochlorothiazide (Additive effect on lowering blood pressure). Products include:
Aldactazide Tablets ... 2556
Aldoril Tablets ... 1644
Apresazide Capsules ... 824
Capozide Tablets ... 744
Dyazide Capsules ... 2653
Esidrix Tablets ... 839
Esimil Tablets ... 840
HydroDIURIL Tablets ... 1716
Hydropres Tablets ... 1718
Hyzaar Tablets ... 1720
Inderide Tablets ... 2838
Inderide LA Long Acting Capsules ... 2840
Lopressor HCT Tablets ... 850
Lotensin HCT Tablets ... 855
Moduretic Tablets ... 1748
Oretic Tablets ... 450
Prinzide Tablets ... 1780
Ser-Ap-Es Tablets ... 867
Timolide Tablets ... 1791
Vaseretic Tablets ... 1810
Zestoretic Tablets ... 2968
Ziac ... 1459

Hydroflumethiazide (Additive effect on lowering blood pressure). Products include:
Diucardin Tablets ... 2824

Indapamide (Additive effect on lowering blood pressure).
No products indexed under this heading.

Isoflurane (Excessive cardiovascular depression).
No products indexed under this heading.

Labetalol Hydrochloride (Additive negative effects on heart rate, AV conduction and/or cardiac contractility; additive hypotensive effect). Products include:
Normodyne Injection ... 2519
Normodyne Tablets ... 2522
Trandate ... 1158

Levobunolol Hydrochloride (Additive negative effects on heart rate, AV conduction and/or cardiac contractility; additive hypotensive effect). Products include:
Betagan ... 230

Lisinopril (Additive effect on lowering blood pressure). Products include:
Prinivil Tablets ... 1776
Prinzide Tablets ... 1780
Zestoretic Tablets ... 2968
Zestril Tablets ... 2972

Lithium Carbonate (May result in lowering of serum lithium levels and increased sensitivity to the effects of lithium). Products include:
Eskalith ... 2658
Lithium Carbonate Capsules & Tablets ... 2352
Lithonate/Lithotabs/Lithobid ... 2721

Lithium Citrate (May result in lowering of serum lithium levels and increased sensitivity to the effects of lithium).
No products indexed under this heading.

Mecamylamine Hydrochloride (Additive effect on lowering blood pressure). Products include:
Inversine Tablets ... 1729

Methoxyflurane (Excessive cardiovascular depression).
No products indexed under this heading.

Methyclothiazide (Additive effect on lowering blood pressure). Products include:
Enduron Tablets ... 424

Methyldopa (Additive effect on lowering blood pressure). Products include:
Aldoclor Tablets ... 1638
Aldomet Oral ... 1640
Aldoril Tablets ... 1644

Methyldopate Hydrochloride (Additive effect on lowering blood pressure). Products include:
Aldomet Ester HCl Injection ... 1642

Metipranolol Hydrochloride (Additive negative effects on heart rate, AV conduction and/or cardiac contractility; additive hypotensive effect). Products include:
OptiPranolol (Metipranolol 0.3%) Sterile Ophthalmic Solution ... 256

Metocurine Iodide (Activity of neuromuscular blocking agents potentiated). Products include:
Metubine Iodide Vials ... 932

Metolazone (Additive effect on lowering blood pressure). Products include:
Mykrox Tablets ... 1617
Zaroxolyn Tablets ... 1625

Metoprolol Succinate (Additive negative effects on heart rate, AV conduction and/or cardiac contractility; additive hypotensive effect). Products include:
Toprol-XL Tablets ... 560

Metoprolol Tartrate (Additive negative effects on heart rate, AV conduction and/or cardiac contractility; additive hypotensive effect; decrease in metoprolol clearance). Products include:
Lopressor ... 848
Lopressor HCT Tablets ... 850

Metyrosine (Additive effect on lowering blood pressure). Products include:
Demser Capsules ... 1690

Minoxidil (Additive effect on lowering blood pressure).
No products indexed under this heading.

Mivacurium Chloride (Activity of neuromuscular blocking agents potentiated). Products include:
Mivacron ... 1125

Moexipril Hydrochloride (Additive effect on lowering blood pressure). Products include:
Univasc Tablets ... 2553

Nadolol (Additive negative effects on heart rate, AV conduction and/or cardiac contractility; additive hypotensive effect).
No products indexed under this heading.

Pancuronium Bromide (Activity of neuromuscular blocking agents potentiated).
No products indexed under this heading.

Pargyline Hydrochloride (Additive effect on lowering blood pressure).
No products indexed under this heading.

IMPORTANT NOTE: Always consult each drug listing in the patient's regimen for possible interactions.

Calan Tablets — Interactions Index — 148

Penbutolol Sulfate (Additive negative effects on heart rate, AV conduction, and/or cardiac contractility; additive hypotensive effect). Products include:
- Levatol Tablets 2547

Phenobarbital (Verapamil clearance may be increased). Products include:
- Arco-Lase Plus Tablets 513
- Bellergal-S Tablets 2375
- Donnatal 2234
- Donnatal Extentabs 2234
- Donnatal Tablets 2234
- Phenobarbital Elixir and Tablets .. 1523
- Quadrinal Tablets 1398

Phenoxybenzamine Hydrochloride (Additive effect on lowering blood pressure). Products include:
- Dibenzyline Capsules 2650

Phentolamine Mesylate (Additive effect on lowering blood pressure). Products include:
- Regitine Vials 864

Pindolol (Additive negative effects on heart rate, AV conduction and/or cardiac contractility; additive hypotensive effect). Products include:
- Visken Tablets 2428

Polythiazide (Additive effect on lowering blood pressure). Products include:
- Minizide Capsules 2016

Prazosin Hydrochloride (May result in a reduction in blood pressure that is excessive in some patients). Products include:
- Minipress Capsules 2015
- Minizide Capsules 2016

Propranolol Hydrochloride (Additive negative effects on heart rate, AV conduction and/or cardiac contractility; additive hypotensive effect; decrease in propranolol clearance). Products include:
- Inderal 2834
- Inderal LA Long Acting Capsules .. 2836
- Inderide Tablets 2838
- Inderide LA Long Acting Capsules .. 2840

Quinapril Hydrochloride (Additive effect on lowering blood pressure). Products include:
- Accupril Tablets 1950

Quinidine Gluconate (Hypotension in patients with hypertrophic cardiomyopathy; increased quinidine levels). Products include:
- Quinaglute Dura-Tabs Tablets 644

Quinidine Polygalacturonate (Hypotension in patients with hypertrophic cardiomyopathy; increased quinidine levels). Products include:
- Cardioquin Tablets 2146

Quinidine Sulfate (Hypotension in patients with hypertrophic cardiomyopathy; increased quinidine levels). Products include:
- Quinidex Extentabs 2240

Ramipril (Additive effect on lowering blood pressure). Products include:
- Altace Capsules 1238

Rifampin (Bioavailability of oral verapamil may be markedly reduced). Products include:
- Rifadin 1276
- Rifamate Capsules 1278
- Rifater 1280
- Rimactane Capsules 865

Rocuronium Bromide (Activity of neuromuscular blocking agents potentiated). Products include:
- Zemuron Injection 1885

Sotalol Hydrochloride (Additive negative effects on heart rate, AV conduction and/or cardiac contractility; additive hypotensive effect). Products include:
- Betapace Tablets 637

Spirapril Hydrochloride (Additive effect on lowering blood pressure).
No products indexed under this heading.

Spironolactone (Additive effect on lowering blood pressure). Products include:
- Aldactazide Tablets 2556
- Aldactone Tablets 2558

Succinylcholine Chloride (Potentiation of neuromuscular blockers). Products include:
- Anectine 1062

Terazosin Hydrochloride (May result in a reduction in blood pressure that is excessive in some patients). Products include:
- Hytrin Capsules 434

Theophylline (Verapamil may inhibit the clearance and increase the plasma levels of theophylline). Products include:
- Marax Tablets & DF Syrup 2015
- Quibron 2227

Theophylline Anhydrous (Verapamil may inhibit the clearance and increase the plasma levels of theophylline). Products include:
- Aerolate 1003
- Primatene Tablets 844
- Respbid Tablets 687
- Slo-bid Gyrocaps 2201
- Theo-24 Extended Release Capsules 2753
- Theo-Dur Extended-Release Tablets 1367
- Theo-X Extended-Release Tablets .. 793
- Uni-Dur Extended-Release Tablets .. 1374
- Uniphyl 400 mg and 600 mg Tablets 2157

Theophylline Calcium Salicylate (Verapamil may inhibit the clearance and increase the plasma levels of theophylline). Products include:
- Quadrinal Tablets 1398

Theophylline Sodium Glycinate (Verapamil may inhibit the clearance and increase the plasma levels of theophylline).
No products indexed under this heading.

Timolol Hemihydrate (Additive negative effects on heart rate, AV conduction and/or cardiac contractility; additive hypotensive effect). Products include:
- Betimol 0.25%, 0.5% 259

Timolol Maleate (Additive negative effects on heart rate, AV conduction and/or cardiac contractility; additive hypotensive effect). Products include:
- Blocadren Tablets 1654
- Timolide Tablets 1791
- Timoptic in Ocudose 1796
- Timoptic Sterile Ophthalmic Solution 1794
- Timoptic-XE 1798

Torsemide (Additive effect on lowering blood pressure). Products include:
- Demadex Tablets and Injection ... 691

Trandolapril (Additive effect on lowering blood pressure). Products include:
- Mavik Tablets 1407

Triamterene (Additive effect on lowering blood pressure). Products include:
- Dyazide Capsules 2653
- Dyrenium Capsules 2655

Vecuronium Bromide (Activity of neuromuscular blocking agents potentiated). Products include:
- Norcuron for Injection 1875

CALCI-CHEW TABLETS
(Calcium Carbonate) 2168
None cited in PDR database.

CALCIJEX INJECTION
(Calcitriol) 412
May interact with:

Magnesium Carbonate (Co-administration with magnesium-containing antacids may lead to the development of hypermagnesemia; concurrent use should be avoided). Products include:
- Bufferin Analgesic Tablets 636
- Arthritis Strength Bufferin Analgesic Caplets 637
- Extra Strength Bufferin Analgesic Tablets 637
- Gaviscon Extra Strength Relief Formula Antacid Tablets 778
- Gaviscon Extra Strength Relief Formula Liquid Antacid 779
- Gaviscon Liquid Antacid 779
- Maalox Antacid Caplets 657
- Maalox Heartburn Relief Suspension 658
- Mag-Carb Capsules 2168
- Marblen 671
- One-A-Day Calcium Plus 625

Magnesium Hydroxide (Co-administration with magnesium-containing antacids may lead to the development of hypermagnesemia; concurrent use should be avoided). Products include:
- Aludrox Oral Suspension 850
- Ascriptin 650
- Di-Gel Antacid/Anti-Gas 762
- Gelusil Antacid-Anti-gas Liquid ... 819
- Gelusil Antacid-Anti-gas Tablets .. 819
- Maalox Antacid/Anti-Gas Tablets . 889
- Maalox Antacid Liquid 888
- Extra Strength Maalox Antacid/Anti-Gas Liquid and Tablets 888
- Mylanta Fast-Acting 1359
- Mylanta Gelcaps Antacid 678
- Fast-Acting Mylanta Liquid Antacid 1359
- Mylanta Tablets 677
- Maximum-Strength Fast-Acting Mylanta Liquid Antacid 1359
- Mylanta Double Strength Tablets . 677
- Phillips' Milk of Magnesia Liquid .. 627
- Rolaids Antacid Tablets 807
- Tempo Soft Antacid 799

CALCIMAR INJECTION, SYNTHETIC
(Calcitonin, Synthetic) 2176
None cited in PDR database.

CALCI-MIX CAPSULES
(Calcium Carbonate) 2168
None cited in PDR database.

CALCIUM DISODIUM VERSENATE INJECTION
(Calcium Disodium Edetate) 1548
May interact with:

Insulin, Human, Zinc Suspension (Interference with the action of zinc insulin by chelating the zinc). Products include:
- Humulin L, 100 Units 1494
- Humulin U, 100 Units 1498
- Novolin L Human Insulin 10 ml Vials 1846

Insulin, Zinc Crystals (Interference with the action of zinc insulin by chelating the zinc). Products include:
- NPH, 100 Units 1502

Insulin, Zinc Suspension (Interference with the action of zinc insulin by chelating the zinc). Products include:
- Iletin I 1501
- Lente, 100 Units 1501
- Iletin II 1504
- Pork Lente, 100 Units 1504
- Purified Pork Lente Insulin 1852

Steroids, unspecified (Enhances renal toxicity of edetate calcium disodium in animals).
No products indexed under this heading.

CALDECORT ANTI-ITCH HYDROCORTISONE CREAM
(Hydrocortisone Acetate) 651
None cited in PDR database.

CALDESENE MEDICATED OINTMENT
(Petrolatum, White, Zinc Oxide) ... 652
None cited in PDR database.

CALDESENE MEDICATED POWDER
(Calcium Undecylenate) 652
None cited in PDR database.

CALPHOSAN INJECTION
(Calcium Glycerophosphate, Calcium Lactate) 1234
None cited in PDR database.

CALTRATE 600
(Calcium Carbonate) 681
None cited in PDR database.

CALTRATE PLUS
(Calcium Carbonate, Vitamin D) ... 681
None cited in PDR database.

CALTRATE 600 + D
(Calcium Carbonate, Vitamin D) ... 681
None cited in PDR database.

CAMA ARTHRITIS PAIN RELIEVER
(Aspirin, Aluminum Hydroxide, Magnesium Oxide) 748
May interact with oral hypoglycemic agents, oral anticoagulants, and antigout agents. Compounds in these categories include:

Acarbose (Do not use concomitantly). Products include:
- Precose 604

Allopurinol (Do not use concomitantly). Products include:
- Zyloprim Tablets 1194

Chlorpropamide (Do not use concomitantly). Products include:
- Diabinese Tablets 2002

Dicumarol (Do not use concomitantly).
No products indexed under this heading.

Glimepiride (Do not use concomitantly). Products include:
- Amaryl Tablets 1241

Glipizide (Do not use concomitantly). Products include:
- Glucotrol Tablets 2011
- Glucotrol XL Extended Release Tablets 2012

Glyburide (Do not use concomitantly). Products include:
- DiaBeta Tablets 1265
- Glynase PresTab Tablets 2091
- Micronase Tablets 2099

Metformin Hydrochloride (Do not use concomitantly). Products include:
- Glucophage Tablets 754

Probenecid (Do not use concomitantly). Products include:
- Benemid Tablets 1651
- ColBENEMID Tablets 1662

Sulfinpyrazone (Do not use concomitantly). Products include:
- Anturane 823

Tolazamide (Do not use concomitantly).
No products indexed under this heading.

Tolbutamide (Do not use concomitantly).
No products indexed under this heading.

(Described in PDR For Nonprescription Drugs)   (Described in PDR For Ophthalmology)

Warfarin Sodium (Do not use concomitantly). Products include:
Coumadin 941

CAPASTAT SULFATE INJECTION
(Capreomycin Sulfate) 968
May interact with aminoglycosides, antituberculosis drugs, and certain other agents. Compounds in these categories include:

Amikacin Sulfate (Additive ototoxicity and/or nephrotoxicity). Products include:
Amikacin Sulfate Injection, USP ... 523
Amikacin Sulfate Injection, USP ... 981
Amikin Injectable 502

Aminosalicylic Acid (Potential for febrile reactions and abnormal liver function tests). Products include:
PASER Granules 1333

p-Aminosalicylic Acid (Potential for febrile reactions and abnormal liver function tests).
No products indexed under this heading.

Colistin Sulfate (Additive ototoxicity and/or nephrotoxicity). Products include:
Coly-Mycin S Otic w/Neomycin & Hydrocortisone 1965

Cycloserine (Potential for febrile reactions and abnormal liver function tests). Products include:
Seromycin Capsules 975

Ethambutol Hydrochloride (Potential for febrile reactions and abnormal liver function tests). Products include:
Myambutol Tablets 1432

Ether (Neuromuscular block enhanced).

Gentamicin Sulfate (Additive ototoxicity and/or nephrotoxicity). Products include:
Garamycin Cream 0.1% 2501
Garamycin Injectable 2502
Garamycin Ointment 0.1% 2501
Garamycin Ophthalmic 2501
Genoptic Sterile Ophthalmic Solution 241
Genoptic Sterile Ophthalmic Ointment 241
Gentak 209
Pred-G Liquifilm Sterile Ophthalmic Suspension 248
Pred-G S.O.P. Sterile Ophthalmic Ointment 249

Isoniazid (Potential for febrile reactions and abnormal liver function tests). Products include:
Nydrazid Injection 509
Rifamate Capsules 1278
Rifater 1280

Kanamycin Sulfate (Additive ototoxicity and/or nephrotoxicity).
No products indexed under this heading.

Neomycin, oral (Additive ototoxicity and/or nephrotoxicity).

Paromomycin Sulfate (Additive ototoxicity and/or nephrotoxicity).
No products indexed under this heading.

Polymyxin B Sulfate (Additive ototoxicity and/or nephrotoxicity). Products include:
AK-Spore 205
AK-Trol Ointment & Suspension ... 205
Betadine Brand First Aid Antibiotics & Moisturizer Ointment 2144
Cortisporin Cream 1073
Cortisporin Ointment 1074
Cortisporin Ophthalmic Ointment Sterile 1074
Cortisporin Ophthalmic Suspension Sterile 1075
Cortisporin Otic Solution Sterile ... 1076
Cortisporin Otic Suspension Sterile 1077

Maxitrol Ophthalmic Ointment and Suspension 222
Mycitracin 803
Neosporin G.U. Irrigant Sterile 1130
Neosporin Ointment 821
Neosporin Plus Maximum Strength Cream 821
Neosporin Plus Maximum Strength Ointment 822
Neosporin Ophthalmic Ointment Sterile 1130
Neosporin Ophthalmic Solution Sterile 1131
Pediotic Suspension Sterile 1140
Poly-Pred Liquifilm 246
Polysporin Ointment 822
Polysporin Ophthalmic Ointment Sterile 1140
Polysporin Powder 823
Polytrim Ophthalmic Solution Sterile 479
TERAK Ointment 210
Terramycin with Polymyxin B Sulfate Ophthalmic Ointment 2035

Pyrazinamide (Potential for febrile reactions and abnormal liver function tests). Products include:
Pyrazinamide Tablets 1442
Rifater 1280

Rifampin (Potential for febrile reactions and abnormal liver function tests). Products include:
Rifadin 1276
Rifamate Capsules 1278
Rifater 1280
Rimactane Capsules 865

Streptomycin Sulfate (Additive ototoxicity and/or nephrotoxicity). Products include:
Streptomycin Sulfate Injection 2031

Tobramycin (Additive ototoxicity and/or nephrotoxicity). Products include:
AKTOB 207
TobraDex Ophthalmic Suspension and Ointment 469
Tobrex Ophthalmic Ointment and Solution 226

Tobramycin Sulfate (Additive ototoxicity and/or nephrotoxicity). Products include:
Nebcin Vials, Hyporets & ADD-Vantage 1518

Vancomycin Hydrochloride (Additive ototoxicity and/or nephrotoxicity). Products include:
Vancocin HCl, Oral Solution & Pulvules 1536
Vancocin HCl, Vials & ADD-Vantage 1534

Viomycin (Additive ototoxicity and/or nephrotoxicity).

CAPITROL SHAMPOO
(Chloroxine) 2791
None cited in PDR database.

CAPOTEN TABLETS
(Captopril) 740
May interact with diuretics, thiazides, ganglionic blocking agents, peripheral adrenergic blockers, potassium sparing diuretics, potassium preparations, non-steroidal anti-inflammatory agents, beta blockers, vasodilators, lithium preparations, nitrates and nitrites, agents causing renin release, inhibitors of endogenous prostaglandin synthesis, and certain other agents. Compounds in these categories include:

Acebutolol Hydrochloride (Less than additive antihypertensive effect). Products include:
Sectral Capsules 2914

Amiloride Hydrochloride (Hypotension; increased serum potassium). Products include:
Midamor Tablets 1746
Moduretic Tablets 1748

Amyl Nitrite (Discontinue before starting captopril; if resumed administer at lower dosage).
No products indexed under this heading.

Aspirin (Antihypertensive effects of captopril reduced). Products include:
Alka-Seltzer Cherry Effervescent Antacid and Pain Reliever 609
Alka-Seltzer Extra Strength Effervescent Antacid and Pain Reliever 609
Alka-Seltzer Lemon Lime Effervescent Antacid and Pain Reliever 609
Alka-Seltzer Original Effervescent Antacid and Pain Reliever 609
Alka-Seltzer Plus 611
Alka-Seltzer Plus Sinus Medicine .. 611
Ascriptin 650
Arthritis Strength BC Powder 631
BC Cold Powder Multi-Symptom Formula (Cold-Sinus-Allergy) 631
BC Cold Powder Non-Drowsy Formula (Cold-Sinus) 631
BC Powder 631
Genuine Bayer Aspirin Tablets & Caplets 618
Extra Strength Bayer Arthritis Pain Regimen Formula 615
Extra Strength Bayer Aspirin Caplets & Tablets 617
Extended-Release Bayer 8-Hour Aspirin 616
Extra Strength Bayer Plus Aspirin Caplets 617
Extra Strength Bayer PM Aspirin Plus Sleep Aid 617
Aspirin Regimen Bayer 81 mg Tablets with Calcium 615
Aspirin Regimen Bayer Adult Low Strength 81 mg Tablets 613
Aspirin Regimen Bayer Children's Chewable Aspirin 616
Aspirin Regimen Bayer Regular Strength 325 mg Caplets 613
Bufferin Analgesic Tablets 636
Arthritis Strength Bufferin Analgesic Caplets 637
Extra Strength Bufferin Analgesic Tablets 637
Cama Arthritis Pain Reliever 748
Darvon Compound-65 Pulvules ... 1475
Easprin 1971
Ecotrin 2625
Ecotrin Enteric Coated Aspirin Maximum Strength Tablets and Caplets 775
Ecotrin Enteric Coated Aspirin Regular Strength Tablets 2625
Empirin Aspirin Tablets 818
Excedrin Extra-Strength Analgesic Tablets, Caplets, and Geltabs 734
Fiorinal Capsules 2388
Fiorinal with Codeine Capsules .. 2390
Fiorinal Tablets 2388
Goody's Extra Strength Headache Powders 632
Goody's Extra Strength Pain Relief Tablets 632
Halfprin Tablets 1413
Norgesic 1554
Percodan Tablets 955
Percodan-Demi Tablets 956
Robaxisal Tablets 2246
Soma Compound w/Codeine Tablets 2784
Soma Compound Tablets 2783
St. Joseph Adult Chewable Aspirin (81 mg.) 768
Talwin Compound 2466
Vanquish Analgesic Caplets 627

Atenolol (Less than additive antihypertensive effect). Products include:
Tenoretic Tablets 2963
Tenormin Tablets and I.V. Injection 2965

Bendroflumethiazide (Captopril's effect will be augmented).
No products indexed under this heading.

Betaxolol Hydrochloride (Less than additive antihypertensive effect). Products include:
Betoptic Ophthalmic Solution 465
Betoptic S Ophthalmic Suspension 467
Kerlone Tablets 2588

Bisoprolol Fumarate (Less than additive antihypertensive effect). Products include:
Zebeta Tablets 1457
Ziac 1459

Bumetanide (Captopril's effect will be augmented; hypotension). Products include:
Bumex 2260

Carteolol Hydrochloride (Less than additive antihypertensive effect). Products include:
Cartrol Tablets 413
Ocupress Ophthalmic Solution, 1% Sterile 297

Chlorothiazide (Captopril's effect will be augmented). Products include:
Aldoclor Tablets 1638
Diupres Tablets 1691
Diuril Oral 1694

Chlorothiazide Sodium (Captopril's effect will be augmented). Products include:
Diuril Sodium Intravenous 1693

Chlorthalidone (Captopril's effect will be augmented; hypotension; increased serum potassium). Products include:
Combipres Tablets 682
Tenoretic Tablets 2963
Thalitone 1293

Deserpidine (Use with caution).
No products indexed under this heading.

Diazoxide (Drugs having vasodilator activity should, if possible, be discontinued before starting Capoten). Products include:
Hyperstat I.V. Injection 2504
Proglycem 575

Diclofenac Potassium (Antihypertensive effects of captopril reduced). Products include:
Cataflam Tablets 833

Diclofenac Sodium (Antihypertensive effects of captopril reduced). Products include:
Voltaren Ophthalmic Sterile Ophthalmic Solution 264
Cataflam/Voltaren/Voltaren-XR .. 833

Epoprostenol Sodium (Drugs having vasodilator activity should, if possible, be discontinued before starting Capoten). Products include:
Flolan for Injection 1085

Erythrityl Tetranitrate (Discontinue before starting captopril; if resumed administer at lower dosage).
No products indexed under this heading.

Esmolol Hydrochloride (Less than additive antihypertensive effect). Products include:
Brevibloc (esmolol HCl) Injection .. 1860

Ethacrynic Acid (Captopril's effect will be augmented; hypotension). Products include:
Edecrin Tablets 1698

Etodolac (Antihypertensive effects of captopril reduced). Products include:
Lodine Capsules and Tablets 2849

Fenoprofen Calcium (Antihypertensive effects of captopril reduced). Products include:
Nalfon 200 Pulvules & Nalfon Tablets 933

Flurbiprofen (Antihypertensive effects of captopril reduced).
No products indexed under this heading.

Furosemide (Captopril's effect will be augmented; hypotension). Products include:
Lasix Injection, Oral Solution and Tablets 1267

IMPORTANT NOTE: Always consult each drug listing in the patient's regimen for possible interactions.

Capoten Interactions Index 150

Guanethidine Monosulfate (Use with caution). Products include:
- Esimil Tablets ... 840
- Ismelin Tablets ... 845

Hydralazine Hydrochloride (Drugs having vasodilator activity should, if possible, be discontinued before starting Capoten). Products include:
- Apresazide Capsules ... 824
- Apresoline Hydrochloride Tablets .. 826
- Hydralazine Hydrochloride Injection USP ... 2712
- Ser-Ap-Es Tablets ... 867

Hydrochlorothiazide (Captopril's effect will be augmented). Products include:
- Aldactazide Tablets ... 2556
- Aldoril Tablets ... 1644
- Apresazide Capsules ... 824
- Capozide Tablets ... 744
- Dyazide Capsules ... 2653
- Esidrix Tablets ... 839
- Esimil Tablets ... 840
- HydroDIURIL Tablets ... 1716
- Hydropres Tablets ... 1718
- Hyzaar Tablets ... 1720
- Inderide Tablets ... 2838
- Inderide LA Long Acting Capsules ... 2840
- Lopressor HCT Tablets ... 850
- Lotensin HCT Tablets ... 855
- Moduretic Tablets ... 1748
- Oretic Tablets ... 450
- Prinzide Tablets ... 1780
- Ser-Ap-Es Tablets ... 867
- Timolide Tablets ... 1791
- Vaseretic Tablets ... 1810
- Zestoretic Tablets ... 2968
- Ziac ... 1459

Hydroflumethiazide (Captopril's effect will be augmented). Products include:
- Diucardin Tablets ... 2824

Ibuprofen (Antihypertensive effects of captopril reduced). Products include:
- Advil Cold and Sinus Caplets and Tablets ... ▣ 837
- Advil Ibuprofen Tablets, Caplets and Gel Caplets ... ▣ 836
- Children's Motrin Ibuprofen Oral Suspension ... 1558
- IBU Tablets ... 1389
- Ibuprohm ... ▣ 713
- Motrin IB Caplets, Tablets, and Gelcaps ... ▣ 802
- Motrin Ibuprofen Suspension, Oral Drops, Chewable Tablets, Caplets ... 1563
- Nuprin Ibuprofen/Analgesic Tablets & Caplets ... ▣ 645
- Vicks DayQuil SINUS Pressure & PAIN Relief with IBUPROFEN ... ▣ 735

Indapamide (Captopril's effect will be augmented; hypotension).
- No products indexed under this heading.

Indomethacin (Antihypertensive effects of captopril reduced). Products include:
- Indocin ... 1723

Indomethacin Sodium Trihydrate (Antihypertensive effects of captopril reduced). Products include:
- Indocin I.V. ... 1727

Isosorbide Dinitrate (Discontinue before starting captopril; if resumed administer at lower dosage). Products include:
- Dilatrate-SR Capsules ... 2542
- Isordil Sublingual Tablets ... 2845
- Isordil Tembids ... 2847
- Isordil Titradose Tablets ... 2848
- Sorbitrate ... 2959

Isosorbide Mononitrate (Discontinue before starting captopril; if resumed administer at lower dosage). Products include:
- Imdur ... 1362
- Ismo Tablets ... 2844
- Monoket Tablets ... 2550

Ketoprofen (Antihypertensive effects of captopril reduced). Products include:
- Actron Caplets and Tablets ... ▣ 608
- Orudis Capsules ... 2874
- Orudis KT ... ▣ 842
- Oruvail Capsules ... 2874

Ketorolac Tromethamine (Antihypertensive effects of captopril reduced). Products include:
- Acular Sterile Ophthalmic Solution 470
- Toradol ... 2319

Labetalol Hydrochloride (Less than additive antihypertensive effect). Products include:
- Normodyne Injection ... 2519
- Normodyne Tablets ... 2522
- Trandate ... 1158

Levobunolol Hydrochloride (Less than additive antihypertensive effect). Products include:
- Betagan ... ⊙ 230

Lithium Carbonate (Increased serum lithium levels and symptoms of lithium toxicity). Products include:
- Eskalith ... 2658
- Lithium Carbonate Capsules & Tablets ... 2352
- Lithonate/Lithotabs/Lithobid ... 2721

Lithium Citrate (Increased serum lithium levels and symptoms of lithium toxicity).
- No products indexed under this heading.

Mecamylamine Hydrochloride (Use with caution). Products include:
- Inversine Tablets ... 1729

Meclofenamate Sodium (Antihypertensive effects of captopril reduced).
- No products indexed under this heading.

Mefenamic Acid (Antihypertensive effects of captopril reduced). Products include:
- Ponstel ... 1982

Methyclothiazide (Captopril's effect will be augmented). Products include:
- Enduron Tablets ... 424

Metipranolol Hydrochloride (Less than additive antihypertensive effect). Products include:
- OptiPranolol (Metipranolol 0.3%) Sterile Ophthalmic Solution ... ⊙ 256

Metolazone (Captopril's effect will be augmented; hypotension). Products include:
- Mykrox Tablets ... 1617
- Zaroxolyn Tablets ... 1625

Metoprolol Succinate (Less than additive antihypertensive effect). Products include:
- Toprol-XL Tablets ... 560

Metoprolol Tartrate (Less than additive antihypertensive effect). Products include:
- Lopressor ... 848
- Lopressor HCT Tablets ... 850

Minoxidil (Drugs having vasodilator activity should, if possible, be discontinued before starting Capoten).
- No products indexed under this heading.

Nabumetone (Antihypertensive effects of captopril reduced). Products include:
- Relafen Tablets ... 2688

Nadolol (Less than additive antihypertensive effect).
- No products indexed under this heading.

Naproxen (Antihypertensive effects of captopril reduced). Products include:
- Anaprox/Naprosyn ... 2277

Naproxen Sodium (Antihypertensive effects of captopril reduced). Products include:
- Aleve ... 2124
- Anaprox/Naprosyn ... 2277
- Naprelan Tablets ... 2861

Nitroglycerin (Discontinue before starting captopril; if resumed administer at lower dosage). Products include:
- Deponit NTG Transdermal Delivery System ... 2541
- Nitro-Bid IV ... 1270
- Nitro-Bid Ointment ... 1272
- Nitro-Dur (nitroglycerin) Transdermal Infusion System ... 1365
- Nitrolingual Spray ... 2193
- Nitrostat Tablets ... 1981
- Transderm-Nitro Transdermal Therapeutic System ... 878

Oxaprozin (Antihypertensive effects of captopril reduced). Products include:
- Daypro Caplets ... 2578

Penbutolol Sulfate (Less than additive antihypertensive effect). Products include:
- Levatol Tablets ... 2547

Pentaerythritol Tetranitrate (Discontinue before starting captopril; if resumed administer at lower dosage).
- No products indexed under this heading.

Phenylbutazone (Antihypertensive effects of captopril reduced).
- No products indexed under this heading.

Pindolol (Less than additive antihypertensive effect). Products include:
- Visken Tablets ... 2428

Piroxicam (Antihypertensive effects of captopril reduced). Products include:
- Feldene Capsules ... 2008

Polythiazide (Captopril's effect will be augmented). Products include:
- Minizide Capsules ... 2016

Potassium Acid Phosphate (Potential for significant increase in serum potassium). Products include:
- K-Phos Original Formula 'Sodium Free' Tablets ... 633

Potassium Bicarbonate (Potential for significant increase in serum potassium). Products include:
- Alka-Seltzer Gold Effervescent Antacid ... ▣ 611

Potassium Chloride (Potential for significant increase in serum potassium). Products include:
- Chlor-3 Condiment ... 1003
- Colyte and Colyte-flavored ... 2540
- GoLYTELY ... 694
- K-Dur Microburst Release System (potassium chloride, USP) E.R. Tablets ... 1364
- K-Lor Powder Packets ... 438
- K-Norm Capsules ... 1615
- K-Tab Filmtab ... 439
- Micro-K ... 2237
- Micro-K LS Packets ... 2238
- NuLYTELY ... 694
- Cherry Flavor NuLYTELY ... 694
- Rum-K Syrup ... 1004
- Slow-K Extended-Release Tablets ... 869

Potassium Citrate (Potential for significant increase in serum potassium). Products include:
- Polycitra Syrup ... 574
- Polycitra-K Crystals ... 574
- Polycitra-K Oral Solution ... 575
- Polycitra-LC ... 574
- Urocit-K Tablets ... 1828

Potassium Gluconate (Potential for significant increase in serum potassium).
- No products indexed under this heading.

Potassium Phosphate, Dibasic (Potential for significant increase in serum potassium).
- No products indexed under this heading.

Potassium Phosphate, Monobasic (Potential for significant increase in serum potassium). Products include:
- K-Phos Neutral Tablets ... 633
- K-Phos Original Formula 'Sodium Free' Tablets ... 633

Prazosin Hydrochloride (Use with caution). Products include:
- Minipress Capsules ... 2015
- Minizide Capsules ... 2016

Propranolol Hydrochloride (Less than additive antihypertensive effect). Products include:
- Inderal ... 2834
- Inderal LA Long Acting Capsules ... 2836
- Inderide Tablets ... 2838
- Inderide LA Long Acting Capsules .. 2840

Reserpine (Use with caution). Products include:
- Diupres Tablets ... 1691
- Hydropres Tablets ... 1718
- Ser-Ap-Es Tablets ... 867

Sotalol Hydrochloride (Less than additive antihypertensive effect). Products include:
- Betapace Tablets ... 637

Spironolactone (Captopril's effect will be augmented; hypotension; increased serum potassium). Products include:
- Aldactazide Tablets ... 2556
- Aldactone Tablets ... 2558

Sulindac (Antihypertensive effects of captopril reduced). Products include:
- Clinoril Tablets ... 1658

Terazosin Hydrochloride (Use with caution). Products include:
- Hytrin Capsules ... 434

Timolol Hemihydrate (Less than additive antihypertensive effect). Products include:
- Betimol 0.25%, 0.5% ... ⊙ 259

Timolol Maleate (Less than additive antihypertensive effect). Products include:
- Blocadren Tablets ... 1654
- Timolide Tablets ... 1791
- Timoptic in Ocudose ... 1796
- Timoptic Sterile Ophthalmic Solution ... 1794
- Timoptic-XE ... 1798

Tolmetin Sodium (Antihypertensive effects of captopril reduced). Products include:
- Tolectin (200, 400 and 600 mg) .. 1591

Torsemide (Captopril's effect will be augmented; hypotension). Products include:
- Demadex Tablets and Injection ... 691

Triamterene (Captopril's effect will be augmented; hypotension; increased serum potassium). Products include:
- Dyazide Capsules ... 2653
- Dyrenium Capsules ... 2655

Trimethaphan Camsylate (Use with caution).
- No products indexed under this heading.

Food Interactions

Food, unspecified (Reduces absorption by about 30% to 40%; should be given one hour before meals).

CAPOZIDE TABLETS

(Captopril, Hydrochlorothiazide) ... 744

May interact with diuretics, thiazides, ganglionic blocking agents, peripheral adrenergic blockers, lithium preparations, potassium sparing diuretics, potassium preparations, oral anticoagulants, calcium prepara-

(▣ Described in PDR For Nonprescription Drugs) (⊙ Described in PDR For Ophthalmology)

Interactions Index

tions, cardiac glycosides, non-steroidal anti-inflammatory agents, barbiturates, agents causing renin release, inhibitors of endogenous prostaglandin synthesis, narcotic analgesics, antihypertensives, corticosteroids, preanesthetic medications, general anesthetics, nondepolarizing neuromuscular blocking agents, oral hypoglycemic agents, insulin, monoamine oxidase inhibitors, antigout agents, and certain other agents. Compounds in these categories include:

Acarbose (Thiazide-induced hyperglycemia may require dosage adjustment of antidiabetic drugs). Products include:

Precose	604

Acebutolol Hydrochloride (Potential for additive or potentiative effects). Products include:

Sectral Capsules	2914

ACTH (Co-administration with thiazides may intensify electrolyte imbalance, particularly hypokalemia).
No products indexed under this heading.

Alfentanil Hydrochloride (Potentiation of orthostatic hypotension). Products include:

Alfenta Injection	1334

Allopurinol (Dosage adjustment may be necessary since hydrochlorothiazide may have hyperuricemic effect). Products include:

Zyloprim Tablets	1194

Amiloride Hydrochloride (Increased risk of hyperkalemia and increased potential for precipitous reduction in blood pressure). Products include:

Midamor Tablets	1746
Moduretic Tablets	1748

Amlodipine Besylate (Potential for additive or potentiative effects). Products include:

Lotrel Capsules	858
Norvasc Tablets	2020

Amphotericin B (Co-administration with thiazides may intensify electrolyte imbalance, particularly hypokalemia). Products include:

Abelcet Injection	1540
Fungizone Intravenous	507
Fungizone Oral Suspension	704

Aprobarbital (Potentiation of orthostatic hypotension).
No products indexed under this heading.

Aspirin (Co-administration with inhibitors of endogenous prostaglandin synthesis may reduce the antihypertensive effects of captopril). Products include:

Alka-Seltzer Cherry Effervescent Antacid and Pain Reliever	◼ 609
Alka-Seltzer Extra Strength Effervescent Antacid and Pain Reliever	◼ 609
Alka-Seltzer Lemon Lime Effervescent Antacid and Pain Reliever	◼ 609
Alka-Seltzer Original Effervescent Antacid and Pain Reliever	◼ 609
Alka-Seltzer Plus	◼ 611
Alka-Seltzer Plus Sinus Medicine	◼ 611
Ascriptin	◼ 650
Arthritis Strength BC Powder	◼ 631
BC Cold Powder Multi-Symptom Formula (Cold-Sinus-Allergy)	◼ 631
BC Cold Powder Non-Drowsy Formula (Cold-Sinus)	◼ 631
BC Powder	◼ 631
Genuine Bayer Aspirin Tablets & Caplets	◼ 618
Extra Strength Bayer Arthritis Pain Regimen Formula	◼ 615
Extra Strength Bayer Aspirin Caplets & Tablets	◼ 617
Extended-Release Bayer 8-Hour Aspirin	◼ 616
Extra Strength Bayer Plus Aspirin Caplets	◼ 617
Extra Strength Bayer PM Aspirin Plus Sleep Aid	◼ 617
Aspirin Regimen Bayer 81 mg Tablets with Calcium	◼ 615
Aspirin Regimen Bayer Adult Low Strength 81 mg Tablets	◼ 613
Aspirin Regimen Bayer Children's Chewable Aspirin	◼ 616
Aspirin Regimen Bayer Regular Strength 325 mg Caplets	◼ 613
Bufferin Analgesic Tablets	◼ 636
Arthritis Strength Bufferin Analgesic Caplets	◼ 637
Extra Strength Bufferin Analgesic Tablets	◼ 637
Cama Arthritis Pain Reliever	◼ 748
Darvon Compound-65 Pulvules	1475
Easprin	1971
Ecotrin	2625
Ecotrin Enteric Coated Aspirin Maximum Strength Tablets and Caplets	◼ 775
Ecotrin Enteric Coated Aspirin Regular Strength Tablets	2625
Empirin Aspirin Tablets	◼ 818
Excedrin Extra-Strength Analgesic Tablets, Caplets, and Geltabs	734
Fiorinal Tablets	2388
Fiorinal with Codeine Capsules	2390
Fiorinal Tablets	2388
Goody's Extra Strength Headache Powders	632
Goody's Extra Strength Pain Relief Tablets	632
Halfprin Tablets	1413
Norgesic	1554
Percodan Tablets	955
Percodan-Demi Tablets	956
Robaxisal Tablets	2246
Soma Compound w/Codeine Tablets	2784
Soma Compound Tablets	2783
St. Joseph Adult Chewable Aspirin (81 mg.)	◼ 768
Talwin Compound	2466
Vanquish Analgesic Caplets	◼ 627

Atenolol (Potential for additive or potentiative effects). Products include:

Tenoretic Tablets	2963
Tenormin Tablets and I.V. Injection	2965

Atracurium Besylate (Effects of nondepolarizing muscle relaxants may be potentiated). Products include:

Tracrium Injection	1155

Benazepril Hydrochloride (Potential for additive or potentiative effects). Products include:

Lotensin Tablets	852
Lotensin HCT Tablets	855
Lotrel Capsules	858

Bendroflumethiazide (Potential for precipitous reduction in blood pressure).
No products indexed under this heading.

Betamethasone Acetate (Co-administration with thiazides may intensify electrolyte imbalance, particularly hypokalemia). Products include:

Celestone Soluspan Suspension	2484

Betamethasone Sodium Phosphate (Co-administration with thiazides may intensify electrolyte imbalance, particularly hypokalemia). Products include:

Celestone Soluspan Suspension	2484

Betaxolol Hydrochloride (Potential for additive or potentiative effects). Products include:

Betoptic Ophthalmic Solution	465
Betoptic S Ophthalmic Suspension	467
Kerlone Tablets	2588

Bisoprolol Fumarate (Potential for additive or potentiative effects). Products include:

Zebeta Tablets	1457
Ziac	1459

Bumetanide (Potential for precipitous reduction in blood pressure). Products include:

Bumex	2260

Buprenorphine (Potentiation of orthostatic hypotension). Products include:

Buprenex Injectable	2170

Butabarbital (Potentiation of orthostatic hypotension).
No products indexed under this heading.

Butalbital (Potentiation of orthostatic hypotension). Products include:

Axocet Capsules	2469
Esgic-plus Capsules	1012
Esgic-plus Tablets	1012
Fioricet Tablets	2386
Fioricet with Codeine Capsules	2387
Fiorinal Capsules	2388
Fiorinal with Codeine Capsules	2390
Fiorinal Tablets	2388
Phrenilin	790
Sedapap Tablets 50 mg/650 mg	1826

Calcium Carbonate (Potential for hypercalcemia). Products include:

Alka-Mints Chewable Antacid	◼ 609
Alka-Seltzer Fast Relief Caplets	◼ 610
Ascriptin	◼ 650
Extra Strength Bayer Plus Aspirin Caplets	◼ 617
Aspirin Regimen Bayer 81 mg Tablets with Calcium	◼ 615
Bufferin Analgesic Tablets	◼ 636
Arthritis Strength Bufferin Analgesic Caplets	◼ 637
Extra Strength Bufferin Analgesic Tablets	◼ 637
Calci-Chew Tablets	2168
Calci-Mix Capsules	2168
Caltrate 600	◼ 681
Caltrate PLUS	◼ 681
Caltrate 600 + D	◼ 681
Cotazym Capsules	1866
Di-Gel Antacid/Anti-Gas	◼ 762
Florical Capsules and Tablets	1825
Gerimed Tablets	1000
Maalox Antacid Caplets	◼ 657
Marblen	◼ 671
Materna Tablets	1427
Monocal Tablets	1825
Mylanta Fast-Acting	1359
Mylanta Gelcaps Antacid	◼ 678
Mylanta Soothing Lozenges	1360
Mylanta Tablets	◼ 677
Mylanta Double Strength Tablets	◼ 677
Nephro-Calci Tablets	2168
One-A-Day Calcium Plus	◼ 625
Rolaids Antacid Tablets	◼ 807
Rolaids Antacid Calcium Rich/Sodium Free Tablets	◼ 807
Tempo Soft Antacid	◼ 799
Titralac	◼ 686
Titralac Plus	◼ 687
Tums Antacid/Calcium Supplement Tablets	◼ 787
Tums Anti-gas/Antacid Formula Tablets, Assorted Fruit	◼ 788
Tums E-X Antacid/Calcium Supplement Tablets	◼ 787
Tums 500 Calcium Supplement	◼ 788
Tums ULTRA Antacid/Calcium Supplement Tablets	◼ 787
TYLENOL Headache Plus Pain Reliever with Antacid, Extra Strength Caplets	◼ 705

Calcium Chloride (Potential for hypercalcemia).
No products indexed under this heading.

Calcium Citrate (Potential for hypercalcemia). Products include:

Citracal Tablets	1828

Calcium Glubionate (Potential for hypercalcemia).
No products indexed under this heading.

Carteolol Hydrochloride (Potential for additive or potentiative effects). Products include:

Cartrol Tablets	413
Ocupress Ophthalmic Solution, 1% Sterile	◎ 297

Chlorothiazide (Potential for precipitous reduction in blood pressure). Products include:

Aldoclor Tablets	1638
Diupres Tablets	1691
Diuril Oral	1694

Chlorothiazide Sodium (Potential for precipitous reduction in blood pressure). Products include:

Diuril Sodium Intravenous	1693

Chlorpropamide (Thiazide-induced hyperglycemia may require dosage adjustment of antidiabetic drugs). Products include:

Diabinese Tablets	2002

Chlorthalidone (Potential for precipitous reduction in blood pressure). Products include:

Combipres Tablets	682
Tenoretic Tablets	2963
Thalitone	1293

Cholestyramine (Delays or decreases absorption of hydrochlorothiazide). Products include:

Questran	774

Cisatracurium Besylate (Effects of nondepolarizing muscle relaxants may be potentiated). Products include:

Nimbex Injection	1131

Clonidine (Potential for additive or potentiative effects). Products include:

Catapres-TTS	680

Clonidine Hydrochloride (Potential for additive or potentiative effects). Products include:

Catapres Tablets	679
Combipres Tablets	682

Codeine Phosphate (Potentiation of orthostatic hypotension). Products include:

Brontex	2130
Dimetane-DC Cough Syrup	2232
Fioricet with Codeine Capsules	2387
Fiorinal with Codeine Capsules	2390
Nucofed	2225
Phenergan with Codeine	2883
Phenergan VC with Codeine	2888
Robitussin A-C Syrup	2248
Robitussin-DAC Syrup	2249
Ryna	◼ 804
Soma Compound w/Codeine Tablets	2784
Tylenol with Codeine	1592

Colestipol Hydrochloride (Delays or decreases absorption of hydrochlorothiazide). Products include:

Colestid	2073

Cortisone Acetate (Co-administration with thiazides may intensify electrolyte imbalance, particularly hypokalemia). Products include:

Cortone Acetate Sterile Suspension	1663
Cortone Acetate Tablets	1664

Deserpidine (Potential for additive or potentiative effects).
No products indexed under this heading.

Deslanoside (Thiazide-induced hypokalemia may enhance the possibility of digitalis toxicity).
No products indexed under this heading.

Dexamethasone (Co-administration with thiazides may intensify electrolyte imbalance, particularly hypokalemia). Products include:

AK-Trol Ointment & Suspension	◎ 205
Decadron Elixir	1676
Decadron Tablets	1678
Decaspray Topical Aerosol	1689
Maxitrol Ophthalmic Ointment and Suspension	◎ 222
TobraDex Ophthalmic Suspension and Ointment	469

IMPORTANT NOTE: Always consult each drug listing in the patient's regimen for possible interactions.

Capozide Interactions Index 152

Dexamethasone Acetate (Co-administration with thiazides may intensify electrolyte imbalance, particularly hypokalemia). Products include:
- Dalalone D.P. Injectable ... 1009
- Decadron-LA Sterile Suspension ... 1687

Dexamethasone Sodium Phosphate (Co-administration with thiazides may intensify electrolyte imbalance, particularly hypokalemia). Products include:
- Decadron Phosphate Injection ... 1680
- Decadron Phosphate Sterile Ophthalmic Ointment ... 1684
- Decadron Phosphate Sterile Ophthalmic Solution ... 1685
- Decadron Phosphate Topical Cream ... 1686
- Decadron Phosphate with Xylocaine Injection, Sterile ... 1683
- Dexacort Phosphate in Respihaler .. 1606
- Dexacort Phosphate in Turbinaire .. 1607
- NeoDecadron Sterile Ophthalmic Ointment ... 1755
- NeoDecadron Sterile Ophthalmic Solution ... 1756
- NeoDecadron Topical Cream ... 1757

Dezocine (Potentiation of orthostatic hypotension). Products include:
- Dalgan Injection ... 529

Diazepam (Effects of preanesthetic agents may be potentiated). Products include:
- Dizac (diazepam injectable emulsion) CIV ... 1862
- Valium Injectable ... 2336
- Valium Tablets ... 2335

Diazoxide (Potential for additive or potentiative effects). Products include:
- Hyperstat I.V. Injection ... 2504
- Proglycem ... 575

Diclofenac Potassium (Reduces antihypertensive, natriuretic, and diuretic effects). Products include:
- Cataflam Tablets ... 833

Diclofenac Sodium (Reduces antihypertensive, natriuretic, and diuretic effects). Products include:
- Voltaren Ophthalmic Sterile Ophthalmic Solution ... ⊙ 264
- Cataflam/Voltaren/Voltaren-XR ... 833

Dicumarol (Hydrochlorothiazide may decrease effects of anticoagulant; dosage adjustment may be necessary).
- No products indexed under this heading.

Digitoxin (Thiazide-induced hypokalemia may enhance the possibility of digitalis toxicity). Products include:
- Crystodigin Tablets ... 1472

Digoxin (Thiazide-induced hypokalemia may enhance the possibility of digitalis toxicity). Products include:
- Lanoxicaps ... 1110
- Lanoxin Elixir Pediatric ... 1113
- Lanoxin Injection ... 1116
- Lanoxin Injection Pediatric ... 1119
- Lanoxin Tablets ... 1121

Diltiazem Hydrochloride (Potential for additive or potentiative effects). Products include:
- Cardizem CD Capsules ... 1251
- Cardizem SR Capsules ... 1255
- Cardizem Injectable ... 1253
- Cardizem Tablets ... 1257
- Dilacor XR Extended-release Capsules ... 2183
- Tiazac Capsules ... 1019

Dopamine Hydrochloride (Decreased reponse to pressor amines).
- No products indexed under this heading.

Doxazosin Mesylate (Potential for additive or potentiative effects). Products include:
- Cardura Tablets ... 1993

Droperidol (Effects of preanesthetic agents may be potentiated). Products include:
- Inapsine Injection ... 462

Enalapril Maleate (Potential for additive or potentiative effects). Products include:
- Vaseretic Tablets ... 1810
- Vasotec Tablets ... 1816

Enalaprilat (Potential for additive or potentiative effects). Products include:
- Vasotec I.V. ... 1814

Enflurane (Effects of anesthetic agents may be potentiated).
- No products indexed under this heading.

Epinephrine Hydrochloride (Decreased reponse to pressor amines). Products include:
- Ana-Kit Anaphylaxis Emergency Treatment Kit ... 611

Erythrityl Tetranitrate (Discontinue before starting captopril; if resumed administer at lower dosage).
- No products indexed under this heading.

Esmolol Hydrochloride (Potential for additive or potentiative effects). Products include:
- Brevibloc (esmolol HCl) Injection ... 1860

Ethacrynic Acid (Potential for precipitous reduction in blood pressure). Products include:
- Edecrin Tablets ... 1698

Etodolac (Reduces antihypertensive, natriuretic, and diuretic effects). Products include:
- Lodine Capsules and Tablets ... 2849

Felodipine (Potential for additive or potentiative effects). Products include:
- Plendil Extended-Release Tablets ... 514

Fenoprofen Calcium (Reduces antihypertensive, natriuretic, and diuretic effects). Products include:
- Nalfon 200 Pulvules & Nalfon Tablets ... 933

Fentanyl (Potentiation of orthostatic hypotension). Products include:
- Duragesic Transdermal System ... 1336

Fentanyl Citrate (Potentiation of orthostatic hypotension). Products include:
- Sublimaze Injection ... 463

Fludrocortisone Acetate (Co-administration with thiazides may intensify electrolyte imbalance, particularly hypokalemia). Products include:
- Florinef Acetate Tablets ... 506

Flurbiprofen (Reduces antihypertensive, natriuretic, and diuretic effects).
- No products indexed under this heading.

Fosinopril Sodium (Potential for additive or potentiative effects). Products include:
- Monopril Tablets ... 762

Furazolidone (Enhanced hypotensive effects; dosage adjustments of one or both agents may be necessary). Products include:
- Furoxone ... 2221

Furosemide (Potential for precipitous reduction in blood pressure). Products include:
- Lasix Injection, Oral Solution and Tablets ... 1267

Gallamine (Effects of gallamine may be potentiated).

Glimepiride (Thiazide-induced hyperglycemia may require dosage adjustment of antidiabetic drugs). Products include:
- Amaryl Tablets ... 1241

Glipizide (Thiazide-induced hyperglycemia may require dosage adjustment of antidiabetic drugs). Products include:
- Glucotrol Tablets ... 2011
- Glucotrol XL Extended Release Tablets ... 2012

Glyburide (Thiazide-induced hyperglycemia may require dosage adjustment of antidiabetic drugs). Products include:
- DiaBeta Tablets ... 1265
- Glynase PresTab Tablets ... 2091
- Micronase Tablets ... 2099

Guanabenz Acetate (Potential for additive or potentiative effects).
- No products indexed under this heading.

Guanethidine Monosulfate (Potential for additive or potentiative effects). Products include:
- Esimil Tablets ... 840
- Ismelin Tablets ... 845

Hydralazine Hydrochloride (Potential for additive or potentiative effects). Products include:
- Apresazide Capsules ... 824
- Apresoline Hydrochloride Tablets .. 826
- Hydralazine Hydrochloride Injection USP ... 2712
- Ser-Ap-Es Tablets ... 867

Hydrocodone Bitartrate (Potentiation of orthostatic hypotension). Products include:
- Codiclear DH Syrup ... 808
- Duratuss HD Elixir ... 2750
- Histussin D Liquid ... 670
- Hycodan Tablets and Syrup ... 946
- Hycomine Compound Tablets ... 948
- Hycomine ... 947
- Hycotuss Expectorant Syrup ... 950
- Hydrocet Capsules ... 787
- Lorcet 10/650 Tablets ... 1016
- Lortab ... 2751
- Tussend ... 1830
- Tussend Expectorant ... 1831
- Vicodin Tablets ... 1404
- Vicodin ES Tablets ... 1405
- Vicodin HP Tablets ... 1403
- Vicodin Tuss Expectorant ... 1406
- Zydone Capsules ... 967

Hydrocodone Polistirex (Potentiation of orthostatic hypotension). Products include:
- Tussionex Pennkinetic Extended-Release Suspension ... 1624

Hydrocortisone (Co-administration with thiazides may intensify electrolyte imbalance, particularly hypokalemia). Products include:
- Anusol-HC Cream 2.5% ... 1953
- Aquanil HC Lotion ... 1989
- Maximum Strength Cortaid Spray ▣ 800
- CORTENEMA ... 2713
- Cortisporin Ointment ... 1074
- Cortisporin Ophthalmic Ointment Sterile ... 1074
- Cortisporin Ophthalmic Suspension Sterile ... 1075
- Cortisporin Otic Solution Sterile ... 1076
- Cortisporin Otic Suspension Sterile 1077
- Cortizone-5 ... ▣ 795
- Cortizone-10 ... ▣ 795
- Hydrocortone Tablets ... 1715
- Hytone ... 922
- Hytone Ointment 2 ½% ... 923
- Massengill Medicated Soft Cloth Towelettes ... 2628
- Pediotic Suspension Sterile ... 1140
- Preparation H Hydrocortisone 1% Cream ... ▣ 843
- ProctoCream-HC 2.5% ... 2552
- VōSoL HC Otic Solution ... 2786

Hydrocortisone Acetate (Co-administration with thiazides may intensify electrolyte imbalance, particularly hypokalemia). Products include:
- Analpram-HC Rectal Cream 1% and 2.5% ... 993
- Anusol HC-1 Hydrocortisone Anti-Itch Ointment ... ▣ 810
- Anusol-HC Suppositories ... 1954
- Caldecort Anti-Itch Hydrocortisone Cream ... ▣ 651
- Coly-Mycin S Otic w/Neomycin & Hydrocortisone ... 1965
- Cortaid ... ▣ 800
- Cortifoam ... 2540
- Cortisporin Cream ... 1073
- Epifoam ... 2543
- Hydrocortone Acetate Sterile Suspension ... 1712
- Mantadil Cream ... 1124
- Nupercainal Hydrocortisone 1% Cream ... ▣ 661
- Pramosone Cream, Lotion & Ointment ... 995
- ProctoFoam-HC ... 2552
- Terra-Cortril Ophthalmic Suspension ... 2033

Hydrocortisone Sodium Phosphate (Co-administration with thiazides may intensify electrolyte imbalance, particularly hypokalemia). Products include:
- Hydrocortone Phosphate Injection, Sterile ... 1713

Hydrocortisone Sodium Succinate (Co-administration with thiazides may intensify electrolyte imbalance, particularly hypokalemia).
- No products indexed under this heading.

Hydroflumethiazide (Potential for precipitous reduction in blood pressure). Products include:
- Diucardin Tablets ... 2824

Hydromorphone Hydrochloride (Potentiation of orthostatic hypotension). Products include:
- Dilaudid Ampules ... 1382
- Dilaudid Cough Syrup ... 1383
- Dilaudid-HP Injection ... 1384
- Dilaudid-HP Lyophilized Powder 250 mg ... 1384
- Dilaudid ... 1382
- Dilaudid Oral Liquid ... 1386
- Dilaudid ... 1382
- Dilaudid Tablets - 8 mg ... 1386

Hydroxyzine Hydrochloride (Effects of preanesthetic agents may be potentiated). Products include:
- Atarax Tablets & Syrup ... 1992
- Marax Tablets & DF Syrup ... 2015
- Vistaril Intramuscular Solution ... 2042

Ibuprofen (Reduces antihypertensive, natriuretic, and diuretic effects). Products include:
- Advil Cold and Sinus Caplets and Tablets ... ▣ 837
- Advil Ibuprofen Tablets, Caplets and Gel Caplets ... ▣ 836
- Children's Motrin Ibuprofen Oral Suspension ... 1558
- IBU Tablets ... 1389
- Ibuprohm ... ▣ 713
- Motrin IB Caplets, Tablets, and Gelcaps ... ▣ 802
- Motrin Ibuprofen Suspension, Oral Drops, Chewable Tablets, Caplets ... 1563
- Nuprin Ibuprofen/Analgesic Tablets & Caplets ... ▣ 645
- Vicks DayQuil SINUS Pressure & PAIN Relief with IBUPROFEN ... ▣ 735

Indapamide (Potential for precipitous reduction in blood pressure).
- No products indexed under this heading.

Indomethacin (Reduces antihypertensive, natriuretic, and diuretic effects). Products include:
- Indocin ... 1723

(▣ Described in PDR For Nonprescription Drugs) (⊙ Described in PDR For Ophthalmology)

Interactions Index — Capozide

Indomethacin Sodium Trihydrate (Reduces antihypertensive, natriuretic, and diuretic effects). Products include:
- Indocin I.V. 1727

Insulin, Human (Thiazide-induced hyperglycemia may require dosage adjustment of antidiabetic drugs).
- No products indexed under this heading.

Insulin, Human Isophane Suspension (Thiazide-induced hyperglycemia may require dosage adjustment of antidiabetic drugs). Products include:
- Novolin N Human Insulin 10 ml Vials 1846

Insulin, Human NPH (Thiazide-induced hyperglycemia may require dosage adjustment of antidiabetic drugs). Products include:
- Humulin N, 100 Units 1495
- Novolin N PenFill 1.5 ml Cartridges Durable Insulin Delivery System 1849
- Novolin N Prefilled Syringe Disposable Insulin Delivery System 1850

Insulin, Human Regular (Thiazide-induced hyperglycemia may require dosage adjustment of antidiabetic drugs). Products include:
- Humulin R, 100 Units 1497
- Novolin R Human Insulin 10 ml Vials 1846
- Novolin R PenFill 1.5 ml Cartridges Durable Insulin Delivery System 1849
- Novolin R Prefilled Syringe Disposable Insulin Delivery System 1850
- Velosulin BR Human Insulin 10 ml Vials 1847

Insulin, Human, Zinc Suspension (Thiazide-induced hyperglycemia may require dosage adjustment of antidiabetic drugs). Products include:
- Humulin L, 100 Units 1494
- Humulin U, 100 Units 1498
- Novolin L Human Insulin 10 ml Vials 1846

Insulin Lispro, Human (Thiazide-induced hyperglycemia may require dosage adjustment of antidiabetic drugs). Products include:
- Humalog Injection 1488

Insulin, NPH (Thiazide-induced hyperglycemia may require dosage adjustment of antidiabetic drugs). Products include:
- NPH, 100 Units 1502
- Pork NPH, 100 Units 1506
- Purified Pork NPH Isophane Insulin 1852

Insulin, Regular (Thiazide-induced hyperglycemia may require dosage adjustment of antidiabetic drugs). Products include:
- Regular, 100 Units 1503
- Pork Regular, 100 Units 1507
- Pork Regular (Concentrated), 500 Units 1508
- Purified Pork Regular Insulin 1852

Insulin, Zinc Crystals (Thiazide-induced hyperglycemia may require dosage adjustment of antidiabetic drugs). Products include:
- NPH, 100 Units 1502

Insulin, Zinc Suspension (Thiazide-induced hyperglycemia may require dosage adjustment of antidiabetic drugs). Products include:
- Iletin I 1501
- Lente, 100 Units 1501
- Iletin II 1504
- Pork Lente, 100 Units 1504
- Purified Pork Lente Insulin 1852

Isocarboxazid (Enhanced hypotensive effects; dosage adjustments of one or both agents may be necessary).
- No products indexed under this heading.

Isoflurane (Effects of anesthetic agents may be potentiated).
- No products indexed under this heading.

Isosorbide Dinitrate (Data on concomitant use are not available; nitrates should be discontinued, if possible, or administer cautiously at lower dosage). Products include:
- Dilatrate-SR Capsules 2542
- Isordil Sublingual Tablets 2845
- Isordil Tembids 2847
- Isordil Titradose Tablets 2848
- Sorbitrate 2959

Isosorbide Mononitrate (Data on concomitant use are not available; nitrates should be discontinued, if possible, or administer cautiously at lower dosage). Products include:
- Imdur 1362
- Ismo Tablets 2844
- Monoket Tablets 2550

Isradipine (Potential for additive or potentiative effects). Products include:
- DynaCirc Capsules 2381
- DynaCirc CR Tablets 2383

Ketamine Hydrochloride (Effects of anesthetic agents may be potentiated).
- No products indexed under this heading.

Ketoprofen (Reduces antihypertensive, natriuretic, and diuretic effects). Products include:
- Actron Caplets and Tablets 608
- Orudis Capsules 2874
- Orudis KT 842
- Oruvail Capsules 2874

Ketorolac Tromethamine (Reduces antihypertensive, natriuretic, and diuretic effects). Products include:
- Acular Sterile Ophthalmic Solution 470
- Toradol 2319

Labetalol Hydrochloride (Potential for additive or potentiative effects). Products include:
- Normodyne Injection 2519
- Normodyne Tablets 2522
- Trandate 1158

Levorphanol Tartrate (Potentiation of orthostatic hypotension). Products include:
- Levo-Dromoran 2297

Lisinopril (Potential for additive or potentiative effects). Products include:
- Prinivil Tablets 1776
- Prinzide Tablets 1780
- Zestoretic Tablets 2968
- Zestril Tablets 2972

Lithium Carbonate (Co-administration may result in reduction in renal clearance with resultant increase in serum lithium levels; increased potential for lithium toxicity). Products include:
- Eskalith 2658
- Lithium Carbonate Capsules & Tablets 2352
- Lithonate/Lithotabs/Lithobid 2721

Lithium Citrate (Co-administration may result in reduction in renal clearance with resultant increase in serum lithium levels; increased potential for lithium toxicity).
- No products indexed under this heading.

Lorazepam (Effects of preanesthetic agents may be potentiated). Products include:
- Ativan Injection 2805
- Ativan Tablets 2807

Losartan Potassium (Potential for additive or potentiative effects). Products include:
- Cozaar Tablets 1668
- Hyzaar Tablets 1720

Mecamylamine Hydrochloride (Potential for additive or potentiative effects). Products include:
- Inversine Tablets 1729

Meclofenamate Sodium (Reduces antihypertensive, natriuretic, and diuretic effects).
- No products indexed under this heading.

Mefenamic Acid (Reduces antihypertensive, natriuretic, and diuretic effects). Products include:
- Ponstel 1982

Meperidine Hydrochloride (Potentiation of orthostatic hypotension). Products include:
- Demerol 2438
- Mepergan Injection 2859

Mephobarbital (Potentiation of orthostatic hypotension). Products include:
- Mebaral Tablets 2452

Metaraminol Bitartrate (Decreased response to pressor amines). Products include:
- Aramine Injection 1649

Metformin Hydrochloride (Thiazide-induced hyperglycemia may require dosage adjustment of antidiabetic drugs). Products include:
- Glucophage Tablets 754

Methadone Hydrochloride (Potentiation of orthostatic hypotension). Products include:
- Methadone Hydrochloride Oral Concentrate 2356
- Methadone Hydrochloride Oral Solution & Tablets 2357

Methenamine (Possible decreased effectiveness due to alkalinization of urine). Products include:
- Urised Tablets 2123

Methohexital Sodium (Effects of anesthetic agents may be potentiated).
- No products indexed under this heading.

Methoxamine Hydrochloride (Effects of anesthetic agents may be potentiated). Products include:
- Vasoxyl Injection 1169

Methoxyflurane (Effects of anesthetic agents may be potentiated).
- No products indexed under this heading.

Methyclothiazide (Potential for precipitous reduction in blood pressure). Products include:
- Enduron Tablets 424

Methyldopa (Potential for additive or potentiative effects). Products include:
- Aldoclor Tablets 1638
- Aldomet Oral 1640
- Aldoril Tablets 1644

Methyldopate Hydrochloride (Potential for additive or potentiative effects). Products include:
- Aldomet Ester HCl Injection 1642

Methylprednisolone Acetate (Co-administration with thiazides may intensify electrolyte imbalance, particularly hypokalemia).
- No products indexed under this heading.

Methylprednisolone Sodium Succinate (Co-administration with thiazides may intensify electrolyte imbalance, particularly hypokalemia).
- No products indexed under this heading.

Metocurine Iodide (Effects of nondepolarizing muscle relaxants may be potentiated). Products include:
- Metubine Iodide Vials 932

Metolazone (Potential for precipitous reduction in blood pressure). Products include:
- Mykrox Tablets 1617
- Zaroxolyn Tablets 1625

Metoprolol Succinate (Potential for additive or potentiative effects). Products include:
- Toprol-XL Tablets 560

Metoprolol Tartrate (Potential for additive or potentiative effects). Products include:
- Lopressor 848
- Lopressor HCT Tablets 850

Metyrosine (Potential for additive or potentiative effects). Products include:
- Demser Capsules 1690

Minoxidil (Potential for additive or potentiative effects).
- No products indexed under this heading.

Mivacurium Chloride (Effects of nondepolarizing muscle relaxants may be potentiated). Products include:
- Mivacron 1125

Moexipril Hydrochloride (Potential for additive or potentiative effects). Products include:
- Univasc Tablets 2553

Morphine Sulfate (Potentiation of orthostatic hypotension). Products include:
- Astramorph/PF Injection, USP (Preservative-Free) 526
- Duramorph Injection 983
- Infumorph 200 and Infumorph 500 Sterile Solutions 985
- Kadian Capsules 2948
- MS Contin Tablets 2149
- MSIR 2152
- Oramorph SR (Morphine Sulfate Sustained Release Tablets) 2359
- RMS Suppositories CII 2766
- Roxanol 2365

Nabumetone (Reduces antihypertensive, natriuretic, and diuretic effects). Products include:
- Relafen Tablets 2688

Nadolol (Potential for additive or potentiative effects).
- No products indexed under this heading.

Naproxen (Reduces antihypertensive, natriuretic, and diuretic effects). Products include:
- Anaprox/Naprosyn 2277

Naproxen Sodium (Reduces antihypertensive, natriuretic, and diuretic effects). Products include:
- Aleve 2124
- Anaprox/Naprosyn 2277
- Naprelan Tablets 2861

Nicardipine Hydrochloride (Potential for additive or potentiative effects). Products include:
- Cardene Capsules 2261
- Cardene I.V. 2815
- Cardene SR Capsules 2264

Nifedipine (Potential for additive or potentiative effects). Products include:
- Adalat Capsules (10 mg and 20 mg) 580
- Adalat CC 582
- Procardia Capsules 2024
- Procardia XL Extended Release Tablets 2026

Nisoldipine (Potential for additive or potentiative effects). Products include:
- Sular Tablets 2961

IMPORTANT NOTE: Always consult each drug listing in the patient's regimen for possible interactions.

Capozide — Interactions Index

Nitroglycerin (Data on concomitant use are not available; nitrates should be discontinued, if possible, or administer cautiously at lower dosage). Products include:
- Deponit NTG Transdermal Delivery System ... 2541
- Nitro-Bid IV ... 1270
- Nitro-Bid Ointment ... 1272
- Nitro-Dur (nitroglycerin) Transdermal Infusion System ... 1365
- Nitrolingual Spray ... 2193
- Nitrostat Tablets ... 1981
- Transderm-Nitro Transdermal Therapeutic System ... 878

Norepinephrine Bitartrate (Possible decreased response to pressor amines). Products include:
- Levophed Bitartrate Injection ... 2445

Opium Alkaloids (Potentiation of orthostatic hypotension).
No products indexed under this heading.

Oxaprozin (Reduces antihypertensive, natriuretic, and diuretic effects). Products include:
- Daypro Caplets ... 2578

Oxycodone Hydrochloride (Potentiation of orthostatic hypotension). Products include:
- OxyContin Tablets ... 2163
- OxyIR Capsules ... 2167
- Percocet Tablets ... 955
- Percodan Tablets ... 955
- Percodan-Demi Tablets ... 956
- Roxicodone Tablets, Oral Solution & Intensol (Oxycodone) ... 2366
- Tylox Capsules ... 1593

Pancuronium Bromide (Effects of nondepolarizing muscle relaxants may be potentiated).
No products indexed under this heading.

Penbutolol Sulfate (Potential for additive or potentiative effects). Products include:
- Levatol Tablets ... 2547

Pentaerythritol Tetranitrate (Discontinue before starting captopril; if resumed administer at lower dosage).
No products indexed under this heading.

Pentobarbital Sodium (Potentiation of orthostatic hypotension). Products include:
- Nembutal Sodium Capsules ... 440
- Nembutal Sodium Solution ... 442
- Nembutal Sodium Suppositories ... 444

Phenelzine Sulfate (Enhanced hypotensive effects; dosage adjustments of one or both agents may be necessary). Products include:
- Nardil ... 1977

Phenobarbital (Potentiation of orthostatic hypotension). Products include:
- Arco-Lase Plus Tablets ... 513
- Bellergal-S Tablets ... 2375
- Donnatal ... 2234
- Donnatal Extentabs ... 2234
- Donnatal Tablets ... 2234
- Phenobarbital Elixir and Tablets ... 1523
- Quadrinal Tablets ... 1398

Phenoxybenzamine Hydrochloride (Potential for additive or potentiative effects). Products include:
- Dibenzyline Capsules ... 2650

Phentolamine Mesylate (Potential for additive or potentiative effects). Products include:
- Regitine Vials ... 864

Phenylbutazone (Reduces antihypertensive, natriuretic, and diuretic effects).
No products indexed under this heading.

Phenylephrine Hydrochloride (Decreased response to pressor amines). Products include:
- Atrohist Plus Tablets ... 1605

- Cerose DM ... ⊞ 853
- D.A. II Tablets ... 972
- D.A. Chewable Tablets ... 970
- Dura-Vent/DA Tablets ... 972
- Extendryl ... 1003
- 4-Way Fast Acting Nasal Spray (regular & mentholated) ... ⊞ 644
- Hemoroid ... ⊞ 797
- Hycomine Compound Tablets ... 948
- Neo-Synephrine Hydrochloride 1% Carpuject ... 2455
- Neo-Synephrine Hydrochloride 1% Injection ... 2455
- Neo-Synephrine Hydrochloride (Ophthalmic) ... 2456
- Neo-Synephrine ... ⊞ 624
- Novahistine Elixir ... ⊞ 782
- Phenergan VC ... 2886
- Phenergan VC with Codeine ... 2888
- Preparation H ... ⊞ 842
- Tympagesic Ear Drops ... 2476
- Vicks Sinex Nasal Spray and Ultra Fine Mist ... ⊞ 738

Pindolol (Potential for additive or potentiative effects). Products include:
- Visken Tablets ... 2428

Piroxicam (Reduces antihypertensive, natriuretic, and diuretic effects). Products include:
- Feldene Capsules ... 2008

Polythiazide (Potential for precipitous reduction in blood pressure). Products include:
- Minizide Capsules ... 2016

Potassium Acid Phosphate (Potential for significant increase in serum potassium levels). Products include:
- K-Phos Original Formula 'Sodium Free' Tablets ... 633

Potassium Bicarbonate (Potential for significant increase in serum potassium levels). Products include:
- Alka-Seltzer Gold Effervescent Antacid ... ⊞ 611

Potassium Chloride (Potential for significant increase in serum potassium levels). Products include:
- Chlor-3 Condiment ... 1003
- Colyte and Colyte-flavored ... 2540
- GoLYTELY ... 694
- K-Dur Microburst Release System (potassium chloride, USP) E.R. Tablets ... 1364
- K-Lor Powder Packets ... 438
- K-Norm Capsules ... 1615
- K-Tab Filmtab ... 439
- Micro-K ... 2237
- Micro-K LS Packets ... 2238
- NuLYTELY ... 694
- Cherry Flavor NuLYTELY ... 694
- Rum-K Syrup ... 1004
- Slow-K Extended-Release Tablets ... 869

Potassium Citrate (Potential for significant increase in serum potassium levels). Products include:
- Polycitra Syrup ... 574
- Polycitra-K Crystals ... 574
- Polycitra-K Oral Solution ... 575
- Polycitra-LC ... 574
- Urocit-K Tablets ... 1828

Potassium Gluconate (Potential for significant increase in serum potassium levels).
No products indexed under this heading.

Potassium Phosphate, Dibasic (Potential for significant increase in serum potassium levels).
No products indexed under this heading.

Potassium Phosphate, Monobasic (Potential for significant increase in serum potassium levels). Products include:
- K-Phos Neutral Tablets ... 633
- K-Phos Original Formula 'Sodium Free' Tablets ... 633

Prazosin Hydrochloride (Potential for additive or potentiative effects). Products include:
- Minipress Capsules ... 2015

- Minizide Capsules ... 2016

Prednisolone Acetate (Co-administration with thiazides may intensify electrolyte imbalance, particularly hypokalemia). Products include:
- AK-CIDE ... ⊙ 203
- AK-CIDE Ointment ... ⊙ 203
- Blephamide Liquifilm Sterile Ophthalmic Suspension ... 472
- Blephamide Ointment ... ⊙ 234
- Econopred & Econopred Plus Ophthalmic Suspensions ... ⊙ 216
- Poly-Pred Liquifilm ... ⊙ 246
- Pred Forte ... ⊙ 247
- Pred Mild ... ⊙ 250
- Pred-G Liquifilm Sterile Ophthalmic Suspension ... ⊙ 248
- Pred-G S.O.P. Sterile Ophthalmic Ointment ... ⊙ 249

Prednisolone Sodium Phosphate (Co-administration with thiazides may intensify electrolyte imbalance, particularly hypokalemia). Products include:
- AK-PRED ... ⊙ 204
- Hydeltrasol Injection, Sterile ... 1708
- Pediapred Oral Solution ... 1618

Prednisolone Tebutate (Co-administration with thiazides may intensify electrolyte imbalance, particularly hypokalemia). Products include:
- Hydeltra-T.B.A. Sterile Suspension ... 1710

Prednisone (Co-administration with thiazides may intensify electrolyte imbalance, particularly hypokalemia).
No products indexed under this heading.

Probenecid (Dosage adjustment may be necessary since hydrochlorothiazide may have hyperuricemic effect). Products include:
- Benemid Tablets ... 1651
- ColBENEMID Tablets ... 1662

Promethazine Hydrochloride (Effects of preanesthetic agents may be potentiated). Products include:
- Mepergan Injection ... 2859
- Phenergan with Codeine ... 2883
- Phenergan with Dextromethorphan ... 2885
- Phenergan Injection ... 2880
- Phenergan Suppositories ... 2882
- Phenergan Syrup ... 2881
- Phenergan Tablets ... 2882
- Phenergan VC ... 2886
- Phenergan VC with Codeine ... 2888

Propofol (Effects of anesthetic agents may be potentiated). Products include:
- Diprivan Injectable Emulsion ... 2939

Propoxyphene Hydrochloride (Potentiation of orthostatic hypotension). Products include:
- Darvon ... 1475
- Wygesic Tablets ... 2930

Propoxyphene Napsylate (Potentiation of orthostatic hypotension). Products include:
- Darvon-N/Darvocet-N ... 1473

Propranolol Hydrochloride (Potential for additive or potentiative effects). Products include:
- Inderal ... 2834
- Inderal LA Long Acting Capsules ... 2836
- Inderide Tablets ... 2838
- Inderide LA Long Acting Capsules ... 2840

Quinapril Hydrochloride (Potential for additive or potentiative effects). Products include:
- Accupril Tablets ... 1950

Ramipril (Potential for additive or potentiative effects). Products include:
- Altace Capsules ... 1238

Rauwolfia Serpentina (Potential for additive or potentiative effects).
No products indexed under this heading.

Rescinnamine (Potential for additive or potentiative effects).
No products indexed under this heading.

Reserpine (Potential for additive or potentiative effects). Products include:
- Diupres Tablets ... 1691
- Hydropres Tablets ... 1718
- Ser-Ap-Es Tablets ... 867

Rocuronium Bromide (Effects of nondepolarizing muscle relaxants may be potentiated). Products include:
- Zemuron Injection ... 1885

Secobarbital Sodium (Potentiation of orthostatic hypotension). Products include:
- Seconal Sodium Pulvules ... 1529

Selegiline Hydrochloride (Enhanced hypotensive effects; dosage adjustments of one or both agents may be necessary). Products include:
- Eldepryl Capsules ... 2729

Sevoflurane (Effects of anesthetic agents may be potentiated).
No products indexed under this heading.

Sodium Nitroprusside (Potential for additive or potentiative effects).
No products indexed under this heading.

Sotalol Hydrochloride (Potential for additive or potentiative effects). Products include:
- Betapace Tablets ... 637

Spirapril Hydrochloride (Potential for additive or potentiative effects).
No products indexed under this heading.

Spironolactone (Increased risk of hyperkalemia and increased potential for precipitous reduction in blood pressure). Products include:
- Aldactazide Tablets ... 2556
- Aldactone Tablets ... 2558

Sufentanil Citrate (Potentiation of orthostatic hypotension). Products include:
- Sufenta Injection ... 1355

Sulfinpyrazone (Dosage adjustment may be necessary since hydrochlorothiazide may have hyperuricemic effect). Products include:
- Anturane ... 823

Sulindac (Reduces antihypertensive, natriuretic, and diuretic effects). Products include:
- Clinoril Tablets ... 1658

Terazosin Hydrochloride (Potential for additive or potentiative effects). Products include:
- Hytrin Capsules ... 434

Thiamylal Sodium (Potentiation of orthostatic hypotension).
No products indexed under this heading.

Timolol Maleate (Potential for additive or potentiative effects). Products include:
- Blocadren Tablets ... 1654
- Timolide Tablets ... 1791
- Timoptic in Ocudose ... 1796
- Timoptic Sterile Ophthalmic Solution ... 1794
- Timoptic-XE ... 1798

Tolazamide (Thiazide-induced hyperglycemia may require dosage adjustment of antidiabetic drugs).
No products indexed under this heading.

Tolbutamide (Thiazide-induced hyperglycemia may require dosage adjustment of antidiabetic drugs).
No products indexed under this heading.

(⊞ Described in PDR For Nonprescription Drugs)   (⊙ Described in PDR For Ophthalmology)

Tolmetin Sodium (Reduces antihypertensive, natriuretic, and diuretic effects). Products include:

- Tolectin (200, 400 and 600 mg) .. 1591

Torsemide (Potential for precipitous reduction in blood pressure). Products include:

- Demadex Tablets and Injection 691

Tranylcypromine Sulfate (Enhanced hypotensive effects; dosage adjustments of one or both agents may be necessary). Products include:

- Parnate Tablets 2679

Triamcinolone (Co-administration with thiazides may intensify electrolyte imbalance, particularly hypokalemia).

No products indexed under this heading.

Triamcinolone Acetonide (Co-administration with thiazides may intensify electrolyte imbalance, particularly hypokalemia). Products include:

- Azmacort Oral Inhaler 2175
- Nasacort AQ Nasal Spray 2191
- Nasacort Nasal Inhaler 2189

Triamcinolone Diacetate (Co-administration with thiazides may intensify electrolyte imbalance, particularly hypokalemia).

No products indexed under this heading.

Triamcinolone Hexacetonide (Co-administration with thiazides may intensify electrolyte imbalance, particularly hypokalemia).

No products indexed under this heading.

Triamterene (Increased risk of hyperkalemia and increased potential for precipitous reduction in blood pressure). Products include:

- Dyazide Capsules 2653
- Dyrenium Capsules 2655

Trimethaphan Camsylate (Potential for additive or potentiative effects).

No products indexed under this heading.

Tubocurarine Chloride (Effects of tubocurarine may be potentiated).

No products indexed under this heading.

Vecuronium Bromide (Effects of nondepolarizing muscle relaxants may be potentiated). Products include:

- Norcuron for Injection 1875

Verapamil Hydrochloride (Potential for additive or potentiative effects). Products include:

- Calan SR Caplets 2571
- Calan Tablets 2568
- Covera-HS Tablets 2573
- Isoptin Injectable 1391
- Isoptin Oral Tablets 1393
- Isoptin SR Tablets 1395
- Verelan Capsules 1455

Warfarin Sodium (Hydrochlorothiazide may decrease effects of anticoagulant; dosage adjustment may be necessary). Products include:

- Coumadin 941

Food Interactions

Alcohol (Potentation of orthostatic hypotension).

Food, unspecified (Reduces captopril's absorption by about 30% to 40%; should be given one hour before meals).

CAPSAGEL

(Capsaicin) .... ■D 674

None cited in PDR database.

CAPZASIN-P

(Capsaicin) .... ■D 794

None cited in PDR database.

CARAFATE SUSPENSION

(Sucralfate) 1250

May interact with fluoroquinolone antibiotics, quinidine, xanthine bronchodilators, and certain other agents. Compounds in these categories include:

Aluminum Carbonate (Simultaneous administration within one-half hour before or after sucralfate should be avoided; may increase the total body burden of aluminum). Products include:

- Basaljel Capsules 2810
- Basaljel Suspension 2810
- Basaljel Tablets 2810

Aluminum Hydroxide (Simultaneous administration within one-half hour before or after sucralfate should be avoided; may increase the total body burden of aluminum). Products include:

- ALternaGEL Liquid 1358
- Maximum Strength Ascriptin .... ■D 650
- Cama Arthritis Pain Reliever .... ■D 748
- Gaviscon Extra Strength Relief Formula Antacid Tablets .... ■D 778
- Gaviscon Extra Strength Relief Formula Liquid Antacid .... ■D 779
- Gaviscon Liquid Antacid .... ■D 779
- Gelusil Antacid-Anti-gas Liquid .... ■D 819
- Gelusil Antacid-Anti-gas Tablets .... ■D 819
- Maalox Antacid/Anti-Gas Tablets 889
- Maalox Heartburn Relief Suspension .... ■D 658
- Maalox Antacid Liquid 888
- Extra Strength Maalox Antacid/Anti-Gas Liquid and Tablets 888
- Mylanta 1359
- Tempo Soft Antacid .... ■D 799

Aluminum Hydroxide Gel (Simultaneous administration within one-half hour before or after sucralfate should be avoided; may increase the total body burden of aluminum). Products include:

- ALternaGEL Liquid .... ■D 675
- Aludrox Oral Suspension .... ■D 850
- Amphojel Suspension 2802
- Amphojel Suspension without Flavor 2802
- Amphojel Tablets 2802
- Ascriptin .... ■D 650
- Gaviscon Antacid Tablets .... ■D 778
- Gaviscon-2 Antacid Tablets .... ■D 779
- Mylanta Liquid .... ■D 676
- Mylanta Double Strength Liquid .... ■D 676
- Nephrox Suspension .... ■D 671

Aminophylline (Simultaneous administration results in reduced oral absorption of theophylline).

No products indexed under this heading.

Cimetidine (Simultaneous administration results in reduced oral absorption of oral cimetidine; dosing the concomitant medication 2 hours before sucralfate eliminates the interaction). Products include:

- Tagamet HB Tablets .... ■D 786
- Tagamet Tablets 2694

Cimetidine Hydrochloride (Simultaneous administration results in reduced oral absorption of oral cimetidine; dosing the concomitant medication 2 hours before sucralfate eliminates the interaction). Products include:

- Tagamet 2694

Ciprofloxacin (Potential for reduced extent of absorption (bioavailability) with concomitant oral administration; dosing the concomitant medication 2 hours before sucralfate eliminates the interaction). Products include:

- Cipro I.V. 587
- Cipro I.V. Pharmacy Bulk Package .. 590

Ciprofloxacin Hydrochloride (Potential for reduced extent of absorption (bioavailability) with concomitant oral administration; dosing the concomitant medication 2 hours before sucralfate eliminates the interaction). Products include:

- Ciloxan Ophthalmic Solution 468
- Cipro Tablets 584

Digoxin (Simultaneous administration results in reduced oral absorption of oral digoxin; dosing the concomitant medication 2 hours before sucralfate eliminates the interaction). Products include:

- Lanoxicaps 1110
- Lanoxin Elixir Pediatric 1113
- Lanoxin Injection 1116
- Lanoxin Injection Pediatric 1119
- Lanoxin Tablets 1121

Dyphylline (Simultaneous administration results in reduced oral absorption of theophylline). Products include:

- Lufyllin & Lufyllin-400 Tablets 2778
- Lufyllin-GG Elixir & Tablets 2779

Enoxacin (Potential for reduced extent of absorption (bioavailability) with concomitant oral administration; dosing the concomitant medication 2 hours before sucralfate eliminates the interaction). Products include:

- Penetrex Tablets 2196

Ketoconazole (Simultaneous administration results in reduced oral absorption of oral ketoconazole). Products include:

- Nizoral 2% Cream 1344
- Nizoral 2% Shampoo 1344
- Nizoral Tablets 1345

Levothyroxine Sodium (Potential for reduced extent of absorption (bioavailability) with concomitant oral administration). Products include:

- Eltroxin Tablets 2214
- Levothroid Tablets 1015
- Levothyroxine Sodium, USP for Injection 546
- Levoxyl Tablets 918
- Synthroid 1410

Lomefloxacin Hydrochloride (Potential for reduced extent of absorption (bioavailability) with concomitant oral administration; dosing the concomitant medication 2 hours before sucralfate eliminates the interaction). Products include:

- Maxaquin Tablets 2593

Magnesium Hydroxide (Simultaneous administration within one-half hour before or after sucralfate should be avoided; may increase the total body burden of aluminum). Products include:

- Aludrox Oral Suspension .... ■D 850
- Ascriptin .... ■D 650
- Di-Gel Antacid/Anti-Gas .... ■D 762
- Gelusil Antacid-Anti-gas Liquid .... ■D 819
- Gelusil Antacid-Anti-gas Tablets .... ■D 819
- Maalox Antacid/Anti-Gas Tablets 889
- Maalox Antacid Liquid 888
- Extra Strength Maalox Antacid/Anti-Gas Liquid and Tablets 888
- Mylanta Fast-Acting 1359
- Mylanta Gelcaps Antacid .... ■D 678
- Fast-Acting Mylanta Liquid Antacid 1359
- Mylanta Tablets .... ■D 677
- Maximum-Strength Fast-Acting Mylanta Liquid Antacid 1359
- Mylanta Double Strength Tablets .. ■D 677
- Phillips' Milk of Magnesia Liquid .... ■D 627
- Rolaids Antacid Tablets .... ■D 807
- Tempo Soft Antacid .... ■D 799

Magnesium Oxide (Simultaneous administration within one-half hour before or after sucralfate should be avoided; may increase the total body burden of aluminum). Products include:

- Beelith Tablets 632
- Bufferin Analgesic Tablets .... ■D 636
- Arthritis Strength Bufferin Analgesic Caplets .... ■D 637
- Extra Strength Bufferin Analgesic Tablets .... ■D 637
- Caltrate PLUS .... ■D 681
- Cama Arthritis Pain Reliever .... ■D 748
- Mag-Ox 400 666
- Uro-Mag 666

Norfloxacin (Potential for reduced extent of absorption (bioavailability) with concomitant oral administration; dosing the concomitant medication 2 hours before sucralfate eliminates the interaction). Products include:

- Chibroxin Sterile Ophthalmic Solution 1657
- Noroxin Tablets 1758
- Noroxin Tablets 2222

Ofloxacin (Potential for reduced extent of absorption (bioavailability) with concomitant oral administration; dosing the concomitant medication 2 hours before sucralfate eliminates the interaction). Products include:

- Floxin I.V. 1580
- Floxin Tablets (200 mg, 300 mg, 400 mg) 1577
- Ocuflox Ophthalmic Solution 478
- Ocuflox .... ⊙ 242

Phenytoin (Simultaneous administration results in reduced oral absorption of oral phenytoin). Products include:

- Dilantin Infatabs 1967
- Dilantin-125 Suspension 1969

Phenytoin Sodium (Simultaneous administration results in reduced oral absorption of oral phenytoin). Products include:

- Dilantin Kapseals 1965

Quinidine Gluconate (Potential for reduced extent of absorption (bioavailability) with concomitant oral administration). Products include:

- Quinaglute Dura-Tabs Tablets 644

Quinidine Polygalacturonate (Potential for reduced extent of absorption (bioavailability) with concomitant oral administration). Products include:

- Cardioquin Tablets 2146

Quinidine Sulfate (Potential for reduced extent of absorption (bioavailability) with concomitant oral administration). Products include:

- Quinidex Extentabs 2240

Ranitidine Hydrochloride (Simultaneous administration results in reduced oral absorption of oral ranitidine; dosing the concomitant medication 2 hours before sucralfate eliminates the interaction). Products include:

- Zantac 1182
- Zantac Injection 1180
- Zantac Syrup 1182

Tetracycline Hydrochloride (Simultaneous administration results in reduced oral absorption of oral tetracycline). Products include:

- Achromycin V Capsules 1417
- Helidac Therapy 2135

Theophylline (Simultaneous administration results in reduced oral absorption of theophylline). Products include:

- Marax Tablets & DF Syrup 2015
- Quibron 2227

Theophylline Anhydrous (Simultaneous administration results in reduced oral absorption of theophylline). Products include:

- Aerolate 1003
- Primatene Tablets .... ■D 844
- Respbid Tablets 687
- Slo-bid Gyrocaps 2201

IMPORTANT NOTE: Always consult each drug listing in the patient's regimen for possible interactions.

Carafate Suspension — Interactions Index

Theo-24 Extended Release Capsules 2753
Theo-Dur Extended-Release Tablets 1367
Theo-X Extended-Release Tablets .. 793
Uni-Dur Extended-Release Tablets .. 1374
Uniphyl 400 mg and 600 mg Tablets 2157

Theophylline Calcium Salicylate (Simultaneous administration results in reduced oral absorption of theophylline). Products include:
Quadrinal Tablets 1398

Theophylline Sodium Glycinate (Simultaneous administration results in reduced oral absorption of theophylline).
No products indexed under this heading.

Warfarin Sodium (Subtherapeutic prothrombin times with concomitant warfarin and sucralfate have been reported in spontaneous and published reports; clinical studies have demonstrated no changes in the prothrombin time with the addition of sucralfate to chronic warfarin therapy). Products include:
Coumadin 941

CARAFATE TABLETS
(Sucralfate) 1249
May interact with fluoroquinolone antibiotics, xanthine bronchodilators, quinidine, and certain other agents. Compounds in these categories include:

Aluminum Carbonate (Simultaneous administration within one-half hour before or after sucralfate should be avoided; may increase the total body burden of aluminum). Products include:
Basaljel Capsules 2810
Basaljel Suspension 2810
Basaljel Tablets 2810

Aluminum Hydroxide (Simultaneous administration within one-half hour before or after sucralfate should be avoided; may increase the total body burden of aluminum). Products include:
ALternaGEL Liquid 1358
Maximum Strength Ascriptin 650
Cama Arthritis Pain Reliever............ 748
Gaviscon Extra Strength Relief Formula Antacid Tablets............ 778
Gaviscon Extra Strength Relief Formula Liquid Antacid 779
Gaviscon Liquid Antacid 779
Gelusil Antacid-Anti-gas Liquid 819
Gelusil Antacid-Anti-gas Tablets 819
Maalox Antacid/Anti-Gas Tablets 889
Maalox Heartburn Relief Suspension 658
Maalox Antacid Liquid 888
Extra Strength Maalox Antacid/Anti-Gas Liquid and Tablets 888
Mylanta 1359
Tempo Soft Antacid 799

Aluminum Hydroxide Gel (Simultaneous administration within one-half hour before or after sucralfate should be avoided; may increase the total body burden of aluminum). Products include:
ALternaGEL Liquid 675
Aludrox Oral Suspension 850
Amphojel Suspension 2802
Amphojel Suspension without Flavor 2802
Amphojel Tablets 2802
Ascriptin 650
Gaviscon Antacid Tablets............ 778
Gaviscon-2 Antacid Tablets 779
Mylanta Liquid 676
Mylanta Double Strength Liquid ... 676
Nephrox Suspension 671

Aminophylline (Simultaneous administration results in reduced oral absorption of theophylline).
No products indexed under this heading.

Cimetidine (Simultaneous administration results in reduced oral absorption of oral cimetidine; dosing the concomitant medication 2 hours before sucralfate eliminates the interaction). Products include:
Tagamet HB Tablets............ 786
Tagamet Tablets 2694

Cimetidine Hydrochloride (Simultaneous administration results in reduced oral absorption of oral cimetidine; dosing the concomitant medication 2 hours before sucralfate eliminates the interaction). Products include:
Tagamet 2694

Ciprofloxacin (Potential for reduced extent of absorption (bioavailability) with concomitant oral administration; dosing the concomitant medication 2 hours before sucralfate eliminates the interaction). Products include:
Cipro I.V. 587
Cipro I.V. Pharmacy Bulk Package.. 590

Ciprofloxacin Hydrochloride (Potential for reduced extent of absorption (bioavailability) with concomitant oral administration; dosing the concomitant medication 2 hours before sucralfate eliminates the interaction). Products include:
Ciloxan Ophthalmic Solution............ 468
Cipro Tablets 584

Digoxin (Simultaneous administration results in reduced oral absorption of oral digoxin; dosing the concomitant medication 2 hours before sucralfate eliminates the interaction). Products include:
Lanoxicaps 1110
Lanoxin Elixir Pediatric 1113
Lanoxin Injection 1116
Lanoxin Injection Pediatric............ 1119
Lanoxin Tablets 1121

Dyphylline (Simultaneous administration results in reduced oral absorption of theophylline). Products include:
Lufyllin & Lufyllin-400 Tablets 2778
Lufyllin-GG Elixir & Tablets 2779

Enoxacin (Potential for reduced extent of absorption (bioavailability) with concomitant oral administration; dosing the concomitant medication 2 hours before sucralfate eliminates the interaction). Products include:
Penetrex Tablets 2196

Ketoconazole (Simultaneous administration results in reduced oral absorption of oral ketoconazole). Products include:
Nizoral 2% Cream 1344
Nizoral 2% Shampoo............ 1344
Nizoral Tablets 1345

Levothyroxine Sodium (Potential for reduced extent of absorption (bioavailability) with concomitant oral administration). Products include:
Eltroxin Tablets 2214
Levothroid Tablets 1015
Levothyroxine Sodium, USP for Injection 546
Levoxyl Tablets 918
Synthroid 1410

Lomefloxacin Hydrochloride (Potential for reduced extent of absorption (bioavailability) with concomitant oral administration; dosing the concomitant medication 2 hours before sucralfate eliminates the interaction). Products include:
Maxaquin Tablets 2593

Magnesium Hydroxide (Simultaneous administration within one-half hour before or after sucralfate should be avoided; may increase the total body burden of aluminum). Products include:
Aludrox Oral Suspension 850
Ascriptin 650
Di-Gel Antacid/Anti-Gas 762
Gelusil Antacid-Anti-gas Liquid 819
Gelusil Antacid-Anti-gas Tablets 819
Maalox Antacid/Anti-Gas Tablets 889
Maalox Antacid Liquid 888
Extra Strength Maalox Antacid/Anti-Gas Liquid and Tablets 888
Mylanta Fast-Acting 1359
Mylanta Gelcaps Antacid 678
Fast-Acting Mylanta Liquid Antacid 1359
Mylanta Tablets 677
Maximum-Strength Fast-Acting Mylanta Liquid Antacid 1359
Mylanta Double Strength Tablets .. 677
Phillips' Milk of Magnesia Liquid.... 627
Rolaids Antacid Tablets 807
Tempo Soft Antacid 799

Magnesium Oxide (Simultaneous administration within one-half hour before or after sucralfate should be avoided; may increase the total body burden of aluminum). Products include:
Beelith Tablets 632
Bufferin Analgesic Tablets 636
Arthritis Strength Bufferin Analgesic Caplets 637
Extra Strength Bufferin Analgesic Tablets 637
Caltrate PLUS 681
Cama Arthritis Pain Reliever............ 748
Mag-Ox 400 666
Uro-Mag 666

Norfloxacin (Potential for reduced extent of absorption (bioavailability) with concomitant oral administration; dosing the concomitant medication 2 hours before sucralfate eliminates the interaction). Products include:
Chibroxin Sterile Ophthalmic Solution............ 1657
Noroxin Tablets 1758
Noroxin Tablets 2222

Ofloxacin (Potential for reduced extent of absorption (bioavailability) with concomitant oral administration; dosing the concomitant medication 2 hours before sucralfate eliminates the interaction). Products include:
Floxin I.V. 1580
Floxin Tablets (200 mg, 300 mg, 400 mg) 1577
Ocuflox Ophthalmic Solution 478
Ocuflox............ 242

Phenytoin (Simultaneous administration results in reduced oral absorption of oral phenytoin). Products include:
Dilantin Infatabs............ 1967
Dilantin-125 Suspension 1969

Phenytoin Sodium (Simultaneous administration results in reduced oral absorption of oral phenytoin). Products include:
Dilantin Kapseals 1965

Quinidine Gluconate (Potential for reduced extent of absorption (bioavailability) with concomitant oral administration. Products include:
Quinaglute Dura-Tabs Tablets 644

Quinidine Polygalacturonate (Potential for reduced extent of absorption (bioavailability) with concomitant oral administration). Products include:
Cardioquin Tablets 2146

Quinidine Sulfate (Potential for reduced extent of absorption (bioavailability) with concomitant oral administration). Products include:
Quinidex Extentabs 2240

Ranitidine Hydrochloride (Simultaneous administration results in reduced oral absorption of oral ranitidine; dosing the concomitant medication 2 hours before sucralfate eliminates the interaction). Products include:
Zantac 1182
Zantac Injection 1180
Zantac Syrup............ 1182

Tetracycline Hydrochloride (Simultaneous administration results in reduced oral absorption of oral tetracycline). Products include:
Achromycin V Capsules 1417
Helidac Therapy 2135

Theophylline (Simultaneous administration results in reduced oral absorption of theophylline). Products include:
Marax Tablets & DF Syrup............ 2015
Quibron 2227

Theophylline Anhydrous (Simultaneous administration results in reduced oral absorption of theophylline). Products include:
Aerolate 1003
Primatene Tablets 844
Respbid Tablets 687
Slo-bid Gyrocaps 2201
Theo-24 Extended Release Capsules 2753
Theo-Dur Extended-Release Tablets 1367
Theo-X Extended-Release Tablets .. 793
Uni-Dur Extended-Release Tablets .. 1374
Uniphyl 400 mg and 600 mg Tablets 2157

Theophylline Calcium Salicylate (Simultaneous administration results in reduced oral absorption of theophylline). Products include:
Quadrinal Tablets 1398

Theophylline Sodium Glycinate (Simultaneous administration results in reduced oral absorption of theophylline).
No products indexed under this heading.

Warfarin Sodium (Subtherapeutic prothrombin times with concomitant warfarin and sucralfate have been reported in spontaneous and published reports; clinical studies have demonstrated no changes in the prothrombin time with the addition of sucralfate to chronic warfarin therapy). Products include:
Coumadin 941

CARBASTAT INTRAOCULAR SOLUTION
(Carbachol) 260
None cited in PDR database.

CARBOCAINE INJECTION
(Mepivacaine Hydrochloride Injection) 2432
None cited in PDR database.

CARDENE CAPSULES
(Nicardipine Hydrochloride) 2261
May interact with:

Cimetidine (Co-administration increases nicardipine plasma levels). Products include:
Tagamet HB Tablets............ 786
Tagamet Tablets 2694

Cimetidine Hydrochloride (Co-administration increases nicardipine plasma levels). Products include:
Tagamet............ 2694

Cyclosporine (Concomitant administration results in elevated plasma cyclosporine levels). Products include:
Neoral 2405
Sandimmune 2416

(▣ Described in PDR For Nonprescription Drugs)   (⊙ Described in PDR For Ophthalmology)

Fentanyl (Severe hypotension has been reported during fentanyl anesthesia with concomitant use of a beta blocker and a calcium channel blocker). Products include:
Duragesic Transdermal System......... 1336

Fentanyl Citrate (Severe hypotension has been reported during fentanyl anesthesia with concomitant use of a beta blocker and a calcium channel blocker). Products include:
Sublimaze Injection.............................. 463

CARDENE I.V.
(Nicardipine Hydrochloride)................2815
May interact with beta blockers and certain other agents. Compounds in these categories include:

Acebutolol Hydrochloride (In vitro and in some patients a negative inotropic effect has been observed with Cardene I.V., therefore, caution should be exercised when co-administered with beta blocker in patients with CHF or significant left ventricular dysfunction). Products include:
Sectral Capsules 2914

Atenolol (In vitro and in some patients a negative inotropic effect has been observed with Cardene I.V., therefore, caution should be exercised when co-administered with beta blocker in patients with CHF or significant left ventricular dysfunction). Products include:
Tenoretic Tablets 2963
Tenormin Tablets and I.V. Injection 2965

Betaxolol Hydrochloride (In vitro and in some patients a negative inotropic effect has been observed with Cardene I.V., therefore, caution should be exercised when co-administered with beta blocker in patients with CHF or significant left ventricular dysfunction). Products include:
Betoptic Ophthalmic Solution........... 465
Betoptic S Ophthalmic Suspension 467
Kerlone Tablets 2588

Bisoprolol Fumarate (In vitro and in some patients a negative inotropic effect has been observed with Cardene I.V., therefore, caution should be exercised when co-administered with beta blocker in patients with CHF or significant left ventricular dysfunction). Products include:
Zebeta Tablets 1457
Ziac 1459

Carteolol Hydrochloride (In vitro and in some patients a negative inotropic effect has been observed with Cardene I.V., therefore, caution should be exercised when co-administered with beta blocker in patients with CHF or significant left ventricular dysfunction). Products include:
Cartrol Tablets 413
Ocupress Ophthalmic Solution, 1% Sterile.. 297

Cimetidine (Co-administration of cimetidine with Cardene Capsules increases nicardipine plasma concentration). Products include:
Tagamet HB Tablets........................... 786
Tagamet Tablets 2694

Cimetidine Hydrochloride (Co-administration of cimetidine with Cardene Capsules increases nicardipine plasma concentration). Products include:
Tagamet... 2694

Cyclosporine (Co-administration of Cardene Capsules and cyclosporine results in elevated plasma cyclosporine levels). Products include:
Neoral 2405
Sandimmune 2416

Digoxin (No alteration in digoxin plasma levels, however, as a precaution, digoxin levels should be evaluated when concomitant therapy is initiated). Products include:
Lanoxicaps 1110
Lanoxin Elixir Pediatric 1113
Lanoxin Injection 1116
Lanoxin Injection Pediatric................. 1119
Lanoxin Tablets 1121

Esmolol Hydrochloride (In vitro and in some patients a negative inotropic effect has been observed with Cardene I.V., therefore, caution should be exercised when co-administered with beta blocker in patients with CHF or significant left ventricular dysfunction). Products include:
Brevibloc (esmolol HCl) Injection 1860

Fentanyl (Potential for hypotension with fentanyl anesthesia when used with calcium channel blocker and beta blocker; such reaction has not been observed with Cardene I.V. during clinical trials). Products include:
Duragesic Transdermal System......... 1336

Fentanyl Citrate (Potential for hypotension with fentanyl anesthesia when used with calcium channel blocker and beta blocker; such reaction has not been observed with Cardene I.V. during clinical trials). Products include:
Sublimaze Injection............................. 463

Labetalol Hydrochloride (In vitro and in some patients a negative inotropic effect has been observed with Cardene I.V., therefore, caution should be exercised when co-administered with beta blocker in patients with CHF or significant left ventricular dysfunction). Products include:
Normodyne Injection 2519
Normodyne Tablets 2522
Trandate 1158

Levobunolol Hydrochloride (In vitro and in some patients a negative inotropic effect has been observed with Cardene I.V., therefore, caution should be exercised when co-administered with beta blocker in patients with CHF or significant left ventricular dysfunction). Products include:
Betagan 230

Metipranolol Hydrochloride (In vitro and in some patients a negative inotropic effect has been observed with Cardene I.V., therefore, caution should be exercised when co-administered with beta blocker in patients with CHF or significant left ventricular dysfunction). Products include:
OptiPranolol (Metipranolol 0.3%) Sterile Ophthalmic Solution......... 256

Metoprolol Succinate (In vitro and in some patients a negative inotropic effect has been observed with Cardene I.V., therefore, caution should be exercised when co-administered with beta blocker in patients with CHF or significant left ventricular dysfunction). Products include:
Toprol-XL Tablets 560

Metoprolol Tartrate (In vitro and in some patients a negative inotropic effect has been observed with Cardene I.V., therefore, caution should be exercised when co-administered with beta blocker in patients with CHF or significant left ventricular dysfunction). Products include:
Lopressor 848
Lopressor HCT Tablets 850

Nadolol (In vitro and in some patients a negative inotropic effect has been observed with Cardene I.V., therefore, caution should be exercised when co-administered with beta blocker in patients with CHF or significant left ventricular dysfunction).
No products indexed under this heading.

Penbutolol Sulfate (In vitro and in some patients a negative inotropic effect has been observed with Cardene I.V., therefore, caution should be exercised when co-administered with beta blocker in patients with CHF or significant left ventricular dysfunction). Products include:
Levatol Tablets 2547

Pindolol (In vitro and in some patients a negative inotropic effect has been observed with Cardene I.V., therefore, caution should be exercised when co-administered with beta blocker in patients with CHF or significant left ventricular dysfunction). Products include:
Visken Tablets 2428

Propranolol Hydrochloride (In vitro and in some patients a negative inotropic effect has been observed with Cardene I.V., therefore, caution should be exercised when co-administered with beta blocker in patients with CHF or significant left ventricular dysfunction). Products include:
Inderal 2834
Inderal LA Long Acting Capsules 2836
Inderide Tablets 2838
Inderide LA Long Acting Capsules .. 2840

Sotalol Hydrochloride (In vitro and in some patients a negative inotropic effect has been observed with Cardene I.V., therefore, caution should be exercised when co-administered with beta blocker in patients with CHF or significant left ventricular dysfunction). Products include:
Betapace Tablets 637

Timolol Hemihydrate (In vitro and in some patients a negative inotropic effect has been observed with Cardene I.V., therefore, caution should be exercised when co-administered with beta blocker in patients with CHF or significant left ventricular dysfunction). Products include:
Betimol 0.25%, 0.5% 259

Timolol Maleate (In vitro and in some patients a negative inotropic effect has been observed with Cardene I.V., therefore, caution should be exercised when co-administered with beta blocker in patients with CHF or significant left ventricular dysfunction). Products include:
Blocadren Tablets 1654
Timolide Tablets 1791
Timoptic in Ocudose 1796
Timoptic Sterile Ophthalmic Solution.. 1794
Timoptic-XE 1798

CARDENE SR CAPSULES
(Nicardipine Hydrochloride)................2264
May interact with:

Cimetidine (Increases plasma levels). Products include:
Tagamet HB Tablets........................... 786
Tagamet Tablets 2694

Cimetidine Hydrochloride (Increases plasma levels). Products include:
Tagamet... 2694

Cyclosporine (Elevated plasma cyclosporine levels). Products include:
Neoral 2405
Sandimmune 2416

Digoxin (Serum digoxin levels should be evaluated after concomitant therapy with Cardene is initiated because of the potential of increased digoxin serum concentrations). Products include:
Lanoxicaps 1110
Lanoxin Elixir Pediatric 1113
Lanoxin Injection 1116
Lanoxin Injection Pediatric................. 1119
Lanoxin Tablets 1121

Fentanyl (Potential for severe hypotension). Products include:
Duragesic Transdermal System......... 1336

Fentanyl Citrate (Potential for severe hypotension). Products include:
Sublimaze Injection............................. 463

Food Interactions
Diet, high-lipid (Results in lower C_{max} and AUC; higher trough levels).

CARDIOQUIN TABLETS
(Quinidine Polygalacturonate)............2146
May interact with carbonic anhydrase inhibitors, thiazides, anticholinergics, vasodilators, negative inotropic agents, neuromuscular blocking agents, phenothiazines, tricyclic antidepressants, and certain other agents. Compounds in these categories include:

Acebutolol Hydrochloride (Quinidine's negative inotropic actions may be additive to those of other similar drugs). Products include:
Sectral Capsules 2914

Acetazolamide (Reduces renal elimination of quinidine by alkalinizing urine). Products include:
Diamox Sequels (Sustained Release) 318
Diamox Tablets 317

Amiodarone Hydrochloride (Co-administration may increase quinidine levels). Products include:
Cordarone Intravenous 2821
Cordarone Tablets.............................. 2818

Amitriptyline Hydrochloride (Therapeutic serum levels of quinidine inhibit the action of cytochrome P450IID6 and most polycyclic antidepressants are metabolized by this enzyme; caution should be exercised). Products include:
Elavil 2945
Etrafon 2495
Limbitrol 2333
Triavil Tablets 1800

Amoxapine (Therapeutic serum levels of quinidine inhibit the action of cytochrome P450IID6 and most polycyclic antidepressants are metabolized by this enzyme; caution should be exercised). Products include:
Asendin Tablets 1419

Atenolol (Quinidine's negative inotropic actions may be additive to those of other similar drugs). Products include:
Tenoretic Tablets 2963
Tenormin Tablets and I.V. Injection 2965

Atracurium Besylate (Quinidine potentiates the action of neuromuscular blocking agents). Products include:
Tracrium Injection 1155

Atropine Sulfate (Quinidine's anticholinergic actions may be additive to those of other anticholinergic drugs). Products include:
Arco-Lase Plus Tablets 513
Atrohist Plus Tablets 1605
Donnatal 2234
Donnatal Extentabs........................... 2234
Donnatal Tablets 2234

IMPORTANT NOTE: Always consult each drug listing in the patient's regimen for possible interactions.

Lomotil ... 2591
Motofen Tablets ... 789
Urised Tablets ... 2123

Belladonna Alkaloids (Quinidine's anticholinergic actions may be additive to those of other anticholinergic drugs). Products include:

Bellergal-S Tablets ... 2375
Hyland's Bedwetting Tablets ... ▣ 788
Hyland's EnurAid Tablets ... ▣ 789
Hyland's Headache Tablets ... ▣ 790
Hyland's Teething Tablets ... ▣ 790
Similasan Eye Drops #1 ... ▣ 769

Bendroflumethiazide (Reduces renal elimination of quinidine by alkalinizing urine).

No products indexed under this heading.

Benztropine Mesylate (Quinidine's anticholinergic actions may be additive to those of other anticholinergic drugs). Products include:

Cogentin ... 1661

Betaxolol Hydrochloride (Quinidine's negative inotropic actions may be additive to those of other similar drugs). Products include:

Betoptic Ophthalmic Solution ... 465
Betoptic S Ophthalmic Suspension ... 467
Kerlone Tablets ... 2588

Biperiden Hydrochloride (Quinidine's anticholinergic actions may be additive to those of other anticholinergic drugs). Products include:

Akineton ... 1380

Carteolol Hydrochloride (Quinidine's negative inotropic actions may be additive to those of other similar drugs). Products include:

Cartrol Tablets ... 413
Ocupress Ophthalmic Solution, 1% Sterile ... ◉ 297

Chlorothiazide (Reduces renal elimination of quinidine by alkalinizing urine). Products include:

Aldoclor Tablets ... 1638
Diupres Tablets ... 1691
Diuril Oral ... 1694

Chlorothiazide Sodium (Reduces renal elimination of quinidine by alkalinizing urine). Products include:

Diuril Sodium Intravenous ... 1693

Chlorpromazine (Therapeutic serum levels of quinidine inhibit the action of cytochrome P450IID6 and certain unspecified phenothiazines are metabolized by this enzyme; caution should be exercised). Products include:

Thorazine Suppositories ... 2701

Chlorpromazine Hydrochloride (Therapeutic serum levels of quinidine inhibit the action of cytochrome P450IID6 and certain unspecified phenothiazines are metabolized by this enzyme; caution should be exercised). Products include:

Thorazine ... 2701

Cimetidine (Co-administration may increase quinidine levels). Products include:

Tagamet HB Tablets ... ▣ 786
Tagamet Tablets ... 2694

Cimetidine Hydrochloride (Co-administration may increase quinidine levels). Products include:

Tagamet ... 2694

Cisatracurium Besylate (Quinidine potentiates the action of neuromuscular blocking agents). Products include:

Nimbex Injection ... 1131

Clidinium Bromide (Quinidine's anticholinergic actions may be additive to those of other anticholinergic drugs). Products include:

Librax Capsules ... 2330

Clomipramine Hydrochloride (Therapeutic serum levels of quinidine inhibit the action of cytochrome P450IID6 and most polycyclic antidepressants are metabolized by this enzyme; caution should be exercised). Products include:

Anafranil Capsules ... 819

Desipramine Hydrochloride (Therapeutic serum levels of quinidine inhibit the action of cytochrome P450IID6 and most polycyclic antidepressants are metabolized by this enzyme; caution should be exercised). Products include:

Norpramin Tablets ... 1273

Diazoxide (Quinidine's vasodilating actions may be additive to those of other vasodilators). Products include:

Hyperstat I.V. Injection ... 2504
Proglycem ... 575

Dichlorphenamide (Reduces renal elimination of quinidine by alkalinizing urine). Products include:

Daranide Tablets ... 1676

Dicyclomine Hydrochloride (Quinidine's anticholinergic actions may be additive to those of other anticholinergic drugs). Products include:

Bentyl ... 1246

Digitoxin (Increased serum digitoxin levels). Products include:

Crystodigin Tablets ... 1472

Digoxin (Quinidine slows the elimination of digoxin and simultaneously reduces digoxin's apparent volume distribution, thereby increasing serum digoxin levels as much as twofold). Products include:

Lanoxicaps ... 1110
Lanoxin Elixir Pediatric ... 1113
Lanoxin Injection ... 1116
Lanoxin Injection Pediatric ... 1119
Lanoxin Tablets ... 1121

Dorzolamide Hydrochloride (Reduces renal elimination of quinidine by alkalinizing urine). Products include:

Trusopt Sterile Ophthalmic Solution ... 1803

Doxacurium Chloride (Quinidine potentiates the action of neuromuscular blocking agents). Products include:

Nuromax Injection ... 1136

Doxepin Hydrochloride (Therapeutic serum levels of quinidine inhibit the action of cytochrome P450IID6 and most polycyclic antidepressants are metabolized by this enzyme; caution should be exercised). Products include:

Adapin Capsules ... 1542
Sinequan ... 2028
Zonalon Cream ... 1042

Epoprostenol Sodium (Quinidine's vasodilating actions may be additive to those of other vasodilators). Products include:

Flolan for Injection ... 1085

Esmolol Hydrochloride (Quinidine's negative inotropic actions may be additive to those of other similar drugs). Products include:

Brevibloc (esmolol HCl) Injection ... 1860

Felodipine (Potential for variable slowing of the metabolism of felodipine). Products include:

Plendil Extended-Release Tablets ... 514

Fluphenazine Decanoate (Therapeutic serum levels of quinidine inhibit the action of cytochrome P450IID6 and certain unspecified phenothiazines are metabolized by this enzyme; caution should be exercised). Products include:

Prolixin Decanoate ... 510

Fluphenazine Enanthate (Therapeutic serum levels of quinidine inhibit the action of cytochrome P450IID6 and certain unspecified phenothiazines are metabolized by this enzyme; caution should be exercised). Products include:

Prolixin Enanthate ... 510

Fluphenazine Hydrochloride (Therapeutic serum levels of quinidine inhibit the action of cytochrome P450IID6 and certain unspecified phenothiazines are metabolized by this enzyme; caution should be exercised). Products include:

Prolixin ... 510

Glycopyrrolate (Quinidine's anticholinergic actions may be additive to those of other anticholinergic drugs). Products include:

Robinul Forte Tablets ... 2247
Robinul Injectable ... 2247
Robinul Tablets ... 2247

Haloperidol (Co-administration increases serum levels of haloperidol). Products include:

Haldol Injection, Tablets and Concentrate ... 1585

Haloperidol Decanoate (Co-administration increases serum levels of haloperidol). Products include:

Haldol Decanoate ... 1587

Hydralazine Hydrochloride (Quinidine's vasodilating actions may be additive to those of other vasodilators). Products include:

Apresazide Capsules ... 824
Apresoline Hydrochloride Tablets ... 826
Hydralazine Hydrochloride Injection USP ... 2712
Ser-Ap-Es Tablets ... 867

Hydrochlorothiazide (Reduces renal elimination of quinidine by alkalinizing urine). Products include:

Aldactazide Tablets ... 2556
Aldoril Tablets ... 1644
Apresazide Capsules ... 824
Capozide Tablets ... 744
Dyazide Capsules ... 2653
Esidrix Tablets ... 839
Esimil Tablets ... 840
HydroDIURIL Tablets ... 1716
Hydropres Tablets ... 1718
Hyzaar Tablets ... 1720
Inderide Tablets ... 2838
Inderide LA Long Acting Capsules ... 2840
Lopressor HCT Tablets ... 850
Lotensin HCT Tablets ... 855
Moduretic Tablets ... 1748
Oretic Tablets ... 450
Prinzide Tablets ... 1780
Ser-Ap-Es Tablets ... 867
Timolide Tablets ... 1791
Vaseretic Tablets ... 1810
Zestoretic Tablets ... 2968
Ziac ... 1459

Hydroflumethiazide (Reduces renal elimination of quinidine by alkalinizing urine). Products include:

Diucardin Tablets ... 2824

Hyoscyamine (Quinidine's anticholinergic actions may be additive to those of other anticholinergic drugs). Products include:

Cystospaz Tablets ... 2123
Urised Tablets ... 2123

Hyoscyamine Sulfate (Quinidine's anticholinergic actions may be additive to those of other anticholinergic drugs). Products include:

Arco-Lase Plus Tablets ... 513
Atrohist Plus Tablets ... 1605
Cystospaz-M Capsules ... 2123
Donnatal ... 2234
Donnatal Extentabs ... 2234
Donnatal Tablets ... 2234
Kutrase Capsules ... 2546
Levsin/Levsinex/Levbid ... 2549

Imipramine Hydrochloride (Therapeutic serum levels of quinidine inhibit the action of cytochrome P450IID6 and most polycyclic antidepressants are metabolized by this enzyme; caution should be exercised). Products include:

Tofranil Ampuls ... 873
Tofranil Tablets ... 875

Imipramine Pamoate (Therapeutic serum levels of quinidine inhibit the action of cytochrome P450IID6 and most polycyclic antidepressants are metabolized by this enzyme; caution should be exercised). Products include:

Tofranil-PM Capsules ... 876

Ipratropium Bromide (Quinidine's anticholinergic actions may be additive to those of other anticholinergic drugs). Products include:

Atrovent Inhalation Aerosol ... 674
Atrovent Inhalation Solution ... 675
Atrovent Nasal Spray 0.03% ... 676
Atrovent Nasal Spray 0.06% ... 678

Ketoconazole (Co-administration may increase quinidine levels through competition for the P450IIIA4 metabolic pathway). Products include:

Nizoral 2% Cream ... 1344
Nizoral 2% Shampoo ... 1344
Nizoral Tablets ... 1345

Labetalol Hydrochloride (Quinidine's negative inotropic actions may be additive to those of other similar drugs). Products include:

Normodyne Injection ... 2519
Normodyne Tablets ... 2522
Trandate ... 1158

Maprotiline Hydrochloride (Therapeutic serum levels of quinidine inhibit the action of cytochrome P450IID6 and most polycyclic antidepressants are metabolized by this enzyme; caution should be exercised). Products include:

Ludiomil Tablets ... 861

Mepenzolate Bromide (Quinidine's anticholinergic actions may be additive to those of other anticholinergic drugs).

No products indexed under this heading.

Mesoridazine Besylate (Therapeutic serum levels of quinidine inhibit the action of cytochrome P450IID6 and certain unspecified phenothiazines are metabolized by this enzyme; caution should be exercised). Products include:

Serentil ... 689

Methazolamide (Reduces renal elimination of quinidine by alkalinizing urine). Products include:

GlaucTabs ... ◉ 209
Neptazane Tablets ... ◉ 320

Methotrimeprazine (Therapeutic serum levels of quinidine inhibit the action of cytochrome P450IID6 and certain unspecified phenothiazines are metabolized by this enzyme; caution should be exercised). Products include:

Levoprome ... 1321

Methyclothiazide (Reduces renal elimination of quinidine by alkalinizing urine). Products include:

Enduron Tablets ... 424

Metocurine Iodide (Quinidine potentiates the action of neuromuscular blocking agents). Products include:

Metubine Iodide Vials ... 932

(▣ Described in PDR For Nonprescription Drugs) (◉ Described in PDR For Ophthalmology)

Metoprolol Tartrate (Quinidine's negative inotropic actions may be additive to those of other similar drugs). Products include:
Lopressor ... 848
Lopressor HCT Tablets ... 850

Mexiletine Hydrochloride (Therapeutic serum levels of quinidine inhibit the action of cytochrome P450IID6 and mexiletine is metabolized by this enzyme; caution should be exercised). Products include:
Mexitil Capsules ... 684

Minoxidil (Quinidine's vasodilating actions may be additive to those of other vasodilators).
No products indexed under this heading.

Mivacurium Chloride (Quinidine potentiates the action of neuromuscular blocking agents). Products include:
Mivacron ... 1125

Nadolol (Quinidine's negative inotropic actions may be additive to those of other similar drugs).
No products indexed under this heading.

Nicardipine Hydrochloride (Potential for variable slowing of the metabolism of nicardipine). Products include:
Cardene Capsules ... 2261
Cardene I.V. ... 2815
Cardene SR Capsules ... 2264

Nifedipine (Very rarely, co-administration may decrease quinidine levels; variable slowing of the metabolism of nifedipine). Products include:
Adalat Capsules (10 mg and 20 mg) ... 580
Adalat CC ... 582
Procardia Capsules ... 2024
Procardia XL Extended Release Tablets ... 2026

Nimodipine (Potential for variable slowing of the metabolism of nimodipine). Products include:
Nimotop Capsules ... 603

Nortriptyline Hydrochloride (Therapeutic serum levels of quinidine inhibit the action of cytochrome P450IID6 and most polycyclic antidepressants are metabolized by this enzyme; caution should be exercised). Products include:
Pamelor ... 2409

Oxybutynin Chloride (Quinidine's anticholinergic actions may be additive to those of other anticholinergic drugs). Products include:
Ditropan ... 1267

Pancuronium Bromide (Quinidine potentiates the action of neuromuscular blocking agents).
No products indexed under this heading.

Penbutolol Sulfate (Quinidine's negative inotropic actions may be additive to those of other similar drugs). Products include:
Levatol Tablets ... 2547

Perphenazine (Therapeutic serum levels of quinidine inhibit the action of cytochrome P450IID6 and certain unspecified phenothiazines are metabolized by this enzyme; caution should be exercised). Products include:
Etrafon ... 2495
Triavil Tablets ... 1800
Trilafon ... 2532

Phenobarbital (Hepatic elimination of quinidine is accelerated by co-administration with phenobarbital). Products include:
Arco-Lase Plus Tablets ... 513
Bellergal-S Tablets ... 2375
Donnatal ... 2234
Donnatal Extentabs ... 2234
Donnatal Tablets ... 2234
Phenobarbital Elixir and Tablets ... 1523
Quadrinal Tablets ... 1398

Phenytoin (Hepatic elimination of quinidine is accelerated by co-administration with phenytoin). Products include:
Dilantin Infatabs ... 1967
Dilantin-125 Suspension ... 1969

Phenytoin Sodium (Hepatic elimination of quinidine is accelerated by co-administration with phenytoin). Products include:
Dilantin Kapseals ... 1965

Pindolol (Quinidine's negative inotropic actions may be additive to those of other similar drugs). Products include:
Visken Tablets ... 2428

Polythiazide (Reduces renal elimination of quinidine by alkalinizing urine). Products include:
Minizide Capsules ... 2016

Procainamide Hydrochloride (Increased serum levels of procainamide through competition for pathways of renal clearance). Products include:
Procanbid Extended-Release Tablets ... 1983

Prochlorperazine (Therapeutic serum levels of quinidine inhibit the action of cytochrome P450IID6 and certain unspecified phenothiazines are metabolized by this enzyme; caution should be exercised). Products include:
Compazine ... 2644

Procyclidine Hydrochloride (Quinidine's anticholinergic actions may be additive to those of other anticholinergic drugs). Products include:
Kemadrin Tablets ... 1105

Promethazine Hydrochloride (Therapeutic serum levels of quinidine inhibit the action of cytochrome P450IID6 and certain unspecified phenothiazines are metabolized by this enzyme; caution should be exercised). Products include:
Mepergan Injection ... 2859
Phenergan with Codeine ... 2883
Phenergan with Dextromethorphan 2885
Phenergan Injection ... 2880
Phenergan Suppositories ... 2882
Phenergan Syrup ... 2881
Phenergan Tablets ... 2882
Phenergan VC ... 2886
Phenergan VC with Codeine ... 2888

Propantheline Bromide (Quinidine's anticholinergic actions may be additive to those of other anticholinergic drugs). Products include:
Pro-Banthine Tablets ... 2226

Propranolol Hydrochloride (Co-administration in some patients may increase the peak serum levels, decrease the volume of distribution, and decrease the total quinidine clearance; quinidine's negative inotropic actions may be additive to those of other similar drugs). Products include:
Inderal ... 2834
Inderal LA Long Acting Capsules ... 2836
Inderide Tablets ... 2838
Inderide LA Long Acting Capsules .. 2840

Protriptyline Hydrochloride (Therapeutic serum levels of quinidine inhibit the action of cytochrome P450IID6 and most polycyclic antidepressants are metabolized by this enzyme; caution should be exercised). Products include:
Vivactil Tablets ... 1820

Rifampin (Hepatic elimination of quinidine is accelerated by co-administration with rifampin). Products include:
Rifadin ... 1276
Rifamate Capsules ... 1278
Rifater ... 1280
Rimactane Capsules ... 865

Rocuronium Bromide (Quinidine potentiates the action of neuromuscular blocking agents). Products include:
Zemuron Injection ... 1885

Scopolamine (Quinidine's anticholinergic actions may be additive to those of other anticholinergic drugs). Products include:
Transderm Scōp Transdermal Therapeutic System ... 890

Scopolamine Hydrobromide (Quinidine's anticholinergic actions may be additive to those of other anticholinergic drugs). Products include:
Atrohist Plus Tablets ... 1605
Donnatal ... 2234
Donnatal Extentabs ... 2234
Donnatal Tablets ... 2234

Sodium Bicarbonate (Reduces renal elimination of quinidine by alkalinizing urine). Products include:
Alka-Seltzer Cherry Effervescent Antacid and Pain Reliever ... 609
Alka-Seltzer Extra Strength Effervescent Antacid and Pain Reliever ... 609
Alka-Seltzer Gold Effervescent Antacid ... 611
Alka-Seltzer Lemon Lime Effervescent Antacid and Pain Reliever ... 609
Alka-Seltzer Original Effervescent Antacid and Pain Reliever ... 609
Arm & Hammer Pure Baking Soda ... 648
Colyte and Colyte-flavored ... 2540
GoLYTELY ... 694
Massengill Disposable Douches ... 780
Massengill Liquid Concentrate ... 780
NuLYTELY ... 694
Cherry Flavor NuLYTELY ... 694

Succinylcholine Chloride (Quinidine potentiates the action of neuromuscular blocking agents). Products include:
Anectine ... 1062

Thioridazine Hydrochloride (Therapeutic serum levels of quinidine inhibit the action of cytochrome P450IID6 and certain unspecified phenothiazines are metabolized by this enzyme; caution should be exercised). Products include:
Mellaril ... 2398

Timolol Maleate (Quinidine's negative inotropic actions may be additive to those of other similar drugs). Products include:
Blocadren Tablets ... 1654
Timolide Tablets ... 1791
Timoptic in Ocudose ... 1796
Timoptic Sterile Ophthalmic Solution ... 1794
Timoptic-XE ... 1798

Tridihexethyl Chloride (Quinidine's anticholinergic actions may be additive to those of other anticholinergic drugs).
No products indexed under this heading.

Trifluoperazine Hydrochloride (Therapeutic serum levels of quinidine inhibit the action of cytochrome P450IID6 and certain unspecified phenothiazines are metabolized by this enzyme; caution should be exercised). Products include:
Stelazine ... 2692

Trihexyphenidyl Hydrochloride (Quinidine's anticholinergic actions may be additive to those of other anticholinergic drugs). Products include:
Artane ... 1418

Trimipramine Maleate (Therapeutic serum levels of quinidine inhibit the action of cytochrome P450IID6 and most polycyclic antidepressants are metabolized by this enzyme; caution should be exercised). Products include:
Surmontil Capsules ... 2917

Tubocurarine Chloride (Quinidine potentiates the action of neuromuscular blocking agents).
No products indexed under this heading.

Vecuronium Bromide (Quinidine potentiates the action of neuromuscular blocking agents). Products include:
Norcuron for Injection ... 1875

Verapamil Hydrochloride (Significantly reduces hepatic clearance with corresponding increases in serum levels and half-life; additive peripheral alpha- blockade may produce hypotension). Products include:
Calan SR Caplets ... 2571
Calan Tablets ... 2568
Covera-HS Tablets ... 2573
Isoptin Injectable ... 1391
Isoptin Oral Tablets ... 1393
Isoptin SR Tablets ... 1395
Verelan Capsules ... 1455

Warfarin Sodium (Quinidine potentiates the anticoagulatory action of warfarin). Products include:
Coumadin ... 941

Food Interactions

Food, unspecified (Food delays absorption, but not the extent).

CARDIZEM CD CAPSULES

(Diltiazem Hydrochloride) ... 1251
May interact with cardiac glycosides, anesthetics, beta blockers, and certain other agents. Compounds in these categories include:

Acebutolol Hydrochloride (Possible additive effects on cardiac conduction (prolonged AV conduction)). Products include:
Sectral Capsules ... 2914

Alfentanil Hydrochloride (Depression of cardiac contractility, conductivity, automaticity, and vasodilation associated with anesthetic may be potentiated). Products include:
Alfenta Injection ... 1334

Atenolol (Possible additive effects on cardiac conduction (prolonged AV conduction)). Products include:
Tenoretic Tablets ... 2963
Tenormin Tablets and I.V. Injection 2965

Betaxolol Hydrochloride (Possible additive effects on cardiac conduction (prolonged AV conduction)). Products include:
Betoptic Ophthalmic Solution ... 465
Betoptic S Ophthalmic Suspension 467
Kerlone Tablets ... 2588

Bisoprolol Fumarate (Possible additive effects on cardiac conduction (prolonged AV conduction)). Products include:
Zebeta Tablets ... 1457
Ziac ... 1459

Carbamazepine (Potential for elevated serum levels of carbamazepine (40% to 72% increase), resulting in toxicity in some cases). Products include:
Atretol Tablets ... 569
Tegretol/Tegretol-XR ... 870

IMPORTANT NOTE: Always consult each drug listing in the patient's regimen for possible interactions.

Cardizem CD

Carteolol Hydrochloride (Possible additive effects on cardiac conduction (prolonged AV conduction)). Products include:
- Cartrol Tablets 413
- Ocupress Ophthalmic Solution, 1% Sterile .... ⓞ 297

Cimetidine (Potential for significant increase in peak plasma levels (58%) and AUC (53%); an adjustment in diltiazem dosage may be warranted). Products include:
- Tagamet HB Tablets .... 🅱 786
- Tagamet Tablets 2694

Cimetidine Hydrochloride (Potential for significant increase in peak plasma levels (58%) and AUC (53%); an adjustment in diltiazem dosage may be warranted). Products include:
- Tagamet 2694

Cyclosporine (A pharmacokinetic interaction between diltiazem and cyclosporine has been observed in renal and cardiac transplant patients requiring a reduction of cyclosporine dose). Products include:
- Neoral 2405
- Sandimmune 2416

Deslanoside (Possible additive effects on cardiac conduction).
No products indexed under this heading.

Digitoxin (Possible additive effects on cardiac conduction). Products include:
- Crystodigin Tablets 1472

Digoxin (Possible increase in digoxin levels; possible additive effects on cardiac conduction). Products include:
- Lanoxicaps 1110
- Lanoxin Elixir Pediatric 1113
- Lanoxin Injection 1116
- Lanoxin Injection Pediatric 1119
- Lanoxin Tablets 1121

Drugs which undergo biotransformation by cytochrome P-450 mixed function oxidase (May result in competitive inhibition of metabolism).

Enflurane (Depression of cardiac contractility, conductivity, automaticity, and vasodilation may be potentiated with anesthetic may be potentiated).
No products indexed under this heading.

Esmolol Hydrochloride (Possible additive effects on cardiac conduction (prolonged AV conduction)). Products include:
- Brevibloc (esmolol HCl) Injection ... 1860

Fentanyl Citrate (Depression of cardiac contractility, conductivity, automaticity, and vasodilation associated with anesthetic may be potentiated). Products include:
- Sublimaze Injection 463

Halothane (Depression of cardiac contractility, conductivity, automaticity, and vasodilation associated with anesthetic may be potentiated). Products include:
- Fluothane 2830

Isoflurane (Depression of cardiac contractility, conductivity, automaticity, and vasodilation associated with anesthetic may be potentiated).
No products indexed under this heading.

Ketamine Hydrochloride (Depression of cardiac contractility, conductivity, automaticity, and vasodilation associated with anesthetic may be potentiated).
No products indexed under this heading.

Labetalol Hydrochloride (Possible additive effects on cardiac conduction (prolonged AV conduction)). Products include:
- Normodyne Injection 2519
- Normodyne Tablets 2522
- Trandate 1158

Levobunolol Hydrochloride (Possible additive effects on cardiac conduction (prolonged AV conduction)). Products include:
- Betagan .... ⓞ 230

Methohexital Sodium (Depression of cardiac contractility, conductivity, automaticity, and vasodilation associated with anesthetic may be potentiated).
No products indexed under this heading.

Metipranolol Hydrochloride (Possible additive effects on cardiac conduction (prolonged AV conduction)). Products include:
- OptiPranolol (Metipranolol 0.3%) Sterile Ophthalmic Solution ... ⓞ 256

Metoprolol Succinate (Possible additive effects on cardiac conduction (prolonged AV conduction)). Products include:
- Toprol-XL Tablets 560

Metoprolol Tartrate (Possible additive effects on cardiac conduction (prolonged AV conduction)). Products include:
- Lopressor 848
- Lopressor HCT Tablets 850

Midazolam Hydrochloride (Depression of cardiac contractility, conductivity, automaticity, and vasodilation associated with anesthetic may be potentiated). Products include:
- Versed Injection 2324

Nadolol (Possible additive effects on cardiac conduction (prolonged AV conduction)).
No products indexed under this heading.

Penbutolol Sulfate (Possible additive effects on cardiac conduction (prolonged AV conduction)). Products include:
- Levatol Tablets 2547

Pindolol (Possible additive effects on cardiac conduction (prolonged AV conduction)). Products include:
- Visken Tablets 2428

Propofol (Depression of cardiac contractility, conductivity, automaticity, and vasodilation associated with anesthetic may be potentiated). Products include:
- Diprivan Injectable Emulsion 2939

Propranolol Hydrochloride (Increased levels and bioavailability of propranolol; dosage of propranolol may need to be adjusted; possible additive effects on cardiac conduction (prolonged AV conduction)). Products include:
- Inderal 2834
- Inderal LA Long Acting Capsules . 2836
- Inderide Tablets 2838
- Inderide LA Long Acting Capsules .. 2840

Ranitidine Hydrochloride (Produces smaller, nonsignificant increase in diltiazem plasma levels). Products include:
- Zantac 1182
- Zantac Injection 1180
- Zantac Syrup 1182

Sotalol Hydrochloride (Possible additive effects on cardiac conduction (prolonged AV conduction)). Products include:
- Betapace Tablets 637

Interactions Index

Sufentanil Citrate (Depression of cardiac contractility, conductivity, automaticity, and vasodilation associated with anesthetic may be potentiated). Products include:
- Sufenta Injection 1355

Thiamylal Sodium (Depression of cardiac contractility, conductivity, automaticity, and vasodilation associated with anesthetic may be potentiated).
No products indexed under this heading.

Timolol Hemihydrate (Possible additive effects on cardiac conduction (prolonged AV conduction)). Products include:
- Betimol 0.25%, 0.5% .... ⓞ 259

Timolol Maleate (Possible additive effects on cardiac conduction (prolonged AV conduction)). Products include:
- Blocadren Tablets 1654
- Timolide Tablets 1791
- Timoptic in Ocudose 1796
- Timoptic Sterile Ophthalmic Solution 1794
- Timoptic-XE 1798

CARDIZEM SR CAPSULES
(Diltiazem Hydrochloride) 1255
May interact with beta blockers, cardiac glycosides, general anesthetics, drugs which undergo biotransformation by cytochrome p-450 mixed function oxidase, and certain other agents. Compounds in these categories include:

Acebutolol Hydrochloride (Concomitant administration may result in additive effects in prolonging AV conduction). Products include:
- Sectral Capsules 2914

Atenolol (Concomitant administration may result in additive effects in prolonging AV conduction). Products include:
- Tenoretic Tablets 2963
- Tenormin Tablets and I.V. Injection 2965

Betaxolol Hydrochloride (Concomitant administration may result in additive effects in prolonging AV conduction). Products include:
- Betoptic Ophthalmic Solution 465
- Betoptic S Ophthalmic Suspension . 467
- Kerlone Tablets 2588

Bisoprolol Fumarate (Concomitant administration may result in additive effects in prolonging AV conduction). Products include:
- Zebeta Tablets 1457
- Ziac 1459

Carbamazepine (Potential for elevated serum levels of carbamazepine (40% to 72% increase), resulting in toxicity in some cases). Products include:
- Atretol Tablets 569
- Tegretol/Tegretol-XR 870

Carteolol Hydrochloride (Concomitant administration may result in additive effects in prolonging AV conduction). Products include:
- Cartrol Tablets 413
- Ocupress Ophthalmic Solution, 1% Sterile .... ⓞ 297

Cimetidine (Increases peak diltiazem plasma levels (58%) and AUC (53%)). Products include:
- Tagamet HB Tablets .... 🅱 786
- Tagamet Tablets 2694

Cimetidine Hydrochloride (Increases peak diltiazem plasma levels (58%) and AUC (53%)). Products include:
- Tagamet 2694

Cyclosporine (A pharmacokinetic interaction between diltiazem and cyclosporine has been observed in renal and cardiac transplant patients requiring a reduction of cyclosporine dose). Products include:
- Neoral 2405
- Sandimmune 2416

Deslanoside (Additive effects on cardiac conduction; variable effect on plasma digoxin).
No products indexed under this heading.

Digitoxin (Additive effects on cardiac conduction; variable effect on plasma digoxin). Products include:
- Crystodigin Tablets 1472

Digoxin (Additive effects on cardiac conduction; variable effect on plasma digoxin). Products include:
- Lanoxicaps 1110
- Lanoxin Elixir Pediatric 1113
- Lanoxin Injection 1116
- Lanoxin Injection Pediatric 1119
- Lanoxin Tablets 1121

Drugs which undergo biotransformation by cytochrome P-450 mixed function oxidase (Coadministration may result in the competitive inhibition of metabolism).

Enflurane (Depression of cardiac contractility, conductivity, automaticity, and vasodilation may be potentiated).
No products indexed under this heading.

Esmolol Hydrochloride (Concomitant administration may result in additive effects in prolonging AV conduction). Products include:
- Brevibloc (esmolol HCl) Injection . 1860

Isoflurane (Depression of cardiac contractility, conductivity, automaticity, and vasodilation may be potentiated).
No products indexed under this heading.

Ketamine Hydrochloride (Depression of cardiac contractility, conductivity, automaticity, and vasodilation may be potentiated).
No products indexed under this heading.

Labetalol Hydrochloride (Concomitant administration may result in additive effects in prolonging AV conduction). Products include:
- Normodyne Injection 2519
- Normodyne Tablets 2522
- Trandate 1158

Levobunolol Hydrochloride (Concomitant administration may result in additive effects in prolonging AV conduction). Products include:
- Betagan .... ⓞ 230

Methohexital Sodium (Depression of cardiac contractility, conductivity, automaticity, and vasodilation may be potentiated).
No products indexed under this heading.

Methoxyflurane (Depression of cardiac contractility, conductivity, automaticity, and vasodilation may be potentiated).
No products indexed under this heading.

Metipranolol Hydrochloride (Concomitant administration may result in additive effects in prolonging AV conduction). Products include:
- OptiPranolol (Metipranolol 0.3%) Sterile Ophthalmic Solution ... ⓞ 256

(🅱 Described in PDR For Nonprescription Drugs)   (ⓞ Described in PDR For Ophthalmology)

Metoprolol Succinate (Concomitant administration may result in additive effects in prolonging AV conduction). Products include:
Toprol-XL Tablets 560

Metoprolol Tartrate (Concomitant administration may result in additive effects in prolonging AV conduction). Products include:
Lopressor 848
Lopressor HCT Tablets 850

Nadolol (Concomitant administration may result in additive effects in prolonging AV conduction).
No products indexed under this heading.

Penbutolol Sulfate (Concomitant administration may result in additive effects in prolonging AV conduction). Products include:
Levatol Tablets 2547

Pindolol (Concomitant administration may result in additive effects in prolonging AV conduction). Products include:
Visken Tablets 2428

Propofol (Depression of cardiac contractility, conductivity, automaticity, and vasodilation may be potentiated). Products include:
Diprivan Injectable Emulsion 2939

Propranolol Hydrochloride (Concomitant administration may result in additive effects in prolonging AV conduction; increased bioavailability of propranolol by 50%). Products include:
Inderal 2834
Inderal LA Long Acting Capsules 2836
Inderide Tablets 2838
Inderide LA Long Acting Capsules .. 2840

Ranitidine Hydrochloride (Produces smaller, nonsignificant increase in plasma levels). Products include:
Zantac 1182
Zantac Injection 1180
Zantac Syrup 1182

Sevoflurane (Depression of cardiac contractility, conductivity, automaticity, and vasodilation may be potentiated).
No products indexed under this heading.

Sotalol Hydrochloride (Concomitant administration may result in additive effects in prolonging AV conduction). Products include:
Betapace Tablets 637

Timolol Hemihydrate (Concomitant administration may result in additive effects in prolonging AV conduction). Products include:
Betimol 0.25%, 0.5% .... ⊚ 259

Timolol Maleate (Concomitant administration may result in additive effects in prolonging AV conduction). Products include:
Blocadren Tablets 1654
Timolide Tablets 1791
Timoptic in Ocudose 1796
Timoptic Sterile Ophthalmic Solution 1794
Timoptic-XE 1798

CARDIZEM INJECTABLE
(Diltiazem Hydrochloride)....................1253
May interact with beta blockers, intravenous beta-blockers, cardiac glycosides, anesthetics, agents known affect cardiac contractility and/or sa or av node conduction (selected), and certain other agents.

Compounds in these categories include:

Acebutolol Hydrochloride (Potential for bradycardia, AV block, and/or depression of contractility in patients receiving chronic oral beta-blockers). Products include:
Sectral Capsules 2914

Alfentanil Hydrochloride (Potential for additive effects; potential for the increased depression of cardiac contractility, conductivity and automaticity). Products include:
Alfenta Injection 1334

Atenolol (Concurrent intravenous administration should not be undertaken together or in close proximity; potential for bradycardia, AV block, and/or depression of contractility in patients receiving chronic oral beta-blockers). Products include:
Tenoretic Tablets 2963
Tenormin Tablets and I.V. Injection 2965

Betaxolol Hydrochloride (Potential for bradycardia, AV block, and/or depression of contractility in patients receiving chronic oral beta-blockers). Products include:
Betoptic Ophthalmic Solution........... 465
Betoptic S Ophthalmic Suspension 467
Kerlone Tablets 2588

Bisoprolol Fumarate (Potential for bradycardia, AV block, and/or depression of contractility in patients receiving chronic oral beta-blockers). Products include:
Zebeta Tablets 1457
Ziac 1459

Carbamazepine (Potential for elevated serum levels of carbamazepine (40% to 72% increase), resulting in toxicity in some cases). Products include:
Atretol Tablets 569
Tegretol/Tegretol-XR 870

Carteolol Hydrochloride (Potential for bradycardia, AV block, and/or depression of contractility in patients receiving chronic oral beta-blockers). Products include:
Cartrol Tablets 413
Ocupress Ophthalmic Solution, 1% Sterile... ⊚ 297

Cyclosporine (A pharmacokinetic interaction between diltiazem and cyclosporine has been observed in renal and cardiac transplant patients requiring a reduction of cyclosporine dose). Products include:
Neoral 2405
Sandimmune 2416

Deslanoside (Potential for additive effects; potential for excessive slowing of the heart rate and/or AV block).
No products indexed under this heading.

Digitoxin (Potential for additive effects; potential for excessive slowing of the heart rate and/or AV block). Products include:
Crystodigin Tablets.............................. 1472

Digoxin (Potential for additive effects; potential for excessive slowing of the heart rate and/or AV block). Products include:
Lanoxicaps 1110
Lanoxin Elixir Pediatric 1113
Lanoxin Injection 1116
Lanoxin Injection Pediatric 1119
Lanoxin Tablets 1121

Enflurane (Potential for additive effects; potential for the increased depression of cardiac contractility, conductivity and automaticity).
No products indexed under this heading.

Esmolol Hydrochloride (Concurrent intravenous administration should not be undertaken together or in close proximity; potential for bradycardia, AV block, and/or depression of contractility in patients receiving chronic oral beta-blockers). Products include:
Brevibloc (esmolol HCl) Injection 1860

Fentanyl Citrate (Potential for additive effects; potential for the increased depression of cardiac contractility, conductivity and automaticity). Products include:
Sublimaze Injection............................. 463

Halothane (Potential for additive effects; potential for the increased depression of cardiac contractility, conductivity and automaticity). Products include:
Fluothane 2830

Isoflurane (Potential for additive effects; potential for the increased depression of cardiac contractility, conductivity and automaticity).
No products indexed under this heading.

Ketamine Hydrochloride (Potential for additive effects; potential for the increased depression of cardiac contractility, conductivity and automaticity).
No products indexed under this heading.

Labetalol Hydrochloride (Concurrent intravenous administration should not be undertaken together or in close proximity; potential for bradycardia, AV block, and/or depression of contractility in patients receiving chronic oral beta-blockers). Products include:
Normodyne Injection 2519
Normodyne Tablets 2522
Trandate 1158

Levobunolol Hydrochloride (Potential for bradycardia, AV block, and/or depression of contractility in patients receiving chronic oral beta-blockers). Products include:
Betagan .... ⊚ 230

Methohexital Sodium (Potential for additive effects; potential for the increased depression of cardiac contractility, conductivity and automaticity).
No products indexed under this heading.

Metipranolol Hydrochloride (Potential for bradycardia, AV block, and/or depression of contractility in patients receiving chronic oral beta-blockers). Products include:
OptiPranolol (Metipranolol 0.3%) Sterile Ophthalmic Solution......... ⊚ 256

Metoprolol Succinate (Potential for bradycardia, AV block, and/or depression of contractility in patients receiving chronic oral beta-blockers). Products include:
Toprol-XL Tablets 560

Metoprolol Tartrate (Concurrent intravenous administration should not be undertaken together or in close proximity; potential for bradycardia, AV block, and/or depression of contractility in patients receiving chronic oral beta-blockers). Products include:
Lopressor 848
Lopressor HCT Tablets 850

Midazolam Hydrochloride (Potential for additive effects; potential for the increased depression of cardiac contractility, conductivity and automaticity). Products include:
Versed Injection 2324

Nadolol (Potential for bradycardia, AV block, and/or depression of contractility in patients receiving chronic oral beta-blockers).
No products indexed under this heading.

Penbutolol Sulfate (Potential for bradycardia, AV block, and/or depression of contractility in patients receiving chronic oral beta-blockers). Products include:
Levatol Tablets 2547

Pindolol (Potential for bradycardia, AV block, and/or depression of contractility in patients receiving chronic oral beta-blockers). Products include:
Visken Tablets 2428

Propofol (Potential for additive effects; potential for the increased depression of cardiac contractility, conductivity and automaticity). Products include:
Diprivan Injectable Emulsion 2939

Propranolol Hydrochloride (Concurrent intravenous administration should not be undertaken together or in close proximity; potential for bradycardia, AV block, and/or depression of contractility in patients receiving chronic oral beta-blockers). Products include:
Inderal 2834
Inderal LA Long Acting Capsules 2836
Inderide Tablets 2838
Inderide LA Long Acting Capsules .. 2840

Sotalol Hydrochloride (Potential for bradycardia, AV block, and/or depression of contractility in patients receiving chronic oral beta-blockers). Products include:
Betapace Tablets 637

Sufentanil Citrate (Potential for additive effects; potential for the increased depression of cardiac contractility, conductivity and automaticity). Products include:
Sufenta Injection 1355

Thiamylal Sodium (Potential for additive effects; potential for the increased depression of cardiac contractility, conductivity and automaticity).
No products indexed under this heading.

Timolol Hemihydrate (Potential for bradycardia, AV block, and/or depression of contractility in patients receiving chronic oral beta-blockers). Products include:
Betimol 0.25%, 0.5% .... ⊚ 259

Timolol Maleate (Potential for bradycardia, AV block, and/or depression of contractility in patients receiving chronic oral beta-blockers). Products include:
Blocadren Tablets 1654
Timolide Tablets 1791
Timoptic in Ocudose 1796
Timoptic Sterile Ophthalmic Solution 1794
Timoptic-XE 1798

CARDIZEM LYO-JECT SYRINGE
(Diltiazem Hydrochloride)....................1253
See **Cardizem Injectable**

CARDIZEM TABLETS
(Diltiazem Hydrochloride)....................1257
May interact with beta blockers, cardiac glycosides, anesthetics, and certain other agents. Compounds in these categories include:

Acebutolol Hydrochloride (Potential for additive effects on cardiac conduction). Products include:
Sectral Capsules 2914

IMPORTANT NOTE: Always consult each drug listing in the patient's regimen for possible interactions.

Alfentanil Hydrochloride (Depression of cardiac contractility, conductivity, automaticity, and vasodilation associated with anesthetic may be potentiated). Products include:
- Alfenta Injection 1334

Atenolol (Potential for additive effects on cardiac conduction). Products include:
- Tenoretic Tablets 2963
- Tenormin Tablets and I.V. Injection 2965

Betaxolol Hydrochloride (Potential for additive effects on cardiac conduction). Products include:
- Betoptic Ophthalmic Solution 465
- Betoptic S Ophthalmic Suspension 467
- Kerlone Tablets 2588

Bisoprolol Fumarate (Potential for additive effects on cardiac conduction). Products include:
- Zebeta Tablets 1457
- Ziac 1459

Carbamazepine (Co-administration results in elevated serum levels of carbamazepine (40% to 72%) resulting in toxicity in some cases). Products include:
- Atretol Tablets 569
- Tegretol/Tegretol-XR 870

Carteolol Hydrochloride (Potential for additive effects on cardiac conduction). Products include:
- Cartrol Tablets 413
- Ocupress Ophthalmic Solution, 1% Sterile .... ◉ 297

Cimetidine (May increase peak plasma levels and AUC when administered concurrently; an adjustment in the diltiazem dose may be warranted). Products include:
- Tagamet HB Tablets .... ▣ 786
- Tagamet Tablets 2694

Cimetidine Hydrochloride (May increase peak plasma levels and AUC when administered concurrently; an adjustment in the diltiazem dose may be warranted). Products include:
- Tagamet 2694

Cyclosporine (In renal and cardiac transplant recipients, a reduction of cyclosporine dose ranging from 15% to 48% may be necessary; monitor cyclosporine levels). Products include:
- Neoral 2405
- Sandimmune 2416

Deslanoside (Potential for additive effects on cardiac conduction; variable effect on plasma digoxin concentrations).
- No products indexed under this heading.

Digitoxin (Potential for additive effects on cardiac conduction; variable effect on plasma digoxin concentrations). Products include:
- Crystodigin Tablets 1472

Digoxin (Potential for additive effects on cardiac conduction; variable effect on plasma digoxin concentrations). Products include:
- Lanoxicaps 1110
- Lanoxin Elixir Pediatric 1113
- Lanoxin Injection 1116
- Lanoxin Injection Pediatric 1119
- Lanoxin Tablets 1121

Drugs which undergo biotransformation by cytochrome P-450 mixed function oxidase (Co-administration may result in the competitive inhibition of metabolism).

Enflurane (Depression of cardiac contractility, conductivity, automaticity, and vasodilation associated with anesthetic may be potentiated).
- No products indexed under this heading.

Esmolol Hydrochloride (Potential for additive effects on cardiac conduction). Products include:
- Brevibloc (esmolol HCl) Injection 1860

Fentanyl Citrate (Depression of cardiac contractility, conductivity, automaticity, and vasodilation associated with anesthetic may be potentiated). Products include:
- Sublimaze Injection 463

Halothane (Depression of cardiac contractility, conductivity, automaticity, and vasodilation associated with anesthetic may be potentiated). Products include:
- Fluothane 2830

Isoflurane (Depression of cardiac contractility, conductivity, automaticity, and vasodilation associated with anesthetic may be potentiated).
- No products indexed under this heading.

Ketamine Hydrochloride (Depression of cardiac contractility, conductivity, automaticity, and vasodilation associated with anesthetic may be potentiated).
- No products indexed under this heading.

Labetalol Hydrochloride (Potential for additive effects on cardiac conduction). Products include:
- Normodyne Injection 2519
- Normodyne Tablets 2522
- Trandate 1158

Levobunolol Hydrochloride (Potential for additive effects on cardiac conduction). Products include:
- Betagan .... ◉ 230

Methohexital Sodium (Depression of cardiac contractility, conductivity, automaticity, and vasodilation associated with anesthetic may be potentiated).
- No products indexed under this heading.

Metipranolol Hydrochloride (Potential for additive effects on cardiac conduction). Products include:
- OptiPranolol (Metipranolol 0.3%) Sterile Ophthalmic Solution .... ◉ 256

Metoprolol Succinate (Potential for additive effects on cardiac conduction). Products include:
- Toprol-XL Tablets 560

Metoprolol Tartrate (Potential for additive effects on cardiac conduction). Products include:
- Lopressor 848
- Lopressor HCT Tablets 850

Midazolam Hydrochloride (Depression of cardiac contractility, conductivity, automaticity, and vasodilation associated with anesthetic may be potentiated). Products include:
- Versed Injection 2324

Nadolol (Potential for additive effects on cardiac conduction).
- No products indexed under this heading.

Penbutolol Sulfate (Potential for additive effects on cardiac conduction). Products include:
- Levatol Tablets 2547

Pindolol (Potential for additive effects on cardiac conduction). Products include:
- Visken Tablets 2428

Propofol (Depression of cardiac contractility, conductivity, automaticity, and vasodilation associated with anesthetic may be potentiated). Products include:
- Diprivan Injectable Emulsion 2939

Propranolol Hydrochloride (Potential for additive effects on cardiac conduction; increased propranolol levels, in vitro propranolol appears to be displaced from its binding sites by diltiazem). Products include:
- Inderal 2834
- Inderal LA Long Acting Capsules 2836
- Inderide Tablets 2838
- Inderide LA Long Acting Capsules .. 2840

Ranitidine Hydrochloride (Produces smaller increases in plasma levels). Products include:
- Zantac 1182
- Zantac Injection 1180
- Zantac Syrup 1182

Sotalol Hydrochloride (Potential for additive effects on cardiac conduction). Products include:
- Betapace Tablets 637

Sufentanil Citrate (Depression of cardiac contractility, conductivity, automaticity, and vasodilation associated with anesthetic may be potentiated). Products include:
- Sufenta Injection 1355

Thiamylal Sodium (Depression of cardiac contractility, conductivity, automaticity, and vasodilation associated with anesthetic may be potentiated).
- No products indexed under this heading.

Timolol Hemihydrate (Potential for additive effects on cardiac conduction). Products include:
- Betimol 0.25%, 0.5% .... ◉ 259

Timolol Maleate (Potential for additive effects on cardiac conduction). Products include:
- Blocadren Tablets 1654
- Timolide Tablets 1791
- Timoptic in Ocudose 1796
- Timoptic Sterile Ophthalmic Solution 1794
- Timoptic-XE 1798

CARDURA TABLETS
(Doxazosin Mesylate) 1993
May interact with:

Cimetidine (Co-administration with oral cimetidine has resulted in a 10% increase in mean AUC of doxazosin and a slight but statistically insignificant increase in mean C_{max} and mean half-life of doxazosin). Products include:
- Tagamet HB Tablets .... ▣ 786
- Tagamet Tablets 2694

Cimetidine Hydrochloride (Co-administration with oral cimetidine has resulted in a 10% increase in mean AUC of doxazosin and a slight but statistically insignificant increase in mean C_{max} and mean half-life of doxazosin). Products include:
- Tagamet 2694

Food Interactions

Food, unspecified (Reduction of 18% in mean maximum plasma concentration and 12% in the AUC occurred when Cardura was administered with food; neither of these differences were statistically or clinically significant).

CARE CREME ANTIMICROBIAL CREAM
(Chloroxylenol) .... ▣ 646
None cited in PDR database.

L-CARNITINE 250MG, 500MG TABLETS AND 500MG CHEWABLE WAFERS
(Levocarnitine) 2767
None cited in PDR database.

CARNITOR INJECTION
(Levocarnitine) 2623
None cited in PDR database.

CARNITOR TABLETS AND SOLUTION
(Levocarnitine) 2624
None cited in PDR database.

CARTROL TABLETS
(Carteolol Hydrochloride) 413
May interact with calcium channel blockers, insulin, oral hypoglycemic agents, non-steroidal anti-inflammatory agents, sympathomimetic bronchodilators, catecholamine depleting drugs, and general anesthetics. Compounds in these categories include:

Acarbose (Concomitant administration may result in hypo- or hyperglycemia). Products include:
- Precose 604

Albuterol (Diminished response to therapy with a beta-receptor agonist). Products include:
- Proventil Inhalation Aerosol 2524
- Ventolin Inhalation Aerosol and Refill 1170

Albuterol Sulfate (Diminished response to therapy with a beta-receptor agonist). Products include:
- Airet Albuterol Sulfate Inhalation Solution 1602
- Albuterol Sulfate, USP Solution for Inhalation, Arm-a-Med 522
- Proventil Inhalation Solution 0.083% 2527
- Proventil Repetabs Tablets 2529
- Proventil Solution for Inhalation 0.5% 2525
- Proventil Syrup 2528
- Proventil Tablets 2529
- Ventolin Inhalation Solution 1171
- Ventolin Nebules Inhalation Solution 1172
- Ventolin Rotacaps for Inhalation 1173
- Ventolin Syrup 1175
- Ventolin Tablets 1176
- Volmax Extended-Release Tablets .. 1835

Amlodipine Besylate (Potential for hypotension, AV conduction disturbances and LVF in some patients). Products include:
- Lotrel Capsules 858
- Norvasc Tablets 2020

Bepridil Hydrochloride (Potential for hypotension, AV conduction disturbances and LVF in some patients). Products include:
- Vascor Tablets (200 and 300 mg) 1597

Bitolterol Mesylate (Diminished response to therapy with a beta-receptor agonist). Products include:
- Tornalate Solution for Inhalation, 0.2% 976
- Tornalate Metered Dose Inhaler 978

Chlorpropamide (Concomitant administration may result in hypo- or hyperglycemia). Products include:
- Diabinese Tablets 2002

Deserpidine (Possible additive effect).
- No products indexed under this heading.

Diclofenac Potassium (Possible blunting of the antihypertensive effect). Products include:
- Cataflam Tablets 833

Diclofenac Sodium (Possible blunting of the antihypertensive effect). Products include:
- Voltaren Ophthalmic Sterile Ophthalmic Solution .... ◉ 264

(▣ Described in PDR For Nonprescription Drugs) (◉ Described in PDR For Ophthalmology)

Cataflam/Voltaren/Voltaren-XR 833

Diltiazem Hydrochloride (Potential for hypotension, AV conduction disturbances and LVF in some patients). Products include:
Cardizem CD Capsules 1251
Cardizem SR Capsules 1255
Cardizem Injectable 1253
Cardizem Tablets 1257
Dilacor XR Extended-release Capsules 2183
Tiazac Capsules 1019

Enflurane (Possible exaggeration of hypotension).
No products indexed under this heading.

Ephedrine Hydrochloride (Diminished response to therapy with a beta-receptor agonist). Products include:
Primatene Tablets 844
Quadrinal Tablets 1398

Ephedrine Sulfate (Diminished response to therapy with a beta-receptor agonist). Products include:
Marax Tablets & DF Syrup 2015

Ephedrine Tannate (Diminished response to therapy with a beta-receptor agonist). Products include:
Rynatuss 2782

Epinephrine (Diminished response to therapy with a beta-receptor agonist). Products include:
EPIFRIN 237
EpiPen 808
Marcaine with Epinephrine 2446
Primatene Mist 843
Sensorcaine with Epinephrine Injection 554
Sus-Phrine Injection 1017
Xylocaine with Epinephrine Injections 562

Epinephrine Hydrochloride (Diminished response to therapy with a beta-receptor agonist). Products include:
Ana-Kit Anaphylaxis Emergency Treatment Kit 611

Ethylnorepinephrine Hydrochloride (Diminished response to therapy with a beta-receptor agonist).
No products indexed under this heading.

Etodolac (Possible blunting of the antihypertensive effect). Products include:
Lodine Capsules and Tablets 2849

Felodipine (Potential for hypotension, AV conduction disturbances and LVF in some patients). Products include:
Plendil Extended-Release Tablets 514

Fenoprofen Calcium (Possible blunting of the antihypertensive effect). Products include:
Nalfon 200 Pulvules & Nalfon Tablets 933

Flurbiprofen (Possible blunting of the antihypertensive effect).
No products indexed under this heading.

Glimepiride (Concomitant administration may result in hypo- or hyperglycemia). Products include:
Amaryl Tablets 1241

Glipizide (Concomitant administration may result in hypo- or hyperglycemia). Products include:
Glucotrol Tablets 2011
Glucotrol XL Extended Release Tablets 2012

Glyburide (Concomitant administration may result in hypo- or hyperglycemia). Products include:
DiaBeta Tablets 1265
Glynase PresTab Tablets 2091
Micronase Tablets 2099

Guanethidine Monosulfate (Possible additive effect). Products include:
Esimil Tablets 840
Ismelin Tablets 845

Ibuprofen (Possible blunting of the antihypertensive effect). Products include:
Advil Cold and Sinus Caplets and Tablets 837
Advil Ibuprofen Tablets, Caplets and Gel Caplets 836
Children's Motrin Ibuprofen Oral Suspension 1558
IBU Tablets 1389
Ibuprohm 713
Motrin IB Caplets, Tablets, and Gelcaps 802
Motrin Ibuprofen Suspension, Oral Drops, Chewable Tablets, Caplets 1563
Nuprin Ibuprofen/Analgesic Tablets & Caplets 645
Vicks DayQuil SINUS Pressure & PAIN Relief with IBUPROFEN 735

Indomethacin (Possible blunting of the antihypertensive effect). Products include:
Indocin 1723

Indomethacin Sodium Trihydrate (Possible blunting of the antihypertensive effect). Products include:
Indocin I.V. 1727

Insulin, Human (Concomitant administration may result in hypo- or hyperglycemia).
No products indexed under this heading.

Insulin, Human Isophane Suspension (Concomitant administration may result in hypo- or hyperglycemia). Products include:
Novolin N Human Insulin 10 ml Vials 1846

Insulin, Human NPH (Concomitant administration may result in hypo- or hyperglycemia). Products include:
Humulin N, 100 Units 1495
Novolin N PenFill 1.5 ml Cartridges Durable Insulin Delivery System 1849
Novolin N Prefilled Syringe Disposable Insulin Delivery System 1850

Insulin, Human Regular (Concomitant administration may result in hypo- or hyperglycemia). Products include:
Humulin R, 100 Units 1497
Novolin R Human Insulin 10 ml Vials 1846
Novolin R PenFill 1.5 ml Cartridges Durable Insulin Delivery System 1849
Novolin R Prefilled Syringe Disposable Insulin Delivery System 1850
Velosulin BR Human Insulin 10 ml Vials 1847

Insulin, Human, Zinc Suspension (Concomitant administration may result in hypo- or hyperglycemia). Products include:
Humulin L, 100 Units 1494
Humulin U, 100 Units 1498
Novolin L Human Insulin 10 ml Vials 1846

Insulin Lispro, Human (Concomitant administration may result in hypo- or hyperglycemia). Products include:
Humalog Injection 1488

Insulin, NPH (Concomitant administration may result in hypo- or hyperglycemia). Products include:
NPH, 100 Units 1502
Pork NPH, 100 Units 1506
Purified Pork NPH Isophane Insulin 1852

Insulin, Regular (Concomitant administration may result in hypo- or hyperglycemia). Products include:
Regular, 100 Units 1503
Pork Regular, 100 Units 1507
Pork Regular (Concentrated), 500 Units 1508
Purified Pork Regular Insulin 1852

Insulin, Zinc Crystals (Concomitant administration may result in hypo- or hyperglycemia). Products include:
NPH, 100 Units 1502

Insulin, Zinc Suspension (Concomitant administration may result in hypo- or hyperglycemia). Products include:
Iletin I 1501
Lente, 100 Units 1501
Iletin II 1504
Pork Lente, 100 Units 1504
Purified Pork Lente Insulin 1852

Isoetharine (Diminished response to therapy with a beta-receptor agonist). Products include:
Bronkometer Aerosol 2432
Bronkosol Solution 2432
Isoetharine Inhalation Solution, USP, Arm-a-Med 545

Isoflurane (Possible exaggeration of hypotension).
No products indexed under this heading.

Isoproterenol Hydrochloride (Diminished response to therapy with a beta-receptor agonist). Products include:
Isuprel Hydrochloride Solution 2443
Isuprel Injection 2441
Isuprel Mistometer 2442

Isoproterenol Sulfate (Diminished response to therapy with a beta-receptor agonist). Products include:
Norisodrine with Calcium Iodide Syrup 446

Isradipine (Potential for hypotension, AV conduction disturbances and LVF in some patients). Products include:
DynaCirc Capsules 2381
DynaCirc CR Tablets 2383

Ketamine Hydrochloride (Possible exaggeration of hypotension).
No products indexed under this heading.

Ketoprofen (Possible blunting of the antihypertensive effect). Products include:
Actron Caplets and Tablets 608
Orudis Capsules 2874
Orudis KT 842
Oruvail Capsules 2874

Ketorolac Tromethamine (Possible blunting of the antihypertensive effect). Products include:
Acular Sterile Ophthalmic Solution 470
Toradol 2319

Meclofenamate Sodium (Possible blunting of the antihypertensive effect).
No products indexed under this heading.

Mefenamic Acid (Possible blunting of the antihypertensive effect). Products include:
Ponstel 1982

Metaproterenol Sulfate (Diminished response to therapy with a beta-receptor agonist). Products include:
Alupent 672
Metaproterenol Sulfate Inhalation Solution, USP, Arm-a-Med 547

Metformin Hydrochloride (Concomitant administration may result in hypo- or hyperglycemia). Products include:
Glucophage Tablets 754

Methohexital Sodium (Possible exaggeration of hypotension).
No products indexed under this heading.

Methoxyflurane (Possible exaggeration of hypotension).
No products indexed under this heading.

Nabumetone (Possible blunting of the antihypertensive effect). Products include:
Relafen Tablets 2688

Naproxen (Possible blunting of the antihypertensive effect). Products include:
Anaprox/Naprosyn 2277

Naproxen Sodium (Possible blunting of the antihypertensive effect). Products include:
Aleve 2124
Anaprox/Naprosyn 2277
Naprelan Tablets 2861

Nicardipine Hydrochloride (Potential for hypotension, AV conduction disturbances and LVF in some patients). Products include:
Cardene Capsules 2261
Cardene I.V. 2815
Cardene SR Capsules 2264

Nifedipine (Potential for hypotension, AV conduction disturbances and LVF in some patients). Products include:
Adalat Capsules (10 mg and 20 mg) 580
Adalat CC 582
Procardia Capsules 2024
Procardia XL Extended Release Tablets 2026

Nimodipine (Potential for hypotension, AV conduction disturbances and LVF in some patients). Products include:
Nimotop Capsules 603

Nisoldipine (Potential for hypotension, AV conduction disturbances and LVF in some patients). Products include:
Sular Tablets 2961

Oxaprozin (Possible blunting of the antihypertensive effect). Products include:
Daypro Caplets 2578

Phenylbutazone (Possible blunting of the antihypertensive effect).
No products indexed under this heading.

Pirbuterol Acetate (Diminished response to therapy with a beta-receptor agonist). Products include:
Maxair Autohaler 1550
Maxair Inhaler 1552

Piroxicam (Possible blunting of the antihypertensive effect). Products include:
Feldene Capsules 2008

Propofol (Possible exaggeration of hypotension). Products include:
Diprivan Injectable Emulsion 2939

Rauwolfia Serpentina (Possible additive effect).
No products indexed under this heading.

Rescinnamine (Possible additive effect).
No products indexed under this heading.

Reserpine (Possible additive effect). Products include:
Diupres Tablets 1691
Hydropres Tablets 1718
Ser-Ap-Es Tablets 867

Salmeterol Xinafoate (Diminished response to therapy with a beta-receptor agonist). Products include:
Serevent Inhalation Aerosol 1149

IMPORTANT NOTE: Always consult each drug listing in the patient's regimen for possible interactions.

Cartrol **Interactions Index** 164

Sevoflurane (Possible exaggeration of hypotension).
No products indexed under this heading.

Sulindac (Possible blunting of the antihypertensive effect). Products include:
Clinoril Tablets ... 1658

Terbutaline Sulfate (Diminished response to therapy with a beta-receptor agonist). Products include:
Brethaire Inhaler ... 830
Brethine Ampuls ... 832
Brethine Tablets ... 831
Bricanyl Subcutaneous Injection ... 1247
Bricanyl Tablets ... 1248

Tolazamide (Concomitant administration may result in hypo- or hyperglycemia).
No products indexed under this heading.

Tolbutamide (Concomitant administration may result in hypo- or hyperglycemia).
No products indexed under this heading.

Tolmetin Sodium (Possible blunting of the antihypertensive effect). Products include:
Tolectin (200, 400 and 600 mg) .. 1591

Verapamil Hydrochloride (Potential for hypotension, AV conduction disturbances and LVF in some patients). Products include:
Calan SR Caplets ... 2571
Calan Tablets ... 2568
Covera-HS Tablets ... 2573
Isoptin Injectable ... 1391
Isoptin Oral Tablets ... 1393
Isoptin SR Tablets ... 1395
Verelan Capsules ... 1455

CASODEX TABLETS
(Bicalutamide) ... 2934
May interact with oral anticoagulants. Compounds in this category include:

Dicumarol (Bicalutamide can displace coumarin anticoagulants from their protein-binding sites as shown in *in vitro* studies; close monitoring of prothrombin time is advised).
No products indexed under this heading.

Warfarin Sodium (Bicalutamide can displace coumarin anticoagulants from their protein-binding sites as shown in *in vitro* studies; close monitoring of prothrombin time is advised). Products include:
Coumadin ... 941

CATAFLAM TABLETS
(Diclofenac Potassium) ... 833
See **Voltaren Tablets**

CATAPRES TABLETS
(Clonidine Hydrochloride) ... 679
May interact with tricyclic antidepressants, barbiturates, hypnotics and sedatives, cardiac glycosides, beta blockers, calcium channel blockers, and certain other agents. Compounds in these categories include:

Acebutolol Hydrochloride (Co-administration with agents known to affect sinus node function or AV nodal conduction, such as beta blockers, may result in additive effects such as bradycardia and AV block). Products include:
Sectral Capsules ... 2914

Amitriptyline Hydrochloride (Co-administration may reduce the hypotensive effects; dosage adjustment may be necessary; concurrent use has resulted in corneal lesions in rats within 5 days). Products include:
Elavil ... 2945
Etrafon ... 2495
Limbitrol ... 2333
Triavil Tablets ... 1800

Amlodipine Besylate (Co-administration with agents known to affect sinus node function or AV nodal conduction, such as calcium channel blockers, may result in additive effects such as bradycardia and AV block). Products include:
Lotrel Capsules ... 858
Norvasc Tablets ... 2020

Amoxapine (Co-administration may reduce the hypotensive effects; dosage adjustment may be necessary). Products include:
Asendin Tablets ... 1419

Aprobarbital (Clonidine may potentiate the CNS-depressive effects).
No products indexed under this heading.

Atenolol (Co-administration with agents known to affect sinus node function or AV nodal conduction, such as beta blockers, may result in additive effects such as bradycardia and AV block). Products include:
Tenoretic Tablets ... 2963
Tenormin Tablets and I.V. Injection 2965

Bepridil Hydrochloride (Co-administration with agents known to affect sinus node function or AV nodal conduction, such as calcium channel blockers, may result in additive effects such as bradycardia and AV block). Products include:
Vascor Tablets (200 and 300 mg) 1597

Betaxolol Hydrochloride (Co-administration with agents known to affect sinus node function or AV nodal conduction, such as beta blockers, may result in additive effects such as bradycardia and AV block). Products include:
Betoptic Ophthalmic Solution ... 465
Betoptic S Ophthalmic Suspension 467
Kerlone Tablets ... 2588

Bisoprolol Fumarate (Co-administration with agents known to affect sinus node function or AV nodal conduction, such as beta blockers, may result in additive effects such as bradycardia and AV block). Products include:
Zebeta Tablets ... 1457
Ziac ... 1459

Butabarbital (Clonidine may potentiate the CNS-depressive effects).
No products indexed under this heading.

Butalbital (Clonidine may potentiate the CNS-depressive effects). Products include:
Axocet Capsules ... 2469
Esgic-plus Capsules ... 1012
Esgic-plus Tablets ... 1012
Fioricet Tablets ... 2386
Fioricet with Codeine Capsules ... 2387
Fiorinal Capsules ... 2388
Fiorinal with Codeine Capsules ... 2390
Fiorinal Tablets ... 2388
Phrenilin ... 790
Sedapap Tablets 50 mg/650 mg .. 1826

Carteolol Hydrochloride (Co-administration with agents known to affect sinus node function or AV nodal conduction, such as beta blockers, may result in additive effects such as bradycardia and AV block). Products include:
Cartrol Tablets ... 413
Ocupress Ophthalmic Solution, 1% Sterile ... ⊚ 297

Clomipramine Hydrochloride (Co-administration may reduce the hypotensive effects; dosage adjustment may be necessary). Products include:
Anafranil Capsules ... 819

Desipramine Hydrochloride (Co-administration may reduce the hypotensive effects; dosage adjustment may be necessary). Products include:
Norpramin Tablets ... 1273

Deslanoside (Co-administration with agents known to affect sinus node function or AV nodal conduction, such as digitalis, may result in additive effects such as bradycardia and AV block).
No products indexed under this heading.

Digitoxin (Co-administration with agents known to affect sinus node function or AV nodal conduction, such as digitalis, may result in additive effects such as bradycardia and AV block). Products include:
Crystodigin Tablets ... 1472

Digoxin (Co-administration with agents known to affect sinus node function or AV nodal conduction, such as digitalis, may result in additive effects such as bradycardia and AV block). Products include:
Lanoxicaps ... 1110
Lanoxin Elixir Pediatric ... 1113
Lanoxin Injection ... 1116
Lanoxin Injection Pediatric ... 1119
Lanoxin Tablets ... 1121

Diltiazem Hydrochloride (Co-administration with agents known to affect sinus node function or AV nodal conduction, such as calcium channel blockers, may result in additive effects such as bradycardia and AV block). Products include:
Cardizem CD Capsules ... 1251
Cardizem SR Capsules ... 1255
Cardizem Injectable ... 1253
Cardizem Tablets ... 1257
Dilacor XR Extended-release Capsules ... 2183
Tiazac Capsules ... 1019

Doxepin Hydrochloride (Co-administration may reduce the hypotensive effects; dosage adjustment may be necessary). Products include:
Adapin Capsules ... 1542
Sinequan ... 2028
Zonalon Cream ... 1042

Esmolol Hydrochloride (Co-administration with agents known to affect sinus node function or AV nodal conduction, such as beta blockers, may result in additive effects such as bradycardia and AV block). Products include:
Brevibloc (esmolol HCl) Injection ... 1860

Estazolam (Clonidine may potentiate the CNS-depressive effects). Products include:
ProSom Tablets ... 457

Ethchlorvynol (Clonidine may potentiate the CNS-depressive effects). Products include:
Placidyl Capsules ... 456

Ethinamate (Clonidine may potentiate the CNS-depressive effects).
No products indexed under this heading.

Felodipine (Co-administration with agents known to affect sinus node function or AV nodal conduction, such as calcium channel blockers, may result in additive effects such as bradycardia and AV block). Products include:
Plendil Extended-Release Tablets 514

Flurazepam Hydrochloride (Clonidine may potentiate the CNS-depressive effects). Products include:
Dalmane Capsules ... 2329

Glutethimide (Clonidine may potentiate the CNS-depressive effects).
No products indexed under this heading.

Imipramine Hydrochloride (Co-administration may reduce the hypotensive effects; dosage adjustment may be necessary). Products include:
Tofranil Ampuls ... 873
Tofranil Tablets ... 875

Imipramine Pamoate (Co-administration may reduce the hypotensive effects; dosage adjustment may be necessary). Products include:
Tofranil-PM Capsules ... 876

Isradipine (Co-administration with agents known to affect sinus node function or AV nodal conduction, such as calcium channel blockers, may result in additive effects such as bradycardia and AV block). Products include:
DynaCirc Capsules ... 2381
DynaCirc CR Tablets ... 2383

Labetalol Hydrochloride (Co-administration with agents known to affect sinus node function or AV nodal conduction, such as beta blockers, may result in additive effects such as bradycardia and AV block). Products include:
Normodyne Injection ... 2519
Normodyne Tablets ... 2522
Trandate ... 1158

Levobunolol Hydrochloride (Co-administration with agents known to affect sinus node function or AV nodal conduction, such as beta blockers, may result in additive effects such as bradycardia and AV block). Products include:
Betagan ... ⊚ 230

Lorazepam (Clonidine may potentiate the CNS-depressive effects). Products include:
Ativan Injection ... 2805
Ativan Tablets ... 2807

Maprotiline Hydrochloride (Co-administration may reduce the hypotensive effects; dosage adjustment may be necessary). Products include:
Ludiomil Tablets ... 861

Mephobarbital (Clonidine may potentiate the CNS-depressive effects). Products include:
Mebaral Tablets ... 2452

Metipranolol Hydrochloride (Co-administration with agents known to affect sinus node function or AV nodal conduction, such as beta blockers, may result in additive effects such as bradycardia and AV block). Products include:
OptiPranolol (Metipranolol 0.3%) Sterile Ophthalmic Solution ... ⊚ 256

Metoprolol Succinate (Co-administration with agents known to affect sinus node function or AV nodal conduction, such as beta blockers, may result in additive effects such as bradycardia and AV block). Products include:
Toprol-XL Tablets ... 560

(▣ Described in PDR For Nonprescription Drugs) (⊚ Described in PDR For Ophthalmology)

Metoprolol Tartrate (Co-administration with agents known to affect sinus node function or AV nodal conduction, such as beta blockers, may result in additive effects such as bradycardia and AV block). Products include:
- Lopressor 848
- Lopressor HCT Tablets 850

Midazolam Hydrochloride (Clonidine may potentiate the CNS-depressive effects). Products include:
- Versed Injection 2324

Nadolol (Co-administration with agents known to affect sinus node function or AV nodal conduction, such as beta blockers, may result in additive effects such as bradycardia and AV block).
No products indexed under this heading.

Nicardipine Hydrochloride (Co-administration with agents known to affect sinus node function or AV nodal conduction, such as calcium channel blockers, may result in additive effects such as bradycardia and AV block). Products include:
- Cardene Capsules 2261
- Cardene I.V. 2815
- Cardene SR Capsules 2264

Nifedipine (Co-administration with agents known to affect sinus node function or AV nodal conduction, such as calcium channel blockers, may result in additive effects such as bradycardia and AV block). Products include:
- Adalat Capsules (10 mg and 20 mg) 580
- Adalat CC 582
- Procardia Capsules 2024
- Procardia XL Extended Release Tablets 2026

Nimodipine (Co-administration with agents known to affect sinus node function or AV nodal conduction, such as calcium channel blockers, may result in additive effects such as bradycardia and AV block). Products include:
- Nimotop Capsules 603

Nisoldipine (Co-administration with agents known to affect sinus node function or AV nodal conduction, such as calcium channel blockers, may result in additive effects such as bradycardia and AV block). Products include:
- Sular Tablets 2961

Nortriptyline Hydrochloride (Co-administration may reduce the hypotensive effects; dosage adjustment may be necessary). Products include:
- Pamelor 2409

Penbutolol Sulfate (Co-administration with agents known to affect sinus node function or AV nodal conduction, such as beta blockers, may result in additive effects such as bradycardia and AV block). Products include:
- Levatol Tablets 2547

Pentobarbital Sodium (Clonidine may potentiate the CNS-depressive effects). Products include:
- Nembutal Sodium Capsules 440
- Nembutal Sodium Solution 442
- Nembutal Sodium Suppositories...... 444

Phenobarbital (Clonidine may potentiate the CNS-depressive effects). Products include:
- Arco-Lase Plus Tablets 513
- Bellergal-S Tablets 2375
- Donnatal 2234
- Donnatal Extentabs 2234
- Donnatal Tablets 2234
- Phenobarbital Elixir and Tablets 1523
- Quadrinal Tablets 1398

Pindolol (Co-administration with agents known to affect sinus node function or AV nodal conduction, such as beta blockers, may result in additive effects such as bradycardia and AV block). Products include:
- Visken Tablets 2428

Propofol (Clonidine may potentiate the CNS-depressive effects). Products include:
- Diprivan Injectable Emulsion 2939

Propranolol Hydrochloride (Co-administration with agents known to affect sinus node function or AV nodal conduction, such as beta blockers, may result in additive effects such as bradycardia and AV block). Products include:
- Inderal 2834
- Inderal LA Long Acting Capsules 2836
- Inderide Tablets 2838
- Inderide LA Long Acting Capsules .. 2840

Protriptyline Hydrochloride (Co-administration may reduce the hypotensive effects; dosage adjustment may be necessary). Products include:
- Vivactil Tablets 1820

Quazepam (Clonidine may potentiate the CNS-depressive effects). Products include:
- Doral Tablets 2773

Secobarbital Sodium (Clonidine may potentiate the CNS-depressive effects). Products include:
- Seconal Sodium Pulvules 1529

Sotalol Hydrochloride (Co-administration with agents known to affect sinus node function or AV nodal conduction, such as beta blockers, may result in additive effects such as bradycardia and AV block). Products include:
- Betapace Tablets 637

Temazepam (Clonidine may potentiate the CNS-depressive effects). Products include:
- Restoril Capsules 2413

Thiamylal Sodium (Clonidine may potentiate the CNS-depressive effects).
No products indexed under this heading.

Timolol Hemihydrate (Co-administration with agents known to affect sinus node function or AV nodal conduction, such as beta blockers, may result in additive effects such as bradycardia and AV block). Products include:
- Betimol 0.25%, 0.5% .... ⓢ 259

Timolol Maleate (Co-administration with agents known to affect sinus node function or AV nodal conduction, such as beta blockers, may result in additive effects such as bradycardia and AV block). Products include:
- Blocadren Tablets 1654
- Timolide Tablets 1791
- Timoptic in Ocudose 1796
- Timoptic Sterile Ophthalmic Solution 1794
- Timoptic-XE 1798

Triazolam (Clonidine may potentiate the CNS-depressive effects). Products include:
- Halcion Tablets 2093

Trimipramine Maleate (Co-administration may reduce the hypotensive effects; dosage adjustment may be necessary). Products include:
- Surmontil Capsules 2917

Verapamil Hydrochloride (Co-administration with agents known to affect sinus node function or AV nodal conduction, such as calcium channel blockers, may result in additive effects such as bradycardia and AV block). Products include:
- Calan SR Caplets 2571
- Calan Tablets 2568
- Covera-HS Tablets 2573
- Isoptin Injectable 1391
- Isoptin Oral Tablets 1393
- Isoptin SR Tablets 1395
- Verelan Capsules 1455

Zolpidem Tartrate (Clonidine may potentiate the CNS-depressive effects). Products include:
- Ambien Tablets 2559

Food Interactions

Alcohol (Clonidine may potentiate the CNS-depressive effects).

CATAPRES-TTS
(Clonidine) 680

May interact with tricyclic antidepressants, barbiturates, hypnotics and sedatives, cardiac glycosides, calcium channel blockers, beta blockers, and certain other agents. Compounds in these categories include:

Acebutolol Hydrochloride (Co-administration with agents known to affect sinus node function or AV nodal conduction, such as beta blockers, may result in additive effects such as bradycardia and AV block). Products include:
- Sectral Capsules 2914

Amitriptyline Hydrochloride (Co-administration may reduce the hypotensive effects; dosage adjustment may be necessary; concurrent use has resulted in corneal lesions in rats within 5 days). Products include:
- Elavil 2945
- Etrafon 2495
- Limbitrol 2333
- Triavil Tablets 1800

Amlodipine Besylate (Co-administration with agents known to affect sinus node function or AV nodal conduction, such as calcium channel blockers, may result in additive effects such as bradycardia and AV block). Products include:
- Lotrel Capsules 858
- Norvasc Tablets 2020

Amoxapine (Co-administration may reduce the hypotensive effects; dosage adjustment may be necessary). Products include:
- Asendin Tablets 1419

Aprobarbital (Clonidine may potentiate the CNS-depressive effects).
No products indexed under this heading.

Atenolol (Co-administration with agents known to affect sinus node function or AV nodal conduction, such as beta blockers, may result in additive effects such as bradycardia and AV block). Products include:
- Tenoretic Tablets 2963
- Tenormin Tablets and I.V. Injection 2965

Bepridil Hydrochloride (Co-administration with agents known to affect sinus node function or AV nodal conduction, such as calcium channel blockers, may result in additive effects such as bradycardia and AV block). Products include:
- Vascor Tablets (200 and 300 mg) 1597

Betaxolol Hydrochloride (Co-administration with agents known to affect sinus node function or AV nodal conduction, such as beta blockers, may result in additive effects such as bradycardia and AV block). Products include:
- Betoptic Ophthalmic Solution 465
- Betoptic S Ophthalmic Suspension 467
- Kerlone Tablets 2588

Bisoprolol Fumarate (Co-administration with agents known to affect sinus node function or AV nodal conduction, such as beta blockers, may result in additive effects such as bradycardia and AV block). Products include:
- Zebeta Tablets 1457
- Ziac 1459

Butabarbital (Clonidine may potentiate the CNS-depressive effects).
No products indexed under this heading.

Butalbital (Clonidine may potentiate the CNS-depressive effects). Products include:
- Axocet Capsules 2469
- Esgic-plus Capsules 1012
- Esgic-plus Tablets 1012
- Fioricet Tablets 2386
- Fioricet with Codeine Capsules 2387
- Fiorinal Capsules 2388
- Fiorinal with Codeine Capsules 2390
- Fiorinal Tablets 2388
- Phrenilin 790
- Sedapap Tablets 50 mg/650 mg .. 1826

Carteolol Hydrochloride (Co-administration with agents known to affect sinus node function or AV nodal conduction, such as beta blockers, may result in additive effects such as bradycardia and AV block). Products include:
- Cartrol Tablets 413
- Ocupress Ophthalmic Solution, 1% Sterile .... ⓢ 297

Clomipramine Hydrochloride (Co-administration may reduce the hypotensive effects; dosage adjustment may be necessary). Products include:
- Anafranil Capsules 819

Desipramine Hydrochloride (Co-administration may reduce the hypotensive effects; dosage adjustment may be necessary). Products include:
- Norpramin Tablets 1273

Deslanoside (Co-administration with agents known to affect sinus node function or AV nodal conduction, such as digitalis, may result in additive effects such as bradycardia and AV block).
No products indexed under this heading.

Digitoxin (Co-administration with agents known to affect sinus node function or AV nodal conduction, such as digitalis, may result in additive effects such as bradycardia and AV block). Products include:
- Crystodigin Tablets 1472

Digoxin (Co-administration with agents known to affect sinus node function or AV nodal conduction, such as digitalis, may result in additive effects such as bradycardia and AV block). Products include:
- Lanoxicaps 1110
- Lanoxin Elixir Pediatric 1113
- Lanoxin Injection 1116
- Lanoxin Injection Pediatric 1119
- Lanoxin Tablets 1121

IMPORTANT NOTE: Always consult each drug listing in the patient's regimen for possible interactions.

Catapres-TTS — Interactions Index

Diltiazem Hydrochloride (Co-administration with agents known to affect sinus node function or AV nodal conduction, such as calcium channel blockers, may result in additive effects such as bradycardia and AV block). Products include:
- Cardizem CD Capsules 1251
- Cardizem SR Capsules 1255
- Cardizem Injectable 1253
- Cardizem Tablets 1257
- Dilacor XR Extended-release Capsules 2183
- Tiazac Capsules 1019

Doxepin Hydrochloride (Co-administration may reduce the hypotensive effects; dosage adjustment may be necessary). Products include:
- Adapin Capsules 1542
- Sinequan 2028
- Zonalon Cream 1042

Esmolol Hydrochloride (Co-administration with agents known to affect sinus node function or AV nodal conduction, such as beta blockers, may result in additive effects such as bradycardia and AV block). Products include:
- Brevibloc (esmolol HCl) Injection 1860

Estazolam (Clonidine may potentiate the CNS-depressive effects). Products include:
- ProSom Tablets 457

Ethchlorvynol (Clonidine may potentiate the CNS-depressive effects). Products include:
- Placidyl Capsules 456

Ethinamate (Clonidine may potentiate the CNS-depressive effects).
No products indexed under this heading.

Felodipine (Co-administration with agents known to affect sinus node function or AV nodal conduction, such as calcium channel blockers, may result in additive effects such as bradycardia and AV block). Products include:
- Plendil Extended-Release Tablets 514

Flurazepam Hydrochloride (Clonidine may potentiate the CNS-depressive effects). Products include:
- Dalmane Capsules 2329

Glutethimide (Clonidine may potentiate the CNS-depressive effects).
No products indexed under this heading.

Imipramine Hydrochloride (Co-administration may reduce the hypotensive effects; dosage adjustment may be necessary). Products include:
- Tofranil Ampuls 873
- Tofranil Tablets 875

Imipramine Pamoate (Co-administration may reduce the hypotensive effects; dosage adjustment may be necessary). Products include:
- Tofranil-PM Capsules 876

Isradipine (Co-administration with agents known to affect sinus node function or AV nodal conduction, such as calcium channel blockers, may result in additive effects such as bradycardia and AV block). Products include:
- DynaCirc Capsules 2381
- DynaCirc CR Tablets 2383

Labetalol Hydrochloride (Co-administration with agents known to affect sinus node function or AV nodal conduction, such as beta blockers, may result in additive effects such as bradycardia and AV block). Products include:
- Normodyne Injection 2519
- Normodyne Tablets 2522
- Trandate 1158

Levobunolol Hydrochloride (Co-administration with agents known to affect sinus node function or AV nodal conduction, such as beta blockers, may result in additive effects such as bradycardia and AV block). Products include:
- Betagan .... ⓞ 230

Lorazepam (Clonidine may potentiate the CNS-depressive effects). Products include:
- Ativan Injection 2805
- Ativan Tablets 2807

Maprotiline Hydrochloride (Co-administration may reduce the hypotensive effects; dosage adjustment may be necessary). Products include:
- Ludiomil Tablets 861

Mephobarbital (Clonidine may potentiate the CNS-depressive effects). Products include:
- Mebaral Tablets 2452

Metipranolol Hydrochloride (Co-administration with agents known to affect sinus node function or AV nodal conduction, such as beta blockers, may result in additive effects such as bradycardia and AV block). Products include:
- OptiPranolol (Metipranolol 0.3%) Sterile Ophthalmic Solution .... ⓞ 256

Metoprolol Succinate (Co-administration with agents known to affect sinus node function or AV nodal conduction, such as beta blockers, may result in additive effects such as bradycardia and AV block). Products include:
- Toprol-XL Tablets 560

Metoprolol Tartrate (Co-administration with agents known to affect sinus node function or AV nodal conduction, such as beta blockers, may result in additive effects such as bradycardia and AV block). Products include:
- Lopressor 848
- Lopressor HCT Tablets 850

Midazolam Hydrochloride (Clonidine may potentiate the CNS-depressive effects). Products include:
- Versed Injection 2324

Nadolol (Co-administration with agents known to affect sinus node function or AV nodal conduction, such as beta blockers, may result in additive effects such as bradycardia and AV block).
No products indexed under this heading.

Nicardipine Hydrochloride (Co-administration with agents known to affect sinus node function or AV nodal conduction, such as calcium channel blockers, may result in additive effects such as bradycardia and AV block). Products include:
- Cardene Capsules 2261
- Cardene I.V. 2815
- Cardene SR Capsules 2264

Nifedipine (Co-administration with agents known to affect sinus node function or AV nodal conduction, such as calcium channel blockers, may result in additive effects such as bradycardia and AV block). Products include:
- Adalat Capsules (10 mg and 20 mg) 580
- Adalat CC 582
- Procardia Capsules 2024
- Procardia XL Extended Release Tablets 2026

Nimodipine (Co-administration with agents known to affect sinus node function or AV nodal conduction, such as calcium channel blockers, may result in additive effects such as bradycardia and AV block). Products include:
- Nimotop Capsules 603

Nisoldipine (Co-administration with agents known to affect sinus node function or AV nodal conduction, such as calcium channel blockers, may result in additive effects such as bradycardia and AV block). Products include:
- Sular Tablets 2961

Nortriptyline Hydrochloride (Co-administration may reduce the hypotensive effects; dosage adjustment may be necessary). Products include:
- Pamelor 2409

Penbutolol Sulfate (Co-administration with agents known to affect sinus node function or AV nodal conduction, such as beta blockers, may result in additive effects such as bradycardia and AV block). Products include:
- Levatol Tablets 2547

Pentobarbital Sodium (Clonidine may potentiate the CNS-depressive effects). Products include:
- Nembutal Sodium Capsules 440
- Nembutal Sodium Solution 442
- Nembutal Sodium Suppositories .. 444

Phenobarbital (Clonidine may potentiate the CNS-depressive effects). Products include:
- Arco-Lase Plus Tablets 513
- Bellergal-S Tablets 2375
- Donnatal 2234
- Donnatal Extentabs 2234
- Donnatal Tablets 2234
- Phenobarbital Elixir and Tablets 1523
- Quadrinal Tablets 1398

Pindolol (Co-administration with agents known to affect sinus node function or AV nodal conduction, such as beta blockers, may result in additive effects such as bradycardia and AV block). Products include:
- Visken Tablets 2428

Propofol (Clonidine may potentiate the CNS-depressive effects). Products include:
- Diprivan Injectable Emulsion 2939

Propranolol Hydrochloride (Co-administration with agents known to affect sinus node function or AV nodal conduction, such as beta blockers, may result in additive effects such as bradycardia and AV block). Products include:
- Inderal 2834
- Inderal LA Long Acting Capsules 2836
- Inderide Tablets 2838
- Inderide LA Long Acting Capsules .. 2840

Protriptyline Hydrochloride (Co-administration may reduce the hypotensive effects; dosage adjustment may be necessary). Products include:
- Vivactil Tablets 1820

Quazepam (Clonidine may potentiate the CNS-depressive effects). Products include:
- Doral Tablets 2773

Secobarbital Sodium (Clonidine may potentiate the CNS-depressive effects). Products include:
- Seconal Sodium Pulvules 1529

Sotalol Hydrochloride (Co-administration with agents known to affect sinus node function or AV nodal conduction, such as beta blockers, may result in additive effects such as bradycardia and AV block). Products include:
- Betapace Tablets 637

Temazepam (Clonidine may potentiate the CNS-depressive effects). Products include:
- Restoril Capsules 2413

Thiamylal Sodium (Clonidine may potentiate the CNS-depressive effects).
No products indexed under this heading.

Timolol Hemihydrate (Co-administration with agents known to affect sinus node function or AV nodal conduction, such as beta blockers, may result in additive effects such as bradycardia and AV block). Products include:
- Betimol 0.25%, 0.5% .... ⓞ 259

Timolol Maleate (Co-administration with agents known to affect sinus node function or AV nodal conduction, such as beta blockers, may result in additive effects such as bradycardia and AV block). Products include:
- Blocadren Tablets 1654
- Timolide Tablets 1791
- Timoptic in Ocudose 1796
- Timoptic Sterile Ophthalmic Solution 1794
- Timoptic-XE 1798

Triazolam (Clonidine may potentiate the CNS-depressive effects). Products include:
- Halcion Tablets 2093

Trimipramine Maleate (Co-administration may reduce the hypotensive effects; dosage adjustment may be necessary). Products include:
- Surmontil Capsules 2917

Verapamil Hydrochloride (Co-administration with agents known to affect sinus node function or AV nodal conduction, such as calcium channel blockers, may result in additive effects such as bradycardia and AV block). Products include:
- Calan SR Caplets 2571
- Calan Tablets 2568
- Covera-HS Tablets 2573
- Isoptin Injectable 1391
- Isoptin Oral Tablets 1393
- Isoptin SR Tablets 1395
- Verelan Capsules 1455

Zolpidem Tartrate (Clonidine may potentiate the CNS-depressive effects). Products include:
- Ambien Tablets 2559

Food Interactions

Alcohol (Clonidine may potentiate the CNS-depressive effects).

CATEMINE ENTERIC TABLETS (TYROSINE)
(L-Tyrosine) 2750
None cited in PDR database.

CAVERJECT INJECTION
(Alprostadil) 2064
May interact with anticoagulants. Compounds in this category include:

Dalteparin Sodium (Increased propensity for bleeding after intracavernosal injections). Products include:
- Fragmin Injection 2088

(ⓝ Described in PDR For Nonprescription Drugs)   (ⓞ Described in PDR For Ophthalmology)

Dicumarol (Increased propensity for bleeding after intracavernosal injections).
  No products indexed under this heading.
Enoxaparin (Increased propensity for bleeding after intracavernosal injections). Products include:
  Lovenox Injection 2187
Heparin Calcium (Increased propensity for bleeding after intracavernosal injections).
  No products indexed under this heading.
Heparin Sodium (Increased propensity for bleeding after intracavernosal injections). Products include:
  Heparin Lock Flush Solution 2831
  Heparin Sodium Injection 2832
  Heparin Sodium Vials 1486
Warfarin Sodium (Increased propensity for bleeding after intracavernosal injections). Products include:
  Coumadin 941

CECLOR PULVULES & SUSPENSION
(Cefaclor) 1470
May interact with:

Probenecid (Inhibits renal excretion of cefaclor). Products include:
  Benemid Tablets 1651
  ColBENEMID Tablets 1662
Warfarin Sodium (Rare reports of increased prothrombin time—with or without clinical bleeding—with concomitant use). Products include:
  Coumadin 941

CEDAX CAPSULES
(Ceftibuten Dihydrate) 2480
May interact with:

Ranitidine Hydrochloride (Ranitidine increases the ceftibuten C_{max} by 23% and AUC by 16%; clinical relevance in this interaction is not known). Products include:
  Zantac 1182
  Zantac Injection 1180
  Zantac Syrup 1182

Food Interactions
Food, unspecified (Food delays the time of C_{max}, decreases the C_{max}, and the extent of absorption (AUC); cefibuten oral suspension should be taken at least 2 hours before meal or at least 1 hour after meal).

CEDAX ORAL SUSPENSION
(Ceftibuten Dihydrate) 2480
  See Cedax Capsules

CEENU CAPSULES
(Lomustine (CCNU)) 699
None cited in PDR database.

CEFIZOX FOR INTRAMUSCULAR OR INTRAVENOUS USE
(Ceftizoxime Sodium) 1025
May interact with aminoglycosides. Compounds in this category include:

Amikacin Sulfate (Co-administration of other cephalosporins with aminoglycosides has resulted in nephrotoxicity). Products include:
  Amikacin Sulfate Injection, USP 523
  Amikacin Sulfate Injection, USP 981
  Amikin Injectable 502
Gentamicin Sulfate (Co-administration of other cephalosporins with aminoglycosides has resulted in nephrotoxicity). Products include:
  Garamycin Cream 0.1% 2501
  Garamycin Injectable 2502
  Garamycin Ointment 0.1% 2501
  Genoptic Sterile Ophthalmic Solution .... ⊙ 241
  Genoptic Sterile Ophthalmic Ointment .... ⊙ 241
  Gentak .... ⊙ 209
  Pred-G Liquifilm Sterile Ophthalmic Suspension .... ⊙ 248
  Pred-G S.O.P. Sterile Ophthalmic Ointment .... ⊙ 249
Kanamycin Sulfate (Co-administration of other cephalosporins with aminoglycosides has resulted in nephrotoxicity).
  No products indexed under this heading.
Streptomycin Sulfate (Co-administration of other cephalosporins with aminoglycosides has resulted in nephrotoxicity). Products include:
  Streptomycin Sulfate Injection 2031
Tobramycin (Co-administration of other cephalosporins with aminoglycosides has resulted in nephrotoxicity). Products include:
  AKTOB .... ⊙ 207
  TobraDex Ophthalmic Suspension and Ointment 469
  Tobrex Ophthalmic Ointment and Solution .... ⊙ 226
Tobramycin Sulfate (Co-administration of other cephalosporins with aminoglycosides has resulted in nephrotoxicity). Products include:
  Nebcin Vials, Hyporets & ADD-Vantage 1518

CEFOBID INTRAVENOUS/INTRAMUSCULAR
(Cefoperazone Sodium) 1996
May interact with aminoglycosides and certain other agents. Compounds in these categories include:

Amikacin Sulfate (Nephrotoxicity). Products include:
  Amikacin Sulfate Injection, USP 523
  Amikacin Sulfate Injection, USP 981
  Amikin Injectable 502
Gentamicin Sulfate (Nephrotoxicity). Products include:
  Garamycin Cream 0.1% 2501
  Garamycin Injectable 2502
  Garamycin Ointment 0.1% 2501
  Garamycin Ophthalmic 2501
  Genoptic Sterile Ophthalmic Solution .... ⊙ 241
  Genoptic Sterile Ophthalmic Ointment .... ⊙ 241
  Gentak .... ⊙ 209
  Pred-G Liquifilm Sterile Ophthalmic Suspension .... ⊙ 248
  Pred-G S.O.P. Sterile Ophthalmic Ointment .... ⊙ 249
Kanamycin Sulfate (Nephrotoxicity).
  No products indexed under this heading.
Streptomycin Sulfate (Nephrotoxicity). Products include:
  Streptomycin Sulfate Injection 2031
Tobramycin (Nephrotoxicity). Products include:
  AKTOB .... ⊙ 207
  TobraDex Ophthalmic Suspension and Ointment 469
  Tobrex Ophthalmic Ointment and Solution .... ⊙ 226
Tobramycin Sulfate (Nephrotoxicity). Products include:
  Nebcin Vials, Hyporets & ADD-Vantage 1518

Food Interactions
Alcohol (When ingested within 72 hours, flushing, sweating, headache, and tachycardia have been reported).

CEFOBID PHARMACY BULK PACKAGE - NOT FOR DIRECT INFUSION
(Cefoperazone Sodium) 1999
May interact with aminoglycosides and certain other agents. Compounds in these categories include:

Amikacin Sulfate (Potential for nephrotoxicity). Products include:
  Amikacin Sulfate Injection, USP 523
  Amikacin Sulfate Injection, USP 981
  Amikin Injectable 502
Gentamicin Sulfate (Potential for nephrotoxicity). Products include:
  Garamycin Cream 0.1% 2501
  Garamycin Injectable 2502
  Garamycin Ointment 0.1% 2501
  Garamycin Ophthalmic 2501
  Genoptic Sterile Ophthalmic Solution .... ⊙ 241
  Genoptic Sterile Ophthalmic Ointment .... ⊙ 241
  Gentak .... ⊙ 209
  Pred-G Liquifilm Sterile Ophthalmic Suspension .... ⊙ 248
  Pred-G S.O.P. Sterile Ophthalmic Ointment .... ⊙ 249
Kanamycin Sulfate (Potential for nephrotoxicity).
  No products indexed under this heading.
Streptomycin Sulfate (Potential for nephrotoxicity). Products include:
  Streptomycin Sulfate Injection 2031
Tobramycin (Potential for nephrotoxicity). Products include:
  AKTOB .... ⊙ 207
  TobraDex Ophthalmic Suspension and Ointment 469
  Tobrex Ophthalmic Ointment and Solution .... ⊙ 226
Tobramycin Sulfate (Potential for nephrotoxicity). Products include:
  Nebcin Vials, Hyporets & ADD-Vantage 1518

Food Interactions
Alcohol (A disulfiram-like reaction characterized by flushing, sweating, headache, and tachycardia has been reported when alcohol was ingested within 72 hours after Cefobid administration).

CEFOL FILMTAB
(Vitamin B Complex With Vitamin C, Vitamin E, Folic Acid) 415
None cited in PDR database.

CEFOTAN FOR INJECTION
(Cefotetan) 2936
May interact with aminoglycosides and certain other agents. Compounds in these categories include:

Amikacin Sulfate (Cefotetan increases serum creatinine; concurrent use may lead to potentiation of nephrotoxicity). Products include:
  Amikacin Sulfate Injection, USP 523
  Amikacin Sulfate Injection, USP 981
  Amikin Injectable 502
Gentamicin Sulfate (Cefotetan increases serum creatinine; concurrent use may lead to potentiation of nephrotoxicity). Products include:
  Garamycin Cream 0.1% 2501
  Garamycin Injectable 2502
  Garamycin Ointment 0.1% 2501
  Garamycin Ophthalmic 2501
  Genoptic Sterile Ophthalmic Solution .... ⊙ 241
  Genoptic Sterile Ophthalmic Ointment .... ⊙ 241
  Gentak .... ⊙ 209
  Pred-G Liquifilm Sterile Ophthalmic Suspension .... ⊙ 248
  Pred-G S.O.P. Sterile Ophthalmic Ointment .... ⊙ 249
Kanamycin Sulfate (Cefotetan increases serum creatinine; concurrent use may lead to potentiation of nephrotoxicity).
  No products indexed under this heading.
Streptomycin Sulfate (Cefotetan increases serum creatinine; concurrent use may lead to potentiation of nephrotoxicity). Products include:
  Streptomycin Sulfate Injection 2031
Tobramycin (Cefotetan increases serum creatinine; concurrent use may lead to potentiation of nephrotoxicity). Products include:
  AKTOB .... ⊙ 207
  TobraDex Ophthalmic Suspension and Ointment 469
  Tobrex Ophthalmic Ointment and Solution .... ⊙ 226
Tobramycin Sulfate (Cefotetan increases serum creatinine; concurrent use may lead to potentiation of nephrotoxicity). Products include:
  Nebcin Vials, Hyporets & ADD-Vantage 1518

Food Interactions
Alcohol (When ingested within 72 hours after Cefotan administration may cause disulfiram-like reactions, including flushing, headache, sweating and tachycardia).

CEFOTAN INJECTION
(Cefotetan) 2936
  See Cefotan for Injection

CEFTIN FOR ORAL SUSPENSION
(Cefuroxime Axetil) 1067
  See Ceftin Tablets

CEFTIN TABLETS
(Cefuroxime Axetil) 1067
May interact with:

Amiloride Hydrochloride (Concurrent treatment with unspecified potent diuretics may adversely affect renal function; caution is advised). Products include:
  Midamor Tablets 1746
  Moduretic Tablets 1748
Bendroflumethiazide (Concurrent treatment with unspecified potent diuretics may adversely affect renal function; caution is advised).
  No products indexed under this heading.
Bumetanide (Concurrent treatment with unspecified potent diuretics may adversely affect renal function; caution is advised). Products include:
  Bumex 2260
Chlorothiazide (Concurrent treatment with unspecified potent diuretics may adversely affect renal function; caution is advised). Products include:
  Aldoclor Tablets 1638
  Diupres Tablets 1691
  Diuril Oral 1694
Chlorothiazide Sodium (Concurrent treatment with unspecified potent diuretics may adversely affect renal function; caution is advised). Products include:
  Diuril Sodium Intravenous 1693
Chlorthalidone (Concurrent treatment with unspecified potent diuretics may adversely affect renal function; caution is advised). Products include:
  Combipres Tablets 682
  Tenoretic Tablets 2963
  Thalitone 1293

IMPORTANT NOTE: Always consult each drug listing in the patient's regimen for possible interactions.

Ethacrynic Acid (Concurrent treatment with unspecified potent diuretics may adversely affect renal function; caution is advised). Products include:

- Edecrin Tablets 1698

Furosemide (Concurrent treatment with unspecified potent diuretics may adversely affect renal function; caution is advised). Products include:

- Lasix Injection, Oral Solution and Tablets 1267

Hydrochlorothiazide (Concurrent treatment with unspecified potent diuretics may adversely affect renal function; caution is advised). Products include:

- Aldactazide Tablets 2556
- Aldoril Tablets 1644
- Apresazide Capsules 824
- Capozide Tablets 744
- Dyazide Capsules 2653
- Esidrix Tablets 839
- Esimil Tablets 840
- HydroDIURIL Tablets 1716
- Hydropres Tablets 1718
- Hyzaar Tablets 1720
- Inderide Tablets 2838
- Inderide LA Long Acting Capsules .. 2840
- Lopressor HCT Tablets 850
- Lotensin HCT Tablets 855
- Moduretic Tablets 1748
- Oretic Tablets 450
- Prinzide Tablets 1780
- Ser-Ap-Es Tablets 867
- Timolide Tablets 1791
- Vaseretic Tablets 1810
- Zestoretic Tablets 2968
- Ziac 1459

Hydroflumethiazide (Concurrent treatment with unspecified potent diuretics may adversely affect renal function; caution is advised). Products include:

- Diucardin Tablets 2824

Indapamide (Concurrent treatment with unspecified potent diuretics may adversely affect renal function; caution is advised).

No products indexed under this heading.

Methyclothiazide (Concurrent treatment with unspecified potent diuretics may adversely affect renal function; caution is advised). Products include:

- Enduron Tablets 424

Metolazone (Concurrent treatment with unspecified potent diuretics may adversely affect renal function; caution is advised). Products include:

- Mykrox Tablets 1617
- Zaroxolyn Tablets 1625

Polythiazide (Concurrent treatment with unspecified potent diuretics may adversely affect renal function; caution is advised). Products include:

- Minizide Capsules 2016

Probenecid (Increases serum concentration of cefuroxime). Products include:

- Benemid Tablets 1651
- ColBENEMID Tablets 1662

Spironolactone (Concurrent treatment with unspecified potent diuretics may adversely affect renal function; caution is advised). Products include:

- Aldactazide Tablets 2556
- Aldactone Tablets 2558

Torsemide (Concurrent treatment with unspecified potent diuretics may adversely affect renal function; caution is advised). Products include:

- Demadex Tablets and Injection 691

Triamterene (Concurrent treatment with unspecified potent diuretics may adversely affect renal function; caution is advised). Products include:

- Dyazide Capsules 2653
- Dyrenium Capsules 2655

Food Interactions

Food, unspecified (Absorption is greater when taken after food).

CEFZIL TABLETS AND ORAL SUSPENSION

(Cefprozil) 747

May interact with aminoglycosides and certain other agents. Compounds in these categories include:

Amikacin Sulfate (Potential for nephrotoxicity). Products include:

- Amikacin Sulfate Injection, USP 523
- Amikacin Sulfate Injection, USP 981
- Amikin Injectable 502

Gentamicin Sulfate (Potential for nephrotoxicity). Products include:

- Garamycin Cream 0.1% 2501
- Garamycin Injectable 2502
- Garamycin Ointment 0.1% 2501
- Garamycin Ophthalmic 2501
- Genoptic Sterile Ophthalmic Solution .... ◉ 241
- Genoptic Sterile Ophthalmic Ointment .... ◉ 241
- Gentak .... ◉ 209
- Pred-G Liquifilm Sterile Ophthalmic Suspension .... ◉ 248
- Pred-G S.O.P. Sterile Ophthalmic Ointment .... ◉ 249

Kanamycin Sulfate (Potential for nephrotoxicity).

No products indexed under this heading.

Probenecid (Doubles the AUC for cefprozil). Products include:

- Benemid Tablets 1651
- ColBENEMID Tablets 1662

Streptomycin Sulfate (Potential for nephrotoxicity). Products include:

- Streptomycin Sulfate Injection 2031

Tobramycin (Potential for nephrotoxicity). Products include:

- AKTOB .... ◉ 207
- TobraDex Ophthalmic Suspension and Ointment 469
- Tobrex Ophthalmic Ointment and Solution .... ◉ 226

Tobramycin Sulfate (Potential for nephrotoxicity). Products include:

- Nebcin Vials, Hyporets & ADD-Vantage 1518

CELESTIAL SEASONINGS SOOTHERS HERBAL THROAT DROPS

(Menthol, Pectin) .... ▣ 805

None cited in PDR database.

CELESTONE SOLUSPAN SUSPENSION

(Betamethasone Sodium Phosphate, Betamethasone Acetate) 2484

May interact with oral hypoglycemic agents, insulin, and certain other agents. Compounds in these categories include:

Acarbose (Increased requirements for oral hypoglycemic agents in diabetes). Products include:

- Precose 604

Aspirin (Concurrent use in hypoprothrombinemia may be undertaken with caution). Products include:

- Alka-Seltzer Cherry Effervescent Antacid and Pain Reliever .... ▣ 609
- Alka-Seltzer Extra Strength Effervescent Antacid and Pain Reliever .... ▣ 609
- Alka-Seltzer Lemon Lime Effervescent Antacid and Pain Reliever .... ▣ 609
- Alka-Seltzer Original Effervescent Antacid and Pain Reliever .... ▣ 609
- Alka-Seltzer Plus .... ▣ 611
- Alka-Seltzer Plus Sinus Medicine .. ▣ 611
- Ascriptin .... ▣ 650
- Arthritis Strength BC Powder .... ▣ 631
- BC Cold Powder Multi-Symptom Formula (Cold-Sinus-Allergy) .... ▣ 631
- BC Cold Powder Non-Drowsy Formula (Cold-Sinus) .... ▣ 631
- BC Powder .... ▣ 631
- Genuine Bayer Aspirin Tablets & Caplets .... ▣ 618
- Extra Strength Bayer Arthritis Pain Regimen Formula .... ▣ 615
- Extra Strength Bayer Aspirin Caplets & Tablets .... ▣ 617
- Extended-Release Bayer 8-Hour Aspirin .... ▣ 616
- Extra Strength Bayer Plus Aspirin Caplets .... ▣ 617
- Extra Strength Bayer PM Aspirin Plus Sleep Aid .... ▣ 617
- Aspirin Regimen Bayer 81 mg Tablets with Calcium .... ▣ 615
- Aspirin Regimen Bayer Adult Low Strength 81 mg Tablets .... ▣ 613
- Aspirin Regimen Bayer Children's Chewable Aspirin .... ▣ 616
- Aspirin Regimen Bayer Regular Strength 325 mg Caplets .... ▣ 613
- Bufferin Analgesic Tablets .... ▣ 636
- Arthritis Strength Bufferin Analgesic Caplets .... ▣ 637
- Extra Strength Bufferin Analgesic Tablets .... ▣ 637
- Cama Arthritis Pain Reliever .... ▣ 748
- Darvon Compound-65 Pulvules 1475
- Easprin 1971
- Ecotrin 2625
- Ecotrin Enteric Coated Aspirin Maximum Strength Tablets and Caplets .... ▣ 775
- Ecotrin Enteric Coated Aspirin Regular Strength Tablets 2625
- Empirin Aspirin Tablets .... ▣ 818
- Excedrin Extra-Strength Analgesic Tablets, Caplets, and Geltabs 734
- Fiorinal Capsules 2388
- Fiorinal with Codeine Capsules 2390
- Fiorinal Tablets 2388
- Goody's Extra Strength Headache Powders .... ▣ 632
- Goody's Extra Strength Pain Relief Tablets .... ▣ 632
- Halfprin Tablets 1413
- Norgesic 1554
- Percodan Tablets 955
- Percodan-Demi Tablets 956
- Robaxisal Tablets 2246
- Soma Compound w/Codeine Tablets 2784
- Soma Compound Tablets 2783
- St. Joseph Adult Chewable Aspirin (81 mg.) .... ▣ 768
- Talwin Compound 2466
- Vanquish Analgesic Caplets .... ▣ 627

Chlorpropamide (Increased requirements for oral hypoglycemic agents in diabetes). Products include:

- Diabinese Tablets 2002

Glimepiride (Increased requirements for oral hypoglycemic agents in diabetes). Products include:

- Amaryl Tablets 1241

Glipizide (Increased requirements for oral hypoglycemic agents in diabetes). Products include:

- Glucotrol Tablets 2011
- Glucotrol XL Extended Release Tablets 2012

Glyburide (Increased requirements for oral hypoglycemic agents in diabetes). Products include:

- DiaBeta Tablets 1265
- Glynase PresTab Tablets 2091
- Micronase Tablets 2099

Immunization (Neurological complications).

Insulin, Human (Increased requirements for insulin in diabetes).

No products indexed under this heading.

Insulin, Human Isophane Suspension (Increased requirements for insulin in diabetes). Products include:

- Novolin N Human Insulin 10 ml Vials 1846

Insulin, Human NPH (Increased requirements for insulin in diabetes). Products include:

- Humulin N, 100 Units 1495
- Novolin N PenFill 1.5 ml Cartridges Durable Insulin Delivery System 1849
- Novolin N Prefilled Syringe Disposable Insulin Delivery System 1850

Insulin, Human Regular (Increased requirements for insulin in diabetes). Products include:

- Humulin R, 100 Units 1497
- Novolin R Human Insulin 10 ml Vials 1846
- Novolin R PenFill 1.5 ml Cartridges Durable Insulin Delivery System 1849
- Novolin R Prefilled Syringe Disposable Insulin Delivery System 1850
- Velosulin BR Human Insulin 10 ml Vials 1847

Insulin, Human, Zinc Suspension (Increased requirements for insulin in diabetes). Products include:

- Humulin L, 100 Units 1494
- Humulin U, 100 Units 1498
- Novolin L Human Insulin 10 ml Vials 1846

Insulin Lispro, Human (Increased requirements for insulin in diabetes). Products include:

- Humalog Injection 1488

Insulin, NPH (Increased requirements for insulin in diabetes). Products include:

- NPH, 100 Units 1502
- Pork NPH, 100 Units 1506
- Purified Pork NPH Isophane Insulin 1852

Insulin, Regular (Increased requirements for insulin in diabetes). Products include:

- Regular, 100 Units 1503
- Pork Regular, 100 Units 1507
- Pork Regular (Concentrated), 500 Units 1508
- Purified Pork Regular Insulin 1852

Insulin, Zinc Crystals (Increased requirements for insulin in diabetes). Products include:

- NPH, 100 Units 1502

Insulin, Zinc Suspension (Increased requirements for insulin in diabetes). Products include:

- Iletin I 1501
- Lente, 100 Units 1501
- Iletin II 1504
- Pork Lente, 100 Units 1504
- Purified Pork Lente Insulin 1852

Metformin Hydrochloride (Increased requirements for oral hypoglycemic agents in diabetes). Products include:

- Glucophage Tablets 754

Tolazamide (Increased requirements for oral hypoglycemic agents in diabetes).

No products indexed under this heading.

Tolbutamide (Increased requirements for oral hypoglycemic agents in diabetes).

No products indexed under this heading.

CELLCEPT CAPSULES

(Mycophenolate Mofetil) 2265

May interact with oral contraceptives

(▣ Described in PDR For Nonprescription Drugs) (◉ Described in PDR For Ophthalmology)

and certain other agents. Compounds in these categories include:

Acyclovir (Potential for these two drugs to compete for tubular secretion further increasing the concentrations of both drugs; AUCs were increased 10.6% for phenolic glucuronide of mycophenolate mofetil and 21.9% for acyclovir). Products include:
- Zovirax Capsules 1187
- Zovirax Ointment 5% 1190
- Zovirax 1187

Acyclovir Sodium (Potential for these two drugs to compete for tubular secretion further increasing the concentrations of both drugs; AUCs were increased 10.6% for phenolic glucuronide of mycophenolate mofetil and 21.9% for acyclovir). Products include:
- Zovirax Sterile Powder 1191

Aluminum Hydroxide (Potential for decreased absorption when CellCept is administered with the antacids containing aluminum and magnesium hydroxide; avoid simultaneous administration). Products include:
- ALternaGEL Liquid 1358
- Maximum Strength Ascriptin 650
- Cama Arthritis Pain Reliever 748
- Gaviscon Extra Strength Relief Formula Antacid Tablets 778
- Gaviscon Extra Strength Relief Formula Liquid Antacid 779
- Gaviscon Liquid Antacid 779
- Gelusil Antacid-Anti-gas Liquid 819
- Gelusil Antacid-Anti-gas Tablets ... 819
- Maalox Antacid/Anti-Gas Tablets ... 889
- Maalox Heartburn Relief Suspension 658
- Maalox Antacid Liquid 888
- Extra Strength Maalox Antacid/Anti-Gas Liquid and Tablets 888
- Mylanta 1359
- Tempo Soft Antacid 799

Aluminum Hydroxide Gel (Potential for decreased absorption when CellCept is administered with the antacids containing aluminum and magnesium hydroxide; avoid simultaneous administration). Products include:
- ALternaGEL Liquid 675
- Aludrox Oral Suspension 850
- Amphojel Suspension 2802
- Amphojel Suspension without Flavor 2802
- Amphojel Tablets 2802
- Ascriptin 650
- Gaviscon Antacid Tablets 778
- Gaviscon-2 Antacid Tablets 779
- Mylanta Liquid 676
- Mylanta Double Strength Liquid 676
- Nephrox Suspension 671

Antibiotics, unspecified (Drugs that alter gastrointestinal flora may interact with mycophenolate mofetil by disrupting enterohepatic recirculation).

Azathioprine (Concomitant administration is not recommended because such co-administration has not been studied clinically). Products include:
- Azathioprine Tablets 2349
- Imuran 1103

Azathioprine Sodium (Concomitant administration is not recommended because such co-administration has not been studied clinically).
No products indexed under this heading.

Cholestyramine (Decreased AUC of mycophenolate mofetil by approximately 40%; concomitant use with agents that may interfere with enterohepatic circulation should be avoided). Products include:
- Questran 774

Desogestrel (Possibility of changes in the pharmacokinetics of the oral contraceptives under long term dosing conditions with CellCept which might adversely affect the efficacy of the oral contraceptive). Products include:
- Desogen Tablets 1867
- Ortho-Cept 1907

Ethinyl Estradiol (Possibility of changes in the pharmacokinetics of the oral contraceptives under long term dosing conditions with CellCept which might adversely affect the efficacy of the oral contraceptive). Products include:
- Brevicon 2563
- Demulen 2580
- Desogen Tablets 1867
- Levlen/Tri-Levlen 646
- Lo/Ovral Tablets 2852
- Lo/Ovral-28 Tablets 2857
- Modicon 1928
- Nordette-21 Tablets 2863
- Nordette-28 Tablets 2866
- Norinyl 2563
- Ortho-Cept 1907
- Ortho-Cyclen/Ortho-Tri-Cyclen ... 1914
- Ortho-Novum 1928
- Ortho-Cyclen/Ortho Tri-Cyclen ... 1914
- Ovcon 765
- Ovral Tablets 2877
- Ovral-28 Tablets 2878
- Levlen/Tri-Levlen 646
- Tri-Norinyl 2607
- Triphasil-21 Tablets 2919
- Triphasil-28 Tablets 2924

Ethynodiol Diacetate (Possibility of changes in the pharmacokinetics of the oral contraceptives under long term dosing conditions with CellCept which might adversely affect the efficacy of the oral contraceptive). Products include:
- Demulen 2580

Ganciclovir Sodium (Potential for these two drugs to compete for tubular secretion further increasing the concentrations of both drugs). Products include:
- Cytovene-IV 2270

Levonorgestrel (Possibility of changes in the pharmacokinetics of the oral contraceptives under long term dosing conditions with CellCept which might adversely affect the efficacy of the oral contraceptive). Products include:
- Levlen/Tri-Levlen 646
- Nordette-21 Tablets 2863
- Nordette-28 Tablets 2866
- Norplant System 2868
- Levlen/Tri-Levlen 646
- Triphasil-21 Tablets 2919
- Triphasil-28 Tablets 2924

Magnesium Hydroxide (Potential for decreased absorption when CellCept is administered with the antacids containing aluminum and magnesium hydroxide; avoid simultaneous administration). Products include:
- Aludrox Oral Suspension 850
- Ascriptin 650
- Di-Gel Antacid/Anti-Gas 762
- Gelusil Antacid-Anti-gas Liquid 819
- Gelusil Antacid-Anti-gas Tablets ... 819
- Maalox Antacid/Anti-Gas Tablets ... 889
- Maalox Antacid Liquid 888
- Extra Strength Maalox Antacid/Anti-Gas Liquid and Tablets 888
- Mylanta Fast-Acting 1359
- Mylanta Gelcaps Antacid 678
- Fast-Acting Mylanta Liquid Antacid 1359
- Mylanta Tablets 677
- Maximum-Strength Fast-Acting Mylanta Liquid Antacid 1359
- Mylanta Double Strength Tablets .. 677
- Phillips' Milk of Magnesia Liquid .. 627
- Rolaids Antacid Tablets 807
- Tempo Soft Antacid 799

Mestranol (Possibility of changes in the pharmacokinetics of the oral contraceptives under long term dosing conditions with CellCept which might adversely affect the efficacy of the oral contraceptive). Products include:
- Norinyl 2563
- Ortho-Novum 1928

Norethindrone (Possibility of changes in the pharmacokinetics of the oral contraceptives under long term dosing conditions with CellCept which might adversely affect the efficacy of the oral contraceptive). Products include:
- Brevicon 2563
- Micronor Tablets 1903
- Modicon 1928
- Norinyl 2563
- Nor-Q D Tablets 2598
- Ortho-Novum 1928
- Ovcon 765
- Tri-Norinyl 2607

Norethynodrel (Possibility of changes in the pharmacokinetics of the oral contraceptives under long term dosing conditions with CellCept which might adversely affect the efficacy of the oral contraceptive).
No products indexed under this heading.

Norgestimate (Possibility of changes in the pharmacokinetics of the oral contraceptives under long term dosing conditions with CellCept which might adversely affect the efficacy of the oral contraceptive). Products include:
- Ortho-Cyclen/Ortho-Tri-Cyclen ... 1914
- Ortho-Cyclen/Ortho Tri-Cyclen ... 1914

Norgestrel (Possibility of changes in the pharmacokinetics of the oral contraceptives under long term dosing conditions with CellCept which might adversely affect the efficacy of the oral contraceptive). Products include:
- Lo/Ovral Tablets 2852
- Lo/Ovral-28 Tablets 2857
- Ovral Tablets 2877
- Ovral-28 Tablets 2878
- Ovrette Tablets 2878

Probenecid (Potential for increased plasma concentration of MPA). Products include:
- Benemid Tablets 1651
- ColBENEMID Tablets 1662

Food Interactions

Food, unspecified (Decreased Cmax of mycophenolate mofetil by 40% in the presence of food; no effect on the extent of absorption).

CELLUVISC LUBRICANT EYE DROPS
(Carboxymethylcellulose Sodium) .. 236
None cited in PDR database.

CELONTIN KAPSEALS
(Methsuximide) 1955
May interact with anticonvulsants. Compounds in this category include:

Carbamazepine (Effect not specified; periodic serum level determination may be necessary). Products include:
- Atretol Tablets 569
- Tegretol/Tegretol-XR 870

Divalproex Sodium (Effect not specified; periodic serum level determination may be necessary). Products include:
- Depakote Tablets 418

Ethosuximide (Effect not specified; periodic serum level determination may be necessary). Products include:
- Zarontin Capsules 1986
- Zarontin Syrup 1986

Ethotoin (Effect not specified; periodic serum level determination may be necessary). Products include:
- Peganone Tablets 455

Felbamate (Effect not specified; periodic serum level determination may be necessary). Products include:
- Felbatol 2774

Lamotrigine (Effect not specified; periodic serum level determination may be necessary). Products include:
- Lamictal Tablets 1105

Mephenytoin (Effect not specified; periodic serum level determination may be necessary). Products include:
- Mesantoin Tablets 2400

Paramethadione (Effect not specified; periodic serum level determination may be necessary).
No products indexed under this heading.

Phenacemide (Effect not specified; periodic serum level determination may be necessary). Products include:
- Phenurone Tablets 455

Phenobarbital (Increased plasma concentration of phenobarbital). Products include:
- Arco-Lase Plus Tablets 513
- Bellergal-S Tablets 2375
- Donnatal 2234
- Donnatal Extentabs 2234
- Donnatal Tablets 2234
- Phenobarbital Elixir and Tablets .. 1523
- Quadrinal Tablets 1398

Phensuximide (Effect not specified; periodic serum level determination may be necessary).
No products indexed under this heading.

Phenytoin (Increased plasma concentration of phenytoin). Products include:
- Dilantin Infatabs 1967
- Dilantin-125 Suspension 1969

Phenytoin Sodium (Increased plasma concentration of phenytoin). Products include:
- Dilantin Kapseals 1965

Primidone (Effect not specified; periodic serum level determination may be necessary). Products include:
- Mysoline 2860

Trimethadione (Effect not specified; periodic serum level determination may be necessary).
No products indexed under this heading.

Valproic Acid (Effect not specified; periodic serum level determination may be necessary). Products include:
- Depakene 416

CENTRUM
(Vitamins with Minerals) 682
None cited in PDR database.

CENTRUM, JR. (CHILDREN'S CHEWABLE) + EXTRA C
(Vitamins with Minerals) 682
None cited in PDR database.

IMPORTANT NOTE: Always consult each drug listing in the patient's regimen for possible interactions.

Centrum, Jr. | Interactions Index | 170

CENTRUM, JR. (CHILDREN'S CHEWABLE) + EXTRA CALCIUM
(Vitamins with Minerals) ▣ 682
None cited in PDR database.

CENTRUM, JR. (CHILDREN'S CHEWABLE) + IRON
(Vitamins with Minerals) ▣ 683
None cited in PDR database.

CENTRUM SILVER
(Vitamins with Minerals) ▣ 683
None cited in PDR database.

CēPACOL/CēPACOL MINT ANTISEPTIC MOUTHWASH/GARGLE
(Cetylpyridinium Chloride) ▣ 849
None cited in PDR database.

CēPACOL MAXIMUM STRENGTH SORE THROAT LOZENGES, CHERRY FLAVOR
(Benzocaine, Menthol) ▣ 850
None cited in PDR database.

CēPACOL MAXIMUM STRENGTH SORE THROAT LOZENGES, ORIGINAL MINT FLAVOR
(Benzocaine, Menthol) ▣ 850
None cited in PDR database.

CēPACOL REGULAR STRENGTH SORE THROAT LOZENGES, CHERRY FLAVOR
(Menthol) ▣ 850
None cited in PDR database.

CēPACOL REGULAR STRENGTH SORE THROAT LOZENGES, ORIGINAL MINT FLAVOR
(Menthol) ▣ 850
None cited in PDR database.

CēPACOL MAXIMUM STRENGTH SORE THROAT SPRAY, CHERRY FLAVOR
(Dyclonine Hydrochloride) ▣ 849
None cited in PDR database.

CēPACOL MAXIMUM STRENGTH SORE THROAT SPRAY, COOL MENTHOL FLAVOR
(Dyclonine Hydrochloride) ▣ 849
None cited in PDR database.

CEPASTAT CHERRY FLAVOR SORE THROAT LOZENGES
(Phenol) ▣ 770
None cited in PDR database.

CEPASTAT EXTRA STRENGTH SORE THROAT LOZENGES
(Phenol) ▣ 770
None cited in PDR database.

CEPTAZ
(Ceftazidime) 1070
May interact with aminoglycosides and certain other agents. Compounds in these categories include:

Amikacin Sulfate (Potential for nephrotoxicity following concomitant administration). Products include:
- Amikacin Sulfate Injection, USP 523
- Amikacin Sulfate Injection, USP 981
- Amikin Injectable 502

Chloramphenicol (Possible antagonism in vivo). Products include:
- Chloromycetin Ophthalmic Ointment, 1% ⊙ 298
- Chloromycetin Ophthalmic Solution ⊙ 299
- Chloroptic S.O.P. ⊙ 236
- Chloroptic Sterile Ophthalmic Solution ⊙ 236

Chloramphenicol Palmitate (Possible antagonism in vivo).
No products indexed under this heading.

Chloramphenicol Sodium Succinate (Possible antagonism in vivo). Products include:
- Chloromycetin Sodium Succinate 1960

Furosemide (Potential for nephrotoxicity following concomitant administration). Products include:
- Lasix Injection, Oral Solution and Tablets 1267

Gentamicin Sulfate (Potential for nephrotoxicity following concomitant administration). Products include:
- Garamycin Cream 0.1% 2501
- Garamycin Injectable 2502
- Garamycin Ointment 0.1% 2501
- Garamycin Ophthalmic 2501
- Genoptic Sterile Ophthalmic Solution ⊙ 241
- Genoptic Sterile Ophthalmic Ointment ⊙ 241
- Gentak ⊙ 209
- Pred-G Liquifilm Sterile Ophthalmic Suspension ⊙ 248
- Pred-G S.O.P. Sterile Ophthalmic Ointment ⊙ 249

Kanamycin Sulfate (Potential for nephrotoxicity following concomitant administration).
No products indexed under this heading.

Streptomycin Sulfate (Potential for nephrotoxicity following concomitant administration). Products include:
- Streptomycin Sulfate Injection 2031

Tobramycin (Potential for nephrotoxicity following concomitant administration). Products include:
- AKTOB ⊙ 207
- TobraDex Ophthalmic Suspension and Ointment 469
- Tobrex Ophthalmic Ointment and Solution ⊙ 226

Tobramycin Sulfate (Potential for nephrotoxicity following concomitant administration). Products include:
- Nebcin Vials, Hyporets & ADD-Vantage 1518

CEREBYX INJECTION
(Fosphenytoin Sodium) 1956
May interact with oral contraceptives, estrogens, histamine h2-receptor antagonists, phenothiazines, salicylates, succinimides, sulfonamides, oral anticoagulants, tricyclic antidepressants, corticosteroids, quinidine, xanthine bronchodilators, and certain other agents. Compounds in these categories include:

Aminophylline (Efficacy of theophylline is impaired by phenytoin).
No products indexed under this heading.

Amiodarone Hydrochloride (Co-administration may increase plasma phenytoin concentration). Products include:
- Cordarone Intravenous 2821
- Cordarone Tablets 2818

Amitriptyline Hydrochloride (Tricyclic antidepressants may precipitate seizures in susceptible patients; Cerebyx dosage may need to be adjusted). Products include:
- Elavil 2945
- Etrafon 2495
- Limbitrol 2333
- Triavil Tablets 1800

Amoxapine (Tricyclic antidepressants may precipitate seizures in susceptible patients; Cerebyx dosage may need to be adjusted). Products include:
- Asendin Tablets 1419

Aspirin (Co-administration may increase plasma phenytoin concentration). Products include:
- Alka-Seltzer Cherry Effervescent Antacid and Pain Reliever ▣ 609
- Alka-Seltzer Extra Strength Effervescent Antacid and Pain Reliever ▣ 609
- Alka-Seltzer Lemon Lime Effervescent Antacid and Pain Reliever ▣ 609
- Alka-Seltzer Original Effervescent Antacid and Pain Reliever ▣ 609
- Alka-Seltzer Plus ▣ 611
- Alka-Seltzer Plus Sinus Medicine ▣ 611
- Ascriptin ▣ 650
- Arthritis Strength BC Powder ▣ 631
- BC Cold Powder Multi-Symptom Formula (Cold-Sinus-Allergy) ▣ 631
- BC Cold Powder Non-Drowsy Formula (Cold-Sinus) ▣ 631
- BC Powder ▣ 631
- Genuine Bayer Aspirin Tablets & Caplets ▣ 618
- Extra Strength Bayer Arthritis Pain Regimen Formula ▣ 615
- Extra Strength Bayer Aspirin Caplets & Tablets ▣ 617
- Extended-Release Bayer 8-Hour Aspirin ▣ 616
- Extra Strength Bayer Plus Aspirin Caplets ▣ 617
- Extra Strength Bayer PM Aspirin Plus Sleep Aid ▣ 617
- Aspirin Regimen Bayer 81 mg Tablets with Calcium ▣ 615
- Aspirin Regimen Bayer Adult Low Strength 81 mg Tablets ▣ 613
- Aspirin Regimen Bayer Children's Chewable Aspirin ▣ 616
- Aspirin Regimen Bayer Regular Strength 325 mg Caplets ▣ 613
- Bufferin Analgesic Tablets ▣ 636
- Arthritis Strength Bufferin Analgesic Caplets ▣ 637
- Extra Strength Bufferin Analgesic Tablets ▣ 637
- Cama Arthritis Pain Reliever ▣ 748
- Darvon Compound-65 Pulvules 1475
- Easprin 1971
- Ecotrin 2625
- Ecotrin Enteric Coated Aspirin Maximum Strength Tablets and Caplets ▣ 775
- Ecotrin Enteric Coated Aspirin Regular Strength Tablets 2625
- Empirin Aspirin Tablets ▣ 818
- Excedrin Extra-Strength Analgesic Tablets, Caplets, and Geltabs 734
- Fiorinal Capsules 2388
- Fiorinal with Codeine Capsules 2390
- Fiorinal Tablets 2388
- Goody's Extra Strength Headache Powders ▣ 632
- Goody's Extra Strength Pain Relief Tablets ▣ 632
- Halfprin Tablets 1413
- Norgesic 1554
- Percodan Tablets 955
- Percodan-Demi Tablets 956
- Robaxisal Tablets 2246
- Soma Compound w/Codeine Tablets 2784
- Soma Compound Tablets 2783
- St. Joseph Adult Chewable Aspirin (81 mg.) ▣ 768
- Talwin Compound 2466
- Vanquish Analgesic Caplets ▣ 627

Bendroflumethiazide (Co-administration with sulfonamides may increase plasma phenytoin concentration).
No products indexed under this heading.

Betamethasone Acetate (Efficacy of corticosteroids is impaired by phenytoin). Products include:
- Celestone Soluspan Suspension 2484

Betamethasone Sodium Phosphate (Efficacy of corticosteroids is impaired by phenytoin). Products include:
- Celestone Soluspan Suspension 2484

Carbamazepine (Co-administration may decrease plasma phenytoin concentration). Products include:
- Atretol Tablets 569
- Tegretol/Tegretol-XR 870

Chloramphenicol (Co-administration may increase plasma phenytoin concentration). Products include:
- Chloromycetin Ophthalmic Ointment, 1% ⊙ 298
- Chloromycetin Ophthalmic Solution ⊙ 299
- Chloroptic S.O.P. ⊙ 236
- Chloroptic Sterile Ophthalmic Solution ⊙ 236

Chloramphenicol Palmitate (Co-administration may increase plasma phenytoin concentration).
No products indexed under this heading.

Chloramphenicol Sodium Succinate (Co-administration may increase plasma phenytoin concentration). Products include:
- Chloromycetin Sodium Succinate 1960

Chlordiazepoxide (Co-administration may increase plasma phenytoin concentration). Products include:
- Limbitrol 2333

Chlordiazepoxide Hydrochloride (Co-administration amy increase plasma phenytoin concentration). Products include:
- Librax Capsules 2330
- Librium Capsules 2331
- Librium Injectable 2332

Chlorothiazide (Co-administration with sulfonamides may increase plasma phenytoin concentration). Products include:
- Aldoclor Tablets 1638
- Diupres Tablets 1691
- Diuril Oral 1694

Chlorothiazide Sodium (Co-administration with sulfonamides may increase plasma phenytoin concentration). Products include:
- Diuril Sodium Intravenous 1693

Chlorotrianisene (Co-administration with estrogens may increase plasma phenytoin concentration; efficacy of estrogens is impaired by phenytoin).
No products indexed under this heading.

Chlorpromazine (Co-administration with phenothiazines may increase plasma phenytoin concentration). Products include:
- Thorazine Suppositories 2701

Chlorpromazine Hydrochloride (Co-administration with phenothiazines may increase plasma phenytoin concentration). Products include:
- Thorazine 2701

Chlorpropamide (Co-administration with sulfonamides may increase plasma phenytoin concentration). Products include:
- Diabinese Tablets 2002

Choline Magnesium Trisalicylate (Co-administration may increase plasma phenytoin concentration). Products include:
- Trilisate 2155

Cimetidine (Co-administration may increase plasma phenytoin concentration). Products include:
- Tagamet HB Tablets ▣ 786
- Tagamet Tablets 2694

(▣ Described in PDR For Nonprescription Drugs) (⊙ Described in PDR For Ophthalmology)

171 Interactions Index Cerebyx

Cimetidine Hydrochloride (Co-administration may increase plasma phenytoin concentration). Products include:
Tagamet ... 2694

Clomipramine Hydrochloride (Tricyclic antidepressants may precipitate seizures in susceptible patients; Cerebyx dosage may need to be adjusted). Products include:
Anafranil Capsules ... 819

Cortisone Acetate (Efficacy of corticosteroids is impaired by phenytoin). Products include:
Cortone Acetate Sterile Suspension ... 1663
Cortone Acetate Tablets ... 1664

Desipramine Hydrochloride (Tricyclic antidepressants may precipitate seizures in susceptible patients; Cerebyx dosage may need to be adjusted). Products include:
Norpramin Tablets ... 1273

Desogestrel (Efficacy of oral contraceptives impaired by phenytoin). Products include:
Desogen Tablets ... 1867
Ortho-Cept ... 1907

Dexamethasone (Efficacy of corticosteroids is impaired by phenytoin). Products include:
AK-Trol Ointment & Suspension ... ◎ 205
Decadron Elixir ... 1676
Decadron Tablets ... 1678
Decaspray Topical Aerosol ... 1689
Maxitrol Ophthalmic Ointment and Suspension ... ◎ 222
TobraDex Ophthalmic Suspension and Ointment ... 469

Dexamethasone Acetate (Efficacy of corticosteroids is impaired by phenytoin). Products include:
Dalalone D.P. Injectable ... 1009
Decadron-LA Sterile Suspension ... 1687

Dexamethasone Sodium Phosphate (Efficacy of corticosteroids is impaired by phenytoin). Products include:
Decadron Phosphate Injection ... 1680
Decadron Phosphate Sterile Ophthalmic Ointment ... 1684
Decadron Phosphate Sterile Ophthalmic Solution ... 1685
Decadron Phosphate Topical Cream ... 1686
Decadron Phosphate with Xylocaine Injection, Sterile ... 1683
Dexacort Phosphate in Respihaler .. 1606
Dexacort Phosphate in Turbinaire .. 1607
NeoDecadron Sterile Ophthalmic Ointment ... 1755
NeoDecadron Sterile Ophthalmic Solution ... 1756
NeoDecadron Topical Cream ... 1757

Diazepam (Co-administration may increase plasma phenytoin concentration). Products include:
Dizac (diazepam injectable emulsion) CIV ... 1862
Valium Injectable ... 2336
Valium Tablets ... 2335

Dicumarol (Co-administration may increase plasma phenytoin concentration; efficacy of coumarin is impaired by phenytoin).
No products indexed under this heading.

Dienestrol (Co-administration with estrogens may increase plasma phenytoin concentration; efficacy of estrogens is impaired by phenytoin). Products include:
Ortho Dienestrol Cream ... 1922

Diethylstilbestrol (Co-administration with estrogens may increase plasma phenytoin concentration; efficacy of estrogens is impaired by phenytoin). Products include:
Diethylstilbestrol Tablets ... 1477

Diflunisal (Co-administration may increase plasma phenytoin concentration). Products include:
Dolobid Tablets ... 1695

Digitoxin (Efficacy of digitoxin is impaired by phenytoin). Products include:
Crystodigin Tablets ... 1472

Disulfiram (Co-administration may increase plasma phenytoin concentration). Products include:
Antabuse Tablets ... 2802

Divalproex Sodium (Co-administration may result in either decrease or increase in plasma phenytoin concentrations; unpredictable effect of phenytoin on valproate plasma concentrations). Products include:
Depakote Tablets ... 418

Doxepin Hydrochloride (Tricyclic antidepressants may precipitate seizures in susceptible patients; Cerebyx dosage may need to be adjusted). Products include:
Adapin Capsules ... 1542
Sinequan ... 2028
Zonalon Cream ... 1042

Doxycycline Calcium (Efficacy of doxycycline is impaired by phenytoin). Products include:
Vibramycin Calcium Oral Suspension Syrup ... 2038

Doxycycline Hyclate (Efficacy of doxycycline is impaired by phenytoin). Products include:
Doryx Capsules ... 1970
Vibramycin Hyclate Capsules ... 2038
Vibramycin Hyclate Intravenous ... 2040
Vibra-Tabs Film Coated Tablets ... 2038

Doxycycline Monohydrate (Efficacy of doxycycline is impaired by phenytoin). Products include:
Monodox Capsules ... 1858
Vibramycin Monohydrate for Oral Suspension ... 2038

Dyphylline (Efficacy of theophylline is impaired by phenytoin). Products include:
Lufyllin & Lufyllin-400 Tablets ... 2778
Lufyllin-GG Elixir & Tablets ... 2779

Estradiol (Co-administration with estrogens may increase plasma phenytoin concentration; efficacy of estrogens is impaired by phenytoin). Products include:
Climara Transdermal System ... 640
Estrace Cream and Tablets ... 751
Estraderm Transdermal System ... 842
Estring Vaginal Ring ... 2086
Vivelle Transdermal System ... 880

Estrogens, Conjugated (Co-administration with estrogens may increase plasma phenytoin concentration; efficacy of estrogens is impaired by phenytoin). Products include:
PMB 200 and PMB 400 ... 2890
Premarin Intravenous ... 2893
Premarin Tablets ... 2896
Premarin Vaginal Cream ... 2898
Premphase ... 2900
Prempro ... 2905

Estrogens, Esterified (Co-administration with estrogens may increase plasma phenytoin concentration; efficacy of estrogens is impaired by phenytoin). Products include:
ESTRATAB Tablets (0.3, 0.625, 1.25, 2.5 mg) ... 2715
Estratest ... 2718
Menest Tablets ... 2671

Estropipate (Co-administration with estrogens may increase plasma phenytoin concentration; efficacy of estrogens is impaired by phenytoin). Products include:
Ogen Tablets ... 2103
Ogen Vaginal Cream ... 2106
Ortho-Est ... 1925

Ethinyl Estradiol (Co-administration with estrogens may increase plasma phenytoin concentration; efficacy of estrogens is impaired by phenytoin). Products include:
Brevicon ... 2563
Demulen ... 2580
Desogen Tablets ... 1867
Levlen/Tri-Levlen ... 646
Lo/Ovral Tablets ... 2852
Lo/Ovral-28 Tablets ... 2857
Modicon ... 1928
Nordette-21 Tablets ... 2863
Nordette-28 Tablets ... 2866
Norinyl ... 2563
Ortho-Cept ... 1907
Ortho-Cyclen/Ortho-Tri-Cyclen ... 1914
Ortho-Novum ... 1928
Ortho-Cyclen/Ortho Tri-Cyclen ... 1914
Ovcon ... 765
Ovral Tablets ... 2877
Ovral-28 Tablets ... 2878
Levlen/Tri-Levlen ... 646
Tri-Norinyl ... 2607
Triphasil-21 Tablets ... 2919
Triphasil-28 Tablets ... 2924

Ethosuximide (Co-administration may increase plasma phenytoin concentration). Products include:
Zarontin Capsules ... 1986
Zarontin Syrup ... 1986

Ethynodiol Diacetate (Efficacy of oral contraceptives impaired by phenytoin). Products include:
Demulen ... 2580

Famotidine (Co-administration may increase plasma phenytoin concentration). Products include:
Pepcid AC Acid Controller ... 1360
Pepcid Injection ... 1765
Pepcid ... 1763

Fludrocortisone Acetate (Efficacy of corticosteroids is impaired by phenytoin). Products include:
Florinef Acetate Tablets ... 506

Fluoxetine Hydrochloride (Co-administration may increase plasma phenytoin concentration). Products include:
Prozac Pulvules & Liquid, Oral Solution ... 935

Fluphenazine Decanoate (Co-administration with phenothiazines may increase plasma phenytoin concentration). Products include:
Prolixin Decanoate ... 510

Fluphenazine Enanthate (Co-administration with phenothiazines may increase plasma phenytoin concentration). Products include:
Prolixin Enanthate ... 510

Fluphenazine Hydrochloride (Co-administration with phenothiazines may increase plasma phenytoin concentration). Products include:
Prolixin ... 510

Furosemide (Efficacy of furosemide is impaired by phenytoin). Products include:
Lasix Injection, Oral Solution and Tablets ... 1267

Glipizide (Co-administration with sulfonamides may increase plasma phenytoin concentration). Products include:
Glucotrol Tablets ... 2011
Glucotrol XL Extended Release Tablets ... 2012

Glyburide (Co-administration with sulfonamides may increase plasma phenytoin concentration). Products include:
DiaBeta Tablets ... 1265
Glynase PresTab Tablets ... 2091
Micronase Tablets ... 2099

Halothane (Co-administration may increase plasma phenytoin concentration). Products include:
Fluothane ... 2830

Hydrochlorothiazide (Co-administration with sulfonamides may increase plasma phenytoin concentration). Products include:
Aldactazide Tablets ... 2556
Aldoril Tablets ... 1644
Apresazide Capsules ... 824
Capozide Tablets ... 744
Dyazide Capsules ... 2653
Esidrix Tablets ... 839
Esimil Tablets ... 840
HydroDIURIL Tablets ... 1716
Hydropres Tablets ... 1718
Hyzaar Tablets ... 1720
Inderide Tablets ... 2838
Inderide LA Long Acting Capsules .. 2840
Lopressor HCT Tablets ... 850
Lotensin HCT Tablets ... 855
Moduretic Tablets ... 1748
Oretic Tablets ... 450
Prinzide Tablets ... 1780
Ser-Ap-Es Tablets ... 867
Timolide Tablets ... 1791
Vaseretic Tablets ... 1810
Zestoretic Tablets ... 2968
Ziac ... 1459

Hydrocortisone (Efficacy of corticosteroids is impaired by phenytoin). Products include:
Anusol-HC Cream 2.5% ... 1953
Aquanil HC Lotion ... 1989
Maximum Strength Cortaid Spray ▣ 800
CORTENEMA ... 2713
Cortisporin Ointment ... 1074
Cortisporin Ophthalmic Ointment Sterile ... 1074
Cortisporin Ophthalmic Suspension Sterile ... 1075
Cortisporin Otic Solution Sterile ... 1076
Cortisporin Otic Suspension Sterile 1077
Cortizone-5 ... ▣ 795
Cortizone-10 ... ▣ 795
Hydrocortone Tablets ... 1715
Hytone ... 922
Hytone Ointment 2 ½% ... 923
Massengill Medicated Soft Cloth Towelettes ... 2628
Pediotic Suspension Sterile ... 1140
Preparation H Hydrocortisone 1% Cream ... ▣ 843
ProctoCream-HC 2.5% ... 2552
VōSoL HC Otic Solution ... 2786

Hydrocortisone Acetate (Efficacy of corticosteroids is impaired by phenytoin). Products include:
Analpram-HC Rectal Cream 1% and 2.5% ... 993
Anusol HC-1 Hydrocortisone Anti-Itch Ointment ... ▣ 810
Anusol-HC Suppositories ... 1954
Caldecort Anti-Itch Hydrocortisone Cream ... ▣ 651
Coly-Mycin S Otic w/Neomycin & Hydrocortisone ... 1965
Cortaid ... ▣ 800
Cortifoam ... 2540
Cortisporin Cream ... 1073
Epifoam ... 2543
Hydrocortone Acetate Sterile Suspension ... 1712
Mantadil Cream ... 1124
Nupercainal Hydrocortisone 1% Cream ... ▣ 661
Pramosone Cream, Lotion & Ointment ... 995
ProctoFoam-HC ... 2552
Terra-Cortril Ophthalmic Suspension ... 2033

Hydrocortisone Sodium Phosphate (Efficacy of corticosteroids is impaired by phenytoin). Products include:
Hydrocortone Phosphate Injection, Sterile ... 1713

Hydrocortisone Sodium Succinate (Efficacy of corticosteroids is impaired by phenytoin).
No products indexed under this heading.

Hydroflumethiazide (Co-administration with sulfonamides may increase plasma phenytoin concentration). Products include:
Diucardin Tablets ... 2824

IMPORTANT NOTE: Always consult each drug listing in the patient's regimen for possible interactions.

Cerebyx — Interactions Index

Imipramine Hydrochloride (Tricyclic antidepressants may precipitate seizures in susceptible patients; Cerebyx dosage may need to be adjusted). Products include:
- Tofranil Ampuls 873
- Tofranil Tablets 875

Imipramine Pamoate (Tricyclic antidepressants may precipitate seizures in susceptible patients; Cerebyx dosage may need to be adjusted). Products include:
- Tofranil-PM Capsules 876

Isoniazid (Co-administration may increase plasma phenytoin concentration). Products include:
- Nydrazid Injection 509
- Rifamate Capsules 1278
- Rifater 1280

Levonorgestrel (Efficacy of oral contraceptives impaired by phenytoin). Products include:
- Levlen/Tri-Levlen 646
- Nordette-21 Tablets 2863
- Nordette-28 Tablets 2866
- Norplant System 2868
- Levlen/Tri-Levlen 646
- Triphasil-21 Tablets 2919
- Triphasil-28 Tablets 2924

Magnesium Salicylate (Co-administration may increase plasma phenytoin concentration). Products include:
- Backache Caplets 635
- Doan's Extra-Strength Analgesic 653
- Extra Strength Doan's P.M. 653
- Doan's Regular Strength Analgesic 654
- Mobigesic Tablets 607

Maprotiline Hydrochloride (Tricyclic antidepressants may precipitate seizures in susceptible patients; Cerebyx dosage may need to be adjusted). Products include:
- Ludiomil Tablets 861

Mesoridazine Besylate (Co-administration with phenothiazines may increase plasma phenytoin concentration). Products include:
- Serentil 689

Mestranol (Efficacy of oral contraceptives impaired by phenytoin). Products include:
- Norinyl 2563
- Ortho-Novum 1928

Methotrimeprazine (Co-administration with phenothiazines may increase plasma phenytoin concentration). Products include:
- Levoprome 1321

Methsuximide (Co-administration may increase plasma phenytoin concentration). Products include:
- Celontin Kapseals 1955

Methyclothiazide (Co-administration with sulfonamides may increase plasma phenytoin concentration). Products include:
- Enduron Tablets 424

Methylphenidate Hydrochloride (Co-administration may increase plasma phenytoin concentration). Products include:
- Ritalin 866

Methylprednisolone Acetate (Efficacy of corticosteroids is impaired by phenytoin).
No products indexed under this heading.

Methylprednisolone Sodium Succinate (Efficacy of corticosteroids is impaired by phenytoin).
No products indexed under this heading.

Nizatidine (Co-administration may increase plasma phenytoin concentration). Products include:
- Axid Pulvules 1468

Norethindrone (Efficacy of oral contraceptives impaired by phenytoin). Products include:
- Brevicon 2563
- Micronor Tablets 1903
- Modicon 1928
- Norinyl 2563
- Nor-Q D Tablets 2598
- Ortho-Novum 1928
- Ovcon 765
- Tri-Norinyl 2607

Norethynodrel (Efficacy of oral contraceptives impaired by phenytoin).
No products indexed under this heading.

Norgestimate (Efficacy of oral contraceptives impaired by phenytoin). Products include:
- Ortho-Cyclen/Ortho Tri-Cyclen 1914
- Ortho-Cyclen/Ortho Tri-Cyclen 1914

Norgestrel (Efficacy of oral contraceptives impaired by phenytoin). Products include:
- Lo/Ovral Tablets 2852
- Lo/Ovral-28 Tablets 2857
- Ovral Tablets 2877
- Ovral-28 Tablets 2878
- Ovrette Tablets 2878

Nortriptyline Hydrochloride (Tricyclic antidepressants may precipitate seizures in susceptible patients; Cerebyx dosage may need to be adjusted). Products include:
- Pamelor 2409

Perphenazine (Co-administration with phenothiazines may increase plasma phenytoin concentration). Products include:
- Etrafon 2495
- Triavil Tablets 1800
- Trilafon 2532

Phenobarbital (Co-administration may result in either decrease or increase in plasma phenytoin concentrations; unpredictable effect of phenytoin on phenobarbital plasma concentrations). Products include:
- Arco-Lase Plus Tablets 513
- Bellergal-S Tablets 2375
- Donnatal 2234
- Donnatal Extentabs 2234
- Donnatal Tablets 2234
- Phenobarbital Elixir and Tablets 1523
- Quadrinal Tablets 1398

Phensuximide (Co-administration may increase plasma phenytoin concentration).
No products indexed under this heading.

Phenylbutazone (Co-administration may increase plasma phenytoin concentration).
No products indexed under this heading.

Polyestradiol Phosphate (Co-administration with estrogens may increase plasma phenytoin concentration; efficacy of estrogens is impaired by phenytoin).
No products indexed under this heading.

Polythiazide (Co-administration with sulfonamides may increase plasma phenytoin concentration). Products include:
- Minizide Capsules 2016

Prednisolone Acetate (Efficacy of corticosteroids is impaired by phenytoin). Products include:
- AK-CIDE .... ⊚ 203
- AK-CIDE Ointment .... ⊚ 203
- Blephamide Liquifilm Sterile Ophthalmic Suspension 472
- Blephamide Ointment .... ⊚ 234
- Econopred & Econopred Plus Ophthalmic Suspensions .... ⊚ 216
- Poly-Pred Liquifilm .... ⊚ 246
- Pred Forte .... ⊚ 247
- Pred Mild .... ⊚ 250
- Pred-G Liquifilm Sterile Ophthalmic Suspension .... ⊚ 248
- Pred-G S.O.P. Sterile Ophthalmic Ointment .... ⊚ 249

Prednisolone Sodium Phosphate (Efficacy of corticosteroids is impaired by phenytoin). Products include:
- AK-PRED .... ⊚ 204
- Hydeltrasol Injection, Sterile 1708
- Pediapred Oral Solution 1618

Prednisolone Tebutate (Efficacy of corticosteroids is impaired by phenytoin). Products include:
- Hydeltra-T.B.A. Sterile Suspension 1710

Prednisone (Efficacy of corticosteroids is impaired by phenytoin).
No products indexed under this heading.

Prochlorperazine (Co-administration with phenothiazines may increase plasma phenytoin concentration). Products include:
- Compazine 2644

Promethazine Hydrochloride (Co-administration with phenothiazines may increase plasma phenytoin concentration). Products include:
- Meperganic Injection 2859
- Phenergan with Codeine 2883
- Phenergan with Dextromethorphan 2885
- Phenergan Injection 2880
- Phenergan Suppositories 2882
- Phenergan Syrup 2881
- Phenergan Tablets 2882
- Phenergan VC 2886
- Phenergan VC with Codeine 2888

Protriptyline Hydrochloride (Tricyclic antidepressants may precipitate seizures in susceptible patients; Cerebyx dosage may need to be adjusted). Products include:
- Vivactil Tablets 1820

Quinestrol (Co-administration with estrogens may increase plasma phenytoin concentration; efficacy of estrogens is impaired by phenytoin).
No products indexed under this heading.

Quinidine Gluconate (Efficacy of quinidine is impaired by phenytoin). Products include:
- Quinaglute Dura-Tabs Tablets 644

Quinidine Polygalacturonate (Efficacy of quinidine is impaired by phenytoin). Products include:
- Cardioquin Tablets 2146

Quinidine Sulfate (Efficacy of quinidine is impaired by phenytoin). Products include:
- Quinidex Extentabs 2240

Ranitidine Hydrochloride (Co-administration may increase plasma phenytoin concentration). Products include:
- Zantac 1182
- Zantac Injection 1180
- Zantac Syrup 1182

Reserpine (Co-administration may decrease plasma phenytoin concentration). Products include:
- Diupres Tablets 1691
- Hydropres Tablets 1718
- Ser-Ap-Es Tablets 867

Rifampin (Efficacy of rifampin is impaired by phenytoin). Products include:
- Rifadin 1276
- Rifamate Capsules 1278
- Rifater 1280
- Rimactane Capsules 865

Salsalate (Co-administration may increase plasma phenytoin concentration). Products include:
- Disalcid 1549
- Mono-Gesic Tablets 810
- Salflex Tablets 791

Sulfacytine (Co-administration with sulfonamides may increase plasma phenytoin concentration).

Sulfamethizole (Co-administration with sulfonamides may increase plasma phenytoin concentration). Products include:
- Urobiotic-250 Capsules 2038

Sulfamethoxazole (Co-administration with sulfonamides may increase plasma phenytoin concentration). Products include:
- Bactrim DS Tablets 2257
- Bactrim I.V. Infusion 2255
- Bactrim 2257
- Gantanol Tablets 2285
- Septra 1146
- Septra I.V. Infusion 1142
- Septra I.V. Infusion ADD-Vantage Vials 1144
- Septra 1146

Sulfasalazine (Co-administration with sulfonamides may increase plasma phenytoin concentration). Products include:
- Azulfidine 2059

Sulfinpyrazone (Co-administration with sulfonamides may increase plasma phenytoin concentration). Products include:
- Anturane 823

Sulfisoxazole (Co-administration with sulfonamides may increase plasma phenytoin concentration). Products include:
- Gantrisin Tablets 2286

Sulfisoxazole Diolamine (Co-administration with sulfonamides may increase plasma phenytoin concentration).
No products indexed under this heading.

Theophylline (Efficacy of theophylline is impaired by phenytoin). Products include:
- Marax Tablets & DF Syrup 2015
- Quibron 2227

Theophylline Anhydrous (Efficacy of theophylline is impaired by phenytoin). Products include:
- Aerolate 1003
- Primatene Tablets 844
- Respbid Tablets 687
- Slo-bid Gyrocaps 2201
- Theo-24 Extended Release Capsules 2753
- Theo-Dur Extended-Release Tablets 1367
- Theo-X Extended-Release Tablets 793
- Uni-Dur Extended-Release Tablets 1374
- Uniphyl 400 mg and 600 mg Tablets 2157

Theophylline Calcium Salicylate (Efficacy of theophylline is impaired by phenytoin). Products include:
- Quadrinal Tablets 1398

Theophylline Sodium Glycinate (Efficacy of theophylline is impaired by phenytoin).
No products indexed under this heading.

Thioridazine Hydrochloride (Co-administration with phenothiazines may increase plasma phenytoin concentration). Products include:
- Mellaril 2398

Tolazamide (Co-administration with sulfonamides may increase plasma phenytoin concentration).
No products indexed under this heading.

Tolbutamide (Co-administration may increase plasma phenytoin concentration).
No products indexed under this heading.

Trazodone Hydrochloride (Co-administration may increase plasma phenytoin concentration). Products include:
- Desyrel and Desyrel Dividose 504

(▣ Described in PDR For Nonprescription Drugs)   (⊚ Described in PDR For Ophthalmology)

Interactions Index

Triamcinolone (Efficacy of corticosteroids is impaired by phenytoin).
No products indexed under this heading.

Triamcinolone Acetonide (Efficacy of corticosteroids is impaired by phenytoin). Products include:
Azmacort Oral Inhaler 2175
Nasacort AQ Nasal Spray........... 2191
Nasacort Nasal Inhaler 2189

Triamcinolone Diacetate (Efficacy of corticosteroids is impaired by phenytoin).
No products indexed under this heading.

Triamcinolone Hexacetonide (Efficacy of corticosteroids is impaired by phenytoin).
No products indexed under this heading.

Trifluoperazine Hydrochloride (Co-administration with phenothiazines may increase plasma phenytoin concentration). Products include:
Stelazine 2692

Trimipramine Maleate (Tricyclic antidepressants may precipitate seizures in susceptible patients; Cerebyx dosage may need to be adjusted). Products include:
Surmontil Capsules..................... 2917

Valproic Acid (Co-administration may result in either decrease or increase in plasma phenytoin concentrations; unpredictable effect of phenytoin on valproic acid plasma concentrations). Products include:
Depakene 416

Vitamin D (Efficacy of vitamin D is impaired by phenytoin). Products include:
Caltrate PLUS 681
Caltrate 600 + D 681
Dical-D Tablets & Wafers 424
Materna Tablets 1427
Megadose 513
One-A-Day Calcium Plus............ 625

Warfarin Sodium (Efficacy of coumarin is impaired by phenytoin). Products include:
Coumadin 941

Food Interactions
Alcohol (Acute alcohol intake may increase plasma phenytoin concentration; chronic alcohol abuse may decrease plasma phenytoin concentration).

CEREDASE
(Alglucerase)................................1055
None cited in PDR database.

CEREZYME
(Imiglucerase).............................1056
None cited in PDR database.

CEROSE DM
(Chlorpheniramine Maleate, Dextromethorphan Hydrobromide, Phenylephrine Hydrochloride)......... 853
May interact with monoamine oxidase inhibitors, hypnotics and sedatives, tranquilizers, and certain other agents. Compounds in these categories include:

Alprazolam (May increase drowsiness effect). Products include:
Xanax Tablets 2115

Buspirone Hydrochloride (May increase drowsiness effect). Products include:
BuSpar Tablets 738

Chlordiazepoxide (May increase drowsiness effect). Products include:
Limbitrol 2333

Chlordiazepoxide Hydrochloride (May increase drowsiness effect). Products include:
Librax Capsules 2330
Librium Capsules........................ 2331
Librium Injectable 2332

Chlorpromazine (May increase drowsiness effect). Products include:
Thorazine Suppositories 2701

Chlorpromazine Hydrochloride (May increase drowsiness effect). Products include:
Thorazine 2701

Chlorprothixene (May increase drowsiness effect).
No products indexed under this heading.

Chlorprothixene Hydrochloride (May increase drowsiness effect).
No products indexed under this heading.

Clorazepate Dipotassium (May increase drowsiness effect). Products include:
Tranxene 459

Diazepam (May increase drowsiness effect). Products include:
Dizac (diazepam injectable emulsion) CIV 1862
Valium Injectable 2336
Valium Tablets 2335

Droperidol (May increase drowsiness effect). Products include:
Inapsine Injection....................... 462

Estazolam (May increase drowsiness effect). Products include:
ProSom Tablets 457

Ethchlorvynol (May increase drowsiness effect). Products include:
Placidyl Capsules 456

Ethinamate (May increase drowsiness effect).
No products indexed under this heading.

Fluphenazine Decanoate (May increase drowsiness effect). Products include:
Prolixin Decanoate 510

Fluphenazine Enanthate (May increase drowsiness effect). Products include:
Prolixin Enanthate 510

Fluphenazine Hydrochloride (May increase drowsiness effect). Products include:
Prolixin 510

Flurazepam Hydrochloride (May increase drowsiness effect). Products include:
Dalmane Capsules...................... 2329

Furazolidone (Concurrent and/or sequential use is not recommended). Products include:
Furoxone 2221

Glutethimide (May increase drowsiness effect).
No products indexed under this heading.

Haloperidol (May increase drowsiness effect). Products include:
Haldol Injection, Tablets and Concentrate 1585

Haloperidol Decanoate (May increase drowsiness effect). Products include:
Haldol Decanoate 1587

Hydroxyzine Hydrochloride (May increase drowsiness effect). Products include:
Atarax Tablets & Syrup 1992
Marax Tablets & DF Syrup....... 2015
Vistaril Intramuscular Solution........ 2042

Isocarboxazid (Concurrent and/or sequential use is not recommended).
No products indexed under this heading.

Lorazepam (May increase drowsiness effect). Products include:
Ativan Injection.......................... 2805
Ativan Tablets 2807

Loxapine Hydrochloride (May increase drowsiness effect). Products include:
Loxitane 1426

Loxapine Succinate (May increase drowsiness effect). Products include:
Loxitane Capsules 1426

Meprobamate (May increase drowsiness effect). Products include:
Miltown Tablets 2780
PMB 200 and PMB 400 2890

Mesoridazine Besylate (May increase drowsiness effect). Products include:
Serentil.. 689

Midazolam Hydrochloride (May increase drowsiness effect). Products include:
Versed Injection 2324

Molindone Hydrochloride (May increase drowsiness effect). Products include:
Moban Tablets and Concentrate...... 1036

Oxazepam (May increase drowsiness effect). Products include:
Serax Capsules 2916
Serax Tablets 2916

Perphenazine (May increase drowsiness effect). Products include:
Etrafon 2495
Triavil Tablets 1800
Trilafon 2532

Phenelzine Sulfate (Concurrent and/or sequential use is not recommended). Products include:
Nardil 1977

Prazepam (May increase drowsiness effect).
No products indexed under this heading.

Prochlorperazine (May increase drowsiness effect). Products include:
Compazine 2644

Promethazine Hydrochloride (May increase drowsiness effect). Products include:
Mepergan Injection 2859
Phenergan with Codeine 2883
Phenergan with Dextromethorphan 2885
Phenergan Injection 2880
Phenergan Suppositories 2882
Phenergan Syrup 2881
Phenergan Tablets 2882
Phenergan VC 2886
Phenergan VC with Codeine 2888

Propofol (May increase drowsiness effect). Products include:
Diprivan Injectable Emulsion ... 2939

Quazepam (May increase drowsiness effect). Products include:
Doral Tablets 2773

Secobarbital Sodium (May increase drowsiness effect). Products include:
Seconal Sodium Pulvules 1529

Selegiline Hydrochloride (Concurrent and/or sequential use is not recommended). Products include:
Eldepryl Capsules 2729

Temazepam (May increase drowsiness effect). Products include:
Restoril Capsules 2413

Thioridazine Hydrochloride (May increase drowsiness effect). Products include:
Mellaril 2398

Thiothixene (May increase drowsiness effect). Products include:
Navane Capsules and Concentrate 2018
Navane Intramuscular 2019

Tranylcypromine Sulfate (Concurrent and/or sequential use is not recommended). Products include:
Parnate Tablets 2679

Triazolam (May increase drowsiness effect). Products include:
Halcion Tablets 2093

Trifluoperazine Hydrochloride (May increase drowsiness effect). Products include:
Stelazine 2692

Zolpidem Tartrate (May increase drowsiness effect). Products include:
Ambien Tablets........................... 2559

Food Interactions
Alcohol (May increase drowsiness effect).

CERUBIDINE FOR INJECTION
(Daunorubicin Hydrochloride) 634
May interact with:

Bone Marrow Depressants, unspecified (Therapy with Cerubidine should not be started in patients with pre-existing drug-induced myelosuppression).

CERUMENEX DROPS
(Triethanolamine Polypeptide Oleate-Condensate) 2148
None cited in PDR database.

CERVIDIL
(Dinoprostone) 1008
May interact with oxytocic drugs. Compounds in this category include:

Ergonovine Maleate (Dinoprostone may augment the activity of oxytocic agents and concomitant use is not recommended; a dosing interval of at least 30 minutes is recommended for sequential use).
No products indexed under this heading.

Methylergonovine Maleate (Dinoprostone may augment the activity of oxytocic agents and concomitant use is not recommended; a dosing interval of at least 30 minutes is recommended for sequential use). Products include:
Methergine 2401

Oxytocin (Dinoprostone may augment the activity of oxytocic agents and concomitant use is not recommended; a dosing interval of at least 30 minutes is recommended for sequential use). Products include:
Syntocinon Injection 2425

CETACAINE TOPICAL ANESTHETIC
(Benzocaine, Tetracaine Hydrochloride, Butyl Aminobenzoate) 812
None cited in PDR database.

CETAPHIL GENTLE CLEANSING BAR
(Cleanser) 1032
None cited in PDR database.

CETAPHIL MOISTURIZING CREAM
(Moisturizing formula) 1032
None cited in PDR database.

CETAPHIL MOISTURIZING LOTION
(Moisturizing formula) 1032
None cited in PDR database.

CETAPHIL SKIN CLEANSER
(Cetyl Alcohol) 1032
None cited in PDR database.

CHARCOAID 2000
(Charcoal, Activated) 740
None cited in PDR database.

IMPORTANT NOTE: Always consult each drug listing in the patient's regimen for possible interactions.

CHARCOCAPS
(Sulfur, Charcoal, Activated, Cinchona Officinalis, Lycopodium Clavatum)......................... 740
None cited in PDR database.

CHEMET CAPSULES
(Succimer) 666
May interact with:

Calcium Disodium Edetate (Concomitant administration is not recommended). Products include:
Calcium Disodium Versenate Injection.................................... 1548

CHERACOL D COUGH FORMULA
(Dextromethorphan Hydrobromide, Guaifenesin).......................... 740
May interact with monoamine oxidase inhibitors. Compounds in this category include:

Furazolidone (Concurrent and/or sequential use is not recommended). Products include:
Furoxone 2221

Isocarboxazid (Concurrent and/or sequential use is not recommended).
No products indexed under this heading.

Phenelzine Sulfate (Concurrent and/or sequential use is not recommended). Products include:
Nardil 1977

Selegiline Hydrochloride (Concurrent and/or sequential use is not recommended). Products include:
Eldepryl Capsules 2729

Tranylcypromine Sulfate (Concurrent and/or sequential use is not recommended). Products include:
Parnate Tablets 2679

CHERACOL PLUS HEAD COLD/COUGH FORMULA
(Phenylpropanolamine Hydrochloride, Dextromethorphan Hydrobromide, Chlorpheniramine Maleate) 741
May interact with monoamine oxidase inhibitors. Compounds in this category include:

Furazolidone (Concurrent and/or sequential administration is not recommended). Products include:
Furoxone 2221

Isocarboxazid (Concurrent and/or sequential administration is not recommended).
No products indexed under this heading.

Phenelzine Sulfate (Concurrent and/or sequential administration is not recommended). Products include:
Nardil 1977

Selegiline Hydrochloride (Concurrent and/or sequential administration is not recommended). Products include:
Eldepryl Capsules 2729

Tranylcypromine Sulfate (Concurrent and/or sequential administration is not recommended). Products include:
Parnate Tablets 2679

CHIBROXIN STERILE OPHTHALMIC SOLUTION
(Norfloxacin)........................... 1657
May interact with oral anticoagulants

and certain other agents. Compounds in these categories include:

Aminophylline (Potential elevation of serum theophylline concentrations).
No products indexed under this heading.

Caffeine (Interferes with the metabolism of caffeine). Products include:
Arthritis Strength BC Powder.......... 631
BC Powder 631
Cafergot 2376
DHCplus Capsules 2148
Darvon Compound-65 Pulvules ... 1475
Esgic-plus Capsules 1012
Esgic-plus Tablets 1012
Aspirin Free Excedrin Analgesic Caplets and Geltabs 734
Excedrin Extra-Strength Analgesic Tablets, Caplets, and Geltabs ... 734
Fioricet Tablets 2386
Fioricet with Codeine Capsules ... 2387
Fiorinal Capsules 2388
Fiorinal with Codeine Capsules ... 2390
Fiorinal Tablets 2388
Goody's Extra Strength Headache Powders 632
Goody's Extra Strength Pain Relief Tablets 632
Maximum Strength Multi-Symptom Formula Midol 621
No Doz Maximum Strength Caplets 644
Norgesic 1554
Vanquish Analgesic Caplets 627
Wigraine Tablets 1884

Cyclosporine (Elevated serum levels of cyclosporine). Products include:
Neoral 2405
Sandimmune 2416

Dicumarol (Enhanced effects of anticoagulant).
No products indexed under this heading.

Dyphylline (Potential elevation of serum theophylline concentrations). Products include:
Lufyllin & Lufyllin-400 Tablets 2778
Lufyllin-GG Elixir & Tablets 2779

Theophylline (Potential elevation of serum theophylline concentrations). Products include:
Marax Tablets & DF Syrup........ 2015
Quibron 2227

Theophylline Anhydrous (Potential elevation of serum theophylline concentrations). Products include:
Aerolate 1003
Primatene Tablets 844
Respbid Tablets 687
Slo-bid Gyrocaps 2201
Theo-24 Extended Release Capsules 2753
Theo-Dur Extended-Release Tablets 1367
Theo-X Extended-Release Tablets .. 793
Uni-Dur Extended-Release Tablets... 1374
Uniphyl 400 mg and 600 mg Tablets 2157

Theophylline Calcium Salicylate (Potential elevation of serum theophylline concentrations). Products include:
Quadrinal Tablets 1398

Theophylline Sodium Glycinate (Potential elevation of serum theophylline concentrations).
No products indexed under this heading.

Warfarin Sodium (Enhanced effects of anticoagulant). Products include:
Coumadin 941

CHILDREN'S MOTRIN IBUPROFEN ORAL SUSPENSION
(Ibuprofen) 1558
None cited in PDR database.

CHILDREN'S TYLENOL ACETAMINOPHEN CHEWABLE TABLETS, ELIXIR, SUSPENSION LIQUID, AND SUSPENSION DROPS
(Acetaminophen) 1559
None cited in PDR database.

CHILDREN'S TYLENOL COLD MULTI-SYMPTOM CHEWABLE TABLETS AND LIQUID
(Acetaminophen, Chlorpheniramine Maleate, Pseudoephedrine Hydrochloride).................... 1559
May interact with hypnotics and sedatives, tranquilizers, and monoamine oxidase inhibitors. Compounds in these categories include:

Alprazolam (Increases drowsiness effect). Products include:
Xanax Tablets 2115

Buspirone Hydrochloride (Increases drowsiness effect). Products include:
BuSpar Tablets 738

Chlordiazepoxide (Increases drowsiness effect). Products include:
Limbitrol 2333

Chlordiazepoxide Hydrochloride (Increases drowsiness effect). Products include:
Librax Capsules 2330
Librium Capsules 2331
Librium Injectable 2332

Chlorpromazine (Increases drowsiness effect). Products include:
Thorazine Suppositories 2701

Chlorpromazine Hydrochloride (Increases drowsiness effect). Products include:
Thorazine 2701

Chlorprothixene (Increases drowsiness effect).
No products indexed under this heading.

Chlorprothixene Hydrochloride (Increases drowsiness effect).
No products indexed under this heading.

Clorazepate Dipotassium (Increases drowsiness effect). Products include:
Tranxene 459

Diazepam (Increases drowsiness effect). Products include:
Dizac (diazepam injectable emulsion) CIV 1862
Valium Injectable 2336
Valium Tablets 2335

Droperidol (Increases drowsiness effect). Products include:
Inapsine Injection 462

Estazolam (Increases drowsiness effect). Products include:
ProSom Tablets 457

Ethchlorvynol (Increases drowsiness effect). Products include:
Placidyl Capsules 456

Ethinamate (Increases drowsiness effect).
No products indexed under this heading.

Fluphenazine Decanoate (Increases drowsiness effect). Products include:
Prolixin Decanoate 510

Fluphenazine Enanthate (Increases drowsiness effect). Products include:
Prolixin Enanthate 510

Fluphenazine Hydrochloride (Increases drowsiness effect). Products include:
Prolixin 510

Flurazepam Hydrochloride (Increases drowsiness effect). Products include:
Dalmane Capsules 2329

Furazolidone (Concurrent and/or sequential administration is not recommended). Products include:
Furoxone 2221

Glutethimide (Increases drowsiness effect).
No products indexed under this heading.

Haloperidol (Increases drowsiness effect). Products include:
Haldol Injection, Tablets and Concentrate 1585

Haloperidol Decanoate (Increases drowsiness effect). Products include:
Haldol Decanoate 1587

Hydroxyzine Hydrochloride (Increases drowsiness effect). Products include:
Atarax Tablets & Syrup 1992
Marax Tablets & DF Syrup 2015
Vistaril Intramuscular Solution .. 2042

Isocarboxazid (Concurrent and/or sequential administration is not recommended).
No products indexed under this heading.

Lorazepam (Increases drowsiness effect). Products include:
Ativan Injection 2805
Ativan Tablets 2807

Loxapine Hydrochloride (Increases drowsiness effect). Products include:
Loxitane 1426

Loxapine Succinate (Increases drowsiness effect). Products include:
Loxitane Capsules 1426

Meprobamate (Increases drowsiness effect). Products include:
Miltown Tablets 2780
PMB 200 and PMB 400 2890

Mesoridazine Besylate (Increases drowsiness effect). Products include:
Serentil 689

Midazolam Hydrochloride (Increases drowsiness effect). Products include:
Versed Injection 2324

Molindone Hydrochloride (Increases drowsiness effect). Products include:
Moban Tablets and Concentrate ... 1036

Oxazepam (Increases drowsiness effect). Products include:
Serax Capsules 2916
Serax Tablets 2916

Perphenazine (Increases drowsiness effect). Products include:
Etrafon 2495
Triavil Tablets 1800
Trilafon 2532

Phenelzine Sulfate (Concurrent and/or sequential administration is not recommended). Products include:
Nardil 1977

Prazepam (Increases drowsiness effect).
No products indexed under this heading.

Prochlorperazine (Increases drowsiness effect). Products include:
Compazine 2644

Promethazine Hydrochloride (Increases drowsiness effect). Products include:
Mepergan Injection 2859
Phenergan with Codeine 2883
Phenergan with Dextromethorphan ... 2885
Phenergan Injection 2880
Phenergan Suppositories 2882
Phenergan Syrup 2881
Phenergan Tablets 2882

175 Interactions Index Tylenol Flu Children's

Phenergan VC 2886
Phenergan VC with Codeine 2888

Propofol (Increases drowsiness effect). Products include:
Diprivan Injectable Emulsion 2939

Quazepam (Increases drowsiness effect). Products include:
Doral Tablets 2773

Secobarbital Sodium (Increases drowsiness effect). Products include:
Seconal Sodium Pulvules 1529

Selegiline Hydrochloride (Concurrent and/or sequential administration is not recommended). Products include:
Eldepryl Capsules 2729

Temazepam (Increases drowsiness effect). Products include:
Restoril Capsules 2413

Thioridazine Hydrochloride (Increases drowsiness effect). Products include:
Mellaril 2398

Thiothixene (Increases drowsiness effect). Products include:
Navane Capsules and Concentrate 2018
Navane Intramuscular 2019

Tranylcypromine Sulfate (Concurrent and/or sequential administration is not recommended). Products include:
Parnate Tablets 2679

Triazolam (Increases drowsiness effect). Products include:
Halcion Tablets 2093

Trifluoperazine Hydrochloride (Increases drowsiness effect). Products include:
Stelazine 2692

Zolpidem Tartrate (Increases drowsiness effect). Products include:
Ambien Tablets 2559

CHILDREN'S TYLENOL COLD PLUS COUGH MULTI SYMPTOM CHEWABLE TABLETS AND LIQUID

(Acetaminophen, Chlorpheniramine Maleate, Dextromethorphan Hydrobromide, Pseudoephedrine Hydrochloride) 1560

May interact with monoamine oxidase inhibitors, hypnotics and sedatives, tranquilizers, and certain other agents. Compounds in these categories include:

Alprazolam (May increase drowsiness effect). Products include:
Xanax Tablets 2115

Buspirone Hydrochloride (May increase drowsiness effect). Products include:
BuSpar Tablets 738

Chlordiazepoxide (May increase drowsiness effect). Products include:
Limbitrol 2333

Chlordiazepoxide Hydrochloride (May increase drowsiness effect). Products include:
Librax Capsules 2330
Librium Capsules 2331
Librium Injectable 2332

Chlorpromazine (May increase drowsiness effect). Products include:
Thorazine Suppositories 2701

Chlorpromazine Hydrochloride (May increase drowsiness effect). Products include:
Thorazine 2701

Chlorprothixene (May increase drowsiness effect).
No products indexed under this heading.

Chlorprothixene Hydrochloride (May increase drowsiness effect).
No products indexed under this heading.

Clorazepate Dipotassium (May increase drowsiness effect). Products include:
Tranxene 459

Diazepam (May increase drowsiness effect). Products include:
Dizac (diazepam injectable emulsion) CIV 1862
Valium Injectable 2336
Valium Tablets 2335

Droperidol (May increase drowsiness effect). Products include:
Inapsine Injection 462

Estazolam (May increase drowsiness effect). Products include:
ProSom Tablets 457

Ethchlorvynol (May increase drowsiness effect). Products include:
Placidyl Capsules 456

Ethinamate (May increase drowsiness effect).
No products indexed under this heading.

Fluphenazine Decanoate (May increase drowsiness effect). Products include:
Prolixin Decanoate 510

Fluphenazine Enanthate (May increase drowsiness effect). Products include:
Prolixin Enanthate 510

Fluphenazine Hydrochloride (May increase drowsiness effect). Products include:
Prolixin 510

Flurazepam Hydrochloride (May increase drowsiness effect). Products include:
Dalmane Capsules 2329

Furazolidone (Concurrent and/or sequential use is not recommended). Products include:
Furoxone 2221

Glutethimide (May increase drowsiness effect).
No products indexed under this heading.

Haloperidol (May increase drowsiness effect). Products include:
Haldol Injection, Tablets and Concentrate 1585

Haloperidol Decanoate (May increase drowsiness effect). Products include:
Haldol Decanoate 1587

Hydroxyzine Hydrochloride (May increase drowsiness effect). Products include:
Atarax Tablets & Syrup 1992
Marax Tablets & DF Syrup 2015
Vistaril Intramuscular Solution 2042

Isocarboxazid (Concurrent and/or sequential use is not recommended).
No products indexed under this heading.

Lorazepam (May increase drowsiness effect). Products include:
Ativan Injection 2805
Ativan Tablets 2807

Loxapine Hydrochloride (May increase drowsiness effect). Products include:
Loxitane 1426

Loxapine Succinate (May increase drowsiness effect). Products include:
Loxitane Capsules 1426

Meprobamate (May increase drowsiness effect). Products include:
Miltown Tablets 2780
PMB 200 and PMB 400 2890

Mesoridazine Besylate (May increase drowsiness effect). Products include:
Serentil 689

Midazolam Hydrochloride (May increase drowsiness effect). Products include:
Versed Injection 2324

Molindone Hydrochloride (May increase drowsiness effect). Products include:
Moban Tablets and Concentrate 1036

Oxazepam (May increase drowsiness effect). Products include:
Serax Capsules 2916
Serax Tablets 2916

Perphenazine (May increase drowsiness effect). Products include:
Etrafon 2495
Triavil Tablets 1800
Trilafon 2532

Phenelzine Sulfate (Concurrent and/or sequential use is not recommended). Products include:
Nardil 1977

Prazepam (May increase drowsiness effect).
No products indexed under this heading.

Prochlorperazine (May increase drowsiness effect). Products include:
Compazine 2644

Promethazine Hydrochloride (May increase drowsiness effect). Products include:
Mepergan Injection 2859
Phenergan with Codeine 2883
Phenergan with Dextromethorphan 2885
Phenergan Injection 2880
Phenergan Suppositories 2882
Phenergan Syrup 2881
Phenergan Tablets 2882
Phenergan VC 2886
Phenergan VC with Codeine 2888

Propofol (May increase drowsiness effect). Products include:
Diprivan Injectable Emulsion 2939

Quazepam (May increase drowsiness effect). Products include:
Doral Tablets 2773

Secobarbital Sodium (May increase drowsiness effect). Products include:
Seconal Sodium Pulvules 1529

Selegiline Hydrochloride (Concurrent and/or sequential use is not recommended). Products include:
Eldepryl Capsules 2729

Temazepam (May increase drowsiness effect). Products include:
Restoril Capsules 2413

Thioridazine Hydrochloride (May increase drowsiness effect). Products include:
Mellaril 2398

Thiothixene (May increase drowsiness effect). Products include:
Navane Capsules and Concentrate 2018
Navane Intramuscular 2019

Tranylcypromine Sulfate (Concurrent and/or sequential use is not recommended). Products include:
Parnate Tablets 2679

Triazolam (May increase drowsiness effect). Products include:
Halcion Tablets 2093

Trifluoperazine Hydrochloride (May increase drowsiness effect). Products include:
Stelazine 2692

Zolpidem Tartrate (May increase drowsiness effect). Products include:
Ambien Tablets 2559

CHILDREN'S TYLENOL FLU SUSPENSION LIQUID

(Acetaminophen, Chlorpheniramine Maleate, Dextromethorphan Hydrobromide, Pseudoephedrine Hydrochloride) 1560

May interact with monoamine oxidase inhibitors, hypnotics and sedatives, and tranquilizers. Compounds in these categories include:

Alprazolam (May increase the drowsiness effect). Products include:
Xanax Tablets 2115

Buspirone Hydrochloride (May increase the drowsiness effect). Products include:
BuSpar Tablets 738

Chlordiazepoxide (May increase the drowsiness effect). Products include:
Limbitrol 2333

Chlordiazepoxide Hydrochloride (May increase the drowsiness effect). Products include:
Librax Capsules 2330
Librium Capsules 2331
Librium Injectable 2332

Chlorpromazine (May increase the drowsiness effect). Products include:
Thorazine Suppositories 2701

Chlorpromazine Hydrochloride (May increase the drowsiness effect). Products include:
Thorazine 2701

Chlorprothixene (May increase the drowsiness effect).
No products indexed under this heading.

Chlorprothixene Hydrochloride (May increase the drowsiness effect).
No products indexed under this heading.

Clorazepate Dipotassium (May increase the drowsiness effect). Products include:
Tranxene 459

Diazepam (May increase the drowsiness effect). Products include:
Dizac (diazepam injectable emulsion) CIV 1862
Valium Injectable 2336
Valium Tablets 2335

Droperidol (May increase the drowsiness effect). Products include:
Inapsine Injection 462

Estazolam (May increase the drowsiness effect). Products include:
ProSom Tablets 457

Ethchlorvynol (May increase the drowsiness effect). Products include:
Placidyl Capsules 456

Ethinamate (May increase the drowsiness effect).
No products indexed under this heading.

Fluphenazine Decanoate (May increase the drowsiness effect). Products include:
Prolixin Decanoate 510

Fluphenazine Enanthate (May increase the drowsiness effect). Products include:
Prolixin Enanthate 510

Fluphenazine Hydrochloride (May increase the drowsiness effect). Products include:
Prolixin 510

Flurazepam Hydrochloride (May increase the drowsiness effect). Products include:
Dalmane Capsules 2329

Furazolidone (Concurrent and/or sequential use is not recommended). Products include:
Furoxone 2221

Glutethimide (May increase the drowsiness effect).
No products indexed under this heading.

Haloperidol (May increase the drowsiness effect). Products include:
Haldol Injection, Tablets and Concentrate 1585

IMPORTANT NOTE: Always consult each drug listing in the patient's regimen for possible interactions.

Tylenol Flu Children's — Interactions Index — 176

Haloperidol Decanoate (May increase the drowsiness effect). Products include:
- Haldol Decanoate ... 1587

Hydroxyzine Hydrochloride (May increase the drowsiness effect). Products include:
- Atarax Tablets & Syrup ... 1992
- Marax Tablets & DF Syrup ... 2015
- Vistaril Intramuscular Solution ... 2042

Isocarboxazid (Concurrent and/or sequential use is not recommended).
- No products indexed under this heading.

Lorazepam (May increase the drowsiness effect). Products include:
- Ativan Injection ... 2805
- Ativan Tablets ... 2807

Loxapine Hydrochloride (May increase the drowsiness effect). Products include:
- Loxitane ... 1426

Loxapine Succinate (May increase the drowsiness effect). Products include:
- Loxitane Capsules ... 1426

Meprobamate (May increase the drowsiness effect). Products include:
- Miltown Tablets ... 2780
- PMB 200 and PMB 400 ... 2890

Mesoridazine Besylate (May increase the drowsiness effect). Products include:
- Serentil ... 689

Midazolam Hydrochloride (May increase the drowsiness effect). Products include:
- Versed Injection ... 2324

Molindone Hydrochloride (May increase the drowsiness effect). Products include:
- Moban Tablets and Concentrate ... 1036

Oxazepam (May increase the drowsiness effect). Products include:
- Serax Capsules ... 2916
- Serax Tablets ... 2916

Perphenazine (May increase the drowsiness effect). Products include:
- Etrafon ... 2495
- Triavil Tablets ... 1800
- Trilafon ... 2532

Phenelzine Sulfate (Concurrent and/or sequential use is not recommended). Products include:
- Nardil ... 1977

Prazepam (May increase the drowsiness effect).
- No products indexed under this heading.

Prochlorperazine (May increase the drowsiness effect). Products include:
- Compazine ... 2644

Promethazine Hydrochloride (May increase the drowsiness effect). Products include:
- Mepergan Injection ... 2859
- Phenergan with Codeine ... 2883
- Phenergan with Dextromethorphan 2885
- Phenergan Injection ... 2880
- Phenergan Suppositories ... 2882
- Phenergan Syrup ... 2881
- Phenergan Tablets ... 2882
- Phenergan VC ... 2886
- Phenergan VC with Codeine ... 2888

Propofol (May increase the drowsiness effect). Products include:
- Diprivan Injectable Emulsion ... 2939

Quazepam (May increase the drowsiness effect). Products include:
- Doral Tablets ... 2773

Secobarbital Sodium (May increase the drowsiness effect). Products include:
- Seconal Sodium Pulvules ... 1529

Selegiline Hydrochloride (Concurrent and/or sequential use is not recommended). Products include:
- Eldepryl Capsules ... 2729

Temazepam (May increase the drowsiness effect). Products include:
- Restoril Capsules ... 2413

Thioridazine Hydrochloride (May increase the drowsiness effect). Products include:
- Mellaril ... 2398

Thiothixene (May increase the drowsiness effect). Products include:
- Navane Capsules and Concentrate 2018
- Navane Intramuscular ... 2019

Tranylcypromine Sulfate (Concurrent and/or sequential use is not recommended). Products include:
- Parnate Tablets ... 2679

Triazolam (May increase the drowsiness effect). Products include:
- Halcion Tablets ... 2093

Trifluoperazine Hydrochloride (May increase the drowsiness effect). Products include:
- Stelazine ... 2692

Zolpidem Tartrate (May increase the drowsiness effect). Products include:
- Ambien Tablets ... 2559

CHLOR-3 CONDIMENT

(Potassium Chloride) ... 1003
None cited in PDR database.

CHILDREN'S VICKS CHLORASEPTIC SORE THROAT LOZENGES

(Benzocaine) ... ◘ 730
None cited in PDR database.

CHILDREN'S VICKS CHLORASEPTIC SORE THROAT SPRAY

(Phenol) ... ◘ 730
None cited in PDR database.

CHILDREN'S VICKS DAYQUIL ALLERGY RELIEF

(Chlorpheniramine Maleate, Pseudoephedrine Hydrochloride) ... ◘ 730
May interact with tranquilizers, hypnotics and sedatives, monoamine oxidase inhibitors, and certain other agents. Compounds in these categories include:

Alprazolam (May increase drowsiness effect). Products include:
- Xanax Tablets ... 2115

Buspirone Hydrochloride (May increase drowsiness effect). Products include:
- BuSpar Tablets ... 738

Chlordiazepoxide (May increase drowsiness effect). Products include:
- Limbitrol ... 2333

Chlordiazepoxide Hydrochloride (May increase drowsiness effect). Products include:
- Librax Capsules ... 2330
- Librium Capsules ... 2331
- Librium Injectable ... 2332

Chlorpromazine (May increase drowsiness effect). Products include:
- Thorazine Suppositories ... 2701

Chlorpromazine Hydrochloride (May increase drowsiness effect). Products include:
- Thorazine ... 2701

Chlorprothixene (May increase drowsiness effect).
- No products indexed under this heading.

Chlorprothixene Hydrochloride (May increase drowsiness effect).
- No products indexed under this heading.

Clorazepate Dipotassium (May increase drowsiness effect). Products include:
- Tranxene ... 459

Diazepam (May increase drowsiness effect). Products include:
- Dizac (diazepam injectable emulsion) CIV ... 1862
- Valium Injectable ... 2336
- Valium Tablets ... 2335

Droperidol (May increase drowsiness effect). Products include:
- Inapsine Injection ... 462

Estazolam (May increase drowsiness effect). Products include:
- ProSom Tablets ... 457

Ethchlorvynol (May increase drowsiness effect). Products include:
- Placidyl Capsules ... 456

Ethinamate (May increase drowsiness effect).
- No products indexed under this heading.

Fluphenazine Decanoate (May increase drowsiness effect). Products include:
- Prolixin Decanoate ... 510

Fluphenazine Enanthate (May increase drowsiness effect). Products include:
- Prolixin Enanthate ... 510

Fluphenazine Hydrochloride (May increase drowsiness effect). Products include:
- Prolixin ... 510

Flurazepam Hydrochloride (May increase drowsiness effect). Products include:
- Dalmane Capsules ... 2329

Furazolidone (Concurrent and/or sequential use is not recommended). Products include:
- Furoxone ... 2221

Glutethimide (May increase drowsiness effect).
- No products indexed under this heading.

Haloperidol (May increase drowsiness effect). Products include:
- Haldol Injection, Tablets and Concentrate ... 1585

Haloperidol Decanoate (May increase drowsiness effect). Products include:
- Haldol Decanoate ... 1587

Hydroxyzine Hydrochloride (May increase drowsiness effect). Products include:
- Atarax Tablets & Syrup ... 1992
- Marax Tablets & DF Syrup ... 2015
- Vistaril Intramuscular Solution ... 2042

Isocarboxazid (Concurrent and/or sequential use is not recommended).
- No products indexed under this heading.

Lorazepam (May increase drowsiness effect). Products include:
- Ativan Injection ... 2805
- Ativan Tablets ... 2807

Loxapine Hydrochloride (May increase drowsiness effect). Products include:
- Loxitane ... 1426

Loxapine Succinate (May increase drowsiness effect). Products include:
- Loxitane Capsules ... 1426

Meprobamate (May increase drowsiness effect). Products include:
- Miltown Tablets ... 2780
- PMB 200 and PMB 400 ... 2890

Mesoridazine Besylate (May increase drowsiness effect). Products include:
- Serentil ... 689

Midazolam Hydrochloride (May increase drowsiness effect). Products include:
- Versed Injection ... 2324

Molindone Hydrochloride (May increase drowsiness effect). Products include:
- Moban Tablets and Concentrate ... 1036

Oxazepam (May increase drowsiness effect). Products include:
- Serax Capsules ... 2916
- Serax Tablets ... 2916

Perphenazine (May increase drowsiness effect). Products include:
- Etrafon ... 2495
- Triavil Tablets ... 1800
- Trilafon ... 2532

Phenelzine Sulfate (Concurrent and/or sequential use is not recommended). Products include:
- Nardil ... 1977

Prazepam (May increase drowsiness effect).
- No products indexed under this heading.

Prochlorperazine (May increase drowsiness effect). Products include:
- Compazine ... 2644

Promethazine Hydrochloride (May increase drowsiness effect). Products include:
- Mepergan Injection ... 2859
- Phenergan with Codeine ... 2883
- Phenergan with Dextromethorphan 2885
- Phenergan Injection ... 2880
- Phenergan Suppositories ... 2882
- Phenergan Syrup ... 2881
- Phenergan Tablets ... 2882
- Phenergan VC ... 2886
- Phenergan VC with Codeine ... 2888

Propofol (May increase drowsiness effect). Products include:
- Diprivan Injectable Emulsion ... 2939

Quazepam (May increase drowsiness effect). Products include:
- Doral Tablets ... 2773

Secobarbital Sodium (May increase drowsiness effect). Products include:
- Seconal Sodium Pulvules ... 1529

Selegiline Hydrochloride (Concurrent and/or sequential use is not recommended). Products include:
- Eldepryl Capsules ... 2729

Temazepam (May increase drowsiness effect). Products include:
- Restoril Capsules ... 2413

Thioridazine Hydrochloride (May increase drowsiness effect). Products include:
- Mellaril ... 2398

Thiothixene (May increase drowsiness effect). Products include:
- Navane Capsules and Concentrate 2018
- Navane Intramuscular ... 2019

Tranylcypromine Sulfate (Concurrent and/or sequential use is not recommended). Products include:
- Parnate Tablets ... 2679

Triazolam (May increase drowsiness effect). Products include:
- Halcion Tablets ... 2093

Trifluoperazine Hydrochloride (May increase drowsiness effect). Products include:
- Stelazine ... 2692

Zolpidem Tartrate (May increase drowsiness effect). Products include:
- Ambien Tablets ... 2559

Food Interactions

Alcohol (May increase drowsiness effect).

(◘ Described in PDR For Nonprescription Drugs) (◉ Described in PDR For Ophthalmology)

CHILDREN'S VICKS NYQUIL COLD/COUGH RELIEF
(Chlorpheniramine Maleate, Dextromethorphan Hydrobromide, Pseudoephedrine Hydrochloride) 731
May interact with hypnotics and sedatives, tranquilizers, monoamine oxidase inhibitors, and certain other agents. Compounds in these categories include:

Alprazolam (May increase drowsiness effect). Products include:
- Xanax Tablets 2115

Buspirone Hydrochloride (May increase drowsiness effect). Products include:
- BuSpar Tablets 738

Chlordiazepoxide (May increase drowsiness effect). Products include:
- Limbitrol 2333

Chlordiazepoxide Hydrochloride (May increase drowsiness effect). Products include:
- Librax Capsules 2330
- Librium Capsules 2331
- Librium Injectable 2332

Chlorpromazine (May increase drowsiness effect). Products include:
- Thorazine Suppositories 2701

Chlorpromazine Hydrochloride (May increase drowsiness effect). Products include:
- Thorazine 2701

Chlorprothixene (May increase drowsiness effect).
No products indexed under this heading.

Chlorprothixene Hydrochloride (May increase drowsiness effect).
No products indexed under this heading.

Clorazepate Dipotassium (May increase drowsiness effect). Products include:
- Tranxene 459

Diazepam (May increase drowsiness effect). Products include:
- Dizac (diazepam injectable emulsion) CIV 1862
- Valium Injectable 2336
- Valium Tablets 2335

Droperidol (May increase drowsiness effect). Products include:
- Inapsine Injection 462

Estazolam (May increase drowsiness effect). Products include:
- ProSom Tablets 457

Ethchlorvynol (May increase drowsiness effect). Products include:
- Placidyl Capsules 456

Ethinamate (May increase drowsiness effect).
No products indexed under this heading.

Fluphenazine Decanoate (May increase drowsiness effect). Products include:
- Prolixin Decanoate 510

Fluphenazine Enanthate (May increase drowsiness effect). Products include:
- Prolixin Enanthate 510

Fluphenazine Hydrochloride (May increase drowsiness effect). Products include:
- Prolixin 510

Flurazepam Hydrochloride (May increase drowsiness effect). Products include:
- Dalmane Capsules 2329

Furazolidone (Concurrent and/or sequential use is not recommended). Products include:
- Furoxone 2221

Glutethimide (May increase drowsiness effect).
No products indexed under this heading.

Haloperidol (May increase drowsiness effect). Products include:
- Haldol Injection, Tablets and Concentrate 1585

Haloperidol Decanoate (May increase drowsiness effect). Products include:
- Haldol Decanoate 1587

Hydroxyzine Hydrochloride (May increase drowsiness effect). Products include:
- Atarax Tablets & Syrup 1992
- Marax Tablets & DF Syrup 2015
- Vistaril Intramuscular Solution 2042

Isocarboxazid (Concurrent and/or sequential use is not recommended).
No products indexed under this heading.

Lorazepam (May increase drowsiness effect). Products include:
- Ativan Injection 2805
- Ativan Tablets 2807

Loxapine Hydrochloride (May increase drowsiness effect). Products include:
- Loxitane 1426

Loxapine Succinate (May increase drowsiness effect). Products include:
- Loxitane Capsules 1426

Meprobamate (May increase drowsiness effect). Products include:
- Miltown Tablets 2780
- PMB 200 and PMB 400 2890

Mesoridazine Besylate (May increase drowsiness effect). Products include:
- Serentil 689

Midazolam Hydrochloride (May increase drowsiness effect). Products include:
- Versed Injection 2324

Molindone Hydrochloride (May increase drowsiness effect). Products include:
- Moban Tablets and Concentrate ... 1036

Oxazepam (May increase drowsiness effect). Products include:
- Serax Capsules 2916
- Serax Tablets 2916

Perphenazine (May increase drowsiness effect). Products include:
- Etrafon 2495
- Triavil Tablets 1800
- Trilafon 2532

Phenelzine Sulfate (Concurrent and/or sequential use is not recommended). Products include:
- Nardil 1977

Prazepam (May increase drowsiness effect).
No products indexed under this heading.

Prochlorperazine (May increase drowsiness effect). Products include:
- Compazine 2644

Promethazine Hydrochloride (May increase drowsiness effect). Products include:
- Mepergan Injection 2859
- Phenergan with Codeine 2883
- Phenergan with Dextromethorphan 2885
- Phenergan Injection 2880
- Phenergan Suppositories 2882
- Phenergan Syrup 2881
- Phenergan Tablets 2882
- Phenergan VC 2886
- Phenergan VC with Codeine 2888

Propofol (May increase drowsiness effect). Products include:
- Diprivan Injectable Emulsion 2939

Quazepam (May increase drowsiness effect). Products include:
- Doral Tablets 2773

Secobarbital Sodium (May increase drowsiness effect). Products include:
- Seconal Sodium Pulvules 1529

Selegiline Hydrochloride (Concurrent and/or sequential use is not recommended). Products include:
- Eldepryl Capsules 2729

Temazepam (May increase drowsiness effect). Products include:
- Restoril Capsules 2413

Thioridazine Hydrochloride (May increase drowsiness effect). Products include:
- Mellaril 2398

Thiothixene (May increase drowsiness effect). Products include:
- Navane Capsules and Concentrate 2018
- Navane Intramuscular 2019

Tranylcypromine Sulfate (Concurrent and/or sequential use is not recommended). Products include:
- Parnate Tablets 2679

Triazolam (May increase drowsiness effect). Products include:
- Halcion Tablets 2093

Trifluoperazine Hydrochloride (May increase drowsiness effect). Products include:
- Stelazine 2692

Zolpidem Tartrate (May increase drowsiness effect). Products include:
- Ambien Tablets 2559

Food Interactions
Alcohol (May increase drowsiness effect).

CHLORESIUM OINTMENT
(Chlorophyllin Copper Complex) 2371
None cited in PDR database.

CHLORESIUM SOLUTION
(Chlorophyllin Copper Complex) 2371
None cited in PDR database.

CHLOROMYCETIN OPHTHALMIC OINTMENT, 1%
(Chloramphenicol) 298
None cited in PDR database.

CHLOROMYCETIN OPHTHALMIC SOLUTION
(Chloramphenicol) 299
None cited in PDR database.

CHLOROMYCETIN SODIUM SUCCINATE
(Chloramphenicol Sodium Succinate) 1960
May interact with:

Bone Marrow Depressants, unspecified (Concurrent therapy should be avoided).

CHLOROPTIC S.O.P.
(Chloramphenicol) 236
None cited in PDR database.

CHLOROPTIC STERILE OPHTHALMIC SOLUTION
(Chloramphenicol) 236
None cited in PDR database.

CHLOR-TRIMETON ALLERGY DECONGESTANT TABLETS
(Chlorpheniramine Maleate, Pseudoephedrine Sulfate) 759
May interact with monoamine oxidase inhibitors, hypnotics and sedatives, tranquilizers, and certain other agents. Compounds in these categories include:

Alprazolam (May increase drowsiness effect). Products include:
- Xanax Tablets 2115

Buspirone Hydrochloride (May increase drowsiness effect). Products include:
- BuSpar Tablets 738

Chlordiazepoxide (May increase drowsiness effect). Products include:
- Limbitrol 2333

Chlordiazepoxide Hydrochloride (May increase drowsiness effect). Products include:
- Librax Capsules 2330
- Librium Capsules 2331
- Librium Injectable 2332

Chlorpromazine (May increase drowsiness effect). Products include:
- Thorazine Suppositories 2701

Chlorpromazine Hydrochloride (May increase drowsiness effect). Products include:
- Thorazine 2701

Chlorprothixene (May increase drowsiness effect).
No products indexed under this heading.

Chlorprothixene Hydrochloride (May increase drowsiness effect).
No products indexed under this heading.

Clorazepate Dipotassium (May increase drowsiness effect). Products include:
- Tranxene 459

Diazepam (May increase drowsiness effect). Products include:
- Dizac (diazepam injectable emulsion) CIV 1862
- Valium Injectable 2336
- Valium Tablets 2335

Droperidol (May increase drowsiness effect). Products include:
- Inapsine Injection 462

Estazolam (May increase drowsiness effect). Products include:
- ProSom Tablets 457

Ethchlorvynol (May increase drowsiness effect). Products include:
- Placidyl Capsules 456

Ethinamate (May increase drowsiness effect).
No products indexed under this heading.

Fluphenazine Decanoate (May increase drowsiness effect). Products include:
- Prolixin Decanoate 510

Fluphenazine Enanthate (May increase drowsiness effect). Products include:
- Prolixin Enanthate 510

Fluphenazine Hydrochloride (May increase drowsiness effect). Products include:
- Prolixin 510

Flurazepam Hydrochloride (May increase drowsiness effect). Products include:
- Dalmane Capsules 2329

Furazolidone (Concurrent and/or sequential use is not recommended). Products include:
- Furoxone 2221

Glutethimide (May increase drowsiness effect).
No products indexed under this heading.

Haloperidol (May increase drowsiness effect). Products include:
- Haldol Injection, Tablets and Concentrate 1585

Haloperidol Decanoate (May increase drowsiness effect). Products include:
- Haldol Decanoate 1587

Hydroxyzine Hydrochloride (May increase drowsiness effect). Products include:
- Atarax Tablets & Syrup 1992

IMPORTANT NOTE: Always consult each drug listing in the patient's regimen for possible interactions.

Chlor-Trimeton Allergy Decongestant · Interactions Index

Marax Tablets & DF Syrup............... 2015
Vistaril Intramuscular Solution 2042
Isocarboxazid (Concurrent and/or sequential use is not recommended).
 No products indexed under this heading.
Lorazepam (May increase drowsiness effect). Products include:
 Ativan Injection 2805
 Ativan Tablets 2807
Loxapine Hydrochloride (May increase drowsiness effect). Products include:
 Loxitane 1426
Loxapine Succinate (May increase drowsiness effect). Products include:
 Loxitane Capsules 1426
Meprobamate (May increase drowsiness effect). Products include:
 Miltown Tablets 2780
 PMB 200 and PMB 400 2890
Mesoridazine Besylate (May increase drowsiness effect). Products include:
 Serentil 689
Midazolam Hydrochloride (May increase drowsiness effect). Products include:
 Versed Injection 2324
Molindone Hydrochloride (May increase drowsiness effect). Products include:
 Moban Tablets and Concentrate ... 1036
Oxazepam (May increase drowsiness effect). Products include:
 Serax Capsules 2916
 Serax Tablets 2916
Perphenazine (May increase drowsiness effect). Products include:
 Etrafon 2495
 Triavil Tablets 1800
 Trilafon 2532
Phenelzine Sulfate (Concurrent and/or sequential use is not recommended). Products include:
 Nardil 1977
Prazepam (May increase drowsiness effect).
 No products indexed under this heading.
Prochlorperazine (May increase drowsiness effect). Products include:
 Compazine 2644
Promethazine Hydrochloride (May increase drowsiness effect). Products include:
 Mepergan Injection 2859
 Phenergan with Codeine 2883
 Phenergan with Dextromethorphan .. 2885
 Phenergan Injection 2880
 Phenergan Suppositories 2882
 Phenergan Syrup 2881
 Phenergan Tablets 2882
 Phenergan VC 2886
 Phenergan VC with Codeine 2888
Propofol (May increase drowsiness effect). Products include:
 Diprivan Injectable Emulsion 2939
Quazepam (May increase drowsiness effect). Products include:
 Doral Tablets 2773
Secobarbital Sodium (May increase drowsiness effect). Products include:
 Seconal Sodium Pulvules 1529
Selegiline Hydrochloride (Concurrent and/or sequential use is not recommended). Products include:
 Eldepryl Capsules 2729
Temazepam (May increase drowsiness effect). Products include:
 Restoril Capsules 2413
Thioridazine Hydrochloride (May increase drowsiness effect). Products include:
 Mellaril 2398
Thiothixene (May increase drowsiness effect). Products include:
 Navane Capsules and Concentrate .. 2018
 Navane Intramuscular 2019
Tranylcypromine Sulfate (Concurrent and/or sequential use is not recommended). Products include:
 Parnate Tablets 2679
Triazolam (May increase drowsiness effect). Products include:
 Halcion Tablets 2093
Trifluoperazine Hydrochloride (May increase drowsiness effect). Products include:
 Stelazine 2692
Zolpidem Tartrate (May increase drowsiness effect). Products include:
 Ambien Tablets 2559

Food Interactions
Alcohol (May increase drowsiness effect).

CHLOR-TRIMETON ALLERGY TABLETS
(Chlorpheniramine Maleate) 758
May interact with hypnotics and sedatives, tranquilizers, and certain other agents. Compounds in these categories include:

Alprazolam (Do not use concomitantly). Products include:
 Xanax Tablets 2115
Buspirone Hydrochloride (Do not use concomitantly). Products include:
 BuSpar Tablets 738
Chlordiazepoxide (Do not use concomitantly). Products include:
 Limbitrol 2333
Chlordiazepoxide Hydrochloride (Do not use concomitantly). Products include:
 Librax Capsules 2330
 Librium Capsules 2331
 Librium Injectable 2332
Chlorpromazine (Do not use concomitantly). Products include:
 Thorazine Suppositories 2701
Chlorpromazine Hydrochloride (Do not use concomitantly). Products include:
 Thorazine 2701
Chlorprothixene (Do not use concomitantly).
 No products indexed under this heading.
Chlorprothixene Hydrochloride (Do not use concomitantly).
 No products indexed under this heading.
Clorazepate Dipotassium (Do not use concomitantly). Products include:
 Tranxene 459
Diazepam (Do not use concomitantly). Products include:
 Dizac (diazepam injectable emulsion) CIV 1862
 Valium Injectable 2336
 Valium Tablets 2335
Droperidol (Do not use concomitantly). Products include:
 Inapsine Injection 462
Estazolam (Do not use concomitantly). Products include:
 ProSom Tablets 457
Ethchlorvynol (Do not use concomitantly). Products include:
 Placidyl Capsules 456
Ethinamate (Do not use concomitantly).
 No products indexed under this heading.
Fluphenazine Decanoate (Do not use concomitantly). Products include:
 Prolixin Decanoate 510
Fluphenazine Enanthate (Do not use concomitantly). Products include:
 Prolixin Enanthate 510
Fluphenazine Hydrochloride (Do not use concomitantly). Products include:
 Prolixin 510
Flurazepam Hydrochloride (Do not use concomitantly). Products include:
 Dalmane Capsules 2329
Glutethimide (Do not use concomitantly).
 No products indexed under this heading.
Haloperidol (Do not use concomitantly). Products include:
 Haldol Injection, Tablets and Concentrate 1585
Haloperidol Decanoate (Do not use concomitantly). Products include:
 Haldol Decanoate 1587
Hydroxyzine Hydrochloride (Do not use concomitantly). Products include:
 Atarax Tablets & Syrup 1992
 Marax Tablets & DF Syrup 2015
 Vistaril Intramuscular Solution ... 2042
Lorazepam (Do not use concomitantly). Products include:
 Ativan Injection 2805
 Ativan Tablets 2807
Loxapine Hydrochloride (Do not use concomitantly). Products include:
 Loxitane 1426
Loxapine Succinate (Do not use concomitantly). Products include:
 Loxitane Capsules 1426
Meprobamate (Do not use concomitantly). Products include:
 Miltown Tablets 2780
 PMB 200 and PMB 400 2890
Mesoridazine Besylate (Do not use concomitantly). Products include:
 Serentil 689
Midazolam Hydrochloride (Do not use concomitantly). Products include:
 Versed Injection 2324
Molindone Hydrochloride (Do not use concomitantly). Products include:
 Moban Tablets and Concentrate ... 1036
Oxazepam (Do not use concomitantly). Products include:
 Serax Capsules 2916
 Serax Tablets 2916
Perphenazine (Do not use concomitantly). Products include:
 Etrafon 2495
 Triavil Tablets 1800
 Trilafon 2532
Prazepam (Do not use concomitantly).
 No products indexed under this heading.
Prochlorperazine (Do not use concomitantly). Products include:
 Compazine 2644
Promethazine Hydrochloride (Do not use concomitantly). Products include:
 Mepergan Injection 2859
 Phenergan with Codeine 2883
 Phenergan with Dextromethorphan .. 2885
 Phenergan Injection 2880
 Phenergan Suppositories 2882
 Phenergan Syrup 2881
 Phenergan Tablets 2882
 Phenergan VC 2886
 Phenergan VC with Codeine 2888
Propofol (Do not use concomitantly). Products include:
 Diprivan Injectable Emulsion 2939
Quazepam (Do not use concomitantly). Products include:
 Doral Tablets 2773
Secobarbital Sodium (Do not use concomitantly). Products include:
 Seconal Sodium Pulvules 1529
Temazepam (Do not use concomitantly). Products include:
 Restoril Capsules 2413
Thioridazine Hydrochloride (Do not use concomitantly). Products include:
 Mellaril 2398
Thiothixene (Do not use concomitantly). Products include:
 Navane Capsules and Concentrate .. 2018
 Navane Intramuscular 2019
Triazolam (Do not use concomitantly). Products include:
 Halcion Tablets 2093
Trifluoperazine Hydrochloride (Do not use concomitantly). Products include:
 Stelazine 2692
Zolpidem Tartrate (Do not use concomitantly). Products include:
 Ambien Tablets 2559

Food Interactions
Alcohol (Do not use concomitantly).

CHOLERA VACCINE
(Cholera Vaccine) 2818
None cited in PDR database.

CHOLESTIN CAPSULES
(Homeopathic Medications) 2985

Food Interactions
Alcohol (Concurrent use in patients consuming more than 3 drinks per day is not recommended.)

CHROMAGEN CAPSULES
(Ferrous Fumarate, Vitamin C, Vitamin B_{12}) 2470
None cited in PDR database.

CHROMAGEN FA
(Ascorbic Acid, Cyanocobalamin, Ferrous Fumarate, Folic Acid) 2471
None cited in PDR database.

CHROMAGEN FORTE
(Ascorbic Acid, Cyanocobalamin, Ferrous Fumarate, Folic Acid) 2471
None cited in PDR database.

CILOXAN OPHTHALMIC SOLUTION
(Ciprofloxacin Hydrochloride) 468
May interact with xanthine bronchodilators, oral anticoagulants, and certain other agents. Compounds in these categories include:

Aminophylline (Systemic administration of quinolones elevates plasma concentrations of theophylline.)
 No products indexed under this heading.
Caffeine-containing medications (Interference with caffeine metabolism with systemic quinolones).
Cyclosporine (Concomitant administration with systemic quinolones may result in transient elevations in serum creatinine). Products include:
 Neoral 2405
 Sandimmune 2416

(▣ Described in PDR For Nonprescription Drugs)   (⊚ Described in PDR For Ophthalmology)

Dicumarol (Enhanced anticoagulant effect with systemic quinolones).
No products indexed under this heading.

Dyphylline (Systemic administration of quinolones elevates plasma concentrations of theophylline). Products include:
Lufyllin & Lufyllin-400 Tablets 2778
Lufyllin-GG Elixir & Tablets 2779

Theophylline (Systemic administration of quinolones elevates plasma concentrations of theophylline). Products include:
Marax Tablets & DF Syrup 2015
Quibron 2227

Theophylline Anhydrous (Systemic administration of quinolones elevates plasma concentrations of theophylline). Products include:
Aerolate 1003
Primatene Tablets 844
Respbid Tablets 687
Slo-bid Gyrocaps 2201
Theo-24 Extended Release Capsules 2753
Theo-Dur Extended-Release Tablets 1367
Theo-X Extended-Release Tablets .. 793
Uni-Dur Extended-Release Tablets .. 1374
Uniphyl 400 mg and 600 mg Tablets 2157

Theophylline Calcium Salicylate (Systemic administration of quinolones elevates plasma concentrations of theophylline). Products include:
Quadrinal Tablets 1398

Theophylline Sodium Glycinate (Systemic administration of quinolones elevates plasma concentrations of theophylline).
No products indexed under this heading.

Warfarin Sodium (Enhanced anticoagulant effect with systemic quinolones). Products include:
Coumadin 941

CIPRO I.V.
(Ciprofloxacin) **587**
May interact with oral anticoagulants and certain other agents. Compounds in these categories include:

Aminophylline (Potential for severe and fatal reactions including cardiac arrest, seizures, respiratory failure and status epilepticus; concurrent use should be avoided or serum levels of theophylline should be monitored carefully).
No products indexed under this heading.

Caffeine (Reduced clearance of caffeine and prolongation of its serum half-life). Products include:
Arthritis Strength BC Powder 631
BC Powder 631
Cafergot 2376
DHCplus Capsules 2148
Darvon Compound-65 Pulvules 1475
Esgic-plus Capsules 1012
Esgic-plus Tablets 1012
Aspirin Free Excedrin Analgesic Caplets and Geltabs 734
Excedrin Extra-Strength Analgesic Tablets, Caplets, and Geltabs 734
Fioricet Tablets 2386
Fioricet with Codeine Capsules 2387
Fiorinal Capsules 2388
Fiorinal with Codeine Capsules 2390
Fiorinal Tablets 2388
Goody's Extra Strength Headache Powders 632
Goody's Extra Strength Pain Relief Tablets 632
Maximum Strength Multi-Symptom Formula Midol 621
No Doz Maximum Strength Caplets 644
Norgesic 1554
Vanquish Analgesic Caplets 627
Wigraine Tablets 1884

Cyclosporine (Potential for transient elevations in serum creatinine). Products include:
Neoral 2405
Sandimmune 2416

Dicumarol (Enhanced effects of anticoagulant).
No products indexed under this heading.

Dyphylline (Potential for severe and fatal reactions including cardiac arrest, seizures, respiratory failure and status epilepticus; concurrent use should be avoided or serum levels of theophylline should be monitored carefully). Products include:
Lufyllin & Lufyllin-400 Tablets 2778
Lufyllin-GG Elixir & Tablets 2779

Probenecid (Interferes with renal tubular secretion and produces an increase in the level of ciprofloxacin). Products include:
Benemid Tablets 1651
ColBENEMID Tablets 1662

Theophylline (Potential for severe and fatal reactions including cardiac arrest, seizures, respiratory failure and status epilepticus; concurrent use should be avoided or serum levels of theophylline should be monitored carefully). Products include:
Marax Tablets & DF Syrup 2015
Quibron 2227

Theophylline Anhydrous (Potential for severe and fatal reactions including cardiac arrest, seizures, respiratory failure and status epilepticus; concurrent use should be avoided or serum levels of theophylline should be monitored carefully). Products include:
Aerolate 1003
Primatene Tablets 844
Respbid Tablets 687
Slo-bid Gyrocaps 2201
Theo-24 Extended Release Capsules 2753
Theo-Dur Extended-Release Tablets 1367
Theo-X Extended-Release Tablets .. 793
Uni-Dur Extended-Release Tablets .. 1374
Uniphyl 400 mg and 600 mg Tablets 2157

Theophylline Calcium Salicylate (Potential for severe and fatal reactions including cardiac arrest, seizures, respiratory failure and status epilepticus; concurrent use should be avoided or serum levels of theophylline should be monitored carefully). Products include:
Quadrinal Tablets 1398

Theophylline Sodium Glycinate (Potential for severe and fatal reactions including cardiac arrest, seizures, respiratory failure and status epilepticus; concurrent use should be avoided or serum levels of theophylline should be monitored carefully).
No products indexed under this heading.

Warfarin Sodium (Enhanced effects of anticoagulant). Products include:
Coumadin 941

CIPRO I.V. PHARMACY BULK PACKAGE
(Ciprofloxacin) **590**
May interact with oral anticoagulants and certain other agents. Compounds in these categories include:

Aminophylline (Potential for severe and fatal reactions including cardiac arrest, seizures, respiratory failure and status epilepticus; concurrent use should be avoided or serum levels of theophylline should be monitored carefully).
No products indexed under this heading.

Caffeine (Reduced clearance of caffeine and a prolongation of serum half-life). Products include:
Arthritis Strength BC Powder 631
BC Powder 631
Cafergot 2376
DHCplus Capsules 2148
Darvon Compound-65 Pulvules 1475
Esgic-plus Capsules 1012
Esgic-plus Tablets 1012
Aspirin Free Excedrin Analgesic Caplets and Geltabs 734
Excedrin Extra-Strength Analgesic Tablets, Caplets, and Geltabs 734
Fioricet Tablets 2386
Fioricet with Codeine Capsules 2387
Fiorinal Capsules 2388
Fiorinal with Codeine Capsules 2390
Fiorinal Tablets 2388
Goody's Extra Strength Headache Powders 632
Goody's Extra Strength Pain Relief Tablets 632
Maximum Strength Multi-Symptom Formula Midol 621
No Doz Maximum Strength Caplets 644
Norgesic 1554
Vanquish Analgesic Caplets 627
Wigraine Tablets 1884

Cyclosporine (Concomitant use may produce transient elevations in serum creatinine). Products include:
Neoral 2405
Sandimmune 2416

Dicumarol (Enhanced effects of oral anticoagulant).
No products indexed under this heading.

Dyphylline (Potential for severe and fatal reactions including cardiac arrest, seizures, respiratory failure and status epilepticus; concurrent use should be avoided or serum levels of theophylline should be monitored carefully). Products include:
Lufyllin & Lufyllin-400 Tablets 2778
Lufyllin-GG Elixir & Tablets 2779

Probenecid (Interferes with renal tubular secretion of ciprofloxacin). Products include:
Benemid Tablets 1651
ColBENEMID Tablets 1662

Theophylline (Potential for severe and fatal reactions including cardiac arrest, seizures, respiratory failure and status epilepticus; concurrent use should be avoided or serum levels of theophylline should be monitored carefully). Products include:
Marax Tablets & DF Syrup 2015
Quibron 2227

Theophylline Anhydrous (Potential for severe and fatal reactions including cardiac arrest, seizures, respiratory failure and status epilepticus; concurrent use should be avoided or serum levels of theophylline should be monitored carefully). Products include:
Aerolate 1003
Primatene Tablets 844
Respbid Tablets 687
Slo-bid Gyrocaps 2201
Theo-24 Extended Release Capsules 2753
Theo-Dur Extended-Release Tablets 1367
Theo-X Extended-Release Tablets .. 793
Uni-Dur Extended-Release Tablets .. 1374
Uniphyl 400 mg and 600 mg Tablets 2157

Theophylline Calcium Salicylate (Potential for severe and fatal reactions including cardiac arrest, seizures, respiratory failure and status epilepticus; concurrent use should be avoided or serum levels of theophylline should be monitored carefully). Products include:
Quadrinal Tablets 1398

Theophylline Sodium Glycinate (Potential for severe and fatal reactions including cardiac arrest, seizures, respiratory failure and status epilepticus; concurrent use should be avoided or serum levels of theophylline should be monitored carefully).
No products indexed under this heading.

Warfarin Sodium (Enhanced effects of oral anticoagulant). Products include:
Coumadin 941

CIPRO TABLETS
(Ciprofloxacin Hydrochloride) **584**
May interact with xanthine bronchodilators, antacids containing aluminium, calcium and magnesium, oral anticoagulants, iron containing oral preparations, and certain other agents. Compounds in these categories include:

Aluminum Carbonate (Concurrant administration of these antacids may substantially interfere with the oral absorption of ciprofloxacin; antacids may be administered either 2 hours after or 6 hours before ciprofloxacin dosing without a significant decrease in bioavailability). Products include:
Basaljel Capsules 2810
Basaljel Suspension 2810
Basaljel Tablets 2810

Aluminum Hydroxide (Concurrent administration of these antacids may substantially interfere with the oral absorption of ciprofloxacin; antacids may be administered either 2 hours after or 6 hours before ciprofloxacin dosing without a significant decrease in bioavailability). Products include:
ALternaGEL Liquid 1358
Maximum Strength Ascriptin 650
Cama Arthritis Pain Reliever 748
Gaviscon Extra Strength Relief Formula Antacid Tablets 778
Gaviscon Extra Strength Relief Formula Liquid Antacid 779
Gaviscon Liquid Antacid 779
Gelusil Antacid-Anti-gas Liquid 819
Gelusil Antacid-Anti-gas Tablets 819
Maalox Antacid/Anti-Gas Tablets 889
Maalox Heartburn Relief Suspension 658
Maalox Antacid Liquid 888
Extra Strength Maalox Antacid/Anti-Gas Liquid and Tablets 888
Mylanta 1359
Tempo Soft Antacid 799

Aluminum Hydroxide Gel (Concurrent administration of these antacids may substantially interfere with the oral absorption of ciprofloxacin; antacids may be administered either 2 hours after or 6 hours before ciprofloxacin dosing without a significant decrease in bioavailability). Products include:
ALternaGEL Liquid 675
Aludrox Oral Suspension 850
Amphojel Suspension 2802
Amphojel Suspension without Flavor 2802
Amphojel Tablets 2802
Ascriptin 650
Gaviscon Antacid Tablets 778
Gaviscon-2 Antacid Tablets 779
Mylanta Liquid 676
Mylanta Double Strength Liquid 676

IMPORTANT NOTE: Always consult each drug listing in the patient's regimen for possible interactions.

Nephrox Suspension ▣ 671

Aminophylline (Potential for severe and fatal reactions including cardiac arrest, seizures, respiratory failure and status epilepticus; concurrent use should be avoided or serum levels of theophylline should be monitored carefully).

No products indexed under this heading.

Caffeine (Reduced clearance of caffeine and a prolongation of its serum half-life). Products include:

Arthritis Strength BC Powder ▣ 631
BC Powder ▣ 631
Cafergot 2376
DHCplus Capsules 2148
Darvon Compound-65 Pulvules 1475
Esgic-plus Capsules 1012
Esgic-plus Tablets 1012
Aspirin Free Excedrin Analgesic Caplets and Geltabs 734
Excedrin Extra-Strength Analgesic Tablets, Caplets, and Geltabs 734
Fioricet Tablets 2386
Fioricet with Codeine Capsules 2387
Fiorinal Capsules 2388
Fiorinal with Codeine Capsules 2390
Fiorinal Tablets 2388
Goody's Extra Strength Headache Powders ▣ 632
Goody's Extra Strength Pain Relief Tablets ▣ 632
Maximum Strength Multi-Symptom Formula Midol ▣ 621
No Doz Maximum Strength Caplets ▣ 644
Norgesic 1554
Vanquish Analgesic Caplets ▣ 627
Wigraine Tablets 1884

Cyclosporine (Transient elevations in serum creatinine). Products include:

Neoral 2405
Sandimmune 2416

Dicumarol (Enhanced effects of anticoagulant).

No products indexed under this heading.

Dyphylline (Potential for severe and fatal reactions including cardiac arrest, seizures, respiratory failure and status epilepticus; concurrent use should be avoided or serum levels of theophylline should be monitored carefully). Products include:

Lufyllin & Lufyllin-400 Tablets 2778
Lufyllin-GG Elixir & Tablets 2779

Ferrous Fumarate (Concurrent administration of iron-containing products may substantially interfere with the oral absorption of ciprofloxacin). Products include:

Chromagen Capsules 2470
Chromagen FA 2471
Chromagen Forte 2471
Ferro-Sequels ▣ 684
Nephro-Fer Tablets 2168
Nephro-Fer Rx Tablets 2168
Nephro-Vite + Fe Tablets 2170
Stresstabs + Iron ▣ 685
Trinsicon Capsules 2759
Vitron-C Tablets ▣ 667

Ferrous Gluconate (Concurrent administration of iron-containing products may substantially interfere with the oral absorption of ciprofloxacin). Products include:

Megadose 513

Ferrous Sulfate (Concurrent administration of iron-containing products may substantially interfere with the oral absorption of ciprofloxacin). Products include:

Feosol Capsules ▣ 777
Feosol Elixir 2627
Feosol Tablets 2627
Fero-Folic-500 Filmtab 433
Fero-Grad-500 Filmtab 434
Fero-Gradumet Filmtab 434
Iberet Tablets 437
Iberet-500 Liquid 438
Iberet-Folic-500 Filmtab 433
Iberet-Liquid 438
Irospan 1000
Slow Fe Tablets 889
Slow Fe with Folic Acid 890

Fosphenytoin Sodium (Potential for change in serum phenytoin levels). Products include:

Cerebyx Injection 1956

Glyburide (Co-administration, on rare occasions, has resulted in severe hypoglycemia). Products include:

DiaBeta Tablets 1265
Glynase PresTab Tablets 2091
Micronase Tablets 2099

Magaldrate (Concurrent administration of these antacids may substantially interfere with the oral absorption of ciprofloxacin; antacids may be administered either 2 hours after or 6 hours before ciprofloxacin dosing without a significant decrease in bioavailability).

No products indexed under this heading.

Magnesium Hydroxide (Concurrent administration of these antacids may substantially interfere with the oral absorption of ciprofloxacin; antacids may be administered either 2 hours after or 6 hours before ciprofloxacin dosing without a significant decrease in bioavailability). Products include:

Aludrox Oral Suspension ▣ 850
Ascriptin ▣ 650
Di-Gel Antacid/Anti-Gas ▣ 762
Gelusil Antacid-Anti-gas Liquid ▣ 819
Gelusil Antacid-Anti-gas Tablets ▣ 819
Maalox Antacid/Anti-Gas Tablets 889
Maalox Antacid Liquid 888
Extra Strength Maalox Antacid/Anti-Gas Liquid and Tablets 888
Mylanta Fast-Acting 1359
Mylanta Gelcaps Antacid ▣ 678
Fast-Acting Mylanta Liquid Antacid 1359
Mylanta Tablets ▣ 677
Maximum-Strength Fast-Acting Mylanta Liquid Antacid 1359
Mylanta Double Strength Tablets ▣ 677
Phillips' Milk of Magnesia Liquid ▣ 627
Rolaids Antacid Tablets ▣ 807
Tempo Soft Antacid ▣ 799

Magnesium Oxide (Concurrent administration of these antacids may substantially interfere with the oral absorption of ciprofloxacin; antacids may be administered either 2 hours after or 6 hours before ciprofloxacin dosing without a significant decrease in bioavailability). Products include:

Beelith Tablets 632
Bufferin Analgesic Tablets ▣ 636
Arthritis Strength Bufferin Analgesic Caplets ▣ 637
Extra Strength Bufferin Analgesic Tablets ▣ 637
Caltrate PLUS ▣ 681
Cama Arthritis Pain Reliever ▣ 748
Mag-Ox 400 666
Uro-Mag 666

Phenytoin (Potential for change in serum phenytoin levels). Products include:

Dilantin Infatabs 1967
Dilantin-125 Suspension 1969

Phenytoin Sodium (Potential for change in serum phenytoin levels). Products include:

Dilantin Kapseals 1965

Polysaccharide-Iron Complex (Concurrent administration of iron-containing products may substantially interfere with the oral absorption of ciprofloxacin). Products include:

Niferex-150 Capsules 811
Niferex Elixir 811
Niferex-150 Forte Capsules 811
Niferex 811
Niferex-PN Tablets 811
Nu-Iron 150 Capsules 1826
Nu-Iron Elixir 1826

Probenecid (Interferes with renal tubular secretion of ciprofloxacin). Products include:

Benemid Tablets 1651
ColBENEMID Tablets 1662

Sucralfate (Substantially interferes with absorption of ciprofloxacin). Products include:

Carafate Suspension 1250
Carafate Tablets 1249

Theophylline (Potential for severe and fatal reactions including cardiac arrest, seizures, respiratory failure and status epilepticus; concurrent use should be avoided or serum levels of theophylline should be monitored carefully). Products include:

Marax Tablets & DF Syrup 2015
Quibron 2227

Theophylline Anhydrous (Potential for severe and fatal reactions including cardiac arrest, seizures, respiratory failure and status epilepticus; concurrent use should be avoided or serum levels of theophylline should be monitored carefully). Products include:

Aerolate 1003
Primatene Tablets ▣ 844
Respbid Tablets 687
Slo-bid Gyrocaps 2201
Theo-24 Extended Release Capsules 2753
Theo-Dur Extended-Release Tablets 1367
Theo-X Extended-Release Tablets 793
Uni-Dur Extended-Release Tablets 1374
Uniphyl 400 mg and 600 mg Tablets 2157

Theophylline Calcium Salicylate (Potential for severe and fatal reactions including cardiac arrest, seizures, respiratory failure and status epilepticus; concurrent use should be avoided or serum levels of theophylline should be monitored carefully). Products include:

Quadrinal Tablets 1398

Theophylline Sodium Glycinate (Potential for severe and fatal reactions including cardiac arrest, seizures, respiratory failure and status epilepticus; concurrent use should be avoided or serum levels of theophylline should be monitored carefully).

No products indexed under this heading.

Warfarin Sodium (Enhanced effects of anticoagulant). Products include:

Coumadin 941

Zinc Sulfate (Zinc-containing multivitamin preparations interfere with absorption of ciprofloxacin). Products include:

Clear Eyes ACR Astringent/Lubricant Eye Redness Reliever Eye Drops ◎ 314
Visine A.C. Seasonal Relief From Pollen and Dust ◎ 301

Food Interactions

Food, unspecified (Delays the absorption of the drug resulting in peak concentrations that are closer to 2 hours after dosing).

CITRACAL TABLETS

(Calcium Citrate) 1828
None cited in PDR database.

CITRUCEL ORANGE FLAVOR

(Methylcellulose) ▣ 770
None cited in PDR database.

CITRUCEL SUGAR FREE ORANGE FLAVOR

(Methylcellulose) ▣ 770
None cited in PDR database.

CLAFORAN STERILE AND INJECTION

(Cefotaxime Sodium) 1259
May interact with aminoglycosides. Compounds in this category include:

Amikacin Sulfate (Increased nephrotoxicity). Products include:

Amikacin Sulfate Injection, USP 523
Amikacin Sulfate Injection, USP 981
Amikin Injectable 502

Gentamicin Sulfate (Increased nephrotoxicity). Products include:

Garamycin Cream 0.1% 2501
Garamycin Injectable 2502
Garamycin Ointment 0.1% 2501
Garamycin Ophthalmic 2501
Genoptic Sterile Ophthalmic Solution ◎ 241
Genoptic Sterile Ophthalmic Ointment ◎ 241
Gentak ◎ 209
Pred-G Liquifilm Sterile Ophthalmic Suspension ◎ 248
Pred-G S.O.P. Sterile Ophthalmic Ointment ◎ 249

Kanamycin Sulfate (Increased nephrotoxicity).

No products indexed under this heading.

Streptomycin Sulfate (Increased nephrotoxicity). Products include:

Streptomycin Sulfate Injection 2031

Tobramycin (Increased nephrotoxicity). Products include:

AKTOB ◎ 207
TobraDex Ophthalmic Suspension and Ointment 469
Tobrex Ophthalmic Ointment and Solution ◎ 226

Tobramycin Sulfate (Increased nephrotoxicity). Products include:

Nebcin Vials, Hyporets & ADD-Vantage 1518

CLARITIN TABLETS

(Loratadine) 2485
May interact with drugs affecting hepatic drug metabolizing enzyme systems, xanthine bronchodilators, and certain other agents. Compounds in these categories include:

Aminophylline (The number of subjects who concomitantly received these drugs in the clinical trials is too small to rule out possible drug-drug interactions).

No products indexed under this heading.

Carbamazepine (Co-administration should be undertaken with caution until definitive interaction studies are completed). Products include:

Atretol Tablets 569
Tegretol/Tegretol-XR 870

Cimetidine (Increased plasma concentrations (AUC_{0-24} hours) of loratadine and/or decarboethoxyloratadine have been reported following co-administration; no clinically relevant changes in the safety profile of loratadine have been observed). Products include:

Tagamet HB Tablets ▣ 786
Tagamet Tablets 2694

Cimetidine Hydrochloride (Increased plasma concentrations (AUC_{0-24} hours) of loratadine and/or decarboethoxyloratadine have been reported following co-administration; no clinically relevant changes in the safety profile of loratadine have been observed). Products include:

Tagamet 2694

(▣ Described in PDR For Nonprescription Drugs) (◎ Described in PDR For Ophthalmology)

Dyphylline (The number of subjects who concomitantly received these drugs in the clinical trials is too small to rule out possible drug-drug interactions). Products include:
- Lufyllin & Lufyllin-400 Tablets 2778
- Lufyllin-GG Elixir & Tablets 2779

Erythromycin (Increased plasma concentrations (AUC$_{0-24}$ hours) of loratadine and/or decarboethoxyloratadine have been reported following co-administration; no clinically relevant changes in the safety profile of loratadine have been observed). Products include:
- A/T/S 2% Acne Topical Gel 1244
- A/T/S 2% Acne Topical Solution 1244
- Benzamycin Topical Gel 919
- E-Mycin Tablets 1388
- Emgel 2% Topical Gel 1081
- ERYC 1972
- Erycette (erythromycin 2%) Topical Solution 1943
- Ery-Tab Tablets 426
- Erythromycin Base Filmtab 430
- Erythromycin Delayed-Release Capsules, USP 431
- Ilotycin Ophthalmic Ointment............. 928
- PCE Dispertab Tablets 453
- T-Stat 2.0% Topical Solution and Pads 2797
- THERAMYCIN Z 2% Solution........... 1629

Erythromycin Estolate (Increased plasma concentrations (AUC$_{0-24}$ hours) of loratadine and/or decarboethoxyloratadine have been reported following co-administration; no clinically relevant changes in the safety profile of loratadine have been observed). Products include:
- Ilosone 927

Erythromycin Ethylsuccinate (Increased plasma concentrations (AUC$_{0-24}$ hours) of loratadine and/or decarboethoxyloratadine have been reported following co-administration; no clinically relevant changes in the safety profile of loratadine have been observed). Products include:
- E.E.S. 427
- EryPed 425
- Pediazole Suspension 2340

Erythromycin Gluceptate (Increased plasma concentrations (AUC$_{0-24}$ hours) of loratadine and/or decarboethoxyloratadine have been reported following co-administration; no clinically relevant changes in the safety profile of loratadine have been observed). Products include:
- Ilotycin Gluceptate, IV, Vials 929

Erythromycin Stearate (Increased plasma concentrations (AUC$_{0-24}$ hours) of loratadine and/or decarboethoxyloratadine have been reported following co-administration; no clinically relevant changes in the safety profile of loratadine have been observed). Products include:
- Erythrocin Stearate Filmtab 429

Fosphenytoin Sodium (Co-administration should be undertaken with caution until definitive interaction studies are completed). Products include:
- Cerebyx Injection 1956

Ketoconazole (Increased plasma concentrations (AUC$_{0-24}$ hours) of loratadine and/or decarboethoxyloratadine have been reported following co-administration; no clinically relevant changes in the safety profile of loratadine have been observed). Products include:
- Nizoral 2% Cream 1344
- Nizoral 2% Shampoo 1344
- Nizoral Tablets 1345

Phenobarbital (Co-administration should be undertaken with caution until definitive interaction studies are completed). Products include:
- Arco-Lase Plus Tablets 513
- Bellergal-S Tablets 2375
- Donnatal 2234
- Donnatal Extentabs 2234
- Donnatal Tablets 2234
- Phenobarbital Elixir and Tablets 1523
- Quadrinal Tablets 1398

Phenytoin (Co-administration should be undertaken with caution until definitive interaction studies are completed). Products include:
- Dilantin Infatabs 1967
- Dilantin-125 Suspension 1969

Phenytoin Sodium (Co-administration should be undertaken with caution until definitive interaction studies are completed). Products include:
- Dilantin Kapseals 1965

Ranitidine Hydrochloride (The number of subjects who concomitantly received these drugs in the clinical trials is too small to rule out possible drug-drug interactions). Products include:
- Zantac 1182
- Zantac Injection 1180
- Zantac Syrup 1182

Theophylline (The number of subjects who concomitantly received these drugs in the clinical trials is too small to rule out possible drug-drug interactions). Products include:
- Marax Tablets & DF Syrup............... 2015
- Quibron 2227

Theophylline Anhydrous (The number of subjects who concomitantly received these drugs in the clinical trials is too small to rule out possible drug-drug interactions). Products include:
- Aerolate 1003
- Primatene Tablets 844
- Respbid Tablets 687
- Slo-bid Gyrocaps 2201
- Theo-24 Extended Release Capsules 2753
- Theo-Dur Extended-Release Tablets 1367
- Theo-X Extended-Release Tablets .. 793
- Uni-Dur Extended-Release Tablets.. 1374
- Uniphyl 400 mg and 600 mg Tablets 2157

Theophylline Calcium Salicylate (The number of subjects who concomitantly received these drugs in the clinical trials is too small to rule out possible drug-drug interactions). Products include:
- Quadrinal Tablets 1398

Theophylline Sodium Glycinate (The number of subjects who concomitantly received these drugs in the clinical trials is too small to rule out possible drug-drug interactions).
No products indexed under this heading.

Food Interactions

Meal, unspecified (Food increases the AUC by approximately 73%, the time to peak plasma concentration is delayed by one-hour).

CLARITIN-D TABLETS
(Loratadine, Pseudoephedrine Sulfate) 2487
May interact with monoamine oxidase inhibitors, beta blockers, veratrum alkaloids, and cardiac glycosides. Compounds in these categories include:

Acebutolol Hydrochloride (Antihypertensive effects may be reduced by sympathomimetics). Products include:
- Sectral Capsules 2914

Atenolol (Antihypertensive effects may be reduced by sympathomimetics). Products include:
- Tenoretic Tablets............................. 2963
- Tenormin Tablets and I.V. Injection 2965

Betaxolol Hydrochloride (Antihypertensive effects may be reduced by sympathomimetics). Products include:
- Betoptic Ophthalmic Solution 465
- Betoptic S Ophthalmic Suspension 467
- Kerlone Tablets 2588

Bisoprolol Fumarate (Antihypertensive effects may be reduced by sympathomimetics). Products include:
- Zebeta Tablets 1457
- Ziac 1459

Carteolol Hydrochloride (Antihypertensive effects may be reduced by sympathomimetics). Products include:
- Cartrol Tablets 413
- Ocupress Ophthalmic Solution, 1% Sterile 297

Cimetidine (Increased plasma concentrations (AUC$_{0-24}$ hours) of loratadine and/or decarboethoxyloratadine have been reported following co-administration; no clinically relevant changes in the safety profile of loratadine have been observed). Products include:
- Tagamet HB Tablets.......................... 786
- Tagamet Tablets 2694

Cimetidine Hydrochloride (Increased plasma concentrations (AUC$_{0-24}$ hours) of loratadine and/or decarboethoxyloratadine have been reported following co-administration; no clinically relevant changes in the safety profile of loratadine have been observed). Products include:
- Tagamet.. 2694

Cryptenamine Preparations (Antihypertensive effects may be reduced by sympathomimetics).

Deslanoside (Increased ectopic pacemaker activity can occur when pseudoephedrine is used concomitantly with digitalis).
No products indexed under this heading.

Digitoxin (Increased ectopic pacemaker activity can occur when pseudoephedrine is used concomitantly with digitalis). Products include:
- Crystodigin Tablets.......................... 1472

Digoxin (Increased ectopic pacemaker activity can occur when pseudoephedrine is used concomitantly with digitalis). Products include:
- Lanoxicaps 1110
- Lanoxin Elixir Pediatric 1113
- Lanoxin Injection 1116
- Lanoxin Injection Pediatric.............. 1119
- Lanoxin Tablets 1121

Erythromycin (Increased plasma concentrations (AUC$_{0-24}$ hours) of loratadine and/or decarboethoxyloratadine have been reported following co-administration; plasma concentrations (AUC$_{0-24}$ hours) of eryhromycin decreased 15% with co-administration; no clinically relevant changes in the safety profile of loratadine have been observed). Products include:
- A/T/S 2% Acne Topical Gel 1244
- A/T/S 2% Acne Topical Solution.... 1244
- Benzamycin Topical Gel 919
- E-Mycin Tablets 1388
- Emgel 2% Topical Gel 1081
- ERYC 1972
- Erycette (erythromycin 2%) Topical Solution 1943
- Ery-Tab Tablets 426
- Erythromycin Base Filmtab 430
- Erythromycin Delayed-Release Capsules, USP 431
- Ilotycin Ophthalmic Ointment............. 928
- PCE Dispertab Tablets 453
- T-Stat 2.0% Topical Solution and Pads 2797
- THERAMYCIN Z 2% Solution........... 1629

Erythromycin Estolate (Increased plasma concentrations (AUC$_{0-24}$ hours) of loratadine and/or decarboethoxyloratadine have been reported following co-administration; plasma concentrations (AUC$_{0-24}$ hours) of eryhromycin decreased 15% with co-administration; no clinically relevant changes in the safety profile of loratadine have been observed). Products include:
- Ilosone 927

Erythromycin Ethylsuccinate (Increased plasma concentrations (AUC$_{0-24}$ hours) of loratadine and/or decarboethoxyloratadine have been reported following co-administration; plasma concentrations (AUC$_{0-24}$ hours) of eryhromycin decreased 15% with co-administration; no clinically relevant changes in the safety profile of loratadine have been observed). Products include:
- E.E.S. 427
- EryPed 425
- Pediazole Suspension 2340

Erythromycin Gluceptate (Increased plasma concentrations (AUC$_{0-24}$ hours) of loratadine and/or decarboethoxyloratadine have been reported following co-administration; plasma concentrations (AUC$_{0-24}$ hours) of eryhromycin decreased 15% with co-administration; no clinically relevant changes in the safety profile of loratadine have been observed). Products include:
- Ilotycin Gluceptate, IV, Vials 929

Erythromycin Stearate (Increased plasma concentrations (AUC$_{0-24}$ hours) of loratadine and/or decarboethoxyloratadine have been reported following co-administration; plasma concentrations (AUC$_{0-24}$ hours) of eryhromycin decreased 15% with co-administration; no clinically relevant changes in the safety profile of loratadine have been observed). Products include:
- Erythrocin Stearate Filmtab 429

Esmolol Hydrochloride (Antihypertensive effects may be reduced by sympathomimetics). Products include:
- Brevibloc (esmolol HCl) Injection 1860

Furazolidone (Concurrent and/or sequential use is contraindicated). Products include:
- Furoxone 2221

Isocarboxazid (Concurrent and/or sequential use is contraindicated).
No products indexed under this heading.

Ketoconazole (Increased plasma concentrations (AUC$_{0-24}$ hours) of loratadine and/or decarboethoxyloratadine have been reported following co-administration; no clinically relevant changes in the safety profile of loratadine have been observed). Products include:
- Nizoral 2% Cream 1344
- Nizoral 2% Shampoo 1344
- Nizoral Tablets 1345

IMPORTANT NOTE: Always consult each drug listing in the patient's regimen for possible interactions.

Interactions Index

Labetalol Hydrochloride (Antihypertensive effects may be reduced by sympathomimetics). Products include:
- Normodyne Injection 2519
- Normodyne Tablets 2522
- Trandate 1158

Levobunolol Hydrochloride (Antihypertensive effects may be reduced by sympathomimetics). Products include:
- Betagan .... ⊚ 230

Mecamylamine Hydrochloride (Antihypertensive effects may be reduced by sympathomimetics). Products include:
- Inversine Tablets 1729

Methyldopa (Antihypertensive effects may be reduced by sympathomimetics). Products include:
- Aldoclor Tablets 1638
- Aldomet Oral 1640
- Aldoril Tablets 1644

Methyldopate Hydrochloride (Antihypertensive effects may be reduced by sympathomimetics). Products include:
- Aldomet Ester HCl Injection .. 1642

Metipranolol Hydrochloride (Antihypertensive effects may be reduced by sympathomimetics). Products include:
- OptiPranolol (Metipranolol 0.3%) Sterile Ophthalmic Solution .... ⊚ 256

Metoprolol Succinate (Antihypertensive effects may be reduced by sympathomimetics). Products include:
- Toprol-XL Tablets 560

Metoprolol Tartrate (Antihypertensive effects may be reduced by sympathomimetics). Products include:
- Lopressor 848
- Lopressor HCT Tablets 850

Nadolol (Antihypertensive effects may be reduced by sympathomimetics).
No products indexed under this heading.

Penbutolol Sulfate (Antihypertensive effects may be reduced by sympathomimetics). Products include:
- Levatol Tablets 2547

Phenelzine Sulfate (Concurrent and/or sequential use is contraindicated). Products include:
- Nardil 1977

Pindolol (Antihypertensive effects may be reduced by sympathomimetics). Products include:
- Visken Tablets 2428

Propranolol Hydrochloride (Antihypertensive effects may be reduced by sympathomimetics). Products include:
- Inderal 2834
- Inderal LA Long Acting Capsules 2836
- Inderide Tablets 2838
- Inderide LA Long Acting Capsules .. 2840

Selegiline Hydrochloride (Concurrent and/or sequential use is contraindicated). Products include:
- Eldepryl Capsules 2729

Sotalol Hydrochloride (Antihypertensive effects may be reduced by sympathomimetics). Products include:
- Betapace Tablets 637

Timolol Hemihydrate (Antihypertensive effects may be reduced by sympathomimetics). Products include:
- Betimol 0.25%, 0.5% .... ⊚ 259

Timolol Maleate (Antihypertensive effects may be reduced by sympathomimetics). Products include:
- Blocadren Tablets 1654
- Timolide Tablets 1791
- Timoptic in Ocudose 1796
- Timoptic Sterile Ophthalmic Solution 1794
- Timoptic-XE 1798

Tranylcypromine Sulfate (Concurrent and/or sequential use is contraindicated). Products include:
- Parnate Tablets 2679

Food Interactions

Meal, unspecified (Food increases the AUC of loratadine by approximately 40% and of decarboethoxyloratadine by approximately 15%; the time of peak plasma concentration (T_{max}) of loratadine and decarboethoxyloratadine was delayed by 1 hour with meal.)

CLEAR EYES ACR ASTRINGENT/LUBRICANT EYE REDNESS RELIEVER EYE DROPS
(Zinc Sulfate, Naphazoline Hydrochloride) .... ⊚ 314
None cited in PDR database.

CLEAR EYES CLR SOOTHING DROPS
(Hydroxypropyl Methylcellulose) .... ⊚ 315
None cited in PDR database.

CLEAR EYES LUBRICANT EYE REDNESS RELIEVER
(Glycerin, Naphazoline Hydrochloride) .... ⊚ 314
None cited in PDR database.

CLEOCIN PHOSPHATE IV SOLUTION
(Clindamycin Phosphate) 2068
See **Cleocin Phosphate Sterile Solution**

CLEOCIN PHOSPHATE STERILE SOLUTION
(Clindamycin Phosphate) 2068
May interact with neuromuscular blocking agents, erythromycin, and certain other agents. Compounds in these categories include:

Atracurium Besylate (Clindamycin has been shown to have neuromuscular blocking properties that may enhance the action of other neuromuscular blocking agents). Products include:
- Tracrium Injection 1155

Cisatracurium Besylate (Clindamycin has been shown to have neuromuscular blocking properties that may enhance the action of other neuromuscular blocking agents). Products include:
- Nimbex Injection 1131

Diphenoxylate Hydrochloride (May prolong and/or worsen colitis). Products include:
- Lomotil 2591

Doxacurium Chloride (Clindamycin has been shown to have neuromuscular blocking properties that may enhance the action of other neuromuscular blocking agents). Products include:
- Nuromax Injection 1136

Erythromycin (Antagonism has been demonstrated between clindamycin and erythromycin in vitro; because of possible clinical significance, these two drugs should not be administered concurrently). Products include:
- A/T/S 2% Acne Topical Gel 1244
- A/T/S 2% Acne Topical Solution ... 1244
- Benzamycin Topical Gel 919
- E-Mycin Tablets 1388
- Emgel 2% Topical Gel 1081
- ERYC 1972
- Erycette (erythromycin 2%) Topical Solution 1943
- Ery-Tab Tablets 426
- Erythromycin Base Filmtab 430
- Erythromycin Delayed-Release Capsules, USP 431
- Ilotycin Ophthalmic Ointment..... 928
- PCE Dispertab Tablets 453
- T-Stat 2.0% Topical Solution and Pads 2797
- THERAMYCIN Z 2% Solution...... 1629

Erythromycin Estolate (Antagonism has been demonstrated between clindamycin and erythromycin in vitro; because of possible clinical significance, these two drugs should not be administered concurrently). Products include:
- Ilosone 927

Erythromycin Ethylsuccinate (Antagonism has been demonstrated between clindamycin and erythromycin in vitro; because of possible clinical significance, these two drugs should not be administered concurrently). Products include:
- E.E.S. 427
- EryPed 425
- Pediazole Suspension 2340

Erythromycin Gluceptate (Antagonism has been demonstrated between clindamycin and erythromycin in vitro; because of possible clinical significance, these two drugs should not be administered concurrently). Products include:
- Ilotycin Gluceptate, IV, Vials 929

Erythromycin Stearate (Antagonism has been demonstrated between clindamycin and erythromycin in vitro; because of possible clinical significance, these two drugs should not be administered concurrently). Products include:
- Erythrocin Stearate Filmtab 429

Metocurine Iodide (Clindamycin has been shown to have neuromuscular blocking properties that may enhance the action of other neuromuscular blocking agents). Products include:
- Metubine Iodide Vials 932

Mivacurium Chloride (Clindamycin has been shown to have neuromuscular blocking properties that may enhance the action of other neuromuscular blocking agents). Products include:
- Mivacron 1125

Pancuronium Bromide (Clindamycin has been shown to have neuromuscular blocking properties that may enhance the action of other neuromuscular blocking agents).
No products indexed under this heading.

Rocuronium Bromide (Clindamycin has been shown to have neuromuscular blocking properties that may enhance the action of other neuromuscular blocking agents). Products include:
- Zemuron Injection 1885

Succinylcholine Chloride (Clindamycin has been shown to have neuromuscular blocking properties that may enhance the action of other neuromuscular blocking agents). Products include:
- Anectine 1062

Vecuronium Bromide (Clindamycin has been shown to have neuromuscular blocking properties that may enhance the action of other neuromuscular blocking agents). Products include:
- Norcuron for Injection 1875

CLEOCIN T TOPICAL GEL
(Clindamycin Phosphate) 2072
May interact with neuromuscular blocking agents. Compounds in this category include:

Atracurium Besylate (Clindamycin has neuromuscular blocking properties that may enhance the action of other neuromuscular blocking agents). Products include:
- Tracrium Injection 1155

Cisatracurium Besylate (Clindamycin has neuromuscular blocking properties that may enhance the action of other neuromuscular blocking agents). Products include:
- Nimbex Injection 1131

Doxacurium Chloride (Clindamycin has neuromuscular blocking properties that may enhance the action of other neuromuscular blocking agents). Products include:
- Nuromax Injection 1136

Metocurine Iodide (Clindamycin has neuromuscular blocking properties that may enhance the action of other neuromuscular blocking agents). Products include:
- Metubine Iodide Vials 932

Mivacurium Chloride (Clindamycin has neuromuscular blocking properties that may enhance the action of other neuromuscular blocking agents). Products include:
- Mivacron 1125

Pancuronium Bromide (Clindamycin has neuromuscular blocking properties that may enhance the action of other neuromuscular blocking agents).
No products indexed under this heading.

Rocuronium Bromide (Clindamycin has neuromuscular blocking properties that may enhance the action of other neuromuscular blocking agents). Products include:
- Zemuron Injection 1885

Succinylcholine Chloride (Clindamycin has neuromuscular blocking properties that may enhance the action of other neuromuscular blocking agents). Products include:
- Anectine 1062

Vecuronium Bromide (Clindamycin has neuromuscular blocking properties that may enhance the action of other neuromuscular blocking agents). Products include:
- Norcuron for Injection 1875

CLEOCIN T TOPICAL LOTION
(Clindamycin Phosphate) 2072
See **Cleocin T Topical Gel**

CLEOCIN T TOPICAL SOLUTION
(Clindamycin Phosphate) 2072
See **Cleocin T Topical Gel**

CLIMARA TRANSDERMAL SYSTEM
(Estradiol) 640
May interact with progestins. Compounds in this category include:

Desogestrel (Potential for adverse effects on carbohydrate and lipid metabolism). Products include:
- Desogen Tablets 1867
- Ortho-Cept 1907

Medroxyprogesterone Acetate (Potential for adverse effects on carbohydrate and lipid metabolism). Products include:
- Amen Tablets 785
- Cycrin Tablets 991

(⊞ Described in PDR For Nonprescription Drugs)   (⊚ Described in PDR For Ophthalmology)

Interactions Index — Clinoril

Depo-Provera Contraceptive Injection 2079
Depo-Provera Sterile Aqueous Suspension 2083
Premphase 2900
Prempro 2905
Provera Tablets 2110

Megestrol Acetate (Potential for adverse effects on carbohydrate and lipid metabolism). Products include:
Megace Oral Suspension 708
Megace Tablets 710

Norgestimate (Potential for adverse effects on carbohydrate and lipid metabolism). Products include:
Ortho-Cyclen/Ortho-Tri-Cyclen 1914
Ortho-Cyclen/Ortho Tri-Cyclen 1914

CLEOCIN VAGINAL CREAM
(Clindamycin Phosphate) 2070
May interact with neuromuscular blocking agents. Compounds in this category include:

Atracurium Besylate (Enhanced action of neuromuscular blocking agents; caution is advised when co-administered). Products include:
Tracrium Injection 1155

Cisatracurium Besylate (Enhanced action of neuromuscular blocking agents; caution is advised when co-administered). Products include:
Nimbex Injection 1131

Doxacurium Chloride (Enhanced action of neuromuscular blocking agents; caution is advised when co-administered). Products include:
Nuromax Injection 1136

Metocurine Iodide (Enhanced action of neuromuscular blocking agents; caution is advised when co-administered). Products include:
Metubine Iodide Vials 932

Mivacurium Chloride (Enhanced action of neuromuscular blocking agents; caution is advised when co-administered). Products include:
Mivacron 1125

Pancuronium Bromide (Enhanced action of neuromuscular blocking agents; caution is advised when co-administered).
No products indexed under this heading.

Rocuronium Bromide (Enhanced action of neuromuscular blocking agents; caution is advised when co-administered). Products include:
Zemuron Injection 1885

Rubber or latex products (Use of such products within 72 hours following treatment with Cleocin Vaginal Cream is not recommended).

Succinylcholine Chloride (Enhanced action of neuromuscular blocking agents; caution is advised when co-administered). Products include:
Anectine 1062

Vecuronium Bromide (Enhanced action of neuromuscular blocking agents; caution is advised when co-administered). Products include:
Norcuron for Injection 1875

CLINICAL CARE DERMAL WOUND CLEANSER
(Benzethonium Chloride) 646
None cited in PDR database.

CLINORIL TABLETS
(Sulindac) 1658
May interact with oral anticoagulants, oral hypoglycemic agents, non-steroidal anti-inflammatory agents, and certain other agents.

Compounds in these categories include:

Acarbose (Special attention should be paid to patients taking higher doses than those recommended and to patients with renal or metabolic impairment). Products include:
Precose 604

Aspirin (Increased gastrointestinal reactions). Products include:
Alka-Seltzer Cherry Effervescent Antacid and Pain Reliever 609
Alka-Seltzer Extra Strength Effervescent Antacid and Pain Reliever 609
Alka-Seltzer Lemon Lime Effervescent Antacid and Pain Reliever 609
Alka-Seltzer Original Effervescent Antacid and Pain Reliever 609
Alka-Seltzer Plus 611
Alka-Seltzer Plus Sinus Medicine 611
Ascriptin 650
Arthritis Strength BC Powder 618
BC Cold Powder Multi-Symptom Formula (Cold-Sinus-Allergy) 631
BC Cold Powder Non-Drowsy Formula (Cold-Sinus) 631
BC Powder 631
Genuine Bayer Aspirin Tablets & Caplets 618
Extra Strength Bayer Arthritis Pain Regimen Formula 615
Extra Strength Bayer Aspirin Caplets & Tablets 617
Extended-Release Bayer 8-Hour Aspirin 616
Extra Strength Bayer Plus Aspirin Caplets 617
Extra Strength Bayer PM Aspirin Plus Sleep Aid 617
Aspirin Regimen Bayer 81 mg Tablets with Calcium 615
Aspirin Regimen Bayer Adult Low Strength 81 mg Tablets 613
Aspirin Regimen Bayer Children's Chewable Aspirin 616
Aspirin Regimen Bayer Regular Strength 325 mg Caplets 613
Bufferin Analgesic Tablets 636
Arthritis Strength Bufferin Analgesic Caplets 637
Extra Strength Bufferin Analgesic Tablets 637
Cama Arthritis Pain Reliever 748
Darvon Compound-65 Pulvules 1475
Easprin 1971
Ecotrin 2625
Ecotrin Enteric Coated Aspirin Maximum Strength Tablets and Caplets 775
Ecotrin Enteric Coated Aspirin Regular Strength Tablets 2625
Empirin Aspirin Tablets 818
Excedrin Extra-Strength Analgesic Tablets, Caplets, and Geltabs 734
Fiorinal Capsules 2388
Fiorinal with Codeine Capsules 2390
Fiorinal Tablets 2388
Goody's Extra Strength Headache Powders 632
Goody's Extra Strength Pain Relief Tablets 632
Halfprin Tablets 1413
Norgesic 1554
Percodan Tablets 955
Percodan-Demi Tablets 956
Robaxisal Tablets 2246
Soma Compound w/Codeine Tablets 2784
Soma Compound Tablets 2783
St. Joseph Adult Chewable Aspirin (81 mg.) 768
Talwin Compound 2466
Vanquish Analgesic Caplets 627

Aspirin, Enteric Coated (Increased gastrointestinal reactions).
No products indexed under this heading.

Chlorpropamide (Special attention should be paid to patients taking higher doses than those recommended and to patients with renal or metabolic impairment). Products include:
Diabinese Tablets 2002

Cyclosporine (Increased cyclosporine-induced toxicity). Products include:
Neoral 2405
Sandimmune 2416

DMSO (Reduced efficacy of sulindac; peripheral neuropathy).

Diclofenac Potassium (Concomitant use is not recommended due to the increased possibility of gastrointestinal toxicity, with little or no increase in efficacy). Products include:
Cataflam Tablets 833

Diclofenac Sodium (Concomitant use is not recommended due to the increased possibility of gastrointestinal toxicity, with little or no increase in efficacy). Products include:
Voltaren Ophthalmic Sterile Ophthalmic Solution 264
Cataflam/Voltaren/Voltaren-XR 833

Dicumarol (Special attention should be paid to patients taking higher doses than those recommended and to patients with renal or metabolic impairment).
No products indexed under this heading.

Diflunisal (Decreased plasma levels of sulindac). Products include:
Dolobid Tablets 1695

Etodolac (Concomitant use is not recommended due to the increased possibility of gastrointestinal toxicity, with little or no increase in efficacy). Products include:
Lodine Capsules and Tablets 2849

Fenoprofen Calcium (Concomitant use is not recommended due to the increased possibility of gastrointestinal toxicity, with little or no increase in efficacy). Products include:
Nalfon 200 Pulvules & Nalfon Tablets 933

Flurbiprofen (Concomitant use is not recommended due to the increased possibility of gastrointestinal toxicity, with little or no increase in efficacy).
No products indexed under this heading.

Furosemide (Clinoril may blunt the renal response to I.V. furosemide). Products include:
Lasix Injection, Oral Solution and Tablets 1267

Glimepiride (Special attention should be paid to patients taking higher doses than those recommended and to patients with renal or metabolic impairment). Products include:
Amaryl Tablets 1241

Glipizide (Special attention should be paid to patients taking higher doses than those recommended and to patients with renal or metabolic impairment). Products include:
Glucotrol Tablets 2011
Glucotrol XL Extended Release Tablets 2012

Glyburide (Special attention should be paid to patients taking higher doses than those recommended and to patients with renal or metabolic impairment). Products include:
DiaBeta Tablets 1265
Glynase PresTab Tablets 2091
Micronase Tablets 2099

Ibuprofen (Concomitant use is not recommended due to the increased possibility of gastrointestinal toxicity, with little or no increase in efficacy). Products include:
Advil Cold and Sinus Caplets and Tablets 837
Advil Ibuprofen Tablets, Caplets, and Gel Caplets 836

Children's Motrin Ibuprofen Oral Suspension 1558
IBU Tablets 1389
Ibuprohm 713
Motrin IB Caplets, Tablets, and Gelcaps 802
Motrin Ibuprofen Suspension, Oral Drops, Chewable Tablets, Caplets 1563
Nuprin Ibuprofen/Analgesic Tablets & Caplets 645
Vicks DayQuil SINUS Pressure & PAIN Relief with IBUPROFEN 735

Indomethacin (Concomitant use is not recommended due to the increased possibility of gastrointestinal toxicity, with little or no increase in efficacy). Products include:
Indocin 1723

Indomethacin Sodium Trihydrate (Concomitant use is not recommended due to the increased possibility of gastrointestinal toxicity, with little or no increase in efficacy). Products include:
Indocin I.V. 1727

Ketoprofen (Concomitant use is not recommended due to the increased possibility of gastrointestinal toxicity, with little or no increase in efficacy). Products include:
Actron Caplets and Tablets 608
Orudis Capsules 2874
Orudis KT 842
Oruvail Capsules 2874

Ketorolac Tromethamine (Concomitant use is not recommended due to the increased possibility of gastrointestinal toxicity, with little or no increase in efficacy). Products include:
Acular Sterile Ophthalmic Solution 470
Toradol 2319

Meclofenamate Sodium (Concomitant use is not recommended due to the increased possibility of gastrointestinal toxicity, with little or no increase in efficacy).
No products indexed under this heading.

Mefenamic Acid (Concomitant use is not recommended due to the increased possibility of gastrointestinal toxicity, with little or no increase in efficacy). Products include:
Ponstel 1982

Metformin Hydrochloride (Special attention should be paid to patients taking higher doses than those recommended and to patients with renal or metabolic impairment). Products include:
Glucophage Tablets 754

Methotrexate Sodium (Decreased tubular secretion of methotrexate and potentiation of its toxicity). Products include:
Methotrexate Sodium Tablets, Injection, for Injection and LPF Injection 1322

Nabumetone (Concomitant use is not recommended due to the increased possibility of gastrointestinal toxicity, with little or no increase in efficacy). Products include:
Relafen Tablets 2688

Naproxen (Concomitant use is not recommended due to the increased possibility of gastrointestinal toxicity, with little or no increase in efficacy). Products include:
Anaprox/Naprosyn 2277

Naproxen Sodium (Concomitant use is not recommended due to the increased possibility of gastrointestinal toxicity, with little or no increase in efficacy). Products include:
Aleve 2124
Anaprox/Naprosyn 2277
Naprelan Tablets 2861

IMPORTANT NOTE: Always consult each drug listing in the patient's regimen for possible interactions.

Clinoril / Interactions Index

Oxaprozin (Concomitant use is not recommended due to the increased possibility of gastrointestinal toxicity, with little or no increase in efficacy). Products include:
- Daypro Caplets 2578

Phenylbutazone (Concomitant use is not recommended due to the increased possibility of gastrointestinal toxicity, with little or no increase in efficacy).
- No products indexed under this heading.

Piroxicam (Concomitant use is not recommended due to the increased possibility of gastrointestinal toxicity, with little or no increase in efficacy). Products include:
- Feldene Capsules 2008

Probenecid (Increased plasma levels of sulindac; modest reduction in uricosuric action of probenecid). Products include:
- Benemid Tablets 1651
- ColBENEMID Tablets 1662

Tolazamide (Special attention should be paid to patients taking higher doses than those recommended and to patients with renal or metabolic impairment).
- No products indexed under this heading.

Tolbutamide (Special attention should be paid to patients taking higher doses than those recommended and to patients with renal or metabolic impairment).
- No products indexed under this heading.

Tolmetin Sodium (Concomitant use is not recommended due to the increased possibility of gastrointestinal toxicity, with little or no increase in efficacy). Products include:
- Tolectin (200, 400 and 600 mg) .. 1591

Warfarin Sodium (Special attention should be paid to patients taking higher doses than those recommended and to patients with renal or metabolic impairment). Products include:
- Coumadin 941

Food Interactions
Food, unspecified (The peak plasma concentrations of biologically active sulfide metabolite is delayed slightly in the presence of food).

CLOMID
(Clomiphene Citrate) 1262
None cited in PDR database.

CLORPACTIN WCS-90
(Sodium Oxychlorosene) 1236
None cited in PDR database.

CLOZARIL TABLETS
(Clozapine) 2377
May interact with antihypertensives, belladona products, benzodiazepines, antidepressant drugs, phenothiazines, selective serotonin reuptake inhibitors, and certain other agents. Compounds in these categories include:

Acebutolol Hydrochloride (Hypotensive effects potentiated). Products include:
- Sectral Capsules 2914

Alprazolam (Potential for profound collapse and respiratory depression). Products include:
- Xanax Tablets 2115

Amitriptyline Hydrochloride (Concomitant use of clozapine with other drugs metabolized by cytochrome P$_{450}$IID$_6$ may require lower than usual doses prescribed for either drug). Products include:
- Elavil 2945
- Etrafon 2495
- Limbitrol 2333
- Triavil Tablets 1800

Amlodipine Besylate (Hypotensive effects potentiated). Products include:
- Lotrel Capsules 858
- Norvasc Tablets 2020

Amoxapine (Concomitant use of clozapine with other drugs metabolized by cytochrome P$_{450}$IID$_6$ may require lower than usual doses prescribed for either drug). Products include:
- Asendin Tablets 1419

Atenolol (Hypotensive effects potentiated). Products include:
- Tenoretic Tablets 2963
- Tenormin Tablets and I.V. Injection 2965

Atropine Sulfate (Anticholinergic effects potentiated). Products include:
- Arco-Lase Plus Tablets 513
- Atrohist Plus Tablets 1605
- Donnatal 2234
- Donnatal Extentabs 2234
- Donnatal Tablets 2234
- Lomotil 2591
- Motofen Tablets 789
- Urised Tablets 2123

Belladonna Alkaloids (Anticholinergic effects potentiated). Products include:
- Bellergal-S Tablets 2375
- Hyland's Bedwetting Tablets 788
- Hyland's EnurAid Tablets 789
- Hyland's Headache Tablets... 790
- Hyland's Teething Tablets 790
- Similasan Eye Drops # 1 769

Benazepril Hydrochloride (Hypotensive effects potentiated). Products include:
- Lotensin Tablets 852
- Lotensin HCT Tablets 855
- Lotrel Capsules 858

Bendroflumethiazide (Hypotensive effects potentiated).
- No products indexed under this heading.

Betaxolol Hydrochloride (Hypotensive effects potentiated). Products include:
- Betoptic Ophthalmic Solution........... 465
- Betoptic S Ophthalmic Suspension ... 467
- Kerlone Tablets 2588

Bisoprolol Fumarate (Hypotensive effects potentiated). Products include:
- Zebeta Tablets 1457
- Ziac 1459

Bone Marrow Depressants, unspecified (Increases the risk and/or severity of bone marrow suppression).

Bupropion Hydrochloride (Concomitant use of clozapine with other drugs metabolized by cytochrome P$_{450}$IID$_6$ may require lower than usual doses prescribed for either drug). Products include:
- Wellbutrin Tablets 1177

Captopril (Hypotensive effects potentiated). Products include:
- Capoten Tablets 740
- Capozide Tablets 744

Carbamazepine (Concomitant use is not recommended; discontinuation of concomitant carbamazepine administration may result in increase in clozapine levels). Products include:
- Atretol Tablets 569
- Tegretol/Tegretol-XR 870

Carteolol Hydrochloride (Hypotensive effects potentiated). Products include:
- Cartrol Tablets 413
- Ocupress Ophthalmic Solution, 1% Sterile........................... 297

Chlordiazepoxide (Potential for profound collapse and respiratory depression). Products include:
- Limbitrol 2333

Chlordiazepoxide Hydrochloride (Potential for profound collapse and respiratory depression). Products include:
- Librax Capsules 2330
- Librium Capsules 2331
- Librium Injectable 2332

Chlorothiazide (Hypotensive effects potentiated). Products include:
- Aldoclor Tablets 1638
- Diupres Tablets 1691
- Diuril Oral 1694

Chlorothiazide Sodium (Hypotensive effects potentiated). Products include:
- Diuril Sodium Intravenous 1693

Chlorpromazine (Concomitant use of clozapine with other drugs metabolized by cytochrome P$_{450}$IID$_6$ may require lower than usual doses prescribed for either drug). Products include:
- Thorazine Suppositories 2701

Chlorpromazine Hydrochloride (Concomitant use of clozapine with other drugs metabolized by cytochrome P$_{450}$IID$_6$ may require lower than usual doses prescribed for either drug). Products include:
- Thorazine 2701

Chlorthalidone (Hypotensive effects potentiated). Products include:
- Combipres Tablets 682
- Tenoretic Tablets 2963
- Thalitone 1293

Cimetidine (May increase plasma levels of clozapine, potentially resulting in adverse effects). Products include:
- Tagamet HB Tablets............ 786
- Tagamet Tablets 2694

Cimetidine Hydrochloride (May increase levels of clozapine potentially resulting in adverse effects). Products include:
- Tagamet 2694

Clonidine (Hypotensive effects potentiated). Products include:
- Catapres-TTS 680

Clonidine Hydrochloride (Hypotensive effects potentiated). Products include:
- Catapres Tablets 679
- Combipres Tablets 682

Clorazepate Dipotassium (Potential for profound collapse and respiratory depression). Products include:
- Tranxene 459

CNS-Active Drugs, unspecified (Caution is advised).

Deserpidine (Hypotensive effects potentiated).
- No products indexed under this heading.

Desipramine Hydrochloride (Concomitant use of clozapine with other drugs metabolized by cytochrome P$_{450}$IID$_6$ may require lower than usual doses prescribed for either drug). Products include:
- Norpramin Tablets 1273

Diazepam (Potential for profound collapse and respiratory depression). Products include:
- Dizac (diazepam injectable emulsion) CIV 1862

Valium Injectable 2336
Valium Tablets 2335

Diazoxide (Hypotensive effects potentiated). Products include:
- Hyperstat I.V. Injection 2504
- Proglycem 575

Digitoxin (Potential for increased plasma levels and adverse effects). Products include:
- Crystodigin Tablets 1472

Digoxin (Increase in plasma concentrations resulting in adverse affects). Products include:
- Lanoxicaps 1110
- Lanoxin Elixir Pediatric 1113
- Lanoxin Injection 1116
- Lanoxin Injection Pediatric.... 1119
- Lanoxin Tablets 1121

Diltiazem Hydrochloride (Hypotensive effects potentiated). Products include:
- Cardizem CD Capsules 1251
- Cardizem SR Capsules 1255
- Cardizem Injectable 1253
- Cardizem Tablets 1257
- Dilacor XR Extended-release Capsules 2183
- Tiazac Capsules 1019

Doxazosin Mesylate (Hypotensive effects potentiated). Products include:
- Cardura Tablets 1993

Doxepin Hydrochloride (Concomitant use of clozapine with other drugs metabolized by cytochrome P$_{450}$IID$_6$ may require lower than usual doses prescribed for either drug). Products include:
- Adapin Capsules 1542
- Sinequan 2028
- Zonalon Cream 1042

Enalapril Maleate (Hypotensive effects potentiated). Products include:
- Vaseretic Tablets 1810
- Vasotec Tablets 1816

Enalaprilat (Hypotensive effects potentiated). Products include:
- Vasotec I.V. 1814

Encainide Hydrochloride (Concomitant use of clozapine with other drugs metabolized by cytochrome P$_{450}$IID$_6$ may require lower than usual doses.
- No products indexed under this heading.

Epinephrine Hydrochloride (Possible reverse epinephrine effect). Products include:
- Ana-Kit Anaphylaxis Emergency Treatment Kit 611

Esmolol Hydrochloride (Hypotensive effects potentiated). Products include:
- Brevibloc (esmolol HCl) Injection 1860

Estazolam (Potential for profound collapse and respiratory depression). Products include:
- ProSom Tablets 457

Felodipine (Hypotensive effects potentiated). Products include:
- Plendil Extended-Release Tablets ... 514

Flecainide Acetate (Concomitant use of clozapine with other drugs metabolized by cytochrome P$_{450}$IID$_6$ may require lower than usual doses prescribed for either drug). Products include:
- Tambocor Tablets 1555

Fluoxetine Hydrochloride (Concomitant use of clozapine with other drugs metabolized by cytochrome P$_{450}$IID$_6$ may require lower than usual doses prescribed for either drug). Products include:
- Prozac Pulvules & Liquid, Oral Solution 935

(▣ Described in PDR For Nonprescription Drugs) (◉ Described in PDR For Ophthalmology)

Fluphenazine Decanoate (Concomitant use of clozapine with other drugs metabolized by cytochrome P$_{450}$IID$_6$ may require lower than usual doses prescribed for either drug). Products include:
- Prolixin Decanoate 510

Fluphenazine Enanthate (Concomitant use of clozapine with other drugs metabolized by cytochrome P$_{450}$IID$_6$ may require lower than usual doses prescribed for either drug). Products include:
- Prolixin Enanthate 510

Fluphenazine Hydrochloride (Concomitant use of clozapine with other drugs metabolized by cytochrome P$_{450}$IID$_6$ may require lower than usual doses prescribed for either drug). Products include:
- Prolixin 510

Flurazepam Hydrochloride (Potential for profound collapse and respiratory depression). Products include:
- Dalmane Capsules 2329

Fluvoxamine Maleate (Concomitant use of clozapine with other drugs metabolized by cytochrome P$_{450}$IID$_6$ may require lower than usual doses prescribed for either drug). Products include:
- LUVOX Tablets 2723

Fosinopril Sodium (Hypotensive effects potentiated). Products include:
- Monopril Tablets 762

Furosemide (Hypotensive effects potentiated). Products include:
- Lasix Injection, Oral Solution and Tablets 1267

Guanabenz Acetate (Hypotensive effects potentiated).
No products indexed under this heading.

Guanethidine Monosulfate (Hypotensive effects potentiated). Products include:
- Esimil Tablets 840
- Ismelin Tablets 845

Halazepam (Potential for profound collapse and respiratory depression).
No products indexed under this heading.

Hydralazine Hydrochloride (Hypotensive effects potentiated). Products include:
- Apresazide Capsules 824
- Apresoline Hydrochloride Tablets .. 826
- Hydralazine Hydrochloride Injection USP 2712
- Ser-Ap-Es Tablets 867

Hydrochlorothiazide (Hypotensive effects potentiated). Products include:
- Aldactazide Tablets 2556
- Aldoril Tablets 1644
- Apresazide Capsules 824
- Capozide Tablets 744
- Dyazide Capsules 2653
- Esidrix Tablets 839
- Esimil Tablets 840
- HydroDIURIL Tablets 1716
- Hydropres Tablets 1718
- Hyzaar Tablets 1720
- Inderide Tablets 2838
- Inderide LA Long Acting Capsules .. 2840
- Lopressor HCT Tablets 850
- Lotensin HCT Tablets 855
- Moduretic Tablets 1748
- Oretic Tablets 450
- Prinzide Tablets 1780
- Ser-Ap-Es Tablets 867
- Timolide Tablets 1791
- Vaseretic Tablets 1810
- Zestoretic Tablets 2968
- Ziac 1459

Hydroflumethiazide (Hypotensive effects potentiated). Products include:
- Diucardin Tablets 2824

Hyoscyamine (Anticholinergic effects potentiated). Products include:
- Cystospaz Tablets 2123
- Urised Tablets 2123

Hyoscyamine Sulfate (Anticholinergic effects potentiated). Products include:
- Arco-Lase Plus Tablets 513
- Atrohist Plus Tablets 1605
- Cystospaz-M Capsules 2123
- Donnatal 2234
- Donnatal Extentabs 2234
- Donnatal Tablets 2234
- Kutrase Capsules 2546
- Levsin/Levsinex/Levbid 2549

Imipramine Hydrochloride (Concomitant use of clozapine with other drugs metabolized by cytochrome P$_{450}$IID$_6$ may require lower than usual doses prescribed for either drug). Products include:
- Tofranil Ampuls 873
- Tofranil Tablets 875

Imipramine Pamoate (Concomitant use of clozapine with other drugs metabolized by cytochrome P$_{450}$IID$_6$ may require lower than usual doses prescribed for either drug). Products include:
- Tofranil-PM Capsules 876

Indapamide (Hypotensive effects potentiated).
No products indexed under this heading.

Isocarboxazid (Concomitant use of clozapine with other drugs metabolized by cytochrome P$_{450}$IID$_6$ may require lower than usual doses prescribed for either drug).
No products indexed under this heading.

Isradipine (Hypotensive effects potentiated). Products include:
- DynaCirc Capsules 2381
- DynaCirc CR Tablets 2383

Labetalol Hydrochloride (Hypotensive effects potentiated). Products include:
- Normodyne Injection 2519
- Normodyne Tablets 2522
- Trandate 1158

Lisinopril (Hypotensive effects potentiated). Products include:
- Prinivil Tablets 1776
- Prinzide Tablets 1780
- Zestoretic Tablets 2968
- Zestril Tablets 2972

Lorazepam (Potential for profound collapse and respiratory depression). Products include:
- Ativan Injection 2805
- Ativan Tablets 2807

Losartan Potassium (Hypotensive effects potentiated). Products include:
- Cozaar Tablets 1668
- Hyzaar Tablets 1720

Maprotiline Hydrochloride (Concomitant use of clozapine with other drugs metabolized by cytochrome P$_{450}$IID$_6$ may require lower than usual doses prescribed for either drug). Products include:
- Ludiomil Tablets 861

Mecamylamine Hydrochloride (Hypotensive effects potentiated). Products include:
- Inversine Tablets 1729

Mesoridazine Besylate (Concomitant use of clozapine with other drugs metabolized by cytochrome P$_{450}$IID$_6$ may require lower than usual doses prescribed for either drug). Products include:
- Serentil 689

Methotrimeprazine (Concomitant use of clozapine with other drugs metabolized by cytochrome P$_{450}$IID$_6$ may require lower than usual doses prescribed for either drug). Products include:
- Levoprome 1321

Methyclothiazide (Hypotensive effects potentiated). Products include:
- Enduron Tablets 424

Methyldopa (Hypotensive effects potentiated). Products include:
- Aldoclor Tablets 1638
- Aldomet Oral 1640
- Aldoril Tablets 1644

Methyldopate Hydrochloride (Hypotensive effects potentiated). Products include:
- Aldomet Ester HCl Injection 1642

Metolazone (Hypotensive effects potentiated). Products include:
- Mykrox Tablets 1617
- Zaroxolyn Tablets 1625

Metoprolol Succinate (Hypotensive effects potentiated). Products include:
- Toprol-XL Tablets 560

Metoprolol Tartrate (Hypotensive effects potentiated). Products include:
- Lopressor 848
- Lopressor HCT Tablets 850

Metyrosine (Hypotensive effects potentiated). Products include:
- Demser Capsules 1690

Midazolam Hydrochloride (Potential for profound collapse and respiratory depression). Products include:
- Versed Injection 2324

Minoxidil (Hypotensive effects potentiated).
No products indexed under this heading.

Moexipril Hydrochloride (Hypotensive effects potentiated). Products include:
- Univasc Tablets 2553

Nadolol (Hypotensive effects potentiated).
No products indexed under this heading.

Nefazodone Hydrochloride (Concomitant use of clozapine with other drugs metabolized by cytochrome P$_{450}$IID$_6$ may require lower than usual doses prescribed for either drug). Products include:
- Serzone Tablets 776

Nicardipine Hydrochloride (Hypotensive effects potentiated). Products include:
- Cardene Capsules 2261
- Cardene I.V. 2815
- Cardene SR Capsules 2264

Nifedipine (Hypotensive effects potentiated). Products include:
- Adalat Capsules (10 mg and 20 mg) 580
- Adalat CC 582
- Procardia Capsules 2024
- Procardia XL Extended Release Tablets 2026

Nisoldipine (Hypotensive effects potentiated). Products include:
- Sular Tablets 2961

Nitroglycerin (Hypotensive effects potentiated). Products include:
- Deponit NTG Transdermal Delivery System 2541
- Nitro-Bid IV 1270
- Nitro-Bid Ointment 1272
- Nitro-Dur (nitroglycerin) Transdermal Infusion System 1365
- Nitrolingual Spray 2193
- Nitrostat Tablets 1981
- Transderm-Nitro Transdermal Therapeutic System 878

Norepinephrine Bitartrate (Possible reverse epinephrine effect). Products include:
- Levophed Bitartrate Injection 2445

Nortriptyline Hydrochloride (Concomitant use of clozapine with other drugs metabolized by cytochrome P$_{450}$IID$_6$ may require lower than usual doses prescribed for either drug). Products include:
- Pamelor 2409

Oxazepam (Potential for profound collapse and respiratory depression). Products include:
- Serax Capsules 2916
- Serax Tablets 2916

Paroxetine Hydrochloride (Concomitant use of clozapine with other drugs metabolized by cytochrome P$_{450}$IID$_6$ may require lower than usual doses prescribed for either drug). Products include:
- Paxil Tablets 2681

Penbutolol Sulfate (Hypotensive effects potentiated). Products include:
- Levatol Tablets 2547

Perphenazine (Concomitant use of clozapine with other drugs metabolized by cytochrome P$_{450}$IID$_6$ may require lower than usual doses prescribed for either drug). Products include:
- Etrafon 2495
- Triavil Tablets 1800
- Trilafon 2532

Phenelzine Sulfate (Concomitant use of clozapine with other drugs metabolized by cytochrome P$_{450}$IID$_6$ may require lower than usual doses prescribed for either drug). Products include:
- Nardil 1977

Phenoxybenzamine Hydrochloride (Hypotensive effects potentiated). Products include:
- Dibenzyline Capsules 2650

Phentolamine Mesylate (Hypotensive effects potentiated). Products include:
- Regitine Vials 864

Phenytoin (May decrease clozapine plasma levels, a decrease in effectiveness of a previously effective clozapine dose). Products include:
- Dilantin Infatabs 1967
- Dilantin-125 Suspension 1969

Phenytoin Sodium (May decrease clozapine plasma levels, a decrease in effectiveness of a previously effective clozapine dose). Products include:
- Dilantin Kapseals 1965

Pindolol (Hypotensive effects potentiated). Products include:
- Visken Tablets 2428

Polythiazide (Hypotensive effects potentiated). Products include:
- Minizide Capsules 2016

Prazepam (Potential for profound collapse and respiratory depression).
No products indexed under this heading.

Prazosin Hydrochloride (Hypotensive effects potentiated). Products include:
- Minipress Capsules 2015
- Minizide Capsules 2016

Prochlorperazine (Concomitant use of clozapine with other drugs metabolized by cytochrome P$_{450}$IID$_6$ may require lower than usual doses prescribed for either drug). Products include:
- Compazine 2644

IMPORTANT NOTE: Always consult each drug listing in the patient's regimen for possible interactions.

Clozaril / Interactions Index

Promethazine Hydrochloride (Concomitant use of clozapine with other drugs metabolized by cytochrome $P_{450}IID_6$ may require lower than usual doses prescribed for either drug). Products include:
- Mepergan Injection 2859
- Phenergan with Codeine 2883
- Phenergan with Dextromethorphan 2885
- Phenergan Injection 2880
- Phenergan Suppositories 2882
- Phenergan Syrup 2881
- Phenergan Tablets 2882
- Phenergan VC 2886
- Phenergan VC with Codeine 2888

Propafenone Hydrochloride (Concomitant use of clozapine with other drugs metabolized by cytochrome $P_{450}IID_6$ may require lower than usual doses prescribed for either drug). Products include:
- Rythmol Tablets–150mg, 225mg, 300mg 1399

Propranolol Hydrochloride (Hypotensive effects potentiated). Products include:
- Inderal 2834
- Inderal LA Long Acting Capsules 2836
- Inderide 2838
- Inderide LA Long Acting Capsules 2840

Protriptyline Hydrochloride (Concomitant use of clozapine with other drugs metabolized by cytochrome $P_{450}IID_6$ may require lower than usual doses prescribed for either drug). Products include:
- Vivactil Tablets 1820

Quazepam (Potential for profound collapse and respiratory depression). Products include:
- Doral Tablets 2773

Quinapril Hydrochloride (Hypotensive effects potentiated). Products include:
- Accupril Tablets 1950

Quinidine Gluconate (Concomitant use of clozapine with quinidine which inhibits cytochrome $P_{450}IID_6$ should be approached with caution). Products include:
- Quinaglute Dura-Tabs Tablets 644

Quinidine Polygalacturonate (Concomitant use of clozapine with quinidine which inhibits cytochrome $P_{450}IID_6$ should be approached with caution). Products include:
- Cardioquin Tablets 2146

Quinidine Sulfate (Concomitant use of clozapine with quinidine which inhibits cytochrome $P_{450}IID_6$ should be approached with caution). Products include:
- Quinidex Extentabs 2240

Ramipril (Hypotensive effects potentiated). Products include:
- Altace Capsules 1238

Rauwolfia Serpentina (Hypotensive effects potentiated).
No products indexed under this heading.

Rescinnamine (Hypotensive effects potentiated).
No products indexed under this heading.

Reserpine (Hypotensive effects potentiated). Products include:
- Diupres Tablets 1691
- Hydropres Tablets 1718
- Ser-Ap-Es Tablets 867

Scopolamine (Anticholinergic effects potentiated). Products include:
- Transderm Scōp Transdermal Therapeutic System 890

Scopolamine Hydrobromide (Anticholinergic effects potentiated). Products include:
- Atrohist Plus Tablets 1605
- Donnatal 2234
- Donnatal Extentabs 2234
- Donnatal Tablets 2234

Sertraline Hydrochloride (Concomitant use of clozapine with other drugs metabolized by cytochrome $P_{450}IID_6$ may require lower than usual doses prescribed for either drug). Products include:
- Zoloft Tablets 2051

Sodium Nitroprusside (Hypotensive effects potentiated).
No products indexed under this heading.

Sotalol Hydrochloride (Hypotensive effects potentiated). Products include:
- Betapace Tablets 637

Spirapril Hydrochloride (Hypotensive effects potentiated).
No products indexed under this heading.

Temazepam (Potential for profound collapse and respiratory depression). Products include:
- Restoril Capsules 2413

Terazosin Hydrochloride (Hypotensive effects potentiated). Products include:
- Hytrin Capsules 434

Thioridazine Hydrochloride (Concomitant use of clozapine with other drugs metabolized by cytochrome $P_{450}IID_6$ may require lower than usual doses prescribed for either drug). Products include:
- Mellaril 2398

Timolol Maleate (Hypotensive effects potentiated). Products include:
- Blocadren Tablets 1654
- Timolide Tablets 1791
- Timoptic in Ocudose 1796
- Timoptic Sterile Ophthalmic Solution 1794
- Timoptic-XE 1798

Torsemide (Hypotensive effects potentiated). Products include:
- Demadex Tablets and Injection 691

Tranylcypromine Sulfate (Concomitant use of clozapine with other drugs metabolized by cytochrome $P_{450}IID_6$ may require lower than usual doses prescribed for either drug). Products include:
- Parnate Tablets 2679

Trazodone Hydrochloride (Concomitant use of clozapine with other drugs metabolized by cytochrome $P_{450}IID_6$ may require lower than usual doses prescribed for either drug). Products include:
- Desyrel and Desyrel Dividose 504

Triazolam (Potential for profound collapse and respiratory depression). Products include:
- Halcion Tablets 2093

Trifluoperazine Hydrochloride (Concomitant use of clozapine with other drugs metabolized by cytochrome $P_{450}IID_6$ may require lower than usual doses prescribed for either drug). Products include:
- Stelazine 2692

Trimethaphan Camsylate (Hypotensive effects potentiated).
No products indexed under this heading.

Trimipramine Maleate (Concomitant use of clozapine with other drugs metabolized by cytochrome $P_{450}IID_6$ may require lower than usual doses prescribed for either drug). Products include:
- Surmontil Capsules 2917

Venlafaxine Hydrochloride (Concomitant use of clozapine with other drugs metabolized by cytochrome $P_{450}IID_6$ may require lower than usual doses prescribed for either drug). Products include:
- Effexor 2825

Verapamil Hydrochloride (Hypotensive effects potentiated). Products include:
- Calan SR Caplets 2571
- Calan Tablets 2568
- Covera-HS Tablets 2573
- Isoptin Injectable 1391
- Isoptin Oral Tablets 1393
- Isoptin SR Tablets 1395
- Verelan Capsules 1455

Warfarin Sodium (Potential for increased plasma levels and adverse effects). Products include:
- Coumadin 941

Food Interactions

Alcohol (Caution is advised with concomitant use).

COCAINE HYDROCHLORIDE TOPICAL SOLUTIONS
(Cocaine Hydrochloride) 529
None cited in PDR database.

CODICLEAR DH SYRUP
(Guaifenesin, Hydrocodone Bitartrate) 808
May interact with narcotic analgesics, hypnotics and sedatives, tranquilizers, central nervous system depressants, and certain other agents. Compounds in these categories include:

Alfentanil Hydrochloride (Additive CNS depression). Products include:
- Alfenta Injection 1334

Alprazolam (Additive CNS depression). Products include:
- Xanax Tablets 2115

Aprobarbital (Additive CNS depression).
No products indexed under this heading.

Buprenorphine (Additive CNS depression). Products include:
- Buprenex Injectable 2170

Buspirone Hydrochloride (Additive CNS depression). Products include:
- BuSpar Tablets 738

Butabarbital (Additive CNS depression).
No products indexed under this heading.

Butalbital (Additive CNS depression). Products include:
- Axocet Capsules 2469
- Esgic-plus Capsules 1012
- Esgic-plus Tablets 1012
- Fioricet Tablets 2386
- Fioricet with Codeine Capsules 2387
- Fiorinal Capsules 2388
- Fiorinal with Codeine Capsules 2390
- Fiorinal Tablets 2388
- Phrenilin 790
- Sedapap Tablets 50 mg/650 mg .. 1826

Chlordiazepoxide (Additive CNS depression). Products include:
- Limbitrol 2333

Chlordiazepoxide Hydrochloride (Additive CNS depression). Products include:
- Librax Capsules 2330
- Librium Capsules 2331
- Librium Injectable 2332

Chlorpromazine (Additive CNS depression). Products include:
- Thorazine Suppositories 2701

Chlorprothixene (Additive CNS depression).
No products indexed under this heading.

Chlorprothixene Hydrochloride (Additive CNS depression).
No products indexed under this heading.

Chlorprothixene Lactate (Additive CNS depression).
No products indexed under this heading.

Clorazepate Dipotassium (Additive CNS depression). Products include:
- Tranxene 459

Clozapine (Additive CNS depression). Products include:
- Clozaril Tablets 2377

Codeine Phosphate (Additive CNS depression). Products include:
- Brontex 2130
- Dimetane-DC Cough Syrup 2232
- Fioricet with Codeine Capsules 2387
- Fiorinal with Codeine Capsules 2390
- Nucofed 2225
- Phenergan with Codeine 2883
- Phenergan VC with Codeine 2888
- Robitussin A-C Syrup 2248
- Robitussin-DAC Syrup 2249
- Ryna 804
- Soma Compound w/Codeine Tablets 2784
- Tylenol with Codeine 1592

Desflurane (Additive CNS depression). Products include:
- Suprane (desflurane, USP) 1865

Dezocine (Additive CNS depression). Products include:
- Dalgan Injection 529

Diazepam (Additive CNS depression). Products include:
- Dizac (diazepam injectable emulsion) CIV 1862
- Valium Injectable 2336
- Valium Tablets 2335

Droperidol (Additive CNS depression). Products include:
- Inapsine Injection 462

Enflurane (Additive CNS depression).
No products indexed under this heading.

Estazolam (Additive CNS depression). Products include:
- ProSom Tablets 457

Ethchlorvynol (Additive CNS depression). Products include:
- Placidyl Capsules 456

Ethinamate (Additive CNS depression).
No products indexed under this heading.

Fentanyl (Additive CNS depression). Products include:
- Duragesic Transdermal System 1336

Fentanyl Citrate (Additive CNS depression). Products include:
- Sublimaze Injection 463

Fluphenazine Decanoate (Additive CNS depression). Products include:
- Prolixin Decanoate 510

Fluphenazine Enanthate (Additive CNS depression). Products include:
- Prolixin Enanthate 510

Fluphenazine Hydrochloride (Additive CNS depression). Products include:
- Prolixin 510

Flurazepam Hydrochloride (Additive CNS depression). Products include:
- Dalmane Capsules 2329

Glutethimide (Additive CNS depression).
No products indexed under this heading.

(⊞ Described in PDR For Nonprescription Drugs)   (⊙ Described in PDR For Ophthalmology)

Interactions Index — Cogentin

Haloperidol (Additive CNS depression). Products include:
- Haldol Injection, Tablets and Concentrate ... 1585

Haloperidol Decanoate (Additive CNS depression). Products include:
- Haldol Decanoate ... 1587

Hydrocodone Polistirex (Additive CNS depression). Products include:
- Tussionex Pennkinetic Extended-Release Suspension ... 1624

Hydromorphone Hydrochloride (Additive CNS depression). Products include:
- Dilaudid Ampules ... 1382
- Dilaudid Cough Syrup ... 1383
- Dilaudid-HP Injection ... 1384
- Dilaudid-HP Lyophilized Powder 250 mg ... 1384
- Dilaudid ... 1382
- Dilaudid Oral Liquid ... 1386
- Dilaudid ... 1382
- Dilaudid Tablets - 8 mg ... 1386

Hydroxyzine Hydrochloride (Additive CNS depression). Products include:
- Atarax Tablets & Syrup ... 1992
- Marax Tablets & DF Syrup ... 2015
- Vistaril Intramuscular Solution ... 2042

Isoflurane (Additive CNS depression).
- No products indexed under this heading.

Ketamine Hydrochloride (Additive CNS depression).
- No products indexed under this heading.

Levomethadyl Acetate Hydrochloride (Additive CNS depression). Products include:
- Orlaam Oral Solution ... 2361

Levorphanol Tartrate (Additive CNS depression). Products include:
- Levo-Dromoran ... 2297

Lorazepam (Additive CNS depression). Products include:
- Ativan Injection ... 2805
- Ativan Tablets ... 2807

Loxapine Hydrochloride (Additive CNS depression). Products include:
- Loxitane ... 1426

Loxapine Succinate (Additive CNS depression). Products include:
- Loxitane Capsules ... 1426

Meperidine Hydrochloride (Additive CNS depression). Products include:
- Demerol ... 2438
- Mepergan Injection ... 2859

Mephobarbital (Additive CNS depression). Products include:
- Mebaral Tablets ... 2452

Meprobamate (Additive CNS depression). Products include:
- Miltown Tablets ... 2780
- PMB 200 and PMB 400 ... 2890

Mesoridazine Besylate (Additive CNS depression). Products include:
- Serentil ... 689

Methadone Hydrochloride (Additive CNS depression). Products include:
- Methadone Hydrochloride Oral Concentrate ... 2356
- Methadone Hydrochloride Oral Solution & Tablets ... 2357

Methohexital Sodium (Additive CNS depression).
- No products indexed under this heading.

Methotrimeprazine (Additive CNS depression). Products include:
- Levoprome ... 1321

Methoxyflurane (Additive CNS depression).
- No products indexed under this heading.

Midazolam Hydrochloride (Additive CNS depression). Products include:
- Versed Injection ... 2324

Molindone Hydrochloride (Additive CNS depression). Products include:
- Moban Tablets and Concentrate ... 1036

Morphine Sulfate (Additive CNS depression). Products include:
- Astramorph/PF Injection, USP (Preservative-Free) ... 526
- Duramorph Injection ... 983
- Infumorph 200 and Infumorph 500 Sterile Solutions ... 985
- Kadian Capsules ... 2948
- MS Contin Tablets ... 2149
- MSIR ... 2152
- Oramorph SR (Morphine Sulfate Sustained Release Tablets) ... 2359
- RMS Suppositories CII ... 2766
- Roxanol ... 2365

Opium Alkaloids (Additive CNS depression).
- No products indexed under this heading.

Oxazepam (Additive CNS depression). Products include:
- Serax Capsules ... 2916
- Serax Tablets ... 2916

Oxycodone Hydrochloride (Additive CNS depression). Products include:
- OxyContin Tablets ... 2163
- OxyIR Capsules ... 2167
- Percocet Tablets ... 955
- Percodan Tablets ... 955
- Percodan-Demi Tablets ... 956
- Roxicodone Tablets, Oral Solution & Intensol (Oxycodone) ... 2366
- Tylox Capsules ... 1593

Pentobarbital Sodium (Additive CNS depression). Products include:
- Nembutal Sodium Capsules ... 440
- Nembutal Sodium Solution ... 442
- Nembutal Sodium Suppositories ... 444

Perphenazine (Additive CNS depression). Products include:
- Etrafon ... 2495
- Triavil Tablets ... 1800
- Trilafon ... 2532

Phenobarbital (Additive CNS depression). Products include:
- Arco-Lase Plus Tablets ... 513
- Bellergal-S Tablets ... 2375
- Donnatal ... 2234
- Donnatal Extentabs ... 2234
- Donnatal Tablets ... 2234
- Phenobarbital Elixir and Tablets ... 1523
- Quadrinal Tablets ... 1398

Prazepam (Additive CNS depression).
- No products indexed under this heading.

Prochlorperazine (Additive CNS depression). Products include:
- Compazine ... 2644

Promethazine Hydrochloride (Additive CNS depression). Products include:
- Mepergan Injection ... 2859
- Phenergan with Codeine ... 2883
- Phenergan with Dextromethorphan ... 2885
- Phenergan Injection ... 2880
- Phenergan Suppositories ... 2882
- Phenergan Syrup ... 2881
- Phenergan Tablets ... 2882
- Phenergan VC ... 2886
- Phenergan VC with Codeine ... 2888

Propofol (Additive CNS depression). Products include:
- Diprivan Injectable Emulsion ... 2939

Propoxyphene Hydrochloride (Additive CNS depression). Products include:
- Darvon ... 1475
- Wygesic Tablets ... 2930

Propoxyphene Napsylate (Additive CNS depression). Products include:
- Darvon-N/Darvocet-N ... 1473

Quazepam (Additive CNS depression). Products include:
- Doral Tablets ... 2773

Risperidone (Additive CNS depression). Products include:
- Risperdal Tablets ... 1348

Secobarbital Sodium (Additive CNS depression). Products include:
- Seconal Sodium Pulvules ... 1529

Sevoflurane (Additive CNS depression).
- No products indexed under this heading.

Sufentanil Citrate (Additive CNS depression). Products include:
- Sufenta Injection ... 1355

Temazepam (Additive CNS depression). Products include:
- Restoril Capsules ... 2413

Thiamylal Sodium (Additive CNS depression).
- No products indexed under this heading.

Thiothixene (Additive CNS depression). Products include:
- Navane Capsules and Concentrate ... 2018
- Navane Intramuscular ... 2019

Triazolam (Additive CNS depression). Products include:
- Halcion Tablets ... 2093

Trifluoperazine Hydrochloride (Additive CNS depression). Products include:
- Stelazine ... 2692

Zolpidem Tartrate (Additive CNS depression). Products include:
- Ambien Tablets ... 2559

Food Interactions

Alcohol (Additive CNS depression).

COENZYME Q10 200MG, 100MG & 60MG CHEWABLE WAFERS, AND 200MG, 60MG & 25MG TABLETS
(Coenzyme Q-10) ... 2768
None cited in PDR database.

COGENTIN INJECTION
(Benztropine Mesylate) ... 1661
May interact with phenothiazines, tricyclic antidepressants, belladona products, anticholinergics, butyrophenones, and dopamine antagonists. Compounds in these categories include:

Amitriptyline Hydrochloride (Potential for paralytic ileus, hyperthermia and heat stroke). Products include:
- Elavil ... 2945
- Etrafon ... 2495
- Limbitrol ... 2333
- Triavil Tablets ... 1800

Amoxapine (Potential for paralytic ileus, hyperthermia and heat stroke). Products include:
- Asendin Tablets ... 1419

Atropine Sulfate (Potential for paralytic ileus, hyperthermia and heat stroke). Products include:
- Arco-Lase Plus Tablets ... 513
- Atrohist Plus Tablets ... 1605
- Donnatal ... 2234
- Donnatal Extentabs ... 2234
- Donnatal Tablets ... 2234
- Lomotil ... 2591
- Motofen Tablets ... 789
- Urised Tablets ... 2123

Belladonna Alkaloids (Potential for paralytic ileus, hyperthermia and heat stroke). Products include:
- Bellergal-S Tablets ... 2375
- Hyland's Bedwetting Tablets ... ⊡ 788
- Hyland's EnurAid Tablets ... ⊡ 789
- Hyland's Headache Tablets ... ⊡ 790
- Hyland's Teething Tablets ... ⊡ 790
- Similasan Eye Drops #1 ... ⊡ 769

Biperiden Hydrochloride (Potential for paralytic ileus, hyperthermia and heat stroke). Products include:
- Akineton ... 1380

Chlorpromazine (Potential for paralytic ileus, hyperthermia and heat stroke). Products include:
- Thorazine Suppositories ... 2701

Clidinium Bromide (Potential for paralytic ileus, hyperthermia and heat stroke). Products include:
- Librax Capsules ... 2330

Clomipramine Hydrochloride (Potential for paralytic ileus, hyperthermia and heat stroke). Products include:
- Anafranil Capsules ... 819

Clozapine (Potential for paralytic ileus, hyperthermia and heat stroke). Products include:
- Clozaril Tablets ... 2377

Desipramine Hydrochloride (Potential for paralytic ileus, hyperthermia and heat stroke). Products include:
- Norpramin Tablets ... 1273

Dicyclomine Hydrochloride (Potential for paralytic ileus, hyperthermia and heat stroke). Products include:
- Bentyl ... 1246

Doxepin Hydrochloride (Potential for paralytic ileus, hyperthermia and heat stroke). Products include:
- Adapin Capsules ... 1542
- Sinequan ... 2028
- Zonalon Cream ... 1042

Fluphenazine Decanoate (Potential for paralytic ileus, hyperthermia and heat stroke). Products include:
- Prolixin Decanoate ... 510

Fluphenazine Enanthate (Potential for paralytic ileus, hyperthermia and heat stroke). Products include:
- Prolixin Enanthate ... 510

Fluphenazine Hydrochloride (Potential for paralytic ileus, hyperthermia and heat stroke). Products include:
- Prolixin ... 510

Glycopyrrolate (Potential for paralytic ileus, hyperthermia and heat stroke). Products include:
- Robinul Forte Tablets ... 2247
- Robinul Injectable ... 2247
- Robinul Tablets ... 2247

Haloperidol (Potential for paralytic ileus, hyperthermia and heat stroke). Products include:
- Haldol Injection, Tablets and Concentrate ... 1585

Haloperidol Decanoate (Potential for paralytic ileus, hyperthermia and heat stroke). Products include:
- Haldol Decanoate ... 1587

Hyoscyamine (Potential for paralytic ileus, hyperthermia and heat stroke). Products include:
- Cystospaz Tablets ... 2123
- Urised Tablets ... 2123

Hyoscyamine Sulfate (Potential for paralytic ileus, hyperthermia and heat stroke). Products include:
- Arco-Lase Plus Tablets ... 513
- Atrohist Plus Tablets ... 1605
- Cystospaz-M Capsules ... 2123
- Donnatal ... 2234
- Donnatal Extentabs ... 2234
- Donnatal Tablets ... 2234
- Kutrase Capsules ... 2546
- Levsin/Levsinex/Levbid ... 2549

Imipramine Hydrochloride (Potential for paralytic ileus, hyperthermia and heat stroke). Products include:
- Tofranil Ampuls ... 873
- Tofranil Tablets ... 875

IMPORTANT NOTE: Always consult each drug listing in the patient's regimen for possible interactions.

Cogentin | **Interactions Index** | **188**

Imipramine Pamoate (Potential for paralytic ileus, hyperthermia and heat stroke). Products include:

Tofranil-PM Capsules 876

Ipratropium Bromide (Potential for paralytic ileus, hyperthermia and heat stroke). Products include:

Atrovent Inhalation Aerosol 674
Atrovent Inhalation Solution 675
Atrovent Nasal Spray 0.03% 676
Atrovent Nasal Spray 0.06% 678

Maprotiline Hydrochloride (Potential for paralytic ileus, hyperthermia and heat stroke). Products include:

Ludiomil Tablets 861

Mepenzolate Bromide (Potential for paralytic ileus, hyperthermia and heat stroke).

No products indexed under this heading.

Mesoridazine Besylate (Potential for paralytic ileus, hyperthermia and heat stroke). Products include:

Serentil 689

Methotrimeprazine (Potential for paralytic ileus, hyperthermia and heat stroke). Products include:

Levoprome 1321

Metoclopramide Hydrochloride (Potential for paralytic ileus, hyperthermia and heat stroke). Products include:

Reglan 2243

Nortriptyline Hydrochloride (Potential for paralytic ileus, hyperthermia and heat stroke). Products include:

Pamelor 2409

Oxybutynin Chloride (Potential for paralytic ileus, hyperthermia and heat stroke). Products include:

Ditropan 1267

Perphenazine (Potential for paralytic ileus, hyperthermia and heat stroke). Products include:

Etrafon 2495
Triavil Tablets 1800
Trilafon 2532

Pimozide (Potential for paralytic ileus, hyperthermia and heat stroke). Products include:

Orap Tablets 1037

Prochlorperazine (Potential for paralytic ileus, hyperthermia and heat stroke). Products include:

Compazine 2644

Procyclidine Hydrochloride (Potential for paralytic ileus, hyperthermia and heat stroke). Products include:

Kemadrin Tablets 1105

Promethazine Hydrochloride (Potential for paralytic ileus, hyperthermia and heat stroke). Products include:

Mepergan Injection 2859
Phenergan with Codeine 2883
Phenergan with Dextromethorphan 2885
Phenergan Injection 2880
Phenergan Suppositories 2882
Phenergan Syrup 2881
Phenergan Tablets 2882
Phenergan VC 2886
Phenergan VC with Codeine 2888

Propantheline Bromide (Potential for paralytic ileus, hyperthermia and heat stroke). Products include:

Pro-Banthine Tablets 2226

Protriptyline Hydrochloride (Potential for paralytic ileus, hyperthermia and heat stroke). Products include:

Vivactil Tablets 1820

Scopolamine (Potential for paralytic ileus, hyperthermia and heat stroke). Products include:

Transderm Scōp Transdermal Therapeutic System 890

Scopolamine Hydrobromide (Potential for paralytic ileus, hyperthermia and heat stroke). Products include:

Atrohist Plus Tablets 1605
Donnatal 2234
Donnatal Extentabs 2234
Donnatal Tablets 2234

Thioridazine Hydrochloride (Potential for paralytic ileus, hyperthermia and heat stroke). Products include:

Mellaril 2398

Tridihexethyl Chloride (Potential for paralytic ileus, hyperthermia and heat stroke).

No products indexed under this heading.

Trifluoperazine Hydrochloride (Potential for paralytic ileus, hyperthermia and heat stroke). Products include:

Stelazine 2692

Trihexyphenidyl Hydrochloride (Potential for paralytic ileus, hyperthermia and heat stroke). Products include:

Artane 1418

Trimipramine Maleate (Potential for paralytic ileus, hyperthermia and heat stroke). Products include:

Surmontil Capsules 2917

COGENTIN TABLETS

(Benztropine Mesylate) 1661

See **Cogentin Injection**

COGNEX CAPSULES

(Tacrine Hydrochloride) 1961

May interact with xanthine bronchodilators, non-steroidal anti-inflammatory agents, cholinergic agents, anticholinergics, and certain other agents. Compounds in these categories include:

Aminophylline (Co-administration increases theophylline elimination half-life and average plasma theophylline concentrations by approximately 2-fold).

No products indexed under this heading.

Atropine Sulfate (Tacrine has potential to interfere with the activity of anticholinergic drugs). Products include:

Arco-Lase Plus Tablets 513
Atrohist Plus Tablets 1605
Donnatal 2234
Donnatal Extentabs 2234
Donnatal Tablets 2234
Lomotil 2591
Motofen Tablets 789
Urised Tablets 2123

Belladonna Alkaloids (Tacrine has potential to interfere with the activity of anticholinergic drugs). Products include:

Bellergal-S Tablets 2375
Hyland's Bedwetting Tablets ..... ◼ 788
Hyland's EnurAid Tablets ..... ◼ 789
Hyland's Headache Tablets ..... ◼ 790
Hyland's Teething Tablets ..... ◼ 790
Similasan Eye Drops #1 ..... ◼ 769

Benztropine Mesylate (Tacrine has potential to interfere with the activity of anticholinergic drugs). Products include:

Cogentin 1661

Bethanechol Chloride (Concurrent administration with cholinergic agonist may result in synergistic effect). Products include:

Urecholine 1804

Biperiden Hydrochloride (Tacrine has potential to interfere with the activity of anticholinergic drugs). Products include:

Akineton 1380

Cimetidine (Increases C_{max} and AUC of tacrine by approximately 54% and 64% respectively). Products include:

Tagamet HB Tablets ..... ◼ 786
Tagamet Tablets 2694

Cimetidine Hydrochloride (Increases C_{max} and AUC of tacrine by approximately 54% and 64% respectively). Products include:

Tagamet 2694

Clidinium Bromide (Tacrine has potential to interfere with the activity of anticholinergic drugs). Products include:

Librax Capsules 2330

Diclofenac Potassium (Patients receiving concurrent nonsteroidal anti-inflammatory agents are at increased risk for developing ulcers since tacrine may be expected to increase gastric acid secretion due to increased cholinergic activity). Products include:

Cataflam Tablets 833

Diclofenac Sodium (Patients receiving concurrent nonsteroidal anti-inflammatory agents are at increased risk for developing ulcers since tacrine may be expected to increase gastric acid secretion due to increased cholinergic activity). Products include:

Voltaren Ophthalmic Sterile Ophthalmic Solution ..... ◉ 264
Cataflam/Voltaren/Voltaren-XR 833

Dicyclomine Hydrochloride (Tacrine has potential to interfere with the activity of anticholinergic drugs). Products include:

Bentyl 1246

Dyphylline (Co-administration increases theophylline elimination half-life and average plasma theophylline concentrations by approximately 2-fold). Products include:

Lufyllin & Lufyllin-400 Tablets 2778
Lufyllin-GG Elixir & Tablets 2779

Edrophonium Chloride (Concurrent administration may result in synergistic effect). Products include:

Tensilon Injectable 1307

Etodolac (Patients receiving concurrent nonsteroidal anti-inflammatory agents are at increased risk for developing ulcers since tacrine may be expected to increase gastric acid secretion due to increased cholinergic activity). Products include:

Lodine Capsules and Tablets 2849

Fenoprofen Calcium (Patients receiving concurrent nonsteroidal anti-inflammatory agents are at increased risk for developing ulcers since tacrine may be expected to increase gastric acid secretion due to increased cholinergic activity). Products include:

Nalfon 200 Pulvules & Nalfon Tablets 933

Flurbiprofen (Patients receiving concurrent nonsteroidal anti-inflammatory agents are at increased risk for developing ulcers since tacrine may be expected to increase gastric acid secretion due to increased cholinergic activity).

No products indexed under this heading.

Glycopyrrolate (Tacrine has potential to interfere with the activity of anticholinergic drugs). Products include:

Robinul Forte Tablets 2247
Robinul Injectable 2247
Robinul Tablets 2247

Hyoscyamine (Tacrine has potential to interfere with the activity of anticholinergic drugs). Products include:

Cystospaz Tablets 2123
Urised Tablets 2123

Hyoscyamine Sulfate (Tacrine has potential to interfere with the activity of anticholinergic drugs). Products include:

Arco-Lase Plus Tablets 513
Atrohist Plus Tablets 1605
Cystospaz-M Capsules 2123
Donnatal 2234
Donnatal Extentabs 2234
Donnatal Tablets 2234
Kutrase Capsules 2546
Levsin/Levsinex/Levbid 2549

Ibuprofen (Patients receiving concurrent nonsteroidal anti-inflammatory agents are at increased risk for developing ulcers since tacrine may be expected to increase gastric acid secretion due to increased cholinergic activity). Products include:

Advil Cold and Sinus Caplets and Tablets ..... ◼ 837
Advil Ibuprofen Tablets, Caplets and Gel Caplets ..... ◼ 836
Children's Motrin Ibuprofen Oral Suspension 1558
IBU Tablets 1389
Ibuprohm ..... ◼ 713
Motrin IB Caplets, Tablets, and Gelcaps ..... ◼ 802
Motrin Ibuprofen Suspension, Oral Drops, Chewable Tablets, Caplets 1563
Nuprin Ibuprofen/Analgesic Tablets & Caplets ..... ◼ 645
Vicks DayQuil SINUS Pressure & PAIN Relief with IBUPROFEN ..... ◼ 735

Indomethacin (Patients receiving concurrent nonsteroidal anti-inflammatory agents are at increased risk for developing ulcers since tacrine may be expected to increase gastric acid secretion due to increased cholinergic activity). Products include:

Indocin 1723

Indomethacin Sodium Trihydrate (Patients receiving concurrent nonsteroidal anti-inflammatory agents are at increased risk for developing ulcers since tacrine may be expected to increase gastric acid secretion due to increased cholinergic activity). Products include:

Indocin I.V. 1727

Ipratropium Bromide (Tacrine has potential to interfere with the activity of anticholinergic drugs). Products include:

Atrovent Inhalation Aerosol 674
Atrovent Inhalation Solution 675
Atrovent Nasal Spray 0.03% 676
Atrovent Nasal Spray 0.06% 678

Ketoprofen (Patients receiving concurrent nonsteroidal anti-inflammatory agents are at increased risk for developing ulcers since tacrine may be expected to increase gastric acid secretion due to increased cholinergic activity). Products include:

Actron Caplets and Tablets ..... ◼ 608
Orudis Capsules 2874
Orudis KT ..... ◼ 842
Oruvail Capsules 2874

Ketorolac Tromethamine (Patients receiving concurrent nonsteroidal anti-inflammatory agents are at increased risk for developing ulcers since tacrine may be expected to increase gastric acid secretion due to increased cholinergic activity). Products include:

Acular Sterile Ophthalmic Solution 470
Toradol 2319

(◼ Described in PDR For Nonprescription Drugs) (◉ Described in PDR For Ophthalmology)

189 **Interactions Index** **ColBENEMID**

Meclofenamate Sodium (Patients receiving concurrent nonsteroidal anti-inflammatory agents are at increased risk for developing ulcers since tacrine may be expected to increase gastric acid secretion due to increased cholinergic activity).
- No products indexed under this heading.

Mefenamic Acid (Patients receiving concurrent nonsteroidal anti-inflammatory agents are at increased risk for developing ulcers since tacrine may be expected to increase gastric acid secretion due to increased cholinergic activity). Products include:
- Ponstel ... 1982

Mepenzolate Bromide (Tacrine has potential to interfere with the activity of anticholinergic drugs).
- No products indexed under this heading.

Nabumetone (Patients receiving concurrent nonsteroidal anti-inflammatory agents are at increased risk for developing ulcers since tacrine may be expected to increase gastric acid secretion due to increased cholinergic activity). Products include:
- Relafen Tablets ... 2688

Naproxen (Patients receiving concurrent nonsteroidal anti-inflammatory agents are at increased risk for developing ulcers since tacrine may be expected to increase gastric acid secretion due to increased cholinergic activity). Products include:
- Anaprox/Naprosyn ... 2277

Naproxen Sodium (Patients receiving concurrent nonsteroidal anti-inflammatory agents are at increased risk for developing ulcers since tacrine may be expected to increase gastric acid secretion due to increased cholinergic activity). Products include:
- Aleve ... 2124
- Anaprox/Naprosyn ... 2277
- Naprelan Tablets ... 2861

Neostigmine Bromide (Concurrent administration may result in synergistic effect). Products include:
- Prostigmin Tablets ... 1306

Neostigmine Methylsulfate (Concurrent administration may result in synergistic effect). Products include:
- Prostigmin Injectable ... 1305

Oxaprozin (Patients receiving concurrent nonsteroidal anti-inflammatory agents are at increased risk for developing ulcers since tacrine may be expected to increase gastric acid secretion due to increased cholinergic activity). Products include:
- Daypro Caplets ... 2578

Oxybutynin Chloride (Tacrine has potential to interfere with the activity of anticholinergic drugs). Products include:
- Ditropan ... 1267

Phenylbutazone (Patients receiving concurrent nonsteroidal anti-inflammatory agents are at increased risk for developing ulcers since tacrine may be expected to increase gastric acid secretion due to increased cholinergic activity).
- No products indexed under this heading.

Piroxicam (Patients receiving concurrent nonsteroidal anti-inflammatory agents are at increased risk for developing ulcers since tacrine may be expected to increase gastric acid secretion due to increased cholinergic activity). Products include:
- Feldene Capsules ... 2008

Procyclidine Hydrochloride (Tacrine has potential to interfere with the activity of anticholinergic drugs). Products include:
- Kemadrin Tablets ... 1105

Propantheline Bromide (Tacrine has potential to interfere with the activity of anticholinergic drugs). Products include:
- Pro-Banthine Tablets ... 2226

Pyridostigmine Bromide (Concurrent administration may result in synergistic effect). Products include:
- Mestinon Injectable ... 1300
- Mestinon ... 1300

Scopolamine (Tacrine has potential to interfere with the activity of anticholinergic drugs). Products include:
- Transderm Scōp Transdermal Therapeutic System ... 890

Scopolamine Hydrobromide (Tacrine has potential to interfere with the activity of anticholinergic drugs). Products include:
- Atrohist Plus Tablets ... 1605
- Donnatal ... 2234
- Donnatal Extentabs ... 2234
- Donnatal Tablets ... 2234

Succinylcholine Chloride (Tacrine, as a cholinesterase inhibitor, may exaggerate succinylcholine-type muscle relaxation during anesthesia). Products include:
- Anectine ... 1062

Sulindac (Patients receiving concurrent nonsteroidal anti-inflammatory agents are at increased risk for developing ulcers since tacrine may be expected to increase gastric acid secretion due to increased cholinergic activity). Products include:
- Clinoril Tablets ... 1658

Theophylline (Co-administration increases theophylline elimination half-life and average plasma theophylline concentrations by approximately 2-fold). Products include:
- Marax Tablets & DF Syrup ... 2015
- Quibron ... 2227

Theophylline Anhydrous (Co-administration increases theophylline elimination half-life and average plasma theophylline concentrations by approximately 2-fold). Products include:
- Aerolate ... 1003
- Primatene Tablets ... 844
- Respbid Tablets ... 687
- Slo-bid Gyrocaps ... 2201
- Theo-24 Extended Release Capsules ... 2753
- Theo-Dur Extended-Release Tablets ... 1367
- Theo-X Extended-Release Tablets .. 793
- Uni-Dur Extended-Release Tablets .. 1374
- Uniphyl 400 mg and 600 mg Tablets ... 2157

Theophylline Calcium Salicylate (Co-administration increases theophylline elimination half-life and average plasma theophylline concentrations by approximately 2-fold). Products include:
- Quadrinal Tablets ... 1398

Theophylline Sodium Glycinate (Co-administration increases theophylline elimination half-life and average plasma theophylline concentrations by approximately 2-fold).
- No products indexed under this heading.

Tolmetin Sodium (Patients receiving concurrent nonsteroidal anti-inflammatory agents are at increased risk for developing ulcers since tacrine may be expected to increase gastric acid secretion due to increased cholinergic activity). Products include:
- Tolectin (200, 400 and 600 mg) .. 1591

Tridihexethyl Chloride (Tacrine has potential to interfere with the activity of anticholinergic drugs).
- No products indexed under this heading.

Trihexyphenidyl Hydrochloride (Tacrine has potential to interfere with the activity of anticholinergic drugs). Products include:
- Artane ... 1418

Food Interactions

Food, unspecified (Food reduces tacrine bioavailability by approximately 30% to 40%; no effect if tacrine is administered at least one hour before meals).

COLACE CAPSULES, SYRUP, LIQUID
(Docusate Sodium) ... 2212
None cited in PDR database.

COLACE MICROENEMA
(Docusate Sodium) ... 2213
None cited in PDR database.

COLACE-T 50 MG TABLETS
(Docusate Sodium) ... 2213
None cited in PDR database.

COLACE-T 100 MG TABLETS
(Docusate Sodium) ... 2213
None cited in PDR database.

COLBENEMID TABLETS
(Probenecid, Colchicine) ... 1662
May interact with salicylates, sulfonamides, sulfonylureas, and certain other agents. Compounds in these categories include:

Acetaminophen (Co-administration increases the mean plasma elimination half-life of acetaminophen which can lead to increased plasma concentrations). Products include:
- Actifed Cold & Sinus Caplets and Tablets ... 808
- Actifed Sinus Daytime/Nighttime Tablets and Caplets ... 809
- Alka-Seltzer Fast Relief Caplets ... 610
- Alka-Seltzer Plus Liqui-Gels ... 612
- Alka-Seltzer Plus Flu & Body Aches Effervescent Tablets ... 612
- Alka-Seltzer Plus Flu & Body Aches Liqui-Gels Non-Drowsy Formula ... 613
- Alka-Seltzer Plus Night-Time Cold Medicine Liqui-Gels ... 612
- Allerest No Drowsiness ... 649
- Allerest Sinus Pain Formula ... 649
- Axocet Capsules ... 2469
- Benadryl Allergy/Cold Tablets ... 811
- Benadryl Allergy Sinus Headache Caplets ... 813
- Children's TYLENOL acetaminophen Chewable Tablets, Elixir, Suspension Liquid, and Suspension Drops ... 1559
- Children's TYLENOL Cold Multi-Symptom Chewable Tablets and Liquid ... 1559
- Children's TYLENOL Cold Plus Cough Multi Symptom Chewable Tablets and Liquid ... 1560
- Children's TYLENOL Flu Suspension Liquid ... 1560
- Allergy-Sinus Comtrex Multi-Symptom Allergy-Sinus Formula Tablets and Caplets ... 639
- Comtrex Multi-Symptom ... 638
- Comtrex Non-Drowsy ... 640
- Contac Day Allergy/Sinus Caplets ... 771
- Contac Day & Night ... 772
- Contac Night Allergy/Sinus Caplets ... 771
- Contac Severe Cold and Flu Formula Caplets ... 773
- Contac Severe Cold & Flu Non-Drowsy ... 774
- Coricidin Cold + Flu Tablets ... 760
- Coricidin 'D' Decongestant Tablets ... 760
- DHCplus Capsules ... 2148
- Darvon-N/Darvocet-N ... 1473
- Dimetapp Allergy Sinus Caplets ... 838
- Dimetapp Cold & Fever Suspension ... 839
- Drixoral Cold and Flu Extended-Release Tablets ... 764
- Drixoral Cough + Sore Throat Liquid Caps ... 763
- Drixoral Allergy/Sinus Extended Release Tablets ... 765
- Esgic-plus Capsules ... 1012
- Esgic-plus Tablets ... 1012
- Aspirin Free Excedrin Analgesic Caplets and Geltabs ... 734
- Excedrin Extra-Strength Analgesic Tablets, Caplets, and Geltabs ... 734
- Excedrin P.M. Analgesic/Sleeping Aid Tablets, Caplets, Liquigels ... 735
- Fioricet Tablets ... 2386
- Fioricet with Codeine Capsules ... 2387
- Goody's Extra Strength Headache Powders ... 632
- Goody's Extra Strength Pain Relief Tablets ... 632
- Hycomine Compound Tablets ... 948
- Hydrocet Capsules ... 787
- Infants' TYLENOL acetaminophen Suspension Drops ... 1559
- Infants' TYLENOL Cold Decongestant & Fever-Reducer Drops ... 1561
- Junior Strength TYLENOL acetaminophen Coated Caplets and Chewable Tablets ... 1562
- Lorcet 10/650 Tablets ... 1016
- Lortab ... 2751
- Lurline PMS Tablets ... 1000
- Maximum Strength Multi-Symptom Formula Midol ... 621
- PMS Multi-Symptom Formula Midol ... 622
- Maximum Strength Midol Teen Multi-Symptom Formula ... 621
- Midrin Capsules ... 788
- Panodol Tablets and Caplets ... 783
- Children's Panadol Chewable Tablets, Liquid, Infant's Drops ... 783
- Percocet Tablets ... 955
- Percogesic Analgesic Tablets ... 727
- Phrenilin ... 790
- Pyrroxate Caplets ... 742
- Robitussin Cold, Cough & Flu Liqui-Gels ... 844
- Robitussin Night-Time Cold Formula ... 847
- Sedapap Tablets 50 mg/650 mg .. 1826
- Sinarest ... 663
- Sine-Aid Maximum Strength Sinus Headache Gelcaps, Caplets and Tablets ... 1570
- Sine-Off No Drowsiness Formula Caplets ... 784
- Sine-Off Sinus Medicine ... 784
- Singlet Tablets ... 785
- Sinulin Tablets ... 792
- Sinutab Sinus Allergy Medication, Maximum Strength Tablets and Caplets ... 823
- Sinutab Sinus Medication, Maximum Strength Without Drowsiness Formula, Tablets & Caplets ... 824
- Sudafed Cold and Cough Liquid Caps ... 826
- Sudafed Severe Cold Formula Caplets ... 828
- Sudafed Severe Cold Formula Tablets ... 828
- Sudafed Sinus Caplets ... 829
- Sudafed Sinus Tablets ... 829
- Talacen Caplets ... 2464
- TheraFlu Flu and Cold Medicine ... 750
- Theraflu Maximum Strength Flu and Cold Medicine For Sore Throat ... 751
- TheraFlu Flu, Cold and Cough Medicine ... 750
- TheraFlu Maximum Strength Nighttime Flu, Cold & Cough Medicine ... 751

IMPORTANT NOTE: Always consult each drug listing in the patient's regimen for possible interactions.

ColBENEMID Interactions Index 190

TheraFlu Maximum Strength Non-Drowsy Formula Flu, Cold & Cough Medicine ▣ 751
TheraFlu Maximum Strength, Non-Drowsy Formula Flu, Cold and Cough Caplets ▣ 752
Theraflu Maximum Strength Sinus Non-Drowsy Formula Caplets ▣ 752
Triaminic Sore Throat Formula ▣ 755
Triaminicin Tablets ▣ 756
TYLENOL acetaminophen Extended Relief Caplets 1570
TYLENOL acetaminophen, Extra Strength Adult Liquid Pain Reliever 1570
TYLENOL acetaminophen, Extra Strength Gelcaps, Geltabs, Caplets, Tablets 1570
TYLENOL acetaminophen, Regular Strength Caplets and Tablets 1570
TYLENOL Allergy Sinus, Maximum Strength Caplets and Gelcaps 1571
TYLENOL Allergy Sinus NightTime, Maximum Strength Caplets 1571
TYLENOL Cold Medication, Multi-Symptom Formula Tablets and Caplets 1572
TYLENOL Cold Medication, Multi-Symptom Hot Liquid Packets 1572
TYLENOL Cold Medication, No Drowsiness Formula Caplets and Gelcaps 1572
TYLENOL Cold Severe Congestion Caplets 1573
TYLENOL Cough Medication, Multi Symptom 1574
TYLENOL Cough Medication with Decongestant, Multi Symptom 1574
TYLENOL Flu No Drowsiness Formula, Maximum Strength Gelcaps 1575
TYLENOL Flu NightTime, Maximum Strength Gelcaps 1575
TYLENOL Flu NightTime, Maximum Strength Hot Medication Packets 1575
TYLENOL Headache Plus Pain Reliever with Antacid, Extra Strength Caplets ▣ 705
TYLENOL PM Pain Reliever/Sleep Aid, Extra Strength Gelcaps, Caplets, Geltabs 1576
TYLENOL Severe Allergy Medication Caplets 1571
TYLENOL Sinus, Maximum Strength Geltabs, Gelcaps, Caplets and Tablets 1576
Tylenol with Codeine 1592
Tylox Capsules 1593
Unisom With Pain Relief-Nighttime Sleep Aid and Pain Reliever 1991
Vanquish Analgesic Caplets ▣ 627
Vicks 44 LiquiCaps Cough, Cold & Flu Relief ▣ 728
Vicks 44M Cough, Cold & Flu Relief ▣ 729
Vicks DayQuil LiquiCaps/Liquid Multi-Symptom Cold/Flu Relief ▣ 734
Vicks Nyquil Hot Therapy ▣ 735
Vicks NyQuil LiquiCaps/Liquid Multi-Symptom Cold/Flu Relief, Original and Cherry Flavors ▣ 736
Vicodin Tablets 1404
Vicodin ES Tablets 1405
Vicodin HP Tablets 1403
Wygesic Tablets 2930
Zydone Capsules 967

Aminosalicylic Acid (Probenecid inhibits renal transport of aminosalicylic acid). Products include:
PASER Granules 1333

Aminohippurate Sodium (Probenecid inhibits renal transport of amino hippuric acid). Products include:
Aminohippurate Sodium Injection 1646

Amoxicillin Trihydrate (Concurrent use of therapeutic dose of probenecid and penicillin or other beta-lactams results in higher plasma concentrations of penicillin or beta-lactam antibiotics resulting in increased side effects such as psychic disturbances). Products include:
Amoxil 2631
Augmentin 2637
Augmentin Tablets 2640

Ampicillin (Concurrent use of therapeutic dose of probenecid and penicillin or other beta-lactams results in higher plasma concentrations of penicillin or beta-lactam antibiotics resulting in increased side effects such as psychic disturbances). Products include:
Omnipen Capsules 2872
Omnipen for Oral Suspension 2873

Ampicillin Sodium (Concurrent use of therapeutic dose of probenecid and penicillin or other beta-lactams results in higher plasma concentrations of penicillin or beta-lactam antibiotics resulting in increased side effects such as psychic disturbances). Products include:
Unasyn 2035

Ampicillin Trihydrate (Concurrent use of therapeutic dose of probenecid and penicillin or other beta-lactams results in higher plasma concentrations of penicillin or beta-lactam antibiotics resulting in increased side effects such as psychic disturbances).
No products indexed under this heading.

Aspirin (Concurrent use with salicylates is contraindicated because salicylates antagonize the uricosuric action of probenecid). Products include:
Alka-Seltzer Cherry Effervescent Antacid and Pain Reliever ▣ 609
Alka-Seltzer Extra Strength Effervescent Antacid and Pain Reliever ▣ 609
Alka-Seltzer Lemon Lime Effervescent Antacid and Pain Reliever ▣ 609
Alka-Seltzer Original Effervescent Antacid and Pain Reliever ▣ 609
Alka-Seltzer Plus ▣ 611
Alka-Seltzer Plus Sinus Medicine ▣ 611
Ascriptin ▣ 650
Arthritis Strength BC Powder ▣ 631
BC Cold Powder Multi-Symptom Formula (Cold-Sinus-Allergy) ▣ 631
BC Cold Powder Non-Drowsy Formula (Cold-Sinus) ▣ 631
BC Powder ▣ 631
Genuine Bayer Aspirin Tablets & Caplets ▣ 618
Extra Strength Bayer Arthritis Pain Regimen Formula ▣ 615
Extra Strength Bayer Aspirin Caplets & Tablets ▣ 617
Extended-Release Bayer 8-Hour Aspirin ▣ 616
Extra Strength Bayer Plus Aspirin Caplets ▣ 617
Extra Strength Bayer PM Aspirin Plus Sleep Aid ▣ 617
Aspirin Regimen Bayer 81 mg Tablets with Calcium ▣ 615
Aspirin Regimen Bayer Adult Low Strength 81 mg Tablets ▣ 613
Aspirin Regimen Bayer Children's Chewable Aspirin ▣ 616
Aspirin Regimen Bayer Regular Strength 325 mg Caplets ▣ 613
Bufferin Analgesic Tablets ▣ 636
Arthritis Strength Bufferin Analgesic Caplets ▣ 637
Extra Strength Bufferin Analgesic Tablets ▣ 637
Cama Arthritis Pain Reliever ▣ 748
Darvon Compound-65 Pulvules 1475
Easprin 1971
Ecotrin 2625
Ecotrin Enteric Coated Aspirin Maximum Strength Tablets and Caplets ▣ 775
Ecotrin Enteric Coated Aspirin Regular Strength Tablets 2625
Empirin Aspirin Tablets ▣ 818
Excedrin Extra-Strength Analgesic Tablets, Caplets, and Geltabs 734
Fiorinal Capsules 2388
Fiorinal with Codeine Capsules 2390
Fiorinal Tablets 2388
Goody's Extra Strength Headache Powders ▣ 632
Goody's Extra Strength Pain Relief Tablets ▣ 632
Halfprin Tablets 1413
Norgesic 1554
Percodan Tablets 955
Percodan-Demi Tablets 956
Robaxisal Tablets 2246
Soma Compound w/Codeine Tablets 2784
Soma Compound Tablets 2783
St. Joseph Adult Chewable Aspirin (81 mg.) ▣ 768
Talwin Compound 2466
Vanquish Analgesic Caplets ▣ 627

Azlocillin Sodium (Concurrent use of therapeutic dose of probenecid and penicillin or other beta-lactams results in higher plasma concentrations of penicillin or beta-lactam antibiotics resulting in increased side effects such as psychic disturbances).
No products indexed under this heading.

Aztreonam (Concurrent use of therapeutic dose of probenecid and penicillin or other beta-lactams results in higher plasma concentrations of penicillin or beta-lactam antibiotics resulting in increased side effects such as psychic disturbances). Products include:
Azactam for Injection 736

Bacampicillin Hydrochloride (Concurrent use of therapeutic dose of probenecid and penicillin or other beta-lactams results in higher plasma concentrations of penicillin or beta-lactam antibiotics resulting in increased side effects such as psychic disturbances). Products include:
Spectrobid Tablets 2030

Bendroflumethiazide (Probenecid produces insignificant increase in free sulfonamide plasma concentrations but a significant increase in total sulfonamide plasma levels).
No products indexed under this heading.

Carbenicillin Disodium (Concurrent use of therapeutic dose of probenecid and penicillin or other beta-lactams results in higher plasma concentrations of penicillin or beta-lactam antibiotics resulting in increased side effects such as psychic disturbances).
No products indexed under this heading.

Carbenicillin Indanyl Sodium (Concurrent use of therapeutic dose of probenecid and penicillin or other beta-lactams results in higher plasma concentrations of penicillin or beta-lactam antibiotics resulting in increased side effects such as psychic disturbances). Products include:
Geocillin Tablets 2009

Cefaclor (Concurrent use of therapeutic dose of probenecid and penicillin or other beta-lactams results in higher plasma concentrations of penicillin or beta-lactam antibiotics resulting in increased side effects such as psychic disturbances). Products include:
Ceclor Pulvules & Suspension 1470

Cefadroxil (Concurrent use of therapeutic dose of probenecid and penicillin or other beta-lactams results in higher plasma concentrations of penicillin or beta-lactam antibiotics resulting in increased side effects such as psychic disturbances). Products include:
Duricef Capsules, Tablets, and Oral Suspension 750

Cefamandole Nafate (Concurrent use of therapeutic dose of probenecid and penicillin or other beta-lactams results in higher plasma concentrations of penicillin or beta-lactam antibiotics resulting in increased side effects such as psychic disturbances). Products include:
Mandol Vials, Faspak & ADD-Vantage 1516

Cefazolin Sodium (Concurrent use of therapeutic dose of probenecid and penicillin or other beta-lactams results in higher plasma concentrations of penicillin or beta-lactam antibiotics resulting in increased side effects such as psychic disturbances). Products include:
Ancef Injection 2632
Kefzol Vials, Faspak & ADD-Vantage 1511

Cefixime (Concurrent use of therapeutic dose of probenecid and penicillin or other beta-lactams results in higher plasma concentrations of penicillin or beta-lactam antibiotics resulting in increased side effects such as psychic disturbances). Products include:
Suprax 1443

Cefmetazole Sodium (Concurrent use of therapeutic dose of probenecid and penicillin or other beta-lactams results in higher plasma concentrations of penicillin or beta-lactam antibiotics resulting in increased side effects such as psychic disturbances).
No products indexed under this heading.

Cefonicid Sodium (Concurrent use of therapeutic dose of probenecid and penicillin or other beta-lactams results in higher plasma concentrations of penicillin or beta-lactam antibiotics resulting in increased side effects such as psychic disturbances). Products include:
Monocid Injection 2674

Cefoperazone Sodium (Concurrent use of therapeutic dose of probenecid and penicillin or other beta-lactams results in higher plasma concentrations of penicillin or beta-lactam antibiotics resulting in increased side effects such as psychic disturbances). Products include:
Cefobid Intravenous/Intramuscular 1996
Cefobid Pharmacy Bulk Package - Not for Direct Infusion 1999

Ceforanide (Concurrent use of therapeutic dose of probenecid and penicillin or other beta-lactams results in higher plasma concentrations of penicillin or beta-lactam antibiotics resulting in increased side effects such as psychic disturbances).
No products indexed under this heading.

Cefotaxime Sodium (Concurrent use of therapeutic dose of probenecid and penicillin or other beta-lactams results in higher plasma concentrations of penicillin or beta-lactam antibiotics resulting in increased side effects such as psychic disturbances). Products include:
Claforan Sterile and Injection 1259

Cefotetan (Concurrent use of therapeutic dose of probenecid and penicillin or other beta-lactams results in higher plasma concentrations of penicillin or beta-lactam antibiotics resulting in increased side effects such as psychic disturbances). Products include:
Cefotan 2936

(▣ Described in PDR For Nonprescription Drugs) (◉ Described in PDR For Ophthalmology)

Cefoxitin Sodium (Concurrent use of therapeutic dose of probenecid and penicillin or other beta-lactams results in higher plasma concentrations of penicillin or beta-lactam antibiotics resulting in increased side effects such as psychic disturbances). Products include:
- Mefoxin 1734
- Mefoxin Premixed Intravenous Solution 1737

Cefpodoxime Proxetil (Concurrent use of therapeutic dose of probenecid and penicillin or other beta-lactams results in higher plasma concentrations of penicillin or beta-lactam antibiotics resulting in increased side effects such as psychic disturbances). Products include:
- Vantin for Oral Suspension and Vantin Tablets 2112

Cefprozil (Concurrent use of therapeutic dose of probenecid and penicillin or other beta-lactams results in higher plasma concentrations of penicillin or beta-lactam antibiotics resulting in increased side effects such as psychic disturbances). Products include:
- Cefzil Tablets and Oral Suspension 747

Ceftazidime (Concurrent use of therapeutic dose of probenecid and penicillin or other beta-lactams results in higher plasma concentrations of penicillin or beta-lactam antibiotics resulting in increased side effects such as psychic disturbances). Products include:
- Ceptaz 1070
- Fortaz 1092
- Tazicef for Injection 2697
- Tazidime Vials, Faspak & ADD-Vantage 1531

Ceftizoxime Sodium (Concurrent use of therapeutic dose of probenecid and penicillin or other beta-lactams results in higher plasma concentrations of penicillin or beta-lactam antibiotics resulting in increased side effects such as psychic disturbances). Products include:
- Cefizox for Intramuscular or Intravenous Use 1025

Ceftriaxone Sodium (Concurrent use of therapeutic dose of probenecid and penicillin or other beta-lactams results in higher plasma concentrations of penicillin or beta-lactam antibiotics resulting in increased side effects such as psychic disturbances). Products include:
- Rocephin Injectable Vials, ADD-Vantage, Galaxy Container........ 2305

Cefuroxime Axetil (Concurrent use of therapeutic dose of probenecid and penicillin or other beta-lactams results in higher plasma concentrations of penicillin or beta-lactam antibiotics resulting in increased side effects such as psychic disturbances). Products include:
- Ceftin 1067

Cefuroxime Sodium (Concurrent use of therapeutic dose of probenecid and penicillin or other beta-lactams results in higher plasma concentrations of penicillin or beta-lactam antibiotics resulting in increased side effects such as psychic disturbances). Products include:
- Kefurox Vials, Faspak & ADD-Vantage 1509
- Zinacef 1184

Cephalexin (Concurrent use of therapeutic dose of probenecid and penicillin or other beta-lactams results in higher plasma concentrations of penicillin or beta-lactam antibiotics resulting in increased side effects such as psychic disturbances). Products include:
- Keflex Pulvules & Oral Suspension 930

Cephalothin Sodium (Concurrent use of therapeutic dose of probenecid and penicillin or other beta-lactams results in higher plasma concentrations of penicillin or beta-lactam antibiotics resulting in increased side effects such as psychic disturbances).

Cephapirin Sodium (Concurrent use of therapeutic dose of probenecid and penicillin or other beta-lactams results in higher plasma concentrations of penicillin or beta-lactam antibiotics resulting in increased side effects such as psychic disturbances).
- No products indexed under this heading.

Cephradine (Concurrent use of therapeutic dose of probenecid and penicillin or other beta-lactams results in higher plasma concentrations of penicillin or beta-lactam antibiotics resulting in increased side effects such as psychic disturbances).
- No products indexed under this heading.

Chlorothiazide (Probenecid produces insignificant increase in free sulfonamide plasma concentrations but a significant increase in total sulfonamide plasma levels). Products include:
- Aldoclor Tablets 1638
- Diupres Tablets 1691
- Diuril Oral 1694

Chlorothiazide Sodium (Probenecid produces insignificant increase in free sulfonamide plasma concentrations but a significant increase in total sulfonamide plasma levels). Products include:
- Diuril Sodium Intravenous 1693

Chlorpropamide (Probenecid may prolong or enhance the action of oral sulfonylureas and thereby increase the risk of hypoglycemia). Products include:
- Diabinese Tablets 2002

Choline Magnesium Trisalicylate (Concurrent use with salicylates is contraindicated because salicylates antagonize the uricosuric action of probenecid). Products include:
- Trilisate 2155

Cilastatin Sodium (Concurrent use of therapeutic dose of probenecid and penicillin or other beta-lactams results in higher plasma concentrations of penicillin or beta-lactam antibiotics resulting in increased side effects such as psychic disturbances). Products include:
- Primaxin I.M. 1770
- Primaxin I.V. 1772

Dicloxacillin Sodium (Concurrent use of therapeutic dose of probenecid and penicillin or other beta-lactams results in higher plasma concentrations of penicillin or beta-lactam antibiotics resulting in increased side effects such as psychic disturbances).
- No products indexed under this heading.

Diflunisal (Concurrent use with salicylates is contraindicated because salicylates antagonize the uricosuric action of probenecid). Products include:
- Dolobid Tablets 1695

Glimepiride (Probenecid may prolong or enhance the action of oral sulfonylureas and thereby increase the risk of hypoglycemia). Products include:
- Amaryl Tablets 1241

Glipizide (Probenecid may prolong or enhance the action of oral sulfonylureas and thereby increase the risk of hypoglycemia). Products include:
- Glucotrol Tablets 2011
- Glucotrol XL Extended Release Tablets 2012

Glyburide (Probenecid may prolong or enhance the action of oral sulfonylureas and thereby increase the risk of hypoglycemia). Products include:
- DiaBeta Tablets 1265
- Glynase PresTab Tablets 2091
- Micronase Tablets 2099

Hydrochlorothiazide (Probenecid produces insignificant increase in free sulfonamide plasma concentrations but a significant increase in total sulfonamide plasma levels). Products include:
- Aldactazide Tablets 2556
- Aldoril Tablets 1644
- Apresazide Capsules 824
- Capozide Tablets 744
- Dyazide Capsules 2653
- Esidrix Tablets 839
- Esimil Tablets 840
- HydroDIURIL Tablets 1716
- Hydropres Tablets 1718
- Hyzaar Tablets 1720
- Inderide Tablets 2838
- Inderide LA Long Acting Capsules .. 2840
- Lopressor HCT Tablets 850
- Lotensin HCT Tablets 855
- Moduretic Tablets 1748
- Oretic Tablets 450
- Prinzide Tablets 1780
- Ser-Ap-Es Tablets 867
- Timolide Tablets 1791
- Vaseretic Tablets 1810
- Zestoretic Tablets 2968
- Ziac 1459

Hydroflumethiazide (Probenecid produces insignificant increase in free sulfonamide plasma concentrations but a significant increase in total sulfonamide plasma levels). Products include:
- Diucardin Tablets 2824

Imipenem (Concurrent use of therapeutic dose of probenecid and penicillin or other beta-lactams results in higher plasma concentrations of penicillin or beta-lactam antibiotics resulting in increased side effects such as psychic disturbances). Products include:
- Primaxin I.M. 1770
- Primaxin I.V. 1772

Indomethacin (Co-administration increases the mean plasma elimination half-life of indomethacin which can lead to increased plasma concentrations). Products include:
- Indocin 1723

Indomethacin Sodium Trihydrate (Co-administration increases the mean plasma elimination half-life of indomethacin which can lead to increased plasma concentrations). Products include:
- Indocin I.V. 1727

Ketamine Hydrochloride (Potential for prolonged anesthesia based on animal data).
- No products indexed under this heading.

Ketoprofen (Co-administration increases the mean plasma elimination half-life of ketoprofen which can lead to increased plasma concentrations). Products include:
- Actron Caplets and Tablets 608
- Orudis Capsules 2874
- Orudis KT 842
- Oruvail Capsules 2874

Loracarbef (Concurrent use of therapeutic dose of probenecid and penicillin or other beta-lactams results in higher plasma concentrations of penicillin or beta-lactam antibiotics resulting in increased side effects such as psychic disturbances). Products include:
- Lorabid Suspension and Pulvules.... 1513

Lorazepam (Co-administration increases the mean plasma elimination half-life of lorazepam which can lead to increased plasma concentrations). Products include:
- Ativan Injection 2805
- Ativan Tablets 2807

Magnesium Salicylate (Concurrent use with salicylates is contraindicated because salicylates antagonize the uricosuric action of probenecid). Products include:
- Backache Caplets 635
- Doan's Extra-Strength Analgesic.... 653
- Extra Strength Doan's P.M. 653
- Doan's Regular Strength Analgesic 654
- Mobigesic Tablets 607

Meclofenamate Sodium (Co-administration increases the mean plasma elimination half-life of meclofenamate which can lead to increased plasma concentrations).
- No products indexed under this heading.

Methotrexate Sodium (Increased plasma concentrations of methotrexate which may result in methotrexate toxicity; dosage of methotrexate may need to be reduced and serum levels may need to be monitored if given concurrently). Products include:
- Methotrexate Sodium Tablets, Injection, for Injection and LPF Injection 1322

Methyclothiazide (Probenecid produces insignificant increase in free sulfonamide plasma concentrations but a significant increase in total sulfonamide plasma levels). Products include:
- Enduron Tablets 424

Mezlocillin Sodium (Concurrent use of therapeutic dose of probenecid and penicillin or other beta-lactams results in higher plasma concentrations of penicillin or beta-lactam antibiotics resulting in increased side effects such as psychic disturbances). Products include:
- Mezlin 594
- Mezlin Pharmacy Bulk Package........ 597

Nafcillin Sodium (Concurrent use of therapeutic dose of probenecid and penicillin or other beta-lactams results in higher plasma concentrations of penicillin or beta-lactam antibiotics resulting in increased side effects such as psychic disturbances).
- No products indexed under this heading.

Naproxen (Co-administration increases the mean plasma elimination half-life of naproxen which can lead to increased plasma concentrations). Products include:
- Anaprox/Naprosyn 2277

IMPORTANT NOTE: Always consult each drug listing in the patient's regimen for possible interactions.

Naproxen Sodium (Co-administration increases the mean plasma elimination half-life of naproxen which can lead to increased plasma concentrations). Products include:
- Aleve 2124
- Anaprox/Naprosyn 2277
- Naprelan Tablets 2861

Penicillin G Benzathine (Concurrent use of therapeutic dose of probenecid and penicillin or other beta-lactams results in higher plasma concentrations of penicillin or beta-lactam antibiotics resulting in increased side effects such as psychic disturbances). Products include:
- Bicillin C-R Injection 2810
- Bicillin C-R 900/300 Injection 2812
- Bicillin L-A Injection 2813

Penicillin G Potassium (Concurrent use of therapeutic dose of probenecid and penicillin or other beta-lactams results in higher plasma concentrations of penicillin or beta-lactam antibiotics resulting in increased side effects such as psychic disturbances). Products include:
- Pfizerpen for Injection 2022

Penicillin G Procaine (Concurrent use of therapeutic dose of probenecid and penicillin or other beta-lactams results in higher plasma concentrations of penicillin or beta-lactam antibiotics resulting in increased side effects such as psychic disturbances). Products include:
- Bicillin C-R Injection 2810
- Bicillin C-R 900/300 Injection 2812

Penicillin G Sodium (Concurrent use of therapeutic dose of probenecid and penicillin or other beta-lactams results in higher plasma concentrations of penicillin or beta-lactam antibiotics resulting in increased side effects such as psychic disturbances).

No products indexed under this heading.

Penicillin V Potassium (Concurrent use of therapeutic dose of probenecid and penicillin or other beta-lactams results in higher plasma concentrations of penicillin or beta-lactam antibiotics resulting in increased side effects such as psychic disturbances). Products include:
- Pen•Vee K........ 2879

Polythiazide (Probenecid produces insignificant increase in free sulfonamide plasma concentrations but a significant increase in total sulfonamide plasma levels). Products include:
- Minizide Capsules 2016

Pyrazinamide (Pyrazinamide antagonizes the uricosuric action of probenecid). Products include:
- Pyrazinamide Tablets 1442
- Rifater........ 1280

Rifampin (Co-administration increases the mean plasma elimination half-life of rifampin which can lead to increased plasma concentrations). Products include:
- Rifadin 1276
- Rifamate Capsules 1278
- Rifater........ 1280
- Rimactane Capsules 865

Salsalate (Concurrent use with salicylates is contraindicated because salicylates antagonize the uricosuric action of probenecid). Products include:
- Disalcid 1549
- Mono-Gesic Tablets 810
- Salflex Tablets........ 791

Sodium Thiopental (Patients receiving probenecid require less thiopental for induction of anesthesia).

No products indexed under this heading.

Sulfacytine (Probenecid produces insignificant increase in free sulfonamide plasma concentrations but a significant increase in total sulfonamide plasma levels).

Sulfamethizole (Probenecid produces insignificant increase in free sulfonamide plasma concentrations but a significant increase in total sulfonamide plasma levels). Products include:
- Urobiotic-250 Capsules 2038

Sulfamethoxazole (Probenecid produces insignificant increase in free sulfonamide plasma concentrations but a significant increase in total sulfonamide plasma levels). Products include:
- Bactrim DS Tablets........ 2257
- Bactrim I.V. Infusion........ 2255
- Bactrim 2257
- Gantanol Tablets 2285
- Septra........ 1146
- Septra I.V. Infusion 1142
- Septra I.V. Infusion ADD-Vantage Vials........ 1144
- Septra........ 1146

Sulfasalazine (Probenecid produces insignificant increase in free sulfonamide plasma concentrations but a significant increase in total sulfonamide plasma levels). Products include:
- Azulfidine 2059

Sulfinpyrazone (Probenecid produces insignificant increase in free sulfonamide plasma concentrations but a significant increase in total sulfonamide plasma levels). Products include:
- Anturane 823

Sulfisoxazole (Probenecid produces insignificant increase in free sulfonamide plasma concentrations but a significant increase in total sulfonamide plasma levels). Products include:
- Gantrisin Tablets 2286

Sulfisoxazole Diolamine (Probenecid produces insignificant increase in free sulfonamide plasma concentrations but a significant increase in total sulfonamide plasma levels).

No products indexed under this heading.

Sulindac (Co-administration has slight effect on plasma sulfide levels but plasma levels of sulindac and sulfone are increased; modest reduction in uricosuric action of probenecid). Products include:
- Clinoril Tablets 1658

Ticarcillin Disodium (Concurrent use of therapeutic dose of probenecid and penicillin or other beta-lactams results in higher plasma concentrations of penicillin or beta-lactam antibiotics resulting in increased side effects such as psychic disturbances). Products include:
- Ticar for Injection 2704
- Timentin for Injection........ 2706

Tolazamide (Probenecid may prolong or enhance the action of oral sulfonylureas and thereby increase the risk of hypoglycemia).

No products indexed under this heading.

Tolbutamide (Probenecid may prolong or enhance the action of oral sulfonylureas and thereby increase the risk of hypoglycemia).

No products indexed under this heading.

COLESTID GRANULES

(Colestipol Hydrochloride) 2073

May interact with tetracyclines, cardiac glycosides, and certain other agents. Compounds in these categories include:

Chlorothiazide (The absorption of chlorothiazide as reflected in urinary excretion is markedly decreased even when administered one hour before colestipol). Products include:
- Aldoclor Tablets 1638
- Diupres Tablets 1691
- Diuril Oral 1694

Demeclocycline Hydrochloride (Simultaneous administration results in decreased absorption of oral tetracyclines). Products include:
- Declomycin Tablets........ 1421

Deslanoside (Potential for binding of digitalis glycosides).

No products indexed under this heading.

Digitoxin (Potential for binding of digitalis glycosides). Products include:
- Crystodigin Tablets........ 1472

Digoxin (Potential for binding of digitalis glycosides). Products include:
- Lanoxicaps 1110
- Lanoxin Elixir Pediatric 1113
- Lanoxin Injection 1116
- Lanoxin Injection Pediatric........ 1119
- Lanoxin Tablets 1121

Doxycycline Calcium (Simultaneous administration results in decreased absorption of oral tetracyclines). Products include:
- Vibramycin Calcium Oral Suspension Syrup........ 2038

Doxycycline Hyclate (Simultaneous administration results in decreased absorption of oral tetracyclines). Products include:
- Doryx Capsules........ 1970
- Vibramycin Hyclate Capsules 2038
- Vibramycin Hyclate Intravenous 2040
- Vibra-Tabs Film Coated Tablets 2038

Doxycycline Monohydrate (Simultaneous administration results in decreased absorption of oral tetracyclines). Products include:
- Monodox Capsules 1858
- Vibramycin Monohydrate for Oral Suspension........ 2038

Folic Acid (Colestipol may reduce absorption of oral folic acid). Products include:
- Cefol Filmtab 415
- Chromagen FA 2471
- Chromagen Forte........ 2471
- Fero-Folic-500 Filmtab 433
- Iberet-Folic-500 Filmtab........ 433
- Materna Tablets 1427
- Mega-B 513
- Megadose 513
- Nephro-Fer Rx Tablets........ 2168
- Nephro-Vite + Fe Tablets 2170
- Nephro-Vite Rx Tablets 2170
- Niferex-150 Forte Capsules 811
- Slow Fe with Folic Acid 890
- Trinsicon Capsules 2759

Furosemide (Simultaneous administration results in decreased absorption of oral furosemide). Products include:
- Lasix Injection, Oral Solution and Tablets 1267

Gamma Globulin (Simultaneous administration results in decreased absorption of oral furosemide).

No products indexed under this heading.

Gemfibrozil (Simultaneous administration results in decreased absorption of gemfibrozil). Products include:
- Lopid Tablets........ 1974

Hydrochlorothiazide (Simultaneous administration results in decreased absorption of hydrochlorothiazide). Products include:
- Aldactazide Tablets 2556
- Aldoril Tablets........ 1644
- Apresazide Capsules 824
- Capozide Tablets 744
- Dyazide Capsules........ 2653
- Esidrix Tablets 839
- Esimil Tablets 840
- HydroDIURIL Tablets 1716
- Hydropres Tablets........ 1718
- Hyzaar Tablets 1720
- Inderide Tablets 2838
- Inderide LA Long Acting Capsules .. 2840
- Lopressor HCT Tablets 850
- Lotensin HCT Tablets 855
- Moduretic Tablets 1748
- Oretic Tablets 450
- Prinzide Tablets 1780
- Ser-Ap-Es Tablets 867
- Timolide Tablets........ 1791
- Vaseretic Tablets 1810
- Zestoretic Tablets 2968
- Ziac 1459

Hydrocortisone (Bile acid binding agents may interfere with the absorption of oral hydrocortisone). Products include:
- Anusol-HC Cream 2.5% 1953
- Aquanil HC Lotion 1989
- Maximum Strength Cortaid Spray ▣ 800
- CORTENEMA........ 2713
- Cortisporin Ointment........ 1074
- Cortisporin Ophthalmic Ointment Sterile 1074
- Cortisporin Ophthalmic Suspension Sterile 1075
- Cortisporin Otic Solution Sterile 1076
- Cortisporin Otic Suspension Sterile 1077
- Cortizone-5 .... ▣ 795
- Cortizone-10 .... ▣ 795
- Hydrocortone Tablets 1715
- Hytone 922
- Hytone Ointment 2 ½% 923
- Massengill Medicated Soft Cloth Towelettes........ 2628
- Pediotic Suspension Sterile........ 1140
- Preparation H Hydrocortisone 1% Cream .... ▣ 843
- ProctoCream-HC 2.5%........ 2552
- VōSoL HC Otic Solution........ 2786

Methacycline Hydrochloride (Simultaneous administration results in decreased absorption of oral tetracyclines).

No products indexed under this heading.

Minocycline Hydrochloride (Simultaneous administration results in decreased absorption of oral tetracyclines). Products include:
- DYNACIN Capsules........ 1627
- Minocin Intravenous........ 1428
- Minocin Oral Suspension 1431
- Minocin Pellet-Filled Capsules 1429

Oxytetracycline Hydrochloride (Simultaneous administration results in decreased absorption of oral tetracyclines). Products include:
- TERAK Ointment .... ⊙ 210
- Terra-Cortril Ophthalmic Suspension 2033
- Terramycin with Polymyxin B Sulfate Ophthalmic Ointment........ 2035
- Urobiotic-250 Capsules 2038

Penicillin G Potassium (Simultaneous administration results in decreased absorption of oral penicillin G). Products include:
- Pfizerpen for Injection........ 2022

Phytonadione (Colestipol may reduce absorption of oral fat soluble vitamins).

No products indexed under this heading.

(▣ Described in PDR For Nonprescription Drugs) (⊙ Described in PDR For Ophthalmology)

Interactions Index — Combipres

Potassium Phosphate, Monobasic (Bile acid binding agents may interfere with the absorption of oral phosphate supplements). Products include:
- K-Phos Neutral Tablets 633
- K-Phos Original Formula 'Sodium Free' Tablets 633

Propranolol Hydrochloride (Repeated doses of colestipol given prior to a single dose of propranolol has resulted in decreased propranolol absorption; statistically significant effect on the rate of absorption has been noted). Products include:
- Inderal 2834
- Inderal LA Long Acting Capsules 2836
- Inderide Tablets 2838
- Inderide LA Long Acting Capsules 2840

Tetracycline Hydrochloride (Simultaneous administration results in decreased absorption of oral tetracyclines). Products include:
- Achromycin V Capsules 1417
- Helidac Therapy 2135

Vitamin A (Colestipol may reduce absorption of oral fat soluble vitamins). Products include:
- Aquasol A Vitamin A Capsules, USP 525
- Aquasol A Parenteral 526
- Breath + Plus 603
- Materna Tablets 1427
- Megadose 513
- One-A-Day Antioxidant Plus 625

Vitamin D (Colestipol may reduce absorption of oral fat soluble vitamins). Products include:
- Caltrate PLUS 681
- Caltrate 600 + D 681
- Dical-D Tablets & Wafers 424
- Materna Tablets 1427
- Megadose 513
- One-A-Day Calcium Plus 625

Vitamin K (Colestipol may reduce absorption of oral fat soluble vitamins).
No products indexed under this heading.

FLAVORED COLESTID GRANULES
(Colestipol Hydrochloride) 2073
See **Colestid Granules**

COLLAGEN PLUGS (INTRACANALICULAR)
(Collagen, bovine) 275
None cited in PDR database.

COLLAGENASE SANTYL OINTMENT
(Collagenase) 1381
May interact with:

Cortisone Acetate (Chronic concurrent use may result in systemic manifestations of hypersensitivity to collagenase). Products include:
- Cortone Acetate Sterile Suspension 1663
- Cortone Acetate Tablets 1664

COLLYRIUM FOR FRESH EYES
(Boric Acid, Sodium Borate) 316
May interact with:

Polyvinyl Alcohol (Avoid concurrent use). Products include:
- Hypotears 262
- Murine Tears Lubricant Eye Drops 744
- Murine Tears Plus Lubricant Redness Reliever Eye Drops 744
- Murine Tears Lubricant Eye Drops 315
- Murine Tears Plus Lubricant Redness Reliever Eye Drops 315

COLLYRIUM FRESH
(Tetrahydrozoline Hydrochloride, Glycerin) 316
None cited in PDR database.

COLY-MYCIN S OTIC W/NEOMYCIN & HYDROCORTISONE
(Colistin Sulfate, Neomycin Sulfate, Hydrocortisone Acetate) 1965
None cited in PDR database.

COLYTE AND COLYTE-FLAVORED
(Polyethylene Glycol) 2540
May interact with:

Oral Medications, unspecified (Those administered within one hour of Colyte usage may be flushed from the gastrointestinal tract and not absorbed).

COMBIPRES TABLETS
(Clonidine Hydrochloride, Chlorthalidone) 682
May interact with tricyclic antidepressants, barbiturates, hypnotics and sedatives, antihypertensives, insulin, oral hypoglycemic agents, lithium preparations, narcotic analgesics, and certain other agents. Compounds in these categories include:

Acarbose (Higher dosage of oral hypoglycemic agents may be required). Products include:
- Precose 604

Acebutolol Hydrochloride (Chlorthalidone may add to or potentiate the action of other antihypertensive drugs). Products include:
- Sectral Capsules 2914

Alfentanil Hydrochloride (Orthostatic hypotension produced by chlorthalidone may be aggravated by narcotics). Products include:
- Alfenta Injection 1334

Amitriptyline Hydrochloride (Amitriptyline in combination with clonidine enhances the manifestation of corneal lesions in rats; co-administration therapy may result in reduced effect of clonidine, thus necessitating an increase in dosage). Products include:
- Elavil 2945
- Etrafon 2495
- Limbitrol 2333
- Triavil Tablets 1800

Amlodipine Besylate (Chlorthalidone may add to or potentiate the action of other antihypertensive drugs). Products include:
- Lotrel Capsules 858
- Norvasc Tablets 2020

Amoxapine (Co-administration results in reduced effect of clonidine, thus necessitating an increase in dosage). Products include:
- Asendin Tablets 1419

Aprobarbital (Orthostatic hypotension produced by chlorthalidone may be aggravated by barbiturates; potential for enhanced CNS-depressive effects).
No products indexed under this heading.

Atenolol (Chlorthalidone may add to or potentiate the action of other antihypertensive drugs). Products include:
- Tenoretic Tablets 2963
- Tenormin Tablets and I.V. Injection 2965

Benazepril Hydrochloride (Chlorthalidone may add to or potentiate the action of other antihypertensive drugs). Products include:
- Lotensin Tablets 852
- Lotensin HCT Tablets 855
- Lotrel Capsules 858

Bendroflumethiazide (Chlorthalidone may add to or potentiate the action of other antihypertensive drugs).
No products indexed under this heading.

Betaxolol Hydrochloride (Chlorthalidone may add to or potentiate the action of other antihypertensive drugs). Products include:
- Betoptic Ophthalmic Solution 465
- Betoptic S Ophthalmic Suspension 467
- Kerlone Tablets 2588

Bisoprolol Fumarate (Chlorthalidone may add to or potentiate the action of other antihypertensive drugs). Products include:
- Zebeta Tablets 1457
- Ziac 1459

Buprenorphine (Orthostatic hypotension produced by chlorthalidone may be aggravated by narcotics). Products include:
- Buprenex Injectable 2170

Butabarbital (Orthostatic hypotension produced by chlorthalidone may be aggravated by barbiturates; potential for enhanced CNS-depressive effects).
No products indexed under this heading.

Butalbital (Orthostatic hypotension produced by chlorthalidone may be aggravated by barbiturates; potential for enhanced CNS-depressive effects). Products include:
- Axocet Capsules 2469
- Esgic-plus Capsules 1012
- Esgic-plus Tablets 1012
- Fioricet Tablets 2386
- Fioricet with Codeine Capsules 2387
- Fiorinal Capsules 2388
- Fiorinal with Codeine Capsules 2390
- Fiorinal Tablets 2388
- Phrenilin 790
- Sedapap Tablets 50 mg/650 mg 1826

Captopril (Chlorthalidone may add to or potentiate the action of other antihypertensive drugs). Products include:
- Capoten Tablets 740
- Capozide Tablets 744

Carteolol Hydrochloride (Chlorthalidone may add to or potentiate the action of other antihypertensive drugs). Products include:
- Cartrol Tablets 413
- Ocupress Ophthalmic Solution, 1% Sterile 297

Chlorothiazide (Chlorthalidone may add to or potentiate the action of other antihypertensive drugs). Products include:
- Aldoclor Tablets 1638
- Diupres Tablets 1691
- Diuril Oral 1694

Chlorothiazide Sodium (Chlorthalidone may add to or potentiate the action of other antihypertensive drugs). Products include:
- Diuril Sodium Intravenous 1693

Chlorpropamide (Higher dosage of oral hypoglycemic agents may be required). Products include:
- Diabinese Tablets 2002

Clomipramine Hydrochloride (Co-administration results in reduced effect of clonidine, thus necessitating an increase in dosage). Products include:
- Anafranil Capsules 819

Clonidine (Chlorthalidone may add to or potentiate the action of other antihypertensive drugs). Products include:
- Catapres-TTS 680

Codeine Phosphate (Orthostatic hypotension produced by chlorthalidone may be aggravated by narcotics). Products include:
- Brontex 2130
- Dimetane-DC Cough Syrup 2232
- Fioricet with Codeine Capsules 2387
- Fiorinal with Codeine Capsules 2390
- Nucofed 2225
- Phenergan with Codeine 2883
- Phenergan VC with Codeine 2888
- Robitussin A-C Syrup 2248
- Robitussin-DAC Syrup 2249
- Ryna 804
- Soma Compound w/Codeine Tablets 2784
- Tylenol with Codeine 1592

Deserpidine (Chlorthalidone may add to or potentiate the action of other antihypertensive drugs).
No products indexed under this heading.

Desipramine Hydrochloride (Co-administration results in reduced effect of clonidine, thus necessitating an increase in dosage). Products include:
- Norpramin Tablets 1273

Dezocine (Orthostatic hypotension produced by chlorthalidone may be aggravated by narcotics). Products include:
- Dalgan Injection 529

Diazoxide (Chlorthalidone may add to or potentiate the action of other antihypertensive drugs). Products include:
- Hyperstat I.V. Injection 2504
- Proglycem 575

Diltiazem Hydrochloride (Chlorthalidone may add to or potentiate the action of other antihypertensive drugs). Products include:
- Cardizem CD Capsules 1251
- Cardizem SR Capsules 1255
- Cardizem Injectable 1253
- Cardizem Tablets 1257
- Dilacor XR Extended-release Capsules 2183
- Tiazac Capsules 1019

Doxazosin Mesylate (Chlorthalidone may add to or potentiate the action of other antihypertensive drugs). Products include:
- Cardura Tablets 1993

Doxepin Hydrochloride (Co-administration results in reduced effect of clonidine, thus necessitating an increase in dosage). Products include:
- Adapin Capsules 1542
- Sinequan 2028
- Zonalon Cream 1042

Enalapril Maleate (Chlorthalidone may add to or potentiate the action of other antihypertensive drugs). Products include:
- Vaseretic Tablets 1810
- Vasotec Tablets 1816

Enalaprilat (Chlorthalidone may add to or potentiate the action of other antihypertensive drugs). Products include:
- Vasotec I.V. 1814

Esmolol Hydrochloride (Chlorthalidone may add to or potentiate the action of other antihypertensive drugs). Products include:
- Brevibloc (esmolol HCl) Injection 1860

Estazolam (Enhanced CNS-depressive effects). Products include:
- ProSom Tablets 457

Ethchlorvynol (Enhanced CNS-depressive effects). Products include:
- Placidyl Capsules 456

Ethinamate (Enhanced CNS-depressive effects).
No products indexed under this heading.

IMPORTANT NOTE: Always consult each drug listing in the patient's regimen for possible interactions.

Combipres — Interactions Index — 194

Felodipine (Chlorthalidone may add to or potentiate the action of other antihypertensive drugs). Products include:
- Plendil Extended-Release Tablets.... 514

Fentanyl (Orthostatic hypotension produced by chlorthalidone may be aggravated by narcotics). Products include:
- Duragesic Transdermal System........ 1336

Fentanyl Citrate (Orthostatic hypotension produced by chlorthalidone may be aggravated by narcotics). Products include:
- Sublimaze Injection.............................. 463

Flurazepam Hydrochloride (Enhanced CNS-depressive effects). Products include:
- Dalmane Capsules............................. 2329

Fosinopril Sodium (Chlorthalidone may add to or potentiate the action of other antihypertensive drugs). Products include:
- Monopril Tablets................................. 762

Furosemide (Chlorthalidone may add to or potentiate the action of other antihypertensive drugs). Products include:
- Lasix Injection, Oral Solution and Tablets 1267

Glimepiride (Higher dosage of oral hypoglycemic agents may be required). Products include:
- Amaryl Tablets 1241

Glipizide (Higher dosage of oral hypoglycemic agents may be required). Products include:
- Glucotrol Tablets 2011
- Glucotrol XL Extended Release Tablets 2012

Glutethimide (Enhanced CNS-depressive effects).
No products indexed under this heading.

Glyburide (Higher dosage of oral hypoglycemic agents may be required). Products include:
- DiaBeta Tablets 1265
- Glynase PresTab Tablets 2091
- Micronase Tablets 2099

Guanabenz Acetate (Chlorthalidone may add to or potentiate the action of other antihypertensive drugs).
No products indexed under this heading.

Guanethidine Monosulfate (Chlorthalidone may add to or potentiate the action of other antihypertensive drugs). Products include:
- Esimil Tablets 840
- Ismelin Tablets 845

Hydralazine Hydrochloride (Chlorthalidone may add to or potentiate the action of other antihypertensive drugs). Products include:
- Apresazide Capsules 824
- Apresoline Hydrochloride Tablets .. 826
- Hydralazine Hydrochloride Injection USP.. 2712
- Ser-Ap-Es Tablets 867

Hydrochlorothiazide (Chlorthalidone may add to or potentiate the action of other antihypertensive drugs). Products include:
- Aldactazide Tablets 2556
- Aldoril Tablets 1644
- Apresazide Capsules 824
- Capozide Tablets 744
- Dyazide Capsules 2653
- Esidrix Tablets 839
- Esimil Tablets 840
- HydroDIURIL Tablets 1716
- Hydropres Tablets 1718
- Hyzaar Tablets 1720
- Inderide Tablets 2838
- Inderide LA Long Acting Capsules .. 2840
- Lopressor HCT Tablets 850
- Lotensin HCT Tablets 855
- Moduretic Tablets 1748
- Oretic Tablets 450
- Prinzide Tablets 1780
- Ser-Ap-Es Tablets 867
- Timolide Tablets 1791
- Vaseretic Tablets 1810
- Zestoretic Tablets 2968
- Ziac 1459

Hydrocodone Bitartrate (Orthostatic hypotension produced by chlorthalidone may be aggravated by narcotics). Products include:
- Codiclear DH Syrup 808
- Duratuss HD Elixir 2750
- Histussin D Liquid 670
- Hycodan Tablets and Syrup 946
- Hycomine Compound Tablets 948
- Hycomine 947
- Hycotuss Expectorant Syrup 950
- Hydrocet Capsules 787
- Lorcet 10/650 Tablets 1016
- Lortab 2751
- Tussend 1830
- Tussend Expectorant 1831
- Vicodin Tablets 1404
- Vicodin ES Tablets 1405
- Vicodin HP Tablets 1403
- Vicodin Tuss Expectorant 1406
- Zydone Capsules 967

Hydrocodone Polistirex (Orthostatic hypotension produced by chlorthalidone may be aggravated by narcotics). Products include:
- Tussionex Pennkinetic Extended-Release Suspension 1624

Hydroflumethiazide (Chlorthalidone may add to or potentiate the action of other antihypertensive drugs). Products include:
- Diucardin Tablets 2824

Hydromorphone Hydrochloride (Orthostatic hypotension produced by chlorthalidone may be aggravated by narcotics). Products include:
- Dilaudid Ampules 1382
- Dilaudid Cough Syrup 1383
- Dilaudid-HP Injection 1384
- Dilaudid-HP Lyophilized Powder 250 mg 1384
- Dilaudid 1382
- Dilaudid Oral Liquid 1386
- Dilaudid 1382
- Dilaudid Tablets - 8 mg.................... 1386

Imipramine Hydrochloride (Co-administration results in reduced effect of clonidine, thus necessitating an increase in dosage). Products include:
- Tofranil Ampuls 873
- Tofranil Tablets 875

Imipramine Pamoate (Co-administration results in reduced effect of clonidine, thus necessitating an increase in dosage). Products include:
- Tofranil-PM Capsules........................ 876

Indapamide (Chlorthalidone may add to or potentiate the action of other antihypertensive drugs).
No products indexed under this heading.

Insulin, Human (Insulin requirements in diabetic patients may be increased, decreased or unchanged).
No products indexed under this heading.

Insulin, Human Isophane Suspension (Insulin requirements in diabetic patients may be increased, decreased or unchanged). Products include:
- Novolin N Human Insulin 10 ml Vials.. 1846

Insulin, Human NPH (Insulin requirements in diabetic patients may be increased, decreased or unchanged). Products include:
- Humulin N, 100 Units 1495
- Novolin N PenFill 1.5 ml Cartridges Durable Insulin Delivery System 1849
- Novolin N Prefilled Syringe Disposable Insulin Delivery System 1850

Insulin, Human Regular (Insulin requirements in diabetic patients may be increased, decreased or unchanged). Products include:
- Humulin R, 100 Units 1497
- Novolin R Human Insulin 10 ml Vials.. 1846
- Novolin R PenFill 1.5 ml Cartridges Durable Insulin Delivery System 1849
- Novolin R Prefilled Syringe Disposable Insulin Delivery System 1850
- Velosulin BR Human Insulin 10 ml Vials.. 1847

Insulin, Human, Zinc Suspension (Insulin requirements in diabetic patients may be increased, decreased or unchanged). Products include:
- Humulin L, 100 Units 1494
- Humulin U, 100 Units 1498
- Novolin L Human Insulin 10 ml Vials.. 1846

Insulin Lispro, Human (Insulin requirements in diabetic patients may be increased, decreased or unchanged). Products include:
- Humalog Injection 1488

Insulin, NPH (Insulin requirements in diabetic patients may be increased, decreased or unchanged). Products include:
- NPH, 100 Units 1502
- Pork NPH, 100 Units 1506
- Purified Pork NPH Isophane Insulin 1852

Insulin, Regular (Insulin requirements in diabetic patients may be increased, decreased or unchanged). Products include:
- Regular, 100 Units 1503
- Pork Regular, 100 Units 1507
- Pork Regular (Concentrated), 500 Units 1508
- Purified Pork Regular Insulin 1852

Insulin, Zinc Crystals (Insulin requirements in diabetic patients may be increased, decreased or unchanged). Products include:
- NPH, 100 Units 1502

Insulin, Zinc Suspension (Insulin requirements in diabetic patients may be increased, decreased or unchanged). Products include:
- Iletin I 1501
- Lente, 100 Units 1501
- Iletin II 1504
- Pork Lente, 100 Units....................... 1504
- Purified Pork Lente Insulin 1852

Isradipine (Chlorthalidone may add to or potentiate the action of other antihypertensive drugs). Products include:
- DynaCirc Capsules 2381
- DynaCirc CR Tablets 2383

Labetalol Hydrochloride (Chlorthalidone may add to or potentiate the action of other antihypertensive drugs). Products include:
- Normodyne Injection 2519
- Normodyne Tablets 2522
- Trandate 1158

Levorphanol Tartrate (Orthostatic hypotension produced by chlorthalidone may be aggravated by narcotics). Products include:
- Levo-Dromoran 2297

Lisinopril (Chlorthalidone may add to or potentiate the action of other antihypertensive drugs). Products include:
- Prinivil Tablets 1776
- Prinzide Tablets 1780
- Zestoretic Tablets 2968
- Zestril Tablets 2972

Lithium Carbonate (Reduced renal lithium clearance and increased risk of lithium toxicity). Products include:
- Eskalith 2658

Lithium Carbonate Capsules & Tablets 2352
Lithonate/Lithotabs/Lithobid 2721

Lithium Citrate (Reduced renal lithium clearance and increased risk of lithium toxicity).
No products indexed under this heading.

Lorazepam (Enhanced CNS-depressive effects). Products include:
- Ativan Injection 2805
- Ativan Tablets 2807

Losartan Potassium (Chlorthalidone may add to or potentiate the action of other antihypertensive drugs). Products include:
- Cozaar Tablets 1668
- Hyzaar Tablets 1720

Maprotiline Hydrochloride (Co-administration results in reduced effect of clonidine, thus necessitating an increase in dosage). Products include:
- Ludiomil Tablets 861

Mecamylamine Hydrochloride (Chlorthalidone may add to or potentiate the action of other antihypertensive drugs). Products include:
- Inversine Tablets 1729

Meperidine Hydrochloride (Orthostatic hypotension produced by chlorthalidone may be aggravated by narcotics). Products include:
- Demerol 2438
- Mepergan Injection 2859

Mephobarbital (Orthostatic hypotension produced by chlorthalidone may be aggravated by barbiturates; potential for enhanced CNS-depressive effects). Products include:
- Mebaral Tablets 2452

Metformin Hydrochloride (Higher dosage of oral hypoglycemic agents may be required). Products include:
- Glucophage Tablets 754

Methadone Hydrochloride (Orthostatic hypotension produced by chlorthalidone may be aggravated by narcotics). Products include:
- Methadone Hydrochloride Oral Concentrate 2356
- Methadone Hydrochloride Oral Solution & Tablets 2357

Methyclothiazide (Chlorthalidone may add to or potentiate the action of other antihypertensive drugs). Products include:
- Enduron Tablets 424

Methyldopa (Chlorthalidone may add to or potentiate the action of other antihypertensive drugs). Products include:
- Aldoclor Tablets 1638
- Aldomet Oral 1640
- Aldoril Tablets 1644

Methyldopate Hydrochloride (Chlorthalidone may add to or potentiate the action of other antihypertensive drugs). Products include:
- Aldomet Ester HCl Injection 1642

Metolazone (Chlorthalidone may add to or potentiate the action of other antihypertensive drugs). Products include:
- Mykrox Tablets 1617
- Zaroxolyn Tablets 1625

Metoprolol Succinate (Chlorthalidone may add to or potentiate the action of other antihypertensive drugs). Products include:
- Toprol-XL Tablets 560

Metoprolol Tartrate (Chlorthalidone may add to or potentiate the action of other antihypertensive drugs). Products include:
- Lopressor 848
- Lopressor HCT Tablets 850

(◘ Described in PDR For Nonprescription Drugs)   (⊙ Described in PDR For Ophthalmology)

Metyrosine (Chlorthalidone may add to or potentiate the action of other antihypertensive drugs). Products include:
- Demser Capsules 1690

Midazolam Hydrochloride (Enhanced CNS-depressive effects). Products include:
- Versed Injection 2324

Minoxidil (Chlorthalidone may add to or potentiate the action of other antihypertensive drugs).
- No products indexed under this heading.

Moexipril Hydrochloride (Chlorthalidone may add to or potentiate the action of other antihypertensive drugs). Products include:
- Univasc Tablets 2553

Morphine Sulfate (Orthostatic hypotension produced by chlorthalidone may be aggravated by narcotics). Products include:
- Astramorph/PF Injection, USP (Preservative-Free) 526
- Duramorph Injection 983
- Infumorph 200 and Infumorph 500 Sterile Solutions 985
- Kadian Capsules 2948
- MS Contin Tablets 2149
- MSIR 2152
- Oramorph SR (Morphine Sulfate Sustained Release Tablets) 2359
- RMS Suppositories CII 2766
- Roxanol 2365

Nadolol (Chlorthalidone may add to or potentiate the action of other antihypertensive drugs).
- No products indexed under this heading.

Nicardipine Hydrochloride (Chlorthalidone may add to or potentiate the action of other antihypertensive drugs). Products include:
- Cardene Capsules 2261
- Cardene I.V. 2815
- Cardene SR Capsules 2264

Nifedipine (Chlorthalidone may add to or potentiate the action of other antihypertensive drugs). Products include:
- Adalat Capsules (10 mg and 20 mg) 580
- Adalat CC 582
- Procardia Capsules 2024
- Procardia XL Extended Release Tablets 2026

Nisoldipine (Chlorthalidone may add to or potentiate the action of other antihypertensive drugs). Products include:
- Sular Tablets 2961

Nitroglycerin (Chlorthalidone may add to or potentiate the action of other antihypertensive drugs). Products include:
- Deponit NTG Transdermal Delivery System 2541
- Nitro-Bid IV 1270
- Nitro-Bid Ointment 1272
- Nitro-Dur (nitroglycerin) Transdermal Infusion System 1365
- Nitrolingual Spray 2193
- Nitrostat Tablets 1981
- Transderm-Nitro Transdermal Therapeutic System 878

Norepinephrine Bitartrate (Decreased arterial responsiveness to norepinephrine). Products include:
- Levophed Bitartrate Injection 2445

Nortriptyline Hydrochloride (Co-administration results in reduced effect of clonidine, thus necessitating an increase in dosage). Products include:
- Pamelor 2409

Opium Alkaloids (Orthostatic hypotension produced by chlorthalidone may be aggravated by narcotics).
- No products indexed under this heading.

Oxycodone Hydrochloride (Orthostatic hypotension produced by chlorthalidone may be aggravated by narcotics). Products include:
- OxyContin Tablets 2163
- OxyIR Capsules 2167
- Percocet Tablets 955
- Percodan Tablets 955
- Percodan-Demi Tablets 956
- Roxicodone Tablets, Oral Solution & Intensol (Oxycodone) 2366
- Tylox Capsules 1593

Papaverine (Drug-induced hepatitis (one case)).

Penbutolol Sulfate (Chlorthalidone may add to or potentiate the action of other antihypertensive drugs). Products include:
- Levatol Tablets 2547

Pentobarbital Sodium (Orthostatic hypotension produced by chlorthalidone may be aggravated by barbiturates; potential for enhanced CNS-depressive effects). Products include:
- Nembutal Sodium Capsules 440
- Nembutal Sodium Solution 442
- Nembutal Sodium Suppositories 444

Phenobarbital (Orthostatic hypotension produced by chlorthalidone may be aggravated by barbiturates; potential for enhanced CNS-depressive effects). Products include:
- Arco-Lase Plus Tablets 513
- Bellergal-S Tablets 2375
- Donnatal 2234
- Donnatal Extentabs 2234
- Donnatal Tablets 2234
- Phenobarbital Elixir and Tablets 1523
- Quadrinal Tablets 1398

Phenoxybenzamine Hydrochloride (Chlorthalidone may add to or potentiate the action of other antihypertensive drugs). Products include:
- Dibenzyline Capsules 2650

Phentolamine Mesylate (Chlorthalidone may add to or potentiate the action of other antihypertensive drugs). Products include:
- Regitine Vials 864

Pindolol (Chlorthalidone may add to or potentiate the action of other antihypertensive drugs). Products include:
- Visken Tablets 2428

Polythiazide (Chlorthalidone may add to or potentiate the action of other antihypertensive drugs). Products include:
- Minizide Capsules 2016

Prazosin Hydrochloride (Chlorthalidone may add to or potentiate the action of other antihypertensive drugs). Products include:
- Minipress Capsules 2015
- Minizide Capsules 2016

Propofol (Enhanced CNS-depressive effects). Products include:
- Diprivan Injectable Emulsion 2939

Propoxyphene Hydrochloride (Orthostatic hypotension produced by chlorthalidone may be aggravated by narcotics). Products include:
- Darvon 1475
- Wygesic Tablets 2930

Propoxyphene Napsylate (Orthostatic hypotension produced by chlorthalidone may be aggravated by narcotics). Products include:
- Darvon-N/Darvocet-N 1473

Propranolol Hydrochloride (Chlorthalidone may add to or potentiate the action of other antihypertensive drugs). Products include:
- Inderal 2834
- Inderal LA Long Acting Capsules 2836
- Inderide Tablets 2838
- Inderide LA Long Acting Capsules 2840

Protriptyline Hydrochloride (Co-administration results in reduced effect of clonidine, thus necessitating an increase in dosage). Products include:
- Vivactil Tablets 1820

Quazepam (Enhanced CNS-depressive effects). Products include:
- Doral Tablets 2773

Quinapril Hydrochloride (Chlorthalidone may add to or potentiate the action of other antihypertensive drugs). Products include:
- Accupril Tablets 1950

Ramipril (Chlorthalidone may add to or potentiate the action of other antihypertensive drugs). Products include:
- Altace Capsules 1238

Rauwolfia Serpentina (Chlorthalidone may add to or potentiate the action of other antihypertensive drugs).
- No products indexed under this heading.

Rescinnamine (Chlorthalidone may add to or potentiate the action of other antihypertensive drugs).
- No products indexed under this heading.

Reserpine (Chlorthalidone may add to or potentiate the action of other antihypertensive drugs). Products include:
- Diupres Tablets 1691
- Hydropres Tablets 1718
- Ser-Ap-Es Tablets 867

Secobarbital Sodium (Orthostatic hypotension produced by chlorthalidone may be aggravated by barbiturates; potential for enhanced CNS-depressive effects). Products include:
- Seconal Sodium Pulvules 1529

Sodium Nitroprusside (Chlorthalidone may add to or potentiate the action of other antihypertensive drugs).
- No products indexed under this heading.

Sotalol Hydrochloride (Chlorthalidone may add to or potentiate the action of other antihypertensive drugs). Products include:
- Betapace Tablets 637

Spirapril Hydrochloride (Chlorthalidone may add to or potentiate the action of other antihypertensive drugs).
- No products indexed under this heading.

Sufentanil Citrate (Orthostatic hypotension produced by chlorthalidone may be aggravated by narcotics). Products include:
- Sufenta Injection 1355

Temazepam (Enhanced CNS-depressive effects). Products include:
- Restoril Capsules 2413

Terazosin Hydrochloride (Chlorthalidone may add to or potentiate the action of other antihypertensive drugs). Products include:
- Hytrin Capsules 434

Thiamylal Sodium (Orthostatic hypotension produced by chlorthalidone may be aggravated by barbiturates; potential for enhanced CNS-depressive effects).
- No products indexed under this heading.

Timolol Maleate (Chlorthalidone may add to or potentiate the action of other antihypertensive drugs). Products include:
- Blocadren Tablets 1654
- Timolide Tablets 1791
- Timoptic in Ocudose 1796
- Timoptic Sterile Ophthalmic Solution 1794
- Timoptic-XE 1798

Tolazamide (Higher dosage of oral hypoglycemic agents may be required).
- No products indexed under this heading.

Tolbutamide (Higher dosage of oral hypoglycemic agents may be required).
- No products indexed under this heading.

Torsemide (Chlorthalidone may add to or potentiate the action of other antihypertensive drugs). Products include:
- Demadex Tablets and Injection 691

Triazolam (Enhanced CNS-depressive effects). Products include:
- Halcion Tablets 2093

Trimethaphan Camsylate (Chlorthalidone may add to or potentiate the action of other antihypertensive drugs).
- No products indexed under this heading.

Trimipramine Maleate (Co-administration results in reduced effect of clonidine, thus necessitating an increase in dosage). Products include:
- Surmontil Capsules 2917

Tubocurarine Chloride (Increased responsiveness to tubocurarine).
- No products indexed under this heading.

Verapamil Hydrochloride (Chlorthalidone may add to or potentiate the action of other antihypertensive drugs). Products include:
- Calan SR Caplets 2571
- Calan Tablets 2568
- Covera-HS Tablets 2573
- Isoptin Injectable 1391
- Isoptin Oral Tablets 1393
- Isoptin SR Tablets 1395
- Verelan Capsules 1455

Zolpidem Tartrate (Enhanced CNS-depressive effects). Products include:
- Ambien Tablets 2559

Food Interactions

Alcohol (Orthostatic hypotension produced by chlorthalidone may be aggravated by alcohol; potential for enhanced CNS-depressive effects).

COMPAZINE INJECTION
(Prochlorperazine) 2644
See **Compazine Tablets**

COMPAZINE MULTI-DOSE VIALS
(Prochlorperazine) 2644
See **Compazine Tablets**

COMPAZINE SPANSULE CAPSULES
(Prochlorperazine) 2644
See **Compazine Tablets**

IMPORTANT NOTE: Always consult each drug listing in the patient's regimen for possible interactions.

COMPAZINE SUPPOSITORIES
(Prochlorperazine)....2644
See **Compazine Tablets**

COMPAZINE SYRUP
(Prochlorperazine)....2644
See **Compazine Tablets**

COMPAZINE TABLETS
(Prochlorperazine)....2644
May interact with central nervous system depressants, narcotic analgesics, general anesthetics, antihistamines, barbiturates, oral anticoagulants, thiazides, anticonvulsants, antineoplastics, and certain other agents. Compounds in these categories include:

Acrivastine (Phenothiazines may intensify or prolong the action of other central nervous system depressants). Products include:
Semprex-D Capsules 1620

Alfentanil Hydrochloride (Phenothiazines may intensify or prolong the action of other central nervous system depressants). Products include:
Alfenta Injection 1334

Alprazolam (Phenothiazines may intensify or prolong the action of other central nervous system depressants). Products include:
Xanax Tablets 2115

Altretamine (Vomiting as a sign of toxicity of antineoplastic agents may be obscured by the antiemetic effect of Compazine). Products include:
Hexalen Capsules 2760

Anastrozole (Vomiting as a sign of toxicity of antineoplastic agents may be obscured by the antiemetic effect of Compazine). Products include:
Arimidex Tablets 2932

Aprobarbital (Phenothiazines may intensify or prolong the action of other central nervous system depressants).
No products indexed under this heading.

Asparaginase (Vomiting as a sign of toxicity of antineoplastic agents may be obscured by the antiemetic effect of Compazine). Products include:
Elspar 1700

Astemizole (Phenothiazines may intensify or prolong the action of other central nervous system depressants). Products include:
Hismanal Tablets 1341

Atropine Sulfate (Phenothiazines may intensify or prolong the action of atropine). Products include:
Arco-Lase Plus Tablets 513
Atrohist Plus Tablets 1605
Donnatal 2234
Donnatal Extentabs 2234
Donnatal Tablets 2234
Lomotil 2591
Motofen Tablets 789
Urised Tablets 2123

Azatadine Maleate (Phenothiazines may intensify or prolong the action of other central nervous system depressants). Products include:
Trinalin Repetabs Tablets 1373

Bendroflumethiazide (Accentuates the orthostatic hypotension that may occur with phenothiazines).
No products indexed under this heading.

Bicalutamide (Vomiting as a sign of toxicity of antineoplastic agents may be obscured by the antiemetic effect of Compazine). Products include:
Casodex Tablets 2934

Bleomycin Sulfate (Vomiting as a sign of toxicity of antineoplastic agents may be obscured by the antiemetic effect of Compazine). Products include:
Blenoxane 697

Bromodiphenhydramine Hydrochloride (Phenothiazines may intensify or prolong the action of other central nervous system depressants).
No products indexed under this heading.

Brompheniramine Maleate (Phenothiazines may intensify or prolong the action of other central nervous system depressants). Products include:
Alka-Seltzer Plus Sinus Medicine .. ▣ 611
Bromfed Capsules (Extended-Release) 1832
Bromfed Syrup .... ▣ 712
Bromfed Tablets 1832
Bromfed-DM Cough Syrup.... 1832
Bromfed-PD Capsules (Extended-Release) 1832
Dimetane-DC Cough Syrup 2232
Dimetane-DX Cough Syrup 2233
Dimetapp Allergy Dye-Free Elixir.... ▣ 838
Dimetapp Allergy Sinus Caplets .... ▣ 838
Dimetapp Cold & Allergy Chewable Tablets .... ▣ 838
Dimetapp Cold & Cough Liqui-Gels .... ▣ 839
Dimetapp Cold & Fever Suspension .... ▣ 839
Dimetapp DM Elixir .... ▣ 840
Dimetapp Elixir .... ▣ 840
Dimetapp Extentabs .... ▣ 841
Dimetapp Tablets/Liqui-Gels .... ▣ 841
Rondec Chewable Tablets 974
Vicks DayQuil Allergy Relief 12-Hour Extended Release Tablets.. ▣ 733
Vicks DayQuil Allergy Relief 4-Hour Tablets .... ▣ 733

Buprenorphine (Phenothiazines may intensify or prolong the action of other central nervous system depressants). Products include:
Buprenex Injectable 2170

Buspirone Hydrochloride (Phenothiazines may intensify or prolong the action of other central nervous system depressants). Products include:
BuSpar Tablets 738

Busulfan (Vomiting as a sign of toxicity of antineoplastic agents may be obscured by the antiemetic effect of Compazine). Products include:
Myleran Tablets 1209

Butabarbital (Phenothiazines may intensify or prolong the action of other central nervous system depressants).
No products indexed under this heading.

Butalbital (Phenothiazines may intensify or prolong the action of other central nervous system depressants). Products include:
Axocet Capsules 2469
Esgic-plus Capsules 1012
Esgic-plus Tablets 1012
Fioricet Tablets 2386
Fioricet with Codeine Capsules 2387
Fiorinal Capsules 2388
Fiorinal with Codeine Capsules 2390
Fiorinal Tablets 2388
Phrenilin 790
Sedapap Tablets 50 mg/650 mg .. 1826

Carbamazepine (Phenothiazines may lower convulsive threshold; dosage adjustments of anticonvulsant may be necessary). Products include:
Atretol Tablets 569
Tegretol/Tegretol-XR 870

Carboplatin (Vomiting as a sign of toxicity of antineoplastic agents may be obscured by the antiemetic effect of Compazine). Products include:
Paraplatin for Injection 713

Carmustine (BCNU) (Vomiting as a sign of toxicity of antineoplastic agents may be obscured by the antiemetic effect of Compazine). Products include:
BiCNU 696

Cetirizine Hydrochloride (Phenothiazines may intensify or prolong the action of other central nervous system depressants). Products include:
Zyrtec Tablets 2053

Chlorambucil (Vomiting as a sign of toxicity of antineoplastic agents may be obscured by the antiemetic effect of Compazine). Products include:
Leukeran Tablets 1205

Chlordiazepoxide (Phenothiazines may intensify or prolong the action of other central nervous system depressants). Products include:
Limbitrol 2333

Chlordiazepoxide Hydrochloride (Phenothiazines may intensify or prolong the action of other central nervous system depressants). Products include:
Librax Capsules 2330
Librium Capsules 2331
Librium Injectable 2332

Chlorothiazide (Accentuates the orthostatic hypotension that may occur with phenothiazines). Products include:
Aldoclor Tablets 1638
Diupres Tablets 1691
Diuril Oral 1694

Chlorothiazide Sodium (Accentuates the orthostatic hypotension that may occur with phenothiazines). Products include:
Diuril Sodium Intravenous 1693

Chlorpheniramine Maleate (Phenothiazines may intensify or prolong the action of other central nervous system depressants). Products include:
Alka-Seltzer Plus Cold Medicine .... ▣ 611
Alka-Seltzer Plus Cold Medicine Liqui-Gels .... ▣ 612
Alka-Seltzer Plus Cold & Cough Medicine .... ▣ 611
Alka-Seltzer Plus Cold & Cough Medicine Liqui-Gels.... ▣ 612
Alka-Seltzer Plus Flu & Body Aches Effervescent Tablets .... ▣ 612
Allerest Maximum Strength.... ▣ 649
Allerest Sinus Pain Formula .... ▣ 649
Ana-Kit Anaphylaxis Emergency Treatment Kit 611
Atrohist Pediatric Capsules 1603
Atrohist Plus Tablets 1605
BC Cold Powder Multi-Symptom Formula (Cold-Sinus-Allergy) .... ▣ 631
Cerose DM .... ▣ 853
Cheracol Plus Head Cold/Cough Formula .... ▣ 741
Children's TYLENOL Cold Multi-Symptom Chewable Tablets and Liquid 1559
Children's TYLENOL Cold Plus Cough Multi Symptom Chewable Tablets and Liquid 1560
Children's TYLENOL Flu Suspension Liquid 1560
Children's Vicks DayQuil Allergy Relief .... ▣ 730
Children's Vicks NyQuil Cold/Cough Relief .... ▣ 731
Chlor-Trimeton Allergy Decongestant Tablets .... ▣ 759
Chlor-Trimeton Allergy Tablets .... ▣ 758
Allergy-Sinus Comtrex Multi-Symptom Allergy-Sinus Formula Tablets and Caplets .... ▣ 639
Comtrex Multi-Symptom .... ▣ 638
Contac Continuous Action Nasal Decongestant/Antihistamine 12 Hour Capsules .... ▣ 773
Contac Maximum Strength Continuous Action Decongestant/Antihistamine 12 Hour Caplets.. ▣ 772
Contac Severe Cold and Flu Formula Caplets .... ▣ 773
Coricidin Cold + Flu Tablets .... ▣ 760
Coricidin Cough + Cold Tablets .... ▣ 760
Coricidin 'D' Decongestant Tablets .... ▣ 760
D.A. II Tablets 972
D.A. Chewable Tablets 970
Dura-Tap/PD Capsules 970
Dura-Vent/DA Tablets 972
Efidac 24 Chlorpheniramine .... ▣ 655
Extendryl 1003
Fedahist Gyrocaps 2545
Hycomine Compound Tablets 948
Kronofed-A 994
Nolamine Timed-Release Tablets 790
Novahistine Elixir .... ▣ 782
Ornade Spansule Capsules 2678
PediaCare Cough-Cold Chewable Tablets and Liquid 1569
PediaCare NightRest Cough-Cold Liquid 1569
Pediatric Vicks 44m Cough & Cold Relief .... ▣ 737
Pyrroxate Caplets .... ▣ 742
Ryna .... ▣ 804
Sinarest .... ▣ 663
Sine-Off Sinus Medicine .... ▣ 784
Singlet Tablets .... ▣ 785
Sinulin Tablets 792
Sinutab Sinus Allergy Medication, Maximum Strength Tablets and Caplets .... ▣ 823
Sudafed Cold & Allergy Tablets .... ▣ 826
Teldrin 12 Hour Antihistamine/Nasal Decongestant Allergy Relief Capsules .... ▣ 786
TheraFlu Flu and Cold Medicine .... ▣ 750
Theraflu Maximum Strength Flu and Cold Medicine For Sore Throat .... ▣ 751
TheraFlu Flu, Cold and Cough Medicine .... ▣ 750
TheraFlu Maximum Strength Nighttime Flu, Cold & Cough Medicine .... ▣ 751
Triaminic Night Time .... ▣ 754
Triaminic Syrup .... ▣ 755
Triaminic Triaminicol Cold & Cough .... ▣ 756
Triaminicin Tablets .... ▣ 756
Tussend 1830
TYLENOL Allergy Sinus, Maximum Strength Caplets and Gelcaps 1571
TYLENOL Cold Medication, Multi-Symptom Formula Tablets and Caplets 1572
TYLENOL Cold Medication, Multi-Symptom Hot Liquid Packets 1572
Vicks 44 LiquiCaps Cough, Cold & Flu Relief .... ▣ 728
Vicks 44M Cough, Cold & Flu Relief .... ▣ 729

Chlorpheniramine Polistirex (Phenothiazines may intensify or prolong the action of other central nervous system depressants). Products include:
Tussionex Pennkinetic Extended-Release Suspension 1624

Chlorpheniramine Tannate (Phenothiazines may intensify or prolong the action of other central nervous system depressants). Products include:
Atrohist Pediatric Suspension 1604
Atrohist Pediatric Suspension Dye-Free 1604
Rynatan 2781
Rynatuss 2782

Chlorpromazine (Phenothiazines may intensify or prolong the action of other central nervous system depressants). Products include:
Thorazine Suppositories 2701

Chlorpromazine Hydrochloride (Phenothiazines may intensify or prolong the action of other central nervous system depressants). Products include:
Thorazine 2701

(▣ Described in PDR For Nonprescription Drugs) (◉ Described in PDR For Ophthalmology)

Chlorprothixene (Phenothiazines may intensify or prolong the action of other central nervous system depressants).
   No products indexed under this heading.

Chlorprothixene Hydrochloride (Phenothiazines may intensify or prolong the action of other central nervous system depressants).
   No products indexed under this heading.

Chlorprothixene Lactate (Phenothiazines may intensify or prolong the action of other central nervous system depressants).
   No products indexed under this heading.

Cisplatin (Vomiting as a sign of toxicity of antineoplastic agents may be obscured by the antiemetic effect of Compazine). Products include:
   Platinol for Injection 717
   Platinol-AQ Injection 719

Clemastine Fumarate (Phenothiazines may intensify or prolong the action of other central nervous system depressants). Products include:
   Tavist Syrup 2426
   Tavist Tablets 2427
   Tavist-1 12 Hour Relief Tablets ... 749
   Tavist-D 12 Hour Relief Tablets ... 750

Clorazepate Dipotassium (Phenothiazines may intensify or prolong the action of other central nervous system depressants). Products include:
   Tranxene 459

Clozapine (Phenothiazines may intensify or prolong the action of other central nervous system depressants). Products include:
   Clozaril Tablets 2377

Codeine Phosphate (Phenothiazines may intensify or prolong the action of other central nervous system depressants). Products include:
   Brontex 2130
   Dimetane-DC Cough Syrup 2232
   Fioricet with Codeine Capsules ... 2387
   Fiorinal with Codeine Capsules ... 2390
   Nucofed 2225
   Phenergan with Codeine 2883
   Phenergan VC with Codeine 2888
   Robitussin A-C Syrup 2248
   Robitussin-DAC Syrup 2249
   Ryna 804
   Soma Compound w/Codeine Tablets 2784
   Tylenol with Codeine 1592

Cyclophosphamide (Vomiting as a sign of toxicity of antineoplastic agents may be obscured by the antiemetic effect of Compazine). Products include:
   Cytoxan 700

Cyproheptadine Hydrochloride (Phenothiazines may intensify or prolong the action of other central nervous system depressants). Products include:
   Periactin 1767

Dacarbazine (Vomiting as a sign of toxicity of antineoplastic agents may be obscured by the antiemetic effect of Compazine). Products include:
   DTIC-Dome 593

Daunorubicin Citrate (Vomiting as a sign of toxicity of antineoplastic agents may be obscured by the antiemetic effect of Compazine). Products include:
   DaunoXome 1842

Daunorubicin Hydrochloride (Vomiting as a sign of toxicity of antineoplastic agents may be obscured by the antiemetic effect of Compazine). Products include:
   Cerubidine for Injection 634

Desflurane (Phenothiazines may intensify or prolong the action of other central nervous system depressants). Products include:
   Suprane (desflurane, USP) 1865

Dexchlorpheniramine Maleate (Phenothiazines may intensify or prolong the action of other central nervous system depressants).
   No products indexed under this heading.

Dezocine (Phenothiazines may intensify or prolong the action of other central nervous system depressants). Products include:
   Dalgan Injection 529

Diazepam (Phenothiazines may intensify or prolong the action of other central nervous system depressants). Products include:
   Dizac (diazepam injectable emulsion) CIV 1862
   Valium Injectable 2336
   Valium Tablets 2335

Dicumarol (Diminished effect of oral anticoagulants).
   No products indexed under this heading.

Diphenhydramine Citrate (Phenothiazines may intensify or prolong the action of other central nervous system depressants). Products include:
   Excedrin P.M. Analgesic/Sleeping Aid Tablets, Caplets, Liquigels ... 735

Diphenhydramine Hydrochloride (Phenothiazines may intensify or prolong the action of other central nervous system depressants). Products include:
   Actifed Allergy Daytime/Nighttime Caplets 808
   Actifed Sinus Daytime/Nighttime Tablets and Caplets 809
   Extra Strength Bayer PM Aspirin Plus Sleep Aid 617
   Benadryl Allergy Chewables 811
   Benadryl Allergy/Cold Tablets ... 811
   Benadryl Allergy Decongestant Liquid Medication 812
   Benadryl Allergy Decongestant Tablets 812
   Benadryl Allergy Liquid Medication 813
   Benadryl Allergy 811
   Benadryl Allergy Sinus Headache Caplets 813
   Benadryl Dye-Free Allergy Liquigel Softgels 813
   Benadryl Dye-Free Allergy Liquid Medication 814
   Benadryl Itch Relief Stick Extra Strength 814
   Benadryl Cream 814
   Benadryl Gel 815
   Benadryl Spray 815
   Benadryl Injection 1955
   Contac Day & Night Cold/Flu Night Caplets 772
   Contac Night Allergy/Sinus Caplets 771
   Extra Strength Doan's P.M. 653
   Excedrin P.M. Analgesic/Sleeping Aid Tablets, Caplets, Liquigels 643
   Nytol QuickCaps Caplets 632
   Sleepinal Night-time Sleep Aid Capsules and Softgels 798
   TYLENOL Allergy Sinus NightTime, Maximum Strength Caplets 1571
   TYLENOL Flu NightTime, Maximum Strength Gelcaps 1575
   TYLENOL Flu NightTime, Maximum Strength Hot Medication Packets 1575
   TYLENOL PM Pain Reliever/Sleep Aid, Extra Strength Gelcaps, Caplets, Geltabs 1576
   TYLENOL Severe Allergy Medication Caplets 1571
   Maximum Strength Unisom Sleepgels 1990
   Unisom With Pain Relief-Nighttime Sleep Aid and Pain Reliever 1991

Divalproex Sodium (Phenothiazines may lower convulsive threshold; dosage adjustments of anticonvulsant may be necessary). Products include:
   Depakote Tablets 418

Docetaxel (Vomiting as a sign of toxicity of antineoplastic agents may be obscured by the antiemetic effect of Compazine). Products include:
   Taxotere for Injection Concentrate 2204

Doxorubicin Hydrochloride (Vomiting as a sign of toxicity of antineoplastic agents may be obscured by the antiemetic effect of Compazine). Products include:
   Adriamycin PFS 2056
   Adriamycin RDF 2056
   Doxil 2613
   Doxorubicin Astra 531
   Rubex for Injection 721

Droperidol (Phenothiazines may intensify or prolong the action of other central nervous system depressants). Products include:
   Inapsine Injection 462

Enflurane (Phenothiazines may intensify or prolong the action of other central nervous system depressants).
   No products indexed under this heading.

Epinephrine (Potential for paradoxical lowering of blood pressure). Products include:
   EPIFRIN 237
   EpiPen 808
   Marcaine with Epinephrine 2446
   Primatene Mist 843
   Sensorcaine with Epinephrine Injection 554
   Sus-Phrine Injection 1017
   Xylocaine with Epinephrine Injections 562

Epinephrine Hydrochloride (Potential for paradoxical lowering of blood pressure). Products include:
   Ana-Kit Anaphylaxis Emergency Treatment Kit 611

Estazolam (Phenothiazines may intensify or prolong the action of other central nervous system depressants). Products include:
   ProSom Tablets 457

Estramustine Phosphate Sodium (Vomiting as a sign of toxicity of antineoplastic agents may be obscured by the antiemetic effect of Compazine). Products include:
   Emcyt Capsules 2085

Ethchlorvynol (Phenothiazines may intensify or prolong the action of other central nervous system depressants). Products include:
   Placidyl Capsules 456

Ethinamate (Phenothiazines may intensify or prolong the action of other central nervous system depressants).
   No products indexed under this heading.

Ethosuximide (Phenothiazines may lower convulsive threshold; dosage adjustments of anticonvulsant may be necessary). Products include:
   Zarontin Capsules 1986
   Zarontin Syrup 1986

Ethotoin (Phenothiazines may lower convulsive threshold; dosage adjustments of anticonvulsant may be necessary). Products include:
   Peganone Tablets 455

Etoposide (Vomiting as a sign of toxicity of antineoplastic agents may be obscured by the antiemetic effect of Compazine). Products include:
   Etoposide Injection 539

   VePesid Capsules and Injection 727

Felbamate (Phenothiazines may lower convulsive threshold; dosage adjustments of anticonvulsant may be necessary). Products include:
   Felbatol 2774

Fentanyl (Phenothiazines may intensify or prolong the action of other central nervous system depressants). Products include:
   Duragesic Transdermal System ... 1336

Fentanyl Citrate (Phenothiazines may intensify or prolong the action of other central nervous system depressants). Products include:
   Sublimaze Injection 463

Floxuridine (Vomiting as a sign of toxicity of antineoplastic agents may be obscured by the antiemetic effect of Compazine). Products include:
   Sterile FUDR 2284

Fluorouracil (Vomiting as a sign of toxicity of antineoplastic agents may be obscured by the antiemetic effect of Compazine). Products include:
   Efudex 2280
   Fluoroplex Topical Solution & Cream 1% 475
   Fluorouracil Injection 2282

Fluphenazine Decanoate (Phenothiazines may intensify or prolong the action of other central nervous system depressants). Products include:
   Prolixin Decanoate 510

Fluphenazine Enanthate (Phenothiazines may intensify or prolong the action of other central nervous system depressants). Products include:
   Prolixin Enanthate 510

Fluphenazine Hydrochloride (Phenothiazines may intensify or prolong the action of other central nervous system depressants). Products include:
   Prolixin 510

Flurazepam Hydrochloride (Phenothiazines may intensify or prolong the action of other central nervous system depressants). Products include:
   Dalmane Capsules 2329

Flutamide (Vomiting as a sign of toxicity of antineoplastic agents may be obscured by the antiemetic effect of Compazine). Products include:
   Eulexin Capsules 2498

Gemcitabine Hydrochloride (Vomiting as a sign of toxicity of antineoplastic agents may be obscured by the antiemetic effect of Compazine). Products include:
   Gemzar for Injection 1482

Glutethimide (Phenothiazines may intensify or prolong the action of other central nervous system depressants).
   No products indexed under this heading.

Guanadrel Sulfate (Co-administration may counteract antihypertensive effects of guanadrel). Products include:
   Hylorel Tablets 1613

Guanethidine Monosulfate (Co-administration may counteract antihypertensive effects of guanethidine). Products include:
   Esimil Tablets 840
   Ismelin Tablets 845

Haloperidol (Phenothiazines may intensify or prolong the action of other central nervous system depressants). Products include:
   Haldol Injection, Tablets and Concentrate 1585

IMPORTANT NOTE: Always consult each drug listing in the patient's regimen for possible interactions.

Compazine | Interactions Index | 198

Haloperidol Decanoate (Phenothiazines may intensify or prolong the action of other central nervous system depressants). Products include:
- Haldol Decanoate 1587

Hydrochlorothiazide (Accentuates the orthostatic hypotension that may occur with phenothiazines). Products include:
- Aldactazide Tablets 2556
- Aldoril Tablets 1644
- Apresazide Capsules 824
- Capozide Tablets 744
- Dyazide Capsules 2653
- Esidrix Tablets 839
- Esimil Tablets 840
- HydroDIURIL Tablets 1716
- Hydropres Tablets 1718
- Hyzaar Tablets 1720
- Inderide Tablets 2838
- Inderide LA Long Acting Capsules .. 2840
- Lopressor HCT Tablets 850
- Lotensin HCT Tablets 855
- Moduretic Tablets 1748
- Oretic Tablets 450
- Prinzide Tablets 1780
- Ser-Ap-Es Tablets 867
- Timolide Tablets 1791
- Vaseretic Tablets 1810
- Zestoretic Tablets 2968
- Ziac 1459

Hydrocodone Bitartrate (Phenothiazines may intensify or prolong the action of other central nervous system depressants). Products include:
- Codiclear DH Syrup 808
- Duratuss HD Elixir 2750
- Histussin D Liquid 670
- Hycodan Tablets and Syrup .. 946
- Hycomine Compound Tablets .. 948
- Hycomine 947
- Hycotuss Expectorant Syrup .. 950
- Hydrocet Capsules 787
- Lorcet 10/650 Tablets 1016
- Lortab 2751
- Tussend 1830
- Tussend Expectorant 1831
- Vicodin Tablets 1404
- Vicodin ES Tablets 1405
- Vicodin HP Tablets 1403
- Vicodin Tuss Expectorant 1406
- Zydone Capsules 967

Hydrocodone Polistirex (Phenothiazines may intensify or prolong the action of other central nervous system depressants). Products include:
- Tussionex Pennkinetic Extended-Release Suspension 1624

Hydroflumethiazide (Accentuates the orthostatic hypotension that may occur with phenothiazines). Products include:
- Diucardin Tablets 2824

Hydromorphone Hydrochloride (Phenothiazines may intensify or prolong the action of other central nervous system depressants). Products include:
- Dilaudid Ampules 1382
- Dilaudid Cough Syrup 1383
- Dilaudid-HP Injection 1384
- Dilaudid-HP Lyophilized Powder 250 mg 1384
- Dilaudid 1382
- Dilaudid Oral Liquid 1386
- Dilaudid 1382
- Dilaudid Tablets - 8 mg 1386

Hydroxyurea (Vomiting as a sign of toxicity of antineoplastic agents may be obscured by the antiemetic effect of Compazine). Products include:
- Hydrea Capsules 705

Hydroxyzine Hydrochloride (Phenothiazines may intensify or prolong the action of other central nervous system depressants). Products include:
- Atarax Tablets & Syrup 1992
- Marax Tablets & DF Syrup ... 2015
- Vistaril Intramuscular Solution 2042

Idarubicin Hydrochloride (Vomiting as a sign of toxicity of antineoplastic agents may be obscured by the antiemetic effect of Compazine). Products include:
- Idamycin Injection 2096

Ifosfamide (Vomiting as a sign of toxicity of antineoplastic agents may be obscured by the antiemetic effect of Compazine). Products include:
- IFEX 706

Interferon alfa-2A, Recombinant (Vomiting as a sign of toxicity of antineoplastic agents may be obscured by the antiemetic effect of Compazine). Products include:
- Roferon-A Injection 2308

Interferon alfa-2B, Recombinant (Vomiting as a sign of toxicity of antineoplastic agents may be obscured by the antiemetic effect of Compazine). Products include:
- Intron A for Injection 2506

Irinotecan Hydrochloride (Vomiting as a sign of toxicity of antineoplastic agents may be obscured by the antiemetic effect of Compazine).
No products indexed under this heading.

Isoflurane (Phenothiazines may intensify or prolong the action of other central nervous system depressants).
No products indexed under this heading.

Ketamine Hydrochloride (Phenothiazines may intensify or prolong the action of other central nervous system depressants).
No products indexed under this heading.

Lamotrigine (Phenothiazines may lower convulsive threshold; dosage adjustments of anticonvulsant may be necessary). Products include:
- Lamictal Tablets 1105

Levamisole Hydrochloride (Vomiting as a sign of toxicity of antineoplastic agents may be obscured by the antiemetic effect of Compazine). Products include:
- Ergamisol Tablets 1340

Levomethadyl Acetate Hydrochloride (Phenothiazines may intensify or prolong the action of other central nervous system depressants). Products include:
- Orlaam Oral Solution 2361

Levorphanol Tartrate (Phenothiazines may intensify or prolong the action of other central nervous system depressants). Products include:
- Levo-Dromoran 2297

Lomustine (CCNU) (Vomiting as a sign of toxicity of antineoplastic agents may be obscured by the antiemetic effect of Compazine). Products include:
- CeeNU Capsules 699

Loratadine (Phenothiazines may intensify or prolong the action of other central nervous system depressants). Products include:
- Claritin Tablets 2485
- Claritin-D Tablets 2487

Lorazepam (Phenothiazines may intensify or prolong the action of other central nervous system depressants). Products include:
- Ativan Injection 2805
- Ativan Tablets 2807

Loxapine Hydrochloride (Phenothiazines may intensify or prolong the action of other central nervous system depressants). Products include:
- Loxitane 1426

Loxapine Succinate (Phenothiazines may intensify or prolong the action of other central nervous system depressants). Products include:
- Loxitane Capsules 1426

Mechlorethamine Hydrochloride (Vomiting as a sign of toxicity of antineoplastic agents may be obscured by the antiemetic effect of Compazine). Products include:
- Mustargen 1752

Megestrol Acetate (Vomiting as a sign of toxicity of antineoplastic agents may be obscured by the antiemetic effect of Compazine). Products include:
- Megace Oral Suspension 708
- Megace Tablets 710

Melphalan (Vomiting as a sign of toxicity of antineoplastic agents may be obscured by the antiemetic effect of Compazine). Products include:
- Alkeran Tablets 1198

Meperidine Hydrochloride (Phenothiazines may intensify or prolong the action of other central nervous system depressants). Products include:
- Demerol 2438
- Mepergan Injection 2859

Mephenytoin (Phenothiazines may lower convulsive threshold; dosage adjustments of anticonvulsant may be necessary). Products include:
- Mesantoin Tablets 2400

Mephobarbital (Phenothiazines may intensify or prolong the action of other central nervous system depressants). Products include:
- Mebaral Tablets 2452

Meprobamate (Phenothiazines may intensify or prolong the action of other central nervous system depressants). Products include:
- Miltown Tablets 2780
- PMB 200 and PMB 400 2890

Mercaptopurine (Vomiting as a sign of toxicity of antineoplastic agents may be obscured by the antiemetic effect of Compazine). Products include:
- Purinethol Tablets 1214

Mesoridazine Besylate (Phenothiazines may intensify or prolong the action of other central nervous system depressants). Products include:
- Serentil 689

Methadone Hydrochloride (Phenothiazines may intensify or prolong the action of other central nervous system depressants). Products include:
- Methadone Hydrochloride Oral Concentrate 2356
- Methadone Hydrochloride Oral Solution & Tablets 2357

Methdilazine Hydrochloride (Phenothiazines may intensify or prolong the action of other central nervous system depressants).
No products indexed under this heading.

Methohexital Sodium (Phenothiazines may intensify or prolong the action of other central nervous system depressants).
No products indexed under this heading.

Methotrexate Sodium (Vomiting as a sign of toxicity of antineoplastic agents may be obscured by the antiemetic effect of Compazine). Products include:
- Methotrexate Sodium Tablets, Injection, for Injection and LPF Injection 1322

Methotrimeprazine (Phenothiazines may intensify or prolong the action of other central nervous system depressants). Products include:
- Levoprome 1321

Methoxyflurane (Phenothiazines may intensify or prolong the action of other central nervous system depressants).
No products indexed under this heading.

Methsuximide (Phenothiazines may lower convulsive threshold; dosage adjustments of anticonvulsant may be necessary). Products include:
- Celontin Kapseals 1955

Methyclothiazide (Accentuates the orthostatic hypotension that may occur with phenothiazines). Products include:
- Enduron Tablets 424

Metrizamide (Concurrent use is not recommended; Compazine should be discontinued at least 48 hours before myelography and should not be resumed for at least 24 hours).

Midazolam Hydrochloride (Phenothiazines may intensify or prolong the action of other central nervous system depressants). Products include:
- Versed Injection 2324

Mitomycin (Mitomycin-C) (Vomiting as a sign of toxicity of antineoplastic agents may be obscured by the antiemetic effect of Compazine). Products include:
- Mutamycin for Injection 712

Mitotane (Vomiting as a sign of toxicity of antineoplastic agents may be obscured by the antiemetic effect of Compazine). Products include:
- Lysodren Tablets 707

Mitoxantrone Hydrochloride (Vomiting as a sign of toxicity of antineoplastic agents may be obscured by the antiemetic effect of Compazine). Products include:
- Novantrone for Injection 1327

Molindone Hydrochloride (Phenothiazines may intensify or prolong the action of other central nervous system depressants). Products include:
- Moban Tablets and Concentrate 1036

Morphine Sulfate (Phenothiazines may intensify or prolong the action of other central nervous system depressants). Products include:
- Astramorph/PF Injection, USP (Preservative-Free) 526
- Duramorph Injection 983
- Infumorph 200 and Infumorph 500 Sterile Solutions 985
- Kadian Capsules 2948
- MS Contin Tablets 2149
- MSIR 2152
- Oramorph SR (Morphine Sulfate Sustained Release Tablets) ... 2359
- RMS Suppositories CII 2766
- Roxanol 2365

Oxazepam (Phenothiazines may intensify or prolong the action of other central nervous system depressants). Products include:
- Serax Capsules 2916
- Serax Tablets 2916

Oxycodone Hydrochloride (Phenothiazines may intensify or prolong the action of other central nervous system depressants). Products include:
- OxyContin Tablets 2163
- OxyIR Capsules 2167
- Percocet Tablets 955
- Percodan Tablets 955
- Percodan-Demi Tablets 956

(⊞ Described in PDR For Nonprescription Drugs)   (⊚ Described in PDR For Ophthalmology)

Interactions Index

Roxicodone Tablets, Oral Solution & Intensol (Oxycodone) ... 2366
Tylox Capsules ... 1593

Paclitaxel (Vomiting as a sign of toxicity of antineoplastic agents may be obscured by the antiemetic effect of Compazine). Products include:
Taxol Injection ... 723

Paramethadione (Phenothiazines may lower convulsive threshold; dosage adjustments of anticonvulsant may be necessary).
No products indexed under this heading.

Pentobarbital Sodium (Phenothiazines may intensify or prolong the action of other central nervous system depressants). Products include:
Nembutal Sodium Capsules ... 440
Nembutal Sodium Solution ... 442
Nembutal Sodium Suppositories ... 444

Perphenazine (Phenothiazines may intensify or prolong the action of other central nervous system depressants). Products include:
Etrafon ... 2495
Triavil Tablets ... 1800
Trilafon ... 2532

Phenacemide (Phenothiazines may lower convulsive threshold; dosage adjustments of anticonvulsant may be necessary). Products include:
Phenurone Tablets ... 455

Phenobarbital (Phenothiazines may lower convulsive threshold; dosage adjustments of anticonvulsant may be necessary; phenothiazines may intensify or prolong the action of other central nervous system depressants). Products include:
Arco-Lase Plus Tablets ... 513
Bellergal-S Tablets ... 2375
Donnatal ... 2234
Donnatal Extentabs ... 2234
Donnatal Tablets ... 2234
Phenobarbital Elixir and Tablets ... 1523
Quadrinal Tablets ... 1398

Phensuximide (Phenothiazines may lower convulsive threshold; dosage adjustments of anticonvulsant may be necessary).
No products indexed under this heading.

Phenytoin (Phenothiazines may lower convulsive threshold; dosage adjustments of anticonvulsant may be necessary; interference with the metabolism of phenytoin precipitating in the phenytoin toxicity). Products include:
Dilantin Infatabs ... 1967
Dilantin-125 Suspension ... 1969

Phenytoin Sodium (Phenothiazines may lower convulsive threshold; dosage adjustments of anticonvulsant may be necessary; interference with the metabolism of phenytoin precipitating in the phenytoin toxicity). Products include:
Dilantin Kapseals ... 1965

Polythiazide (Accentuates the orthostatic hypotension that may occur with phenothiazines). Products include:
Minizide Capsules ... 2016

Prazepam (Phenothiazines may intensify or prolong the action of other central nervous system depressants).
No products indexed under this heading.

Primidone (Phenothiazines may lower convulsive threshold; dosage adjustments of anticonvulsant may be necessary). Products include:
Mysoline ... 2860

Procarbazine Hydrochloride (Vomiting as a sign of toxicity of antineoplastic agents may be obscured by the antiemetic effect of Compazine). Products include:
Matulane Capsules ... 2300

Promethazine Hydrochloride (Phenothiazines may intensify or prolong the action of other central nervous system depressants). Products include:
Mepergan Injection ... 2859
Phenergan with Codeine ... 2883
Phenergan with Dextromethorphan ... 2885
Phenergan Injection ... 2880
Phenergan Suppositories ... 2882
Phenergan Syrup ... 2881
Phenergan Tablets ... 2882
Phenergan VC ... 2886
Phenergan VC with Codeine ... 2888

Propofol (Phenothiazines may intensify or prolong the action of other central nervous system depressants). Products include:
Diprivan Injectable Emulsion ... 2939

Propoxyphene Hydrochloride (Phenothiazines may intensify or prolong the action of other central nervous system depressants). Products include:
Darvon ... 1475
Wygesic Tablets ... 2930

Propoxyphene Napsylate (Phenothiazines may intensify or prolong the action of other central nervous system depressants). Products include:
Darvon-N/Darvocet-N ... 1473

Propranolol Hydrochloride (Co-administration results in increased plasma levels of both drugs). Products include:
Inderal ... 2834
Inderal LA Long Acting Capsules ... 2836
Inderide Tablets ... 2838
Inderide LA Long Acting Capsules ... 2840

Pyrilamine Maleate (Phenothiazines may intensify or prolong the action of other central nervous system depressants). Products include:
4-Way Fast Acting Nasal Spray (regular & mentholated) ... 644
Maximum Strength Multi-Symptom Formula Midol ... 621
PMS Multi-Symptom Formula Midol ... 622

Pyrilamine Tannate (Phenothiazines may intensify or prolong the action of other central nervous system depressants). Products include:
Atrohist Pediatric Suspension ... 1604
Atrohist Pediatric Suspension Dye-Free ... 1604
Rynatan ... 2781

Quazepam (Phenothiazines may intensify or prolong the action of other central nervous system depressants). Products include:
Doral Tablets ... 2773

Risperidone (Phenothiazines may intensify or prolong the action of other central nervous system depressants). Products include:
Risperdal Tablets ... 1348

Secobarbital Sodium (Phenothiazines may intensify or prolong the action of other central nervous system depressants). Products include:
Seconal Sodium Pulvules ... 1529

Sevoflurane (Phenothiazines may intensify or prolong the action of other central nervous system depressants).
No products indexed under this heading.

Streptozocin (Vomiting as a sign of toxicity of antineoplastic agents may be obscured by the antiemetic effect of Compazine). Products include:
Zanosar Sterile Powder ... 2119

Sufentanil Citrate (Phenothiazines may intensify or prolong the action of other central nervous system depressants). Products include:
Sufenta Injection ... 1355

Tamoxifen Citrate (Vomiting as a sign of toxicity of antineoplastic agents may be obscured by the antiemetic effect of Compazine). Products include:
Nolvadex Tablets ... 2957

Temazepam (Phenothiazines may intensify or prolong the action of other central nervous system depressants). Products include:
Restoril Capsules ... 2413

Teniposide (Vomiting as a sign of toxicity of antineoplastic agents may be obscured by the antiemetic effect of Compazine). Products include:
Vumon for Injection ... 729

Terfenadine (Phenothiazines may intensify or prolong the action of other central nervous system depressants). Products include:
Seldane Tablets ... 1284
Seldane-D Extended-Release Tablets ... 1286

Thiamylal Sodium (Phenothiazines may intensify or prolong the action of other central nervous system depressants).
No products indexed under this heading.

Thioguanine (Vomiting as a sign of toxicity of antineoplastic agents may be obscured by the antiemetic effect of Compazine). Products include:
Thioguanine Tablets, Tabloid Brand ... 1225

Thioridazine Hydrochloride (Phenothiazines may intensify or prolong the action of other central nervous system depressants). Products include:
Mellaril ... 2398

Thiotepa (Vomiting as a sign of toxicity of antineoplastic agents may be obscured by the antiemetic effect of Compazine). Products include:
Thioplex (Thiotepa For Injection) ... 1329

Thiothixene (Phenothiazines may intensify or prolong the action of other central nervous system depressants). Products include:
Navane Capsules and Concentrate ... 2018
Navane Intramuscular ... 2019

Topotecan Hydrochloride (Vomiting as a sign of toxicity of antineoplastic agents may be obscured by the antiemetic effect of Compazine). Products include:
Hycamtin for Injection ... 2665

Triazolam (Phenothiazines may intensify or prolong the action of other central nervous system depressants). Products include:
Halcion Tablets ... 2093

Trifluoperazine Hydrochloride (Phenothiazines may intensify or prolong the action of other central nervous system depressants). Products include:
Stelazine ... 2692

Trimeprazine Tartrate (Phenothiazines may intensify or prolong the action of other central nervous system depressants).
No products indexed under this heading.

Trimethadione (Phenothiazines may lower convulsive threshold; dosage adjustments of anticonvulsant may be necessary).
No products indexed under this heading.

Tripelennamine Hydrochloride (Phenothiazines may intensify or prolong the action of other central nervous system depressants). Products include:
PBZ Tablets ... 863
PBZ-SR Tablets ... 862

Triprolidine Hydrochloride (Phenothiazines may intensify or prolong the action of other central nervous system depressants). Products include:
Actifed Cold & Allergy Tablets ... 807
Actifed Cold & Sinus Caplets and Tablets ... 808

Valproic Acid (Phenothiazines may lower convulsive threshold; dosage adjustments of anticonvulsant may be necessary). Products include:
Depakene ... 416

Vincristine Sulfate (Vomiting as a sign of toxicity of antineoplastic agents may be obscured by the antiemetic effect of Compazine). Products include:
Oncovin Solution Vials & Hyporets ... 1521

Vinorelbine Tartrate (Vomiting as a sign of toxicity of antineoplastic agents may be obscured by the antiemetic effect of Compazine). Products include:
Navelbine Injection ... 1212

Warfarin Sodium (Diminished effect of oral anticoagulants). Products include:
Coumadin ... 941

Zolpidem Tartrate (Phenothiazines may intensify or prolong the action of other central nervous system depressants). Products include:
Ambien Tablets ... 2559

Food Interactions

Alcohol (Phenothiazines may intensify or prolong the action of other central nervous system depressants).

COMPLETE FOR MEN (Vitamins with Minerals) ... 603
None cited in PDR database.

COMPLETE FOR WOMEN (Vitamins with Minerals) ... 603
None cited in PDR database.

COMMON SENSE COMPLETE (Vitamins with Minerals) ... 604
None cited in PDR database.

COMMON SENSE COMPLETE WITH EXTRA CALCIUM AND IRON (Vitamins with Minerals) ... 604
None cited in PDR database.

NATURAL MD COMPLETE RX (Vitamins with Minerals) ... 605
None cited in PDR database.

ALLERGY-SINUS COMTREX MULTI-SYMPTOM ALLERGY-SINUS FORMULA TABLETS AND CAPLETS
(Acetaminophen, Chlorpheniramine Maleate, Pseudoephedrine Hydrochloride) ... 639
May interact with:

IMPORTANT NOTE: Always consult each drug listing in the patient's regimen for possible interactions.

Comtrex Allergy-Sinus / Interactions Index

Alprazolam (Increases drowsiness effect). Products include:
  Xanax Tablets 2115
Antidepressant Medications, unspecified (Effect not specified).
Blood Pressure Medications, unspecified (Effect not specified).
  No products indexed under this heading.
Buspirone Hydrochloride (Increases drowsiness effect). Products include:
  BuSpar Tablets 738
Chlordiazepoxide (Increases drowsiness effect). Products include:
  Limbitrol 2333
Chlordiazepoxide Hydrochloride (Increases drowsiness effect). Products include:
  Librax Capsules 2330
  Librium Capsules 2331
  Librium Injectable 2332
Chlorpromazine (Increases drowsiness effect). Products include:
  Thorazine Suppositories 2701
Chlorprothixene (Increases drowsiness effect).
  No products indexed under this heading.
Chlorprothixene Hydrochloride (Increases drowsiness effect).
  No products indexed under this heading.
Clorazepate Dipotassium (Increases drowsiness effect). Products include:
  Tranxene 459
Diazepam (Increases drowsiness effect). Products include:
  Dizac (diazepam injectable emulsion) CIV 1862
  Valium Injectable 2336
  Valium Tablets 2335
Droperidol (Increases drowsiness effect). Products include:
  Inapsine Injection 462
Estazolam (Increases drowsiness effect). Products include:
  ProSom Tablets 457
Ethchlorvynol (Increases drowsiness effect). Products include:
  Placidyl Capsules 456
Ethinamate (Increases drowsiness effect).
  No products indexed under this heading.
Fluphenazine Decanoate (Increases drowsiness effect). Products include:
  Prolixin Decanoate 510
Fluphenazine Enanthate (Increases drowsiness effect). Products include:
  Prolixin Enanthate 510
Fluphenazine Hydrochloride (Increases drowsiness effect). Products include:
  Prolixin 510
Flurazepam Hydrochloride (Increases drowsiness effect). Products include:
  Dalmane Capsules 2329
Glutethimide (Increases drowsiness effect).
  No products indexed under this heading.
Haloperidol (Increases drowsiness effect). Products include:
  Haldol Injection, Tablets and Concentrate 1585
Haloperidol Decanoate (Increases drowsiness effect). Products include:
  Haldol Decanoate 1587

Hydroxyzine Hydrochloride (Increases drowsiness effect). Products include:
  Atarax Tablets & Syrup 1992
  Marax Tablets & DF Syrup 2015
  Vistaril Intramuscular Solution ... 2042
Lorazepam (Increases drowsiness effect). Products include:
  Ativan Injection 2805
  Ativan Tablets 2807
Loxapine Hydrochloride (Increases drowsiness effect). Products include:
  Loxitane 1426
Loxapine Succinate (Increases drowsiness effect). Products include:
  Loxitane Capsules 1426
Meprobamate (Increases drowsiness effect). Products include:
  Miltown Tablets 2780
  PMB 200 and PMB 400 2890
Mesoridazine Besylate (Increases drowsiness effect). Products include:
  Serentil 689
Midazolam Hydrochloride (Increases drowsiness effect). Products include:
  Versed Injection 2324
Molindone Hydrochloride (Increases drowsiness effect). Products include:
  Moban Tablets and Concentrate ... 1036
Oxazepam (Increases drowsiness effect). Products include:
  Serax Capsules 2916
  Serax Tablets 2916
Perphenazine (Increases drowsiness effect). Products include:
  Etrafon 2495
  Triavil Tablets 1800
  Trilafon 2532
Prazepam (Increases drowsiness effect).
  No products indexed under this heading.
Prochlorperazine (Increases drowsiness effect). Products include:
  Compazine 2644
Promethazine Hydrochloride (Increases drowsiness effect). Products include:
  Mepergan Injection 2859
  Phenergan with Codeine 2883
  Phenergan with Dextromethorphan ... 2885
  Phenergan Injection 2880
  Phenergan Suppositories 2882
  Phenergan Syrup 2881
  Phenergan Tablets 2882
  Phenergan VC 2886
  Phenergan VC with Codeine 2888
Propofol (Increases drowsiness effect). Products include:
  Diprivan Injectable Emulsion ... 2939
Quazepam (Increases drowsiness effect). Products include:
  Doral Tablets 2773
Secobarbital Sodium (Increases drowsiness effect). Products include:
  Seconal Sodium Pulvules 1529
Temazepam (Increases drowsiness effect). Products include:
  Restoril Capsules 2413
Thioridazine Hydrochloride (Increases drowsiness effect). Products include:
  Mellaril 2398
Thiothixene (Increases drowsiness effect). Products include:
  Navane Capsules and Concentrate ... 2018
  Navane Intramuscular 2019
Triazolam (Increases drowsiness effect). Products include:
  Halcion Tablets 2093
Trifluoperazine Hydrochloride (Increases drowsiness effect). Products include:
  Stelazine 2692

Zolpidem Tartrate (Increases drowsiness effect). Products include:
  Ambien Tablets 2559

Food Interactions
Alcohol (Increases drowsiness effect).

COMTREX MULTI-SYMPTOM COLD RELIEVER LIQUID
(Acetaminophen, Chlorpheniramine Maleate, Dextromethorphan Hydrobromide, Pseudoephedrine Hydrochloride) ▣ 638
See Comtrex Multi-Symptom Cold Reliever Tablets and Caplets

COMTREX MULTI-SYMPTOM COLD RELIEVER LIQUI-GELS
(Acetaminophen, Chlorpheniramine Maleate, Dextromethorphan Hydrobromide, Pseudoephedrine Hydrochloride) ▣ 638
See Comtrex Multi-Symptom Cold Reliever Tablets and Caplets

COMTREX MULTI-SYMPTOM COLD RELIEVER TABLETS AND CAPLETS
(Acetaminophen, Chlorpheniramine Maleate, Dextromethorphan Hydrobromide, Pseudoephedrine Hydrochloride) ▣ 638
May interact with monoamine oxidase inhibitors, hypnotics and sedatives, tranquilizers, and certain other agents. Compounds in these categories include:

Alprazolam (May increase drowsiness effect). Products include:
  Xanax Tablets 2115
Buspirone Hydrochloride (May increase drowsiness effect). Products include:
  BuSpar Tablets 738
Chlordiazepoxide (May increase drowsiness effect). Products include:
  Limbitrol 2333
Chlordiazepoxide Hydrochloride (May increase drowsiness effect). Products include:
  Librax Capsules 2330
  Librium Capsules 2331
  Librium Injectable 2332
Chlorpromazine (May increase drowsiness effect). Products include:
  Thorazine Suppositories 2701
Chlorpromazine Hydrochloride (May increase drowsiness effect). Products include:
  Thorazine 2701
Chlorprothixene (May increase drowsiness effect).
  No products indexed under this heading.
Chlorprothixene Hydrochloride (May increase drowsiness effect).
  No products indexed under this heading.
Clorazepate Dipotassium (May increase drowsiness effect). Products include:
  Tranxene 459
Diazepam (May increase drowsiness effect). Products include:
  Dizac (diazepam injectable emulsion) CIV 1862
  Valium Injectable 2336
  Valium Tablets 2335
Droperidol (May increase drowsiness effect). Products include:
  Inapsine Injection 462
Estazolam (May increase drowsiness effect). Products include:
  ProSom Tablets 457

Ethchlorvynol (May increase drowsiness effect). Products include:
  Placidyl Capsules 456
Ethinamate (May increase drowsiness effect).
  No products indexed under this heading.
Fluphenazine Decanoate (May increase drowsiness effect). Products include:
  Prolixin Decanoate 510
Fluphenazine Enanthate (May increase drowsiness effect). Products include:
  Prolixin Enanthate 510
Fluphenazine Hydrochloride (May increase drowsiness effect). Products include:
  Prolixin 510
Flurazepam Hydrochloride (May increase drowsiness effect). Products include:
  Dalmane Capsules 2329
Furazolidone (Concurrent and/or sequential use is not recommended). Products include:
  Furoxone 2221
Glutethimide (May increase drowsiness effect).
  No products indexed under this heading.
Haloperidol (May increase drowsiness effect). Products include:
  Haldol Injection, Tablets and Concentrate 1585
Haloperidol Decanoate (May increase drowsiness effect). Products include:
  Haldol Decanoate 1587
Hydroxyzine Hydrochloride (May increase drowsiness effect). Products include:
  Atarax Tablets & Syrup 1992
  Marax Tablets & DF Syrup 2015
  Vistaril Intramuscular Solution ... 2042
Isocarboxazid (Concurrent and/or sequential use is not recommended).
  No products indexed under this heading.
Lorazepam (May increase drowsiness effect). Products include:
  Ativan Injection 2805
  Ativan Tablets 2807
Loxapine Hydrochloride (May increase drowsiness effect). Products include:
  Loxitane 1426
Loxapine Succinate (May increase drowsiness effect). Products include:
  Loxitane Capsules 1426
Meprobamate (May increase drowsiness effect). Products include:
  Miltown Tablets 2780
  PMB 200 and PMB 400 2890
Mesoridazine Besylate (May increase drowsiness effect). Products include:
  Serentil 689
Midazolam Hydrochloride (May increase drowsiness effect). Products include:
  Versed Injection 2324
Molindone Hydrochloride (May increase drowsiness effect). Products include:
  Moban Tablets and Concentrate ... 1036
Oxazepam (May increase drowsiness effect). Products include:
  Serax Capsules 2916
  Serax Tablets 2916
Perphenazine (May increase drowsiness effect). Products include:
  Etrafon 2495
  Triavil Tablets 1800
  Trilafon 2532

(▣ Described in PDR For Nonprescription Drugs)   (◎ Described in PDR For Ophthalmology)

Interactions Index / Contac Continuous Capsules

Phenelzine Sulfate (Concurrent and/or sequential use is not recommended). Products include:
Nardil 1977
Prazepam (May increase drowsiness effect).
No products indexed under this heading.
Prochlorperazine (May increase drowsiness effect). Products include:
Compazine 2644
Promethazine Hydrochloride (May increase drowsiness effect). Products include:
Mepergan Injection 2859
Phenergan with Codeine 2883
Phenergan with Dextromethorphan 2885
Phenergan Injection 2880
Phenergan Suppositories 2882
Phenergan Syrup 2881
Phenergan Tablets 2882
Phenergan VC 2886
Phenergan VC with Codeine 2888
Propofol (May increase drowsiness effect). Products include:
Diprivan Injectable Emulsion 2939
Quazepam (May increase drowsiness effect). Products include:
Doral Tablets 2773
Secobarbital Sodium (May increase drowsiness effect). Products include:
Seconal Sodium Pulvules 1529
Selegiline Hydrochloride (Concurrent and/or sequential use is not recommended). Products include:
Eldepryl Capsules 2729
Temazepam (May increase drowsiness effect). Products include:
Restoril Capsules 2413
Thioridazine Hydrochloride (May increase drowsiness effect). Products include:
Mellaril 2398
Thiothixene (May increase drowsiness effect). Products include:
Navane Capsules and Concentrate 2018
Navane Intramuscular 2019
Tranylcypromine Sulfate (Concurrent and/or sequential use is not recommended). Products include:
Parnate Tablets 2679
Triazolam (May increase drowsiness effect). Products include:
Halcion Tablets 2093
Trifluoperazine Hydrochloride (May increase drowsiness effect). Products include:
Stelazine 2692
Zolpidem Tartrate (May increase drowsiness effect). Products include:
Ambien Tablets 2559

Food Interactions
Alcohol (May increase drowsiness effect).

COMTREX MULTI-SYMPTOM NON-DROWSY CAPLETS
(Acetaminophen, Dextromethorphan Hydrobromide, Pseudoephedrine Hydrochloride) 640
May interact with monoamine oxidase inhibitors. Compounds in this category include:

Furazolidone (Concurrent and/or sequential use is not recommended). Products include:
Furoxone 2221
Isocarboxazid (Concurrent and/or sequential use is not recommended).
No products indexed under this heading.
Phenelzine Sulfate (Concurrent and/or sequential use is not recommended). Products include:
Nardil 1977

Selegiline Hydrochloride (Concurrent and/or sequential use is not recommended). Products include:
Eldepryl Capsules 2729
Tranylcypromine Sulfate (Concurrent and/or sequential use is not recommended). Products include:
Parnate Tablets 2679

COMTREX MULTI-SYMPTOM NON-DROWSY LIQUI-GELS
(Acetaminophen, Dextromethorphan Hydrobromide, Phenylpropanolamine Hydrochloride) 640
See Comtrex Multi-Symptom Non-Drowsy Caplets

CONCEPT ANTIMICROBIAL SKIN CLEANSER
(Chloroxylenol) 646
None cited in PDR database.

CONDYLOX TOPICAL SOLUTION
(Podofilox) 1853
None cited in PDR database.

CONGESS JR. T.D. CAPSULES
(Guaifenesin, Pseudoephedrine Hydrochloride) 1003
May interact with monoamine oxidase inhibitors. Compounds in this category include:

Furazolidone (Concurrent administration is contraindicated). Products include:
Furoxone 2221
Isocarboxazid (Concurrent administration is contraindicated).
No products indexed under this heading.
Phenelzine Sulfate (Concurrent administration is contraindicated). Products include:
Nardil 1977
Selegiline Hydrochloride (Concurrent administration is contraindicated). Products include:
Eldepryl Capsules 2729
Tranylcypromine Sulfate (Concurrent administration is contraindicated). Products include:
Parnate Tablets 2679

CONGESS SR. T.D. CAPSULES
(Guaifenesin, Pseudoephedrine Hydrochloride) 1003
May interact with monoamine oxidase inhibitors. Compounds in this category include:

Furazolidone (Concurrent administration is contraindicated). Products include:
Furoxone 2221
Isocarboxazid (Concurrent administration is contraindicated).
No products indexed under this heading.
Phenelzine Sulfate (Concurrent administration is contraindicated). Products include:
Nardil 1977
Selegiline Hydrochloride (Concurrent administration is contraindicated). Products include:
Eldepryl Capsules 2729
Tranylcypromine Sulfate (Concurrent administration is contraindicated). Products include:
Parnate Tablets 2679

CONTAC CONTINUOUS ACTION NASAL DECONGESTANT/ANTIHISTAMINE 12 HOUR CAPSULES
(Chlorpheniramine Maleate, Phenylpropanolamine Hydrochloride) 773
May interact with monoamine oxidase inhibitors, tranquilizers, hypnotics and sedatives, and certain other agents. Compounds in these categories include:

Alprazolam (May increase drowsiness effect; concurrent use should be avoided). Products include:
Xanax Tablets 2115
Buspirone Hydrochloride (May increase drowsiness effect; concurrent use should be avoided). Products include:
BuSpar Tablets 738
Chlordiazepoxide (May increase drowsiness effect; concurrent use should be avoided). Products include:
Limbitrol 2333
Chlordiazepoxide Hydrochloride (May increase drowsiness effect; concurrent use should be avoided). Products include:
Librax Capsules 2330
Librium Capsules 2331
Librium Injectable 2332
Chlorpromazine (May increase drowsiness effect; concurrent use should be avoided). Products include:
Thorazine Suppositories 2701
Chlorpromazine Hydrochloride (May increase drowsiness effect; concurrent use should be avoided). Products include:
Thorazine 2701
Chlorprothixene (May increase drowsiness effect; concurrent use should be avoided).
No products indexed under this heading.
Chlorprothixene Hydrochloride (May increase drowsiness effect; concurrent use should be avoided).
No products indexed under this heading.
Clorazepate Dipotassium (May increase drowsiness effect; concurrent use should be avoided). Products include:
Tranxene 459
Diazepam (May increase drowsiness effect; concurrent use should be avoided). Products include:
Dizac (diazepam injectable emulsion) CIV 1862
Valium Injectable 2336
Valium Tablets 2335
Droperidol (May increase drowsiness effect; concurrent use should be avoided). Products include:
Inapsine Injection 462
Estazolam (May increase drowsiness effect; concurrent use should be avoided). Products include:
ProSom Tablets 457
Ethchlorvynol (May increase drowsiness effect; concurrent use should be avoided). Products include:
Placidyl Capsules 456
Ethinamate (May increase drowsiness effect; concurrent use should be avoided).
No products indexed under this heading.

Fluphenazine Decanoate (May increase drowsiness effect; concurrent use should be avoided). Products include:
Prolixin Decanoate 510
Fluphenazine Enanthate (May increase drowsiness effect; concurrent use should be avoided). Products include:
Prolixin Enanthate 510
Fluphenazine Hydrochloride (May increase drowsiness effect; concurrent use should be avoided). Products include:
Prolixin 510
Flurazepam Hydrochloride (May increase drowsiness effect; concurrent use should be avoided). Products include:
Dalmane Capsules 2329
Furazolidone (Concurrent and/or sequential use is not recommended unless directed by a doctor). Products include:
Furoxone 2221
Glutethimide (May increase drowsiness effect; concurrent use should be avoided).
No products indexed under this heading.
Haloperidol (May increase drowsiness effect; concurrent use should be avoided). Products include:
Haldol Injection, Tablets and Concentrate 1585
Haloperidol Decanoate (May increase drowsiness effect; concurrent use should be avoided). Products include:
Haldol Decanoate 1587
Hydroxyzine Hydrochloride (May increase drowsiness effect; concurrent use should be avoided). Products include:
Atarax Tablets & Syrup 1992
Marax Tablets & DF Syrup 2015
Vistaril Intramuscular Solution 2042
Isocarboxazid (Concurrent and/or sequential use is not recommended unless directed by a doctor).
No products indexed under this heading.
Lorazepam (May increase drowsiness effect; concurrent use should be avoided). Products include:
Ativan Injection 2805
Ativan Tablets 2807
Loxapine Hydrochloride (May increase drowsiness effect; concurrent use should be avoided). Products include:
Loxitane 1426
Loxapine Succinate (May increase drowsiness effect; concurrent use should be avoided). Products include:
Loxitane Capsules 1426
Meprobamate (May increase drowsiness effect; concurrent use should be avoided). Products include:
Miltown Tablets 2780
PMB 200 and PMB 400 2890
Mesoridazine Besylate (May increase drowsiness effect; concurrent use should be avoided). Products include:
Serentil 689
Midazolam Hydrochloride (May increase drowsiness effect; concurrent use should be avoided). Products include:
Versed Injection 2324
Molindone Hydrochloride (May increase drowsiness effect; concurrent use should be avoided). Products include:
Moban Tablets and Concentrate 1036

IMPORTANT NOTE: Always consult each drug listing in the patient's regimen for possible interactions.

Contac Continuous Capsules

Oxazepam (May increase drowsiness effect; concurrent use should be avoided). Products include:
Serax Capsules 2916
Serax Tablets 2916

Perphenazine (May increase drowsiness effect; concurrent use should be avoided). Products include:
Etrafon 2495
Triavil Tablets 1800
Trilafon 2532

Phenelzine Sulfate (Concurrent and/or sequential use is not recommended unless directed by a doctor). Products include:
Nardil 1977

Prazepam (May increase drowsiness effect; concurrent use should be avoided).
No products indexed under this heading.

Prochlorperazine (May increase drowsiness effect; concurrent use should be avoided). Products include:
Compazine 2644

Promethazine Hydrochloride (May increase drowsiness effect; concurrent use should be avoided). Products include:
Mepergan Injection 2859
Phenergan with Codeine 2883
Phenergan with Dextromethorphan 2885
Phenergan Injection 2880
Phenergan Suppositories 2882
Phenergan Syrup 2881
Phenergan Tablets 2882
Phenergan VC 2886
Phenergan VC with Codeine 2888

Propofol (May increase drowsiness effect; concurrent use should be avoided). Products include:
Diprivan Injectable Emulsion 2939

Quazepam (May increase drowsiness effect; concurrent use should be avoided). Products include:
Doral Tablets 2773

Secobarbital Sodium (May increase drowsiness effect; concurrent use should be avoided). Products include:
Seconal Sodium Pulvules 1529

Selegiline Hydrochloride (Concurrent and/or sequential use is not recommended unless directed by a doctor). Products include:
Eldepryl Capsules 2729

Temazepam (May increase drowsiness effect; concurrent use should be avoided). Products include:
Restoril Capsules 2413

Thioridazine Hydrochloride (May increase drowsiness effect; concurrent use should be avoided). Products include:
Mellaril 2398

Thiothixene (May increase drowsiness effect; concurrent use should be avoided). Products include:
Navane Capsules and Concentrate 2018
Navane Intramuscular 2019

Tranylcypromine Sulfate (Concurrent and/or sequential use is not recommended unless directed by a doctor). Products include:
Parnate Tablets 2679

Triazolam (May increase drowsiness effect; concurrent use should be avoided). Products include:
Halcion Tablets 2093

Trifluoperazine Hydrochloride (May increase drowsiness effect; concurrent use should be avoided). Products include:
Stelazine 2692

Zolpidem Tartrate (May increase drowsiness effect; concurrent use should be avoided). Products include:
Ambien Tablets 2559

Food Interactions
Alcohol (May increase drowsiness effect; concurrent use should be avoided).

CONTAC DAY ALLERGY/SINUS CAPLETS
(Acetaminophen) .... ⊞ 771
See **Contac Night Allergy/Sinus Caplets**

CONTAC DAY & NIGHT COLD/FLU CAPLETS
(Acetaminophen, Pseudoephedrine Hydrochloride, Dextromethorphan Hydrobromide) .... ⊞ 772
See **Contac Day & Night Cold/Flu Night Caplets**

CONTAC DAY & NIGHT COLD/FLU NIGHT CAPLETS
(Acetaminophen, Pseudoephedrine Hydrochloride, Diphenhydramine Hydrochloride) .... ⊞ 772
May interact with monoamine oxidase inhibitors, tranquilizers, hypnotics and sedatives, and certain other agents. Compounds in these categories include:

Alprazolam (May increase the drowsiness effect). Products include:
Xanax Tablets 2115

Buspirone Hydrochloride (May increase the drowsiness effect). Products include:
BuSpar Tablets 738

Chlordiazepoxide (May increase the drowsiness effect). Products include:
Limbitrol 2333

Chlordiazepoxide Hydrochloride (May increase the drowsiness effect). Products include:
Librax Capsules 2330
Librium Capsules 2331
Librium Injectable 2332

Chlorpromazine (May increase the drowsiness effect). Products include:
Thorazine Suppositories 2701

Chlorpromazine Hydrochloride (May increase the drowsiness effect). Products include:
Thorazine 2701

Chlorprothixene (May increase the drowsiness effect).
No products indexed under this heading.

Chlorprothixene Hydrochloride (May increase the drowsiness effect).
No products indexed under this heading.

Clorazepate Dipotassium (May increase the drowsiness effect). Products include:
Tranxene 459

Diazepam (May increase the drowsiness effect). Products include:
Dizac (diazepam injectable emulsion) CIV 1862
Valium Injectable 2336
Valium Tablets 2335

Droperidol (May increase the drowsiness effect). Products include:
Inapsine Injection 462

Estazolam (May increase the drowsiness effect). Products include:
ProSom Tablets 457

Ethchlorvynol (May increase the drowsiness effect). Products include:
Placidyl Capsules 456

Ethinamate (May increase the drowsiness effect).
No products indexed under this heading.

Fluphenazine Decanoate (May increase the drowsiness effect). Products include:
Prolixin Decanoate 510

Fluphenazine Enanthate (May increase the drowsiness effect). Products include:
Prolixin Enanthate 510

Fluphenazine Hydrochloride (May increase the drowsiness effect). Products include:
Prolixin 510

Flurazepam Hydrochloride (May increase the drowsiness effect). Products include:
Dalmane Capsules 2329

Furazolidone (Concurrent and/or sequential use is not recommended). Products include:
Furoxone 2221

Glutethimide (May increase the drowsiness effect).
No products indexed under this heading.

Haloperidol (May increase the drowsiness effect). Products include:
Haldol Injection, Tablets and Concentrate 1585

Haloperidol Decanoate (May increase the drowsiness effect). Products include:
Haldol Decanoate 1587

Hydroxyzine Hydrochloride (May increase the drowsiness effect). Products include:
Atarax Tablets & Syrup 1992
Marax Tablets & DF Syrup 2015
Vistaril Intramuscular Solution... 2042

Isocarboxazid (Concurrent and/or sequential use is not recommended).
No products indexed under this heading.

Lorazepam (May increase the drowsiness effect). Products include:
Ativan Injection 2805
Ativan Tablets 2807

Loxapine Hydrochloride (May increase the drowsiness effect). Products include:
Loxitane 1426

Loxapine Succinate (May increase the drowsiness effect). Products include:
Loxitane Capsules 1426

Meprobamate (May increase the drowsiness effect). Products include:
Miltown Tablets 2780
PMB 200 and PMB 400 2890

Mesoridazine Besylate (May increase the drowsiness effect). Products include:
Serentil 689

Midazolam Hydrochloride (May increase the drowsiness effect). Products include:
Versed Injection 2324

Molindone Hydrochloride (May increase the drowsiness effect). Products include:
Moban Tablets and Concentrate... 1036

Oxazepam (May increase the drowsiness effect). Products include:
Serax Capsules 2916
Serax Tablets 2916

Perphenazine (May increase the drowsiness effect). Products include:
Etrafon 2495
Triavil Tablets 1800
Trilafon 2532

Phenelzine Sulfate (Concurrent and/or sequential use is not recommended). Products include:
Nardil 1977

Prazepam (May increase the drowsiness effect).
No products indexed under this heading.

Prochlorperazine (May increase the drowsiness effect). Products include:
Compazine 2644

Promethazine Hydrochloride (May increase the drowsiness effect). Products include:
Mepergan Injection 2859
Phenergan with Codeine 2883
Phenergan with Dextromethorphan 2885
Phenergan Injection 2880
Phenergan Suppositories 2882
Phenergan Syrup 2881
Phenergan Tablets 2882
Phenergan VC 2886
Phenergan VC with Codeine 2888

Propofol (May increase the drowsiness effect). Products include:
Diprivan Injectable Emulsion 2939

Quazepam (May increase the drowsiness effect). Products include:
Doral Tablets 2773

Secobarbital Sodium (May increase the drowsiness effect). Products include:
Seconal Sodium Pulvules 1529

Selegiline Hydrochloride (Concurrent and/or sequential use is not recommended). Products include:
Eldepryl Capsules 2729

Temazepam (May increase the drowsiness effect). Products include:
Restoril Capsules 2413

Thioridazine Hydrochloride (May increase the drowsiness effect). Products include:
Mellaril 2398

Thiothixene (May increase the drowsiness effect). Products include:
Navane Capsules and Concentrate 2018
Navane Intramuscular 2019

Tranylcypromine Sulfate (Concurrent and/or sequential use is not recommended). Products include:
Parnate Tablets 2679

Triazolam (May increase the drowsiness effect). Products include:
Halcion Tablets 2093

Trifluoperazine Hydrochloride (May increase the drowsiness effect). Products include:
Stelazine 2692

Zolpidem Tartrate (May increase the drowsiness effect). Products include:
Ambien Tablets 2559

Food Interactions
Alcohol (Increases drowsiness effect).

CONTAC MAXIMUM STRENGTH CONTINUOUS ACTION DECONGESTANT/ANTIHISTAMINE 12 HOUR CAPLETS
(Chlorpheniramine Maleate, Phenylpropanolamine Hydrochloride) .... ⊞ 772
May interact with monoamine oxidase inhibitors, tranquilizers, hypnotics and sedatives, and certain other agents. Compounds in these categories include:

Alprazolam (May increase drowsiness effect; concurrent use should be avoided). Products include:
Xanax Tablets 2115

Buspirone Hydrochloride (May increase drowsiness effect; concurrent use should be avoided). Products include:
BuSpar Tablets 738

(⊞ Described in PDR For Nonprescription Drugs) (⊙ Described in PDR For Ophthalmology)

Chlordiazepoxide (May increase drowsiness effect; concurrent use should be avoided). Products include:
Limbitrol 2333

Chlordiazepoxide Hydrochloride (May increase drowsiness effect; concurrent use should be avoided). Products include:
Librax Capsules 2330
Librium Capsules 2331
Librium Injectable 2332

Chlorpromazine (May increase drowsiness effect; concurrent use should be avoided). Products include:
Thorazine Suppositories 2701

Chlorpromazine Hydrochloride (May increase drowsiness effect; concurrent use should be avoided). Products include:
Thorazine 2701

Chlorprothixene (May increase drowsiness effect; concurrent use should be avoided).
No products indexed under this heading.

Chlorprothixene Hydrochloride (May increase drowsiness effect; concurrent use should be avoided).
No products indexed under this heading.

Clorazepate Dipotassium (May increase drowsiness effect; concurrent use should be avoided). Products include:
Tranxene 459

Diazepam (May increase drowsiness effect; concurrent use should be avoided). Products include:
Dizac (diazepam injectable emulsion) CIV 1862
Valium Injectable 2336
Valium Tablets 2335

Droperidol (May increase drowsiness effect; concurrent use should be avoided). Products include:
Inapsine Injection 462

Estazolam (May increase drowsiness effect; concurrent use should be avoided). Products include:
ProSom Tablets 457

Ethchlorvynol (May increase drowsiness effect; concurrent use should be avoided). Products include:
Placidyl Capsules 456

Ethinamate (May increase drowsiness effect; concurrent use should be avoided).
No products indexed under this heading.

Fluphenazine Decanoate (May increase drowsiness effect; concurrent use should be avoided). Products include:
Prolixin Decanoate 510

Fluphenazine Enanthate (May increase drowsiness effect; concurrent use should be avoided). Products include:
Prolixin Enanthate 510

Fluphenazine Hydrochloride (May increase drowsiness effect; concurrent use should be avoided). Products include:
Prolixin 510

Flurazepam Hydrochloride (May increase drowsiness effect; concurrent use should be avoided). Products include:
Dalmane Capsules 2329

Furazolidone (Concurrent and/or sequential use is not recommended unless directed by a doctor). Products include:
Furoxone 2221

Glutethimide (May increase drowsiness effect; concurrent use should be avoided).
No products indexed under this heading.

Haloperidol (May increase drowsiness effect; concurrent use should be avoided). Products include:
Haldol Injection, Tablets and Concentrate 1585

Haloperidol Decanoate (May increase drowsiness effect; concurrent use should be avoided). Products include:
Haldol Decanoate 1587

Hydroxyzine Hydrochloride (May increase drowsiness effect; concurrent use should be avoided). Products include:
Atarax Tablets & Syrup 1992
Marax Tablets & DF Syrup 2015
Vistaril Intramuscular Solution 2042

Isocarboxazid (Concurrent and/or sequential use is not recommended unless directed by a doctor).
No products indexed under this heading.

Lorazepam (May increase drowsiness effect; concurrent use should be avoided). Products include:
Ativan Injection 2805
Ativan Tablets 2807

Loxapine Hydrochloride (May increase drowsiness effect; concurrent use should be avoided). Products include:
Loxitane 1426

Loxapine Succinate (May increase drowsiness effect; concurrent use should be avoided). Products include:
Loxitane Capsules 1426

Meprobamate (May increase drowsiness effect; concurrent use should be avoided). Products include:
Miltown Tablets 2780
PMB 200 and PMB 400 2890

Mesoridazine Besylate (May increase drowsiness effect; concurrent use should be avoided). Products include:
Serentil 689

Midazolam Hydrochloride (May increase drowsiness effect; concurrent use should be avoided). Products include:
Versed Injection 2324

Molindone Hydrochloride (May increase drowsiness effect; concurrent use should be avoided). Products include:
Moban Tablets and Concentrate 1036

Oxazepam (May increase drowsiness effect; concurrent use should be avoided). Products include:
Serax Capsules 2916
Serax Tablets 2916

Perphenazine (May increase drowsiness effect; concurrent use should be avoided). Products include:
Etrafon 2495
Triavil Tablets 1800
Trilafon 2532

Phenelzine Sulfate (Concurrent and/or sequential use is not recommended unless directed by a doctor). Products include:
Nardil 1977

Prazepam (May increase drowsiness effect; concurrent use should be avoided).
No products indexed under this heading.

Prochlorperazine (May increase drowsiness effect; concurrent use should be avoided). Products include:
Compazine 2644

Promethazine Hydrochloride (May increase drowsiness effect; concurrent use should be avoided). Products include:
Mepergan Injection 2859
Phenergan with Codeine 2883
Phenergan with Dextromethorphan 2885
Phenergan Injection 2880
Phenergan Suppositories 2882
Phenergan Syrup 2881
Phenergan Tablets 2882
Phenergan VC 2886
Phenergan VC with Codeine 2888

Propofol (May increase drowsiness effect; concurrent use should be avoided). Products include:
Diprivan Injectable Emulsion 2939

Quazepam (May increase drowsiness effect; concurrent use should be avoided). Products include:
Doral Tablets 2773

Secobarbital Sodium (May increase drowsiness effect; concurrent use should be avoided). Products include:
Seconal Sodium Pulvules 1529

Selegiline Hydrochloride (Concurrent and/or sequential use is not recommended unless directed by a doctor). Products include:
Eldepryl Capsules 2729

Temazepam (May increase drowsiness effect; concurrent use should be avoided). Products include:
Restoril Capsules 2413

Thioridazine Hydrochloride (May increase drowsiness effect; concurrent use should be avoided). Products include:
Mellaril 2398

Thiothixene (May increase drowsiness effect; concurrent use should be avoided). Products include:
Navane Capsules and Concentrate 2018
Navane Intramuscular 2019

Tranylcypromine Sulfate (Concurrent and/or sequential use is not recommended unless directed by a doctor). Products include:
Parnate Tablets 2679

Triazolam (May increase drowsiness effect; concurrent use should be avoided). Products include:
Halcion Tablets 2093

Trifluoperazine Hydrochloride (May increase drowsiness effect; concurrent use should be avoided). Products include:
Stelazine 2692

Zolpidem Tartrate (May increase drowsiness effect; concurrent use should be avoided). Products include:
Ambien Tablets 2559

Food Interactions

Alcohol (May increase drowsiness effect; concurrent use should be avoided).

CONTAC NIGHT ALLERGY/SINUS CAPLETS

(Acetaminophen, Pseudoephedrine Hydrochloride, Diphenhydramine Hydrochloride) ..... ▣ 771
May interact with monoamine oxidase inhibitors, hypnotics and sedatives, tranquilizers, and certain other agents. Compounds in these categories include:

Alprazolam (May increase the drowsiness effect; avoid concurrent use). Products include:
Xanax Tablets 2115

Buspirone Hydrochloride (May increase the drowsiness effect; avoid concurrent use). Products include:
BuSpar Tablets 738

Chlordiazepoxide (May increase the drowsiness effect; avoid concurrent use). Products include:
Limbitrol 2333

Chlordiazepoxide Hydrochloride (May increase the drowsiness effect; avoid concurrent use). Products include:
Librax Capsules 2330
Librium Capsules 2331
Librium Injectable 2332

Chlorpromazine (May increase the drowsiness effect; avoid concurrent use). Products include:
Thorazine Suppositories 2701

Chlorpromazine Hydrochloride (May increase the drowsiness effect; avoid concurrent use). Products include:
Thorazine 2701

Chlorprothixene (May increase the drowsiness effect; avoid concurrent use).
No products indexed under this heading.

Chlorprothixene Hydrochloride (May increase the drowsiness effect; avoid concurrent use).
No products indexed under this heading.

Clorazepate Dipotassium (May increase the drowsiness effect; avoid concurrent use). Products include:
Tranxene 459

Diazepam (May increase the drowsiness effect; avoid concurrent use). Products include:
Dizac (diazepam injectable emulsion) CIV 1862
Valium Injectable 2336
Valium Tablets 2335

Droperidol (May increase the drowsiness effect; avoid concurrent use). Products include:
Inapsine Injection 462

Estazolam (May increase the drowsiness effect; avoid concurrent use). Products include:
ProSom Tablets 457

Ethchlorvynol (May increase the drowsiness effect; avoid concurrent use). Products include:
Placidyl Capsules 456

Ethinamate (May increase the drowsiness effect; avoid concurrent use).
No products indexed under this heading.

Fluphenazine Decanoate (May increase the drowsiness effect; avoid concurrent use). Products include:
Prolixin Decanoate 510

Fluphenazine Enanthate (May increase the drowsiness effect; avoid concurrent use). Products include:
Prolixin Enanthate 510

Fluphenazine Hydrochloride (May increase the drowsiness effect; avoid concurrent use). Products include:
Prolixin 510

Flurazepam Hydrochloride (May increase the drowsiness effect; avoid concurrent use). Products include:
Dalmane Capsules 2329

Furazolidone (Concurrent and/or sequential use is not recommended). Products include:
Furoxone 2221

Glutethimide (May increase the drowsiness effect; avoid concurrent use).
No products indexed under this heading.

IMPORTANT NOTE: Always consult each drug listing in the patient's regimen for possible interactions.

Haloperidol (May increase the drowsiness effect; avoid concurrent use). Products include:
Haldol Injection, Tablets and Concentrate 1585
Haloperidol Decanoate (May increase the drowsiness effect; avoid concurrent use). Products include:
Haldol Decanoate 1587
Hydroxyzine Hydrochloride (May increase the drowsiness effect; avoid concurrent use). Products include:
Atarax Tablets & Syrup 1992
Marax Tablets & DF Syrup 2015
Vistaril Intramuscular Solution 2042
Isocarboxazid (Concurrent and/or sequential use is not recommended). No products indexed under this heading.
Lorazepam (May increase the drowsiness effect; avoid concurrent use). Products include:
Ativan Injection 2805
Ativan Tablets 2807
Loxapine Hydrochloride (May increase the drowsiness effect; avoid concurrent use). Products include:
Loxitane 1426
Loxapine Succinate (May increase drowsiness effect; avoid concurrent use). Products include:
Loxitane Capsules 1426
Meprobamate (May increase the drowsiness effect; avoid concurrent use). Products include:
Miltown Tablets 2780
PMB 200 and PMB 400 2890
Mesoridazine Besylate (May increase the drowsiness effect; avoid concurrent use). Products include:
Serentil 689
Midazolam Hydrochloride (May increase the drowsiness effect; avoid concurrent use). Products include:
Versed Injection 2324
Molindone Hydrochloride (May increase the drowsiness effect; avoid concurrent use). Products include:
Moban Tablets and Concentrate .. 1036
Oxazepam (May increase the drowsiness effect; avoid concurrent use). Products include:
Serax Capsules 2916
Serax Tablets 2916
Perphenazine (May increase the drowsiness effect; avoid concurrent use). Products include:
Etrafon 2495
Triavil Tablets 1800
Trilafon 2532
Phenelzine Sulfate (Concurrent and/or sequential use is not recommended). Products include:
Nardil 1977
Prazepam (May increase the drowsiness effect; avoid concurrent use). No products indexed under this heading.
Prochlorperazine (May increase the drowsiness effect; avoid concurrent use). Products include:
Compazine 2644
Promethazine Hydrochloride (May increase the drowsiness effect; avoid concurrent use). Products include:
Mepergan Injection 2859
Phenergan with Codeine 2883
Phenergan with Dextromethorphan 2885
Phenergan Injection 2880
Phenergan Suppositories 2882
Phenergan Syrup 2881
Phenergan Tablets 2882
Phenergan VC 2886
Phenergan VC with Codeine 2888

Propofol (May increase the drowsiness effect; avoid concurrent use). Products include:
Diprivan Injectable Emulsion 2939
Quazepam (May increase the drowsiness effect; avoid concurrent use). Products include:
Doral Tablets 2773
Secobarbital Sodium (May increase the drowsiness effect; avoid concurrent use). Products include:
Seconal Sodium Pulvules 1529
Selegiline Hydrochloride (Concurrent and/or sequential use is not recommended). Products include:
Eldepryl Capsules 2729
Temazepam (May increase the drowsiness effect; avoid concurrent use). Products include:
Restoril Capsules 2413
Thioridazine Hydrochloride (May increase the drowsiness effect; avoid concurrent use). Products include:
Mellaril 2398
Thiothixene (May increase the drowsiness effect; avoid concurrent use). Products include:
Navane Capsules and Concentrate 2018
Navane Intramuscular 2019
Tranylcypromine Sulfate (Concurrent and/or sequential use is not recommended). Products include:
Parnate Tablets 2679
Triazolam (May increase the drowsiness effect; avoid concurrent use). Products include:
Halcion Tablets 2093
Trifluoperazine Hydrochloride (May increase the drowsiness effect; avoid concurrent use). Products include:
Stelazine 2692
Zolpidem Tartrate (May increase the drowsiness effect; avoid concurrent use). Products include:
Ambien Tablets 2559

Food Interactions
Alcohol (May increase the drowsiness effect; avoid concurrent use).

CONTAC SEVERE COLD AND FLU FORMULA CAPLETS
(Acetaminophen, Chlorpheniramine Maleate, Dextromethorphan Hydrobromide, Phenylpropanolamine Hydrochloride) 773
May interact with monoamine oxidase inhibitors, tranquilizers, hypnotics and sedatives, and certain other agents. Compounds in these categories include:

Alprazolam (May increase drowsiness effect; concurrent use should be avoided). Products include:
Xanax Tablets 2115
Buspirone Hydrochloride (May increase drowsiness effect; concurrent use should be avoided). Products include:
BuSpar Tablets 738
Chlordiazepoxide (May increase drowsiness effect; concurrent use should be avoided). Products include:
Limbitrol 2333
Chlordiazepoxide Hydrochloride (May increase drowsiness effect; concurrent use should be avoided). Products include:
Librax Capsules 2330
Librium Capsules 2331
Librium Injectable 2332

Chlorpromazine (May increase drowsiness effect; concurrent use should be avoided). Products include:
Thorazine Suppositories 2701
Chlorpromazine Hydrochloride (May increase drowsiness effect; concurrent use should be avoided). Products include:
Thorazine 2701
Chlorprothixene (May increase drowsiness effect; concurrent use should be avoided). No products indexed under this heading.
Chlorprothixene Hydrochloride (May increase drowsiness effect; concurrent use should be avoided). No products indexed under this heading.
Clorazepate Dipotassium (May increase drowsiness effect; concurrent use should be avoided). Products include:
Tranxene 459
Diazepam (May increase drowsiness effect; concurrent use should be avoided). Products include:
Dizac (diazepam injectable emulsion) CIV 1862
Valium Injectable 2336
Valium Tablets 2335
Droperidol (May increase drowsiness effect; concurrent use should be avoided). Products include:
Inapsine Injection 462
Estazolam (May increase drowsiness effect; concurrent use should be avoided). Products include:
ProSom Tablets 457
Ethchlorvynol (May increase drowsiness effect; concurrent use should be avoided). Products include:
Placidyl Capsules 456
Ethinamate (May increase drowsiness effect; concurrent use should be avoided). No products indexed under this heading.
Fluphenazine Decanoate (May increase drowsiness effect; concurrent use should be avoided). Products include:
Prolixin Decanoate 510
Fluphenazine Enanthate (May increase drowsiness effect; concurrent use should be avoided). Products include:
Prolixin Enanthate 510
Fluphenazine Hydrochloride (May increase drowsiness effect; concurrent use should be avoided). Products include:
Prolixin 510
Flurazepam Hydrochloride (May increase drowsiness effect; concurrent use should be avoided). Products include:
Dalmane Capsules 2329
Furazolidone (Concurrent and/or sequential use is not recommended unless directed by a doctor). Products include:
Furoxone 2221
Glutethimide (May increase drowsiness effect; concurrent use should be avoided). No products indexed under this heading.
Haloperidol (May increase drowsiness effect; concurrent use should be avoided). Products include:
Haldol Injection, Tablets and Concentrate 1585

Haloperidol Decanoate (May increase drowsiness effect; concurrent use should be avoided). Products include:
Haldol Decanoate 1587
Hydroxyzine Hydrochloride (May increase drowsiness effect; concurrent use should be avoided). Products include:
Atarax Tablets & Syrup 1992
Marax Tablets & DF Syrup 2015
Vistaril Intramuscular Solution 2042
Isocarboxazid (Concurrent and/or sequential use is not recommended unless directed by a doctor). No products indexed under this heading.
Lorazepam (May increase drowsiness effect; concurrent use should be avoided). Products include:
Ativan Injection 2805
Ativan Tablets 2807
Loxapine Hydrochloride (May increase drowsiness effect; concurrent use should be avoided). Products include:
Loxitane 1426
Loxapine Succinate (May increase drowsiness effect; concurrent use should be avoided). Products include:
Loxitane Capsules 1426
Meprobamate (May increase drowsiness effect; concurrent use should be avoided). Products include:
Miltown Tablets 2780
PMB 200 and PMB 400 2890
Mesoridazine Besylate (May increase drowsiness effect; concurrent use should be avoided). Products include:
Serentil 689
Midazolam Hydrochloride (May increase drowsiness effect; concurrent use should be avoided). Products include:
Versed Injection 2324
Molindone Hydrochloride (May increase drowsiness effect; concurrent use should be avoided). Products include:
Moban Tablets and Concentrate . 1036
Oxazepam (May increase drowsiness effect; concurrent use should be avoided). Products include:
Serax Capsules 2916
Serax Tablets 2916
Perphenazine (May increase drowsiness effect; concurrent use should be avoided). Products include:
Etrafon 2495
Triavil Tablets 1800
Trilafon 2532
Phenelzine Sulfate (Concurrent and/or sequential use is not recommended unless directed by a doctor). Products include:
Nardil 1977
Prazepam (May increase drowsiness effect; concurrent use should be avoided). No products indexed under this heading.
Prochlorperazine (May increase drowsiness effect; concurrent use should be avoided). Products include:
Compazine 2644
Promethazine Hydrochloride (May increase drowsiness effect; concurrent use should be avoided). Products include:
Mepergan Injection 2859
Phenergan with Codeine 2883
Phenergan with Dextromethorphan 2885
Phenergan Injection 2880
Phenergan Suppositories 2882

(■ Described in PDR For Nonprescription Drugs)   (◉ Described in PDR For Ophthalmology)

205 **Interactions Index** **Cordarone Intravenous**

Phenergan Syrup 2881
Phenergan Tablets 2882
Phenergan VC 2886
Phenergan VC with Codeine 2888

Propofol (May increase drowsiness effect; concurrent use should be avoided). Products include:
Diprivan Injectable Emulsion 2939

Quazepam (May increase drowsiness effect; concurrent use should be avoided). Products include:
Doral Tablets 2773

Secobarbital Sodium (May increase drowsiness effect; concurrent use should be avoided). Products include:
Seconal Sodium Pulvules 1529

Selegiline Hydrochloride (Concurrent and/or sequential use is not recommended unless directed by a doctor). Products include:
Eldepryl Capsules 2729

Temazepam (May increase drowsiness effect; concurrent use should be avoided). Products include:
Restoril Capsules 2413

Thioridazine Hydrochloride (May increase drowsiness effect; concurrent use should be avoided). Products include:
Mellaril 2398

Thiothixene (May increase drowsiness effect; concurrent use should be avoided). Products include:
Navane Capsules and Concentrate 2018
Navane Intramuscular 2019

Tranylcypromine Sulfate (Concurrent and/or sequential use is not recommended unless directed by a doctor). Products include:
Parnate Tablets 2679

Triazolam (May increase drowsiness effect; concurrent use should be avoided). Products include:
Halcion Tablets 2093

Trifluoperazine Hydrochloride (May increase drowsiness effect; concurrent use should be avoided). Products include:
Stelazine 2692

Zolpidem Tartrate (May increase drowsiness effect; concurrent use should be avoided). Products include:
Ambien Tablets 2559

Food Interactions

Alcohol (May increase drowsiness effect; concurrent use should be avoided).

CONTAC SEVERE COLD & FLU NON-DROWSY
(Acetaminophen, Dextromethorphan Hydrobromide, Pseudoephedrine Hydrochloride) 774
May interact with monoamine oxidase inhibitors. Compounds in this category include:

Furazolidone (Concurrent and/or sequential use is not recommended). Products include:
Furoxone 2221

Isocarboxazid (Concurrent and/or sequential use is not recommended).
No products indexed under this heading.

Phenelzine Sulfate (Concurrent and/or sequential use is not recommended). Products include:
Nardil 1977

Selegiline Hydrochloride (Concurrent and/or sequential use is not recommended). Products include:
Eldepryl Capsules 2729

Tranylcypromine Sulfate (Concurrent and/or sequential use is not recommended). Products include:
Parnate Tablets 2679

COPPERTONE SKIN SELECTS SUNSCREEN LOTION SPF 15 FOR DRY SKIN
(Ethylhexyl p-Methoxycinnamate, Oxybenzone) 759
None cited in PDR database.

COPPERTONE SKIN SELECTS SUNSCREEN LOTION SPF 15 FOR OILY SKIN
(Ethylhexyl p-Methoxycinnamate, Oxybenzone) 760
None cited in PDR database.

COPPERTONE SKIN SELECTS SUNSCREEN LOTION SPF 15 FOR SENSITIVE SKIN
(Ethylhexyl p-Methoxycinnamate, Titanium Dioxide) 760
None cited in PDR database.

CORDARONE INTRAVENOUS
(Amiodarone Hydrochloride) 2821
May interact with beta blockers, calcium channel blockers, and certain other agents. Compounds in these categories include:

Acebutolol Hydrochloride (Increased risk of hypotension and bradycardia). Products include:
Sectral Capsules 2914

Amlodipine Besylate (Increased risk of AV block and hypotension). Products include:
Lotrel Capsules 858
Norvasc Tablets 2020

Atenolol (Increased risk of hypotension and bradycardia). Products include:
Tenoretic Tablets 2963
Tenormin Tablets and I.V. Injection 2965

Bepridil Hydrochloride (Increased risk of AV block and hypotension). Products include:
Vascor Tablets (200 and 300 mg) 1597

Betaxolol Hydrochloride (Increased risk of hypotension and bradycardia). Products include:
Betoptic Ophthalmic Solution 465
Betoptic S Ophthalmic Suspension 467
Kerlone Tablets 2588

Bisoprolol Fumarate (Increased risk of hypotension and bradycardia). Products include:
Zebeta Tablets 1457
Ziac 1459

Carteolol Hydrochloride (Increased risk of hypotension and bradycardia). Products include:
Cartrol Tablets 413
Ocupress Ophthalmic Solution, 1% Sterile .... ◉ 297

Cholestyramine (Increases enterohepatic elimination of amiodarone and may reduce serum levels and t½). Products include:
Questran 774

Cimetidine (Increases serum amiodarone levels). Products include:
Tagamet HB Tablets 786
Tagamet Tablets 2694

Cimetidine Hydrochloride (Increases serum amiodarone levels). Products include:
Tagamet 2694

Cyclosporine (Elevated plasma concentrations of cyclosporine resulting in elevated creatinine, despite reduction in dose of cyclosporine). Products include:
Neoral 2405
Sandimmune 2416

Dextromethorphan Hydrobromide (Chronic oral amiodarone administration impairs metabolism of dextromethorphan). Products include:
Alka-Seltzer Plus Cold & Cough Medicine 611
Alka-Seltzer Plus Cold & Cough Medicine Liqui-Gels 612
Alka-Seltzer Plus Flu & Body Aches Effervescent Tablets 612
Alka-Seltzer Plus Flu & Body Aches Liqui-Gels Non-Drowsy Formula 613
Alka-Seltzer Plus Night-Time Cold Medicine 611
Alka-Seltzer Plus Night-Time Cold Medicine Liqui-Gels 612
Benylin Adult Formula Cough Suppressant 817
Benylin Expectorant 816
Benylin Multisymptom 816
Benylin Pediatric Cough Suppressant 817
Bromfed-DM Cough Syrup 1832
Cerose DM 853
Cheracol D Cough Formula 740
Cheracol Plus Head Cold/Cough Formula 741
Children's TYLENOL Cold Plus Cough Multi Symptom Chewable Tablets and Liquid 1560
Children's TYLENOL Flu Suspension Liquid 1560
Children's Vicks NyQuil Cold/Cough Relief 731
Comtrex Multi-Symptom 638
Comtrex Non-Drowsy 640
Contac Day & Night Cold/Flu Caplets 772
Contac Severe Cold and Flu Formula Caplets 773
Contac Severe Cold & Flu Non-Drowsy 774
Coricidin Cough + Cold Tablets 760
Cough-X Lozenges 606
Diabe-Tuss DM Syrup 1948
Dimetane-DX Cough Syrup 2233
Dimetapp Cold & Cough Liqui-Gels 839
Dimetapp DM Elixir 840
Dorcol Children's Cough Syrup 748
Drixoral Cough Liquid Caps 762
Drixoral Cough + Congestion Liquid Caps 763
Drixoral Cough + Sore Throat Liquid Caps 763
Humibid DM Tablets 1612
Novahistine DMX 782
PediaCare Cough-Cold Chewable Tablets and Liquid 1569
PediaCare Infants' Drops Decongestant Plus Cough 1569
PediaCare NightRest Cough-Cold Liquid 1569
Pediatric Vicks 44d Cough & Head Congestion Relief 736
Pediatric Vicks 44e Cough & Chest Congestion Relief 737
Pediatric Vicks 44m Cough & Cold Relief 737
Pertussin Adult Extra Strength 630
Pertussin Children's Strength 630
Phenergan with Dextromethorphan 2885
Robitussin Cold & Cough Liqui-Gels 844
Robitussin Cold, Cough & Flu Liqui-Gels 844
Robitussin Maximum Strength Cough Suppressant 847
Robitussin Maximum Strength Cough & Cold 847
Robitussin Night-Time Cold Formula 847
Robitussin Pediatric Cough & Cold Formula 848
Robitussin Pediatric Cough Suppressant 848
Robitussin Pediatric Drops 849
Robitussin-CF 846
Robitussin-DM 846
Safe Tussin 30 Liquid 1413
Sucrets 4-Hour Cough Suppressant 785
Sudafed Children's Cold & Cough Liquid Medication 825
Sudafed Cold and Cough Liquid Caps 826
Sudafed Severe Cold Formula Caplets 828
Sudafed Severe Cold Formula Tablets 828
Syn-Rx DM Tablets 1623
TheraFlu Flu, Cold and Cough Medicine 750
TheraFlu Maximum Strength Nighttime Flu, Cold & Cough Medicine 751
TheraFlu Maximum Strength Non-Drowsy Formula Flu, Cold & Cough Medicine 751
TheraFlu Maximum Strength, Non-Drowsy Formula Flu, Cold and Cough Caplets 752
Triaminic AM Cough and Decongestant Formula 753
Triaminic Night Time 754
Triaminic Sore Throat Formula 755
Triaminic Triaminicol Cold & Cough 756
Triaminic DM Syrup 756
Tussi-Organidin DM NR Liquid and DM-S NR Liquid 2786
TYLENOL Cold Medication, Multi-Symptom Formula Tablets and Caplets 1572
TYLENOL Cold Medication, Multi-Symptom Hot Liquid Packets 1572
TYLENOL Cold Medication, No Drowsiness Formula Caplets and Gelcaps 1572
TYLENOL Cold Severe Congestion Caplets 1573
TYLENOL Cough Medication, Multi Symptom 1574
TYLENOL Cough Medication with Decongestant, Multi Symptom 1574
TYLENOL Flu No Drowsiness Formula, Maximum Strength Gelcaps 1575
Vicks 44 Cough Relief 728
Vicks 44 LiquiCaps Cough, Cold & Flu Relief 728
Vicks 44 LiquiCaps Non-Drowsy Cough & Cold Relief 729
Vicks 44D Cough & Head Congestion Relief 728
Vicks 44E Cough & Chest Congestion Relief 729
Vicks 44M Cough, Cold & Flu Relief 729
Vicks DayQuil LiquiCaps/Liquid Multi-Symptom Cold/Flu Relief 734
Vicks Nyquil Hot Therapy 735
Vicks NyQuil LiquiCaps/Liquid Multi-Symptom Cold/Flu Relief, Original and Cherry Flavors 736

Digoxin (Amiodarone increases serum concentration and effects of digoxin). Products include:
Lanoxicaps 1110
Lanoxin Elixir Pediatric 1113
Lanoxin Injection 1116
Lanoxin Injection Pediatric 1119
Lanoxin Tablets 1121

Diltiazem Hydrochloride (Increased risk of AV block and hypotension). Products include:
Cardizem CD Capsules 1251
Cardizem SR Capsules 1255
Cardizem Injectable 1253
Cardizem Tablets 1257
Dilacor XR Extended-release Capsules 2183
Tiazac Capsules 1019

Disopyramide Phosphate (Increased QT prolongation which would cause arrhythmia). Products include:
Norpace 2596

Esmolol Hydrochloride (Increased risk of hypotension and bradycardia). Products include:
Brevibloc (esmolol HCl) Injection 1860

Felodipine (Increased risk of AV block and hypotension). Products include:
Plendil Extended-Release Tablets 514

Fentanyl (Potential for hypotension, bradycardia, decreased cardiac output). Products include:
Duragesic Transdermal System 1336

Fentanyl Citrate (Potential for hypotension, bradycardia, decreased cardiac output). Products include:
Sublimaze Injection 463

IMPORTANT NOTE: Always consult each drug listing in the patient's regimen for possible interactions.

Cordarone Intravenous — **Interactions Index** — **206**

Flecainide Acetate (Increased effects of flecainide; reduces the dose of flecainide needed to maintain therapeutic plasma concentrations). Products include:
Tambocor Tablets 1555
Isradipine (Increased risk of AV block and hypotension). Products include:
DynaCirc Capsules 2381
DynaCirc CR Tablets 2383
Labetalol Hydrochloride (Increased risk of hypotension and bradycardia). Products include:
Normodyne Injection 2519
Normodyne Tablets 2522
Trandate 1158
Levobunolol Hydrochloride (Increased risk of hypotension and bradycardia). Products include:
Betagan .... ⊙ 230
Lidocaine Hydrochloride (Potential for seizure associated with increased lidocaine concentrations; sinus bradycardia has been observed with oral amiodarone and lidocaine for anesthesia). Products include:
Decadron Phosphate with Xylocaine Injection, Sterile 1683
Unguentine Plus .... ▣ 712
Xylocaine Injections 562
Methotrexate Sodium (Chronic oral amiodarone administration impairs metabolism of methotrexate). Products include:
Methotrexate Sodium Tablets, Injection, for Injection and LPF Injection 1322
Metipranolol Hydrochloride (Increased risk of hypotension and bradycardia). Products include:
OptiPranolol (Metipranolol 0.3%) Sterile Ophthalmic Solution .... ⊙ 256
Metoprolol Succinate (Increased risk of hypotension and bradycardia). Products include:
Toprol-XL Tablets 560
Metoprolol Tartrate (Increased risk of hypotension and bradycardia). Products include:
Lopressor 848
Lopressor HCT Tablets 850
Nadolol (Increased risk of hypotension and bradycardia).
No products indexed under this heading.
Nicardipine Hydrochloride (Increased risk of AV block and hypotension). Products include:
Cardene Capsules 2261
Cardene I.V. 2815
Cardene SR Capsules 2264
Nifedipine (Increased risk of AV block and hypotension). Products include:
Adalat Capsules (10 mg and 20 mg) 580
Adalat CC 582
Procardia Capsules 2024
Procardia XL Extended Release Tablets 2026
Nimodipine (Increased risk of AV block and hypotension). Products include:
Nimotop Capsules 603
Nisoldipine (Increased risk of AV block and hypotension). Products include:
Sular Tablets 2961
Penbutolol Sulfate (Increased risk of hypotension and bradycardia). Products include:
Levatol Tablets 2547
Phenytoin (Decreases serum amiodarone levels; chronic oral amiodarone administration impairs metabolism of phenytoin). Products include:
Dilantin Infatabs 1967
Dilantin-125 Suspension 1969
Phenytoin Sodium (Decreases serum amiodarone levels; chronic oral amiodarone administration impairs metabolism of phenytoin). Products include:
Dilantin Kapseals 1965
Pindolol (Increased risk of hypotension and bradycardia). Products include:
Visken Tablets 2428
Procainamide Hydrochloride (Amiodarone increases serum concentration of procainamide and N-acetylprocainamide; increased effects of procainamide). Products include:
Procanbid Extended-Release Tablets 1983
Propranolol Hydrochloride (Increased risk of hypotension and bradycardia). Products include:
Inderal 2834
Inderal LA Long Acting Capsules 2836
Inderide Tablets 2838
Inderide LA Long Acting Capsules 2840
Quinidine Gluconate (Amiodarone increases serum concentration and effects of quinidine). Products include:
Quinaglute Dura-Tabs Tablets 644
Quinidine Polygalacturonate (Amiodarone increases serum concentration and effects of quinidine). Products include:
Cardioquin Tablets 2146
Quinidine Sulfate (Amiodarone increases serum concentration and effects of quinidine). Products include:
Quinidex Extentabs 2240
Sotalol Hydrochloride (Increased risk of hypotension and bradycardia). Products include:
Betapace Tablets 637
Timolol Hemihydrate (Increased risk of hypotension and bradycardia). Products include:
Betimol 0.25%, 0.5% .... ⊙ 259
Timolol Maleate (Increased risk of hypotension and bradycardia). Products include:
Blocadren Tablets 1654
Timolide Tablets 1791
Timoptic in Ocudose 1796
Timoptic Sterile Ophthalmic Solution 1794
Timoptic-XE 1798
Verapamil Hydrochloride (Increased risk of AV block and hypotension). Products include:
Calan SR Caplets 2571
Calan Tablets 2568
Covera-HS Tablets 2573
Isoptin Injectable 1391
Isoptin Oral Tablets 1393
Isoptin SR Tablets 1395
Verelan Capsules 1455
Warfarin Sodium (Increased prothrombin time; amiodarone increases effects of warfarin). Products include:
Coumadin 941

CORDARONE TABLETS
(Amiodarone Hydrochloride) 2818
May interact with oral anticoagulants, antiarrhythmics, beta blockers, calcium channel blockers, cardiac glycosides, and certain other agents. Compounds in these categories include:

Acebutolol Hydrochloride (Possible potentiation of bradycardia, sinus arrest and AV block). Products include:
Sectral Capsules 2914
Adenosine (Possible increase in serious toxicity when amiodarone is used with other antiarrhythmics). Products include:
Adenocard Injection 1021
Adenoscan 1022
Amlodipine Besylate (Possible potentiation of bradycardia, sinus arrest and AV block). Products include:
Lotrel Capsules 858
Norvasc Tablets 2020
Atenolol (Possible potentiation of bradycardia, sinus arrest and AV block). Products include:
Tenoretic Tablets 2963
Tenormin Tablets and I.V. Injection 2965
Bepridil Hydrochloride (Possible potentiation of bradycardia, sinus arrest and AV block). Products include:
Vascor Tablets (200 and 300 mg) 1597
Betaxolol Hydrochloride (Possible potentiation of bradycardia, sinus arrest and AV block). Products include:
Betoptic Ophthalmic Solution 465
Betoptic S Ophthalmic Suspension 467
Kerlone Tablets 2588
Bisoprolol Fumarate (Possible potentiation of bradycardia, sinus arrest and AV block). Products include:
Zebeta Tablets 1457
Ziac 1459
Bretylium Tosylate (Possible increase in serious toxicity when amiodarone is used with other antiarrhythmics).
No products indexed under this heading.
Carteolol Hydrochloride (Possible potentiation of bradycardia, sinus arrest and AV block). Products include:
Cartrol Tablets 413
Ocupress Ophthalmic Solution, 1% Sterile .... ⊙ 297
Cyclosporine (Concomitant use has reported to produce persistently elevated plasma concentrations of cyclosporine resulting in elevated creatinine, despite reduction in dose of cyclosporine). Products include:
Neoral 2405
Sandimmune 2416
Deslanoside (Co-administration results in an increase in serum cardiac glycosides concentration that may reach toxic levels with resultant clinical toxicity; discontinue or reduce dose of digitalis by approximately 50%).
No products indexed under this heading.
Dicumarol (Potentiation of warfarin-type anticoagulant resulting in serious or fatal bleeding; the dose of anticoagulant should be reduced by 1/3 to 1/2; monitor prothrombin time closely).
No products indexed under this heading.
Digitoxin (Co-administration results in an increase in serum cardiac glycosides concentration that may reach toxic levels with resultant clinical toxicity; discontinue or reduce dose of digitalis by approximately 50%). Products include:
Crystodigin Tablets 1472
Digoxin (Co-administration results in an increase in serum digoxin concentration by 70% with resultant clinical toxicity; discontinue or reduce dose of digoxin by approximately 50%). Products include:
Lanoxicaps 1110
Lanoxin Elixir Pediatric 1113
Lanoxin Injection 1116
Lanoxin Injection Pediatric 1119
Lanoxin Tablets 1121
Diltiazem Hydrochloride (Possible potentiation of bradycardia, sinus arrest and AV block). Products include:
Cardizem CD Capsules 1251
Cardizem SR Capsules 1255
Cardizem Injectable 1253
Cardizem Tablets 1257
Dilacor XR Extended-release Capsules 2183
Tiazac Capsules 1019
Disopyramide Phosphate (Possible increase in serious toxicity when amiodarone is used with other antiarrhythmics). Products include:
Norpace 2596
Esmolol Hydrochloride (Possible potentiation of bradycardia, sinus arrest and AV block). Products include:
Brevibloc (esmolol HCl) Injection 1860
Felodipine (Possible potentiation of bradycardia, sinus arrest and AV block). Products include:
Plendil Extended-Release Tablets 514
Flecainide Acetate (Possible increase in serious toxicity when amiodarone is used with other antiarrhythmics). Products include:
Tambocor Tablets 1555
Isradipine (Possible potentiation of bradycardia, sinus arrest and AV block). Products include:
DynaCirc Capsules 2381
DynaCirc CR Tablets 2383
Labetalol Hydrochloride (Possible potentiation of bradycardia, sinus arrest and AV block). Products include:
Normodyne Injection 2519
Normodyne Tablets 2522
Trandate 1158
Levobunolol Hydrochloride (Possible potentiation of bradycardia, sinus arrest and AV block). Products include:
Betagan .... ⊙ 230
Lidocaine Hydrochloride (Possible increase in serious toxicity when amiodarone is used with other antiarrhythmics). Products include:
Decadron Phosphate with Xylocaine Injection, Sterile 1683
Unguentine Plus .... ▣ 712
Xylocaine Injections 562
Metipranolol Hydrochloride (Possible potentiation of bradycardia, sinus arrest and AV block). Products include:
OptiPranolol (Metipranolol 0.3%) Sterile Ophthalmic Solution .... ⊙ 256
Metoprolol Succinate (Possible potentiation of bradycardia, sinus arrest and AV block). Products include:
Toprol-XL Tablets 560
Metoprolol Tartrate (Possible potentiation of bradycardia, sinus arrest and AV block). Products include:
Lopressor 848
Lopressor HCT Tablets 850
Mexiletine Hydrochloride (Possible increase in serious toxicity when amiodarone is used with other antiarrhythmics). Products include:
Mexitil Capsules 684
Moricizine Hydrochloride (Possible increase in serious toxicity when amiodarone is used with other antiarrhythmics). Products include:
Ethmozine Tablets 2217

(▣ Described in PDR For Nonprescription Drugs) (⊙ Described in PDR For Ophthalmology)

Interactions Index — Coricidin/Coricidin 'D'

Nadolol (Possible potentiation of bradycardia, sinus arrest and AV block).
    No products indexed under this heading.

Nicardipine Hydrochloride (Possible potentiation of bradycardia, sinus arrest and AV block). Products include:
- Cardene Capsules 2261
- Cardene I.V. 2815
- Cardene SR Capsules 2264

Nifedipine (Possible potentiation of bradycardia, sinus arrest and AV block). Products include:
- Adalat Capsules (10 mg and 20 mg) 580
- Adalat CC 582
- Procardia Capsules 2024
- Procardia XL Extended Release Tablets 2026

Nimodipine (Possible potentiation of bradycardia, sinus arrest and AV block). Products include:
- Nimotop Capsules 603

Nisoldipine (Possible potentiation of bradycardia, sinus arrest and AV block). Products include:
- Sular Tablets 2961

Penbutolol Sulfate (Possible potentiation of bradycardia, sinus arrest and AV block). Products include:
- Levatol Tablets 2547

Pindolol (Possible potentiation of bradycardia, sinus arrest and AV block). Products include:
- Visken Tablets 2428

Procainamide Hydrochloride (Increased plasma concentration of procainamide by 55%, n-acetyl procainamide concentration by 33%; discontinue or reduce quinidine dose by 1/3). Products include:
- Procanbid Extended-Release Tablets 1983

Propafenone Hydrochloride (Possible increase in serious toxicity when amiodarone is used with other antiarrhythmics). Products include:
- Rythmol Tablets—150mg, 225mg, 300mg 1399

Propranolol Hydrochloride (Possible potentiation of bradycardia, sinus arrest and AV block). Products include:
- Inderal 2834
- Inderal LA Long Acting Capsules 2836
- Inderide Tablets 2838
- Inderide LA Long Acting Capsules .. 2840

Quinidine Gluconate (Increased steady-state levels of quinidine by 33%; discontinue or reduce quinidine dose by 1/3 to 1/2). Products include:
- Quinaglute Dura-Tabs Tablets 644

Quinidine Polygalacturonate (Increased steady-state levels of quinidine by 33%; discontinue or reduce quinidine dose by 1/3 to 1/2). Products include:
- Cardioquin Tablets 2146

Quinidine Sulfate (Increased steady-state levels of quinidine by 33%; discontinue or reduce quinidine dose by 1/3 to 1/2). Products include:
- Quinidex Extentabs 2240

Sotalol Hydrochloride (Possible potentiation of bradycardia, sinus arrest and AV block). Products include:
- Betapace Tablets 637

Timolol Hemihydrate (Possible potentiation of bradycardia, sinus arrest and AV block). Products include:
- Betimol 0.25%, 0.5% 259

Timolol Maleate (Possible potentiation of bradycardia, sinus arrest and AV block). Products include:
- Blocadren Tablets 1654
- Timolide Tablets 1791
- Timoptic in Ocudose 1796
- Timoptic Sterile Ophthalmic Solution 1794
- Timoptic-XE 1798

Tocainide Hydrochloride (Possible increase in serious toxicity when amiodarone is used with other antiarrhythmics). Products include:
- Tonocard Tablets 519

Verapamil Hydrochloride (Possible potentiation of bradycardia, sinus arrest and AV block). Products include:
- Calan SR Caplets 2571
- Calan Tablets 2568
- Covera-HS Tablets 2573
- Isoptin Injectable 1391
- Isoptin Oral Tablets 1393
- Isoptin SR Tablets 1395
- Verelan Capsules 1455

Warfarin Sodium (Increased prothrombin time by 100%; potentiation of warfarin-type anticoagulant resulting in serious or fatal bleeding; the dose of anticoagulant should be reduced by 1/3 to 1/2; monitor prothrombin time closely). Products include:
- Coumadin 941

CORDRAN LOTION
(Flurandrenolide) 1854
None cited in PDR database.

CORDRAN TAPE
(Flurandrenolide) 1855
None cited in PDR database.

CORDYMAX CS-4 CAPSULES
(Dietary Supplement) 2985
None cited in PDR database.

CORICIDIN COLD + FLU TABLETS
(Acetaminophen, Chlorpheniramine Maleate) 760
See **Coricidin 'D' Decongestant Tablets**

CORICIDIN COUGH + COLD TABLETS
(Chlorpheniramine Maleate, Dextromethorphan Hydrobromide) 760
See **Coricidin 'D' Decongestant Tablets**

CORICIDIN 'D' DECONGESTANT TABLETS
(Acetaminophen, Chlorpheniramine Maleate, Phenylpropanolamine Hydrochloride) 760
May interact with hypnotics and sedatives, tranquilizers, monoamine oxidase inhibitors, and certain other agents. Compounds in these categories include:

Alprazolam (May increase drowsiness effect). Products include:
- Xanax Tablets 2115

Buspirone Hydrochloride (May increase drowsiness effect). Products include:
- BuSpar Tablets 738

Chlordiazepoxide (May increase drowsiness effect). Products include:
- Limbitrol 2333

Chlordiazepoxide Hydrochloride (May increase drowsiness effect). Products include:
- Librax Capsules 2330
- Librium Capsules 2331
- Librium Injectable 2332

Chlorpromazine (May increase drowsiness effect). Products include:
- Thorazine Suppositories 2701

Chlorpromazine Hydrochloride (May increase drowsiness effect). Products include:
- Thorazine 2701

Chlorprothixene (May increase drowsiness effect).
    No products indexed under this heading.

Chlorprothixene Hydrochloride (May increase drowsiness effect).
    No products indexed under this heading.

Clorazepate Dipotassium (May increase drowsiness effect). Products include:
- Tranxene 459

Diazepam (May increase drowsiness effect). Products include:
- Dizac (diazepam injectable emulsion) CIV 1862
- Valium Injectable 2336
- Valium Tablets 2335

Droperidol (May increase drowsiness effect). Products include:
- Inapsine Injection 462

Estazolam (May increase drowsiness effect). Products include:
- ProSom Tablets 457

Ethchlorvynol (May increase drowsiness effect). Products include:
- Placidyl Capsules 456

Ethinamate (May increase drowsiness effect).
    No products indexed under this heading.

Fluphenazine Decanoate (May increase drowsiness effect). Products include:
- Prolixin Decanoate 510

Fluphenazine Enanthate (May increase drowsiness effect). Products include:
- Prolixin Enanthate 510

Fluphenazine Hydrochloride (May increase drowsiness effect). Products include:
- Prolixin 510

Flurazepam Hydrochloride (May increase drowsiness effect). Products include:
- Dalmane Capsules 2329

Furazolidone (Concurrent and/or sequential use is not recommended). Products include:
- Furoxone 2221

Glutethimide (May increase drowsiness effect).
    No products indexed under this heading.

Haloperidol (May increase drowsiness effect). Products include:
- Haldol Injection, Tablets and Concentrate 1585

Haloperidol Decanoate (May increase drowsiness effect). Products include:
- Haldol Decanoate 1587

Hydroxyzine Hydrochloride (May increase drowsiness effect). Products include:
- Atarax Tablets & Syrup 1992
- Marax Tablets & DF Syrup 2015
- Vistaril Intramuscular Solution 2042

Isocarboxazid (Concurrent and/or sequential use is not recommended).
    No products indexed under this heading.

Lorazepam (May increase drowsiness effect). Products include:
- Ativan Injection 2805
- Ativan Tablets 2807

Loxapine Hydrochloride (May increase drowsiness effect). Products include:
- Loxitane 1426

Loxapine Succinate (May increase drowsiness effect). Products include:
- Loxitane Capsules 1426

Meprobamate (May increase drowsiness effect). Products include:
- Miltown Tablets 2780
- PMB 200 and PMB 400 2890

Mesoridazine Besylate (May increase drowsiness effect). Products include:
- Serentil 689

Midazolam Hydrochloride (May increase drowsiness effect). Products include:
- Versed Injection 2324

Molindone Hydrochloride (May increase drowsiness effect). Products include:
- Moban Tablets and Concentrate 1036

Oxazepam (May increase drowsiness effect). Products include:
- Serax Capsules 2916
- Serax Tablets 2916

Perphenazine (May increase drowsiness effect). Products include:
- Etrafon 2495
- Triavil Tablets 1800
- Trilafon 2532

Phenelzine Sulfate (Concurrent and/or sequential use is not recommended). Products include:
- Nardil 1977

Phenylpropanolamine Containing Anorectics (Concurrent use with appetite-controlling medication containing phenylpropanolamine is not recommended).

Prazepam (May increase drowsiness effect).
    No products indexed under this heading.

Prochlorperazine (May increase drowsiness effect). Products include:
- Compazine 2644

Promethazine Hydrochloride (May increase drowsiness effect). Products include:
- Mepergan Injection 2859
- Phenergan with Codeine 2883
- Phenergan with Dextromethorphan 2885
- Phenergan Injection 2880
- Phenergan Suppositories ... 2882
- Phenergan Syrup 2881
- Phenergan Tablets 2882
- Phenergan VC 2886
- Phenergan VC with Codeine 2888

Propofol (May increase drowsiness effect). Products include:
- Diprivan Injectable Emulsion 2939

Quazepam (May increase drowsiness effect). Products include:
- Doral Tablets 2773

Secobarbital Sodium (May increase drowsiness effect). Products include:
- Seconal Sodium Pulvules ... 1529

Selegiline Hydrochloride (Concurrent and/or sequential use is not recommended). Products include:
- Eldepryl Capsules 2729

Temazepam (May increase drowsiness effect). Products include:
- Restoril Capsules 2413

Thioridazine Hydrochloride (May increase drowsiness effect). Products include:
- Mellaril 2398

Thiothixene (May increase drowsiness effect). Products include:
- Navane Capsules and Concentrate 2018
- Navane Intramuscular 2019

Tranylcypromine Sulfate (Concurrent and/or sequential use is not recommended). Products include:
- Parnate Tablets 2679

IMPORTANT NOTE: Always consult each drug listing in the patient's regimen for possible interactions.

Coricidin/Coricidin 'D' — Interactions Index — 208

Triazolam (May increase drowsiness effect). Products include:
- Halcion Tablets 2093

Trifluoperazine Hydrochloride (May increase drowsiness effect). Products include:
- Stelazine 2692

Zolpidem Tartrate (May increase drowsiness effect). Products include:
- Ambien Tablets 2559

Food Interactions

Alcohol (May increase drowsiness effect).

CORMAX OINTMENT
(Clobetasol Propionate) 1856
None cited in PDR database.

CORMAX SCALP APPLICATION
(Clobetasol Propionate) 1857
None cited in PDR database.

CORRECTOL EXTRA GENTLE STOOL SOFTENER
(Docusate Sodium) .... ▣ 762
May interact with:

Mineral Oil (Concurrent use with oral mineral oil is not recommended, unless directed by a doctor). Products include:
- Alpha Keri Moisture Rich Body Oil ▣ 635
- Anusol Hemorrhoidal Ointment .... ▣ 810
- Aquaphor Healing Ointment 636
- Aquaphor Healing Ointment, Original Formula 636
- Eucerin Original Moisturizing Creme (Unscented) 636
- Eucerin Original Moisturizing Lotion 636
- Eucerin Plus Dry Skin Care Moisturizing Lotion 636
- Eucerin Plus Moisturizing Creme ... 636
- Fleet Mineral Oil Enema 1001
- Hemorid .... ▣ 797
- HypoTears Ointment .... ◉ 262
- Keri Lotion - Original Formula ..... ▣ 644
- Kondremul .... ▣ 656
- Lubriderm Bath and Shower Oil ... ▣ 821
- Nephrox Suspension .... ▣ 671
- Preparation H Hemorrhoidal Ointment .... ▣ 842
- Refresh PM Lubricant Eye Ointment .... ◉ 252
- Replens Vaginal Moisturizer .... ▣ 823
- Tears Renewed Ointment .... ◉ 210

CORRECTOL HERBAL TEA LAXATIVE
(Senna Concentrates) .... ▣ 761
None cited in PDR database.

CORRECTOL LAXATIVE TABLETS & CAPLETS
(Bisacodyl) .... ▣ 761
May interact with antacids and certain other agents. Compounds in these categories include:

Aluminum Carbonate (Concurrent use within one hour after taking antacid is not recommended). Products include:
- Basaljel Capsules 2810
- Basaljel Suspension 2810
- Basaljel Tablets 2810

Aluminum Hydroxide (Concurrent use within one hour after taking antacid is not recommended). Products include:
- ALternaGEL Liquid 1358
- Maximum Strength Ascriptin ...... ▣ 650
- Cama Arthritis Pain Reliever .... ▣ 748
- Gaviscon Extra Strength Relief Formula Antacid Tablets ...... ▣ 778
- Gaviscon Extra Strength Relief Formula Liquid Antacid 779
- Gaviscon Antacid Liquid .... ▣ 779
- Gelusil Antacid-Anti-gas Liquid ... ▣ 819
- Gelusil Antacid-Anti-gas Tablets ... ▣ 819
- Maalox Antacid/Anti-Gas Tablets 889
- Maalox Heartburn Relief Suspension .... ▣ 658
- Maalox Antacid Liquid 888
- Extra Strength Maalox Antacid/Anti-Gas Liquid and Tablets 888
- Mylanta 1359
- Tempo Soft Antacid .... ▣ 799

Aluminum Hydroxide Gel (Concurrent use within one hour after taking antacid is not recommended). Products include:
- ALternaGEL Liquid .... ▣ 675
- Aludrox Oral Suspension .... ▣ 850
- Amphojel Suspension 2802
- Amphojel Suspension without Flavor 2802
- Amphojel Tablets 2802
- Ascriptin .... ▣ 650
- Gaviscon Antacid Tablets .... ▣ 778
- Gaviscon-2 Antacid Tablets .... ▣ 779
- Mylanta Liquid .... ▣ 676
- Mylanta Double Strength Liquid ... ▣ 676
- Nephrox Suspension .... ▣ 671

Magaldrate (Concurrent use within one hour after taking antacid is not recommended).
No products indexed under this heading.

Magnesium Hydroxide (Concurrent use within one hour after taking antacid is not recommended). Products include:
- Aludrox Oral Suspension .... ▣ 850
- Ascriptin .... ▣ 650
- Di-Gel Antacid/Anti-Gas .... ▣ 762
- Gelusil Antacid-Anti-gas Liquid ... ▣ 819
- Gelusil Antacid-Anti-gas Tablets ... ▣ 819
- Maalox Antacid/Anti-Gas Tablets 889
- Maalox Antacid Liquid 888
- Extra Strength Maalox Antacid/Anti-Gas Liquid and Tablets 888
- Mylanta Fast-Acting 1359
- Mylanta Gelcaps Antacid .... ▣ 678
- Fast-Acting Mylanta Liquid Antacid 1359
- Mylanta Tablets .... ▣ 677
- Maximum-Strength Fast-Acting Mylanta Liquid Antacid 1359
- Mylanta Double Strength Tablets .. ▣ 677
- Phillips' Milk of Magnesia Liquid .... ▣ 627
- Rolaids Antacid Tablets .... ▣ 807
- Tempo Soft Antacid .... ▣ 799

Magnesium Oxide (Concurrent use within one hour after taking antacid is not recommended). Products include:
- Beelith Tablets 632
- Bufferin Analgesic Tablets .... ▣ 636
- Arthritis Strength Bufferin Analgesic Caplets .... ▣ 637
- Extra Strength Bufferin Analgesic Tablets .... ▣ 637
- Caltrate PLUS .... ▣ 681
- Cama Arthritis Pain Reliever .... ▣ 748
- Mag-Ox 400 666
- Uro-Mag 666

Sodium Bicarbonate (Concurrent use within one hour after taking antacid is not recommended). Products include:
- Alka-Seltzer Cherry Effervescent Antacid and Pain Reliever .... ▣ 609
- Alka-Seltzer Extra Strength Effervescent Antacid and Pain Reliever .... ▣ 609
- Alka-Seltzer Gold Effervescent Antacid .... ▣ 611
- Alka-Seltzer Lemon Lime Effervescent Antacid and Pain Reliever .... ▣ 609
- Alka-Seltzer Original Effervescent Antacid and Pain Reliever .... ▣ 609
- Arm & Hammer Pure Baking Soda .... ▣ 648
- Colyte and Colyte-flavored 2540
- GoLYTELY 694
- Massengill Disposable Douches ... ▣ 780
- Massengill Liquid Concentrate .... ▣ 780
- NuLYTELY 694
- Cherry Flavor NuLYTELY 694

Food Interactions

Dairy products (Concurrent use within one hour after taking milk is not recommended).

CORTAID SENSITIVE SKIN CREAM WITH ALOE
(Hydrocortisone Acetate) .... ▣ 800
None cited in PDR database.

CORTAID SENSITIVE SKIN OINTMENT WITH ALOE
(Hydrocortisone Acetate) .... ▣ 800
None cited in PDR database.

MAXIMUM STRENGTH CORTAID CREAM
(Hydrocortisone Acetate) .... ▣ 800
None cited in PDR database.

MAXIMUM STRENGTH CORTAID FASTSTICK
(Hydrocortisone Acetate) .... ▣ 800
None cited in PDR database.

MAXIMUM STRENGTH CORTAID OINTMENT
(Hydrocortisone Acetate) .... ▣ 800
None cited in PDR database.

MAXIMUM STRENGTH CORTAID SPRAY
(Hydrocortisone) .... ▣ 800
None cited in PDR database.

CORTENEMA
(Hydrocortisone) 2713
May interact with:

Aspirin (Concurrent use requires caution in hypoprothrombinemia). Products include:
- Alka-Seltzer Cherry Effervescent Antacid and Pain Reliever .... ▣ 609
- Alka-Seltzer Extra Strength Effervescent Antacid and Pain Reliever .... ▣ 609
- Alka-Seltzer Lemon Lime Effervescent Antacid and Pain Reliever .... ▣ 609
- Alka-Seltzer Original Effervescent Antacid and Pain Reliever .... ▣ 609
- Alka-Seltzer Plus .... ▣ 611
- Alka-Seltzer Plus Sinus Medicine .. ▣ 611
- Ascriptin .... ▣ 650
- Arthritis Strength BC Powder ...... ▣ 631
- BC Cold Powder Multi-Symptom Formula (Cold-Sinus-Allergy) .... ▣ 631
- BC Cold Powder Non-Drowsy Formula (Cold-Sinus) .... ▣ 631
- BC Powder .... ▣ 631
- Genuine Bayer Aspirin Tablets & Caplets .... ▣ 618
- Extra Strength Bayer Arthritis Pain Regimen Formula .... ▣ 615
- Extra Strength Bayer Aspirin Caplets & Tablets .... ▣ 617
- Extended-Release Bayer 8-Hour Aspirin .... ▣ 616
- Extra Strength Bayer Plus Aspirin Caplets .... ▣ 617
- Extra Strength Bayer PM Aspirin Plus Sleep Aid .... ▣ 617
- Aspirin Regimen Bayer 81 mg Tablets with Calcium .... ▣ 615
- Aspirin Regimen Bayer Adult Low Strength 81 mg Tablets .... ▣ 613
- Aspirin Regimen Bayer Children's Chewable Aspirin .... ▣ 616
- Aspirin Regimen Bayer Regular Strength 325 mg Caplets .... ▣ 613
- Bufferin Analgesic Tablets .... ▣ 636
- Arthritis Strength Bufferin Analgesic Caplets .... ▣ 637
- Extra Strength Bufferin Analgesic Tablets .... ▣ 637
- Cama Arthritis Pain Reliever .... ▣ 748
- Darvon Compound-65 Pulvules 1475
- Easprin 1971
- Ecotrin 2625
- Ecotrin Enteric Coated Aspirin Maximum Strength Tablets and Caplets .... ▣ 775
- Ecotrin Enteric Coated Aspirin Regular Strength Tablets 2625
- Empirin Aspirin Tablets .... ▣ 818
- Excedrin Extra-Strength Analgesic Tablets, Caplets, and Geltabs 734
- Fiorinal Capsules 2388
- Fiorinal with Codeine Capsules 2390
- Fiorinal Tablets 2388
- Goody's Extra Strength Headache Powders .... ▣ 632
- Goody's Extra Strength Pain Relief Tablets .... ▣ 632
- Halfprin Tablets 1413
- Norgesic 1554
- Percodan Tablets 955
- Percodan-Demi Tablets 956
- Robaxisal Tablets 2246
- Soma Compound w/Codeine Tablets 2784
- Soma Compound Tablets 2783
- St. Joseph Adult Chewable Aspirin (81 mg.) .... ▣ 768
- Talwin Compound 2466
- Vanquish Analgesic Caplets .... ▣ 627

Immunization (Possible hazards of neurological complications and a lack of antibody response, especially in patients on high dose of corticosteroid).

Smallpox Vaccine (Possible hazards of neurological complications and a lack of antibody response, especially in patients on high dose of corticosteroid).

CORTIFOAM
(Hydrocortisone Acetate) 2540
None cited in PDR database.

CORTISPORIN CREAM
(Polymyxin B Sulfate, Neomycin Sulfate, Hydrocortisone Acetate) 1073
None cited in PDR database.

CORTISPORIN OINTMENT
(Polymyxin B Sulfate, Bacitracin Zinc, Neomycin Sulfate, Hydrocortisone) 1074
None cited in PDR database.

CORTISPORIN OPHTHALMIC OINTMENT STERILE
(Polymyxin B Sulfate, Bacitracin Zinc, Neomycin Sulfate, Hydrocortisone) 1074
None cited in PDR database.

CORTISPORIN OPHTHALMIC SUSPENSION STERILE
(Hydrocortisone, Polymyxin B Sulfate, Neomycin Sulfate) 1075
None cited in PDR database.

CORTISPORIN OTIC SOLUTION STERILE
(Polymyxin B Sulfate, Neomycin Sulfate, Hydrocortisone) 1076
None cited in PDR database.

CORTISPORIN OTIC SUSPENSION STERILE
(Polymyxin B Sulfate, Neomycin Sulfate, Hydrocortisone) 1077
None cited in PDR database.

CORTIZONE FOR KIDS
(Hydrocortisone) .... ▣ 795
None cited in PDR database.

CORTIZONE-5 CREME AND OINTMENT
(Hydrocortisone) .... ▣ 795
None cited in PDR database.

CORTIZONE-10 CREME AND OINTMENT
(Hydrocortisone) .... ▣ 795
None cited in PDR database.

CORTIZONE-10 EXTERNAL ANAL ITCH RELIEF
(Hydrocortisone) .... ▣ 795

(▣ Described in PDR For Nonprescription Drugs)   (◉ Described in PDR For Ophthalmology)

CORTIZONE-10 SCALP ITCH FORMULA
(Hydrocortisone) 795
None cited in PDR database.

CORTONE ACETATE STERILE SUSPENSION
(Cortisone Acetate) 1663
May interact with oral anticoagulants, potassium-depleting diuretics, oral hypoglycemic agents, insulin, and certain other agents. Compounds in these categories include:

Acarbose (Potential for increased requirements of oral hypoglycemic agents). Products include:
- Precose 604

Aspirin (Aspirin should be used cautiously in conjunction with corticosteroids in hypoprothrombinemia). Products include:
- Alka-Seltzer Cherry Effervescent Antacid and Pain Reliever 609
- Alka-Seltzer Extra Strength Effervescent Antacid and Pain Reliever 609
- Alka-Seltzer Lemon Lime Effervescent Antacid and Pain Reliever 609
- Alka-Seltzer Original Effervescent Antacid and Pain Reliever 609
- Alka-Seltzer Plus 611
- Alka-Seltzer Plus Sinus Medicine 611
- Ascriptin 650
- Arthritis Strength BC Powder 631
- BC Cold Powder Multi-Symptom Formula (Cold-Sinus-Allergy) 631
- BC Cold Powder Non-Drowsy Formula (Cold-Sinus) 631
- BC Powder 631
- Genuine Bayer Aspirin Tablets & Caplets 618
- Extra Strength Bayer Arthritis Pain Regimen Formula 615
- Extra Strength Bayer Aspirin Caplets & Tablets 617
- Extended-Release Bayer 8-Hour Aspirin 616
- Extra Strength Bayer Plus Aspirin Caplets 617
- Extra Strength Bayer PM Aspirin Plus Sleep Aid 617
- Aspirin Regimen Bayer 81 mg Tablets with Calcium 615
- Aspirin Regimen Bayer Adult Low Strength 81 mg Tablets 613
- Aspirin Regimen Bayer Children's Chewable Aspirin 616
- Aspirin Regimen Bayer Regular Strength 325 mg Caplets 613
- Bufferin Analgesic Tablets 636
- Arthritis Strength Bufferin Analgesic Caplets 637
- Extra Strength Bufferin Analgesic Tablets 637
- Cama Arthritis Pain Reliever 748
- Darvon Compound-65 Pulvules 1475
- Easprin 1971
- Ecotrin 2625
- Ecotrin Enteric Coated Aspirin Maximum Strength Tablets and Caplets 775
- Ecotrin Enteric Coated Aspirin Regular Strength Tablets 2625
- Empirin Aspirin Tablets 818
- Excedrin Extra-Strength Analgesic Tablets, Caplets, and Geltabs 734
- Fiorinal Capsules 2388
- Fiorinal with Codeine Capsules 2390
- Fiorinal Tablets 2388
- Goody's Extra Strength Headache Powders 632
- Goody's Extra Strength Pain Relief Tablets 632
- Halfprin Tablets 1413
- Norgesic 1554
- Percodan Tablets 955
- Percodan-Demi Tablets 956
- Robaxisal Tablets 2246
- Soma Compound w/Codeine Tablets 2784
- Soma Compound Tablets 2783
- St. Joseph Adult Chewable Aspirin (81 mg.) 768
- Talwin Compound 2466
- Vanquish Analgesic Caplets 627

Bendroflumethiazide (Co-administration may result in hypokalemia).
- No products indexed under this heading.

Chlorothiazide (Co-administration may result in hypokalemia). Products include:
- Aldoclor Tablets 1638
- Diupres Tablets 1691
- Diuril Oral 1694

Chlorothiazide Sodium (Co-administration may result in hypokalemia). Products include:
- Diuril Sodium Intravenous 1693

Chlorpropamide (Potential for increased requirements of oral hypoglycemic agents). Products include:
- Diabinese Tablets 2002

Dicumarol (Potential for altered response to coumarin anticoagulants).
- No products indexed under this heading.

Ephedrine Hydrochloride (Enhanced metabolic clearance of corticosteroids). Products include:
- Primatene Tablets 844
- Quadrinal Tablets 1398

Ephedrine Sulfate (Enhanced metabolic clearance of corticosteroids). Products include:
- Marax Tablets & DF Syrup 2015

Ephedrine Tannate (Enhanced metabolic clearance of corticosteroids). Products include:
- Rynatuss 2782

Fosphenytoin Sodium (Enhanced metabolic clearance of corticosteroids). Products include:
- Cerebyx Injection 1956

Glimepiride (Potential for increased requirements of oral hypoglycemic agents). Products include:
- Amaryl Tablets 1241

Glipizide (Potential for increased requirements of oral hypoglycemic agents). Products include:
- Glucotrol Tablets 2011
- Glucotrol XL Extended Release Tablets 2012

Glyburide (Potential for increased requirements of oral hypoglycemic agents). Products include:
- DiaBeta Tablets 1265
- Glynase PresTab Tablets 2091
- Micronase Tablets 2099

Hydrochlorothiazide (Co-administration may result in hypokalemia). Products include:
- Aldactazide Tablets 2556
- Aldoril Tablets 1644
- Apresazide Capsules 824
- Capozide Tablets 744
- Dyazide Capsules 2653
- Esidrix Tablets 839
- Esimil Tablets 840
- HydroDIURIL Tablets 1716
- Hydropres Tablets 1718
- Hyzaar Tablets 1720
- Inderide Tablets 2838
- Inderide LA Long Acting Capsules 2840
- Lopressor HCT Tablets 850
- Lotensin HCT Tablets 855
- Moduretic Tablets 1748
- Oretic Tablets 450
- Prinzide Tablets 1780
- Ser-Ap-Es Tablets 867
- Timolide Tablets 1791
- Vaseretic Tablets 1810
- Zestoretic Tablets 2968
- Ziac 1459

Hydroflumethiazide (Co-administration may result in hypokalemia). Products include:
- Diucardin Tablets 2824

Insulin, Human (Potential for increased requirements of insulin).
- No products indexed under this heading.

Insulin, Human Isophane Suspension (Potential for increased requirements of insulin). Products include:
- Novolin N Human Insulin 10 ml Vials 1846

Insulin, Human NPH (Potential for increased requirements of insulin). Products include:
- Humulin N, 100 Units 1495
- Novolin N PenFill 1.5 ml Cartridges Durable Insulin Delivery System 1849
- Novolin N Prefilled Syringe Disposable Insulin Delivery System 1850

Insulin, Human Regular (Potential for increased requirements of insulin). Products include:
- Humulin R, 100 Units 1497
- Novolin R Human Insulin 10 ml Vials 1846
- Novolin R PenFill 1.5 ml Cartridges Durable Insulin Delivery System 1849
- Novolin R Prefilled Syringe Disposable Insulin Delivery System 1850
- Velosulin BR Human Insulin 10 ml Vials 1847

Insulin, Human, Zinc Suspension (Potential for increased requirements of insulin). Products include:
- Humulin L, 100 Units 1494
- Humulin U, 100 Units 1498
- Novolin L Human Insulin 10 ml Vials 1846

Insulin Lispro, Human (Potential for increased requirements of insulin). Products include:
- Humalog Injection 1488

Insulin, NPH (Potential for increased requirements of insulin). Products include:
- NPH, 100 Units 1502
- Pork NPH, 100 Units 1506
- Purified Pork NPH Isophane Insulin 1852

Insulin, Regular (Potential for increased requirements of insulin). Products include:
- Regular, 100 Units 1503
- Pork Regular, 100 Units 1507
- Pork Regular (Concentrated), 500 Units 1508
- Purified Pork Regular Insulin 1852

Insulin, Zinc Crystals (Potential for increased requirements of insulin). Products include:
- NPH, 100 Units 1502

Insulin, Zinc Suspension (Potential for increased requirements of insulin). Products include:
- Iletin I 1501
- Lente, 100 Units 1501
- Iletin II 1504
- Pork Lente, 100 Units 1504
- Purified Pork Lente Insulin 1852

Live Virus Vaccines (Co-administration is contraindicated in patients receiving immunosuppressive doses of corticosteroids).

Metformin Hydrochloride (Potential for increased requirements of oral hypoglycemic agents). Products include:
- Glucophage Tablets 754

Methyclothiazide (Co-administration may result in hypokalemia). Products include:
- Enduron Tablets 424

Phenobarbital (Enhanced metabolic clearance of corticosteroids). Products include:
- Arco-Lase Plus Tablets 513
- Bellergal-S Tablets 2375
- Donnatal 2234
- Donnatal Extentabs 2234
- Donnatal Tablets 2234
- Phenobarbital Elixir and Tablets 1523
- Quadrinal Tablets 1398

Phenytoin (Enhanced metabolic clearance of corticosteroids). Products include:
- Dilantin Infatabs 1967
- Dilantin-125 Suspension 1969

Phenytoin Sodium (Enhanced metabolic clearance of corticosteroids). Products include:
- Dilantin Kapseals 1965

Polythiazide (Co-administration may result in hypokalemia). Products include:
- Minizide Capsules 2016

Rifampin (Enhanced metabolic clearance of corticosteroids). Products include:
- Rifadin 1276
- Rifamate Capsules 1278
- Rifater 1280
- Rimactane Capsules 865

Tolazamide (Potential for increased requirements of oral hypoglycemic agents).
- No products indexed under this heading.

Tolbutamide (Potential for increased requirements of oral hypoglycemic agents).
- No products indexed under this heading.

Warfarin Sodium (Potential for altered response to coumarin anticoagulants). Products include:
- Coumadin 941

CORTONE ACETATE TABLETS
(Cortisone Acetate) 1664
May interact with potassium-depleting diuretics, oral anticoagulants, oral hypoglycemic agents, insulin, and certain other agents. Compounds in these categories include:

Acarbose (Potential for increased requirements of oral hypoglycemic agents). Products include:
- Precose 604

Aspirin (Aspirin should be used cautiously in conjunction with corticosteroids in hypoprothrombinemia). Products include:
- Alka-Seltzer Cherry Effervescent Antacid and Pain Reliever 609
- Alka-Seltzer Extra Strength Effervescent Antacid and Pain Reliever 609
- Alka-Seltzer Lemon Lime Effervescent Antacid and Pain Reliever 609
- Alka-Seltzer Original Effervescent Antacid and Pain Reliever 609
- Alka-Seltzer Plus 611
- Alka-Seltzer Plus Sinus Medicine 611
- Ascriptin 650
- Arthritis Strength BC Powder 631
- BC Cold Powder Multi-Symptom Formula (Cold-Sinus-Allergy) 631
- BC Cold Powder Non-Drowsy Formula (Cold-Sinus) 631
- BC Powder 631
- Genuine Bayer Aspirin Tablets & Caplets 618
- Extra Strength Bayer Arthritis Pain Regimen Formula 615
- Extra Strength Bayer Aspirin Caplets & Tablets 617
- Extended-Release Bayer 8-Hour Aspirin 616
- Extra Strength Bayer Plus Aspirin Caplets 617
- Extra Strength Bayer PM Aspirin Plus Sleep Aid 617
- Aspirin Regimen Bayer 81 mg Tablets with Calcium 615
- Aspirin Regimen Bayer Adult Low Strength 81 mg Tablets 613
- Aspirin Regimen Bayer Children's Chewable Aspirin 616
- Aspirin Regimen Bayer Regular Strength 325 mg Caplets 613
- Bufferin Analgesic Tablets 636
- Arthritis Strength Bufferin Analgesic Caplets 637

IMPORTANT NOTE: Always consult each drug listing in the patient's regimen for possible interactions.

Cortone Acetate Tablets — Interactions Index

Extra Strength Bufferin Analgesic Tablets 637
Cama Arthritis Pain Reliever 748
Darvon Compound-65 Pulvules 1475
Easprin 1971
Ecotrin 2625
Ecotrin Enteric Coated Aspirin Maximum Strength Tablets and Caplets 775
Ecotrin Enteric Coated Aspirin Regular Strength Tablets 2625
Empirin Aspirin Tablets 818
Excedrin Extra-Strength Analgesic Tablets, Caplets, and Geltabs 734
Fiorinal Capsules 2388
Fiorinal with Codeine Capsules 2390
Fiorinal Tablets 2388
Goody's Extra Strength Headache Powders 632
Goody's Extra Strength Pain Relief Tablets 632
Halfprin Tablets 1413
Norgesic 1554
Percodan Tablets 955
Percodan-Demi Tablets 956
Robaxisal Tablets 2246
Soma Compound w/Codeine Tablets 2784
Soma Compound Tablets 2783
St. Joseph Adult Chewable Aspirin (81 mg.) 768
Talwin Compound 2466
Vanquish Analgesic Caplets 627

Bendroflumethiazide (Co-administration may result in hypokalemia).
No products indexed under this heading.

Chlorothiazide (Co-administration may result in hypokalemia). Products include:
Aldoclor Tablets 1638
Diupres Tablets 1691
Diuril Oral 1694

Chlorothiazide Sodium (Co-administration may result in hypokalemia). Products include:
Diuril Sodium Intravenous 1693

Chlorpropamide (Potential for increased requirements of oral hypoglycemic agents). Products include:
Diabinese Tablets 2002

Dicumarol (Potential for altered response to coumarin anticoagulants).
No products indexed under this heading.

Ephedrine Hydrochloride (Enhanced metabolic clearance of corticosteroids). Products include:
Primatene Tablets 844
Quadrinal Tablets 1398

Ephedrine Sulfate (Enhanced metabolic clearance of corticosteroids). Products include:
Marax Tablets & DF Syrup 2015

Ephedrine Tannate (Enhanced metabolic clearance of corticosteroids). Products include:
Rynatuss 2782

Fosphenytoin Sodium (Enhanced metabolic clearance of corticosteroids). Products include:
Cerebyx Injection 1956

Glimepiride (Potential for increased requirements of oral hypoglycemic agents). Products include:
Amaryl Tablets 1241

Glipizide (Potential for increased requirements of oral hypoglycemic agents). Products include:
Glucotrol Tablets 2011
Glucotrol XL Extended Release Tablets 2012

Glyburide (Potential for increased requirements of oral hypoglycemic agents). Products include:
DiaBeta Tablets 1265
Glynase PresTab Tablets 2091
Micronase Tablets 2099

Hydrochlorothiazide (Co-administration may result in hypokalemia). Products include:
Aldactazide Tablets 2556
Aldoril Tablets 1644
Apresazide Capsules 824
Capozide Tablets 744
Dyazide Capsules 2653
Esidrix Tablets 839
Esimil Tablets 840
HydroDIURIL Tablets 1716
Hydropres Tablets 1718
Hyzaar Tablets 1720
Inderide Tablets 2838
Inderide LA Long Acting Capsules .. 2840
Lopressor HCT Tablets 850
Lotensin HCT Tablets 855
Moduretic Tablets 1748
Oretic Tablets 450
Prinzide Tablets 1780
Ser-Ap-Es Tablets 867
Timolide Tablets 1791
Vaseretic Tablets 1810
Zestoretic Tablets 2968
Ziac 1459

Hydroflumethiazide (Co-administration may result in hypokalemia). Products include:
Diucardin Tablets 2824

Insulin, Human (Potential for increased requirements of insulin).
No products indexed under this heading.

Insulin, Human Isophane Suspension (Potential for increased requirements of insulin). Products include:
Novolin N Human Insulin 10 ml Vials 1846

Insulin, Human NPH (Potential for increased requirements of insulin). Products include:
Humulin N, 100 Units 1495
Novolin N PenFill 1.5 ml Cartridges Durable Insulin Delivery System 1849
Novolin N Prefilled Syringe Disposable Insulin Delivery System 1850

Insulin, Human Regular (Potential for increased requirements of insulin). Products include:
Humulin R, 100 Units 1497
Novolin R Human Insulin 10 ml Vials 1846
Novolin R PenFill 1.5 ml Cartridges Durable Insulin Delivery System 1849
Novolin R Prefilled Syringe Disposable Insulin Delivery System 1850
Velosulin BR Human Insulin 10 ml Vials 1847

Insulin, Human, Zinc Suspension (Potential for increased requirements of insulin). Products include:
Humulin L, 100 Units 1494
Humulin U, 100 Units 1498
Novolin L Human Insulin 10 ml Vials 1846

Insulin Lispro, Human (Potential for increased requirements of insulin). Products include:
Humalog Injection 1488

Insulin, NPH (Potential for increased requirements of insulin). Products include:
NPH, 100 Units 1502
Pork NPH, 100 Units 1506
Purified Pork NPH Isophane Insulin 1852

Insulin, Regular (Potential for increased requirements of insulin). Products include:
Regular, 100 Units 1503
Pork Regular, 100 Units 1507
Pork Regular (Concentrated), 500 Units 1508
Purified Pork Regular Insulin 1852

Insulin, Zinc Crystals (Potential for increased requirements of insulin). Products include:
NPH, 100 Units 1502

Insulin, Zinc Suspension (Potential for increased requirements of insulin). Products include:
Iletin I 1501
Lente, 100 Units 1501
Iletin II 1504
Pork Lente, 100 Units 1504
Purified Pork Lente Insulin 1852

Metformin Hydrochloride (Potential for increased requirements of oral hypoglycemic agents). Products include:
Glucophage Tablets 754

Methylclothiazide (Co-administration may result in hypokalemia). Products include:
Enduron Tablets 424

Phenobarbital (Enhanced metabolic clearance of corticosteroids). Products include:
Arco-Lase Plus Tablets 513
Bellergal-S Tablets 2375
Donnatal 2234
Donnatal Extentabs 2234
Donnatal Tablets 2234
Phenobarbital Elixir and Tablets 1523
Quadrinal Tablets 1398

Phenytoin (Enhanced metabolic clearance of corticosteroids). Products include:
Dilantin Infatabs 1967
Dilantin-125 Suspension 1969

Phenytoin Sodium (Enhanced metabolic clearance of corticosteroids). Products include:
Dilantin Kapseals 1965

Polythiazide (Co-administration may result in hypokalemia). Products include:
Minizide Capsules 2016

Rifampin (Enhanced metabolic clearance of corticosteroids). Products include:
Rifadin 1276
Rifamate Capsules 1278
Rifater 1280
Rimactane Capsules 865

Tolazamide (Potential for increased requirements of oral hypoglycemic agents).
No products indexed under this heading.

Tolbutamide (Potential for increased requirements of oral hypoglycemic agents).
No products indexed under this heading.

Warfarin Sodium (Potential for altered response to coumarin anticoagulants). Products include:
Coumadin 941

CORVERT INJECTION
(Ibutilide Fumarate) 2075
May interact with drugs that prolong the qt interval, quinidine, and certain other agents. Compounds in these categories include:

Amiodarone Hydrochloride (Potential for prolonged refractoriness; amiodarone should not be given concomitantly or within 4 hours postinfusion). Products include:
Cordarone Intravenous 2821
Cordarone Tablets 2818

Amitriptyline Hydrochloride (The potential for proarrhythmia may increase with co-administration of ibutilide to patients who are being treated with drugs that prolong the QT interval). Products include:
Elavil 2945
Etrafon 2495
Limbitrol 2333
Triavil Tablets 1800

Amoxapine (The potential for proarrhythmia may increase with co-administration of ibutilide to patients who are being treated with drugs that prolong the QT interval). Products include:
Asendin Tablets 1419

Astemizole (The potential for proarrhythmia may increase with co-administration of ibutilide to patients who are being treated with drugs that prolong the QT interval). Products include:
Hismanal Tablets 1341

Bretylium Tosylate (The potential for proarrhythmia may increase with co-administration of ibutilide to patients who are being treated with drugs that prolong the QT interval).
No products indexed under this heading.

Chlorpromazine (The potential for proarrhythmia may increase with co-administration of ibutilide to patients who are being treated with drugs that prolong the QT interval). Products include:
Thorazine Suppositories 2701

Chlorpromazine Hydrochloride (The potential for proarrhythmia may increase with co-administration of ibutilide to patients who are being treated with drugs that prolong the QT interval). Products include:
Thorazine 2701

Clomipramine Hydrochloride (The potential for proarrhythmia may increase with co-administration of ibutilide to patients who are being treated with drugs that prolong the QT interval). Products include:
Anafranil Capsules 819

Desipramine Hydrochloride (The potential for proarrhythmia may increase with co-administration of ibutilide to patients who are being treated with drugs that prolong the QT interval). Products include:
Norpramin Tablets 1273

Digoxin (Supraventricular arrhythmias may mask the cardiotoxicity associated with excessive digoxin levels; caution is advised in patients whose plasma digoxin levels are above or suspected to be above the therapeutic range; co-administration did not have effects on the safety or efficacy of ibutilide). Products include:
Lanoxicaps 1110
Lanoxin Elixir Pediatric 1113
Lanoxin Injection 1116
Lanoxin Injection Pediatric 1119
Lanoxin Tablets 1121

Disopyramide Phosphate (Potential for prolonged refractoriness; disopyramide should not be given concomitantly or within 4 hours postinfusion). Products include:
Norpace 2596

Doxepin Hydrochloride (The potential for proarrhythmia may increase with co-administration of ibutilide to patients who are being treated with drugs that prolong the QT interval). Products include:
Adapin Capsules 1542
Sinequan 2028
Zonalon Cream 1042

Flecainide Acetate (The potential for proarrhythmia may increase with co-administration of ibutilide to patients who are being treated with drugs that prolong the QT interval). Products include:
Tambocor Tablets 1555

(■ Described in PDR For Nonprescription Drugs)   (◉ Described in PDR For Ophthalmology)

211 **Interactions Index** **Coumadin**

Fluphenazine Decanoate (The potential for proarrhythmia may increase with co-administration of ibutilide to patients who are being treated with drugs that prolong the QT interval). Products include:

Prolixin Decanoate 510

Fluphenazine Enanthate (The potential for proarrhythmia may increase with co-administration of ibutilide to patients who are being treated with drugs that prolong the QT interval). Products include:

Prolixin Enanthate 510

Fluphenazine Hydrochloride (The potential for proarrhythmia may increase with co-administration of ibutilide to patients who are being treated with drugs that prolong the QT interval). Products include:

Prolixin 510

Imipramine Hydrochloride (The potential for proarrhythmia may increase with co-administration of ibutilide to patients who are being treated with drugs that prolong the QT interval). Products include:

Tofranil Ampuls 873
Tofranil Tablets 875

Imipramine Pamoate (The potential for proarrhythmia may increase with co-administration of ibutilide to patients who are being treated with drugs that prolong the QT interval). Products include:

Tofranil-PM Capsules 876

Lidocaine Hydrochloride (The potential for proarrhythmia may increase with co-administration of ibutilide to patients who are being treated with drugs that prolong the QT interval). Products include:

Decadron Phosphate with Xylocaine Injection, Sterile 1683
Unguentine Plus 712
Xylocaine Injections 562

Maprotiline Hydrochloride (The potential for proarrhythmia may increase with co-administration of ibutilide to patients who are being treated with drugs that prolong the QT interval). Products include:

Ludiomil Tablets 861

Mesoridazine (The potential for proarrhythmia may increase with co-administration of ibutilide to patients who are being treated with drugs that prolong the QT interval).

Mexiletine Hydrochloride (The potential for proarrhythmia may increase with co-administration of ibutilide to patients who are being treated with drugs that prolong the QT interval). Products include:

Mexitil Capsules 684

Nortriptyline Hydrochloride (The potential for proarrhythmia may increase with co-administration of ibutilide to patients who are being treated with drugs that prolong the QT interval). Products include:

Pamelor 2409

Perphenazine (The potential for proarrhythmia may increase with co-administration of ibutilide to patients who are being treated with drugs that prolong the QT interval). Products include:

Etrafon 2495
Triavil Tablets 1800
Trilafon 2532

Procainamide Hydrochloride (Potential for prolonged refractoriness; procainamide should not be given concomitantly or within 4 hours postinfusion). Products include:

Procanbid Extended-Release Tablets 1983

Prochlorperazine (The potential for proarrhythmia may increase with co-administration of ibutilide to patients who are being treated with drugs that prolong the QT interval). Products include:

Compazine 2644

Promethazine Hydrochloride (The potential for proarrhythmia may increase with co-administration of ibutilide to patients who are being treated with drugs that prolong the QT interval). Products include:

Mepergan Injection 2859
Phenergan with Codeine 2883
Phenergan with Dextromethorphan 2885
Phenergan Injection 2880
Phenergan Suppositories 2882
Phenergan Syrup 2881
Phenergan Tablets 2882
Phenergan VC 2886
Phenergan VC with Codeine 2888

Propafenone Hydrochloride (The potential for proarrhythmia may increase with co-administration of ibutilide to patients who are being treated with drugs that prolong the QT interval). Products include:

Rythmol Tablets–150mg, 225mg, 300mg 1399

Protriptyline Hydrochloride (The potential for proarrhythmia may increase with co-administration of ibutilide to patients who are being treated with drugs that prolong the QT interval). Products include:

Vivactil Tablets 1820

Quinidine Gluconate (Potential for prolonged refractoriness; quinidine should not be given concomitantly or within 4 hours postinfusion). Products include:

Quinaglute Dura-Tabs Tablets 644

Quinidine Polygalacturonate (Potential for prolonged refractoriness; quinidine should not be given concomitantly or within 4 hours postinfusion). Products include:

Cardioquin Tablets 2146

Quinidine Sulfate (Potential for prolonged refractoriness; quinidine should not be given concomitantly or within 4 hours postinfusion). Products include:

Quinidex Extentabs 2240

Sotalol Hydrochloride (Potential for prolonged refractoriness; sotalol should not be given concomitantly or within 4 hours postinfusion). Products include:

Betapace Tablets 637

Terfenadine (The potential for proarrhythmia may increase with co-administration of ibutilide to patients who are being treated with drugs that prolong the QT interval). Products include:

Seldane Tablets 1284
Seldane-D Extended-Release Tablets 1286

Thioridazine Hydrochloride (The potential for proarrhythmia may increase with co-administration of ibutilide to patients who are being treated with drugs that prolong the QT interval). Products include:

Mellaril 2398

Tocainide Hydrochloride (The potential for proarrhythmia may increase with co-administration of ibutilide to patients who are being treated with drugs that prolong the QT interval). Products include:

Tonocard Tablets 519

Trifluoperazine Hydrochloride (The potential for proarrhythmia may increase with co-administration of ibutilide to patients who are being treated with drugs that prolong the QT interval). Products include:

Stelazine 2692

Trimipramine Maleate (The potential for proarrhythmia may increase with co-administration of ibutilide to patients who are being treated with drugs that prolong the QT interval). Products include:

Surmontil Capsules 2917

COSMEGEN INJECTION
(Dactinomycin) 1666
None cited in PDR database.

COTAZYM CAPSULES
(Pancrelipase) 1866
None cited in PDR database.

COUGH-X LOZENGES
(Dextromethorphan Hydrobromide, Benzocaine) 606
May interact with monoamine oxidase inhibitors. Compounds in this category include:

Furazolidone (Concurrent use is not recommended). Products include:

Furoxone 2221

Isocarboxazid (Concurrent use is not recommended).

No products indexed under this heading.

Phenelzine Sulfate (Concurrent use is not recommended). Products include:

Nardil 1977

Selegiline Hydrochloride (Concurrent use is not recommended). Products include:

Eldepryl Capsules 2729

Tranylcypromine Sulfate (Concurrent use is not recommended). Products include:

Parnate Tablets 2679

COUMADIN FOR INJECTION
(Warfarin Sodium) 941
See **Coumadin Tablets**

COUMADIN TABLETS
(Warfarin Sodium) 941
May interact with antihistamines, diuretics, androgens, monoamine oxidase inhibitors, salicylates, sulfonamides, thyroid preparations, barbiturates, non-steroidal anti-inflammatory agents, oral contraceptives, inhalant anesthetics, corticosteroids, narcotic analgesics, antacids, fluoroquinolone antibiotics, pyrazolon derivatives, oral aminoglycosides, erythromycin, and certain other agents. Compounds in these categories include:

Acetaminophen (May be responsible for increased prothrombin time response). Products include:

Actifed Cold & Sinus Caplets and Tablets 808
Actifed Sinus Daytime/Nighttime Tablets and Caplets 809
Alka-Seltzer Fast Relief Caplets 610
Alka-Seltzer Plus Liqui-Gels 612
Alka-Seltzer Plus Flu & Body Aches Effervescent Tablets 612
Alka-Seltzer Plus Flu & Body Aches Liqui-Gels Non-Drowsy Formula 613
Alka-Seltzer Plus Night-Time Cold Medicine Liqui-Gels 612
Allerest No Drowsiness 649
Allerest Sinus Pain Formula 649
Axocet Capsules 2469
Benadryl Allergy/Cold Tablets 811
Benadryl Allergy Sinus Headache Caplets 813
Children's TYLENOL acetaminophen Chewable Tablets, Elixir, Suspension Liquid, and Suspension Drops 1559
Children's TYLENOL Cold Multi-Symptom Chewable Tablets and Liquid 1559
Children's TYLENOL Cold Plus Cough Multi Symptom Chewable Tablets and Liquid 1560
Children's TYLENOL Flu Suspension Liquid 1560
Allergy-Sinus Comtrex Multi-Symptom Allergy-Sinus Formula Tablets and Caplets 639
Comtrex Multi-Symptom 638
Comtrex Non-Drowsy 640
Contac Day Allergy/Sinus Caplets 771
Contac Day & Night 772
Contac Night Allergy/Sinus Caplets 771
Contac Severe Cold and Flu Formula Caplets 773
Contac Severe Cold & Flu Non-Drowsy 774
Coricidin Cold + Flu Tablets 760
Coricidin 'D' Decongestant Tablets 760
DHCplus Capsules 2148
Darvon-N/Darvocet-N 1473
Dimetapp Allergy Sinus Caplets 838
Dimetapp Cold & Fever Suspension 839
Drixoral Cold and Flu Extended-Release Tablets 764
Drixoral Cough + Sore Throat Liquid Caps 763
Drixoral Allergy/Sinus Extended Release Tablets 765
Esgic-plus Capsules 1012
Esgic-plus Tablets 1012
Aspirin Free Excedrin Analgesic Caplets and Geltabs 734
Excedrin Extra-Strength Analgesic Tablets, Caplets, and Geltabs 734
Excedrin P.M. Analgesic/Sleeping Aid Tablets, Caplets, Liquigels 735
Fioricet Tablets 2386
Fioricet with Codeine Capsules 2387
Goody's Extra Strength Headache Powders 632
Goody's Extra Strength Pain Relief Tablets 632
Hycomine Compound Tablets 948
Hydrocet Capsules 787
Infants' TYLENOL acetaminophen Suspension Drops 1559
Infants' TYLENOL Cold Decongestant & Fever-Reducer Drops 1561
Junior Strength TYLENOL acetaminophen Coated Caplets and Chewable Tablets 1562
Lorcet 10/650 Tablets 1016
Lortab 2751
Lurline PMS Tablets 1000
Maximum Strength Multi-Symptom Formula Midol 621
PMS Multi-Symptom Formula Midol 622
Maximum Strength Midol Teen Multi-Symptom Formula 621
Midrin Capsules 788
Panodol Tablets and Caplets 783
Children's Panadol Chewable Tablets, Liquid, Infant's Drops 783
Percocet Tablets 955
Percogesic Analgesic Tablets 727
Phrenilin 790
Pyrroxate Caplets 742
Robitussin Cold, Cough & Flu Liqui-Gels 844
Robitussin Night-Time Cold Formula 847
Sedapap Tablets 50 mg/650 mg .. 1826
Sinarest 663
Sine-Aid Maximum Strength Sinus Headache Gelcaps, Caplets and Tablets 1570
Sine-Off No Drowsiness Formula Caplets 784

IMPORTANT NOTE: Always consult each drug listing in the patient's regimen for possible interactions.

Coumadin **Interactions Index** **212**

Sine-Off Sinus Medicine ■ 784
Singlet Tablets ■ 785
Sinulin Tablets 792
Sinutab Sinus Allergy Medication, Maximum Strength Tablets and Caplets ■ 823
Sinutab Sinus Medication, Maximum Strength Without Drowsiness Formula, Tablets & Caplets ■ 824
Sudafed Cold and Cough Liquid Caps ■ 826
Sudafed Severe Cold Formula Caplets ■ 828
Sudafed Severe Cold Formula Tablets ■ 828
Sudafed Sinus Caplets ■ 829
Sudafed Sinus Tablets ■ 829
Talacen Caplets 2464
TheraFlu Flu and Cold Medicine ■ 750
Theraflu Maximum Strength Flu and Cold Medicine For Sore Throat ■ 751
TheraFlu Flu, Cold and Cough Medicine ■ 750
TheraFlu Maximum Strength Nighttime Flu, Cold & Cough Medicine ■ 751
TheraFlu Maximum Strength Non-Drowsy Formula Flu, Cold & Cough Medicine ■ 751
TheraFlu Maximum Strength, Non-Drowsy Formula Flu, Cold and Cough Caplets ■ 752
Theraflu Maximum Strength Sinus Non-Drowsy Formula Caplets ■ 752
Triaminic Sore Throat Formula ■ 755
Triaminicin Tablets ■ 756
TYLENOL acetaminophen Extended Relief Caplets 1570
TYLENOL acetaminophen, Extra Strength Adult Liquid Pain Reliever 1570
TYLENOL acetaminophen, Extra Strength Gelcaps, Geltabs, Caplets, Tablets 1570
TYLENOL acetaminophen, Regular Strength Caplets and Tablets 1570
TYLENOL Allergy Sinus, Maximum Strength Caplets and Gelcaps 1571
TYLENOL Allergy Sinus NightTime, Maximum Strength Caplets 1571
TYLENOL Cold Medication, Multi-Symptom Formula Tablets and Caplets 1572
TYLENOL Cold Medication, Multi-Symptom Hot Liquid Packets 1572
TYLENOL Cold Medication, No Drowsiness Formula Caplets and Gelcaps 1572
TYLENOL Cold Severe Congestion Caplets 1573
TYLENOL Cough Medication, Multi Symptom 1574
TYLENOL Cough Medication with Decongestant, Multi Symptom 1574
TYLENOL Flu No Drowsiness Formula, Maximum Strength Gelcaps 1575
TYLENOL Flu NightTime, Maximum Strength Gelcaps 1575
TYLENOL Flu NightTime, Maximum Strength Hot Medication Packets 1575
TYLENOL Headache Plus Pain Reliever with Antacid, Extra Strength Caplets ■ 705
TYLENOL PM Pain Reliever/Sleep Aid, Extra Strength Gelcaps, Caplets, Geltabs 1576
TYLENOL Severe Allergy Medication Caplets 1571
TYLENOL Sinus, Maximum Strength Geltabs, Gelcaps, Caplets and Tablets 1576
Tylenol with Codeine 1592
Tylox Capsules 1593
Unisom With Pain Relief-Nighttime Sleep Aid and Pain Reliever 1991
Vanquish Analgesic Caplets ■ 627
Vicks 44 LiquiCaps Cough, Cold & Flu Relief ■ 728
Vicks 44M Cough, Cold & Flu Relief ■ 729
Vicks DayQuil LiquiCaps/Liquid Multi-Symptom Cold/Flu Relief ■ 734
Vicks Nyquil Hot Therapy ■ 735
Vicks NyQuil LiquiCaps/Liquid Multi-Symptom Cold/Flu Relief, Original and Cherry Flavors ■ 736
Vicodin Tablets 1404
Vicodin ES Tablets 1405
Vicodin HP Tablets 1403
Wygesic Tablets 2930
Zydone Capsules 967

Acrivastine (Decreased prothrombin time response). Products include:
Semprex-D Capsules 1620

ACTH (Decreased prothrombin time response).
No products indexed under this heading.

Alfentanil Hydrochloride (Increased prothrombin time response with prolonged use). Products include:
Alfenta Injection 1334

Allopurinol (Increased prothrombin time response). Products include:
Zyloprim Tablets 1194

Alteplase, Recombinant (Increased prothrombin time response). Products include:
Activase 1045

Aluminum Carbonate (Decreased prothrombin time response). Products include:
Basaljel Capsules 2810
Basaljel Suspension 2810
Basaljel Tablets 2810

Aluminum Hydroxide (Decreased prothrombin response). Products include:
ALternaGEL Liquid 1358
Maximum Strength Ascriptin ■ 650
Cama Arthritis Pain Reliever ■ 748
Gaviscon Extra Strength Relief Formula Antacid Tablets ■ 778
Gaviscon Extra Strength Relief Formula Liquid Antacid ■ 779
Gaviscon Liquid Antacid ■ 779
Gelusil Antacid-Anti-gas Liquid ■ 819
Gelusil Antacid-Anti-gas Tablets ■ 819
Maalox Antacid/Anti-Gas Tablets 889
Maalox Heartburn Relief Suspension ■ 658
Maalox Antacid Liquid 888
Extra Strength Maalox Antacid/Anti-Gas Liquid and Tablets 888
Mylanta 1359
Tempo Soft Antacid ■ 799

Aluminum Hydroxide Gel (Decreased prothrombin time response). Products include:
ALternaGEL Liquid ■ 675
Aludrox Oral Suspension ■ 850
Amphojel Suspension 2802
Amphojel Suspension without Flavor 2802
Amphojel Tablets 2802
Ascriptin ■ 650
Gaviscon Antacid Tablets ■ 778
Gaviscon-2 Antacid Tablets ■ 779
Mylanta Liquid ■ 676
Mylanta Double Strength Liquid ■ 676
Nephrox Suspension ■ 671

Amiloride Hydrochloride (Decreased or increased prothrombin time response). Products include:
Midamor Tablets 1746
Moduretic Tablets 1748

Aminoglutethimide (Decreased prothrombin time response). Products include:
Cytadren Tablets 837

p-Aminosalicylic Acid (Increased prothrombin time response).
No products indexed under this heading.

Amiodarone Hydrochloride (Increased prothrombin time response). Products include:
Cordarone Intravenous 2821
Cordarone Tablets 2818

Amobarbital (Decreased prothrombin time response).

Anistreplase (Increased prothrombin time response). Products include:
Eminase 2215

Antibiotics, unspecified (Decreased or increased prothrombin time response).

Antipyrine (Increased prothrombin time response). Products include:
Auralgan Otic Solution 2810
Tympagesic Ear Drops 2476

Aprobarbital (Decreased prothrombin time response).
No products indexed under this heading.

Aspirin (Increased prothrombin time response). Products include:
Alka-Seltzer Cherry Effervescent Antacid and Pain Reliever ■ 609
Alka-Seltzer Extra Strength Effervescent Antacid and Pain Reliever ■ 609
Alka-Seltzer Lemon Lime Effervescent Antacid and Pain Reliever ■ 609
Alka-Seltzer Original Effervescent Antacid and Pain Reliever ■ 609
Alka-Seltzer Plus ■ 611
Alka-Seltzer Plus Sinus Medicine ■ 611
Ascriptin ■ 650
Arthritis Strength BC Powder ■ 631
BC Cold Powder Multi-Symptom Formula (Cold-Sinus-Allergy) ■ 631
BC Cold Powder Non-Drowsy Formula (Cold-Sinus) ■ 631
BC Powder ■ 631
Genuine Bayer Aspirin Tablets & Caplets ■ 618
Extra Strength Bayer Arthritis Pain Regimen Formula ■ 615
Extra Strength Bayer Aspirin Caplets & Tablets ■ 617
Extended-Release Bayer 8-Hour Aspirin ■ 616
Extra Strength Bayer Plus Aspirin Caplets ■ 617
Extra Strength Bayer PM Aspirin Plus Sleep Aid ■ 617
Aspirin Regimen Bayer 81 mg Tablets with Calcium ■ 615
Aspirin Regimen Bayer Adult Low Strength 81 mg Tablets ■ 613
Aspirin Regimen Bayer Children's Chewable Aspirin ■ 616
Aspirin Regimen Bayer Regular Strength 325 mg Caplets ■ 613
Bufferin Analgesic Tablets ■ 636
Arthritis Strength Bufferin Analgesic Caplets ■ 637
Extra Strength Bufferin Analgesic Tablets ■ 637
Cama Arthritis Pain Reliever ■ 748
Darvon Compound-65 Pulvules 1475
Easprin 1971
Ecotrin 2625
Ecotrin Enteric Coated Aspirin Maximum Strength Tablets and Caplets ■ 775
Ecotrin Enteric Coated Aspirin Regular Strength Tablets 2625
Empirin Aspirin Tablets ■ 818
Excedrin Extra-Strength Analgesic Tablets, Caplets, and Geltabs 734
Fiorinal Capsules 2388
Fiorinal with Codeine Capsules 2390
Fiorinal Tablets 2388
Goody's Extra Strength Headache Powders ■ 632
Goody's Extra Strength Pain Relief Tablets ■ 632
Halfprin Tablets 1413
Norgesic 1554
Percodan Tablets 955
Percodan-Demi Tablets 956
Robaxisal Tablets 2246
Soma Compound w/Codeine Tablets 2784
Soma Compound Tablets 2783
St. Joseph Adult Chewable Aspirin (81 mg.) ■ 768
Talwin Compound 2466
Vanquish Analgesic Caplets ■ 627

Astemizole (Decreased prothrombin time response). Products include:
Hismanal Tablets 1341

Azatadine Maleate (Decreased prothrombin time response). Products include:
Trinalin Repetabs Tablets 1373

Azathioprine (Decreased prothrombin time response). Products include:
Azathioprine Tablets 2349
Imuran 1103

Bendroflumethiazide (Decreased or increased prothrombin time response).
No products indexed under this heading.

Betamethasone Acetate (Decreased or increased prothrombin time response). Products include:
Celestone Soluspan Suspension 2484

Betamethasone Sodium Phosphate (Decreased or increased prothrombin time response). Products include:
Celestone Soluspan Suspension 2484

Bromelains (Increased prothrombin time response).
No products indexed under this heading.

Bromodiphenhydramine Hydrochloride (Decreased prothrombin time response).
No products indexed under this heading.

Brompheniramine Maleate (Decreased prothrombin time response). Products include:
Alka-Seltzer Plus Sinus Medicine ■ 611
Bromfed Capsules (Extended-Release) 1832
Bromfed Syrup ■ 712
Bromfed Tablets 1832
Bromfed-DM Cough Syrup 1832
Bromfed-PD Capsules (Extended-Release) 1832
Dimetane-DC Cough Syrup 2232
Dimetane-DX Cough Syrup 2233
Dimetapp Allergy Dye-Free Elixir ■ 838
Dimetapp Allergy Sinus Caplets ■ 838
Dimetapp Cold & Allergy Chewable Tablets ■ 838
Dimetapp Cold & Cough Liqui-Gels ■ 839
Dimetapp Cold & Fever Suspension ■ 839
Dimetapp DM Elixir ■ 840
Dimetapp Elixir ■ 840
Dimetapp Extentabs ■ 841
Dimetapp Tablets/Liqui-Gels ■ 841
Rondec Chewable Tablets 974
Vicks DayQuil Allergy Relief 12-Hour Extended Release Tablets ■ 733
Vicks DayQuil Allergy Relief 4-Hour Tablets ■ 733

Bumetanide (Decreased or increased prothrombin time response). Products include:
Bumex 2260

Buprenorphine (Increased prothrombin time response with prolonged use). Products include:
Buprenex Injectable 2170

Butabarbital (Decreased prothrombin time response).
No products indexed under this heading.

Butalbital (Decreased prothrombin time response). Products include:
Axocet Capsules 2469
Esgic-plus Capsules 1012
Esgic-plus Tablets 1012
Fioricet Tablets 2386
Fioricet with Codeine Capsules 2387
Fiorinal Capsules 2388
Fiorinal with Codeine Capsules 2390
Fiorinal Tablets 2388
Phrenilin 790
Sedapap Tablets 50 mg/650 mg 1826

Carbamazepine (Decreased prothrombin time response). Products include:
Atretol Tablets 569
Tegretol/Tegretol-XR 870

Cefamandole Nafate (Increased prothrombin time response). Products include:
Mandol Vials, Faspak & ADD-Vantage 1516

(■ Described in PDR For Nonprescription Drugs) (◉ Described in PDR For Ophthalmology)

Cefazolin Sodium (Increased prothrombin time response). Products include:
Ancef Injection 2632
Kefzol Vials, Faspak & ADD-Vantage 1511

Cefoperazone Sodium (Increased prothrombin time response). Products include:
Cefobid Intravenous/Intramuscular 1996
Cefobid Pharmacy Bulk Package - Not for Direct Infusion 1999

Cefotetan (Increased prothrombin time response). Products include:
Cefotan 2936

Cefoxitin Sodium (Increased prothrombin time response). Products include:
Mefoxin 1734
Mefoxin Premixed Intravenous Solution 1737

Ceftriaxone Sodium (Increased prothrombin time response). Products include:
Rocephin Injectable Vials, ADD-Vantage, Galaxy Container 2305

Cetirizine Hydrochloride (Decreased prothrombin time response). Products include:
Zyrtec Tablets 2053

Chenodiol (Increased prothrombin time response).
No products indexed under this heading.

Chloral Hydrate (Decreased or increased prothrombin time response).
No products indexed under this heading.

Chloramphenicol (Increased prothrombin time response). Products include:
Chloromycetin Ophthalmic Ointment, 1% .... ⓓ 298
Chloromycetin Ophthalmic Solution .... ⓓ 299
Chloroptic S.O.P. .... ⓓ 236
Chloroptic Sterile Ophthalmic Solution .... ⓓ 236

Chloramphenicol Palmitate (Increased prothrombin time response).
No products indexed under this heading.

Chloramphenicol Sodium Succinate (Increased prothrombin time response). Products include:
Chloromycetin Sodium Succinate 1960

Chlordiazepoxide (Decreased prothrombin time response). Products include:
Limbitrol 2333

Chlordiazepoxide Hydrochloride (Decreased prothrombin time response). Products include:
Librax Capsules 2330
Librium Capsules 2331
Librium Injectable 2332

Chlorothiazide (Decreased or increased prothrombin time response). Products include:
Aldoclor Tablets 1638
Diupres Tablets 1691
Diuril Oral 1694

Chlorothiazide Sodium (Decreased or increased prothrombin time response). Products include:
Diuril Sodium Intravenous 1693

Chlorpheniramine Maleate (Decreased prothrombin time response). Products include:
Alka-Seltzer Plus Cold Medicine .... ⓓ 611
Alka-Seltzer Plus Cold Medicine Liqui-Gels .... ⓓ 612
Alka-Seltzer Plus Cold & Cough Medicine .... ⓓ 611
Alka-Seltzer Plus Cold & Cough Medicine Liqui-Gels .... ⓓ 612
Alka-Seltzer Plus Flu & Body Aches Effervescent Tablets ...... ⓓ 612

Allerest Maximum Strength .... ⓓ 649
Allerest Sinus Pain Formula .... ⓓ 649
Ana-Kit Anaphylaxis Emergency Treatment Kit 611
Atrohist Pediatric Capsules 1603
Atrohist Plus Tablets 1605
BC Cold Powder Multi-Symptom Formula (Cold-Sinus-Allergy) .... ⓓ 631
Cerose DM 853
Cheracol Plus Head Cold/Cough Formula .... ⓓ 741
Children's TYLENOL Cold Multi-Symptom Chewable Tablets and Liquid 1559
Children's TYLENOL Cold Plus Cough Multi Symptom Chewable Tablets and Liquid 1560
Children's TYLENOL Flu Suspension Liquid 1560
Children's Vicks DayQuil Allergy Relief .... ⓓ 730
Children's Vicks NyQuil Cold/Cough Relief .... ⓓ 731
Chlor-Trimeton Allergy Decongestant Tablets .... ⓓ 759
Chlor-Trimeton Allergy Tablets ...... ⓓ 758
Allergy-Sinus Comtrex Multi-Symptom Allergy-Sinus Formula Tablets and Caplets .... ⓓ 639
Comtrex Multi-Symptom .... ⓓ 638
Contac Continuous Action Nasal Decongestant/Antihistamine 12 Hour Capsules .... ⓓ 773
Contac Maximum Strength Continuous Action Decongestant/Antihistamine 12 Hour Caplets .. ⓓ 772
Contac Severe Cold and Flu Formula Caplets .... ⓓ 773
Coricidin Cold + Flu Tablets ...... ⓓ 760
Coricidin Cough + Cold Tablets .. ⓓ 760
Coricidin 'D' Decongestant Tablets .... ⓓ 760
D.A. II Tablets 972
D.A. Chewable Tablets 970
Dura-Tap/PD Capsules 970
Dura-Vent/DA Tablets 972
Efidac 24 Chlorpheniramine .... ⓓ 655
Extendryl 1003
Fedahist Gyrocaps 2545
Hycomine Compound Tablets 948
Kronofed-A 994
Nolamine Timed-Release Tablets ... 790
Novahistine Elixir .... ⓓ 782
Ornade Spansule Capsules 2678
PediaCare Cough-Cold Chewable Tablets and Liquid 1569
PediaCare NightRest Cough-Cold Liquid 1569
Pediatric Vicks 44m Cough & Cold Relief .... ⓓ 737
Pyrroxate Caplets .... ⓓ 742
Ryna .... ⓓ 804
Sinarest .... ⓓ 663
Sine-Off Sinus Medicine .... ⓓ 784
Singlet Tablets .... ⓓ 785
Sinulin Tablets 792
Sinutab Sinus Allergy Medication, Maximum Strength Tablets and Caplets .... ⓓ 823
Sudafed Cold & Allergy Tablets ... ⓓ 826
Teldrin 12 Hour Antihistamine/Nasal Decongestant Allergy Relief Capsules .... ⓓ 786
TheraFlu Flu and Cold Medicine ... ⓓ 750
Theraflu Maximum Strength Flu and Cold Medicine For Sore Throat .... ⓓ 751
TheraFlu Flu, Cold and Cough Medicine .... ⓓ 750
TheraFlu Maximum Strength Nighttime Flu, Cold & Cough Medicine .... ⓓ 751
Triaminic Night Time .... ⓓ 754
Triaminic Syrup .... ⓓ 755
Triaminic Triaminicol Cold & Cough .... ⓓ 756
Triaminicin Tablets .... ⓓ 756
Tussend 1830
TYLENOL Allergy Sinus, Maximum Strength Caplets and Gelcaps ... 1571
TYLENOL Cold Medication, Multi-Symptom Formula Tablets and Caplets 1572
TYLENOL Cold Medication, Multi-Symptom Hot Liquid Packets ... 1572
Vicks 44 LiquiCaps Cough, Cold & Flu Relief .... ⓓ 728
Vicks 44M Cough, Cold & Flu Relief .... ⓓ 729

Chlorpheniramine Polistirex (Decreased prothrombin time response). Products include:
Tussionex Pennkinetic Extended-Release Suspension 1624

Chlorpheniramine Tannate (Decreased prothrombin time response). Products include:
Atrohist Pediatric Suspension 1604
Atrohist Pediatric Suspension Dye-Free 1604
Rynatan 2781
Rynatuss 2782

Chlorpropamide (Increased prothrombin time response; accumulation of chlorpropamide). Products include:
Diabinese Tablets 2002

Chlorthalidone (Decreased or increased prothrombin time response). Products include:
Combipres Tablets 682
Tenoretic Tablets 2963
Thalitone 1293

Cholestyramine (Decreased or increased prothrombin time response). Products include:
Questran 774

Choline Magnesium Trisalicylate (Increased prothrombin time response). Products include:
Trilisate 2155

Cimetidine (Increased prothrombin time response). Products include:
Tagamet HB Tablets .... ⓓ 786
Tagamet Tablets 2694

Cimetidine Hydrochloride (Increased prothrombin time response). Products include:
Tagamet 2694

Ciprofloxacin (Increased prothrombin time response). Products include:
Cipro I.V. 587
Cipro I.V. Pharmacy Bulk Package .. 590

Ciprofloxacin Hydrochloride (Increased prothrombin time response). Products include:
Ciloxan Ophthalmic Solution 468
Cipro Tablets 584

Clarithromycin (Increased prothrombin time response). Products include:
Biaxin 406

Clemastine Fumarate (Decreased prothrombin time response). Products include:
Tavist Syrup 2426
Tavist Tablets 2427
Tavist-1 12 Hour Relief Tablets ... ⓓ 749
Tavist-D 12 Hour Relief Tablets ... ⓓ 750

Clofibrate (Increased prothrombin time response). Products include:
Atromid-S Capsules 2808

Codeine Phosphate (Increased prothrombin time response with prolonged use). Products include:
Brontex 2130
Dimetane-DC Cough Syrup 2232
Fioricet with Codeine Capsules 2387
Fiorinal with Codeine Capsules ... 2390
Nucofed 2225
Phenergan with Codeine 2883
Phenergan VC with Codeine 2888
Robitussin A-C Syrup 2248
Robitussin-DAC Syrup 2249
Ryna .... ⓓ 804
Soma Compound w/Codeine Tablets 2784
Tylenol with Codeine 1592

Cortisone Acetate (Decreased or increased prothrombin time response). Products include:
Cortone Acetate Sterile Suspension 1663
Cortone Acetate Tablets 1664

Cyclophosphamide (Increased or decreased prothrombin time response). Products include:
Cytoxan 700

Cyproheptadine Hydrochloride (Decreased prothrombin time response). Products include:
Periactin 1767

Danazol (Increased prothrombin time response). Products include:
Danocrine Capsules 2437

Desflurane (Increased prothrombin time response). Products include:
Suprane (desflurane, USP) 1865

Desogestrel (Decreased prothrombin time response). Products include:
Desogen Tablets 1867
Ortho-Cept 1907

Dexamethasone (Decreased or increased prothrombin time response). Products include:
AK-Trol Ointment & Suspension .... ⓓ 205
Decadron Elixir 1676
Decadron Tablets 1678
Decaspray Topical Aerosol 1689
Maxitrol Ophthalmic Ointment and Suspension .... ⓓ 222
TobraDex Ophthalmic Suspension and Ointment 469

Dexamethasone Acetate (Decreased or increased prothrombin time response). Products include:
Dalalone D.P. Injectable 1009
Decadron-LA Sterile Suspension 1687

Dexamethasone Sodium Phosphate (Decreased or increased prothrombin time response). Products include:
Decadron Phosphate Injection 1680
Decadron Phosphate Sterile Ophthalmic Ointment 1684
Decadron Phosphate Sterile Ophthalmic Solution 1685
Decadron Phosphate Topical Cream 1686
Decadron Phosphate with Xylocaine Injection, Sterile 1683
Dexacort Phosphate in Respihaler .. 1606
Dexacort Phosphate in Turbinaire ... 1607
NeoDecadron Sterile Ophthalmic Ointment 1755
NeoDecadron Sterile Ophthalmic Solution 1756
NeoDecadron Topical Cream 1757

Dexchlorpheniramine Maleate (Decreased prothrombin time response).
No products indexed under this heading.

Dextrans (Low Molecular Weight) (Increased prothrombin time response).
No products indexed under this heading.

Dextrothyroxine Sodium (Increased prothrombin time response).
No products indexed under this heading.

Dezocine (Increased prothrombin time response with prolonged use). Products include:
Dalgan Injection 529

Diazoxide (Increased prothrombin time response). Products include:
Hyperstat I.V. Injection 2504
Proglycem 575

Diclofenac Potassium (Increased prothrombin time response; caution should be observed when used concurrently). Products include:
Cataflam Tablets 833

Diclofenac Sodium (Increased prothrombin time response; caution should be observed when used concurrently). Products include:
Voltaren Ophthalmic Sterile Ophthalmic Solution .... ⓓ 264
Cataflam/Voltaren/Voltaren-XR ... 833

IMPORTANT NOTE: Always consult each drug listing in the patient's regimen for possible interactions.

Coumadin | Interactions Index | 214

Dicloxacillin Sodium (Decreased prothrombin time response).
No products indexed under this heading.

Diflunisal (Increased prothrombin time response). Products include:
Dolobid Tablets ... 1695

Diphenhydramine Citrate (Decreased prothrombin time response). Products include:
Excedrin P.M. Analgesic/Sleeping Aid Tablets, Caplets, Liquigels ... 735

Diphenhydramine Hydrochloride (Decreased prothrombin time response). Products include:
Actifed Allergy Daytime/Nighttime Caplets ... ▣ 808
Actifed Sinus Daytime/Nighttime Tablets and Caplets ... ▣ 809
Extra Strength Bayer PM Aspirin Plus Sleep Aid ... ▣ 617
Benadryl Allergy Chewables ... ▣ 811
Benadryl Allergy/Cold Tablets ... ▣ 811
Benadryl Allergy Decongestant Liquid Medication ... ▣ 812
Benadryl Allergy Decongestant Tablets ... ▣ 812
Benadryl Allergy Liquid Medication ... ▣ 813
Benadryl Allergy ... ▣ 811
Benadryl Allergy Sinus Headache Caplets ... ▣ 813
Benadryl Dye-Free Allergy Liquigel Softgels ... ▣ 813
Benadryl Dye-Free Allergy Liquid Medication ... ▣ 814
Benadryl Itch Relief Stick Extra Strength ... ▣ 814
Benadryl Cream ... ▣ 814
Benadryl Gel ... ▣ 815
Benadryl Spray ... ▣ 815
Benadryl Injection ... 1955
Contac Day & Night Cold/Flu Night Caplets ... ▣ 772
Contac Night Allergy/Sinus Caplets ... ▣ 771
Extra Strength Doan's P.M. ... ▣ 653
Excedrin P.M. Analgesic/Sleeping Aid Tablets, Caplets, Liquigels ... ▣ 643
Nytol QuickCaps Caplets ... ▣ 632
Sleepinal Night-time Sleep Aid Capsules and Softgels ... ▣ 798
TYLENOL Allergy Sinus NightTime, Maximum Strength Caplets ... 1571
TYLENOL Flu NightTime, Maximum Strength Gelcaps ... 1575
TYLENOL Flu NightTime, Maximum Strength Hot Medication Packets ... 1575
TYLENOL PM Pain Reliever/Sleep Aid, Extra Strength Gelcaps, Caplets, Geltabs ... 1576
TYLENOL Severe Allergy Medication Caplets ... 1571
Maximum Strength Unisom Sleepgels ... 1990
Unisom With Pain Relief-Nighttime Sleep Aid and Pain Reliever ... 1991

Diphenylpyraline Hydrochloride (Decreased prothrombin time response).
No products indexed under this heading.

Disulfiram (Increased prothrombin time response). Products include:
Antabuse Tablets ... 2802

Divalproex Sodium (Increased prothrombin time response). Products include:
Depakote Tablets ... 418

Doxycycline Calcium (Increased prothrombin time response). Products include:
Vibramycin Calcium Oral Suspension Syrup ... 2038

Doxycycline Hyclate (Increased prothrombin time response). Products include:
Doryx Capsules ... 1970
Vibramycin Hyclate Capsules ... 2038
Vibramycin Hyclate Intravenous ... 2040
Vibra-Tabs Film Coated Tablets ... 2038

Doxycycline Monohydrate (Increased prothrombin time response). Products include:
Monodox Capsules ... 1858
Vibramycin Monohydrate for Oral Suspension ... 2038

Enflurane (Increased prothrombin time response).
No products indexed under this heading.

Enoxacin (Increased prothrombin time response). Products include:
Penetrex Tablets ... 2196

Erythromycin (Increased prothrombin time response). Products include:
A/T/S 2% Acne Topical Gel ... 1244
A/T/S 2% Acne Topical Solution ... 1244
Benzamycin Topical Gel ... 919
E-Mycin Tablets ... 1388
Emgel 2% Topical Gel ... 1081
ERYC ... 1972
Erycette (erythromycin 2%) Topical Solution ... 1943
Ery-Tab Tablets ... 426
Erythromycin Base Filmtab ... 430
Erythromycin Delayed-Release Capsules, USP ... 431
Ilotycin Ophthalmic Ointment ... 928
PCE Dispertab Tablets ... 453
T-Stat 2.0% Topical Solution and Pads ... 2797
THERAMYCIN Z 2% Solution ... 1629

Erythromycin Estolate (Increased prothrombin time response). Products include:
Ilosone ... 927

Erythromycin Ethylsuccinate (Increased prothrombin time response). Products include:
E.E.S. ... 427
EryPed ... 425
Pediazole Suspension ... 2340

Erythromycin Gluceptate (Increased prothrombin time response). Products include:
Ilotycin Gluceptate, IV, Vials ... 929

Erythromycin Stearate (Increased prothrombin time response). Products include:
Erythrocin Stearate Filmtab ... 429

Ethacrynic Acid (Decreased or increased prothrombin time response). Products include:
Edecrin Tablets ... 1698

Ethchlorvynol (Decreased prothrombin time response). Products include:
Placidyl Capsules ... 456

Ethinyl Estradiol (Decreased prothrombin time response). Products include:
Brevicon ... 2563
Demulen ... 2580
Desogen Tablets ... 1867
Levlen/Tri-Levlen ... 646
Lo/Ovral Tablets ... 2852
Lo/Ovral-28 Tablets ... 2857
Modicon ... 1928
Nordette-21 Tablets ... 2863
Nordette-28 Tablets ... 2866
Norinyl ... 2563
Ortho-Cept ... 1907
Ortho-Cyclen/Ortho-Tri-Cyclen ... 1914
Ortho-Novum ... 1928
Ortho-Cyclen/Ortho Tri-Cyclen ... 1914
Ovcon ... 765
Ovral Tablets ... 2877
Ovral-28 Tablets ... 2878
Levlen/Tri-Levlen ... 646
Tri-Norinyl ... 2607
Triphasil-21 Tablets ... 2919
Triphasil-28 Tablets ... 2924

Ethynodiol Diacetate (Decreased prothrombin time response). Products include:
Demulen ... 2580

Etodolac (Increased prothrombin time response; caution should be observed when used concurrently). Products include:
Lodine Capsules and Tablets ... 2849

Fenoprofen Calcium (Increased prothrombin time response; caution should be observed when used concurrently). Products include:
Nalfon 200 Pulvules & Nalfon Tablets ... 933

Fentanyl (Increased prothrombin time response with prolonged use). Products include:
Duragesic Transdermal System ... 1336

Fentanyl Citrate (Increased prothrombin time response with prolonged use). Products include:
Sublimaze Injection ... 463

Fluconazole (Increased prothrombin time response). Products include:
Diflucan Tablets, Injection, and Oral Suspension ... 2003

Fludrocortisone Acetate (Decreased or increased prothrombin time response). Products include:
Florinef Acetate Tablets ... 506

Fluorouracil (Increased prothrombin time response). Products include:
Efudex ... 2280
Fluoroplex Topical Solution & Cream 1% ... 475
Fluorouracil Injection ... 2282

Fluoxymesterone (Increased prothrombin time response). Products include:
Halotestin Tablets ... 2095

Flurbiprofen (Increased prothrombin time response; caution should be observed when used concurrently).
No products indexed under this heading.

Fosphenytoin Sodium (Accumulation of phenytoin; decreased or increased prothrombin time response). Products include:
Cerebyx Injection ... 1956

Furazolidone (Increased prothrombin time response). Products include:
Furoxone ... 2221

Furosemide (Decreased or increased prothrombin time response). Products include:
Lasix Injection, Oral Solution and Tablets ... 1267

Glipizide (Increased prothrombin time response). Products include:
Glucotrol Tablets ... 2011
Glucotrol XL Extended Release Tablets ... 2012

Glucagon (Increased prothrombin time response). Products include:
Glucagon for Injection Vials and Emergency Kit ... 1485

Glutethimide (Decreased prothrombin time response).
No products indexed under this heading.

Glyburide (Increased prothrombin time response). Products include:
DiaBeta Tablets ... 1265
Glynase PresTab Tablets ... 2091
Micronase Tablets ... 2099

Griseofulvin (Decreased prothrombin time response). Products include:
Fulvicin P/G Tablets ... 2499
Fulvicin P/G 165 & 330 Tablets ... 2500
Grifulvin V (griseofulvin tablets) Microsize (griseofulvin oral suspension) Microsize ... 1944
Gris-PEG Tablets, 125 mg & 250 mg ... 476

Haloperidol (Decreased prothrombin time response). Products include:
Haldol Injection, Tablets and Concentrate ... 1585

Haloperidol Decanoate (Decreased prothrombin time response). Products include:
Haldol Decanoate ... 1587

Halothane (Increased prothrombin time response). Products include:
Fluothane ... 2830

Heparin Calcium (Concomitant administration prolongs one-stage prothrombin time response).
No products indexed under this heading.

Heparin Sodium (Concomitant administration prolongs one-stage prothrombin time response). Products include:
Heparin Lock Flush Solution ... 2831
Heparin Sodium Injection ... 2832
Heparin Sodium Vials ... 1486

Hepatotoxic Drugs, unspecified (Increased prothrombin time response).

Hydrochlorothiazide (Decreased or increased prothrombin time response). Products include:
Aldactazide Tablets ... 2556
Aldoril Tablets ... 1644
Apresazide Capsules ... 824
Capozide Tablets ... 744
Dyazide Capsules ... 2653
Esidrix Tablets ... 839
Esimil Tablets ... 840
HydroDIURIL Tablets ... 1716
Hydropres Tablets ... 1718
Hyzaar Tablets ... 1720
Inderide Tablets ... 2838
Inderide LA Long Acting Capsules ... 2840
Lopressor HCT Tablets ... 850
Lotensin HCT Tablets ... 855
Moduretic Tablets ... 1748
Oretic Tablets ... 450
Prinzide Tablets ... 1780
Ser-Ap-Es Tablets ... 867
Timolide Tablets ... 1791
Vaseretic Tablets ... 1810
Zestoretic Tablets ... 2968
Ziac ... 1459

Hydrocodone Bitartrate (Increased prothrombin time response with prolonged use). Products include:
Codiclear DH Syrup ... 808
Duratuss HD Elixir ... 2750
Histussin D Liquid ... 670
Hycodan Tablets and Syrup ... 946
Hycomine Compound Tablets ... 948
Hycomine ... 947
Hycotuss Expectorant Syrup ... 950
Hydrocet Capsules ... 787
Lorcet 10/650 Tablets ... 1016
Lortab ... 2751
Tussend ... 1830
Tussend Expectorant ... 1831
Vicodin Tablets ... 1404
Vicodin ES Tablets ... 1405
Vicodin HP Tablets ... 1403
Vicodin Tuss Expectorant ... 1406
Zydone Capsules ... 967

Hydrocodone Polistirex (Increased prothrombin time response with prolonged use). Products include:
Tussionex Pennkinetic Extended-Release Suspension ... 1624

Hydrocortisone (Decreased or increased prothrombin time response). Products include:
Anusol-HC Cream 2.5% ... 1953
Aquanil HC Lotion ... 1989
Maximum Strength Cortaid Spray ▣ 800
CORTENEMA ... 2713
Cortisporin Ointment ... 1074
Cortisporin Ophthalmic Ointment Sterile ... 1074
Cortisporin Ophthalmic Suspension Sterile ... 1075
Cortisporin Otic Solution Sterile ... 1076
Cortisporin Otic Suspension Sterile 1077
Cortizone-5 ... ▣ 795
Cortizone-10 ... ▣ 795
Hydrocortone Tablets ... 1715
Hytone ... 922
Hytone Ointment 2½% ... 923
Massengill Medicated Soft Cloth Towelettes ... 2628

(▣ Described in PDR For Nonprescription Drugs) (◉ Described in PDR For Ophthalmology)

Pediotic Suspension Sterile 1140
Preparation H Hydrocortisone 1% Cream 843
ProctoCream-HC 2.5% 2552
VōSoL HC Otic Solution 2786

Hydrocortisone Acetate (Decreased or increased prothrombin time response). Products include:
Analpram-HC Rectal Cream 1% and 2.5% 993
Anusol HC-1 Hydrocortisone Anti-Itch Ointment 810
Anusol-HC Suppositories 1954
Caldecort Anti-Itch Hydrocortisone Cream 651
Coly-Mycin S Otic w/Neomycin & Hydrocortisone 1965
Cortaid 800
Cortifoam 2540
Cortisporin Cream 1073
Epifoam 2543
Hydrocortone Acetate Sterile Suspension 1712
Mantadil Cream 1124
Nupercainal Hydrocortisone 1% Cream 661
Pramosone Cream, Lotion & Ointment 995
ProctoFoam-HC 2552
Terra-Cortril Ophthalmic Suspension 2033

Hydrocortisone Sodium Phosphate (Decreased or increased prothrombin time response). Products include:
Hydrocortone Phosphate Injection, Sterile 1713

Hydrocortisone Sodium Succinate (Decreased or increased prothrombin time response).
No products indexed under this heading.

Hydroflumethiazide (Decreased or increased prothrombin time response). Products include:
Diucardin Tablets 2824

Hydromorphone Hydrochloride (Increased prothrombin time response with prolonged use). Products include:
Dilaudid Ampules 1382
Dilaudid Cough Syrup 1383
Dilaudid-HP Injection 1384
Dilaudid-HP Lyophilized Powder 250 mg 1384
Dilaudid 1382
Dilaudid Oral Liquid 1386
Dilaudid 1382
Dilaudid Tablets - 8 mg 1386

Ibuprofen (Increased prothrombin time response; caution should be observed when used concurrently). Products include:
Advil Cold and Sinus Caplets and Tablets 837
Advil Ibuprofen Tablets, Caplets and Gel Caplets 836
Children's Motrin Ibuprofen Oral Suspension 1558
IBU Tablets 1389
Ibuprohm 713
Motrin IB Caplets, Tablets, and Gelcaps 802
Motrin Ibuprofen Suspension, Oral Drops, Chewable Tablets, Caplets 1563
Nuprin Ibuprofen/Analgesic Tablets & Caplets 645
Vicks DayQuil SINUS Pressure & PAIN Relief with IBUPROFEN 735

Ifosfamide (Increased prothrombin time response). Products include:
IFEX 706

Indapamide (Decreased or increased prothrombin time response).
No products indexed under this heading.

Indomethacin (Increased prothrombin time response; caution should be observed when used concurrently). Products include:
Indocin 1723

Indomethacin Sodium Trihydrate (Increased prothrombin time response; caution should be observed when used concurrently). Products include:
Indocin I.V. 1727

Influenza Virus Vaccine (Increased prothrombin time response). Products include:
Fluvirin (Influenza Virus Vaccine) 1608
Influenza Virus Vaccine, Trivalent, Types A and B (chromatograph- and filter-purified subviron antigen) FluShield, 1996-1997 Formula 2842

Isocarboxazid (Increased prothrombin time response).
No products indexed under this heading.

Isoflurane (Increased prothrombin time response).
No products indexed under this heading.

Itraconazole (Increased prothrombin time response). Products include:
Sporanox Capsules 1352

Kanamycin Sulfate (Increased prothrombin time response with oral aminoglycosides).
No products indexed under this heading.

Ketoprofen (Increased prothrombin time response; caution should be observed when used concurrently). Products include:
Actron Caplets and Tablets 608
Orudis Capsules 2874
Orudis KT 842
Oruvail Capsules 2874

Ketorolac Tromethamine (Increased prothrombin time response; caution should be observed when used concurrently). Products include:
Acular Sterile Ophthalmic Solution 470
Toradol 2319

Levamisole Hydrochloride (Increased prothrombin time response). Products include:
Ergamisol Tablets 1340

Levonorgestrel (Decreased prothrombin time response). Products include:
Levlen/Tri-Levlen 646
Nordette-21 Tablets 2863
Nordette-28 Tablets 2866
Norplant System 2868
Levlen/Tri-Levlen 646
Triphasil-21 Tablets 2919
Triphasil-28 Tablets 2924

Levorphanol Tartrate (Increased prothrombin response with prolonged use). Products include:
Levo-Dromoran 2297

Levothyroxine Sodium (Decreased or increased prothrombin time response). Products include:
Eltroxin Tablets 2214
Levothroid Tablets 1015
Levothyroxine Sodium, USP for Injection 546
Levoxyl Tablets 918
Synthroid 1410

Liothyronine Sodium (Decreased or increased prothrombin time response). Products include:
Cytomel Tablets 2647
Triostat Injection 2708

Liotrix (Decreased or increased prothrombin time response).
No products indexed under this heading.

Lomefloxacin Hydrochloride (Increased prothrombin time response). Products include:
Maxaquin Tablets 2593

Loratadine (Decreased prothrombin time response). Products include:
Claritin Tablets 2485
Claritin-D Tablets 2487

Lovastatin (Increased prothrombin time response). Products include:
Mevacor Tablets 1742

Magaldrate (Decreased prothrombin time response).
No products indexed under this heading.

Magnesium Hydroxide (Decreased prothrombin time response). Products include:
Aludrox Oral Suspension 850
Ascriptin 650
Di-Gel Antacid/Anti-Gas 762
Gelusil Antacid-Anti-gas Liquid 819
Gelusil Antacid-Anti-gas Tablets 819
Maalox Antacid/Anti-Gas Tablets 889
Maalox Antacid Liquid 888
Extra Strength Maalox Antacid/Anti-Gas Liquid and Tablets 888
Mylanta Fast-Acting 1359
Mylanta Gelcaps Antacid 678
Fast-Acting Mylanta Liquid Antacid 1359
Mylanta Tablets 677
Maximum-Strength Fast-Acting Mylanta Liquid Antacid 1359
Mylanta Double Strength Tablets 677
Phillips' Milk of Magnesia Liquid 627
Rolaids Antacid Tablets 807
Tempo Soft Antacid 799

Magnesium Oxide (Decreased prothrombin time response). Products include:
Beelith Tablets 632
Bufferin Analgesic Tablets 636
Arthritis Strength Bufferin Analgesic Caplets 637
Extra Strength Bufferin Analgesic Tablets 637
Caltrate PLUS 681
Cama Arthritis Pain Reliever 748
Mag-Ox 400 666
Uro-Mag 666

Magnesium Salicylate (Increased prothrombin time response). Products include:
Backache Caplets 635
Doan's Extra-Strength Analgesic 653
Extra Strength Doan's P.M. 653
Doan's Regular Strength Analgesic 654
Mobigesic Tablets 607

Meclofenamate Sodium (Increased prothrombin time response; caution should be observed when used concurrently).
No products indexed under this heading.

Mefenamic Acid (Increased prothrombin time response; caution should be observed when used concurrently). Products include:
Ponstel 1982

Meperidine Hydrochloride (Increased prothrombin time response with prolonged use). Products include:
Demerol 2438
Mepergan Injection 2859

Mephobarbital (Decreased prothrombin time response). Products include:
Mebaral Tablets 2452

Meprobamate (Decreased prothrombin time response). Products include:
Miltown Tablets 2780
PMB 200 and PMB 400 2890

Mestranol (Decreased prothrombin time response). Products include:
Norinyl 2563
Ortho-Novum 1928

Methadone Hydrochloride (Increased prothrombin time response with prolonged use). Products include:
Methadone Hydrochloride Oral Concentrate 2356
Methadone Hydrochloride Oral Solution & Tablets 2357

Methdilazine Hydrochloride (Decreased prothrombin time response).
No products indexed under this heading.

Methimazole (Increased or decreased prothrombin time response). Products include:
Tapazole Tablets 1361

Methoxyflurane (Increased prothrombin time response).
No products indexed under this heading.

Methyclothiazide (Decreased or increased prothrombin time response). Products include:
Enduron Tablets 424

Methyl Salicylate (Increased prothrombin time response with topical methyl salicylate ointment). Products include:
ArthriCare Triple Medicated Rub 667
BenGay External Analgesic Products 714
Listerine Antiseptic 820
Cool Mint Listerine 820
FreshBurst Listerine 820
Mentholatum Deep Heating Extra Strength Formula Rub 710
Thera-Gesic 1830

Methyldopa (Increased prothrombin time response). Products include:
Aldoclor Tablets 1638
Aldomet Oral 1640
Aldoril Tablets 1644

Methyldopate Hydrochloride (Increased prothrombin time response). Products include:
Aldomet Ester HCl Injection 1642

Methylphenidate Hydrochloride (Increased prothrombin time response). Products include:
Ritalin 866

Methylprednisolone Acetate (Decreased or increased prothrombin time response).
No products indexed under this heading.

Methylprednisolone Sodium Succinate (Decreased or increased prothrombin time response).
No products indexed under this heading.

Methyltestosterone (Increased prothrombin time response). Products include:
Android Capsules, 10 mg 1297
Estratest 2718
Testred Capsules, 10 mg 1308

Metolazone (Decreased or increased prothrombin time response). Products include:
Mykrox Tablets 1617
Zaroxolyn Tablets 1625

Metronidazole (Increased prothrombin time response). Products include:
Flagyl 375 Capsules 2587
Flagyl I.V. RTU 2373
Helidac Therapy 2135
MetroCream 1034
MetroGel 1034
MetroGel-Vaginal 917
Protostat Tablets 1939

Metronidazole Hydrochloride (Increased prothrombin time response). Products include:
Flagyl I.V. 2373

Miconazole (Increased prothrombin time response).
No products indexed under this heading.

IMPORTANT NOTE: Always consult each drug listing in the patient's regimen for possible interactions.

Coumadin **Interactions Index** **216**

Moricizine Hydrochloride (Decreased or increased prothrombin time response). Products include:
Ethmozine Tablets.......... 2217

Morphine Sulfate (Increased prothrombin time response with prolonged use). Products include:
Astramorph/PF Injection, USP (Preservative-Free).......... 526
Duramorph Injection.......... 983
Infumorph 200 and Infumorph 500 Sterile Solutions.......... 985
Kadian Capsules.......... 2948
MS Contin Tablets.......... 2149
MSIR.......... 2152
Oramorph SR (Morphine Sulfate Sustained Release Tablets).......... 2359
RMS Suppositories CII.......... 2766
Roxanol.......... 2365

Nabumetone (Increased prothrombin time response; caution should be observed when used concurrently). Products include:
Relafen Tablets.......... 2688

Nafcillin Sodium (Decreased prothrombin time response).
No products indexed under this heading.

Nalidixic Acid (Increased prothrombin time response). Products include:
NegGram.......... 2453

Naproxen (Increased prothrombin time response; caution should be observed when used concurrently). Products include:
Anaprox/Naprosyn.......... 2277

Naproxen Sodium (Increased prothrombin time response; caution should be observed when used concurrently). Products include:
Aleve.......... 2124
Anaprox/Naprosyn.......... 2277
Naprelan Tablets.......... 2861

Neomycin, oral (Increased prothrombin time response with oral aminoglycosides).

Norethindrone (Decreased prothrombin time response). Products include:
Brevicon.......... 2563
Micronor Tablets.......... 1903
Modicon.......... 1928
Norinyl.......... 2563
Nor-Q D Tablets.......... 2598
Ortho-Novum.......... 1928
Ovcon.......... 765
Tri-Norinyl.......... 2607

Norethynodrel (Decreased prothrombin time response).
No products indexed under this heading.

Norfloxacin (Increased prothrombin time response). Products include:
Chibroxin Sterile Ophthalmic Solution.......... 1657
Noroxin Tablets.......... 1758
Noroxin Tablets.......... 2222

Norgestimate (Decreased prothrombin time response). Products include:
Ortho-Cyclen/Ortho-Tri-Cyclen.......... 1914
Ortho-Cyclen/Ortho Tri-Cyclen.......... 1914

Norgestrel (Decreased prothrombin time response). Products include:
Lo/Ovral Tablets.......... 2852
Lo/Ovral-28 Tablets.......... 2857
Ovral Tablets.......... 2877
Ovral-28 Tablets.......... 2878
Ovrette Tablets.......... 2878

Ofloxacin (Increased prothrombin time response). Products include:
Floxin I.V.......... 1580
Floxin Tablets (200 mg, 300 mg, 400 mg).......... 1577
Ocuflox Ophthalmic Solution.......... 478
Ocuflox.......... ⊙ 242

Olsalazine Sodium (Increased prothrombin time response). Products include:
Dipentum Capsules.......... 2084

Opium Alkaloids (Increased prothrombin time response with prolonged use).
No products indexed under this heading.

Oxandrolone (Increased prothrombin time response). Products include:
Oxandrin.......... 783

Oxaprozin (Increased prothrombin time response; caution should be observed when used concurrently). Products include:
Daypro Caplets.......... 2578

Oxycodone Hydrochloride (Increased prothrombin time response with prolonged use). Products include:
OxyContin Tablets.......... 2163
OxyIR Capsules.......... 2167
Percocet Tablets.......... 955
Percodan Tablets.......... 955
Percodan-Demi Tablets.......... 956
Roxicodone Tablets, Oral Solution & Intensol (Oxycodone).......... 2366
Tylox Capsules.......... 1593

Oxymetholone (Increased prothrombin time response).
No products indexed under this heading.

Oxyphenbutazone (Increased prothrombin time response).

Paraldehyde (Decreased prothrombin time response).

Paromomycin Sulfate (Increased prothrombin time response with oral aminoglycosides).
No products indexed under this heading.

Paroxetine Hydrochloride (Increased prothrombin time response). Products include:
Paxil Tablets.......... 2681

Penicillin G Potassium (Increased prothrombin time response with intravenous penicillin G). Products include:
Pfizerpen for Injection.......... 2022

Penicillin G Sodium (Increased prothrombin time response with intravenous penicillin G).
No products indexed under this heading.

Pentobarbital Sodium (Decreased prothrombin time response). Products include:
Nembutal Sodium Capsules.......... 440
Nembutal Sodium Solution.......... 442
Nembutal Sodium Suppositories.......... 444

Pentoxifylline (Increased prothrombin time response). Products include:
Trental Tablets.......... 1291

Phenelzine Sulfate (Increased prothrombin time response). Products include:
Nardil.......... 1977

Phenobarbital (Decreased prothrombin time response; accumulation of phenobarbital). Products include:
Arco-Lase Plus Tablets.......... 513
Bellergal-S Tablets.......... 2375
Donnatal.......... 2234
Donnatal Extentabs.......... 2234
Donnatal Tablets.......... 2234
Phenobarbital Elixir and Tablets.......... 1523
Quadrinal Tablets.......... 1398

Phenylbutazone (Increased prothrombin time response; caution should be observed when used concurrently).
No products indexed under this heading.

Phenytoin (Accumulation of phenytoin; decreased or increased prothrombin time response). Products include:
Dilantin Infatabs.......... 1967
Dilantin-125 Suspension.......... 1969

Phenytoin Sodium (Accumulation of phenytoin; decreased or increased prothrombin time response). Products include:
Dilantin Kapseals.......... 1965

Piperacillin Sodium (Increased prothrombin time response). Products include:
Pipracil.......... 1435
Zosyn.......... 1463

Piroxicam (Increased prothrombin time response; caution should be observed when used concurrently). Products include:
Feldene Capsules.......... 2008

Polythiazide (Decreased or increased prothrombin time response). Products include:
Minizide Capsules.......... 2016

Prednisolone Acetate (Decreased or increased prothrombin time response). Products include:
AK-CIDE.......... ⊙ 203
AK-CIDE Ointment.......... ⊙ 203
Blephamide Liquifilm Sterile Ophthalmic Suspension.......... 472
Blephamide Ointment.......... ⊙ 234
Econopred & Econopred Plus Ophthalmic Suspensions.......... ⊙ 216
Poly-Pred Liquifilm.......... ⊙ 246
Pred Forte.......... ⊙ 247
Pred Mild.......... ⊙ 250
Pred-G Liquifilm Sterile Ophthalmic Suspension.......... ⊙ 248
Pred-G S.O.P. Sterile Ophthalmic Ointment.......... ⊙ 249

Prednisolone Sodium Phosphate (Decreased or increased prothrombin time response). Products include:
AK-PRED.......... ⊙ 204
Hydeltrasol Injection, Sterile.......... 1708
Pediapred Oral Solution.......... 1618

Prednisolone Tebutate (Decreased or increased prothrombin time response). Products include:
Hydeltra-T.B.A. Sterile Suspension 1710

Prednisone (Decreased or increased prothrombin time response).
No products indexed under this heading.

Primidone (Decreased prothrombin time response). Products include:
Mysoline.......... 2860

Promethazine Hydrochloride (Decreased prothrombin time response). Products include:
Mepergan Injection.......... 2859
Phenergan with Codeine.......... 2883
Phenergan with Dextromethorphan 2885
Phenergan Injection.......... 2880
Phenergan Suppositories.......... 2882
Phenergan Syrup.......... 2881
Phenergan Tablets.......... 2882
Phenergan VC.......... 2886
Phenergan VC with Codeine.......... 2888

Propafenone Hydrochloride (Increased prothrombin time response). Products include:
Rythmol Tablets–150mg, 225mg, 300mg.......... 1399

Propoxyphene Hydrochloride (Increased prothrombin time response with prolonged use). Products include:
Darvon.......... 1475
Wygesic Tablets.......... 2930

Propoxyphene Napsylate (Increased prothrombin time response with prolonged use). Products include:
Darvon-N/Darvocet-N.......... 1473

Propranolol Hydrochloride (Increased prothrombin time response). Products include:
Inderal.......... 2834
Inderal LA Long Acting Capsules.......... 2836
Inderide Tablets.......... 2838
Inderide LA Long Acting Capsules.......... 2840

Propylthiouracil (Increased prothrombin time response).
No products indexed under this heading.

Pyrazolones (Increased prothrombin time response).

Pyrilamine Maleate (Decreased prothrombin time response). Products include:
4-Way Fast Acting Nasal Spray (regular & mentholated).......... ▣ 644
Maximum Strength Multi-Symptom Formula Midol.......... ▣ 621
PMS Multi-Symptom Formula Midol.......... ▣ 622

Pyrilamine Tannate (Decreased prothrombin time response). Products include:
Atrohist Pediatric Suspension.......... 1604
Atrohist Pediatric Suspension Dye-Free.......... 1604
Rynatan.......... 2781

Quinidine Gluconate (Increased prothrombin time response). Products include:
Quinaglute Dura-Tabs Tablets.......... 644

Quinidine Polygalacturonate (Increased prothrombin time response). Products include:
Cardioquin Tablets.......... 2146

Quinidine Sulfate (Increased prothrombin time response). Products include:
Quinidex Extentabs.......... 2240

Quinine Sulfate (Increased prothrombin time response).
No products indexed under this heading.

Ranitidine Hydrochloride (Decreased or increased prothrombin time response). Products include:
Zantac.......... 1182
Zantac Injection.......... 1180
Zantac Syrup.......... 1182

Rifampin (Decreased prothrombin time response). Products include:
Rifadin.......... 1276
Rifamate Capsules.......... 1278
Rifater.......... 1280
Rimactane Capsules.......... 865

Salsalate (Increased prothrombin time response). Products include:
Disalcid.......... 1549
Mono-Gesic Tablets.......... 810
Salflex Tablets.......... 791

Secobarbital Sodium (Decreased prothrombin time response). Products include:
Seconal Sodium Pulvules.......... 1529

Selegiline Hydrochloride (Increased prothrombin time response). Products include:
Eldepryl Capsules.......... 2729

Sertraline Hydrochloride (Increased prothrombin time response). Products include:
Zoloft Tablets.......... 2051

Simvastatin (Increased prothrombin time response). Products include:
Zocor Tablets.......... 1821

Sodium Bicarbonate (Decreased prothrombin time response). Products include:
Alka-Seltzer Cherry Effervescent Antacid and Pain Reliever.......... ▣ 609
Alka-Seltzer Extra Strength Effervescent Antacid and Pain Reliever.......... ▣ 609
Alka-Seltzer Gold Effervescent Antacid.......... ▣ 611

(▣ Described in PDR For Nonprescription Drugs) (⊙ Described in PDR For Ophthalmology)

Alka-Seltzer Lemon Lime Effervescent Antacid and Pain Reliever 609
Alka-Seltzer Original Effervescent Antacid and Pain Reliever 609
Arm & Hammer Pure Baking Soda 648
Colyte and Colyte-flavored 2540
GoLYTELY 694
Massengill Disposable Douches 780
Massengill Liquid Concentrate 780
NuLYTELY 694
Cherry Flavor NuLYTELY 694

Spironolactone (Decreased or increased prothrombin time response). Products include:
Aldactazide Tablets 2556
Aldactone Tablets 2558

Stanozolol (Increased prothrombin time response). Products include:
Winstrol Tablets 2468

Streptokinase (Concurrent use is not recommended and may be hazardous; increased prothrombin time response). Products include:
Streptase for Infusion 557

Sucralfate (Decreased prothrombin time response). Products include:
Carafate Suspension 1250
Carafate Tablets 1249

Sufentanil Citrate (Increased prothrombin time response with prolonged use). Products include:
Sufenta Injection 1355

Sulfacytine (Increased prothrombin time response).

Sulfamethizole (Increased prothrombin time response). Products include:
Urobiotic-250 Capsules 2038

Sulfamethoxazole (Increased prothrombin time response). Products include:
Bactrim DS Tablets 2257
Bactrim I.V. Infusion 2255
Bactrim 2257
Gantanol Tablets 2285
Septra 1146
Septra I.V. Infusion 1142
Septra I.V. Infusion ADD-Vantage Vials 1144
Septra 1146

Sulfasalazine (Increased prothrombin time response). Products include:
Azulfidine 2059

Sulfinpyrazone (Increased prothrombin time response). Products include:
Anturane 823

Sulfisoxazole (Increased prothrombin time response). Products include:
Gantrisin Tablets 2286

Sulfisoxazole Diolamine (Increased prothrombin time response).
No products indexed under this heading.

Sulindac (Increased prothrombin time response; caution should be observed when used concurrently). Products include:
Clinoril Tablets 1658

Tamoxifen Citrate (Increased prothrombin time response). Products include:
Nolvadex Tablets 2957

Terfenadine (Decreased prothrombin time response). Products include:
Seldane Tablets 1284
Seldane-D Extended-Release Tablets 1286

Tetracycline Hydrochloride (Increased prothrombin time response). Products include:
Achromycin V Capsules 1417
Helidac Therapy 2135

Thiamylal Sodium (Decreased prothrombin time response).
No products indexed under this heading.

Thyroglobulin (Decreased or increased prothrombin time response).
No products indexed under this heading.

Thyroid (Decreased or increased prothrombin time response).
No products indexed under this heading.

Thyroxine (Decreased or increased prothrombin time response).
No products indexed under this heading.

Thyroxine Sodium (Decreased or increased prothrombin time response).
No products indexed under this heading.

Ticarcillin Disodium (Increased prothrombin time response). Products include:
Ticar for Injection 2704
Timentin for Injection 2706

Ticlopidine Hydrochloride (Concomitant administration may be associated with cholestatic hepatitis; increased prothrombin time). Products include:
Ticlid Tablets 2317

Tolazamide (Increased prothrombin time response).
No products indexed under this heading.

Tolbutamide (Increased prothrombin time response; accumulation of tolbutamide).
No products indexed under this heading.

Tolmetin Sodium (Increased prothrombin time response; caution should be observed when used concurrently). Products include:
Tolectin (200, 400 and 600 mg) .. 1591

Torsemide (Decreased or increased prothrombin time response). Products include:
Demadex Tablets and Injection 691

Tranylcypromine Sulfate (Increased prothrombin time response). Products include:
Parnate Tablets 2679

Trazodone Hydrochloride (Decreased prothrombin time response). Products include:
Desyrel and Desyrel Dividose 504

Triamcinolone (Decreased or increased prothrombin time response).
No products indexed under this heading.

Triamcinolone Acetonide (Decreased or increased prothrombin time response). Products include:
Azmacort Oral Inhaler 2175
Nasacort AQ Nasal Spray 2191
Nasacort Nasal Inhaler 2189

Triamcinolone Diacetate (Decreased or increased prothrombin time response).
No products indexed under this heading.

Triamcinolone Hexacetonide (Decreased or increased prothrombin time response).
No products indexed under this heading.

Triamterene (Decreased or increased prothrombin time response). Products include:
Dyazide Capsules 2653
Dyrenium Capsules 2655

Trimeprazine Tartrate (Decreased prothrombin time response).
No products indexed under this heading.

Trimethoprim (Increased prothrombin time response). Products include:
Bactrim DS Tablets 2257
Bactrim I.V. Infusion 2255
Bactrim 2257
Proloprim Tablets 1141
Septra 1146
Septra I.V. Infusion 1142
Septra I.V. Infusion ADD-Vantage Vials 1144
Septra 1146
Trimpex Tablets 2323

Tripelennamine Hydrochloride (Decreased prothrombin time response). Products include:
PBZ Tablets 863
PBZ-SR Tablets 862

Triprolidine Hydrochloride (Decreased prothrombin time response). Products include:
Actifed Cold & Allergy Tablets 807
Actifed Cold & Sinus Caplets and Tablets 808

Urokinase (Concurrent use is not recommended and may be hazardous). Products include:
Abbokinase 403
Abbokinase Open-Cath 405

Valproic Acid (Increased prothrombin time response). Products include:
Depakene 416

Vitamin C (Decreased prothrombin time response (with high dose)). Products include:
ACES Antioxidant Soft Gels 647
Chromagen Capsules 2470
Chromagen FA 2471
Chromagen Forte 2471
Dexatrim Maximum Strength Plus Vitamin C/Caffeine-Free Caplets 795
Ester-C Mineral Ascorbates Powder 673
Fero-Folic-500 Filmtab 433
Fero-Grad-500 Filmtab 434
Halls Vitamin C Drops 807
Irospan 1000
Materna Tablets 1427
Niferex w/Vitamin C Tablets 811
One-A-Day Antioxidant Plus 625
Protegra Antioxidant Vitamin & Mineral Supplement 685
Sunkist Children's Chewable Multivitamins - Plus Extra C 665
Sunkist Vitamin C 666
Trinsicon Capsules 2759
Venolax 686
Vitron-C Tablets 667

Vitamin E (Increased prothrombin time response). Products include:
ACES Antioxidant Soft Gels 647
Breath + Plus 603
Cefol Filmtab 415
Materna Tablets 1427
Megadose 513
Nutr-E-Sol 461
One-A-Day Antioxidant Plus 625
Protegra Antioxidant Vitamin & Mineral Supplement 685
StePHan Essential 834
StePHan Feminine 834
Stresstabs 685
Unique E Vitamin E Capsules 1236

Food Interactions

Alcohol (Decreased or increased prothrombin time response).

Diet high in vitamin K (Decreased prothrombin time).

Vegetables, green leafy (Large amounts of green leafy vegetables may affect Coumadin therapy).

COVERA-HS TABLETS

(Verapamil Hydrochloride) 2573

May interact with antihypertensives, ACE inhibitors, vasodilators, diuretics, cardiac glycosides, beta blockers, lithium preparations, xanthine bronchodilators, inhalant anesthetics, nondepolarizing neuromuscular blocking agents, and certain other agents. Compounds in these categories include:

Acebutolol Hydrochloride (Concomitant therapy may result in additive negative effects on heart rate, atrioventricular conduction and/or cardiac contractility; excessive bradycardia and AV block, including complete heart block). Products include:
Sectral Capsules 2914

Amiloride Hydrochloride (Possible additive effect on lowering of blood pressure). Products include:
Midamor Tablets 1746
Moduretic Tablets 1748

Aminophylline (Verapamil may inhibit the clearance and increase plasma levels of theophylline).
No products indexed under this heading.

Amlodipine Besylate (Possible additive effect on lowering of blood pressure). Products include:
Lotrel Capsules 858
Norvasc Tablets 2020

Atenolol (Concomitant therapy may result in additive negative effects on heart rate, atrioventricular conduction and/or cardiac contractility; excessive bradycardia and AV block, including complete heart block; a variable effect on atenolol clearance has been observed with concomitant use). Products include:
Tenoretic Tablets 2963
Tenormin Tablets and I.V. Injection 2965

Atracurium Besylate (Verapamil may potentiate the activity of neuromuscular blocking agents). Products include:
Tracrium Injection 1155

Benazepril Hydrochloride (Possible additive effect on lowering of blood pressure). Products include:
Lotensin Tablets 852
Lotensin HCT Tablets 855
Lotrel Capsules 858

Bendroflumethiazide (Possible additive effect on lowering of blood pressure).
No products indexed under this heading.

Betaxolol Hydrochloride (Concomitant therapy may result in additive negative effects on heart rate, atrioventricular conduction and/or cardiac contractility; excessive bradycardia and AV block, including complete heart block). Products include:
Betoptic Ophthalmic Solution 465
Betoptic S Ophthalmic Suspension 467
Kerlone Tablets 2588

Bisoprolol Fumarate (Concomitant therapy may result in additive negative effects on heart rate, atrioventricular conduction and/or cardiac contractility; excessive bradycardia and AV block, including complete heart block). Products include:
Zebeta Tablets 1457
Ziac 1459

Bumetanide (Possible additive effect on lowering of blood pressure). Products include:
Bumex 2260

Captopril (Possible additive effect on lowering of blood pressure). Products include:
Capoten Tablets 740
Capozide Tablets 744

IMPORTANT NOTE: Always consult each drug listing in the patient's regimen for possible interactions.

Covera-HS — Interactions Index

Carbamazepine (Co-administration may increase carbamazepine concentrations and this may produce side effects such as diplopia, headache, ataxia, or dizziness). Products include:
- Atretol Tablets 569
- Tegretol/Tegretol-XR 870

Carteolol Hydrochloride (Concomitant therapy may result in additive negative effects on heart rate, atrioventricular conduction and/or cardiac contractility; excessive bradycardia and AV block, including complete heart block). Products include:
- Cartrol Tablets 413
- Ocupress Ophthalmic Solution, 1% Sterile .... ◉ 297

Chlorothiazide (Possible additive effect on lowering of blood pressure). Products include:
- Aldoclor Tablets 1638
- Diupres Tablets 1691
- Diuril Oral 1694

Chlorothiazide Sodium (Possible additive effect on lowering of blood pressure). Products include:
- Diuril Sodium Intravenous 1693

Chlorthalidone (Possible additive effect on lowering of blood pressure). Products include:
- Combipres Tablets 682
- Tenoretic Tablets 2963
- Thalitone 1293

Cimetidine (Variable results on verapamil clearance). Products include:
- Tagamet HB Tablets .... ▣ 786
- Tagamet Tablets 2694

Cimetidine Hydrochloride (Variable results on verapamil clearance). Products include:
- Tagamet 2694

Cisatracurium Besylate (Verapamil may potentiate the activity of neuromuscular blocking agents). Products include:
- Nimbex Injection 1131

Clonidine (Possible additive effect on lowering of blood pressure). Products include:
- Catapres-TTS 680

Clonidine Hydrochloride (Possible additive effect on lowering of blood pressure). Products include:
- Catapres Tablets 679
- Combipres Tablets 682

Cyclosporine (Increased serum levels of cyclosporine). Products include:
- Neoral 2405
- Sandimmune 2416

Deserpidine (Possible additive effect on lowering of blood pressure).
No products indexed under this heading.

Desflurane (Potential for excessive cardiovascular depression). Products include:
- Suprane (desflurane, USP) 1865

Deslanoside (Chronic verapamil treatment can increase serum digoxin levels by 50% to 75% and this can result in digitalis toxicity).
No products indexed under this heading.

Diazoxide (Possible additive effect on lowering of blood pressure). Products include:
- Hyperstat I.V. Injection 2504
- Proglycem 575

Digitoxin (Chronic verapamil treatment can increase serum digitoxin levels by 50% to 75% and this can result in digitalis toxicity). Products include:
- Crystodigin Tablets 1472

Digoxin (Chronic verapamil treatment can increase serum digoxin levels by 50% to 75% and this can result in digitalis toxicity). Products include:
- Lanoxicaps 1110
- Lanoxin Elixir Pediatric 1113
- Lanoxin Injection 1116
- Lanoxin Injection Pediatric 1119
- Lanoxin Tablets 1121

Diltiazem Hydrochloride (Possible additive effect on lowering of blood pressure). Products include:
- Cardizem CD Capsules 1251
- Cardizem SR Capsules 1255
- Cardizem Injectable 1253
- Cardizem Tablets 1257
- Dilacor XR Extended-release Capsules 2183
- Tiazac Capsules 1019

Disopyramide Phosphate (Concurrent use within 48 hours before or 24 hours after verapamil administration is not recommended). Products include:
- Norpace 2596

Doxazosin Mesylate (Possible additive effect on lowering of blood pressure). Products include:
- Cardura Tablets 1993

Dyphylline (Verapamil may inhibit the clearance and increase plasma levels of theophylline). Products include:
- Lufyllin & Lufyllin-400 Tablets .. 2778
- Lufyllin-GG Elixir & Tablets 2779

Enalapril Maleate (Possible additive effect on lowering of blood pressure). Products include:
- Vaseretic Tablets 1810
- Vasotec Tablets 1816

Enalaprilat (Possible additive effect on lowering of blood pressure). Products include:
- Vasotec I.V. 1814

Enflurane (Potential for excessive cardiovascular depression).
No products indexed under this heading.

Epoprostenol Sodium (Possible additive effect on lowering of blood pressure). Products include:
- Flolan for Injection 1085

Esmolol Hydrochloride (Concomitant therapy may result in additive negative effects on heart rate, atrioventricular conduction and/or cardiac contractility; excessive bradycardia and AV block, including complete heart block). Products include:
- Brevibloc (esmolol HCl) Injection 1860

Ethacrynic Acid (Possible additive effect on lowering of blood pressure). Products include:
- Edecrin Tablets 1698

Felodipine (Possible additive effect on lowering of blood pressure). Products include:
- Plendil Extended-Release Tablets 514

Flecainide Acetate (Potential for additive effects on myocardial contractility, AV conduction, and repolarization). Products include:
- Tambocor Tablets 1555

Fosinopril Sodium (Possible additive effect on lowering of blood pressure). Products include:
- Monopril Tablets 762

Furosemide (Possible additive effect on lowering of blood pressure). Products include:
- Lasix Injection, Oral Solution and Tablets 1267

Guanabenz Acetate (Possible additive effect on lowering of blood pressure).
No products indexed under this heading.

Guanethidine Monosulfate (Possible additive effect on lowering of blood pressure). Products include:
- Esimil Tablets 840
- Ismelin Tablets 845

Halothane (Potential for excessive cardiovascular depression). Products include:
- Fluothane 2830

Hydralazine Hydrochloride (Possible additive effect on lowering of blood pressure). Products include:
- Apresazide Capsules 824
- Apresoline Hydrochloride Tablets .. 826
- Hydralazine Hydrochloride Injection USP 2712
- Ser-Ap-Es Tablets 867

Hydrochlorothiazide (Possible additive effect on lowering of blood pressure). Products include:
- Aldactazide Tablets 2556
- Aldoril Tablets 1644
- Apresazide Capsules 824
- Capozide Tablets 744
- Dyazide Capsules 2653
- Esidrix Tablets 839
- Esimil Tablets 840
- HydroDIURIL Tablets 1716
- Hydropres Tablets 1718
- Hyzaar Tablets 1720
- Inderide Tablets 2838
- Inderide LA Long Acting Capsules ... 2840
- Lopressor HCT Tablets 850
- Lotensin HCT Tablets 855
- Moduretic Tablets 1748
- Oretic Tablets 450
- Prinzide Tablets 1780
- Ser-Ap-Es Tablets 867
- Timolide Tablets 1791
- Vaseretic Tablets 1810
- Zestoretic Tablets 2968
- Ziac 1459

Hydroflumethiazide (Possible additive effect on lowering of blood pressure). Products include:
- Diucardin Tablets 2824

Indapamide (Possible additive effect on lowering of blood pressure).
No products indexed under this heading.

Isoflurane (Potential for excessive cardiovascular depression).
No products indexed under this heading.

Isradipine (Possible additive effect on lowering of blood pressure). Products include:
- DynaCirc Capsules 2381
- DynaCirc CR Tablets 2383

Labetalol Hydrochloride (Concomitant therapy may result in additive negative effects on heart rate, atrioventricular conduction and/or cardiac contractility; excessive bradycardia and AV block, including complete heart block). Products include:
- Normodyne Injection 2519
- Normodyne Tablets 2522
- Trandate 1158

Levobunolol Hydrochloride (Concomitant therapy may result in additive negative effects on heart rate, atrioventricular conduction and/or cardiac contractility; excessive bradycardia and AV block, including complete heart block). Products include:
- Betagan .... ◉ 230

Lisinopril (Possible additive effect on lowering of blood pressure). Products include:
- Prinivil Tablets 1776
- Prinzide Tablets 1780
- Zestoretic Tablets 2968
- Zestril Tablets 2972

Lithium Carbonate (Increased sensitivity to the effects of lithium (neurotoxicity); the addition of verapamil also results in the lowering of lithium levels in patients receiving chronic stable oral lithium). Products include:
- Eskalith 2658
- Lithium Carbonate Capsules & Tablets 2352
- Lithonate/Lithotabs/Lithobid 2721

Lithium Citrate (Increased sensitivity to the effects of lithium (neurotoxicity); the addition of verapamil also results in the lowering of lithium levels in patients receiving chronic stable oral lithium).
No products indexed under this heading.

Losartan Potassium (Possible additive effect on lowering of blood pressure). Products include:
- Cozaar Tablets 1668
- Hyzaar Tablets 1720

Mecamylamine Hydrochloride (Possible additive effect on lowering of blood pressure). Products include:
- Inversine Tablets 1729

Methoxyflurane (Potential for excessive cardiovascular depression).
No products indexed under this heading.

Methyclothiazide (Possible additive effect on lowering of blood pressure). Products include:
- Enduron Tablets 424

Methyldopa (Possible additive effect on lowering of blood pressure). Products include:
- Aldoclor Tablets 1638
- Aldomet Oral 1640
- Aldoril Tablets 1644

Methyldopate Hydrochloride (Possible additive effect on lowering of blood pressure). Products include:
- Aldomet Ester HCl Injection ... 1642

Metipranolol Hydrochloride (Concomitant therapy may result in additive negative effects on heart rate, atrioventricular conduction and/or cardiac contractility; excessive bradycardia and AV block, including complete heart block). Products include:
- OptiPranolol (Metipranolol 0.3%) Sterile Ophthalmic Solution ..... ◉ 256

Metocurine Iodide (Verapamil may potentiate the activity of neuromuscular blocking agents). Products include:
- Metubine Iodide Vials 932

Metolazone (Possible additive effect on lowering of blood pressure). Products include:
- Mykrox Tablets 1617
- Zaroxolyn Tablets 1625

Metoprolol Succinate (Concomitant therapy may result in additive negative effects on heart rate, atrioventricular conduction and/or cardiac contractility; excessive bradycardia and AV block, including complete heart block; a decrease in metoprolol clearance has been observed with concomitant use). Products include:
- Toprol-XL Tablets 560

(▣ Described in PDR For Nonprescription Drugs) (◉ Described in PDR For Ophthalmology)

Metoprolol Tartrate (Concomitant therapy may result in additive negative effects on heart rate, atrioventricular conduction and/or cardiac contractility; excessive bradycardia and AV block, including complete heart block; a decrease in metoprolol clearance has been observed with concomitant use). Products include:
Lopressor 848
Lopressor HCT Tablets 850

Metyrosine (Possible additive effect on lowering of blood pressure). Products include:
Demser Capsules 1690

Minoxidil (Possible additive effect on lowering of blood pressure).
No products indexed under this heading.

Mivacurium Chloride (Verapamil may potentiate the activity of neuromuscular blocking agents). Products include:
Mivacron 1125

Moexipril Hydrochloride (Possible additive effect on lowering of blood pressure). Products include:
Univasc Tablets 2553

Nadolol (Concomitant therapy may result in additive negative effects on heart rate, atrioventricular conduction and/or cardiac contractility; excessive bradycardia and AV block, including complete heart block).
No products indexed under this heading.

Nicardipine Hydrochloride (Possible additive effect on lowering of blood pressure). Products include:
Cardene Capsules 2261
Cardene I.V. 2815
Cardene SR Capsules 2264

Nifedipine (Possible additive effect on lowering of blood pressure). Products include:
Adalat Capsules (10 mg and 20 mg) 580
Adalat CC 582
Procardia Capsules 2024
Procardia XL Extended Release Tablets 2026

Nisoldipine (Possible additive effect on lowering of blood pressure). Products include:
Sular Tablets 2961

Nitroglycerin (Possible additive effect on lowering of blood pressure). Products include:
Deponit NTG Transdermal Delivery System 2541
Nitro-Bid IV 1270
Nitro-Bid Ointment 1272
Nitro-Dur (nitroglycerin) Transdermal Infusion System 1365
Nitrolingual Spray 2193
Nitrostat Tablets 1981
Transderm-Nitro Transdermal Therapeutic System 878

Pancuronium Bromide (Verapamil may potentiate the activity of neuromuscular blocking agents).
No products indexed under this heading.

Penbutolol Sulfate (Concomitant therapy may result in additive negative effects on heart rate, atrioventricular conduction and/or cardiac contractility; excessive bradycardia and AV block, including complete heart block). Products include:
Levatol Tablets 2547

Phenobarbital (May increase verapamil clearance). Products include:
Arco-Lase Plus Tablets 513

Bellergal-S Tablets 2375
Donnatal 2234
Donnatal Extentabs 2234
Donnatal Tablets 2234
Phenobarbital Elixir and Tablets 1523
Quadrinal Tablets 1398

Phenoxybenzamine Hydrochloride (Possible additive effect on lowering of blood pressure). Products include:
Dibenzyline Capsules 2650

Phentolamine Mesylate (Possible additive effect on lowering of blood pressure). Products include:
Regitine Vials 864

Pindolol (Concomitant therapy may result in additive negative effects on heart rate, atrioventricular conduction and/or cardiac contractility; excessive bradycardia and AV block, including complete heart block). Products include:
Visken Tablets 2428

Polythiazide (Possible additive effect on lowering of blood pressure). Products include:
Minizide Capsules 2016

Prazosin Hydrochloride (Possible additive effect on lowering of blood pressure). Products include:
Minipress Capsules 2015
Minizide Capsules 2016

Propranolol Hydrochloride (Concomitant therapy may result in additive negative effects on heart rate, atrioventricular conduction and/or cardiac contractility; excessive bradycardia and AV block, including complete heart block; a decrease in propranolol clearance has been observed with concomitant use). Products include:
Inderal 2834
Inderal LA Long Acting Capsules ... 2836
Inderide Tablets 2838
Inderide LA Long Acting Capsules .. 2840

Quinapril Hydrochloride (Possible additive effect on lowering of blood pressure). Products include:
Accupril Tablets 1950

Quinidine Gluconate (Concomitant use may result in significant hypotension; verapamil significantly counteracts the effects of quinidine on AV conduction; potential for increased quinidine levels with co-administration). Products include:
Quinaglute Dura-Tabs Tablets 644

Quinidine Polygalacturonate (Concomitant use may result in significant hypotension; verapamil significantly counteracts the effects of quinidine on AV conduction; potential for increased quinidine levels with co-administration). Products include:
Cardioquin Tablets 2146

Quinidine Sulfate (Concomitant use may result in significant hypotension; verapamil significantly counteracts the effects of quinidine on AV conduction; potential for increased quinidine levels with co-administration). Products include:
Quinidex Extentabs 2240

Ramipril (Possible additive effect on lowering of blood pressure). Products include:
Altace Capsules 1238

Rauwolfia Serpentina (Possible additive effect on lowering of blood pressure).
No products indexed under this heading.

Rescinnamine (Possible additive effect on lowering of blood pressure).
No products indexed under this heading.

Reserpine (Possible additive effect on lowering of blood pressure). Products include:
Diupres Tablets 1691
Hydropres Tablets 1718
Ser-Ap-Es Tablets 867

Rifampin (Therapy with rifampin may markedly reduce oral verapamil bioavailability). Products include:
Rifadin 1276
Rifamate Capsules 1278
Rifater 1280
Rimactane Capsules 865

Rocuronium Bromide (Verapamil may potentiate the activity of neuromuscular blocking agents). Products include:
Zemuron Injection 1885

Sodium Nitroprusside (Possible additive effect on lowering of blood pressure).
No products indexed under this heading.

Sotalol Hydrochloride (Concomitant therapy may result in additive negative effects on heart rate, atrioventricular conduction and/or cardiac contractility; excessive bradycardia and AV block, including complete heart block). Products include:
Betapace Tablets 637

Spirapril Hydrochloride (Possible additive effect on lowering of blood pressure).
No products indexed under this heading.

Spironolactone (Possible additive effect on lowering of blood pressure). Products include:
Aldactazide Tablets 2556
Aldactone Tablets 2558

Terazosin Hydrochloride (Possible additive effect on lowering of blood pressure). Products include:
Hytrin Capsules 434

Theophylline (Verapamil may inhibit the clearance and increase plasma levels of theophylline). Products include:
Marax Tablets & DF Syrup 2015
Quibron 2227

Theophylline Anhydrous (Verapamil may inhibit the clearance and increase plasma levels of theophylline). Products include:
Aerolate 1003
Primatene Tablets 844
Respbid Tablets 687
Slo-bid Gyrocaps 2201
Theo-24 Extended Release Capsules 2753
Theo-Dur Extended-Release Tablets 1367
Theo-X Extended-Release Tablets .. 793
Uni-Dur Extended-Release Tablets .. 1374
Uniphyl 400 mg and 600 mg Tablets 2157

Theophylline Calcium Salicylate (Verapamil may inhibit the clearance and increase plasma levels of theophylline). Products include:
Quadrinal Tablets 1398

Theophylline Sodium Glycinate (Verapamil may inhibit the clearance and increase plasma levels of theophylline).
No products indexed under this heading.

Timolol Hemihydrate (Concomitant therapy may result in additive negative effects on heart rate, atrioventricular conduction and/or cardiac contractility; excessive bradycardia and AV block, including complete heart block; one case of asymptomatic bradycardia with a wandering atrial pacemaker has been observed with timolol eye drops and oral verapamil). Products include:
Betimol 0.25%, 0.5% 259

Timolol Maleate (Concomitant therapy may result in additive negative effects on heart rate, atrioventricular conduction and/or cardiac contractility; excessive bradycardia and AV block, including complete heart block; one case of asymptomatic bradycardia with a wandering atrial pacemaker has been observed with timolol eye drops and oral verapamil). Products include:
Blocadren Tablets 1654
Timolide Tablets 1791
Timoptic in Ocudose 1796
Timoptic Sterile Ophthalmic Solution 1794
Timoptic-XE 1798

Torsemide (Possible additive effect on lowering of blood pressure). Products include:
Demadex Tablets and Injection 691

Trandolapril (Possible additive effect on lowering of blood pressure). Products include:
Mavik Tablets 1407

Triamterene (Possible additive effect on lowering of blood pressure). Products include:
Dyazide Capsules 2653
Dyrenium Capsules 2655

Trimethaphan Camsylate (Possible additive effect on lowering of blood pressure).
No products indexed under this heading.

Vecuronium Bromide (Verapamil may potentiate the activity of neuromuscular blocking agents). Products include:
Norcuron for Injection 1875

Food Interactions

Alcohol (Verapamil may increase blood alcohol concentrations and prolong its effect).

COVERLET EYE OCCLUSOR
(Eye Occlusor) 257
None cited in PDR database.

COZAAR TABLETS
(Losartan Potassium) 1668
May interact with:

Cimetidine (Co-administration leads to an increase of about 18% in AUC of losartan with no effect on pharmacokinetics of its active metabolites). Products include:
Tagamet HB Tablets 786
Tagamet Tablets 2694

Cimetidine Hydrochloride (Co-administration leads to an increase of about 18% in AUC of losartan with no effect on pharmacokinetics of its active metabolites). Products include:
Tagamet 2694

IMPORTANT NOTE: Always consult each drug listing in the patient's regimen for possible interactions.

Gestodene (*In Vitro* studies show significant inhibition of the formation of the active metabolite by inhibitors of P450 3A4 such as gestodene; pharmacodynamic consequences of concomitant use is undefined).
No products indexed under this heading.

Ketoconazole (*In Vitro* studies show significant inhibition of the formation of the active metabolite by inhibitors of P450 3A4 such as ketoconazole or complete inhibition by the combination of ketoconazole and sulfaphenazole; pharmacodynamic consequences of concomitant use is undefined). Products include:
- Nizoral 2% Cream 1344
- Nizoral 2% Shampoo 1344
- Nizoral Tablets 1345

Phenobarbital (Co-administration leads to a reduction of about 20% in AUC of losartan and that of its active metabolites). Products include:
- Arco-Lase Plus Tablets 513
- Bellergal-S Tablets 2375
- Donnatal 2234
- Donnatal Extentabs 2234
- Donnatal Tablets 2234
- Phenobarbital Elixir and Tablets 1523
- Quadrinal Tablets 1398

Sulfaphenazole (*In Vitro* studies show significant inhibition of the formation of the active metabolite by inhibitors of P450 3A4 such as sulfaphenazole; pharmacodynamic consequences of concomitant use is undefined).
No products indexed under this heading.

Troleandomycin (*In Vitro* studies show significant inhibition of the formation of the active metabolite by inhibitors of P450 3A4 such as troleandomycin; pharmacodynamic consequences of concomitant use is undefined). Products include:
- Tao Capsules 2033

Food Interactions

Meal, unspecified (Meal slows absorption and decreases C_{max} but has minor effects on losartan AUC or on the AUC of the metabolite).

CREON 5 CAPSULES
(Pancrelipase) 2714

Food Interactions

Food having a pH greater than 5.5 (Can dissolve the protective coating resulting in early release of enzymes, irritation of oral mucosa, and/or loss of enzyme activity).

CREON 10 CAPSULES
(Pancrelipase) 2714
See **CREON 5 Capsules**

CREON 20 CAPSULES
(Pancrelipase) 2714
See **CREON 5 Capsules**

CREST SENSITIVITY PROTECTION TOOTHPASTE
(Potassium Nitrate, Sodium Fluoride) .... ▣ 723
None cited in PDR database.

CRIXIVAN CAPSULES
(Indinavir Sulfate) 1670
May interact with:

Astemizole (Competition for CYP3A4 by indinavir could result in inhibition of the metabolism of astemizole and create the potential for serious and/or life-threatening events; concurrent use is not recommended). Products include:
- Hismanal Tablets 1341

Cisapride (Competition for CYP3A4 by indinavir could result in inhibition of the metabolism of cisapride and create the potential for serious and/or life-threatening events; concurrent use is not recommended). Products include:
- Propulsid 1346

Clarithromycin (Co-administration has resulted in a 29% +/- 42% increase in indinavir AUC and a 53% +/- 36% increase in clarithromycin AUC). Products include:
- Biaxin 406

Didanosine (Gastric acid rapidly degrades didanosine and a normal (acidic) gastric pH may be necessary for optimum absorption of indinavir; if administered concomitantly, they should be administered at least 1 hour apart on an empty stomach). Products include:
- Videx Tablets, Powder for Oral Solution, & Pediatric Powder for Oral Solution 2980

Ethinyl Estradiol (Co-administration with Ortho-Novum 1/35 has resulted in an increase in ethinyl estradiol AUC). Products include:
- Brevicon 2563
- Demulen 2580
- Desogen Tablets 1867
- Levlen/Tri-Levlen 646
- Lo/Ovral Tablets 2852
- Lo/Ovral-28 Tablets 2857
- Modicon 1928
- Nordette-21 Tablets 2863
- Nordette-28 Tablets 2866
- Norinyl 2563
- Ortho-Cept 1907
- Ortho-Cyclen/Ortho-Tri-Cyclen 1914
- Ortho-Novum 1928
- Ortho-Cyclen/Ortho Tri-Cyclen 1914
- Ovcon 765
- Ovral Tablets 2877
- Ovral-28 Tablets 2878
- Levlen/Tri-Levlen 646
- Tri-Norinyl 2607
- Triphasil-21 Tablets 2919
- Triphasil-28 Tablets 2924

Fluconazole (Co-administration has resulted in a 19% +/- 33% decrease in indinavir AUC). Products include:
- Diflucan Tablets, Injection, and Oral Suspension 2003

Isoniazid (Co-administration has resulted in a 13% +/- 15% increase in isoniazid AUC). Products include:
- Nydrazid Injection 509
- Rifamate Capsules 1278
- Rifater 1280

Ketoconazole (Co-administration results in an increase in the plasma concentrations of indinavir; a dosage reduction of indinavir may be necessary). Products include:
- Nizoral 2% Cream 1344
- Nizoral 2% Shampoo 1344
- Nizoral Tablets 1345

Midazolam Hydrochloride (Competition for CYP3A4 by indinavir could result in inhibition of the metabolism of midazolam and create the potential for serious and/or life-threatening events; concurrent use is not recommended). Products include:
- Versed Injection 2324

Norethindrone (Co-administration with Ortho-Novum 1/35 has resulted in an increase in norethindrone AUC). Products include:
- Brevicon 2563
- Micronor Tablets 1903
- Modicon 1928
- Norinyl 2563
- Nor-Q D Tablets 2598
- Ortho-Novum 1928
- Ovcon 765
- Tri-Norinyl 2607

Quinidine Sulfate (Potential for increase in indinavir AUC). Products include:
- Quinidex Extentabs 2240

Rifabutin (Co-administration results in an increase in the plasma concentrations of rifabutin; a dosage reduction of rifabutin may be necessary). Products include:
- Mycobutin Capsules 2101

Rifampin (Because rifampin is a potent inducer of P4503A4 which could markedly diminish plasma concentrations of indinavir; co-administration is not recommended). Products include:
- Rifadin 1276
- Rifamate Capsules 1278
- Rifater 1280
- Rimactane Capsules 865

Terfenadine (Competition for CYP3A4 by indinavir could result in inhibition of the metabolism of terfenadine and create the potential for serious and/or life-threatening events; concurrent use is not recommended). Products include:
- Seldane Tablets 1284
- Seldane-D Extended-Release Tablets 1286

Triazolam (Competition for CYP3A4 by indinavir could result in inhibition of the metabolism of triazolam and create the potential for serious and/or life-threatening events; concurrent use is not recommended). Products include:
- Halcion Tablets 2093

Trimethoprim (Co-administration with trimethoprim/sulfamethoxazole tablet has resulted in a 19% +/- 31% increase in trimethoprim AUC). Products include:
- Bactrim DS Tablets 2257
- Bactrim I.V. Infusion 2255
- Bactrim 2257
- Proloprim Tablets 1141
- Septra 1146
- Septra I.V. Infusion 1142
- Septra I.V. Infusion ADD-Vantage Vials 1144
- Septra 1146
- Trimpex Tablets 2323

Food Interactions

Food, unspecified (Co-administration with a meal high in calories, fat, and protein has resulted in a 77% +/- 8% reduction in AUC and an 84% +/- 7% reduction in C_{max}; administer without food 1 hour before or 2 hours after a meal).

Grapefruit Juice (Potential for decrease in indinavir AUC).

CROLOM
(Cromolyn Sodium) .... ◉ 254
None cited in PDR database.

CRUEX ANTIFUNGAL CREAM
(Undecylenic Acid, Zinc Undecylenate) .... ▣ 652
None cited in PDR database.

CRUEX ANTIFUNGAL POWDER
(Calcium Undecylenate) .... ▣ 652
None cited in PDR database.

CRUEX ANTIFUNGAL SPRAY POWDER
(Undecylenic Acid, Zinc Undecylenate) .... ▣ 652
None cited in PDR database.

CRYSTODIGIN TABLETS
(Digitoxin) 1472
May interact with antihistamines, anticonvulsants, barbiturates, oral hypoglycemic agents, diuretics, and certain other agents. Compounds in these categories include:

Acarbose (Digitoxin metabolism stimulated). Products include:
- Precose 604

Acrivastine (Digitoxin metabolism stimulated). Products include:
- Semprex-D Capsules 1620

Amphotericin B (Increased potassium excretion). Products include:
- Abelcet Injection 1540
- Fungizone Intravenous 507
- Fungizone Oral Suspension 704

Aprobarbital (Digitoxin metabolism stimulated).
No products indexed under this heading.

Astemizole (Digitoxin metabolism stimulated). Products include:
- Hismanal Tablets 1341

Azatadine Maleate (Digitoxin metabolism stimulated). Products include:
- Trinalin Repetabs Tablets 1373

Bendroflumethiazide (Hypokalemia).
No products indexed under this heading.

Bromodiphenhydramine Hydrochloride (Digitoxin metabolism stimulated).
No products indexed under this heading.

Brompheniramine Maleate (Digitoxin metabolism stimulated). Products include:
- Alka-Seltzer Plus Sinus Medicine .... ▣ 611
- Bromfed Capsules (Extended-Release) 1832
- Bromfed Syrup .... ▣ 712
- Bromfed Tablets 1832
- Bromfed-DM Cough Syrup 1832
- Bromfed-PD Capsules (Extended-Release) 1832
- Dimetane-DC Cough Syrup 2232
- Dimetane-DX Cough Syrup 2233
- Dimetapp Allergy Dye-Free Elixir .... ▣ 838
- Dimetapp Allergy Sinus Caplets .... ▣ 838
- Dimetapp Cold & Allergy Chewable Tablets .... ▣ 838
- Dimetapp Cold & Cough Liqui-Gels .... ▣ 839
- Dimetapp Cold & Fever Suspension .... ▣ 839
- Dimetapp DM Elixir .... ▣ 840
- Dimetapp Elixir .... ▣ 840
- Dimetapp Extentabs .... ▣ 841
- Dimetapp Tablets/Liqui-Gels .... ▣ 841
- Rondec Chewable Tablets 974
- Vicks DayQuil Allergy Relief 12-Hour Extended Release Tablets .... ▣ 733
- Vicks DayQuil Allergy Relief 4-Hour Tablets .... ▣ 733

Bumetanide (Hypokalemia). Products include:
- Bumex 2260

Butabarbital (Digitoxin metabolism stimulated).
No products indexed under this heading.

Butalbital (Digitoxin metabolism stimulated). Products include:
- Axocet Capsules 2469
- Esgic-plus Capsules 1012
- Esgic-plus Tablets 1012
- Fioricet Tablets 2386
- Fioricet with Codeine Capsules 2387
- Fiorinal Capsules 2388
- Fiorinal with Codeine Capsules 2390
- Fiorinal Tablets 2388
- Phrenilin 790

(▣ Described in PDR For Nonprescription Drugs) (◉ Described in PDR For Ophthalmology)

221 Interactions Index Crystodigin

Sedapap Tablets 50 mg/650 mg .. 1826

Calcium, intravenous (Concurrent use is contraindicated).
No products indexed under this heading.

Carbamazepine (Digitoxin metabolism stimulated). Products include:
Atretol Tablets ... 569
Tegretol/Tegretol-XR ... 870

Cetirizine Hydrochloride (Digitoxin metabolism stimulated). Products include:
Zyrtec Tablets ... 2053

Chlorothiazide (Hypokalemia). Products include:
Aldoclor Tablets ... 1638
Diupres Tablets ... 1691
Diuril Oral ... 1694

Chlorothiazide Sodium (Hypokalemia). Products include:
Diuril Sodium Intravenous ... 1693

Chlorpheniramine Maleate (Digitoxin metabolism stimulated). Products include:
Alka-Seltzer Plus Cold Medicine ... 611
Alka-Seltzer Plus Cold Medicine Liqui-Gels ... 612
Alka-Seltzer Plus Cold & Cough Medicine ... 611
Alka-Seltzer Plus Cold & Cough Medicine Liqui-Gels ... 612
Alka-Seltzer Plus Flu & Body Aches Effervescent Tablets ... 612
Allerest Maximum Strength ... 649
Allerest Sinus Pain Formula ... 649
Ana-Kit Anaphylaxis Emergency Treatment Kit ... 611
Atrohist Pediatric Capsules ... 1603
Atrohist Plus Tablets ... 1605
BC Cold Powder Multi-Symptom Formula (Cold-Sinus-Allergy) ... 631
Cerose DM ... 853
Cheracol Plus Head Cold/Cough Formula ... 741
Children's TYLENOL Cold Multi-Symptom Chewable Tablets and Liquid ... 1559
Children's TYLENOL Cold Plus Cough Multi Symptom Chewable Tablets and Liquid ... 1560
Children's TYLENOL Flu Suspension Liquid ... 1560
Children's Vicks DayQuil Allergy Relief ... 730
Children's Vicks NyQuil Cold/Cough Relief ... 731
Chlor-Trimeton Allergy Decongestant Tablets ... 759
Chlor-Trimeton Allergy Tablets ... 758
Allergy-Sinus Comtrex Multi-Symptom Allergy-Sinus Formula Tablets and Caplets ... 639
Comtrex Multi-Symptom ... 638
Contac Continuous Action Nasal Decongestant/Antihistamine 12 Hour Capsules ... 773
Contac Maximum Strength Continuous Action Decongestant/Antihistamine 12 Hour Caplets ... 772
Contac Severe Cold and Flu Formula Caplets ... 773
Coricidin Cold + Flu Tablets ... 760
Coricidin Cough + Cold Tablets ... 760
Coricidin 'D' Decongestant Tablets ... 760
D.A. II Tablets ... 972
D.A. Chewable Tablets ... 970
Dura-Tap/PD Capsules ... 970
Dura-Vent/DA Tablets ... 972
Efidac 24 Chlorpheniramine ... 655
Extendryl ... 1003
Fedahist Gyrocaps ... 2545
Hycomine Compound Tablets ... 948
Kronofed-A ... 994
Nolamine Timed-Release Tablets ... 790
Novahistine Elixir ... 782
Ornade Spansule Capsules ... 2678
PediaCare Cough-Cold Chewable Tablets and Liquid ... 1569
PediaCare NightRest Cough-Cold Liquid ... 1569
Pediatric Vicks 44m Cough & Cold Relief ... 737
Pyrroxate Caplets ... 742
Ryna ... 804
Sinarest ... 663
Sine-Off Sinus Medicine ... 784
Singlet Tablets ... 785
Sinulin Tablets ... 792
Sinutab Sinus Allergy Medication, Maximum Strength Tablets and Caplets ... 823
Sudafed Cold & Allergy Tablets ... 826
Teldrin 12 Hour Antihistamine/Nasal Decongestant Allergy Relief Capsules ... 786
TheraFlu Flu and Cold Medicine ... 750
Theraflu Maximum Strength Flu and Cold Medicine For Sore Throat ... 751
TheraFlu Flu, Cold and Cough Medicine ... 750
TheraFlu Maximum Strength Nighttime Flu, Cold & Cough Medicine ... 751
Triaminic Night Time ... 754
Triaminic Syrup ... 755
Triaminic Triaminicol Cold & Cough ... 756
Triaminicin Tablets ... 756
Tussend ... 1830
TYLENOL Allergy Sinus, Maximum Strength Caplets and Gelcaps ... 1571
TYLENOL Cold Medication, Multi-Symptom Formula Tablets and Caplets ... 1572
TYLENOL Cold Medication, Multi-Symptom Hot Liquid Packets ... 1572
Vicks 44 LiquiCaps Cough, Cold & Flu Relief ... 728
Vicks 44M Cough, Cold & Flu Relief ... 729

Chlorpheniramine Polistirex (Digitoxin metabolism stimulated). Products include:
Tussionex Pennkinetic Extended-Release Suspension ... 1624

Chlorpheniramine Tannate (Digitoxin metabolism stimulated). Products include:
Atrohist Pediatric Suspension ... 1604
Atrohist Pediatric Suspension Dye-Free ... 1604
Rynatan ... 2781
Rynatuss ... 2782

Chlorpropamide (Digitoxin metabolism stimulated). Products include:
Diabinese Tablets ... 2002

Chlorthalidone (Hypokalemia). Products include:
Combipres Tablets ... 682
Tenoretic Tablets ... 2963
Thalitone ... 1293

Clemastine Fumarate (Digitoxin metabolism stimulated). Products include:
Tavist Syrup ... 2426
Tavist Tablets ... 2427
Tavist-1 12 Hour Relief Tablets ... 749
Tavist-D 12 Hour Relief Tablets ... 750

Cyproheptadine Hydrochloride (Digitoxin metabolism stimulated). Products include:
Periactin ... 1767

Dexchlorpheniramine Maleate (Digitoxin metabolism stimulated).
No products indexed under this heading.

Diphenhydramine Citrate (Digitoxin metabolism stimulated). Products include:
Excedrin P.M. Analgesic/Sleeping Aid Tablets, Caplets, Liquigels ... 735

Diphenylpyraline Hydrochloride (Digitoxin metabolism stimulated).
No products indexed under this heading.

Divalproex Sodium (Digitoxin metabolism stimulated). Products include:
Depakote Tablets ... 418

Ethacrynic Acid (Hypokalemia). Products include:
Edecrin Tablets ... 1698

Ethosuximide (Digitoxin metabolism stimulated). Products include:
Zarontin Capsules ... 1986
Zarontin Syrup ... 1986

Ethotoin (Digitoxin metabolism stimulated). Products include:
Peganone Tablets ... 455

Felbamate (Digitoxin metabolism stimulated). Products include:
Felbatol ... 2774

Furosemide (Hypokalemia). Products include:
Lasix Injection, Oral Solution and Tablets ... 1267

Glimepiride (Digitoxin metabolism stimulated). Products include:
Amaryl Tablets ... 1241

Glipizide (Digitoxin metabolism stimulated). Products include:
Glucotrol Tablets ... 2011
Glucotrol XL Extended Release Tablets ... 2012

Glyburide (Digitoxin metabolism stimulated). Products include:
DiaBeta Tablets ... 1265
Glynase PresTab Tablets ... 2091
Micronase Tablets ... 2099

Hydrochlorothiazide (Hypokalemia). Products include:
Aldactazide Tablets ... 2556
Aldoril Tablets ... 1644
Apresazide Capsules ... 824
Capozide Tablets ... 744
Dyazide Capsules ... 2653
Esidrix Tablets ... 839
Esimil Tablets ... 840
HydroDIURIL Tablets ... 1716
Hydropres Tablets ... 1718
Hyzaar Tablets ... 1720
Inderide Tablets ... 2838
Inderide LA Long Acting Capsules .. 2840
Lopressor HCT Tablets ... 850
Lotensin HCT Tablets ... 855
Moduretic Tablets ... 1748
Oretic Tablets ... 450
Prinzide Tablets ... 1780
Ser-Ap-Es Tablets ... 867
Timolide Tablets ... 1791
Vaseretic Tablets ... 1810
Zestoretic Tablets ... 2968
Ziac ... 1459

Hydroflumethiazide (Hypokalemia). Products include:
Diucardin Tablets ... 2824

Indapamide (Hypokalemia).
No products indexed under this heading.

Lamotrigine (Digitoxin metabolism stimulated). Products include:
Lamictal Tablets ... 1105

Loratadine (Digitoxin metabolism stimulated). Products include:
Claritin Tablets ... 2485
Claritin-D Tablets ... 2487

Mephenytoin (Digitoxin metabolism stimulated). Products include:
Mesantoin Tablets ... 2400

Mephobarbital (Digitoxin metabolism stimulated). Products include:
Mebaral Tablets ... 2452

Metformin Hydrochloride (Digitoxin metabolism stimulated). Products include:
Glucophage Tablets ... 754

Methdilazine Hydrochloride (Digitoxin metabolism stimulated).
No products indexed under this heading.

Methsuximide (Digitoxin metabolism stimulated). Products include:
Celontin Kapseals ... 1955

Methyclothiazide (Hypokalemia). Products include:
Enduron Tablets ... 424

Metolazone (Hypokalemia). Products include:
Mykrox Tablets ... 1617
Zaroxolyn Tablets ... 1625

Paramethadione (Digitoxin metabolism stimulated).
No products indexed under this heading.

Pentobarbital Sodium (Digitoxin metabolism stimulated). Products include:
Nembutal Sodium Capsules ... 440
Nembutal Sodium Solution ... 442
Nembutal Sodium Suppositories ... 444

Phenacemide (Digitoxin metabolism stimulated). Products include:
Phenurone Tablets ... 455

Phenobarbital (Increases rate of metabolism of digitoxin). Products include:
Arco-Lase Plus Tablets ... 513
Bellergal-S Tablets ... 2375
Donnatal ... 2234
Donnatal Extentabs ... 2234
Donnatal Tablets ... 2234
Phenobarbital Elixir and Tablets ... 1523
Quadrinal Tablets ... 1398

Phensuximide (Digitoxin metabolism stimulated).
No products indexed under this heading.

Phenylbutazone (Increased rate of digitoxin metabolism).
No products indexed under this heading.

Phenytoin (Increased rate of digitoxin metabolism). Products include:
Dilantin Infatabs ... 1967
Dilantin-125 Suspension ... 1969

Phenytoin Sodium (Increased rate of digitoxin metabolism). Products include:
Dilantin Kapseals ... 1965

Polythiazide (Hypokalemia). Products include:
Minizide Capsules ... 2016

Prednisone (Increased potassium excretion).
No products indexed under this heading.

Primidone (Digitoxin metabolism stimulated). Products include:
Mysoline ... 2860

Promethazine Hydrochloride (Digitoxin metabolism stimulated). Products include:
Mepergan Injection ... 2859
Phenergan with Codeine ... 2883
Phenergan with Dextromethorphan 2885
Phenergan Injection ... 2880
Phenergan Suppositories ... 2882
Phenergan Syrup ... 2881
Phenergan Tablets ... 2882
Phenergan VC ... 2886
Phenergan VC with Codeine ... 2888

Pyrilamine Maleate (Digitoxin metabolism stimulated). Products include:
4-Way Fast Acting Nasal Spray (regular & mentholated) ... 644
Maximum Strength Multi-Symptom Formula Midol ... 621
PMS Multi-Symptom Formula Midol ... 622

Pyrilamine Tannate (Digitoxin metabolism stimulated). Products include:
Atrohist Pediatric Suspension ... 1604
Atrohist Pediatric Suspension Dye-Free ... 1604
Rynatan ... 2781

Secobarbital Sodium (Digitoxin metabolism stimulated). Products include:
Seconal Sodium Pulvules ... 1529

Terfenadine (Digitoxin metabolism stimulated). Products include:
Seldane Tablets ... 1284
Seldane-D Extended-Release Tablets ... 1286

Thiamylal Sodium (Digitoxin metabolism stimulated).
No products indexed under this heading.

Tolazamide (Digitoxin metabolism stimulated).
No products indexed under this heading.

Tolbutamide (Digitoxin metabolism stimulated).
No products indexed under this heading.

IMPORTANT NOTE: Always consult each drug listing in the patient's regimen for possible interactions.

Crystodigin — Interactions Index

Torsemide (Hypokalemia). Products include:
Demadex Tablets and Injection 691

Trimeprazine Tartrate (Digitoxin metabolism stimulated).
No products indexed under this heading.

Trimethadione (Digitoxin metabolism stimulated).
No products indexed under this heading.

Tripelennamine Hydrochloride (Digitoxin metabolism stimulated). Products include:
PBZ Tablets 863
PBZ-SR Tablets 862

Triprolidine Hydrochloride (Digitoxin metabolism stimulated). Products include:
Actifed Cold & Allergy Tablets ..... ⊞ 807
Actifed Cold & Sinus Caplets and Tablets ..... ⊞ 808

Valproic Acid (Digitoxin metabolism stimulated). Products include:
Depakene 416

CUPRIMINE CAPSULES
(Penicillamine) 1673
May interact with cytotoxic drugs, antimalarials, and certain other agents. Compounds in these categories include:

Auranofin (Concurrent use not recommended). Products include:
Ridaura Capsules 2691

Aurothioglucose (Concurrent use not recommended). Products include:
Solganal Suspension 2530

Bleomycin Sulfate (Concurrent use not recommended). Products include:
Blenoxane 697

Chloroquine Hydrochloride (Concurrent use not recommended). Products include:
Aralen Hydrochloride Injection 2430

Chloroquine Phosphate (Concurrent use not recommended). Products include:
Aralen Phosphate Tablets 2431

Daunorubicin Hydrochloride (Concurrent use not recommended). Products include:
Cerubidine for Injection 634

Doxorubicin Hydrochloride (Concurrent use not recommended). Products include:
Adriamycin PFS 2056
Adriamycin RDF 2056
Doxil 2613
Doxorubicin Astra 531
Rubex for Injection 721

Fluorouracil (Concurrent use not recommended). Products include:
Efudex 2280
Fluoroplex Topical Solution & Cream 1% 475
Fluorouracil Injection 2282

Hydroxychloroquine Sulfate (Concurrent use not recommended). Products include:
Plaquenil Sulfate Tablets 2459

Hydroxyurea (Concurrent use not recommended). Products include:
Hydrea Capsules 705

Mefloquine Hydrochloride (Concurrent use not recommended). Products include:
Lariam Tablets 2295

Methotrexate Sodium (Concurrent use not recommended). Products include:
Methotrexate Sodium Tablets, Injection, for Injection and LPF Injection 1322

Mineral Supplements (Block response).

Mitotane (Concurrent use not recommended). Products include:
Lysodren Tablets 707

Mitoxantrone Hydrochloride (Concurrent use not recommended). Products include:
Novantrone for Injection 1327

Oxyphenbutazone (Concurrent use not recommended).

Phenylbutazone (Concurrent use not recommended).
No products indexed under this heading.

Procarbazine Hydrochloride (Concurrent use not recommended). Products include:
Matulane Capsules 2300

Pyridoxine (Penicillamine increases pyridoxine requirement).

Pyrimethamine (Concurrent use not recommended). Products include:
Daraprim Tablets 1199
Fansidar Tablets 2281

Tamoxifen Citrate (Concurrent use not recommended). Products include:
Nolvadex Tablets 2957

Vincristine Sulfate (Concurrent use not recommended). Products include:
Oncovin Solution Vials & Hyporets 1521

CUREL LOTION AND CREAM
(Moisturizing formula) ..... ⊞ 608
None cited in PDR database.

CUTIVATE CREAM
(Fluticasone Propionate) 1078
None cited in PDR database.

CUTIVATE OINTMENT
(Fluticasone Propionate) 1078
None cited in PDR database.

CYCRIN TABLETS
(Medroxyprogesterone Acetate) 991
May interact with estrogens and certain other agents. Compounds in these categories include:

Aminoglutethimide (Concomitant administration may depress the bioavailability of Amen). Products include:
Cytadren Tablets 837

Chlorotrianisene (Potential for adverse effects on carbohydrate and lipid metabolism).
No products indexed under this heading.

Dienestrol (Potential for adverse effects on carbohydrate and lipid metabolism). Products include:
Ortho Dienestrol Cream 1922

Diethylstilbestrol (Potential for adverse effects on carbohydrate and lipid metabolism). Products include:
Diethylstilbestrol Tablets 1477

Estradiol (Potential for adverse effects on carbohydrate and lipid metabolism). Products include:
Climara Transdermal System 640
Estrace Cream and Tablets 751
Estraderm Transdermal System 842
Estring Vaginal Ring 2086
Vivelle Transdermal System 880

Estrogens, Conjugated (Potential for adverse effects on carbohydrate and lipid metabolism). Products include:
PMB 200 and PMB 400 2890
Premarin Intravenous 2893
Premarin Tablets 2896
Premarin Vaginal Cream 2898
Premphase 2900
Prempro 2905

Estrogens, Esterified (Potential for adverse effects on carbohydrate and lipid metabolism). Products include:
ESTRATAB Tablets (0.3, 0.625, 1.25, 2.5 mg) 2715
Estratest 2718
Menest Tablets 2671

Estropipate (Potential for adverse effects on carbohydrate and lipid metabolism). Products include:
Ogen Tablets 2103
Ogen Vaginal Cream 2106
Ortho-Est 1925

Ethinyl Estradiol (Potential for adverse effects on carbohydrate and lipid metabolism). Products include:
Brevicon 2563
Demulen 2580
Desogen Tablets 1867
Levlen/Tri-Levlen 646
Lo/Ovral Tablets 2852
Lo/Ovral-28 Tablets 2857
Modicon 1928
Nordette-21 Tablets 2863
Nordette-28 Tablets 2866
Norinyl 2563
Ortho-Cept 1907
Ortho-Cyclen/Ortho-Tri-Cyclen 1914
Ortho-Novum 1928
Ortho-Cyclen/Ortho Tri-Cyclen 1914
Ovcon 765
Ovral Tablets 2877
Ovral-28 Tablets 2878
Levlen/Tri-Levlen 646
Tri-Norinyl 2607
Triphasil-21 Tablets 2919
Triphasil-28 Tablets 2924

Polyestradiol Phosphate (Potential for adverse effects on carbohydrate and lipid metabolism).
No products indexed under this heading.

Quinestrol (Potential for adverse effects on carbohydrate and lipid metabolism).
No products indexed under this heading.

CYLERT CHEWABLE TABLETS
(Pemoline) 415
See **Cylert Tablets**

CYLERT TABLETS
(Pemoline) 415
May interact with anticonvulsants and certain other agents. Compounds in these categories include:

Carbamazepine (Co-administration with antiepileptic medications results in decreased seizure threshold). Products include:
Atretol Tablets 569
Tegretol/Tegretol-XR 870

Clonazepam (Co-administration with antiepileptic medications results in decreased seizure threshold). Products include:
Klonopin Tablets 2294

CNS-Active Drugs, unspecified (Patients receiving Cylert concurrently with other drugs with CNS activity should be monitored carefully).

Divalproex Sodium (Co-administration with antiepileptic medications results in decreased seizure threshold). Products include:
Depakote Tablets 418

Ethosuximide (Co-administration with antiepileptic medications results in decreased seizure threshold). Products include:
Zarontin Capsules 1986
Zarontin Syrup 1986

Ethotoin (Co-administration with antiepileptic medications results in decreased seizure threshold). Products include:
Peganone Tablets 455

Felbamate (Co-administration with antiepileptic medications results in decreased seizure threshold). Products include:
Felbatol 2774

Lamotrigine (Co-administration with antiepileptic medications results in decreased seizure threshold). Products include:
Lamictal Tablets 1105

Mephenytoin (Co-administration with antiepileptic medications results in decreased seizure threshold). Products include:
Mesantoin Tablets 2400

Methsuximide (Co-administration with antiepileptic medications results in decreased seizure threshold). Products include:
Celontin Kapseals 1955

Paramethadione (Co-administration with antiepileptic medications results in decreased seizure threshold).
No products indexed under this heading.

Phenacemide (Co-administration with antiepileptic medications results in decreased seizure threshold). Products include:
Phenurone Tablets 455

Phenobarbital (Co-administration with antiepileptic medications results in decreased seizure threshold). Products include:
Arco-Lase Plus Tablets 513
Bellergal-S Tablets 2375
Donnatal 2234
Donnatal Extentabs 2234
Donnatal Tablets 2234
Phenobarbital Elixir and Tablets 1523
Quadrinal Tablets 1398

Phensuximide (Co-administration with antiepileptic medications results in decreased seizure threshold).
No products indexed under this heading.

Phenytoin (Co-administration with antiepileptic medications results in decreased seizure threshold). Products include:
Dilantin Infatabs 1967
Dilantin-125 Suspension 1969

Phenytoin Sodium (Co-administration with antiepileptic medications results in decreased seizure threshold). Products include:
Dilantin Kapseals 1965

Primidone (Co-administration with antiepileptic medications results in decreased seizure threshold). Products include:
Mysoline 2860

Trimethadione (Co-administration with antiepileptic medications results in decreased seizure threshold).
No products indexed under this heading.

Valproic Acid (Co-administration with antiepileptic medications results in decreased seizure threshold). Products include:
Depakene 416

CYSTOSPAZ TABLETS
(Hyoscyamine) 2123
May interact with phenothiazines, monoamine oxidase inhibitors, tricyclic antidepressants, antihistamines, antimuscarinic drugs, antacids, and certain other agents. Compounds in these categories include:

Acrivastine (Additive adverse effects resulting from cholinergic blockade). Products include:
Semprex-D Capsules 1620

(⊞ Described in PDR For Nonprescription Drugs)   (⊙ Described in PDR For Ophthalmology)

223 **Interactions Index** **Cystospaz**

Aluminum Carbonate (Interferes with absorption). Products include:
Basaljel Capsules 2810
Basaljel Suspension 2810
Basaljel Tablets 2810

Aluminum Hydroxide (Interferes with absorption). Products include:
ALternaGEL Liquid 1358
Maximum Strength Ascriptin 650
Cama Arthritis Pain Reliever 748
Gaviscon Extra Strength Relief Formula Antacid Tablets 778
Gaviscon Extra Strength Relief Formula Liquid Antacid 779
Gaviscon Liquid Antacid 779
Gelusil Antacid-Anti-gas Liquid 819
Gelusil Antacid-Anti-gas Tablets 819
Maalox Antacid/Anti-Gas Tablets 889
Maalox Heartburn Relief Suspension 658
Maalox Antacid Liquid 888
Extra Strength Maalox Antacid/Anti-Gas Liquid and Tablets 888
Mylanta 1359
Tempo Soft Antacid 799

Aluminum Hydroxide Gel (Interferes with absorption). Products include:
ALternaGEL Liquid 675
Aludrox Oral Suspension 850
Amphojel Suspension 2802
Amphojel Suspension without Flavor 2802
Amphojel Tablets 2802
Ascriptin 650
Gaviscon Antacid Tablets 778
Gaviscon-2 Antacid Tablets 779
Mylanta Liquid 676
Mylanta Double Strength Liquid 676
Nephrox Suspension 671

Amantadine Hydrochloride (Additive adverse effects resulting from cholinergic blockade). Products include:
Symmetrel Capsules 965
Symmetrel Syrup 963

Amitriptyline Hydrochloride (Additive adverse effects resulting from cholinergic blockade). Products include:
Elavil 2945
Etrafon 2495
Limbitrol 2333
Triavil Tablets 1800

Amoxapine (Additive adverse effects resulting from cholinergic blockade). Products include:
Asendin Tablets 1419

Astemizole (Additive adverse effects resulting from cholinergic blockade). Products include:
Hismanal Tablets 1341

Atropine Sulfate (Additive adverse effects resulting from cholinergic blockade). Products include:
Arco-Lase Plus Tablets 513
Atrohist Plus Tablets 1605
Donnatal 2234
Donnatal Extentabs 2234
Donnatal Tablets 2234
Lomotil 2591
Motofen Tablets 789
Urised Tablets 2123

Azatadine Maleate (Additive adverse effects resulting from cholinergic blockade). Products include:
Trinalin Repetabs Tablets 1373

Belladonna Alkaloids (Additive adverse effects resulting from cholinergic blockade). Products include:
Bellergal-S Tablets 2375
Hyland's Bedwetting Tablets 788
Hyland's EnurAid Tablets 789
Hyland's Headache Tablets 790
Hyland's Teething Tablets 790
Similasan Eye Drops #1 769

Bromodiphenhydramine Hydrochloride (Additive adverse effects resulting from cholinergic blockade).
No products indexed under this heading.

Brompheniramine Maleate (Additive adverse effects resulting from cholinergic blockade). Products include:
Alka-Seltzer Plus Sinus Medicine 611
Bromfed Capsules (Extended-Release) 1832
Bromfed Syrup 712
Bromfed Tablets 1832
Bromfed-DM Cough Syrup 1832
Bromfed-PD Capsules (Extended-Release) 1832
Dimetane-DC Cough Syrup 2232
Dimetane-DX Cough Syrup 2233
Dimetapp Allergy Dye-Free Elixir 838
Dimetapp Allergy Sinus Caplets 838
Dimetapp Cold & Allergy Chewable Tablets 838
Dimetapp Cold & Cough Liqui-Gels 839
Dimetapp Cold & Fever Suspension 839
Dimetapp DM Elixir 840
Dimetapp Elixir 840
Dimetapp Extentabs 841
Dimetapp Tablets/Liqui-Gels 841
Rondec Chewable Tablets 974
Vicks DayQuil Allergy Relief 12-Hour Extended Release Tablets 733
Vicks DayQuil Allergy Relief 4-Hour Tablets 733

Cetirizine Hydrochloride (Additive adverse effects resulting from cholinergic blockade). Products include:
Zyrtec Tablets 2053

Chlorpheniramine Maleate (Additive adverse effects resulting from cholinergic blockade). Products include:
Alka-Seltzer Plus Cold Medicine 611
Alka-Seltzer Plus Cold Medicine Liqui-Gels 612
Alka-Seltzer Plus Cold & Cough Medicine 611
Alka-Seltzer Plus Cold & Cough Medicine Liqui-Gels 612
Alka-Seltzer Plus Flu & Body Aches Effervescent Tablets 612
Allerest Maximum Strength 649
Allerest Sinus Pain Formula 649
Ana-Kit Anaphylaxis Emergency Treatment Kit 611
Atrohist Pediatric Capsules 1603
Atrohist Plus Tablets 1605
BC Cold Powder Multi-Symptom Formula (Cold-Sinus-Allergy) 631
Cerose DM 853
Cheracol Plus Head Cold/Cough Formula 741
Children's TYLENOL Cold Multi-Symptom Chewable Tablets and Liquid 1559
Children's TYLENOL Cold Plus Cough Multi Symptom Chewable Tablets and Liquid 1560
Children's TYLENOL Flu Suspension Liquid 1560
Children's Vicks DayQuil Allergy Relief 730
Children's Vicks NyQuil Cold/Cough Relief 731
Chlor-Trimeton Allergy Decongestant Tablets 759
Chlor-Trimeton Allergy Tablets 758
Allergy-Sinus Comtrex Multi-Symptom Allergy-Sinus Formula Tablets and Caplets 639
Comtrex Multi-Symptom 638
Contac Continuous Action Nasal Decongestant/Antihistamine 12 Hour Capsules 773
Contac Maximum Strength Continuous Action Decongestant/Antihistamine 12 Hour Caplets 772
Contac Severe Cold and Flu Formula Caplets 773
Coricidin Cold + Flu Tablets 760
Coricidin Cough + Cold Tablets 760
Coricidin 'D' Decongestant Tablets 760
D.A. II Tablets 972
D.A. Chewable Tablets 970
Dura-Tap/PD Capsules 970
Dura-Vent/DA Tablets 972
Efidac 24 Chlorpheniramine 655
Extendryl 1003
Fedahist Gyrocaps 2545
Hycomine Compound Tablets 948
Kronofed-A 994
Nolamine Timed-Release Tablets 790
Novahistine Elixir 782
Ornade Spansule Capsules 2678
PediaCare Cough-Cold Chewable Tablets and Liquid 1569
PediaCare NightRest Cough-Cold Liquid 1569
Pediatric Vicks 44m Cough & Cold Relief 737
Pyrroxate Caplets 742
Ryna 804
Sinarest 663
Sine-Off Sinus Medicine 784
Singlet Tablets 785
Sinulin Tablets 792
Sinutab Sinus Allergy Medication, Maximum Strength Tablets and Caplets 823
Sudafed Cold & Allergy Tablets 826
Teldrin 12 Hour Antihistamine/Nasal Decongestant Allergy Relief Capsules 786
TheraFlu Flu and Cold Medicine 750
Theraflu Maximum Strength Flu and Cold Medicine For Sore Throat 751
TheraFlu Flu, Cold and Cough Medicine 750
TheraFlu Maximum Strength Nighttime Flu, Cold & Cough Medicine 751
Triaminic Night Time 754
Triaminic Syrup 755
Triaminic Triaminicol Cold & Cough 756
Triaminicin Tablets 756
Tussend 1830
TYLENOL Allergy Sinus, Maximum Strength Caplets and Gelcaps 1571
TYLENOL Cold Medication, Multi-Symptom Formula Tablets and Caplets 1572
TYLENOL Cold Medication, Multi-Symptom Hot Liquid Packets 1572
Vicks 44 LiquiCaps Cough, Cold & Flu Relief 728
Vicks 44M Cough, Cold & Flu Relief 729

Chlorpheniramine Polistirex (Additive adverse effects resulting from cholinergic blockade). Products include:
Tussionex Pennkinetic Extended-Release Suspension 1624

Chlorpheniramine Tannate (Additive adverse effects resulting from cholinergic blockade). Products include:
Atrohist Pediatric Suspension 1604
Atrohist Pediatric Suspension Dye-Free 1604
Rynatan 2781
Rynatuss 2782

Chlorpromazine (Additive adverse effects resulting from cholinergic blockade). Products include:
Thorazine Suppositories 2701

Chlorpromazine Hydrochloride (Additive adverse effects resulting from cholinergic blockade). Products include:
Thorazine 2701

Clemastine Fumarate (Additive adverse effects resulting from cholinergic blockade). Products include:
Tavist Syrup 2426
Tavist Tablets 2427
Tavist-1 12 Hour Relief Tablets 749
Tavist-D 12 Hour Relief Tablets 750

Clidinium Bromide (Additive adverse effects resulting from cholinergic blockade). Products include:
Librax Capsules 2330

Clomipramine Hydrochloride (Additive adverse effects resulting from cholinergic blockade). Products include:
Anafranil Capsules 819

Cyproheptadine Hydrochloride (Additive adverse effects resulting from cholinergic blockade). Products include:
Periactin 1767

Desipramine Hydrochloride (Additive adverse effects resulting from cholinergic blockade). Products include:
Norpramin Tablets 1273

Dexchlorpheniramine Maleate (Additive adverse effects resulting from cholinergic blockade).
No products indexed under this heading.

Dicyclomine Hydrochloride (Additive adverse effects resulting from cholinergic blockade). Products include:
Bentyl 1246

Diphenhydramine Citrate (Additive adverse effects resulting from cholinergic blockade). Products include:
Excedrin P.M. Analgesic/Sleeping Aid Tablets, Caplets, Liquigels 735

Diphenhydramine Hydrochloride (Additive adverse effects resulting from cholinergic blockade). Products include:
Actifed Allergy Daytime/Nighttime Caplets 808
Actifed Sinus Daytime/Nighttime Tablets and Caplets 809
Extra Strength Bayer PM Aspirin Plus Sleep Aid 617
Benadryl Allergy Chewables 811
Benadryl Allergy/Cold Tablets 811
Benadryl Allergy Decongestant Liquid Medication 812
Benadryl Allergy Decongestant Tablets 812
Benadryl Allergy Liquid Medication 813
Benadryl Allergy 811
Benadryl Allergy Sinus Headache Caplets 813
Benadryl Dye-Free Allergy Liqui-gel Softgels 813
Benadryl Dye-Free Allergy Liquid Medication 814
Benadryl Itch Relief Stick Extra Strength 814
Benadryl Cream 814
Benadryl Gel 815
Benadryl Spray 815
Benadryl Injection 1955
Contac Day & Night Cold/Flu Night Caplets 772
Contac Night Allergy/Sinus Caplets 771
Extra Strength Doan's P.M. 653
Excedrin P.M. Analgesic/Sleeping Aid Tablets, Caplets, Liquigels 643
Nytol QuickCaps Caplets 632
Sleepinal Night-time Sleep Aid Capsules and Softgels 798
TYLENOL Allergy Sinus NightTime, Maximum Strength Caplets 1571
TYLENOL Flu NightTime, Maximum Strength Gelcaps 1575
TYLENOL Flu NightTime, Maximum Strength Hot Medication Packets 1575
TYLENOL PM Pain Reliever/Sleep Aid, Extra Strength Gelcaps, Caplets, Geltabs 1576
TYLENOL Severe Allergy Medication Caplets 1571
Maximum Strength Unisom Sleepgels 1990
Unisom With Pain Relief-Nighttime Sleep Aid and Pain Reliever 1991

Diphenylpyraline Hydrochloride (Additive adverse effects resulting from cholinergic blockade).
No products indexed under this heading.

Doxepin Hydrochloride (Additive adverse effects resulting from cholinergic blockade). Products include:
Adapin Capsules 1542
Sinequan 2028
Zonalon Cream 1042

Fluphenazine Decanoate (Additive adverse effects resulting from cholinergic blockade). Products include:
Prolixin Decanoate 510

IMPORTANT NOTE: Always consult each drug listing in the patient's regimen for possible interactions.

Cystospaz | Interactions Index | 224

Fluphenazine Enanthate (Additive adverse effects resulting from cholinergic blockade). Products include:
- Prolixin Enanthate 510

Fluphenazine Hydrochloride (Additive adverse effects resulting from cholinergic blockade). Products include:
- Prolixin 510

Furazolidone (Additive adverse effects resulting from cholinergic blockade). Products include:
- Furoxone 2221

Glycopyrrolate (Additive adverse effects resulting from cholinergic blockade). Products include:
- Robinul Forte Tablets 2247
- Robinul Injectable 2247
- Robinul Tablets 2247

Haloperidol (Additive adverse effects resulting from cholinergic blockade). Products include:
- Haldol Injection, Tablets and Concentrate 1585

Haloperidol Decanoate (Additive adverse effects resulting from cholinergic blockade). Products include:
- Haldol Decanoate 1587

Hyoscyamine Sulfate (Additive adverse effects resulting from cholinergic blockade). Products include:
- Arco-Lase Plus Tablets 513
- Atrohist Plus Tablets 1605
- Cystospaz-M Capsules 2123
- Donnatal 2234
- Donnatal Extentabs 2234
- Donnatal Tablets 2234
- Kutrase Capsules 2546
- Levsin/Levsinex/Levbid 2549

Imipramine Hydrochloride (Additive adverse effects resulting from cholinergic blockade). Products include:
- Tofranil Ampuls 873
- Tofranil Tablets 875

Imipramine Pamoate (Additive adverse effects resulting from cholinergic blockade). Products include:
- Tofranil-PM Capsules 876

Ipratropium Bromide (Additive adverse effects resulting from cholinergic blockade). Products include:
- Atrovent Inhalation Aerosol 674
- Atrovent Inhalation Solution 675
- Atrovent Nasal Spray 0.03% 676
- Atrovent Nasal Spray 0.06% 678

Isocarboxazid (Additive adverse effects resulting from cholinergic blockade).
- No products indexed under this heading.

Loratadine (Additive adverse effects resulting from cholinergic blockade). Products include:
- Claritin Tablets 2485
- Claritin-D Tablets 2487

Magaldrate (Interferes with absorption).
- No products indexed under this heading.

Magnesium Hydroxide (Interferes with absorption). Products include:
- Aludrox Oral Suspension .... ▣ 850
- Ascriptin .... ▣ 650
- Di-Gel Antacid/Anti-Gas .... ▣ 762
- Gelusil Antacid-Anti-gas Liquid .... ▣ 819
- Gelusil Antacid-Anti-gas Tablets .... ▣ 819
- Maalox Antacid/Anti-Gas Tablets 889
- Maalox Antacid Liquid 888
- Extra Strength Maalox Antacid/Anti-Gas Liquid and Tablets 888
- Mylanta Fast-Acting 1359
- Mylanta Gelcaps Antacid .... ▣ 678
- Fast-Acting Mylanta Liquid Antacid 1359
- Mylanta Tablets .... ▣ 677
- Maximum-Strength Fast-Acting Mylanta Liquid Antacid 1359
- Mylanta Double Strength Tablets .... ▣ 677
- Phillips' Milk of Magnesia Liquid .... ▣ 627
- Rolaids Antacid Tablets .... ▣ 807
- Tempo Soft Antacid .... ▣ 799

Magnesium Oxide (Interferes with absorption). Products include:
- Beelith Tablets 632
- Bufferin Analgesic Tablets .... ▣ 636
- Arthritis Strength Bufferin Analgesic Caplets .... ▣ 637
- Extra Strength Bufferin Analgesic Tablets .... ▣ 637
- Caltrate PLUS .... ▣ 681
- Cama Arthritis Pain Reliever 748
- Mag-Ox 400 666
- Uro-Mag 666

Maprotiline Hydrochloride (Additive adverse effects resulting from cholinergic blockade). Products include:
- Ludiomil Tablets 861

Mepenzolate Bromide (Additive adverse effects resulting from cholinergic blockade).
- No products indexed under this heading.

Mesoridazine Besylate (Additive adverse effects resulting from cholinergic blockade). Products include:
- Serentil 689

Methdilazine Hydrochloride (Additive adverse effects resulting from cholinergic blockade). Products include:
- No products indexed under this heading.

Methotrimeprazine (Additive adverse effects resulting from cholinergic blockade). Products include:
- Levoprome 1321

Nortriptyline Hydrochloride (Additive adverse effects resulting from cholinergic blockade). Products include:
- Pamelor 2409

Oxyphenonium Bromide (Additive adverse effects resulting from cholinergic blockade).

Perphenazine (Additive adverse effects resulting from cholinergic blockade). Products include:
- Etrafon 2495
- Triavil Tablets 1800
- Trilafon 2532

Phenelzine Sulfate (Additive adverse effects resulting from cholinergic blockade). Products include:
- Nardil 1977

Prochlorperazine (Additive adverse effects resulting from cholinergic blockade). Products include:
- Compazine 2644

Promethazine Hydrochloride (Additive adverse effects resulting from cholinergic blockade). Products include:
- Mepergan Injection 2859
- Phenergan with Codeine 2883
- Phenergan with Dextromethorphan 2885
- Phenergan Injection 2880
- Phenergan Suppositories 2882
- Phenergan Syrup 2881
- Phenergan Tablets 2882
- Phenergan VC 2886
- Phenergan VC with Codeine 2888

Propantheline Bromide (Additive adverse effects resulting from cholinergic blockade). Products include:
- Pro-Banthine Tablets 2226

Protriptyline Hydrochloride (Additive adverse effects resulting from cholinergic blockade). Products include:
- Vivactil Tablets 1820

Pyrilamine Maleate (Additive adverse effects resulting from cholinergic blockade). Products include:
- 4-Way Fast Acting Nasal Spray (regular & mentholated) .... ▣ 644

Maximum Strength Multi-Symptom Formula Midol .... ▣ 621
PMS Multi-Symptom Formula Midol .... ▣ 622

Pyrilamine Tannate (Additive adverse effects resulting from cholinergic blockade). Products include:
- Atrohist Pediatric Suspension 1604
- Atrohist Pediatric Suspension Dye-Free 1604
- Rynatan 2781

Scopolamine (Additive adverse effects resulting from cholinergic blockade). Products include:
- Transderm Scōp Transdermal Therapeutic System 890

Scopolamine Hydrobromide (Additive adverse effects resulting from cholinergic blockade). Products include:
- Atrohist Plus Tablets 1605
- Donnatal 2234
- Donnatal Extentabs 2234
- Donnatal Tablets 2234

Selegiline Hydrochloride (Additive adverse effects resulting from cholinergic blockade). Products include:
- Eldepryl Capsules 2729

Sodium Bicarbonate (Interferes with absorption). Products include:
- Alka-Seltzer Cherry Effervescent Antacid and Pain Reliever .... ▣ 609
- Alka-Seltzer Extra Strength Effervescent Antacid and Pain Reliever .... ▣ 609
- Alka-Seltzer Gold Effervescent Antacid .... ▣ 611
- Alka-Seltzer Lemon Lime Effervescent Antacid and Pain Reliever .... ▣ 609
- Alka-Seltzer Original Effervescent Antacid and Pain Reliever .... ▣ 609
- Arm & Hammer Pure Baking Soda .... ▣ 648
- Colyte and Colyte-flavored 2540
- GoLYTELY 694
- Massengill Disposable Douches .... ▣ 780
- Massengill Liquid Concentrate .... ▣ 780
- NuLYTELY 694
- Cherry Flavor NuLYTELY 694

Terfenadine (Additive adverse effects resulting from cholinergic blockade). Products include:
- Seldane Tablets 1284
- Seldane-D Extended-Release Tablets 1286

Thioridazine Hydrochloride (Additive adverse effects resulting from cholinergic blockade). Products include:
- Mellaril 2398

Tranylcypromine Sulfate (Additive adverse effects resulting from cholinergic blockade). Products include:
- Parnate Tablets 2679

Tridihexethyl Chloride (Additive adverse effects resulting from cholinergic blockade).
- No products indexed under this heading.

Trifluoperazine Hydrochloride (Additive adverse effects resulting from cholinergic blockade). Products include:
- Stelazine 2692

Trimeprazine Tartrate (Additive adverse effects resulting from cholinergic blockade). Products include:
- No products indexed under this heading.

Trimipramine Maleate (Additive adverse effects resulting from cholinergic blockade). Products include:
- Surmontil Capsules 2917

Tripelennamine Hydrochloride (Additive adverse effects resulting from cholinergic blockade). Products include:
- PBZ Tablets 863

- PBZ-SR Tablets 862

Triprolidine Hydrochloride (Additive adverse effects resulting from cholinergic blockade). Products include:
- Actifed Cold & Allergy Tablets .... ▣ 807
- Actifed Cold & Sinus Caplets and Tablets .... ▣ 808

CYSTOSPAZ-M CAPSULES (Hyoscyamine Sulfate) 2123
See **Cystospaz Tablets**

CYTADREN TABLETS
(Aminoglutethimide) 837
May interact with oral anticoagulants and certain other agents. Compounds in these categories include:

Dexamethasone (Accelerates metabolism of dexamethasone). Products include:
- AK-Trol Ointment & Suspension .... ⊙ 205
- Decadron Elixir 1676
- Decadron Tablets 1678
- Decaspray Topical Aerosol 1689
- Maxitrol Ophthalmic Ointment and Suspension .... ⊙ 222
- TobraDex Ophthalmic Suspension and Ointment 469

Dexamethasone Acetate (Accelerates metabolism of dexamethasone). Products include:
- Dalalone D.P. Injectable 1009
- Decadron-LA Sterile Suspension 1687

Dexamethasone Phosphate (Accelerates metabolism of dexamethasone).
- No products indexed under this heading.

Dexamethasone Sodium Phosphate (Accelerates metabolism of dexamethasone). Products include:
- Decadron Phosphate Injection 1680
- Decadron Phosphate Sterile Ophthalmic Ointment 1684
- Decadron Phosphate Sterile Ophthalmic Solution 1685
- Decadron Phosphate Topical Cream 1686
- Decadron Phosphate with Xylocaine Injection, Sterile 1683
- Dexacort Phosphate in Respihaler 1606
- Dexacort Phosphate in Turbinaire 1607
- NeoDecadron Sterile Ophthalmic Ointment 1755
- NeoDecadron Sterile Ophthalmic Solution 1756
- NeoDecadron Topical Cream 1757

Dicumarol (Diminishes anticoagulant effect).
- No products indexed under this heading.

Warfarin Sodium (Diminishes anticoagulant effect). Products include:
- Coumadin 941

Food Interactions
Alcohol (Effects of alcohol potentiated).

CYTOGAM
(Cytomegalovirus Immune Globulin) 1630
May interact with:

Measles, Mumps & Rubella Virus Vaccine Live (May interfere with the immune response to live virus vaccine). Products include:
- M-M-R II 1730

CYTOMEL TABLETS
(Liothyronine Sodium) 2647
May interact with oral anticoagulants, insulin, oral hypoglycemic agents, estrogens, oral contraceptives, tricyclic antidepressants, cardiac glycosides, and certain other

(▣ Described in PDR For Nonprescription Drugs) (⊙ Described in PDR For Ophthalmology)

225 **Interactions Index** **Cytosar-U**

agents. Compounds in these categories include:

Acarbose (Possible increase in oral hypoglycemic requirements). Products include:
- Precose ... 604

Amitriptyline Hydrochloride (Enhanced antidepressant and thyroid activities). Products include:
- Elavil ... 2945
- Etrafon ... 2495
- Limbitrol ... 2333
- Triavil Tablets ... 1800

Amoxapine (Enhanced antidepressant and thyroid activities). Products include:
- Asendin Tablets ... 1419

Chlorpropamide (Possible increase in oral hypoglycemic requirements). Products include:
- Diabinese Tablets ... 2002

Cholestyramine (Impaired absorption of T4 and T3). Products include:
- Questran ... 774

Clomipramine Hydrochloride (Enhanced antidepressant and thyroid activities). Products include:
- Anafranil Capsules ... 819

Desipramine Hydrochloride (Enhanced antidepressant and thyroid activities). Products include:
- Norpramin Tablets ... 1273

Deslanoside (Toxic effects of digitalis glycosides potentiated).
- No products indexed under this heading.

Desogestrel (Increases thyroid requirements). Products include:
- Desogen Tablets ... 1867
- Ortho-Cept ... 1907

Dicumarol (Reduction of anticoagulant dosage may be necessary).
- No products indexed under this heading.

Dienestrol (Increases thyroid requirements). Products include:
- Ortho Dienestrol Cream ... 1922

Diethylstilbestrol (Increases thyroid requirements). Products include:
- Diethylstilbestrol Tablets ... 1477

Digitoxin (Toxic effects of digitalis glycosides potentiated). Products include:
- Crystodigin Tablets ... 1472

Digoxin (Toxic effects of digitalis glycosides potentiated). Products include:
- Lanoxicaps ... 1110
- Lanoxin Elixir Pediatric ... 1113
- Lanoxin Injection ... 1116
- Lanoxin Injection Pediatric ... 1119
- Lanoxin Tablets ... 1121

Doxepin Hydrochloride (Enhanced antidepressant and thyroid activities). Products include:
- Adapin Capsules ... 1542
- Sinequan ... 2028
- Zonalon Cream ... 1042

Epinephrine (Increased adrenergic effect; increased risk of precipitating coronary insufficiency). Products include:
- EPIFRIN ... ◉ 237
- EpiPen ... 808
- Marcaine with Epinephrine ... 2446
- Primatene Mist ... 843
- Sensorcaine with Epinephrine Injection ... 554
- Sus-Phrine Injection ... 1017
- Xylocaine with Epinephrine Injections ... 562

Epinephrine Bitartrate (Increased adrenergic effect; increased risk of precipitating coronary insufficiency). Products include:
- Sensorcaine-MPF with Epinephrine Injection ... 554

Estradiol (Increases thyroid requirements). Products include:
- Climara Transdermal System ... 640
- Estrace Cream and Tablets ... 751
- Estraderm Transdermal System ... 842
- Estring Vaginal Ring ... 2086
- Vivelle Transdermal System ... 880

Estrogens, Conjugated (Increases thyroid requirements). Products include:
- PMB 200 and PMB 400 ... 2890
- Premarin Intravenous ... 2893
- Premarin Tablets ... 2896
- Premarin Vaginal Cream ... 2898
- Premphase ... 2900
- Prempro ... 2905

Estrogens, Esterified (Increases thyroid requirements). Products include:
- ESTRATAB Tablets (0.3, 0.625, 1.25, 2.5 mg) ... 2715
- Estratest ... 2718
- Menest Tablets ... 2671

Estropipate (Increases thyroid requirements). Products include:
- Ogen Tablets ... 2103
- Ogen Vaginal Cream ... 2106
- Ortho-Est ... 1925

Ethinyl Estradiol (Increases thyroid requirements). Products include:
- Brevicon ... 2563
- Demulen ... 2580
- Desogen Tablets ... 1867
- Levlen/Tri-Levlen ... 646
- Lo/Ovral Tablets ... 2852
- Lo/Ovral-28 Tablets ... 2857
- Modicon ... 1928
- Nordette-21 Tablets ... 2863
- Nordette-28 Tablets ... 2866
- Norinyl ... 2563
- Ortho-Cept ... 1907
- Ortho-Cyclen/Ortho-Tri-Cyclen ... 1914
- Ortho-Novum ... 1928
- Ortho-Cyclen/Ortho Tri-Cyclen ... 1914
- Ovcon ... 765
- Ovral Tablets ... 2877
- Ovral-28 Tablets ... 2878
- Levlen/Tri-Levlen ... 646
- Tri-Norinyl ... 2607
- Triphasil-21 Tablets ... 2919
- Triphasil-28 Tablets ... 2924

Ethynodiol Diacetate (Increases thyroid requirements). Products include:
- Demulen ... 2580

Glimepiride (Possible increase in oral hypoglycemic requirements). Products include:
- Amaryl Tablets ... 1241

Glipizide (Possible increase in oral hypoglycemic requirements). Products include:
- Glucotrol Tablets ... 2011
- Glucotrol XL Extended Release Tablets ... 2012

Glyburide (Possible increase in oral hypoglycemic requirements). Products include:
- DiaBeta Tablets ... 1265
- Glynase PresTab Tablets ... 2091
- Micronase Tablets ... 2099

Imipramine Hydrochloride (Enhanced antidepressant and thyroid activities). Products include:
- Tofranil Ampuls ... 873
- Tofranil Tablets ... 875

Imipramine Pamoate (Enhanced antidepressant and thyroid activities). Products include:
- Tofranil-PM Capsules ... 876

Insulin, Human (Possible increase in insulin requirements).
- No products indexed under this heading.

Insulin, Human Isophane Suspension (Possible increase in insulin requirements). Products include:
- Novolin N Human Insulin 10 ml Vials ... 1846

Insulin, Human NPH (Possible increase in insulin requirements). Products include:
- Humulin N, 100 Units ... 1495
- Novolin N PenFill 1.5 ml Cartridges Durable Insulin Delivery System ... 1849
- Novolin N Prefilled Syringe Disposable Insulin Delivery System ... 1850

Insulin, Human Regular (Possible increase in insulin requirements). Products include:
- Humulin R, 100 Units ... 1497
- Novolin R Human Insulin 10 ml Vials ... 1846
- Novolin R PenFill 1.5 ml Cartridges Durable Insulin Delivery System ... 1849
- Novolin R Prefilled Syringe Disposable Insulin Delivery System ... 1850
- Velosulin BR Human Insulin 10 ml Vials ... 1847

Insulin, Human, Zinc Suspension (Possible increase in insulin requirements). Products include:
- Humulin L, 100 Units ... 1494
- Humulin U, 100 Units ... 1498
- Novolin L Human Insulin 10 ml Vials ... 1846

Insulin Lispro, Human (Possible increase in insulin requirements). Products include:
- Humalog Injection ... 1488

Insulin, NPH (Possible increase in insulin requirements). Products include:
- NPH, 100 Units ... 1502
- Pork NPH, 100 Units ... 1506
- Purified Pork NPH Isophane Insulin ... 1852

Insulin, Regular (Possible increase in insulin requirements). Products include:
- Regular, 100 Units ... 1503
- Pork Regular, 100 Units ... 1507
- Pork Regular (Concentrated), 500 Units ... 1508
- Purified Pork Regular Insulin ... 1852

Insulin, Zinc Crystals (Possible increase in insulin requirements). Products include:
- NPH, 100 Units ... 1502

Insulin, Zinc Suspension (Possible increase in insulin requirements). Products include:
- Iletin I ... 1501
- Lente, 100 Units ... 1501
- Iletin II ... 1504
- Pork Lente, 100 Units ... 1504
- Purified Pork Lente Insulin ... 1852

Ketamine Hydrochloride (May cause hypertension, and tachycardia).
- No products indexed under this heading.

Levonorgestrel (Increases thyroid requirements). Products include:
- Levlen/Tri-Levlen ... 646
- Nordette-21 Tablets ... 2863
- Nordette-28 Tablets ... 2866
- Norplant System ... 2868
- Levlen/Tri-Levlen ... 646
- Triphasil-21 Tablets ... 2919
- Triphasil-28 Tablets ... 2924

Maprotiline Hydrochloride (Enhanced antidepressant and thyroid activities). Products include:
- Ludiomil Tablets ... 861

Mestranol (Increases thyroid requirements). Products include:
- Norinyl ... 2563
- Ortho-Novum ... 1928

Metformin Hydrochloride (Possible increase in oral hypoglycemic requirements). Products include:
- Glucophage Tablets ... 754

Norepinephrine Bitartrate (Increased adrenergic effect; increased risk of precipitating coronary insufficiency). Products include:
- Levophed Bitartrate Injection ... 2445

Norethindrone (Increases thyroid requirements). Products include:
- Brevicon ... 2563
- Micronor Tablets ... 1903
- Modicon ... 1928
- Norinyl ... 2563
- Nor-Q D Tablets ... 2598
- Ortho-Novum ... 1928
- Ovcon ... 765
- Tri-Norinyl ... 2607

Norethynodrel (Increases thyroid requirements).
- No products indexed under this heading.

Norgestimate (Increases thyroid requirements). Products include:
- Ortho-Cyclen/Ortho-Tri-Cyclen ... 1914
- Ortho-Cyclen/Ortho Tri-Cyclen ... 1914

Norgestrel (Increases thyroid requirements). Products include:
- Lo/Ovral Tablets ... 2852
- Lo/Ovral-28 Tablets ... 2857
- Ovral Tablets ... 2877
- Ovral-28 Tablets ... 2878
- Ovrette Tablets ... 2878

Nortriptyline Hydrochloride (Enhanced antidepressant and thyroid activities). Products include:
- Pamelor ... 2409

Polyestradiol Phosphate (Increases thyroid requirements).
- No products indexed under this heading.

Protriptyline Hydrochloride (Enhanced antidepressant and thyroid activities). Products include:
- Vivactil Tablets ... 1820

Quinestrol (Increases thyroid requirements).
- No products indexed under this heading.

Tolazamide (Possible increase in oral hypoglycemic requirements).
- No products indexed under this heading.

Tolbutamide (Possible increase in oral hypoglycemic requirements).
- No products indexed under this heading.

Trimipramine Maleate (Enhanced antidepressant and thyroid activities). Products include:
- Surmontil Capsules ... 2917

Warfarin Sodium (Reduction of anticoagulant dosage may be necessary). Products include:
- Coumadin ... 941

CYTOSAR-U STERILE POWDER
(Cytarabine) ... 2077

May interact with:

Asparaginase (May result in acute pancreatitis). Products include:
- Elspar ... 1700

Cyclophosphamide (Increased cardiomyopathy). Products include:
- Cytoxan ... 700

Digoxin (A reversible decrease in steady-state plasma digoxin concentrations and renal glycoside excretion in patients receiving beta-acetyl-digoxin and combination chemotherapy regimens). Products include:
- Lanoxicaps ... 1110
- Lanoxin Elixir Pediatric ... 1113
- Lanoxin Injection ... 1116
- Lanoxin Injection Pediatric ... 1119
- Lanoxin Tablets ... 1121

Flucytosine (Possible inhibition of flucytosine efficacy). Products include:
- Ancobon Capsules ... 2254

Gentamicin Sulfate (Possible lack of antibacterial therapeutic response). Products include:
- Garamycin Cream 0.1% ... 2501
- Garamycin Injectable ... 2502

IMPORTANT NOTE: Always consult each drug listing in the patient's regimen for possible interactions.

Garamycin Ointment 0.1% 2501
Garamycin Ophthalmic 2501
Genoptic Sterile Ophthalmic Solution .... ⊙ 241
Genoptic Sterile Ophthalmic Ointment .... ⊙ 241
Gentak .... ⊙ 209
Pred-G Liquifilm Sterile Ophthalmic Suspension .... ⊙ 248
Pred-G S.O.P. Sterile Ophthalmic Ointment .... ⊙ 249

CYTOTEC

(Misoprostol) 2576

May interact with antacids containing aluminium, calcium and magnesium. Compounds in this category include:

Aluminum Carbonate (Total availability of misoprostol is reduced by use of concomitant antacid). Products include:

Basaljel Capsules 2810
Basaljel Suspension 2810
Basaljel Tablets 2810

Aluminum Hydroxide (Total availability of misoprostol is reduced by use of concomitant antacid). Products include:

ALternaGEL Liquid 1358
Maximum Strength Ascriptin .... ▣ 650
Cama Arthritis Pain Reliever .... ▣ 748
Gaviscon Extra Strength Relief Formula Antacid Tablets .... ▣ 778
Gaviscon Extra Strength Relief Formula Liquid Antacid .... ▣ 779
Gaviscon Liquid Antacid .... ▣ 779
Gelusil Antacid-Anti-gas Liquid .... ▣ 819
Gelusil Antacid-Anti-gas Tablets .... ▣ 819
Maalox Antacid/Anti-Gas Tablets 889
Maalox Heartburn Relief Suspension .... ▣ 658
Maalox Antacid Liquid 888
Extra Strength Maalox Antacid/Anti-Gas Liquid and Tablets 888
Mylanta 1359
Tempo Soft Antacid .... ▣ 799

Aluminum Hydroxide Gel (Total availability of misoprostol is reduced by use of concomitant antacid). Products include:

ALternaGEL Liquid .... ▣ 675
Aludrox Oral Suspension .... ▣ 850
Amphojel Suspension 2802
Amphojel Suspension without Flavor 2802
Amphojel Tablets 2802
Ascriptin .... ▣ 650
Gaviscon Antacid Tablets .... ▣ 778
Gaviscon-2 Antacid Tablets .... ▣ 779
Mylanta Liquid .... ▣ 676
Mylanta Double Strength Liquid .... ▣ 676
Nephrox Suspension .... ▣ 671

Magaldrate (Avoid co-administration with magnesium-containing antacids; total availability of misoprostol is reduced by use of concomitant antacid).

No products indexed under this heading.

Magnesium Carbonate (Avoid co-administration with magnesium-containing antacids). Products include:

Bufferin Analgesic Tablets .... ▣ 636
Arthritis Strength Bufferin Analgesic Caplets .... ▣ 637
Extra Strength Bufferin Analgesic Tablets .... ▣ 637
Gaviscon Extra Strength Relief Formula Antacid Tablets .... ▣ 778
Gaviscon Extra Strength Relief Formula Liquid Antacid .... ▣ 779
Gaviscon Liquid Antacid .... ▣ 779
Maalox Antacid Caplets .... ▣ 657
Maalox Heartburn Relief Suspension .... ▣ 658
Mag-Carb Capsules 2168
Marblen .... ▣ 671
One-A-Day Calcium Plus .... ▣ 625

Magnesium Hydroxide (Avoid co-administration with magnesium-containing antacids; total availability of misoprostol is reduced by use of concomitant antacid). Products include:

Aludrox Oral Suspension .... ▣ 850
Ascriptin .... ▣ 650
Di-Gel Antacid/Anti-Gas .... ▣ 762
Gelusil Antacid-Anti-gas Liquid .... ▣ 819
Gelusil Antacid-Anti-gas Tablets .... ▣ 819
Maalox Antacid/Anti-Gas Tablets 889
Maalox Antacid Liquid 888
Extra Strength Maalox Antacid/Anti-Gas Liquid and Tablets 888
Mylanta Fast-Acting 1359
Mylanta Gelcaps Antacid .... ▣ 678
Fast-Acting Mylanta Liquid Antacid 1359
Mylanta Tablets .... ▣ 677
Maximum-Strength Fast-Acting Mylanta Liquid Antacid 1359
Mylanta Double Strength Tablets .... ▣ 677
Phillips' Milk of Magnesia Liquid .... ▣ 627
Rolaids Antacid Tablets .... ▣ 807
Tempo Soft Antacid .... ▣ 799

Magnesium Oxide (Total availability of misoprostol is reduced by use of concomitant antacid). Products include:

Beelith Tablets 632
Bufferin Analgesic Tablets .... ▣ 636
Arthritis Strength Bufferin Analgesic Caplets .... ▣ 637
Extra Strength Bufferin Analgesic Tablets .... ▣ 637
Caltrate PLUS .... ▣ 681
Cama Arthritis Pain Reliever .... ▣ 748
Mag-Ox 400 666
Uro-Mag 666

Food Interactions

Food, unspecified (Diminishes maximum plasma concentrations).

CYTOVENE CAPSULES

(Ganciclovir Sodium) 2270

May interact with drugs inhibiting replication of cell populations of bone marrow, spermatogonia, and germinal layers of skin and gi mucosa, nucleoside analogues, and certain other agents. Compounds in these categories include:

Acyclovir (Potential for additive toxicity). Products include:

Zovirax Capsules 1187
Zovirax Ointment 5% 1190
Zovirax 1187

Acyclovir Sodium (Potential for additive toxicity). Products include:

Zovirax Sterile Powder 1191

Amphotericin B (Potential for additive toxicity; increases in serum creatinine and may result in increased nephrotoxicity). Products include:

Abelcet Injection 1540
Fungizone Intravenous 507
Fungizone Oral Suspension 704

Cilastatin Sodium (Co-administration results in generalized seizures). Products include:

Primaxin I.M. 1770
Primaxin I.V. 1772

Cyclosporine (Increases in serum creatinine and may result in increased nephrotoxicity). Products include:

Neoral 2405
Sandimmune 2416

Dapsone (Potential for additive toxicity). Products include:

Dapsone Tablets USP 1331

Didanosine (When administered concurrently or 2 hours prior to oral Cytovene, the steady-state didanosine AUC$_{0-12}$ increased 111 +/- 114%; a decrease in ganciclovir steady-state AUC of 21 +/- 17%). Products include:

Videx Tablets, Powder for Oral Solution, & Pediatric Powder for Oral Solution 2980

Doxorubicin Hydrochloride (Potential for additive toxicity). Products include:

Adriamycin PFS 2056
Adriamycin RDF 2056
Doxil 2613
Doxorubicin Astra 531
Rubex for Injection 721

Flucytosine (Potential for additive toxicity). Products include:

Ancobon Capsules 2254

Imipenem (Co-administration results in generalized seizures). Products include:

Primaxin I.M. 1770
Primaxin I.V. 1772

Pentamidine Isethionate (Potential for additive toxicity).

No products indexed under this heading.

Probenecid (Increases AUC$_{0-8}$ 53 +/- 91%, decreases renal clearance 22 +/- 20%). Products include:

Benemid Tablets 1651
ColBENEMID Tablets 1662

Sulfamethoxazole (Potential for additive toxicity). Products include:

Bactrim DS Tablets 2257
Bactrim I.V. Infusion 2255
Bactrim 2257
Gantanol Tablets 2285
Septra 1146
Septra I.V. Infusion 1142
Septra I.V. Infusion ADD-Vantage Vials 1144
Septra 1146

Trimethoprim (Potential for additive toxicity). Products include:

Bactrim DS Tablets 2257
Bactrim I.V. Infusion 2255
Bactrim 2257
Proloprim Tablets 1141
Septra 1146
Septra I.V. Infusion 1142
Septra I.V. Infusion ADD-Vantage Vials 1144
Septra 1146
Trimpex Tablets 2323

Vinblastine Sulfate (Potential for additive toxicity). Products include:

Velban Vials 1537

Vincristine Sulfate (Potential for additive toxicity). Products include:

Oncovin Solution Vials & Hyporets 1521

Zidovudine (Man steady-state ganciclovir AUC$_{0-8}$ decreases 17 +/- 25% in presence of zidovudine; steady-state zidovudine AUC$_{0-4}$ increases 19 +/- 27%; both have potential to cause anemia and neutropenia). Products include:

Retrovir Capsules 1216
Retrovir I.V. Infusion 1221
Retrovir Syrup 1216

Food Interactions

Meal, unspecified (Meal containing 46.5% fat increases the steady-state AUC of oral Cytovene by 22% +/- 22% and significant prolongation of time T_{max} and a higher C_{max}).

CYTOVENE-IV

(Ganciclovir Sodium) 2270

See **Cytovene Capsules**

CYTOXAN FOR INJECTION

(Cyclophosphamide) 700

May interact with cytotoxic drugs, general anesthetics, and certain other agents. Compounds in these categories include:

Bleomycin Sulfate (Concurrent use may require reduction in dose of Cytoxan as well as that of other cytotoxic drugs). Products include:

Blenoxane 697

Daunorubicin Hydrochloride (Concurrent use may require reduction in dose of Cytoxan as well as that of other cytotoxic drugs). Products include:

Cerubidine for Injection 634

Doxorubicin Hydrochloride (Potentiation of doxorubicin-induced cardiotoxicity; concurrent use may require reduction in dose of Cytoxan as well as that of other cytotoxic drugs). Products include:

Adriamycin PFS 2056
Adriamycin RDF 2056
Doxil 2613
Doxorubicin Astra 531
Rubex for Injection 721

Enflurane (Anesthesiologist should be alerted if patient has been treated with cyclophosphamide within 10 days).

No products indexed under this heading.

Fluorouracil (Concurrent use may require reduction in dose of Cytoxan as well as that of other cytotoxic drugs). Products include:

Efudex 2280
Fluoroplex Topical Solution & Cream 1% 475
Fluorouracil Injection 2282

Hydroxyurea (Concurrent use may require reduction in dose of Cytoxan as well as that of other cytotoxic drugs). Products include:

Hydrea Capsules 705

Isoflurane (Anesthesiologist should be alerted if patient has been treated with cyclophosphamide within 10 days).

No products indexed under this heading.

Ketamine Hydrochloride (Anesthesiologist should be alerted if patient has been treated with cyclophosphamide within 10 days).

No products indexed under this heading.

Methohexital Sodium (Anesthesiologist should be alerted if patient has been treated with cyclophosphamide within 10 days).

No products indexed under this heading.

Methotrexate Sodium (Concurrent use may require reduction in dose of Cytoxan as well as that of other cytotoxic drugs). Products include:

Methotrexate Sodium Tablets, Injection, for Injection and LPF Injection 1322

Methoxyflurane (Anesthesiologist should be alerted if patient has been treated with cyclophosphamide within 10 days).

No products indexed under this heading.

Mitotane (Concurrent use may require reduction in dose of Cytoxan as well as that of other cytotoxic drugs). Products include:

Lysodren Tablets 707

Mitoxantrone Hydrochloride (Concurrent use may require reduction in dose of Cytoxan as well as that of other cytotoxic drugs). Products include:

Novantrone for Injection 1327

(▣ Described in PDR For Nonprescription Drugs) (⊙ Described in PDR For Ophthalmology)

Interactions Index

Phenobarbital (Increased rate of metabolism and leukopenic activity of cyclophosphamide). Products include:
- Arco-Lase Plus Tablets ... 513
- Bellergal-S Tablets ... 2375
- Donnatal ... 2234
- Donnatal Extentabs ... 2234
- Donnatal Tablets ... 2234
- Phenobarbital Elixir and Tablets ... 1523
- Quadrinal Tablets ... 1398

Procarbazine Hydrochloride (Concurrent use may require reduction in dose of Cytoxan as well as that of other cytotoxic drugs). Products include:
- Matulane Capsules ... 2300

Propofol (Anesthesiologist should be alerted if patient has been treated with cyclophosphamide within 10 days). Products include:
- Diprivan Injectable Emulsion ... 2939

Sevoflurane (Anesthesiologist should be alerted if patient has been treated with cyclophosphamide within 10 days).
- No products indexed under this heading.

Succinylcholine Chloride (Inhibition of cholinesterase activity and potentiation of succinylcholine chloride's effect). Products include:
- Anectine ... 1062

Tamoxifen Citrate (Concurrent use may require reduction in dose of Cytoxan as well as that of other cytotoxic drugs). Products include:
- Nolvadex Tablets ... 2957

Vincristine Sulfate (Concurrent use may require reduction in dose of Cytoxan as well as that of other cytotoxic drugs). Products include:
- Oncovin Solution Vials & Hyporets ... 1521

CYTOXAN TABLETS
(Cyclophosphamide) ... 700
See **Cytoxan for Injection**

D.A. II TABLETS
(Chlorpheniramine Maleate, Methscopolamine Nitrate, Phenylephrine Hydrochloride) ... 972
See **Dura-Vent/DA Tablets**

D.A. CHEWABLE TABLETS
(Chlorpheniramine Maleate, Phenylephrine Hydrochloride, Methscopolamine Nitrate) ... 970
May interact with monoamine oxidase inhibitors, beta blockers, hypnotics and sedatives, tricyclic antidepressants, barbiturates, central nervous system depressants, tranquilizers, and certain other agents. Compounds in these categories include:

Acebutolol Hydrochloride (Increases the effects of sympathomimetics). Products include:
- Sectral Capsules ... 2914

Alfentanil Hydrochloride (Potential for additive effects). Products include:
- Alfenta Injection ... 1334

Alprazolam (Potential for additive effects). Products include:
- Xanax Tablets ... 2115

Amitriptyline Hydrochloride (Potential for additive effects). Products include:
- Elavil ... 2945
- Etrafon ... 2495
- Limbitrol ... 2333
- Triavil Tablets ... 1800

Amoxapine (Potential for additive effects). Products include:
- Asendin Tablets ... 1419

Aprobarbital (Potential for additive effects).
- No products indexed under this heading.

Atenolol (Increases the effects of sympathomimetics). Products include:
- Tenoretic Tablets ... 2963
- Tenormin Tablets and I.V. Injection ... 2965

Betaxolol Hydrochloride (Increases the effects of sympathomimetics). Products include:
- Betoptic Ophthalmic Solution ... 465
- Betoptic S Ophthalmic Suspension ... 467
- Kerlone Tablets ... 2588

Bisoprolol Fumarate (Increases the effects of sympathomimetics). Products include:
- Zebeta Tablets ... 1457
- Ziac ... 1459

Buprenorphine (Potential for additive effects). Products include:
- Buprenex Injectable ... 2170

Buspirone Hydrochloride (Potential for additive effects). Products include:
- BuSpar Tablets ... 738

Butabarbital (Potential for additive effects).
- No products indexed under this heading.

Butalbital (Potential for additive effects). Products include:
- Axocet Capsules ... 2469
- Esgic-plus Capsules ... 1012
- Esgic-plus Tablets ... 1012
- Fioricet Tablets ... 2386
- Fioricet with Codeine Capsules ... 2387
- Fiorinal Capsules ... 2388
- Fiorinal with Codeine Capsules ... 2390
- Fiorinal Tablets ... 2388
- Phrenilin ... 790
- Sedapap Tablets 50 mg/650 mg ... 1826

Carteolol Hydrochloride (Increases the effects of sympathomimetics). Products include:
- Cartrol Tablets ... 413
- Ocupress Ophthalmic Solution, 1% Sterile ... ⊙ 297

Chlordiazepoxide (Potential for additive effects). Products include:
- Limbitrol ... 2333

Chlordiazepoxide Hydrochloride (Potential for additive effects). Products include:
- Librax Capsules ... 2330
- Librium Capsules ... 2331
- Librium Injectable ... 2332

Chlorpromazine (Potential for additive effects). Products include:
- Thorazine Suppositories ... 2701

Chlorpromazine Hydrochloride (Potential for additive effects). Products include:
- Thorazine ... 2701

Chlorprothixene (Potential for additive effects).
- No products indexed under this heading.

Chlorprothixene Hydrochloride (Potential for additive effects).
- No products indexed under this heading.

Chlorprothixene Lactate (Potential for additive effects).
- No products indexed under this heading.

Clomipramine Hydrochloride (Potential for additive effects). Products include:
- Anafranil Capsules ... 819

Clorazepate Dipotassium (Potential for additive effects). Products include:
- Tranxene ... 459

Clozapine (Potential for additive effects). Products include:
- Clozaril Tablets ... 2377

Codeine Phosphate (Potential for additive effects). Products include:
- Brontex ... 2130
- Dimetane-DC Cough Syrup ... 2232
- Fioricet with Codeine Capsules ... 2387
- Fiorinal with Codeine Capsules ... 2390
- Nucofed ... 2225
- Phenergan with Codeine ... 2883
- Phenergan VC with Codeine ... 2888
- Robitussin A-C Syrup ... 2248
- Robitussin-DAC Syrup ... 2249
- Ryna ... ⊙ 804
- Soma Compound w/Codeine Tablets ... 2784
- Tylenol with Codeine ... 1592

Desflurane (Potential for additive effects). Products include:
- Suprane (desflurane, USP) ... 1865

Desipramine Hydrochloride (Potential for additive effects). Products include:
- Norpramin Tablets ... 1273

Dezocine (Potential for additive effects). Products include:
- Dalgan Injection ... 529

Diazepam (Potential for additive effects). Products include:
- Dizac (diazepam injectable emulsion) CIV ... 1862
- Valium Injectable ... 2336
- Valium Tablets ... 2335

Doxepin Hydrochloride (Potential for additive effects). Products include:
- Adapin Capsules ... 1542
- Sinequan ... 2028
- Zonalon Cream ... 1042

Droperidol (Potential for additive effects). Products include:
- Inapsine Injection ... 462

Enflurane (Potential for additive effects).
- No products indexed under this heading.

Esmolol Hydrochloride (Increases the effects of sympathomimetics). Products include:
- Brevibloc (esmolol HCl) Injection ... 1860

Estazolam (Potential for additive effects). Products include:
- ProSom Tablets ... 457

Ethchlorvynol (Potential for additive effects). Products include:
- Placidyl Capsules ... 456

Ethinamate (Potential for additive effects).
- No products indexed under this heading.

Fentanyl (Potential for additive effects). Products include:
- Duragesic Transdermal System ... 1336

Fentanyl Citrate (Potential for additive effects). Products include:
- Sublimaze Injection ... 463

Fluphenazine Decanoate (Potential for additive effects). Products include:
- Prolixin Decanoate ... 510

Fluphenazine Enanthate (Potential for additive effects). Products include:
- Prolixin Enanthate ... 510

Fluphenazine Hydrochloride (Potential for additive effects). Products include:
- Prolixin ... 510

Flurazepam Hydrochloride (Potential for additive effects). Products include:
- Dalmane Capsules ... 2329

Furazolidone (Increases the effects of sympathomimetics; concurrent and/or sequential use is contraindicated). Products include:
- Furoxone ... 2221

Glutethimide (Potential for additive effects).
- No products indexed under this heading.

Haloperidol (Potential for additive effects). Products include:
- Haldol Injection, Tablets and Concentrate ... 1585

Haloperidol Decanoate (Potential for additive effects). Products include:
- Haldol Decanoate ... 1587

Hydrocodone Bitartrate (Potential for additive effects). Products include:
- Codiclear DH Syrup ... 808
- Duratuss HD Elixir ... 2750
- Histussin D Liquid ... 670
- Hycodan Tablets and Syrup ... 946
- Hycomine Compound Tablets ... 948
- Hycomine ... 947
- Hycotuss Expectorant Syrup ... 950
- Hydrocet Capsules ... 787
- Lorcet 10/650 Tablets ... 1016
- Lortab ... 2751
- Tussend ... 1830
- Tussend Expectorant ... 1831
- Vicodin Tablets ... 1404
- Vicodin ES Tablets ... 1405
- Vicodin HP Tablets ... 1403
- Vicodin Tuss Expectorant ... 1406
- Zydone Capsules ... 967

Hydrocodone Polistirex (Potential for additive effects). Products include:
- Tussionex Pennkinetic Extended-Release Suspension ... 1624

Hydroxyzine Hydrochloride (Potential for additive effects). Products include:
- Atarax Tablets & Syrup ... 1992
- Marax Tablets & DF Syrup ... 2015
- Vistaril Intramuscular Solution ... 2042

Imipramine Hydrochloride (Potential for additive effects). Products include:
- Tofranil Ampuls ... 873
- Tofranil Tablets ... 875

Imipramine Pamoate (Potential for additive effects). Products include:
- Tofranil-PM Capsules ... 876

Isocarboxazid (Increases the effects of sympathomimetics; concurrent and/or sequential use is contraindicated).
- No products indexed under this heading.

Isoflurane (Potential for additive effects).
- No products indexed under this heading.

Ketamine Hydrochloride (Potential for additive effects).
- No products indexed under this heading.

Labetalol Hydrochloride (Increases the effects of sympathomimetics). Products include:
- Normodyne Injection ... 2519
- Normodyne Tablets ... 2522
- Trandate ... 1158

Levobunolol Hydrochloride (Increases the effects of sympathomimetics). Products include:
- Betagan ... ⊙ 230

Levorphanol Tartrate (Potential for additive effects). Products include:
- Levo-Dromoran ... 2297

Lorazepam (Potential for additive effects). Products include:
- Ativan Injection ... 2805
- Ativan Tablets ... 2807

Loxapine Hydrochloride (Potential for additive effects). Products include:
- Loxitane ... 1426

Loxapine Succinate (Potential for additive effects). Products include:
- Loxitane Capsules ... 1426

IMPORTANT NOTE: Always consult each drug listing in the patient's regimen for possible interactions.

D.A. Chewable Interactions Index 228

Maprotiline Hydrochloride (Potential for additive effects). Products include:
- Ludiomil Tablets ... 861

Mecamylamine Hydrochloride (Sympathomimetic may reduce the antihypertensive effects). Products include:
- Inversine Tablets ... 1729

Meperidine Hydrochloride (Potential for additive effects). Products include:
- Demerol ... 2438
- Mepergan Injection ... 2859

Mephobarbital (Potential for additive effects). Products include:
- Mebaral Tablets ... 2452

Meprobamate (Potential for additive effects). Products include:
- Miltown Tablets ... 2780
- PMB 200 and PMB 400 ... 2890

Mesoridazine Besylate (Potential for additive effects). Products include:
- Serentil ... 689

Methadone Hydrochloride (Potential for additive effects). Products include:
- Methadone Hydrochloride Oral Concentrate ... 2356
- Methadone Hydrochloride Oral Solution & Tablets ... 2357

Methohexital Sodium (Potential for additive effects).
- No products indexed under this heading.

Methotrimeprazine (Potential for additive effects). Products include:
- Levoprome ... 1321

Methoxyflurane (Potential for additive effects).
- No products indexed under this heading.

Methyldopa (Sympathomimetic may reduce the antihypertensive effects). Products include:
- Aldoclor Tablets ... 1638
- Aldomet Oral ... 1640
- Aldoril Tablets ... 1644

Methyldopate Hydrochloride (Sympathomimetic may reduce the antihypertensive effects). Products include:
- Aldomet Ester HCl Injection ... 1642

Metipranolol Hydrochloride (Increases the effects of sympathomimetics). Products include:
- OptiPranolol (Metipranolol 0.3%) Sterile Ophthalmic Solution ... ⊙ 256

Metoprolol Succinate (Increases the effects of sympathomimetics). Products include:
- Toprol-XL Tablets ... 560

Metoprolol Tartrate (Increases the effects of sympathomimetics). Products include:
- Lopressor ... 848
- Lopressor HCT Tablets ... 850

Midazolam Hydrochloride (Potential for additive effects). Products include:
- Versed Injection ... 2324

Molindone Hydrochloride (Potential for additive effects). Products include:
- Moban Tablets and Concentrate ... 1036

Morphine Sulfate (Potential for additive effects). Products include:
- Astramorph/PF Injection, USP (Preservative-Free) ... 526
- Duramorph Injection ... 983
- Infumorph 200 and Infumorph 500 Sterile Solutions ... 985
- Kadian Capsules ... 2948
- MS Contin Tablets ... 2149
- MSIR ... 2152
- Oramorph SR (Morphine Sulfate Sustained Release Tablets) ... 2359
- RMS Suppositories CII ... 2766
- Roxanol ... 2365

Nadolol (Increases the effects of sympathomimetics).
- No products indexed under this heading.

Nortriptyline Hydrochloride (Potential for additive effects). Products include:
- Pamelor ... 2409

Opium Alkaloids (Potential for additive effects).
- No products indexed under this heading.

Oxazepam (Potential for additive effects). Products include:
- Serax Capsules ... 2916
- Serax Tablets ... 2916

Oxycodone Hydrochloride (Potential for additive effects). Products include:
- OxyContin Tablets ... 2163
- OxyIR Capsules ... 2167
- Percocet Tablets ... 955
- Percodan Tablets ... 955
- Percodan-Demi Tablets ... 956
- Roxicodone Tablets, Oral Solution & Intensol (Oxycodone) ... 2366
- Tylox Capsules ... 1593

Penbutolol Sulfate (Increases the effects of sympathomimetics). Products include:
- Levatol Tablets ... 2547

Pentobarbital Sodium (Potential for additive effects). Products include:
- Nembutal Sodium Capsules ... 440
- Nembutal Sodium Solution ... 442
- Nembutal Sodium Suppositories ... 444

Perphenazine (Potential for additive effects). Products include:
- Etrafon ... 2495
- Triavil Tablets ... 1800
- Trilafon ... 2532

Phenelzine Sulfate (Increases the effects of sympathomimetics; concurrent and/or sequential use is contraindicated). Products include:
- Nardil ... 1977

Phenobarbital (Potential for additive effects). Products include:
- Arco-Lase Plus Tablets ... 513
- Bellergal-S Tablets ... 2375
- Donnatal ... 2234
- Donnatal Extentabs ... 2234
- Donnatal Tablets ... 2234
- Phenobarbital Elixir and Tablets ... 1523
- Quadrinal Tablets ... 1398

Pindolol (Increases the effects of sympathomimetics). Products include:
- Visken Tablets ... 2428

Prazepam (Potential for additive effects).
- No products indexed under this heading.

Prochlorperazine (Potential for additive effects). Products include:
- Compazine ... 2644

Promethazine Hydrochloride (Potential for additive effects). Products include:
- Mepergan Injection ... 2859
- Phenergan with Codeine ... 2883
- Phenergan with Dextromethorphan ... 2885
- Phenergan Injection ... 2880
- Phenergan Suppositories ... 2882
- Phenergan Syrup ... 2881
- Phenergan Tablets ... 2882
- Phenergan VC ... 2886
- Phenergan VC with Codeine ... 2888

Propofol (Potential for additive effects). Products include:
- Diprivan Injectable Emulsion ... 2939

Propoxyphene Hydrochloride (Potential for additive effects). Products include:
- Darvon ... 1475
- Wygesic Tablets ... 2930

Propoxyphene Napsylate (Potential for additive effects). Products include:
- Darvon-N/Darvocet-N ... 1473

Propranolol Hydrochloride (Increases the effects of sympathomimetics). Products include:
- Inderal ... 2834
- Inderal LA Long Acting Capsules ... 2836
- Inderide Tablets ... 2838
- Inderide LA Long Acting Capsules ... 2840

Protriptyline Hydrochloride (Potential for additive effects). Products include:
- Vivactil Tablets ... 1820

Quazepam (Potential for additive effects). Products include:
- Doral Tablets ... 2773

Reserpine (Sympathomimetic may reduce the antihypertensive effects). Products include:
- Diupres Tablets ... 1691
- Hydropres Tablets ... 1718
- Ser-Ap-Es Tablets ... 867

Risperidone (Potential for additive effects). Products include:
- Risperdal Tablets ... 1348

Secobarbital Sodium (Potential for additive effects). Products include:
- Seconal Sodium Pulvules ... 1529

Selegiline Hydrochloride (Increases the effects of sympathomimetics; concurrent and/or sequential use is contraindicated). Products include:
- Eldepryl Capsules ... 2729

Sevoflurane (Potential for additive effects).
- No products indexed under this heading.

Sotalol Hydrochloride (Increases the effects of sympathomimetics). Products include:
- Betapace Tablets ... 637

Sufentanil Citrate (Potential for additive effects). Products include:
- Sufenta Injection ... 1355

Temazepam (Potential for additive effects). Products include:
- Restoril Capsules ... 2413

Thiamylal Sodium (Potential for additive effects).
- No products indexed under this heading.

Thioridazine Hydrochloride (Potential for additive effects). Products include:
- Mellaril ... 2398

Thiothixene (Potential for additive effects). Products include:
- Navane Capsules and Concentrate ... 2018
- Navane Intramuscular ... 2019

Timolol Maleate (Increases the effects of sympathomimetics). Products include:
- Blocadren Tablets ... 1654
- Timolide Tablets ... 1791
- Timoptic in Ocudose ... 1796
- Timoptic Sterile Ophthalmic Solution ... 1794
- Timoptic-XE ... 1798

Tranylcypromine Sulfate (Increases the effects of sympathomimetics; concurrent and/or sequential use is contraindicated). Products include:
- Parnate Tablets ... 2679

Triazolam (Potential for additive effects). Products include:
- Halcion Tablets ... 2093

Trifluoperazine Hydrochloride (Potential for additive effects). Products include:
- Stelazine ... 2692

Trimipramine Maleate (Potential for additive effects). Products include:
- Surmontil Capsules ... 2917

Zolpidem Tartrate (Potential for additive effects). Products include:
- Ambien Tablets ... 2559

Food Interactions

Alcohol (Potential for additive effects).

DDAVP INJECTION

(Desmopressin Acetate) ... 2178

May interact with vasopressors. Compounds in this category include:

Dopamine Hydrochloride (Possible additive effects; use only with careful monitoring).
- No products indexed under this heading.

Epinephrine Hydrochloride (Possible additive effects; use only with careful monitoring). Products include:
- Ana-Kit Anaphylaxis Emergency Treatment Kit ... 611

Metaraminol Bitartrate (Possible additive effects; use only with careful monitoring). Products include:
- Aramine Injection ... 1649

Methoxamine Hydrochloride (Possible additive effects; use only with careful monitoring). Products include:
- Vasoxyl Injection ... 1169

Norepinephrine Bitartrate (Possible additive effects; use only with careful monitoring). Products include:
- Levophed Bitartrate Injection ... 2445

Phenylephrine Hydrochloride (Possible additive effects; use only with careful monitoring). Products include:
- Atrohist Plus Tablets ... 1605
- Cerose DM ... ▣ 853
- D.A. II Tablets ... 972
- D.A. Chewable Tablets ... 970
- Dura-Vent/DA Tablets ... 972
- Extendryl ... 1003
- 4-Way Fast Acting Nasal Spray (regular & mentholated) ... ▣ 644
- Hemorid ... ▣ 797
- Hycomine Compound Tablets ... 948
- Neo-Synephrine Hydrochloride 1% Carpuject ... 2455
- Neo-Synephrine Hydrochloride 1% Injection ... 2455
- Neo-Synephrine Hydrochloride (Ophthalmic) ... 2456
- Neo-Synephrine ... ▣ 624
- Novahistine Elixir ... ▣ 782
- Phenergan VC ... 2886
- Phenergan VC with Codeine ... 2888
- Preparation H ... ▣ 842
- Tympagesic Ear Drops ... 2476
- Vicks Sinex Nasal Spray and Ultra Fine Mist ... ▣ 738

DDAVP INJECTION 15 MCG/ML

(Desmopressin Acetate) ... 2179

May interact with vasopressors. Compounds in this category include:

Dopamine Hydrochloride (Use of doses as large as 0.3ug/kg of DDAVP with other vasopressor agents should be done only with careful patient monitoring).
- No products indexed under this heading.

Epinephrine Bitartrate (Use of doses as large as 0.3ug/kg of DDAVP with other vasopressor agents should be done only with careful patient monitoring). Products include:
- Sensorcaine-MPF with Epinephrine Injection ... 554

Epinephrine Hydrochloride (Use of doses as large as 0.3ug/kg of DDAVP with other vasopressor agents should be done only with careful patient monitoring). Products include:
- Ana-Kit Anaphylaxis Emergency Treatment Kit ... 611

(▣ Described in PDR For Nonprescription Drugs) (⊙ Described in PDR For Ophthalmology)

Metaraminol Bitartrate (Use of doses as large as 0.3ug/kg of DDAVP with other vasopressor agents should be done only with careful patient monitoring). Products include:

Aramine Injection 1649

Methoxamine Hydrochloride (Use of doses as large as 0.3ug/kg of DDAVP with other vasopressor agents should be done only with careful patient monitoring). Products include:

Vasoxyl Injection 1169

Norepinephrine Bitartrate (Use of doses as large as 0.3ug/kg of DDAVP with other vasopressor agents should be done only with careful patient monitoring). Products include:

Levophed Bitartrate Injection 2445

Phenylephrine Hydrochloride (Use of doses as large as 0.3ug/kg of DDAVP with other vasopressor agents should be done only with careful patient monitoring). Products include:

Atrohist Plus Tablets 1605
Cerose DM 853
D.A. II Tablets 972
D.A. Chewable Tablets 970
Dura-Vent/DA Tablets 972
Extendryl 1003
4-Way Fast Acting Nasal Spray (regular & mentholated) 644
Hemorid 797
Hycomine Compound Tablets 948
Neo-Synephrine Hydrochloride 1% Carpuject 2455
Neo-Synephrine Hydrochloride 1% Injection 2455
Neo-Synephrine Hydrochloride (Ophthalmic) 2456
Neo-Synephrine 624
Novahistine Elixir 782
Phenergan VC 2886
Phenergan VC with Codeine 2888
Preparation H 842
Tympagesic Ear Drops 2476
Vicks Sinex Nasal Spray and Ultra Fine Mist 738

DDAVP NASAL SPRAY

(Desmopressin Acetate) 2180
See **DDAVP Rhinal Tube**

DDAVP RHINAL TUBE

(Desmopressin Acetate) 2180
May interact with vasopressors. Compounds in this category include:

Dopamine Hydrochloride (Possible additive effects; use only with careful monitoring).

No products indexed under this heading.

Epinephrine Hydrochloride (Possible additive effects; use only with careful monitoring). Products include:

Ana-Kit Anaphylaxis Emergency Treatment Kit 611

Metaraminol Bitartrate (Possible additive effects; use only with careful monitoring). Products include:

Aramine Injection 1649

Methoxamine Hydrochloride (Possible additive effects; use only with careful monitoring). Products include:

Vasoxyl Injection 1169

Norepinephrine Bitartrate (Possible additive effects; use only with careful monitoring). Products include:

Levophed Bitartrate Injection 2445

Phenylephrine Hydrochloride (Possible additive effects; use only with careful monitoring). Products include:

Atrohist Plus Tablets 1605
Cerose DM 853
D.A. II Tablets 972
D.A. Chewable Tablets 970
Dura-Vent/DA Tablets 972
Extendryl 1003
4-Way Fast Acting Nasal Spray (regular & mentholated) 644
Hemorid 797
Hycomine Compound Tablets 948
Neo-Synephrine Hydrochloride 1% Carpuject 2455
Neo-Synephrine Hydrochloride 1% Injection 2455
Neo-Synephrine Hydrochloride (Ophthalmic) 2456
Neo-Synephrine 624
Novahistine Elixir 782
Phenergan VC 2886
Phenergan VC with Codeine 2888
Preparation H 842
Tympagesic Ear Drops 2476
Vicks Sinex Nasal Spray and Ultra Fine Mist 738

DDAVP TABLETS

(Desmopressin Acetate) 2182
May interact with vasopressors. Compounds in this category include:

Dopamine Hydrochloride (Although the pressor activity of DDAVP is very low, large doses of DDAVP tablets should be used with other vasopressor agents only with careful patient monitoring).

No products indexed under this heading.

Epinephrine Bitartrate (Although the pressor activity of DDAVP is very low, large doses of DDAVP tablets should be used with other vasopressor agents only with careful patient monitoring). Products include:

Sensorcaine-MPF with Epinephrine Injection 554

Epinephrine Hydrochloride (Although the pressor activity of DDAVP is very low, large doses of DDAVP tablets should be used with other vasopressor agents only with careful patient monitoring). Products include:

Ana-Kit Anaphylaxis Emergency Treatment Kit 611

Metaraminol Bitartrate (Although the pressor activity of DDAVP is very low, large doses of DDAVP tablets should be used with other vasopressor agents only with careful patient monitoring). Products include:

Aramine Injection 1649

Methoxamine Hydrochloride (Although the pressor activity of DDAVP is very low, large doses of DDAVP tablets should be used with other vasopressor agents only with careful patient monitoring). Products include:

Vasoxyl Injection 1169

Norepinephrine Bitartrate (Although the pressor activity of DDAVP is very low, large doses of DDAVP tablets should be used with other vasopressor agents only with careful patient monitoring). Products include:

Levophed Bitartrate Injection 2445

Phenylephrine Hydrochloride (Although the pressor activity of DDAVP is very low, large doses of DDAVP tablets should be used with other vasopressor agents only with careful patient monitoring). Products include:

Atrohist Plus Tablets 1605
Cerose DM 853
D.A. II Tablets 972
D.A. Chewable Tablets 970
Dura-Vent/DA Tablets 972
Extendryl 1003
4-Way Fast Acting Nasal Spray (regular & mentholated) 644
Hemorid 797
Hycomine Compound Tablets 948
Neo-Synephrine Hydrochloride 1% Carpuject 2455
Neo-Synephrine Hydrochloride 1% Injection 2455
Neo-Synephrine Hydrochloride (Ophthalmic) 2456
Neo-Synephrine 624
Novahistine Elixir 782
Phenergan VC 2886
Phenergan VC with Codeine 2888
Preparation H 842
Tympagesic Ear Drops 2476
Vicks Sinex Nasal Spray and Ultra Fine Mist 738

DDS-ACIDOPHILUS

(Lactobacillus Acidophilus) 800
None cited in PDR database.

DHC PLUS CAPSULES

(Dihydrocodeine Bitartrate, Acetaminophen, Caffeine) 2148
May interact with central nervous system depressants, beta-adrenergic stimulating agents, fluoroquinolone antibiotics, and certain other agents. Compounds in these categories include:

Albuterol (Caffeine may enhance the cardiac inotropic effects of beta-adrenergic stimulating agents). Products include:

Proventil Inhalation Aerosol 2524
Ventolin Inhalation Aerosol and Refill 1170

Albuterol Sulfate (Caffeine may enhance the cardiac inotropic effects of beta-adrenergic stimulating agents). Products include:

Airet Albuterol Sulfate Inhalation Solution 1602
Albuterol Sulfate, USP Solution for Inhalation, Arm-a-Med 522
Proventil Inhalation Solution 0.083% 2527
Proventil Repetabs Tablets 2529
Proventil Solution for Inhalation 0.5% 2525
Proventil Syrup 2528
Proventil Tablets 2529
Ventolin Inhalation Solution 1171
Ventolin Nebules Inhalation Solution 1172
Ventolin Rotacaps for Inhalation 1173
Ventolin Syrup 1175
Ventolin Tablets 1176
Volmax Extended-Release Tablets 1835

Alfentanil Hydrochloride (Potential for additive CNS depression). Products include:

Alfenta Injection 1334

Alprazolam (Potential for additive CNS depression). Products include:

Xanax Tablets 2115

Aprobarbital (Potential for additive CNS depression).

No products indexed under this heading.

Aspirin (Caffeine may increase the metabolism of aspirin). Products include:

Alka-Seltzer Cherry Effervescent Antacid and Pain Reliever 609
Alka-Seltzer Extra Strength Effervescent Antacid and Pain Reliever 609
Alka-Seltzer Lemon Lime Effervescent Antacid and Pain Reliever 609
Alka-Seltzer Original Effervescent Antacid and Pain Reliever 609
Alka-Seltzer Plus 611
Alka-Seltzer Plus Sinus Medicine 611
Ascriptin 650
Arthritis Strength BC Powder 631
BC Cold Powder Multi-Symptom Formula (Cold-Sinus-Allergy) 631
BC Cold Powder Non-Drowsy Formula (Cold-Sinus) 631
BC Powder 631
Genuine Bayer Aspirin Tablets & Caplets 618
Extra Strength Bayer Arthritis Pain Regimen Formula 615
Extra Strength Bayer Aspirin Caplets & Tablets 617
Extended-Release Bayer 8-Hour Aspirin 616
Extra Strength Bayer Plus Aspirin Caplets 617
Extra Strength Bayer PM Aspirin Plus Sleep Aid 617
Aspirin Regimen Bayer 81 mg Tablets with Calcium 615
Aspirin Regimen Bayer Adult Low Strength 81 mg Tablets 613
Aspirin Regimen Bayer Children's Chewable Aspirin 616
Aspirin Regimen Bayer Regular Strength 325 mg Caplets 613
Bufferin Analgesic Tablets 636
Arthritis Strength Bufferin Analgesic Caplets 637
Extra Strength Bufferin Analgesic Tablets 637
Cama Arthritis Pain Reliever 748
Darvon Compound-65 Pulvules 1475
Easprin 1971
Ecotrin 2625
Ecotrin Enteric Coated Aspirin Maximum Strength Tablets and Caplets 775
Ecotrin Enteric Coated Aspirin Regular Strength Tablets 2625
Empirin Aspirin Tablets 818
Excedrin Extra-Strength Analgesic Tablets, Caplets, and Geltabs 734
Fiorinal Capsules 2388
Fiorinal with Codeine Capsules 2390
Fiorinal Tablets 2388
Goody's Extra Strength Headache Powders 632
Goody's Extra Strength Pain Relief Tablets 632
Halfprin Tablets 1413
Norgesic 1554
Percodan Tablets 955
Percodan-Demi Tablets 956
Robaxisal Tablets 2246
Soma Compound w/Codeine Tablets 2784
Soma Compound Tablets 2783
St. Joseph Adult Chewable Aspirin (81 mg.) 768
Talwin Compound 2466
Vanquish Analgesic Caplets 627

Bitolterol Mesylate (Caffeine may enhance the cardiac inotropic effects of beta-adrenergic stimulating agents). Products include:

Tornalate Solution for Inhalation, 0.2% 976
Tornalate Metered Dose Inhaler 978

Buprenorphine (Potential for additive CNS depression). Products include:

Buprenex Injectable 2170

Buspirone Hydrochloride (Potential for additive CNS depression). Products include:

BuSpar Tablets 738

Butabarbital (Potential for additive CNS depression).

No products indexed under this heading.

Butalbital (Potential for additive CNS depression). Products include:

Axocet Capsules 2469
Esgic-plus Capsules 1012
Esgic-plus Tablets 1012
Fioricet Tablets 2386
Fioricet with Codeine Capsules 2387
Fiorinal Capsules 2388
Fiorinal with Codeine Capsules 2390
Fiorinal Tablets 2388
Phrenilin 790
Sedapap Tablets 50 mg/650 mg 1826

Chlordiazepoxide (Potential for additive CNS depression). Products include:

Limbitrol 2333

Chlordiazepoxide Hydrochloride (Potential for additive CNS depression). Products include:

Librax Capsules 2330
Librium Capsules 2331
Librium Injectable 2332

IMPORTANT NOTE: Always consult each drug listing in the patient's regimen for possible interactions.

DHC Plus | Interactions Index | 230

Chlorpromazine (Potential for additive CNS depression). Products include:
- Thorazine Suppositories 2701

Chlorpromazine Hydrochloride (Potential for additive CNS depression). Products include:
- Thorazine 2701

Chlorprothixene (Potential for additive CNS depression).
- No products indexed under this heading.

Chlorprothixene Hydrochloride (Potential for additive CNS depression).
- No products indexed under this heading.

Chlorprothixene Lactate (Potential for additive CNS depression).
- No products indexed under this heading.

Ciprofloxacin (Concomitant use may result in caffeine accumulation when DHC Plus is consumed with quinolones). Products include:
- Cipro I.V. 587
- Cipro I.V. Pharmacy Bulk Package .. 590

Ciprofloxacin Hydrochloride (Concomitant use may result in caffeine accumulation when DHC Plus is consumed with quinolones). Products include:
- Ciloxan Ophthalmic Solution 468
- Cipro Tablets 584

Clorazepate Dipotassium (Potential for additive CNS depression). Products include:
- Tranxene 459

Clozapine (Potential for additive CNS depression). Products include:
- Clozaril Tablets 2377

Codeine Phosphate (Potential for additive CNS depression). Products include:
- Brontex 2130
- Dimetane-DC Cough Syrup 2232
- Fioricet with Codeine Capsules 2387
- Fiorinal with Codeine Capsules 2390
- Nucofed 2225
- Phenergan with Codeine 2883
- Phenergan VC with Codeine 2888
- Robitussin A-C Syrup 2248
- Robitussin-DAC Syrup 2249
- Ryna ..... ⊞ 804
- Soma Compound w/Codeine Tablets 2784
- Tylenol with Codeine 1592

Desflurane (Potential for additive CNS depression). Products include:
- Suprane (desflurane, USP) 1865

Dezocine (Potential for additive CNS depression). Products include:
- Dalgan Injection 529

Diazepam (Potential for additive CNS depression). Products include:
- Dizac (diazepam injectable emulsion) CIV 1862
- Valium Injectable 2336
- Valium Tablets 2335

Disulfiram (Co-administration may lead to a substantial decrease in caffeine clearance). Products include:
- Antabuse Tablets 2802

Droperidol (Potential for additive CNS depression). Products include:
- Inapsine Injection 462

Enflurane (Potential for additive CNS depression).
- No products indexed under this heading.

Enoxacin (Concomitant use may result in caffeine accumulation when DHC Plus is consumed with quinolones). Products include:
- Penetrex Tablets 2196

Ephedrine Hydrochloride (Caffeine may enhance the cardiac inotropic effects of beta-adrenergic stimulating agents). Products include:
- Primatene Tablets ..... ⊞ 844
- Quadrinal Tablets 1398

Ephedrine Sulfate (Caffeine may enhance the cardiac inotropic effects of beta-adrenergic stimulating agents). Products include:
- Marax Tablets & DF Syrup 2015

Ephedrine Tannate (Caffeine may enhance the cardiac inotropic effects of beta-adrenergic stimulating agents). Products include:
- Rynatuss 2782

Epinephrine (Caffeine may enhance the cardiac inotropic effects of beta-adrenergic stimulating agents). Products include:
- EPIFRIN ..... ⊙ 237
- EpiPen 808
- Marcaine with Epinephrine 2446
- Primatene Mist ..... ⊞ 843
- Sensorcaine with Epinephrine Injection 554
- Sus-Phrine Injection 1017
- Xylocaine with Epinephrine Injections 562

Epinephrine Hydrochloride (Caffeine may enhance the cardiac inotropic effects of beta-adrenergic stimulating agents). Products include:
- Ana-Kit Anaphylaxis Emergency Treatment Kit 611

Estazolam (Potential for additive CNS depression). Products include:
- ProSom Tablets 457

Ethchlorvynol (Potential for additive CNS depression). Products include:
- Placidyl Capsules 456

Ethinamate (Potential for additive CNS depression).
- No products indexed under this heading.

Ethylnorepinephrine Hydrochloride (Caffeine may enhance the cardiac inotropic effects of beta-adrenergic stimulating agents).
- No products indexed under this heading.

Fentanyl (Potential for additive CNS depression). Products include:
- Duragesic Transdermal System 1336

Fentanyl Citrate (Potential for additive CNS depression). Products include:
- Sublimaze Injection 463

Fluphenazine Decanoate (Potential for additive CNS depression). Products include:
- Prolixin Decanoate 510

Fluphenazine Enanthate (Potential for additive CNS depression). Products include:
- Prolixin Enanthate 510

Fluphenazine Hydrochloride (Potential for additive CNS depression). Products include:
- Prolixin 510

Flurazepam Hydrochloride (Potential for additive CNS depression). Products include:
- Dalmane Capsules 2329

Glutethimide (Potential for additive CNS depression).
- No products indexed under this heading.

Haloperidol (Potential for additive CNS depression). Products include:
- Haldol Injection, Tablets and Concentrate 1585

Haloperidol Decanoate (Potential for additive CNS depression). Products include:
- Haldol Decanoate 1587

Hydrocodone Bitartrate (Potential for additive CNS depression). Products include:
- Codiclear DH Syrup 808
- Duratuss HD Elixir 2750
- Histussin D Liquid 670
- Hycodan Tablets and Syrup 946
- Hycomine Compound Tablets 948
- Hycomine 947
- Hycotuss Expectorant Syrup 950
- Hydrocet Capsules 787
- Lorcet 10/650 Tablets 1016
- Lortab 2751
- Tussend 1830
- Tussend Expectorant 1831
- Vicodin Tablets 1404
- Vicodin ES Tablets 1405
- Vicodin HP Tablets 1403
- Vicodin Tuss Expectorant 1406
- Zydone Capsules 967

Hydrocodone Polistirex (Potential for additive CNS depression). Products include:
- Tussionex Pennkinetic Extended-Release Suspension 1624

Hydromorphone Hydrochloride (Potential for additive CNS depression). Products include:
- Dilaudid Ampules 1382
- Dilaudid Cough Syrup 1383
- Dilaudid-HP Injection 1384
- Dilaudid-HP Lyophilized Powder 250 mg 1384
- Dilaudid 1382
- Dilaudid Oral Liquid 1386
- Dilaudid 1382
- Dilaudid Tablets - 8 mg 1386

Hydroxyzine Hydrochloride (Potential for additive CNS depression). Products include:
- Atarax Tablets & Syrup 1992
- Marax Tablets & DF Syrup 2015
- Vistaril Intramuscular Solution 2042

Isoetharine (Caffeine may enhance the cardiac inotropic effects of beta-adrenergic stimulating agents). Products include:
- Bronkometer Aerosol 2432
- Bronkosol Solution 2432
- Isoetharine Inhalation Solution, USP, Arm-a-Med 545

Isoflurane (Potential for additive CNS depression).
- No products indexed under this heading.

Isoproterenol Hydrochloride (Caffeine may enhance the cardiac inotropic effects of beta-adrenergic stimulating agents). Products include:
- Isuprel Hydrochloride Solution 2443
- Isuprel Injection 2441
- Isuprel Mistometer 2442

Isoproterenol Sulfate (Caffeine may enhance the cardiac inotropic effects of beta-adrenergic stimulating agents). Products include:
- Norisodrine with Calcium Iodide Syrup 446

Ketamine Hydrochloride (Potential for additive CNS depression).
- No products indexed under this heading.

Levomethadyl Acetate Hydrochloride (Potential for additive CNS depression). Products include:
- Orlaam Oral Solution 2361

Levorphanol Tartrate (Potential for additive CNS depression). Products include:
- Levo-Dromoran 2297

Lomefloxacin Hydrochloride (Concomitant use may result in caffeine accumulation when DHC Plus is consumed with quinolones). Products include:
- Maxaquin Tablets 2593

Lorazepam (Potential for additive CNS depression). Products include:
- Ativan Injection 2805
- Ativan Tablets 2807

Loxapine Hydrochloride (Potential for additive CNS depression). Products include:
- Loxitane 1426

Loxapine Succinate (Potential for additive CNS depression). Products include:
- Loxitane Capsules 1426

Meperidine Hydrochloride (Potential for additive CNS depression). Products include:
- Demerol 2438
- Mepergan Injection 2859

Mephobarbital (Potential for additive CNS depression). Products include:
- Mebaral Tablets 2452

Meprobamate (Potential for additive CNS depression). Products include:
- Miltown Tablets 2780
- PMB 200 and PMB 400 2890

Mesoridazine Besylate (Potential for additive CNS depression). Products include:
- Serentil 689

Metaproterenol Sulfate (Caffeine may enhance the cardiac inotropic effects of beta-adrenergic stimulating agents). Products include:
- Alupent 672
- Metaproterenol Sulfate Inhalation Solution, USP, Arm-a-Med 547

Methadone Hydrochloride (Potential for additive CNS depression). Products include:
- Methadone Hydrochloride Oral Concentrate 2356
- Methadone Hydrochloride Oral Solution & Tablets 2357

Methohexital Sodium (Potential for additive CNS depression).
- No products indexed under this heading.

Methotrimeprazine (Potential for additive CNS depression). Products include:
- Levoprome 1321

Methoxyflurane (Potential for additive CNS depression).
- No products indexed under this heading.

Midazolam Hydrochloride (Potential for additive CNS depression). Products include:
- Versed Injection 2324

Molindone Hydrochloride (Potential for additive CNS depression). Products include:
- Moban Tablets and Concentrate 1036

Morphine Sulfate (Potential for additive CNS depression). Products include:
- Astramorph/PF Injection, USP (Preservative-Free) 526
- Duramorph Injection 983
- Infumorph 200 and Infumorph 500 Sterile Solutions 985
- Kadian Capsules 2948
- MS Contin Tablets 2149
- MSIR 2152
- Oramorph SR (Morphine Sulfate Sustained Release Tablets) 2359
- RMS Suppositories CII 2766
- Roxanol 2365

Norfloxacin (Concomitant use may result in caffeine accumulation when DHC Plus is consumed with quinolones). Products include:
- Chibroxin Sterile Ophthalmic Solution 1657
- Noroxin Tablets 1758
- Noroxin Tablets 2222

(⊞ Described in PDR For Nonprescription Drugs) (⊙ Described in PDR For Ophthalmology)

Ofloxacin (Concomitant use may result in caffeine accumulation when DHC Plus is consumed with quinolones). Products include:
Floxin I.V. ... 1580
Floxin Tablets (200 mg, 300 mg, 400 mg) ... 1577
Ocuflox Ophthalmic Solution ... 478
Ocuflox ... ◉ 242

Opium Alkaloids (Potential for additive CNS depression).
No products indexed under this heading.

Oxazepam (Potential for additive CNS depression). Products include:
Serax Capsules ... 2916
Serax Tablets ... 2916

Oxycodone Hydrochloride (Potential for additive CNS depression). Products include:
OxyContin Tablets ... 2163
OxyIR Capsules ... 2167
Percocet Tablets ... 955
Percodan Tablets ... 955
Percodan-Demi Tablets ... 956
Roxicodone Tablets, Oral Solution & Intensol (Oxycodone) ... 2366
Tylox Capsules ... 1593

Pentobarbital Sodium (Potential for additive CNS depression). Products include:
Nembutal Sodium Capsules ... 440
Nembutal Sodium Solution ... 442
Nembutal Sodium Suppositories ... 444

Perphenazine (Potential for additive CNS depression). Products include:
Etrafon ... 2495
Triavil Tablets ... 1800
Trilafon ... 2532

Phenobarbital (Potential for additive CNS depression; caffeine may increase the metabolism of phenobarbital). Products include:
Arco-Lase Plus Tablets ... 513
Bellergal-S Tablets ... 2375
Donnatal ... 2234
Donnatal Extentabs ... 2234
Donnatal Tablets ... 2234
Phenobarbital Elixir and Tablets ... 1523
Quadrinal Tablets ... 1398

Pirbuterol Acetate (Caffeine may enhance the cardiac inotropic effects of beta-adrenergic stimulating agents). Products include:
Maxair Autohaler ... 1550
Maxair Inhaler ... 1552

Prazepam (Potential for additive CNS depression).
No products indexed under this heading.

Prochlorperazine (Potential for additive CNS depression). Products include:
Compazine ... 2644

Promethazine Hydrochloride (Potential for additive CNS depression). Products include:
Mepergan Injection ... 2859
Phenergan with Codeine ... 2883
Phenergan with Dextromethorphan 2885
Phenergan Injection ... 2880
Phenergan Suppositories ... 2882
Phenergan Syrup ... 2881
Phenergan Tablets ... 2882
Phenergan VC ... 2886
Phenergan VC with Codeine ... 2888

Propofol (Potential for additive CNS depression). Products include:
Diprivan Injectable Emulsion ... 2939

Propoxyphene Hydrochloride (Potential for additive CNS depression). Products include:
Darvon ... 1475
Wygesic Tablets ... 2930

Propoxyphene Napsylate (Potential for additive CNS depression). Products include:
Darvon-N/Darvocet-N ... 1473

Quazepam (Potential for additive CNS depression). Products include:
Doral Tablets ... 2773

Risperidone (Potential for additive CNS depression). Products include:
Risperdal Tablets ... 1348

Salmeterol Xinafoate (Caffeine may enhance the cardiac inotropic effects of beta-adrenergic stimulating agents). Products include:
Serevent Inhalation Aerosol ... 1149

Secobarbital Sodium (Potential for additive CNS depression). Products include:
Seconal Sodium Pulvules ... 1529

Sevoflurane (Potential for additive CNS depression).
No products indexed under this heading.

Sufentanil Citrate (Potential for additive CNS depression). Products include:
Sufenta Injection ... 1355

Temazepam (Potential for additive CNS depression). Products include:
Restoril Capsules ... 2413

Terbutaline Sulfate (Caffeine may enhance the cardiac inotropic effects of beta-adrenergic stimulating agents). Products include:
Brethaire Inhaler ... 830
Brethine Ampuls ... 832
Brethine Tablets ... 831
Bricanyl Subcutaneous Injection ... 1247
Bricanyl Tablets ... 1248

Thiamylal Sodium (Potential for additive CNS depression).
No products indexed under this heading.

Thioridazine Hydrochloride (Potential for additive CNS depression). Products include:
Mellaril ... 2398

Thiothixene (Potential for additive CNS depression). Products include:
Navane Capsules and Concentrate 2018
Navane Intramuscular ... 2019

Triazolam (Potential for additive CNS depression). Products include:
Halcion Tablets ... 2093

Trifluoperazine Hydrochloride (Potential for additive CNS depression). Products include:
Stelazine ... 2692

Zolpidem Tartrate (Potential for additive CNS depression). Products include:
Ambien Tablets ... 2559

Food Interactions

Alcohol (Potential for additive CNS depression).

Food, caffeine containing (Concomitant use may result in caffeine accumulation when DHC Plus is consumed with caffeine-containing foods).

D.H.E. 45 INJECTION

(Dihydroergotamine Mesylate) ... 2381
May interact with vasopressors, macrolide antibiotics, and certain other agents. Compounds in these categories include:

Azithromycin (Potential for increased plasma levels of unchanged alkaloids and peripheral vasoconstriction; vasospastic reactions may result from concurrent use). Products include:
Zithromax ... 2043
Zithromax Tablets ... 2046

Clarithromycin (Potential for increased plasma levels of unchanged alkaloids and peripheral vasoconstriction; vasospastic reactions may result from concurrent use). Products include:
Biaxin ... 406

Dirithromycin (Potential for increased plasma levels of unchanged alkaloids and peripheral vasoconstriction; vasospastic reactions may result from concurrent use). Products include:
Dynabac ... 668

Dopamine Hydrochloride (Concurrent administration may cause extreme elevation of blood pressure).
No products indexed under this heading.

Epinephrine Bitartrate (Concurrent administration may cause extreme elevation of blood pressure). Products include:
Sensorcaine-MPF with Epinephrine Injection ... 554

Epinephrine Hydrochloride (Concurrent administration may cause extreme elevation of blood pressure). Products include:
Ana-Kit Anaphylaxis Emergency Treatment Kit ... 611

Erythromycin (Potential for increased plasma levels of unchanged alkaloids and peripheral vasoconstriction; vasospastic reactions may result from concurrent use). Products include:
A/T/S 2% Acne Topical Gel ... 1244
A/T/S 2% Acne Topical Solution ... 1244
Benzamycin Topical Gel ... 919
E-Mycin Tablets ... 1388
Emgel 2% Topical Gel ... 1081
ERYC ... 1972
Erycette (erythromycin 2%) Topical Solution ... 1943
Ery-Tab Tablets ... 426
Erythromycin Base Filmtab ... 430
Erythromycin Delayed-Release Capsules, USP ... 431
Ilotycin Ophthalmic Ointment ... 928
PCE Dispertab Tablets ... 453
T-Stat 2.0% Topical Solution and Pads ... 2797
THERAMYCIN Z 2% Solution ... 1629

Erythromycin Estolate (Potential for increased plasma levels of unchanged alkaloids and peripheral vasoconstriction; vasospastic reactions may result from concurrent use). Products include:
Ilosone ... 927

Erythromycin Ethylsuccinate (Potential for increased plasma levels of unchanged alkaloids and peripheral vasoconstriction; vasospastic reactions may result from concurrent use). Products include:
E.E.S. ... 427
EryPed ... 425
Pediazole Suspension ... 2340

Erythromycin Gluceptate (Potential for increased plasma levels of unchanged alkaloids and peripheral vasoconstriction; vasospastic reactions may result from concurrent use). Products include:
Ilotycin Gluceptate, IV, Vials ... 929

Erythromycin Stearate (Potential for increased plasma levels of unchanged alkaloids and peripheral vasoconstriction; vasospastic reactions may result from concurrent use). Products include:
Erythrocin Stearate Filmtab ... 429

Metaraminol Bitartrate (Concurrent administration may cause extreme elevation of blood pressure). Products include:
Aramine Injection ... 1649

Methoxamine Hydrochloride (Concurrent administration may cause extreme elevation of blood pressure). Products include:
Vasoxyl Injection ... 1169

Nicotine (Nicotine may provoke vasoconstriction in some patients, predisposing to a greater ischemic response to ergot therapy). Products include:
Habitrol Nicotine Transdermal System ... 884
Nicotrol NS Nicotine Nasal Spray ... 1565
Nicotrol Nicotine Transdermal System ... 1568
Prostep (nicotine transdermal system) ... 1439

Nicotine Polacrilex (Nicotine may provoke vasoconstriction in some patients, predisposing to a greater ischemic response to ergot therapy).
No products indexed under this heading.

Norepinephrine Bitartrate (Concurrent administration may cause extreme elevation of blood pressure). Products include:
Levophed Bitartrate Injection ... 2445

Phenylephrine Hydrochloride (Concurrent administration may cause extreme elevation of blood pressure). Products include:
Atrohist Plus Tablets ... 1605
Cerose DM ... ▣ 853
D.A. II Tablets ... 972
D.A. Chewable Tablets ... 970
Dura-Vent/DA Tablets ... 972
Extendryl ... 1003
4-Way Fast Acting Nasal Spray (regular & mentholated) ... ▣ 644
Hemorid ... ▣ 797
Hycomine Compound Tablets ... 948
Neo-Synephrine Hydrochloride 1% Carpuject ... 2455
Neo-Synephrine Hydrochloride 1% Injection ... 2455
Neo-Synephrine Hydrochloride (Ophthalmic) ... 2456
Neo-Synephrine ... ▣ 624
Novahistine Elixir ... ▣ 782
Phenergan VC ... 2886
Phenergan VC with Codeine ... 2888
Preparation H ... ▣ 842
Tympagesic Ear Drops ... 2476
Vicks Sinex Nasal Spray and Ultra Fine Mist ... ▣ 738

Propranolol Hydrochloride (Potentiates the vasoconstrictive action of ergotamine). Products include:
Inderal ... 2834
Inderal LA Long Acting Capsules ... 2836
Inderide Tablets ... 2838
Inderide LA Long Acting Capsules .. 2840

Troleandomycin (Potential for increased plasma levels of unchanged alkaloids and peripheral vasoconstriction; vasospastic reactions may result from concurrent use). Products include:
Tao Capsules ... 2033

DHS TAR GEL SHAMPOO

(Coal Tar) ... 1989
None cited in PDR database.

DHS TAR SHAMPOO

(Coal Tar) ... 1989
None cited in PDR database.

DHS ZINC DANDRUFF SHAMPOO

(Pyrithione Zinc) ... 1989
None cited in PDR database.

DHT (DIHYDROTACHYSTEROL) TABLETS & INTENSOL

(Dihydrotachysterol) ... 2351
May interact with thiazides. Compounds in this category include:

Bendroflumethiazide (May cause hypercalcemia in hypoparathyroid patients).
No products indexed under this heading.

IMPORTANT NOTE: Always consult each drug listing in the patient's regimen for possible interactions.

DHT Tablets & Intensol

Chlorothiazide (May cause hypercalcemia in hypoparathyroid patients). Products include:
- Aldoclor Tablets 1638
- Diupres Tablets 1691
- Diuril Oral 1694

Chlorothiazide Sodium (May cause hypercalcemia in hypoparathyroid patients. Products include:
- Diuril Sodium Intravenous ... 1693

Hydrochlorothiazide (May cause hypercalcemia in hypoparathyroid patients. Products include:
- Aldactazide Tablets 2556
- Aldoril Tablets 1644
- Apresazide Capsules 824
- Capozide Tablets 744
- Dyazide Capsules 2653
- Esidrix Tablets 839
- Esimil Tablets 840
- HydroDIURIL Tablets 1716
- Hydropres Tablets 1718
- Hyzaar Tablets 1720
- Inderide Tablets 2838
- Inderide LA Long Acting Capsules .. 2840
- Lopressor HCT Tablets 850
- Lotensin HCT Tablets 855
- Moduretic Tablets 1748
- Oretic Tablets 450
- Prinzide Tablets 1780
- Ser-Ap-Es Tablets 867
- Timolide Tablets 1791
- Vaseretic Tablets 1810
- Zestoretic Tablets 2968
- Ziac 1459

Hydroflumethiazide (May cause hypercalcemia in hypoparathyroid patients. Products include:
- Diucardin Tablets 2824

Methyclothiazide (May cause hypercalcemia in hypoparathyroid patients. Products include:
- Enduron Tablets 424

Polythiazide (May cause hypercalcemia in hypoparathyroid patients. Products include:
- Minizide Capsules 2016

DML FACIAL MOISTURIZER WITH SUNSCREEN
(Glycerin, Hyaluronic Acid, Octyl Methoxycinnamate, Oxybenzone) 1989
None cited in PDR database.

DTIC-DOME
(Dacarbazine) 593
May interact with antineoplastics. Compounds in this category include:

Altretamine (Hepatic toxicity). Products include:
- Hexalen Capsules 2760

Anastrozole (Hepatic toxicity). Products include:
- Arimidex Tablets 2932

Asparaginase (Hepatic toxicity). Products include:
- Elspar 1700

Bicalutamide (Hepatic toxicity). Products include:
- Casodex Tablets 2934

Bleomycin Sulfate (Hepatic toxicity). Products include:
- Blenoxane 697

Busulfan (Hepatic toxicity). Products include:
- Myleran Tablets 1209

Carboplatin (Hepatic toxicity). Products include:
- Paraplatin for Injection 713

Carmustine (BCNU) (Hepatic toxicity). Products include:
- BiCNU 696

Chlorambucil (Hepatic toxicity). Products include:
- Leukeran Tablets 1205

Cisplatin (Hepatic toxicity). Products include:
- Platinol for Injection 717
- Platinol-AQ Injection 719

Cyclophosphamide (Hepatic toxicity). Products include:
- Cytoxan 700

Daunorubicin Citrate (Hepatic toxicity). Products include:
- DaunoXome 1842

Daunorubicin Hydrochloride (Hepatic toxicity). Products include:
- Cerubidine for Injection 634

Docetaxel (Hepatic toxicity). Products include:
- Taxotere for Injection Concentrate ... 2204

Doxorubicin Hydrochloride (Hepatic toxicity). Products include:
- Adriamycin PFS 2056
- Adriamycin RDF 2056
- Doxil 2613
- Doxorubicin Astra 531
- Rubex for Injection 721

Estramustine Phosphate Sodium (Hepatic toxicity). Products include:
- Emcyt Capsules 2085

Etoposide (Hepatic toxicity). Products include:
- Etoposide Injection 539
- VePesid Capsules and Injection 727

Floxuridine (Hepatic toxicity). Products include:
- Sterile FUDR 2284

Fluorouracil (Hepatic toxicity). Products include:
- Efudex 2280
- Fluoroplex Topical Solution & Cream 1% 475
- Fluorouracil Injection 2282

Flutamide (Hepatic toxicity). Products include:
- Eulexin Capsules 2498

Gemcitabine Hydrochloride (Hepatic toxicity). Products include:
- Gemzar for Injection 1482

Hydroxyurea (Hepatic toxicity). Products include:
- Hydrea Capsules 705

Idarubicin Hydrochloride (Hepatic toxicity). Products include:
- Idamycin Injection 2096

Ifosfamide (Hepatic toxicity). Products include:
- IFEX 706

Interferon alfa-2A, Recombinant (Hepatic toxicity). Products include:
- Roferon-A Injection 2308

Interferon alfa-2B, Recombinant (Hepatic toxicity). Products include:
- Intron A for Injection 2506

Irinotecan Hydrochloride (Hepatic toxicity). Products include:
No products indexed under this heading.

Levamisole Hydrochloride (Hepatic toxicity). Products include:
- Ergamisol Tablets 1340

Lomustine (CCNU) (Hepatic toxicity). Products include:
- CeeNU Capsules 699

Mechlorethamine Hydrochloride (Hepatic toxicity). Products include:
- Mustargen 1752

Megestrol Acetate (Hepatic toxicity). Products include:
- Megace Oral Suspension 708
- Megace Tablets 710

Melphalan (Hepatic toxicity). Products include:
- Alkeran Tablets 1198

Mercaptopurine (Hepatic toxicity). Products include:
- Purinethol Tablets 1214

Methotrexate Sodium (Hepatic toxicity). Products include:
- Methotrexate Sodium Tablets, Injection, for Injection and LPF Injection 1322

Mitomycin (Mitomycin-C) (Hepatic toxicity). Products include:
- Mutamycin for Injection 712

Mitotane (Hepatic toxicity). Products include:
- Lysodren Tablets 707

Mitoxantrone Hydrochloride (Hepatic Toxicity). Products include:
- Novantrone for Injection 1327

Paclitaxel (Hepatic toxicity). Products include:
- Taxol Injection 723

Procarbazine Hydrochloride (Hepatic toxicity). Products include:
- Matulane Capsules 2300

Streptozocin (Hepatic toxicity). Products include:
- Zanosar Sterile Powder 2119

Tamoxifen Citrate (Hepatic toxicity). Products include:
- Nolvadex Tablets 2957

Teniposide (Hepatic toxicity). Products include:
- Vumon for Injection 729

Thioguanine (Hepatic toxicity). Products include:
- Thioguanine Tablets, Tabloid Brand 1225

Thiotepa (Hepatic toxicity). Products include:
- Thioplex (Thiotepa For Injection) 1329

Topotecan Hydrochloride (Hepatic toxicity). Products include:
- Hycamtin for Injection 2665

Vincristine Sulfate (Hepatic toxicity). Products include:
- Oncovin Solution Vials & Hyporets ... 1521

Vinorelbine Tartrate (Hepatic toxicity). Products include:
- Navelbine Injection 1212

DAILY CARE FROM DESITIN
(Zinc Oxide) .... ▣ 715
None cited in PDR database.

DALALONE D.P. INJECTABLE
(Dexamethasone Acetate) 1009
May interact with oral anticoagulants, potassium-depleting diuretics, and certain other agents. Compounds in these categories include:

Bendroflumethiazide (Potential for hypokalemia).
No products indexed under this heading.

Chlorothiazide (Potential for hypokalemia). Products include:
- Aldoclor Tablets 1638
- Diupres Tablets 1691
- Diuril Oral 1694

Chlorothiazide Sodium (Potential for hypokalemia). Products include:
- Diuril Sodium Intravenous ... 1693

Dicumarol (Corticosteroids may alter the response to this anticoagulant).
No products indexed under this heading.

Ephedrine (May alter cortisol metabolism).

Ephedrine Hydrochloride (May alter cortisol metabolism). Products include:
- Primatene Tablets .... ▣ 844
- Quadrinal Tablets 1398

Ephedrine Sulfate (May alter cortisol metabolism). Products include:
- Marax Tablets & DF Syrup 2015

Ephedrine Tannate (May alter cortisol metabolism). Products include:
- Rynatuss 2782

Flucytosine (Neurological complications and lack of antibody response). Products include:
- Ancobon Capsules 2254

Hydrochlorothiazide (Potential for hypokalemia). Products include:
- Aldactazide Tablets 2556
- Aldoril Tablets 1644
- Apresazide Capsules 824
- Capozide Tablets 744
- Dyazide Capsules 2653
- Esidrix Tablets 839
- Esimil Tablets 840
- HydroDIURIL Tablets 1716
- Hydropres Tablets 1718
- Hyzaar Tablets 1720
- Inderide Tablets 2838
- Inderide LA Long Acting Capsules .. 2840
- Lopressor HCT Tablets 850
- Lotensin HCT Tablets 855
- Moduretic Tablets 1748
- Oretic Tablets 450
- Prinzide Tablets 1780
- Ser-Ap-Es Tablets 867
- Timolide Tablets 1791
- Vaseretic Tablets 1810
- Zestoretic Tablets 2968
- Ziac 1459

Hydroflumethiazide (Potential for hypokalemia). Products include:
- Diucardin Tablets 2824

Live Virus Vaccines (Potential for neurological complications and loss of antibody response).

Methyclothiazide (Potential for hypokalemia). Products include:
- Enduron Tablets 424

Phenobarbital (May enhance the metabolic clearance of corticosteroids resulting in decreased blood levels and lessened physiologic activity). Products include:
- Arco-Lase Plus Tablets 513
- Bellergal-S Tablets 2375
- Donnatal 2234
- Donnatal Extentabs 2234
- Donnatal Tablets 2234
- Phenobarbital Elixir and Tablets .. 1523
- Quadrinal Tablets 1398

Phenytoin (May enhance the metabolic clearance of corticosteroids resulting in decreased blood levels and lessened physiologic activity). Products include:
- Dilantin Infatabs 1967
- Dilantin-125 Suspension 1969

Phenytoin Sodium (May enhance the metabolic clearance of corticosteroids resulting in decreased blood levels and lessened physiologic activity). Products include:
- Dilantin Kapseals 1965

Polythiazide (Potential for hypokalemia). Products include:
- Minizide Capsules 2016

Rifampin (May enhance the metabolic cleearance of corticosteroids resulting in decreased blood levels and lessened physiologic activity). Products include:
- Rifadin 1276
- Rifamate Capsules 1278
- Rifater 1280
- Rimactane Capsules 865

Smallpox Vaccine (Neurological complications and lack of antibody response).

Warfarin Sodium (Corticosteroids may alter the response to this anticoagulant). Products include:
- Coumadin 941

DALGAN INJECTION
(Dezocine) 529
May interact with central nervous system depressants, general anesthetics, hypnotics and sedatives,

(▣ Described in PDR For Nonprescription Drugs)   (◉ Described in PDR For Ophthalmology)

tranquilizers, narcotic analgesics, and certain other agents. Compounds in these categories include:

Alfentanil Hydrochloride (Concomitant administration may have an additive effect). Products include:
- Alfenta Injection ... 1334

Alprazolam (Concomitant administration may have an additive effect). Products include:
- Xanax Tablets ... 2115

Aprobarbital (Concomitant administration may have an additive effect).
- No products indexed under this heading.

Buprenorphine (Concomitant administration may have an additive effect). Products include:
- Buprenex Injectable ... 2170

Buspirone Hydrochloride (Concomitant administration may have an additive effect). Products include:
- BuSpar Tablets ... 738

Butabarbital (Concomitant administration may have an additive effect).
- No products indexed under this heading.

Butalbital (Concomitant administration may have an additive effect). Products include:
- Axocet Capsules ... 2469
- Esgic-plus Capsules ... 1012
- Esgic-plus Tablets ... 1012
- Fioricet Tablets ... 2386
- Fioricet with Codeine Capsules ... 2387
- Fiorinal Capsules ... 2388
- Fiorinal with Codeine Capsules ... 2390
- Fiorinal Tablets ... 2388
- Phrenilin ... 790
- Sedapap Tablets 50 mg/650 mg .. 1826

Chlordiazepoxide (Concomitant administration may have an additive effect). Products include:
- Limbitrol ... 2333

Chlordiazepoxide Hydrochloride (Concomitant administration may have an additive effect). Products include:
- Librax Capsules ... 2330
- Librium Capsules ... 2331
- Librium Injectable ... 2332

Chlorpromazine (Concomitant administration may have an additive effect). Products include:
- Thorazine Suppositories ... 2701

Chlorprothixene (Concomitant administration may have an additive effect).
- No products indexed under this heading.

Chlorprothixene Hydrochloride (Concomitant administration may have an additive effect).
- No products indexed under this heading.

Chlorprothixene Lactate (Concomitant administration may have an additive effect).
- No products indexed under this heading.

Clorazepate Dipotassium (Concomitant administration may have an additive effect). Products include:
- Tranxene ... 459

Clozapine (Concomitant administration may have an additive effect). Products include:
- Clozaril Tablets ... 2377

Codeine Phosphate (Concomitant administration may have an additive effect). Products include:
- Brontex ... 2130
- Dimetane-DC Cough Syrup ... 2232
- Fioricet with Codeine Capsules ... 2387
- Fiorinal with Codeine Capsules ... 2390
- Nucofed ... 2225
- Phenergan with Codeine ... 2883
- Phenergan VC with Codeine ... 2888
- Robitussin A-C Syrup ... 2248
- Robitussin-DAC Syrup ... 2249
- Ryna ... 804
- Soma Compound w/Codeine Tablets ... 2784
- Tylenol with Codeine ... 1592

Desflurane (Concomitant administration may have an additive effect). Products include:
- Suprane (desflurane, USP) ... 1865

Diazepam (Concomitant administration may have an additive effect). Products include:
- Dizac (diazepam injectable emulsion) CIV ... 1862
- Valium Injectable ... 2336
- Valium Tablets ... 2335

Droperidol (Concomitant administration may have an additive effect). Products include:
- Inapsine Injection ... 462

Enflurane (Concomitant administration may have an additive effect).
- No products indexed under this heading.

Estazolam (Concomitant administration may have an additive effect). Products include:
- ProSom Tablets ... 457

Ethchlorvynol (Concomitant administration may have an additive effect). Products include:
- Placidyl Capsules ... 456

Ethinamate (Concomitant administration may have an additive effect).
- No products indexed under this heading.

Fentanyl (Concomitant administration may have an additive effect). Products include:
- Duragesic Transdermal System ... 1336

Fentanyl Citrate (Concomitant administration may have an additive effect). Products include:
- Sublimaze Injection ... 463

Fluphenazine Decanoate (Concomitant administration may have an additive effect). Products include:
- Prolixin Decanoate ... 510

Fluphenazine Enanthate (Concomitant administration may have an additive effect). Products include:
- Prolixin Enanthate ... 510

Fluphenazine Hydrochloride (Concomitant administration may have an additive effect). Products include:
- Prolixin ... 510

Flurazepam Hydrochloride (Concomitant administration may have an additive effect). Products include:
- Dalmane Capsules ... 2329

Glutethimide (Concomitant administration may have an additive effect).
- No products indexed under this heading.

Haloperidol (Concomitant administration may have an additive effect). Products include:
- Haldol Injection, Tablets and Concentrate ... 1585

Haloperidol Decanoate (Concomitant administration may have an additive effect). Products include:
- Haldol Decanoate ... 1587

Hydrocodone Bitartrate (Concomitant administration may have an additive effect). Products include:
- Codiclear DH Syrup ... 808
- Duratuss HD Elixir ... 2750
- Histussin D Liquid ... 670
- Hycodan Tablets and Syrup ... 946
- Hycomine Compound Tablets ... 948
- Hycomine ... 947
- Hycotuss Expectorant Syrup ... 950
- Hydrocet Capsules ... 787
- Lorcet 10/650 Tablets ... 1016
- Lortab ... 2751
- Tussend ... 1830
- Tussend Expectorant ... 1831
- Vicodin Tablets ... 1404
- Vicodin ES Tablets ... 1405
- Vicodin HP Tablets ... 1403
- Vicodin Tuss Expectorant ... 1406
- Zydone Capsules ... 967

Hydrocodone Polistirex (Concomitant administration may have an additive effect). Products include:
- Tussionex Pennkinetic Extended-Release Suspension ... 1624

Hydromorphone Hydrochloride (Concomitant administration may have an additive effect). Products include:
- Dilaudid Ampules ... 1382
- Dilaudid Cough Syrup ... 1383
- Dilaudid-HP Injection ... 1384
- Dilaudid-HP Lyophilized Powder 250 mg ... 1384
- Dilaudid ... 1382
- Dilaudid Oral Liquid ... 1386
- Dilaudid ... 1382
- Dilaudid Tablets - 8 mg ... 1386

Hydroxyzine Hydrochloride (Concomitant administration may have an additive effect). Products include:
- Atarax Tablets & Syrup ... 1992
- Marax Tablets & DF Syrup ... 2015
- Vistaril Intramuscular Solution ... 2042

Isoflurane (Concomitant administration may have an additive effect).
- No products indexed under this heading.

Ketamine Hydrochloride (Concomitant administration may have an additive effect).
- No products indexed under this heading.

Levomethadyl Acetate Hydrochloride (Concomitant administration may have an additive effect). Products include:
- Orlaam Oral Solution ... 2361

Levorphanol Tartrate (Concomitant administration may have an additive effect). Products include:
- Levo-Dromoran ... 2297

Lorazepam (Concomitant administration may have an additive effect). Products include:
- Ativan Injection ... 2805
- Ativan Tablets ... 2807

Loxapine Hydrochloride (Concomitant administration may have an additive effect). Products include:
- Loxitane ... 1426

Loxapine Succinate (Concomitant administration may have an additive effect). Products include:
- Loxitane Capsules ... 1426

Meperidine Hydrochloride (Concomitant administration may have an additive effect). Products include:
- Demerol ... 2438
- Mepergan Injection ... 2859

Mephobarbital (Concomitant administration may have an additive effect). Products include:
- Mebaral Tablets ... 2452

Meprobamate (Concomitant administration may have an additive effect). Products include:
- Miltown Tablets ... 2780
- PMB 200 and PMB 400 ... 2890

Mesoridazine Besylate (Concomitant administration may have an additive effect). Products include:
- Serentil ... 689

Methadone Hydrochloride (Concomitant administration may have an additive effect). Products include:
- Methadone Hydrochloride Oral Concentrate ... 2356
- Methadone Hydrochloride Oral Solution & Tablets ... 2357

Methohexital Sodium (Concomitant administration may have an additive effect).
- No products indexed under this heading.

Methotrimeprazine (Concomitant administration may have an additive effect). Products include:
- Levoprome ... 1321

Methoxyflurane (Concomitant administration may have an additive effect).
- No products indexed under this heading.

Midazolam Hydrochloride (Concomitant administration may have an additive effect). Products include:
- Versed Injection ... 2324

Molindone Hydrochloride (Concomitant administration may have an additive effect). Products include:
- Moban Tablets and Concentrate ... 1036

Morphine Sulfate (Concomitant administration may have an additive effect). Products include:
- Astramorph/PF Injection, USP (Preservative-Free) ... 526
- Duramorph Injection ... 983
- Infumorph 200 and Infumorph 500 Sterile Solutions ... 985
- Kadian Capsules ... 2948
- MS Contin Tablets ... 2149
- MSIR ... 2152
- Oramorph SR (Morphine Sulfate Sustained Release Tablets) ... 2359
- RMS Suppositories CII ... 2766
- Roxanol ... 2365

Opium Alkaloids (Concomitant administration may have an additive effect).
- No products indexed under this heading.

Oxazepam (Concomitant administration may have an additive effect). Products include:
- Serax Capsules ... 2916
- Serax Tablets ... 2916

Oxycodone Hydrochloride (Concomitant administration may have an additive effect). Products include:
- OxyContin Tablets ... 2163
- OxyIR Capsules ... 2167
- Percocet Tablets ... 955
- Percodan Tablets ... 955
- Percodan-Demi Tablets ... 956
- Roxicodone Tablets, Oral Solution & Intensol (Oxycodone) ... 2366
- Tylox Capsules ... 1593

Pentobarbital Sodium (Concomitant administration may have an additive effect). Products include:
- Nembutal Sodium Capsules ... 440
- Nembutal Sodium Solution ... 442
- Nembutal Sodium Suppositories ... 444

Perphenazine (Concomitant administration may have an additive effect). Products include:
- Etrafon ... 2495
- Triavil Tablets ... 1800
- Trilafon ... 2532

Phenobarbital (Concomitant administration may have an additive effect). Products include:
- Arco-Lase Plus Tablets ... 513
- Bellergal-S Tablets ... 2375
- Donnatal ... 2234
- Donnatal Extentabs ... 2234
- Donnatal Tablets ... 2234
- Phenobarbital Elixir and Tablets ... 1523
- Quadrinal Tablets ... 1398

Prazepam (Concomitant administration may have an additive effect).
- No products indexed under this heading.

Prochlorperazine (Concomitant administration may have an additive effect). Products include:
- Compazine ... 2644

IMPORTANT NOTE: Always consult each drug listing in the patient's regimen for possible interactions.

Dalgan — Interactions Index

Promethazine Hydrochloride (Concomitant administration may have an additive effect). Products include:
- Mepergan Injection ... 2859
- Phenergan with Codeine ... 2883
- Phenergan with Dextromethorphan ... 2885
- Phenergan Injection ... 2880
- Phenergan Suppositories ... 2882
- Phenergan Syrup ... 2881
- Phenergan Tablets ... 2882
- Phenergan VC ... 2886
- Phenergan VC with Codeine ... 2888

Propofol (Concomitant administration may have an additive effect). Products include:
- Diprivan Injectable Emulsion ... 2939

Propoxyphene Hydrochloride (Concomitant administration may have an additive effect). Products include:
- Darvon ... 1475
- Wygesic Tablets ... 2930

Propoxyphene Napsylate (Concomitant administration may have an additive effect). Products include:
- Darvon-N/Darvocet-N ... 1473

Quazepam (Concomitant administration may have an additive effect). Products include:
- Doral Tablets ... 2773

Risperidone (Concomitant administration may have an additive effect). Products include:
- Risperdal Tablets ... 1348

Secobarbital Sodium (Concomitant administration may have an additive effect). Products include:
- Seconal Sodium Pulvules ... 1529

Sevoflurane (Concomitant administration may have an additive effect).
- No products indexed under this heading.

Sufentanil Citrate (Concomitant administration may have an additive effect). Products include:
- Sufenta Injection ... 1355

Temazepam (Concomitant administration may have an additive effect). Products include:
- Restoril Capsules ... 2413

Thiamylal Sodium (Concomitant administration may have an additive effect).
- No products indexed under this heading.

Thioridazine Hydrochloride (Concomitant administration may have an additive effect). Products include:
- Mellaril ... 2398

Thiothixene (Concomitant administration may have an additive effect). Products include:
- Navane Capsules and Concentrate ... 2018
- Navane Intramuscular ... 2019

Triazolam (Concomitant administration may have an additive effect). Products include:
- Halcion Tablets ... 2093

Trifluoperazine Hydrochloride (Concomitant administration may have an additive effect). Products include:
- Stelazine ... 2692

Zolpidem Tartrate (Concomitant administration may have an additive effect). Products include:
- Ambien Tablets ... 2559

Food Interactions
Alcohol (Concomitant administration may have an additive effect).

DALMANE CAPSULES
(Flurazepam Hydrochloride) ... 2329
May interact with central nervous system depressants and certain other agents. Compounds in these categories include:

Alfentanil Hydrochloride (Additive effects). Products include:
- Alfenta Injection ... 1334

Alprazolam (Additive effects). Products include:
- Xanax Tablets ... 2115

Aprobarbital (Additive effects).
- No products indexed under this heading.

Buprenorphine (Additive effects). Products include:
- Buprenex Injectable ... 2170

Buspirone Hydrochloride (Additive effects). Products include:
- BuSpar Tablets ... 738

Butabarbital (Additive effects).
- No products indexed under this heading.

Butalbital (Additive effects). Products include:
- Axocet Capsules ... 2469
- Esgic-plus Capsules ... 1012
- Esgic-plus Tablets ... 1012
- Fioricet Tablets ... 2386
- Fioricet with Codeine Capsules ... 2387
- Fiorinal Capsules ... 2388
- Fiorinal with Codeine Capsules ... 2390
- Fiorinal Tablets ... 2388
- Phrenilin ... 790
- Sedapap Tablets 50 mg/650 mg ... 1826

Chlordiazepoxide (Additive effects). Products include:
- Limbitrol ... 2333

Chlordiazepoxide Hydrochloride (Additive effects). Products include:
- Librax Capsules ... 2330
- Librium Capsules ... 2331
- Librium Injectable ... 2332

Chlorpromazine (Additive effects). Products include:
- Thorazine Suppositories ... 2701

Chlorprothixene (Additive effects).
- No products indexed under this heading.

Chlorprothixene Hydrochloride (Additive effects).
- No products indexed under this heading.

Chlorprothixene Lactate (Additive effects).
- No products indexed under this heading.

Clorazepate Dipotassium (Additive effects). Products include:
- Tranxene ... 459

Clozapine (Additive effects). Products include:
- Clozaril Tablets ... 2377

Codeine Phosphate (Additive effects). Products include:
- Brontex ... 2130
- Dimetane-DC Cough Syrup ... 2232
- Fioricet with Codeine Capsules ... 2387
- Fiorinal with Codeine Capsules ... 2390
- Nucofed ... 2225
- Phenergan with Codeine ... 2883
- Phenergan VC with Codeine ... 2888
- Robitussin A-C Syrup ... 2248
- Robitussin-DAC Syrup ... 2249
- Ryna ... 804
- Soma Compound w/Codeine Tablets ... 2784
- Tylenol with Codeine ... 1592

Desflurane (Additive effects). Products include:
- Suprane (desflurane, USP) ... 1865

Dezocine (Additive effects). Products include:
- Dalgan Injection ... 529

Diazepam (Additive effects). Products include:
- Dizac (diazepam injectable emulsion) CIV ... 1862
- Valium Injectable ... 2336
- Valium Tablets ... 2335

Droperidol (Additive effects). Products include:
- Inapsine Injection ... 462

Enflurane (Additive effects).
- No products indexed under this heading.

Estazolam (Additive effects). Products include:
- ProSom Tablets ... 457

Ethchlorvynol (Additive effects). Products include:
- Placidyl Capsules ... 456

Ethinamate (Additive effects).
- No products indexed under this heading.

Fentanyl (Additive effects). Products include:
- Duragesic Transdermal System ... 1336

Fentanyl Citrate (Additive effects). Products include:
- Sublimaze Injection ... 463

Fluphenazine Decanoate (Additive effects). Products include:
- Prolixin Decanoate ... 510

Fluphenazine Enanthate (Additive effects). Products include:
- Prolixin Enanthate ... 510

Fluphenazine Hydrochloride (Additive effects). Products include:
- Prolixin ... 510

Glutethimide (Additive effects).
- No products indexed under this heading.

Haloperidol (Additive effects). Products include:
- Haldol Injection, Tablets and Concentrate ... 1585

Haloperidol Decanoate (Additive effects). Products include:
- Haldol Decanoate ... 1587

Hydrocodone Bitartrate (Additive effects). Products include:
- Codiclear DH Syrup ... 808
- Duratuss HD Elixir ... 2750
- Histussin D Liquid ... 670
- Hycodan Tablets and Syrup ... 946
- Hycomine Compound Tablets ... 948
- Hycomine ... 947
- Hycotuss Expectorant Syrup ... 950
- Hydrocet Capsules ... 787
- Lorcet 10/650 Tablets ... 1016
- Lortab ... 2751
- Tussend ... 1830
- Tussend Expectorant ... 1831
- Vicodin Tablets ... 1404
- Vicodin ES Tablets ... 1405
- Vicodin HP Tablets ... 1403
- Vicodin Tuss Expectorant ... 1406
- Zydone Capsules ... 967

Hydrocodone Polistirex (Additive effects). Products include:
- Tussionex Pennkinetic Extended-Release Suspension ... 1624

Hydroxyzine Hydrochloride (Additive effects). Products include:
- Atarax Tablets & Syrup ... 1992
- Marax Tablets & DF Syrup ... 2015
- Vistaril Intramuscular Solution ... 2042

Isoflurane (Additive effects).
- No products indexed under this heading.

Ketamine Hydrochloride (Additive effects).
- No products indexed under this heading.

Levomethadyl Acetate Hydrochloride (Additive effects). Products include:
- Orlaam Oral Solution ... 2361

Levorphanol Tartrate (Additive effects). Products include:
- Levo-Dromoran ... 2297

Lorazepam (Additive effects). Products include:
- Ativan Injection ... 2805
- Ativan Tablets ... 2807

Loxapine Hydrochloride (Additive effects). Products include:
- Loxitane ... 1426

Loxapine Succinate (Additive effects). Products include:
- Loxitane Capsules ... 1426

Meperidine Hydrochloride (Additive effects). Products include:
- Demerol ... 2438
- Mepergan Injection ... 2859

Mephobarbital (Additive effects). Products include:
- Mebaral Tablets ... 2452

Meprobamate (Additive effects). Products include:
- Miltown Tablets ... 2780
- PMB 200 and PMB 400 ... 2890

Mesoridazine Besylate (Additive effects). Products include:
- Serentil ... 689

Methadone Hydrochloride (Additive effects). Products include:
- Methadone Hydrochloride Oral Concentrate ... 2356
- Methadone Hydrochloride Oral Solution & Tablets ... 2357

Methohexital Sodium (Additive effects).
- No products indexed under this heading.

Methotrimeprazine (Additive effects). Products include:
- Levoprome ... 1321

Methoxyflurane (Additive effects).
- No products indexed under this heading.

Midazolam Hydrochloride (Additive effects). Products include:
- Versed Injection ... 2324

Molindone Hydrochloride (Additive effects). Products include:
- Moban Tablets and Concentrate ... 1036

Morphine Sulfate (Additive effects). Products include:
- Astramorph/PF Injection, USP (Preservative-Free) ... 526
- Duramorph Injection ... 983
- Infumorph 200 and Infumorph 500 Sterile Solutions ... 985
- Kadian Capsules ... 2948
- MS Contin Tablets ... 2149
- MSIR ... 2152
- Oramorph SR (Morphine Sulfate Sustained Release Tablets) ... 2359
- RMS Suppositories CII ... 2766
- Roxanol ... 2365

Opium Alkaloids (Additive effects).
- No products indexed under this heading.

Oxazepam (Additive effects). Products include:
- Serax Capsules ... 2916
- Serax Tablets ... 2916

Oxycodone Hydrochloride (Additive effects). Products include:
- OxyContin Tablets ... 2163
- OxyIR Capsules ... 2167
- Percocet Tablets ... 955
- Percodan Tablets ... 955
- Percodan-Demi Tablets ... 956
- Roxicodone Tablets, Oral Solution & Intensol (Oxycodone) ... 2366
- Tylox Capsules ... 1593

Pentobarbital Sodium (Additive effects). Products include:
- Nembutal Sodium Capsules ... 440
- Nembutal Sodium Solution ... 442
- Nembutal Sodium Suppositories ... 444

Perphenazine (Additive effects). Products include:
- Etrafon ... 2495
- Triavil Tablets ... 1800
- Trilafon ... 2532

Phenobarbital (Additive effects). Products include:
- Arco-Lase Plus Tablets ... 513
- Bellergal-S Tablets ... 2375
- Donnatal ... 2234
- Donnatal Extentabs ... 2234
- Donnatal Tablets ... 2234
- Phenobarbital Elixir and Tablets ... 1523
- Quadrinal Tablets ... 1398

(▣ Described in PDR For Nonprescription Drugs)   (◉ Described in PDR For Ophthalmology)

235 Interactions Index Dantrium Intravenous

Prazepam (Additive effects).
No products indexed under this heading.
Prochlorperazine (Additive effects). Products include:
Compazine ... 2644
Promethazine Hydrochloride (Additive effects). Products include:
Mepergan Injection ... 2859
Phenergan with Codeine ... 2883
Phenergan with Dextromethorphan 2885
Phenergan Injection ... 2880
Phenergan Suppositories ... 2882
Phenergan Syrup ... 2881
Phenergan Tablets ... 2882
Phenergan VC ... 2886
Phenergan VC with Codeine ... 2888
Propofol (Additive effects). Products include:
Diprivan Injectable Emulsion ... 2939
Propoxyphene Hydrochloride (Additive effects). Products include:
Darvon ... 1475
Wygesic Tablets ... 2930
Propoxyphene Napsylate (Additive effects). Products include:
Darvon-N/Darvocet-N ... 1473
Quazepam (Additive effects). Products include:
Doral Tablets ... 2773
Risperidone (Additive effects). Products include:
Risperdal Tablets ... 1348
Secobarbital Sodium (Additive effects). Products include:
Seconal Sodium Pulvules ... 1529
Sevoflurane (Additive effects).
No products indexed under this heading.
Sufentanil Citrate (Additive effects). Products include:
Sufenta Injection ... 1355
Temazepam (Additive effects). Products include:
Restoril Capsules ... 2413
Thiamylal Sodium (Additive effects).
No products indexed under this heading.
Thioridazine Hydrochloride (Additive effects). Products include:
Mellaril ... 2398
Thiothixene (Additive effects). Products include:
Navane Capsules and Concentrate 2018
Navane Intramuscular ... 2019
Triazolam (Additive effects). Products include:
Halcion Tablets ... 2093
Trifluoperazine Hydrochloride (Additive effects). Products include:
Stelazine ... 2692
Zolpidem Tartrate (Additive effects). Products include:
Ambien Tablets ... 2559

Food Interactions

Alcohol (Additive effects; potential for continuation of interaction after discontinuance of flurazepam).

DANOCRINE CAPSULES
(Danazol) ... 2437
May interact with insulin and certain other agents. Compounds in these categories include:

Carbamazepine (May result in increased carbamazepine levels). Products include:
Atretol Tablets ... 569
Tegretol/Tegretol-XR ... 870
Insulin, Human (Insulin requirement may be increased in diabetic patients).
No products indexed under this heading.
Insulin, Human Isophane Suspension (Insulin requirement may be increased in diabetic patients). Products include:
Novolin N Human Insulin 10 ml Vials ... 1846
Insulin, Human NPH (Insulin requirement may be increased in diabetic patients). Products include:
Humulin N, 100 Units ... 1495
Novolin N PenFill 1.5 ml Cartridges Durable Insulin Delivery System ... 1849
Novolin N Prefilled Syringe Disposable Insulin Delivery System ... 1850
Insulin, Human Regular (Insulin requirement may be increased in diabetic patients). Products include:
Humulin R, 100 Units ... 1497
Novolin R Human Insulin 10 ml Vials ... 1846
Novolin R PenFill 1.5 ml Cartridges Durable Insulin Delivery System ... 1849
Novolin R Prefilled Syringe Disposable Insulin Delivery System ... 1850
Velosulin BR Human Insulin 10 ml Vials ... 1847
Insulin, Human, Zinc Suspension (Insulin requirement may be increased in diabetic patients). Products include:
Humulin L, 100 Units ... 1494
Humulin U, 100 Units ... 1498
Novolin L Human Insulin 10 ml Vials ... 1846
Insulin Lispro, Human (Insulin requirement may be increased in diabetic patients). Products include:
Humalog Injection ... 1488
Insulin, NPH (Insulin requirement may be increased in diabetic patients). Products include:
NPH, 100 Units ... 1502
Pork NPH, 100 Units ... 1506
Purified Pork NPH Isophane Insulin ... 1852
Insulin, Regular (Insulin requirement may be increased in diabetic patients). Products include:
Regular, 100 Units ... 1503
Pork Regular, 100 Units ... 1507
Pork Regular (Concentrated), 500 Units ... 1508
Purified Pork Regular Insulin ... 1852
Insulin, Zinc Crystals (Insulin requirement may be increased in diabetic patients). Products include:
NPH, 100 Units ... 1502
Insulin, Zinc Suspension (Insulin requirement may be increased in diabetic patients). Products include:
Iletin I ... 1501
Lente, 100 Units ... 1501
Iletin II ... 1504
Pork Lente, 100 Units ... 1504
Purified Pork Lente Insulin ... 1852
Warfarin Sodium (Prolongation of prothrombin time in patients stabilized on warfarin). Products include:
Coumadin ... 941

DANTRIUM CAPSULES
(Dantrolene Sodium) ... 2131
May interact with estrogens and certain other agents. Compounds in these categories include:

Chlorotrianisene (Hepatotoxicity has occurred more often in women over 35 years of age receiving concomitant estrogen therapy).
No products indexed under this heading.
Dienestrol (Hepatotoxicity has occurred more often in women over 35 years of age receiving concomitant estrogen therapy). Products include:
Ortho Dienestrol Cream ... 1922
Diethylstilbestrol (Hepatotoxicity has occurred more often in women over 35 years of age receiving concomitant estrogen therapy). Products include:
Diethylstilbestrol Tablets ... 1477
Estradiol (Hepatotoxicity has occurred more often in women over 35 years of age receiving concomitant estrogen therapy). Products include:
Climara Transdermal System ... 640
Estrace Cream and Tablets ... 751
Estraderm Transdermal System ... 842
Estring Vaginal Ring ... 2086
Vivelle Transdermal System ... 880
Estrogens, Conjugated (Hepatotoxicity has occurred more often in women over 35 years of age receiving concomitant estrogen therapy). Products include:
PMB 200 and PMB 400 ... 2890
Premarin Intravenous ... 2893
Premarin Tablets ... 2896
Premarin Vaginal Cream ... 2898
Premphase ... 2900
Prempro ... 2905
Estrogens, Esterified (Hepatotoxicity has occurred more often in women over 35 years of age receiving concomitant estrogen therapy). Products include:
ESTRATAB Tablets (0.3, 0.625, 1.25, 2.5 mg) ... 2715
Estratest ... 2718
Menest Tablets ... 2671
Estropipate (Hepatotoxicity has occurred more often in women over 35 years of age receiving concomitant estrogen therapy). Products include:
Ogen Tablets ... 2103
Ogen Vaginal Cream ... 2106
Ortho-Est ... 1925
Ethinyl Estradiol (Hepatotoxicity has occurred more often in women over 35 years of age receiving concomitant estrogen therapy). Products include:
Brevicon ... 2563
Demulen ... 2580
Desogen Tablets ... 1867
Levlen/Tri-Levlen ... 646
Lo/Ovral Tablets ... 2852
Lo/Ovral-28 Tablets ... 2857
Modicon ... 1928
Nordette-21 Tablets ... 2863
Nordette-28 Tablets ... 2866
Norinyl ... 2563
Ortho-Cept ... 1907
Ortho-Cyclen/Ortho-Tri-Cyclen ... 1914
Ortho-Novum ... 1928
Ortho-Cyclen/Ortho Tri-Cyclen ... 1914
Ovcon ... 765
Ovral Tablets ... 2877
Ovral-28 Tablets ... 2878
Levlen/Tri-Levlen ... 646
Tri-Norinyl ... 2607
Triphasil-21 Tablets ... 2919
Triphasil-28 Tablets ... 2924
Polyestradiol Phosphate (Hepatotoxicity has occurred more often in women over 35 years of age receiving concomitant estrogen therapy).
No products indexed under this heading.
Quinestrol (Hepatotoxicity has occurred more often in women over 35 years of age receiving concomitant estrogen therapy).
No products indexed under this heading.
Verapamil Hydrochloride (The combination of therapeutic doses of intravenous dantrolene sodium and verapamil in halothane anesthetized subjects has resulted in ventricular fibrillation and cardiovascular collapse; this combination is not recommended during the management of malignant hyperthermia). Products include:
Calan SR Caplets ... 2571
Calan Tablets ... 2568
Covera-HS Tablets ... 2573
Isoptin Injectable ... 1391
Isoptin Oral Tablets ... 1393
Isoptin SR Tablets ... 1395
Verelan Capsules ... 1455

DANTRIUM INTRAVENOUS
(Dantrolene Sodium) ... 2132
May interact with hepatic microsomal emzyme inducers and certain other agents. Compounds in these categories include:

Carbamazepine (Theoretical possibility that the metabolism of dantrolene may be enhanced by drugs known to induce hepatic microsomal enzymes). Products include:
Atretol Tablets ... 569
Tegretol/Tegretol-XR ... 870
Chlorpropamide (Theoretical possibility that the metabolism of dantrolene may be enhanced by drugs known to induce hepatic microsomal enzymes). Products include:
Diabinese Tablets ... 2002
Clofibrate (Reduces binding of dantrolene to plasma proteins). Products include:
Atromid-S Capsules ... 2808
Fosphenytoin Sodium (Theoretical possibility that the metabolism of dantrolene may be enhanced by drugs known to induce hepatic microsomal enzyme). Products include:
Cerebyx Injection ... 1956
Glipizide (Theoretical possibility that the metabolism of dantrolene may be enhanced by drugs known to induce hepatic microsomal enzymes). Products include:
Glucotrol Tablets ... 2011
Glucotrol XL Extended Release Tablets ... 2012
Glyburide (Theoretical possibility that the metabolism of dantrolene may be enhanced by drugs known to induce hepatic microsomal enzymes). Products include:
DiaBeta Tablets ... 1265
Glynase PresTab Tablets ... 2091
Micronase Tablets ... 2099
Phenobarbital (Theoretical possibility that the metabolism of dantrolene may be enhanced by drugs known to induce hepatic microsomal enzymes; phenobarbital does not appear to affect Dantrium metabolism). Products include:
Arco-Lase Plus Tablets ... 513
Bellergal-S Tablets ... 2375
Donnatal ... 2234
Donnatal Extentabs ... 2234
Donnatal Tablets ... 2234
Phenobarbital Elixir and Tablets ... 1523
Quadrinal Tablets ... 1398
Phenylbutazone (Theoretical possibility that the metabolism of dantrolene may be enhanced by drugs known to induce hepatic microsomal enzymes).
No products indexed under this heading.
Phenytoin (Theoretical possibility that the metabolism of dantrolene may be enhanced by drugs known to induce hepatic microsomal enzymes). Products include:
Dilantin Infatabs ... 1967
Dilantin-125 Suspension ... 1969
Phenytoin Sodium (Theoretical possibility that the metabolism of dantrolene may be enhanced by drugs known to induce hepatic microsomal enzymes). Products include:
Dilantin Kapseals ... 1965

IMPORTANT NOTE: Always consult each drug listing in the patient's regimen for possible interactions.

Rifampin (Theoretical possibility that the metabolism of dantrolene may be enhanced by drugs known to induce hepatic microsomal enzymes). Products include:

Rifadin 1276
Rifamate Capsules 1278
Rifater 1280
Rimactane Capsules 865

Tolazamide (Theoretical possibility that the metabolism of dantrolene may be enhanced by drugs known to induce hepatic microsomal enzymes).

No products indexed under this heading.

Tolbutamide (Increases binding of dantrolene to plasma proteins).

No products indexed under this heading.

Verapamil Hydrochloride (The combination of therapeutic doses of intravenous dantrolene sodium and verapamil in halothane/alpha-chloralose anesthetized swine has resulted in ventricular collapse in association with marked hyperkalemia; this combination should not be used during the management of malignant hyperthermia crisis). Products include:

Calan SR Caplets 2571
Calan Tablets 2568
Covera-HS Tablets 2573
Isoptin Injectable 1391
Isoptin Oral Tablets 1393
Isoptin SR Tablets 1395
Verelan Capsules 1455

Warfarin Sodium (Reduces binding of dantrolene to plasma proteins). Products include:

Coumadin 941

DAPSONE TABLETS USP

(Dapsone) 1331
May interact with:

Pyrimethamine (Agranulocytosis; increased likelihood of hematological reactions). Products include:

Daraprim Tablets 1199
Fansidar Tablets 2281

Rifampin (Lowered Dapsone levels). Products include:

Rifadin 1276
Rifamate Capsules 1278
Rifater 1280
Rimactane Capsules 865

Trimethoprim (Mutual interaction between Dapsone and trimethoprim in which each raises the level of the other about 1.5 times). Products include:

Bactrim DS Tablets 2257
Bactrim I.V. Infusion 2255
Bactrim 2257
Proloprim Tablets 1141
Septra 1146
Septra I.V. Infusion 1142
Septra I.V. Infusion ADD-Vantage Vials 1144
Septra 1146
Trimpex Tablets 2323

DARANIDE TABLETS

(Dichlorphenamide) 1676
May interact with corticosteroids and certain other agents. Compounds in these categories include:

ACTH (Hypokalemia may develop).

No products indexed under this heading.

Aspirin (Concomitant high-dose aspirin may produce anorexia, tachypnea, lethargy and coma). Products include:

Alka-Seltzer Cherry Effervescent Antacid and Pain Reliever .... ▣ 609
Alka-Seltzer Extra Strength Effervescent Antacid and Pain Reliever .... ▣ 609
Alka-Seltzer Lemon Lime Effervescent Antacid and Pain Reliever .... ▣ 609
Alka-Seltzer Original Effervescent Antacid and Pain Reliever .... ▣ 609
Alka-Seltzer Plus .... ▣ 611
Alka-Seltzer Plus Sinus Medicine .. ▣ 611
Ascriptin .... ▣ 650
Arthritis Strength BC Powder .... ▣ 631
BC Cold Powder Multi-Symptom Formula (Cold-Sinus-Allergy) .... ▣ 631
BC Cold Powder Non-Drowsy Formula (Cold-Sinus) .... ▣ 631
BC Powder .... ▣ 631
Genuine Bayer Aspirin Tablets & Caplets .... ▣ 618
Extra Strength Bayer Arthritis Pain Regimen Formula .... ▣ 615
Extra Strength Bayer Aspirin Caplets & Tablets .... ▣ 617
Extended-Release Bayer 8-Hour Aspirin .... ▣ 616
Extra Strength Bayer Plus Aspirin Caplets .... ▣ 617
Extra Strength Bayer PM Aspirin Plus Sleep Aid .... ▣ 617
Aspirin Regimen Bayer 81 mg Tablets with Calcium .... ▣ 615
Aspirin Regimen Bayer Adult Low Strength 81 mg Tablets .... ▣ 613
Aspirin Regimen Bayer Children's Chewable Aspirin .... ▣ 616
Aspirin Regimen Bayer Regular Strength 325 mg Caplets .... ▣ 613
Bufferin Analgesic Tablets .... ▣ 636
Arthritis Strength Bufferin Analgesic Caplets .... ▣ 637
Extra Strength Bufferin Analgesic Tablets .... ▣ 637
Cama Arthritis Pain Reliever .... ▣ 748
Darvon Compound-65 Pulvules 1475
Easprin 1971
Ecotrin 2625
Ecotrin Enteric Coated Aspirin Maximum Strength Tablets and Caplets .... ▣ 775
Ecotrin Enteric Coated Aspirin Regular Strength Tablets 2625
Empirin Aspirin Tablets .... ▣ 818
Excedrin Extra-Strength Analgesic Tablets, Caplets, and Geltabs 734
Fiorinal Capsules 2388
Fiorinal with Codeine Capsules 2390
Fiorinal Tablets 2388
Goody's Extra Strength Headache Powders .... ▣ 632
Goody's Extra Strength Pain Relief Tablets .... ▣ 632
Halfprin Tablets 1413
Norgesic 1554
Percodan Tablets 955
Percodan-Demi Tablets 956
Robaxisal Tablets 2246
Soma Compound w/Codeine Tablets 2784
Soma Compound Tablets 2783
St. Joseph Adult Chewable Aspirin (81 mg.) .... ▣ 768
Talwin Compound 2466
Vanquish Analgesic Caplets .... ▣ 627

Aspirin, Enteric Coated (Concomitant high-dose aspirin may produce anorexia, tachypnea, lethargy and coma).

No products indexed under this heading.

Betamethasone Acetate (Hypokalemia may develop). Products include:

Celestone Soluspan Suspension 2484

Betamethasone Sodium Phosphate (Hypokalemia may develop). Products include:

Celestone Soluspan Suspension 2484

Cortisone Acetate (Hypokalemia may develop). Products include:

Cortone Acetate Sterile Suspension 1663
Cortone Acetate Tablets 1664

Dexamethasone (Hypokalemia may develop). Products include:

AK-Trol Ointment & Suspension .... ⊙ 205
Decadron Elixir 1676
Decadron Tablets 1678
Decaspray Topical Aerosol 1689
Maxitrol Ophthalmic Ointment and Suspension .... ⊙ 222
TobraDex Ophthalmic Suspension and Ointment 469

Dexamethasone Acetate (Hypokalemia may develop). Products include:

Dalalone D.P. Injectable 1009
Decadron-LA Sterile Suspension 1687

Dexamethasone Sodium Phosphate (Hypokalemia may develop). Products include:

Decadron Phosphate Injection 1680
Decadron Phosphate Sterile Ophthalmic Ointment 1684
Decadron Phosphate Sterile Ophthalmic Solution 1685
Decadron Phosphate Topical Cream 1686
Decadron Phosphate with Xylocaine Injection, Sterile 1683
Dexacort Phosphate in Respihaler .. 1606
Dexacort Phosphate in Turbinaire .. 1607
NeoDecadron Sterile Ophthalmic Ointment 1755
NeoDecadron Sterile Ophthalmic Solution 1756
NeoDecadron Topical Cream 1757

Fludrocortisone Acetate (Hypokalemia may develop). Products include:

Florinef Acetate Tablets 506

Hydrocortisone (Hypokalemia may develop). Products include:

Anusol-HC Cream 2.5% 1953
Aquanil HC Lotion 1989
Maximum Strength Cortaid Spray ▣ 800
CORTENEMA 2713
Cortisporin Ointment 1074
Cortisporin Ophthalmic Ointment Sterile 1074
Cortisporin Ophthalmic Suspension Sterile 1075
Cortisporin Otic Solution Sterile 1076
Cortisporin Otic Suspension Sterile 1077
Cortizone-5 .... ▣ 795
Cortizone-10 .... ▣ 795
Hydrocortone Tablets 1715
Hytone 922
Hytone Ointment 2 ½% 923
Massengill Medicated Soft Cloth Towelettes 2628
Pediotic Suspension Sterile 1140
Preparation H Hydrocortisone 1% Cream .... ▣ 843
ProctoCream-HC 2.5% 2552
VōSoL HC Otic Solution 2786

Hydrocortisone Acetate (Hypokalemia may develop). Products include:

Analpram-HC Rectal Cream 1% and 2.5% 993
Anusol HC-1 Hydrocortisone Anti-Itch Ointment .... ▣ 810
Anusol-HC Suppositories 1954
Caldecort Anti-Itch Hydrocortisone Cream .... ▣ 651
Coly-Mycin S Otic w/Neomycin & Hydrocortisone 1965
Cortaid .... ▣ 800
Cortifoam 2540
Cortisporin Cream 1073
Epifoam 2543
Hydrocortone Acetate Sterile Suspension 1712
Mantadil Cream 1124
Nupercainal Hydrocortisone 1% Cream .... ▣ 661
Pramosone Cream, Lotion & Ointment 995
ProctoFoam-HC 2552
Terra-Cortril Ophthalmic Suspension 2033

Hydrocortisone Sodium Phosphate (Hypokalemia may develop). Products include:

Hydrocortone Phosphate Injection, Sterile 1713

Hydrocortisone Sodium Succinate (Hypokalemia may develop).

No products indexed under this heading.

Methylprednisolone Acetate (Hypokalemia may develop).

No products indexed under this heading.

Methylprednisolone Sodium Succinate (Hypokalemia may develop).

No products indexed under this heading.

Prednisolone Acetate (Hypokalemia may develop). Products include:

AK-CIDE .... ⊙ 203
AK-CIDE Ointment .... ⊙ 203
Blephamide Liquifilm Sterile Ophthalmic Suspension 472
Blephamide Ointment .... ⊙ 234
Econopred & Econopred Plus Ophthalmic Suspensions .... ⊙ 216
Poly-Pred Liquifilm .... ⊙ 246
Pred Forte .... ⊙ 247
Pred Mild .... ⊙ 250
Pred-G Liquifilm Sterile Ophthalmic Suspension .... ⊙ 248
Pred-G S.O.P. Sterile Ophthalmic Ointment .... ⊙ 249

Prednisolone Sodium Phosphate (Hypokalemia may develop). Products include:

AK-PRED .... ⊙ 204
Hydeltrasol Injection, Sterile 1708
Pediapred Oral Solution 1618

Prednisolone Tebutate (Hypokalemia may develop). Products include:

Hydeltra-T.B.A. Sterile Suspension 1710

Prednisone (Hypokalemia may develop).

No products indexed under this heading.

Triamcinolone (Hypokalemia may develop).

No products indexed under this heading.

Triamcinolone Acetonide (Hypokalemia may develop). Products include:

Azmacort Oral Inhaler 2175
Nasacort AQ Nasal Spray 2191
Nasacort Nasal Inhaler 2189

Triamcinolone Diacetate (Hypokalemia may develop).

No products indexed under this heading.

Triamcinolone Hexacetonide (Hypokalemia may develop).

No products indexed under this heading.

DARAPRIM TABLETS

(Pyrimethamine) 1199
May interact with sulfonamides and certain other agents. Compounds in these categories include:

Lorazepam (Concomitant therapy may result in mild hepatotoxicity). Products include:

Ativan Injection 2805
Ativan Tablets 2807

Phenytoin (Daraprim should be used with caution). Products include:

Dilantin Infatabs 1967
Dilantin-125 Suspension 1969

Phenytoin Sodium (Daraprim should be used with caution). Products include:

Dilantin Kapseals 1965

Sulfamethizole (Increased risk of bone marrow suppression and hypersensitivity reactions). Products include:

Urobiotic-250 Capsules 2038

Sulfamethoxazole (Increased risk of bone marrow suppression and hypersensitivity reactions). Products include:

Bactrim DS Tablets 2257
Bactrim I.V. Infusion 2255
Bactrim 2257
Gantanol Tablets 2285
Septra 1146
Septra I.V. Infusion 1142
Septra I.V. Infusion ADD-Vantage Vials 1144
Septra 1146

(▣ Described in PDR For Nonprescription Drugs) (⊙ Described in PDR For Ophthalmology)

Sulfasalazine (Increased risk of bone marrow suppression and hypersensitivity reactions). Products include:
Azulfidine 2059

Sulfinpyrazone (Increased risk of bone marrow suppression and hypersensitivity reactions). Products include:
Anturane 823

Sulfisoxazole (Increased risk of bone marrow suppression and hypersensitivity reactions). Products include:
Gantrisin Tablets 2286

Sulfisoxazole Diolamine (Increased risk of bone marrow suppression and hypersensitivity reactions).
No products indexed under this heading.

Trimethoprim (Increased risk of bone marrow suppression and hypersensitivity reactions). Products include:
Bactrim DS Tablets 2257
Bactrim I.V. Infusion 2255
Bactrim 2257
Proloprim Tablets 1141
Septra 1146
Septra I.V. Infusion 1142
Septra I.V. Infusion ADD-Vantage Vials 1144
Septra 1146
Trimpex Tablets 2323

DARVOCET-N 50 TABLETS
(Propoxyphene Napsylate, Acetaminophen) 1473
May interact with central nervous system depressants, tricyclic antidepressants, anticonvulsants, oral anticoagulants, and certain other agents. Compounds in these categories include:

Alfentanil Hydrochloride (Additive CNS depression). Products include:
Alfenta Injection 1334

Alprazolam (Additive CNS depression). Products include:
Xanax Tablets 2115

Amitriptyline Hydrochloride (Propoxyphene may slow metabolism). Products include:
Elavil 2945
Etrafon 2495
Limbitrol 2333
Triavil Tablets 1800

Amoxapine (Propoxyphene may slow metabolism). Products include:
Asendin Tablets 1419

Aprobarbital (Additive CNS depression).
No products indexed under this heading.

Buprenorphine (Additive CNS depression). Products include:
Buprenex Injectable 2170

Buspirone Hydrochloride (Additive CNS depression). Products include:
BuSpar Tablets 738

Butabarbital (Additive CNS depression).
No products indexed under this heading.

Butalbital (Additive CNS depression). Products include:
Axocet Capsules 2469
Esgic-plus Capsules 1012
Esgic-plus Tablets 1012
Fioricet Tablets 2386
Fioricet with Codeine Capsules ... 2387
Fiorinal Capsules 2388
Fiorinal with Codeine Capsules ... 2390
Fiorinal Tablets 2388
Phrenilin 790
Sedapap Tablets 50 mg/650 mg .. 1826

Carbamazepine (Concurrent use may result in severe neurological signs, including coma). Products include:
Atretol Tablets 569
Tegretol/Tegretol-XR 870

Chlordiazepoxide (Additive CNS depression). Products include:
Limbitrol 2333

Chlordiazepoxide Hydrochloride (Additive CNS depression). Products include:
Librax Capsules 2330
Librium Capsules 2331
Librium Injectable 2332

Chlorpromazine (Additive CNS depression). Products include:
Thorazine Suppositories 2701

Chlorprothixene (Additive CNS depression).
No products indexed under this heading.

Chlorprothixene Hydrochloride (Additive CNS depression).
No products indexed under this heading.

Chlorprothixene Lactate (Additive CNS depression).
No products indexed under this heading.

Clomipramine Hydrochloride (Propoxyphene may slow metabolism). Products include:
Anafranil Capsules 819

Clorazepate Dipotassium (Additive CNS depression). Products include:
Tranxene 459

Clozapine (Additive CNS depression). Products include:
Clozaril Tablets 2377

Codeine Phosphate (Additive CNS depression). Products include:
Brontex 2130
Dimetane-DC Cough Syrup 2232
Fioricet with Codeine Capsules .. 2387
Fiorinal with Codeine Capsules .. 2390
Nucofed 2225
Phenergan with Codeine 2883
Phenergan VC with Codeine ... 2888
Robitussin A-C Syrup 2248
Robitussin-DAC Syrup 2249
Ryna 804
Soma Compound w/Codeine Tablets 2784
Tylenol with Codeine 1592

Desflurane (Additive CNS depression). Products include:
Suprane (desflurane, USP) 1865

Desipramine Hydrochloride (Propoxyphene may slow metabolism). Products include:
Norpramin Tablets 1273

Dezocine (Additive CNS depression). Products include:
Dalgan Injection 529

Diazepam (Additive CNS depression). Products include:
Dizac (diazepam injectable emulsion) CIV 1862
Valium Injectable 2336
Valium Tablets 2335

Dicumarol (Propoxyphene may slow metabolism).
No products indexed under this heading.

Divalproex Sodium (Propoxyphene may slow metabolism). Products include:
Depakote Tablets 418

Doxepin Hydrochloride (Propoxyphene may slow metabolism). Products include:
Adapin Capsules 1542
Sinequan 2028
Zonalon Cream 1042

Droperidol (Additive CNS depression). Products include:
Inapsine Injection 462

Enflurane (Additive CNS depression).
No products indexed under this heading.

Estazolam (Additive CNS depression). Products include:
ProSom Tablets 457

Ethchlorvynol (Additive CNS depression). Products include:
Placidyl Capsules 456

Ethinamate (Additive CNS depression).
No products indexed under this heading.

Ethosuximide (Propoxyphene may slow metabolism). Products include:
Zarontin Capsules 1986
Zarontin Syrup 1986

Ethotoin (Propoxyphene may slow metabolism). Products include:
Peganone Tablets 455

Felbamate (Concurrent use may result in severe neurological signs, including coma). Products include:
Felbatol 2774

Fentanyl (Additive CNS depression). Products include:
Duragesic Transdermal System .. 1336

Fentanyl Citrate (Additive CNS depression). Products include:
Sublimaze Injection 463

Fluphenazine Decanoate (Additive CNS depression). Products include:
Prolixin Decanoate 510

Fluphenazine Enanthate (Additive CNS depression). Products include:
Prolixin Enanthate 510

Fluphenazine Hydrochloride (Additive CNS depression). Products include:
Prolixin 510

Flurazepam Hydrochloride (Additive CNS depression). Products include:
Dalmane Capsules 2329

Glutethimide (Additive CNS depression).
No products indexed under this heading.

Haloperidol (Additive CNS depression). Products include:
Haldol Injection, Tablets and Concentrate 1585

Haloperidol Decanoate (Additive CNS depression). Products include:
Haldol Decanoate 1587

Hydrocodone Bitartrate (Additive CNS depression). Products include:
Codiclear DH Syrup 808
Duratuss HD Elixir 2750
Histussin D Liquid 670
Hycodan Tablets and Syrup 946
Hycomine Compound Tablets .. 948
Hycomine 947
Hycotuss Expectorant Syrup 950
Hydrocet Capsules 787
Lorcet 10/650 Tablets 1016
Lortab 2751
Tussend 1830
Tussend Expectorant 1831
Vicodin Tablets 1404
Vicodin ES Tablets 1405
Vicodin HP Tablets 1403
Vicodin Tuss Expectorant 1406
Zydone Capsules 967

Hydrocodone Polistirex (Additive CNS depression). Products include:
Tussionex Pennkinetic Extended-Release Suspension 1624

Hydroxyzine Hydrochloride (Additive CNS depression). Products include:
Atarax Tablets & Syrup 1992
Marax Tablets & DF Syrup 2015
Vistaril Intramuscular Solution .. 2042

Imipramine Hydrochloride (Propoxyphene may slow metabolism). Products include:
Tofranil Ampuls 873
Tofranil Tablets 875

Imipramine Pamoate (Propoxyphene may slow metabolism). Products include:
Tofranil-PM Capsules 876

Isoflurane (Additive CNS depression).
No products indexed under this heading.

Ketamine Hydrochloride (Additive CNS depression).
No products indexed under this heading.

Lamotrigine (Propoxyphene may slow the metabolism of anticonvulsants). Products include:
Lamictal Tablets 1105

Levomethadyl Acetate Hydrochloride (Additive CNS depression). Products include:
Orlaam Oral Solution 2361

Levorphanol Tartrate (Additive CNS depression). Products include:
Levo-Dromoran 2297

Lorazepam (Additive CNS depression). Products include:
Ativan Injection 2805
Ativan Tablets 2807

Loxapine Hydrochloride (Additive CNS depression). Products include:
Loxitane 1426

Loxapine Succinate (Additive CNS depression). Products include:
Loxitane Capsules 1426

Maprotiline Hydrochloride (Propoxyphene may slow metabolism). Products include:
Ludiomil Tablets 861

Meperidine Hydrochloride (Additive CNS depression). Products include:
Demerol 2438
Mepergan Injection 2859

Mephenytoin (Propoxyphene may slow metabolism). Products include:
Mesantoin Tablets 2400

Mephobarbital (Additive CNS depression). Products include:
Mebaral Tablets 2452

Meprobamate (Additive CNS depression). Products include:
Miltown Tablets 2780
PMB 200 and PMB 400 2890

Mesoridazine Besylate (Additive CNS depression). Products include:
Serentil 689

Methadone Hydrochloride (Additive CNS depression). Products include:
Methadone Hydrochloride Oral Concentrate 2356
Methadone Hydrochloride Oral Solution & Tablets 2357

Methohexital Sodium (Additive CNS depression).
No products indexed under this heading.

Methotrimeprazine (Additive CNS depression). Products include:
Levoprome 1321

Methoxyflurane (Additive CNS depression).
No products indexed under this heading.

Methsuximide (Propoxyphene may slow metabolism). Products include:
Celontin Kapseals 1955

Midazolam Hydrochloride (Additive CNS depression). Products include:
Versed Injection 2324

IMPORTANT NOTE: Always consult each drug listing in the patient's regimen for possible interactions.

Darvon-N/Darvocet-N — Interactions Index — 238

Molindone Hydrochloride (Additive CNS depression). Products include:
- Moban Tablets and Concentrate 1036

Morphine Sulfate (Additive CNS depression). Products include:
- Astramorph/PF Injection, USP (Preservative-Free) 526
- Duramorph Injection 983
- Infumorph 200 and Infumorph 500 Sterile Solutions 985
- Kadian Capsules 2948
- MS Contin Tablets 2149
- MSIR 2152
- Oramorph SR (Morphine Sulfate Sustained Release Tablets) 2359
- RMS Suppositories CII 2766
- Roxanol 2365

Nortriptyline Hydrochloride (Propoxyphene may slow metabolism). Products include:
- Pamelor 2409

Opium Alkaloids (Additive CNS depression).
- No products indexed under this heading.

Oxazepam (Additive CNS depression). Products include:
- Serax Capsules 2916
- Serax Tablets 2916

Oxycodone Hydrochloride (Additive CNS depression). Products include:
- OxyContin Tablets 2163
- OxyIR Capsules 2167
- Percocet Tablets 955
- Percodan Tablets 955
- Percodan-Demi Tablets 956
- Roxicodone Tablets, Oral Solution & Intensol (Oxycodone) 2366
- Tylox Capsules 1593

Paramethadione (Propoxyphene may slow metabolism).
- No products indexed under this heading.

Pentobarbital Sodium (Additive CNS depression). Products include:
- Nembutal Sodium Capsules 440
- Nembutal Sodium Solution 442
- Nembutal Sodium Suppositories 444

Perphenazine (Additive CNS depression). Products include:
- Etrafon 2495
- Triavil Tablets 1800
- Trilafon 2532

Phenacemide (Propoxyphene may slow metabolism). Products include:
- Phenurone Tablets 455

Phenobarbital (Additive CNS depression; propoxyphene may slow metabolism). Products include:
- Arco-Lase Plus Tablets 513
- Bellergal-S Tablets 2375
- Donnatal 2234
- Donnatal Extentabs 2234
- Donnatal Tablets 2234
- Phenobarbital Elixir and Tablets 1523
- Quadrinal Tablets 1398

Phensuximide (Propoxyphene may slow metabolism).
- No products indexed under this heading.

Phenytoin (Propoxyphene may slow metabolism). Products include:
- Dilantin Infatabs 1967
- Dilantin-125 Suspension 1969

Phenytoin Sodium (Propoxyphene may slow metabolism). Products include:
- Dilantin Kapseals 1965

Prazepam (Additive CNS depression).
- No products indexed under this heading.

Primidone (Propoxyphene may slow metabolism). Products include:
- Mysoline 2860

Prochlorperazine (Additive CNS depression). Products include:
- Compazine 2644

Promethazine Hydrochloride (Additive CNS depression). Products include:
- Mepergan Injection 2859
- Phenergan with Codeine 2883
- Phenergan with Dextromethorphan 2885
- Phenergan Injection 2880
- Phenergan Suppositories 2882
- Phenergan Syrup 2881
- Phenergan Tablets 2882
- Phenergan VC 2886
- Phenergan VC with Codeine 2888

Propofol (Additive CNS depression). Products include:
- Diprivan Injectable Emulsion 2939

Propoxyphene Hydrochloride (Additive CNS depression). Products include:
- Darvon 1475
- Wygesic Tablets 2930

Protriptyline Hydrochloride (Propoxyphene may slow metabolism). Products include:
- Vivactil Tablets 1820

Quazepam (Additive CNS depression). Products include:
- Doral Tablets 2773

Risperidone (Additive CNS depression). Products include:
- Risperdal Tablets 1348

Secobarbital Sodium (Additive CNS depression). Products include:
- Seconal Sodium Pulvules 1529

Sevoflurane (Additive CNS depression).
- No products indexed under this heading.

Sufentanil Citrate (Additive CNS depression). Products include:
- Sufenta Injection 1355

Temazepam (Additive CNS depression). Products include:
- Restoril Capsules 2413

Thiamylal Sodium (Additive CNS depression).
- No products indexed under this heading.

Thioridazine Hydrochloride (Additive CNS depression). Products include:
- Mellaril 2398

Thiothixene (Additive CNS depression). Products include:
- Navane Capsules and Concentrate 2018
- Navane Intramuscular 2019

Triazolam (Additive CNS depression). Products include:
- Halcion Tablets 2093

Trifluoperazine Hydrochloride (Additive CNS depression). Products include:
- Stelazine 2692

Trimethadione (Propoxyphene may slow metabolism).
- No products indexed under this heading.

Trimipramine Maleate (Propoxyphene may slow metabolism). Products include:
- Surmontil Capsules 2917

Valproic Acid (Propoxyphene may slow metabolism). Products include:
- Depakene 416

Warfarin Sodium (Propoxyphene may slow metabolism). Products include:
- Coumadin 941

Zolpidem Tartrate (Additive CNS depression). Products include:
- Ambien Tablets 2559

Food Interactions
Alcohol (Additive CNS depression).

DARVOCET-N 100 TABLETS
(Propoxyphene Napsylate, Acetaminophen) 1473
See **Darvocet-N 50 Tablets**

DARVON COMPOUND-65 PULVULES
(Propoxyphene Hydrochloride, Aspirin, Caffeine) 1475
May interact with central nervous system depressants, oral anticoagulants, antigout agents, antidepressant drugs, anticonvulsants, and certain other agents. Compounds in these categories include:

Alfentanil Hydrochloride (The CNS-depressant effect of propoxyphene is additive with that of other CNS depressants). Products include:
- Alfenta Injection 1334

Allopurinol (Salicylates may inhibit the uricosuric effect of uricosuric agents). Products include:
- Zyloprim Tablets 1194

Alprazolam (The CNS-depressant effect of propoxyphene is additive with that of other CNS depressants). Products include:
- Xanax Tablets 2115

Amitriptyline Hydrochloride (Propoxyphene may slow the metabolism of antidepressants). Products include:
- Elavil 2945
- Etrafon 2495
- Limbitrol 2333
- Triavil Tablets 1800

Amoxapine (Propoxyphene may slow the metabolism of antidepressants). Products include:
- Asendin Tablets 1419

Aprobarbital (The CNS-depressant effect of propoxyphene is additive with that of other CNS depressants).
- No products indexed under this heading.

Buprenorphine (The CNS-depressant effect of propoxyphene is additive with that of other CNS depressants). Products include:
- Buprenex Injectable 2170

Bupropion Hydrochloride (Propoxyphene may slow the metabolism of antidepressants). Products include:
- Wellbutrin Tablets 1177

Buspirone Hydrochloride (The CNS-depressant effect of propoxyphene is additive with that of other CNS depressants). Products include:
- BuSpar Tablets 738

Butabarbital (The CNS-depressant effect of propoxyphene is additive with that of other CNS depressants).
- No products indexed under this heading.

Butalbital (The CNS-depressant effect of propoxyphene is additive with that of other CNS depressants). Products include:
- Axocet Capsules 2469
- Esgic-plus Capsules 1012
- Esgic-plus Tablets 1012
- Fioricet Tablets 2386
- Fioricet with Codeine Tablets 2387
- Fiorinal Capsules 2388
- Fiorinal with Codeine Capsules 2390
- Fiorinal Tablets 2388
- Phrenilin 790
- Sedapap Tablets 50 mg/650 mg 1826

Carbamazepine (Co-administration has resulted in severe neurological signs, including coma). Products include:
- Atretol Tablets 569
- Tegretol/Tegretol-XR 870

Chlordiazepoxide (The CNS-depressant effect of propoxyphene is additive with that of other CNS depressants). Products include:
- Limbitrol 2333

Chlordiazepoxide Hydrochloride (The CNS-depressant effect of propoxyphene is additive with that of other CNS depressants). Products include:
- Librax Capsules 2330
- Librium Capsules 2331
- Librium Injectable 2332

Chlorpromazine (The CNS-depressant effect of propoxyphene is additive with that of other CNS depressants). Products include:
- Thorazine Suppositories 2701

Chlorpromazine Hydrochloride (The CNS-depressant effect of propoxyphene is additive with that of other CNS depressants). Products include:
- Thorazine 2701

Chlorprothixene (The CNS-depressant effect of propoxyphene is additive with that of other CNS depressants).
- No products indexed under this heading.

Chlorprothixene Hydrochloride (The CNS-depressant effect of propoxyphene is additive with that of other CNS depressants).
- No products indexed under this heading.

Chlorprothixene Lactate (The CNS-depressant effect of propoxyphene is additive with that of other CNS depressants).
- No products indexed under this heading.

Clorazepate Dipotassium (The CNS-depressant effect of propoxyphene is additive with that of other CNS depressants). Products include:
- Tranxene 459

Clozapine (The CNS-depressant effect of propoxyphene is additive with that of other CNS depressants). Products include:
- Clozaril Tablets 2377

Codeine Phosphate (The CNS-depressant effect of propoxyphene is additive with that of other CNS depressants). Products include:
- Brontex 2130
- Dimetane-DC Cough Syrup 2232
- Fioricet with Codeine Capsules 2387
- Fiorinal with Codeine Capsules 2390
- Nucofed 2225
- Phenergan with Codeine 2883
- Phenergan VC with Codeine 2888
- Robitussin A-C Syrup 2248
- Robitussin-DAC Syrup 2249
- Ryna ...... [ℝ] 804
- Soma Compound w/Codeine Tablets 2784
- Tylenol with Codeine 1592

Desflurane (The CNS-depressant effect of propoxyphene is additive with that of other CNS depressants). Products include:
- Suprane (desflurane, USP) 1865

Desipramine Hydrochloride (Propoxyphene may slow the metabolism of antidepressants). Products include:
- Norpramin Tablets 1273

Dezocine (The CNS-depressant effect of propoxyphene is additive with that of other CNS depressants). Products include:
- Dalgan Injection 529

Diazepam (The CNS-depressant effect of propoxyphene is additive with that of other CNS depressants). Products include:
- Dizac (diazepam injectable emulsion) CIV 1862
- Valium Injectable 2336
- Valium Tablets 2335

([ℝ] Described in PDR For Nonprescription Drugs)   (⊙ Described in PDR For Ophthalmology)

Dicumarol (Salicylates may enhance the effect of anticoagulants; propoxyphene may slow the metabolism of warfarin-like drugs).
No products indexed under this heading.

Divalproex Sodium (Propoxyphene may slow the metabolism of anticonvulsants). Products include:
Depakote Tablets ... 418

Doxepin Hydrochloride (Propoxyphene may slow the metabolism of antidepressants). Products include:
Adapin Capsules ... 1542
Sinequan ... 2028
Zonalon Cream ... 1042

Droperidol (The CNS-depressant effect of propoxyphene is additive with that of other CNS depressants). Products include:
Inapsine Injection ... 462

Enflurane (The CNS-depressant effect of propoxyphene is additive with that of other CNS depressants).
No products indexed under this heading.

Estazolam (The CNS-depressant effect of propoxyphene is additive with that of other CNS depressants). Products include:
ProSom Tablets ... 457

Ethchlorvynol (The CNS-depressant effect of propoxyphene is additive with that of other CNS depressants). Products include:
Placidyl Capsules ... 456

Ethinamate (The CNS-depressant effect of propoxyphene is additive with that of other CNS depressants).
No products indexed under this heading.

Ethosuximide (Propoxyphene may slow the metabolism of anticonvulsants). Products include:
Zarontin Capsules ... 1986
Zarontin Syrup ... 1986

Ethotoin (Propoxyphene may slow the metabolism of anticonvulsants). Products include:
Peganone Tablets ... 455

Felbamate (Propoxyphene may slow the metabolism of anticonvulsants). Products include:
Felbatol ... 2774

Fentanyl (The CNS-depressant effect of propoxyphene is additive with that of other CNS depressants). Products include:
Duragesic Transdermal System ... 1336

Fentanyl Citrate (The CNS-depressant effect of propoxyphene is additive with that of other CNS depressants). Products include:
Sublimaze Injection ... 463

Fluoxetine Hydrochloride (Propoxyphene may slow the metabolism of antidepressants). Products include:
Prozac Pulvules & Liquid, Oral Solution ... 935

Fluphenazine Decanoate (The CNS-depressant effect of propoxyphene is additive with that of other CNS depressants). Products include:
Prolixin Decanoate ... 510

Fluphenazine Enanthate (The CNS-depressant effect of propoxyphene is additive with that of other CNS depressants). Products include:
Prolixin Enanthate ... 510

Fluphenazine Hydrochloride (The CNS-depressant effect of propoxyphene is additive with that of other CNS depressants). Products include:
Prolixin ... 510

Flurazepam Hydrochloride (The CNS-depressant effect of propoxyphene is additive with that of other CNS depressants). Products include:
Dalmane Capsules ... 2329

Fosphenytoin Sodium (Propoxyphene may slow the metabolism of anticonvulsants). Products include:
Cerebyx Injection ... 1956

Glutethimide (The CNS-depressant effect of propoxyphene is additive with that of other CNS depressants).
No products indexed under this heading.

Haloperidol (The CNS-depressant effect of propoxyphene is additive with that of other CNS depressants). Products include:
Haldol Injection, Tablets and Concentrate ... 1585

Haloperidol Decanoate (The CNS-depressant effect of propoxyphene is additive with that of other CNS depressants). Products include:
Haldol Decanoate ... 1587

Hydrocodone Bitartrate (The CNS-depressant effect of propoxyphene is additive with that of other CNS depressants). Products include:
Codiclear DH Syrup ... 808
Duratuss HD Elixir ... 2750
Histussin D Liquid ... 670
Hycodan Tablets and Syrup ... 946
Hycomine Compound Tablets ... 948
Hycomine ... 947
Hycotuss Expectorant Syrup ... 950
Hydrocet Capsules ... 787
Lorcet 10/650 Tablets ... 1016
Lortab ... 2751
Tussend ... 1830
Tussend Expectorant ... 1831
Vicodin Tablets ... 1404
Vicodin ES Tablets ... 1405
Vicodin HP Tablets ... 1403
Vicodin Tuss Expectorant ... 1406
Zydone Capsules ... 967

Hydrocodone Polistirex (The CNS-depressant effect of propoxyphene is additive with that of other CNS depressants). Products include:
Tussionex Pennkinetic Extended-Release Suspension ... 1624

Hydromorphone Hydrochloride (The CNS-depressant effect of propoxyphene is additive with that of other CNS depressants). Products include:
Dilaudid Ampules ... 1382
Dilaudid Cough Syrup ... 1383
Dilaudid-HP Injection ... 1384
Dilaudid-HP Lyophilized Powder 250 mg ... 1384
Dilaudid ... 1382
Dilaudid Oral Liquid ... 1386
Dilaudid ... 1382
Dilaudid Tablets - 8 mg ... 1386

Hydroxyzine Hydrochloride (The CNS-depressant effect of propoxyphene is additive with that of other CNS depressants). Products include:
Atarax Tablets & Syrup ... 1992
Marax Tablets & DF Syrup ... 2015
Vistaril Intramuscular Solution ... 2042

Imipramine Hydrochloride (Propoxyphene may slow the metabolism of antidepressants). Products include:
Tofranil Ampuls ... 873
Tofranil Tablets ... 875

Imipramine Pamoate (Propoxyphene may slow the metabolism of antidepressants). Products include:
Tofranil-PM Capsules ... 876

Isocarboxazid (Propoxyphene may slow the metabolism of antidepressants).
No products indexed under this heading.

Isoflurane (The CNS-depressant effect of propoxyphene is additive with that of other CNS depressants).
No products indexed under this heading.

Ketamine Hydrochloride (The CNS-depressant effect of propoxyphene is additive with that of other CNS depressants).
No products indexed under this heading.

Lamotrigine (Propoxyphene may slow the metabolism of anticonvulsants). Products include:
Lamictal Tablets ... 1105

Levomethadyl Acetate Hydrochloride (The CNS-depressant effect of propoxyphene is additive with that of other CNS depressants). Products include:
Orlaam Oral Solution ... 2361

Levorphanol Tartrate (The CNS-depressant effect of propoxyphene is additive with that of other CNS depressants). Products include:
Levo-Dromoran ... 2297

Lorazepam (The CNS-depressant effect of propoxyphene is additive with that of other CNS depressants). Products include:
Ativan Injection ... 2805
Ativan Tablets ... 2807

Loxapine Hydrochloride (The CNS-depressant effect of propoxyphene is additive with that of other CNS depressants). Products include:
Loxitane ... 1426

Loxapine Succinate (The CNS-depressant effect of propoxyphene is additive with that of other CNS depressants). Products include:
Loxitane Capsules ... 1426

Maprotiline Hydrochloride (Propoxyphene may slow the metabolism of antidepressants). Products include:
Ludiomil Tablets ... 861

Meperidine Hydrochloride (The CNS-depressant effect of propoxyphene is additive with that of other CNS depressants). Products include:
Demerol ... 2438
Mepergan Injection ... 2859

Mephenytoin (Propoxyphene may slow the metabolism of anticonvulsants). Products include:
Mesantoin Tablets ... 2400

Mephobarbital (The CNS-depressant effect of propoxyphene is additive with that of other CNS depressants). Products include:
Mebaral Tablets ... 2452

Meprobamate (The CNS-depressant effect of propoxyphene is additive with that of other CNS depressants). Products include:
Miltown Tablets ... 2780
PMB 200 and PMB 400 ... 2890

Mesoridazine Besylate (The CNS-depressant effect of propoxyphene is additive with that of other CNS depressants). Products include:
Serentil ... 689

Methadone Hydrochloride (The CNS-depressant effect of propoxyphene is additive with that of other CNS depressants). Products include:
Methadone Hydrochloride Oral Concentrate ... 2356
Methadone Hydrochloride Oral Solution & Tablets ... 2357

Methohexital Sodium (The CNS-depressant effect of propoxyphene is additive with that of other CNS depressants).
No products indexed under this heading.

Methotrimeprazine (The CNS-depressant effect of propoxyphene is additive with that of other CNS depressants). Products include:
Levoprome ... 1321

Methoxyflurane (The CNS-depressant effect of propoxyphene is additive with that of other CNS depressants).
No products indexed under this heading.

Methsuximide (Propoxyphene may slow the metabolism of anticonvulsants). Products include:
Celontin Kapseals ... 1955

Midazolam Hydrochloride (The CNS-depressant effect of propoxyphene is additive with that of other CNS depressants). Products include:
Versed Injection ... 2324

Mirtazapine (Propoxyphene may slow the metabolism of antidepressants). Products include:
Remeron Tablets ... 1878

Molindone Hydrochloride (The CNS-depressant effect of propoxyphene is additive with that of other CNS depressants). Products include:
Moban Tablets and Concentrate ... 1036

Morphine Sulfate (The CNS-depressant effect of propoxyphene is additive with that of other CNS depressants). Products include:
Astramorph/PF Injection, USP (Preservative-Free) ... 526
Duramorph Injection ... 983
Infumorph 200 and Infumorph 500 Sterile Solutions ... 985
Kadian Capsules ... 2948
MS Contin Tablets ... 2149
MSIR ... 2152
Oramorph SR (Morphine Sulfate Sustained Release Tablets) ... 2359
RMS Suppositories CII ... 2766
Roxanol ... 2365

Nefazodone Hydrochloride (Propoxyphene may slow the metabolism of antidepressants). Products include:
Serzone Tablets ... 776

Nortriptyline Hydrochloride (Propoxyphene may slow the metabolism of antidepressants). Products include:
Pamelor ... 2409

Opium Alkaloids (The CNS-depressant effect of propoxyphene is additive with that of other CNS depressants).
No products indexed under this heading.

Oxazepam (The CNS-depressant effect of propoxyphene is additive with that of other CNS depressants). Products include:
Serax Capsules ... 2916
Serax Tablets ... 2916

Oxycodone Hydrochloride (The CNS-depressant effect of propoxyphene is additive with that of other CNS depressants). Products include:
OxyContin Tablets ... 2163
OxyIR Capsules ... 2167
Percocet Tablets ... 955
Percodan Tablets ... 955
Percodan-Demi Tablets ... 956
Roxicodone Tablets, Oral Solution & Intensol (Oxycodone) ... 2366
Tylox Capsules ... 1593

Paramethadione (Propoxyphene may slow the metabolism of anticonvulsants).
No products indexed under this heading.

Paroxetine Hydrochloride (Propoxyphene may slow the metabolism of antidepressants). Products include:
Paxil Tablets ... 2681

IMPORTANT NOTE: Always consult each drug listing in the patient's regimen for possible interactions.

Pentobarbital Sodium (The CNS-depressant effect of propoxyphene is additive with that of other CNS depressants). Products include:
- Nembutal Sodium Capsules 440
- Nembutal Sodium Solution 442
- Nembutal Sodium Suppositories 444

Perphenazine (The CNS-depressant effect of propoxyphene is additive with that of other CNS depressants). Products include:
- Etrafon 2495
- Triavil Tablets 1800
- Trilafon 2532

Phenacemide (Propoxyphene may slow the metabolism of anticonvulsants). Products include:
- Phenurone Tablets 455

Phenelzine Sulfate (Propoxyphene may slow the metabolism of antidepressants). Products include:
- Nardil 1977

Phenobarbital (Propoxyphene may slow the metabolism of anticonvulsants). Products include:
- Arco-Lase Plus Tablets 513
- Bellergal-S Tablets 2375
- Donnatal 2234
- Donnatal Extentabs 2234
- Donnatal Tablets 2234
- Phenobarbital Elixir and Tablets 1523
- Quadrinal Tablets 1398

Phensuximide (Propoxyphene may slow the metabolism of anticonvulsants).
- No products indexed under this heading.

Phenytoin (Propoxyphene may slow the metabolism of anticonvulsants). Products include:
- Dilantin Infatabs 1967
- Dilantin-125 Suspension 1969

Phenytoin Sodium (Propoxyphene may slow the metabolism of anticonvulsants). Products include:
- Dilantin Kapseals 1965

Prazepam (The CNS-depressant effect of propoxyphene is additive with that of other CNS depressants).
- No products indexed under this heading.

Primidone (Propoxyphene may slow the metabolism of anticonvulsants). Products include:
- Mysoline 2860

Probenecid (Salicylates may inhibit the uricosuric effect of uricosuric agents). Products include:
- Benemid Tablets 1651
- ColBENEMID Tablets 1662

Prochlorperazine (The CNS-depressant effect of propoxyphene is additive with that of other CNS depressants). Products include:
- Compazine 2644

Promethazine Hydrochloride (The CNS-depressant effect of propoxyphene is additive with that of other CNS depressants). Products include:
- Mepergan Injection 2859
- Phenergan with Codeine 2883
- Phenergan with Dextromethorphan 2885
- Phenergan Injection 2880
- Phenergan Suppositories 2882
- Phenergan Syrup 2881
- Phenergan Tablets 2882
- Phenergan VC 2886
- Phenergan VC with Codeine 2888

Propofol (The CNS-depressant effect of propoxyphene is additive with that of other CNS depressants). Products include:
- Diprivan Injectable Emulsion 2939

Propoxyphene Napsylate (The CNS-depressant effect of propoxyphene is additive with that of other CNS depressants). Products include:
- Darvon-N/Darvocet-N 1473

Protriptyline Hydrochloride (Propoxyphene may slow the metabolism of antidepressants). Products include:
- Vivactil Tablets 1820

Quazepam (The CNS-depressant effect of propoxyphene is additive with that of other CNS depressants). Products include:
- Doral Tablets 2773

Risperidone (The CNS-depressant effect of propoxyphene is additive with that of other CNS depressants). Products include:
- Risperdal Tablets 1348

Secobarbital Sodium (The CNS-depressant effect of propoxyphene is additive with that of other CNS depressants). Products include:
- Seconal Sodium Pulvules 1529

Sertraline Hydrochloride (Propoxyphene may slow the metabolism of antidepressants). Products include:
- Zoloft Tablets 2051

Sevoflurane (The CNS-depressant effect of propoxyphene is additive with that of other CNS depressants).
- No products indexed under this heading.

Sufentanil Citrate (The CNS-depressant effect of propoxyphene is additive with that of other CNS depressants). Products include:
- Sufenta Injection 1355

Sulfinpyrazone (Salicylates may inhibit the uricosuric effect of uricosuric agents). Products include:
- Anturane 823

Temazepam (The CNS-depressant effect of propoxyphene is additive with that of other CNS depressants). Products include:
- Restoril Capsules 2413

Thiamylal Sodium (The CNS-depressant effect of propoxyphene is additive with that of other CNS depressants).
- No products indexed under this heading.

Thioridazine Hydrochloride (The CNS-depressant effect of propoxyphene is additive with that of other CNS depressants). Products include:
- Mellaril 2398

Thiothixene (The CNS-depressant effect of propoxyphene is additive with that of other CNS depressants). Products include:
- Navane Capsules and Concentrate 2018
- Navane Intramuscular 2019

Tranylcypromine Sulfate (Propoxyphene may slow the metabolism of antidepressants). Products include:
- Parnate Tablets 2679

Trazodone Hydrochloride (Propoxyphene may slow the metabolism of antidepressants). Products include:
- Desyrel and Desyrel Dividose 504

Triazolam (The CNS-depressant effect of propoxyphene is additive with that of other CNS depressants). Products include:
- Halcion Tablets 2093

Trifluoperazine Hydrochloride (The CNS-depressant effect of propoxyphene is additive with that of other CNS depressants). Products include:
- Stelazine 2692

Trimethadione (Propoxyphene may slow the metabolism of anticonvulsants).
- No products indexed under this heading.

Trimipramine Maleate (Propoxyphene may slow the metabolism of antidepressants). Products include:
- Surmontil Capsules 2917

Valproic Acid (Propoxyphene may slow the metabolism of anticonvulsants). Products include:
- Depakene 416

Venlafaxine Hydrochloride (Propoxyphene may slow the metabolism of antidepressants). Products include:
- Effexor 2825

Warfarin Sodium (Salicylates may enhance the effect of anticoagulants; propoxyphene may slow the metabolism of warfarin-like drugs). Products include:
- Coumadin 941

Zolpidem Tartrate (The CNS-depressant effect of propoxyphene is additive with that of other CNS depressants). Products include:
- Ambien Tablets 2559

Food Interactions

Alcohol (The CNS-depressant effect of propoxyphene is additive with that of other CNS depressants).

DARVON PULVULES
(Propoxyphene Hydrochloride) 1475

See **Darvon Compound-65 Pulvules**

DARVON-N SUSPENSION & TABLETS
(Propoxyphene Napsylate) 1473

See **Darvocet-N 50 Tablets**

DAUNOXOME
(Daunorubicin Citrate) 1842

May interact with:

Daunorubicin Hydrochloride (Special attention must be given to the potential cardiac toxicity of DaunoXome, particularly in patients who have received prior anthracyclines). Products include:
- Cerubidine for Injection 634

Doxorubicin Hydrochloride (Special attention must be given to the potential cardiac toxicity of DaunoXome, particularly in patients who have received prior anthracyclines). Products include:
- Adriamycin PFS 2056
- Adriamycin RDF 2056
- Doxil 2613
- Doxorubicin Astra 531
- Rubex for Injection 721

Idarubicin Hydrochloride (Special attention must be given to the potential cardiac toxicity of DaunoXome, particularly in patients who have received prior anthracyclines). Products include:
- Idamycin Injection 2096

DAYPRO CAPLETS
(Oxaprozin) 2578

May interact with oral anticoagulants and certain other agents. Compounds in these categories include:

Aspirin (Co-administration is not recommended because oxaprozin displaces salicylates from binding sites resulting in increased risk of salicylate toxicity). Products include:
- Alka-Seltzer Cherry Effervescent Antacid and Pain Reliever .... ▣ 609
- Alka-Seltzer Extra Strength Effervescent Antacid and Pain Reliever .... ▣ 609
- Alka-Seltzer Lemon Lime Effervescent Antacid and Pain Reliever .... ▣ 609
- Alka-Seltzer Original Effervescent Antacid and Pain Reliever .... ▣ 609
- Alka-Seltzer Plus .... ▣ 611
- Alka-Seltzer Plus Sinus Medicine .... ▣ 611
- Ascriptin .... ▣ 650
- Arthritis Strength BC Powder .... ▣ 631
- BC Cold Powder Multi-Symptom Formula (Cold-Sinus-Allergy) .... ▣ 631
- BC Cold Powder Non-Drowsy Formula (Cold-Sinus) .... ▣ 631
- BC Powder .... ▣ 631
- Genuine Bayer Aspirin Tablets & Caplets .... ▣ 618
- Extra Strength Bayer Arthritis Pain Regimen Formula .... ▣ 615
- Extra Strength Bayer Aspirin Caplets & Tablets .... ▣ 617
- Extended-Release Bayer 8-Hour Aspirin .... ▣ 616
- Extra Strength Bayer Plus Aspirin Caplets .... ▣ 617
- Extra Strength Bayer PM Aspirin Plus Sleep Aid .... ▣ 617
- Aspirin Regimen Bayer 81 mg Tablets with Calcium .... ▣ 615
- Aspirin Regimen Bayer Adult Low Strength 81 mg Tablets .... ▣ 613
- Aspirin Regimen Bayer Children's Chewable Aspirin .... ▣ 616
- Aspirin Regimen Bayer Regular Strength 325 mg Caplets .... ▣ 613
- Bufferin Analgesic Tablets .... ▣ 636
- Arthritis Strength Bufferin Analgesic Caplets .... ▣ 637
- Extra Strength Bufferin Analgesic Tablets .... ▣ 637
- Cama Arthritis Pain Reliever .... ▣ 748
- Darvon Compound-65 Pulvules 1475
- Easprin 1971
- Ecotrin 2625
- Ecotrin Enteric Coated Aspirin Maximum Strength Tablets and Caplets .... ▣ 775
- Ecotrin Enteric Coated Aspirin Regular Strength Tablets 2625
- Empirin Aspirin Tablets .... ▣ 818
- Excedrin Extra-Strength Analgesic Tablets, Caplets, and Geltabs 734
- Fiorinal Capsules 2388
- Fiorinal with Codeine Capsules 2390
- Fiorinal Tablets 2388
- Goody's Extra Strength Headache Powders .... ▣ 632
- Goody's Extra Strength Pain Relief Tablets .... ▣ 632
- Halfprin Tablets 1413
- Norgesic 1554
- Percodan Tablets 955
- Percodan-Demi Tablets 956
- Robaxisal Tablets 2246
- Soma Compound w/Codeine Tablets 2784
- Soma Compound Tablets 2783
- St. Joseph Adult Chewable Aspirin (81 mg.) .... ▣ 768
- Talwin Compound 2466
- Vanquish Analgesic Caplets .... ▣ 627

Cimetidine (Concurrent use may reduce the total body clearance of oxaprozin). Products include:
- Tagamet HB Tablets .... ▣ 786
- Tagamet Tablets 2694

Cimetidine Hydrochloride (Concurrent use may reduce the total body clearance of oxaprozin). Products include:
- Tagamet 2694

Dicumarol (Co-administration with 1200 mg/day of Daypro does not affect anticoagulant effects of warfarin; however, caution should be exercised).
- No products indexed under this heading.

Metoprolol Succinate (Concurrent use of 1200 mg Daypro q.d. and 100 mg metoprolol b.i.d. exhibits statistically significant but transient increase in sitting and standing blood pressure). Products include:
- Toprol-XL Tablets 560

(▣ Described in PDR For Nonprescription Drugs) (◉ Described in PDR For Ophthalmology)

241 Interactions Index Decadron Injection

Metoprolol Tartrate (Concurrent use of 1200 mg Daypro q.d. and 100 mg metoprolol b.i.d. exhibits statistically significant but transient increase in sitting and standing blood pressure). Products include:

- Lopressor ... 848
- Lopressor HCT Tablets ... 850

Ranitidine Hydrochloride (Concurrent use may reduce the total body clearance of oxaprozin). Products include:

- Zantac ... 1182
- Zantac Injection ... 1180
- Zantac Syrup ... 1182

Warfarin Sodium (Co-administration with 1200 mg/day of Daypro does not affect anticoagulant effects of warfarin; however, caution should be exercised). Products include:

- Coumadin ... 941

Food Interactions

Food, unspecified (Reduces the rate of absorption of oxaprozin, but the extent of absorption is unchanged).

DEBROX DROPS

(Carbamide Peroxide) ... 775
None cited in PDR database.

DECADRON ELIXIR

(Dexamethasone) ... 1676
May interact with potassium-depleting diuretics, oral anticoagulants, oral hypoglycemic agents, insulin, and certain other agents. Compounds in these categories include:

Acarbose (Potential for increased requirements of oral hypoglycemic agents). Products include:

- Precose ... 604

Aspirin (Aspirin should be used cautiously in conjunction with corticosteroids in hypoprothrombinemia). Products include:

- Alka-Seltzer Cherry Effervescent Antacid and Pain Reliever ... 609
- Alka-Seltzer Extra Strength Effervescent Antacid and Pain Reliever ... 609
- Alka-Seltzer Lemon Lime Effervescent Antacid and Pain Reliever ... 609
- Alka-Seltzer Original Effervescent Antacid and Pain Reliever ... 609
- Alka-Seltzer Plus ... 611
- Alka-Seltzer Plus Sinus Medicine ... 611
- Ascriptin ... 650
- Arthritis Strength BC Powder ... 631
- BC Cold Powder Multi-Symptom Formula (Cold-Sinus-Allergy) ... 631
- BC Cold Powder Non-Drowsy Formula (Cold-Sinus) ... 631
- BC Powder ... 631
- Genuine Bayer Aspirin Tablets & Caplets ... 618
- Extra Strength Bayer Arthritis Pain Regimen Formula ... 615
- Extra Strength Bayer Aspirin Caplets & Tablets ... 617
- Extended-Release Bayer 8-Hour Aspirin ... 616
- Extra Strength Bayer Plus Aspirin Caplets ... 617
- Extra Strength Bayer PM Aspirin Plus Sleep Aid ... 617
- Aspirin Regimen Bayer 81 mg Tablets with Calcium ... 615
- Aspirin Regimen Bayer Adult Low Strength 81 mg Tablets ... 613
- Aspirin Regimen Bayer Children's Chewable Aspirin ... 616
- Aspirin Regimen Bayer Regular Strength 325 mg Caplets ... 613
- Bufferin Analgesic Tablets ... 636
- Arthritis Strength Bufferin Analgesic Caplets ... 637
- Extra Strength Bufferin Analgesic Tablets ... 637
- Cama Arthritis Pain Reliever ... 748
- Darvon Compound-65 Pulvules ... 1475
- Easprin ... 1971
- Ecotrin ... 2625
- Ecotrin Enteric Coated Aspirin Maximum Strength Tablets and Caplets ... 775
- Ecotrin Enteric Coated Aspirin Regular Strength Tablets ... 2625
- Empirin Aspirin Tablets ... 818
- Excedrin Extra-Strength Analgesic Tablets, Caplets, and Geltabs ... 734
- Fiorinal Capsules ... 2388
- Fiorinal with Codeine Capsules ... 2390
- Fiorinal Tablets ... 2388
- Goody's Extra Strength Headache Powders ... 632
- Goody's Extra Strength Pain Relief Tablets ... 632
- Halfprin Tablets ... 1413
- Norgesic ... 1554
- Percodan Tablets ... 955
- Percodan-Demi Tablets ... 956
- Robaxisal Tablets ... 2246
- Soma Compound w/Codeine Tablets ... 2784
- Soma Compound Tablets ... 2783
- St. Joseph Adult Chewable Aspirin (81 mg.) ... 768
- Talwin Compound ... 2466
- Vanquish Analgesic Caplets ... 627

Bendroflumethiazide (Co-administration may result in hypokalemia).

No products indexed under this heading.

Chlorothiazide (Co-administration may result in hypokalemia). Products include:

- Aldoclor Tablets ... 1638
- Diupres Tablets ... 1691
- Diuril Oral ... 1694

Chlorothiazide Sodium (Co-administration may result in hypokalemia). Products include:

- Diuril Sodium Intravenous ... 1693

Chlorpropamide (Potential for increased requirements of oral hypoglycemic agents). Products include:

- Diabinese Tablets ... 2002

Dicumarol (Potential for altered response to coumarin anticoagulants).

No products indexed under this heading.

Ephedrine (Enhanced metabolic clearance of corticosteroids).

Ephedrine Hydrochloride (Enhanced metabolic clearance of corticosteroids). Products include:

- Primatene Tablets ... 844
- Quadrinal Tablets ... 1398

Ephedrine Sulfate (Enhanced metabolic clearance of corticosteroids). Products include:

- Marax Tablets & DF Syrup ... 2015

Ephedrine Tannate (Enhanced metabolic clearance of corticosteroids). Products include:

- Rynatuss ... 2782

Fosphenytoin Sodium (Enhanced metabolic clearance of corticosteroids). Products include:

- Cerebyx Injection ... 1956

Glimepiride (Potential for increased requirements of oral hypoglycemic agents). Products include:

- Amaryl Tablets ... 1241

Glipizide (Potential for increased requirements of oral hypoglycemic agents). Products include:

- Glucotrol Tablets ... 2011
- Glucotrol XL Extended Release Tablets ... 2012

Glyburide (Potential for increased requirements of oral hypoglycemic agents). Products include:

- DiaBeta Tablets ... 1265
- Glynase PresTab Tablets ... 2091
- Micronase Tablets ... 2099

Hydrochlorothiazide (Co-administration may result in hypokalemia). Products include:

- Aldactazide Tablets ... 2556
- Aldoril Tablets ... 1644
- Apresazide Capsules ... 824
- Capozide Tablets ... 744
- Dyazide Capsules ... 2653
- Esidrix Tablets ... 839
- Esimil Tablets ... 840
- HydroDIURIL Tablets ... 1716
- Hydropres Tablets ... 1718
- Hyzaar Tablets ... 1720
- Inderide Tablets ... 2838
- Inderide LA Long Acting Capsules ... 2840
- Lopressor HCT Tablets ... 850
- Lotensin HCT Tablets ... 855
- Moduretic Tablets ... 1748
- Oretic Tablets ... 450
- Prinzide Tablets ... 1780
- Ser-Ap-Es Tablets ... 867
- Timolide Tablets ... 1791
- Vaseretic Tablets ... 1810
- Zestoretic Tablets ... 2968
- Ziac ... 1459

Hydroflumethiazide (Co-administration may result in hypokalemia). Products include:

- Diucardin Tablets ... 2824

Insulin, Human (Potential for increased requirements of insulin).

No products indexed under this heading.

Insulin, Human Isophane Suspension (Potential for increased requirements of insulin). Products include:

- Novolin N Human Insulin 10 ml Vials ... 1846

Insulin, Human NPH (Potential for increased requirements of insulin). Products include:

- Humulin N, 100 Units ... 1495
- Novolin N PenFill 1.5 ml Cartridges Durable Insulin Delivery System ... 1849
- Novolin N Prefilled Syringe Disposable Insulin Delivery System ... 1850

Insulin, Human Regular (Potential for increased requirements of insulin). Products include:

- Humulin R, 100 Units ... 1497
- Novolin R Human Insulin 10 ml Vials ... 1846
- Novolin R PenFill 1.5 ml Cartridges Durable Insulin Delivery System ... 1849
- Novolin R Prefilled Syringe Disposable Insulin Delivery System ... 1850
- Velosulin BR Human Insulin 10 ml Vials ... 1847

Insulin, Human, Zinc Suspension (Potential for increased requirements of insulin). Products include:

- Humulin L, 100 Units ... 1494
- Humulin U, 100 Units ... 1498
- Novolin L Human Insulin 10 ml Vials ... 1846

Insulin Lispro, Human (Potential for increased requirements of insulin). Products include:

- Humalog Injection ... 1488

Insulin, NPH (Potential for increased requirements of insulin). Products include:

- NPH, 100 Units ... 1502
- Pork NPH, 100 Units ... 1506
- Purified Pork NPH Isophane Insulin ... 1852

Insulin, Regular (Potential for increased requirements of insulin). Products include:

- Regular, 100 Units ... 1503
- Pork Regular, 100 Units ... 1507
- Pork Regular (Concentrated), 500 Units ... 1508
- Purified Pork Regular Insulin ... 1852

Insulin, Zinc Crystals (Potential for increased requirements of insulin). Products include:

- NPH, 100 Units ... 1502

Insulin, Zinc Suspension (Potential for increased requirements of insulin). Products include:

- Iletin I ... 1501
- Lente, 100 Units ... 1501
- Iletin II ... 1504
- Pork Lente, 100 Units ... 1504
- Purified Pork Lente Insulin ... 1852

Live Virus Vaccines (Co-administration is contraindicated in patients receiving immunosuppressive doses of corticosteroids).

Metformin Hydrochloride (Potential for increased requirements of oral hypoglycemic agents). Products include:

- Glucophage Tablets ... 754

Methyclothiazide (Co-administration may result in hypokalemia). Products include:

- Enduron Tablets ... 424

Phenobarbital (Enhanced metabolic clearance of corticosteroids). Products include:

- Arco-Lase Plus Tablets ... 513
- Bellergal-S Tablets ... 2375
- Donnatal ... 2234
- Donnatal Extentabs ... 2234
- Donnatal Tablets ... 2234
- Phenobarbital Elixir and Tablets ... 1523
- Quadrinal Tablets ... 1398

Phenytoin (Enhanced metabolic clearance of corticosteroids). Products include:

- Dilantin Infatabs ... 1967
- Dilantin-125 Suspension ... 1969

Phenytoin Sodium (Enhanced metabolic clearance of corticosteroids). Products include:

- Dilantin Kapseals ... 1965

Polythiazide (Co-administration may result in hypokalemia). Products include:

- Minizide Capsules ... 2016

Rifampin (Enhanced metabolic clearance of corticosteroids). Products include:

- Rifadin ... 1276
- Rifamate Capsules ... 1278
- Rifater ... 1280
- Rimactane Capsules ... 865

Tolazamide (Potential for increased requirements of oral hypoglycemic agents).

No products indexed under this heading.

Tolbutamide (Potential for increased requirements of oral hypoglycemic agents).

No products indexed under this heading.

Warfarin Sodium (Potential for altered response to coumarin anticoagulants). Products include:

- Coumadin ... 941

DECADRON PHOSPHATE INJECTION

(Dexamethasone Sodium Phosphate) 1680
May interact with potassium-depleting diuretics, oral anticoagulants, oral hypoglycemic agents, insulin, and certain other agents. Compounds in these categories include:

Acarbose (Potential for increased requirements of oral hypoglycemic agents). Products include:

- Precose ... 604

Aspirin (Aspirin should be used cautiously in conjunction with corticosteroids in hypoprothrombinemia). Products include:

- Alka-Seltzer Cherry Effervescent Antacid and Pain Reliever ... 609
- Alka-Seltzer Extra Strength Effervescent Antacid and Pain Reliever ... 609
- Alka-Seltzer Lemon Lime Effervescent Antacid and Pain Reliever ... 609
- Alka-Seltzer Original Effervescent Antacid and Pain Reliever ... 609
- Alka-Seltzer Plus ... 611
- Alka-Seltzer Plus Sinus Medicine ... 611
- Ascriptin ... 650
- Arthritis Strength BC Powder ... 631
- BC Cold Powder Multi-Symptom Formula (Cold-Sinus-Allergy) ... 631

IMPORTANT NOTE: Always consult each drug listing in the patient's regimen for possible interactions.

Decadron Injection / Interactions Index

BC Cold Powder Non-Drowsy Formula (Cold-Sinus) 631
BC Powder 631
Genuine Bayer Aspirin Tablets & Caplets 618
Extra Strength Bayer Arthritis Pain Regimen Formula 615
Extra Strength Bayer Aspirin Caplets & Tablets 617
Extended-Release Bayer 8-Hour Aspirin 616
Extra Strength Bayer Plus Aspirin Caplets 617
Extra Strength Bayer PM Aspirin Plus Sleep Aid 617
Aspirin Regimen Bayer 81 mg Tablets with Calcium 615
Aspirin Regimen Bayer Adult Low Strength 81 mg Tablets 613
Aspirin Regimen Bayer Children's Chewable Aspirin 616
Aspirin Regimen Bayer Regular Strength 325 mg Caplets 613
Bufferin Analgesic Tablets 636
Arthritis Strength Bufferin Analgesic Caplets 637
Extra Strength Bufferin Analgesic Tablets 637
Cama Arthritis Pain Reliever 748
Darvon Compound-65 Pulvules 1475
Easprin 1971
Ecotrin 2625
Ecotrin Enteric Coated Aspirin Maximum Strength Tablets and Caplets 775
Ecotrin Enteric Coated Aspirin Regular Strength Tablets 2625
Empirin Aspirin Tablets 818
Excedrin Extra-Strength Analgesic Tablets, Caplets, and Geltabs 734
Fiorinal Capsules 2388
Fiorinal with Codeine Capsules 2390
Fiorinal Tablets 2388
Goody's Extra Strength Headache Powders 632
Goody's Extra Strength Pain Relief Tablets 632
Halfprin Tablets 1413
Norgesic 1554
Percodan Tablets 955
Percodan-Demi Tablets 956
Robaxisal Tablets 2246
Soma Compound w/Codeine Tablets 2784
Soma Compound Tablets 2783
St. Joseph Adult Chewable Aspirin (81 mg.) 768
Talwin Compound 2466
Vanquish Analgesic Caplets 627

Bendroflumethiazide (Co-administration may result in hypokalemia).
No products indexed under this heading.

Chlorothiazide (Co-administration may result in hypokalemia). Products include:
Aldoclor Tablets 1638
Diupres Tablets 1691
Diuril Oral 1694

Chlorothiazide Sodium (Co-administration may result in hypokalemia). Products include:
Diuril Sodium Intravenous 1693

Chlorpropamide (Potential for increased requirements of oral hypoglycemic agents). Products include:
Diabinese Tablets 2002

Dicumarol (Potential for altered response to coumarin anticoagulants).
No products indexed under this heading.

Ephedrine (Enhanced metabolic clearance of corticosteroids).

Ephedrine Hydrochloride (Enhanced metabolic clearance of corticosteroids). Products include:
Primatene Tablets 844
Quadrinal Tablets 1398

Ephedrine Sulfate (Enhanced metabolic clearance of corticosteroids). Products include:
Marax Tablets & DF Syrup 2015

Ephedrine Tannate (Enhanced metabolic clearance of corticosteroids). Products include:
Rynatuss 2782

Fosphenytoin Sodium (Enhanced metabolic clearance of corticosteroids). Products include:
Cerebyx Injection 1956

Glimepiride (Potential for increased requirements of oral hypoglycemic agents). Products include:
Amaryl Tablets 1241

Glipizide (Potential for increased requirements of oral hypoglycemic agents). Products include:
Glucotrol Tablets 2011
Glucotrol XL Extended Release Tablets 2012

Glyburide (Potential for increased requirements of oral hypoglycemic agents). Products include:
DiaBeta Tablets 1265
Glynase PresTab Tablets 2091
Micronase Tablets 2099

Hydrochlorothiazide (Co-administration may result in hypokalemia). Products include:
Aldactazide Tablets 2556
Aldoril Tablets 1644
Apresazide Capsules 824
Capozide Tablets 744
Dyazide Capsules 2653
Esidrix Tablets 839
Esimil Tablets 840
HydroDIURIL Tablets 1716
Hydropres Tablets 1718
Hyzaar Tablets 1720
Inderide Tablets 2838
Inderide LA Long Acting Capsules 2840
Lopressor HCT Tablets 850
Lotensin HCT Tablets 855
Moduretic Tablets 1748
Oretic Tablets 450
Prinzide Tablets 1780
Ser-Ap-Es Tablets 867
Timolide Tablets 1791
Vaseretic Tablets 1810
Zestoretic Tablets 2968
Ziac 1459

Hydroflumethiazide (Co-administration may result in hypokalemia). Products include:
Diucardin Tablets 2824

Insulin, Human (Potential for increased requirements of insulin).
No products indexed under this heading.

Insulin, Human Isophane Suspension (Potential for increased requirements of insulin). Products include:
Novolin N Human Insulin 10 ml Vials 1846

Insulin, Human NPH (Potential for increased requirements of insulin). Products include:
Humulin N, 100 Units 1495
Novolin N PenFill 1.5 ml Cartridges Durable Insulin Delivery System 1849
Novolin N Prefilled Syringe Disposable Insulin Delivery System 1850

Insulin, Human Regular (Potential for increased requirements of insulin). Products include:
Humulin R, 100 Units 1497
Novolin R Human Insulin 10 ml Vials 1846
Novolin R PenFill 1.5 ml Cartridges Durable Insulin Delivery System 1849
Novolin R Prefilled Syringe Disposable Insulin Delivery System 1850
Velosulin BR Human Insulin 10 ml Vials 1847

Insulin, Human, Zinc Suspension (Potential for increased requirements of insulin). Products include:
Humulin L, 100 Units 1494
Humulin U, 100 Units 1498
Novolin L Human Insulin 10 ml Vials 1846

Insulin Lispro, Human (Potential for increased requirements of insulin). Products include:
Humalog Injection 1488

Insulin, NPH (Potential for increased requirements of insulin). Products include:
NPH, 100 Units 1502
Pork NPH, 100 Units 1506
Purified Pork NPH Isophane Insulin 1852

Insulin, Regular (Potential for increased requirements of insulin). Products include:
Regular, 100 Units 1503
Pork Regular, 100 Units 1507
Pork Regular (Concentrated), 500 Units 1508
Purified Pork Regular Insulin 1852

Insulin, Zinc Crystals (Potential for increased requirements of insulin). Products include:
NPH, 100 Units 1502

Insulin, Zinc Suspension (Potential for increased requirements of insulin). Products include:
Iletin I 1501
Lente, 100 Units 1501
Iletin II 1504
Pork Lente, 100 Units 1504
Purified Pork Lente Insulin 1852

Live Virus Vaccines (Co-administration is contraindicated in patients receiving immunosuppressive doses of corticosteroids).

Metformin Hydrochloride (Potential for increased requirements of oral hypoglycemic agents). Products include:
Glucophage Tablets 754

Methyclothiazide (Co-administration may result in hypokalemia). Products include:
Enduron Tablets 424

Phenobarbital (Enhanced metabolic clearance of corticosteroids). Products include:
Arco-Lase Plus Tablets 513
Bellergal-S Tablets 2375
Donnatal 2234
Donnatal Extentabs 2234
Donnatal Tablets 2234
Phenobarbital Elixir and Tablets 1523
Quadrinal Tablets 1398

Phenytoin (Enhanced metabolic clearance of corticosteroids). Products include:
Dilantin Infatabs 1967
Dilantin-125 Suspension 1969

Phenytoin Sodium (Enhanced metabolic clearance of corticosteroids). Products include:
Dilantin Kapseals 1965

Polythiazide (Co-administration may result in hypokalemia). Products include:
Minizide Capsules 2016

Rifampin (Enhanced metabolic clearance of corticosteroids). Products include:
Rifadin 1276
Rifamate Capsules 1278
Rifater 1280
Rimactane Capsules 865

Tolazamide (Potential for increased requirements of oral hypoglycemic agents).
No products indexed under this heading.

Tolbutamide (Potential for increased requirements of oral hypoglycemic agents).
No products indexed under this heading.

Warfarin Sodium (Potential for altered response to coumarin anticoagulants). Products include:
Coumadin 941

DECADRON PHOSPHATE STERILE OPHTHALMIC OINTMENT
(Dexamethasone Sodium Phosphate) 1684
None cited in PDR database.

DECADRON PHOSPHATE STERILE OPHTHALMIC SOLUTION
(Dexamethasone Sodium Phosphate) 1685
None cited in PDR database.

DECADRON PHOSPHATE TOPICAL CREAM
(Dexamethasone Sodium Phosphate) 1686
None cited in PDR database.

DECADRON PHOSPHATE WITH XYLOCAINE INJECTION, STERILE
(Dexamethasone Sodium Phosphate, Lidocaine Hydrochloride) 1683
May interact with oral anticoagulants, potassium-depleting diuretics, insulin, oral hypoglycemic agents, and certain other agents. Compounds in these categories include:

Acarbose (Potential for increased requirements of oral hypoglycemic agents). Products include:
Precose 604

Aspirin (Aspirin should be used cautiously in conjunction with corticosteroids in hypoprothrombinemia). Products include:
Alka-Seltzer Cherry Effervescent Antacid and Pain Reliever 609
Alka-Seltzer Extra Strength Effervescent Antacid and Pain Reliever 609
Alka-Seltzer Lemon Lime Effervescent Antacid and Pain Reliever 609
Alka-Seltzer Original Effervescent Antacid and Pain Reliever 609
Alka-Seltzer Plus 611
Alka-Seltzer Plus Sinus Medicine 611
Ascriptin 650
Arthritis Strength BC Powder 631
BC Cold Powder Multi-Symptom Formula (Cold-Sinus-Allergy) 631
BC Cold Powder Non-Drowsy Formula (Cold-Sinus) 631
BC Powder 631
Genuine Bayer Aspirin Tablets & Caplets 618
Extra Strength Bayer Arthritis Pain Regimen Formula 615
Extra Strength Bayer Aspirin Caplets & Tablets 617
Extended-Release Bayer 8-Hour Aspirin 616
Extra Strength Bayer Plus Aspirin Caplets 617
Extra Strength Bayer PM Aspirin Plus Sleep Aid 617
Aspirin Regimen Bayer 81 mg Tablets with Calcium 615
Aspirin Regimen Bayer Adult Low Strength 81 mg Tablets 613
Aspirin Regimen Bayer Children's Chewable Aspirin 616
Aspirin Regimen Bayer Regular Strength 325 mg Caplets 613
Bufferin Analgesic Tablets 636
Arthritis Strength Bufferin Analgesic Caplets 637
Extra Strength Bufferin Analgesic Tablets 637
Cama Arthritis Pain Reliever 748
Darvon Compound-65 Pulvules 1475
Easprin 1971
Ecotrin 2625
Ecotrin Enteric Coated Aspirin Maximum Strength Tablets and Caplets 775
Ecotrin Enteric Coated Aspirin Regular Strength Tablets 2625
Empirin Aspirin Tablets 818
Excedrin Extra-Strength Analgesic Tablets, Caplets, and Geltabs 734
Fiorinal Capsules 2388
Fiorinal with Codeine Capsules 2390
Fiorinal Tablets 2388

(Described in PDR For Nonprescription Drugs)   (Described in PDR For Ophthalmology)

Goody's Extra Strength Headache Powders ... 632
Goody's Extra Strength Pain Relief Tablets ... 632
Halfprin Tablets ... 1413
Norgesic ... 1554
Percodan Tablets ... 955
Percodan-Demi Tablets ... 956
Robaxisal Tablets ... 2246
Soma Compound w/Codeine Tablets ... 2784
Soma Compound Tablets ... 2783
St. Joseph Adult Chewable Aspirin (81 mg.) ... 768
Talwin Compound ... 2466
Vanquish Analgesic Caplets ... 627

Bendroflumethiazide (Co-administration may result in hypokalemia).
No products indexed under this heading.

Chlorothiazide (Co-administration may result in hypokalemia). Products include:
Aldoclor Tablets ... 1638
Diupres Tablets ... 1691
Diuril Oral ... 1694

Chlorothiazide Sodium (Co-administration may result in hypokalemia). Products include:
Diuril Sodium Intravenous ... 1693

Chlorpropamide (Potential for increased requirements of oral hypoglycemic agents). Products include:
Diabinese Tablets ... 2002

Dicumarol (Potential for altered response to coumarin anticoagulants).
No products indexed under this heading.

Ephedrine (Enhances metabolic clearance of corticosteroids resulting in decreased blood levels and lessened physiological activity).

Ephedrine Hydrochloride (Enhances metabolic clearance of corticosteroids resulting in decreased blood levels and lessened physiological activity). Products include:
Primatene Tablets ... 844
Quadrinal Tablets ... 1398

Ephedrine Sulfate (Enhances metabolic clearance of corticosteroids resulting in decreased blood levels and lessened physiological activity). Products include:
Marax Tablets & DF Syrup ... 2015

Ephedrine Tannate (Enhances metabolic clearance of corticosteroids resulting in decreased blood levels and lessened physiological activity). Products include:
Rynatuss ... 2782

Fosphenytoin Sodium (Enhances metabolic clearance of corticosteroids resulting in decreased blood levels and lessened physiological activity). Products include:
Cerebyx Injection ... 1956

Glimepiride (Potential for increased requirements of oral hypoglycemic agents). Products include:
Amaryl Tablets ... 1241

Glipizide (Potential for increased requirements of oral hypoglycemic agents). Products include:
Glucotrol Tablets ... 2011
Glucotrol XL Extended Release Tablets ... 2012

Glyburide (Potential for increased requirements of oral hypoglycemic agents). Products include:
DiaBeta Tablets ... 1265
Glynase PresTab Tablets ... 2091
Micronase Tablets ... 2099

Hydrochlorothiazide (Co-administration may result in hypokalemia). Products include:
Aldactazide Tablets ... 2556
Aldoril Tablets ... 1644
Apresazide Capsules ... 824
Capozide Tablets ... 744
Dyazide Capsules ... 2653
Esidrix Tablets ... 839
Esimil Tablets ... 840
HydroDIURIL Tablets ... 1716
Hydropres Tablets ... 1718
Hyzaar Tablets ... 1720
Inderide Tablets ... 2838
Inderide LA Long Acting Capsules ... 2840
Lopressor HCT Tablets ... 850
Lotensin HCT Tablets ... 855
Moduretic Tablets ... 1748
Oretic Tablets ... 450
Prinzide Tablets ... 1780
Ser-Ap-Es Tablets ... 867
Timolide Tablets ... 1791
Vaseretic Tablets ... 1810
Zestoretic Tablets ... 2968
Ziac ... 1459

Hydroflumethiazide (Co-administration may result in hypokalemia). Products include:
Diucardin Tablets ... 2824

Insulin, Human (Potential for increased requirements of insulin).
No products indexed under this heading.

Insulin, Human Isophane Suspension (Potential for increased requirements of insulin). Products include:
Novolin N Human Insulin 10 ml Vials ... 1846

Insulin, Human NPH (Potential for increased requirements of insulin). Products include:
Humulin N, 100 Units ... 1495
Novolin N PenFill 1.5 ml Cartridges Durable Insulin Delivery System ... 1849
Novolin N Prefilled Syringe Disposable Insulin Delivery System ... 1850

Insulin, Human Regular (Potential for increased requirements of insulin). Products include:
Humulin R, 100 Units ... 1497
Novolin R Human Insulin 10 ml Vials ... 1846
Novolin R PenFill 1.5 ml Cartridges Durable Insulin Delivery System ... 1849
Novolin R Prefilled Syringe Disposable Insulin Delivery System ... 1850
Velosulin BR Human Insulin 10 ml Vials ... 1847

Insulin, Human, Zinc Suspension (Potential for increased requirements of insulin). Products include:
Humulin L, 100 Units ... 1494
Humulin U, 100 Units ... 1498
Novolin L Human Insulin 10 ml Vials ... 1846

Insulin Lispro, Human (Potential for increased requirements of insulin). Products include:
Humalog Injection ... 1488

Insulin, NPH (Potential for increased requirements of insulin). Products include:
NPH, 100 Units ... 1502
Pork NPH, 100 Units ... 1506
Purified Pork NPH Isophane Insulin ... 1852

Insulin, Regular (Potential for increased requirements of insulin). Products include:
Regular, 100 Units ... 1503
Pork Regular, 100 Units ... 1507
Pork Regular (Concentrated), 500 Units ... 1508
Purified Pork Regular Insulin ... 1852

Insulin, Zinc Crystals (Potential for increased requirements of insulin). Products include:
NPH, 100 Units ... 1502

Insulin, Zinc Suspension (Potential for increased requirements of insulin). Products include:
Iletin I ... 1501
Lente, 100 Units ... 1501
Iletin II ... 1504
Pork Lente, 100 Units ... 1504
Purified Pork Lente Insulin ... 1852

Live Virus Vaccines (Co-administration is contraindicated in patients receiving immunosuppressive doses of corticosteroids).

Metformin Hydrochloride (Potential for increased requirements of oral hypoglycemic agents). Products include:
Glucophage Tablets ... 754

Methyclothiazide (Co-administration may result in hypokalemia). Products include:
Enduron Tablets ... 424

Phenobarbital (Enhances metabolic clearance of corticosteroids resulting in decreased blood levels and lessened physiological activity). Products include:
Arco-Lase Plus Tablets ... 513
Bellergal-S Tablets ... 2375
Donnatal ... 2234
Donnatal Extentabs ... 2234
Donnatal Tablets ... 2234
Phenobarbital Elixir and Tablets ... 1523
Quadrinal Tablets ... 1398

Phenytoin (Enhances metabolic clearance of corticosteroids resulting in decreased blood levels and lessened physiological activity). Products include:
Dilantin Infatabs ... 1967
Dilantin-125 Suspension ... 1969

Phenytoin Sodium (Enhances metabolic clearance of corticosteroids resulting in decreased blood levels and lessened physiological activity). Products include:
Dilantin Kapseals ... 1965

Polythiazide (Co-administration may result in hypokalemia). Products include:
Minizide Capsules ... 2016

Rifampin (Enhances metabolic clearance of corticosteroids resulting in decreased blood levels and lessened physiological activity). Products include:
Rifadin ... 1276
Rifamate Capsules ... 1278
Rifater ... 1280
Rimactane Capsules ... 865

Tolazamide (Potential for increased requirements of oral hypoglycemic agents).
No products indexed under this heading.

Tolbutamide (Potential for increased requirements of oral hypoglycemic agents).
No products indexed under this heading.

Warfarin Sodium (Potential for altered response to coumarin anticoagulants). Products include:
Coumadin ... 941

DECADRON TABLETS

(Dexamethasone) ... 1678
May interact with potassium-depleting diuretics, oral anticoagulants, oral hypoglycemic agents, insulin, and certain other agents. Compounds in these categories include:

Acarbose (Increased requirements for oral hypoglycemic agents in diabetes). Products include:
Precose ... 604

Aspirin (Aspirin should be used cautiously in conjunction with corticosteroids in hypoprothrombinemia). Products include:
Alka-Seltzer Cherry Effervescent Antacid and Pain Reliever ... 609
Alka-Seltzer Extra Strength Effervescent Antacid and Pain Reliever ... 609
Alka-Seltzer Lemon Lime Effervescent Antacid and Pain Reliever ... 609
Alka-Seltzer Original Effervescent Antacid and Pain Reliever ... 609
Alka-Seltzer Plus ... 611
Alka-Seltzer Plus Sinus Medicine ... 611
Ascriptin ... 650
Arthritis Strength BC Powder ... 631
BC Cold Powder Multi-Symptom Formula (Cold-Sinus-Allergy) ... 631
BC Cold Powder Non-Drowsy Formula (Cold-Sinus) ... 631
BC Powder ... 631
Genuine Bayer Aspirin Tablets & Caplets ... 618
Extra Strength Bayer Arthritis Pain Regimen Formula ... 615
Extra Strength Bayer Aspirin Caplets & Tablets ... 617
Extended-Release Bayer 8-Hour Aspirin ... 616
Extra Strength Bayer Plus Aspirin Caplets ... 617
Extra Strength Bayer PM Aspirin Plus Sleep Aid ... 617
Aspirin Regimen Bayer 81 mg Tablets with Calcium ... 615
Aspirin Regimen Bayer Adult Low Strength 81 mg Tablets ... 613
Aspirin Regimen Bayer Children's Chewable Aspirin ... 616
Aspirin Regimen Bayer Regular Strength 325 mg Caplets ... 613
Bufferin Analgesic Tablets ... 636
Arthritis Strength Bufferin Analgesic Caplets ... 637
Extra Strength Bufferin Analgesic Tablets ... 637
Cama Arthritis Pain Reliever ... 748
Darvon Compound-65 Pulvules ... 1475
Easprin ... 1971
Ecotrin ... 2625
Ecotrin Enteric Coated Aspirin Maximum Strength Tablets and Caplets ... 775
Ecotrin Enteric Coated Aspirin Regular Strength Tablets ... 2625
Empirin Aspirin Tablets ... 818
Excedrin Extra-Strength Analgesic Tablets, Caplets, and Geltabs ... 734
Fiorinal Capsules ... 2388
Fiorinal with Codeine Capsules ... 2390
Fiorinal Tablets ... 2388
Goody's Extra Strength Headache Powders ... 632
Goody's Extra Strength Pain Relief Tablets ... 632
Halfprin Tablets ... 1413
Norgesic ... 1554
Percodan Tablets ... 955
Percodan-Demi Tablets ... 956
Robaxisal Tablets ... 2246
Soma Compound w/Codeine Tablets ... 2784
Soma Compound Tablets ... 2783
St. Joseph Adult Chewable Aspirin (81 mg.) ... 768
Talwin Compound ... 2466
Vanquish Analgesic Caplets ... 627

Bendroflumethiazide (Co-administration may result in hypokalemia).
No products indexed under this heading.

Chlorothiazide (Co-administration may result in hypokalemia). Products include:
Aldoclor Tablets ... 1638
Diupres Tablets ... 1691
Diuril Oral ... 1694

Chlorothiazide Sodium (Co-administration may result in hypokalemia). Products include:
Diuril Sodium Intravenous ... 1693

Chlorpropamide (Increased requirements for oral hypoglycemic agents in diabetes). Products include:
Diabinese Tablets ... 2002

Dicumarol (Potential for altered response to coumarin anticoagulants).
No products indexed under this heading.

Ephedrine (Enhanced metabolic clearance of corticosteroids).

IMPORTANT NOTE: Always consult each drug listing in the patient's regimen for possible interactions.

Decadron Tablets — Interactions Index — 244

Ephedrine Hydrochloride (Enhanced metabolic clearance of corticosteroids). Products include:
- Primatene Tablets ▣ 844
- Quadrinal Tablets 1398

Ephedrine Sulfate (Enhanced metabolic clearance of corticosteroids). Products include:
- Marax Tablets & DF Syrup 2015

Ephedrine Tannate (Enhanced metabolic clearance of corticosteroids). Products include:
- Rynatuss 2782

Fosphenytoin Sodium (Enhanced metabolic clearance of corticosteroids). Products include:
- Cerebyx Injection 1956

Glimepiride (Increased requirements for oral hypoglycemic agents in diabetes). Products include:
- Amaryl Tablets 1241

Glipizide (Increased requirements for oral hypoglycemic agents in diabetes). Products include:
- Glucotrol Tablets 2011
- Glucotrol XL Extended Release Tablets 2012

Glyburide (Increased requirements for oral hypoglycemic agents in diabetes). Products include:
- DiaBeta Tablets 1265
- Glynase PresTab Tablets 2091
- Micronase Tablets 2099

Hydrochlorothiazide (Co-administration may result in hypokalemia). Products include:
- Aldactazide Tablets 2556
- Aldoril Tablets 1644
- Apresazide Capsules 824
- Capozide Tablets 744
- Dyazide Capsules 2653
- Esidrix Tablets 839
- Esimil Tablets 840
- HydroDIURIL Tablets 1716
- Hydropres Tablets 1718
- Hyzaar Tablets 1720
- Inderide Tablets 2838
- Inderide LA Long Acting Capsules 2840
- Lopressor HCT Tablets 850
- Lotensin HCT Tablets 855
- Moduretic Tablets 1748
- Oretic Tablets 450
- Prinzide Tablets 1780
- Ser-Ap-Es Tablets 867
- Timolide Tablets 1791
- Vaseretic Tablets 1810
- Zestoretic Tablets 2968
- Ziac 1459

Hydroflumethiazide (Co-administration may result in hypokalemia). Products include:
- Diucardin Tablets 2824

Insulin, Human (Increased requirements for insulin in diabetes).
- No products indexed under this heading.

Insulin, Human Isophane Suspension (Increased requirements for insulin in diabetes). Products include:
- Novolin N Human Insulin 10 ml Vials 1846

Insulin, Human NPH (Increased requirements for insulin in diabetes). Products include:
- Humulin N, 100 Units 1495
- Novolin N PenFill 1.5 ml Cartridges Durable Insulin Delivery System 1849
- Novolin N Prefilled Syringe Disposable Insulin Delivery System 1850

Insulin, Human Regular (Increased requirements for insulin in diabetes). Products include:
- Humulin R, 100 Units 1497
- Novolin R Human Insulin 10 ml Vials 1846
- Novolin R PenFill 1.5 ml Cartridges Durable Insulin Delivery System 1849
- Novolin R Prefilled Syringe Disposable Insulin Delivery System 1850
- Velosulin BR Human Insulin 10 ml Vials 1847

Insulin, Human, Zinc Suspension (Increased requirements for insulin in diabetes). Products include:
- Humulin L, 100 Units 1494
- Humulin U, 100 Units 1498
- Novolin L Human Insulin 10 ml Vials 1846

Insulin Lispro, Human (Increased requirements for insulin in diabetes). Products include:
- Humalog Injection 1488

Insulin, NPH (Increased requirements for insulin in diabetes). Products include:
- NPH, 100 Units 1502
- Pork NPH, 100 Units 1506
- Purified Pork NPH Isophane Insulin 1852

Insulin, Regular (Increased requirements for insulin in diabetes). Products include:
- Regular, 100 Units 1503
- Pork Regular, 100 Units 1507
- Pork Regular (Concentrated), 500 Units 1508
- Purified Pork Regular Insulin 1852

Insulin, Zinc Crystals (Increased requirements for insulin in diabetes). Products include:
- NPH, 100 Units 1502

Insulin, Zinc Suspension (Increased requirements for insulin in diabetes). Products include:
- Iletin I 1501
- Lente, 100 Units 1501
- Iletin II 1504
- Pork Lente, 100 Units 1504
- Purified Pork Lente Insulin 1852

Live Virus Vaccines (Co-administration is contraindicated in patients receiving immunosuppressive doses of corticosteroids).

Metformin Hydrochloride (Increased requirements for oral hypoglycemic agents in diabetes). Products include:
- Glucophage Tablets 754

Methyclothiazide (Co-administration may result in hypokalemia). Products include:
- Enduron Tablets 424

Phenobarbital (Enhanced metabolic clearance of corticosteroids). Products include:
- Arco-Lase Plus Tablets 513
- Bellergal-S Tablets 2375
- Donnatal 2234
- Donnatal Extentabs 2234
- Donnatal Tablets 2234
- Phenobarbital Elixir and Tablets 1523
- Quadrinal Tablets 1398

Phenytoin (Enhanced metabolic clearance of corticosteroids). Products include:
- Dilantin Infatabs 1967
- Dilantin-125 Suspension 1969

Phenytoin Sodium (Enhanced metabolic clearance of corticosteroids). Products include:
- Dilantin Kapseals 1965

Polythiazide (Co-administration may result in hypokalemia). Products include:
- Minizide Capsules 2016

Rifampin (Enhanced metabolic clearance of corticosteroids). Products include:
- Rifadin 1276
- Rifamate Capsules 1278
- Rifater 1280
- Rimactane Capsules 865

Tolazamide (Increased requirements for oral hypoglycemic agents in diabetes).
- No products indexed under this heading.

Tolbutamide (Increased requirements for oral hypoglycemic agents in diabetes).
- No products indexed under this heading.

Warfarin Sodium (Potential for altered response to coumarin anticoagulants). Products include:
- Coumadin 941

DECADRON-LA STERILE SUSPENSION

(Dexamethasone Acetate) 1687

May interact with potassium-depleting diuretics, oral anticoagulants, oral hypoglycemic agents, insulin, and certain other agents. Compounds in these categories include:

Acarbose (Potential for increased requirements of oral hypoglycemic agents). Products include:
- Precose 604

Aspirin (Aspirin should be used cautiously in conjunction with corticosteroids in hypoprothrombinemia). Products include:
- Alka-Seltzer Cherry Effervescent Antacid and Pain Reliever ▣ 609
- Alka-Seltzer Extra Strength Effervescent Antacid and Pain Reliever ▣ 609
- Alka-Seltzer Lemon Lime Effervescent Antacid and Pain Reliever ▣ 609
- Alka-Seltzer Original Effervescent Antacid and Pain Reliever ▣ 609
- Alka-Seltzer Plus ▣ 611
- Alka-Seltzer Plus Sinus Medicine ▣ 611
- Ascriptin ▣ 650
- Arthritis Strength BC Powder ▣ 631
- BC Cold Powder Multi-Symptom Formula (Cold-Sinus-Allergy) ▣ 631
- BC Cold Powder Non-Drowsy Formula (Cold-Sinus) ▣ 631
- BC Powder ▣ 631
- Genuine Bayer Aspirin Tablets & Caplets ▣ 618
- Extra Strength Bayer Arthritis Pain Regimen Formula ▣ 615
- Extra Strength Bayer Aspirin Caplets & Tablets ▣ 617
- Extended-Release Bayer 8-Hour Aspirin ▣ 616
- Extra Strength Bayer Plus Aspirin Caplets ▣ 617
- Extra Strength Bayer PM Aspirin Plus Sleep Aid ▣ 617
- Aspirin Regimen Bayer 81 mg Tablets with Calcium ▣ 615
- Aspirin Regimen Bayer Adult Low Strength 81 mg Tablets ▣ 613
- Aspirin Regimen Bayer Children's Chewable Aspirin ▣ 616
- Aspirin Regimen Bayer Regular Strength 325 mg Caplets ▣ 613
- Bufferin Analgesic Tablets ▣ 636
- Arthritis Strength Bufferin Analgesic Caplets ▣ 637
- Extra Strength Bufferin Analgesic Tablets ▣ 637
- Cama Arthritis Pain Reliever ▣ 748
- Darvon Compound-65 Pulvules 1475
- Easprin 1971
- Ecotrin 2625
- Ecotrin Enteric Coated Aspirin Maximum Strength Tablets and Caplets ▣ 775
- Ecotrin Enteric Coated Aspirin Regular Strength Tablets 2625
- Empirin Aspirin Tablets ▣ 818
- Excedrin Extra-Strength Analgesic Tablets, Caplets, and Geltabs 734
- Fiorinal Capsules 2388
- Fiorinal with Codeine Capsules 2390
- Fiorinal Tablets 2388
- Goody's Extra Strength Headache Powders ▣ 632
- Goody's Extra Strength Pain Relief Tablets ▣ 632
- Halfprin Tablets 1413
- Norgesic 1554
- Percodan Tablets 955
- Percodan-Demi Tablets 956
- Robaxisal Tablets 2246
- Soma Compound w/Codeine Tablets 2784
- Soma Compound Tablets 2783
- St. Joseph Adult Chewable Aspirin (81 mg.) ▣ 768
- Talwin Compound 2466
- Vanquish Analgesic Caplets ▣ 627

Bendroflumethiazide (Co-administration may result in hypokalemia).
- No products indexed under this heading.

Chlorothiazide (Co-administration may result in hypokalemia). Products include:
- Aldoclor Tablets 1638
- Diupres Tablets 1691
- Diuril Oral 1694

Chlorothiazide Sodium (Co-administration may result in hypokalemia). Products include:
- Diuril Sodium Intravenous 1693

Chlorpropamide (Potential for increased requirements of oral hypoglycemic agents). Products include:
- Diabinese Tablets 2002

Dicumarol (Potential for altered response to coumarin anticoagulants).
- No products indexed under this heading.

Ephedrine (Enhanced metabolic clearance of corticosteroids).

Ephedrine Hydrochloride (Enhanced metabolic clearance of corticosteroids). Products include:
- Primatene Tablets ▣ 844
- Quadrinal Tablets 1398

Ephedrine Sulfate (Enhanced metabolic clearance of corticosteroids). Products include:
- Marax Tablets & DF Syrup 2015

Ephedrine Tannate (Enhanced metabolic clearance of corticosteroids). Products include:
- Rynatuss 2782

Glimepiride (Potential for increased requirements of oral hypoglycemic agents). Products include:
- Amaryl Tablets 1241

Glipizide (Potential for increased requirements of oral hypoglycemic agents). Products include:
- Glucotrol Tablets 2011
- Glucotrol XL Extended Release Tablets 2012

Glyburide (Potential for increased requirements of oral hypoglycemic agents). Products include:
- DiaBeta Tablets 1265
- Glynase PresTab Tablets 2091
- Micronase Tablets 2099

Hydrochlorothiazide (Co-administration may result in hypokalemia). Products include:
- Aldactazide Tablets 2556
- Aldoril Tablets 1644
- Apresazide Capsules 824
- Capozide Tablets 744
- Dyazide Capsules 2653
- Esidrix Tablets 839
- Esimil Tablets 840
- HydroDIURIL Tablets 1716
- Hydropres Tablets 1718
- Hyzaar Tablets 1720
- Inderide Tablets 2838
- Inderide LA Long Acting Capsules 2840
- Lopressor HCT Tablets 850
- Lotensin HCT Tablets 855
- Moduretic Tablets 1748
- Oretic Tablets 450
- Prinzide Tablets 1780
- Ser-Ap-Es Tablets 867
- Timolide Tablets 1791
- Vaseretic Tablets 1810
- Zestoretic Tablets 2968
- Ziac 1459

Hydroflumethiazide (Co-administration may result in hypokalemia). Products include:
- Diucardin Tablets 2824

Insulin, Human (Potential for increased requirements of insulin).
- No products indexed under this heading.

(▣ Described in PDR For Nonprescription Drugs) (◉ Described in PDR For Ophthalmology)

Interactions Index — Declomycin

Insulin, Human Isophane Suspension (Potential for increased requirements of insulin). Products include:
- Novolin N Human Insulin 10 ml Vials ... 1846

Insulin, Human NPH (Potential for increased requirements of insulin). Products include:
- Humulin N, 100 Units ... 1495
- Novolin N PenFill 1.5 ml Cartridges Durable Insulin Delivery System ... 1849
- Novolin N Prefilled Syringe Disposable Insulin Delivery System ... 1850

Insulin, Human Regular (Potential for increased requirements of insulin). Products include:
- Humulin R, 100 Units ... 1497
- Novolin R Human Insulin 10 ml Vials ... 1846
- Novolin R PenFill 1.5 ml Cartridges Durable Insulin Delivery System ... 1849
- Novolin R Prefilled Syringe Disposable Insulin Delivery System ... 1850
- Velosulin BR Human Insulin 10 ml Vials ... 1847

Insulin, Human, Zinc Suspension (Potential for increased requirements of insulin). Products include:
- Humulin L, 100 Units ... 1494
- Humulin U, 100 Units ... 1498
- Novolin L Human Insulin 10 ml Vials ... 1846

Insulin Lispro, Human (Potential for increased requirements of insulin). Products include:
- Humalog Injection ... 1488

Insulin, NPH (Potential for increased requirements of insulin). Products include:
- NPH, 100 Units ... 1502
- Pork NPH, 100 Units ... 1506
- Purified Pork NPH Isophane Insulin ... 1852

Insulin, Regular (Potential for increased requirements of insulin). Products include:
- Regular, 100 Units ... 1503
- Pork Regular, 100 Units ... 1507
- Pork Regular (Concentrated), 500 Units ... 1508
- Purified Pork Regular Insulin ... 1852

Insulin, Zinc Crystals (Potential for increased requirements of insulin). Products include:
- NPH, 100 Units ... 1502

Insulin, Zinc Suspension (Potential for increased requirements of insulin). Products include:
- Iletin I ... 1501
- Lente, 100 Units ... 1501
- Iletin II ... 1504
- Pork Lente, 100 Units ... 1504
- Purified Pork Lente Insulin ... 1852

Live Virus Vaccines (Co-administration is contraindicated in patients receiving immunosuppressive doses of corticosteroids).

Metformin Hydrochloride (Potential for increased requirements of oral hypoglycemic agents). Products include:
- Glucophage Tablets ... 754

Methyclothiazide (Co-administration may result in hypokalemia). Products include:
- Enduron Tablets ... 424

Phenobarbital (Enhanced metabolic clearance of corticosteroids). Products include:
- Arco-Lase Plus Tablets ... 513
- Bellergal-S Tablets ... 2375
- Donnatal ... 2234
- Donnatal Extentabs ... 2234
- Donnatal Tablets ... 2234
- Phenobarbital Elixir and Tablets ... 1523
- Quadrinal Tablets ... 1398

Phenytoin (Enhanced metabolic clearance of corticosteroids). Products include:
- Dilantin Infatabs ... 1967
- Dilantin-125 Suspension ... 1969

Phenytoin Sodium (Enhanced metabolic clearance of corticosteroids). Products include:
- Dilantin Kapseals ... 1965

Polythiazide (Co-administration may result in hypokalemia). Products include:
- Minizide Capsules ... 2016

Rifampin (Enhanced metabolic clearance of corticosteroids). Products include:
- Rifadin ... 1276
- Rifamate Capsules ... 1278
- Rifater ... 1280
- Rimactane Capsules ... 865

Tolazamide (Potential for increased requirements of oral hypoglycemic agents).
No products indexed under this heading.

Tolbutamide (Potential for increased requirements of oral hypoglycemic agents).
No products indexed under this heading.

Warfarin Sodium (Potential for altered response to coumarin anticoagulants). Products include:
- Coumadin ... 941

DECASPRAY TOPICAL AEROSOL
(Dexamethasone) ... 1689
None cited in PDR database.

DECLOMYCIN TABLETS
(Demeclocycline Hydrochloride) ... 1421
May interact with anticoagulants, penicillins, antacids, oral contraceptives, and certain other agents. Compounds in these categories include:

Aluminum Carbonate (Tetracycline absorption impaired). Products include:
- Basaljel Capsules ... 2810
- Basaljel Suspension ... 2810
- Basaljel Tablets ... 2810

Aluminum Hydroxide (Tetracycline absorption impaired). Products include:
- ALternaGEL Liquid ... 1358
- Maximum Strength Ascriptin ... 650
- Cama Arthritis Pain Reliever ... 748
- Gaviscon Extra Strength Relief Formula Antacid Tablets ... 778
- Gaviscon Extra Strength Relief Formula Liquid Antacid ... 779
- Gaviscon Liquid Antacid ... 779
- Gelusil Antacid-Anti-gas Liquid ... 819
- Gelusil Antacid-Anti-gas Tablets ... 819
- Maalox Antacid/Anti-Gas Tablets ... 889
- Maalox Heartburn Relief Suspension ... 658
- Maalox Antacid Liquid ... 888
- Extra Strength Maalox Antacid/Anti-Gas Liquid and Tablets ... 888
- Mylanta ... 1359
- Tempo Soft Antacid ... 799

Aluminum Hydroxide Gel (Tetracycline absorption impaired). Products include:
- ALternaGEL Liquid ... 675
- Aludrox Oral Suspension ... 850
- Amphojel Suspension ... 2802
- Amphojel Suspension without Flavor ... 2802
- Amphojel Tablets ... 2802
- Ascriptin ...
- Gaviscon Antacid Tablets ... 778
- Gaviscon-2 Antacid Tablets ... 779
- Mylanta Liquid ... 676
- Mylanta Double Strength Liquid ... 676
- Nephrox Suspension ... 671

Amoxicillin Trihydrate (Interference with bactericidal action of penicillin). Products include:
- Amoxil ... 2631
- Augmentin ... 2637
- Augmentin Tablets ... 2640

Ampicillin Sodium (Interference with bactericidal action of penicillin). Products include:
- Unasyn ... 2035

Azlocillin Sodium (Interference with bactericidal action of penicillin).
No products indexed under this heading.

Bacampicillin Hydrochloride (Interference with bactericidal action of penicillin). Products include:
- Spectrobid Tablets ... 2030

Carbenicillin Disodium (Interference with bactericidal action of penicillin).
No products indexed under this heading.

Carbenicillin Indanyl Sodium (Interference with bactericidal action of penicillin). Products include:
- Geocillin Tablets ... 2009

Dalteparin Sodium (Plasma prothrombin activity depressed; downward adjustment of anticoagulant dosage may be necessary). Products include:
- Fragmin Injection ... 2088

Desogestrel (Reduced efficacy and increased breakthrough bleeding). Products include:
- Desogen Tablets ... 1867
- Ortho-Cept ... 1907

Dicloxacillin Sodium (Interference with bactericidal action of penicillin).
No products indexed under this heading.

Dicumarol (Plasma prothrombin activity depressed; downward adjustment of anticoagulant dosage may be necessary).
No products indexed under this heading.

Enoxaparin (Plasma prothrombin activity depressed; downward adjustment of anticoagulant dosage may be necessary). Products include:
- Lovenox Injection ... 2187

Ethinyl Estradiol (Reduced efficacy and increased breakthrough bleeding). Products include:
- Brevicon ... 2563
- Demulen ... 2580
- Desogen Tablets ... 1867
- Levlen/Tri-Levlen ... 646
- Lo/Ovral Tablets ... 2852
- Lo/Ovral-28 Tablets ... 2857
- Modicon ... 1928
- Nordette-21 Tablets ... 2863
- Nordette-28 Tablets ... 2866
- Norinyl ... 2563
- Ortho-Cept ... 1907
- Ortho-Cyclen/Ortho-Tri-Cyclen ... 1914
- Ortho-Novum ... 1928
- Ortho-Cyclen/Ortho Tri-Cyclen ... 1914
- Ovcon ... 765
- Ovral Tablets ... 2877
- Ovral-28 Tablets ... 2878
- Levlen/Tri-Levlen ... 646
- Tri-Norinyl ... 2607
- Triphasil-21 Tablets ... 2919
- Triphasil-28 Tablets ... 2924

Ethynodiol Diacetate (Reduced efficacy and increased breakthrough bleeding). Products include:
- Demulen ... 2580

Heparin Calcium (Plasma prothrombin activity depressed; downward adjustment of anticoagulant dosage may be necessary).
No products indexed under this heading.

Heparin Sodium (Plasma prothrombin activity depressed; downward adjustment of anticoagulant dosage may be necessary). Products include:
- Heparin Lock Flush Solution ... 2831
- Heparin Sodium Injection ... 2832
- Heparin Sodium Vials ... 1486

Levonorgestrel (Reduced efficacy and increased breakthrough bleeding). Products include:
- Levlen/Tri-Levlen ... 646
- Nordette-21 Tablets ... 2863
- Nordette-28 Tablets ... 2866
- Norplant System ... 2868
- Levlen/Tri-Levlen ... 646
- Triphasil-21 Tablets ... 2919
- Triphasil-28 Tablets ... 2924

Magaldrate (Tetracycline absorption impaired).
No products indexed under this heading.

Magnesium Hydroxide (Tetracycline absorption impaired). Products include:
- Aludrox Oral Suspension ... 850
- Ascriptin ... 650
- Di-Gel Antacid/Anti-Gas ... 762
- Gelusil Antacid-Anti-gas Liquid ... 819
- Gelusil Antacid-Anti-gas Tablets ... 819
- Maalox Antacid/Anti-Gas Tablets ... 889
- Maalox Antacid Liquid ... 888
- Extra Strength Maalox Antacid/Anti-Gas Liquid and Tablets ... 888
- Mylanta Fast-Acting ... 1359
- Mylanta Gelcaps Antacid ... 678
- Fast-Acting Mylanta Liquid Antacid ... 1359
- Mylanta Tablets ... 677
- Maximum-Strength Fast-Acting Mylanta Liquid Antacid ... 1359
- Mylanta Double Strength Tablets ... 677
- Phillips' Milk of Magnesia Liquid ... 627
- Rolaids Antacid Tablets ... 807
- Tempo Soft Antacid ... 799

Magnesium Oxide (Tetracycline absorption impaired). Products include:
- Beelith Tablets ... 632
- Bufferin Analgesic Tablets ... 636
- Arthritis Strength Bufferin Analgesic Caplets ... 637
- Extra Strength Bufferin Analgesic Tablets ... 637
- Caltrate PLUS ... 681
- Cama Arthritis Pain Reliever ... 748
- Mag-Ox 400 ... 666
- Uro-Mag ... 666

Mestranol (Reduced efficacy and increased breakthrough bleeding). Products include:
- Norinyl ... 2563
- Ortho-Novum ... 1928

Mezlocillin Sodium (Interference with bactericidal action of penicillin). Products include:
- Mezlin ... 594
- Mezlin Pharmacy Bulk Package ... 597

Nafcillin Sodium (Interference with bactericidal action of penicillin).
No products indexed under this heading.

Norethindrone (Reduced efficacy and increased breakthrough bleeding). Products include:
- Brevicon ... 2563
- Micronor Tablets ... 1903
- Modicon ... 1928
- Norinyl ... 2563
- Nor-Q D Tablets ... 2598
- Ortho-Novum ... 1928
- Ovcon ... 765
- Tri-Norinyl ... 2607

Norethynodrel (Reduced efficacy and increased breakthrough bleeding).
No products indexed under this heading.

Norgestimate (Reduced efficacy and increased breakthrough bleeding). Products include:
- Ortho-Cyclen/Ortho-Tri-Cyclen ... 1914
- Ortho-Cyclen/Ortho Tri-Cyclen ... 1914

IMPORTANT NOTE: Always consult each drug listing in the patient's regimen for possible interactions.

Declomycin — Interactions Index

Norgestrel (Reduced efficacy and increased breakthrough bleeding). Products include:
- Lo/Ovral Tablets 2852
- Lo/Ovral-28 Tablets 2857
- Ovral Tablets 2877
- Ovral-28 Tablets 2878
- Ovrette Tablets 2878

Penicillin G Benzathine (Interference with bactericidal action of penicillin). Products include:
- Bicillin C-R Injection 2810
- Bicillin C-R 900/300 Injection ... 2812
- Bicillin L-A Injection 2813

Penicillin G Potassium (Interference with bactericidal action of penicillin). Products include:
- Pfizerpen for Injection 2022

Penicillin G Procaine (Interference with bactericidal action of penicillin). Products include:
- Bicillin C-R Injection 2810
- Bicillin C-R 900/300 Injection ... 2812

Penicillin V Potassium (Interference with bactericidal action of penicillin). Products include:
- Pen•Vee K 2879

Ticarcillin Disodium (Interference with bactericidal action of penicillin). Products include:
- Ticar for Injection 2704
- Timentin for Injection 2706

Warfarin Sodium (Plasma prothrombin activity depressed; downward adjustment of anticoagulant dosage may be necessary). Products include:
- Coumadin 941

Food Interactions

Dairy products (Interferes with absorption).

Food, unspecified (Interferes with absorption).

DECONSAL II TABLETS
(Pseudoephedrine Hydrochloride, Guaifenesin) 1605

May interact with monoamine oxidase inhibitors, beta blockers, cardiac glycosides, veratrum alkaloids, tricyclic antidepressants, and certain other agents. Compounds in these categories include:

Acebutolol Hydrochloride (Potentiates the pressor effect of sympathomimetic amines). Products include:
- Sectral Capsules 2914

Amitriptyline Hydrochloride (Antagonizes the effects of sympathomimetic amines). Products include:
- Elavil 2945
- Etrafon 2495
- Limbitrol 2333
- Triavil Tablets 1800

Amoxapine (Antagonizes the effects of sympathomimetic amines). Products include:
- Asendin Tablets 1419

Atenolol (Potentiates the pressor effect of sympathomimetic amines). Products include:
- Tenoretic Tablets 2963
- Tenormin Tablets and I.V. Injection ... 2965

Betaxolol Hydrochloride (Potentiates the pressor effect of sympathomimetic amines). Products include:
- Betoptic Ophthalmic Solution ... 465
- Betoptic S Ophthalmic Suspension ... 467
- Kerlone Tablets 2588

Bisoprolol Fumarate (Potentiates the pressor effect of sympathomimetic amines). Products include:
- Zebeta Tablets 1457

- Ziac 1459

Carteolol Hydrochloride (Potentiates the pressor effect of sympathomimetic amines). Products include:
- Cartrol Tablets 413
- Ocupress Ophthalmic Solution, 1% Sterile .... ⊙ 297

Clomipramine Hydrochloride (Antagonizes the effects of sympathomimetic amines). Products include:
- Anafranil Capsules 819

Cryptenamine Preparations (Reduced hypotensive effect).

Deserpidine (Reduced hypotensive effect).
No products indexed under this heading.

Desipramine Hydrochloride (Antagonizes the effects of sympathomimetic amines). Products include:
- Norpramin Tablets 1273

Deslanoside (Increased possibility of cardiac arrhythmias).
No products indexed under this heading.

Digitoxin (Increased possibility of cardiac arrhythmias). Products include:
- Crystodigin Tablets 1472

Digoxin (Increased possibility of cardiac arrhythmias). Products include:
- Lanoxicaps 1110
- Lanoxin Elixir Pediatric 1113
- Lanoxin Injection 1116
- Lanoxin Injection Pediatric . 1119
- Lanoxin Tablets 1121

Doxepin Hydrochloride (Antagonizes the effects of sympathomimetic amines). Products include:
- Adapin Capsules 1542
- Sinequan 2028
- Zonalon Cream 1042

Esmolol Hydrochloride (Potentiates the pressor effect of sympathomimetic amines). Products include:
- Brevibloc (esmolol HCl) Injection ... 1860

Furazolidone (Potentiates the pressor effect of sympathomimetic amines; concurrent use is contraindicated). Products include:
- Furoxone 2221

Guanethidine Monosulfate (Reduced hypotensive effect). Products include:
- Esimil Tablets 840
- Ismelin Tablets 845

Imipramine Hydrochloride (Antagonizes the effects of sympathomimetic amines). Products include:
- Tofranil Ampuls 873
- Tofranil Tablets 875

Imipramine Pamoate (Antagonizes the effects of sympathomimetic amines). Products include:
- Tofranil-PM Capsules 876

Isocarboxazid (Potentiates the pressor effect of sympathomimetic amines; concurrent use is contraindicated).
No products indexed under this heading.

Labetalol Hydrochloride (Potentiates the pressor effect of sympathomimetic amines). Products include:
- Normodyne Injection 2519
- Normodyne Tablets 2522
- Trandate 1158

Levobunolol Hydrochloride (Potentiates the pressor effect of sympathomimetic amines). Products include:
- Betagan .... ⊙ 230

Maprotiline Hydrochloride (Antagonizes the effects of sympathomimetic amines). Products include:
- Ludiomil Tablets 861

Mecamylamine Hydrochloride (Reduced hypotensive effect). Products include:
- Inversine Tablets 1729

Methyldopa (Reduced hypotensive effect). Products include:
- Aldoclor Tablets 1638
- Aldomet Oral 1640
- Aldoril Tablets 1644

Methyldopate Hydrochloride (Reduced hypotensive effect). Products include:
- Aldomet Ester HCl Injection . 1642

Metipranolol Hydrochloride (Potentiates the pressor effect of sympathomimetic amines). Products include:
- OptiPranolol (Metipranolol 0.3%) Sterile Ophthalmic Solution .... ⊙ 256

Metoprolol Succinate (Potentiates the pressor effect of sympathomimetic amines). Products include:
- Toprol-XL Tablets 560

Metoprolol Tartrate (Potentiates the pressor effect of sympathomimetic amines). Products include:
- Lopressor 848
- Lopressor HCT Tablets 850

Nadolol (Potentiates the pressor effect of sympathomimetic amines).
No products indexed under this heading.

Nortriptyline Hydrochloride (Antagonizes the effects of sympathomimetic amines). Products include:
- Pamelor 2409

Penbutolol Sulfate (Potentiates the pressor effect of sympathomimetic amines). Products include:
- Levatol Tablets 2547

Phenelzine Sulfate (Potentiates the pressor effect of sympathomimetic amines; concurrent use is contraindicated). Products include:
- Nardil 1977

Pindolol (Potentiates the pressor effect of sympathomimetic amines). Products include:
- Visken Tablets 2428

Propranolol Hydrochloride (Potentiates the pressor effect of sympathomimetic amines). Products include:
- Inderal 2834
- Inderal LA Long Acting Capsules ... 2836
- Inderide Tablets 2838
- Inderide LA Long Acting Capsules ... 2840

Protriptyline Hydrochloride (Antagonizes the effects of sympathomimetic amines). Products include:
- Vivactil Tablets 1820

Rauwolfia Serpentina (Reduced hypotensive effect).
No products indexed under this heading.

Rescinnamine (Reduced hypotensive effect).
No products indexed under this heading.

Reserpine (Reduced hypotensive effect). Products include:
- Diupres Tablets 1691
- Hydropres Tablets 1718
- Ser-Ap-Es Tablets 867

Selegiline Hydrochloride (Potentiates the pressor effect of sympathomimetic amines; concurrent use is contraindicated). Products include:
- Eldepryl Capsules 2729

Sotalol Hydrochloride (Potentiates the pressor effect of sympathomimetic amines). Products include:
- Betapace Tablets 637

Timolol Hemihydrate (Potentiates the pressor effect of sympathomimetic amines). Products include:
- Betimol 0.25%, 0.5% .... ⊙ 259

Timolol Maleate (Potentiates the pressor effect of sympathomimetic amines). Products include:
- Blocadren Tablets 1654
- Timolide Tablets 1791
- Timoptic in Ocudose 1796
- Timoptic Sterile Ophthalmic Solution ... 1794
- Timoptic-XE 1798

Tranylcypromine Sulfate (Potentiates the pressor effect of sympathomimetic amines; concurrent use is contraindicated). Products include:
- Parnate Tablets 2679

Trimipramine Maleate (Antagonizes the effects of sympathomimetic amines). Products include:
- Surmontil Capsules 2917

DELSYM EXTENDED-RELEASE SUSPENSION
(Dextromethorphan Polistirex) ...... ⊡ 670

May interact with monoamine oxidase inhibitors. Compounds in this category include:

Furazolidone (Concurrent and/or sequential use is not recommended). Products include:
- Furoxone 2221

Isocarboxazid (Concurrent and/or sequential use is not recommended).
No products indexed under this heading.

Phenelzine Sulfate (Concurrent and/or sequential use is not recommended). Products include:
- Nardil 1977

Selegiline Hydrochloride (Concurrent and/or sequential use is not recommended). Products include:
- Eldepryl Capsules 2729

Tranylcypromine Sulfate (Concurrent and/or sequential use is not recommended). Products include:
- Parnate Tablets 2679

DEMADEX TABLETS AND INJECTION
(Torsemide) 691

May interact with aminoglycosides, salicylates, non-steroidal anti-inflammatory agents, and certain other agents. Compounds in these categories include:

Amikacin Sulfate (Co-administration of other diuretics has been reported to increase the ototoxic potential of aminoglycoside antibiotics, especially in the presence of impaired renal function; concurrent use of aminoglycoside and torsemide has not been studied, however, such combined therapy should be undertaken with great caution). Products include:
- Amikacin Sulfate Injection, USP ... 523
- Amikacin Sulfate Injection, USP ... 981
- Amikin Injectable 502

Aspirin (Co-administration in patients receiving high dose of salicylates may be associated with salicylate toxicity due to competition for secretion by renal tubule). Products include:
- Alka-Seltzer Cherry Effervescent Antacid and Pain Reliever ..... ⊡ 609

(⊡ Described in PDR For Nonprescription Drugs)   (⊙ Described in PDR For Ophthalmology)

Interactions Index — Demadex

Alka-Seltzer Extra Strength Effervescent Antacid and Pain Reliever 609
Alka-Seltzer Lemon Lime Effervescent Antacid and Pain Reliever 609
Alka-Seltzer Original Effervescent Antacid and Pain Reliever 609
Alka-Seltzer Plus 611
Alka-Seltzer Plus Sinus Medicine .. 611
Ascriptin 650
Arthritis Strength BC Powder......... 631
BC Cold Powder Multi-Symptom Formula (Cold-Sinus-Allergy) 631
BC Cold Powder Non-Drowsy Formula (Cold-Sinus) 631
BC Powder 631
Genuine Bayer Aspirin Tablets & Caplets 618
Extra Strength Bayer Arthritis Pain Regimen Formula 615
Extra Strength Bayer Aspirin Caplets & Tablets 617
Extended-Release Bayer 8-Hour Aspirin 616
Extra Strength Bayer Plus Aspirin Caplets 617
Extra Strength Bayer PM Aspirin Plus Sleep Aid 617
Aspirin Regimen Bayer 81 mg Tablets with Calcium 615
Aspirin Regimen Bayer Adult Low Strength 81 mg Tablets 613
Aspirin Regimen Bayer Children's Chewable Aspirin 616
Aspirin Regimen Bayer Regular Strength 325 mg Caplets 613
Bufferin Analgesic Tablets............ 636
Arthritis Strength Bufferin Analgesic Caplets 637
Extra Strength Bufferin Analgesic Tablets 637
Cama Arthritis Pain Reliever............ 748
Darvon Compound-65 Pulvules ... 1475
Easprin 1971
Ecotrin 2625
Ecotrin Enteric Coated Aspirin Maximum Strength Tablets and Caplets 775
Ecotrin Enteric Coated Aspirin Regular Strength Tablets 2625
Empirin Aspirin Tablets 818
Excedrin Extra-Strength Analgesic Tablets, Caplets, and Geltabs......... 734
Fiorinal Capsules 2388
Fiorinal with Codeine Capsules 2390
Fiorinal Tablets 2388
Goody's Extra Strength Headache Powders............ 632
Goody's Extra Strength Pain Relief Tablets 632
Halfprin Tablets 1413
Norgesic 1554
Percodan Tablets............ 955
Percodan-Demi Tablets 956
Robaxisal Tablets............ 2246
Soma Compound w/Codeine Tablets 2784
Soma Compound Tablets............ 2783
St. Joseph Adult Chewable Aspirin (81 mg.) 768
Talwin Compound 2466
Vanquish Analgesic Caplets 627

Cholestyramine (Possibility of decreased oral absorption of torsemide; simultaneous administration is not recommended). Products include:
Questran 774

Choline Magnesium Trisalicylate (Co-administration in patients receiving high dose of salicylates may be associated with salicylate toxicity due to competition for secretion by renal tubule). Products include:
Trilisate 2155

Diclofenac Potassium (Co-administration of another loop diuretic and nonsteroidal anti-inflammatory agents has been associated with renal dysfunction; concurrent use of torsemide and these agents has not been studied, however, such combined therapy should be undertaken with great caution). Products include:
Cataflam Tablets 833

Diclofenac Sodium (Co-administration of another loop diuretic and nonsteroidal anti-inflammatory agents has been associated with renal dysfunction; concurrent use of torsemide and these agents has not been studied, however, such combined therapy should be undertaken with great caution). Products include:
Voltaren Ophthalmic Sterile Ophthalmic Solution 264
Cataflam/Voltaren/Voltaren-XR 833

Diflunisal (Co-administration in patients receiving high dose of salicylates may be associated with salicylate toxicity due to competition for secretion by renal tubule). Products include:
Dolobid Tablets............ 1695

Digoxin (Co-administration of digoxin is reported to increase the AUC for torsemide by 50%). Products include:
Lanoxicaps 1110
Lanoxin Elixir Pediatric 1113
Lanoxin Injection 1116
Lanoxin Injection Pediatric............ 1119
Lanoxin Tablets 1121

Etodolac (Co-administration of another loop diuretic and nonsteroidal anti-inflammatory agents has been associated with renal dysfunction; concurrent use of torsemide and these agents has not been studied, however, such combined therapy should be undertaken with great caution). Products include:
Lodine Capsules and Tablets 2849

Fenoprofen Calcium (Co-administration of another loop diuretic and nonsteroidal anti-inflammatory agents has been associated with renal dysfunction; concurrent use of torsemide and these agents has not been studied, however, such combined therapy should be undertaken with great caution). Products include:
Nalfon 200 Pulvules & Nalfon Tablets 933

Flurbiprofen (Co-administration of another loop diuretic and nonsteroidal anti-inflammatory agents has been associated with renal dysfunction; concurrent use of torsemide and these agents has not been studied, however, such combined therapy should be undertaken with great caution).
No products indexed under this heading.

Gentamicin Sulfate (Co-administration of other diuretics has been reported to increase the ototoxic potential of aminoglycoside antibiotics, especially in the presence of impaired renal function; concurrent use of aminoglycoside and torsemide has not been studied, however, such combined therapy should be undertaken with great caution). Products include:
Garamycin Cream 0.1% 2501
Garamycin Injectable 2502
Garamycin Ointment 0.1% 2501
Garamycin Ophthalmic 2501
Genoptic Sterile Ophthalmic Solution............ 241
Genoptic Sterile Ophthalmic Ointment............ 241
Gentak 209
Pred-G Liquifilm Sterile Ophthalmic Suspension 248
Pred-G S.O.P. Sterile Ophthalmic Ointment 249

Ibuprofen (Co-administration of another loop diuretic and nonsteroidal anti-inflammatory agents has been associated with renal dysfunction; concurrent use of torsemide and these agents has not been studied, however, such combined therapy should be undertaken with great caution). Products include:
Advil Cold and Sinus Caplets and Tablets 837
Advil Ibuprofen Tablets, Caplets and Gel Caplets 836
Children's Motrin Ibuprofen Oral Suspension 1558
IBU Tablets 1389
Ibuprohm............ 713
Motrin IB Caplets, Tablets, and Gelcaps 802
Motrin Ibuprofen Suspension, Oral Drops, Chewable Tablets, Caplets 1563
Nuprin Ibuprofen/Analgesic Tablets & Caplets 645
Vicks DayQuil SINUS Pressure & PAIN Relief with IBUPROFEN 735

Indomethacin (The natriuretic effect of torsemide is partially inhibited by the co-administration). Products include:
Indocin 1723

Indomethacin Sodium Trihydrate (The natriuretic effect of torsemide is partially inhibited by the co-administration). Products include:
Indocin I.V. 1727

Kanamycin Sulfate (Co-administration of other diuretics has been reported to increase the ototoxic potential of aminoglycoside antibiotics, especially in the presence of impaired renal function; concurrent use of aminoglycoside and torsemide has not been studied, however, such combined therapy should be undertaken with great caution).
No products indexed under this heading.

Ketoprofen (Co-administration of another loop diuretic and nonsteroidal anti-inflammatory agents has been associated with renal dysfunction; concurrent use of torsemide and these agents has not been studied, however, such combined therapy should be undertaken with great caution). Products include:
Actron Caplets and Tablets............ 608
Orudis Capsules 2874
Orudis KT 842
Oruvail Capsules 2874

Ketorolac Tromethamine (Co-administration of another loop diuretic and nonsteroidal anti-inflammatory agents has been associated with renal dysfunction; concurrent use of torsemide and these agents has not been studied, however, such combined therapy should be undertaken with great caution). Products include:
Acular Sterile Ophthalmic Solution 470
Toradol 2319

Lithium Carbonate (Co-administration of other diuretics are known to reduce the renal clearance of lithium, inducing a high risk of lithium toxicity; concurrent use of lithium and torsemide has not been studied, however, such combined therapy should be undertaken with great caution). Products include:
Eskalith 2658
Lithium Carbonate Capsules & Tablets 2352
Lithonate/Lithotabs/Lithobid 2721

Lithium Citrate (Co-administration of other diuretics are known to reduce the renal clearance of lithium, inducing a high risk of lithium toxicity; concurrent use of lithium and torsemide has not been studied, however, such combined therapy should be undertaken with great caution).
No products indexed under this heading.

Magnesium Salicylate (Co-administration in patients receiving high dose of salicylates may be associated with salicylate toxicity due to competition for secretion by renal tubule). Products include:
Backache Caplets 635
Doan's Extra-Strength Analgesic..... 653
Extra Strength Doan's P.M. 653
Doan's Regular Strength Analgesic............ 654
Mobigesic Tablets 607

Meclofenamate Sodium (Co-administration of another loop diuretic and nonsteroidal anti-inflammatory agents has been associated with renal dysfunction; concurrent use of torsemide and these agents has not been studied, however, such combined therapy should be undertaken with great caution).
No products indexed under this heading.

Mefenamic Acid (Co-administration of another loop diuretic and nonsteroidal anti-inflammatory agents has been associated with renal dysfunction; concurrent use of torsemide and these agents has not been studied, however, such combined therapy should be undertaken with great caution). Products include:
Ponstel 1982

Nabumetone (Co-administration of another loop diuretic and nonsteroidal anti-inflammatory agents has been associated with renal dysfunction; concurrent use of torsemide and these agents has not been studied, however, such combined therapy should be undertaken with great caution). Products include:
Relafen Tablets............ 2688

Naproxen (Co-administration of another loop diuretic and nonsteroidal anti-inflammatory agents has been associated with renal dysfunction; concurrent use of torsemide and these agents has not been studied, however, such combined therapy should be undertaken with great caution). Products include:
Anaprox/Naprosyn 2277

Naproxen Sodium (Co-administration of another loop diuretic and nonsteroidal anti-inflammatory agents has been associated with renal dysfunction; concurrent use of torsemide and these agents has not been studied, however, such combined therapy should be undertaken with great caution). Products include:
Aleve 2124
Anaprox/Naprosyn 2277
Naprelan Tablets 2861

IMPORTANT NOTE: Always consult each drug listing in the patient's regimen for possible interactions.

Oxaprozin (Co-administration of another loop diuretic and nonsteroidal anti-inflammatory agents has been associated with renal dysfunction; concurrent use of torsemide and these agents has not been studied, however, such combined therapy should be undertaken with great caution). Products include:
- Daypro Caplets ... 2578

Phenylbutazone (Co-administration of another loop diuretic and nonsteroidal anti-inflammatory agents has been associated with renal dysfunction; concurrent use of torsemide and these agents has not been studied, however, such combined therapy should be undertaken with great caution).
- No products indexed under this heading.

Piroxicam (Co-administration of another loop diuretic and nonsteroidal anti-inflammatory agents has been associated with renal dysfunction; concurrent use of torsemide and these agents has not been studied, however, such combined therapy should be undertaken with great caution). Products include:
- Feldene Capsules ... 2008

Probenecid (Reduces secretion of torsemide into the proximal tubule and thereby decreases diuretic effect). Products include:
- Benemid Tablets ... 1651
- ColBENEMID Tablets ... 1662

Salsalate (Co-administration in patients receiving high dose of salicylates may be associated with salicylate toxicity due to competition for secretion by renal tubule). Products include:
- Disalcid ... 1549
- Mono-Gesic Tablets ... 810
- Salflex Tablets ... 791

Spironolactone (Co-administration may be associated with significant reduction in the renal clearance of spironolactone, with corresponding increase in the AUC). Products include:
- Aldactazide Tablets ... 2556
- Aldactone Tablets ... 2558

Streptomycin Sulfate (Co-administration of other diuretics has been reported to increase the ototoxic potential of aminoglycoside antibiotics, especially in the presence of impaired renal function; concurrent use of aminoglycoside and torsemide has not been studied, however, such combined therapy should be undertaken with great caution). Products include:
- Streptomycin Sulfate Injection ... 2031

Sulindac (Co-administration of another loop diuretic and nonsteroidal anti-inflammatory agents has been associated with renal dysfunction; concurrent use of torsemide and these agents has not been studied, however, such combined therapy should be undertaken with great caution). Products include:
- Clinoril Tablets ... 1658

Tobramycin (Co-administration of other diuretics has been reported to increase the ototoxic potential of aminoglycoside antibiotics, especially in the presence of impaired renal function; concurrent use of aminoglycoside and torsemide has not been studied, however, such combined therapy should be undertaken with great caution). Products include:
- AKTOB ... ◉ 207
- TobraDex Ophthalmic Suspension and Ointment ... 469
- Tobrex Ophthalmic Ointment and Solution ... ◉ 226

Tobramycin Sulfate (Co-administration of other diuretics has been reported to increase the ototoxic potential of aminoglycoside antibiotics, especially in the presence of impaired renal function; concurrent use of aminoglycoside and torsemide has not been studied, however, such combined therapy should be undertaken with great caution). Products include:
- Nebcin Vials, Hyporets & ADD-Vantage ... 1518

Tolmetin Sodium (Co-administration of another loop diuretic and nonsteroidal anti-inflammatory agents has been associated with renal dysfunction; concurrent use of torsemide and these agents has not been studied, however, such combined therapy should be undertaken with great caution). Products include:
- Tolectin (200, 400 and 600 mg) .. 1591

Food Interactions

Food, unspecified (Simultaneous food intake delays the time to C_{max} by about 30 minutes, but overall bioavailability (AUC) and diuretic activity are unchanged).

DEMEROL CARPUJECT
(Meperidine Hydrochloride) ... 2438
See **Demerol Tablets**

DEMEROL INJECTION
(Meperidine Hydrochloride) ... 2438
See **Demerol Tablets**

DEMEROL SYRUP
(Meperidine Hydrochloride) ... 2438
See **Demerol Tablets**

DEMEROL TABLETS
(Meperidine Hydrochloride) ... 2438
May interact with narcotic analgesics, general anesthetics, phenothiazines, tranquilizers, hypnotics and sedatives, barbiturates, tricyclic antidepressants, antihistamines, central nervous system depressants, monoamine oxidase inhibitors, and certain other agents. Compounds in these categories include:

Acrivastine (Co-administration may result in respiratory depression, hypotension, and profound sedation or coma; reduced dosage of meperidine may be required if given concurrently). Products include:
- Semprex-D Capsules ... 1620

Alfentanil Hydrochloride (Co-administration may result in respiratory depression, hypotension, and profound sedation or coma; reduced dosage of meperidine may be required if given concurrently). Products include:
- Alfenta Injection ... 1334

Alprazolam (Co-administration may result in respiratory depression, hypotension, and profound sedation or coma; reduced dosage of meperidine may be required if given concurrently). Products include:
- Xanax Tablets ... 2115

Amitriptyline Hydrochloride (Co-administration may result in respiratory depression, hypotension, and profound sedation or coma; reduced dosage of meperidine may be required if given concurrently). Products include:
- Elavil ... 2945
- Etrafon ... 2495
- Limbitrol ... 2333
- Triavil Tablets ... 1800

Amoxapine (Co-administration may result in respiratory depression, hypotension, and profound sedation or coma; reduced dosage of meperidine may be required if given concurrently). Products include:
- Asendin Tablets ... 1419

Aprobarbital (Co-administration may result in respiratory depression, hypotension, and profound sedation or coma; reduced dosage of meperidine may be required if given concurrently).
- No products indexed under this heading.

Astemizole (Co-administration may result in respiratory depression, hypotension, and profound sedation or coma; reduced dosage of meperidine may be required if given concurrently). Products include:
- Hismanal Tablets ... 1341

Azatadine Maleate (Co-administration may result in respiratory depression, hypotension, and profound sedation or coma; reduced dosage of meperidine may be required if given concurrently). Products include:
- Trinalin Repetabs Tablets ... 1373

Bromodiphenhydramine Hydrochloride (Co-administration may result in respiratory depression, hypotension, and profound sedation or coma; reduced dosage of meperidine may be required if given concurrently).
- No products indexed under this heading.

Brompheniramine Maleate (Co-administration may result in respiratory depression, hypotension, and profound sedation or coma; reduced dosage of meperidine may be required if given concurrently). Products include:
- Alka-Seltzer Plus Sinus Medicine .. ▣ 611
- Bromfed Capsules (Extended-Release) ... 1832
- Bromfed Syrup ... ▣ 712
- Bromfed Tablets ... 1832
- Bromfed-DM Cough Syrup ... 1832
- Bromfed-PD Capsules (Extended-Release) ... 1832
- Dimetane-DC Cough Syrup ... 2232
- Dimetane-DX Cough Syrup ... 2233
- Dimetapp Allergy Dye-Free Elixir ... ▣ 838
- Dimetapp Allergy Sinus Caplets ... ▣ 838
- Dimetapp Cold & Allergy Chewable Tablets ... ▣ 838
- Dimetapp Cold & Cough Liqui-Gels ... ▣ 839
- Dimetapp Cold & Fever Suspension ... ▣ 839
- Dimetapp DM Elixir ... ▣ 840
- Dimetapp Elixir ... ▣ 840
- Dimetapp Extentabs ... ▣ 841
- Dimetapp Tablets/Liqui-Gels ... ▣ 841
- Rondec Chewable Tablets ... 974
- Vicks DayQuil Allergy Relief 12-Hour Extended Release Tablets.. ▣ 733
- Vicks DayQuil Allergy Relief 4-Hour Tablets ... ▣ 733

Buprenorphine (Co-administration may result in respiratory depression, hypotension, and profound sedation or coma; reduced dosage of meperidine may be required if given concurrently). Products include:
- Buprenex Injectable ... 2170

Buspirone Hydrochloride (Co-administration may result in respiratory depression, hypotension, and profound sedation or coma; reduced dosage of meperidine may be required if given concurrently). Products include:
- BuSpar Tablets ... 738

Butabarbital (Co-administration may result in respiratory depression, hypotension, and profound sedation or coma; reduced dosage of meperidine may be required if given concurrently).
- No products indexed under this heading.

Butalbital (Co-administration may result in respiratory depression, hypotension, and profound sedation or coma; reduced dosage of meperidine may be required if given concurrently). Products include:
- Axocet Capsules ... 2469
- Esgic-plus Capsules ... 1012
- Esgic-plus Tablets ... 1012
- Fioricet Tablets ... 2386
- Fioricet with Codeine Capsules ... 2387
- Fiorinal Capsules ... 2388
- Fiorinal with Codeine Capsules ... 2390
- Fiorinal Tablets ... 2388
- Phrenilin ... 790
- Sedapap Tablets 50 mg/650 mg .. 1826

Cetirizine Hydrochloride (Co-administration may result in respiratory depression, hypotension, and profound sedation or coma; reduced dosage of meperidine may be required if given concurrently). Products include:
- Zyrtec Tablets ... 2053

Chlordiazepoxide (Co-administration may result in respiratory depression, hypotension, and profound sedation or coma; reduced dosage of meperidine may be required if given concurrently). Products include:
- Limbitrol ... 2333

Chlordiazepoxide Hydrochloride (Co-administration may result in respiratory depression, hypotension, and profound sedation or coma; reduced dosage of meperidine may be required if given concurrently). Products include:
- Librax Capsules ... 2330
- Librium Capsules ... 2331
- Librium Injectable ... 2332

Chlorpheniramine Maleate (Co-administration may result in respiratory depression, hypotension, and profound sedation or coma; reduced dosage of meperidine may be required if given concurrently). Products include:
- Alka-Seltzer Plus Cold Medicine ... ▣ 611
- Alka-Seltzer Plus Cold Medicine Liqui-Gels ... ▣ 612
- Alka-Seltzer Plus Cold & Cough Medicine ... ▣ 611
- Alka-Seltzer Plus Cold & Cough Medicine Liqui-Gels ... ▣ 612
- Alka-Seltzer Plus Flu & Body Aches Effervescent Tablets ... ▣ 612
- Allerest Maximum Strength ... ▣ 649
- Allerest Sinus Pain Formula ... ▣ 649
- Ana-Kit Anaphylaxis Emergency Treatment Kit ... 611
- Atrohist Pediatric Capsules ... 1603
- Atrohist Plus Tablets ... 1605
- BC Cold Powder Multi-Symptom Formula (Cold-Sinus-Allergy) ... ▣ 631
- Cerose DM ... ▣ 853
- Cheracol Plus Head Cold/Cough Formula ... ▣ 741
- Children's TYLENOL Cold Multi-Symptom Chewable Tablets and Liquid ... 1559
- Children's TYLENOL Cold Plus Cough Multi Symptom Chewable Tablets and Liquid ... 1560
- Children's TYLENOL Flu Suspension Liquid ... 1560
- Children's Vicks DayQuil Allergy Relief ... ▣ 730
- Children's Vicks NyQuil Cold/Cough Relief ... ▣ 731
- Chlor-Trimeton Allergy Decongestant Tablets ... ▣ 759
- Chlor-Trimeton Allergy Tablets ... ▣ 758
- Allergy-Sinus Comtrex Multi-Symptom Allergy-Sinus Formula Tablets and Caplets ... ▣ 639

(▣ Described in PDR For Nonprescription Drugs) (◉ Described in PDR For Ophthalmology)

Comtrex Multi-Symptom............... 638	**Chlorpromazine Hydrochloride** (Co-administration may result in respiratory depression, hypotension, and profound sedation or coma; reduced dosage of meperidine may be required if given concurrently). Products include:	**Desflurane** (Co-administration may result in respiratory depression, hypotension, and profound sedation or coma; reduced dosage of meperidine may be required if given concurrently). Products include:	Sleepinal Night-time Sleep Aid Capsules and Softgels.......... 798
Contac Continuous Action Nasal Decongestant/Antihistamine 12 Hour Capsules............................ 773			TYLENOL Allergy Sinus NightTime, Maximum Strength Caplets 1571
Contac Maximum Strength Continuous Action Decongestant/Antihistamine 12 Hour Caplets... 772			TYLENOL Flu NightTime, Maximum Strength Gelcaps.............. 1575
Contac Severe Cold and Flu Formula Caplets 773	Thorazine 2701	Suprane (desflurane, USP)......... 1865	TYLENOL Flu NightTime, Maximum Strength Hot Medication Packets.............................. 1575
Coricidin Cold + Flu Tablets......... 760	**Chlorprothixene** (Co-administration may result in respiratory depression, hypotension, and profound sedation or coma; reduced dosage of meperidine may be required if given concurrently).	**Desipramine Hydrochloride** (Co-administration may result in respiratory depression, hypotension, and profound sedation or coma; reduced dosage of meperidine may be required if given concurrently). Products include:	
Coricidin Cough + Cold Tablets 760			TYLENOL PM Pain Reliever/Sleep Aid, Extra Strength Gelcaps, Caplets, Geltabs 1576
Coricidin 'D' Decongestant Tablets 760			
D.A. II Tablets 972			TYLENOL Severe Allergy Medication Caplets 1571
D.A. Chewable Tablets................. 970	No products indexed under this heading.	Norpramin Tablets 1273	Maximum Strength Unisom Sleepgels 1990
Dura-Tap/PD Capsules 970		**Dexchlorpheniramine Maleate** (Co-administration may result in respiratory depression, hypotension, and profound sedation or coma; reduced dosage of meperidine may be required if given concurrently).	
Dura-Vent/DA Tablets.................. 972	**Chlorprothixene Hydrochloride** (Co-administration may result in respiratory depression, hypotension, and profound sedation or coma; reduced dosage of meperidine may be required if given concurrently).		Unisom With Pain Relief-Nighttime Sleep Aid and Pain Reliever....... 1991
Efidac 24 Chlorpheniramine........... 655			**Diphenylpyraline Hydrochloride** (Co-administration may result in respiratory depression, hypotension, and profound sedation or coma; reduced dosage of meperidine may be required if given concurrently).
Extendryl 1003			
Fedahist Gyrocaps 2545			
Hycomine Compound Tablets 948		No products indexed under this heading.	
Kronofed-A................................. 994		**Dezocine** (Co-administration may result in respiratory depression, hypotension, and profound sedation or coma; reduced dosage of meperidine may be required if given concurrently). Products include:	
Nolamine Timed-Release Tablets 790	No products indexed under this heading.		
Novahistine Elixir 782			No products indexed under this heading.
Ornade Spansule Capsules 2678	**Chlorprothixene Lactate** (Co-administration may result in respiratory depression, hypotension, and profound sedation or coma; reduced dosage of meperidine may be required if given concurrently).		**Doxepin Hydrochloride** (Co-administration may result in respiratory depression, hypotension, and profound sedation or coma; reduced dosage of meperidine may be required if given concurrently). Products include:
PediaCare Cough-Cold Chewable Tablets and Liquid 1569			
PediaCare NightRest Cough-Cold Liquid 1569		Dalgan Injection 529	
Pediatric Vicks 44m Cough & Cold Relief 737		**Diazepam** (Co-administration may result in respiratory depression, hypotension, and profound sedation or coma; reduced dosage of meperidine may be required if given concurrently). Products include:	
Pyrroxate Caplets 742	No products indexed under this heading.		
Ryna 804	**Clemastine Fumarate** (Co-administration may result in respiratory depression, hypotension, and profound sedation or coma; reduced dosage of meperidine may be required if given concurrently). Products include:		Adapin Capsules 1542
Sinarest 663			Sinequan 2028
Sine-Off Sinus Medicine 784			Zonalon Cream 1042
Singlet Tablets 785			**Droperidol** (Co-administration may result in respiratory depression, hypotension, and profound sedation or coma; reduced dosage of meperidine may be required if given concurrently). Products include:
Sinulin Tablets 792		Dizac (diazepam injectable emulsion) CIV 1862	
Sinutab Sinus Allergy Medication, Maximum Strength Tablets and Caplets 823			
	Tavist Syrup 2426	Valium Injectable 2336	
Sudafed Cold & Allergy Tablets...... 826	Tavist Tablets 2427	Valium Tablets 2335	
Teldrin 12 Hour Antihistamine/Nasal Decongestant Allergy Relief Capsules 786	Tavist-1 12 Hour Relief Tablets 749	**Diphenhydramine Citrate** (Co-administration may result in respiratory depression, hypotension, and profound sedation or coma; reduced dosage of meperidine may be required if given concurrently). Products include:	Inapsine Injection 462
	Tavist-D 12 Hour Relief Tablets 750		**Enflurane** (Co-administration may result in respiratory depression, hypotension, and profound sedation or coma; reduced dosage of meperidine may be required if given concurrently).
TheraFlu Flu and Cold Medicine 750	**Clomipramine Hydrochloride** (Co-administration may result in respiratory depression, hypotension, and profound sedation or coma; reduced dosage of meperidine may be required if given concurrently). Products include:		
Theraflu Maximum Strength Flu and Cold Medicine For Sore Throat 751			
		Excedrin P.M. Analgesic/Sleeping Aid Tablets, Caplets, Liquigels 735	
TheraFlu Flu, Cold and Cough Medicine 750		**Diphenhydramine Hydrochloride** (Co-administration may result in respiratory depression, hypotension, and profound sedation or coma; reduced dosage of meperidine may be required if given concurrently). Products include:	No products indexed under this heading.
			Estazolam (Co-administration may result in respiratory depression, hypotension, and profound sedation or coma; reduced dosage of meperidine may be required if given concurrently). Products include:
TheraFlu Maximum Strength Nighttime Flu, Cold & Cough Medicine 751	Anafranil Capsules 819		
	Clorazepate Dipotassium (Co-administration may result in respiratory depression, hypotension, and profound sedation or coma; reduced dosage of meperidine may be required if given concurrently). Products include:		
Triaminic Night Time 754			
Triaminic Syrup 755		Actifed Allergy Daytime/Nighttime Caplets....................... 808	
Triaminic Triaminicol Cold & Cough 756			ProSom Tablets 457
		Actifed Sinus Daytime/Nighttime Tablets and Caplets............. 809	**Ethchlorvynol** (Co-administration may result in respiratory depression, hypotension, and profound sedation or coma; reduced dosage of meperidine may be required if given concurrently). Products include:
Triaminicin Tablets 756			
Tussend 1830	Tranxene 459	Extra Strength Bayer PM Aspirin Plus Sleep Aid 617	
TYLENOL Allergy Sinus, Maximum Strength Caplets and Gelcaps ... 1571	**Codeine Phosphate** (Co-administration may result in respiratory depression, hypotension, and profound sedation or coma; reduced dosage of meperidine may be required if given concurrently). Products include:		
		Benadryl Allergy Chewables 811	
TYLENOL Cold Medication, Multi-Symptom Formula Tablets and Caplets 1572		Benadryl Allergy/Cold Tablets..... 811	
		Benadryl Allergy Decongestant Liquid Medication 812	Placidyl Capsules 456
TYLENOL Cold Medication, Multi-Symptom Hot Liquid Packets....... 1572			**Ethinamate** (Co-administration may result in respiratory depression, hypotension, and profound sedation or coma; reduced dosage of meperidine may be required if given concurrently).
	Brontex 2130	Benadryl Allergy Decongestant Tablets.............................. 812	
Vicks 44 LiquiCaps Cough, Cold & Flu Relief 728	Dimetane-DC Cough Syrup 2232		
	Fioricet with Codeine Capsules 2387	Benadryl Allergy Liquid Medication................................... 813	
Vicks 44M Cough, Cold & Flu Relief 729	Fiorinal with Codeine Capsules 2390		
Chlorpheniramine Polistirex (Co-administration may result in respiratory depression, hypotension, and profound sedation or coma; reduced dosage of meperidine may be required if given concurrently). Products include:	Nucofed 2225	Benadryl Allergy........................ 811	No products indexed under this heading.
	Phenergan with Codeine 2883	Benadryl Allergy Sinus Headache Caplets............................... 813	**Fentanyl** (Co-administration may result in respiratory depression, hypotension, and profound sedation or coma; reduced dosage of meperidine may be required if given concurrently). Products include:
	Phenergan VC with Codeine 2888		
	Robitussin A-C Syrup................ 2248	Benadryl Dye-Free Allergy Liquigel Softgels........................ 813	
	Robitussin-DAC Syrup............... 2249		
Tussionex Pennkinetic Extended-Release Suspension................. 1624	Ryna 804	Benadryl Dye-Free Allergy Liquid Medication........................... 814	
	Soma Compound w/Codeine Tablets...................................... 2784		Durageisic Transdermal System.... 1336
Chlorpheniramine Tannate (Co-administration may result in respiratory depression, hypotension, and profound sedation or coma; reduced dosage of meperidine may be required if given concurrently). Products include:		Benadryl Itch Relief Stick Extra Strength............................. 814	**Fentanyl Citrate** (Co-administration may result in respiratory depression, hypotension, and profound sedation or coma; reduced dosage of meperidine may be required if given concurrently). Products include:
	Tylenol with Codeine 1592	Benadryl Cream 814	
	Cyproheptadine Hydrochloride (Co-administration may result in respiratory depression, hypotension, and profound sedation or coma; reduced dosage of meperidine may be required if given concurrently). Products include:	Benadryl Gel 815	
		Benadryl Spray 815	
Atrohist Pediatric Suspension 1604		Benadryl Injection 1955	
Atrohist Pediatric Suspension Dye-Free 1604		Contac Day & Night Cold/Flu Night Caplets....................... 772	
Rynatan 2781			
Rynatuss 2782		Contac Night Allergy/Sinus Caplets.................................... 771	
Chlorpromazine (Co-administration may result in respiratory depression, hypotension, and profound sedation or coma; reduced dosage of meperidine may be required if given concurrently). Products include:	Periactin................................. 1767	Extra Strength Doan's P.M. 653	
		Excedrin P.M. Analgesic/Sleeping Aid Tablets, Caplets, Liquigels 643	Sublimaze Injection 463
Thorazine Suppositories............ 2701		Nytol QuickCaps Caplets 632	

IMPORTANT NOTE: Always consult each drug listing in the patient's regimen for possible interactions.

Demerol / Interactions Index

Fluphenazine Decanoate (Co-administration may result in respiratory depression, hypotension, and profound sedation or coma; reduced dosage of meperidine may be required if given concurrently). Products include:
- Prolixin Decanoate 510

Fluphenazine Enanthate (Co-administration may result in respiratory depression, hypotension, and profound sedation or coma; reduced dosage of meperidine may be required if given concurrently). Products include:
- Prolixin Enanthate 510

Fluphenazine Hydrochloride (Co-administration may result in respiratory depression, hypotension, and profound sedation or coma; reduced dosage of meperidine may be required if given concurrently). Products include:
- Prolixin 510

Flurazepam Hydrochloride (Co-administration may result in respiratory depression, hypotension, and profound sedation or coma; reduced dosage of meperidine may be required if given concurrently). Products include:
- Dalmane Capsules 2329

Furazolidone (Co-administration with the therapeutic doses of meperidine and MAO inhibitors has occasionally precipitated unpredictable, severe, and sometimes fatal reactions; concurrent and/or sequential use is contraindicated. Products include:
- Furoxone 2221

Glutethimide (Co-administration may result in respiratory depression, hypotension, and profound sedation or coma; reduced dosage of meperidine may be required if given concurrently).
- No products indexed under this heading.

Haloperidol (Co-administration may result in respiratory depression, hypotension, and profound sedation or coma; reduced dosage of meperidine may be required if given concurrently). Products include:
- Haldol Injection, Tablets and Concentrate 1585

Haloperidol Decanoate (Co-administration may result in respiratory depression, hypotension, and profound sedation or coma; reduced dosage of meperidine may be required if given concurrently). Products include:
- Haldol Decanoate 1587

Hydrocodone Bitartrate (Co-administration may result in respiratory depression, hypotension, and profound sedation or coma; reduced dosage of meperidine may be required if given concurrently). Products include:
- Codiclear DH Syrup 808
- Duratuss HD Elixir 2750
- Histussin D Liquid 670
- Hycodan Tablets and Syrup 946
- Hycomine Compound Tablets 948
- Hycomine 947
- Hycotuss Expectorant Syrup 950
- Hydrocet Capsules 787
- Lorcet 10/650 Tablets 1016
- Lortab 2751
- Tussend 1830
- Tussend Expectorant 1831
- Vicodin Tablets 1404
- Vicodin ES Tablets 1405
- Vicodin HP Tablets 1403
- Vicodin Tuss Expectorant 1406
- Zydone 967

Hydrocodone Polistirex (Co-administration may result in respiratory depression, hypotension, and profound sedation or coma; reduced dosage of meperidine may be required if given concurrently). Products include:
- Tussionex Pennkinetic Extended-Release Suspension 1624

Hydromorphone Hydrochloride (Co-administration may result in respiratory depression, hypotension, and profound sedation or coma; reduced dosage of meperidine may be required if given concurrently). Products include:
- Dilaudid Ampules 1382
- Dilaudid Cough Syrup 1383
- Dilaudid-HP Injection 1384
- Dilaudid-HP Lyophilized Powder 250 mg 1384
- Dilaudid 1382
- Dilaudid Oral Liquid 1386
- Dilaudid 1382
- Dilaudid Tablets - 8 mg 1386

Hydroxyzine Hydrochloride (Co-administration may result in respiratory depression, hypotension, and profound sedation or coma; reduced dosage of meperidine may be required if given concurrently). Products include:
- Atarax Tablets & Syrup 1992
- Marax Tablets & DF Syrup 2015
- Vistaril Intramuscular Solution 2042

Imipramine Hydrochloride (Co-administration may result in respiratory depression, hypotension, and profound sedation or coma; reduced dosage of meperidine may be required if given concurrently). Products include:
- Tofranil Ampuls 873
- Tofranil Tablets 875

Imipramine Pamoate (Co-administration may result in respiratory depression, hypotension, and profound sedation or coma; reduced dosage of meperidine may be required if given concurrently). Products include:
- Tofranil-PM Capsules 876

Isocarboxazid (Co-administration with the therapeutic doses of meperidine and MAO inhibitors has occasionally precipitated unpredictable, severe, and sometimes fatal reactions; concurrent and/or sequential use is contraindicated.
- No products indexed under this heading.

Isoflurane (Co-administration may result in respiratory depression, hypotension, and profound sedation or coma; reduced dosage of meperidine may be required if given concurrently).
- No products indexed under this heading.

Ketamine Hydrochloride (Co-administration may result in respiratory depression, hypotension, and profound sedation or coma; reduced dosage of meperidine may be required if given concurrently).
- No products indexed under this heading.

Levomethadyl Acetate Hydrochloride (Co-administration may result in respiratory depression, hypotension, and profound sedation or coma; reduced dosage of meperidine may be required if given concurrently). Products include:
- Orlaam Oral Solution 2361

Levorphanol Tartrate (Co-administration may result in respiratory depression, hypotension, and profound sedation or coma; reduced dosage of meperidine may be required if given concurrently). Products include:
- Levo-Dromoran 2297

Loratadine (Co-administration may result in respiratory depression, hypotension, and profound sedation or coma; reduced dosage of meperidine may be required if given concurrently). Products include:
- Claritin Tablets 2485
- Claritin-D Tablets 2487

Lorazepam (Co-administration may result in respiratory depression, hypotension, and profound sedation or coma; reduced dosage of meperidine may be required if given concurrently). Products include:
- Ativan Injection 2805
- Ativan Tablets 2807

Loxapine Hydrochloride (Co-administration may result in respiratory depression, hypotension, and profound sedation or coma; reduced dosage of meperidine may be required if given concurrently). Products include:
- Loxitane 1426

Loxapine Succinate (Co-administration may result in respiratory depression, hypotension, and profound sedation or coma; reduced dosage of meperidine may be required if given concurrently). Products include:
- Loxitane Capsules 1426

Maprotiline Hydrochloride (Co-administration may result in respiratory depression, hypotension, and profound sedation or coma; reduced dosage of meperidine may be required if given concurrently). Products include:
- Ludiomil Tablets 861

Mephobarbital (Co-administration may result in respiratory depression, hypotension, and profound sedation or coma; reduced dosage of meperidine may be required if given concurrently). Products include:
- Mebaral Tablets 2452

Meprobamate (Co-administration may result in respiratory depression, hypotension, and profound sedation or coma; reduced dosage of meperidine may be required if given concurrently). Products include:
- Miltown Tablets 2780
- PMB 200 and PMB 400 2890

Mesoridazine Besylate (Co-administration may result in respiratory depression, hypotension, and profound sedation or coma; reduced dosage of meperidine may be required if given concurrently). Products include:
- Serentil 689

Methadone Hydrochloride (Co-administration may result in respiratory depression, hypotension, and profound sedation or coma; reduced dosage of meperidine may be required if given concurrently). Products include:
- Methadone Hydrochloride Oral Concentrate 2356
- Methadone Hydrochloride Oral Solution & Tablets 2357

Methdilazine Hydrochloride (Co-administration may result in respiratory depression, hypotension, and profound sedation or coma; reduced dosage of meperidine may be required if given concurrently).
- No products indexed under this heading.

Methohexital Sodium (Co-administration may result in respiratory depression, hypotension, and profound sedation or coma; reduced dosage of meperidine may be required if given concurrently).
- No products indexed under this heading.

Methotrimeprazine (Co-administration may result in respiratory depression, hypotension, and profound sedation or coma; reduced dosage of meperidine may be required if given concurrently). Products include:
- Levoprome 1321

Methoxyflurane (Co-administration may result in respiratory depression, hypotension, and profound sedation or coma; reduced dosage of meperidine may be required if given concurrently).
- No products indexed under this heading.

Midazolam Hydrochloride (Co-administration may result in respiratory depression, hypotension, and profound sedation or coma; reduced dosage of meperidine may be required if given concurrently). Products include:
- Versed Injection 2324

Mirtazapine (Co-administration may result in respiratory depression, hypotension, and profound sedation or coma; reduced dosage of meperidine may be required if given concurrently). Products include:
- Remeron Tablets 1878

Molindone Hydrochloride (Co-administration may result in respiratory depression, hypotension, and profound sedation or coma; reduced dosage of meperidine may be required if given concurrently). Products include:
- Moban Tablets and Concentrate 1036

Morphine Sulfate (Co-administration may result in respiratory depression, hypotension, and profound sedation or coma; reduced dosage of meperidine may be required if given concurrently). Products include:
- Astramorph/PF Injection, USP (Preservative-Free) 526
- Duramorph Injection 983
- Infumorph 200 and Infumorph 500 Sterile Solutions 985
- Kadian Capsules 2948
- MS Contin Tablets 2149
- MSIR 2152
- Oramorph SR (Morphine Sulfate Sustained Release Tablets) 2359
- RMS Suppositories CII 2766
- Roxanol 2365

Nortriptyline Hydrochloride (Co-administration may result in respiratory depression, hypotension, and profound sedation or coma; reduced dosage of meperidine may be required if given concurrently). Products include:
- Pamelor 2409

Opium Alkaloids (Co-administration may result in respiratory depression, hypotension, and profound sedation or coma; reduced dosage of meperidine may be required if given concurrently).
- No products indexed under this heading.

(⊞ Described in PDR For Nonprescription Drugs)   (⊙ Described in PDR For Ophthalmology)

251 Interactions Index Demser

Oxazepam (Co-administration may result in respiratory depression, hypotension, and profound sedation or coma; reduced dosage of meperidine may be required if given concurrently). Products include:
Serax Capsules ... 2916
Serax Tablets ... 2916

Oxycodone Hydrochloride (Co-administration may result in respiratory depression, hypotension, and profound sedation or coma; reduced dosage of meperidine may be required if given concurrently). Products include:
OxyContin Tablets ... 2163
OxyIR Capsules ... 2167
Percocet Tablets ... 955
Percodan Tablets ... 955
Percodan-Demi Tablets ... 956
Roxicodone Tablets, Oral Solution & Intensol (Oxycodone) ... 2366
Tylox Capsules ... 1593

Pentobarbital Sodium (Co-administration may result in respiratory depression, hypotension, and profound sedation or coma; reduced dosage of meperidine may be required if given concurrently). Products include:
Nembutal Sodium Capsules ... 440
Nembutal Sodium Solution ... 442
Nembutal Sodium Suppositories ... 444

Perphenazine (Co-administration may result in respiratory depression, hypotension, and profound sedation or coma; reduced dosage of meperidine may be required if given concurrently). Products include:
Etrafon ... 2495
Triavil Tablets ... 1800
Trilafon ... 2532

Phenelzine Sulfate (Co-administration with the therapeutic doses of meperidine and MAO inhibitors has occasionally precipitated unpredictable, severe, and sometimes fatal reactions; concurrent and/or sequential use is contraindicated). Products include:
Nardil ... 1977

Phenobarbital (Co-administration may result in respiratory depression, hypotension, and profound sedation or coma; reduced dosage of meperidine may be required if given concurrently). Products include:
Arco-Lase Plus Tablets ... 513
Bellergal-S Tablets ... 2375
Donnatal ... 2234
Donnatal Extentabs ... 2234
Donnatal Tablets ... 2234
Phenobarbital Elixir and Tablets ... 1523
Quadrinal Tablets ... 1398

Prazepam (Co-administration may result in respiratory depression, hypotension, and profound sedation or coma; reduced dosage of meperidine may be required if given concurrently).
No products indexed under this heading.

Prochlorperazine (Co-administration may result in respiratory depression, hypotension, and profound sedation or coma; reduced dosage of meperidine may be required if given concurrently). Products include:
Compazine ... 2644

Promethazine Hydrochloride (Co-administration may result in respiratory depression, hypotension, and profound sedation or coma; reduced dosage of meperidine may be required if given concurrently). Products include:
Mepergan Injection ... 2859
Phenergan with Codeine ... 2883
Phenergan with Dextromethorphan ... 2885
Phenergan Injection ... 2880
Phenergan Suppositories ... 2882
Phenergan Syrup ... 2881
Phenergan Tablets ... 2882
Phenergan VC ... 2886
Phenergan VC with Codeine ... 2888

Propofol (Co-administration may result in respiratory depression, hypotension, and profound sedation or coma; reduced dosage of meperidine may be required if given concurrently). Products include:
Diprivan Injectable Emulsion ... 2939

Propoxyphene Hydrochloride (Co-administration may result in respiratory depression, hypotension, and profound sedation or coma; reduced dosage of meperidine may be required if given concurrently). Products include:
Darvon ... 1475
Wygesic Tablets ... 2930

Propoxyphene Napsylate (Co-administration may result in respiratory depression, hypotension, and profound sedation or coma; reduced dosage of meperidine may be required if given concurrently). Products include:
Darvon-N/Darvocet-N ... 1473

Protriptyline Hydrochloride (Co-administration may result in respiratory depression, hypotension, and profound sedation or coma; reduced dosage of meperidine may be required if given concurrently). Products include:
Vivactil Tablets ... 1820

Pyrilamine Maleate (Co-administration may result in respiratory depression, hypotension, and profound sedation or coma; reduced dosage of meperidine may be required if given concurrently). Products include:
4-Way Fast Acting Nasal Spray (regular & mentholated) ... 644
Maximum Strength Multi-Symptom Formula Midol ... 621
PMS Multi-Symptom Formula Midol ... 622

Pyrilamine Tannate (Co-administration may result in respiratory depression, hypotension, and profound sedation or coma; reduced dosage of meperidine may be required if given concurrently). Products include:
Atrohist Pediatric Suspension ... 1604
Atrohist Pediatric Suspension Dye-Free ... 1604
Rynatan ... 2781

Quazepam (Co-administration may result in respiratory depression, hypotension, and profound sedation or coma; reduced dosage of meperidine may be required if given concurrently). Products include:
Doral Tablets ... 2773

Risperidone (Co-administration may result in respiratory depression, hypotension, and profound sedation or coma; reduced dosage of meperidine may be required if given concurrently). Products include:
Risperdal Tablets ... 1348

Secobarbital Sodium (Co-administration may result in respiratory depression, hypotension, and profound sedation or coma; reduced dosage of meperidine may be required if given concurrently). Products include:
Seconal Sodium Pulvules ... 1529

Selegiline Hydrochloride (Co-administration with the therapeutic doses of meperidine and MAO inhibitors has occasionally precipitated unpredictable, severe, and sometimes fatal reactions; concurrent and/or sequential use is contraindicated). Products include:
Eldepryl Capsules ... 2729

Sevoflurane (Co-administration may result in respiratory depression, hypotension, and profound sedation or coma; reduced dosage of meperidine may be required if given concurrently).
No products indexed under this heading.

Sufentanil Citrate (Co-administration may result in respiratory depression, hypotension, and profound sedation or coma; reduced dosage of meperidine may be required if given concurrently). Products include:
Sufenta Injection ... 1355

Temazepam (Co-administration may result in respiratory depression, hypotension, and profound sedation or coma; reduced dosage of meperidine may be required if given concurrently). Products include:
Restoril Capsules ... 2413

Terfenadine (Co-administration may result in respiratory depression, hypotension, and profound sedation or coma; reduced dosage of meperidine may be required if given concurrently). Products include:
Seldane Tablets ... 1284
Seldane-D Extended-Release Tablets ... 1286

Thiamylal Sodium (Co-administration may result in respiratory depression, hypotension, and profound sedation or coma; reduced dosage of meperidine may be required if given concurrently).
No products indexed under this heading.

Thioridazine Hydrochloride (Co-administration may result in respiratory depression, hypotension, and profound sedation or coma; reduced dosage of meperidine may be required if given concurrently). Products include:
Mellaril ... 2398

Thiothixene (Co-administration may result in respiratory depression, hypotension, and profound sedation or coma; reduced dosage of meperidine may be required if given concurrently). Products include:
Navane Capsules and Concentrate ... 2018
Navane Intramuscular ... 2019

Tranylcypromine Sulfate (Co-administration with the therapeutic doses of meperidine and MAO inhibitors has occasionally precipitated unpredictable, severe, and sometimes fatal reactions; concurrent and/or sequential use is contraindicated). Products include:
Parnate Tablets ... 2679

Triazolam (Co-administration may result in respiratory depression, hypotension, and profound sedation or coma; reduced dosage of meperidine may be required if given concurrently). Products include:
Halcion Tablets ... 2093

Trifluoperazine Hydrochloride (Co-administration may result in respiratory depression, hypotension, and profound sedation or coma; reduced dosage of meperidine may be required if given concurrently). Products include:
Stelazine ... 2692

Trimeprazine Tartrate (Co-administration may result in respiratory depression, hypotension, and profound sedation or coma; reduced dosage of meperidine may be required if given concurrently).
No products indexed under this heading.

Trimipramine Maleate (Co-administration may result in respiratory depression, hypotension, and profound sedation or coma; reduced dosage of meperidine may be required if given concurrently). Products include:
Surmontil Capsules ... 2917

Tripelennamine Hydrochloride (Co-administration may result in respiratory depression, hypotension, and profound sedation or coma; reduced dosage of meperidine may be required if given concurrently). Products include:
PBZ Tablets ... 863
PBZ-SR Tablets ... 862

Triprolidine Hydrochloride (Co-administration may result in respiratory depression, hypotension, and profound sedation or coma; reduced dosage of meperidine may be required if given concurrently). Products include:
Actifed Cold & Allergy Tablets ... 807
Actifed Cold & Sinus Caplets and Tablets ... 808

Zolpidem Tartrate (Co-administration may result in respiratory depression, hypotension, and profound sedation or coma; reduced dosage of meperidine may be required if given concurrently). Products include:
Ambien Tablets ... 2559

Food Interactions

Alcohol (Concurrent use may result in respiratory depression, hypotension, and profound sedation or coma).

DEMEROL UNI-AMP
(Meperidine Hydrochloride) ... 2438
See **Demerol Tablets**

DEMSER CAPSULES
(Metyrosine) ... 1690
May interact with central nervous system depressants, phenothiazines, and certain other agents. Compounds in these categories include:

Alfentanil Hydrochloride (Additive sedative effects). Products include:
Alfenta Injection ... 1334

Alprazolam (Additive sedative effects). Products include:
Xanax Tablets ... 2115

Aprobarbital (Additive sedative effects).
No products indexed under this heading.

Buprenorphine (Additive sedative effects). Products include:
Buprenex Injectable ... 2170

Buspirone Hydrochloride (Additive sedative effects). Products include:
BuSpar Tablets ... 738

Butabarbital (Additive sedative effects).
No products indexed under this heading.

Butalbital (Additive sedative effects). Products include:
Axocet Capsules ... 2469
Esgic-plus Capsules ... 1012
Esgic-plus Tablets ... 1012
Fioricet Tablets ... 2386
Fioricet with Codeine Capsules ... 2387
Fiorinal Capsules ... 2388

IMPORTANT NOTE: Always consult each drug listing in the patient's regimen for possible interactions.

Demser

Interactions Index

Fiorinal with Codeine Capsules 2390
Fiorinal Tablets 2388
Phrenilin 790
Sedapap Tablets 50 mg/650 mg .. 1826

Chlordiazepoxide (Additive sedative effects). Products include:
Limbitrol 2333

Chlordiazepoxide Hydrochloride (Additive sedative effects). Products include:
Librax Capsules 2330
Librium Capsules 2331
Librium Injectable 2332

Chlorpromazine (Possible potentiation of extrapyramidal effects; additive sedative effects). Products include:
Thorazine Suppositories 2701

Chlorpromazine Hydrochloride (Possible potentiation of extrapyramidal effects; additive sedative effects). Products include:
Thorazine 2701

Chlorprothixene (Additive sedative effects).
No products indexed under this heading.

Chlorprothixene Hydrochloride (Additive sedative effects).
No products indexed under this heading.

Chlorprothixene Lactate (Additive sedative effects).
No products indexed under this heading.

Clorazepate Dipotassium (Additive sedative effects). Products include:
Tranxene 459

Clozapine (Additive sedative effects). Products include:
Clozaril Tablets 2377

Codeine Phosphate (Additive sedative effects). Products include:
Brontex 2130
Dimetane-DC Cough Syrup 2232
Fioricet with Codeine Capsules .. 2387
Fiorinal with Codeine Capsules .. 2390
Nucofed 2225
Phenergan with Codeine 2883
Phenergan VC with Codeine 2888
Robitussin A-C Syrup 2248
Robitussin-DAC Syrup 2249
Ryna ....☒ 804
Soma Compound w/Codeine Tablets 2784
Tylenol with Codeine 1592

Desflurane (Additive sedative effects). Products include:
Suprane (desflurane, USP) 1865

Dezocine (Additive sedative effects). Products include:
Dalgan Injection 529

Diazepam (Additive sedative effects). Products include:
Dizac (diazepam injectable emulsion) CIV 1862
Valium Injectable 2336
Valium Tablets 2335

Droperidol (Additive sedative effects). Products include:
Inapsine Injection 462

Enflurane (Additive sedative effects).
No products indexed under this heading.

Estazolam (Additive sedative effects). Products include:
ProSom Tablets 457

Ethchlorvynol (Additive sedative effects). Products include:
Placidyl Capsules 456

Ethinamate (Additive sedative effects).
No products indexed under this heading.

Fentanyl (Additive sedative effects). Products include:
Duragesic Transdermal System ... 1336

Fentanyl Citrate (Additive sedative effects). Products include:
Sublimaze Injection 463

Fluphenazine Decanoate (Possible potentiation of extrapyramidal effects; additive sedative effects). Products include:
Prolixin Decanoate 510

Fluphenazine Enanthate (Possible potentiation of extrapyramidal effects; additive sedative effects). Products include:
Prolixin Enanthate 510

Fluphenazine Hydrochloride (Possible potentiation of extrapyramidal effects; additive sedative effects). Products include:
Prolixin 510

Flurazepam Hydrochloride (Additive sedative effects). Products include:
Dalmane Capsules 2329

Glutethimide (Additive sedative effects).
No products indexed under this heading.

Haloperidol (Possible potentiation of extrapyramidal effects; additive sedative effects). Products include:
Haldol Injection, Tablets and Concentrate 1585

Haloperidol Decanoate (Possible potentiation of extrapyramidal effects; additive sedative effects). Products include:
Haldol Decanoate 1587

Hydrocodone Bitartrate (Additive sedative effects). Products include:
Codiclear DH Syrup 808
Duratuss HD Elixir 2750
Histussin D Liquid 670
Hycodan Tablets and Syrup 946
Hycomine Compound Tablets ... 948
Hycomine 947
Hycotuss Expectorant Syrup 950
Hydrocet Capsules 787
Lorcet 10/650 Tablets 1016
Lortab 2751
Tussend 1830
Tussend Expectorant 1831
Vicodin Tablets 1404
Vicodin ES Tablets 1405
Vicodin HP Tablets 1403
Vicodin Tuss Expectorant 1406
Zydone Capsules 967

Hydrocodone Polistirex (Additive sedative effects). Products include:
Tussionex Pennkinetic Extended-Release Suspension 1624

Hydroxyzine Hydrochloride (Additive sedative effects). Products include:
Atarax Tablets & Syrup 1992
Marax Tablets & DF Syrup 2015
Vistaril Intramuscular Solution .. 2042

Isoflurane (Additive sedative effects).
No products indexed under this heading.

Ketamine Hydrochloride (Additive sedative effects).
No products indexed under this heading.

Levomethadyl Acetate Hydrochloride (Additive sedative effects). Products include:
Orlaam Oral Solution 2361

Levorphanol Tartrate (Additive sedative effects). Products include:
Levo-Dromoran 2297

Lorazepam (Additive sedative effects). Products include:
Ativan Injection 2805

Ativan Tablets 2807

Loxapine Hydrochloride (Additive sedative effects). Products include:
Loxitane 1426

Loxapine Succinate (Additive sedative effects). Products include:
Loxitane Capsules 1426

Meperidine Hydrochloride (Additive sedative effects). Products include:
Demerol 2438
Mepergan Injection 2859

Mephobarbital (Additive sedative effects). Products include:
Mebaral Tablets 2452

Meprobamate (Additive sedative effects). Products include:
Miltown Tablets 2780
PMB 200 and PMB 400 2890

Mesoridazine Besylate (Possible potentiation of extrapyramidal effects; additive sedative effects). Products include:
Serentil 689

Methadone Hydrochloride (Additive sedative effects). Products include:
Methadone Hydrochloride Oral Concentrate 2356
Methadone Hydrochloride Oral Solution & Tablets 2357

Methohexital Sodium (Additive sedative effects).
No products indexed under this heading.

Methotrimeprazine (Possible potentiation of extrapyramidal effects; additive sedative effects). Products include:
Levoprome 1321

Methoxyflurane (Additive sedative effects).
No products indexed under this heading.

Midazolam Hydrochloride (Additive sedative effects). Products include:
Versed Injection 2324

Molindone Hydrochloride (Additive sedative effects). Products include:
Moban Tablets and Concentrate ... 1036

Morphine Sulfate (Additive sedative effects). Products include:
Astramorph/PF Injection, USP (Preservative-Free) 526
Duramorph Injection 983
Infumorph 200 and Infumorph 500 Sterile Solutions 985
Kadian Capsules 2948
MS Contin Tablets 2149
MSIR 2152
Oramorph SR (Morphine Sulfate Sustained Release Tablets) 2359
RMS Suppositories CII 2766
Roxanol 2365

Opium Alkaloids (Additive sedative effects).
No products indexed under this heading.

Oxazepam (Additive sedative effects). Products include:
Serax Capsules 2916
Serax Tablets 2916

Oxycodone Hydrochloride (Additive sedative effects). Products include:
OxyContin Tablets 2163
OxyIR Capsules 2167
Percocet Tablets 955
Percodan Tablets 955
Percodan-Demi Tablets 956
Roxicodone Tablets, Oral Solution & Intensol (Oxycodone) 2366
Tylox Capsules 1593

Pentobarbital Sodium (Additive sedative effects). Products include:
Nembutal Sodium Capsules 440

Nembutal Sodium Solution 442
Nembutal Sodium Suppositories .. 444

Perphenazine (Possible potentiation of extrapyramidal effects; additive sedative effects). Products include:
Etrafon 2495
Triavil Tablets 1800
Trilafon 2532

Phenobarbital (Additive sedative effects). Products include:
Arco-Lase Plus Tablets 513
Bellergal-S Tablets 2375
Donnatal 2234
Donnatal Extentabs 2234
Donnatal Tablets 2234
Phenobarbital Elixir and Tablets ... 1523
Quadrinal Tablets 1398

Prazepam (Additive sedative effects).
No products indexed under this heading.

Prochlorperazine (Possible potentiation of extrapyramidal effects; additive sedative effects). Products include:
Compazine 2644

Promethazine Hydrochloride (Possible potentiation of extrapyramidal effects; additive sedative effects). Products include:
Mepergan Injection 2859
Phenergan with Codeine 2883
Phenergan with Dextromethorphan .. 2885
Phenergan Injection 2880
Phenergan Suppositories 2882
Phenergan Syrup 2881
Phenergan Tablets 2882
Phenergan VC 2886
Phenergan VC with Codeine 2888

Propofol (Additive sedative effects). Products include:
Diprivan Injectable Emulsion 2939

Propoxyphene Hydrochloride (Additive sedative effects). Products include:
Darvon 1475
Wygesic Tablets 2930

Propoxyphene Napsylate (Additive sedative effects). Products include:
Darvon-N/Darvocet-N 1473

Quazepam (Additive sedative effects). Products include:
Doral Tablets 2773

Risperidone (Additive sedative effects). Products include:
Risperdal Tablets 1348

Secobarbital Sodium (Additive sedative effects). Products include:
Seconal Sodium Pulvules 1529

Sevoflurane (Additive sedative effects).
No products indexed under this heading.

Sufentanil Citrate (Additive sedative effects). Products include:
Sufenta Injection 1355

Temazepam (Additive sedative effects). Products include:
Restoril Capsules 2413

Thiamylal Sodium (Additive sedative effects).
No products indexed under this heading.

Thioridazine Hydrochloride (Possible potentiation of extrapyramidal effects; additive sedative effects). Products include:
Mellaril 2398

Thiothixene (Additive sedative effects). Products include:
Navane Capsules and Concentrate .. 2018
Navane Intramuscular 2019

Triazolam (Additive sedative effects). Products include:
Halcion Tablets 2093

(☒ Described in PDR For Nonprescription Drugs)   (⊙ Described in PDR For Ophthalmology)

Trifluoperazine Hydrochloride (Possible potentiation of extrapyramidal effects; additive sedative effects). Products include:

- Stelazine 2692

Zolpidem Tartrate (Additive sedative effects). Products include:

- Ambien Tablets 2559

Food Interactions

Alcohol (Additive sedative effects).

DEMULEN 1/35-21

(Ethynodiol Diacetate, Ethinyl Estradiol) 2580

May interact with barbiturates, tetracyclines, and certain other agents. Compounds in these categories include:

Ampicillin Sodium (Reduces efficacy and increased incidence of breakthrough bleeding and menstrual irregularities). Products include:

- Unasyn 2035

Aprobarbital (Reduces efficacy and increased incidence of breakthrough bleeding and menstrual irregularities).

No products indexed under this heading.

Butabarbital (Reduces efficacy and increased incidence of breakthrough bleeding and menstrual irregularities).

No products indexed under this heading.

Butalbital (Reduces efficacy and increased incidence of breakthrough bleeding and menstrual irregularities). Products include:

- Axocet Capsules 2469
- Esgic-plus Capsules 1012
- Esgic-plus Tablets 1012
- Fioricet Tablets 2386
- Fioricet with Codeine Capsules 2387
- Fiorinal Capsules 2388
- Fiorinal with Codeine Capsules 2390
- Fiorinal Tablets 2388
- Phrenilin 790
- Sedapap Tablets 50 mg/650 mg 1826

Demeclocycline Hydrochloride (Reduces efficacy and increased incidence of breakthrough bleeding and menstrual irregularities). Products include:

- Declomycin Tablets 1421

Doxycycline Calcium (Reduces efficacy and increased incidence of breakthrough bleeding and menstrual irregularities). Products include:

- Vibramycin Calcium Oral Suspension Syrup 2038

Doxycycline Hyclate (Reduces efficacy and increased incidence of breakthrough bleeding and menstrual irregularities). Products include:

- Doryx Capsules 1970
- Vibramycin Hyclate Capsules 2038
- Vibramycin Hyclate Intravenous 2040
- Vibra-Tabs Film Coated Tablets 2038

Doxycycline Monohydrate (Reduces efficacy and increased incidence of breakthrough bleeding and menstrual irregularities). Products include:

- Monodox Capsules 1858
- Vibramycin Monohydrate for Oral Suspension 2038

Griseofulvin (Reduces efficacy and increased incidence of breakthrough bleeding and menstrual irregularities). Products include:

- Fulvicin P/G Tablets 2499
- Fulvicin P/G 165 & 330 Tablets 2500
- Grifulvin V (griseofulvin tablets) Microsize (griseofulvin oral suspension) Microsize 1944
- Gris-PEG Tablets, 125 mg & 250 mg 476

Mephobarbital (Reduces efficacy and increased incidence of breakthrough bleeding and menstrual irregularities). Products include:

- Mebaral Tablets 2452

Methacycline Hydrochloride (Reduces efficacy and increased incidence of breakthrough bleeding and menstrual irregularities).

No products indexed under this heading.

Minocycline Hydrochloride (Reduces efficacy and increased incidence of breakthrough bleeding and menstrual irregularities). Products include:

- DYNACIN Capsules 1627
- Minocin Intravenous 1428
- Minocin Oral Suspension 1431
- Minocin Pellet-Filled Capsules 1429

Oxytetracycline Hydrochloride (Reduces efficacy and increased incidence of breakthrough bleeding and menstrual irregularities). Products include:

- TERAK Ointment ◉ 210
- Terra-Cortril Ophthalmic Suspension 2033
- Terramycin with Polymyxin B Sulfate Ophthalmic Ointment 2035
- Urobiotic-250 Capsules 2038

Pentobarbital Sodium (Reduces efficacy and increased incidence of breakthrough bleeding and menstrual irregularities). Products include:

- Nembutal Sodium Capsules 440
- Nembutal Sodium Solution 442
- Nembutal Sodium Suppositories 444

Phenobarbital (Reduces efficacy and increased incidence of breakthrough bleeding and menstrual irregularities). Products include:

- Arco-Lase Plus Tablets 513
- Bellergal-S Tablets 2375
- Donnatal 2234
- Donnatal Extentabs 2234
- Donnatal Tablets 2234
- Phenobarbital Elixir and Tablets 1523
- Quadrinal Tablets 1398

Phenylbutazone (Reduces efficacy and increased incidence of breakthrough bleeding and menstrual irregularities).

No products indexed under this heading.

Phenytoin (Reduces efficacy and increased incidence of breakthrough bleeding and menstrual irregularities). Products include:

- Dilantin Infatabs 1967
- Dilantin-125 Suspension 1969

Phenytoin Sodium (Reduces efficacy and increased incidence of breakthrough bleeding and menstrual irregularities). Products include:

- Dilantin Kapseals 1965

Rifampin (Reduces efficacy and increased incidence of breakthrough bleeding and menstrual irregularities). Products include:

- Rifadin 1276
- Rifamate Capsules 1278
- Rifater 1280
- Rimactane Capsules 865

Secobarbital Sodium (Reduces efficacy and increased incidence of breakthrough bleeding and menstrual irregularities). Products include:

- Seconal Sodium Pulvules 1529

Tetracycline Hydrochloride (Reduces efficacy and increased incidence of breakthrough bleeding and menstrual irregularities). Products include:

- Achromycin V Capsules 1417
- Helidac Therapy 2135

Thiamylal Sodium (Reduces efficacy and increased incidence of breakthrough bleeding and menstrual irregularities).

No products indexed under this heading.

DEMULEN 1/35-28

(Ethynodiol Diacetate, Ethinyl Estradiol) 2580

See **Demulen 1/35-21**

DEMULEN 1/50-21

(Ethynodiol Diacetate, Ethinyl Estradiol) 2580

See **Demulen 1/35-21**

DEMULEN 1/50-28

(Ethynodiol Diacetate, Ethinyl Estradiol) 2580

See **Demulen 1/35-21**

DEPAKENE CAPSULES

(Valproic Acid) 416

May interact with central nervous system depressants, benzodiazepines, oral contraceptives, and certain other agents. Compounds in these categories include:

Alfentanil Hydrochloride (Valproate may potentiate the action of CNS depressants). Products include:

- Alfenta Injection 1334

Alprazolam (Valproate may potentiate the action of CNS depressants). Products include:

- Xanax Tablets 2115

Aprobarbital (Valproate may potentiate the action of CNS depressants).

No products indexed under this heading.

Aspirin (Co-administration of valproate with drugs that exhibit extensive protein binding e.g., aspirin, may result in alteration of serum drug concentration). Products include:

- Alka-Seltzer Cherry Effervescent Antacid and Pain Reliever ◘ 609
- Alka-Seltzer Extra Strength Effervescent Antacid and Pain Reliever ◘ 609
- Alka-Seltzer Lemon Lime Effervescent Antacid and Pain Reliever ◘ 609
- Alka-Seltzer Original Effervescent Antacid and Pain Reliever ◘ 609
- Alka-Seltzer Plus ◘ 611
- Alka-Seltzer Plus Sinus Medicine ◘ 611
- Ascriptin ◘ 650
- Arthritis Strength BC Powder ◘ 631
- BC Cold Powder Multi-Symptom Formula (Cold-Sinus-Allergy) ◘ 631
- BC Cold Powder Non-Drowsy Formula (Cold-Sinus) ◘ 631
- BC Powder ◘ 631
- Genuine Bayer Aspirin Tablets & Caplets ◘ 618
- Extra Strength Bayer Arthritis Pain Regimen Formula ◘ 615
- Extra Strength Bayer Aspirin Caplets & Tablets ◘ 617
- Extended-Release Bayer 8-Hour Aspirin ◘ 616
- Extra Strength Bayer Plus Aspirin Caplets ◘ 617
- Extra Strength Bayer PM Aspirin Plus Sleep Aid ◘ 617
- Aspirin Regimen Bayer 81 mg Tablets with Calcium ◘ 615
- Aspirin Regimen Bayer Adult Low Strength 81 mg Tablets ◘ 613
- Aspirin Regimen Bayer Children's Chewable Aspirin ◘ 616
- Aspirin Regimen Bayer Regular Strength 325 mg Caplets ◘ 613
- Bufferin Analgesic Tablets ◘ 636
- Arthritis Strength Bufferin Analgesic Caplets ◘ 637
- Extra Strength Bufferin Analgesic Tablets ◘ 637
- Cama Arthritis Pain Reliever ◘ 748
- Darvon Compound-65 Pulvules 1475
- Easprin 1971
- Ecotrin 2625
- Ecotrin Enteric Coated Aspirin Maximum Strength Tablets and Caplets ◘ 775
- Ecotrin Enteric Coated Aspirin Regular Strength Tablets 2625
- Empirin Aspirin Tablets ◘ 818
- Excedrin Extra-Strength Analgesic Tablets, Caplets, and Geltabs 734
- Fiorinal Capsules 2388
- Fiorinal with Codeine Capsules 2390
- Fiorinal Tablets 2388
- Goody's Extra Strength Headache Powders ◘ 632
- Goody's Extra Strength Pain Relief Tablets ◘ 632
- Halfprin Tablets 1413
- Norgesic 1554
- Percodan Tablets 955
- Percodan-Demi Tablets 956
- Robaxisal Tablets 2246
- Soma Compound w/Codeine Tablets 2784
- Soma Compound Tablets 2783
- St. Joseph Adult Chewable Aspirin (81 mg.) ◘ 768
- Talwin Compound 2466
- Vanquish Analgesic Caplets ◘ 627

Buprenorphine (Valproate may potentiate the action of CNS depressants). Products include:

- Buprenex Injectable 2170

Buspirone Hydrochloride (Valproate may potentiate the action of CNS depressants). Products include:

- BuSpar Tablets 738

Butabarbital (Valproate may potentiate the action of CNS depressants).

No products indexed under this heading.

Butalbital (Valproate may potentiate the action of CNS depressants). Products include:

- Axocet Capsules 2469
- Esgic-plus Capsules 1012
- Esgic-plus Tablets 1012
- Fioricet Tablets 2386
- Fioricet with Codeine Capsules 2387
- Fiorinal Capsules 2388
- Fiorinal with Codeine Capsules 2390
- Fiorinal Tablets 2388
- Phrenilin 790
- Sedapap Tablets 50 mg/650 mg 1826

Carbamazepine (Co-administration of valproate with drugs that exhibit extensive protein binding e.g., carbamazepine, may result in alteration of serum drug concentration). Products include:

- Atretol Tablets 569
- Tegretol/Tegretol-XR 870

Chlordiazepoxide (Valproate may potentiate the action of CNS depressants). Products include:

- Limbitrol 2333

Chlordiazepoxide Hydrochloride (Valproate may potentiate the action of CNS depressants). Products include:

- Librax Capsules 2330
- Librium Capsules 2331
- Librium Injectable 2332

Chlorpromazine (Valproate may potentiate the action of CNS depressants). Products include:

- Thorazine Suppositories 2701

Chlorprothixene (Valproate may potentiate the action of CNS depressants).

No products indexed under this heading.

Chlorprothixene Hydrochloride (Valproate may potentiate the action of CNS depressants).

No products indexed under this heading.

Chlorprothixene Lactate (Valproate may potentiate the action of CNS depressants).

No products indexed under this heading.

IMPORTANT NOTE: Always consult each drug listing in the patient's regimen for possible interactions.

Depakene — Interactions Index

Clonazepam (Concomitant use may produce absence status in patients with a history of absence type seizures). Products include:
- Klonopin Tablets 2294

Clorazepate Dipotassium (Valproate may potentiate the action of CNS depressants). Products include:
- Tranxene 459

Clozapine (Valproate may potentiate the action of CNS depressants). Products include:
- Clozaril Tablets 2377

Codeine Phosphate (Valproate may potentiate the action of CNS depressants). Products include:
- Brontex 2130
- Dimetane-DC Cough Syrup 2232
- Fioricet with Codeine Capsules 2387
- Fiorinal with Codeine Capsules 2390
- Nucofed 2225
- Phenergan with Codeine 2883
- Phenergan VC with Codeine 2888
- Robitussin A-C Syrup 2248
- Robitussin-DAC Syrup 2249
- Ryna ..... ⊞ 804
- Soma Compound w/Codeine Tablets 2784
- Tylenol with Codeine 1592

Desflurane (Valproate may potentiate the action of CNS depressants). Products include:
- Suprane (desflurane, USP) 1865

Desogestrel (Possible oral contraceptive failure). Products include:
- Desogen Tablets 1867
- Ortho-Cept 1907

Dezocine (Valproate may potentiate the action of CNS depressants). Products include:
- Dalgan Injection 529

Diazepam (Valproate may potentiate the action of CNS depressants). Products include:
- Dizac (diazepam injectable emulsion) CIV 1862
- Valium Injectable 2336
- Valium Tablets 2335

Dicumarol (Co-administration of valproate with drugs that exhibit extensive protein binding e.g., dicumarol, may result in alteration of serum drug concentration).
- No products indexed under this heading.

Droperidol (Valproate may potentiate the action of CNS depressants). Products include:
- Inapsine Injection 462

Enflurane (Valproate may potentiate the action of CNS depressants).
- No products indexed under this heading.

Estazolam (Valproate may potentiate the action of CNS depressants). Products include:
- ProSom Tablets 457

Ethchlorvynol (Valproate may potentiate the action of CNS depressants). Products include:
- Placidyl Capsules 456

Ethinamate (Valproate may potentiate the action of CNS depressants).
- No products indexed under this heading.

Ethinyl Estradiol (Possible oral contraceptive failure). Products include:
- Brevicon 2563
- Demulen 2580
- Desogen Tablets 1867
- Levlen/Tri-Levlen 646
- Lo/Ovral Tablets 2852
- Lo/Ovral-28 Tablets 2857
- Modicon 1928
- Nordette-21 Tablets 2863
- Nordette-28 Tablets 2866
- Norinyl 2563
- Ortho-Cept 1907
- Ortho-Cyclen/Ortho Tri-Cyclen 1914
- Ortho-Novum 1928

- Ortho-Cyclen/Ortho Tri-Cyclen 1914
- Ovcon 765
- Ovral Tablets 2877
- Ovral-28 Tablets 2878
- Levlen/Tri-Levlen 646
- Tri-Norinyl 2607
- Triphasil-21 Tablets 2919
- Triphasil-28 Tablets 2924

Ethosuximide (Altered serum concentrations of both drugs). Products include:
- Zarontin Capsules 1986
- Zarontin Syrup 1986

Ethynodiol Diacetate (Possible oral contraceptive failure). Products include:
- Demulen 2580

Fentanyl (Valproate may potentiate the action of CNS depressants). Products include:
- Duragesic Transdermal System 1336

Fentanyl Citrate (Valproate may potentiate the action of CNS depressants). Products include:
- Sublimaze Injection 463

Fluphenazine Decanoate (Valproate may potentiate the action of CNS depressants). Products include:
- Prolixin Decanoate 510

Fluphenazine Enanthate (Valproate may potentiate the action of CNS depressants). Products include:
- Prolixin Enanthate 510

Fluphenazine Hydrochloride (Valproate may potentiate the action of CNS depressants). Products include:
- Prolixin 510

Flurazepam Hydrochloride (Valproate may potentiate the action of CNS depressants). Products include:
- Dalmane Capsules 2329

Glutethimide (Valproate may potentiate the action of CNS depressants).
- No products indexed under this heading.

Halazepam (Valproate may potentiate the action of CNS depressants).
- No products indexed under this heading.

Haloperidol (Valproate may potentiate the action of CNS depressants). Products include:
- Haldol Injection, Tablets and Concentrate 1585

Haloperidol Decanoate (Valproate may potentiate the action of CNS depressants). Products include:
- Haldol Decanoate 1587

Hydrocodone Bitartrate (Valproate may potentiate the action of CNS depressants). Products include:
- Codiclear DH Syrup 808
- Duratuss HD Elixir 2750
- Histussin D Liquid 670
- Hycodan Tablets and Syrup 946
- Hycomine Compound Tablets 948
- Hycomine 947
- Hycotuss Expectorant Syrup 950
- Hydrocet Capsules 787
- Lorcet 10/650 Tablets 1016
- Lortab 2751
- Tussend 1830
- Tussend Expectorant 1831
- Vicodin Tablets 1404
- Vicodin ES Tablets 1405
- Vicodin HP Tablets 1403
- Vicodin Tuss Expectorant 1406
- Zydone Capsules 967

Hydrocodone Polistirex (Valproate may potentiate the action of CNS depressants). Products include:
- Tussionex Pennkinetic Extended-Release Suspension 1624

Hydroxyzine Hydrochloride (Valproate may potentiate the action of CNS depressants). Products include:
- Atarax Tablets & Syrup 1992
- Marax Tablets & DF Syrup 2015

- Vistaril Intramuscular Solution 2042

Isoflurane (Valproate may potentiate the action of CNS depressants).
- No products indexed under this heading.

Ketamine Hydrochloride (Valproate may potentiate the action of CNS depressants).
- No products indexed under this heading.

Levomethadyl Acetate Hydrochloride (Valproate may potentiate the action of CNS depressants). Products include:
- Orlaam Oral Solution 2361

Levonorgestrel (Possible oral contraceptive failure). Products include:
- Levlen/Tri-Levlen 646
- Nordette-21 Tablets 2863
- Nordette-28 Tablets 2866
- Norplant System 2868
- Levlen/Tri-Levlen 646
- Triphasil-21 Tablets 2919
- Triphasil-28 Tablets 2924

Levorphanol Tartrate (Valproate may potentiate the action of CNS depressants). Products include:
- Levo-Dromoran 2297

Lorazepam (Valproate may potentiate the action of CNS depressants). Products include:
- Ativan Injection 2805
- Ativan Tablets 2807

Loxapine Hydrochloride (Valproate may potentiate the action of CNS depressants). Products include:
- Loxitane 1426

Loxapine Succinate (Valproate may potentiate the action of CNS depressants). Products include:
- Loxitane Capsules 1426

Meperidine Hydrochloride (Valproate may potentiate the action of CNS depressants). Products include:
- Demerol 2438
- Mepergan Injection 2859

Mephobarbital (Valproate may potentiate the action of CNS depressants). Products include:
- Mebaral Tablets 2452

Meprobamate (Valproate may potentiate the action of CNS depressants). Products include:
- Miltown Tablets 2780
- PMB 200 and PMB 400 2890

Mesoridazine Besylate (Valproate may potentiate the action of CNS depressants). Products include:
- Serentil 689

Mestranol (Possible oral contraceptive failure). Products include:
- Norinyl 2563
- Ortho-Novum 1928

Methadone Hydrochloride (Valproate may potentiate the action of CNS depressants). Products include:
- Methadone Hydrochloride Oral Concentrate 2356
- Methadone Hydrochloride Oral Solution & Tablets 2357

Methohexital Sodium (Valproate may potentiate the action of CNS depressants).
- No products indexed under this heading.

Methotrimeprazine (Valproate may potentiate the action of CNS depressants). Products include:
- Levoprome 1321

Methoxyflurane (Valproate may potentiate the action of CNS depressants).
- No products indexed under this heading.

Midazolam Hydrochloride (Valproate may potentiate the action of CNS depressants). Products include:
- Versed Injection 2324

Molindone Hydrochloride (Valproate may potentiate the action of CNS depressants). Products include:
- Moban Tablets and Concentrate 1036

Morphine Sulfate (Valproate may potentiate the action of CNS depressants). Products include:
- Astramorph/PF Injection, USP (Preservative-Free) 526
- Duramorph Injection 983
- Infumorph 200 and Infumorph 500 Sterile Solutions 985
- Kadian Capsules 2948
- MS Contin Tablets 2149
- MSIR 2152
- Oramorph SR (Morphine Sulfate Sustained Release Tablets) 2359
- RMS Suppositories CII 2766
- Roxanol 2365

Norethindrone (Possible oral contraceptive failure). Products include:
- Brevicon 2563
- Micronor Tablets 1903
- Modicon 1928
- Norinyl 2563
- Nor-Q D Tablets 2598
- Ortho-Novum 1928
- Ovcon 765
- Tri-Norinyl 2607

Norethynodrel (Possible oral contraceptive failure).
- No products indexed under this heading.

Norgestimate (Possible oral contraceptive failure). Products include:
- Ortho-Cyclen/Ortho Tri-Cyclen 1914
- Ortho-Cyclen/Ortho Tri-Cyclen 1914

Norgestrel (Possible oral contraceptive failure). Products include:
- Lo/Ovral Tablets 2852
- Lo/Ovral-28 Tablets 2857
- Ovral Tablets 2877
- Ovral-28 Tablets 2878
- Ovrette Tablets 2878

Opium Alkaloids (Valproate may potentiate the action of CNS depressants).
- No products indexed under this heading.

Oxazepam (Valproate may potentiate the action of CNS depressants). Products include:
- Serax Capsules 2916
- Serax Tablets 2916

Oxycodone Hydrochloride (Valproate may potentiate the action of CNS depressants). Products include:
- OxyContin Tablets 2163
- OxyIR Capsules 2167
- Percocet Tablets 955
- Percodan Tablets 955
- Percodan-Demi Tablets 956
- Roxicodone Tablets, Oral Solution & Intensol (Oxycodone) 2366
- Tylox Capsules 1593

Pentobarbital Sodium (Valproate may potentiate the action of CNS depressants). Products include:
- Nembutal Sodium Capsules 440
- Nembutal Sodium Solution 442
- Nembutal Sodium Suppositories 444

Perphenazine (Valproate may potentiate the action of CNS depressants). Products include:
- Etrafon 2495
- Triavil Tablets 1800
- Trilafon 2532

Phenobarbital (Increased serum phenobarbital levels; potential for increased CNS depression; monitor for neurological toxicity). Products include:
- Arco-Lase Plus Tablets 513
- Bellergal-S Tablets 2375
- Donnatal 2234
- Donnatal Extentabs 2234
- Donnatal Tablets 2234
- Phenobarbital Elixir and Tablets 1523
- Quadrinal Tablets 1398

(⊞ Described in PDR For Nonprescription Drugs)   (⊙ Described in PDR For Ophthalmology)

Phenytoin (Co-administration of valproate with drugs that exhibit extensive protein binding e.g., phenytoin, may result in alteration of serum drug concentration; potential for breakthrough seizures). Products include:
- Dilantin Infatabs 1967
- Dilantin-125 Suspension 1969

Phenytoin Sodium (Co-administration of valproate with drugs that exhibit extensive protein binding e.g., phenytoin, may result in alteration of serum drug concentration; potential for breakthrough seizures). Products include:
- Dilantin Kapseals 1965

Prazepam (Valproate may potentiate the action of CNS depressants).
No products indexed under this heading.

Primidone (Potential for neurological toxicity). Products include:
- Mysoline 2860

Prochlorperazine (Valproate may potentiate the action of CNS depressants). Products include:
- Compazine 2644

Promethazine Hydrochloride (Valproate may potentiate the action of CNS depressants). Products include:
- Mepergan Injection 2859
- Phenergan with Codeine 2883
- Phenergan with Dextromethorphan .. 2885
- Phenergan Injection 2880
- Phenergan Suppositories 2882
- Phenergan Syrup 2881
- Phenergan Tablets 2882
- Phenergan VC 2886
- Phenergan VC with Codeine 2888

Propofol (Valproate may potentiate the action of CNS depressants). Products include:
- Diprivan Injectable Emulsion 2939

Propoxyphene Hydrochloride (Valproate may potentiate the action of CNS depressants). Products include:
- Darvon 1475
- Wygesic Tablets 2930

Propoxyphene Napsylate (Valproate may potentiate the action of CNS depressants). Products include:
- Darvon-N/Darvocet-N 1473

Quazepam (Valproate may potentiate the action of CNS depressants). Products include:
- Doral Tablets 2773

Risperidone (Valproate may potentiate the action of CNS depressants). Products include:
- Risperdal Tablets 1348

Secobarbital Sodium (Valproate may potentiate the action of CNS depressants). Products include:
- Seconal Sodium Pulvules 1529

Sevoflurane (Valproate may potentiate the action of CNS depressants).
No products indexed under this heading.

Sufentanil Citrate (Valproate may potentiate the action of CNS depressants). Products include:
- Sufenta Injection 1355

Temazepam (Valproate may potentiate the action of CNS depressants). Products include:
- Restoril Capsules 2413

Thiamylal Sodium (Valproate may potentiate the action of CNS depressants).
No products indexed under this heading.

Thioridazine Hydrochloride (Valproate may potentiate the action of CNS depressants). Products include:
- Mellaril 2398

Thiothixene (Valproate may potentiate the action of CNS depressants). Products include:
- Navane Capsules and Concentrate ... 2018
- Navane Intramuscular 2019

Triazolam (Valproate may potentiate the action of CNS depressants). Products include:
- Halcion Tablets 2093

Trifluoperazine Hydrochloride (Valproate may potentiate the action of CNS depressants). Products include:
- Stelazine 2692

Warfarin Sodium (Valproate affects the secondary phase of platelet aggregation which may be reflected in altered bleeding time; co-administration requires caution). Products include:
- Coumadin 941

Zolpidem Tartrate (Valproate may potentiate the action of CNS depressants). Products include:
- Ambien Tablets 2559

Food Interactions

Alcohol (Depakene may potentiate CNS depressant activity).

DEPAKENE SYRUP
(Valproic Acid) 416
See **Depakene Capsules**

DEPAKOTE TABLETS
(Divalproex Sodium) 418
May interact with central nervous system depressants and certain other agents. Compounds in these categories include:

Alfentanil Hydrochloride (Co-administration may result in additive CNS depression). Products include:
- Alfenta Injection 1334

Alprazolam (Co-administration may result in additive CNS depression). Products include:
- Xanax Tablets 2115

Amitriptyline Hydrochloride (Decreased plasma clearance of amitriptyline). Products include:
- Elavil 2945
- Etrafon 2495
- Limbitrol 2333
- Triavil Tablets 1800

Aprobarbital (Co-administration may result in additive CNS depression).
No products indexed under this heading.

Aspirin (Co-administration with aspirin at antipyretic doses has resulted in a decrease in protein binding and inhibition of metabolism of valproate). Products include:
- Alka-Seltzer Cherry Effervescent Antacid and Pain Reliever 609
- Alka-Seltzer Extra Strength Effervescent Antacid and Pain Reliever 609
- Alka-Seltzer Lemon Lime Effervescent Antacid and Pain Reliever 609
- Alka-Seltzer Original Effervescent Antacid and Pain Reliever 609
- Alka-Seltzer Plus 611
- Alka-Seltzer Plus Sinus Medicine 611
- Ascriptin 650
- Arthritis Strength BC Powder 631
- BC Cold Powder Multi-Symptom Formula (Cold-Sinus-Allergy) 631
- BC Cold Powder Non-Drowsy Formula (Cold-Sinus) 631
- BC Powder 631
- Genuine Bayer Aspirin Tablets & Caplets 618
- Extra Strength Bayer Arthritis Pain Regimen Formula 615
- Extra Strength Bayer Aspirin Caplets & Tablets 617
- Extended-Release Bayer 8-Hour Aspirin 616
- Extra Strength Bayer Plus Aspirin Caplets 617
- Extra Strength Bayer PM Aspirin Plus Sleep Aid 617
- Aspirin Regimen Bayer 81 mg Tablets with Calcium 615
- Aspirin Regimen Bayer Adult Low Strength 81 mg Tablets 613
- Aspirin Regimen Bayer Children's Chewable Aspirin 616
- Aspirin Regimen Bayer Regular Strength 325 mg Caplets 613
- Bufferin Analgesic Tablets 636
- Arthritis Strength Bufferin Analgesic Caplets 637
- Extra Strength Bufferin Analgesic Tablets 637
- Cama Arthritis Pain Reliever 748
- Darvon Compound-65 Pulvules 1475
- Easprin 1971
- Ecotrin 2625
- Ecotrin Enteric Coated Aspirin Maximum Strength Tablets and Caplets 775
- Ecotrin Enteric Coated Aspirin Regular Strength Tablets 2625
- Empirin Aspirin Tablets 818
- Excedrin Extra-Strength Analgesic Tablets, Caplets, and Geltabs 734
- Fiorinal Capsules 2388
- Fiorinal with Codeine Capsules 2390
- Fiorinal Tablets 2388
- Goody's Extra Strength Headache Powders 632
- Goody's Extra Strength Pain Relief Tablets 632
- Halfprin Tablets 1413
- Norgesic 1554
- Percodan Tablets 955
- Percodan-Demi Tablets 956
- Robaxisal Tablets 2246
- Soma Compound w/Codeine Tablets 2784
- Soma Compound Tablets 2783
- St. Joseph Adult Chewable Aspirin (81 mg.) 768
- Talwin Compound 2466
- Vanquish Analgesic Caplets 627

Buprenorphine (Co-administration may result in additive CNS depression). Products include:
- Buprenex Injectable 2170

Buspirone Hydrochloride (Co-administration may result in additive CNS depression). Products include:
- BuSpar Tablets 738

Butabarbital (Co-administration may result in additive CNS depression).
No products indexed under this heading.

Butalbital (Co-administration may result in additive CNS depression). Products include:
- Axocet Capsules 2469
- Esgic-plus Capsules 1012
- Esgic-plus Tablets 1012
- Fioricet Tablets 2386
- Fioricet with Codeine Capsules 2387
- Fiorinal Capsules 2388
- Fiorinal with Codeine Capsules 2390
- Fiorinal Tablets 2388
- Phrenilin 790
- Sedapap Tablets 50 mg/650 mg 1826

Carbamazepine (Co-administration results in decrease in serum carbamazepine levels and increase in carbamazepine epoxide levels; carbamazepine may increase the clearance of valproate through elevation of glucuronosyl transferases). Products include:
- Atretol Tablets 569
- Tegretol/Tegretol-XR 870

Chlordiazepoxide (Co-administration may result in additive CNS depression). Products include:
- Limbitrol 2333

Chlordiazepoxide Hydrochloride (Co-administration may result in additive CNS depression). Products include:
- Librax Capsules 2330
- Librium Capsules 2331
- Librium Injectable 2332

Chlorpromazine (Co-administration in schizophrenic patients has resulted in 15%, clinically insignificant, increase in trough plasma levels of valproate; concurrent use may result in additive CNS depression). Products include:
- Thorazine Suppositories 2701

Chlorpromazine Hydrochloride (Co-administration in schizophrenic patients has resulted in 15%, clinically insignificant, increase in trough plasma levels of valproate; concurrent use may result in additive CNS depression). Products include:
- Thorazine 2701

Chlorprothixene (Co-administration may result in additive CNS depression).
No products indexed under this heading.

Chlorprothixene Hydrochloride (Co-administration may result in additive CNS depression).
No products indexed under this heading.

Chlorprothixene Lactate (Co-administration may result in additive CNS depression).
No products indexed under this heading.

Clonazepam (Co-administration may induce absence of status in patients with a history of absence type seizures). Products include:
- Klonopin Tablets 2294

Clorazepate Dipotassium (Co-administration may result in additive CNS depression). Products include:
- Tranxene 459

Clozapine (Co-administration may result in additive CNS depression). Products include:
- Clozaril Tablets 2377

Codeine Phosphate (Co-administration may result in additive CNS depression). Products include:
- Brontex 2130
- Dimetane-DC Cough Syrup 2232
- Fioricet with Codeine Capsules 2387
- Fiorinal with Codeine Capsules 2390
- Nucofed 2225
- Phenergan with Codeine 2883
- Phenergan VC with Codeine 2888
- Robitussin A-C Syrup 2248
- Robitussin-DAC Syrup 2249
- Ryna 804
- Soma Compound w/Codeine Tablets 2784
- Tylenol with Codeine 1592

Desflurane (Co-administration may result in additive CNS depression). Products include:
- Suprane (desflurane, USP) 1865

Dezocine (Co-administration may result in additive CNS depression). Products include:
- Dalgan Injection 529

Diazepam (Valproate displaces diazepam from its plasma binding sites and inhibits its metabolism; plasma clearance and volume of distribution for free diazepam is reduced). Products include:
- Dizac (diazepam injectable emulsion) CIV 1862
- Valium Injectable 2336
- Valium Tablets 2335

Droperidol (Co-administration may result in additive CNS depression). Products include:
- Inapsine Injection 462

Enflurane (Co-administration may result in additive CNS depression).
No products indexed under this heading.

IMPORTANT NOTE: Always consult each drug listing in the patient's regimen for possible interactions.

Depakote | Interactions Index | 256

Estazolam (Co-administration may result in additive CNS depression). Products include:
- ProSom Tablets ... 457

Ethchlorvynol (Co-administration may result in additive CNS depression). Products include:
- Placidyl Capsules ... 456

Ethinamate (Co-administration may result in additive CNS depression).
- No products indexed under this heading.

Ethosuximide (Co-administration results in the inhibition of ethosuximide metabolism, increase in elimination half-life of ethosuximide and decrease in its total clearance). Products include:
- Zarontin Capsules ... 1986
- Zarontin Syrup ... 1986

Felbamate (Co-administration in epileptic patients has resulted in an increase in mean valproate peak concentration; a reduction in valproate dosage may be necessary). Products include:
- Felbatol ... 2774

Fentanyl (Co-administration may result in additive CNS depression). Products include:
- Duragesic Transdermal System ... 1336

Fentanyl Citrate (Co-administration may result in additive CNS depression). Products include:
- Sublimaze Injection ... 463

Fluphenazine Decanoate (Co-administration may result in additive CNS depression). Products include:
- Prolixin Decanoate ... 510

Fluphenazine Enanthate (Co-administration may result in additive CNS depression). Products include:
- Prolixin Enanthate ... 510

Fluphenazine Hydrochloride (Co-administration may result in additive CNS depression). Products include:
- Prolixin ... 510

Flurazepam Hydrochloride (Co-administration may result in additive CNS depression). Products include:
- Dalmane Capsules ... 2329

Fosphenytoin Sodium (Valproate displaces phenytoin from its plasma albumin binding sites and inhibits its hepatic metabolism; phenytoin may increase the clearance of valproate through elevation of glucuronosyl transferases; co-administration has resulted in breakthrough seizures in epileptic patients). Products include:
- Cerebyx Injection ... 1956

Glutethimide (Co-administration may result in additive CNS depression).
- No products indexed under this heading.

Haloperidol (Co-administration may result in additive CNS depression). Products include:
- Haldol Injection, Tablets and Concentrate ... 1585

Haloperidol Decanoate (Co-administration may result in additive CNS depression). Products include:
- Haldol Decanoate ... 1587

Hydrocodone Bitartrate (Co-administration may result in additive CNS depression). Products include:
- Codiclear DH Syrup ... 808
- Duratuss HD Elixir ... 2750
- Histussin D Liquid ... 670
- Hycodan Tablets and Syrup ... 946
- Hycomine Compound Tablets ... 948
- Hycomine ... 947
- Hycotuss Expectorant Syrup ... 950
- Hydrocet Capsules ... 787
- Lorcet 10/650 Tablets ... 1016
- Lortab ... 2751
- Tussend ... 1830
- Tussend Expectorant ... 1831
- Vicodin Tablets ... 1404
- Vicodin ES Tablets ... 1405
- Vicodin HP Tablets ... 1403
- Vicodin Tuss Expectorant ... 1406
- Zydone Capsules ... 967

Hydrocodone Polistirex (Co-administration may result in additive CNS depression). Products include:
- Tussionex Pennkinetic Extended-Release Suspension ... 1624

Hydromorphone Hydrochloride (Co-administration may result in additive CNS depression). Products include:
- Dilaudid Ampules ... 1382
- Dilaudid Cough Syrup ... 1383
- Dilaudid-HP Injection ... 1384
- Dilaudid-HP Lyophilized Powder 250 mg ... 1384
- Dilaudid ... 1382
- Dilaudid Oral Liquid ... 1386
- Dilaudid ... 1382
- Dilaudid Tablets - 8 mg ... 1386

Hydroxyzine Hydrochloride (Co-administration may result in additive CNS depression). Products include:
- Atarax Tablets & Syrup ... 1992
- Marax Tablets & DF Syrup ... 2015
- Vistaril Intramuscular Solution ... 2042

Isoflurane (Co-administration may result in additive CNS depression).
- No products indexed under this heading.

Ketamine Hydrochloride (Co-administration may result in additive CNS depression).
- No products indexed under this heading.

Lamotrigine (Co-administration has resulted in an increase in elimination half-life of lamotrigine; a reduction in lamotrigine dosage should be considered). Products include:
- Lamictal Tablets ... 1105

Levomethadyl Acetate Hydrochloride (Co-administration may result in additive CNS depression). Products include:
- Orlaam Oral Solution ... 2361

Levorphanol Tartrate (Co-administration may result in additive CNS depression). Products include:
- Levo-Dromoran ... 2297

Lorazepam (Co-administration has resulted in decreased plasma clearance of lorazepam; concurrent use may result in additive CNS depression). Products include:
- Ativan Injection ... 2805
- Ativan Tablets ... 2807

Loxapine Hydrochloride (Co-administration may result in additive CNS depression). Products include:
- Loxitane ... 1426

Loxapine Succinate (Co-administration may result in additive CNS depression). Products include:
- Loxitane Capsules ... 1426

Meperidine Hydrochloride (Co-administration may result in additive CNS depression). Products include:
- Demerol ... 2438
- Mepergan Injection ... 2859

Mephobarbital (Co-administration may result in additive CNS depression). Products include:
- Mebaral Tablets ... 2452

Meprobamate (Co-administration may result in additive CNS depression). Products include:
- Miltown Tablets ... 2780
- PMB 200 and PMB 400 ... 2890

Mesoridazine Besylate (Co-administration may result in additive CNS depression). Products include:
- Serentil ... 689

Methadone Hydrochloride (Co-administration may result in additive CNS depression). Products include:
- Methadone Hydrochloride Oral Concentrate ... 2356
- Methadone Hydrochloride Oral Solution & Tablets ... 2357

Methohexital Sodium (Co-administration may result in additive CNS depression).
- No products indexed under this heading.

Methotrimeprazine (Co-administration may result in additive CNS depression). Products include:
- Levoprome ... 1321

Methoxyflurane (Co-administration may result in additive CNS depression).
- No products indexed under this heading.

Midazolam Hydrochloride (Co-administration may result in additive CNS depression). Products include:
- Versed Injection ... 2324

Molindone Hydrochloride (Co-administration may result in additive CNS depression). Products include:
- Moban Tablets and Concentrate ... 1036

Morphine Sulfate (Co-administration may result in additive CNS depression). Products include:
- Astramorph/PF Injection, USP (Preservative-Free) ... 526
- Duramorph Injection ... 983
- Infumorph 200 and Infumorph 500 Sterile Solutions ... 985
- Kadian Capsules ... 2948
- MS Contin Tablets ... 2149
- MSIR ... 2152
- Oramorph SR (Morphine Sulfate Sustained Release Tablets) ... 2359
- RMS Suppositories CII ... 2766
- Roxanol ... 2365

Nortriptyline Hydrochloride (Decrease in net clearance of nortriptyline). Products include:
- Pamelor ... 2409

Opium Alkaloids (Co-administration may result in additive CNS depression).
- No products indexed under this heading.

Oxazepam (Co-administration may result in additive CNS depression). Products include:
- Serax Capsules ... 2916
- Serax Tablets ... 2916

Oxycodone Hydrochloride (Co-administration may result in additive CNS depression). Products include:
- OxyContin Tablets ... 2163
- OxyIR Capsules ... 2167
- Percocet Tablets ... 955
- Percodan Tablets ... 955
- Percodan-Demi Tablets ... 956
- Roxicodone Tablets, Oral Solution & Intensol (Oxycodone) ... 2366
- Tylox Capsules ... 1593

Pentobarbital Sodium (Co-administration may result in additive CNS depression). Products include:
- Nembutal Sodium Capsules ... 440
- Nembutal Sodium Solution ... 442
- Nembutal Sodium Suppositories ... 444

Perphenazine (Co-administration may result in additive CNS depression). Products include:
- Etrafon ... 2495
- Triavil Tablets ... 1800
- Trilafon ... 2532

Phenobarbital (Valproate inhibits phenobarbital metabolism; phenobarbital may increase the clearance of valproate through elevation of glucuronosyl transferases; co-administration may result in severe CNS depression). Products include:
- Arco-Lase Plus Tablets ... 513
- Bellergal-S Tablets ... 2375
- Donnatal ... 2234
- Donnatal Extentabs ... 2234
- Donnatal Tablets ... 2234
- Phenobarbital Elixir and Tablets ... 1523
- Quadrinal Tablets ... 1398

Phenytoin (Valproate displaces phenytoin from its plasma albumin binding sites and inhibits its hepatic metabolism; phenytoin may increase the clearance of valproate through elevation of glucuronosyl transferases; co-administration has resulted in breakthrough seizures in epileptic patients). Products include:
- Dilantin Infatabs ... 1967
- Dilantin-125 Suspension ... 1969

Phenytoin Sodium (Valproate displaces phenytoin from its plasma albumin binding sites and inhibits its hepatic metabolism; phenytoin may increase the clearance of valproate through elevation of glucuronosyl transferases; co-administration has resulted in breakthrough seizures in epileptic patients). Products include:
- Dilantin Kapseals ... 1965

Prazepam (Co-administration may result in additive CNS depression).
- No products indexed under this heading.

Primidone (Primidone is metabolized to barbiturate and valproate inhibits barbiturate metabolism; primidone may increase the clearance of valproate through elevation of glucuronosyl transferases). Products include:
- Mysoline ... 2860

Prochlorperazine (Co-administration may result in additive CNS depression). Products include:
- Compazine ... 2644

Promethazine Hydrochloride (Co-administration may result in additive CNS depression). Products include:
- Mepergan Injection ... 2859
- Phenergan with Codeine ... 2883
- Phenergan with Dextromethorphan ... 2885
- Phenergan Injection ... 2880
- Phenergan Suppositories ... 2882
- Phenergan Syrup ... 2881
- Phenergan Tablets ... 2882
- Phenergan VC ... 2886
- Phenergan VC with Codeine ... 2888

Propofol (Co-administration may result in additive CNS depression). Products include:
- Diprivan Injectable Emulsion ... 2939

Propoxyphene Hydrochloride (Co-administration may result in additive CNS depression). Products include:
- Darvon ... 1475
- Wygesic Tablets ... 2930

Propoxyphene Napsylate (Co-administration may result in additive CNS depression). Products include:
- Darvon-N/Darvocet-N ... 1473

Quazepam (Co-administration may result in additive CNS depression). Products include:
- Doral Tablets ... 2773

Rifampin (Co-administration has resulted in a 40% increase in oral clearance of valproate; valproate dosage adjustment may be necessary). Products include:
- Rifadin ... 1276
- Rifamate Capsules ... 1278
- Rifater ... 1280

(Described in PDR For Nonprescription Drugs) (◉ Described in PDR For Ophthalmology)

Rimactane Capsules 865
Risperidone (Co-administration may result in additive CNS depression). Products include:
  Risperdal Tablets 1348
Secobarbital Sodium (Co-administration may result in additive CNS depression). Products include:
  Seconal Sodium Pulvules 1529
Sevoflurane (Co-administration may result in additive CNS depression).
  No products indexed under this heading.
Sufentanil Citrate (Co-administration may result in additive CNS depression). Products include:
  Sufenta Injection 1355
Temazepam (Co-administration may result in additive CNS depression). Products include:
  Restoril Capsules 2413
Thiamylal Sodium (Co-administration may result in additive CNS depression).
  No products indexed under this heading.
Thioridazine Hydrochloride (Co-administration may result in additive CNS depression). Products include:
  Mellaril 2398
Thiothixene (Co-administration may result in additive CNS depression). Products include:
  Navane Capsules and Concentrate 2018
  Navane Intramuscular 2019
Tolbutamide (Potential for increased unbound fraction of tolbutamide based on *in vitro* studies; clinical relevance is unknown).
  No products indexed under this heading.
Triazolam (Co-administration may result in additive CNS depression). Products include:
  Halcion Tablets 2093
Trifluoperazine Hydrochloride (Co-administration may result in additive CNS depression). Products include:
  Stelazine 2692
Warfarin Sodium (Potential for increased unbound fraction of warfarin based on *in vitro* studies; clinical relevance is unknown). Products include:
  Coumadin 941
Zidovudine (Co-administration has resulted in decreased zidovudine clearance, however, the half-life of zidovudine was unaffected). Products include:
  Retrovir Capsules 1216
  Retrovir I.V. Infusion 1221
  Retrovir Syrup 1216
Zolpidem Tartrate (Co-administration may result in additive CNS depression). Products include:
  Ambien Tablets 2559

Food Interactions
Alcohol (Co-administration may result in additive CNS depression).

DEPEN TITRATABLE TABLETS
(Penicillamine) 2770
May interact with cytotoxic drugs, antimalarials, and certain other agents. Compounds in these categories include:

Auranofin (Serious hematologic and/or renal adverse reactions). Products include:
  Ridaura Capsules 2691
Aurothioglucose (Serious hematologic and/or renal adverse reactions). Products include:
  Solganal Suspension 2530
Bleomycin Sulfate (Hematologic and renal reactions). Products include:
  Blenoxane 697
Chloroquine Hydrochloride (Serious hematologic and/or renal adverse reactions). Products include:
  Aralen Hydrochloride Injection 2430
Chloroquine Phosphate (Serious hematologic and/or renal adverse reactions). Products include:
  Aralen Phosphate Tablets 2431
Daunorubicin Hydrochloride (Hematologic and renal reactions). Products include:
  Cerubidine for Injection 634
Doxorubicin Hydrochloride (Hematologic and renal reactions). Products include:
  Adriamycin PFS 2056
  Adriamycin RDF 2056
  Doxil 2613
  Doxorubicin Astra 531
  Rubex for Injection 721
Fluorouracil (Hematologic and renal reactions). Products include:
  Efudex 2280
  Fluoroplex Topical Solution & Cream 1% 475
  Fluorouracil Injection 2282
Gold Sodium Thiomalate (Serious hematologic and/or renal adverse reactions). Products include:
  Myochrysine Injection 1754
Hydroxyurea (Hematologic and renal reactions). Products include:
  Hydrea Capsules 705
Iron Supplements (Reduced effects of penicillamine with orally administered iron).
Mefloquine Hydrochloride (Serious hematologic and/or renal adverse reactions). Products include:
  Lariam Tablets 2295
Methotrexate Sodium (Hematologic and renal reactions). Products include:
  Methotrexate Sodium Tablets, Injection, for Injection and LPF Injection 1322
Mineral Supplements (Blocked response to penicillamine).
Mitotane (Hematologic and renal reactions). Products include:
  Lysodren Tablets 707
Mitoxantrone Hydrochloride (Hematologic and renal reactions). Products include:
  Novantrone for Injection 1327
Oxyphenbutazone (Hematologic and renal reactions).
Phenylbutazone (Hematologic and renal reactions).
  No products indexed under this heading.
Primaquine Phosphate (Serious hematologic and/or renal adverse reactions).
  No products indexed under this heading.
Procarbazine Hydrochloride (Hematologic and renal reactions). Products include:
  Matulane Capsules 2300
Pyrimethamine (Serious hematologic and/or renal adverse reactions). Products include:
  Daraprim Tablets 1199
  Fansidar Tablets 2281
Tamoxifen Citrate (Hematologic and renal reactions). Products include:
  Nolvadex Tablets 2957

Vincristine Sulfate (Hematologic and renal reactions). Products include:
  Oncovin Solution Vials & Hyporets 1521

Food Interactions
Meal, unspecified (Potential for reduced absorption and the likelihood of inactivation by metal binding in the GI tract; Depen should be given on an empty stomach).

DEPO-PROVERA CONTRACEPTIVE INJECTION
(Medroxyprogesterone Acetate) 2079
May interact with:

Aminoglutethimide (Significantly depresses the serum concentrations of medroxyprogesterone acetate). Products include:
  Cytadren Tablets 837

DEPO-PROVERA STERILE AQUEOUS SUSPENSION
(Medroxyprogesterone Acetate) 2083
May interact with:

Aminoglutethimide (Significantly depresses the bioavailability of Depo-Provera). Products include:
  Cytadren Tablets 837

DEPONIT NTG TRANSDERMAL DELIVERY SYSTEM
(Nitroglycerin) 2541
May interact with vasodilators and certain other agents. Compounds in these categories include:

Diazoxide (Additive vasodilating effects). Products include:
  Hyperstat I.V. Injection 2504
  Proglycem 575
Epoprostenol Sodium (Additive vasodilating effects). Products include:
  Flolan for Injection 1085
Hydralazine Hydrochloride (Additive vasodilating effects). Products include:
  Apresazide Capsules 824
  Apresoline Hydrochloride Tablets .. 826
  Hydralazine Hydrochloride Injection USP 2712
  Ser-Ap-Es Tablets 867
Minoxidil (Additive vasodilating effects).
  No products indexed under this heading.

Food Interactions
Alcohol (Additive vasodilating effects).

DERIFIL TABLETS
(Chlorophyllin Copper Complex) 2371
None cited in PDR database.

DERMATOP EMOLLIENT CREAM 0.1%
(Prednicarbate) 1264
None cited in PDR database.

DESENEX ANTIFUNGAL OINTMENT
(Undecylenic Acid, Zinc Undecylenate) 652
None cited in PDR database.

DESENEX ANTIFUNGAL POWDER
(Undecylenic Acid, Zinc Undecylenate) 652
None cited in PDR database.

DESENEX ANTIFUNGAL SPRAY POWDER
(Undecylenic Acid, Zinc Undecylenate) 652
None cited in PDR database.

DESENEX FOOT & SNEAKER DEODORANT SPRAY
(Aluminum Chlorhydrate) 653
None cited in PDR database.

PRESCRIPTION STRENGTH DESENEX AF CREAM
(Clotrimazole) 653
None cited in PDR database.

PRESCRIPTION STRENGTH DESENEX SPRAY POWDER AND SPRAY LIQUID
(Mineral Supplements) 653
None cited in PDR database.

DESFERAL VIALS
(Deferoxamine Mesylate) 838
None cited in PDR database.

DESITIN CORNSTARCH BABY POWDER
(Zinc Oxide, Corn Starch) 715
None cited in PDR database.

DESITIN OINTMENT
(Cod Liver Oil, Zinc Oxide) 715
None cited in PDR database.

DESMOPRESSIN ACETATE INJECTION
(Desmopressin Acetate) 996
May interact with vasopressors. Compounds in this category include:

Dopamine Hydrochloride (Although the pressor activity of desmopressin is very low, use of doses as large as 0.3 mcg/kg of desmopressin with other vasopressors should be undertaken with caution).
  No products indexed under this heading.
Epinephrine Bitartrate (Although the pressor activity of desmopressin is very low, use of doses as large as 0.3 mcg/kg of desmopressin with other vasopressors should be undertaken with caution). Products include:
  Sensorcaine-MPF with Epinephrine Injection 554
Epinephrine Hydrochloride (Although the pressor activity of desmopressin is very low, use of doses as large as 0.3 mcg/kg of desmopressin with other vasopressors should be undertaken with caution). Products include:
  Ana-Kit Anaphylaxis Emergency Treatment Kit 611
Metaraminol Bitartrate (Although the pressor activity of desmopressin is very low, use of doses as large as 0.3 mcg/kg of desmopressin with other vasopressors should be undertaken with caution). Products include:
  Aramine Injection 1649
Methoxamine Hydrochloride (Although the pressor activity of desmopressin is very low, use of doses as large as 0.3 mcg/kg of desmopressin with other vasopressors should be undertaken with caution). Products include:
  Vasoxyl Injection 1169

IMPORTANT NOTE: Always consult each drug listing in the patient's regimen for possible interactions.

Norepinephrine Bitartrate (Although the pressor activity of desmopressin is very low, use of doses as large as 0.3 mcg/kg of desmopressin with other vasopressors should be undertaken with caution). Products include:

- Levophed Bitartrate Injection ... 2445

Phenylephrine Hydrochloride (Although the pressor activity of desmopressin is very low, use of doses as large as 0.3 mcg/kg of desmopressin with other vasopressors should be undertaken with caution). Products include:

- Atrohist Plus Tablets ... 1605
- Cerose DM ... ▣ 853
- D.A. II Tablets ... 972
- D.A. Chewable Tablets ... 970
- Dura-Vent/DA Tablets ... 972
- Extendryl ... 1003
- 4-Way Fast Acting Nasal Spray (regular & mentholated) ... ▣ 644
- Hemorid ... ▣ 797
- Hycomine Compound Tablets ... 948
- Neo-Synephrine Hydrochloride 1% Carpuject ... 2455
- Neo-Synephrine Hydrochloride 1% Injection ... 2455
- Neo-Synephrine Hydrochloride (Ophthalmic) ... 2456
- Neo-Synephrine ... ▣ 624
- Novahistine Elixir ... ▣ 782
- Phenergan VC ... 2886
- Phenergan VC with Codeine ... 2888
- Preparation H ... ▣ 842
- Tympagesic Ear Drops ... 2476
- Vicks Sinex Nasal Spray and Ultra Fine Mist ... ▣ 738

DESMOPRESSIN ACETATE RHINAL TUBE

(Desmopressin Acetate) ... 997

May interact with vasopressors and certain other agents. Compounds in these categories include:

Dopamine Hydrochloride (The pressor activity of desmopressin is very low, use of large doses of desmopressin with pressor agents should only be done with careful monitoring).

No products indexed under this heading.

Epinephrine Bitartrate (The pressor activity of desmopressin is very low, use of large doses of desmopressin with pressor agents should only be done with careful monitoring). Products include:

- Sensorcaine-MPF with Epinephrine Injection ... 554

Epinephrine Hydrochloride (The pressor activity of desmopressin is very low, use of large doses of desmopressin with pressor agents should only be done with careful monitoring). Products include:

- Ana-Kit Anaphylaxis Emergency Treatment Kit ... 611

Metaraminol Bitartrate (The pressor activity of desmopressin is very low, use of large doses of desmopressin with pressor agents should only be done with careful monitoring). Products include:

- Aramine Injection ... 1649

Methoxamine Hydrochloride (The pressor activity of desmopressin is very low, use of large doses of desmopressin with pressor agents should only be done with careful monitoring). Products include:

- Vasoxyl Injection ... 1169

Norepinephrine Bitartrate (The pressor activity of desmopressin is very low, use of large doses of desmopressin with pressor agents should only be done with careful monitoring). Products include:

- Levophed Bitartrate Injection ... 2445

Phenylephrine Hydrochloride (The pressor activity of desmopressin is very low, use of large doses of desmopressin with pressor agents should only be done with careful monitoring). Products include:

- Atrohist Plus Tablets ... 1605
- Cerose DM ... ▣ 853
- D.A. II Tablets ... 972
- D.A. Chewable Tablets ... 970
- Dura-Vent/DA Tablets ... 972
- Extendryl ... 1003
- 4-Way Fast Acting Nasal Spray (regular & mentholated) ... ▣ 644
- Hemorid ... ▣ 797
- Hycomine Compound Tablets ... 948
- Neo-Synephrine Hydrochloride 1% Carpuject ... 2455
- Neo-Synephrine Hydrochloride 1% Injection ... 2455
- Neo-Synephrine Hydrochloride (Ophthalmic) ... 2456
- Neo-Synephrine ... ▣ 624
- Novahistine Elixir ... ▣ 782
- Phenergan VC ... 2886
- Phenergan VC with Codeine ... 2888
- Preparation H ... ▣ 842
- Tympagesic Ear Drops ... 2476
- Vicks Sinex Nasal Spray and Ultra Fine Mist ... ▣ 738

DESOGEN TABLETS

(Desogestrel, Ethinyl Estradiol) ... 1867

May interact with barbiturates and tetracyclines. Compounds in these categories include:

Ampicillin (Potential for reduced efficacy and increased incidence of breakthrough bleeding and menstrual irregularities). Products include:

- Omnipen Capsules ... 2872
- Omnipen for Oral Suspension ... 2873

Ampicillin Sodium (Potential for reduced efficacy and increased incidence of breakthrough bleeding and menstrual irregularities). Products include:

- Unasyn ... 2035

Aprobarbital (Potential for reduced efficacy and increased incidence of breakthrough bleeding and menstrual irregularities).

No products indexed under this heading.

Butabarbital (Potential for reduced efficacy and increased incidence of breakthrough bleeding and menstrual irregularities).

No products indexed under this heading.

Butalbital (Potential for reduced efficacy and increased incidence of breakthrough bleeding and menstrual irregularities). Products include:

- Axocet Capsules ... 2459
- Esgic-plus Capsules ... 1012
- Esgic-plus Tablets ... 1012
- Fioricet Tablets ... 2386
- Fioricet with Codeine Capsules ... 2387
- Fiorinal Capsules ... 2388
- Fiorinal with Codeine Capsules ... 2390
- Fiorinal Tablets ... 2388
- Phrenilin ... 790
- Sedapap Tablets 50 mg/650 mg ... 1826

Demeclocycline Hydrochloride (Potential for reduced efficacy and increased incidence of breakthrough bleeding and menstrual irregularities). Products include:

- Declomycin Tablets ... 1421

Doxycycline Calcium (Potential for reduced efficacy and increased incidence of breakthrough bleeding and menstrual irregularities). Products include:

- Vibramycin Calcium Oral Suspension Syrup ... 2038

Doxycycline Hyclate (Potential for reduced efficacy and increased incidence of breakthrough bleeding and menstrual irregularities). Products include:

- Doryx Capsules ... 1970
- Vibramycin Hyclate Capsules ... 2038
- Vibramycin Hyclate Intravenous ... 2040
- Vibra-Tabs Film Coated Tablets ... 2038

Doxycycline Monohydrate (Potential for reduced efficacy and increased incidence of breakthrough bleeding and menstrual irregularities). Products include:

- Monodox Capsules ... 1858
- Vibramycin Monohydrate for Oral Suspension ... 2038

Griseofulvin (Potential for reduced efficacy and increased incidence of breakthrough bleeding and menstrual irregularities). Products include:

- Fulvicin P/G Tablets ... 2499
- Fulvicin P/G 165 & 330 Tablets ... 2500
- Grifulvin V (griseofulvin tablets) Microsize (griseofulvin oral suspension) Microsize ... 1944
- Gris-PEG Tablets, 125 mg & 250 mg ... 476

Mephobarbital (Potential for reduced efficacy and increased incidence of breakthrough bleeding and menstrual irregularities). Products include:

- Mebaral Tablets ... 2452

Methacycline Hydrochloride (Potential for reduced efficacy and increased incidence of breakthrough bleeding and menstrual irregularities).

No products indexed under this heading.

Minocycline Hydrochloride (Potential for reduced efficacy and increased incidence of breakthrough bleeding and menstrual irregularities). Products include:

- DYNACIN Capsules ... 1627
- Minocin Intravenous ... 1428
- Minocin Oral Suspension ... 1431
- Minocin Pellet-Filled Capsules ... 1429

Oxytetracycline Hydrochloride (Potential for reduced efficacy and increased incidence of breakthrough bleeding and menstrual irregularities). Products include:

- TERAK Ointment ... ◉ 210
- Terra-Cortril Ophthalmic Suspension ... 2033
- Terramycin with Polymyxin B Sulfate Ophthalmic Ointment ... 2035
- Urobiotic-250 Capsules ... 2038

Pentobarbital Sodium (Potential for reduced efficacy and increased incidence of breakthrough bleeding and menstrual irregularities). Products include:

- Nembutal Sodium Capsules ... 440
- Nembutal Sodium Solution ... 442
- Nembutal Sodium Suppositories ... 444

Phenobarbital (Potential for reduced efficacy and increased incidence of breakthrough bleeding and menstrual irregularities). Products include:

- Arco-Lase Plus Tablets ... 513
- Bellergal-S Tablets ... 2375
- Donnatal ... 2234
- Donnatal Extentabs ... 2234
- Donnatal Tablets ... 2234
- Phenobarbital Elixir and Tablets ... 1523
- Quadrinal Tablets ... 1398

Phenylbutazone (Potential for reduced efficacy and increased incidence of breakthrough bleeding and menstrual irregularities).

No products indexed under this heading.

Phenytoin Sodium (Potential for reduced efficacy and increased incidence of breakthrough bleeding and menstrual irregularities). Products include:

- Dilantin Kapseals ... 1965

Rifampin (Potential for reduced efficacy and increased incidence of breakthrough bleeding and menstrual irregularities). Products include:

- Rifadin ... 1276
- Rifamate Capsules ... 1278
- Rifater ... 1280
- Rimactane Capsules ... 865

Secobarbital Sodium (Potential for reduced efficacy and increased incidence of breakthrough bleeding and menstrual irregularities). Products include:

- Seconal Sodium Pulvules ... 1529

Tetracycline Hydrochloride (Potential for reduced efficacy and increased incidence of breakthrough bleeding and menstrual irregularities). Products include:

- Achromycin V Capsules ... 1417
- Helidac Therapy ... 2135

Thiamylal Sodium (Potential for reduced efficacy and increased incidence of breakthrough bleeding and menstrual irregularities).

No products indexed under this heading.

DESOWEN CREAM, OINTMENT AND LOTION

(Desonide) ... 1032

None cited in PDR database.

DESOXYN GRADUMET TABLETS

(Methamphetamine Hydrochloride) ... 422

May interact with insulin, monoamine oxidase inhibitors, phenothiazines, tricyclic antidepressants, and certain other agents. Compounds in these categories include:

Amitriptyline Hydrochloride (Co-administration of tricyclic antidepressants and indirect-acting sympathomimetic amines such as amphetamines should be closely supervised and dosage carefully adjusted). Products include:

- Elavil ... 2945
- Etrafon ... 2495
- Limbitrol ... 2333
- Triavil Tablets ... 1800

Amoxapine (Co-administration of tricyclic antidepressants and indirect-acting sympathomimetic amines such as amphetamines should be closely supervised and dosage carefully adjusted). Products include:

- Asendin Tablets ... 1419

Chlorpromazine (May antagonize the CNS stimulant action of the amphetamine). Products include:

- Thorazine Suppositories ... 2701

Clomipramine Hydrochloride (Co-administration of tricyclic antidepressants and indirect-acting sympathomimetic amines such as amphetamines should be closely supervised and dosage carefully adjusted). Products include:

- Anafranil Capsules ... 819

Desipramine Hydrochloride (Co-administration of tricyclic antidepressants and indirect-acting sympathomimetic amines such as amphetamines should be closely supervised and dosage carefully adjusted). Products include:

- Norpramin Tablets ... 1273

(▣ Described in PDR For Nonprescription Drugs) (◉ Described in PDR For Ophthalmology)

Doxepin Hydrochloride (Co-administration of tricyclic antidepressants and indirect-acting sympathomimetic amines such as amphetamines should be closely supervised and dosage carefully adjusted). Products include:
  Adapin Capsules 1542
  Sinequan 2028
  Zonalon Cream 1042

Fluphenazine Decanoate (May antagonize the CNS stimulant action of the amphetamine). Products include:
  Prolixin Decanoate 510

Fluphenazine Enanthate (May antagonize the CNS stimulant action of the amphetamine). Products include:
  Prolixin Enanthate 510

Fluphenazine Hydrochloride (May antagonize the CNS stimulant action of the amphetamine). Products include:
  Prolixin 510

Furazolidone (Co-administration may result in hypertensive crises; concurrent and/or sequential use is contraindicated). Products include:
  Furoxone 2221

Guanethidine Monosulfate (Decreased hypotensive effect). Products include:
  Esimil Tablets 840
  Ismelin Tablets 845

Imipramine Hydrochloride (Co-administration of tricyclic antidepressants and indirect-acting sympathomimetic amines such as amphetamines should be closely supervised and dosage carefully adjusted). Products include:
  Tofranil Ampuls 873
  Tofranil Tablets 875

Imipramine Pamoate (Co-administration of tricyclic antidepressants and indirect-acting sympathomimetic amines such as amphetamines should be closely supervised and dosage carefully adjusted). Products include:
  Tofranil-PM Capsules 876

Insulin, Human (Insulin requirement in diabetics may be altered).
  No products indexed under this heading.

Insulin, Human Isophane Suspension (Insulin requirement in diabetics may be altered). Products include:
  Novolin N Human Insulin 10 ml Vials 1846

Insulin, Human NPH (Insulin requirement in diabetics may be altered). Products include:
  Humulin N, 100 Units 1495
  Novolin N PenFill 1.5 ml Cartridges Durable Insulin Delivery System 1849
  Novolin N Prefilled Syringe Disposable Insulin Delivery System ... 1850

Insulin, Human Regular (Insulin requirement in diabetics may be altered). Products include:
  Humulin R, 100 Units 1497
  Novolin R Human Insulin 10 ml Vials 1846
  Novolin R PenFill 1.5 ml Cartridges Durable Insulin Delivery System 1849
  Novolin R Prefilled Syringe Disposable Insulin Delivery System ... 1850
  Velosulin BR Human Insulin 10 ml Vials 1847

Insulin, Human, Zinc Suspension (Insulin requirement in diabetics may be altered). Products include:
  Humulin L, 100 Units 1494
  Humulin U, 100 Units 1498
  Novolin L Human Insulin 10 ml Vials 1846

Insulin Lispro, Human (Insulin requirement in diabetics may be altered). Products include:
  Humalog Injection 1488

Insulin, NPH (Insulin requirement in diabetics may be altered). Products include:
  NPH, 100 Units 1502
  Pork NPH, 100 Units 1506
  Purified Pork NPH Isophane Insulin 1852

Insulin, Regular (Insulin requirement in diabetics may be altered). Products include:
  Regular, 100 Units 1503
  Pork Regular, 100 Units 1507
  Pork Regular (Concentrated), 500 Units 1508
  Purified Pork Regular Insulin .. 1852

Insulin, Zinc Crystals (Insulin requirement in diabetics may be altered). Products include:
  NPH, 100 Units 1502

Insulin, Zinc Suspension (Insulin requirement in diabetics may be altered). Products include:
  Iletin I 1501
  Lente, 100 Units 1501
  Iletin II 1504
  Pork Lente, 100 Units 1504
  Purified Pork Lente Insulin 1852

Isocarboxazid (Co-administration may result in hypertensive crises; concurrent and/or sequential use is contraindicated).
  No products indexed under this heading.

Maprotiline Hydrochloride (Co-administration of tricyclic antidepressants and indirect-acting sympathomimetic amines such as amphetamines should be closely supervised and dosage carefully adjusted). Products include:
  Ludiomil Tablets 861

Mesoridazine Besylate (May antagonize the CNS stimulant action of the amphetamine). Products include:
  Serentil 689

Methotrimeprazine (May antagonize the CNS stimulant action of the amphetamine). Products include:
  Levoprome 1321

Nortriptyline Hydrochloride (Co-administration of tricyclic antidepressants and indirect-acting sympathomimetic amines such as amphetamines should be closely supervised and dosage carefully adjusted). Products include:
  Pamelor 2409

Perphenazine (May antagonize the CNS stimulant action of the amphetamine). Products include:
  Etrafon 2495
  Triavil Tablets 1800
  Trilafon 2532

Phenelzine Sulfate (Co-administration may result in hypertensive crises; concurrent and/or sequential use is contraindicated). Products include:
  Nardil 1977

Prochlorperazine (May antagonize the CNS stimulant action of the amphetamine). Products include:
  Compazine 2644

Promethazine Hydrochloride (May antagonize the CNS stimulant action of the amphetamine). Products include:
  Mepergan Injection 2859
  Phenergan with Codeine 2883
  Phenergan with Dextromethorphan 2885
  Phenergan Injection 2880
  Phenergan Suppositories 2882
  Phenergan Syrup 2881
  Phenergan Tablets 2882
  Phenergan VC 2886
  Phenergan VC with Codeine .. 2888

Protriptyline Hydrochloride (Co-administration of tricyclic antidepressants and indirect-acting sympathomimetic amines such as amphetamines should be closely supervised and dosage carefully adjusted). Products include:
  Vivactil Tablets 1820

Selegiline Hydrochloride (Co-administration may result in hypertensive crises; concurrent and/or sequential use is contraindicated). Products include:
  Eldepryl Capsules 2729

Thioridazine Hydrochloride (May antagonize the CNS stimulant action of the amphetamine). Products include:
  Mellaril 2398

Tranylcypromine Sulfate (Co-administration may result in hypertensive crises; concurrent and/or sequential use is contraindicated). Products include:
  Parnate Tablets 2679

Trifluoperazine Hydrochloride (May antagonize the CNS stimulant action of the amphetamine). Products include:
  Stelazine 2692

Trimipramine Maleate (Co-administration of tricyclic antidepressants and indirect-acting sympathomimetic amines such as amphetamines should be closely supervised and dosage carefully adjusted). Products include:
  Surmontil Capsules 2917

DESQUAM-E 2.5 EMOLLIENT GEL
(Benzoyl Peroxide) 2792
May interact with:

Octyl Dimethyl PABA (Concurrent use with PABA-containing sunscreens may result in transient discoloration of the skin).
  No products indexed under this heading.

DESQUAM-E 5 EMOLLIENT GEL
(Benzoyl Peroxide) 2792
See **Desquam-E 2.5 Emollient Gel**

DESQUAM-E 10 EMOLLIENT GEL
(Benzoyl Peroxide) 2792
See **Desquam-E 2.5 Emollient Gel**

DESQUAM-X 5 GEL
(Benzoyl Peroxide) 2792
See **Desquam-E 2.5 Emollient Gel**

DESQUAM-X 10 GEL
(Benzoyl Peroxide) 2792
See **Desquam-E 2.5 Emollient Gel**

DESQUAM-X 10 BAR
(Benzoyl Peroxide) 2792
See **Desquam-E 2.5 Emollient Gel**

DESQUAM-X 5 WASH
(Benzoyl Peroxide) 2792
See **Desquam-E 2.5 Emollient Gel**

DESQUAM-X 10 WASH
(Benzoyl Peroxide) 2792
See **Desquam-E 2.5 Emollient Gel**

DESYREL AND DESYREL DIVIDOSE
(Trazodone Hydrochloride) 504
May interact with monoamine oxidase inhibitors, central nervous system depressants, antihypertensives, oral anticoagulants, and certain other agents. Compounds in these categories include:

Acebutolol Hydrochloride (Concomitant administration may require a reduction in the dose of the antihypertensive). Products include:
  Sectral Capsules 2914

Alfentanil Hydrochloride (Enhanced response to CNS depressants). Products include:
  Alfenta Injection 1334

Alprazolam (Enhanced response to CNS depressants). Products include:
  Xanax Tablets 2115

Amlodipine Besylate (Concomitant administration may require a reduction in the dose of the antihypertensive). Products include:
  Lotrel Capsules 858
  Norvasc Tablets 2020

Aprobarbital (Enhanced response to CNS depressants).
  No products indexed under this heading.

Atenolol (Concomitant administration may require a reduction in the dose of the antihypertensive). Products include:
  Tenoretic Tablets 2963
  Tenormin Tablets and I.V. Injection 2965

Benazepril Hydrochloride (Concomitant administration may require a reduction in the dose of the antihypertensive). Products include:
  Lotensin Tablets 852
  Lotensin HCT Tablets 855
  Lotrel Capsules 858

Bendroflumethiazide (Concomitant administration may require a reduction in the dose of the antihypertensive).
  No products indexed under this heading.

Betaxolol Hydrochloride (Concomitant administration may require a reduction in the dose of the antihypertensive). Products include:
  Betoptic Ophthalmic Solution ... 465
  Betoptic S Ophthalmic Suspension 467
  Kerlone Tablets 2588

Bisoprolol Fumarate (Concomitant administration may require a reduction in the dose of the antihypertensive). Products include:
  Zebeta Tablets 1457
  Ziac 1459

Buprenorphine (Enhanced response to CNS depressants). Products include:
  Buprenex Injectable 2170

Buspirone Hydrochloride (Enhanced response to CNS depressants). Products include:
  BuSpar Tablets 738

Butabarbital (Enhanced response to CNS depressants).
  No products indexed under this heading.

Butalbital (Enhanced response to CNS depressants). Products include:
  Axocet Capsules 2469
  Esgic-plus Capsules 1012
  Esgic-plus Tablets 1012
  Fioricet Tablets 2386
  Fioricet with Codeine Capsules 2387
  Fiorinal Capsules 2388
  Fiorinal with Codeine Capsules 2390
  Fiorinal Tablets 2388
  Phrenilin 790
  Sedapap Tablets 50 mg/650 mg 1826

Captopril (Concomitant administration may require a reduction in the dose of the antihypertensive). Products include:
  Capoten Tablets 740
  Capozide Tablets 744

IMPORTANT NOTE: Always consult each drug listing in the patient's regimen for possible interactions.

Desyrel **Interactions Index** 260

Carteolol Hydrochloride (Concomitant administration may require a reduction in the dose of the antihypertensive). Products include:
- Cartrol Tablets ... 413
- Ocupress Ophthalmic Solution, 1% Sterile ... ⊙ 297

Chlordiazepoxide (Enhanced response to CNS depressants). Products include:
- Limbitrol ... 2333

Chlordiazepoxide Hydrochloride (Enhanced response to CNS depressants). Products include:
- Librax Capsules ... 2330
- Librium Capsules ... 2331
- Librium Injectable ... 2332

Chlorothiazide (Concomitant administration may require a reduction in the dose of the antihypertensive). Products include:
- Aldoclor Tablets ... 1638
- Diupres Tablets ... 1691
- Diuril Oral ... 1694

Chlorothiazide Sodium (Concomitant administration may require a reduction in the dose of the antihypertensive). Products include:
- Diuril Sodium Intravenous ... 1693

Chlorpromazine (Enhanced response to CNS depressants). Products include:
- Thorazine Suppositories ... 2701

Chlorpromazine Hydrochloride (Enhanced response to CNS depressants). Products include:
- Thorazine ... 2701

Chlorprothixene (Enhanced response to CNS depressants).
- No products indexed under this heading.

Chlorprothixene Hydrochloride (Enhanced response to CNS depressants).
- No products indexed under this heading.

Chlorprothixene Lactate (Enhanced response to CNS depressants).
- No products indexed under this heading.

Chlorthalidone (Concomitant administration may require a reduction in the dose of the antihypertensive). Products include:
- Combipres Tablets ... 682
- Tenoretic Tablets ... 2963
- Thalitone ... 1293

Clonidine (Concomitant administration may require a reduction in the dose of the antihypertensive). Products include:
- Catapres-TTS ... 680

Clonidine Hydrochloride (Concomitant administration may require a reduction in the dose of the antihypertensive). Products include:
- Catapres Tablets ... 679
- Combipres Tablets ... 682

Clorazepate Dipotassium (Enhanced response to CNS depressants). Products include:
- Tranxene ... 459

Clozapine (Enhanced response to CNS depressants). Products include:
- Clozaril Tablets ... 2377

Codeine Phosphate (Enhanced response to CNS depressants). Products include:
- Brontex ... 2130
- Dimetane-DC Cough Syrup ... 2232
- Fioricet with Codeine Capsules ... 2387
- Fiorinal with Codeine Capsules ... 2390
- Nucofed ... 2225
- Phenergan with Codeine ... 2883
- Phenergan VC with Codeine ... 2888
- Robitussin A-C Syrup ... 2248
- Robitussin-DAC Syrup ... 2249
- Ryna ... ▣ 804
- Soma Compound w/Codeine Tablets ... 2784
- Tylenol with Codeine ... 1592

Deserpidine (Concomitant administration may require a reduction in the dose of the antihypertensive).
- No products indexed under this heading.

Desflurane (Enhanced response to CNS depressants). Products include:
- Suprane (desflurane, USP) ... 1865

Dezocine (Enhanced response to CNS depressants). Products include:
- Dalgan Injection ... 529

Diazepam (Enhanced response to CNS depressants). Products include:
- Dizac (diazepam injectable emulsion) CIV ... 1862
- Valium Injectable ... 2336
- Valium Tablets ... 2335

Diazoxide (Concomitant administration may require a reduction in the dose of the antihypertensive). Products include:
- Hyperstat I.V. Injection ... 2504
- Proglycem ... 575

Dicumarol (Increased or decreased prothrombin time).
- No products indexed under this heading.

Digoxin (Increased serum levels of digoxin). Products include:
- Lanoxicaps ... 1110
- Lanoxin Elixir Pediatric ... 1113
- Lanoxin Injection ... 1116
- Lanoxin Injection Pediatric ... 1119
- Lanoxin Tablets ... 1121

Diltiazem Hydrochloride (Concomitant administration may require a reduction in the dose of the antihypertensive). Products include:
- Cardizem CD Capsules ... 1251
- Cardizem SR Capsules ... 1255
- Cardizem Injectable ... 1253
- Cardizem Tablets ... 1257
- Dilacor XR Extended-release Capsules ... 2183
- Tiazac Capsules ... 1019

Doxazosin Mesylate (Concomitant administration may require a reduction in the dose of the antihypertensive). Products include:
- Cardura Tablets ... 1993

Droperidol (Enhanced response to CNS depressants). Products include:
- Inapsine Injection ... 462

Enalapril Maleate (Concomitant administration may require a reduction in the dose of the antihypertensive). Products include:
- Vaseretic Tablets ... 1810
- Vasotec Tablets ... 1816

Enalaprilat (Concomitant administration may require a reduction in the dose of the antihypertensive). Products include:
- Vasotec I.V. ... 1814

Enflurane (Enhanced response to CNS depressants).
- No products indexed under this heading.

Esmolol Hydrochloride (Concomitant administration may require a reduction in the dose of the antihypertensive). Products include:
- Brevibloc (esmolol HCl) Injection ... 1860

Estazolam (Enhanced response to CNS depressants). Products include:
- ProSom Tablets ... 457

Ethchlorvynol (Enhanced response to CNS depressants). Products include:
- Placidyl Capsules ... 456

Ethinamate (Enhanced response to CNS depressants).
- No products indexed under this heading.

Felodipine (Concomitant administration may require a reduction in the dose of the antihypertensive). Products include:
- Plendil Extended-Release Tablets ... 514

Fentanyl (Enhanced response to CNS depressants). Products include:
- Duragesic Transdermal System ... 1336

Fentanyl Citrate (Enhanced response to CNS depressants). Products include:
- Sublimaze Injection ... 463

Fluphenazine Decanoate (Enhanced response to CNS depressants). Products include:
- Prolixin Decanoate ... 510

Fluphenazine Enanthate (Enhanced response to CNS depressants). Products include:
- Prolixin Enanthate ... 510

Fluphenazine Hydrochloride (Enhanced response to CNS depressants). Products include:
- Prolixin ... 510

Flurazepam Hydrochloride (Enhanced response to CNS depressants). Products include:
- Dalmane Capsules ... 2329

Fosinopril Sodium (Concomitant administration may require a reduction in the dose of the antihypertensive). Products include:
- Monopril Tablets ... 762

Furazolidone (Initiate Desyrel cautiously). Products include:
- Furoxone ... 2221

Furosemide (Concomitant administration may require a reduction in the dose of the antihypertensive). Products include:
- Lasix Injection, Oral Solution and Tablets ... 1267

Glutethimide (Enhanced response to CNS depressants).
- No products indexed under this heading.

Guanabenz Acetate (Concomitant administration may require a reduction in the dose of the antihypertensive).
- No products indexed under this heading.

Guanethidine Monosulfate (Concomitant administration may require a reduction in the dose of the antihypertensive). Products include:
- Esimil Tablets ... 840
- Ismelin Tablets ... 845

Haloperidol (Enhanced response to CNS depressants). Products include:
- Haldol Injection, Tablets and Concentrate ... 1585

Haloperidol Decanoate (Enhanced response to CNS depressants). Products include:
- Haldol Decanoate ... 1587

Hydralazine Hydrochloride (Concomitant administration may require a reduction in the dose of the antihypertensive). Products include:
- Apresazide Capsules ... 824
- Apresoline Hydrochloride Tablets ... 826
- Hydralazine Hydrochloride Injection USP ... 2712
- Ser-Ap-Es Tablets ... 867

Hydrochlorothiazide (Concomitant administration may require a reduction in the dose of the antihypertensive). Products include:
- Aldactazide Tablets ... 2556
- Aldoril Tablets ... 1644
- Apresazide Capsules ... 824
- Capozide Tablets ... 744
- Dyazide Capsules ... 2653
- Esidrix Tablets ... 839
- Esimil Tablets ... 840
- HydroDIURIL Tablets ... 1716
- Hydropres Tablets ... 1718
- Hyzaar Tablets ... 1720
- Inderide Tablets ... 2838
- Inderide LA Long Acting Capsules ... 2840
- Lopressor HCT Tablets ... 850
- Lotensin HCT Tablets ... 855
- Moduretic Tablets ... 1748
- Oretic Tablets ... 450
- Prinzide Tablets ... 1780
- Ser-Ap-Es Tablets ... 867
- Timolide Tablets ... 1791
- Vaseretic Tablets ... 1810
- Zestoretic Tablets ... 2968
- Ziac ... 1459

Hydrocodone Bitartrate (Enhanced response to CNS depressants). Products include:
- Codiclear DH Syrup ... 808
- Duratuss HD Elixir ... 2750
- Histussin D Liquid ... 670
- Hycodan Tablets and Syrup ... 946
- Hycomine Compound Tablets ... 948
- Hycomine ... 947
- Hycotuss Expectorant Syrup ... 950
- Hydrocet Capsules ... 787
- Lorcet 10/650 Tablets ... 1016
- Lortab ... 2751
- Tussend ... 1830
- Tussend Expectorant ... 1831
- Vicodin Tablets ... 1404
- Vicodin ES Tablets ... 1405
- Vicodin HP Tablets ... 1403
- Vicodin Tuss Expectorant ... 1406
- Zydone Capsules ... 967

Hydrocodone Polistirex (Enhanced response to CNS depressants). Products include:
- Tussionex Pennkinetic Extended-Release Suspension ... 1624

Hydroflumethiazide (Concomitant administration may require a reduction in the dose of the antihypertensive). Products include:
- Diucardin Tablets ... 2824

Hydroxyzine Hydrochloride (Enhanced response to CNS depressants). Products include:
- Atarax Tablets & Syrup ... 1992
- Marax Tablets & DF Syrup ... 2015
- Vistaril Intramuscular Solution ... 2042

Indapamide (Concomitant administration may require a reduction in the dose of the antihypertensive).
- No products indexed under this heading.

Isocarboxazid (Initiate Desyrel cautiously).
- No products indexed under this heading.

Isoflurane (Enhanced response to CNS depressants).
- No products indexed under this heading.

Isradipine (Concomitant administration may require a reduction in the dose of the antihypertensive). Products include:
- DynaCirc Capsules ... 2381
- DynaCirc CR Tablets ... 2383

Ketamine Hydrochloride (Enhanced response to CNS depressants).
- No products indexed under this heading.

Labetalol Hydrochloride (Concomitant administration may require a reduction in the dose of the antihypertensive). Products include:
- Normodyne Injection ... 2519
- Normodyne Tablets ... 2522
- Trandate ... 1158

Levomethadyl Acetate Hydrochloride (Enhanced response to CNS depressants). Products include:
- Orlaam Oral Solution ... 2361

Levorphanol Tartrate (Enhanced response to CNS depressants). Products include:
- Levo-Dromoran ... 2297

(▣ Described in PDR For Nonprescription Drugs) (⊙ Described in PDR For Ophthalmology)

261 **Interactions Index** **Desyrel**

Lisinopril (Concomitant administration may require a reduction in the dose of the antihypertensive). Products include:
Prinivil Tablets ... 1776
Prinzide Tablets ... 1780
Zestoretic Tablets ... 2968
Zestril Tablets ... 2972

Lorazepam (Enhanced response to CNS depressants). Products include:
Ativan Injection ... 2805
Ativan Tablets ... 2807

Losartan Potassium (Concomitant administration may require a reduction in the dose of the antihypertensive). Products include:
Cozaar Tablets ... 1668
Hyzaar Tablets ... 1720

Loxapine Hydrochloride (Enhanced response to CNS depressants). Products include:
Loxitane ... 1426

Loxapine Succinate (Enhanced response to CNS depressants). Products include:
Loxitane Capsules ... 1426

Mecamylamine Hydrochloride (Concomitant administration may require a reduction in the dose of the antihypertensive). Products include:
Inversine Tablets ... 1729

Meperidine Hydrochloride (Enhanced response to CNS depressants). Products include:
Demerol ... 2438
Mepergan Injection ... 2859

Mephobarbital (Enhanced response to CNS depressants). Products include:
Mebaral Tablets ... 2452

Meprobamate (Enhanced response to CNS depressants). Products include:
Miltown Tablets ... 2780
PMB 200 and PMB 400 ... 2890

Mesoridazine Besylate (Enhanced response to CNS depressants). Products include:
Serentil ... 689

Methadone Hydrochloride (Enhanced response to CNS depressants). Products include:
Methadone Hydrochloride Oral Concentrate ... 2356
Methadone Hydrochloride Oral Solution & Tablets ... 2357

Methohexital Sodium (Enhanced response to CNS depressants).
No products indexed under this heading.

Methotrimeprazine (Enhanced response to CNS depressants). Products include:
Levoprome ... 1321

Methoxyflurane (Enhanced response to CNS depressants).
No products indexed under this heading.

Methyclothiazide (Concomitant administration may require a reduction in the dose of the antihypertensive). Products include:
Enduron Tablets ... 424

Methyldopa (Concomitant administration may require a reduction in the dose of the antihypertensive). Products include:
Aldoclor Tablets ... 1638
Aldomet Oral ... 1640
Aldoril Tablets ... 1644

Methyldopate Hydrochloride (Concomitant administration may require a reduction in the dose of the antihypertensive). Products include:
Aldomet Ester HCl Injection ... 1642

Metolazone (Concomitant administration may require a reduction in the dose of the antihypertensive). Products include:
Mykrox Tablets ... 1617
Zaroxolyn Tablets ... 1625

Metoprolol Succinate (Concomitant administration may require a reduction in the dose of the antihypertensive). Products include:
Toprol-XL Tablets ... 560

Metoprolol Tartrate (Concomitant administration may require a reduction in the dose of the antihypertensive). Products include:
Lopressor ... 848
Lopressor HCT Tablets ... 850

Metyrosine (Concomitant administration may require a reduction in the dose of the antihypertensive). Products include:
Demser Capsules ... 1690

Midazolam Hydrochloride (Enhanced response to CNS depressants). Products include:
Versed Injection ... 2324

Minoxidil (Concomitant administration may require a reduction in the dose of the antihypertensive).
No products indexed under this heading.

Moexipril Hydrochloride (Concomitant administration may require a reduction in the dose of the antihypertensive). Products include:
Univasc Tablets ... 2553

Molindone Hydrochloride (Enhanced response to CNS depressants). Products include:
Moban Tablets and Concentrate ... 1036

Morphine Sulfate (Enhanced response to CNS depressants). Products include:
Astramorph/PF Injection, USP (Preservative-Free) ... 526
Duramorph Injection ... 983
Infumorph 200 and Infumorph 500 Sterile Solutions ... 985
Kadian Capsules ... 2948
MS Contin Tablets ... 2149
MSIR ... 2152
Oramorph SR (Morphine Sulfate Sustained Release Tablets) ... 2359
RMS Suppositories CII ... 2766
Roxanol ... 2365

Nadolol (Concomitant administration may require a reduction in the dose of the antihypertensive).
No products indexed under this heading.

Nicardipine Hydrochloride (Concomitant administration may require a reduction in the dose of the antihypertensive). Products include:
Cardene Capsules ... 2261
Cardene I.V. ... 2815
Cardene SR Capsules ... 2264

Nifedipine (Concomitant administration may require a reduction in the dose of the antihypertensive). Products include:
Adalat Capsules (10 mg and 20 mg) ... 580
Adalat CC ... 582
Procardia Capsules ... 2024
Procardia XL Extended Release Tablets ... 2026

Nisoldipine (Concomitant administration may require a reduction in the dose of the antihypertensive). Products include:
Sular Tablets ... 2961

Nitroglycerin (Concomitant administration may require a reduction in the dose of the antihypertensive). Products include:
Deponit NTG Transdermal Delivery System ... 2541
Nitro-Bid IV ... 1270
Nitro-Bid Ointment ... 1272
Nitro-Dur (nitroglycerin) Transdermal Infusion System ... 1365
Nitrolingual Spray ... 2193
Nitrostat Tablets ... 1981
Transderm-Nitro Transdermal Therapeutic System ... 878

Opium Alkaloids (Enhanced response to CNS depressants).
No products indexed under this heading.

Oxazepam (Enhanced response to CNS depressants). Products include:
Serax Capsules ... 2916
Serax Tablets ... 2916

Oxycodone Hydrochloride (Enhanced response to CNS depressants). Products include:
OxyContin Tablets ... 2163
OxyIR Capsules ... 2167
Percocet Tablets ... 955
Percodan Tablets ... 955
Percodan-Demi Tablets ... 956
Roxicodone Tablets, Oral Solution & Intensol (Oxycodone) ... 2366
Tylox Capsules ... 1593

Penbutolol Sulfate (Concomitant administration may require a reduction in the dose of the antihypertensive). Products include:
Levatol Tablets ... 2547

Pentobarbital Sodium (Enhanced response to CNS depressants). Products include:
Nembutal Sodium Capsules ... 440
Nembutal Sodium Solution ... 442
Nembutal Sodium Suppositories ... 444

Perphenazine (Enhanced response to CNS depressants). Products include:
Etrafon ... 2495
Triavil Tablets ... 1800
Trilafon ... 2532

Phenelzine Sulfate (Initiate Desyrel cautiously). Products include:
Nardil ... 1977

Phenobarbital (Enhanced response to CNS depressants). Products include:
Arco-Lase Plus Tablets ... 513
Bellergal-S Tablets ... 2375
Donnatal ... 2234
Donnatal Extentabs ... 2234
Donnatal Tablets ... 2234
Phenobarbital Elixir and Tablets ... 1523
Quadrinal Tablets ... 1398

Phenoxybenzamine Hydrochloride (Concomitant administration may require a reduction in the dose of the antihypertensive). Products include:
Dibenzyline Capsules ... 2650

Phentolamine Mesylate (Concomitant administration may require a reduction in the dose of the antihypertensive). Products include:
Regitine Vials ... 864

Phenytoin (Increased serum levels of phenytoin). Products include:
Dilantin Infatabs ... 1967
Dilantin-125 Suspension ... 1969

Phenytoin Sodium (Increased serum levels of phenytoin). Products include:
Dilantin Kapseals ... 1965

Pindolol (Concomitant administration may require a reduction in the dose of the antihypertensive). Products include:
Visken Tablets ... 2428

Polythiazide (Concomitant administration may require a reduction in the dose of the antihypertensive). Products include:
Minizide Capsules ... 2016

Prazepam (Enhanced response to CNS depressants).
No products indexed under this heading.

Prazosin Hydrochloride (Concomitant administration may require a reduction in the dose of the antihypertensive). Products include:
Minipress Capsules ... 2015
Minizide Capsules ... 2016

Prochlorperazine (Enhanced response to CNS depressants). Products include:
Compazine ... 2644

Promethazine Hydrochloride (Enhanced response to CNS depressants). Products include:
Mepergan Injection ... 2859
Phenergan with Codeine ... 2883
Phenergan with Dextromethorphan 2885
Phenergan Injection ... 2880
Phenergan Suppositories ... 2882
Phenergan Syrup ... 2881
Phenergan Tablets ... 2882
Phenergan VC ... 2886
Phenergan VC with Codeine ... 2888

Propofol (Enhanced response to CNS depressants). Products include:
Diprivan Injectable Emulsion ... 2939

Propoxyphene Hydrochloride (Enhanced response to CNS depressants). Products include:
Darvon ... 1475
Wygesic Tablets ... 2930

Propoxyphene Napsylate (Enhanced response to CNS depressants). Products include:
Darvon-N/Darvocet-N ... 1473

Propranolol Hydrochloride (Concomitant administration may require a reduction in the dose of the antihypertensive). Products include:
Inderal ... 2834
Inderal LA Long Acting Capsules ... 2836
Inderide Tablets ... 2838
Inderide LA Long Acting Capsules .. 2840

Quazepam (Enhanced response to CNS depressants). Products include:
Doral Tablets ... 2773

Quinapril Hydrochloride (Concomitant administration may require a reduction in the dose of the antihypertensive). Products include:
Accupril Tablets ... 1950

Ramipril (Concomitant administration may require a reduction in the dose of the antihypertensive). Products include:
Altace Capsules ... 1238

Rauwolfia Serpentina (Concomitant administration may require a reduction in the dose of the antihypertensive).
No products indexed under this heading.

Rescinnamine (Concomitant administration may require a reduction in the dose of the antihypertensive).
No products indexed under this heading.

Reserpine (Concomitant administration may require a reduction in the dose of the antihypertensive). Products include:
Diupres Tablets ... 1691
Hydropres Tablets ... 1718
Ser-Ap-Es Tablets ... 867

Risperidone (Enhanced response to CNS depressants). Products include:
Risperdal Tablets ... 1348

Secobarbital Sodium (Enhanced response to CNS depressants). Products include:
Seconal Sodium Pulvules ... 1529

Selegiline Hydrochloride (Initiate Desyrel cautiously). Products include:
Eldepryl Capsules ... 2729

Sevoflurane (Enhanced response to CNS depressants).
No products indexed under this heading.

IMPORTANT NOTE: Always consult each drug listing in the patient's regimen for possible interactions.

Sodium Nitroprusside (Concomitant administration may require a reduction in the dose of the antihypertensive).
No products indexed under this heading.

Sotalol Hydrochloride (Concomitant administration may require a reduction in the dose of the antihypertensive). Products include:
Betapace Tablets 637

Spirapril Hydrochloride (Concomitant administration may require a reduction in the dose of the antihypertensive).
No products indexed under this heading.

Sufentanil Citrate (Enhanced response to CNS depressants). Products include:
Sufenta Injection 1355

Temazepam (Enhanced response to CNS depressants). Products include:
Restoril Capsules 2413

Terazosin Hydrochloride (Concomitant administration may require a reduction in the dose of the antihypertensive). Products include:
Hytrin Capsules 434

Thiamylal Sodium (Enhanced response to CNS depressants).
No products indexed under this heading.

Thioridazine Hydrochloride (Enhanced response to CNS depressants). Products include:
Mellaril 2398

Thiothixene (Enhanced response to CNS depressants). Products include:
Navane Capsules and Concentrate 2018
Navane Intramuscular 2019

Timolol Maleate (Concomitant administration may require a reduction in the dose of the antihypertensive). Products include:
Blocadren Tablets 1654
Timolide Tablets 1791
Timoptic in Ocudose 1796
Timoptic Sterile Ophthalmic Solution 1794
Timoptic-XE 1798

Torsemide (Concomitant administration may require a reduction in the dose of the antihypertensive). Products include:
Demadex Tablets and Injection 691

Tranylcypromine Sulfate (Initiate Desyrel cautiously). Products include:
Parnate Tablets 2679

Triazolam (Enhanced response to CNS depressants). Products include:
Halcion Tablets 2093

Trifluoperazine Hydrochloride (Enhanced response to CNS depressants). Products include:
Stelazine 2692

Trimethaphan Camsylate (Concomitant administration may require a reduction in the dose of the antihypertensive).
No products indexed under this heading.

Verapamil Hydrochloride (Concomitant administration may require a reduction in the dose of the antihypertensive). Products include:
Calan SR Caplets 2571
Calan Tablets 2568
Covera-HS Tablets 2573
Isoptin Injectable 1391
Isoptin Oral Tablets 1393
Isoptin SR Tablets 1395
Verelan Capsules 1455

Warfarin Sodium (Increased or decreased prothrombin time). Products include:
Coumadin 941

Zolpidem Tartrate (Enhanced response to CNS depressants). Products include:
Ambien Tablets 2559

Food Interactions

Alcohol (Enhanced response to alcohol).

Food, unspecified (Total drug absorption may be up to 20% higher when the drug is taken with food rather than on an empty stomach; the risk of dizziness, lightheadedness may increase under fasting conditions).

DEVROM CHEWABLE TABLETS
(Bismuth Subgallate) .... ▣ 714
None cited in PDR database.

DEXACORT PHOSPHATE IN RESPIHALER
(Dexamethasone Sodium Phosphate) 1606
May interact with oral anticoagulants, potassium sparing diuretics, and certain other agents. Compounds in these categories include:

Amiloride Hydrochloride (Potential for hypokalemia). Products include:
Midamor Tablets 1746
Moduretic Tablets 1748

Aspirin (Aspirin should be used cautiously in conjunction with Dexacort in hypoprothrombinemia). Products include:
Alka-Seltzer Cherry Effervescent Antacid and Pain Reliever .... ▣ 609
Alka-Seltzer Extra Strength Effervescent Antacid and Pain Reliever .... ▣ 609
Alka-Seltzer Lemon Lime Effervescent Antacid and Pain Reliever .... ▣ 609
Alka-Seltzer Original Effervescent Antacid and Pain Reliever .... ▣ 609
Alka-Seltzer Plus .... ▣ 611
Alka-Seltzer Plus Sinus Medicine .. ▣ 611
Ascriptin .... ▣ 650
Arthritis Strength BC Powder .... ▣ 631
BC Cold Powder Multi-Symptom Formula (Cold-Sinus-Allergy) .... ▣ 631
BC Cold Powder Non-Drowsy Formula (Cold-Sinus) .... ▣ 631
BC Powder .... ▣ 631
Genuine Bayer Aspirin Tablets & Caplets .... ▣ 618
Extra Strength Bayer Arthritis Pain Regimen Formula .... ▣ 615
Extra Strength Bayer Aspirin Caplets & Tablets .... ▣ 617
Extended-Release Bayer 8-Hour Aspirin .... ▣ 616
Extra Strength Bayer Plus Aspirin Caplets .... ▣ 617
Extra Strength Bayer PM Aspirin Plus Sleep Aid .... ▣ 617
Aspirin Regimen Bayer 81 mg Tablets with Calcium .... ▣ 615
Aspirin Regimen Bayer Adult Low Strength 81 mg Tablets .... ▣ 613
Aspirin Regimen Bayer Children's Chewable Aspirin .... ▣ 616
Aspirin Regimen Bayer Regular Strength 325 mg Caplets .... ▣ 613
Bufferin Analgesic Tablets .... ▣ 636
Arthritis Strength Bufferin Analgesic Caplets .... ▣ 637
Extra Strength Bufferin Analgesic Tablets .... ▣ 637
Cama Arthritis Pain Reliever .... ▣ 748
Darvon Compound-65 Pulvules 1475
Easprin 1971
Ecotrin 2625
Ecotrin Enteric Coated Aspirin Maximum Strength Tablets and Caplets .... ▣ 775
Ecotrin Enteric Coated Aspirin Regular Strength Tablets 2625
Empirin Aspirin Tablets .... ▣ 818
Excedrin Extra-Strength Analgesic Tablets, Caplets, and Geltabs 734
Fiorinal Capsules 2388
Fiorinal with Codeine Capsules 2390
Fiorinal Tablets 2388
Goody's Extra Strength Headache Powders .... ▣ 632
Goody's Extra Strength Pain Relief Tablets .... ▣ 632
Halfprin Tablets 1413
Norgesic 1554
Percodan Tablets 955
Percodan-Demi Tablets 956
Robaxisal Tablets 2246
Soma Compound w/Codeine Tablets 2784
Soma Compound Tablets 2783
St. Joseph Adult Chewable Aspirin (81 mg.) .... ▣ 768
Talwin Compound 2466
Vanquish Analgesic Caplets .... ▣ 627

Dicumarol (Corticosteroid may alter the response to coumarin anticoagulant).
No products indexed under this heading.

Ephedrine (May enhance the metabolic clearance of dexamethasone, resulting in decreased blood levels and lessened physiologic activity).

Ephedrine Hydrochloride (May enhance the metabolic clearance of dexamethasone, resulting in decreased blood levels and lessened physiologic activity). Products include:
Primatene Tablets .... ▣ 844
Quadrinal Tablets 1398

Ephedrine Sulfate (May enhance the metabolic clearance of dexamethasone, resulting in decreased blood levels and lessened physiologic activity). Products include:
Marax Tablets & DF Syrup 2015

Phenobarbital (May enhance the metabolic clearance of dexamethasone, resulting in decreased blood levels and lessened physiologic activity). Products include:
Arco-Lase Plus Tablets 513
Bellergal-S Tablets 2375
Donnatal 2234
Donnatal Extentabs 2234
Donnatal Tablets 2234
Phenobarbital Elixir and Tablets 1523
Quadrinal Tablets 1398

Phenytoin (May enhance the metabolic clearance of dexamethasone, resulting in decreased blood levels and lessened physiologic activity). Products include:
Dilantin Infatabs 1967
Dilantin-125 Suspension 1969

Phenytoin Sodium (May enhance the metabolic clearance of dexamethasone, resulting in decreased blood levels and lessened physiologic activity). Products include:
Dilantin Kapseals 1965

Rifampin (May enhance the metabolic clearance of dexamethasone, resulting in decreased blood levels and lessened physiologic activity). Products include:
Rifadin 1276
Rifamate Capsules 1278
Rifater 1280
Rimactane Capsules 865

Smallpox Vaccine (The expected serum antibody response may not be obtained in individuals receiving immunosuppressive doses of corticosteroid).

Spironolactone (Potential for hypokalemia). Products include:
Aldactazide Tablets 2556
Aldactone Tablets 2558

Triamterene (Potential for hypokalemia). Products include:
Dyazide Capsules 2653
Dyrenium Capsules 2655

Warfarin Sodium (Corticosteroid may alter the response to coumarin anticoagulant). Products include:
Coumadin 941

DEXACORT PHOSPHATE IN TURBINAIRE
(Dexamethasone Sodium Phosphate) 1607
May interact with oral anticoagulants, potassium sparing diuretics, and certain other agents. Compounds in these categories include:

Amiloride Hydrochloride (Potential for hypokalemia). Products include:
Midamor Tablets 1746
Moduretic Tablets 1748

Aspirin (Aspirin should be used cautiously in conjunction with Dexacort in hypoprothrombinemia). Products include:
Alka-Seltzer Cherry Effervescent Antacid and Pain Reliever .... ▣ 609
Alka-Seltzer Extra Strength Effervescent Antacid and Pain Reliever .... ▣ 609
Alka-Seltzer Lemon Lime Effervescent Antacid and Pain Reliever .... ▣ 609
Alka-Seltzer Original Effervescent Antacid and Pain Reliever .... ▣ 609
Alka-Seltzer Plus .... ▣ 611
Alka-Seltzer Plus Sinus Medicine .. ▣ 611
Ascriptin .... ▣ 650
Arthritis Strength BC Powder .... ▣ 631
BC Cold Powder Multi-Symptom Formula (Cold-Sinus-Allergy) .... ▣ 631
BC Cold Powder Non-Drowsy Formula (Cold-Sinus) .... ▣ 631
BC Powder .... ▣ 631
Genuine Bayer Aspirin Tablets & Caplets .... ▣ 618
Extra Strength Bayer Arthritis Pain Regimen Formula .... ▣ 615
Extra Strength Bayer Aspirin Caplets & Tablets .... ▣ 617
Extended-Release Bayer 8-Hour Aspirin .... ▣ 616
Extra Strength Bayer Plus Aspirin Caplets .... ▣ 617
Extra Strength Bayer PM Aspirin Plus Sleep Aid .... ▣ 617
Aspirin Regimen Bayer 81 mg Tablets with Calcium .... ▣ 615
Aspirin Regimen Bayer Adult Low Strength 81 mg Tablets .... ▣ 613
Aspirin Regimen Bayer Children's Chewable Aspirin .... ▣ 616
Aspirin Regimen Bayer Regular Strength 325 mg Caplets .... ▣ 613
Bufferin Analgesic Tablets .... ▣ 636
Arthritis Strength Bufferin Analgesic Caplets .... ▣ 637
Extra Strength Bufferin Analgesic Tablets .... ▣ 637
Cama Arthritis Pain Reliever .... ▣ 748
Darvon Compound-65 Pulvules 1475
Easprin 1971
Ecotrin 2625
Ecotrin Enteric Coated Aspirin Maximum Strength Tablets and Caplets .... ▣ 775
Ecotrin Enteric Coated Aspirin Regular Strength Tablets 2625
Empirin Aspirin Tablets .... ▣ 818
Excedrin Extra-Strength Analgesic Tablets, Caplets, and Geltabs 734
Fiorinal Capsules 2388
Fiorinal with Codeine Capsules 2390
Fiorinal Tablets 2388
Goody's Extra Strength Headache Powders .... ▣ 632
Goody's Extra Strength Pain Relief Tablets .... ▣ 632
Halfprin Tablets 1413
Norgesic 1554
Percodan Tablets 955
Percodan-Demi Tablets 956
Robaxisal Tablets 2246
Soma Compound w/Codeine Tablets 2784
Soma Compound Tablets 2783
St. Joseph Adult Chewable Aspirin (81 mg.) .... ▣ 768
Talwin Compound 2466
Vanquish Analgesic Caplets .... ▣ 627

(▣ Described in PDR For Nonprescription Drugs) (⊙ Described in PDR For Ophthalmology)

Dicumarol (Corticosteroid may alter the response to coumarin anticoagulant).

No products indexed under this heading.

Ephedrine (May enhance the metabolic clearance of dexamethasone, resulting in decreased blood levels and lessened physiologic activity).

Ephedrine Hydrochloride (May enhance the metabolic clearance of dexamethasone, resulting in decreased blood levels and lessened physiologic activity). Products include:

Primatene Tablets ... 844
Quadrinal Tablets ... 1398

Ephedrine Sulfate (May enhance the metabolic clearance of dexamethasone, resulting in decreased blood levels and lessened physiologic activity). Products include:

Marax Tablets & DF Syrup ... 2015

Phenobarbital (May enhance the metabolic clearance of dexamethasone, resulting in decreased blood levels and lessened physiologic activity). Products include:

Arco-Lase Plus Tablets ... 513
Bellergal-S Tablets ... 2375
Donnatal ... 2234
Donnatal Extentabs ... 2234
Donnatal Tablets ... 2234
Phenobarbital Elixir and Tablets ... 1523
Quadrinal Tablets ... 1398

Phenytoin (May enhance the metabolic clearance of dexamethasone, resulting in decreased blood levels and lessened physiologic activity). Products include:

Dilantin Infatabs ... 1967
Dilantin-125 Suspension ... 1969

Phenytoin Sodium (May enhance the metabolic clearance of dexamethasone, resulting in decreased blood levels and lessened physiologic activity). Products include:

Dilantin Kapseals ... 1965

Rifampin (May enhance the metabolic clearance of dexamethasone, resulting in decreased blood levels and lessened physiologic activity). Products include:

Rifadin ... 1276
Rifamate Capsules ... 1278
Rifater ... 1280
Rimactane Capsules ... 865

Smallpox Vaccine (The expected serum antibody response may not be obtained in individuals receiving immunosuppressive doses of corticosteroid).

Spironolactone (Potential for hypokalemia). Products include:

Aldactazide Tablets ... 2556
Aldactone Tablets ... 2558

Triamterene (Potential for hypokalemia). Products include:

Dyazide Capsules ... 2653
Dyrenium Capsules ... 2655

Warfarin Sodium (Corticosteroid may alter the response to coumarin anticoagulant). Products include:

Coumadin ... 941

DEXATRIM MAXIMUM STRENGTH CAFFEINE-FREE CAPLETS

(Phenylpropanolamine Hydrochloride) ... 795

May interact with monoamine oxidase inhibitors. Compounds in this category include:

Furazolidone (Concurrent and/or sequential use is not recommended). Products include:

Furoxone ... 2221

Isocarboxazid (Concurrent and/or sequential use is not recommended).

No products indexed under this heading.

Phenelzine Sulfate (Concurrent and/or sequential use is not recommended). Products include:

Nardil ... 1977

Phenylpropanolamine Containing Anorectics (Concurrent use with phenylpropanolamine-containing products should be avoided).

Selegiline Hydrochloride (Concurrent and/or sequential use is not recommended). Products include:

Eldepryl Capsules ... 2729

Tranylcypromine Sulfate (Concurrent and/or sequential use is not recommended). Products include:

Parnate Tablets ... 2679

DEXATRIM MAXIMUM STRENGTH EXTENDED DURATION TIME TABLETS

(Phenylpropanolamine Hydrochloride) ... 795

See **Dexatrim Maximum Strength Caffeine-Free Caplets**

DEXATRIM MAXIMUM STRENGTH PLUS VITAMIN C/CAFFEINE-FREE CAPLETS

(Phenylpropanolamine Hydrochloride, Vitamin C) ... 795

See **Dexatrim Maximum Strength Caffeine-Free Caplets**

DEXATRIM PLUS VITAMINS CAPLETS

(Phenylpropanolamine Hydrochloride, Vitamins with Minerals) ... 796

May interact with monoamine oxidase inhibitors and certain other agents. Compounds in these categories include:

Furazolidone (Concurrent and/or sequential use is not recommended). Products include:

Furoxone ... 2221

Isocarboxazid (Concurrent and/or sequential use is not recommended).

No products indexed under this heading.

Phenelzine Sulfate (Concurrent and/or sequential use is not recommended). Products include:

Nardil ... 1977

Phenylpropanolamine (Concurrent use with any form of phenylpropanolamine is not recommended).

Selegiline Hydrochloride (Concurrent and/or sequential use is not recommended). Products include:

Eldepryl Capsules ... 2729

Tranylcypromine Sulfate (Concurrent and/or sequential use is not recommended). Products include:

Parnate Tablets ... 2679

DEXEDRINE SPANSULE CAPSULES

(Dextroamphetamine Sulfate) ... 2648

May interact with monoamine oxidase inhibitors, tricyclic antidepressants, antihistamines, antihypertensives, beta blockers, veratrum alkaloids, thiazides, urinary alkalizing agents, and certain other agents. Compounds in these categories include:

Acebutolol Hydrochloride (Amphetamine may antagonize the hypotensive effects of antihypertensives; adrenergic blockers are inhibited by amphetamines). Products include:

Sectral Capsules ... 2914

Acetazolamide (Increases the concentration of the non-ionized species of the amphetamine molecule, thereby decreasing urinary excretion; increases amphetamines blood levels and thereby potentiates the actions of amphetamines). Products include:

Diamox Sequels (Sustained Release) ... ◉ 318
Diamox Tablets ... ◉ 317

Acetazolamide Sodium (Increases the concentration of the non-ionized species of the amphetamine molecule, thereby decreasing urinary excretion; increases amphetamines blood levels and thereby potentiates the actions of amphetamines). Products include:

Diamox Intravenous ... ◉ 317

Acrivastine (Amphetamines may counteract the sedative effect of antihistamine). Products include:

Semprex-D Capsules ... 1620

Amitriptyline Hydrochloride (Enhanced activity of tricyclic or sympathomimetics; possible increases in the brain concentration of d-amphetamine in the brain; cardiovascular effect may be potentiated). Products include:

Elavil ... 2945
Etrafon ... 2495
Limbitrol ... 2333
Triavil Tablets ... 1800

Amlodipine Besylate (Amphetamine may antagonize the hypotensive effects of antihypertensives). Products include:

Lotrel Capsules ... 858
Norvasc Tablets ... 2020

Ammonium Chloride (Increases the concentration of the ionized species of the amphetamine molecule, thereby increasing urinary excretion; lowers amphetamines blood levels and efficacy).

No products indexed under this heading.

Amoxapine (Enhanced activity of tricyclic or sympathomimetics; possible increases in the brain concentration of d-amphetamine in the brain; cardiovascular effect may be potentiated). Products include:

Asendin Tablets ... 1419

Astemizole (Amphetamines may counteract the sedative effect of antihistamine). Products include:

Hismanal Tablets ... 1341

Atenolol (Amphetamine may antagonize the hypotensive effects of antihypertensives; adrenergic blockers are inhibited by amphetamines). Products include:

Tenoretic Tablets ... 2963
Tenormin Tablets and I.V. Injection 2965

Azatadine Maleate (Amphetamines may counteract the sedative effect of antihistamine). Products include:

Trinalin Repetabs Tablets ... 1373

Benazepril Hydrochloride (Amphetamine may antagonize the hypotensive effects of antihypertensives). Products include:

Lotensin Tablets ... 852
Lotensin HCT Tablets ... 855
Lotrel Capsules ... 858

Bendroflumethiazide (Increases the concentration of the non-ionized species of the amphetamine molecule, thereby decreasing urinary excretion; increases amphetamines blood levels and thereby potentiates the actions of amphetamines).

No products indexed under this heading.

Betaxolol Hydrochloride (Amphetamine may antagonize the hypotensive effects of antihypertensives; adrenergic blockers are inhibited by amphetamines). Products include:

Betoptic Ophthalmic Solution ... 465
Betoptic S Ophthalmic Suspension 467
Kerlone Tablets ... 2588

Bisoprolol Fumarate (Amphetamine may antagonize the hypotensive effects of antihypertensives; adrenergic blockers are inhibited by amphetamines). Products include:

Zebeta Tablets ... 1457
Ziac ... 1459

Bromodiphenhydramine Hydrochloride (Amphetamines may counteract the sedative effect of antihistamine).

No products indexed under this heading.

Brompheniramine Maleate (Amphetamines may counteract the sedative effect of antihistamine). Products include:

Alka-Seltzer Plus Sinus Medicine ... 611
Bromfed Capsules (Extended-Release) ... 1832
Bromfed Syrup ... 712
Bromfed Tablets ... 1832
Bromfed-DM Cough Syrup ... 1832
Bromfed-PD Capsules (Extended-Release) ... 1832
Dimetane-DC Cough Syrup ... 2232
Dimetane-DX Cough Syrup ... 2233
Dimetapp Allergy Dye-Free Elixir ... 838
Dimetapp Allergy Sinus Caplets ... 838
Dimetapp Cold & Allergy Chewable Tablets ... 838
Dimetapp Cold & Cough Liqui-Gels ... 839
Dimetapp Cold & Fever Suspension ... 839
Dimetapp DM Elixir ... 840
Dimetapp Elixir ... 840
Dimetapp Extentabs ... 841
Dimetapp Tablets/Liqui-Gels ... 841
Rondec Chewable Tablets ... 974
Vicks DayQuil Allergy Relief 12-Hour Extended Release Tablets ... 733
Vicks DayQuil Allergy Relief 4-Hour Tablets ... 733

Captopril (Amphetamine may antagonize the hypotensive effects of antihypertensives). Products include:

Capoten Tablets ... 740
Capozide Tablets ... 744

Carteolol Hydrochloride (Amphetamine may antagonize the hypotensive effects of antihypertensives; adrenergic blockers are inhibited by amphetamines). Products include:

Cartrol Tablets ... 413
Ocupress Ophthalmic Solution, 1% Sterile ... ◉ 297

Cetirizine Hydrochloride (Amphetamines may counteract the sedative effect of antihistamine). Products include:

Zyrtec Tablets ... 2053

Chlorothiazide (Increases the concentration of the non-ionized species of the amphetamine molecule, thereby decreasing urinary excretion; increases amphetamines blood levels and thereby potentiates the actions of amphetamines). Products include:

Aldoclor Tablets ... 1638
Diupres Tablets ... 1691
Diuril Oral ... 1694

IMPORTANT NOTE: Always consult each drug listing in the patient's regimen for possible interactions.

Chlorothiazide Sodium (Increases the concentration of the non-ionized species of the amphetamine molecule, thereby decreasing urinary excretion; increases amphetamines blood levels and thereby potentiates the actions of amphetamines). Products include:

- Diuril Sodium Intravenous ... 1693

Chlorpheniramine Maleate (Amphetamines may counteract the sedative effect of antihistamine). Products include:

- Alka-Seltzer Plus Cold Medicine ... ▣ 611
- Alka-Seltzer Plus Cold Medicine Liqui-Gels ... ▣ 612
- Alka-Seltzer Plus Cold & Cough Medicine ... ▣ 611
- Alka-Seltzer Plus Cold & Cough Medicine Liqui-Gels ... ▣ 612
- Alka-Seltzer Plus Flu & Body Aches Effervescent Tablets ... ▣ 612
- Allerest Maximum Strength ... ▣ 649
- Allerest Sinus Pain Formula ... ▣ 649
- Ana-Kit Anaphylaxis Emergency Treatment Kit ... 611
- Atrohist Pediatric Capsules ... 1603
- Atrohist Plus Tablets ... 1605
- BC Cold Powder Multi-Symptom Formula (Cold-Sinus-Allergy) ... ▣ 631
- Cerose DM ... ▣ 853
- Cheracol Plus Head Cold/Cough Formula ... ▣ 741
- Children's TYLENOL Cold Multi-Symptom Chewable Tablets and Liquid ... 1559
- Children's TYLENOL Cold Plus Cough Multi Symptom Chewable Tablets and Liquid ... 1560
- Children's TYLENOL Flu Suspension Liquid ... 1560
- Children's Vicks DayQuil Allergy Relief ... ▣ 730
- Children's Vicks NyQuil Cold/Cough Relief ... ▣ 731
- Chlor-Trimeton Allergy Decongestant Tablets ... ▣ 759
- Chlor-Trimeton Allergy Tablets ... ▣ 758
- Allergy-Sinus Comtrex Multi-Symptom Allergy-Sinus Formula Tablets and Caplets ... ▣ 639
- Comtrex Multi-Symptom ... ▣ 638
- Contac Continuous Action Nasal Decongestant/Antihistamine 12 Hour Capsules ... ▣ 773
- Contac Maximum Strength Continuous Action Decongestant/Antihistamine 12 Hour Caplets ... ▣ 772
- Contac Severe Cold and Flu Formula Caplets ... ▣ 773
- Coricidin Cold + Flu Tablets ... ▣ 760
- Coricidin Cough + Cold Tablets ... ▣ 760
- Coricidin 'D' Decongestant Tablets ... ▣ 760
- D.A. II Tablets ... 972
- D.A. Chewable Tablets ... 970
- Dura-Tap/PD Capsules ... 970
- Dura-Vent/DA Tablets ... 972
- Efidac 24 Chlorpheniramine ... ▣ 655
- Extendryl ... 1003
- Fedahist Gyrocaps ... 2545
- Hycomine Compound Tablets ... 948
- Kronofed-A ... 994
- Nolamine Timed-Release Tablets ... 790
- Novahistine Elixir ... ▣ 782
- Ornade Spansule Capsules ... 2678
- PediaCare Cough-Cold Chewable Tablets and Liquid ... 1569
- PediaCare NightRest Cough-Cold Liquid ... 1569
- Pediatric Vicks 44m Cough & Cold Relief ... ▣ 737
- Pyrroxate Caplets ... ▣ 742
- Ryna ... ▣ 804
- Sinarest ... ▣ 663
- Sine-Off Sinus Medicine ... ▣ 784
- Singlet Tablets ... ▣ 785
- Sinulin Tablets ... 792
- Sinutab Sinus Allergy Medication, Maximum Strength Tablets and Caplets ... ▣ 823
- Sudafed Cold & Allergy Tablets ... ▣ 826
- Teldrin 12 Hour Antihistamine/Nasal Decongestant Allergy Relief Capsules ... ▣ 786
- TheraFlu Flu and Cold Medicine ... ▣ 750
- Theraflu Maximum Strength Flu and Cold Medicine For Sore Throat ... ▣ 751
- TheraFlu Flu, Cold and Cough Medicine ... ▣ 750
- TheraFlu Maximum Strength Nighttime Flu, Cold & Cough Medicine ... ▣ 751
- Triaminic Night Time ... ▣ 754
- Triaminic Syrup ... ▣ 755
- Triaminic Triaminicol Cold & Cough ... ▣ 756
- Triaminicin Tablets ... ▣ 756
- Tussend ... 1830
- TYLENOL Allergy Sinus, Maximum Strength Caplets and Gelcaps ... 1571
- TYLENOL Cold Medication, Multi-Symptom Formula Tablets and Caplets ... 1572
- TYLENOL Cold Medication, Multi-Symptom Hot Liquid Packets ... 1572
- Vicks 44 LiquiCaps Cough, Cold & Flu Relief ... ▣ 728
- Vicks 44M Cough, Cold & Flu Relief ... ▣ 729

Chlorpheniramine Polistirex (Amphetamines may counteract the sedative effect of antihistamine). Products include:

- Tussionex Pennkinetic Extended-Release Suspension ... 1624

Chlorpheniramine Tannate (Amphetamines may counteract the sedative effect of antihistamine). Products include:

- Atrohist Pediatric Suspension ... 1604
- Atrohist Pediatric Suspension Dye-Free ... 1604
- Rynatan ... 2781
- Rynatuss ... 2782

Chlorpromazine (Blocks dopamine and norepinephrine reuptake resulting in inhibition of central stimulating effects). Products include:

- Thorazine Suppositories ... 2701

Chlorpromazine Hydrochloride (Blocks dopamine and norepinephrine reuptake resulting in inhibition of central stimulating effects). Products include:

- Thorazine ... 2701

Chlorthalidone (Amphetamine may antagonize the hypotensive effects of antihypertensives). Products include:

- Combipres Tablets ... 682
- Tenoretic Tablets ... 2963
- Thalitone ... 1293

Clemastine Fumarate (Amphetamines may counteract the sedative effect of antihistamine). Products include:

- Tavist Syrup ... 2426
- Tavist Tablets ... 2427
- Tavist-1 12 Hour Relief Tablets ... ▣ 749
- Tavist-D 12 Hour Relief Tablets ... ▣ 750

Clomipramine Hydrochloride (Enhanced activity of tricyclic or sympathomimetics; possible increases in the brain concentration of d-amphetamine in the brain; cardiovascular effect may be potentiated). Products include:

- Anafranil Capsules ... 819

Clonidine (Amphetamine may antagonize the hypotensive effects of antihypertensives). Products include:

- Catapres-TTS ... 680

Clonidine Hydrochloride (Amphetamine may antagonize the hypotensive effects of antihypertensives). Products include:

- Catapres Tablets ... 679
- Combipres Tablets ... 682

Cryptenamine Preparations (Amphetamines inhibit the hypotensive effect of veratrum alkaloids).

Cyproheptadine Hydrochloride (Amphetamines may counteract the sedative effect of antihistamine). Products include:

- Periactin ... 1767

Deserpidine (Amphetamine may antagonize the hypotensive effects of antihypertensives).

No products indexed under this heading.

Desipramine Hydrochloride (Enhanced activity of tricyclic or sympathomimetics; possible increases in the brain concentration of d-amphetamine in the brain; cardiovascular effect may be potentiated). Products include:

- Norpramin Tablets ... 1273

Dexchlorpheniramine Maleate (Amphetamines may counteract the sedative effect of antihistamine).

No products indexed under this heading.

Diazoxide (Amphetamine may antagonize the hypotensive effects of antihypertensives). Products include:

- Hyperstat I.V. Injection ... 2504
- Proglycem ... 575

Diltiazem Hydrochloride (Amphetamine may antagonize the hypotensive effects of antihypertensives). Products include:

- Cardizem CD Capsules ... 1251
- Cardizem SR Capsules ... 1255
- Cardizem Injectable ... 1253
- Cardizem Tablets ... 1257
- Dilacor XR Extended-release Capsules ... 2183
- Tiazac Capsules ... 1019

Diphenhydramine Citrate (Amphetamines may counteract the sedative effect of antihistamine). Products include:

- Excedrin P.M. Analgesic/Sleeping Aid Tablets, Caplets, Liquigels ... 735

Diphenhydramine Hydrochloride (Amphetamines may counteract the sedative effect of antihistamine). Products include:

- Actifed Allergy Daytime/Nighttime Caplets ... ▣ 808
- Actifed Sinus Daytime/Nighttime Tablets and Caplets ... ▣ 809
- Extra Strength Bayer PM Aspirin Plus Sleep Aid ... ▣ 617
- Benadryl Allergy Chewables ... ▣ 811
- Benadryl Allergy/Cold Tablets ... ▣ 811
- Benadryl Allergy Decongestant Liquid Medication ... ▣ 812
- Benadryl Allergy Decongestant Tablets ... ▣ 812
- Benadryl Allergy Liquid Medication ... ▣ 813
- Benadryl Allergy ... ▣ 811
- Benadryl Allergy Sinus Headache Caplets ... ▣ 813
- Benadryl Dye-Free Allergy Liqui-gel Softgels ... ▣ 813
- Benadryl Dye-Free Allergy Liquid Medication ... ▣ 814
- Benadryl Itch Relief Stick Extra Strength ... ▣ 814
- Benadryl Cream ... ▣ 814
- Benadryl Gel ... ▣ 815
- Benadryl Spray ... ▣ 815
- Benadryl Injection ... 1955
- Contac Day & Night Cold/Flu Night Caplets ... ▣ 772
- Contac Night Allergy/Sinus Caplets ... ▣ 771
- Extra Strength Doan's P.M. ... ▣ 653
- Excedrin P.M. Analgesic/Sleeping Aid Tablets, Caplets, Liquigels ... ▣ 643
- Nytol QuickCaps Caplets ... ▣ 632
- Sleepinal Night-time Sleep Aid Capsules and Softgels ... ▣ 798
- TYLENOL Allergy Sinus NightTime, Maximum Strength Caplets ... 1571
- TYLENOL Flu NightTime, Maximum Strength Gelcaps ... 1575
- TYLENOL Flu NightTime, Maximum Strength Hot Medication Packets ... 1575
- TYLENOL PM Pain Reliever/Sleep Aid, Extra Strength Gelcaps, Caplets, Geltabs ... 1576
- TYLENOL Severe Allergy Medication Caplets ... 1571
- Maximum Strength Unisom Sleepgels ... 1990
- Unisom With Pain Relief-Nighttime Sleep Aid and Pain Reliever ... 1991

Diphenylpyraline Hydrochloride (Amphetamines may counteract the sedative effect of antihistamine).

No products indexed under this heading.

Doxazosin Mesylate (Amphetamine may antagonize the hypotensive effects of antihypertensives). Products include:

- Cardura Tablets ... 1993

Doxepin Hydrochloride (Enhanced activity of tricyclic or sympathomimetics; possible increases in the brain concentration of d-amphetamine in the brain; cardiovascular effect may be potentiated). Products include:

- Adapin Capsules ... 1542
- Sinequan ... 2028
- Zonalon Cream ... 1042

Enalapril Maleate (Amphetamine may antagonize the hypotensive effects of antihypertensives). Products include:

- Vaseretic Tablets ... 1810
- Vasotec Tablets ... 1816

Enalaprilat (Amphetamine may antagonize the hypotensive effects of antihypertensives). Products include:

- Vasotec I.V. ... 1814

Esmolol Hydrochloride (Amphetamine may antagonize the hypotensive effects of antihypertensives; adrenergic blockers are inhibited by amphetamines). Products include:

- Brevibloc (esmolol HCl) Injection ... 1860

Ethosuximide (Amphetamine may delay intestinal absorption of ethosuximide). Products include:

- Zarontin Capsules ... 1986
- Zarontin Syrup ... 1986

Felodipine (Amphetamine may antagonize the hypotensive effects of antihypertensives). Products include:

- Plendil Extended-Release Tablets ... 514

Fosinopril Sodium (Amphetamine may antagonize the hypotensive effects of antihypertensives). Products include:

- Monopril Tablets ... 762

Furazolidone (Concurrent and/or sequential use is contraindicated; hypertensive crisis may result). Products include:

- Furoxone ... 2221

Furosemide (Amphetamine may antagonize the hypotensive effects of antihypertensives). Products include:

- Lasix Injection, Oral Solution and Tablets ... 1267

Glutamic Acid Hydrochloride (Lowers absorption of amphetamines).

No products indexed under this heading.

Guanabenz Acetate (Amphetamine may antagonize the hypotensive effects of antihypertensives).

No products indexed under this heading.

Guanethidine Monosulfate (Lowers absorption of amphetamines). Products include:

- Esimil Tablets ... 840
- Ismelin Tablets ... 845

Haloperidol (Blocks dopamine and norepinephrine reuptake resulting in inhibition of central stimulating effects). Products include:

- Haldol Injection, Tablets and Concentrate ... 1585

(▣ Described in PDR For Nonprescription Drugs) (◉ Described in PDR For Ophthalmology)

Haloperidol Decanoate (Blocks dopamine and norepinephrine reuptake resulting in inhibition of central stimulating effects). Products include:
Haldol Decanoate 1587

Hydralazine Hydrochloride (Amphetamine may antagonize the hypotensive effects of antihypertensives). Products include:
Apresazide Capsules 824
Apresoline Hydrochloride Tablets .. 826
Hydralazine Hydrochloride Injection USP 2712
Ser-Ap-Es Tablets 867

Hydrochlorothiazide (Increases the concentration of the non-ionized species of the amphetamine molecule, thereby decreasing urinary excretion; increases amphetamines blood levels and thereby potentiates the actions of amphetamines). Products include:
Aldactazide Tablets 2556
Aldoril Tablets 1644
Apresazide Capsules 824
Capozide Tablets 744
Dyazide Capsules 2653
Esidrix Tablets 839
Esimil Tablets 840
HydroDIURIL Tablets 1716
Hydropres Tablets 1718
Hyzaar Tablets 1720
Inderide Tablets 2838
Inderide LA Long Acting Capsules .. 2840
Lopressor HCT Tablets 850
Lotensin HCT Tablets 855
Moduretic Tablets 1748
Oretic Tablets 450
Prinzide Tablets 1780
Ser-Ap-Es Tablets 867
Timolide Tablets 1791
Vaseretic Tablets 1810
Zestoretic Tablets 2968
Ziac 1459

Hydroflumethiazide (Increases the concentration of the non-ionized species of the amphetamine molecule, thereby decreasing urinary excretion; increases amphetamines blood levels and thereby potentiates the actions of amphetamines). Products include:
Diucardin Tablets 2824

Imipramine Hydrochloride (Enhanced activity of tricyclic or sympathomimetics; possible increases in the brain concentration of d-amphetamine in the brain; cardiovascular effect may be potentiated). Products include:
Tofranil Ampuls 873
Tofranil Tablets 875

Imipramine Pamoate (Enhanced activity of tricyclic or sympathomimetics; possible increases in the brain concentration of d-amphetamine in the brain; cardiovascular effect may be potentiated). Products include:
Tofranil-PM Capsules 876

Indapamide (Amphetamine may antagonize the hypotensive effects of antihypertensives).
No products indexed under this heading.

Isocarboxazid (Concurrent and/or sequential use is contraindicated; hypertensive crisis may result).
No products indexed under this heading.

Isradipine (Amphetamine may antagonize the hypotensive effects of antihypertensives). Products include:
DynaCirc Capsules 2381
DynaCirc CR Tablets 2383

Labetalol Hydrochloride (Amphetamine may antagonize the hypotensive effects of antihypertensives; adrenergic blockers are inhibited by amphetamines). Products include:
Normodyne Injection 2519
Normodyne Tablets 2522
Trandate 1158

Levobunolol Hydrochloride (Amphetamine may antagonize the hypotensive effects of antihypertensives; adrenergic blockers are inhibited by amphetamines). Products include:
Betagan ⊙ 230

Lisinopril (Amphetamine may antagonize the hypotensive effects of antihypertensives). Products include:
Prinivil Tablets 1776
Prinzide Tablets 1780
Zestoretic Tablets 2968
Zestril Tablets 2972

Lithium Carbonate (Inhibits antiobesity and stimulatory effects of amphetamines). Products include:
Eskalith 2658
Lithium Carbonate Capsules & Tablets 2352
Lithonate/Lithotabs/Lithobid 2721

Loratadine (Amphetamines may counteract the sedative effect of antihistamine). Products include:
Claritin Tablets 2485
Claritin-D Tablets 2487

Losartan Potassium (Amphetamine may antagonize the hypotensive effects of antihypertensives). Products include:
Cozaar Tablets 1668
Hyzaar Tablets 1720

Maprotiline Hydrochloride (Enhanced activity of tricyclic or sympathomimetics; possible increases in the brain concentration of d-amphetamine in the brain; cardiovascular effect may be potentiated). Products include:
Ludiomil Tablets 861

Mecamylamine Hydrochloride (Amphetamine may antagonize the hypotensive effects of antihypertensives). Products include:
Inversine Tablets 1729

Meperidine Hydrochloride (Amphetamine potentiates the analgesic effect of meperidine). Products include:
Demerol 2438
Mepergan Injection 2859

Methdilazine Hydrochloride (Amphetamines may counteract the sedative effect of antihistamine).
No products indexed under this heading.

Methenamine (Acidifying agents used in methenamine therapy increases the urinary excretion and reduces the efficacy of amphetamine). Products include:
Urised Tablets 2123

Methenamine Hippurate (Acidifying agents used in methenamine therapy increases the urinary excretion and reduces the efficacy of amphetamine).
No products indexed under this heading.

Methenamine Mandelate (Acidifying agents used in methenamine therapy increases the urinary excretion and reduces the efficacy of amphetamine). Products include:
Uroqid-Acid No. 2 Tablets 633

Methyclothiazide (Increases the concentration of the non-ionized species of the amphetamine molecule, thereby decreasing urinary excretion; increases amphetamines blood levels and thereby potentiates the actions of amphetamines). Products include:
Enduron Tablets 424

Methyldopa (Amphetamine may antagonize the hypotensive effects of antihypertensives). Products include:
Aldoclor Tablets 1638
Aldomet Oral 1640
Aldoril Tablets 1644

Methyldopate Hydrochloride (Amphetamine may antagonize the hypotensive effects of antihypertensives). Products include:
Aldomet Ester HCl Injection 1642

Metipranolol Hydrochloride (Amphetamine may antagonize the hypotensive effects of antihypertensives; adrenergic blockers are inhibited by amphetamines). Products include:
OptiPranolol (Metipranolol 0.3%) Sterile Ophthalmic Solution ⊙ 256

Metolazone (Amphetamine may antagonize the hypotensive effects of antihypertensives). Products include:
Mykrox Tablets 1617
Zaroxolyn Tablets 1625

Metoprolol Succinate (Amphetamine may antagonize the hypotensive effects of antihypertensives; adrenergic blockers are inhibited by amphetamines). Products include:
Toprol-XL Tablets 560

Metoprolol Tartrate (Amphetamine may antagonize the hypotensive effects of antihypertensives; adrenergic blockers are inhibited by amphetamines). Products include:
Lopressor 848
Lopressor HCT Tablets 850

Metyrosine (Amphetamine may antagonize the hypotensive effects of antihypertensives). Products include:
Demser Capsules 1690

Minoxidil (Amphetamine may antagonize the hypotensive effects of antihypertensives).
No products indexed under this heading.

Moexipril Hydrochloride (Amphetamine may antagonize the hypotensive effects of antihypertensives). Products include:
Univasc Tablets 2553

Nadolol (Amphetamine may antagonize the hypotensive effects of antihypertensives; adrenergic blockers are inhibited by amphetamines).
No products indexed under this heading.

Nicardipine Hydrochloride (Amphetamine may antagonize the hypotensive effects of antihypertensives). Products include:
Cardene Capsules 2261
Cardene I.V. 2815
Cardene SR Capsules 2264

Nifedipine (Amphetamine may antagonize the hypotensive effects of antihypertensives). Products include:
Adalat Capsules (10 mg and 20 mg) 580
Adalat CC 582
Procardia Capsules 2024
Procardia XL Extended Release Tablets 2026

Nisoldipine (Amphetamine may antagonize the hypotensive effects of antihypertensives). Products include:
Sular Tablets 2961

Nitroglycerin (Amphetamine may antagonize the hypotensive effects of antihypertensives). Products include:
Deponit NTG Transdermal Delivery System 2541
Nitro-Bid IV 1270
Nitro-Bid Ointment 1272
Nitro-Dur (nitroglycerin) Transdermal Infusion System 1365
Nitrolingual Spray 2193
Nitrostat Tablets 1981
Transderm-Nitro Transdermal Therapeutic System 878

Norepinephrine Hydrochloride (Enhances adrenergic effect of norepinephrine).

Nortriptyline Hydrochloride (Enhanced activity of tricyclic or sympathomimetics; possible increases in the brain concentration of d-amphetamine in the brain; cardiovascular effect may be potentiated). Products include:
Pamelor 2409

Penbutolol Sulfate (Amphetamine may antagonize the hypotensive effects of antihypertensives; adrenergic blockers are inhibited by amphetamines). Products include:
Levatol Tablets 2547

Phenelzine Sulfate (Concurrent and/or sequential use is contraindicated; hypertensive crisis may result). Products include:
Nardil 1977

Phenobarbital (Amphetamine delays intestinal absorption of phenobarbital; co-administration may produce synergistic anticonvulsant action). Products include:
Arco-Lase Plus Tablets 513
Bellergal-S Tablets 2375
Donnatal 2234
Donnatal Extentabs 2234
Donnatal Tablets 2234
Phenobarbital Elixir and Tablets 1523
Quadrinal Tablets 1398

Phenoxybenzamine Hydrochloride (Amphetamine may antagonize the hypotensive effects of antihypertensives). Products include:
Dibenzyline Capsules 2650

Phentolamine Mesylate (Amphetamine may antagonize the hypotensive effects of antihypertensives). Products include:
Regitine Vials 864

Phenytoin (Amphetamine delays intestinal absorption of phenytoin; co-administration may produce synergistic anticonvulsant action). Products include:
Dilantin Infatabs 1967
Dilantin-125 Suspension 1969

Phenytoin Sodium (Amphetamine delays intestinal absorption of phenytoin; co-administration may produce synergistic anticonvulsant action). Products include:
Dilantin Kapseals 1965

Pindolol (Amphetamine may antagonize the hypotensive effects of antihypertensives; adrenergic blockers are inhibited by amphetamines). Products include:
Visken Tablets 2428

IMPORTANT NOTE: Always consult each drug listing in the patient's regimen for possible interactions.

Dexedrine **Interactions Index** **266**

Polythiazide (Increases the concentration of the non-ionized species of the amphetamine molecule, thereby decreasing urinary excretion; increases amphetamines blood levels and thereby potentiates the actions of amphetamines). Products include:
- Minizide Capsules 2016

Potassium Citrate (Increases the concentration of the non-ionized species of the amphetamine molecule, thereby decreasing urinary excretion; increases amphetamines blood levels and thereby potentiates the actions of amphetamines). Products include:
- Polycitra Syrup 574
- Polycitra-K Crystals 574
- Polycitra-K Oral Solution 575
- Polycitra-LC 574
- Urocit-K Tablets 1828

Prazosin Hydrochloride (Amphetamine may antagonize the hypotensive effects of antihypertensives). Products include:
- Minipress Capsules 2015
- Minizide Capsules 2016

Promethazine Hydrochloride (Amphetamines may counteract the sedative effect of antihistamine). Products include:
- Mepergan Injection 2859
- Phenergan with Codeine 2883
- Phenergan with Dextromethorphan 2885
- Phenergan Injection 2880
- Phenergan Suppositories 2882
- Phenergan Syrup 2881
- Phenergan Tablets 2882
- Phenergan VC 2886
- Phenergan VC with Codeine 2888

Propoxyphene Hydrochloride (In cases of propoxyphene overdosage, amphetamine CNS stimulation is potentiated and fatal convulsions can occur). Products include:
- Darvon 1475
- Wygesic Tablets 2930

Propoxyphene Napsylate (In cases of propoxyphene overdosage, amphetamine CNS stimulation is potentiated and fatal convulsions can occur). Products include:
- Darvon-N/Darvocet-N 1473

Propranolol Hydrochloride (Amphetamine may antagonize the hypotensive effects of antihypertensives; adrenergic blockers are inhibited by amphetamines). Products include:
- Inderal 2834
- Inderal LA Long Acting Capsules 2836
- Inderide Tablets 2838
- Inderide LA Long Acting Capsules .. 2840

Protriptyline Hydrochloride (Enhanced activity of tricyclic or sympathomimetics; possible increases in the brain concentration of d-amphetamine in the brain; cardiovascular effect may be potentiated). Products include:
- Vivactil Tablets 1820

Pyrilamine Maleate (Amphetamines may counteract the sedative effect of antihistamine). Products include:
- 4-Way Fast Acting Nasal Spray (regular & mentholated) ..... ND 644
- Maximum Strength Multi-Symptom Formula Midol ..... ND 621
- PMS Multi-Symptom Formula Midol ..... ND 622

Pyrilamine Tannate (Amphetamines may counteract the sedative effect of antihistamine). Products include:
- Atrohist Pediatric Suspension 1604
- Atrohist Pediatric Suspension Dye-Free 1604
- Rynatan 2781

Quinapril Hydrochloride (Amphetamine may antagonize the hypotensive effects of antihypertensives). Products include:
- Accupril Tablets 1950

Ramipril (Amphetamine may antagonize the hypotensive effects of antihypertensives). Products include:
- Altace Capsules 1238

Rauwolfia Serpentina (Amphetamine may antagonize the hypotensive effects of antihypertensives).
- No products indexed under this heading.

Rescinnamine (Amphetamine may antagonize the hypotensive effects of antihypertensives).
- No products indexed under this heading.

Reserpine (Lowers absorption of amphetamines). Products include:
- Diupres Tablets 1691
- Hydropres Tablets 1718
- Ser-Ap-Es Tablets 867

Selegiline Hydrochloride (Concurrent and/or sequential use is contraindicated; hypertensive crisis may result). Products include:
- Eldepryl Capsules 2729

Sodium Acid Phosphate (Increases the concentration of the ionized species of the amphetamine molecule, thereby increasing urinary excretion; lowers amphetamines blood levels and efficacy). Products include:
- Uroqid-Acid No. 2 Tablets 633

Sodium Bicarbonate (Increases absorption of amphetamines). Products include:
- Alka-Seltzer Cherry Effervescent Antacid and Pain Reliever ..... ND 609
- Alka-Seltzer Extra Strength Effervescent Antacid and Pain Reliever ..... ND 609
- Alka-Seltzer Gold Effervescent Antacid ..... ND 611
- Alka-Seltzer Lemon Lime Effervescent Antacid and Pain Reliever ..... ND 609
- Alka-Seltzer Original Effervescent Antacid and Pain Reliever ..... ND 609
- Arm & Hammer Pure Baking Soda ..... ND 648
- Colyte and Colyte-flavored 2540
- GoLYTELY 694
- Massengill Disposable Douches ..... ND 780
- Massengill Liquid Concentrate ..... ND 780
- NuLYTELY 694
- Cherry Flavor NuLYTELY 694

Sodium Citrate (Increases the concentration of the non-ionized species of the amphetamine molecule, thereby decreasing urinary excretion; increases amphetamines blood levels and thereby potentiates the actions of amphetamines). Products include:
- Bicitra 573
- Polycitra 574
- Salix SST Lozenges Saliva Stimulant ..... ND 757

Sodium Nitroprusside (Amphetamine may antagonize the hypotensive effects of antihypertensives).
- No products indexed under this heading.

Sotalol Hydrochloride (Amphetamine may antagonize the hypotensive effects of antihypertensives; adrenergic blockers are inhibited by amphetamines). Products include:
- Betapace Tablets 637

Spirapril Hydrochloride (Amphetamine may antagonize the hypotensive effects of antihypertensives).
- No products indexed under this heading.

Terazosin Hydrochloride (Amphetamine may antagonize the hypotensive effects of antihypertensives). Products include:
- Hytrin Capsules 434

Terfenadine (Amphetamines may counteract the sedative effect of antihistamine). Products include:
- Seldane Tablets 1284
- Seldane-D Extended-Release Tablets 1286

Timolol Hemihydrate (Amphetamine may antagonize the hypotensive effects of antihypertensives; adrenergic blockers are inhibited by amphetamines). Products include:
- Betimol 0.25%, 0.5% ..... ⊙ 259

Timolol Maleate (Amphetamine may antagonize the hypotensive effects of antihypertensives; adrenergic blockers are inhibited by amphetamines). Products include:
- Blocadren Tablets 1654
- Timolide Tablets 1791
- Timoptic in Ocudose 1796
- Timoptic Sterile Ophthalmic Solution 1794
- Timoptic-XE 1798

Torsemide (Amphetamine may antagonize the hypotensive effects of antihypertensives). Products include:
- Demadex Tablets and Injection 691

Tranylcypromine Sulfate (Concurrent and/or sequential use is contraindicated; hypertensive crisis may result). Products include:
- Parnate Tablets 2679

Trimeprazine Tartrate (Amphetamines may counteract the sedative effect of antihistamine).
- No products indexed under this heading.

Trimethaphan Camsylate (Amphetamine may antagonize the hypotensive effects of antihypertensives).
- No products indexed under this heading.

Trimipramine Maleate (Enhanced activity of tricyclic or sympathomimetics; possible increases in the brain concentration of d-amphetamine in the brain; cardiovascular effect may be potentiated). Products include:
- Surmontil Capsules 2917

Tripelennamine Hydrochloride (Amphetamines may counteract the sedative effect of antihistamine). Products include:
- PBZ Tablets 863
- PBZ-SR Tablets 862

Triprolidine Hydrochloride (Amphetamines may counteract the sedative effect of antihistamine). Products include:
- Actifed Cold & Allergy Tablets ..... ND 807
- Actifed Cold & Sinus Caplets and Tablets ..... ND 808

Verapamil Hydrochloride (Amphetamine may antagonize the hypotensive effects of antihypertensives). Products include:
- Calan SR Caplets 2571
- Calan Tablets 2568
- Covera-HS Tablets 2573
- Isoptin Injectable 1391
- Isoptin Oral Tablets 1393
- Isoptin SR Tablets 1395
- Verelan Capsules 1455

Vitamin C (Lowers absorption of amphetamines). Products include:
- ACES Antioxidant Soft Gels ..... ND 647
- Chromagen Capsules 2470
- Chromagen FA 2471
- Chromagen Forte 2471
- Dexatrim Maximum Strength Plus Vitamin C/Caffeine-Free Caplets ..... ND 795
- Ester-C Mineral Ascorbates Powder ..... ND 673
- Fero-Folic-500 Filmtab 433
- Fero-Grad-500 Filmtab 434
- Halls Vitamin C Drops ..... ND 807
- Irospan 1000
- Materna Tablets 1427
- Niferex w/Vitamin C Tablets 811
- One-A-Day Antioxidant Plus ..... ND 625
- Protegra Antioxidant Vitamin & Mineral Supplement ..... ND 685
- Sunkist Children's Chewable Multivitamins - Plus Extra C ..... ND 665
- Sunkist Vitamin C ..... ND 666
- Trinsicon Capsules 2759
- Venolax ..... ND 686
- Vitron-C Tablets ..... ND 667

Food Interactions

Fruit juices, unspecified (Lowers absorption of amphetamines).

DEXEDRINE TABLETS
(Dextroamphetamine Sulfate) 2648
See **Dexedrine Spansule Capsules**

DEXTROSTAT-DEXTROAMPHETAMINE SULFATE TABLETS
(Dextroamphetamine Sulfate) 2211
May interact with monoamine oxidase inhibitors, antihypertensives, beta blockers, alpha adrenergic blockers, urinary alkalizing agents, thiazides, tricyclic antidepressants, sympathomimetics, antihistamines, veratrum alkaloids, and certain other agents. Compounds in these categories include:

Acebutolol Hydrochloride (Adrenergic blockers are inhibited by amphetamines; amphetamines may antagonize the hypotensive effects of antihypertensives). Products include:
- Sectral Capsules 2914

Acetazolamide (Increases the concentration of the non-ionized species of the amphetamine molecule thereby decreasing urinary excretion; increases blood levels and potentiates the action of amphetamines). Products include:
- Diamox Sequels (Sustained Release) ..... ⊙ 318
- Diamox Tablets ..... ⊙ 317

Acetazolamide Sodium (Increases the concentration of the non-ionized species of the amphetamine molecule thereby decreasing urinary excretion; increases blood levels and potentiates the action of amphetamines). Products include:
- Diamox Intravenous ..... ⊙ 317

Acrivastine (Amphetamines may counteract the sedative effect of antihistamines). Products include:
- Semprex-D Capsules 1620

Albuterol (Enhanced activity of sympathomimetics). Products include:
- Proventil Inhalation Aerosol 2524
- Ventolin Inhalation Aerosol and Refill 1170

Albuterol Sulfate (Enhanced activity of sympathomimetics). Products include:
- Airet Albuterol Sulfate Inhalation Solution 1602
- Albuterol Sulfate, USP Solution for Inhalation, Arm-a-Med 522
- Proventil Inhalation Solution 0.083% 2527
- Proventil Repetabs Tablets 2529
- Proventil Solution for Inhalation 0.5% 2525
- Proventil Syrup 2528
- Proventil Tablets 2529
- Ventolin Inhalation Solution 1171
- Ventolin Nebules Inhalation Solution 1172
- Ventolin Rotacaps for Inhalation 1173
- Ventolin Syrup 1175

(ND Described in PDR For Nonprescription Drugs) (⊙ Described in PDR For Ophthalmology)

Ventolin Tablets 1176
Volmax Extended-Release Tablets .. 1835

Amitriptyline Hydrochloride (Enhanced activity of tricyclic antidepressants; cardiovascular effects can be potentiated). Products include:
Elavil 2945
Etrafon 2495
Limbitrol 2333
Triavil Tablets 1800

Amlodipine Besylate (Amphetamines may antagonize the hypotensive effects of antihypertensives). Products include:
Lotrel Capsules 858
Norvasc Tablets 2020

Ammonium Chloride (Increases the concentration of ionized species of the amphetamine molecule thereby increasing urinary excretion; lowers blood levels and efficacy of amphetamines).
No products indexed under this heading.

Amoxapine (Enhanced activity of tricyclic antidepressants; cardiovascular effects can be potentiated). Products include:
Asendin Tablets 1419

Astemizole (Amphetamines may counteract the sedative effect of antihistamines). Products include:
Hismanal Tablets 1341

Atenolol (Adrenergic blockers are inhibited by amphetamines; amphetamines may antagonize the hypotensive effects of antihypertensives). Products include:
Tenoretic Tablets 2963
Tenormin Tablets and I.V. Injection 2965

Azatadine Maleate (Amphetamines may counteract the sedative effect of antihistamines). Products include:
Trinalin Repetabs Tablets 1373

Benazepril Hydrochloride (Amphetamines may antagonize the hypotensive effects of antihypertensives). Products include:
Lotensin Tablets 852
Lotensin HCT Tablets 855
Lotrel Capsules 858

Bendroflumethiazide (Some thiazide diuretics increase concentration of the non-ionized species of the amphetamine molecule thereby decreasing urinary excretion; increases blood levels and potentiates the action of amphetamines; amphetamines may antagonize the hypotensive effects of antihypertensives).
No products indexed under this heading.

Betaxolol Hydrochloride (Adrenergic blockers are inhibited by amphetamines; amphetamines may antagonize the hypotensive effects of antihypertensives). Products include:
Betoptic Ophthalmic Solution........ 465
Betoptic S Ophthalmic Suspension 467
Kerlone Tablets........ 2588

Bisoprolol Fumarate (Adrenergic blockers are inhibited by amphetamines; amphetamines may antagonize the hypotensive effects of antihypertensives). Products include:
Zebeta Tablets 1457
Ziac 1459

Bromodiphenhydramine Hydrochloride (Amphetamines may counteract the sedative effect of antihistamines).
No products indexed under this heading.

Brompheniramine Maleate (Amphetamines may counteract the sedative effect of antihistamines). Products include:
Alka-Seltzer Plus Sinus Medicine .. 611
Bromfed Capsules (Extended-Release) 1832
Bromfed Syrup 712
Bromfed Tablets 1832
Bromfed-DM Cough Syrup........ 1832
Bromfed-PD Capsules (Extended-Release) 1832
Dimetane-DC Cough Syrup 2232
Dimetane-DX Cough Syrup 2233
Dimetapp Allergy Dye-Free Elixir.... 838
Dimetapp Allergy Sinus Caplets 838
Dimetapp Cold & Allergy Chewable Tablets 838
Dimetapp Cold & Cough Liqui-Gels 839
Dimetapp Cold & Fever Suspension 839
Dimetapp DM Elixir........ 840
Dimetapp Elixir........ 840
Dimetapp Extentabs 841
Dimetapp Tablets/Liqui-Gels 841
Rondec Chewable Tablets 974
Vicks DayQuil Allergy Relief 12-Hour Extended Release Tablets.. 733
Vicks DayQuil Allergy Relief 4-Hour Tablets 733

Captopril (Amphetamines may antagonize the hypotensive effects of antihypertensives). Products include:
Capoten Tablets 740
Capozide Tablets 744

Carteolol Hydrochloride (Adrenergic blockers are inhibited by amphetamines; amphetamines may antagonize the hypotensive effects of antihypertensives). Products include:
Cartrol Tablets 413
Ocupress Ophthalmic Solution, 1% Sterile........ ⊙ 297

Cetirizine Hydrochloride (Amphetamines may counteract the sedative effect of antihistamines). Products include:
Zyrtec Tablets 2053

Chlorothiazide (Some thiazide diuretics increase concentration of the non-ionized species of the amphetamine molecule thereby decreasing urinary excretion; increases blood levels and potentiates the action of amphetamines; amphetamines may antagonize the hypotensive effects of antihypertensives). Products include:
Aldoclor Tablets 1638
Diupres Tablets 1691
Diuril Oral 1694

Chlorothiazide Sodium (Some thiazide diuretics increase concentration of the non-ionized species of the amphetamine molecule thereby decreasing urinary excretion; increases blood levels and potentiates the action of amphetamines; amphetamines may antagonize the hypotensive effects of antihypertensives). Products include:
Diuril Sodium Intravenous 1693

Chlorpheniramine Maleate (Amphetamines may counteract the sedative effect of antihistamines). Products include:
Alka-Seltzer Plus Cold Medicine 611
Alka-Seltzer Plus Cold Medicine Liqui-Gels 612
Alka-Seltzer Plus Cold & Cough Medicine 611
Alka-Seltzer Plus Cold & Cough Medicine Liqui-Gels........ 612
Alka-Seltzer Plus Flu & Body Aches Effervescent Tablets........ 612
Allerest Maximum Strength........ 649
Allerest Sinus Pain Formula 649
Ana-Kit Anaphylaxis Emergency Treatment Kit 611
Atrohist Pediatric Capsules........ 1603
Atrohist Plus Tablets 1605
BC Cold Powder Multi-Symptom Formula (Cold-Sinus-Allergy) 631
Cerose DM 853
Cheracol Plus Head Cold/Cough Formula 741
Children's TYLENOL Cold Multi-Symptom Chewable Tablets and Liquid 1559
Children's TYLENOL Cold Plus Cough Multi Symptom Chewable Tablets and Liquid........ 1560
Children's TYLENOL Flu Suspension Liquid 1560
Children's Vicks DayQuil Allergy Relief........ 730
Children's Vicks NyQuil Cold/Cough Relief........ 731
Chlor-Trimeton Allergy Decongestant Tablets 759
Chlor-Trimeton Allergy Tablets 758
Allergy-Sinus Comtrex Multi-Symptom Allergy-Sinus Formula Tablets and Caplets 639
Comtrex Multi-Symptom........ 638
Contac Continuous Action Nasal Decongestant/Antihistamine 12 Hour Capsules........ 773
Contac Maximum Strength Continuous Action Decongestant/Antihistamine 12 Hour Caplets.. 772
Contac Severe Cold and Flu Formula Caplets 773
Coricidin Cold + Flu Tablets........ 760
Coricidin Cough + Cold Tablets 760
Coricidin 'D' Decongestant Tablets 760
D.A. II Tablets 972
D.A. Chewable Tablets........ 970
Dura-Tap/PD Capsules 970
Dura-Vent/DA Tablets 972
Efidac 24 Chlorpheniramine........ 655
Extendryl 1003
Fedahist Gyrocaps........ 2545
Hycomine Compound Tablets 948
Kronofed-A 994
Nolamine Timed-Release Tablets 790
Novahistine Elixir 782
Ornade Spansule Capsules 2678
PediaCare Cough-Cold Chewable Tablets and Liquid........ 1569
PediaCare NightRest Cough-Cold Liquid 1569
Pediatric Vicks 44m Cough & Cold Relief 737
Pyrroxate Caplets 742
Ryna 804
Sinarest 663
Sine-Off Sinus Medicine 784
Singlet Tablets 785
Sinulin Tablets 792
Sinutab Sinus Allergy Medication, Maximum Strength Tablets and Caplets 823
Sudafed Cold & Allergy Tablets........ 826
Teldrin 12 Hour Antihistamine/Nasal Decongestant Allergy Relief Capsules 786
TheraFlu Flu and Cold Medicine 750
Theraflu Maximum Strength Flu and Cold Medicine For Sore Throat 751
TheraFlu Flu, Cold and Cough Medicine 750
TheraFlu Maximum Strength Nighttime Flu, Cold & Cough Medicine 751
Triaminic Night Time 754
Triaminic Syrup 755
Triaminic Triaminicol Cold & Cough 756
Triaminicin Tablets 756
Tussend 1830
TYLENOL Allergy Sinus, Maximum Strength Caplets and Gelcaps 1571
TYLENOL Cold Medication, Multi-Symptom Formula Tablets and Caplets 1572
TYLENOL Cold Medication, Multi-Symptom Hot Liquid Packets........ 1572
Vicks 44 LiquiCaps Cough, Cold & Flu Relief........ 728
Vicks 44M Cough, Cold & Flu Relief........ 729

Chlorpheniramine Polistirex (Amphetamines may counteract the sedative effect of antihistamines). Products include:
Tussionex Pennkinetic Extended-Release Suspension 1624

Chlorpheniramine Tannate (Amphetamines may counteract the sedative effect of antihistamines). Products include:
Atrohist Pediatric Suspension 1604
Atrohist Pediatric Suspension Dye-Free 1604
Rynatan 2781
Rynatuss 2782

Chlorpromazine (Inhibits central stimulant effects of amphetamines). Products include:
Thorazine Suppositories........ 2701

Chlorpromazine Hydrochloride (Inhibits central stimulant effects of amphetamines). Products include:
Thorazine 2701

Chlorthalidone (Amphetamines may antagonize the hypotensive effects of antihypertensives). Products include:
Combipres Tablets 682
Tenoretic Tablets........ 2963
Thalitone 1293

Clemastine Fumarate (Amphetamines may counteract the sedative effect of antihistamines). Products include:
Tavist Syrup........ 2426
Tavist Tablets 2427
Tavist-1 12 Hour Relief Tablets 749
Tavist-D 12 Hour Relief Tablets 750

Clomipramine Hydrochloride (Enhanced activity of tricyclic antidepressants; cardiovascular effects can be potentiated). Products include:
Anafranil Capsules 819

Clonidine (Amphetamines may antagonize the hypotensive effects of antihypertensives). Products include:
Catapres-TTS........ 680

Clonidine Hydrochloride (Amphetamines may antagonize the hypotensive effects of antihypertensives). Products include:
Catapres Tablets 679
Combipres Tablets 682

Cryptenamine Preparations (Amphetamines may inhibit the hypotensive effects of veratrum alkaloids).

Cyproheptadine Hydrochloride (Amphetamines may counteract the sedative effect of antihistamines). Products include:
Periactin 1767

Deserpidine (Amphetamines may antagonize the hypotensive effects of antihypertensives).
No products indexed under this heading.

Desipramine Hydrochloride (Enhanced activity of tricyclic antidepressants; cardiovascular effects can be potentiated). Products include:
Norpramin Tablets 1273

Dexchlorpheniramine Maleate (Amphetamines may counteract the sedative effect of antihistamines).
No products indexed under this heading.

Diazoxide (Amphetamines may antagonize the hypotensive effects of antihypertensives). Products include:
Hyperstat I.V. Injection 2504
Proglycem........ 575

Diltiazem Hydrochloride (Amphetamines may antagonize the hypotensive effects of antihypertensives). Products include:
Cardizem CD Capsules 1251
Cardizem SR Capsules 1255
Cardizem Injectable 1253
Cardizem Tablets........ 1257
Dilacor XR Extended-release Capsules 2183
Tiazac Capsules 1019

IMPORTANT NOTE: Always consult each drug listing in the patient's regimen for possible interactions.

DextroStat Interactions Index 268

Diphenhydramine Citrate (Amphetamines may counteract the sedative effect of antihistamines). Products include:
- Excedrin P.M. Analgesic/Sleeping Aid Tablets, Caplets, Liquigels 735

Diphenhydramine Hydrochloride (Amphetamines may counteract the sedative effect of antihistamines). Products include:
- Actifed Allergy Daytime/Nighttime Caplets ▣ 808
- Actifed Sinus Daytime/Nighttime Tablets and Caplets ▣ 809
- Extra Strength Bayer PM Aspirin Plus Sleep Aid ▣ 617
- Benadryl Allergy Chewables ▣ 811
- Benadryl Allergy/Cold Tablets ▣ 811
- Benadryl Allergy Decongestant Liquid Medication ▣ 812
- Benadryl Allergy Decongestant Tablets ▣ 812
- Benadryl Allergy Liquid Medication ▣ 813
- Benadryl Allergy ▣ 811
- Benadryl Allergy Sinus Headache Caplets ▣ 813
- Benadryl Dye-Free Allergy Liqui-gel Softgels ▣ 813
- Benadryl Dye-Free Allergy Liquid Medication ▣ 814
- Benadryl Itch Relief Stick Extra Strength ▣ 814
- Benadryl Cream ▣ 814
- Benadryl Gel ▣ 815
- Benadryl Spray ▣ 815
- Benadryl Injection 1955
- Contac Day & Night Cold/Flu Night Caplets ▣ 772
- Contac Night Allergy/Sinus Caplets ▣ 771
- Extra Strength Doan's P.M. ▣ 653
- Excedrin P.M. Analgesic/Sleeping Aid Tablets, Caplets, Liquigels ▣ 643
- Nytol QuickCaps Caplets ▣ 632
- Sleepinal Night-time Sleep Aid Capsules and Softgels ▣ 798
- TYLENOL Allergy Sinus NightTime, Maximum Strength Caplets 1571
- TYLENOL Flu NightTime, Maximum Strength Gelcaps 1575
- TYLENOL Flu NightTime, Maximum Strength Hot Medication Packets 1575
- TYLENOL PM Pain Reliever/Sleep Aid, Extra Strength Gelcaps, Caplets, Geltabs 1576
- TYLENOL Severe Allergy Medication Caplets 1571
- Maximum Strength Unisom Sleepgels 1990
- Unisom With Pain Relief-Nighttime Sleep Aid and Pain Reliever 1991

Diphenylpyraline Hydrochloride (Amphetamines may counteract the sedative effect of antihistamines).
- No products indexed under this heading.

Dobutamine Hydrochloride (Enhanced activity of sympathomimetics). Products include:
- Dobutrex Solution Vials 1480

Dopamine Hydrochloride (Enhanced activity of sympathomimetics).
- No products indexed under this heading.

Doxazosin Mesylate (Adrenergic blockers are inhibited by amphetamines; amphetamines may antagonize the hypotensive effects of antihypertensives). Products include:
- Cardura Tablets 1993

Doxepin Hydrochloride (Enhanced activity of tricyclic antidepressants; cardiovascular effects can be potentiated). Products include:
- Adapin Capsules 1542
- Sinequan 2028
- Zonalon Cream 1042

Enalapril Maleate (Amphetamines may antagonize the hypotensive effects of antihypertensives). Products include:
- Vaseretic Tablets 1810
- Vasotec Tablets 1816

Enalaprilat (Amphetamines may antagonize the hypotensive effects of antihypertensives). Products include:
- Vasotec I.V. 1814

Ephedrine Hydrochloride (Enhanced activity of sympathomimetics). Products include:
- Primatene Tablets ▣ 844
- Quadrinal Tablets 1398

Ephedrine Sulfate (Enhanced activity of sympathomimetics). Products include:
- Marax Tablets & DF Syrup 2015

Ephedrine Tannate (Enhanced activity of sympathomimetics). Products include:
- Rynatuss 2782

Epinephrine (Enhanced activity of sympathomimetics). Products include:
- EPIFRIN ⊙ 237
- EpiPen 808
- Marcaine with Epinephrine 2446
- Primatene Mist ▣ 843
- Sensorcaine with Epinephrine Injection 554
- Sus-Phrine Injection 1017
- Xylocaine with Epinephrine Injections 562

Epinephrine Bitartrate (Enhanced activity of sympathomimetics). Products include:
- Sensorcaine-MPF with Epinephrine Injection 554

Epinephrine Hydrochloride (Enhanced activity of sympathomimetics). Products include:
- Ana-Kit Anaphylaxis Emergency Treatment Kit 611

Esmolol Hydrochloride (Adrenergic blockers are inhibited by amphetamines; amphetamines may antagonize the hypotensive effects of antihypertensives). Products include:
- Brevibloc (esmolol HCl) Injection 1860

Ethosuximide (Delayed intestinal absorption of ethosuximide). Products include:
- Zarontin Capsules 1986
- Zarontin Syrup 1986

Felodipine (Amphetamines may antagonize the hypotensive effects of antihypertensives). Products include:
- Plendil Extended-Release Tablets 514

Fosinopril Sodium (Amphetamines may antagonize the hypotensive effects of antihypertensives). Products include:
- Monopril Tablets 762

Fosphenytoin Sodium (Co-administration may produce synergistic anticonvulsant action). Products include:
- Cerebyx Injection 1956

Furazolidone (Potential for hypertensive crisis; slows amphetamine metabolism; concurrent and/or sequential use is contraindicated). Products include:
- Furoxone 2221

Furosemide (Amphetamines may antagonize the hypotensive effects of antihypertensives). Products include:
- Lasix Injection, Oral Solution and Tablets 1267

Glutamic Acid Hydrochloride (Lowers absorption of amphetamines by acting as gastrointestinal acidifying agent).
- No products indexed under this heading.

Guanabenz Acetate (Amphetamines may antagonize the hypotensive effects of antihypertensives).
- No products indexed under this heading.

Guanethidine Monosulfate (Lowers absorption of amphetamines by acting as gastrointestinal acidifying agent; amphetamines may antagonize the hypotensive effects of antihypertensives). Products include:
- Esimil Tablets 840
- Ismelin Tablets 845

Haloperidol (Inhibits central stimulant effects of amphetamines). Products include:
- Haldol Injection, Tablets and Concentrate 1585

Haloperidol Decanoate (Inhibits central stimulant effects of amphetamines). Products include:
- Haldol Decanoate 1587

Hydralazine Hydrochloride (Amphetamines may antagonize the hypotensive effects of antihypertensives). Products include:
- Apresazide Capsules 824
- Apresoline Hydrochloride Tablets 826
- Hydralazine Hydrochloride Injection USP 2712
- Ser-Ap-Es Tablets 867

Hydrochlorothiazide (Some thiazide diuretics increase concentration of the non-ionized species of the amphetamine molecule thereby decreasing urinary excretion; increases blood levels and potentiates the action of amphetamines; amphetamines may antagonize the hypotensive effects of antihypertensives). Products include:
- Aldactazide Tablets 2556
- Aldoril Tablets 1644
- Apresazide Capsules 824
- Capozide Tablets 744
- Dyazide Capsules 2653
- Esidrix Tablets 839
- Esimil Tablets 840
- HydroDIURIL Tablets 1716
- Hydropres Tablets 1718
- Hyzaar Tablets 1720
- Inderide Tablets 2838
- Inderide LA Long Acting Capsules 2840
- Lopressor HCT Tablets 850
- Lotensin HCT Tablets 855
- Moduretic Tablets 1748
- Oretic Tablets 450
- Prinzide Tablets 1780
- Ser-Ap-Es Tablets 867
- Timolide Tablets 1791
- Vaseretic Tablets 1810
- Zestoretic Tablets 2968
- Ziac 1459

Hydroflumethiazide (Some thiazide diuretics increase concentration of the non-ionized species of the amphetamine molecule thereby decreasing urinary excretion; increases blood levels and potentiates the action of amphetamines; amphetamines may antagonize the hypotensive effects of antihypertensives). Products include:
- Diucardin Tablets 2824

Imipramine Hydrochloride (Enhanced activity of tricyclic antidepressants; cardiovascular effects can be potentiated). Products include:
- Tofranil Ampuls 873
- Tofranil Tablets 875

Imipramine Pamoate (Enhanced activity of tricyclic antidepressants; cardiovascular effects can be potentiated). Products include:
- Tofranil-PM Capsules 876

Indapamide (Amphetamines may antagonize the hypotensive effects of antihypertensives).
- No products indexed under this heading.

Isocarboxazid (Potential for hypertensive crisis; slows amphetamine metabolism; concurrent and/or sequential use is contraindicated).
- No products indexed under this heading.

Isoproterenol Hydrochloride (Enhanced activity of sympathomimetics). Products include:
- Isuprel Hydrochloride Solution 2443
- Isuprel Injection 2441
- Isuprel Mistometer 2442

Isoproterenol Sulfate (Enhanced activity of sympathomimetics). Products include:
- Norisodrine with Calcium Iodide Syrup 446

Isradipine (Amphetamines may antagonize the hypotensive effects of antihypertensives). Products include:
- DynaCirc Capsules 2381
- DynaCirc CR Tablets 2383

Labetalol Hydrochloride (Adrenergic blockers are inhibited by amphetamines; amphetamines may antagonize the hypotensive effects of antihypertensives). Products include:
- Normodyne Injection 2519
- Normodyne Tablets 2522
- Trandate 1158

Levobunolol Hydrochloride (Adrenergic blockers are inhibited by amphetamines; amphetamines may antagonize the hypotensive effects of antihypertensives). Products include:
- Betagan ⊙ 230

Lisinopril (Amphetamines may antagonize the hypotensive effects of antihypertensives). Products include:
- Prinivil Tablets 1776
- Prinzide Tablets 1780
- Zestoretic Tablets 2968
- Zestril Tablets 2972

Lithium Carbonate (Inhibits anti-obesity and stimulatory effects). Products include:
- Eskalith 2658
- Lithium Carbonate Capsules & Tablets 2352
- Lithonate/Lithotabs/Lithobid 2721

Loratadine (Amphetamines may counteract the sedative effect of antihistamines). Products include:
- Claritin Tablets 2485
- Claritin-D Tablets 2487

Losartan Potassium (Amphetamines may antagonize the hypotensive effects of antihypertensives). Products include:
- Cozaar Tablets 1668
- Hyzaar Tablets 1720

Maprotiline Hydrochloride (Enhanced activity of tricyclic antidepressants; cardiovascular effects can be potentiated). Products include:
- Ludiomil Tablets 861

Mecamylamine Hydrochloride (Amphetamines may antagonize the hypotensive effects of antihypertensives). Products include:
- Inversine Tablets 1729

Meperidine Hydrochloride (Analgesic effect of meperidine potentiated). Products include:
- Demerol 2438
- Mepergan Injection 2859

Metaproterenol Sulfate (Enhanced activity of sympathomimetics). Products include:
- Alupent 672

(▣ Described in PDR For Nonprescription Drugs) (⊙ Described in PDR For Ophthalmology)

Interactions Index

Metaproterenol Sulfate Inhalation Solution, USP, Arm-a-Med 547

Metaraminol Bitartrate (Enhanced activity of sympathomimetics). Products include:
Aramine Injection 1649

Methdilazine Hydrochloride (Amphetamines may counteract the sedative effect of antihistamines).
No products indexed under this heading.

Methenamine (Increases urinary excretion and efficacy is reduced by acidifying agents used in methenamine therapy). Products include:
Urised Tablets 2123

Methenamine Hippurate (Increases urinary excretion and efficacy is reduced by acidifying agents used in methenamine therapy).
No products indexed under this heading.

Methenamine Mandelate (Increases urinary excretion and efficacy is reduced by acidifying agents used in methenamine therapy). Products include:
Uroqid-Acid No. 2 Tablets 633

Methoxamine Hydrochloride (Enhanced activity of sympathomimetics). Products include:
Vasoxyl Injection 1169

Methyclothiazide (Some thiazide diuretics increase concentration of the non-ionized species of the amphetamine molecule thereby decreasing urinary excretion; increases blood levels and potentiates the action of amphetamines; amphetamines may antagonize the hypotensive effects of antihypertensives). Products include:
Enduron Tablets 424

Methyldopa (Amphetamines may antagonize the hypotensive effects of antihypertensives). Products include:
Aldoclor Tablets 1638
Aldomet Oral 1640
Aldoril Tablets 1644

Methyldopate Hydrochloride (Amphetamines may antagonize the hypotensive effects of antihypertensives). Products include:
Aldomet Ester HCl Injection 1642

Metipranolol Hydrochloride (Adrenergic blockers are inhibited by amphetamines; amphetamines may antagonize the hypotensive effects of antihypertensives). Products include:
OptiPranolol (Metipranolol 0.3%) Sterile Ophthalmic Solution .... © 256

Metolazone (Amphetamines may antagonize the hypotensive effects of antihypertensives). Products include:
Mykrox Tablets 1617
Zaroxolyn Tablets 1625

Metoprolol Succinate (Adrenergic blockers are inhibited by amphetamines; amphetamines may antagonize the hypotensive effects of antihypertensives). Products include:
Toprol-XL Tablets 560

Metoprolol Tartrate (Adrenergic blockers are inhibited by amphetamines; amphetamines may antagonize the hypotensive effects of antihypertensives). Products include:
Lopressor 848
Lopressor HCT Tablets 850

Metyrosine (Amphetamines may antagonize the hypotensive effects of antihypertensives). Products include:
Demser Capsules 1690

Minoxidil (Amphetamines may antagonize the hypotensive effects of antihypertensives).
No products indexed under this heading.

Moexipril Hydrochloride (Amphetamines may antagonize the hypotensive effects of antihypertensives). Products include:
Univasc Tablets 2553

Nadolol (Adrenergic blockers are inhibited by amphetamines; amphetamines may antagonize the hypotensive effects of antihypertensives).
No products indexed under this heading.

Nicardipine Hydrochloride (Amphetamines may antagonize the hypotensive effects of antihypertensives). Products include:
Cardene Capsules 2261
Cardene I.V. 2815
Cardene SR Capsules 2264

Nifedipine (Amphetamines may antagonize the hypotensive effects of antihypertensives). Products include:
Adalat Capsules (10 mg and 20 mg) 580
Adalat CC 582
Procardia Capsules 2024
Procardia XL Extended Release Tablets 2026

Nisoldipine (Amphetamines may antagonize the hypotensive effects of antihypertensives). Products include:
Sular Tablets 2961

Nitroglycerin (Amphetamines may antagonize the hypotensive effects of antihypertensives). Products include:
Deponit NTG Transdermal Delivery System 2541
Nitro-Bid IV 1270
Nitro-Bid Ointment 1272
Nitro-Dur (nitroglycerin) Transdermal Infusion System 1365
Nitrolingual Spray 2193
Nitrostat Tablets 1981
Transderm-Nitro Transdermal Therapeutic System 878

Norepinephrine Bitartrate (Enhanced activity of sympathomimetics). Products include:
Levophed Bitartrate Injection 2445

Norepinephrine Hydrochloride (Enhanced adrenergic effect of norepinephrine).

Nortriptyline Hydrochloride (Enhanced activity of tricyclic antidepressants; cardiovascular effects can be potentiated). Products include:
Pamelor 2409

Penbutolol Sulfate (Adrenergic blockers are inhibited by amphetamines; amphetamines may antagonize the hypotensive effects of antihypertensives). Products include:
Levatol Tablets 2547

Phenelzine Sulfate (Potential for hypertensive crisis; slows amphetamine metabolism; concurrent and/or sequential use is contraindicated). Products include:
Nardil 1977

Phenobarbital (Delayed intestinal absorption of phenobarbital; synergistic anticonvulsant action may be produced). Products include:
Arco-Lase Plus Tablets 513
Bellergal-S Tablets 2375
Donnatal 2234
Donnatal Extentabs 2234
Donnatal Tablets 2234
Phenobarbital Elixir and Tablets 1523
Quadrinal Tablets 1398

Phenoxybenzamine Hydrochloride (Amphetamines may antagonize the hypotensive effects of antihypertensives). Products include:
Dibenzyline Capsules 2650

Phentolamine Mesylate (Amphetamines may antagonize the hypotensive effects of antihypertensives). Products include:
Regitine Vials 864

Phenylephrine Bitartrate (Enhanced activity of sympathomimetics).
No products indexed under this heading.

Phenylephrine Hydrochloride (Enhanced activity of sympathomimetics). Products include:
Atrohist Plus Tablets 1605
Cerose DM 853
D.A. II Tablets 972
D.A. Chewable Tablets 970
Dura-Vent/DA Tablets 972
Extendryl 1003
4-Way Fast Acting Nasal Spray (regular & mentholated) 644
Hemoril 797
Hycomine Compound Tablets 948
Neo-Synephrine Hydrochloride 1% Carpuject 2455
Neo-Synephrine Hydrochloride 1% Injection 2455
Neo-Synephrine Hydrochloride (Ophthalmic) 2456
Neo-Synephrine 624
Novahistine Elixir 782
Phenergan VC 2886
Phenergan VC with Codeine 2888
Preparation H 842
Tympagesic Ear Drops 2476
Vicks Sinex Nasal Spray and Ultra Fine Mist 738

Phenylephrine Tannate (Enhanced activity of sympathomimetics). Products include:
Atrohist Pediatric Suspension 1604
Atrohist Pediatric Suspension Dye-Free 1604
Rynatan 2781
Rynatuss 2782

Phenylpropanolamine Hydrochloride (Enhanced activity of sympathomimetics). Products include:
Acutrim 648
Atrohist Plus Tablets 1605
BC Cold Powder Multi-Symptom Formula (Cold-Sinus-Allergy) 631
BC Cold Powder Non-Drowsy Formula (Cold-Sinus) 631
Cheracol Plus Head Cold/Cough Formula 741
Comtrex Multi-Symptom Cold Reliever Liqui-Gels 638
Comtrex Multi-Symptom Non-Drowsy Liqui-gels 640
Contac Continuous Action Nasal Decongestant/Antihistamine 12 Hour Capsules 773
Contac Maximum Strength Continuous Action Decongestant/Antihistamine 12 Hour Caplets 772
Contac Severe Cold and Flu Formula Caplets 773
Coricidin 'D' Decongestant Tablets 760
Dexatrim 795
Dexatrim Plus Vitamins Caplets 796
Dimetane-DC Cough Syrup 2232
Dimetapp Allergy Sinus Caplets 838
Dimetapp Cold & Allergy Chewable Tablets 838
Dimetapp Cold & Cough Liqui-Gels 839
Dimetapp DM Elixir 840
Dimetapp Elixir 840
Dimetapp Extentabs 841
Dimetapp Tablets/Liqui-Gels 841
Dura-Vent Tablets 971
Entex LA Tablets 972
Exgest LA Tablets 787
Hycomine 947
Nolamine Timed-Release Tablets 790
Ornade Spansule Capsules 2678
Propagest Tablets 791
Pyrroxate Caplets 742

Robitussin-CF 846
Sinulin Tablets 792
Tavist-D 12 Hour Relief Tablets 750
Teldrin 12 Hour Antihistamine/Nasal Decongestant Allergy Relief Capsules 786
Triaminic Expectorant 753
Triaminic Syrup 755
Triaminic Triaminicol Cold & Cough 756
Triaminic DM Syrup 756
Triaminicin Tablets 756
Vicks DayQuil Allergy Relief 12-Hour Extended Release Tablets 733
Vicks DayQuil Allergy Relief 4-Hour Tablets 733
Vicks DayQuil SINUS Pressure & CONGESTION Relief 734

Phenytoin (Delayed intestinal absorption of phenobarbital; synergistic anticonvulsant action may be produced). Products include:
Dilantin Infatabs 1967
Dilantin-125 Suspension 1969

Phenytoin Sodium (Delayed intestinal absorption of phenobarbital; synergistic anticonvulsant action may be produced). Products include:
Dilantin Kapseals 1965

Pindolol (Adrenergic blockers are inhibited by amphetamines; amphetamines may antagonize the hypotensive effects of antihypertensives). Products include:
Visken Tablets 2428

Pirbuterol Acetate (Enhanced activity of sympathomimetics). Products include:
Maxair Autohaler 1550
Maxair Inhaler 1552

Polythiazide (Some thiazide diuretics increase concentration of the non-ionized species of the amphetamine molecule thereby decreasing urinary excretion; increases blood levels and potentiates the action of amphetamines; amphetamines may antagonize the hypotensive effects of antihypertensives). Products include:
Minizide Capsules 2016

Potassium Citrate (Increases the concentration of the non-ionized species of the amphetamine molecule thereby decreasing urinary excretion; increases blood levels and potentiates the action of amphetamines). Products include:
Polycitra Syrup 574
Polycitra-K Crystals 574
Polycitra-K Oral Solution 575
Polycitra-LC 574
Urocit-K Tablets 1828

Prazosin Hydrochloride (Adrenergic blockers are inhibited by amphetamines; amphetamines may antagonize the hypotensive effects of antihypertensives). Products include:
Minipress Capsules 2015
Minizide Capsules 2016

Promethazine Hydrochloride (Amphetamines may counteract the sedative effect of antihistamines). Products include:
Mepergan Injection 2859
Phenergan with Codeine 2883
Phenergan with Dextromethorphan 2885
Phenergan Injection 2880
Phenergan Suppositories 2882
Phenergan Syrup 2881
Phenergan Tablets 2882
Phenergan VC 2886
Phenergan VC with Codeine 2888

Propoxyphene Hydrochloride (In cases of propoxyphene overdosage, amphetamine CNS stimulation is potentiated and fatal convulsions can occur). Products include:
Darvon 1475
Wygesic Tablets 2930

IMPORTANT NOTE: Always consult each drug listing in the patient's regimen for possible interactions.

DextroStat | Interactions Index | 270

Propoxyphene Napsylate (In cases of propoxyphene overdosage, amphetamine CNS stimulation is potentiated and fatal convulsions can occur). Products include:

Darvon-N/Darvocet-N ... 1473

Propranolol Hydrochloride (Adrenergic blockers are inhibited by amphetamines; amphetamines may antagonize the hypotensive effects of antihypertensives). Products include:

Inderal ... 2834
Inderal LA Long Acting Capsules ... 2836
Inderide Tablets ... 2838
Inderide LA Long Acting Capsules ... 2840

Protriptyline Hydrochloride (Enhanced activity of tricyclic antidepressants; cardiovascular effects can be potentiated). Products include:

Vivactil Tablets ... 1820

Pseudoephedrine Hydrochloride (Enhanced activity of sympathomimetics). Products include:

Actifed Allergy Daytime/Nighttime Caplets ... ◼ 808
Actifed Cold & Allergy Tablets ... ◼ 807
Actifed Cold & Sinus Caplets and Tablets ... ◼ 808
Actifed Sinus Daytime/Nighttime Tablets and Caplets ... ◼ 809
Advil Cold and Sinus Caplets and Tablets ... ◼ 837
Alka-Seltzer Plus Liqui-Gels ... ◼ 612
Alka-Seltzer Plus Flu & Body Aches Liqui-Gels Non-Drowsy Formula ... ◼ 613
Alka-Seltzer Plus Night-Time Cold Medicine Liqui-Gels ... ◼ 612
Allerest Maximum Strength ... ◼ 649
Allerest No Drowsiness ... ◼ 649
Allerest Sinus Pain Formula ... ◼ 649
Atrohist Pediatric Capsules ... 1603
Benadryl Allergy/Cold Tablets ... ◼ 811
Benadryl Allergy Decongestant Liquid Medication ... ◼ 812
Benadryl Allergy Decongestant Tablets ... ◼ 812
Benadryl Allergy Sinus Headache Caplets ... ◼ 813
Benylin Multisymptom ... ◼ 816
Bromfed Capsules (Extended-Release) ... 1832
Bromfed Syrup ... ◼ 712
Bromfed Tablets ... 1832
Bromfed-DM Cough Syrup ... 1832
Bromfed-PD Capsules (Extended-Release) ... 1832
Children's TYLENOL Cold Multi-Symptom Chewable Tablets and Liquid ... 1559
Children's TYLENOL Cold Plus Cough Multi Symptom Chewable Tablets and Liquid ... 1560
Children's TYLENOL Flu Suspension Liquid ... 1560
Children's Vicks DayQuil Allergy Relief ... ◼ 730
Children's Vicks NyQuil Cold/Cough Relief ... ◼ 731
Allergy-Sinus Comtrex Multi-Symptom Allergy-Sinus Formula Tablets and Caplets ... ◼ 639
Comtrex Multi-Symptom ... ◼ 638
Comtrex Multi-Symptom Non-Drowsy Caplets ... ◼ 640
Congess ... 1003
Contac Day Allergy/Sinus Caplets ◼ 771
Contac Day & Night ... ◼ 772
Contac Night Allergy/Sinus Caplets ... ◼ 771
Contac Severe Cold & Flu Non-Drowsy ... ◼ 774
Deconsal II Tablets ... 1605
Dimetane-DX Cough Syrup ... 2233
Dimetapp Cold & Fever Suspension ... ◼ 839
Dimetapp Decongestant Pediatric Drops ... ◼ 840
Dorcol Children's Cough Syrup ... ◼ 748
Drixoral Cough + Congestion Liquid Caps ... ◼ 763
Dura-Tap/PD Capsules ... 970
Duratuss Tablets ... 2750
Duratuss HD Elixir ... 2750
Efidac/24 ... ◼ 655
Entex PSE Tablets ... 973
Fedahist Gyrocaps ... 2545
Guaifed ... 1833
Guaifed Syrup ... ◼ 712
Guaimax-D Tablets ... 809
Histussin D Liquid ... 670
Infants' TYLENOL Cold Decongestant & Fever-Reducer Drops ... 1561
Kronofed-A ... 994
Novahistine DMX ... ◼ 782
Nucofed ... 2225
PediaCare Cough-Cold Chewable Tablets and Liquid ... 1569
PediaCare Infants' Decongestant Drops ... 1569
PediaCare Infants' Drops Decongestant Plus Cough ... 1569
PediaCare NightRest Cough-Cold Liquid ... 1569
Pediatric Vicks 44d Cough & Head Congestion Relief ... ◼ 736
Pediatric Vicks 44m Cough & Cold Relief ... ◼ 737
Robitussin Cold & Cough Liqui-Gels ... ◼ 844
Robitussin Cold, Cough & Flu Liqui-Gels ... ◼ 844
Robitussin Maximum Strength Cough & Cold ... ◼ 847
Robitussin Night-Time Cold Formula ... ◼ 847
Robitussin Pediatric Cough & Cold Formula ... ◼ 848
Robitussin Pediatric Drops ... ◼ 849
Robitussin Severe Congestion Liqui-Gels ... ◼ 845
Robitussin-DAC Syrup ... 2249
Robitussin-PE ... ◼ 846
Rondec Oral Drops ... 974
Rondec Syrup ... 974
Rondec Tablet ... 974
Rondec Chewable Tablets ... 974
Rondec-TR Tablet ... 974
Ryna ... ◼ 804
Seldane-D Extended-Release Tablets ... 1286
Semprex-D Capsules ... 1620
Sinarest ... ◼ 663
Sine-Aid Maximum Strength Sinus Headache Gelcaps, Caplets and Tablets ... 1570
Sine-Off No Drowsiness Formula Caplets ... ◼ 784
Sine-Off Sinus Medicine ... ◼ 784
Singlet Tablets ... ◼ 785
Sinutab Non-Drying Liquid Caps ... ◼ 823
Sinutab Sinus Allergy Medication, Maximum Strength Tablets and Caplets ... ◼ 823
Sinutab Sinus Medication, Maximum Strength Without Drowsiness Formula, Tablets & Caplets ... ◼ 824
Sudafed Children's Cold & Cough Liquid Medication ... ◼ 825
Sudafed Children's Nasal Decongestant Liquid Medication ... ◼ 826
Sudafed Cold & Allergy Tablets ... ◼ 826
Sudafed Cold and Cough Liquid Caps ... ◼ 826
Sudafed Nasal Decongestant Tablets, 30 mg ... ◼ 825
Sudafed Nasal Decongestant Tablets, 60 mg ... ◼ 825
Sudafed Non-Drying Sinus Liquid Caps ... ◼ 827
Sudafed Pediatric Nasal Decongestant Liquid Oral Drops ... ◼ 827
Sudafed Severe Cold Formula Caplets ... ◼ 828
Sudafed Severe Cold Formula Tablets ... ◼ 828
Sudafed Sinus Caplets ... ◼ 829
Sudafed Sinus Tablets ... ◼ 829
Sudafed 12 Hour Caplets ... ◼ 824
Syn-Rx Tablets ... 1622
Syn-Rx DM Tablets ... 1623
TheraFlu Flu and Cold Medicine ... ◼ 750
Theraflu Maximum Strength Flu and Cold Medicine For Sore Throat ... ◼ 751
TheraFlu Flu, Cold and Cough Medicine ... ◼ 750
TheraFlu Maximum Strength Nighttime Flu, Cold & Cough Medicine ... ◼ 751
TheraFlu Maximum Strength Non-Drowsy Formula Flu, Cold & Cough Medicine ... ◼ 751
TheraFlu Maximum Strength, Non-Drowsy Formula Flu, Cold and Cough Caplets ... ◼ 752
Theraflu Maximum Strength Sinus Non-Drowsy Formula Caplets ... ◼ 752
Triaminic AM Cough and Decongestant Formula ... ◼ 753
Triaminic AM Decongestant Formula ... ◼ 753
Triaminic Infant Oral Decongestant Drops ... ◼ 754
Triaminic Night Time ... ◼ 754
Triaminic Sore Throat Formula ... ◼ 755
Tussend ... 1830
Tussend Expectorant ... 1831
TYLENOL Allergy Sinus, Maximum Strength Caplets and Gelcaps ... 1571
TYLENOL Allergy Sinus NightTime, Maximum Strength Caplets ... 1571
TYLENOL Cold Medication, Multi-Symptom Formula Tablets and Caplets ... 1572
TYLENOL Cold Medication, Multi-Symptom Hot Liquid Packets ... 1572
TYLENOL Cold Medication, No Drowsiness Formula Caplets and Gelcaps ... 1572
TYLENOL Cold Severe Congestion Caplets ... 1573
TYLENOL Cough Medication with Decongestant, Multi Symptom ... 1574
TYLENOL Flu No Drowsiness Formula, Maximum Strength Gelcaps ... 1575
TYLENOL Flu NightTime, Maximum Strength Gelcaps ... 1575
TYLENOL Flu NightTime, Maximum Strength Hot Medication Packets ... 1575
TYLENOL Sinus, Maximum Strength Geltabs, Gelcaps, Caplets and Tablets ... 1576
Vicks 44 LiquiCaps Cough, Cold & Flu Relief ... ◼ 728
Vicks 44 LiquiCaps Non-Drowsy Cough & Cold Relief ... ◼ 729
Vicks 44D Cough & Head Congestion Relief ... ◼ 728
Vicks 44M Cough, Cold & Flu Relief ... ◼ 729
Vicks DayQuil LiquiCaps/Liquid Multi-Symptom Cold/Flu Relief ... ◼ 734
Vicks DayQuil SINUS Pressure & PAIN Relief with IBUPROFEN ... ◼ 735
Vicks Nyquil Hot Therapy ... ◼ 735
Vicks NyQuil LiquiCaps/Liquid Multi-Symptom Cold/Flu Relief, Original and Cherry Flavors ... ◼ 736

Pseudoephedrine Sulfate (Enhanced activity of sympathomimetics). Products include:

Chlor-Trimeton Allergy Decongestant Tablets ... ◼ 759
Claritin-D Tablets ... 2487
Drixoral Cold and Allergy Sustained-Action Tablets ... ◼ 763
Drixoral Cold and Flu Extended-Release Tablets ... ◼ 764
Drixoral Non-Drowsy Formula Extended-Release Tablets ... ◼ 764
Drixoral Allergy/Sinus Extended Release Tablets ... ◼ 765
Trinalin Repetabs Tablets ... 1373

Pyrilamine Maleate (Amphetamines may counteract the sedative effect of antihistamines). Products include:

4-Way Fast Acting Nasal Spray (regular & mentholated) ... ◼ 644
Maximum Strength Multi-Symptom Formula Midol ... ◼ 621
PMS Multi-Symptom Formula Midol ... ◼ 622

Pyrilamine Tannate (Amphetamines may counteract the sedative effect of antihistamines). Products include:

Atrohist Pediatric Suspension ... 1604
Atrohist Pediatric Suspension Dye-Free ... 1604
Rynatan ... 2781

Quinapril Hydrochloride (Amphetamines may antagonize the hypotensive effects of antihypertensives). Products include:

Accupril Tablets ... 1950

Ramipril (Amphetamines may antagonize the hypotensive effects of antihypertensives). Products include:

Altace Capsules ... 1238

Rauwolfia Serpentina (Amphetamines may antagonize the hypotensive effects of antihypertensives).

No products indexed under this heading.

Rescinnamine (Amphetamines may antagonize the hypotensive effects of antihypertensives).

No products indexed under this heading.

Reserpine (Lowers absorption of amphetamines by acting as gastrointestinal acidifying agent; amphetamines may antagonize the hypotensive effects of antihypertensives). Products include:

Diupres Tablets ... 1691
Hydropres Tablets ... 1718
Ser-Ap-Es Tablets ... 867

Salmeterol Xinafoate (Enhanced activity of sympathomimetics). Products include:

Serevent Inhalation Aerosol ... 1149

Selegiline Hydrochloride (Potential for hypertensive crisis; slows amphetamine metabolism; concurrent and/or sequential use is contraindicated). Products include:

Eldepryl Capsules ... 2729

Sodium Acid Phosphate (Increases the concentration of ionized species of the amphetamine molecule thereby increasing urinary excretion; lowers blood levels and efficacy of amphetamines). Products include:

Uroqid-Acid No. 2 Tablets ... 633

Sodium Bicarbonate (Increases absorption of amphetamines; increases blood levels and potentiates the action of amphetamines). Products include:

Alka-Seltzer Cherry Effervescent Antacid and Pain Reliever ... ◼ 609
Alka-Seltzer Extra Strength Effervescent Antacid and Pain Reliever ... ◼ 609
Alka-Seltzer Gold Effervescent Antacid ... ◼ 611
Alka-Seltzer Lemon Lime Effervescent Antacid and Pain Reliever ... ◼ 609
Alka-Seltzer Original Effervescent Antacid and Pain Reliever ... ◼ 609
Arm & Hammer Pure Baking Soda ... ◼ 648
Colyte and Colyte-flavored ... 2540
GoLYTELY ... 694
Massengill Disposable Douches ... ◼ 780
Massengill Liquid Concentrate ... ◼ 780
NuLYTELY ... 694
Cherry Flavor NuLYTELY ... 694

Sodium Citrate (Increases the concentration of the non-ionized species of the amphetamine molecule thereby decreasing urinary excretion; increases blood levels and potentiates the action of amphetamines). Products include:

Bicitra ... 573
Polycitra ... 574
Salix SST Lozenges Saliva Stimulant ... ◼ 757

Sodium Nitroprusside (Amphetamines may antagonize the hypotensive effects of antihypertensives).

No products indexed under this heading.

Sotalol Hydrochloride (Adrenergic blockers are inhibited by amphetamines; amphetamines may antagonize the hypotensive effects of antihypertensives). Products include:

Betapace Tablets ... 637

Spirapril Hydrochloride (Amphetamines may antagonize the hypotensive effects of antihypertensives).

No products indexed under this heading.

(◼ Described in PDR For Nonprescription Drugs) (⊙ Described in PDR For Ophthalmology)

271 Interactions Index DiaBeta

Terazosin Hydrochloride (Adrenergic blockers are inhibited by amphetamines; amphetamines may antagonize the hypotensive effects of antihypertensives). Products include:
- Hytrin Capsules ... 434

Terbutaline Sulfate (Enhanced activity of sympathomimetics). Products include:
- Brethaire Inhaler ... 830
- Brethine Ampuls ... 832
- Brethine Tablets ... 831
- Bricanyl Subcutaneous Injection ... 1247
- Bricanyl Tablets ... 1248

Terfenadine (Amphetamines may counteract the sedative effect of antihistamines). Products include:
- Seldane Tablets ... 1284
- Seldane-D Extended-Release Tablets ... 1286

Timolol Hemihydrate (Adrenergic blockers are inhibited by amphetamines; amphetamines may antagonize the hypotensive effects of antihypertensives). Products include:
- Betimol 0.25%, 0.5% ... ◉ 259

Timolol Maleate (Adrenergic blockers are inhibited by amphetamines; amphetamines may antagonize the hypotensive effects of antihypertensives). Products include:
- Blocadren Tablets ... 1654
- Timolide Tablets ... 1791
- Timoptic in Ocudose ... 1796
- Timoptic Sterile Ophthalmic Solution ... 1794
- Timoptic-XE ... 1798

Torsemide (Amphetamines may antagonize the hypotensive effects of antihypertensives). Products include:
- Demadex Tablets and Injection ... 691

Tranylcypromine Sulfate (Potential for hypertensive crisis; slows amphetamine metabolism; concurrent and/or sequential use is contraindicated). Products include:
- Parnate Tablets ... 2679

Trimeprazine Tartrate (Amphetamines may counteract the sedative effect of antihistamines).
- No products indexed under this heading.

Trimethaphan Camsylate (Amphetamines may antagonize the hypotensive effects of antihypertensives).
- No products indexed under this heading.

Trimipramine Maleate (Enhanced activity of tricyclic antidepressants; cardiovascular effects can be potentiated). Products include:
- Surmontil Capsules ... 2917

Tripelennamine Hydrochloride (Amphetamines may counteract the sedative effect of antihistamines). Products include:
- PBZ Tablets ... 863
- PBZ-SR Tablets ... 862

Triprolidine Hydrochloride (Amphetamines may counteract the sedative effect of antihistamines). Products include:
- Actifed Cold & Allergy Tablets ... ▣ 807
- Actifed Cold & Sinus Caplets and Tablets ... ▣ 808

Verapamil Hydrochloride (Amphetamines may antagonize the hypotensive effects of antihypertensives). Products include:
- Calan SR Caplets ... 2571
- Calan Tablets ... 2568
- Covera-HS Tablets ... 2573
- Isoptin Injectable ... 1391
- Isoptin Oral Tablets ... 1393
- Isoptin SR Tablets ... 1395
- Verelan Capsules ... 1455

Vitamin C (Lowers absorption of amphetamines by acting as gastrointestinal acidifying agent). Products include:
- ACES Antioxidant Soft Gels ... ▣ 647
- Chromagen Capsules ... 2470
- Chromagen FA ... 2471
- Chromagen Forte ... 2471
- Dexatrim Maximum Strength Plus Vitamin C/Caffeine-Free Caplets ... ▣ 795
- Ester-C Mineral Ascorbates Powder ... ▣ 673
- Fero-Folic-500 Filmtab ... 433
- Fero-Grad-500 Filmtab ... 434
- Halls Vitamin C Drops ... ▣ 807
- Irospan ... 1000
- Materna Tablets ... 1427
- Niferex w/Vitamin C Tablets ... 811
- One-A-Day Antioxidant Plus ... ▣ 625
- Protegra Antioxidant Vitamin & Mineral Supplement ... ▣ 685
- Sunkist Children's Chewable Multivitamins - Plus Extra C ... ▣ 665
- Sunkist Vitamin C ... ▣ 666
- Trinsicon Capsules ... 2759
- Venolax ... ▣ 686
- Vitron-C Tablets ... ▣ 667

Food Interactions

Fruit juices, unspecified (Lowers absorption of amphetamines by acting as gastrointestinal acidifying agent).

DIA-RELIEVER TABLETS
(Nutritional Supplement) ... 461
None cited in PDR database.

DIABETA TABLETS
(Glyburide) ... 1265
May interact with salicylates, sulfonamides, oral anticoagulants, monoamine oxidase inhibitors, beta blockers, thiazides, diuretics, corticosteroids, phenothiazines, thyroid preparations, estrogens, oral contraceptives, sympathomimetics, calcium channel blockers, non-steroidal anti-inflammatory agents, highly protein bound drugs (selected), fluoroquinolone antibiotics, and certain other agents. Compounds in these categories include:

Acebutolol Hydrochloride (Co-administration with beta blockers may result in hypoglycemia). Products include:
- Sectral Capsules ... 2914

Albuterol (Sympathomimetics tend to produce hyperglycemia and concurrent use may lead to loss of control). Products include:
- Proventil Inhalation Aerosol ... 2524
- Ventolin Inhalation Aerosol and Refill ... 1170

Albuterol Sulfate (Sympathomimetics tend to produce hyperglycemia and concurrent use may lead to loss of control). Products include:
- Airet Albuterol Sulfate Inhalation Solution ... 1602
- Albuterol Sulfate, USP Solution for Inhalation, Arm-a-Med ... 522
- Proventil Inhalation Solution 0.083% ... 2527
- Proventil Repetabs Tablets ... 2529
- Proventil Solution for Inhalation 0.5% ... 2525
- Proventil Syrup ... 2528
- Proventil Tablets ... 2529
- Ventolin Inhalation Solution ... 1171
- Ventolin Nebules Inhalation Solution ... 1172
- Ventolin Rotacaps for Inhalation ... 1173
- Ventolin Syrup ... 1175
- Ventolin Tablets ... 1176
- Volmax Extended-Release Tablets .. 1835

Amiloride Hydrochloride (Diuretics tend to produce hyperglycemia and concurrent use may lead to loss of control). Products include:
- Midamor Tablets ... 1746
- Moduretic Tablets ... 1748

Amiodarone Hydrochloride (Co-administration with drugs that are highly protein bound may result in hypoglycemia). Products include:
- Cordarone Intravenous ... 2821
- Cordarone Tablets ... 2818

Amitriptyline Hydrochloride (Co-administration with drugs that are highly protein bound may result in hypoglycemia). Products include:
- Elavil ... 2945
- Etrafon ... 2495
- Limbitrol ... 2333
- Triavil Tablets ... 1800

Amlodipine Besylate (Calcium channel blockers tend to produce hyperglycemia and concurrent use may lead to loss of control). Products include:
- Lotrel Capsules ... 858
- Norvasc Tablets ... 2020

Aspirin (Co-administration with salicylates may result in hypoglycemia). Products include:
- Alka-Seltzer Cherry Effervescent Antacid and Pain Reliever ... ▣ 609
- Alka-Seltzer Extra Strength Effervescent Antacid and Pain Reliever ... ▣ 609
- Alka-Seltzer Lemon Lime Effervescent Antacid and Pain Reliever ... ▣ 609
- Alka-Seltzer Original Effervescent Antacid and Pain Reliever ... ▣ 609
- Alka-Seltzer Plus ... ▣ 611
- Alka-Seltzer Plus Sinus Medicine .. ▣ 611
- Ascriptin ... ▣ 650
- Arthritis Strength BC Powder ... ▣ 631
- BC Cold Powder Multi-Symptom Formula (Cold-Sinus-Allergy) ... ▣ 631
- BC Cold Powder Non-Drowsy Formula (Cold-Sinus) ... ▣ 631
- BC Powder ... ▣ 631
- Genuine Bayer Aspirin Tablets & Caplets ... ▣ 618
- Extra Strength Bayer Arthritis Pain Regimen Formula ... ▣ 615
- Extra Strength Bayer Aspirin Caplets & Tablets ... ▣ 617
- Extended-Release Bayer 8-Hour Aspirin ... ▣ 616
- Extra Strength Bayer Plus Aspirin Caplets ... ▣ 617
- Extra Strength Bayer PM Aspirin Plus Sleep Aid ... ▣ 617
- Aspirin Regimen Bayer 81 mg Tablets with Calcium ... ▣ 615
- Aspirin Regimen Bayer Adult Low Strength 81 mg Tablets ... ▣ 613
- Aspirin Regimen Bayer Children's Chewable Aspirin ... ▣ 616
- Aspirin Regimen Bayer Regular Strength 325 mg Caplets ... ▣ 613
- Bufferin Analgesic Tablets ... ▣ 636
- Arthritis Strength Bufferin Analgesic Caplets ... ▣ 637
- Extra Strength Bufferin Analgesic Tablets ... ▣ 637
- Cama Arthritis Pain Reliever ... ▣ 748
- Darvon Compound-65 Pulvules ... 1475
- Easprin ... 1971
- Ecotrin ... 2625
- Ecotrin Enteric Coated Aspirin Maximum Strength Tablets and Caplets ... ▣ 775
- Ecotrin Enteric Coated Aspirin Regular Strength Tablets ... 2625
- Empirin Aspirin Tablets ... ▣ 818
- Excedrin Extra-Strength Analgesic Tablets, Caplets, and Geltabs ... 734
- Fiorinal Capsules ... 2388
- Fiorinal with Codeine Capsules ... 2390
- Fiorinal Tablets ... 2388
- Goody's Extra Strength Headache Powders ... ▣ 632
- Goody's Extra Strength Pain Relief Tablets ... ▣ 632
- Halfprin Tablets ... 1413
- Norgesic ... 1554
- Percodan Tablets ... 955
- Percodan-Demi Tablets ... 956
- Robaxisal Tablets ... 2246
- Soma Compound w/Codeine Tablets ... 2784
- Soma Compound Tablets ... 2783
- St. Joseph Adult Chewable Aspirin (81 mg.) ... ▣ 768
- Talwin Compound ... 2466
- Vanquish Analgesic Caplets ... ▣ 627

Atenolol (Co-administration with beta blockers may result in hypoglycemia). Products include:
- Tenoretic Tablets ... 2963
- Tenormin Tablets and I.V. Injection 2965

Atovaquone (Co-administration with drugs that are highly protein bound may result in hypoglycemia). Products include:
- Mepron Suspension ... 1206

Bendroflumethiazide (Thiazides tend to produce hperglycemia and concurrent use may lead to loss of control).
- No products indexed under this heading.

Bepridil Hydrochloride (Calcium channel blockers tend to produce hyperglycemia and concurrent use may lead to loss of control). Products include:
- Vascor Tablets (200 and 300 mg) 1597

Betamethasone Acetate (Corticosteroids tend to produce hyperglycemia and concurrent use may lead to loss of control). Products include:
- Celestone Soluspan Suspension ... 2484

Betamethasone Sodium Phosphate (Corticosteroids tend to produce hyperglycemia and concurrent use may lead to loss of control). Products include:
- Celestone Soluspan Suspension ... 2484

Betaxolol Hydrochloride (Co-administration with beta blockers may result in hypoglycemia). Products include:
- Betoptic Ophthalmic Solution ... 465
- Betoptic S Ophthalmic Suspension 467
- Kerlone Tablets ... 2588

Bisoprolol Fumarate (Co-administration with beta blockers may result in hypoglycemia). Products include:
- Zebeta Tablets ... 1457
- Ziac ... 1459

Bumetanide (Diuretics tend to produce hyperglycemia and concurrent use may lead to loss of control). Products include:
- Bumex ... 2260

Carteolol Hydrochloride (Co-administration with beta blockers may result in hypoglycemia). Products include:
- Cartrol Tablets ... 413
- Ocupress Ophthalmic Solution, 1% Sterile ... ◉ 297

Cefonicid Sodium (Co-administration with drugs that are highly protein bound may result in hypoglycemia). Products include:
- Monocid Injection ... 2674

Chloramphenicol Palmitate (Co-administration with chloramphenicol may result in hypoglycemia).
- No products indexed under this heading.

Chloramphenicol Sodium Succinate (Co-administration with chloramphenicol may result in hypoglycemia). Products include:
- Chloromycetin Sodium Succinate ... 1960

Chlordiazepoxide (Co-administration with drugs that are highly protein bound may result in hypoglycemia). Products include:
- Limbitrol ... 2333

Chlordiazepoxide Hydrochloride (Co-administration with drugs that are highly protein bound may result in hypoglycemia). Products include:
- Librax Capsules ... 2330
- Librium Capsules ... 2331
- Librium Injectable ... 2332

IMPORTANT NOTE: Always consult each drug listing in the patient's regimen for possible interactions.

DiaBeta — Interactions Index

Chlorothiazide (Thiazides tend to produce hperglycemia and concurrent use may lead to loss of control). Products include:
- Aldoclor Tablets 1638
- Diupres Tablets 1691
- Diuril Oral 1694

Chlorothiazide Sodium (Thiazides tend to produce hperglycemia and concurrent use may lead to loss of control). Products include:
- Diuril Sodium Intravenous 1693

Chlorotrianisene (Estrogens tend to produce hyperglycemia and concurrent use may lead to loss of control).
- No products indexed under this heading.

Chlorpromazine (Phenothiazines tend to produce hyperglycemia and concurrent use may lead to loss of control). Products include:
- Thorazine Suppositories 2701

Chlorpromazine Hydrochloride (Phenothiazines tend to produce hyperglycemia and concurrent use may lead to loss of control). Products include:
- Thorazine 2701

Chlorpropamide (Co-administration with sulfonamides may result in hypoglycemia). Products include:
- Diabinese Tablets 2002

Chlorthalidone (Diuretics tend to produce hyperglycemia and concurrent use may lead to loss of control). Products include:
- Combipres Tablets 682
- Tenoretic Tablets 2963
- Thalitone 1293

Choline Magnesium Trisalicylate (Co-administration with salicylates may result in hypoglycemia). Products include:
- Trilisate 2155

Ciprofloxacin (Co-administration has resulted in a potentiation of the hypoglycemic action of glyburide). Products include:
- Cipro I.V. 587
- Cipro I.V. Pharmacy Bulk Package 590

Ciprofloxacin Hydrochloride (Co-administration has resulted in a potentiation of the hypoglycemic action of glyburide). Products include:
- Ciloxan Ophthalmic Solution 468
- Cipro Tablets 584

Clomipramine Hydrochloride (Co-administration with drugs that are highly protein bound may result in hypoglycemia). Products include:
- Anafranil Capsules 819

Clozapine (Co-administration with drugs that are highly protein bound may result in hypoglycemia). Products include:
- Clozaril Tablets 2377

Cortisone Acetate (Corticosteroids tend to produce hyperglycemia and concurrent use may lead to loss of control). Products include:
- Cortone Acetate Sterile Suspension 1663
- Cortone Acetate Tablets 1664

Cyclosporine (Co-administration with drugs that are highly protein bound may result in hypoglycemia). Products include:
- Neoral 2405
- Sandimmune 2416

Desogestrel (Oral contraceptives tend to produce hyperglycemia and concurrent use may lead to loss of control). Products include:
- Desogen Tablets 1867
- Ortho-Cept 1907

Dexamethasone (Corticosteroids tend to produce hyperglycemia and concurrent use may lead to loss of control). Products include:
- AK-Trol Ointment & Suspension .... ⊙ 205
- Decadron Elixir 1676
- Decadron Tablets 1678
- Decaspray Topical Aerosol 1689
- Maxitrol Ophthalmic Ointment and Suspension .... ⊙ 222
- TobraDex Ophthalmic Suspension and Ointment 469

Dexamethasone Acetate (Corticosteroids tend to produce hyperglycemia and concurrent use may lead to loss of control). Products include:
- Dalalone D.P. Injectable 1009
- Decadron-LA Sterile Suspension 1687

Dexamethasone Sodium Phosphate (Corticosteroids tend to produce hyperglycemia and concurrent use may lead to loss of control). Products include:
- Decadron Phosphate Injection 1680
- Decadron Phosphate Sterile Ophthalmic Ointment 1684
- Decadron Phosphate Sterile Ophthalmic Solution 1685
- Decadron Phosphate Topical Cream 1686
- Decadron Phosphate with Xylocaine Injection, Sterile 1683
- Dexacort Phosphate in Respihaler 1606
- Dexacort Phosphate in Turbinaire 1607
- NeoDecadron Sterile Ophthalmic Ointment 1755
- NeoDecadron Sterile Ophthalmic Solution 1756
- NeoDecadron Topical Cream 1757

Diazepam (Co-administration with drugs that are highly protein bound may result in hypoglycemia). Products include:
- Dizac (diazepam injectable emulsion) CIV 1862
- Valium Injectable 2336
- Valium Tablets 2335

Diclofenac Potassium (Co-administration with nonsteroidal anti-inflammatory agents may result in hypoglycemia). Products include:
- Cataflam Tablets 833

Diclofenac Sodium (Co-administration with nonsteroidal anti-inflammatory agents may result in hypoglycemia). Products include:
- Voltaren Ophthalmic Sterile Ophthalmic Solution .... ⊙ 264
- Cataflam/Voltaren/Voltaren-XR 833

Dicumarol (Co-administration with coumarins may result in hypoglycemia).
- No products indexed under this heading.

Dienestrol (Estrogens tend to produce hyperglycemia and concurrent use may lead to loss of control). Products include:
- Ortho Dienestrol Cream 1922

Diethylstilbestrol (Estrogens tend to produce hyperglycemia and concurrent use may lead to loss of control). Products include:
- Diethylstilbestrol Tablets 1477

Diflunisal (Co-administration with salicylates may result in hypoglycemia). Products include:
- Dolobid Tablets 1695

Diltiazem Hydrochloride (Calcium channel blockers tend to produce hyperglycemia and concurrent use may lead to loss of control). Products include:
- Cardizem CD Capsules 1251
- Cardizem SR Capsules 1255
- Cardizem Injectable 1253
- Cardizem Tablets 1257
- Dilacor XR Extended-release Capsules 2183
- Tiazac Capsules 1019

Dipyridamole (Co-administration with drugs that are highly protein bound may result in hypoglycemia). Products include:
- Persantine Tablets 686

Dobutamine Hydrochloride (Sympathomimetics tend to produce hyperglycemia and concurrent use may lead to loss of control). Products include:
- Dobutrex Solution Vials 1480

Dopamine Hydrochloride (Sympathomimetics tend to produce hyperglycemia and concurrent use may lead to loss of control).
- No products indexed under this heading.

Enoxacin (Potentiates the hypoglycemic action). Products include:
- Penetrex Tablets 2196

Ephedrine Hydrochloride (Sympathomimetics tend to produce hyperglycemia and concurrent use may lead to loss of control). Products include:
- Primatene Tablets .... ⊞ 844
- Quadrinal Tablets 1398

Ephedrine Sulfate (Sympathomimetics tend to produce hyperglycemia and concurrent use may lead to loss of control). Products include:
- Marax Tablets & DF Syrup 2015

Ephedrine Tannate (Sympathomimetics tend to produce hyperglycemia and concurrent use may lead to loss of control). Products include:
- Rynatuss 2782

Epinephrine (Sympathomimetics tend to produce hyperglycemia and concurrent use may lead to loss of control). Products include:
- EPIFRIN .... ⊙ 237
- EpiPen 808
- Marcaine with Epinephrine 2446
- Primatene Mist .... ⊞ 843
- Sensorcaine with Epinephrine Injection 554
- Sus-Phrine Injection 1017
- Xylocaine with Epinephrine Injections 562

Epinephrine Bitartrate (Sympathomimetics tend to produce hyperglycemia and concurrent use may lead to loss of control). Products include:
- Sensorcaine-MPF with Epinephrine Injection 554

Epinephrine Hydrochloride (Sympathomimetics tend to produce hyperglycemia and concurrent use may lead to loss of control). Products include:
- Ana-Kit Anaphylaxis Emergency Treatment Kit 611

Esmolol Hydrochloride (Co-administration with beta blockers may result in hypoglycemia). Products include:
- Brevibloc (esmolol HCl) Injection 1860

Estradiol (Estrogens tend to produce hyperglycemia and concurrent use may lead to loss of control). Products include:
- Climara Transdermal System 640
- Estrace Cream and Tablets 751
- Estraderm Transdermal System 842
- Estring Vaginal Ring 2086
- Vivelle Transdermal System 880

Estrogens, Conjugated (Estrogens tend to produce hyperglycemia and concurrent use may lead to loss of control). Products include:
- PMB 200 and PMB 400 2890
- Premarin Intravenous 2893
- Premarin Tablets 2896
- Premarin Vaginal Cream 2898
- Premphase 2900
- Prempro 2905

Estrogens, Esterified (Estrogens tend to produce hyperglycemia and concurrent use may lead to loss of control). Products include:
- ESTRATAB Tablets (0.3, 0.625, 1.25, 2.5 mg) 2715
- Estratest 2718
- Menest Tablets 2671

Estropipate (Estrogens tend to produce hyperglycemia and concurrent use may lead to loss of control). Products include:
- Ogen Tablets 2103
- Ogen Vaginal Cream 2106
- Ortho-Est 1925

Ethacrynic Acid (Diuretics tend to produce hyperglycemia and concurrent use may lead to loss of control). Products include:
- Edecrin Tablets 1698

Ethinyl Estradiol (Estrogens tend to produce hyperglycemia and concurrent use may lead to loss of control). Products include:
- Brevicon 2563
- Demulen 2580
- Desogen Tablets 1867
- Levlen/Tri-Levlen 646
- Lo/Ovral Tablets 2852
- Lo/Ovral-28 Tablets 2857
- Modicon 1928
- Nordette-21 Tablets 2863
- Nordette-28 Tablets 2866
- Norinyl 2563
- Ortho-Cept 1907
- Ortho-Cyclen/Ortho-Tri-Cyclen 1914
- Ortho-Novum 1928
- Ortho-Cyclen/Ortho Tri-Cyclen 1914
- Ovcon 765
- Ovral Tablets 2877
- Ovral-28 Tablets 2878
- Levlen/Tri-Levlen 646
- Tri-Norinyl 2607
- Triphasil-21 Tablets 2919
- Triphasil-28 Tablets 2924

Ethynodiol Diacetate (Oral contraceptives tend to produce hyperglycemia and concurrent use may lead to loss of control). Products include:
- Demulen 2580

Etodolac (Co-administration with nonsteroidal anti-inflammatory agents may result in hypoglycemia). Products include:
- Lodine Capsules and Tablets 2849

Felodipine (Calcium channel blockers tend to produce hyperglycemia and concurrent use may lead to loss of control). Products include:
- Plendil Extended-Release Tablets 514

Fenoprofen Calcium (Co-administration with nonsteroidal anti-inflammatory agents may result in hypoglycemia). Products include:
- Nalfon 200 Pulvules & Nalfon Tablets 933

Fludrocortisone Acetate (Corticosteroids tend to produce hyperglycemia and concurrent use may lead to loss of control). Products include:
- Florinef Acetate Tablets 506

Fluphenazine Decanoate (Phenothiazines tend to produce hyperglycemia and concurrent use may lead to loss of control). Products include:
- Prolixin Decanoate 510

Fluphenazine Enanthate (Phenothiazines tend to produce hyperglycemia and concurrent use may lead to loss of control). Products include:
- Prolixin Enanthate 510

Fluphenazine Hydrochloride (Phenothiazines tend to produce hyperglycemia and concurrent use may lead to loss of control). Products include:
- Prolixin 510

(⊞ Described in PDR For Nonprescription Drugs) (⊙ Described in PDR For Ophthalmology)

Flurazepam Hydrochloride (Co-administration with drugs that are highly protein bound may result in hypoglycemia). Products include:
- Dalmane Capsules 2329

Flurbiprofen (Co-administration with nonsteroidal anti-inflammatory agents may result in hypoglycemia).
- No products indexed under this heading.

Fosphenytoin Sodium (Phenytoin tends to produce hyperglycemia and concurrent use may lead to loss of control). Products include:
- Cerebyx Injection 1956

Furazolidone (Co-administration with monamine oxidase inhibitors may result in hypoglycemia). Products include:
- Furoxone 2221

Furosemide (Diuretics tend to produce hyperglycemia and concurrent use may lead to loss of control). Products include:
- Lasix Injection, Oral Solution and Tablets 1267

Glipizide (Co-administration with sulfonamides may result in hypoglycemia). Products include:
- Glucotrol Tablets 2011
- Glucotrol XL Extended Release Tablets 2012

Hydrochlorothiazide (Thiazides tend to produce hperglycemia and concurrent use may lead to loss of control). Products include:
- Aldactazide Tablets 2556
- Aldoril Tablets 1644
- Apresazide Capsules 824
- Capozide Tablets 744
- Dyazide Capsules 2653
- Esidrix Tablets 839
- Esimil Tablets 840
- HydroDIURIL Tablets 1716
- Hydropres Tablets 1718
- Hyzaar Tablets 1720
- Inderide Tablets 2838
- Inderide LA Long Acting Capsules .. 2840
- Lopressor HCT Tablets 850
- Lotensin HCT Tablets 855
- Moduretic Tablets 1748
- Oretic Tablets 450
- Prinzide Tablets 1780
- Ser-Ap-Es Tablets 867
- Timolide Tablets 1791
- Vaseretic Tablets 1810
- Zestoretic Tablets 2968
- Ziac 1459

Hydrocortisone (Corticosteroids tend to produce hyperglycemia and concurrent use may lead to loss of control). Products include:
- Anusol-HC Cream 2.5% 1953
- Aquanil HC Lotion 1989
- Maximum Strength Cortaid Spray ◘ 800
- CORTENEMA 2713
- Cortisporin Ointment 1074
- Cortisporin Ophthalmic Ointment Sterile 1074
- Cortisporin Ophthalmic Suspension Sterile 1075
- Cortisporin Otic Solution Sterile 1076
- Cortisporin Otic Suspension Sterile 1077
- Cortizone-5 .... ◘ 795
- Cortizone-10 .... ◘ 795
- Hydrocortone Tablets 1715
- Hytone 922
- Hytone Ointment 2 ½% 923
- Massengill Medicated Soft Cloth Towelettes 2628
- Pediotic Suspension Sterile 1140
- Preparation H Hydrocortisone 1% Cream .... ◘ 843
- ProctoCream-HC 2.5% 2552
- VōSoL HC Otic Solution 2786

Hydrocortisone Acetate (Corticosteroids tend to produce hyperglycemia and concurrent use may lead to loss of control). Products include:
- Analpram-HC Rectal Cream 1% and 2.5% 993
- Anusol HC-1 Hydrocortisone Anti-Itch Ointment .... ◘ 810
- Anusol-HC Suppositories 1954
- Caldecort Anti-Itch Hydrocortisone Cream .... ◘ 651
- Coly-Mycin S Otic w/Neomycin & Hydrocortisone 1965
- Cortaid .... ◘ 800
- Cortifoam 2540
- Cortisporin Cream 1073
- Epifoam 2543
- Hydrocortone Acetate Sterile Suspension 1712
- Mantadil Cream 1124
- Nupercainal Hydrocortisone 1% Cream .... ◘ 661
- Pramosone Cream, Lotion & Ointment 995
- ProctoFoam-HC 2552
- Terra-Cortril Ophthalmic Suspension 2033

Hydrocortisone Sodium Phosphate (Corticosteroids tend to produce hyperglycemia and concurrent use may lead to loss of control). Products include:
- Hydrocortone Phosphate Injection, Sterile 1713

Hydrocortisone Sodium Succinate (Corticosteroids tend to produce hyperglycemia and concurrent use may lead to loss of control).
- No products indexed under this heading.

Hydroflumethiazide (Thiazides tend to produce hperglycemia and concurrent use may lead to loss of control). Products include:
- Diucardin Tablets 2824

Ibuprofen (Co-administration with nonsteroidal anti-inflammatory agents may result in hypoglycemia). Products include:
- Advil Cold and Sinus Caplets and Tablets .... ◘ 837
- Advil Ibuprofen Tablets, Caplets and Gel Caplets .... ◘ 836
- Children's Motrin Ibuprofen Oral Suspension 1558
- IBU Tablets 1389
- Ibuprohm .... ◘ 713
- Motrin IB Caplets, Tablets, and Gelcaps .... ◘ 802
- Motrin Ibuprofen Suspension, Oral Drops, Chewable Tablets, Caplets 1563
- Nuprin Ibuprofen/Analgesic Tablets & Caplets .... ◘ 645
- Vicks DayQuil SINUS Pressure & PAIN Relief with IBUPROFEN .... ◘ 735

Imipramine Hydrochloride (Co-administration with drugs that are highly protein bound may result in hypoglycemia). Products include:
- Tofranil Ampuls 873
- Tofranil Tablets 875

Imipramine Pamoate (Co-administration with drugs that are highly protein bound may result in hypoglycemia). Products include:
- Tofranil-PM Capsules 876

Indapamide (Diuretics tend to produce hyperglycemia and concurrent use may lead to loss of control).
- No products indexed under this heading.

Indomethacin (Co-administration with nonsteroidal anti-inflammatory agents may result in hypoglycemia). Products include:
- Indocin 1723

Indomethacin Sodium Trihydrate (Co-administration with nonsteroidal anti-inflammatory agents may result in hypoglycemia). Products include:
- Indocin I.V. 1727

Isocarboxazid (Co-administration with monamine oxidase inhibitors may result in hypoglycemia).
- No products indexed under this heading.

Isoniazid (Isoniazid tends to produce hyperglycemia and concurrent use may lead to loss of control). Products include:
- Nydrazid Injection 509
- Rifamate Capsules 1278
- Rifater 1280

Isoproterenol Hydrochloride (Sympathomimetics tend to produce hyperglycemia and concurrent use may lead to loss of control). Products include:
- Isuprel Hydrochloride Solution 2443
- Isuprel Injection 2441
- Isuprel Mistometer 2442

Isoproterenol Sulfate (Sympathomimetics tend to produce hyperglycemia and concurrent use may lead to loss of control). Products include:
- Norisodrine with Calcium Iodide Syrup 446

Isradipine (Calcium channel blockers tend to produce hyperglycemia and concurrent use may lead to loss of control). Products include:
- DynaCirc Capsules 2381
- DynaCirc CR Tablets 2383

Ketoprofen (Co-administration with nonsteroidal anti-inflammatory agents may result in hypoglycemia). Products include:
- Actron Caplets and Tablets .... ◘ 608
- Orudis Capsules 2874
- Orudis KT .... ◘ 842
- Oruvail Capsules 2874

Ketorolac Tromethamine (Co-administration with nonsteroidal anti-inflammatory agents may result in hypoglycemia). Products include:
- Acular Sterile Ophthalmic Solution 470
- Toradol 2319

Labetalol Hydrochloride (Co-administration with beta blockers may result in hypoglycemia). Products include:
- Normodyne Injection 2519
- Normodyne Tablets 2522
- Trandate 1158

Levobunolol Hydrochloride (Co-administration with beta blockers may result in hypoglycemia). Products include:
- Betagan .... ◉ 230

Levonorgestrel (Oral contraceptives tend to produce hyperglycemia and concurrent use may lead to loss of control). Products include:
- Levlen/Tri-Levlen 646
- Nordette-21 Tablets 2863
- Nordette-28 Tablets 2866
- Norplant System 2868
- Levlen/Tri-Levlen 646
- Triphasil-21 Tablets 2919
- Triphasil-28 Tablets 2924

Levothyroxine Sodium (Thyroid products tend to produce hyperglycemia and concurrent use may lead to loss of control). Products include:
- Eltroxin Tablets 2214
- Levothroid Tablets 1015
- Levothyroxine Sodium, USP for Injection 546
- Levoxyl Tablets 918
- Synthroid 1410

Liothyronine Sodium (Thyroid products tend to produce hyperglycemia and concurrent use may lead to loss of control). Products include:
- Cytomel Tablets 2647
- Triostat Injection 2708

Liotrix (Thyroid products tend to produce hyperglycemia and concurrent use may lead to loss of control).
- No products indexed under this heading.

Lomefloxacin Hydrochloride (Potentiates the hypoglycemic action). Products include:
- Maxaquin Tablets 2593

Magnesium Salicylate (Co-administration with salicylates may result in hypoglycemia). Products include:
- Backache Caplets .... ◘ 635
- Doan's Extra-Strength Analgesic .... ◘ 653
- Extra Strength Doan's P.M. .... ◘ 653
- Doan's Regular Strength Analgesic .... ◘ 654
- Mobigesic Tablets .... ◘ 607

Meclofenamate Sodium (Co-administration with nonsteroidal anti-inflammatory agents may result in hypoglycemia).
- No products indexed under this heading.

Mefenamic Acid (Co-administration with nonsteroidal anti-inflammatory agents may result in hypoglycemia). Products include:
- Ponstel 1982

Mesoridazine Besylate (Phenothiazines tend to produce hyperglycemia and concurrent use may lead to loss of control). Products include:
- Serentil 689

Mestranol (Oral contraceptives tend to produce hyperglycemia and concurrent use may lead to loss of control). Products include:
- Norinyl 2563
- Ortho-Novum 1928

Metaproterenol Sulfate (Sympathomimetics tend to produce hyperglycemia and concurrent use may lead to loss of control). Products include:
- Alupent 672
- Metaproterenol Sulfate Inhalation Solution, USP, Arm-a-Med 547

Metaraminol Bitartrate (Sympathomimetics tend to produce hyperglycemia and concurrent use may lead to loss of control). Products include:
- Aramine Injection 1649

Methotrimeprazine (Phenothiazines tend to produce hyperglycemia and concurrent use may lead to loss of control). Products include:
- Levoprome 1321

Methoxamine Hydrochloride (Sympathomimetics tend to produce hyperglycemia and concurrent use may lead to loss of control). Products include:
- Vasoxyl Injection 1169

Methyclothiazide (Thiazides tend to produce hperglycemia and concurrent use may lead to loss of control). Products include:
- Enduron Tablets 424

Methylprednisolone Acetate (Corticosteroids tend to produce hyperglycemia and concurrent use may lead to loss of control).
- No products indexed under this heading.

Methylprednisolone Sodium Succinate (Corticosteroids tend to produce hyperglycemia and concurrent use may lead to loss of control).
- No products indexed under this heading.

Metipranolol Hydrochloride (Co-administration with beta blockers may result in hypoglycemia). Products include:
- OptiPranolol (Metipranolol 0.3%) Sterile Ophthalmic Solution .... ◉ 256

Metolazone (Diuretics tend to produce hyperglycemia and concurrent use may lead to loss of control). Products include:
- Mykrox Tablets 1617
- Zaroxolyn Tablets 1625

IMPORTANT NOTE: Always consult each drug listing in the patient's regimen for possible interactions.

DiaBeta Interactions Index 274

Metoprolol Succinate (Co-administration with beta blockers may result in hypoglycemia). Products include:
Toprol-XL Tablets ... 560
Metoprolol Tartrate (Co-administration with beta blockers may result in hypoglycemia). Products include:
Lopressor ... 848
Lopressor HCT Tablets ... 850
Miconazole (Co-administration with oral miconazole and oral hypoglycemic agents has resulted in severe hypoglycemia).
No products indexed under this heading.
Midazolam Hydrochloride (Co-administration with drugs that are highly protein bound may result in hypoglycemia). Products include:
Versed Injection ... 2324
Nabumetone (Co-administration with nonsteroidal anti-inflammatory agents may result in hypoglycemia). Products include:
Relafen Tablets ... 2688
Nadolol (Co-administration with beta blockers may result in hypoglycemia).
No products indexed under this heading.
Naproxen (Co-administration with nonsteroidal anti-inflammatory agents may result in hypoglycemia). Products include:
Anaprox/Naprosyn ... 2277
Naproxen Sodium (Co-administration with nonsteroidal anti-inflammatory agents may result in hypoglycemia). Products include:
Aleve ... 2124
Anaprox/Naprosyn ... 2277
Naprelan Tablets ... 2861
Nicardipine Hydrochloride (Calcium channel blockers tend to produce hyperglycemia and concurrent use may lead to loss of control). Products include:
Cardene Capsules ... 2261
Cardene I.V. ... 2815
Cardene SR Capsules ... 2264
Nicotinic Acid (Nicotinic acid tends to produce hyperglycemia and concurrent use may lead to loss of control).
No products indexed under this heading.
Nifedipine (Calcium channel blockers tend to produce hyperglycemia and concurrent use may lead to loss of control). Products include:
Adalat Capsules (10 mg and 20 mg) ... 580
Adalat CC ... 582
Procardia Capsules ... 2024
Procardia XL Extended Release Tablets ... 2026
Nimodipine (Calcium channel blockers tend to produce hyperglycemia and concurrent use may lead to loss of control). Products include:
Nimotop Capsules ... 603
Nisoldipine (Calcium channel blockers tend to produce hyperglycemia and concurrent use may lead to loss of control). Products include:
Sular Tablets ... 2961
Norepinephrine Bitartrate (Sympathomimetics tend to produce hyperglycemia and concurrent use may lead to loss of control). Products include:
Levophed Bitartrate Injection ... 2445
Norethindrone (Oral contraceptives tend to produce hyperglycemia and concurrent use may lead to loss of control). Products include:
Brevicon ... 2563
Micronor Tablets ... 1903
Modicon ... 1928
Norinyl ... 2563
Nor-Q D Tablets ... 2598
Ortho-Novum ... 1928
Ovcon ... 765
Tri-Norinyl ... 2607
Norethynodrel (Oral contraceptives tend to produce hyperglycemia and concurrent use may lead to loss of control).
No products indexed under this heading.
Norfloxacin (Potentiates the hypoglycemic action). Products include:
Chibroxin Sterile Ophthalmic Solution ... 1657
Noroxin Tablets ... 1758
Noroxin Tablets ... 2222
Norgestimate (Oral contraceptives tend to produce hyperglycemia and concurrent use may lead to loss of control). Products include:
Ortho-Cyclen/Ortho-Tri-Cyclen ... 1914
Ortho-Cyclen/Ortho Tri-Cyclen ... 1914
Norgestrel (Oral contraceptives tend to produce hyperglycemia and concurrent use may lead to loss of control). Products include:
Lo/Ovral Tablets ... 2852
Lo/Ovral-28 Tablets ... 2857
Ovral Tablets ... 2877
Ovral-28 Tablets ... 2878
Ovrette Tablets ... 2878
Nortriptyline Hydrochloride (Co-administration with drugs that are highly protein bound may result in hypoglycemia). Products include:
Pamelor ... 2409
Ofloxacin (Potentiates the hypoglycemic action). Products include:
Floxin I.V. ... 1580
Floxin Tablets (200 mg, 300 mg, 400 mg) ... 1577
Ocuflox Ophthalmic Solution ... 478
Ocuflox ... ⊙ 242
Oxaprozin (Co-administration with nonsteroidal anti-inflammatory agents may result in hypoglycemia). Products include:
Daypro Caplets ... 2578
Oxazepam (Co-administration with drugs that are highly protein bound may result in hypoglycemia). Products include:
Serax Capsules ... 2916
Serax Tablets ... 2916
Penbutolol Sulfate (Co-administration with beta blockers may result in hypoglycemia). Products include:
Levatol Tablets ... 2547
Perphenazine (Phenothiazines tend to produce hyperglycemia and concurrent use may lead to loss of control). Products include:
Etrafon ... 2495
Triavil Tablets ... 1800
Trilafon ... 2532
Phenelzine Sulfate (Co-administration with monamine oxidase inhibitors may result in hypoglycemia). Products include:
Nardil ... 1977
Phenylbutazone (Co-administration with nonsteroidal anti-inflammatory agents may result in hypoglycemia).
No products indexed under this heading.
Phenylephrine Bitartrate (Sympathomimetics tend to produce hyperglycemia and concurrent use may lead to loss of control).
No products indexed under this heading.
Phenylephrine Hydrochloride (Sympathomimetics tend to produce hyperglycemia and concurrent use may lead to loss of control). Products include:
Atrohist Plus Tablets ... 1605
Cerose DM ... ▣ 853
D.A. II Tablets ... 972
D.A. Chewable Tablets ... 970
Dura-Vent/DA Tablets ... 1003
Extendryl ... 1003
4-Way Fast Acting Nasal Spray (regular & mentholated) ... ▣ 644
Hemorid ... ▣ 797
Hycomine Compound Tablets ... 948
Neo-Synephrine Hydrochloride 1% Carpuject ... 2455
Neo-Synephrine Hydrochloride 1% Injection ... 2455
Neo-Synephrine Hydrochloride (Ophthalmic) ... 2456
Neo-Synephrine ... ▣ 624
Novahistine Elixir ... ▣ 782
Phenergan VC ... 2886
Phenergan VC with Codeine ... 2888
Preparation H ... ▣ 842
Tympagesic Ear Drops ... 2476
Vicks Sinex Nasal Spray and Ultra Fine Mist ... ▣ 738
Phenylephrine Tannate (Sympathomimetics tend to produce hyperglycemia and concurrent use may lead to loss of control). Products include:
Atrohist Pediatric Suspension ... 1604
Atrohist Pediatric Suspension Dye-Free ... 1604
Rynatan ... 2781
Rynatuss ... 2782
Phenylpropanolamine Hydrochloride (Sympathomimetics tend to produce hyperglycemia and concurrent use may lead to loss of control). Products include:
Acutrim ... ▣ 648
Atrohist Plus Tablets ... 1605
BC Cold Powder Multi-Symptom Formula (Cold-Sinus-Allergy) ... ▣ 631
BC Cold Powder Non-Drowsy Formula (Cold-Sinus) ... ▣ 631
Cheracol Plus Head Cold/Cough Formula ... ▣ 741
Comtrex Multi-Symptom Cold Reliever Liqui-Gels ... ▣ 638
Comtrex Multi-Symptom Non-Drowsy Liqui-gels ... ▣ 640
Contac Continuous Action Nasal Decongestant/Antihistamine 12 Hour Capsules ... ▣ 773
Contac Maximum Strength Continuous Action Decongestant/Antihistamine 12 Hour Caplets ... ▣ 772
Contac Severe Cold and Flu Formula Caplets ... ▣ 773
Coricidin 'D' Decongestant Tablets ... ▣ 760
Dexatrim ... ▣ 795
Dexatrim Plus Vitamins Caplets ... ▣ 796
Dimetane-DC Cough Syrup ... 2232
Dimetapp Allergy Sinus Caplets ... ▣ 838
Dimetapp Cold & Allergy Chewable Tablets ... ▣ 838
Dimetapp Cold & Cough Liqui-Gels ... ▣ 839
Dimetapp DM Elixir ... ▣ 840
Dimetapp Elixir ... ▣ 840
Dimetapp Extentabs ... ▣ 841
Dimetapp Tablets/Liqui-Gels ... ▣ 841
Dura-Vent Tablets ... 971
Entex LA Tablets ... 972
Exgest LA Tablets ... 787
Hycomine ... 947
Nolamine Timed-Release Tablets ... 790
Ornade Spansule Capsules ... 2678
Propagest Tablets ... 791
Pyrroxate Caplets ... ▣ 742
Robitussin-CF ... ▣ 846
Sinulin Tablets ... 792
Tavist-D 12 Hour Relief Tablets ... ▣ 750
Teldrin 12 Hour Antihistamine/Nasal Decongestant Allergy Relief Capsules ... ▣ 786
Triaminic Expectorant ... ▣ 753
Triaminic Syrup ... ▣ 755
Triaminic Triaminicol Cold & Cough ... ▣ 756
Triaminic DM Syrup ... ▣ 756
Triaminicin Tablets ... ▣ 756
Vicks DayQuil Allergy Relief 12-Hour Extended Release Tablets ... ▣ 733
Vicks DayQuil Allergy Relief 4-Hour Tablets ... ▣ 733
Vicks DayQuil SINUS Pressure & CONGESTION Relief ... ▣ 734
Phenytoin (Phenytoin tends to produce hyperglycemia and concurrent use may lead to loss of control). Products include:
Dilantin Infatabs ... 1967
Dilantin-125 Suspension ... 1969
Phenytoin Sodium (Phenytoin tends to produce hyperglycemia and concurrent use may lead to loss of control). Products include:
Dilantin Kapseals ... 1965
Pindolol (Co-administration with beta blockers may result in hypoglycemia). Products include:
Visken Tablets ... 2428
Pirbuterol Acetate (Sympathomimetics tend to produce hyperglycemia and concurrent use may lead to loss of control). Products include:
Maxair Autohaler ... 1550
Maxair Inhaler ... 1552
Piroxicam (Co-administration with nonsteroidal anti-inflammatory agents may result in hypoglycemia). Products include:
Feldene Capsules ... 2008
Polyestradiol Phosphate (Estrogens tend to produce hyperglycemia and concurrent use may lead to loss of control).
No products indexed under this heading.
Polythiazide (Thiazides tend to produce hperglycemia and concurrent use may lead to loss of control). Products include:
Minizide Capsules ... 2016
Prednisolone Acetate (Corticosteroids tend to produce hyperglycemia and concurrent use may lead to loss of control). Products include:
AK-CIDE ... ⊙ 203
AK-CIDE Ointment ... ⊙ 203
Blephamide Liquifilm Sterile Ophthalmic Suspension ... 472
Blephamide Ointment ... ⊙ 234
Econopred & Econopred Plus Ophthalmic Suspensions ... ⊙ 216
Poly-Pred Liquifilm ... ⊙ 246
Pred Forte ... ⊙ 247
Pred Mild ... ⊙ 250
Pred-G Liquifilm Sterile Ophthalmic Suspension ... ⊙ 248
Pred-G S.O.P. Sterile Ophthalmic Ointment ... ⊙ 249
Prednisolone Sodium Phosphate (Corticosteroids tend to produce hyperglycemia and concurrent use may lead to loss of control). Products include:
AK-PRED ... ⊙ 204
Hydeltrasol Injection, Sterile ... 1708
Pediapred Oral Solution ... 1618
Prednisolone Tebutate (Corticosteroids tend to produce hyperglycemia and concurrent use may lead to loss of control). Products include:
Hydeltra-T.B.A. Sterile Suspension ... 1710
Prednisone (Corticosteroids tend to produce hyperglycemia and concurrent use may lead to loss of control).
No products indexed under this heading.
Probenecid (Co-administration with probenecid may result in hypoglycemia). Products include:
Benemid Tablets ... 1651
ColBENEMID Tablets ... 1662
Prochlorperazine (Phenothiazines tend to produce hyperglycemia and concurrent use may lead to loss of control). Products include:
Compazine ... 2644
Promethazine Hydrochloride (Phenothiazines tend to produce hyperglycemia and concurrent use may lead to loss of control). Products include:
Mepergan Injection ... 2859

(▣ Described in PDR For Nonprescription Drugs) (⊙ Described in PDR For Ophthalmology)

Phenergan with Codeine 2883
Phenergan with Dextromethorphan 2885
Phenergan Injection 2880
Phenergan Suppositories 2882
Phenergan Syrup 2881
Phenergan Tablets 2882
Phenergan VC 2886
Phenergan VC with Codeine 2888

Propranolol Hydrochloride (Co-administration with beta blockers may result in hypoglycemia). Products include:

Inderal 2834
Inderal LA Long Acting Capsules 2836
Inderide Tablets 2838
Inderide LA Long Acting Capsules .. 2840

Pseudoephedrine Hydrochloride (Sympathomimetics tend to produce hyperglycemia and concurrent use may lead to loss of control). Products include:

Actifed Allergy Daytime/Nighttime Caplets .... PD 808
Actifed Cold & Allergy Tablets .... PD 807
Actifed Cold & Sinus Caplets and Tablets .... PD 808
Actifed Sinus Daytime/Nighttime Tablets and Caplets .... PD 809
Advil Cold and Sinus Caplets and Tablets .... PD 837
Alka-Seltzer Plus Liqui-Gels .... PD 612
Alka-Seltzer Plus Flu & Body Aches Liqui-Gels Non-Drowsy Formula .... PD 613
Alka-Seltzer Plus Night-Time Cold Medicine Liqui-Gels .... PD 612
Allerest Maximum Strength .... PD 649
Allerest No Drowsiness .... PD 649
Allerest Sinus Pain Formula .... PD 649
Atrohist Pediatric Capsules 1603
Benadryl Allergy/Cold Tablets .... PD 811
Benadryl Allergy Decongestant Liquid Medication .... PD 812
Benadryl Allergy Decongestant Tablets .... PD 812
Benadryl Allergy Sinus Headache Caplets .... PD 813
Benylin Multisymptom .... PD 816
Bromfed Capsules (Extended-Release) 1832
Bromfed Syrup .... PD 712
Bromfed Tablets 1832
Bromfed-DM Cough Syrup 1832
Bromfed-PD Capsules (Extended-Release) 1832
Children's TYLENOL Cold Multi-Symptom Chewable Tablets and Liquid 1559
Children's TYLENOL Cold Plus Cough Multi Symptom Chewable Tablets and Liquid 1560
Children's TYLENOL Flu Suspension Liquid 1560
Children's Vicks DayQuil Allergy Relief .... PD 730
Children's Vicks NyQuil Cold/Cough Relief .... PD 731
Allergy-Sinus Comtrex Multi-Symptom Allergy-Sinus Formula Tablets and Caplets .... PD 639
Comtrex Multi-Symptom .... PD 638
Comtrex Multi-Symptom Non-Drowsy Caplets .... PD 640
Congess 1003
Contac Day Allergy/Sinus Caplets PD 771
Contac Day & Night .... PD 772
Contac Night Allergy/Sinus Caplets .... PD 771
Contac Severe Cold & Flu Non-Drowsy .... PD 774
Deconsal II Tablets 1605
Dimetane-DX Cough Syrup 2233
Dimetapp Cold & Fever Suspension .... PD 839
Dimetapp Decongestant Pediatric Drops .... PD 840
Dorcol Children's Cough Syrup .... PD 748
Drixoral Cough + Congestion Liquid Caps .... PD 763
Dura-Tap/PD Capsules 970
Duratuss Tablets 2750
Duratuss HD Elixir 2750
Efidac/24 .... PD 655
Entex PSE Tablets 973
Fedahist Gyrocaps 2545
Guaifed 1833
Guaifed Syrup .... PD 712
Guaimax-D Tablets 809
Histussin D Liquid 670
Infants' TYLENOL Cold Decongestant & Fever-Reducer Drops 1561
Kronofed-A 994
Novahistine DMX .... PD 782
Nucofed 2225
PediaCare Cough-Cold Chewable Tablets and Liquid 1569
PediaCare Infants' Decongestant Drops 1569
PediaCare Infants' Drops Decongestant Plus Cough 1569
PediaCare NightRest Cough-Cold Liquid 1569
Pediatric Vicks 44d Cough & Head Congestion Relief .... PD 736
Pediatric Vicks 44m Cough & Cold Relief .... PD 737
Robitussin Cold & Cough Liqui-Gels .... PD 844
Robitussin Cold, Cough & Flu Liqui-Gels .... PD 844
Robitussin Maximum Strength Cough & Cold .... PD 847
Robitussin Night-Time Cold Formula .... PD 847
Robitussin Pediatric Cough & Cold Formula .... PD 848
Robitussin Pediatric Drops .... PD 849
Robitussin Severe Congestion Liqui-Gels .... PD 845
Robitussin-DAC Syrup 2249
Robitussin-PE .... PD 846
Rondec Oral Drops 974
Rondec Syrup 974
Rondec Tablet 974
Rondec Chewable Tablets 974
Rondec-TR Tablet 974
Ryna .... PD 804
Seldane-D Extended-Release Tablets 1286
Semprex-D Capsules 1620
Sinarest .... PD 663
Sine-Aid Maximum Strength Sinus Headache Gelcaps, Caplets and Tablets 1570
Sine-Off No Drowsiness Formula Caplets .... PD 784
Sine-Off Sinus Medicine .... PD 784
Singlet Tablets .... PD 785
Sinutab Non-Drying Liquid Caps .... PD 823
Sinutab Sinus Allergy Medication, Maximum Strength Tablets and Caplets .... PD 823
Sinutab Sinus Medication, Maximum Strength Without Drowsiness Formula, Tablets & Caplets .... PD 824
Sudafed Children's Cold & Cough Liquid Medication .... PD 825
Sudafed Children's Nasal Decongestant Liquid Medication .... PD 826
Sudafed Cold & Allergy Tablets .... PD 826
Sudafed Cold and Cough Liquid Caps .... PD 826
Sudafed Nasal Decongestant Tablets, 30 mg .... PD 825
Sudafed Nasal Decongestant Tablets, 60 mg .... PD 825
Sudafed Non-Drying Sinus Liquid Caps .... PD 827
Sudafed Pediatric Nasal Decongestant Liquid Oral Drops .... PD 827
Sudafed Severe Cold Formula Caplets .... PD 828
Sudafed Severe Cold Formula Tablets .... PD 828
Sudafed Sinus Caplets .... PD 829
Sudafed Sinus Tablets .... PD 829
Sudafed 12 Hour Caplets .... PD 824
Syn-Rx Tablets 1622
Syn-Rx DM Tablets 1623
TheraFlu Flu and Cold Medicine .... PD 750
Theraflu Maximum Strength Flu and Cold Medicine For Sore Throat .... PD 751
TheraFlu Flu, Cold and Cough Medicine .... PD 750
TheraFlu Maximum Strength Nighttime Flu, Cold & Cough Medicine .... PD 751
TheraFlu Maximum Strength Non-Drowsy Formula Flu, Cold & Cough Medicine .... PD 751
TheraFlu Maximum Strength, Non-Drowsy Formula Flu, Cold and Cough Caplets .... PD 752
Theraflu Maximum Strength Sinus Non-Drowsy Formula Caplets .... PD 752
Triaminic AM Cough and Decongestant Formula .... PD 753
Triaminic AM Decongestant Formula .... PD 753
Triaminic Infant Oral Decongestant Drops .... PD 754
Triaminic Night Time .... PD 754
Triaminic Sore Throat Formula .... PD 755
Tussend 1830
Tussend Expectorant 1831
TYLENOL Allergy Sinus, Maximum Strength Caplets and Gelcaps 1571
TYLENOL Allergy Sinus NightTime, Maximum Strength Caplets 1571
TYLENOL Cold Medication, Multi-Symptom Formula Tablets and Caplets 1572
TYLENOL Cold Medication, Multi-Symptom Hot Liquid Packets 1572
TYLENOL Cold Medication, No Drowsiness Formula Caplets and Gelcaps 1572
TYLENOL Cold Severe Congestion Caplets 1573
TYLENOL Cough Medication with Decongestant, Multi Symptom 1574
TYLENOL Flu No Drowsiness Formula, Maximum Strength Gelcaps 1575
TYLENOL Flu NightTime, Maximum Strength Gelcaps 1575
TYLENOL Flu NightTime, Maximum Strength Hot Medication Packets 1575
TYLENOL Sinus, Maximum Strength Geltabs, Gelcaps, Caplets and Tablets 1576
Vicks 44 LiquiCaps Cough, Cold & Flu Relief .... PD 728
Vicks 44 LiquiCaps Non-Drowsy Cough & Cold Relief .... PD 729
Vicks 44D Cough & Head Congestion Relief .... PD 728
Vicks 44M Cough, Cold & Flu Relief .... PD 729
Vicks DayQuil LiquiCaps/Liquid Multi-Symptom Cold/Flu Relief .. PD 734
Vicks DayQuil SINUS Pressure & PAIN Relief with IBUPROFEN .... PD 735
Vicks Nyquil Hot Therapy .... PD 735
Vicks NyQuil LiquiCaps/Liquid Multi-Symptom Cold/Flu Relief, Original and Cherry Flavors .... PD 736

Pseudoephedrine Sulfate (Sympathomimetics tend to produce hyperglycemia and concurrent use may lead to loss of control). Products include:

Chlor-Trimeton Allergy Decongestant Tablets .... PD 759
Claritin-D Tablets 2487
Drixoral Cold and Allergy Sustained-Action Tablets .... PD 763
Drixoral Cold and Flu Extended-Release Tablets .... PD 764
Drixoral Non-Drowsy Formula Extended-Release Tablets .... PD 764
Drixoral Allergy/Sinus Extended Release Tablets .... PD 765
Trinalin Repetabs Tablets 1373

Quinestrol (Estrogens tend to produce hyperglycemia and concurrent use may lead to loss of control).

No products indexed under this heading.

Salmeterol Xinafoate (Sympathomimetics tend to produce hyperglycemia and concurrent use may lead to loss of control). Products include:

Serevent Inhalation Aerosol 1149

Salsalate (Co-administration with salicylates may result in hypoglycemia). Products include:

Disalcid 1549
Mono-Gesic Tablets 810
Salflex Tablets 791

Selegiline Hydrochloride (Co-administration with monamine oxidase inhibitors may result in hypoglycemia). Products include:

Eldepryl Capsules 2729

Sotalol Hydrochloride (Co-administration with beta blockers may result in hypoglycemia). Products include:

Betapace Tablets 637

Spironolactone (Diuretics tend to produce hyperglycemia and concurrent use may lead to loss of control). Products include:

Aldactazide Tablets 2556
Aldactone Tablets 2558

Sulfacytine (Co-administration with sulfonamides may result in hypoglycemia).

Sulfamethizole (Co-administration with sulfonamides may result in hypoglycemia). Products include:

Urobiotic-250 Capsules 2038

Sulfamethoxazole (Co-administration with sulfonamides may result in hypoglycemia). Products include:

Bactrim DS Tablets 2257
Bactrim I.V. Infusion 2255
Bactrim 2257
Gantanol Tablets 2285
Septra 1146
Septra I.V. Infusion 1142
Septra I.V. Infusion ADD-Vantage Vials 1144
Septra 1146

Sulfasalazine (Co-administration with sulfonamides may result in hypoglycemia). Products include:

Azulfidine 2059

Sulfinpyrazone (Co-administration with sulfonamides may result in hypoglycemia). Products include:

Anturane 823

Sulfisoxazole (Co-administration with sulfonamides may result in hypoglycemia). Products include:

Gantrisin Tablets 2286

Sulfisoxazole Diolamine (Co-administration with sulfonamides may result in hypoglycemia).

No products indexed under this heading.

Sulindac (Co-administration with nonsteroidal anti-inflammatory agents may result in hypoglycemia). Products include:

Clinoril Tablets 1658

Temazepam (Co-administration with drugs that are highly protein bound may result in hypoglycemia). Products include:

Restoril Capsules 2413

Terbutaline Sulfate (Sympathomimetics tend to produce hyperglycemia and concurrent use may lead to loss of control). Products include:

Brethaire Inhaler 830
Brethine Ampuls 832
Brethine Tablets 831
Bricanyl Subcutaneous Injection 1247
Bricanyl Tablets 1248

Thioridazine Hydrochloride (Phenothiazines tend to produce hyperglycemia and concurrent use may lead to loss of control). Products include:

Mellaril 2398

Thyroglobulin (Thyroid products tend to produce hyperglycemia and concurrent use may lead to loss of control).

No products indexed under this heading.

Thyroid (Thyroid products tend to produce hyperglycemia and concurrent use may lead to loss of control).

No products indexed under this heading.

Thyroxine (Thyroid products tend to produce hyperglycemia and concurrent use may lead to loss of control).

No products indexed under this heading.

IMPORTANT NOTE: Always consult each drug listing in the patient's regimen for possible interactions.

Thyroxine Sodium (Thyroid products tend to produce hyperglycemia and concurrent use may lead to loss of control).
No products indexed under this heading.

Timolol Hemihydrate (Co-administration with beta blockers may result in hypoglycemia). Products include:
Betimol 0.25%, 0.5% .... ◉ 259

Timolol Maleate (Co-administration with beta blockers may result in hypoglycemia). Products include:
Blocadren Tablets 1654
Timolide Tablets..................... 1791
Timoptic in Ocudose 1796
Timoptic Sterile Ophthalmic Solution.................................. 1794
Timoptic-XE 1798

Tolazamide (Co-administration with sulfonamides may result in hypoglycemia).
No products indexed under this heading.

Tolbutamide (Co-administration with sulfonamides may result in hypoglycemia).
No products indexed under this heading.

Tolmetin Sodium (Co-administration with nonsteroidal anti-inflammatory agents may result in hypoglycemia). Products include:
Tolectin (200, 400 and 600 mg) .. 1591

Torsemide (Diuretics tend to produce hyperglycemia and concurrent use may lead to loss of control). Products include:
Demadex Tablets and Injection 691

Tranylcypromine Sulfate (Co-administration with monamine oxidase inhibitors may result in hypoglycemia). Products include:
Parnate Tablets 2679

Triamcinolone (Corticosteroids tend to produce hyperglycemia and concurrent use may lead to loss of control).
No products indexed under this heading.

Triamcinolone Acetonide (Corticosteroids tend to produce hyperglycemia and concurrent use may lead to loss of control). Products include:
Azmacort Oral Inhaler 2175
Nasacort AQ Nasal Spray.................. 2191
Nasacort Nasal Inhaler 2189

Triamcinolone Diacetate (Corticosteroids tend to produce hyperglycemia and concurrent use may lead to loss of control).
No products indexed under this heading.

Triamcinolone Hexacetonide (Corticosteroids tend to produce hyperglycemia and concurrent use may lead to loss of control).
No products indexed under this heading.

Triamterene (Diuretics tend to produce hyperglycemia and concurrent use may lead to loss of control). Products include:
Dyazide Capsules.......................... 2653
Dyrenium Capsules........................ 2655

Trifluoperazine Hydrochloride (Phenothiazines tend to produce hyperglycemia and concurrent use may lead to loss of control). Products include:
Stelazine 2692

Trimipramine Maleate (Co-administration with drugs that are highly protein bound may result in hypoglycemia). Products include:
Surmontil Capsules........................ 2917

Verapamil Hydrochloride (Calcium channel blockers tend to produce hyperglycemia and concurrent use may lead to loss of control). Products include:
Calan SR Caplets 2571
Calan Tablets.............................. 2568
Covera-HS Tablets 2573
Isoptin Injectable 1391
Isoptin Oral Tablets 1393
Isoptin SR Tablets 1395
Verelan Capsules 1455

Warfarin Sodium (Co-administration with coumarins may result in hypoglycemia). Products include:
Coumadin 941

Food Interactions

Alcohol (Potential for hypoglycemia).

DIABE-TUSS DM SYRUP

(Dextromethorphan Hydrobromide) ..1948
None cited in PDR database.

DIABEVITE TABLETS

(Vitamins with Minerals).....................2168
None cited in PDR database.

DIABINESE TABLETS

(Chlorpropamide) 2002
May interact with highly protein bound drugs (selected), non-steroidal anti-inflammatory agents, salicylates, sulfonamides, monoamine oxidase inhibitors, beta blockers, oral anticoagulants, diuretics, thiazides, corticosteroids, phenothiazines, thyroid preparations, oral contraceptives, estrogens, calcium channel blockers, sympathomimetics, barbiturates, and certain other agents. Compounds in these categories include:

Acebutolol Hydrochloride (The hypoglycemic action of sulfonylureas may be potentiated by beta adrenergic blockers). Products include:
Sectral Capsules 2914

Albuterol (Sympathomimetics tend to produce hyperglycemia and concurrent use may lead to loss of control). Products include:
Proventil Inhalation Aerosol 2524
Ventolin Inhalation Aerosol and Refill 1170

Albuterol Sulfate (Sympathomimetics tend to produce hyperglycemia and concurrent use may lead to loss of control). Products include:
Airet Albuterol Sulfate Inhalation Solution 1602
Albuterol Sulfate, USP Solution for Inhalation, Arm-a-Med 522
Proventil Inhalation Solution 0.083%...................................... 2527
Proventil Repetabs Tablets 2529
Proventil Solution for Inhalation 0.5%.. 2525
Proventil Syrup............................. 2528
Proventil Tablets 2529
Ventolin Inhalation Solution............... 1171
Ventolin Nebules Inhalation Solution.. 1172
Ventolin Rotacaps for Inhalation...... 1173
Ventolin Syrup.............................. 1175
Ventolin Tablets 1176
Volmax Extended-Release Tablets .. 1835

Amiloride Hydrochloride (Diuretics tend to produce hyperglycemia and concurrent use may lead to loss of control). Products include:
Midamor Tablets 1746
Moduretic Tablets 1748

Amiodarone Hydrochloride (The hypoglycemic action of sulfonylureas may be potentiated by drugs that are highly protein bound). Products include:
Cordarone Intravenous 2821
Cordarone Tablets......................... 2818

Amitriptyline Hydrochloride (The hypoglycemic action of sulfonylureas may be potentiated by drugs that are highly protein bound). Products include:
Elavil 2945
Etrafon 2495
Limbitrol 2333
Triavil Tablets 1800

Amlodipine Besylate (Calcium channel blockers tend to produce hyperglycemia and concurrent use may lead to loss of control). Products include:
Lotrel Capsules............................. 858
Norvasc Tablets 2020

Aprobarbital (The action of barbiturates may be prolonged by therapy with chlorpropamide; barbiturates should be employed with caution).
No products indexed under this heading.

Aspirin (The hypoglycemic action of sulfonylureas may be potentiated by salicylates). Products include:
Alka-Seltzer Cherry Effervescent Antacid and Pain Reliever .... ▣ 609
Alka-Seltzer Extra Strength Effervescent Antacid and Pain Reliever .... ▣ 609
Alka-Seltzer Lemon Lime Effervescent Antacid and Pain Reliever .... ▣ 609
Alka-Seltzer Original Effervescent Antacid and Pain Reliever .... ▣ 609
Alka-Seltzer Plus .... ▣ 611
Alka-Seltzer Plus Sinus Medicine .. ▣ 611
Ascriptin .... ▣ 650
Arthritis Strength BC Powder.......... ▣ 631
BC Cold Powder Multi-Symptom Formula (Cold-Sinus-Allergy) ...... ▣ 631
BC Cold Powder Non-Drowsy Formula (Cold-Sinus) .... ▣ 631
BC Powder .... ▣ 631
Genuine Bayer Aspirin Tablets & Caplets .... ▣ 618
Extra Strength Bayer Arthritis Pain Regimen Formula .... ▣ 615
Extra Strength Bayer Aspirin Caplets & Tablets .... ▣ 617
Extended-Release Bayer 8-Hour Aspirin .... ▣ 616
Extra Strength Bayer Plus Aspirin Caplets .... ▣ 617
Extra Strength Bayer PM Aspirin Plus Sleep Aid .... ▣ 617
Aspirin Regimen Bayer 81 mg Tablets with Calcium .... ▣ 615
Aspirin Regimen Bayer Adult Low Strength 81 mg Tablets .... ▣ 613
Aspirin Regimen Bayer Children's Chewable Aspirin.......................... ▣ 616
Aspirin Regimen Bayer Regular Strength 325 mg Caplets .... ▣ 613
Bufferin Analgesic Tablets.............. ▣ 636
Arthritis Strength Bufferin Analgesic Caplets .... ▣ 637
Extra Strength Bufferin Analgesic Tablets .... ▣ 637
Cama Arthritis Pain Reliever........... ▣ 748
Darvon Compound-65 Pulvules 1475
Easprin 1971
Ecotrin 2625
Ecotrin Enteric Coated Aspirin Maximum Strength Tablets and Caplets .... ▣ 775
Ecotrin Enteric Coated Aspirin Regular Strength Tablets 2625
Empirin Aspirin Tablets .... ▣ 818
Excedrin Extra-Strength Analgesic Tablets, Caplets, and Geltabs......... 734
Fiorinal Capsules 2388
Fiorinal with Codeine Capsules 2390
Fiorinal Tablets............................ 2388
Goody's Extra Strength Headache Powders...................................... ▣ 632
Goody's Extra Strength Pain Relief Tablets .... ▣ 632
Halfprin Tablets 1413
Norgesic.................................... 1554
Percodan Tablets.......................... 955
Percodan-Demi Tablets.................... 956
Robaxisal Tablets.......................... 2246
Soma Compound w/Codeine Tablets 2784
Soma Compound Tablets................. 2783
St. Joseph Adult Chewable Aspirin (81 mg.) .... ▣ 768
Talwin Compound 2466
Vanquish Analgesic Caplets .... ▣ 627

Atenolol (The hypoglycemic action of sulfonylureas may be potentiated by beta adrenergic blockers). Products include:
Tenoretic Tablets.......................... 2963
Tenormin Tablets and I.V. Injection 2965

Atovaquone (The hypoglycemic action of sulfonylureas may be potentiated by drugs that are highly protein bound). Products include:
Mepron Suspension 1206

Bendroflumethiazide (Thiazides tend to produce hyperglycemia and concurrent use may lead to loss of control).
No products indexed under this heading.

Bepridil Hydrochloride (Calcium channel blockers tend to produce hyperglycemia and concurrent use may lead to loss of control). Products include:
Vascor Tablets (200 and 300 mg) 1597

Betamethasone Acetate (Corticosteroids tend to produce hyperglycemia and concurrent use may lead to loss of control). Products include:
Celestone Soluspan Suspension 2484

Betamethasone Sodium Phosphate (Corticosteroids tend to produce hyperglycemia and concurrent use may lead to loss of control). Products include:
Celestone Soluspan Suspension 2484

Betaxolol Hydrochloride (The hypoglycemic action of sulfonylureas may be potentiated by beta adrenergic blockers). Products include:
Betoptic Ophthalmic Solution........... 465
Betoptic S Ophthalmic Suspension 467
Kerlone Tablets............................ 2588

Bisoprolol Fumarate (The hypoglycemic action of sulfonylureas may be potentiated by beta adrenergic blockers). Products include:
Zebeta Tablets 1457
Ziac 1459

Bumetanide (Diuretics tend to produce hyperglycemia and concurrent use may lead to loss of control). Products include:
Bumex 2260

Butabarbital (The action of barbiturates may be prolonged by therapy with chlorpropamide; barbiturates should be employed with caution).
No products indexed under this heading.

Butalbital (The action of barbiturates may be prolonged by therapy with chlorpropamide; barbiturates should be employed with caution). Products include:
Axocet Capsules............................ 2469
Esgic-plus Capsules 1012
Esgic-plus Tablets 1012
Fioricet Tablets............................ 2386
Fioricet with Codeine Capsules 2387
Fiorinal Capsules 2388
Fiorinal with Codeine Capsules 2390
Fiorinal Tablets............................ 2388
Phrenilin 790
Sedapap Tablets 50 mg/650 mg .. 1826

Carteolol Hydrochloride (The hypoglycemic action of sulfonylureas may be potentiated by beta adrenergic blockers). Products include:
Cartrol Tablets 413
Ocupress Ophthalmic Solution, 1% Sterile................................ ◉ 297

Cefonicid Sodium (The hypoglycemic action of sulfonylureas may be potentiated by drugs that are highly protein bound). Products include:
Monocid Injection 2674

(▣ Described in PDR For Nonprescription Drugs) (◉ Described in PDR For Ophthalmology)

277 **Interactions Index** Diabinese

Chloramphenicol (The hypoglycemic action of sulfonylureas may be potentiated by chloramphenicol). Products include:

Chloromycetin Ophthalmic Ointment, 1% ◉ 298
Chloromycetin Ophthalmic Solution ◉ 299
Chloroptic S.O.P. ◉ 236
Chloroptic Sterile Ophthalmic Solution ◉ 236

Chloramphenicol Palmitate (The hypoglycemic action of sulfonylureas may be potentiated by chloramphenicol).

No products indexed under this heading.

Chloramphenicol Sodium Succinate (The hypoglycemic action of sulfonylureas may be potentiated by chloramphenicol). Products include:

Chloromycetin Sodium Succinate 1960

Chlordiazepoxide (The hypoglycemic action of sulfonylureas may be potentiated by drugs that are highly protein bound). Products include:

Limbitrol 2333

Chlordiazepoxide Hydrochloride (The hypoglycemic action of sulfonylureas may be potentiated by drugs that are highly protein bound). Products include:

Librax Capsules 2330
Librium Capsules 2331
Librium Injectable 2332

Chlorothiazide (Thiazides tend to produce hyperglycemia and concurrent use may lead to loss of control). Products include:

Aldoclor Tablets 1638
Diupres Tablets 1691
Diuril Oral 1694

Chlorothiazide Sodium (Thiazides tend to produce hyperglycemia and concurrent use may lead to loss of control). Products include:

Diuril Sodium Intravenous 1693

Chlorotrianisene (Estrogens tend to produce hyperglycemia and concurrent use may lead to loss of control).

No products indexed under this heading.

Chlorpromazine (Phenothiazines tend to produce hyperglycemia and concurrent use may lead to loss of control). Products include:

Thorazine Suppositories 2701

Chlorpromazine Hydrochloride (Phenothiazines tend to produce hyperglycemia and concurrent use may lead to loss of control). Products include:

Thorazine 2701

Chlorthalidone (Diuretics tend to produce hyperglycemia and concurrent use may lead to loss of control). Products include:

Combipres Tablets 682
Tenoretic Tablets 2963
Thalitone 1293

Choline Magnesium Trisalicylate (The hypoglycemic action of sulfonylureas may be potentiated by salicylates). Products include:

Trilisate 2155

Clomipramine Hydrochloride (The hypoglycemic action of sulfonylureas may be potentiated by drugs that are highly protein bound). Products include:

Anafranil Capsules 819

Clozapine (The hypoglycemic action of sulfonylureas may be potentiated by drugs that are highly protein bound). Products include:

Clozaril Tablets 2377

Cortisone Acetate (Corticosteroids tend to produce hyperglycemia and concurrent use may lead to loss of control). Products include:

Cortone Acetate Sterile Suspension 1663
Cortone Acetate Tablets 1664

Cyclosporine (The hypoglycemic action of sulfonylureas may be potentiated by drugs that are highly protein bound). Products include:

Neoral 2405
Sandimmune 2416

Desogestrel (Oral contraceptives tend to produce hyperglycemia and concurrent use may lead to loss of control). Products include:

Desogen Tablets 1867
Ortho-Cept 1907

Dexamethasone (Corticosteroids tend to produce hyperglycemia and concurrent use may lead to loss of control). Products include:

AK-Trol Ointment & Suspension ◉ 205
Decadron Elixir 1676
Decadron Tablets 1678
Decaspray Topical Aerosol 1689
Maxitrol Ophthalmic Ointment and Suspension ◉ 222
TobraDex Ophthalmic Suspension and Ointment 469

Dexamethasone Acetate (Corticosteroids tend to produce hyperglycemia and concurrent use may lead to loss of control). Products include:

Dalalone D.P. Injectable 1009
Decadron-LA Sterile Suspension 1687

Dexamethasone Sodium Phosphate (Corticosteroids tend to produce hyperglycemia and concurrent use may lead to loss of control). Products include:

Decadron Phosphate Injection 1680
Decadron Phosphate Sterile Ophthalmic Ointment 1684
Decadron Phosphate Sterile Ophthalmic Solution 1685
Decadron Phosphate Topical Cream 1686
Decadron Phosphate with Xylocaine Injection, Sterile 1683
Dexacort Phosphate in Respihaler 1606
Dexacort Phosphate in Turbinaire 1607
NeoDecadron Sterile Ophthalmic Ointment 1755
NeoDecadron Sterile Ophthalmic Solution 1756
NeoDecadron Topical Cream 1757

Diazepam (The hypoglycemic action of sulfonylureas may be potentiated by drugs that are highly protein bound). Products include:

Dizac (diazepam injectable emulsion) CIV 1862
Valium Injectable 2336
Valium Tablets 2335

Diclofenac Potassium (The hypoglycemic action of sulfonylureas may be potentiated by nonsteroidal anti-inflammatory agents). Products include:

Cataflam Tablets 833

Diclofenac Sodium (The hypoglycemic action of sulfonylureas may be potentiated by nonsteroidal anti-inflammatory agents). Products include:

Voltaren Ophthalmic Sterile Ophthalmic Solution ◉ 264
Cataflam/Voltaren/Voltaren-XR 833

Dicumarol (The hypoglycemic action of sulfonylureas may be potentiated by coumarins).

No products indexed under this heading.

Dienestrol (Estrogens tend to produce hyperglycemia and concurrent use may lead to loss of control). Products include:

Ortho Dienestrol Cream 1922

Diethylstilbestrol (Estrogens tend to produce hyperglycemia and concurrent use may lead to loss of control). Products include:

Diethylstilbestrol Tablets 1477

Diflunisal (The hypoglycemic action of sulfonylureas may be potentiated by salicylates). Products include:

Dolobid Tablets 1695

Diltiazem Hydrochloride (Calcium channel blockers tend to produce hyperglycemia and concurrent use may lead to loss of control). Products include:

Cardizem CD Capsules 1251
Cardizem SR Capsules 1255
Cardizem Injectable 1253
Cardizem Tablets 1257
Dilacor XR Extended-release Capsules 2183
Tiazac Capsules 1019

Dipyridamole (The hypoglycemic action of sulfonylureas may be potentiated by drugs that are highly protein bound). Products include:

Persantine Tablets 686

Dobutamine Hydrochloride (Sympathomimetics tend to produce hyperglycemia and concurrent use may lead to loss of control). Products include:

Dobutrex Solution Vials 1480

Dopamine Hydrochloride (Sympathomimetics tend to produce hyperglycemia and concurrent use may lead to loss of control).

No products indexed under this heading.

Ephedrine Hydrochloride (Sympathomimetics tend to produce hyperglycemia and concurrent use may lead to loss of control). Products include:

Primatene Tablets ▣ 844
Quadrinal Tablets 1398

Ephedrine Sulfate (Sympathomimetics tend to produce hyperglycemia and concurrent use may lead to loss of control). Products include:

Marax Tablets & DF Syrup 2015

Ephedrine Tannate (Sympathomimetics tend to produce hyperglycemia and concurrent use may lead to loss of control). Products include:

Rynatuss 2782

Epinephrine (Sympathomimetics tend to produce hyperglycemia and concurrent use may lead to loss of control). Products include:

EPIFRIN ◉ 237
EpiPen 808
Marcaine with Epinephrine 2446
Primatene Mist ▣ 843
Sensorcaine with Epinephrine Injection 554
Sus-Phrine Injection 1017
Xylocaine with Epinephrine Injections 562

Epinephrine Bitartrate (Sympathomimetics tend to produce hyperglycemia and concurrent use may lead to loss of control). Products include:

Sensorcaine-MPF with Epinephrine Injection 554

Epinephrine Hydrochloride (Sympathomimetics tend to produce hyperglycemia and concurrent use may lead to loss of control). Products include:

Ana-Kit Anaphylaxis Emergency Treatment Kit 611

Esmolol Hydrochloride (The hypoglycemic action of sulfonylureas may be potentiated by beta adrenergic blockers). Products include:

Brevibloc (esmolol HCl) Injection 1860

Estradiol (Estrogens tend to produce hyperglycemia and concurrent use may lead to loss of control). Products include:

Climara Transdermal System 640
Estrace Cream and Tablets 751
Estraderm Transdermal System 842
Estring Vaginal Ring 2086
Vivelle Transdermal System 880

Estrogens, Conjugated (Estrogens tend to produce hyperglycemia and concurrent use may lead to loss of control). Products include:

PMB 200 and PMB 400 2890
Premarin Intravenous 2893
Premarin Tablets 2896
Premarin Vaginal Cream 2898
Premphase 2900
Prempro 2905

Estrogens, Esterified (Estrogens tend to produce hyperglycemia and concurrent use may lead to loss of control). Products include:

ESTRATAB Tablets (0.3, 0.625, 1.25, 2.5 mg) 2715
Estratest 2718
Menest Tablets 2671

Estropipate (Estrogens tend to produce hyperglycemia and concurrent use may lead to loss of control). Products include:

Ogen Tablets 2103
Ogen Vaginal Cream 2106
Ortho-Est 1925

Ethacrynic Acid (Diuretics tend to produce hyperglycemia and concurrent use may lead to loss of control). Products include:

Edecrin Tablets 1698

Ethinyl Estradiol (Estrogens tend to produce hyperglycemia and concurrent use may lead to loss of control). Products include:

Brevicon 2563
Demulen 2580
Desogen Tablets 1867
Levlen/Tri-Levlen 646
Lo/Ovral Tablets 2852
Lo/Ovral-28 Tablets 2857
Modicon 1928
Nordette-21 Tablets 2863
Nordette-28 Tablets 2866
Norinyl 2563
Ortho-Cept 1907
Ortho-Cyclen/Ortho-Tri-Cyclen 1914
Ortho-Novum 1928
Ortho-Cyclen/Ortho Tri-Cyclen 1914
Ovcon 765
Ovral Tablets 2877
Ovral-28 Tablets 2878
Levlen/Tri-Levlen 646
Tri-Norinyl 2607
Triphasil-21 Tablets 2919
Triphasil-28 Tablets 2924

Ethynodiol Diacetate (Oral contraceptives tend to produce hyperglycemia and concurrent use may lead to loss of control). Products include:

Demulen 2580

Etodolac (The hypoglycemic action of sulfonylureas may be potentiated by nonsteroidal anti-inflammatory agents). Products include:

Lodine Capsules and Tablets 2849

Felodipine (Calcium channel blockers tend to produce hyperglycemia and concurrent use may lead to loss of control). Products include:

Plendil Extended-Release Tablets 514

Fenoprofen Calcium (The hypoglycemic action of sulfonylureas may be potentiated by nonsteroidal anti-inflammatory agents). Products include:

Nalfon 200 Pulvules & Nalfon Tablets 933

Fludrocortisone Acetate (Corticosteroids tend to produce hyperglycemia and concurrent use may lead to loss of control). Products include:

Florinef Acetate Tablets 506

IMPORTANT NOTE: Always consult each drug listing in the patient's regimen for possible interactions.

Diabinese — Interactions Index

Fluphenazine Decanoate (Phenothiazines tend to produce hyperglycemia and concurrent use may lead to loss of control). Products include:
- Prolixin Decanoate 510

Fluphenazine Enanthate (Phenothiazines tend to produce hyperglycemia and concurrent use may lead to loss of control). Products include:
- Prolixin Enanthate 510

Fluphenazine Hydrochloride (Phenothiazines tend to produce hyperglycemia and concurrent use may lead to loss of control). Products include:
- Prolixin 510

Flurazepam Hydrochloride (The hypoglycemic action of sulfonylureas may be potentiated by drugs that are highly protein bound). Products include:
- Dalmane Capsules 2329

Flurbiprofen (The hypoglycemic action of sulfonylureas may be potentiated by nonsteroidal anti-inflammatory agents).
- No products indexed under this heading.

Furazolidone (The hypoglycemic action of sulfonylureas may be potentiated by monoamine oxidase inhibitors). Products include:
- Furoxone 2221

Furosemide (Diuretics tend to produce hyperglycemia and concurrent use may lead to loss of control). Products include:
- Lasix Injection, Oral Solution and Tablets 1267

Glipizide (The hypoglycemic action of sulfonylureas may be potentiated by sulfonamides). Products include:
- Glucotrol Tablets 2011
- Glucotrol XL Extended Release Tablets 2012

Glyburide (The hypoglycemic action of sulfonylureas may be potentiated by sulfonamides). Products include:
- DiaBeta Tablets 1265
- Glynase PresTab Tablets 2091
- Micronase Tablets 2099

Hydrochlorothiazide (Thiazides tend to produce hyperglycemia and concurrent use may lead to loss of control). Products include:
- Aldactazide Tablets 2556
- Aldoril Tablets 1644
- Apresazide Capsules 824
- Capozide Tablets 744
- Dyazide Capsules 2653
- Esidrix Tablets 839
- Esimil Tablets 840
- HydroDIURIL Tablets 1716
- Hydropres Tablets 1718
- Hyzaar Tablets 1720
- Inderide Tablets 2838
- Inderide LA Long Acting Capsules .. 2840
- Lopressor HCT Tablets 850
- Lotensin HCT Tablets 855
- Moduretic Tablets 1748
- Oretic Tablets 450
- Prinzide Tablets 1780
- Ser-Ap-Es Tablets 867
- Timolide Tablets 1791
- Vaseretic Tablets 1810
- Zestoretic Tablets 2968
- Ziac 1459

Hydrocortisone (Corticosteroids tend to produce hyperglycemia and concurrent use may lead to loss of control). Products include:
- Anusol-HC Cream 2.5% 1953
- Aquanil HC Lotion 1989
- Maximum Strength Cortaid Spray ⊞ 800
- CORTENEMA 2713
- Cortisporin Ointment 1074
- Cortisporin Ophthalmic Ointment Sterile 1074
- Cortisporin Ophthalmic Suspension Sterile 1075
- Cortisporin Otic Solution Sterile 1076
- Cortisporin Otic Suspension Sterile 1077
- Cortizone-5 .... ⊞ 795
- Cortizone-10 .... ⊞ 795
- Hydrocortone Tablets 1715
- Hytone 922
- Hytone Ointment 2 ½ % 923
- Massengill Medicated Soft Cloth Towelettes 2628
- Pediotic Suspension Sterile 1140
- Preparation H Hydrocortisone 1% Cream .... ⊞ 843
- ProctoCream-HC 2.5% 2552
- VōSol HC Otic Solution 2786

Hydrocortisone Acetate (Corticosteroids tend to produce hyperglycemia and concurrent use may lead to loss of control). Products include:
- Analpram-HC Rectal Cream 1% and 2.5% 993
- Anusol HC-1 Hydrocortisone Anti-Itch Ointment .... ⊞ 810
- Anusol-HC Suppositories 1954
- Caldecort Anti-Itch Hydrocortisone Cream .... ⊞ 651
- Coly-Mycin S Otic w/Neomycin & Hydrocortisone 1965
- Cortaid .... ⊞ 800
- Cortifoam 2540
- Cortisporin Cream 1073
- Epifoam 2543
- Hydrocortone Acetate Sterile Suspension 1712
- Mantadil Cream 1124
- Nupercainal Hydrocortisone 1% Cream .... ⊞ 661
- Pramosone Cream, Lotion & Ointment 995
- ProctoFoam-HC 2552
- Terra-Cortril Ophthalmic Suspension 2033

Hydrocortisone Sodium Phosphate (Corticosteroids tend to produce hyperglycemia and concurrent use may lead to loss of control). Products include:
- Hydrocortone Phosphate Injection, Sterile 1713

Hydrocortisone Sodium Succinate (Corticosteroids tend to produce hyperglycemia and concurrent use may lead to loss of control).
- No products indexed under this heading.

Hydroflumethiazide (Thiazides tend to produce hyperglycemia and concurrent use may lead to loss of control). Products include:
- Diucardin Tablets 2824

Ibuprofen (The hypoglycemic action of sulfonylureas may be potentiated by nonsteroidal anti-inflammatory agents). Products include:
- Advil Cold and Sinus Caplets and Tablets .... ⊞ 837
- Advil Ibuprofen Tablets, Caplets and Gel Caplets .... ⊞ 836
- Children's Motrin Ibuprofen Oral Suspension 1558
- IBU Tablets 1389
- Ibuprohm 713
- Motrin IB Caplets, Tablets, and Gelcaps .... ⊞ 802
- Motrin Ibuprofen Suspension, Oral Drops, Chewable Tablets, Caplets 1563
- Nuprin Ibuprofen/Analgesic Tablets & Caplets .... ⊞ 645
- Vicks DayQuil SINUS Pressure & PAIN Relief with IBUPROFEN ...... ⊞ 735

Imipramine Hydrochloride (The hypoglycemic action of sulfonylureas may be potentiated by drugs that are highly protein bound). Products include:
- Tofranil Ampuls 873
- Tofranil Tablets 875

Imipramine Pamoate (The hypoglycemic action of sulfonylureas may be potentiated by drugs that are highly protein bound). Products include:
- Tofranil-PM Capsules 876

Indapamide (Diuretics tend to produce hyperglycemia and concurrent use may lead to loss of control).
- No products indexed under this heading.

Indomethacin (The hypoglycemic action of sulfonylureas may be potentiated by nonsteroidal anti-inflammatory agents). Products include:
- Indocin 1723

Indomethacin Sodium Trihydrate (The hypoglycemic action of sulfonylureas may be potentiated by nonsteroidal anti-inflammatory agents). Products include:
- Indocin I.V. 1727

Isocarboxazid (The hypoglycemic action of sulfonylureas may be potentiated by monoamine oxidase inhibitors).
- No products indexed under this heading.

Isoniazid (Isoniazid tend to produce hyperglycemia and concurrent use may lead to loss of control). Products include:
- Nydrazid Injection 509
- Rifamate Capsules 1278
- Rifater 1280

Isoproterenol Hydrochloride (Sympathomimetics tend to produce hyperglycemia and concurrent use may lead to loss of control). Products include:
- Isuprel Hydrochloride Solution 2443
- Isuprel Injection 2441
- Isuprel Mistometer 2442

Isoproterenol Sulfate (Sympathomimetics tend to produce hyperglycemia and concurrent use may lead to loss of control). Products include:
- Norisodrine with Calcium Iodide Syrup 446

Isradipine (Calcium channel blockers tend to produce hyperglycemia and concurrent use may lead to loss of control). Products include:
- DynaCirc Capsules 2381
- DynaCirc CR Tablets 2383

Ketoprofen (The hypoglycemic action of sulfonylureas may be potentiated by nonsteroidal anti-inflammatory agents). Products include:
- Actron Caplets and Tablets .... ⊞ 608
- Orudis Capsules 2874
- Orudis KT .... ⊞ 842
- Oruvail Capsules 2874

Ketorolac Tromethamine (The hypoglycemic action of sulfonylureas may be potentiated by nonsteroidal anti-inflammatory agents). Products include:
- Acular Sterile Ophthalmic Solution 470
- Toradol 2319

Labetalol Hydrochloride (The hypoglycemic action of sulfonylureas may be potentiated by beta adrenergic blockers). Products include:
- Normodyne Injection 2519
- Normodyne Tablets 2522
- Trandate 1158

Levobunolol Hydrochloride (The hypoglycemic action of sulfonylureas may be potentiated by beta adrenergic blockers). Products include:
- Betagan .... ⊙ 230

Levonorgestrel (Oral contraceptives tend to produce hyperglycemia and concurrent use may lead to loss of control). Products include:
- Levlen/Tri-Levlen 646
- Nordette-21 Tablets 2863
- Nordette-28 Tablets 2866
- Norplant System 2868
- Levlen/Tri-Levlen 646
- Triphasil-21 Tablets 2919
- Triphasil-28 Tablets 2924

Levothyroxine Sodium (Thyroid products tend to produce hyperglycemia and concurrent use may lead to loss of control). Products include:
- Eltroxin Tablets 2214
- Levothroid Tablets 1015
- Levothyroxine Sodium, USP for Injection 546
- Levoxyl Tablets 918
- Synthroid 1410

Liothyronine Sodium (Thyroid products tend to produce hyperglycemia and concurrent use may lead to loss of control). Products include:
- Cytomel Tablets 2647
- Triostat Injection 2708

Liotrix (Thyroid products tend to produce hyperglycemia and concurrent use may lead to loss of control).
- No products indexed under this heading.

Magnesium Salicylate (The hypoglycemic action of sulfonylureas may be potentiated by salicylates). Products include:
- Backache Caplets .... ⊞ 635
- Doan's Extra-Strength Analgesic ... ⊞ 653
- Extra Strength Doan's P.M. .... ⊞ 653
- Doan's Regular Strength Analgesic .... ⊞ 654
- Mobigesic Tablets .... ⊞ 607

Meclofenamate Sodium (The hypoglycemic action of sulfonylureas may be potentiated by nonsteroidal anti-inflammatory agents).
- No products indexed under this heading.

Mefenamic Acid (The hypoglycemic action of sulfonylureas may be potentiated by nonsteroidal anti-inflammatory agents). Products include:
- Ponstel 1982

Mephobarbital (The action of barbiturates may be prolonged by therapy with chlorpropamide; barbiturates should be employed with caution). Products include:
- Mebaral Tablets 2452

Mesoridazine Besylate (Phenothiazines tend to produce hyperglycemia and concurrent use may lead to loss of control). Products include:
- Serentil 689

Mestranol (Oral contraceptives tend to produce hyperglycemia and concurrent use may lead to loss of control). Products include:
- Norinyl 2563
- Ortho-Novum 1928

Metaproterenol Sulfate (Sympathomimetics tend to produce hyperglycemia and concurrent use may lead to loss of control). Products include:
- Alupent 672
- Metaproterenol Sulfate Inhalation Solution, USP, Arm-a-Med 547

Metaraminol Bitartrate (Sympathomimetics tend to produce hyperglycemia and concurrent use may lead to loss of control). Products include:
- Aramine Injection 1649

Methotrimeprazine (Phenothiazines tend to produce hyperglycemia and concurrent use may lead to loss of control). Products include:
- Levoprome 1321

Methoxamine Hydrochloride (Sympathomimetics tend to produce hyperglycemia and concurrent use may lead to loss of control). Products include:
- Vasoxyl Injection 1169

(⊞ Described in PDR For Nonprescription Drugs)   (⊙ Described in PDR For Ophthalmology)

Methyclothiazide (Thiazides tend to produce hyperglycemia and concurrent use may lead to loss of control). Products include:
- Enduron Tablets ... 424

Methylprednisolone Acetate (Corticosteroids tend to produce hyperglycemia and concurrent use may lead to loss of control).
- No products indexed under this heading.

Methylprednisolone Sodium Succinate (Corticosteroids tend to produce hyperglycemia and concurrent use may lead to loss of control).
- No products indexed under this heading.

Metipranolol Hydrochloride (The hypoglycemic action of sulfonylureas may be potentiated by beta adrenergic blockers). Products include:
- OptiPranolol (Metipranolol 0.3%) Sterile Ophthalmic Solution ... ◉ 256

Metolazone (Diuretics tend to produce hyperglycemia and concurrent use may lead to loss of control). Products include:
- Mykrox Tablets ... 1617
- Zaroxolyn Tablets ... 1625

Metoprolol Succinate (The hypoglycemic action of sulfonylureas may be potentiated by beta adrenergic blockers). Products include:
- Toprol-XL Tablets ... 560

Metoprolol Tartrate (The hypoglycemic action of sulfonylureas may be potentiated by beta adrenergic blockers). Products include:
- Lopressor ... 848
- Lopressor HCT Tablets ... 850

Miconazole (Co-administration with oral miconazole and oral hypoglycemic agents has resulted in severe hypoglycemia).
- No products indexed under this heading.

Midazolam Hydrochloride (The hypoglycemic action of sulfonylureas may be potentiated by drugs that are highly protein bound). Products include:
- Versed Injection ... 2324

Nabumetone (The hypoglycemic action of sulfonylureas may be potentiated by nonsteroidal anti-inflammatory agents). Products include:
- Relafen Tablets ... 2688

Nadolol (The hypoglycemic action of sulfonylureas may be potentiated by beta adrenergic blockers).
- No products indexed under this heading.

Naproxen (The hypoglycemic action of sulfonylureas may be potentiated by nonsteroidal anti-inflammatory agents). Products include:
- Anaprox/Naprosyn ... 2277

Naproxen Sodium (The hypoglycemic action of sulfonylureas may be potentiated by nonsteroidal anti-inflammatory agents). Products include:
- Aleve ... 2124
- Anaprox/Naprosyn ... 2277
- Naprelan Tablets ... 2861

Niacin (Nicotinic acid tend to produce hyperglycemia and concurrent use may lead to loss of control). Products include:
- Kyo-Chrome ... 680
- Nicotinex Elixir ... 671
- Slo-Niacin Tablets ... 2767

Nicardipine Hydrochloride (Calcium channel blockers tend to produce hyperglycemia and concurrent use may lead to loss of control). Products include:
- Cardene Capsules ... 2261
- Cardene I.V. ... 2815
- Cardene SR Capsules ... 2264

Nifedipine (Calcium channel blockers tend to produce hyperglycemia and concurrent use may lead to loss of control). Products include:
- Adalat Capsules (10 mg and 20 mg) ... 580
- Adalat CC ... 582
- Procardia Capsules ... 2024
- Procardia XL Extended Release Tablets ... 2026

Nimodipine (Calcium channel blockers tend to produce hyperglycemia and concurrent use may lead to loss of control). Products include:
- Nimotop Capsules ... 603

Nisoldipine (Calcium channel blockers tend to produce hyperglycemia and concurrent use may lead to loss of control). Products include:
- Sular Tablets ... 2961

Norepinephrine Bitartrate (Sympathomimetics tend to produce hyperglycemia and concurrent use may lead to loss of control). Products include:
- Levophed Bitartrate Injection ... 2445

Norethindrone (Oral contraceptives tend to produce hyperglycemia and concurrent use may lead to loss of control). Products include:
- Brevicon ... 2563
- Micronor Tablets ... 1903
- Modicon ... 1928
- Norinyl ... 2563
- Nor-Q D Tablets ... 2598
- Ortho-Novum ... 1928
- Ovcon ... 765
- Tri-Norinyl ... 2607

Norethynodrel (Oral contraceptives tend to produce hyperglycemia and concurrent use may lead to loss of control).
- No products indexed under this heading.

Norgestimate (Oral contraceptives tend to produce hyperglycemia and concurrent use may lead to loss of control). Products include:
- Ortho-Cyclen/Ortho-Tri-Cyclen ... 1914
- Ortho-Cyclen/Ortho Tri-Cyclen ... 1914

Norgestrel (Oral contraceptives tend to produce hyperglycemia and concurrent use may lead to loss of control). Products include:
- Lo/Ovral Tablets ... 2852
- Lo/Ovral-28 Tablets ... 2857
- Ovral Tablets ... 2877
- Ovral-28 Tablets ... 2878
- Ovrette Tablets ... 2878

Nortriptyline Hydrochloride (The hypoglycemic action of sulfonylureas may be potentiated by drugs that are highly protein bound). Products include:
- Pamelor ... 2409

Oxaprozin (The hypoglycemic action of sulfonylureas may be potentiated by nonsteroidal anti-inflammatory agents). Products include:
- Daypro Caplets ... 2578

Oxazepam (The hypoglycemic action of sulfonylureas may be potentiated by drugs that are highly protein bound). Products include:
- Serax Capsules ... 2916
- Serax Tablets ... 2916

Penbutolol Sulfate (The hypoglycemic action of sulfonylureas may be potentiated by beta adrenergic blockers). Products include:
- Levatol Tablets ... 2547

Pentobarbital Sodium (The action of barbiturates may be prolonged by therapy with chlorpropamide; barbiturates should be employed with caution). Products include:
- Nembutal Sodium Capsules ... 440
- Nembutal Sodium Solution ... 442
- Nembutal Sodium Suppositories ... 444

Perphenazine (Phenothiazines tend to produce hyperglycemia and concurrent use may lead to loss of control). Products include:
- Etrafon ... 2495
- Triavil Tablets ... 1800
- Trilafon ... 2532

Phenelzine Sulfate (The hypoglycemic action of sulfonylureas may be potentiated by monoamine oxidase inhibitors). Products include:
- Nardil ... 1977

Phenobarbital (The action of barbiturates may be prolonged by therapy with chlorpropamide; barbiturates should be employed with caution). Products include:
- Arco-Lase Plus Tablets ... 513
- Bellergal-S Tablets ... 2375
- Donnatal ... 2234
- Donnatal Extentabs ... 2234
- Donnatal Tablets ... 2234
- Phenobarbital Elixir and Tablets ... 1523
- Quadrinal Tablets ... 1398

Phenylbutazone (The hypoglycemic action of sulfonylureas may be potentiated by nonsteroidal anti-inflammatory agents).
- No products indexed under this heading.

Phenylephrine Bitartrate (Sympathomimetics tend to produce hyperglycemia and concurrent use may lead to loss of control).
- No products indexed under this heading.

Phenylephrine Hydrochloride (Sympathomimetics tend to produce hyperglycemia and concurrent use may lead to loss of control). Products include:
- Atrohist Plus Tablets ... 1605
- Cerose DM ... 853
- D.A. II Tablets ... 972
- D.A. Chewable Tablets ... 970
- Dura-Vent/DA Tablets ... 972
- Extendryl ... 1003
- 4-Way Fast Acting Nasal Spray (regular & mentholated) ... 644
- Hemorid ... 797
- Hycomine Compound Tablets ... 948
- Neo-Synephrine Hydrochloride 1% Carpuject ... 2455
- Neo-Synephrine Hydrochloride 1% Injection ... 2455
- Neo-Synephrine Hydrochloride (Ophthalmic) ... 2456
- Neo-Synephrine ... 624
- Novahistine Elixir ... 782
- Phenergan VC ... 2886
- Phenergan VC with Codeine ... 2888
- Preparation H ... 842
- Tympagesic Ear Drops ... 2476
- Vicks Sinex Nasal Spray and Ultra Fine Mist ... 738

Phenylephrine Tannate (Sympathomimetics tend to produce hyperglycemia and concurrent use may lead to loss of control). Products include:
- Atrohist Pediatric Suspension ... 1604
- Atrohist Pediatric Suspension Dye-Free ... 1604
- Rynatan ... 2781
- Rynatuss ... 2782

Phenylpropanolamine Hydrochloride (Sympathomimetics tend to produce hyperglycemia and concurrent use may lead to loss of control). Products include:
- Acutrim ... 648
- Atrohist Plus Tablets ... 1605
- BC Cold Powder Multi-Symptom Formula (Cold-Sinus-Allergy) ... 631
- BC Cold Powder Non-Drowsy Formula (Cold-Sinus) ... 631
- Cheracol Plus Head Cold/Cough Formula ... 741
- Comtrex Multi-Symptom Cold Reliever Liqui-Gels ... 638
- Comtrex Multi-Symptom Non-Drowsy Liqui-gels ... 640
- Contac Continuous Action Nasal Decongestant/Antihistamine 12 Hour Capsules ... 773
- Contac Maximum Strength Continuous Action Decongestant/Antihistamine 12 Hour Caplets ... 772
- Contac Severe Cold and Flu Formula Caplets ... 773
- Coricidin 'D' Decongestant Tablets ... 760
- Dexatrim ... 795
- Dexatrim Plus Vitamins Caplets ... 796
- Dimetane-DC Cough Syrup ... 2232
- Dimetapp Allergy Sinus Caplets ... 838
- Dimetapp Cold & Allergy Chewable Tablets ... 838
- Dimetapp Cold & Cough Liqui-Gels ... 839
- Dimetapp DM Elixir ... 840
- Dimetapp Elixir ... 840
- Dimetapp Extentabs ... 841
- Dimetapp Tablets/Liqui-Gels ... 841
- Dura-Vent Tablets ... 971
- Entex LA Tablets ... 972
- Exgest LA Tablets ... 787
- Hycomine ... 947
- Nolamine Timed-Release Tablets ... 790
- Ornade Spansule Capsules ... 2678
- Propagest Tablets ... 791
- Pyrroxate Caplets ... 742
- Robitussin-CF ... 846
- Sinulin Tablets ... 792
- Tavist-D 12 Hour Relief Tablets ... 750
- Teldrin 12 Hour Antihistamine/Nasal Decongestant Allergy Relief Capsules ... 786
- Triaminic Expectorant ... 753
- Triaminic Syrup ... 755
- Triaminic Triaminicol Cold & Cough ... 756
- Triaminic DM Syrup ... 756
- Triaminicin Tablets ... 756
- Vicks DayQuil Allergy Relief 12-Hour Extended Release Tablets ... 733
- Vicks DayQuil Allergy Relief 4-Hour Tablets ... 733
- Vicks DayQuil SINUS Pressure & CONGESTION Relief ... 734

Phenytoin (Phenytoin tend to produce hyperglycemia and concurrent use may lead to loss of control). Products include:
- Dilantin Infatabs ... 1967
- Dilantin-125 Suspension ... 1969

Phenytoin Sodium (Phenytoin tend to produce hyperglycemia and concurrent use may lead to loss of control). Products include:
- Dilantin Kapseals ... 1965

Pindolol (The hypoglycemic action of sulfonylureas may be potentiated by beta adrenergic blockers). Products include:
- Visken Tablets ... 2428

Pirbuterol Acetate (Sympathomimetics tend to produce hyperglycemia and concurrent use may lead to loss of control). Products include:
- Maxair Autohaler ... 1550
- Maxair Inhaler ... 1552

Piroxicam (The hypoglycemic action of sulfonylureas may be potentiated by nonsteroidal anti-inflammatory agents). Products include:
- Feldene Capsules ... 2008

Polyestradiol Phosphate (Estrogens tend to produce hyperglycemia and concurrent use may lead to loss of control).
- No products indexed under this heading.

Polythiazide (Thiazides tend to produce hyperglycemia and concurrent use may lead to loss of control). Products include:
- Minizide Capsules ... 2016

IMPORTANT NOTE: Always consult each drug listing in the patient's regimen for possible interactions.

Diabinese — Interactions Index

Prednisolone Acetate (Corticosteroids tend to produce hyperglycemia and concurrent use may lead to loss of control). Products include:

AK-CIDE	⊙ 203
AK-CIDE Ointment	⊙ 203
Blephamide Liquifilm Sterile Ophthalmic Suspension	472
Blephamide Ointment	⊙ 234
Econopred & Econopred Plus Ophthalmic Suspensions	⊙ 216
Poly-Pred Liquifilm	⊙ 246
Pred Forte	⊙ 247
Pred Mild	⊙ 250
Pred-G Liquifilm Sterile Ophthalmic Suspension	⊙ 248
Pred-G S.O.P. Sterile Ophthalmic Ointment	⊙ 249

Prednisolone Sodium Phosphate (Corticosteroids tend to produce hyperglycemia and concurrent use may lead to loss of control). Products include:

AK-PRED	⊙ 204
Hydeltrasol Injection, Sterile	1708
Pediapred Oral Solution	1618

Prednisolone Tebutate (Corticosteroids tend to produce hyperglycemia and concurrent use may lead to loss of control). Products include:

Hydeltra-T.B.A. Sterile Suspension	1710

Prednisone (Corticosteroids tend to produce hyperglycemia and concurrent use may lead to loss of control).
No products indexed under this heading.

Probenecid (The hypoglycemic action of sulfonylureas may be potentiated by probenecid). Products include:

Benemid Tablets	1651
ColBENEMID Tablets	1662

Prochlorperazine (Phenothiazines tend to produce hyperglycemia and concurrent use may lead to loss of control). Products include:

Compazine	2644

Promethazine Hydrochloride (Phenothiazines tend to produce hyperglycemia and concurrent use may lead to loss of control). Products include:

Mepergan Injection	2859
Phenergan with Codeine	2883
Phenergan with Dextromethorphan	2885
Phenergan Injection	2880
Phenergan Suppositories	2882
Phenergan Syrup	2881
Phenergan Tablets	2882
Phenergan VC	2886
Phenergan VC with Codeine	2888

Propranolol Hydrochloride (The hypoglycemic action of sulfonylureas may be potentiated by beta adrenergic blockers). Products include:

Inderal	2834
Inderal LA Long Acting Capsules	2836
Inderide Tablets	2838
Inderide LA Long Acting Capsules	2840

Pseudoephedrine Hydrochloride (Sympathomimetics tend to produce hyperglycemia and concurrent use may lead to loss of control). Products include:

Actifed Allergy Daytime/Nighttime Caplets	⊡ 808
Actifed Cold & Allergy Tablets	⊡ 807
Actifed Cold & Sinus Caplets and Tablets	⊡ 808
Actifed Sinus Daytime/Nighttime Tablets and Caplets	⊡ 809
Advil Cold and Sinus Caplets and Tablets	⊡ 837
Alka-Seltzer Plus Liqui-Gels	⊡ 612
Alka-Seltzer Plus Flu & Body Aches Liqui-Gels Non-Drowsy Formula	⊡ 613
Alka-Seltzer Plus Night-Time Cold Medicine Liqui-Gels	⊡ 612
Allerest Maximum Strength	⊡ 649
Allerest No Drowsiness	⊡ 649
Allerest Sinus Pain Formula	⊡ 649
Atrohist Pediatric Capsules	1603
Benadryl Allergy/Cold Tablets	⊡ 811
Benadryl Allergy Decongestant Liquid Medication	⊡ 812
Benadryl Allergy Decongestant Tablets	⊡ 812
Benadryl Allergy Sinus Headache Caplets	⊡ 813
Benylin Multisymptom	⊡ 816
Bromfed Capsules (Extended-Release)	1832
Bromfed Syrup	⊡ 712
Bromfed Tablets	1832
Bromfed-DM Cough Syrup	1832
Bromfed-PD Capsules (Extended-Release)	1832
Children's TYLENOL Cold Multi-Symptom Chewable Tablets and Liquid	1559
Children's TYLENOL Cold Plus Cough Multi Symptom Chewable Tablets and Liquid	1560
Children's TYLENOL Flu Suspension Liquid	1560
Children's Vicks DayQuil Allergy Relief	⊡ 730
Children's Vicks NyQuil Cold/Cough Relief	⊡ 731
Allergy-Sinus Comtrex Multi-Symptom Allergy-Sinus Formula Tablets and Caplets	⊡ 639
Comtrex Multi-Symptom	⊡ 638
Comtrex Multi-Symptom Non-Drowsy Caplets	⊡ 640
Congess	1003
Contac Day Allergy/Sinus Caplets	⊡ 771
Contac Day & Night	⊡ 772
Contac Night Allergy/Sinus Caplets	⊡ 771
Contac Severe Cold & Flu Non-Drowsy	⊡ 774
Deconsal II Tablets	1605
Dimetane-DX Cough Syrup	2233
Dimetapp Cold & Fever Suspension	⊡ 839
Dimetapp Decongestant Pediatric Drops	⊡ 840
Dorcol Children's Cough Syrup	⊡ 748
Drixoral Cough + Congestion Liquid Caps	⊡ 763
Dura-Tap/PD Capsules	970
Duratuss Tablets	2750
Duratuss HD Elixir	2750
Efidac/24	⊡ 655
Entex PSE Tablets	973
Fedahist Gyrocaps	2545
Guaifed	1833
Guaifed Syrup	⊡ 712
Guaimax-D Tablets	809
Histussin D Liquid	670
Infants' TYLENOL Cold Decongestant & Fever-Reducer Drops	1561
Kronofed-A	994
Novahistine DMX	782
Nucofed	2225
PediaCare Cough-Cold Chewable Tablets and Liquid	1569
PediaCare Infants' Decongestant Drops	1569
PediaCare Infants' Drops Decongestant Plus Cough	1569
PediaCare NightRest Cough-Cold Liquid	1569
Pediatric Vicks 44d Cough & Head Congestion Relief	⊡ 736
Pediatric Vicks 44m Cough & Cold Relief	⊡ 737
Robitussin Cold & Cough Liqui-Gels	⊡ 844
Robitussin Cold, Cough & Flu Liqui-Gels	⊡ 844
Robitussin Maximum Strength Cough & Cold	⊡ 847
Robitussin Night-Time Cold Formula	⊡ 847
Robitussin Pediatric Cough & Cold Formula	⊡ 848
Robitussin Pediatric Drops	⊡ 849
Robitussin Severe Congestion Liqui-Gels	⊡ 845
Robitussin-DAC Syrup	2249
Robitussin-PE	⊡ 846
Rondec Oral Drops	974
Rondec Syrup	974
Rondec Tablet	974
Rondec Chewable Tablets	974
Rondec-TR Tablet	974
Ryna	⊡ 804
Seldane-D Extended-Release Tablets	1286
Semprex-D Capsules	1620
Sinarest	⊡ 663
Sine-Aid Maximum Strength Sinus Headache Gelcaps, Caplets and Tablets	1570
Sine-Off No Drowsiness Formula Caplets	⊡ 784
Sine-Off Sinus Medicine	⊡ 784
Singlet Tablets	⊡ 785
Sinutab Non-Drying Liquid Caps	⊡ 823
Sinutab Sinus Allergy Medication, Maximum Strength Tablets and Caplets	⊡ 823
Sinutab Sinus Medication, Maximum Strength Without Drowsiness Formula, Tablets & Caplets	⊡ 824
Sudafed Children's Cold & Cough Liquid Medication	⊡ 825
Sudafed Children's Nasal Decongestant Liquid Medication	⊡ 826
Sudafed Cold & Allergy Tablets	⊡ 826
Sudafed Cold and Cough Liquid Caps	⊡ 826
Sudafed Nasal Decongestant Tablets, 30 mg.	⊡ 825
Sudafed Nasal Decongestant Tablets, 60 mg.	⊡ 825
Sudafed Non-Drying Sinus Liquid Caps	⊡ 827
Sudafed Pediatric Nasal Decongestant Liquid Oral Drops	⊡ 827
Sudafed Severe Cold Formula Caplets	⊡ 828
Sudafed Severe Cold Formula Tablets	⊡ 828
Sudafed Sinus Caplets	⊡ 829
Sudafed Sinus Tablets	⊡ 829
Sudafed 12 Hour Caplets	⊡ 824
Syn-Rx Tablets	1622
Syn-Rx DM Tablets	1623
TheraFlu Flu and Cold Medicine	⊡ 750
Theraflu Maximum Strength Flu and Cold Medicine For Sore Throat	⊡ 751
TheraFlu Flu, Cold and Cough Medicine	⊡ 750
TheraFlu Maximum Strength Nighttime Flu, Cold & Cough Medicine	⊡ 751
TheraFlu Maximum Strength Non-Drowsy Formula Flu, Cold & Cough Medicine	⊡ 751
TheraFlu Maximum Strength, Non-Drowsy Formula Flu, Cold and Cough Caplets	⊡ 752
Theraflu Maximum Strength Sinus Non-Drowsy Formula Caplets	⊡ 752
Triaminic AM Cough and Decongestant Formula	⊡ 753
Triaminic AM Decongestant Formula	⊡ 753
Triaminic Infant Oral Decongestant Drops	⊡ 754
Triaminic Night Time	⊡ 754
Triaminic Sore Throat Formula	⊡ 755
Tussend	1830
Tussend Expectorant	1831
TYLENOL Allergy Sinus, Maximum Strength Caplets and Gelcaps	1571
TYLENOL Allergy Sinus NightTime, Maximum Strength Caplets	1571
TYLENOL Cold Medication, Multi-Symptom Formula Tablets and Caplets	1572
TYLENOL Cold Medication, Multi-Symptom Hot Liquid Packets	1572
TYLENOL Cold Medication, No Drowsiness Formula Caplets and Gelcaps	1572
TYLENOL Cold Severe Congestion Caplets	1573
TYLENOL Cough Medication with Decongestant, Multi Symptom	1574
TYLENOL Flu No Drowsiness Formula, Maximum Strength Gelcaps	1575
TYLENOL Flu NightTime, Maximum Strength Gelcaps	1575
TYLENOL Flu NightTime, Maximum Strength Hot Medication Packets	1575
TYLENOL Sinus, Maximum Strength Geltabs, Gelcaps, Caplets and Tablets	1576
Vicks 44 LiquiCaps Cough, Cold & Flu Relief	⊡ 728
Vicks 44 LiquiCaps Non-Drowsy Cough & Cold Relief	⊡ 729
Vicks 44D Cough & Head Congestion Relief	⊡ 728
Vicks 44M Cough, Cold & Flu Relief	⊡ 729
Vicks DayQuil LiquiCaps/Liquid Multi-Symptom Cold/Flu Relief	⊡ 734
Vicks DayQuil SINUS Pressure & PAIN Relief with IBUPROFEN	⊡ 735
Vicks Nyquil Hot Therapy	⊡ 735
Vicks NyQuil LiquiCaps/Liquid Multi-Symptom Cold/Flu Relief, Original and Cherry Flavors	⊡ 736

Pseudoephedrine Sulfate (Sympathomimetics tend to produce hyperglycemia and concurrent use may lead to loss of control). Products include:

Chlor-Trimeton Allergy Decongestant Tablets	⊡ 759
Claritin-D Tablets	2487
Drixoral Cold and Allergy Sustained-Action Tablets	⊡ 763
Drixoral Cold and Flu Extended-Release Tablets	⊡ 764
Drixoral Non-Drowsy Formula Extended-Release Tablets	⊡ 764
Drixoral Allergy/Sinus Extended Release Tablets	⊡ 765
Trinalin Repetabs Tablets	1373

Quinestrol (Estrogens tend to produce hyperglycemia and concurrent use may lead to loss of control).
No products indexed under this heading.

Salmeterol Xinafoate (Sympathomimetics tend to produce hyperglycemia and concurrent use may lead to loss of control). Products include:

Serevent Inhalation Aerosol	1149

Salsalate (The hypoglycemic action of sulfonylureas may be potentiated by salicylates). Products include:

Disalcid	1549
Mono-Gesic Tablets	810
Salflex Tablets	791

Secobarbital Sodium (The action of barbiturates may be prolonged by therapy with chlorpropamide; barbiturates should be employed with caution). Products include:

Seconal Sodium Pulvules	1529

Selegiline Hydrochloride (The hypoglycemic action of sulfonylureas may be potentiated by monoamine oxidase inhibitors). Products include:

Eldepryl Capsules	2729

Sotalol Hydrochloride (The hypoglycemic action of sulfonylureas may be potentiated by beta adrenergic blockers). Products include:

Betapace Tablets	637

Spironolactone (Diuretics tend to produce hyperglycemia and concurrent use may lead to loss of control). Products include:

Aldactazide Tablets	2556
Aldactone Tablets	2558

Sulfacytine (The hypoglycemic action of sulfonylureas may be potentiated by sulfonamides).

Sulfamethizole (The hypoglycemic action of sulfonylureas may be potentiated by sulfonamides). Products include:

Urobiotic-250 Capsules	2038

Sulfamethoxazole (The hypoglycemic action of sulfonylureas may be potentiated by sulfonamides). Products include:

Bactrim DS Tablets	2257
Bactrim I.V. Infusion	2255
Bactrim	2257
Gantanol Tablets	2285
Septra	1146
Septra I.V. Infusion	1142
Septra I.V. Infusion ADD-Vantage Vials	1144
Septra	1146

(⊡ Described in PDR For Nonprescription Drugs)   (⊙ Described in PDR For Ophthalmology)

281 **Interactions Index** **Diamox**

Sulfasalazine (The hypoglycemic action of sulfonylureas may be potentiated by sulfonamides). Products include:
- Azulfidine ... 2059

Sulfinpyrazone (The hypoglycemic action of sulfonylureas may be potentiated by sulfonamides). Products include:
- Anturane ... 823

Sulfisoxazole (The hypoglycemic action of sulfonylureas may be potentiated by sulfonamides). Products include:
- Gantrisin Tablets ... 2286

Sulfisoxazole Diolamine (The hypoglycemic action of sulfonylureas may be potentiated by sulfonamides).
- No products indexed under this heading.

Sulindac (The hypoglycemic action of sulfonylureas may be potentiated by nonsteroidal anti-inflammatory agents). Products include:
- Clinoril Tablets ... 1658

Temazepam (The hypoglycemic action of sulfonylureas may be potentiated by drugs that are highly protein bound). Products include:
- Restoril Capsules ... 2413

Terbutaline Sulfate (Sympathomimetics tend to produce hyperglycemia and concurrent use may lead to loss of control). Products include:
- Brethaire Inhaler ... 830
- Brethine Ampuls ... 832
- Brethine Tablets ... 831
- Bricanyl Subcutaneous Injection ... 1247
- Bricanyl Tablets ... 1248

Thiamylal Sodium (The action of barbiturates may be prolonged by therapy with chlorpropamide; barbiturates should be employed with caution).
- No products indexed under this heading.

Thioridazine Hydrochloride (Phenothiazines tend to produce hyperglycemia and concurrent use may lead to loss of control). Products include:
- Mellaril ... 2398

Thyroglobulin (Thyroid products tend to produce hyperglycemia and concurrent use may lead to loss of control).
- No products indexed under this heading.

Thyroid (Thyroid products tend to produce hyperglycemia and concurrent use may lead to loss of control).
- No products indexed under this heading.

Thyroxine (Thyroid products tend to produce hyperglycemia and concurrent use may lead to loss of control).
- No products indexed under this heading.

Thyroxine Sodium (Thyroid products tend to produce hyperglycemia and concurrent use may lead to loss of control).
- No products indexed under this heading.

Timolol Hemihydrate (The hypoglycemic action of sulfonylureas may be potentiated by beta adrenergic blockers). Products include:
- Betimol 0.25%, 0.5% ... ◉ 259

Timolol Maleate (The hypoglycemic action of sulfonylureas may be potentiated by beta adrenergic blockers). Products include:
- Blocadren Tablets ... 1654
- Timolide Tablets ... 1791
- Timoptic in Ocudose ... 1796
- Timoptic Sterile Ophthalmic Solution ... 1794
- Timoptic-XE ... 1798

Tolazamide (The hypoglycemic action of sulfonylureas may be potentiated by sulfonamides).
- No products indexed under this heading.

Tolbutamide (The hypoglycemic action of sulfonylureas may be potentiated by sulfonamides).
- No products indexed under this heading.

Tolmetin Sodium (The hypoglycemic action of sulfonylureas may be potentiated by nonsteroidal anti-inflammatory agents). Products include:
- Tolectin (200, 400 and 600 mg) .. 1591

Torsemide (Diuretics tend to produce hyperglycemia and concurrent use may lead to loss of control). Products include:
- Demadex Tablets and Injection ... 691

Tranylcypromine Sulfate (The hypoglycemic action of sulfonylureas may be potentiated by monoamine oxidase inhibitors). Products include:
- Parnate Tablets ... 2679

Triamcinolone (Corticosteroids tend to produce hyperglycemia and concurrent use may lead to loss of control).
- No products indexed under this heading.

Triamcinolone Acetonide (Corticosteroids tend to produce hyperglycemia and concurrent use may lead to loss of control). Products include:
- Azmacort Oral Inhaler ... 2175
- Nasacort AQ Nasal Spray ... 2191
- Nasacort Nasal Inhaler ... 2189

Triamcinolone Diacetate (Corticosteroids tend to produce hyperglycemia and concurrent use may lead to loss of control).
- No products indexed under this heading.

Triamcinolone Hexacetonide (Corticosteroids tend to produce hyperglycemia and concurrent use may lead to loss of control).
- No products indexed under this heading.

Triamterene (Diuretics tend to produce hyperglycemia and concurrent use may lead to loss of control). Products include:
- Dyazide Capsules ... 2653
- Dyrenium Capsules ... 2655

Trifluoperazine Hydrochloride (Phenothiazines tend to produce hyperglycemia and concurrent use may lead to loss of control). Products include:
- Stelazine ... 2692

Trimipramine Maleate (The hypoglycemic action of sulfonylureas may be potentiated by drugs that are highly protein bound). Products include:
- Surmontil Capsules ... 2917

Verapamil Hydrochloride (Calcium channel blockers tend to produce hyperglycemia and concurrent use may lead to loss of control). Products include:
- Calan SR Caplets ... 2571
- Calan Tablets ... 2568
- Covera-HS Tablets ... 2573
- Isoptin Injectable ... 1391
- Isoptin Oral Tablets ... 1393
- Isoptin SR Tablets ... 1395
- Verelan Capsules ... 1455

Warfarin Sodium (The hypoglycemic action of sulfonylureas may be potentiated by coumarins). Products include:
- Coumadin ... 941

Food Interactions

Alcohol (In some patients disulfiram-like reaction may be produced by the ingestion of alcohol).

DIALOSE TABLETS
(Docusate Sodium) ... 1358
May interact with:

Mineral Oil (Effect not specified). Products include:
- Alpha Keri Moisture Rich Body Oil ... 635
- Anusol Hemorrhoidal Ointment ... 810
- Aquaphor Healing Ointment ... 636
- Aquaphor Healing Ointment, Original Formula ... 636
- Eucerin Original Moisturizing Creme (Unscented) ... 636
- Eucerin Original Moisturizing Lotion ... 636
- Eucerin Plus Dry Skin Care Moisturizing Lotion ... 636
- Eucerin Plus Moisturizing Creme ... 636
- Fleet Mineral Oil Enema ... 1001
- Hemorid ... 797
- HypoTears Ointment ... ◉ 262
- Keri Lotion - Original Formula ... 644
- Kondremul ... 656
- Lubriderm Bath and Shower Oil ... 821
- Nephrox Suspension ... 671
- Preparation H Hemorrhoidal Ointment ... 842
- Refresh PM Lubricant Eye Ointment ... ◉ 252
- Replens Vaginal Moisturizer ... 823
- Tears Renewed Ointment ... ◉ 210

Prescription Drugs, unspecified (Effect not specified).

DIALOSE PLUS TABLETS
(Docusate Sodium, Phenolphthalein) 1358
May interact with:

Mineral Oil (Effect not specified). Products include:
- Alpha Keri Moisture Rich Body Oil ... 635
- Anusol Hemorrhoidal Ointment ... 810
- Aquaphor Healing Ointment ... 636
- Aquaphor Healing Ointment, Original Formula ... 636
- Eucerin Original Moisturizing Creme (Unscented) ... 636
- Eucerin Original Moisturizing Lotion ... 636
- Eucerin Plus Dry Skin Care Moisturizing Lotion ... 636
- Eucerin Plus Moisturizing Creme ... 636
- Fleet Mineral Oil Enema ... 1001
- Hemorid ... 797
- HypoTears Ointment ... ◉ 262
- Keri Lotion - Original Formula ... 644
- Kondremul ... 656
- Lubriderm Bath and Shower Oil ... 821
- Nephrox Suspension ... 671
- Preparation H Hemorrhoidal Ointment ... 842
- Refresh PM Lubricant Eye Ointment ... ◉ 252
- Replens Vaginal Moisturizer ... 823
- Tears Renewed Ointment ... ◉ 210

Prescription Drugs, unspecified (Effect not specified).

DIAMOX INTRAVENOUS
(Acetazolamide Sodium) ... ◉ 317
See **Diamox Tablets**

DIAMOX SEQUELS (SUSTAINED RELEASE)
(Acetazolamide) ... ◉ 318
May interact with:

Aspirin (Concomitant administration with high-dose aspirin may result in anorexia, tachypnea, lethargy, coma and death). Products include:
- Alka-Seltzer Cherry Effervescent Antacid and Pain Reliever ... 609
- Alka-Seltzer Extra Strength Effervescent Antacid and Pain Reliever ... 609
- Alka-Seltzer Lemon Lime Effervescent Antacid and Pain Reliever ... 609
- Alka-Seltzer Original Effervescent Antacid and Pain Reliever ... 609
- Alka-Seltzer Plus ... 611
- Alka-Seltzer Plus Sinus Medicine .. 611
- Ascriptin ... 650
- Arthritis Strength BC Powder ... 631
- BC Cold Powder Multi-Symptom Formula (Cold-Sinus-Allergy) ... 631
- BC Cold Powder Non-Drowsy Formula (Cold-Sinus) ... 631
- BC Powder ... 631
- Genuine Bayer Aspirin Tablets & Caplets ... 618
- Extra Strength Bayer Arthritis Pain Regimen Formula ... 615
- Extra Strength Bayer Aspirin Caplets & Tablets ... 617
- Extended-Release Bayer 8-Hour Aspirin ... 616
- Extra Strength Bayer Plus Aspirin Caplets ... 617
- Extra Strength Bayer PM Aspirin Plus Sleep Aid ... 617
- Aspirin Regimen Bayer 81 mg Tablets with Calcium ... 615
- Aspirin Regimen Bayer Adult Low Strength 81 mg Tablets ... 613
- Aspirin Regimen Bayer Children's Chewable Aspirin ... 616
- Aspirin Regimen Bayer Regular Strength 325 mg Caplets ... 613
- Bufferin Analgesic Tablets ... 636
- Arthritis Strength Bufferin Analgesic Caplets ... 637
- Extra Strength Bufferin Analgesic Tablets ... 637
- Cama Arthritis Pain Reliever ... 748
- Darvon Compound-65 Pulvules ... 1475
- Easprin ... 1971
- Ecotrin ... 2625
- Ecotrin Enteric Coated Aspirin Maximum Strength Tablets and Caplets ... 775
- Ecotrin Enteric Coated Aspirin Regular Strength Tablets ... 2625
- Empirin Aspirin Tablets ... 818
- Excedrin Extra-Strength Analgesic Tablets, Caplets, and Geltabs ... 734
- Fiorinal Capsules ... 2388
- Fiorinal with Codeine Capsules ... 2390
- Fiorinal Tablets ... 2388
- Goody's Extra Strength Headache Powders ... 632
- Goody's Extra Strength Pain Relief Tablets ... 632
- Halfprin Tablets ... 1413
- Norgesic ... 1554
- Percodan Tablets ... 955
- Percodan-Demi Tablets ... 956
- Robaxisal Tablets ... 2246
- Soma Compound w/Codeine Tablets ... 2784
- Soma Compound Tablets ... 2783
- St. Joseph Adult Chewable Aspirin (81 mg.) ... 768
- Talwin Compound ... 2466
- Vanquish Analgesic Caplets ... 627

DIAMOX TABLETS
(Acetazolamide) ... ◉ 317
May interact with:

Aspirin (Concomitant administration with high-dose aspirin may result in anorexia, tachypnea, lethargy, coma and death). Products include:
- Alka-Seltzer Cherry Effervescent Antacid and Pain Reliever ... 609
- Alka-Seltzer Extra Strength Effervescent Antacid and Pain Reliever ... 609
- Alka-Seltzer Lemon Lime Effervescent Antacid and Pain Reliever ... 609
- Alka-Seltzer Original Effervescent Antacid and Pain Reliever ... 609
- Alka-Seltzer Plus ... 611
- Alka-Seltzer Plus Sinus Medicine .. 611
- Ascriptin ... 650
- Arthritis Strength BC Powder ... 631
- BC Cold Powder Multi-Symptom Formula (Cold-Sinus-Allergy) ... 631
- BC Cold Powder Non-Drowsy Formula (Cold-Sinus) ... 631
- BC Powder ... 631
- Genuine Bayer Aspirin Tablets & Caplets ... 618
- Extra Strength Bayer Arthritis Pain Regimen Formula ... 615
- Extra Strength Bayer Aspirin Caplets & Tablets ... 617

IMPORTANT NOTE: Always consult each drug listing in the patient's regimen for possible interactions.

Diamox | Interactions Index | 282

Extended-Release Bayer 8-Hour Aspirin ◘ 616
Extra Strength Bayer Plus Aspirin Caplets ◘ 617
Extra Strength Bayer PM Aspirin Plus Sleep Aid ◘ 617
Aspirin Regimen Bayer 81 mg Tablets with Calcium ◘ 615
Aspirin Regimen Bayer Adult Low Strength 81 mg Tablets ◘ 613
Aspirin Regimen Bayer Children's Chewable Aspirin ◘ 616
Aspirin Regimen Bayer Regular Strength 325 mg Caplets ◘ 613
Bufferin Analgesic Tablets ◘ 636
Arthritis Strength Bufferin Analgesic Caplets ◘ 637
Extra Strength Bufferin Analgesic Tablets ◘ 637
Cama Arthritis Pain Reliever ◘ 748
Darvon Compound-65 Pulvules 1475
Easprin 1971
Ecotrin 2625
Ecotrin Enteric Coated Aspirin Maximum Strength Tablets and Caplets ◘ 775
Ecotrin Enteric Coated Aspirin Regular Strength Tablets 2625
Empirin Aspirin Tablets ◘ 818
Excedrin Extra-Strength Analgesic Tablets, Caplets, and Geltabs 734
Fiorinal Capsules 2388
Fiorinal with Codeine Capsules 2390
Fiorinal Tablets 2388
Goody's Extra Strength Headache Powders ◘ 632
Goody's Extra Strength Pain Relief Tablets ◘ 632
Halfprin Tablets 1413
Norgesic 1554
Percodan Tablets 955
Percodan-Demi Tablets 956
Robaxisal Tablets 2246
Soma Compound w/Codeine Tablets 2784
Soma Compound Tablets 2783
St. Joseph Adult Chewable Aspirin (81 mg.) ◘ 768
Talwin Compound 2466
Vanquish Analgesic Caplets ◘ 627

DIBENZYLINE CAPSULES
(Phenoxybenzamine Hydrochloride) 2650
May interact with:

Alpha and Beta Adrenergic Stimulators (Exaggerated hypotensive response; tachycardia).

Epinephrine (Exaggerated hypotensive response; tachycardia). Products include:
EPIFRIN ⊙ 237
EpiPen 808
Marcaine with Epinephrine 2446
Primatene Mist ◘ 843
Sensorcaine with Epinephrine Injection 554
Sus-Phrine Injection 1017
Xylocaine with Epinephrine Injections 562

Epinephrine Bitartrate (Exaggerated hypotensive response; tachycardia). Products include:
Sensorcaine-MPF with Epinephrine Injection 554

Norepinephrine Bitartrate (Hyperthermia production of levarterenol blocked by dibenzyline). Products include:
Levophed Bitartrate Injection 2445

Reserpine (Hypothermia production of reserpine blocked by dibenzyline). Products include:
Diupres Tablets 1691
Hydropres Tablets 1718
Ser-Ap-Es Tablets 867

DICAL-D TABLETS & WAFERS
(Calcium Phosphate, Dibasic, Vitamin D) 424
None cited in PDR database.

DIDRONEL I.V. INFUSION
(Etidronate Disodium (Biphosphonate)) 1545
May interact with:

Nephrotoxic Drugs (Potential for excessive depression of renal function).

DIDRONEL TABLETS
(Etidronate Disodium (Diphosphonate)) 2133
May interact with:

Warfarin Sodium (Co-administration has resulted in isolated reports of increase in prothrombin time without clinically significant sequelae). Products include:
Coumadin 941

DIETHYLSTILBESTROL TABLETS
(Diethylstilbestrol) 1477
None cited in PDR database.

DIFFERIN GEL
(Adapalene) 1033
May interact with:

Resorcinol (Increased potential for local irritation). Products include:
BiCozene Creme ◘ 747

Salicylic Acid (Increased potential for local irritation). Products include:
DHS Sal Shampoo 1989
DuoFilm Liquid Wart Remover ◘ 765
DuoFilm Patch Wart Remover ◘ 765
DuoPlant Gel Plantar Wart Remover ◘ 765
Exact Pore Treatment Gel ◘ 722
MG 217 ◘ 800
Occlusal-HP 1041
SalAc 1042
Wart-Off Wart Remover ◘ 720

Sulfur (Increased potential for local irritation). Products include:
CharcoCaps ◘ 740
MG 217 Medicated Tar-Free Shampoo ◘ 800
Novacet Lotion 1041
Sulfacet-R Lotion 925
Sulfacet-R Tint Free Lotion 925

DIFLUCAN TABLETS, INJECTION, AND ORAL SUSPENSION
(Fluconazole) 2003
May interact with sulfonylureas, oral anticoagulants, xanthine bronchodilators, and certain other agents. Compounds in these categories include:

Aminophylline (Increased serum concentrations of theophylline).
No products indexed under this heading.

Astemizole (Potential for elevation in serum levels of astemizole). Products include:
Hismanal Tablets 1341

Chlorpropamide (Co-administration with sulfonylurea oral hypoglycemic agent may precipitate clinically significant hypoglycemia). Products include:
Diabinese Tablets 2002

Cimetidine (Potential for a significant decrease in fluconazole AUC (13% +/- 11%) and C_{max} (19% +/- 14%) after oral dose). Products include:
Tagamet HB Tablets ◘ 786
Tagamet Tablets 2694

Cimetidine Hydrochloride (Potential for a significant decrease in fluconazole AUC (13% +/- 11%) and C_{max} (19% +/- 14%) after oral dose). Products include:
Tagamet 2694

Cisapride (Potential for elevation in serum levels of cisapride). Products include:
Propulsid 1346

Cyclosporine (Fluconazole may significantly increase cyclosporine levels in renal transplant patients with or without renal impairment). Products include:
Neoral 2405
Sandimmune 2416

Dicumarol (Increased prothrombin time; monitoring of prothrombin time is recommended).
No products indexed under this heading.

Dyphylline (Increased serum concentrations of theophylline). Products include:
Lufyllin & Lufyllin-400 Tablets 2778
Lufyllin-GG Elixir & Tablets 2779

Ethinyl Estradiol (Co-administration with ethinyl estradiol and levonorgestrel-containing oral contraceptive produces an overall mean increase in ethinyl estradiol and levonorgestrel levels; however, in some patients there may be a decrease in these levels; clinical significance unknown). Products include:
Brevicon 2563
Demulen 2580
Desogen Tablets 1867
Levlen/Tri-Levlen 646
Lo/Ovral Tablets 2852
Lo/Ovral-28 Tablets 2857
Modicon 1928
Nordette-21 Tablets 2863
Nordette-28 Tablets 2866
Norinyl 2563
Ortho-Cept 1907
Ortho-Cyclen/Ortho-Tri-Cyclen 1914
Ortho-Novum 1928
Ortho-Cyclen/Ortho Tri-Cyclen 1914
Ovcon 765
Ovral Tablets 2877
Ovral-28 Tablets 2878
Levlen/Tri-Levlen 646
Tri-Norinyl 2607
Triphasil-21 Tablets 2919
Triphasil-28 Tablets 2924

Glimepiride (Co-administration with sulfonylurea oral hypoglycemic agent may precipitate clinically significant hypoglycemia). Products include:
Amaryl Tablets 1241

Glipizide (Co-administration with sulfonylurea oral hypoglycemic agent may precipitate clinically significant hypoglycemia; reduced metabolism of glipizide). Products include:
Glucotrol Tablets 2011
Glucotrol XL Extended Release Tablets 2012

Glyburide (Co-administration with sulfonylurea oral hypoglycemic agent may precipitate clinically significant hypoglycemia; one fatality has been reported with combined use due to hypoglycemia; reduced metabolism of glyburide). Products include:
DiaBeta Tablets 1265
Glynase PresTab Tablets 2091
Micronase Tablets 2099

Hydrochlorothiazide (Potential for a significant increase in fluconazole AUC (45% +/- 31%) and C_{max} (43% +/- 31%) attributable to reduction in renal clearance of 30% +/- 12%). Products include:
Aldactazide Tablets 2556
Aldoril Tablets 1644
Apresazide Capsules 824
Capozide Tablets 744
Dyazide Capsules 2653
Esidrix Tablets 839
Esimil Tablets 840
HydroDIURIL Tablets 1716
Hydropres Tablets 1718
Hyzaar Tablets 1720
Inderide Tablets 2838
Inderide LA Long Acting Capsules 2840
Lopressor HCT Tablets 850
Lotensin HCT Tablets 855
Moduretic Tablets 1748
Oretic Tablets 450
Prinzide Tablets 1780
Ser-Ap-Es Tablets 867
Timolide Tablets 1791
Vaseretic Tablets 1810
Zestoretic Tablets 2968
Ziac 1459

Isoniazid (The incidence of abnormally elevated serum transaminase was greater in patients taking Diflucan concomitantly with isoniazid). Products include:
Nydrazid Injection 509
Rifamate Capsules 1278
Rifater 1280

Levonorgestrel (Co-administration with ethinyl estradiol and levonorgestrel-containing oral contraceptive produces an overall mean increase in ethinyl estradiol and levonorgestrel levels; however, in some patients there may be a decrease in these levels; clinical significance unknown). Products include:
Levlen/Tri-Levlen 646
Nordette-21 Tablets 2863
Nordette-28 Tablets 2866
Norplant System 2868
Levlen/Tri-Levlen 646
Triphasil-21 Tablets 2919
Triphasil-28 Tablets 2924

Phenytoin (Increased plasma concentrations of phenytoin; monitor phenytoin concentration). Products include:
Dilantin Infatabs 1967
Dilantin-125 Suspension 1969

Phenytoin Sodium (Increased plasma concentrations of phenytoin; monitor phenytoin concentration). Products include:
Dilantin Kapseals 1965

Rifampin (Enhances the metabolism of concurrently administered fluconazole and decreases fluconazole AUC significantly). Products include:
Rifadin 1276
Rifamate Capsules 1278
Rifater 1280
Rimactane Capsules 865

Terfenadine (Potential for increase in terfenadine acid metabolite AUC (36%) from day 8 to day 15 with concomitant fluconazole administration; no change in cardiac repolarization as measured by Holter QTc interval). Products include:
Seldane Tablets 1284
Seldane-D Extended-Release Tablets 1286

Theophylline (Increased serum concentrations of theophylline). Products include:
Marax Tablets & DF Syrup 2015
Quibron 2227

Theophylline Anhydrous (Increased serum concentrations of theophylline). Products include:
Aerolate 1003
Primatene Tablets ◘ 844
Respbid Tablets 687
Slo-bid Gyrocaps 2201
Theo-24 Extended Release Capsules 2753
Theo-Dur Extended-Release Tablets 1367
Theo-X Extended-Release Tablets 793
Uni-Dur Extended-Release Tablets 1374
Uniphyl 400 mg and 600 mg Tablets 2157

Theophylline Calcium Salicylate (Increased serum concentrations of theophylline). Products include:
Quadrinal Tablets 1398

Theophylline Sodium Glycinate (Increased serum concentrations of theophylline).
  No products indexed under this heading.

Tolazamide (Co-administration with sulfonylurea oral hypoglycemic agent may precipitate clinically significant hypoglycemia).
  No products indexed under this heading.

Tolbutamide (Co-administration with sulfonylurea oral hypoglycemic agent may precipitate clinically significant hypoglycemia; reduced metabolism of tolbutamide).
  No products indexed under this heading.

Valproic Acid (The incidence of abnormally elevated serum transaminase was greater in patients taking Diflucan concomitantly with isoniazid). Products include:
  Depakene 416

Warfarin Sodium (Co-administration has resulted in a significant increase in prothrombin time response (area under the prothrombin time-time curve); monitoring of prothrombin time is recommended). Products include:
  Coumadin 941

Zidovudine (Potential for a significant increase in zidovudine AUC (20% +/- 32%) following the administration of fluconazole). Products include:
  Retrovir Capsules 1216
  Retrovir I.V. Infusion 1221
  Retrovir Syrup 1216

DI-GEL ANTACID/ANTI-GAS
(Calcium Carbonate, Magnesium Hydroxide, Simethicone) 762
May interact with tetracyclines. Compounds in this category include:

Demeclocycline Hydrochloride (Concurrent use with Di-Gel Liquid is not recommended). Products include:
  Declomycin Tablets 1421

Doxycycline Calcium (Concurrent use with Di-Gel Liquid is not recommended). Products include:
  Vibramycin Calcium Oral Suspension Syrup 2038

Doxycycline Hyclate (Concurrent use with Di-Gel Liquid is not recommended). Products include:
  Doryx Capsules 1970
  Vibramycin Hyclate Capsules 2038
  Vibramycin Hyclate Intravenous 2040
  Vibra-Tabs Film Coated Tablets 2038

Doxycycline Monohydrate (Concurrent use with Di-Gel Liquid is not recommended). Products include:
  Monodox Capsules 1858
  Vibramycin Monohydrate for Oral Suspension 2038

Methacycline Hydrochloride (Concurrent use with Di-Gel Liquid is not recommended).
  No products indexed under this heading.

Minocycline Hydrochloride (Concurrent use with Di-Gel Liquid is not recommended). Products include:
  DYNACIN Capsules 1627
  Minocin Intravenous 1428
  Minocin Oral Suspension 1431
  Minocin Pellet-Filled Capsules 1429

Oxytetracycline Hydrochloride (Concurrent use with Di-Gel Liquid is not recommended). Products include:
  TERAK Ointment 210
  Terra-Cortril Ophthalmic Suspension 2033
  Terramycin with Polymyxin B Sulfate Ophthalmic Ointment 2035
  Urobiotic-250 Capsules 2038

Tetracycline Hydrochloride (Concurrent use with Di-Gel Liquid is not recommended). Products include:
  Achromycin V Capsules 1417
  Helidac Therapy 2135

DIGIBIND
(Digoxin Immune Fab (Ovine)) 1079
None cited in PDR database.

DILACOR XR EXTENDED-RELEASE CAPSULES
(Diltiazem Hydrochloride) 2183
May interact with beta blockers, cardiac glycosides, anesthetics, and certain other agents. Compounds in these categories include:

Acebutolol Hydrochloride (Possible additive effects in prolonging AV conduction). Products include:
  Sectral Capsules 2914

Alfentanil Hydrochloride (Depression of cardiac contractility, conductivity, automaticity, and vasodilation associated with anesthetic may be potentiated). Products include:
  Alfenta Injection 1334

Atenolol (Possible additive effects in prolonging AV conduction). Products include:
  Tenoretic Tablets 2963
  Tenormin Tablets and I.V. Injection 2965

Betaxolol Hydrochloride (Possible additive effects in prolonging AV conduction). Products include:
  Betoptic Ophthalmic Solution 465
  Betoptic S Ophthalmic Suspension 467
  Kerlone Tablets 2588

Bisoprolol Fumarate (Possible additive effects in prolonging AV conduction). Products include:
  Zebeta Tablets 1457
  Ziac 1459

Carteolol Hydrochloride (Possible additive effects in prolonging AV conduction). Products include:
  Cartrol Tablets 413
  Ocupress Ophthalmic Solution, 1% Sterile 297

Cimetidine (Significant increase in peak diltiazem plasma levels and area under the curve). Products include:
  Tagamet HB Tablets 786
  Tagamet Tablets 2694

Cimetidine Hydrochloride (Significant increase in peak diltiazem plasma levels and area under the curve). Products include:
  Tagamet 2694

Cyclosporine (May result in competitive inhibition of metabolism; dosage of cyclosporin may need to be adjusted). Products include:
  Neoral 2405
  Sandimmune 2416

Deslanoside (Possible additive effects in prolonging AV conduction; potential for increased digoxin serum levels).
  No products indexed under this heading.

Digitoxin (Possible additive effects in prolonging AV conduction; potential for increased digoxin serum levels). Products include:
  Crystodigin Tablets 1472

Digoxin (Possible additive effects in prolonging AV conduction; potential for increased digoxin serum levels). Products include:
  Lanoxicaps 1110
  Lanoxin Elixir Pediatric 1113
  Lanoxin Injection 1116
  Lanoxin Injection Pediatric 1119
  Lanoxin Tablets 1121

Drugs which undergo biotransformation by cytochrome P-450 mixed function oxidase (Coadministration may result in the competitive inhibition of metabolism).

Enflurane (Depression of cardiac contractility, conductivity, automaticity, and vasodilation associated with anesthetic may be potentiated).
  No products indexed under this heading.

Esmolol Hydrochloride (Possible additive effects in prolonging AV conduction). Products include:
  Brevibloc (esmolol HCl) Injection 1860

Fentanyl Citrate (Depression of cardiac contractility, conductivity, automaticity, and vasodilation associated with anesthetic may be potentiated). Products include:
  Sublimaze Injection 463

Halothane (Depression of cardiac contractility, conductivity, automaticity, and vasodilation associated with anesthetic may be potentiated). Products include:
  Fluothane 2830

Isoflurane (Depression of cardiac contractility, conductivity, automaticity, and vasodilation associated with anesthetic may be potentiated).
  No products indexed under this heading.

Ketamine Hydrochloride (Depression of cardiac contractility, conductivity, automaticity, and vasodilation associated with anesthetic may be potentiated).
  No products indexed under this heading.

Labetalol Hydrochloride (Possible additive effects in prolonging AV conduction). Products include:
  Normodyne Injection 2519
  Normodyne Tablets 2522
  Trandate 1158

Levobunolol Hydrochloride (Possible additive effects in prolonging AV conduction). Products include:
  Betagan 230

Methohexital Sodium (Depression of cardiac contractility, conductivity, automaticity, and vasodilation associated with anesthetic may be potentiated).
  No products indexed under this heading.

Metipranolol Hydrochloride (Possible additive effects in prolonging AV conduction). Products include:
  OptiPranolol (Metipranolol 0.3%) Sterile Ophthalmic Solution 256

Metoprolol Succinate (Possible additive effects in prolonging AV conduction). Products include:
  Toprol-XL Tablets 560

Metoprolol Tartrate (Possible additive effects in prolonging AV conduction). Products include:
  Lopressor 848

Lopressor HCT Tablets 850

Midazolam Hydrochloride (Depression of cardiac contractility, conductivity, automaticity, and vasodilation associated with anesthetic may be potentiated). Products include:
  Versed Injection 2324

Nadolol (Possible additive effects in prolonging AV conduction).
  No products indexed under this heading.

Penbutolol Sulfate (Possible additive effects in prolonging AV conduction). Products include:
  Levatol Tablets 2547

Pindolol (Possible additive effects in prolonging AV conduction). Products include:
  Visken Tablets 2428

Propofol (Depression of cardiac contractility, conductivity, automaticity, and vasodilation associated with anesthetic may be potentiated). Products include:
  Diprivan Injectable Emulsion 2939

Propranolol Hydrochloride (Possible additive effects in prolonging AV conduction). Products include:
  Inderal 2834
  Inderal LA Long Acting Capsules 2836
  Inderide Tablets 2838
  Inderide LA Long Acting Capsules ... 2840

Ranitidine Hydrochloride (Produces smaller, nonsignificant increase in diltiazem plasma levels). Products include:
  Zantac 1182
  Zantac Injection 1180
  Zantac Syrup 1182

Sotalol Hydrochloride (Possible additive effects in prolonging AV conduction). Products include:
  Betapace Tablets 637

Sufentanil Citrate (Depression of cardiac contractility, conductivity, automaticity, and vasodilation associated with anesthetic may be potentiated). Products include:
  Sufenta Injection 1355

Thiamylal Sodium (Depression of cardiac contractility, conductivity, automaticity, and vasodilation associated with anesthetic may be potentiated).
  No products indexed under this heading.

Timolol Hemihydrate (Possible additive effects in prolonging AV conduction). Products include:
  Betimol 0.25%, 0.5% 259

Timolol Maleate (Possible additive effects in prolonging AV conduction). Products include:
  Blocadren Tablets 1654
  Timolide Tablets 1791
  Timoptic in Ocudose 1796
  Timoptic Sterile Ophthalmic Solution 1794
  Timoptic-XE 1798

Food Interactions
Diet, high-lipid (Simultaneous administration of Dilacor XR with a high-fat breakfast has a modest effect on diltiazem bioavailability).

DILANTIN INFATABS
(Phenytoin) 1967
May interact with histamine h2-receptor antagonists, oral anticoagulants, oral contraceptives, estrogens, phenothiazines, salicylates, succinimides, sulfonamides, tricyclic antidepressants, corticosteroids, xanthine bronchodilators, and certain other

---
IMPORTANT NOTE: Always consult each drug listing in the patient's regimen for possible interactions.

Dilantin Infatabs | Interactions Index | 284

agents. Compounds in these categories include:

Aminophylline (Phenytoin impairs efficacy of theophylline).
No products indexed under this heading.

Amiodarone Hydrochloride (May increase serum phenytoin levels). Products include:
Cordarone Intravenous ... 2821
Cordarone Tablets ... 2818

Amitriptyline Hydrochloride (Tricyclic antidepressants may precipitate seizures in susceptible patients and phenytoin dosage may need to be adjusted). Products include:
Elavil ... 2945
Etrafon ... 2495
Limbitrol ... 2333
Triavil Tablets ... 1800

Amoxapine (Tricyclic antidepressants may precipitate seizures in susceptible patients and phenytoin dosage may need to be adjusted). Products include:
Asendin Tablets ... 1419

Aspirin (May increase serum phenytoin levels). Products include:
Alka-Seltzer Cherry Effervescent Antacid and Pain Reliever ... ▣ 609
Alka-Seltzer Extra Strength Effervescent Antacid and Pain Reliever ... ▣ 609
Alka-Seltzer Lemon Lime Effervescent Antacid and Pain Reliever ... ▣ 609
Alka-Seltzer Original Effervescent Antacid and Pain Reliever ... ▣ 609
Alka-Seltzer Plus ... ▣ 611
Alka-Seltzer Plus Sinus Medicine ... ▣ 611
Ascriptin ... ▣ 650
Arthritis Strength BC Powder ... ▣ 631
BC Cold Powder Multi-Symptom Formula (Cold-Sinus-Allergy) ... ▣ 631
BC Cold Powder Non-Drowsy Formula (Cold-Sinus) ... ▣ 631
BC Powder ... ▣ 631
Genuine Bayer Aspirin Tablets & Caplets ... ▣ 618
Extra Strength Bayer Arthritis Pain Regimen Formula ... ▣ 615
Extra Strength Bayer Aspirin Caplets & Tablets ... ▣ 617
Extended-Release Bayer 8-Hour Aspirin ... ▣ 616
Extra Strength Bayer Plus Aspirin Caplets ... ▣ 617
Extra Strength Bayer PM Aspirin Plus Sleep Aid ... ▣ 617
Aspirin Regimen Bayer 81 mg Tablets with Calcium ... ▣ 615
Aspirin Regimen Bayer Adult Low Strength 81 mg Tablets ... ▣ 613
Aspirin Regimen Bayer Children's Chewable Aspirin ... ▣ 616
Aspirin Regimen Bayer Regular Strength 325 mg Caplets ... ▣ 613
Bufferin Analgesic Tablets ... ▣ 636
Arthritis Strength Bufferin Analgesic Caplets ... ▣ 637
Extra Strength Bufferin Analgesic Tablets ... ▣ 637
Cama Arthritis Pain Reliever ... ▣ 748
Darvon Compound-65 Pulvules ... 1475
Easprin ... 1971
Ecotrin ... 2625
Ecotrin Enteric Coated Aspirin Maximum Strength Tablets and Caplets ... ▣ 775
Ecotrin Enteric Coated Aspirin Regular Strength Tablets ... 2625
Empirin Aspirin Tablets ... ▣ 818
Excedrin Extra-Strength Analgesic Tablets, Caplets, and Geltabs ... 734
Fiorinal Capsules ... 2388
Fiorinal with Codeine Capsules ... 2390
Fiorinal Tablets ... 2388
Goody's Extra Strength Headache Powders ... ▣ 632
Goody's Extra Strength Pain Relief Tablets ... ▣ 632
Halfprin Tablets ... 1413
Norgesic ... 1554
Percodan Tablets ... 955
Percodan-Demi Tablets ... 956
Robaxisal Tablets ... 2246
Soma Compound w/Codeine Tablets ... 2784
Soma Compound Tablets ... 2783
St. Joseph Adult Chewable Aspirin (81 mg.) ... ▣ 768
Talwin Compound ... 2466
Vanquish Analgesic Caplets ... ▣ 627

Bendroflumethiazide (May increase serum phenytoin levels).
No products indexed under this heading.

Betamethasone Acetate (Phenytoin impairs efficacy of corticosteroids). Products include:
Celestone Soluspan Suspension ... 2484

Betamethasone Sodium Phosphate (Phenytoin impairs efficacy of corticosteroids). Products include:
Celestone Soluspan Suspension ... 2484

Calcium Carbonate (Calcium ions interfere with the absorption of phenytoin; ingestion times of phenytoin and antacids containing calcium should be staggered in patients with low phenytoin levels). Products include:
Alka-Mints Chewable Antacid ... ▣ 609
Alka-Seltzer Fast Relief Caplets ... ▣ 610
Ascriptin ... ▣ 650
Extra Strength Bayer Plus Aspirin Caplets ... ▣ 617
Aspirin Regimen Bayer 81 mg Tablets with Calcium ... ▣ 615
Bufferin Analgesic Tablets ... ▣ 636
Arthritis Strength Bufferin Analgesic Caplets ... ▣ 637
Extra Strength Bufferin Analgesic Tablets ... ▣ 637
Calci-Chew Tablets ... 2168
Calci-Mix Capsules ... 2168
Caltrate 600 ... ▣ 681
Caltrate PLUS ... ▣ 681
Caltrate 600 + D ... ▣ 681
Cotazym Capsules ... 1866
Di-Gel Antacid/Anti-Gas ... ▣ 762
Florical Capsules and Tablets ... 1825
Gerimed Tablets ... 1000
Maalox Antacid Caplets ... ▣ 657
Marblen ... ▣ 671
Materna Tablets ... 1427
Monocal Tablets ... 1825
Mylanta Fast-Acting ... 1359
Mylanta Gelcaps Antacid ... ▣ 678
Mylanta Soothing Lozenges ... 1360
Mylanta Tablets ... ▣ 677
Mylanta Double Strength Tablets ... ▣ 677
Nephro-Calci Tablets ... 2168
One-A-Day Calcium Plus ... ▣ 625
Rolaids Antacid Tablets ... ▣ 807
Rolaids Antacid Calcium Rich/Sodium Free Tablets ... ▣ 807
Tempo Soft Antacid ... ▣ 799
Titralac ... ▣ 686
Titralac Plus ... ▣ 687
Tums Antacid/Calcium Supplement Tablets ... ▣ 787
Tums Anti-gas/Antacid Formula Tablets, Assorted Fruit ... ▣ 788
Tums E-X Antacid/Calcium Supplement Tablets ... ▣ 787
Tums 500 Calcium Supplement ... ▣ 788
Tums ULTRA Antacid/Calcium Supplement Tablets ... ▣ 787
TYLENOL Headache Plus Pain Reliever with Antacid, Extra Strength Caplets ... ▣ 705

Carbamazepine (May decrease serum phenytoin levels). Products include:
Atretol Tablets ... 569
Tegretol/Tegretol-XR ... 870

Chloramphenicol (May increase serum phenytoin levels). Products include:
Chloromycetin Ophthalmic Ointment, 1% ... ⊙ 298
Chloromycetin Ophthalmic Solution ... ⊙ 299
Chloroptic S.O.P. ... ⊙ 236
Chloroptic Sterile Ophthalmic Solution ... ⊙ 236

Chloramphenicol Palmitate (May increase serum phenytoin levels).
No products indexed under this heading.

Chloramphenicol Sodium Succinate (May increase serum phenytoin levels). Products include:
Chloromycetin Sodium Succinate ... 1960

Chlordiazepoxide (May increase serum phenytoin levels). Products include:
Limbitrol ... 2333

Chlordiazepoxide Hydrochloride (May increase serum phenytoin levels). Products include:
Librax Capsules ... 2330
Librium Capsules ... 2331
Librium Injectable ... 2332

Chlorothiazide (May increase serum phenytoin levels). Products include:
Aldoclor Tablets ... 1638
Diupres Tablets ... 1691
Diuril Oral ... 1694

Chlorothiazide Sodium (May increase serum phenytoin levels). Products include:
Diuril Sodium Intravenous ... 1693

Chlorotrianisene (May increase serum phenytoin levels; phenytoin impairs efficacy of estrogens).
No products indexed under this heading.

Chlorpromazine (May increase serum phenytoin levels). Products include:
Thorazine Suppositories ... 2701

Chlorpromazine Hydrochloride (May increase serum phenytoin levels). Products include:
Thorazine ... 2701

Chlorpropamide (May increase serum phenytoin levels). Products include:
Diabinese Tablets ... 2002

Choline Magnesium Trisalicylate (May increase serum phenytoin levels). Products include:
Trilisate ... 2155

Cimetidine (May increase serum phenytoin levels). Products include:
Tagamet HB Tablets ... ▣ 786
Tagamet Tablets ... 2694

Cimetidine Hydrochloride (May increase serum phenytoin levels). Products include:
Tagamet ... 2694

Clomipramine Hydrochloride (Tricyclic antidepressants may precipitate seizures in susceptible patients and phenytoin dosage may need to be adjusted). Products include:
Anafranil Capsules ... 819

Cortisone Acetate (Phenytoin impairs efficacy of corticosteroids). Products include:
Cortone Acetate Sterile Suspension ... 1663
Cortone Acetate Tablets ... 1664

Desipramine Hydrochloride (Tricyclic antidepressants may precipitate seizures in susceptible patients and phenytoin dosage may need to be adjusted). Products include:
Norpramin Tablets ... 1273

Desogestrel (Phenytoin impairs efficacy of oral contraceptives). Products include:
Desogen Tablets ... 1867
Ortho-Cept ... 1907

Dexamethasone (Phenytoin impairs efficacy of corticosteroids). Products include:
AK-Trol Ointment & Suspension ... ⊙ 205
Decadron Elixir ... 1676
Decadron Tablets ... 1678
Decaspray Topical Aerosol ... 1689
Maxitrol Ophthalmic Ointment and Suspension ... ⊙ 222
TobraDex Ophthalmic Suspension and Ointment ... 469

Dexamethasone Acetate (Phenytoin impairs efficacy of corticosteroids). Products include:
Dalalone D.P. Injectable ... 1009
Decadron-LA Sterile Suspension ... 1687

Dexamethasone Sodium Phosphate (Phenytoin impairs efficacy of corticosteroids). Products include:
Decadron Phosphate Injection ... 1680
Decadron Phosphate Sterile Ophthalmic Ointment ... 1684
Decadron Phosphate Sterile Ophthalmic Solution ... 1685
Decadron Phosphate Topical Cream ... 1686
Decadron Phosphate with Xylocaine Injection, Sterile ... 1683
Dexacort Phosphate in Respihaler ... 1606
Dexacort Phosphate in Turbinaire ... 1607
NeoDecadron Sterile Ophthalmic Ointment ... 1755
NeoDecadron Sterile Ophthalmic Solution ... 1756
NeoDecadron Topical Cream ... 1757

Diazepam (May increase serum phenytoin levels). Products include:
Dizac (diazepam injectable emulsion) CIV ... 1862
Valium Injectable ... 2336
Valium Tablets ... 2335

Dicumarol (May increase serum phenytoin levels; phenytoin impairs efficacy of coumarin anticoagulants).
No products indexed under this heading.

Dienestrol (May increase serum phenytoin levels; phenytoin impairs efficacy of estrogens). Products include:
Ortho Dienestrol Cream ... 1922

Diethylstilbestrol (May increase serum phenytoin levels; phenytoin impairs efficacy of estrogens). Products include:
Diethylstilbestrol Tablets ... 1477

Diflunisal (May increase serum phenytoin levels). Products include:
Dolobid Tablets ... 1695

Digitoxin (Phenytoin impairs efficacy of digitoxin). Products include:
Crystodigin Tablets ... 1472

Disulfiram (May increase serum phenytoin levels). Products include:
Antabuse Tablets ... 2802

Divalproex Sodium (May increase or decrease phenytoin serum levels; unpredictable effect on valproate serum levels). Products include:
Depakote Tablets ... 418

Doxepin Hydrochloride (Tricyclic antidepressants may precipitate seizures in susceptible patients and phenytoin dosage may need to be adjusted). Products include:
Adapin Capsules ... 1542
Sinequan ... 2028
Zonalon Cream ... 1042

Doxycycline Calcium (Phenytoin impairs efficacy of doxycycline). Products include:
Vibramycin Calcium Oral Suspension Syrup ... 2038

Doxycycline Hyclate (Phenytoin impairs efficacy of doxycycline). Products include:
Doryx Capsules ... 1970
Vibramycin Hyclate Capsules ... 2038
Vibramycin Hyclate Intravenous ... 2040
Vibra-Tabs Film Coated Tablets ... 2038

Doxycycline Monohydrate (Phenytoin impairs efficacy of doxycycline). Products include:
Monodox Capsules ... 1858
Vibramycin Monohydrate for Oral Suspension ... 2038

Dyphylline (Phenytoin impairs efficacy of theophylline). Products include:
Lufyllin & Lufyllin-400 Tablets ... 2778
Lufyllin-GG Elixir & Tablets ... 2779

(▣ Described in PDR For Nonprescription Drugs) (⊙ Described in PDR For Ophthalmology)

Estradiol (May increase serum phenytoin levels; phenytoin impairs efficacy of estrogens). Products include:
- Climara Transdermal System ... 640
- Estrace Cream and Tablets ... 751
- Estraderm Transdermal System ... 842
- Estring Vaginal Ring ... 2086
- Vivelle Transdermal System ... 880

Estrogens, Conjugated (May increase serum phenytoin levels; phenytoin impairs efficacy of estrogens). Products include:
- PMB 200 and PMB 400 ... 2890
- Premarin Intravenous ... 2893
- Premarin Tablets ... 2896
- Premarin Vaginal Cream ... 2898
- Premphase ... 2900
- Prempro ... 2905

Estrogens, Esterified (May increase serum phenytoin levels; phenytoin impairs efficacy of estrogens). Products include:
- ESTRATAB Tablets (0.3, 0.625, 1.25, 2.5 mg) ... 2715
- Estratest ... 2718
- Menest Tablets ... 2671

Estropipate (May increase serum phenytoin levels; phenytoin impairs efficacy of estrogens). Products include:
- Ogen Tablets ... 2103
- Ogen Vaginal Cream ... 2106
- Ortho-Est ... 1925

Ethinyl Estradiol (May increase serum phenytoin levels; phenytoin impairs efficacy of estrogens). Products include:
- Brevicon ... 2563
- Demulen ... 2580
- Desogen Tablets ... 1867
- Levlen/Tri-Levlen ... 646
- Lo/Ovral Tablets ... 2852
- Lo/Ovral-28 Tablets ... 2857
- Modicon ... 1928
- Nordette-21 Tablets ... 2863
- Nordette-28 Tablets ... 2866
- Norinyl ... 2563
- Ortho-Cept ... 1907
- Ortho-Cyclen/Ortho-Tri-Cyclen ... 1914
- Ortho-Novum ... 1928
- Ortho-Cyclen/Ortho Tri-Cyclen ... 1914
- Ovcon ... 765
- Ovral Tablets ... 2877
- Ovral-28 Tablets ... 2878
- Levlen/Tri-Levlen ... 646
- Tri-Norinyl ... 2607
- Triphasil-21 Tablets ... 2919
- Triphasil-28 Tablets ... 2924

Ethosuximide (May increase serum phenytoin levels). Products include:
- Zarontin Capsules ... 1986
- Zarontin Syrup ... 1986

Ethynodiol Diacetate (Phenytoin impairs efficacy of oral contraceptives). Products include:
- Demulen ... 2580

Famotidine (May increase serum phenytoin levels). Products include:
- Pepcid AC Acid Controller ... 1360
- Pepcid Injection ... 1765
- Pepcid ... 1763

Fludrocortisone Acetate (Phenytoin impairs efficacy of corticosteroids). Products include:
- Florinef Acetate Tablets ... 506

Fluphenazine Decanoate (May increase serum phenytoin levels). Products include:
- Prolixin Decanoate ... 510

Fluphenazine Enanthate (May increase serum phenytoin levels). Products include:
- Prolixin Enanthate ... 510

Fluphenazine Hydrochloride (May increase serum phenytoin levels). Products include:
- Prolixin ... 510

Furosemide (Phenytoin impairs efficacy of furosemide). Products include:
- Lasix Injection, Oral Solution and Tablets ... 1267

Glipizide (May increase serum phenytoin levels). Products include:
- Glucotrol Tablets ... 2011
- Glucotrol XL Extended Release Tablets ... 2012

Glyburide (May increase serum phenytoin levels). Products include:
- DiaBeta Tablets ... 1265
- Glynase PresTab Tablets ... 2091
- Micronase Tablets ... 2099

Halothane (May increase serum phenytoin levels). Products include:
- Fluothane ... 2830

Hydrochlorothiazide (May increase serum phenytoin levels). Products include:
- Aldactazide Tablets ... 2556
- Aldoril Tablets ... 1644
- Apresazide Capsules ... 824
- Capozide Tablets ... 744
- Dyazide Capsules ... 2653
- Esidrix Tablets ... 839
- Esimil Tablets ... 840
- HydroDIURIL Tablets ... 1716
- Hydropres Tablets ... 1718
- Hyzaar Tablets ... 1720
- Inderide Tablets ... 2838
- Inderide LA Long Acting Capsules .. 2840
- Lopressor HCT Tablets ... 850
- Lotensin HCT Tablets ... 855
- Moduretic Tablets ... 1748
- Oretic Tablets ... 450
- Prinzide Tablets ... 1780
- Ser-Ap-Es Tablets ... 867
- Timolide Tablets ... 1791
- Vaseretic Tablets ... 1810
- Zestoretic Tablets ... 2968
- Ziac ... 1459

Hydrocortisone (Phenytoin impairs efficacy of corticosteroids). Products include:
- Anusol-HC Cream 2.5% ... 1953
- Aquanil HC Lotion ... 1989
- Maximum Strength Cortaid Spray ... 800
- CORTENEMA ... 2713
- Cortisporin Ointment ... 1074
- Cortisporin Ophthalmic Ointment Sterile ... 1074
- Cortisporin Ophthalmic Suspension Sterile ... 1075
- Cortisporin Otic Solution Sterile ... 1076
- Cortisporin Otic Suspension Sterile 1077
- Cortizone-5 ... 795
- Cortizone-10 ... 795
- Hydrocortone Tablets ... 1715
- Hytone ... 922
- Hytone Ointment 2 ½% ... 923
- Massengill Medicated Soft Cloth Towelettes ... 2628
- Pediotic Suspension Sterile ... 1140
- Preparation H Hydrocortisone 1% Cream ... 843
- ProctoCream-HC 2.5% ... 2552
- VōSoL HC Otic Solution ... 2786

Hydrocortisone Acetate (Phenytoin impairs efficacy of corticosteroids). Products include:
- Analpram-HC Rectal Cream 1% and 2.5% ... 993
- Anusol HC-1 Hydrocortisone Anti-Itch Ointment ... 810
- Anusol-HC Suppositories ... 1954
- Caldecort Anti-Itch Hydrocortisone Cream ... 651
- Coly-Mycin S Otic w/Neomycin & Hydrocortisone ... 1965
- Cortaid ... 800
- Cortifoam ... 2540
- Cortisporin Cream ... 1073
- Epifoam ... 2543
- Hydrocortone Acetate Sterile Suspension ... 1712
- Mantadil Cream ... 1124
- Nupercainal Hydrocortisone 1% Cream ... 661
- Pramosone Cream, Lotion & Ointment ... 995
- ProctoFoam-HC ... 2552
- Terra-Cortril Ophthalmic Suspension ... 2033

Hydrocortisone Sodium Phosphate (Phenytoin impairs efficacy of corticosteroids). Products include:
- Hydrocortone Phosphate Injection, Sterile ... 1713

Hydrocortisone Sodium Succinate (Phenytoin impairs efficacy of corticosteroids).
- No products indexed under this heading.

Hydroflumethiazide (May increase serum phenytoin levels). Products include:
- Diucardin Tablets ... 2824

Imipramine Hydrochloride (Tricyclic antidepressants may precipitate seizures in susceptible patients and phenytoin dosage may need to be adjusted). Products include:
- Tofranil Ampuls ... 873
- Tofranil Tablets ... 875

Imipramine Pamoate (Tricyclic antidepressants may precipitate seizures in susceptible patients and phenytoin dosage may need to be adjusted). Products include:
- Tofranil-PM Capsules ... 876

Isoniazid (May increase serum phenytoin levels). Products include:
- Nydrazid Injection ... 509
- Rifamate Capsules ... 1278
- Rifater ... 1280

Levonorgestrel (Phenytoin impairs efficacy of oral contraceptives). Products include:
- Levlen/Tri-Levlen ... 646
- Nordette-21 Tablets ... 2863
- Nordette-28 Tablets ... 2866
- Norplant System ... 2868
- Levlen/Tri-Levlen ... 646
- Triphasil-21 Tablets ... 2919
- Triphasil-28 Tablets ... 2924

Magnesium Salicylate (May increase serum phenytoin levels). Products include:
- Backache Caplets ... 635
- Doan's Extra-Strength Analgesic ... 653
- Extra Strength Doan's P.M. ... 653
- Doan's Regular Strength Analgesic ... 654
- Mobigesic Tablets ... 607

Maprotiline Hydrochloride (Tricyclic antidepressants may precipitate seizures in susceptible patients and phenytoin dosage may need to be adjusted). Products include:
- Ludiomil Tablets ... 861

Mesoridazine Besylate (May increase serum phenytoin levels). Products include:
- Serentil ... 689

Mestranol (Phenytoin impairs efficacy of oral contraceptives). Products include:
- Norinyl ... 2563
- Ortho-Novum ... 1928

Methotrimeprazine (May increase serum phenytoin levels). Products include:
- Levoprome ... 1321

Methsuximide (May increase serum phenytoin levels). Products include:
- Celontin Kapseals ... 1955

Methyclothiazide (May increase serum phenytoin levels). Products include:
- Enduron Tablets ... 424

Methylphenidate Hydrochloride (May increase serum phenytoin levels). Products include:
- Ritalin ... 866

Methylprednisolone Acetate (Phenytoin impairs efficacy of corticosteroids).
- No products indexed under this heading.

Methylprednisolone Sodium Succinate (Phenytoin impairs efficacy of corticosteroids).
- No products indexed under this heading.

Molindone Hydrochloride (Moban brand of molindone contains calcium ions which interfere with the absorption of phenytoin). Products include:
- Moban Tablets and Concentrate ... 1036

Nizatidine (May increase serum phenytoin levels). Products include:
- Axid Pulvules ... 1468

Norethindrone (Phenytoin impairs efficacy of oral contraceptives). Products include:
- Brevicon ... 2563
- Micronor Tablets ... 1903
- Modicon ... 1928
- Norinyl ... 2563
- Nor-Q D Tablets ... 2598
- Ortho-Novum ... 1928
- Ovcon ... 765
- Tri-Norinyl ... 2607

Norethynodrel (Phenytoin impairs efficacy of oral contraceptives).
- No products indexed under this heading.

Norgestimate (Phenytoin impairs efficacy of oral contraceptives). Products include:
- Ortho-Cyclen/Ortho-Tri-Cyclen ... 1914
- Ortho-Cyclen/Ortho Tri-Cyclen ... 1914

Norgestrel (Phenytoin impairs efficacy of oral contraceptives). Products include:
- Lo/Ovral Tablets ... 2852
- Lo/Ovral-28 Tablets ... 2857
- Ovral Tablets ... 2877
- Ovral-28 Tablets ... 2878
- Ovrette Tablets ... 2878

Nortriptyline Hydrochloride (Tricyclic antidepressants may precipitate seizures in susceptible patients and phenytoin dosage may need to be adjusted). Products include:
- Pamelor ... 2409

Perphenazine (May increase serum phenytoin levels). Products include:
- Etrafon ... 2495
- Triavil Tablets ... 1800
- Trilafon ... 2532

Phenobarbital (May increase or decrease phenytoin serum levels; unpredictable effect on phenobarbital serum levels). Products include:
- Arco-Lase Plus Tablets ... 513
- Bellergal-S Tablets ... 2375
- Donnatal ... 2234
- Donnatal Extentabs ... 2234
- Donnatal Tablets ... 2234
- Phenobarbital Elixir and Tablets ... 1523
- Quadrinal Tablets ... 1398

Phensuximide (May increase serum phenytoin levels).
- No products indexed under this heading.

Phenylbutazone (May increase serum phenytoin levels).
- No products indexed under this heading.

Polyestradiol Phosphate (May increase serum phenytoin levels; phenytoin impairs efficacy of estrogens).
- No products indexed under this heading.

Polythiazide (May increase serum phenytoin levels). Products include:
- Minizide Capsules ... 2016

Prednisolone Acetate (Phenytoin impairs efficacy of corticosteroids). Products include:
- AK-CIDE ... ◎ 203
- AK-CIDE Ointment ... ◎ 203
- Blephamide Liquifilm Sterile Ophthalmic Suspension ... 472
- Blephamide Ointment ... ◎ 234

IMPORTANT NOTE: Always consult each drug listing in the patient's regimen for possible interactions.

Dilantin Infatabs | **Interactions Index** | **286**

Econopred & Econopred Plus Ophthalmic Suspensions ⊙ 216
Poly-Pred Liquifilm ⊙ 246
Pred Forte ⊙ 247
Pred Mild ⊙ 250
Pred-G Liquifilm Sterile Ophthalmic Suspension ⊙ 248
Pred-G S.O.P. Sterile Ophthalmic Ointment ⊙ 249

Prednisolone Sodium Phosphate (Phenytoin impairs efficacy of corticosteroids). Products include:
AK-PRED ⊙ 204
Hydeltrasol Injection, Sterile 1708
Pediapred Oral Solution 1618

Prednisolone Tebutate (Phenytoin impairs efficacy of corticosteroids). Products include:
Hydeltra-T.B.A. Sterile Suspension 1710

Prednisone (Phenytoin impairs efficacy of corticosteroids).
No products indexed under this heading.

Prochlorperazine (May increase serum phenytoin levels). Products include:
Compazine 2644

Promethazine Hydrochloride (May increase serum phenytoin levels). Products include:
Mepergan Injection 2859
Phenergan with Codeine 2883
Phenergan with Dextromethorphan 2885
Phenergan Injection 2880
Phenergan Suppositories 2882
Phenergan Syrup 2881
Phenergan Tablets 2882
Phenergan VC 2886
Phenergan VC with Codeine 2888

Protriptyline Hydrochloride (Tricyclic antidepressants may precipitate seizures in susceptible patients and phenytoin dosage may need to be adjusted). Products include:
Vivactil Tablets 1820

Quinestrol (May increase serum phenytoin levels; phenytoin impairs efficacy of estrogens).
No products indexed under this heading.

Quinidine Gluconate (Phenytoin impairs efficacy of quinidine). Products include:
Quinaglute Dura-Tabs Tablets 644

Quinidine Polygalacturonate (Phenytoin impairs efficacy of quinidine). Products include:
Cardioquin Tablets 2146

Quinidine Sulfate (Phenytoin impairs efficacy of quinidine). Products include:
Quinidex Extentabs 2240

Ranitidine Hydrochloride (May increase serum phenytoin levels). Products include:
Zantac 1182
Zantac Injection 1180
Zantac Syrup 1182

Reserpine (May decrease serum phenytoin levels). Products include:
Diupres Tablets 1691
Hydropres Tablets 1718
Ser-Ap-Es Tablets 867

Rifampin (Phenytoin impairs efficacy of rifampin). Products include:
Rifadin 1276
Rifamate Capsules 1278
Rifater 1280
Rimactane Capsules 865

Salsalate (May increase serum phenytoin levels). Products include:
Disalcid 1549
Mono-Gesic Tablets 810
Salflex Tablets 791

Sucralfate (May decrease serum phenytoin levels). Products include:
Carafate Suspension 1250
Carafate Tablets 1249

Sulfacytine (May increase serum phenytoin levels).

Sulfamethizole (May increase serum phenytoin levels). Products include:
Urobiotic-250 Capsules 2038

Sulfamethoxazole (May increase serum phenytoin levels). Products include:
Bactrim DS Tablets 2257
Bactrim I.V. Infusion 2255
Bactrim 2257
Gantanol Tablets 2285
Septra 1146
Septra I.V. Infusion 1142
Septra I.V. Infusion ADD-Vantage Vials 1144
Septra 1146

Sulfasalazine (May increase serum phenytoin levels). Products include:
Azulfidine 2059

Sulfinpyrazone (May increase serum phenytoin levels). Products include:
Anturane 823

Sulfisoxazole (May increase serum phenytoin levels). Products include:
Gantrisin Tablets 2286

Sulfisoxazole Diolamine (May increase serum phenytoin levels).
No products indexed under this heading.

Theophylline (Phenytoin impairs efficacy of theophylline). Products include:
Marax Tablets & DF Syrup 2015
Quibron 2227

Theophylline Anhydrous (Phenytoin impairs efficacy of theophylline). Products include:
Aerolate 1003
Primatene Tablets ▣ 844
Respbid Tablets 687
Slo-bid Gyrocaps 2201
Theo-24 Extended Release Capsules 2753
Theo-Dur Extended-Release Tablets 1367
Theo-X Extended-Release Tablets 793
Uni-Dur Extended-Release Tablets 1374
Uniphyl 400 mg and 600 mg Tablets 2157

Theophylline Calcium Salicylate (Phenytoin impairs efficacy of theophylline). Products include:
Quadrinal Tablets 1398

Theophylline Sodium Glycinate (Phenytoin impairs efficacy of theophylline).
No products indexed under this heading.

Thioridazine Hydrochloride (May increase serum phenytoin levels). Products include:
Mellaril 2398

Tolazamide (May increase serum phenytoin levels).
No products indexed under this heading.

Tolbutamide (May increase serum phenytoin levels).
No products indexed under this heading.

Trazodone Hydrochloride (May increase serum phenytoin levels). Products include:
Desyrel and Desyrel Dividose 504

Triamcinolone (Phenytoin impairs efficacy of corticosteroids).
No products indexed under this heading.

Triamcinolone Acetonide (Phenytoin impairs efficacy of corticosteroids). Products include:
Azmacort Oral Inhaler 2175
Nasacort AQ Nasal Spray 2191
Nasacort Nasal Inhaler 2189

Triamcinolone Diacetate (Phenytoin impairs efficacy of corticosteroids).
No products indexed under this heading.

Triamcinolone Hexacetonide (Phenytoin impairs efficacy of corticosteroids).
No products indexed under this heading.

Trifluoperazine Hydrochloride (May increase serum phenytoin levels). Products include:
Stelazine 2692

Trimipramine Maleate (Tricyclic antidepressants may precipitate seizures in susceptible patients and phenytoin dosage may need to be adjusted). Products include:
Surmontil Capsules 2917

Valproic Acid (May increase or decrease phenytoin serum levels; unpredictable effect on valproic serum levels). Products include:
Depakene 416

Vitamin D (Phenytoin impairs efficacy of vitamin D). Products include:
Caltrate PLUS ▣ 681
Caltrate 600 + D ▣ 681
Dical-D Tablets & Wafers 424
Materna Tablets 1427
Megadose 513
One-A-Day Calcium Plus ▣ 625

Warfarin Sodium (Phenytoin impairs efficacy of coumarin anticoagulants). Products include:
Coumadin 941

Food Interactions

Alcohol (Acute alcohol intake increases serum phenytoin levels; chronic alcohol intake decreases serum phenytoin levels).

DILANTIN KAPSEALS

(Phenytoin Sodium) 1965
May interact with histamine h2-receptor antagonists, oral anticoagulants, oral contraceptives, estrogens, phenothiazines, salicylates, succinimides, sulfonamides, tricyclic antidepressants, corticosteroids, xanthine bronchodilators, and certain other agents. Compounds in these categories include:

Aminophylline (Phenytoin impairs efficacy of theophylline).
No products indexed under this heading.

Amiodarone Hydrochloride (May increase serum phenytoin levels). Products include:
Cordarone Intravenous 2821
Cordarone Tablets 2818

Amitriptyline Hydrochloride (Tricyclic antidepressants may precipitate seizures in susceptible patients and phenytoin dosage may need to be adjusted). Products include:
Elavil 2945
Etrafon 2495
Limbitrol 2333
Triavil Tablets 1800

Amoxapine (Tricyclic antidepressants may precipitate seizures in susceptible patients and phenytoin dosage may need to be adjusted). Products include:
Asendin Tablets 1419

Aspirin (May increase serum phenytoin levels). Products include:
Alka-Seltzer Cherry Effervescent Antacid and Pain Reliever ▣ 609
Alka-Seltzer Extra Strength Effervescent Antacid and Pain Reliever ▣ 609
Alka-Seltzer Lemon Lime Effervescent Antacid and Pain Reliever ▣ 609
Alka-Seltzer Original Effervescent Antacid and Pain Reliever ▣ 609
Alka-Seltzer Plus ▣ 611
Alka-Seltzer Plus Sinus Medicine ▣ 611
Ascriptin ▣ 650
Arthritis Strength BC Powder ▣ 631
BC Cold Powder Multi-Symptom Formula (Cold-Sinus-Allergy) ▣ 631
BC Cold Powder Non-Drowsy Formula (Cold-Sinus) ▣ 631
BC Powder ▣ 631
Genuine Bayer Aspirin Tablets & Caplets ▣ 618
Extra Strength Bayer Arthritis Pain Regimen Formula ▣ 615
Extra Strength Bayer Aspirin Caplets & Tablets ▣ 617
Extended-Release Bayer 8-Hour Aspirin ▣ 616
Extra Strength Bayer Plus Aspirin Caplets ▣ 617
Extra Strength Bayer PM Aspirin Plus Sleep Aid ▣ 617
Aspirin Regimen Bayer 81 mg Tablets with Calcium ▣ 615
Aspirin Regimen Bayer Adult Low Strength 81 mg Tablets ▣ 613
Aspirin Regimen Bayer Children's Chewable Aspirin ▣ 616
Aspirin Regimen Bayer Regular Strength 325 mg Caplets ▣ 613
Bufferin Analgesic Tablets ▣ 636
Arthritis Strength Bufferin Analgesic Caplets ▣ 637
Extra Strength Bufferin Analgesic Tablets ▣ 637
Cama Arthritis Pain Reliever ▣ 748
Darvon Compound-65 Pulvules 1475
Easprin 1971
Ecotrin 2625
Ecotrin Enteric Coated Aspirin Maximum Strength Tablets and Caplets ▣ 775
Ecotrin Enteric Coated Aspirin Regular Strength Tablets 2625
Empirin Aspirin Tablets ▣ 818
Excedrin Extra-Strength Analgesic Tablets, Caplets, and Geltabs 734
Fiorinal Capsules 2388
Fiorinal with Codeine Capsules 2390
Fiorinal Tablets 2388
Goody's Extra Strength Headache Powders ▣ 632
Goody's Extra Strength Pain Relief Tablets ▣ 632
Halfprin Tablets 1413
Norgesic 1554
Percodan Tablets 955
Percodan-Demi Tablets 956
Robaxisal Tablets 2246
Soma Compound w/Codeine Tablets 2784
Soma Compound Tablets 2783
St. Joseph Adult Chewable Aspirin (81 mg.) ▣ 768
Talwin Compound 2466
Vanquish Analgesic Caplets ▣ 627

Bendroflumethiazide (May increase serum phenytoin levels).
No products indexed under this heading.

Betamethasone Acetate (Phenytoin impairs efficacy of corticosteroids). Products include:
Celestone Soluspan Suspension 2484

Betamethasone Sodium Phosphate (Phenytoin impairs efficacy of corticosteroids). Products include:
Celestone Soluspan Suspension 2484

Calcium Carbonate (Calcium ions interfere with the absorption of phenytoin; ingestion times of phenytoin and antacids containing calcium should be staggered in patients with low phenytoin levels). Products include:
Alka-Mints Chewable Antacid ▣ 609
Alka-Seltzer Fast Relief Caplets ▣ 610
Ascriptin ▣ 650
Extra Strength Bayer Plus Aspirin Caplets ▣ 617
Aspirin Regimen Bayer 81 mg Tablets with Calcium ▣ 615
Bufferin Analgesic Tablets ▣ 636
Arthritis Strength Bufferin Analgesic Caplets ▣ 637
Extra Strength Bufferin Analgesic Tablets ▣ 637
Calci-Chew Tablets 2168
Calci-Mix Capsules 2168

(▣ Described in PDR For Nonprescription Drugs) (⊙ Described in PDR For Ophthalmology)

Caltrate 600 ... 681
Caltrate PLUS ... 681
Caltrate 600 + D ... 681
Cotazym Capsules ... 1866
Di-Gel Antacid/Anti-Gas ... 762
Florical Capsules and Tablets ... 1825
Gerimed Tablets ... 1000
Maalox Antacid Caplets ... 657
Marblen ... 671
Materna Tablets ... 1427
Monocal Tablets ... 1825
Mylanta Fast-Acting ... 1359
Mylanta Gelcaps Antacid ... 678
Mylanta Soothing Lozenges ... 1360
Mylanta Tablets ... 677
Mylanta Double Strength Tablets ... 677
Nephro-Calci Tablets ... 2168
One-A-Day Calcium Plus ... 625
Rolaids Antacid Tablets ... 807
Rolaids Antacid Calcium Rich/Sodium Free Tablets ... 807
Tempo Soft Antacid ... 799
Titralac ... 686
Titralac Plus ... 687
Tums Antacid/Calcium Supplement Tablets ... 787
Tums Anti-gas/Antacid Formula Tablets, Assorted Fruit ... 788
Tums E-X Antacid/Calcium Supplement Tablets ... 787
Tums 500 Calcium Supplement ... 788
Tums ULTRA Antacid/Calcium Supplement Tablets ... 787
TYLENOL Headache Plus Pain Reliever with Antacid, Extra Strength Caplets ... 705

Carbamazepine (May decrease serum phenytoin levels). Products include:
Atretol Tablets ... 569
Tegretol/Tegretol-XR ... 870

Chloramphenicol (May increase serum phenytoin levels). Products include:
Chloromycetin Ophthalmic Ointment, 1% ... ⊙ 298
Chloromycetin Ophthalmic Solution ... ⊙ 299
Chloroptic S.O.P. ... ⊙ 236
Chloroptic Sterile Ophthalmic Solution ... ⊙ 236

Chloramphenicol Palmitate (May increase serum phenytoin levels).
No products indexed under this heading.

Chloramphenicol Sodium Succinate (May increase serum phenytoin levels). Products include:
Chloromycetin Sodium Succinate ... 1960

Chlordiazepoxide (May increase serum phenytoin levels). Products include:
Limbitrol ... 2333

Chlordiazepoxide Hydrochloride (May increase serum phenytoin levels). Products include:
Librax Capsules ... 2330
Librium Capsules ... 2331
Librium Injectable ... 2332

Chlorothiazide (May increase serum phenytoin levels). Products include:
Aldoclor Tablets ... 1638
Diupres Tablets ... 1691
Diuril Oral ... 1694

Chlorothiazide Sodium (May increase serum phenytoin levels). Products include:
Diuril Sodium Intravenous ... 1693

Chlorotrianisene (May increase serum phenytoin levels; phenytoin impairs efficacy of estrogens).
No products indexed under this heading.

Chlorpromazine (May increase serum phenytoin levels). Products include:
Thorazine Suppositories ... 2701

Chlorpromazine Hydrochloride (May increase serum phenytoin levels). Products include:
Thorazine ... 2701

Chlorpropamide (May increase serum phenytoin levels). Products include:
Diabinese Tablets ... 2002

Choline Magnesium Trisalicylate (May increase serum phenytoin levels). Products include:
Trilisate ... 2155

Cimetidine (May increase serum phenytoin levels). Products include:
Tagamet HB Tablets ... 786
Tagamet Tablets ... 2694

Cimetidine Hydrochloride (May increase serum phenytoin levels). Products include:
Tagamet ... 2694

Clomipramine Hydrochloride (Tricyclic antidepressants may precipitate seizures in susceptible patients and phenytoin dosage may need to be adjusted). Products include:
Anafranil Capsules ... 819

Cortisone Acetate (Phenytoin impairs efficacy of corticosteroids). Products include:
Cortone Acetate Sterile Suspension ... 1663
Cortone Acetate Tablets ... 1664

Desipramine Hydrochloride (Tricyclic antidepressants may precipitate seizures in susceptible patients and phenytoin dosage may need to be adjusted). Products include:
Norpramin Tablets ... 1273

Desogestrel (Phenytoin impairs efficacy of oral contraceptives). Products include:
Desogen Tablets ... 1867
Ortho-Cept ... 1907

Dexamethasone (Phenytoin impairs efficacy of corticosteroids). Products include:
AK-Trol Ointment & Suspension ... ⊙ 205
Decadron Elixir ... 1676
Decadron Tablets ... 1678
Decaspray Topical Aerosol ... 1689
Maxitrol Ophthalmic Ointment and Suspension ... ⊙ 222
TobraDex Ophthalmic Suspension and Ointment ... 469

Dexamethasone Acetate (Phenytoin impairs efficacy of corticosteroids). Products include:
Dalalone D.P. Injectable ... 1009
Decadron-LA Sterile Suspension ... 1687

Dexamethasone Sodium Phosphate (Phenytoin impairs efficacy of corticosteroids). Products include:
Decadron Phosphate Injection ... 1680
Decadron Phosphate Sterile Ophthalmic Ointment ... 1684
Decadron Phosphate Sterile Ophthalmic Solution ... 1685
Decadron Phosphate Topical Cream ... 1686
Decadron Phosphate with Xylocaine Injection, Sterile ... 1683
Dexacort Phosphate in Respihaler ... 1606
Dexacort Phosphate in Turbinaire ... 1607
NeoDecadron Sterile Ophthalmic Ointment ... 1755
NeoDecadron Sterile Ophthalmic Solution ... 1756
NeoDecadron Topical Cream ... 1757

Diazepam (May increase serum phenytoin levels). Products include:
Dizac (diazepam injectable emulsion) CIV ... 1862
Valium Injectable ... 2336
Valium Tablets ... 2335

Dicumarol (May increase serum phenytoin levels; phenytoin impairs efficacy of coumarin anticoagulants).
No products indexed under this heading.

Dienestrol (May increase serum phenytoin levels; phenytoin impairs efficacy of estrogens). Products include:
Ortho Dienestrol Cream ... 1922

Diethylstilbestrol (May increase serum phenytoin levels; phenytoin impairs efficacy of estrogens). Products include:
Diethylstilbestrol Tablets ... 1477

Diflunisal (May increase serum phenytoin levels). Products include:
Dolobid Tablets ... 1695

Digitoxin (Phenytoin impairs efficacy of digitoxin). Products include:
Crystodigin Tablets ... 1472

Disulfiram (May increase serum phenytoin levels). Products include:
Antabuse Tablets ... 2802

Divalproex Sodium (May increase or decrease phenytoin serum levels; unpredictable effect on valproate serum levels). Products include:
Depakote Tablets ... 418

Doxepin Hydrochloride (Tricyclic antidepressants may precipitate seizures in susceptible patients and phenytoin dosage may need to be adjusted). Products include:
Adapin Capsules ... 1542
Sinequan ... 2028
Zonalon Cream ... 1042

Doxycycline Calcium (Phenytoin impairs efficacy of doxycycline). Products include:
Vibramycin Calcium Oral Suspension Syrup ... 2038

Doxycycline Hyclate (Phenytoin impairs efficacy of doxycycline). Products include:
Doryx Capsules ... 1970
Vibramycin Hyclate Capsules ... 2038
Vibramycin Hyclate Intravenous ... 2040
Vibra-Tabs Film Coated Tablets ... 2038

Doxycycline Monohydrate (Phenytoin impairs efficacy of doxycycline). Products include:
Monodox Capsules ... 1858
Vibramycin Monohydrate for Oral Suspension ... 2038

Dyphylline (Phenytoin impairs efficacy of theophylline). Products include:
Lufyllin & Lufyllin-400 Tablets ... 2778
Lufyllin-GG Elixir & Tablets ... 2779

Estradiol (May increase serum phenytoin levels; phenytoin impairs efficacy of estrogens). Products include:
Climara Transdermal System ... 640
Estrace Cream and Tablets ... 751
Estraderm Transdermal System ... 842
Estring Vaginal Ring ... 2086
Vivelle Transdermal System ... 880

Estrogens, Conjugated (May increase serum phenytoin levels; phenytoin impairs efficacy of estrogens). Products include:
PMB 200 and PMB 400 ... 2890
Premarin Intravenous ... 2893
Premarin Tablets ... 2896
Premarin Vaginal Cream ... 2898
Premphase ... 2900
Prempro ... 2905

Estrogens, Esterified (May increase serum phenytoin levels; phenytoin impairs efficacy of estrogens). Products include:
ESTRATAB Tablets (0.3, 0.625, 1.25, 2.5 mg) ... 2715
Estratest ... 2718
Menest Tablets ... 2671

Estropipate (May increase serum phenytoin levels; phenytoin impairs efficacy of estrogens). Products include:
Ogen Tablets ... 2103
Ogen Vaginal Cream ... 2106
Ortho-Est ... 1925

Ethinyl Estradiol (May increase serum phenytoin levels; phenytoin impairs efficacy of estrogens). Products include:
Brevicon ... 2563
Demulen ... 2580
Desogen Tablets ... 1867
Levlen/Tri-Levlen ... 646
Lo/Ovral Tablets ... 2852
Lo/Ovral-28 Tablets ... 2857
Modicon ... 1928
Nordette-21 Tablets ... 2863
Nordette-28 Tablets ... 2866
Norinyl ... 2563
Ortho-Cept ... 1907
Ortho-Cyclen/Ortho-Tri-Cyclen ... 1914
Ortho-Novum ... 1928
Ortho-Cyclen/Ortho Tri-Cyclen ... 1914
Ovcon ... 765
Ovral Tablets ... 2877
Ovral-28 Tablets ... 2878
Levlen/Tri-Levlen ... 646
Tri-Norinyl ... 2607
Triphasil-21 Tablets ... 2919
Triphasil-28 Tablets ... 2924

Ethosuximide (May increase serum phenytoin levels). Products include:
Zarontin Capsules ... 1986
Zarontin Syrup ... 1986

Ethynodiol Diacetate (Phenytoin impairs efficacy of oral contraceptives). Products include:
Demulen ... 2580

Famotidine (May increase serum phenytoin levels). Products include:
Pepcid AC Acid Controller ... 1360
Pepcid Injection ... 1765
Pepcid ... 1763

Fludrocortisone Acetate (Phenytoin impairs efficacy of corticosteroids). Products include:
Florinef Acetate Tablets ... 506

Fluphenazine Decanoate (May increase serum phenytoin levels). Products include:
Prolixin Decanoate ... 510

Fluphenazine Enanthate (May increase serum phenytoin levels). Products include:
Prolixin Enanthate ... 510

Fluphenazine Hydrochloride (May increase serum phenytoin levels). Products include:
Prolixin ... 510

Furosemide (Phenytoin impairs efficacy of furosemide). Products include:
Lasix Injection, Oral Solution and Tablets ... 1267

Glipizide (May increase serum phenytoin levels). Products include:
Glucotrol Tablets ... 2011
Glucotrol XL Extended Release Tablets ... 2012

Glyburide (May increase serum phenytoin levels). Products include:
DiaBeta Tablets ... 1265
Glynase PresTab Tablets ... 2091
Micronase Tablets ... 2099

Halothane (May increase serum phenytoin levels). Products include:
Fluothane ... 2830

Hydrochlorothiazide (May increase serum phenytoin levels). Products include:
Aldactazide Tablets ... 2556
Aldoril Tablets ... 1644
Apresazide Capsules ... 824
Capozide Tablets ... 744
Dyazide Capsules ... 2653
Esidrix Tablets ... 839
Esimil Tablets ... 840
HydroDIURIL Tablets ... 1716
Hydropres Tablets ... 1718
Hyzaar Tablets ... 1720
Inderide Tablets ... 2838
Inderide LA Long Acting Capsules ... 2840
Lopressor HCT Tablets ... 850
Lotensin HCT Tablets ... 855
Moduretic Tablets ... 1748
Oretic Tablets ... 450
Prinzide Tablets ... 1780

IMPORTANT NOTE: Always consult each drug listing in the patient's regimen for possible interactions.

Dilantin Kapseals — Interactions Index — 288

Ser-Ap-Es Tablets 867
Timolide Tablets 1791
Vaseretic Tablets 1810
Zestoretic Tablets 2968
Ziac 1459

Hydrocortisone (Phenytoin impairs efficacy of corticosteroids). Products include:
Anusol-HC Cream 2.5% 1953
Aquanil HC Lotion 1989
Maximum Strength Cortaid Spray ▣ 800
CORTENEMA 2713
Cortisporin Ointment 1074
Cortisporin Ophthalmic Ointment Sterile 1074
Cortisporin Ophthalmic Suspension Sterile 1075
Cortisporin Otic Solution Sterile 1076
Cortisporin Otic Suspension Sterile 1077
Cortizone-5 .... ▣ 795
Cortizone-10 .... ▣ 795
Hydrocortone Tablets 1715
Hytone 922
Hytone Ointment 2 ½% 923
Massengill Medicated Soft Cloth Towelettes 2628
Pediotic Suspension Sterile 1140
Preparation H Hydrocortisone 1% Cream .... ▣ 843
ProctoCream-HC 2.5% 2552
VōSoL HC Otic Solution 2786

Hydrocortisone Acetate (Phenytoin impairs efficacy of corticosteroids). Products include:
Analpram-HC Rectal Cream 1% and 2.5% 993
Anusol HC-1 Hydrocortisone Anti-Itch Ointment .... ▣ 810
Anusol-HC Suppositories 1954
Caldecort Anti-Itch Hydrocortisone Cream .... ▣ 651
Coly-Mycin S Otic w/Neomycin & Hydrocortisone 1965
Cortaid .... ▣ 800
Cortifoam 2540
Cortisporin Cream 1073
Epifoam 2543
Hydrocortone Acetate Sterile Suspension 1712
Mantadil Cream 1124
Nupercainal Hydrocortisone 1% Cream .... ▣ 661
Pramosone Cream, Lotion & Ointment 995
ProctoFoam-HC 2552
Terra-Cortril Ophthalmic Suspension 2033

Hydrocortisone Sodium Phosphate (Phenytoin impairs efficacy of corticosteroids). Products include:
Hydrocortone Phosphate Injection, Sterile 1713

Hydrocortisone Sodium Succinate (Phenytoin impairs efficacy of corticosteroids).
No products indexed under this heading.

Hydroflumethiazide (May increase serum phenytoin levels). Products include:
Diucardin Tablets 2824

Imipramine Hydrochloride (Tricyclic antidepressants may precipitate seizures in susceptible patients and phenytoin dosage may need to be adjusted). Products include:
Tofranil Ampuls 873
Tofranil Tablets 875

Imipramine Pamoate (Tricyclic antidepressants may precipitate seizures in susceptible patients and phenytoin dosage may need to be adjusted). Products include:
Tofranil-PM Capsules 876

Isoniazid (May increase serum phenytoin levels). Products include:
Nydrazid Injection 509
Rifamate Capsules 1278
Rifater 1280

Levonorgestrel (Phenytoin impairs efficacy of oral contraceptives). Products include:
Levlen/Tri-Levlen 646
Nordette-21 Tablets 2863
Nordette-28 Tablets 2866
Norplant System 2868
Levlen/Tri-Levlen 646
Triphasil-21 Tablets 2919
Triphasil-28 Tablets 2924

Magnesium Salicylate (May increase serum phenytoin levels). Products include:
Backache Caplets .... ▣ 635
Doan's Extra-Strength Analgesic .... ▣ 653
Extra Strength Doan's P.M. .... ▣ 653
Doan's Regular Strength Analgesic .... ▣ 654
Mobigesic Tablets .... ▣ 607

Maprotiline Hydrochloride (Tricyclic antidepressants may precipitate seizures in susceptible patients and phenytoin dosage may need to be adjusted). Products include:
Ludiomil Tablets 861

Mesoridazine Besylate (May increase serum phenytoin levels). Products include:
Serentil 689

Mestranol (Phenytoin impairs efficacy of oral contraceptives). Products include:
Norinyl 2563
Ortho-Novum 1928

Methotrimeprazine (May increase serum phenytoin levels). Products include:
Levoprome 1321

Methsuximide (May increase serum phenytoin levels). Products include:
Celontin Kapseals 1955

Methyclothiazide (May increase serum phenytoin levels). Products include:
Enduron Tablets 424

Methylphenidate Hydrochloride (May increase serum phenytoin levels). Products include:
Ritalin 866

Methylprednisolone Acetate (Phenytoin impairs efficacy of corticosteroids).
No products indexed under this heading.

Methylprednisolone Sodium Succinate (Phenytoin impairs efficacy of corticosteroids).
No products indexed under this heading.

Molindone Hydrochloride (Moban brand of molindone contains calcium ions which interfere with the absorption of phenytoin). Products include:
Moban Tablets and Concentrate 1036

Nizatidine (May increase serum phenytoin levels). Products include:
Axid Pulvules 1468

Norethindrone (Phenytoin impairs efficacy of oral contraceptives). Products include:
Brevicon 2563
Micronor Tablets 1903
Modicon 1928
Norinyl 2563
Nor-Q D Tablets 2598
Ortho-Novum 1928
Ovcon 765
Tri-Norinyl 2607

Norethynodrel (Phenytoin impairs efficacy of oral contraceptives).
No products indexed under this heading.

Norgestimate (Phenytoin impairs efficacy of oral contraceptives). Products include:
Ortho-Cyclen/Ortho-Tri-Cyclen 1914
Ortho-Cyclen/Ortho Tri-Cyclen 1914

Norgestrel (Phenytoin impairs efficacy of oral contraceptives). Products include:
Lo/Ovral Tablets 2852
Lo/Ovral-28 Tablets 2857
Ovral Tablets 2877
Ovral-28 Tablets 2878
Ovrette Tablets 2878

Nortriptyline Hydrochloride (Tricyclic antidepressants may precipitate seizures in susceptible patients and phenytoin dosage may need to be adjusted). Products include:
Pamelor 2409

Perphenazine (May increase serum phenytoin levels). Products include:
Etrafon 2495
Triavil Tablets 1800
Trilafon 2532

Phenobarbital (May increase or decrease phenytoin serum levels; unpredictable effect on phenobarbital serum levels). Products include:
Arco-Lase Plus Tablets 513
Bellergal-S Tablets 2375
Donnatal 2234
Donnatal Extentabs 2234
Donnatal Tablets 2234
Phenobarbital Elixir and Tablets 1523
Quadrinal Tablets 1398

Phensuximide (May increase serum phenytoin levels).
No products indexed under this heading.

Phenylbutazone (May increase serum phenytoin levels).
No products indexed under this heading.

Polyestradiol Phosphate (May increase serum phenytoin levels; phenytoin impairs efficacy of estrogens).
No products indexed under this heading.

Polythiazide (May increase serum phenytoin levels). Products include:
Minizide Capsules 2016

Prednisolone Acetate (Phenytoin impairs efficacy of corticosteroids). Products include:
AK-CIDE .... ⊙ 203
AK-CIDE Ointment .... ⊙ 203
Blephamide Liquifilm Sterile Ophthalmic Suspension 472
Blephamide Ointment .... ⊙ 234
Econopred & Econopred Plus Ophthalmic Suspensions .... ⊙ 216
Poly-Pred Liquifilm .... ⊙ 246
Pred Forte .... ⊙ 247
Pred Mild .... ⊙ 250
Pred-G Liquifilm Sterile Ophthalmic Suspension .... ⊙ 248
Pred-G S.O.P. Sterile Ophthalmic Ointment .... ⊙ 249

Prednisolone Sodium Phosphate (Phenytoin impairs efficacy of corticosteroids). Products include:
AK-PRED .... ⊙ 204
Hydeltrasol Injection, Sterile 1708
Pediapred Oral Solution 1618

Prednisolone Tebutate (Phenytoin impairs efficacy of corticosteroids). Products include:
Hydeltra-T.B.A. Sterile Suspension 1710

Prednisone (Phenytoin impairs efficacy of corticosteroids).
No products indexed under this heading.

Prochlorperazine (May increase serum phenytoin levels). Products include:
Compazine 2644

Promethazine Hydrochloride (May increase serum phenytoin levels). Products include:
Mepergan Injection 2859
Phenergan with Codeine 2883
Phenergan with Dextromethorphan 2885
Phenergan Injection 2880
Phenergan Suppositories 2882
Phenergan Syrup 2881
Phenergan Tablets 2882
Phenergan VC 2886
Phenergan VC with Codeine 2888

Protriptyline Hydrochloride (Tricyclic antidepressants may precipitate seizures in susceptible patients and phenytoin dosage may need to be adjusted). Products include:
Vivactil Tablets 1820

Quinestrol (May increase serum phenytoin levels; phenytoin impairs efficacy of estrogens).
No products indexed under this heading.

Quinidine Gluconate (Phenytoin impairs efficacy of quinidine). Products include:
Quinaglute Dura-Tabs Tablets 644

Quinidine Polygalacturonate (Phenytoin impairs efficacy of quinidine). Products include:
Cardioquin Tablets 2146

Quinidine Sulfate (Phenytoin impairs efficacy of quinidine). Products include:
Quinidex Extentabs 2240

Ranitidine Hydrochloride (May increase serum phenytoin levels). Products include:
Zantac 1182
Zantac Injection 1180
Zantac Syrup 1182

Reserpine (May decrease serum phenytoin levels). Products include:
Diupres Tablets 1691
Hydropres Tablets 1718
Ser-Ap-Es Tablets 867

Rifampin (Phenytoin impairs efficacy of rifampin). Products include:
Rifadin 1276
Rifamate Capsules 1278
Rifater 1280
Rimactane Capsules 865

Salsalate (May increase serum phenytoin levels). Products include:
Disalcid 1549
Mono-Gesic Tablets 810
Salflex Tablets 791

Sucralfate (May decrease serum phenytoin levels). Products include:
Carafate Suspension 1250
Carafate Tablets 1249

Sulfacytine (May increase serum phenytoin levels).

Sulfamethizole (May increase serum phenytoin levels). Products include:
Urobiotic-250 Capsules 2038

Sulfamethoxazole (May increase serum phenytoin levels). Products include:
Bactrim DS Tablets 2257
Bactrim I.V. Infusion 2255
Bactrim 2257
Gantanol Tablets 2285
Septra 1146
Septra I.V. Infusion 1142
Septra I.V. Infusion ADD-Vantage Vials 1144
Septra 1146

Sulfasalazine (May increase serum phenytoin levels). Products include:
Azulfidine 2059

Sulfinpyrazone (May increase serum phenytoin levels). Products include:
Anturane 823

Sulfisoxazole (May increase serum phenytoin levels). Products include:
Gantrisin Tablets 2286

Sulfisoxazole Diolamine (May increase serum phenytoin levels).
No products indexed under this heading.

Theophylline (Phenytoin impairs efficacy of theophylline). Products include:
Marax Tablets & DF Syrup 2015
Quibron 2227

(▣ Described in PDR For Nonprescription Drugs) (⊙ Described in PDR For Ophthalmology)

289 **Interactions Index** **Dilantin Suspension**

Theophylline Anhydrous (Phenytoin impairs efficacy of theophylline). Products include:
Aerolate ... 1003
Primatene Tablets ... 844
Respbid Tablets ... 687
Slo-bid Gyrocaps ... 2201
Theo-24 Extended Release Capsules ... 2753
Theo-Dur Extended-Release Tablets ... 1367
Theo-X Extended-Release Tablets ... 793
Uni-Dur Extended-Release Tablets ... 1374
Uniphyl 400 mg and 600 mg Tablets ... 2157

Theophylline Calcium Salicylate (Phenytoin impairs efficacy of theophylline). Products include:
Quadrinal Tablets ... 1398

Theophylline Sodium Glycinate (Phenytoin impairs efficacy of theophylline).
No products indexed under this heading.

Thioridazine Hydrochloride (May increase serum phenytoin levels). Products include:
Mellaril ... 2398

Tolazamide (May increase serum phenytoin levels).
No products indexed under this heading.

Tolbutamide (May increase serum phenytoin levels).
No products indexed under this heading.

Trazodone Hydrochloride (May increase serum phenytoin levels). Products include:
Desyrel and Desyrel Dividose ... 504

Triamcinolone (Phenytoin impairs efficacy of corticosteroids).
No products indexed under this heading.

Triamcinolone Acetonide (Phenytoin impairs efficacy of corticosteroids). Products include:
Azmacort Oral Inhaler ... 2175
Nasacort AQ Nasal Spray ... 2191
Nasacort Nasal Inhaler ... 2189

Triamcinolone Diacetate (Phenytoin impairs efficacy of corticosteroids).
No products indexed under this heading.

Triamcinolone Hexacetonide (Phenytoin impairs efficacy of corticosteroids).
No products indexed under this heading.

Trifluoperazine Hydrochloride (May increase serum phenytoin levels). Products include:
Stelazine ... 2692

Trimipramine Maleate (Tricyclic antidepressants may precipitate seizures in susceptible patients and phenytoin dosage may need to be adjusted). Products include:
Surmontil Capsules ... 2917

Valproic Acid (May increase or decrease phenytoin serum levels; unpredictable effect on valproic serum levels). Products include:
Depakene ... 416

Vitamin D (Phenytoin impairs efficacy of vitamin D). Products include:
Caltrate PLUS ... 681
Caltrate 600 + D ... 681
Dical-D Tablets & Wafers ... 424
Materna Tablets ... 1427
Megadose ... 513
One-A-Day Calcium Plus ... 625

Warfarin Sodium (Phenytoin impairs efficacy of coumarin anticoagulants). Products include:
Coumadin ... 941

Food Interactions

Alcohol (Acute alcohol intake increases serum phenytoin levels; chronic alcohol intake decreases serum phenytoin levels).

DILANTIN-125 SUSPENSION
(Phenytoin) ... 1969
May interact with histamine h2-receptor antagonists, oral anticoagulants, oral contraceptives, estrogens, phenothiazines, salicylates, succinimides, sulfonamides, tricyclic antidepressants, corticosteroids, xanthine bronchodilators, and certain other agents. Compounds in these categories include:

Aminophylline (Phenytoin impairs efficacy of theophylline).
No products indexed under this heading.

Amiodarone Hydrochloride (May increase serum phenytoin levels). Products include:
Cordarone Intravenous ... 2821
Cordarone Tablets ... 2818

Amitriptyline Hydrochloride (Tricyclic antidepressants may precipitate seizures in susceptible patients and phenytoin dosage may need to be adjusted). Products include:
Elavil ... 2945
Etrafon ... 2495
Limbitrol ... 2333
Triavil Tablets ... 1800

Amoxapine (Tricyclic antidepressants may precipitate seizures in susceptible patients and phenytoin dosage may need to be adjusted). Products include:
Asendin Tablets ... 1419

Aspirin (May increase serum phenytoin levels). Products include:
Alka-Seltzer Cherry Effervescent Antacid and Pain Reliever ... 609
Alka-Seltzer Extra Strength Effervescent Antacid and Pain Reliever ... 609
Alka-Seltzer Lemon Lime Effervescent Antacid and Pain Reliever ... 609
Alka-Seltzer Original Effervescent Antacid and Pain Reliever ... 609
Alka-Seltzer Plus ... 611
Alka-Seltzer Plus Sinus Medicine ... 611
Ascriptin ... 650
Arthritis Strength BC Powder ... 631
BC Cold Powder Multi-Symptom Formula (Cold-Sinus-Allergy) ... 631
BC Cold Powder Non-Drowsy Formula (Cold-Sinus) ... 631
BC Powder ... 631
Genuine Bayer Aspirin Tablets & Caplets ... 618
Extra Strength Bayer Arthritis Pain Regimen Formula ... 615
Extra Strength Bayer Aspirin Caplets & Tablets ... 617
Extended-Release Bayer 8-Hour Aspirin ... 616
Extra Strength Bayer Plus Aspirin Caplets ... 617
Extra Strength Bayer PM Aspirin Plus Sleep Aid ... 617
Aspirin Regimen Bayer 81 mg Tablets with Calcium ... 615
Aspirin Regimen Bayer Adult Low Strength 81 mg Tablets ... 613
Aspirin Regimen Bayer Children's Chewable Aspirin ... 616
Aspirin Regimen Bayer Regular Strength 325 mg Caplets ... 613
Bufferin Analgesic Tablets ... 636
Arthritis Strength Bufferin Analgesic Caplets ... 637
Extra Strength Bufferin Analgesic Tablets ... 637
Cama Arthritis Pain Reliever ... 748
Darvon Compound-65 Pulvules ... 1475
Easprin ... 1971
Ecotrin ... 2625
Ecotrin Enteric Coated Aspirin Maximum Strength Tablets and Caplets ... 775
Ecotrin Enteric Coated Aspirin Regular Strength Tablets ... 2625
Empirin Aspirin Tablets ... 818
Excedrin Extra-Strength Analgesic Tablets, Caplets, and Geltabs ... 734
Fiorinal Capsules ... 2388
Fiorinal with Codeine Capsules ... 2390
Fiorinal Tablets ... 2388
Goody's Extra Strength Headache Powders ... 632
Goody's Extra Strength Pain Relief Tablets ... 632
Halfprin Tablets ... 1413
Norgesic ... 1554
Percodan Tablets ... 955
Percodan-Demi Tablets ... 956
Robaxisal Tablets ... 2246
Soma Compound w/Codeine Tablets ... 2784
Soma Compound Tablets ... 2783
St. Joseph Adult Chewable Aspirin (81 mg.) ... 768
Talwin Compound ... 2466
Vanquish Analgesic Caplets ... 627

Bendroflumethiazide (May increase serum phenytoin levels).
No products indexed under this heading.

Betamethasone Acetate (Phenytoin impairs efficacy of corticosteroids). Products include:
Celestone Soluspan Suspension ... 2484

Betamethasone Sodium Phosphate (Phenytoin impairs efficacy of corticosteroids). Products include:
Celestone Soluspan Suspension ... 2484

Calcium Carbonate (Calcium ions interfere with the absorption of phenytoin; ingestion times of phenytoin and antacids containing calcium should be staggered in patients with low phenytoin levels). Products include:
Alka-Mints Chewable Antacid ... 609
Alka-Seltzer Fast Relief Caplets ... 610
Ascriptin ... 650
Extra Strength Bayer Plus Aspirin Caplets ... 617
Aspirin Regimen Bayer 81 mg Tablets with Calcium ... 615
Bufferin Analgesic Tablets ... 636
Arthritis Strength Bufferin Analgesic Caplets ... 637
Extra Strength Bufferin Analgesic Tablets ... 637
Calci-Chew Tablets ... 2168
Calci-Mix Capsules ... 2168
Caltrate 600 ... 681
Caltrate PLUS ... 681
Caltrate 600 + D ... 681
Cotazym Capsules ... 1866
Di-Gel Antacid/Anti-Gas ... 762
Florical Capsules and Tablets ... 1825
Gerimed Tablets ... 1000
Maalox Antacid Caplets ... 657
Marblen ... 671
Materna Tablets ... 1427
Monocal Tablets ... 1825
Mylanta Fast-Acting ... 1359
Mylanta Gelcaps Antacid ... 678
Mylanta Soothing Lozenges ... 1360
Mylanta Tablets ... 677
Mylanta Double Strength Tablets ... 677
Nephro-Calci Tablets ... 2168
One-A-Day Calcium Plus ... 625
Rolaids Antacid Tablets ... 807
Rolaids Antacid Calcium Rich/Sodium Free Tablets ... 807
Tempo Soft Antacid ... 799
Titralac ... 686
Titralac Plus ... 687
Tums Antacid/Calcium Supplement Tablets ... 787
Tums Anti-gas/Antacid Formula Tablets, Assorted Fruit ... 788
Tums E-X Antacid/Calcium Supplement Tablets ... 787
Tums 500 Calcium Supplement ... 788
Tums ULTRA Antacid/Calcium Supplement Tablets ... 787
TYLENOL Headache Plus Pain Reliever with Antacid, Extra Strength Caplets ... 705

Carbamazepine (May decrease serum phenytoin levels). Products include:
Atretol Tablets ... 569
Tegretol/Tegretol-XR ... 870

Chloramphenicol (May increase serum phenytoin levels). Products include:
Chloromycetin Ophthalmic Ointment, 1% ... 298
Chloromycetin Ophthalmic Solution ... 299
Chloroptic S.O.P. ... 236
Chloroptic Sterile Ophthalmic Solution ... 236

Chloramphenicol Palmitate (May increase serum phenytoin levels).
No products indexed under this heading.

Chloramphenicol Sodium Succinate (May increase serum phenytoin levels). Products include:
Chloromycetin Sodium Succinate ... 1960

Chlordiazepoxide (May increase serum phenytoin levels). Products include:
Limbitrol ... 2333

Chlordiazepoxide Hydrochloride (May increase serum phenytoin levels). Products include:
Librax Capsules ... 2330
Librium Capsules ... 2331
Librium Injectable ... 2332

Chlorothiazide (May increase serum phenytoin levels). Products include:
Aldoclor Tablets ... 1638
Diupres Tablets ... 1691
Diuril Oral ... 1694

Chlorothiazide Sodium (May increase serum phenytoin levels). Products include:
Diuril Sodium Intravenous ... 1693

Chlorotrianisene (May increase serum phenytoin levels; phenytoin impairs efficacy of estrogens).
No products indexed under this heading.

Chlorpromazine (May increase serum phenytoin levels). Products include:
Thorazine Suppositories ... 2701

Chlorpromazine Hydrochloride (May increase serum phenytoin levels). Products include:
Thorazine ... 2701

Chlorpropamide (May increase serum phenytoin levels). Products include:
Diabinese Tablets ... 2002

Choline Magnesium Trisalicylate (May increase serum phenytoin levels). Products include:
Trilisate ... 2155

Cimetidine (May increase serum phenytoin levels). Products include:
Tagamet HB Tablets ... 786
Tagamet Tablets ... 2694

Cimetidine Hydrochloride (May increase serum phenytoin levels). Products include:
Tagamet ... 2694

Clomipramine Hydrochloride (Tricyclic antidepressants may precipitate seizures in susceptible patients and phenytoin dosage may need to be adjusted). Products include:
Anafranil Capsules ... 819

Cortisone Acetate (Phenytoin impairs efficacy of corticosteroids). Products include:
Cortone Acetate Sterile Suspension ... 1663
Cortone Acetate Tablets ... 1664

Desipramine Hydrochloride (Tricyclic antidepressants may precipitate seizures in susceptible patients and phenytoin dosage may need to be adjusted). Products include:
Norpramin Tablets ... 1273

IMPORTANT NOTE: Always consult each drug listing in the patient's regimen for possible interactions.

Desogestrel (Phenytoin impairs efficacy of oral contraceptives). Products include:
- Desogen Tablets ... 1867
- Ortho-Cept ... 1907

Dexamethasone (Phenytoin impairs efficacy of corticosteroids). Products include:
- AK-Trol Ointment & Suspension ... ◉ 205
- Decadron Elixir ... 1676
- Decadron Tablets ... 1678
- Decaspray Topical Aerosol ... 1689
- Maxitrol Ophthalmic Ointment and Suspension ... ◉ 222
- TobraDex Ophthalmic Suspension and Ointment ... 469

Dexamethasone Acetate (Phenytoin impairs efficacy of corticosteroids). Products include:
- Dalalone D.P. Injectable ... 1009
- Decadron-LA Sterile Suspension ... 1687

Dexamethasone Sodium Phosphate (Phenytoin impairs efficacy of corticosteroids). Products include:
- Decadron Phosphate Injection ... 1680
- Decadron Phosphate Sterile Ophthalmic Ointment ... 1684
- Decadron Phosphate Sterile Ophthalmic Solution ... 1685
- Decadron Phosphate Topical Cream ... 1686
- Decadron Phosphate with Xylocaine Injection, Sterile ... 1683
- Dexacort Phosphate in Respihaler ... 1606
- Dexacort Phosphate in Turbinaire ... 1607
- NeoDecadron Sterile Ophthalmic Ointment ... 1755
- NeoDecadron Sterile Ophthalmic Solution ... 1756
- NeoDecadron Topical Cream ... 1757

Diazepam (May increase serum phenytoin levels). Products include:
- Dizac (diazepam injectable emulsion) CIV ... 1862
- Valium Injectable ... 2336
- Valium Tablets ... 2335

Dicumarol (May increase serum phenytoin levels; phenytoin impairs efficacy of coumarin anticoagulants).
- No products indexed under this heading.

Dienestrol (May increase serum phenytoin levels; phenytoin impairs efficacy of estrogens). Products include:
- Ortho Dienestrol Cream ... 1922

Diethylstilbestrol (May increase serum phenytoin levels; phenytoin impairs efficacy of estrogens). Products include:
- Diethylstilbestrol Tablets ... 1477

Diflunisal (May increase serum phenytoin levels). Products include:
- Dolobid Tablets ... 1695

Digitoxin (Phenytoin impairs efficacy of digitoxin). Products include:
- Crystodigin Tablets ... 1472

Disulfiram (May increase serum phenytoin levels). Products include:
- Antabuse Tablets ... 2802

Divalproex Sodium (May increase or decrease phenytoin serum levels; unpredictable effect on valproate serum levels). Products include:
- Depakote Tablets ... 418

Doxepin Hydrochloride (Tricyclic antidepressants may precipitate seizures in susceptible patients and phenytoin dosage may need to be adjusted). Products include:
- Adapin Capsules ... 1542
- Sinequan ... 2028
- Zonalon Cream ... 1042

Doxycycline Calcium (Phenytoin impairs efficacy of doxycycline). Products include:
- Vibramycin Calcium Oral Suspension Syrup ... 2038

Doxycycline Hyclate (Phenytoin impairs efficacy of doxycycline). Products include:
- Doryx Capsules ... 1970
- Vibramycin Hyclate Capsules ... 2038
- Vibramycin Hyclate Intravenous ... 2040
- Vibra-Tabs Film Coated Tablets ... 2038

Doxycycline Monohydrate (Phenytoin impairs efficacy of doxycycline). Products include:
- Monodox Capsules ... 1858
- Vibramycin Monohydrate for Oral Suspension ... 2038

Dyphylline (Phenytoin impairs efficacy of theophylline). Products include:
- Lufyllin & Lufyllin-400 Tablets ... 2778
- Lufyllin-GG Elixir & Tablets ... 2779

Estradiol (May increase serum phenytoin levels; phenytoin impairs efficacy of estrogens). Products include:
- Climara Transdermal System ... 640
- Estrace Cream and Tablets ... 751
- Estraderm Transdermal System ... 842
- Estring Vaginal Ring ... 2086
- Vivelle Transdermal System ... 880

Estrogens, Conjugated (May increase serum phenytoin levels; phenytoin impairs efficacy of estrogens). Products include:
- PMB 200 and PMB 400 ... 2890
- Premarin Intravenous ... 2893
- Premarin Tablets ... 2896
- Premarin Vaginal Cream ... 2898
- Premphase ... 2900
- Prempro ... 2905

Estrogens, Esterified (May increase serum phenytoin levels; phenytoin impairs efficacy of estrogens). Products include:
- ESTRATAB Tablets (0.3, 0.625, 1.25, 2.5 mg) ... 2715
- Estratest ... 2718
- Menest Tablets ... 2671

Estropipate (May increase serum phenytoin levels; phenytoin impairs efficacy of estrogens). Products include:
- Ogen Tablets ... 2103
- Ogen Vaginal Cream ... 2106
- Ortho-Est ... 1925

Ethinyl Estradiol (May increase serum phenytoin levels; phenytoin impairs efficacy of estrogens). Products include:
- Brevicon ... 2563
- Demulen ... 2580
- Desogen Tablets ... 1867
- Levlen/Tri-Levlen ... 646
- Lo/Ovral Tablets ... 2852
- Lo/Ovral-28 Tablets ... 2857
- Modicon ... 1928
- Nordette-21 Tablets ... 2863
- Nordette-28 Tablets ... 2866
- Norinyl ... 2563
- Ortho-Cept ... 1907
- Ortho-Cyclen/Ortho-Tri-Cyclen ... 1914
- Ortho-Novum ... 1928
- Ortho-Cyclen/Ortho Tri-Cyclen ... 1914
- Ovcon ... 765
- Ovral Tablets ... 2877
- Ovral-28 Tablets ... 2878
- Levlen/Tri-Levlen ... 646
- Tri-Norinyl ... 2607
- Triphasil-21 Tablets ... 2919
- Triphasil-28 Tablets ... 2924

Ethosuximide (May increase serum phenytoin levels). Products include:
- Zarontin Capsules ... 1986
- Zarontin Syrup ... 1986

Ethynodiol Diacetate (Phenytoin impairs efficacy of oral contraceptives). Products include:
- Demulen ... 2580

Famotidine (May increase serum phenytoin levels). Products include:
- Pepcid AC Acid Controller ... 1360
- Pepcid Injection ... 1765
- Pepcid ... 1763

Fludrocortisone Acetate (Phenytoin impairs efficacy of corticosteroids). Products include:
- Florinef Acetate Tablets ... 506

Fluphenazine Decanoate (May increase serum phenytoin levels). Products include:
- Prolixin Decanoate ... 510

Fluphenazine Enanthate (May increase serum phenytoin levels). Products include:
- Prolixin Enanthate ... 510

Fluphenazine Hydrochloride (May increase serum phenytoin levels). Products include:
- Prolixin ... 510

Furosemide (Phenytoin impairs efficacy of furosemide). Products include:
- Lasix Injection, Oral Solution and Tablets ... 1267

Glipizide (May increase serum phenytoin levels). Products include:
- Glucotrol Tablets ... 2011
- Glucotrol XL Extended Release Tablets ... 2012

Glyburide (May increase serum phenytoin levels). Products include:
- DiaBeta Tablets ... 1265
- Glynase PresTab Tablets ... 2091
- Micronase Tablets ... 2099

Halothane (May increase serum phenytoin levels). Products include:
- Fluothane ... 2830

Hydrochlorothiazide (May increase serum phenytoin levels). Products include:
- Aldactazide Tablets ... 2556
- Aldoril Tablets ... 1644
- Apresazide Capsules ... 824
- Capozide Tablets ... 744
- Dyazide Capsules ... 2653
- Esidrix Tablets ... 839
- Esimil Tablets ... 840
- HydroDIURIL Tablets ... 1716
- Hydropres Tablets ... 1718
- Hyzaar Tablets ... 1720
- Inderide Tablets ... 2838
- Inderide LA Long Acting Capsules ... 2840
- Lopressor HCT Tablets ... 850
- Lotensin HCT Tablets ... 855
- Moduretic Tablets ... 1748
- Oretic Tablets ... 450
- Prinzide Tablets ... 1780
- Ser-Ap-Es Tablets ... 867
- Timolide Tablets ... 1791
- Vaseretic Tablets ... 1810
- Zestoretic Tablets ... 2968
- Ziac ... 1459

Hydrocortisone (Phenytoin impairs efficacy of corticosteroids). Products include:
- Anusol-HC Cream 2.5% ... 1953
- Aquanil HC Lotion ... 1989
- Maximum Strength Cortaid Spray ND 800
- CORTENEMA ... 2713
- Cortisporin Ointment ... 1074
- Cortisporin Ophthalmic Ointment Sterile ... 1074
- Cortisporin Ophthalmic Suspension Sterile ... 1075
- Cortisporin Otic Solution Sterile ... 1076
- Cortisporin Otic Suspension Sterile ... 1077
- Cortizone-5 ... ND 795
- Cortizone-10 ... ND 795
- Hydrocortone Tablets ... 1715
- Hytone ... 922
- Hytone Ointment 2 ½% ... 923
- Massengill Medicated Soft Cloth Towelettes ... 2628
- Pediotic Suspension Sterile ... 1140
- Preparation H Hydrocortisone 1% Cream ... ND 843
- ProctoCream-HC 2.5% ... 2552
- VōSoL HC Otic Solution ... 2786

Hydrocortisone Acetate (Phenytoin impairs efficacy of corticosteroids). Products include:
- Analpram-HC Rectal Cream 1% and 2.5% ... 993
- Anusol HC-1 Hydrocortisone Anti-Itch Ointment ... ND 810
- Anusol-HC Suppositories ... 1954
- Caldecort Anti-Itch Hydrocortisone Cream ... ND 651
- Coly-Mycin S Otic w/Neomycin & Hydrocortisone ... 1965
- Cortaid ... ND 800
- Cortifoam ... 2540
- Cortisporin Cream ... 1073
- Epifoam ... 2543
- Hydrocortone Acetate Sterile Suspension ... 1712
- Mantadil Cream ... 1124
- Nupercainal Hydrocortisone 1% Cream ... ND 661
- Pramosone Cream, Lotion & Ointment ... 995
- ProctoFoam-HC ... 2552
- Terra-Cortril Ophthalmic Suspension ... 2033

Hydrocortisone Sodium Phosphate (Phenytoin impairs efficacy of corticosteroids). Products include:
- Hydrocortone Phosphate Injection, Sterile ... 1713

Hydrocortisone Sodium Succinate (Phenytoin impairs efficacy of corticosteroids).
- No products indexed under this heading.

Hydroflumethiazide (May increase serum phenytoin levels). Products include:
- Diucardin Tablets ... 2824

Imipramine Hydrochloride (Tricyclic antidepressants may precipitate seizures in susceptible patients and phenytoin dosage may need to be adjusted). Products include:
- Tofranil Ampuls ... 873
- Tofranil Tablets ... 875

Imipramine Pamoate (Tricyclic antidepressants may precipitate seizures in susceptible patients and phenytoin dosage may need to be adjusted). Products include:
- Tofranil-PM Capsules ... 876

Isoniazid (May increase serum phenytoin levels). Products include:
- Nydrazid Injection ... 509
- Rifamate Capsules ... 1278
- Rifater ... 1280

Levonorgestrel (Phenytoin impairs efficacy of oral contraceptives). Products include:
- Levlen/Tri-Levlen ... 646
- Nordette-21 Tablets ... 2863
- Nordette-28 Tablets ... 2866
- Norplant System ... 2868
- Levlen/Tri-Levlen ... 646
- Triphasil-21 Tablets ... 2919
- Triphasil-28 Tablets ... 2924

Magnesium Salicylate (May increase serum phenytoin levels). Products include:
- Backache Caplets ... ND 635
- Doan's Extra-Strength Analgesic ... ND 653
- Extra Strength Doan's P.M. ... ND 653
- Doan's Regular Strength Analgesic ... ND 654
- Mobigesic Tablets ... ND 607

Maprotiline Hydrochloride (Tricyclic antidepressants may precipitate seizures in susceptible patients and phenytoin dosage may need to be adjusted). Products include:
- Ludiomil Tablets ... 861

Mesoridazine Besylate (May increase serum phenytoin levels). Products include:
- Serentil ... 689

Mestranol (Phenytoin impairs efficacy of oral contraceptives). Products include:
- Norinyl ... 2563
- Ortho-Novum ... 1928

Methotrimeprazine (May increase serum phenytoin levels). Products include:
- Levoprome ... 1321

(ND Described in PDR For Nonprescription Drugs) (◉ Described in PDR For Ophthalmology)

Methsuximide (May increase serum phenytoin levels). Products include:
Celontin Kapseals 1955

Methyclothiazide (May increase serum phenytoin levels). Products include:
Enduron Tablets 424

Methylphenidate Hydrochloride (May increase serum phenytoin levels). Products include:
Ritalin 866

Methylprednisolone Acetate (Phenytoin impairs efficacy of corticosteroids).
No products indexed under this heading.

Methylprednisolone Sodium Succinate (Phenytoin impairs efficacy of corticosteroids).
No products indexed under this heading.

Molindone Hydrochloride (Moban brand of molindone contains calcium ions which interfere with the absorption of phenytoin). Products include:
Moban Tablets and Concentrate 1036

Nizatidine (May increase serum phenytoin levels). Products include:
Axid Pulvules 1468

Norethindrone (Phenytoin impairs efficacy of oral contraceptives). Products include:
Brevicon 2563
Micronor Tablets 1903
Modicon 1928
Norinyl 2563
Nor-Q D Tablets 2598
Ortho-Novum 1928
Ovcon 765
Tri-Norinyl 2607

Norethynodrel (Phenytoin impairs efficacy of oral contraceptives).
No products indexed under this heading.

Norgestimate (Phenytoin impairs efficacy of oral contraceptives). Products include:
Ortho-Cyclen/Ortho Tri-Cyclen 1914
Ortho-Cyclen/Ortho Tri-Cyclen 1914

Norgestrel (Phenytoin impairs efficacy of oral contraceptives). Products include:
Lo/Ovral Tablets 2852
Lo/Ovral-28 Tablets 2857
Ovral Tablets 2877
Ovral-28 Tablets 2878
Ovrette Tablets 2878

Nortriptyline Hydrochloride (Tricyclic antidepressants may precipitate seizures in susceptible patients and phenytoin dosage may need to be adjusted). Products include:
Pamelor 2409

Perphenazine (May increase serum phenytoin levels). Products include:
Etrafon 2495
Triavil Tablets 1800
Trilafon 2532

Phenobarbital (May increase or decrease phenytoin serum levels; unpredictable effect on phenobarbital serum levels). Products include:
Arco-Lase Plus Tablets 513
Bellergal-S Tablets 2375
Donnatal 2234
Donnatal Extentabs 2234
Donnatal Tablets 2234
Phenobarbital Elixir and Tablets 1523
Quadrinal Tablets 1398

Phensuximide (May increase serum phenytoin levels).
No products indexed under this heading.

Phenylbutazone (May increase serum phenytoin levels).
No products indexed under this heading.

Polyestradiol Phosphate (May increase serum phenytoin levels; phenytoin impairs efficacy of estrogens).
No products indexed under this heading.

Polythiazide (May increase serum phenytoin levels). Products include:
Minizide Capsules 2016

Prednisolone Acetate (Phenytoin impairs efficacy of corticosteroids). Products include:
AK-CIDE 203
AK-CIDE Ointment 203
Blephamide Liquifilm Sterile Ophthalmic Suspension 472
Blephamide Ointment 234
Econopred & Econopred Plus Ophthalmic Suspensions 216
Poly-Pred Liquifilm 246
Pred Forte 247
Pred Mild 250
Pred-G Liquifilm Sterile Ophthalmic Suspension 248
Pred-G S.O.P. Sterile Ophthalmic Ointment 249

Prednisolone Sodium Phosphate (Phenytoin impairs efficacy of corticosteroids). Products include:
AK-PRED 204
Hydeltrasol Injection, Sterile ... 1708
Pediapred Oral Solution 1618

Prednisolone Tebutate (Phenytoin impairs efficacy of corticosteroids). Products include:
Hydeltra-T.B.A. Sterile Suspension 1710

Prednisone (Phenytoin impairs efficacy of corticosteroids).
No products indexed under this heading.

Prochlorperazine (May increase serum phenytoin levels). Products include:
Compazine 2644

Promethazine Hydrochloride (May increase serum phenytoin levels). Products include:
Mepergan Injection 2859
Phenergan with Codeine 2883
Phenergan with Dextromethorphan 2885
Phenergan Injection 2880
Phenergan Suppositories 2882
Phenergan Syrup 2881
Phenergan Tablets 2882
Phenergan VC 2886
Phenergan VC with Codeine ... 2888

Protriptyline Hydrochloride (Tricyclic antidepressants may precipitate seizures in susceptible patients and phenytoin dosage may need to be adjusted). Products include:
Vivactil Tablets 1820

Quinestrol (May increase serum phenytoin levels; phenytoin impairs efficacy of estrogens).
No products indexed under this heading.

Quinidine Gluconate (Phenytoin impairs efficacy of quinidine). Products include:
Quinaglute Dura-Tabs Tablets ... 644

Quinidine Polygalacturonate (Phenytoin impairs efficacy of quinidine). Products include:
Cardioquin Tablets 2146

Quinidine Sulfate (Phenytoin impairs efficacy of quinidine). Products include:
Quinidex Extentabs 2240

Ranitidine Hydrochloride (May increase serum phenytoin levels). Products include:
Zantac 1182
Zantac Injection 1180
Zantac Syrup 1182

Reserpine (May decrease serum phenytoin levels). Products include:
Diupres Tablets 1691
Hydropres Tablets 1718
Ser-Ap-Es Tablets 867

Rifampin (Phenytoin impairs efficacy of rifampin). Products include:
Rifadin 1276
Rifamate Capsules 1278
Rifater 1280
Rimactane Capsules 865

Salsalate (May increase serum phenytoin levels). Products include:
Disalcid 1549
Mono-Gesic Tablets 810
Salflex Tablets 791

Sucralfate (May decrease serum phenytoin levels). Products include:
Carafate Suspension 1250
Carafate Tablets 1249

Sulfacytine (May increase serum phenytoin levels).

Sulfamethizole (May increase serum phenytoin levels). Products include:
Urobiotic-250 Capsules 2038

Sulfamethoxazole (May increase serum phenytoin levels). Products include:
Bactrim DS Tablets 2257
Bactrim I.V. Infusion 2255
Bactrim 2257
Gantanol Tablets 2285
Septra 1146
Septra I.V. Infusion 1142
Septra I.V. Infusion ADD-Vantage Vials 1144
Septra 1146

Sulfasalazine (May increase serum phenytoin levels). Products include:
Azulfidine 2059

Sulfinpyrazone (May increase serum phenytoin levels). Products include:
Anturane 823

Sulfisoxazole (May increase serum phenytoin levels). Products include:
Gantrisin Tablets 2286

Sulfisoxazole Diolamine (May increase serum phenytoin levels).
No products indexed under this heading.

Theophylline (Phenytoin impairs efficacy of theophylline). Products include:
Marax Tablets & DF Syrup 2015
Quibron 2227

Theophylline Anhydrous (Phenytoin impairs efficacy of theophylline). Products include:
Aerolate 1003
Primatene Tablets 844
Respbid Tablets 687
Slo-bid Gyrocaps 2201
Theo-24 Extended Release Capsules 2753
Theo-Dur Extended-Release Tablets 1367
Theo-X Extended-Release Tablets .. 793
Uni-Dur Extended-Release Tablets .. 1374
Uniphyl 400 mg and 600 mg Tablets 2157

Theophylline Calcium Salicylate (Phenytoin impairs efficacy of theophylline). Products include:
Quadrinal Tablets 1398

Theophylline Sodium Glycinate (Phenytoin impairs efficacy of theophylline).
No products indexed under this heading.

Thioridazine Hydrochloride (May increase serum phenytoin levels). Products include:
Mellaril 2398

Tolazamide (May increase serum phenytoin levels).
No products indexed under this heading.

Tolbutamide (May increase serum phenytoin levels).
No products indexed under this heading.

Trazodone Hydrochloride (May increase serum phenytoin levels). Products include:
Desyrel and Desyrel Dividose ... 504

Triamcinolone (Phenytoin impairs efficacy of corticosteroids).
No products indexed under this heading.

Triamcinolone Acetonide (Phenytoin impairs efficacy of corticosteroids). Products include:
Azmacort Oral Inhaler 2175
Nasacort AQ Nasal Spray 2191
Nasacort Nasal Inhaler 2189

Triamcinolone Diacetate (Phenytoin impairs efficacy of corticosteroids).
No products indexed under this heading.

Triamcinolone Hexacetonide (Phenytoin impairs efficacy of corticosteroids).
No products indexed under this heading.

Trifluoperazine Hydrochloride (May increase serum phenytoin levels). Products include:
Stelazine 2692

Trimipramine Maleate (Tricyclic antidepressants may precipitate seizures in susceptible patients and phenytoin dosage may need to be adjusted). Products include:
Surmontil Capsules 2917

Valproic Acid (May increase or decrease phenytoin serum levels; unpredictable effect on valproic serum levels). Products include:
Depakene 416

Vitamin D (Phenytoin impairs efficacy of vitamin D). Products include:
Caltrate PLUS 681
Caltrate 600 + D 681
Dical-D Tablets & Wafers 424
Materna Tablets 1427
Megadose 513
One-A-Day Calcium Plus 625

Warfarin Sodium (Phenytoin impairs efficacy of coumarin anticoagulants). Products include:
Coumadin 941

Food Interactions

Alcohol (Acute alcohol intake increases serum phenytoin levels; chronic alcohol intake decreases serum phenytoin levels).

DILATRATE-SR CAPSULES
(Isosorbide Dinitrate) 2542
May interact with vasodilators and certain other agents. Compounds in these categories include:

Diazoxide (Vasodilating effects of isosorbide dinitrate may be additive with those of other vasodilators). Products include:
Hyperstat I.V. Injection 2504
Proglycem 575

Epoprostenol Sodium (Vasodilating effects of isosorbide dinitrate may be additive with those of other vasodilators). Products include:
Flolan for Injection 1085

Hydralazine Hydrochloride (Vasodilating effects of isosorbide dinitrate may be additive with those of other vasodilators). Products include:
Apresazide Capsules 824
Apresoline Hydrochloride Tablets .. 826
Hydralazine Hydrochloride Injection USP 2712
Ser-Ap-Es Tablets 867

IMPORTANT NOTE: Always consult each drug listing in the patient's regimen for possible interactions.

Dilatrate-SR

Minoxidil (Vasodilating effects of isosorbide dinitrate may be additive with those of other vasodilators).
No products indexed under this heading.

Food Interactions
Alcohol (Alcohol has been found to exhibit additive vasodilating effects).

DILAUDID AMPULES
(Hydromorphone Hydrochloride) 1382
May interact with central nervous system depressants, tricyclic antidepressants, and certain other agents. Compounds in these categories include:

Alfentanil Hydrochloride (Additive CNS depression). Products include:
Alfenta Injection 1334

Alprazolam (Additive CNS depression). Products include:
Xanax Tablets 2115

Amitriptyline Hydrochloride (Additive CNS depression). Products include:
Elavil 2945
Etrafon 2495
Limbitrol 2333
Triavil Tablets 1800

Amoxapine (Additive CNS depression). Products include:
Asendin Tablets 1419

Aprobarbital (Additive CNS depression).
No products indexed under this heading.

Buprenorphine (Additive CNS depression). Products include:
Buprenex Injectable 2170

Buspirone Hydrochloride (Additive CNS depression). Products include:
BuSpar Tablets 738

Butabarbital (Additive CNS depression).
No products indexed under this heading.

Butalbital (Additive CNS depression). Products include:
Axocet Capsules 2469
Esgic-plus Capsules 1012
Esgic-plus Tablets 1012
Fioricet Tablets 2386
Fioricet with Codeine Capsules ... 2387
Fiorinal Capsules 2388
Fiorinal with Codeine Capsules .. 2390
Fiorinal Tablets 2388
Phrenilin 790
Sedapap Tablets 50 mg/650 mg .. 1826

Chlordiazepoxide (Additive CNS depression). Products include:
Limbitrol 2333

Chlordiazepoxide Hydrochloride (Additive CNS depression). Products include:
Librax Capsules 2330
Librium Capsules 2331
Librium Injectable 2332

Chlorpromazine (Additive CNS depression). Products include:
Thorazine Suppositories 2701

Chlorprothixene (Additive CNS depression).
No products indexed under this heading.

Chlorprothixene Hydrochloride (Additive CNS depression).
No products indexed under this heading.

Chlorprothixene Lactate (Additive CNS depression).
No products indexed under this heading.

Clomipramine Hydrochloride (Additive CNS depression). Products include:
Anafranil Capsules 819

Interactions Index

Clorazepate Dipotassium (Additive CNS depression). Products include:
Tranxene 459

Clozapine (Additive CNS depression). Products include:
Clozaril Tablets 2377

Codeine Phosphate (Additive CNS depression). Products include:
Brontex 2130
Dimetane-DC Cough Syrup 2232
Fioricet with Codeine Capsules ... 2387
Fiorinal with Codeine Capsules .. 2390
Nucofed 2225
Phenergan with Codeine 2883
Phenergan VC with Codeine .. 2888
Robitussin A-C Syrup 2248
Robitussin-DAC Syrup 2249
Ryna 804
Soma Compound w/Codeine Tablets 2784
Tylenol with Codeine 1592

Desflurane (Additive CNS depression). Products include:
Suprane (desflurane, USP) 1865

Desipramine Hydrochloride (Additive CNS depression). Products include:
Norpramin Tablets 1273

Dezocine (Additive CNS depression). Products include:
Dalgan Injection 529

Diazepam (Additive CNS depression). Products include:
Dizac (diazepam injectable emulsion) CIV 1862
Valium Injectable 2336
Valium Tablets 2335

Doxepin Hydrochloride (Additive CNS depression). Products include:
Adapin Capsules 1542
Sinequan 2028
Zonalon Cream 1042

Droperidol (Additive CNS depression). Products include:
Inapsine Injection 462

Enflurane (Additive CNS depression).
No products indexed under this heading.

Estazolam (Additive CNS depression). Products include:
ProSom Tablets 457

Ethchlorvynol (Additive CNS depression). Products include:
Placidyl Capsules 456

Ethinamate (Additive CNS depression).
No products indexed under this heading.

Fentanyl (Additive CNS depression). Products include:
Duragesic Transdermal System 1336

Fentanyl Citrate (Additive CNS depression). Products include:
Sublimaze Injection 463

Fluphenazine Decanoate (Additive CNS depression). Products include:
Prolixin Decanoate 510

Fluphenazine Enanthate (Additive CNS depression). Products include:
Prolixin Enanthate 510

Fluphenazine Hydrochloride (Additive CNS depression). Products include:
Prolixin 510

Flurazepam Hydrochloride (Additive CNS depression). Products include:
Dalmane Capsules 2329

Glutethimide (Additive CNS depression).
No products indexed under this heading.

Haloperidol (Additive CNS depression). Products include:
Haldol Injection, Tablets and Concentrate 1585

Haloperidol Decanoate (Additive CNS depression). Products include:
Haldol Decanoate 1587

Hydrocodone Bitartrate (Additive CNS depression). Products include:
Codiclear DH Syrup 808
Duratuss HD Elixir 2750
Histussin D Liquid 670
Hycodan Tablets and Syrup .. 946
Hycomine Compound Tablets .. 948
Hycomine 947
Hycotuss Expectorant Syrup .. 950
Hydrocet Capsules 787
Lorcet 10/650 Tablets 1016
Lortab 2751
Tussend 1830
Tussend Expectorant 1831
Vicodin Tablets 1404
Vicodin ES Tablets 1405
Vicodin HP Tablets 1403
Vicodin Tuss Expectorant 1406
Zydone Tablets 967

Hydrocodone Polistirex (Additive CNS depression). Products include:
Tussionex Pennkinetic Extended-Release Suspension 1624

Hydroxyzine Hydrochloride (Additive CNS depression). Products include:
Atarax Tablets & Syrup 1992
Marax Tablets & DF Syrup 2015
Vistaril Intramuscular Solution .. 2042

Imipramine Hydrochloride (Additive CNS depression). Products include:
Tofranil Ampuls 873
Tofranil Tablets 875

Imipramine Pamoate (Additive CNS depression). Products include:
Tofranil-PM Capsules 876

Isoflurane (Additive CNS depression).
No products indexed under this heading.

Ketamine Hydrochloride (Additive CNS depression).
No products indexed under this heading.

Levomethadyl Acetate Hydrochloride (Additive CNS depression). Products include:
Orlaam Oral Solution 2361

Levorphanol Tartrate (Additive CNS depression). Products include:
Levo-Dromoran 2297

Lorazepam (Additive CNS depression). Products include:
Ativan Injection 2805
Ativan Tablets 2807

Loxapine Hydrochloride (Additive CNS depression). Products include:
Loxitane 1426

Loxapine Succinate (Additive CNS depression). Products include:
Loxitane Capsules 1426

Maprotiline Hydrochloride (Additive CNS depression). Products include:
Ludiomil Tablets 861

Meperidine Hydrochloride (Additive CNS depression). Products include:
Demerol 2438
Mepergan Injection 2859

Mephobarbital (Additive CNS depression). Products include:
Mebaral Tablets 2452

Meprobamate (Additive CNS depression). Products include:
Miltown Tablets 2780
PMB 200 and PMB 400 2890

Mesoridazine Besylate (Additive CNS depression). Products include:
Serentil 689

Methadone Hydrochloride (Additive CNS depression). Products include:
Methadone Hydrochloride Oral Concentrate 2356
Methadone Hydrochloride Oral Solution & Tablets 2357

Methohexital Sodium (Additive CNS depression).
No products indexed under this heading.

Methotrimeprazine (Additive CNS depression). Products include:
Levoprome 1321

Methoxyflurane (Additive CNS depression).
No products indexed under this heading.

Midazolam Hydrochloride (Additive CNS depression). Products include:
Versed Injection 2324

Molindone Hydrochloride (Additive CNS depression). Products include:
Moban Tablets and Concentrate 1036

Morphine Sulfate (Additive CNS depression). Products include:
Astramorph/PF Injection, USP (Preservative-Free) 526
Duramorph Injection 983
Infumorph 200 and Infumorph 500 Sterile Solutions 985
Kadian Capsules 2948
MS Contin Tablets 2149
MSIR 2152
Oramorph SR (Morphine Sulfate Sustained Release Tablets) .. 2359
RMS Suppositories CII 2766
Roxanol 2365

Nortriptyline Hydrochloride (Additive CNS depression). Products include:
Pamelor 2409

Opium Alkaloids (Additive CNS depression).
No products indexed under this heading.

Oxazepam (Additive CNS depression). Products include:
Serax Capsules 2916
Serax Tablets 2916

Oxycodone Hydrochloride (Additive CNS depression). Products include:
OxyContin Tablets 2163
OxyIR Capsules 2167
Percocet Tablets 955
Percodan Tablets 955
Percodan-Demi Tablets 956
Roxicodone Tablets, Oral Solution & Intensol (Oxycodone) .. 2366
Tylox Capsules 1593

Pentobarbital Sodium (Additive CNS depression). Products include:
Nembutal Sodium Capsules .. 440
Nembutal Sodium Solution 442
Nembutal Sodium Suppositories .. 444

Perphenazine (Additive CNS depression). Products include:
Etrafon 2495
Triavil Tablets 1800
Trilafon 2532

Phenobarbital (Additive CNS depression). Products include:
Arco-Lase Plus Tablets 513
Bellergal-S Tablets 2375
Donnatal 2234
Donnatal Extentabs 2234
Donnatal Tablets 2234
Phenobarbital Elixir and Tablets .. 1523
Quadrinal Tablets 1398

Prazepam (Additive CNS depression).
No products indexed under this heading.

(◨ Described in PDR For Nonprescription Drugs)   (◉ Described in PDR For Ophthalmology)

293 Interactions Index Dilaudid Cough Syrup

Prochlorperazine (Additive CNS depression). Products include:
Compazine ... 2644
Promethazine Hydrochloride (Additive CNS depression). Products include:
Mepergan Injection ... 2859
Phenergan with Codeine ... 2883
Phenergan with Dextromethorphan 2885
Phenergan Injection ... 2880
Phenergan Suppositories ... 2882
Phenergan Syrup ... 2881
Phenergan Tablets ... 2882
Phenergan VC ... 2886
Phenergan VC with Codeine ... 2888
Propofol (Additive CNS depression). Products include:
Diprivan Injectable Emulsion ... 2939
Propoxyphene Hydrochloride (Additive CNS depression). Products include:
Darvon ... 1475
Wygesic Tablets ... 2930
Propoxyphene Napsylate (Additive CNS depression). Products include:
Darvon-N/Darvocet-N ... 1473
Protriptyline Hydrochloride (Additive CNS depression). Products include:
Vivactil Tablets ... 1820
Quazepam (Additive CNS depression). Products include:
Doral Tablets ... 2773
Risperidone (Additive CNS depression). Products include:
Risperdal Tablets ... 1348
Secobarbital Sodium (Additive CNS depression). Products include:
Seconal Sodium Pulvules ... 1529
Sevoflurane (Additive CNS depression).
No products indexed under this heading.
Sufentanil Citrate (Additive CNS depression). Products include:
Sufenta Injection ... 1355
Temazepam (Additive CNS depression). Products include:
Restoril Capsules ... 2413
Thiamylal Sodium (Additive CNS depression).
No products indexed under this heading.
Thioridazine Hydrochloride (Additive CNS depression). Products include:
Mellaril ... 2398
Thiothixene (Additive CNS depression). Products include:
Navane Capsules and Concentrate 2018
Navane Intramuscular 2019
Triazolam (Additive CNS depression). Products include:
Halcion Tablets ... 2093
Trifluoperazine Hydrochloride (Additive CNS depression). Products include:
Stelazine ... 2692
Trimipramine Maleate (Additive CNS depression). Products include:
Surmontil Capsules ... 2917
Zolpidem Tartrate (Additive CNS depression). Products include:
Ambien Tablets ... 2559

Food Interactions

Alcohol (Additive CNS depression).

DILAUDID COUGH SYRUP
(Hydromorphone Hydrochloride) 1383
May interact with central nervous system depressants, tricyclic antidepressants, and certain other agents. Compounds in these categories include:

Alfentanil Hydrochloride (Additive CNS depression). Products include:
Alfenta Injection ... 1334
Alprazolam (Additive CNS depression). Products include:
Xanax Tablets ... 2115
Amitriptyline Hydrochloride (Additive CNS depression). Products include:
Elavil ... 2945
Etrafon ... 2495
Limbitrol ... 2333
Triavil Tablets ... 1800
Amoxapine (Additive CNS depression). Products include:
Asendin Tablets ... 1419
Aprobarbital (Additive CNS depression).
No products indexed under this heading.
Buprenorphine (Additive CNS depression). Products include:
Buprenex Injectable ... 2170
Buspirone Hydrochloride (Additive CNS depression). Products include:
BuSpar Tablets ... 738
Butabarbital (Additive CNS depression).
No products indexed under this heading.
Butalbital (Additive CNS depression). Products include:
Axocet Capsules ... 2469
Esgic-plus Capsules ... 1012
Esgic-plus Tablets ... 1012
Fioricet Tablets ... 2386
Fioricet with Codeine Capsules ... 2387
Fiorinal Capsules ... 2388
Fiorinal with Codeine Capsules ... 2390
Fiorinal Tablets ... 2388
Phrenilin ... 790
Sedapap Tablets 50 mg/650 mg .. 1826
Chlordiazepoxide (Additive CNS depression). Products include:
Limbitrol ... 2333
Chlordiazepoxide Hydrochloride (Additive CNS depression). Products include:
Librax Capsules ... 2330
Librium Capsules ... 2331
Librium Injectable ... 2332
Chlorpromazine (Additive CNS depression). Products include:
Thorazine Suppositories ... 2701
Chlorprothixene (Additive CNS depression).
No products indexed under this heading.
Chlorprothixene Hydrochloride (Additive CNS depression).
No products indexed under this heading.
Chlorprothixene Lactate (Additive CNS depression).
No products indexed under this heading.
Clomipramine Hydrochloride (Additive CNS depression). Products include:
Anafranil Capsules ... 819
Clorazepate Dipotassium (Additive CNS depression). Products include:
Tranxene ... 459
Clozapine (Additive CNS depression). Products include:
Clozaril Tablets ... 2377
Codeine Phosphate (Additive CNS depression). Products include:
Brontex ... 2130
Dimetane-DC Cough Syrup ... 2232
Fioricet with Codeine Capsules ... 2387
Fiorinal with Codeine Capsules ... 2390
Nucofed ... 2225
Phenergan with Codeine ... 2883
Phenergan VC with Codeine ... 2888
Robitussin A-C Syrup ... 2248
Robitussin-DAC Syrup ... 2249
Ryna ... 804
Soma Compound w/Codeine Tablets ... 2784
Tylenol with Codeine ... 1592
Desflurane (Additive CNS depression). Products include:
Suprane (desflurane, USP) ... 1865
Desipramine Hydrochloride (Additive CNS depression). Products include:
Norpramin Tablets ... 1273
Dezocine (Additive CNS depression). Products include:
Dalgan Injection ... 529
Diazepam (Additive CNS depression). Products include:
Dizac (diazepam injectable emulsion) CIV ... 1862
Valium Injectable ... 2336
Valium Tablets ... 2335
Doxepin Hydrochloride (Additive CNS depression). Products include:
Adapin Capsules ... 1542
Sinequan ... 2028
Zonalon Cream ... 1042
Droperidol (Additive CNS depression). Products include:
Inapsine Injection ... 462
Enflurane (Additive CNS depression).
No products indexed under this heading.
Estazolam (Additive CNS depression). Products include:
ProSom Tablets ... 457
Ethchlorvynol (Additive CNS depression). Products include:
Placidyl Capsules ... 456
Ethinamate (Additive CNS depression).
No products indexed under this heading.
Fentanyl (Additive CNS depression). Products include:
Duragesic Transdermal System ... 1336
Fentanyl Citrate (Additive CNS depression). Products include:
Sublimaze Injection ... 463
Fluphenazine Decanoate (Additive CNS depression). Products include:
Prolixin Decanoate ... 510
Fluphenazine Enanthate (Additive CNS depression). Products include:
Prolixin Enanthate ... 510
Fluphenazine Hydrochloride (Additive CNS depression). Products include:
Prolixin ... 510
Flurazepam Hydrochloride (Additive CNS depression). Products include:
Dalmane Capsules ... 2329
Glutethimide (Additive CNS depression).
No products indexed under this heading.
Haloperidol (Additive CNS depression). Products include:
Haldol Injection, Tablets and Concentrate ... 1585
Haloperidol Decanoate (Additive CNS depression). Products include:
Haldol Decanoate ... 1587
Hydrocodone Bitartrate (Additive CNS depression). Products include:
Codiclear DH Syrup ... 808
Duratuss HD Elixir ... 2750
Histussin D Liquid ... 670
Hycodan Tablets and Syrup ... 946
Hycomine Compound Tablets ... 948
Hycomine ... 947
Hycotuss Expectorant Syrup ... 950
Hydrocet Capsules ... 787
Lorcet 10/650 Tablets ... 1016
Lortab ... 2751
Tussend ... 1830
Tussend Expectorant ... 1831
Vicodin Tablets ... 1404
Vicodin ES Tablets ... 1405
Vicodin HP Tablets ... 1403
Vicodin Tuss Expectorant ... 1406
Zydone Capsules ... 967
Hydrocodone Polistirex (Additive CNS depression). Products include:
Tussionex Pennkinetic Extended-Release Suspension ... 1624
Hydroxyzine Hydrochloride (Additive CNS depression). Products include:
Atarax Tablets & Syrup ... 1992
Marax Tablets & DF Syrup ... 2015
Vistaril Intramuscular Solution ... 2042
Imipramine Hydrochloride (Additive CNS depression). Products include:
Tofranil Ampuls ... 873
Tofranil Tablets ... 875
Imipramine Pamoate (Additive CNS depression). Products include:
Tofranil-PM Capsules ... 876
Isoflurane (Additive CNS depression).
No products indexed under this heading.
Ketamine Hydrochloride (Additive CNS depression).
No products indexed under this heading.
Levomethadyl Acetate Hydrochloride (Additive CNS depression). Products include:
Orlaam Oral Solution ... 2361
Levorphanol Tartrate (Additive CNS depression). Products include:
Levo-Dromoran ... 2297
Lorazepam (Additive CNS depression). Products include:
Ativan Injection ... 2805
Ativan Tablets ... 2807
Loxapine Hydrochloride (Additive CNS depression). Products include:
Loxitane ... 1426
Loxapine Succinate (Additive CNS depression). Products include:
Loxitane Capsules ... 1426
Maprotiline Hydrochloride (Additive CNS depression). Products include:
Ludiomil Tablets ... 861
Meperidine Hydrochloride (Additive CNS depression). Products include:
Demerol ... 2438
Mepergan Injection ... 2859
Mephobarbital (Additive CNS depression). Products include:
Mebaral Tablets ... 2452
Meprobamate (Additive CNS depression). Products include:
Miltown Tablets ... 2780
PMB 200 and PMB 400 ... 2890
Mesoridazine Besylate (Additive CNS depression). Products include:
Serentil ... 689
Methadone Hydrochloride (Additive CNS depression). Products include:
Methadone Hydrochloride Oral Concentrate ... 2356
Methadone Hydrochloride Oral Solution & Tablets ... 2357
Methohexital Sodium (Additive CNS depression).
No products indexed under this heading.
Methotrimeprazine (Additive CNS depression). Products include:
Levoprome ... 1321

IMPORTANT NOTE: Always consult each drug listing in the patient's regimen for possible interactions.

Dilaudid Cough Syrup / Interactions Index

Methoxyflurane (Additive CNS depression).
No products indexed under this heading.

Midazolam Hydrochloride (Additive CNS depression). Products include:
Versed Injection 2324

Molindone Hydrochloride (Additive CNS depression). Products include:
Moban Tablets and Concentrate 1036

Morphine Sulfate (Additive CNS depression). Products include:
Astramorph/PF Injection, USP (Preservative-Free) 526
Duramorph Injection 983
Infumorph 200 and Infumorph 500 Sterile Solutions 985
Kadian Capsules 2948
MS Contin Tablets 2149
MSIR 2152
Oramorph SR (Morphine Sulfate Sustained Release Tablets) 2359
RMS Suppositories CII 2766
Roxanol 2365

Nortriptyline Hydrochloride (Additive CNS depression). Products include:
Pamelor 2409

Opium Alkaloids (Additive CNS depression).
No products indexed under this heading.

Oxazepam (Additive CNS depression). Products include:
Serax Capsules 2916
Serax Tablets 2916

Oxycodone Hydrochloride (Additive CNS depression). Products include:
OxyContin Tablets 2163
OxyIR Capsules 2167
Percocet Tablets 955
Percodan Tablets 955
Percodan-Demi Tablets 956
Roxicodone Tablets, Oral Solution & Intensol (Oxycodone) 2366
Tylox Capsules 1593

Pentobarbital Sodium (Additive CNS depression). Products include:
Nembutal Sodium Capsules 440
Nembutal Sodium Solution 442
Nembutal Sodium Suppositories 444

Perphenazine (Additive CNS depression). Products include:
Etrafon 2495
Triavil Tablets 1800
Trilafon 2532

Phenobarbital (Additive CNS depression). Products include:
Arco-Lase Plus Tablets 513
Bellergal-S Tablets 2375
Donnatal 2234
Donnatal Extentabs 2234
Donnatal Tablets 2234
Phenobarbital Elixir and Tablets 1523
Quadrinal Tablets 1398

Prazepam (Additive CNS depression).
No products indexed under this heading.

Prochlorperazine (Additive CNS depression). Products include:
Compazine 2644

Promethazine Hydrochloride (Additive CNS depression). Products include:
Mepergan Injection 2859
Phenergan with Codeine 2883
Phenergan with Dextromethorphan 2885
Phenergan Injection 2880
Phenergan Suppositories 2882
Phenergan Syrup 2881
Phenergan Tablets 2882
Phenergan VC 2886
Phenergan VC with Codeine 2888

Propofol (Additive CNS depression). Products include:
Diprivan Injectable Emulsion 2939

Propoxyphene Hydrochloride (Additive CNS depression). Products include:
Darvon 1475
Wygesic Tablets 2930

Propoxyphene Napsylate (Additive CNS depression). Products include:
Darvon-N/Darvocet-N 1473

Protriptyline Hydrochloride (Additive CNS depression). Products include:
Vivactil Tablets 1820

Quazepam (Additive CNS depression). Products include:
Doral Tablets 2773

Risperidone (Additive CNS depression). Products include:
Risperdal Tablets 1348

Secobarbital Sodium (Additive CNS depression). Products include:
Seconal Sodium Pulvules 1529

Sevoflurane (Additive CNS depression).
No products indexed under this heading.

Sufentanil Citrate (Additive CNS depression). Products include:
Sufenta Injection 1355

Temazepam (Additive CNS depression). Products include:
Restoril Capsules 2413

Thiamylal Sodium (Additive CNS depression).
No products indexed under this heading.

Thioridazine Hydrochloride (Additive CNS depression). Products include:
Mellaril 2398

Thiothixene (Additive CNS depression). Products include:
Navane Capsules and Concentrate 2018
Navane Intramuscular 2019

Triazolam (Additive CNS depression). Products include:
Halcion Tablets 2093

Trifluoperazine Hydrochloride (Additive CNS depression). Products include:
Stelazine 2692

Trimipramine Maleate (Additive CNS depression). Products include:
Surmontil Capsules 2917

Zolpidem Tartrate (Additive CNS depression). Products include:
Ambien Tablets 2559

Food Interactions

Alcohol (Additive CNS depression).

DILAUDID-HP INJECTION
(Hydromorphone Hydrochloride) 1384
May interact with central nervous system depressants, nondepolarizing neuromuscular blocking agents, general anesthetics, tranquilizers, phenothiazines, hypnotics and sedatives, and certain other agents. Compounds in these categories include:

Alfentanil Hydrochloride (Additive depressant effects). Products include:
Alfenta Injection 1334

Alprazolam (Additive depressant effects). Products include:
Xanax Tablets 2115

Aprobarbital (Additive depressant effects).
No products indexed under this heading.

Atracurium Besylate (Increased respiratory depression; enhanced action of neuromuscular blocking agents). Products include:
Tracrium Injection 1155

Buprenorphine (Additive depressant effects). Products include:
Buprenex Injectable 2170

Buspirone Hydrochloride (Additive depressant effects). Products include:
BuSpar Tablets 738

Butabarbital (Additive depressant effects).
No products indexed under this heading.

Butalbital (Additive depressant effects). Products include:
Axocet Capsules 2469
Esgic-plus Capsules 1012
Esgic-plus Tablets 1012
Fioricet Tablets 2386
Fioricet with Codeine Capsules 2387
Fiorinal Capsules 2388
Fiorinal with Codeine Capsules 2390
Fiorinal Tablets 2388
Phrenilin 790
Sedapap Tablets 50 mg/650 mg .. 1826

Chlordiazepoxide (Additive depressant effects). Products include:
Limbitrol 2333

Chlordiazepoxide Hydrochloride (Additive depressant effects). Products include:
Librax Capsules 2330
Librium Capsules 2331
Librium Injectable 2332

Chlorpromazine (Additive depressant effects). Products include:
Thorazine Suppositories 2701

Chlorpromazine Hydrochloride (Additive depressant effects). Products include:
Thorazine 2701

Chlorprothixene (Additive depressant effects).
No products indexed under this heading.

Chlorprothixene Hydrochloride (Additive depressant effects).
No products indexed under this heading.

Chlorprothixene Lactate (Additive depressant effects).
No products indexed under this heading.

Cisatracurium Besylate (Increased respiratory depression; enhanced action of neuromuscular blocking agents). Products include:
Nimbex Injection 1131

Clorazepate Dipotassium (Additive depressant effects). Products include:
Tranxene 459

Clozapine (Additive depressant effects). Products include:
Clozaril Tablets 2377

Codeine Phosphate (Additive depressant effects). Products include:
Brontex 2130
Dimetane-DC Cough Syrup 2232
Fioricet with Codeine Capsules 2387
Fiorinal with Codeine Capsules 2390
Nucofed 2225
Phenergan with Codeine 2883
Phenergan VC with Codeine 2888
Robitussin A-C Syrup 2248
Robitussin-DAC Syrup 2249
Ryna 804
Soma Compound w/Codeine Tablets 2784
Tylenol with Codeine 1592

Desflurane (Additive depressant effects). Products include:
Suprane (desflurane, USP) 1865

Dezocine (Additive depressant effects). Products include:
Dalgan Injection 529

Diazepam (Additive depressant effects). Products include:
Dizac (diazepam injectable emulsion) CIV 1862

Valium Injectable 2336
Valium Tablets 2335

Droperidol (Additive depressant effects). Products include:
Inapsine Injection 462

Enflurane (Additive depressant effects).
No products indexed under this heading.

Estazolam (Additive depressant effects). Products include:
ProSom Tablets 457

Ethchlorvynol (Additive depressant effects). Products include:
Placidyl Capsules 456

Ethinamate (Additive depressant effects).
No products indexed under this heading.

Fentanyl (Additive depressant effects). Products include:
Duragesic Transdermal System 1336

Fentanyl Citrate (Additive depressant effects). Products include:
Sublimaze Injection 463

Fluphenazine Decanoate (Additive depressant effects). Products include:
Prolixin Decanoate 510

Fluphenazine Enanthate (Additive depressant effects). Products include:
Prolixin Enanthate 510

Fluphenazine Hydrochloride (Additive depressant effects). Products include:
Prolixin 510

Flurazepam Hydrochloride (Additive depressant effects). Products include:
Dalmane Capsules 2329

Glutethimide (Additive depressant effects).
No products indexed under this heading.

Haloperidol (Additive depressant effects). Products include:
Haldol Injection, Tablets and Concentrate 1585

Haloperidol Decanoate (Additive depressant effects). Products include:
Haldol Decanoate 1587

Hydrocodone Bitartrate (Additive depressant effects). Products include:
Codiclear DH Syrup 808
Duratuss HD Elixir 2750
Histussin D Liquid 670
Hycodan Tablets and Syrup 946
Hycomine Compound Tablets 948
Hycomine 947
Hycotuss Expectorant Syrup 950
Hydrocet Capsules 787
Lorcet 10/650 Tablets 1016
Lortab 2751
Tussend 1830
Tussend Expectorant 1831
Vicodin Tablets 1404
Vicodin ES Tablets 1405
Vicodin HP Tablets 1403
Vicodin Tuss Expectorant 1406
Zydone Capsules 967

Hydrocodone Polistirex (Additive depressant effects). Products include:
Tussionex Pennkinetic Extended-Release Suspension 1624

Hydroxyzine Hydrochloride (Additive depressant effects). Products include:
Atarax Tablets & Syrup 1992
Marax Tablets & DF Syrup 2015
Vistaril Intramuscular Solution 2042

Isoflurane (Additive depressant effects).
No products indexed under this heading.

(▣ Described in PDR For Nonprescription Drugs)   (⊚ Described in PDR For Ophthalmology)

Interactions Index / Dilaudid Tablets and Liquid

Ketamine Hydrochloride (Additive depressant effects).
  No products indexed under this heading.
Levomethadyl Acetate Hydrochloride (Additive depressant effects). Products include:
  Orlaam Oral Solution 2361
Levorphanol Tartrate (Additive depressant effects). Products include:
  Levo-Dromoran 2297
Lorazepam (Additive depressant effects). Products include:
  Ativan Injection 2805
  Ativan Tablets 2807
Loxapine Hydrochloride (Additive depressant effects). Products include:
  Loxitane 1426
Loxapine Succinate (Additive depressant effects). Products include:
  Loxitane Capsules 1426
Meperidine Hydrochloride (Additive depressant effects). Products include:
  Demerol 2438
  Mepergan Injection 2859
Mephobarbital (Additive depressant effects). Products include:
  Mebaral Tablets 2452
Meprobamate (Additive depressant effects). Products include:
  Miltown Tablets 2780
  PMB 200 and PMB 400 2890
Mesoridazine Besylate (Additive depressant effects). Products include:
  Serentil 689
Methadone Hydrochloride (Additive depressant effects). Products include:
  Methadone Hydrochloride Oral Concentrate 2356
  Methadone Hydrochloride Oral Solution & Tablets 2357
Methohexital Sodium (Additive depressant effects).
  No products indexed under this heading.
Methotrimeprazine (Additive depressant effects). Products include:
  Levoprome 1321
Methoxyflurane (Additive depressant effects).
  No products indexed under this heading.
Metocurine Iodide (Increased respiratory depression; enhanced action of neuromuscular blocking agents). Products include:
  Metubine Iodide Vials 932
Midazolam Hydrochloride (Additive depressant effects). Products include:
  Versed Injection 2324
Mivacurium Chloride (Increased respiratory depression; enhanced action of neuromuscular blocking agents). Products include:
  Mivacron 1125
Molindone Hydrochloride (Additive depressant effects). Products include:
  Moban Tablets and Concentrate 1036
Morphine Sulfate (Additive depressant effects). Products include:
  Astramorph/PF Injection, USP (Preservative-Free) 526
  Duramorph Injection 983
  Infumorph 200 and Infumorph 500 Sterile Solutions 985
  Kadian Capsules 2948
  MS Contin Tablets 2149
  MSIR 2152
  Oramorph SR (Morphine Sulfate Sustained Release Tablets) 2359
  RMS Suppositories CII 2766
  Roxanol 2365
Opium Alkaloids (Additive depressant effects).
  No products indexed under this heading.
Oxazepam (Additive depressant effects). Products include:
  Serax Capsules 2916
  Serax Tablets 2916
Oxycodone Hydrochloride (Additive depressant effects). Products include:
  OxyContin Tablets 2163
  OxyIR Capsules 2167
  Percocet Tablets 955
  Percodan Tablets 955
  Percodan-Demi Tablets 956
  Roxicodone Tablets, Oral Solution & Intensol (Oxycodone) 2366
  Tylox Capsules 1593
Pancuronium Bromide (Increased respiratory depression; enhanced action of neuromuscular blocking agents).
  No products indexed under this heading.
Pentobarbital Sodium (Additive depressant effects). Products include:
  Nembutal Sodium Capsules 440
  Nembutal Sodium Solution 442
  Nembutal Sodium Suppositories 444
Perphenazine (Additive depressant effects). Products include:
  Etrafon 2495
  Triavil Tablets 1800
  Trilafon 2532
Phenobarbital (Additive depressant effects). Products include:
  Arco-Lase Plus Tablets 513
  Bellergal-S Tablets 2375
  Donnatal 2234
  Donnatal Extentabs 2234
  Donnatal 2234
  Phenobarbital Elixir and Tablets 1523
  Quadrinal Tablets 1398
Prazepam (Additive depressant effects).
  No products indexed under this heading.
Prochlorperazine (Additive depressant effects). Products include:
  Compazine 2644
Promethazine Hydrochloride (Additive depressant effects). Products include:
  Mepergan Injection 2859
  Phenergan with Codeine 2883
  Phenergan with Dextromethorphan 2885
  Phenergan Injection 2880
  Phenergan Suppositories 2882
  Phenergan Syrup 2881
  Phenergan Tablets 2882
  Phenergan VC 2886
  Phenergan VC with Codeine 2888
Propofol (Additive depressant effects). Products include:
  Diprivan Injectable Emulsion 2939
Propoxyphene Hydrochloride (Additive depressant effects). Products include:
  Darvon 1475
  Wygesic Tablets 2930
Propoxyphene Napsylate (Additive depressant effects). Products include:
  Darvon-N/Darvocet-N 1473
Quazepam (Additive depressant effects). Products include:
  Doral Tablets 2773
Risperidone (Additive depressant effects). Products include:
  Risperdal Tablets 1348
Rocuronium Bromide (Increased respiratory depression; enhanced action of neuromuscular blocking agents). Products include:
  Zemuron Injection 1885
Secobarbital Sodium (Additive depressant effects). Products include:
  Seconal Sodium Pulvules 1529
Sevoflurane (Additive depressant effects).
  No products indexed under this heading.
Sufentanil Citrate (Additive depressant effects). Products include:
  Sufenta Injection 1355
Temazepam (Additive depressant effects). Products include:
  Restoril Capsules 2413
Thiamylal Sodium (Additive depressant effects).
  No products indexed under this heading.
Thioridazine Hydrochloride (Additive depressant effects). Products include:
  Mellaril 2398
Thiothixene (Additive depressant effects). Products include:
  Navane Capsules and Concentrate 2018
  Navane Intramuscular 2019
Triazolam (Additive depressant effects). Products include:
  Halcion Tablets 2093
Trifluoperazine Hydrochloride (Additive depressant effects). Products include:
  Stelazine 2692
Vecuronium Bromide (Increased respiratory depression; enhanced action of neuromuscular blocking agents). Products include:
  Norcuron for Injection 1875
Zolpidem Tartrate (Additive depressant effects). Products include:
  Ambien Tablets 2559

Food Interactions
Alcohol (Additive depressant effects).

DILAUDID-HP LYOPHILIZED POWDER 250 MG
(Hydromorphone Hydrochloride) 1384
See **Dilaudid-HP Injection**

DILAUDID INJECTION
(Hydromorphone Hydrochloride) 1382
See **Dilaudid Ampules**

DILAUDID MULTIPLE DOSE VIALS (STERILE SOLUTION)
(Hydromorphone Hydrochloride) 1382
See **Dilaudid Ampules**

DILAUDID ORAL LIQUID
(Hydromorphone Hydrochloride) 1386
May interact with central nervous system depressants, hypnotics and sedatives, general anesthetics, phenothiazines, tranquilizers, neuromuscular blocking agents, and certain other agents. Compounds in these categories include:

Alfentanil Hydrochloride (May produce additive depressant effects; respiratory depression, hypotension and profound sedation or coma may occur; the dose of one or both agents should be reduced). Products include:
  Alfenta Injection 1334
Alprazolam (May produce additive depressant effects; respiratory depression, hypotension and profound sedation or coma may occur; the dose of one or both agents should be reduced). Products include:
  Xanax Tablets 2115
Aprobarbital (May produce additive depressant effects; respiratory depression, hypotension and profound sedation or coma may occur; the dose of one or both agents should be reduced).
  No products indexed under this heading.
Atracurium Besylate (Enhanced action of neuromuscular blocking agents and produce an excessive degree of respiratory depression). Products include:
  Tracrium Injection 1155
Buprenorphine (May produce additive depressant effects; respiratory depression, hypotension and profound sedation or coma may occur; the dose of one or both agents should be reduced). Products include:
  Buprenex Injectable 2170
Buspirone Hydrochloride (May produce additive depressant effects; respiratory depression, hypotension and profound sedation or coma may occur; the dose of one or both agents should be reduced). Products include:
  BuSpar Tablets 738
Butabarbital (May produce additive depressant effects; respiratory depression, hypotension and profound sedation or coma may occur; the dose of one or both agents should be reduced).
  No products indexed under this heading.
Butalbital (May produce additive depressant effects; respiratory depression, hypotension and profound sedation or coma may occur; the dose of one or both agents should be reduced). Products include:
  Axocet Capsules 2469
  Esgic-plus Capsules 1012
  Esgic-plus Tablets 1012
  Fioricet Tablets 2386
  Fioricet with Codeine Capsules 2387
  Fiorinal Capsules 2388
  Fiorinal with Codeine Capsules 2390
  Fiorinal Tablets 2388
  Phrenilin 790
  Sedapap Tablets 50 mg/650 mg 1826
Chlordiazepoxide (May produce additive depressant effects; respiratory depression, hypotension and profound sedation or coma may occur; the dose of one or both agents should be reduced). Products include:
  Limbitrol 2333
Chlordiazepoxide Hydrochloride (May produce additive depressant effects; respiratory depression, hypotension and profound sedation or coma may occur; the dose of one or both agents should be reduced). Products include:
  Librax Capsules 2330
  Librium Capsules 2331
  Librium Injectable 2332
Chlorpromazine (May produce additive depressant effects; respiratory depression, hypotension and profound sedation or coma may occur; the dose of one or both agents should be reduced). Products include:
  Thorazine Suppositories 2701
Chlorpromazine Hydrochloride (May produce additive depressant effects; respiratory depression, hypotension and profound sedation or coma may occur; the dose of one or both agents should be reduced). Products include:
  Thorazine 2701

IMPORTANT NOTE: Always consult each drug listing in the patient's regimen for possible interactions.

Dilaudid Tablets and Liquid / Interactions Index

Chlorprothixene (May produce additive depressant effects; respiratory depression, hypotension and profound sedation or coma may occur; the dose of one or both agents should be reduced.
 No products indexed under this heading.
Chlorprothixene Hydrochloride (May produce additive depressant effects; respiratory depression, hypotension and profound sedation or coma may occur; the dose of one or both agents should be reduced).
 No products indexed under this heading.
Chlorprothixene Lactate (May produce additive depressant effects; respiratory depression, hypotension and profound sedation or coma may occur; the dose of one or both agents should be reduced).
 No products indexed under this heading.
Cisatracurium Besylate (Enhanced action of neuromuscular blocking agents and produce an excessive degree of respiratory depression). Products include:
 Nimbex Injection 1131
Clorazepate Dipotassium (May produce additive depressant effects; respiratory depression, hypotension and profound sedation or coma may occur; the dose of one or both agents should be reduced). Products include:
 Tranxene 459
Clozapine (May produce additive depressant effects; respiratory depression, hypotension and profound sedation or coma may occur; the dose of one or both agents should be reduced). Products include:
 Clozaril Tablets 2377
Codeine Phosphate (May produce additive depressant effects; respiratory depression, hypotension and profound sedation or coma may occur; the dose of one or both agents should be reduced). Products include:
 Brontex 2130
 Dimetane-DC Cough Syrup 2232
 Fioricet with Codeine Tablets 2387
 Fiorinal with Codeine Capsules 2390
 Nucofed 2225
 Phenergan with Codeine 2883
 Phenergan VC with Codeine 2888
 Robitussin A-C Syrup 2248
 Robitussin-DAC Syrup 2249
 Ryna .... ◼ 804
 Soma Compound w/Codeine Tablets 2784
 Tylenol with Codeine 1592
Desflurane (May produce additive depressant effects; respiratory depression, hypotension and profound sedation or coma may occur; the dose of one or both agents should be reduced). Products include:
 Suprane (desflurane, USP) 1865
Dezocine (May produce additive depressant effects; respiratory depression, hypotension and profound sedation or coma may occur; the dose of one or both agents should be reduced). Products include:
 Dalgan Injection 529
Diazepam (May produce additive depressant effects; respiratory depression, hypotension and profound sedation or coma may occur; the dose of one or both agents should be reduced). Products include:
 Dizac (diazepam injectable emulsion) CIV 1862
 Valium Injectable 2336
 Valium Tablets 2335

Doxacurium Chloride (Enhanced action of neuromuscular blocking agents and produce an excessive degree of respiratory depression). Products include:
 Nuromax Injection 1136
Droperidol (May produce additive depressant effects; respiratory depression, hypotension and profound sedation or coma may occur; the dose of one or both agents should be reduced). Products include:
 Inapsine Injection 462
Enflurane (May produce additive depressant effects; respiratory depression, hypotension and profound sedation or coma may occur; the dose of one or both agents should be reduced).
 No products indexed under this heading.
Estazolam (May produce additive depressant effects; respiratory depression, hypotension and profound sedation or coma may occur; the dose of one or both agents should be reduced). Products include:
 ProSom Tablets 457
Ethchlorvynol (May produce additive depressant effects; respiratory depression, hypotension and profound sedation or coma may occur; the dose of one or both agents should be reduced). Products include:
 Placidyl Capsules 456
Ethinamate (May produce additive depressant effects; respiratory depression, hypotension and profound sedation or coma may occur; the dose of one or both agents should be reduced).
 No products indexed under this heading.
Fentanyl (May produce additive depressant effects; respiratory depression, hypotension and profound sedation or coma may occur; the dose of one or both agents should be reduced). Products include:
 Duragesic Transdermal System 1336
Fentanyl Citrate (May produce additive depressant effects; respiratory depression, hypotension and profound sedation or coma may occur; the dose of one or both agents should be reduced). Products include:
 Sublimaze Injection 463
Fluphenazine Decanoate (May produce additive depressant effects; respiratory depression, hypotension and profound sedation or coma may occur; the dose of one or both agents should be reduced). Products include:
 Prolixin Decanoate 510
Fluphenazine Enanthate (May produce additive depressant effects; respiratory depression, hypotension and profound sedation or coma may occur; the dose of one or both agents should be reduced). Products include:
 Prolixin Enanthate 510
Fluphenazine Hydrochloride (May produce additive depressant effects; respiratory depression, hypotension and profound sedation or coma may occur; the dose of one or both agents should be reduced). Products include:
 Prolixin 510

Flurazepam Hydrochloride (May produce additive depressant effects; respiratory depression, hypotension and profound sedation or coma may occur; the dose of one or both agents should be reduced). Products include:
 Dalmane Capsules 2329
Glutethimide (May produce additive depressant effects; respiratory depression, hypotension and profound sedation or coma may occur; the dose of one or both agents should be reduced).
 No products indexed under this heading.
Haloperidol (May produce additive depressant effects; respiratory depression, hypotension and profound sedation or coma may occur; the dose of one or both agents should be reduced). Products include:
 Haldol Injection, Tablets and Concentrate 1585
Haloperidol Decanoate (May produce additive depressant effects; respiratory depression, hypotension and profound sedation or coma may occur; the dose of one or both agents should be reduced). Products include:
 Haldol Decanoate 1587
Hydrocodone Bitartrate (May produce additive depressant effects; respiratory depression, hypotension and profound sedation or coma may occur; the dose of one or both agents should be reduced). Products include:
 Codiclear DH Syrup 808
 Duratuss HD Elixir 2750
 Histussin D Liquid 670
 Hycodan Tablets and Syrup 946
 Hycomine Compound Tablets 948
 Hycomine 947
 Hycotuss Expectorant Syrup 950
 Hydrocet Capsules 787
 Lorcet 10/650 Tablets 1016
 Lortab 2751
 Tussend 1830
 Tussend Expectorant 1831
 Vicodin Tablets 1404
 Vicodin ES Tablets 1405
 Vicodin HP Tablets 1403
 Vicodin Tuss Expectorant 1406
 Zydone Capsules 967
Hydrocodone Polistirex (May produce additive depressant effects; respiratory depression, hypotension and profound sedation or coma may occur; the dose of one or both agents should be reduced). Products include:
 Tussionex Pennkinetic Extended-Release Suspension 1624
Hydroxyzine Hydrochloride (May produce additive depressant effects; respiratory depression, hypotension and profound sedation or coma may occur; the dose of one or both agents should be reduced). Products include:
 Atarax Tablets & Syrup 1992
 Marax Tablets & DF Syrup 2015
 Vistaril Intramuscular Solution 2042
Isoflurane (May produce additive depressant effects; respiratory depression, hypotension and profound sedation or coma may occur; the dose of one or both agents should be reduced).
 No products indexed under this heading.
Ketamine Hydrochloride (May produce additive depressant effects; respiratory depression, hypotension and profound sedation or coma may occur; the dose of one or both agents should be reduced).
 No products indexed under this heading.

Levomethadyl Acetate Hydrochloride (May produce additive depressant effects; respiratory depression, hypotension and profound sedation or coma may occur; the dose of one or both agents should be reduced). Products include:
 Orlaam Oral Solution 2361
Levorphanol Tartrate (May produce additive depressant effects; respiratory depression, hypotension and profound sedation or coma may occur; the dose of one or both agents should be reduced). Products include:
 Levo-Dromoran 2297
Lorazepam (May produce additive depressant effects; respiratory depression, hypotension and profound sedation or coma may occur; the dose of one or both agents should be reduced). Products include:
 Ativan Injection 2805
 Ativan Tablets 2807
Loxapine Hydrochloride (May produce additive depressant effects; respiratory depression, hypotension and profound sedation or coma may occur; the dose of one or both agents should be reduced). Products include:
 Loxitane 1426
Loxapine Succinate (May produce additive depressant effects; respiratory depression, hypotension and profound sedation or coma may occur; the dose of one or both agents should be reduced). Products include:
 Loxitane Capsules 1426
Meperidine Hydrochloride (May produce additive depressant effects; respiratory depression, hypotension and profound sedation or coma may occur; the dose of one or both agents should be reduced). Products include:
 Demerol 2438
 Mepergan Injection 2859
Mephobarbital (May produce additive depressant effects; respiratory depression, hypotension and profound sedation or coma may occur; the dose of one or both agents should be reduced). Products include:
 Mebaral Tablets 2452
Meprobamate (May produce additive depressant effects; respiratory depression, hypotension and profound sedation or coma may occur; the dose of one or both agents should be reduced). Products include:
 Miltown Tablets 2780
 PMB 200 and PMB 400 2890
Mesoridazine Besylate (May produce additive depressant effects; respiratory depression, hypotension and profound sedation or coma may occur; the dose of one or both agents should be reduced). Products include:
 Serentil 689
Methadone Hydrochloride (May produce additive depressant effects; respiratory depression, hypotension and profound sedation or coma may occur; the dose of one or both agents should be reduced). Products include:
 Methadone Hydrochloride Oral Concentrate 2356
 Methadone Hydrochloride Oral Solution & Tablets 2357

(◼ Described in PDR For Nonprescription Drugs) (◉ Described in PDR For Ophthalmology)

Interactions Index

Methohexital Sodium (May produce additive depressant effects; respiratory depression, hypotension and profound sedation or coma may occur; the dose of one or both agents should be reduced).
   No products indexed under this heading.

Methotrimeprazine (May produce additive depressant effects; respiratory depression, hypotension and profound sedation or coma may occur; the dose of one or both agents should be reduced). Products include:
   Levoprome 1321

Methoxyflurane (May produce additive depressant effects; respiratory depression, hypotension and profound sedation or coma may occur; the dose of one or both agents should be reduced).
   No products indexed under this heading.

Metocurine Iodide (Enhanced action of neuromuscular blocking agents and produce an excessive degree of respiratory depression). Products include:
   Metubine Iodide Vials 932

Midazolam Hydrochloride (May produce additive depressant effects; respiratory depression, hypotension and profound sedation or coma may occur; the dose of one or both agents should be reduced). Products include:
   Versed Injection 2324

Mivacurium Chloride (Enhanced action of neuromuscular blocking agents and produce an excessive degree of respiratory depression). Products include:
   Mivacron 1125

Molindone Hydrochloride (May produce additive depressant effects; respiratory depression, hypotension and profound sedation or coma may occur; the dose of one or both agents should be reduced). Products include:
   Moban Tablets and Concentrate 1036

Morphine Sulfate (May produce additive depressant effects; respiratory depression, hypotension and profound sedation or coma may occur; the dose of one or both agents should be reduced). Products include:
   Astramorph/PF Injection, USP (Preservative-Free) 526
   Duramorph Injection 983
   Infumorph 200 and Infumorph 500 Sterile Solutions 985
   Kadian Capsules 2948
   MS Contin Tablets 2149
   MSIR 2152
   Oramorph SR (Morphine Sulfate Sustained Release Tablets) 2359
   RMS Suppositories CII 2766
   Roxanol 2365

Opium Alkaloids (May produce additive depressant effects; respiratory depression, hypotension and profound sedation or coma may occur; the dose of one or both agents should be reduced).
   No products indexed under this heading.

Oxazepam (May produce additive depressant effects; respiratory depression, hypotension and profound sedation or coma may occur; the dose of one or both agents should be reduced). Products include:
   Serax Capsules 2916
   Serax Tablets 2916

Oxycodone Hydrochloride (May produce additive depressant effects; respiratory depression, hypotension and profound sedation or coma may occur; the dose of one or both agents should be reduced). Products include:
   OxyContin Tablets 2163
   OxyIR Capsules 2167
   Percocet Tablets 955
   Percodan Tablets 955
   Percodan-Demi Tablets 956
   Roxicodone Tablets, Oral Solution & Intensol (Oxycodone) 2366
   Tylox Capsules 1593

Pancuronium Bromide (Enhanced action of neuromuscular blocking agents and produce an excessive degree of respiratory depression).
   No products indexed under this heading.

Pentobarbital Sodium (May produce additive depressant effects; respiratory depression, hypotension and profound sedation or coma may occur; the dose of one or both agents should be reduced). Products include:
   Nembutal Sodium Capsules 440
   Nembutal Sodium Solution 442
   Nembutal Sodium Suppositories 444

Perphenazine (May produce additive depressant effects; respiratory depression, hypotension and profound sedation or coma may occur; the dose of one or both agents should be reduced). Products include:
   Etrafon 2495
   Triavil Tablets 1800
   Trilafon 2532

Phenobarbital (May produce additive depressant effects; respiratory depression, hypotension and profound sedation or coma may occur; the dose of one or both agents should be reduced). Products include:
   Arco-Lase Plus Tablets 513
   Bellergal-S Tablets 2375
   Donnatal 2234
   Donnatal Extentabs 2234
   Donnatal Tablets 2234
   Phenobarbital Elixir and Tablets 1523
   Quadrinal Tablets 1398

Prazepam (May produce additive depressant effects; respiratory depression, hypotension and profound sedation or coma may occur; the dose of one or both agents should be reduced).
   No products indexed under this heading.

Prochlorperazine (May produce additive depressant effects; respiratory depression, hypotension and profound sedation or coma may occur; the dose of one or both agents should be reduced). Products include:
   Compazine 2644

Promethazine Hydrochloride (May produce additive depressant effects; respiratory depression, hypotension and profound sedation or coma may occur; the dose of one or both agents should be reduced). Products include:
   Mepergan Injection 2859
   Phenergan with Codeine 2883
   Phenergan with Dextromethorphan ... 2885
   Phenergan Injection 2880
   Phenergan Suppositories 2882
   Phenergan Syrup 2881
   Phenergan Tablets 2882
   Phenergan VC 2886
   Phenergan VC with Codeine 2888

Propofol (May produce additive depressant effects; respiratory depression, hypotension and profound sedation or coma may occur; the dose of one or both agents should be reduced). Products include:
   Diprivan Injectable Emulsion 2939

Propoxyphene Hydrochloride (May produce additive depressant effects; respiratory depression, hypotension and profound sedation or coma may occur; the dose of one or both agents should be reduced). Products include:
   Darvon 1475
   Wygesic Tablets 2930

Propoxyphene Napsylate (May produce additive depressant effects; respiratory depression, hypotension and profound sedation or coma may occur; the dose of one or both agents should be reduced). Products include:
   Darvon-N/Darvocet-N 1473

Quazepam (May produce additive depressant effects; respiratory depression, hypotension and profound sedation or coma may occur; the dose of one or both agents should be reduced). Products include:
   Doral Tablets 2773

Risperidone (May produce additive depressant effects; respiratory depression, hypotension and profound sedation or coma may occur; the dose of one or both agents should be reduced). Products include:
   Risperdal Tablets 1348

Rocuronium Bromide (Enhanced action of neuromuscular blocking agents and produce an excessive degree of respiratory depression). Products include:
   Zemuron Injection 1885

Secobarbital Sodium (May produce additive depressant effects; respiratory depression, hypotension and profound sedation or coma may occur; the dose of one or both agents should be reduced). Products include:
   Seconal Sodium Pulvules 1529

Sevoflurane (May produce additive depressant effects; respiratory depression, hypotension and profound sedation or coma may occur; the dose of one or both agents should be reduced).
   No products indexed under this heading.

Succinylcholine Chloride (Enhanced action of neuromuscular blocking agents and produce an excessive degree of respiratory depression). Products include:
   Anectine 1062

Sufentanil Citrate (May produce additive depressant effects; respiratory depression, hypotension and profound sedation or coma may occur; the dose of one or both agents should be reduced). Products include:
   Sufenta Injection 1355

Temazepam (May produce additive depressant effects; respiratory depression, hypotension and profound sedation or coma may occur; the dose of one or both agents should be reduced). Products include:
   Restoril Capsules 2413

Thiamylal Sodium (May produce additive depressant effects; respiratory depression, hypotension and profound sedation or coma may occur; the dose of one or both agents should be reduced).
   No products indexed under this heading.

Thioridazine Hydrochloride (May produce additive depressant effects; respiratory depression, hypotension and profound sedation or coma may occur; the dose of one or both agents should be reduced). Products include:
   Mellaril 2398

Thiothixene (May produce additive depressant effects; respiratory depression, hypotension and profound sedation or coma may occur; the dose of one or both agents should be reduced). Products include:
   Navane Capsules and Concentrate ... 2018
   Navane Intramuscular 2019

Triazolam (May produce additive depressant effects; respiratory depression, hypotension and profound sedation or coma may occur; the dose of one or both agents should be reduced). Products include:
   Halcion Tablets 2093

Trifluoperazine Hydrochloride (May produce additive depressant effects; respiratory depression, hypotension and profound sedation or coma may occur; the dose of one or both agents should be reduced). Products include:
   Stelazine 2692

Vecuronium Bromide (Enhanced action of neuromuscular blocking agents and produce an excessive degree of respiratory depression). Products include:
   Norcuron for Injection 1875

Zolpidem Tartrate (May produce additive depressant effects; respiratory depression, hypotension and profound sedation or coma may occur; the dose of one or both agents should be reduced). Products include:
   Ambien Tablets 2559

Food Interactions

Alcohol (May exhibit an additive CNS depression).

DILAUDID POWDER
(Hydromorphone Hydrochloride) 1382
See **Dilaudid Ampules**

DILAUDID RECTAL SUPPOSITORIES
(Hydromorphone Hydrochloride) 1382
See **Dilaudid Ampules**

DILAUDID TABLETS 2 MG AND 4 MG
(Hydromorphone Hydrochloride) 1382
See **Dilaudid Ampules**

DILAUDID TABLETS - 8 MG
(Hydromorphone Hydrochloride) 1386
See **Dilaudid Oral Liquid**

DIMETANE-DC COUGH SYRUP
(Brompheniramine Maleate, Phenylpropanolamine Hydrochloride, Codeine Phosphate) 2232
May interact with monoamine oxidase inhibitors, tranquilizers, hypnotics and sedatives, central nervous system depressants, antihyperten-

IMPORTANT NOTE: Always consult each drug listing in the patient's regimen for possible interactions.

Dimetane-DC Interactions Index 298

sives, and certain other agents. Compounds in these categories include:

Acebutolol Hydrochloride (Sympathomimetics may reduce the effects of antihypertensive drugs). Products include:
Sectral Capsules 2914

Alfentanil Hydrochloride (Antihistamines have additive effects with CNS depressants). Products include:
Alfenta Injection 1334

Alprazolam (Antihistamines have additive effects with CNS depressants). Products include:
Xanax Tablets 2115

Amlodipine Besylate (Sympathomimetics may reduce the effects of antihypertensive drugs). Products include:
Lotrel Capsules 858
Norvasc Tablets 2020

Aprobarbital (Antihistamines have additive effects with CNS depressants).
No products indexed under this heading.

Atenolol (Sympathomimetics may reduce the effects of antihypertensive drugs). Products include:
Tenoretic Tablets 2963
Tenormin Tablets and I.V. Injection 2965

Benazepril Hydrochloride (Sympathomimetics may reduce the effects of antihypertensive drugs). Products include:
Lotensin Tablets 852
Lotensin HCT Tablets 855
Lotrel Capsules 858

Bendroflumethiazide (Sympathomimetics may reduce the effects of antihypertensive drugs).
No products indexed under this heading.

Betaxolol Hydrochloride (Sympathomimetics may reduce the effects of antihypertensive drugs). Products include:
Betoptic Ophthalmic Solution 465
Betoptic S Ophthalmic Suspension 467
Kerlone Tablets 2588

Bisoprolol Fumarate (Sympathomimetics may reduce the effects of antihypertensive drugs). Products include:
Zebeta Tablets 1457
Ziac 1459

Buprenorphine (Antihistamines have additive effects with CNS depressants). Products include:
Buprenex Injectable 2170

Buspirone Hydrochloride (Antihistamines have additive effects with CNS depressants). Products include:
BuSpar Tablets 738

Butabarbital (Antihistamines have additive effects with CNS depressants).
No products indexed under this heading.

Butalbital (Antihistamines have additive effects with CNS depressants). Products include:
Axocet Capsules 2469
Esgic-plus Capsules 1012
Esgic-plus Tablets 1012
Fioricet Tablets 2386
Fioricet with Codeine Capsules 2387
Fiorinal Capsules 2388
Fiorinal with Codeine Capsules 2390
Fiorinal Tablets 2388
Phrenilin 790
Sedapap Tablets 50 mg/650 mg .. 1826

Captopril (Sympathomimetics may reduce the effects of antihypertensive drugs). Products include:
Capoten Tablets 740
Capozide Tablets 744

Carteolol Hydrochloride (Sympathomimetics may reduce the effects of antihypertensive drugs). Products include:
Cartrol Tablets 413
Ocupress Ophthalmic Solution, 1% Sterile ..... ◉ 297

Chlordiazepoxide (Antihistamines have additive effects with CNS depressants). Products include:
Limbitrol 2333

Chlordiazepoxide Hydrochloride (Antihistamines have additive effects with CNS depressants). Products include:
Librax Capsules 2330
Librium Capsules 2331
Librium Injectable 2332

Chlorothiazide (Sympathomimetics may reduce the effects of antihypertensive drugs). Products include:
Aldoclor Tablets 1638
Diupres Tablets 1691
Diuril Oral 1694

Chlorothiazide Sodium (Sympathomimetics may reduce the effects of antihypertensive drugs). Products include:
Diuril Sodium Intravenous 1693

Chlorpromazine (Antihistamines have additive effects with CNS depressants). Products include:
Thorazine Suppositories 2701

Chlorpromazine Hydrochloride (Antihistamines have additive effects with CNS depressants). Products include:
Thorazine 2701

Chlorprothixene (Antihistamines have additive effects with CNS depressants).
No products indexed under this heading.

Chlorprothixene Hydrochloride (Antihistamines have additive effects with CNS depressants).
No products indexed under this heading.

Chlorprothixene Lactate (Antihistamines have additive effects with CNS depressants).
No products indexed under this heading.

Chlorthalidone (Sympathomimetics may reduce the effects of antihypertensive drugs). Products include:
Combipres Tablets 682
Tenoretic Tablets 2963
Thalitone 1293

Clonidine (Sympathomimetics may reduce the effects of antihypertensive drugs). Products include:
Catapres-TTS 680

Clonidine Hydrochloride (Sympathomimetics may reduce the effects of antihypertensive drugs). Products include:
Catapres Tablets 679
Combipres Tablets 682

Clorazepate Dipotassium (Antihistamines have additive effects with CNS depressants). Products include:
Tranxene 459

Clozapine (Antihistamines have additive effects with CNS depressants). Products include:
Clozaril Tablets 2377

Deserpidine (Sympathomimetics may reduce the effects of antihypertensive drugs).
No products indexed under this heading.

Desflurane (Antihistamines have additive effects with CNS depressants). Products include:
Suprane (desflurane, USP) 1865

Dezocine (Antihistamines have additive effects with CNS depressants). Products include:
Dalgan Injection 529

Diazepam (Antihistamines have additive effects with CNS depressants). Products include:
Dizac (diazepam injectable emulsion) CIV 1862
Valium Injectable 2336
Valium Tablets 2335

Diazoxide (Sympathomimetics may reduce the effects of antihypertensive drugs). Products include:
Hyperstat I.V. Injection 2504
Proglycem 575

Diltiazem Hydrochloride (Sympathomimetics may reduce the effects of antihypertensive drugs). Products include:
Cardizem CD Capsules 1251
Cardizem SR Capsules 1255
Cardizem Injectable 1253
Cardizem Tablets 1257
Dilacor XR Extended-release Capsules 2183
Tiazac Capsules 1019

Doxazosin Mesylate (Sympathomimetics may reduce the effects of antihypertensive drugs). Products include:
Cardura Tablets 1993

Droperidol (Antihistamines have additive effects with CNS depressants). Products include:
Inapsine Injection 462

Enalapril Maleate (Sympathomimetics may reduce the effects of antihypertensive drugs). Products include:
Vaseretic Tablets 1810
Vasotec Tablets 1816

Enalaprilat (Sympathomimetics may reduce the effects of antihypertensive drugs). Products include:
Vasotec I.V. 1814

Enflurane (Antihistamines have additive effects with CNS depressants).
No products indexed under this heading.

Esmolol Hydrochloride (Sympathomimetics may reduce the effects of antihypertensive drugs). Products include:
Brevibloc (esmolol HCl) Injection 1860

Estazolam (Antihistamines have additive effects with CNS depressants). Products include:
ProSom Tablets 457

Ethchlorvynol (Antihistamines have additive effects with CNS depressants). Products include:
Placidyl Capsules 456

Ethinamate (Antihistamines have additive effects with CNS depressants).
No products indexed under this heading.

Felodipine (Sympathomimetics may reduce the effects of antihypertensive drugs). Products include:
Plendil Extended-Release Tablets 514

Fentanyl (Antihistamines have additive effects with CNS depressants). Products include:
Duragesic Transdermal System 1336

Fentanyl Citrate (Antihistamines have additive effects with CNS depressants). Products include:
Sublimaze Injection 463

Fluphenazine Decanoate (Antihistamines have additive effects with CNS depressants). Products include:
Prolixin Decanoate 510

Fluphenazine Enanthate (Antihistamines have additive effects with CNS depressants). Products include:
Prolixin Enanthate 510

Fluphenazine Hydrochloride (Antihistamines have additive effects with CNS depressants). Products include:
Prolixin 510

Flurazepam Hydrochloride (Antihistamines have additive effects with CNS depressants). Products include:
Dalmane Capsules 2329

Fosinopril Sodium (Sympathomimetics may reduce the effects of antihypertensive drugs). Products include:
Monopril Tablets 762

Furazolidone (Prolongs and intensifies the anticholinergic effects of antihistamines; may enhance the effect of phenylpropanolamine; concurrent and/or sequential use is contraindicated). Products include:
Furoxone 2221

Furosemide (Sympathomimetics may reduce the effects of antihypertensive drugs). Products include:
Lasix Injection, Oral Solution and Tablets 1267

Glutethimide (Antihistamines have additive effects with CNS depressants).
No products indexed under this heading.

Guanabenz Acetate (Sympathomimetics may reduce the effects of antihypertensive drugs).
No products indexed under this heading.

Guanethidine Monosulfate (Sympathomimetics may reduce the effects of antihypertensive drugs). Products include:
Esimil Tablets 840
Ismelin Tablets 845

Haloperidol (Antihistamines have additive effects with CNS depressants). Products include:
Haldol Injection, Tablets and Concentrate 1585

Haloperidol Decanoate (Antihistamines have additive effects with CNS depressants). Products include:
Haldol Decanoate 1587

Hydralazine Hydrochloride (Sympathomimetics may reduce the effects of antihypertensive drugs). Products include:
Apresazide Capsules 824
Apresoline Hydrochloride Tablets .. 826
Hydralazine Hydrochloride Injection USP 2712
Ser-Ap-Es Tablets 867

Hydrochlorothiazide (Sympathomimetics may reduce the effects of antihypertensive drugs). Products include:
Aldactazide Tablets 2556
Aldoril Tablets 1644
Apresazide Capsules 824
Capozide Tablets 744
Dyazide Capsules 2653
Esidrix Tablets 839
Esimil Tablets 840
HydroDIURIL Tablets 1716
Hydropres Tablets 1718
Hyzaar Tablets 1720
Inderide Tablets 2838
Inderide LA Long Acting Capsules .. 2840
Lopressor HCT Tablets 850
Lotensin HCT Tablets 855
Moduretic Tablets 1748
Oretic Tablets 450
Prinzide Tablets 1780
Ser-Ap-Es Tablets 867
Timolide Tablets 1791
Vaseretic Tablets 1810
Zestoretic Tablets 2968
Ziac 1459

(▣ Described in PDR For Nonprescription Drugs) (◉ Described in PDR For Ophthalmology)

Hydrocodone Bitartrate (Antihistamines have additive effects with CNS depressants). Products include:
- Codiclear DH Syrup ... 808
- Duratuss HD Elixir ... 2750
- Histussin D Liquid ... 670
- Hycodan Tablets and Syrup ... 946
- Hycomine Compound Tablets ... 948
- Hycomine ... 947
- Hycotuss Expectorant Syrup ... 950
- Hydrocet Capsules ... 787
- Lorcet 10/650 Tablets ... 1016
- Lortab ... 2751
- Tussend ... 1830
- Tussend Expectorant ... 1831
- Vicodin Tablets ... 1404
- Vicodin ES Tablets ... 1405
- Vicodin HP Tablets ... 1403
- Vicodin Tuss Expectorant ... 1406
- Zydone Capsules ... 967

Hydrocodone Polistirex (Antihistamines have additive effects with CNS depressants). Products include:
- Tussionex Pennkinetic Extended-Release Suspension ... 1624

Hydroflumethiazide (Sympathomimetics may reduce the effects of antihypertensive drugs). Products include:
- Diucardin Tablets ... 2824

Hydroxyzine Hydrochloride (Antihistamines have additive effects with CNS depressants). Products include:
- Atarax Tablets & Syrup ... 1992
- Marax Tablets & DF Syrup ... 2015
- Vistaril Intramuscular Solution ... 2042

Indapamide (Sympathomimetics may reduce the effects of antihypertensive drugs).
No products indexed under this heading.

Isocarboxazid (Prolongs and intensifies the anticholinergic effects of antihistamines; may enhance the effect of phenylpropanolamine; concurrent and/or sequential use is contraindicated).
No products indexed under this heading.

Isoflurane (Antihistamines have additive effects with CNS depressants).
No products indexed under this heading.

Isradipine (Sympathomimetics may reduce the effects of antihypertensive drugs). Products include:
- DynaCirc Capsules ... 2381
- DynaCirc CR Tablets ... 2383

Ketamine Hydrochloride (Antihistamines have additive effects with CNS depressants).
No products indexed under this heading.

Labetalol Hydrochloride (Sympathomimetics may reduce the effects of antihypertensive drugs). Products include:
- Normodyne Injection ... 2519
- Normodyne Tablets ... 2522
- Trandate ... 1158

Levomethadyl Acetate Hydrochloride (Antihistamines have additive effects with CNS depressants). Products include:
- Orlaam Oral Solution ... 2361

Levorphanol Tartrate (Antihistamines have additive effects with CNS depressants). Products include:
- Levo-Dromoran ... 2297

Lisinopril (Sympathomimetics may reduce the effects of antihypertensive drugs). Products include:
- Prinivil Tablets ... 1776
- Prinzide Tablets ... 1780
- Zestoretic Tablets ... 2968
- Zestril Tablets ... 2972

Lorazepam (Antihistamines have additive effects with CNS depressants). Products include:
- Ativan Injection ... 2805
- Ativan Tablets ... 2807

Losartan Potassium (Sympathomimetics may reduce the effects of antihypertensive drugs). Products include:
- Cozaar Tablets ... 1668
- Hyzaar Tablets ... 1720

Loxapine Hydrochloride (Antihistamines have additive effects with CNS depressants). Products include:
- Loxitane ... 1426

Loxapine Succinate (Antihistamines have additive effects with CNS depressants). Products include:
- Loxitane Capsules ... 1426

Mecamylamine Hydrochloride (Sympathomimetics may reduce the effects of antihypertensive drugs). Products include:
- Inversine Tablets ... 1729

Meperidine Hydrochloride (Antihistamines have additive effects with CNS depressants). Products include:
- Demerol ... 2438
- Mepergan Injection ... 2859

Mephobarbital (Antihistamines have additive effects with CNS depressants). Products include:
- Mebaral Tablets ... 2452

Meprobamate (Antihistamines have additive effects with CNS depressants). Products include:
- Miltown Tablets ... 2780
- PMB 200 and PMB 400 ... 2890

Mesoridazine Besylate (Antihistamines have additive effects with CNS depressants). Products include:
- Serentil ... 689

Methadone Hydrochloride (Antihistamines have additive effects with CNS depressants). Products include:
- Methadone Hydrochloride Oral Concentrate ... 2356
- Methadone Hydrochloride Oral Solution & Tablets ... 2357

Methohexital Sodium (Antihistamines have additive effects with CNS depressants).
No products indexed under this heading.

Methotrimeprazine (Antihistamines have additive effects with CNS depressants). Products include:
- Levoprome ... 1321

Methoxyflurane (Antihistamines have additive effects with CNS depressants).
No products indexed under this heading.

Methyclothiazide (Sympathomimetics may reduce the effects of antihypertensive drugs). Products include:
- Enduron Tablets ... 424

Methyldopa (Sympathomimetics may reduce the effects of antihypertensive drugs). Products include:
- Aldoclor Tablets ... 1638
- Aldomet Oral ... 1640
- Aldoril Tablets ... 1644

Methyldopate Hydrochloride (Sympathomimetics may reduce the effects of antihypertensive drugs). Products include:
- Aldomet Ester HCl Injection ... 1642

Metolazone (Sympathomimetics may reduce the effects of antihypertensive drugs). Products include:
- Mykrox Tablets ... 1617
- Zaroxolyn Tablets ... 1625

Metoprolol Succinate (Sympathomimetics may reduce the effects of antihypertensive drugs). Products include:
- Toprol-XL Tablets ... 560

Metoprolol Tartrate (Sympathomimetics may reduce the effects of antihypertensive drugs). Products include:
- Lopressor ... 848
- Lopressor HCT Tablets ... 850

Metyrosine (Sympathomimetics may reduce the effects of antihypertensive drugs). Products include:
- Demser Capsules ... 1690

Midazolam Hydrochloride (Antihistamines have additive effects with CNS depressants). Products include:
- Versed Injection ... 2324

Minoxidil (Sympathomimetics may reduce the effects of antihypertensive drugs).
No products indexed under this heading.

Moexipril Hydrochloride (Sympathomimetics may reduce the effects of antihypertensive drugs). Products include:
- Univasc Tablets ... 2553

Molindone Hydrochloride (Antihistamines have additive effects with CNS depressants). Products include:
- Moban Tablets and Concentrate ... 1036

Morphine Sulfate (Antihistamines have additive effects with CNS depressants). Products include:
- Astramorph/PF Injection, USP (Preservative-Free) ... 526
- Duramorph Injection ... 983
- Infumorph 200 and Infumorph 500 Sterile Solutions ... 985
- Kadian Capsules ... 2948
- MS Contin Tablets ... 2149
- MSIR ... 2152
- Oramorph SR (Morphine Sulfate Sustained Release Tablets) ... 2359
- RMS Suppositories CII ... 2766
- Roxanol ... 2365

Nadolol (Sympathomimetics may reduce the effects of antihypertensive drugs).
No products indexed under this heading.

Nicardipine Hydrochloride (Sympathomimetics may reduce the effects of antihypertensive drugs). Products include:
- Cardene Capsules ... 2261
- Cardene I.V. ... 2815
- Cardene SR Capsules ... 2264

Nifedipine (Sympathomimetics may reduce the effects of antihypertensive drugs). Products include:
- Adalat Capsules (10 mg and 20 mg) ... 580
- Adalat CC ... 582
- Procardia Capsules ... 2024
- Procardia XL Extended Release Tablets ... 2026

Nisoldipine (Sympathomimetics may reduce the effects of antihypertensive drugs). Products include:
- Sular Tablets ... 2961

Nitroglycerin (Sympathomimetics may reduce the effects of antihypertensive drugs). Products include:
- Deponit NTG Transdermal Delivery System ... 2541
- Nitro-Bid IV ... 1270
- Nitro-Bid Ointment ... 1272
- Nitro-Dur (nitroglycerin) Transdermal Infusion System ... 1365
- Nitrolingual Spray ... 2193
- Nitrostat Tablets ... 1981
- Transderm-Nitro Transdermal Therapeutic System ... 878

Opium Alkaloids (Antihistamines have additive effects with CNS depressants).
No products indexed under this heading.

Oxazepam (Antihistamines have additive effects with CNS depressants). Products include:
- Serax Capsules ... 2916
- Serax Tablets ... 2916

Oxycodone Hydrochloride (Antihistamines have additive effects with CNS depressants). Products include:
- OxyContin Tablets ... 2163
- OxyIR Capsules ... 2167
- Percocet Tablets ... 955
- Percodan Tablets ... 955
- Percodan-Demi Tablets ... 956
- Roxicodone Tablets, Oral Solution & Intensol (Oxycodone) ... 2366
- Tylox Capsules ... 1593

Penbutolol Sulfate (Sympathomimetics may reduce the effects of antihypertensive drugs). Products include:
- Levatol Tablets ... 2547

Pentobarbital Sodium (Antihistamines have additive effects with CNS depressants). Products include:
- Nembutal Sodium Capsules ... 440
- Nembutal Sodium Solution ... 442
- Nembutal Sodium Suppositories ... 444

Perphenazine (Antihistamines have additive effects with CNS depressants). Products include:
- Etrafon ... 2495
- Triavil Tablets ... 1800
- Trilafon ... 2532

Phenelzine Sulfate (Prolongs and intensifies the anticholinergic effects of antihistamines; may enhance the effect of phenylpropanolamine; concurrent and/or sequential use is contraindicated). Products include:
- Nardil ... 1977

Phenobarbital (Antihistamines have additive effects with CNS depressants). Products include:
- Arco-Lase Plus Tablets ... 513
- Bellergal-S Tablets ... 2375
- Donnatal ... 2234
- Donnatal Extentabs ... 2234
- Donnatal Tablets ... 2234
- Phenobarbital Elixir and Tablets ... 1523
- Quadrinal Tablets ... 1398

Phenoxybenzamine Hydrochloride (Sympathomimetics may reduce the effects of antihypertensive drugs). Products include:
- Dibenzyline Capsules ... 2650

Phentolamine Mesylate (Sympathomimetics may reduce the effects of antihypertensive drugs). Products include:
- Regitine Vials ... 864

Pindolol (Sympathomimetics may reduce the effects of antihypertensive drugs). Products include:
- Visken Tablets ... 2428

Polythiazide (Sympathomimetics may reduce the effects of antihypertensive drugs). Products include:
- Minizide Capsules ... 2016

Prazepam (Antihistamines have additive effects with CNS depressants).
No products indexed under this heading.

Prazosin Hydrochloride (Sympathomimetics may reduce the effects of antihypertensive drugs). Products include:
- Minipress Capsules ... 2015
- Minizide Capsules ... 2016

Prochlorperazine (Antihistamines have additive effects with CNS depressants). Products include:
- Compazine ... 2644

Promethazine Hydrochloride (Antihistamines have additive effects with CNS depressants). Products include:
- Mepergan Injection ... 2859
- Phenergan with Codeine ... 2883
- Phenergan with Dextromethorphan ... 2885

IMPORTANT NOTE: Always consult each drug listing in the patient's regimen for possible interactions.

Dimetane-DC Interactions Index 300

Phenergan Injection 2880
Phenergan Suppositories 2882
Phenergan Syrup 2881
Phenergan Tablets 2882
Phenergan VC 2886
Phenergan VC with Codeine 2888

Propofol (Antihistamines have additive effects with CNS depressants). Products include:
Diprivan Injectable Emulsion 2939

Propoxyphene Hydrochloride (Antihistamines have additive effects with CNS depressants). Products include:
Darvon 1475
Wygesic Tablets 2930

Propoxyphene Napsylate (Antihistamines have additive effects with CNS depressants). Products include:
Darvon-N/Darvocet-N 1473

Propranolol Hydrochloride (Sympathomimetics may reduce the effects of antihypertensive drugs). Products include:
Inderal 2834
Inderal LA Long Acting Capsules 2836
Inderide Tablets 2838
Inderide LA Long Acting Capsules 2840

Quazepam (Antihistamines have additive effects with CNS depressants). Products include:
Doral Tablets 2773

Quinapril Hydrochloride (Sympathomimetics may reduce the effects of antihypertensive drugs). Products include:
Accupril Tablets 1950

Ramipril (Sympathomimetics may reduce the effects of antihypertensive drugs). Products include:
Altace Capsules 1238

Rauwolfia Serpentina (Sympathomimetics may reduce the effects of antihypertensive drugs).
No products indexed under this heading.

Rescinnamine (Sympathomimetics may reduce the effects of antihypertensive drugs).
No products indexed under this heading.

Reserpine (Sympathomimetics may reduce the effects of antihypertensive drugs). Products include:
Diupres Tablets 1691
Hydropres Tablets 1718
Ser-Ap-Es Tablets 867

Risperidone (Antihistamines have additive effects with CNS depressants). Products include:
Risperdal Tablets 1348

Secobarbital Sodium (Antihistamines have additive effects with CNS depressants). Products include:
Seconal Sodium Pulvules 1529

Selegiline Hydrochloride (Prolongs and intensifies the anticholinergic effects of antihistamines; may enhance the effect of phenylpropanolamine; concurrent and/or sequential use is contraindicated). Products include:
Eldepryl Capsules 2729

Sevoflurane (Antihistamines have additive effects with CNS depressants).
No products indexed under this heading.

Sodium Nitroprusside (Sympathomimetics may reduce the effects of antihypertensive drugs).
No products indexed under this heading.

Sotalol Hydrochloride (Sympathomimetics may reduce the effects of antihypertensive drugs). Products include:
Betapace Tablets 637

Spirapril Hydrochloride (Sympathomimetics may reduce the effects of antihypertensive drugs).
No products indexed under this heading.

Sufentanil Citrate (Antihistamines have additive effects with CNS depressants). Products include:
Sufenta Injection 1355

Temazepam (Antihistamines have additive effects with CNS depressants). Products include:
Restoril Capsules 2413

Terazosin Hydrochloride (Sympathomimetics may reduce the effects of antihypertensive drugs). Products include:
Hytrin Capsules 434

Thiamylal Sodium (Antihistamines have additive effects with CNS depressants).
No products indexed under this heading.

Thioridazine Hydrochloride (Antihistamines have additive effects with CNS depressants). Products include:
Mellaril 2398

Thiothixene (Antihistamines have additive effects with CNS depressants). Products include:
Navane Capsules and Concentrate 2018
Navane Intramuscular 2019

Timolol Maleate (Sympathomimetics may reduce the effects of antihypertensive drugs). Products include:
Blocadren Tablets 1654
Timolide Tablets 1791
Timoptic in Ocudose 1796
Timoptic Sterile Ophthalmic Solution 1794
Timoptic-XE 1798

Torsemide (Sympathomimetics may reduce the effects of antihypertensive drugs). Products include:
Demadex Tablets and Injection 691

Tranylcypromine Sulfate (Prolongs and intensifies the anticholinergic effects of antihistamines; may enhance the effect of phenylpropanolamine; concurrent and/or sequential use is contraindicated). Products include:
Parnate Tablets 2679

Triazolam (Antihistamines have additive effects with CNS depressants). Products include:
Halcion Tablets 2093

Trifluoperazine Hydrochloride (Antihistamines have additive effects with CNS depressants). Products include:
Stelazine 2692

Trimethaphan Camsylate (Sympathomimetics may reduce the effects of antihypertensive drugs).
No products indexed under this heading.

Verapamil Hydrochloride (Sympathomimetics may reduce the effects of antihypertensive drugs). Products include:
Calan SR Caplets 2571
Calan Tablets 2568
Covera-HS Tablets 2573
Isoptin Injectable 1391
Isoptin Oral Tablets 1393
Isoptin SR Tablets 1395
Verelan Capsules 1455

Zolpidem Tartrate (Antihistamines have additive effects with CNS depressants). Products include:
Ambien Tablets 2559

Food Interactions

Alcohol (Antihistamines have additive effects with alcohol).

DIMETANE-DX COUGH SYRUP
(Brompheniramine Maleate, Pseudoephedrine Hydrochloride, Dextromethorphan Hydrobromide) 2233
May interact with monoamine oxidase inhibitors, central nervous system depressants, and antihypertensives. Compounds in these categories include:

Acebutolol Hydrochloride (Decreased antihypertensive effect). Products include:
Sectral Capsules 2914

Alfentanil Hydrochloride (Additive effect). Products include:
Alfenta Injection 1334

Alprazolam (Additive effect). Products include:
Xanax Tablets 2115

Amlodipine Besylate (Decreased antihypertensive effect). Products include:
Lotrel Capsules 858
Norvasc Tablets 2020

Aprobarbital (Additive effect).
No products indexed under this heading.

Atenolol (Decreased antihypertensive effect). Products include:
Tenoretic Tablets 2963
Tenormin Tablets and I.V. Injection 2965

Benazepril Hydrochloride (Decreased antihypertensive effect). Products include:
Lotensin Tablets 852
Lotensin HCT Tablets 855
Lotrel Capsules 858

Bendroflumethiazide (Decreased antihypertensive effect).
No products indexed under this heading.

Betaxolol Hydrochloride (Decreased antihypertensive effect). Products include:
Betoptic Ophthalmic Solution 465
Betoptic S Ophthalmic Suspension 467
Kerlone Tablets 2588

Bisoprolol Fumarate (Decreased antihypertensive effect). Products include:
Zebeta Tablets 1457
Ziac 1459

Buprenorphine (Additive effect). Products include:
Buprenex Injectable 2170

Buspirone Hydrochloride (Additive effect). Products include:
BuSpar Tablets 738

Butabarbital (Additive effect).
No products indexed under this heading.

Butalbital (Additive effect). Products include:
Axocet Capsules 2469
Esgic-plus Capsules 1012
Esgic-plus Tablets 1012
Fioricet Tablets 2386
Fioricet with Codeine Capsules 2387
Fiorinal Capsules 2388
Fiorinal with Codeine Capsules 2390
Fiorinal Tablets 2388
Phrenilin 790
Sedapap Tablets 50 mg/650 mg 1826

Captopril (Decreased antihypertensive effect). Products include:
Capoten Tablets 740
Capozide Tablets 744

Carteolol Hydrochloride (Decreased antihypertensive effect). Products include:
Cartrol Tablets 413
Ocupress Ophthalmic Solution, 1% Sterile ..... ⊛ 297

Chlordiazepoxide (Additive effect). Products include:
Limbitrol 2333

Chlordiazepoxide Hydrochloride (Additive effect). Products include:
Librax Capsules 2330
Librium Capsules 2331
Librium Injectable 2332

Chlorothiazide (Decreased antihypertensive effect). Products include:
Aldoclor Tablets 1638
Diupres Tablets 1691
Diuril Oral 1694

Chlorothiazide Sodium (Decreased antihypertensive effect). Products include:
Diuril Sodium Intravenous 1693

Chlorpromazine (Additive effect). Products include:
Thorazine Suppositories 2701

Chlorprothixene (Additive effect).
No products indexed under this heading.

Chlorprothixene Hydrochloride (Additive effect).
No products indexed under this heading.

Chlorprothixene Lactate (Additive effect).
No products indexed under this heading.

Chlorthalidone (Decreased antihypertensive effect). Products include:
Combipres Tablets 682
Tenoretic Tablets 2963
Thalitone 1293

Clonidine (Decreased antihypertensive effect). Products include:
Catapres-TTS 680

Clonidine Hydrochloride (Decreased antihypertensive effect). Products include:
Catapres Tablets 679
Combipres Tablets 682

Clorazepate Dipotassium (Additive effect). Products include:
Tranxene 459

Clozapine (Additive effect). Products include:
Clozaril Tablets 2377

Codeine Phosphate (Additive effect). Products include:
Brontex 2130
Dimetane-DC Cough Syrup 2232
Fioricet with Codeine Capsules 2387
Fiorinal with Codeine Capsules 2390
Nucofed 2225
Phenergan with Codeine 2883
Phenergan VC with Codeine 2888
Robitussin A-C Syrup 2248
Robitussin-DAC Syrup 2249
Ryna ..... ▣ 804
Soma Compound w/Codeine Tablets 2784
Tylenol with Codeine 1592

Deserpidine (Decreased antihypertensive effect).
No products indexed under this heading.

Desflurane (Additive effect). Products include:
Suprane (desflurane, USP) 1865

Dezocine (Additive effect). Products include:
Dalgan Injection 529

Diazepam (Additive effect). Products include:
Dizac (diazepam injectable emulsion) CIV 1862
Valium Injectable 2336
Valium Tablets 2335

Diazoxide (Decreased antihypertensive effect). Products include:
Hyperstat I.V. Injection 2504
Proglycem 575

Diltiazem Hydrochloride (Decreased antihypertensive effect). Products include:
Cardizem CD Capsules 1251
Cardizem SR Capsules 1255
Cardizem Injectable 1253
Cardizem Tablets 1257

(▣ Described in PDR For Nonprescription Drugs) (⊛ Described in PDR For Ophthalmology)

Interactions Index

Dilacor XR Extended-release Capsules 2183
Tiazac Capsules 1019

Doxazosin Mesylate (Decreased antihypertensive effect). Products include:
Cardura Tablets 1993

Droperidol (Additive effect). Products include:
Inapsine Injection 462

Enalapril Maleate (Decreased antihypertensive effect). Products include:
Vaseretic Tablets 1810
Vasotec Tablets 1816

Enalaprilat (Decreased antihypertensive effect). Products include:
Vasotec I.V. 1814

Enflurane (Additive effect).
No products indexed under this heading.

Esmolol Hydrochloride (Decreased antihypertensive effect). Products include:
Brevibloc (esmolol HCl) Injection 1860

Estazolam (Additive effect). Products include:
ProSom Tablets 457

Ethchlorvynol (Additive effect). Products include:
Placidyl Capsules 456

Ethinamate (Additive effect).
No products indexed under this heading.

Felodipine (Decreased antihypertensive effect). Products include:
Plendil Extended-Release Tablets 514

Fentanyl (Additive effect). Products include:
Duragesic Transdermal System 1336

Fentanyl Citrate (Additive effect). Products include:
Sublimaze Injection 463

Fluphenazine Decanoate (Additive effect). Products include:
Prolixin Decanoate 510

Fluphenazine Enanthate (Additive effect). Products include:
Prolixin Enanthate 510

Fluphenazine Hydrochloride (Additive effect). Products include:
Prolixin 510

Flurazepam Hydrochloride (Additive effect). Products include:
Dalmane Capsules 2329

Fosinopril Sodium (Decreased antihypertensive effect). Products include:
Monopril Tablets 762

Furazolidone (Prolonged anticholinergic effect). Products include:
Furoxone 2221

Furosemide (Decreased antihypertensive effect). Products include:
Lasix Injection, Oral Solution and Tablets 1267

Glutethimide (Additive effect).
No products indexed under this heading.

Guanabenz Acetate (Decreased antihypertensive effect).
No products indexed under this heading.

Guanethidine Monosulfate (Decreased antihypertensive effect). Products include:
Esimil Tablets 840
Ismelin Tablets 845

Haloperidol (Additive effect). Products include:
Haldol Injection, Tablets and Concentrate 1585

Haloperidol Decanoate (Additive effect). Products include:
Haldol Decanoate 1587

Hydralazine Hydrochloride (Decreased antihypertensive effect). Products include:
Apresazide Capsules 824
Apresoline Hydrochloride Tablets 826
Hydralazine Hydrochloride Injection USP 2712
Ser-Ap-Es Tablets 867

Hydrochlorothiazide (Decreased antihypertensive effect). Products include:
Aldactazide Tablets 2556
Aldoril Tablets 1644
Apresazide Capsules 824
Capozide Tablets 744
Dyazide Capsules 2653
Esidrix Tablets 839
Esimil Tablets 840
HydroDIURIL Tablets 1716
Hydropres Tablets 1718
Hyzaar Tablets 1720
Inderide Tablets 2838
Inderide LA Long Acting Capsules 2840
Lopressor HCT Tablets 850
Lotensin HCT Tablets 855
Moduretic Tablets 1748
Oretic Tablets 450
Prinzide Tablets 1780
Ser-Ap-Es Tablets 867
Timolide Tablets 1791
Vaseretic Tablets 1810
Zestoretic Tablets 2968
Ziac 1459

Hydrocodone Bitartrate (Additive effect). Products include:
Codiclear DH Syrup 808
Duratuss HD Elixir 2750
Histussin D Liquid 670
Hycodan Tablets and Syrup 946
Hycomine Compound Tablets 948
Hycomine 947
Hycotuss Expectorant Syrup 950
Hydrocet Capsules 787
Lorcet 10/650 Tablets 1016
Lortab 2751
Tussend 1830
Tussend Expectorant 1831
Vicodin Tablets 1404
Vicodin ES Tablets 1405
Vicodin HP Tablets 1403
Vicodin Tuss Expectorant 1406
Zydone Capsules 967

Hydrocodone Polistirex (Additive effect). Products include:
Tussionex Pennkinetic Extended-Release Suspension 1624

Hydroflumethiazide (Decreased antihypertensive effect). Products include:
Diucardin Tablets 2824

Hydroxyzine Hydrochloride (Additive effect). Products include:
Atarax Tablets & Syrup 1992
Marax Tablets & DF Syrup 2015
Vistaril Intramuscular Solution 2042

Indapamide (Decreased antihypertensive effect).
No products indexed under this heading.

Isocarboxazid (Prolonged anticholinergic effect).
No products indexed under this heading.

Isoflurane (Additive effect).
No products indexed under this heading.

Isradipine (Decreased antihypertensive effect). Products include:
DynaCirc Capsules 2381
DynaCirc CR Tablets 2383

Ketamine Hydrochloride (Additive effect).
No products indexed under this heading.

Labetalol Hydrochloride (Decreased antihypertensive effect). Products include:
Normodyne Injection 2519
Normodyne Tablets 2522
Trandate 1158

Levomethadyl Acetate Hydrochloride (Additive effect). Products include:
Orlaam Oral Solution 2361

Levorphanol Tartrate (Additive effect). Products include:
Levo-Dromoran 2297

Lisinopril (Decreased antihypertensive effect). Products include:
Prinivil Tablets 1776
Prinzide Tablets 1780
Zestoretic Tablets 2968
Zestril Tablets 2972

Lorazepam (Additive effect). Products include:
Ativan Injection 2805
Ativan Tablets 2807

Losartan Potassium (Decreased antihypertensive effect). Products include:
Cozaar Tablets 1668
Hyzaar Tablets 1720

Loxapine Hydrochloride (Additive effect). Products include:
Loxitane 1426

Loxapine Succinate (Additive effect). Products include:
Loxitane Capsules 1426

Mecamylamine Hydrochloride (Decreased antihypertensive effect). Products include:
Inversine Tablets 1729

Meperidine Hydrochloride (Additive effect). Products include:
Demerol 2438
Mepergan Injection 2859

Mephobarbital (Additive effect). Products include:
Mebaral Tablets 2452

Meprobamate (Additive effect). Products include:
Miltown Tablets 2780
PMB 200 and PMB 400 2890

Mesoridazine Besylate (Additive effect). Products include:
Serentil 689

Methadone Hydrochloride (Additive effect). Products include:
Methadone Hydrochloride Oral Concentrate 2356
Methadone Hydrochloride Oral Solution & Tablets 2357

Methohexital Sodium (Additive effect).
No products indexed under this heading.

Methotrimeprazine (Additive effect). Products include:
Levoprome 1321

Methoxyflurane (Additive effect).
No products indexed under this heading.

Methyclothiazide (Decreased antihypertensive effect). Products include:
Enduron Tablets 424

Methyldopa (Decreased antihypertensive effect). Products include:
Aldoclor Tablets 1638
Aldomet Oral 1640
Aldoril Tablets 1644

Methyldopate Hydrochloride (Decreased antihypertensive effect). Products include:
Aldomet Ester HCl Injection 1642

Metolazone (Decreased antihypertensive effect). Products include:
Mykrox Tablets 1617
Zaroxolyn Tablets 1625

Metoprolol Succinate (Decreased antihypertensive effect). Products include:
Toprol-XL Tablets 560

Metoprolol Tartrate (Decreased antihypertensive effect). Products include:
Lopressor 848
Lopressor HCT Tablets 850

Metyrosine (Decreased antihypertensive effect). Products include:
Demser Capsules 1690

Midazolam Hydrochloride (Additive effect). Products include:
Versed Injection 2324

Minoxidil (Decreased antihypertensive effect).
No products indexed under this heading.

Moexipril Hydrochloride (Decreased antihypertensive effect). Products include:
Univasc Tablets 2553

Molindone Hydrochloride (Additive effect). Products include:
Moban Tablets and Concentrate 1036

Morphine Sulfate (Additive effect). Products include:
Astramorph/PF Injection, USP (Preservative-Free) 526
Duramorph Injection 983
Infumorph 200 and Infumorph 500 Sterile Solutions 985
Kadian Capsules 2948
MS Contin Tablets 2149
MSIR 2152
Oramorph SR (Morphine Sulfate Sustained Release Tablets) 2359
RMS Suppositories CII 2766
Roxanol 2365

Nadolol (Decreased antihypertensive effect).
No products indexed under this heading.

Nicardipine Hydrochloride (Decreased antihypertensive effect). Products include:
Cardene Capsules 2261
Cardene I.V. 2815
Cardene SR Capsules 2264

Nifedipine (Decreased antihypertensive effect). Products include:
Adalat Capsules (10 mg and 20 mg) 580
Adalat CC 582
Procardia Capsules 2024
Procardia XL Extended Release Tablets 2026

Nisoldipine (Decreased antihypertensive effect). Products include:
Sular Tablets 2961

Nitroglycerin (Decreased antihypertensive effect). Products include:
Deponit NTG Transdermal Delivery System 2541
Nitro-Bid IV 1270
Nitro-Bid Ointment 1272
Nitro-Dur (nitroglycerin) Transdermal Infusion System 1365
Nitrolingual Spray 2193
Nitrostat Tablets 1981
Transderm-Nitro Transdermal Therapeutic System 878

Opium Alkaloids (Additive effect).
No products indexed under this heading.

Oxazepam (Additive effect). Products include:
Serax Capsules 2916
Serax Tablets 2916

Oxycodone Hydrochloride (Additive effect). Products include:
OxyContin Tablets 2163
OxyIR Capsules 2167
Percocet Tablets 955
Percodan Tablets 955
Percodan-Demi Tablets 956
Roxicodone Tablets, Oral Solution & Intensol (Oxycodone) 2366
Tylox Capsules 1593

Penbutolol Sulfate (Decreased antihypertensive effect). Products include:
Levatol Tablets 2547

Pentobarbital Sodium (Additive effect). Products include:
Nembutal Sodium Capsules 440
Nembutal Sodium Solution 442
Nembutal Sodium Suppositories 444

Perphenazine (Additive effect). Products include:
Etrafon 2495
Triavil Tablets 1800
Trilafon 2532

IMPORTANT NOTE: Always consult each drug listing in the patient's regimen for possible interactions.

Dimetane-DX | Interactions Index | 302

Phenelzine Sulfate (Prolonged anticholinergic effect). Products include:
Nardil 1977

Phenobarbital (Additive effect). Products include:
Arco-Lase Plus Tablets 513
Bellergal-S Tablets 2375
Donnatal 2234
Donnatal Extentabs 2234
Donnatal Tablets 2234
Phenobarbital Elixir and Tablets 1523
Quadrinal Tablets 1398

Phenoxybenzamine Hydrochloride (Decreased antihypertensive effect). Products include:
Dibenzyline Capsules 2650

Phentolamine Mesylate (Decreased antihypertensive effect). Products include:
Regitine Vials 864

Pindolol (Decreased antihypertensive effect). Products include:
Visken Tablets 2428

Polythiazide (Decreased antihypertensive effect). Products include:
Minizide Capsules 2016

Prazepam (Additive effect).
No products indexed under this heading.

Prazosin Hydrochloride (Decreased antihypertensive effect). Products include:
Minipress Capsules 2015
Minizide Capsules 2016

Prochlorperazine (Additive effect). Products include:
Compazine 2644

Promethazine Hydrochloride (Additive effect). Products include:
Mepergan Injection 2859
Phenergan with Codeine 2883
Phenergan with Dextromethorphan 2885
Phenergan Injection 2880
Phenergan Suppositories 2882
Phenergan Syrup 2881
Phenergan Tablets 2882
Phenergan VC 2886
Phenergan VC with Codeine 2888

Propofol (Additive effect). Products include:
Diprivan Injectable Emulsion 2939

Propoxyphene Hydrochloride (Additive effect). Products include:
Darvon 1475
Wygesic Tablets 2930

Propoxyphene Napsylate (Additive effect). Products include:
Darvon-N/Darvocet-N 1473

Propranolol Hydrochloride (Decreased antihypertensive effect). Products include:
Inderal 2834
Inderal LA Long Acting Capsules 2836
Inderide Tablets 2838
Inderide LA Long Acting Capsules 2840

Quazepam (Additive effect). Products include:
Doral Tablets 2773

Quinapril Hydrochloride (Decreased antihypertensive effect). Products include:
Accupril Tablets 1950

Ramipril (Decreased antihypertensive effect). Products include:
Altace Capsules 1238

Rauwolfia Serpentina (Decreased antihypertensive effect).
No products indexed under this heading.

Rescinnamine (Decreased antihypertensive effect).
No products indexed under this heading.

Reserpine (Decreased antihypertensive effect). Products include:
Diupres Tablets 1691
Hydropres Tablets 1718
Ser-Ap-Es Tablets 867

Risperidone (Additive effect). Products include:
Risperdal Tablets 1348

Secobarbital Sodium (Additive effect). Products include:
Seconal Sodium Pulvules 1529

Selegiline Hydrochloride (Prolonged anticholinergic effect). Products include:
Eldepryl Capsules 2729

Sevoflurane (Additive effect).
No products indexed under this heading.

Sodium Nitroprusside (Decreased antihypertensive effect).
No products indexed under this heading.

Sotalol Hydrochloride (Decreased antihypertensive effect). Products include:
Betapace Tablets 637

Spirapril Hydrochloride (Decreased antihypertensive effect).
No products indexed under this heading.

Sufentanil Citrate (Additive effect). Products include:
Sufenta Injection 1355

Temazepam (Additive effect). Products include:
Restoril Capsules 2413

Terazosin Hydrochloride (Decreased antihypertensive effect). Products include:
Hytrin Capsules 434

Thiamylal Sodium (Additive effect).
No products indexed under this heading.

Thioridazine Hydrochloride (Additive effect). Products include:
Mellaril 2398

Thiothixene (Additive effect). Products include:
Navane Capsules and Concentrate 2018
Navane Intramuscular 2019

Timolol Maleate (Decreased antihypertensive effect). Products include:
Blocadren Tablets 1654
Timolide Tablets 1791
Timoptic in Ocudose 1796
Timoptic Sterile Ophthalmic Solution 1794
Timoptic-XE 1798

Torsemide (Decreased antihypertensive effect). Products include:
Demadex Tablets and Injection 691

Tranylcypromine Sulfate (Prolonged anticholinergic effect). Products include:
Parnate Tablets 2679

Triazolam (Additive effect). Products include:
Halcion Tablets 2093

Trifluoperazine Hydrochloride (Additive effect). Products include:
Stelazine 2692

Trimethaphan Camsylate (Decreased antihypertensive effect).
No products indexed under this heading.

Verapamil Hydrochloride (Decreased antihypertensive effect). Products include:
Calan SR Caplets 2571
Calan Tablets 2568
Covera-HS Tablets 2573
Isoptin Injectable 1391
Isoptin Oral Tablets 1393
Isoptin SR Tablets 1395
Verelan Capsules 1455

Zolpidem Tartrate (Additive effect). Products include:
Ambien Tablets 2559

Food Interactions

Alcohol (Additive effect).

DIMETAPP ALLERGY DYE-FREE ELIXIR
(Brompheniramine Maleate) ▣ 838
May interact with hypnotics and sedatives, tranquilizers, and certain other agents. Compounds in these categories include:

Alprazolam (May increase drowsiness effect). Products include:
Xanax Tablets 2115

Buspirone Hydrochloride (May increase drowsiness effect). Products include:
BuSpar Tablets 738

Chlordiazepoxide (May increase drowsiness effect). Products include:
Limbitrol 2333

Chlordiazepoxide Hydrochloride (May increase drowsiness effect). Products include:
Librax Capsules 2330
Librium Capsules 2331
Librium Injectable 2332

Chlorpromazine (May increase drowsiness effect). Products include:
Thorazine Suppositories 2701

Chlorpromazine Hydrochloride (May increase drowsiness effect). Products include:
Thorazine 2701

Chlorprothixene (May increase drowsiness effect).
No products indexed under this heading.

Chlorprothixene Hydrochloride (May increase drowsiness effect).
No products indexed under this heading.

Clorazepate Dipotassium (May increase drowsiness effect). Products include:
Tranxene 459

Diazepam (May increase drowsiness effect). Products include:
Dizac (diazepam injectable emulsion) CIV 1862
Valium Injectable 2336
Valium Tablets 2335

Droperidol (May increase drowsiness effect). Products include:
Inapsine Injection 462

Estazolam (May increase drowsiness effect). Products include:
ProSom Tablets 457

Ethchlorvynol (May increase drowsiness effect). Products include:
Placidyl Capsules 456

Ethinamate (May increase drowsiness effect).
No products indexed under this heading.

Fluphenazine Decanoate (May increase drowsiness effect). Products include:
Prolixin Decanoate 510

Fluphenazine Enanthate (May increase drowsiness effect). Products include:
Prolixin Enanthate 510

Fluphenazine Hydrochloride (May increase drowsiness effect). Products include:
Prolixin 510

Flurazepam Hydrochloride (May increase drowsiness effect). Products include:
Dalmane Capsules 2329

Glutethimide (May increase drowsiness effect).
No products indexed under this heading.

Haloperidol (May increase drowsiness effect). Products include:
Haldol Injection, Tablets and Concentrate 1585

Haloperidol Decanoate (May increase drowsiness effect). Products include:
Haldol Decanoate 1587

Hydroxyzine Hydrochloride (May increase drowsiness effect). Products include:
Atarax Tablets & Syrup 1992
Marax Tablets & DF Syrup 2015
Vistaril Intramuscular Solution 2042

Lorazepam (May increase drowsiness effect). Products include:
Ativan Injection 2805
Ativan Tablets 2807

Loxapine Hydrochloride (May increase drowsiness effect). Products include:
Loxitane 1426

Loxapine Succinate (May increase drowsiness effect). Products include:
Loxitane Capsules 1426

Meprobamate (May increase drowsiness effect). Products include:
Miltown Tablets 2780
PMB 200 and PMB 400 2890

Mesoridazine Besylate (May increase drowsiness effect). Products include:
Serentil 689

Midazolam Hydrochloride (May increase drowsiness effect). Products include:
Versed Injection 2324

Molindone Hydrochloride (May increase drowsiness effect). Products include:
Moban Tablets and Concentrate 1036

Oxazepam (May increase drowsiness effect). Products include:
Serax Capsules 2916
Serax Tablets 2916

Perphenazine (May increase drowsiness effect). Products include:
Etrafon 2495
Triavil Tablets 1800
Trilafon 2532

Prazepam (May increase drowsiness effect).
No products indexed under this heading.

Prochlorperazine (May increase drowsiness effect). Products include:
Compazine 2644

Promethazine Hydrochloride (May increase drowsiness effect). Products include:
Mepergan Injection 2859
Phenergan with Codeine 2883
Phenergan with Dextromethorphan 2885
Phenergan Injection 2880
Phenergan Suppositories 2882
Phenergan Syrup 2881
Phenergan Tablets 2882
Phenergan VC 2886
Phenergan VC with Codeine 2888

Propofol (May increase drowsiness effect). Products include:
Diprivan Injectable Emulsion 2939

Quazepam (May increase drowsiness effect). Products include:
Doral Tablets 2773

Secobarbital Sodium (May increase drowsiness effect). Products include:
Seconal Sodium Pulvules 1529

Temazepam (May increase drowsiness effect). Products include:
Restoril Capsules 2413

Thioridazine Hydrochloride (May increase drowsiness effect). Products include:
Mellaril 2398

Thiothixene (May increase drowsiness effect). Products include:
Navane Capsules and Concentrate 2018
Navane Intramuscular 2019

(▣ Described in PDR For Nonprescription Drugs) (◉ Described in PDR For Ophthalmology)

Triazolam (May increase drowsiness effect). Products include:
Halcion Tablets ... 2093
Trifluoperazine Hydrochloride (May increase drowsiness effect). Products include:
Stelazine ... 2692
Zolpidem Tartrate (May increase drowsiness effect). Products include:
Ambien Tablets ... 2559

Food Interactions

Alcohol (May increase drowsiness effect).

DIMETAPP ALLERGY SINUS CAPLETS

(Acetaminophen, Brompheniramine Maleate, Phenylpropanolamine Hydrochloride) ... 838
May interact with monoamine oxidase inhibitors, tranquilizers, hypnotics and sedatives, and certain other agents. Compounds in these categories include:

Alprazolam (May increase drowsiness effect). Products include:
Xanax Tablets ... 2115
Buspirone Hydrochloride (May increase drowsiness effect). Products include:
BuSpar Tablets ... 738
Chlordiazepoxide (May increase drowsiness effect). Products include:
Limbitrol ... 2333
Chlordiazepoxide Hydrochloride (May increase drowsiness effect). Products include:
Librax Capsules ... 2330
Librium Capsules ... 2331
Librium Injectable ... 2332
Chlorpromazine (May increase drowsiness effect). Products include:
Thorazine Suppositories ... 2701
Chlorpromazine Hydrochloride (May increase drowsiness effect). Products include:
Thorazine ... 2701
Chlorprothixene (May increase drowsiness effect).
No products indexed under this heading.
Chlorprothixene Hydrochloride (May increase drowsiness effect).
No products indexed under this heading.
Clorazepate Dipotassium (May increase drowsiness effect). Products include:
Tranxene ... 459
Diazepam (May increase drowsiness effect). Products include:
Dizac (diazepam injectable emulsion) CIV ... 1862
Valium Injectable ... 2336
Valium Tablets ... 2335
Droperidol (May increase drowsiness effect). Products include:
Inapsine Injection ... 462
Estazolam (May increase drowsiness effect). Products include:
ProSom Tablets ... 457
Ethchlorvynol (May increase drowsiness effect). Products include:
Placidyl Capsules ... 456
Ethinamate (May increase drowsiness effect).
No products indexed under this heading.
Fluphenazine Decanoate (May increase drowsiness effect). Products include:
Prolixin Decanoate ... 510
Fluphenazine Enanthate (May increase drowsiness effect). Products include:
Prolixin Enanthate ... 510
Fluphenazine Hydrochloride (May increase drowsiness effect). Products include:
Prolixin ... 510
Flurazepam Hydrochloride (May increase drowsiness effect). Products include:
Dalmane Capsules ... 2329
Furazolidone (Concurrent and/or sequential use is not recommended). Products include:
Furoxone ... 2221
Glutethimide (May increase drowsiness effect).
No products indexed under this heading.
Haloperidol (May increase drowsiness effect). Products include:
Haldol Injection, Tablets and Concentrate ... 1585
Haloperidol Decanoate (May increase drowsiness effect). Products include:
Haldol Decanoate ... 1587
Hydroxyzine Hydrochloride (May increase drowsiness effect). Products include:
Atarax Tablets & Syrup ... 1992
Marax Tablets & DF Syrup ... 2015
Vistaril Intramuscular Solution ... 2042
Isocarboxazid (Concurrent and/or sequential use is not recommended).
No products indexed under this heading.
Lorazepam (May increase drowsiness effect). Products include:
Ativan Injection ... 2805
Ativan Tablets ... 2807
Loxapine Hydrochloride (May increase drowsiness effect). Products include:
Loxitane ... 1426
Loxapine Succinate (May increase drowsiness effect). Products include:
Loxitane Capsules ... 1426
Meprobamate (May increase drowsiness effect). Products include:
Miltown Tablets ... 2780
PMB 200 and PMB 400 ... 2890
Mesoridazine Besylate (May increase drowsiness effect). Products include:
Serentil ... 689
Midazolam Hydrochloride (May increase drowsiness effect). Products include:
Versed Injection ... 2324
Molindone Hydrochloride (May increase drowsiness effect). Products include:
Moban Tablets and Concentrate ... 1036
Oxazepam (May increase drowsiness effect). Products include:
Serax Capsules ... 2916
Serax Tablets ... 2916
Perphenazine (May increase drowsiness effect). Products include:
Etrafon ... 2495
Triavil Tablets ... 1800
Trilafon ... 2532
Phenelzine Sulfate (Concurrent and/or sequential use is not recommended). Products include:
Nardil ... 1977
Prazepam (May increase drowsiness effect).
No products indexed under this heading.
Prochlorperazine (May increase drowsiness effect). Products include:
Compazine ... 2644
Promethazine Hydrochloride (May increase drowsiness effect). Products include:
Mepergan Injection ... 2859
Phenergan with Codeine ... 2883
Phenergan with Dextromethorphan 2885
Phenergan Injection ... 2880
Phenergan Suppositories ... 2882
Phenergan Syrup ... 2881
Phenergan Tablets ... 2882
Phenergan VC ... 2886
Phenergan VC with Codeine ... 2888
Propofol (May increase drowsiness effect). Products include:
Diprivan Injectable Emulsion ... 2939
Quazepam (May increase drowsiness effect). Products include:
Doral Tablets ... 2773
Secobarbital Sodium (May increase drowsiness effect). Products include:
Seconal Sodium Pulvules ... 1529
Selegiline Hydrochloride (Concurrent and/or sequential use is not recommended). Products include:
Eldepryl Capsules ... 2729
Temazepam (May increase drowsiness effect). Products include:
Restoril Capsules ... 2413
Thioridazine Hydrochloride (May increase drowsiness effect). Products include:
Mellaril ... 2398
Thiothixene (May increase drowsiness effect). Products include:
Navane Capsules and Concentrate 2018
Navane Intramuscular ... 2019
Tranylcypromine Sulfate (Concurrent and/or sequential use is not recommended). Products include:
Parnate Tablets ... 2679
Triazolam (May increase drowsiness effect). Products include:
Halcion Tablets ... 2093
Trifluoperazine Hydrochloride (May increase drowsiness effect). Products include:
Stelazine ... 2692
Zolpidem Tartrate (May increase drowsiness effect). Products include:
Ambien Tablets ... 2559

Food Interactions

Alcohol (May increase drowsiness effect).

DIMETAPP COLD & ALLERGY CHEWABLE TABLETS

(Brompheniramine Maleate, Phenylpropanolamine Hydrochloride) ... 838
May interact with hypnotics and sedatives, monoamine oxidase inhibitors, and tranquilizers. Compounds in these categories include:

Alprazolam (May increase drowsiness effect). Products include:
Xanax Tablets ... 2115
Buspirone Hydrochloride (May increase drowsiness effect). Products include:
BuSpar Tablets ... 738
Chlordiazepoxide (May increase drowsiness effect). Products include:
Limbitrol ... 2333
Chlordiazepoxide Hydrochloride (May increase drowsiness effect). Products include:
Librax Capsules ... 2330
Librium Capsules ... 2331
Librium Injectable ... 2332
Chlorpromazine (May increase drowsiness effect). Products include:
Thorazine Suppositories ... 2701
Chlorpromazine Hydrochloride (May increase drowsiness effect). Products include:
Thorazine ... 2701
Chlorprothixene (May increase drowsiness effect).
No products indexed under this heading.
Chlorprothixene Hydrochloride (May increase drowsiness effect).
No products indexed under this heading.
Clorazepate Dipotassium (May increase drowsiness effect). Products include:
Tranxene ... 459
Diazepam (May increase drowsiness effect). Products include:
Dizac (diazepam injectable emulsion) CIV ... 1862
Valium Injectable ... 2336
Valium Tablets ... 2335
Droperidol (May increase drowsiness effect). Products include:
Inapsine Injection ... 462
Estazolam (May increase drowsiness effect). Products include:
ProSom Tablets ... 457
Ethchlorvynol (May increase drowsiness effect). Products include:
Placidyl Capsules ... 456
Ethinamate (May increase drowsiness effect).
No products indexed under this heading.
Fluphenazine Decanoate (May increase drowsiness effect). Products include:
Prolixin Decanoate ... 510
Fluphenazine Enanthate (May increase drowsiness effect). Products include:
Prolixin Enanthate ... 510
Fluphenazine Hydrochloride (May increase drowsiness effect). Products include:
Prolixin ... 510
Flurazepam Hydrochloride (May increase drowsiness effect). Products include:
Dalmane Capsules ... 2329
Furazolidone (Concurrent and/or sequential use is not recommended). Products include:
Furoxone ... 2221
Glutethimide (May increase drowsiness effect).
No products indexed under this heading.
Haloperidol (May increase drowsiness effect). Products include:
Haldol Injection, Tablets and Concentrate ... 1585
Haloperidol Decanoate (May increase drowsiness effect). Products include:
Haldol Decanoate ... 1587
Hydroxyzine Hydrochloride (May increase drowsiness effect). Products include:
Atarax Tablets & Syrup ... 1992
Marax Tablets & DF Syrup ... 2015
Vistaril Intramuscular Solution ... 2042
Isocarboxazid (Concurrent and/or sequential use is not recommended).
No products indexed under this heading.
Lorazepam (May increase drowsiness effect). Products include:
Ativan Injection ... 2805
Ativan Tablets ... 2807
Loxapine Hydrochloride (May increase drowsiness effect). Products include:
Loxitane ... 1426
Loxapine Succinate (May increase drowsiness effect). Products include:
Loxitane Capsules ... 1426
Meprobamate (May increase drowsiness effect). Products include:
Miltown Tablets ... 2780
PMB 200 and PMB 400 ... 2890

IMPORTANT NOTE: Always consult each drug listing in the patient's regimen for possible interactions.

Mesoridazine Besylate (May increase drowsiness effect). Products include:
- Serentil ... 689

Midazolam Hydrochloride (May increase drowsiness effect). Products include:
- Versed Injection ... 2324

Molindone Hydrochloride (May increase drowsiness effect). Products include:
- Moban Tablets and Concentrate ... 1036

Oxazepam (May increase drowsiness effect). Products include:
- Serax Capsules ... 2916
- Serax Tablets ... 2916

Perphenazine (May increase drowsiness effect). Products include:
- Etrafon ... 2495
- Triavil Tablets ... 1800
- Trilafon ... 2532

Phenelzine Sulfate (Concurrent and/or sequential use is not recommended). Products include:
- Nardil ... 1977

Prazepam (May increase drowsiness effect).
- No products indexed under this heading.

Prochlorperazine (May increase drowsiness effect). Products include:
- Compazine ... 2644

Promethazine Hydrochloride (May increase drowsiness effect). Products include:
- Mepergan Injection ... 2859
- Phenergan with Codeine ... 2883
- Phenergan with Dextromethorphan 2885
- Phenergan Injection ... 2880
- Phenergan Suppositories ... 2882
- Phenergan Syrup ... 2881
- Phenergan Tablets ... 2882
- Phenergan VC ... 2886
- Phenergan VC with Codeine ... 2888

Propofol (May increase drowsiness effect). Products include:
- Diprivan Injectable Emulsion ... 2939

Quazepam (May increase drowsiness effect). Products include:
- Doral Tablets ... 2773

Secobarbital Sodium (May increase drowsiness effect). Products include:
- Seconal Sodium Pulvules ... 1529

Selegiline Hydrochloride (Concurrent and/or sequential use is not recommended). Products include:
- Eldepryl Capsules ... 2729

Temazepam (May increase drowsiness effect). Products include:
- Restoril Capsules ... 2413

Thioridazine Hydrochloride (May increase drowsiness effect). Products include:
- Mellaril ... 2398

Thiothixene (May increase drowsiness effect). Products include:
- Navane Capsules and Concentrate 2018
- Navane Intramuscular ... 2019

Tranylcypromine Sulfate (Concurrent and/or sequential use is not recommended). Products include:
- Parnate Tablets ... 2679

Triazolam (May increase drowsiness effect). Products include:
- Halcion Tablets ... 2093

Trifluoperazine Hydrochloride (May increase drowsiness effect). Products include:
- Stelazine ... 2692

Zolpidem Tartrate (May increase drowsiness effect). Products include:
- Ambien Tablets ... 2559

DIMETAPP COLD & COUGH LIQUI-GELS

(Brompheniramine Maleate, Dextromethorphan Hydrobromide, Phenylpropanolamine Hydrochloride) ... ⊞ 839

May interact with monoamine oxidase inhibitors, tranquilizers, hypnotics and sedatives, and certain other agents. Compounds in these categories include:

Alprazolam (May increase drowsiness effect). Products include:
- Xanax Tablets ... 2115

Buspirone Hydrochloride (May increase drowsiness effect). Products include:
- BuSpar Tablets ... 738

Chlordiazepoxide (May increase drowsiness effect). Products include:
- Limbitrol ... 2333

Chlordiazepoxide Hydrochloride (May increase drowsiness effect). Products include:
- Librax Capsules ... 2330
- Librium Capsules ... 2331
- Librium Injectable ... 2332

Chlorpromazine (May increase drowsiness effect). Products include:
- Thorazine Suppositories ... 2701

Chlorpromazine Hydrochloride (May increase drowsiness effect). Products include:
- Thorazine ... 2701

Chlorprothixene (May increase drowsiness effect).
- No products indexed under this heading.

Chlorprothixene Hydrochloride (May increase drowsiness effect).
- No products indexed under this heading.

Clorazepate Dipotassium (May increase drowsiness effect). Products include:
- Tranxene ... 459

Diazepam (May increase drowsiness effect). Products include:
- Dizac (diazepam injectable emulsion) CIV ... 1862
- Valium Injectable ... 2336
- Valium Tablets ... 2335

Droperidol (May increase drowsiness effect). Products include:
- Inapsine Injection ... 462

Estazolam (May increase drowsiness effect). Products include:
- ProSom Tablets ... 457

Ethchlorvynol (May increase drowsiness effect). Products include:
- Placidyl Capsules ... 456

Ethinamate (May increase drowsiness effect).
- No products indexed under this heading.

Fluphenazine Decanoate (May increase drowsiness effect). Products include:
- Prolixin Decanoate ... 510

Fluphenazine Enanthate (May increase drowsiness effect). Products include:
- Prolixin Enanthate ... 510

Fluphenazine Hydrochloride (May increase drowsiness effect). Products include:
- Prolixin ... 510

Flurazepam Hydrochloride (May increase drowsiness effect). Products include:
- Dalmane Capsules ... 2329

Furazolidone (Concurrent and/or sequential use is not recommended). Products include:
- Furoxone ... 2221

Glutethimide (May increase drowsiness effect).
- No products indexed under this heading.

Haloperidol (May increase drowsiness effect). Products include:
- Haldol Injection, Tablets and Concentrate ... 1585

Haloperidol Decanoate (May increase drowsiness effect). Products include:
- Haldol Decanoate ... 1587

Hydroxyzine Hydrochloride (May increase drowsiness effect). Products include:
- Atarax Tablets & Syrup ... 1992
- Marax Tablets & DF Syrup ... 2015
- Vistaril Intramuscular Solution ... 2042

Isocarboxazid (Concurrent and/or sequential use is not recommended).
- No products indexed under this heading.

Lorazepam (May increase drowsiness effect). Products include:
- Ativan Injection ... 2805
- Ativan Tablets ... 2807

Loxapine Hydrochloride (May increase drowsiness effect). Products include:
- Loxitane ... 1426

Loxapine Succinate (May increase drowsiness effect). Products include:
- Loxitane Capsules ... 1426

Meprobamate (May increase drowsiness effect). Products include:
- Miltown Tablets ... 2780
- PMB 200 and PMB 400 ... 2890

Mesoridazine Besylate (May increase drowsiness effect). Products include:
- Serentil ... 689

Midazolam Hydrochloride (May increase drowsiness effect). Products include:
- Versed Injection ... 2324

Molindone Hydrochloride (May increase drowsiness effect). Products include:
- Moban Tablets and Concentrate ... 1036

Oxazepam (May increase drowsiness effect). Products include:
- Serax Capsules ... 2916
- Serax Tablets ... 2916

Perphenazine (May increase drowsiness effect). Products include:
- Etrafon ... 2495
- Triavil Tablets ... 1800
- Trilafon ... 2532

Phenelzine Sulfate (Concurrent and/or sequential use is not recommended). Products include:
- Nardil ... 1977

Prazepam (May increase drowsiness effect).
- No products indexed under this heading.

Prochlorperazine (May increase drowsiness effect). Products include:
- Compazine ... 2644

Promethazine Hydrochloride (May increase drowsiness effect). Products include:
- Mepergan Injection ... 2859
- Phenergan with Codeine ... 2883
- Phenergan with Dextromethorphan 2885
- Phenergan Injection ... 2880
- Phenergan Suppositories ... 2882
- Phenergan Syrup ... 2881
- Phenergan Tablets ... 2882
- Phenergan VC ... 2886
- Phenergan VC with Codeine ... 2888

Propofol (May increase drowsiness effect). Products include:
- Diprivan Injectable Emulsion ... 2939

Quazepam (May increase drowsiness effect). Products include:
- Doral Tablets ... 2773

Secobarbital Sodium (May increase drowsiness effect). Products include:
- Seconal Sodium Pulvules ... 1529

Selegiline Hydrochloride (Concurrent and/or sequential use is not recommended). Products include:
- Eldepryl Capsules ... 2729

Temazepam (May increase drowsiness effect). Products include:
- Restoril Capsules ... 2413

Thioridazine Hydrochloride (May increase drowsiness effect). Products include:
- Mellaril ... 2398

Thiothixene (May increase drowsiness effect). Products include:
- Navane Capsules and Concentrate 2018
- Navane Intramuscular ... 2019

Tranylcypromine Sulfate (Concurrent and/or sequential use is not recommended). Products include:
- Parnate Tablets ... 2679

Triazolam (May increase drowsiness effect). Products include:
- Halcion Tablets ... 2093

Trifluoperazine Hydrochloride (May increase drowsiness effect). Products include:
- Stelazine ... 2692

Zolpidem Tartrate (May increase drowsiness effect). Products include:
- Ambien Tablets ... 2559

Food Interactions

Alcohol (May increase drowsiness effect).

DIMETAPP COLD & FEVER SUSPENSION

(Acetaminophen, Brompheniramine Maleate, Pseudoephedrine Hydrochloride) ... ⊞ 839

May interact with monoamine oxidase inhibitors, hypnotics and sedatives, tranquilizers, and certain other agents. Compounds in these categories include:

Alprazolam (May increase drowsiness effect). Products include:
- Xanax Tablets ... 2115

Buspirone Hydrochloride (May increase drowsiness effect). Products include:
- BuSpar Tablets ... 738

Chlordiazepoxide (May increase drowsiness effect). Products include:
- Limbitrol ... 2333

Chlordiazepoxide Hydrochloride (May increase drowsiness effect). Products include:
- Librax Capsules ... 2330
- Librium Capsules ... 2331
- Librium Injectable ... 2332

Chlorpromazine (May increase drowsiness effect). Products include:
- Thorazine Suppositories ... 2701

Chlorpromazine Hydrochloride (May increase drowsiness effect). Products include:
- Thorazine ... 2701

Chlorprothixene (May increase drowsiness effect).
- No products indexed under this heading.

Chlorprothixene Hydrochloride (May increase drowsiness effect).
- No products indexed under this heading.

Clorazepate Dipotassium (May increase drowsiness effect). Products include:
- Tranxene ... 459

Diazepam (May increase drowsiness effect). Products include:
- Dizac (diazepam injectable emulsion) CIV ... 1862
- Valium Injectable ... 2336

(⊞ Described in PDR For Nonprescription Drugs) (◉ Described in PDR For Ophthalmology)

305 **Interactions Index** **Dimetapp DM**

Valium Tablets ... 2335

Droperidol (May increase drowsiness effect). Products include:

Inapsine Injection ... 462

Estazolam (May increase drowsiness effect). Products include:

ProSom Tablets ... 457

Ethchlorvynol (May increase drowsiness effect). Products include:

Placidyl Capsules ... 456

Ethinamate (May increase drowsiness effect).

No products indexed under this heading.

Fluphenazine Decanoate (May increase drowsiness effect). Products include:

Prolixin Decanoate ... 510

Fluphenazine Enanthate (May increase drowsiness effect). Products include:

Prolixin Enanthate ... 510

Fluphenazine Hydrochloride (May increase drowsiness effect). Products include:

Prolixin ... 510

Flurazepam Hydrochloride (May increase drowsiness effect). Products include:

Dalmane Capsules ... 2329

Furazolidone (Concurrent and/or sequential use is not recommended). Products include:

Furoxone ... 2221

Glutethimide (May increase drowsiness effect).

No products indexed under this heading.

Haloperidol (May increase drowsiness effect). Products include:

Haldol Injection, Tablets and Concentrate ... 1585

Haloperidol Decanoate (May increase drowsiness effect). Products include:

Haldol Decanoate ... 1587

Hydroxyzine Hydrochloride (May increase drowsiness effect). Products include:

Atarax Tablets & Syrup ... 1992
Marax Tablets & DF Syrup ... 2015
Vistaril Intramuscular Solution ... 2042

Isocarboxazid (Concurrent and/or sequential use is not recommended).

No products indexed under this heading.

Lorazepam (May increase drowsiness effect). Products include:

Ativan Injection ... 2805
Ativan Tablets ... 2807

Loxapine Hydrochloride (May increase drowsiness effect). Products include:

Loxitane ... 1426

Loxapine Succinate (May increase drowsiness effect). Products include:

Loxitane Capsules ... 1426

Meprobamate (May increase drowsiness effect). Products include:

Miltown Tablets ... 2780
PMB 200 and PMB 400 ... 2890

Mesoridazine Besylate (May increase drowsiness effect). Products include:

Serentil ... 689

Midazolam Hydrochloride (May increase drowsiness effect). Products include:

Versed Injection ... 2324

Molindone Hydrochloride (May increase drowsiness effect). Products include:

Moban Tablets and Concentrate ... 1036

Oxazepam (May increase drowsiness effect). Products include:

Serax Capsules ... 2916
Serax Tablets ... 2916

Perphenazine (May increase drowsiness effect). Products include:

Etrafon ... 2495
Triavil Tablets ... 1800
Trilafon ... 2532

Phenelzine Sulfate (Concurrent and/or sequential use is not recommended). Products include:

Nardil ... 1977

Prazepam (May increase drowsiness effect).

No products indexed under this heading.

Prochlorperazine (May increase drowsiness effect). Products include:

Compazine ... 2644

Promethazine Hydrochloride (May increase drowsiness effect). Products include:

Mepergan Injection ... 2859
Phenergan with Codeine ... 2883
Phenergan with Dextromethorphan ... 2885
Phenergan Injection ... 2880
Phenergan Suppositories ... 2882
Phenergan Syrup ... 2881
Phenergan Tablets ... 2882
Phenergan VC ... 2886
Phenergan VC with Codeine ... 2888

Propofol (May increase drowsiness effect). Products include:

Diprivan Injectable Emulsion ... 2939

Quazepam (May increase drowsiness effect). Products include:

Doral Tablets ... 2773

Secobarbital Sodium (May increase drowsiness effect). Products include:

Seconal Sodium Pulvules ... 1529

Selegiline Hydrochloride (Concurrent and/or sequential use is not recommended). Products include:

Eldepryl Capsules ... 2729

Temazepam (May increase drowsiness effect). Products include:

Restoril Capsules ... 2413

Thioridazine Hydrochloride (May increase drowsiness effect). Products include:

Mellaril ... 2398

Thiothixene (May increase drowsiness effect). Products include:

Navane Capsules and Concentrate ... 2018
Navane Intramuscular ... 2019

Tranylcypromine Sulfate (Concurrent and/or sequential use is not recommended). Products include:

Parnate Tablets ... 2679

Triazolam (May increase drowsiness effect). Products include:

Halcion Tablets ... 2093

Trifluoperazine Hydrochloride (May increase drowsiness effect). Products include:

Stelazine ... 2692

Zolpidem Tartrate (May increase drowsiness effect). Products include:

Ambien Tablets ... 2559

Food Interactions

Alcohol (May increase drowsiness effect).

DIMETAPP DECONGESTANT PEDIATRIC DROPS

(Pseudoephedrine Hydrochloride) .. ⊞ 840

May interact with monoamine oxidase inhibitors. Compounds in this category include:

Furazolidone (Concurrent and/or sequential use is not recommended). Products include:

Furoxone ... 2221

Isocarboxazid (Concurrent and/or sequential use is not recommended).

No products indexed under this heading.

Phenelzine Sulfate (Concurrent and/or sequential use is not recommended). Products include:

Nardil ... 1977

Selegiline Hydrochloride (Concurrent and/or sequential use is not recommended). Products include:

Eldepryl Capsules ... 2729

Tranylcypromine Sulfate (Concurrent and/or sequential use is not recommended). Products include:

Parnate Tablets ... 2679

DIMETAPP DM ELIXIR

(Brompheniramine Maleate, Dextromethorphan Hydrobromide) ⊞ 840

May interact with monoamine oxidase inhibitors, tranquilizers, hypnotics and sedatives, and certain other agents. Compounds in these categories include:

Alprazolam (Increases drowsiness effect). Products include:

Xanax Tablets ... 2115

Buspirone Hydrochloride (Increases drowsiness effect). Products include:

BuSpar Tablets ... 738

Chlordiazepoxide (Increases drowsiness effect). Products include:

Limbitrol ... 2333

Chlordiazepoxide Hydrochloride (Increases drowsiness effect). Products include:

Librax Capsules ... 2330
Librium Capsules ... 2331
Librium Injectable ... 2332

Chlorpromazine (Increases drowsiness effect). Products include:

Thorazine Suppositories ... 2701

Chlorpromazine Hydrochloride (Increases drowsiness effect). Products include:

Thorazine ... 2701

Chlorprothixene (Increases drowsiness effect).

No products indexed under this heading.

Chlorprothixene Hydrochloride (Increases drowsiness effect).

No products indexed under this heading.

Clorazepate Dipotassium (Increases drowsiness effect). Products include:

Tranxene ... 459

Diazepam (Increases drowsiness effect). Products include:

Dizac (diazepam injectable emulsion) CIV ... 1862
Valium Injectable ... 2336
Valium Tablets ... 2335

Droperidol (Increases drowsiness effect). Products include:

Inapsine Injection ... 462

Estazolam (Increases drowsiness effect). Products include:

ProSom Tablets ... 457

Ethchlorvynol (Increases drowsiness effect). Products include:

Placidyl Capsules ... 456

Ethinamate (Increases drowsiness effect).

No products indexed under this heading.

Fluphenazine Decanoate (Increases drowsiness effect). Products include:

Prolixin Decanoate ... 510

Fluphenazine Enanthate (Increases drowsiness effect). Products include:

Prolixin Enanthate ... 510

Fluphenazine Hydrochloride (Increases drowsiness effect). Products include:

Prolixin ... 510

Flurazepam Hydrochloride (Increases drowsiness effect). Products include:

Dalmane Capsules ... 2329

Furazolidone (Concurrent and/or sequential use is contraindicated). Products include:

Furoxone ... 2221

Glutethimide (Increases drowsiness effect).

No products indexed under this heading.

Haloperidol (Increases drowsiness effect). Products include:

Haldol Injection, Tablets and Concentrate ... 1585

Haloperidol Decanoate (Increases drowsiness effect). Products include:

Haldol Decanoate ... 1587

Hydroxyzine Hydrochloride (Increases drowsiness effect). Products include:

Atarax Tablets & Syrup ... 1992
Marax Tablets & DF Syrup ... 2015
Vistaril Intramuscular Solution ... 2042

Isocarboxazid (Concurrent and/or sequential use is contraindicated).

No products indexed under this heading.

Lorazepam (Increases drowsiness effect). Products include:

Ativan Injection ... 2805
Ativan Tablets ... 2807

Loxapine Hydrochloride (Increases drowsiness effect). Products include:

Loxitane ... 1426

Loxapine Succinate (Increases drowsiness effect). Products include:

Loxitane Capsules ... 1426

Meprobamate (Increases drowsiness effect). Products include:

Miltown Tablets ... 2780
PMB 200 and PMB 400 ... 2890

Mesoridazine Besylate (Increases drowsiness effect). Products include:

Serentil ... 689

Midazolam Hydrochloride (Increases drowsiness effect). Products include:

Versed Injection ... 2324

Molindone Hydrochloride (Increases drowsiness effect). Products include:

Moban Tablets and Concentrate ... 1036

Oxazepam (Increases drowsiness effect). Products include:

Serax Capsules ... 2916
Serax Tablets ... 2916

Perphenazine (Increases drowsiness effect). Products include:

Etrafon ... 2495
Triavil Tablets ... 1800
Trilafon ... 2532

Phenelzine Sulfate (Concurrent and/or sequential use is contraindicated). Products include:

Nardil ... 1977

Prazepam (Increases drowsiness effect).

No products indexed under this heading.

Prochlorperazine (Increases drowsiness effect). Products include:

Compazine ... 2644

Promethazine Hydrochloride (Increases drowsiness effect). Products include:

Mepergan Injection ... 2859
Phenergan with Codeine ... 2883
Phenergan with Dextromethorphan ... 2885
Phenergan Injection ... 2880
Phenergan Suppositories ... 2882
Phenergan Syrup ... 2881
Phenergan Tablets ... 2882
Phenergan VC ... 2886
Phenergan VC with Codeine ... 2888

IMPORTANT NOTE: Always consult each drug listing in the patient's regimen for possible interactions.

Propofol (Increases drowsiness effect). Products include:
- Diprivan Injectable Emulsion 2939

Quazepam (Increases drowsiness effect). Products include:
- Doral Tablets 2773

Secobarbital Sodium (Increases drowsiness effect). Products include:
- Seconal Sodium Pulvules 1529

Selegiline Hydrochloride (Concurrent and/or sequential use is contraindicated). Products include:
- Eldepryl Capsules 2729

Temazepam (Increases drowsiness effect). Products include:
- Restoril Capsules 2413

Thioridazine Hydrochloride (Increases drowsiness effect). Products include:
- Mellaril 2398

Thiothixene (Increases drowsiness effect). Products include:
- Navane Capsules and Concentrate 2018
- Navane Intramuscular 2019

Tranylcypromine Sulfate (Concurrent and/or sequential use is contraindicated). Products include:
- Parnate Tablets 2679

Triazolam (Increases drowsiness effect). Products include:
- Halcion Tablets 2093

Trifluoperazine Hydrochloride (Increases drowsiness effect). Products include:
- Stelazine 2692

Zolpidem Tartrate (Increases drowsiness effect). Products include:
- Ambien Tablets 2559

Food Interactions

Alcohol (Increases drowsiness effect; avoid concurrent use).

DIMETAPP ELIXIR
(Brompheniramine Maleate, Phenylpropanolamine Hydrochloride) .... ▣ 840
May interact with monoamine oxidase inhibitors, hypnotics and sedatives, tranquilizers, and certain other agents. Compounds in these categories include:

Alprazolam (May increase drowsiness effect). Products include:
- Xanax Tablets 2115

Buspirone Hydrochloride (May increase drowsiness effect). Products include:
- BuSpar Tablets 738

Chlordiazepoxide (May increase drowsiness effect). Products include:
- Limbitrol 2333

Chlordiazepoxide Hydrochloride (May increase drowsiness effect). Products include:
- Librax Capsules 2330
- Librium Capsules 2331
- Librium Injectable 2332

Chlorpromazine (May increase drowsiness effect). Products include:
- Thorazine Suppositories 2701

Chlorpromazine Hydrochloride (May increase drowsiness effect). Products include:
- Thorazine 2701

Chlorprothixene (May increase drowsiness effect).
- No products indexed under this heading.

Chlorprothixene Hydrochloride (May increase drowsiness effect).
- No products indexed under this heading.

Clorazepate Dipotassium (May increase drowsiness effect). Products include:
- Tranxene 459

Diazepam (May increase drowsiness effect). Products include:
- Dizac (diazepam injectable emulsion) CIV 1862
- Valium Injectable 2336
- Valium Tablets 2335

Droperidol (May increase drowsiness effect). Products include:
- Inapsine Injection 462

Estazolam (May increase drowsiness effect). Products include:
- ProSom Tablets 457

Ethchlorvynol (May increase drowsiness effect). Products include:
- Placidyl Capsules 456

Ethinamate (May increase drowsiness effect).
- No products indexed under this heading.

Fluphenazine Decanoate (May increase drowsiness effect). Products include:
- Prolixin Decanoate 510

Fluphenazine Enanthate (May increase drowsiness effect). Products include:
- Prolixin Enanthate 510

Fluphenazine Hydrochloride (May increase drowsiness effect). Products include:
- Prolixin 510

Flurazepam Hydrochloride (May increase drowsiness effect). Products include:
- Dalmane Capsules 2329

Furazolidone (Concurrent and/or sequential use is not recommended). Products include:
- Furoxone 2221

Glutethimide (May increase drowsiness effect).
- No products indexed under this heading.

Haloperidol (May increase drowsiness effect). Products include:
- Haldol Injection, Tablets and Concentrate 1585

Haloperidol Decanoate (May increase drowsiness effect). Products include:
- Haldol Decanoate 1587

Hydroxyzine Hydrochloride (May increase drowsiness effect). Products include:
- Atarax Tablets & Syrup 1992
- Marax Tablets & DF Syrup 2015
- Vistaril Intramuscular Solution 2042

Isocarboxazid (Concurrent and/or sequential use is not recommended).
- No products indexed under this heading.

Lorazepam (May increase drowsiness effect). Products include:
- Ativan Injection 2805
- Ativan Tablets 2807

Loxapine Hydrochloride (May increase drowsiness effect). Products include:
- Loxitane 1426

Loxapine Succinate (May increase drowsiness effect). Products include:
- Loxitane Capsules 1426

Meprobamate (May increase drowsiness effect). Products include:
- Miltown Tablets 2780
- PMB 200 and PMB 400 2890

Mesoridazine Besylate (May increase drowsiness effect). Products include:
- Serentil 689

Midazolam Hydrochloride (May increase drowsiness effect). Products include:
- Versed Injection 2324

Molindone Hydrochloride (May increase drowsiness effect). Products include:
- Moban Tablets and Concentrate 1036

Oxazepam (May increase drowsiness effect). Products include:
- Serax Capsules 2916
- Serax Tablets 2916

Perphenazine (May increase drowsiness effect). Products include:
- Etrafon 2495
- Triavil Tablets 1800
- Trilafon 2532

Phenelzine Sulfate (Concurrent and/or sequential use is not recommended). Products include:
- Nardil 1977

Prazepam (May increase drowsiness effect).
- No products indexed under this heading.

Prochlorperazine (May increase drowsiness effect). Products include:
- Compazine 2644

Promethazine Hydrochloride (May increase drowsiness effect). Products include:
- Mepergan Injection 2859
- Phenergan with Codeine 2883
- Phenergan with Dextromethorphan 2885
- Phenergan Injection 2880
- Phenergan Suppositories 2882
- Phenergan Syrup 2881
- Phenergan Tablets 2882
- Phenergan VC 2886
- Phenergan VC with Codeine 2888

Propofol (May increase drowsiness effect). Products include:
- Diprivan Injectable Emulsion 2939

Quazepam (May increase drowsiness effect). Products include:
- Doral Tablets 2773

Secobarbital Sodium (May increase drowsiness effect). Products include:
- Seconal Sodium Pulvules 1529

Selegiline Hydrochloride (Concurrent and/or sequential use is not recommended). Products include:
- Eldepryl Capsules 2729

Temazepam (May increase drowsiness effect). Products include:
- Restoril Capsules 2413

Thioridazine Hydrochloride (May increase drowsiness effect). Products include:
- Mellaril 2398

Thiothixene (May increase drowsiness effect). Products include:
- Navane Capsules and Concentrate 2018
- Navane Intramuscular 2019

Tranylcypromine Sulfate (Concurrent and/or sequential use is not recommended). Products include:
- Parnate Tablets 2679

Triazolam (May increase drowsiness effect). Products include:
- Halcion Tablets 2093

Trifluoperazine Hydrochloride (May increase drowsiness effect). Products include:
- Stelazine 2692

Zolpidem Tartrate (May increase drowsiness effect). Products include:
- Ambien Tablets 2559

Food Interactions

Alcohol (May increase drowsiness effect).

DIMETAPP EXTENTABS
(Brompheniramine Maleate, Phenylpropanolamine Hydrochloride) .... ▣ 841
May interact with monoamine oxidase inhibitors, hypnotics and sedatives, tranquilizers, and certain other agents. Compounds in these categories include:

Alprazolam (May increase drowsiness effect). Products include:
- Xanax Tablets 2115

Buspirone Hydrochloride (May increase drowsiness effect). Products include:
- BuSpar Tablets 738

Chlordiazepoxide (May increase drowsiness effect). Products include:
- Limbitrol 2333

Chlordiazepoxide Hydrochloride (May increase drowsiness effect). Products include:
- Librax Capsules 2330
- Librium Capsules 2331
- Librium Injectable 2332

Chlorpromazine (May increase drowsiness effect). Products include:
- Thorazine Suppositories 2701

Chlorpromazine Hydrochloride (May increase drowsiness effect). Products include:
- Thorazine 2701

Chlorprothixene (May increase drowsiness effect).
- No products indexed under this heading.

Chlorprothixene Hydrochloride (May increase drowsiness effect).
- No products indexed under this heading.

Clorazepate Dipotassium (May increase drowsiness effect). Products include:
- Tranxene 459

Diazepam (May increase drowsiness effect). Products include:
- Dizac (diazepam injectable emulsion) CIV 1862
- Valium Injectable 2336
- Valium Tablets 2335

Droperidol (May increase drowsiness effect). Products include:
- Inapsine Injection 462

Estazolam (May increase drowsiness effect). Products include:
- ProSom Tablets 457

Ethchlorvynol (May increase drowsiness effect). Products include:
- Placidyl Capsules 456

Ethinamate (May increase drowsiness effect).
- No products indexed under this heading.

Fluphenazine Decanoate (May increase drowsiness effect). Products include:
- Prolixin Decanoate 510

Fluphenazine Enanthate (May increase drowsiness effect). Products include:
- Prolixin Enanthate 510

Fluphenazine Hydrochloride (May increase drowsiness effect). Products include:
- Prolixin 510

Flurazepam Hydrochloride (May increase drowsiness effect). Products include:
- Dalmane Capsules 2329

Furazolidone (Concurrent and/or sequential use is not recommended). Products include:
- Furoxone 2221

Glutethimide (May increase drowsiness effect).
- No products indexed under this heading.

Haloperidol (May increase drowsiness effect). Products include:
- Haldol Injection, Tablets and Concentrate 1585

(▣ Described in PDR For Nonprescription Drugs) (◉ Described in PDR For Ophthalmology)

307 **Interactions Index** **Dipentum**

Haloperidol Decanoate (May increase drowsiness effect). Products include:

Haldol Decanoate ... 1587

Hydroxyzine Hydrochloride (May increase drowsiness effect). Products include:

Atarax Tablets & Syrup ... 1992
Marax Tablets & DF Syrup ... 2015
Vistaril Intramuscular Solution ... 2042

Isocarboxazid (Concurrent and/or sequential use is not recommended).

No products indexed under this heading.

Lorazepam (May increase drowsiness effect). Products include:

Ativan Injection ... 2805
Ativan Tablets ... 2807

Loxapine Hydrochloride (May increase drowsiness effect). Products include:

Loxitane ... 1426

Loxapine Succinate (May increase drowsiness effect). Products include:

Loxitane Capsules ... 1426

Meprobamate (May increase drowsiness effect). Products include:

Miltown Tablets ... 2780
PMB 200 and PMB 400 ... 2890

Mesoridazine Besylate (May increase drowsiness effect). Products include:

Serentil ... 689

Midazolam Hydrochloride (May increase drowsiness effect). Products include:

Versed Injection ... 2324

Molindone Hydrochloride (May increase drowsiness effect). Products include:

Moban Tablets and Concentrate ... 1036

Oxazepam (May increase drowsiness effect). Products include:

Serax Capsules ... 2916
Serax Tablets ... 2916

Perphenazine (May increase drowsiness effect). Products include:

Etrafon ... 2495
Triavil Tablets ... 1800
Trilafon ... 2532

Phenelzine Sulfate (Concurrent and/or sequential use is not recommended). Products include:

Nardil ... 1977

Prazepam (May increase drowsiness effect).

No products indexed under this heading.

Prochlorperazine (May increase drowsiness effect). Products include:

Compazine ... 2644

Promethazine Hydrochloride (May increase drowsiness effect). Products include:

Mepergan Injection ... 2859
Phenergan with Codeine ... 2883
Phenergan with Dextromethorphan 2885
Phenergan Injection ... 2880
Phenergan Suppositories ... 2882
Phenergan Syrup ... 2881
Phenergan Tablets ... 2882
Phenergan VC ... 2886
Phenergan VC with Codeine ... 2888

Propofol (May increase drowsiness effect). Products include:

Diprivan Injectable Emulsion ... 2939

Quazepam (May increase drowsiness effect). Products include:

Doral Tablets ... 2773

Secobarbital Sodium (May increase drowsiness effect). Products include:

Seconal Sodium Pulvules ... 1529

Selegiline Hydrochloride (Concurrent and/or sequential use is not recommended). Products include:

Eldepryl Capsules ... 2729

Temazepam (May increase drowsiness effect). Products include:

Restoril Capsules ... 2413

Thioridazine Hydrochloride (May increase drowsiness effect). Products include:

Mellaril ... 2398

Thiothixene (May increase drowsiness effect). Products include:

Navane Capsules and Concentrate 2018
Navane Intramuscular ... 2019

Tranylcypromine Sulfate (Concurrent and/or sequential use is not recommended). Products include:

Parnate Tablets ... 2679

Triazolam (May increase drowsiness effect). Products include:

Halcion Tablets ... 2093

Trifluoperazine Hydrochloride (May increase drowsiness effect). Products include:

Stelazine ... 2692

Zolpidem Tartrate (May increase drowsiness effect). Products include:

Ambien Tablets ... 2559

Food Interactions

Alcohol (May increase drowsiness effect).

DIMETAPP LIQUI-GELS

(Brompheniramine Maleate, Phenylpropanolamine Hydrochloride) ... 841

May interact with hypnotics and sedatives, tranquilizers, monoamine oxidase inhibitors, and certain other agents. Compounds in these categories include:

Alprazolam (Increases drowsiness effect). Products include:

Xanax Tablets ... 2115

Buspirone Hydrochloride (Increases drowsiness effect). Products include:

BuSpar Tablets ... 738

Chlordiazepoxide (Increases drowsiness effect). Products include:

Limbitrol ... 2333

Chlordiazepoxide Hydrochloride (Increases drowsiness effect). Products include:

Librax Capsules ... 2330
Librium Capsules ... 2331
Librium Injectable ... 2332

Chlorpromazine (Increases drowsiness effect). Products include:

Thorazine Suppositories ... 2701

Chlorpromazine Hydrochloride (Increases drowsiness effect). Products include:

Thorazine ... 2701

Chlorprothixene (Increases drowsiness effect).

No products indexed under this heading.

Chlorprothixene Hydrochloride (Increases drowsiness effect).

No products indexed under this heading.

Clorazepate Dipotassium (Increases drowsiness effect). Products include:

Tranxene ... 459

Diazepam (Increases drowsiness effect). Products include:

Dizac (diazepam injectable emulsion) CIV ... 1862
Valium Injectable ... 2336
Valium Tablets ... 2335

Droperidol (Increases drowsiness effect). Products include:

Inapsine Injection ... 462

Estazolam (Increases drowsiness effect). Products include:

ProSom Tablets ... 457

Ethchlorvynol (Increases drowsiness effect). Products include:

Placidyl Capsules ... 456

Ethinamate (Increases drowsiness effect).

No products indexed under this heading.

Fluphenazine Decanoate (Increases drowsiness effect). Products include:

Prolixin Decanoate ... 510

Fluphenazine Enanthate (Increases drowsiness effect). Products include:

Prolixin Enanthate ... 510

Fluphenazine Hydrochloride (Increases drowsiness effect). Products include:

Prolixin ... 510

Flurazepam Hydrochloride (Increases drowsiness effect). Products include:

Dalmane Capsules ... 2329

Furazolidone (Concurrent and/or sequential use is contraindicated). Products include:

Furoxone ... 2221

Glutethimide (Increases drowsiness effect).

No products indexed under this heading.

Haloperidol (Increases drowsiness effect). Products include:

Haldol Injection, Tablets and Concentrate ... 1585

Haloperidol Decanoate (Increases drowsiness effect). Products include:

Haldol Decanoate ... 1587

Hydroxyzine Hydrochloride (Increases drowsiness effect). Products include:

Atarax Tablets & Syrup ... 1992
Marax Tablets & DF Syrup ... 2015
Vistaril Intramuscular Solution ... 2042

Isocarboxazid (Concurrent and/or sequential use is contraindicated).

No products indexed under this heading.

Lorazepam (Increases drowsiness effect). Products include:

Ativan Injection ... 2805
Ativan Tablets ... 2807

Loxapine Hydrochloride (Increases drowsiness effect). Products include:

Loxitane ... 1426

Loxapine Succinate (Increases drowsiness effect). Products include:

Loxitane Capsules ... 1426

Meprobamate (Increases drowsiness effect). Products include:

Miltown Tablets ... 2780
PMB 200 and PMB 400 ... 2890

Mesoridazine Besylate (Increases drowsiness effect). Products include:

Serentil ... 689

Midazolam Hydrochloride (Increases drowsiness effect). Products include:

Versed Injection ... 2324

Molindone Hydrochloride (Increases drowsiness effect). Products include:

Moban Tablets and Concentrate ... 1036

Oxazepam (Increases drowsiness effect). Products include:

Serax Capsules ... 2916
Serax Tablets ... 2916

Perphenazine (Increases drowsiness effect). Products include:

Etrafon ... 2495
Triavil Tablets ... 1800
Trilafon ... 2532

Phenelzine Sulfate (Concurrent and/or sequential use is contraindicated). Products include:

Nardil ... 1977

Prazepam (Increases drowsiness effect).

No products indexed under this heading.

Prochlorperazine (Increases drowsiness effect). Products include:

Compazine ... 2644

Promethazine Hydrochloride (Increases drowsiness effect). Products include:

Mepergan Injection ... 2859
Phenergan with Codeine ... 2883
Phenergan with Dextromethorphan 2885
Phenergan Injection ... 2880
Phenergan Suppositories ... 2882
Phenergan Syrup ... 2881
Phenergan Tablets ... 2882
Phenergan VC ... 2886
Phenergan VC with Codeine ... 2888

Propofol (Increases drowsiness effect). Products include:

Diprivan Injectable Emulsion ... 2939

Quazepam (Increases drowsiness effect). Products include:

Doral Tablets ... 2773

Secobarbital Sodium (Increases drowsiness effect). Products include:

Seconal Sodium Pulvules ... 1529

Selegiline Hydrochloride (Concurrent and/or sequential use is contraindicated). Products include:

Eldepryl Capsules ... 2729

Temazepam (Increases drowsiness effect). Products include:

Restoril Capsules ... 2413

Thioridazine Hydrochloride (Increases drowsiness effect). Products include:

Mellaril ... 2398

Thiothixene (Increases drowsiness effect). Products include:

Navane Capsules and Concentrate 2018
Navane Intramuscular ... 2019

Tranylcypromine Sulfate (Concurrent and/or sequential use is contraindicated). Products include:

Parnate Tablets ... 2679

Triazolam (Increases drowsiness effect). Products include:

Halcion Tablets ... 2093

Trifluoperazine Hydrochloride (Increases drowsiness effect). Products include:

Stelazine ... 2692

Zolpidem Tartrate (Increases drowsiness effect). Products include:

Ambien Tablets ... 2559

Food Interactions

Alcohol (Increases drowsiness effect; avoid concurrent use).

DIMETAPP TABLETS

(Brompheniramine Maleate, Phenylpropanolamine Hydrochloride) ... 841

See Dimetapp Liqui-Gels

DIPENTUM CAPSULES

(Olsalazine Sodium) ... 2084

May interact with oral anticoagulants. Compounds in this category include:

Dicumarol (Potential for increased prothrombin time).

No products indexed under this heading.

Warfarin Sodium (Potential for increased prothrombin time). Products include:

Coumadin ... 941

IMPORTANT NOTE: Always consult each drug listing in the patient's regimen for possible interactions.

DIPHTHERIA & TETANUS TOXOIDS ADSORBED PUROGENATED
(Diphtheria & Tetanus Toxoids Adsorbed, (For Pediatric Use)) 1422
None cited in PDR database.

DIPHTHERIA AND TETANUS TOXOIDS AND PERTUSSIS VACCINE ADSORBED
(Diphtheria & Tetanus Toxoids and Pertussis Vaccine Adsorbed) 2650
May interact with immunosuppressive agents, corticosteroids, cytotoxic drugs, alkylating agents, anticoagulants, and certain other agents. Compounds in these categories include:

Azathioprine (Reduces response to active immunization procedure). Products include:
Azathioprine Tablets 2349
Imuran 1103

Betamethasone Acetate (Reduces response to active immunization procedure). Products include:
Celestone Soluspan Suspension 2484

Betamethasone Sodium Phosphate (Reduces response to active immunization procedure). Products include:
Celestone Soluspan Suspension 2484

Bleomycin Sulfate (Reduces response to active immunization procedure). Products include:
Blenoxane 697

Busulfan (Reduces response to active immunization procedure). Products include:
Myleran Tablets 1209

Carmustine (BCNU) (Reduces response to active immunization procedure). Products include:
BiCNU 696

Chlorambucil (Reduces response to active immunization procedure). Products include:
Leukeran Tablets 1205

Cortisone Acetate (Reduces response to active immunization procedure). Products include:
Cortone Acetate Sterile Suspension 1663
Cortone Acetate Tablets 1664

Cyclophosphamide (Reduces response to active immunization procedure). Products include:
Cytoxan 700

Cyclosporine (Reduces response to active immunization procedure). Products include:
Neoral 2405
Sandimmune 2416

Dacarbazine (Reduces response to active immunization procedure). Products include:
DTIC-Dome 593

Dalteparin Sodium (Caution should be exercised). Products include:
Fragmin Injection 2088

Daunorubicin Hydrochloride (Reduces response to active immunization procedure). Products include:
Cerubidine for Injection 634

Dexamethasone (Reduces response to active immunization procedure). Products include:
AK-Trol Ointment & Suspension .... ⊙ 205
Decadron Elixir 1676
Decadron Tablets 1678
Decaspray Topical Aerosol 1689
Maxitrol Ophthalmic Ointment and Suspension .... ⊙ 222
TobraDex Ophthalmic Suspension and Ointment 469

Dexamethasone Acetate (Reduces response to active immunization procedure). Products include:
Dalalone D.P. Injectable 1009
Decadron-LA Sterile Suspension 1687

Dexamethasone Sodium Phosphate (Reduces response to active immunization procedure). Products include:
Decadron Phosphate Injection 1680
Decadron Phosphate Sterile Ophthalmic Ointment 1684
Decadron Phosphate Sterile Ophthalmic Solution 1685
Decadron Phosphate Topical Cream 1686
Decadron Phosphate with Xylocaine Injection, Sterile 1683
Dexacort Phosphate in Respihaler .. 1606
Dexacort Phosphate in Turbinaire .. 1607
NeoDecadron Sterile Ophthalmic Ointment 1755
NeoDecadron Sterile Ophthalmic Solution 1756
NeoDecadron Topical Cream 1757

Dicumarol (Caution should be exercised).
No products indexed under this heading.

Doxorubicin Hydrochloride (Reduces response to active immunization procedure). Products include:
Adriamycin PFS 2056
Adriamycin RDF 2056
Doxil 2613
Doxorubicin Astra 531
Rubex for Injection 721

Enoxaparin (Caution should be exercised). Products include:
Lovenox Injection 2187

Fludrocortisone Acetate (Reduces response to active immunization procedure). Products include:
Florinef Acetate Tablets 506

Fluorouracil (Reduces response to active immunization procedure). Products include:
Efudex 2280
Fluoroplex Topical Solution & Cream 1% 475
Fluorouracil Injection 2282

Heparin Calcium (Caution should be exercised).
No products indexed under this heading.

Heparin Sodium (Caution should be exercised). Products include:
Heparin Lock Flush Solution 2831
Heparin Sodium Injection 2832
Heparin Sodium Vials 1486

Hydrocortisone (Reduces response to active immunization procedure). Products include:
Anusol-HC Cream 2.5% 1953
Aquanil HC Lotion 1989
Maximum Strength Cortaid Spray .... ◘ 800
CORTENEMA 2713
Cortisporin Ointment 1074
Cortisporin Ophthalmic Ointment Sterile 1074
Cortisporin Ophthalmic Suspension Sterile 1075
Cortisporin Otic Solution Sterile 1076
Cortisporin Otic Suspension Sterile 1077
Cortizone-5 .... ◘ 795
Cortizone-10 .... ◘ 795
Hydrocortone Tablets 1715
Hytone 922
Hytone Ointment 2½% 923
Massengill Medicated Soft Cloth Towelettes 2628
Pediotic Suspension Sterile 1140
Preparation H Hydrocortisone 1% Cream .... ◘ 843
ProctoCream-HC 2.5% 2552
VōSoL HC Otic Solution 2786

Hydrocortisone Acetate (Reduces response to active immunization procedure). Products include:
Analpram-HC Rectal Cream 1% and 2.5% 993
Anusol HC-1 Hydrocortisone Anti-Itch Ointment .... ◘ 810
Anusol-HC Suppositories 1954
Caldecort Anti-Itch Hydrocortisone Cream .... ◘ 651
Coly-Mycin S Otic w/Neomycin & Hydrocortisone 1965
Cortaid .... ◘ 800
Cortifoam 2540
Cortisporin Cream 1073
Epifoam 2543
Hydrocortone Acetate Sterile Suspension 1712
Mantadil Cream 1124
Nupercainal Hydrocortisone 1% Cream .... ◘ 661
Pramosone Cream, Lotion & Ointment 995
ProctoFoam-HC 2552
Terra-Cortril Ophthalmic Suspension 2033

Hydrocortisone Sodium Phosphate (Reduces response to active immunization procedure). Products include:
Hydrocortone Phosphate Injection, Sterile 1713

Hydrocortisone Sodium Succinate (Reduces response to active immunization procedure).
No products indexed under this heading.

Hydroxyurea (Reduces response to active immunization procedure). Products include:
Hydrea Capsules 705

Immune Globulin (Human) (Reduces response to active immunization procedure).
No products indexed under this heading.

Influenza Virus Vaccine (Influenza Virus Vaccine should not be given within 3 days of immunization). Products include:
Fluvirin (Influenza Virus Vaccine) 1608
Influenza Virus Vaccine, Trivalent, Types A and B (chromatograph- and filter-purified subviron antigen) FluShield, 1996-1997 Formula 2842

Lomustine (CCNU) (Reduces response to active immunization procedure). Products include:
CeeNU Capsules 699

Mechlorethamine Hydrochloride (Reduces response to active immunization procedure). Products include:
Mustargen 1752

Melphalan (Reduces response to active immunization procedure). Products include:
Alkeran Tablets 1198

Methotrexate Sodium (Reduces response to active immunization procedure). Products include:
Methotrexate Sodium Tablets, Injection, for Injection and LPF Injection 1322

Methylprednisolone Acetate (Reduces response to active immunization procedure).
No products indexed under this heading.

Methylprednisolone Sodium Succinate (Reduces response to active immunization procedure).
No products indexed under this heading.

Mitotane (Reduces response to active immunization procedure). Products include:
Lysodren Tablets 707

Mitoxantrone Hydrochloride (Reduces response to active immunization procedure). Products include:
Novantrone for Injection 1327

Muromonab-CD3 (Reduces response to active immunization procedure). Products include:
Orthoclone OKT3 Sterile Solution .. 1892

Mycophenolate Mofetil (Reduces response to active immunization procedure). Products include:
CellCept Capsules 2265

Prednisolone Acetate (Reduces response to active immunization procedure). Products include:
AK-CIDE .... ⊙ 203
AK-CIDE Ointment .... ⊙ 203
Blephamide Liquifilm Sterile Ophthalmic Suspension 472
Blephamide Ointment .... ⊙ 234
Econopred & Econopred Plus Ophthalmic Suspensions .... ⊙ 216
Poly-Pred Liquifilm .... ⊙ 246
Pred Forte .... ⊙ 247
Pred Mild .... ⊙ 250
Pred-G Liquifilm Sterile Ophthalmic Suspension .... ⊙ 248
Pred-G S.O.P. Sterile Ophthalmic Ointment .... ⊙ 249

Prednisolone Sodium Phosphate (Reduces response to active immunization procedure). Products include:
AK-PRED .... ⊙ 204
Hydeltrasol Injection, Sterile 1708
Pediapred Oral Solution 1618

Prednisolone Tebutate (Reduces response to active immunization procedure). Products include:
Hydeltra-T.B.A. Sterile Suspension 1710

Prednisone (Reduces response to active immunization procedure).
No products indexed under this heading.

Procarbazine Hydrochloride (Reduces response to active immunization procedure). Products include:
Matulane Capsules 2300

Tacrolimus (Reduces response to active immunization procedure). Products include:
Prograf 1028

Tamoxifen Citrate (Reduces response to active immunization procedure). Products include:
Nolvadex Tablets 2957

Thiotepa (Reduces response to active immunization procedure). Products include:
Thioplex (Thiotepa For Injection) 1329

Triamcinolone (Reduces response to active immunization procedure).
No products indexed under this heading.

Triamcinolone Acetonide (Reduces response to active immunization procedure). Products include:
Azmacort Oral Inhaler 2175
Nasacort AQ Nasal Spray 2191
Nasacort Nasal Inhaler 2189

Triamcinolone Diacetate (Reduces response to active immunization procedure).
No products indexed under this heading.

Triamcinolone Hexacetonide (Reduces response to active immunization procedure).
No products indexed under this heading.

Vincristine Sulfate (Reduces response to active immunization procedure). Products include:
Oncovin Solution Vials & Hyporets 1521

Warfarin Sodium (Caution should be exercised). Products include:
Coumadin 941

DIPRIVAN INJECTABLE EMULSION
(Propofol) 2939
May interact with narcotic analgesics, hypnotics and sedatives, benzodiazepines, barbiturates, inhalant anesthetics, and certain other

(◘ Described in PDR For Nonprescription Drugs) (⊙ Described in PDR For Ophthalmology)

309 **Interactions Index** **Diprivan**

agents. Compounds in these categories include:

Alfentanil Hydrochloride (Increases anesthetic or sedative effects; may also result in pronounced decreases in systolic, diastolic, and mean arterial pressure and cardiac output). Products include:

- Alfenta Injection ... 1334

Alprazolam (Increases anesthetic or sedative effects; may also result in pronounced decreases in systolic, diastolic, and mean arterial pressure and cardiac output). Products include:

- Xanax Tablets ... 2115

Aprobarbital (Increases anesthetic or sedative effects; may also result in pronounced decreases in systolic, diastolic, and mean arterial pressure and cardiac output).

No products indexed under this heading.

Buprenorphine (Increases anesthetic or sedative effects; may also result in pronounced decreases in systolic, diastolic, and mean arterial pressure and cardiac output). Products include:

- Buprenex Injectable ... 2170

Butabarbital (Increases anesthetic or sedative effects; may also result in pronounced decreases in systolic, diastolic, and mean arterial pressure and cardiac output).

No products indexed under this heading.

Butalbital (Increases anesthetic or sedative effects; may also result in pronounced decreases in systolic, diastolic, and mean arterial pressure and cardiac output). Products include:

- Axocet Capsules ... 2469
- Esgic-plus Capsules ... 1012
- Esgic-plus Tablets ... 1012
- Fioricet Tablets ... 2386
- Fioricet with Codeine Capsules ... 2387
- Fiorinal Capsules ... 2388
- Fiorinal with Codeine Capsules ... 2390
- Fiorinal Tablets ... 2388
- Phrenilin ... 790
- Sedapap Tablets 50 mg/650 mg .. 1826

Chloral Hydrate (Increases anesthetic or sedative effects; may also result in pronounced decreases in systolic, diastolic, and mean arterial pressure and cardiac output).

No products indexed under this heading.

Chlordiazepoxide (Increases anesthetic or sedative effects; may also result in pronounced decreases in systolic, diastolic, and mean arterial pressure and cardiac output). Products include:

- Limbitrol ... 2333

Chlordiazepoxide Hydrochloride (Increases anesthetic or sedative effects; may also result in pronounced decreases in systolic, diastolic, and mean arterial pressure and cardiac output). Products include:

- Librax Capsules ... 2330
- Librium Capsules ... 2331
- Librium Injectable ... 2332

Clonazepam (Increases anesthetic or sedative effects; may also result in pronounced decreases in systolic, diastolic, and mean arterial pressure and cardiac output). Products include:

- Klonopin Tablets ... 2294

Clorazepate Dipotassium (Increases anesthetic or sedative effects; may also result in pronounced decreases in systolic, diastolic, and mean arterial pressure and cardiac output). Products include:

- Tranxene ... 459

Codeine Phosphate (Increases anesthetic or sedative effects; may also result in pronounced decreases in systolic, diastolic, and mean arterial pressure and cardiac output). Products include:

- Brontex ... 2130
- Dimetane-DC Cough Syrup ... 2232
- Fioricet with Codeine Capsules ... 2387
- Fiorinal with Codeine Capsules ... 2390
- Nucofed ... 2225
- Phenergan with Codeine ... 2883
- Phenergan VC with Codeine ... 2888
- Robitussin A-C Syrup ... 2248
- Robitussin-DAC Syrup ... 2249
- Ryna ... 804
- Soma Compound w/Codeine Tablets ... 2784
- Tylenol with Codeine ... 1592

Desflurane (Increases anesthetic or sedative and cardiorespiratory effects). Products include:

- Suprane (desflurane, USP) ... 1865

Dezocine (Increases anesthetic or sedative effects; may also result in pronounced decreases in systolic, diastolic, and mean arterial pressure and cardiac output). Products include:

- Dalgan Injection ... 529

Diazepam (Increases anesthetic or sedative effects; may also result in pronounced decreases in systolic, diastolic, and mean arterial pressure and cardiac output). Products include:

- Dizac (diazepam injectable emulsion) CIV ... 1862
- Valium Injectable ... 2336
- Valium Tablets ... 2335

Droperidol (Increases anesthetic or sedative effects; may also result in pronounced decreases in systolic, diastolic, and mean arterial pressure and cardiac output). Products include:

- Inapsine Injection ... 462

Enflurane (Increases anesthetic or sedative and cardiorespiratory effects).

No products indexed under this heading.

Estazolam (Increases anesthetic or sedative effects; may also result in pronounced decreases in systolic, diastolic, and mean arterial pressure and cardiac output). Products include:

- ProSom Tablets ... 457

Ethchlorvynol (Increases anesthetic or sedative effects; may also result in pronounced decreases in systolic, diastolic, and mean arterial pressure and cardiac output). Products include:

- Placidyl Capsules ... 456

Ethinamate (Increases anesthetic or sedative effects; may also result in pronounced decreases in systolic, diastolic, and mean arterial pressure and cardiac output).

No products indexed under this heading.

Fentanyl (Increases anesthetic or sedative effects; may also result in pronounced decreases in systolic, diastolic, and mean arterial pressure and cardiac output). Products include:

- Duragesic Transdermal System ... 1336

Fentanyl Citrate (Increases anesthetic or sedative effects; may also result in pronounced decreases in systolic, diastolic, and mean arterial pressure and cardiac output). Products include:

- Sublimaze Injection ... 463

Flurazepam Hydrochloride (Increases anesthetic or sedative effects; may also result in pronounced decreases in systolic, diastolic, and mean arterial pressure and cardiac output). Products include:

- Dalmane Capsules ... 2329

Glutethimide (Increases anesthetic or sedative effects; may also result in pronounced decreases in systolic, diastolic, and mean arterial pressure and cardiac output).

No products indexed under this heading.

Halazepam (Increases anesthetic or sedative effects; may also result in pronounced decreases in systolic, diastolic, and mean arterial pressure and cardiac output).

No products indexed under this heading.

Halothane (Increases anesthetic or sedative and cardiorespiratory effects). Products include:

- Fluothane ... 2830

Hydrocodone Bitartrate (Increases anesthetic or sedative effects; may also result in pronounced decreases in systolic, diastolic, and mean arterial pressure and cardiac output). Products include:

- Codiclear DH Syrup ... 808
- Duratuss HD Elixir ... 2750
- Histussin D Liquid ... 670
- Hycodan Tablets and Syrup ... 946
- Hycomine Compound Tablets ... 948
- Hycomine ... 947
- Hycotuss Expectorant Syrup ... 950
- Hydrocet Capsules ... 787
- Lorcet 10/650 Tablets ... 1016
- Lortab ... 2751
- Tussend ... 1830
- Tussend Expectorant ... 1831
- Vicodin Tablets ... 1404
- Vicodin ES Tablets ... 1405
- Vicodin HP Tablets ... 1403
- Vicodin Tuss Expectorant ... 1406
- Zydone Capsules ... 967

Hydrocodone Polistirex (Increases anesthetic or sedative effects; may also result in pronounced decreases in systolic, diastolic, and mean arterial pressure and cardiac output). Products include:

- Tussionex Pennkinetic Extended-Release Suspension ... 1624

Hydromorphone Hydrochloride (Increases anesthetic or sedative effects; may also result in pronounced decreases in systolic, diastolic, and mean arterial pressure and cardiac output). Products include:

- Dilaudid Ampules ... 1382
- Dilaudid Cough Syrup ... 1383
- Dilaudid-HP Injection ... 1384
- Dilaudid-HP Lyophilized Powder 250 mg ... 1384
- Dilaudid ... 1382
- Dilaudid Oral Liquid ... 1386
- Dilaudid ... 1382
- Dilaudid Tablets - 8 mg ... 1386

Isoflurane (Increases anesthetic or sedative and cardiorespiratory effects).

No products indexed under this heading.

Levorphanol Tartrate (Increases anesthetic or sedative effects; may also result in pronounced decreases in systolic, diastolic, and mean arterial pressure and cardiac output). Products include:

- Levo-Dromoran ... 2297

Lorazepam (Increases anesthetic or sedative effects; may also result in pronounced decreases in systolic, diastolic, and mean arterial pressure and cardiac output). Products include:

- Ativan Injection ... 2805
- Ativan Tablets ... 2807

Meperidine Hydrochloride (Increases anesthetic or sedative effects; may also result in pronounced decreases in systolic, diastolic, and mean arterial pressure and cardiac output). Products include:

- Demerol ... 2438
- Mepergan Injection ... 2859

Mephobarbital (Increases anesthetic or sedative effects; may also result in pronounced decreases in systolic, diastolic, and mean arterial pressure and cardiac output). Products include:

- Mebaral Tablets ... 2452

Methadone Hydrochloride (Increases anesthetic or sedative effects; may also result in pronounced decreases in systolic, diastolic, and mean arterial pressure and cardiac output). Products include:

- Methadone Hydrochloride Oral Concentrate ... 2356
- Methadone Hydrochloride Oral Solution & Tablets ... 2357

Methoxyflurane (Increases anesthetic or sedative and cardiorespiratory effects).

No products indexed under this heading.

Midazolam Hydrochloride (Increases anesthetic or sedative effects; may also result in pronounced decreases in systolic, diastolic, and mean arterial pressure and cardiac output). Products include:

- Versed Injection ... 2324

Morphine Sulfate (Increases anesthetic or sedative effects; may also result in pronounced decreases in systolic, diastolic, and mean arterial pressure and cardiac output). Products include:

- Astramorph/PF Injection, USP (Preservative-Free) ... 526
- Duramorph Injection ... 983
- Infumorph 200 and Infumorph 500 Sterile Solutions ... 985
- Kadian Capsules ... 2948
- MS Contin Tablets ... 2149
- MSIR ... 2152
- Oramorph SR (Morphine Sulfate Sustained Release Tablets) ... 2359
- RMS Suppositories CII ... 2766
- Roxanol ... 2365

Nitrous Oxide (Rate of administration requires adjustment).

Opium Alkaloids (Increases anesthetic or sedative effects; may also result in pronounced decreases in systolic, diastolic, and mean arterial pressure and cardiac output).

No products indexed under this heading.

Oxazepam (Increases anesthetic or sedative effects; may also result in pronounced decreases in systolic, diastolic, and mean arterial pressure and cardiac output). Products include:

- Serax Capsules ... 2916
- Serax Tablets ... 2916

Oxycodone Hydrochloride (Increases anesthetic or sedative effects; may also result in pronounced decreases in systolic, diastolic, and mean arterial pressure and cardiac output). Products include:

- OxyContin Tablets ... 2163
- OxyIR Capsules ... 2167
- Percocet Tablets ... 955
- Percodan Tablets ... 955

IMPORTANT NOTE: Always consult each drug listing in the patient's regimen for possible interactions.

Diprivan   Interactions Index

Percodan-Demi Tablets 956
Roxicodone Tablets, Oral Solution
 & Intensol (Oxycodone) 2366
Tylox Capsules 1593

Pentobarbital Sodium (Increases anesthetic or sedative effects; may also result in pronounced decreases in systolic, diastolic, and mean arterial pressure and cardiac output). Products include:
Nembutal Sodium Capsules 440
Nembutal Sodium Solution 442
Nembutal Sodium Suppositories..... 444

Phenobarbital (Increases anesthetic or sedative effects; may also result in pronounced decreases in systolic, diastolic, and mean arterial pressure and cardiac output). Products include:
Arco-Lase Plus Tablets 513
Bellergal-S Tablets 2375
Donnatal 2234
Donnatal Extentabs 2234
Donnatal Tablets 2234
Phenobarbital Elixir and Tablets .. 1523
Quadrinal Tablets 1398

Prazepam (Increases anesthetic or sedative effects; may also result in pronounced decreases in systolic, diastolic, and mean arterial pressure and cardiac output).
No products indexed under this heading.

Propoxyphene Hydrochloride (Increases anesthetic or sedative effects; may also result in pronounced decreases in systolic, diastolic, and mean arterial pressure and cardiac output). Products include:
Darvon 1475
Wygesic Tablets 2930

Propoxyphene Napsylate (Increases anesthetic or sedative effects; may also result in pronounced decreases in systolic, diastolic, and mean arterial pressure and cardiac output). Products include:
Darvon-N/Darvocet-N 1473

Quazepam (Increases anesthetic or sedative effects; may also result in pronounced decreases in systolic, diastolic, and mean arterial pressure and cardiac output). Products include:
Doral Tablets 2773

Secobarbital Sodium (Increases anesthetic or sedative effects; may also result in pronounced decreases in systolic, diastolic, and mean arterial pressure and cardiac output). Products include:
Seconal Sodium Pulvules 1529

Sufentanil Citrate (Increases anesthetic or sedative effects; may also result in pronounced decreases in systolic, diastolic, and mean arterial pressure and cardiac output). Products include:
Sufenta Injection 1355

Temazepam (Increases anesthetic or sedative effects; may also result in pronounced decreases in systolic, diastolic, and mean arterial pressure and cardiac output). Products include:
Restoril Capsules 2413

Thiamylal Sodium (Increases anesthetic or sedative effects; may also result in pronounced decreases in systolic, diastolic, and mean arterial pressure and cardiac output).
No products indexed under this heading.

Triazolam (Increases anesthetic or sedative effects; may also result in pronounced decreases in systolic, diastolic, and mean arterial pressure and cardiac output). Products include:
Halcion Tablets 2093

Zolpidem Tartrate (Increases anesthetic or sedative effects; may also result in pronounced decreases in systolic, diastolic, and mean arterial pressure and cardiac output). Products include:
Ambien Tablets 2559

DIPROLENE AF CREAM 0.05%
(Betamethasone Dipropionate) 2489
None cited in PDR database.

DIPROLENE GEL 0.05%
(Betamethasone Dipropionate) 2490
None cited in PDR database.

DIPROLENE LOTION 0.05%
(Betamethasone Dipropionate) 2491
None cited in PDR database.

DIPROLENE OINTMENT 0.05%
(Betamethasone Dipropionate) 2491
None cited in PDR database.

DISALCID CAPSULES
(Salsalate) 1549
May interact with anticoagulants, sulfonylureas, penicillins, corticosteroids, antacids, and certain other agents. Compounds in these categories include:

Acetazolamide (Co-administration with drugs that raise urine pH, such as acetazolamide, will increase renal clearance and urinary excretion of salicylic acid, thus lowering plasma levels). Products include:
Diamox Sequels (Sustained Release) .... ⊙ 318
Diamox Tablets .... ⊙ 317

Acetazolamide Sodium (Co-administration with drugs that raise urine pH, such as acetazolamide, will increase renal clearance and urinary excretion of salicylic acid, thus lowering plasma levels). Products include:
Diamox Intravenous .... ⊙ 317

Aluminum Carbonate (Co-administration with drugs that raise urine pH secondary to their pharmacological effect, such as antacids, will increase renal clearance and urinary excretion of salicylic acid, thus lowering plasma levels). Products include:
Basaljel Capsules 2810
Basaljel Suspension 2810
Basaljel Tablets 2810

Aluminum Hydroxide (Co-administration with drugs that raise urine pH secondary to their pharmacological effect, such as antacids, will increase renal clearance and urinary excretion of salicylic acid, thus lowering plasma levels). Products include:
ALternaGEL Liquid 1358
Maximum Strength Ascriptin ...... ▣ 650
Cama Arthritis Pain Reliever .... ▣ 748
Gaviscon Extra Strength Relief Formula Antacid Tablets .... ▣ 778
Gaviscon Extra Strength Relief Formula Liquid Antacid .... ▣ 779
Gaviscon Liquid Antacid .... ▣ 779
Gelusil Antacid-Anti-gas Liquid ... ▣ 819
Gelusil Antacid-Anti-gas Tablets .. ▣ 819

Maalox Antacid/Anti-Gas Tablets ... 889
Maalox Heartburn Relief Suspension .... ▣ 658
Maalox Antacid Liquid 888
Extra Strength Maalox Antacid/Anti-Gas Liquid and Tablets 888
Mylanta 1359
Tempo Soft Antacid .... ▣ 799

Aluminum Hydroxide Gel (Co-administration with drugs that raise urine pH secondary to their pharmacological effect, such as antacids, will increase renal clearance and urinary excretion of salicylic acid, thus lowering plasma levels). Products include:
ALternaGEL Liquid .... ▣ 675
Aludrox Oral Suspension .... ▣ 850
Amphojel Suspension 2802
Amphojel Suspension without Flavor 2802
Amphojel Tablets 2802
Ascriptin .... ▣ 650
Gaviscon Antacid Tablets .... ▣ 778
Gaviscon-2 Antacid Tablets .... ▣ 779
Mylanta Liquid .... ▣ 676
Mylanta Double Strength Liquid .. ▣ 676
Nephrox Suspension .... ▣ 671

Amoxicillin Trihydrate (Salicylates compete for protein binding sites). Products include:
Amoxil 2631
Augmentin 2637
Augmentin Tablets 2640

Ampicillin (Salicylates compete for protein binding sites). Products include:
Omnipen Capsules 2872
Omnipen for Oral Suspension 2873

Ampicillin Sodium (Salicylates compete for protein binding sites). Products include:
Unasyn 2035

Ampicillin Trihydrate (Salicylates compete for protein binding sites).
No products indexed under this heading.

Azlocillin Sodium (Salicylates compete for protein binding sites).
No products indexed under this heading.

Bacampicillin Hydrochloride (Salicylates compete for protein binding sites). Products include:
Spectrobid Tablets 2030

Betamethasone Acetate (Salicylates, possibly, compete for protein binding sites). Products include:
Celestone Soluspan Suspension ... 2484

Betamethasone Sodium Phosphate (Salicylates, possibly, compete for protein binding sites). Products include:
Celestone Soluspan Suspension ... 2484

Carbenicillin Disodium (Salicylates compete for protein binding sites).
No products indexed under this heading.

Carbenicillin Indanyl Sodium (Salicylates compete for protein binding sites). Products include:
Geocillin Tablets 2009

Chlorpropamide (Salicylates enhance hypoglycemic effect of sulfonylureas). Products include:
Diabinese Tablets 2002

Cortisone Acetate (Salicylates, possibly, compete for protein binding sites). Products include:
Cortone Acetate Sterile Suspension 1663
Cortone Acetate Tablets 1664

Dalteparin Sodium (Salicylates given concomitantly with anticoagulant drugs may predispose to systemic bleeding). Products include:
Fragmin Injection 2088

Dexamethasone (Salicylates, possibly, compete for protein binding sites). Products include:
AK-Trol Ointment & Suspension ... ⊙ 205
Decadron Elixir 1676
Decadron Tablets 1678
Decaspray Topical Aerosol 1689
Maxitrol Ophthalmic Ointment and Suspension .... ⊙ 222
TobraDex Ophthalmic Suspension and Ointment 469

Dexamethasone Acetate (Salicylates, possibly, compete for protein binding sites). Products include:
Dalalone D.P. Injectable 1009
Decadron-LA Sterile Suspension .. 1687

Dexamethasone Sodium Phosphate (Salicylates, possibly, compete for protein binding sites). Products include:
Decadron Phosphate Injection 1680
Decadron Phosphate Sterile Ophthalmic Ointment 1684
Decadron Phosphate Sterile Ophthalmic Solution 1685
Decadron Phosphate Topical Cream 1686
Decadron Phosphate with Xylocaine Injection, Sterile 1683
Dexacort Phosphate in Respihaler .. 1606
Dexacort Phosphate in Turbinaire .. 1607
NeoDecadron Sterile Ophthalmic Ointment 1755
NeoDecadron Sterile Ophthalmic Solution 1756
NeoDecadron Topical Cream 1757

Dicloxacillin Sodium (Salicylates compete for protein binding sites).
No products indexed under this heading.

Dicumarol (Salicylates given concomitantly with anticoagulant drugs may predispose to systemic bleeding).
No products indexed under this heading.

Enoxaparin (Salicylates given concomitantly with anticoagulant drugs may predispose to systemic bleeding). Products include:
Lovenox Injection 2187

Fludrocortisone Acetate (Salicylates, possibly, compete for protein binding sites). Products include:
Florinef Acetate Tablets 506

Fosphenytoin Sodium (Salicylates compete for protein binding sites). Products include:
Cerebyx Injection 1956

Glimepiride (Salicylates enhance hypoglycemic effect of sulfonylureas). Products include:
Amaryl Tablets 1241

Glipizide (Salicylates enhance hypoglycemic effect of sulfonylureas). Products include:
Glucotrol Tablets 2011
Glucotrol XL Extended Release Tablets 2012

Glyburide (Salicylates enhance hypoglycemic effect of sulfonylureas). Products include:
DiaBeta Tablets 1265
Glynase PresTab Tablets 2091
Micronase Tablets 2099

Heparin Calcium (Salicylates given concomitantly with anticoagulant drugs may predispose to systemic bleeding).
No products indexed under this heading.

Heparin Sodium (Salicylates given concomitantly with anticoagulant drugs may predispose to systemic bleeding). Products include:
Heparin Lock Flush Solution 2831
Heparin Sodium Injection 2832
Heparin Sodium Vials 1486

(▣ Described in PDR For Nonprescription Drugs)   (⊙ Described in PDR For Ophthalmology)

Hydrocortisone (Salicylates, possibly, compete for protein binding sites). Products include:
Anusol-HC Cream 2.5% 1953
Aquanil HC Lotion 1989
Maximum Strength Cortaid Spray ⊞ 800
CORTENEMA 2713
Cortisporin Ointment 1074
Cortisporin Ophthalmic Ointment Sterile 1074
Cortisporin Ophthalmic Suspension Sterile 1075
Cortisporin Otic Solution Sterile 1076
Cortisporin Otic Suspension Sterile 1077
Cortizone-5 .... ⊞ 795
Cortizone-10 .... ⊞ 795
Hydrocortone Tablets 1715
Hytone 922
Hytone Ointment 2 ½ % 923
Massengill Medicated Soft Cloth Towelettes 2628
Pediotic Suspension Sterile 1140
Preparation H Hydrocortisone 1% Cream .... ⊞ 843
ProctoCream-HC 2.5% 2552
VōSoL HC Otic Solution 2786

Hydrocortisone Acetate (Salicylates, possibly, compete for protein binding sites). Products include:
Analpram-HC Rectal Cream 1% and 2.5% 993
Anusol HC-1 Hydrocortisone Anti-Itch Ointment .... ⊞ 810
Anusol-HC Suppositories 1954
Caldecort Anti-Itch Hydrocortisone Cream .... ⊞ 651
Coly-Mycin S Otic w/Neomycin & Hydrocortisone 1965
Cortaid .... ⊞ 800
Cortifoam 2540
Cortisporin Cream 1073
Epifoam 2543
Hydrocortone Acetate Sterile Suspension 1712
Mantadil Cream 1124
Nupercainal Hydrocortisone 1% Cream .... ⊞ 661
Pramosone Cream, Lotion & Ointment 995
ProctoFoam-HC 2552
Terra-Cortril Ophthalmic Suspension 2033

Hydrocortisone Sodium Phosphate (Salicylates, possibly, compete for protein binding sites). Products include:
Hydrocortone Phosphate Injection, Sterile 1713

Hydrocortisone Sodium Succinate (Salicylates, possibly, compete for protein binding sites).
No products indexed under this heading.

Levothyroxine Sodium (Salicylates compete for protein binding sites). Products include:
Eltroxin Tablets 2214
Levothroid Tablets 1015
Levothyroxine Sodium, USP for Injection 546
Levoxyl Tablets 918
Synthroid 1410

Magaldrate (Co-administration with drugs that raise urine pH secondary to their pharmacological effect, such as antacids, will increase renal clearance and urinary excretion of salicylic acid, thus lowering plasma levels).
No products indexed under this heading.

Magnesium Hydroxide (Co-administration with drugs that raise urine pH secondary to their pharmacological effect, such as antacids, will increase renal clearance and urinary excretion of salicylic acid, thus lowering plasma levels). Products include:
Aludrox Oral Suspension .... ⊞ 850
Ascriptin .... ⊞ 650
Di-Gel Antacid/Anti-Gas .... ⊞ 762
Gelusil Antacid-Anti-gas Liquid .... ⊞ 819
Gelusil Antacid-Anti-gas Tablets .... ⊞ 819
Maalox Antacid/Anti-Gas Tablets 889
Maalox Antacid Liquid 888
Extra Strength Maalox Antacid/Anti-Gas Liquid and Tablets 888
Mylanta Fast-Acting 1359
Mylanta Gelcaps Antacid .... ⊞ 678
Fast-Acting Mylanta Liquid Antacid 1359
Mylanta Tablets .... ⊞ 677
Maximum-Strength Fast-Acting Mylanta Liquid Antacid 1359
Mylanta Double Strength Tablets .. ⊞ 677
Phillips' Milk of Magnesia Liquid ... ⊞ 627
Rolaids Antacid Tablets .... ⊞ 807
Tempo Soft Antacid .... ⊞ 799

Magnesium Oxide (Co-administration with drugs that raise urine pH secondary to their pharmacological effect, such as antacids, will increase renal clearance and urinary excretion of salicylic acid, thus lowering plasma levels). Products include:
Beelith Tablets 632
Bufferin Analgesic Tablets .... ⊞ 636
Arthritis Strength Bufferin Analgesic Caplets .... ⊞ 637
Extra Strength Bufferin Analgesic Tablets .... ⊞ 637
Caltrate PLUS .... ⊞ 681
Cama Arthritis Pain Reliever .... ⊞ 748
Mag-Ox 400 666
Uro-Mag 666

Methotrexate Sodium (Salicylates compete for protein binding sites). Products include:
Methotrexate Sodium Tablets, Injection, for Injection and LPF Injection 1322

Methylprednisolone Acetate (Salicylates, possibly, compete for protein binding sites).
No products indexed under this heading.

Methylprednisolone Sodium Succinate (Salicylates, possibly, compete for protein binding sites).
No products indexed under this heading.

Mezlocillin Sodium (Salicylates compete for protein binding sites). Products include:
Mezlin 594
Mezlin Pharmacy Bulk Package ... 597

Nafcillin Sodium (Salicylates compete for protein binding sites).
No products indexed under this heading.

Naproxen (Salicylates compete for protein binding sites). Products include:
Anaprox/Naprosyn 2277

Naproxen Sodium (Salicylates compete for protein binding sites). Products include:
Aleve 2124
Anaprox/Naprosyn 2277
Naprelan Tablets 2861

Penicillin G Benzathine (Salicylates compete for protein binding sites). Products include:
Bicillin C-R Injection 2810
Bicillin C-R 900/300 Injection 2812
Bicillin L-A Injection 2813

Penicillin G Potassium (Salicylates compete for protein binding sites). Products include:
Pfizerpen for Injection 2022

Penicillin G Procaine (Salicylates compete for protein binding sites). Products include:
Bicillin C-R Injection 2810
Bicillin C-R 900/300 Injection 2812

Penicillin G Sodium (Salicylates compete for protein binding sites).
No products indexed under this heading.

Penicillin V Potassium (Salicylates compete for protein binding sites). Products include:
Pen•Vee K 2879

Phenytoin (Salicylates compete for protein binding sites). Products include:
Dilantin Infatabs 1967
Dilantin-125 Suspension 1969

Phenytoin Sodium (Salicylates compete for protein binding sites). Products include:
Dilantin Kapseals 1965

Prednisolone Acetate (Salicylates, possibly, compete for protein binding sites). Products include:
AK-CIDE .... ⓡ 203
AK-CIDE Ointment .... ⓡ 203
Blephamide Liquifilm Sterile Ophthalmic Suspension 472
Blephamide Ointment .... ⓡ 234
Econopred & Econopred Plus Ophthalmic Suspensions .... ⓡ 216
Poly-Pred Liquifilm .... ⓡ 246
Pred Forte .... ⓡ 247
Pred Mild .... ⓡ 250
Pred-G Liquifilm Sterile Ophthalmic Suspension .... ⓡ 248
Pred-G S.O.P. Sterile Ophthalmic Ointment .... ⓡ 249

Prednisolone Sodium Phosphate (Salicylates, possibly, compete for protein binding sites). Products include:
AK-PRED .... ⓡ 204
Hydeltrasol Injection, Sterile 1708
Pediapred Oral Solution 1618

Prednisolone Tebutate (Salicylates, possibly, compete for protein binding sites). Products include:
Hydeltra-T.B.A. Sterile Suspension 1710

Prednisone (Salicylates, possibly, compete for protein binding sites).
No products indexed under this heading.

Probenecid (Co-administration has been reported to result in antagonism of uricosuric effect of probenecid to treat gout). Products include:
Benemid Tablets 1651
ColBENEMID Tablets 1662

Sodium Acid Phosphate (Co-administration with drugs that lower urine pH, such as sodium acid phosphate, will decrease renal clearance and urinary excretion of salicylic acid, thus increase plasma levels). Products include:
Uroqid-Acid No. 2 Tablets 633

Sodium Bicarbonate (Co-administration with drugs that raise urine pH secondary to their pharmacological effect, such as antacids, will increase renal clearance and urinary excretion of salicylic acid, thus lowering plasma levels). Products include:
Alka-Seltzer Cherry Effervescent Antacid and Pain Reliever .... ⊞ 609
Alka-Seltzer Extra Strength Effervescent Antacid and Pain Reliever .... ⊞ 609
Alka-Seltzer Gold Effervescent Antacid .... ⊞ 611
Alka-Seltzer Lemon Lime Effervescent Antacid and Pain Reliever .... ⊞ 609
Alka-Seltzer Original Effervescent Antacid and Pain Reliever .... ⊞ 609
Arm & Hammer Pure Baking Soda .... ⊞ 648
Colyte and Colyte-flavored 2540
GoLYTELY 694
Massengill Disposable Douches . ⊞ 780
Massengill Liquid Concentrate .. ⊞ 780
NuLYTELY 694
Cherry Flavor NuLYTELY 694

Sodium Thiopental (Salicylates compete for protein binding sites).
No products indexed under this heading.

Sulfinpyrazone (Co-administration has been reported to result in antagonism of uricosuric effect of sulfinpyrazone to treat gout; salicylates compete for protein binding sites). Products include:
Anturane 823

Ticarcillin Disodium (Salicylates compete for protein binding sites). Products include:
Ticar for Injection 2704
Timentin for Injection 2706

Tolazamide (Salicylates enhance hypoglycemic effect of sulfonylureas).
No products indexed under this heading.

Tolbutamide (Salicylates enhance hypoglycemic effect of sulfonylureas).
No products indexed under this heading.

Triamcinolone (Salicylates, possibly, compete for protein binding sites).
No products indexed under this heading.

Triamcinolone Acetonide (Salicylates, possibly, compete for protein binding sites). Products include:
Azmacort Oral Inhaler 2175
Nasacort AQ Nasal Spray 2191
Nasacort Nasal Inhaler 2189

Triamcinolone Diacetate (Salicylates, possibly, compete for protein binding sites).
No products indexed under this heading.

Triamcinolone Hexacetonide (Salicylates, possibly, compete for protein binding sites).
No products indexed under this heading.

l-Triiodothyronine (Salicylates compete for protein binding sites).
No products indexed under this heading.

Warfarin Sodium (Salicylates given concomitantly with anticoagulant drugs may predispose to systemic bleeding; salicylates compete for protein binding sites). Products include:
Coumadin 941

Food Interactions

Food that lowers urinary pH (Co-administration with food that lowers urine pH will decrease renal clearance and urinary excretion of salicylic acid, thus increase plasma levels).

Food that raises urinary pH (Co-administration with food that raises urine pH will increase renal clearance and urinary excretion of salicylic acid, thus lowering plasma levels).

DISALCID TABLETS
(Salsalate) 1549
See **Disalcid Capsules**

DITROPAN SYRUP
(Oxybutynin Chloride) 1267
See **Ditropan Tablets**

DITROPAN TABLETS
(Oxybutynin Chloride) 1267
May interact with hypnotics and sedatives and certain other agents. Compounds in these categories include:

Estazolam (Enhances the drowsiness effect). Products include:
ProSom Tablets 457

Ethchlorvynol (Enhances the drowsiness effect). Products include:
Placidyl Capsules 456

IMPORTANT NOTE: Always consult each drug listing in the patient's regimen for possible interactions.

Ethinamate (Enhances the drowsiness effect).
No products indexed under this heading.

Flurazepam Hydrochloride (Enhances the drowsiness effect). Products include:
Dalmane Capsules 2329

Glutethimide (Enhances the drowsiness effect).
No products indexed under this heading.

Lorazepam (Enhances the drowsiness effect). Products include:
Ativan Injection 2805
Ativan Tablets 2807

Midazolam Hydrochloride (Enhances the drowsiness effect). Products include:
Versed Injection 2324

Propofol (Enhances the drowsiness effect). Products include:
Diprivan Injectable Emulsion 2939

Quazepam (Enhances the drowsiness effect). Products include:
Doral Tablets 2773

Secobarbital Sodium (Enhances the drowsiness effect). Products include:
Seconal Sodium Pulvules 1529

Temazepam (Enhances the drowsiness effect). Products include:
Restoril Capsules 2413

Triazolam (Enhances the drowsiness effect). Products include:
Halcion Tablets 2093

Zolpidem Tartrate (Enhances the drowsiness effect). Products include:
Ambien Tablets 2559

Food Interactions

Alcohol (Enhances the drowsiness effect).

DIUCARDIN TABLETS

(Hydroflumethiazide) 2824

May interact with oral hypoglycemic agents, insulin, corticosteroids, lithium preparations, oral anticoagulants, antigout agents, antihypertensives, general anesthetics, barbiturates, narcotic analgesics, cardiac glycosides, non-steroidal anti-inflammatory agents, and certain other agents. Compounds in these categories include:

Acarbose (Hyperglycemia may occur with thiazide diuretics; dosage adjustment of the oral antidiabetic drug may be required). Products include:
Precose 604

ACTH (Intensified electrolyte depletion, particularly hypokalemia).
No products indexed under this heading.

Alfentanil Hydrochloride (Thiazide-induced orthostatic hypotension may be potentiated). Products include:
Alfenta Injection 1334

Allopurinol (Thiazide diuretics may raise the levels of blood uric acid; dosage adjustment of antigout medication may be necessary to control gout and hyperuricemia). Products include:
Zyloprim Tablets 1194

Amphotericin B (Intensified electrolyte depletion, particularly hypokalemia). Products include:
Abelcet Injection 1540
Fungizone Intravenous 507
Fungizone Oral Suspension 704

Aprobarbital (Thiazide-induced orthostatic hypotension may be potentiated).
No products indexed under this heading.

Betamethasone Acetate (Intensified electrolyte depletion, particularly hypokalemia). Products include:
Celestone Soluspan Suspension 2484

Betamethasone Sodium Phosphate (Intensified electrolyte depletion, particularly hypokalemia). Products include:
Celestone Soluspan Suspension 2484

Buprenorphine (Thiazide-induced orthostatic hypotension may be potentiated). Products include:
Buprenex Injectable 2170

Butabarbital (Thiazide-induced orthostatic hypotension may be potentiated).
No products indexed under this heading.

Butalbital (Thiazide-induced orthostatic hypotension may be potentiated). Products include:
Axocet Capsules 2469
Esgic-plus Capsules 1012
Esgic-plus Tablets 1012
Fioricet Tablets 2386
Fioricet with Codeine Capsules 2387
Fiorinal Capsules 2388
Fiorinal with Codeine Capsules 2390
Fiorinal Tablets 2388
Phrenilin 790
Sedapap Tablets 50 mg/650 mg .. 1826

Captopril (Antihypertensive effects may be potentiated when used concurrently with thiazide diuretics; dosage adjustment may be necessary). Products include:
Capoten Tablets 740
Capozide Tablets 744

Chlorpropamide (Hyperglycemia may occur with thiazide diuretics; dosage adjustment of the oral antidiabetic drug may be required). Products include:
Diabinese Tablets 2002

Chlorthalidone (Antihypertensive effects may be potentiated when used concurrently with thiazide diuretics; dosage adjustment may be necessary). Products include:
Combipres Tablets 682
Tenoretic Tablets 2963
Thalitone 1293

Clonidine (Antihypertensive effects may be potentiated when used concurrently with thiazide diuretics; dosage adjustment may be necessary). Products include:
Catapres-TTS 680

Clonidine Hydrochloride (Antihypertensive effects may be potentiated when used concurrently with thiazide diuretics; dosage adjustment may be necessary). Products include:
Catapres Tablets 679
Combipres Tablets 682

Codeine Phosphate (Thiazide-induced orthostatic hypotension may be potentiated). Products include:
Brontex 2130
Dimetane-DC Cough Syrup 2232
Fioricet with Codeine Capsules 2387
Fiorinal with Codeine Capsules 2390
Nucofed 2225
Phenergan with Codeine 2883
Phenergan VC with Codeine 2888
Robitussin A-C Syrup 2248
Robitussin-DAC Syrup 2249
Ryna .... ◘ 804
Soma Compound w/Codeine Tablets 2784
Tylenol with Codeine 1592

Colestipol Hydrochloride (May inhibit gastrointestinal absorption of the thiazide diuretics; administration 1 hour before or 4 hours after colestipol is recommended). Products include:
Colestid 2073

Cortisone Acetate (Intensified electrolyte depletion, particularly hypokalemia). Products include:
Cortone Acetate Sterile Suspension 1663
Cortone Acetate Tablets 1664

Deslanoside (Thiazide-induced hypokalemia may exaggerate or sensitize the response of heart to the toxic effect of digitalis).
No products indexed under this heading.

Dexamethasone (Intensified electrolyte depletion, particularly hypokalemia). Products include:
AK-Trol Ointment & Suspension .... ◉ 205
Decadron Elixir 1676
Decadron Tablets 1678
Decaspray Topical Aerosol 1689
Maxitrol Ophthalmic Ointment and Suspension .... ◉ 222
TobraDex Ophthalmic Suspension and Ointment 469

Dexamethasone Acetate (Intensified electrolyte depletion, particularly hypokalemia). Products include:
Dalalone D.P. Injectable 1009
Decadron-LA Sterile Suspension 1687

Dexamethasone Sodium Phosphate (Intensified electrolyte depletion, particularly hypokalemia). Products include:
Decadron Phosphate Injection 1680
Decadron Phosphate Sterile Ophthalmic Ointment 1684
Decadron Phosphate Sterile Ophthalmic Solution 1685
Decadron Phosphate Topical Cream 1686
Decadron Phosphate with Xylocaine Injection, Sterile 1683
Dexacort Phosphate in Respihaler .. 1606
Dexacort Phosphate in Turbinaire .. 1607
NeoDecadron Sterile Ophthalmic Ointment 1755
NeoDecadron Sterile Ophthalmic Solution 1756
NeoDecadron Topical Cream 1757

Dezocine (Thiazide-induced orthostatic hypotension may be potentiated). Products include:
Dalgan Injection 529

Diclofenac Potassium (Concurrent use of nonsteroidal anti-inflammatory agents in some patients may reduce the diuretic, natriuretic and antihypertensive effects of thiazide diuretics). Products include:
Cataflam Tablets 833

Diclofenac Sodium (Concurrent use of nonsteroidal anti-inflammatory agents in some patients may reduce the diuretic, natriuretic and antihypertensive effects of thiazide diuretics). Products include:
Voltaren Ophthalmic Sterile Ophthalmic Solution .... ◉ 264
Cataflam/Voltaren/Voltaren-XR 833

Dicumarol (Thiazide diuretics may decrease the effects of oral anticoagulants).
No products indexed under this heading.

Digitoxin (Thiazide-induced hypokalemia may exaggerate or sensitize the response of heart to the toxic effect of digitalis). Products include:
Crystodigin Tablets 1472

Digoxin (Thiazide-induced hypokalemia may exaggerate or sensitize the response of heart to the toxic effect of digitalis). Products include:
Lanoxicaps 1110
Lanoxin Elixir Pediatric 1113
Lanoxin Injection 1116
Lanoxin Injection Pediatric 1119
Lanoxin Tablets 1121

Enalapril Maleate (Antihypertensive effects may be potentiated when used concurrently with thiazide diuretics; dosage adjustment may be necessary). Products include:
Vaseretic Tablets 1810
Vasotec Tablets 1816

Enalaprilat (Antihypertensive effects may be potentiated when used concurrently with thiazide diuretics; dosage adjustment may be necessary). Products include:
Vasotec I.V. 1814

Enflurane (Effects may be potentiated when used concurrently with thiazide diuretics; dosage adjustment may be necessary).
No products indexed under this heading.

Etodolac (Concurrent use of nonsteroidal anti-inflammatory agents in some patients may reduce the diuretic, natriuretic and antihypertensive effects of thiazide diuretics). Products include:
Lodine Capsules and Tablets 2849

Fenoprofen Calcium (Concurrent use of nonsteroidal anti-inflammatory agents in some patients may reduce the diuretic, natriuretic and antihypertensive effects of thiazide diuretics). Products include:
Nalfon 200 Pulvules & Nalfon Tablets 933

Fentanyl (Thiazide-induced orthostatic hypotension may be potentiated). Products include:
Duragesic Transdermal System 1336

Fentanyl Citrate (Thiazide-induced orthostatic hypotension may be potentiated). Products include:
Sublimaze Injection 463

Fludrocortisone Acetate (Intensified electrolyte depletion, particularly hypokalemia). Products include:
Florinef Acetate Tablets 506

Flurbiprofen (Concurrent use of nonsteroidal anti-inflammatory agents in some patients may reduce the diuretic, natriuretic and antihypertensive effects of thiazide diuretics).
No products indexed under this heading.

Furosemide (Antihypertensive effects may be potentiated when used concurrently with thiazide diuretics dosage adjustment may be necessary). Products include:
Lasix Injection, Oral Solution and Tablets 1267

Glimepiride (Hyperglycemia may occur with thiazide diuretics; dosage adjustment of the oral antidiabetic drug may be required). Products include:
Amaryl Tablets 1241

Glipizide (Hyperglycemia may occur with thiazide diuretics; dosage adjustment of the oral antidiabetic drug may be required). Products include:
Glucotrol Tablets 2011
Glucotrol XL Extended Release Tablets 2012

Glyburide (Hyperglycemia may occur with thiazide diuretics; dosage adjustment of the oral antidiabetic drug may be required). Products include:
DiaBeta Tablets 1265
Glynase PresTab Tablets 2091
Micronase Tablets 2099

(◘ Described in PDR For Nonprescription Drugs) (◉ Described in PDR For Ophthalmology)

Interactions Index — Diucardin

Guanabenz Acetate (Antihypertensive effects may be potentiated when used concurrently with thiazide diuretics; dosage adjustment may be necessary).
No products indexed under this heading.

Guanethidine Monosulfate (Antihypertensive effects may be potentiated when used concurrently with thiazide diuretics; dosage adjustment may be necessary). Products include:
- Esimil Tablets 840
- Ismelin Tablets 845

Hydralazine Hydrochloride (Antihypertensive effects may be potentiated when used concurrently with thiazide diuretics; dosage adjustment may be necessary). Products include:
- Apresazide Capsules 824
- Apresoline Hydrochloride Tablets 826
- Hydralazine Hydrochloride Injection USP 2712
- Ser-Ap-Es Tablets 867

Hydrocodone Bitartrate (Thiazide-induced orthostatic hypotension may be potentiated). Products include:
- Codiclear DH Syrup 808
- Duratuss HD Elixir 2750
- Histussin D Liquid 670
- Hycodan Tablets and Syrup 946
- Hycomine Compound Tablets 948
- Hycomine 947
- Hycotuss Expectorant Syrup 950
- Hydrocet Capsules 787
- Lorcet 10/650 Tablets 1016
- Lortab 2751
- Tussend 1830
- Tussend Expectorant 1831
- Vicodin Tablets 1404
- Vicodin ES Tablets 1405
- Vicodin HP Tablets 1403
- Vicodin Tuss Expectorant 1406
- Zydone Capsules 967

Hydrocodone Polistirex (Thiazide-induced orthostatic hypotension may be potentiated). Products include:
- Tussionex Pennkinetic Extended-Release Suspension 1624

Hydrocortisone (Intensified electrolyte depletion, particularly hypokalemia). Products include:
- Anusol-HC Cream 2.5% 1953
- Aquanil HC Lotion 1989
- Maximum Strength Cortaid Spray 800
- CORTENEMA 2713
- Cortisporin Ointment 1074
- Cortisporin Ophthalmic Ointment Sterile 1074
- Cortisporin Ophthalmic Suspension Sterile 1075
- Cortisporin Otic Solution Sterile 1076
- Cortisporin Otic Suspension Sterile 1077
- Cortizone-5 795
- Cortizone-10 795
- Hydrocortone Tablets 1715
- Hytone 922
- Hytone Ointment 2 ½% 923
- Massengill Medicated Soft Cloth Towelettes 2628
- Pediotic Suspension Sterile 1140
- Preparation H Hydrocortisone 1% Cream 843
- ProctoCream-HC 2.5% 2552
- VōSoL HC Otic Solution 2786

Hydrocortisone Acetate (Intensified electrolyte depletion, particularly hypokalemia). Products include:
- Analpram-HC Rectal Cream 1% and 2.5% 993
- Anusol HC-1 Hydrocortisone Anti-Itch Ointment 810
- Anusol-HC Suppositories 1954
- Caldecort Anti-Itch Hydrocortisone Cream 651
- Coly-Mycin S Otic w/Neomycin & Hydrocortisone 1965
- Cortaid 800
- Cortifoam 2540
- Cortisporin Cream 1073
- Epifoam 2543
- Hydrocortone Acetate Sterile Suspension 1712
- Mantadil Cream 1124
- Nupercainal Hydrocortisone 1% Cream 661
- Pramosone Cream, Lotion & Ointment 995
- ProctoFoam-HC 2552
- Terra-Cortril Ophthalmic Suspension 2033

Hydrocortisone Sodium Phosphate (Intensified electrolyte depletion, particularly hypokalemia). Products include:
- Hydrocortone Phosphate Injection, Sterile 1713

Hydrocortisone Sodium Succinate (Intensified electrolyte depletion, particularly hypokalemia).
No products indexed under this heading.

Hydromorphone Hydrochloride (Thiazide-induced orthostatic hypotension may be potentiated). Products include:
- Dilaudid Ampules 1382
- Dilaudid Cough Syrup 1383
- Dilaudid-HP Injection 1384
- Dilaudid-HP Lyophilized Powder 250 mg 1384
- Dilaudid 1382
- Dilaudid Oral Liquid 1386
- Dilaudid 1382
- Dilaudid Tablets - 8 mg 1386

Ibuprofen (Concurrent use of nonsteroidal anti-inflammatory agents in some patients may reduce the diuretic, natriuretic and antihypertensive effects of thiazide diuretics). Products include:
- Advil Cold and Sinus Caplets and Tablets 837
- Advil Ibuprofen Tablets, Caplets and Gel Caplets 836
- Children's Motrin Ibuprofen Oral Suspension 1558
- IBU Tablets 1389
- Ibuprohm 713
- Motrin IB Caplets, Tablets, and Gelcaps 802
- Motrin Ibuprofen Suspension, Oral Drops, Chewable Tablets, Caplets 1563
- Nuprin Ibuprofen/Analgesic Tablets & Caplets 645
- Vicks DayQuil SINUS Pressure & PAIN Relief with IBUPROFEN 735

Indapamide (Antihypertensive effects may be potentiated when used concurrently with thiazide diuretics; dosage adjustment may be necessary).
No products indexed under this heading.

Indomethacin (Concurrent use of nonsteroidal anti-inflammatory agents in some patients may reduce the diuretic, natriuretic and antihypertensive effects of thiazide diuretics). Products include:
- Indocin 1723

Indomethacin Sodium Trihydrate (Concurrent use of nonsteroidal anti-inflammatory agents in some patients may reduce the diuretic, natriuretic and antihypertensive effects of thiazide diuretics). Products include:
- Indocin I.V. 1727

Insulin, Human (Hyperglycemia may occur with thiazide diuretics; dosage adjustment of insulin may be required).
No products indexed under this heading.

Insulin, Human Isophane Suspension (Hyperglycemia may occur with thiazide diuretics; dosage adjustment of insulin may be required). Products include:
- Novolin N Human Insulin 10 ml Vials 1846

Insulin, Human NPH (Hyperglycemia may occur with thiazide diuretics; dosage adjustment of insulin may be required). Products include:
- Humulin N, 100 Units 1495
- Novolin N PenFill 1.5 ml Cartridges Durable Insulin Delivery System 1849
- Novolin N Prefilled Syringe Disposable Insulin Delivery System 1850

Insulin, Human Regular (Hyperglycemia may occur with thiazide diuretics; dosage adjustment of insulin may be required). Products include:
- Humulin R, 100 Units 1497
- Novolin R Human Insulin 10 ml Vials 1846
- Novolin R PenFill 1.5 ml Cartridges Durable Insulin Delivery System 1849
- Novolin R Prefilled Syringe Disposable Insulin Delivery System 1850
- Velosulin BR Human Insulin 10 ml Vials 1847

Insulin, Human, Zinc Suspension (Hyperglycemia may occur with thiazide diuretics; dosage adjustment of insulin may be required). Products include:
- Humulin L, 100 Units 1494
- Humulin U, 100 Units 1498
- Novolin L Human Insulin 10 ml Vials 1846

Insulin Lispro, Human (Hyperglycemia may occur with thiazide diuretics; dosage adjustment of insulin may be required). Products include:
- Humalog Injection 1488

Insulin, NPH (Hyperglycemia may occur with thiazide diuretics; dosage adjustment of insulin may be required). Products include:
- NPH, 100 Units 1502
- Pork NPH, 100 Units 1506
- Purified Pork NPH Isophane Insulin 1852

Insulin, Regular (Hyperglycemia may occur with thiazide diuretics; dosage adjustment of insulin may be required). Products include:
- Regular, 100 Units 1503
- Pork Regular, 100 Units 1507
- Pork Regular (Concentrated), 500 Units 1508
- Purified Pork Regular Insulin 1852

Insulin, Zinc Crystals (Hyperglycemia may occur with thiazide diuretics; dosage adjustment of insulin may be required). Products include:
- NPH, 100 Units 1502

Insulin, Zinc Suspension (Hyperglycemia may occur with thiazide diuretics; dosage adjustment of insulin may be required). Products include:
- Iletin I 1501
- Lente, 100 Units 1501
- Iletin II 1504
- Pork Lente, 100 Units 1504
- Purified Pork Lente Insulin 1852

Isoflurane (Effects may be potentiated when used concurrently with thiazide diuretics; dosage adjustment may be necessary).
No products indexed under this heading.

Ketamine Hydrochloride (Effects may be potentiated when used concurrently with thiazide diuretics; dosage adjustment may be necessary).
No products indexed under this heading.

Ketoprofen (Concurrent use of nonsteroidal anti-inflammatory agents in some patients may reduce the diuretic, natriuretic and antihypertensive effects of thiazide diuretics). Products include:
- Actron Caplets and Tablets 608
- Orudis Capsules 2874
- Orudis KT 842
- Oruvail Capsules 2874

Ketorolac Tromethamine (Concurrent use of nonsteroidal anti-inflammatory agents in some patients may reduce the diuretic, natriuretic and antihypertensive effects of thiazide diuretics). Products include:
- Acular Sterile Ophthalmic Solution 470
- Toradol 2319

Levorphanol Tartrate (Thiazide-induced orthostatic hypotension may be potentiated). Products include:
- Levo-Dromoran 2297

Lisinopril (Antihypertensive effects may be potentiated when used concurrently with thiazide diuretics; dosage adjustment may be necessary). Products include:
- Prinivil Tablets 1776
- Prinzide Tablets 1780
- Zestoretic Tablets 2968
- Zestril Tablets 2972

Lithium Carbonate (Diuretics reduce the renal clearance of lithium and add a high risk of lithium toxicity). Products include:
- Eskalith 2658
- Lithium Carbonate Capsules & Tablets 2352
- Lithonate/Lithotabs/Lithobid 2721

Lithium Citrate (Diuretics reduce the renal clearance of lithium and add a high risk of lithium toxicity).
No products indexed under this heading.

Mecamylamine Hydrochloride (Antihypertensive effects may be potentiated when used concurrently with thiazide diuretics; dosage adjustment may be necessary). Products include:
- Inversine Tablets 1729

Meclofenamate Sodium (Concurrent use of nonsteroidal anti-inflammatory agents in some patients may reduce the diuretic, natriuretic and antihypertensive effects of thiazide diuretics).
No products indexed under this heading.

Mefenamic Acid (Concurrent use of nonsteroidal anti-inflammatory agents in some patients may reduce the diuretic, natriuretic and antihypertensive effects of thiazide diuretics). Products include:
- Ponstel 1982

Meperidine Hydrochloride (Thiazide-induced orthostatic hypotension may be potentiated). Products include:
- Demerol 2438
- Mepergan Injection 2859

Mephobarbital (Thiazide-induced orthostatic hypotension may be potentiated). Products include:
- Mebaral Tablets 2452

Metformin Hydrochloride (Hyperglycemia may occur with thiazide diuretics; dosage adjustment of the oral antidiabetic drug may be required). Products include:
- Glucophage Tablets 754

Methadone Hydrochloride (Thiazide-induced orthostatic hypotension may be potentiated). Products include:
- Methadone Hydrochloride Oral Concentrate 2356
- Methadone Hydrochloride Oral Solution & Tablets 2357

Methenamine (Effectiveness of methenamine may be decreased when used concurrently with thiazide diuretics because of alkalinization of the urine). Products include:
- Urised Tablets 2123

IMPORTANT NOTE: Always consult each drug listing in the patient's regimen for possible interactions.

Methenamine Hippurate (Effectiveness of methenamine may be decreased when used concurrently with thiazide diuretics because of alkalinization of the urine).
No products indexed under this heading.

Methenamine Mandelate (Effectiveness of methenamine may be decreased when used concurrently with thiazide diuretics because of alkalinization of the urine). Products include:
Uroqid-Acid No. 2 Tablets ... 633

Methohexital Sodium (Effects may be potentiated when used concurrently with thiazide diuretics; dosage adjustment may be necessary).
No products indexed under this heading.

Methoxyflurane (Effects may be potentiated when used concurrently with thiazide diuretics; dosage adjustment may be necessary).
No products indexed under this heading.

Methyldopa (Antihypertensive effects may be potentiated when used concurrently with thiazide diuretics; dosage adjustment may be necessary). Products include:
Aldoclor Tablets ... 1638
Aldomet Oral ... 1640
Aldoril Tablets ... 1644

Methyldopate Hydrochloride (Antihypertensive effects may be potentiated when used concurrently with thiazide diuretics; dosage adjustment may be necessary). Products include:
Aldomet Ester HCl Injection ... 1642

Methylprednisolone Acetate (Intensified electrolyte depletion, particularly hypokalemia).
No products indexed under this heading.

Methylprednisolone Sodium Succinate (Intensified electrolyte depletion, particularly hypokalemia).
No products indexed under this heading.

Metolazone (Antihypertensive effects may be potentiated when used concurrently with thiazide diuretics; dosage adjustment may be necessary). Products include:
Mykrox Tablets ... 1617
Zaroxolyn Tablets ... 1625

Metyrosine (Antihypertensive effects may be potentiated when used concurrently with thiazide diuretics; dosage adjustment may be necessary). Products include:
Demser Capsules ... 1690

Minoxidil (Antihypertensive effects may be potentiated when used concurrently with thiazide diuretics; dosage adjustment may be necessary).
No products indexed under this heading.

Morphine Sulfate (Thiazide-induced orthostatic hypotension may be potentiated). Products include:
Astramorph/PF Injection, USP (Preservative-Free) ... 526
Duramorph Injection ... 983
Infumorph 200 and Infumorph 500 Sterile Solutions ... 985
Kadian Capsules ... 2948
MS Contin Tablets ... 2149
MSIR ... 2152
Oramorph SR (Morphine Sulfate Sustained Release Tablets) ... 2359
RMS Suppositories CII ... 2766
Roxanol ... 2365

Nabumetone (Concurrent use of nonsteroidal anti-inflammatory agents in some patients may reduce the diuretic, natriuretic and antihypertensive effects of thiazide diuretics). Products include:
Relafen Tablets ... 2688

Naproxen (Concurrent use of nonsteroidal anti-inflammatory agents in some patients may reduce the diuretic, natriuretic and antihypertensive effects of thiazide diuretics). Products include:
Anaprox/Naprosyn ... 2277

Naproxen Sodium (Concurrent use of nonsteroidal anti-inflammatory agents in some patients may reduce the diuretic, natriuretic and antihypertensive effects of thiazide diuretics). Products include:
Aleve ... 2124
Anaprox/Naprosyn ... 2277
Naprelan Tablets ... 2861

Nicardipine Hydrochloride (Antihypertensive effects may be potentiated when used concurrently with thiazide diuretics; dosage adjustment may be necessary). Products include:
Cardene Capsules ... 2261
Cardene I.V. ... 2815
Cardene SR Capsules ... 2264

Nitroglycerin (Antihypertensive effects may be potentiated when used concurrently with thiazide diuretics; dosage adjustment may be necessary). Products include:
Deponit NTG Transdermal Delivery System ... 2541
Nitro-Bid IV ... 1270
Nitro-Bid Ointment ... 1272
Nitro-Dur (nitroglycerin) Transdermal Infusion System ... 1365
Nitrolingual Spray ... 2193
Nitrostat Tablets ... 1981
Transderm-Nitro Transdermal Therapeutic System ... 878

Norepinephrine Bitartrate (Thiazides may decrease the arterial responsiveness to norepinephrine). Products include:
Levophed Bitartrate Injection ... 2445

Opium Alkaloids (Thiazide-induced orthostatic hypotension may be potentiated).
No products indexed under this heading.

Oxaprozin (Concurrent use of nonsteroidal anti-inflammatory agents in some patients may reduce the diuretic, natriuretic and antihypertensive effects of thiazide diuretics). Products include:
Daypro Caplets ... 2578

Oxycodone Hydrochloride (Thiazide-induced orthostatic hypotension may be potentiated). Products include:
OxyContin Tablets ... 2163
OxyIR Capsules ... 2167
Percocet Tablets ... 955
Percodan Tablets ... 955
Percodan-Demi Tablets ... 956
Roxicodone Tablets, Oral Solution & Intensol (Oxycodone) ... 2366
Tylox Capsules ... 1593

Pentobarbital Sodium (Thiazide-induced orthostatic hypotension may be potentiated). Products include:
Nembutal Sodium Capsules ... 440
Nembutal Sodium Solution ... 442
Nembutal Sodium Suppositories ... 444

Phenobarbital (Thiazide-induced orthostatic hypotension may be potentiated). Products include:
Arco-Lase Plus Tablets ... 513
Bellergal-S Tablets ... 2375
Donnatal ... 2234
Donnatal Extentabs ... 2234
Donnatal Tablets ... 2234
Phenobarbital Elixir and Tablets ... 1523
Quadrinal Tablets ... 1398

Phenoxybenzamine Hydrochloride (Antihypertensive effects may be potentiated when used concurrently with thiazide diuretics; dosage adjustment may be necessary). Products include:
Dibenzyline Capsules ... 2650

Phentolamine Mesylate (Antihypertensive effects may be potentiated when used concurrently with thiazide diuretics; dosage adjustment may be necessary). Products include:
Regitine Vials ... 864

Phenylbutazone (Concurrent use of nonsteroidal anti-inflammatory agents in some patients may reduce the diuretic, natriuretic and antihypertensive effects of thiazide diuretics).
No products indexed under this heading.

Piroxicam (Concurrent use of nonsteroidal anti-inflammatory agents in some patients may reduce the diuretic, natriuretic and antihypertensive effects of thiazide diuretics). Products include:
Feldene Capsules ... 2008

Prazosin Hydrochloride (Antihypertensive effects may be potentiated when used concurrently with thiazide diuretics; dosage adjustment may be necessary). Products include:
Minipress Capsules ... 2015
Minizide Capsules ... 2016

Prednisolone Acetate (Intensified electrolyte depletion, particularly hypokalemia). Products include:
AK-CIDE ... ◉ 203
AK-CIDE Ointment ... ◉ 203
Blephamide Liquifilm Sterile Ophthalmic Suspension ... 472
Blephamide Ointment ... ◉ 234
Econopred & Econopred Plus Ophthalmic Suspensions ... ◉ 216
Poly-Pred Liquifilm ... ◉ 246
Pred Forte ... ◉ 247
Pred Mild ... ◉ 250
Pred-G Liquifilm Sterile Ophthalmic Suspension ... ◉ 248
Pred-G S.O.P. Sterile Ophthalmic Ointment ... ◉ 249

Prednisolone Sodium Phosphate (Intensified electrolyte depletion, particularly hypokalemia). Products include:
AK-PRED ... ◉ 204
Hydeltrasol Injection, Sterile ... 1708
Pediapred Oral Solution ... 1618

Prednisolone Tebutate (Intensified electrolyte depletion, particularly hypokalemia). Products include:
Hydeltra-T.B.A. Sterile Suspension 1710

Prednisone (Intensified electrolyte depletion, particularly hypokalemia).
No products indexed under this heading.

Probenecid (Thiazide diuretics may raise the levels of blood uric acid; dosage adjustment of antigout medication may be necessary to control gout and hyperuricemia). Products include:
Benemid Tablets ... 1651
ColBENEMID Tablets ... 1662

Propofol (Effects may be potentiated when used concurrently with thiazide diuretics; dosage adjustment may be necessary). Products include:
Diprivan Injectable Emulsion ... 2939

Propoxyphene Hydrochloride (Thiazide-induced orthostatic hypotension may be potentiated). Products include:
Darvon ... 1475
Wygesic Tablets ... 2930

Propoxyphene Napsylate (Thiazide-induced orthostatic hypotension may be potentiated). Products include:
Darvon-N/Darvocet-N ... 1473

Secobarbital Sodium (Thiazide-induced orthostatic hypotension may be potentiated). Products include:
Seconal Sodium Pulvules ... 1529

Sevoflurane (Effects may be potentiated when used concurrently with thiazide diuretics; dosage adjustment may be necessary).
No products indexed under this heading.

Sodium Nitroprusside (Antihypertensive effects may be potentiated when used concurrently with thiazide diuretics; dosage adjustment may be necessary).
No products indexed under this heading.

Sufentanil Citrate (Thiazide-induced orthostatic hypotension may be potentiated). Products include:
Sufenta Injection ... 1355

Sulfinpyrazone (Thiazide diuretics may raise the levels of blood uric acid; dosage adjustment of antigout medication may be necessary to control gout and hyperuricemia). Products include:
Anturane ... 823

Sulindac (Concurrent use of nonsteroidal anti-inflammatory agents in some patients may reduce the diuretic, natriuretic and antihypertensive effects of thiazide diuretics). Products include:
Clinoril Tablets ... 1658

Terazosin Hydrochloride (Antihypertensive effects may be potentiated when used concurrently with thiazide diuretics; dosage adjustment may be necessary). Products include:
Hytrin Capsules ... 434

Thiamylal Sodium (Thiazide-induced orthostatic hypotension may be potentiated).
No products indexed under this heading.

Tolazamide (Hyperglycemia may occur with thiazide diuretics; dosage adjustment of the oral antidiabetic drug may be required).
No products indexed under this heading.

Tolbutamide (Hyperglycemia may occur with thiazide diuretics; dosage adjustment of the oral antidiabetic drug may be required).
No products indexed under this heading.

Tolmetin Sodium (Concurrent use of nonsteroidal anti-inflammatory agents in some patients may reduce the diuretic, natriuretic and antihypertensive effects of thiazide diuretics). Products include:
Tolectin (200, 400 and 600 mg) .. 1591

Trandolapril (Antihypertensive effects may be potentiated when used concurrently with thiazide diuretics; dosage adjustment may be necessary). Products include:
Mavik Tablets ... 1407

Triamcinolone (Intensified electrolyte depletion, particularly hypokalemia).
No products indexed under this heading.

Triamcinolone Acetonide (Intensified electrolyte depletion, particularly hypokalemia). Products include:
Azmacort Oral Inhaler ... 2175
Nasacort AQ Nasal Spray ... 2191

(▣ Described in PDR For Nonprescription Drugs) (◉ Described in PDR For Ophthalmology)

315 **Interactions Index** **Diupres**

Nasacort Nasal Inhaler 2189

Triamcinolone Diacetate (Intensified electrolyte depletion, particularly hypokalemia).
No products indexed under this heading.

Triamcinolone Hexacetonide (Intensified electrolyte depletion, particularly hypokalemia).
No products indexed under this heading.

Trimethaphan Camsylate (Antihypertensive effects may be potentiated when used concurrently with thiazide diuretics; dosage adjustment may be necessary).
No products indexed under this heading.

Tubocurarine Chloride (Thiazides may increase the responsiveness to tubocurarine).
No products indexed under this heading.

Warfarin Sodium (Thiazide diuretics may decrease the effects of oral anticoagulants). Products include:
Coumadin 941

Food Interactions

Alcohol (Thiazide-induced orthostatic hypotension may be potentiated).

DIUPRES TABLETS

(Reserpine, Chlorothiazide) 1691
May interact with antihypertensives, lithium preparations, cardiac glycosides, corticosteroids, insulin, nonsteroidal anti-inflammatory agents, barbiturates, monoamine oxidase inhibitors, narcotic analgesics, oral hypoglycemic agents, general anesthetics, and certain other agents. Compounds in these categories include:

Acarbose (Hyperglycemia may occur; dosage adjustment of the antidiabetic drug may be required). Products include:
Precose 604

ACTH (Potential for intensified electrolyte depletion, particularly hypokalemia).
No products indexed under this heading.

Alfentanil Hydrochloride (Orthostatic hypotension may be aggravated). Products include:
Alfenta Injection 1334

Amlodipine Besylate (Potentiated; additive effects). Products include:
Lotrel Capsules 858
Norvasc Tablets 2020

Aprobarbital (Potentiation of orthostatic hypotension produced by thiazides; enhances CNS depressant effects of reserpine).
No products indexed under this heading.

Atenolol (Potentiated; additive effects). Products include:
Tenoretic Tablets 2963
Tenormin Tablets and I.V. Injection 2965

Benazepril Hydrochloride (Potentiated; additive effects). Products include:
Lotensin Tablets 852
Lotensin HCT Tablets 855
Lotrel Capsules 858

Bendroflumethiazide (Potentiated; additive effects).
No products indexed under this heading.

Betamethasone Acetate (Potential for intensified electrolyte depletion, particularly hypokalemia). Products include:
Celestone Soluspan Suspension 2484

Betamethasone Sodium Phosphate (Potential for intensified electrolyte depletion, particularly hypokalemia). Products include:
Celestone Soluspan Suspension 2484

Betaxolol Hydrochloride (Potentiated; additive effects). Products include:
Betoptic Ophthalmic Solution 465
Betoptic S Ophthalmic Suspension 467
Kerlone Tablets 2588

Bisoprolol Fumarate (Potentiated; additive effects). Products include:
Zebeta Tablets 1457
Ziac 1459

Buprenorphine (Orthostatic hypotension may be aggravated). Products include:
Buprenex Injectable 2170

Butabarbital (Potentiation of orthostatic hypotension produced by thiazides; enhances CNS depressant effects of reserpine).
No products indexed under this heading.

Butalbital (Potentiation of orthostatic hypotension produced by thiazides; enhances CNS depressant effects of reserpine). Products include:
Axocet Capsules 2469
Esgic-plus Capsules 1012
Esgic-plus Tablets 1012
Fioricet Tablets 2386
Fioricet with Codeine Capsules 2387
Fiorinal Capsules 2388
Fiorinal with Codeine Capsules 2390
Fiorinal Tablets 2388
Phrenilin 790
Sedapap Tablets 50 mg/650 mg .. 1826

Captopril (Potentiated; additive effects). Products include:
Capoten Tablets 740
Capozide Tablets 744

Carteolol Hydrochloride (Potentiated; additive effects). Products include:
Cartrol Tablets 413
Ocupress Ophthalmic Solution, 1% Sterile .... ⊚ 297

Chlorothiazide Sodium (Potentiated; additive effects). Products include:
Diuril Sodium Intravenous 1693

Chlorpropamide (Hyperglycemia may occur; dosage adjustment of the antidiabetic drug may be required). Products include:
Diabinese Tablets 2002

Chlorthalidone (Potentiated; additive effects). Products include:
Combipres Tablets 682
Tenoretic Tablets 2963
Thalitone 1293

Cholestyramine (Cholestyramine resin has potential of binding thiazide diuretics and reducing diuretic absorption from the GI tract). Products include:
Questran 774

Clonidine (Potentiated; additive effects). Products include:
Catapres-TTS 680

Clonidine Hydrochloride (Potentiated; additive effects). Products include:
Catapres Tablets 679
Combipres Tablets 682

Codeine Phosphate (Orthostatic hypotension may be aggravated). Products include:
Brontex 2130
Dimetane-DC Cough Syrup 2232
Fioricet with Codeine Capsules 2387
Fiorinal with Codeine Capsules 2390
Nucofed 2225
Phenergan with Codeine 2883
Phenergan VC with Codeine 2888
Robitussin A-C Syrup 2248
Robitussin-DAC Syrup 2249
Ryna .... ▣ 804
Soma Compound w/Codeine Tablets 2784
Tylenol with Codeine 1592

Colestipol Hydrochloride (Colestipol resin has potential of binding thiazide diuretics and reducing diuretic absorption from the GI tract). Products include:
Colestid 2073

Cortisone Acetate (Potential for intensified electrolyte depletion, particularly hypokalemia). Products include:
Cortone Acetate Sterile Suspension 1663
Cortone Acetate Tablets 1664

Deserpidine (Potentiated; additive effects).
No products indexed under this heading.

Deslanoside (Thiazide-induced hypokalemia may exaggerate or sensitize the response of the heart to toxic effects of digitalis, e.g., increased ventricular irritability; reserpine causes cardiac arrhythmia, use cautiously with digitalis).
No products indexed under this heading.

Dexamethasone (Potential for intensified electrolyte depletion, particularly hypokalemia). Products include:
AK-Trol Ointment & Suspension .... ⊚ 205
Decadron Elixir 1676
Decadron Tablets 1678
Decaspray Topical Aerosol 1689
Maxitrol Ophthalmic Ointment and Suspension .... ⊚ 222
TobraDex Ophthalmic Suspension and Ointment 469

Dexamethasone Acetate (Potential for intensified electrolyte depletion, particularly hypokalemia). Products include:
Dalalone D.P. Injectable 1009
Decadron-LA Sterile Suspension 1687

Dexamethasone Sodium Phosphate (Potential for intensified electrolyte depletion, particularly hypokalemia). Products include:
Decadron Phosphate Injection 1680
Decadron Phosphate Sterile Ophthalmic Ointment 1684
Decadron Phosphate Sterile Ophthalmic Solution 1685
Decadron Phosphate Topical Cream 1686
Decadron Phosphate with Xylocaine Injection, Sterile 1683
Dexacort Phosphate in Respihaler .. 1606
Dexacort Phosphate in Turbinaire .. 1607
NeoDecadron Sterile Ophthalmic Ointment 1755
NeoDecadron Sterile Ophthalmic Solution 1756
NeoDecadron Topical Cream 1757

Dezocine (Orthostatic hypotension may be aggravated). Products include:
Dalgan Injection 529

Diazoxide (Potentiated; additive effects). Products include:
Hyperstat I.V. Injection 2504
Proglycem 575

Diclofenac Potassium (Reduced diuretic, natriuretic, and antihypertensive effects of chlorothiazide). Products include:
Cataflam Tablets 833

Diclofenac Sodium (Reduced diuretic, natriuretic, and antihypertensive effects of chlorothiazide). Products include:
Voltaren Ophthalmic Sterile Ophthalmic Solution .... ⊚ 264
Cataflam/Voltaren/Voltaren-XR 833

Digitoxin (Thiazide-induced hypokalemia may exaggerate or sensitize the response of the heart to toxic effects of digitalis, e.g., increased ventricular irritability; reserpine causes cardiac arrhythmia, use cautiously with digitalis). Products include:
Crystodigin Tablets 1472

Digoxin (Thiazide-induced hypokalemia may exaggerate or sensitize the response of the heart to toxic effects of digitalis, e.g., increased ventricular irritability; reserpine causes cardiac arrhythmia, use cautiously with digitalis). Products include:
Lanoxicaps 1110
Lanoxin Elixir Pediatric 1113
Lanoxin Injection 1116
Lanoxin Injection Pediatric 1119
Lanoxin Tablets 1121

Diltiazem Hydrochloride (Potentiated; additive effects). Products include:
Cardizem CD Capsules 1251
Cardizem SR Capsules 1255
Cardizem Injectable 1253
Cardizem Tablets 1257
Dilacor XR Extended-release Capsules 2183
Tiazac Capsules 1019

Doxazosin Mesylate (Potentiated; additive effects). Products include:
Cardura Tablets 1993

Enalapril Maleate (Potentiated; additive effects). Products include:
Vaseretic Tablets 1810
Vasotec Tablets 1816

Enalaprilat (Potentiation of antihypertensive effect). Products include:
Vasotec I.V. 1814

Enflurane (Significant hypotension; bradycardia).
No products indexed under this heading.

Esmolol Hydrochloride (Potentiated; additive effects). Products include:
Brevibloc (esmolol HCl) Injection ... 1860

Etodolac (Reduced diuretic, natriuretic, and antihypertensive effects of chlorothiazide). Products include:
Lodine Capsules and Tablets 2849

Felodipine (Potentiated; additive effects). Products include:
Plendil Extended-Release Tablets 514

Fenoprofen Calcium (Reduced diuretic, natriuretic, and antihypertensive effects of chlorothiazide). Products include:
Nalfon 200 Pulvules & Nalfon Tablets 933

Fentanyl (Orthostatic hypotension may be aggravated). Products include:
Duragesic Transdermal System 1336

Fentanyl Citrate (Orthostatic hypotension may be aggravated). Products include:
Sublimaze Injection 463

Fludrocortisone Acetate (Potential for intensified electrolyte depletion, particularly hypokalemia). Products include:
Florinef Acetate Tablets 506

Flurbiprofen (Reduced diuretic, natriuretic, and antihypertensive effects of chlorothiazide).
No products indexed under this heading.

Fosinopril Sodium (Potentiated; additive effects). Products include:
Monopril Tablets 762

Furazolidone (Concurrent use is contraindicated). Products include:
Furoxone 2221

IMPORTANT NOTE: Always consult each drug listing in the patient's regimen for possible interactions.

Diupres | Interactions Index | 316

Furosemide (Potentiated; additive effects). Products include:
- Lasix Injection, Oral Solution and Tablets 1267

Glimepiride (Hyperglycemia may occur; dosage adjustment of the antidiabetic drug may be required). Products include:
- Amaryl Tablets 1241

Glipizide (Hyperglycemia may occur; dosage adjustment of the antidiabetic drug may be required). Products include:
- Glucotrol Tablets 2011
- Glucotrol XL Extended Release Tablets 2012

Glyburide (Hyperglycemia may occur; dosage adjustment of the antidiabetic drug may be required). Products include:
- DiaBeta Tablets 1265
- Glynase PresTab Tablets 2091
- Micronase Tablets 2099

Guanabenz Acetate (Potentiated; additive effects).
No products indexed under this heading.

Guanethidine Monosulfate (Potentiated; additive effects). Products include:
- Esimil Tablets 840
- Ismelin Tablets 845

Hydralazine Hydrochloride (Potentiated; additive effects). Products include:
- Apresazide Capsules 824
- Apresoline Hydrochloride Tablets 826
- Hydralazine Hydrochloride Injection USP 2712
- Ser-Ap-Es Tablets 867

Hydrochlorothiazide (Potentiated; additive effects). Products include:
- Aldactazide Tablets 2556
- Aldoril Tablets 1644
- Apresazide Capsules 824
- Capozide Tablets 744
- Dyazide Capsules 2653
- Esidrix Tablets 839
- Esimil Tablets 840
- HydroDIURIL Tablets 1716
- Hydropres Tablets 1718
- Hyzaar Tablets 1720
- Inderide Tablets 2838
- Inderide LA Long Acting Capsules 2840
- Lopressor HCT Tablets 850
- Lotensin HCT Tablets 855
- Moduretic Tablets 1748
- Oretic Tablets 450
- Prinzide Tablets 1780
- Ser-Ap-Es Tablets 867
- Timolide Tablets 1791
- Vaseretic Tablets 1810
- Zestoretic Tablets 2968
- Ziac 1459

Hydrocodone Bitartrate (Orthostatic hypotension may be aggravated). Products include:
- Codiclear DH Syrup 808
- Duratuss HD Elixir 2750
- Histussin D Liquid 670
- Hycodan Tablets and Syrup 946
- Hycomine Compound Tablets 948
- Hycomine 947
- Hycotuss Expectorant Syrup 950
- Hydrocet Capsules 787
- Lorcet 10/650 Tablets 1016
- Lortab 2751
- Tussend 1830
- Tussend Expectorant 1831
- Vicodin Tablets 1404
- Vicodin ES Tablets 1405
- Vicodin HP Tablets 1403
- Vicodin Tuss Expectorant 1406
- Zydone Capsules 967

Hydrocodone Polistirex (Orthostatic hypotension may be aggravated). Products include:
- Tussionex Pennkinetic Extended-Release Suspension 1624

Hydrocortisone (Potential for intensified electrolyte depletion, particularly hypokalemia. Products include:
- Anusol-HC Cream 2.5% 1953
- Aquanil HC Lotion 1989
- Maximum Strength Cortaid Spray 800
- CORTENEMA 2713
- Cortisporin Ointment 1074
- Cortisporin Ophthalmic Ointment Sterile 1074
- Cortisporin Ophthalmic Suspension Sterile 1075
- Cortisporin Otic Solution Sterile 1076
- Cortisporin Otic Suspension Sterile 1077
- Cortizone-5 795
- Cortizone-10 795
- Hydrocortone Tablets 1715
- Hytone 922
- Hytone Ointment 2 ½% 923
- Massengill Medicated Soft Cloth Towelettes 2628
- Pediotic Suspension Sterile 1140
- Preparation H Hydrocortisone 1% Cream 843
- ProctoCream-HC 2.5% 2552
- VōSoL HC Otic Solution 2786

Hydrocortisone Acetate (Potential for intensified electrolyte depletion, particularly hypokalemia). Products include:
- Analpram-HC Rectal Cream 1% and 2.5% 993
- Anusol HC-1 Hydrocortisone Anti-Itch Ointment 810
- Anusol-HC Suppositories 1954
- Caldecort Anti-Itch Hydrocortisone Cream 651
- Coly-Mycin S Otic w/Neomycin & Hydrocortisone 1965
- Cortaid 800
- Cortifoam 2540
- Cortisporin Cream 1073
- Cortifoam 2543
- Epifoam 2543
- Hydrocortone Acetate Sterile Suspension 1712
- Mantadil Cream 1124
- Nupercainal Hydrocortisone 1% Cream 661
- Pramosone Cream, Lotion & Ointment 995
- ProctoFoam-HC 2552
- Terra-Cortril Ophthalmic Suspension 2033

Hydrocortisone Sodium Phosphate (Potential for intensified electrolyte depletion, particularly hypokalemia). Products include:
- Hydrocortone Phosphate Injection, Sterile 1713

Hydrocortisone Sodium Succinate (Potential for intensified electrolyte depletion, particularly hypokalemia).
No products indexed under this heading.

Hydroflumethiazide (Potentiated; additive effects). Products include:
- Diucardin Tablets 2824

Hydromorphone Hydrochloride (Orthostatic hypotension may be aggravated). Products include:
- Dilaudid Ampules 1382
- Dilaudid Cough Syrup 1383
- Dilaudid-HP Injection 1384
- Dilaudid-HP Lyophilized Powder 250 mg 1384
- Dilaudid 1382
- Dilaudid Oral Liquid 1386
- Dilaudid 1382
- Dilaudid Tablets - 8 mg 1386

Ibuprofen (Reduced diuretic, natriuretic, and antihypertensive effects of chlorothiazide). Products include:
- Advil Cold and Sinus Caplets and Tablets 837
- Advil Ibuprofen Tablets, Caplets and Gel Caplets 836
- Children's Motrin Ibuprofen Oral Suspension 1558
- IBU Tablets 1389
- Ibuprohm 713
- Motrin IB Caplets, Tablets, and Gelcaps 802
- Motrin Ibuprofen Suspension, Oral Drops, Chewable Tablets, Caplets 1563
- Nuprin Ibuprofen/Analgesic Tablets & Caplets 645
- Vicks DayQuil SINUS Pressure & PAIN Relief with IBUPROFEN 735

Indapamide (Potentiated; additive effects).
No products indexed under this heading.

Indomethacin (Reduced diuretic, natriuretic, and antihypertensive effects of chlorothiazide). Products include:
- Indocin 1723

Indomethacin Sodium Trihydrate (Reduced diuretic, natriuretic, and antihypertensive effects of chlorothiazide). Products include:
- Indocin I.V. 1727

Insulin, Human (Hyperglycemia may occur; dosage adjustment of insulin may be required).
No products indexed under this heading.

Insulin, Human Isophane Suspension (Hyperglycemia may occur; dosage adjustment of insulin may be required). Products include:
- Novolin N Human Insulin 10 ml Vials 1846

Insulin, Human NPH (Hyperglycemia may occur; dosage adjustment of insulin may be required). Products include:
- Humulin N, 100 Units 1495
- Novolin N PenFill 1.5 ml Cartridges Durable Insulin Delivery System 1849
- Novolin N Prefilled Syringe Disposable Insulin Delivery System 1850

Insulin, Human Regular (Hyperglycemia may occur; dosage adjustment of insulin may be required). Products include:
- Humulin R, 100 Units 1497
- Novolin R Human Insulin 10 ml Vials 1846
- Novolin R PenFill 1.5 ml Cartridges Durable Insulin Delivery System 1849
- Novolin R Prefilled Syringe Disposable Insulin Delivery System 1850
- Velosulin BR Human Insulin 10 ml Vials 1847

Insulin, Human, Zinc Suspension (Hyperglycemia may occur; dosage adjustment of insulin may be required). Products include:
- Humulin L, 100 Units 1494
- Humulin U, 100 Units 1498
- Novolin L Human Insulin 10 ml Vials 1846

Insulin Lispro, Human (Hyperglycemia may occur; dosage adjustment of insulin may be required). Products include:
- Humalog Injection 1488

Insulin, NPH (Hyperglycemia may occur; dosage adjustment of insulin may be required). Products include:
- NPH, 100 Units 1502
- Pork NPH, 100 Units 1506
- Purified Pork NPH Isophane Insulin 1852

Insulin, Regular (Hyperglycemia may occur; dosage adjustment of insulin may be required). Products include:
- Regular, 100 Units 1503
- Pork Regular, 100 Units 1507
- Pork Regular (Concentrated), 500 Units 1508
- Purified Pork Regular Insulin 1852

Insulin, Zinc Crystals (Hyperglycemia may occur; dosage adjustment of insulin may be required). Products include:
- NPH, 100 Units 1502

Insulin, Zinc Suspension (Hyperglycemia may occur; dosage adjustment of insulin may be required). Products include:
- Iletin I 1501
- Lente, 100 Units 1501
- Iletin II 1504
- Pork Lente, 100 Units 1504
- Purified Pork Lente Insulin 1852

Isocarboxazid (Concurrent use is contraindicated).
No products indexed under this heading.

Isoflurane (Significant hypotension; bradycardia).
No products indexed under this heading.

Isradipine (Potentiated; additive effects). Products include:
- DynaCirc Capsules 2381
- DynaCirc CR Tablets 2383

Ketamine Hydrochloride (May require reduced dose of anesthetics).
No products indexed under this heading.

Ketoprofen (Reduced diuretic, natriuretic, and antihypertensive effects of chlorothiazide). Products include:
- Actron Caplets and Tablets 608
- Orudis Capsules 2874
- Orudis KT 842
- Oruvail Capsules 2874

Ketorolac Tromethamine (Reduced diuretic, natriuretic, and antihypertensive effects of chlorothiazide). Products include:
- Acular Sterile Ophthalmic Solution 470
- Toradol 2319

Labetalol Hydrochloride (Potentiated; additive effects). Products include:
- Normodyne Injection 2519
- Normodyne Tablets 2522
- Trandate 1158

Levorphanol Tartrate (Orthostatic hypotension may be aggravated). Products include:
- Levo-Dromoran 2297

Lisinopril (Potentiation of antihypertensive effect). Products include:
- Prinivil Tablets 1776
- Prinzide Tablets 1780
- Zestoretic Tablets 2968
- Zestril Tablets 2972

Lithium Carbonate (Reduced renal clearance of lithium with resultant risk of lithium toxicity). Products include:
- Eskalith 2658
- Lithium Carbonate Capsules & Tablets 2352
- Lithonate/Lithotabs/Lithobid 2721

Lithium Citrate (Reduced renal clearance of lithium with resultant risk of lithium toxicity).
No products indexed under this heading.

Losartan Potassium (Potentiated; additive effects). Products include:
- Cozaar Tablets 1668
- Hyzaar Tablets 1720

Mecamylamine Hydrochloride (Potentiated; additive effects). Products include:
- Inversine Tablets 1729

Meclofenamate Sodium (Reduced diuretic, natriuretic, and antihypertensive effects of chlorothiazide).
No products indexed under this heading.

Mefenamic Acid (Reduced diuretic, natriuretic, and antihypertensive effects of chlorothiazide). Products include:
- Ponstel 1982

(Described in PDR For Nonprescription Drugs)   (Described in PDR For Ophthalmology)

Meperidine Hydrochloride (Orthostatic hypotension may be aggravated). Products include:
- Demerol 2438
- Mepergan Injection 2859

Mephobarbital (Potentiation of orthostatic hypotension produced by thiazides; enhances CNS depressant effects of reserpine). Products include:
- Mebaral Tablets 2452

Metformin Hydrochloride (Hyperglycemia may occur; dosage adjustment of the antidiabetic drug may be required). Products include:
- Glucophage Tablets 754

Methadone Hydrochloride (Orthostatic hypotension may be aggravated). Products include:
- Methadone Hydrochloride Oral Concentrate 2356
- Methadone Hydrochloride Oral Solution & Tablets 2357

Methohexital Sodium (Significant hypotension; bradycardia).
No products indexed under this heading.

Methoxyflurane (Significant hypotension; bradycardia).
No products indexed under this heading.

Methyclothiazide (Potentiated; additive effects). Products include:
- Enduron Tablets 424

Methyldopa (Potentiated; additive effects). Products include:
- Aldoclor Tablets 1638
- Aldomet Oral 1640
- Aldoril Tablets 1644

Methyldopate Hydrochloride (Potentiated; additive effects). Products include:
- Aldomet Ester HCl Injection 1642

Methylprednisolone Acetate (Potential for intensified electrolyte depletion, particularly hypokalemia).
No products indexed under this heading.

Methylprednisolone Sodium Succinate (Potential for intensified electrolyte depletion, particularly hypokalemia).
No products indexed under this heading.

Metolazone (Potentiated; additive effects). Products include:
- Mykrox Tablets 1617
- Zaroxolyn Tablets 1625

Metoprolol Succinate (Potentiated; additive effects). Products include:
- Toprol-XL Tablets 560

Metoprolol Tartrate (Potentiated; additive effects). Products include:
- Lopressor 848
- Lopressor HCT Tablets 850

Metyrosine (Potentiated; additive effects). Products include:
- Demser Capsules 1690

Minoxidil (Potentiated; additive effects).
No products indexed under this heading.

Moexipril Hydrochloride (Potentiated; additive effects). Products include:
- Univasc Tablets 2553

Morphine Sulfate (Orthostatic hypotension may be aggravated). Products include:
- Astramorph/PF Injection, USP (Preservative-Free) 526
- Duramorph Injection 983
- Infumorph 200 and Infumorph 500 Sterile Solutions 985
- Kadian Capsules 2948
- MS Contin Tablets 2149
- MSIR 2152

Oramorph SR (Morphine Sulfate Sustained Release Tablets) 2359
- RMS Suppositories CII 2766
- Roxanol 2365

Nabumetone (Reduced diuretic, natriuretic, and antihypertensive effects of chlorothiazide). Products include:
- Relafen Tablets 2688

Nadolol (Potentiated; additive effects).
No products indexed under this heading.

Naproxen (Reduced diuretic natriuretic, and antihypertensive effects of chlorothiazide). Products include:
- Anaprox/Naprosyn 2277

Naproxen Sodium (Reduced diuretic, natriuretic, and antihypertensive effects of chlorothiazide). Products include:
- Aleve 2124
- Anaprox/Naprosyn 2277
- Naprelan Tablets 2861

Nicardipine Hydrochloride (Potentiated; additive effects). Products include:
- Cardene Capsules 2261
- Cardene I.V. 2815
- Cardene SR Capsules 2264

Nifedipine (Potentiated; additive effects). Products include:
- Adalat Capsules (10 mg and 20 mg) 580
- Adalat CC 582
- Procardia Capsules 2024
- Procardia XL Extended Release Tablets 2026

Nisoldipine (Potentiated; additive effects). Products include:
- Sular Tablets 2961

Nitroglycerin (Potentiated; additive effects). Products include:
- Deponit NTG Transdermal Delivery System 2541
- Nitro-Bid IV 1270
- Nitro-Bid Ointment 1272
- Nitro-Dur (nitroglycerin) Transdermal Infusion System 1365
- Nitrolingual Spray 2193
- Nitrostat Tablets 1981
- Transderm-Nitro Transdermal Therapeutic System 878

Norepinephrine Bitartrate (Decreased arterial responsiveness to norepinephrine). Products include:
- Levophed Bitartrate Injection 2445

Opium Alkaloids (Orthostatic hypotension may be aggravated).
No products indexed under this heading.

Oxaprozin (Reduced diuretic, natriuretic, and antihypertensive effects of chlorothiazide). Products include:
- Daypro Caplets 2578

Oxycodone Hydrochloride (Orthostatic hypotension may be aggravated). Products include:
- OxyContin Tablets 2163
- OxyIR Capsules 2167
- Percocet Tablets 955
- Percodan Tablets 955
- Percodan-Demi Tablets 956
- Roxicodone Tablets, Oral Solution & Intensol (Oxycodone) 2366
- Tylox Capsules 1593

Penbutolol Sulfate (Potentiated; additive effects). Products include:
- Levatol Tablets 2547

Pentobarbital Sodium (Potentiation of orthostatic hypotension produced by thiazides; enhances CNS depressant effects of reserpine). Products include:
- Nembutal Sodium Capsules 440
- Nembutal Sodium Solution 442
- Nembutal Sodium Suppositories... 444

Phenelzine Sulfate (Concurrent use is contraindicated). Products include:
- Nardil 1977

Phenobarbital (Potentiation of orthostatic hypotension produced by thiazides; enhances CNS depressant effects of reserpine). Products include:
- Arco-Lase Plus Tablets 513
- Bellergal-S Tablets 2375
- Donnatal 2234
- Donnatal Extentabs 2234
- Donnatal Tablets 2234
- Phenobarbital Elixir and Tablets 1523
- Quadrinal Tablets 1398

Phenoxybenzamine Hydrochloride (Potentiated; additive effects). Products include:
- Dibenzyline Capsules 2650

Phentolamine Mesylate (Potentiated; additive effects). Products include:
- Regitine Vials 864

Phenylbutazone (Reduced diuretic, natriuretic, and antihypertensive effects of chlorothiazide).
No products indexed under this heading.

Pindolol (Potentiated; additive effects). Products include:
- Visken Tablets 2428

Piroxicam (Reduced diuretic, natriuretic, and antihypertensive effects of chlorothiazide). Products include:
- Feldene Capsules 2008

Polythiazide (Potentiated; additive effects). Products include:
- Minizide Capsules 2016

Prazosin Hydrochloride (Potentiated; additive effects). Products include:
- Minipress Capsules 2015
- Minizide Capsules 2016

Prednisolone Acetate (Potential for intensified electrolyte depletion, particularly hypokalemia). Products include:
- AK-CIDE .... ⦿ 203
- AK-CIDE Ointment .... ⦿ 203
- Blephamide Liquifilm Sterile Ophthalmic Suspension 472
- Blephamide Ointment .... ⦿ 234
- Econopred & Econopred Plus Ophthalmic Suspensions ...... ⦿ 216
- Poly-Pred Liquifilm .... ⦿ 246
- Pred Forte .... ⦿ 247
- Pred Mild .... ⦿ 250
- Pred-G Liquifilm Sterile Ophthalmic Suspension .... ⦿ 248
- Pred-G S.O.P. Sterile Ophthalmic Ointment .... ⦿ 249

Prednisolone Sodium Phosphate (Potential for intensified electrolyte depletion, particularly hypokalemia). Products include:
- AK-PRED .... ⦿ 204
- Hydeltrasol Injection, Sterile 1708
- Pediapred Oral Solution 1618

Prednisolone Tebutate (Potential for intensified electrolyte depletion, particularly hypokalemia). Products include:
- Hydeltra-T.B.A. Sterile Suspension 1710

Prednisone (Potential for intensified electrolyte depletion, particularly hypokalemia).
No products indexed under this heading.

Propofol (Significant hypotension; bradycardia). Products include:
- Diprivan Injectable Emulsion ... 2939

Propoxyphene Hydrochloride (Orthostatic hypotension may be aggravated). Products include:
- Darvon 1475
- Wygesic Tablets 2930

Propoxyphene Napsylate (Orthostatic hypotension may be aggravated). Products include:
- Darvon-N/Darvocet-N 1473

Propranolol Hydrochloride (Potentiated; additive effects). Products include:
- Inderal 2834
- Inderal LA Long Acting Capsules 2836
- Inderide Tablets 2838
- Inderide LA Long Acting Capsules .. 2840

Quinapril Hydrochloride (Potentiated; additive effects). Products include:
- Accupril Tablets 1950

Quinidine Gluconate (Reserpine causes cardiac arrhythmia, use cautiously with quinidine). Products include:
- Quinaglute Dura-Tabs Tablets 644

Quinidine Polygalacturonate (Reserpine causes cardiac arrhythmia, use cautiously with quinidine). Products include:
- Cardioquin Tablets 2146

Quinidine Sulfate (Reserpine causes cardiac arrhythmia, use cautiously with quinidine). Products include:
- Quinidex Extentabs 2240

Ramipril (Potentiated; additive effects). Products include:
- Altace Capsules 1238

Rauwolfia Serpentina (Potentiated; additive effects).
No products indexed under this heading.

Rescinnamine (Potentiated; additive effects).
No products indexed under this heading.

Secobarbital Sodium (Potentiation of orthostatic hypotension produced by thiazides; enhances CNS depressant effects of reserpine). Products include:
- Seconal Sodium Pulvules 1529

Selegiline Hydrochloride (Concurrent use is contraindicated). Products include:
- Eldepryl Capsules 2729

Sevoflurane (Significant hypotension; bradycardia).
No products indexed under this heading.

Sodium Nitroprusside (Potentiated; additive effects).
No products indexed under this heading.

Sotalol Hydrochloride (Potentiated; additive effects). Products include:
- Betapace Tablets 637

Spirapril Hydrochloride (Potentiated; additive effects).
No products indexed under this heading.

Sufentanil Citrate (Orthostatic hypotension may be aggravated). Products include:
- Sufenta Injection 1355

Sulindac (Reduced diuretic, natriuretic, and antihypertensive effects of chlorothiazide). Products include:
- Clinoril Tablets 1658

Terazosin Hydrochloride (Potentiated; additive effects). Products include:
- Hytrin Capsules 434

Thiamylal Sodium (Potentiation of orthostatic hypotension produced by thiazides; enhances CNS depressant effects of reserpine).
No products indexed under this heading.

Timolol Maleate (Potentiated; additive effects). Products include:
- Blocadren Tablets 1654
- Timolide Tablets 1791
- Timoptic in Ocudose 1796
- Timoptic Sterile Ophthalmic Solution 1794

IMPORTANT NOTE: Always consult each drug listing in the patient's regimen for possible interactions.

Timoptic-XE 1798

Tolazamide (Hyperglycemia may occur; dosage adjustment of the antidiabetic drug may be required).
No products indexed under this heading.

Tolbutamide (Hyperglycemia may occur; dosage adjustment of the antidiabetic drug may be required).
No products indexed under this heading.

Tolmetin Sodium (Reduced diuretic, natriuretic, and antihypertensive effects of chlorothiazide). Products include:
Tolectin (200, 400 and 600 mg) .. 1591

Torsemide (Potentiated; additive effects). Products include:
Demadex Tablets and Injection 691

Tranylcypromine Sulfate (Concurrent use is contraindicated). Products include:
Parnate Tablets 2679

Triamcinolone (Potential for intensified electrolyte depletion, particularly hypokalemia).
No products indexed under this heading.

Triamcinolone Acetonide (Potential for intensified electrolyte depletion, particularly hypokalemia). Products include:
Azmacort Oral Inhaler 2175
Nasacort AQ Nasal Spray........ 2191
Nasacort Nasal Inhaler 2189

Triamcinolone Diacetate (Potential for intensified electrolyte depletion, particularly hypokalemia).
No products indexed under this heading.

Triamcinolone Hexacetonide (Potential for intensified electrolyte depletion, particularly hypokalemia).
No products indexed under this heading.

Trimethaphan Camsylate (Potentiated; additive effects).
No products indexed under this heading.

Tubocurarine Chloride (Increased responsiveness to tubocurarine).
No products indexed under this heading.

Verapamil Hydrochloride (Potentiated; additive effects). Products include:
Calan SR Caplets 2571
Calan Tablets........ 2568
Covera-HS Tablets 2573
Isoptin Injectable 1391
Isoptin Oral Tablets 1393
Isoptin SR Tablets 1395
Verelan Capsules 1455

Food Interactions

Alcohol (Orthostatic hypotension may be aggravated).

DIURIL ORAL SUSPENSION

(Chlorothiazide) 1694
May interact with antihypertensives, barbiturates, narcotic analgesics, insulin, oral hypoglycemic agents, corticosteroids, lithium preparations, non-steroidal anti-inflammatory agents, cardiac glycosides, nondepolarizing neuromuscular blocking agents, bile acid sequestering agents, and certain other agents. Compounds in these categories include:

Acarbose (Thiazide-induced hyperglycemia may require dosage adjustment of hypoglycemic agents). Products include:
Precose 604

Acebutolol Hydrochloride (Concurrent use with other antihypertensive agents may result in additive effect or potentiation). Products include:
Sectral Capsules 2914

ACTH (Intensified electrolyte depletion particularly hypokalemia).
No products indexed under this heading.

Alfentanil Hydrochloride (Potentiation of orthostatic hypotension may occur). Products include:
Alfenta Injection 1334

Amlodipine Besylate (Concurrent use with other antihypertensive agents may result in additive effect or potentiation). Products include:
Lotrel Capsules........ 858
Norvasc Tablets 2020

Aprobarbital (Potentiation of orthostatic hypotension may occur).
No products indexed under this heading.

Atenolol (Concurrent use with other antihypertensive agents may result in additive effect or potentiation). Products include:
Tenoretic Tablets........ 2963
Tenormin Tablets and I.V. Injection 2965

Atracurium Besylate (Possible increased responsiveness to the muscle relaxants). Products include:
Tracrium Injection 1155

Benazepril Hydrochloride (Concurrent use with other antihypertensive agents may result in additive effect or potentiation). Products include:
Lotensin Tablets........ 852
Lotensin HCT Tablets 855
Lotrel Capsules........ 858

Bendroflumethiazide (Concurrent use with other antihypertensive agents may result in additive effect or potentiation).
No products indexed under this heading.

Betamethasone Acetate (Intensified electrolyte depletion particularly hypokalemia). Products include:
Celestone Soluspan Suspension 2484

Betamethasone Sodium Phosphate (Intensified electrolyte depletion particularly hypokalemia). Products include:
Celestone Soluspan Suspension 2484

Betaxolol Hydrochloride (Concurrent use with other antihypertensive agents may result in additive effect or potentiation). Products include:
Betoptic Ophthalmic Solution........ 465
Betoptic S Ophthalmic Suspension 467
Kerlone Tablets........ 2588

Bisoprolol Fumarate (Concurrent use with other antihypertensive agents may result in additive effect or potentiation). Products include:
Zebeta Tablets 1457
Ziac 1459

Buprenorphine (Potentiation of orthostatic hypotension may occur). Products include:
Buprenex Injectable 2170

Butabarbital (Potentiation of orthostatic hypotension may occur).
No products indexed under this heading.

Butalbital (Potentiation of orthostatic hypotension may occur). Products include:
Axocet Capsules........ 2469
Esgic-plus Capsules 1012
Esgic-plus Tablets 1012
Fioricet Tablets........ 2386
Fioricet with Codeine Capsules 2387
Fiorinal Capsules 2388
Fiorinal with Codeine Capsules 2390
Fiorinal Tablets 2388
Phrenilin 790
Sedapap Tablets 50 mg/650 mg .. 1826

Captopril (Concurrent use with other antihypertensive agents may result in additive effect or potentiation). Products include:
Capoten Tablets........ 740
Capozide Tablets 744

Carteolol Hydrochloride (Concurrent use with other antihypertensive agents may result in additive effect or potentiation). Products include:
Cartrol Tablets 413
Ocupress Ophthalmic Solution, 1% Sterile........ ⊙ 297

Chlorothiazide Sodium (Concurrent use with other antihypertensive agents may result in additive effect or potentiation). Products include:
Diuril Sodium Intravenous 1693

Chlorpropamide (Thiazide-induced hyperglycemia may require dosage adjustment of hypoglycemic agents). Products include:
Diabinese Tablets 2002

Chlorthalidone (Concurrent use with other antihypertensive agents may result in additive effect or potentiation). Products include:
Combipres Tablets 682
Tenoretic Tablets........ 2963
Thalitone 1293

Cholestyramine (Resins have potential to bind thiazide diuretics and reduce their absorption from the gastrointestinal tract). Products include:
Questran 774

Cisatracurium Besylate (Possible increased responsiveness to the muscle relaxants). Products include:
Nimbex Injection 1131

Clonidine (Concurrent use with other antihypertensive agents may result in additive effect or potentiation). Products include:
Catapres-TTS........ 680

Clonidine Hydrochloride (Concurrent use with other antihypertensive agents may result in additive effect or potentiation). Products include:
Catapres Tablets 679
Combipres Tablets 682

Codeine Phosphate (Potentiation of orthostatic hypotension may occur). Products include:
Brontex 2130
Dimetane-DC Cough Syrup 2232
Fioricet with Codeine Capsules 2387
Fiorinal with Codeine Capsules 2390
Nucofed 2225
Phenergan with Codeine........ 2883
Phenergan VC with Codeine 2888
Robitussin A-C Syrup........ 2248
Robitussin-DAC Syrup........ 2249
Ryna .... ▣ 804
Soma Compound w/Codeine Tablets........ 2784
Tylenol with Codeine 1592

Colestipol Hydrochloride (Resins have potential to bind thiazide diuretics and reduce their absorption from the gastrointestinal tract). Products include:
Colestid 2073

Cortisone Acetate (Intensified electrolyte depletion particularly hypokalemia). Products include:
Cortone Acetate Sterile Suspension 1663
Cortone Acetate Tablets........ 1664

Deserpidine (Concurrent use with other antihypertensive agents may result in additive effect or potentiation).
No products indexed under this heading.

Deslanoside (Thiazide-induced hypokalemia may sensitize or exaggerate the response of the heart to the toxic effects of digitalis).
No products indexed under this heading.

Dexamethasone (Intensified electrolyte depletion particularly hypokalemia). Products include:
AK-Trol Ointment & Suspension .... ⊙ 205
Decadron Elixir 1676
Decadron Tablets........ 1678
Decaspray Topical Aerosol 1689
Maxitrol Ophthalmic Ointment and Suspension .... ⊙ 222
TobraDex Ophthalmic Suspension and Ointment........ 469

Dexamethasone Acetate (Intensified electrolyte depletion particularly hypokalemia). Products include:
Dalalone D.P. Injectable 1009
Decadron-LA Sterile Suspension........ 1687

Dexamethasone Sodium Phosphate (Intensified electrolyte depletion particularly hypokalemia). Products include:
Decadron Phosphate Injection........ 1680
Decadron Phosphate Sterile Ophthalmic Ointment........ 1684
Decadron Phosphate Sterile Ophthalmic Solution 1685
Decadron Phosphate Topical Cream........ 1686
Decadron Phosphate with Xylocaine Injection, Sterile 1683
Dexacort Phosphate in Respihaler .. 1606
Dexacort Phosphate in Turbinaire .. 1607
NeoDecadron Sterile Ophthalmic Ointment 1755
NeoDecadron Sterile Ophthalmic Solution 1756
NeoDecadron Topical Cream 1757

Dezocine (Potentiation of orthostatic hypotension may occur). Products include:
Dalgan Injection 529

Diazoxide (Concurrent use with other antihypertensive agents may result in additive effect or potentiation). Products include:
Hyperstat I.V. Injection 2504
Proglycem........ 575

Diclofenac Potassium (Reduces diuretic, natriuretic, and antihypertensive effects). Products include:
Cataflam Tablets 833

Diclofenac Sodium (Reduces diuretic, natriuretic, and antihypertensive effects). Products include:
Voltaren Ophthalmic Sterile Ophthalmic Solution .... ⊙ 264
Cataflam/Voltaren/Voltaren-XR 833

Digitoxin (Thiazide-induced hypokalemia may sensitize or exaggerate the response of the heart to the toxic effects of digitalis). Products include:
Crystodigin Tablets........ 1472

Digoxin (Thiazide-induced hypokalemia may sensitize or exaggerate the response of the heart to the toxic effects of digitalis). Products include:
Lanoxicaps 1110
Lanoxin Elixir Pediatric 1113
Lanoxin Injection 1116
Lanoxin Injection Pediatric........ 1119
Lanoxin Tablets 1121

Diltiazem Hydrochloride (Concurrent use with other antihypertensive agents may result in additive effect or potentiation). Products include:
Cardizem CD Capsules 1251
Cardizem SR Capsules 1255
Cardizem Injectable 1253
Cardizem Tablets........ 1257
Dilacor XR Extended-release Capsules 2183
Tiazac Capsules 1019

(▣ Described in PDR For Nonprescription Drugs) (⊙ Described in PDR For Ophthalmology)

319 **Interactions Index** **Diuril Oral**

Doxazosin Mesylate (Concurrent use with other antihypertensive agents may result in additive effect or potentiation). Products include:
- Cardura Tablets ... 1993

Enalapril Maleate (Concurrent use with other antihypertensive agents may result in additive effect or potentiation). Products include:
- Vaseretic Tablets ... 1810
- Vasotec Tablets ... 1816

Enalaprilat (Concurrent use with other antihypertensive agents may result in additive effect or potentiation). Products include:
- Vasotec I.V. ... 1814

Esmolol Hydrochloride (Concurrent use with other antihypertensive agents may result in additive effect or potentiation). Products include:
- Brevibloc (esmolol HCl) Injection ... 1860

Etodolac (Reduces diuretic, natriuretic, and antihypertensive effects). Products include:
- Lodine Capsules and Tablets ... 2849

Felodipine (Concurrent use with other antihypertensive agents may result in additive effect or potentiation). Products include:
- Plendil Extended-Release Tablets ... 514

Fenoprofen Calcium (Reduces diuretic, natriuretic, and antihypertensive effects). Products include:
- Nalfon 200 Pulvules & Nalfon Tablets ... 933

Fentanyl (Potentiation of orthostatic hypotension may occur). Products include:
- Duragesic Transdermal System ... 1336

Fentanyl Citrate (Potentiation of orthostatic hypotension may occur). Products include:
- Sublimaze Injection ... 463

Fludrocortisone Acetate (Intensified electrolyte depletion particularly hypokalemia). Products include:
- Florinef Acetate Tablets ... 506

Flurbiprofen (Reduces diuretic, natriuretic, and antihypertensive effects).
- No products indexed under this heading.

Fosinopril Sodium (Concurrent use with other antihypertensive agents may result in additive effect or potentiation). Products include:
- Monopril Tablets ... 762

Furosemide (Concurrent use with other antihypertensive agents may result in additive effect or potentiation). Products include:
- Lasix Injection, Oral Solution and Tablets ... 1267

Glimepiride (Thiazide-induced hyperglycemia may require dosage adjustment of hypoglycemic agents). Products include:
- Amaryl Tablets ... 1241

Glipizide (Thiazide-induced hyperglycemia may require dosage adjustment of hypoglycemic agents). Products include:
- Glucotrol Tablets ... 2011
- Glucotrol XL Extended Release Tablets ... 2012

Glyburide (Thiazide-induced hyperglycemia may require dosage adjustment of hypoglycemic agents). Products include:
- DiaBeta Tablets ... 1265
- Glynase PresTab Tablets ... 2091
- Micronase Tablets ... 2099

Guanabenz Acetate (Concurrent use with other antihypertensive agents may result in additive effect or potentiation).
- No products indexed under this heading.

Guanethidine Monosulfate (Concurrent use with other antihypertensive agents may result in additive effect or potentiation). Products include:
- Esimil Tablets ... 840
- Ismelin Tablets ... 845

Hydralazine Hydrochloride (Concurrent use with other antihypertensive agents may result in additive effect or potentiation). Products include:
- Apresazide Capsules ... 824
- Apresoline Hydrochloride Tablets ... 826
- Hydralazine Hydrochloride Injection USP ... 2712
- Ser-Ap-Es Tablets ... 867

Hydrochlorothiazide (Concurrent use with other antihypertensive agents may result in additive effect or potentiation). Products include:
- Aldactazide Tablets ... 2556
- Aldoril Tablets ... 1644
- Apresazide Capsules ... 824
- Capozide Tablets ... 744
- Dyazide Capsules ... 2653
- Esidrix Tablets ... 839
- Esimil Tablets ... 840
- HydroDIURIL Tablets ... 1716
- Hydropres Tablets ... 1718
- Hyzaar Tablets ... 1720
- Inderide Tablets ... 2838
- Inderide LA Long Acting Capsules ... 2840
- Lopressor HCT Tablets ... 850
- Lotensin HCT Tablets ... 855
- Moduretic Tablets ... 1748
- Oretic Tablets ... 450
- Prinzide Tablets ... 1780
- Ser-Ap-Es Tablets ... 867
- Timolide Tablets ... 1791
- Vaseretic Tablets ... 1810
- Zestoretic Tablets ... 2968
- Ziac ... 1459

Hydrocodone Bitartrate (Potentiation of orthostatic hypotension may occur). Products include:
- Codiclear DH Syrup ... 808
- Duratuss HD Elixir ... 2750
- Histussin D Liquid ... 670
- Hycodan Tablets and Syrup ... 946
- Hycomine Compound Tablets ... 948
- Hycomine ... 947
- Hycotuss Expectorant Syrup ... 950
- Hydrocet Capsules ... 787
- Lorcet 10/650 Tablets ... 1016
- Lortab ... 2751
- Tussend ... 1830
- Tussend Expectorant ... 1831
- Vicodin Tablets ... 1404
- Vicodin ES Tablets ... 1405
- Vicodin HP Tablets ... 1403
- Vicodin Tuss Expectorant ... 1406
- Zydone Capsules ... 967

Hydrocodone Polistirex (Potentiation of orthostatic hypotension may occur). Products include:
- Tussionex Pennkinetic Extended-Release Suspension ... 1624

Hydrocortisone (Intensified electrolyte depletion particularly hypokalemia). Products include:
- Anusol-HC Cream 2.5% ... 1953
- Aquanil HC Lotion ... 1989
- Maximum Strength Cortaid Spray ... 800
- CORTENEMA ... 2713
- Cortisporin Ointment ... 1074
- Cortisporin Ophthalmic Ointment Sterile ... 1074
- Cortisporin Ophthalmic Suspension Sterile ... 1075
- Cortisporin Otic Solution Sterile ... 1076
- Cortisporin Otic Suspension Sterile 1077
- Cortizone-5 ... 795
- Cortizone-10 ... 795
- Hydrocortone Tablets ... 1715
- Hytone ... 922
- Hytone Ointment 2 ½% ... 923
- Massengill Medicated Soft Cloth Towelettes ... 2628
- Pediotic Suspension Sterile ... 1140
- Preparation H Hydrocortisone 1% Cream ... 843
- ProctoCream-HC 2.5% ... 2552
- VōSoL HC Otic Solution ... 2786

Hydrocortisone Acetate (Intensified electrolyte depletion particularly hypokalemia). Products include:
- Analpram-HC Rectal Cream 1% and 2.5% ... 993
- Anusol HC-1 Hydrocortisone Anti-Itch Ointment ... 810
- Anusol-HC Suppositories ... 1954
- Caldecort Anti-Itch Hydrocortisone Cream ... 651
- Coly-Mycin S Otic w/Neomycin & Hydrocortisone ... 1965
- Cortaid ... 800
- Cortifoam ... 2540
- Cortisporin Cream ... 1073
- Epifoam ... 2543
- Hydrocortone Acetate Sterile Suspension ... 1712
- Mantadil Cream ... 1124
- Nupercainal Hydrocortisone 1% Cream ... 661
- Pramosone Cream, Lotion & Ointment ... 995
- ProctoFoam-HC ... 2552
- Terra-Cortril Ophthalmic Suspension ... 2033

Hydrocortisone Sodium Phosphate (Intensified electrolyte depletion particularly hypokalemia). Products include:
- Hydrocortone Phosphate Injection, Sterile ... 1713

Hydrocortisone Sodium Succinate (Intensified electrolyte depletion particularly hypokalemia).
- No products indexed under this heading.

Hydroflumethiazide (Concurrent use with other antihypertensive agents may result in additive effect or potentiation). Products include:
- Diucardin Tablets ... 2824

Hydromorphone Hydrochloride (Potentiation of orthostatic hypotension may occur). Products include:
- Dilaudid Ampules ... 1382
- Dilaudid Cough Syrup ... 1383
- Dilaudid-HP Injection ... 1384
- Dilaudid-HP Lyophilized Powder 250 mg ... 1384
- Dilaudid ... 1382
- Dilaudid Oral Liquid ... 1386
- Dilaudid ... 1382
- Dilaudid Tablets - 8 mg ... 1386

Ibuprofen (Reduces diuretic, natriuretic, and antihypertensive effects). Products include:
- Advil Cold and Sinus Caplets and Tablets ... 837
- Advil Ibuprofen Tablets, Caplets and Gel Caplets ... 836
- Children's Motrin Ibuprofen Oral Suspension ... 1558
- IBU Tablets ... 1389
- Ibuprohm ... 713
- Motrin IB Caplets, Tablets, and Gelcaps ... 802
- Motrin Ibuprofen Suspension, Oral Drops, Chewable Tablets, Caplets ... 1563
- Nuprin Ibuprofen/Analgesic Tablets & Caplets ... 645
- Vicks DayQuil SINUS Pressure & PAIN Relief with IBUPROFEN ... 735

Indapamide (Concurrent use with other antihypertensive agents may result in additive effect or potentiation).
- No products indexed under this heading.

Indomethacin (Reduces diuretic, natriuretic, and antihypertensive effects). Products include:
- Indocin ... 1723

Indomethacin Sodium Trihydrate (Reduces diuretic, natriuretic, and antihypertensive effects). Products include:
- Indocin I.V. ... 1727

Insulin, Human (Thiazide-induced hyperglycemia may require dosage adjustment of hypoglycemic agents).
- No products indexed under this heading.

Insulin, Human Isophane Suspension (Thiazide-induced hyperglycemia may require dosage adjustment of hypoglycemic agents). Products include:
- Novolin N Human Insulin 10 ml Vials ... 1846

Insulin, Human NPH (Thiazide-induced hyperglycemia may require dosage adjustment of hypoglycemic agents). Products include:
- Humulin N, 100 Units ... 1495
- Novolin N PenFill 1.5 ml Cartridges Durable Insulin Delivery System ... 1849
- Novolin N Prefilled Syringe Disposable Insulin Delivery System ... 1850

Insulin, Human Regular (Thiazide-induced hyperglycemia may require dosage adjustment of hypoglycemic agents). Products include:
- Humulin R, 100 Units ... 1497
- Novolin R Human Insulin 10 ml Vials ... 1846
- Novolin R PenFill 1.5 ml Cartridges Durable Insulin Delivery System ... 1849
- Novolin R Prefilled Syringe Disposable Insulin Delivery System ... 1850
- Velosulin BR Human Insulin 10 ml Vials ... 1847

Insulin, Human, Zinc Suspension (Thiazide-induced hyperglycemia may require dosage adjustment of hypoglycemic agents). Products include:
- Humulin L, 100 Units ... 1494
- Humulin U, 100 Units ... 1498
- Novolin L Human Insulin 10 ml Vials ... 1846

Insulin Lispro, Human (Thiazide-induced hyperglycemia may require dosage adjustment of hypoglycemic agents). Products include:
- Humalog Injection ... 1488

Insulin, NPH (Thiazide-induced hyperglycemia may require dosage adjustment of hypoglycemic agents). Products include:
- NPH, 100 Units ... 1502
- Pork NPH, 100 Units ... 1506
- Purified Pork NPH Isophane Insulin ... 1852

Insulin, Regular (Thiazide-induced hyperglycemia may require dosage adjustment of hypoglycemic agents). Products include:
- Regular, 100 Units ... 1503
- Pork Regular, 100 Units ... 1507
- Pork Regular (Concentrated), 500 Units ... 1508
- Purified Pork Regular Insulin ... 1852

Insulin, Zinc Crystals (Thiazide-induced hyperglycemia may require dosage adjustment of hypoglycemic agents). Products include:
- NPH, 100 Units ... 1502

Insulin, Zinc Suspension (Thiazide-induced hyperglycemia may require dosage adjustment of hypoglycemic agents). Products include:
- Iletin I ... 1501
- Lente, 100 Units ... 1501
- Iletin II ... 1504
- Pork Lente, 100 Units ... 1504
- Purified Pork Lente Insulin ... 1852

Isradipine (Concurrent use with other antihypertensive agents may result in additive effect or potentiation). Products include:
- DynaCirc Capsules ... 2381
- DynaCirc CR Tablets ... 2383

Ketoprofen (Reduces diuretic, natriuretic, and antihypertensive effects). Products include:
- Actron Caplets and Tablets ... 608
- Orudis Capsules ... 2874
- Orudis KT ... 842
- Oruvail Capsules ... 2874

IMPORTANT NOTE: Always consult each drug listing in the patient's regimen for possible interactions.

Diuril Oral — Interactions Index — 320

Ketorolac Tromethamine (Reduces diuretic, natriuretic, and antihypertensive effects). Products include:
- Acular Sterile Ophthalmic Solution ... 470
- Toradol ... 2319

Labetalol Hydrochloride (Concurrent use with other antihypertensive agents may result in additive effect or potentiation). Products include:
- Normodyne Injection ... 2519
- Normodyne Tablets ... 2522
- Trandate ... 1158

Levorphanol Tartrate (Potentiation of orthostatic hypotension may occur). Products include:
- Levo-Dromoran ... 2297

Lisinopril (Concurrent use with other antihypertensive agents may result in additive effect or potentiation). Products include:
- Prinivil Tablets ... 1776
- Prinzide Tablets ... 1780
- Zestoretic Tablets ... 2968
- Zestril Tablets ... 2972

Lithium Carbonate (Diuretics reduce the renal clearance of lithium and this may lead to lithium toxicity). Products include:
- Eskalith ... 2658
- Lithium Carbonate Capsules & Tablets ... 2352
- Lithonate/Lithotabs/Lithobid ... 2721

Lithium Citrate (Diuretics reduce the renal clearance of lithium and this may lead to lithium toxicity).
  No products indexed under this heading.

Losartan Potassium (Concurrent use with other antihypertensive agents may result in additive effect or potentiation). Products include:
- Cozaar Tablets ... 1668
- Hyzaar Tablets ... 1720

Mecamylamine Hydrochloride (Concurrent use with other antihypertensive agents may result in additive effect or potentiation). Products include:
- Inversine Tablets ... 1729

Meclofenamate Sodium (Reduces diuretic, natriuretic, and antihypertensive effects).
  No products indexed under this heading.

Mefenamic Acid (Reduces diuretic, natriuretic, and antihypertensive effects). Products include:
- Ponstel ... 1982

Meperidine Hydrochloride (Potentiation of orthostatic hypotension may occur). Products include:
- Demerol ... 2438
- Mepergan Injection ... 2859

Mephobarbital (Potentiation of orthostatic hypotension may occur). Products include:
- Mebaral Tablets ... 2452

Metformin Hydrochloride (Thiazide-induced hyperglycemia may require dosage adjustment of hypoglycemic agents). Products include:
- Glucophage Tablets ... 754

Methadone Hydrochloride (Potentiation of orthostatic hypotension may occur). Products include:
- Methadone Hydrochloride Oral Concentrate ... 2356
- Methadone Hydrochloride Oral Solution & Tablets ... 2357

Methyclothiazide (Concurrent use with other antihypertensive agents may result in additive effect or potentiation). Products include:
- Enduron Tablets ... 424

Methyldopa (Concurrent use with other antihypertensive agents may result in additive effect or potentiation). Products include:
- Aldoclor Tablets ... 1638
- Aldomet Oral ... 1640
- Aldoril Tablets ... 1644

Methyldopate Hydrochloride (Concurrent use with other antihypertensive agents may result in additive effect or potentiation). Products include:
- Aldomet Ester HCl Injection ... 1642

Methylprednisolone Acetate (Intensified electrolyte depletion particularly hypokalemia).
  No products indexed under this heading.

Methylprednisolone Sodium Succinate (Intensified electrolyte depletion particularly hypokalemia).
  No products indexed under this heading.

Metocurine Iodide (Possible increased responsiveness to the muscle relaxants). Products include:
- Metubine Iodide Vials ... 932

Metolazone (Concurrent use with other antihypertensive agents may result in additive effect or potentiation). Products include:
- Mykrox Tablets ... 1617
- Zaroxolyn Tablets ... 1625

Metoprolol Succinate (Concurrent use with other antihypertensive agents may result in additive effect or potentiation). Products include:
- Toprol-XL Tablets ... 560

Metoprolol Tartrate (Concurrent use with other antihypertensive agents may result in additive effect or potentiation). Products include:
- Lopressor ... 848
- Lopressor HCT Tablets ... 850

Metyrosine (Concurrent use with other antihypertensive agents may result in additive effect or potentiation). Products include:
- Demser Capsules ... 1690

Minoxidil (Concurrent use with other antihypertensive agents may result in additive effect or potentiation).
  No products indexed under this heading.

Mivacurium Chloride (Possible increased responsiveness to the muscle relaxants). Products include:
- Mivacron ... 1125

Moexipril Hydrochloride (Concurrent use with other antihypertensive agents may result in additive effect or potentiation). Products include:
- Univasc Tablets ... 2553

Morphine Sulfate (Potentiation of orthostatic hypotension may occur). Products include:
- Astramorph/PF Injection, USP (Preservative-Free) ... 526
- Duramorph Injection ... 983
- Infumorph 200 and Infumorph 500 Sterile Solutions ... 985
- Kadian Capsules ... 2948
- MS Contin Tablets ... 2149
- MSIR ... 2152
- Oramorph SR (Morphine Sulfate Sustained Release Tablets) ... 2359
- RMS Suppositories CII ... 2766
- Roxanol ... 2365

Nabumetone (Reduces diuretic, natriuretic, and antihypertensive effects). Products include:
- Relafen Tablets ... 2688

Nadolol (Concurrent use with other antihypertensive agents may result in additive effect or potentiation).
  No products indexed under this heading.

Naproxen (Reduces diuretic, natriuretic, and antihypertensive effects). Products include:
- Anaprox/Naprosyn ... 2277

Naproxen Sodium (Reduces diuretic, natriuretic, and antihypertensive effects). Products include:
- Aleve ... 2124
- Anaprox/Naprosyn ... 2277
- Naprelan Tablets ... 2861

Nicardipine Hydrochloride (Concurrent use with other antihypertensive agents may result in additive effect or potentiation). Products include:
- Cardene Capsules ... 2261
- Cardene I.V. ... 2815
- Cardene SR Capsules ... 2264

Nifedipine (Concurrent use with other antihypertensive agents may result in additive effect or potentiation). Products include:
- Adalat Capsules (10 mg and 20 mg) ... 580
- Adalat CC ... 582
- Procardia Capsules ... 2024
- Procardia XL Extended Release Tablets ... 2026

Nisoldipine (Concurrent use with other antihypertensive agents may result in additive effect or potentiation). Products include:
- Sular Tablets ... 2961

Nitroglycerin (Concurrent use with other antihypertensive agents may result in additive effect or potentiation). Products include:
- Deponit NTG Transdermal Delivery System ... 2541
- Nitro-Bid IV ... 1270
- Nitro-Bid Ointment ... 1272
- Nitro-Dur (nitroglycerin) Transdermal Infusion System ... 1365
- Nitrolingual Spray ... 2193
- Nitrostat Tablets ... 1981
- Transderm-Nitro Transdermal Therapeutic System ... 878

Norepinephrine Hydrochloride (Decreased arterial responsiveness to pressor amine).

Opium Alkaloids (Potentiation of orthostatic hypotension may occur).
  No products indexed under this heading.

Oxaprozin (Reduces diuretic, natriuretic, and antihypertensive effects). Products include:
- Daypro Caplets ... 2578

Oxycodone Hydrochloride (Potentiation of orthostatic hypotension may occur). Products include:
- OxyContin Tablets ... 2163
- OxyIR Capsules ... 2167
- Percocet Tablets ... 955
- Percodan Tablets ... 955
- Percodan-Demi Tablets ... 956
- Roxicodone Tablets, Oral Solution & Intensol (Oxycodone) ... 2366
- Tylox Capsules ... 1593

Pancuronium Bromide (Possible increased responsiveness to the muscle relaxants).
  No products indexed under this heading.

Penbutolol Sulfate (Concurrent use with other antihypertensive agents may result in additive effect or potentiation). Products include:
- Levatol Tablets ... 2547

Pentobarbital Sodium (Potentiation of orthostatic hypotension may occur). Products include:
- Nembutal Sodium Capsules ... 440
- Nembutal Sodium Solution ... 442
- Nembutal Sodium Suppositories ... 444

Phenobarbital (Potentiation of orthostatic hypotension may occur). Products include:
- Arco-Lase Plus Tablets ... 513
- Bellergal-S Tablets ... 2375
- Donnatal ... 2234
- Donnatal Extentabs ... 2234
- Donnatal Tablets ... 2234
- Phenobarbital Elixir and Tablets ... 1523
- Quadrinal Tablets ... 1398

Phenoxybenzamine Hydrochloride (Concurrent use with other antihypertensive agents may result in additive effect or potentiation). Products include:
- Dibenzyline Capsules ... 2650

Phentolamine Mesylate (Concurrent use with other antihypertensive agents may result in additive effect or potentiation). Products include:
- Regitine Vials ... 864

Phenylbutazone (Reduces diuretic, natriuretic, and antihypertensive effects).
  No products indexed under this heading.

Pindolol (Concurrent use with other antihypertensive agents may result in additive effect or potentiation). Products include:
- Visken Tablets ... 2428

Piroxicam (Reduces diuretic, natriuretic, and antihypertensive effects). Products include:
- Feldene Capsules ... 2008

Polythiazide (Concurrent use with other antihypertensive agents may result in additive effect or potentiation). Products include:
- Minizide Capsules ... 2016

Prazosin Hydrochloride (Concurrent use with other antihypertensive agents may result in additive effect or potentiation). Products include:
- Minipress Capsules ... 2015
- Minizide Capsules ... 2016

Prednisolone Acetate (Intensified electrolyte depletion particularly hypokalemia). Products include:
- AK-CIDE ... ⊚ 203
- AK-CIDE Ointment ... ⊚ 203
- Blephamide Liquifilm Sterile Ophthalmic Suspension ... 472
- Blephamide Ointment ... ⊚ 234
- Econopred & Econopred Plus Ophthalmic Suspensions ... ⊚ 216
- Poly-Pred Liquifilm ... ⊚ 246
- Pred Forte ... ⊚ 247
- Pred Mild ... ⊚ 250
- Pred-G Liquifilm Sterile Ophthalmic Suspension ... ⊚ 248
- Pred-G S.O.P. Sterile Ophthalmic Ointment ... ⊚ 249

Prednisolone Sodium Phosphate (Intensified electrolyte depletion particularly hypokalemia). Products include:
- AK-PRED ... ⊚ 204
- Hydeltrasol Injection, Sterile ... 1708
- Pediapred Oral Solution ... 1618

Prednisolone Tebutate (Intensified electrolyte depletion particularly hypokalemia). Products include:
- Hydeltra-T.B.A. Sterile Suspension ... 1710

Prednisone (Intensified electrolyte depletion particularly hypokalemia).
  No products indexed under this heading.

Propoxyphene Hydrochloride (Potentiation of orthostatic hypotension may occur). Products include:
- Darvon ... 1475
- Wygesic Tablets ... 2930

Propoxyphene Napsylate (Potentiation of orthostatic hypotension may occur). Products include:
- Darvon-N/Darvocet-N ... 1473

Propranolol Hydrochloride (Concurrent use with other antihypertensive agents may result in additive effect or potentiation). Products include:
- Inderal ... 2834
- Inderal LA Long Acting Capsules ... 2836

(▣ Described in PDR For Nonprescription Drugs)   (⊚ Described in PDR For Ophthalmology)

Inderide Tablets ... 2838
Inderide LA Long Acting Capsules .. 2840

Quinapril Hydrochloride (Concurrent use with other antihypertensive agents may result in additive effect or potentiation). Products include:
Accupril Tablets ... 1950

Ramipril (Concurrent use with other antihypertensive agents may result in additive effect or potentiation). Products include:
Altace Capsules ... 1238

Rauwolfia Serpentina (Concurrent use with other antihypertensive agents may result in additive effect or potentiation).
No products indexed under this heading.

Rescinnamine (Concurrent use with other antihypertensive agents may result in additive effect or potentiation).
No products indexed under this heading.

Reserpine (Concurrent use with other antihypertensive agents may result in additive effect or potentiation). Products include:
Diupres Tablets ... 1691
Hydropres Tablets ... 1718
Ser-Ap-Es Tablets ... 867

Rocuronium Bromide (Possible increased responsiveness to the muscle relaxants). Products include:
Zemuron Injection ... 1885

Secobarbital Sodium (Potentiation of orthostatic hypotension may occur). Products include:
Seconal Sodium Pulvules ... 1529

Sodium Nitroprusside (Concurrent use with other antihypertensive agents may result in additive effect or potentiation).
No products indexed under this heading.

Sotalol Hydrochloride (Concurrent use with other antihypertensive agents may result in additive effect or potentiation). Products include:
Betapace Tablets ... 637

Spirapril Hydrochloride (Concurrent use with other antihypertensive agents may result in additive effect or potentiation).
No products indexed under this heading.

Sufentanil Citrate (Potentiation of orthostatic hypotension may occur). Products include:
Sufenta Injection ... 1355

Sulindac (Reduces diuretic, natriuretic, and antihypertensive effects). Products include:
Clinoril Tablets ... 1658

Terazosin Hydrochloride (Concurrent use with other antihypertensive agents may result in additive effect or potentiation). Products include:
Hytrin Capsules ... 434

Thiamylal Sodium (Potentiation of orthostatic hypotension may occur).
No products indexed under this heading.

Timolol Maleate (Concurrent use with other antihypertensive agents may result in additive effect or potentiation). Products include:
Blocadren Tablets ... 1654
Timolide Tablets ... 1791
Timoptic in Ocudose ... 1796
Timoptic Sterile Ophthalmic Solution ... 1794
Timoptic-XE ... 1798

Tolazamide (Thiazide-induced hyperglycemia may require dosage adjustment of hypoglycemic agents).
No products indexed under this heading.

Tolbutamide (Thiazide-induced hyperglycemia may require dosage adjustment of hypoglycemic agents).
No products indexed under this heading.

Tolmetin Sodium (Reduces diuretic, natriuretic, and antihypertensive effects). Products include:
Tolectin (200, 400 and 600 mg) .. 1591

Torsemide (Concurrent use with other antihypertensive agents may result in additive effect or potentiation). Products include:
Demadex Tablets and Injection ... 691

Triamcinolone (Intensified electrolyte depletion particularly hypokalemia).
No products indexed under this heading.

Triamcinolone Acetonide (Intensified electrolyte depletion particularly hypokalemia). Products include:
Azmacort Oral Inhaler ... 2175
Nasacort AQ Nasal Spray ... 2191
Nasacort Nasal Inhaler ... 2189

Triamcinolone Diacetate (Intensified electrolyte depletion particularly hypokalemia).
No products indexed under this heading.

Triamcinolone Hexacetonide (Intensified electrolyte depletion particularly hypokalemia).
No products indexed under this heading.

Trimethaphan Camsylate (Concurrent use with other antihypertensive agents may result in additive effect or potentiation).
No products indexed under this heading.

Tubocurarine Chloride (Possible increased responsiveness to the muscle relaxants).
No products indexed under this heading.

Vecuronium Bromide (Possible increased responsiveness to the muscle relaxants). Products include:
Norcuron Injection ... 1875

Verapamil Hydrochloride (Concurrent use with other antihypertensive agents may result in additive effect or potentiation). Products include:
Calan SR Caplets ... 2571
Calan Tablets ... 2568
Covera-HS Tablets ... 2573
Isoptin Injectable ... 1391
Isoptin Oral Tablets ... 1393
Isoptin SR Tablets ... 1395
Verelan Capsules ... 1455

Food Interactions

Alcohol (Potentiation of orthostatic hypotension may occur).

DIURIL SODIUM INTRAVENOUS

(Chlorothiazide Sodium) ... 1693

May interact with antihypertensives, barbiturates, narcotic analgesics, insulin, oral hypoglycemic agents, corticosteroids, lithium preparations, non-steroidal anti-inflammatory agents, cardiac glycosides, nondepolarizing neuromuscular blocking agents, and certain other agents. Compounds in these categories include:

Acarbose (Thiazide-induced hyperglycemia may require dosage adjustment of hypoglycemic agents). Products include:
Precose ... 604

Acebutolol Hydrochloride (Concurrent use with other antihypertensive agents may result in additive effect or potentiation). Products include:
Sectral Capsules ... 2914

ACTH (Intensified electrolyte depletion particularly hypokalemia).
No products indexed under this heading.

Alfentanil Hydrochloride (Potentiation of orthostatic hypotension may occur). Products include:
Alfenta Injection ... 1334

Amlodipine Besylate (Concurrent use with other antihypertensive agents may result in additive effect or potentiation). Products include:
Lotrel Capsules ... 858
Norvasc Tablets ... 2020

Aprobarbital (Potentiation of orthostatic hypotension may occur).
No products indexed under this heading.

Atenolol (Concurrent use with other antihypertensive agents may result in additive effect or potentiation). Products include:
Tenoretic Tablets ... 2963
Tenormin Tablets and I.V. Injection 2965

Atracurium Besylate (Possible increased responsiveness to the muscle relaxants). Products include:
Tracrium Injection ... 1155

Benazepril Hydrochloride (Concurrent use with other antihypertensive agents may result in additive effect or potentiation). Products include:
Lotensin Tablets ... 852
Lotensin HCT Tablets ... 855
Lotrel Capsules ... 858

Bendroflumethiazide (Concurrent use with other antihypertensive agents may result in additive effect or potentiation).
No products indexed under this heading.

Betamethasone Acetate (Intensified electrolyte depletion particularly hypokalemia). Products include:
Celestone Soluspan Suspension ... 2484

Betamethasone Sodium Phosphate (Intensified electrolyte depletion particularly hypokalemia). Products include:
Celestone Soluspan Suspension ... 2484

Betaxolol Hydrochloride (Concurrent use with other antihypertensive agents may result in additive effect or potentiation). Products include:
Betoptic Ophthalmic Solution ... 465
Betoptic S Ophthalmic Suspension 467
Kerlone Tablets ... 2588

Bisoprolol Fumarate (Concurrent use with other antihypertensive agents may result in additive effect or potentiation). Products include:
Zebeta Tablets ... 1457
Ziac ... 1459

Buprenorphine (Potentiation of orthostatic hypotension may occur). Products include:
Buprenex Injectable ... 2170

Butabarbital (Potentiation of orthostatic hypotension may occur).
No products indexed under this heading.

Butalbital (Potentiation of orthostatic hypotension may occur). Products include:
Axocet Capsules ... 2469
Esgic-plus Capsules ... 1012
Esgic-plus Tablets ... 1012
Fioricet Tablets ... 2386
Fioricet with Codeine Capsules ... 2387
Fiorinal Capsules ... 2388
Fiorinal with Codeine Capsules ... 2390
Fiorinal Tablets ... 2388
Phrenilin ... 790
Sedapap Tablets 50 mg/650 mg .. 1826

Captopril (Concurrent use with other antihypertensive agents may result in additive effect or potentiation). Products include:
Capoten Tablets ... 740
Capozide Tablets ... 744

Carteolol Hydrochloride (Concurrent use with other antihypertensive agents may result in additive effect or potentiation). Products include:
Cartrol Tablets ... 413
Ocupress Ophthalmic Solution, 1% Sterile ... ⊛ 297

Chlorothiazide (Concurrent use with other antihypertensive agents may result in additive effect or potentiation). Products include:
Aldoclor Tablets ... 1638
Diupres Tablets ... 1691
Diuril Oral ... 1694

Chlorpropamide (Thiazide-induced hyperglycemia may require dosage adjustment of hypoglycemic agents). Products include:
Diabinese Tablets ... 2002

Chlorthalidone (Concurrent use with other antihypertensive agents may result in additive effect or potentiation). Products include:
Combipres Tablets ... 682
Tenoretic Tablets ... 2963
Thalitone ... 1293

Cisatracurium Besylate (Possible increased responsiveness to the muscle relaxants). Products include:
Nimbex Injection ... 1131

Clonidine (Concurrent use with other antihypertensive agents may result in additive effect or potentiation). Products include:
Catapres-TTS ... 680

Clonidine Hydrochloride (Concurrent use with other antihypertensive agents may result in additive effect or potentiation). Products include:
Catapres Tablets ... 679
Combipres Tablets ... 682

Codeine Phosphate (Potentiation of orthostatic hypotension may occur). Products include:
Brontex ... 2130
Dimetane-DC Cough Syrup ... 2232
Fioricet with Codeine Capsules ... 2387
Fiorinal with Codeine Capsules ... 2390
Nucofed ... 2225
Phenergan with Codeine ... 2883
Phenergan VC with Codeine ... 2888
Robitussin A-C Syrup ... 2248
Robitussin-DAC Syrup ... 2249
Ryna ... 804
Soma Compound w/Codeine Tablets ... 2784
Tylenol with Codeine ... 1592

Cortisone Acetate (Intensified electrolyte depletion particularly hypokalemia). Products include:
Cortone Acetate Sterile Suspension ... 1663
Cortone Acetate Tablets ... 1664

Deserpidine (Concurrent use with other antihypertensive agents may result in additive effect or potentiation).
No products indexed under this heading.

IMPORTANT NOTE: Always consult each drug listing in the patient's regimen for possible interactions.

Diuril Intravenous — Interactions Index — 322

Deslanoside (Thiazide-induced hypokalemia may sensitize or exaggerate the response of the heart to the toxic effects of digitalis).
No products indexed under this heading.

Dexamethasone (Intensified electrolyte depletion particularly hypokalemia). Products include:
- AK-Trol Ointment & Suspension ... ⊙ 205
- Decadron Elixir ... 1676
- Decadron Tablets ... 1678
- Decaspray Topical Aerosol ... 1689
- Maxitrol Ophthalmic Ointment and Suspension ... ⊙ 222
- TobraDex Ophthalmic Suspension and Ointment ... 469

Dexamethasone Acetate (Intensified electrolyte depletion particularly hypokalemia). Products include:
- Dalalone D.P. Injectable ... 1009
- Decadron-LA Sterile Suspension ... 1687

Dexamethasone Sodium Phosphate (Intensified electrolyte depletion particularly hypokalemia). Products include:
- Decadron Phosphate Injection ... 1680
- Decadron Phosphate Sterile Ophthalmic Ointment ... 1684
- Decadron Phosphate Sterile Ophthalmic Solution ... 1685
- Decadron Phosphate Topical Cream ... 1686
- Decadron Phosphate with Xylocaine Injection, Sterile ... 1683
- Dexacort Phosphate in Respihaler ... 1606
- Dexacort Phosphate in Turbinaire ... 1607
- NeoDecadron Sterile Ophthalmic Ointment ... 1755
- NeoDecadron Sterile Ophthalmic Solution ... 1756
- NeoDecadron Topical Cream ... 1757

Dezocine (Potentiation of orthostatic hypotension may occur). Products include:
- Dalgan Injection ... 529

Diazoxide (Concurrent use with other antihypertensive agents may result in additive effect or potentiation). Products include:
- Hyperstat I.V. Injection ... 2504
- Proglycem ... 575

Diclofenac Potassium (Reduces diuretic, natriuretic, and antihypertensive effects). Products include:
- Cataflam Tablets ... 833

Diclofenac Sodium (Reduces diuretic, natriuretic, and antihypertensive effects). Products include:
- Voltaren Ophthalmic Sterile Ophthalmic Solution ... ⊙ 264
- Cataflam/Voltaren/Voltaren-XR ... 833

Digitoxin (Thiazide-induced hypokalemia may sensitize or exaggerate the response of the heart to the toxic effects of digitalis). Products include:
- Crystodigin Tablets ... 1472

Digoxin (Thiazide-induced hypokalemia may sensitize or exaggerate the response of the heart to the toxic effects of digitalis). Products include:
- Lanoxicaps ... 1110
- Lanoxin Elixir Pediatric ... 1113
- Lanoxin Injection ... 1116
- Lanoxin Injection Pediatric ... 1119
- Lanoxin Tablets ... 1121

Diltiazem Hydrochloride (Concurrent use with other antihypertensive agents may result in additive effect or potentiation). Products include:
- Cardizem CD Capsules ... 1251
- Cardizem SR Capsules ... 1255
- Cardizem Injectable ... 1253
- Cardizem Tablets ... 1257
- Dilacor XR Extended-release Capsules ... 2183
- Tiazac Capsules ... 1019

Doxazosin Mesylate (Concurrent use with other antihypertensive agents may result in additive effect or potentiation). Products include:
- Cardura Tablets ... 1993

Enalapril Maleate (Concurrent use with other antihypertensive agents may result in additive effect or potentiation). Products include:
- Vaseretic Tablets ... 1810
- Vasotec Tablets ... 1816

Enalaprilat (Concurrent use with other antihypertensive agents may result in additive effect or potentiation). Products include:
- Vasotec I.V. ... 1814

Esmolol Hydrochloride (Concurrent use with other antihypertensive agents may result in additive effect or potentiation). Products include:
- Brevibloc (esmolol HCl) Injection ... 1860

Etodolac (Reduces diuretic, natriuretic, and antihypertensive effects). Products include:
- Lodine Capsules and Tablets ... 2849

Felodipine (Concurrent use with other antihypertensive agents may result in additive effect or potentiation). Products include:
- Plendil Extended-Release Tablets ... 514

Fenoprofen Calcium (Reduces diuretic, natriuretic, and antihypertensive effects). Products include:
- Nalfon 200 Pulvules & Nalfon Tablets ... 933

Fentanyl (Potentiation of orthostatic hypotension may occur). Products include:
- Duragesic Transdermal System ... 1336

Fentanyl Citrate (Potentiation of orthostatic hypotension may occur). Products include:
- Sublimaze Injection ... 463

Fludrocortisone Acetate (Intensified electrolyte depletion particularly hypokalemia). Products include:
- Florinef Acetate Tablets ... 506

Flurbiprofen (Reduces diuretic, natriuretic, and antihypertensive effects).
No products indexed under this heading.

Fosinopril Sodium (Concurrent use with other antihypertensive agents may result in additive effect or potentiation). Products include:
- Monopril Tablets ... 762

Furosemide (Concurrent use with other antihypertensive agents may result in additive effect or potentiation). Products include:
- Lasix Injection, Oral Solution and Tablets ... 1267

Glimepiride (Thiazide-induced hyperglycemia may require dosage adjustment of hypoglycemic agents). Products include:
- Amaryl Tablets ... 1241

Glipizide (Thiazide-induced hyperglycemia may require dosage adjustment of hypoglycemic agents). Products include:
- Glucotrol Tablets ... 2011
- Glucotrol XL Extended Release Tablets ... 2012

Glyburide (Thiazide-induced hyperglycemia may require dosage adjustment of hypoglycemic agents). Products include:
- DiaBeta Tablets ... 1265
- Glynase PresTab Tablets ... 2091
- Micronase Tablets ... 2099

Guanabenz Acetate (Concurrent use with other antihypertensive agents may result in additive effect or potentiation).
No products indexed under this heading.

Guanethidine Monosulfate (Concurrent use with other antihypertensive agents may result in additive effect or potentiation). Products include:
- Esimil Tablets ... 840
- Ismelin Tablets ... 845

Hydralazine Hydrochloride (Concurrent use with other antihypertensive agents may result in additive effect or potentiation). Products include:
- Apresazide Capsules ... 824
- Apresoline Hydrochloride Tablets ... 826
- Hydralazine Hydrochloride Injection USP ... 2712
- Ser-Ap-Es Tablets ... 867

Hydrochlorothiazide (Concurrent use with other antihypertensive agents may result in additive effect or potentiation). Products include:
- Aldactazide Tablets ... 2556
- Aldoril Tablets ... 1644
- Apresazide Capsules ... 824
- Capozide Tablets ... 744
- Dyazide Capsules ... 2653
- Esidrix Tablets ... 839
- Esimil Tablets ... 840
- HydroDIURIL Tablets ... 1716
- Hydropres Tablets ... 1718
- Hyzaar Tablets ... 1720
- Inderide Tablets ... 2838
- Inderide LA Long Acting Capsules ... 2840
- Lopressor HCT Tablets ... 850
- Lotensin HCT Tablets ... 855
- Moduretic Tablets ... 1748
- Oretic Tablets ... 450
- Prinzide Tablets ... 1780
- Ser-Ap-Es Tablets ... 867
- Timolide Tablets ... 1791
- Vaseretic Tablets ... 1810
- Zestoretic Tablets ... 2968
- Ziac ... 1459

Hydrocodone Bitartrate (Potentiation of orthostatic hypotension may occur). Products include:
- Codiclear DH Syrup ... 808
- Duratuss HD Elixir ... 2750
- Histussin D Liquid ... 670
- Hycodan Tablets and Syrup ... 946
- Hycomine Compound Tablets ... 948
- Hycomine ... 947
- Hycotuss Expectorant Syrup ... 950
- Hydrocet Capsules ... 787
- Lorcet 10/650 Tablets ... 1016
- Lortab ... 2751
- Tussend ... 1830
- Tussend Expectorant ... 1831
- Vicodin Tablets ... 1404
- Vicodin ES Tablets ... 1405
- Vicodin HP Tablets ... 1403
- Vicodin Tuss Expectorant ... 1406
- Zydone Capsules ... 967

Hydrocodone Polistirex (Potentiation of orthostatic hypotension may occur). Products include:
- Tussionex Pennkinetic Extended-Release Suspension ... 1624

Hydrocortisone (Intensified electrolyte depletion particularly hypokalemia). Products include:
- Anusol-HC Cream 2.5% ... 1953
- Aquanil HC Lotion ... 1989
- Maximum Strength Cortaid Spray ... ▣ 800
- CORTENEMA ... 2713
- Cortisporin Ointment ... 1074
- Cortisporin Ophthalmic Ointment Sterile ... 1074
- Cortisporin Ophthalmic Suspension Sterile ... 1075
- Cortisporin Otic Solution Sterile ... 1076
- Cortisporin Otic Suspension Sterile ... 1077
- Cortizone-5 ... ▣ 795
- Cortizone-10 ... ▣ 795
- Hydrocortone Tablets ... 1715
- Hytone ... 922
- Hytone Ointment 2 ½% ... 923
- Massengill Medicated Soft Cloth Towelettes ... 2628
- Pediotic Suspension Sterile ... 1140
- Preparation H Hydrocortisone 1% Cream ... ▣ 843
- ProctoCream-HC 2.5% ... 2552
- VōSoL HC Otic Solution ... 2786

Hydrocortisone Acetate (Intensified electrolyte depletion particularly hypokalemia). Products include:
- Analpram-HC Rectal Cream 1% and 2.5% ... 993
- Anusol HC-1 Hydrocortisone Anti-Itch Ointment ... ▣ 810
- Anusol-HC Suppositories ... 1954
- Caldecort Anti-Itch Hydrocortisone Cream ... ▣ 651
- Coly-Mycin S Otic w/Neomycin & Hydrocortisone ... 1965
- Cortaid ... ▣ 800
- Cortifoam ... 2540
- Cortisporin Cream ... 1073
- Epifoam ... 2543
- Hydrocortone Acetate Sterile Suspension ... 1712
- Mantadil Cream ... 1124
- Nupercainal Hydrocortisone 1% Cream ... ▣ 661
- Pramosone Cream, Lotion & Ointment ... 995
- ProctoFoam-HC ... 2552
- Terra-Cortril Ophthalmic Suspension ... 2033

Hydrocortisone Sodium Phosphate (Intensified electrolyte depletion particularly hypokalemia). Products include:
- Hydrocortone Phosphate Injection, Sterile ... 1713

Hydrocortisone Sodium Succinate (Intensified electrolyte depletion particularly hypokalemia).
No products indexed under this heading.

Hydroflumethiazide (Concurrent use with other antihypertensive agents may result in additive effect or potentiation). Products include:
- Diucardin Tablets ... 2824

Hydromorphone Hydrochloride (Potentiation of orthostatic hypotension may occur). Products include:
- Dilaudid Ampules ... 1382
- Dilaudid Cough Syrup ... 1383
- Dilaudid-HP Injection ... 1384
- Dilaudid-HP Lyophilized Powder 250 mg ... 1384
- Dilaudid ... 1382
- Dilaudid Oral Liquid ... 1386
- Dilaudid ... 1382
- Dilaudid Tablets - 8 mg. ... 1386

Ibuprofen (Reduces diuretic, natriuretic, and antihypertensive effects). Products include:
- Advil Cold and Sinus Caplets and Tablets ... ▣ 837
- Advil Ibuprofen Tablets, Caplets and Gel Caplets ... ▣ 836
- Children's Motrin Ibuprofen Oral Suspension ... 1558
- IBU Tablets ... 1389
- Ibuprohm ... ▣ 713
- Motrin IB Caplets, Tablets, and Gelcaps ... ▣ 802
- Motrin Ibuprofen Suspension, Oral Drops, Chewable Tablets, Caplets ... 1563
- Nuprin Ibuprofen/Analgesic Tablets & Caplets ... ▣ 645
- Vicks DayQuil SINUS Pressure & PAIN Relief with IBUPROFEN ... ▣ 735

Indapamide (Concurrent use with other antihypertensive agents may result in additive effect or potentiation).
No products indexed under this heading.

Indomethacin (Reduces diuretic, natriuretic, and antihypertensive effects). Products include:
- Indocin ... 1723

Indomethacin Sodium Trihydrate (Reduces diuretic, natriuretic, and antihypertensive effects). Products include:
- Indocin I.V. ... 1727

Insulin, Human (Thiazide-induced hyperglycemia may require dosage adjustment of hypoglycemic agents).
No products indexed under this heading.

(▣ Described in PDR For Nonprescription Drugs)   (⊙ Described in PDR For Ophthalmology)

Insulin, Human Isophane Suspension (Thiazide-induced hyperglycemia may require dosage adjustment of hypoglycemic agents). Products include:
- Novolin N Human Insulin 10 ml Vials ... 1846

Insulin, Human NPH (Thiazide-induced hyperglycemia may require dosage adjustment of hypoglycemic agents). Products include:
- Humulin N, 100 Units ... 1495
- Novolin N PenFill 1.5 ml Cartridges Durable Insulin Delivery System ... 1849
- Novolin N Prefilled Syringe Disposable Insulin Delivery System ... 1850

Insulin, Human Regular (Thiazide-induced hyperglycemia may require dosage adjustment of hypoglycemic agents). Products include:
- Humulin R, 100 Units ... 1497
- Novolin R Human Insulin 10 ml Vials ... 1846
- Novolin R PenFill 1.5 ml Cartridges Durable Insulin Delivery System ... 1849
- Novolin R Prefilled Syringe Disposable Insulin Delivery System ... 1850
- Velosulin BR Human Insulin 10 ml Vials ... 1847

Insulin, Human, Zinc Suspension (Thiazide-induced hyperglycemia may require dosage adjustment of hypoglycemic agents). Products include:
- Humulin L, 100 Units ... 1494
- Humulin U, 100 Units ... 1498
- Novolin L Human Insulin 10 ml Vials ... 1846

Insulin Lispro, Human (Thiazide-induced hyperglycemia may require dosage adjustment of hypoglycemic agents). Products include:
- Humalog Injection ... 1488

Insulin, NPH (Thiazide-induced hyperglycemia may require dosage adjustment of hypoglycemic agents). Products include:
- NPH, 100 Units ... 1502
- Pork NPH, 100 Units ... 1506
- Purified Pork NPH Isophane Insulin ... 1852

Insulin, Regular (Thiazide-induced hyperglycemia may require dosage adjustment of hypoglycemic agents). Products include:
- Regular, 100 Units ... 1503
- Pork Regular, 100 Units ... 1507
- Pork Regular (Concentrated), 500 Units ... 1508
- Purified Pork Regular Insulin ... 1852

Insulin, Zinc Crystals (Thiazide-induced hyperglycemia may require dosage adjustment of hypoglycemic agents). Products include:
- NPH, 100 Units ... 1502

Insulin, Zinc Suspension (Thiazide-induced hyperglycemia may require dosage adjustment of hypoglycemic agents). Products include:
- Iletin I ... 1501
- Lente, 100 Units ... 1501
- Iletin II ... 1504
- Pork Lente, 100 Units ... 1504
- Purified Pork Lente Insulin ... 1852

Isradipine (Concurrent use with other antihypertensive agents may result in additive effect or potentiation). Products include:
- DynaCirc Capsules ... 2381
- DynaCirc CR Tablets ... 2383

Ketoprofen (Reduces diuretic, natriuretic, and antihypertensive effects). Products include:
- Actron Caplets and Tablets ... 608
- Orudis Capsules ... 2874
- Orudis KT ... 842
- Oruvail Capsules ... 2874

Ketorolac Tromethamine (Reduces diuretic, natriuretic, and antihypertensive effects). Products include:
- Acular Sterile Ophthalmic Solution 470
- Toradol ... 2319

Labetalol Hydrochloride (Concurrent use with other antihypertensive agents may result in additive effect or potentiation). Products include:
- Normodyne Injection ... 2519
- Normodyne Tablets ... 2522
- Trandate ... 1158

Levorphanol Tartrate (Potentiation of orthostatic hypotension may occur). Products include:
- Levo-Dromoran ... 2297

Lisinopril (Concurrent use with other antihypertensive agents may result in additive effect or potentiation). Products include:
- Prinivil Tablets ... 1776
- Prinzide Tablets ... 1780
- Zestoretic Tablets ... 2968
- Zestril Tablets ... 2972

Lithium Carbonate (Diuretics reduce the renal clearance of lithium and this may lead to lithium toxicity). Products include:
- Eskalith ... 2658
- Lithium Carbonate Capsules & Tablets ... 2352
- Lithonate/Lithotabs/Lithobid ... 2721

Lithium Citrate (Diuretics reduce the renal clearance of lithium and this may lead to lithium toxicity).
- No products indexed under this heading.

Losartan Potassium (Concurrent use with other antihypertensive agents may result in additive effect or potentiation). Products include:
- Cozaar Tablets ... 1668
- Hyzaar Tablets ... 1720

Mecamylamine Hydrochloride (Concurrent use with other antihypertensive agents may result in additive effect or potentiation). Products include:
- Inversine Tablets ... 1729

Meclofenamate Sodium (Reduces diuretic, natriuretic, and antihypertensive effects).
- No products indexed under this heading.

Mefenamic Acid (Reduces diuretic, natriuretic, and antihypertensive effects). Products include:
- Ponstel ... 1982

Meperidine Hydrochloride (Potentiation of orthostatic hypotension may occur). Products include:
- Demerol ... 2438
- Mepergan Injection ... 2859

Mephobarbital (Potentiation of orthostatic hypotension may occur). Products include:
- Mebaral Tablets ... 2452

Metformin Hydrochloride (Thiazide-induced hyperglycemia may require dosage adjustment of hypoglycemic agents). Products include:
- Glucophage Tablets ... 754

Methadone Hydrochloride (Potentiation of orthostatic hypotension may occur). Products include:
- Methadone Hydrochloride Oral Concentrate ... 2356
- Methadone Hydrochloride Oral Solution & Tablets ... 2357

Methyclothiazide (Concurrent use with other antihypertensive agents may result in additive effect or potentiation). Products include:
- Enduron Tablets ... 424

Methyldopa (Concurrent use with other antihypertensive agents may result in additive effect or potentiation). Products include:
- Aldoclor Tablets ... 1638
- Aldomet Oral ... 1640
- Aldoril Tablets ... 1644

Methyldopate Hydrochloride (Concurrent use with other antihypertensive agents may result in additive effect or potentiation). Products include:
- Aldomet Ester HCl Injection ... 1642

Methylprednisolone Acetate (Intensified electrolyte depletion particularly hypokalemia).
- No products indexed under this heading.

Methylprednisolone Sodium Succinate (Intensified electrolyte depletion particularly hypokalemia).
- No products indexed under this heading.

Metocurine Iodide (Possible increased responsiveness to the muscle relaxants). Products include:
- Metubine Iodide Vials ... 932

Metolazone (Concurrent use with other antihypertensive agents may result in additive effect or potentiation). Products include:
- Mykrox Tablets ... 1617
- Zaroxolyn Tablets ... 1625

Metoprolol Succinate (Concurrent use with other antihypertensive agents may result in additive effect or potentiation). Products include:
- Toprol-XL Tablets ... 560

Metoprolol Tartrate (Concurrent use with other antihypertensive agents may result in additive effect or potentiation). Products include:
- Lopressor ... 848
- Lopressor HCT Tablets ... 850

Metyrosine (Concurrent use with other antihypertensive agents may result in additive effect or potentiation). Products include:
- Demser Capsules ... 1690

Minoxidil (Concurrent use with other antihypertensive agents may result in additive effect or potentiation).
- No products indexed under this heading.

Mivacurium Chloride (Possible increased responsiveness to the muscle relaxants). Products include:
- Mivacron ... 1125

Moexipril Hydrochloride (Concurrent use with other antihypertensive agents may result in additive effect or potentiation). Products include:
- Univasc Tablets ... 2553

Morphine Sulfate (Potentiation of orthostatic hypotension may occur). Products include:
- Astramorph/PF Injection, USP (Preservative-Free) ... 526
- Duramorph Injection ... 983
- Infumorph 200 and Infumorph 500 Sterile Solutions ... 985
- Kadian Capsules ... 2948
- MS Contin Tablets ... 2149
- MSIR ... 2152
- Oramorph SR (Morphine Sulfate Sustained Release Tablets) ... 2359
- RMS Suppositories CII ... 2766
- Roxanol ... 2365

Nabumetone (Reduces diuretic, natriuretic, and antihypertensive effects). Products include:
- Relafen Tablets ... 2688

Nadolol (Concurrent use with other antihypertensive agents may result in additive effect or potentiation).
- No products indexed under this heading.

Naproxen (Reduces diuretic, natriuretic, and antihypertensive effects). Products include:
- Anaprox/Naprosyn ... 2277

Naproxen Sodium (Reduces diuretic, natriuretic, and antihypertensive effects). Products include:
- Aleve ... 2124
- Anaprox/Naprosyn ... 2277
- Naprelan Tablets ... 2861

Nicardipine Hydrochloride (Concurrent use with other antihypertensive agents may result in additive effect or potentiation). Products include:
- Cardene Capsules ... 2261
- Cardene I.V. ... 2815
- Cardene SR Capsules ... 2264

Nifedipine (Concurrent use with other antihypertensive agents may result in additive effect or potentiation). Products include:
- Adalat Capsules (10 mg and 20 mg) ... 580
- Adalat CC ... 582
- Procardia Capsules ... 2024
- Procardia XL Extended Release Tablets ... 2026

Nisoldipine (Concurrent use with other antihypertensive agents may result in additive effect or potentiation). Products include:
- Sular Tablets ... 2961

Nitroglycerin (Concurrent use with other antihypertensive agents may result in additive effect or potentiation). Products include:
- Deponit NTG Transdermal Delivery System ... 2541
- Nitro-Bid IV ... 1270
- Nitro-Bid Ointment ... 1272
- Nitro-Dur (nitroglycerin) Transdermal Infusion System ... 1365
- Nitrolingual Spray ... 2193
- Nitrostat Tablets ... 1981
- Transderm-Nitro Transdermal Therapeutic System ... 878

Norepinephrine Hydrochloride (Decreased arterial responsiveness to pressor amine).

Opium Alkaloids (Potentiation of orthostatic hypotension may occur).
- No products indexed under this heading.

Oxaprozin (Reduces diuretic, natriuretic, and antihypertensive effects). Products include:
- Daypro Caplets ... 2578

Oxycodone Hydrochloride (Potentiation of orthostatic hypotension may occur). Products include:
- OxyContin Tablets ... 2163
- OxyIR Capsules ... 2167
- Percocet Tablets ... 955
- Percodan Tablets ... 955
- Percodan-Demi Tablets ... 956
- Roxicodone Tablets, Oral Solution & Intensol (Oxycodone) ... 2366
- Tylox Capsules ... 1593

Pancuronium Bromide (Possible increased responsiveness to the muscle relaxants).
- No products indexed under this heading.

Penbutolol Sulfate (Concurrent use with other antihypertensive agents may result in additive effect or potentiation). Products include:
- Levatol Tablets ... 2547

Pentobarbital Sodium (Potentiation of orthostatic hypotension may occur). Products include:
- Nembutal Sodium Capsules ... 440
- Nembutal Sodium Solution ... 442
- Nembutal Sodium Suppositories ... 444

Phenobarbital (Potentiation of orthostatic hypotension may occur). Products include:
- Arco-Lase Plus Tablets ... 513
- Bellergal-S Tablets ... 2375
- Donnatal ... 2234

IMPORTANT NOTE: Always consult each drug listing in the patient's regimen for possible interactions.

Diuril Intravenous

Donnatal Extentabs 2234
Donnatal Tablets 2234
Phenobarbital Elixir and Tablets 1523
Quadrinal Tablets 1398

Phenoxybenzamine Hydrochloride (Concurrent use with other antihypertensive agents may result in additive effect or potentiation). Products include:
Dibenzyline Capsules 2650

Phentolamine Mesylate (Concurrent use with other antihypertensive agents may result in additive effect or potentiation). Products include:
Regitine Vials 864

Phenylbutazone (Reduces diuretic, natriuretic, and antihypertensive effects).
No products indexed under this heading.

Pindolol (Concurrent use with other antihypertensive agents may result in additive effect or potentiation). Products include:
Visken Tablets 2428

Piroxicam (Reduces diuretic, natriuretic, and antihypertensive effects). Products include:
Feldene Capsules 2008

Polythiazide (Concurrent use with other antihypertensive agents may result in additive effect or potentiation). Products include:
Minizide Capsules 2016

Prazosin Hydrochloride (Concurrent use with other antihypertensive agents may result in additive effect or potentiation). Products include:
Minipress Capsules 2015
Minizide Capsules 2016

Prednisolone Acetate (Intensified electrolyte depletion particularly hypokalemia). Products include:
AK-CIDE .... ⊚ 203
AK-CIDE Ointment .... ⊚ 203
Blephamide Liquifilm Sterile Ophthalmic Suspension 472
Blephamide Ointment .... ⊚ 234
Econopred & Econopred Plus Ophthalmic Suspensions .... ⊚ 216
Poly-Pred Liquifilm .... ⊚ 246
Pred Forte .... ⊚ 247
Pred Mild .... ⊚ 250
Pred-G Liquifilm Sterile Ophthalmic Suspension .... ⊚ 248
Pred-G S.O.P. Sterile Ophthalmic Ointment .... ⊚ 249

Prednisolone Sodium Phosphate (Intensified electrolyte depletion particularly hypokalemia). Products include:
AK-PRED .... ⊚ 204
Hydeltrasol Injection, Sterile 1708
Pediapred Oral Solution 1618

Prednisolone Tebutate (Intensified electrolyte depletion particularly hypokalemia). Products include:
Hydeltra-T.B.A. Sterile Suspension ... 1710

Prednisone (Intensified electrolyte depletion particularly hypokalemia).
No products indexed under this heading.

Propoxyphene Hydrochloride (Potentiation of orthostatic hypotension may occur). Products include:
Darvon 1475
Wygesic Tablets 2930

Propoxyphene Napsylate (Potentiation of orthostatic hypotension may occur). Products include:
Darvon-N/Darvocet-N 1473

Propranolol Hydrochloride (Concurrent use with other antihypertensive agents may result in additive effect or potentiation). Products include:
Inderal 2834
Inderal LA Long Acting Capsules 2836

Inderide Tablets 2838
Inderide LA Long Acting Capsules .. 2840

Quinapril Hydrochloride (Concurrent use with other antihypertensive agents may result in additive effect or potentiation). Products include:
Accupril Tablets 1950

Ramipril (Concurrent use with other antihypertensive agents may result in additive effect or potentiation). Products include:
Altace Capsules 1238

Rauwolfia Serpentina (Concurrent use with other antihypertensive agents may result in additive effect or potentiation).
No products indexed under this heading.

Rescinnamine (Concurrent use with other antihypertensive agents may result in additive effect or potentiation).
No products indexed under this heading.

Reserpine (Concurrent use with other antihypertensive agents may result in additive effect or potentiation). Products include:
Diupres Tablets 1691
Hydropres Tablets 1718
Ser-Ap-Es Tablets 867

Rocuronium Bromide (Possible increased responsiveness to the muscle relaxants). Products include:
Zemuron Injection 1885

Secobarbital Sodium (Potentiation of orthostatic hypotension may occur). Products include:
Seconal Sodium Pulvules 1529

Sodium Nitroprusside (Concurrent use with other antihypertensive agents may result in additive effect or potentiation).
No products indexed under this heading.

Sotalol Hydrochloride (Concurrent use with other antihypertensive agents may result in additive effect or potentiation). Products include:
Betapace Tablets 637

Spirapril Hydrochloride (Concurrent use with other antihypertensive agents may result in additive effect or potentiation).
No products indexed under this heading.

Sufentanil Citrate (Potentiation of orthostatic hypotension may occur). Products include:
Sufenta Injection 1355

Sulindac (Reduces diuretic, natriuretic, and antihypertensive effects). Products include:
Clinoril Tablets 1658

Terazosin Hydrochloride (Concurrent use with other antihypertensive agents may result in additive effect or potentiation). Products include:
Hytrin Capsules 434

Thiamylal Sodium (Potentiation of orthostatic hypotension may occur).
No products indexed under this heading.

Timolol Maleate (Concurrent use with other antihypertensive agents may result in additive effect or potentiation). Products include:
Blocadren Tablets 1654
Timolide Tablets 1791
Timoptic in Ocudose 1796
Timoptic Sterile Ophthalmic Solution 1794
Timoptic-XE 1798

Interactions Index

Tolazamide (Thiazide-induced hyperglycemia may require dosage adjustment of hypoglycemic agents).
No products indexed under this heading.

Tolbutamide (Thiazide-induced hyperglycemia may require dosage adjustment of hypoglycemic agents).
No products indexed under this heading.

Tolmetin Sodium (Reduces diuretic, natriuretic, and antihypertensive effects). Products include:
Tolectin (200, 400 and 600 mg) .. 1591

Torsemide (Concurrent use with other antihypertensive agents may result in additive effect or potentiation). Products include:
Demadex Tablets and Injection 691

Triamcinolone (Intensified electrolyte depletion particularly hypokalemia).
No products indexed under this heading.

Triamcinolone Acetonide (Intensified electrolyte depletion particularly hypokalemia). Products include:
Azmacort Oral Inhaler 2175
Nasacort AQ Nasal Spray 2191
Nasacort Nasal Inhaler 2189

Triamcinolone Diacetate (Intensified electrolyte depletion particularly hypokalemia).
No products indexed under this heading.

Triamcinolone Hexacetonide (Intensified electrolyte depletion particularly hypokalemia).
No products indexed under this heading.

Trimethaphan Camsylate (Concurrent use with other antihypertensive agents may result in additive effect or potentiation).
No products indexed under this heading.

Tubocurarine Chloride (Possible increased responsiveness to the muscle relaxants).
No products indexed under this heading.

Vecuronium Bromide (Possible increased responsiveness to the muscle relaxants). Products include:
Norcuron for Injection 1875

Verapamil Hydrochloride (Concurrent use with other antihypertensive agents may result in additive effect or potentiation). Products include:
Calan SR Caplets 2571
Calan Tablets 2568
Covera-HS Tablets 2573
Isoptin Injectable 1391
Isoptin Oral Tablets 1393
Isoptin SR Tablets 1395
Verelan Capsules 1455

Food Interactions

Alcohol (Potentiation of orthostatic hypotension may occur).

DIURIL TABLETS
(Chlorothiazide) 1694
See **Diuril Oral Suspension**

DIZAC (DIAZEPAM INJECTABLE EMULSION) CIV
(Diazepam) 1862
May interact with central nervous system depressants, barbiturates, narcotic analgesics, phenothiazines, monoamine oxidase inhibitors, antidepressant drugs, and certain other

agents. Compounds in these categories include:

Alfentanil Hydrochloride (Concomitant use increases depression with increased risk of apnea; dosage of narcotic analgesic should be reduced by at least one-third and administered in small increments; potentiates the action of diazepam). Products include:
Alfenta Injection 1334

Alprazolam (Concomitant use increases depression with increased risk of apnea). Products include:
Xanax Tablets 2115

Amitriptyline Hydrochloride (Potentiates the action of diazepam). Products include:
Elavil 2945
Etrafon 2495
Limbitrol 2333
Triavil Tablets 1800

Amoxapine (Potentiates the action of diazepam). Products include:
Asendin Tablets 1419

Aprobarbital (Concomitant use increases depression with increased risk of apnea; potentiates the action of diazepam).
No products indexed under this heading.

Buprenorphine (Concomitant use increases depression with increased risk of apnea; dosage of narcotic analgesic should be reduced by at least one-third and administered in small increments; potentiates the action of diazepam). Products include:
Buprenex Injectable 2170

Bupropion Hydrochloride (Potentiates the action of diazepam). Products include:
Wellbutrin Tablets 1177

Buspirone Hydrochloride (Concomitant use increases depression with increased risk of apnea). Products include:
BuSpar Tablets 738

Butabarbital (Concomitant use increases depression with increased risk of apnea; potentiates the action of diazepam).
No products indexed under this heading.

Butalbital (Concomitant use increases depression with increased risk of apnea; potentiates the action of diazepam). Products include:
Axocet Capsules 2469
Esgic-plus Capsules 1012
Esgic-plus Tablets 1012
Fioricet Tablets 2386
Fioricet with Codeine Capsules 2387
Fiorinal Capsules 2388
Fiorinal with Codeine Capsules 2390
Fiorinal Tablets 2388
Phrenilin 790
Sedapap Tablets 50 mg/650 mg .. 1826

Chlordiazepoxide (Concomitant use increases depression with increased risk of apnea). Products include:
Limbitrol 2333

Chlordiazepoxide Hydrochloride (Concomitant use increases depression with increased risk of apnea). Products include:
Librax Capsules 2330
Librium Capsules 2331
Librium Injectable 2332

Chlorpromazine (Potentiates the action of diazepam). Products include:
Thorazine Suppositories 2701

Chlorpromazine Hydrochloride (Potentiates the action of diazepam). Products include:
Thorazine 2701

(⌑ Described in PDR For Nonprescription Drugs)   (⊚ Described in PDR For Ophthalmology)

Chlorprothixene (Concomitant use increases depression with increased risk of apnea).
　No products indexed under this heading.

Chlorprothixene Hydrochloride (Concomitant use increases depression with increased risk of apnea).
　No products indexed under this heading.

Chlorprothixene Lactate (Concomitant use increases depression with increased risk of apnea; dosage of narcotic analgesic should be reduced by at least one-third and administered in small increments; potentiates the action of diazepam).
　No products indexed under this heading.

Cimetidine (The clearance of diazepam is delayed by concurrent use of cimetidine; clinical significance is unknown). Products include:
　Tagamet HB Tablets 786
　Tagamet Tablets 2694

Cimetidine Hydrochloride (The clearance of diazepam is delayed by concurrent use of cimetidine; clinical significance is unknown). Products include:
　Tagamet 2694

Clorazepate Dipotassium (Concomitant use increases depression with increased risk of apnea). Products include:
　Tranxene 459

Clozapine (Concomitant use increases depression with increased risk of apnea). Products include:
　Clozaril Tablets 2377

Codeine Phosphate (Concomitant use increases depression with increased risk of apnea; dosage of narcotic analgesic should be reduced by at least one-third and administered in small increments; potentiates the action of diazepam). Products include:
　Brontex 2130
　Dimetane-DC Cough Syrup 2232
　Fioricet with Codeine Capsules .. 2387
　Fiorinal with Codeine Capsules .. 2390
　Nucofed 2225
　Phenergan with Codeine 2883
　Phenergan VC with Codeine ... 2888
　Robitussin A-C Syrup 2248
　Robitussin-DAC Syrup 2249
　Ryna 804
　Soma Compound w/Codeine Tablets 2784
　Tylenol with Codeine 1592

Desflurane (Concomitant use increases depression with increased risk of apnea). Products include:
　Suprane (desflurane, USP) 1865

Desipramine Hydrochloride (Potentiates the action of diazepam). Products include:
　Norpramin Tablets 1273

Dezocine (Concomitant use increases depression with increased risk of apnea; dosage of narcotic analgesic should be reduced by at least one-third and administered in small increments; potentiates the action of diazepam). Products include:
　Dalgan Injection 529

Doxepin Hydrochloride (Potentiates the action of diazepam). Products include:
　Adapin Capsules 1542
　Sinequan 2028
　Zonalon Cream 1042

Droperidol (Concomitant use increases depression with increased risk of apnea). Products include:
　Inapsine Injection 462

Enflurane (Concomitant use increases depression with increased risk of apnea).
　No products indexed under this heading.

Estazolam (Concomitant use increases depression with increased risk of apnea). Products include:
　ProSom Tablets 457

Ethchlorvynol (Concomitant use increases depression with increased risk of apnea). Products include:
　Placidyl Capsules 456

Ethinamate (Concomitant use increases depression with increased risk of apnea).
　No products indexed under this heading.

Fentanyl (Concomitant use increases depression with increased risk of apnea; dosage of narcotic analgesic should be reduced by at least one-third and administered in small increments; potentiates the action of diazepam). Products include:
　Duragesic Transdermal System 1336

Fentanyl Citrate (Concomitant use increases depression with increased risk of apnea; dosage of narcotic analgesic should be reduced by at least one-third and administered in small increments; potentiates the action of diazepam). Products include:
　Sublimaze Injection 463

Fluoxetine Hydrochloride (Potentiates the action of diazepam). Products include:
　Prozac Pulvules & Liquid, Oral Solution 935

Fluphenazine Decanoate (Potentiates the action of diazepam). Products include:
　Prolixin Decanoate 510

Fluphenazine Enanthate (Potentiates the action of diazepam). Products include:
　Prolixin Enanthate 510

Fluphenazine Hydrochloride (Potentiates the action of diazepam). Products include:
　Prolixin 510

Flurazepam Hydrochloride (Concomitant use increases depression with increased risk of apnea). Products include:
　Dalmane Capsules 2329

Furazolidone (Potentiates the action of diazepam). Products include:
　Furoxone 2221

Glutethimide (Concomitant use increases depression with increased risk of apnea).
　No products indexed under this heading.

Haloperidol (Concomitant use increases depression with increased risk of apnea). Products include:
　Haldol Injection, Tablets and Concentrate 1585

Haloperidol Decanoate (Concomitant use increases depression with increased risk of apnea). Products include:
　Haldol Decanoate 1587

Hydrocodone Bitartrate (Concomitant use increases depression with increased risk of apnea; dosage of narcotic analgesic should be reduced by at least one-third and administered in small increments; potentiates the action of diazepam). Products include:
　Codiclear DH Syrup 808
　Duratuss HD Elixir 2750
　Histussin D Liquid 670
　Hycodan Tablets and Syrup ... 946
　Hycomine Compound Tablets .. 948
　Hycomine 947
　Hycotuss Expectorant Syrup .. 950
　Hydrocet Capsules 787
　Lorcet 10/650 Tablets 1016
　Lortab 2751
　Tussend 1830
　Tussend Expectorant 1831
　Vicodin Tablets 1404
　Vicodin ES Tablets 1405
　Vicodin HP Tablets 1403
　Vicodin Tuss Expectorant 1406
　Zydone Capsules 967

Hydrocodone Polistirex (Concomitant use increases depression with increased risk of apnea; dosage of narcotic analgesic should be reduced by at least one-third and administered in small increments; potentiates the action of diazepam). Products include:
　Tussionex Pennkinetic Extended-Release Suspension 1624

Hydromorphone Hydrochloride (Concomitant use increases depression with increased risk of apnea; dosage of narcotic analgesic should be reduced by at least one-third and administered in small increments; potentiates the action of diazepam). Products include:
　Dilaudid Ampules 1382
　Dilaudid Cough Syrup 1383
　Dilaudid-HP Injection 1384
　Dilaudid-HP Lyophilized Powder 250 mg 1384
　Dilaudid 1382
　Dilaudid Oral Liquid 1386
　Dilaudid 1382
　Dilaudid Tablets - 8 mg 1386

Hydroxyzine Hydrochloride (Concomitant use increases depression with increased risk of apnea). Products include:
　Atarax Tablets & Syrup 1992
　Marax Tablets & DF Syrup 2015
　Vistaril Intramuscular Solution 2042

Imipramine Hydrochloride (Potentiates the action of diazepam). Products include:
　Tofranil Ampuls 873
　Tofranil Tablets 875

Imipramine Pamoate (Potentiates the action of diazepam). Products include:
　Tofranil-PM Capsules 876

Isocarboxazid (Potentiates the action of diazepam).
　No products indexed under this heading.

Isoflurane (Concomitant use increases depression with increased risk of apnea).
　No products indexed under this heading.

Ketamine Hydrochloride (Concomitant use increases depression with increased risk of apnea).
　No products indexed under this heading.

Levomethadyl Acetate Hydrochloride (Concomitant use increases depression with increased risk of apnea). Products include:
　Orlaam Oral Solution 2361

Levorphanol Tartrate (Concomitant use increases depression with increased risk of apnea; dosage of narcotic analgesic should be reduced by at least one-third and administered in small increments; potentiates the action of diazepam). Products include:
　Levo-Dromoran 2297

Lorazepam (Concomitant use increases depression with increased risk of apnea). Products include:
　Ativan Injection 2805
　Ativan Tablets 2807

Loxapine Hydrochloride (Concomitant use increases depression with increased risk of apnea). Products include:
　Loxitane 1426

Loxapine Succinate (Concomitant use increases depression with increased risk of apnea). Products include:
　Loxitane Capsules 1426

Maprotiline Hydrochloride (Potentiates the action of diazepam). Products include:
　Ludiomil Tablets 861

Meperidine Hydrochloride (Concomitant use increases depression with increased risk of apnea; dosage of narcotic analgesic should be reduced by at least one-third and administered in small increments; potentiates the action of diazepam). Products include:
　Demerol 2438
　Mepergan Injection 2859

Mephobarbital (Concomitant use increases depression with increased risk of apnea; potentiates the action of diazepam). Products include:
　Mebaral Tablets 2452

Meprobamate (Concomitant use increases depression with increased risk of apnea). Products include:
　Miltown Tablets 2780
　PMB 200 and PMB 400 2890

Mesoridazine Besylate (Potentiates the action of diazepam). Products include:
　Serentil 689

Methadone Hydrochloride (Concomitant use increases depression with increased risk of apnea; dosage of narcotic analgesic should be reduced by at least one-third and administered in small increments; potentiates the action of diazepam). Products include:
　Methadone Hydrochloride Oral Concentrate 2356
　Methadone Hydrochloride Oral Solution & Tablets 2357

Methohexital Sodium (Concomitant use increases depression with increased risk of apnea).
　No products indexed under this heading.

Methotrimeprazine (Potentiates the action of diazepam). Products include:
　Levoprome 1321

Methoxyflurane (Concomitant use increases depression with increased risk of apnea).
　No products indexed under this heading.

Midazolam Hydrochloride (Concomitant use increases depression with increased risk of apnea). Products include:
　Versed Injection 2324

Mirtazapine (Potentiates the action of diazepam). Products include:
　Remeron Tablets 1878

Molindone Hydrochloride (Concomitant use increases depression with increased risk of apnea). Products include:
　Moban Tablets and Concentrate 1036

Morphine Sulfate (Concomitant use increases depression with increased risk of apnea; dosage of narcotic analgesic should be reduced by at least one-third and administered in small increments; potentiates the action of diazepam). Products include:
　Astramorph/PF Injection, USP (Preservative-Free) 526
　Duramorph Injection 983

IMPORTANT NOTE: Always consult each drug listing in the patient's regimen for possible interactions.

Dizac | Interactions Index | 326

Infumorph 200 and Infumorph 500 Sterile Solutions ... 985
Kadian Capsules ... 2948
MS Contin Tablets ... 2149
MSIR ... 2152
Oramorph SR (Morphine Sulfate Sustained Release Tablets) ... 2359
RMS Suppositories CII ... 2766
Roxanol ... 2365

Nefazodone Hydrochloride (Potentiates the action of diazepam). Products include:
Serzone Tablets ... 776

Nortriptyline Hydrochloride (Potentiates the action of diazepam). Products include:
Pamelor ... 2409

Opium Alkaloids (Concomitant use increases depression with increased risk of apnea; dosage of narcotic analgesic should be reduced by at least one-third and administered in small increments; potentiates the action of diazepam).
No products indexed under this heading.

Oxazepam (Concomitant use increases depression with increased risk of apnea). Products include:
Serax Capsules ... 2916
Serax Tablets ... 2916

Oxycodone Hydrochloride (Concomitant use increases depression with increased risk of apnea; dosage of narcotic analgesic should be reduced by at least one-third and administered in small increments; potentiates the action of diazepam). Products include:
OxyContin Tablets ... 2163
OxyIR Capsules ... 2167
Percocet Tablets ... 955
Percodan Tablets ... 955
Percodan-Demi Tablets ... 956
Roxicodone Tablets, Oral Solution & Intensol (Oxycodone) ... 2366
Tylox Capsules ... 1593

Paroxetine Hydrochloride (Potentiates the action of diazepam). Products include:
Paxil Tablets ... 2681

Pentobarbital Sodium (Concomitant use increases depression with increased risk of apnea; potentiates the action of diazepam). Products include:
Nembutal Sodium Capsules ... 440
Nembutal Sodium Solution ... 442
Nembutal Sodium Suppositories ... 444

Perphenazine (Potentiates the action of diazepam). Products include:
Etrafon ... 2495
Triavil Tablets ... 1800
Trilafon ... 2532

Phenelzine Sulfate (Potentiates the action of diazepam). Products include:
Nardil ... 1977

Phenobarbital (Concomitant use increases depression with increased risk of apnea; potentiates the action of diazepam). Products include:
Arco-Lase Plus Tablets ... 513
Bellergal-S Tablets ... 2375
Donnatal ... 2234
Donnatal Extentabs ... 2234
Donnatal Tablets ... 2234
Phenobarbital Elixir and Tablets ... 1523
Quadrinal Tablets ... 1398

Prazepam (Concomitant use increases depression with increased risk of apnea).
No products indexed under this heading.

Prochlorperazine (Potentiates the action of diazepam). Products include:
Compazine ... 2644

Promethazine Hydrochloride (Potentiates the action of diazepam). Products include:
Mepergan Injection ... 2859
Phenergan with Codeine ... 2883
Phenergan with Dextromethorphan ... 2885
Phenergan Injection ... 2880
Phenergan Suppositories ... 2882
Phenergan Syrup ... 2881
Phenergan Tablets ... 2882
Phenergan VC ... 2886
Phenergan VC with Codeine ... 2888

Propofol (Concomitant use increases depression with increased risk of apnea). Products include:
Diprivan Injectable Emulsion ... 2939

Propoxyphene Hydrochloride (Concomitant use increases depression with increased risk of apnea; dosage of narcotic analgesic should be reduced by at least one-third and administered in small increments; potentiates the action of diazepam). Products include:
Darvon ... 1475
Wygesic Tablets ... 2930

Propoxyphene Napsylate (Concomitant use increases depression with increased risk of apnea; dosage of narcotic analgesic should be reduced by at least one-third and administered in small increments; potentiates the action of diazepam). Products include:
Darvon-N/Darvocet-N ... 1473

Protriptyline Hydrochloride (Potentiates the action of diazepam). Products include:
Vivactil Tablets ... 1820

Quazepam (Concomitant use increases depression with increased risk of apnea). Products include:
Doral Tablets ... 2773

Risperidone (Concomitant use increases depression with increased risk of apnea). Products include:
Risperdal Tablets ... 1348

Secobarbital Sodium (Concomitant use increases depression with increased risk of apnea; potentiates the action of diazepam). Products include:
Seconal Sodium Pulvules ... 1529

Selegiline Hydrochloride (Potentiates the action of diazepam). Products include:
Eldepryl Capsules ... 2729

Sertraline Hydrochloride (Potentiates the action of diazepam). Products include:
Zoloft Tablets ... 2051

Sevoflurane (Concomitant use increases depression with increased risk of apnea; dosage of narcotic analgesic should be reduced by at least one-third and administered in small increments; potentiates the action of diazepam).
No products indexed under this heading.

Sufentanil Citrate (Concomitant use increases depression with increased risk of apnea; dosage of narcotic analgesic should be reduced by at least one-third and administered in small increments; potentiates the action of diazepam). Products include:
Sufenta Injection ... 1355

Temazepam (Concomitant use increases depression with increased risk of apnea). Products include:
Restoril Capsules ... 2413

Thiamylal Sodium (Concomitant use increases depression with increased risk of apnea; potentiates the action of diazepam).
No products indexed under this heading.

Thioridazine Hydrochloride (Potentiates the action of diazepam). Products include:
Mellaril ... 2398

Thiothixene (Concomitant use increases depression with increased risk of apnea). Products include:
Navane Capsules and Concentrate ... 2018
Navane Intramuscular ... 2019

Tranylcypromine Sulfate (Potentiates the action of diazepam). Products include:
Parnate Tablets ... 2679

Trazodone Hydrochloride (Potentiates the action of diazepam). Products include:
Desyrel and Desyrel Dividose ... 504

Triazolam (Concomitant use increases depression with increased risk of apnea). Products include:
Halcion Tablets ... 2093

Trifluoperazine Hydrochloride (Potentiates the action of diazepam). Products include:
Stelazine ... 2692

Trimipramine Maleate (Potentiates the action of diazepam). Products include:
Surmontil Capsules ... 2917

Venlafaxine Hydrochloride (Potentiates the action of diazepam). Products include:
Effexor ... 2825

Zolpidem Tartrate (Concomitant use increases depression with increased risk of apnea). Products include:
Ambien Tablets ... 2559

Food Interactions

Alcohol (Potentiates the action of diazepam; concomitant use increases depression with increased risk of apnea).

DOAN'S EXTRA-STRENGTH ANALGESIC
(Magnesium Salicylate) ... ⊞ 653
May interact with oral anticoagulants and certain other agents. Compounds in these categories include:

Antiarthritic Drugs, unspecified (Concurrent use is not recommended).

Antidiabetic Drugs, unspecified (Concurrent use is not recommended).

Antigout Drugs, unspecified (Concurrent use is not recommended).

Dicumarol (Concurrent use is not recommended).
No products indexed under this heading.

Warfarin Sodium (Concurrent use is not recommended). Products include:
Coumadin ... 941

EXTRA STRENGTH DOAN'S P.M.
(Magnesium Salicylate, Diphenhydramine Hydrochloride) ... ⊞ 653
May interact with hypnotics and sedatives, tranquilizers, and certain other agents. Compounds in these categories include:

Alprazolam (Effect not specified). Products include:
Xanax Tablets ... 2115

Antiarthritic Drugs, unspecified (Concurrent use is not recommended).

Antidiabetic Drugs, unspecified (Concurrent use is not recommended).

Antigout Drugs, unspecified (Concurrent use is not recommended).

Buspirone Hydrochloride (Effect not specified). Products include:
BuSpar Tablets ... 738

Chlordiazepoxide (Effect not specified). Products include:
Limbitrol ... 2333

Chlordiazepoxide Hydrochloride (Effect not specified). Products include:
Librax Capsules ... 2330
Librium Capsules ... 2331
Librium Injectable ... 2332

Chlorpromazine (Effect not specified). Products include:
Thorazine Suppositories ... 2701

Chlorprothixene (Effect not specified).
No products indexed under this heading.

Chlorprothixene Hydrochloride (Effect not specified).
No products indexed under this heading.

Clorazepate Dipotassium (Effect not specified). Products include:
Tranxene ... 459

Diazepam (Effect not specified). Products include:
Dizac (diazepam injectable emulsion) CIV ... 1862
Valium Injectable ... 2336
Valium Tablets ... 2335

Dicumarol (Concurrent use is not recommended).
No products indexed under this heading.

Droperidol (Effect not specified). Products include:
Inapsine Injection ... 462

Estazolam (Effect not specified). Products include:
ProSom Tablets ... 457

Ethchlorvynol (Effect not specified). Products include:
Placidyl Capsules ... 456

Ethinamate (Effect not specified).
No products indexed under this heading.

Fluphenazine Decanoate (Effect not specified). Products include:
Prolixin Decanoate ... 510

Fluphenazine Enanthate (Effect not specified). Products include:
Prolixin Enanthate ... 510

Fluphenazine Hydrochloride (Effect not specified). Products include:
Prolixin ... 510

Flurazepam Hydrochloride (Effect not specified). Products include:
Dalmane Capsules ... 2329

Glutethimide (Effect not specified).
No products indexed under this heading.

Haloperidol (Effect not specified). Products include:
Haldol Injection, Tablets and Concentrate ... 1585

Haloperidol Decanoate (Effect not specified). Products include:
Haldol Decanoate ... 1587

Hydroxyzine Hydrochloride (Effect not specified). Products include:
Atarax Tablets & Syrup ... 1992
Marax Tablets & DF Syrup ... 2015
Vistaril Intramuscular Solution ... 2042

Lorazepam (Effect not specified). Products include:
Ativan Injection ... 2805
Ativan Tablets ... 2807

Loxapine Hydrochloride (Effect not specified). Products include:
Loxitane ... 1426

(⊞ Described in PDR For Nonprescription Drugs) (⊚ Described in PDR For Ophthalmology)

327 **Interactions Index** **Dolobid**

Loxapine Succinate (Effect not specified). Products include:
- Loxitane Capsules ... 1426

Meprobamate (Effect not specified). Products include:
- Miltown Tablets ... 2780
- PMB 200 and PMB 400 ... 2890

Mesoridazine Besylate (Effect not specified). Products include:
- Serentil ... 689

Midazolam Hydrochloride (Effect not specified). Products include:
- Versed Injection ... 2324

Molindone Hydrochloride (Effect not specified). Products include:
- Moban Tablets and Concentrate ... 1036

Oxazepam (Effect not specified). Products include:
- Serax Capsules ... 2916
- Serax Tablets ... 2916

Perphenazine (Effect not specified). Products include:
- Etrafon ... 2495
- Triavil Tablets ... 1800
- Trilafon ... 2532

Prazepam (Effect not specified).
- No products indexed under this heading.

Prochlorperazine (Effect not specified). Products include:
- Compazine ... 2644

Promethazine Hydrochloride (Effect not specified). Products include:
- Mepergan Injection ... 2859
- Phenergan with Codeine ... 2883
- Phenergan with Dextromethorphan 2885
- Phenergan Injection ... 2880
- Phenergan Suppositories ... 2882
- Phenergan Syrup ... 2881
- Phenergan Tablets ... 2882
- Phenergan VC ... 2886
- Phenergan VC with Codeine ... 2888

Propofol (Effect not specified). Products include:
- Diprivan Injectable Emulsion ... 2939

Quazepam (Effect not specified). Products include:
- Doral Tablets ... 2773

Secobarbital Sodium (Effect not specified). Products include:
- Seconal Sodium Pulvules ... 1529

Temazepam (Effect not specified). Products include:
- Restoril Capsules ... 2413

Thioridazine Hydrochloride (Effect not specified). Products include:
- Mellaril ... 2398

Thiothixene (Effect not specified). Products include:
- Navane Capsules and Concentrate 2018
- Navane Intramuscular ... 2019

Triazolam (Effect not specified). Products include:
- Halcion Tablets ... 2093

Trifluoperazine Hydrochloride (Effect not specified). Products include:
- Stelazine ... 2692

Warfarin Sodium (Concurrent use is not recommended). Products include:
- Coumadin ... 941

Zolpidem Tartrate (Effect not specified). Products include:
- Ambien Tablets ... 2559

Food Interactions

Alcohol (Avoid concomitant use).

DOAN'S REGULAR STRENGTH ANALGESIC

(Magnesium Salicylate) ... ▣ 654

May interact with oral anticoagulants and certain other agents. Compounds in these categories include:

Antiarthritic Drugs, unspecified (Concurrent use is not recommended unless directed by a doctor).

Antidiabetic Drugs, unspecified (Concurrent use is not recommended unless directed by a doctor).

Antigout Drugs, unspecified (Concurrent use is not recommended unless directed by a doctor).

Dicumarol (Concurrent use is not recommended unless directed by a doctor).
- No products indexed under this heading.

Warfarin Sodium (Concurrent use is not recommended unless directed by a doctor). Products include:
- Coumadin ... 941

DOBUTREX SOLUTION VIALS

(Dobutamine Hydrochloride) ... 1480

May interact with beta blockers and certain other agents. Compounds in these categories include:

Acebutolol Hydrochloride (Based on animal studies, dobutamine may be ineffective in patients recently on beta blocker; potential for increased peripheral vascular resistance). Products include:
- Sectral Capsules ... 2914

Atenolol (Based on animal studies, dobutamine may be ineffective in patients recently on beta blocker; potential for increased peripheral vascular resistance). Products include:
- Tenoretic Tablets ... 2963
- Tenormin Tablets and I.V. Injection 2965

Betaxolol Hydrochloride (Based on animal studies, dobutamine may be ineffective in patients recently on beta blocker; potential for increased peripheral vascular resistance). Products include:
- Betoptic Ophthalmic Solution ... 465
- Betoptic S Ophthalmic Suspension 467
- Kerlone Tablets ... 2588

Bisoprolol Fumarate (Based on animal studies, dobutamine may be ineffective in patients recently on beta blocker; potential for increased peripheral vascular resistance). Products include:
- Zebeta Tablets ... 1457
- Ziac ... 1459

Carteolol Hydrochloride (Based on animal studies, dobutamine may be ineffective in patients recently on beta blocker; potential for increased peripheral vascular resistance). Products include:
- Cartrol Tablets ... 413
- Ocupress Ophthalmic Solution, 1% Sterile ... ⊙ 297

Esmolol Hydrochloride (Based on animal studies, dobutamine may be ineffective in patients recently on beta blocker; potential for increased peripheral vascular resistance). Products include:
- Brevibloc (esmolol HCl) Injection ... 1860

Labetalol Hydrochloride (Based on animal studies, dobutamine may be ineffective in patients recently on beta blocker; potential for increased peripheral vascular resistance). Products include:
- Normodyne Injection ... 2519
- Normodyne Tablets ... 2522
- Trandate ... 1158

Levobunolol Hydrochloride (Based on animal studies, dobutamine may be ineffective in patients recently on beta blocker; potential for increased peripheral vascular resistance). Products include:
- Betagan ... ⊙ 230

Metipranolol Hydrochloride (Based on animal studies, dobutamine may be ineffective in patients recently on beta blocker; potential for increased peripheral vascular resistance). Products include:
- OptiPranolol (Metipranolol 0.3%) Sterile Ophthalmic Solution ... ⊙ 256

Metoprolol Succinate (Based on animal studies, dobutamine may be ineffective in patients recently on beta blocker; potential for increased peripheral vascular resistance). Products include:
- Toprol-XL Tablets ... 560

Metoprolol Tartrate (Based on animal studies, dobutamine may be ineffective in patients recently on beta blocker; potential for increased peripheral vascular resistance). Products include:
- Lopressor ... 848
- Lopressor HCT Tablets ... 850

Nadolol (Based on animal studies, dobutamine may be ineffective in patients recently on beta blocker; potential for increased peripheral vascular resistance).
- No products indexed under this heading.

Penbutolol Sulfate (Based on animal studies, dobutamine may be ineffective in patients recently on beta blocker; potential for increased peripheral vascular resistance). Products include:
- Levatol Tablets ... 2547

Pindolol (Based on animal studies, dobutamine may be ineffective in patients recently on beta blocker; potential for increased peripheral vascular resistance). Products include:
- Visken Tablets ... 2428

Propranolol Hydrochloride (Based on animal studies, dobutamine may be ineffective in patients recently on beta blocker; potential for increased peripheral vascular resistance). Products include:
- Inderal ... 2834
- Inderal LA Long Acting Capsules ... 2836
- Inderide Tablets ... 2838
- Inderide LA Long Acting Capsules .. 2840

Sodium Nitroprusside (Concomitant use results in a higher cardiac output and, usually, a lower pulmonary wedge pressure).
- No products indexed under this heading.

Sotalol Hydrochloride (Based on animal studies, dobutamine may be ineffective in patients recently on beta blocker; potential for increased peripheral vascular resistance). Products include:
- Betapace Tablets ... 637

Timolol Hemihydrate (Based on animal studies, dobutamine may be ineffective in patients recently on beta blocker; potential for increased peripheral vascular resistance). Products include:
- Betimol 0.25%, 0.5% ... ⊙ 259

Timolol Maleate (Based on animal studies, dobutamine may be ineffective in patients recently on beta blocker; potential for increased peripheral vascular resistance). Products include:
- Blocadren Tablets ... 1654
- Timolide Tablets ... 1791
- Timoptic in Ocudose ... 1796
- Timoptic Sterile Ophthalmic Solution ... 1794
- Timoptic-XE ... 1798

DOLOBID TABLETS

(Diflunisal) ... 1695

May interact with oral anticoagulants, antacids, non-steroidal anti-inflammatory agents, and certain other agents. Compounds in these categories include:

Acetaminophen (Increased plasma levels of acetaminophen). Products include:
- Actifed Cold & Sinus Caplets and Tablets ... ▣ 808
- Actifed Sinus Daytime/Nighttime Tablets and Caplets ... ▣ 809
- Alka-Seltzer Fast Relief Caplets ... ▣ 610
- Alka-Seltzer Plus Liqui-Gels ... ▣ 612
- Alka-Seltzer Plus Flu & Body Aches Effervescent Tablets ... ▣ 612
- Alka-Seltzer Plus Flu & Body Aches Liqui-Gels Non-Drowsy Formula ... ▣ 613
- Alka-Seltzer Plus Night-Time Cold Medicine Liqui-Gels ... ▣ 612
- Allerest No Drowsiness ... ▣ 649
- Allerest Sinus Pain Formula ... ▣ 649
- Axocet Capsules ... 2469
- Benadryl Allergy/Cold Tablets ... ▣ 811
- Benadryl Allergy Sinus Headache Caplets ... ▣ 813
- Children's TYLENOL acetaminophen Chewable Tablets, Elixir, Suspension Liquid, and Suspension Drops ... 1559
- Children's TYLENOL Cold Multi-Symptom Chewable Tablets and Liquid ... 1559
- Children's TYLENOL Cold Plus Cough Multi Symptom Chewable Tablets and Liquid ... 1560
- Children's TYLENOL Flu Suspension Liquid ... 1560
- Allergy-Sinus Comtrex Multi-Symptom Allergy-Sinus Formula Tablets and Caplets ... ▣ 639
- Comtrex Multi-Symptom ... ▣ 638
- Comtrex Non-Drowsy ... ▣ 640
- Contac Day Allergy/Sinus Caplets ▣ 771
- Contac Day & Night ... ▣ 772
- Contac Night Allergy/Sinus Caplets ... ▣ 771
- Contac Severe Cold and Flu Formula Caplets ... ▣ 773
- Contac Severe Cold & Flu Non-Drowsy ... ▣ 774
- Coricidin Cold + Flu Tablets ... ▣ 760
- Coricidin 'D' Decongestant Tablets ... ▣ 760
- DHCplus Capsules ... 2148
- Darvon-N/Darvocet-N ... 1473
- Dimetapp Allergy Sinus Caplets ... ▣ 838
- Dimetapp Cold & Fever Suspension ... ▣ 839
- Drixoral Cold and Flu Extended-Release Tablets ... ▣ 764
- Drixoral Cough + Sore Throat Liquid Caps ... ▣ 763
- Drixoral Allergy/Sinus Extended Release Tablets ... ▣ 765
- Esgic-plus Capsules ... 1012
- Esgic-plus Tablets ... 1012
- Aspirin Free Excedrin Analgesic Caplets and Geltabs ... 734
- Excedrin Extra-Strength Analgesic Tablets, Caplets, and Geltabs ... 734
- Excedrin P.M. Analgesic/Sleeping Aid Tablets, Caplets, Liquigels ... 735
- Fioricet Tablets ... 2386
- Fioricet with Codeine Capsules ... 2387
- Goody's Extra Strength Headache Powders ... ▣ 632
- Goody's Extra Strength Pain Relief Tablets ... ▣ 632
- Hycomine Compound Tablets ... 948
- Hydrocet Capsules ... 787
- Infants' TYLENOL acetaminophen Suspension Drops ... 1559
- Infants' TYLENOL Cold Decongestant & Fever-Reducer Drops ... 1561
- Junior Strength TYLENOL acetaminophen Coated Caplets and Chewable Tablets ... 1562
- Lorcet 10/650 Tablets ... 1016
- Lortab ... 2751
- Lurline PMS Tablets ... 1000

IMPORTANT NOTE: Always consult each drug listing in the patient's regimen for possible interactions.

Dolobid

Entry	Page
Maximum Strength Multi-Symptom Formula Midol	▣ 621
PMS Multi-Symptom Formula Midol	▣ 622
Maximum Strength Midol Teen Multi-Symptom Formula	▣ 621
Midrin Capsules	788
Panodol Tablets and Caplets	▣ 783
Children's Panadol Chewable Tablets, Liquid, Infant's Drops	▣ 783
Percocet Tablets	955
Percogesic Analgesic Tablets	▣ 727
Phrenilin	790
Pyrroxate Caplets	▣ 742
Robitussin Cold, Cough & Flu Liqui-Gels	▣ 844
Robitussin Night-Time Cold Formula	▣ 847
Sedapap Tablets 50 mg/650 mg	1826
Sinarest	663
Sine-Aid Maximum Strength Sinus Headache Gelcaps, Caplets and Tablets	1570
Sine-Off No Drowsiness Formula Caplets	▣ 784
Sine-Off Sinus Medicine	▣ 784
Singlet Tablets	▣ 785
Sinulin Tablets	792
Sinutab Sinus Allergy Medication, Maximum Strength Tablets and Caplets	▣ 823
Sinutab Sinus Medication, Maximum Strength Without Drowsiness Formula, Tablets & Caplets	▣ 824
Sudafed Cold and Cough Liquid Caps	▣ 826
Sudafed Severe Cold Formula Caplets	▣ 828
Sudafed Severe Cold Formula Tablets	▣ 828
Sudafed Sinus Caplets	▣ 829
Sudafed Sinus Tablets	▣ 829
Talacen Caplets	2464
TheraFlu Flu and Cold Medicine	▣ 750
TheraFlu Maximum Strength Flu and Cold Medicine For Sore Throat	▣ 751
TheraFlu Flu, Cold and Cough Medicine	▣ 750
TheraFlu Maximum Strength Nighttime Flu, Cold & Cough Medicine	▣ 751
TheraFlu Maximum Strength Non-Drowsy Formula Flu, Cold & Cough Medicine	▣ 751
TheraFlu Maximum Strength, Non-Drowsy Formula Flu, Cold and Cough Caplets	▣ 752
TheraFlu Maximum Strength Sinus Non-Drowsy Formula Caplets	▣ 752
Triaminic Sore Throat Formula	▣ 755
Triaminicin Tablets	▣ 756
TYLENOL acetaminophen Extended Relief Caplets	1570
TYLENOL acetaminophen, Extra Strength Adult Liquid Pain Reliever	1570
TYLENOL acetaminophen, Extra Strength Gelcaps, Geltabs, Caplets, Tablets	1570
TYLENOL acetaminophen, Regular Strength Caplets and Tablets	1570
TYLENOL Allergy Sinus, Maximum Strength Caplets and Gelcaps	1571
TYLENOL Allergy Sinus NightTime, Maximum Strength Caplets	1571
TYLENOL Cold Medication, Multi-Symptom Formula Tablets and Caplets	1572
TYLENOL Cold Medication, Multi-Symptom Hot Liquid Packets	1572
TYLENOL Cold Medication, No Drowsiness Formula Caplets and Gelcaps	1572
TYLENOL Cold Severe Congestion Caplets	1573
TYLENOL Cough Medication, Multi Symptom	1574
TYLENOL Cough Medication with Decongestant, Multi Symptom	1574
TYLENOL Flu No Drowsiness Formula, Maximum Strength Gelcaps	1575
TYLENOL Flu NightTime, Maximum Strength Gelcaps	1575
TYLENOL Flu NightTime, Maximum Strength Hot Medication Packets	1575
TYLENOL Headache Plus Pain Reliever with Antacid, Extra Strength Caplets	▣ 705
TYLENOL PM Pain Reliever/Sleep Aid, Extra Strength Gelcaps, Caplets, Geltabs	1576
TYLENOL Severe Allergy Medication Caplets	1571
TYLENOL Sinus, Maximum Strength Geltabs, Gelcaps, Caplets and Tablets	1576
Tylenol with Codeine	1592
Tylox Capsules	1593
Unisom With Pain Relief-Nighttime Sleep Aid and Pain Reliever	1991
Vanquish Analgesic Caplets	▣ 627
Vicks 44 LiquiCaps Cough, Cold & Flu Relief	▣ 728
Vicks 44M Cough, Cold & Flu Relief	▣ 729
Vicks DayQuil LiquiCaps/Liquid Multi-Symptom Cold/Flu Relief	▣ 734
Vicks Nyquil Hot Therapy	▣ 735
Vicks NyQuil LiquiCaps/Liquid Multi-Symptom Cold/Flu Relief, Original and Cherry Flavors	▣ 736
Vicodin Tablets	1404
Vicodin ES Tablets	1405
Vicodin HP Tablets	1403
Wygesic Tablets	2930
Zydone Capsules	967

Aluminum Carbonate (Reduced plasma levels of Dolobid). Products include:

Basaljel Capsules	2810
Basaljel Suspension	2810
Basaljel Tablets	2810

Aluminum Hydroxide (Reduced plasma levels of Dolobid). Products include:

ALternaGEL Liquid	1358
Maximum Strength Ascriptin	▣ 650
Cama Arthritis Pain Reliever	▣ 748
Gaviscon Extra Strength Relief Formula Antacid Tablets	▣ 778
Gaviscon Extra Strength Relief Formula Liquid Antacid	▣ 779
Gaviscon Liquid Antacid	▣ 779
Gelusil Antacid-Anti-gas Liquid	▣ 819
Gelusil Antacid-Anti-gas Tablets	▣ 819
Maalox Antacid/Anti-Gas Tablets	889
Maalox Heartburn Relief Suspension	▣ 658
Maalox Antacid Liquid	888
Extra Strength Maalox Antacid/Anti-Gas Liquid and Tablets	888
Mylanta	1359
Tempo Soft Antacid	▣ 799

Aluminum Hydroxide Gel (Reduced plasma levels of Dolobid). Products include:

ALternaGEL Liquid	▣ 675
Aludrox Oral Suspension	▣ 850
Amphojel Suspension	2802
Amphojel Suspension without Flavor	2802
Amphojel Tablets	2802
Ascriptin	▣ 650
Gaviscon Antacid Tablets	▣ 778
Gaviscon-2 Antacid Tablets	▣ 779
Mylanta Liquid	▣ 676
Mylanta Double Strength Liquid	▣ 676
Nephrox Suspension	▣ 671

Aspirin (Small decrease in diflunisal levels). Products include:

Alka-Seltzer Cherry Effervescent Antacid and Pain Reliever	▣ 609
Alka-Seltzer Extra Strength Effervescent Antacid and Pain Reliever	▣ 609
Alka-Seltzer Lemon Lime Effervescent Antacid and Pain Reliever	▣ 609
Alka-Seltzer Original Effervescent Antacid and Pain Reliever	▣ 609
Alka-Seltzer Plus	▣ 611
Alka-Seltzer Plus Sinus Medicine	▣ 611
Ascriptin	▣ 650
Arthritis Strength BC Powder	▣ 631
BC Cold Powder Multi-Symptom Formula (Cold-Sinus-Allergy)	▣ 631
BC Cold Powder Non-Drowsy Formula (Cold-Sinus)	▣ 631
BC Powder	▣ 631
Genuine Bayer Aspirin Tablets & Caplets	▣ 618
Extra Strength Bayer Arthritis Pain Regimen Formula	▣ 615
Extra Strength Bayer Aspirin Caplets & Tablets	▣ 617
Extended-Release Bayer 8-Hour Aspirin	▣ 616
Extra Strength Bayer Plus Aspirin Caplets	▣ 617
Extra Strength Bayer PM Aspirin Plus Sleep Aid	▣ 617
Aspirin Regimen Bayer 81 mg Tablets with Calcium	▣ 615
Aspirin Regimen Bayer Adult Low Strength 81 mg Tablets	▣ 613
Aspirin Regimen Bayer Children's Chewable Aspirin	▣ 616
Aspirin Regimen Bayer Regular Strength 325 mg Caplets	▣ 613
Bufferin Analgesic Tablets	▣ 636
Arthritis Strength Bufferin Analgesic Caplets	▣ 637
Extra Strength Bufferin Analgesic Tablets	▣ 637
Cama Arthritis Pain Reliever	▣ 748
Darvon Compound-65 Pulvules	1475
Easprin	1971
Ecotrin	2625
Ecotrin Enteric Coated Aspirin Maximum Strength Tablets and Caplets	▣ 775
Ecotrin Enteric Coated Aspirin Regular Strength Tablets	2625
Empirin Aspirin Tablets	▣ 818
Excedrin Extra-Strength Analgesic Tablets, Caplets, and Geltabs	734
Fiorinal Capsules	2388
Fiorinal with Codeine Capsules	2390
Fiorinal Tablets	2388
Goody's Extra Strength Headache Powders	▣ 632
Goody's Extra Strength Pain Relief Tablets	▣ 632
Halfprin Tablets	1413
Norgesic	1554
Percodan Tablets	955
Percodan-Demi Tablets	956
Robaxisal Tablets	2246
Soma Compound w/Codeine Tablets	2784
Soma Compound Tablets	2783
St. Joseph Adult Chewable Aspirin (81 mg.)	▣ 768
Talwin Compound	2466
Vanquish Analgesic Caplets	▣ 627

Cyclosporine (Increased cyclosporine-induced toxicity). Products include:

Neoral	2405
Sandimmune	2416

Diclofenac Potassium (Concomitant use with other NSAIDs is not recommended due to the increased possibility of gastrointestinal toxicity, with little or no increase in efficacy). Products include:

Cataflam Tablets	833

Diclofenac Sodium (Concomitant use with other NSAIDs is not recommended due to the increased possibility of gastrointestinal toxicity, with little or no increase in efficacy). Products include:

Voltaren Ophthalmic Sterile Ophthalmic Solution	◉ 264
Cataflam/Voltaren/Voltaren-XR	833

Dicumarol (Prolonged prothrombin time; adjustment of dosage of oral anticoagulants may be required).
No products indexed under this heading.

Etodolac (Concomitant use with other NSAIDs is not recommended due to the increased possibility of gastrointestinal toxicity, with little or no increase in efficacy). Products include:

Lodine Capsules and Tablets	2849

Fenoprofen Calcium (Concomitant use with other NSAIDs is not recommended due to the increased possibility of gastrointestinal toxicity, with little or no increase in efficacy). Products include:

Nalfon 200 Pulvules & Nalfon Tablets	933

Interactions Index

Flurbiprofen (Concomitant use with other NSAIDs is not recommended due to the increased possibility of gastrointestinal toxicity, with little or no increase in efficacy).
No products indexed under this heading.

Furosemide (Decreased hyperuricemic effect). Products include:

Lasix Injection, Oral Solution and Tablets	1267

Hydrochlorothiazide (Decreased hyperuricemic effect; increased plasma levels). Products include:

Aldactazide Tablets	2556
Aldoril Tablets	1644
Apresazide Capsules	824
Capozide Tablets	744
Dyazide Capsules	2653
Esidrix Tablets	839
Esimil Tablets	840
HydroDIURIL Tablets	1716
Hydropres Tablets	1718
Hyzaar Tablets	1720
Inderide Tablets	2838
Inderide LA Long Acting Capsules	2840
Lopressor HCT Tablets	850
Lotensin HCT Tablets	855
Moduretic Tablets	1748
Oretic Tablets	450
Prinzide Tablets	1780
Ser-Ap-Es Tablets	867
Timolide Tablets	1791
Vaseretic Tablets	1810
Zestoretic Tablets	2968
Ziac	1459

Ibuprofen (Concomitant use with other NSAIDs is not recommended due to the increased possibility of gastrointestinal toxicity, with little or no increase in efficacy). Products include:

Advil Cold and Sinus Caplets and Tablets	▣ 837
Advil Ibuprofen Tablets, Caplets and Gel Caplets	▣ 836
Children's Motrin Ibuprofen Oral Suspension	1558
IBU Tablets	1389
Ibuprohm	▣ 713
Motrin IB Caplets, Tablets, and Gelcaps	▣ 802
Motrin Ibuprofen Suspension, Oral Drops, Chewable Tablets, Caplets	1563
Nuprin Ibuprofen/Analgesic Tablets & Caplets	▣ 645
Vicks DayQuil SINUS Pressure & PAIN Relief with IBUPROFEN	▣ 735

Indomethacin (Decreased renal clearance and significantly increased plasma levels of indomethacin; potential for fatal gastrointestinal hemorrhage; concomitant use with indomethacin is not recommended). Products include:

Indocin	1723

Indomethacin Sodium Trihydrate (Decreased renal clearance and significantly increased plasma levels of indomethacin; potential for fatal gastrointestinal hemorrhage; concomitant use with indomethacin is not recommended). Products include:

Indocin I.V.	1727

Ketoprofen (Concomitant use with other NSAIDs is not recommended due to the increased possibility of gastrointestinal toxicity, with little or no increase in efficacy). Products include:

Actron Caplets and Tablets	▣ 608
Orudis Capsules	2874
Orudis KT	▣ 842
Oruvail Capsules	2874

Ketorolac Tromethamine (Concomitant use with other NSAIDs is not recommended due to the increased possibility of gastrointestinal toxicity, with little or no increase in efficacy). Products include:

Acular Sterile Ophthalmic Solution	470

(▣ Described in PDR For Nonprescription Drugs)   (◉ Described in PDR For Ophthalmology)

Toradol 2319
Magaldrate (Reduced plasma levels of Dolobid).
   No products indexed under this heading.
Magnesium Hydroxide (Reduced plasma levels of Dolobid). Products include:
   Aludrox Oral Suspension 850
   Ascriptin 650
   Di-Gel Antacid/Anti-Gas 762
   Gelusil Antacid-Anti-gas Liquid ... 819
   Gelusil Antacid-Anti-gas Tablets ... 819
   Maalox Antacid/Anti-Gas Tablets ... 889
   Maalox Antacid Liquid 888
   Extra Strength Maalox Antacid/ Anti-Gas Liquid and Tablets 888
   Mylanta Fast-Acting 1359
   Mylanta Gelcaps Antacid 678
   Fast-Acting Mylanta Liquid Antacid 1359
   Mylanta Tablets 677
   Maximum-Strength Fast-Acting Mylanta Liquid Antacid 1359
   Mylanta Double Strength Tablets ... 677
   Phillips' Milk of Magnesia Liquid ... 627
   Rolaids Antacid Tablets 807
   Tempo Soft Antacid 799
Magnesium Oxide (Reduced plasma levels of Dolobid). Products include:
   Beelith Tablets 632
   Bufferin Analgesic Tablets 636
   Arthritis Strength Bufferin Analgesic Caplets 637
   Extra Strength Bufferin Analgesic Tablets 637
   Caltrate PLUS 681
   Cama Arthritis Pain Reliever 748
   Mag-Ox 400 666
   Uro-Mag 666
Meclofenamate Sodium (Concomitant use with other NSAIDs is not recommended due to the increased possibility of gastrointestinal toxicity, with little or no increase in efficacy).
   No products indexed under this heading.
Mefenamic Acid (Concomitant use with other NSAIDs is not recommended due to the increased possibility of gastrointestinal toxicity, with little or no increase in efficacy). Products include:
   Ponstel 1982
Methotrexate Sodium (Decreased tubular secretion of methotrexate and potentiation of its toxicity). Products include:
   Methotrexate Sodium Tablets, Injection, for Injection and LPF Injection 1322
Nabumetone (Concomitant use with other NSAIDs is not recommended due to the increased possibility of gastrointestinal toxicity, with little or no increase in efficacy). Products include:
   Relafen Tablets 2688
Naproxen (Significant decrease in urinary excretion of naproxen and its glucuronide metabolite; concomitant use with other NSAIDs is not recommended due to the increased possibility of gastrointestinal toxicity, with little or no increase in efficacy). Products include:
   Anaprox/Naprosyn 2277
Naproxen Sodium (Significant decrease in urinary excretion of naproxen and its glucuronide metabolite; concomitant use with other NSAIDs is not recommended due to the increased possibility of gastrointestinal toxicity, with little or no increase in efficacy). Products include:
   Aleve 2124
   Anaprox/Naprosyn 2277
   Naprelan Tablets 2861

Nephrotoxic Drugs (Overt renal decompensation).
Oxaprozin (Concomitant use with other NSAIDs is not recommended due to the increased possibility of gastrointestinal toxicity, with little or no increase in efficacy). Products include:
   Daypro Caplets 2578
Phenprocoumon (Prolonged prothrombin time).
Phenylbutazone (Concomitant use with other NSAIDs is not recommended due to the increased possibility of gastrointestinal toxicity, with little or no increase in efficacy).
   No products indexed under this heading.
Piroxicam (Concomitant use with other NSAIDs is not recommended due to the increased possibility of gastrointestinal toxicity, with little or no increase in efficacy). Products include:
   Feldene Capsules 2008
Sulindac (Lowering of the plasma levels of active sulindac sulfide metabolite by approximately one-third; concomitant use with other NSAIDs is not recommended due to the increased possibility of gastrointestinal toxicity, with little or no increase in efficacy). Products include:
   Clinoril Tablets 1658
Tolmetin Sodium (Concomitant use with other NSAIDs is not recommended due to the increased possibility of gastrointestinal toxicity, with little or no increase in efficacy). Products include:
   Tolectin (200, 400 and 600 mg) ... 1591
Warfarin Sodium (Prolonged prothrombin time; adjustment of dosage of oral anticoagulants may be required). Products include:
   Coumadin 941

DOLORAC CREAM (Capsaicin) 1041
None cited in PDR database.

DOMEBORO ASTRINGENT SOLUTION EFFERVESCENT TABLETS (Aluminum Acetate, Calcium Acetate) 620
None cited in PDR database.

DOMEBORO ASTRINGENT SOLUTION POWDER PACKETS (Aluminum Acetate, Calcium Acetate) 620
None cited in PDR database.

DONNAGEL LIQUID AND DONNAGEL CHEWABLE TABLETS (Attapulgite) 854
None cited in PDR database.

DONNATAL CAPSULES (Phenobarbital, Belladonna Alkaloids) 2234
May interact with oral anticoagulants. Compounds in this category include:
Dicumarol (Decreased phenobarbital effect).
   No products indexed under this heading.
Warfarin Sodium (Decreased phenobarbital effect). Products include:
   Coumadin 941

DONNATAL ELIXIR (Phenobarbital, Belladonna Alkaloids) 2234
   See **Donnatal Capsules**

DONNATAL EXTENTABS (Phenobarbital, Belladonna Alkaloids) 2234
May interact with oral anticoagulants. Compounds in this category include:
Dicumarol (Decreased phenobarbital effect).
   No products indexed under this heading.
Warfarin Sodium (Decreased phenobarbital effect). Products include:
   Coumadin 941

DONNATAL TABLETS (Phenobarbital, Belladonna Alkaloids) 2234
   See **Donnatal Capsules**

DONNAZYME TABLETS (Pancreatin) 2235
None cited in PDR database.

DOPRAM INJECTABLE (Doxapram Hydrochloride) 2235
May interact with sympathomimetics, monoamine oxidase inhibitors, muscle relaxants, inhalant anesthetics, and certain other agents. Compounds in these categories include:
Albuterol (Additive pressor effect). Products include:
   Proventil Inhalation Aerosol 2524
   Ventolin Inhalation Aerosol and Refill 1170
Albuterol Sulfate (Additive pressor effect). Products include:
   Airet Albuterol Sulfate Inhalation Solution 1602
   Albuterol Sulfate, USP Solution for Inhalation, Arm-a-Med 522
   Proventil Inhalation Solution 0.083% 2527
   Proventil Repetabs Tablets 2529
   Proventil Solution for Inhalation 0.5% 2525
   Proventil Syrup 2528
   Proventil Tablets 2529
   Ventolin Inhalation Solution 1171
   Ventolin Nebules Inhalation Solution 1172
   Ventolin Rotacaps for Inhalation 1173
   Ventolin Syrup 1175
   Ventolin Tablets 1175
   Volmax Extended-Release Tablets .. 1835
Atracurium Besylate (Residual effects masked by Dopram). Products include:
   Tracrium Injection 1155
Baclofen (Residual effects masked by Dopram). Products include:
   Lioresal Intrathecal 1634
   Lioresal Tablets 847
Carisoprodol (Residual effects masked by Dopram). Products include:
   Soma Compound w/Codeine Tablets 2784
   Soma Compound Tablets 2783
   Soma Tablets 2782
Chlorzoxazone (Residual effects masked by Dopram). Products include:
   Parafon Forte DSC Caplets 1590
Cisatracurium Besylate (Residual effects masked by Dopram). Products include:
   Nimbex Injection 1131
Cyclobenzaprine Hydrochloride (Residual effects masked by Dopram). Products include:
   Flexeril Tablets 1701

Dantrolene Sodium (Residual effects masked by Dopram). Products include:
   Dantrium Capsules 2131
   Dantrium Intravenous 2132
Desflurane (Increased epinephrine release). Products include:
   Suprane (desflurane, USP) 1865
Dobutamine Hydrochloride (Additive pressor effect). Products include:
   Dobutrex Solution Vials 1480
Dopamine Hydrochloride (Additive pressor effect).
   No products indexed under this heading.
Doxacurium Chloride (Residual effects masked by Dopram). Products include:
   Nuromax Injection 1136
Enflurane (Increased epinephrine release).
   No products indexed under this heading.
Ephedrine Hydrochloride (Additive pressor effect). Products include:
   Primatene Tablets 844
   Quadrinal Tablets 1398
Ephedrine Sulfate (Additive pressor effect). Products include:
   Marax Tablets & DF Syrup 2015
Ephedrine Tannate (Additive pressor effect). Products include:
   Rynatuss 2782
Epinephrine (Additive pressor effect). Products include:
   EPIFRIN 237
   EpiPen 808
   Marcaine with Epinephrine 2446
   Primatene Mist 843
   Sensorcaine with Epinephrine Injection 554
   Sus-Phrine Injection 1017
   Xylocaine with Epinephrine Injections 562
Epinephrine Bitartrate (Additive pressor effect). Products include:
   Sensorcaine-MPF with Epinephrine Injection 554
Epinephrine Hydrochloride (Additive pressor effect). Products include:
   Ana-Kit Anaphylaxis Emergency Treatment Kit 611
Furazolidone (Additive pressor effect). Products include:
   Furoxone 2221
Halothane (Increased epinephrine release). Products include:
   Fluothane 2830
Isocarboxazid (Additive pressor effect).
   No products indexed under this heading.
Isoflurane (Increased epinephrine release).
   No products indexed under this heading.
Isoproterenol Hydrochloride (Additive pressor effect). Products include:
   Isuprel Hydrochloride Solution ... 2443
   Isuprel Injection 2441
   Isuprel Mistometer 2442
Isoproterenol Sulfate (Additive pressor effect). Products include:
   Norisodrine with Calcium Iodide Syrup 446
Metaproterenol Sulfate (Additive pressor effect). Products include:
   Alupent 672
   Metaproterenol Sulfate Inhalation Solution, USP, Arm-a-Med 547
Metaraminol Bitartrate (Additive pressor effect). Products include:
   Aramine Injection 1649

IMPORTANT NOTE: Always consult each drug listing in the patient's regimen for possible interactions.

Dopram | **Interactions Index** | **330**

Metaxalone (Residual effects masked by Dopram). Products include:
Skelaxin Tablets ... 793

Methocarbamol (Residual effects masked by Dopram). Products include:
Robaxin Injectable ... 2245
Robaxin Tablets ... 2246
Robaxisal Tablets ... 2246

Methoxamine Hydrochloride (Additive pressor effect). Products include:
Vasoxyl Injection ... 1169

Methoxyflurane (Increased epinephrine release).
No products indexed under this heading.

Metocurine Iodide (Residual effects masked by Dopram). Products include:
Metubine Iodide Vials ... 932

Norepinephrine Bitartrate (Additive pressor effect). Products include:
Levophed Bitartrate Injection ... 2445

Orphenadrine Citrate (Residual effects masked by Dopram). Products include:
Norflex ... 1554
Norgesic ... 1554

Pancuronium Bromide (Residual effects masked by Dopram).
No products indexed under this heading.

Phenelzine Sulfate (Additive pressor effect). Products include:
Nardil ... 1977

Phenylephrine Bitartrate (Additive pressor effect).
No products indexed under this heading.

Phenylephrine Hydrochloride (Additive pressor effect). Products include:
Atrohist Plus Tablets ... 1605
Cerose DM ... ◘ 853
D.A. II Tablets ... 972
D.A. Chewable Tablets ... 970
Dura-Vent/DA Tablets ... 972
Extendryl ... 1003
4-Way Fast Acting Nasal Spray (regular & mentholated) ... ◘ 644
Hemorid ... ◘ 797
Hycomine Compound Tablets ... 948
Neo-Synephrine Hydrochloride 1% Carpuject ... 2455
Neo-Synephrine Hydrochloride 1% Injection ... 2455
Neo-Synephrine Hydrochloride (Ophthalmic) ... 2456
Neo-Synephrine ... ◘ 624
Novahistine Elixir ... ◘ 782
Phenergan VC ... 2886
Phenergan VC with Codeine ... 2888
Preparation H ... ◘ 842
Tympagesic Ear Drops ... 2476
Vicks Sinex Nasal Spray and Ultra Fine Mist ... ◘ 738

Phenylephrine Tannate (Additive pressor effect). Products include:
Atrohist Pediatric Suspension ... 1604
Atrohist Pediatric Suspension Dye-Free ... 1604
Rynatan ... 2781
Rynatuss ... 2782

Phenylpropanolamine Hydrochloride (Additive pressor effect). Products include:
Acutrim ... ◘ 648
Atrohist Plus Tablets ... 1605
BC Cold Powder Multi-Symptom Formula (Cold-Sinus-Allergy) ... ◘ 631
BC Cold Powder Non-Drowsy Formula (Cold-Sinus) ... ◘ 631
Cheracol Plus Head Cold/Cough Formula ... ◘ 741
Comtrex Multi-Symptom Cold Reliever Liqui-Gels ... ◘ 638
Comtrex Multi-Symptom Non-Drowsy Liqui-gels ... ◘ 640
Contac Continuous Action Nasal Decongestant/Antihistamine 12 Hour Capsules ... ◘ 773
Contac Maximum Strength Continuous Action Decongestant/Antihistamine 12 Hour Caplets ... ◘ 772
Contac Severe Cold and Flu Formula Caplets ... ◘ 773
Coricidin 'D' Decongestant Tablets ... ◘ 760
Dexatrim ... ◘ 795
Dexatrim Plus Vitamins Caplets ... ◘ 796
Dimetane-DC Cough Syrup ... 2232
Dimetapp Allergy Sinus Caplets ... ◘ 838
Dimetapp Cold & Allergy Chewable Tablets ... ◘ 838
Dimetapp Cold & Cough Liqui-Gels ... ◘ 839
Dimetapp DM Elixir ... ◘ 840
Dimetapp Elixir ... ◘ 840
Dimetapp Extentabs ... ◘ 841
Dimetapp Tablets/Liqui-Gels ... ◘ 841
Dura-Vent Tablets ... 971
Entex LA Tablets ... 972
Exgest LA Tablets ... 787
Hycomine ... 947
Nolamine Timed-Release Tablets ... 790
Ornade Spansule Capsules ... 2678
Propagest Tablets ... 791
Pyrroxate Caplets ... ◘ 742
Robitussin-CF ... ◘ 846
Sinulin Tablets ... 792
Tavist-D 12 Hour Relief Tablets ... ◘ 750
Teldrin 12 Hour Antihistamine/Nasal Decongestant Allergy Relief Capsules ... ◘ 786
Triaminic Expectorant ... ◘ 753
Triaminic Syrup ... ◘ 755
Triaminic Triaminicol Cold & Cough ... ◘ 756
Triaminic DM Syrup ... ◘ 756
Triaminicin Tablets ... ◘ 756
Vicks DayQuil Allergy Relief 12-Hour Extended Release Tablets ... ◘ 733
Vicks DayQuil Allergy Relief 4-Hour Tablets ... ◘ 733
Vicks DayQuil SINUS Pressure & CONGESTION Relief ... ◘ 734

Pirbuterol Acetate (Additive pressor effect). Products include:
Maxair Autohaler ... 1550
Maxair Inhaler ... 1552

Pseudoephedrine Hydrochloride (Additive pressor effect). Products include:
Actifed Allergy Daytime/Nighttime Caplets ... ◘ 808
Actifed Cold & Allergy Tablets ... ◘ 807
Actifed Cold & Sinus Caplets and Tablets ... ◘ 808
Actifed Sinus Daytime/Nighttime Tablets and Caplets ... ◘ 809
Advil Cold and Sinus Caplets and Tablets ... ◘ 837
Alka-Seltzer Plus Liqui-Gels ... ◘ 612
Alka-Seltzer Plus Flu & Body Aches Liqui-Gels Non-Drowsy Formula ... ◘ 613
Alka-Seltzer Plus Night-Time Cold Medicine Liqui-Gels ... ◘ 612
Allerest Maximum Strength ... ◘ 649
Allerest No Drowsiness ... ◘ 649
Allerest Sinus Pain Formula ... ◘ 649
Atrohist Pediatric Capsules ... 1603
Benadryl Allergy/Cold Tablets ... ◘ 811
Benadryl Allergy Decongestant Liquid Medication ... ◘ 812
Benadryl Allergy Decongestant Tablets ... ◘ 812
Benadryl Allergy Sinus Headache Caplets ... ◘ 813
Benylin Multisymptom ... ◘ 816
Bromfed Capsules (Extended-Release) ... 1832
Bromfed Syrup ... ◘ 712
Bromfed Tablets ... 1832
Bromfed-DM Cough Syrup ... 1832
Bromfed-PD Capsules (Extended-Release) ... 1832
Children's TYLENOL Cold Multi-Symptom Chewable Tablets and Liquid ... 1559
Children's TYLENOL Cold Plus Cough Multi Symptom Chewable Tablets and Liquid ... 1560
Children's TYLENOL Flu Suspension Liquid ... 1560
Children's Vicks DayQuil Allergy Relief ... ◘ 730
Children's Vicks NyQuil Cold/Cough Relief ... ◘ 731
Allergy-Sinus Comtrex Multi-Symptom Allergy-Sinus Formula Tablets and Caplets ... ◘ 639
Comtrex Multi-Symptom ... ◘ 638
Comtrex Multi-Symptom Non-Drowsy Caplets ... ◘ 640
Congess ... 1003
Contac Day Allergy/Sinus Caplets ◘ 771
Contac Day & Night ... ◘ 772
Contac Night Allergy/Sinus Caplets ... ◘ 771
Contac Severe Cold & Flu Non-Drowsy ... ◘ 774
Deconsal II Tablets ... 1605
Dimetane-DX Cough Syrup ... 2233
Dimetapp Cold & Fever Suspension ... ◘ 839
Dimetapp Decongestant Pediatric Drops ... ◘ 840
Dorcol Children's Cough Syrup ... ◘ 748
Drixoral Cough + Congestion Liquid Caps ... ◘ 763
Dura-Tap/PD Capsules ... 970
Duratuss Tablets ... 2750
Duratuss HD Elixir ... 2750
Efidac/24 ... ◘ 655
Entex PSE Tablets ... 973
Fedahist Gyrocaps ... 2545
Guaifed ... 1833
Guaifed Syrup ... ◘ 712
Guaimax-D Tablets ... 809
Histussin D Liquid ... 670
Infants' TYLENOL Cold Decongestant & Fever-Reducer Drops ... 1561
Kronofed-A ... 994
Novahistine DMX ... ◘ 782
Nucofed ... 2225
PediaCare Cough-Cold Chewable Tablets and Liquid ... 1569
PediaCare Infants' Decongestant Drops ... 1569
PediaCare Infants' Drops Decongestant Plus Cough ... 1569
PediaCare NightRest Cough-Cold Liquid ... 1569
Pediatric Vicks 44d Cough & Head Congestion Relief ... ◘ 736
Pediatric Vicks 44m Cough & Cold Relief ... ◘ 737
Robitussin Cold & Cough Liqui-Gels ... ◘ 844
Robitussin Cold, Cough & Flu Liqui-Gels ... ◘ 844
Robitussin Maximum Strength Cough & Cold ... ◘ 847
Robitussin Night-Time Cold Formula ... ◘ 847
Robitussin Pediatric Cough & Cold Formula ... ◘ 848
Robitussin Pediatric Drops ... ◘ 849
Robitussin Severe Congestion Liqui-Gels ... ◘ 845
Robitussin-DAC Syrup ... 2249
Robitussin-PE ... ◘ 846
Rondec Oral Drops ... 974
Rondec Syrup ... 974
Rondec Tablet ... 974
Rondec Chewable Tablets ... 974
Rondec-TR Tablet ... 974
Ryna ... ◘ 804
Seldane-D Extended-Release Tablets ... 1286
Semprex-D Capsules ... 1620
Sinarest ... ◘ 663
Sine-Aid Maximum Strength Sinus Headache Gelcaps, Caplets and Tablets ... 1570
Sine-Off No Drowsiness Formula Caplets ... ◘ 784
Sine-Off Sinus Medicine ... ◘ 784
Singlet Tablets ... ◘ 785
Sinutab Non-Drying Liquid Caps ... ◘ 823
Sinutab Sinus Allergy Medication, Maximum Strength Tablets and Caplets ... ◘ 823
Sinutab Sinus Medication, Maximum Strength Without Drowsiness Formula, Tablets & Caplets ... ◘ 824
Sudafed Children's Cold & Cough Liquid Medication ... ◘ 825
Sudafed Children's Nasal Decongestant Liquid Medication ... ◘ 826
Sudafed Cold & Allergy Tablets ... ◘ 826
Sudafed Cold and Cough Liquid Caps ... ◘ 826
Sudafed Nasal Decongestant Tablets, 30 mg ... ◘ 825
Sudafed Nasal Decongestant Tablets, 60 mg ... ◘ 825
Sudafed Non-Drying Sinus Liquid Caps ... ◘ 827
Sudafed Pediatric Nasal Decongestant Liquid Oral Drops ... ◘ 827
Sudafed Severe Cold Formula Caplets ... ◘ 828
Sudafed Severe Cold Formula Tablets ... ◘ 828
Sudafed Sinus Caplets ... ◘ 829
Sudafed Sinus Tablets ... ◘ 829
Sudafed 12 Hour Caplets ... ◘ 824
Syn-Rx Tablets ... 1622
Syn-Rx DM Tablets ... 1623
TheraFlu Flu and Cold Medicine ... ◘ 750
Theraflu Maximum Strength Flu and Cold Medicine For Sore Throat ... ◘ 751
TheraFlu Flu, Cold and Cough Medicine ... ◘ 750
TheraFlu Maximum Strength Nighttime Flu, Cold & Cough Medicine ... ◘ 751
TheraFlu Maximum Strength Non-Drowsy Formula Flu, Cold & Cough Medicine ... ◘ 751
TheraFlu Maximum Strength, Non-Drowsy Formula Flu, Cold and Cough Caplets ... ◘ 752
Theraflu Maximum Strength Sinus Non-Drowsy Formula Caplets ... ◘ 752
Triaminic AM Cough and Decongestant Formula ... ◘ 753
Triaminic AM Decongestant Formula ... ◘ 753
Triaminic Infant Oral Decongestant Drops ... ◘ 754
Triaminic Night Time ... ◘ 754
Triaminic Sore Throat Formula ... ◘ 755
Tussend ... 1830
Tussend Expectorant ... 1831
TYLENOL Allergy Sinus, Maximum Strength Caplets and Gelcaps ... 1571
TYLENOL Allergy Sinus NightTime, Maximum Strength Caplets ... 1571
TYLENOL Cold Medication, Multi-Symptom Formula Tablets and Caplets ... 1572
TYLENOL Cold Medication, Multi-Symptom Hot Liquid Packets ... 1572
TYLENOL Cold Medication, No Drowsiness Formula Caplets and Gelcaps ... 1572
TYLENOL Cold Severe Congestion Caplets ... 1573
TYLENOL Cough Medication with Decongestant, Multi Symptom ... 1574
TYLENOL Flu No Drowsiness Formula, Maximum Strength Gelcaps ... 1575
TYLENOL Flu NightTime, Maximum Strength Gelcaps ... 1575
TYLENOL Flu NightTime, Maximum Strength Hot Medication Packets ... 1575
TYLENOL Sinus, Maximum Strength Geltabs, Gelcaps, Caplets and Tablets ... 1576
Vicks 44 LiquiCaps Cough, Cold & Flu Relief ... ◘ 728
Vicks 44 LiquiCaps Non-Drowsy Cough & Cold Relief ... ◘ 729
Vicks 44D Cough & Head Congestion Relief ... ◘ 728
Vicks 44M Cough, Cold & Flu Relief ... ◘ 729
Vicks DayQuil LiquiCaps/Liquid Multi-Symptom Cold/Flu Relief ... ◘ 734
Vicks DayQuil SINUS Pressure & PAIN Relief with IBUPROFEN ... ◘ 735
Vicks Nyquil Hot Therapy ... ◘ 735
Vicks NyQuil LiquiCaps/Liquid Multi-Symptom Cold/Flu Relief, Original and Cherry Flavors ... ◘ 736

Pseudoephedrine Sulfate (Additive pressor effect). Products include:
Chlor-Trimeton Allergy Decongestant Tablets ... ◘ 759
Claritin-D Tablets ... 2487
Drixoral Cold and Allergy Sustained-Action Tablets ... ◘ 763
Drixoral Cold and Flu Extended-Release Tablets ... ◘ 764
Drixoral Non-Drowsy Formula Extended-Release Tablets ... ◘ 764
Drixoral Allergy/Sinus Extended Release Tablets ... ◘ 765
Trinalin Repetabs Tablets ... 1373

(◘ Described in PDR For Nonprescription Drugs) (◉ Described in PDR For Ophthalmology)

Rocuronium Bromide (Residual effects masked by Dopram). Products include:
  Zemuron Injection 1885
Salmeterol Xinafoate (Additive pressor effect). Products include:
  Serevent Inhalation Aerosol............ 1149
Selegiline Hydrochloride (Additive pressor effect). Products include:
  Eldepryl Capsules 2729
Succinylcholine Chloride (Residual effects masked by Dopram). Products include:
  Anectine 1062
Terbutaline Sulfate (Additive pressor effect). Products include:
  Brethaire Inhaler 830
  Brethine Ampuls 832
  Brethine Tablets 831
  Bricanyl Subcutaneous Injection 1247
  Bricanyl Tablets 1248
Tranylcypromine Sulfate (Additive pressor effect). Products include:
  Parnate Tablets 2679
Vecuronium Bromide (Residual effects masked by Dopram). Products include:
  Norcuron for Injection 1875

DORAL TABLETS
(Quazepam) 2773
May interact with central nervous system depressants, anticonvulsants, psychotropics, antihistamines, and certain other agents. Compounds in these categories include:

Acrivastine (Additive CNS depressant effects). Products include:
  Semprex-D Capsules 1620
Alfentanil Hydrochloride (Additive CNS depressant effects). Products include:
  Alfenta Injection 1334
Alprazolam (Additive CNS depressant effects). Products include:
  Xanax Tablets 2115
Amitriptyline Hydrochloride (Additive CNS depressant effects). Products include:
  Elavil 2945
  Etrafon 2495
  Limbitrol 2333
  Triavil Tablets 1800
Amoxapine (Additive CNS depressant effects). Products include:
  Asendin Tablets 1419
Aprobarbital (Additive CNS depressant effects).
  No products indexed under this heading.
Astemizole (Additive CNS depressant effects). Products include:
  Hismanal Tablets 1341
Azatadine Maleate (Additive CNS depressant effects). Products include:
  Trinalin Repetabs Tablets 1373
Bromodiphenhydramine Hydrochloride (Additive CNS depressant effects).
  No products indexed under this heading.
Brompheniramine Maleate (Additive CNS depressant effects). Products include:
  Alka-Seltzer Plus Sinus Medicine .. ◨611
  Bromfed Capsules (Extended-Release) 1832
  Bromfed Syrup .... ◨712
  Bromfed Tablets 1832
  Bromfed-DM Cough Syrup 1832
  Bromfed-PD Capsules (Extended-Release) 1832
  Dimetane-DC Cough Syrup 2232
  Dimetane-DX Cough Syrup 2233
  Dimetapp Allergy Dye-Free Elixir.... ◨838
  Dimetapp Allergy Sinus Caplets 838

Dimetapp Cold & Allergy Chewable Tablets .... ◨838
Dimetapp Cold & Cough Liqui-Gels .... ◨839
Dimetapp Cold & Fever Suspension .... ◨839
Dimetapp DM Elixir .... ◨840
Dimetapp Elixir .... ◨840
Dimetapp Extentabs .... ◨841
Dimetapp Tablets/Liqui-Gels .... ◨841
Rondec Chewable Tablets 974
Vicks DayQuil Allergy Relief 12-Hour Extended Release Tablets.. ◨733
Vicks DayQuil Allergy Relief 4-Hour Tablets .... ◨733
Buprenorphine (Additive CNS depressant effects). Products include:
  Buprenex Injectable 2170
Buspirone Hydrochloride (Additive CNS depressant effects). Products include:
  BuSpar Tablets 738
Butabarbital (Additive CNS depressant effects).
  No products indexed under this heading.
Butalbital (Additive CNS depressant effects). Products include:
  Axocet Capsules 2469
  Esgic-plus Capsules 1012
  Esgic-plus Tablets 1012
  Fioricet Tablets 2386
  Fioricet with Codeine Capsules 2387
  Fiorinal Capsules 2388
  Fiorinal with Codeine Capsules 2390
  Fiorinal Tablets 2388
  Phrenilin 790
  Sedapap Tablets 50 mg/650 mg .. 1826
Carbamazepine (Additive CNS depressant effects). Products include:
  Atretol Tablets 569
  Tegretol/Tegretol-XR 870
Cetirizine Hydrochloride (Additive CNS depressant effects). Products include:
  Zyrtec Tablets 2053
Chlordiazepoxide (Additive CNS depressant effects). Products include:
  Limbitrol 2333
Chlordiazepoxide Hydrochloride (Additive CNS depressant effects). Products include:
  Librax Capsules 2330
  Librium Capsules 2331
  Librium Injectable 2332
Chlorpheniramine Maleate (Additive CNS depressant effects). Products include:
  Alka-Seltzer Plus Cold Medicine .... ◨611
  Alka-Seltzer Plus Cold Medicine Liqui-Gels .... ◨612
  Alka-Seltzer Plus Cold & Cough Medicine .... ◨611
  Alka-Seltzer Plus Cold & Cough Medicine Liqui-Gels .... ◨612
  Alka-Seltzer Plus Flu & Body Aches Effervescent Tablets......... ◨612
  Allerest Maximum Strength............. ◨649
  Allerest Sinus Pain Formula .... ◨649
  Ana-Kit Anaphylaxis Emergency Treatment Kit 611
  Atrohist Pediatric Capsules.............. 1603
  Atrohist Plus Tablets 1605
  BC Cold Powder Multi-Symptom Formula (Cold-Sinus-Allergy) .... ◨631
  Cerose DM .... ◨853
  Cheracol Plus Head Cold/Cough Formula .... ◨741
  Children's TYLENOL Cold Multi-Symptom Chewable Tablets and Liquid 1559
  Children's TYLENOL Cold Plus Cough Multi Symptom Chewable Tablets and Liquid 1560
  Children's TYLENOL Flu Suspension Liquid 1560
  Children's Vicks DayQuil Allergy Relief .... ◨730
  Children's Vicks NyQuil Cold/Cough Relief .... ◨731
  Chlor-Trimeton Allergy Decongestant Tablets .... ◨759

Chlor-Trimeton Allergy Tablets ...... ◨758
Allergy-Sinus Comtrex Multi-Symptom Allergy-Sinus Formula Tablets and Caplets .... ◨639
Comtrex Multi-Symptom.................. ◨638
Contac Continuous Action Nasal Decongestant/Antihistamine 12 Hour Capsules .... ◨773
Contac Maximum Strength Continuous Action Decongestant/Antihistamine 12 Hour Caplets.. ◨772
Contac Severe Cold and Flu Formula Caplets .... ◨773
Coricidin Cold + Flu Tablets............ ◨760
Coricidin Cough + Cold Tablets ...... ◨760
Coricidin 'D' Decongestant Tablets .... ◨760
D.A. II Tablets 972
D.A. Chewable Tablets 970
Dura-Tap/PD Capsules 970
Dura-Vent/DA Tablets 972
Efidac 24 Chlorpheniramine........... ◨655
Extendryl 1003
Fedahist Gyrocaps 2545
Hycomine Compound Tablets 948
Kronofed-A 994
Nolamine Timed-Release Tablets 790
Novahistine Elixir .... ◨782
Ornade Spansule Capsules 2678
PediaCare Cough-Cold Chewable Tablets and Liquid 1569
PediaCare NightRest Cough-Cold Liquid 1569
Pediatric Vicks 44m Cough & Cold Relief .... ◨737
Pyrroxate Caplets .... ◨742
Ryna .... ◨804
Sinarest .... ◨663
Sine-Off Sinus Medicine .... ◨784
Singlet Tablets .... ◨785
Sinulin Tablets 792
Sinutab Sinus Allergy Medication, Maximum Strength Tablets and Caplets .... ◨823
Sudafed Cold & Allergy Tablets...... ◨826
Teldrin 12 Hour Antihistamine/Nasal Decongestant Allergy Relief Capsules .... ◨786
TheraFlu Flu and Cold Medicine .... ◨750
Theraflu Maximum Strength Flu and Cold Medicine For Sore Throat .... ◨751
TheraFlu Flu, Cold and Cough Medicine .... ◨750
TheraFlu Maximum Strength Nighttime Flu, Cold & Cough Medicine .... ◨751
Triaminic Night Time .... ◨754
Triaminic Syrup .... ◨755
Triaminic Triaminicol Cold & Cough .... ◨756
Triaminicin Tablets .... ◨756
Tussend 1830
TYLENOL Allergy Sinus, Maximum Strength Caplets and Gelcaps 1571
TYLENOL Cold Medication, Multi-Symptom Formula Tablets and Caplets 1572
TYLENOL Cold Medication, Multi-Symptom Hot Liquid Packets 1572
Vicks 44 LiquiCaps Cough, Cold & Flu Relief .... ◨728
Vicks 44M Cough, Cold & Flu Relief .... ◨729
Chlorpheniramine Polistirex (Additive CNS depressant effects). Products include:
  Tussionex Pennkinetic Extended-Release Suspension 1624
Chlorpheniramine Tannate (Additive CNS depressant effects). Products include:
  Atrohist Pediatric Suspension 1604
  Atrohist Pediatric Suspension Dye-Free 1604
  Rynatan 2781
  Rynatuss 2782
Chlorpromazine (Additive CNS depressant effects). Products include:
  Thorazine Suppositories 2701
Chlorprothixene (Additive CNS depressant effects).
  No products indexed under this heading.
Chlorprothixene Hydrochloride (Additive CNS depressant effects).
  No products indexed under this heading.

Chlorprothixene Lactate (Additive CNS depressant effects).
  No products indexed under this heading.
Clemastine Fumarate (Additive CNS depressant effects). Products include:
  Tavist Syrup 2426
  Tavist Tablets 2427
  Tavist-1 12 Hour Relief Tablets ..... ◨749
  Tavist-D 12 Hour Relief Tablets .... ◨750
Clonazepam (Additive CNS depressant effects). Products include:
  Klonopin Tablets 2294
Clorazepate Dipotassium (Additive CNS depressant effects). Products include:
  Tranxene 459
Clozapine (Additive CNS depressant effects). Products include:
  Clozaril Tablets 2377
Codeine Phosphate (Additive CNS depressant effects). Products include:
  Brontex 2130
  Dimetane-DC Cough Syrup 2232
  Fioricet with Codeine Capsules 2387
  Fiorinal with Codeine Capsules 2390
  Nucofed 2225
  Phenergan with Codeine 2883
  Phenergan VC with Codeine 2888
  Robitussin A-C Syrup 2248
  Robitussin-DAC Syrup 2249
  Ryna .... ◨804
  Soma Compound w/Codeine Tablets 2784
  Tylenol with Codeine 1592
Cyproheptadine Hydrochloride (Additive CNS depressant effects). Products include:
  Periactin 1767
Desflurane (Additive CNS depressant effects). Products include:
  Suprane (desflurane, USP) 1865
Desipramine Hydrochloride (Additive CNS depressant effects). Products include:
  Norpramin Tablets 1273
Dexchlorpheniramine Maleate (Additive CNS depressant effects).
  No products indexed under this heading.
Dezocine (Additive CNS depressant effects). Products include:
  Dalgan Injection 529
Diazepam (Additive CNS depressant effects). Products include:
  Dizac (diazepam injectable emulsion) CIV 1862
  Valium Injectable 2336
  Valium Tablets 2335
Diphenhydramine Citrate (Additive CNS depressant effects). Products include:
  Excedrin P.M. Analgesic/Sleeping Aid Tablets, Caplets, Liquigels 735
Diphenhydramine Hydrochloride (Additive CNS depressant effects). Products include:
  Actifed Allergy Daytime/Nighttime Caplets .... ◨808
  Actifed Sinus Daytime/Nighttime Tablets and Caplets .... ◨809
  Extra Strength Bayer PM Aspirin Plus Sleep Aid .... ◨617
  Benadryl Allergy Chewables .... ◨811
  Benadryl Allergy/Cold Tablets .... ◨811
  Benadryl Allergy Decongestant Liquid Medication .... ◨812
  Benadryl Allergy Decongestant Tablets .... ◨812
  Benadryl Allergy Liquid Medication .... ◨813
  Benadryl Allergy .... ◨811
  Benadryl Allergy Sinus Headache Caplets .... ◨813
  Benadryl Dye-Free Allergy Liquigel Softgels .... ◨813
  Benadryl Dye-Free Allergy Liquid Medication .... ◨814
  Benadryl Itch Relief Stick Extra Strength .... ◨814
  Benadryl Cream .... ◨814

IMPORTANT NOTE: Always consult each drug listing in the patient's regimen for possible interactions.

Doral **Interactions Index** 332

Benadryl Gel ▣ 815
Benadryl Spray ▣ 815
Benadryl Injection 1955
Contac Day & Night Cold/Flu Night Caplets ▣ 772
Contac Night Allergy/Sinus Caplets ▣ 771
Extra Strength Doan's P.M. ▣ 653
Excedrin P.M. Analgesic/Sleeping Aid Tablets, Caplets, Liquigels ▣ 643
Nytol QuickCaps Caplets ▣ 632
Sleepinal Night-time Sleep Aid Capsules and Softgels ▣ 798
TYLENOL Allergy Sinus NightTime, Maximum Strength Caplets 1571
TYLENOL Flu NightTime, Maximum Strength Gelcaps 1575
TYLENOL Flu NightTime, Maximum Strength Hot Medication Packets 1575
TYLENOL PM Pain Reliever/Sleep Aid, Extra Strength Gelcaps, Caplets, Geltabs 1576
TYLENOL Severe Allergy Medication Caplets 1571
Maximum Strength Unisom Sleepgels 1990
Unisom With Pain Relief-Nighttime Sleep Aid and Pain Reliever 1991

Diphenylpyraline Hydrochloride (Additive CNS depressant effects).
No products indexed under this heading.

Divalproex Sodium (Additive CNS depressant effects). Products include:
Depakote Tablets 418

Doxepin Hydrochloride (Additive CNS depressant effects). Products include:
Adapin Capsules 1542
Sinequan 2028
Zonalon Cream 1042

Droperidol (Additive CNS depressant effects). Products include:
Inapsine Injection 462

Enflurane (Additive CNS depressant effects).
No products indexed under this heading.

Estazolam (Additive CNS depressant effects). Products include:
ProSom Tablets 457

Ethchlorvynol (Additive CNS depressant effects). Products include:
Placidyl Capsules 456

Ethinamate (Additive CNS depressant effects).
No products indexed under this heading.

Ethosuximide (Additive CNS depressant effects). Products include:
Zarontin Capsules 1986
Zarontin Syrup 1986

Ethotoin (Additive CNS depressant effects). Products include:
Peganone Tablets 455

Felbamate (Additive CNS depressant effects). Products include:
Felbatol 2774

Fentanyl (Additive CNS depressant effects). Products include:
Duragesic Transdermal System 1336

Fentanyl Citrate (Additive CNS depressant effects). Products include:
Sublimaze Injection 463

Fluphenazine Decanoate (Additive CNS depressant effects). Products include:
Prolixin Decanoate 510

Fluphenazine Enanthate (Additive CNS depressant effects). Products include:
Prolixin Enanthate 510

Fluphenazine Hydrochloride (Additive CNS depressant effects). Products include:
Prolixin 510

Flurazepam Hydrochloride (Additive CNS depressant effects). Products include:
Dalmane Capsules 2329

Fosphenytoin Sodium (Additive CNS depressant effects). Products include:
Cerebyx Injection 1956

Glutethimide (Additive CNS depressant effects).
No products indexed under this heading.

Haloperidol (Additive CNS depressant effects). Products include:
Haldol Injection, Tablets and Concentrate 1585

Haloperidol Decanoate (Additive CNS depressant effects). Products include:
Haldol Decanoate 1587

Hydrocodone Bitartrate (Additive CNS depressant effects). Products include:
Codiclear DH Syrup 808
Duratuss HD Elixir 2750
Histussin D Liquid 670
Hycodan Tablets and Syrup 946
Hycomine Compound Tablets 948
Hycomine 947
Hycotuss Expectorant Syrup 950
Hydrocet Capsules 787
Lorcet 10/650 Tablets 1016
Lortab 2751
Tussend 1830
Tussend Expectorant 1831
Vicodin Tablets 1404
Vicodin ES Tablets 1405
Vicodin HP Tablets 1403
Vicodin Tuss Expectorant 1406
Zydone Capsules 967

Hydrocodone Polistirex (Additive CNS depressant effects). Products include:
Tussionex Pennkinetic Extended-Release Suspension 1624

Hydromorphone Hydrochloride (Additive CNS depressant effects). Products include:
Dilaudid Ampules 1382
Dilaudid Cough Syrup 1383
Dilaudid-HP Injection 1384
Dilaudid-HP Lyophilized Powder 250 mg 1384
Dilaudid 1382
Dilaudid Oral Liquid 1386
Dilaudid 1382
Dilaudid Tablets - 8 mg 1386

Hydroxyzine Hydrochloride (Additive CNS depressant effects). Products include:
Atarax Tablets & Syrup 1992
Marax Tablets & DF Syrup 2015
Vistaril Intramuscular Solution 2042

Imipramine Hydrochloride (Additive CNS depressant effects). Products include:
Tofranil Ampuls 873
Tofranil Tablets 875

Imipramine Pamoate (Additive CNS depressant effects). Products include:
Tofranil-PM Capsules 876

Isocarboxazid (Additive CNS depressant effects).
No products indexed under this heading.

Isoflurane (Additive CNS depressant effects).
No products indexed under this heading.

Ketamine Hydrochloride (Additive CNS depressant effects).
No products indexed under this heading.

Lamotrigine (Additive CNS depressant effects). Products include:
Lamictal Tablets 1105

Levomethadyl Acetate Hydrochloride (Additive CNS depressant effects). Products include:
Orlaam Oral Solution 2361

Levorphanol Tartrate (Additive CNS depressant effects). Products include:
Levo-Dromoran 2297

Lithium Carbonate (Additive CNS depressant effects). Products include:
Eskalith 2658
Lithium Carbonate Capsules & Tablets 2352
Lithonate/Lithotabs/Lithobid 2721

Lithium Citrate (Additive CNS depressant effects).
No products indexed under this heading.

Loratadine (Additive CNS depressant effects). Products include:
Claritin Tablets 2485
Claritin-D Tablets 2487

Lorazepam (Additive CNS depressant effects). Products include:
Ativan Injection 2805
Ativan Tablets 2807

Loxapine Hydrochloride (Additive CNS depressant effects). Products include:
Loxitane 1426

Loxapine Succinate (Additive CNS depressant effects). Products include:
Loxitane Capsules 1426

Maprotiline Hydrochloride (Additive CNS depressant effects). Products include:
Ludiomil Tablets 861

Meperidine Hydrochloride (Additive CNS depressant effects). Products include:
Demerol 2438
Mepergan Injection 2859

Mephenytoin (Additive CNS depressant effects). Products include:
Mesantoin Tablets 2400

Mephobarbital (Additive CNS depressant effects). Products include:
Mebaral Tablets 2452

Meprobamate (Additive CNS depressant effects). Products include:
Miltown Tablets 2780
PMB 200 and PMB 400 2890

Mesoridazine Besylate (Additive CNS depressant effects). Products include:
Serentil 689

Methadone Hydrochloride (Additive CNS depressant effects). Products include:
Methadone Hydrochloride Oral Concentrate 2356
Methadone Hydrochloride Oral Solution & Tablets 2357

Methdilazine Hydrochloride (Additive CNS depressant effects).
No products indexed under this heading.

Methohexital Sodium (Additive CNS depressant effects).
No products indexed under this heading.

Methotrimeprazine (Additive CNS depressant effects). Products include:
Levoprome 1321

Methoxyflurane (Additive CNS depressant effects).
No products indexed under this heading.

Methsuximide (Additive CNS depressant effects). Products include:
Celontin Kapseals 1955

Midazolam Hydrochloride (Additive CNS depressant effects). Products include:
Versed Injection 2324

Mirtazapine (Additive CNS depressant effects). Products include:
Remeron Tablets 1878

Molindone Hydrochloride (Additive CNS depressant effects). Products include:
Moban Tablets and Concentrate 1036

Morphine Sulfate (Additive CNS depressant effects). Products include:
Astramorph/PF Injection, USP (Preservative-Free) 526
Duramorph Injection 983
Infumorph 200 and Infumorph 500 Sterile Solutions 985
Kadian Capsules 2948
MS Contin Tablets 2149
MSIR 2152
Oramorph SR (Morphine Sulfate Sustained Release Tablets) 2359
RMS Suppositories CII 2766
Roxanol 2365

Nortriptyline Hydrochloride (Additive CNS depressant effects). Products include:
Pamelor 2409

Opium Alkaloids (Additive CNS depressant effects).
No products indexed under this heading.

Oxazepam (Additive CNS depressant effects). Products include:
Serax Capsules 2916
Serax Tablets 2916

Oxycodone Hydrochloride (Additive CNS depressant effects). Products include:
OxyContin Tablets 2163
OxyIR Capsules 2167
Percocet Tablets 955
Percodan Tablets 955
Percodan-Demi Tablets 956
Roxicodone Tablets, Oral Solution & Intensol (Oxycodone) 2366
Tylox Capsules 1593

Paramethadione (Additive CNS depressant effects).
No products indexed under this heading.

Pentobarbital Sodium (Additive CNS depressant effects). Products include:
Nembutal Sodium Capsules 440
Nembutal Sodium Solution 442
Nembutal Sodium Suppositories 444

Perphenazine (Additive CNS depressant effects). Products include:
Etrafon 2495
Triavil Tablets 1800
Trilafon 2532

Phenacemide (Additive CNS depressant effects). Products include:
Phenurone Tablets 455

Phenelzine Sulfate (Additive CNS depressant effects). Products include:
Nardil 1977

Phenobarbital (Additive CNS depressant effects). Products include:
Arco-Lase Plus Tablets 513
Bellergal-S Tablets 2375
Donnatal 2234
Donnatal Extentabs 2234
Donnatal Tablets 2234
Phenobarbital Elixir and Tablets 1523
Quadrinal Tablets 1398

Phensuximide (Additive CNS depressant effects).
No products indexed under this heading.

Phenytoin (Additive CNS depressant effects). Products include:
Dilantin Infatabs 1967
Dilantin-125 Suspension 1969

Phenytoin Sodium (Additive CNS depressant effects). Products include:
Dilantin Kapseals 1965

Prazepam (Additive CNS depressant effects).
No products indexed under this heading.

(▣ Described in PDR For Nonprescription Drugs) (◉ Described in PDR For Ophthalmology)

Primidone (Additive CNS depressant effects). Products include:
Mysoline 2860

Prochlorperazine (Additive CNS depressant effects). Products include:
Compazine 2644

Promethazine Hydrochloride (Additive CNS depressant effects). Products include:
Mepergan Injection 2859
Phenergan with Codeine 2883
Phenergan with Dextromethorphan 2885
Phenergan Injection 2880
Phenergan Suppositories 2882
Phenergan Syrup 2881
Phenergan Tablets 2882
Phenergan VC 2886
Phenergan VC with Codeine 2888

Propofol (Additive CNS depressant effects). Products include:
Diprivan Injectable Emulsion 2939

Propoxyphene Hydrochloride (Additive CNS depressant effects). Products include:
Darvon 1475
Wygesic Tablets 2930

Propoxyphene Napsylate (Additive CNS depressant effects). Products include:
Darvon-N/Darvocet-N 1473

Protriptyline Hydrochloride (Additive CNS depressant effects). Products include:
Vivactil Tablets 1820

Pyrilamine Maleate (Additive CNS depressant effects). Products include:
4-Way Fast Acting Nasal Spray (regular & mentholated) 644
Maximum Strength Multi-Symptom Formula Midol 621
PMS Multi-Symptom Formula Midol 622

Pyrilamine Tannate (Additive CNS depressant effects). Products include:
Atrohist Pediatric Suspension 1604
Atrohist Pediatric Suspension Dye-Free 1604
Rynatan 2781

Risperidone (Additive CNS depressant effects). Products include:
Risperdal Tablets 1348

Secobarbital Sodium (Additive CNS depressant effects). Products include:
Seconal Sodium Pulvules 1529

Sevoflurane (Additive CNS depressant effects).
No products indexed under this heading.

Sufentanil Citrate (Additive CNS depressant effects). Products include:
Sufenta Injection 1355

Temazepam (Additive CNS depressant effects). Products include:
Restoril Capsules 2413

Terfenadine (Additive CNS depressant effects). Products include:
Seldane Tablets 1284
Seldane-D Extended-Release Tablets 1286

Thiamylal Sodium (Additive CNS depressant effects).
No products indexed under this heading.

Thioridazine Hydrochloride (Additive CNS depressant effects). Products include:
Mellaril 2398

Thiothixene (Additive CNS depressant effects). Products include:
Navane Capsules and Concentrate 2018
Navane Intramuscular 2019

Tranylcypromine Sulfate (Additive CNS depressant effects). Products include:
Parnate Tablets 2679

Triazolam (Additive CNS depressant effects). Products include:
Halcion Tablets 2093

Trifluoperazine Hydrochloride (Additive CNS depressant effects). Products include:
Stelazine 2692

Trimeprazine Tartrate (Additive CNS depressant effects).
No products indexed under this heading.

Trimethadione (Additive CNS depressant effects).
No products indexed under this heading.

Trimipramine Maleate (Additive CNS depressant effects). Products include:
Surmontil Capsules 2917

Tripelennamine Hydrochloride (Additive CNS depressant effects). Products include:
PBZ Tablets 863
PBZ-SR Tablets 862

Triprolidine Hydrochloride (Additive CNS depressant effects). Products include:
Actifed Cold & Allergy Tablets 807
Actifed Cold & Sinus Caplets and Tablets 808

Valproic Acid (Additive CNS depressant effects). Products include:
Depakene 416

Zolpidem Tartrate (Additive CNS depressant effects). Products include:
Ambien Tablets 2559

Food Interactions

Alcohol (Additive CNS depressant effects).

DORCOL CHILDREN'S COUGH SYRUP

(Pseudoephedrine Hydrochloride, Guaifenesin, Dextromethorphan Hydrobromide) 748
May interact with monoamine oxidase inhibitors. Compounds in this category include:

Furazolidone (Concurrent and/or sequential use is not recommended). Products include:
Furoxone 2221

Isocarboxazid (Concurrent and/or sequential use is not recommended).
No products indexed under this heading.

Phenelzine Sulfate (Concurrent and/or sequential use is not recommended). Products include:
Nardil 1977

Selegiline Hydrochloride (Concurrent and/or sequential use is not recommended). Products include:
Eldepryl Capsules 2729

Tranylcypromine Sulfate (Concurrent and/or sequential use is not recommended). Products include:
Parnate Tablets 2679

DORYX CAPSULES

(Doxycycline Hyclate) 1970
May interact with penicillins, antacids, anticoagulants, iron containing oral preparations, and certain other agents. Compounds in these categories include:

Aluminum Carbonate (Should not be given concurrently). Products include:
Basaljel Capsules 2810
Basaljel Suspension 2810
Basaljel Tablets 2810

Aluminum Hydroxide (Should not be given concurrently). Products include:
ALternaGEL Liquid 1358
Maximum Strength Ascriptin 650
Cama Arthritis Pain Reliever 748
Gaviscon Extra Strength Relief Formula Antacid Tablets 778
Gaviscon Extra Strength Relief Formula Liquid Antacid 779
Gaviscon Liquid Antacid 779
Gelusil Antacid-Anti-gas Liquid 819
Gelusil Antacid-Anti-gas Tablets 819
Maalox Antacid/Anti-Gas Tablets 889
Maalox Heartburn Relief Suspension 658
Maalox Antacid Liquid 888
Extra Strength Maalox Antacid/Anti-Gas Liquid and Tablets 888
Mylanta 1359
Tempo Soft Antacid 799

Aluminum Hydroxide Gel (Should not be given concurrently). Products include:
ALternaGEL Liquid 675
Aludrox Oral Suspension 850
Amphojel Suspension 2802
Amphojel Suspension without Flavor 2802
Amphojel Tablets 2802
Ascriptin 650
Gaviscon Antacid Tablets 778
Gaviscon-2 Antacid Tablets 779
Mylanta Liquid 676
Mylanta Double Strength Liquid 676
Nephrox Suspension 671

Amoxicillin Trihydrate (Interference with bactericidal action of penicillins). Products include:
Amoxil 2631
Augmentin 2637
Augmentin Tablets 2640

Ampicillin (Interference with bactericidal action of penicillins). Products include:
Omnipen Capsules 2872
Omnipen for Oral Suspension 2873

Ampicillin Sodium (Interference with bactericidal action of penicillins). Products include:
Unasyn 2035

Azlocillin Sodium (Interference with bactericidal action of penicillins).
No products indexed under this heading.

Bacampicillin Hydrochloride (Interference with bactericidal action of penicillins). Products include:
Spectrobid Tablets 2030

Carbenicillin Disodium (Interference with bactericidal action of penicillins).
No products indexed under this heading.

Carbenicillin Indanyl Sodium (Interference with bactericidal action of penicillins). Products include:
Geocillin Tablets 2009

Dalteparin Sodium (Downward adjustment of anticoagulant dosage may be necessary). Products include:
Fragmin Injection 2088

Dicloxacillin Sodium (Interference with bactericidal action of penicillins).
No products indexed under this heading.

Dicumarol (Downward adjustment of anticoagulant dosage may be necessary).
No products indexed under this heading.

Enoxaparin (Downward adjustment of anticoagulant dosage may be necessary). Products include:
Lovenox Injection 2187

Ferrous Fumarate (Should not be given concurrently). Products include:
Chromagen Capsules 2470
Chromagen FA 2471
Chromagen Forte 2471
Ferro-Sequels 684
Nephro-Fer Tablets 2168
Nephro-Fer Rx Tablets 2168
Nephro-Vite + Fe Tablets 2170
Stresstabs + Iron 685
Trinsicon Capsules 2759
Vitron-C Tablets 667

Ferrous Gluconate (Should not be given concurrently). Products include:
Megadose 513

Ferrous Sulfate (Should not be given concurrently). Products include:
Feosol Capsules 777
Feosol Elixir 2627
Feosol Tablets 2627
Fero-Folic-500 Filmtab 433
Fero-Grad-500 Filmtab 434
Fero-Gradumet Filmtab 434
Iberet Tablets 437
Iberet-500 Liquid 438
Iberet-Folic-500 Filmtab 433
Iberet-Liquid 438
Irospan 1000
Slow Fe Tablets 889
Slow Fe with Folic Acid 890

Heparin Calcium (Downward adjustment of anticoagulant dosage may be necessary).
No products indexed under this heading.

Heparin Sodium (Downward adjustment of anticoagulant dosage may be necessary). Products include:
Heparin Lock Flush Solution 2831
Heparin Sodium Injection 2832
Heparin Sodium Vials 1486

Magaldrate (Should not be given concurrently).
No products indexed under this heading.

Magnesium Hydroxide (Should not be given concurrently). Products include:
Aludrox Oral Suspension 850
Ascriptin 650
Di-Gel Antacid/Anti-Gas 762
Gelusil Antacid-Anti-gas Liquid 819
Gelusil Antacid-Anti-gas Tablets 819
Maalox Antacid/Anti-Gas Tablets 889
Maalox Antacid Liquid 888
Extra Strength Maalox Antacid/Anti-Gas Liquid and Tablets 888
Mylanta Fast-Acting 1359
Mylanta Gelcaps Antacid 678
Fast-Acting Mylanta Liquid Antacid 1359
Mylanta Tablets 677
Maximum-Strength Fast-Acting Mylanta Liquid Antacid 1359
Mylanta Double Strength Tablets 677
Phillips' Milk of Magnesia Liquid 627
Rolaids Antacid Tablets 807
Tempo Soft Antacid 799

Magnesium Oxide (Should not be given concurrently). Products include:
Beelith Tablets 632
Bufferin Analgesic Tablets 636
Arthritis Strength Bufferin Analgesic Caplets 637
Extra Strength Bufferin Analgesic Tablets 637
Caltrate PLUS 681
Cama Arthritis Pain Reliever 748
Mag-Ox 400 666
Uro-Mag 666

Mezlocillin Sodium (Interference with bactericidal action of penicillins). Products include:
Mezlin 594
Mezlin Pharmacy Bulk Package 597

Nafcillin Sodium (Interference with bactericidal action of penicillins).
No products indexed under this heading.

Penicillin G Benzathine (Interference with bactericidal action of penicillin). Products include:
Bicillin C-R Injection 2810
Bicillin C-R 900/300 Injection 2812
Bicillin L-A Injection 2813

IMPORTANT NOTE: Always consult each drug listing in the patient's regimen for possible interactions.

Interactions Index

Doryx

Penicillin G Potassium (Interference with bactericidal action of penicillin). Products include:
- Pfizerpen for Injection 2022

Penicillin G Procaine (Interference with bactericidal action of penicillin). Products include:
- Bicillin C-R Injection 2810
- Bicillin C-R 900/300 Injection 2812

Penicillin G Sodium (Interference with bactericidal action of penicillin).
No products indexed under this heading.

Penicillin V Potassium (Interference with bactericidal action of penicillin). Products include:
- Pen•Vee K 2879

Polysaccharide-Iron Complex (Should not be given concurrently). Products include:
- Niferex-150 Capsules 811
- Niferex Elixir 811
- Niferex-150 Forte Capsules 811
- Niferex 811
- Niferex-PN Tablets 811
- Nu-Iron 150 Capsules 1826
- Nu-Iron Elixir 1826

Ticarcillin Disodium (Interference with bactericidal action of penicillins). Products include:
- Ticar for Injection 2704
- Timentin for Injection 2706

Warfarin Sodium (Downward adjustment of anticoagulant dosage may be necessary). Products include:
- Coumadin 941

DOVE BAR (ORIGINAL, UNSCENTED, AND SENSITIVE SKIN FORMULA)
(Sodium Tallowate) 686
None cited in PDR database.

DOVE MOISTURIZING BODY WASH
(Sodium Cocoyl Isethionate) 686
None cited in PDR database.

LIQUID DOVE BEAUTY WASH
(Sodium Tallowate) 686
None cited in PDR database.

DOVONEX CREAM 0.005%
(Calcipotriene) 2792
None cited in PDR database.

DOVONEX OINTMENT 0.005%
(Calcipotriene) 2793
None cited in PDR database.

DOXIDAN LIQUI-GELS
(Docusate Calcium, Phenolphthalein) 801
May interact with:

Mineral Oil (Concurrent use with oral mineral oil is not recommended unless directed by a doctor). Products include:
- Alpha Keri Moisture Rich Body Oil 635
- Anusol Hemorrhoidal Ointment 810
- Aquaphor Healing Ointment 636
- Aquaphor Healing Ointment, Original Formula 636
- Eucerin Original Moisturizing Creme (Unscented) 636
- Eucerin Original Moisturizing Lotion 636
- Eucerin Plus Dry Skin Care Moisturizing Lotion 636
- Eucerin Plus Moisturizing Creme 636
- Fleet Mineral Oil Enema 1001
- Hemorid 797
- HypoTears Ointment 262
- Keri Lotion - Original Formula 644
- Kondremul 656
- Lubriderm Bath and Shower Oil 821
- Nephrox Suspension 671
- Preparation H Hemorrhoidal Ointment 842
- Refresh PM Lubricant Eye Ointment 252
- Replens Vaginal Moisturizer 823
- Tears Renewed Ointment 210

DOXIL
(Doxorubicin Hydrochloride) 2613
May interact with antineoplastics and certain other agents. Compounds in these categories include:

Altretamine (Co-administration with the conventional formulation of doxorubicin results in potentiation of the toxicity of other anticancer therapies; this interaction may occur with Doxil). Products include:
- Hexalen Capsules 2760

Anastrozole (Co-administration with the conventional formulation of doxorubicin results in potentiation of the toxicity of other anticancer therapies; this interaction may occur with Doxil). Products include:
- Arimidex Tablets 2932

Asparaginase (Co-administration with the conventional formulation of doxorubicin results in potentiation of the toxicity of other anticancer therapies; this interaction may occur with Doxil). Products include:
- Elspar 1700

Bicalutamide (Co-administration with the conventional formulation of doxorubicin results in potentiation of the toxicity of other anticancer therapies; this interaction may occur with Doxil). Products include:
- Casodex Tablets 2934

Bleomycin Sulfate (Co-administration with the conventional formulation of doxorubicin results in potentiation of the toxicity of other anticancer therapies; this interaction may occur with Doxil). Products include:
- Blenoxane 697

Busulfan (Co-administration with the conventional formulation of doxorubicin results in potentiation of the toxicity of other anticancer therapies; this interaction may occur with Doxil). Products include:
- Mylleran Tablets 1209

Carboplatin (Co-administration with the conventional formulation of doxorubicin results in potentiation of the toxicity of other anticancer therapies; this interaction may occur with Doxil). Products include:
- Paraplatin for Injection 713

Carmustine (BCNU) (Co-administration with the conventional formulation of doxorubicin results in potentiation of the toxicity of other anticancer therapies; this interaction may occur with Doxil). Products include:
- BiCNU 696

Chlorambucil (Co-administration with the conventional formulation of doxorubicin results in potentiation of the toxicity of other anticancer therapies; this interaction may occur with Doxil). Products include:
- Leukeran Tablets 1205

Cisplatin (Co-administration with the conventional formulation of doxorubicin results in potentiation of the toxicity of other anticancer therapies; this interaction may occur with Doxil). Products include:
- Platinol for Injection 717
- Platinol-AQ Injection 719

Cyclophosphamide (Cardiac toxicity may occur at lower cumulative doses in patients who are receiving cyclophosphamide). Products include:
- Cytoxan 700

Cyclosporine (Co-administration with the conventional formulation of doxorubicin results in coma and/or seizures; this interaction may occur with Doxil). Products include:
- Neoral 2405
- Sandimmune 2416

Dacarbazine (Co-administration with the conventional formulation of doxorubicin results in potentiation of the toxicity of other anticancer therapies; this interaction may occur with Doxil). Products include:
- DTIC-Dome 593

Daunorubicin Citrate (Co-administration with the conventional formulation of doxorubicin results in potentiation of the toxicity of other anticancer therapies; this interaction may occur with Doxil). Products include:
- DaunoXome 1842

Daunorubicin Hydrochloride (Co-administration with the conventional formulation of doxorubicin results in potentiation of the toxicity of other anticancer therapies; this interaction may occur with Doxil). Products include:
- Cerubidine for Injection 634

Docetaxel (Co-administration with the conventional formulation of doxorubicin results in potentiation of the toxicity of other anticancer therapies; this interaction may occur with Doxil). Products include:
- Taxotere for Injection Concentrate 2204

Estramustine Phosphate Sodium (Co-administration with the conventional formulation of doxorubicin results in potentiation of the toxicity of other anticancer therapies; this interaction may occur with Doxil). Products include:
- Emcyt Capsules 2085

Etoposide (Co-administration with the conventional formulation of doxorubicin results in potentiation of the toxicity of other anticancer therapies; this interaction may occur with Doxil). Products include:
- Etoposide Injection 539
- VePesid Capsules and Injection 727

Floxuridine (Co-administration with the conventional formulation of doxorubicin results in potentiation of the toxicity of other anticancer therapies; this interaction may occur with Doxil). Products include:
- Sterile FUDR 2284

Fluorouracil (Co-administration with the conventional formulation of doxorubicin results in potentiation of the toxicity of other anticancer therapies; this interaction may occur with Doxil). Products include:
- Efudex 2280
- Fluoroplex Topical Solution & Cream 1% 475
- Fluorouracil Injection 2282

Flutamide (Co-administration with the conventional formulation of doxorubicin results in potentiation of the toxicity of other anticancer therapies; this interaction may occur with Doxil). Products include:
- Eulexin Capsules 2498

Gemcitabine Hydrochloride (Co-administration with the conventional formulation of doxorubicin results in potentiation of the toxicity of other anticancer therapies; this interaction may occur with Doxil). Products include:
- Gemzar for Injection 1482

Hydroxyurea (Co-administration with the conventional formulation of doxorubicin results in potentiation of the toxicity of other anticancer therapies; this interaction may occur with Doxil). Products include:
- Hydrea Capsules 705

Idarubicin Hydrochloride (Co-administration with the conventional formulation of doxorubicin results in potentiation of the toxicity of other anticancer therapies; this interaction may occur with Doxil). Products include:
- Idamycin Injection 2096

Ifosfamide (Co-administration with the conventional formulation of doxorubicin results in potentiation of the toxicity of other anticancer therapies; this interaction may occur with Doxil). Products include:
- IFEX 706

Interferon alfa-2A, Recombinant (Co-administration with the conventional formulation of doxorubicin results in potentiation of the toxicity of other anticancer therapies; this interaction may occur with Doxil). Products include:
- Roferon-A Injection 2308

Interferon alfa-2B, Recombinant (Co-administration with the conventional formulation of doxorubicin results in potentiation of the toxicity of other anticancer therapies; this interaction may occur with Doxil). Products include:
- Intron A for Injection 2506

Irinotecan Hydrochloride (Co-administration with the conventional formulation of doxorubicin results in potentiation of the toxicity of other anticancer therapies; this interaction may occur with Doxil).
No products indexed under this heading.

Levamisole Hydrochloride (Co-administration with the conventional formulation of doxorubicin results in potentiation of the toxicity of other anticancer therapies; this interaction may occur with Doxil). Products include:
- Ergamisol Tablets 1340

Lomustine (CCNU) (Co-administration with the conventional formulation of doxorubicin results in potentiation of the toxicity of other anticancer therapies; this interaction may occur with Doxil). Products include:
- CeeNU Capsules 699

Mechlorethamine Hydrochloride (Co-administration with the conventional formulation of doxorubicin results in potentiation of the toxicity of other anticancer therapies; this interaction may occur with Doxil). Products include:
- Mustargen 1752

Megestrol Acetate (Co-administration with the conventional formulation of doxorubicin results in potentiation of the toxicity of other anticancer therapies; this interaction may occur with Doxil). Products include:
- Megace Oral Suspension 708
- Megace Tablets 710

(Described in PDR For Nonprescription Drugs) (Described in PDR For Ophthalmology)

335 Interactions Index Doxorubicin Astra

Melphalan (Co-administration with the conventional formulation of doxorubicin results in potentiation of the toxicity of other anticancer therapies; this interaction may occur with Doxil). Products include:
Alkeran Tablets ... 1198
Mercaptopurine (Co-administration with the conventional formulation of doxorubicin results in potentiation of the toxicity of other anticancer therapies; this interaction may occur with Doxil). Products include:
Purinethol Tablets ... 1214
Methotrexate Sodium (Co-administration with the conventional formulation of doxorubicin results in potentiation of the toxicity of other anticancer therapies; this interaction may occur with Doxil). Products include:
Methotrexate Sodium Tablets, Injection, for Injection and LPF Injection ... 1322
Mitomycin (Mitomycin-C) (Co-administration with the conventional formulation of doxorubicin results in potentiation of the toxicity of other anticancer therapies; this interaction may occur with Doxil). Products include:
Mutamycin for Injection ... 712
Mitotane (Co-administration with the conventional formulation of doxorubicin results in potentiation of the toxicity of other anticancer therapies; this interaction may occur with Doxil). Products include:
Lysodren Tablets ... 707
Mitoxantrone Hydrochloride (Co-administration with the conventional formulation of doxorubicin results in potentiation of the toxicity of other anticancer therapies; this interaction may occur with Doxil). Products include:
Novantrone for Injection ... 1327
Paclitaxel (Co-administration with the conventional formulation of doxorubicin results in potentiation of the toxicity of other anticancer therapies; this interaction may occur with Doxil). Products include:
Taxol Injection ... 723
Phenobarbital (Co-administration with the conventional formulation of doxorubicin results in increased elimination of doxorubicin; this interaction may occur with Doxil). Products include:
Arco-Lase Plus Tablets ... 513
Bellergal-S Tablets ... 2375
Donnatal ... 2234
Donnatal Extentabs ... 2234
Donnatal Tablets ... 2234
Phenobarbital Elixir and Tablets ... 1523
Quadrinal Tablets ... 1398
Phenytoin (Co-administration with the conventional formulation of doxorubicin results in decreased phenytoin levels; this interaction may occur with Doxil). Products include:
Dilantin Infatabs ... 1967
Dilantin-125 Suspension ... 1969
Phenytoin Sodium (Co-administration with the conventional formulation of doxorubicin results in decreased phenytoin levels; this interaction may occur with Doxil). Products include:
Dilantin Kapseals ... 1965
Procarbazine Hydrochloride (Co-administration with the conventional formulation of doxorubicin results in potentiation of the toxicity of other anticancer therapies; this interaction may occur with Doxil). Products include:
Matulane Capsules ... 2300
Streptozocin (Co-administration with the conventional formulation of doxorubicin results in inhibition of hepatic metabolism; this interaction may occur with Doxil). Products include:
Zanosar Sterile Powder ... 2119
Tamoxifen Citrate (Co-administration with the conventional formulation of doxorubicin results in potentiation of the toxicity of other anticancer therapies; this interaction may occur with Doxil). Products include:
Nolvadex Tablets ... 2957
Teniposide (Co-administration with the conventional formulation of doxorubicin results in potentiation of the toxicity of other anticancer therapies; this interaction may occur with Doxil). Products include:
Vumon for Injection ... 729
Thioguanine (Co-administration with the conventional formulation of doxorubicin results in potentiation of the toxicity of other anticancer therapies; this interaction may occur with Doxil). Products include:
Thioguanine Tablets, Tabloid Brand ... 1225
Thiotepa (Co-administration with the conventional formulation of doxorubicin results in potentiation of the toxicity of other anticancer therapies; this interaction may occur with Doxil). Products include:
Thioplex (Thiotepa For Injection) ... 1329
Topotecan Hydrochloride (Co-administration with the conventional formulation of doxorubicin results in potentiation of the toxicity of other anticancer therapies; this interaction may occur with Doxil). Products include:
Hycamtin for Injection ... 2665
Vincristine Sulfate (Co-administration with the conventional formulation of doxorubicin results in potentiation of the toxicity of other anticancer therapies; this interaction may occur with Doxil). Products include:
Oncovin Solution Vials & Hyporets 1521
Vinorelbine Tartrate (Co-administration with the conventional formulation of doxorubicin results in potentiation of the toxicity of other anticancer therapies; this interaction may occur with Doxil). Products include:
Navelbine Injection ... 1212

DOXORUBICIN HYDROCHLORIDE INJECTION, USP
(Doxorubicin Hydrochloride) ... 531
See **Doxorubicin Hydrochloride for Injection, USP**

DOXORUBICIN HYDROCHLORIDE FOR INJECTION, USP
(Doxorubicin Hydrochloride) ... 531
May interact with antineoplastics and certain other agents. Compounds in these categories include:

Altretamine (Toxicity of other anticancer therapies potentiated). Products include:
Hexalen Capsules ... 2760
Anastrozole (Toxicity of other anticancer therapies potentiated). Products include:
Arimidex Tablets ... 2932
Asparaginase (Toxicity of other anticancer therapies potentiated). Products include:
Elspar ... 1700
Bicalutamide (Toxicity of other anticancer therapies potentiated). Products include:
Casodex Tablets ... 2934
Bleomycin Sulfate (Toxicity of other anticancer therapies potentiated). Products include:
Blenoxane ... 697
Busulfan (Toxicity of other anticancer therapies potentiated). Products include:
Myleran Tablets ... 1209
Carboplatin (Toxicity of other anticancer therapies potentiated). Products include:
Paraplatin for Injection ... 713
Carmustine (BCNU) (Toxicity of other anticancer therapies potentiated). Products include:
BiCNU ... 696
Chlorambucil (Toxicity of other anticancer therapies potentiated). Products include:
Leukeran Tablets ... 1205
Cisplatin (Toxicity of other anticancer therapies potentiated). Products include:
Platinol for Injection ... 717
Platinol-AQ Injection ... 719
Cyclophosphamide (Toxicity of other anticancer therapies potentiated; exacerbation of cyclophosphamide-induced hemorrhagic cystitis). Products include:
Cytoxan ... 700
Dacarbazine (Toxicity of other anticancer therapies potentiated). Products include:
DTIC-Dome ... 593
Daunorubicin Citrate (Toxicity of other anticancer therapies potentiated). Products include:
DaunoXome ... 1842
Daunorubicin Hydrochloride (Toxicity of other anticancer therapies potentiated). Products include:
Cerubidine for Injection ... 634
Docetaxel (Toxicity of other anticancer therapies potentiated). Products include:
Taxotere for Injection Concentrate 2204
Estramustine Phosphate Sodium (Toxicity of other anticancer therapies potentiated). Products include:
Emcyt Capsules ... 2085
Etoposide (Toxicity of other anticancer therapies potentiated). Products include:
Etoposide Injection ... 539
VePesid Capsules and Injection ... 727
Floxuridine (Toxicity of other anticancer therapies potentiated). Products include:
Sterile FUDR ... 2284
Fluorouracil (Toxicity of other anticancer therapies potentiated). Products include:
Efudex ... 2280
Fluoroplex Topical Solution & Cream 1% ... 475
Fluorouracil Injection ... 2282
Flutamide (Toxicity of other anticancer therapies potentiated). Products include:
Eulexin Capsules ... 2498
Gemcitabine Hydrochloride (Toxicity of other anticancer therapies potentiated). Products include:
Gemzar for Injection ... 1482
Hydroxyurea (Toxicity of other anticancer therapies potentiated). Products include:
Hydrea Capsules ... 705
Idarubicin Hydrochloride (Toxicity of other anticancer therapies potentiated). Products include:
Idamycin Injection ... 2096
Ifosfamide (Toxicity of other anticancer therapies potentiated). Products include:
IFEX ... 706
Interferon alfa-2A, Recombinant (Toxicity of other anticancer therapies potentiated). Products include:
Roferon-A Injection ... 2308
Interferon alfa-2B, Recombinant (Toxicity of other anticancer therapies potentiated). Products include:
Intron A for Injection ... 2506
Irinotecan Hydrochloride (Toxicity of other anticancer therapies potentiated).
No products indexed under this heading.
Levamisole Hydrochloride (Toxicity of other anticancer therapies potentiated). Products include:
Ergamisol Tablets ... 1340
Lomustine (CCNU) (Toxicity of other anticancer therapies potentiated). Products include:
CeeNU Capsules ... 699
Mechlorethamine Hydrochloride (Toxicity of other anticancer therapies potentiated). Products include:
Mustargen ... 1752
Megestrol Acetate (Toxicity of other anticancer therapies potentiated). Products include:
Megace Oral Suspension ... 708
Megace Tablets ... 710
Melphalan (Toxicity of other anticancer therapies potentiated). Products include:
Alkeran Tablets ... 1198
Mercaptopurine (Toxicity of other anticancer therapies potentiated; enhancement of the hepatotoxicity of 6-mercaptopurine). Products include:
Purinethol Tablets ... 1214
Methotrexate Sodium (Toxicity of other anticancer therapies potentiated). Products include:
Methotrexate Sodium Tablets, Injection, for Injection and LPF Injection ... 1322
Mitomycin (Mitomycin-C) (Toxicity of other anticancer therapies potentiated). Products include:
Mutamycin for Injection ... 712
Mitotane (Toxicity of other anticancer therapies potentiated). Products include:
Lysodren Tablets ... 707
Mitoxantrone Hydrochloride (Toxicity of other anticancer therapies potentiated). Products include:
Novantrone for Injection ... 1327
Paclitaxel (Toxicity of other anticancer therapies potentiated). Products include:
Taxol Injection ... 723

IMPORTANT NOTE: Always consult each drug listing in the patient's regimen for possible interactions.

Doxorubicin Astra

Procarbazine Hydrochloride (Toxicity of other anticancer therapies potentiated). Products include:
Matulane Capsules 2300

Streptozocin (Toxicity of other anticancer therapies potentiated). Products include:
Zanosar Sterile Powder 2119

Tamoxifen Citrate (Toxicity of other anticancer therapies potentiated). Products include:
Nolvadex Tablets 2957

Teniposide (Toxicity of other anticancer therapies potentiated). Products include:
Vumon for Injection 729

Thioguanine (Toxicity of other anticancer therapies potentiated). Products include:
Thioguanine Tablets, Tabloid Brand 1225

Thiotepa (Toxicity of other anticancer therapies potentiated). Products include:
Thioplex (Thiotepa For Injection) 1329

Topotecan Hydrochloride (Toxicity of other anticancer therapies potentiated). Products include:
Hycamtin for Injection 2665

Vincristine Sulfate (Toxicity of other anticancer therapies potentiated). Products include:
Oncovin Solution Vials & Hyporets ... 1521

Vinorelbine Tartrate (Toxicity of other anticancer therapies potentiated). Products include:
Navelbine Injection 1212

DRAMAMINE CHEWABLE TABLETS
(Dimenhydrinate) 801
See Dramamine Tablets

CHILDREN'S DRAMAMINE LIQUID
(Dimenhydrinate) 801
See Dramamine Tablets

DRAMAMINE TABLETS
(Dimenhydrinate) 801
May interact with hypnotics and sedatives, tranquilizers, and certain other agents. Compounds in these categories include:

Alprazolam (May increase drowsiness effect). Products include:
Xanax Tablets 2115

Buspirone Hydrochloride (May increase drowsiness effect). Products include:
BuSpar Tablets 738

Chlordiazepoxide (May increase drowsiness effect). Products include:
Limbitrol 2333

Chlordiazepoxide Hydrochloride (May increase drowsiness effect). Products include:
Librax Capsules 2330
Librium Capsules 2331
Librium Injectable 2332

Chlorpromazine (May increase drowsiness effect). Products include:
Thorazine Suppositories 2701

Chlorpromazine Hydrochloride (May increase drowsiness effect). Products include:
Thorazine 2701

Chlorprothixene (May increase drowsiness effect).
No products indexed under this heading.

Chlorprothixene Hydrochloride (May increase drowsiness effect).
No products indexed under this heading.

Clorazepate Dipotassium (May increase drowsiness effect). Products include:
Tranxene 459

Diazepam (May increase drowsiness effect). Products include:
Dizac (diazepam injectable emulsion) CIV 1862
Valium Injectable 2336
Valium Tablets 2335

Droperidol (May increase drowsiness effect). Products include:
Inapsine Injection 462

Estazolam (May increase drowsiness effect). Products include:
ProSom Tablets 457

Ethchlorvynol (May increase drowsiness effect). Products include:
Placidyl Capsules 456

Ethinamate (May increase drowsiness effect).
No products indexed under this heading.

Fluphenazine Decanoate (May increase drowsiness effect). Products include:
Prolixin Decanoate 510

Fluphenazine Enanthate (May increase drowsiness effect). Products include:
Prolixin Enanthate 510

Fluphenazine Hydrochloride (May increase drowsiness effect). Products include:
Prolixin 510

Flurazepam Hydrochloride (May increase drowsiness effect). Products include:
Dalmane Capsules 2329

Glutethimide (May increase drowsiness effect).
No products indexed under this heading.

Haloperidol (May increase drowsiness effect). Products include:
Haldol Injection, Tablets and Concentrate 1585

Haloperidol Decanoate (May increase drowsiness effect). Products include:
Haldol Decanoate 1587

Hydroxyzine Hydrochloride (May increase drowsiness effect). Products include:
Atarax Tablets & Syrup 1992
Marax Tablets & DF Syrup 2015
Vistaril Intramuscular Solution 2042

Lorazepam (May increase drowsiness effect). Products include:
Ativan Injection 2805
Ativan Tablets 2807

Loxapine Hydrochloride (May increase drowsiness effect). Products include:
Loxitane 1426

Loxapine Succinate (May increase drowsiness effect). Products include:
Loxitane Capsules 1426

Meprobamate (May increase drowsiness effect). Products include:
Miltown Tablets 2780
PMB 200 and PMB 400 2890

Mesoridazine Besylate (May increase drowsiness effect). Products include:
Serentil 689

Midazolam Hydrochloride (May increase drowsiness effect). Products include:
Versed Injection 2324

Molindone Hydrochloride (May increase drowsiness effect). Products include:
Moban Tablets and Concentrate ... 1036

Interactions Index

Oxazepam (May increase drowsiness effect). Products include:
Serax Capsules 2916
Serax Tablets 2916

Perphenazine (May increase drowsiness effect). Products include:
Etrafon 2495
Triavil Tablets 1800
Trilafon 2532

Prazepam (May increase drowsiness effect).
No products indexed under this heading.

Prochlorperazine (May increase drowsiness effect). Products include:
Compazine 2644

Promethazine Hydrochloride (May increase drowsiness effect). Products include:
Mepergan Injection 2859
Phenergan with Codeine 2883
Phenergan with Dextromethorphan .. 2885
Phenergan Injection 2880
Phenergan Suppositories 2882
Phenergan Syrup 2881
Phenergan Tablets 2882
Phenergan VC 2886
Phenergan VC with Codeine 2888

Propofol (May increase drowsiness effect). Products include:
Diprivan Injectable Emulsion 2939

Quazepam (May increase drowsiness effect). Products include:
Doral Tablets 2773

Secobarbital Sodium (May increase drowsiness effect). Products include:
Seconal Sodium Pulvules 1529

Temazepam (May increase drowsiness effect). Products include:
Restoril Capsules 2413

Thioridazine Hydrochloride (May increase drowsiness effect). Products include:
Mellaril 2398

Thiothixene (May increase drowsiness effect). Products include:
Navane Capsules and Concentrate .. 2018
Navane Intramuscular 2019

Triazolam (May increase drowsiness effect). Products include:
Halcion Tablets 2093

Trifluoperazine Hydrochloride (May increase drowsiness effect). Products include:
Stelazine 2692

Zolpidem Tartrate (May increase drowsiness effect). Products include:
Ambien Tablets 2559

Food Interactions
Alcohol (May increase drowsiness effect).

DRAMAMINE II TABLETS
(Meclizine Hydrochloride) 801
May interact with hypnotics and sedatives, tranquilizers, and certain other agents. Compounds in these categories include:

Alprazolam (May increase drowsiness effect). Products include:
Xanax Tablets 2115

Buspirone Hydrochloride (May increase drowsiness effect). Products include:
BuSpar Tablets 738

Chlordiazepoxide (May increase drowsiness effect). Products include:
Limbitrol 2333

Chlordiazepoxide Hydrochloride (May increase drowsiness effect). Products include:
Librax Capsules 2330
Librium Capsules 2331
Librium Injectable 2332

Chlorpromazine (May increase drowsiness effect). Products include:
Thorazine Suppositories 2701

Chlorpromazine Hydrochloride (May increase drowsiness effect). Products include:
Thorazine 2701

Chlorprothixene (May increase drowsiness effect).
No products indexed under this heading.

Chlorprothixene Hydrochloride (May increase drowsiness effect).
No products indexed under this heading.

Clorazepate Dipotassium (May increase drowsiness effect). Products include:
Tranxene 459

Diazepam (May increase drowsiness effect). Products include:
Dizac (diazepam injectable emulsion) CIV 1862
Valium Injectable 2336
Valium Tablets 2335

Droperidol (May increase drowsiness effect). Products include:
Inapsine Injection 462

Estazolam (May increase drowsiness effect). Products include:
ProSom Tablets 457

Ethchlorvynol (May increase drowsiness effect). Products include:
Placidyl Capsules 456

Ethinamate (May increase drowsiness effect).
No products indexed under this heading.

Fluphenazine Decanoate (May increase drowsiness effect). Products include:
Prolixin Decanoate 510

Fluphenazine Enanthate (May increase drowsiness effect). Products include:
Prolixin Enanthate 510

Fluphenazine Hydrochloride (May increase drowsiness effect). Products include:
Prolixin 510

Flurazepam Hydrochloride (May increase drowsiness effect). Products include:
Dalmane Capsules 2329

Glutethimide (May increase drowsiness effect).
No products indexed under this heading.

Haloperidol (May increase drowsiness effect). Products include:
Haldol Injection, Tablets and Concentrate 1585

Haloperidol Decanoate (May increase drowsiness effect). Products include:
Haldol Decanoate 1587

Hydroxyzine Hydrochloride (May increase drowsiness effect). Products include:
Atarax Tablets & Syrup 1992
Marax Tablets & DF Syrup 2015
Vistaril Intramuscular Solution 2042

Lorazepam (May increase drowsiness effect). Products include:
Ativan Injection 2805
Ativan Tablets 2807

Loxapine Hydrochloride (May increase drowsiness effect). Products include:
Loxitane 1426

Loxapine Succinate (May increase drowsiness effect). Products include:
Loxitane Capsules 1426

Meprobamate (May increase drowsiness effect). Products include:
Miltown Tablets 2780
PMB 200 and PMB 400 2890

(▣ Described in PDR For Nonprescription Drugs)   (⊙ Described in PDR For Ophthalmology)

Mesoridazine Besylate (May increase drowsiness effect). Products include:
　Serentil 689

Midazolam Hydrochloride (May increase drowsiness effect). Products include:
　Versed Injection 2324

Molindone Hydrochloride (May increase drowsiness effect). Products include:
　Moban Tablets and Concentrate 1036

Oxazepam (May increase drowsiness effect). Products include:
　Serax Capsules 2916
　Serax Tablets 2916

Perphenazine (May increase drowsiness effect). Products include:
　Etrafon 2495
　Triavil Tablets 1800
　Trilafon 2532

Prazepam (May increase drowsiness effect).
　No products indexed under this heading.

Prochlorperazine (May increase drowsiness effect). Products include:
　Compazine 2644

Promethazine Hydrochloride (May increase drowsiness effect). Products include:
　Mepergan Injection 2859
　Phenergan with Codeine 2883
　Phenergan with Dextromethorphan 2885
　Phenergan Injection 2880
　Phenergan Suppositories 2882
　Phenergan Syrup 2881
　Phenergan Tablets 2882
　Phenergan VC 2886
　Phenergan VC with Codeine 2888

Propofol (May increase drowsiness effect). Products include:
　Diprivan Injectable Emulsion 2939

Quazepam (May increase drowsiness effect). Products include:
　Doral Tablets 2773

Secobarbital Sodium (May increase drowsiness effect). Products include:
　Seconal Sodium Pulvules 1529

Temazepam (May increase drowsiness effect). Products include:
　Restoril Capsules 2413

Thioridazine Hydrochloride (May increase drowsiness effect). Products include:
　Mellaril 2398

Thiothixene (May increase drowsiness effect). Products include:
　Navane Capsules and Concentrate 2018
　Navane Intramuscular 2019

Triazolam (May increase drowsiness effect). Products include:
　Halcion Tablets 2093

Trifluoperazine Hydrochloride (May increase drowsiness effect). Products include:
　Stelazine 2692

Zolpidem Tartrate (May increase drowsiness effect). Products include:
　Ambien Tablets 2559

Food Interactions
Alcohol (May increase drowsiness effect).

DRITHOCREME 0.1%, 0.25%, 0.5%, 1.0% (HP)
(Anthralin) 920
May interact with:

Corticosteroids, Topical, Unspecified (Withdrawal of topical corticosteroids may give rise to a "rebound" phenomenon, an interval of at least one week should be allowed between the discontinuance of such steroids and the commencement of Drithocreme).
　No products indexed under this heading.

DRITHO-SCALP 0.25%, 0.5%
(Anthralin) 921
May interact with:

Corticosteroids, Topical, Unspecified (Withdrawal of topical corticosteroids may give rise to a "rebound" phenomenon, an interval of at least one week should be allowed between the discontinuance of such steroids and the commencement of Drithocreme).
　No products indexed under this heading.

DRIXORAL COLD AND ALLERGY SUSTAINED-ACTION TABLETS
(Dexbrompheniramine Maleate, Pseudoephedrine Sulfate) 763
May interact with monoamine oxidase inhibitors, hypnotics and sedatives, tranquilizers, and certain other agents. Compounds in these categories include:

Alprazolam (May increase drowsiness effect). Products include:
　Xanax Tablets 2115

Buspirone Hydrochloride (May increase drowsiness effect). Products include:
　BuSpar Tablets 738

Chlordiazepoxide (May increase drowsiness effect). Products include:
　Limbitrol 2333

Chlordiazepoxide Hydrochloride (May increase drowsiness effect). Products include:
　Librax Capsules 2330
　Librium Capsules 2331
　Librium Injectable 2332

Chlorpromazine (May increase drowsiness effect). Products include:
　Thorazine Suppositories 2701

Chlorpromazine Hydrochloride (May increase drowsiness effect). Products include:
　Thorazine 2701

Chlorprothixene (May increase drowsiness effect).
　No products indexed under this heading.

Chlorprothixene Hydrochloride (May increase drowsiness effect).
　No products indexed under this heading.

Clorazepate Dipotassium (May increase drowsiness effect). Products include:
　Tranxene 459

Diazepam (May increase drowsiness effect). Products include:
　Dizac (diazepam injectable emulsion) CIV 1862
　Valium Injectable 2336
　Valium Tablets 2335

Droperidol (May increase drowsiness effect). Products include:
　Inapsine Injection 462

Estazolam (May increase drowsiness effect). Products include:
　ProSom Tablets 457

Ethchlorvynol (May increase drowsiness effect). Products include:
　Placidyl Capsules 456

Ethinamate (May increase drowsiness effect).
　No products indexed under this heading.

Fluphenazine Decanoate (May increase drowsiness effect). Products include:
　Prolixin Decanoate 510

Fluphenazine Enanthate (May increase drowsiness effect). Products include:
　Prolixin Enanthate 510

Fluphenazine Hydrochloride (May increase drowsiness effect). Products include:
　Prolixin 510

Flurazepam Hydrochloride (May increase drowsiness effect). Products include:
　Dalmane Capsules 2329

Furazolidone (Concurrent and/or sequential use is not recommended). Products include:
　Furoxone 2221

Glutethimide (May increase drowsiness effect).
　No products indexed under this heading.

Haloperidol (May increase drowsiness effect). Products include:
　Haldol Injection, Tablets and Concentrate 1585

Haloperidol Decanoate (May increase drowsiness effect). Products include:
　Haldol Decanoate 1587

Hydroxyzine Hydrochloride (May increase drowsiness effect). Products include:
　Atarax Tablets & Syrup 1992
　Marax Tablets & DF Syrup . 2015
　Vistaril Intramuscular Solution .. 2042

Isocarboxazid (Concurrent and/or sequential use is not recommended).
　No products indexed under this heading.

Lorazepam (May increase drowsiness effect). Products include:
　Ativan Injection 2805
　Ativan Tablets 2807

Loxapine Hydrochloride (May increase drowsiness effect). Products include:
　Loxitane 1426

Loxapine Succinate (May increase drowsiness effect). Products include:
　Loxitane Capsules 1426

Meprobamate (May increase drowsiness effect). Products include:
　Miltown Tablets 2780
　PMB 200 and PMB 400 2890

Mesoridazine Besylate (May increase drowsiness effect). Products include:
　Serentil 689

Midazolam Hydrochloride (May increase drowsiness effect). Products include:
　Versed Injection 2324

Molindone Hydrochloride (May increase drowsiness effect). Products include:
　Moban Tablets and Concentrate 1036

Oxazepam (May increase drowsiness effect). Products include:
　Serax Capsules 2916
　Serax Tablets 2916

Perphenazine (May increase drowsiness effect). Products include:
　Etrafon 2495
　Triavil Tablets 1800
　Trilafon 2532

Phenelzine Sulfate (Concurrent and/or sequential use is not recommended). Products include:
　Nardil 1977

Prazepam (May increase drowsiness effect).
　No products indexed under this heading.

Prochlorperazine (May increase drowsiness effect). Products include:
　Compazine 2644

Promethazine Hydrochloride (May increase drowsiness effect). Products include:
　Mepergan Injection 2859
　Phenergan with Codeine 2883
　Phenergan with Dextromethorphan 2885
　Phenergan Injection 2880
　Phenergan Suppositories 2882
　Phenergan Syrup 2881
　Phenergan Tablets 2882
　Phenergan VC 2886
　Phenergan VC with Codeine 2888

Propofol (May increase drowsiness effect). Products include:
　Diprivan Injectable Emulsion 2939

Quazepam (May increase drowsiness effect). Products include:
　Doral Tablets 2773

Secobarbital Sodium (May increase drowsiness effect). Products include:
　Seconal Sodium Pulvules 1529

Selegiline Hydrochloride (Concurrent and/or sequential use is not recommended). Products include:
　Eldepryl Capsules 2729

Temazepam (May increase drowsiness effect). Products include:
　Restoril Capsules 2413

Thioridazine Hydrochloride (May increase drowsiness effect). Products include:
　Mellaril 2398

Thiothixene (May increase drowsiness effect). Products include:
　Navane Capsules and Concentrate 2018
　Navane Intramuscular 2019

Tranylcypromine Sulfate (Concurrent and/or sequential use is not recommended). Products include:
　Parnate Tablets 2679

Triazolam (May increase drowsiness effect). Products include:
　Halcion Tablets 2093

Trifluoperazine Hydrochloride (May increase drowsiness effect). Products include:
　Stelazine 2692

Zolpidem Tartrate (May increase drowsiness effect). Products include:
　Ambien Tablets 2559

Food Interactions
Alcohol (May increase drowsiness effect).

DRIXORAL COLD AND FLU EXTENDED-RELEASE TABLETS
(Acetaminophen, Dexbrompheniramine Maleate, Pseudoephedrine Sulfate) 764
May interact with hypnotics and sedatives, tranquilizers, monoamine oxidase inhibitors, and certain other agents. Compounds in these categories include:

Alprazolam (May increase drowsiness effect). Products include:
　Xanax Tablets 2115

Buspirone Hydrochloride (May increase drowsiness effect). Products include:
　BuSpar Tablets 738

IMPORTANT NOTE: Always consult each drug listing in the patient's regimen for possible interactions.

Drixoral Cold and Flu — Interactions Index

Chlordiazepoxide (May increase drowsiness effect). Products include:
- Limbitrol 2333

Chlordiazepoxide Hydrochloride (May increase drowsiness effect). Products include:
- Librax Capsules 2330
- Librium Capsules 2331
- Librium Injectable 2332

Chlorpromazine (May increase drowsiness effect). Products include:
- Thorazine Suppositories 2701

Chlorpromazine Hydrochloride (May increase drowsiness effect). Products include:
- Thorazine 2701

Chlorprothixene (May increase drowsiness effect).
- No products indexed under this heading.

Chlorprothixene Hydrochloride (May increase drowsiness effect).
- No products indexed under this heading.

Clorazepate Dipotassium (May increase drowsiness effect). Products include:
- Tranxene 459

Diazepam (May increase drowsiness effect). Products include:
- Dizac (diazepam injectable emulsion) CIV 1862
- Valium Injectable 2336
- Valium Tablets 2335

Droperidol (May increase drowsiness effect). Products include:
- Inapsine Injection 462

Estazolam (May increase drowsiness effect). Products include:
- ProSom Tablets 457

Ethchlorvynol (May increase drowsiness effect). Products include:
- Placidyl Capsules 456

Ethinamate (May increase drowsiness effect).
- No products indexed under this heading.

Fluphenazine Decanoate (May increase drowsiness effect). Products include:
- Prolixin Decanoate 510

Fluphenazine Enanthate (May increase drowsiness effect). Products include:
- Prolixin Enanthate 510

Fluphenazine Hydrochloride (May increase drowsiness effect). Products include:
- Prolixin 510

Flurazepam Hydrochloride (May increase drowsiness effect). Products include:
- Dalmane Capsules 2329

Furazolidone (Concurrent and/or sequential use is not recommended). Products include:
- Furoxone 2221

Glutethimide (May increase drowsiness effect).
- No products indexed under this heading.

Haloperidol (May increase drowsiness effect). Products include:
- Haldol Injection, Tablets and Concentrate 1585

Haloperidol Decanoate (May increase drowsiness effect). Products include:
- Haldol Decanoate 1587

Hydroxyzine Hydrochloride (May increase drowsiness effect). Products include:
- Atarax Tablets & Syrup 1992
- Marax Tablets & DF Syrup 2015
- Vistaril Intramuscular Solution 2042

Isocarboxazid (Concurrent and/or sequential use is not recommended).
- No products indexed under this heading.

Lorazepam (May increase drowsiness effect). Products include:
- Ativan Injection 2805
- Ativan Tablets 2807

Loxapine Hydrochloride (May increase drowsiness effect). Products include:
- Loxitane 1426

Loxapine Succinate (May increase drowsiness effect). Products include:
- Loxitane Capsules 1426

Meprobamate (May increase drowsiness effect). Products include:
- Miltown Tablets 2780
- PMB 200 and PMB 400 2890

Mesoridazine Besylate (May increase drowsiness effect). Products include:
- Serentil 689

Midazolam Hydrochloride (May increase drowsiness effect). Products include:
- Versed Injection 2324

Molindone Hydrochloride (May increase drowsiness effect). Products include:
- Moban Tablets and Concentrate 1036

Oxazepam (May increase drowsiness effect). Products include:
- Serax Capsules 2916
- Serax Tablets 2916

Perphenazine (May increase drowsiness effect). Products include:
- Etrafon 2495
- Triavil Tablets 1800
- Trilafon 2532

Phenelzine Sulfate (Concurrent and/or sequential use is not recommended). Products include:
- Nardil 1977

Prazepam (May increase drowsiness effect).
- No products indexed under this heading.

Prochlorperazine (May increase drowsiness effect). Products include:
- Compazine 2644

Promethazine Hydrochloride (May increase drowsiness effect). Products include:
- Mepergan Injection 2859
- Phenergan with Codeine 2883
- Phenergan with Dextromethorphan 2885
- Phenergan Injection 2880
- Phenergan Suppositories 2882
- Phenergan Syrup 2881
- Phenergan Tablets 2882
- Phenergan VC 2886
- Phenergan VC with Codeine 2888

Propofol (May increase drowsiness effect). Products include:
- Diprivan Injectable Emulsion 2939

Quazepam (May increase drowsiness effect). Products include:
- Doral Tablets 2773

Secobarbital Sodium (May increase drowsiness effect). Products include:
- Seconal Sodium Pulvules 1529

Selegiline Hydrochloride (Concurrent and/or sequential use is not recommended). Products include:
- Eldepryl Capsules 2729

Temazepam (May increase drowsiness effect). Products include:
- Restoril Capsules 2413

Thioridazine Hydrochloride (May increase drowsiness effect). Products include:
- Mellaril 2398

Thiothixene (May increase drowsiness effect). Products include:
- Navane Capsules and Concentrate 2018
- Navane Intramuscular 2019

Tranylcypromine Sulfate (Concurrent and/or sequential use is not recommended). Products include:
- Parnate Tablets 2679

Triazolam (May increase drowsiness effect). Products include:
- Halcion Tablets 2093

Trifluoperazine Hydrochloride (May increase drowsiness effect). Products include:
- Stelazine 2692

Zolpidem Tartrate (May increase drowsiness effect). Products include:
- Ambien Tablets 2559

Food Interactions

Alcohol (May increase drowsiness effect).

DRIXORAL COUGH LIQUID CAPS
(Dextromethorphan Hydrobromide) .... ▣ 762
May interact with monoamine oxidase inhibitors. Compounds in this category include:

Furazolidone (Concurrent and/or sequential use is not recommended). Products include:
- Furoxone 2221

Isocarboxazid (Concurrent and/or sequential use is not recommended).
- No products indexed under this heading.

Phenelzine Sulfate (Concurrent and/or sequential use is not recommended). Products include:
- Nardil 1977

Selegiline Hydrochloride (Concurrent and/or sequential use is not recommended). Products include:
- Eldepryl Capsules 2729

Tranylcypromine Sulfate (Concurrent and/or sequential use is not recommended). Products include:
- Parnate Tablets 2679

DRIXORAL COUGH + CONGESTION LIQUID CAPS
(Dextromethorphan Hydrobromide, Pseudoephedrine Hydrochloride) .... ▣ 763
May interact with monoamine oxidase inhibitors. Compounds in this category include:

Furazolidone (Concurrent and/or sequential use is not recommended). Products include:
- Furoxone 2221

Isocarboxazid (Concurrent and/or sequential use is not recommended).
- No products indexed under this heading.

Phenelzine Sulfate (Concurrent and/or sequential use is not recommended). Products include:
- Nardil 1977

Selegiline Hydrochloride (Concurrent and/or sequential use is not recommended). Products include:
- Eldepryl Capsules 2729

Tranylcypromine Sulfate (Concurrent and/or sequential use is not recommended). Products include:
- Parnate Tablets 2679

DRIXORAL COUGH + SORE THROAT LIQUID CAPS
(Dextromethorphan Hydrobromide, Acetaminophen) .... ▣ 763
May interact with monoamine oxidase inhibitors. Compounds in this category include:

Furazolidone (Concurrent and/or sequential use is not recommended). Products include:
- Furoxone 2221

Isocarboxazid (Concurrent and/or sequential use is not recommended).
- No products indexed under this heading.

Phenelzine Sulfate (Concurrent and/or sequential use is not recommended). Products include:
- Nardil 1977

Selegiline Hydrochloride (Concurrent and/or sequential use is not recommended). Products include:
- Eldepryl Capsules 2729

Tranylcypromine Sulfate (Concurrent and/or sequential use is not recommended). Products include:
- Parnate Tablets 2679

DRIXORAL NON-DROWSY FORMULA EXTENDED-RELEASE TABLETS
(Pseudoephedrine Sulfate) .... ▣ 764
May interact with monoamine oxidase inhibitors. Compounds in this category include:

Furazolidone (Concurrent and/or sequential use is not recommended). Products include:
- Furoxone 2221

Isocarboxazid (Concurrent and/or sequential use is not recommended).
- No products indexed under this heading.

Phenelzine Sulfate (Concurrent and/or sequential use is not recommended). Products include:
- Nardil 1977

Selegiline Hydrochloride (Concurrent and/or sequential use is not recommended). Products include:
- Eldepryl Capsules 2729

Tranylcypromine Sulfate (Concurrent and/or sequential use is not recommended). Products include:
- Parnate Tablets 2679

DRIXORAL ALLERGY/SINUS EXTENDED RELEASE TABLETS
(Acetaminophen, Pseudoephedrine Sulfate, Dexbrompheniramine Maleate) .... ▣ 765
May interact with hypnotics and sedatives, tranquilizers, monoamine oxidase inhibitors, and certain other agents. Compounds in these categories include:

Alprazolam (May increase the drowsiness effect). Products include:
- Xanax Tablets 2115

Buspirone Hydrochloride (May increase the drowsiness effect). Products include:
- BuSpar Tablets 738

Chlordiazepoxide (May increase the drowsiness effect). Products include:
- Limbitrol 2333

Chlordiazepoxide Hydrochloride (May increase the drowsiness effect). Products include:
- Librax Capsules 2330
- Librium Capsules 2331
- Librium Injectable 2332

Chlorpromazine (May increase the drowsiness effect). Products include:
- Thorazine Suppositories 2701

(▣ Described in PDR For Nonprescription Drugs)   (⊙ Described in PDR For Ophthalmology)

Chlorpromazine Hydrochloride (May increase the drowsiness effect). Products include:
- Thorazine 2701

Chlorprothixene (May increase the drowsiness effect).
- No products indexed under this heading.

Chlorprothixene Hydrochloride (May increase the drowsiness effect).
- No products indexed under this heading.

Clorazepate Dipotassium (May increase the drowsiness effect). Products include:
- Tranxene 459

Diazepam (May increase the drowsiness effect). Products include:
- Dizac (diazepam injectable emulsion) CIV 1862
- Valium Injectable 2336
- Valium Tablets 2335

Droperidol (May increase the drowsiness effect). Products include:
- Inapsine Injection 462

Estazolam (May increase the drowsiness effect). Products include:
- ProSom Tablets 457

Ethchlorvynol (May increase the drowsiness effect). Products include:
- Placidyl Capsules 456

Ethinamate (May increase the drowsiness effect).
- No products indexed under this heading.

Fluphenazine Decanoate (May increase the drowsiness effect). Products include:
- Prolixin Decanoate 510

Fluphenazine Enanthate (May increase the drowsiness effect). Products include:
- Prolixin Enanthate 510

Fluphenazine Hydrochloride (May increase the drowsiness effect). Products include:
- Prolixin 510

Flurazepam Hydrochloride (May increase the drowsiness effect). Products include:
- Dalmane Capsules 2329

Furazolidone (Concurrent and/or sequential use is not recommended). Products include:
- Furoxone 2221

Glutethimide (May increase the drowsiness effect).
- No products indexed under this heading.

Haloperidol (May increase the drowsiness effect). Products include:
- Haldol Injection, Tablets and Concentrate 1585

Haloperidol Decanoate (May increase the drowsiness effect). Products include:
- Haldol Decanoate 1587

Hydroxyzine Hydrochloride (May increase the drowsiness effect). Products include:
- Atarax Tablets & Syrup 1992
- Marax Tablets & DF Syrup 2015
- Vistaril Intramuscular Solution .. 2042

Isocarboxazid (Concurrent and/or sequential use is not recommended).
- No products indexed under this heading.

Lorazepam (May increase the drowsiness effect). Products include:
- Ativan Injection 2805
- Ativan Tablets 2807

Loxapine Hydrochloride (May increase the drowsiness effect). Products include:
- Loxitane 1426

Loxapine Succinate (May increase the drowsiness effect). Products include:
- Loxitane Capsules 1426

Meprobamate (May increase the drowsiness effect). Products include:
- Miltown Tablets 2780
- PMB 200 and PMB 400 2890

Mesoridazine Besylate (May increase the drowsiness effect). Products include:
- Serentil 689

Midazolam Hydrochloride (May increase the drowsiness effect). Products include:
- Versed Injection 2324

Molindone Hydrochloride (May increase the drowsiness effect). Products include:
- Moban Tablets and Concentrate 1036

Oxazepam (May increase the drowsiness effect). Products include:
- Serax Capsules 2916
- Serax Tablets 2916

Perphenazine (May increase the drowsiness effect). Products include:
- Etrafon 2495
- Triavil Tablets 1800
- Trilafon 2532

Phenelzine Sulfate (Concurrent and/or sequential use is not recommended). Products include:
- Nardil 1977

Prazepam (May increase the drowsiness effect).
- No products indexed under this heading.

Prochlorperazine (May increase the drowsiness effect). Products include:
- Compazine 2644

Promethazine Hydrochloride (May increase the drowsiness effect). Products include:
- Mepergan Injection 2859
- Phenergan with Codeine 2883
- Phenergan with Dextromethorphan ... 2885
- Phenergan Injection 2880
- Phenergan Suppositories 2882
- Phenergan Syrup 2881
- Phenergan Tablets 2882
- Phenergan VC 2886
- Phenergan VC with Codeine ... 2888

Propofol (May increase the drowsiness effect). Products include:
- Diprivan Injectable Emulsion .. 2939

Quazepam (May increase the drowsiness effect). Products include:
- Doral Tablets 2773

Secobarbital Sodium (May increase the drowsiness effect). Products include:
- Seconal Sodium Pulvules 1529

Selegiline Hydrochloride (Concurrent and/or sequential use is not recommended). Products include:
- Eldepryl Capsules 2729

Temazepam (May increase the drowsiness effect). Products include:
- Restoril Capsules 2413

Thioridazine Hydrochloride (May increase the drowsiness effect). Products include:
- Mellaril 2398

Thiothixene (May increase the drowsiness effect). Products include:
- Navane Capsules and Concentrate ... 2018
- Navane Intramuscular 2019

Tranylcypromine Sulfate (Concurrent and/or sequential use is not recommended). Products include:
- Parnate Tablets 2679

Triazolam (May increase the drowsiness effect). Products include:
- Halcion Tablets 2093

Trifluoperazine Hydrochloride (May increase the drowsiness effect). Products include:
- Stelazine 2692

Zolpidem Tartrate (May increase the drowsiness effect). Products include:
- Ambien Tablets 2559

Food Interactions

Alcohol (May increase the drowsiness effect).

DRYSOL SOLUTION
(Aluminum Chloride) 1989
None cited in PDR database.

DULCOLAX SUPPOSITORIES
(Bisacodyl) 883
None cited in PDR database.

DULCOLAX TABLETS
(Bisacodyl) 883
None cited in PDR database.

DUOFILM LIQUID WART REMOVER
(Salicylic Acid) 765
None cited in PDR database.

DUOFILM PATCH WART REMOVER
(Salicylic Acid) 765
None cited in PDR database.

DUOPLANT GEL PLANTAR WART REMOVER
(Salicylic Acid) 765
None cited in PDR database.

DUPHALAC SOLUTION
(Lactulose) 2714
May interact with nonabsorbable antacids. Compounds in this category include:

Aluminum Carbonate (Concurrent use with nonabsorbable antacids may inhibit the desired lactulose-induced drop in colonic pH resulting in possible lack of desired therapeutic effect). Products include:
- Basaljel Capsules 2810
- Basaljel Suspension 2810
- Basaljel Tablets 2810

Aluminum Hydroxide (Concurrent use with nonabsorbable antacids may inhibit the desired lactulose-induced drop in colonic pH resulting in possible lack of desired therapeutic effect). Products include:
- ALternaGEL Liquid 1358
- Maximum Strength Ascriptin .. 650
- Cama Arthritis Pain Reliever .. 748
- Gaviscon Extra Strength Relief Formula Antacid Tablets 778
- Gaviscon Extra Strength Relief Formula Liquid Antacid 779
- Gaviscon Liquid Antacid 779
- Gelusil Antacid-Anti-gas Liquid .. 819
- Gelusil Antacid-Anti-gas Tablets .. 819
- Maalox Antacid/Anti-Gas Tablets .. 889
- Maalox Heartburn Relief Suspension 658
- Maalox Antacid Liquid 888
- Extra Strength Maalox Antacid/Anti-Gas Liquid and Tablets ... 888
- Mylanta 1359
- Tempo Soft Antacid 799

Aluminum Hydroxide Gel (Concurrent use with nonabsorbable antacids may inhibit the desired lactulose-induced drop in colonic pH resulting in possible lack of desired therapeutic effect). Products include:
- ALternaGEL Liquid 675
- Aludrox Oral Suspension 850
- Amphojel Suspension 2802
- Amphojel Suspension without Flavor 2802

- Amphojel Tablets 2802
- Ascriptin 650
- Gaviscon Antacid Tablets 778
- Gaviscon-2 Antacid Tablets 779
- Mylanta Liquid 676
- Mylanta Double Strength Liquid 676
- Nephrox Suspension 671

Calcium Carbonate (Concurrent use with nonabsorbable antacids may inhibit the desired lactulose-induced drop in colonic pH resulting in possible lack of desired therapeutic effect). Products include:
- Alka-Mints Chewable Antacid .. 609
- Alka-Seltzer Fast Relief Caplets .. 610
- Ascriptin 650
- Extra Strength Bayer Plus Aspirin Caplets 617
- Aspirin Regimen Bayer 81 mg Tablets with Calcium 615
- Bufferin Analgesic Tablets 636
- Arthritis Strength Bufferin Analgesic Caplets 637
- Extra Strength Bufferin Analgesic Tablets 637
- Calci-Chew Tablets 2168
- Calci-Mix Capsules 2168
- Caltrate 600 681
- Caltrate PLUS 681
- Caltrate 600 + D 681
- Cotazym Capsules 1866
- Di-Gel Antacid/Anti-Gas 762
- Florical Capsules and Tablets .. 1825
- Gerimed Tablets 1000
- Maalox Antacid Caplets 657
- Marblen 671
- Materna Tablets 1427
- Monocal Tablets 1825
- Mylanta Fast-Acting 1359
- Mylanta Gelcaps Antacid 678
- Mylanta Soothing Lozenges ... 1360
- Mylanta Tablets 677
- Mylanta Double Strength Tablets .. 677
- Nephro-Calci Tablets 2168
- One-A-Day Calcium Plus 625
- Rolaids Antacid Tablets 807
- Rolaids Antacid Calcium Rich/Sodium Free Tablets 807
- Tempo Soft Antacid 799
- Titralac 686
- Titralac Plus 687
- Tums Antacid/Calcium Supplement Tablets 787
- Tums Anti-gas/Antacid Formula Tablets, Assorted Fruit ... 788
- Tums E-X Antacid/Calcium Supplement Tablets 787
- Tums 500 Calcium Supplement .. 788
- Tums ULTRA Antacid/Calcium Supplement Tablets 787
- TYLENOL Headache Plus Pain Reliever with Antacid, Extra Strength Caplets 705

Magnesium Carbonate (Concurrent use with nonabsorbable antacids may inhibit the desired lactulose-induced drop in colonic pH resulting in possible lack of desired therapeutic effect). Products include:
- Bufferin Analgesic Tablets 636
- Arthritis Strength Bufferin Analgesic Caplets 637
- Extra Strength Bufferin Analgesic Tablets 637
- Gaviscon Extra Strength Relief Formula Antacid Tablets 778
- Gaviscon Extra Strength Relief Formula Liquid Antacid 779
- Gaviscon Liquid Antacid 779
- Maalox Antacid Caplets 657
- Maalox Heartburn Relief Suspension 658
- Mag-Carb Capsules 2168
- Marblen 671
- One-A-Day Calcium Plus 625

Magnesium Oxide (Concurrent use with nonabsorbable antacids may inhibit the desired lactulose-induced drop in colonic pH resulting in possible lack of desired therapeutic effect). Products include:
- Beelith Tablets 632
- Bufferin Analgesic Tablets 636
- Arthritis Strength Bufferin Analgesic Caplets 637
- Extra Strength Bufferin Analgesic Tablets 637
- Caltrate PLUS 681

IMPORTANT NOTE: Always consult each drug listing in the patient's regimen for possible interactions.

Duphalac **Interactions Index** 340

Cama Arthritis Pain Reliever ▣ 748
Mag-Ox 400 666
Uro-Mag 666

DURAGESIC TRANSDERMAL SYSTEM
(Fentanyl) 1336
May interact with central nervous system depressants, narcotic analgesics, hypnotics and sedatives, tranquilizers, phenothiazines, antihistamines, and certain other agents. Compounds in these categories include:

Acrivastine (May produce additive depressant effects, hypoventilation, hypotension and profound sedation or coma may occur). Products include:
Semprex-D Capsules 1620

Alfentanil Hydrochloride (May produce additive depressant effects, hypoventilation, hypotension and profound sedation or coma may occur). Products include:
Alfenta Injection 1334

Alprazolam (May produce additive depressant effects, hypoventilation, hypotension and profound sedation or coma may occur). Products include:
Xanax Tablets 2115

Aprobarbital (May produce additive depressant effects, hypoventilation, hypotension and profound sedation or coma may occur).
No products indexed under this heading.

Astemizole (May produce additive depressant effects, hypoventilation, hypotension and profound sedation or coma may occur). Products include:
Hismanal Tablets 1341

Azatadine Maleate (May produce additive depressant effects, hypoventilation, hypotension and profound sedation or coma may occur). Products include:
Trinalin Repetabs Tablets 1373

Bromodiphenhydramine Hydrochloride (May produce additive depressant effects, hypoventilation, hypotension and profound sedation or coma may occur).
No products indexed under this heading.

Brompheniramine Maleate (May produce additive depressant effects, hypoventilation, hypotension and profound sedation or coma may occur). Products include:
Alka-Seltzer Plus Sinus Medicine ▣ 611
Bromfed Capsules (Extended-Release) 1832
Bromfed Syrup ▣ 712
Bromfed Tablets 1832
Bromfed-DM Cough Syrup 1832
Bromfed-PD Capsules (Extended-Release) 1832
Dimetane-DC Cough Syrup 2232
Dimetane-DX Cough Syrup 2233
Dimetapp Allergy Dye-Free Elixir ▣ 838
Dimetapp Allergy Sinus Caplets ▣ 838
Dimetapp Cold & Allergy Chewable Tablets ▣ 838
Dimetapp Cold & Cough Liqui-Gels ▣ 839
Dimetapp Cold & Fever Suspension ▣ 839
Dimetapp DM Elixir ▣ 840
Dimetapp Elixir ▣ 840
Dimetapp Extentabs ▣ 841
Dimetapp Tablets/Liqui-Gels ▣ 841
Rondec Chewable Tablets 974
Vicks DayQuil Allergy Relief 12-Hour Extended Release Tablets ▣ 733
Vicks DayQuil Allergy Relief 4-Hour Tablets ▣ 733

Buprenorphine (May produce additive depressant effects, hypoventilation, hypotension and profound sedation or coma may occur). Products include:
Buprenex Injectable 2170

Buspirone Hydrochloride (May produce additive depressant effects, hypoventilation, hypotension and profound sedation or coma may occur). Products include:
BuSpar Tablets 738

Butabarbital (May produce additive depressant effects, hypoventilation, hypotension and profound sedation or coma may occur).
No products indexed under this heading.

Butalbital (May produce additive depressant effects, hypoventilation, hypotension and profound sedation or coma may occur). Products include:
Axocet Capsules 2469
Esgic-plus Capsules 1012
Esgic-plus Tablets 1012
Fioricet Tablets 2386
Fioricet with Codeine Capsules 2387
Fiorinal Capsules 2388
Fiorinal with Codeine Capsules 2390
Fiorinal Tablets 2388
Phrenilin 790
Sedapap Tablets 50 mg/650 mg 1826

Cetirizine Hydrochloride (May produce additive depressant effects, hypoventilation, hypotension and profound sedation or coma may occur). Products include:
Zyrtec Tablets 2053

Chlordiazepoxide (May produce additive depressant effects, hypoventilation, hypotension and profound sedation or coma may occur). Products include:
Limbitrol 2333

Chlordiazepoxide Hydrochloride (May produce additive depressant effects, hypoventilation, hypotension and profound sedation or coma may occur). Products include:
Librax Capsules 2330
Librium Capsules 2331
Librium Injectable 2332

Chlorpheniramine Maleate (May produce additive depressant effects, hypoventilation, hypotension and profound sedation or coma may occur). Products include:
Alka-Seltzer Plus Cold Medicine ▣ 611
Alka-Seltzer Plus Cold Medicine Liqui-Gels ▣ 612
Alka-Seltzer Plus Cold & Cough Medicine ▣ 611
Alka-Seltzer Plus Cold & Cough Medicine Liqui-Gels ▣ 612
Alka-Seltzer Plus Flu & Body Aches Effervescent Tablets ▣ 612
Allerest Maximum Strength ▣ 649
Allerest Sinus Pain Formula ▣ 649
Ana-Kit Anaphylaxis Emergency Treatment Kit 611
Atrohist Pediatric Capsules 1603
Atrohist Plus Tablets 1605
BC Cold Powder Multi-Symptom Formula (Cold-Sinus-Allergy) ▣ 631
Cerose DM ▣ 853
Cheracol Plus Head Cold/Cough Formula ▣ 741
Children's TYLENOL Cold Multi-Symptom Chewable Tablets and Liquid 1559
Children's TYLENOL Cold Plus Cough Multi Symptom Chewable Tablets and Liquid 1560
Children's TYLENOL Flu Suspension Liquid 1560
Children's Vicks DayQuil Allergy Relief ▣ 730
Children's Vicks NyQuil Cold/Cough Relief ▣ 731
Chlor-Trimeton Allergy Decongestant Tablets ▣ 759
Chlor-Trimeton Allergy Tablets ▣ 758
Allergy-Sinus Comtrex Multi-Symptom Allergy-Sinus Formula Tablets and Caplets ▣ 639
Comtrex Multi-Symptom ▣ 638
Contac Continuous Action Nasal Decongestant/Antihistamine 12 Hour Capsules ▣ 773
Contac Maximum Strength Continuous Action Decongestant/Antihistamine 12 Hour Caplets ▣ 772
Contac Severe Cold and Flu Formula Caplets ▣ 773
Coricidin Cold + Flu Tablets ▣ 760
Coricidin Cough + Cold Tablets ▣ 760
Coricidin 'D' Decongestant Tablets ▣ 760
D.A. II Tablets 972
D.A. Chewable Tablets 970
Dura-Tap/PD Capsules 970
Dura-Vent/DA Tablets 972
Efidac 24 Chlorpheniramine ▣ 655
Extendryl 1003
Fedahist Gyrocaps 2545
Hycomine Compound Tablets 948
Kronofed-A 994
Nolamine Timed-Release Tablets 790
Novahistine Elixir ▣ 782
Ornade Spansule Capsules 2678
PediaCare Cough-Cold Chewable Tablets and Liquid 1569
PediaCare NightRest Cough-Cold Liquid 1569
Pediatric Vicks 44m Cough & Cold Relief ▣ 737
Pyrroxate Caplets ▣ 742
Ryna ▣ 804
Sinarest ▣ 663
Sine-Off Sinus Medicine ▣ 784
Singlet Tablets ▣ 785
Sinulin Tablets 792
Sinutab Sinus Allergy Medication, Maximum Strength Tablets and Caplets ▣ 823
Sudafed Cold & Allergy Tablets ▣ 826
Teldrin 12 Hour Antihistamine/Nasal Decongestant Allergy Relief Capsules ▣ 786
TheraFlu Flu and Cold Medicine ▣ 750
Theraflu Maximum Strength Flu and Cold Medicine For Sore Throat ▣ 751
TheraFlu Flu, Cold and Cough Medicine ▣ 750
TheraFlu Maximum Strength Nighttime Flu, Cold & Cough Medicine ▣ 751
Triaminic Night Time ▣ 754
Triaminic Syrup ▣ 755
Triaminic Triaminicol Cold & Cough ▣ 756
Triaminicin Tablets ▣ 756
Tussend 1830
TYLENOL Allergy Sinus, Maximum Strength Caplets and Gelcaps 1571
TYLENOL Cold Medication, Multi-Symptom Formula Tablets and Caplets 1572
TYLENOL Cold Medication, Multi-Symptom Hot Liquid Packets 1572
Vicks 44 LiquiCaps Cough, Cold & Flu Relief ▣ 728
Vicks 44M Cough, Cold & Flu Relief ▣ 729

Chlorpheniramine Polistirex (May produce additive depressant effects, hypoventilation, hypotension and profound sedation or coma may occur). Products include:
Tussionex Pennkinetic Extended-Release Suspension 1624

Chlorpheniramine Tannate (May produce additive depressant effects, hypoventilation, hypotension and profound sedation or coma may occur). Products include:
Atrohist Pediatric Suspension 1604
Atrohist Pediatric Suspension Dye-Free 1604
Rynatan 2781
Rynatuss 2782

Chlorpromazine (May produce additive depressant effects, hypoventilation, hypotension and profound sedation or coma may occur). Products include:
Thorazine Suppositories 2701

Chlorprothixene (May produce additive depressant effects, hypoventilation, hypotension and profound sedation or coma may occur).
No products indexed under this heading.

Chlorprothixene Hydrochloride (May produce additive depressant effects, hypoventilation, hypotension and profound sedation or coma may occur).
No products indexed under this heading.

Chlorprothixene Lactate (May produce additive depressant effects, hypoventilation, hypotension and profound sedation or coma may occur).
No products indexed under this heading.

Clemastine Fumarate (May produce additive depressant effects, hypoventilation, hypotension and profound sedation or coma may occur). Products include:
Tavist Syrup 2426
Tavist Tablets 2427
Tavist-1 12 Hour Relief Tablets ▣ 749
Tavist-D 12 Hour Relief Tablets ▣ 750

Clorazepate Dipotassium (May produce additive depressant effects, hypoventilation, hypotension and profound sedation or coma may occur). Products include:
Tranxene 459

Clozapine (May produce additive depressant effects, hypoventilation, hypotension and profound sedation or coma may occur). Products include:
Clozaril Tablets 2377

Codeine Phosphate (May produce additive depressant effects, hypoventilation, hypotension and profound sedation or coma may occur). Products include:
Brontex 2130
Dimetane-DC Cough Syrup 2232
Fioricet with Codeine Capsules 2387
Fiorinal with Codeine Capsules 2390
Nucofed 2225
Phenergan with Codeine 2883
Phenergan VC with Codeine 2888
Robitussin A-C Syrup 2248
Robitussin-DAC Syrup 2249
Ryna ▣ 804
Soma Compound w/Codeine Tablets 2784
Tylenol with Codeine 1592

Cyproheptadine Hydrochloride (May produce additive depressant effects, hypoventilation, hypotension and profound sedation or coma may occur). Products include:
Periactin 1767

Desflurane (May produce additive depressant effects, hypoventilation, hypotension and profound sedation or coma may occur). Products include:
Suprane (desflurane, USP) 1865

Dexchlorpheniramine Maleate (May produce additive depressant effects, hypoventilation, hypotension and profound sedation or coma may occur).
No products indexed under this heading.

Dezocine (May produce additive depressant effects, hypoventilation, hypotension and profound sedation or coma may occur). Products include:
Dalgan Injection 529

(▣ Described in PDR For Nonprescription Drugs) (◉ Described in PDR For Ophthalmology)

Diazepam (May produce additive depressant effects, hypoventilation, hypotension and profound sedation or coma may occur). Products include:
- Dizac (diazepam injectable emulsion) CIV 1862
- Valium Injectable 2336
- Valium Tablets 2335

Diphenhydramine Citrate (May produce additive depressant effects, hypoventilation, hypotension and profound sedation or coma may occur). Products include:
- Excedrin P.M. Analgesic/Sleeping Aid Tablets, Caplets, Liquigels 735

Diphenhydramine Hydrochloride (May produce additive depressant effects, hypoventilation, hypotension and profound sedation or coma may occur). Products include:
- Actifed Allergy Daytime/Nighttime Caplets 808
- Actifed Sinus Daytime/Nighttime Tablets and Caplets 809
- Extra Strength Bayer PM Aspirin Plus Sleep Aid 617
- Benadryl Allergy Chewables 811
- Benadryl Allergy/Cold Tablets 811
- Benadryl Allergy Decongestant Liquid Medication 812
- Benadryl Allergy Decongestant Tablets 812
- Benadryl Allergy Liquid Medication 813
- Benadryl Allergy 811
- Benadryl Allergy Sinus Headache Caplets 813
- Benadryl Dye-Free Allergy Liquigel Softgels 813
- Benadryl Dye-Free Allergy Liquid Medication 814
- Benadryl Itch Relief Stick Extra Strength 814
- Benadryl Cream 814
- Benadryl Gel 815
- Benadryl Spray 815
- Benadryl Injection 1955
- Contac Day & Night Cold/Flu Night Caplets 772
- Contac Night Allergy/Sinus Caplets 771
- Extra Strength Doan's P.M. 653
- Excedrin P.M. Analgesic/Sleeping Aid Tablets, Caplets, Liquigels 643
- Nytol QuickCaps Caplets 632
- Sleepinal Night-time Sleep Aid Capsules and Softgels 798
- TYLENOL Allergy Sinus NightTime, Maximum Strength Caplets 1571
- TYLENOL Flu NightTime, Maximum Strength Gelcaps 1575
- TYLENOL Flu NightTime, Maximum Strength Hot Medication Packets 1575
- TYLENOL PM Pain Reliever/Sleep Aid, Extra Strength Gelcaps, Caplets, Geltabs 1576
- TYLENOL Severe Allergy Medication Caplets 1571
- Maximum Strength Unisom Sleepgels 1990
- Unisom With Pain Relief-Nighttime Sleep Aid and Pain Reliever 1991

Droperidol (May produce additive depressant effects, hypoventilation, hypotension and profound sedation or coma may occur). Products include:
- Inapsine Injection 462

Enflurane (May produce additive depressant effects, hypoventilation, hypotension and profound sedation or coma may occur).
- No products indexed under this heading.

Estazolam (May produce additive depressant effects, hypoventilation, hypotension and profound sedation or coma may occur). Products include:
- ProSom Tablets 457

Ethchlorvynol (May produce additive depressant effects, hypoventilation, hypotension and profound sedation or coma may occur). Products include:
- Placidyl Capsules 456

Ethinamate (May produce additive depressant effects, hypoventilation, hypotension and profound sedation or coma may occur).
- No products indexed under this heading.

Fentanyl Citrate (May produce additive depressant effects, hypoventilation, hypotension and profound sedation or coma may occur). Products include:
- Sublimaze Injection 463

Fluphenazine Decanoate (May produce additive depressant effects, hypoventilation, hypotension and profound sedation or coma may occur). Products include:
- Prolixin Decanoate 510

Fluphenazine Enanthate (May produce additive depressant effects, hypoventilation, hypotension and profound sedation or coma may occur). Products include:
- Prolixin Enanthate 510

Fluphenazine Hydrochloride (May produce additive depressant effects, hypoventilation, hypotension and profound sedation or coma may occur). Products include:
- Prolixin 510

Flurazepam Hydrochloride (May produce additive depressant effects, hypoventilation, hypotension and profound sedation or coma may occur). Products include:
- Dalmane Capsules 2329

Glutethimide (May produce additive depressant effects, hypoventilation, hypotension and profound sedation or coma may occur).
- No products indexed under this heading.

Haloperidol (May produce additive depressant effects, hypoventilation, hypotension and profound sedation or coma may occur). Products include:
- Haldol Injection, Tablets and Concentrate 1585

Haloperidol Decanoate (May produce additive depressant effects, hypoventilation, hypotension and profound sedation or coma may occur). Products include:
- Haldol Decanoate 1587

Hydrocodone Bitartrate (May produce additive depressant effects, hypoventilation, hypotension and profound sedation or coma may occur). Products include:
- Codiclear DH Syrup 808
- Duratuss HD Elixir 2750
- Histussin D Liquid 670
- Hycodan Tablets and Syrup 946
- Hycomine Compound Tablets 948
- Hycomine 947
- Hycotuss Expectorant Syrup 950
- Hydrocet Capsules 787
- Lorcet 10/650 Tablets 1016
- Lortab 2751
- Tussend 1830
- Tussend Expectorant 1831
- Vicodin Tablets 1404
- Vicodin ES Tablets 1405
- Vicodin HP Tablets 1403
- Vicodin Tuss Expectorant 1406
- Zydone Capsules 967

Hydrocodone Polistirex (May produce additive depressant effects, hypoventilation, hypotension and profound sedation or coma may occur). Products include:
- Tussionex Pennkinetic Extended-Release Suspension 1624

Hydromorphone Hydrochloride (May produce additive depressant effects, hypoventilation, hypotension and profound sedation or coma may occur). Products include:
- Dilaudid Ampules 1382
- Dilaudid Cough Syrup 1383
- Dilaudid-HP Injection 1384
- Dilaudid-HP Lyophilized Powder 250 mg 1384
- Dilaudid 1382
- Dilaudid Oral Liquid 1386
- Dilaudid 1382
- Dilaudid Tablets - 8 mg 1386

Hydroxyzine Hydrochloride (May produce additive depressant effects, hypoventilation, hypotension and profound sedation or coma may occur). Products include:
- Atarax Tablets & Syrup 1992
- Marax Tablets & DF Syrup 2015
- Vistaril Intramuscular Solution 2042

Isoflurane (May produce additive depressant effects, hypoventilation, hypotension and profound sedation or coma may occur).
- No products indexed under this heading.

Ketamine Hydrochloride (May produce additive depressant effects, hypoventilation, hypotension and profound sedation or coma may occur).
- No products indexed under this heading.

Levomethadyl Acetate Hydrochloride (May produce additive depressant effects, hypoventilation, hypotension and profound sedation or coma may occur). Products include:
- Orlaam Oral Solution 2361

Levorphanol Tartrate (May produce additive depressant effects, hypoventilation, hypotension and profound sedation or coma may occur). Products include:
- Levo-Dromoran 2297

Loratadine (May produce additive depressant effects, hypoventilation, hypotension and profound sedation or coma may occur). Products include:
- Claritin Tablets 2485
- Claritin-D Tablets 2487

Lorazepam (May produce additive depressant effects, hypoventilation, hypotension and profound sedation or coma may occur). Products include:
- Ativan Injection 2805
- Ativan Tablets 2807

Loxapine Hydrochloride (May produce additive depressant effects, hypoventilation, hypotension and profound sedation or coma may occur). Products include:
- Loxitane 1426

Loxapine Succinate (May produce additive depressant effects, hypoventilation, hypotension and profound sedation or coma may occur). Products include:
- Loxitane Capsules 1426

Meperidine Hydrochloride (May produce additive depressant effects, hypoventilation, hypotension and profound sedation or coma may occur). Products include:
- Demerol 2438
- Mepergan Injection 2859

Mephobarbital (May produce additive depressant effects, hypoventilation, hypotension and profound sedation or coma may occur). Products include:
- Mebaral Tablets 2452

Meprobamate (May produce additive depressant effects, hypoventilation, hypotension and profound sedation or coma may occur). Products include:
- Miltown Tablets 2780
- PMB 200 and PMB 400 2890

Mesoridazine Besylate (May produce additive depressant effects, hypoventilation, hypotension and profound sedation or coma may occur). Products include:
- Serentil 689

Methadone Hydrochloride (May produce additive depressant effects, hypoventilation, hypotension and profound sedation or coma may occur). Products include:
- Methadone Hydrochloride Oral Concentrate 2356
- Methadone Hydrochloride Oral Solution & Tablets 2357

Methdilazine Hydrochloride (May produce additive depressant effects, hypoventilation, hypotension and profound sedation or coma may occur).
- No products indexed under this heading.

Methohexital Sodium (May produce additive depressant effects, hypoventilation, hypotension and profound sedation or coma may occur).
- No products indexed under this heading.

Methotrimeprazine (May produce additive depressant effects, hypoventilation, hypotension and profound sedation or coma may occur). Products include:
- Levoprome 1321

Methoxyflurane (May produce additive depressant effects, hypoventilation, hypotension and profound sedation or coma may occur).
- No products indexed under this heading.

Midazolam Hydrochloride (May produce additive depressant effects, hypoventilation, hypotension and profound sedation or coma may occur). Products include:
- Versed Injection 2324

Molindone Hydrochloride (May produce additive depressant effects, hypoventilation, hypotension and profound sedation or coma may occur). Products include:
- Moban Tablets and Concentrate 1036

Morphine Sulfate (May produce additive depressant effects, hypoventilation, hypotension and profound sedation or coma may occur). Products include:
- Astramorph/PF Injection, USP (Preservative-Free) 526
- Duramorph Injection 983
- Infumorph 200 and Infumorph 500 Sterile Solutions 985
- Kadian Capsules 2948
- MS Contin Tablets 2149
- MSIR 2152
- Oramorph SR (Morphine Sulfate Sustained Release Tablets) 2359
- RMS Suppositories CII 2766
- Roxanol 2365

Opium Alkaloids (May produce additive depressant effects, hypoventilation, hypotension and profound sedation or coma may occur).
- No products indexed under this heading.

Oxazepam (May produce additive depressant effects, hypoventilation, hypotension and profound sedation or coma may occur). Products include:
- Serax Capsules 2916
- Serax Tablets 2916

IMPORTANT NOTE: Always consult each drug listing in the patient's regimen for possible interactions.

Duragesic | Interactions Index | 342

Oxycodone Hydrochloride (May produce additive depressant effects, hypoventilation, hypotension and profound sedation or coma may occur). Products include:
- OxyContin Tablets ... 2163
- OxyIR Capsules ... 2167
- Percocet Tablets ... 955
- Percodan Tablets ... 955
- Percodan-Demi Tablets ... 956
- Roxicodone Tablets, Oral Solution & Intensol (Oxycodone) ... 2366
- Tylox Capsules ... 1593

Pentobarbital Sodium (May produce additive depressant effects, hypoventilation, hypotension and profound sedation or coma may occur). Products include:
- Nembutal Sodium Capsules ... 440
- Nembutal Sodium Solution ... 442
- Nembutal Sodium Suppositories ... 444

Perphenazine (May produce additive depressant effects, hypoventilation, hypotension and profound sedation or coma may occur). Products include:
- Etrafon ... 2495
- Triavil Tablets ... 1800
- Trilafon ... 2532

Phenobarbital (May produce additive depressant effects, hypoventilation, hypotension and profound sedation or coma may occur). Products include:
- Arco-Lase Plus Tablets ... 513
- Bellergal-S Tablets ... 2375
- Donnatal ... 2234
- Donnatal Extentabs ... 2234
- Donnatal Tablets ... 2234
- Phenobarbital Elixir and Tablets ... 1523
- Quadrinal Tablets ... 1398

Prazepam (May produce additive depressant effects, hypoventilation, hypotension and profound sedation or coma may occur).
- No products indexed under this heading.

Prochlorperazine (May produce additive depressant effects, hypoventilation, hypotension and profound sedation or coma may occur). Products include:
- Compazine ... 2644

Promethazine Hydrochloride (May produce additive depressant effects, hypoventilation, hypotension and profound sedation or coma may occur). Products include:
- Mepergan Injection ... 2859
- Phenergan with Codeine ... 2883
- Phenergan with Dextromethorphan 2885
- Phenergan Injection ... 2880
- Phenergan Suppositories ... 2882
- Phenergan Syrup ... 2881
- Phenergan Tablets ... 2882
- Phenergan VC ... 2886
- Phenergan VC with Codeine ... 2888

Propofol (May produce additive depressant effects, hypoventilation, hypotension and profound sedation or coma may occur). Products include:
- Diprivan Injectable Emulsion ... 2939

Propoxyphene Hydrochloride (May produce additive depressant effects, hypoventilation, hypotension and profound sedation or coma may occur). Products include:
- Darvon ... 1475
- Wygesic Tablets ... 2930

Propoxyphene Napsylate (May produce additive depressant effects, hypoventilation, hypotension and profound sedation or coma may occur). Products include:
- Darvon-N/Darvocet-N ... 1473

Pyrilamine Maleate (May produce additive depressant effects, hypoventilation, hypotension and profound sedation or coma may occur). Products include:
- 4-Way Fast Acting Nasal Spray (regular & mentholated) ... ◘ 644
- Maximum Strength Multi-Symptom Formula Midol ... ◘ 621
- PMS Multi-Symptom Formula Midol ... ◘ 622

Pyrilamine Tannate (May produce additive depressant effects, hypoventilation, hypotension and profound sedation or coma may occur). Products include:
- Atrohist Pediatric Suspension ... 1604
- Atrohist Pediatric Suspension Dye-Free ... 1604
- Rynatan ... 2781

Quazepam (May produce additive depressant effects, hypoventilation, hypotension and profound sedation or coma may occur). Products include:
- Doral Tablets ... 2773

Risperidone (May produce additive depressant effects, hypoventilation, hypotension and profound sedation or coma may occur). Products include:
- Risperdal Tablets ... 1348

Secobarbital Sodium (May produce additive depressant effects, hypoventilation, hypotension and profound sedation or coma may occur). Products include:
- Seconal Sodium Pulvules ... 1529

Sevoflurane (May produce additive depressant effects, hypoventilation, hypotension and profound sedation or coma may occur).
- No products indexed under this heading.

Sufentanil Citrate (May produce additive depressant effects, hypoventilation, hypotension and profound sedation or coma may occur). Products include:
- Sufenta Injection ... 1355

Temazepam (May produce additive depressant effects, hypoventilation, hypotension and profound sedation or coma may occur). Products include:
- Restoril Capsules ... 2413

Terfenadine (May produce additive depressant effects, hypoventilation, hypotension and profound sedation or coma may occur). Products include:
- Seldane Tablets ... 1284
- Seldane-D Extended-Release Tablets ... 1286

Thiamylal Sodium (May produce additive depressant effects, hypoventilation, hypotension and profound sedation or coma may occur).
- No products indexed under this heading.

Thioridazine Hydrochloride (May produce additive depressant effects, hypoventilation, hypotension and profound sedation or coma may occur). Products include:
- Mellaril ... 2398

Thiothixene (May produce additive depressant effects, hypoventilation, hypotension and profound sedation or coma may occur). Products include:
- Navane Capsules and Concentrate 2018
- Navane Intramuscular ... 2019

Triazolam (May produce additive depressant effects, hypoventilation, hypotension and profound sedation or coma may occur). Products include:
- Halcion Tablets ... 2093

Trifluoperazine Hydrochloride (May produce additive depressant effects, hypoventilation, hypotension and profound sedation or coma may occur). Products include:
- Stelazine ... 2692

Trimeprazine Tartrate (May produce additive depressant effects, hypoventilation, hypotension and profound sedation or coma may occur).
- No products indexed under this heading.

Tripelennamine Hydrochloride (May produce additive depressant effects, hypoventilation, hypotension and profound sedation or coma may occur). Products include:
- PBZ Tablets ... 863
- PBZ-SR Tablets ... 862

Triprolidine Hydrochloride (May produce additive depressant effects, hypoventilation, hypotension and profound sedation or coma may occur). Products include:
- Actifed Cold & Allergy Tablets ... ◘ 807
- Actifed Cold & Sinus Caplets and Tablets ... ◘ 808

Zolpidem Tartrate (May produce additive depressant effects, hypoventilation, hypotension and profound sedation or coma may occur). Products include:
- Ambien Tablets ... 2559

Food Interactions

Alcohol (May produce additive depressant effects).

DURAMORPH INJECTION (Morphine Sulfate) ... 983

May interact with hypnotics and sedatives, monoamine oxidase inhibitors, tricyclic antidepressants, butyrophenones, anticoagulants, antihistamines, psychotropics, phenothiazines, antipsychotic agents, and certain other agents. Compounds in these categories include:

Acrivastine (Potentiation of depressant effect). Products include:
- Semprex-D Capsules ... 1620

Alfentanil Hydrochloride (Potentiation of depressant effect). Products include:
- Alfenta Injection ... 1334

Alprazolam (Potentiation of depressant effect). Products include:
- Xanax Tablets ... 2115

Amitriptyline Hydrochloride (Potentiation of depressant effect). Products include:
- Elavil ... 2945
- Etrafon ... 2495
- Limbitrol ... 2333
- Triavil Tablets ... 1800

Amoxapine (Potentiation of depressant effect). Products include:
- Asendin Tablets ... 1419

Aprobarbital (Potentiation of depressant effect).
- No products indexed under this heading.

Astemizole (Potentiation of depressant effect). Products include:
- Hismanal Tablets ... 1341

Azatadine Maleate (Potentiation of depressant effect). Products include:
- Trinalin Repetabs Tablets ... 1373

Bromodiphenhydramine Hydrochloride (Potentiation of depressant effect).
- No products indexed under this heading.

Brompheniramine Maleate (Potentiation of depressant effect). Products include:
- Alka-Seltzer Plus Sinus Medicine .. ◘ 611
- Bromfed Capsules (Extended-Release) ... 1832
- Bromfed Syrup ... ◘ 712
- Bromfed Tablets ... 1832
- Bromfed-DM Cough Syrup ... 1832
- Bromfed-PD Capsules (Extended-Release) ... 1832
- Dimetane-DC Cough Syrup ... 2232
- Dimetane-DX Cough Syrup ... 2233
- Dimetapp Allergy Dye-Free Elixir ... ◘ 838
- Dimetapp Allergy Sinus Caplets ... ◘ 838
- Dimetapp Cold & Allergy Chewable Tablets ... ◘ 838
- Dimetapp Cold & Cough Liqui-Gels ... ◘ 839
- Dimetapp Cold & Fever Suspension ... ◘ 839
- Dimetapp DM Elixir ... ◘ 840
- Dimetapp Elixir ... ◘ 840
- Dimetapp Extentabs ... ◘ 841
- Dimetapp Tablets/Liqui-Gels ... ◘ 841
- Rondec Chewable Tablets ... 974
- Vicks DayQuil Allergy Relief 12-Hour Extended Release Tablets .. ◘ 733
- Vicks DayQuil Allergy Relief 4-Hour Tablets ... ◘ 733

Buprenorphine (Potentiation of depressant effect). Products include:
- Buprenex Injectable ... 2170

Buspirone Hydrochloride (Potentiation of depressant effect). Products include:
- BuSpar Tablets ... 738

Butabarbital (Potentiation of depressant effect).
- No products indexed under this heading.

Butalbital (Potentiation of depressant effect). Products include:
- Axocet Capsules ... 2469
- Esgic-plus Capsules ... 1012
- Esgic-plus Tablets ... 1012
- Fioricet Tablets ... 2386
- Fioricet with Codeine Capsules ... 2387
- Fiorinal Capsules ... 2388
- Fiorinal with Codeine Capsules ... 2390
- Fiorinal Tablets ... 2388
- Phrenilin ... 790
- Sedapap Tablets 50 mg/650 mg .. 1826

Cetirizine Hydrochloride (Potentiation of depressant effect). Products include:
- Zyrtec Tablets ... 2053

Chlordiazepoxide (Potentiation of depressant effect). Products include:
- Limbitrol ... 2333

Chlordiazepoxide Hydrochloride (Potentiation of depressant effect). Products include:
- Librax Capsules ... 2330
- Librium Capsules ... 2331
- Librium Injectable ... 2332

Chlorpheniramine Maleate (Potentiation of depressant effect). Products include:
- Alka-Seltzer Plus Cold Medicine ... ◘ 611
- Alka-Seltzer Plus Cold Medicine Liqui-Gels ... ◘ 612
- Alka-Seltzer Plus Cold & Cough Medicine ... ◘ 611
- Alka-Seltzer Plus Cold & Cough Medicine Liqui-Gels ... ◘ 612
- Alka-Seltzer Plus Flu & Body Aches Effervescent Tablets ... ◘ 612
- Allerest Maximum Strength ... ◘ 649
- Allerest Sinus Pain Formula ... ◘ 649
- Ana-Kit Anaphylaxis Emergency Treatment Kit ... 611
- Atrohist Pediatric Capsules ... 1603
- Atrohist Plus Tablets ... 1605
- BC Cold Powder Multi-Symptom Formula (Cold-Sinus-Allergy) ... ◘ 631
- Cerose DM ... ◘ 853
- Cheracol Plus Head Cold/Cough Formula ... ◘ 741
- Children's TYLENOL Cold Multi-Symptom Chewable Tablets and Liquid ... 1559
- Children's TYLENOL Cold Plus Cough Multi Symptom Chewable Tablets and Liquid ... 1560
- Children's TYLENOL Flu Suspension Liquid ... 1560
- Children's Vicks DayQuil Allergy Relief ... ◘ 730

(◘ Described in PDR For Nonprescription Drugs) (◉ Described in PDR For Ophthalmology)

Interactions Index

Children's Vicks NyQuil Cold/Cough Relief ... 731
Chlor-Trimeton Allergy Decongestant Tablets ... 759
Chlor-Trimeton Allergy Tablets ... 758
Allergy-Sinus Comtrex Multi-Symptom Allergy-Sinus Formula Tablets and Caplets ... 639
Comtrex Multi-Symptom ... 638
Contac Continuous Action Nasal Decongestant/Antihistamine 12 Hour Capsules ... 773
Contac Maximum Strength Continuous Action Decongestant/Antihistamine 12 Hour Caplets ... 772
Contac Severe Cold and Flu Formula Caplets ... 773
Coricidin Cold + Flu Tablets ... 760
Coricidin Cough + Cold Tablets ... 760
Coricidin 'D' Decongestant Tablets ... 760
D.A. II Tablets ... 972
D.A. Chewable Tablets ... 970
Dura-Tap/PD Capsules ... 970
Dura-Vent/DA Tablets ... 972
Efidac 24 Chlorpheniramine ... 655
Extendryl ... 1003
Fedahist Gyrocaps ... 2545
Hycomine Compound Tablets ... 948
Kronofed-A ... 994
Nolamine Timed-Release Tablets ... 790
Novahistine Elixir ... 782
Ornade Spansule Capsules ... 2678
PediaCare Cough-Cold Chewable Tablets and Liquid ... 1569
PediaCare NightRest Cough-Cold Liquid ... 1569
Pediatric Vicks 44m Cough & Cold Relief ... 737
Pyrroxate Caplets ... 742
Ryna ... 804
Sinarest ... 663
Sine-Off Sinus Medicine ... 784
Singlet Tablets ... 785
Sinulin Tablets ... 792
Sinutab Sinus Allergy Medication, Maximum Strength Tablets and Caplets ... 823
Sudafed Cold & Allergy Tablets ... 826
Teldrin 12 Hour Antihistamine/Nasal Decongestant Allergy Relief Capsules ... 786
TheraFlu Flu and Cold Medicine ... 750
TheraFlu Maximum Strength Flu and Cold Medicine For Sore Throat ... 751
TheraFlu Flu, Cold and Cough Medicine ... 750
TheraFlu Maximum Strength Nighttime Flu, Cold & Cough Medicine ... 751
Triaminic Night Time ... 754
Triaminic Syrup ... 755
Triaminic Triaminicol Cold & Cough ... 756
Triaminicin Tablets ... 756
Tussend ... 1830
TYLENOL Allergy Sinus, Maximum Strength Caplets and Gelcaps ... 1571
TYLENOL Cold Medication, Multi-Symptom Formula Tablets and Caplets ... 1572
TYLENOL Cold Medication, Multi-Symptom Hot Liquid Packets ... 1572
Vicks 44 LiquiCaps Cough, Cold & Flu Relief ... 728
Vicks 44M Cough, Cold & Flu Relief ... 729

Chlorpheniramine Polistirex (Potentiation of depressant effect). Products include:
Tussionex Pennkinetic Extended-Release Suspension ... 1624

Chlorpheniramine Tannate (Potentiation of depressant effect). Products include:
Atrohist Pediatric Suspension ... 1604
Atrohist Pediatric Suspension Dye-Free ... 1604
Rynatan ... 2781
Rynatuss ... 2782

Chlorpromazine (Potentiation of depressant effect; increased risk of respiratory depression). Products include:
Thorazine Suppositories ... 2701

Chlorpromazine Hydrochloride (Potentiation of depressant effect; increased risk of respiratory depression). Products include:
Thorazine ... 2701

Chlorprothixene (Potentiation of depressant effect; increased risk of respiratory depression).
No products indexed under this heading.

Chlorprothixene Hydrochloride (Potentiation of depressant effect; increased risk of respiratory depression).
No products indexed under this heading.

Clemastine Fumarate (Potentiation of depressant effect). Products include:
Tavist Syrup ... 2426
Tavist Tablets ... 2427
Tavist-1 12 Hour Relief Tablets ... 749
Tavist-D 12 Hour Relief Tablets ... 750

Clomipramine Hydrochloride (Potentiation of depressant effect). Products include:
Anafranil Capsules ... 819

Clorazepate Dipotassium (Potentiation of depressant effect). Products include:
Tranxene ... 459

Clozapine (Potentiation of depressant effect; increased risk of respiratory depression). Products include:
Clozaril Tablets ... 2377

Codeine Phosphate (Potentiation of depressant effect). Products include:
Brontex ... 2130
Dimetane-DC Cough Syrup ... 2232
Fioricet with Codeine Capsules ... 2387
Fiorinal with Codeine Capsules ... 2390
Nucofed ... 2225
Phenergan with Codeine ... 2883
Phenergan VC with Codeine ... 2888
Robitussin A-C Syrup ... 2248
Robitussin-DAC Syrup ... 2249
Ryna ... 804
Soma Compound w/Codeine Tablets ... 2784
Tylenol with Codeine ... 1592

Cyproheptadine Hydrochloride (Potentiation of depressant effect). Products include:
Periactin ... 1767

Dalteparin Sodium (Concurrent use by epidural or intrathecal route is contraindicated with anticoagulant therapy). Products include:
Fragmin Injection ... 2088

Desipramine Hydrochloride (Potentiation of depressant effect). Products include:
Norpramin Tablets ... 1273

Dexchlorpheniramine Maleate (Potentiation of depressant effect).
No products indexed under this heading.

Diazepam (Potentiation of depressant effect). Products include:
Dizac (diazepam injectable emulsion) CIV ... 1862
Valium Injectable ... 2336
Valium Tablets ... 2335

Dicumarol (Concurrent use by epidural or intrathecal route is contraindicated with anticoagulant therapy).
No products indexed under this heading.

Diphenhydramine Citrate (Potentiation of depressant effect). Products include:
Excedrin P.M. Analgesic/Sleeping Aid Tablets, Caplets, Liquigels ... 735

Diphenhydramine Hydrochloride (Potentiation of depressant effect). Products include:
Actifed Allergy Daytime/Nighttime Caplets ... 808
Actifed Sinus Daytime/Nighttime Tablets and Caplets ... 809
Extra Strength Bayer PM Aspirin Plus Sleep Aid ... 617
Benadryl Allergy Chewables ... 811
Benadryl Allergy/Cold Tablets ... 811
Benadryl Allergy Decongestant Liquid Medication ... 812
Benadryl Allergy Decongestant Tablets ... 812
Benadryl Allergy Liquid Medication ... 813
Benadryl Allergy ... 811
Benadryl Allergy Sinus Headache Caplets ... 813
Benadryl Dye-Free Allergy Liquigel Softgels ... 813
Benadryl Dye-Free Allergy Liquid Medication ... 814
Benadryl Itch Relief Stick Extra Strength ... 814
Benadryl Cream ... 814
Benadryl Gel ... 815
Benadryl Spray ... 815
Benadryl Injection ... 1955
Contac Day & Night Cold/Flu Night Caplets ... 772
Contac Night Allergy/Sinus Caplets ... 771
Extra Strength Doan's P.M. ... 653
Excedrin P.M. Analgesic/Sleeping Aid Tablets, Caplets, Liquigels ... 643
Nytol QuickCaps Caplets ... 632
Sleepinal Night-time Sleep Aid Capsules and Softgels ... 798
TYLENOL Allergy Sinus NightTime, Maximum Strength Caplets ... 1571
TYLENOL Flu NightTime, Maximum Strength Gelcaps ... 1575
TYLENOL Flu NightTime, Maximum Strength Hot Medication Packets ... 1575
TYLENOL PM Pain Reliever/Sleep Aid, Extra Strength Gelcaps, Caplets, Geltabs ... 1576
TYLENOL Severe Allergy Medication Caplets ... 1571
Maximum Strength Unisom Sleepgels ... 1990
Unisom With Pain Relief-Nighttime Sleep Aid and Pain Reliever ... 1991

Diphenylpyraline Hydrochloride (Potentiation of depressant effect).
No products indexed under this heading.

Doxepin Hydrochloride (Potentiation of depressant effect). Products include:
Adapin Capsules ... 1542
Sinequan ... 2028
Zonalon Cream ... 1042

Droperidol (Potentiation of depressant effect). Products include:
Inapsine Injection ... 462

Enflurane (Potentiation of depressant effect).
No products indexed under this heading.

Enoxaparin (Concurrent use by epidural or intrathecal route is contraindicated with anticoagulant therapy). Products include:
Lovenox Injection ... 2187

Estazolam (Potentiation of depressant effect). Products include:
ProSom Tablets ... 457

Ethchlorvynol (Potentiation of depressant effect). Products include:
Placidyl Capsules ... 456

Ethinamate (Potentiation of depressant effect).
No products indexed under this heading.

Fentanyl Citrate (Potentiation of depressant effect). Products include:
Sublimaze Injection ... 463

Fluphenazine Decanoate (Potentiation of depressant effect; increased risk of respiratory depression). Products include:
Prolixin Decanoate ... 510

Fluphenazine Enanthate (Potentiation of depressant effect; increased risk of respiratory depression). Products include:
Prolixin Enanthate ... 510

Fluphenazine Hydrochloride (Potentiation of depressant effect; increased risk of respiratory depression). Products include:
Prolixin ... 510

Flurazepam Hydrochloride (Potentiation of depressant effect). Products include:
Dalmane Capsules ... 2329

Furazolidone (Potentiation of depressant effect). Products include:
Furoxone ... 2221

Glutethimide (Potentiation of depressant effect).
No products indexed under this heading.

Haloperidol (Potentiation of depressant effect; increased risk of respiratory depression). Products include:
Haldol Injection, Tablets and Concentrate ... 1585

Haloperidol Decanoate (Potentiation of depressant effect; increased risk of respiratory depression). Products include:
Haldol Decanoate ... 1587

Heparin Calcium (Concurrent use by epidural or intrathecal route is contraindicated with anticoagulant therapy).
No products indexed under this heading.

Heparin Sodium (Concurrent use by epidural or intrathecal route is contraindicated with anticoagulant therapy). Products include:
Heparin Lock Flush Solution ... 2831
Heparin Sodium Injection ... 2832
Heparin Sodium Vials ... 1486

Hydrocodone Bitartrate (Potentiation of depressant effect). Products include:
Codiclear DH Syrup ... 808
Duratuss HD Elixir ... 2750
Histussin D Liquid ... 670
Hycodan Tablets and Syrup ... 946
Hycomine Compound Tablets ... 948
Hycomine ... 947
Hycotuss Expectorant Syrup ... 950
Hydrocet Capsules ... 787
Lorcet 10/650 Tablets ... 1016
Lortab ... 2751
Tussend ... 1830
Tussend Expectorant ... 1831
Vicodin Tablets ... 1404
Vicodin ES Tablets ... 1405
Vicodin HP Tablets ... 1403
Vicodin Tuss Expectorant ... 1406
Zydone Capsules ... 967

Hydrocodone Polistirex (Potentiation of depressant effect). Products include:
Tussionex Pennkinetic Extended-Release Suspension ... 1624

Hydroxyzine Hydrochloride (Potentiation of depressant effect). Products include:
Atarax Tablets & Syrup ... 1992
Marax Tablets & DF Syrup ... 2015
Vistaril Intramuscular Solution ... 2042

Imipramine Hydrochloride (Potentiation of depressant effect). Products include:
Tofranil Ampuls ... 873
Tofranil Tablets ... 875

Imipramine Pamoate (Potentiation of depressant effect). Products include:
Tofranil-PM Capsules ... 876

Isocarboxazid (Potentiation of depressant effect).
No products indexed under this heading.

IMPORTANT NOTE: Always consult each drug listing in the patient's regimen for possible interactions.

Duramorph — **Interactions Index** — 344

Isoflurane (Potentiation of depressant effect).
  No products indexed under this heading.
Ketamine Hydrochloride (Potentiation of depressant effect).
  No products indexed under this heading.
Levorphanol Tartrate (Potentiation of depressant effect). Products include:
  Levo-Dromoran 2297
Lithium Carbonate (Potentiation of depressant effect; increased risk of respiratory depression). Products include:
  Eskalith 2658
  Lithium Carbonate Capsules & Tablets 2352
  Lithonate/Lithotabs/Lithobid 2721
Lithium Citrate (Potentiation of depressant effect; increased risk of respiratory depression).
  No products indexed under this heading.
Loratadine (Potentiation of depressant effect). Products include:
  Claritin Tablets 2485
  Claritin-D Tablets 2487
Lorazepam (Potentiation of depressant effect). Products include:
  Ativan Injection 2805
  Ativan Tablets 2807
Loxapine Hydrochloride (Potentiation of depressant effect; increased risk of respiratory depression). Products include:
  Loxitane 1426
Loxapine Succinate (Potentiation of depressant effect; increased risk of respiratory depression). Products include:
  Loxitane Capsules 1426
Maprotiline Hydrochloride (Potentiation of depressant effect). Products include:
  Ludiomil Tablets 861
Meperidine Hydrochloride (Potentiation of depressant effect). Products include:
  Demerol 2438
  Mepergan Injection 2859
Mephobarbital (Potentiation of depressant effect). Products include:
  Mebaral Tablets 2452
Meprobamate (Potentiation of depressant effect). Products include:
  Miltown Tablets 2780
  PMB 200 and PMB 400 2890
Mesoridazine Besylate (Potentiation of depressant effect; increased risk of respiratory depression). Products include:
  Serentil 689
Methadone Hydrochloride (Potentiation of depressant effect). Products include:
  Methadone Hydrochloride Oral Concentrate 2356
  Methadone Hydrochloride Oral Solution & Tablets 2357
Methdilazine Hydrochloride (Potentiation of depressant effect).
  No products indexed under this heading.
Methohexital Sodium (Potentiation of depressant effect).
  No products indexed under this heading.
Methotrimeprazine (Potentiation of depressant effect; increased risk of respiratory depression). Products include:
  Levoprome 1321
Methoxyflurane (Potentiation of depressant effect).
  No products indexed under this heading.

Midazolam Hydrochloride (Potentiation of depressant effect). Products include:
  Versed Injection 2324
Molindone Hydrochloride (Potentiation of depressant effect; increased risk of respiratory depression). Products include:
  Moban Tablets and Concentrate 1036
Nortriptyline Hydrochloride (Potentiation of depressant effect). Products include:
  Pamelor 2409
Opium Alkaloids (Potentiation of depressant effect).
  No products indexed under this heading.
Oxazepam (Potentiation of depressant effect). Products include:
  Serax Capsules 2916
  Serax Tablets 2916
Oxycodone Hydrochloride (Potentiation of depressant effect). Products include:
  OxyContin Tablets 2163
  OxyIR Capsules 2167
  Percocet Tablets 955
  Percodan Tablets 955
  Percodan-Demi Tablets 956
  Roxicodone Tablets, Oral Solution & Intensol (Oxycodone) 2366
  Tylox Capsules 1593
Pentobarbital Sodium (Potentiation of depressant effect). Products include:
  Nembutal Sodium Capsules 440
  Nembutal Sodium Solution 442
  Nembutal Sodium Suppositories ... 444
Perphenazine (Potentiation of depressant effect; increased risk of respiratory depression). Products include:
  Etrafon 2495
  Triavil Tablets 1800
  Trilafon 2532
Phenelzine Sulfate (Potentiation of depressant effect). Products include:
  Nardil 1977
Phenobarbital (Potentiation of depressant effect). Products include:
  Arco-Lase Plus Tablets 513
  Bellergal-S Tablets 2375
  Donnatal 2234
  Donnatal Extentabs 2234
  Donnatal Tablets 2234
  Phenobarbital Elixir and Tablets 1523
  Quadrinal Tablets 1398
Pimozide (Potentiation of depressant effect; increased risk of respiratory depression). Products include:
  Orap Tablets 1037
Prazepam (Potentiation of depressant effect).
  No products indexed under this heading.
Prochlorperazine (Potentiation of depressant effect; increased risk of respiratory depression). Products include:
  Compazine 2644
Promethazine Hydrochloride (Potentiation of depressant effect; increased risk of respiratory depression). Products include:
  Mepergan Injection 2859
  Phenergan with Codeine 2883
  Phenergan with Dextromethorphan ... 2885
  Phenergan Injection 2880
  Phenergan Suppositories 2882
  Phenergan Syrup 2881
  Phenergan Tablets 2882
  Phenergan VC 2886
  Phenergan VC with Codeine 2888
Propofol (Potentiation of depressant effect). Products include:
  Diprivan Injectable Emulsion 2939

Propoxyphene Hydrochloride (Potentiation of depressant effect). Products include:
  Darvon 1475
  Wygesic Tablets 2930
Propoxyphene Napsylate (Potentiation of depressant effect). Products include:
  Darvon-N/Darvocet-N 1473
Protriptyline Hydrochloride (Potentiation of depressant effect). Products include:
  Vivactil Tablets 1820
Pyrilamine Maleate (Potentiation of depressant effect). Products include:
  4-Way Fast Acting Nasal Spray (regular & mentholated) .... ⊠ 644
  Maximum Strength Multi-Symptom Formula Midol .... ⊠ 621
  PMS Multi-Symptom Formula Midol .... ⊠ 622
Pyrilamine Tannate (Potentiation of depressant effect). Products include:
  Atrohist Pediatric Suspension 1604
  Atrohist Pediatric Suspension Dye-Free 1604
  Rynatan 2781
Quazepam (Potentiation of depressant effect). Products include:
  Doral Tablets 2773
Risperidone (Potentiation of depressant effect; increased risk of respiratory depression). Products include:
  Risperdal Tablets 1348
Secobarbital Sodium (Potentiation of depressant effect). Products include:
  Seconal Sodium Pulvules 1529
Selegiline Hydrochloride (Potentiation of depressant effect). Products include:
  Eldepryl Capsules 2729
Sufentanil Citrate (Potentiation of depressant effect). Products include:
  Sufenta Injection 1355
Temazepam (Potentiation of depressant effect). Products include:
  Restoril Capsules 2413
Terfenadine (Potentiation of depressant effect). Products include:
  Seldane Tablets 1284
  Seldane-D Extended-Release Tablets 1286
Thiamylal Sodium (Potentiation of depressant effect).
  No products indexed under this heading.
Thioridazine Hydrochloride (Potentiation of depressant effect; increased risk of respiratory depression). Products include:
  Mellaril 2398
Thiothixene (Potentiation of depressant effect; increased risk of respiratory depression). Products include:
  Navane Capsules and Concentrate ... 2018
  Navane Intramuscular 2019
Tranylcypromine Sulfate (Potentiation of depressant effect). Products include:
  Parnate Tablets 2679
Triazolam (Potentiation of depressant effect). Products include:
  Halcion Tablets 2093
Trifluoperazine Hydrochloride (Potentiation of depressant effect; increased risk of respiratory depression). Products include:
  Stelazine 2692
Trimeprazine Tartrate (Potentiation of depressant effect).
  No products indexed under this heading.

Trimipramine Maleate (Potentiation of depressant effect). Products include:
  Surmontil Capsules 2917
Tripelennamine Hydrochloride (Potentiation of depressant effect). Products include:
  PBZ Tablets 863
  PBZ-SR Tablets 862
Triprolidine Hydrochloride (Potentiation of depressant effect). Products include:
  Actifed Cold & Allergy Tablets ..... ⊠ 807
  Actifed Cold & Sinus Caplets and Tablets .... ⊠ 808
Warfarin Sodium (Concurrent use by epidural or intrathecal route is contraindicated with anticoagulant therapy). Products include:
  Coumadin 941
Zolpidem Tartrate (Potentiation of depressant effect). Products include:
  Ambien Tablets 2559

Food Interactions

Alcohol (Potentiation of depressant effect).

DURANEST INJECTIONS
(Etidocaine Hydrochloride) 533
May interact with monoamine oxidase inhibitors, tricyclic antidepressants, phenothiazines, and ergot-type oxytocic drugs. Compounds in these categories include:

Amitriptyline Hydrochloride (Concurrent use of Duranest Injection containing epinephrine with tricyclic antidepressant may produce severe, prolonged hypotension or hypertension; concurrent use should be avoided). Products include:
  Elavil 2945
  Etrafon 2495
  Limbitrol 2333
  Triavil Tablets 1800
Amoxapine (Concurrent use of Duranest Injection containing epinephrine with tricyclic antidepressant may produce severe, prolonged hypotension or hypertension; concurrent use should be avoided). Products include:
  Asendin Tablets 1419
Chlorpromazine (Concurrent use of Duranest Injection containing epinephrine with phenothiazine may produce severe, prolonged hypotension or hypertension; concurrent use should be avoided). Products include:
  Thorazine Suppositories 2701
Chlorpromazine Hydrochloride (Concurrent use of Duranest Injection containing epinephrine with phenothiazine may produce severe, prolonged hypotension or hypertension; concurrent use should be avoided). Products include:
  Thorazine 2701
Clomipramine Hydrochloride (Concurrent use of Duranest Injection containing epinephrine with tricyclic antidepressant may produce severe, prolonged hypotension or hypertension; concurrent use should be avoided). Products include:
  Anafranil Capsules 819
Desipramine Hydrochloride (Concurrent use of Duranest Injection containing epinephrine with tricyclic antidepressant may produce severe, prolonged hypotension or hypertension; concurrent use should be avoided). Products include:
  Norpramin Tablets 1273

(⊠ Described in PDR For Nonprescription Drugs)   (⊙ Described in PDR For Ophthalmology)

Doxepin Hydrochloride (Concurrent use of Duranest Injection containing epinephrine with tricyclic antidepressant may produce severe, prolonged hypotension or hypertension; concurrent use should be avoided). Products include:
- Adapin Capsules 1542
- Sinequan 2028
- Zonalon Cream 1042

Fluphenazine Decanoate (Concurrent use of Duranest Injection containing epinephrine with phenothiazine may produce severe, prolonged hypotension or hypertension; concurrent use should be avoided). Products include:
- Prolixin Decanoate 510

Fluphenazine Enanthate (Concurrent use of Duranest Injection containing epinephrine with phenothiazine may produce severe, prolonged hypotension or hypertension; concurrent use should be avoided). Products include:
- Prolixin Enanthate 510

Fluphenazine Hydrochloride (Concurrent use of Duranest Injection containing epinephrine with phenothiazine may produce severe, prolonged hypotension or hypertension; concurrent use should be avoided). Products include:
- Prolixin 510

Furazolidone (Concurrent use of Duranest Injection containing epinephrine with MAOI may produce severe, prolonged hypotension or hypertension; concurrent use should be avoided). Products include:
- Furoxone 2221

Imipramine Hydrochloride (Concurrent use of Duranest Injection containing epinephrine with tricyclic antidepressant may produce severe, prolonged hypotension or hypertension; concurrent use should be avoided). Products include:
- Tofranil Ampuls 873
- Tofranil Tablets 875

Imipramine Pamoate (Concurrent use of Duranest Injection containing epinephrine with tricyclic antidepressant may produce severe, prolonged hypotension or hypertension; concurrent use should be avoided). Products include:
- Tofranil-PM Capsules 876

Isocarboxazid (Concurrent use of Duranest Injection containing epinephrine with MAOI may produce severe, prolonged hypotension or hypertension; concurrent use should be avoided). Products include:
- No products indexed under this heading.

Maprotiline Hydrochloride (Concurrent use of Duranest Injection containing epinephrine with tricyclic antidepressant may produce severe, prolonged hypotension or hypertension; concurrent use should be avoided). Products include:
- Ludiomil Tablets 861

Mesoridazine Besylate (Concurrent use of Duranest Injection containing epinephrine with phenothiazine may produce severe, prolonged hypotension or hypertension; concurrent use should be avoided). Products include:
- Serentil 689

Methotrimeprazine (Concurrent use of Duranest Injection containing epinephrine with phenothiazine may produce severe, prolonged hypotension or hypertension; concurrent use should be avoided). Products include:
- Levoprome 1321

Methylergonovine Maleate (Concurrent use of vasopressor drugs, for the treatment of hypotension related to epidural blocks, and ergot-type oxytocic drugs may cause severe, persistent hypertension or cerebrovascular accidents). Products include:
- Methergine 2401

Nortriptyline Hydrochloride (Concurrent use of Duranest Injection containing epinephrine with tricyclic antidepressant may produce severe, prolonged hypotension or hypertension; concurrent use should be avoided). Products include:
- Pamelor 2409

Perphenazine (Concurrent use of Duranest Injection containing epinephrine with phenothiazine may produce severe, prolonged hypotension or hypertension; concurrent use should be avoided). Products include:
- Etrafon 2495
- Triavil Tablets 1800
- Trilafon 2532

Phenelzine Sulfate (Concurrent use of Duranest Injection containing epinephrine with MAOI may produce severe, prolonged hypotension or hypertension; concurrent use should be avoided). Products include:
- Nardil 1977

Prochlorperazine (Concurrent use of Duranest Injection containing epinephrine with phenothiazine may produce severe, prolonged hypotension or hypertension; concurrent use should be avoided). Products include:
- Compazine 2644

Promethazine Hydrochloride (Concurrent use of Duranest Injection containing epinephrine with phenothiazine may produce severe, prolonged hypotension or hypertension; concurrent use should be avoided). Products include:
- Mepergan Injection 2859
- Phenergan with Codeine 2883
- Phenergan with Dextromethorphan 2885
- Phenergan Injection 2880
- Phenergan Suppositories 2882
- Phenergan Syrup 2881
- Phenergan Tablets 2882
- Phenergan VC 2886
- Phenergan VC with Codeine ... 2888

Protriptyline Hydrochloride (Concurrent use of Duranest Injection containing epinephrine with tricyclic antidepressant may produce severe, prolonged hypotension or hypertension; concurrent use should be avoided). Products include:
- Vivactil Tablets 1820

Selegiline Hydrochloride (Concurrent use of Duranest Injection containing epinephrine with MAOI may produce severe, prolonged hypotension or hypertension; concurrent use should be avoided). Products include:
- Eldepryl Capsules 2729

Thioridazine Hydrochloride (Concurrent use of Duranest Injection containing epinephrine with phenothiazine may produce severe, prolonged hypotension or hypertension; concurrent use should be avoided). Products include:
- Mellaril 2398

Tranylcypromine Sulfate (Concurrent use of Duranest Injection containing epinephrine with MAOI may produce severe, prolonged hypotension or hypertension; concurrent use should be avoided). Products include:
- Parnate Tablets 2679

Trifluoperazine Hydrochloride (Concurrent use of Duranest Injection containing epinephrine with phenothiazine may produce severe, prolonged hypotension or hypertension; concurrent use should be avoided). Products include:
- Stelazine 2692

Trimipramine Maleate (Concurrent use of Duranest Injection containing epinephrine with tricyclic antidepressant may produce severe, prolonged hypotension or hypertension; concurrent use should be avoided). Products include:
- Surmontil Capsules 2917

DURA-TAP/PD CAPSULES
(Chlorpheniramine Maleate, Pseudoephedrine Hydrochloride) 970
May interact with monoamine oxidase inhibitors, beta blockers, hypnotics and sedatives, tricyclic antidepressants, barbiturates, central nervous system depressants, tranquilizers, and certain other agents. Compounds in these categories include:

Acebutolol Hydrochloride (Increases the effects of sympathomimetics). Products include:
- Sectral Capsules 2914

Alfentanil Hydrochloride (Potential for additive effects). Products include:
- Alfenta Injection 1334

Alprazolam (Potential for additive effects). Products include:
- Xanax Tablets 2115

Amitriptyline Hydrochloride (Potential for additive effects). Products include:
- Elavil 2945
- Etrafon 2495
- Limbitrol 2333
- Triavil Tablets 1800

Amoxapine (Potential for additive effects). Products include:
- Asendin Tablets 1419

Aprobarbital (Potential for additive effects).
- No products indexed under this heading.

Atenolol (Increases the effects of sympathomimetics). Products include:
- Tenoretic Tablets 2963
- Tenormin Tablets and I.V. Injection 2965

Betaxolol Hydrochloride (Increases the effects of sympathomimetics). Products include:
- Betoptic Ophthalmic Solution 465
- Betoptic S Ophthalmic Suspension 467
- Kerlone Tablets 2588

Bisoprolol Fumarate (Increases the effects of sympathomimetics). Products include:
- Zebeta Tablets 1457
- Ziac 1459

Buprenorphine (Potential for additive effects). Products include:
- Buprenex Injectable 2170

Buspirone Hydrochloride (Potential for additive effects). Products include:
- BuSpar Tablets 738

Butabarbital (Potential for additive effects).
- No products indexed under this heading.

Butalbital (Potential for additive effects). Products include:
- Axocet Capsules 2469
- Esgic-plus Capsules 1012
- Esgic-plus Tablets 1012
- Fioricet Tablets 2386
- Fioricet with Codeine Capsules 2387
- Fiorinal Capsules 2388
- Fiorinal with Codeine Capsules 2390
- Fiorinal Tablets 2388
- Phrenilin 790
- Sedapap Tablets 50 mg/650 mg .. 1826

Carteolol Hydrochloride (Increases the effects of sympathomimetics). Products include:
- Cartrol Tablets 413
- Ocupress Ophthalmic Solution, 1% Sterile 297

Chlordiazepoxide (Potential for additive effects). Products include:
- Limbitrol 2333

Chlordiazepoxide Hydrochloride (Potential for additive effects). Products include:
- Librax Capsules 2330
- Librium Capsules 2331
- Librium Injectable 2332

Chlorpromazine (Potential for additive effects). Products include:
- Thorazine Suppositories 2701

Chlorpromazine Hydrochloride (Potential for additive effects). Products include:
- Thorazine 2701

Chlorprothixene (Potential for additive effects).
- No products indexed under this heading.

Chlorprothixene Hydrochloride (Potential for additive effects).
- No products indexed under this heading.

Chlorprothixene Lactate (Potential for additive effects).
- No products indexed under this heading.

Clomipramine Hydrochloride (Potential for additive effects). Products include:
- Anafranil Capsules 819

Clorazepate Dipotassium (Potential for additive effects). Products include:
- Tranxene 459

Clozapine (Potential for additive effects). Products include:
- Clozaril Tablets 2377

Codeine Phosphate (Potential for additive effects). Products include:
- Brontex 2130
- Dimetane-DC Cough Syrup ... 2232
- Fioricet with Codeine Capsules 2387
- Fiorinal with Codeine Capsules 2390
- Nucofed 2225
- Phenergan with Codeine 2883
- Phenergan VC with Codeine .. 2888
- Robitussin A-C Syrup 2248
- Robitussin-DAC Syrup 2249
- Ryna 804
- Soma Compound w/Codeine Tablets 2784
- Tylenol with Codeine 1592

Desflurane (Potential for additive effects). Products include:
- Suprane (desflurane, USP) ... 1865

Desipramine Hydrochloride (Potential for additive effects). Products include:
- Norpramin Tablets 1273

Dezocine (Potential for additive effects). Products include:
- Dalgan Injection 529

IMPORTANT NOTE: Always consult each drug listing in the patient's regimen for possible interactions.

Dura-Tap/PD Interactions Index 346

Diazepam (Potential for additive effects). Products include:
- Dizac (diazepam injectable emulsion) CIV ... 1862
- Valium Injectable ... 2336
- Valium Tablets ... 2335

Doxepin Hydrochloride (Potential for additive effects). Products include:
- Adapin Capsules ... 1542
- Sinequan ... 2028
- Zonalon Cream ... 1042

Droperidol (Potential for additive effects). Products include:
- Inapsine Injection ... 462

Enflurane (Potential for additive effects).
- No products indexed under this heading.

Esmolol Hydrochloride (Increases the effects of sympathomimetics). Products include:
- Brevibloc (esmolol HCl) Injection ... 1860

Estazolam (Potential for additive effects). Products include:
- ProSom Tablets ... 457

Ethchlorvynol (Potential for additive effects). Products include:
- Placidyl Capsules ... 456

Ethinamate (Potential for additive effects).
- No products indexed under this heading.

Fentanyl (Potential for additive effects). Products include:
- Duragesic Transdermal System ... 1336

Fentanyl Citrate (Potential for additive effects). Products include:
- Sublimaze Injection ... 463

Fluphenazine Decanoate (Potential for additive effects). Products include:
- Prolixin Decanoate ... 510

Fluphenazine Enanthate (Potential for additive effects). Products include:
- Prolixin Enanthate ... 510

Fluphenazine Hydrochloride (Potential for additive effects). Products include:
- Prolixin ... 510

Flurazepam Hydrochloride (Potential for additive effects). Products include:
- Dalmane Capsules ... 2329

Furazolidone (Increases the effects of sympathomimetics; concurrent and/or sequential use is contraindicated). Products include:
- Furoxone ... 2221

Glutethimide (Potential for additive effects).
- No products indexed under this heading.

Haloperidol (Potential for additive effects). Products include:
- Haldol Injection, Tablets and Concentrate ... 1585

Haloperidol Decanoate (Potential for additive effects). Products include:
- Haldol Decanoate ... 1587

Hydrocodone Bitartrate (Potential for additive effects). Products include:
- Codiclear DH Syrup ... 808
- Duratuss HD Elixir ... 2750
- Histussin D Liquid ... 670
- Hycodan Tablets and Syrup ... 946
- Hycomine Compound Tablets ... 948
- Hycomine ... 947
- Hycotuss Expectorant Syrup ... 950
- Hydrocet Capsules ... 787
- Lorcet 10/650 Tablets ... 1016
- Lortab ... 2751
- Tussend ... 1830
- Tussend Expectorant ... 1831
- Vicodin Tablets ... 1404
- Vicodin ES Tablets ... 1405
- Vicodin HP Tablets ... 1403
- Vicodin Tuss Expectorant ... 1406
- Zydone Capsules ... 967

Hydrocodone Polistirex (Potential for additive effects). Products include:
- Tussionex Pennkinetic Extended-Release Suspension ... 1624

Hydroxyzine Hydrochloride (Potential for additive effects). Products include:
- Atarax Tablets & Syrup ... 1992
- Marax Tablets & DF Syrup ... 2015
- Vistaril Intramuscular Solution ... 2042

Imipramine Hydrochloride (Potential for additive effects). Products include:
- Tofranil Ampuls ... 873
- Tofranil Tablets ... 875

Imipramine Pamoate (Potential for additive effects). Products include:
- Tofranil-PM Capsules ... 876

Isocarboxazid (Increases the effects of sympathomimetics; concurrent and/or sequential use is contraindicated).
- No products indexed under this heading.

Isoflurane (Potential for additive effects).
- No products indexed under this heading.

Ketamine Hydrochloride (Potential for additive effects).
- No products indexed under this heading.

Labetalol Hydrochloride (Increases the effects of sympathomimetics). Products include:
- Normodyne Injection ... 2519
- Normodyne Tablets ... 2522
- Trandate ... 1158

Levobunolol Hydrochloride (Increases the effects of sympathomimetics). Products include:
- Betagan ... ⊙ 230

Levomethadyl Acetate Hydrochloride (Potential for additive effects). Products include:
- Orlaam Oral Solution ... 2361

Levorphanol Tartrate (Potential for additive effects). Products include:
- Levo-Dromoran ... 2297

Lorazepam (Potential for additive effects). Products include:
- Ativan Injection ... 2805
- Ativan Tablets ... 2807

Loxapine Hydrochloride (Potential for additive effects). Products include:
- Loxitane ... 1426

Loxapine Succinate (Potential for additive effects). Products include:
- Loxitane Capsules ... 1426

Maprotiline Hydrochloride (Potential for additive effects). Products include:
- Ludiomil Tablets ... 861

Mecamylamine Hydrochloride (Sympathomimetic may reduce the antihypertensive effects). Products include:
- Inversine Tablets ... 1729

Meperidine Hydrochloride (Potential for additive effects). Products include:
- Demerol ... 2438
- Mepergan Injection ... 2859

Mephobarbital (Potential for additive effects). Products include:
- Mebaral Tablets ... 2452

Meprobamate (Potential for additive effects). Products include:
- Miltown Tablets ... 2780
- PMB 200 and PMB 400 ... 2890

Mesoridazine Besylate (Potential for additive effects). Products include:
- Serentil ... 689

Methadone Hydrochloride (Potential for additive effects). Products include:
- Methadone Hydrochloride Oral Concentrate ... 2356
- Methadone Hydrochloride Oral Solution & Tablets ... 2357

Methohexital Sodium (Potential for additive effects).
- No products indexed under this heading.

Methotrimeprazine (Potential for additive effects). Products include:
- Levoprome ... 1321

Methoxyflurane (Potential for additive effects).
- No products indexed under this heading.

Methyldopa (Sympathomimetic may reduce the antihypertensive effects). Products include:
- Aldoclor Tablets ... 1638
- Aldomet Oral ... 1640
- Aldoril Tablets ... 1644

Methyldopate Hydrochloride (Sympathomimetic may reduce the antihypertensive effects). Products include:
- Aldomet Ester HCl Injection ... 1642

Metipranolol Hydrochloride (Increases the effects of sympathomimetics). Products include:
- OptiPranolol (Metipranolol 0.3%) Sterile Ophthalmic Solution ... ⊙ 256

Metoprolol Succinate (Increases the effects of sympathomimetics). Products include:
- Toprol-XL Tablets ... 560

Metoprolol Tartrate (Increases the effects of sympathomimetics). Products include:
- Lopressor ... 848
- Lopressor HCT Tablets ... 850

Midazolam Hydrochloride (Potential for additive effects). Products include:
- Versed Injection ... 2324

Molindone Hydrochloride (Potential for additive effects). Products include:
- Moban Tablets and Concentrate ... 1036

Morphine Sulfate (Potential for additive effects). Products include:
- Astramorph/PF Injection, USP (Preservative-Free) ... 526
- Duramorph Injection ... 983
- Infumorph 200 and Infumorph 500 Sterile Solutions ... 985
- Kadian Capsules ... 2948
- MS Contin Tablets ... 2149
- MSIR ... 2152
- Oramorph SR (Morphine Sulfate Sustained Release Tablets) ... 2359
- RMS Suppositories CII ... 2766
- Roxanol ... 2365

Nadolol (Increases the effects of sympathomimetics).
- No products indexed under this heading.

Nortriptyline Hydrochloride (Potential for additive effects). Products include:
- Pamelor ... 2409

Opium Alkaloids (Potential for additive effects).
- No products indexed under this heading.

Oxazepam (Potential for additive effects). Products include:
- Serax Capsules ... 2916
- Serax Tablets ... 2916

Oxycodone Hydrochloride (Potential for additive effects). Products include:
- OxyContin Tablets ... 2163
- OxyIR Capsules ... 2167
- Percocet Tablets ... 955
- Percodan Tablets ... 955
- Percodan-Demi Tablets ... 956
- Roxicodone Tablets, Oral Solution & Intensol (Oxycodone) ... 2366
- Tylox Capsules ... 1593

Penbutolol Sulfate (Increases the effects of sympathomimetics). Products include:
- Levatol Tablets ... 2547

Pentobarbital Sodium (Potential for additive effects). Products include:
- Nembutal Sodium Capsules ... 440
- Nembutal Sodium Solution ... 442
- Nembutal Sodium Suppositories ... 444

Perphenazine (Potential for additive effects). Products include:
- Etrafon ... 2495
- Triavil Tablets ... 1800
- Trilafon ... 2532

Phenelzine Sulfate (Increases the effects of sympathomimetics; concurrent and/or sequential use is contraindicated). Products include:
- Nardil ... 1977

Phenobarbital (Potential for additive effects). Products include:
- Arco-Lase Plus Tablets ... 513
- Bellergal-S Tablets ... 2375
- Donnatal ... 2234
- Donnatal Extentabs ... 2234
- Donnatal Tablets ... 2234
- Phenobarbital Elixir and Tablets ... 1523
- Quadrinal Tablets ... 1398

Pindolol (Increases the effects of sympathomimetics). Products include:
- Visken Tablets ... 2428

Prazepam (Potential for additive effects).
- No products indexed under this heading.

Prochlorperazine (Potential for additive effects). Products include:
- Compazine ... 2644

Promethazine Hydrochloride (Potential for additive effects). Products include:
- Mepergan Injection ... 2859
- Phenergan with Codeine ... 2883
- Phenergan with Dextromethorphan 2885
- Phenergan Injection ... 2880
- Phenergan Suppositories ... 2882
- Phenergan Syrup ... 2881
- Phenergan Tablets ... 2882
- Phenergan VC ... 2886
- Phenergan VC with Codeine ... 2888

Propofol (Potential for additive effects). Products include:
- Diprivan Injectable Emulsion ... 2939

Propoxyphene Hydrochloride (Potential for additive effects). Products include:
- Darvon ... 1475
- Wygesic Tablets ... 2930

Propoxyphene Napsylate (Potential for additive effects). Products include:
- Darvon-N/Darvocet-N ... 1473

Propranolol Hydrochloride (Increases the effects of sympathomimetics). Products include:
- Inderal ... 2834
- Inderal LA Long Acting Capsules ... 2836
- Inderide Tablets ... 2838
- Inderide LA Long Acting Capsules .. 2840

Protriptyline Hydrochloride (Potential for additive effects). Products include:
- Vivactil Tablets ... 1820

Quazepam (Potential for additive effects). Products include:
- Doral Tablets ... 2773

Reserpine (Sympathomimetic may reduce the antihypertensive effects). Products include:
- Diupres Tablets ... 1691
- Hydropres Tablets ... 1718
- Ser-Ap-Es Tablets ... 867

(▣ Described in PDR For Nonprescription Drugs) (⊙ Described in PDR For Ophthalmology)

Risperidone (Potential for additive effects). Products include:
- Risperdal Tablets 1348

Secobarbital Sodium (Potential for additive effects). Products include:
- Seconal Sodium Pulvules 1529

Selegiline Hydrochloride (Increases the effects of sympathomimetics; concurrent and/or sequential use is contraindicated). Products include:
- Eldepryl Capsules 2729

Sevoflurane (Potential for additive effects).
- No products indexed under this heading.

Sotalol Hydrochloride (Increases the effects of sympathomimetics). Products include:
- Betapace Tablets 637

Sufentanil Citrate (Potential for additive effects). Products include:
- Sufenta Injection 1355

Temazepam (Potential for additive effects). Products include:
- Restoril Capsules 2413

Thiamylal Sodium (Potential for additive effects).
- No products indexed under this heading.

Thioridazine Hydrochloride (Potential for additive effects). Products include:
- Mellaril 2398

Thiothixene (Potential for additive effects). Products include:
- Navane Capsules and Concentrate 2018
- Navane Intramuscular 2019

Timolol Hemihydrate (Increases the effects of sympathomimetics). Products include:
- Betimol 0.25%, 0.5% 259

Timolol Maleate (Increases the effects of sympathomimetics). Products include:
- Blocadren Tablets 1654
- Timolide Tablets 1791
- Timoptic in Ocudose 1796
- Timoptic Sterile Ophthalmic Solution 1794
- Timoptic-XE 1798

Tranylcypromine Sulfate (Increases the effects of sympathomimetics; concurrent and/or sequential use is contraindicated). Products include:
- Parnate Tablets 2679

Triazolam (Potential for additive effects). Products include:
- Halcion Tablets 2093

Trifluoperazine Hydrochloride (Potential for additive effects). Products include:
- Stelazine 2692

Trimipramine Maleate (Potential for additive effects). Products include:
- Surmontil Capsules 2917

Zolpidem Tartrate (Potential for additive effects). Products include:
- Ambien Tablets 2559

Food Interactions
Alcohol (Potential for additive effects).

DURATION 12 HOUR NASAL SPRAY
(Oxymetazoline Hydrochloride) 766
None cited in PDR database.

DURATUSS TABLETS
(Pseudoephedrine Hydrochloride, Guaifenesin) 2750

May interact with monoamine oxidase inhibitors. Compounds in this category include:

Furazolidone (Concurrent use is contraindicated). Products include:
- Furoxone 2221

Isocarboxazid (Concurrent use is contraindicated).
- No products indexed under this heading.

Phenelzine Sulfate (Concurrent use is contraindicated). Products include:
- Nardil 1977

Selegiline Hydrochloride (Concurrent use is contraindicated). Products include:
- Eldepryl Capsules 2729

Tranylcypromine Sulfate (Concurrent use is contraindicated). Products include:
- Parnate Tablets 2679

DURA-VENT/DA TABLETS
(Chlorpheniramine Maleate, Phenylephrine Hydrochloride, Methscopolamine Nitrate) 972

May interact with monoamine oxidase inhibitors, beta blockers, hypnotics and sedatives, tricyclic antidepressants, barbiturates, central nervous system depressants, tranquilizers, and certain other agents. Compounds in these categories include:

Acebutolol Hydrochloride (Increases the effects of sympathomimetics). Products include:
- Sectral Capsules 2914

Alfentanil Hydrochloride (Potential for additive effects). Products include:
- Alfenta Injection 1334

Alprazolam (Potential for additive effects). Products include:
- Xanax Tablets 2115

Amitriptyline Hydrochloride (Potential for additive effects). Products include:
- Elavil 2945
- Etrafon 2495
- Limbitrol 2333
- Triavil Tablets 1800

Amoxapine (Potential for additive effects). Products include:
- Asendin Tablets 1419

Aprobarbital (Potential for additive effects).
- No products indexed under this heading.

Atenolol (Increases the effects of sympathomimetics). Products include:
- Tenoretic Tablets 2963
- Tenormin Tablets and I.V. Injection 2965

Betaxolol Hydrochloride (Increases the effects of sympathomimetics). Products include:
- Betoptic Ophthalmic Solution 465
- Betoptic S Ophthalmic Suspension 467
- Kerlone Tablets 2588

Bisoprolol Fumarate (Increases the effects of sympathomimetics). Products include:
- Zebeta Tablets 1457
- Ziac 1459

Buprenorphine (Potential for additive effects). Products include:
- Buprenex Injectable 2170

Buspirone Hydrochloride (Potential for additive effects). Products include:
- BuSpar Tablets 738

Butabarbital (Potential for additive effects).
- No products indexed under this heading.

Butalbital (Potential for additive effects). Products include:
- Axocet Capsules 2469
- Esgic-plus Capsules 1012
- Esgic-plus Tablets 1012
- Fioricet Tablets 2386
- Fioricet with Codeine Capsules 2387
- Fiorinal Capsules 2388
- Fiorinal with Codeine Capsules 2390
- Fiorinal Tablets 2388
- Phrenilin 790
- Sedapap Tablets 50 mg/650 mg .. 1826

Carteolol Hydrochloride (Increases the effects of sympathomimetics). Products include:
- Cartrol Tablets 413
- Ocupress Ophthalmic Solution, 1% Sterile 297

Chlordiazepoxide (Potential for additive effects). Products include:
- Limbitrol 2333

Chlordiazepoxide Hydrochloride (Potential for additive effects). Products include:
- Librax Capsules 2330
- Librium Capsules 2331
- Librium Injectable 2332

Chlorpromazine (Potential for additive effects). Products include:
- Thorazine Suppositories 2701

Chlorpromazine Hydrochloride (Potential for additive effects). Products include:
- Thorazine 2701

Chlorprothixene (Potential for additive effects).
- No products indexed under this heading.

Chlorprothixene Hydrochloride (Potential for additive effects).
- No products indexed under this heading.

Chlorprothixene Lactate (Potential for additive effects).
- No products indexed under this heading.

Clomipramine Hydrochloride (Potential for additive effects). Products include:
- Anafranil Capsules 819

Clorazepate Dipotassium (Potential for additive effects). Products include:
- Tranxene 459

Clozapine (Potential for additive effects). Products include:
- Clozaril Tablets 2377

Codeine Phosphate (Potential for additive effects). Products include:
- Brontex 2130
- Dimetane-DC Cough Syrup 2232
- Fioricet with Codeine Capsules 2387
- Fiorinal with Codeine Capsules 2390
- Nucofed 2225
- Phenergan with Codeine 2883
- Phenergan VC with Codeine 2888
- Robitussin A-C Syrup 2248
- Robitussin-DAC Syrup 2249
- Ryna 804
- Soma Compound w/Codeine Tablets 2784
- Tylenol with Codeine 1592

Desflurane (Potential for additive effects). Products include:
- Suprane (desflurane, USP) 1865

Desipramine Hydrochloride (Potential for additive effects). Products include:
- Norpramin Tablets 1273

Dezocine (Potential for additive effects). Products include:
- Dalgan Injection 529

Diazepam (Potential for additive effects). Products include:
- Dizac (diazepam injectable emulsion) CIV 1862
- Valium Injectable 2336
- Valium Tablets 2335

Doxepin Hydrochloride (Potential for additive effects). Products include:
- Adapin Capsules 1542
- Sinequan 2028
- Zonalon Cream 1042

Droperidol (Potential for additive effects). Products include:
- Inapsine Injection 462

Enflurane (Potential for additive effects).
- No products indexed under this heading.

Esmolol Hydrochloride (Increases the effects of sympathomimetics). Products include:
- Brevibloc (esmolol HCl) Injection 1860

Estazolam (Potential for additive effects). Products include:
- ProSom Tablets 457

Ethchlorvynol (Potential for additive effects). Products include:
- Placidyl Capsules 456

Ethinamate (Potential for additive effects).
- No products indexed under this heading.

Fentanyl (Potential for additive effects). Products include:
- Duragesic Transdermal System ... 1336

Fentanyl Citrate (Potential for additive effects). Products include:
- Sublimaze Injection 463

Fluphenazine Decanoate (Potential for additive effects). Products include:
- Prolixin Decanoate 510

Fluphenazine Enanthate (Potential for additive effects). Products include:
- Prolixin Enanthate 510

Fluphenazine Hydrochloride (Potential for additive effects). Products include:
- Prolixin 510

Flurazepam Hydrochloride (Potential for additive effects). Products include:
- Dalmane Capsules 2329

Furazolidone (Increases the effects of sympathomimetics; concurrent and/or sequential use is contraindicated). Products include:
- Furoxone 2221

Glutethimide (Potential for additive effects).
- No products indexed under this heading.

Haloperidol (Potential for additive effects). Products include:
- Haldol Injection, Tablets and Concentrate 1585

Haloperidol Decanoate (Potential for additive effects). Products include:
- Haldol Decanoate 1587

Hydrocodone Bitartrate (Potential for additive effects). Products include:
- Codiclear DH Syrup 808
- Duratuss HD Elixir 2750
- Histussin D Liquid 670
- Hycodan Tablets and Syrup 946
- Hycomine Compound Tablets 948
- Hycomine 947
- Hycotuss Expectorant Syrup 950
- Hydrocet Capsules 787
- Lorcet 10/650 Tablets 1016
- Lortab 2751
- Tussend 1830
- Tussend Expectorant 1831
- Vicodin Tablets 1404
- Vicodin ES Tablets 1405
- Vicodin HP Tablets 1403
- Vicodin Tuss Expectorant 1406
- Zydone Capsules 967

IMPORTANT NOTE: Always consult each drug listing in the patient's regimen for possible interactions.

Hydrocodone Polistirex (Potential for additive effects). Products include:
Tussionex Pennkinetic Extended-Release Suspension ... 1624
Hydromorphone Hydrochloride (Potential for additive effects). Products include:
Dilaudid Ampules ... 1382
Dilaudid Cough Syrup ... 1383
Dilaudid-HP Injection ... 1384
Dilaudid-HP Lyophilized Powder 250 mg ... 1384
Dilaudid ... 1382
Dilaudid Oral Liquid ... 1386
Dilaudid ... 1382
Dilaudid Tablets - 8 mg ... 1386
Hydroxyzine Hydrochloride (Potential for additive effects). Products include:
Atarax Tablets & Syrup ... 1992
Marax Tablets & DF Syrup ... 2015
Vistaril Intramuscular Solution ... 2042
Imipramine Hydrochloride (Potential for additive effects). Products include:
Tofranil Ampuls ... 873
Tofranil Tablets ... 875
Imipramine Pamoate (Potential for additive effects). Products include:
Tofranil-PM Capsules ... 876
Isocarboxazid (Increases the effects of sympathomimetics; concurrent and/or sequential use is contraindicated).
No products indexed under this heading.
Isoflurane (Potential for additive effects).
No products indexed under this heading.
Ketamine Hydrochloride (Potential for additive effects).
No products indexed under this heading.
Labetalol Hydrochloride (Increases the effects of sympathomimetics). Products include:
Normodyne Injection ... 2519
Normodyne Tablets ... 2522
Trandate ... 1158
Levobunolol Hydrochloride (Increases the effects of sympathomimetics). Products include:
Betagan ... ◉ 230
Levomethadyl Acetate Hydrochloride (Potential for additive effects). Products include:
Orlaam Oral Solution ... 2361
Levorphanol Tartrate (Potential for additive effects). Products include:
Levo-Dromoran ... 2297
Lorazepam (Potential for additive effects). Products include:
Ativan Injection ... 2805
Ativan Tablets ... 2807
Loxapine Hydrochloride (Potential for additive effects). Products include:
Loxitane ... 1426
Loxapine Succinate (Potential for additive effects). Products include:
Loxitane Capsules ... 1426
Maprotiline Hydrochloride (Potential for additive effects). Products include:
Ludiomil Tablets ... 861
Mecamylamine Hydrochloride (Sympathomimetic may reduce the antihypertensive effects). Products include:
Inversine Tablets ... 1729
Meperidine Hydrochloride (Potential for additive effects). Products include:
Demerol ... 2438
Mepergan Injection ... 2859
Mephobarbital (Potential for additive effects). Products include:
Mebaral Tablets ... 2452
Meprobamate (Potential for additive effects). Products include:
Miltown Tablets ... 2780
PMB 200 and PMB 400 ... 2890
Mesoridazine Besylate (Potential for additive effects). Products include:
Serentil ... 689
Methadone Hydrochloride (Potential for additive effects). Products include:
Methadone Hydrochloride Oral Concentrate ... 2356
Methadone Hydrochloride Oral Solution & Tablets ... 2357
Methohexital Sodium (Potential for additive effects).
No products indexed under this heading.
Methotrimeprazine (Potential for additive effects). Products include:
Levoprome ... 1321
Methoxyflurane (Potential for additive effects).
No products indexed under this heading.
Methyldopa (Sympathomimetic may reduce the antihypertensive effects). Products include:
Aldoclor Tablets ... 1638
Aldomet Oral ... 1640
Aldoril Tablets ... 1644
Methyldopate Hydrochloride (Sympathomimetic may reduce the antihypertensive effects). Products include:
Aldomet Ester HCl Injection ... 1642
Metipranolol Hydrochloride (Increases the effects of sympathomimetics). Products include:
OptiPranolol (Metipranolol 0.3%) Sterile Ophthalmic Solution ... ◉ 256
Metoprolol Succinate (Increases the effects of sympathomimetics). Products include:
Toprol-XL Tablets ... 560
Metoprolol Tartrate (Increases the effects of sympathomimetics). Products include:
Lopressor ... 848
Lopressor HCT Tablets ... 850
Midazolam Hydrochloride (Potential for additive effects). Products include:
Versed Injection ... 2324
Molindone Hydrochloride (Potential for additive effects). Products include:
Moban Tablets and Concentrate ... 1036
Morphine Sulfate (Potential for additive effects). Products include:
Astramorph/PF Injection, USP (Preservative-Free) ... 526
Duramorph Injection ... 983
Infumorph 200 and Infumorph 500 Sterile Solutions ... 985
Kadian Capsules ... 2948
MS Contin Tablets ... 2149
MSIR ... 2152
Oramorph SR (Morphine Sulfate Sustained Release Tablets) ... 2359
RMS Suppositories CII ... 2766
Roxanol ... 2365
Nadolol (Increases the effects of sympathomimetics).
No products indexed under this heading.
Nortriptyline Hydrochloride (Potential for additive effects). Products include:
Pamelor ... 2409
Opium Alkaloids (Potential for additive effects).
No products indexed under this heading.
Oxazepam (Potential for additive effects). Products include:
Serax Capsules ... 2916
Serax Tablets ... 2916
Oxycodone Hydrochloride (Potential for additive effects). Products include:
OxyContin Tablets ... 2163
OxyIR Capsules ... 2167
Percocet Tablets ... 955
Percodan Tablets ... 955
Percodan-Demi Tablets ... 956
Roxicodone Tablets, Oral Solution & Intensol (Oxycodone) ... 2366
Tylox Capsules ... 1593
Penbutolol Sulfate (Increases the effects of sympathomimetics). Products include:
Levatol Tablets ... 2547
Pentobarbital Sodium (Potential for additive effects). Products include:
Nembutal Sodium Capsules ... 440
Nembutal Sodium Solution ... 442
Nembutal Sodium Suppositories ... 444
Perphenazine (Potential for additive effects). Products include:
Etrafon ... 2495
Triavil Tablets ... 1800
Trilafon ... 2532
Phenelzine Sulfate (Increases the effects of sympathomimetics; concurrent and/or sequential use is contraindicated). Products include:
Nardil ... 1977
Phenobarbital (Potential for additive effects). Products include:
Arco-Lase Plus Tablets ... 513
Bellergal-S Tablets ... 2375
Donnatal ... 2234
Donnatal Extentabs ... 2234
Donnatal Tablets ... 2234
Phenobarbital Elixir and Tablets ... 1523
Quadrinal Tablets ... 1398
Pindolol (Increases the effects of sympathomimetics). Products include:
Visken Tablets ... 2428
Prazepam (Potential for additive effects).
No products indexed under this heading.
Prochlorperazine (Potential for additive effects). Products include:
Compazine ... 2644
Promethazine Hydrochloride (Potential for additive effects). Products include:
Mepergan Injection ... 2859
Phenergan with Codeine ... 2883
Phenergan with Dextromethorphan 2885
Phenergan Injection ... 2880
Phenergan Suppositories ... 2882
Phenergan Syrup ... 2881
Phenergan Tablets ... 2882
Phenergan VC ... 2886
Phenergan VC with Codeine ... 2888
Propofol (Potential for additive effects). Products include:
Diprivan Injectable Emulsion ... 2939
Propoxyphene Hydrochloride (Potential for additive effects). Products include:
Darvon ... 1475
Wygesic Tablets ... 2930
Propoxyphene Napsylate (Potential for additive effects). Products include:
Darvon-N/Darvocet-N ... 1473
Propranolol Hydrochloride (Increases the effects of sympathomimetics). Products include:
Inderal ... 2834
Inderal LA Long Acting Capsules ... 2836
Inderide Tablets ... 2838
Inderide LA Long Acting Capsules .. 2840
Protriptyline Hydrochloride (Potential for additive effects). Products include:
Vivactil Tablets ... 1820
Quazepam (Potential for additive effects). Products include:
Doral Tablets ... 2773
Reserpine (Sympathomimetic may reduce the antihypertensive effects). Products include:
Diupres Tablets ... 1691
Hydropres Tablets ... 1718
Ser-Ap-Es Tablets ... 867
Risperidone (Potential for additive effects). Products include:
Risperdal Tablets ... 1348
Secobarbital Sodium (Potential for additive effects). Products include:
Seconal Sodium Pulvules ... 1529
Selegiline Hydrochloride (Increases the effects of sympathomimetics; concurrent and/or sequential use is contraindicated). Products include:
Eldepryl Capsules ... 2729
Sevoflurane (Potential for additive effects).
No products indexed under this heading.
Sotalol Hydrochloride (Increases the effects of sympathomimetics). Products include:
Betapace Tablets ... 637
Sufentanil Citrate (Potential for additive effects). Products include:
Sufenta Injection ... 1355
Temazepam (Potential for additive effects). Products include:
Restoril Capsules ... 2413
Thiamylal Sodium (Potential for additive effects).
No products indexed under this heading.
Thioridazine Hydrochloride (Potential for additive effects). Products include:
Mellaril ... 2398
Thiothixene (Potential for additive effects). Products include:
Navane Capsules and Concentrate 2018
Navane Intramuscular ... 2019
Timolol Hemihydrate (Increases the effects of sympathomimetics). Products include:
Betimol 0.25%, 0.5% ... ◉ 259
Timolol Maleate (Increases the effects of sympathomimetics). Products include:
Blocadren Tablets ... 1654
Timolide Tablets ... 1791
Timoptic in Ocudose ... 1796
Timoptic Sterile Ophthalmic Solution ... 1794
Timoptic-XE ... 1798
Tranylcypromine Sulfate (Increases the effects of sympathomimetics; concurrent and/or sequential use is contraindicated). Products include:
Parnate Tablets ... 2679
Triazolam (Potential for additive effects). Products include:
Halcion Tablets ... 2093
Trifluoperazine Hydrochloride (Potential for additive effects). Products include:
Stelazine ... 2692
Trimipramine Maleate (Potential for additive effects). Products include:
Surmontil Capsules ... 2917
Zolpidem Tartrate (Potential for additive effects). Products include:
Ambien Tablets ... 2559

Food Interactions

Alcohol (Potential for additive effects).

DURATUSS HD ELIXIR
(Hydrocodone Bitartrate, Pseudoephedrine Hydrochloride, Guaifenesin) 2750
May interact with central nervous system depressants, narcotic analgesics, general anesthetics, hypnotics and sedatives, tranquilizers, tricyclic antidepressants, monoamine oxidase inhibitors, beta blockers, veratrum alkaloids, and certain other agents. Compounds in these categories include:

Acebutolol Hydrochloride (Potentiation of sympathomimetic effects of pseudoephedrine). Products include:
   Sectral Capsules 2914

Alfentanil Hydrochloride (Potentiation of central nervous system effects). Products include:
   Alfenta Injection 1334

Alprazolam (Potentiation of central nervous system effects). Products include:
   Xanax Tablets 2115

Amitriptyline Hydrochloride (Potentiation of central nervous system effects). Products include:
   Elavil 2945
   Etrafon 2495
   Limbitrol 2333
   Triavil Tablets 1800

Amoxapine (Potentiation of central nervous system effects). Products include:
   Asendin Tablets 1419

Aprobarbital (Potentiation of central nervous system effects).
   No products indexed under this heading.

Atenolol (Potentiation of sympathomimetic effects of pseudoephedrine). Products include:
   Tenoretic Tablets 2963
   Tenormin Tablets and I.V. Injection 2965

Betaxolol Hydrochloride (Potentiation of sympathomimetic effects of pseudoephedrine). Products include:
   Betoptic Ophthalmic Solution 465
   Betoptic S Ophthalmic Suspension 467
   Kerlone Tablets 2588

Bisoprolol Fumarate (Potentiation of sympathomimetic effects of pseudoephedrine). Products include:
   Zebeta Tablets 1457
   Ziac 1459

Buprenorphine (Potentiation of central nervous system effects). Products include:
   Buprenex Injectable 2170

Buspirone Hydrochloride (Potentiation of central nervous system effects). Products include:
   BuSpar Tablets 738

Butabarbital (Potentiation of central nervous system effects).
   No products indexed under this heading.

Butalbital (Potentiation of central nervous system effects). Products include:
   Axocet Capsules 2469
   Esgic-plus Capsules 1012
   Esgic-plus Tablets 1012
   Fioricet Tablets 2386
   Fioricet with Codeine Capsules 2387
   Fiorinal Capsules 2388
   Fiorinal with Codeine Capsules 2390
   Fiorinal Tablets 2388
   Phrenilin 790
   Sedapap Tablets 50 mg/650 mg . 1826

Carteolol Hydrochloride (Potentiation of sympathomimetic effects of pseudoephedrine). Products include:
   Cartrol Tablets 413
   Ocupress Ophthalmic Solution, 1% Sterile .... ⊙ 297

Chlordiazepoxide (Potentiation of central nervous system effects). Products include:
   Limbitrol 2333

Chlordiazepoxide Hydrochloride (Potentiation of central nervous system effects). Products include:
   Librax Capsules 2330
   Librium Capsules 2331
   Librium Injectable 2332

Chlorpromazine (Potentiation of central nervous system effects). Products include:
   Thorazine Suppositories 2701

Chlorpromazine Hydrochloride (Potentiation of central nervous system effects). Products include:
   Thorazine 2701

Chlorprothixene (Potentiation of central nervous system effects).
   No products indexed under this heading.

Chlorprothixene Hydrochloride (Potentiation of central nervous system effects).
   No products indexed under this heading.

Chlorprothixene Lactate (Potentiation of central nervous system effects).
   No products indexed under this heading.

Clomipramine Hydrochloride (Potentiation of central nervous system effects). Products include:
   Anafranil Capsules 819

Clorazepate Dipotassium (Potentiation of central nervous system effects). Products include:
   Tranxene 459

Clozapine (Potentiation of central nervous system effects). Products include:
   Clozaril Tablets 2377

Codeine Phosphate (Potentiation of central nervous system effects). Products include:
   Brontex 2130
   Dimetane-DC Cough Syrup 2232
   Fioricet with Codeine Capsules 2387
   Fiorinal with Codeine Capsules 2390
   Nucofed 2225
   Phenergan with Codeine 2883
   Phenergan VC with Codeine 2888
   Robitussin A-C Syrup 2248
   Robitussin-DAC Syrup 2249
   Ryna .... ⊙ 804
   Soma Compound w/Codeine Tablets 2784
   Tylenol with Codeine 1592

Cryptenamine Preparations (Reduced antihypertensive effects).

Desflurane (Potentiation of central nervous system effects). Products include:
   Suprane (desflurane, USP) 1865

Desipramine Hydrochloride (Potentiation of central nervous system effects). Products include:
   Norpramin Tablets 1273

Dezocine (Potentiation of central nervous system effects). Products include:
   Dalgan Injection 529

Diazepam (Potentiation of central nervous system effects). Products include:
   Dizac (diazepam injectable emulsion) CIV 1862
   Valium Injectable 2336
   Valium Tablets 2335

Doxepin Hydrochloride (Potentiation of central nervous system effects). Products include:
   Adapin Capsules 1542
   Sinequan 2028
   Zonalon Cream 1042

Droperidol (Potentiation of central nervous system effects). Products include:
   Inapsine Injection 462

Enflurane (Potentiation of central nervous system effects).
   No products indexed under this heading.

Esmolol Hydrochloride (Potentiation of sympathomimetic effects of pseudoephedrine). Products include:
   Brevibloc (esmolol HCl) Injection 1860

Estazolam (Potentiation of central nervous system effects). Products include:
   ProSom Tablets 457

Ethchlorvynol (Potentiation of central nervous system effects). Products include:
   Placidyl Capsules 456

Ethinamate (Potentiation of central nervous system effects).
   No products indexed under this heading.

Fentanyl (Potentiation of central nervous system effects). Products include:
   Duragesic Transdermal System 1336

Fentanyl Citrate (Potentiation of central nervous system effects). Products include:
   Sublimaze Injection 463

Fluphenazine Decanoate (Potentiation of central nervous system effects). Products include:
   Prolixin Decanoate 510

Fluphenazine Enanthate (Potentiation of central nervous system effects). Products include:
   Prolixin Enanthate 510

Fluphenazine Hydrochloride (Potentiation of central nervous system effects). Products include:
   Prolixin 510

Flurazepam Hydrochloride (Potentiation of central nervous system effects). Products include:
   Dalmane Capsules 2329

Furazolidone (Concurrent use is contraindicated; potentiation of central nervous system effects of hydrocodone and potentiation of sympathomimetic effects of pseudoephedrine). Products include:
   Furoxone 2221

Glutethimide (Potentiation of central nervous system effects).
   No products indexed under this heading.

Haloperidol (Potentiation of central nervous system effects). Products include:
   Haldol Injection, Tablets and Concentrate 1585

Haloperidol Decanoate (Potentiation of central nervous system effects). Products include:
   Haldol Decanoate 1587

Hydrocodone Polistirex (Potentiation of central nervous system effects). Products include:
   Tussionex Pennkinetic Extended-Release Suspension 1624

Hydromorphone Hydrochloride (Potentiation of central nervous system effects). Products include:
   Dilaudid Ampules 1382
   Dilaudid Cough Syrup 1383
   Dilaudid-HP Injection 1384
   Dilaudid-HP Lyophilized Powder 250 mg 1384
   Dilaudid 1382
   Dilaudid Oral Liquid 1386
   Dilaudid 1382
   Dilaudid Tablets - 8 mg 1386

Hydroxyzine Hydrochloride (Potentiation of central nervous system effects). Products include:
   Atarax Tablets & Syrup 1992
   Marax Tablets & DF Syrup 2015
   Vistaril Intramuscular Solution 2042

Imipramine Hydrochloride (Potentiation of central nervous system effects). Products include:
   Tofranil Ampuls 873
   Tofranil Tablets 875

Imipramine Pamoate (Potentiation of central nervous system effects). Products include:
   Tofranil-PM Capsules 876

Isocarboxazid (Concurrent use is contraindicated; potentiation of central nervous system effects of hydrocodone and potentiation of sympathomimetic effects of pseudoephedrine).
   No products indexed under this heading.

Isoflurane (Potentiation of central nervous system effects).
   No products indexed under this heading.

Ketamine Hydrochloride (Potentiation of central nervous system effects).
   No products indexed under this heading.

Labetalol Hydrochloride (Potentiation of sympathomimetic effects of pseudoephedrine). Products include:
   Normodyne Injection 2519
   Normodyne Tablets 2522
   Trandate 1158

Levobunolol Hydrochloride (Potentiation of sympathomimetic effects of pseudoephedrine). Products include:
   Betagan .... ⊙ 230

Levomethadyl Acetate Hydrochloride (Potentiation of central nervous system effects). Products include:
   Orlaam Oral Solution 2361

Levorphanol Tartrate (Potentiation of central nervous system effects). Products include:
   Levo-Dromoran 2297

Lorazepam (Potentiation of central nervous system effects). Products include:
   Ativan Injection 2805
   Ativan Tablets 2807

Loxapine Hydrochloride (Potentiation of central nervous system effects). Products include:
   Loxitane 1426

Loxapine Succinate (Potentiation of central nervous system effects). Products include:
   Loxitane Capsules 1426

Maprotiline Hydrochloride (Potentiation of central nervous system effects). Products include:
   Ludiomil Tablets 861

Mecamylamine Hydrochloride (Reduced antihypertensive effects). Products include:
   Inversine Tablets 1729

Meperidine Hydrochloride (Potentiation of central nervous system effects). Products include:
   Demerol 2438
   Mepergan Injection 2859

Mephobarbital (Potentiation of central nervous system effects). Products include:
   Mebaral Tablets 2452

Meprobamate (Potentiation of central nervous system effects). Products include:
   Miltown Tablets 2780
   PMB 200 and PMB 400 2890

IMPORTANT NOTE: Always consult each drug listing in the patient's regimen for possible interactions.

Mesoridazine Besylate (Potentiation of central nervous system effects). Products include:
   Serentil 689

Methadone Hydrochloride (Potentiation of central nervous system effects). Products include:
   Methadone Hydrochloride Oral Concentrate 2356
   Methadone Hydrochloride Oral Solution & Tablets 2357

Methohexital Sodium (Potentiation of central nervous system effects).
   No products indexed under this heading.

Methotrimeprazine (Potentiation of central nervous system effects). Products include:
   Levoprome 1321

Methoxyflurane (Potentiation of central nervous system effects).
   No products indexed under this heading.

Methyldopa (Reduced antihypertensive effects). Products include:
   Aldoclor Tablets 1638
   Aldomet Oral 1640
   Aldoril Tablets 1644

Methyldopate Hydrochloride (Reduced antihypertensive effects). Products include:
   Aldomet Ester HCl Injection 1642

Metipranolol Hydrochloride (Potentiation of sympathomimetic effects of pseudoephedrine). Products include:
   OptiPranolol (Metipranolol 0.3%) Sterile Ophthalmic Solution...... ⊙ 256

Metoprolol Succinate (Potentiation of sympathomimetic effects of pseudoephedrine). Products include:
   Toprol-XL Tablets 560

Metoprolol Tartrate (Potentiation of sympathomimetic effects of pseudoephedrine). Products include:
   Lopressor 848
   Lopressor HCT Tablets 850

Midazolam Hydrochloride (Potentiation of central nervous system effects). Products include:
   Versed Injection 2324

Molindone Hydrochloride (Potentiation of central nervous system effects). Products include:
   Moban Tablets and Concentrate 1036

Morphine Sulfate (Potentiation of central nervous system effects). Products include:
   Astramorph/PF Injection, USP (Preservative-Free) 526
   Duramorph Injection 983
   Infumorph 200 and Infumorph 500 Sterile Solutions 985
   Kadian Capsules 2948
   MS Contin Tablets 2149
   MSIR 2152
   Oramorph SR (Morphine Sulfate Sustained Release Tablets) 2359
   RMS Suppositories CII 2766
   Roxanol 2365

Nadolol (Potentiation of sympathomimetic effects of pseudoephedrine).
   No products indexed under this heading.

Nortriptyline Hydrochloride (Potentiation of central nervous system effects). Products include:
   Pamelor 2409

Opium Alkaloids (Potentiation of central nervous system effects).
   No products indexed under this heading.

Oxazepam (Potentiation of central nervous system effects). Products include:
   Serax Capsules 2916

Serax Tablets 2916

Oxycodone Hydrochloride (Potentiation of central nervous system effects). Products include:
   OxyContin Tablets 2163
   OxyIR Capsules 2167
   Percocet Tablets 955
   Percodan Tablets 955
   Percodan-Demi Tablets 956
   Roxicodone Tablets, Oral Solution & Intensol (Oxycodone) 2366
   Tylox Capsules 1593

Penbutolol Sulfate (Potentiation of sympathomimetic effects of pseudoephedrine). Products include:
   Levatol Tablets 2547

Pentobarbital Sodium (Potentiation of central nervous system effects). Products include:
   Nembutal Sodium Capsules 440
   Nembutal Sodium Solution 442
   Nembutal Sodium Suppositories 444

Perphenazine (Potentiation of central nervous system effects). Products include:
   Etrafon 2495
   Triavil Tablets 1800
   Trilafon 2532

Phenelzine Sulfate (Concurrent use is contraindicated; potentiation of central nervous system effects of hydrocodone and potentiation of sympathomimetic effects of pseudoephedrine). Products include:
   Nardil 1977

Phenobarbital (Potentiation of central nervous system effects). Products include:
   Arco-Lase Plus Tablets 513
   Bellergal-S Tablets 2375
   Donnatal 2234
   Donnatal Extentabs 2234
   Donnatal Tablets 2234
   Phenobarbital Elixir and Tablets 1523
   Quadrinal Tablets 1398

Pindolol (Potentiation of sympathomimetic effects of pseudoephedrine). Products include:
   Visken Tablets 2428

Prazepam (Potentiation of central nervous system effects).
   No products indexed under this heading.

Prochlorperazine (Potentiation of central nervous system effects). Products include:
   Compazine 2644

Promethazine Hydrochloride (Potentiation of central nervous system effects). Products include:
   Mepergan Injection 2859
   Phenergan with Codeine 2883
   Phenergan with Dextromethorphan 2885
   Phenergan Injection 2880
   Phenergan Suppositories 2882
   Phenergan Syrup 2881
   Phenergan Tablets 2882
   Phenergan VC 2886
   Phenergan VC with Codeine 2888

Propofol (Potentiation of central nervous system effects). Products include:
   Diprivan Injectable Emulsion 2939

Propoxyphene Hydrochloride (Potentiation of central nervous system effects). Products include:
   Darvon 1475
   Wygesic Tablets 2930

Propoxyphene Napsylate (Potentiation of central nervous system effects). Products include:
   Darvon-N/Darvocet-N 1473

Propranolol Hydrochloride (Potentiation of sympathomimetic effects of pseudoephedrine). Products include:
   Inderal 2834
   Inderal LA Long Acting Capsules .. 2836
   Inderide Tablets 2838

Inderide LA Long Acting Capsules .. 2840

Protriptyline Hydrochloride (Potentiation of central nervous system effects). Products include:
   Vivactil Tablets 1820

Quazepam (Potentiation of central nervous system effects). Products include:
   Doral Tablets 2773

Reserpine (Reduced antihypertensive effects). Products include:
   Diupres Tablets 1691
   Hydropres Tablets 1718
   Ser-Ap-Es Tablets 867

Risperidone (Potentiation of central nervous system effects). Products include:
   Risperdal Tablets 1348

Secobarbital Sodium (Potentiation of central nervous system effects). Products include:
   Seconal Sodium Pulvules 1529

Selegiline Hydrochloride (Concurrent use is contraindicated; potentiation of central nervous system effects of hydrocodone and potentiation of sympathomimetic effects of pseudoephedrine). Products include:
   Eldepryl Capsules 2729

Sevoflurane (Potentiation of central nervous system effects).
   No products indexed under this heading.

Sotalol Hydrochloride (Potentiation of sympathomimetic effects of pseudoephedrine). Products include:
   Betapace Tablets 637

Sufentanil Citrate (Potentiation of central nervous system effects). Products include:
   Sufenta Injection 1355

Temazepam (Potentiation of central nervous system effects). Products include:
   Restoril Capsules 2413

Thiamylal Sodium (Potentiation of central nervous system effects).
   No products indexed under this heading.

Thioridazine Hydrochloride (Potentiation of central nervous system effects). Products include:
   Mellaril 2398

Thiothixene (Potentiation of central nervous system effects). Products include:
   Navane Capsules and Concentrate 2018
   Navane Intramuscular 2019

Timolol Hemihydrate (Potentiation of sympathomimetic effects of pseudoephedrine). Products include:
   Betimol 0.25%, 0.5% .... ⊙ 259

Timolol Maleate (Potentiation of sympathomimetic effects of pseudoephedrine). Products include:
   Blocadren Tablets 1654
   Timolide Tablets 1791
   Timoptic in Ocudose 1796
   Timoptic Sterile Ophthalmic Solution 1794
   Timoptic-XE 1798

Tranylcypromine Sulfate (Concurrent use is contraindicated; potentiation of central nervous system effects of hydrocodone and potentiation of sympathomimetic effects of pseudoephedrine). Products include:
   Parnate Tablets 2679

Triazolam (Potentiation of central nervous system effects). Products include:
   Halcion Tablets 2093

Trifluoperazine Hydrochloride (Potentiation of central nervous system effects). Products include:
   Stelazine 2692

Trimipramine Maleate (Potentiation of central nervous system effects). Products include:
   Surmontil Capsules 2917

Zolpidem Tartrate (Potentiation of central nervous system effects). Products include:
   Ambien Tablets 2559

Food Interactions

Alcohol (Potentiation of central nervous system effects).

DURA-VENT TABLETS
(Phenylpropanolamine Hydrochloride, Guaifenesin) 971
May interact with monoamine oxidase inhibitors, beta blockers, and certain other agents. Compounds in these categories include:

Acebutolol Hydrochloride (Increases the effects of sympathomimetics). Products include:
   Sectral Capsules 2914

Atenolol (Increases the effects of sympathomimetics). Products include:
   Tenoretic Tablets 2963
   Tenormin Tablets and I.V. Injection 2965

Betaxolol Hydrochloride (Increases the effects of sympathomimetics). Products include:
   Betoptic Ophthalmic Solution 465
   Betoptic S Ophthalmic Suspension 467
   Kerlone Tablets 2588

Bisoprolol Fumarate (Increases the effects of sympathomimetics). Products include:
   Zebeta Tablets 1457
   Ziac 1459

Carteolol Hydrochloride (Increases the effects of sympathomimetics). Products include:
   Cartrol Tablets 413
   Ocupress Ophthalmic Solution, 1% Sterile .... ⊙ 297

Esmolol Hydrochloride (Increases the effects of sympathomimetics). Products include:
   Brevibloc (esmolol HCl) Injection 1860

Furazolidone (Co-administration with monoamine oxidase inhibitors results in increased effect of sympathomimetics; concurrent and/or sequential use is contraindicated). Products include:
   Furoxone 2221

Isocarboxazid (Co-administration with monoamine oxidase inhibitors results in increased effect of sympathomimetics; concurrent and/or sequential use is contraindicated).
   No products indexed under this heading.

Labetalol Hydrochloride (Increases the effects of sympathomimetics). Products include:
   Normodyne Injection 2519
   Normodyne Tablets 2522
   Trandate 1158

Levobunolol Hydrochloride (Increases the effects of sympathomimetics). Products include:
   Betagan .... ⊙ 230

Mecamylamine Hydrochloride (Sympathomimetic may reduce the antihypertensive effects). Products include:
   Inversine Tablets 1729

Methyldopa (Sympathomimetic may reduce the antihypertensive effects). Products include:
   Aldoclor Tablets 1638
   Aldomet Oral 1640
   Aldoril Tablets 1644

351 **Interactions Index** **Dyazide**

Methyldopate Hydrochloride (Sympathomimetic may reduce the antihypertensive effects). Products include:
Aldomet Ester HCl Injection 1642
Metipranolol Hydrochloride (Increases the effects of sympathomimetics). Products include:
OptiPranolol (Metipranolol 0.3%) Sterile Ophthalmic Solution.......... ◉ 256
Metoprolol Succinate (Increases the effects of sympathomimetics). Products include:
Toprol-XL Tablets 560
Metoprolol Tartrate (Increases the effects of sympathomimetics). Products include:
Lopressor 848
Lopressor HCT Tablets 850
Nadolol (Increases the effects of sympathomimetics).
No products indexed under this heading.
Penbutolol Sulfate (Increases the effects of sympathomimetics). Products include:
Levatol Tablets 2547
Phenelzine Sulfate (Co-administration with monoamine oxidase inhibitors results in increased effect of sympathomimetics; concurrent and/or sequential use is contraindicated). Products include:
Nardil 1977
Pindolol (Increases the effects of sympathomimetics). Products include:
Visken Tablets........................ 2428
Propranolol Hydrochloride (Increases the effects of sympathomimetics). Products include:
Inderal 2834
Inderal LA Long Acting Capsules 2836
Inderide Tablets 2838
Inderide LA Long Acting Capsules .. 2840
Reserpine (Sympathomimetic may reduce the antihypertensive effects). Products include:
Diupres Tablets 1691
Hydropres Tablets........................ 1718
Ser-Ap-Es Tablets 867
Selegiline Hydrochloride (Co-administration with monoamine oxidase inhibitors results in increased effect of sympathomimetics; concurrent and/or sequential use is contraindicated). Products include:
Eldepryl Capsules 2729
Sotalol Hydrochloride (Increases the effects of sympathomimetics). Products include:
Betapace Tablets........................ 637
Timolol Hemihydrate (Increases the effects of sympathomimetics). Products include:
Betimol 0.25%, 0.5% .... ◉ 259
Timolol Maleate (Increases the effects of sympathomimetics). Products include:
Blocadren Tablets 1654
Timolide Tablets........................ 1791
Timoptic in Ocudose 1796
Timoptic Sterile Ophthalmic Solution........................ 1794
Timoptic-XE 1798
Tranylcypromine Sulfate (Co-administration with monoamine oxidase inhibitors results in increased effect of sympathomimetics; concurrent and/or sequential use is contraindicated). Products include:
Parnate Tablets 2679

DURICEF CAPSULES, TABLETS, AND ORAL SUSPENSION
(Cefadroxil)........................ 750
None cited in PDR database.

DYAZIDE CAPSULES
(Triamterene, Hydrochlorothiazide) ..2653
May interact with potassium sparing diuretics, potassium preparations, ACE inhibitors, non-steroidal anti-inflammatory agents, lithium preparations, corticosteroids, antihypertensives, oral anticoagulants, antigout agents, nondepolarizing neuromuscular blocking agents, and certain other agents. Compounds in these categories include:

Acarbose (Increased risk of severe hyponatremia). Products include:
Precose 604
Acebutolol Hydrochloride (May add to potentiate the action of other hypertensives). Products include:
Sectral Capsules 2914
ACTH (May intensify electrolyte imbalance, particularly hypokalemia).
No products indexed under this heading.
Allopurinol (Dyazide may raise the level of blood uric acid; may require dosage adjustment of antigout agent). Products include:
Zyloprim Tablets 1194
Amiloride Hydrochloride (Concurrent use is contraindicated). Products include:
Midamor Tablets 1746
Moduretic Tablets 1748
Amlodipine Besylate (May add to potentiate the action of other hypertensives). Products include:
Lotrel Capsules........................ 858
Norvasc Tablets 2020
Amphotericin B (May intensify electrolyte imbalance, particularly hypokalemia). Products include:
Abelcet Injection........................ 1540
Fungizone Intravenous 507
Fungizone Oral Suspension 704
Atenolol (May add to potentiate the action of other hypertensives). Products include:
Tenoretic Tablets........................ 2963
Tenormin Tablets and I.V. Injection 2965
Atracurium Besylate (Increased paralyzing effect). Products include:
Tracrium Injection........................ 1155
Benazepril Hydrochloride (May add to potentiate the action of other hypertensives; increased risk of hyperkalemia). Products include:
Lotensin Tablets........................ 852
Lotensin HCT Tablets 855
Lotrel Capsules........................ 858
Bendroflumethiazide (May add to potentiate the action of other hypertensives).
No products indexed under this heading.
Betamethasone Acetate (May intensify electrolyte imbalance, particularly hypokalemia). Products include:
Celestone Soluspan Suspension 2484
Betamethasone Sodium Phosphate (May intensify electrolyte imbalance, particularly hypokalemia). Products include:
Celestone Soluspan Suspension 2484
Betaxolol Hydrochloride (May add to potentiate the action of other hypertensives). Products include:
Betoptic Ophthalmic Solution........... 465
Betoptic S Ophthalmic Suspension 467
Kerlone Tablets........................ 2588
Bisoprolol Fumarate (May add to potentiate the action of other hypertensives). Products include:
Zebeta Tablets 1457
Ziac 1459
Blood, whole (Concurrent use of whole blood from blood bank with triamterene may result in hyperkalemia, especially in patients with renal insufficiency).
No products indexed under this heading.
Captopril (May add to potentiate the action of other hypertensives; increased risk of hyperkalemia). Products include:
Capoten Tablets 740
Capozide Tablets 744
Carteolol Hydrochloride (May add to potentiate the action of other hypertensives). Products include:
Cartrol Tablets 413
Ocupress Ophthalmic Solution, 1% Sterile........................ ◉ 297
Chlorothiazide (May add to potentiate the action of other hypertensives). Products include:
Aldoclor Tablets........................ 1638
Diupres Tablets 1691
Diuril Oral 1694
Chlorothiazide Sodium (May add to potentiate the action of other hypertensives). Products include:
Diuril Sodium Intravenous 1693
Chlorpropamide (Increased risk of severe hyponatremia). Products include:
Diabinese Tablets 2002
Chlorthalidone (May add to potentiate the action of other hypertensives). Products include:
Combipres Tablets 682
Tenoretic Tablets........................ 2963
Thalitone 1293
Cisatracurium Besylate (Increased paralyzing effect). Products include:
Nimbex Injection 1131
Clonidine (May add to potentiate the action of other hypertensives). Products include:
Catapres-TTS........................ 680
Clonidine Hydrochloride (May add to potentiate the action of other hypertensives). Products include:
Catapres Tablets 679
Combipres Tablets 682
Cortisone Acetate (May intensify electrolyte imbalance, particularly hypokalemia). Products include:
Cortone Acetate Sterile Suspension 1663
Cortone Acetate Tablets........................ 1664
Deserpidine (May add to potentiate the action of other hypertensives).
No products indexed under this heading.
Dexamethasone (May intensify electrolyte imbalance, particularly hypokalemia). Products include:
AK-Trol Ointment & Suspension .... ◉ 205
Decadron Elixir 1676
Decadron Tablets........................ 1678
Decaspray Topical Aerosol 1689
Maxitrol Ophthalmic Ointment and Suspension .... ◉ 222
TobraDex Ophthalmic Suspension and Ointment........................ 469
Dexamethasone Acetate (May intensify electrolyte imbalance, particularly hypokalemia). Products include:
Dalalone D.P. Injectable 1009
Decadron-LA Sterile Suspension...... 1687
Dexamethasone Sodium Phosphate (May intensify electrolyte imbalance, particularly hypokalemia). Products include:
Decadron Phosphate Injection......... 1680
Decadron Phosphate Sterile Ophthalmic Ointment........................ 1684
Decadron Phosphate Sterile Ophthalmic Solution 1685
Decadron Phosphate Topical Cream........................ 1686
Decadron Phosphate with Xylocaine Injection, Sterile 1683
Dexacort Phosphate in Respihaler .. 1606
Dexacort Phosphate in Turbinaire .. 1607
NeoDecadron Sterile Ophthalmic Ointment 1755
NeoDecadron Sterile Ophthalmic Solution 1756
NeoDecadron Topical Cream 1757
Diazoxide (May add to potentiate the action of other hypertensives). Products include:
Hyperstat I.V. Injection 2504
Proglycem........................ 575
Diclofenac Potassium (Potential for acute renal failure). Products include:
Cataflam Tablets 833
Diclofenac Sodium (Potential for acute renal failure). Products include:
Voltaren Ophthalmic Sterile Ophthalmic Solution .... ◉ 264
Cataflam/Voltaren/Voltaren-XR 833
Dicumarol (Effects of oral anticoagulants may be decreased).
No products indexed under this heading.
Diltiazem Hydrochloride (May add to potentiate the action of other hypertensives). Products include:
Cardizem CD Capsules 1251
Cardizem SR Capsules 1255
Cardizem Injectable 1253
Cardizem Tablets........................ 1257
Dilacor XR Extended-release Capsules 2183
Tiazac Capsules 1019
Doxazosin Mesylate (May add to potentiate the action of other hypertensives). Products include:
Cardura Tablets 1993
Enalapril Maleate (May add to potentiate the action of other hypertensives; increased risk of hyperkalemia). Products include:
Vaseretic Tablets 1810
Vasotec Tablets 1816
Enalaprilat (May add to potentiate the action of other hypertensives; increased risk of hyperkalemia). Products include:
Vasotec I.V........................ 1814
Esmolol Hydrochloride (May add to potentiate the action of other hypertensives). Products include:
Brevibloc (esmolol HCl) Injection 1860
Etodolac (Potential for acute renal failure). Products include:
Lodine Capsules and Tablets 2849
Felodipine (May add to potentiate the action of other hypertensives). Products include:
Plendil Extended-Release Tablets.... 514
Fenoprofen Calcium (Potential for acute renal failure). Products include:
Nalfon 200 Pulvules & Nalfon Tablets 933
Fludrocortisone Acetate (May intensify electrolyte imbalance, particularly hypokalemia). Products include:
Florinef Acetate Tablets 506
Flurbiprofen (Potential for acute renal failure).
No products indexed under this heading.
Fosinopril Sodium (May add to potentiate the action of other hypertensives; increased risk of hyperkalemia). Products include:
Monopril Tablets 762
Furosemide (May add to potentiate the action of other hypertensives). Products include:
Lasix Injection, Oral Solution and Tablets 1267

IMPORTANT NOTE: Always consult each drug listing in the patient's regimen for possible interactions.

Dyazide **Interactions Index** **352**

Guanabenz Acetate (May add to potentiate the action of other hypertensives).
- No products indexed under this heading.

Guanethidine Monosulfate (May add to potentiate the action of other hypertensives). Products include:
- Esimil Tablets 840
- Ismelin Tablets 845

Hydralazine Hydrochloride (May add to potentiate the action of other hypertensives). Products include:
- Apresazide Capsules 824
- Apresoline Hydrochloride Tablets .. 826
- Hydralazine Hydrochloride Injection USP 2712
- Ser-Ap-Es Tablets 867

Hydrocortisone (May intensify electrolyte imbalance, particularly hypokalemia). Products include:
- Anusol-HC Cream 2.5% 1953
- Aquanil HC Lotion 1989
- Maximum Strength Cortaid Spray BD 800
- CORTENEMA 2713
- Cortisporin Ointment 1074
- Cortisporin Ophthalmic Ointment Sterile 1074
- Cortisporin Ophthalmic Suspension Sterile 1075
- Cortisporin Otic Solution Sterile 1076
- Cortisporin Otic Suspension Sterile 1077
- Cortizone-5 .... BD 795
- Cortizone-10 .... BD 795
- Hydrocortone Tablets 1715
- Hytone 922
- Hytone Ointment 2 ½% 923
- Massengill Medicated Soft Cloth Towelettes 2628
- Pediotic Suspension Sterile 1140
- Preparation H Hydrocortisone 1% Cream .... BD 843
- ProctoCream-HC 2.5% 2552
- VōSoL HC Otic Solution 2786

Hydrocortisone Acetate (May intensify electrolyte imbalance, particularly hypokalemia). Products include:
- Analpram-HC Rectal Cream 1% and 2.5% 993
- Anusol HC-1 Hydrocortisone Anti-Itch Ointment .... BD 810
- Anusol-HC Suppositories 1954
- Caldecort Anti-Itch Hydrocortisone Cream .... BD 651
- Coly-Mycin S Otic w/Neomycin & Hydrocortisone 1965
- Cortaid .... BD 800
- Cortifoam 2540
- Cortisporin Cream 1073
- Epifoam 2543
- Hydrocortone Acetate Sterile Suspension 1712
- Mantadil Cream 1124
- Nupercainal Hydrocortisone 1% Cream .... BD 661
- Pramosone Cream, Lotion & Ointment 995
- ProctoFoam-HC 2552
- Terra-Cortril Ophthalmic Suspension 2033

Hydrocortisone Sodium Phosphate (May intensify electrolyte imbalance, particularly hypokalemia). Products include:
- Hydrocortone Phosphate Injection, Sterile 1713

Hydrocortisone Sodium Succinate (May intensify electrolyte imbalance, particularly hypokalemia).
- No products indexed under this heading.

Hydroflumethiazide (May add to potentiate the action of other hypertensives). Products include:
- Diucardin Tablets 2824

Ibuprofen (Potential for acute renal failure). Products include:
- Advil Cold and Sinus Caplets and Tablets .... BD 837
- Advil Ibuprofen Tablets, Caplets and Gel Caplets .... BD 836
- Children's Motrin Ibuprofen Oral Suspension 1558
- IBU Tablets 1389
- Ibuprohm .... BD 713
- Motrin IB Caplets, Tablets, and Gelcaps .... BD 802
- Motrin Ibuprofen Suspension, Oral Drops, Chewable Tablets, Caplets 1563
- Nuprin Ibuprofen/Analgesic Tablets & Caplets .... BD 645
- Vicks DayQuil SINUS Pressure & PAIN Relief with IBUPROFEN ...... BD 735

Indapamide (May add to potentiate the action of other hypertensives).
- No products indexed under this heading.

Indomethacin (Potential for acute renal failure). Products include:
- Indocin 1723

Indomethacin Sodium Trihydrate (Potential for acute renal failure). Products include:
- Indocin I.V. 1727

Isradipine (May add to potentiate the action of other hypertensives). Products include:
- DynaCirc Capsules 2381
- DynaCirc CR Tablets 2383

Ketoprofen (Potential for acute renal failure). Products include:
- Actron Caplets and Tablets .... BD 608
- Orudis Capsules 2874
- Orudis KT .... BD 842
- Oruvail Capsules 2874

Ketorolac Tromethamine (Potential for acute renal failure). Products include:
- Acular Sterile Ophthalmic Solution 470
- Toradol 2319

Labetalol Hydrochloride (May add to potentiate the action of other hypertensives). Products include:
- Normodyne Injection 2519
- Normodyne Tablets 2522
- Trandate 1158

Laxatives, unspecified (Interferes with the potassium-retaining effects of triamterene; chronic or overuse of laxatives may reduce serum potassium).
- No products indexed under this heading.

Lisinopril (May add to potentiate the action of other hypertensives; increased risk of hyperkalemia). Products include:
- Prinivil Tablets 1776
- Prinzide Tablets 1780
- Zestoretic Tablets 2968
- Zestril Tablets 2972

Lithium Carbonate (Reduced renal clearance and increased risk of lithium toxicity). Products include:
- Eskalith 2658
- Lithium Carbonate Capsules & Tablets 2352
- Lithonate/Lithotabs/Lithobid 2721

Lithium Citrate (Reduced renal clearance and increased risk of lithium toxicity).
- No products indexed under this heading.

Losartan Potassium (May add to potentiate the action of other hypertensives). Products include:
- Cozaar Tablets 1668
- Hyzaar Tablets 1720

Mecamylamine Hydrochloride (May add to potentiate the action of other hypertensives). Products include:
- Inversine Tablets 1729

Meclofenamate Sodium (Potential for acute renal failure).
- No products indexed under this heading.

Mefenamic Acid (Potential for acute renal failure). Products include:
- Ponstel 1982

Metformin Hydrochloride (Increased risk of severe hyponatremia). Products include:
- Glucophage Tablets 754

Methenamine (Decreased effectiveness of methenamine due to alkalinization of urine). Products include:
- Urised Tablets 2123

Methenamine Hippurate (Decreased effectiveness of methenamine due to alkalinization of urine).
- No products indexed under this heading.

Methenamine Mandelate (Decreased effectiveness of methenamine due to alkalinization of urine). Products include:
- Uroqid-Acid No. 2 Tablets 633

Methyclothiazide (May add to potentiate the action of other hypertensives). Products include:
- Enduron Tablets 424

Methyldopa (May add to potentiate the action of other hypertensives). Products include:
- Aldoclor Tablets 1638
- Aldomet Oral 1640
- Aldoril Tablets 1644

Methyldopate Hydrochloride (May add to potentiate the action of other hypertensives). Products include:
- Aldomet Ester HCl Injection 1642

Methylprednisolone Acetate (May intensify electrolyte imbalance, particularly hypokalemia).
- No products indexed under this heading.

Methylprednisolone Sodium Succinate (May intensify electrolyte imbalance, particularly hypokalemia).
- No products indexed under this heading.

Metocurine Iodide (Increased paralyzing effect). Products include:
- Metubine Iodide Vials 932

Metolazone (May add to potentiate the action of other hypertensives). Products include:
- Mykrox Tablets 1617
- Zaroxolyn Tablets 1625

Metoprolol Succinate (May add to potentiate the action of other hypertensives). Products include:
- Toprol-XL Tablets 560

Metoprolol Tartrate (May add to potentiate the action of other hypertensives). Products include:
- Lopressor 848
- Lopressor HCT Tablets 850

Metyrosine (May add to potentiate the action of other hypertensives). Products include:
- Demser Capsules 1690

Minoxidil (May add to potentiate the action of other hypertensives).
- No products indexed under this heading.

Mivacurium Chloride (Increased paralyzing effect). Products include:
- Mivacron 1125

Moexipril Hydrochloride (May add to potentiate the action of other hypertensives; increased risk of hyperkalemia). Products include:
- Univasc Tablets 2553

Nabumetone (Potential for acute renal failure). Products include:
- Relafen Tablets 2688

Nadolol (May add to potentiate the action of other hypertensives).
- No products indexed under this heading.

Naproxen (Potential for acute renal failure). Products include:
- Anaprox/Naprosyn 2277

Naproxen Sodium (Potential for acute renal failure). Products include:
- Aleve 2124
- Anaprox/Naprosyn 2277
- Naprelan Tablets 2861

Nicardipine Hydrochloride (May add to potentiate the action of other hypertensives). Products include:
- Cardene Capsules 2261
- Cardene I.V. 2815
- Cardene SR Capsules 2264

Nifedipine (May add to potentiate the action of other hypertensives). Products include:
- Adalat Capsules (10 mg and 20 mg) 580
- Adalat CC 582
- Procardia Capsules 2024
- Procardia XL Extended Release Tablets 2026

Nisoldipine (May add to potentiate the action of other hypertensives). Products include:
- Sular Tablets 2961

Nitroglycerin (May add to potentiate the action of other hypertensives). Products include:
- Deponit NTG Transdermal Delivery System 2541
- Nitro-Bid IV 1270
- Nitro-Bid Ointment 1272
- Nitro-Dur (nitroglycerin) Transdermal Infusion System 1365
- Nitrolingual Spray 2193
- Nitrostat Tablets 1981
- Transderm-Nitro Transdermal Therapeutic System 878

Norepinephrine Bitartrate (Decreased arterial responsiveness to norepinephrine). Products include:
- Levophed Bitartrate Injection 2445

Oxaprozin (Potential for acute renal failure). Products include:
- Daypro Caplets 2578

Pancuronium Bromide (Increased paralyzing effect).
- No products indexed under this heading.

Penbutolol Sulfate (May add to potentiate the action of other hypertensives). Products include:
- Levatol Tablets 2547

Penicillin G Potassium (Concurrent use of parenteral penicillin G potassium with triamterene may result in hyperkalemia, especially in patients with renal insufficiency). Products include:
- Pfizerpen for Injection 2022

Phenoxybenzamine Hydrochloride (May add to potentiate the action of other hypertensives). Products include:
- Dibenzyline Capsules 2650

Phentolamine Mesylate (May add to potentiate the action of other hypertensives). Products include:
- Regitine Vials 864

Phenylbutazone (Potential for acute renal failure).
- No products indexed under this heading.

Pindolol (May add to potentiate the action of other hypertensives). Products include:
- Visken Tablets 2428

Piroxicam (Potential for acute renal failure). Products include:
- Feldene Capsules 2008

Polythiazide (May add to potentiate the action of other hypertensives). Products include:
- Minizide Capsules 2016

(BD Described in PDR For Nonprescription Drugs) (◉ Described in PDR For Ophthalmology)

Interactions Index

Potassium Acid Phosphate (Potential for hyperkalemia; concomitant use should be avoided). Products include:
K-Phos Original Formula 'Sodium Free' Tablets 633

Potassium Bicarbonate (Potential for hyperkalemia; concomitant use should be avoided). Products include:
Alka-Seltzer Gold Effervescent Antacid 611

Potassium Chloride (Potential for hyperkalemia; concomitant use should be avoided). Products include:
Chlor-3 Condiment 1003
Colyte and Colyte-flavored 2540
GoLYTELY 694
K-Dur Microburst Release System (potassium chloride, USP) E.R. Tablets 1364
K-Lor Powder Packets 438
K-Norm Capsules 1615
K-Tab Filmtab 439
Micro-K 2237
Micro-K LS Packets 2238
NuLYTELY 694
Cherry Flavor NuLYTELY 694
Rum-K Syrup 1004
Slow-K Extended-Release Tablets 869

Potassium Citrate (Potential for hyperkalemia; concomitant use should be avoided). Products include:
Polycitra Syrup 574
Polycitra-K Crystals 574
Polycitra-K Oral Solution 575
Polycitra-LC 574
Urocit-K Tablets 1828

Potassium Gluconate (Potential for hyperkalemia; concomitant use should be avoided).
No products indexed under this heading.

Potassium Phosphate, Dibasic (Potential for hyperkalemia; concomitant use should be avoided).
No products indexed under this heading.

Potassium Phosphate, Monobasic (Potential for hyperkalemia; concomitant use should be avoided). Products include:
K-Phos Neutral Tablets 633
K-Phos Original Formula 'Sodium Free' Tablets 633

Prazosin Hydrochloride (May add to potentiate the action of other hypertensives). Products include:
Minipress Capsules 2015
Minizide Capsules 2016

Prednisolone Acetate (May intensify electrolyte imbalance, particularly hypokalemia). Products include:
AK-CIDE 203
AK-CIDE Ointment 203
Blephamide Liquifilm Sterile Ophthalmic Suspension 472
Blephamide Ointment 234
Econopred & Econopred Plus Ophthalmic Suspensions 216
Poly-Pred Liquifilm 246
Pred Forte 247
Pred Mild 250
Pred-G Liquifilm Sterile Ophthalmic Suspension 248
Pred-G S.O.P. Sterile Ophthalmic Ointment 249

Prednisolone Sodium Phosphate (May intensify electrolyte imbalance, particularly hypokalemia). Products include:
AK-PRED 204
Hydeltrasol Injection, Sterile 1708
Pediapred Oral Solution 1618

Prednisolone Tebutate (May intensify electrolyte imbalance, particularly hypokalemia). Products include:
Hydeltra-T.B.A. Sterile Suspension 1710

Prednisone (May intensify electrolyte imbalance, particularly hypokalemia).
No products indexed under this heading.

Probenecid (Dyazide may raise the level of blood uric acid; may require dosage adjustment of antigout agent). Products include:
Benemid Tablets 1651
ColBENEMID Tablets 1662

Propranolol Hydrochloride (May add to potentiate the action of other hypertensives). Products include:
Inderal 2834
Inderal LA Long Acting Capsules 2836
Inderide Tablets 2838
Inderide LA Long Acting Capsules 2840

Quinapril Hydrochloride (May add to potentiate the action of other hypertensives; increased risk of hyperkalemia). Products include:
Accupril Tablets 1950

Ramipril (May add to potentiate the action of other hypertensives; increased risk of hyperkalemia). Products include:
Altace Capsules 1238

Rauwolfia Serpentina (May add to potentiate the action of other hypertensives).
No products indexed under this heading.

Rescinnamine (May add to potentiate the action of other hypertensives).
No products indexed under this heading.

Reserpine (May add to potentiate the action of other hypertensives). Products include:
Diupres Tablets 1691
Hydropres Tablets 1718
Ser-Ap-Es Tablets 867

Rocuronium Bromide (Increased paralyzing effect). Products include:
Zemuron Injection 1885

Salt Substitutes (Concurrent use of salt substitutes with triamterene may result in hyperkalemia, especially in patients with renal insufficiency).
No products indexed under this heading.

Sodium Nitroprusside (May add to potentiate the action of other hypertensives).
No products indexed under this heading.

Sodium Polystyrene Sulfonate (May result in fluid retention). Products include:
Kayexalate 2444
Sodium Polystyrene Sulfonate Suspension 2367

Sotalol Hydrochloride (May add to potentiate the action of other hypertensives). Products include:
Betapace Tablets 637

Spirapril Hydrochloride (May add to potentiate the action of other hypertensives; increased risk of hyperkalemia).
No products indexed under this heading.

Spironolactone (Concurrent use is contraindicated). Products include:
Aldactazide Tablets 2556
Aldactone Tablets 2558

Sulfinpyrazone (Dyazide may raise the level of blood uric acid; may require dosage adjustment of antigout agent). Products include:
Anturane 823

Sulindac (Potential for acute renal failure). Products include:
Clinoril Tablets 1658

Terazosin Hydrochloride (May add to potentiate the action of other hypertensives). Products include:
Hytrin Capsules 434

Timolol Maleate (May add to potentiate the action of other hypertensives). Products include:
Blocadren Tablets 1654
Timolide Tablets 1791
Timoptic in Ocudose 1796
Timoptic Sterile Ophthalmic Solution 1794
Timoptic-XE 1798

Tolmetin Sodium (Potential for acute renal failure). Products include:
Tolectin (200, 400 and 600 mg) .. 1591

Torsemide (May add to potentiate the action of other hypertensives). Products include:
Demadex Tablets and Injection 691

Trandolapril (May add to potentiate the action of other hypertensives; increased risk of hyperkalemia). Products include:
Mavik Tablets 1407

Triamcinolone (May intensify electrolyte imbalance, particularly hypokalemia).
No products indexed under this heading.

Triamcinolone Acetonide (May intensify electrolyte imbalance, particularly hypokalemia). Products include:
Azmacort Oral Inhaler 2175
Nasacort AQ Nasal Spray 2191
Nasacort Nasal Inhaler 2189

Triamcinolone Diacetate (May intensify electrolyte imbalance, particularly hypokalemia).
No products indexed under this heading.

Triamcinolone Hexacetonide (May intensify electrolyte imbalance, particularly hypokalemia).
No products indexed under this heading.

Trimethaphan Camsylate (May add to potentiate the action of other hypertensives).
No products indexed under this heading.

Tubocurarine Chloride (Increased paralyzing effect).
No products indexed under this heading.

Vecuronium Bromide (Increased paralyzing effect). Products include:
Norcuron for Injection 1875

Verapamil Hydrochloride (May add to potentiate the action of other hypertensives). Products include:
Calan SR Caplets 2571
Calan Tablets 2568
Covera-HS Tablets 2573
Isoptin Injectable 1391
Isoptin Oral Tablets 1393
Isoptin SR Tablets 1395
Verelan Capsules 1455

Warfarin Sodium (Effects of oral anticoagulants may be decreased). Products include:
Coumadin 941

Food Interactions
Milk, low fat (Concurrent use of low-salt milk with triamterene may result in hyperkalemia, especially in patients with renal insufficiency).

DYCLONE 0.5% AND 1% TOPICAL SOLUTIONS, USP
(Dyclonine Hydrochloride) 535

Food Interactions
Food, unspecified (Topical anesthesia may impair swallowing and thus enhance the danger of aspiration; food should not be ingested for 60 minutes).

DYNABAC
(Dirithromycin) 668
May interact with xanthine bronchodilators, antacids containing aluminium, calcium and magnesium, histamine h2-receptor antagonists, oral anticoagulants, and certain other agents. Compounds in these categories include:

Alfentanil Hydrochloride (Caution is advised since erythromycin, a macrolide antibiotic, and alfentanil co-administration is associated with elevation in alfentanil serum levels). Products include:
Alfenta Injection 1334

Aluminum Carbonate (When dirithromycin is administered immediately following antacids, the absorption of dirithromycin is slightly enhanced). Products include:
Basaljel Capsules 2810
Basaljel Suspension 2810
Basaljel Tablets 2810

Aluminum Hydroxide (When dirithromycin is administered immediately following antacids, the absorption of dirithromycin is slightly enhanced). Products include:
ALternaGEL Liquid 1358
Maximum Strength Ascriptin 650
Cama Arthritis Pain Reliever 748
Gaviscon Extra Strength Relief Formula Antacid Tablets 778
Gaviscon Extra Strength Relief Formula Liquid Antacid 779
Gaviscon Liquid Antacid 779
Gelusil Antacid-Anti-gas Liquid 819
Gelusil Antacid-Anti-gas Tablets 819
Maalox Antacid/Anti-Gas Tablets 889
Maalox Heartburn Relief Suspension 658
Maalox Antacid Liquid 888
Extra Strength Maalox Antacid/Anti-Gas Liquid and Tablets 888
Mylanta 1359
Tempo Soft Antacid 799

Aluminum Hydroxide Gel (When dirithromycin is administered immediately following antacids, the absorption of dirithromycin is slightly enhanced). Products include:
ALternaGEL Liquid 675
Aludrox Oral Suspension 850
Amphojel Suspension 2802
Amphojel Suspension without Flavor 2802
Amphojel Tablets 2802
Ascriptin 650
Gaviscon Antacid Tablets 778
Gaviscon-2 Antacid Tablets 779
Mylanta Liquid 676
Mylanta Double Strength Liquid 676
Nephrox Suspension 671

Aminophylline (Steady-state plasma concentration is not significantly affected, however, patients with theophylline concentrations at the higher end of the therapeutic range should be monitored for dosage adjustment).
No products indexed under this heading.

Bromocriptine Mesylate (Caution is advised since erythromycin, a macrolide antibiotic, and bromocriptine co-administration is associated with elevation in bromocriptine serum levels). Products include:
Parlodel 2411

Carbamazepine (Caution is advised since erythromycin, a macrolide antibiotic, and carbamazepine co-administration is associated with elevation in carbamazepine serum levels). Products include:
Atretol Tablets 569
Tegretol/Tegretol-XR 870

IMPORTANT NOTE: Always consult each drug listing in the patient's regimen for possible interactions.

Cimetidine (When dirithromycin is administered immediately following H_2-receptor antagonists, the absorption of dirithromycin is slightly enhanced). Products include:

Tagamet HB Tablets ▣ 786
Tagamet Tablets 2694

Cimetidine Hydrochloride (When dirithromycin is administered immediately following H_2-receptor antagonists, the absorption of dirithromycin is slightly enhanced). Products include:

Tagamet 2694

Cyclosporine (Caution is advised since erythromcyin, a macrolide antibiotic, and cyclosporine co-administration is associated with elevation in cyclosporine serum levels). Products include:

Neoral 2405
Sandimmune 2416

Dicumarol (Caution is advised since erythromcyin, a macrolide antibiotic, increases anticoagulant effect).

No products indexed under this heading.

Digoxin (Caution is advised since erythromycin, a macrolide antibiotic, elevates digoxin serum levels). Products include:

Lanoxicaps 1110
Lanoxin Elixir Pediatric 1113
Lanoxin Injection 1116
Lanoxin Injection Pediatric 1119
Lanoxin Tablets 1121

Dihydroergotamine Mesylate (Caution is advised since erythromycin, a macrolide antibiotic, and ergotamine co-administration is associated with acute ergot toxicity). Products include:

D.H.E. 45 Injection 2381

Disopyramide Phosphate (Caution is advised since erythromycin, a macrolide antibiotic, and disopyramide co-administration is associated with elevation in disopyramide serum levels). Products include:

Norpace 2596

Dyphylline (Steady-state plasma concentration is not significantly affected, however, patients with theophylline concentrations at the higher end of the therapeutic range should be monitored for dosage adjustment). Products include:

Lufyllin & Lufyllin-400 Tablets 2778
Lufyllin-GG Elixir & Tablets 2779

Ergotamine Tartrate (Caution is advised since erythromycin, a macrolide antibiotic, and ergotamine co-administration is associated with acute ergot toxicity). Products include:

Bellergal-S Tablets 2375
Cafergot 2376
Ergomar Tablets 1543
Wigraine Tablets 1884

Famotidine (When dirithromycin is administered immediately following H_2-receptor antagonists, the absorption of dirithromycin is slightly enhanced). Products include:

Pepcid AC Acid Controller 1360
Pepcid Injection 1765
Pepcid 1763

Hexobarbital (Caution is advised since erythromycin, a macrolide antibiotic, and hexobarbital co-administration is associated with elevation in hexobarbital serum levels).

Lovastatin (Caution is advised since erythromycin, a macrolide antibiotic, and lovastatin co-administration is associated with elevation in lovastatin serum levels). Products include:

Mevacor Tablets 1742

Magaldrate (When dirithromycin is administered immediately following antacids, the absorption of dirithromycin is slightly enhanced).

No products indexed under this heading.

Magnesium Hydroxide (When dirithromycin is administered immediately following antacids, the absorption of dirithromycin is slightly enhanced). Products include:

Aludrox Oral Suspension ▣ 850
Ascriptin ▣ 650
Di-Gel Antacid/Anti-Gas ▣ 762
Gelusil Antacid-Anti-gas Liquid ▣ 819
Gelusil Antacid-Anti-gas Tablets ▣ 819
Maalox Antacid/Anti-Gas Tablets 889
Maalox Antacid Liquid 888
Extra Strength Maalox Antacid/Anti-Gas Liquid and Tablets 888
Mylanta Fast-Acting 1359
Mylanta Gelcaps Antacid ▣ 678
Fast-Acting Mylanta Liquid Antacid 1359
Mylanta Tablets ▣ 677
Maximum-Strength Fast-Acting Mylanta Liquid Antacid 1359
Mylanta Double Strength Tablets ▣ 677
Phillips' Milk of Magnesia Liquid ▣ 627
Rolaids Antacid Tablets ▣ 807
Tempo Soft Antacid ▣ 799

Magnesium Oxide (When dirithromycin is administered immediately following antacids, the absorption of dirithromycin is slightly enhanced). Products include:

Beelith Tablets 632
Bufferin Analgesic Tablets ▣ 636
Arthritis Strength Bufferin Analgesic Caplets ▣ 637
Extra Strength Bufferin Analgesic Tablets ▣ 637
Caltrate PLUS ▣ 681
Cama Arthritis Pain Reliever ▣ 748
Mag-Ox 400 666
Uro-Mag 666

Nizatidine (When dirithromycin is administered immediately following H_2-receptor antagonists, the absorption of dirithromycin is slightly enhanced). Products include:

Axid Pulvules 1468

Phenytoin (Caution is advised since erythromycin, a macrolide antibiotic, and phenytoin co-administration is associated with elevation in phenytoin serum levels). Products include:

Dilantin Infatabs 1967
Dilantin-125 Suspension 1969

Phenytoin Sodium (Caution is advised since erythromycin, a macrolide antibiotic, and phenytoin co-administration is associated with elevation in phenytoin serum levels). Products include:

Dilantin Kapseals 1965

Ranitidine Hydrochloride (When dirithromycin is administered immediately following H_2-receptor antagonists, the absorption of dirithromycin is slightly enhanced). Products include:

Zantac 1182
Zantac Injection 1180
Zantac Syrup 1182

Terfenadine (Until further use data are available, it is prudent to monitor the terfenadine levels when both drugs are co-administered; most macrolide antibiotics are contraindicated in patients receiving terfenadine; in one study dirithromycin did not affect terfenadine's metabolism). Products include:

Seldane Tablets 1284
Seldane-D Extended-Release Tablets 1286

Theophylline (Steady-state plasma concentration is not significantly affected, however, patients with theophylline concentrations at the higher end of the therapeutic range should be monitored for dosage adjustment). Products include:

Marax Tablets & DF Syrup 2015
Quibron 2227

Theophylline Anhydrous (Steady-state plasma concentration is not significantly affected, however, patients with theophylline concentrations at the higher end of the therapeutic range should be monitored for dosage adjustment). Products include:

Aerolate 1003
Primatene Tablets ▣ 844
Respbid Tablets 687
Slo-bid Gyrocaps 2201
Theo-24 Extended Release Capsules 2753
Theo-Dur Extended-Release Tablets 1367
Theo-X Extended-Release Tablets 793
Uni-Dur Extended-Release Tablets 1374
Uniphyl 400 mg and 600 mg Tablets 2157

Theophylline Calcium Salicylate (Steady-state plasma concentration is not significantly affected, however, patients with theophylline concentrations at the higher end of the therapeutic range should be monitored for dosage adjustment). Products include:

Quadrinal Tablets 1398

Theophylline Sodium Glycinate (Steady-state plasma concentration is not significantly affected, however, patients with theophylline concentrations at the higher end of the therapeutic range should be monitored for dosage adjustment).

No products indexed under this heading.

Triazolam (Caution is advised since erythromycin, a macrolide antibiotic, decreases the clearance of triazolam and thereby increasing the pharmacologic effect of triazolam). Products include:

Halcion Tablets 2093

Warfarin Sodium (Caution is advised since erythromcyin, a macrolide antibiotic, increases anticoagulant effect). Products include:

Coumadin 941

Food Interactions

Food, unspecified (Slight increase in the absorption of erythromycylamine when dirithromycin tablets were administered after food; significant decrease in C_{max} (33%) and AUC (31%) occurs when administered one hour before food; administer with food or within an hour of having eaten).

DYNACIN CAPSULES
(Minocycline Hydrochloride) 1627
May interact with oral anticoagulants, penicillins, antacids containing aluminium, calcium and magnesium, iron containing oral preparations, oral contraceptives, and certain other agents. Compounds in these categories include:

Aluminum Carbonate (Absorption of tetracyclines is impaired by antacids). Products include:

Basaljel Capsules 2810
Basaljel Suspension 2810
Basaljel Tablets 2810

Aluminum Hydroxide (Absorption of tetracyclines is impaired by antacids). Products include:

ALternaGEL Liquid 1358
Maximum Strength Ascriptin ▣ 650
Cama Arthritis Pain Reliever ▣ 748
Gaviscon Extra Strength Relief Formula Antacid Tablets ▣ 778
Gaviscon Extra Strength Relief Formula Liquid Antacid ▣ 779
Gaviscon Liquid Antacid ▣ 779
Gelusil Antacid-Anti-gas Liquid ▣ 819
Gelusil Antacid-Anti-gas Tablets ▣ 819
Maalox Antacid/Anti-Gas Tablets 889
Maalox Heartburn Relief Suspension ▣ 658
Maalox Antacid Liquid 888
Extra Strength Maalox Antacid/Anti-Gas Liquid and Tablets 888
Mylanta 1359
Tempo Soft Antacid ▣ 799

Aluminum Hydroxide Gel (Absorption of tetracyclines is impaired by antacids). Products include:

ALternaGEL Liquid ▣ 675
Aludrox Oral Suspension ▣ 850
Amphojel Suspension 2802
Amphojel Suspension without Flavor 2802
Amphojel Tablets 2802
Ascriptin ▣ 650
Gaviscon Antacid Tablets ▣ 778
Gaviscon-2 Antacid Tablets ▣ 779
Mylanta Liquid ▣ 676
Mylanta Double Strength Liquid ▣ 676
Nephrox Suspension ▣ 671

Amoxicillin Trihydrate (Interference with bactericidal action of penicillin; avoid giving tetracycline-class drugs in conjunction with penicillin). Products include:

Amoxil 2631
Augmentin 2637
Augmentin Tablets 2640

Ampicillin (Interference with bactericidal action of penicillin; avoid giving tetracycline-class drugs in conjunction with penicillin). Products include:

Omnipen Capsules 2872
Omnipen for Oral Suspension 2873

Ampicillin Sodium (Interference with bactericidal action of penicillin; avoid giving tetracycline-class drugs in conjunction with penicillin). Products include:

Unasyn 2035

Ampicillin Trihydrate (Interference with bactericidal action of penicillin; avoid giving tetracycline-class drugs in conjunction with penicillin).

No products indexed under this heading.

Azlocillin Sodium (Interference with bactericidal action of penicillin; avoid giving tetracycline-class drugs in conjunction with penicillin).

No products indexed under this heading.

Bacampicillin Hydrochloride (Interference with bactericidal action of penicillin; avoid giving tetracycline-class drugs in conjunction with penicillin). Products include:

Spectrobid Tablets 2030

Carbenicillin Disodium (Interference with bactericidal action of penicillin; avoid giving tetracycline-class drugs in conjunction with penicillin).

No products indexed under this heading.

(▣ Described in PDR For Nonprescription Drugs) (⊚ Described in PDR For Ophthalmology)

355 **Interactions Index** **DynaCirc CR**

Carbenicillin Indanyl Sodium (Interference with bactericidal action of penicillin; avoid giving tetracycline-class drugs in conjunction with penicillin). Products include:
Geocillin Tablets 2009

Desogestrel (Concurrent use of tetracyclines may render oral contraceptives less effective). Products include:
Desogen Tablets 1867
Ortho-Cept 1907

Dicloxacillin Sodium (Interference with bactericidal action of penicillin; avoid giving tetracycline-class drugs in conjunction with penicillin).
No products indexed under this heading.

Dicumarol (Tetracyclines have shown to depress plasma prothrombin activity; patients on anticoagulant may require downward adjustments of their anticoagulant dosage).
No products indexed under this heading.

Ethinyl Estradiol (Concurrent use of tetracyclines may render oral contraceptives less effective). Products include:
Brevicon 2563
Demulen 2580
Desogen Tablets 1867
Levlen/Tri-Levlen 646
Lo/Ovral Tablets 2852
Lo/Ovral-28 Tablets 2857
Modicon 1928
Nordette-21 Tablets 2863
Nordette-28 Tablets 2866
Norinyl 2563
Ortho-Cept 1907
Ortho-Cyclen/Ortho-Tri-Cyclen 1914
Ortho-Novum 1928
Ortho-Cyclen/Ortho Tri-Cyclen 1914
Ovcon 765
Ovral Tablets 2877
Ovral-28 Tablets 2878
Levlen/Tri-Levlen 646
Tri-Norinyl 2607
Triphasil-21 Tablets 2919
Triphasil-28 Tablets 2924

Ethynodiol Diacetate (Concurrent use of tetracyclines may render oral contraceptives less effective). Products include:
Demulen 2580

Ferrous Fumarate (Absorption of tetracyclines is impaired by iron-containing preparations). Products include:
Chromagen Capsules 2470
Chromagen FA 2471
Chromagen Forte 2471
Ferro-Sequels 684
Nephro-Fer Tablets 2168
Nephro-Fer Rx Tablets 2168
Nephro-Vite + Fe Tablets 2170
Stresstabs + Iron 685
Trinsicon Capsules 2759
Vitron-C Tablets 667

Ferrous Gluconate (Absorption of tetracyclines is impaired by iron-containing preparations). Products include:
Megadose 513

Ferrous Sulfate (Absorption of tetracyclines is impaired by iron-containing preparations). Products include:
Feosol Capsules 777
Feosol Elixir 2627
Feosol Tablets 2627
Fero-Folic-500 Filmtab 433
Fero-Grad-500 Filmtab 434
Fero-Gradumet Filmtab 434
Iberet Tablets 437
Iberet-500 Liquid 438
Iberet-Folic-500 Filmtab 433
Iberet-Liquid 438
Irospan 1000
Slow Fe Tablets 889
Slow Fe with Folic Acid 890

Levonorgestrel (Concurrent use of tetracyclines may render oral contraceptives less effective). Products include:
Levlen/Tri-Levlen 646
Nordette-21 Tablets 2863
Nordette-28 Tablets 2866
Norplant System 2868
Levlen/Tri-Levlen 646
Triphasil-21 Tablets 2919
Triphasil-28 Tablets 2924

Magaldrate (Absorption of tetracyclines is impaired by antacids).
No products indexed under this heading.

Magnesium Hydroxide (Absorption of tetracyclines is impaired by antacids). Products include:
Aludrox Oral Suspension 850
Ascriptin 650
Di-Gel Antacid/Anti-Gas 762
Gelusil Antacid-Anti-gas Liquid 819
Gelusil Antacid-Anti-gas Tablets 819
Maalox Antacid/Anti-Gas Tablets 889
Maalox Antacid Liquid 888
Extra Strength Maalox Antacid/Anti-Gas Liquid and Tablets 888
Mylanta Fast-Acting 1359
Mylanta Gelcaps Antacid 678
Fast-Acting Mylanta Liquid Antacid 1359
Mylanta Tablets 677
Maximum-Strength Fast-Acting Mylanta Liquid Antacid 1359
Mylanta Double Strength Tablets 677
Phillips' Milk of Magnesia Liquid 627
Rolaids Antacid Tablets 807
Tempo Soft Antacid 799

Magnesium Oxide (Absorption of tetracyclines is impaired by antacids). Products include:
Beelith Tablets 632
Bufferin Analgesic Tablets 636
Arthritis Strength Bufferin Analgesic Caplets 637
Extra Strength Bufferin Analgesic Tablets 637
Caltrate PLUS 681
Cama Arthritis Pain Reliever 748
Mag-Ox 400 666
Uro-Mag 666

Mestranol (Concurrent use of tetracyclines may render oral contraceptives less effective). Products include:
Norinyl 2563
Ortho-Novum 1928

Methoxyflurane (Potential for fatal renal toxicity).
No products indexed under this heading.

Mezlocillin Sodium (Interference with bactericidal action of penicillin; avoid giving tetracycline-class drugs in conjunction with penicillin). Products include:
Mezlin 594
Mezlin Pharmacy Bulk Package 597

Nafcillin Sodium (Interference with bactericidal action of penicillin; avoid giving tetracycline-class drugs in conjunction with penicillin).
No products indexed under this heading.

Norethindrone (Concurrent use of tetracyclines may render oral contraceptives less effective). Products include:
Brevicon 2563
Micronor Tablets 1903
Modicon 1928
Norinyl 2563
Nor-Q D Tablets 2598
Ortho-Novum 1928
Ovcon 765
Tri-Norinyl 2607

Norethynodrel (Concurrent use of tetracyclines may render oral contraceptives less effective).
No products indexed under this heading.

Norgestimate (Concurrent use of tetracyclines may render oral contraceptives less effective). Products include:
Ortho-Cyclen/Ortho-Tri-Cyclen 1914
Ortho-Cyclen/Ortho Tri-Cyclen 1914

Norgestrel (Concurrent use of tetracyclines may render oral contraceptives less effective). Products include:
Lo/Ovral Tablets 2852
Lo/Ovral-28 Tablets 2857
Ovral Tablets 2877
Ovral-28 Tablets 2878
Ovrette Tablets 2878

Penicillin G Benzathine (Interference with bactericidal action of penicillin; avoid giving tetracycline-class drugs in conjunction with penicillin). Products include:
Bicillin C-R Injection 2810
Bicillin C-R 900/300 Injection 2812
Bicillin L-A Injection 2813

Penicillin G Potassium (Interference with bactericidal action of penicillin; avoid giving tetracycline-class drugs in conjunction with penicillin). Products include:
Pfizerpen for Injection 2022

Penicillin G Procaine (Interference with bactericidal action of penicillin; avoid giving tetracycline-class drugs in conjunction with penicillin). Products include:
Bicillin C-R Injection 2810
Bicillin C-R 900/300 Injection 2812

Penicillin G Sodium (Interference with bactericidal action of penicillin; avoid giving tetracycline-class drugs in conjunction with penicillin).
No products indexed under this heading.

Penicillin V Potassium (Interference with bactericidal action of penicillin; avoid giving tetracycline-class drugs in conjunction with penicillin). Products include:
Pen•Vee K 2879

Polysaccharide-Iron Complex (Absorption of tetracyclines is impaired by iron-containing preparations). Products include:
Niferex-150 Capsules 811
Niferex Elixir 811
Niferex-150 Forte Capsules 811
Niferex 811
Niferex-PN Tablets 811
Nu-Iron 150 Capsules 1826
Nu-Iron Elixir 1826

Ticarcillin Disodium (Interference with bactericidal action of penicillin; avoid giving tetracycline-class drugs in conjunction with penicillin). Products include:
Ticar for Injection 2704
Timentin for Injection 2706

Warfarin Sodium (Tetracyclines have shown to depress plasma prothrombin activity; patients on anticoagulant may require downward adjustments of their anticoagulant dosage). Products include:
Coumadin 941

Food Interactions

Food, unspecified (The peak plasma concentrations were slightly decreased and delayed by one hour when administered with a meal which included dairy products; extent of absorption was not noticeably influenced).

DYNACIRC CAPSULES
(Isradipine) 2381
May interact with:

Cimetidine (Potential for increase in isradipine mean peak plasma concentration and significant increase in the AUC). Products include:
Tagamet HB Tablets 786
Tagamet Tablets 2694

Cimetidine Hydrochloride (Potential for increase in isradipine mean peak plasma concentration and significant increase in the AUC). Products include:
Tagamet 2694

Fentanyl (Severe hypotension has been reported during fentanyl anesthesia with concomitant use of beta blocker and calcium channel blocker). Products include:
Duragesic Transdermal System 1336

Fentanyl Citrate (Severe hypotension has been reported during fentanyl anesthesia with concomitant use of beta blocker and calcium channel blocker). Products include:
Sublimaze Injection 463

Hydrochlorothiazide (Co-administration does not alter pharmacokinetic of either drug; isradipine has an additional antihypertensive effect with combined therapy). Products include:
Aldactazide Tablets 2556
Aldoril Tablets 1644
Apresazide Capsules 824
Capozide Tablets 744
Dyazide Capsules 2653
Esidrix Tablets 839
Esimil Tablets 840
HydroDIURIL Tablets 1716
Hydropres Tablets 1718
Hyzaar Tablets 1720
Inderide Tablets 2838
Inderide LA Long Acting Capsules 2840
Lopressor HCT Tablets 850
Lotensin HCT Tablets 855
Moduretic Tablets 1748
Oretic Tablets 450
Prinzide Tablets 1780
Ser-Ap-Es Tablets 867
Timolide Tablets 1791
Vaseretic Tablets 1810
Zestoretic Tablets 2968
Ziac 1459

Propranolol Hydrochloride (Variable effect on either drug's bioavailability with concurrent administration). Products include:
Inderal 2834
Inderal LA Long Acting Capsules 2836
Inderide Tablets 2838
Inderide LA Long Acting Capsules 2840

Rifampin (Increased metabolism and higher clearance of isradipine leading to reduction in its levels below detectable limit and therapeutic effects are likely to be abolished or markedly reduced). Products include:
Rifadin 1276
Rifamate Capsules 1278
Rifater 1280
Rimactane Capsules 865

Food Interactions

Food, unspecified (Coadministration significantly increases the time to peak by about an hour with no effect on AUC).

DYNACIRC CR TABLETS
(Isradipine) 2383
May interact with:

Fentanyl (Severe hypotension has been reported during fentanyl anesthesia with concomitant use of beta blocker and calcium channel blocker). Products include:
Duragesic Transdermal System 1336

IMPORTANT NOTE: Always consult each drug listing in the patient's regimen for possible interactions.

DynaCirc CR / Interactions Index

Fentanyl Citrate (Severe hypotension has been reported during fentanyl anesthesia with concomitant use of beta blocker and calcium channel blocker). Products include:
- Sublimaze Injection ... 463

Hydrochlorothiazide (Co-administration does not alter pharmacokinetics of either drug; isradipine has an additional antihypertensive effect with combined therapy). Products include:
- Aldactazide Tablets ... 2556
- Aldoril Tablets ... 1644
- Apresazide Capsules ... 824
- Capozide Tablets ... 744
- Dyazide Capsules ... 2653
- Esidrix Tablets ... 839
- Esimil Tablets ... 840
- HydroDIURIL Tablets ... 1716
- Hydropres Tablets ... 1718
- Hyzaar Tablets ... 1720
- Inderide Tablets ... 2838
- Inderide LA Long Acting Capsules ... 2840
- Lopressor HCT Tablets ... 850
- Lotensin HCT Tablets ... 855
- Moduretic Tablets ... 1748
- Oretic Tablets ... 450
- Prinzide Tablets ... 1780
- Ser-Ap-Es Tablets ... 867
- Timolide Tablets ... 1791
- Vaseretic Tablets ... 1810
- Zestoretic Tablets ... 2968
- Ziac ... 1459

Propranolol Hydrochloride (Variable effect on either drug's bioavailability with concurrent administration). Products include:
- Inderal ... 2834
- Inderal LA Long Acting Capsules ... 2836
- Inderide Tablets ... 2838
- Inderide LA Long Acting Capsules ... 2840

Food Interactions
Food, unspecified (Food has been shown to decrease the extent of bioavailability of DynaCirc CR by up to 25%).

DYRENIUM CAPSULES
(Triamterene) ... 2655

May interact with potassium preparations, lithium preparations, nonsteroidal anti-inflammatory agents, antihypertensives, diuretics, preanesthetic medications, general anesthetics, nondepolarizing neuromuscular blocking agents, ACE inhibitors, oral hypoglycemic agents, potassium sparing diuretics, and certain other agents. Compounds in these categories include:

Acarbose (Triamterene may raise blood glucose levels; for adult-onset diabetes, dosage adjustments of hypoglycemic agents may be necessary). Products include:
- Precose ... 604

Acebutolol Hydrochloride (Potentiation of antihypertensive effect). Products include:
- Sectral Capsules ... 2914

Amiloride Hydrochloride (Potentiation of diuretic effect; concomitant administration is contraindicated). Products include:
- Midamor Tablets ... 1746
- Moduretic Tablets ... 1748

Amlodipine Besylate (Potentiation of antihypertensive effect). Products include:
- Lotrel Capsules ... 858
- Norvasc Tablets ... 2020

Atenolol (Potentiation of antihypertensive effect). Products include:
- Tenoretic Tablets ... 2963
- Tenormin Tablets and I.V. Injection ... 2965

Atracurium Besylate (The effects of nondepolarizing skeletal muscle relaxants may be potentiated). Products include:
- Tracrium Injection ... 1155

Benazepril Hydrochloride (Potential for antihypertensive effect and increased risk of hyperkalemia). Products include:
- Lotensin Tablets ... 852
- Lotensin HCT Tablets ... 855
- Lotrel Capsules ... 858

Bendroflumethiazide (Potentiation of diuretic effect).
No products indexed under this heading.

Betaxolol Hydrochloride (Potentiation of antihypertensive effect). Products include:
- Betoptic Ophthalmic Solution ... 465
- Betoptic S Ophthalmic Suspension ... 467
- Kerlone Tablets ... 2588

Bisoprolol Fumarate (Potentiation of antihypertensive effect). Products include:
- Zebeta Tablets ... 1457
- Ziac ... 1459

Blood, whole (Co-administration with blood from blood bank may promote serum potassium accumulation and possibly resulting in hyperkalemia).
No products indexed under this heading.

Bumetanide (Potentiation of diuretic effect). Products include:
- Bumex ... 2260

Captopril (Potential for antihypertensive effect and increased risk of hyperkalemia). Products include:
- Capoten Tablets ... 740
- Capozide Tablets ... 744

Carteolol Hydrochloride (Potentiation of antihypertensive effect). Products include:
- Cartrol Tablets ... 413
- Ocupress Ophthalmic Solution, 1% Sterile ... ⊙ 297

Chlorothiazide (Potentiation of diuretic effect). Products include:
- Aldoclor Tablets ... 1638
- Diupres Tablets ... 1691
- Diuril Oral ... 1694

Chlorothiazide Sodium (Potentiation of antihypertensive and/or diuretic effect). Products include:
- Diuril Sodium Intravenous ... 1693

Chlorpropamide (Concurrent use may increase the risk of severe hyponatremia; triamterene may raise blood glucose levels; for adult-onset diabetes, dosage adjustments of hypoglycemic agents may be necessary). Products include:
- Diabinese Tablets ... 2002

Chlorthalidone (Potentiation of antihypertensive and/or diuretic effect). Products include:
- Combipres Tablets ... 682
- Tenoretic Tablets ... 2963
- Thalitone ... 1293

Cisatracurium Besylate (The effects of nondepolarizing skeletal muscle relaxants may be potentiated). Products include:
- Nimbex Injection ... 1131

Clonidine (Potentiation of antihypertensive effect). Products include:
- Catapres-TTS ... 680

Clonidine Hydrochloride (Potentiation of antihypertensive effect). Products include:
- Catapres Tablets ... 679
- Combipres Tablets ... 682

Deserpidine (Potentiation of antihypertensive effect).
No products indexed under this heading.

Diazepam (The effects of preanesthetic agents may be potentiated). Products include:
- Dizac (diazepam injectable emulsion) CIV ... 1862
- Valium Tablets ... 2336

Valium Tablets ... 2335

Diazoxide (Potentiation of antihypertensive effect). Products include:
- Hyperstat I.V. Injection ... 2504
- Proglycem ... 575

Diclofenac Potassium (Possibility for acute renal failure). Products include:
- Cataflam Tablets ... 833

Diclofenac Sodium (Possibility for acute renal failure). Products include:
- Voltaren Ophthalmic Sterile Ophthalmic Solution ... ⊙ 264
- Cataflam/Voltaren/Voltaren-XR ... 833

Diltiazem Hydrochloride (Potentiation of antihypertensive effect). Products include:
- Cardizem CD Capsules ... 1251
- Cardizem SR Capsules ... 1255
- Cardizem Injectable ... 1253
- Cardizem Tablets ... 1257
- Dilacor XR Extended-release Capsules ... 2183
- Tiazac Capsules ... 1019

Doxazosin Mesylate (Potentiation of antihypertensive effect). Products include:
- Cardura Tablets ... 1993

Droperidol (The effects of preanesthetic agents may be potentiated). Products include:
- Inapsine Injection ... 462

Enalapril Maleate (Potential for increased antihypertensive effect and risk of hyperkalemia). Products include:
- Vaseretic Tablets ... 1810
- Vasotec Tablets ... 1816

Enalaprilat (Potential for increased antihypertensive effect and risk of hyperkalemia). Products include:
- Vasotec I.V. ... 1814

Enflurane (The effects of anesthetic agents may be potentiated).
No products indexed under this heading.

Esmolol Hydrochloride (Potentiation of antihypertensive effect). Products include:
- Brevibloc (esmolol HCl) Injection ... 1860

Ethacrynic Acid (Potentiation of diuretic effect). Products include:
- Edecrin Tablets ... 1698

Etodolac (Possibility for acute renal failure). Products include:
- Lodine Capsules and Tablets ... 2849

Felodipine (Potentiation of antihypertensive effect). Products include:
- Plendil Extended-Release Tablets ... 514

Fenoprofen Calcium (Possibility for acute renal failure). Products include:
- Nalfon 200 Pulvules & Nalfon Tablets ... 933

Fentanyl Citrate (The effects of preanesthetic agents may be potentiated). Products include:
- Sublimaze Injection ... 463

Flurbiprofen (Possibility for acute renal failure).
No products indexed under this heading.

Fosinopril Sodium (Potential for antihypertensive effect and increased risk of hyperkalemia). Products include:
- Monopril Tablets ... 762

Furosemide (Potentiation of antihypertensive and/or diuretic effect). Products include:
- Lasix Injection, Oral Solution and Tablets ... 1267

Glimepiride (Triamterene may raise blood glucose levels; for adult-onset diabetes, dosage adjustments of hypoglycemic agents may be necessary). Products include:
- Amaryl Tablets ... 1241

Glipizide (Triamterene may raise blood glucose levels; for adult-onset diabetes, dosage adjustments of hypoglycemic agents may be necessary). Products include:
- Glucotrol Tablets ... 2011
- Glucotrol XL Extended Release Tablets ... 2012

Glyburide (Triamterene may raise blood glucose levels; for adult-onset diabetes, dosage adjustments of hypoglycemic agents may be necessary). Products include:
- DiaBeta Tablets ... 1265
- Glynase PresTab Tablets ... 2091
- Micronase Tablets ... 2099

Guanabenz Acetate (Potentiation of antihypertensive effect).
No products indexed under this heading.

Guanethidine Monosulfate (Potentiation of antihypertensive effect). Products include:
- Esimil Tablets ... 840
- Ismelin Tablets ... 845

Hydralazine Hydrochloride (Potentiation of antihypertensive effect). Products include:
- Apresazide Capsules ... 824
- Apresoline Hydrochloride Tablets ... 826
- Hydralazine Hydrochloride Injection USP ... 2712
- Ser-Ap-Es Tablets ... 867

Hydrochlorothiazide (Potentiation of antihypertensive and/or diuretic effect). Products include:
- Aldactazide Tablets ... 2556
- Aldoril Tablets ... 1644
- Apresazide Capsules ... 824
- Capozide Tablets ... 744
- Dyazide Capsules ... 2653
- Esidrix Tablets ... 839
- Esimil Tablets ... 840
- HydroDIURIL Tablets ... 1716
- Hydropres Tablets ... 1718
- Hyzaar Tablets ... 1720
- Inderide Tablets ... 2838
- Inderide LA Long Acting Capsules ... 2840
- Lopressor HCT Tablets ... 850
- Lotensin HCT Tablets ... 855
- Moduretic Tablets ... 1748
- Oretic Tablets ... 450
- Prinzide Tablets ... 1780
- Ser-Ap-Es Tablets ... 867
- Timolide Tablets ... 1791
- Vaseretic Tablets ... 1810
- Zestoretic Tablets ... 2968
- Ziac ... 1459

Hydroflumethiazide (Potentiation of antihypertensive and/or diuretic effect). Products include:
- Diucardin Tablets ... 2824

Hydroxyzine Hydrochloride (The effects of preanesthetic agents may be potentiated). Products include:
- Atarax Tablets & Syrup ... 1992
- Marax Tablets & DF Syrup ... 2015
- Vistaril Intramuscular Solution ... 2042

Ibuprofen (Possibility for acute renal failure). Products include:
- Advil Cold and Sinus Caplets and Tablets ... ▣ 837
- Advil Ibuprofen Tablets, Caplets and Gel Caplets ... ▣ 836
- Children's Motrin Ibuprofen Oral Suspension ... 1558
- IBU Tablets ... 1389
- Ibuprohm ... ▣ 713
- Motrin IB Caplets, Tablets, and Gelcaps ... ▣ 802
- Motrin Ibuprofen Suspension, Oral Drops, Chewable Tablets, Caplets ... 1563
- Nuprin Ibuprofen/Analgesic Tablets & Caplets ... ▣ 645
- Vicks DayQuil SINUS Pressure & PAIN Relief with IBUPROFEN ... ▣ 735

(▣ Described in PDR For Nonprescription Drugs)   (⊙ Described in PDR For Ophthalmology)

357 **Interactions Index** **Dyrenium**

Indapamide (Potentiation of antihypertensive and/or diuretic effect).
No products indexed under this heading.

Indomethacin (Possibility for acute renal failure). Products include:
Indocin 1723

Indomethacin Sodium Trihydrate (Possibility for acute renal failure). Products include:
Indocin I.V. 1727

Isoflurane (The effects of anesthetic agents may be potentiated).
No products indexed under this heading.

Isradipine (Potentiation of antihypertensive effect). Products include:
DynaCirc Capsules 2381
DynaCirc CR Tablets 2383

Ketamine Hydrochloride (The effects of anesthetic agents may be potentiated).
No products indexed under this heading.

Ketoprofen (Possibility for acute renal failure). Products include:
Actron Caplets and Tablets 608
Orudis Capsules 2874
Orudis KT 842
Oruvail Capsules 2874

Ketorolac Tromethamine (Possibility for acute renal failure). Products include:
Acular Sterile Ophthalmic Solution 470
Toradol 2319

Labetalol Hydrochloride (Potentiation of antihypertensive effect). Products include:
Normodyne Injection 2519
Normodyne Tablets 2522
Trandate 1158

Lisinopril (Potential for antihypertensive effect and increased risk of hyperkalemia). Products include:
Prinivil Tablets 1776
Prinzide Tablets 1780
Zestoretic Tablets 2968
Zestril Tablets 2972

Lithium Carbonate (Diuretic-induced sodium loss may reduce the renal clearance of lithium and increase serum lithium levels with the risk of lithium toxicity). Products include:
Eskalith 2658
Lithium Carbonate Capsules & Tablets 2352
Lithonate/Lithotabs/Lithobid 2721

Lithium Citrate (Diuretic-induced sodium loss may reduce the renal clearance of lithium and increase serum lithium levels with the risk of lithium toxicity).
No products indexed under this heading.

Lorazepam (The effects of preanesthetic agents may be potentiated). Products include:
Ativan Injection 2805
Ativan Tablets 2807

Losartan Potassium (Potentiation of antihypertensive effect). Products include:
Cozaar Tablets 1668
Hyzaar Tablets 1720

Mecamylamine Hydrochloride (Potentiation of antihypertensive effect). Products include:
Inversine Tablets 1729

Meclofenamate Sodium (Possibility for acute renal failure).
No products indexed under this heading.

Mefenamic Acid (Possibility for acute renal failure). Products include:
Ponstel 1982

Meperidine Hydrochloride (The effects of preanesthetic agents may be potentiated). Products include:
Demerol 2438
Mepergan Injection 2859

Metformin Hydrochloride (Triamterene may raise blood glucose levels; for adult-onset diabetes, dosage adjustments of hypoglycemic agents may be necessary). Products include:
Glucophage Tablets 754

Methohexital Sodium (The effects of anesthetic agents may be potentiated).
No products indexed under this heading.

Methoxyflurane (The effects of anesthetic agents may be potentiated).
No products indexed under this heading.

Methyclothiazide (Potentiation of antihypertensive and/or diuretic effect). Products include:
Enduron Tablets 424

Methyldopa (Potentiation of antihypertensive effect). Products include:
Aldoclor Tablets 1638
Aldomet Oral 1640
Aldoril Tablets 1644

Methyldopate Hydrochloride (Potentiation of antihypertensive effect). Products include:
Aldomet Ester HCl Injection 1642

Metocurine Iodide (The effects of nondepolarizing skeletal muscle relaxants may be potentiated). Products include:
Metubine Iodide Vials 932

Metolazone (Potentiation of antihypertensive and/or diuretic effect). Products include:
Mykrox Tablets 1617
Zaroxolyn Tablets 1625

Metoprolol Succinate (Potentiation of antihypertensive effect). Products include:
Toprol-XL Tablets 560

Metoprolol Tartrate (Potentiation of antihypertensive effect). Products include:
Lopressor 848
Lopressor HCT Tablets 850

Metyrosine (Potentiation of antihypertensive effect). Products include:
Demser Capsules 1690

Minoxidil (Potentiation of antihypertensive effect).
No products indexed under this heading.

Mivacurium Chloride (The effects of nondepolarizing skeletal muscle relaxants may be potentiated). Products include:
Mivacron 1125

Moexipril Hydrochloride (Potential for antihypertensive effect and increased risk of hyperkalemia). Products include:
Univasc Tablets 2553

Morphine Sulfate (The effects of preanesthetic agents may be potentiated). Products include:
Astramorph/PF Injection, USP (Preservative-Free) 526
Duramorph Injection 983
Infumorph 200 and Infumorph 500 Sterile Solutions 985
Kadian Capsules 2948
MS Contin Tablets 2149
MSIR 2152
Oramorph SR (Morphine Sulfate Sustained Release Tablets) 2359
RMS Suppositories CII 2766
Roxanol 2365

Nabumetone (Possibility for acute renal failure). Products include:
Relafen Tablets 2688

Nadolol (Potentiation of antihypertensive effect).
No products indexed under this heading.

Naproxen (Possibility for acute renal failure). Products include:
Anaprox/Naprosyn 2277

Naproxen Sodium (Possibility for acute renal failure). Products include:
Aleve 2124
Anaprox/Naprosyn 2277
Naprelan Tablets 2861

Nicardipine Hydrochloride (Potentiation of antihypertensive effect). Products include:
Cardene Capsules 2261
Cardene I.V. 2815
Cardene SR Capsules 2264

Nifedipine (Potentiation of antihypertensive effect). Products include:
Adalat Capsules (10 mg and 20 mg) 580
Adalat CC 582
Procardia Capsules 2024
Procardia XL Extended Release Tablets 2026

Nisoldipine (Potentiation of antihypertensive effect). Products include:
Sular Tablets 2961

Nitroglycerin (Potentiation of antihypertensive effect). Products include:
Deponit NTG Transdermal Delivery System 2541
Nitro-Bid IV 1270
Nitro-Bid Ointment 1272
Nitro-Dur (nitroglycerin) Transdermal Infusion System 1365
Nitrolingual Spray 2193
Nitrostat Tablets 1981
Transderm-Nitro Transdermal Therapeutic System 878

Oxaprozin (Possibility for acute renal failure). Products include:
Daypro Caplets 2578

Pancuronium Bromide (The effects of nondepolarizing skeletal muscle relaxants may be potentiated).
No products indexed under this heading.

Penbutolol Sulfate (Potentiation of antihypertensive effect). Products include:
Levatol Tablets 2547

Penicillin G Potassium (Co-administration may promote serum potassium accumulation and possibly resulting in hyperkalemia). Products include:
Pfizerpen for Injection 2022

Pentobarbital Sodium (The effects of preanesthetic agents may be potentiated). Products include:
Nembutal Sodium Capsules 440
Nembutal Sodium Solution 442
Nembutal Sodium Suppositories 444

Phenoxybenzamine Hydrochloride (Potentiation of antihypertensive effect). Products include:
Dibenzyline Capsules 2650

Phentolamine Mesylate (Potentiation of antihypertensive effect). Products include:
Regitine Vials 864

Phenylbutazone (Possibility for acute renal failure).
No products indexed under this heading.

Pindolol (Potentiation of antihypertensive effect). Products include:
Visken Tablets 2428

Piroxicam (Possibility for acute renal failure). Products include:
Feldene Capsules 2008

Polythiazide (Potentiation of antihypertensive and/or diuretic effect). Products include:
Minizide Capsules 2016

Potassium Acid Phosphate (Concomitant administration is contraindicated). Products include:
K-Phos Original Formula 'Sodium Free' Tablets 633

Potassium Bicarbonate (Concomitant administration is contraindicated). Products include:
Alka-Seltzer Gold Effervescent Antacid 611

Potassium Chloride (Concomitant administration is contraindicated). Products include:
Chlor-3 Condiment 1003
Colyte and Colyte-flavored 2540
GoLYTELY 694
K-Dur Microburst Release System (potassium chloride, USP) E.R. Tablets 1364
K-Lor Powder Packets 438
K-Norm Capsules 1615
K-Tab Filmtab 439
Micro-K 2237
Micro-K LS Packets 2238
NuLYTELY 694
Cherry Flavor NuLYTELY 694
Rum-K Syrup 1004
Slow-K Extended-Release Tablets 869

Potassium Citrate (Concomitant administration is contraindicated). Products include:
Polycitra Syrup 574
Polycitra-K Crystals 574
Polycitra-K Oral Solution 575
Polycitra-LC 574
Urocit-K Tablets 1828

Potassium Gluconate (Concomitant administration is contraindicated).
No products indexed under this heading.

Potassium Phosphate, Dibasic (Concomitant administration is contraindicated).
No products indexed under this heading.

Potassium Phosphate, Monobasic (Concomitant administration is contraindicated). Products include:
K-Phos Neutral Tablets 633
K-Phos Original Formula 'Sodium Free' Tablets 633

Prazosin Hydrochloride (Potentiation of antihypertensive effect). Products include:
Minipress Capsules 2015
Minizide Capsules 2016

Promethazine Hydrochloride (The effects of preanesthetic agents may be potentiated). Products include:
Mepergan Injection 2859
Phenergan with Codeine 2883
Phenergan with Dextromethorphan 2885
Phenergan Injection 2880
Phenergan Suppositories 2882
Phenergan Syrup 2881
Phenergan Tablets 2882
Phenergan VC 2886
Phenergan VC with Codeine 2888

Propofol (The effects of anesthetic agents may be potentiated). Products include:
Diprivan Injectable Emulsion 2939

Propranolol Hydrochloride (Potentiation of antihypertensive effect). Products include:
Inderal 2834
Inderal LA Long Acting Capsules 2836
Inderide Tablets 2838
Inderide LA Long Acting Capsules .. 2840

Quinapril Hydrochloride (Potential for antihypertensive effect and increased risk of hyperkalemia). Products include:
Accupril Tablets 1950

IMPORTANT NOTE: Always consult each drug listing in the patient's regimen for possible interactions.

Ramipril (Potential for increased risk of hyperkalemia). Products include:
Altace Capsules 1238

Rauwolfia Serpentina (Potentiation of antihypertensive effect).
No products indexed under this heading.

Rescinnamine (Potentiation of antihypertensive effect).
No products indexed under this heading.

Reserpine (Potentiation of antihypertensive effect). Products include:
Diupres Tablets 1691
Hydropres Tablets 1718
Ser-Ap-Es Tablets 867

Rocuronium Bromide (The effects of nondepolarizing skeletal muscle relaxants may be potentiated). Products include:
Zemuron Injection 1885

Secobarbital Sodium (The effects of preanesthetic agents may be potentiated). Products include:
Seconal Sodium Pulvules 1529

Sevoflurane (The effects of anesthetic agents may be potentiated).
No products indexed under this heading.

Sodium Nitroprusside (Potentiation of antihypertensive effect).
No products indexed under this heading.

Sotalol Hydrochloride (Potentiation of antihypertensive effect). Products include:
Betapace Tablets 637

Spirapril Hydrochloride (Potential for antihypertensive effect and increased risk of hyperkalemia).
No products indexed under this heading.

Spironolactone (Concomitant use has resulted in fatalities; co-administration is contraindicated). Products include:
Aldactazide Tablets 2556
Aldactone Tablets 2558

Sulindac (Possibility for acute renal failure). Products include:
Clinoril Tablets 1658

Terazosin Hydrochloride (Potentiation of antihypertensive effect). Products include:
Hytrin Capsules 434

Timolol Maleate (Potentiation of antihypertensive effect). Products include:
Blocadren Tablets 1654
Timolide Tablets 1791
Timoptic in Ocudose 1796
Timoptic Sterile Ophthalmic Solution 1794
Timoptic-XE 1798

Tolazamide (Triamterene may raise blood glucose levels; for adult-onset diabetes, dosage adjustments of hypoglycemic agents may be necessary).
No products indexed under this heading.

Tolbutamide (Triamterene may raise blood glucose levels; for adult-onset diabetes, dosage adjustments of hypoglycemic agents may be necessary).
No products indexed under this heading.

Tolmetin Sodium (Possibility for acute renal failure). Products include:
Tolectin (200, 400 and 600 mg) .. 1591

Torsemide (Potentiation of diuretic effect). Products include:
Demadex Tablets and Injection 691

Trandolapril (Potential for increased antihypertensive effect and increased risk of hyperkalemia). Products include:
Mavik Tablets 1407

Trimethaphan Camsylate (Potentiation of antihypertensive effect).
No products indexed under this heading.

Vecuronium Bromide (The effects of nondepolarizing skeletal muscle relaxants may be potentiated). Products include:
Norcuron for Injection 1875

Verapamil Hydrochloride (Potentiation of antihypertensive effect). Products include:
Calan SR Caplets 2571
Calan Tablets 2568
Covera-HS Tablets 2573
Isoptin Injectable 1391
Isoptin Oral Tablets 1393
Isoptin SR Tablets 1395
Verelan Capsules 1455

Food Interactions

Milk, low salt (Co-administration may promote serum potassium accumulation and possibly resulting in hyperkalemia).

E.E.S. 400 FILMTAB
(Erythromycin Ethylsuccinate) 427
May interact with xanthine bronchodilators, oral anticoagulants, and certain other agents. Compounds in these categories include:

Aminophylline (Concomitant administration with high doses of theophylline may be associated with increased theophylline levels and potential toxicity).
No products indexed under this heading.

Carbamazepine (Elevations in serum erythromycin and carbamazepine concentration). Products include:
Atretol Tablets 569
Tegretol/Tegretol-XR 870

Cyclosporine (Elevations in serum erythromycin and cyclosporine concentration). Products include:
Neoral 2405
Sandimmune 2416

Dicumarol (Increased anticoagulant effects).
No products indexed under this heading.

Digoxin (Elevated digoxin serum levels). Products include:
Lanoxicaps 1110
Lanoxin Elixir Pediatric 1113
Lanoxin Injection 1116
Lanoxin Injection Pediatric 1119
Lanoxin Tablets 1121

Dihydroergotamine Mesylate (Potential for acute ergot toxicity characterized by severe peripheral vasospasm and dysesthesia). Products include:
D.H.E. 45 Injection 2381

Dyphylline (Concomitant administration with high doses of theophylline may be associated with increased theophylline levels and potential toxicity). Products include:
Lufyllin & Lufyllin-400 Tablets 2778
Lufyllin-GG Elixir & Tablets 2779

Ergotamine Tartrate (Potential for acute ergot toxicity characterized by severe peripheral vasospasm and dysesthesia). Products include:
Bellergal-S Tablets 2375
Cafergot 2376
Ergomar Tablets 1543
Wigraine Tablets 1884

Hexobarbital (Elevations in serum erythromycin and hexobarbital concentration).

Lovastatin (Potential for rhabdomyolysis in seriously ill patients). Products include:
Mevacor Tablets 1742

Phenytoin (Elevations in serum erythromycin and phenytoin concentration). Products include:
Dilantin Infatabs 1967
Dilantin-125 Suspension 1969

Phenytoin Sodium (Elevations in serum erythromycin and phenytoin concentration). Products include:
Dilantin Kapseals 1965

Terfenadine (Potential for altered terfenadine metabolism). Products include:
Seldane Tablets 1284
Seldane-D Extended-Release Tablets 1286

Theophylline (Concomitant administration with high doses of theophylline may be associated with increased theophylline levels and potential toxicity). Products include:
Marax Tablets & DF Syrup 2015
Quibron 2227

Theophylline Anhydrous (Concomitant administration with high doses of theophylline may be associated with increased theophylline levels and potential toxicity). Products include:
Aerolate 1003
Primatene Tablets 844
Respbid Tablets 687
Slo-bid Gyrocaps 2201
Theo-24 Extended Release Capsules 2753
Theo-Dur Extended-Release Tablets 1367
Theo-X Extended-Release Tablets .. 793
Uni-Dur Extended-Release Tablets .. 1374
Uniphyl 400 mg and 600 mg Tablets 2157

Theophylline Calcium Salicylate (Concomitant administration with high doses of theophylline may be associated with increased theophylline levels and potential toxicity). Products include:
Quadrinal Tablets 1398

Theophylline Sodium Glycinate (Concomitant administration with high doses of theophylline may be associated with increased theophylline levels and potential toxicity).
No products indexed under this heading.

Triazolam (Decreased clearance of triazolam and increased the pharmacologic effect of triazolam). Products include:
Halcion Tablets 2093

Warfarin Sodium (Increased anticoagulant effects). Products include:
Coumadin 941

E.E.S. GRANULES
(Erythromycin Ethylsuccinate) 427
See E.E.S. 400 Filmtab

E.E.S. 200 LIQUID
(Erythromycin Ethylsuccinate) 427
See E.E.S. 400 Filmtab

E.E.S. 400 LIQUID
(Erythromycin Ethylsuccinate) 427
See E.E.S. 400 Filmtab

E-MYCIN TABLETS
(Erythromycin) 1388
May interact with xanthine bronchodilators, oral anticoagulants, drugs which undergo biotransformation by cytochrome p-450 mixed function oxidase, and certain other agents.

Compounds in these categories include:

Alfentanil Hydrochloride (Concurrent use may be associated with elevation in serum level of alfentanil; monitor serum levels closely). Products include:
Alfenta Injection 1334

Aminophylline (Co-administration with high doses of theophylline may be associated with increased serum theophylline levels and potential theophylline toxicity).
No products indexed under this heading.

Bromocriptine Mesylate (Concurrent use may be associated with elevation in serum level of bromocriptine; monitor serum levels closely). Products include:
Parlodel 2411

Carbamazepine (Concurrent use may be associated with elevation in serum level of carbamazepine; monitor serum levels closely). Products include:
Atretol Tablets 569
Tegretol/Tegretol-XR 870

Cyclosporine (Concurrent use may be associated with elevation in serum level of cyclosporine; monitor serum levels closely). Products include:
Neoral 2405
Sandimmune 2416

Dicumarol (Concomitant therapy may result in increased anticoagulant effects).
No products indexed under this heading.

Digoxin (Co-administration may result in elevated digoxin serum levels). Products include:
Lanoxicaps 1110
Lanoxin Elixir Pediatric 1113
Lanoxin Injection 1116
Lanoxin Injection Pediatric 1119
Lanoxin Tablets 1121

Dihydroergotamine Mesylate (Concurrent use has been associated with acute ergot toxicity characterized by severe peripheral vasospasm and dysesthesia). Products include:
D.H.E. 45 Injection 2381

Disopyramide Phosphate (Concurrent use may be associated with elevation in serum level of disopyramide; monitor serum levels closely). Products include:
Norpace 2596

Drugs which undergo biotransformation by cytochrome P-450 mixed function oxidase (Concurrent use may be associated with elevation in serum level of drugs metabolized by the cytochrome P450 system).

Dyphylline (Co-administration with high doses of theophylline may be associated with increased serum theophylline levels and potential theophylline toxicity). Products include:
Lufyllin & Lufyllin-400 Tablets 2778
Lufyllin-GG Elixir & Tablets 2779

Ergotamine Tartrate (Concurrent use has been associated with acute ergot toxicity characterized by severe peripheral vasospasm and dysesthesia). Products include:
Bellergal-S Tablets 2375
Cafergot 2376
Ergomar Tablets 1543
Wigraine Tablets 1884

Hexobarbital (Concurrent use may be associated with elevation in serum level of hexobarbital; monitor serum levels closely).

359 **Interactions Index** **Easprin**

Lovastatin (Potential for rhabdomyolysis with or without renal impairment in seriously ill patients; concurrent use may be associated with elevation in serum level of lovastatin; monitor serum levels closely). Products include:
- Mevacor Tablets 1742

Midazolam Hydrochloride (Decrease clearance of midazolam; potential for increased pharmacologic effect of midazolam). Products include:
- Versed Injection 2324

Phenytoin (Concurrent use may be associated with elevation in serum level of phenytoin; monitor serum levels closely). Products include:
- Dilantin Infatabs 1967
- Dilantin-125 Suspension 1969

Phenytoin Sodium (Concurrent use may be associated with elevation in serum level of phenytoin; monitor serum levels closely). Products include:
- Dilantin Kapseals 1965

Terfenadine (Concomitant use may significantly alter the metabolism of terfenadine; rare cases of serious cardiovascular adverse events, including death, cardiac arrest, torsades de pointes and other ventricular arrhythmias have been reported; concurrent use is contraindicated). Products include:
- Seldane Tablets 1284
- Seldane-D Extended-Release Tablets 1286

Theophylline (Co-administration with high doses of theophylline may be associated with increased serum theophylline levels and potential theophylline toxicity). Products include:
- Marax Tablets & DF Syrup 2015
- Quibron 2227

Theophylline Anhydrous (Co-administration with high doses of theophylline may be associated with increased serum theophylline levels and potential theophylline toxicity). Products include:
- Aerolate 1003
- Primatene Tablets 844
- Respbid Tablets 687
- Slo-bid Gyrocaps 2201
- Theo-24 Extended Release Capsules 2753
- Theo-Dur Extended-Release Tablets 1367
- Theo-X Extended-Release Tablets .. 793
- Uni-Dur Extended-Release Tablets .. 1374
- Uniphyl 400 mg and 600 mg Tablets 2157

Theophylline Calcium Salicylate (Co-administration with high doses of theophylline may be associated with increased serum theophylline levels and potential theophylline toxicity). Products include:
- Quadrinal Tablets 1398

Theophylline Sodium Glycinate (Co-administration with high doses of theophylline may be associated with increased serum theophylline levels and potential theophylline toxicity).
- No products indexed under this heading.

Triazolam (Decrease clearance of triazolam; potential for increased pharmacologic effect of triazolam). Products include:
- Halcion Tablets 2093

Warfarin Sodium (Concomitant therapy may result in increased anticoagulant effects). Products include:
- Coumadin 941

E.P.T. PREGNANCY TEST
(HCG Monoclonal Antibody) 818
None cited in PDR database.

EASPRIN
(Aspirin) 1971
May interact with anticoagulants, oral hypoglycemic agents, corticosteroids, insulin, urinary alkalizing agents, antacids, pyrazolon derivatives, and certain other agents. Compounds in these categories include:

Acarbose (Large doses of salicylates have a hypoglycemic action and may enhance the effect of oral hypoglycemics). Products include:
- Precose 604

Aluminum Carbonate (Increases stomach pH; affects enteric coating of tablets). Products include:
- Basaljel Capsules 2810
- Basaljel Suspension 2810
- Basaljel Tablets 2810

Aluminum Hydroxide (Increases stomach pH; affects enteric coating of tablets). Products include:
- ALternaGEL Liquid 1358
- Maximum Strength Ascriptin 650
- Cama Arthritis Pain Reliever 748
- Gaviscon Extra Strength Relief Formula Antacid Tablets 778
- Gaviscon Extra Strength Relief Formula Liquid Antacid 779
- Gaviscon Liquid Antacid 779
- Gelusil Antacid-Anti-gas Liquid 819
- Gelusil Antacid-Anti-gas Tablets 819
- Maalox Antacid/Anti-Gas Tablets 889
- Maalox Heartburn Relief Suspension 658
- Maalox Antacid Liquid 888
- Extra Strength Maalox Antacid/Anti-Gas Liquid and Tablets 888
- Mylanta 1359
- Tempo Soft Antacid 799

Aluminum Hydroxide Gel (Increases stomach pH; affects enteric coating of tablets). Products include:
- ALternaGEL Liquid 675
- Aludrox Oral Suspension 850
- Amphojel Suspension 2802
- Amphojel Suspension without Flavor 2802
- Amphojel Tablets 2802
- Ascriptin 650
- Gaviscon Antacid Tablets 778
- Gaviscon-2 Antacid Tablets 779
- Mylanta Liquid 676
- Mylanta Double Strength Liquid 676
- Nephrox Suspension 671

Antipyrine (Increased risk of gastrointestinal ulceration). Products include:
- Auralgan Otic Solution 2810
- Tympagesic Ear Drops 2476

Betamethasone Acetate (Increased risk of gastrointestinal ulceration; may reduce serum salicylate levels). Products include:
- Celestone Soluspan Suspension 2484

Betamethasone Sodium Phosphate (Increased risk of gastrointestinal ulceration; may reduce serum salicylate levels). Products include:
- Celestone Soluspan Suspension 2484

Chlorpropamide (Large doses of salicylates have a hypoglycemic action and may enhance the effect of oral hypoglycemics). Products include:
- Diabinese Tablets 2002

Cortisone Acetate (Increased risk of gastrointestinal ulceration; may reduce serum salicylate levels). Products include:
- Cortone Acetate Sterile Suspension 1663
- Cortone Acetate Tablets 1664

Dalteparin Sodium (Increased bleeding time). Products include:
- Fragmin Injection 2088

Dexamethasone (Increased risk of gastrointestinal ulceration; may reduce serum salicylate levels). Products include:
- AK-Trol Ointment & Suspension ..... ◉ 205
- Decadron Elixir 1676
- Decadron Tablets 1678
- Decaspray Topical Aerosol 1689
- Maxitrol Ophthalmic Ointment and Suspension ..... ◉ 222
- TobraDex Ophthalmic Suspension and Ointment 469

Dexamethasone Acetate (Increased risk of gastrointestinal ulceration; may reduce serum salicylate levels). Products include:
- Dalalone D.P. Injectable 1009
- Decadron-LA Sterile Suspension 1687

Dexamethasone Sodium Phosphate (Increased risk of gastrointestinal ulceration; may reduce serum salicylate levels). Products include:
- Decadron Phosphate Injection 1680
- Decadron Phosphate Sterile Ophthalmic Ointment 1684
- Decadron Phosphate Sterile Ophthalmic Solution 1685
- Decadron Phosphate Topical Cream 1686
- Decadron Phosphate with Xylocaine Injection, Sterile 1683
- Dexacort Phosphate in Respihaler .. 1606
- Dexacort Phosphate in Turbinaire .. 1607
- NeoDecadron Sterile Ophthalmic Ointment 1755
- NeoDecadron Sterile Ophthalmic Solution 1756
- NeoDecadron Topical Cream 1757

Dicumarol (Increased bleeding time).
- No products indexed under this heading.

Dipyrone (Possible increase in gastrointestinal ulceration).

Enoxaparin (Increased bleeding time). Products include:
- Lovenox Injection 2187

Fludrocortisone Acetate (Increased risk of gastrointestinal ulceration; may reduce serum salicylate levels). Products include:
- Florinef Acetate Tablets 506

Glimepiride (Large doses of salicylates have a hypoglycemic action and may enhance the effect of oral hypoglycemics). Products include:
- Amaryl Tablets 1241

Glipizide (Large doses of salicylates have a hypoglycemic action and may enhance the effect of oral hypoglycemics). Products include:
- Glucotrol Tablets 2011
- Glucotrol XL Extended Release Tablets 2012

Glyburide (Large doses of salicylates have a hypoglycemic action and may enhance the effect of oral hypoglycemics). Products include:
- DiaBeta Tablets 1265
- Glynase PresTab Tablets 2091
- Micronase Tablets 2099

Heparin Calcium (Increased bleeding time).
- No products indexed under this heading.

Heparin Sodium (Increased bleeding time). Products include:
- Heparin Lock Flush Solution 2831
- Heparin Sodium Injection 2832
- Heparin Sodium Vials 1486

Hydrocortisone (Increased risk of gastrointestinal ulceration; may reduce serum salicylate levels). Products include:
- Anusol-HC Cream 2.5% 1953
- Aquanil HC Lotion 1989
- Maximum Strength Cortaid Spray 800
- CORTENEMA 2713
- Cortisporin Ointment 1074
- Cortisporin Ophthalmic Ointment Sterile 1074
- Cortisporin Ophthalmic Suspension Sterile 1075
- Cortisporin Otic Solution Sterile 1076
- Cortisporin Otic Suspension Sterile 1077
- Cortizone-5 795
- Cortizone-10 795
- Hydrocortone Tablets 1715
- Hytone 922
- Hytone Ointment 2 ½% 923
- Massengill Medicated Soft Cloth Towelettes 2628
- Pediotic Suspension Sterile 1140
- Preparation H Hydrocortisone 1% Cream 843
- ProctoCream-HC 2.5% 2552
- VōSoL HC Otic Solution 2786

Hydrocortisone Acetate (Increased risk of gastrointestinal ulceration; may reduce serum salicylate levels). Products include:
- Analpram-HC Rectal Cream 1% and 2.5% 993
- Anusol HC-1 Hydrocortisone Anti-Itch Ointment 810
- Anusol-HC Suppositories 1954
- Caldecort Anti-Itch Hydrocortisone Cream 651
- Coly-Mycin S Otic w/Neomycin & Hydrocortisone 1965
- Cortaid 800
- Cortifoam 2540
- Cortisporin Cream 1073
- Epifoam 2543
- Hydrocortone Acetate Sterile Suspension 1712
- Mantadil Cream 1124
- Nupercainal Hydrocortisone 1% Cream 661
- Pramosone Cream, Lotion & Ointment 995
- ProctoFoam-HC 2552
- Terra-Cortril Ophthalmic Suspension 2033

Hydrocortisone Sodium Phosphate (Increased risk of gastrointestinal ulceration; may reduce serum salicylate levels). Products include:
- Hydrocortone Phosphate Injection, Sterile 1713

Hydrocortisone Sodium Succinate (Increased risk of gastrointestinal ulceration; may reduce serum salicylate levels).
- No products indexed under this heading.

Insulin, Human (Altered insulin requirements).
- No products indexed under this heading.

Insulin, Human Isophane Suspension (Altered insulin requirements). Products include:
- Novolin N Human Insulin 10 ml Vials 1846

Insulin, Human NPH (Altered insulin requirements). Products include:
- Humulin N, 100 Units 1495
- Novolin N PenFill 1.5 ml Cartridges Durable Insulin Delivery System 1849
- Novolin N Prefilled Syringe Disposable Insulin Delivery System 1850

Insulin, Human Regular (Altered insulin requirements). Products include:
- Humulin R, 100 Units 1497
- Novolin R Human Insulin 10 ml Vials 1846
- Novolin R PenFill 1.5 ml Cartridges Durable Insulin Delivery System 1849
- Novolin R Prefilled Syringe Disposable Insulin Delivery System 1850
- Velosulin BR Human Insulin 10 ml Vials 1847

Insulin, Human, Zinc Suspension (Altered insulin requirements). Products include:
- Humulin L, 100 Units 1494
- Humulin U, 100 Units 1498
- Novolin L Human Insulin 10 ml Vials 1846

IMPORTANT NOTE: Always consult each drug listing in the patient's regimen for possible interactions.

Insulin Lispro, Human (Altered insulin requirements). Products include:

- Humalog Injection 1488

Insulin, NPH (Altered insulin requirements). Products include:

- NPH, 100 Units 1502
- Pork NPH, 100 Units 1506
- Purified Pork NPH Isophane Insulin 1852

Insulin, Regular (Altered insulin requirements). Products include:

- Regular, 100 Units 1503
- Pork Regular, 100 Units 1507
- Pork Regular (Concentrated), 500 Units 1508
- Purified Pork Regular Insulin 1852

Insulin, Zinc Crystals (Altered insulin requirements). Products include:

- NPH, 100 Units 1502

Insulin, Zinc Suspension (Altered insulin requirements). Products include:

- Iletin I 1501
- Lente, 100 Units 1501
- Iletin II 1504
- Pork Lente, 100 Units 1504
- Purified Pork Lente Insulin 1852

Magaldrate (Increases stomach pH; affects enteric coating of tablets).

- No products indexed under this heading.

Magnesium Hydroxide (Increases stomach pH; affects enteric coating of tablets). Products include:

- Aludrox Oral Suspension .... ▣ 850
- Ascriptin .... ▣ 650
- Di-Gel Antacid/Anti-Gas .... ▣ 762
- Gelusil Antacid-Anti-gas Liquid .... ▣ 819
- Gelusil Antacid-Anti-gas Tablets .... ▣ 819
- Maalox Antacid/Anti-Gas Tablets 889
- Maalox Antacid Liquid 888
- Extra Strength Maalox Antacid/Anti-Gas Liquid and Tablets 888
- Mylanta Fast-Acting 1359
- Mylanta Gelcaps Antacid .... ▣ 678
- Fast-Acting Mylanta Liquid Antacid 1359
- Mylanta Tablets .... ▣ 677
- Maximum-Strength Fast-Acting Mylanta Liquid Antacid 1359
- Mylanta Double Strength Tablets .. ▣ 677
- Phillips' Milk of Magnesia Liquid .... ▣ 627
- Rolaids Antacid Tablets .... ▣ 807
- Tempo Soft Antacid .... ▣ 799

Magnesium Oxide (Increases stomach pH; affects enteric coating of tablets). Products include:

- Beelith Tablets 632
- Bufferin Analgesic Tablets .... ▣ 636
- Arthritis Strength Bufferin Analgesic Caplets .... ▣ 637
- Extra Strength Bufferin Analgesic Tablets .... ▣ 637
- Caltrate PLUS .... ▣ 681
- Cama Arthritis Pain Reliever .... ▣ 748
- Mag-Ox 400 666
- Uro-Mag 666

Metformin Hydrochloride (Large doses of salicylates have a hypoglycemic action and may enhance the effect of oral hypoglycemics). Products include:

- Glucophage Tablets 754

Methylprednisolone Acetate (Increased risk of gastrointestinal ulceration; may reduce serum salicylate levels).

- No products indexed under this heading.

Methylprednisolone Sodium Succinate (Increased risk of gastrointestinal ulceration; may reduce serum salicylate levels).

- No products indexed under this heading.

Oxyphenbutazone (Increased risk of gastrointestinal ulceration).

Phenobarbital (Decreases aspirin effectiveness by enzyme induction). Products include:

- Arco-Lase Plus Tablets 513
- Bellergal-S Tablets 2375
- Donnatal 2234
- Donnatal Extentabs 2234
- Donnatal Tablets 2234
- Phenobarbital Elixir and Tablets 1523
- Quadrinal Tablets 1398

Phenylbutazone (Decreased effects of phenylbutazone; increased risk of gastrointestinal ulceration).

- No products indexed under this heading.

Phenytoin (Increased serum phenytoin levels). Products include:

- Dilantin Infatabs 1967
- Dilantin-125 Suspension 1969

Phenytoin Sodium (Increased phenytoin levels). Products include:

- Dilantin Kapseals 1965

Potassium Citrate (Decreased aspirin effectiveness). Products include:

- Polycitra Syrup 574
- Polycitra-K Crystals 574
- Polycitra-K Oral Solution 575
- Polycitra-LC 574
- Urocit-K Tablets 1828

Prednisolone Acetate (Increased risk of gastrointestinal ulceration; may reduce serum salicylate levels). Products include:

- AK-CIDE .... ⊙ 203
- AK-CIDE Ointment .... ⊙ 203
- Blephamide Liquifilm Sterile Ophthalmic Suspension 472
- Blephamide Ointment .... ⊙ 234
- Econopred & Econopred Plus Ophthalmic Suspensions .... ⊙ 216
- Poly-Pred Liquifilm .... ⊙ 246
- Pred Forte .... ⊙ 247
- Pred Mild .... ⊙ 250
- Pred-G Liquifilm Sterile Ophthalmic Suspension .... ⊙ 248
- Pred-G S.O.P. Sterile Ophthalmic Ointment .... ⊙ 249

Prednisolone Sodium Phosphate (Increased risk of gastrointestinal ulceration; may reduce serum salicylate levels). Products include:

- AK-PRED .... ⊙ 204
- Hydeltrasol Injection, Sterile 1708
- Pediapred Oral Solution 1618

Prednisolone Tebutate (Increased risk of gastrointestinal ulceration; may reduce serum salicylate levels). Products include:

- Hydeltra-T.B.A. Sterile Suspension 1710

Prednisone (Increased risk of gastrointestinal ulceration; may reduce serum salicylate levels).

- No products indexed under this heading.

Probenecid (Decreased effects of uricosuric agent probenecid). Products include:

- Benemid Tablets 1651
- ColBENEMID Tablets 1662

Propranolol Hydrochloride (Decreases anti-inflammatory action of aspirin). Products include:

- Inderal 2834
- Inderal LA Long Acting Capsules 2836
- Inderide Tablets 2838
- Inderide LA Long Acting Capsules .. 2840

Sodium Bicarbonate (Increases stomach pH affects enteric coating of tablets). Products include:

- Alka-Seltzer Cherry Effervescent Antacid and Pain Reliever .... ▣ 609
- Alka-Seltzer Extra Strength Effervescent Antacid and Pain Reliever .... ▣ 609
- Alka-Seltzer Gold Effervescent Antacid .... ▣ 611
- Alka-Seltzer Lemon Lime Effervescent Antacid and Pain Reliever .... ▣ 609
- Alka-Seltzer Original Effervescent Antacid and Pain Reliever .... ▣ 609
- Arm & Hammer Pure Baking Soda .... ▣ 648
- Colyte and Colyte-flavored 2540
- GoLYTELY 694
- Massengill Disposable Douches .... ▣ 780
- Massengill Liquid Concentrate .... ▣ 780
- NuLYTELY 694
- Cherry Flavor NuLYTELY 694

Sodium Citrate (Decreased aspirin effectiveness). Products include:

- Bicitra 573
- Polycitra 574
- Salix SST Lozenges Saliva Stimulant .... ▣ 757

Spironolactone (Decreased sodium excretion). Products include:

- Aldactazide Tablets 2556
- Aldactone Tablets 2558

Sulfinpyrazone (Decreased effects of uricosuric agent sulfinpyrazone). Products include:

- Anturane 823

Tolazamide (Large doses of salicylates have a hypoglycemic action and may enhance the effect of oral hypoglycemics).

- No products indexed under this heading.

Tolbutamide (Large doses of salicylates have a hypoglycemic action and may enhance the effect of oral hypoglycemics).

- No products indexed under this heading.

Triamcinolone (Increased risk of gastrointestinal ulceration; may reduce serum salicylate levels).

- No products indexed under this heading.

Triamcinolone Acetonide (Increased risk of gastrointestinal ulceration; may reduce serum salicylate levels). Products include:

- Azmacort Oral Inhaler 2175
- Nasacort AQ Nasal Spray 2191
- Nasacort Nasal Inhaler 2189

Triamcinolone Diacetate (Increased risk of gastrointestinal ulceration; may reduce serum salicylate levels).

- No products indexed under this heading.

Triamcinolone Hexacetonide (Increased risk of gastrointestinal ulceration; may reduce serum salicylate levels).

- No products indexed under this heading.

Warfarin Sodium (Increased bleeding time). Products include:

- Coumadin 941

Food Interactions

Alcohol (Alcohol has a synergistic effect with aspirin in causing gastrointestinal bleeding).

EC-NAPROSYN DELAYED-RELEASE TABLETS

(Naproxen) 2277

May interact with oral anticoagulants, sulfonamides, oral hypoglycemic agents, hydantoin anticonvulsants, lithium preparations, beta blockers, histamine h2-receptor antagonists, antacids containing aluminium, calcium and magnesium, ACE inhibitors, sulfonylureas, and certain other agents. Compounds in these categories include:

Acebutolol Hydrochloride (Reduced antihypertensive effect of beta blockers). Products include:

- Sectral Capsules 2914

Aluminum Carbonate (Due to the gastric pH elevating effects of intensive antacids therapy, concomitant administration of EC-Naprosyn is not recommended). Products include:

- Basaljel Capsules 2810
- Basaljel Suspension 2810
- Basaljel Tablets 2810

Aluminum Hydroxide (Due to the gastric pH elevating effects of intensive antacids therapy, concomitant administration of EC-Naprosyn is not recommended). Products include:

- ALternaGEL Liquid 1358
- Maximum Strength Ascriptin .... ▣ 650
- Cama Arthritis Pain Reliever .... ▣ 748
- Gaviscon Extra Strength Relief Formula Antacid Tablets .... ▣ 778
- Gaviscon Extra Strength Relief Formula Liquid Antacid .... ▣ 779
- Gaviscon Liquid Antacid .... ▣ 779
- Gelusil Antacid-Anti-gas Liquid .... ▣ 819
- Gelusil Antacid-Anti-gas Tablets .... ▣ 819
- Maalox Antacid/Anti-Gas Tablets 889
- Maalox Heartburn Relief Suspension .... ▣ 658
- Maalox Antacid Liquid 888
- Extra Strength Maalox Antacid/Anti-Gas Liquid and Tablets 888
- Mylanta 1359
- Tempo Soft Antacid .... ▣ 799

Aluminum Hydroxide Gel (Due to the gastric pH elevating effects of intensive antacids therapy, concomitant administration of EC-Naprosyn is not recommended). Products include:

- ALternaGEL Liquid .... ▣ 675
- Aludrox Oral Suspension .... ▣ 850
- Amphojel Suspension 2802
- Amphojel Suspension without Flavor 2802
- Amphojel Tablets 2802
- Ascriptin .... ▣ 650
- Gaviscon Antacid Tablets .... ▣ 778
- Gaviscon-2 Antacid Tablets .... ▣ 779
- Mylanta Liquid .... ▣ 676
- Mylanta Double Strength Liquid .... ▣ 676
- Nephrox Suspension .... ▣ 671

Aspirin (Naproxen is displaced from its binding sites during the concomitant administration of aspirin resulting in lower plasma concentrations and peak plasma levels; concurrent use is not recommended). Products include:

- Alka-Seltzer Cherry Effervescent Antacid and Pain Reliever .... ▣ 609
- Alka-Seltzer Extra Strength Effervescent Antacid and Pain Reliever .... ▣ 609
- Alka-Seltzer Lemon Lime Effervescent Antacid and Pain Reliever .... ▣ 609
- Alka-Seltzer Original Effervescent Antacid and Pain Reliever .... ▣ 609
- Alka-Seltzer Plus .... ▣ 611
- Alka-Seltzer Plus Sinus Medicine .. ▣ 611
- Ascriptin .... ▣ 650
- Arthritis Strength BC Powder .... ▣ 631
- BC Cold Powder Multi-Symptom Formula (Cold-Sinus-Allergy) .... ▣ 631
- BC Cold Powder Non-Drowsy Formula (Cold-Sinus) .... ▣ 631
- BC Powder .... ▣ 631
- Genuine Bayer Aspirin Tablets & Caplets .... ▣ 618
- Extra Strength Bayer Arthritis Pain Regimen Formula .... ▣ 615
- Extra Strength Bayer Aspirin Caplets & Tablets .... ▣ 617
- Extended-Release Bayer 8-Hour Aspirin .... ▣ 616
- Extra Strength Bayer Plus Aspirin Caplets .... ▣ 617
- Extra Strength Bayer PM Aspirin Plus Sleep Aid .... ▣ 617
- Aspirin Regimen Bayer 81 mg Tablets with Calcium .... ▣ 615
- Aspirin Regimen Bayer Adult Low Strength 81 mg Tablets .... ▣ 613
- Aspirin Regimen Bayer Children's Chewable Aspirin .... ▣ 616
- Aspirin Regimen Bayer Regular Strength 325 mg Caplets .... ▣ 613
- Bufferin Analgesic Tablets .... ▣ 636

(▣ Described in PDR For Nonprescription Drugs) (⊙ Described in PDR For Ophthalmology)

Interactions Index — Anaprox/Naprosyn

Arthritis Strength Bufferin Analgesic Caplets ... 637
Extra Strength Bufferin Analgesic Tablets ... 637
Cama Arthritis Pain Reliever ... 748
Darvon Compound-65 Pulvules ... 1475
Easprin ... 1971
Ecotrin ... 2625
Ecotrin Enteric Coated Aspirin Maximum Strength Tablets and Caplets ... 775
Ecotrin Enteric Coated Aspirin Regular Strength Tablets ... 2625
Empirin Aspirin Tablets ... 818
Excedrin Extra-Strength Analgesic Tablets, Caplets, and Geltabs ... 734
Fiorinal Capsules ... 2388
Fiorinal with Codeine Capsules ... 2390
Fiorinal Tablets ... 2388
Goody's Extra Strength Headache Powders ... 632
Goody's Extra Strength Pain Relief Tablets ... 632
Halfprin Tablets ... 1413
Norgesic ... 1554
Percodan Tablets ... 955
Percodan-Demi Tablets ... 956
Robaxisal Tablets ... 2246
Soma Compound w/Codeine Tablets ... 2784
Soma Compound Tablets ... 2783
St. Joseph Adult Chewable Aspirin (81 mg.) ... 768
Talwin Compound ... 2466
Vanquish Analgesic Caplets ... 627

Atenolol (Reduced antihypertensive effect of beta blockers). Products include:
Tenoretic Tablets ... 2963
Tenormin Tablets and I.V. Injection ... 2965

Benazepril Hydrochloride (Co-administration of NSAIDs and ACE inhibitors may potentiate renal disease states). Products include:
Lotensin Tablets ... 852
Lotensin HCT Tablets ... 855
Lotrel Capsules ... 858

Betaxolol Hydrochloride (Reduced antihypertensive effect of beta blockers). Products include:
Betoptic Ophthalmic Solution ... 465
Betoptic S Ophthalmic Suspension ... 467
Kerlone Tablets ... 2588

Bisoprolol Fumarate (Reduced antihypertensive effect of beta blockers). Products include:
Zebeta Tablets ... 1457
Ziac ... 1459

Captopril (Co-administration of NSAIDs and ACE inhibitors may potentiate renal disease states). Products include:
Capoten Tablets ... 740
Capozide Tablets ... 744

Carteolol Hydrochloride (Reduced antihypertensive effect of beta blockers). Products include:
Cartrol Tablets ... 413
Ocupress Ophthalmic Solution, 1% Sterile ... 297

Chlorpropamide (Potential for sulfonylurea toxicity). Products include:
Diabinese Tablets ... 2002

Cimetidine (Due to the gastric pH elevating effects of H$_2$-blockers concomitant administration of EC-Naprosyn is not recommended). Products include:
Tagamet HB Tablets ... 786
Tagamet Tablets ... 2694

Cimetidine Hydrochloride (Due to the gastric pH elevating effects of H$_2$-blockers concomitant administration of EC-Naprosyn is not recommended). Products include:
Tagamet ... 2694

Dicumarol (Short-term studies have failed to show any significant effect of concurrent use on prothrombin time; caution is advised since interactions have been seen with other NSAIDs).
No products indexed under this heading.

Enalapril Maleate (Co-administration of NSAIDs and ACE inhibitors may potentiate renal disease states). Products include:
Vaseretic Tablets ... 1810
Vasotec Tablets ... 1816

Enalaprilat (Co-administration of NSAIDs and ACE inhibitors may potentiate renal disease states). Products include:
Vasotec I.V. ... 1814

Esmolol Hydrochloride (Reduced antihypertensive effect of beta blockers). Products include:
Brevibloc (esmolol HCl) Injection ... 1860

Ethotoin (Potential for hydantoin toxicity). Products include:
Peganone Tablets ... 455

Famotidine (Due to the gastric pH elevating effects of H$_2$-blockers concomitant administration of EC-Naprosyn is not recommended). Products include:
Pepcid AC Acid Controller ... 1360
Pepcid Injection ... 1765
Pepcid ... 1763

Fosinopril Sodium (Co-administration of NSAIDs and ACE inhibitors may potentiate renal disease states). Products include:
Monopril Tablets ... 762

Fosphenytoin Sodium (Potential for hydantoin toxicity). Products include:
Cerebyx Injection ... 1956

Furosemide (Inhibition of natriuretic effect of furosemide). Products include:
Lasix Injection, Oral Solution and Tablets ... 1267

Glimepiride (Potential for sulfonylurea toxicity). Products include:
Amaryl Tablets ... 1241

Glipizide (Potential for sulfonylurea toxicity). Products include:
Glucotrol Tablets ... 2011
Glucotrol XL Extended Release Tablets ... 2012

Glyburide (Potential for sulfonylurea toxicity). Products include:
DiaBeta Tablets ... 1265
Glynase PresTab Tablets ... 2091
Micronase Tablets ... 2099

Labetalol Hydrochloride (Reduced antihypertensive effect of beta blockers). Products include:
Normodyne Injection ... 2519
Normodyne Tablets ... 2522
Trandate ... 1158

Lisinopril (Co-administration of NSAIDs and ACE inhibitors may potentiate renal disease states). Products include:
Prinivil Tablets ... 1776
Prinzide Tablets ... 1780
Zestoretic Tablets ... 2968
Zestril Tablets ... 2972

Lithium Carbonate (Inhibition of lithium renal clearance leading to increase in plasma lithium concentrations). Products include:
Eskalith ... 2658
Lithium Carbonate Capsules & Tablets ... 2352
Lithonate/Lithotabs/Lithobid ... 2721

Lithium Citrate (Inhibition of lithium renal clearance leading to increase in plasma lithium concentrations).
No products indexed under this heading.

Magaldrate (Due to the gastric pH elevating effects of intensive antacids therapy, concomitant administration of EC-Naprosyn is not recommended).
No products indexed under this heading.

Magnesium Hydroxide (Due to the gastric pH elevating effects of intensive antacids therapy, concomitant administration of EC-Naprosyn is not recommended). Products include:
Aludrox Oral Suspension ... 850
Ascriptin ... 650
Di-Gel Antacid/Anti-Gas ... 762
Gelusil Antacid-Anti-gas Liquid ... 819
Gelusil Antacid-Anti-gas Tablets ... 819
Maalox Antacid/Anti-Gas Tablets ... 889
Maalox Antacid Liquid ... 888
Extra Strength Maalox Antacid/Anti-Gas Liquid and Tablets ... 888
Mylanta Fast-Acting ... 1359
Mylanta Gelcaps Antacid ... 678
Fast-Acting Mylanta Liquid Antacid ... 1359
Mylanta Tablets ... 677
Maximum-Strength Fast-Acting Mylanta Liquid Antacid ... 1359
Mylanta Double Strength Tablets ... 677
Phillips' Milk of Magnesia Liquid ... 627
Rolaids Antacid Tablets ... 807
Tempo Soft Antacid ... 799

Magnesium Oxide (Due to the gastric pH elevating effects of intensive antacids therapy, concomitant administration of EC-Naprosyn is not recommended). Products include:
Beelith Tablets ... 632
Bufferin Analgesic Tablets ... 636
Arthritis Strength Bufferin Analgesic Caplets ... 637
Extra Strength Bufferin Analgesic Tablets ... 637
Caltrate PLUS ... 681
Cama Arthritis Pain Reliever ... 748
Mag-Ox 400 ... 666
Uro-Mag ... 666

Mephenytoin (Potential for hydantoin toxicity). Products include:
Mesantoin Tablets ... 2400

Methotrexate Sodium (Potential for reduced tubular secretion of methotrexate and possible increased methotrexate toxicity as shown in animal model; caution is recommended). Products include:
Methotrexate Sodium Tablets, Injection, for Injection and LPF Injection ... 1322

Metoprolol Succinate (Reduced antihypertensive effect of beta blockers). Products include:
Toprol-XL Tablets ... 560

Metoprolol Tartrate (Reduced antihypertensive effect of beta blockers). Products include:
Lopressor ... 848
Lopressor HCT Tablets ... 850

Moexipril Hydrochloride (Co-administration of NSAIDs and ACE inhibitors may potentiate renal disease states). Products include:
Univasc Tablets ... 2553

Nadolol (Reduced antihypertensive effect of beta blockers).
No products indexed under this heading.

Naproxen Sodium (Concurrent use of naproxen or naproxen sodium in any dosage form is not recommended since they all circulate in the plasma as the naproxen anion). Products include:
Aleve ... 2124
Anaprox/Naprosyn ... 2277
Naprelan Tablets ... 2861

Nizatidine (Due to the gastric pH elevating effects of H$_2$-blockers concomitant administration of EC-Naprosyn is not recommended). Products include:
Axid Pulvules ... 1468

Penbutolol Sulfate (Reduced antihypertensive effect of beta blockers). Products include:
Levatol Tablets ... 2547

Phenytoin (Potential for hydantoin toxicity). Products include:
Dilantin Infatabs ... 1967
Dilantin-125 Suspension ... 1969

Phenytoin Sodium (Potential for hydantoin toxicity). Products include:
Dilantin Kapseals ... 1965

Pindolol (Reduced antihypertensive effect of beta blockers). Products include:
Visken Tablets ... 2428

Probenecid (Probenecid given concurrently increases naproxen anion plasma levels and extends its plasma half-life significantly). Products include:
Benemid Tablets ... 1651
ColBENEMID Tablets ... 1662

Propranolol Hydrochloride (Reduced antihypertensive effect of beta blockers). Products include:
Inderal ... 2834
Inderal LA Long Acting Capsules ... 2836
Inderide Tablets ... 2838
Inderide LA Long Acting Capsules ... 2840

Quinapril Hydrochloride (Co-administration of NSAIDs and ACE inhibitors may potentiate renal disease states). Products include:
Accupril Tablets ... 1950

Ramipril (Co-administration of NSAIDs and ACE inhibitors may potentiate renal disease states). Products include:
Altace Capsules ... 1238

Ranitidine Hydrochloride (Due to the gastric pH elevating effects of H$_2$-blockers concomitant administration of EC-Naprosyn is not recommended). Products include:
Zantac ... 1182
Zantac Injection ... 1180
Zantac Syrup ... 1182

Sotalol Hydrochloride (Reduced antihypertensive effect of beta blockers). Products include:
Betapace Tablets ... 637

Spirapril Hydrochloride (Co-administration of NSAIDs and ACE inhibitors may potentiate renal disease states).
No products indexed under this heading.

Sucralfate (Due to the gastric pH elevating effects of sucralfate concomitant administration of EC-Naprosyn is not recommended). Products include:
Carafate Suspension ... 1250
Carafate Tablets ... 1249

Sulfacytine (Potential for sulfonamide toxicity).

Sulfamethizole (Potential for sulfonamide toxicity). Products include:
Urobiotic-250 Capsules ... 2038

Sulfamethoxazole (Potential for sulfonamide toxicity). Products include:
Bactrim DS Tablets ... 2257
Bactrim I.V. Infusion ... 2255
Bactrim ... 2257
Gantanol Tablets ... 2285
Septra ... 1146
Septra I.V. Infusion ... 1142
Septra I.V. Infusion ADD-Vantage Vials ... 1144
Septra ... 1146

Sulfasalazine (Potential for sulfonamide toxicity). Products include:
Azulfidine ... 2059

Sulfinpyrazone (Potential for sulfonamide toxicity). Products include:
Anturane ... 823

IMPORTANT NOTE: Always consult each drug listing in the patient's regimen for possible interactions.

Sulfisoxazole (Potential for sulfonamide toxicity). Products include:
- Gantrisin Tablets ... 2286

Sulfisoxazole Diolamine (Potential for sulfonamide toxicity).
- No products indexed under this heading.

Timolol Hemihydrate (Reduced antihypertensive effect of beta blockers). Products include:
- Betimol 0.25%, 0.5% ... ⊙ 259

Timolol Maleate (Reduced antihypertensive effect of beta blockers). Products include:
- Blocadren Tablets ... 1654
- Timolide Tablets ... 1791
- Timoptic in Ocudose ... 1796
- Timoptic Sterile Ophthalmic Solution ... 1794
- Timoptic-XE ... 1798

Tolazamide (Potential for sulfonylurea toxicity).
- No products indexed under this heading.

Tolbutamide (Potential for sulfonylurea toxicity).
- No products indexed under this heading.

Trandolapril (Co-administration of NSAIDs and ACE inhibitors may potentiate renal disease states). Products include:
- Mavik Tablets ... 1407

Warfarin Sodium (Short-term studies have failed to show any significant effect of concurrent use on prothrombin time; caution is advised since interactions have been seen with other NSAIDs). Products include:
- Coumadin ... 941

Food Interactions

Food, unspecified (The presence of food prolonged the time the EC-Naprosyn remained in the stomach, time to first detectable serum naproxen levels, and time to maximal naproxen levels (T_{max}), but did not affect peak naproxen levels (C_{max})).

ECONOPRED & ECONOPRED PLUS OPHTHALMIC SUSPENSIONS

(Prednisolone Acetate) ... ⊙ 216

None cited in PDR database.

ECOTRIN ENTERIC COATED ASPIRIN LOW STRENGTH TABLETS

(Aspirin) ... 2625

See Ecotrin Enteric Coated Aspirin Maximum Strength Tablets and Caplets

ECOTRIN ENTERIC COATED ASPIRIN MAXIMUM STRENGTH TABLETS AND CAPLETS

(Aspirin) ... 2625

May interact with antacids containing aluminium, calcium and magnesium, oral hypoglycemic agents, non-steroidal anti-inflammatory agents, and certain other agents. Compounds in these categories include:

Acarbose (Concurrent use with hypoglycemic agents is not recommended). Products include:
- Precose ... 604

Aluminum Carbonate (Co-administration of nonabsorbable antacids may alter the rate of absorption of aspirin thereby resulting in a decreased acetylsalicylic acid/salicylic acid ratio in plasma). Products include:
- Basaljel Capsules ... 2810
- Basaljel Suspension ... 2810
- Basaljel Tablets ... 2810

Aluminum Hydroxide (Co-administration of nonabsorbable antacids may alter the rate of absorption of aspirin thereby resulting in a decreased acetylsalicylic acid/salicylic acid ratio in plasma). Products include:
- ALternaGEL Liquid ... 1358
- Maximum Strength Ascriptin ... ■ 650
- Cama Arthritis Pain Reliever ... ■ 748
- Gaviscon Extra Strength Relief Formula Antacid Tablets ... ■ 778
- Gaviscon Extra Strength Relief Formula Liquid Antacid ... ■ 779
- Gaviscon Liquid Antacid ... ■ 779
- Gelusil Antacid-Anti-gas Liquid ... ■ 819
- Gelusil Antacid-Anti-gas Tablets ... ■ 819
- Maalox Antacid/Anti-Gas Tablets ... 889
- Maalox Heartburn Relief Suspension ... ■ 658
- Maalox Antacid Liquid ... 888
- Extra Strength Maalox Antacid/Anti-Gas Liquid and Tablets ... 888
- Mylanta ... 1359
- Tempo Soft Antacid ... ■ 799

Aluminum Hydroxide Gel (Co-administration of nonabsorbable antacids may alter the rate of absorption of aspirin thereby resulting in a decreased acetylsalicylic acid/salicylic acid ratio in plasma). Products include:
- ALternaGEL Liquid ... ■ 675
- Aludrox Oral Suspension ... ■ 850
- Amphojel Suspension ... 2802
- Amphojel Suspension without Flavor ... 2802
- Amphojel Tablets ... 2802
- Ascriptin ... ■ 650
- Gaviscon Antacid Tablets ... ■ 778
- Gaviscon-2 Antacid Tablets ... ■ 779
- Mylanta Liquid ... ■ 676
- Mylanta Double Strength Liquid ... ■ 676
- Nephrox Suspension ... ■ 671

Chlorpropamide (Concurrent use with hypoglycemic agents is not recommended). Products include:
- Diabinese Tablets ... 2002

Diclofenac Potassium (Concurrent use with antiarthritic drugs is not recommended). Products include:
- Cataflam Tablets ... 833

Diclofenac Sodium (Concurrent use with antiarthritic drugs is not recommended). Products include:
- Voltaren Ophthalmic Sterile Ophthalmic Solution ... ⊙ 264
- Cataflam/Voltaren/Voltaren-XR ... 833

Dicumarol (Concurrent use with anticoagulants is not recommended).
- No products indexed under this heading.

Etodolac (Concurrent use with antiarthritic drugs is not recommended). Products include:
- Lodine Capsules and Tablets ... 2849

Fenoprofen Calcium (Concurrent use with antiarthritic drugs is not recommended). Products include:
- Nalfon 200 Pulvules & Nalfon Tablets ... 933

Flurbiprofen (Concurrent use with antiarthritic drugs is not recommended).
- No products indexed under this heading.

Glimepiride (Concurrent use with hypoglycemic agents is not recommended). Products include:
- Amaryl Tablets ... 1241

Glipizide (Concurrent use with hypoglycemic agents is not recommended). Products include:
- Glucotrol Tablets ... 2011
- Glucotrol XL Extended Release Tablets ... 2012

Glyburide (Concurrent use with hypoglycemic agents is not recommended). Products include:
- DiaBeta Tablets ... 1265
- Glynase PresTab Tablets ... 2091
- Micronase Tablets ... 2099

Ibuprofen (Concurrent use with antiarthritic drugs is not recommended). Products include:
- Advil Cold and Sinus Caplets and Tablets ... ■ 837
- Advil Ibuprofen Tablets, Caplets and Gel Caplets ... ■ 836
- Children's Motrin Ibuprofen Oral Suspension ... 1558
- IBU Tablets ... 1389
- Ibuprohm ... ■ 713
- Motrin IB Caplets, Tablets, and Gelcaps ... ■ 802
- Motrin Ibuprofen Suspension, Oral Drops, Chewable Tablets, Caplets ... 1563
- Nuprin Ibuprofen/Analgesic Tablets & Caplets ... ■ 645
- Vicks DayQuil SINUS Pressure & PAIN Relief with IBUPROFEN ... ■ 735

Indomethacin (Concurrent use with antiarthritic drugs is not recommended). Products include:
- Indocin ... 1723

Indomethacin Sodium Trihydrate (Concurrent use with antiarthritic drugs is not recommended). Products include:
- Indocin I.V. ... 1727

Ketoprofen (Concurrent use with antiarthritic drugs is not recommended). Products include:
- Actron Caplets and Tablets ... ■ 608
- Orudis Capsules ... 2874
- Orudis KT ... ■ 842
- Oruvail Capsules ... 2874

Ketorolac Tromethamine (Concurrent use with antiarthritic drugs is not recommended). Products include:
- Acular Sterile Ophthalmic Solution ... 470
- Toradol ... 2319

Magaldrate (Co-administration of nonabsorbable antacids may alter the rate of absorption of aspirin thereby resulting in a decreased acetylsalicylic acid/salicylic acid ratio in plasma).
- No products indexed under this heading.

Magnesium Hydroxide (Co-administration of nonabsorbable antacids may alter the rate of absorption of aspirin thereby resulting in a decreased acetylsalicylic acid/salicylic acid ratio in plasma). Products include:
- Aludrox Oral Suspension ... ■ 850
- Ascriptin ... ■ 650
- Di-Gel Antacid/Anti-Gas ... ■ 762
- Gelusil Antacid-Anti-gas Liquid ... ■ 819
- Gelusil Antacid-Anti-gas Tablets ... ■ 819
- Maalox Antacid/Anti-Gas Tablets ... 889
- Maalox Antacid Liquid ... 888
- Extra Strength Maalox Antacid/Anti-Gas Liquid and Tablets ... 888
- Mylanta Fast-Acting ... 1359
- Mylanta Gelcaps Antacid ... ■ 678
- Fast-Acting Mylanta Liquid Antacid ... 1359
- Mylanta Tablets ... ■ 677
- Maximum-Strength Fast-Acting Mylanta Liquid Antacid ... 1359
- Mylanta Double Strength Tablets ... ■ 677
- Phillips' Milk of Magnesia Liquid ... ■ 627
- Rolaids Antacid Tablets ... ■ 807
- Tempo Soft Antacid ... ■ 799

Magnesium Oxide (Co-administration of nonabsorbable antacids may alter the rate of absorption of aspirin thereby resulting in a decreased acetylsalicylic acid/salicylic acid ratio in plasma). Products include:
- Beelith Tablets ... 632
- Bufferin Analgesic Tablets ... ■ 636
- Arthritis Strength Bufferin Analgesic Caplets ... ■ 637
- Extra Strength Bufferin Analgesic Tablets ... ■ 637
- Caltrate PLUS ... ■ 681
- Cama Arthritis Pain Reliever ... ■ 748
- Mag-Ox 400 ... 666
- Uro-Mag ... 666

Meclofenamate Sodium (Concurrent use with antiarthritic drugs is not recommended).
- No products indexed under this heading.

Mefenamic Acid (Concurrent use with antiarthritic drugs is not recommended). Products include:
- Ponstel ... 1982

Metformin Hydrochloride (Concurrent use with hypoglycemic agents is not recommended). Products include:
- Glucophage Tablets ... 754

Nabumetone (Concurrent use with antiarthritic drugs is not recommended). Products include:
- Relafen Tablets ... 2688

Naproxen (Concurrent use with antiarthritic drugs is not recommended). Products include:
- Anaprox/Naprosyn ... 2277

Naproxen Sodium (Concurrent use with antiarthritic drugs is not recommended). Products include:
- Aleve ... 2124
- Anaprox/Naprosyn ... 2277
- Naprelan Tablets ... 2861

Oxaprozin (Concurrent use with antiarthritic drugs is not recommended). Products include:
- Daypro Caplets ... 2578

Phenylbutazone (Concurrent use with antiarthritic drugs is not recommended).
- No products indexed under this heading.

Piroxicam (Concurrent use with antiarthritic drugs is not recommended). Products include:
- Feldene Capsules ... 2008

Probenecid (Concurrent use with antigout agents is not recommended). Products include:
- Benemid Tablets ... 1651
- ColBENEMID Tablets ... 1662

Sodium Bicarbonate (Concurrent administration with absorbable antacids may increase the clearance of salicylates). Products include:
- Alka-Seltzer Cherry Effervescent Antacid and Pain Reliever ... ■ 609
- Alka-Seltzer Extra Strength Effervescent Antacid and Pain Reliever ... ■ 609
- Alka-Seltzer Gold Effervescent Antacid ... ■ 611
- Alka-Seltzer Lemon Lime Effervescent Antacid and Pain Reliever ... ■ 609
- Alka-Seltzer Original Effervescent Antacid and Pain Reliever ... ■ 609
- Arm & Hammer Pure Baking Soda ... ■ 648
- Colyte and Colyte-flavored ... 2540
- GoLYTELY ... 694
- Massengill Disposable Douches ... ■ 780
- Massengill Liquid Concentrate ... ■ 780
- NuLYTELY ... 694
- Cherry Flavor NuLYTELY ... 694

Sulfinpyrazone (Concurrent use with antigout agents is not recommended). Products include:
- Anturane ... 823

(■ Described in PDR For Nonprescription Drugs) (⊙ Described in PDR For Ophthalmology)

Sulindac (Concurrent use with antiarthritic drugs is not recommended). Products include:
Clinoril Tablets ... 1658

Tolazamide (Concurrent use with hypoglycemic agents is not recommended).
No products indexed under this heading.

Tolbutamide (Concurrent use with hypoglycemic agents is not recommended).
No products indexed under this heading.

Tolmetin Sodium (Concurrent use with antiarthritic drugs is not recommended). Products include:
Tolectin (200, 400 and 600 mg) .. 1591

Warfarin Sodium (Concurrent use with anticoagulants is not recommended). Products include:
Coumadin ... 941

ECOTRIN ENTERIC COATED ASPIRIN REGULAR STRENGTH TABLETS
(Aspirin) ... 2625
See **Ecotrin Enteric Coated Aspirin Maximum Strength Tablets and Caplets**

EDECRIN SODIUM INTRAVENOUS
(Ethacrynate Sodium) ... 1698
May interact with aminoglycosides, cephalosporins, non-steroidal anti-inflammatory agents, cardiac glycosides, and certain other agents. Compounds in these categories include:

Amikacin Sulfate (Increased ototoxic potential of aminoglycosides). Products include:
Amikacin Sulfate Injection, USP ... 523
Amikacin Sulfate Injection, USP ... 981
Amikin Injectable ... 502

Cefaclor (Increased ototoxic potential of cephalosporins). Products include:
Ceclor Pulvules & Suspension ... 1470

Cefadroxil (Increased ototoxic potential of cephalosporins). Products include:
Duricef Capsules, Tablets, and Oral Suspension ... 750

Cefamandole Nafate (Increased ototoxic potential of cephalosporins). Products include:
Mandol Vials, Faspak & ADD-Vantage ... 1516

Cefazolin Sodium (Increased ototoxic potential of cephalosporins). Products include:
Ancef Injection ... 2632
Kefzol Vials, Faspak & ADD-Vantage ... 1511

Cefixime (Increased ototoxic potential of cephalosporins). Products include:
Suprax ... 1443

Cefmetazole Sodium (Increased ototoxic potential of cephalosporins).
No products indexed under this heading.

Cefonicid Sodium (Increased ototoxic potential of cephalosporins). Products include:
Monocid Injection ... 2674

Cefoperazone Sodium (Increased ototoxic potential of cephalosporins). Products include:
Cefobid Intravenous/Intramuscular 1996
Cefobid Pharmacy Bulk Package - Not for Direct Infusion ... 1999

Ceforanide (Increased ototoxic potential of cephalosporins).
No products indexed under this heading.

Cefotaxime Sodium (Increased ototoxic potential of cephalosporins). Products include:
Claforan Sterile and Injection ... 1259

Cefotetan (Increased ototoxic potential of cephalosporins). Products include:
Cefotan ... 2936

Cefoxitin Sodium (Increased ototoxic potential of cephalosporins). Products include:
Mefoxin ... 1734
Mefoxin Premixed Intravenous Solution ... 1737

Cefpodoxime Proxetil (Increased ototoxic potential of cephalosporins). Products include:
Vantin for Oral Suspension and Vantin Tablets ... 2112

Cefprozil (Increased ototoxic potential of cephalosporins). Products include:
Cefzil Tablets and Oral Suspension 747

Ceftazidime (Increased ototoxic potential of cephalosporins). Products include:
Ceptaz ... 1070
Fortaz ... 1092
Tazicef for Injection ... 2697
Tazidime Vials, Faspak & ADD-Vantage ... 1531

Ceftizoxime Sodium (Increased ototoxic potential of cephalosporins). Products include:
Cefizox for Intramuscular or Intravenous Use ... 1025

Ceftriaxone Sodium (Increased ototoxic potential of cephalosporins). Products include:
Rocephin Injectable Vials, ADD-Vantage, Galaxy Container ... 2305

Cefuroxime Axetil (Increased ototoxic potential of cephalosporins). Products include:
Ceftin ... 1067

Cefuroxime Sodium (Increased ototoxic potential of cephalosporins). Products include:
Kefurox Vials, Faspak & ADD-Vantage ... 1509
Zinacef ... 1184

Cephalexin (Increased ototoxic potential of cephalosporins). Products include:
Keflex Pulvules & Oral Suspension 930

Cephalothin Sodium (Increased ototoxic potential of cephalosporins).

Cephapirin Sodium (Increased ototoxic potential of cephalosporins).
No products indexed under this heading.

Cephradine (Increased ototoxic potential of cephalosporins).
No products indexed under this heading.

Deslanoside (Excessive potassium loss may precipitate digitalis toxicity).
No products indexed under this heading.

Diclofenac Potassium (Reduces diuretic, natriuretic, and antihypertensive effects). Products include:
Cataflam Tablets ... 833

Diclofenac Sodium (Reduces diuretic, natriuretic, and antihypertensive effects). Products include:
Voltaren Ophthalmic Sterile Ophthalmic Solution ... ⊙ 264
Cataflam/Voltaren/Voltaren-XR ... 833

Digitoxin (Excessive potassium loss may precipitate digitalis toxicity). Products include:
Crystodigin Tablets ... 1472

Digoxin (Excessive potassium loss may precipitate digitalis toxicity). Products include:
Lanoxicaps ... 1110
Lanoxin Elixir Pediatric ... 1113
Lanoxin Injection ... 1116
Lanoxin Injection Pediatric ... 1119
Lanoxin Tablets ... 1121

Etodolac (Reduces diuretic, natriuretic, and antihypertensive effects). Products include:
Lodine Capsules and Tablets ... 2849

Fenoprofen Calcium (Reduces diuretic, natriuretic, and antihypertensive effects). Products include:
Nalfon 200 Pulvules & Nalfon Tablets ... 933

Flurbiprofen (Reduces diuretic, natriuretic, and antihypertensive effects).
No products indexed under this heading.

Gentamicin Sulfate (Increased ototoxic potential of aminoglycosides). Products include:
Garamycin Cream 0.1% ... 2501
Garamycin Injectable ... 2502
Garamycin Ointment 0.1% ... 2501
Garamycin Ophthalmic ... 2501
Genoptic Sterile Ophthalmic Solution ... ⊙ 241
Genoptic Sterile Ophthalmic Ointment ... ⊙ 241
Gentak ... ⊙ 209
Pred-G Liquifilm Sterile Ophthalmic Suspension ... ⊙ 248
Pred-G S.O.P. Sterile Ophthalmic Ointment ... ⊙ 249

Ibuprofen (Reduces diuretic, natriuretic, and antihypertensive effects). Products include:
Advil Cold and Sinus Caplets and Tablets ... [PD] 837
Advil Ibuprofen Tablets, Caplets and Gel Caplets ... [PD] 836
Children's Motrin Ibuprofen Oral Suspension ... 1558
IBU Tablets ... 1389
Ibuprohm ... [PD] 713
Motrin IB Caplets, Tablets, and Gelcaps ... [PD] 802
Motrin Ibuprofen Suspension, Oral Drops, Chewable Tablets, Caplets ... 1563
Nuprin Ibuprofen/Analgesic Tablets & Caplets ... [PD] 645
Vicks DayQuil SINUS Pressure & PAIN Relief with IBUPROFEN ... [PD] 735

Indomethacin (Reduces diuretic, natriuretic, and antihypertensive effects). Products include:
Indocin ... 1723

Indomethacin Sodium Trihydrate (Reduces diuretic, natriuretic, and antihypertensive effects). Products include:
Indocin I.V. ... 1727

Isoproterenol Hydrochloride (Careful adjustment of dosages required). Products include:
Isuprel Hydrochloride Solution ... 2443
Isuprel Injection ... 2441
Isuprel Mistometer ... 2442

Kanamycin Sulfate (Increased ototoxic potential of aminoglycosides).
No products indexed under this heading.

Ketoprofen (Reduces diuretic, natriuretic, and antihypertensive effects). Products include:
Actron Caplets and Tablets ... [PD] 608
Orudis Capsules ... 2874
Orudis KT ... [PD] 842
Oruvail Capsules ... 2874

Ketorolac Tromethamine (Reduces diuretic, natriuretic, and antihypertensive effects). Products include:
Acular Sterile Ophthalmic Solution 470
Toradol ... 2319

Lithium Carbonate (High risk of lithium toxicity). Products include:
Eskalith ... 2658
Lithium Carbonate Capsules & Tablets ... 2352
Lithonate/Lithotabs/Lithobid ... 2721

Lithium Citrate (High risk of lithium toxicity).
No products indexed under this heading.

Loracarbef (Increased ototoxic potential of cephalosporins). Products include:
Lorabid Suspension and Pulvules ... 1513

Meclofenamate Sodium (Reduces diuretic, natriuretic, and antihypertensive effects).
No products indexed under this heading.

Mefenamic Acid (Reduces diuretic, natriuretic, and antihypertensive effects). Products include:
Ponstel ... 1982

Nabumetone (Reduces diuretic, natriuretic, and antihypertensive effects). Products include:
Relafen Tablets ... 2688

Naproxen (Reduces diuretic, natriuretic, and antihypertensive effects). Products include:
Anaprox/Naprosyn ... 2277

Naproxen Sodium (Reduces diuretic, natriuretic, and antihypertensive effects). Products include:
Aleve ... 2124
Anaprox/Naprosyn ... 2277
Naprelan Tablets ... 2861

Oxaprozin (Reduces diuretic, natriuretic, and antihypertensive effects). Products include:
Daypro Caplets ... 2578

Phenylbutazone (Reduces diuretic, natriuretic, and antihypertensive effects).
No products indexed under this heading.

Piroxicam (Reduces diuretic, natriuretic, and antihypertensive effects). Products include:
Feldene Capsules ... 2008

Streptomycin Sulfate (Increased ototoxic potential of aminoglycosides). Products include:
Streptomycin Sulfate Injection ... 2031

Sulindac (Reduces diuretic, natriuretic, and antihypertensive effects). Products include:
Clinoril Tablets ... 1658

Tobramycin Sulfate (Increased ototoxic potential of aminoglycosides). Products include:
Nebcin Vials, Hyporets & ADD-Vantage ... 1518

Tolmetin Sodium (Reduces diuretic, natriuretic, and antihypertensive effects). Products include:
Tolectin (200, 400 and 600 mg) .. 1591

Warfarin Sodium (Warfarin displaced from plasma protein; reduction in warfarin dosage may be required). Products include:
Coumadin ... 941

EDECRIN TABLETS
(Ethacrynic Acid) ... 1698
See **Edecrin Sodium Intravenous**

EFFEXOR
(Venlafaxine Hydrochloride) ... 2825
May interact with monoamine oxidase inhibitors and certain other

IMPORTANT NOTE: Always consult each drug listing in the patient's regimen for possible interactions.

agents. Compounds in these categories include:

Cimetidine (Inhibition of first-pass metabolism of venlafaxine; reduces the oral clearance by 43% and the AUC and C_{max} of venlafaxine were increased by about 60%). Products include:

Tagamet HB Tablets .... ◙ 786
Tagamet Tablets 2694

Cimetidine Hydrochloride (Inhibition of first-pass metabolism of venlafaxine; reduces the oral clearance by 43% and the AUC and C_{max} of venlafaxine were increased by about 60%). Products include:

Tagamet 2694

Furazolidone (Potential for serious, sometimes fatal reactions including hyperthermia, rigidity, myoclonus, autonomic instability; concurrent and or sequential use within 14 days is contraindicated). Products include:

Furoxone 2221

Isocarboxazid (Potential for serious, sometimes fatal reactions including hyperthermia, rigidity, myoclonus, autonomic instability; concurrent and or sequential use within 14 days is contraindicated).

No products indexed under this heading.

Phenelzine Sulfate (Potential for serious, sometimes fatal reactions including hyperthermia, rigidity, myoclonus, autonomic instability; concurrent and or sequential use within 14 days is contraindicated). Products include:

Nardil 1977

Selegiline Hydrochloride (Potential for serious, sometimes fatal reactions including hyperthermia, rigidity, myoclonus, autonomic instability; concurrent and or sequential use within 14 days is contraindicated). Products include:

Eldepryl Capsules 2729

Tranylcypromine Sulfate (Potential for serious, sometimes fatal reactions including hyperthermia, rigidity, myoclonus, autonomic instability; concurrent and or sequential use within 14 days is contraindicated). Products include:

Parnate Tablets 2679

Food Interactions

Alcohol (Concurrent use should be avoided).

EFIDAC/24

(Pseudoephedrine Hydrochloride) .. ◙ 655
May interact with antihypertensives, antidepressant drugs, and certain other agents. Compounds in these categories include:

Acebutolol Hydrochloride (Concurrent use is not recommended; consult your doctor). Products include:

Sectral Capsules 2914

Amitriptyline Hydrochloride (Concurrent use is not recommended; consult your doctor). Products include:

Elavil 2945
Etrafon 2495
Limbitrol 2333
Triavil Tablets 1800

Amlodipine Besylate (Concurrent use is not recommended; consult your doctor). Products include:

Lotrel Capsules 858
Norvasc Tablets 2020

Amoxapine (Concurrent use is not recommended; consult your doctor). Products include:

Asendin Tablets 1419

Atenolol (Concurrent use is not recommended; consult your doctor). Products include:

Tenoretic Tablets 2963
Tenormin Tablets and I.V. Injection 2965

Benazepril Hydrochloride (Concurrent use is not recommended; consult your doctor). Products include:

Lotensin Tablets 852
Lotensin HCT Tablets 855
Lotrel Capsules 858

Bendroflumethiazide (Concurrent use is not recommended; consult your doctor).

No products indexed under this heading.

Betaxolol Hydrochloride (Concurrent use is not recommended; consult your doctor). Products include:

Betoptic Ophthalmic Solution 465
Betoptic S Ophthalmic Suspension 467
Kerlone Tablets 2588

Bisoprolol Fumarate (Concurrent use is not recommended; consult your doctor). Products include:

Zebeta Tablets 1457
Ziac 1459

Bupropion Hydrochloride (Concurrent use is not recommended; consult your doctor). Products include:

Wellbutrin Tablets 1177

Captopril (Concurrent use is not recommended; consult your doctor). Products include:

Capoten Tablets 740
Capozide Tablets 744

Carteolol Hydrochloride (Concurrent use is not recommended; consult your doctor). Products include:

Cartrol Tablets 413
Ocupress Ophthalmic Solution, 1% Sterile .... ⊙ 297

Chlorothiazide (Concurrent use is not recommended; consult your doctor). Products include:

Aldoclor Tablets 1638
Diupres Tablets 1691
Diuril Oral 1694

Chlorothiazide Sodium (Concurrent use is not recommended; consult your doctor). Products include:

Diuril Sodium Intravenous 1693

Chlorthalidone (Concurrent use is not recommended; consult your doctor). Products include:

Combipres Tablets 682
Tenoretic Tablets 2963
Thalitone 1293

Clonidine (Concurrent use is not recommended; consult your doctor). Products include:

Catapres-TTS 680

Clonidine Hydrochloride (Concurrent use is not recommended; consult your doctor). Products include:

Catapres Tablets 679
Combipres Tablets 682

Deserpidine (Concurrent use is not recommended; consult your doctor).

No products indexed under this heading.

Desipramine Hydrochloride (Concurrent use is not recommended; consult your doctor). Products include:

Norpramin Tablets 1273

Diazoxide (Concurrent use is not recommended; consult your doctor). Products include:

Hyperstat I.V. Injection 2504
Proglycem 575

Diltiazem Hydrochloride (Concurrent use is not recommended; consult your doctor). Products include:

Cardizem CD Capsules 1251
Cardizem SR Capsules 1255
Cardizem Injectable 1253
Cardizem Tablets 1257
Dilacor XR Extended-release Capsules 2183
Tiazac Capsules 1019

Doxazosin Mesylate (Concurrent use is not recommended; consult your doctor). Products include:

Cardura Tablets 1993

Doxepin Hydrochloride (Concurrent use is not recommended; consult your doctor). Products include:

Adapin Capsules 1542
Sinequan 2028
Zonalon Cream 1042

Enalapril Maleate (Concurrent use is not recommended; consult your doctor). Products include:

Vaseretic Tablets 1810
Vasotec Tablets 1816

Enalaprilat (Concurrent use is not recommended; consult your doctor). Products include:

Vasotec I.V. 1814

Esmolol Hydrochloride (Concurrent use is not recommended; consult your doctor). Products include:

Brevibloc (esmolol HCl) Injection 1860

Felodipine (Concurrent use is not recommended; consult your doctor). Products include:

Plendil Extended-Release Tablets 514

Fluoxetine Hydrochloride (Concurrent use is not recommended; consult your doctor). Products include:

Prozac Pulvules & Liquid, Oral Solution 935

Fosinopril Sodium (Concurrent use is not recommended; consult your doctor). Products include:

Monopril Tablets 762

Furosemide (Concurrent use is not recommended; consult your doctor). Products include:

Lasix Injection, Oral Solution and Tablets 1267

Guanabenz Acetate (Concurrent use is not recommended; consult your doctor).

No products indexed under this heading.

Guanethidine Monosulfate (Concurrent use is not recommended; consult your doctor). Products include:

Esimil Tablets 840
Ismelin Tablets 845

Hydralazine Hydrochloride (Concurrent use is not recommended; consult your doctor). Products include:

Apresazide Capsules 824
Apresoline Hydrochloride Tablets .. 826
Hydralazine Hydrochloride Injection USP 2712
Ser-Ap-Es Tablets 867

Hydrochlorothiazide (Concurrent use is not recommended; consult your doctor). Products include:

Aldactazide Tablets 2556
Aldoril Tablets 1644
Apresazide Capsules 824
Capozide Tablets 744
Dyazide Capsules 2653
Esidrix Tablets 839
Esimil Tablets 840
HydroDIURIL Tablets 1716
Hydropres Tablets 1718
Hyzaar Tablets 1720
Inderide Tablets 2838
Inderide LA Long Acting Capsules .. 2840
Lopressor HCT Tablets 850
Lotensin HCT Tablets 855
Moduretic Tablets 1748
Oretic Tablets 450
Prinzide Tablets 1780
Ser-Ap-Es Tablets 867
Timolide Tablets 1791
Vaseretic Tablets 1810
Zestoretic Tablets 2968
Ziac 1459

Hydroflumethiazide (Concurrent use is not recommended; consult your doctor). Products include:

Diucardin Tablets 2824

Imipramine Hydrochloride (Concurrent use is not recommended; consult your doctor). Products include:

Tofranil Ampuls 873
Tofranil Tablets 875

Imipramine Pamoate (Concurrent use is not recommended; consult your doctor). Products include:

Tofranil-PM Capsules 876

Indapamide (Concurrent use is not recommended; consult your doctor).

No products indexed under this heading.

Isocarboxazid (Concurrent use is not recommended; consult your doctor).

No products indexed under this heading.

Isradipine (Concurrent use is not recommended; consult your doctor). Products include:

DynaCirc Capsules 2381
DynaCirc CR Tablets 2383

Labetalol Hydrochloride (Concurrent use is not recommended; consult your doctor). Products include:

Normodyne Injection 2519
Normodyne Tablets 2522
Trandate 1158

Lisinopril (Concurrent use is not recommended; consult your doctor). Products include:

Prinivil Tablets 1776
Prinzide Tablets 1780
Zestoretic Tablets 2968
Zestril Tablets 2972

Losartan Potassium (Concurrent use is not recommended; consult your doctor). Products include:

Cozaar Tablets 1668
Hyzaar Tablets 1720

Maprotiline Hydrochloride (Concurrent use is not recommended; consult your doctor). Products include:

Ludiomil Tablets 861

Mecamylamine Hydrochloride (Concurrent use is not recommended; consult your doctor). Products include:

Inversine Tablets 1729

Methyclothiazide (Concurrent use is not recommended; consult your doctor). Products include:

Enduron Tablets 424

Methyldopa (Concurrent use is not recommended; consult your doctor). Products include:

Aldoclor Tablets 1638
Aldomet Oral 1640
Aldoril Tablets 1644

Methyldopate Hydrochloride (Concurrent use is not recommended; consult your doctor). Products include:

Aldomet Ester HCl Injection 1642

Metolazone (Concurrent use is not recommended; consult your doctor). Products include:

Mykrox Tablets 1617
Zaroxolyn Tablets 1625

(◙ Described in PDR For Nonprescription Drugs) (⊙ Described in PDR For Ophthalmology)

365 Interactions Index Efidac 24 Chlorpheniramine

Metoprolol Succinate (Concurrent use is not recommended; consult your doctor). Products include:
Toprol-XL Tablets ... 560
Metoprolol Tartrate (Concurrent use is not recommended; consult your doctor). Products include:
Lopressor ... 848
Lopressor HCT Tablets ... 850
Metyrosine (Concurrent use is not recommended; consult your doctor). Products include:
Demser Capsules ... 1690
Minoxidil (Concurrent use is not recommended; consult your doctor).
No products indexed under this heading.
Moexipril Hydrochloride (Concurrent use is not recommended; consult your doctor). Products include:
Univasc Tablets ... 2553
Nadolol (Concurrent use is not recommended; consult your doctor).
No products indexed under this heading.
Nefazodone Hydrochloride (Concurrent use is not recommended; consult your doctor). Products include:
Serzone Tablets ... 776
Nicardipine Hydrochloride (Concurrent use is not recommended; consult your doctor). Products include:
Cardene Capsules ... 2261
Cardene I.V. ... 2815
Cardene SR Capsules ... 2264
Nifedipine (Concurrent use is not recommended; consult your doctor). Products include:
Adalat Capsules (10 mg and 20 mg) ... 580
Adalat CC ... 582
Procardia Capsules ... 2024
Procardia XL Extended Release Tablets ... 2026
Nisoldipine (Concurrent use is not recommended; consult your doctor). Products include:
Sular Tablets ... 2961
Nitroglycerin (Concurrent use is not recommended; consult your doctor). Products include:
Deponit NTG Transdermal Delivery System ... 2541
Nitro-Bid IV ... 1270
Nitro-Bid Ointment ... 1272
Nitro-Dur (nitroglycerin) Transdermal Infusion System ... 1365
Nitrolingual Spray ... 2193
Nitrostat Tablets ... 1981
Transderm-Nitro Transdermal Therapeutic System ... 878
Nortriptyline Hydrochloride (Concurrent use is not recommended; consult your doctor). Products include:
Pamelor ... 2409
Paroxetine Hydrochloride (Concurrent use is not recommended; consult your doctor). Products include:
Paxil Tablets ... 2681
Penbutolol Sulfate (Concurrent use is not recommended; consult your doctor). Products include:
Levatol Tablets ... 2547
Phenelzine Sulfate (Concurrent use is not recommended; consult your doctor). Products include:
Nardil ... 1977
Phenoxybenzamine Hydrochloride (Concurrent use is not recommended; consult your doctor). Products include:
Dibenzyline Capsules ... 2650
Phentolamine Mesylate (Concurrent use is not recommended; consult your doctor). Products include:
Regitine Vials ... 864
Pindolol (Concurrent use is not recommended; consult your doctor). Products include:
Visken Tablets ... 2428
Polythiazide (Concurrent use is not recommended; consult your doctor). Products include:
Minizide Capsules ... 2016
Prazosin Hydrochloride (Concurrent use is not recommended; consult your doctor). Products include:
Minipress Capsules ... 2015
Minizide Capsules ... 2016
Propranolol Hydrochloride (Concurrent use is not recommended; consult your doctor). Products include:
Inderal ... 2834
Inderal LA Long Acting Capsules ... 2836
Inderide Tablets ... 2838
Inderide LA Long Acting Capsules ... 2840
Protriptyline Hydrochloride (Concurrent use is not recommended; consult your doctor). Products include:
Vivactil Tablets ... 1820
Quinapril Hydrochloride (Concurrent use is not recommended; consult your doctor). Products include:
Accupril Tablets ... 1950
Ramipril (Concurrent use is not recommended; consult your doctor). Products include:
Altace Capsules ... 1238
Rauwolfia Serpentina (Concurrent use is not recommended; consult your doctor).
No products indexed under this heading.
Rescinnamine (Concurrent use is not recommended; consult your doctor).
No products indexed under this heading.
Reserpine (Concurrent use is not recommended; consult your doctor). Products include:
Diupres Tablets ... 1691
Hydropres Tablets ... 1718
Ser-Ap-Es Tablets ... 867
Sertraline Hydrochloride (Concurrent use is not recommended; consult your doctor). Products include:
Zoloft Tablets ... 2051
Sodium Nitroprusside (Concurrent use is not recommended; consult your doctor).
No products indexed under this heading.
Sotalol Hydrochloride (Concurrent use is not recommended; consult your doctor). Products include:
Betapace Tablets ... 637
Spirapril Hydrochloride (Concurrent use is not recommended; consult your doctor).
No products indexed under this heading.
Terazosin Hydrochloride (Concurrent use is not recommended; consult your doctor). Products include:
Hytrin Capsules ... 434
Timolol Maleate (Concurrent use is not recommended; consult your doctor). Products include:
Blocadren Tablets ... 1654
Timolide Tablets ... 1791
Timoptic in Ocudose ... 1796
Timoptic Sterile Ophthalmic Solution ... 1794
Timoptic-XE ... 1798
Torsemide (Concurrent use is not recommended; consult your doctor). Products include:
Demadex Tablets and Injection ... 691
Tranylcypromine Sulfate (Concurrent use is not recommended; consult your doctor). Products include:
Parnate Tablets ... 2679
Trazodone Hydrochloride (Concurrent use is not recommended; consult your doctor). Products include:
Desyrel and Desyrel Dividose ... 504
Trimethaphan Camsylate (Concurrent use is not recommended; consult your doctor).
No products indexed under this heading.
Trimipramine Maleate (Concurrent use is not recommended; consult your doctor). Products include:
Surmontil Capsules ... 2917
Venlafaxine Hydrochloride (Concurrent use is not recommended; consult your doctor). Products include:
Effexor ... 2825
Verapamil Hydrochloride (Concurrent use is not recommended; consult your doctor). Products include:
Calan SR Caplets ... 2571
Calan Tablets ... 2568
Covera-HS Tablets ... 2573
Isoptin Injectable ... 1391
Isoptin Oral Tablets ... 1393
Isoptin SR Tablets ... 1395
Verelan Capsules ... 1455

EFIDAC 24 CHLORPHENIRAMINE
(Chlorpheniramine Maleate) ... 655
May interact with hypnotics and sedatives, tranquilizers, and certain other agents. Compounds in these categories include:

Alprazolam (May increase drowsiness effect). Products include:
Xanax Tablets ... 2115
Buspirone Hydrochloride (May increase drowsiness effect). Products include:
BuSpar Tablets ... 738
Chlordiazepoxide (May increase drowsiness effect). Products include:
Limbitrol ... 2333
Chlordiazepoxide Hydrochloride (May increase drowsiness effect). Products include:
Librax Capsules ... 2330
Librium Capsules ... 2331
Librium Injectable ... 2332
Chlorpromazine (May increase drowsiness effect). Products include:
Thorazine Suppositories ... 2701
Chlorpromazine Hydrochloride (May increase drowsiness effect). Products include:
Thorazine ... 2701
Chlorprothixene (May increase drowsiness effect).
No products indexed under this heading.
Chlorprothixene Hydrochloride (May increase drowsiness effect).
No products indexed under this heading.
Clorazepate Dipotassium (May increase drowsiness effect). Products include:
Tranxene ... 459
Diazepam (May increase drowsiness effect). Products include:
Dizac (diazepam injectable emulsion) CIV ... 1862
Valium Injectable ... 2336
Valium Tablets ... 2335
Droperidol (May increase drowsiness effect). Products include:
Inapsine Injection ... 462
Estazolam (May increase drowsiness effect). Products include:
ProSom Tablets ... 457
Ethchlorvynol (May increase drowsiness effect). Products include:
Placidyl Capsules ... 456
Ethinamate (May increase drowsiness effect).
No products indexed under this heading.
Fluphenazine Decanoate (May increase drowsiness effect). Products include:
Prolixin Decanoate ... 510
Fluphenazine Enanthate (May increase drowsiness effect). Products include:
Prolixin Enanthate ... 510
Fluphenazine Hydrochloride (May increase drowsiness effect). Products include:
Prolixin ... 510
Flurazepam Hydrochloride (May increase drowsiness effect). Products include:
Dalmane Capsules ... 2329
Glutethimide (May increase drowsiness effect).
No products indexed under this heading.
Haloperidol (May increase drowsiness effect). Products include:
Haldol Injection, Tablets and Concentrate ... 1585
Haloperidol Decanoate (May increase drowsiness effect). Products include:
Haldol Decanoate ... 1587
Hydroxyzine Hydrochloride (May increase drowsiness effect). Products include:
Atarax Tablets & Syrup ... 1992
Marax Tablets & DF Syrup ... 2015
Vistaril Intramuscular Solution ... 2042
Lorazepam (May increase drowsiness effect). Products include:
Ativan Injection ... 2805
Ativan Tablets ... 2807
Loxapine Hydrochloride (May increase drowsiness effect). Products include:
Loxitane ... 1426
Loxapine Succinate (May increase drowsiness effect). Products include:
Loxitane Capsules ... 1426
Meprobamate (May increase drowsiness effect). Products include:
Miltown Tablets ... 2780
PMB 200 and PMB 400 ... 2890
Mesoridazine Besylate (May increase drowsiness effect). Products include:
Serentil ... 689
Midazolam Hydrochloride (May increase drowsiness effect). Products include:
Versed Injection ... 2324
Molindone Hydrochloride (May increase drowsiness effect). Products include:
Moban Tablets and Concentrate ... 1036
Oxazepam (May increase drowsiness effect). Products include:
Serax Capsules ... 2916
Serax Tablets ... 2916
Perphenazine (May increase drowsiness effect). Products include:
Etrafon ... 2495
Triavil Tablets ... 1800
Trilafon ... 2532

IMPORTANT NOTE: Always consult each drug listing in the patient's regimen for possible interactions.

Prazepam (May increase drowsiness effect).
No products indexed under this heading.

Prochlorperazine (May increase drowsiness effect). Products include:
Compazine 2644

Promethazine Hydrochloride (May increase drowsiness effect). Products include:
Mepergan Injection 2859
Phenergan with Codeine 2883
Phenergan with Dextromethorphan 2885
Phenergan Injection 2880
Phenergan Suppositories 2882
Phenergan Syrup 2881
Phenergan Tablets 2882
Phenergan VC 2886
Phenergan VC with Codeine 2888

Propofol (May increase drowsiness effect). Products include:
Diprivan Injectable Emulsion 2939

Quazepam (May increase drowsiness effect). Products include:
Doral Tablets 2773

Secobarbital Sodium (May increase drowsiness effect). Products include:
Seconal Sodium Pulvules 1529

Temazepam (May increase drowsiness effect). Products include:
Restoril Capsules 2413

Thioridazine Hydrochloride (May increase drowsiness effect). Products include:
Mellaril 2398

Thiothixene (May increase drowsiness effect). Products include:
Navane Capsules and Concentrate 2018
Navane Intramuscular 2019

Triazolam (May increase drowsiness effect). Products include:
Halcion Tablets 2093

Trifluoperazine Hydrochloride (May increase drowsiness effect). Products include:
Stelazine 2692

Zolpidem Tartrate (May increase drowsiness effect). Products include:
Ambien Tablets 2559

Food Interactions

Alcohol (May increase drowsiness effect).

EFLONE STERILE OPHTHALMIC SUSPENSION

(Fluorometholone Acetate) .... ⊙ 261
None cited in PDR database.

EFUDEX CREAM

(Fluorouracil) 2280
None cited in PDR database.

EFUDEX TOPICAL SOLUTIONS

(Fluorouracil) 2280
None cited in PDR database.

ELAVIL INJECTION

(Amitriptyline Hydrochloride) 2945
May interact with barbiturates, central nervous system depressants, anticholinergics, phenothiazines, quinidine, antidepressant drugs, selective serotonin reuptake inhibitors, monoamine oxidase inhibitors, sympathomimetics, thyroid preparations, and certain other agents. Compounds in these categories include:

Albuterol (Effects of concurrent use not specified; careful adjustment of dosage and close supervision are required). Products include:
Proventil Inhalation Aerosol 2524
Ventolin Inhalation Aerosol and Refill 1170

Albuterol Sulfate (Effects of concurrent use not specified; careful adjustment of dosage and close supervision are required). Products include:
Airet Albuterol Sulfate Inhalation Solution 1602
Albuterol Sulfate, USP Solution for Inhalation, Arm-a-Med 522
Proventil Inhalation Solution 0.083% 2527
Proventil Repetabs Tablets 2529
Proventil Solution for Inhalation 0.5% 2525
Proventil Syrup 2528
Proventil Tablets 2529
Ventolin Inhalation Solution 1171
Ventolin Nebules Inhalation Solution 1172
Ventolin Rotacaps for Inhalation 1173
Ventolin Syrup 1175
Ventolin Tablets 1176
Volmax Extended-Release Tablets .. 1835

Alfentanil Hydrochloride (Co-administration results in enhanced response to CNS depressants). Products include:
Alfenta Injection 1334

Alprazolam (Co-administration results in enhanced response to CNS depressants). Products include:
Xanax Tablets 2115

Amoxapine (Co-administration with cytochrome P4502D6 inhibitors, such as antidepressants, may make normal metabolizer resemble poor metabolizer leading to higher than expected plasma concentration of TCA with resultant toxicity; lower than usual doses of either drug may be required). Products include:
Asendin Tablets 1419

Aprobarbital (Co-administration results in enhanced response to CNS depressants).
No products indexed under this heading.

Atropine Sulfate (Co-administration may result in paralytic ileus; hyperpyrexia has been reported with concurrent use, particularly during hot weather). Products include:
Arco-Lase Plus Tablets 513
Atrohist Plus Tablets 1605
Donnatal 2234
Donnatal Extentabs 2234
Donnatal Tablets 2234
Lomotil 2591
Motofen Tablets 789
Urised Tablets 2123

Belladonna Alkaloids (Co-administration may result in paralytic ileus; hyperpyrexia has been reported with concurrent use, particularly during hot weather). Products include:
Bellergal-S Tablets 2375
Hyland's Bedwetting Tablets .... ◘ 788
Hyland's EnurAid Tablets .... ◘ 789
Hyland's Headache Tablets .... ◘ 790
Hyland's Teething Tablets .... ◘ 790
Similasan Eye Drops #1 .... ◘ 769

Benztropine Mesylate (Co-administration may result in paralytic ileus; hyperpyrexia has been reported with concurrent use, particularly during hot weather). Products include:
Cogentin 1661

Biperiden Hydrochloride (Co-administration may result in paralytic ileus; hyperpyrexia has been reported with concurrent use, particularly during hot weather). Products include:
Akineton 1380

Buprenorphine (Co-administration results in enhanced response to CNS depressants). Products include:
Buprenex Injectable 2170

Bupropion Hydrochloride (Co-administration with cytochrome P4502D6 inhibitors, such as antidepressants, may make normal metabolizer resemble poor metabolizer leading to higher than expected plasma concentration of TCA with resultant toxicity; lower than usual doses of either drug may be required). Products include:
Wellbutrin Tablets 1177

Buspirone Hydrochloride (Co-administration results in enhanced response to CNS depressants). Products include:
BuSpar Tablets 738

Butabarbital (Co-administration results in enhanced response to CNS depressants).
No products indexed under this heading.

Butalbital (Co-administration results in enhanced response to CNS depressants). Products include:
Axocet Capsules 2469
Esgic-plus Capsules 1012
Esgic-plus Tablets 1012
Fioricet Tablets 2386
Fioricet with Codeine Capsules 2387
Fiorinal Capsules 2388
Fiorinal with Codeine Capsules 2390
Fiorinal Tablets 2388
Phrenilin 790
Sedapap Tablets 50 mg/650 mg .. 1826

Chlordiazepoxide (Co-administration results in enhanced response to CNS depressants). Products include:
Limbitrol 2333

Chlordiazepoxide Hydrochloride (Co-administration results in enhanced response to CNS depressants). Products include:
Librax Capsules 2330
Librium Capsules 2331
Librium Injectable 2332

Chlorpromazine (Co-administration with cytochrome P4502D6 inhibitors, such as phenothiazines, may make normal metabolizer resemble poor metabolizer leading to higher than expected plasma concentration of TCA with resultant toxicity; lower than usual doses of either drug may be required; co-administration results in enhanced response to CNS depressants). Products include:
Thorazine Suppositories 2701

Chlorpromazine Hydrochloride (Co-administration with cytochrome P4502D6 inhibitors, such as phenothiazines, may make normal metabolizer resemble poor metabolizer leading to higher than expected plasma concentration of TCA with resultant toxicity; lower than usual doses of either drug may be required; co-administration results in enhanced response to CNS depressants). Products include:
Thorazine 2701

Chlorprothixene (Co-administration results in enhanced response to CNS depressants).
No products indexed under this heading.

Chlorprothixene Hydrochloride (Co-administration results in enhanced response to CNS depressants).
No products indexed under this heading.

Chlorprothixene Lactate (Co-administration results in enhanced response to CNS depressants).
No products indexed under this heading.

Cimetidine (Co-administration has been reported to reduce hepatic metabolism of certain tricyclic antidepressants, thereby delaying elimination and increasing steady-state concentrations of TCA resulting in the frequency and severity of side effects, particularly anticholinergic). Products include:
Tagamet HB Tablets .... ◘ 786
Tagamet Tablets 2694

Cimetidine Hydrochloride (Co-administration has been reported to reduce hepatic metabolism of certain tricyclic antidepressants, thereby delaying elimination and increasing steady-state concentrations of TCA resulting in the frequency and severity of side effects, particularly anticholinergic). Products include:
Tagamet 2694

Clidinium Bromide (Co-administration may result in paralytic ileus; hyperpyrexia has been reported with concurrent use, particularly during hot weather). Products include:
Librax Capsules 2330

Clorazepate Dipotassium (Co-administration results in enhanced response to CNS depressants). Products include:
Tranxene 459

Clozapine (Co-administration results in enhanced response to CNS depressants). Products include:
Clozaril Tablets 2377

Codeine Phosphate (Co-administration results in enhanced response to CNS depressants). Products include:
Brontex 2130
Dimetane-DC Cough Syrup 2232
Fioricet with Codeine Capsules 2387
Fiorinal with Codeine Capsules 2390
Nucofed 2225
Phenergan with Codeine 2883
Phenergan VC with Codeine 2888
Robitussin A-C Syrup 2248
Robitussin-DAC Syrup 2249
Ryna .... ◘ 804
Soma Compound w/Codeine Tablets 2784
Tylenol with Codeine 1592

Desflurane (Co-administration results in enhanced response to CNS depressants). Products include:
Suprane (desflurane, USP) 1865

Desipramine Hydrochloride (Co-administration with cytochrome P4502D6 inhibitors, such as antidepressants, may make normal metabolizer resemble poor metabolizer leading to higher than expected plasma concentration of TCA with resultant toxicity; lower than usual doses of either drug may be required). Products include:
Norpramin Tablets 1273

Dezocine (Co-administration results in enhanced response to CNS depressants). Products include:
Dalgan Injection 529

Diazepam (Co-administration results in enhanced response to CNS depressants). Products include:
Dizac (diazepam injectable emulsion) CIV 1862
Valium Injectable 2336
Valium Tablets 2335

Dicyclomine Hydrochloride (Co-administration may result in paralytic ileus; hyperpyrexia has been reported with concurrent use, particularly during hot weather). Products include:
Bentyl 1246

(◘ Described in PDR For Nonprescription Drugs) (⊙ Described in PDR For Ophthalmology)

367 **Interactions Index** **Elavil**

Disulfiram (Concurrent use has resulted in delirium). Products include:
Antabuse Tablets ... 2802

Dobutamine Hydrochloride (Effects of concurrent use not specified; careful adjustment of dosage and close supervision are required). Products include:
Dobutrex Solution Vials ... 1480

Dopamine Hydrochloride (Effects of concurrent use not specified; careful adjustment of dosage and close supervision are required).
No products indexed under this heading.

Doxepin Hydrochloride (Co-administration with cytochrome P4502D6 inhibitors, such as antidepressants, may make normal metabolizer resemble poor metabolizer leading to higher than expected plasma concentration of TCA with resultant toxicity; lower than usual doses of either drug may be required). Products include:
Adapin Capsules ... 1542
Sinequan ... 2028
Zonalon Cream ... 1042

Droperidol (Co-administration results in enhanced response to CNS depressants). Products include:
Inapsine Injection ... 462

Enflurane (Co-administration results in enhanced response to CNS depressants).
No products indexed under this heading.

Ephedrine Hydrochloride (Effects of concurrent use not specified; careful adjustment of dosage and close supervision are required). Products include:
Primatene Tablets ... 844
Quadrinal Tablets ... 1398

Ephedrine Sulfate (Effects of concurrent use not specified; careful adjustment of dosage and close supervision are required). Products include:
Marax Tablets & DF Syrup ... 2015

Ephedrine Tannate (Effects of concurrent use not specified; careful adjustment of dosage and close supervision are required). Products include:
Rynatuss ... 2782

Epinephrine (Effects of concurrent use not specified; careful adjustment of dosage and close supervision are required). Products include:
EPIFRIN ... 237
EpiPen ... 808
Marcaine with Epinephrine ... 2446
Primatene Mist ... 843
Sensorcaine with Epinephrine Injection ... 554
Sus-Phrine Injection ... 1017
Xylocaine with Epinephrine Injections ... 562

Epinephrine Bitartrate (Effects of concurrent use not specified; careful adjustment of dosage and close supervision are required). Products include:
Sensorcaine-MPF with Epinephrine Injection ... 554

Epinephrine Hydrochloride (Effects of concurrent use not specified; careful adjustment of dosage and close supervision are required). Products include:
Ana-Kit Anaphylaxis Emergency Treatment Kit ... 611

Estazolam (Co-administration results in enhanced response to CNS depressants). Products include:
ProSom Tablets ... 457

Ethchlorvynol (Concurrent use with large doses of ethchlorvynol has resulted in transient delirium). Products include:
Placidyl Capsules ... 456

Ethinamate (Co-administration results in enhanced response to CNS depressants).
No products indexed under this heading.

Fentanyl (Co-administration results in enhanced response to CNS depressants). Products include:
Duragesic Transdermal System ... 1336

Fentanyl Citrate (Co-administration results in enhanced response to CNS depressants). Products include:
Sublimaze Injection ... 463

Flecainide Acetate (Co-administration with cytochrome P4502D6 inhibitors, such as flecainide, may make normal metabolizer resemble poor metabolizer leading to higher than expected plasma concentration of TCA with resultant toxicity; lower than usual doses of either drug may be required). Products include:
Tambocor Tablets ... 1555

Fluoxetine Hydrochloride (Co-administration with cytochrome P4502D6 inhibitors, such as antidepressants, may make normal metabolizer resemble poor metabolizer leading to higher than expected plasma concentration of TCA with resultant toxicity; due to variation in the extent of inhibition of P4502D6 and long half-life of fluoxetine, sufficient time, at least 5 weeks, should elapse in switching to TCA). Products include:
Prozac Pulvules & Liquid, Oral Solution ... 935

Fluphenazine Decanoate (Co-administration with cytochrome P4502D6 inhibitors, such as phenothiazines, may make normal metabolizer resemble poor metabolizer leading to higher than expected plasma concentration of TCA with resultant toxicity; lower than usual doses of either drug may be required; co-administration results in enhanced response to CNS depressants). Products include:
Prolixin Decanoate ... 510

Fluphenazine Enanthate (Co-administration with cytochrome P4502D6 inhibitors, such as phenothiazines, may make normal metabolizer resemble poor metabolizer leading to higher than expected plasma concentration of TCA with resultant toxicity; lower than usual doses of either drug may be required; co-administration results in enhanced response to CNS depressants). Products include:
Prolixin Enanthate ... 510

Fluphenazine Hydrochloride (Co-administration with cytochrome P4502D6 inhibitors, such as phenothiazines, may make normal metabolizer resemble poor metabolizer leading to higher than expected plasma concentration of TCA with resultant toxicity; lower than usual doses of either drug may be required; co-administration results in enhanced response to CNS depressants). Products include:
Prolixin ... 510

Flurazepam Hydrochloride (Co-administration results in enhanced response to CNS depressants). Products include:
Dalmane Capsules ... 2329

Fluvoxamine Maleate (Co-administration with cytochrome P4502D6 inhibitors, such as antidepressants, may make normal metabolizer resemble poor metabolizer leading to higher than expected plasma concentration of TCA with resultant toxicity; due to variation in the extent of inhibition of P4502D6, sufficient time should elapse in switching from one class to the other). Products include:
LUVOX Tablets ... 2723

Furazolidone (Co-administration of tricyclic antidepressants and MAO inhibitors has resulted in hyperpyretic crises, severe convulsions, and death; concurrent and/or sequential use is contraindicated). Products include:
Furoxone ... 2221

Glutethimide (Co-administration results in enhanced response to CNS depressants).
No products indexed under this heading.

Glycopyrrolate (Co-administration may result in paralytic ileus; hyperpyrexia has been reported with concurrent use, particularly during hot weather). Products include:
Robinul Forte Tablets ... 2247
Robinul Injectable ... 2247
Robinul Tablets ... 2247

Guanadrel Sulfate (Amitriptyline may block the antihypertensive action). Products include:
Hylorel Tablets ... 1613

Guanethidine Monosulfate (Amitriptyline may block the antihypertensive action of guanethidine). Products include:
Esimil Tablets ... 840
Ismelin Tablets ... 845

Haloperidol (Co-administration results in enhanced response to CNS depressants). Products include:
Haldol Injection, Tablets and Concentrate ... 1585

Haloperidol Decanoate (Co-administration results in enhanced response to CNS depressants). Products include:
Haldol Decanoate ... 1587

Hydrocodone Bitartrate (Co-administration results in enhanced response to CNS depressants). Products include:
Codiclear DH Syrup ... 808
Duratuss HD Elixir ... 2750
Histussin D Liquid ... 670
Hycodan Tablets and Syrup ... 946
Hycomine Compound Tablets ... 948
Hycomine ... 947
Hycotuss Expectorant Syrup ... 950
Hydrocet Capsules ... 787
Lorcet 10/650 Tablets ... 1016
Lortab ... 2751
Tussend ... 1830
Tussend Expectorant ... 1831
Vicodin Tablets ... 1404
Vicodin ES Tablets ... 1405
Vicodin HP Tablets ... 1403
Vicodin Tuss Expectorant ... 1406
Zydone Capsules ... 967

Hydrocodone Polistirex (Co-administration results in enhanced response to CNS depressants). Products include:
Tussionex Pennkinetic Extended-Release Suspension ... 1624

Hydromorphone Hydrochloride (Co-administration results in enhanced response to CNS depressants). Products include:
Dilaudid Ampules ... 1382
Dilaudid Cough Syrup ... 1383
Dilaudid-HP Injection ... 1384
Dilaudid-HP Lyophilized Powder 250 mg ... 1384
Dilaudid ... 1382
Dilaudid Oral Liquid ... 1386
Dilaudid ... 1382
Dilaudid Tablets - 8 mg ... 1386

Hydroxyzine Hydrochloride (Co-administration results in enhanced response to CNS depressants). Products include:
Atarax Tablets & Syrup ... 1992
Marax Tablets & DF Syrup ... 2015
Vistaril Intramuscular Solution ... 2042

Hyoscyamine (Co-administration may result in paralytic ileus; hyperpyrexia has been reported with concurrent use, particularly during hot weather). Products include:
Cystospaz Tablets ... 2123
Urised Tablets ... 2123

Hyoscyamine Sulfate (Co-administration may result in paralytic ileus; hyperpyrexia has been reported with concurrent use, particularly during hot weather). Products include:
Arco-Lase Plus Tablets ... 513
Atrohist Plus Tablets ... 1605
Cystospaz-M Capsules ... 2123
Donnatal ... 2234
Donnatal Extentabs ... 2234
Donnatal Tablets ... 2234
Kutrase Capsules ... 2546
Levsin/Levsinex/Levbid ... 2549

Imipramine Hydrochloride (Co-administration with cytochrome P4502D6 inhibitors, such as antidepressants, may make normal metabolizer resemble poor metabolizer leading to higher than expected plasma concentration of TCA with resultant toxicity; lower than usual doses of either drug may be required). Products include:
Tofranil Ampuls ... 873
Tofranil Tablets ... 875

Imipramine Pamoate (Co-administration with cytochrome P4502D6 inhibitors, such as antidepressants, may make normal metabolizer resemble poor metabolizer leading to higher than expected plasma concentration of TCA with resultant toxicity; lower than usual doses of either drug may be required). Products include:
Tofranil-PM Capsules ... 876

Ipratropium Bromide (Co-administration may result in paralytic ileus; hyperpyrexia has been reported with concurrent use, particularly during hot weather). Products include:
Atrovent Inhalation Aerosol ... 674
Atrovent Inhalation Solution ... 675
Atrovent Nasal Spray 0.03% ... 676
Atrovent Nasal Spray 0.06% ... 678

Isocarboxazid (Co-administration of tricyclic antidepressants and MAO inhibitors has resulted in hyperpyretic crises, severe convulsions, and death; concurrent and/or sequential use is contraindicated).
No products indexed under this heading.

Isoflurane (Co-administration results in enhanced response to CNS depressants).
No products indexed under this heading.

Isoproterenol Hydrochloride (Effects of concurrent use not specified; careful adjustment of dosage and close supervision are required). Products include:
Isuprel Hydrochloride Solution ... 2443
Isuprel Injection ... 2441
Isuprel Mistometer ... 2442

Isoproterenol Sulfate (Effects of concurrent use not specified; careful adjustment of dosage and close supervision are required). Products include:
Norisodrine with Calcium Iodide Syrup ... 446

IMPORTANT NOTE: Always consult each drug listing in the patient's regimen for possible interactions.

Elavil **Interactions Index** 368

Ketamine Hydrochloride (Co-administration results in enhanced response to CNS depressants).
No products indexed under this heading.

Levomethadyl Acetate Hydrochloride (Co-administration results in enhanced response to CNS depressants). Products include:
Orlaam Oral Solution 2361

Levorphanol Tartrate (Co-administration results in enhanced response to CNS depressants). Products include:
Levo-Dromoran 2297

Levothyroxine Sodium (Effects of concurrent use not specified; close supervision is required). Products include:
Eltroxin Tablets 2214
Levothroid Tablets 1015
Levothyroxine Sodium, USP for Injection 546
Levoxyl Tablets 918
Synthroid 1410

Liothyronine Sodium (Effects of concurrent use not specified; close supervision is required). Products include:
Cytomel Tablets 2647
Triostat Injection 2708

Liotrix (Effects of concurrent use not specified; close supervision is required).
No products indexed under this heading.

Lorazepam (Co-administration results in enhanced response to CNS depressants). Products include:
Ativan Injection 2805
Ativan Tablets 2807

Loxapine Hydrochloride (Co-administration results in enhanced response to CNS depressants). Products include:
Loxitane 1426

Loxapine Succinate (Co-administration results in enhanced response to CNS depressants). Products include:
Loxitane Capsules 1426

Maprotiline Hydrochloride (Co-administration with cytochrome P4502D6 inhibitors, such as antidepressants, may make normal metabolizer resemble poor metabolizer leading to higher than expected plasma concentration of TCA with resultant toxicity; lower than usual doses of either drug may be required). Products include:
Ludiomil Tablets 861

Mepenzolate Bromide (Co-administration may result in paralytic ileus; hyperpyrexia has been reported with concurrent use, particularly during hot weather).
No products indexed under this heading.

Meperidine Hydrochloride (Co-administration results in enhanced response to CNS depressants). Products include:
Demerol 2438
Mepergan Injection 2859

Mephobarbital (Co-administration results in enhanced response to CNS depressants). Products include:
Mebaral Tablets 2452

Meprobamate (Co-administration results in enhanced response to CNS depressants). Products include:
Miltown Tablets 2780
PMB 200 and PMB 400 2890

Mesoridazine Besylate (Co-administration with cytochrome P4502D6 inhibitors, such as phenothiazines, may make normal metabolizer resemble poor metabolizer leading to higher than expected plasma concentration of TCA with resultant toxicity; lower than usual doses of either drug may be required; co-administration results in enhanced response to CNS depressants). Products include:
Serentil 689

Metaproterenol Sulfate (Effects of concurrent use not specified; careful adjustment of dosage and close supervision are required). Products include:
Alupent 672
Metaproterenol Sulfate Inhalation Solution, USP, Arm-a-Med 547

Metaraminol Bitartrate (Effects of concurrent use not specified; careful adjustment of dosage and close supervision are required). Products include:
Aramine Injection 1649

Methadone Hydrochloride (Co-administration results in enhanced response to CNS depressants). Products include:
Methadone Hydrochloride Oral Concentrate 2356
Methadone Hydrochloride Oral Solution & Tablets 2357

Methohexital Sodium (Co-administration results in enhanced response to CNS depressants).
No products indexed under this heading.

Methotrimeprazine (Co-administration with cytochrome P4502D6 inhibitors, such as phenothiazines, may make normal metabolizer resemble poor metabolizer leading to higher than expected plasma concentration of TCA with resultant toxicity; lower than usual doses of either drug may be required; co-administration results in enhanced response to CNS depressants). Products include:
Levoprome 1321

Methoxamine Hydrochloride (Effects of concurrent use not specified; careful adjustment of dosage and close supervision are required). Products include:
Vasoxyl Injection 1169

Methoxyflurane (Co-administration results in enhanced response to CNS depressants).
No products indexed under this heading.

Midazolam Hydrochloride (Co-administration results in enhanced response to CNS depressants). Products include:
Versed Injection 2324

Mirtazapine (Co-administration with cytochrome P4502D6 inhibitors, such as antidepressants, may make normal metabolizer resemble poor metabolizer leading to higher than expected plasma concentration of TCA with resultant toxicity; lower than usual doses of either drug may be required). Products include:
Remeron Tablets 1878

Molindone Hydrochloride (Co-administration results in enhanced response to CNS depressants). Products include:
Moban Tablets and Concentrate 1036

Morphine Sulfate (Co-administration results in enhanced response to CNS depressants). Products include:
Astramorph/PF Injection, USP (Preservative-Free) 526
Duramorph Injection 983
Infumorph 200 and Infumorph 500 Sterile Solutions 985
Kadian Capsules 2948
MS Contin Tablets 2149
MSIR 2152
Oramorph SR (Morphine Sulfate Sustained Release Tablets) 2359
RMS Suppositories CII 2766
Roxanol 2365

Nefazodone Hydrochloride (Co-administration with cytochrome P4502D6 inhibitors, such as antidepressants, may make normal metabolizer resemble poor metabolizer leading to higher than expected plasma concentration of TCA with resultant toxicity; lower than usual doses of either drug may be required). Products include:
Serzone Tablets 776

Norepinephrine Bitartrate (Effects of concurrent use not specified; careful adjustment of dosage and close supervision are required). Products include:
Levophed Bitartrate Injection 2445

Nortriptyline Hydrochloride (Co-administration with cytochrome P4502D6 inhibitors, such as antidepressants, may make normal metabolizer resemble poor metabolizer leading to higher than expected plasma concentration of TCA with resultant toxicity; lower than usual doses of either drug may be required). Products include:
Pamelor 2409

Opium Alkaloids (Co-administration results in enhanced response to CNS depressants).
No products indexed under this heading.

Oxazepam (Co-administration results in enhanced response to CNS depressants). Products include:
Serax Capsules 2916
Serax Tablets 2916

Oxybutynin Chloride (Co-administration may result in paralytic ileus; hyperpyrexia has been reported with concurrent use, particularly during hot weather). Products include:
Ditropan 1267

Oxycodone Hydrochloride (Co-administration results in enhanced response to CNS depressants). Products include:
OxyContin Tablets 2163
OxyIR Capsules 2167
Percocet Tablets 955
Percodan Tablets 955
Percodan-Demi Tablets 956
Roxicodone Tablets, Oral Solution & Intensol (Oxycodone) 2366
Tylox Capsules 1593

Paroxetine Hydrochloride (Co-administration with cytochrome P4502D6 inhibitors, such as antidepressants, may make normal metabolizer resemble poor metabolizer leading to higher than expected plasma concentration of TCA with resultant toxicity; due to variation in the extent of inhibition of P4502D6, sufficient time should elapse in switching from one class to the other). Products include:
Paxil Tablets 2681

Pentobarbital Sodium (Co-administration results in enhanced response to CNS depressants). Products include:
Nembutal Sodium Capsules 440
Nembutal Sodium Solution 442
Nembutal Sodium Suppositories 444

Perphenazine (Co-administration with cytochrome P4502D6 inhibitors, such as phenothiazines, may make normal metabolizer resemble poor metabolizer leading to higher than expected plasma concentration of TCA with resultant toxicity; lower than usual doses of either drug may be required; co-administration results in enhanced response to CNS depressants). Products include:
Etrafon 2495
Triavil Tablets 1800
Trilafon 2532

Phenelzine Sulfate (Co-administration of tricyclic antidepressants and MAO inhibitors has resulted in hyperpyretic crises, severe convulsions, and death; concurrent and/or sequential use is contraindicated). Products include:
Nardil 1977

Phenobarbital (Co-administration results in enhanced response to CNS depressants). Products include:
Arco-Lase Plus Tablets 513
Bellergal-S Tablets 2375
Donnatal 2234
Donnatal Extentabs 2234
Donnatal Tablets 2234
Phenobarbital Elixir and Tablets 1523
Quadrinal Tablets 1398

Phenylephrine Bitartrate (Effects of concurrent use not specified; careful adjustment of dosage and close supervision are required).
No products indexed under this heading.

Phenylephrine Hydrochloride (Effects of concurrent use not specified; careful adjustment of dosage and close supervision are required). Products include:
Atrohist Plus Tablets 1605
Cerose DM .... ■ 853
D.A. II Tablets 972
D.A. Chewable Tablets 970
Dura-Vent/DA Tablets 972
Extendryl 1003
4-Way Fast Acting Nasal Spray (regular & mentholated) .... ■ 644
Hemorid .... ■ 797
Hycomine Compound Tablets 948
Neo-Synephrine Hydrochloride 1% Carpuject 2455
Neo-Synephrine Hydrochloride 1% Injection 2455
Neo-Synephrine Hydrochloride (Ophthalmic) 2456
Neo-Synephrine .... ■ 624
Novahistine Elixir .... ■ 782
Phenergan VC 2886
Phenergan VC with Codeine 2888
Preparation H .... ■ 842
Tympagesic Ear Drops 2476
Vicks Sinex Nasal Spray and Ultra Fine Mist .... ■ 738

Phenylephrine Tannate (Effects of concurrent use not specified; careful adjustment of dosage and close supervision are required). Products include:
Atrohist Pediatric Suspension 1604
Atrohist Pediatric Suspension Dye-Free 1604
Rynatan 2781
Rynatuss 2782

Phenylpropanolamine Hydrochloride (Effects of concurrent use not specified; careful adjustment of dosage and close supervision are required). Products include:
Acutrim .... ■ 648
Atrohist Plus Tablets 1605
BC Cold Powder Multi-Symptom Formula (Cold-Sinus-Allergy) .... ■ 631
BC Cold Powder Non-Drowsy Formula (Cold-Sinus) .... ■ 631
Cheracol Plus Head Cold/Cough Formula .... ■ 741
Comtrex Multi-Symptom Cold Reliever Liqui-Gels .... ■ 638

(■ Described in PDR For Nonprescription Drugs) (◉ Described in PDR For Ophthalmology)

Comtrex Multi-Symptom Non-Drowsy Liqui-gels ... 640
Contac Continuous Action Nasal Decongestant/Antihistamine 12 Hour Capsules ... 773
Contac Maximum Strength Continuous Action Decongestant/Antihistamine 12 Hour Caplets ... 772
Contac Severe Cold and Flu Formula Caplets ... 773
Coricidin 'D' Decongestant Tablets ... 760
Dexatrim ... 795
Dexatrim Plus Vitamins Caplets ... 796
Dimetane-DC Cough Syrup ... 2232
Dimetapp Allergy Sinus Caplets ... 838
Dimetapp Cold & Allergy Chewable Tablets ... 838
Dimetapp Cold & Cough Liqui-Gels ... 839
Dimetapp DM Elixir ... 840
Dimetapp Elixir ... 840
Dimetapp Extentabs ... 841
Dimetapp Tablets/Liqui-Gels ... 841
Dura-Vent Tablets ... 971
Entex LA Tablets ... 972
Exgest LA Tablets ... 787
Hycomine ... 947
Nolamine Timed-Release Tablets ... 790
Ornade Spansule Capsules ... 2678
Propagest Tablets ... 791
Pyrroxate Caplets ... 742
Robitussin-CF ... 846
Sinulin Tablets ... 792
Tavist-D 12 Hour Relief Tablets ... 750
Teldrin 12 Hour Antihistamine/Nasal Decongestant Allergy Relief Capsules ... 786
Triaminic Expectorant ... 753
Triaminic Syrup ... 755
Triaminic Triaminicol Cold & Cough ... 756
Triaminic DM Syrup ... 756
Triaminicin Tablets ... 756
Vicks DayQuil Allergy Relief 12-Hour Extended Release Tablets ... 733
Vicks DayQuil Allergy Relief 4-Hour Tablets ... 733
Vicks DayQuil SINUS Pressure & CONGESTION Relief ... 734

Pirbuterol Acetate (Effects of concurrent use not specified; careful adjustment of dosage and close supervision are required). Products include:
Maxair Autohaler ... 1550
Maxair Inhaler ... 1552

Prazepam (Co-administration results in enhanced response to CNS depressants).
No products indexed under this heading.

Prochlorperazine (Co-administration with cytochrome P4502D6 inhibitors, such as phenothiazines, may make normal metabolizer resemble poor metabolizer leading to higher than expected plasma concentration of TCA with resultant toxicity; lower than usual doses of either drug may be required; co-administration results in enhanced response to CNS depressants). Products include:
Compazine ... 2644

Procyclidine Hydrochloride (Co-administration may result in paralytic ileus; hyperpyrexia has been reported with concurrent use, particularly during hot weather). Products include:
Kemadrin Tablets ... 1105

Promethazine Hydrochloride (Co-administration with cytochrome P4502D6 inhibitors, such as phenothiazines, may make normal metabolizer resemble poor metabolizer leading to higher than expected plasma concentration of TCA with resultant toxicity; lower than usual doses of either drug may be required; co-administration results in enhanced response to CNS depressants). Products include:
Mepergan Injection ... 2859
Phenergan with Codeine ... 2883
Phenergan with Dextromethorphan ... 2885
Phenergan Injection ... 2880
Phenergan Suppositories ... 2882
Phenergan Syrup ... 2881
Phenergan Tablets ... 2882
Phenergan VC ... 2886
Phenergan VC with Codeine ... 2888

Propafenone Hydrochloride (Co-administration with cytochrome P4502D6 inhibitors, such as propafenone, may make normal metabolizer resemble poor metabolizer leading to higher than expected plasma concentration of TCA with resultant toxicity; lower than usual doses of either drug may be required). Products include:
Rythmol Tablets–150mg, 225mg, 300mg ... 1399

Propantheline Bromide (Co-administration may result in paralytic ileus; hyperpyrexia has been reported with concurrent use, particularly during hot weather). Products include:
Pro-Banthine Tablets ... 2226

Propofol (Co-administration results in enhanced response to CNS depressants). Products include:
Diprivan Injectable Emulsion ... 2939

Propoxyphene Hydrochloride (Co-administration results in enhanced response to CNS depressants). Products include:
Darvon ... 1475
Wygesic Tablets ... 2930

Propoxyphene Napsylate (Co-administration results in enhanced response to CNS depressants). Products include:
Darvon-N/Darvocet-N ... 1473

Protriptyline Hydrochloride (Co-administration with cytochrome P4502D6 inhibitors, such as antidepressants, may make normal metabolizer resemble poor metabolizer leading to higher than expected plasma concentration of TCA with resultant toxicity; lower than usual doses of either drug may be required). Products include:
Vivactil Tablets ... 1820

Pseudoephedrine Hydrochloride (Effects of concurrent use not specified; careful adjustment of dosage and close supervision are required). Products include:
Actifed Allergy Daytime/Nighttime Caplets ... 808
Actifed Cold & Allergy Tablets ... 807
Actifed Cold & Sinus Caplets and Tablets ... 808
Actifed Sinus Daytime/Nighttime Tablets and Caplets ... 809
Advil Cold and Sinus Caplets and Tablets ... 837
Alka-Seltzer Plus Liqui-Gels ... 612
Alka-Seltzer Plus Flu & Body Aches Liqui-Gels Non-Drowsy Formula ... 613
Alka-Seltzer Plus Night-Time Cold Medicine Liqui-Gels ... 612
Allerest Maximum Strength ... 649
Allerest No Drowsiness ... 649
Allerest Sinus Pain Formula ... 649
Atrohist Pediatric Capsules ... 1603
Benadryl Allergy/Cold Tablets ... 811
Benadryl Allergy Decongestant Liquid Medication ... 812
Benadryl Allergy Decongestant Tablets ... 812
Benadryl Allergy Sinus Headache Caplets ... 813
Benylin Multisymptom ... 816
Bromfed Capsules (Extended-Release) ... 1832
Bromfed Syrup ... 712
Bromfed Tablets ... 1832
Bromfed-DM Cough Syrup ... 1832
Bromfed-PD Capsules (Extended-Release) ... 1832
Children's TYLENOL Cold Multi-Symptom Chewable Tablets and Liquid ... 1559
Children's TYLENOL Cold Plus Cough Multi Symptom Chewable Tablets and Liquid ... 1560
Children's TYLENOL Flu Suspension Liquid ... 1560
Children's Vicks DayQuil Allergy Relief ... 730
Children's Vicks NyQuil Cold/Cough Relief ... 731
Allergy-Sinus Comtrex Multi-Symptom Allergy-Sinus Formula Tablets and Caplets ... 639
Comtrex Multi-Symptom ... 638
Comtrex Multi-Symptom Non-Drowsy Caplets ... 640
Congess ... 1003
Contac Day Allergy/Sinus Caplets ... 771
Contac Day & Night ... 772
Contac Night Allergy/Sinus Caplets ... 771
Contac Severe Cold & Flu Non-Drowsy ... 774
Deconsal II Tablets ... 1605
Dimetane-DX Cough Syrup ... 2233
Dimetapp Cold & Fever Suspension ... 839
Dimetapp Decongestant Pediatric Drops ... 840
Dorcol Children's Cough Syrup ... 748
Drixoral Cough + Congestion Liquid Caps ... 763
Dura-Tap/PD Capsules ... 970
Duratuss Tablets ... 2750
Duratuss HD Elixir ... 2750
Efidac/24 ... 655
Entex PSE Tablets ... 973
Fedahist Gyrocaps ... 2545
Guaifed ... 1833
Guaifed Syrup ... 712
Guaimax-D Tablets ... 809
Histussin D Liquid ... 670
Infants' TYLENOL Cold Decongestant & Fever-Reducer Drops ... 1561
Kronofed-A ... 994
Novahistine DMX ... 782
Nucofed ... 2225
PediaCare Cough-Cold Chewable Tablets and Liquid ... 1569
PediaCare Infants' Decongestant Drops ... 1569
PediaCare Infants' Drops Decongestant Plus Cough ... 1569
PediaCare NightRest Cough-Cold Liquid ... 1569
Pediatric Vicks 44d Cough & Head Congestion Relief ... 736
Pediatric Vicks 44m Cough & Cold Relief ... 737
Robitussin Cold & Cough Liqui-Gels ... 844
Robitussin Cold, Cough & Flu Liqui-Gels ... 844
Robitussin Maximum Strength Cough & Cold ... 847
Robitussin Night-Time Cold Formula ... 847
Robitussin Pediatric Cough & Cold Formula ... 848
Robitussin Pediatric Drops ... 849
Robitussin Severe Congestion Liqui-Gels ... 845
Robitussin-DAC Syrup ... 2249
Robitussin-PE ... 846
Rondec Oral Drops ... 974
Rondec Syrup ... 974
Rondec Tablet ... 974
Rondec Chewable Tablets ... 974
Rondec-TR Tablet ... 974
Ryna ... 804
Seldane-D Extended-Release Tablets ... 1286
Semprex-D Capsules ... 1620
Sinarest ... 663
Sine-Aid Maximum Strength Sinus Headache Gelcaps, Caplets and Tablets ... 1570
Sine-Off No Drowsiness Formula Caplets ... 784
Sine-Off Sinus Medicine ... 784
Singlet Tablets ... 785
Sinutab Non-Drying Liquid Caps ... 823
Sinutab Sinus Allergy Medication, Maximum Strength Tablets and Caplets ... 823
Sinutab Sinus Medication, Maximum Strength Without Drowsiness Formula, Tablets & Caplets ... 824
Sudafed Children's Cold & Cough Liquid Medication ... 825
Sudafed Children's Nasal Decongestant Liquid Medication ... 826
Sudafed Cold & Allergy Tablets ... 826
Sudafed Cold and Cough Liquid Caps ... 826
Sudafed Nasal Decongestant Tablets, 30 mg ... 825
Sudafed Nasal Decongestant Tablets, 60 mg ... 825
Sudafed Non-Drying Sinus Liquid Caps ... 827
Sudafed Pediatric Nasal Decongestant Liquid Oral Drops ... 827
Sudafed Severe Cold Formula Caplets ... 828
Sudafed Severe Cold Formula Tablets ... 828
Sudafed Sinus Caplets ... 829
Sudafed Sinus Tablets ... 829
Sudafed 12 Hour Caplets ... 824
Syn-Rx Tablets ... 1622
Syn-Rx DM Tablets ... 1623
TheraFlu Flu and Cold Medicine ... 750
Theraflu Maximum Strength Flu and Cold Medicine For Sore Throat ... 751
TheraFlu Flu, Cold and Cough Medicine ... 750
TheraFlu Maximum Strength Nighttime Flu, Cold & Cough Medicine ... 751
TheraFlu Maximum Strength Non-Drowsy Formula Flu, Cold & Cough Medicine ... 751
TheraFlu Maximum Strength, Non-Drowsy Formula Flu, Cold and Cough Caplets ... 752
Theraflu Maximum Strength Sinus Non-Drowsy Formula Caplets ... 752
Triaminic AM Cough and Decongestant Formula ... 753
Triaminic AM Decongestant Formula ... 753
Triaminic Infant Oral Decongestant Drops ... 754
Triaminic Night Time ... 754
Triaminic Sore Throat Formula ... 755
Tussend ... 1830
Tussend Expectorant ... 1831
TYLENOL Allergy Sinus, Maximum Strength Caplets and Gelcaps ... 1571
TYLENOL Allergy Sinus NightTime, Maximum Strength Caplets ... 1571
TYLENOL Cold Medication, Multi-Symptom Formula Tablets and Caplets ... 1572
TYLENOL Cold Medication, Multi-Symptom Hot Liquid Packets ... 1572
TYLENOL Cold Medication, No Drowsiness Formula Caplets and Gelcaps ... 1572
TYLENOL Cold Severe Congestion Caplets ... 1573
TYLENOL Cough Medication with Decongestant, Multi Symptom ... 1574
TYLENOL Flu No Drowsiness Formula, Maximum Strength Gelcaps ... 1575
TYLENOL Flu NightTime, Maximum Strength Gelcaps ... 1575
TYLENOL Flu NightTime, Maximum Strength Hot Medication Packets ... 1575
TYLENOL Sinus, Maximum Strength Geltabs, Gelcaps, Caplets and Tablets ... 1576
Vicks 44 LiquiCaps Cough, Cold & Flu Relief ... 728
Vicks 44 LiquiCaps Non-Drowsy Cough & Cold Relief ... 729
Vicks 44D Cough & Head Congestion Relief ... 728
Vicks 44M Cough, Cold & Flu Relief ... 729
Vicks DayQuil LiquiCaps/Liquid Multi-Symptom Cold/Flu Relief ... 734
Vicks DayQuil SINUS Pressure & PAIN Relief with IBUPROFEN ... 735
Vicks Nyquil Hot Therapy ... 735
Vicks NyQuil LiquiCaps/Liquid Multi-Symptom Cold/Flu Relief, Original and Cherry Flavors ... 736

IMPORTANT NOTE: Always consult each drug listing in the patient's regimen for possible interactions.

Elavil — Interactions Index

Pseudoephedrine Sulfate (Effects of concurrent use not specified; careful adjustment of dosage and close supervision are required). Products include:
- Chlor-Trimeton Allergy Decongestant Tablets 759
- Claritin-D Tablets 2487
- Drixoral Cold and Allergy Sustained-Action Tablets 763
- Drixoral Cold and Flu Extended-Release Tablets 764
- Drixoral Non-Drowsy Formula Extended-Release Tablets 764
- Drixoral Allergy/Sinus Extended Release Tablets 765
- Trinalin Repetabs Tablets 1373

Quazepam (Co-administration results in enhanced response to CNS depressants). Products include:
- Doral Tablets 2773

Quinidine Gluconate (Co-administration with cytochrome P4502D6 inhibitors, such as quinidine, may make normal metabolizer resemble poor metabolizer leading to higher than expected plasma concentration of TCA with resultant toxicity; lower than usual doses of either drug may be required). Products include:
- Quinaglute Dura-Tabs Tablets 644

Quinidine Polygalacturonate (Co-administration with cytochrome P4502D6 inhibitors, such as quinidine, may make normal metabolizer resemble poor metabolizer leading to higher than expected plasma concentration of TCA with resultant toxicity; lower than usual doses of either drug may be required). Products include:
- Cardioquin Tablets 2146

Quinidine Sulfate (Co-administration with cytochrome P4502D6 inhibitors, such as quinidine, may make normal metabolizer resemble poor metabolizer leading to higher than expected plasma concentration of TCA with resultant toxicity; lower than usual doses of either drug may be required). Products include:
- Quinidex Extentabs 2240

Risperidone (Co-administration results in enhanced response to CNS depressants). Products include:
- Risperdal Tablets 1348

Salmeterol Xinafoate (Effects of concurrent use not specified; careful adjustment of dosage and close supervision are required). Products include:
- Serevent Inhalation Aerosol 1149

Scopolamine (Co-administration may result in paralytic ileus; hyperpyrexia has been reported with concurrent use, particularly during hot weather). Products include:
- Transderm Scōp Transdermal Therapeutic System 890

Scopolamine Hydrobromide (Co-administration may result in paralytic ileus; hyperpyrexia has been reported with concurrent use, particularly during hot weather). Products include:
- Atrohist Plus Tablets 1605
- Donnatal 2234
- Donnatal Extentabs 2234
- Donnatal Tablets 2234

Secobarbital Sodium (Co-administration results in enhanced response to CNS depressants). Products include:
- Seconal Sodium Pulvules 1529

Selegiline Hydrochloride (Co-administration of tricyclic antidepressants and MAO inhibitors has resulted in hyperpyretic crises, severe convulsions, and death; concurrent and/or sequential use is contraindicated). Products include:
- Eldepryl Capsules 2729

Sertraline Hydrochloride (Co-administration with cytochrome P4502D6 inhibitors, such as antidepressants, may make normal metabolizer resemble poor metabolizer leading to higher than expected plasma concentration of TCA with resultant toxicity; due to variation in the extent of inhibition of P4502D6, sufficient time should elapse in switching from one class to the other). Products include:
- Zoloft Tablets 2051

Sevoflurane (Co-administration results in enhanced response to CNS depressants).
- No products indexed under this heading.

Sufentanil Citrate (Co-administration results in enhanced response to CNS depressants). Products include:
- Sufenta Injection 1355

Temazepam (Co-administration results in enhanced response to CNS depressants). Products include:
- Restoril Capsules 2413

Terbutaline Sulfate (Effects of concurrent use not specified; careful adjustment of dosage and close supervision are required). Products include:
- Brethaire Inhaler 830
- Brethine Ampuls 832
- Brethine Tablets 831
- Bricanyl Subcutaneous Injection 1247
- Bricanyl Tablets 1248

Thiamylal Sodium (Co-administration results in enhanced response to CNS depressants).
- No products indexed under this heading.

Thioridazine Hydrochloride (Co-administration with cytochrome P4502D6 inhibitors, such as phenothiazines, may make normal metabolizer resemble poor metabolizer leading to higher than expected plasma concentration of TCA with resultant toxicity; lower than usual doses of either drug may be required; co-administration results in enhanced response to CNS depressants). Products include:
- Mellaril 2398

Thiothixene (Co-administration results in enhanced response to CNS depressants). Products include:
- Navane Capsules and Concentrate 2018
- Navane Intramuscular 2019

Thyroglobulin (Effects of concurrent use not specified; close supervision is required).
- No products indexed under this heading.

Thyroid (Effects of concurrent use not specified; close supervision is required).
- No products indexed under this heading.

Thyroxine (Effects of concurrent use not specified; close supervision is required).
- No products indexed under this heading.

Thyroxine Sodium (Effects of concurrent use not specified; close supervision is required).
- No products indexed under this heading.

Tranylcypromine Sulfate (Co-administration of tricyclic antidepressants and MAO inhibitors has resulted in hyperpyretic crises, severe convulsions, and death; concurrent and/or sequential use is contraindicated). Products include:
- Parnate Tablets 2679

Trazodone Hydrochloride (Co-administration with cytochrome P4502D6 inhibitors, such as antidepressants, may make normal metabolizer resemble poor metabolizer leading to higher than expected plasma concentration of TCA with resultant toxicity; lower than usual doses of either drug may be required). Products include:
- Desyrel and Desyrel Dividose 504

Triazolam (Co-administration results in enhanced response to CNS depressants). Products include:
- Halcion Tablets 2093

Tridihexethyl Chloride (Co-administration may result in paralytic ileus; hyperpyrexia has been reported with concurrent use, particularly during hot weather).
- No products indexed under this heading.

Trifluoperazine Hydrochloride (Co-administration with cytochrome P4502D6 inhibitors, such as phenothiazines, may make normal metabolizer resemble poor metabolizer leading to higher than expected plasma concentration of TCA with resultant toxicity; lower than usual doses of either drug may be required; co-administration results in enhanced response to CNS depressants). Products include:
- Stelazine 2692

Trihexyphenidyl Hydrochloride (Co-administration may result in paralytic ileus; hyperpyrexia has been reported with concurrent use, particularly during hot weather). Products include:
- Artane 1418

Trimipramine Maleate (Co-administration with cytochrome P4502D6 inhibitors, such as antidepressants, may make normal metabolizer resemble poor metabolizer leading to higher than expected plasma concentration of TCA with resultant toxicity; lower than usual doses of either drug may be required). Products include:
- Surmontil Tablets 2917

Venlafaxine Hydrochloride (Co-administration with cytochrome P4502D6 inhibitors, such as antidepressants, may make normal metabolizer resemble poor metabolizer leading to higher than expected plasma concentration of TCA with resultant toxicity; due to variation in the extent of inhibition of P4502D6, sufficient time should elapse in switching from one class to the other). Products include:
- Effexor 2825

Zolpidem Tartrate (Co-administration results in enhanced response to CNS depressants). Products include:
- Ambien Tablets 2559

Food Interactions

Alcohol (Co-administration results in enhanced response to alcohol).

ELAVIL TABLETS
(Amitriptyline Hydrochloride) 2945
See **Elavil Injection**

ELDEPRYL CAPSULES
(Selegiline Hydrochloride) 2729
May interact with narcotic analgesics, selective serotonin reuptake inhibitors, tricyclic antidepressants, and certain other agents. Compounds in these categories include:

Alfentanil Hydrochloride (Contraindication warning for meperidine is extended to other opioids). Products include:
- Alfenta Injection 1334

Amitriptyline Hydrochloride (Co-administration has resulted in severe CNS toxicity associated with hyperpyrexia and fatality; concurrent use in some patients may result in hypertension, syncope, asystole, diaphoresis seizures, changes in behavioral and mental status, and muscular rigidity; concurrent and/or sequential use is not recommended). Products include:
- Elavil 2945
- Etrafon 2495
- Limbitrol 2333
- Triavil Tablets 1800

Amoxapine (Co-administration may result in hypertension, syncope, asystole, diaphoresis seizures, changes in behavioral and mental status, and muscular rigidity; concurrent and/or sequential use is not recommended). Products include:
- Asendin Tablets 1419

Buprenorphine (Contraindication warning for meperidine is extended to other opioids). Products include:
- Buprenex Injectable 2170

Clomipramine Hydrochloride (Co-administration may result in hypertension, syncope, asystole, diaphoresis seizures, changes in behavioral and mental status, and muscular rigidity; concurrent and/or sequential use is not recommended). Products include:
- Anafranil Capsules 819

Codeine Phosphate (Contraindication warning for meperidine is extended to other opioids). Products include:
- Brontex 2130
- Dimetane-DC Cough Syrup 2232
- Fioricet with Codeine Capsules 2387
- Fiorinal with Codeine Capsules 2390
- Nucofed 2225
- Phenergan with Codeine 2883
- Phenergan VC with Codeine 2888
- Robitussin A-C Syrup 2248
- Robitussin-DAC Syrup 2249
- Ryna 804
- Soma Compound w/Codeine Tablets 2784
- Tylenol with Codeine 1592

Desipramine Hydrochloride (Co-administration may result in hypertension, syncope, asystole, diaphoresis seizures, changes in behavioral and mental status, and muscular rigidity; concurrent and/or sequential use is not recommended). Products include:
- Norpramin Tablets 1273

Dezocine (Contraindication warning for meperidine is extended to other opioids). Products include:
- Dalgan Injection 529

Doxepin Hydrochloride (Co-administration may result in hypertension, syncope, asystole, diaphoresis seizures, changes in behavioral and mental status, and muscular rigidity; concurrent and/or sequential use is not recommended). Products include:
- Adapin Capsules 1542
- Sinequan 2028
- Zonalon Cream 1042

(▣ Described in PDR For Nonprescription Drugs)   (⊙ Described in PDR For Ophthalmology)

Ephedrine Hydrochloride (Co-administration has resulted in one case of hypertensive crisis). Products include:
- Primatene Tablets 844
- Quadrinal Tablets 1398

Ephedrine Sulfate (Co-administration has resulted in one case of hypertensive crisis). Products include:
- Marax Tablets & DF Syrup 2015

Ephedrine Tannate (Co-administration has resulted in one case of hypertensive crisis). Products include:
- Rynatuss 2782

Fentanyl (Contraindication warning for meperidine is extended to other opioids). Products include:
- Duragesic Transdermal System ... 1336

Fentanyl Citrate (Contraindication warning for meperidine is extended to other opioids). Products include:
- Sublimaze Injection 463

Fluoxetine Hydrochloride (Co-administration has resulted in serious, sometimes fatal, reactions including hyperthermia, rigidity, myoclonus, autonomic instability, extreme agitation progressing to delirium and coma; concurrent and/or sequential use is not recommended; because of long half-life of fluoxetine, at least 5 weeks or longer should elapse between discontinuation of fluoxetine and initation of Eldepryl). Products include:
- Prozac Pulvules & Liquid, Oral Solution 935

Fluvoxamine Maleate (Potential for serious, sometimes fatal, reactions including hyperthermia, rigidity, myoclonus, autonomic instability, extreme agitation progressing to delirium and coma; concurrent and/or sequential use is not recommended). Products include:
- LUVOX Tablets 2723

Hydrocodone Bitartrate (Contraindication warning for meperidine is extended to other opioids). Products include:
- Codiclear DH Syrup 808
- Duratuss HD Elixir 2750
- Histussin D Liquid 670
- Hycodan Tablets and Syrup 946
- Hycomine Compound Tablets 948
- Hycomine 947
- Hycotuss Expectorant Syrup 950
- Hydrocet Capsules 787
- Lorcet 10/650 Tablets 1016
- Lortab 2751
- Tussend 1830
- Tussend Expectorant 1831
- Vicodin Tablets 1404
- Vicodin ES Tablets 1405
- Vicodin HP Tablets 1403
- Vicodin Tuss Expectorant 1406
- Zydone Capsules 967

Hydrocodone Polistirex (Contraindication warning for meperidine is extended to other opioids). Products include:
- Tussionex Pennkinetic Extended-Release Suspension 1624

Hydromorphone Hydrochloride (Contraindication warning for meperidine is extended to other opioids). Products include:
- Dilaudid Ampules 1382
- Dilaudid Cough Syrup 1383
- Dilaudid-HP Injection 1384
- Dilaudid-HP Lyophilized Powder 250 mg 1384
- Dilaudid 1382
- Dilaudid Oral Liquid 1386
- Dilaudid 1382
- Dilaudid Tablets - 8 mg 1386

Imipramine Hydrochloride (Co-administration may result in hypertension, syncope, asystole, diaphoresis seizures, changes in behavioral and mental status, and muscular rigidity; concurrent and/or sequential use is not recommended). Products include:
- Tofranil Ampuls 873
- Tofranil Tablets 875

Imipramine Pamoate (Co-administration may result in hypertension, syncope, asystole, diaphoresis seizures, changes in behavioral and mental status, and muscular rigidity; concurrent and/or sequential use is not recommended). Products include:
- Tofranil-PM Capsules 876

Levodopa (Co-administration in some patients may exacerbate levodopa-associated side effects). Products include:
- Atamet Tablets 567
- Larodopa Tablets 2296
- Sinemet Tablets 959
- Sinemet CR Tablets 961

Levorphanol Tartrate (Contraindication warning for meperidine is extended to other opioids). Products include:
- Levo-Dromoran 2297

Maprotiline Hydrochloride (Co-administration may result in hypertension, syncope, asystole, diaphoresis seizures, changes in behavioral and mental status, and muscular rigidity; concurrent and/or sequential use is not recommended). Products include:
- Ludiomil Tablets 861

Meperidine Hydrochloride (Co-administration has resulted in stupor, muscular rigidity, severe agitation, hallucination, and hyperpyrexia; concurrent use is contraindicated). Products include:
- Demerol 2438
- Mepergan Injection 2859

Methadone Hydrochloride (Contraindication warning for meperidine is extended to other opioids). Products include:
- Methadone Hydrochloride Oral Concentrate 2356
- Methadone Hydrochloride Oral Solution & Tablets 2357

Morphine Sulfate (Contraindication warning for meperidine is extended to other opioids). Products include:
- Astramorph/PF Injection, USP (Preservative-Free) 526
- Duramorph Injection 983
- Infumorph 200 and Infumorph 500 Sterile Solutions 985
- Kadian Capsules 2948
- MS Contin Tablets 2149
- MSIR 2152
- Oramorph SR (Morphine Sulfate Sustained Release Tablets) 2359
- RMS Suppositories CII 2766
- Roxanol 2365

Nortriptyline Hydrochloride (Co-administration may result in hypertension, syncope, asystole, diaphoresis seizures, changes in behavioral and mental status, and muscular rigidity; concurrent and/or sequential use is not recommended). Products include:
- Pamelor 2409

Opium Alkaloids (Contraindication warning for meperidine is extended to other opioids).
No products indexed under this heading.

Oxycodone Hydrochloride (Contraindication warning for meperidine is extended to other opioids). Products include:
- OxyContin Tablets 2163
- OxyIR Capsules 2167
- Percocet Tablets 955
- Percodan Tablets 955
- Percodan-Demi Tablets 956
- Roxicodone Tablets, Oral Solution & Intensol (Oxycodone) 2366
- Tylox Capsules 1593

Paroxetine Hydrochloride (Potential for serious, sometimes fatal, reactions including hyperthermia, rigidity, myoclonus, autonomic instability, extreme agitation progressing to delirium and coma; concurrent and/or sequential use is not recommended). Products include:
- Paxil Tablets 2681

Propoxyphene Hydrochloride (Contraindication warning for meperidine is extended to other opioids). Products include:
- Darvon 1475
- Wygesic Tablets 2930

Propoxyphene Napsylate (Contraindication warning for meperidine is extended to other opioids). Products include:
- Darvon-N/Darvocet-N 1473

Protriptyline Hydrochloride (Co-administration has resulted in tremors, agitation, and restlessness followed by unresponsiveness and fatality; concurrent use in some patients may result in hypertension, syncope, asystole, diaphoresis seizures, changes in behavioral and mental status, and muscular rigidity; concurrent and/or sequential use is not recommended). Products include:
- Vivactil Tablets 1820

Sertraline Hydrochloride (Potential for serious, sometimes fatal, reactions including hyperthermia, rigidity, myoclonus, autonomic instability, extreme agitation progressing to delirium and coma; concurrent and/or sequential use is not recommended). Products include:
- Zoloft Tablets 2051

Sufentanil Citrate (Contraindication warning for meperidine is extended to other opioids). Products include:
- Sufenta Injection 1355

Trimipramine Maleate (Co-administration may result in hypertension, syncope, asystole, diaphoresis seizures, changes in behavioral and mental status, and muscular rigidity; concurrent and/or sequential use is not recommended). Products include:
- Surmontil Capsules 2917

Venlafaxine Hydrochloride (Potential for serious, sometimes fatal, reactions including hyperthermia, rigidity, myoclonus, autonomic instability, extreme agitation progressing to delirium and coma; concurrent and/or sequential use is not recommended). Products include:
- Effexor 2825

Food Interactions
Food, unspecified (The bioavailability of selegiline is increased 3 to 4 fold when it is taken with food).

ELDERTONIC
(Vitamins with Minerals) 1826
None cited in PDR database.

ELDOPAQUE FORTE 4% CREAM
(Hydroquinone) 1299
None cited in PDR database.

ELDOQUIN FORTE 4% CREAM
(Hydroquinone) 1299
None cited in PDR database.

ELIMITE (PERMETHRIN) 5% CREAM
(Permethrin) 475
None cited in PDR database.

ELOCON CREAM 0.1%
(Mometasone Furoate) 2492
None cited in PDR database.

ELOCON LOTION 0.1%
(Mometasone Furoate) 2493
None cited in PDR database.

ELOCON OINTMENT 0.1%
(Mometasone Furoate) 2494
None cited in PDR database.

ELSPAR
(Asparaginase) 1700
May interact with:

Methotrexate Sodium (Diminished or abolished effect of methotrexate on malignant cells). Products include:
- Methotrexate Sodium Tablets, Injection, for Injection and LPF Injection 1322

Prednisone (Increased toxicity).
No products indexed under this heading.

Vincristine Sulfate (Increased toxicity). Products include:
- Oncovin Solution Vials & Hyporets 1521

ELTROXIN TABLETS
(Levothyroxine Sodium) 2214
May interact with oral anticoagulants, insulin, oral hypoglycemic agents, estrogens, and certain other agents. Compounds in these categories include:

Acarbose (Requirements of oral antidiabetic agents may be reduced in hypothyroid patients with diabetes and may be subsequently increased with initiation of thyroid hormone therapy). Products include:
- Precose 604

Chlorotrianisene (Estrogens or estrogen-containing oral contraceptives tend to increase serum thyroxine binding; free levothyroxine may be decreased in patients with non-functioning thyroid gland resulting in increased thyroid requirements).
No products indexed under this heading.

Chlorpropamide (Requirements of oral antidiabetic agents may be reduced in hypothyroid patients with diabetes and may be subsequently increased with initiation of thyroid hormone therapy). Products include:
- Diabinese Tablets 2002

Cholestyramine (Binds and decreases absorption of levothyroxine sodium from gastrointestinal tract; four to five hours should elapse between administration of resin and thyroid hormones). Products include:
- Questran 774

IMPORTANT NOTE: Always consult each drug listing in the patient's regimen for possible interactions.

Colestipol Hydrochloride (Binds and decreases absorption of levothyroxine sodium from gastrointestinal tract; four to five hours should elapse between administration of resin and thyroid hormones). Products include:
- Colestid 2073

Dicumarol (Thyroid hormones appear to increase catabolism of vitamin K-dependent clotting factors; co-administration results in impairment of compensatory increases in clotting factor synthesis).
- No products indexed under this heading.

Dienestrol (Estrogens or estrogen-containing oral contraceptives tend to increase serum thyroxine binding; free levothyroxine may be decreased in patients with nonfunctioning thyroid gland resulting in increased thyroid requirements). Products include:
- Ortho Dienestrol Cream 1922

Diethylstilbestrol (Estrogens or estrogen-containing oral contraceptives tend to increase serum thyroxine binding; free levothyroxine may be decreased in patients with nonfunctioning thyroid gland resulting in increased thyroid requirements). Products include:
- Diethylstilbestrol Tablets 1477

Estradiol (Estrogens or estrogen-containing oral contraceptives tend to increase serum thyroxine binding; free levothyroxine may be decreased in patients with nonfunctioning thyroid gland resulting in increased thyroid requirements). Products include:
- Climara Transdermal System 640
- Estrace Cream and Tablets 751
- Estraderm Transdermal System 842
- Estring Vaginal Ring 2086
- Vivelle Transdermal System 880

Estrogens, Conjugated (Estrogens or estrogen-containing oral contraceptives tend to increase serum thyroxine binding; free levothyroxine may be decreased in patients with nonfunctioning thyroid gland resulting in increased thyroid requirements). Products include:
- PMB 200 and PMB 400 2890
- Premarin Intravenous 2893
- Premarin Tablets 2896
- Premarin Vaginal Cream 2898
- Premphase 2900
- Prempro 2905

Estrogens, Esterified (Estrogens or estrogen-containing oral contraceptives tend to increase serum thyroxine binding; free levothyroxine may be decreased in patients with nonfunctioning thyroid gland resulting in increased thyroid requirements). Products include:
- ESTRATAB Tablets (0.3, 0.625, 1.25, 2.5 mg) 2715
- Estratest 2718
- Menest Tablets 2671

Estropipate (Estrogens or estrogen-containing oral contraceptives tend to increase serum thyroxine binding; free levothyroxine may be decreased in patients with nonfunctioning thyroid gland resulting in increased thyroid requirements). Products include:
- Ogen Tablets 2103
- Ogen Vaginal Cream 2106
- Ortho-Est 1925

Ethinyl Estradiol (Estrogens or estrogen-containing oral contraceptives tend to increase serum thyroxine binding; free levothyroxine may be decreased in patients with nonfunctioning thyroid gland resulting in increased thyroid requirements). Products include:
- Brevicon 2563
- Demulen 2580
- Desogen Tablets 1867
- Levlen/Tri-Levlen 646
- Lo/Ovral Tablets 2852
- Lo/Ovral-28 Tablets 2857
- Modicon 1928
- Nordette-21 Tablets 2863
- Nordette-28 Tablets 2866
- Norinyl 2563
- Ortho-Cept 1907
- Ortho-Cyclen/Ortho-Tri-Cyclen 1914
- Ortho-Novum 1928
- Ortho-Cyclen/Ortho Tri-Cyclen 1914
- Ovcon 765
- Ovral Tablets 2877
- Ovral-28 Tablets 2878
- Levlen/Tri-Levlen 646
- Tri-Norinyl 2607
- Triphasil-21 Tablets 2919
- Triphasil-28 Tablets 2924

Glimepiride (Requirements of oral antidiabetic agents may be reduced in hypothyroid patients with diabetes and may be subsequently increased with initiation of thyroid hormone therapy). Products include:
- Amaryl Tablets 1241

Glipizide (Requirements of oral antidiabetic agents may be reduced in hypothyroid patients with diabetes and may be subsequently increased with initiation of thyroid hormone therapy). Products include:
- Glucotrol Tablets 2011
- Glucotrol XL Extended Release Tablets 2012

Glyburide (Requirements of oral antidiabetic agents may be reduced in hypothyroid patients with diabetes and may be subsequently increased with initiation of thyroid hormone therapy). Products include:
- DiaBeta Tablets 1265
- Glynase PresTab Tablets 2091
- Micronase Tablets 2099

Insulin, Human (Requirements of insulin may be reduced in hypothyroid patients with diabetes and may be subsequently increased with initiation of thyroid hormone therapy).
- No products indexed under this heading.

Insulin, Human Isophane Suspension (Requirements of insulin may be reduced in hypothyroid patients with diabetes and may be subsequently increased with initiation of thyroid hormone therapy). Products include:
- Novolin N Human Insulin 10 ml Vials 1846

Insulin, Human NPH (Requirements of insulin may be reduced in hypothyroid patients with diabetes and may be subsequently increased with initiation of thyroid hormone therapy). Products include:
- Humulin N, 100 Units 1495
- Novolin N PenFill 1.5 ml Cartridges Durable Insulin Delivery System 1849
- Novolin N Prefilled Syringe Disposable Insulin Delivery System 1850

Insulin, Human Regular (Requirements of insulin may be reduced in hypothyroid patients with diabetes and may be subsequently increased with initiation of thyroid hormone therapy). Products include:
- Humulin R, 100 Units 1497
- Novolin R Human Insulin 10 ml Vials 1846
- Novolin R PenFill 1.5 ml Cartridges Durable Insulin Delivery System 1849
- Novolin R Prefilled Syringe Disposable Insulin Delivery System 1850
- Velosulin BR Human Insulin 10 ml Vials 1847

Insulin, Human, Zinc Suspension (Requirements of insulin may be reduced in hypothyroid patients with diabetes and may be subsequently increased with initiation of thyroid hormone therapy). Products include:
- Humulin L, 100 Units 1494
- Humulin U, 100 Units 1498
- Novolin L Human Insulin 10 ml Vials 1846

Insulin Lispro, Human (Requirements of insulin may be reduced in hypothyroid patients with diabetes and may be subsequently increased with initiation of thyroid hormone therapy). Products include:
- Humalog Injection 1488

Insulin, NPH (Requirements of insulin may be reduced in hypothyroid patients with diabetes and may be subsequently increased with initiation of thyroid hormone therapy). Products include:
- NPH, 100 Units 1502
- Pork NPH, 100 Units 1506
- Purified Pork NPH Isophane Insulin 1852

Insulin, Regular (Requirements of insulin may be reduced in hypothyroid patients with diabetes and may be subsequently increased with initiation of thyroid hormone therapy). Products include:
- Regular, 100 Units 1503
- Pork Regular, 100 Units 1507
- Pork Regular (Concentrated), 500 Units 1508
- Purified Pork Regular Insulin 1852

Insulin, Zinc Crystals (Requirements of insulin may be reduced in hypothyroid patients with diabetes and may be subsequently increased with initiation of thyroid hormone therapy). Products include:
- NPH, 100 Units 1502

Insulin, Zinc Suspension (Requirements of insulin may be reduced in hypothyroid patients with diabetes and may be subsequently increased with initiation of thyroid hormone therapy). Products include:
- Iletin I 1501
- Lente, 100 Units 1501
- Iletin II 1504
- Pork Lente, 100 Units 1504
- Purified Pork Lente Insulin 1852

Metformin Hydrochloride (Requirements of oral antidiabetic agents may be reduced in hypothyroid patients with diabetes and may be subsequently increased with initiation of thyroid hormone therapy). Products include:
- Glucophage Tablets 754

Polyestradiol Phosphate (Estrogens or estrogen-containing oral contraceptives tend to increase serum thyroxine binding; free levothyroxine may be decreased in patients with nonfunctioning thyroid gland resulting in increased thyroid requirements).
- No products indexed under this heading.

Quinestrol (Estrogens or estrogen-containing oral contraceptives tend to increase serum thyroxine binding; free levothyroxine may be decreased in patients with nonfunctioning thyroid gland resulting in increased thyroid requirements).
- No products indexed under this heading.

Tolazamide (Requirements of oral antidiabetic agents may be reduced in hypothyroid patients with diabetes and may be subsequently increased with initiation of thyroid hormone therapy).
- No products indexed under this heading.

Tolbutamide (Requirements of oral antidiabetic agents may be reduced in hypothyroid patients with diabetes and may be subsequently increased with initiation of thyroid hormone therapy).
- No products indexed under this heading.

Warfarin Sodium (Thyroid hormones appear to increase catabolism of vitamin K-dependent clotting factors; co-administration results in impairment of compensatory increases in clotting factor synthesis). Products include:
- Coumadin 941

EMCYT CAPSULES

(Estramustine Phosphate Sodium) 2085
May interact with calcium preparations. Compounds in this category include:

Calcium Carbonate (Calcium-rich drugs may impair the absorption of estramustine). Products include:
- Alka-Mints Chewable Antacid .... ◼ 609
- Alka-Seltzer Fast Relief Caplets .... ◼ 610
- Ascriptin .... ◼ 650
- Extra Strength Bayer Plus Aspirin Caplets .... ◼ 617
- Aspirin Regimen Bayer 81 mg Tablets with Calcium .... ◼ 615
- Bufferin Analgesic Tablets .... ◼ 636
- Arthritis Strength Bufferin Analgesic Caplets .... ◼ 637
- Extra Strength Bufferin Analgesic Tablets .... ◼ 637
- Calci-Chew Tablets 2168
- Calci-Mix Capsules 2168
- Caltrate 600 .... ◼ 681
- Caltrate PLUS .... ◼ 681
- Caltrate 600 + D .... ◼ 681
- Cotazym Capsules 1866
- Di-Gel Antacid/Anti-Gas .... ◼ 762
- Florical Capsules and Tablets 1825
- Gerimed Tablets 1000
- Maalox Antacid Caplets .... ◼ 657
- Marblen .... ◼ 671
- Materna Tablets 1427
- Monocal Tablets 1825
- Mylanta Fast-Acting 1359
- Mylanta Gelcaps Antacid .... ◼ 678
- Mylanta Soothing Lozenges 1360
- Mylanta Tablets .... ◼ 677
- Mylanta Double Strength Tablets .... ◼ 677
- Nephro-Calci Tablets 2168
- One-A-Day Calcium Plus .... ◼ 625
- Rolaids Antacid Tablets .... ◼ 807
- Rolaids Antacid Calcium Rich/Sodium Free Tablets .... ◼ 807
- Tempo Soft Antacid .... ◼ 799
- Titralac .... ◼ 686
- Titralac Plus .... ◼ 687
- Tums Antacid/Calcium Supplement Tablets .... ◼ 787
- Tums Anti-gas/Antacid Formula Tablets, Assorted Fruit .... ◼ 788
- Tums E-X Antacid/Calcium Supplement Tablets .... ◼ 787
- Tums 500 Calcium Supplement .... ◼ 788
- Tums ULTRA Antacid/Calcium Supplement Tablets .... ◼ 787
- TYLENOL Headache Plus Pain Reliever with Antacid, Extra Strength Caplets .... ◼ 705

(◼ Described in PDR For Nonprescription Drugs) (◉ Described in PDR For Ophthalmology)

Calcium Chloride (Calcium-rich drugs may impair the absorption of estramustine).

No products indexed under this heading.

Calcium Citrate (Calcium-rich drugs may impair the absorption of estramustine). Products include:

Citracal Tablets ... 1828

Calcium Glubionate (Calcium-rich drugs may impair the absorption of estramustine).

No products indexed under this heading.

Food Interactions

Dairy products (Calcium-rich foods may impair the absorption of estramustine).

Food, calcium-rich (Calcium-rich foods may impair the absorption of estramustine).

EMETE-CON INTRAMUSCULAR/INTRAVENOUS

(Benzquinamide Hydrochloride) ... 2007

May interact with vasopressors. Compounds in this category include:

Dopamine Hydrochloride (In patients receiving pressor agents and benzquinamide, the latter should be given in fraction of normal dose due to increased potential for hypertension).

No products indexed under this heading.

Epinephrine Bitartrate (In patients receiving pressor agents and benzquinamide, the latter should be given in fraction of normal dose due to increased potential for hypertension). Products include:

Sensorcaine-MPF with Epinephrine Injection ... 554

Epinephrine Hydrochloride (In patients receiving pressor agents and benzquinamide, the latter should be given in fraction of normal dose due to increased potential for hypertension). Products include:

Ana-Kit Anaphylaxis Emergency Treatment Kit ... 611

Metaraminol Bitartrate (In patients receiving pressor agents and benzquinamide, the latter should be given in fraction of normal dose due to increased potential for hypertension). Products include:

Aramine Injection ... 1649

Methoxamine Hydrochloride (In patients receiving pressor agents and benzquinamide, the latter should be given in fraction of normal dose due to increased potential for hypertension). Products include:

Vasoxyl Injection ... 1169

Norepinephrine Bitartrate (In patients receiving pressor agents and benzquinamide, the latter should be given in fraction of normal dose due to increased potential for hypertension). Products include:

Levophed Bitartrate Injection ... 2445

Phenylephrine Hydrochloride (In patients receiving pressor agents and benzquinamide, the latter should be given in fraction of normal dose due to increased potential for hypertension). Products include:

Atrohist Plus Tablets ... 1605
Cerose DM ... 853
D.A. II Tablets ... 972
D.A. Chewable Tablets ... 970
Dura-Vent/DA Tablets ... 972
Extendryl ... 1003
4-Way Fast Acting Nasal Spray (regular & mentholated) ... 644
Hemorid ... 797
Hycomine Compound Tablets ... 948
Neo-Synephrine Hydrochloride 1% Carpuject ... 2455
Neo-Synephrine Hydrochloride 1% Injection ... 2455
Neo-Synephrine Hydrochloride (Ophthalmic) ... 2456
Neo-Synephrine ... 624
Novahistine Elixir ... 782
Phenergan VC ... 2886
Phenergan VC with Codeine ... 2888
Preparation H ... 842
Tympagesic Ear Drops ... 2476
Vicks Sinex Nasal Spray and Ultra Fine Mist ... 738

EMGEL 2% TOPICAL GEL

(Erythromycin) ... 1081

May interact with:

Concomitant Topical Acne Therapy (Possible cumulative irritancy effect).

EMINASE

(Anistreplase) ... 2215

May interact with anticoagulants, platelet inhibitors, and certain other agents. Compounds in these categories include:

Aspirin (Increases risk of bleeding and bleeding events). Products include:

Alka-Seltzer Cherry Effervescent Antacid and Pain Reliever ... 609
Alka-Seltzer Extra Strength Effervescent Antacid and Pain Reliever ... 609
Alka-Seltzer Lemon Lime Effervescent Antacid and Pain Reliever ... 609
Alka-Seltzer Original Effervescent Antacid and Pain Reliever ... 609
Alka-Seltzer Plus ... 611
Alka-Seltzer Plus Sinus Medicine ... 611
Ascriptin ... 650
Arthritis Strength BC Powder ... 631
BC Cold Powder Multi-Symptom Formula (Cold-Sinus-Allergy) ... 631
BC Cold Powder Non-Drowsy Formula (Cold-Sinus) ... 631
BC Powder ... 631
Genuine Bayer Aspirin Tablets & Caplets ... 618
Extra Strength Bayer Arthritis Pain Regimen Formula ... 615
Extra Strength Bayer Aspirin Caplets & Tablets ... 617
Extended-Release Bayer 8-Hour Aspirin ... 616
Extra Strength Bayer Plus Aspirin Caplets ... 617
Extra Strength Bayer PM Aspirin Plus Sleep Aid ... 617
Aspirin Regimen Bayer 81 mg Tablets with Calcium ... 615
Aspirin Regimen Bayer Adult Low Strength 81 mg Tablets ... 613
Aspirin Regimen Bayer Children's Chewable Aspirin ... 616
Aspirin Regimen Bayer Regular Strength 325 mg Caplets ... 613
Bufferin Analgesic Tablets ... 636
Arthritis Strength Bufferin Analgesic Caplets ... 637
Extra Strength Bufferin Analgesic Tablets ... 637
Cama Arthritis Pain Reliever ... 748
Darvon Compound-65 Pulvules ... 1475
Easprin ... 1971
Ecotrin ... 2625
Ecotrin Enteric Coated Aspirin Maximum Strength Tablets and Caplets ... 775
Ecotrin Enteric Coated Aspirin Regular Strength Tablets ... 2625
Empirin Aspirin Tablets ... 818
Excedrin Extra-Strength Analgesic Tablets, Caplets, and Geltabs ... 734
Fiorinal Capsules ... 2388
Fiorinal with Codeine Capsules ... 2390
Fiorinal Tablets ... 2388
Goody's Extra Strength Headache Powders ... 632
Goody's Extra Strength Pain Relief Tablets ... 632
Halfprin Tablets ... 1413
Norgesic ... 1554
Percodan Tablets ... 955
Percodan-Demi Tablets ... 956
Robaxisal Tablets ... 2246
Soma Compound w/Codeine Tablets ... 2784
Soma Compound Tablets ... 2783
St. Joseph Adult Chewable Aspirin (81 mg.) ... 768
Talwin Compound ... 2466
Vanquish Analgesic Caplets ... 627

Azlocillin Sodium (Increases risk of bleeding and bleeding events).

No products indexed under this heading.

Carbenicillin Indanyl Sodium (Increases risk of bleeding and bleeding events). Products include:

Geocillin Tablets ... 2009

Choline Magnesium Trisalicylate (Increases risk of bleeding and bleeding events). Products include:

Trilisate ... 2155

Dalteparin Sodium (Potential for bleeding and bleeding complications). Products include:

Fragmin Injection ... 2088

Diclofenac Potassium (Increases risk of bleeding and bleeding events). Products include:

Cataflam Tablets ... 833

Diclofenac Sodium (Increases risk of bleeding and bleeding events). Products include:

Voltaren Ophthalmic Sterile Ophthalmic Solution ... ⊙ 264
Cataflam/Voltaren/Voltaren-XR ... 833

Dicumarol (Potential for bleeding and bleeding complications).

No products indexed under this heading.

Diflunisal (Increases risk of bleeding and bleeding events). Products include:

Dolobid Tablets ... 1695

Dipyridamole (Increases risk of bleeding and bleeding events). Products include:

Persantine Tablets ... 686

Enoxaparin (Potential for bleeding and bleeding complications). Products include:

Lovenox Injection ... 2187

Fenoprofen Calcium (Increases risk of bleeding and bleeding events). Products include:

Nalfon 200 Pulvules & Nalfon Tablets ... 933

Flurbiprofen (Increases risk of bleeding and bleeding events).

No products indexed under this heading.

Heparin Calcium (Potential for bleeding and bleeding complications).

No products indexed under this heading.

Heparin Sodium (Potential for bleeding and bleeding complications). Products include:

Heparin Lock Flush Solution ... 2831
Heparin Sodium Injection ... 2832
Heparin Sodium Vials ... 1486

Ibuprofen (Increases risk of bleeding and bleeding events). Products include:

Advil Cold and Sinus Caplets and Tablets ... 837
Advil Ibuprofen Tablets, Caplets and Gel Caplets ... 836
Children's Motrin Ibuprofen Oral Suspension ... 1558
IBU Tablets ... 1389
Ibuprohm ... 713
Motrin IB Caplets, Tablets, and Gelcaps ... 802
Motrin Ibuprofen Suspension, Oral Drops, Chewable Tablets, Caplets ... 1563
Nuprin Ibuprofen/Analgesic Tablets & Caplets ... 645
Vicks DayQuil SINUS Pressure & PAIN Relief with IBUPROFEN ... 735

Indomethacin (Increases risk of bleeding and bleeding events). Products include:

Indocin ... 1723

Indomethacin Sodium Trihydrate (Increases risk of bleeding and bleeding events). Products include:

Indocin I.V. ... 1727

Ketoprofen (Increases risk of bleeding and bleeding events). Products include:

Actron Caplets and Tablets ... 608
Orudis Capsules ... 2874
Orudis KT ... 842
Oruvail Capsules ... 2874

Magnesium Salicylate (Increases risk of bleeding and bleeding events). Products include:

Backache Caplets ... 635
Doan's Extra-Strength Analgesic ... 653
Extra Strength Doan's P.M. ... 653
Doan's Regular Strength Analgesic ... 654
Mobigesic Tablets ... 607

Meclofenamate Sodium (Increases risk of bleeding and bleeding events).

No products indexed under this heading.

Mefenamic Acid (Increases risk of bleeding and bleeding events). Products include:

Ponstel ... 1982

Mezlocillin Sodium (Increases risk of bleeding and bleeding events). Products include:

Mezlin ... 594
Mezlin Pharmacy Bulk Package ... 597

Nafcillin Sodium (Increases risk of bleeding and bleeding events).

No products indexed under this heading.

Naproxen (Increases risk of bleeding and bleeding events). Products include:

Anaprox/Naprosyn ... 2277

Naproxen Sodium (Increases risk of bleeding and bleeding events). Products include:

Aleve ... 2124
Anaprox/Naprosyn ... 2277
Naprelan Tablets ... 2861

Penicillin G Benzathine (Increases risk of bleeding and bleeding events). Products include:

Bicillin C-R Injection ... 2810
Bicillin C-R 900/300 Injection ... 2812
Bicillin L-A Injection ... 2813

Penicillin G Procaine (Increases risk of bleeding and bleeding events). Products include:

Bicillin C-R Injection ... 2810
Bicillin C-R 900/300 Injection ... 2812

Phenylbutazone (Increases risk of bleeding and bleeding events).

No products indexed under this heading.

Piroxicam (Increases risk of bleeding and bleeding events). Products include:

Feldene Capsules ... 2008

Salsalate (Increases risk of bleeding and bleeding events). Products include:

Disalcid ... 1549
Mono-Gesic Tablets ... 810
Salflex Tablets ... 791

Sulindac (Increases risk of bleeding and bleeding events). Products include:

Clinoril Tablets ... 1658

Ticarcillin Disodium (Increases risk of bleeding and bleeding events). Products include:

Ticar for Injection ... 2704
Timentin for Injection ... 2706

Eminase | Interactions Index | 374

Ticlopidine Hydrochloride (Increases risk of bleeding and bleeding events). Products include:
- Ticlid Tablets 2317

Tolmetin Sodium (Increases risk of bleeding and bleeding events). Products include:
- Tolectin (200, 400 and 600 mg) .. 1591

Warfarin Sodium (Potential for bleeding and bleeding complications). Products include:
- Coumadin 941

EMLA CREAM

(Prilocaine, Lidocaine) 536

May interact with methemoglobinemia-inducing drugs and certain other agents. Compounds in these categories include:

Acetaminophen (Potential for greater risk of developing methemoglobinemia). Products include:
- Actifed Cold & Sinus Caplets and Tablets .... ■ 808
- Actifed Sinus Daytime/Nighttime Tablets and Caplets .... ■ 809
- Alka-Seltzer Fast Relief Caplets .... ■ 610
- Alka-Seltzer Plus Liqui-Gels .... ■ 612
- Alka-Seltzer Plus Flu & Body Aches Effervescent Tablets .... ■ 612
- Alka-Seltzer Plus Flu & Body Aches Liqui-Gels Non-Drowsy Formula .... ■ 613
- Alka-Seltzer Plus Night-Time Cold Medicine Liqui-Gels .... ■ 612
- Allerest No Drowsiness .... ■ 649
- Allerest Sinus Pain Formula .... ■ 649
- Axocet Capsules 2469
- Benadryl Allergy/Cold Tablets .... ■ 811
- Benadryl Allergy Sinus Headache Caplets .... ■ 813
- Children's TYLENOL acetaminophen Chewable Tablets, Elixir, Suspension Liquid, and Suspension Drops 1559
- Children's TYLENOL Cold Multi-Symptom Chewable Tablets and Liquid 1559
- Children's TYLENOL Cold Plus Cough Multi Symptom Chewable Tablets and Liquid 1560
- Children's TYLENOL Flu Suspension Liquid 1560
- Allergy-Sinus Comtrex Multi-Symptom Allergy-Sinus Formula Tablets and Caplets .... ■ 639
- Comtrex Multi-Symptom .... ■ 638
- Comtrex Non-Drowsy .... ■ 640
- Contac Day Allergy/Sinus Caplets ■ 771
- Contac Day & Night .... ■ 772
- Contac Night Allergy/Sinus Caplets .... ■ 771
- Contac Severe Cold and Flu Formula Caplets .... ■ 773
- Contac Severe Cold & Flu Non-Drowsy .... ■ 774
- Coricidin Cold + Flu Tablets .... ■ 760
- Coricidin 'D' Decongestant Tablets .... ■ 760
- DHCplus Capsules 2148
- Darvon-N/Darvocet-N 1473
- Dimetapp Allergy Sinus Caplets .... ■ 838
- Dimetapp Cold & Fever Suspension .... ■ 839
- Drixoral Cold and Flu Extended-Release Tablets .... ■ 764
- Drixoral Cough + Sore Throat Liquid Caps .... ■ 763
- Drixoral Allergy/Sinus Extended Release Tablets .... ■ 765
- Esgic-plus Capsules 1012
- Esgic-plus Tablets 1012
- Aspirin Free Excedrin Analgesic Caplets and Geltabs 734
- Excedrin Extra-Strength Analgesic Tablets, Caplets, and Geltabs 734
- Excedrin P.M. Analgesic/Sleeping Aid Tablets, Caplets, Liquigels 735
- Fioricet Tablets 2386
- Fioricet with Codeine Capsules 2387
- Goody's Extra Strength Headache Powders .... ■ 632
- Goody's Extra Strength Pain Relief Tablets .... ■ 632
- Hycomine Compound Tablets 948
- Hydrocet Capsules 787
- Infants' TYLENOL acetaminophen Suspension Drops 1559
- Infants' TYLENOL Cold Decongestant & Fever-Reducer Drops 1561
- Junior Strength TYLENOL acetaminophen Coated Caplets and Chewable Tablets 1562
- Lorcet 10/650 Tablets 1016
- Lortab 2751
- Lurline PMS Tablets 1000
- Maximum Strength Multi-Symptom Formula Midol .... ■ 621
- PMS Multi-Symptom Formula Midol .... ■ 622
- Maximum Strength Midol Teen Multi-Symptom Formula .... ■ 621
- Midrin Capsules 788
- Panodol Tablets and Caplets .... ■ 783
- Children's Panadol Chewable Tablets, Liquid, Infant's Drops .... ■ 783
- Percocet Tablets 955
- Percogesic Analgesic Tablets .... ■ 727
- Phrenilin 790
- Pyrroxate Caplets .... ■ 742
- Robitussin Cold, Cough & Flu Liqui-Gels .... ■ 844
- Robitussin Night-Time Cold Formula .... ■ 847
- Sedapap Tablets 50 mg/650 mg .. 1826
- Sinarest .... ■ 663
- Sine-Aid Maximum Strength Sinus Headache Gelcaps, Caplets and Tablets 1570
- Sine-Off No Drowsiness Formula Caplets .... ■ 784
- Sine-Off Sinus Medicine .... ■ 784
- Singlet Tablets .... ■ 785
- Sinulin Tablets 792
- Sinutab Sinus Allergy Medication, Maximum Strength Tablets and Caplets .... ■ 823
- Sinutab Sinus Medication, Maximum Strength Without Drowsiness Formula, Tablets & Caplets .... ■ 824
- Sudafed Cold and Cough Liquid Caps .... ■ 826
- Sudafed Severe Cold Formula Caplets .... ■ 828
- Sudafed Severe Cold Formula Tablets .... ■ 828
- Sudafed Sinus Caplets .... ■ 829
- Sudafed Sinus Tablets .... ■ 829
- Talacen Caplets 2464
- TheraFlu Flu and Cold Medicine .... ■ 750
- Theraflu Maximum Strength Flu and Cold Medicine For Sore Throat .... ■ 751
- TheraFlu Flu, Cold and Cough Medicine .... ■ 750
- TheraFlu Maximum Strength Nighttime Flu, Cold & Cough Medicine .... ■ 751
- TheraFlu Maximum Strength Non-Drowsy Formula Flu, Cold & Cough Medicine .... ■ 751
- TheraFlu Maximum Strength, Non-Drowsy Formula Flu, Cold and Cough Caplets .... ■ 752
- Theraflu Maximum Strength Sinus Non-Drowsy Formula Caplets .... ■ 752
- Triaminic Sore Throat Formula .... ■ 755
- Triaminicin Tablets .... ■ 756
- TYLENOL acetaminophen Extended Relief Caplets 1570
- TYLENOL acetaminophen, Extra Strength Adult Liquid Pain Reliever 1570
- TYLENOL acetaminophen, Extra Strength Gelcaps, Geltabs, Caplets, Tablets 1570
- TYLENOL acetaminophen, Regular Strength Caplets and Tablets 1570
- TYLENOL Allergy Sinus, Maximum Strength Caplets and Gelcaps 1571
- TYLENOL Allergy Sinus NightTime, Maximum Strength Caplets 1571
- TYLENOL Cold Medication, Multi-Symptom Formula Tablets and Caplets 1572
- TYLENOL Cold Medication, Multi-Symptom Hot Liquid Packets 1572
- TYLENOL Cold Medication, No Drowsiness Formula Caplets and Gelcaps 1572
- TYLENOL Cold Severe Congestion Caplets 1573
- TYLENOL Cough Medication, Multi Symptom 1574
- TYLENOL Cough Medication with Decongestant, Multi Symptom 1574
- TYLENOL Flu No Drowsiness Formula, Maximum Strength Gelcaps 1575
- TYLENOL Flu NightTime, Maximum Strength Gelcaps 1575
- TYLENOL Flu NightTime, Maximum Strength Hot Medication Packets 1575
- TYLENOL Headache Plus Pain Reliever with Antacid, Extra Strength Caplets .... ■ 705
- TYLENOL PM Pain Reliever/Sleep Aid, Extra Strength Gelcaps, Caplets, Geltabs 1576
- TYLENOL Severe Allergy Medication Caplets 1571
- TYLENOL Sinus, Maximum Strength Geltabs, Gelcaps, Caplets and Tablets 1576
- Tylenol with Codeine 1592
- Tylox Capsules 1593
- Unisom With Pain Relief-Nighttime Sleep Aid and Pain Reliever 1991
- Vanquish Analgesic Caplets .... ■ 627
- Vicks 44 LiquiCaps Cough, Cold & Flu Relief .... ■ 728
- Vicks 44M Cough, Cold & Flu Relief .... ■ 729
- Vicks DayQuil LiquiCaps/Liquid Multi-Symptom Cold/Flu Relief .. ■ 734
- Vicks Nyquil Hot Therapy .... ■ 735
- Vicks NyQuil LiquiCaps/Liquid Multi-Symptom Cold/Flu Relief, Original and Cherry Flavors .... ■ 736
- Vicodin Tablets 1404
- Vicodin ES Tablets 1405
- Vicodin HP Tablets 1403
- Wygesic Tablets 2930
- Zydone Capsules 967

Amyl Nitrite (Potential for greater risk of developing methemoglobinemia).
- No products indexed under this heading.

Bendroflumethiazide (Potential for greater risk of developing methemoglobinemia).
- No products indexed under this heading.

Benzocaine (Potential for greater risk of developing methemoglobinemia). Products include:
- Americaine Anesthetic Lubricant 1603
- Americaine Hemorrhoidal Ointment .... ■ 649
- Americaine Otic Topical Anesthetic Ear Drops 1603
- Americaine .... ■ 649
- Auralgan Otic Solution 2810
- BiCozene Creme .... ■ 747
- Cēpacol Maximum Strength Sore Throat Lozenges, Cherry Flavor ■ 850
- Cēpacol Maximum Strength Sore Throat Lozenges, Original Mint Flavor .... ■ 850
- Cetacaine Topical Anesthetic 812
- Children's Vicks Chloraseptic Sore Throat Lozenges .... ■ 730
- Cough-X Lozenges .... ■ 606
- Baby Orajel Teething Pain Medicine .... ■ 667
- Orajel Maximum Strength Toothache Medication .... ■ 668
- Orajel Mouth-Aid for Canker and Cold Sores .... ■ 668
- Tanac No Sting Liquid .... ■ 669
- Tympagesic Ear Drops 2476
- Vicks Chloraseptic Sore Throat Lozenges, Menthol and Cherry Flavors .... ■ 732
- Zilactin-B Medicated Gel with Benzocaine .... ■ 856

Chloroquine (Potential for greater risk of developing methemoglobinemia).

Chloroquine Hydrochloride (Potential for greater risk of developing methemoglobinemia). Products include:
- Aralen Hydrochloride Injection 2430

Chloroquine Phosphate (Potential for greater risk of developing methemoglobinemia). Products include:
- Aralen Phosphate Tablets 2431

Chlorothiazide (Potential for greater risk of developing methemoglobinemia). Products include:
- Aldoclor Tablets 1638
- Diupres Tablets 1691
- Diuril Oral 1694

Chlorothiazide Sodium (Potential for greater risk of developing methemoglobinemia). Products include:
- Diuril Sodium Intravenous 1693

Chlorpropamide (Potential for greater risk of developing methemoglobinemia). Products include:
- Diabinese Tablets 2002

Dapsone (Potential for greater risk of developing methemoglobinemia). Products include:
- Dapsone Tablets USP 1331

Erythrityl Tetranitrate (Potential for greater risk of developing methemoglobinemia).
- No products indexed under this heading.

Fosphenytoin Sodium (Potential for greater risk of developing methemoglobinemia). Products include:
- Cerebyx Injection 1956

Glipizide (Potential for greater risk of developing methemoglobinemia). Products include:
- Glucotrol Tablets 2011
- Glucotrol XL Extended Release Tablets 2012

Glyburide (Potential for greater risk of developing methemoglobinemia). Products include:
- DiaBeta Tablets 1265
- Glynase PresTab Tablets 2091
- Micronase Tablets 2099

Hydrochlorothiazide (Potential for greater risk of developing methemoglobinemia). Products include:
- Aldactazide Tablets 2556
- Aldoril Tablets 1644
- Apresazide Capsules 824
- Capozide Tablets 744
- Dyazide Capsules 2653
- Esidrix Tablets 839
- Esimil Tablets 840
- HydroDIURIL Tablets 1716
- Hydropres Tablets 1718
- Hyzaar Tablets 1720
- Inderide Tablets 2838
- Inderide LA Long Acting Capsules .. 2840
- Lopressor HCT Tablets 850
- Lotensin HCT Tablets 855
- Moduretic Tablets 1748
- Oretic Tablets 450
- Prinzide Tablets 1780
- Ser-Ap-Es Tablets 867
- Timolide Tablets 1791
- Vaseretic Tablets 1810
- Zestoretic Tablets 2968
- Ziac 1459

Hydroflumethiazide (Potential for greater risk of developing methemoglobinemia). Products include:
- Diucardin Tablets 2824

Isosorbide Dinitrate (Potential for greater risk of developing methemoglobinemia). Products include:
- Dilatrate-SR Capsules 2542
- Isordil Sublingual Tablets 2845
- Isordil Tembids 2847
- Isordil Titradose Tablets 2848
- Sorbitrate 2959

Isosorbide Mononitrate (Potential for greater risk of developing methemoglobinemia). Products include:
- Imdur 1362
- Ismo Tablets 2844
- Monoket Tablets 2550

Methyclothiazide (Potential for greater risk of developing methemoglobinemia). Products include:
- Enduron Tablets 424

Mexiletine Hydrochloride (Potential for additive or synergistic toxic effects). Products include:
- Mexitil Capsules ... 684

Nitrofurantoin (Potential for greater risk of developing methemoglobinemia). Products include:
- Macrodantin Capsules ... 2140

Nitrofurantoin Monohydrate (Potential for greater risk of developing methemoglobinemia). Products include:
- Macrobid Capsules ... 2138

Nitroglycerin (Potential for greater risk of developing methemoglobinemia). Products include:
- Deponit NTG Transdermal Delivery System ... 2541
- Nitro-Bid IV ... 1270
- Nitro-Bid Ointment ... 1272
- Nitro-Dur (nitroglycerin) Transdermal Infusion System ... 1365
- Nitrolingual Spray ... 2193
- Nitrostat Tablets ... 1981
- Transderm-Nitro Transdermal Therapeutic System ... 878

Para-Aminosalicylic Acid (Potential for greater risk of developing methemoglobinemia).

Pentaerythritol Tetranitrate (Potential for greater risk of developing methemoglobinemia).
- No products indexed under this heading.

Phenacetin (Potential for greater risk of developing methemoglobinemia).

Phenobarbital (Potential for greater risk of developing methemoglobinemia). Products include:
- Arco-Lase Plus Tablets ... 513
- Bellergal-S Tablets ... 2375
- Donnatal ... 2234
- Donnatal Extentabs ... 2234
- Donnatal Tablets ... 2234
- Phenobarbital Elixir and Tablets ... 1523
- Quadrinal Tablets ... 1398

Phenytoin (Potential for greater risk of developing methemoglobinemia). Products include:
- Dilantin Infatabs ... 1967
- Dilantin-125 Suspension ... 1969

Phenytoin Sodium (Potential for greater risk of developing methemoglobinemia). Products include:
- Dilantin Kapseals ... 1965

Polythiazide (Potential for greater risk of developing methemoglobinemia). Products include:
- Minizide Capsules ... 2016

Primaquine Phosphate (Potential for greater risk of developing methemoglobinemia).
- No products indexed under this heading.

Quinine Sulfate (Potential for greater risk of developing methemoglobinemia).
- No products indexed under this heading.

Sodium Nitroprusside (Potential for greater risk of developing methemoglobinemia).
- No products indexed under this heading.

Sulfacytine (Potential for greater risk of developing methemoglobinemia).

Sulfamethizole (Potential for greater risk of developing methemoglobinemia). Products include:
- Urobiotic-250 Capsules ... 2038

Sulfamethoxazole (Potential for greater risk of developing methemoglobinemia). Products include:
- Bactrim DS Tablets ... 2257
- Bactrim I.V. Infusion ... 2255
- Bactrim ... 2257
- Gantanol Tablets ... 2285
- Septra ... 1146
- Septra I.V. Infusion ... 1142
- Septra I.V. Infusion ADD-Vantage Vials ... 1144
- Septra ... 1146

Sulfasalazine (Potential for greater risk of developing methemoglobinemia). Products include:
- Azulfidine ... 2059

Sulfinpyrazone (Potential for greater risk of developing methemoglobinemia). Products include:
- Anturane ... 823

Sulfisoxazole (Potential for greater risk of developing methemoglobinemia). Products include:
- Gantrisin Tablets ... 2286

Sulfisoxazole Diolamine (Potential for greater risk of developing methemoglobinemia).
- No products indexed under this heading.

Tocainide Hydrochloride (Potential for additive or synergistic toxic effects). Products include:
- Tonocard Tablets ... 519

Tolazamide (Potential for greater risk of developing methemoglobinemia).
- No products indexed under this heading.

Tolbutamide (Potential for greater risk of developing methemoglobinemia).
- No products indexed under this heading.

EMPIRIN ASPIRIN TABLETS

(Aspirin) ... ▣ 818

May interact with oral anticoagulants. Compounds in this category include:

Dicumarol (Concurrent administration is not recommended).
- No products indexed under this heading.

Warfarin Sodium (Concurrent administration is not recommended). Products include:
- Coumadin ... 941

ENCARE VAGINAL CONTRACEPTIVE SUPPOSITORIES

(Nonoxynol-9) ... ▣ 797

None cited in PDR database.

ENDURON TABLETS

(Methyclothiazide) ... 424

May interact with antihypertensives, beta blockers, corticosteroids, insulin, barbiturates, narcotic analgesics, cardiac glycosides, lithium preparations, and certain other agents. Compounds in these categories include:

Acebutolol Hydrochloride (Additive action). Products include:
- Sectral Capsules ... 2914

ACTH (Hypokalemia).
- No products indexed under this heading.

Alfentanil Hydrochloride (Potentiates orthostatic hypotension). Products include:
- Alfenta Injection ... 1334

Amlodipine Besylate (Additive action). Products include:
- Lotrel Capsules ... 858
- Norvasc Tablets ... 2020

Aprobarbital (Potentiates orthostatic hypotension).
- No products indexed under this heading.

Atenolol (Additive action). Products include:
- Tenoretic Tablets ... 2963
- Tenormin Tablets and I.V. Injection ... 2965

Benazepril Hydrochloride (Additive action). Products include:
- Lotensin Tablets ... 852
- Lotensin HCT Tablets ... 855
- Lotrel Capsules ... 858

Bendroflumethiazide (Additive action).
- No products indexed under this heading.

Betamethasone Acetate (Hypokalemia). Products include:
- Celestone Soluspan Suspension ... 2484

Betamethasone Sodium Phosphate (Hypokalemia). Products include:
- Celestone Soluspan Suspension ... 2484

Betaxolol Hydrochloride (Additive action). Products include:
- Betoptic Ophthalmic Solution ... 465
- Betoptic S Ophthalmic Suspension ... 467
- Kerlone Tablets ... 2588

Bisoprolol Fumarate (Additive action). Products include:
- Zebeta Tablets ... 1457
- Ziac ... 1459

Buprenorphine (Potentiates orthostatic hypotension). Products include:
- Buprenex Injectable ... 2170

Butabarbital (Potentiates orthostatic hypotension).
- No products indexed under this heading.

Butalbital (Potentiates orthostatic hypotension). Products include:
- Axocet Capsules ... 2469
- Esgic-plus Capsules ... 1012
- Esgic-plus Tablets ... 1012
- Fioricet Tablets ... 2386
- Fioricet with Codeine Capsules ... 2387
- Fiorinal Capsules ... 2388
- Fiorinal with Codeine Capsules ... 2390
- Fiorinal Tablets ... 2388
- Phrenilin ... 790
- Sedapap Tablets 50 mg/650 mg ... 1826

Captopril (Additive action). Products include:
- Capoten Tablets ... 740
- Capozide Tablets ... 744

Carteolol Hydrochloride (Additive action). Products include:
- Cartrol Tablets ... 413
- Ocupress Ophthalmic Solution, 1% Sterile ... ◉ 297

Chlorothiazide (Additive action). Products include:
- Aldoclor Tablets ... 1638
- Diupres Tablets ... 1691
- Diuril Oral ... 1694

Chlorothiazide Sodium (Additive action). Products include:
- Diuril Sodium Intravenous ... 1693

Chlorthalidone (Additive action). Products include:
- Combipres Tablets ... 682
- Tenoretic Tablets ... 2963
- Thalitone ... 1293

Clonidine (Additive action). Products include:
- Catapres-TTS ... 680

Clonidine Hydrochloride (Additive action). Products include:
- Catapres Tablets ... 679
- Combipres Tablets ... 682

Codeine Phosphate (Potentiates orthostatic hypotension). Products include:
- Brontex ... 2130
- Dimetane-DC Cough Syrup ... 2232
- Fioricet with Codeine Capsules ... 2387
- Fiorinal with Codeine Capsules ... 2390
- Nucofed ... 2225
- Phenergan with Codeine ... 2883
- Phenergan VC with Codeine ... 2888
- Robitussin A-C Syrup ... 2248
- Robitussin-DAC Syrup ... 2249
- Ryna ... ▣ 804
- Soma Compound w/Codeine Tablets ... 2784
- Tylenol with Codeine ... 1592

Cortisone Acetate (Hypokalemia). Products include:
- Cortone Acetate Sterile Suspension ... 1663
- Cortone Acetate Tablets ... 1664

Deserpidine (Additive or potentiative action).
- No products indexed under this heading.

Deslanoside (Thiazide-induced hypokalemia may exaggerate the response of the heart to the toxic effects of digitalis).
- No products indexed under this heading.

Dexamethasone (Hypokalemia). Products include:
- AK-Trol Ointment & Suspension ... ◉ 205
- Decadron Elixir ... 1676
- Decadron Tablets ... 1678
- Decaspray Topical Aerosol ... 1689
- Maxitrol Ophthalmic Ointment and Suspension ... ◉ 222
- TobraDex Ophthalmic Suspension and Ointment ... 469

Dexamethasone Acetate (Hypokalemia). Products include:
- Dalalone D.P. Injectable ... 1009
- Decadron-LA Sterile Suspension ... 1687

Dexamethasone Sodium Phosphate (Hypokalemia). Products include:
- Decadron Phosphate Injection ... 1680
- Decadron Phosphate Sterile Ophthalmic Ointment ... 1684
- Decadron Phosphate Sterile Ophthalmic Solution ... 1685
- Decadron Phosphate Topical Cream ... 1686
- Decadron Phosphate with Xylocaine Injection, Sterile ... 1683
- Dexacort Phosphate in Respihaler .. 1606
- Dexacort Phosphate in Turbinaire .. 1607
- NeoDecadron Sterile Ophthalmic Ointment ... 1755
- NeoDecadron Sterile Ophthalmic Solution ... 1756
- NeoDecadron Topical Cream ... 1757

Dezocine (Potentiates orthostatic hypotension). Products include:
- Dalgan Injection ... 529

Diazoxide (Additive action). Products include:
- Hyperstat I.V. Injection ... 2504
- Proglycem ... 575

Digitoxin (Thiazide-induced hypokalemia may exaggerate the response of the heart to the toxic effects of digitalis). Products include:
- Crystodigin Tablets ... 1472

Digoxin (Thiazide-induced hypokalemia may exaggerate the response of the heart to the toxic effects of digitalis). Products include:
- Lanoxicaps ... 1110
- Lanoxin Elixir Pediatric ... 1113
- Lanoxin Injection ... 1116
- Lanoxin Injection Pediatric ... 1119
- Lanoxin Tablets ... 1121

Diltiazem Hydrochloride (Additive action). Products include:
- Cardizem CD Capsules ... 1251
- Cardizem SR Capsules ... 1255
- Cardizem Injectable ... 1253
- Cardizem Tablets ... 1257
- Dilacor XR Extended-release Capsules ... 2183
- Tiazac Capsules ... 1019

Doxazosin Mesylate (Additive action). Products include:
- Cardura Tablets ... 1993

Enalapril Maleate (Additive action). Products include:
- Vaseretic Tablets ... 1810
- Vasotec Tablets ... 1816

Enalaprilat (Additive action). Products include:
- Vasotec I.V. ... 1814

Esmolol Hydrochloride (Additive action). Products include:
- Brevibloc (esmolol HCl) Injection ... 1860

IMPORTANT NOTE: Always consult each drug listing in the patient's regimen for possible interactions.

Enduron **Interactions Index** **376**

Felodipine (Additive action). Products include:
Plendil Extended-Release Tablets.... 514
Fentanyl (Potentiates orthostatic hypotension). Products include:
Duragesic Transdermal System........ 1336
Fentanyl Citrate (Potentiates orthostatic hypotension). Products include:
Sublimaze Injection.......... 463
Fludrocortisone Acetate (Hypokalemia). Products include:
Florinef Acetate Tablets 506
Fosinopril Sodium (Additive action). Products include:
Monopril Tablets 762
Furosemide (Additive action). Products include:
Lasix Injection, Oral Solution and Tablets 1267
Guanabenz Acetate (Additive action).
No products indexed under this heading.
Guanethidine Monosulfate (Additive or potentiative action). Products include:
Esimil Tablets 840
Ismelin Tablets 845
Hydralazine Hydrochloride (Additive action). Products include:
Apresazide Capsules 824
Apresoline Hydrochloride Tablets .. 826
Hydralazine Hydrochloride Injection USP.......... 2712
Ser-Ap-Es Tablets 867
Hydrochlorothiazide (Additive action). Products include:
Aldactazide Tablets 2556
Aldoril Tablets.......... 1644
Apresazide Capsules 824
Capozide Tablets 744
Dyazide Capsules.......... 2653
Esidrix Tablets 839
Esimil Tablets 840
HydroDIURIL Tablets 1716
Hydropres Tablets.......... 1718
Hyzaar Tablets 1720
Inderide Tablets 2838
Inderide LA Long Acting Capsules .. 2840
Lopressor HCT Tablets 850
Lotensin HCT Tablets 855
Moduretic Tablets 1748
Oretic Tablets 450
Prinzide Tablets 1780
Ser-Ap-Es Tablets 867
Timolide Tablets.......... 1791
Vaseretic Tablets 1810
Zestoretic Tablets 2968
Ziac 1459
Hydrocodone Bitartrate (Potentiates orthostatic hypotension). Products include:
Codiclear DH Syrup 808
Duratuss HD Elixir.......... 2750
Histussin D Liquid 670
Hycodan Tablets and Syrup 946
Hycomine Compound Tablets 948
Hycomine 947
Hycotuss Expectorant Syrup 950
Hydrocet Capsules 787
Lorcet 10/650 Tablets 1016
Lortab.......... 2751
Tussend.......... 1830
Tussend Expectorant.......... 1831
Vicodin Tablets 1404
Vicodin ES Tablets 1405
Vicodin HP Tablets 1403
Vicodin Tuss Expectorant 1406
Zydone Capsules 967
Hydrocodone Polistirex (Potentiates orthostatic hypotension). Products include:
Tussionex Pennkinetic Extended-Release Suspension 1624
Hydrocortisone (Hypokalemia). Products include:
Anusol-HC Cream 2.5%.......... 1953
Aquanil HC Lotion 1989
Maximum Strength Cortaid Spray ▣ 800
CORTENEMA.......... 2713
Cortisporin Ointment.......... 1074
Cortisporin Ophthalmic Ointment Sterile 1074
Cortisporin Ophthalmic Suspension Sterile 1075
Cortisporin Otic Solution Sterile 1076
Cortisporin Otic Suspension Sterile 1077
Cortizone-5 .... ▣ 795
Cortizone-10 .... ▣ 795
Hydrocortone Tablets 1715
Hytone 922
Hytone Ointment 2 ½%.......... 923
Massengill Medicated Soft Cloth Towelettes.......... 2628
Pediotic Suspension Sterile.......... 1140
Preparation H Hydrocortisone 1% Cream .... ▣ 843
ProctoCream-HC 2.5%.......... 2552
VōSoL HC Otic Solution.......... 2786
Hydrocortisone Acetate (Hypokalemia). Products include:
Analpram-HC Rectal Cream 1% and 2.5% 993
Anusol HC-1 Hydrocortisone Anti-Itch Ointment .... ▣ 810
Anusol-HC Suppositories 1954
Caldecort Anti-Itch Hydrocortisone Cream .... ▣ 651
Coly-Mycin S Otic w/Neomycin & Hydrocortisone 1965
Cortaid .... ▣ 800
Cortifoam 2540
Cortisporin Cream.......... 1073
Epifoam 2543
Hydrocortone Acetate Sterile Suspension.......... 1712
Mantadil Cream 1124
Nupercainal Hydrocortisone 1% Cream .... ▣ 661
Pramosone Cream, Lotion & Ointment 995
ProctoFoam-HC 2552
Terra-Cortril Ophthalmic Suspension 2033
Hydrocortisone Sodium Phosphate (Hypokalemia). Products include:
Hydrocortone Phosphate Injection, Sterile 1713
Hydrocortisone Sodium Succinate (Hypokalemia).
No products indexed under this heading.
Hydroflumethiazide (Additive action). Products include:
Diucardin Tablets.......... 2824
Hydromorphone Hydrochloride (Potentiates orthostatic hypotension). Products include:
Dilaudid Ampules.......... 1382
Dilaudid Cough Syrup 1383
Dilaudid-HP Injection 1384
Dilaudid-HP Lyophilized Powder 250 mg 1384
Dilaudid 1382
Dilaudid Oral Liquid 1386
Dilaudid 1382
Dilaudid Tablets - 8 mg.......... 1386
Indapamide (Additive action).
No products indexed under this heading.
Insulin, Human (Changes in insulin requirements).
No products indexed under this heading.
Insulin, Human Isophane Suspension (Changes in insulin requirements). Products include:
Novolin N Human Insulin 10 ml Vials.......... 1846
Insulin, Human NPH (Changes in insulin requirements). Products include:
Humulin N, 100 Units.......... 1495
Novolin N PenFill 1.5 ml Cartridges Durable Insulin Delivery System 1849
Novolin N Prefilled Syringe Disposable Insulin Delivery System 1850
Insulin, Human Regular (Changes in insulin requirements). Products include:
Humulin R, 100 Units.......... 1497
Novolin R Human Insulin 10 ml Vials.......... 1846
Novolin R PenFill 1.5 ml Cartridges Durable Insulin Delivery System 1849
Novolin R Prefilled Syringe Disposable Insulin Delivery System 1850
Velosulin BR Human Insulin 10 ml Vials.......... 1847
Insulin, Human, Zinc Suspension (Changes in insulin requirements). Products include:
Humulin L, 100 Units 1494
Humulin U, 100 Units 1498
Novolin L Human Insulin 10 ml Vials.......... 1846
Insulin Lispro, Human (Changes in insulin requirements). Products include:
Humalog Injection 1488
Insulin, NPH (Changes in insulin requirements). Products include:
NPH, 100 Units 1502
Pork NPH, 100 Units.......... 1506
Purified Pork NPH Isophane Insulin 1852
Insulin, Regular (Changes in insulin requirements). Products include:
Regular, 100 Units 1503
Pork Regular, 100 Units 1507
Pork Regular (Concentrated), 500 Units 1508
Purified Pork Regular Insulin 1852
Insulin, Zinc Crystals (Changes in insulin requirements). Products include:
NPH, 100 Units 1502
Insulin, Zinc Suspension (Changes in insulin requirements). Products include:
Iletin I 1501
Lente, 100 Units 1501
Iletin II.......... 1504
Pork Lente, 100 Units.......... 1504
Purified Pork Lente Insulin 1852
Isradipine (Additive action). Products include:
DynaCirc Capsules 2381
DynaCirc CR Tablets 2383
Labetalol Hydrochloride (Additive action). Products include:
Normodyne Injection 2519
Normodyne Tablets 2522
Trandate 1158
Levobunolol Hydrochloride (Additive action). Products include:
Betagan .... ⊙ 230
Levorphanol Tartrate (Potentiates orthostatic hypotension). Products include:
Levo-Dromoran.......... 2297
Lisinopril (Additive action). Products include:
Prinivil Tablets 1776
Prinzide Tablets 1780
Zestoretic Tablets 2968
Zestril Tablets 2972
Lithium Carbonate (Increased risk of lithium toxicity). Products include:
Eskalith 2658
Lithium Carbonate Capsules & Tablets 2352
Lithonate/Lithotabs/Lithobid 2721
Lithium Citrate (Increased risk of lithium toxicity).
No products indexed under this heading.
Losartan Potassium (Additive action). Products include:
Cozaar Tablets 1668
Hyzaar Tablets 1720
Mecamylamine Hydrochloride (Additive or potentiative action). Products include:
Inversine Tablets 1729
Meperidine Hydrochloride (Potentiates orthostatic hypotension). Products include:
Demerol 2438
Mepergan Injection 2859
Mephobarbital (Potentiates orthostatic hypotension). Products include:
Mebaral Tablets 2452
Methadone Hydrochloride (Potentiates orthostatic hypotension). Products include:
Methadone Hydrochloride Oral Concentrate 2356
Methadone Hydrochloride Oral Solution & Tablets.......... 2357
Methyldopa (Additive action). Products include:
Aldoclor Tablets 1638
Aldomet Oral 1640
Aldoril Tablets.......... 1644
Methyldopate Hydrochloride (Additive action). Products include:
Aldomet Ester HCl Injection 1642
Methylprednisolone (Hypokalemia).
No products indexed under this heading.
Methylprednisolone Acetate (Hypokalemia).
No products indexed under this heading.
Methylprednisolone Sodium Succinate (Hypokalemia).
No products indexed under this heading.
Metipranolol Hydrochloride (Additive action). Products include:
OptiPranolol (Metipranolol 0.3%) Sterile Ophthalmic Solution.......... ⊙ 256
Metolazone (Additive action). Products include:
Mykrox Tablets 1617
Zaroxolyn Tablets 1625
Metoprolol Succinate (Additive action). Products include:
Toprol-XL Tablets 560
Metoprolol Tartrate (Additive action). Products include:
Lopressor 848
Lopressor HCT Tablets 850
Metyrosine (Additive action). Products include:
Demser Capsules.......... 1690
Minoxidil (Additive action).
No products indexed under this heading.
Moexipril Hydrochloride (Additive action). Products include:
Univasc Tablets 2553
Morphine Sulfate (Potentiates orthostatic hypotension). Products include:
Astramorph/PF Injection, USP (Preservative-Free) 526
Duramorph Injection 983
Infumorph 200 and Infumorph 500 Sterile Solutions.......... 985
Kadian Capsules.......... 2948
MS Contin Tablets.......... 2149
MSIR 2152
Oramorph SR (Morphine Sulfate Sustained Release Tablets) 2359
RMS Suppositories CII.......... 2766
Roxanol 2365
Nadolol (Additive action).
No products indexed under this heading.
Nicardipine Hydrochloride (Additive action). Products include:
Cardene Capsules.......... 2261
Cardene I.V. 2815
Cardene SR Capsules.......... 2264
Nifedipine (Additive action). Products include:
Adalat Capsules (10 mg and 20 mg) 580
Adalat CC 582
Procardia Capsules.......... 2024
Procardia XL Extended Release Tablets 2026
Nisoldipine (Additive action). Products include:
Sular Tablets 2961
Nitroglycerin (Additive action). Products include:
Deponit NTG Transdermal Delivery System 2541
Nitro-Bid IV.......... 1270
Nitro-Bid Ointment 1272

(▣ Described in PDR For Nonprescription Drugs) (⊙ Described in PDR For Ophthalmology)

Nitro-Dur (nitroglycerin) Transdermal Infusion System ... 1365
Nitrolingual Spray ... 2193
Nitrostat Tablets ... 1981
Transderm-Nitro Transdermal Therapeutic System ... 878

Norepinephrine Bitartrate (Decreased arterial responsiveness). Products include:
Levophed Bitartrate Injection ... 2445

Opium Alkaloids (Potentiates orthostatic hypotension).
No products indexed under this heading.

Oxycodone Hydrochloride (Potentiates orthostatic hypotension). Products include:
OxyContin Tablets ... 2163
OxyIR Capsules ... 2167
Percocet Tablets ... 955
Percodan Tablets ... 955
Percodan-Demi Tablets ... 956
Roxicodone Tablets, Oral Solution & Intensol (Oxycodone) ... 2366
Tylox Capsules ... 1593

Pancuronium Bromide (Decreased serum levels).
No products indexed under this heading.

Penbutolol Sulfate (Additive action). Products include:
Levatol Tablets ... 2547

Pentobarbital Sodium (Potentiates orthostatic hypotension). Products include:
Nembutal Sodium Capsules ... 440
Nembutal Sodium Solution ... 442
Nembutal Sodium Suppositories ... 444

Phenobarbital (Potentiates orthostatic hypotension). Products include:
Arco-Lase Plus Tablets ... 513
Bellergal-S Tablets ... 2375
Donnatal ... 2234
Donnatal Extentabs ... 2234
Donnatal Tablets ... 2234
Phenobarbital Elixir and Tablets ... 1523
Quadrinal Tablets ... 1398

Phenoxybenzamine Hydrochloride (Additive action). Products include:
Dibenzyline Capsules ... 2650

Phentolamine Mesylate (Additive action). Products include:
Regitine Vials ... 864

Pindolol (Additive action). Products include:
Visken Tablets ... 2428

Polythiazide (Additive action). Products include:
Minizide Capsules ... 2016

Prazosin Hydrochloride (Additive or potentiative action). Products include:
Minipress Capsules ... 2015
Minizide Capsules ... 2016

Prednisolone Acetate (Hypokalemia). Products include:
AK-CIDE ... ⊚ 203
AK-CIDE Ointment ... ⊚ 203
Blephamide Liquifilm Sterile Ophthalmic Suspension ... 472
Blephamide Ointment ... ⊚ 234
Econopred & Econopred Plus Ophthalmic Suspensions ... ⊚ 216
Poly-Pred Liquifilm ... ⊚ 246
Pred Forte ... ⊚ 247
Pred Mild ... ⊚ 250
Pred-G Liquifilm Sterile Ophthalmic Suspension ... ⊚ 248
Pred-G S.O.P. Sterile Ophthalmic Ointment ... ⊚ 249

Prednisolone Sodium Phosphate (Hypokalemia). Products include:
AK-PRED ... ⊚ 204
Hydeltrasol Injection, Sterile ... 1708
Pediapred Oral Solution ... 1618

Prednisolone Tebutate (Hypokalemia). Products include:
Hydeltra-T.B.A. Sterile Suspension ... 1710

Prednisone (Hypokalemia).
No products indexed under this heading.

Propoxyphene Hydrochloride (Potentiates orthostatic hypotension). Products include:
Darvon ... 1475
Wygesic Tablets ... 2930

Propoxyphene Napsylate (Potentiates orthostatic hypotension). Products include:
Darvon-N/Darvocet-N ... 1473

Propranolol Hydrochloride (Additive action). Products include:
Inderal ... 2834
Inderal LA Long Acting Capsules ... 2836
Inderide Tablets ... 2838
Inderide LA Long Acting Capsules ... 2840

Quinapril Hydrochloride (Additive action). Products include:
Accupril Tablets ... 1950

Ramipril (Additive action). Products include:
Altace Capsules ... 1238

Rauwolfia Serpentina (Additive or potentiative action).
No products indexed under this heading.

Rescinnamine (Additive or potentiative action).
No products indexed under this heading.

Reserpine (Additive or potentiative action). Products include:
Diupres Tablets ... 1691
Hydropres Tablets ... 1718
Ser-Ap-Es Tablets ... 867

Secobarbital Sodium (Potentiates orthostatic hypotension). Products include:
Seconal Sodium Pulvules ... 1529

Sodium Nitroprusside (Additive action).
No products indexed under this heading.

Sotalol Hydrochloride (Additive action). Products include:
Betapace Tablets ... 637

Spirapril Hydrochloride (Additive action).
No products indexed under this heading.

Sufentanil Citrate (Potentiates orthostatic hypotension). Products include:
Sufenta Injection ... 1355

Terazosin Hydrochloride (Additive or potentiative action). Products include:
Hytrin Capsules ... 434

Thiamylal Sodium (Potentiates orthostatic hypotension).
No products indexed under this heading.

Timolol Hemihydrate (Additive action). Products include:
Betimol 0.25%, 0.5% ... ⊚ 259

Timolol Maleate (Additive action). Products include:
Blocadren Tablets ... 1654
Timolide Tablets ... 1791
Timoptic in Ocudose ... 1796
Timoptic Sterile Ophthalmic Solution ... 1794
Timoptic-XE ... 1798

Torsemide (Additive action). Products include:
Demadex Tablets and Injection ... 691

Triamcinolone Acetonide (Hypokalemia). Products include:
Azmacort Oral Inhaler ... 2175
Nasacort AQ Nasal Spray ... 2191
Nasacort Nasal Inhaler ... 2189

Triamcinolone Diacetate (Hypokalemia).
No products indexed under this heading.

Triamcinolone Hexacetonide (Hypokalemia).
No products indexed under this heading.

Trimethaphan Camsylate (Additive or potentiative action).
No products indexed under this heading.

Tubocurarine Chloride (Increase responsiveness).
No products indexed under this heading.

Verapamil Hydrochloride (Additive action). Products include:
Calan SR Caplets ... 2571
Calan Tablets ... 2568
Covera-HS Tablets ... 2573
Isoptin Injectable ... 1391
Isoptin Oral Tablets ... 1393
Isoptin SR Tablets ... 1395
Verelan Capsules ... 1455

Food Interactions

Alcohol (Potentiates orthostatic hypotension).

ENGERIX-B UNIT-DOSE VIALS
(Hepatitis B Vaccine) ... 2656
None cited in PDR database.

ENSURE COMPLETE BALANCED NUTRITION
(Nutritional Supplement) ... 2338
None cited in PDR database.

ENSURE HIGH PROTEIN COMPLETE BALANCED NUTRITION
(Nutritional Beverage) ... 2337
None cited in PDR database.

ENSURE LIGHT COMPLETE, BALANCED NUTRITION
(Nutritional Supplement) ... 2338
None cited in PDR database.

ENSURE PLUS HIGH CALORIE COMPLETE NUTRITION
(Nutritional Supplement) ... 2338
None cited in PDR database.

ENSURE WITH FIBER COMPLETE, BALANCED NUTRITION
(Nutritional Supplement) ... 2338
None cited in PDR database.

ENTEX LA TABLETS
(Phenylpropanolamine Hydrochloride, Guaifenesin) ... 972
May interact with monoamine oxidase inhibitors and sympathomimetics. Compounds in these categories include:

Albuterol (Concurrent usage not recommended). Products include:
Proventil Inhalation Aerosol ... 2524
Ventolin Inhalation Aerosol and Refill ... 1170

Albuterol Sulfate (Concurrent usage not recommended). Products include:
Airet Albuterol Sulfate Inhalation Solution ... 1602
Albuterol Sulfate, USP Solution for Inhalation, Arm-a-Med ... 522
Proventil Inhalation Solution 0.083% ... 2527
Proventil Repetabs Tablets ... 2529
Proventil Solution for Inhalation 0.5% ... 2525
Proventil Syrup ... 2528
Proventil Tablets ... 2529
Ventolin Inhalation Solution ... 1171
Ventolin Nebules Inhalation Solution ... 1172
Ventolin Rotacaps for Inhalation ... 1173
Ventolin Syrup ... 1175
Ventolin Tablets ... 1176
Volmax Extended-Release Tablets ... 1835

Dobutamine Hydrochloride (Concurrent usage not recommended). Products include:
Dobutrex Solution Vials ... 1480

Dopamine Hydrochloride (Concurrent usage not recommended).
No products indexed under this heading.

Ephedrine Hydrochloride (Concurrent usage not recommended). Products include:
Primatene Tablets ... ⊚ 844
Quadrinal Tablets ... 1398

Ephedrine Sulfate (Concurrent usage not recommended). Products include:
Marax Tablets & DF Syrup ... 2015

Ephedrine Tannate (Concurrent usage not recommended). Products include:
Rynatuss ... 2782

Epinephrine (Concurrent usage not recommended). Products include:
EPIFRIN ... ⊚ 237
EpiPen ... 808
Marcaine with Epinephrine ... 2446
Primatene Mist ... ⊚ 843
Sensorcaine with Epinephrine Injection ... 554
Sus-Phrine Injection ... 1017
Xylocaine with Epinephrine Injections ... 562

Epinephrine Bitartrate (Concurrent usage not recommended). Products include:
Sensorcaine-MPF with Epinephrine Injection ... 554

Epinephrine Hydrochloride (Concurrent usage not recommended). Products include:
Ana-Kit Anaphylaxis Emergency Treatment Kit ... 611

Furazolidone (Concurrent use is contraindicated). Products include:
Furoxone ... 2221

Isocarboxazid (Concurrent use is contraindicated). Products include:
No products indexed under this heading.

Isoproterenol Hydrochloride (Concurrent usage not recommended). Products include:
Isuprel Hydrochloride Solution ... 2443
Isuprel Injection ... 2441
Isuprel Mistometer ... 2442

Isoproterenol Sulfate (Concurrent usage not recommended). Products include:
Norisodrine with Calcium Iodide Syrup ... 446

Metaproterenol Sulfate (Concurrent usage not recommended). Products include:
Alupent ... 672
Metaproterenol Sulfate Inhalation Solution, USP, Arm-a-Med ... 547

Metaraminol Bitartrate (Concurrent usage not recommended). Products include:
Aramine Injection ... 1649

Methoxamine Hydrochloride (Concurrent usage not recommended). Products include:
Vasoxyl Injection ... 1169

Norepinephrine Bitartrate (Concurrent usage not recommended). Products include:
Levophed Bitartrate Injection ... 2445

Phenelzine Sulfate (Concurrent use is contraindicated). Products include:
Nardil ... 1977

Phenylephrine Bitartrate (Concurrent usage not recommended).
No products indexed under this heading.

IMPORTANT NOTE: Always consult each drug listing in the patient's regimen for possible interactions.

Entex LA — Interactions Index — 378

Phenylephrine Hydrochloride (Concurrent usage not recommended). Products include:

Atrohist Plus Tablets	◨ 1605
Cerose DM	◨ 853
D.A. II Tablets	972
D.A. Chewable Tablets	970
Dura-Vent/DA Tablets	972
Extendryl	1003
4-Way Fast Acting Nasal Spray (regular & mentholated)	◨ 644
Hemoril	797
Hycomine Compound Tablets	948
Neo-Synephrine Hydrochloride 1% Carpuject	2455
Neo-Synephrine Hydrochloride 1% Injection	2455
Neo-Synephrine Hydrochloride (Ophthalmic)	2456
Neo-Synephrine	◨ 624
Novahistine Elixir	◨ 782
Phenergan VC	2886
Phenergan VC with Codeine	2888
Preparation H	◨ 842
Tympagesic Ear Drops	2476
Vicks Sinex Nasal Spray and Ultra Fine Mist	◨ 738

Phenylephrine Tannate (Concurrent usage not recommended). Products include:

Atrohist Pediatric Suspension	1604
Atrohist Pediatric Suspension Dye-Free	1604
Rynatan	2781
Rynatuss	2782

Pirbuterol Acetate (Concurrent usage not recommended). Products include:

Maxair Autohaler	1550
Maxair Inhaler	1552

Pseudoephedrine Hydrochloride (Concurrent usage not recommended). Products include:

Actifed Allergy Daytime/Nighttime Caplets	◨ 808
Actifed Cold & Allergy Tablets	◨ 807
Actifed Cold & Sinus Caplets and Tablets	◨ 808
Actifed Sinus Daytime/Nighttime Tablets and Caplets	◨ 809
Advil Cold and Sinus Caplets and Tablets	◨ 837
Alka-Seltzer Plus Liqui-Gels	◨ 612
Alka-Seltzer Plus Flu & Body Aches Liqui-Gels Non-Drowsy Formula	◨ 613
Alka-Seltzer Plus Night-Time Cold Medicine Liqui-Gels	◨ 612
Allerest Maximum Strength	◨ 649
Allerest No Drowsiness	◨ 649
Allerest Sinus Pain Formula	◨ 649
Atrohist Pediatric Capsules	1603
Benadryl Allergy/Cold Tablets	◨ 811
Benadryl Allergy Decongestant Liquid Medication	◨ 812
Benadryl Allergy Decongestant Tablets	◨ 812
Benadryl Allergy Sinus Headache Caplets	◨ 813
Benylin Multisymptom	◨ 816
Bromfed Capsules (Extended-Release)	1832
Bromfed Syrup	◨ 712
Bromfed Tablets	1832
Bromfed-DM Cough Syrup	1832
Bromfed-PD Capsules (Extended-Release)	1832
Children's TYLENOL Cold Multi-Symptom Chewable Tablets and Liquid	1559
Children's TYLENOL Cold Plus Cough Multi Symptom Chewable Tablets and Liquid	1560
Children's TYLENOL Flu Suspension Liquid	1560
Children's Vicks DayQuil Allergy Relief	◨ 730
Children's Vicks NyQuil Cold/Cough Relief	◨ 731
Allergy-Sinus Comtrex Multi-Symptom Allergy-Sinus Formula Tablets and Caplets	◨ 639
Comtrex Multi-Symptom	◨ 638
Comtrex Multi-Symptom Non-Drowsy Caplets	◨ 640
Congess	1003
Contac Day Allergy/Sinus Caplets	◨ 771
Contac Day & Night	◨ 772
Contac Night Allergy/Sinus Caplets	◨ 771
Contac Severe Cold & Flu Non-Drowsy	◨ 774
Deconsal II Tablets	1605
Dimetane-DX Cough Syrup	2233
Dimetapp Cold & Fever Suspension	◨ 839
Dimetapp Decongestant Pediatric Drops	◨ 840
Dorcol Children's Cough Syrup	◨ 748
Drixoral Cough + Congestion Liquid Caps	◨ 763
Dura-Tap/PD Capsules	970
Duratuss Tablets	2750
Duratuss HD Elixir	2750
Efidac/24	◨ 655
Entex PSE Tablets	973
Fedahist Gyrocaps	2545
Guaifed	1833
Guaifed Syrup	◨ 712
Guaimax-D Tablets	809
Histussin D Liquid	670
Infants' TYLENOL Cold Decongestant & Fever-Reducer Drops	1561
Kronofed-A	994
Novahistine DMX	◨ 782
Nucofed	2225
PediaCare Cough-Cold Chewable Tablets and Liquid	1569
PediaCare Infants' Decongestant Drops	1569
PediaCare Infants' Drops Decongestant Plus Cough	1569
PediaCare NightRest Cough-Cold Liquid	1569
Pediatric Vicks 44d Cough & Head Congestion Relief	◨ 736
Pediatric Vicks 44m Cough & Cold Relief	◨ 737
Robitussin Cold & Cough Liqui-Gels	◨ 844
Robitussin Cold, Cough & Flu Liqui-Gels	◨ 844
Robitussin Maximum Strength Cough & Cold	◨ 847
Robitussin Night-Time Cold Formula	◨ 847
Robitussin Pediatric Cough & Cold Formula	◨ 848
Robitussin Pediatric Drops	◨ 849
Robitussin Severe Congestion Liqui-Gels	◨ 845
Robitussin-DAC Syrup	2249
Robitussin-PE	◨ 846
Rondec Oral Drops	974
Rondec Syrup	974
Rondec Tablet	974
Rondec Chewable Tablets	974
Rondec-TR Tablet	◨ 804
Ryna	◨ 804
Seldane-D Extended-Release Tablets	1286
Semprex-D Capsules	1620
Sinarest	◨ 663
Sine-Aid Maximum Strength Sinus Headache Gelcaps, Caplets and Tablets	1570
Sine-Off No Drowsiness Formula Caplets	◨ 784
Sine-Off Sinus Medicine	◨ 784
Singlet Tablets	◨ 785
Sinutab Non-Drying Liquid Caps	◨ 823
Sinutab Sinus Allergy Medication, Maximum Strength Tablets and Caplets	◨ 823
Sinutab Sinus Medication, Maximum Strength Without Drowsiness Formula, Tablets & Caplets	◨ 824
Sudafed Children's Cold & Cough Liquid Medication	825
Sudafed Children's Nasal Decongestant Liquid Medication	◨ 826
Sudafed Cold & Allergy Tablets	◨ 826
Sudafed Cold and Cough Liquid Caps	◨ 826
Sudafed Nasal Decongestant Tablets, 30 mg	◨ 825
Sudafed Nasal Decongestant Tablets, 60 mg	◨ 825
Sudafed Non-Drying Sinus Liquid Caps	◨ 827
Sudafed Pediatric Nasal Decongestant Liquid Oral Drops	◨ 827
Sudafed Severe Cold Formula Caplets	◨ 828
Sudafed Severe Cold Formula Tablets	◨ 828
Sudafed Sinus Caplets	◨ 829
Sudafed Sinus Tablets	◨ 829
Sudafed 12 Hour Caplets	◨ 824
Syn-Rx Tablets	1622
Syn-Rx DM Tablets	1623
TheraFlu Flu and Cold Medicine	◨ 750
Theraflu Maximum Strength Flu and Cold Medicine For Sore Throat	◨ 751
TheraFlu Flu, Cold and Cough Medicine	◨ 750
TheraFlu Maximum Strength Nighttime Flu, Cold & Cough Medicine	◨ 751
TheraFlu Maximum Strength Non-Drowsy Formula Flu, Cold & Cough Medicine	◨ 751
TheraFlu Maximum Strength, Non-Drowsy Formula Flu, Cold and Cough Caplets	◨ 752
TheraFlu Maximum Strength Sinus Non-Drowsy Formula Caplets	◨ 752
Triaminic AM Cough and Decongestant Formula	◨ 753
Triaminic AM Decongestant Formula	◨ 753
Triaminic Infant Oral Decongestant Drops	◨ 754
Triaminic Night Time	◨ 754
Triaminic Sore Throat Formula	◨ 755
Tussend	1830
Tussend Expectorant	1831
TYLENOL Allergy Sinus, Maximum Strength Caplets and Gelcaps	1571
TYLENOL Allergy Sinus NightTime, Maximum Strength Caplets	1571
TYLENOL Cold Medication, Multi-Symptom Formula Tablets and Caplets	1572
TYLENOL Cold Medication, Multi-Symptom Hot Liquid Packets	1572
TYLENOL Cold Medication, No Drowsiness Formula Caplets and Gelcaps	1572
TYLENOL Cold Severe Congestion Caplets	1573
TYLENOL Cough Medication with Decongestant, Multi Symptom	1574
TYLENOL Flu No Drowsiness Formula, Maximum Strength Gelcaps	1575
TYLENOL Flu NightTime, Maximum Strength Gelcaps	1575
TYLENOL Flu NightTime, Maximum Strength Hot Medication Packets	1575
TYLENOL Sinus, Maximum Strength Geltabs, Gelcaps, Caplets and Tablets	1576
Vicks 44 LiquiCaps Cough, Cold & Flu Relief	◨ 728
Vicks 44 LiquiCaps Non-Drowsy Cough & Cold Relief	◨ 729
Vicks 44D Cough & Head Congestion Relief	◨ 728
Vicks 44M Cough, Cold & Flu Relief	◨ 729
Vicks DayQuil LiquiCaps/Liquid Multi-Symptom Cold/Flu Relief	◨ 734
Vicks DayQuil SINUS Pressure & PAIN Relief with IBUPROFEN	◨ 735
Vicks Nyquil Hot Therapy	◨ 735
Vicks NyQuil LiquiCaps/Liquid Multi-Symptom Cold/Flu Relief, Original and Cherry Flavors	◨ 736

Pseudoephedrine Sulfate (Concurrent usage not recommended). Products include:

Chlor-Trimeton Allergy Decongestant Tablets	◨ 759
Claritin-D Tablets	2487
Drixoral Cold and Allergy Sustained-Action Tablets	◨ 763
Drixoral Cold and Flu Extended-Release Tablets	◨ 764
Drixoral Non-Drowsy Formula Extended-Release Tablets	◨ 764
Drixoral Allergy/Sinus Extended Release Tablets	◨ 765
Trinalin Repetabs Tablets	1373

Salmeterol Xinafoate (Concurrent usage not recommended). Products include:

Serevent Inhalation Aerosol	1149

Selegiline Hydrochloride (Concurrent use is contraindicated). Products include:

Eldepryl Capsules	2729

Terbutaline Sulfate (Concurrent usage not recommended). Products include:

Brethaire Inhaler	830
Brethine Ampuls	832
Brethine Tablets	831
Bricanyl Subcutaneous Injection	1247
Bricanyl Tablets	1248

Tranylcypromine Sulfate (Concurrent use is contraindicated). Products include:

Parnate Tablets	2679

ENTEX PSE TABLETS
(Pseudoephedrine Hydrochloride, Guaifenesin) ... 973
May interact with monoamine oxidase inhibitors, beta blockers, veratrum alkaloids, catecholamine depleting drugs, and certain other agents. Compounds in these categories include:

Acebutolol Hydrochloride (Increases effects of sympathomimetics). Products include:

Sectral Capsules	2914

Atenolol (Increases effects of sympathomimetics). Products include:

Tenoretic Tablets	2963
Tenormin Tablets and I.V. Injection	2965

Betaxolol Hydrochloride (Increases effects of sympathomimetics). Products include:

Betoptic Ophthalmic Solution	465
Betoptic S Ophthalmic Suspension	467
Kerlone Tablets	2588

Bisoprolol Fumarate (Increases effects of sympathomimetics). Products include:

Zebeta Tablets	1457
Ziac	1459

Carteolol Hydrochloride (Increases effects of sympathomimetics). Products include:

Cartrol Tablets	413
Ocupress Ophthalmic Solution, 1% Sterile	⊙ 297

Cryptenamine Preparations (Reduced antihypertensive effects).

Deserpidine (Reduced antihypertensive effects).
No products indexed under this heading.

Esmolol Hydrochloride (Increases effects of sympathomimetics). Products include:

Brevibloc (esmolol HCl) Injection	1860

Furazolidone (Increases effects of sympathomimetics; concurrent administration is contraindicated). Products include:

Furoxone	2221

Guanethidine Monosulfate (Reduced antihypertensive effects). Products include:

Esimil Tablets	840
Ismelin Tablets	845

Isocarboxazid (Increases effects of sympathomimetics; concurrent administration is contraindicated).
No products indexed under this heading.

Labetalol Hydrochloride (Increases effects of sympathomimetics). Products include:

Normodyne Injection	2519
Normodyne Tablets	2522
Trandate	1158

Levobunolol Hydrochloride (Increases effects of sympathomimetics). Products include:

Betagan	⊙ 230

Mecamylamine Hydrochloride (Reduced antihypertensive effects). Products include:

Inversine Tablets	1729

Methyldopa (Reduced antihypertensive effects). Products include:

Aldoclor Tablets	1638

(◨ Described in PDR For Nonprescription Drugs)   (⊙ Described in PDR For Ophthalmology)

Aldomet Oral 1640
Aldoril Tablets 1644
Metipranolol Hydrochloride (Increases effects of sympathomimetics). Products include:
    OptiPranolol (Metipranolol 0.3%) Sterile Ophthalmic Solution ...... ⓔ 256
Metoprolol Succinate (Increases effects of sympathomimetics). Products include:
    Toprol-XL Tablets 560
Metoprolol Tartrate (Increases effects of sympathomimetics). Products include:
    Lopressor 848
    Lopressor HCT Tablets 850
Nadolol (Increases effects of sympathomimetics).
    No products indexed under this heading.
Penbutolol Sulfate (Increases effects of sympathomimetics). Products include:
    Levatol Tablets 2547
Phenelzine Sulfate (Increases effects of sympathomimetics; concurrent administration is contraindicated). Products include:
    Nardil 1977
Pindolol (Increases effects of sympathomimetics). Products include:
    Visken Tablets 2428
Propranolol Hydrochloride (Increases effects of sympathomimetics). Products include:
    Inderal 2834
    Inderal LA Long Acting Capsules 2836
    Inderide Tablets 2838
    Inderide LA Long Acting Capsules .. 2840
Rauwolfia Serpentina (Reduced antihypertensive effects).
    No products indexed under this heading.
Rescinnamine (Reduced antihypertensive effects).
    No products indexed under this heading.
Reserpine (Reduced antihypertensive effects). Products include:
    Diupres Tablets 1691
    Hydropres Tablets 1718
    Ser-Ap-Es Tablets 867
Selegiline Hydrochloride (Increases effects of sympathomimetics; concurrent administration is contraindicated). Products include:
    Eldepryl Capsules 2729
Sotalol Hydrochloride (Increases effects of sympathomimetics). Products include:
    Betapace Tablets 637
Timolol Hemihydrate (Increases effects of sympathomimetics). Products include:
    Betimol 0.25%, 0.5% .... ⓔ 259
Timolol Maleate (Increases effects of sympathomimetics). Products include:
    Blocadren Tablets 1654
    Timolide Tablets 1791
    Timoptic in Ocudose 1796
    Timoptic Sterile Ophthalmic Solution 1794
    Timoptic-XE 1798
Tranylcypromine Sulfate (Increases effects of sympathomimetics; concurrent administration is contraindicated). Products include:
    Parnate Tablets 2679

EPIFOAM
(Hydrocortisone Acetate, Pramoxine Hydrochloride) 2543
None cited in PDR database.

EPIFRIN
(Epinephrine) .... ⓔ 237
None cited in PDR database.

EPIPEN–EPINEPHRINE AUTO-INJECTOR
(Epinephrine) 808
May interact with tricyclic antidepressants, monoamine oxidase inhibitors, cardiac glycosides, and certain other agents. Compounds in these categories include:

Amitriptyline Hydrochloride (Potentiation of epinephrine). Products include:
    Elavil 2945
    Etrafon 2495
    Limbitrol 2333
    Triavil Tablets 1800
Amoxapine (Potentiation of epinephrine). Products include:
    Asendin Tablets 1419
Clomipramine Hydrochloride (Potentiation of epinephrine). Products include:
    Anafranil Capsules 819
Desipramine Hydrochloride (Potentiation of epinephrine). Products include:
    Norpramin Tablets 1273
Deslanoside (Concurrent use is not recommended).
    No products indexed under this heading.
Digitoxin (Concurrent use is not recommended). Products include:
    Crystodigin Tablets 1472
Digoxin (Concurrent use is not recommended). Products include:
    Lanoxicaps 1110
    Lanoxin Elixir Pediatric 1113
    Lanoxin Injection 1116
    Lanoxin Injection Pediatric 1119
    Lanoxin Tablets 1121
Doxepin Hydrochloride (Potentiation of epinephrine). Products include:
    Adapin Capsules 1542
    Sinequan 2028
    Zonalon Cream 1042
Furazolidone (Potentiation of epinephrine). Products include:
    Furoxone 2221
Imipramine Hydrochloride (Potentiation of epinephrine). Products include:
    Tofranil Ampuls 873
    Tofranil Tablets 875
Imipramine Pamoate (Potentiation of epinephrine). Products include:
    Tofranil-PM Capsules 876
Isocarboxazid (Potentiation of epinephrine).
    No products indexed under this heading.
Maprotiline Hydrochloride (Potentiation of epinephrine). Products include:
    Ludiomil Tablets 861
Nortriptyline Hydrochloride (Potentiation of epinephrine). Products include:
    Pamelor 2409
Phenelzine Sulfate (Potentiation of epinephrine). Products include:
    Nardil 1977
Protriptyline Hydrochloride (Potentiation of epinephrine). Products include:
    Vivactil Tablets 1820
Quinidine Gluconate (Concurrent use is not recommended). Products include:
    Quinaglute Dura-Tabs Tablets 644
Quinidine Polygalacturonate (Concurrent use is not recommended). Products include:
    Cardioquin Tablets 2146
Quinidine Sulfate (Concurrent use is not recommended). Products include:
    Quinidex Extentabs 2240
Selegiline Hydrochloride (Potentiation of epinephrine). Products include:
    Eldepryl Capsules 2729
Tranylcypromine Sulfate (Potentiation of epinephrine). Products include:
    Parnate Tablets 2679
Trimipramine Maleate (Potentiation of epinephrine). Products include:
    Surmontil Capsules 2917

EPIPEN JR.- EPINEPHRINE AUTO-INJECTOR
(Epinephrine) 808
See EpiPen–Epinephrine Auto-Injector

EPIVIR ORAL SOLUTION
(Lamivudine) 1200
See Epivir Tablets

EPIVIR TABLETS
(Lamivudine) 1200
May interact with:

Sulfamethoxazole (Co-administration with TMP/SMX results in an increase of 44% +/−23% (mean +/−S.D.) in lamivudine AUC (infinity); decreases oral and clearance). Products include:
    Bactrim DS Tablets 2257
    Bactrim I.V. Infusion 2255
    Bactrim 2257
    Gantanol Tablets 2285
    Septra 1146
    Septra I.V. Infusion 1142
    Septra I.V. Infusion ADD-Vantage Vials 1144
    Septra 1146
Trimethoprim (Co-administration with TMP/SMX results in an increase of 44% +/−23% (mean +/−S.D.) in lamivudine AUC (infinity); decreases oral and clearance). Products include:
    Bactrim DS Tablets 2257
    Bactrim I.V. Infusion 2255
    Bactrim 2257
    Proloprim Tablets 1141
    Septra 1146
    Septra I.V. Infusion 1142
    Septra I.V. Infusion ADD-Vantage Vials 1144
    Septra 1146
    Trimpex Tablets 2323
Zidovudine (Co-administration results in increase of 39% +/−62% (mean +/−S.D.) In C_{max} zidovudine; no significant differences in AUC (infinity) or total clearance for lamivudine or zidovudine). Products include:
    Retrovir Capsules 1216
    Retrovir I.V. Infusion 1221
    Retrovir Syrup 1216

Food Interactions
Food, unspecified (Food slows the absorption; no significant difference in systemic exposure AUC (infinity) in the fed and fasted states).

EPOGEN FOR INJECTION
(Epoetin Alfa) 489
None cited in PDR database.

ERGAMISOL TABLETS
(Levamisole Hydrochloride) 1340
May interact with oral anticoagulants and certain other agents. Compounds in these categories include:

Dicumarol (Prolongation of the prothrombin time beyond the therapeutic range when co-administered; monitor PT and the dose of warfarin or other coumarin-like drugs should be adjusted accordingly).
    No products indexed under this heading.
Fluorouracil (Combination therapy may result in marked elevation in triglyceride levels). Products include:
    Efudex 2280
    Fluoroplex Topical Solution & Cream 1% 475
    Fluorouracil Injection 2282
Fosphenytoin Sodium (Co-administration of phenytoin and levamisole plus fluorouracil has led to increased phenytoin plasma levels). Products include:
    Cerebyx Injection 1956
Phenytoin (Co-administration of phenytoin and levamisole plus fluorouracil has led to increased phenytoin plasma levels). Products include:
    Dilantin Infatabs 1967
    Dilantin-125 Suspension 1969
Phenytoin Sodium (Co-administration of phenytoin and levamisole plus fluorouracil has led to increased phenytoin plasma levels). Products include:
    Dilantin Kapseals 1965
Warfarin Sodium (Prolongation of the prothrombin time beyond the therapeutic range when co-administered; monitor PT and the dose of warfarin or other coumarin-like drugs should be adjusted accordingly). Products include:
    Coumadin 941

Food Interactions
Alcohol (May result in ∎ANTABUSE∎-like side effects).

ERGOMAR TABLETS
(Ergotamine Tartrate) 1543
May interact with vasopressors and certain other agents. Compounds in these categories include:

Dopamine Hydrochloride (The pressor effects of Ergomar and other vasoconstrictor drugs can combine to cause dangerous hypertension).
    No products indexed under this heading.
Epinephrine Bitartrate (The pressor effects of Ergomar and other vasoconstrictor drugs can combine to cause dangerous hypertension). Products include:
    Sensorcaine-MPF with Epinephrine Injection 554
Epinephrine Hydrochloride (The pressor effects of Ergomar and other vasoconstrictor drugs can combine to cause dangerous hypertension). Products include:
    Ana-Kit Anaphylaxis Emergency Treatment Kit 611
Metaraminol Bitartrate (The pressor effects of Ergomar and other vasoconstrictor drugs can combine to cause dangerous hypertension). Products include:
    Aramine Injection 1649
Methoxamine Hydrochloride (The pressor effects of Ergomar and other vasoconstrictor drugs can combine to cause dangerous hypertension). Products include:
    Vasoxyl Injection 1169
Norepinephrine Bitartrate (The pressor effects of Ergomar and other vasoconstrictor drugs can combine to cause dangerous hypertension). Products include:
    Levophed Bitartrate Injection 2445

IMPORTANT NOTE: Always consult each drug listing in the patient's regimen for possible interactions.

Ergomar

Phenylephrine Hydrochloride (The pressor effects of Ergomar and other vasoconstrictor drugs can combine to cause dangerous hypertension). Products include:

Atrohist Plus Tablets	1605
Cerose DM	■ 853
D.A. II Tablets	972
D.A. Chewable Tablets	970
Dura-Vent/DA Tablets	972
Extendryl	1003
4-Way Fast Acting Nasal Spray (regular & mentholated)	■ 644
Hemoril	■ 797
Hycomine Compound Tablets	948
Neo-Synephrine Hydrochloride 1% Carpuject	2455
Neo-Synephrine Hydrochloride 1% Injection	2455
Neo-Synephrine Hydrochloride (Ophthalmic)	2456
Neo-Synephrine	■ 624
Novahistine Elixir	■ 782
Phenergan VC	2886
Phenergan VC with Codeine	2888
Preparation H	■ 842
Tympagesic Ear Drops	2476
Vicks Sinex Nasal Spray and Ultra Fine Mist	■ 738

Troleandomycin (Triacetyloleandomycin inhibits the metabolism of ergotamine; potentiates the effects of Ergomar). Products include:

Tao Capsules	2033

ERYC
(Erythromycin) 1972
May interact with xanthine bronchodilators, oral anticoagulants, drugs which undergo biotransformation by cytochrome p-450 mixed function oxidase, and certain other agents. Compounds in these categories include:

Aminophylline (Co-administration with high doses of theophylline may be associated with increased serum theophylline levels and potential theophylline toxicity).
  No products indexed under this heading.

Carbamazepine (Concurrent use may be associated with elevation in serum level of carbamazepine; monitor serum levels closely). Products include:

Atretol Tablets	569
Tegretol/Tegretol-XR	870

Cyclosporine (Concurrent use may be associated with elevation in serum level of cyclosporine; monitor serum levels closely). Products include:

Neoral	2405
Sandimmune	2416

Dicumarol (Concomitant therapy may result in increased anticoagulant effects).
  No products indexed under this heading.

Digoxin (Co-administration may result in elevated digoxin serum levels). Products include:

Lanoxicaps	1110
Lanoxin Elixir Pediatric	1113
Lanoxin Injection	1116
Lanoxin Injection Pediatric	1119
Lanoxin Tablets	1121

Dihydroergotamine Mesylate (Concurrent use has been associated with acute ergot toxicity characterized by severe peripheral vasospasm and dysesthesia). Products include:

D.H.E. 45 Injection	2381

Drugs which undergo biotransformation by cytochrome P-450 mixed function oxidase (Concurrent use may be associated with elevation in serum level of drugs metabolized by the cytochrome P450 system).

Dyphylline (Co-administration with high doses of theophylline may be associated with increased serum theophylline levels and potential theophylline toxicity). Products include:

Lufyllin & Lufyllin-400 Tablets	2778
Lufyllin-GG Elixir & Tablets	2779

Ergotamine Tartrate (Concurrent use has been associated with acute ergot toxicity characterized by severe peripheral vasospasm and dysesthesia). Products include:

Bellergal-S Tablets	2375
Cafergot	2376
Ergomar Tablets	1543
Wigraine Tablets	1884

Hexobarbital (Concurrent use may be associated with elevation in serum level of hexobarbital; monitor serum levels closely).

Phenytoin (Concurrent use may be associated with elevation in serum level of phenytoin; monitor serum levels closely). Products include:

Dilantin Infatabs	1967
Dilantin-125 Suspension	1969

Phenytoin Sodium (Concurrent use may be associated with elevation in serum level of phenytoin; monitor serum levels closely). Products include:

Dilantin Kapseals	1965

Terfenadine (Erythromycin significantly alters the metabolism of terfenadine when used concomitantly; potential for rare cases of serious cardiovascular adverse events, including death, cardiac arrest, torsade de pointes and other ventricular arrhythmias; concurrent use is contraindicated). Products include:

Seldane Tablets	1284
Seldane-D Extended-Release Tablets	1286

Theophylline (Co-administration with high doses of theophylline may be associated with increased serum theophylline levels and potential theophylline toxicity). Products include:

Marax Tablets & DF Syrup	2015
Quibron	2227

Theophylline Anhydrous (Co-administration with high doses of theophylline may be associated with increased serum theophylline levels and potential theophylline toxicity). Products include:

Aerolate	1003
Primatene Tablets	■ 844
Respbid Tablets	687
Slo-bid Gyrocaps	2201
Theo-24 Extended Release Capsules	2753
Theo-Dur Extended-Release Tablets	1367
Theo-X Extended-Release Tablets	793
Uni-Dur Extended-Release Tablets	1374
Uniphyl 400 mg and 600 mg Tablets	2157

Theophylline Calcium Salicylate (Co-administration with high doses of theophylline may be associated with increased serum theophylline levels and potential theophylline toxicity). Products include:

Quadrinal Tablets	1398

Theophylline Sodium Glycinate (Co-administration with high doses of theophylline may be associated with increased serum theophylline levels and potential theophylline toxicity).
  No products indexed under this heading.

Triazolam (Decrease clearance of triazolam; potential for increased pharmacological effect of triazolam). Products include:

Halcion Tablets	2093

Warfarin Sodium (Concomitant therapy may result in increased anticoagulant effects). Products include:

Coumadin	941

Food Interactions
Meal, unspecified (Optimum blood levels are obtained on a fasting stomach; administration is preferable one-half hour pre- or two hours post-meal).

ERYCETTE (ERYTHROMYCIN 2%) TOPICAL SOLUTION
(Erythromycin) 1943
None cited in PDR database.

ERYPED DROPS AND CHEWABLE TABLETS
(Erythromycin Ethylsuccinate) 425
May interact with xanthine bronchodilators, oral anticoagulants, and certain other agents. Compounds in these categories include:

Aminophylline (Concomitant administration with high doses of theophylline may be associated with increased theophylline levels and potential toxicity).
  No products indexed under this heading.

Carbamazepine (Elevations in serum erythromycin and carbamazepine concentration). Products include:

Atretol Tablets	569
Tegretol/Tegretol-XR	870

Cyclosporine (Elevations in serum erythromycin and cyclosporine concentration). Products include:

Neoral	2405
Sandimmune	2416

Dicumarol (Increased anticoagulant effects).
  No products indexed under this heading.

Digoxin (Elevated digoxin serum levels). Products include:

Lanoxicaps	1110
Lanoxin Elixir Pediatric	1113
Lanoxin Injection	1116
Lanoxin Injection Pediatric	1119
Lanoxin Tablets	1121

Dihydroergotamine Mesylate (Potential for acute ergot toxicity characterized by severe peripheral vasospasm and dysesthesia). Products include:

D.H.E. 45 Injection	2381

Dyphylline (Concomitant administration with high doses of theophylline may be associated with increased theophylline levels and potential toxicity). Products include:

Lufyllin & Lufyllin-400 Tablets	2778
Lufyllin-GG Elixir & Tablets	2779

Ergotamine Tartrate (Potential for acute ergot toxicity characterized by severe peripheral vasospasm and dysesthesia). Products include:

Bellergal-S Tablets	2375
Cafergot	2376
Ergomar Tablets	1543
Wigraine Tablets	1884

Hexobarbital (Elevations in serum erythromycin and hexobarbital concentration).

Lovastatin (Potential for rhabdomyolysis in seriously ill patients). Products include:

Mevacor Tablets	1742

Phenytoin (Elevations in serum erythromycin and phenytoin concentration). Products include:

Dilantin Infatabs	1967
Dilantin-125 Suspension	1969

Phenytoin Sodium (Elevations in serum erythromycin and phenytoin concentration). Products include:

Dilantin Kapseals	1965

Terfenadine (Potential for altered terfenadine metabolism). Products include:

Seldane Tablets	1284
Seldane-D Extended-Release Tablets	1286

Theophylline (Concomitant administration with high doses of theophylline may be associated with increased theophylline levels and potential toxicity). Products include:

Marax Tablets & DF Syrup	2015
Quibron	2227

Theophylline Anhydrous (Concomitant administration with high doses of theophylline may be associated with increased theophylline levels and potential toxicity). Products include:

Aerolate	1003
Primatene Tablets	■ 844
Respbid Tablets	687
Slo-bid Gyrocaps	2201
Theo-24 Extended Release Capsules	2753
Theo-Dur Extended-Release Tablets	1367
Theo-X Extended-Release Tablets	793
Uni-Dur Extended-Release Tablets	1374
Uniphyl 400 mg and 600 mg Tablets	2157

Theophylline Calcium Salicylate (Concomitant administration with high doses of theophylline may be associated with increased theophylline levels and potential toxicity). Products include:

Quadrinal Tablets	1398

Theophylline Sodium Glycinate (Concomitant administration with high doses of theophylline may be associated with increased theophylline levels and potential toxicity).
  No products indexed under this heading.

Triazolam (Decreased clearance of triazolam and increased the pharmacologic effect of triazolam). Products include:

Halcion Tablets	2093

Warfarin Sodium (Increased anticoagulant effects). Products include:

Coumadin	941

ERYPED 200 & ERYPED 400 GRANULES
(Erythromycin Ethylsuccinate) 425
  See ErypPed Drops and Chewable Tablets

ERY-TAB TABLETS
(Erythromycin) 426
May interact with xanthine bronchodilators, oral anticoagulants, and certain other agents. Compounds in these categories include:

Aminophylline (Concomitant administration with high doses of theophylline may be associated with increased theophylline levels and potential toxicity).
  No products indexed under this heading.

Carbamazepine (Elevations in serum erythromycin and carbamazepine concentration). Products include:

Atretol Tablets	569
Tegretol/Tegretol-XR	870

(■ Described in PDR For Nonprescription Drugs)   (◎ Described in PDR For Ophthalmology)

Cyclosporine (Elevations in serum erythromycin and cyclosporine concentration). Products include:
- Neoral 2405
- Sandimmune 2416

Dicumarol (Increased anticoagulant effects).
- No products indexed under this heading.

Digoxin (Elevated digoxin serum levels). Products include:
- Lanoxicaps 1110
- Lanoxin Elixir Pediatric 1113
- Lanoxin Injection 1116
- Lanoxin Injection Pediatric 1119
- Lanoxin Tablets 1121

Dihydroergotamine Mesylate (Potential for acute ergot toxicity characterized by severe peripheral vasospasm and dysesthesia). Products include:
- D.H.E. 45 Injection 2381

Dyphylline (Concomitant administration with high doses of theophylline may be associated with increased theophylline levels and potential toxicity). Products include:
- Lufyllin & Lufyllin-400 Tablets 2778
- Lufyllin-GG Elixir & Tablets 2779

Ergotamine Tartrate (Potential for acute ergot toxicity characterized by severe peripheral vasospasm and dysesthesia). Products include:
- Bellergal-S Tablets 2375
- Cafergot 2376
- Ergomar Tablets 1543
- Wigraine Tablets 1884

Hexobarbital (Elevations in serum erythromycin and hexobarbital concentration).

Lovastatin (Potential for rhabdomyolysis in seriously ill patients). Products include:
- Mevacor Tablets 1742

Phenytoin (Elevations in serum erythromycin and phenytoin concentration). Products include:
- Dilantin Infatabs 1967
- Dilantin-125 Suspension 1969

Phenytoin Sodium (Elevations in serum erythromycin and phenytoin concentration). Products include:
- Dilantin Kapseals 1965

Terfenadine (Potential for altered terfenadine metabolism). Products include:
- Seldane Tablets 1284
- Seldane-D Extended-Release Tablets 1286

Theophylline (Concomitant administration with high doses of theophylline may be associated with increased theophylline levels and potential toxicity). Products include:
- Marax Tablets & DF Syrup 2015
- Quibron 2227

Theophylline Anhydrous (Concomitant administration with high doses of theophylline may be associated with increased theophylline levels and potential toxicity). Products include:
- Aerolate 1003
- Primatene Tablets 844
- Respbid Tablets 687
- Slo-bid Gyrocaps 2201
- Theo-24 Extended Release Capsules 2753
- Theo-Dur Extended-Release Tablets 1367
- Theo-X Extended-Release Tablets 793
- Uni-Dur Extended-Release Tablets 1374
- Uniphyl 400 mg and 600 mg Tablets 2157

Theophylline Calcium Salicylate (Concomitant administration with high doses of theophylline may be associated with increased theophylline levels and potential toxicity). Products include:
- Quadrinal Tablets 1398

Theophylline Sodium Glycinate (Concomitant administration with high doses of theophylline may be associated with increased theophylline levels and potential toxicity).
- No products indexed under this heading.

Triazolam (Decreased clearance of triazolam and increased the pharmacologic effect of triazolam). Products include:
- Halcion Tablets 2093

Warfarin Sodium (Increased anticoagulant effects). Products include:
- Coumadin 941

ERYTHROCIN STEARATE FILMTAB

(Erythromycin Stearate) 429

May interact with xanthine bronchodilators, oral anticoagulants, and certain other agents. Compounds in these categories include:

Aminophylline (Concomitant administration with high doses of theophylline may be associated with increased theophylline levels and potential toxicity).
- No products indexed under this heading.

Carbamazepine (Elevations in serum erythromycin and carbamazepine concentration). Products include:
- Atretol Tablets 569
- Tegretol/Tegretol-XR 870

Cyclosporine (Elevations in serum erythromycin and cyclosporine concentration). Products include:
- Neoral 2405
- Sandimmune 2416

Dicumarol (Increased anticoagulant effects).
- No products indexed under this heading.

Digoxin (Elevated digoxin serum levels). Products include:
- Lanoxicaps 1110
- Lanoxin Elixir Pediatric 1113
- Lanoxin Injection 1116
- Lanoxin Injection Pediatric 1119
- Lanoxin Tablets 1121

Dihydroergotamine Mesylate (Potential for acute ergot toxicity characterized by severe peripheral vasospasm and dysesthesia). Products include:
- D.H.E. 45 Injection 2381

Dyphylline (Concomitant administration with high doses of theophylline may be associated with increased theophylline levels and potential toxicity). Products include:
- Lufyllin & Lufyllin-400 Tablets 2778
- Lufyllin-GG Elixir & Tablets 2779

Ergotamine Tartrate (Potential for acute ergot toxicity characterized by severe peripheral vasospasm and dysesthesia). Products include:
- Bellergal-S Tablets 2375
- Cafergot 2376
- Ergomar Tablets 1543
- Wigraine Tablets 1884

Hexobarbital (Elevations in serum erythromycin and hexobarbital concentration).

Lovastatin (Potential for rhabdomyolysis in seriously ill patients). Products include:
- Mevacor Tablets 1742

Phenytoin (Elevations in serum erythromycin and phenytoin concentration). Products include:
- Dilantin Infatabs 1967
- Dilantin-125 Suspension 1969

Phenytoin Sodium (Elevations in serum erythromycin and phenytoin concentration). Products include:
- Dilantin Kapseals 1965

Terfenadine (Potential for altered terfenadine metabolism). Products include:
- Seldane Tablets 1284
- Seldane-D Extended-Release Tablets 1286

Theophylline (Concomitant administration with high doses of theophylline may be associated with increased theophylline levels and potential toxicity). Products include:
- Marax Tablets & DF Syrup 2015
- Quibron 2227

Theophylline Anhydrous (Concomitant administration with high doses of theophylline may be associated with increased theophylline levels and potential toxicity). Products include:
- Aerolate 1003
- Primatene Tablets 844
- Respbid Tablets 687
- Slo-bid Gyrocaps 2201
- Theo-24 Extended Release Capsules 2753
- Theo-Dur Extended-Release Tablets 1367
- Theo-X Extended-Release Tablets 793
- Uni-Dur Extended-Release Tablets 1374
- Uniphyl 400 mg and 600 mg Tablets 2157

Theophylline Calcium Salicylate (Concomitant administration with high doses of theophylline may be associated with increased theophylline levels and potential toxicity). Products include:
- Quadrinal Tablets 1398

Theophylline Sodium Glycinate (Concomitant administration with high doses of theophylline may be associated with increased theophylline levels and potential toxicity).
- No products indexed under this heading.

Triazolam (Decreased clearance of triazolam and increased the pharmacologic effect of triazolam). Products include:
- Halcion Tablets 2093

Warfarin Sodium (Increased anticoagulant effects). Products include:
- Coumadin 941

ERYTHROMYCIN BASE FILMTAB

(Erythromycin) 430

May interact with xanthine bronchodilators, oral anticoagulants, and certain other agents. Compounds in these categories include:

Aminophylline (Concomitant administration with high doses of theophylline may be associated with increased theophylline levels and potential toxicity).
- No products indexed under this heading.

Carbamazepine (Elevations in serum erythromycin and carbamazepine concentration). Products include:
- Atretol Tablets 569
- Tegretol/Tegretol-XR 870

Cyclosporine (Elevations in serum erythromycin and cyclosporine concentration). Products include:
- Neoral 2405
- Sandimmune 2416

Dicumarol (Increased anticoagulant effects).
- No products indexed under this heading.

Digoxin (Elevated digoxin serum levels). Products include:
- Lanoxicaps 1110
- Lanoxin Elixir Pediatric 1113
- Lanoxin Injection 1116
- Lanoxin Injection Pediatric 1119
- Lanoxin Tablets 1121

Dihydroergotamine Mesylate (Potential for acute ergot toxicity characterized by severe peripheral vasospasm and dysesthesia). Products include:
- D.H.E. 45 Injection 2381

Dyphylline (Concomitant administration with high doses of theophylline may be associated with increased theophylline levels and potential toxicity). Products include:
- Lufyllin & Lufyllin-400 Tablets 2778
- Lufyllin-GG Elixir & Tablets 2779

Ergotamine Tartrate (Potential for acute ergot toxicity characterized by severe peripheral vasospasm and dysesthesia). Products include:
- Bellergal-S Tablets 2375
- Cafergot 2376
- Ergomar Tablets 1543
- Wigraine Tablets 1884

Hexobarbital (Elevations in serum erythromycin and hexobarbital concentration).

Lovastatin (Potential for rhabdomyolysis in seriously ill patients). Products include:
- Mevacor Tablets 1742

Phenytoin (Elevations in serum erythromycin and phenytoin concentration). Products include:
- Dilantin Infatabs 1967
- Dilantin-125 Suspension 1969

Phenytoin Sodium (Elevations in serum erythromycin and phenytoin concentration). Products include:
- Dilantin Kapseals 1965

Terfenadine (Potential for altered terfenadine metabolism). Products include:
- Seldane Tablets 1284
- Seldane-D Extended-Release Tablets 1286

Theophylline (Concomitant administration with high doses of theophylline may be associated with increased theophylline levels and potential toxicity). Products include:
- Marax Tablets & DF Syrup 2015
- Quibron 2227

Theophylline Anhydrous (Concomitant administration with high doses of theophylline may be associated with increased theophylline levels and potential toxicity). Products include:
- Aerolate 1003
- Primatene Tablets 844
- Respbid Tablets 687
- Slo-bid Gyrocaps 2201
- Theo-24 Extended Release Capsules 2753
- Theo-Dur Extended-Release Tablets 1367
- Theo-X Extended-Release Tablets 793
- Uni-Dur Extended-Release Tablets 1374
- Uniphyl 400 mg and 600 mg Tablets 2157

Theophylline Calcium Salicylate (Concomitant administration with high doses of theophylline may be associated with increased theophylline levels and potential toxicity). Products include:
- Quadrinal Tablets 1398

IMPORTANT NOTE: Always consult each drug listing in the patient's regimen for possible interactions.

Theophylline Sodium Glycinate (Concomitant administration with high doses of theophylline may be associated with increased theophylline levels and potential toxicity).
No products indexed under this heading.

Triazolam (Decreased clearance of triazolam and increased the pharmacologic effect of triazolam). Products include:
Halcion Tablets 2093

Warfarin Sodium (Increased anticoagulant effects). Products include:
Coumadin 941

ERYTHROMYCIN DELAYED-RELEASE CAPSULES, USP

(Erythromycin) 431
May interact with xanthine bronchodilators, oral anticoagulants, and certain other agents. Compounds in these categories include:

Aminophylline (Concomitant administration with high doses of theophylline may be associated with increased theophylline levels and potential toxicity).
No products indexed under this heading.

Carbamazepine (Elevations in serum erythromycin and carbamazepine concentration). Products include:
Atretol Tablets 569
Tegretol/Tegretol-XR 870

Cyclosporine (Elevations in serum erythromycin and cyclosporine concentration). Products include:
Neoral 2405
Sandimmune 2416

Dicumarol (Increased anticoagulant effects).
No products indexed under this heading.

Digoxin (Elevated digoxin serum levels). Products include:
Lanoxicaps 1110
Lanoxin Elixir Pediatric 1113
Lanoxin Injection 1116
Lanoxin Injection Pediatric 1119
Lanoxin Tablets 1121

Dihydroergotamine Mesylate (Potential for acute ergot toxicity characterized by severe peripheral vasospasm and dysesthesia). Products include:
D.H.E. 45 Injection 2381

Drugs which undergo biotransformation by cytochrome P-450 mixed function oxidase (Potential for elevation in serum levels).

Dyphylline (Concomitant administration with high doses of theophylline may be associated with increased theophylline levels and potential toxicity). Products include:
Lufyllin & Lufyllin-400 Tablets 2778
Lufyllin-GG Elixir & Tablets 2779

Ergotamine Tartrate (Potential for acute ergot toxicity characterized by severe peripheral vasospasm and dysesthesia). Products include:
Bellergal-S Tablets 2375
Cafergot 2376
Ergomar Tablets 1543
Wigraine Tablets 1884

Hexobarbital (Elevations in serum erythromycin and hexobarbital concentration).

Lovastatin (Potential for rhabdomyolysis in seriously ill patients). Products include:
Mevacor Tablets 1742

Phenytoin (Elevations in serum erythromycin and phenytoin concentration). Products include:
Dilantin Infatabs 1967
Dilantin-125 Suspension 1969

Phenytoin Sodium (Elevations in serum erythromycin and phenytoin concentration). Products include:
Dilantin Kapseals 1965

Terfenadine (Potential for altered terfenadine metabolism). Products include:
Seldane Tablets 1284
Seldane-D Extended-Release Tablets 1286

Theophylline (Concomitant administration with high doses of theophylline may be associated with increased theophylline levels and potential toxicity). Products include:
Marax Tablets & DF Syrup 2015
Quibron 2227

Theophylline Anhydrous (Concomitant administration with high doses of theophylline may be associated with increased theophylline levels and potential toxicity). Products include:
Aerolate 1003
Primatene Tablets .... ▣ 844
Respbid Tablets 687
Slo-bid Gyrocaps 2201
Theo-24 Extended Release Capsules 2753
Theo-Dur Extended-Release Tablets 1367
Theo-X Extended-Release Tablets .. 793
Uni-Dur Extended-Release Tablets .. 1374
Uniphyl 400 mg and 600 mg Tablets 2157

Theophylline Calcium Salicylate (Concomitant administration with high doses of theophylline may be associated with increased theophylline levels and potential toxicity). Products include:
Quadrinal Tablets 1398

Theophylline Sodium Glycinate (Concomitant administration with high doses of theophylline may be associated with increased theophylline levels and potential toxicity).
No products indexed under this heading.

Triazolam (Decreased clearance of triazolam and increased the pharmacologic effect of triazolam). Products include:
Halcion Tablets 2093

Warfarin Sodium (Increased anticoagulant effects). Products include:
Coumadin 941

Food Interactions

Food, unspecified (Lowers the blood levels of systemically available erythromycin).

ESGIC-PLUS CAPSULES

(Butalbital, Acetaminophen, Caffeine) 1012
See **Esgic-plus Tablets**

ESGIC-PLUS TABLETS

(Butalbital, Acetaminophen, Caffeine) 1012
May interact with monoamine oxidase inhibitors, general anesthetics, barbiturates, benzodiazepines, hypnotics and sedatives, central nervous system depressants, narcotic analgesics, tricyclic antidepressants, antihistamines, tranquilizers, and certain other agents. Compounds in these categories include:

Acrivastine (May exhibit additive CNS depressant effects). Products include:
Semprex-D Capsules 1620

Alfentanil Hydrochloride (May exhibit additive CNS depressant effects). Products include:
Alfenta Injection 1334

Alprazolam (May exhibit additive CNS depressant effects). Products include:
Xanax Tablets 2115

Amitriptyline Hydrochloride (May exhibit additive CNS depressant effects). Products include:
Elavil 2945
Etrafon 2495
Limbitrol 2333
Triavil Tablets 1800

Amoxapine (May exhibit additive CNS depressant effects). Products include:
Asendin Tablets 1419

Aprobarbital (May exhibit additive CNS depressant effects).
No products indexed under this heading.

Astemizole (May exhibit additive CNS depressant effects). Products include:
Hismanal Tablets 1341

Azatadine Maleate (May exhibit additive CNS depressant effects). Products include:
Trinalin Repetabs Tablets 1373

Bromodiphenhydramine Hydrochloride (May exhibit additive CNS depressant effects).
No products indexed under this heading.

Brompheniramine Maleate (May exhibit additive CNS depressant effects). Products include:
Alka-Seltzer Plus Sinus Medicine .. ▣ 611
Bromfed Capsules (Extended-Release) 1832
Bromfed Syrup .... ▣ 712
Bromfed Tablets 1832
Bromfed-DM Cough Syrup 1832
Bromfed-PD Capsules (Extended-Release) 1832
Dimetane-DC Cough Syrup 2232
Dimetane-DX Cough Syrup 2233
Dimetapp Allergy Dye-Free Elixir .... ▣ 838
Dimetapp Allergy Sinus Caplets .... ▣ 838
Dimetapp Cold & Allergy Chewable Tablets .... ▣ 838
Dimetapp Cold & Cough Liqui-Gels .... ▣ 839
Dimetapp Cold & Fever Suspension .... ▣ 839
Dimetapp DM Elixir .... ▣ 840
Dimetapp Elixir .... ▣ 840
Dimetapp Extentabs .... ▣ 841
Dimetapp Tablets/Liqui-Gels .... ▣ 841
Rondec Chewable Tablets 974
Vicks DayQuil Allergy Relief 12-Hour Extended Release Tablets .. ▣ 733
Vicks DayQuil Allergy Relief 4-Hour Tablets .... ▣ 733

Buprenorphine (May exhibit additive CNS depressant effects). Products include:
Buprenex Injectable 2170

Buspirone Hydrochloride (May exhibit additive CNS depressant effects). Products include:
BuSpar Tablets 738

Butabarbital (May exhibit additive CNS depressant effects).
No products indexed under this heading.

Cetirizine Hydrochloride (May exhibit additive CNS depressant effects). Products include:
Zyrtec Tablets 2053

Chlordiazepoxide (May exhibit additive CNS depressant effects). Products include:
Limbitrol 2333

Chlordiazepoxide Hydrochloride (May exhibit additive CNS depressant effects). Products include:
Librax Capsules 2330
Librium Capsules 2331
Librium Injectable 2332

Chlorpheniramine Maleate (May exhibit additive CNS depressant effects). Products include:
Alka-Seltzer Plus Cold Medicine .... ▣ 611
Alka-Seltzer Plus Cold Medicine Liqui-Gels .... ▣ 612
Alka-Seltzer Plus Cold & Cough Medicine .... ▣ 611
Alka-Seltzer Plus Cold & Cough Medicine Liqui-Gels .... ▣ 612
Alka-Seltzer Plus Flu & Body Aches Effervescent Tablets .... ▣ 612
Allerest Maximum Strength .... ▣ 649
Allerest Sinus Pain Formula .... ▣ 649
Ana-Kit Anaphylaxis Emergency Treatment Kit 611
Atrohist Pediatric Capsules 1603
Atrohist Plus Tablets 1605
BC Cold Powder Multi-Symptom Formula (Cold-Sinus-Allergy) ...... ▣ 631
Cerose DM .... ▣ 853
Cheracol Plus Head Cold/Cough Formula .... ▣ 741
Children's TYLENOL Cold Multi-Symptom Chewable Tablets and Liquid 1559
Children's TYLENOL Cold Plus Cough Multi Symptom Chewable Tablets and Liquid 1560
Children's TYLENOL Flu Suspension Liquid 1560
Children's Vicks DayQuil Allergy Relief .... ▣ 730
Children's Vicks NyQuil Cold/Cough Relief .... ▣ 731
Chlor-Trimeton Allergy Decongestant Tablets .... ▣ 759
Chlor-Trimeton Allergy Tablets ...... ▣ 758
Allergy-Sinus Comtrex Multi-Symptom Allergy-Sinus Formula Tablets and Caplets .... ▣ 639
Comtrex Multi-Symptom .... ▣ 638
Contac Continuous Action Nasal Decongestant/Antihistamine 12 Hour Capsules .... ▣ 773
Contac Maximum Strength Continuous Action Decongestant/Antihistamine 12 Hour Caplets .. ▣ 772
Contac Severe Cold and Flu Formula Caplets .... ▣ 773
Coricidin Cold + Flu Tablets .... ▣ 760
Coricidin Cough + Cold Tablets ...... ▣ 760
Coricidin 'D' Decongestant Tablets .... ▣ 760
D.A. II Tablets 972
D.A. Chewable Tablets 970
Dura-Tap/PD Capsules 970
Dura-Vent/DA Tablets 972
Efidac 24 Chlorpheniramine .... ▣ 655
Extendryl 1003
Fedahist Gyrocaps 2545
Hycomine Compound Tablets 948
Kronofed-A 994
Nolamine Timed-Release Tablets 790
Novahistine Elixir .... ▣ 782
Ornade Spansule Capsules 2678
PediaCare Cough-Cold Chewable Tablets and Liquid 1569
PediaCare NightRest Cough-Cold Liquid 1569
Pediatric Vicks 44m Cough & Cold Relief .... ▣ 737
Pyrroxate Caplets .... ▣ 742
Ryna .... ▣ 804
Sinarest .... ▣ 663
Sine-Off Sinus Medicine .... ▣ 784
Singlet Tablets .... ▣ 785
Sinulin Tablets 792
Sinutab Sinus Allergy Medication, Maximum Strength Tablets and Caplets .... ▣ 823
Sudafed Cold & Allergy Tablets ...... ▣ 826
Teldrin 12 Hour Antihistamine/Nasal Decongestant Allergy Relief Capsules .... ▣ 786
TheraFlu Flu and Cold Medicine .... ▣ 750
Theraflu Maximum Strength Flu and Cold Medicine For Sore Throat .... ▣ 751
TheraFlu Flu, Cold and Cough Medicine .... ▣ 750
TheraFlu Maximum Strength Nighttime Flu, Cold & Cough Medicine .... ▣ 751
Triaminic Night Time .... ▣ 754
Triaminic Syrup .... ▣ 755
Triaminic Triaminicol Cold & Cough .... ▣ 756
Triaminicin Tablets .... ▣ 756
Tussend 1830

(▣ Described in PDR For Nonprescription Drugs) (◉ Described in PDR For Ophthalmology)

Interactions Index

TYLENOL Allergy Sinus, Maximum Strength Caplets and Gelcaps 1571
TYLENOL Cold Medication, Multi-Symptom Formula Tablets and Caplets 1572
TYLENOL Cold Medication, Multi-Symptom Hot Liquid Packets 1572
Vicks 44 LiquiCaps Cough, Cold & Flu Relief 728
Vicks 44M Cough, Cold & Flu Relief 729

Chlorpheniramine Polistirex (May exhibit additive CNS depressant effects). Products include:
  Tussionex Pennkinetic Extended-Release Suspension 1624

Chlorpheniramine Tannate (May exhibit additive CNS depressant effects). Products include:
  Atrohist Pediatric Suspension 1604
  Atrohist Pediatric Suspension Dye-Free 1604
  Rynatan 2781
  Rynatuss 2782

Chlorpromazine (May exhibit additive CNS depressant effects). Products include:
  Thorazine Suppositories 2701

Chlorpromazine Hydrochloride (May exhibit additive CNS depressant effects). Products include:
  Thorazine 2701

Chlorprothixene (May exhibit additive CNS depressant effects).
  No products indexed under this heading.

Chlorprothixene Hydrochloride (May exhibit additive CNS depressant effects).
  No products indexed under this heading.

Chlorprothixene Lactate (May exhibit additive CNS depressant effects).
  No products indexed under this heading.

Clemastine Fumarate (May exhibit additive CNS depressant effects). Products include:
  Tavist Syrup 2426
  Tavist Tablets 2427
  Tavist-1 12 Hour Relief Tablets 749
  Tavist-D 12 Hour Relief Tablets 750

Clomipramine Hydrochloride (May exhibit additive CNS depressant effects). Products include:
  Anafranil Capsules 819

Clorazepate Dipotassium (May exhibit additive CNS depressant effects). Products include:
  Tranxene 459

Clozapine (May exhibit additive CNS depressant effects). Products include:
  Clozaril Tablets 2377

Codeine Phosphate (May exhibit additive CNS depressant effects). Products include:
  Brontex 2130
  Dimetane-DC Cough Syrup 2232
  Fioricet with Codeine Capsules 2387
  Fiorinal with Codeine Capsules 2390
  Nucofed 2225
  Phenergan with Codeine 2883
  Phenergan VC with Codeine 2888
  Robitussin A-C Syrup 2248
  Robitussin-DAC Syrup 2249
  Ryna 804
  Soma Compound w/Codeine Tablets 2784
  Tylenol with Codeine 1592

Cyproheptadine Hydrochloride (May exhibit additive CNS depressant effects). Products include:
  Periactin 1767

Desflurane (May exhibit additive CNS depressant effects). Products include:
  Suprane (desflurane, USP) 1865

Desipramine Hydrochloride (May exhibit additive CNS depressant effects). Products include:
  Norpramin Tablets 1273

Dexchlorpheniramine Maleate (May exhibit additive CNS depressant effects).
  No products indexed under this heading.

Dezocine (May exhibit additive CNS depressant effects). Products include:
  Dalgan Injection 529

Diazepam (May exhibit additive CNS depressant effects). Products include:
  Dizac (diazepam injectable emulsion) CIV 1862
  Valium Injectable 2336
  Valium Tablets 2335

Diphenhydramine Citrate (May exhibit additive CNS depressant effects). Products include:
  Excedrin P.M. Analgesic/Sleeping Aid Tablets, Caplets, Liquigels 735

Diphenhydramine Hydrochloride (May exhibit additive CNS depressant effects). Products include:
  Actifed Allergy Daytime/Nighttime Caplets 808
  Actifed Sinus Daytime/Nighttime Tablets and Caplets 809
  Extra Strength Bayer PM Aspirin Plus Sleep Aid 617
  Benadryl Allergy Chewables 811
  Benadryl Allergy/Cold Tablets 811
  Benadryl Allergy Decongestant Liquid Medication 812
  Benadryl Allergy Decongestant Tablets 812
  Benadryl Allergy Liquid Medication 813
  Benadryl Allergy Tablets 811
  Benadryl Allergy Sinus Headache Caplets 813
  Benadryl Dye-Free Allergy Liquigel Softgels 813
  Benadryl Dye-Free Allergy Liquid Medication 814
  Benadryl Itch Relief Stick Extra Strength 814
  Benadryl Cream 814
  Benadryl Gel 815
  Benadryl Spray 815
  Benadryl Injection 1955
  Contac Day & Night Cold/Flu Night Caplets 772
  Contac Night Allergy/Sinus Caplets 771
  Extra Strength Doan's P.M. 653
  Excedrin P.M. Analgesic/Sleeping Aid Tablets, Caplets, Liquigels 643
  Nytol QuickCaps Caplets 632
  Sleepinal Night-time Sleep Aid Capsules and Softgels 798
  TYLENOL Allergy Sinus NightTime, Maximum Strength Caplets 1571
  TYLENOL Flu NightTime, Maximum Strength Gelcaps 1575
  TYLENOL Flu NightTime, Maximum Strength Hot Medication Packets 1575
  TYLENOL PM Pain Reliever/Sleep Aid, Extra Strength Gelcaps, Caplets, Geltabs 1576
  TYLENOL Severe Allergy Medication Caplets 1571
  Maximum Strength Unisom Sleepgels 1990
  Unisom With Pain Relief-Nighttime Sleep Aid and Pain Reliever 1991

Diphenylpyraline Hydrochloride (May exhibit additive CNS depressant effects).
  No products indexed under this heading.

Doxepin Hydrochloride (May exhibit additive CNS depressant effects). Products include:
  Adapin Capsules 1542
  Sinequan 2028
  Zonalon Cream 1042

Droperidol (May exhibit additive CNS depressant effects). Products include:
  Inapsine Injection 462

Enflurane (May exhibit additive CNS depressant effects).
  No products indexed under this heading.

Estazolam (May exhibit additive CNS depressant effects). Products include:
  ProSom Tablets 457

Ethchlorvynol (May exhibit additive CNS depressant effects). Products include:
  Placidyl Capsules 456

Ethinamate (May exhibit additive CNS depressant effects).
  No products indexed under this heading.

Fentanyl (May exhibit additive CNS depressant effects). Products include:
  Duragesic Transdermal System 1336

Fentanyl Citrate (May exhibit additive CNS depressant effects). Products include:
  Sublimaze Injection 463

Fluphenazine Decanoate (May exhibit additive CNS depressant effects). Products include:
  Prolixin Decanoate 510

Fluphenazine Enanthate (May exhibit additive CNS depressant effects). Products include:
  Prolixin Enanthate 510

Fluphenazine Hydrochloride (May exhibit additive CNS depressant effects). Products include:
  Prolixin 510

Flurazepam Hydrochloride (May exhibit additive CNS depressant effects). Products include:
  Dalmane Capsules 2329

Furazolidone (CNS effects of butalbital may be enhanced). Products include:
  Furoxone 2221

Glutethimide (May exhibit additive CNS depressant effects).
  No products indexed under this heading.

Halazepam (May exhibit additive CNS depressant effects).
  No products indexed under this heading.

Haloperidol (May exhibit additive CNS depressant effects). Products include:
  Haldol Injection, Tablets and Concentrate 1585

Haloperidol Decanoate (May exhibit additive CNS depressant effects). Products include:
  Haldol Decanoate 1587

Hydrocodone Bitartrate (May exhibit additive CNS depressant effects). Products include:
  Codiclear DH Syrup 808
  Duratuss HD Elixir 2750
  Histussin D Liquid 670
  Hycodan Tablets and Syrup 946
  Hycomine Compound Tablets 948
  Hycomine 947
  Hycotuss Expectorant Syrup 950
  Hydrocet Capsules 787
  Lorcet 10/650 Tablets 1016
  Lortab 2751
  Tussend 1830
  Tussend Expectorant 1831
  Vicodin Tablets 1404
  Vicodin ES Tablets 1405
  Vicodin HP Tablets 1403
  Vicodin Tuss Expectorant 1406
  Zydone Capsules 967

Hydrocodone Polistirex (May exhibit additive CNS depressant effects). Products include:
  Tussionex Pennkinetic Extended-Release Suspension 1624

Hydromorphone Hydrochloride (May exhibit additive CNS depressant effects). Products include:
  Dilaudid Ampules 1382
  Dilaudid Cough Syrup 1383
  Dilaudid-HP Injection 1384
  Dilaudid-HP Lyophilized Powder 250 mg 1384
  Dilaudid 1382
  Dilaudid Oral Liquid 1386
  Dilaudid 1382
  Dilaudid Tablets - 8 mg. 1386

Hydroxyzine Hydrochloride (May exhibit additive CNS depressant effects). Products include:
  Atarax Tablets & Syrup 1992
  Marax Tablets & DF Syrup 2015
  Vistaril Intramuscular Solution 2042

Imipramine Hydrochloride (May exhibit additive CNS depressant effects). Products include:
  Tofranil Ampuls 873
  Tofranil Tablets 875

Imipramine Pamoate (May exhibit additive CNS depressant effects). Products include:
  Tofranil-PM Capsules 876

Isocarboxazid (CNS effects of butalbital may be enhanced).
  No products indexed under this heading.

Isoflurane (May exhibit additive CNS depressant effects).
  No products indexed under this heading.

Ketamine Hydrochloride (May exhibit additive CNS depressant effects).
  No products indexed under this heading.

Levomethadyl Acetate Hydrochloride (May exhibit additive CNS depressant effects). Products include:
  Orlaam Oral Solution 2361

Levorphanol Tartrate (May exhibit additive CNS depressant effects). Products include:
  Levo-Dromoran 2297

Loratadine (May exhibit additive CNS depressant effects). Products include:
  Claritin Tablets 2485
  Claritin-D Tablets 2487

Lorazepam (May exhibit additive CNS depressant effects). Products include:
  Ativan Injection 2805
  Ativan Tablets 2807

Loxapine Hydrochloride (May exhibit additive CNS depressant effects). Products include:
  Loxitane 1426

Loxapine Succinate (May exhibit additive CNS depressant effects). Products include:
  Loxitane Capsules 1426

Maprotiline Hydrochloride (May exhibit additive CNS depressant effects). Products include:
  Ludiomil Tablets 861

Meperidine Hydrochloride (May exhibit additive CNS depressant effects). Products include:
  Demerol 2438
  Mepergan Injection 2859

Mephobarbital (May exhibit additive CNS depressant effects). Products include:
  Mebaral Tablets 2452

Meprobamate (May exhibit additive CNS depressant effects). Products include:
  Miltown Tablets 2780

IMPORTANT NOTE: Always consult each drug listing in the patient's regimen for possible interactions.

PMB 200 and PMB 400 2890

Mesoridazine Besylate (May exhibit additive CNS depressant effects). Products include:
- Serentil 689

Methadone Hydrochloride (May exhibit additive CNS depressant effects). Products include:
- Methadone Hydrochloride Oral Concentrate 2356
- Methadone Hydrochloride Oral Solution & Tablets 2357

Methdilazine Hydrochloride (May exhibit additive CNS depressant effects).
- No products indexed under this heading.

Methohexital Sodium (May exhibit additive CNS depressant effects).
- No products indexed under this heading.

Methotrimeprazine (May exhibit additive CNS depressant effects). Products include:
- Levoprome 1321

Methoxyflurane (May exhibit additive CNS depressant effects).
- No products indexed under this heading.

Midazolam Hydrochloride (May exhibit additive CNS depressant effects). Products include:
- Versed Injection 2324

Molindone Hydrochloride (May exhibit additive CNS depressant effects). Products include:
- Moban Tablets and Concentrate 1036

Morphine Sulfate (May exhibit additive CNS depressant effects). Products include:
- Astramorph/PF Injection, USP (Preservative-Free) 526
- Duramorph Injection 983
- Infumorph 200 and Infumorph 500 Sterile Solutions 985
- Kadian Capsules 2948
- MS Contin Tablets 2149
- MSIR 2152
- Oramorph SR (Morphine Sulfate Sustained Release Tablets) 2359
- RMS Suppositories CII 2766
- Roxanol 2365

Nortriptyline Hydrochloride (May exhibit additive CNS depressant effects). Products include:
- Pamelor 2409

Opium Alkaloids (May exhibit additive CNS depressant effects).
- No products indexed under this heading.

Oxazepam (May exhibit additive CNS depressant effects). Products include:
- Serax Capsules 2916
- Serax Tablets 2916

Oxycodone Hydrochloride (May exhibit additive CNS depressant effects). Products include:
- OxyContin Tablets 2163
- OxyIR Capsules 2167
- Percocet Tablets 955
- Percodan Tablets 955
- Percodan-Demi Tablets 956
- Roxicodone Tablets, Oral Solution & Intensol (Oxycodone) 2366
- Tylox Capsules 1593

Pentobarbital Sodium (May exhibit additive CNS depressant effects). Products include:
- Nembutal Sodium Capsules 440
- Nembutal Sodium Solution 442
- Nembutal Sodium Suppositories 444

Perphenazine (May exhibit additive CNS depressant effects). Products include:
- Etrafon 2495
- Triavil Tablets 1800
- Trilafon 2532

Phenelzine Sulfate (CNS effects of butalbital may be enhanced). Products include:
- Nardil 1977

Phenobarbital (May exhibit additive CNS depressant effects). Products include:
- Arco-Lase Plus Tablets 513
- Bellergal-S Tablets 2375
- Donnatal 2234
- Donnatal Extentabs 2234
- Donnatal Tablets 2234
- Phenobarbital Elixir and Tablets 1523
- Quadrinal Tablets 1398

Prazepam (May exhibit additive CNS depressant effects).
- No products indexed under this heading.

Prochlorperazine (May exhibit additive CNS depressant effects). Products include:
- Compazine 2644

Promethazine Hydrochloride (May exhibit additive CNS depressant effects). Products include:
- Mepergan Injection 2859
- Phenergan with Codeine 2883
- Phenergan with Dextromethorphan 2885
- Phenergan Injection 2880
- Phenergan Suppositories 2882
- Phenergan Syrup 2881
- Phenergan Tablets 2882
- Phenergan VC 2886
- Phenergan VC with Codeine 2888

Propofol (May exhibit additive CNS depressant effects). Products include:
- Diprivan Injectable Emulsion 2939

Propoxyphene Hydrochloride (May exhibit additive CNS depressant effects). Products include:
- Darvon 1475
- Wygesic Tablets 2930

Propoxyphene Napsylate (May exhibit additive CNS depressant effects). Products include:
- Darvon-N/Darvocet-N 1473

Protriptyline Hydrochloride (May exhibit additive CNS depressant effects). Products include:
- Vivactil Tablets 1820

Pyrilamine Maleate (May exhibit additive CNS depressant effects). Products include:
- 4-Way Fast Acting Nasal Spray (regular & mentholated) .... ■□ 644
- Maximum Strength Multi-Symptom Formula Midol .... ■□ 621
- PMS Multi-Symptom Formula Midol .... ■□ 622

Pyrilamine Tannate (May exhibit additive CNS depressant effects). Products include:
- Atrohist Pediatric Suspension 1604
- Atrohist Pediatric Suspension Dye-Free 1604
- Rynatan 2781

Quazepam (May exhibit additive CNS depressant effects). Products include:
- Doral Tablets 2773

Risperidone (May exhibit additive CNS depressant effects). Products include:
- Risperdal Tablets 1348

Secobarbital Sodium (May exhibit additive CNS depressant effects). Products include:
- Seconal Sodium Pulvules 1529

Selegiline Hydrochloride (CNS effects of butalbital may be enhanced). Products include:
- Eldepryl Capsules 2729

Sevoflurane (May exhibit additive CNS depressant effects).
- No products indexed under this heading.

Sufentanil Citrate (May exhibit additive CNS depressant effects). Products include:
- Sufenta Injection 1355

Temazepam (May exhibit additive CNS depressant effects). Products include:
- Restoril Capsules 2413

Terfenadine (May exhibit additive CNS depressant effects). Products include:
- Seldane Tablets 1284
- Seldane-D Extended-Release Tablets 1286

Thiamylal Sodium (May exhibit additive CNS depressant effects).
- No products indexed under this heading.

Thioridazine Hydrochloride (May exhibit additive CNS depressant effects). Products include:
- Mellaril 2398

Thiothixene (May exhibit additive CNS depressant effects). Products include:
- Navane Capsules and Concentrate 2018
- Navane Intramuscular 2019

Tranylcypromine Sulfate (CNS effects of butalbital may be enhanced). Products include:
- Parnate Tablets 2679

Triazolam (May exhibit additive CNS depressant effects). Products include:
- Halcion Tablets 2093

Trifluoperazine Hydrochloride (May exhibit additive CNS depressant effects). Products include:
- Stelazine 2692

Trimeprazine Tartrate (May exhibit additive CNS depressant effects).
- No products indexed under this heading.

Trimipramine Maleate (May exhibit additive CNS depressant effects). Products include:
- Surmontil Capsules 2917

Tripelennamine Hydrochloride (May exhibit additive CNS depressant effects). Products include:
- PBZ Tablets 863
- PBZ-SR Tablets 862

Triprolidine Hydrochloride (May exhibit additive CNS depressant effects). Products include:
- Actifed Cold & Allergy Tablets .... ■□ 807
- Actifed Cold & Sinus Caplets and Tablets .... ■□ 808

Zolpidem Tartrate (May exhibit additive CNS depressant effects). Products include:
- Ambien Tablets 2559

Food Interactions

Alcohol (May exhibit additive CNS depressant effects).

ESIDRIX TABLETS

(Hydrochlorothiazide) 839

May interact with corticosteroids, insulin, antihypertensives, barbiturates, cardiac glycosides, lithium preparations, narcotic analgesics, non-steroidal anti-inflammatory agents, and certain other agents. Compounds in these categories include:

Acebutolol Hydrochloride (Additive or potentiated action). Products include:
- Sectral Capsules 2914

ACTH (Hypokalemia may develop during concomitant use of ACTH).
- No products indexed under this heading.

Alfentanil Hydrochloride (May potentiate orthostatic hypotension). Products include:
- Alfenta Injection 1334

Amlodipine Besylate (Additive or potentiated action). Products include:
- Lotrel Capsules 858
- Norvasc Tablets 2020

Aprobarbital (May potentiate orthostatic hypotension).
- No products indexed under this heading.

Atenolol (Additive or potentiated action). Products include:
- Tenoretic Tablets 2963
- Tenormin Tablets and I.V. Injection 2965

Benazepril Hydrochloride (Additive or potentiated action). Products include:
- Lotensin Tablets 852
- Lotensin HCT Tablets 855
- Lotrel Capsules 858

Bendroflumethiazide (Additive or potentiated action).
- No products indexed under this heading.

Betamethasone Acetate (Hypokalemia may develop during concomitant use of steroid). Products include:
- Celestone Soluspan Suspension 2484

Betamethasone Sodium Phosphate (Hypokalemia may develop during concomitant use of steroid). Products include:
- Celestone Soluspan Suspension 2484

Betaxolol Hydrochloride (Additive or potentiated action). Products include:
- Betoptic Ophthalmic Solution 465
- Betoptic S Ophthalmic Suspension 467
- Kerlone Tablets 2588

Bisoprolol Fumarate (Additive or potentiated action). Products include:
- Zebeta Tablets 1457
- Ziac 1459

Buprenorphine (May potentiate orthostatic hypotension). Products include:
- Buprenex Injectable 2170

Butabarbital (May potentiate orthostatic hypotension).
- No products indexed under this heading.

Butalbital (May potentiate orthostatic hypotension). Products include:
- Axocet Capsules 2469
- Esgic-plus Capsules 1012
- Esgic-plus Tablets 1012
- Fioricet Tablets 2386
- Fioricet with Codeine Capsules 2387
- Fiorinal Capsules 2388
- Fiorinal with Codeine Capsules 2390
- Fiorinal Tablets 2388
- Phrenilin 790
- Sedapap Tablets 50 mg/650 mg .. 1826

Captopril (Additive or potentiated action). Products include:
- Capoten Tablets 740
- Capozide Tablets 744

Carteolol Hydrochloride (Additive or potentiated action). Products include:
- Cartrol Tablets 413
- Ocupress Ophthalmic Solution, 1% Sterile .... ⊙ 297

Chlorothiazide (Additive or potentiated action). Products include:
- Aldoclor Tablets 1638
- Diupres Tablets 1691
- Diuril Oral 1694

Chlorothiazide Sodium (Additive or potentiated action). Products include:
- Diuril Sodium Intravenous 1693

(■□ Described in PDR For Nonprescription Drugs) (⊙ Described in PDR For Ophthalmology)

Chlorthalidone (Additive or potentiated action). Products include:
- Combipres Tablets ... 682
- Tenoretic Tablets ... 2963
- Thalitone ... 1293

Cholestyramine (Impairs the oral absorption of hydrochlorothiazide from gastrointestinal tract by up to 85%). Products include:
- Questran ... 774

Clonidine (Additive or potentiated action). Products include:
- Catapres-TTS ... 680

Clonidine Hydrochloride (Additive or potentiated action). Products include:
- Catapres Tablets ... 679
- Combipres Tablets ... 682

Codeine Phosphate (May potentiate orthostatic hypotension). Products include:
- Brontex ... 2130
- Dimetane-DC Cough Syrup ... 2232
- Fioricet with Codeine Capsules ... 2387
- Fiorinal with Codeine Capsules ... 2390
- Nucofed ... 2225
- Phenergan with Codeine ... 2883
- Phenergan VC with Codeine ... 2888
- Robitussin A-C Syrup ... 2248
- Robitussin-DAC Syrup ... 2249
- Ryna ... [BD] 804
- Soma Compound w/Codeine Tablets ... 2784
- Tylenol with Codeine ... 1592

Colestipol Hydrochloride (Impairs the oral absorption of hydrochlorothiazide from gastrointestinal tract by up to 43%). Products include:
- Colestid ... 2073

Cortisone Acetate (Hypokalemia may develop during concomitant use of steroid). Products include:
- Cortone Acetate Sterile Suspension ... 1663
- Cortone Acetate Tablets ... 1664

Deserpidine (Additive or potentiated action).
- No products indexed under this heading.

Deslanoside (Thiazide-induced hypokalemia can sensitize or exaggerate the response of the heart to the toxic effects of digitalis, e.g., increased ventricular irritability).
- No products indexed under this heading.

Dexamethasone (Hypokalemia may develop during concomitant use of steroid). Products include:
- AK-Trol Ointment & Suspension ... ◉ 205
- Decadron Elixir ... 1676
- Decadron Tablets ... 1678
- Decaspray Topical Aerosol ... 1689
- Maxitrol Ophthalmic Ointment and Suspension ... ◉ 222
- TobraDex Ophthalmic Suspension and Ointment ... 469

Dexamethasone Acetate (Hypokalemia may develop during concomitant use of steroid). Products include:
- Dalalone D.P. Injectable ... 1009
- Decadron-LA Sterile Suspension ... 1687

Dexamethasone Sodium Phosphate (Hypokalemia may develop during concomitant use of steroid). Products include:
- Decadron Phosphate Injection ... 1680
- Decadron Phosphate Sterile Ophthalmic Ointment ... 1684
- Decadron Phosphate Sterile Ophthalmic Solution ... 1685
- Decadron Phosphate Topical Cream ... 1686
- Decadron Phosphate with Xylocaine Injection, Sterile ... 1683
- Dexacort Phosphate in Respihaler .. 1606
- Dexacort Phosphate in Turbinaire .. 1607
- NeoDecadron Sterile Ophthalmic Ointment ... 1755
- NeoDecadron Sterile Ophthalmic Solution ... 1756
- NeoDecadron Topical Cream ... 1757

Dezocine (May potentiate orthostatic hypotension). Products include:
- Dalgan Injection ... 529

Diazoxide (Additive or potentiated action). Products include:
- Hyperstat I.V. Injection ... 2504
- Proglycem ... 575

Diclofenac Potassium (May reduce diuretic, natriuretic, and antihypertensive effects of thiazide diuretics). Products include:
- Cataflam Tablets ... 833

Diclofenac Sodium (May reduce diuretic, natriuretic, and antihypertensive effects of thiazide diuretics). Products include:
- Voltaren Ophthalmic Sterile Ophthalmic Solution ... ◉ 264
- Cataflam/Voltaren/Voltaren-XR ... 833

Digitoxin (Thiazide-induced hypokalemia can sensitize or exaggerate the response of the heart to the toxic effects of digitalis, e.g., increased ventricular irritability). Products include:
- Crystodigin Tablets ... 1472

Digoxin (Thiazide-induced hypokalemia can sensitize or exaggerate the response of the heart to the toxic effects of digitalis, e.g., increased ventricular irritability). Products include:
- Lanoxicaps ... 1110
- Lanoxin Elixir Pediatric ... 1113
- Lanoxin Injection ... 1116
- Lanoxin Injection Pediatric ... 1119
- Lanoxin Tablets ... 1121

Diltiazem Hydrochloride (Additive or potentiated action). Products include:
- Cardizem CD Capsules ... 1251
- Cardizem SR Capsules ... 1255
- Cardizem Injectable ... 1253
- Cardizem Tablets ... 1257
- Dilacor XR Extended-release Capsules ... 2183
- Tiazac Capsules ... 1019

Doxazosin Mesylate (Additive or potentiated action). Products include:
- Cardura Tablets ... 1993

Enalapril Maleate (Additive or potentiated action). Products include:
- Vaseretic Tablets ... 1810
- Vasotec Tablets ... 1816

Enalaprilat (Additive or potentiated action). Products include:
- Vasotec I.V. ... 1814

Esmolol Hydrochloride (Additive or potentiated action). Products include:
- Brevibloc (esmolol HCl) Injection ... 1860

Etodolac (May reduce diuretic, natriuretic, and antihypertensive effects of thiazide diuretics). Products include:
- Lodine Capsules and Tablets ... 2849

Felodipine (Additive or potentiated action). Products include:
- Plendil Extended-Release Tablets ... 514

Fenoprofen Calcium (May reduce diuretic, natriuretic, and antihypertensive effects of thiazide diuretics). Products include:
- Nalfon 200 Pulvules & Nalfon Tablets ... 933

Fentanyl (May potentiate orthostatic hypotension). Products include:
- Duragesic Transdermal System ... 1336

Fentanyl Citrate (May potentiate orthostatic hypotension). Products include:
- Sublimaze Injection ... 463

Fludrocortisone Acetate (Hypokalemia may develop during concomitant use of steroid). Products include:
- Florinef Acetate Tablets ... 506

Flurbiprofen (May reduce diuretic, natriuretic, and antihypertensive effects of thiazide diuretics).
- No products indexed under this heading.

Fosinopril Sodium (Additive or potentiated action). Products include:
- Monopril Tablets ... 762

Furosemide (Additive or potentiated action). Products include:
- Lasix Injection, Oral Solution and Tablets ... 1267

Guanabenz Acetate (Additive or potentiated action).
- No products indexed under this heading.

Guanethidine Monosulfate (Additive or potentiated action). Products include:
- Esimil Tablets ... 840
- Ismelin Tablets ... 845

Hydralazine Hydrochloride (Additive or potentiated action). Products include:
- Apresazide Capsules ... 824
- Apresoline Hydrochloride Tablets .. 826
- Hydralazine Hydrochloride Injection USP ... 2712
- Ser-Ap-Es Tablets ... 867

Hydrocodone Bitartrate (May potentiate orthostatic hypotension). Products include:
- Codiclear DH Syrup ... 808
- Duratuss HD Elixir ... 2750
- Histussin D Liquid ... 670
- Hycodan Tablets and Syrup ... 946
- Hycomine Compound Tablets ... 948
- Hycomine ... 947
- Hycotuss Expectorant Syrup ... 950
- Hydrocet Capsules ... 787
- Lorcet 10/650 Tablets ... 1016
- Lortab ... 2751
- Tussend ... 1830
- Tussend Expectorant ... 1831
- Vicodin Tablets ... 1404
- Vicodin ES Tablets ... 1405
- Vicodin HP Tablets ... 1403
- Vicodin Tuss Expectorant ... 1406
- Zydone Capsules ... 967

Hydrocodone Polistirex (May potentiate orthostatic hypotension). Products include:
- Tussionex Pennkinetic Extended-Release Suspension ... 1624

Hydrocortisone (Hypokalemia may develop during concomitant use of steroid). Products include:
- Anusol-HC Cream 2.5% ... 1953
- Aquanil HC Lotion ... 1989
- Maximum Strength Cortaid Spray [BD] 800
- CORTENEMA ... 2713
- Cortisporin Ointment ... 1074
- Cortisporin Ophthalmic Ointment Sterile ... 1074
- Cortisporin Ophthalmic Suspension Sterile ... 1075
- Cortisporin Otic Solution Sterile ... 1076
- Cortisporin Otic Suspension Sterile 1077
- Cortizone-5 ... [BD] 795
- Cortizone-10 ... [BD] 795
- Hydrocortone Tablets ... 1715
- Hytone ... 922
- Hytone Ointment 2 ½% ... 923
- Massengill Medicated Soft Cloth Towelettes ... 2628
- Pediotic Suspension Sterile ... 1140
- Preparation H Hydrocortisone 1% Cream ... [BD] 843
- ProctoCream-HC 2.5% ... 2552
- VōSoL HC Otic Solution ... 2786

Hydrocortisone Acetate (Hypokalemia may develop during concomitant use of steroid). Products include:
- Analpram-HC Rectal Cream 1% and 2.5% ... 993
- Anusol HC-1 Hydrocortisone Anti-Itch Ointment ... [BD] 810
- Anusol-HC Suppositories ... 1954
- Caldecort Anti-Itch Hydrocortisone Cream ... [BD] 651
- Coly-Mycin S Otic w/Neomycin & Hydrocortisone ... 1965
- Cortaid ... [BD] 800
- Cortifoam ... 2540
- Cortisporin Cream ... 1073
- Epifoam ... 2543
- Hydrocortone Acetate Sterile Suspension ... 1712
- Mantadil Cream ... 1124
- Nupercainal Hydrocortisone 1% Cream ... [BD] 661
- Pramosone Cream, Lotion & Ointment ... 995
- ProctoFoam-HC ... 2552
- Terra-Cortril Ophthalmic Suspension ... 2033

Hydrocortisone Sodium Phosphate (Hypokalemia may develop during concomitant use of steroid). Products include:
- Hydrocortone Phosphate Injection, Sterile ... 1713

Hydrocortisone Sodium Succinate (Hypokalemia may develop during concomitant use of steroid).
- No products indexed under this heading.

Hydroflumethiazide (Additive or potentiated action). Products include:
- Diucardin Tablets ... 2824

Hydromorphone Hydrochloride (May potentiate orthostatic hypotension). Products include:
- Dilaudid Ampules ... 1382
- Dilaudid Cough Syrup ... 1383
- Dilaudid-HP Injection ... 1384
- Dilaudid-HP Lyophilized Powder 250 mg ... 1384
- Dilaudid ... 1382
- Dilaudid Oral Liquid ... 1386
- Dilaudid ... 1382
- Dilaudid Tablets - 8 mg ... 1386

Ibuprofen (May reduce diuretic, natriuretic, and antihypertensive effects of thiazide diuretics). Products include:
- Advil Cold and Sinus Caplets and Tablets ... [BD] 837
- Advil Ibuprofen Tablets, Caplets and Gel Caplets ... [BD] 836
- Children's Motrin Ibuprofen Oral Suspension ... 1558
- IBU Tablets ... 1389
- Ibuprohm ... [BD] 713
- Motrin IB Caplets, Tablets, and Gelcaps ... [BD] 802
- Motrin Ibuprofen Suspension, Oral Drops, Chewable Tablets, Caplets ... 1563
- Nuprin Ibuprofen/Analgesic Tablets & Caplets ... [BD] 645
- Vicks DayQuil SINUS Pressure & PAIN Relief with IBUPROFEN ... [BD] 735

Indapamide (Additive or potentiated action).
- No products indexed under this heading.

Indomethacin (May reduce diuretic, natriuretic, and antihypertensive effects of thiazide diuretics). Products include:
- Indocin ... 1723

Indomethacin Sodium Trihydrate (May reduce diuretic, natriuretic, and antihypertensive effects of thiazide diuretics). Products include:
- Indocin I.V. ... 1727

Insulin, Human (Insulin requirements may be altered).
- No products indexed under this heading.

Insulin, Human Isophane Suspension (Insulin requirements may be altered). Products include:
- Novolin N Human Insulin 10 ml Vials ... 1846

IMPORTANT NOTE: Always consult each drug listing in the patient's regimen for possible interactions.

Esidrix — Interactions Index

Insulin, Human NPH (Insulin requirements may be altered). Products include:
- Humulin N, 100 Units ... 1495
- Novolin N PenFill 1.5 ml Cartridges Durable Insulin Delivery System ... 1849
- Novolin N Prefilled Syringe Disposable Insulin Delivery System ... 1850

Insulin, Human Regular (Insulin requirements may be altered). Products include:
- Humulin R, 100 Units ... 1497
- Novolin R Human Insulin 10 ml Vials ... 1846
- Novolin R PenFill 1.5 ml Cartridges Durable Insulin Delivery System ... 1849
- Novolin R Prefilled Syringe Disposable Insulin Delivery System ... 1850
- Velosulin BR Human Insulin 10 ml Vials ... 1847

Insulin, Human, Zinc Suspension (Insulin requirements may be altered). Products include:
- Humulin L, 100 Units ... 1494
- Humulin U, 100 Units ... 1498
- Novolin L Human Insulin 10 ml Vials ... 1846

Insulin Lispro, Human (Insulin requirements may be altered). Products include:
- Humalog Injection ... 1488

Insulin, NPH (Insulin requirements may be altered). Products include:
- NPH, 100 Units ... 1502
- Pork NPH, 100 Units ... 1506
- Purified Pork NPH Isophane Insulin ... 1852

Insulin, Regular (Insulin requirements may be altered). Products include:
- Regular, 100 Units ... 1503
- Pork Regular, 100 Units ... 1507
- Pork Regular (Concentrated), 500 Units ... 1508
- Purified Pork Regular Insulin ... 1852

Insulin, Zinc Crystals (Insulin requirements may be altered). Products include:
- NPH, 100 Units ... 1502

Insulin, Zinc Suspension (Insulin requirements may be altered). Products include:
- Iletin I ... 1501
- Lente, 100 Units ... 1501
- Iletin II ... 1504
- Pork Lente, 100 Units ... 1504
- Purified Pork Lente Insulin ... 1852

Isradipine (Additive or potentiated action). Products include:
- DynaCirc Capsules ... 2381
- DynaCirc CR Tablets ... 2383

Ketoprofen (May reduce diuretic, natriuretic, and antihypertensive effects of thiazide diuretics). Products include:
- Actron Caplets and Tablets ... ▣ 608
- Orudis Capsules ... 2874
- Orudis KT ... ▣ 842
- Oruvail Capsules ... 2874

Ketorolac Tromethamine (May reduce diuretic, natriuretic, and antihypertensive effects of thiazide diuretics). Products include:
- Acular Sterile Ophthalmic Solution ... 470
- Toradol ... 2319

Labetalol Hydrochloride (Additive or potentiated action). Products include:
- Normodyne Injection ... 2519
- Normodyne Tablets ... 2522
- Trandate ... 1158

Levorphanol Tartrate (May potentiate orthostatic hypotension). Products include:
- Levo-Dromoran ... 2297

Lisinopril (Additive or potentiated action). Products include:
- Prinivil Tablets ... 1776
- Prinzide Tablets ... 1780
- Zestoretic Tablets ... 2968
- Zestril Tablets ... 2972

Lithium Carbonate (Lithium renal clearance is reduced by thiazides, increasing the risk of lithium toxicity). Products include:
- Eskalith ... 2658
- Lithium Carbonate Capsules & Tablets ... 2352
- Lithonate/Lithotabs/Lithobid ... 2721

Lithium Citrate (Lithium renal clearance is reduced by thiazides, increasing the risk of lithium toxicity).
- No products indexed under this heading.

Losartan Potassium (Additive or potentiated action). Products include:
- Cozaar Tablets ... 1668
- Hyzaar Tablets ... 1720

Mecamylamine Hydrochloride (Additive or potentiated action). Products include:
- Inversine Tablets ... 1729

Meclofenamate Sodium (May reduce diuretic, natriuretic, and antihypertensive effects of thiazide diuretics).
- No products indexed under this heading.

Mefenamic Acid (May reduce diuretic, natriuretic, and antihypertensive effects of thiazide diuretics). Products include:
- Ponstel ... 1982

Meperidine Hydrochloride (May potentiate orthostatic hypotension). Products include:
- Demerol ... 2438
- Mepergan Injection ... 2859

Mephobarbital (May potentiate orthostatic hypotension). Products include:
- Mebaral Tablets ... 2452

Methadone Hydrochloride (May potentiate orthostatic hypotension). Products include:
- Methadone Hydrochloride Oral Concentrate ... 2356
- Methadone Hydrochloride Oral Solution & Tablets ... 2357

Methyclothiazide (Additive or potentiated action). Products include:
- Enduron Tablets ... 424

Methyldopa (Co-administration has resulted in rare reports of hemolytic anemia). Products include:
- Aldoclor Tablets ... 1638
- Aldomet Oral ... 1640
- Aldoril Tablets ... 1644

Methyldopate Hydrochloride (Co-administration has resulted in rare reports of hemolytic anemia). Products include:
- Aldomet Ester HCl Injection ... 1642

Methylprednisolone Acetate (Hypokalemia may develop during concomitant use of steroid).
- No products indexed under this heading.

Methylprednisolone Sodium Succinate (Hypokalemia may develop during concomitant use of steroid).
- No products indexed under this heading.

Metolazone (Additive or potentiated action). Products include:
- Mykrox Tablets ... 1617
- Zaroxolyn Tablets ... 1625

Metoprolol Succinate (Additive or potentiated action). Products include:
- Toprol-XL Tablets ... 560

Metoprolol Tartrate (Additive or potentiated action). Products include:
- Lopressor ... 848
- Lopressor HCT Tablets ... 850

Metyrosine (Additive or potentiated action). Products include:
- Demser Capsules ... 1690

Minoxidil (Additive or potentiated action).
- No products indexed under this heading.

Moexipril Hydrochloride (Additive or potentiated action). Products include:
- Univasc Tablets ... 2553

Morphine Sulfate (May potentiate orthostatic hypotension). Products include:
- Astramorph/PF Injection, USP (Preservative-Free) ... 526
- Duramorph Injection ... 983
- Infumorph 200 and Infumorph 500 Sterile Solutions ... 985
- Kadian Capsules ... 2948
- MS Contin Tablets ... 2149
- MSIR ... 2152
- Oramorph SR (Morphine Sulfate Sustained Release Tablets) ... 2359
- RMS Suppositories CII ... 2766
- Roxanol ... 2365

Nabumetone (May reduce diuretic, natriuretic, and antihypertensive effects of thiazide diuretics). Products include:
- Relafen Tablets ... 2688

Nadolol (Additive or potentiated action).
- No products indexed under this heading.

Naproxen (May reduce diuretic, natriuretic, and antihypertensive effects of thiazide diuretics). Products include:
- Anaprox/Naprosyn ... 2277

Naproxen Sodium (May reduce diuretic, natriuretic, and antihypertensive effects of thiazide diuretics). Products include:
- Aleve ... 2124
- Anaprox/Naprosyn ... 2277
- Naprelan Tablets ... 2861

Nicardipine Hydrochloride (Additive or potentiated action). Products include:
- Cardene Capsules ... 2261
- Cardene I.V. ... 2815
- Cardene SR Capsules ... 2264

Nifedipine (Additive or potentiated action). Products include:
- Adalat Capsules (10 mg and 20 mg) ... 580
- Adalat CC ... 582
- Procardia Capsules ... 2024
- Procardia XL Extended Release Tablets ... 2026

Nisoldipine (Additive or potentiated action). Products include:
- Sular Tablets ... 2961

Nitroglycerin (Additive or potentiated action). Products include:
- Deponit NTG Transdermal Delivery System ... 2541
- Nitro-Bid IV ... 1270
- Nitro-Bid Ointment ... 1272
- Nitro-Dur (nitroglycerin) Transdermal Infusion System ... 1365
- Nitrolingual Spray ... 2193
- Nitrostat Tablets ... 1981
- Transderm-Nitro Transdermal Therapeutic System ... 878

Norepinephrine Bitartrate (Decreased arterial response to norepinephrine). Products include:
- Levophed Bitartrate Injection ... 2445

Opium Alkaloids (May potentiate orthostatic hypotension).
- No products indexed under this heading.

Oxaprozin (May reduce diuretic, natriuretic, and antihypertensive effects of thiazide diuretics). Products include:
- Daypro Caplets ... 2578

Oxycodone Hydrochloride (May potentiate orthostatic hypotension). Products include:
- OxyContin Tablets ... 2163
- OxyIR Capsules ... 2167
- Percocet Tablets ... 955
- Percodan Tablets ... 955
- Percodan-Demi Tablets ... 956
- Roxicodone Tablets, Oral Solution & Intensol (Oxycodone) ... 2366
- Tylox Capsules ... 1593

Penbutolol Sulfate (Additive or potentiated action). Products include:
- Levatol Tablets ... 2547

Pentobarbital Sodium (May potentiate orthostatic hypotension). Products include:
- Nembutal Sodium Capsules ... 440
- Nembutal Sodium Solution ... 442
- Nembutal Sodium Suppositories ... 444

Phenobarbital (May potentiate orthostatic hypotension). Products include:
- Arco-Lase Plus Tablets ... 513
- Bellergal-S Tablets ... 2375
- Donnatal ... 2234
- Donnatal Extentabs ... 2234
- Donnatal Tablets ... 2234
- Phenobarbital Elixir and Tablets ... 1523
- Quadrinal Tablets ... 1398

Phenoxybenzamine Hydrochloride (Additive or potentiated action). Products include:
- Dibenzyline Capsules ... 2650

Phentolamine Mesylate (Additive or potentiated action). Products include:
- Regitine Vials ... 864

Phenylbutazone (May reduce diuretic, natriuretic, and antihypertensive effects of thiazide diuretics).
- No products indexed under this heading.

Pindolol (Additive or potentiated action). Products include:
- Visken Tablets ... 2428

Piroxicam (May reduce diuretic, natriuretic, and antihypertensive effects of thiazide diuretics). Products include:
- Feldene Capsules ... 2008

Polythiazide (Additive or potentiated action). Products include:
- Minizide Capsules ... 2016

Prazosin Hydrochloride (Additive or potentiated action). Products include:
- Minipress Capsules ... 2015
- Minizide Capsules ... 2016

Prednisolone Acetate (Hypokalemia may develop during concomitant use of steroid). Products include:
- AK-CIDE ... ◉ 203
- AK-CIDE Ointment ... ◉ 203
- Blephamide Liquifilm Sterile Ophthalmic Suspension ... 472
- Blephamide Ointment ... ◉ 234
- Econopred & Econopred Plus Ophthalmic Suspensions ... ◉ 216
- Poly-Pred Liquifilm ... ◉ 246
- Pred Forte ... ◉ 247
- Pred Mild ... ◉ 250
- Pred-G Liquifilm Sterile Ophthalmic Suspension ... ◉ 248
- Pred-G S.O.P. Sterile Ophthalmic Ointment ... ◉ 249

Prednisolone Sodium Phosphate (Hypokalemia may develop during concomitant use of steroid). Products include:
- AK-PRED ... ◉ 204
- Hydeltrasol Injection, Sterile ... 1708
- Pediapred Oral Solution ... 1618

Prednisolone Tebutate (Hypokalemia may develop during concomitant use of steroid). Products include:
- Hydeltra-T.B.A. Sterile Suspension ... 1710

(▣ Described in PDR For Nonprescription Drugs)   (◉ Described in PDR For Ophthalmology)

Prednisone (Hypokalemia may develop during concomitant use of steroid).
No products indexed under this heading.

Propoxyphene Hydrochloride (May potentiate orthostatic hypotension). Products include:
Darvon 1475
Wygesic Tablets 2930

Propoxyphene Napsylate (May potentiate orthostatic hypotension). Products include:
Darvon-N/Darvocet-N 1473

Propranolol Hydrochloride (Additive or potentiated action). Products include:
Inderal 2834
Inderal LA Long Acting Capsules 2836
Inderide Tablets 2838
Inderide LA Long Acting Capsules .. 2840

Quinapril Hydrochloride (Additive or potentiated action). Products include:
Accupril Tablets 1950

Ramipril (Additive or potentiated action). Products include:
Altace Capsules 1238

Rauwolfia Serpentina (Additive or potentiated action).
No products indexed under this heading.

Rescinnamine (Additive or potentiated action).
No products indexed under this heading.

Reserpine (Additive or potentiated action). Products include:
Diupres Tablets 1691
Hydropres Tablets 1718
Ser-Ap-Es Tablets 867

Secobarbital Sodium (May potentiate orthostatic hypotension). Products include:
Seconal Sodium Pulvules 1529

Sodium Nitroprusside (Additive or potentiated action).
No products indexed under this heading.

Sotalol Hydrochloride (Additive or potentiated action). Products include:
Betapace Tablets 637

Spirapril Hydrochloride (Additive or potentiated action).
No products indexed under this heading.

Sufentanil Citrate (May potentiate orthostatic hypotension). Products include:
Sufenta Injection 1355

Sulindac (May reduce diuretic, natriuretic, and antihypertensive effects of thiazide diuretics). Products include:
Clinoril Tablets 1658

Terazosin Hydrochloride (Additive or potentiated action). Products include:
Hytrin Capsules 434

Thiamylal Sodium (May potentiate orthostatic hypotension).
No products indexed under this heading.

Timolol Maleate (Additive or potentiated action). Products include:
Blocadren Tablets 1654
Timolide Tablets 1791
Timoptic in Ocudose 1796
Timoptic Sterile Ophthalmic Solution 1794
Timoptic-XE 1798

Tolmetin Sodium (May reduce diuretic, natriuretic, and antihypertensive effects of thiazide diuretics). Products include:
Tolectin (200, 400 and 600 mg) .. 1591

Torsemide (Additive or potentiated action). Products include:
Demadex Tablets and Injection 691

Trandolapril (Additive or potentiated action). Products include:
Mavik Tablets 1407

Triamcinolone (Hypokalemia may develop during concomitant use of steroid).
No products indexed under this heading.

Triamcinolone Acetonide (Hypokalemia may develop during concomitant use of steroid). Products include:
Azmacort Oral Inhaler 2175
Nasacort AQ Nasal Spray 2191
Nasacort Nasal Inhaler 2189

Triamcinolone Diacetate (Hypokalemia may develop during concomitant use of steroid).
No products indexed under this heading.

Triamcinolone Hexacetonide (Hypokalemia may develop during concomitant use of steroid).
No products indexed under this heading.

Trimethaphan Camsylate (Additive or potentiated action).
No products indexed under this heading.

Tubocurarine Chloride (Increased responsiveness to tubocurarine).
No products indexed under this heading.

Verapamil Hydrochloride (Additive or potentiated action). Products include:
Calan SR Caplets 2571
Calan Tablets 2568
Covera-HS Tablets 2573
Isoptin Injectable 1391
Isoptin Oral Tablets 1393
Isoptin SR Tablets 1395
Verelan Capsules 1455

Food Interactions

Alcohol (May potentiate orthostatic hypotension).

ESIMIL TABLETS

(Guanethidine Monosulfate, Hydrochlorothiazide) 840

May interact with monoamine oxidase inhibitors, tricyclic antidepressants, phenothiazines, estrogens, corticosteroids, lithium preparations, insulin, non-steroidal anti-inflammatory agents, antihypertensives, oral contraceptives, cardiac glycosides, barbiturates, narcotic analgesics, and certain other agents. Compounds in these categories include:

Acebutolol Hydrochloride (Additive or potentiated action). Products include:
Sectral Capsules 2914

ACTH (Hypokalemia may develop during concomitant use).
No products indexed under this heading.

Alfentanil Hydrochloride (May potentiate orthostatic hypotension). Products include:
Alfenta Injection 1334

Amitriptyline Hydrochloride (Reduces hypotensive effect). Products include:
Elavil 2945
Etrafon 2495
Limbitrol 2333
Triavil Tablets 1800

Amlodipine Besylate (Additive or potentiated action). Products include:
Lotrel Capsules 858
Norvasc Tablets 2020

Amoxapine (Reduces hypotensive effect). Products include:
Asendin Tablets 1419

Aprobarbital (May potentiate orthostatic hypotension).
No products indexed under this heading.

Atenolol (Additive or potentiated action). Products include:
Tenoretic Tablets 2963
Tenormin Tablets and I.V. Injection 2965

Benazepril Hydrochloride (Additive or potentiated action). Products include:
Lotensin Tablets 852
Lotensin HCT Tablets 855
Lotrel Capsules 858

Bendroflumethiazide (Additive or potentiated action).
No products indexed under this heading.

Betamethasone Acetate (Hypokalemia may develop during concomitant use). Products include:
Celestone Soluspan Suspension 2484

Betamethasone Sodium Phosphate (Hypokalemia may develop during concomitant use). Products include:
Celestone Soluspan Suspension 2484

Betaxolol Hydrochloride (Additive or potentiated action). Products include:
Betoptic Ophthalmic Solution 465
Betoptic S Ophthalmic Suspension 467
Kerlone Tablets 2588

Bisoprolol Fumarate (Additive or potentiated action). Products include:
Zebeta Tablets 1457
Ziac 1459

Buprenorphine (May potentiate orthostatic hypotension). Products include:
Buprenex Injectable 2170

Butabarbital (May potentiate orthostatic hypotension).
No products indexed under this heading.

Butalbital (May potentiate orthostatic hypotension). Products include:
Axocet Capsules 2469
Esgic-plus Capsules 1012
Esgic-plus Tablets 1012
Fioricet Tablets 2386
Fioricet with Codeine Capsules 2387
Fiorinal Capsules 2388
Fiorinal with Codeine Capsules 2390
Fiorinal Tablets 2388
Phrenilin 790
Sedapap Tablets 50 mg/650 mg .. 1826

Captopril (Additive or potentiated action). Products include:
Capoten Tablets 740
Capozide Tablets 744

Carteolol Hydrochloride (Additive or potentiated action). Products include:
Cartrol Tablets 413
Ocupress Ophthalmic Solution, 1% Sterile .... ◎ 297

Chlorothiazide (Additive or potentiated action). Products include:
Aldoclor Tablets 1638
Diupres Tablets 1691
Diuril Oral 1694

Chlorothiazide Sodium (Additive or potentiated action). Products include:
Diuril Sodium Intravenous 1693

Chlorotrianisene (Reduces hypotensive effect).
No products indexed under this heading.

Chlorpromazine (Reduces hypotensive effect). Products include:
Thorazine Suppositories 2701

Chlorthalidone (Additive or potentiated action). Products include:
Combipres Tablets 682
Tenoretic Tablets 2963
Thalitone 1293

Cholestyramine (Impairs the oral absorption of hydrochlorothiazide from gastrointestinal tract by up to 85%). Products include:
Questran 774

Clomipramine Hydrochloride (Reduces hypotensive effect). Products include:
Anafranil Capsules 819

Clonidine (Additive or potentiated action). Products include:
Catapres-TTS 680

Clonidine Hydrochloride (Additive or potentiated action). Products include:
Catapres Tablets 679
Combipres Tablets 682

Codeine Phosphate (May potentiate orthostatic hypotension). Products include:
Brontex 2130
Dimetane-DC Cough Syrup 2232
Fioricet with Codeine Capsules 2387
Fiorinal with Codeine Capsules 2390
Nucofed 2225
Phenergan with Codeine 2883
Phenergan VC with Codeine 2888
Robitussin A-C Syrup 2248
Robitussin-DAC Syrup 2249
Ryna .... ▣ 804
Soma Compound w/Codeine Tablets 2784
Tylenol with Codeine 1592

Colestipol Hydrochloride (Impairs the oral absorption of hydrochlorothiazide from gastrointestinal tract by up to 43%). Products include:
Colestid 2073

Cortisone Acetate (Hypokalemia may develop during concomitant use). Products include:
Cortone Acetate Sterile Suspension 1663
Cortone Acetate Tablets 1664

Deserpidine (May result in excessive postural hypotension, bradycardia and mental depression).
No products indexed under this heading.

Desipramine Hydrochloride (Reduces hypotensive effect). Products include:
Norpramin Tablets 1273

Deslanoside (Increased ventricular irritability; slow heart).
No products indexed under this heading.

Desogestrel (Reduces hypotensive effect). Products include:
Desogen Tablets 1867
Ortho-Cept 1907

Dexamethasone (Hypokalemia may develop during concomitant use). Products include:
AK-Trol Ointment & Suspension .... ◎ 205
Decadron Elixir 1676
Decadron Tablets 1678
Decaspray Topical Aerosol 1689
Maxitrol Ophthalmic Ointment and Suspension .... ◎ 222
TobraDex Ophthalmic Suspension and Ointment 469

Dexamethasone Acetate (Hypokalemia may develop during concomitant use). Products include:
Dalalone D.P. Injectable 1009
Decadron-LA Sterile Suspension 1687

Dexamethasone Sodium Phosphate (Hypokalemia may develop during concomitant use). Products include:
Decadron Phosphate Injection 1680
Decadron Phosphate Sterile Ophthalmic Ointment 1684

IMPORTANT NOTE: Always consult each drug listing in the patient's regimen for possible interactions.

Interactions Index

Esimil

Decadron Phosphate Sterile Ophthalmic Solution 1685
Decadron Phosphate Topical Cream 1686
Decadron Phosphate with Xylocaine Injection, Sterile 1683
Dexacort Phosphate in Respihaler .. 1606
Dexacort Phosphate in Turbinaire .. 1607
NeoDecadron Sterile Ophthalmic Ointment 1755
NeoDecadron Sterile Ophthalmic Solution 1756
NeoDecadron Topical Cream 1757

Dezocine (May potentiate orthostatic hypotension). Products include:
Dalgan Injection 529

Diazoxide (Additive or potentiated action). Products include:
Hyperstat I.V. Injection 2504
Proglycem 575

Diclofenac Potassium (May reduce diuretic, natriuretic, and antihypertensive effects of thiazide diuretics). Products include:
Cataflam Tablets 833

Diclofenac Sodium (May reduce diuretic, natriuretic, and antihypertensive effects of thiazide diuretics). Products include:
Voltaren Ophthalmic Sterile Ophthalmic Solution .... ⓒ 264
Cataflam/Voltaren/Voltaren-XR 833

Dienestrol (Reduces hypotensive effect). Products include:
Ortho Dienestrol Cream 1922

Diethylstilbestrol (Reduces hypotensive effect). Products include:
Diethylstilbestrol Tablets 1477

Digitoxin (Increased ventricular irritability; slow heart). Products include:
Crystodigin Tablets 1472

Digoxin (Increased ventricular irritability; slow heart). Products include:
Lanoxicaps 1110
Lanoxin Elixir Pediatric 1113
Lanoxin Injection 1116
Lanoxin Injection Pediatric 1119
Lanoxin Tablets 1121

Diltiazem Hydrochloride (Additive or potentiated action). Products include:
Cardizem CD Capsules 1251
Cardizem SR Capsules 1255
Cardizem Injectable 1253
Cardizem Tablets 1257
Dilacor XR Extended-release Capsules 2183
Tiazac Capsules 1019

Doxazosin Mesylate (Additive or potentiated action). Products include:
Cardura Tablets 1993

Doxepin Hydrochloride (Reduces hypotensive effect). Products include:
Adapin Capsules 1542
Sinequan 2028
Zonalon Cream 1042

Enalapril Maleate (Additive or potentiated action). Products include:
Vaseretic Tablets 1810
Vasotec Tablets 1816

Enalaprilat (Additive or potentiated action). Products include:
Vasotec I.V. 1814

Ephedrine Hydrochloride (Reduces hypotensive effect). Products include:
Primatene Tablets .... ⊞ 844
Quadrinal Tablets 1398

Ephedrine Sulfate (Reduces hypotensive effect). Products include:
Marax Tablets & DF Syrup 2015

Ephedrine Tannate (Reduces hypotensive effect). Products include:
Rynatuss 2782

Esmolol Hydrochloride (Additive or potentiated action). Products include:
Brevibloc (esmolol HCl) Injection 1860

Estradiol (Reduces hypotensive effect). Products include:
Climara Transdermal System 640
Estrace Cream and Tablets 751
Estraderm Transdermal System 842
Estring Vaginal Ring 2086
Vivelle Transdermal System 880

Estrogens, Conjugated (Reduces hypotensive effect). Products include:
PMB 200 and PMB 400 2890
Premarin Intravenous 2893
Premarin Tablets 2896
Premarin Vaginal Cream 2898
Premphase 2900
Prempro 2905

Estrogens, Esterified (Reduces hypotensive effect). Products include:
ESTRATAB Tablets (0.3, 0.625, 1.25, 2.5 mg) 2715
Estratest 2718
Menest Tablets 2671

Estropipate (Reduces hypotensive effect). Products include:
Ogen Tablets 2103
Ogen Vaginal Cream 2106
Ortho-Est 1925

Ethinyl Estradiol (Reduces hypotensive effect). Products include:
Brevicon 2563
Demulen 2580
Desogen Tablets 1867
Levlen/Tri-Levlen 646
Lo/Ovral Tablets 2852
Lo/Ovral-28 Tablets 2857
Modicon 1928
Nordette-21 Tablets 2863
Nordette-28 Tablets 2866
Norinyl 2563
Ortho-Cept 1907
Ortho-Cyclen/Ortho-Tri-Cyclen 1914
Ortho-Novum 1928
Ortho-Cyclen/Ortho Tri-Cyclen 1914
Ovcon 765
Ovral Tablets 2877
Ovral-28 Tablets 2878
Levlen/Tri-Levlen 646
Tri-Norinyl 2607
Triphasil-21 Tablets 2919
Triphasil-28 Tablets 2924

Ethynodiol Diacetate (Reduces hypotensive effect). Products include:
Demulen 2580

Etodolac (May reduce diuretic, natriuretic, and antihypertensive effects of thiazide diuretics). Products include:
Lodine Capsules and Tablets 2849

Felodipine (Additive or potentiated action). Products include:
Plendil Extended-Release Tablets.... 514

Fenoprofen Calcium (May reduce the diuretic, natriuretic, and antihypertensive effects of thiazide diuretics). Products include:
Nalfon 200 Pulvules & Nalfon Tablets 933

Fentanyl (May potentiate orthostatic hypotension). Products include:
Duragesic Transdermal System 1336

Fentanyl Citrate (May potentiate orthostatic hypotension). Products include:
Sublimaze Injection 463

Fludrocortisone Acetate (Hypokalemia may develop during concomitant use). Products include:
Florinef Acetate Tablets 506

Fluphenazine Decanoate (Reduces hypotensive effect). Products include:
Prolixin Decanoate 510

Fluphenazine Enanthate (Reduces hypotensive effect). Products include:
Prolixin Enanthate 510

Fluphenazine Hydrochloride (Reduces hypotensive effect). Products include:
Prolixin 510

Flurbiprofen (May reduce diuretic, natriuretic, and antihypertensive effects of thiazide diuretics).
No products indexed under this heading.

Fosinopril Sodium (Additive or potentiated action). Products include:
Monopril Tablets 762

Furazolidone (Concurrent use contraindicated). Products include:
Furoxone 2221

Furosemide (Additive or potentiated action). Products include:
Lasix Injection, Oral Solution and Tablets 1267

Guanabenz Acetate (Additive or potentiated action).
No products indexed under this heading.

Hydralazine Hydrochloride (Additive or potentiated action). Products include:
Apresazide Capsules 824
Apresoline Hydrochloride Tablets .. 826
Hydralazine Hydrochloride Injection USP 2712
Ser-Ap-Es Tablets 867

Hydrocodone Bitartrate (May potentiate orthostatic hypotension). Products include:
Codiclear DH Syrup 808
Duratuss HD Elixir 2750
Histussin D Liquid 670
Hycodan Tablets and Syrup 946
Hycomine Compound Tablets 948
Hycomine 947
Hycotuss Expectorant Syrup 950
Hydrocet Capsules 787
Lorcet 10/650 Tablets 1016
Lortab 2751
Tussend 1830
Tussend Expectorant 1831
Vicodin Tablets 1404
Vicodin ES Tablets 1405
Vicodin HP Tablets 1403
Vicodin Tuss Expectorant 1406
Zydone Capsules 967

Hydrocodone Polistirex (May potentiate orthostatic hypotension). Products include:
Tussionex Pennkinetic Extended-Release Suspension 1624

Hydrocortisone (Hypokalemia may develop during concomitant use). Products include:
Anusol-HC Cream 2.5% 1953
Aquanil HC Lotion 1989
Maximum Strength Cortaid Spray ⊞ 800
CORTENEMA 2713
Cortisporin Ointment 1074
Cortisporin Ophthalmic Ointment Sterile 1074
Cortisporin Ophthalmic Suspension Sterile 1075
Cortisporin Otic Solution Sterile 1076
Cortisporin Otic Suspension Sterile 1077
Cortizone-5 .... ⊞ 795
Cortizone-10 .... ⊞ 795
Hydrocortone Tablets 1715
Hytone 922
Hytone Ointment 2 ½% 923
Massengill Medicated Soft Cloth Towelettes 2628
Pediotic Suspension Sterile 1140
Preparation H Hydrocortisone 1% Cream .... ⊞ 843
ProctoCream-HC 2.5% 2552
VōSoL HC Otic Solution 2786

Hydrocortisone Acetate (Hypokalemia may develop during concomitant use). Products include:
Analpram-HC Rectal Cream 1% and 2.5% 993
Anusol HC-1 Hydrocortisone Anti-Itch Ointment .... ⊞ 810
Anusol-HC Suppositories 1954
Caldecort Anti-Itch Hydrocortisone Cream .... ⊞ 651
Coly-Mycin S Otic w/Neomycin & Hydrocortisone 1965
Cortaid .... ⊞ 800
Cortifoam 2540
Cortisporin Cream 1073
Epifoam 2543
Hydrocortone Acetate Sterile Suspension 1712
Mantadil Cream 1124
Nupercainal Hydrocortisone 1% Cream .... ⊞ 661
Pramosone Cream, Lotion & Ointment 995
ProctoFoam-HC 2552
Terra-Cortril Ophthalmic Suspension 2033

Hydrocortisone Sodium Phosphate (Hypokalemia may develop during concomitant use). Products include:
Hydrocortone Phosphate Injection, Sterile 1713

Hydrocortisone Sodium Succinate (Hypokalemia may develop during concomitant use).
No products indexed under this heading.

Hydroflumethiazide (Additive or potentiated action). Products include:
Diucardin Tablets 2824

Hydromorphone Hydrochloride (May potentiate orthostatic hypotension). Products include:
Dilaudid Ampules 1382
Dilaudid Cough Syrup 1383
Dilaudid-HP Injection 1384
Dilaudid-HP Lyophilized Powder 250 mg 1384
Dilaudid 1382
Dilaudid Oral Liquid 1386
Dilaudid 1382
Dilaudid Tablets - 8 mg 1386

Ibuprofen (May reduce the diuretic, natriuretic, and antihypertensive effects of thiazide diuretics). Products include:
Advil Cold and Sinus Caplets and Tablets .... ⊞ 837
Advil Ibuprofen Tablets, Caplets and Gel Caplets .... ⊞ 836
Children's Motrin Ibuprofen Oral Suspension 1558
IBU Tablets 1389
Ibuprohm .... ⊞ 713
Motrin IB Caplets, Tablets, and Gelcaps .... ⊞ 802
Motrin Ibuprofen Suspension, Oral Drops, Chewable Tablets, Caplets 1563
Nuprin Ibuprofen/Analgesic Tablets & Caplets .... ⊞ 645
Vicks DayQuil SINUS Pressure & PAIN Relief with IBUPROFEN ...... ⊞ 735

Imipramine Hydrochloride (Reduces hypotensive effect). Products include:
Tofranil Ampuls 873
Tofranil Tablets 875

Imipramine Pamoate (Reduces hypotensive effect). Products include:
Tofranil-PM Capsules 876

Indapamide (Additive or potentiated action).
No products indexed under this heading.

Indomethacin (May reduce the diuretic, natriuretic, and antihypertensive effects of thiazide diuretics). Products include:
Indocin 1723

(⊞ Described in PDR For Nonprescription Drugs)   (ⓒ Described in PDR For Ophthalmology)

Indomethacin Sodium Trihydrate (May reduce the diuretic, natriuretic, and antihypertensive effects of thiazide diuretics). Products include:
- Indocin I.V. 1727

Insulin, Human (Insulin requirements may be altered).
- No products indexed under this heading.

Insulin, Human Isophane Suspension (Insulin requirements may be altered). Products include:
- Novolin N Human Insulin 10 ml Vials 1846

Insulin, Human NPH (Insulin requirements may be altered). Products include:
- Humulin N, 100 Units 1495
- Novolin N PenFill 1.5 ml Cartridges Durable Insulin Delivery System 1849
- Novolin N Prefilled Syringe Disposable Insulin Delivery System 1850

Insulin, Human Regular (Insulin requirements may be altered). Products include:
- Humulin R, 100 Units 1497
- Novolin R Human Insulin 10 ml Vials 1846
- Novolin R PenFill 1.5 ml Cartridges Durable Insulin Delivery System 1849
- Novolin R Prefilled Syringe Disposable Insulin Delivery System 1850
- Velosulin BR Human Insulin 10 ml Vials 1847

Insulin, Human, Zinc Suspension (Insulin requirements may be altered). Products include:
- Humulin L, 100 Units 1494
- Humulin U, 100 Units 1498
- Novolin L Human Insulin 10 ml Vials 1846

Insulin Lispro, Human (Insulin requirements may be altered). Products include:
- Humalog Injection 1488

Insulin, NPH (Insulin requirements may be altered). Products include:
- NPH, 100 Units 1502
- Pork NPH, 100 Units 1506
- Purified Pork NPH Isophane Insulin 1852

Insulin, Regular (Insulin requirements may be altered). Products include:
- Regular, 100 Units 1503
- Pork Regular, 100 Units 1507
- Pork Regular (Concentrated), 500 Units 1508
- Purified Pork Regular Insulin 1852

Insulin, Zinc Crystals (Insulin requirements may be altered). Products include:
- NPH, 100 Units 1502

Insulin, Zinc Suspension (Insulin requirements may be altered). Products include:
- Iletin I 1501
- Lente, 100 Units 1501
- Iletin II 1504
- Pork Lente, 100 Units 1504
- Purified Pork Lente Insulin 1852

Isocarboxazid (Concurrent use contraindicated).
- No products indexed under this heading.

Isradipine (Additive or potentiated action). Products include:
- DynaCirc Capsules 2381
- DynaCirc CR Tablets 2383

Ketoprofen (May reduce the diuretic, natriuretic, and antihypertensive effects of thiazide diuretics). Products include:
- Actron Caplets and Tablets 608
- Orudis Capsules 2874
- Orudis KT 842
- Oruvail Capsules 2874

Ketorolac Tromethamine (May reduce the diuretic, natriuretic, and antihypertensive effects of thiazide diuretics). Products include:
- Acular Sterile Ophthalmic Solution 470
- Toradol 2319

Labetalol Hydrochloride (Additive or potentiated action). Products include:
- Normodyne Injection 2519
- Normodyne Tablets 2522
- Trandate 1158

Levonorgestrel (Reduces hypotensive effect). Products include:
- Levlen/Tri-Levlen 646
- Nordette-21 Tablets 2863
- Nordette-28 Tablets 2866
- Norplant System 2868
- Levlen/Tri-Levlen 646
- Triphasil-21 Tablets 2919
- Triphasil-28 Tablets 2924

Levorphanol Tartrate (May potentiate orthostatic hypotension). Products include:
- Levo-Dromoran 2297

Lisinopril (Additive or potentiated action). Products include:
- Prinivil Tablets 1776
- Prinzide Tablets 1780
- Zestoretic Tablets 2968
- Zestril Tablets 2972

Lithium Carbonate (Increased risk of lithium toxicity). Products include:
- Eskalith 2658
- Lithium Carbonate Capsules & Tablets 2352
- Lithonate/Lithotabs/Lithobid 2721

Lithium Citrate (Increases risk of lithium toxicity).
- No products indexed under this heading.

Losartan Potassium (Additive or potentiated action). Products include:
- Cozaar Tablets 1668
- Hyzaar Tablets 1720

Maprotiline Hydrochloride (Reduces hypotensive effect). Products include:
- Ludiomil Tablets 861

Mecamylamine Hydrochloride (Additive or potentiated action). Products include:
- Inversine Tablets 1729

Meclofenamate Sodium (May reduce the diuretic, natriuretic, and antihypertensive effects of thiazide diuretics).
- No products indexed under this heading.

Mefenamic Acid (May reduce the diuretic, natriuretic, and antihypertensive effects of thiazide diuretics). Products include:
- Ponstel 1982

Meperidine Hydrochloride (May potentiate orthostatic hypotension). Products include:
- Demerol 2438
- Mepergan Injection 2859

Mephobarbital (May potentiate orthostatic hypotension). Products include:
- Mebaral Tablets 2452

Mesoridazine Besylate (Reduces hypotensive effect). Products include:
- Serentil 689

Mestranol (Reduces hypotensive effect). Products include:
- Norinyl 2563
- Ortho-Novum 1928

Methadone Hydrochloride (May potentiate orthostatic hypotension). Products include:
- Methadone Hydrochloride Oral Concentrate 2356
- Methadone Hydrochloride Oral Solution & Tablets 2357

Methotrimeprazine (Reduces hypotensive effect). Products include:
- Levoprome 1321

Methyclothiazide (Additive or potentiated action). Products include:
- Enduron Tablets 424

Methyldopa (Additive or potentiated action; potential for hemolytic anemia with concomitant use of hydrochlorothiazide and methyldopa). Products include:
- Aldoclor Tablets 1638
- Aldomet Oral 1640
- Aldoril Tablets 1644

Methyldopate Hydrochloride (Additive or potentiated action; potential for hemolytic anemia with concomitant use of hydrochlorothiazide and methyldopa). Products include:
- Aldomet Ester HCl Injection 1642

Methylphenidate Hydrochloride (Reduces hypotensive effect). Products include:
- Ritalin 866

Methylprednisolone Acetate (Hypokalemia may develop during concomitant use).
- No products indexed under this heading.

Methylprednisolone Sodium Succinate (Hypokalemia may develop during concomitant use).
- No products indexed under this heading.

Metolazone (Additive or potentiated action). Products include:
- Mykrox Tablets 1617
- Zaroxolyn Tablets 1625

Metoprolol Succinate (Additive or potentiated action). Products include:
- Toprol-XL Tablets 560

Metoprolol Tartrate (Additive or potentiated action). Products include:
- Lopressor 848
- Lopressor HCT Tablets 850

Metyrosine (Additive or potentiated action). Products include:
- Demser Capsules 1690

Minoxidil (Additive or potentiated action).
- No products indexed under this heading.

Moexipril Hydrochloride (Additive or potentiated action). Products include:
- Univasc Tablets 2553

Morphine Sulfate (May potentiate orthostatic hypotension). Products include:
- Astramorph/PF Injection, USP (Preservative-Free) 526
- Duramorph Injection 983
- Infumorph 200 and Infumorph 500 Sterile Solutions 985
- Kadian Capsules 2948
- MS Contin Tablets 2149
- MSIR 2152
- Oramorph SR (Morphine Sulfate Sustained Release Tablets) 2359
- RMS Suppositories CII 2766
- Roxanol 2365

Nabumetone (May reduce diuretic, natriuretic, and antihypertensive effects of thiazide diuretics). Products include:
- Relafen Tablets 2688

Nadolol (Additive or potentiated action).
- No products indexed under this heading.

Naproxen (May reduce the diuretic, natriuretic, and antihypertensive effects of thiazide diuretics). Products include:
- Anaprox/Naprosyn 2277

Naproxen Sodium (May reduce the diuretic, natriuretic, and antihypertensive effects of thiazide diuretics). Products include:
- Aleve 2124
- Anaprox/Naprosyn 2277
- Naprelan Tablets 2861

Nicardipine Hydrochloride (Additive or potentiated action). Products include:
- Cardene Capsules 2261
- Cardene I.V. 2815
- Cardene SR Capsules 2264

Nifedipine (Additive or potentiated action). Products include:
- Adalat Capsules (10 mg and 20 mg) 580
- Adalat CC 582
- Procardia Capsules 2024
- Procardia XL Extended Release Tablets 2026

Nisoldipine (Additive or potentiated action). Products include:
- Sular Tablets 2961

Nitroglycerin (Additive or potentiated action). Products include:
- Deponit NTG Transdermal Delivery System 2541
- Nitro-Bid IV 1270
- Nitro-Bid Ointment 1272
- Nitro-Dur (nitroglycerin) Transdermal Infusion System 1365
- Nitrolingual Spray 2193
- Nitrostat Tablets 1981
- Transderm-Nitro Transdermal Therapeutic System 878

Norepinephrine Bitartrate (Decreased arterial response to norepinephrine). Products include:
- Levophed Bitartrate Injection 2445

Norethindrone (Reduces hypotensive effect). Products include:
- Brevicon 2563
- Micronor Tablets 1903
- Modicon 1928
- Norinyl 2563
- Nor-Q D Tablets 2598
- Ortho-Novum 1928
- Ovcon 765
- Tri-Norinyl 2607

Norethynodrel (Reduces hypotensive effect).
- No products indexed under this heading.

Norgestimate (Reduces hypotensive effect). Products include:
- Ortho-Cyclen/Ortho-Tri-Cyclen 1914
- Ortho-Cyclen/Ortho Tri-Cyclen 1914

Norgestrel (Reduces hypotensive effect). Products include:
- Lo/Ovral Tablets 2852
- Lo/Ovral-28 Tablets 2857
- Ovral Tablets 2877
- Ovral-28 Tablets 2878
- Ovrette Tablets 2878

Nortriptyline Hydrochloride (Reduces hypotensive effect). Products include:
- Pamelor 2409

Opium Alkaloids (May potentiate orthostatic hypotension).
- No products indexed under this heading.

Oxaprozin (May reduce diuretic, natriuretic, and antihypertensive effects of thiazide diuretics). Products include:
- Daypro Caplets 2578

Oxycodone Hydrochloride (May potentiate orthostatic hypotension). Products include:
- OxyContin Tablets 2163
- OxyIR Capsules 2167
- Percocet Tablets 955
- Percodan Tablets 955
- Percodan-Demi Tablets 956

IMPORTANT NOTE: Always consult each drug listing in the patient's regimen for possible interactions.

Roxicodone Tablets, Oral Solution & Intensol (Oxycodone) 2366
Tylox Capsules 1593

Penbutolol Sulfate (Additive or potentiated action). Products include:
Levatol Tablets 2547

Pentobarbital Sodium (May potentiate orthostatic hypotension). Products include:
Nembutal Sodium Capsules 440
Nembutal Sodium Solution 442
Nembutal Sodium Suppositories 444

Perphenazine (Reduces hypotensive effect). Products include:
Etrafon 2495
Triavil Tablets 1800
Trilafon 2532

Phenelzine Sulfate (Concurrent use contraindicated). Products include:
Nardil 1977

Phenobarbital (May potentiate orthostatic hypotension). Products include:
Arco-Lase Plus Tablets 513
Bellergal-S Tablets 2375
Donnatal 2234
Donnatal Extentabs 2234
Donnatal Tablets 2234
Phenobarbital Elixir and Tablets 1523
Quadrinal Tablets 1398

Phenoxybenzamine Hydrochloride (Additive or potentiated action). Products include:
Dibenzyline Capsules 2650

Phentolamine Mesylate (Additive or potentiated action). Products include:
Regitine Vials 864

Phenylbutazone (May reduce the diuretic, natriuretic, and antihypertensive effects of thiazide diuretics).
No products indexed under this heading.

Pindolol (Additive or potentiated action). Products include:
Visken Tablets 2428

Piroxicam (May reduce the diuretic, natriuretic, and antihypertensive effects of thiazide diuretics). Products include:
Feldene Capsules 2008

Polythiazide (Additive or potentiated action). Products include:
Minizide Capsules 2016

Prazosin Hydrochloride (Additive or potentiated action). Products include:
Minipress Capsules 2015
Minizide Capsules 2016

Prednisolone Acetate (Hypokalemia may develop during concomitant use). Products include:
AK-CIDE .... ◉ 203
AK-CIDE Ointment .... ◉ 203
Blephamide Liquifilm Sterile Ophthalmic Suspension 472
Blephamide Ointment .... ◉ 234
Econopred & Econopred Plus Ophthalmic Suspensions .... ◉ 216
Poly-Pred Liquifilm .... ◉ 246
Pred Forte .... ◉ 247
Pred Mild .... ◉ 250
Pred-G Liquifilm Sterile Ophthalmic Suspension .... ◉ 248
Pred-G S.O.P. Sterile Ophthalmic Ointment .... ◉ 249

Prednisolone Sodium Phosphate (Hypokalemia may develop during concomitant use). Products include:
AK-PRED .... ◉ 204
Hydeltrasol Injection, Sterile 1708
Pediapred Oral Solution 1618

Prednisolone Tebutate (Hypokalemia may develop during concomitant use). Products include:
Hydeltra-T.B.A. Sterile Suspension 1710

Prednisone (Hypokalemia may develop during concomitant use).
No products indexed under this heading.

Prochlorperazine (Reduced hypotensive effect). Products include:
Compazine 2644

Promethazine Hydrochloride (Reduces hypotensive effect). Products include:
Mepergan Injection 2859
Phenergan with Codeine 2883
Phenergan with Dextromethorphan 2885
Phenergan Injection 2880
Phenergan Suppositories 2882
Phenergan Syrup 2881
Phenergan Tablets 2882
Phenergan VC 2886
Phenergan VC with Codeine 2888

Propoxyphene Hydrochloride (May potentiate orthostatic hypotension). Products include:
Darvon 1475
Wygesic Tablets 2930

Propoxyphene Napsylate (May potentiate orthostatic hypotension). Products include:
Darvon-N/Darvocet-N 1473

Propranolol Hydrochloride (Additive or potentiated action). Products include:
Inderal 2834
Inderal LA Long Acting Capsules 2836
Inderide Tablets 2838
Inderide LA Long Acting Capsules .. 2840

Protriptyline Hydrochloride (Reduces hypotensive effect). Products include:
Vivactil Tablets 1820

Quinapril Hydrochloride (Additive or potentiated action). Products include:
Accupril Tablets 1950

Quinestrol (Reduces hypotensive effect).
No products indexed under this heading.

Ramipril (Additive or potentiated action). Products include:
Altace Capsules 1238

Rauwolfia Serpentina (May result in excessive postural hypotension, bradycardia and mental depression).
No products indexed under this heading.

Rescinnamine (May result in excessive postural hypotension, bradycardia and mental depression).
No products indexed under this heading.

Reserpine (May result in excessive postural hypotension, bradycardia and mental depression). Products include:
Diupres Tablets 1691
Hydropres Tablets 1718
Ser-Ap-Es Tablets 867

Secobarbital Sodium (May potentiate orthostatic hypotension). Products include:
Seconal Sodium Pulvules 1529

Selegiline Hydrochloride (Concurrent use contraindicated). Products include:
Eldepryl Capsules 2729

Sodium Nitroprusside (Additive or potentiated action).
No products indexed under this heading.

Sotalol Hydrochloride (Additive or potentiated action). Products include:
Betapace Tablets 637

Spirapril Hydrochloride (Additive or potentiated action).
No products indexed under this heading.

Sufentanil Citrate (May potentiate orthostatic hypotension). Products include:
Sufenta Injection 1355

Sulindac (May reduce the diuretic, natriuretic, and antihypertensive effects of thiazide diuretics). Products include:
Clinoril Tablets 1658

Terazosin Hydrochloride (Additive or potentiated action). Products include:
Hytrin Capsules 434

Thiamylal Sodium (May potentiate orthostatic hypotension).
No products indexed under this heading.

Thioridazine Hydrochloride (Reduces hypotensive effect). Products include:
Mellaril 2398

Timolol Maleate (Additive or potentiated action). Products include:
Blocadren Tablets 1654
Timolide Tablets 1791
Timoptic in Ocudose 1796
Timoptic Sterile Ophthalmic Solution 1794
Timoptic-XE 1798

Tolmetin Sodium (May reduce the diuretic, natriuretic, and antihypertensive effects of thiazide diuretics). Products include:
Tolectin (200, 400 and 600 mg) .. 1591

Torsemide (Additive or potentiated action). Products include:
Demadex Tablets and Injection 691

Tranylcypromine Sulfate (Concurrent use contraindicated). Products include:
Parnate Tablets 2679

Triamcinolone (Hypokalemia may develop during concomitant use).
No products indexed under this heading.

Triamcinolone Acetonide (Hypokalemia may develop during concomitant use). Products include:
Azmacort Oral Inhaler 2175
Nasacort AQ Nasal Spray 2191
Nasacort Nasal Inhaler 2189

Triamcinolone Diacetate (Hypokalemia may develop during concomitant use).
No products indexed under this heading.

Triamcinolone Hexacetonide (Hypokalemia may develop during concomitant use).
No products indexed under this heading.

Trifluoperazine Hydrochloride (Reduces hypotensive effect). Products include:
Stelazine 2692

Trimethaphan Camsylate (Additive or potentiated action).
No products indexed under this heading.

Trimipramine Maleate (Reduces hypotensive effect). Products include:
Surmontil Capsules 2917

Tubocurarine Chloride (Increased response to tubocurarine).
No products indexed under this heading.

Verapamil Hydrochloride (Additive or potentiated action). Products include:
Calan SR Caplets 2571
Calan Tablets 2568
Covera-HS Tablets 2573
Isoptin Injectable 1391
Isoptin Oral Tablets 1393
Isoptin SR Tablets 1395
Verelan Capsules 1455

Food Interactions

Alcohol (Orthostatic hypotension aggravated).

Food, unspecified (Enhances gastrointestinal absorption of hydrochlorothiazide).

ESKALITH CAPSULES

(Lithium Carbonate) 2658
May interact with neuromuscular blocking agents, diuretics, urinary alkalizing agents, xanthine bronchodilators, antipsychotic agents, nonsteroidal anti-inflammatory agents, calcium channel blockers, ACE inhibitors, and certain other agents. Compounds in these categories include:

Acetazolamide (Increases urinary lithium excretion). Products include:
Diamox Sequels (Sustained Release) .... ◉ 318
Diamox Tablets .... ◉ 317

Amiloride Hydrochloride (Diuretic-induced sodium loss may reduce the renal clearance of lithium and increase serum lithium levels with risk of lithium toxicity). Products include:
Midamor Tablets 1746
Moduretic Tablets 1748

Aminophylline (Lowers serum lithium concentrations).
No products indexed under this heading.

Amlodipine Besylate (Increases the risk of neurotoxicity). Products include:
Lotrel Capsules 858
Norvasc Tablets 2020

Atracurium Besylate (Lithium may prolong the effect of neuromuscular blocking agents). Products include:
Tracrium Injection 1155

Benazepril Hydrochloride (May substantially increase steady-state plasma lithium levels resulting in lithium toxicity). Products include:
Lotensin Tablets 852
Lotensin HCT Tablets 855
Lotrel Capsules 858

Bendroflumethiazide (Diuretic-induced sodium loss may reduce the renal clearance of lithium and increase serum lithium levels with risk of lithium toxicity).
No products indexed under this heading.

Bepridil Hydrochloride (Increases the risk of neurotoxicity). Products include:
Vascor Tablets (200 and 300 mg) 1597

Bumetanide (Diuretic-induced sodium loss may reduce the renal clearance of lithium and increase serum lithium levels with risk of lithium toxicity). Products include:
Bumex 2260

Captopril (May substantially increase steady-state plasma lithium levels resulting in lithium toxicity). Products include:
Capoten Tablets 740
Capozide Tablets 744

Chlorothiazide (Diuretic-induced sodium loss may reduce the renal clearance of lithium and increase serum lithium levels with risk of lithium toxicity). Products include:
Aldoclor Tablets 1638
Diupres Tablets 1691
Diuril Oral 1694

Chlorothiazide Sodium (Diuretic-induced sodium loss may reduce the renal clearance of lithium and increase serum lithium levels with risk of lithium toxicity). Products include:
Diuril Sodium Intravenous 1693

(▣ Described in PDR For Nonprescription Drugs) (◉ Described in PDR For Ophthalmology)

Chlorpromazine (Potential for an encephalopathic syndrome with possible irreversible brain damage with co-administration of lithium with a neuroleptic). Products include:
Thorazine Suppositories 2701
Chlorpromazine Hydrochloride (Potential for an encephalopathic syndrome with possible irreversible brain damage with co-administration of lithium with a neuroleptic). Products include:
Thorazine 2701
Chlorprothixene (Potential for an encephalopathic syndrome with possible irreversible brain damage with co-administration of lithium with a neuroleptic).
No products indexed under this heading.
Chlorprothixene Hydrochloride (Potential for an encephalopathic syndrome with possible irreversible brain damage with co-administration of lithium with a neuroleptic).
No products indexed under this heading.
Chlorthalidone (Diuretic-induced sodium loss may reduce the renal clearance of lithium and increase serum lithium levels with risk of lithium toxicity). Products include:
Combipres Tablets 682
Tenoretic Tablets 2963
Thalitone 1293
Cisatracurium Besylate (Lithium may prolong the effect of neuromuscular blocking agents). Products include:
Nimbex Injection 1131
Clozapine (Potential for an encephalopathic syndrome with possible irreversible brain damage with co-administration of lithium with a neuroleptic). Products include:
Clozaril Tablets 2377
Diclofenac Potassium (Lithium-indomethacin type interaction may occur with other nonsteroidal anti-inflammatory agents; potential for increase in steady-state plasma lithium levels). Products include:
Cataflam Tablets 833
Diclofenac Sodium (Lithium-indomethacin type interaction may occur with other nonsteroidal anti-inflammatory agents; potential for increase in steady-state plasma lithium levels). Products include:
Voltaren Ophthalmic Sterile Ophthalmic Solution .... ⊙ 264
Cataflam/Voltaren/Voltaren-XR 833
Diltiazem Hydrochloride (Increases the risk of neurotoxicity). Products include:
Cardizem CD Capsules 1251
Cardizem SR Capsules 1255
Cardizem Injectable 1253
Cardizem Tablets 1257
Dilacor XR Extended-release Capsules 2183
Tiazac Capsules 1019
Doxacurium Chloride (Lithium may prolong the effect of neuromuscular blocking agents). Products include:
Nuromax Injection 1136
Dyphylline (Lowers serum lithium concentrations). Products include:
Lufyllin & Lufyllin-400 Tablets 2778
Lufyllin-GG Elixir & Tablets 2779
Enalapril Maleate (May substantially increase steady-state plasma lithium levels resulting in lithium toxicity). Products include:
Vaseretic Tablets 1810
Vasotec Tablets 1816
Enalaprilat (May substantially increase steady-state plasma lithium levels resulting in lithium toxicity). Products include:
Vasotec I.V. 1814
Ethacrynic Acid (Diuretic-induced sodium loss may reduce the renal clearance of lithium and increase serum lithium levels with risk of lithium toxicity). Products include:
Edecrin Tablets 1698
Etodolac (Lithium-indomethacin type interaction may occur with other nonsteroidal anti-inflammatory agents; potential for increase in steady-state plasma lithium levels). Products include:
Lodine Capsules and Tablets 2849
Felodipine (Increases the risk of neurotoxicity). Products include:
Plendil Extended-Release Tablets 514
Fenoprofen Calcium (Lithium-indomethacin type interaction may occur with other nonsteroidal anti-inflammatory agents; potential for increase in steady-state plasma lithium levels). Products include:
Nalfon 200 Pulvules & Nalfon Tablets 933
Fluphenazine Decanoate (Potential for an encephalopathic syndrome with possible irreversible brain damage with co-administration of lithium with a neuroleptic). Products include:
Prolixin Decanoate 510
Fluphenazine Enanthate (Potential for an encephalopathic syndrome with possible irreversible brain damage with co-administration of lithium with a neuroleptic). Products include:
Prolixin Enanthate 510
Fluphenazine Hydrochloride (Potential for an encephalopathic syndrome with possible irreversible brain damage with co-administration of lithium with a neuroleptic). Products include:
Prolixin 510
Flurbiprofen (Lithium-indomethacin type interaction may occur with other nonsteroidal anti-inflammatory agents; potential for increase in steady-state plasma lithium levels).
No products indexed under this heading.
Fosinopril Sodium (May substantially increase steady-state plasma lithium levels resulting in lithium toxicity). Products include:
Monopril Tablets 762
Furosemide (Diuretic-induced sodium loss may reduce the renal clearance of lithium and increase serum lithium levels with risk of lithium toxicity). Products include:
Lasix Injection, Oral Solution and Tablets 1267
Haloperidol (Potential for an encephalopathic syndrome with possible irreversible brain damage with co-administration of lithium with a neuroleptic). Products include:
Haldol Injection, Tablets and Concentrate 1585
Haloperidol Decanoate (Potential for an encephalopathic syndrome with possible irreversible brain damage with co-administration of lithium with a neuroleptic). Products include:
Haldol Decanoate 1587
Hydrochlorothiazide (Diuretic-induced sodium loss may reduce the renal clearance of lithium and increase serum lithium levels with risk of lithium toxicity). Products include:
Aldactazide Tablets 2556
Aldoril Tablets 1644
Apresazide Capsules 824
Capozide Tablets 744
Dyazide Capsules 2653
Esidrix Tablets 839
Esimil Tablets 840
HydroDIURIL Tablets 1716
Hydropres Tablets 1718
Hyzaar Tablets 1720
Inderide Tablets 2838
Inderide LA Long Acting Capsules .. 2840
Lopressor HCT Tablets 850
Lotensin HCT Tablets 855
Moduretic Tablets 1748
Oretic Tablets 450
Prinzide Tablets 1780
Ser-Ap-Es Tablets 867
Timolide Tablets 1791
Vaseretic Tablets 1810
Zestoretic Tablets 2968
Ziac 1459
Hydroflumethiazide (Diuretic-induced sodium loss may reduce the renal clearance of lithium and increase serum lithium levels with risk of lithium toxicity). Products include:
Diucardin Tablets 2824
Ibuprofen (Lithium-indomethacin type interaction may occur with other nonsteroidal anti-inflammatory agents; potential for increase in steady-state plasma lithium levels). Products include:
Advil Cold and Sinus Caplets and Tablets 837
Advil Ibuprofen Tablets, Caplets and Gel Caplets 836
Children's Motrin Ibuprofen Oral Suspension 1558
IBU Tablets 1389
Ibuprohm 713
Motrin IB Caplets, Tablets, and Gelcaps 802
Motrin Ibuprofen Suspension, Oral Drops, Chewable Tablets, Caplets 1563
Nuprin Ibuprofen/Analgesic Tablets & Caplets 645
Vicks DayQuil SINUS Pressure & PAIN Relief with IBUPROFEN 735
Indapamide (Diuretic-induced sodium loss may reduce the renal clearance of lithium and increase serum lithium levels with risk of lithium toxicity).
No products indexed under this heading.
Indomethacin (Co-administration has resulted in significant increase in steady-state plasma lithium levels with risk of lithium toxicity). Products include:
Indocin 1723
Indomethacin Sodium Trihydrate (Co-administration has resulted in significant increase in steady-state plasma lithium levels with risk of lithium toxicity). Products include:
Indocin I.V. 1727
Isradipine (Increases the risk of neurotoxicity). Products include:
DynaCirc Capsules 2381
DynaCirc CR Tablets 2383
Ketoprofen (Lithium-indomethacin type interaction may occur with other nonsteroidal anti-inflammatory agents; potential for increase in steady-state plasma lithium levels). Products include:
Actron Caplets and Tablets 608
Orudis Capsules 2874
Orudis KT 842
Oruvail Capsules 2874
Ketorolac Tromethamine (Lithium-indomethacin type interaction may occur with other nonsteroidal anti-inflammatory agents; potential for increase in steady-state plasma lithium levels). Products include:
Acular Sterile Ophthalmic Solution 470
Toradol 2319
Lisinopril (May substantially increase steady-state plasma lithium levels resulting in lithium toxicity). Products include:
Prinivil Tablets 1776
Prinzide Tablets 1780
Zestoretic Tablets 2968
Zestril Tablets 2972
Lithium Citrate (Potential for an encephalopathic syndrome with possible irreversible brain damage with co-administration of lithium with a neuroleptic).
No products indexed under this heading.
Loxapine Hydrochloride (Potential for an encephalopathic syndrome with possible irreversible brain damage with co-administration of lithium with a neuroleptic). Products include:
Loxitane 1426
Loxapine Succinate (Potential for an encephalopathic syndrome with possible irreversible brain damage with co-administration of lithium with a neuroleptic). Products include:
Loxitane Capsules 1426
Meclofenamate Sodium (Lithium-indomethacin type interaction may occur with other nonsteroidal anti-inflammatory agents; potential for increase in steady-state plasma lithium levels).
No products indexed under this heading.
Mefenamic Acid (Lithium-indomethacin type interaction may occur with other nonsteroidal anti-inflammatory agents; potential for increase in steady-state plasma lithium levels). Products include:
Ponstel 1982
Mesoridazine Besylate (Potential for an encephalopathic syndrome with possible irreversible brain damage with co-administration of lithium with a neuroleptic). Products include:
Serentil 689
Methotrimeprazine (Potential for an encephalopathic syndrome with possible irreversible brain damage with co-administration of lithium with a neuroleptic). Products include:
Levoprome 1321
Methyclothiazide (Diuretic-induced sodium loss may reduce the renal clearance of lithium and increase serum lithium levels with risk of lithium toxicity). Products include:
Enduron Tablets 424
Metocurine Iodide (Lithium may prolong the effect of neuromuscular blocking agents). Products include:
Metubine Iodide Vials 932
Metolazone (Diuretic-induced sodium loss may reduce the renal clearance of lithium and increase serum lithium levels with risk of lithium toxicity). Products include:
Mykrox Tablets 1617
Zaroxolyn Tablets 1625
Metronidazole (May provoke lithium toxicity due to reduced renal clearance). Products include:
Flagyl 375 Capsules 2587
Flagyl I.V. RTU 2373
Helidac Therapy 2135
MetroCream 1034

IMPORTANT NOTE: Always consult each drug listing in the patient's regimen for possible interactions.

MetroGel 1034
MetroGel-Vaginal 917
Protostat Tablets 1939

Metronidazole Hydrochloride (May provoke lithium toxicity due to reduced renal clearance). Products include:
Flagyl I.V. 2373

Mivacurium Chloride (Lithium may prolong the effect of neuromuscular blocking agents). Products include:
Mivacron 1125

Moexipril Hydrochloride (May substantially increase steady-state plasma lithium levels resulting in lithium toxicity). Products include:
Univasc Tablets 2553

Molindone Hydrochloride (Potential for an encephalopathic syndrome with possible irreversible brain damage with co-administration of lithium with a neuroleptic). Products include:
Moban Tablets and Concentrate 1036

Nabumetone (Lithium-indomethacin type interaction may occur with other nonsteroidal anti-inflammatory agents; potential for increase in steady-state plasma lithium levels). Products include:
Relafen Tablets 2688

Naproxen (Lithium-indomethacin type interaction may occur with other nonsteroidal anti-inflammatory agents; potential for increase in steady-state plasma lithium levels). Products include:
Anaprox/Naprosyn 2277

Naproxen Sodium (Lithium-indomethacin type interaction may occur with other nonsteroidal anti-inflammatory agents; potential for increase in steady-state plasma lithium levels). Products include:
Aleve 2124
Anaprox/Naprosyn 2277
Naprelan Tablets 2861

Nicardipine Hydrochloride (Increases the risk of neurotoxicity). Products include:
Cardene Capsules 2261
Cardene I.V. 2815
Cardene SR Capsules 2264

Nifedipine (Increases the risk of neurotoxicity). Products include:
Adalat Capsules (10 mg and 20 mg) 580
Adalat CC 582
Procardia Capsules 2024
Procardia XL Extended Release Tablets 2026

Nimodipine (Increases the risk of neurotoxicity). Products include:
Nimotop Capsules 603

Nisoldipine (Increases the risk of neurotoxicity). Products include:
Sular Tablets 2961

Oxaprozin (Lithium-indomethacin type interaction may occur with other nonsteroidal anti-inflammatory agents; potential for increase in steady-state plasma lithium levels). Products include:
Daypro Caplets 2578

Pancuronium Bromide (Lithium may prolong the effect of neuromuscular blocking agents).
No products indexed under this heading.

Perphenazine (Potential for an encephalopathic syndrome with possible irreversible brain damage with co-administration of lithium with a neuroleptic). Products include:
Etrafon 2495
Triavil Tablets 1800
Trilafon 2532

Phenylbutazone (Lithium-indomethacin type interaction may occur with other nonsteroidal anti-inflammatory agents; potential for increase in steady-state plasma lithium levels).
No products indexed under this heading.

Pimozide (Potential for an encephalopathic syndrome with possible irreversible brain damage with co-administration of lithium with a neuroleptic). Products include:
Orap Tablets 1037

Piroxicam (Co-administration has resulted in significant increase in steady-state plasma lithium levels with risk of lithium toxicity). Products include:
Feldene Capsules 2008

Polythiazide (Diuretic-induced sodium loss may reduce the renal clearance of lithium and increase serum lithium levels with risk of lithium toxicity). Products include:
Minizide Capsules 2016

Potassium Citrate (Increases urinary lithium excretion). Products include:
Polycitra Syrup 574
Polycitra-K Crystals 574
Polycitra-K Oral Solution 575
Polycitra-LC 574
Urocit-K Tablets 1828

Prochlorperazine (Potential for an encephalopathic syndrome with possible irreversible brain damage with co-administration of lithium with a neuroleptic). Products include:
Compazine 2644

Promethazine Hydrochloride (Potential for an encephalopathic syndrome with possible irreversible brain damage with co-administration of lithium with a neuroleptic). Products include:
Mepergan Injection 2859
Phenergan with Codeine 2883
Phenergan with Dextromethorphan 2885
Phenergan Injection 2880
Phenergan Suppositories 2882
Phenergan Syrup 2881
Phenergan Tablets 2882
Phenergan VC 2886
Phenergan VC with Codeine 2888

Quinapril Hydrochloride (May substantially increase steady-state plasma lithium levels resulting in lithium toxicity). Products include:
Accupril Tablets 1950

Ramipril (May substantially increase steady-state plasma lithium levels resulting in lithium toxicity). Products include:
Altace Capsules 1238

Risperidone (Potential for an encephalopathic syndrome with possible irreversible brain damage with co-administration of lithium with a neuroleptic). Products include:
Risperdal Tablets 1348

Rocuronium Bromide (Lithium may prolong the effect of neuromuscular blocking agents). Products include:
Zemuron Injection 1885

Sodium Bicarbonate (Increases urinary lithium excretion). Products include:
Alka-Seltzer Cherry Effervescent Antacid and Pain Reliever .... ▣ 609
Alka-Seltzer Extra Strength Effervescent Antacid and Pain Reliever .... ▣ 609
Alka-Seltzer Gold Effervescent Antacid .... ▣ 611
Alka-Seltzer Lemon Lime Effervescent Antacid and Pain Reliever .... ▣ 609
Alka-Seltzer Original Effervescent Antacid and Pain Reliever .... ▣ 609
Arm & Hammer Pure Baking Soda .... ▣ 648
Colyte and Colyte-flavored 2540
GoLYTELY 694
Massengill Disposable Douches .... ▣ 780
Massengill Liquid Concentrate .... ▣ 780
NuLYTELY 694
Cherry Flavor NuLYTELY 694

Sodium Citrate (Increases urinary lithium excretion). Products include:
Bicitra 573
Polycitra 574
Salix SST Lozenges Saliva Stimulant .... ▣ 757

Spirapril Hydrochloride (May substantially increase steady-state plasma lithium levels resulting in lithium toxicity).
No products indexed under this heading.

Spironolactone (Diuretic-induced sodium loss may reduce the renal clearance of lithium and increase serum lithium levels with risk of lithium toxicity). Products include:
Aldactazide Tablets 2556
Aldactone Tablets 2558

Succinylcholine Chloride (Lithium may prolong the effect of neuromuscular blocking agents). Products include:
Anectine 1062

Sulindac (Lithium-indomethacin type interaction may occur with other nonsteroidal anti-inflammatory agents; potential for increase in steady-state plasma lithium levels). Products include:
Clinoril Tablets 1658

Theophylline (Lowers serum lithium concentrations). Products include:
Marax Tablets & DF Syrup 2015
Quibron 2227

Theophylline Anhydrous (Lowers serum lithium concentrations). Products include:
Aerolate 1003
Primatene Tablets .... ▣ 844
Respbid Tablets 687
Slo-bid Gyrocaps 2201
Theo-24 Extended Release Capsules 2753
Theo-Dur Extended-Release Tablets 1367
Theo-X Extended-Release Tablets 793
Uni-Dur Extended-Release Tablets 1374
Uniphyl 400 mg and 600 mg Tablets 2157

Theophylline Calcium Salicylate (Lowers serum lithium concentrations). Products include:
Quadrinal Tablets 1398

Theophylline Sodium Glycinate (Lowers serum lithium concentrations).
No products indexed under this heading.

Thioridazine Hydrochloride (Potential for an encephalopathic syndrome with possible irreversible brain damage with co-administration of lithium with a neuroleptic). Products include:
Mellaril 2398

Thiothixene (Potential for an encephalopathic syndrome with possible irreversible brain damage with co-administration of lithium with a neuroleptic). Products include:
Navane Capsules and Concentrate 2018
Navane Intramuscular 2019

Tolmetin Sodium (Lithium-indomethacin type interaction may occur with other nonsteroidal anti-inflammatory agents; potential for increase in steady-state plasma lithium levels). Products include:
Tolectin (200, 400 and 600 mg) 1591

Torsemide (Diuretic-induced sodium loss may reduce the renal clearance of lithium and increase serum lithium levels with risk of lithium toxicity). Products include:
Demadex Tablets and Injection 691

Trandolapril (May substantially increase steady-state plasma lithium levels resulting in lithium toxicity). Products include:
Mavik Tablets 1407

Triamterene (Diuretic-induced sodium loss may reduce the renal clearance of lithium and increase serum lithium levels with risk of lithium toxicity). Products include:
Dyazide Capsules 2653
Dyrenium Capsules 2655

Trifluoperazine Hydrochloride (Potential for an encephalopathic syndrome with possible irreversible brain damage with co-administration of lithium with a neuroleptic). Products include:
Stelazine 2692

Urea (Systemic administration of urea with lithium therapy can lower serum lithium concentration by increasing urinary lithium excretion). Products include:
Accuzyme Ointment 1236
Amino-Cerv 1827
Eucerin Plus Dry Skin Care Moisturizing Lotion 636
Eucerin Plus Moisturizing Creme 636
Panafil Ointment 2372
Panafil-White Ointment 2372

Vecuronium Bromide (Lithium may prolong the effect of neuromuscular blocking agents). Products include:
Norcuron for Injection 1875

Verapamil Hydrochloride (Increases the risk of neurotoxicity). Products include:
Calan SR Caplets 2571
Calan Tablets 2568
Covera-HS Tablets 2573
Isoptin Injectable 1391
Isoptin Oral Tablets 1393
Isoptin SR Tablets 1395
Verelan Capsules 1455

ESKALITH CR CONTROLLED RELEASE TABLETS

(Lithium Carbonate) 2658
See **Eskalith Capsules**

ESTER-C MINERAL ASCORBATES POWDER

(Calcium Ascorbate) .... ▣ 673
None cited in PDR database.

ESTRACE CREAM AND TABLETS

(Estradiol) 751
None cited in PDR database.

ESTRADERM TRANSDERMAL SYSTEM

(Estradiol) 842
May interact with progestins. Compounds in this category include:

Desogestrel (Potential for adverse effects on carbohydrate and lipid metabolism). Products include:
Desogen Tablets 1867
Ortho-Cept 1907

Medroxyprogesterone Acetate (Potential for adverse effects on carbohydrate and lipid metabolism). Products include:
Amen Tablets 785
Cycrin Tablets 991
Depo-Provera Contraceptive Injection 2079
Depo-Provera Sterile Aqueous Suspension 2083

(▣ Described in PDR For Nonprescription Drugs) (⊙ Described in PDR For Ophthalmology)

393 **Interactions Index** **Ethyol**

Premphase 2900
Prempro 2905
Provera Tablets 2110

Megestrol Acetate (Potential for adverse effects on carbohydrate and lipid metabolism). Products include:
Megace Oral Suspension 708
Megace Tablets 710

Norgestimate (Potential for adverse effects on carbohydrate and lipid metabolism). Products include:
Ortho-Cyclen/Ortho-Tri-Cyclen 1914
Ortho-Cyclen/Ortho Tri-Cyclen 1914

ESTRATAB TABLETS (0.3, 0.625, 1.25, 2.5 MG)
(Estrogens, Esterified) 2715
May interact with progestins. Compounds in this category include:

Desogestrel (Potential adverse effects on carbohydrate and lipid metabolism). Products include:
Desogen Tablets 1867
Ortho-Cept 1907

Medroxyprogesterone Acetate (Potential adverse effects on carbohydrate and lipid metabolism). Products include:
Amen Tablets 785
Cycrin Tablets 991
Depo-Provera Contraceptive Injection 2079
Depo-Provera Sterile Aqueous Suspension 2083
Premphase 2900
Prempro 2905
Provera Tablets 2110

Megestrol Acetate (Potential adverse effects on carbohydrate and lipid metabolism). Products include:
Megace Oral Suspension 708
Megace Tablets 710

Norgestimate (Potential adverse effects on carbohydrate and lipid metabolism). Products include:
Ortho-Cyclen/Ortho-Tri-Cyclen 1914
Ortho-Cyclen/Ortho Tri-Cyclen 1914

ESTRATEST TABLETS
(Estrogens, Esterified, Methyltestosterone) 2718
See **ESTRATEST H.S. Tablets**

ESTRATEST H.S. TABLETS
(Estrogens, Esterified, Methyltestosterone) 2718
May interact with oral anticoagulants, insulin, and certain other agents. Compounds in these categories include:

Dicumarol (Decreased anticoagulant requirements).
No products indexed under this heading.

Insulin, Human (Decreased blood glucose and insulin requirements).
No products indexed under this heading.

Insulin, Human Isophane Suspension (Decreased blood glucose and insulin requirements). Products include:
Novolin N Human Insulin 10 ml Vials 1846

Insulin, Human NPH (Decreased blood glucose and insulin requirements). Products include:
Humulin N, 100 Units 1495
Novolin N PenFill 1.5 ml Cartridges Durable Insulin Delivery System 1849
Novolin N Prefilled Syringe Disposable Insulin Delivery System 1850

Insulin, Human Regular (Decreased blood glucose and insulin requirements). Products include:
Humulin R, 100 Units 1497
Novolin R Human Insulin 10 ml Vials 1846
Novolin R PenFill 1.5 ml Cartridges Durable Insulin Delivery System 1849
Novolin R Prefilled Syringe Disposable Insulin Delivery System 1850
Velosulin BR Human Insulin 10 ml Vials 1847

Insulin, Human, Zinc Suspension (Decreased blood glucose and insulin requirements). Products include:
Humulin L, 100 Units 1494
Humulin U, 100 Units 1498
Novolin L Human Insulin 10 ml Vials 1846

Insulin Lispro, Human (Decreased blood glucose and insulin requirements). Products include:
Humalog Injection 1488

Insulin, NPH (Decreased blood glucose and insulin requirements). Products include:
NPH, 100 Units 1502
Pork NPH, 100 Units 1506
Purified Pork NPH Isophane Insulin 1852

Insulin, Regular (Decreased blood glucose and insulin requirements). Products include:
Regular, 100 Units 1503
Pork Regular, 100 Units 1507
Pork Regular (Concentrated), 500 Units 1508
Purified Pork Regular Insulin 1852

Insulin, Zinc Crystals (Decreased blood glucose and insulin requirements). Products include:
NPH, 100 Units 1502

Insulin, Zinc Suspension (Decreased blood glucose and insulin requirements). Products include:
Iletin I 1501
Lente, 100 Units 1501
Iletin II 1504
Pork Lente, 100 Units 1504
Purified Pork Lente Insulin 1852

Oxyphenbutazone (Concurrent use may result in elevated serum levels of oxyphenbutazone).

Warfarin Sodium (Decreased anticoagulant requirements). Products include:
Coumadin 941

ESTRING VAGINAL RING
(Estradiol) 2086
May interact with:

Vaginally administered preparations, unspecified (It is recommended that Estring be removed during treatment with other vaginally administered preparations).

ETHAMOLIN INJECTION
(Ethanolamine Oleate) 2544
None cited in PDR database.

ETHIODOL INJECTION
(Ethiodized Oil) 2472
None cited in PDR database.

ETHMOZINE TABLETS
(Moricizine Hydrochloride) 2217
May interact with xanthine bronchodilators and certain other agents. Compounds in these categories include:

Aminophylline (Theophylline clearance and plasma half-life significantly affected).
No products indexed under this heading.

Cimetidine (Concomitant use results in a decrease in Ethmozine clearance of 49% and a 1.4 fold increase in plasma levels). Products include:
Tagamet HB Tablets ◘ 786
Tagamet Tablets 2694

Cimetidine Hydrochloride (Concomitant use results in a decrease in Ethmozine clearance of 49% and a 1.4 fold increase in plasma levels). Products include:
Tagamet 2694

Digoxin (Potential for additive prolongation of the PR interval). Products include:
Lanoxicaps 1110
Lanoxin Elixir Pediatric 1113
Lanoxin Injection 1116
Lanoxin Injection Pediatric 1119
Lanoxin Tablets 1121

Dyphylline (Theophylline clearance and plasma half-life significantly affected). Products include:
Lufyllin & Lufyllin-400 Tablets 2778
Lufyllin-GG Elixir & Tablets 2779

Propranolol Hydrochloride (Small additive increase in the PR interval). Products include:
Inderal 2834
Inderal LA Long Acting Capsules 2836
Inderide Tablets 2838
Inderide LA Long Acting Capsules 2840

Theophylline (Theophylline clearance and plasma half-life significantly affected). Products include:
Marax Tablets & DF Syrup 2015
Quibron 2227

Theophylline Anhydrous (Theophylline clearance and plasma half-life significantly affected). Products include:
Aerolate 1003
Primatene Tablets ◘ 844
Respbid Tablets 687
Slo-bid Gyrocaps 2201
Theo-24 Extended Release Capsules 2753
Theo-Dur Extended-Release Tablets 1367
Theo-X Extended-Release Tablets 793
Uni-Dur Extended-Release Tablets 1374
Uniphyl 400 mg and 600 mg Tablets 2157

Theophylline Calcium Salicylate (Theophylline clearance and plasma half-life significantly affected). Products include:
Quadrinal Tablets 1398

Theophylline Sodium Glycinate (Theophylline clearance and plasma half-life significantly affected).
No products indexed under this heading.

Warfarin Sodium (Isolated reports of the need to either increase or decrease warfarin doses after initiation of Ethmozine; potential for excessive prolongation of prothrombin time following initiation of Ethmozine in patients with stable prothrombin time). Products include:
Coumadin 941

Food Interactions

Meal, unspecified (Administration 30 minutes after a meal delays the rate of absorption but the extent of absorption is not altered).

ETHYL CHLORIDE, U.S.P.
(Chloroethane, Ethyl Chloride) 1040
None cited in PDR database.

ETHYOL (AMIFOSTINE) FOR INJECTION
(Amifostine) 485
May interact with antihypertensives. Compounds in this category include:

Acebutolol Hydrochloride (Amifostine produces transient hypotension; caution is advised if it is used with other antihypertensive agents). Products include:
Sectral Capsules 2914

Amlodipine Besylate (Amifostine produces transient hypotension; caution is advised if it is used with other antihypertensive agents). Products include:
Lotrel Capsules 858
Norvasc Tablets 2020

Atenolol (Amifostine produces transient hypotension; caution is advised if it is used with other antihypertensive agents). Products include:
Tenoretic Tablets 2963
Tenormin Tablets and I.V. Injection 2965

Benazepril Hydrochloride (Amifostine produces transient hypotension; caution is advised if it is used with other antihypertensive agents). Products include:
Lotensin Tablets 852
Lotensin HCT Tablets 855
Lotrel Capsules 858

Bendroflumethiazide (Amifostine produces transient hypotension; caution is advised if it is used with other antihypertensive agents).
No products indexed under this heading.

Betaxolol Hydrochloride (Amifostine produces transient hypotension; caution is advised if it is used with other antihypertensive agents). Products include:
Betoptic Ophthalmic Solution 465
Betoptic S Ophthalmic Suspension 467
Kerlone Tablets 2588

Bisoprolol Fumarate (Amifostine produces transient hypotension; caution is advised if it is used with other antihypertensive agents). Products include:
Zebeta Tablets 1457
Ziac 1459

Captopril (Amifostine produces transient hypotension; caution is advised if it is used with other antihypertensive agents). Products include:
Capoten Tablets 740
Capozide Tablets 744

Carteolol Hydrochloride (Amifostine produces transient hypotension; caution is advised if it is used with other antihypertensive agents). Products include:
Cartrol Tablets 413
Ocupress Ophthalmic Solution, 1% Sterile ⊙ 297

Chlorothiazide (Amifostine produces transient hypotension; caution is advised if it is used with other antihypertensive agents). Products include:
Aldoclor Tablets 1638
Diupres Tablets 1691
Diuril Oral 1694

Chlorothiazide Sodium (Amifostine produces transient hypotension; caution is advised if it is used with other antihypertensive agents). Products include:
Diuril Sodium Intravenous 1693

Chlorthalidone (Amifostine produces transient hypotension; caution is advised if it is used with other antihypertensive agents). Products include:
Combipres Tablets 682
Tenoretic Tablets 2963
Thalitone 1293

Clonidine (Amifostine produces transient hypotension; caution is advised if it is used with other antihypertensive agents). Products include:
Catapres-TTS 680

IMPORTANT NOTE: Always consult each drug listing in the patient's regimen for possible interactions.

Interactions Index

Clonidine Hydrochloride (Amifostine produces transient hypotension; caution is advised if it is used with other antihypertensive agents). Products include:
- Catapres Tablets 679
- Combipres Tablets 682

Deserpidine (Amifostine produces transient hypotension; caution is advised if it is used with other antihypertensive agents).
No products indexed under this heading.

Diazoxide (Amifostine produces transient hypotension; caution is advised if it is used with other antihypertensive agents). Products include:
- Hyperstat I.V. Injection 2504
- Proglycem 575

Diltiazem Hydrochloride (Amifostine produces transient hypotension; caution is advised if it is used with other antihypertensive agents). Products include:
- Cardizem CD Capsules 1251
- Cardizem SR Capsules 1255
- Cardizem Injectable 1253
- Cardizem Tablets 1257
- Dilacor XR Extended-release Capsules 2183
- Tiazac Capsules 1019

Doxazosin Mesylate (Amifostine produces transient hypotension; caution is advised if it is used with other antihypertensive agents). Products include:
- Cardura Tablets 1993

Enalapril Maleate (Amifostine produces transient hypotension; caution is advised if it is used with other antihypertensive agents). Products include:
- Vaseretic Tablets 1810
- Vasotec Tablets 1816

Enalaprilat (Amifostine produces transient hypotension; caution is advised if it is used with other antihypertensive agents). Products include:
- Vasotec I.V. 1814

Esmolol Hydrochloride (Amifostine produces transient hypotension; caution is advised if it is used with other antihypertensive agents). Products include:
- Brevibloc (esmolol HCl) Injection .. 1860

Felodipine (Amifostine produces transient hypotension; caution is advised if it is used with other antihypertensive agents). Products include:
- Plendil Extended-Release Tablets .. 514

Fosinopril Sodium (Amifostine produces transient hypotension; caution is advised if it is used with other antihypertensive agents). Products include:
- Monopril Tablets 762

Furosemide (Amifostine produces transient hypotension; caution is advised if it is used with other antihypertensive agents). Products include:
- Lasix Injection, Oral Solution and Tablets 1267

Guanabenz Acetate (Amifostine produces transient hypotension; caution is advised if it is used with other antihypertensive agents).
No products indexed under this heading.

Guanethidine Monosulfate (Amifostine produces transient hypotension; caution is advised if it is used with other antihypertensive agents). Products include:
- Esimil Tablets 840
- Ismelin Tablets 845

Hydralazine Hydrochloride (Amifostine produces transient hypotension; caution is advised if it is used with other antihypertensive agents). Products include:
- Apresazide Capsules 824
- Apresoline Hydrochloride Tablets .. 826
- Hydralazine Hydrochloride Injection USP 2712
- Ser-Ap-Es Tablets 867

Hydrochlorothiazide (Amifostine produces transient hypotension; caution is advised if it is used with other antihypertensive agents). Products include:
- Aldactazide Tablets 2556
- Aldoril Tablets 1644
- Apresazide Capsules 824
- Capozide Tablets 744
- Dyazide Capsules 2653
- Esidrix Tablets 839
- Esimil Tablets 840
- HydroDIURIL Tablets 1716
- Hydropres Tablets 1718
- Hyzaar Tablets 1720
- Inderide Tablets 2838
- Inderide LA Long Acting Capsules .. 2840
- Lopressor HCT Tablets 850
- Lotensin HCT Tablets 855
- Moduretic Tablets 1748
- Oretic Tablets 450
- Prinzide Tablets 1780
- Ser-Ap-Es Tablets 867
- Timolide Tablets 1791
- Vaseretic Tablets 1810
- Zestoretic Tablets 2968
- Ziac 1459

Hydroflumethiazide (Amifostine produces transient hypotension; caution is advised if it is used with other antihypertensive agents). Products include:
- Diucardin Tablets 2824

Indapamide (Amifostine produces transient hypotension; caution is advised if it is used with other antihypertensive agents).
No products indexed under this heading.

Isradipine (Amifostine produces transient hypotension; caution is advised if it is used with other antihypertensive agents). Products include:
- DynaCirc Capsules 2381
- DynaCirc CR Tablets 2383

Labetalol Hydrochloride (Amifostine produces transient hypotension; caution is advised if it is used with other antihypertensive agents). Products include:
- Normodyne Injection 2519
- Normodyne Tablets 2522
- Trandate 1158

Lisinopril (Amifostine produces transient hypotension; caution is advised if it is used with other antihypertensive agents). Products include:
- Prinivil Tablets 1776
- Prinzide Tablets 1780
- Zestoretic Tablets 2968
- Zestril Tablets 2972

Losartan Potassium (Amifostine produces transient hypotension; caution is advised if it is used with other antihypertensive agents). Products include:
- Cozaar Tablets 1668
- Hyzaar Tablets 1720

Mecamylamine Hydrochloride (Amifostine produces transient hypotension; caution is advised if it is used with other antihypertensive agents). Products include:
- Inversine Tablets 1729

Methyclothiazide (Amifostine produces transient hypotension; caution is advised if it is used with other antihypertensive agents). Products include:
- Enduron Tablets 424

Methyldopa (Amifostine produces transient hypotension; caution is advised if it is used with other antihypertensive agents). Products include:
- Aldoclor Tablets 1638
- Aldomet Oral 1640
- Aldoril Tablets 1644

Methyldopate Hydrochloride (Amifostine produces transient hypotension; caution is advised if it is used with other antihypertensive agents). Products include:
- Aldomet Ester HCl Injection 1642

Metolazone (Amifostine produces transient hypotension; caution is advised if it is used with other antihypertensive agents). Products include:
- Mykrox Tablets 1617
- Zaroxolyn Tablets 1625

Metoprolol Succinate (Amifostine produces transient hypotension; caution is advised if it is used with other antihypertensive agents). Products include:
- Toprol-XL Tablets 560

Metoprolol Tartrate (Amifostine produces transient hypotension; caution is advised if it is used with other antihypertensive agents). Products include:
- Lopressor 848
- Lopressor HCT Tablets 850

Metyrosine (Amifostine produces transient hypotension; caution is advised if it is used with other antihypertensive agents). Products include:
- Demser Capsules 1690

Minoxidil (Amifostine produces transient hypotension; caution is advised if it is used with other antihypertensive agents).
No products indexed under this heading.

Moexipril Hydrochloride (Amifostine produces transient hypotension; caution is advised if it is used with other antihypertensive agents). Products include:
- Univasc Tablets 2553

Nadolol (Amifostine produces transient hypotension; caution is advised if it is used with other antihypertensive agents).
No products indexed under this heading.

Nicardipine Hydrochloride (Amifostine produces transient hypotension; caution is advised if it is used with other antihypertensive agents). Products include:
- Cardene Capsules 2261
- Cardene I.V. 2815
- Cardene SR Capsules 2264

Nifedipine (Amifostine produces transient hypotension; caution is advised if it is used with other antihypertensive agents). Products include:
- Adalat Capsules (10 mg and 20 mg) 580
- Adalat CC 582
- Procardia Capsules 2024
- Procardia XL Extended Release Tablets 2026

Nisoldipine (Amifostine produces transient hypotension; caution is advised if it is used with other antihypertensive agents). Products include:
- Sular Tablets 2961

Nitroglycerin (Amifostine produces transient hypotension; caution is advised if it is used with other antihypertensive agents). Products include:
- Deponit NTG Transdermal Delivery System 2541
- Nitro-Bid IV 1270
- Nitro-Bid Ointment 1272
- Nitro-Dur (nitroglycerin) Transdermal Infusion System 1365
- Nitrolingual Spray 2193
- Nitrostat Tablets 1981
- Transderm-Nitro Transdermal Therapeutic System 878

Penbutolol Sulfate (Amifostine produces transient hypotension; caution is advised if it is used with other antihypertensive agents). Products include:
- Levatol Tablets 2547

Phenoxybenzamine Hydrochloride (Amifostine produces transient hypotension; caution is advised if it is used with other antihypertensive agents). Products include:
- Dibenzyline Capsules 2650

Phentolamine Mesylate (Amifostine produces transient hypotension; caution is advised if it is used with other antihypertensive agents). Products include:
- Regitine Vials 864

Pindolol (Amifostine produces transient hypotension; caution is advised if it is used with other antihypertensive agents). Products include:
- Visken Tablets 2428

Polythiazide (Amifostine produces transient hypotension; caution is advised if it is used with other antihypertensive agents). Products include:
- Minizide Capsules 2016

Prazosin Hydrochloride (Amifostine produces transient hypotension; caution is advised if it is used with other antihypertensive agents). Products include:
- Minipress Capsules 2015
- Minizide Capsules 2016

Propranolol Hydrochloride (Amifostine produces transient hypotension; caution is advised if it is used with other antihypertensive agents). Products include:
- Inderal 2834
- Inderal LA Long Acting Capsules 2836
- Inderide Tablets 2838
- Inderide LA Long Acting Capsules .. 2840

Quinapril Hydrochloride (Amifostine produces transient hypotension; caution is advised if it is used with other antihypertensive agents). Products include:
- Accupril Tablets 1950

Ramipril (Amifostine produces transient hypotension; caution is advised if it is used with other antihypertensive agents). Products include:
- Altace Capsules 1238

Rauwolfia Serpentina (Amifostine produces transient hypotension; caution is advised if it is used with other antihypertensive agents).
No products indexed under this heading.

Rescinnamine (Amifostine produces transient hypotension; caution is advised if it is used with other antihypertensive agents).
No products indexed under this heading.

395 Interactions Index Etrafon

Reserpine (Amifostine produces transient hypotension; caution is advised if it is used with other antihypertensive agents). Products include:
- Diupres Tablets ... 1691
- Hydropres Tablets ... 1718
- Ser-Ap-Es Tablets ... 867

Sodium Nitroprusside (Amifostine produces transient hypotension; caution is advised if it is used with other antihypertensive agents).
- No products indexed under this heading.

Sotalol Hydrochloride (Amifostine produces transient hypotension; caution is advised if it is used with other antihypertensive agents). Products include:
- Betapace Tablets ... 637

Spirapril Hydrochloride (Amifostine produces transient hypotension; caution is advised if it is used with other antihypertensive agents).
- No products indexed under this heading.

Terazosin Hydrochloride (Amifostine produces transient hypotension; caution is advised if it is used with other antihypertensive agents). Products include:
- Hytrin Capsules ... 434

Timolol Maleate (Amifostine produces transient hypotension; caution is advised if it is used with other antihypertensive agents). Products include:
- Blocadren Tablets ... 1654
- Timolide Tablets ... 1791
- Timoptic in Ocudose ... 1796
- Timoptic Sterile Ophthalmic Solution ... 1794
- Timoptic-XE ... 1798

Torsemide (Amifostine produces transient hypotension; caution is advised if it is used with other antihypertensive agents). Products include:
- Demadex Tablets and Injection ... 691

Trimethaphan Camsylate (Amifostine produces transient hypotension; caution is advised if it is used with other antihypertensive agents).
- No products indexed under this heading.

Verapamil Hydrochloride (Amifostine produces transient hypotension; caution is advised if it is used with other antihypertensive agents). Products include:
- Calan SR Caplets ... 2571
- Calan Tablets ... 2568
- Covera-HS Tablets ... 2573
- Isoptin Injectable ... 1391
- Isoptin Oral Tablets ... 1393
- Isoptin SR Tablets ... 1395
- Verelan Capsules ... 1455

ETOPOPHOS FOR INJECTION
(Etoposide Phosphate) ... 701
May interact with:

Cyclosporine (Co-administration with high-dose cyclosporine and oral etoposide has led to an 80% increase in etoposide exposure with a 38% decrease in total body clearance of etoposide compared to etoposide alone). Products include:
- Neoral ... 2405
- Sandimmune ... 2416

Levamisole Hydrochloride (Co-administration with drugs that are known to inhibit phosphatase activities requires caution). Products include:
- Ergamisol Tablets ... 1340

ETOPOSIDE INJECTION
(Etoposide) ... 539
None cited in PDR database.

ETRAFON FORTE TABLETS (4-25)
(Perphenazine, Amitriptyline Hydrochloride) ... 2495
See Etrafon Tablets (2-25)

ETRAFON 2-10 TABLETS (2-10)
(Perphenazine, Amitriptyline Hydrochloride) ... 2495
See Etrafon Tablets (2-25)

ETRAFON TABLETS (2-25)
(Perphenazine, Amitriptyline Hydrochloride) ... 2495
May interact with barbiturates, central nervous system depressants, narcotic analgesics, anticholinergics, antihistamines, sympathomimetics, monoamine oxidase inhibitors, thyroid preparations, drugs that inhibit cytochrome p450iid6, antidepressant drugs, phenothiazines, selective serotonin reuptake inhibitors, and certain other agents. Compounds in these categories include:

Acrivastine (Since phenothiazines and antihistamines are CNS depressants, each can potentiate each other). Products include:
- Semprex-D Capsules ... 1620

Albuterol (Effects of concurrent use not specified; close supervision and careful adjustment of dosages are required). Products include:
- Proventil Inhalation Aerosol ... 2524
- Ventolin Inhalation Aerosol and Refill ... 1170

Albuterol Sulfate (Effects of concurrent use not specified; close supervision and careful adjustment of dosages are required). Products include:
- Airet Albuterol Sulfate Inhalation Solution ... 1602
- Albuterol Sulfate, USP Solution for Inhalation, Arm-a-Med ... 522
- Proventil Inhalation Solution 0.083% ... 2527
- Proventil Repetabs Tablets ... 2529
- Proventil Solution for Inhalation 0.5% ... 2525
- Proventil Syrup ... 2528
- Proventil Tablets ... 2529
- Ventolin Inhalation Solution ... 1171
- Ventolin Nebules Inhalation Solution ... 1172
- Ventolin Rotacaps for Inhalation ... 1173
- Ventolin Syrup ... 1175
- Ventolin Tablets ... 1176
- Volmax Extended-Release Tablets ... 1835

Alfentanil Hydrochloride (Enhanced response to the effects of central nervous system depressants). Products include:
- Alfenta Injection ... 1334

Alprazolam (Enhanced response to the effects of central nervous system depressants). Products include:
- Xanax Tablets ... 2115

Amoxapine (Concurrent use with drugs that are substrate for cytochrome $P_{450}IID_6$ may make normal metabolizer resemble poor metabolizer leading to higher than expected plasma concentrations of TCA with resultant toxicity). Products include:
- Asendin Tablets ... 1419

Aprobarbital (Enhanced response to barbiturates).
- No products indexed under this heading.

Astemizole (Since phenothiazines and antihistamines are CNS depressants, each can potentiate each other). Products include:
- Hismanal Tablets ... 1341

Atropine Sulfate (Concurrent use may result in additive anticholinergic effects including paralytic ileus). Products include:
- Arco-Lase Plus Tablets ... 513
- Atrohist Plus Tablets ... 1605
- Donnatal ... 2234
- Donnatal Extentabs ... 2234
- Donnatal Tablets ... 2234
- Lomotil ... 2591
- Motofen Tablets ... 789
- Urised Tablets ... 2123

Azatadine Maleate (Since phenothiazines and antihistamines are CNS depressants, each can potentiate each other). Products include:
- Trinalin Repetabs Tablets ... 1373

Belladonna Alkaloids (Concurrent use may result in additive anticholinergic effects including paralytic ileus). Products include:
- Bellergal-S Tablets ... 2375
- Hyland's Bedwetting Tablets ... 788
- Hyland's EnurAid Tablets ... 789
- Hyland's Headache Tablets ... 790
- Hyland's Teething Tablets ... 790
- Similasan Eye Drops #1 ... 769

Benztropine Mesylate (Concurrent use may result in additive anticholinergic effects including paralytic ileus). Products include:
- Cogentin ... 1661

Biperiden Hydrochloride (Concurrent use may result in additive anticholinergic effects including paralytic ileus). Products include:
- Akineton ... 1380

Bromodiphenhydramine Hydrochloride (Since phenothiazines and antihistamines are CNS depressants, each can potentiate each other).
- No products indexed under this heading.

Brompheniramine Maleate (Since phenothiazines and antihistamines are CNS depressants, each can potentiate each other). Products include:
- Alka-Seltzer Plus Sinus Medicine ... 611
- Bromfed Capsules (Extended-Release) ... 1832
- Bromfed Syrup ... 712
- Bromfed Tablets ... 1832
- Bromfed-DM Cough Syrup ... 1832
- Bromfed-PD Capsules (Extended-Release) ... 1832
- Dimetane-DC Cough Syrup ... 2232
- Dimetane-DX Cough Syrup ... 2233
- Dimetapp Allergy Dye-Free Elixir ... 838
- Dimetapp Allergy Sinus Caplets ... 838
- Dimetapp Cold & Allergy Chewable Tablets ... 838
- Dimetapp Cold & Cough Liqui-Gels ... 839
- Dimetapp Cold & Fever Suspension ... 839
- Dimetapp DM Elixir ... 840
- Dimetapp Elixir ... 840
- Dimetapp Extentabs ... 841
- Dimetapp Tablets/Liqui-Gels ... 841
- Rondec Chewable Tablets ... 974
- Vicks DayQuil Allergy Relief 12-Hour Extended Release Tablets ... 733
- Vicks DayQuil Allergy Relief 4-Hour Tablets ... 733

Buprenorphine (Enhanced response to the effects of central nervous system depressants). Products include:
- Buprenex Injectable ... 2170

Bupropion Hydrochloride (Concurrent use with drugs that are substrate for cytochrome $P_{450}IID_6$ may make normal metabolizer resemble poor metabolizer leading to higher than expected plasma concentrations of TCA with resultant toxicity). Products include:
- Wellbutrin Tablets ... 1177

Buspirone Hydrochloride (Enhanced response to the effects of central nervous system depressants). Products include:
- BuSpar Tablets ... 738

Butabarbital (Enhanced response to barbiturates).
- No products indexed under this heading.

Butalbital (Enhanced response to barbiturates). Products include:
- Axocet Capsules ... 2469
- Esgic-plus Capsules ... 1012
- Esgic-plus Tablets ... 1012
- Fioricet Tablets ... 2386
- Fioricet with Codeine Capsules ... 2387
- Fiorinal Capsules ... 2388
- Fiorinal with Codeine Capsules ... 2390
- Fiorinal Tablets ... 2388
- Phrenilin ... 790
- Sedapap Tablets 50 mg/650 mg ... 1826

Cetirizine Hydrochloride (Since phenothiazines and antihistamines are CNS depressants, each can potentiate each other). Products include:
- Zyrtec Tablets ... 2053

Chlordiazepoxide (Enhanced response to the effects of central nervous system depressants). Products include:
- Limbitrol ... 2333

Chlordiazepoxide Hydrochloride (Enhanced response to the effects of central nervous system depressants). Products include:
- Librax Capsules ... 2330
- Librium Capsules ... 2331
- Librium Injectable ... 2332

Chlorpheniramine Maleate (Since phenothiazines and antihistamines are CNS depressants, each can potentiate each other). Products include:
- Alka-Seltzer Plus Cold Medicine ... 611
- Alka-Seltzer Plus Cold Medicine Liqui-Gels ... 612
- Alka-Seltzer Plus Cold & Cough Medicine ... 611
- Alka-Seltzer Plus Cold & Cough Medicine Liqui-Gels ... 612
- Alka-Seltzer Plus Flu & Body Aches Effervescent Tablets ... 612
- Allerest Maximum Strength ... 649
- Allerest Sinus Pain Formula ... 649
- Ana-Kit Anaphylaxis Emergency Treatment Kit ... 611
- Atrohist Pediatric Capsules ... 1603
- Atrohist Plus Tablets ... 1605
- BC Cold Powder Multi-Symptom Formula (Cold-Sinus-Allergy) ... 631
- Cerose DM ... 853
- Cheracol Plus Head Cold/Cough Formula ... 741
- Children's TYLENOL Cold Multi-Symptom Chewable Tablets and Liquid ... 1559
- Children's TYLENOL Cold Plus Cough Multi Symptom Chewable Tablets and Liquid ... 1560
- Children's TYLENOL Flu Suspension Liquid ... 1560
- Children's Vicks DayQuil Allergy Relief ... 730
- Children's Vicks NyQuil Cold/Cough Relief ... 731
- Chlor-Trimeton Allergy Decongestant Tablets ... 759
- Chlor-Trimeton Allergy Tablets ... 758
- Allergy-Sinus Comtrex Multi-Symptom Allergy-Sinus Formula Tablets and Caplets ... 639
- Comtrex Multi-Symptom ... 638
- Contac Continuous Action Nasal Decongestant/Antihistamine 12 Hour Capsules ... 773
- Contac Maximum Strength Continuous Action Decongestant/Antihistamine 12 Hour Caplets ... 772
- Contac Severe Cold and Flu Formula Caplets ... 773
- Coricidin Cold + Flu Tablets ... 760
- Coricidin Cough + Cold Tablets ... 760
- Coricidin 'D' Decongestant Tablets ... 760
- D.A. II Tablets ... 972

IMPORTANT NOTE: Always consult each drug listing in the patient's regimen for possible interactions.

D.A. Chewable Tablets ... 970
Dura-Tap/PD Capsules ... 970
Dura-Vent/DA Tablets ... 972
Efidac 24 Chlorpheniramine ... [RD] 655
Extendryl ... 1003
Fedahist Gyrocaps ... 2545
Hycomine Compound Tablets ... 948
Kronofed-A ... 994
Nolamine Timed-Release Tablets ... 790
Novahistine Elixir ... [RD] 782
Ornade Spansule Capsules ... 2678
PediaCare Cough-Cold Chewable Tablets and Liquid ... 1569
PediaCare NightRest Cough-Cold Liquid ... 1569
Pediatric Vicks 44m Cough & Cold Relief ... [RD] 737
Pyrroxate Caplets ... [RD] 742
Ryna ... [RD] 804
Sinarest ... [RD] 663
Sine-Off Sinus Medicine ... [RD] 784
Singlet Tablets ... [RD] 785
Sinulin Tablets ... 792
Sinutab Sinus Allergy Medication, Maximum Strength Tablets and Caplets ... [RD] 823
Sudafed Cold & Allergy Tablets ... [RD] 826
Teldrin 12 Hour Antihistamine/Nasal Decongestant Allergy Relief Capsules ... [RD] 786
TheraFlu Flu and Cold Medicine ... [RD] 750
Theraflu Maximum Strength Flu and Cold Medicine For Sore Throat ... [RD] 751
TheraFlu Flu, Cold and Cough Medicine ... [RD] 750
TheraFlu Maximum Strength Nighttime Flu, Cold & Cough Medicine ... [RD] 751
Triaminic Night Time ... [RD] 754
Triaminic Syrup ... [RD] 755
Triaminic Triaminicol Cold & Cough ... [RD] 756
Triaminicin Tablets ... [RD] 756
Tussend ... 1830
TYLENOL Allergy Sinus, Maximum Strength Caplets and Gelcaps ... 1571
TYLENOL Cold Medication, Multi-Symptom Formula Tablets and Caplets ... 1572
TYLENOL Cold Medication, Multi-Symptom Hot Liquid Packets ... 1572
Vicks 44 LiquiCaps Cough, Cold & Flu Relief ... [RD] 728
Vicks 44M Cough, Cold & Flu Relief ... [RD] 729

Chlorpheniramine Polistirex (Since phenothiazines and antihistamines are CNS depressants, each can potentiate each other). Products include:
Tussionex Pennkinetic Extended-Release Suspension ... 1624

Chlorpheniramine Tannate (Since phenothiazines and antihistamines are CNS depressants, each can potentiate each other). Products include:
Atrohist Pediatric Suspension ... 1604
Atrohist Pediatric Suspension Dye-Free ... 1604
Rynatan ... 2781
Rynatuss ... 2782

Chlorpromazine (Enhanced response to the effects of central nervous system depressants; concurrent use with drugs that are substrate for cytochrome $P_{450}IID_6$ may make normal metabolizer resemble poor metabolizer leading to higher than expected plasma concentrations of TCA with resultant toxicity). Products include:
Thorazine Suppositories ... 2701

Chlorpromazine Hydrochloride (Enhanced response to the effects of central nervous system depressants; concurrent use with drugs that are substrate for cytochrome $P_{450}IID_6$ may make normal metabolizer resemble poor metabolizer leading to higher than expected plasma concentrations of TCA with resultant toxicity). Products include:
Thorazine ... 2701

Chlorprothixene (Enhanced response to the effects of central nervous system depressants).
No products indexed under this heading.

Chlorprothixene Hydrochloride (Enhanced response to the effects of central nervous system depressants).
No products indexed under this heading.

Chlorprothixene Lactate (Enhanced response to the effects of central nervous system depressants).
No products indexed under this heading.

Cimetidine (Co-administration can produce clinically significant increases in plasma concentrations of tricyclic antidepressants resulting in severe anticholinergic symptoms including dry mouth, urinary retention and blurred vision). Products include:
Tagamet HB Tablets ... [RD] 786
Tagamet Tablets ... 2694

Cimetidine Hydrochloride (Co-administration can produce clinically significant increases in plasma concentrations of tricyclic antidepressants resulting in severe anticholinergic symptoms including dry mouth, urinary retention and blurred vision). Products include:
Tagamet ... 2694

Clidinium Bromide (Concurrent use may result in additive anticholinergic effects including paralytic ileus). Products include:
Librax Capsules ... 2330

Clonidine (Amitriptyline may block the antihypertensive effect). Products include:
Catapres-TTS ... 680

Clonidine Hydrochloride (Amitriptyline may block the antihypertensive effect). Products include:
Catapres Tablets ... 679
Combipres Tablets ... 682

Clorazepate Dipotassium (Enhanced response to the effects of central nervous system depressants). Products include:
Tranxene ... 459

Clozapine (Enhanced response to the effects of central nervous system depressants). Products include:
Clozaril Tablets ... 2377

Codeine Phosphate (Enhanced response to the effects of central nervous system depressants; enhanced response to central nervous system depressants). Products include:
Brontex ... 2130
Dimetane-DC Cough Syrup ... 2232
Fioricet with Codeine Capsules ... 2387
Fiorinal with Codeine Capsules ... 2390
Nucofed ... 2225
Phenergan with Codeine ... 2883
Phenergan VC with Codeine ... 2888
Robitussin A-C Syrup ... 2248
Robitussin-DAC Syrup ... 2249
Ryna ... [RD] 804
Soma Compound w/Codeine Tablets ... 2784
Tylenol with Codeine ... 1592

Cyproheptadine Hydrochloride (Since phenothiazines and antihistamines are CNS depressants, each can potentiate each other). Products include:
Periactin ... 1767

Desflurane (Enhanced response to the effects of central nervous system depressants). Products include:
Suprane (desflurane, USP) ... 1865

Desipramine Hydrochloride (Concurrent use with drugs that are substrate for cytochrome $P_{450}IID_6$ may make normal metabolizer resemble poor metabolizer leading to higher than expected plasma concentrations of TCA with resultant toxicity). Products include:
Norpramin Tablets ... 1273

Dexchlorpheniramine Maleate (Since phenothiazines and antihistamines are CNS depressants, each can potentiate each other).
No products indexed under this heading.

Dezocine (Enhanced response to the effects of central nervous system depressants). Products include:
Dalgan Injection ... 529

Diazepam (Enhanced response to the effects of central nervous system depressants). Products include:
Dizac (diazepam injectable emulsion) CIV ... 1862
Valium Injectable ... 2336
Valium Tablets ... 2335

Dicyclomine Hydrochloride (Concurrent use may result in additive anticholinergic effects including paralytic ileus). Products include:
Bentyl ... 1246

Diphenhydramine Citrate (Since phenothiazines and antihistamines are CNS depressants, each can potentiate each other). Products include:
Excedrin P.M. Analgesic/Sleeping Aid Tablets, Caplets, Liquigels ... 735

Diphenhydramine Hydrochloride (Since phenothiazines and antihistamines are CNS depressants, each can potentiate each other). Products include:
Actifed Allergy Daytime/Nighttime Caplets ... [RD] 808
Actifed Sinus Daytime/Nighttime Tablets and Caplets ... [RD] 809
Extra Strength Bayer PM Aspirin Plus Sleep Aid ... [RD] 617
Benadryl Allergy Chewables ... [RD] 811
Benadryl Allergy/Cold Tablets ... [RD] 811
Benadryl Allergy Decongestant Liquid Medication ... [RD] 812
Benadryl Allergy Decongestant Tablets ... [RD] 812
Benadryl Allergy Liquid Medication ... [RD] 813
Benadryl Allergy ... [RD] 811
Benadryl Allergy Sinus Headache Caplets ... [RD] 813
Benadryl Dye-Free Allergy Liqui-gel Softgels ... [RD] 813
Benadryl Dye-Free Allergy Liquid Medication ... [RD] 814
Benadryl Itch Relief Stick Extra Strength ... [RD] 814
Benadryl Cream ... [RD] 814
Benadryl Gel ... [RD] 815
Benadryl Spray ... [RD] 815
Benadryl Injection ... 1955
Contac Day & Night Cold/Flu Night Caplets ... [RD] 772
Contac Night Allergy/Sinus Caplets ... [RD] 771
Extra Strength Doan's P.M. ... [RD] 653
Excedrin P.M. Analgesic/Sleeping Aid Tablets, Caplets, Liquigels ... [RD] 643
Nytol QuickCaps Caplets ... [RD] 632
Sleepinal Night-time Sleep Aid Capsules and Softgels ... [RD] 798
TYLENOL Allergy Sinus NightTime, Maximum Strength Caplets ... 1571
TYLENOL Flu NightTime, Maximum Strength Gelcaps ... 1575
TYLENOL Flu NightTime, Maximum Strength Hot Medication Packets ... 1575
TYLENOL PM Pain Reliever/Sleep Aid, Extra Strength Gelcaps, Caplets, Geltabs ... 1576
TYLENOL Severe Allergy Medication Caplets ... 1571
Maximum Strength Unisom Sleepgels ... 1990
Unisom With Pain Relief-Nighttime Sleep Aid and Pain Reliever ... 1991

Diphenylpyraline Hydrochloride (Since phenothiazines and antihistamines are CNS depressants, each can potentiate each other).
No products indexed under this heading.

Dobutamine Hydrochloride (Effects of concurrent use not specified; close supervision and careful adjustment of dosages are required). Products include:
Dobutrex Solution Vials ... 1480

Dopamine Hydrochloride (Effects of concurrent use not specified; close supervision and careful adjustment of dosages are required).
No products indexed under this heading.

Doxepin Hydrochloride (Concurrent use with drugs that are substrate for cytochrome $P_{450}IID_6$ may make normal metabolizer resemble poor metabolizer leading to higher than expected plasma concentrations of TCA with resultant toxicity). Products include:
Adapin Capsules ... 1542
Sinequan ... 2028
Zonalon Cream ... 1042

Droperidol (Enhanced response to the effects of central nervous system depressants). Products include:
Inapsine Injection ... 462

Enflurane (Enhanced response to the effects of central nervous system depressants).
No products indexed under this heading.

Ephedrine Hydrochloride (Effects of concurrent use not specified; close supervision and careful adjustment of dosages are required). Products include:
Primatene Tablets ... [RD] 844
Quadrinal Tablets ... 1398

Ephedrine Sulfate (Effects of concurrent use not specified; close supervision and careful adjustment of dosages are required). Products include:
Marax Tablets & DF Syrup ... 2015

Ephedrine Tannate (Effects of concurrent use not specified; close supervision and careful adjustment of dosages are required). Products include:
Rynatuss ... 2782

Epinephrine (Effects of concurrent use of epinephrine (combined with local anesthetics) not specified; close supervision and careful adjustment of dosages are required). Products include:
EPIFRIN ... ◉ 237
EpiPen ... 808
Marcaine with Epinephrine ... 2446
Primatene Mist ... [RD] 843
Sensorcaine with Epinephrine Injection ... 554
Sus-Phrine Injection ... 1017
Xylocaine with Epinephrine Injections ... 562

Epinephrine Bitartrate (Effects of concurrent use not specified; close supervision and careful adjustment of dosages are required). Products include:
Sensorcaine-MPF with Epinephrine Injection ... 554

Epinephrine Hydrochloride (Effects of concurrent use of epinephrine (combined with local anesthetics) not specified). Products include:
Ana-Kit Anaphylaxis Emergency Treatment Kit ... 611

([RD] Described in PDR For Nonprescription Drugs) (◉ Described in PDR For Ophthalmology)

Estazolam (Enhanced response to the effects of central nervous system depressants). Products include:
- ProSom Tablets ... 457

Ethchlorvynol (Concurrent use of high dose of ethchlorvynol may produce transient delirium; enhanced response to central nervous system depressants). Products include:
- Placidyl Capsules ... 456

Ethinamate (Enhanced response to the effects of central nervous system depressants).
- No products indexed under this heading.

Fentanyl (Enhanced response to the effects of central nervous system depressants). Products include:
- Duragesic Transdermal System ... 1336

Fentanyl Citrate (Enhanced response to the effects of central nervous system depressants). Products include:
- Sublimaze Injection ... 463

Flecainide Acetate (Concurrent use with drugs that are substrate for cytochrome $P_{450}IID_6$ may make normal metabolizer resemble poor metabolizer leading to higher than expected plasma concentrations of TCA with resultant toxicity). Products include:
- Tambocor Tablets ... 1555

Fluoxetine Hydrochloride (Concurrent use with drugs that are substrate for cytochrome $P_{450}IID_6$ may make normal metabolizer resemble poor metabolizer leading to higher than expected plasma concentrations of TCA with resultant toxicity; due to variation in the extent of inhibition of $P_{450}IID_6$ and long half-life of the parent (fluoxetine) and active metabolite sufficient time must elapse at least 5 weeks before switching to TCA). Products include:
- Prozac Pulvules & Liquid, Oral Solution ... 935

Fluphenazine Decanoate (Enhanced response to the effects of central nervous system depressants; concurrent use with drugs that are substrate for cytochrome $P_{450}IID_6$ may make normal metabolizer resemble poor metabolizer leading to higher than expected plasma concentrations of TCA with resultant toxicity). Products include:
- Prolixin Decanoate ... 510

Fluphenazine Enanthate (Enhanced response to the effects of central nervous system depressants; concurrent use with drugs that are substrate for cytochrome $P_{450}IID_6$ may make normal metabolizer resemble poor metabolizer leading to higher than expected plasma concentrations of TCA with resultant toxicity). Products include:
- Prolixin Enanthate ... 510

Fluphenazine Hydrochloride (Enhanced response to the effects of central nervous system depressants; concurrent use with drugs that are substrate for cytochrome $P_{450}IID_6$ may make normal metabolizer resemble poor metabolizer leading to higher than expected plasma concentrations of TCA with resultant toxicity). Products include:
- Prolixin ... 510

Flurazepam Hydrochloride (Enhanced response to the effects of central nervous system depressants). Products include:
- Dalmane Capsules ... 2329

Fluvoxamine Maleate (Concurrent use with drugs that are substrate for cytochrome $P_{450}IID_6$ may make normal metabolizer resemble poor metabolizer leading to higher than expected plasma concentrations of TCA with resultant toxicity; due to variation in the extent of inhibition of $P_{450}IID_6$ caution is indicated if co-administered sufficient time must elapse). Products include:
- LUVOX Tablets ... 2723

Furazolidone (Potential for hyperpyretic crises, severe convulsions and death; concurrent and/or sequential use is contraindicated). Products include:
- Furoxone ... 2221

Glutethimide (Enhanced response to the effects of central nervous system depressants).
- No products indexed under this heading.

Glycopyrrolate (Concurrent use may result in additive anticholinergic effects including paralytic ileus). Products include:
- Robinul Forte Tablets ... 2247
- Robinul Injectable ... 2247
- Robinul Tablets ... 2247

Guanadrel Sulfate (Amitriptyline may block the antihypertensive effect). Products include:
- Hylorel Tablets ... 1613

Guanethidine Monosulfate (Amitriptyline may block the antihypertensive effect of guanethidine or similarly acting compounds). Products include:
- Esimil Tablets ... 840
- Ismelin Tablets ... 845

Haloperidol (Enhanced response to the effects of central nervous system depressants). Products include:
- Haldol Injection, Tablets and Concentrate ... 1585

Haloperidol Decanoate (Enhanced response to the effects of central nervous system depressants). Products include:
- Haldol Decanoate ... 1587

Hydrocodone Bitartrate (Enhanced response to the effects of central nervous system depressants). Products include:
- Codiclear DH Syrup ... 808
- Duratuss HD Elixir ... 2750
- Histussin D Liquid ... 670
- Hycodan Tablets and Syrup ... 946
- Hycomine Compound Tablets ... 948
- Hycomine ... 947
- Hycotuss Expectorant Syrup ... 950
- Hydrocet Capsules ... 787
- Lorcet 10/650 Tablets ... 1016
- Lortab ... 2751
- Tussend ... 1830
- Tussend Expectorant ... 1831
- Vicodin Tablets ... 1404
- Vicodin ES Tablets ... 1405
- Vicodin HP Tablets ... 1403
- Vicodin Tuss Expectorant ... 1406
- Zydone Capsules ... 967

Hydrocodone Polistirex (Enhanced response to the effects of central nervous system depressants). Products include:
- Tussionex Pennkinetic Extended-Release Suspension ... 1624

Hydromorphone Hydrochloride (Enhanced response to the effects of central nervous system depressants). Products include:
- Dilaudid Ampules ... 1382
- Dilaudid Cough Syrup ... 1383
- Dilaudid-HP Injection ... 1384
- Dilaudid-HP Lyophilized Powder 250 mg ... 1384
- Dilaudid ... 1382
- Dilaudid Oral Liquid ... 1386
- Dilaudid ... 1382
- Dilaudid Tablets - 8 mg ... 1386

Hydroxyzine Hydrochloride (Enhanced response to the effects of central nervous system depressants). Products include:
- Atarax Tablets & Syrup ... 1992
- Marax Tablets & DF Syrup ... 2015
- Vistaril Intramuscular Solution ... 2042

Hyoscyamine (Concurrent use may result in additive anticholinergic effects including paralytic ileus). Products include:
- Cystospaz Tablets ... 2123
- Urised Tablets ... 2123

Hyoscyamine Sulfate (Concurrent use may result in additive anticholinergic effects including paralytic ileus). Products include:
- Arco-Lase Plus Tablets ... 513
- Atrohist Plus Tablets ... 1605
- Cystospaz-M Capsules ... 2123
- Donnatal ... 2234
- Donnatal Extentabs ... 2234
- Donnatal Tablets ... 2234
- Kutrase Capsules ... 2546
- Levsin/Levsinex/Levbid ... 2549

Imipramine Hydrochloride (Concurrent use with drugs that are substrate for cytochrome $P_{450}IID_6$ may make normal metabolizer resemble poor metabolizer leading to higher than expected plasma concentrations of TCA with resultant toxicity). Products include:
- Tofranil Ampuls ... 873
- Tofranil Tablets ... 875

Imipramine Pamoate (Concurrent use with drugs that are substrate for cytochrome $P_{450}IID_6$ may make normal metabolizer resemble poor metabolizer leading to higher than expected plasma concentrations of TCA with resultant toxicity). Products include:
- Tofranil-PM Capsules ... 876

Ipratropium Bromide (Concurrent use may result in additive anticholinergic effects including paralytic ileus). Products include:
- Atrovent Inhalation Aerosol ... 674
- Atrovent Inhalation Solution ... 675
- Atrovent Nasal Spray 0.03% ... 676
- Atrovent Nasal Spray 0.06% ... 678

Isocarboxazid (Potential for hyperpyretic crises, severe convulsions and death; concurrent and/or sequential use is contraindicated).
- No products indexed under this heading.

Isoflurane (Enhanced response to the effects of central nervous system depressants).
- No products indexed under this heading.

Isoproterenol Hydrochloride (Effects of concurrent use not specified; close supervision and careful adjustment of dosages are required). Products include:
- Isuprel Hydrochloride Solution ... 2443
- Isuprel Injection ... 2441
- Isuprel Mistometer ... 2442

Isoproterenol Sulfate (Effects of concurrent use not specified; close supervision and careful adjustment of dosages are required). Products include:
- Norisodrine with Calcium Iodide Syrup ... 446

Ketamine Hydrochloride (Enhanced response to the effects of central nervous system depressants).
- No products indexed under this heading.

Levomethadyl Acetate Hydrochloride (Enhanced response to the effects of central nervous system depressants). Products include:
- Orlaam Oral Solution ... 2361

Levorphanol Tartrate (cnsd; Enhanced response to central nervous system depressants). Products include:
- Levo-Dromoran ... 2297

Levothyroxine Sodium (On rare occasions, co-administration may produce arrhythmias). Products include:
- Eltroxin Tablets ... 2214
- Levothroid Tablets ... 1015
- Levothyroxine Sodium, USP for Injection ... 546
- Levoxyl Tablets ... 918
- Synthroid ... 1410

Liothyronine Sodium (On rare occasions, co-administration may produce arrhythmias). Products include:
- Cytomel Tablets ... 2647
- Triostat Injection ... 2708

Liotrix (On rare occasions, co-administration may produce arrhythmias).
- No products indexed under this heading.

Loratadine (Since phenothiazines and antihistamines are CNS depressants, each can potentiate each other). Products include:
- Claritin Tablets ... 2485
- Claritin-D Tablets ... 2487

Lorazepam (Enhanced response to the effects of central nervous system depressants). Products include:
- Ativan Injection ... 2805
- Ativan Tablets ... 2807

Loxapine Hydrochloride (Enhanced response to the effects of central nervous system depressants). Products include:
- Loxitane ... 1426

Loxapine Succinate (Enhanced response to the effects of central nervous system depressants). Products include:
- Loxitane Capsules ... 1426

Maprotiline Hydrochloride (Concurrent use with drugs that are substrate for cytochrome $P_{450}IID_6$ may make normal metabolizer resemble poor metabolizer leading to higher than expected plasma concentrations of TCA with resultant toxicity). Products include:
- Ludiomil Tablets ... 861

Mepenzolate Bromide (Concurrent use may result in additive anticholinergic effects including paralytic ileus).
- No products indexed under this heading.

Meperidine Hydrochloride (Enhanced response to central nervous system depressants). Products include:
- Demerol ... 2438
- Mepergan Injection ... 2859

Mephobarbital (Enhanced response to barbiturates). Products include:
- Mebaral Tablets ... 2452

Meprobamate (Enhanced response to the effects of central nervous system depressants). Products include:
- Miltown Tablets ... 2780
- PMB 200 and PMB 400 ... 2890

Mesoridazine Besylate (Enhanced response to central nervous system depressants). Products include:
- Serentil ... 689

IMPORTANT NOTE: Always consult each drug listing in the patient's regimen for possible interactions.

Etrafon | Interactions Index | 398

Metaproterenol Sulfate (Effects of concurrent use not specified; close supervision and careful adjustment of dosages are required). Products include:
- Alupent ... 672
- Metaproterenol Sulfate Inhalation Solution, USP, Arm-a-Med ... 547

Metaraminol Bitartrate (Effects of concurrent use not specified; close supervision and careful adjustment of dosages are required). Products include:
- Aramine Injection ... 1649

Methadone Hydrochloride (Enhanced response to central nervous system depressants). Products include:
- Methadone Hydrochloride Oral Concentrate ... 2356
- Methadone Hydrochloride Oral Solution & Tablets ... 2357

Methdilazine Hydrochloride (Since phenothiazines and antihistamines are CNS depressants, each can potentiate each other).
- No products indexed under this heading.

Methohexital Sodium (Enhanced response to the effects of central nervous system depressants).
- No products indexed under this heading.

Methotrimeprazine (Enhanced response to the effects of central nervous system depressants; concurrent use with drugs that are substrate for cytochrome $P_{450}IID_6$ may make normal metabolizer resemble poor metabolizer leading to higher than expected plasma concentrations of TCA with resultant toxicity). Products include:
- Levoprome ... 1321

Methoxamine Hydrochloride (Effects of concurrent use not specified; close supervision and careful adjustment of dosages are required). Products include:
- Vasoxyl Injection ... 1169

Methoxyflurane (Enhanced response to the effects of central nervous system depressants).
- No products indexed under this heading.

Midazolam Hydrochloride (Enhanced response to the effects of central nervous system depressants). Products include:
- Versed Injection ... 2324

Molindone Hydrochloride (Enhanced response to the effects of central nervous system depressants). Products include:
- Moban Tablets and Concentrate ... 1036

Morphine Sulfate (Enhanced response to central nervous system depressants). Products include:
- Astramorph/PF Injection, USP (Preservative-Free) ... 526
- Duramorph Injection ... 983
- Infumorph 200 and Infumorph 500 Sterile Solutions ... 985
- Kadian Capsules ... 2948
- MS Contin Tablets ... 2149
- MSIR ... 2152
- Oramorph SR (Morphine Sulfate Sustained Release Tablets) ... 2359
- RMS Suppositories CII ... 2766
- Roxanol ... 2365

Nefazodone Hydrochloride (Concurrent use with drugs that are substrate for cytochrome $P_{450}IID_6$ may make normal metabolizer resemble poor metabolizer leading to higher than expected plasma concentrations of TCA with resultant toxicity). Products include:
- Serzone Tablets ... 776

Norepinephrine Bitartrate (Effects of concurrent use not specified; close supervision and careful adjustment of dosages are required). Products include:
- Levophed Bitartrate Injection ... 2445

Nortriptyline Hydrochloride (Concurrent use with drugs that are substrate for cytochrome $P_{450}IID_6$ may make normal metabolizer resemble poor metabolizer leading to higher than expected plasma concentrations of TCA with resultant toxicity). Products include:
- Pamelor ... 2409

Opium Alkaloids (Enhanced response to central nervous system depressants).
- No products indexed under this heading.

Oxazepam (Enhanced response to the effects of central nervous system depressants). Products include:
- Serax Capsules ... 2916
- Serax Tablets ... 2916

Oxybutynin Chloride (Concurrent use may result in additive anticholinergic effects including paralytic ileus). Products include:
- Ditropan ... 1267

Oxycodone Hydrochloride (Enhanced response to central nervous system depressants). Products include:
- OxyContin Tablets ... 2163
- OxyIR Capsules ... 2167
- Percocet Tablets ... 955
- Percodan Tablets ... 955
- Percodan-Demi Tablets ... 956
- Roxicodone Tablets, Oral Solution & Intensol (Oxycodone) ... 2366
- Tylox Capsules ... 1593

Paroxetine Hydrochloride (Concurrent use with drugs that are substrate for cytochrome $P_{450}IID_6$ may make normal metabolizer resemble poor metabolizer leading to higher than expected plasma concentrations of TCA with resultant toxicity; due to variation in the extent of inhibition of $P_{450}IID_6$ caution is indicated if co-administered sufficient time must elapse). Products include:
- Paxil Tablets ... 2681

Pentobarbital Sodium (Enhanced response to barbiturates). Products include:
- Nembutal Sodium Capsules ... 440
- Nembutal Sodium Solution ... 442
- Nembutal Sodium Suppositories ... 444

Phenelzine Sulfate (Potential for hyperpyretic crises, severe convulsions and death; concurrent and/or sequential use is contraindicated). Products include:
- Nardil ... 1977

Phenobarbital (Enhanced response to barbiturates). Products include:
- Arco-Lase Plus Tablets ... 513
- Bellergal-S Tablets ... 2375
- Donnatal ... 2234
- Donnatal Extentabs ... 2234
- Donnatal Tablets ... 2234
- Phenobarbital Elixir and Tablets ... 1523
- Quadrinal Tablets ... 1398

Phenylephrine Bitartrate (Effects of concurrent use not specified; close supervision and careful adjustment of dosages are required).
- No products indexed under this heading.

Phenylephrine Hydrochloride (Effects of concurrent use not specified; close supervision and careful adjustment of dosages are required). Products include:
- Atrohist Plus Tablets ... 1605
- Cerose DM ... ▣ 853
- D.A. II Tablets ... 972
- D.A. Chewable Tablets ... 970
- Dura-Vent/DA Tablets ... 972
- Extendryl ... 1003
- 4-Way Fast Acting Nasal Spray (regular & mentholated) ... ▣ 644
- Hemorid ... ▣ 797
- Hycomine Compound Tablets ... 948
- Neo-Synephrine Hydrochloride 1% Carpuject ... 2455
- Neo-Synephrine Hydrochloride 1% Injection ... 2455
- Neo-Synephrine Hydrochloride (Ophthalmic) ... 2456
- Neo-Synephrine ... ▣ 624
- Novahistine Elixir ... ▣ 782
- Phenergan VC ... 2886
- Phenergan VC with Codeine ... 2888
- Preparation H ... ▣ 842
- Tympagesic Ear Drops ... 2476
- Vicks Sinex Nasal Spray and Ultra Fine Mist ... ▣ 738

Phenylephrine Tannate (Effects of concurrent use not specified; close supervision and careful adjustment of dosages are required). Products include:
- Atrohist Pediatric Suspension ... 1604
- Atrohist Pediatric Suspension Dye-Free ... 1604
- Rynatan ... 2781
- Rynatuss ... 2782

Phenylpropanolamine Hydrochloride (Effects of concurrent use not specified; close supervision and careful adjustment of dosages are required). Products include:
- Acutrim ... ▣ 648
- Atrohist Plus Tablets ... 1605
- BC Cold Powder Multi-Symptom Formula (Cold-Sinus-Allergy) ... ▣ 631
- BC Cold Powder Non-Drowsy Formula (Cold-Sinus) ... ▣ 631
- Cheracol Plus Head Cold/Cough Formula ... ▣ 741
- Comtrex Multi-Symptom Cold Reliever Liqui-Gels ... ▣ 638
- Comtrex Multi-Symptom Non-Drowsy Liqui-gels ... ▣ 640
- Contac Continuous Action Nasal Decongestant/Antihistamine 12 Hour Capsules ... ▣ 773
- Contac Maximum Strength Continuous Action Decongestant/Antihistamine 12 Hour Caplets ... ▣ 772
- Contac Severe Cold and Flu Formula Caplets ... ▣ 773
- Coricidin 'D' Decongestant Tablets ... ▣ 760
- Dexatrim ... ▣ 795
- Dexatrim Plus Vitamins Caplets ... ▣ 796
- Dimetane-DC Cough Syrup ... 2232
- Dimetapp Allergy Sinus Caplets ... ▣ 838
- Dimetapp Cold & Allergy Chewable Tablets ... ▣ 838
- Dimetapp Cold & Cough Liqui-Gels ... ▣ 839
- Dimetapp DM Elixir ... ▣ 840
- Dimetapp Elixir ... ▣ 840
- Dimetapp Extentabs ... ▣ 841
- Dimetapp Tablets/Liqui-Gels ... ▣ 841
- Dura-Vent Tablets ... 971
- Entex LA Tablets ... 972
- Exgest LA Tablets ... 787
- Hycomine ... 947
- Nolamine Timed-Release Tablets ... 790
- Ornade Spansule Capsules ... 2678
- Propagest Tablets ... 791
- Pyrroxate Caplets ... ▣ 742
- Robitussin-CF ... ▣ 846
- Sinulin Tablets ... 792
- Tavist-D 12 Hour Relief Tablets ... ▣ 750
- Teldrin 12 Hour Antihistamine/Nasal Decongestant Allergy Relief Capsules ... ▣ 786
- Triaminic Expectorant ... ▣ 753
- Triaminic Syrup ... ▣ 755
- Triaminic Triaminicol Cold & Cough ... ▣ 756
- Triaminic DM Syrup ... ▣ 756
- Triaminicin Tablets ... ▣ 756
- Vicks DayQuil Allergy Relief 12-Hour Extended Release Tablets ... ▣ 733
- Vicks DayQuil Allergy Relief 4-Hour Tablets ... ▣ 733
- Vicks DayQuil SINUS Pressure & CONGESTION Relief ... ▣ 734

Pirbuterol Acetate (Effects of concurrent use not specified; close supervision and careful adjustment of dosages are required). Products include:
- Maxair Autohaler ... 1550
- Maxair Inhaler ... 1552

Prazepam (Enhanced response to the effects of central nervous system depressants).
- No products indexed under this heading.

Prochlorperazine (Enhanced response to the effects of central nervous system depressants; concurrent use with drugs that are substrate for cytochrome $P_{450}IID_6$ may make normal metabolizer resemble poor metabolizer leading to higher than expected plasma concentrations of TCA with resultant toxicity). Products include:
- Compazine ... 2644

Procyclidine Hydrochloride (Concurrent use may result in additive anticholinergic effects including paralytic ileus). Products include:
- Kemadrin Tablets ... 1105

Promethazine Hydrochloride (Enhanced response to the effects of central nervous system depressants; concurrent use with drugs that are substrate for cytochrome $P_{450}IID_6$ may make normal metabolizer resemble poor metabolizer leading to higher than expected plasma concentrations of TCA with resultant toxicity). Products include:
- Mepergan Injection ... 2859
- Phenergan with Codeine ... 2883
- Phenergan with Dextromethorphan ... 2885
- Phenergan Injection ... 2880
- Phenergan Suppositories ... 2882
- Phenergan Syrup ... 2881
- Phenergan Tablets ... 2882
- Phenergan VC ... 2886
- Phenergan VC with Codeine ... 2888

Propafenone Hydrochloride (Concurrent use with drugs that are substrate for cytochrome $P_{450}IID_6$ may make normal metabolizer resemble poor metabolizer leading to higher than expected plasma concentrations of TCA with resultant toxicity). Products include:
- Rythmol Tablets–150mg, 225mg, 300mg ... 1399

Propantheline Bromide (Concurrent use may result in additive anticholinergic effects including paralytic ileus). Products include:
- Pro-Banthine Tablets ... 2226

Propofol (Enhanced response to the effects of central nervous system depressants). Products include:
- Diprivan Injectable Emulsion ... 2939

Propoxyphene Hydrochloride (Enhanced response to central nervous system depressants). Products include:
- Darvon ... 1475
- Wygesic Tablets ... 2930

Propoxyphene Napsylate (Enhanced response to central nervous system depressants). Products include:
- Darvon-N/Darvocet-N ... 1473

Protriptyline Hydrochloride (Concurrent use with drugs that are substrate for cytochrome $P_{450}IID_6$ may make normal metabolizer resemble poor metabolizer leading to higher than expected plasma concentrations of TCA with resultant toxicity). Products include:
- Vivactil Tablets ... 1820

Pseudoephedrine Hydrochloride (Effects of concurrent use not specified; close supervision and careful adjustment of dosages are required). Products include:

Product	Page
Actifed Allergy Daytime/Nighttime Caplets	⬛ 808
Actifed Cold & Allergy Tablets	⬛ 807
Actifed Cold & Sinus Caplets and Tablets	⬛ 808
Actifed Sinus Daytime/Nighttime Tablets and Caplets	⬛ 809
Advil Cold and Sinus Caplets and Tablets	⬛ 837
Alka-Seltzer Plus Liqui-Gels	⬛ 612
Alka-Seltzer Plus Flu & Body Aches Liqui-Gels Non-Drowsy Formula	⬛ 613
Alka-Seltzer Plus Night-Time Cold Medicine Liqui-Gels	⬛ 612
Allerest Maximum Strength	⬛ 649
Allerest No Drowsiness	⬛ 649
Allerest Sinus Pain Formula	⬛ 649
Atrohist Pediatric Capsules	1603
Benadryl Allergy/Cold Tablets	⬛ 811
Benadryl Allergy Decongestant Liquid Medication	⬛ 812
Benadryl Allergy Decongestant Tablets	⬛ 812
Benadryl Allergy Sinus Headache Caplets	⬛ 813
Benylin Multisymptom	⬛ 816
Bromfed Capsules (Extended-Release)	1832
Bromfed Syrup	⬛ 712
Bromfed Tablets	1832
Bromfed-DM Cough Syrup	1832
Bromfed-PD Capsules (Extended-Release)	1832
Children's TYLENOL Cold Multi-Symptom Chewable Tablets and Liquid	1559
Children's TYLENOL Cold Plus Cough Multi Symptom Chewable Tablets and Liquid	1560
Children's TYLENOL Flu Suspension Liquid	1560
Children's Vicks DayQuil Allergy Relief	⬛ 730
Children's Vicks NyQuil Cold/Cough Relief	⬛ 731
Allergy-Sinus Comtrex Multi-Symptom Allergy-Sinus Formula Tablets and Caplets	⬛ 639
Comtrex Multi-Symptom	⬛ 638
Comtrex Multi-Symptom Non-Drowsy Caplets	⬛ 640
Congess	1003
Contac Day Allergy/Sinus Caplets	⬛ 771
Contac Day & Night	⬛ 772
Contac Night Allergy/Sinus Caplets	⬛ 771
Contac Severe Cold & Flu Non-Drowsy	⬛ 774
Deconsal II Tablets	1605
Dimetane-DX Cough Syrup	2233
Dimetapp Cold & Fever Suspension	⬛ 839
Dimetapp Decongestant Pediatric Drops	⬛ 840
Dorcol Children's Cough Syrup	⬛ 748
Drixoral Cough + Congestion Liquid Caps	⬛ 763
Dura-Tap/PD Capsules	970
Duratuss Tablets	2750
Duratuss HD Elixir	2750
Efidac/24	⬛ 655
Entex PSE Tablets	973
Fedahist Gyrocaps	2545
Guaifed	1833
Guaifed Syrup	⬛ 712
Guaimax-D Tablets	809
Histussin D Liquid	670
Infants' TYLENOL Cold Decongestant & Fever-Reducer Drops	1561
Kronofed-A	994
Novahistine DMX	⬛ 782
Nucofed	2225
PediaCare Cough-Cold Chewable Tablets and Liquid	1569
PediaCare Infants' Decongestant Drops	1569
PediaCare Infants' Drops Decongestant Plus Cough	1569
PediaCare NightRest Cough-Cold Liquid	1569
Pediatric Vicks 44d Cough & Head Congestion Relief	⬛ 736
Pediatric Vicks 44m Cough & Cold Relief	⬛ 737
Robitussin Cold & Cough Liqui-Gels	⬛ 844
Robitussin Cold, Cough & Flu Liqui-Gels	⬛ 844
Robitussin Maximum Strength Cough & Cold	⬛ 847
Robitussin Night-Time Cold Formula	⬛ 847
Robitussin Pediatric Cough & Cold Formula	⬛ 848
Robitussin Pediatric Drops	⬛ 849
Robitussin Severe Congestion Liqui-Gels	⬛ 845
Robitussin-DAC Syrup	2249
Robitussin-PE	⬛ 846
Rondec Oral Drops	974
Rondec Syrup	974
Rondec Tablet	974
Rondec Chewable Tablets	974
Rondec-TR Tablet	974
Ryna	⬛ 804
Seldane-D Extended-Release Tablets	1286
Semprex-D Capsules	1620
Sinarest	⬛ 663
Sine-Aid Maximum Strength Sinus Headache Gelcaps, Caplets and Tablets	1570
Sine-Off No Drowsiness Formula Caplets	⬛ 784
Sine-Off Sinus Medicine	⬛ 784
Singlet Tablets	⬛ 785
Sinutab Non-Drying Liquid Caps	⬛ 823
Sinutab Sinus Allergy Medication, Maximum Strength Tablets and Caplets	⬛ 823
Sinutab Sinus Medication, Maximum Strength Without Drowsiness Formula, Tablets & Caplets	⬛ 824
Sudafed Children's Cold & Cough Liquid Medication	⬛ 825
Sudafed Children's Nasal Decongestant Liquid Medication	⬛ 826
Sudafed Cold & Allergy Tablets	⬛ 826
Sudafed Cold and Cough Liquid Caps	⬛ 826
Sudafed Nasal Decongestant Tablets, 30 mg	⬛ 825
Sudafed Nasal Decongestant Tablets, 60 mg	⬛ 825
Sudafed Non-Drying Sinus Liquid Caps	⬛ 827
Sudafed Pediatric Nasal Decongestant Liquid Oral Drops	⬛ 827
Sudafed Severe Cold Formula Caplets	⬛ 828
Sudafed Severe Cold Formula Tablets	⬛ 828
Sudafed Sinus Caplets	⬛ 829
Sudafed Sinus Tablets	⬛ 829
Sudafed 12 Hour Caplets	⬛ 824
Syn-Rx Tablets	1622
Syn-Rx DM Tablets	1623
TheraFlu Flu and Cold Medicine	⬛ 750
Theraflu Maximum Strength Flu and Cold Medicine For Sore Throat	⬛ 751
TheraFlu Flu, Cold and Cough Medicine	⬛ 750
TheraFlu Maximum Strength Nighttime Flu, Cold & Cough Medicine	⬛ 751
TheraFlu Maximum Strength Non-Drowsy Formula Flu, Cold & Cough Medicine	⬛ 751
TheraFlu Maximum Strength, Non-Drowsy Formula Flu, Cold and Cough Caplets	⬛ 752
Theraflu Maximum Strength Sinus Non-Drowsy Formula Caplets	⬛ 752
Triaminic AM Cough and Decongestant Formula	⬛ 753
Triaminic AM Decongestant Formula	⬛ 753
Triaminic Infant Oral Decongestant Drops	⬛ 754
Triaminic Night Time	⬛ 754
Triaminic Sore Throat Formula	⬛ 755
Tussend	1830
Tussend Expectorant	1831
TYLENOL Allergy Sinus, Maximum Strength Caplets and Gelcaps	1571
TYLENOL Allergy Sinus NightTime, Maximum Strength Caplets	1571
TYLENOL Cold Medication, Multi-Symptom Formula Tablets and Caplets	1572
TYLENOL Cold Medication, Multi-Symptom Hot Liquid Packets	1572
TYLENOL Cold Medication, No Drowsiness Formula Caplets and Gelcaps	1572
TYLENOL Cold Severe Congestion Caplets	1573
TYLENOL Cough Medication with Decongestant, Multi Symptom	1574
TYLENOL Flu No Drowsiness Formula, Maximum Strength Gelcaps	1575
TYLENOL Flu NightTime, Maximum Strength Gelcaps	1575
TYLENOL Flu NightTime, Maximum Strength Hot Medication Packets	1575
TYLENOL Sinus, Maximum Strength Geltabs, Gelcaps, Caplets and Tablets	1576
Vicks 44 LiquiCaps Cough, Cold & Flu Relief	⬛ 728
Vicks 44 LiquiCaps Non-Drowsy Cough & Cold Relief	⬛ 728
Vicks 44D Cough & Head Congestion Relief	⬛ 728
Vicks 44M Cough, Cold & Flu Relief	⬛ 729
Vicks DayQuil LiquiCaps/Liquid Multi-Symptom Cold/Flu Relief	⬛ 734
Vicks DayQuil SINUS Pressure & PAIN Relief with IBUPROFEN	⬛ 735
Vicks Nyquil Hot Therapy	⬛ 735
Vicks NyQuil LiquiCaps/Liquid Multi-Symptom Cold/Flu Relief, Original and Cherry Flavors	⬛ 736

Pseudoephedrine Sulfate (Effects of concurrent use not specified; close supervision and careful adjustment of dosages are required). Products include:

Product	Page
Chlor-Trimeton Allergy Decongestant Tablets	⬛ 759
Claritin-D Tablets	2487
Drixoral Cold and Allergy Sustained-Action Tablets	⬛ 763
Drixoral Cold and Flu Extended-Release Tablets	⬛ 764
Drixoral Non-Drowsy Formula Extended-Release Tablets	⬛ 764
Drixoral Allergy/Sinus Extended Release Tablets	⬛ 765
Trinalin Repetabs Tablets	1373

Pyrilamine Maleate (Since phenothiazines and antihistamines are CNS depressants, each can potentiate each other). Products include:

Product	Page
4-Way Fast Acting Nasal Spray (regular & mentholated)	⬛ 644
Maximum Strength Multi-Symptom Formula Midol	⬛ 621
PMS Multi-Symptom Formula Midol	⬛ 622

Pyrilamine Tannate (Since phenothiazines and antihistamines are CNS depressants, each can potentiate each other). Products include:

Product	Page
Atrohist Pediatric Suspension	1604
Atrohist Pediatric Suspension Dye-Free	1604
Rynatan	2781

Quazepam (Enhanced response to the effects of central nervous system depressants). Products include:

Product	Page
Doral Tablets	2773

Quinidine Gluconate (Concurrent use with drugs that inhibit cytochrome $P_{450}IID_6$ may make normal metabolizer resemble poor metabolizer leading to higher than expected plasma concentrations of TCA with resultant toxicity). Products include:

Product	Page
Quinaglute Dura-Tabs Tablets	644

Quinidine Polygalacturonate (Concurrent use with drugs that inhibit cytochrome $P_{450}IID_6$ may make normal metabolizer resemble poor metabolizer leading to higher than expected plasma concentrations of TCA with resultant toxicity). Products include:

Product	Page
Cardioquin Tablets	2146

Quinidine Sulfate (Concurrent use with drugs that inhibit cytochrome $P_{450}IID_6$ may make normal metabolizer resemble poor metabolizer leading to higher than expected plasma concentrations of TCA with resultant toxicity). Products include:

Product	Page
Quinidex Extentabs	2240

Risperidone (Enhanced response to the effects of central nervous system depressants). Products include:

Product	Page
Risperdal Tablets	1348

Salmeterol Xinafoate (Effects of concurrent use not specified; close supervision and careful adjustment of dosages are required). Products include:

Product	Page
Serevent Inhalation Aerosol	1149

Scopolamine (Concurrent use may result in additive anticholinergic effects including paralytic ileus). Products include:

Product	Page
Transderm Scōp Transdermal Therapeutic System	890

Scopolamine Hydrobromide (Concurrent use may result in additive anticholinergic effects including paralytic ileus). Products include:

Product	Page
Atrohist Plus Tablets	1605
Donnatal	2234
Donnatal Extentabs	2234
Donnatal Tablets	2234

Secobarbital Sodium (Enhanced response to barbiturates). Products include:

Product	Page
Seconal Sodium Pulvules	1529

Selegiline Hydrochloride (Potential for hyperpyretic crises, severe convulsions and death; concurrent and/or sequential use is contraindicated). Products include:

Product	Page
Eldepryl Capsules	2729

Sertraline Hydrochloride (Concurrent use with drugs that are substrate for cytochrome $P_{450}IID_6$ may make normal metabolizer resemble poor metabolizer leading to higher than expected plasma concentrations of TCA with resultant toxicity; due to variation in the extent of inhibition of $P_{450}IID_6$ caution is indicated if co-administered sufficient time must elapse). Products include:

Product	Page
Zoloft Tablets	2051

Sevoflurane (Enhanced response to the effects of central nervous system depressants).

No products indexed under this heading.

Sufentanil Citrate (Enhanced response to central nervous system depressants). Products include:

Product	Page
Sufenta Injection	1355

Temazepam (Enhanced response to the effects of central nervous system depressants). Products include:

Product	Page
Restoril Capsules	2413

Terbutaline Sulfate (Effects of concurrent use not specified; close supervision and careful adjustment of dosages are required). Products include:

Product	Page
Brethaire Inhaler	830
Brethine Ampuls	832
Brethine Tablets	831
Bricanyl Subcutaneous Injection	1247
Bricanyl Tablets	1248

Terfenadine (Since phenothiazines and antihistamines are CNS depressants, each can potentiate each other). Products include:

Product	Page
Seldane Tablets	1284
Seldane-D Extended-Release Tablets	1286

IMPORTANT NOTE: Always consult each drug listing in the patient's regimen for possible interactions.

Thiamylal Sodium (Enhanced response to barbiturates).
   No products indexed under this heading.

Thioridazine Hydrochloride (Enhanced response to the effects of central nervous system depressants; concurrent use with drugs that are substrate for cytochrome $P_{450}IID_6$ may make normal metabolizer resemble poor metabolizer leading to higher than expected plasma concentrations of TCA with resultant toxicity). Products include:
   Mellaril 2398

Thiothixene (Enhanced response to the effects of central nervous system depressants). Products include:
   Navane Capsules and Concentrate 2018
   Navane Intramuscular 2019

Thyroglobulin (On rare occasions, co-administration may produce arrhythmias).
   No products indexed under this heading.

Thyroid (On rare occasions, co-administration may produce arrhythmias).
   No products indexed under this heading.

Thyroxine (On rare occasions, co-administration may produce arrhythmias).
   No products indexed under this heading.

Thyroxine Sodium (On rare occasions, co-administration may produce arrhythmias).
   No products indexed under this heading.

Tranylcypromine Sulfate (Potential for hyperpyretic crises, severe convulsions and death; concurrent and/or sequential use is contraindicated). Products include:
   Parnate Tablets 2679

Trazodone Hydrochloride (Concurrent use with drugs that are substrate for cytochrome $P_{450}IID_6$ may make normal metabolizer resemble poor metabolizer leading to higher than expected plasma concentrations of TCA with resultant toxicity). Products include:
   Desyrel and Desyrel Dividose 504

Triazolam (Enhanced response to the effects of central nervous system depressants). Products include:
   Halcion Tablets 2093

Tridihexethyl Chloride (Concurrent use may result in additive anticholinergic effects including paralytic ileus).
   No products indexed under this heading.

Trifluoperazine Hydrochloride (Enhanced response to the effects of central nervous system depressants; concurrent use with drugs that are substrate for cytochrome $P_{450}IID_6$ may make normal metabolizer resemble poor metabolizer leading to higher than expected plasma concentrations of TCA with resultant toxicity). Products include:
   Stelazine 2692

Trihexyphenidyl Hydrochloride (Concurrent use may result in additive anticholinergic effects including paralytic ileus). Products include:
   Artane 1418

Trimeprazine Tartrate (Since phenothiazines and antihistamines are CNS depressants, each can potentiate each other).
   No products indexed under this heading.

Trimipramine Maleate (Concurrent use with drugs that are substrate for cytochrome $P_{450}IID_6$ may make normal metabolizer resemble poor metabolizer leading to higher than expected plasma concentrations of TCA with resultant toxicity). Products include:
   Surmontil Capsules 2917

Tripelennamine Hydrochloride (Since phenothiazines and antihistamines are CNS depressants, each can potentiate each other). Products include:
   PBZ Tablets 863
   PBZ-SR Tablets 862

Triprolidine Hydrochloride (Since phenothiazines and antihistamines are CNS depressants, each can potentiate each other). Products include:
   Actifed Cold & Allergy Tablets 807
   Actifed Cold & Sinus Caplets and Tablets 808

Venlafaxine Hydrochloride (Concurrent use with drugs that are substrate for cytochrome $P_{450}IID_6$ may make normal metabolizer resemble poor metabolizer leading to higher than expected plasma concentrations of TCA with resultant toxicity; due to variation in the extent of inhibition of $P_{450}IID_6$ caution is indicated if co-administered sufficient time must elapse). Products include:
   Effexor 2825

Zolpidem Tartrate (Enhanced response to the effects of central nervous system depressants). Products include:
   Ambien Tablets 2559

Food Interactions

Alcohol (Amitriptyline may enhance the response to alcohol; potential for additive effects and hypotension; concurrent use should be avoided).

EUCALYPTAMINT ARTHRITIS PAIN RELIEVER (EXTERNAL ANALGESIC)
(Menthol) 656
None cited in PDR database.

EUCALYPTAMINT MUSCLE PAIN RELIEF FORMULA
(Menthol) 656
None cited in PDR database.

EUCERIN DRY SKIN THERAPY CLEANSING BAR
(Eucerite) 636
None cited in PDR database.

EUCERIN ORIGINAL MOISTURIZING CREME (UNSCENTED)
(Mineral Oil, Petrolatum) 636
None cited in PDR database.

EUCERIN FACIAL MOISTURIZING LOTION SPF 25
(Phenylbenzimidazole-5-Sulfonic Acid, Titanium Dioxide, 2-Ethylhexyl-p-Methoxycinnamate, 2-Ethylhexyl Salicylate) 636
None cited in PDR database.

EUCERIN ORIGINAL MOISTURIZING LOTION
(Isopropyl Myristate, Mineral Oil) 636
None cited in PDR database.

EUCERIN PLUS DRY SKIN CARE MOISTURIZING LOTION
(Mineral Oil, Urea) 636
None cited in PDR database.

EUCERIN PLUS MOISTURIZING CREME
(Urea, Mineral Oil) 636
None cited in PDR database.

EULEXIN CAPSULES
(Flutamide) 2498
May interact with:

Warfarin Sodium (Increases in prothrombin time have been noted in patients receiving long-term warfarin therapy after flutamide was initiated). Products include:
   Coumadin 941

EURAX CREAM & LOTION
(Crotamiton) 2794
None cited in PDR database.

EXACT ADULT ACNE MEDICATION
(Benzoyl Peroxide) 722
None cited in PDR database.

EXACT PORE TREATMENT GEL
(Salicylic Acid) 722
None cited in PDR database.

EXACT VANISHING AND TINTED CREAMS
(Benzoyl Peroxide) 722
None cited in PDR database.

ASPIRIN FREE EXCEDRIN ANALGESIC CAPLETS AND GELTABS
(Acetaminophen, Caffeine) 734

Food Interactions

Alcohol (Concurrent use should be undertaken with the physician's consultation).

EXCEDRIN EXTRA-STRENGTH ANALGESIC TABLETS, CAPLETS, AND GELTABS
(Acetaminophen, Aspirin, Caffeine) .. 734
May interact with oral anticoagulants, oral hypoglycemic agents, antigout agents, and certain other agents. Compounds in these categories include:

Acarbose (Co-administration is not recommended unless directed by a doctor). Products include:
   Precose 604

Allopurinol (Co-administration is not recommended unless directed by a doctor). Products include:
   Zyloprim Tablets 1194

Chlorpropamide (Co-administration is not recommended unless directed by a doctor). Products include:
   Diabinese Tablets 2002

Dicumarol (Co-administration is not recommended unless directed by a doctor).
   No products indexed under this heading.

Glimepiride (Co-administration is not recommended unless directed by a doctor). Products include:
   Amaryl Tablets 1241

Glipizide (Co-administration is not recommended unless directed by a doctor). Products include:
   Glucotrol Tablets 2011
   Glucotrol XL Extended Release Tablets 2012

Glyburide (Co-administration is not recommended unless directed by a doctor). Products include:
   DiaBeta Tablets 1265
   Glynase PresTab Tablets 2091
   Micronase Tablets 2099

Metformin Hydrochloride (Co-administration is not recommended unless directed by a doctor). Products include:
   Glucophage Tablets 754

Probenecid (Co-administration is not recommended unless directed by a doctor). Products include:
   Benemid Tablets 1651
   ColBENEMID Tablets 1662

Sulfinpyrazone (Co-administration is not recommended unless directed by a doctor). Products include:
   Anturane 823

Tolazamide (Co-administration is not recommended unless directed by a doctor).
   No products indexed under this heading.

Tolbutamide (Co-administration is not recommended unless directed by a doctor).
   No products indexed under this heading.

Warfarin Sodium (Co-administration is not recommended unless directed by a doctor). Products include:
   Coumadin 941

Food Interactions

Alcohol (Concurrent use should be undertaken with the physician's consultation).

EXCEDRIN P.M. ANALGESIC/SLEEPING AID TABLETS, CAPLETS, LIQUIGELS
(Acetaminophen, Diphenhydramine Citrate) 735
May interact with hypnotics and sedatives, tranquilizers, and certain other agents. Compounds in these categories include:

Alprazolam (Concurrent use is not recommended). Products include:
   Xanax Tablets 2115

Buspirone Hydrochloride (Concurrent use is not recommended). Products include:
   BuSpar Tablets 738

Chlordiazepoxide (Concurrent use is not recommended). Products include:
   Limbitrol 2333

Chlordiazepoxide Hydrochloride (Concurrent use is not recommended). Products include:
   Librax Capsules 2330
   Librium Capsules 2331
   Librium Injectable 2332

Chlorpromazine (Concurrent use is not recommended). Products include:
   Thorazine Suppositories 2701

Chlorpromazine Hydrochloride (Concurrent use is not recommended). Products include:
   Thorazine 2701

Chlorprothixene (Concurrent use is not recommended).
   No products indexed under this heading.

Chlorprothixene Hydrochloride (Concurrent use is not recommended).
   No products indexed under this heading.

Interactions Index

Clorazepate Dipotassium (Concurrent use is not recommended). Products include:
- Tranxene 459

Diazepam (Concurrent use is not recommended). Products include:
- Dizac (diazepam injectable emulsion) CIV 1862
- Valium Injectable 2336
- Valium Tablets 2335

Droperidol (Concurrent use is not recommended). Products include:
- Inapsine Injection 462

Estazolam (Concurrent use is not recommended). Products include:
- ProSom Tablets 457

Ethchlorvynol (Concurrent use is not recommended). Products include:
- Placidyl Capsules 456

Ethinamate (Concurrent use is not recommended).
- No products indexed under this heading.

Fluphenazine Decanoate (Concurrent use is not recommended). Products include:
- Prolixin Decanoate 510

Fluphenazine Enanthate (Concurrent use is not recommended). Products include:
- Prolixin Enanthate 510

Fluphenazine Hydrochloride (Concurrent use is not recommended). Products include:
- Prolixin 510

Flurazepam Hydrochloride (Concurrent use is not recommended). Products include:
- Dalmane Capsules 2329

Glutethimide (Concurrent use is not recommended).
- No products indexed under this heading.

Haloperidol (Concurrent use is not recommended). Products include:
- Haldol Injection, Tablets and Concentrate 1585

Haloperidol Decanoate (Concurrent use is not recommended). Products include:
- Haldol Decanoate 1587

Hydroxyzine Hydrochloride (Concurrent use is not recommended). Products include:
- Atarax Tablets & Syrup 1992
- Marax Tablets & DF Syrup .. 2015
- Vistaril Intramuscular Solution .. 2042

Lorazepam (Concurrent use is not recommended). Products include:
- Ativan Injection 2805
- Ativan Tablets 2807

Loxapine Hydrochloride (Concurrent use is not recommended). Products include:
- Loxitane 1426

Loxapine Succinate (Concurrent use is not recommended). Products include:
- Loxitane Capsules 1426

Meprobamate (Concurrent use is not recommended). Products include:
- Miltown Tablets 2780
- PMB 200 and PMB 400 2890

Mesoridazine Besylate (Concurrent use is not recommended). Products include:
- Serentil 689

Midazolam Hydrochloride (Concurrent use is not recommended). Products include:
- Versed Injection 2324

Molindone Hydrochloride (Concurrent use is not recommended). Products include:
- Moban Tablets and Concentrate 1036

Oxazepam (Concurrent use is not recommended). Products include:
- Serax Capsules 2916
- Serax Tablets 2916

Perphenazine (Concurrent use is not recommended). Products include:
- Etrafon 2495
- Triavil Tablets 1800
- Trilafon 2532

Prazepam (Concurrent use is not recommended).
- No products indexed under this heading.

Prochlorperazine (Concurrent use is not recommended). Products include:
- Compazine 2644

Promethazine Hydrochloride (Concurrent use is not recommended). Products include:
- Mepergan Injection 2859
- Phenergan with Codeine 2883
- Phenergan with Dextromethorphan 2885
- Phenergan Injection 2880
- Phenergan Suppositories 2882
- Phenergan Syrup 2881
- Phenergan Tablets 2882
- Phenergan VC 2886
- Phenergan VC with Codeine 2888

Propofol (Concurrent use is not recommended). Products include:
- Diprivan Injectable Emulsion ... 2939

Quazepam (Concurrent use is not recommended). Products include:
- Doral Tablets 2773

Secobarbital Sodium (Concurrent use is not recommended). Products include:
- Seconal Sodium Pulvules 1529

Temazepam (Concurrent use is not recommended). Products include:
- Restoril Capsules 2413

Thioridazine Hydrochloride (Concurrent use is not recommended). Products include:
- Mellaril 2398

Thiothixene (Concurrent use is not recommended). Products include:
- Navane Capsules and Concentrate 2018
- Navane Intramuscular 2019

Triazolam (Concurrent use is not recommended). Products include:
- Halcion Tablets 2093

Trifluoperazine Hydrochloride (Concurrent use is not recommended). Products include:
- Stelazine 2692

Zolpidem Tartrate (Concurrent use is not recommended). Products include:
- Ambien Tablets 2559

Food Interactions

Alcohol (Concurrent use is not recommended; chronic users of alcohol, 3 or more drinks per day should consult their physician for advice before taking this product).

EXELDERM CREAM 1.0% (Sulconazole Nitrate) 2794
None cited in PDR database.

EXELDERM SOLUTION 1.0% (Sulconazole Nitrate) 2795
None cited in PDR database.

EXGEST LA TABLETS (Phenylpropanolamine Hydrochloride, Guaifenesin) 787
May interact with monoamine oxidase inhibitors and sympathomimetics. Compounds in these categories include:

Albuterol (Concurrent use is not recommended). Products include:
- Proventil Inhalation Aerosol ... 2524
- Ventolin Inhalation Aerosol and Refill 1170

Albuterol Sulfate (Concurrent use is not recommended). Products include:
- Airet Albuterol Sulfate Inhalation Solution 1602
- Albuterol Sulfate, USP Solution for Inhalation, Arm-a-Med ... 522
- Proventil Inhalation Solution 0.083% 2527
- Proventil Repetabs Tablets .. 2529
- Proventil Solution for Inhalation 0.5% 2525
- Proventil Syrup 2528
- Proventil Tablets 2529
- Ventolin Inhalation Solution . 1171
- Ventolin Nebules Inhalation Solution 1172
- Ventolin Rotacaps for Inhalation ... 1173
- Ventolin Syrup 1175
- Ventolin Tablets 1176
- Volmax Extended-Release Tablets .. 1835

Dobutamine Hydrochloride (Concurrent use is not recommended). Products include:
- Dobutrex Solution Vials 1480

Dopamine Hydrochloride (Concurrent use is not recommended).
- No products indexed under this heading.

Ephedrine Hydrochloride (Concurrent use is not recommended). Products include:
- Primatene Tablets 844
- Quadrinal Tablets 1398

Ephedrine Sulfate (Concurrent use is not recommended). Products include:
- Marax Tablets & DF Syrup .. 2015

Ephedrine Tannate (Concurrent use is not recommended). Products include:
- Rynatuss 2782

Epinephrine (Concurrent use is not recommended). Products include:
- EPIFRIN 237
- EpiPen 808
- Marcaine with Epinephrine .. 2446
- Primatene Mist 843
- Sensorcaine with Epinephrine Injection 554
- Sus-Phrine Injection 1017
- Xylocaine with Epinephrine Injections 562

Epinephrine Bitartrate (Concurrent use is not recommended). Products include:
- Sensorcaine-MPF with Epinephrine Injection 554

Epinephrine Hydrochloride (Concurrent use is not recommended). Products include:
- Ana-Kit Anaphylaxis Emergency Treatment Kit 611

Furazolidone (Concurrent use is contraindicated). Products include:
- Furoxone 2221

Isocarboxazid (Concurrent use is contraindicated).
- No products indexed under this heading.

Isoproterenol Hydrochloride (Concurrent use is not recommended). Products include:
- Isuprel Hydrochloride Solution ... 2443
- Isuprel Injection 2441
- Isuprel Mistometer 2442

Isoproterenol Sulfate (Concurrent use is not recommended). Products include:
- Norisodrine with Calcium Iodide Syrup 446

Metaproterenol Sulfate (Concurrent use is not recommended). Products include:
- Alupent 672
- Metaproterenol Sulfate Inhalation Solution, USP, Arm-a-Med ... 547

Metaraminol Bitartrate (Concurrent use is not recommended). Products include:
- Aramine Injection 1649

Methoxamine Hydrochloride (Concurrent use is not recommended). Products include:
- Vasoxyl Injection 1169

Norepinephrine Bitartrate (Concurrent use is not recommended). Products include:
- Levophed Bitartrate Injection ... 2445

Phenelzine Sulfate (Concurrent use is contraindicated). Products include:
- Nardil 1977

Phenylephrine Bitartrate (Concurrent use is not recommended).
- No products indexed under this heading.

Phenylephrine Hydrochloride (Concurrent use is not recommended). Products include:
- Atrohist Plus Tablets 1605
- Cerose DM 853
- D.A. II Tablets 972
- D.A. Chewable Tablets 970
- Dura-Vent/DA Tablets 972
- Extendryl 1003
- 4-Way Fast Acting Nasal Spray (regular & mentholated) ... 644
- Hemoril 797
- Hycomine Compound Tablets 948
- Neo-Synephrine Hydrochloride 1% Carpuject 2455
- Neo-Synephrine Hydrochloride 1% Injection 2455
- Neo-Synephrine Hydrochloride (Ophthalmic) 2456
- Neo-Synephrine 624
- Novahistine Elixir 782
- Phenergan VC 2886
- Phenergan VC with Codeine . 2888
- Preparation H 842
- Tympagesic Ear Drops 2476
- Vicks Sinex Nasal Spray and Ultra Fine Mist 738

Phenylephrine Tannate (Concurrent use is not recommended). Products include:
- Atrohist Pediatric Suspension .. 1604
- Atrohist Pediatric Suspension Dye-Free 1604
- Rynatan 2781
- Rynatuss 2782

Pirbuterol Acetate (Concurrent use is not recommended). Products include:
- Maxair Autohaler 1550
- Maxair Inhaler 1552

Pseudoephedrine Hydrochloride (Concurrent use is not recommended). Products include:
- Actifed Allergy Daytime/Nighttime Caplets 808
- Actifed Cold & Allergy Tablets .. 807
- Actifed Cold & Sinus Caplets and Tablets 808
- Actifed Sinus Daytime/Nighttime Tablets and Caplets 809
- Advil Cold and Sinus Caplets and Tablets 837
- Alka-Seltzer Plus Liqui-Gels .. 612
- Alka-Seltzer Plus Flu & Body Aches Liqui-Gels Non-Drowsy Formula 613
- Alka-Seltzer Plus Night-Time Cold Medicine Liqui-Gels 612
- Allerest Maximum Strength .. 649
- Allerest No Drowsiness 649
- Allerest Sinus Pain Formula .. 649
- Atrohist Pediatric Capsules .. 1603
- Benadryl Allergy/Cold Tablets . 811
- Benadryl Allergy Decongestant Liquid Medication 812
- Benadryl Allergy Decongestant Tablets 812
- Benadryl Allergy Sinus Headache Caplets 813
- Benylin Multisymptom 816
- Bromfed Capsules (Extended-Release) 1832
- Bromfed Syrup 712
- Bromfed Tablets 1832
- Bromfed-DM Cough Syrup ... 1832

IMPORTANT NOTE: Always consult each drug listing in the patient's regimen for possible interactions.

Interactions Index

Exgest LA

Bromfed-PD Capsules (Extended-Release) 1832
Children's TYLENOL Cold Multi-Symptom Chewable Tablets and Liquid 1559
Children's TYLENOL Cold Plus Cough Multi Symptom Chewable Tablets and Liquid 1560
Children's TYLENOL Flu Suspension Liquid 1560
Children's Vicks DayQuil Allergy Relief .... ▣ 730
Children's Vicks NyQuil Cold/Cough Relief .... ▣ 731
Allergy-Sinus Comtrex Multi-Symptom Allergy-Sinus Formula Tablets and Caplets .... ▣ 639
Comtrex Multi-Symptom .... ▣ 638
Comtrex Multi-Symptom Non-Drowsy Caplets .... ▣ 640
Congess 1003
Contac Day Allergy/Sinus Caplets .... ▣ 771
Contac Day & Night .... ▣ 772
Contac Night Allergy/Sinus Caplets .... ▣ 771
Contac Severe Cold & Flu Non-Drowsy .... ▣ 774
Deconsal II Tablets 1605
Dimetane-DX Cough Syrup 2233
Dimetapp Cold & Fever Suspension .... ▣ 839
Dimetapp Decongestant Pediatric Drops .... ▣ 840
Dorcol Children's Cough Syrup .... ▣ 748
Drixoral Cough + Congestion Liquid Caps .... ▣ 763
Dura-Tap/PD Capsules 970
Duratuss Tablets 2750
Duratuss HD Elixir 2750
Efidac/24 .... ▣ 655
Entex PSE Tablets 973
Fedahist Gyrocaps 2545
Guaifed 1833
Guaifed Syrup .... ▣ 712
Guaimax-D Tablets 809
Histussin D Liquid 670
Infants' TYLENOL Cold Decongestant & Fever-Reducer Drops 1561
Kronofed-A 994
Novahistine DMX .... ▣ 782
Nucofed 2225
PediaCare Cough-Cold Chewable Tablets and Liquid 1569
PediaCare Infants' Decongestant Drops 1569
PediaCare Infants' Drops Decongestant Plus Cough 1569
PediaCare NightRest Cough-Cold Liquid 1569
Pediatric Vicks 44d Cough & Head Congestion Relief .... ▣ 736
Pediatric Vicks 44m Cough & Cold Relief .... ▣ 737
Robitussin Cold & Cough Liqui-Gels .... ▣ 844
Robitussin Cold, Cough & Flu Liqui-Gels .... ▣ 844
Robitussin Maximum Strength Cough & Cold .... ▣ 847
Robitussin Night-Time Cold Formula .... ▣ 847
Robitussin Pediatric Cough & Cold Formula .... ▣ 848
Robitussin Pediatric Drops .... ▣ 849
Robitussin Severe Congestion Liqui-Gels .... ▣ 845
Robitussin-DAC Syrup 2249
Robitussin-PE .... ▣ 846
Rondec Oral Drops 974
Rondec Syrup 974
Rondec Tablet 974
Rondec Chewable Tablets 974
Rondec-TR Tablet 974
Ryna .... ▣ 804
Seldane-D Extended-Release Tablets 1286
Semprex-D Capsules 1620
Sinarest .... ▣ 663
Sine-Aid Maximum Strength Sinus Headache Gelcaps, Caplets and Tablets 1570
Sine-Off No Drowsiness Formula Caplets .... ▣ 784
Sine-Off Sinus Medicine .... ▣ 784
Singlet Tablets 785
Sinutab Non-Drying Liquid Caps .... ▣ 823
Sinutab Sinus Allergy Medication, Maximum Strength Tablets and Caplets .... ▣ 823
Sinutab Sinus Medication, Maximum Strength Without Drowsiness Formula, Tablets & Caplets .... ▣ 824
Sudafed Children's Cold & Cough Liquid Medication 825
Sudafed Children's Nasal Decongestant Liquid Medication .... ▣ 826
Sudafed Cold & Allergy Tablets .... ▣ 826
Sudafed Cold and Cough Liquid Caps .... ▣ 826
Sudafed Nasal Decongestant Tablets, 30 mg. .... ▣ 825
Sudafed Nasal Decongestant Tablets, 60 mg. .... ▣ 825
Sudafed Non-Drying Sinus Liquid Caps .... ▣ 827
Sudafed Pediatric Nasal Decongestant Liquid Oral Drops .... ▣ 827
Sudafed Severe Cold Formula Caplets .... ▣ 828
Sudafed Severe Cold Formula Tablets .... ▣ 828
Sudafed Sinus Caplets .... ▣ 829
Sudafed Sinus Tablets .... ▣ 829
Sudafed 12 Hour Caplets .... ▣ 824
Syn-Rx Tablets 1622
Syn-Rx DM Tablets 1623
TheraFlu Flu and Cold Medicine .... ▣ 750
Theraflu Maximum Strength Flu and Cold Medicine For Sore Throat .... ▣ 751
TheraFlu Flu, Cold and Cough Medicine .... ▣ 750
TheraFlu Maximum Strength Nighttime Flu, Cold & Cough Medicine .... ▣ 751
TheraFlu Maximum Strength Non-Drowsy Formula Flu, Cold & Cough Medicine .... ▣ 751
TheraFlu Maximum Strength, Non-Drowsy Formula Flu, Cold and Cough Caplets .... ▣ 752
Theraflu Maximum Strength Sinus Non-Drowsy Formula Caplets .... ▣ 752
Triaminic AM Cough and Decongestant Formula .... ▣ 753
Triaminic AM Decongestant Formula .... ▣ 753
Triaminic Infant Oral Decongestant Drops .... ▣ 754
Triaminic Night Time .... ▣ 754
Triaminic Sore Throat Formula .... ▣ 755
Tussend 1830
Tussend Expectorant 1831
TYLENOL Allergy Sinus, Maximum Strength Caplets and Gelcaps 1571
TYLENOL Allergy Sinus NightTime, Maximum Strength Caplets 1571
TYLENOL Cold Medication, Multi-Symptom Formula Tablets and Caplets 1572
TYLENOL Cold Medication, Multi-Symptom Hot Liquid Packets 1572
TYLENOL Cold Medication, No Drowsiness Formula Caplets and Gelcaps 1572
TYLENOL Cold Severe Congestion Caplets 1573
TYLENOL Cough Medication with Decongestant, Multi Symptom 1574
TYLENOL Flu No Drowsiness Formula, Maximum Strength Gelcaps 1575
TYLENOL Flu NightTime, Maximum Strength Gelcaps 1575
TYLENOL Flu NightTime, Maximum Strength Hot Medication Packets 1575
TYLENOL Sinus, Maximum Strength Geltabs, Gelcaps, Caplets and Tablets 1576
Vicks 44 LiquiCaps Cough, Cold & Flu Relief .... ▣ 728
Vicks 44 LiquiCaps Non-Drowsy Cough & Cold Relief .... ▣ 729
Vicks 44D Cough & Head Congestion Relief .... ▣ 728
Vicks 44M Cough, Cold & Flu Relief .... ▣ 729
Vicks DayQuil LiquiCaps/Liquid Multi-Symptom Cold/Flu Relief .... ▣ 734
Vicks DayQuil SINUS Pressure & PAIN Relief with IBUPROFEN .... ▣ 735
Vicks Nyquil Hot Therapy .... ▣ 735
Vicks NyQuil LiquiCaps/Liquid Multi-Symptom Cold/Flu Relief, Original and Cherry Flavors .... ▣ 736

Pseudoephedrine Sulfate (Concurrent use is not recommended). Products include:
Chlor-Trimeton Allergy Decongestant Tablets .... ▣ 759

Claritin-D Tablets 2487
Drixoral Cold and Allergy Sustained-Action Tablets .... ▣ 763
Drixoral Cold and Flu Extended-Release Tablets .... ▣ 764
Drixoral Non-Drowsy Formula Extended-Release Tablets .... ▣ 764
Drixoral Allergy/Sinus Extended Release Tablets .... ▣ 765
Trinalin Repetabs Tablets 1373

Salmeterol Xinafoate (Concurrent use is not recommended). Products include:
Serevent Inhalation Aerosol 1149

Selegiline Hydrochloride (Concurrent use is contraindicated). Products include:
Eldepryl Capsules 2729

Terbutaline Sulfate (Concurrent use is not recommended). Products include:
Brethaire Inhaler 830
Brethine Ampuls 832
Brethine Tablets 831
Bricanyl Subcutaneous Injection 1247
Bricanyl Tablets 1248

Tranylcypromine Sulfate (Concurrent use is contraindicated). Products include:
Parnate Tablets 2679

EX-LAX CHOCOLATED LAXATIVE TABLETS
(Phenolphthalein) .... ▣ 748
None cited in PDR database.

EXTRA GENTLE EX-LAX LAXATIVE PILLS
(Docusate Sodium, Phenolphthalein) .... ▣ 749
None cited in PDR database.

MAXIMUM RELIEF FORMULA EX-LAX LAXATIVE PILLS
(Phenolphthalein) .... ▣ 749
None cited in PDR database.

REGULAR STRENGTH EX-LAX LAXATIVE PILLS
(Phenolphthalein) .... ▣ 749
None cited in PDR database.

EX-LAX GENTLE NATURE LAXATIVE PILLS
(Senna Concentrates) .... ▣ 749
None cited in PDR database.

EXOSURF NEONATAL FOR INTRATRACHEAL SUSPENSION
(Colfosceril Palmitate) 1081
None cited in PDR database.

EXTENDRYL CHEWABLE TABLETS
(Chlorpheniramine Maleate, Methscopolamine Nitrate, Phenylephrine Hydrochloride) 1003
None cited in PDR database.

EXTENDRYL SR. & JR. T.D. CAPSULES
(Chlorpheniramine Maleate, Methscopolamine Nitrate, Phenylephrine Hydrochloride) 1003
None cited in PDR database.

EXTENDRYL SYRUP
(Chlorpheniramine Maleate, Methscopolamine Nitrate, Phenylephrine Hydrochloride) 1003
None cited in PDR database.

EYE-STREAM EYE IRRIGATING SOLUTION
(Balanced Salt Solution) 469
None cited in PDR database.

4-WAY FAST ACTING NASAL SPRAY (REGULAR & MENTHOLATED)
(Naphazoline Hydrochloride, Phenylephrine Hydrochloride, Pyrilamine Maleate) .... ▣ 644
None cited in PDR database.

4-WAY 12 HOUR NASAL SPRAY
(Oxymetazoline Hydrochloride) .... ▣ 644
None cited in PDR database.

FML FORTE LIQUIFILM
(Fluorometholone) .... ◉ 237
None cited in PDR database.

FML LIQUIFILM
(Fluorometholone) .... ◉ 238
None cited in PDR database.

FML S.O.P.
(Fluorometholone) .... ◉ 239
None cited in PDR database.

FML-S LIQUIFILM
(Sulfacetamide Sodium, Fluorometholone) .... ◉ 240
May interact with silver preparations. Compounds in this category include:

Silver Nitrate (Physical incompatibility).
No products indexed under this heading.

FACTREL
(Gonadorelin Hydrochloride) 2996
May interact with androgens, estrogens, progestins, corticosteroids, oral contraceptives, phenothiazines, dopamine antagonists, and certain other agents. Compounds in these categories include:

Betamethasone Acetate (Pituitary secretion of gonadotropins affected). Products include:
Celestone Soluspan Suspension 2484

Betamethasone Sodium Phosphate (Pituitary secretion of gonadotropins affected). Products include:
Celestone Soluspan Suspension 2484

Chlorotrianisene (Pituitary secretion of gonadotropins affected).
No products indexed under this heading.

Chlorpromazine (Rise in prolactin; response to Factrel may be blunted). Products include:
Thorazine Suppositories 2701

Chlorpromazine Hydrochloride (Rise in prolactin; response to Factrel may be blunted). Products include:
Thorazine 2701

Clozapine (Rise in prolactin; response to Factrel may be blunted). Products include:
Clozaril Tablets 2377

Cortisone Acetate (Pituitary secretion of gonadotropins affected). Products include:
Cortone Acetate Sterile Suspension 1663
Cortone Acetate Tablets 1664

Desogestrel (Pituitary secretion of gonadotropins affected; gonadotropin levels suppressed). Products include:
Desogen Tablets 1867
Ortho-Cept 1907

Dexamethasone (Pituitary secretion of gonadotropins affected). Products include:
AK-Trol Ointment & Suspension .... ◉ 205
Decadron Elixir 1676
Decadron Tablets 1678
Decaspray Topical Aerosol 1689

(▣ Described in PDR For Nonprescription Drugs) (◉ Described in PDR For Ophthalmology)

Interactions Index — Factrel

Dexamethasone Acetate (Pituitary secretion of gonadotropins affected). Products include:
- Dalalone D.P. Injectable ... 1009
- Decadron-LA Sterile Suspension ... 1687

Dexamethasone Sodium Phosphate (Pituitary secretion of gonadotropins affected). Products include:
- Decadron Phosphate Injection ... 1680
- Decadron Phosphate Sterile Ophthalmic Ointment ... 1684
- Decadron Phosphate Sterile Ophthalmic Solution ... 1685
- Decadron Phosphate Topical Cream ... 1686
- Decadron Phosphate with Xylocaine Injection, Sterile ... 1683
- Dexacort Phosphate in Respihaler ... 1606
- Dexacort Phosphate in Turbinaire ... 1607
- NeoDecadron Sterile Ophthalmic Ointment ... 1755
- NeoDecadron Sterile Ophthalmic Solution ... 1756
- NeoDecadron Topical Cream ... 1757

Dienestrol (Pituitary secretion of gonadotropins affected). Products include:
- Ortho Dienestrol Cream ... 1922

Diethylstilbestrol (Pituitary secretion of gonadotropins affected). Products include:
- Diethylstilbestrol Tablets ... 1477

Digitoxin (Gonadotropin levels suppressed). Products include:
- Crystodigin Tablets ... 1472

Digoxin (Gonadotropin levels suppressed). Products include:
- Lanoxicaps ... 1110
- Lanoxin Elixir Pediatric ... 1113
- Lanoxin Injection ... 1116
- Lanoxin Injection Pediatric ... 1119
- Lanoxin Tablets ... 1121

Estradiol (Pituitary secretion of gonadotropins affected). Products include:
- Climara Transdermal System ... 640
- Estrace Cream and Tablets ... 751
- Estraderm Transdermal System ... 842
- Estring Vaginal Ring ... 2086
- Vivelle Transdermal System ... 880

Estrogens, Conjugated (Pituitary secretion of gonadotropins affected). Products include:
- PMB 200 and PMB 400 ... 2890
- Premarin Intravenous ... 2893
- Premarin Tablets ... 2896
- Premarin Vaginal Cream ... 2898
- Premphase ... 2900
- Prempro ... 2905

Estrogens, Esterified (Pituitary secretion of gonadotropins affected). Products include:
- ESTRATAB Tablets (0.3, 0.625, 1.25, 2.5 mg) ... 2715
- Estratest ... 2718
- Menest Tablets ... 2671

Estropipate (Pituitary secretion of gonadotropins affected). Products include:
- Ogen Tablets ... 2103
- Ogen Vaginal Cream ... 2106
- Ortho-Est ... 1925

Ethinyl Estradiol (Pituitary secretion of gonadotropins affected; gonadotropin levels suppressed). Products include:
- Brevicon ... 2563
- Demulen ... 2580
- Desogen Tablets ... 1867
- Levlen/Tri-Levlen ... 646
- Lo/Ovral Tablets ... 2852
- Lo/Ovral-28 Tablets ... 2857
- Modicon ... 1928
- Nordette-21 Tablets ... 2863
- Nordette-28 Tablets ... 2866
- Norinyl ... 2563
- Ortho-Cept ... 1907
- Ortho-Cyclen/Ortho-Tri-Cyclen ... 1914
- Ortho-Novum ... 1928
- Ortho-Cyclen/Ortho Tri-Cyclen ... 1914
- Ovcon ... 765
- Ovral Tablets ... 2877
- Ovral-28 Tablets ... 2878
- Levlen/Tri-Levlen ... 646
- Tri-Norinyl ... 2607
- Triphasil-21 Tablets ... 2919
- Triphasil-28 Tablets ... 2924

Ethynodiol Diacetate (Gonadotropin levels suppressed). Products include:
- Demulen ... 2580

Fludrocortisone Acetate (Pituitary secretion of gonadotropins affected). Products include:
- Florinef Acetate Tablets ... 506

Fluoxymesterone (Pituitary secretion of gonadotropins affected). Products include:
- Halotestin Tablets ... 2095

Fluphenazine Decanoate (Rise in prolactin; response to Factrel may be blunted). Products include:
- Prolixin Decanoate ... 510

Fluphenazine Enanthate (Rise in prolactin; response to Factrel may be blunted). Products include:
- Prolixin Enanthate ... 510

Fluphenazine Hydrochloride (Rise in prolactin; response to Factrel may be blunted). Products include:
- Prolixin ... 510

Haloperidol (Rise in prolactin; response to Factrel may be blunted). Products include:
- Haldol Injection, Tablets and Concentrate ... 1585

Haloperidol Decanoate (Rise in prolactin; response to Factrel may be blunted). Products include:
- Haldol Decanoate ... 1587

Hydrocortisone (Pituitary secretion of gonadotropins affected). Products include:
- Anusol-HC Cream 2.5% ... 1953
- Aquanil HC Lotion ... 1989
- Maximum Strength Cortaid Spray ... 800
- CORTENEMA ... 2713
- Cortisporin Ointment ... 1074
- Cortisporin Ophthalmic Ointment Sterile ... 1074
- Cortisporin Ophthalmic Suspension Sterile ... 1075
- Cortisporin Otic Solution Sterile ... 1076
- Cortisporin Otic Suspension Sterile ... 1077
- Cortizone-5 ... 795
- Cortizone-10 ... 795
- Hydrocortone Tablets ... 1715
- Hytone ... 922
- Hytone Ointment 2 ½ % ... 923
- Massengill Medicated Soft Cloth Towelettes ... 2628
- Pediotic Suspension Sterile ... 1140
- Preparation H Hydrocortisone 1% Cream ... 843
- ProctoCream-HC 2.5% ... 2552
- VōSoL HC Otic Solution ... 2786

Hydrocortisone Acetate (Pituitary secretion of gonadotropins affected). Products include:
- Analpram-HC Rectal Cream 1% and 2.5% ... 993
- Anusol HC-1 Hydrocortisone Anti-Itch Ointment ... 810
- Anusol-HC Suppositories ... 1954
- Caldecort Anti-Itch Hydrocortisone Cream ... 651
- Coly-Mycin S Otic w/Neomycin & Hydrocortisone ... 1965
- Cortaid ... 800
- Cortifoam ... 2540
- Cortisporin Cream ... 1073
- Epifoam ... 2543
- Hydrocortone Acetate Sterile Suspension ... 1712
- Mantadil Cream ... 1124
- Nupercainal Hydrocortisone 1% Cream ... 661
- Pramosone Cream, Lotion & Ointment ... 995
- ProctoFoam-HC ... 2552
- Terra-Cortril Ophthalmic Suspension ... 2033

Hydrocortisone Sodium Phosphate (Pituitary secretion of gonadotropins affected). Products include:
- Hydrocortone Phosphate Injection, Sterile ... 1713

Hydrocortisone Sodium Succinate (Pituitary secretion of gonadotropins affected).
No products indexed under this heading.

Levodopa (Minimal elevation of gonadotropin levels). Products include:
- Atamet Tablets ... 567
- Larodopa Tablets ... 2296
- Sinemet Tablets ... 959
- Sinemet CR Tablets ... 961

Levonorgestrel (Gonadotropin levels suppressed). Products include:
- Levlen/Tri-Levlen ... 646
- Nordette-21 Tablets ... 2863
- Nordette-28 Tablets ... 2866
- Norplant System ... 2868
- Levlen/Tri-Levlen ... 646
- Triphasil-21 Tablets ... 2919
- Triphasil-28 Tablets ... 2924

Medroxyprogesterone Acetate (Pituitary secretion of gonadotropins affected). Products include:
- Amen Tablets ... 785
- Cycrin Tablets ... 991
- Depo-Provera Contraceptive Injection ... 2079
- Depo-Provera Sterile Aqueous Suspension ... 2083
- Premphase ... 2900
- Prempro ... 2905
- Provera Tablets ... 2110

Megestrol Acetate (Pituitary secretion of gonadotropins affected). Products include:
- Megace Oral Suspension ... 708
- Megace Tablets ... 710

Mesoridazine Besylate (Rise in prolactin; response to Factrel may be blunted). Products include:
- Serentil ... 689

Mestranol (Gonadotropin levels suppressed). Products include:
- Norinyl ... 2563
- Ortho-Novum ... 1928

Methotrimeprazine (Rise in prolactin; response to Factrel may be blunted). Products include:
- Levoprome ... 1321

Methylprednisolone Acetate (Pituitary secretion of gonadotropins affected).
No products indexed under this heading.

Methylprednisolone Sodium Succinate (Pituitary secretion of gonadotropins affected).
No products indexed under this heading.

Methyltestosterone (Pituitary secretion of gonadotropins affected). Products include:
- Android Capsules, 10 mg ... 1297
- Estratest ... 2718
- Testred Capsules, 10 mg ... 1308

Metoclopramide Hydrochloride (Rise in prolactin; response to Factrel may be blunted). Products include:
- Reglan ... 2243

Norethindrone (Gonadotropin levels suppressed). Products include:
- Brevicon ... 2563
- Micronor Tablets ... 1903
- Modicon ... 1928
- Norinyl ... 2563
- Nor-Q D Tablets ... 2598
- Ortho-Novum ... 1928
- Ovcon ... 765
- Tri-Norinyl ... 2607

Norethynodrel (Gonadotropin levels suppressed).
No products indexed under this heading.

Norgestimate (Pituitary secretion of gonadotropins affected; gonadotropin levels suppressed). Products include:
- Ortho-Cyclen/Ortho-Tri-Cyclen ... 1914
- Ortho-Cyclen/Ortho Tri-Cyclen ... 1914

Norgestrel (Gonadotropin levels suppressed). Products include:
- Lo/Ovral Tablets ... 2852
- Lo/Ovral-28 Tablets ... 2857
- Ovral Tablets ... 2877
- Ovral-28 Tablets ... 2878
- Ovrette Tablets ... 2878

Oxandrolone (Pituitary secretion of gonadotropins affected). Products include:
- Oxandrin ... 783

Oxymetholone (Pituitary secretion of gonadotropins affected).
No products indexed under this heading.

Perphenazine (Rise in prolactin; response to Factrel may be blunted). Products include:
- Etrafon ... 2495
- Triavil Tablets ... 1800
- Trilafon ... 2532

Pimozide (Rise in prolactin; response to Factrel may be blunted). Products include:
- Orap Tablets ... 1037

Polyestradiol Phosphate (Pituitary secretion of gonadotropins affected).
No products indexed under this heading.

Prednisolone Acetate (Pituitary secretion of gonadotropins affected). Products include:
- AK-CIDE ... 203
- AK-CIDE Ointment ... 203
- Blephamide Liquifilm Sterile Ophthalmic Suspension ... 472
- Blephamide Ointment ... 234
- Econopred & Econopred Plus Ophthalmic Suspensions ... 216
- Poly-Pred Liquifilm ... 246
- Pred Forte ... 247
- Pred Mild ... 250
- Pred-G Liquifilm Sterile Ophthalmic Suspension ... 248
- Pred-G S.O.P. Sterile Ophthalmic Ointment ... 249

Prednisolone Sodium Phosphate (Pituitary secretion of gonadotropins affected). Products include:
- AK-PRED ... 204
- Hydeltrasol Injection, Sterile ... 1708
- Pediapred Oral Solution ... 1618

Prednisolone Tebutate (Pituitary secretion of gonadotropins affected). Products include:
- Hydeltra-T.B.A. Sterile Suspension ... 1710

Prednisone (Pituitary secretion of gonadotropins affected).
No products indexed under this heading.

Prochlorperazine (Rise in prolactin; response to Factrel may be blunted). Products include:
- Compazine ... 2644

Promethazine Hydrochloride (Rise in prolactin; response to Factrel may be blunted). Products include:
- Mepergan Injection ... 2859
- Phenergan with Codeine ... 2883
- Phenergan with Dextromethorphan ... 2885
- Phenergan Injection ... 2880
- Phenergan Suppositories ... 2882
- Phenergan Syrup ... 2881
- Phenergan Tablets ... 2882
- Phenergan VC ... 2886
- Phenergan VC with Codeine ... 2888

Maxitrol Ophthalmic Ointment and Suspension ... 222
TobraDex Ophthalmic Suspension and Ointment ... 469

IMPORTANT NOTE: Always consult each drug listing in the patient's regimen for possible interactions.

Quinestrol (Pituitary secretion of gonadotropins affected).
No products indexed under this heading.

Spironolactone (Gonadotropin levels transiently elevated). Products include:
- Aldactazide Tablets 2556
- Aldactone Tablets 2558

Stanozolol (Pituitary secretion of gonadotropins affected). Products include:
- Winstrol Tablets 2468

Thioridazine Hydrochloride (Rise in prolactin; response to Factrel may be blunted). Products include:
- Mellaril 2398

Triamcinolone (Pituitary secretion of gonadotropins affected).
No products indexed under this heading.

Triamcinolone Acetonide (Pituitary secretion of gonadotropins affected). Products include:
- Azmacort Oral Inhaler 2175
- Nasacort AQ Nasal Spray 2191
- Nasacort Nasal Inhaler 2189

Triamcinolone Diacetate (Pituitary secretion of gonadotropins affected).
No products indexed under this heading.

Triamcinolone Hexacetonide (Pituitary secretion of gonadotropins affected).
No products indexed under this heading.

Trifluoperazine Hydrochloride (Rise in prolactin; response to Factrel may be blunted). Products include:
- Stelazine 2692

FAMVIR TABLETS

(Famciclovir) 2660
May interact with xanthine bronchodilators and certain other agents. Compounds in these categories include:

Aminophylline (Potential for increase in penciclovir AUC and C_{max} and decrease in renal clearance; the magnitude of this effect is considered to be of no clinical importance).
No products indexed under this heading.

Cimetidine (Increase in penciclovir AUC and urinary recovery; the magnitude of this effect is considered to be of no clinical importance). Products include:
- Tagamet HB Tablets .... ⊡ 786
- Tagamet Tablets 2694

Cimetidine Hydrochloride (Increase in penciclovir AUC and urinary recovery; the magnitude of this effect is considered to be of no clinical importance). Products include:
- Tagamet 2694

Digoxin (Potential for increase in C_{max} of digoxin). Products include:
- Lanoxicaps 1110
- Lanoxin Elixir Pediatric 1113
- Lanoxin Injection 1116
- Lanoxin Injection Pediatric 1119
- Lanoxin Tablets 1121

Dyphylline (Potential for increase in penciclovir AUC and C_{max} and decrease in renal clearance; the magnitude of this effect is considered to be of no clinical importance). Products include:
- Lufyllin & Lufyllin-400 Tablets 2778
- Lufyllin-GG Elixir & Tablets 2779

Probenecid (Concurrent use may result in increased plasma concentration of penciclovir). Products include:
- Benemid Tablets 1651
- ColBENEMID Tablets 1662

Theophylline (Potential for increase in penciclovir AUC and C_{max} and decrease in renal clearance; the magnitude of this effect is considered to be of no clinical importance). Products include:
- Marax Tablets & DF Syrup 2015
- Quibron 2227

Theophylline Anhydrous (Potential for increase in penciclovir AUC and C_{max} and decrease in renal clearance; the magnitude of this effect is considered to be of no clinical importance). Products include:
- Aerolate 1003
- Primatene Tablets .... ⊡ 844
- Respbid Tablets 687
- Slo-bid Gyrocaps 2201
- Theo-24 Extended Release Capsules 2753
- Theo-Dur Extended-Release Tablets 1367
- Theo-X Extended-Release Tablets .. 793
- Uni-Dur Extended-Release Tablets .. 1374
- Uniphyl 400 mg and 600 mg Tablets 2157

Theophylline Calcium Salicylate (Potential for increase in penciclovir AUC and C_{max} and decrease in renal clearance; the magnitude of this effect is considered to be of no clinical importance). Products include:
- Quadrinal Tablets 1398

Theophylline Sodium Glycinate (Potential for increase in penciclovir AUC and C_{max} and decrease in renal clearance; the magnitude of this effect is considered to be of no clinical importance).
No products indexed under this heading.

Food Interactions

Meal, unspecified (Penciclovir C_{max} decreased approximately 50% and T_{max} was delayed by 1.5 hours when a capsule formulation of famciclovir was administered with food; there is no effect on the extent of availability (AUC) of penciclovir).

FANSIDAR TABLETS

(Sulfadoxine, Pyrimethamine) 2281
May interact with sulfonamides and certain other agents. Compounds in these categories include:

Chloroquine (Increased incidence and severity of adverse reactions).

Sulfamethizole (Interferes with antimalarial prophylaxis). Products include:
- Urobiotic-250 Capsules 2038

Sulfamethoxazole (Interferes with antimalarial prophylaxis). Products include:
- Bactrim DS Tablets 2257
- Bactrim I.V. Infusion 2255
- Bactrim 2257
- Gantanol Tablets 2285
- Septra 1146
- Septra I.V. Infusion 1142
- Septra I.V. Infusion ADD-Vantage Vials 1144
- Septra 1146

Sulfasalazine (Interferes with antimalarial prophylaxis). Products include:
- Azulfidine 2059

Sulfinpyrazone (Interferes with antimalarial prophylaxis). Products include:
- Anturane 823

Sulfisoxazole (Interferes with antimalarial prophylaxis). Products include:
- Gantrisin Tablets 2286

Sulfisoxazole Diolamine (Interferes with antimalarial prophylaxis).
No products indexed under this heading.

FASTIN CAPSULES

(Phentermine Hydrochloride) 2662
May interact with monoamine oxidase inhibitors, insulin, and certain other agents. Compounds in these categories include:

Furazolidone (Hypertensive crises may result). Products include:
- Furoxone 2221

Guanethidine Monosulfate (May decrease hypotensive effect of guanethidine). Products include:
- Esimil Tablets 840
- Ismelin Tablets 845

Insulin, Human (Insulin requirements may be altered).
No products indexed under this heading.

Insulin, Human Isophane Suspension (Insulin requirements may be altered). Products include:
- Novolin N Human Insulin 10 ml Vials 1846

Insulin, Human NPH (Insulin requirements may be altered). Products include:
- Humulin N, 100 Units 1495
- Novolin N PenFill 1.5 ml Cartridges Durable Insulin Delivery System 1849
- Novolin N Prefilled Syringe Disposable Insulin Delivery System 1850

Insulin, Human Regular (Insulin requirements may be altered). Products include:
- Humulin R, 100 Units 1497
- Novolin R Human Insulin 10 ml Vials 1846
- Novolin R PenFill 1.5 ml Cartridges Durable Insulin Delivery System 1849
- Novolin R Prefilled Syringe Disposable Insulin Delivery System 1850
- Velosulin BR Human Insulin 10 ml Vials 1847

Insulin, Human, Zinc Suspension (Insulin requirements may be altered). Products include:
- Humulin L, 100 Units 1494
- Humulin U, 100 Units 1498
- Novolin L Human Insulin 10 ml Vials 1846

Insulin Lispro, Human (Insulin requirements may be altered). Products include:
- Humalog Injection 1488

Insulin, NPH (Insulin requirements may be altered). Products include:
- NPH, 100 Units 1502
- Pork NPH, 100 Units 1506
- Purified Pork NPH Isophane Insulin 1852

Insulin, Regular (Insulin requirements may be altered). Products include:
- Regular, 100 Units 1503
- Pork Regular, 100 Units 1507
- Pork Regular (Concentrated), 500 Units 1508
- Purified Pork Regular Insulin 1852

Insulin, Zinc Crystals (Insulin requirements may be altered). Products include:
- NPH, 100 Units 1502

Insulin, Zinc Suspension (Insulin requirements may be altered). Products include:
- Iletin I 1501
- Lente, 100 Units 1501
- Iletin II 1504
- Pork Lente, 100 Units 1504
- Purified Pork Lente Insulin 1852

Isocarboxazid (Hypertensive crises may result).
No products indexed under this heading.

Phenelzine Sulfate (Hypertensive crises may result). Products include:
- Nardil 1977

Selegiline Hydrochloride (Hypertensive crises may result). Products include:
- Eldepryl Capsules 2729

Tranylcypromine Sulfate (Hypertensive crises may result). Products include:
- Parnate Tablets 2679

Food Interactions

Alcohol (Concomitant use may result in adverse drug interaction).

FAT BURNING FACTORS

(Vitamins, Multiple) .... ⊡ 605
None cited in PDR database.

FEDAHIST GYROCAPS

(Pseudoephedrine Hydrochloride, Chlorpheniramine Maleate) 2545
May interact with monoamine oxidase inhibitors, beta blockers, veratrum alkaloids, tricyclic antidepressants, barbiturates, central nervous system depressants, and certain other agents. Compounds in these categories include:

Acebutolol Hydrochloride (Increases the effect of sympathomimetics). Products include:
- Sectral Capsules 2914

Alfentanil Hydrochloride (May have an additive CNS depressant effect). Products include:
- Alfenta Injection 1334

Alprazolam (May have an additive CNS depressant effect). Products include:
- Xanax Tablets 2115

Amitriptyline Hydrochloride (May have an additive CNS depressant effect). Products include:
- Elavil 2945
- Etrafon 2495
- Limbitrol 2333
- Triavil Tablets 1800

Amoxapine (May have an additive CNS depressant effect). Products include:
- Asendin Tablets 1419

Aprobarbital (May have an additive CNS depressant effect).
No products indexed under this heading.

Atenolol (Increases the effect of sympathomimetics). Products include:
- Tenoretic Tablets 2963
- Tenormin Tablets and I.V. Injection 2965

Betaxolol Hydrochloride (Increases the effect of sympathomimetics). Products include:
- Betoptic Ophthalmic Solution 465
- Betoptic S Ophthalmic Suspension 467
- Kerlone Tablets 2588

Bisoprolol Fumarate (Increases the effect of sympathomimetics). Products include:
- Zebeta Tablets 1457
- Ziac 1459

Buprenorphine (May have an additive CNS depressant effect). Products include:
- Buprenex Injectable 2170

Buspirone Hydrochloride (May have an additive CNS depressant effect). Products include:
- BuSpar Tablets 738

(⊡ Described in PDR For Nonprescription Drugs) (◉ Described in PDR For Ophthalmology)

405 **Interactions Index** **Fedahist GyroCaps/Timecaps**

Butabarbital (May have an additive CNS depressant effect).
No products indexed under this heading.

Butalbital (May have an additive CNS depressant effect). Products include:
Axocet Capsules 2469
Esgic-plus Capsules 1012
Esgic-plus Tablets 1012
Fioricet Tablets 2386
Fioricet with Codeine Capsules 2387
Fiorinal Capsules 2388
Fiorinal with Codeine Capsules 2390
Fiorinal Tablets 2388
Phrenilin 790
Sedapap Tablets 50 mg/650 mg .. 1826

Carteolol Hydrochloride (Increases the effect of sympathomimetics). Products include:
Cartrol Tablets 413
Ocupress Ophthalmic Solution, 1% Sterile .... ⊙ 297

Chlordiazepoxide (May have an additive CNS depressant effect). Products include:
Limbitrol 2333

Chlordiazepoxide Hydrochloride (May have an additive CNS depressant effect). Products include:
Librax Capsules 2330
Librium Capsules 2331
Librium Injectable 2332

Chlorpromazine (May have an additive CNS depressant effect). Products include:
Thorazine Suppositories 2701

Chlorprothixene (May have an additive CNS depressant effect).
No products indexed under this heading.

Chlorprothixene Hydrochloride (May have an additive CNS depressant effect).
No products indexed under this heading.

Chlorprothixene Lactate (May have an additive CNS depressant effect).
No products indexed under this heading.

Clomipramine Hydrochloride (May have an additive CNS depressant effect). Products include:
Anafranil Capsules 819

Clorazepate Dipotassium (May have an additive CNS depressant effect). Products include:
Tranxene 459

Clozapine (May have an additive CNS depressant effect). Products include:
Clozaril Tablets 2377

Codeine Phosphate (May have an additive CNS depressant effect). Products include:
Brontex 2130
Dimetane-DC Cough Syrup 2232
Fioricet with Codeine Capsules 2387
Fiorinal with Codeine Capsules 2390
Nucofed 2225
Phenergan with Codeine 2883
Phenergan VC with Codeine 2888
Robitussin A-C Syrup 2248
Robitussin-DAC Syrup 2249
Ryna 804
Soma Compound w/Codeine Tablets 2784
Tylenol with Codeine 1592

Cryptenamine Preparations (Reduced antihypertensive effect).

Desflurane (May have an additive CNS depressant effect). Products include:
Suprane (desflurane, USP) 1865

Desipramine Hydrochloride (May have an additive CNS depressant effect). Products include:
Norpramin Tablets 1273

Dezocine (May have an additive CNS depressant effect). Products include:
Dalgan Injection 529

Diazepam (May have an additive CNS depressant effect). Products include:
Dizac (diazepam injectable emulsion) CIV 1862
Valium Injectable 2336
Valium Tablets 2335

Doxepin Hydrochloride (May have an additive CNS depressant effect). Products include:
Adapin Capsules 1542
Sinequan 2028
Zonalon Cream 1042

Droperidol (May have an additive CNS depressant effect). Products include:
Inapsine Injection 462

Enflurane (May have an additive CNS depressant effect).
No products indexed under this heading.

Esmolol Hydrochloride (Increases the effect of sympathomimetics). Products include:
Brevibloc (esmolol HCl) Injection 1860

Estazolam (May have an additive CNS depressant effect). Products include:
ProSom Tablets 457

Ethchlorvynol (May have an additive CNS depressant effect). Products include:
Placidyl Capsules 456

Ethinamate (May have an additive CNS depressant effect).
No products indexed under this heading.

Fentanyl (May have an additive CNS depressant effect). Products include:
Duragesic Transdermal System 1336

Fentanyl Citrate (May have an additive CNS depressant effect). Products include:
Sublimaze Injection 463

Fluphenazine Decanoate (May have an additive CNS depressant effect). Products include:
Prolixin Decanoate 510

Fluphenazine Enanthate (May have an additive CNS depressant effect). Products include:
Prolixin Enanthate 510

Fluphenazine Hydrochloride (May have an additive CNS depressant effect). Products include:
Prolixin 510

Flurazepam Hydrochloride (May have an additive CNS depressant effect). Products include:
Dalmane Capsules 2329

Furazolidone (Increases the effect of sympathomimetics; concurrent use is contraindicated). Products include:
Furoxone 2221

Glutethimide (May have an additive CNS depressant effect).
No products indexed under this heading.

Haloperidol (May have an additive CNS depressant effect). Products include:
Haldol Injection, Tablets and Concentrate 1585

Haloperidol Decanoate (May have an additive CNS depressant effect). Products include:
Haldol Decanoate 1587

Hydrocodone Bitartrate (May have an additive CNS depressant effect). Products include:
Codiclear DH Syrup 808
Duratuss HD Elixir 2750
Histussin D Liquid 670
Hycodan Tablets and Syrup 946
Hycomine Compound Tablets 948
Hycomine 947
Hycotuss Expectorant Syrup 950
Hydrocet Capsules 787
Lorcet 10/650 Tablets 1016
Lortab 2751
Tussend 1830
Tussend Expectorant 1831
Vicodin Tablets 1404
Vicodin ES Tablets 1405
Vicodin HP Tablets 1403
Vicodin Tuss Expectorant 1406
Zydone Capsules 967

Hydrocodone Polistirex (May have an additive CNS depressant effect). Products include:
Tussionex Pennkinetic Extended-Release Suspension 1624

Hydroxyzine Hydrochloride (May have an additive CNS depressant effect). Products include:
Atarax Tablets & Syrup 1992
Marax Tablets & DF Syrup 2015
Vistaril Intramuscular Solution 2042

Imipramine Hydrochloride (May have an additive CNS depressant effect). Products include:
Tofranil Ampuls 873
Tofranil Tablets 875

Imipramine Pamoate (May have an additive CNS depressant effect). Products include:
Tofranil-PM Capsules 876

Isocarboxazid (Increases the effect of sympathomimetics; concurrent use is contraindicated).
No products indexed under this heading.

Isoflurane (May have an additive CNS depressant effect).
No products indexed under this heading.

Ketamine Hydrochloride (May have an additive CNS depressant effect).
No products indexed under this heading.

Labetalol Hydrochloride (Increases the effect of sympathomimetics). Products include:
Normodyne Injection 2519
Normodyne Tablets 2522
Trandate 1158

Levobunolol Hydrochloride (Increases the effect of sympathomimetics). Products include:
Betagan .... ⊙ 230

Levomethadyl Acetate Hydrochloride (May have an additive CNS depressant effect). Products include:
Orlaam Oral Solution 2361

Levorphanol Tartrate (May have an additive CNS depressant effect). Products include:
Levo-Dromoran 2297

Lorazepam (May have an additive CNS depressant effect). Products include:
Ativan Injection 2805
Ativan Tablets 2807

Loxapine Hydrochloride (May have an additive CNS depressant effect). Products include:
Loxitane 1426

Loxapine Succinate (May have an additive CNS depressant effect). Products include:
Loxitane Capsules 1426

Maprotiline Hydrochloride (May have an additive CNS depressant effect). Products include:
Ludiomil Tablets 861

Mecamylamine Hydrochloride (Reduced antihypertensive effect). Products include:
Inversine Tablets 1729

Meperidine Hydrochloride (May have an additive CNS depressant effect). Products include:
Demerol 2438
Mepergan Injection 2859

Mephobarbital (May have an additive CNS depressant effect). Products include:
Mebaral Tablets 2452

Meprobamate (May have an additive CNS depressant effect). Products include:
Miltown Tablets 2780
PMB 200 and PMB 400 2890

Mesoridazine Besylate (May have an additive CNS depressant effect). Products include:
Serentil 689

Methadone Hydrochloride (May have an additive CNS depressant effect). Products include:
Methadone Hydrochloride Oral Concentrate 2356
Methadone Hydrochloride Oral Solution & Tablets 2357

Methohexital Sodium (May have an additive CNS depressant effect).
No products indexed under this heading.

Methotrimeprazine (May have an additive CNS depressant effect). Products include:
Levoprome 1321

Methoxyflurane (May have an additive CNS depressant effect).
No products indexed under this heading.

Methyldopa (Reduced antihypertensive effect). Products include:
Aldoclor Tablets 1638
Aldomet Oral 1640
Aldoril Tablets 1644

Methyldopate Hydrochloride (Reduced antihypertensive effect). Products include:
Aldomet Ester HCl Injection 1642

Metipranolol Hydrochloride (Increases the effect of sympathomimetics). Products include:
OptiPranolol (Metipranolol 0.3%) Sterile Ophthalmic Solution .... ⊙ 256

Metoprolol Succinate (Increases the effect of sympathomimetics). Products include:
Toprol-XL Tablets 560

Metoprolol Tartrate (Increases the effect of sympathomimetics). Products include:
Lopressor 848
Lopressor HCT Tablets 850

Midazolam Hydrochloride (May have an additive CNS depressant effect). Products include:
Versed Injection 2324

Molindone Hydrochloride (May have an additive CNS depressant effect). Products include:
Moban Tablets and Concentrate 1036

Morphine Sulfate (May have an additive CNS depressant effect). Products include:
Astramorph/PF Injection, USP (Preservative-Free) 526
Duramorph Injection 983
Infumorph 200 and Infumorph 500 Sterile Solutions 985
Kadian Capsules 2948
MS Contin Tablets 2149
MSIR 2152
Oramorph SR (Morphine Sulfate Sustained Release Tablets) 2359
RMS Suppositories CII 2766
Roxanol 2365

Nadolol (Increases the effect of sympathomimetics).
No products indexed under this heading.

IMPORTANT NOTE: Always consult each drug listing in the patient's regimen for possible interactions.

Fedahist GyroCaps/Timecaps — Interactions Index — 406

Nortriptyline Hydrochloride (May have an additive CNS depressant effect). Products include:
- Pamelor 2409

Opium Alkaloids (May have an additive CNS depressant effect).
- No products indexed under this heading.

Oxazepam (May have an additive CNS depressant effect). Products include:
- Serax Capsules 2916
- Serax Tablets 2916

Oxycodone Hydrochloride (May have an additive CNS depressant effect). Products include:
- OxyContin Tablets 2163
- OxyIR Capsules 2167
- Percocet Tablets 955
- Percodan Tablets 955
- Percodan-Demi Tablets 956
- Roxicodone Tablets, Oral Solution & Intensol (Oxycodone) 2366
- Tylox Capsules 1593

Penbutolol Sulfate (Increases the effect of sympathomimetics). Products include:
- Levatol Tablets 2547

Pentobarbital Sodium (May have an additive CNS depressant effect). Products include:
- Nembutal Sodium Capsules 440
- Nembutal Sodium Solution 442
- Nembutal Sodium Suppositories 444

Perphenazine (May have an additive CNS depressant effect). Products include:
- Etrafon 2495
- Triavil Tablets 1800
- Trilafon 2532

Phenelzine Sulfate (Increases the effect of sympathomimetics; concurrent use is contraindicated). Products include:
- Nardil 1977

Phenobarbital (May have an additive CNS depressant effect). Products include:
- Arco-Lase Plus Tablets 513
- Bellergal-S Tablets 2375
- Donnatal 2234
- Donnatal Extentabs 2234
- Donnatal Tablets 2234
- Phenobarbital Elixir and Tablets 1523
- Quadrinal Tablets 1398

Pindolol (Increases the effect of sympathomimetics). Products include:
- Visken Tablets 2428

Prazepam (May have an additive CNS depressant effect).
- No products indexed under this heading.

Prochlorperazine (May have an additive CNS depressant effect). Products include:
- Compazine 2644

Promethazine Hydrochloride (May have an additive CNS depressant effect). Products include:
- Mepergan Injection 2859
- Phenergan with Codeine 2883
- Phenergan with Dextromethorphan 2885
- Phenergan Injection 2880
- Phenergan Suppositories 2882
- Phenergan Syrup 2881
- Phenergan Tablets 2882
- Phenergan VC 2886
- Phenergan VC with Codeine 2888

Propofol (May have an additive CNS depressant effect). Products include:
- Diprivan Injectable Emulsion 2939

Propoxyphene Hydrochloride (May have an additive CNS depressant effect). Products include:
- Darvon 1475
- Wygesic Tablets 2930

Propoxyphene Napsylate (May have an additive CNS depressant effect). Products include:
- Darvon-N/Darvocet-N 1473

Propranolol Hydrochloride (Increases the effect of sympathomimetics). Products include:
- Inderal 2834
- Inderal LA Long Acting Capsules 2836
- Inderide Tablets 2838
- Inderide LA Long Acting Capsules 2840

Protriptyline Hydrochloride (May have an additive CNS depressant effect). Products include:
- Vivactil Tablets 1820

Quazepam (May have an additive CNS depressant effect). Products include:
- Doral Tablets 2773

Rauwolfia Serpentina (Reduced antihypertensive effect).
- No products indexed under this heading.

Reserpine (Reduced antihypertensive effect). Products include:
- Diupres Tablets 1691
- Hydropres Tablets 1718
- Ser-Ap-Es Tablets 867

Risperidone (May have an additive CNS depressant effect). Products include:
- Risperdal Tablets 1348

Secobarbital Sodium (May have an additive CNS depressant effect). Products include:
- Seconal Sodium Pulvules 1529

Selegiline Hydrochloride (Increases the effect of sympathomimetics; concurrent use is contraindicated). Products include:
- Eldepryl Capsules 2729

Sevoflurane (May have an additive CNS depressant effect).
- No products indexed under this heading.

Sotalol Hydrochloride (Increases the effect of sympathomimetics). Products include:
- Betapace Tablets 637

Sufentanil Citrate (May have an additive CNS depressant effect). Products include:
- Sufenta Injection 1355

Temazepam (May have an additive CNS depressant effect). Products include:
- Restoril Capsules 2413

Thiamylal Sodium (May have an additive CNS depressant effect).
- No products indexed under this heading.

Thioridazine Hydrochloride (May have an additive CNS depressant effect). Products include:
- Mellaril 2398

Thiothixene (May have an additive CNS depressant effect). Products include:
- Navane Capsules and Concentrate 2018
- Navane Intramuscular 2019

Timolol Hemihydrate (Increases the effect of sympathomimetics). Products include:
- Betimol 0.25%, 0.5% ..... ◎ 259

Timolol Maleate (Increases the effect of sympathomimetics). Products include:
- Blocadren Tablets 1654
- Timolide Tablets 1791
- Timoptic in Ocudose 1796
- Timoptic Sterile Ophthalmic Solution 1794
- Timoptic-XE 1798

Tranylcypromine Sulfate (Increases the effect of sympathomimetics; concurrent use is contraindicated). Products include:
- Parnate Tablets 2679

Triazolam (May have an additive CNS depressant effect). Products include:
- Halcion Tablets 2093

Trifluoperazine Hydrochloride (May have an additive CNS depressant effect). Products include:
- Stelazine 2692

Trimipramine Maleate (May have an additive CNS depressant effect). Products include:
- Surmontil Capsules 2917

Zolpidem Tartrate (May have an additive CNS depressant effect). Products include:
- Ambien Tablets 2559

Food Interactions

Alcohol (May have an additive CNS depressant effect).

FELBATOL
(Felbamate) 2774

May interact with:

Carbamazepine (Causes an approximate 50% increase in the clearance of felbamate; decrease in steady-state carbamazepine plasma concentration and an increase in the steady-state carbamazepine epoxide plasma concentration caused by felbamate). Products include:
- Atretol Tablets 569
- Tegretol/Tegretol-XR 870

Divalproex Sodium (Felbamate causes an increase in steady-state valproate concentrations; no significant effect of valproate on the clearance of felbamate). Products include:
- Depakote Tablets 418

Phenytoin (Causes an approximate doubling of the clearance of felbamate; increase in steady-state phenytoin plasma concentration caused by felbamate). Products include:
- Dilantin Infatabs 1967
- Dilantin-125 Suspension 1969

Phenytoin Sodium (Causes an approximate doubling of the clearance of felbamate; increase in steady-state phenytoin plasma concentration caused by felbamate). Products include:
- Dilantin Kapseals 1965

Valproic Acid (Felbamate causes an increase in steady-state valproate concentrations; no significant effect of valproate on the clearance of felbamate). Products include:
- Depakene 416

FELDENE CAPSULES
(Piroxicam) 2008

May interact with oral anticoagulants, lithium preparations, highly protein bound drugs (selected), and certain other agents. Compounds in these categories include:

Amiodarone Hydrochloride (Feldene might displace other highly protein bound drugs). Products include:
- Cordarone Intravenous 2821
- Cordarone Tablets 2818

Amitriptyline Hydrochloride (Feldene might displace other highly protein bound drugs). Products include:
- Elavil 2945
- Etrafon 2495
- Limbitrol 2333
- Triavil Tablets 1800

Aspirin (Aspirin (3900 mg/day) depresses plasma levels of piroxicam). Products include:
- Alka-Seltzer Cherry Effervescent Antacid and Pain Reliever ..... ▣ 609
- Alka-Seltzer Extra Strength Effervescent Antacid and Pain Reliever ..... ▣ 609
- Alka-Seltzer Lemon Lime Effervescent Antacid and Pain Reliever ..... ▣ 609
- Alka-Seltzer Original Effervescent Antacid and Pain Reliever ..... ▣ 609
- Alka-Seltzer Plus ..... ▣ 611
- Alka-Seltzer Plus Sinus Medicine ..... ▣ 611
- Ascriptin 650
- Arthritis Strength BC Powder ..... ▣ 631
- BC Cold Powder Multi-Symptom Formula (Cold-Sinus-Allergy) ..... ▣ 631
- BC Cold Powder Non-Drowsy Formula (Cold-Sinus) ..... ▣ 631
- BC Powder ..... ▣ 631
- Genuine Bayer Aspirin Tablets & Caplets ..... ▣ 618
- Extra Strength Bayer Arthritis Pain Regimen Formula ..... ▣ 615
- Extra Strength Bayer Aspirin Caplets & Tablets ..... ▣ 617
- Extended-Release Bayer 8-Hour Aspirin ..... ▣ 616
- Extra Strength Bayer Plus Aspirin Caplets ..... ▣ 617
- Extra Strength Bayer PM Aspirin Plus Sleep Aid ..... ▣ 617
- Aspirin Regimen Bayer 81 mg Tablets with Calcium ..... ▣ 615
- Aspirin Regimen Bayer Adult Low Strength 81 mg Tablets ..... ▣ 613
- Aspirin Regimen Bayer Children's Chewable Aspirin ..... ▣ 616
- Aspirin Regimen Bayer Regular Strength 325 mg Caplets ..... ▣ 613
- Bufferin Analgesic Tablets ..... ▣ 636
- Arthritis Strength Bufferin Analgesic Caplets ..... ▣ 637
- Extra Strength Bufferin Analgesic Tablets ..... ▣ 637
- Cama Arthritis Pain Reliever ..... ▣ 748
- Darvon Compound-65 Pulvules 1475
- Easprin 1971
- Ecotrin 2625
- Ecotrin Enteric Coated Aspirin Maximum Strength Tablets and Caplets ..... ▣ 775
- Ecotrin Enteric Coated Aspirin Regular Strength Tablets 2625
- Empirin Aspirin Tablets ..... ▣ 818
- Excedrin Extra-Strength Analgesic Tablets, Caplets, and Geltabs 734
- Fiorinal Capsules 2388
- Fiorinal with Codeine Capsules 2390
- Fiorinal Tablets 2388
- Goody's Extra Strength Headache Powders ..... ▣ 632
- Goody's Extra Strength Pain Relief Tablets ..... ▣ 632
- Halfprin Tablets 1413
- Norgesic 1554
- Percodan Tablets 955
- Percodan-Demi Tablets 956
- Robaxisal Tablets 2246
- Soma Compound w/Codeine Tablets 2784
- Soma Compound Tablets 2783
- St. Joseph Adult Chewable Aspirin (81 mg.) ..... ▣ 768
- Talwin Compound 2466
- Vanquish Analgesic Caplets ..... ▣ 627

Aspirin, Enteric Coated (Aspirin (3900 mg/day) depresses plasma levels of piroxicam).
- No products indexed under this heading.

Atovaquone (Feldene might displace other highly protein bound drugs). Products include:
- Mepron Suspension 1206

Cefonicid Sodium (Feldene might displace other highly protein bound drugs). Products include:
- Monocid Injection 2674

Chlordiazepoxide (Feldene might displace other highly protein bound drugs). Products include:
- Limbitrol 2333

Chlordiazepoxide Hydrochloride (Feldene might displace other highly protein bound drugs). Products include:
- Librax Capsules 2330
- Librium Capsules 2331
- Librium Injectable 2332

(▣ Described in PDR For Nonprescription Drugs)   (◎ Described in PDR For Ophthalmology)

Interactions Index

Chlorpromazine (Feldene might displace other highly protein bound drugs). Products include:
- Thorazine Suppositories 2701

Chlorpromazine Hydrochloride (Feldene might displace other highly protein bound drugs). Products include:
- Thorazine 2701

Clomipramine Hydrochloride (Feldene might displace other highly protein bound drugs). Products include:
- Anafranil Capsules 819

Clozapine (Feldene might displace other highly protein bound drugs). Products include:
- Clozaril Tablets 2377

Cyclosporine (Feldene might displace other highly protein bound drugs). Products include:
- Neoral 2405
- Sandimmune 2416

Diazepam (Feldene might displace other highly protein bound drugs). Products include:
- Dizac (diazepam injectable emulsion) CIV 1862
- Valium Injectable 2336
- Valium Tablets 2335

Diclofenac Potassium (Feldene might displace other highly protein bound drugs). Products include:
- Cataflam Tablets 833

Diclofenac Sodium (Feldene might displace other highly protein bound drugs). Products include:
- Voltaren Ophthalmic Sterile Ophthalmic Solution .... ⓔ 264
- Cataflam/Voltaren/Voltaren-XR 833

Dicumarol (Altered dosage requirements).
- No products indexed under this heading.

Dipyridamole (Feldene might displace other highly protein bound drugs). Products include:
- Persantine Tablets 686

Fenoprofen Calcium (Feldene might displace other highly protein bound drugs). Products include:
- Nalfon 200 Pulvules & Nalfon Tablets 933

Flurazepam Hydrochloride (Feldene might displace other highly protein bound drugs). Products include:
- Dalmane Capsules 2329

Flurbiprofen (Feldene might displace other highly protein bound drugs).
- No products indexed under this heading.

Glipizide (Feldene might displace other highly protein bound drugs). Products include:
- Glucotrol Tablets 2011
- Glucotrol XL Extended Release Tablets 2012

Ibuprofen (Feldene might displace other highly protein bound drugs). Products include:
- Advil Cold and Sinus Caplets and Tablets .... ⓔ 837
- Advil Ibuprofen Tablets, Caplets and Gel Caplets .... ⓔ 836
- Children's Motrin Ibuprofen Oral Suspension 1558
- IBU Tablets 1389
- Ibuprohm .... ⓔ 713
- Motrin IB Caplets, Tablets, and Gelcaps .... ⓔ 802
- Motrin Ibuprofen Suspension, Oral Drops, Chewable Tablets, Caplets 1563
- Nuprin Ibuprofen/Analgesic Tablets & Caplets .... ⓔ 645
- Vicks DayQuil SINUS Pressure & PAIN Relief with IBUPROFEN .... ⓔ 735

Imipramine Hydrochloride (Feldene might displace other highly protein bound drugs). Products include:
- Tofranil Ampuls 873
- Tofranil Tablets 875

Imipramine Pamoate (Feldene might displace other highly protein bound drugs). Products include:
- Tofranil-PM Capsules 876

Indomethacin (Feldene might displace other highly protein bound drugs). Products include:
- Indocin 1723

Indomethacin Sodium Trihydrate (Feldene might displace other highly protein bound drugs). Products include:
- Indocin I.V. 1727

Ketoprofen (Feldene might displace other highly protein bound drugs). Products include:
- Actron Caplets and Tablets .... ⓔ 608
- Orudis Capsules 2874
- Orudis KT .... ⓔ 842
- Oruvail Capsules 2874

Ketorolac Tromethamine (Feldene might displace other highly protein bound drugs). Products include:
- Acular Sterile Ophthalmic Solution 470
- Toradol 2319

Lithium Carbonate (Increased plasma lithium levels). Products include:
- Eskalith 2658
- Lithium Carbonate Capsules & Tablets 2352
- Lithonate/Lithotabs/Lithobid 2721

Lithium Citrate (Increased plasma lithium levels).
- No products indexed under this heading.

Meclofenamate Sodium (Feldene might displace other highly protein bound drugs).
- No products indexed under this heading.

Mefenamic Acid (Feldene might displace other highly protein bound drugs). Products include:
- Ponstel 1982

Midazolam Hydrochloride (Feldene might displace other highly protein bound drugs). Products include:
- Versed Injection 2324

Naproxen (Feldene might displace other highly protein bound drugs). Products include:
- Anaprox/Naprosyn 2277

Naproxen Sodium (Feldene might displace other highly protein bound drugs). Products include:
- Aleve 2124
- Anaprox/Naprosyn 2277
- Naprelan Tablets 2861

Nortriptyline Hydrochloride (Feldene might displace other highly protein bound drugs). Products include:
- Pamelor 2409

Oxaprozin (Feldene might displace other highly protein bound drugs). Products include:
- Daypro Caplets 2578

Oxazepam (Feldene might displace other highly protein bound drugs). Products include:
- Serax Capsules 2916
- Serax Tablets 2916

Phenylbutazone (Feldene might displace other highly protein bound drugs).
- No products indexed under this heading.

Propranolol Hydrochloride (Feldene might displace other highly protein bound drugs). Products include:
- Inderal 2834
- Inderal LA Long Acting Capsules 2836
- Inderide Tablets 2838
- Inderide LA Long Acting Capsules 2840

Sulindac (Feldene might displace other highly protein bound drugs). Products include:
- Clinoril Tablets 1658

Temazepam (Feldene might displace other highly protein bound drugs). Products include:
- Restoril Capsules 2413

Tolbutamide (Feldene might displace other highly protein bound drugs).
- No products indexed under this heading.

Tolmetin Sodium (Feldene might displace other highly protein bound drugs). Products include:
- Tolectin (200, 400 and 600 mg) 1591

Trimipramine Maleate (Feldene might displace other highly protein bound drugs). Products include:
- Surmontil Capsules 2917

Warfarin Sodium (Altered dosage requirements; Feldene might displace other highly protein bound drugs). Products include:
- Coumadin 941

FEMSTAT 3
(Butoconazole Nitrate) 2124
None cited in PDR database.

FEOSOL CAPLETS
(Iron) 2626
May interact with tetracyclines. Compounds in this category include:

Demeclocycline Hydrochloride (Oral iron products interfere with absorption of oral tetracyclines; these products should not be taken within two hours of each other). Products include:
- Declomycin Tablets 1421

Doxycycline Calcium (Oral iron products interfere with absorption of oral tetracyclines; these products should not be taken within two hours of each other). Products include:
- Vibramycin Calcium Oral Suspension Syrup 2038

Doxycycline Hyclate (Oral iron products interfere with absorption of oral tetracyclines; these products should not be taken within two hours of each other). Products include:
- Doryx Capsules 1970
- Vibramycin Hyclate Capsules 2038
- Vibramycin Hyclate Intravenous 2040
- Vibra-Tabs Film Coated Tablets 2038

Doxycycline Monohydrate (Oral iron products interfere with absorption of oral tetracyclines; these products should not be taken within two hours of each other). Products include:
- Monodox Capsules 1858
- Vibramycin Monohydrate for Oral Suspension 2038

Methacycline Hydrochloride (Oral iron products interfere with absorption of oral tetracyclines; these products should not be taken within two hours of each other).
- No products indexed under this heading.

Minocycline Hydrochloride (Oral iron products interfere with absorption of oral tetracyclines; these products should not be taken within two hours of each other). Products include:
- DYNACIN Capsules 1627
- Minocin Intravenous 1428
- Minocin Oral Suspension 1431
- Minocin Pellet-Filled Capsules 1429

Oxytetracycline Hydrochloride (Oral iron products interfere with absorption of oral tetracyclines; these products should not be taken within two hours of each other). Products include:
- TERAK Ointment .... ⓔ 210
- Terra-Cortril Ophthalmic Suspension 2033
- Terramycin with Polymyxin B Sulfate Ophthalmic Ointment 2035
- Urobiotic-250 Capsules 2038

Tetracycline Hydrochloride (Oral iron products interfere with absorption of oral tetracyclines; these products should not be taken within two hours of each other). Products include:
- Achromycin V Capsules 1417
- Helidac Therapy 2135

FEOSOL CAPSULES
(Ferrous Sulfate) .... ⓔ 777
May interact with tetracyclines. Compounds in this category include:

Demeclocycline Hydrochloride (Interference with absorption of oral tetracycline products). Products include:
- Declomycin Tablets 1421

Doxycycline Calcium (Interference with absorption of oral tetracycline products). Products include:
- Vibramycin Calcium Oral Suspension Syrup 2038

Doxycycline Hyclate (Interference with absorption of oral tetracycline products). Products include:
- Doryx Capsules 1970
- Vibramycin Hyclate Capsules 2038
- Vibramycin Hyclate Intravenous 2040
- Vibra-Tabs Film Coated Tablets 2038

Doxycycline Monohydrate (Interference with absorption of oral tetracycline products). Products include:
- Monodox Capsules 1858
- Vibramycin Monohydrate for Oral Suspension 2038

Methacycline Hydrochloride (Interference with absorption of oral tetracycline products).
- No products indexed under this heading.

Minocycline Hydrochloride (Interference with absorption of oral tetracycline products). Products include:
- DYNACIN Capsules 1627
- Minocin Intravenous 1428
- Minocin Oral Suspension 1431
- Minocin Pellet-Filled Capsules 1429

Oxytetracycline (Interference with absorption of oral tetracycline products). Products include:
- Terramycin Intramuscular Solution 2034

Oxytetracycline Hydrochloride (Interference with absorption of oral tetracycline products). Products include:
- TERAK Ointment .... ⓔ 210
- Terra-Cortril Ophthalmic Suspension 2033
- Terramycin with Polymyxin B Sulfate Ophthalmic Ointment 2035
- Urobiotic-250 Capsules 2038

Tetracycline Hydrochloride (Interference with absorption of oral tetracycline products). Products include:
- Achromycin V Capsules 1417

IMPORTANT NOTE: Always consult each drug listing in the patient's regimen for possible interactions.

Helidac Therapy ... 2135

FEOSOL ELIXIR
(Ferrous Sulfate) ... 2627
May interact with tetracyclines. Compounds in this category include:

Demeclocycline Hydrochloride (Interference with absorption of oral tetracycline products). Products include:
- Declomycin Tablets ... 1421

Doxycycline Calcium (Interference with absorption of oral tetracycline products). Products include:
- Vibramycin Calcium Oral Suspension Syrup ... 2038

Doxycycline Hyclate (Interference with absorption of oral tetracycline products). Products include:
- Doryx Capsules ... 1970
- Vibramycin Hyclate Capsules ... 2038
- Vibramycin Hyclate Intravenous ... 2040
- Vibra-Tabs Film Coated Tablets ... 2038

Doxycycline Monohydrate (Interference with absorption of oral tetracycline products). Products include:
- Monodox Capsules ... 1858
- Vibramycin Monohydrate for Oral Suspension ... 2038

Methacycline Hydrochloride (Interference with absorption of oral tetracycline products).
- No products indexed under this heading.

Minocycline Hydrochloride (Interference with absorption of oral tetracycline products). Products include:
- DYNACIN Capsules ... 1627
- Minocin Intravenous ... 1428
- Minocin Oral Suspension ... 1431
- Minocin Pellet-Filled Capsules ... 1429

Oxytetracycline (Interference with absorption of oral tetracycline products). Products include:
- Terramycin Intramuscular Solution 2034

Oxytetracycline Hydrochloride (Interference with absorption of oral tetracycline products). Products include:
- TERAK Ointment ... ⊙ 210
- Terra-Cortril Ophthalmic Suspension ... 2033
- Terramycin with Polymyxin B Sulfate Ophthalmic Ointment ... 2035
- Urobiotic-250 Capsules ... 2038

Tetracycline Hydrochloride (Interference with absorption of oral tetracycline products). Products include:
- Achromycin V Capsules ... 1417
- Helidac Therapy ... 2135

FEOSOL TABLETS
(Ferrous Sulfate) ... 2627
May interact with tetracyclines. Compounds in this category include:

Demeclocycline Hydrochloride (Interference with absorption of oral tetracycline products; should not be taken within two hours of each other). Products include:
- Declomycin Tablets ... 1421

Doxycycline Calcium (Interference with absorption of oral tetracycline products; should not be taken within two hours of each other). Products include:
- Vibramycin Calcium Oral Suspension Syrup ... 2038

Doxycycline Hyclate (Interference with absorption of oral tetracycline products; should not be taken within two hours of each other). Products include:
- Doryx Capsules ... 1970
- Vibramycin Hyclate Capsules ... 2038
- Vibramycin Hyclate Intravenous ... 2040
- Vibra-Tabs Film Coated Tablets ... 2038

Doxycycline Monohydrate (Interference with absorption of oral tetracycline products; should not be taken within two hours of each other). Products include:
- Monodox Capsules ... 1858
- Vibramycin Monohydrate for Oral Suspension ... 2038

Methacycline Hydrochloride (Interference with absorption of oral tetracycline products; should not be taken within two hours of each other).
- No products indexed under this heading.

Minocycline Hydrochloride (Interference with absorption of oral tetracycline products; should not be taken within two hours of each other). Products include:
- DYNACIN Capsules ... 1627
- Minocin Intravenous ... 1428
- Minocin Oral Suspension ... 1431
- Minocin Pellet-Filled Capsules ... 1429

Oxytetracycline (Interference with absorption of oral tetracycline products; should not be taken within two hours of each other). Products include:
- Terramycin Intramuscular Solution 2034

Oxytetracycline Hydrochloride (Interference with absorption of oral tetracycline products; should not be taken within two hours of each other). Products include:
- TERAK Ointment ... ⊙ 210
- Terra-Cortril Ophthalmic Suspension ... 2033
- Terramycin with Polymyxin B Sulfate Ophthalmic Ointment ... 2035
- Urobiotic-250 Capsules ... 2038

Tetracycline Hydrochloride (Interference with absorption of oral tetracycline products; should not be taken within two hours of each other). Products include:
- Achromycin V Capsules ... 1417
- Helidac Therapy ... 2135

FERO-FOLIC-500 FILMTAB
(Ferrous Sulfate, Folic Acid, Vitamin C) ... 433
May interact with tetracyclines and certain other agents. Compounds in these categories include:

Calcium Carbonate (Inhibits iron absorption). Products include:
- Alka-Mints Chewable Antacid ... ⊡ 609
- Alka-Seltzer Fast Relief Caplets ... ⊡ 610
- Ascriptin ... ⊡ 650
- Extra Strength Bayer Plus Aspirin Caplets ... ⊡ 617
- Aspirin Regimen Bayer 81 mg Tablets with Calcium ... ⊡ 615
- Bufferin Analgesic Tablets ... ⊡ 636
- Arthritis Strength Bufferin Analgesic Caplets ... ⊡ 637
- Extra Strength Bufferin Analgesic Tablets ... ⊡ 637
- Calci-Chew Tablets ... 2168
- Calci-Mix Capsules ... 2168
- Caltrate 600 ... ⊡ 681
- Caltrate PLUS ... ⊡ 681
- Caltrate 600 + D ... ⊡ 681
- Cotazym Capsules ... 1866
- Di-Gel Antacid/Anti-Gas ... ⊡ 762
- Florical Capsules and Tablets ... 1825
- Gerimed Tablets ... 1000
- Maalox Antacid Caplets ... ⊡ 657
- Marblen ... ⊡ 671
- Materna Tablets ... 1427
- Monocal Tablets ... 1825
- Mylanta Fast-Acting ... 1359
- Mylanta Gelcaps Antacid ... ⊡ 678
- Mylanta Soothing Lozenges ... 1360
- Mylanta Tablets ... ⊡ 677
- Mylanta Double Strength Tablets .. ⊡ 677
- Nephro-Calci Tablets ... 2168
- One-A-Day Calcium Plus ... ⊡ 625
- Rolaids Antacid Tablets ... ⊡ 807
- Rolaids Antacid Calcium Rich/Sodium Free Tablets ... ⊡ 807
- Tempo Soft Antacid ... ⊡ 799
- Titralac ... ⊡ 686
- Titralac Plus ... ⊡ 687
- Tums Antacid/Calcium Supplement Tablets ... ⊡ 787
- Tums Anti-gas/Antacid Formula Tablets, Assorted Fruit ... ⊡ 788
- Tums E-X Antacid/Calcium Supplement Tablets ... ⊡ 787
- Tums 500 Calcium Supplement ... ⊡ 788
- Tums ULTRA Antacid/Calcium Supplement Tablets ... ⊡ 787
- TYLENOL Headache Plus Pain Reliever with Antacid, Extra Strength Caplets ... ⊡ 705

Demeclocycline Hydrochloride (Ferrous sulfate may interfere with absorption of tetracycline). Products include:
- Declomycin Tablets ... 1421

Doxycycline Calcium (Ferrous sulfate may interfere with absorption of tetracycline). Products include:
- Vibramycin Calcium Oral Suspension Syrup ... 2038

Doxycycline Hyclate (Ferrous sulfate may interfere with absorption of tetracycline). Products include:
- Doryx Capsules ... 1970
- Vibramycin Hyclate Capsules ... 2038
- Vibramycin Hyclate Intravenous ... 2040
- Vibra-Tabs Film Coated Tablets ... 2038

Doxycycline Monohydrate (Ferrous sulfate may interfere with absorption of tetracycline). Products include:
- Monodox Capsules ... 1858
- Vibramycin Monohydrate for Oral Suspension ... 2038

Levodopa (Antiparkinsonism effects of levodopa may be reversed by pyridoxine). Products include:
- Atamet Tablets ... 567
- Larodopa Tablets ... 2296
- Sinemet Tablets ... 959
- Sinemet CR Tablets ... 961

Magnesium Trisilicate (Inhibits absorption of iron). Products include:
- Gaviscon Antacid Tablets ... ⊡ 778
- Gaviscon-2 Antacid Tablets ... ⊡ 779

Methacycline Hydrochloride (Ferrous sulfate may interfere with absorption of tetracycline).
- No products indexed under this heading.

Minocycline Hydrochloride (Ferrous sulfate may interfere with absorption of tetracycline). Products include:
- DYNACIN Capsules ... 1627
- Minocin Intravenous ... 1428
- Minocin Oral Suspension ... 1431
- Minocin Pellet-Filled Capsules ... 1429

Oxytetracycline (Ferrous sulfate may interfere with absorption of tetracycline). Products include:
- Terramycin Intramuscular Solution 2034

Oxytetracycline Hydrochloride (Ferrous sulfate may interfere with absorption of tetracycline). Products include:
- TERAK Ointment ... ⊙ 210
- Terra-Cortril Ophthalmic Suspension ... 2033
- Terramycin with Polymyxin B Sulfate Ophthalmic Ointment ... 2035
- Urobiotic-250 Capsules ... 2038

Sodium Bicarbonate (Inhibits iron absorption). Products include:
- Alka-Seltzer Cherry Effervescent Antacid and Pain Reliever ... ⊡ 609
- Alka-Seltzer Extra Strength Effervescent Antacid and Pain Reliever ... ⊡ 609
- Alka-Seltzer Gold Effervescent Antacid ... ⊡ 611
- Alka-Seltzer Lemon Lime Effervescent Antacid and Pain Reliever ... ⊡ 609
- Alka-Seltzer Original Effervescent Antacid and Pain Reliever ... ⊡ 609
- Arm & Hammer Pure Baking Soda ... ⊡ 648
- Colyte and Colyte-flavored ... 2540
- GoLYTELY ... 694
- Massengill Disposable Douches ... ⊡ 780
- Massengill Liquid Concentrate ... ⊡ 780
- NuLYTELY ... 694
- Cherry Flavor NuLYTELY ... 694

Tetracycline Hydrochloride (Ferrous sulfate may interfere with absorption of tetracycline). Products include:
- Achromycin V Capsules ... 1417
- Helidac Therapy ... 2135

Food Interactions

Dairy products (Ingestion of milk inhibits its iron absorption).

Eggs (Ingestion of eggs inhibits iron absorption).

FERO-GRAD-500 FILMTAB
(Ferrous Sulfate, Vitamin C) ... 434
None cited in PDR database.

FERO-GRADUMET FILMTAB
(Ferrous Sulfate) ... 434
None cited in PDR database.

FERRO-SEQUELS
(Ferrous Fumarate) ... ⊡ 684
None cited in PDR database.

FIBERCON CAPLETS
(Calcium Polycarbophil) ... ⊡ 684
May interact with tetracyclines. Compounds in this category include:

Demeclocycline Hydrochloride (Fibercon should be taken at least one hour before or two hours after you have taken any form of tetracycline). Products include:
- Declomycin Tablets ... 1421

Doxycycline Calcium (Fibercon should be taken at least one hour before or two hours after you have taken any form of tetracycline). Products include:
- Vibramycin Calcium Oral Suspension Syrup ... 2038

Doxycycline Hyclate (Fibercon should be taken at least one hour before or two hours after you have taken any form of tetracycline). Products include:
- Doryx Capsules ... 1970
- Vibramycin Hyclate Capsules ... 2038
- Vibramycin Hyclate Intravenous ... 2040
- Vibra-Tabs Film Coated Tablets ... 2038

Doxycycline Monohydrate (Fibercon should be taken at least one hour before or two hours after you have taken any form of tetracycline). Products include:
- Monodox Capsules ... 1858
- Vibramycin Monohydrate for Oral Suspension ... 2038

Methacycline Hydrochloride (Fibercon should be taken at least one hour before or two hours after you have taken any form of tetracycline).
- No products indexed under this heading.

Minocycline Hydrochloride (Fibercon should be taken at least one hour before or two hours after you have taken any form of tetracycline). Products include:
- DYNACIN Capsules ... 1627
- Minocin Intravenous ... 1428
- Minocin Oral Suspension ... 1431
- Minocin Pellet-Filled Capsules ... 1429

Oxytetracycline Hydrochloride (Fibercon should be taken at least one hour before or two hours after you have taken any form of tetracycline). Products include:
- TERAK Ointment ... ⊙ 210
- Terra-Cortril Ophthalmic Suspension ... 2033
- Terramycin with Polymyxin B Sulfate Ophthalmic Ointment ... 2035

(⊡ Described in PDR For Nonprescription Drugs) (⊙ Described in PDR For Ophthalmology)

409 **Interactions Index** **Fioricet**

Urobiotic-250 Capsules 2038

Tetracycline Hydrochloride (Fibercon should be taken at least one hour before or two hours after you have taken any form of tetracycline). Products include:

Achromycin V Capsules 1417
Helidac Therapy 2135

FIORICET TABLETS
(Butalbital, Acetaminophen, Caffeine) 2386

May interact with narcotic analgesics, tranquilizers, central nervous system depressants, monoamine oxidase inhibitors, general anesthetics, hypnotics and sedatives, and certain other agents. Compounds in these categories include:

Acrivastine (Additive CNS depressant effects). Products include:
Semprex-D Capsules 1620

Alfentanil Hydrochloride (Additive CNS depressant effects). Products include:
Alfenta Injection 1334

Alprazolam (Additive CNS depressant effects). Products include:
Xanax Tablets 2115

Aprobarbital (Additive CNS depressant effects).
No products indexed under this heading.

Buprenorphine (Additive CNS depressant effects). Products include:
Buprenex Injectable 2170

Buspirone Hydrochloride (Additive CNS depressant effects). Products include:
BuSpar Tablets 738

Butabarbital (Additive CNS depressant effects).
No products indexed under this heading.

Chlordiazepoxide (Additive CNS depressant effects). Products include:
Limbitrol 2333

Chlordiazepoxide Hydrochloride (Additive CNS depressant effects). Products include:
Librax Capsules 2330
Librium Capsules 2331
Librium Injectable 2332

Chlorpromazine (Additive CNS depressant effects). Products include:
Thorazine Suppositories 2701

Chlorpromazine Hydrochloride (Additive CNS depressant). Products include:
Thorazine 2701

Chlorprothixene (Additive CNS depressant effects).
No products indexed under this heading.

Chlorprothixene Hydrochloride (Additive CNS depressant effects).
No products indexed under this heading.

Chlorprothixene Lactate (Additive CNS depressant effects).
No products indexed under this heading.

Clomipramine Hydrochloride (Decreased blood levels of the antidepressant). Products include:
Anafranil Capsules 819

Clorazepate Dipotassium (Additive CNS depressant effects). Products include:
Tranxene 459

Clozapine (Additive CNS depressant effects). Products include:
Clozaril Tablets 2377

Codeine Phosphate (Additive CNS depressant effects). Products include:
Brontex 2130
Dimetane-DC Cough Syrup 2232
Fioricet with Codeine Capsules 2387
Fiorinal with Codeine Capsules 2390
Nucofed 2225
Phenergan with Codeine 2883
Phenergan VC with Codeine 2888
Robitussin A-C Syrup 2248
Robitussin-DAC Syrup 2249
Ryna 804
Soma Compound w/Codeine Tablets 2784
Tylenol with Codeine 1592

Desflurane (Additive CNS depressant effects). Products include:
Suprane (desflurane, USP) 1865

Dezocine (Additive CNS depressant effects). Products include:
Dalgan Injection 529

Diazepam (Additive CNS depressant effects). Products include:
Dizac (diazepam injectable emulsion) CIV 1862
Valium Injectable 2336
Valium Tablets 2335

Doxepin Hydrochloride (Decreased blood levels of the antidepressant). Products include:
Adapin Capsules 1542
Sinequan 2028
Zonalon Cream 1042

Droperidol (Additive CNS depressant effects). Products include:
Inapsine Injection 462

Enflurane (Additive CNS depressant effects).
No products indexed under this heading.

Estazolam (Additive CNS depressant effects). Products include:
ProSom Tablets 457

Ethchlorvynol (Additive CNS depressant effects). Products include:
Placidyl Capsules 456

Ethinamate (Additive CNS depressant effects).
No products indexed under this heading.

Fentanyl (Additive CNS depressant effects). Products include:
Duragesic Transdermal System 1336

Fentanyl Citrate (Additive CNS depressant effects). Products include:
Sublimaze Injection 463

Fluphenazine Decanoate (Additive CNS depressant effects). Products include:
Prolixin Decanoate 510

Fluphenazine Enanthate (Additive CNS depressant effects). Products include:
Prolixin Enanthate 510

Fluphenazine Hydrochloride (Additive CNS depressant effects). Products include:
Prolixin 510

Flurazepam Hydrochloride (Additive CNS depressant effects). Products include:
Dalmane Capsules 2329

Furazolidone (The CNS effects of butalbital may be enhanced by monoamine oxidase inhibitors). Products include:
Furoxone 2221

Glutethimide (Additive CNS depressant effects).
No products indexed under this heading.

Haloperidol (Additive CNS depressant effects). Products include:
Haldol Injection, Tablets and Concentrate 1585

Haloperidol Decanoate (Additive CNS depressant effects). Products include:
Haldol Decanoate 1587

Hydrocodone Bitartrate (Additive CNS depressant effects). Products include:
Codiclear DH Syrup 808
Duratuss HD Elixir 2750
Histussin D Liquid 670
Hycodan Tablets and Syrup 946
Hycomine Compound Tablets 948
Hycomine 947
Hycotuss Expectorant Syrup 950
Hydrocet Capsules 787
Lorcet 10/650 Tablets 1016
Lortab 2751
Tussend 1830
Tussend Expectorant 1831
Vicodin Tablets 1404
Vicodin ES Tablets 1405
Vicodin HP Tablets 1403
Vicodin Tuss Expectorant 1406
Zydone Capsules 967

Hydrocodone Polistirex (Additive CNS depressant effects). Products include:
Tussionex Pennkinetic Extended-Release Suspension 1624

Hydromorphone Hydrochloride (Additive CNS depressant effects). Products include:
Dilaudid Ampules 1382
Dilaudid Cough Syrup 1383
Dilaudid-HP Injection 1384
Dilaudid-HP Lyophilized Powder 250 mg 1384
Dilaudid 1382
Dilaudid Oral Liquid 1386
Dilaudid 1382
Dilaudid Tablets - 8 mg 1386

Hydroxyzine Hydrochloride (Additive CNS depressant effects). Products include:
Atarax Tablets & Syrup 1992
Marax Tablets & DF Syrup 2015
Vistaril Intramuscular Solution 2042

Isocarboxazid (The CNS effects of butalbital may be enhanced by monoamine oxidase inhibitors).
No products indexed under this heading.

Isoflurane (Additive CNS depressant effects).
No products indexed under this heading.

Ketamine Hydrochloride (Additive CNS depressant effects).
No products indexed under this heading.

Levomethadyl Acetate Hydrochloride (Additive CNS depressant effects). Products include:
Orlaam Oral Solution 2361

Levorphanol Tartrate (Additive CNS depressant effects). Products include:
Levo-Dromoran 2297

Lorazepam (Additive CNS depressant effects). Products include:
Ativan Injection 2805
Ativan Tablets 2807

Loxapine Hydrochloride (Additive CNS depressant effects). Products include:
Loxitane 1426

Loxapine Succinate (Additive CNS depressant effects). Products include:
Loxitane Capsules 1426

Meperidine Hydrochloride (Additive CNS depressant effects). Products include:
Demerol 2438
Mepergan Injection 2859

Mephobarbital (Additive CNS depressant effects). Products include:
Mebaral Tablets 2452

Meprobamate (Additive CNS depressant effects). Products include:
Miltown Tablets 2780
PMB 200 and PMB 400 2890

Mesoridazine Besylate (Additive CNS depressant effects). Products include:
Serentil 689

Methadone Hydrochloride (Additive CNS depressant effects). Products include:
Methadone Hydrochloride Oral Concentrate 2356
Methadone Hydrochloride Oral Solution & Tablets 2357

Methohexital Sodium (Additive CNS depressant effects).
No products indexed under this heading.

Methotrimeprazine (Additive CNS depressant effects). Products include:
Levoprome 1321

Methoxyflurane (Additive CNS depressant effects).
No products indexed under this heading.

Midazolam Hydrochloride (Additive CNS depressant effects). Products include:
Versed Injection 2324

Molindone Hydrochloride (Additive CNS depressant effects). Products include:
Moban Tablets and Concentrate 1036

Morphine Sulfate (Additive CNS depressant effects). Products include:
Astramorph/PF Injection, USP (Preservative-Free) 526
Duramorph Injection 983
Infumorph 200 and Infumorph 500 Sterile Solutions 985
Kadian Capsules 2948
MS Contin Tablets 2149
MSIR 2152
Oramorph SR (Morphine Sulfate Sustained Release Tablets) 2359
RMS Suppositories CII 2766
Roxanol 2365

Opium Alkaloids (Additive CNS depressant effects).
No products indexed under this heading.

Oxazepam (Additive CNS depressant effects). Products include:
Serax Capsules 2916
Serax Tablets 2916

Oxycodone Hydrochloride (Additive CNS depressant effects). Products include:
OxyContin Tablets 2163
OxyIR Capsules 2167
Percocet Tablets 955
Percodan Tablets 955
Percodan-Demi Tablets 956
Roxicodone Tablets, Oral Solution & Intensol (Oxycodone) 2366
Tylox Capsules 1593

Pentobarbital Sodium (Additive CNS depressant effects). Products include:
Nembutal Sodium Capsules 440
Nembutal Sodium Solution 442
Nembutal Sodium Suppositories 444

Perphenazine (Additive CNS depressant effects). Products include:
Etrafon 2495
Triavil Tablets 1800
Trilafon 2532

Phenelzine Sulfate (The CNS effects of butalbital may be enhanced by monoamine oxidase inhibitors). Products include:
Nardil 1977

Phenobarbital (Additive CNS depressant effects). Products include:
Arco-Lase Plus Tablets 513
Bellergal-S Tablets 2375
Donnatal 2234
Donnatal Extentabs 2234

IMPORTANT NOTE: Always consult each drug listing in the patient's regimen for possible interactions.

Donnatal Tablets 2234
Phenobarbital Elixir and Tablets 1523
Quadrinal Tablets 1398

Prazepam (Additive CNS depressant effects).
No products indexed under this heading.

Propofol (Additive CNS depressant effects). Products include:
Diprivan Injectable Emulsion 2939

Propoxyphene Hydrochloride (Additive CNS depressant effects). Products include:
Darvon 1475
Wygesic Tablets 2930

Propoxyphene Napsylate (Additive CNS depressant effects). Products include:
Darvon-N/Darvocet-N 1473

Quazepam (Additive CNS depressant effects). Products include:
Doral Tablets 2773

Risperidone (Additive CNS depressant effects). Products include:
Risperdal Tablets 1348

Secobarbital Sodium (Additive CNS depressant effects). Products include:
Seconal Sodium Pulvules 1529

Selegiline Hydrochloride (The CNS effects of butalbital may be enhanced by monoamine oxidase inhibitors). Products include:
Eldepryl Capsules 2729

Sevoflurane (Additive CNS depressant effects).
No products indexed under this heading.

Sufentanil Citrate (Additive CNS depressant effects). Products include:
Sufenta Injection 1355

Temazepam (Additive CNS depressant effects). Products include:
Restoril Capsules 2413

Thiamylal Sodium (Additive CNS depressant effects).
No products indexed under this heading.

Tranylcypromine Sulfate (The CNS effects of butalbital may be enhanced by monoamine oxidase inhibitors). Products include:
Parnate Tablets 2679

Triazolam (Additive CNS depressant effects). Products include:
Halcion Tablets 2093

Trifluoperazine Hydrochloride (Additive CNS depressant effects). Products include:
Stelazine 2692

Zolpidem Tartrate (Additive CNS depressant effects). Products include:
Ambien Tablets 2559

Food Interactions

Alcohol (Additive CNS depressant effects).

FIORICET WITH CODEINE CAPSULES
(Butalbital, Acetaminophen, Caffeine, Codeine Phosphate) 2387
May interact with central nervous system depressants, narcotic analgesics, hypnotics and sedatives, tranquilizers, general anesthetics, monoamine oxidase inhibitors, and certain other agents. Compounds in these categories include:

Alfentanil Hydrochloride (Increased CNS depression). Products include:
Alfenta Injection 1334

Alprazolam (Increased CNS depression). Products include:
Xanax Tablets 2115

Aprobarbital (Increased CNS depression).
No products indexed under this heading.

Buprenorphine (Increased CNS depression). Products include:
Buprenex Injectable 2170

Buspirone Hydrochloride (Increased CNS depression). Products include:
BuSpar Tablets 738

Butabarbital (Increased CNS depression).
No products indexed under this heading.

Chlordiazepoxide (Increased CNS depression). Products include:
Limbitrol 2333

Chlordiazepoxide Hydrochloride (Increased CNS depression). Products include:
Librax Capsules 2330
Librium Capsules 2331
Librium Injectable 2332

Chlorpromazine (Increased CNS depression). Products include:
Thorazine Suppositories 2701

Chlorpromazine Hydrochloride (Increased CNS depression). Products include:
Thorazine 2701

Chlorprothixene (Increased CNS depression).
No products indexed under this heading.

Chlorprothixene Hydrochloride (Increased CNS depression).
No products indexed under this heading.

Chlorprothixene Lactate (Increased CNS depression).
No products indexed under this heading.

Clorazepate Dipotassium (Increased CNS depression). Products include:
Tranxene 459

Clozapine (Increased CNS depression). Products include:
Clozaril Tablets 2377

Desflurane (Increased CNS depression). Products include:
Suprane (desflurane, USP) 1865

Dezocine (Increased CNS depression). Products include:
Dalgan Injection 529

Diazepam (Increased CNS depression). Products include:
Dizac (diazepam injectable emulsion) CIV 1862
Valium Injectable 2336
Valium Tablets 2335

Droperidol (Increased CNS depression). Products include:
Inapsine Injection 462

Enflurane (Increased CNS depression).
No products indexed under this heading.

Estazolam (Increased CNS depression). Products include:
ProSom Tablets 457

Ethchlorvynol (Increased CNS depression). Products include:
Placidyl Capsules 456

Ethinamate (Increased CNS depression).
No products indexed under this heading.

Fentanyl (Increased CNS depression). Products include:
Duragesic Transdermal System 1336

Fentanyl Citrate (Increased CNS depression). Products include:
Sublimaze Injection 463

Fluphenazine Decanoate (Increased CNS depression). Products include:
Prolixin Decanoate 510

Fluphenazine Enanthate (Increased CNS depression). Products include:
Prolixin Enanthate 510

Fluphenazine Hydrochloride (Increased CNS depression). Products include:
Prolixin 510

Flurazepam Hydrochloride (Increased CNS depression). Products include:
Dalmane Capsules 2329

Furazolidone (The CNS effects of butalbital may be enhanced by monoamine oxidase inhibitors). Products include:
Furoxone 2221

Glutethimide (Increased CNS depression).
No products indexed under this heading.

Haloperidol (Increased CNS depression). Products include:
Haldol Injection, Tablets and Concentrate 1585

Haloperidol Decanoate (Increased CNS depression). Products include:
Haldol Decanoate 1587

Hydrocodone Bitartrate (Increased CNS depression). Products include:
Codiclear DH Syrup 808
Duratuss HD Elixir 2750
Histussin D Liquid 670
Hycodan Tablets and Syrup 946
Hycomine Compound Tablets 948
Hycomine 947
Hycotuss Expectorant Syrup 950
Hydrocet Capsules 787
Lorcet 10/650 Tablets 1016
Lortab 2751
Tussend 1830
Tussend Expectorant 1831
Vicodin Tablets 1404
Vicodin ES Tablets 1405
Vicodin HP Tablets 1403
Vicodin Tuss Expectorant 1406
Zydone Capsules 967

Hydrocodone Polistirex (Increased CNS depression). Products include:
Tussionex Pennkinetic Extended-Release Suspension 1624

Hydromorphone Hydrochloride (Additive CNS depressant effects). Products include:
Dilaudid Ampules 1382
Dilaudid Cough Syrup 1383
Dilaudid-HP Injection 1384
Dilaudid-HP Lyophilized Powder 250 mg 1384
Dilaudid 1382
Dilaudid Oral Liquid 1386
Dilaudid 1382
Dilaudid Tablets - 8 mg 1386

Hydroxyzine Hydrochloride (Increased CNS depression). Products include:
Atarax Tablets & Syrup 1992
Marax Tablets & DF Syrup 2015
Vistaril Intramuscular Solution 2042

Isocarboxazid (The CNS effects of butalbital may be enhanced by monoamine oxidase inhibitors).
No products indexed under this heading.

Isoflurane (Increased CNS depression).
No products indexed under this heading.

Ketamine Hydrochloride (Increased CNS depression).
No products indexed under this heading.

Levomethadyl Acetate Hydrochloride (Increased CNS depression). Products include:
Orlaam Oral Solution 2361

Levorphanol Tartrate (Increased CNS depression). Products include:
Levo-Dromoran 2297

Lorazepam (Increased CNS depression). Products include:
Ativan Injection 2805
Ativan Tablets 2807

Loxapine Hydrochloride (Increased CNS depression). Products include:
Loxitane 1426

Loxapine Succinate (Increased CNS depression). Products include:
Loxitane Capsules 1426

Meperidine Hydrochloride (Increased CNS depression). Products include:
Demerol 2438
Mepergan Injection 2859

Mephobarbital (Increased CNS depression). Products include:
Mebaral Tablets 2452

Meprobamate (Increased CNS depression). Products include:
Miltown Tablets 2780
PMB 200 and PMB 400 2890

Mesoridazine Besylate (Increased CNS depression). Products include:
Serentil 689

Methadone Hydrochloride (Increased CNS depression). Products include:
Methadone Hydrochloride Oral Concentrate 2356
Methadone Hydrochloride Oral Solution & Tablets 2357

Methohexital Sodium (Increased CNS depression).
No products indexed under this heading.

Methotrimeprazine (Increased CNS depression). Products include:
Levoprome 1321

Methoxyflurane (Increased CNS depression).
No products indexed under this heading.

Midazolam Hydrochloride (Increased CNS depression). Products include:
Versed Injection 2324

Molindone Hydrochloride (Increased CNS depression). Products include:
Moban Tablets and Concentrate 1036

Morphine Sulfate (Increased CNS depression). Products include:
Astramorph/PF Injection, USP (Preservative-Free) 526
Duramorph Injection 983
Infumorph 200 and Infumorph 500 Sterile Solutions 985
Kadian Capsules 2948
MS Contin Tablets 2149
MSIR 2152
Oramorph SR (Morphine Sulfate Sustained Release Tablets) 2359
RMS Suppositories CII 2766
Roxanol 2365

Opium Alkaloids (Increased CNS depression).
No products indexed under this heading.

Oxazepam (Increased CNS depression). Products include:
Serax Capsules 2916
Serax Tablets 2916

Oxycodone Hydrochloride (Increased CNS depression). Products include:
OxyContin Tablets 2163
OxyIR Capsules 2167
Percocet Tablets 955
Percodan Tablets 955

(▣ Described in PDR For Nonprescription Drugs) (◉ Described in PDR For Ophthalmology)

Percodan-Demi Tablets 956
Roxicodone Tablets, Oral Solution
& Intensol (Oxycodone) 2366
Tylox Capsules 1593

Pentobarbital Sodium (Increased CNS depression). Products include:
Nembutal Sodium Capsules 440
Nembutal Sodium Solution 442
Nembutal Sodium Suppositories..... 444

Perphenazine (Increased CNS depression). Products include:
Etrafon 2495
Triavil Tablets 1800
Trilafon 2532

Phenelzine Sulfate (The CNS effects of butalbital may be enhanced by monoamine oxidase inhibitors). Products include:
Nardil 1977

Phenobarbital (Increased CNS depression). Products include:
Arco-Lase Plus Tablets 513
Bellergal-S Tablets 2375
Donnatal 2234
Donnatal Extentabs 2234
Donnatal Tablets 2234
Phenobarbital Elixir and Tablets 1523
Quadrinal Tablets 1398

Prazepam (Increased CNS depression). Products include:
No products indexed under this heading.

Prochlorperazine (Increased CNS depression). Products include:
Compazine 2644

Promethazine Hydrochloride (Increased CNS depression). Products include:
Mepergan Injection 2859
Phenergan with Codeine 2883
Phenergan with Dextromethorphan 2885
Phenergan Injection 2880
Phenergan Suppositories 2882
Phenergan Syrup 2881
Phenergan Tablets 2882
Phenergan VC 2886
Phenergan VC with Codeine 2888

Propofol (Increased CNS depression). Products include:
Diprivan Injectable Emulsion 2939

Propoxyphene Hydrochloride (Increased CNS depression). Products include:
Darvon 1475
Wygesic Tablets 2930

Propoxyphene Napsylate (Increased CNS depression). Products include:
Darvon-N/Darvocet-N 1473

Quazepam (Increased CNS depression). Products include:
Doral Tablets 2773

Risperidone (Increased CNS depression). Products include:
Risperdal Tablets 1348

Secobarbital Sodium (Increased CNS depression). Products include:
Seconal Sodium Pulvules 1529

Selegiline Hydrochloride (The CNS effects of butalbital may be enhanced by monoamine oxidase inhibitors). Products include:
Eldepryl Capsules 2729

Sevoflurane (Increased CNS depression).
No products indexed under this heading.

Sufentanil Citrate (Increased CNS depression). Products include:
Sufenta Injection 1355

Temazepam (Increased CNS depression). Products include:
Restoril Capsules 2413

Thiamylal Sodium (Increased CNS depression).
No products indexed under this heading.

Thioridazine Hydrochloride (Increased CNS depression). Products include:
Mellaril 2398

Thiothixene (Increased CNS depression). Products include:
Navane Capsules and Concentrate 2018
Navane Intramuscular 2019

Tranylcypromine Sulfate (The CNS effects of butalbital may be enhanced by monoamine oxidase inhibitors). Products include:
Parnate Tablets 2679

Triazolam (Increased CNS depression). Products include:
Halcion Tablets 2093

Trifluoperazine Hydrochloride (Increased CNS depression). Products include:
Stelazine 2692

Zolpidem Tartrate (Increased CNS depression). Products include:
Ambien Tablets 2559

Food Interactions
Alcohol (Increased CNS depression).

FIORINAL CAPSULES
(Butalbital, Aspirin, Caffeine)..........2388
May interact with monoamine oxidase inhibitors, corticosteroids, oral anticoagulants, oral hypoglycemic agents, insulin, non-steroidal anti-inflammatory agents, narcotic analgesics, general anesthetics, hypnotics and sedatives, tranquilizers, central nervous system depressants, and certain other agents. Compounds in these categories include:

Acarbose (Potential for enhanced effects of oral antidiabetic agents causing hypoglycemia). Products include:
Precose 604

Alfentanil Hydrochloride (Increased CNS depression). Products include:
Alfenta Injection 1334

Alprazolam (Increased CNS depression). Products include:
Xanax Tablets 2115

Aprobarbital (Increased CNS depression).
No products indexed under this heading.

Betamethasone Acetate (Concomitant corticosteroids and chronic use of aspirin may result in salicylism upon withdrawal of corticosteroid because corticosteroids enhance renal clearance of salicylates). Products include:
Celestone Soluspan Suspension 2484

Betamethasone Sodium Phosphate (Concomitant corticosteroids and chronic use of aspirin may result in salicylism upon withdrawal of corticosteroid because corticosteroids enhance renal clearance of salicylates). Products include:
Celestone Soluspan Suspension 2484

Buprenorphine (Increased CNS depression). Products include:
Buprenex Injectable 2170

Buspirone Hydrochloride (Increased CNS depression). Products include:
BuSpar Tablets 738

Butabarbital (Increased CNS depression).
No products indexed under this heading.

Chlordiazepoxide (Increased CNS depression). Products include:
Limbitrol 2333

Chlordiazepoxide Hydrochloride (Increased CNS depression). Products include:
Librax Capsules 2330
Librium Capsules 2331
Librium Injectable 2332

Chlorpromazine (Increased CNS depression). Products include:
Thorazine Suppositories 2701

Chlorpromazine Hydrochloride (Increased CNS depression). Products include:
Thorazine 2701

Chlorpropamide (Potential for enhanced effects of oral antidiabetic agents causing hypoglycemia). Products include:
Diabinese Tablets 2002

Chlorprothixene (Increased CNS depression).
No products indexed under this heading.

Chlorprothixene Hydrochloride (Increased CNS depression).
No products indexed under this heading.

Chlorprothixene Lactate (Increased CNS depression).
No products indexed under this heading.

Clonazepam (Increased CNS depression). Products include:
Klonopin Tablets 2294

Clorazepate Dipotassium (Increased CNS depression). Products include:
Tranxene 459

Clozapine (Increased CNS depression). Products include:
Clozaril Tablets 2377

Codeine Phosphate (Increased CNS depression). Products include:
Brontex 2130
Dimetane-DC Cough Syrup 2232
Fioricet with Codeine Capsules 2387
Fiorinal with Codeine Capsules 2390
Nucofed 2225
Phenergan with Codeine 2883
Phenergan VC with Codeine 2888
Robitussin A-C Syrup 2248
Robitussin-DAC Syrup 2249
Ryna 804
Soma Compound w/Codeine Tablets 2784
Tylenol with Codeine 1592

Cortisone Acetate (Concomitant corticosteroids and chronic use of aspirin may result in salicylism upon withdrawal of corticosteroid because corticosteroids enhance renal clearance of salicylates). Products include:
Cortone Acetate Sterile Suspension 1663
Cortone Acetate Tablets 1664

Desflurane (Increased CNS depression). Products include:
Suprane (desflurane, USP) 1865

Dexamethasone (Concomitant corticosteroids and chronic use of aspirin may result in salicylism upon withdrawal of corticosteroid because corticosteroids enhance renal clearance of salicylates). Products include:
AK-Trol Ointment & Suspension 205
Decadron Elixir 1676
Decadron Tablets 1678
Decaspray Topical Aerosol 1689
Maxitrol Ophthalmic Ointment and Suspension 222
TobraDex Ophthalmic Suspension and Ointment 469

Dexamethasone Acetate (Concomitant corticosteroids and chronic use of aspirin may result in salicylism upon withdrawal of corticosteroid because corticosteroids enhance renal clearance of salicylates). Products include:
Dalalone D.P. Injectable 1009
Decadron-LA Sterile Suspension ... 1687

Dexamethasone Sodium Phosphate (Concomitant corticosteroids and chronic use of aspirin may result in salicylism upon withdrawal of corticosteroid because corticosteroids enhance renal clearance of salicylates). Products include:
Decadron Phosphate Injection 1680
Decadron Phosphate Sterile Ophthalmic Ointment 1684
Decadron Phosphate Sterile Ophthalmic Solution 1685
Decadron Phosphate Topical Cream 1686
Decadron Phosphate with Xylocaine Injection, Sterile 1683
Dexacort Phosphate in Respihaler .. 1606
Dexacort Phosphate in Turbinaire .. 1607
NeoDecadron Sterile Ophthalmic Ointment 1755
NeoDecadron Sterile Ophthalmic Solution 1756
NeoDecadron Topical Cream 1757

Dezocine (Increased CNS depression). Products include:
Dalgan Injection 529

Diazepam (Increased CNS depression). Products include:
Dizac (diazepam injectable emulsion) CIV 1862
Valium Injectable 2336
Valium Tablets 2335

Diclofenac Potassium (Enhanced effects of non-steroidal anti-inflammatory agents thereby increasing the risk of peptic ulceration and bleeding). Products include:
Cataflam Tablets 833

Diclofenac Sodium (Enhanced effects of non-steroidal anti-inflammatory agents thereby increasing the risk of peptic ulceration and bleeding). Products include:
Voltaren Ophthalmic Sterile Ophthalmic Solution 264
Cataflam/Voltaren/Voltaren-XR 833

Dicumarol (Fiorinal may enhance the effects of oral anticoagulants causing bleeding by inhibiting prothrombin formation in the liver and displacing anticoagulants from plasma protein binding sites).
No products indexed under this heading.

Droperidol (Increased CNS depression). Products include:
Inapsine Injection 462

Enflurane (Increased CNS depression).
No products indexed under this heading.

Estazolam (Increased CNS depression). Products include:
ProSom Tablets 457

Ethchlorvynol (Increased CNS depression). Products include:
Placidyl Capsules 456

Ethinamate (Increased CNS depression).
No products indexed under this heading.

Etodolac (Enhanced effects of non-steroidal anti-inflammatory agents thereby increasing the risk of peptic ulceration and bleeding). Products include:
Lodine Capsules and Tablets 2849

IMPORTANT NOTE: Always consult each drug listing in the patient's regimen for possible interactions.

Fenoprofen Calcium (Enhanced effects of non-steroidal anti-inflammatory agents thereby increasing the risk of peptic ulceration and bleeding). Products include:
   Nalfon 200 Pulvules & Nalfon Tablets 933

Fentanyl (Increased CNS depression). Products include:
   Duragesic Transdermal System 1336

Fentanyl Citrate (Increased CNS depression). Products include:
   Sublimaze Injection 463

Fludrocortisone Acetate (Concomitant corticosteroids and chronic use of aspirin may result in salicylism upon withdrawal of corticosteroid because corticosteroids enhance renal clearance of salicylates). Products include:
   Florinef Acetate Tablets 506

Fluphenazine Decanoate (Increased CNS depression). Products include:
   Prolixin Decanoate 510

Fluphenazine Enanthate (Increased CNS depression). Products include:
   Prolixin Enanthate 510

Fluphenazine Hydrochloride (Increased CNS depression). Products include:
   Prolixin 510

Flurazepam Hydrochloride (Increased CNS depression). Products include:
   Dalmane Capsules 2329

Flurbiprofen (Enhanced effects of non-steroidal anti-inflammatory agents thereby increasing the risk of peptic ulceration and bleeding).
   No products indexed under this heading.

Furazolidone (The CNS effects of butalbital may be enhanced by monoamine oxidase inhibitors). Products include:
   Furoxone 2221

Glimepiride (Potential for enhanced effects of oral antidiabetic agents causing hypoglycemia). Products include:
   Amaryl Tablets 1241

Glipizide (Potential for enhanced effects of oral antidiabetic agents causing hypoglycemia). Products include:
   Glucotrol Tablets 2011
   Glucotrol XL Extended Release Tablets 2012

Glutethimide (Increased CNS depression).
   No products indexed under this heading.

Glyburide (Potential for enhanced effects of oral antidiabetic agents causing hypoglycemia). Products include:
   DiaBeta Tablets 1265
   Glynase PresTab Tablets 2091
   Micronase Tablets 2099

Haloperidol (Increased CNS depression). Products include:
   Haldol Injection, Tablets and Concentrate 1585

Haloperidol Decanoate (Increased CNS depression). Products include:
   Haldol Decanoate 1587

Hydrocodone Bitartrate (Increased CNS depression). Products include:
   Codiclear DH Syrup 808
   Duratuss HD Elixir 2750
   Histussin D Liquid 670
   Hycodan Tablets and Syrup 946
   Hycomine Compound Tablets 948
   Hycomine 947
   Hycotuss Expectorant Syrup 950
   Hydrocet Capsules 787
   Lorcet 10/650 Tablets 1016
   Lortab 2751
   Tussend 1830
   Tussend Expectorant 1831
   Vicodin Tablets 1404
   Vicodin ES Tablets 1405
   Vicodin HP Tablets 1403
   Vicodin Tuss Expectorant 1406
   Zydone Capsules 967

Hydrocodone Polistirex (Increased CNS depression). Products include:
   Tussionex Pennkinetic Extended-Release Suspension 1624

Hydrocortisone (Concomitant corticosteroids and chronic use of aspirin may result in salicylism upon withdrawal of corticosteroid because corticosteroids enhance renal clearance of salicylates). Products include:
   Anusol-HC Cream 2.5% 1953
   Aquanil HC Lotion 1989
   Maximum Strength Cortaid Spray 800
   CORTENEMA 2713
   Cortisporin Ointment 1074
   Cortisporin Ophthalmic Ointment Sterile 1074
   Cortisporin Ophthalmic Suspension Sterile 1075
   Cortisporin Otic Solution Sterile 1076
   Cortisporin Otic Suspension Sterile 1077
   Cortizone-5 795
   Cortizone-10 795
   Hydrocortone Tablets 1715
   Hytone 922
   Hytone Ointment 2 ½ % 923
   Massengill Medicated Soft Cloth Towelettes 2628
   Pediotic Suspension Sterile 1140
   Preparation H Hydrocortisone 1% Cream 843
   ProctoCream-HC 2.5% 2552
   VōSoL HC Otic Solution 2786

Hydrocortisone Acetate (Concomitant corticosteroids and chronic use of aspirin may result in salicylism upon withdrawal of corticosteroid because corticosteroids enhance renal clearance of salicylates). Products include:
   Analpram-HC Rectal Cream 1% and 2.5% 993
   Anusol HC-1 Hydrocortisone Anti-Itch Ointment 810
   Anusol-HC Suppositories 1954
   Caldecort Anti-Itch Hydrocortisone Cream 651
   Coly-Mycin S Otic w/Neomycin & Hydrocortisone 1965
   Cortaid 800
   Cortifoam 2540
   Cortisporin Cream 1073
   Epifoam 2543
   Hydrocortone Acetate Sterile Suspension 1712
   Mantadil Cream 1124
   Nupercainal Hydrocortisone 1% Cream 661
   Pramosone Cream, Lotion & Ointment 995
   ProctoFoam-HC 2552
   Terra-Cortril Ophthalmic Suspension 2033

Hydrocortisone Sodium Phosphate (Concomitant corticosteroids and chronic use of aspirin may result in salicylism upon withdrawal of corticosteroid because corticosteroids enhance renal clearance of salicylates). Products include:
   Hydrocortone Phosphate Injection, Sterile 1713

Hydrocortisone Sodium Succinate (Concomitant corticosteroids and chronic use of aspirin may result in salicylism upon withdrawal of corticosteroid because corticosteroids enhance renal clearance of salicylates).
   No products indexed under this heading.

Hydromorphone Hydrochloride (Increased CNS depression). Products include:
   Dilaudid Ampules 1382
   Dilaudid Cough Syrup 1383
   Dilaudid-HP Injection 1384
   Dilaudid-HP Lyophilized Powder 250 mg. 1384
   Dilaudid 1382
   Dilaudid Oral Liquid 1386
   Dilaudid 1382
   Dilaudid Tablets - 8 mg. 1386

Hydroxyzine Hydrochloride (Increased CNS depression). Products include:
   Atarax Tablets & Syrup 1992
   Marax Tablets & DF Syrup 2015
   Vistaril Intramuscular Solution 2042

Ibuprofen (Enhanced effects of non-steroidal anti-inflammatory agents thereby increasing the risk of peptic ulceration and bleeding). Products include:
   Advil Cold and Sinus Caplets and Tablets 837
   Advil Ibuprofen Tablets, Caplets and Gel Caplets 836
   Children's Motrin Ibuprofen Oral Suspension 1558
   IBU Tablets 1389
   Ibuprohm 713
   Motrin IB Caplets, Tablets, and Gelcaps 802
   Motrin Ibuprofen Suspension, Oral Drops, Chewable Tablets, Caplets 1563
   Nuprin Ibuprofen/Analgesic Tablets & Caplets 645
   Vicks DayQuil SINUS Pressure & PAIN Relief with IBUPROFEN 735

Indomethacin (Enhanced effects of non-steroidal anti-inflammatory agents thereby increasing the risk of peptic ulceration and bleeding). Products include:
   Indocin 1723

Indomethacin Sodium Trihydrate (Enhanced effects of non-steroidal anti-inflammatory agents thereby increasing the risk of peptic ulceration and bleeding). Products include:
   Indocin I.V. 1727

Insulin, Human (Potential for enhanced effects of insulin causing hypoglycemia).
   No products indexed under this heading.

Insulin, Human Isophane Suspension (Potential for enhanced effects of insulin causing hypoglycemia). Products include:
   Novolin N Human Insulin 10 ml Vials 1846

Insulin, Human NPH (Potential for enhanced effects of insulin causing hypoglycemia). Products include:
   Humulin N, 100 Units 1495
   Novolin N PenFill 1.5 ml Cartridges Durable Insulin Delivery System 1849
   Novolin N Prefilled Syringe Disposable Insulin Delivery System 1850

Insulin, Human Regular (Potential for enhanced effects of insulin causing hypoglycemia). Products include:
   Humulin R, 100 Units 1497
   Novolin R Human Insulin 10 ml Vials 1846
   Novolin R PenFill 1.5 ml Cartridges Durable Insulin Delivery System 1849
   Novolin R Prefilled Syringe Disposable Insulin Delivery System 1850
   Velosulin BR Human Insulin 10 ml Vials 1847

Insulin, Human, Zinc Suspension (Potential for enhanced effects of insulin causing hypoglycemia). Products include:
   Humulin L, 100 Units 1494

Humulin U, 100 Units 1498
   Novolin L Human Insulin 10 ml Vials 1846

Insulin Lispro, Human (Potential for enhanced effects of insulin causing hypoglycemia). Products include:
   Humalog Injection 1488

Insulin, NPH (Potential for enhanced effects of insulin causing hypoglycemia). Products include:
   NPH, 100 Units 1502
   Pork NPH, 100 Units 1506
   Purified Pork NPH Isophane Insulin 1852

Insulin, Regular (Potential for enhanced effects of insulin causing hypoglycemia). Products include:
   Regular, 100 Units 1503
   Pork Regular, 100 Units 1507
   Pork Regular (Concentrated), 500 Units 1508
   Purified Pork Regular Insulin 1852

Insulin, Zinc Crystals (Potential for enhanced effects of insulin causing hypoglycemia). Products include:
   NPH, 100 Units 1502

Insulin, Zinc Suspension (Potential for enhanced effects of insulin causing hypoglycemia). Products include:
   Iletin I 1501
   Lente, 100 Units 1501
   Iletin II 1504
   Pork Lente, 100 Units 1504
   Purified Pork Lente Insulin 1852

Isocarboxazid (The CNS effects of butalbital may be enhanced by monoamine oxidase inhibitors).
   No products indexed under this heading.

Isoflurane (Increased CNS depression).
   No products indexed under this heading.

Ketamine Hydrochloride (Increased CNS depression).
   No products indexed under this heading.

Ketoprofen (Enhanced effects of non-steroidal anti-inflammatory agents thereby increasing the risk of peptic ulceration and bleeding). Products include:
   Actron Caplets and Tablets 608
   Orudis Capsules 2874
   Orudis KT 842
   Oruvail Capsules 2874

Ketorolac Tromethamine (Enhanced effects of non-steroidal anti-inflammatory agents thereby increasing the risk of peptic ulceration and bleeding). Products include:
   Acular Sterile Ophthalmic Solution 470
   Toradol 2319

Levomethadyl Acetate Hydrochloride (Increased CNS depression). Products include:
   Orlaam Oral Solution 2361

Levorphanol Tartrate (Increased CNS depression). Products include:
   Levo-Dromoran 2297

Lorazepam (Increased CNS depression). Products include:
   Ativan Injection 2805
   Ativan Tablets 2807

Loxapine Hydrochloride (Increased CNS depression). Products include:
   Loxitane 1426

Loxapine Succinate (Increased CNS depression). Products include:
   Loxitane Capsules 1426

Meclofenamate Sodium (Enhanced effects of non-steroidal anti-inflammatory agents thereby increasing the risk of peptic ulceration and bleeding).
   No products indexed under this heading.

(▣ Described in PDR For Nonprescription Drugs)   (⊙ Described in PDR For Ophthalmology)

Mefenamic Acid (Enhanced effects of non-steroidal anti-inflammatory agents thereby increasing the risk of peptic ulceration and bleeding). Products include:
Ponstel 1982

Meperidine Hydrochloride (Increased CNS depression). Products include:
Demerol 2438
Mepergan Injection 2859

Mephobarbital (Increased CNS depression). Products include:
Mebaral Tablets 2452

Meprobamate (Increased CNS depression). Products include:
Miltown Tablets 2780
PMB 200 and PMB 400 2890

Mercaptopurine (Enhanced effects of 6-mercaptopurine causing bone marrow toxicity and blood dyscrasias by displacing it from secondary binding sites). Products include:
Purinethol Tablets 1214

Mesoridazine Besylate (Increased CNS depression). Products include:
Serentil 689

Metformin Hydrochloride (Potential for enhanced effects of oral antidiabetic agents causing hypoglycemia). Products include:
Glucophage Tablets 754

Methadone Hydrochloride (Increased CNS depression). Products include:
Methadone Hydrochloride Oral Concentrate 2356
Methadone Hydrochloride Oral Solution & Tablets 2357

Methohexital Sodium (Increased CNS depression).
No products indexed under this heading.

Methotrexate Sodium (Fiorinal may enhance the effects of methotrexate causing bone marrow toxicity and blood dyscrasias by displacing methotrexate from secondary binding sites and reducing its excretion). Products include:
Methotrexate Sodium Tablets, Injection, for Injection and LPF Injection 1322

Methotrimeprazine (Increased CNS depression). Products include:
Levoprome 1321

Methoxyflurane (Increased CNS depression).
No products indexed under this heading.

Methylprednisolone Acetate (Concomitant corticosteroids and chronic use of aspirin may result in salicylism upon withdrawal of corticosteroid because corticosteroids enhance renal clearance of salicylates).
No products indexed under this heading.

Methylprednisolone Sodium Succinate (Concomitant corticosteroids and chronic use of aspirin may result in salicylism upon withdrawal of corticosteroid because corticosteroids enhance renal clearance of salicylates).
No products indexed under this heading.

Midazolam Hydrochloride (Increased CNS depression). Products include:
Versed Injection 2324

Molindone Hydrochloride (Increased CNS depression). Products include:
Moban Tablets and Concentrate 1036

Morphine Sulfate (Increased CNS depression). Products include:
Astramorph/PF Injection, USP (Preservative-Free) 526
Duramorph Injection 983
Infumorph 200 and Infumorph 500 Sterile Solutions 985
Kadian Capsules 2948
MS Contin Tablets 2149
MSIR 2152
Oramorph SR (Morphine Sulfate Sustained Release Tablets) .. 2359
RMS Suppositories CII 2766
Roxanol 2365

Nabumetone (Enhanced effects of non-steroidal anti-inflammatory agents thereby increasing the risk of peptic ulceration and bleeding). Products include:
Relafen Tablets 2688

Naproxen (Enhanced effects of non-steroidal anti-inflammatory agents thereby increasing the risk of peptic ulceration and bleeding). Products include:
Anaprox/Naprosyn 2277

Naproxen Sodium (Enhanced effects of non-steroidal anti-inflammatory agents thereby increasing the risk of peptic ulceration and bleeding). Products include:
Aleve 2124
Anaprox/Naprosyn 2277
Naprelan Tablets 2861

Opium Alkaloids (Increased CNS depression).
No products indexed under this heading.

Oxaprozin (Enhanced effects of non-steroidal anti-inflammatory agents thereby increasing the risk of peptic ulceration and bleeding). Products include:
Daypro Caplets 2578

Oxazepam (Increased CNS depression). Products include:
Serax Capsules 2916
Serax Tablets 2916

Oxycodone Hydrochloride (Increased CNS depression). Products include:
OxyContin Tablets 2163
OxyIR Capsules 2167
Percocet Tablets 955
Percodan Tablets 955
Percodan-Demi Tablets 956
Roxicodone Tablets, Oral Solution & Intensol (Oxycodone) ... 2366
Tylox Capsules 1593

Pentobarbital Sodium (Increased CNS depression). Products include:
Nembutal Sodium Capsules 440
Nembutal Sodium Solution 442
Nembutal Sodium Suppositories ... 444

Perphenazine (Increased CNS depression). Products include:
Etrafon 2495
Triavil Tablets 1800
Trilafon 2532

Phenelzine Sulfate (The CNS effects of butalbital may be enhanced by monoamine oxidase inhibitors). Products include:
Nardil 1977

Phenobarbital (Increased CNS depression). Products include:
Arco-Lase Plus Tablets 513
Bellergal-S Tablets 2375
Donnatal 2234
Donnatal Extentabs 2234
Donnatal Tablets 2234
Phenobarbital Elixir and Tablets .. 1523
Quadrinal Tablets 1398

Phenylbutazone (Enhanced effects of non-steroidal anti-inflammatory agents thereby increasing the risk of peptic ulceration and bleeding).
No products indexed under this heading.

Piroxicam (Enhanced effects of non-steroidal anti-inflammatory agents thereby increasing the risk of peptic ulceration and bleeding). Products include:
Feldene Capsules 2008

Prazepam (Increased CNS depression).
No products indexed under this heading.

Prednisolone Acetate (Concomitant corticosteroids and chronic use of aspirin may result in salicylism upon withdrawal of corticosteroid because corticosteroids enhance renal clearance of salicylates). Products include:
AK-CIDE .... ⓘ 203
AK-CIDE Ointment .... ⓘ 203
Blephamide Liquifilm Sterile Ophthalmic Suspension 472
Blephamide Ointment .... ⓘ 234
Econopred & Econopred Plus Ophthalmic Suspensions .. ⓘ 216
Poly-Pred Liquifilm .... ⓘ 246
Pred Forte .... ⓘ 247
Pred Mild .... ⓘ 250
Pred-G Liquifilm Sterile Ophthalmic Suspension .... ⓘ 248
Pred-G S.O.P. Sterile Ophthalmic Ointment .... ⓘ 249

Prednisolone Sodium Phosphate (Concomitant corticosteroids and chronic use of aspirin may result in salicylism upon withdrawal of corticosteroid because corticosteroids enhance renal clearance of salicylates). Products include:
AK-PRED .... ⓘ 204
Hydeltrasol Injection, Sterile ... 1708
Pediapred Oral Solution 1618

Prednisolone Tebutate (Concomitant corticosteroids and chronic use of aspirin may result in salicylism upon withdrawal of corticosteroid because corticosteroids enhance renal clearance of salicylates). Products include:
Hydeltra-T.B.A. Sterile Suspension 1710

Prednisone (Concomitant corticosteroids and chronic use of aspirin may result in salicylism upon withdrawal of corticosteroid because corticosteroids enhance renal clearance of salicylates).
No products indexed under this heading.

Probenecid (Diminished effects of uricosuric agent, probenecid, thereby reducing its effectiveness in the treatment of gout). Products include:
Benemid Tablets 1651
ColBENEMID Tablets 1662

Prochlorperazine (Increased CNS depression). Products include:
Compazine 2644

Promethazine Hydrochloride (Increased CNS depression). Products include:
Mepergan Injection 2859
Phenergan with Codeine 2883
Phenergan with Dextromethorphan 2885
Phenergan Injection 2880
Phenergan Suppositories 2882
Phenergan Syrup 2881
Phenergan Tablets 2882
Phenergan VC 2886
Phenergan VC with Codeine .. 2888

Propofol (Increased CNS depression). Products include:
Diprivan Injectable Emulsion .. 2939

Propoxyphene Hydrochloride (Increased CNS depression). Products include:
Darvon 1475
Wygesic Tablets 2930

Propoxyphene Napsylate (Increased CNS depression). Products include:
Darvon-N/Darvocet-N 1473

Quazepam (Increased CNS depression). Products include:
Doral Tablets 2773

Risperidone (Increased CNS depression). Products include:
Risperdal Tablets 1348

Secobarbital Sodium (Increased CNS depression). Products include:
Seconal Sodium Pulvules 1529

Selegiline Hydrochloride (The CNS effects of butalbital may be enhanced by monoamine oxidase inhibitors). Products include:
Eldepryl Capsules 2729

Sevoflurane (Increased CNS depression).
No products indexed under this heading.

Sufentanil Citrate (Increased CNS depression). Products include:
Sufenta Injection 1355

Sulfinpyrazone (Diminished effects of uricosuric agent, sulfinpyrazone, thereby reducing its effectiveness in the treatment of gout). Products include:
Anturane 823

Sulindac (Enhanced effects of non-steroidal anti-inflammatory agents thereby increasing the risk of peptic ulceration and bleeding). Products include:
Clinoril Tablets 1658

Temazepam (Increased CNS depression). Products include:
Restoril Capsules 2413

Thiamylal Sodium (Increased CNS depression).
No products indexed under this heading.

Thioridazine Hydrochloride (Increased CNS depression). Products include:
Mellaril 2398

Thiothixene (Increased CNS depression). Products include:
Navane Capsules and Concentrate 2018
Navane Intramuscular 2019

Tolazamide (Potential for enhanced effects of oral antidiabetic agents causing hypoglycemia).
No products indexed under this heading.

Tolbutamide (Potential for enhanced effects of oral antidiabetic agents causing hypoglycemia).
No products indexed under this heading.

Tolmetin Sodium (Enhanced effects of non-steroidal anti-inflammatory agents thereby increasing the risk of peptic ulceration and bleeding). Products include:
Tolectin (200, 400 and 600 mg) .. 1591

Tranylcypromine Sulfate (The CNS effects of butalbital may be enhanced by monoamine oxidase inhibitors). Products include:
Parnate Tablets 2679

Triamcinolone (Concomitant corticosteroids and chronic use of aspirin may result in salicylism upon withdrawal of corticosteroid because corticosteroids enhance renal clearance of salicylates).
No products indexed under this heading.

Triamcinolone Acetonide (Concomitant corticosteroids and chronic use of aspirin may result in salicylism upon withdrawal of corticosteroid because corticosteroids enhance renal clearance of salicylates). Products include:
Azmacort Oral Inhaler 2175
Nasacort AQ Nasal Spray 2191
Nasacort Nasal Inhaler 2189

IMPORTANT NOTE: Always consult each drug listing in the patient's regimen for possible interactions.

Fiorinal | Interactions Index | 414

Triamcinolone Diacetate (Concomitant corticosteroids and chronic use of aspirin may result in salicylism upon withdrawal of corticosteroid because corticosteroids enhance renal clearance of salicylates).
No products indexed under this heading.
Triamcinolone Hexacetonide (Concomitant corticosteroids and chronic use of aspirin may result in salicylism upon withdrawal of corticosteroid because corticosteroids enhance renal clearance of salicylates).
No products indexed under this heading.
Triazolam (Increased CNS depression). Products include:
Halcion Tablets ... 2093
Trifluoperazine Hydrochloride (Increased CNS depression). Products include:
Stelazine ... 2692
Warfarin Sodium (Fiorinal may enhance the effects of oral anticoagulants causing bleeding by inhibiting prothrombin formation in the liver and displacing anticoagulants from plasma protein binding sites). Products include:
Coumadin ... 941
Zolpidem Tartrate (Increased CNS depression). Products include:
Ambien Tablets ... 2559

Food Interactions
Alcohol (Increased CNS depression).

FIORINAL WITH CODEINE CAPSULES
(Codeine Phosphate, Butalbital, Caffeine, Aspirin) ... 2390
May interact with central nervous system depressants, hypnotics and sedatives, monoamine oxidase inhibitors, corticosteroids, oral anticoagulants, oral hypoglycemic agents, insulin, tranquilizers, narcotic analgesics, non-steroidal anti-inflammatory agents, general anesthetics, and certain other agents. Compounds in these categories include:

Acarbose (Potential for hypoglycemia). Products include:
Precose ... 604
Alfentanil Hydrochloride (Increased CNS depression). Products include:
Alfenta Injection ... 1334
Alprazolam (Increased CNS depression). Products include:
Xanax Tablets ... 2115
Aprobarbital (Increased CNS depression).
No products indexed under this heading.
Betamethasone Acetate (Potential for salicylism when corticosteroids therapy is stopped). Products include:
Celestone Soluspan Suspension ... 2484
Betamethasone Sodium Phosphate (Potential for salicylism when corticosteroids therapy is stopped). Products include:
Celestone Soluspan Suspension ... 2484
Buprenorphine (Increased CNS depression). Products include:
Buprenex Injectable ... 2170
Buspirone Hydrochloride (Increased CNS depression). Products include:
BuSpar Tablets ... 738
Butabarbital (Increased CNS depression).
No products indexed under this heading.
Chlordiazepoxide (Increased CNS depression). Products include:
Limbitrol ... 2333
Chlordiazepoxide Hydrochloride (Increased CNS depression). Products include:
Librax Capsules ... 2330
Librium Capsules ... 2331
Librium Injectable ... 2332
Chlorpromazine (Increased CNS depression). Products include:
Thorazine Suppositories ... 2701
Chlorpromazine Hydrochloride (Increased CNS depression). Products include:
Thorazine ... 2701
Chlorpropamide (Potential for hypoglycemia). Products include:
Diabinese Tablets ... 2002
Chlorprothixene (Increased CNS depression).
No products indexed under this heading.
Chlorprothixene Hydrochloride (Increased CNS depression).
No products indexed under this heading.
Chlorprothixene Lactate (Increased CNS depression).
No products indexed under this heading.
Clorazepate Dipotassium (Increased CNS depression). Products include:
Tranxene ... 459
Clozapine (Increased CNS depression). Products include:
Clozaril Tablets ... 2377
Cortisone Acetate (In patients receiving concomitant corticosteroids and chronic use of aspirin, withdrawal of corticosteroids may result in salicylism). Products include:
Cortone Acetate Sterile Suspension ... 1663
Cortone Acetate Tablets ... 1664
Desflurane (Increased CNS depression). Products include:
Suprane (desflurane, USP) ... 1865
Dexamethasone (In patients receiving concomitant corticosteroids and chronic use of aspirin, withdrawal of corticosteroids may result in salicylism). Products include:
AK-Trol Ointment & Suspension ... ⊙ 205
Decadron Elixir ... 1676
Decadron Tablets ... 1678
Decaspray Topical Aerosol ... 1689
Maxitrol Ophthalmic Ointment and Suspension ... ⊙ 222
TobraDex Ophthalmic Suspension and Ointment ... 469
Dexamethasone Acetate (In patients receiving concomitant corticosteroids and chronic use of aspirin, withdrawal of corticosteroids may result in salicylism). Products include:
Dalalone D.P. Injectable ... 1009
Decadron-LA Sterile Suspension ... 1687
Dexamethasone Sodium Phosphate (In patients receiving concomitant corticosteroids and chronic use of aspirin, withdrawal of corticosteroids may result in salicylism). Products include:
Decadron Phosphate Injection ... 1680
Decadron Phosphate Sterile Ophthalmic Ointment ... 1684
Decadron Phosphate Sterile Ophthalmic Solution ... 1685
Decadron Phosphate Topical Cream ... 1686
Decadron Phosphate with Xylocaine Injection, Sterile ... 1683
Dexacort Phosphate in Respihaler ... 1606
Dexacort Phosphate in Turbinaire ... 1607
NeoDecadron Sterile Ophthalmic Ointment ... 1755
NeoDecadron Sterile Ophthalmic Solution ... 1756
NeoDecadron Topical Cream ... 1757
Dezocine (Increased CNS depression). Products include:
Dalgan Injection ... 529
Diazepam (Increased CNS depression). Products include:
Dizac (diazepam injectable emulsion) CIV ... 1862
Valium Injectable ... 2336
Valium Tablets ... 2335
Diclofenac Potassium (Increased risk of peptic ulceration and bleeding). Products include:
Cataflam Tablets ... 833
Diclofenac Sodium (Increased risk of peptic ulceration and bleeding). Products include:
Voltaren Ophthalmic Sterile Ophthalmic Solution ... ⊙ 264
Cataflam/Voltaren/Voltaren-XR ... 833
Dicumarol (Enhanced effects of anticoagulants).
No products indexed under this heading.
Droperidol (Increased CNS depression). Products include:
Inapsine Injection ... 462
Enflurane (Increased CNS depression).
No products indexed under this heading.
Estazolam (Increased CNS depression). Products include:
ProSom Tablets ... 457
Ethchlorvynol (Increased CNS depression). Products include:
Placidyl Capsules ... 456
Ethinamate (Increased CNS depression).
No products indexed under this heading.
Etodolac (Increased risk of peptic ulceration and bleeding). Products include:
Lodine Capsules and Tablets ... 2849
Fenoprofen Calcium (Increased risk of peptic ulceration and bleeding). Products include:
Nalfon 200 Pulvules & Nalfon Tablets ... 933
Fentanyl (Increased CNS depression). Products include:
Duragesic Transdermal System ... 1336
Fentanyl Citrate (Increased CNS depression). Products include:
Sublimaze Injection ... 463
Fludrocortisone Acetate (In patients receiving concomitant corticosteroids and chronic use of aspirin, withdrawal of corticosteroids may result in salicylism). Products include:
Florinef Acetate Tablets ... 506
Fluphenazine Decanoate (Increased CNS depression). Products include:
Prolixin Decanoate ... 510
Fluphenazine Enanthate (Increased CNS depression). Products include:
Prolixin Enanthate ... 510
Fluphenazine Hydrochloride (Increased CNS depression). Products include:
Prolixin ... 510
Flurazepam Hydrochloride (Increased CNS depression). Products include:
Dalmane Capsules ... 2329
Flurbiprofen (Increased risk of peptic ulceration and bleeding).
No products indexed under this heading.
Furazolidone (The CNS effects of butalbital may be enhanced by monoamine oxidase inhibitors). Products include:
Furoxone ... 2221
Glimepiride (Potential for hypoglycemia). Products include:
Amaryl Tablets ... 1241
Glipizide (Potential for hypoglycemia). Products include:
Glucotrol Tablets ... 2011
Glucotrol XL Extended Release Tablets ... 2012
Glutethimide (Increased CNS depression).
No products indexed under this heading.
Glyburide (Potential for hypoglycemia). Products include:
DiaBeta Tablets ... 1265
Glynase PresTab Tablets ... 2091
Micronase Tablets ... 2099
Haloperidol (Increased CNS depression). Products include:
Haldol Injection, Tablets and Concentrate ... 1585
Haloperidol Decanoate (Increased CNS depression). Products include:
Haldol Decanoate ... 1587
Hydrocodone Bitartrate (Increased CNS depression). Products include:
Codiclear DH Syrup ... 808
Duratuss HD Elixir ... 2750
Histussin D Liquid ... 670
Hycodan Tablets and Syrup ... 946
Hycomine Compound Tablets ... 948
Hycomine ... 947
Hycotuss Expectorant Syrup ... 950
Hydrocet Capsules ... 787
Lorcet 10/650 Tablets ... 1016
Lortab ... 2751
Tussend ... 1830
Tussend Expectorant ... 1831
Vicodin Tablets ... 1404
Vicodin ES Tablets ... 1405
Vicodin HP Tablets ... 1403
Vicodin Tuss Expectorant ... 1406
Zydone Capsules ... 967
Hydrocodone Polistirex (Increased CNS depression). Products include:
Tussionex Pennkinetic Extended-Release Suspension ... 1624
Hydrocortisone (In patients receiving concomitant corticosteroids and chronic use of aspirin, withdrawal of corticosteroids may result in salicylism). Products include:
Anusol-HC Cream 2.5% ... 1953
Aquanil HC Lotion ... 1989
Maximum Strength Cortaid Spray ▣ 800
CORTENEMA ... 2713
Cortisporin Ointment ... 1074
Cortisporin Ophthalmic Ointment Sterile ... 1074
Cortisporin Ophthalmic Suspension Sterile ... 1075
Cortisporin Otic Solution Sterile ... 1076
Cortisporin Otic Suspension Sterile 1077
Cortizone-5 ... ▣ 795
Cortizone-10 ... ▣ 795
Hydrocortone Tablets ... 1715
Hytone ... 922
Hytone Ointment 2 ½% ... 923
Massengill Medicated Soft Cloth Towelettes ... 2628
Pediotic Suspension Sterile ... 1140
Preparation H Hydrocortisone 1% Cream ... ▣ 843
ProctoCream-HC 2.5% ... 2552
VōSoL HC Otic Solution ... 2786
Hydrocortisone Acetate (In patients receiving concomitant corticosteroids and chronic use of aspirin, withdrawal of corticosteroids may result in salicylism). Products include:
Analpram-HC Rectal Cream 1% and 2.5% ... 993
Anusol HC-1 Hydrocortisone Anti-Itch Ointment ... ▣ 810
Anusol-HC Suppositories ... 1954
Caldecort Anti-Itch Hydrocortisone Cream ... ▣ 651
Coly-Mycin S Otic w/Neomycin & Hydrocortisone ... 1965
Cortaid ... ▣ 800

(▣ Described in PDR For Nonprescription Drugs) (⊙ Described in PDR For Ophthalmology)

Cortifoam 2540
Cortisporin Cream 1073
Epifoam 2543
Hydrocortone Acetate Sterile Suspension 1712
Mantadil Cream 1124
Nupercainal Hydrocortisone 1% Cream 661
Pramosone Cream, Lotion & Ointment 995
ProctoFoam-HC 2552
Terra-Cortril Ophthalmic Suspension 2033

Hydrocortisone Sodium Phosphate (In patients receiving concomitant corticosteroids and chronic use of aspirin, withdrawal of corticosteroids may result in salicylism). Products include:
Hydrocortone Phosphate Injection, Sterile 1713

Hydrocortisone Sodium Succinate (In patients receiving concomitant corticosteroids and chronic use of aspirin, withdrawal of corticosteroids may result in salicylism).
No products indexed under this heading.

Hydromorphone Hydrochloride (Increased CNS depressant effects). Products include:
Dilaudid Ampules 1382
Dilaudid Cough Syrup 1383
Dilaudid-HP Injection 1384
Dilaudid-HP Lyophilized Powder 250 mg 1384
Dilaudid 1382
Dilaudid Oral Liquid 1386
Dilaudid 1382
Dilaudid Tablets - 8 mg 1386

Hydroxyzine Hydrochloride (Increased CNS depression). Products include:
Atarax Tablets & Syrup 1992
Marax Tablets & DF Syrup 2015
Vistaril Intramuscular Solution 2042

Ibuprofen (Increased risk of peptic ulceration and bleeding). Products include:
Advil Cold and Sinus Caplets and Tablets 837
Advil Ibuprofen Tablets, Caplets and Gel Caplets 836
Children's Motrin Ibuprofen Oral Suspension 1558
IBU Tablets 1389
Ibuprohm 713
Motrin IB Caplets, Tablets, and Gelcaps 802
Motrin Ibuprofen Suspension, Oral Drops, Chewable Tablets, Caplets 1563
Nuprin Ibuprofen/Analgesic Tablets & Caplets 645
Vicks DayQuil SINUS Pressure & PAIN Relief with IBUPROFEN 735

Indomethacin (Increased risk of peptic ulceration and bleeding). Products include:
Indocin 1723

Indomethacin Sodium Trihydrate (Increased risk of peptic ulceration and bleeding). Products include:
Indocin I.V. 1727

Insulin, Human (Potential for hypoglycemia).
No products indexed under this heading.

Insulin, Human Isophane Suspension (Potential for hypoglycemia). Products include:
Novolin N Human Insulin 10 ml Vials 1846

Insulin, Human NPH (Potential for hypoglycemia). Products include:
Humulin N, 100 Units 1495
Novolin N PenFill 1.5 ml Cartridges Durable Insulin Delivery System 1849
Novolin N Prefilled Syringe Disposable Insulin Delivery System 1850

Insulin, Human Regular (Potential for hypoglycemia). Products include:
Humulin R, 100 Units 1497
Novolin R Human Insulin 10 ml Vials 1846
Novolin R PenFill 1.5 ml Cartridges Durable Insulin Delivery System 1849
Novolin R Prefilled Syringe Disposable Insulin Delivery System 1850
Velosulin BR Human Insulin 10 ml Vials 1847

Insulin, Human, Zinc Suspension (Potential for hypoglycemia). Products include:
Humulin L, 100 Units 1494
Humulin U, 100 Units 1498
Novolin L Human Insulin 10 ml Vials 1846

Insulin Lispro, Human (Potential for hypoglycemia). Products include:
Humalog Injection 1488

Insulin, NPH (Potential for hypoglycemia). Products include:
NPH, 100 Units 1502
Pork NPH, 100 Units 1506
Purified Pork NPH Isophane Insulin 1852

Insulin, Regular (Potential for hypoglycemia). Products include:
Regular, 100 Units 1503
Pork Regular, 100 Units 1507
Pork Regular (Concentrated), 500 Units 1508
Purified Pork Regular Insulin 1852

Insulin, Zinc Crystals (Potential for hypoglycemia). Products include:
NPH, 100 Units 1502

Insulin, Zinc Suspension (Potential for hypoglycemia). Products include:
Iletin I 1501
Lente, 100 Units 1501
Iletin II 1504
Pork Lente, 100 Units 1504
Purified Pork Lente Insulin 1852

Isocarboxazid (The CNS effects of butalbital may be enhanced by monoamine oxidase inhibitors).
No products indexed under this heading.

Isoflurane (Increased CNS depression).
No products indexed under this heading.

Ketamine Hydrochloride (Increased CNS depression).
No products indexed under this heading.

Ketoprofen (Increased risk of peptic ulceration and bleeding). Products include:
Actron Caplets and Tablets 608
Orudis Capsules 2874
Orudis KT 842
Oruvail Capsules 2874

Ketorolac Tromethamine (Increased risk of peptic ulceration and bleeding). Products include:
Acular Sterile Ophthalmic Solution 470
Toradol 2319

Levomethadyl Acetate Hydrochloride (Increased CNS depression). Products include:
Orlaam Oral Solution 2361

Levorphanol Tartrate (Increased CNS depression). Products include:
Levo-Dromoran 2297

Lorazepam (Increased CNS depression). Products include:
Ativan Injection 2805
Ativan Tablets 2807

Loxapine Hydrochloride (Increased CNS depression). Products include:
Loxitane 1426

Loxapine Succinate (Increased CNS depression). Products include:
Loxitane Capsules 1426

Meclofenamate Sodium (Increased risk of peptic ulceration and bleeding).
No products indexed under this heading.

Mefenamic Acid (Increased risk of peptic ulceration and bleeding). Products include:
Ponstel 1982

Meperidine Hydrochloride (Increased CNS depression). Products include:
Demerol 2438
Mepergan Injection 2859

Mephobarbital (Increased CNS depression). Products include:
Mebaral Tablets 2452

Meprobamate (Increased CNS depression). Products include:
Miltown Tablets 2780
PMB 200 and PMB 400 2890

Mercaptopurine (Enhanced effects of 6-mercaptopurine and potential for bone marrow toxicity and blood dyscrasias). Products include:
Purinethol Tablets 1214

Mesoridazine Besylate (Increased CNS depression). Products include:
Serentil 689

Metformin Hydrochloride (Potential for hypoglycemia). Products include:
Glucophage Tablets 754

Methadone Hydrochloride (Increased CNS depression). Products include:
Methadone Hydrochloride Oral Concentrate 2356
Methadone Hydrochloride Oral Solution & Tablets 2357

Methohexital Sodium (Increased CNS depression).
No products indexed under this heading.

Methotrexate Sodium (Enhanced effects of methotrexate and potential for bone marrow toxicity and blood dyscrasias). Products include:
Methotrexate Sodium Tablets, Injection, for Injection and LPF 1322

Methotrimeprazine (Increased CNS depression). Products include:
Levoprome 1321

Methoxyflurane (Increased CNS depression).
No products indexed under this heading.

Methylprednisolone Acetate (In patients receiving concomitant corticosteroids and chronic use of aspirin, withdrawal of corticosteroids may result in salicylism).
No products indexed under this heading.

Methylprednisolone Sodium Succinate (In patients receiving concomitant corticosteroids and chronic use of aspirin, withdrawal of corticosteroids may result in salicylism).
No products indexed under this heading.

Midazolam Hydrochloride (Increased CNS depression). Products include:
Versed Injection 2324

Molindone Hydrochloride (Increased CNS depression). Products include:
Moban Tablets and Concentrate 1036

Morphine Sulfate (Increased CNS depression). Products include:
Astramorph/PF Injection, USP (Preservative-Free) 526
Duramorph Injection 983
Infumorph 200 and Infumorph 500 Sterile Solutions 985
Kadian Capsules 2948
MS Contin Tablets 2149
MSIR 2152
Oramorph SR (Morphine Sulfate Sustained Release Tablets) 2359
RMS Suppositories CII 2766
Roxanol 2365

Nabumetone (Increased risk of peptic ulceration and bleeding). Products include:
Relafen Tablets 2688

Naproxen (Increased risk of peptic ulceration and bleeding). Products include:
Anaprox/Naprosyn 2277

Naproxen Sodium (Increased risk of peptic ulceration and bleeding). Products include:
Aleve 2124
Anaprox/Naprosyn 2277
Naprelan Tablets 2861

Opium Alkaloids (Increased CNS depression).
No products indexed under this heading.

Oxaprozin (Increased risk of peptic ulceration and bleeding). Products include:
Daypro Caplets 2578

Oxazepam (Increased CNS depression). Products include:
Serax Capsules 2916
Serax Tablets 2916

Oxycodone Hydrochloride (Increased CNS depression). Products include:
OxyContin Tablets 2163
OxyIR Capsules 2167
Percocet Tablets 955
Percodan Tablets 955
Percodan-Demi Tablets 956
Roxicodone Tablets, Oral Solution & Intensol (Oxycodone) 2366
Tylox Capsules 1593

Pentobarbital Sodium (Increased CNS depression). Products include:
Nembutal Sodium Capsules 440
Nembutal Sodium Solution 442
Nembutal Sodium Suppositories 444

Perphenazine (Increased CNS depression). Products include:
Etrafon 2495
Triavil Tablets 1800
Trilafon 2532

Phenelzine Sulfate (The CNS effects of butalbital may be enhanced by monoamine oxidase inhibitors). Products include:
Nardil 1977

Phenobarbital (Increased CNS depression). Products include:
Arco-Lase Plus Tablets 513
Bellergal-S Tablets 2375
Donnatal 2234
Donnatal Extentabs 2234
Donnatal Tablets 2234
Phenobarbital Elixir and Tablets 1523
Quadrinal Tablets 1398

Phenylbutazone (Increased risk of peptic ulceration and bleeding).
No products indexed under this heading.

Piroxicam (Increased risk of peptic ulceration and bleeding). Products include:
Feldene Capsules 2008

Potassium Citrate (The renal clearance of aspirin is greatly augmented by an alkaline urine produced by concurrent systemic potassium citrate). Products include:
Polycitra Syrup 574
Polycitra-K Crystals 574
Polycitra-K Oral Solution 575
Polycitra-LC 574
Urocit-K Tablets 1828

IMPORTANT NOTE: Always consult each drug listing in the patient's regimen for possible interactions.

Prazepam (Increased CNS depression).
No products indexed under this heading.

Prednisolone Acetate (In patients receiving concomitant corticosteroids and chronic use of aspirin, withdrawal of corticosteroids may result in salicylism). Products include:
AK-CIDE	⊙ 203
AK-CIDE Ointment	⊙ 203
Blephamide Liquifilm Sterile Ophthalmic Suspension	472
Blephamide Ointment	⊙ 234
Econopred & Econopred Plus Ophthalmic Suspensions	⊙ 216
Poly-Pred Liquifilm	⊙ 246
Pred Forte	⊙ 247
Pred Mild	⊙ 250
Pred-G Liquifilm Sterile Ophthalmic Suspension	⊙ 248
Pred-G S.O.P. Sterile Ophthalmic Ointment	⊙ 249

Prednisolone Sodium Phosphate (In patients receiving concomitant corticosteroids and chronic use of aspirin, withdrawal of corticosteroids may result in salicylism). Products include:
AK-PRED	⊙ 204
Hydeltrasol Injection, Sterile	1708
Pediapred Oral Solution	1618

Prednisolone Tebutate (In patients receiving concomitant corticosteroids and chronic use of aspirin, withdrawal of corticosteroids may result in salicylism). Products include:
Hydeltra-T.B.A. Sterile Suspension	1710

Prednisone (In patients receiving concomitant corticosteroids and chronic use of aspirin, withdrawal of corticosteroids may result in salicylism).
No products indexed under this heading.

Probenecid (Reduced uricosuric effects). Products include:
Benemid Tablets	1651
ColBENEMID Tablets	1662

Prochlorperazine (Increased CNS depression). Products include:
Compazine	2644

Promethazine Hydrochloride (Increased CNS depression). Products include:
Mepergan Injection	2859
Phenergan with Codeine	2883
Phenergan with Dextromethorphan	2885
Phenergan Injection	2880
Phenergan Suppositories	2882
Phenergan Syrup	2881
Phenergan Tablets	2882
Phenergan VC	2886
Phenergan VC with Codeine	2888

Propofol (Increased CNS depression). Products include:
Diprivan Injectable Emulsion	2939

Propoxyphene Hydrochloride (Increased CNS depression). Products include:
Darvon	1475
Wygesic Tablets	2930

Propoxyphene Napsylate (Increased CNS depression). Products include:
Darvon-N/Darvocet-N	1473

Quazepam (Increased CNS depression). Products include:
Doral Tablets	2773

Risperidone (Increased CNS depression). Products include:
Risperdal Tablets	1348

Secobarbital Sodium (Increased CNS depression). Products include:
Seconal Sodium Pulvules	1529

Selegiline Hydrochloride (The CNS effects of butalbital may be enhanced by monoamine oxidase inhibitors). Products include:
Eldepryl Capsules	2729

Sevoflurane (Increased CNS depression).
No products indexed under this heading.

Sodium Bicarbonate (The renal clearance of aspirin is greatly augmented by an alkaline urine produced by concurrent systemic sodium bicarbonate). Products include:
Alka-Seltzer Cherry Effervescent Antacid and Pain Reliever	■□ 609
Alka-Seltzer Extra Strength Effervescent Antacid and Pain Reliever	■□ 609
Alka-Seltzer Gold Effervescent Antacid	■□ 611
Alka-Seltzer Lemon Lime Effervescent Antacid and Pain Reliever	■□ 609
Alka-Seltzer Original Effervescent Antacid and Pain Reliever	■□ 609
Arm & Hammer Pure Baking Soda	■□ 648
Colyte and Colyte-flavored	2540
GoLYTELY	694
Massengill Disposable Douches	■□ 780
Massengill Liquid Concentrate	■□ 780
NuLYTELY	694
Cherry Flavor NuLYTELY	694

Sufentanil Citrate (Increased CNS depression). Products include:
Sufenta Injection	1355

Sulfinpyrazone (Reduced uricosuric effects). Products include:
Anturane	823

Sulindac (Increased risk of peptic ulceration and bleeding). Products include:
Clinoril Tablets	1658

Temazepam (Increased CNS depression). Products include:
Restoril Capsules	2413

Thiamylal Sodium (Increased CNS depression).
No products indexed under this heading.

Thioridazine Hydrochloride (Increased CNS depression). Products include:
Mellaril	2398

Thiothixene (Increased CNS depression). Products include:
Navane Capsules and Concentrate	2018
Navane Intramuscular	2019

Tolazamide (Potential for hypoglycemia).
No products indexed under this heading.

Tolbutamide (Potential for hypoglycemia).
No products indexed under this heading.

Tolmetin Sodium (Increased risk of peptic ulceration and bleeding). Products include:
Tolectin (200, 400 and 600 mg)	1591

Tranylcypromine Sulfate (The CNS effects of butalbital may be enhanced by monoamine oxidase inhibitors). Products include:
Parnate Tablets	2679

Triamcinolone (In patients receiving concomitant corticosteroids and chronic use of aspirin, withdrawal of corticosteroids may result in salicylism).
No products indexed under this heading.

Triamcinolone Acetonide (In patients receiving concomitant corticosteroids and chronic use of aspirin, withdrawal of corticosteroids may result in salicylism). Products include:
Azmacort Oral Inhaler	2175
Nasacort AQ Nasal Spray	2191
Nasacort Nasal Inhaler	2189

Triamcinolone Diacetate (In patients receiving concomitant corticosteroids and chronic use of aspirin, withdrawal of corticosteroids may result in salicylism).
No products indexed under this heading.

Triamcinolone Hexacetonide (In patients receiving concomitant corticosteroids and chronic use of aspirin, withdrawal of corticosteroids may result in salicylism).
No products indexed under this heading.

Triazolam (Increased CNS depression). Products include:
Halcion Tablets	2093

Trifluoperazine Hydrochloride (Increased CNS depression). Products include:
Stelazine	2692

Warfarin Sodium (Enhanced effects of anticoagulants). Products include:
Coumadin	941

Zolpidem Tartrate (Increased CNS depression). Products include:
Ambien Tablets	2559

Food Interactions
Alcohol (Increased CNS depression).

FIORINAL TABLETS
(Butalbital, Aspirin, Caffeine) 2388
See **Fiorinal Capsules**

FLAGYL 375 CAPSULES
(Metronidazole) 2587
May interact with oral anticoagulants, lithium preparations, and certain other agents. Compounds in these categories include:

Cimetidine (May prolong the half-life and decrease plasma clearance of metronidazole). Products include:
Tagamet HB Tablets	■□ 786
Tagamet Tablets	2694

Dicumarol (Metronidazole may potentiate the anticoagulant effect resulting in prolongation of prothrombin time).
No products indexed under this heading.

Disulfiram (Psychotic reactions have been reported in alcoholic patients who are using metronidazole and disulfiram concurrently, do not give metronidazole to patients who have taken disulfiram within the last 2 weeks). Products include:
Antabuse Tablets	2802

Lithium Carbonate (In patients stabilized on relatively high-dose of lithium, short-term metronidazole therapy has been associated with elevation of serum lithium resulting in lithium toxicity). Products include:
Eskalith	2658
Lithium Carbonate Capsules & Tablets	2352
Lithonate/Lithotabs/Lithobid	2721

Lithium Citrate (In patients stabilized on relatively high-dose of lithium, short-term metronidazole therapy has been associated with elevation of serum lithium resulting in lithium toxicity).
No products indexed under this heading.

Phenobarbital (May accelerate the elimination of metronidazole, resulting in reduced plasma levels). Products include:
Arco-Lase Plus Tablets	513
Bellergal-S Tablets	2375
Donnatal	2234
Donnatal Extentabs	2234
Donnatal Tablets	2234
Phenobarbital Elixir and Tablets	1523
Quadrinal Tablets	1398

Phenytoin (May accelerate the elimination of metronidazole, resulting in reduced plasma levels; impaired phenytoin clearance has been reported). Products include:
Dilantin Infatabs	1967
Dilantin-125 Suspension	1969

Phenytoin Sodium (May accelerate the elimination of metronidazole, resulting in reduced plasma levels; impaired phenytoin clearance has been reported). Products include:
Dilantin Kapseals	1965

Warfarin Sodium (Metronidazole may potentiate the anticoagulant effect resulting in prolongation of prothrombin time). Products include:
Coumadin	941

Food Interactions
Alcohol (Alcohol should not be consumed during metronidazole therapy and for at least three days afterward because abdominal cramps, nausea, vomiting, headaches, and flushing may occur).

FLAGYL I.V.
(Metronidazole Hydrochloride) 2373
May interact with oral anticoagulants and certain other agents. Compounds in these categories include:

Cimetidine (Decreases plasma clearance of metronidazole). Products include:
Tagamet HB Tablets	■□ 786
Tagamet Tablets	2694

Cimetidine Hydrochloride (Decreases plasma clearance of metronidazole). Products include:
Tagamet	2694

Dicumarol (Potentiation of anticoagulant effect).
No products indexed under this heading.

Disulfiram (Psychotic reactions have been reported in alcoholic patients who are using metronidazole and disulfiram concurrently). Products include:
Antabuse Tablets	2802

Phenobarbital (Reduces metronidazole plasma levels). Products include:
Arco-Lase Plus Tablets	513
Bellergal-S Tablets	2375
Donnatal	2234
Donnatal Extentabs	2234
Donnatal Tablets	2234
Phenobarbital Elixir and Tablets	1523
Quadrinal Tablets	1398

Phenytoin (Reduces metronidazole plasma levels; impaired clearance of phenytoin). Products include:
Dilantin Infatabs	1967
Dilantin-125 Suspension	1969

Phenytoin Sodium (Reduces metronidazole plasma levels; impaired clearance of phenytoin). Products include:
Dilantin Kapseals	1965

Warfarin Sodium (Potentiation of anticoagulant effect). Products include:
Coumadin	941

Food Interactions
Alcohol (Potential for abdominal cramps, nausea, vomiting, and headaches, and flushing).

FLAGYL I.V. RTU
(Metronidazole) 2373
See **Flagyl I.V.**

(■□ Described in PDR For Nonprescription Drugs) (⊙ Described in PDR For Ophthalmology)

FLAREX OPHTHALMIC SUSPENSION
(Fluorometholone Acetate) .... ⊙ 217
None cited in PDR database.

FLEET BABYLAX
(Glycerin) 1000
None cited in PDR database.

FLEET BISACODYL ENEMA
(Bisacodyl) 1000
None cited in PDR database.

FLEET CHILDREN'S ENEMA
(Sodium Phosphate, Dibasic, Sodium Phosphate, Monobasic) 1001
See **Fleet Enema**

FLEET ENEMA
(Sodium Phosphate, Dibasic, Sodium Phosphate, Monobasic) 1001
May interact with:

Calcium Channel Blockers, Unspecified (Effect not specified).
Diuretics, Unspecified (Effect not specified).

FLEET GLYCERIN LAXATIVE RECTAL APPLICATORS
(Glycerin) 1000
None cited in PDR database.

FLEET MINERAL OIL ENEMA
(Mineral Oil) 1001
None cited in PDR database.

FLEET PAIN RELIEF PADS
(Pramoxine Hydrochloride) 1001
None cited in PDR database.

FLEET PHOSPHO-SODA
(Sodium Phosphate, Dibasic, Sodium Phosphate, Monobasic) 1002
None cited in PDR database.

FLEET PREP KITS
(Sodium Phosphate, Dibasic, Sodium Phosphate, Monobasic) 1002
May interact with antacids and certain other agents. Compounds in these categories include:

Aluminum Carbonate (Concurrent use within one-hour should be avoided). Products include:
Basaljel Capsules 2810
Basaljel Suspension 2810
Basaljel Tablets 2810

Aluminum Hydroxide (Concurrent use within one-hour should be avoided). Products include:
ALternaGEL Liquid 1358
Maximum Strength Ascriptin .... ⊙ 650
Cama Arthritis Pain Reliever .... ⊙ 748
Gaviscon Extra Strength Relief Formula Antacid Tablets .... ⊙ 778
Gaviscon Extra Strength Relief Formula Liquid Antacid .... ⊙ 779
Gaviscon Liquid Antacid .... ⊙ 779
Gelusil Antacid-Anti-gas Liquid ..... ⊙ 819
Gelusil Antacid-Anti-gas Tablets .... ⊙ 819
Maalox Antacid/Anti-Gas Tablets 889
Maalox Heartburn Relief Suspension .... ⊙ 658
Maalox Antacid Liquid 888
Extra Strength Maalox Antacid/Anti-Gas Liquid and Tablets 888
Mylanta 1359
Tempo Soft Antacid .... ⊙ 799

Aluminum Hydroxide Gel (Concurrent use within one-hour should be avoided). Products include:
ALternaGEL Liquid .... ⊙ 675
Aludrox Oral Suspension .... ⊙ 850
Amphojel Suspension 2802
Amphojel Suspension without Flavor 2802

Amphojel Tablets 2802
Ascriptin .... ⊙ 650
Gaviscon Antacid Tablets .... ⊙ 778
Gaviscon-2 Antacid Tablets .... ⊙ 779
Mylanta Liquid 676
Mylanta Double Strength Liquid 676
Nephrox Suspension 671

Magaldrate (Concurrent use within one-hour should be avoided).
No products indexed under this heading.

Magnesium Hydroxide (Concurrent use within one-hour should be avoided). Products include:
Aludrox Oral Suspension .... ⊙ 850
Ascriptin .... ⊙ 650
Di-Gel Antacid/Anti-Gas .... ⊙ 762
Gelusil Antacid-Anti-gas Liquid ..... ⊙ 819
Gelusil Antacid-Anti-gas Tablets .... ⊙ 819
Maalox Antacid/Anti-Gas Tablets 889
Maalox Antacid Liquid 888
Extra Strength Maalox Antacid/Anti-Gas Liquid and Tablets 888
Mylanta Fast-Acting 1359
Mylanta Gelcaps Antacid 678
Fast-Acting Mylanta Liquid Antacid 1359
Mylanta Tablets 677
Maximum-Strength Fast-Acting Mylanta Liquid Antacid 1359
Mylanta Double Strength Tablets .. 677
Phillips' Milk of Magnesia Liquid ..... ⊙ 627
Rolaids Antacid Tablets .... ⊙ 807
Tempo Soft Antacid .... ⊙ 799

Magnesium Oxide (Concurrent use within one-hour should be avoided). Products include:
Beelith Tablets 632
Bufferin Analgesic Tablets .... ⊙ 636
Arthritis Strength Bufferin Analgesic Caplets .... ⊙ 637
Extra Strength Bufferin Analgesic Tablets .... ⊙ 637
Caltrate PLUS .... ⊙ 681
Cama Arthritis Pain Reliever .... ⊙ 748
Mag-Ox 400 666
Uro-Mag 666

Sodium Bicarbonate (Concurrent use within one-hour should be avoided). Products include:
Alka-Seltzer Cherry Effervescent Antacid and Pain Reliever .... ⊙ 609
Alka-Seltzer Extra Strength Effervescent Antacid and Pain Reliever .... ⊙ 609
Alka-Seltzer Gold Effervescent Antacid .... ⊙ 611
Alka-Seltzer Lemon Lime Effervescent Antacid and Pain Reliever .... ⊙ 609
Alka-Seltzer Original Effervescent Antacid and Pain Reliever .... ⊙ 609
Arm & Hammer Pure Baking Soda .... ⊙ 648
Colyte and Colyte-flavored 2540
GoLYTELY 694
Massengill Disposable Douches ..... ⊙ 780
Massengill Liquid Concentrate ..... ⊙ 780
NuLYTELY 694
Cherry Flavor NuLYTELY 694

Food Interactions

Dairy products (Concurrent use within one-hour should be avoided).

FLEET SOF-LAX
(Docusate Sodium) 1003
None cited in PDR database.

FLEET SOF-LAX OVERNIGHT
(Docusate Sodium, Casanthranol) 1003
None cited in PDR database.

FLETCHER'S CASTORIA
(Senna Concentrates) .... ⊙ 709
None cited in PDR database.

FLETCHER'S CHERRY FLAVOR
(Phenolphthalein) .... ⊙ 710
None cited in PDR database.

FLEXERIL TABLETS
(Cyclobenzaprine Hydrochloride) 1701
May interact with monoamine oxidase inhibitors, anticholinergics, barbiturates, central nervous system depressants, and certain other agents. Compounds in these categories include:

Alfentanil Hydrochloride (Co-administration results in enhanced effects). Products include:
Alfenta Injection 1334

Alprazolam (Co-administration results in enhanced effects). Products include:
Xanax Tablets 2115

Aprobarbital (Co-administration results in enhanced effects).
No products indexed under this heading.

Atropine Sulfate (Caution is advised when co-administered due to cyclobenzaprine-induced atropine-like actions). Products include:
Arco-Lase Plus Tablets 513
Atrohist Plus Tablets 1605
Donnatal 2234
Donnatal Extentabs 2234
Donnatal Tablets 2234
Lomotil 2591
Motofen Tablets 789
Urised Tablets 2123

Belladonna Alkaloids (Caution is advised when co-administered due to cyclobenzaprine-induced atropine-like actions). Products include:
Bellergal-S Tablets 2375
Hyland's Bedwetting Tablets ...... ⊙ 788
Hyland's EnurAid Tablets .... ⊙ 789
Hyland's Headache Tablets .... ⊙ 790
Hyland's Teething Tablets .... ⊙ 790
Similasan Eye Drops #1 .... ⊙ 769

Benztropine Mesylate (Caution is advised when co-administered due to cyclobenzaprine-induced atropine-like actions). Products include:
Cogentin 1661

Biperiden Hydrochloride (Caution is advised when co-administered due to cyclobenzaprine-induced atropine-like actions). Products include:
Akineton 1380

Buprenorphine (Co-administration results in enhanced effects). Products include:
Buprenex Injectable 2170

Buspirone Hydrochloride (Co-administration results in enhanced effects). Products include:
BuSpar Tablets 738

Butabarbital (Co-administration results in enhanced effects).
No products indexed under this heading.

Butalbital (Co-administration results in enhanced effects). Products include:
Axocet Capsules 2469
Esgic-plus Capsules 1012
Esgic-plus Tablets 1012
Fioricet Tablets 2386
Fioricet with Codeine Capsules 2387
Fiorinal Capsules 2388
Fiorinal with Codeine Capsules ... 2390
Fiorinal Tablets 2388
Phrenilin 790
Sedapap Tablets 50 mg/650 mg .. 1826

Chlordiazepoxide (Co-administration results in enhanced effects). Products include:
Limbitrol 2333

Chlordiazepoxide Hydrochloride (Co-administration results in enhanced effects). Products include:
Librax Capsules 2330
Librium Capsules 2331
Librium Injectable 2332

Chlorpromazine (Co-administration results in enhanced effects). Products include:
Thorazine Suppositories 2701

Chlorpromazine Hydrochloride (Co-administration results in enhanced effects). Products include:
Thorazine 2701

Chlorprothixene (Co-administration results in enhanced effects).
No products indexed under this heading.

Chlorprothixene Hydrochloride (Co-administration results in enhanced effects).
No products indexed under this heading.

Chlorprothixene Lactate (Co-administration results in enhanced effects).
No products indexed under this heading.

Clidinium Bromide (Caution is advised when co-administered due to cyclobenzaprine-induced atropine-like actions). Products include:
Librax Capsules 2330

Clorazepate Dipotassium (Co-administration results in enhanced effects). Products include:
Tranxene 459

Clozapine (Co-administration results in enhanced effects). Products include:
Clozaril Tablets 2377

Codeine Phosphate (Co-administration results in enhanced effects). Products include:
Brontex 2130
Dimetane-DC Cough Syrup 2232
Fioricet with Codeine Capsules ... 2387
Fiorinal with Codeine Capsules ... 2390
Nucofed 2225
Phenergan with Codeine 2883
Phenergan VC with Codeine 2888
Robitussin A-C Syrup 2248
Robitussin-DAC Syrup 2249
Ryna .... ⊙ 804
Soma Compound w/Codeine Tablets 2784
Tylenol with Codeine 1592

Desflurane (Co-administration results in enhanced effects). Products include:
Suprane (desflurane, USP) 1865

Dezocine (Co-administration results in enhanced effects). Products include:
Dalgan Injection 529

Diazepam (Co-administration results in enhanced effects). Products include:
Dizac (diazepam injectable emulsion) CIV 1862
Valium Injectable 2336
Valium Tablets 2335

Dicyclomine Hydrochloride (Caution is advised when co-administered due to cyclobenzaprine-induced atropine-like actions). Products include:
Bentyl 1246

Droperidol (Co-administration results in enhanced effects). Products include:
Inapsine Injection 462

Enflurane (Co-administration results in enhanced effects).
No products indexed under this heading.

Estazolam (Co-administration results in enhanced effects). Products include:
ProSom Tablets 457

Ethchlorvynol (Co-administration results in enhanced effects). Products include:
Placidyl Capsules 456

Ethinamate (Co-administration results in enhanced effects).
No products indexed under this heading.

IMPORTANT NOTE: Always consult each drug listing in the patient's regimen for possible interactions.

Flexeril | Interactions Index | 418

Fentanyl (Co-administration results in enhanced effects). Products include:
Duragesic Transdermal System 1336

Fentanyl Citrate (Co-administration results in enhanced effects). Products include:
Sublimaze Injection 463

Fluphenazine Decanoate (Co-administration results in enhanced effects). Products include:
Prolixin Decanoate 510

Fluphenazine Enanthate (Co-administration results in enhanced effects). Products include:
Prolixin Enanthate 510

Fluphenazine Hydrochloride (Co-administration results in enhanced effects). Products include:
Prolixin 510

Flurazepam Hydrochloride (Co-administration results in enhanced effects). Products include:
Dalmane Capsules 2329

Furazolidone (Cyclobenzaprine is closely related to tricyclic antidepressants and hyperpyretic crises, severe convulsions and death have occurred in patients taking these agents concurrently; cyclobenzaprine may interact in the same fashion with MAO inhibitors hence concurrent and/or sequential use is contraindicated). Products include:
Furoxone 2221

Glutethimide (Co-administration results in enhanced effects).
No products indexed under this heading.

Glycopyrrolate (Caution is advised when co-administered due to cyclobenzaprine-induced atropine-like actions). Products include:
Robinul Forte Tablets 2247
Robinul Injectable 2247
Robinul Tablets 2247

Guanethidine Monosulfate (Cyclobenzaprine is closely related to tricyclic antidepressants and potential exists for cyclobenzaprine to block antihypertensive effects). Products include:
Esimil Tablets 840
Ismelin Tablets 845

Haloperidol (Co-administration results in enhanced effects). Products include:
Haldol Injection, Tablets and Concentrate 1585

Haloperidol Decanoate (Co-administration results in enhanced effects). Products include:
Haldol Decanoate 1587

Hydrocodone Bitartrate (Co-administration results in enhanced effects). Products include:
Codiclear DH Syrup 808
Duratuss HD Elixir 2750
Histussin D Liquid 670
Hycodan Tablets and Syrup 946
Hycomine Compound Tablets 948
Hycomine 947
Hycotuss Expectorant Syrup 950
Hydrocet Capsules 787
Lorcet 10/650 Tablets 1016
Lortab 2751
Tussend 1830
Tussend Expectorant 1831
Vicodin Tablets 1404
Vicodin ES Tablets 1405
Vicodin HP Tablets 1403
Vicodin Tuss Expectorant 1406
Zydone Capsules 967

Hydrocodone Polistirex (Co-administration results in enhanced effects). Products include:
Tussionex Pennkinetic Extended-Release Suspension 1624

Hydroxyzine Hydrochloride (Co-administration results in enhanced effects). Products include:
Atarax Tablets & Syrup 1992
Marax Tablets & DF Syrup 2015
Vistaril Intramuscular Solution 2042

Hyoscyamine (Caution is advised when co-administered due to cyclobenzaprine-induced atropine-like actions). Products include:
Cystospaz Tablets 2123
Urised Tablets 2123

Hyoscyamine Sulfate (Caution is advised when co-administered due to cyclobenzaprine-induced atropine-like actions). Products include:
Arco-Lase Plus Tablets 513
Atrohist Plus Tablets 1605
Cystospaz-M Capsules 2123
Donnatal 2234
Donnatal Extentabs 2234
Donnatal Tablets 2234
Kutrase Capsules 2546
Levsin/Levsinex/Levbid 2549

Ipratropium Bromide (Caution is advised when co-administered due to cyclobenzaprine-induced atropine-like actions). Products include:
Atrovent Inhalation Aerosol 674
Atrovent Inhalation Solution 675
Atrovent Nasal Spray 0.03% 676
Atrovent Nasal Spray 0.06% 678

Isocarboxazid (Cyclobenzaprine is closely related to tricyclic antidepressants and hyperpyretic crises, severe convulsions and death have occurred in patients taking these agents concurrently; cyclobenzaprine may interact in the same fashion with MAO inhibitors hence concurrent and/or sequential use is contraindicated).
No products indexed under this heading.

Isoflurane (Co-administration results in enhanced effects).
No products indexed under this heading.

Ketamine Hydrochloride (Co-administration results in enhanced effects).
No products indexed under this heading.

Levomethadyl Acetate Hydrochloride (Co-administration results in enhanced effects). Products include:
Orlaam Oral Solution 2361

Levorphanol Tartrate (Co-administration results in enhanced effects). Products include:
Levo-Dromoran 2297

Lorazepam (Co-administration results in enhanced effects). Products include:
Ativan Injection 2805
Ativan Tablets 2807

Loxapine Hydrochloride (Co-administration results in enhanced effects). Products include:
Loxitane 1426

Loxapine Succinate (Co-administration results in enhanced effects). Products include:
Loxitane Capsules 1426

Mepenzolate Bromide (Caution is advised when co-administered due to cyclobenzaprine-induced atropine-like actions).
No products indexed under this heading.

Meperidine Hydrochloride (Co-administration results in enhanced effects). Products include:
Demerol 2438
Mepergan Injection 2859

Mephobarbital (Co-administration results in enhanced effects). Products include:
Mebaral Tablets 2452

Meprobamate (Co-administration results in enhanced effects). Products include:
Miltown Tablets 2780
PMB 200 and PMB 400 2890

Mesoridazine Besylate (Co-administration results in enhanced effects). Products include:
Serentil 689

Methadone Hydrochloride (Co-administration results in enhanced effects). Products include:
Methadone Hydrochloride Oral Concentrate 2356
Methadone Hydrochloride Oral Solution & Tablets 2357

Methohexital Sodium (Co-administration results in enhanced effects).
No products indexed under this heading.

Methotrimeprazine (Co-administration results in enhanced effects). Products include:
Levoprome 1321

Methoxyflurane (Co-administration results in enhanced effects).
No products indexed under this heading.

Midazolam Hydrochloride (Co-administration results in enhanced effects). Products include:
Versed Injection 2324

Molindone Hydrochloride (Co-administration results in enhanced effects). Products include:
Moban Tablets and Concentrate 1036

Morphine Sulfate (Co-administration results in enhanced effects). Products include:
Astramorph/PF Injection, USP (Preservative-Free) 526
Duramorph Injection 983
Infumorph 200 and Infumorph 500 Sterile Solutions 985
Kadian Capsules 2948
MS Contin Tablets 2149
MSIR 2152
Oramorph SR (Morphine Sulfate Sustained Release Tablets) 2359
RMS Suppositories CII 2766
Roxanol 2365

Opium Alkaloids (Co-administration results in enhanced effects).
No products indexed under this heading.

Oxazepam (Co-administration results in enhanced effects). Products include:
Serax Capsules 2916
Serax Tablets 2916

Oxybutynin Chloride (Caution is advised when co-administered due to cyclobenzaprine-induced atropine-like actions). Products include:
Ditropan 1267

Oxycodone Hydrochloride (Co-administration results in enhanced effects). Products include:
OxyContin Tablets 2163
OxyIR Capsules 2167
Percocet Tablets 955
Percodan Tablets 955
Percodan-Demi Tablets 956
Roxicodone Tablets, Oral Solution & Intensol (Oxycodone) 2366
Tylox Capsules 1593

Pentobarbital Sodium (Co-administration results in enhanced effects). Products include:
Nembutal Sodium Capsules 440
Nembutal Sodium Solution 442
Nembutal Sodium Suppositories 444

Perphenazine (Co-administration results in enhanced effects). Products include:
Etrafon 2495
Triavil Tablets 1800
Trilafon 2532

Phenelzine Sulfate (Cyclobenzaprine is closely related to tricyclic antidepressants and hyperpyretic crises, severe convulsions and death have occurred in patients taking these agents concurrently; cyclobenzaprine may interact in the same fashion with MAO inhibitors hence concurrent and/or sequential use is contraindicated). Products include:
Nardil 1977

Phenobarbital (Co-administration results in enhanced effects). Products include:
Arco-Lase Plus Tablets 513
Bellergal-S Tablets 2375
Donnatal 2234
Donnatal Extentabs 2234
Donnatal Tablets 2234
Phenobarbital Elixir and Tablets 1523
Quadrinal Tablets 1398

Prazepam (Co-administration results in enhanced effects).
No products indexed under this heading.

Prochlorperazine (Co-administration results in enhanced effects). Products include:
Compazine 2644

Procyclidine Hydrochloride (Caution is advised when co-administered due to cyclobenzaprine-induced atropine-like actions). Products include:
Kemadrin Tablets 1105

Promethazine Hydrochloride (Co-administration results in enhanced effects). Products include:
Mepergan Injection 2859
Phenergan with Codeine 2883
Phenergan with Dextromethorphan 2885
Phenergan Injection 2880
Phenergan Suppositories 2882
Phenergan Syrup 2881
Phenergan Tablets 2882
Phenergan VC 2886
Phenergan VC with Codeine 2888

Propantheline Bromide (Caution is advised when co-administered due to cyclobenzaprine-induced atropine-like actions). Products include:
Pro-Banthine Tablets 2226

Propofol (Co-administration results in enhanced effects). Products include:
Diprivan Injectable Emulsion 2939

Propoxyphene Hydrochloride (Co-administration results in enhanced effects). Products include:
Darvon 1475
Wygesic Tablets 2930

Propoxyphene Napsylate (Co-administration results in enhanced effects). Products include:
Darvon-N/Darvocet-N 1473

Quazepam (Co-administration results in enhanced effects). Products include:
Doral Tablets 2773

Risperidone (Co-administration results in enhanced effects). Products include:
Risperdal Tablets 1348

Scopolamine (Caution is advised when co-administered due to cyclobenzaprine-induced atropine-like actions). Products include:
Transderm Scōp Transdermal Therapeutic System 890

(▣ Described in PDR For Nonprescription Drugs) (◉ Described in PDR For Ophthalmology)

Scopolamine Hydrobromide
(Caution is advised when co-administered due to cyclobenzaprine-induced atropine-like actions). Products include:
Atrohist Plus Tablets	1605
Donnatal	2234
Donnatal Extentabs	2234
Donnatal Tablets	2234

Secobarbital Sodium (Co-administration results in enhanced effects). Products include:
Seconal Sodium Pulvules	1529

Selegiline Hydrochloride (Cyclobenzaprine is closely related to tricyclic antidepressants and hyperpyretic crises, severe convulsions and death have occurred in patients taking these agents concurrently; cyclobenzaprine may interact in the same fashion with MAO inhibitors hence concurrent and/or sequential use is contraindicated). Products include:
Eldepryl Capsules	2729

Sevoflurane (Co-administration results in enhanced effects).
No products indexed under this heading.

Sufentanil Citrate (Co-administration results in enhanced effects). Products include:
Sufenta Injection	1355

Temazepam (Co-administration results in enhanced effects). Products include:
Restoril Capsules	2413

Thiamylal Sodium (Co-administration results in enhanced effects).
No products indexed under this heading.

Thioridazine Hydrochloride (Co-administration results in enhanced effects). Products include:
Mellaril	2398

Thiothixene (Co-administration results in enhanced effects). Products include:
Navane Capsules and Concentrate	2018
Navane Intramuscular	2019

Tranylcypromine Sulfate (Cyclobenzaprine is closely related to tricyclic antidepressants and hyperpyretic crises, severe convulsions and death have occurred in patients taking these agents concurrently; cyclobenzaprine may interact in the same fashion with MAO inhibitors hence concurrent and/or sequential use is contraindicated). Products include:
Parnate Tablets	2679

Triazolam (Co-administration results in enhanced effects). Products include:
Halcion Tablets	2093

Tridihexethyl Chloride (Caution is advised when co-administered due to cyclobenzaprine-induced atropine-like actions).
No products indexed under this heading.

Trifluoperazine Hydrochloride (Co-administration results in enhanced effects). Products include:
Stelazine	2692

Trihexyphenidyl Hydrochloride (Caution is advised when co-administered due to cyclobenzaprine-induced atropine-like actions). Products include:
Artane	1418

Zolpidem Tartrate (Co-administration results in enhanced effects). Products include:
Ambien Tablets	2559

Food Interactions
Alcohol (Concurrent use results in enhanced effects).

FLINTSTONES CHILDREN'S CHEWABLE VITAMINS
(Vitamins with Minerals) 619
None cited in PDR database.

FLINTSTONES CHILDREN'S CHEWABLE VITAMINS PLUS EXTRA C
(Vitamins with Minerals) 621
None cited in PDR database.

FLINTSTONES CHILDREN'S CHEWABLE VITAMINS PLUS IRON
(Vitamins with Iron) 619
None cited in PDR database.

FLINTSTONES COMPLETE WITH CALCIUM, IRON & MINERALS CHILDREN'S CHEWABLE VITAMINS
(Vitamins with Minerals) 620
None cited in PDR database.

FLINTSTONES PLUS CALCIUM CHILDREN'S CHEWABLE VITAMINS
(Vitamins with Minerals) 620
None cited in PDR database.

FLOLAN FOR INJECTION
(Epoprostenol Sodium) 1085
May interact with diuretics, antihypertensives, vasodilators, platelet inhibitors, and oral anticoagulants. Compounds in these categories include:

Acebutolol Hydrochloride (Additional reductions in blood pressure may occur). Products include:
Sectral Capsules	2914

Amiloride Hydrochloride (Additional reductions in blood pressure may occur). Products include:
Midamor Tablets	1746
Moduretic Tablets	1748

Amlodipine Besylate (Additional reductions in blood pressure may occur). Products include:
Lotrel Capsules	858
Norvasc Tablets	2020

Aspirin (Potential for increased risk of bleeding). Products include:
Alka-Seltzer Cherry Effervescent Antacid and Pain Reliever	609
Alka-Seltzer Extra Strength Effervescent Antacid and Pain Reliever	609
Alka-Seltzer Lemon Lime Effervescent Antacid and Pain Reliever	609
Alka-Seltzer Original Effervescent Antacid and Pain Reliever	609
Alka-Seltzer Plus	611
Alka-Seltzer Plus Sinus Medicine	611
Ascriptin	650
Arthritis Strength BC Powder	631
BC Cold Powder Multi-Symptom Formula (Cold-Sinus-Allergy)	631
BC Cold Powder Non-Drowsy Formula (Cold-Sinus)	631
BC Powder	631
Genuine Bayer Aspirin Tablets & Caplets	618
Extra Strength Bayer Arthritis Pain Regimen Formula	615
Extra Strength Bayer Aspirin Caplets & Tablets	617
Extended-Release Bayer 8-Hour Aspirin	616
Extra Strength Bayer Plus Aspirin Caplets	617
Extra Strength Bayer PM Aspirin Plus Sleep Aid	617
Aspirin Regimen Bayer 81 mg Tablets with Calcium	615
Aspirin Regimen Bayer Adult Low Strength 81 mg Tablets	613
Aspirin Regimen Bayer Children's Chewable Aspirin	616
Aspirin Regimen Bayer Regular Strength 325 mg Caplets	613
Bufferin Analgesic Tablets	636
Arthritis Strength Bufferin Analgesic Caplets	637
Extra Strength Bufferin Analgesic Tablets	637
Cama Arthritis Pain Reliever	748
Darvon Compound-65 Pulvules	1475
Easprin	1971
Ecotrin	2625
Ecotrin Enteric Coated Aspirin Maximum Strength Tablets and Caplets	775
Ecotrin Enteric Coated Aspirin Regular Strength Tablets	2625
Empirin Aspirin Tablets	818
Excedrin Extra-Strength Analgesic Tablets, Caplets, and Geltabs	734
Fiorinal Capsules	2388
Fiorinal with Codeine Capsules	2390
Fiorinal Tablets	2388
Goody's Extra Strength Headache Powders	632
Goody's Extra Strength Pain Relief Tablets	632
Halfprin Tablets	1413
Norgesic	1554
Percodan Tablets	955
Percodan-Demi Tablets	956
Robaxisal Tablets	2246
Soma Compound w/Codeine Tablets	2784
Soma Compound Tablets	2783
St. Joseph Adult Chewable Aspirin (81 mg.)	768
Talwin Compound	2466
Vanquish Analgesic Caplets	627

Atenolol (Additional reductions in blood pressure may occur). Products include:
Tenoretic Tablets	2963
Tenormin Tablets and I.V. Injection	2965

Azlocillin Sodium (Potential for increased risk of bleeding).
No products indexed under this heading.

Benazepril Hydrochloride (Additional reductions in blood pressure may occur). Products include:
Lotensin Tablets	852
Lotensin HCT Tablets	855
Lotrel Capsules	858

Bendroflumethiazide (Additional reductions in blood pressure may occur).
No products indexed under this heading.

Betaxolol Hydrochloride (Additional reductions in blood pressure may occur). Products include:
Betoptic Ophthalmic Solution	465
Betoptic S Ophthalmic Suspension	467
Kerlone Tablets	2588

Bisoprolol Fumarate (Additional reductions in blood pressure may occur). Products include:
Zebeta Tablets	1457
Ziac	1459

Bumetanide (Additional reductions in blood pressure may occur). Products include:
Bumex	2260

Captopril (Additional reductions in blood pressure may occur). Products include:
Capoten Tablets	740
Capozide Tablets	744

Carbenicillin Indanyl Sodium (Potential for increased risk of bleeding). Products include:
Geocillin Tablets	2009

Carteolol Hydrochloride (Additional reductions in blood pressure may occur). Products include:
Cartrol Tablets	413
Ocupress Ophthalmic Solution, 1% Sterile	297

Chlorothiazide (Additional reductions in blood pressure may occur). Products include:
Aldoclor Tablets	1638
Diupres Tablets	1691
Diuril Oral	1694

Chlorothiazide Sodium (Additional reductions in blood pressure may occur). Products include:
Diuril Sodium Intravenous	1693

Chlorthalidone (Additional reductions in blood pressure may occur). Products include:
Combipres Tablets	682
Tenoretic Tablets	2963
Thalitone	1293

Choline Magnesium Trisalicylate (Potential for increased risk of bleeding). Products include:
Trilisate	2155

Clonidine (Additional reductions in blood pressure may occur). Products include:
Catapres-TTS	680

Clonidine Hydrochloride (Additional reductions in blood pressure may occur). Products include:
Catapres Tablets	679
Combipres Tablets	682

Deserpidine (Additional reductions in blood pressure may occur).
No products indexed under this heading.

Diazoxide (Additional reductions in blood pressure may occur). Products include:
Hyperstat I.V. Injection	2504
Proglycem	575

Diclofenac Potassium (Potential for increased risk of bleeding). Products include:
Cataflam Tablets	833

Diclofenac Sodium (Potential for increased risk of bleeding). Products include:
Voltaren Ophthalmic Sterile Ophthalmic Solution	264
Cataflam/Voltaren/Voltaren-XR	833

Dicumarol (Potential for increased risk of bleeding).
No products indexed under this heading.

Diflunisal (Potential for increased risk of bleeding). Products include:
Dolobid Tablets	1695

Diltiazem Hydrochloride (Additional reductions in blood pressure may occur). Products include:
Cardizem CD Capsules	1251
Cardizem SR Capsules	1255
Cardizem Injectable	1253
Cardizem Tablets	1257
Dilacor XR Extended-release Capsules	2183
Tiazac Capsules	1019

Dipyridamole (Potential for increased risk of bleeding). Products include:
Persantine Tablets	686

Doxazosin Mesylate (Additional reductions in blood pressure may occur). Products include:
Cardura Tablets	1993

Enalapril Maleate (Additional reductions in blood pressure may occur). Products include:
Vaseretic Tablets	1810
Vasotec Tablets	1816

Enalaprilat (Additional reductions in blood pressure may occur). Products include:
Vasotec I.V.	1814

Esmolol Hydrochloride (Additional reductions in blood pressure may occur). Products include:
Brevibloc (esmolol HCl) Injection	1860

IMPORTANT NOTE: Always consult each drug listing in the patient's regimen for possible interactions.

Flolan **Interactions Index** **420**

Ethacrynic Acid (Additional reductions in blood pressure may occur). Products include:
- Edecrin Tablets ... 1698

Felodipine (Additional reductions in blood pressure may occur). Products include:
- Plendil Extended-Release Tablets ... 514

Fenoprofen Calcium (Potential for increased risk of bleeding). Products include:
- Nalfon 200 Pulvules & Nalfon Tablets ... 933

Flurbiprofen (Potential for increased risk of bleeding).
- No products indexed under this heading.

Fosinopril Sodium (Additional reductions in blood pressure may occur). Products include:
- Monopril Tablets ... 762

Furosemide (Additional reductions in blood pressure may occur). Products include:
- Lasix Injection, Oral Solution and Tablets ... 1267

Guanabenz Acetate (Additional reductions in blood pressure may occur).
- No products indexed under this heading.

Guanethidine Monosulfate (Additional reductions in blood pressure may occur). Products include:
- Esimil Tablets ... 840
- Ismelin Tablets ... 845

Hydralazine Hydrochloride (Additional reductions in blood pressure may occur). Products include:
- Apresazide Capsules ... 824
- Apresoline Hydrochloride Tablets ... 826
- Hydralazine Hydrochloride Injection USP ... 2712
- Ser-Ap-Es Tablets ... 867

Hydrochlorothiazide (Additional reductions in blood pressure may occur). Products include:
- Aldactazide Tablets ... 2556
- Aldoril Tablets ... 1644
- Apresazide Capsules ... 824
- Capozide Tablets ... 744
- Dyazide Capsules ... 2653
- Esidrix Tablets ... 839
- Esimil Tablets ... 840
- HydroDIURIL Tablets ... 1716
- Hydropres Tablets ... 1718
- Hyzaar Tablets ... 1720
- Inderide Tablets ... 2838
- Inderide LA Long Acting Capsules ... 2840
- Lopressor HCT Tablets ... 850
- Lotensin HCT Tablets ... 855
- Moduretic Tablets ... 1748
- Oretic Tablets ... 450
- Prinzide Tablets ... 1780
- Ser-Ap-Es Tablets ... 867
- Timolide Tablets ... 1791
- Vaseretic Tablets ... 1810
- Zestoretic Tablets ... 2968
- Ziac ... 1459

Hydroflumethiazide (Additional reductions in blood pressure may occur). Products include:
- Diucardin Tablets ... 2824

Ibuprofen (Potential for increased risk of bleeding). Products include:
- Advil Cold and Sinus Caplets and Tablets ... ▣ 837
- Advil Ibuprofen Tablets, Caplets and Gel Caplets ... ▣ 836
- Children's Motrin Ibuprofen Oral Suspension ... 1558
- IBU Tablets ... 1389
- Ibuprohm ... ▣ 713
- Motrin IB Caplets, Tablets, and Gelcaps ... ▣ 802
- Motrin Ibuprofen Suspension, Oral Drops, Chewable Tablets, Caplets ... 1563
- Nuprin Ibuprofen/Analgesic Tablets & Caplets ... ▣ 645
- Vicks DayQuil SINUS Pressure & PAIN Relief with IBUPROFEN ... ▣ 735

Indapamide (Additional reductions in blood pressure may occur).
- No products indexed under this heading.

Indomethacin (Potential for increased risk of bleeding). Products include:
- Indocin ... 1723

Indomethacin Sodium Trihydrate (Potential for increased risk of bleeding). Products include:
- Indocin I.V. ... 1727

Isradipine (Additional reductions in blood pressure may occur). Products include:
- DynaCirc Capsules ... 2381
- DynaCirc CR Tablets ... 2383

Ketoprofen (Potential for increased risk of bleeding). Products include:
- Actron Caplets and Tablets ... ▣ 608
- Orudis Capsules ... 2874
- Orudis KT ... ▣ 842
- Oruvail Capsules ... 2874

Labetalol Hydrochloride (Additional reductions in blood pressure may occur). Products include:
- Normodyne Injection ... 2519
- Normodyne Tablets ... 2522
- Trandate ... 1158

Lisinopril (Additional reductions in blood pressure may occur). Products include:
- Prinivil Tablets ... 1776
- Prinzide Tablets ... 1780
- Zestoretic Tablets ... 2968
- Zestril Tablets ... 2972

Losartan Potassium (Additional reductions in blood pressure may occur). Products include:
- Cozaar Tablets ... 1668
- Hyzaar Tablets ... 1720

Magnesium Salicylate (Potential for increased risk of bleeding). Products include:
- Backache Caplets ... ▣ 635
- Doan's Extra-Strength Analgesic ... ▣ 653
- Extra Strength Doan's P.M. ... ▣ 653
- Doan's Regular Strength Analgesic ... ▣ 654
- Mobigesic Tablets ... ▣ 607

Mecamylamine Hydrochloride (Additional reductions in blood pressure may occur). Products include:
- Inversine Tablets ... 1729

Meclofenamate Sodium (Potential for increased risk of bleeding).
- No products indexed under this heading.

Mefenamic Acid (Potential for increased risk of bleeding). Products include:
- Ponstel ... 1982

Methyclothiazide (Additional reductions in blood pressure may occur). Products include:
- Enduron Tablets ... 424

Methyldopa (Additional reductions in blood pressure may occur). Products include:
- Aldoclor Tablets ... 1638
- Aldomet Oral ... 1640
- Aldoril Tablets ... 1644

Methyldopate Hydrochloride (Additional reductions in blood pressure may occur). Products include:
- Aldomet Ester HCl Injection ... 1642

Metipranolol Hydrochloride (Additional reductions in blood pressure may occur). Products include:
- OptiPranolol (Metipranolol 0.3%) Sterile Ophthalmic Solution ... ◉ 256

Metolazone (Additional reductions in blood pressure may occur). Products include:
- Mykrox Tablets ... 1617
- Zaroxolyn Tablets ... 1625

Metoprolol Succinate (Additional reductions in blood pressure may occur). Products include:
- Toprol-XL Tablets ... 560

Metoprolol Tartrate (Additional reductions in blood pressure may occur). Products include:
- Lopressor ... 848
- Lopressor HCT Tablets ... 850

Metyrosine (Additional reductions in blood pressure may occur). Products include:
- Demser Capsules ... 1690

Mezlocillin Sodium (Potential for increased risk of bleeding). Products include:
- Mezlin ... 594
- Mezlin Pharmacy Bulk Package ... 597

Minoxidil (Additional reductions in blood pressure may occur).
- No products indexed under this heading.

Moexipril Hydrochloride (Additional reductions in blood pressure may occur). Products include:
- Univasc Tablets ... 2553

Nadolol (Additional reductions in blood pressure may occur).
- No products indexed under this heading.

Nafcillin Sodium (Potential for increased risk of bleeding).
- No products indexed under this heading.

Naproxen (Potential for increased risk of bleeding). Products include:
- Anaprox/Naprosyn ... 2277

Naproxen Sodium (Potential for increased risk of bleeding). Products include:
- Aleve ... 2124
- Anaprox/Naprosyn ... 2277
- Naprelan Tablets ... 2861

Nicardipine Hydrochloride (Additional reductions in blood pressure may occur). Products include:
- Cardene Capsules ... 2261
- Cardene I.V. ... 2815
- Cardene SR Capsules ... 2264

Nifedipine (Additional reductions in blood pressure may occur). Products include:
- Adalat Capsules (10 mg and 20 mg) ... 580
- Adalat CC ... 582
- Procardia Capsules ... 2024
- Procardia XL Extended Release Tablets ... 2026

Nisoldipine (Additional reductions in blood pressure may occur). Products include:
- Sular Tablets ... 2961

Nitroglycerin (Additional reductions in blood pressure may occur). Products include:
- Deponit NTG Transdermal Delivery System ... 2541
- Nitro-Bid IV ... 1270
- Nitro-Bid Ointment ... 1272
- Nitro-Dur (nitroglycerin) Transdermal Infusion System ... 1365
- Nitrolingual Spray ... 2193
- Nitrostat Tablets ... 1981
- Transderm-Nitro Transdermal Therapeutic System ... 878

Penbutolol Sulfate (Additional reductions in blood pressure may occur). Products include:
- Levatol Tablets ... 2547

Penicillin G Benzathine (Potential for increased risk of bleeding). Products include:
- Bicillin C-R Injection ... 2810
- Bicillin C-R 900/300 Injection ... 2812
- Bicillin L-A Injection ... 2813

Penicillin G Procaine (Potential for increased risk of bleeding). Products include:
- Bicillin C-R Injection ... 2810
- Bicillin C-R 900/300 Injection ... 2812

Phenoxybenzamine Hydrochloride (Additional reductions in blood pressure may occur). Products include:
- Dibenzyline Capsules ... 2650

Phentolamine Mesylate (Additional reductions in blood pressure may occur). Products include:
- Regitine Vials ... 864

Phenylbutazone (Potential for increased risk of bleeding).
- No products indexed under this heading.

Pindolol (Additional reductions in blood pressure may occur). Products include:
- Visken Tablets ... 2428

Piroxicam (Potential for increased risk of bleeding). Products include:
- Feldene Capsules ... 2008

Polythiazide (Additional reductions in blood pressure may occur). Products include:
- Minizide Capsules ... 2016

Prazosin Hydrochloride (Additional reductions in blood pressure may occur). Products include:
- Minipress Capsules ... 2015
- Minizide Capsules ... 2016

Propranolol Hydrochloride (Additional reductions in blood pressure may occur). Products include:
- Inderal ... 2834
- Inderal LA Long Acting Capsules ... 2836
- Inderide Tablets ... 2838
- Inderide LA Long Acting Capsules ... 2840

Quinapril Hydrochloride (Additional reductions in blood pressure may occur). Products include:
- Accupril Tablets ... 1950

Ramipril (Additional reductions in blood pressure may occur). Products include:
- Altace Capsules ... 1238

Rauwolfia Serpentina (Additional reductions in blood pressure may occur).
- No products indexed under this heading.

Rescinnamine (Additional reductions in blood pressure may occur).
- No products indexed under this heading.

Reserpine (Additional reductions in blood pressure may occur). Products include:
- Diupres Tablets ... 1691
- Hydropres Tablets ... 1718
- Ser-Ap-Es Tablets ... 867

Salsalate (Potential for increased risk of bleeding). Products include:
- Disalcid ... 1549
- Mono-Gesic Tablets ... 810
- Salflex Tablets ... 791

Sodium Nitroprusside (Additional reductions in blood pressure may occur).
- No products indexed under this heading.

Sotalol Hydrochloride (Additional reductions in blood pressure may occur). Products include:
- Betapace Tablets ... 637

Spirapril Hydrochloride (Additional reductions in blood pressure may occur).
- No products indexed under this heading.

Spironolactone (Additional reductions in blood pressure may occur). Products include:
- Aldactazide Tablets ... 2556
- Aldactone Tablets ... 2558

Sulindac (Potential for increased risk of bleeding). Products include:
- Clinoril Tablets ... 1658

421 **Interactions Index** **Florinef Acetate**

Terazosin Hydrochloride (Additional reductions in blood pressure may occur). Products include:
Hytrin Capsules 434
Ticarcillin Disodium (Potential for increased risk of bleeding). Products include:
Ticar for Injection 2704
Timentin for Injection 2706
Ticlopidine Hydrochloride (Potential for increased risk of bleeding). Products include:
Ticlid Tablets 2317
Timolol Maleate (Additional reductions in blood pressure may occur). Products include:
Blocadren Tablets 1654
Timolide Tablets 1791
Timoptic in Ocudose 1796
Timoptic Sterile Ophthalmic Solution 1794
Timoptic-XE 1798
Tolmetin Sodium (Potential for increased risk of bleeding). Products include:
Tolectin (200, 400 and 600 mg) .. 1591
Torsemide (Additional reductions in blood pressure may occur). Products include:
Demadex Tablets and Injection 691
Triamterene (Additional reductions in blood pressure may occur). Products include:
Dyazide Capsules 2653
Dyrenium Capsules 2655
Trimethaphan Camsylate (Additional reductions in blood pressure may occur).
No products indexed under this heading.
Verapamil Hydrochloride (Additional reductions in blood pressure may occur). Products include:
Calan SR Caplets 2571
Calan Tablets 2568
Covera-HS Tablets 2573
Isoptin Injectable 1391
Isoptin Oral Tablets 1393
Isoptin SR Tablets 1395
Verelan Capsules 1455
Warfarin Sodium (Potential for increased risk of bleeding). Products include:
Coumadin 941

FLONASE NASAL SPRAY
(Fluticasone Propionate) 1088
None cited in PDR database.

FLORAJEN
(Lactobacillus Acidophilus) 602
None cited in PDR database.

FLORICAL CAPSULES AND TABLETS
(Sodium Fluoride, Calcium Carbonate) 1825
None cited in PDR database.

FLORINEF ACETATE TABLETS
(Fludrocortisone Acetate) 506
May interact with barbiturates, estrogens, androgens, potassium-depleting diuretics, loop diuretics, cardiac glycosides, oral anticoagulants, oral hypoglycemic agents, insulin, and certain other agents. Compounds in these categories include:

Acarbose (Diminished antidiabetic effect; monitor symptoms of hyperglycemia). Products include:
Precose 604
Amphotericin B (Potential for enhanced hypokalemia; serum potassium levels should be monitored frequently). Products include:
Abelcet Injection 1540
Fungizone Intravenous 507
Fungizone Oral Suspension 704
Aprobarbital (Increased metabolic clearance of fludrocortisone acetate because of the induction of hepatic enzymes).
No products indexed under this heading.
Aspirin (Increased ulcerogenic effect; decreased pharmacologic effect of aspirin). Products include:
Alka-Seltzer Cherry Effervescent Antacid and Pain Reliever 609
Alka-Seltzer Extra Strength Effervescent Antacid and Pain Reliever 609
Alka-Seltzer Lemon Lime Effervescent Antacid and Pain Reliever 609
Alka-Seltzer Original Effervescent Antacid and Pain Reliever 609
Alka-Seltzer Plus 611
Alka-Seltzer Plus Sinus Medicine .. 611
Ascriptin 650
Arthritis Strength BC Powder 631
BC Cold Powder Multi-Symptom Formula (Cold-Sinus-Allergy) 631
BC Cold Powder Non-Drowsy Formula (Cold-Sinus) 631
BC Powder 631
Genuine Bayer Aspirin Tablets & Caplets 618
Extra Strength Bayer Arthritis Pain Regimen Formula 615
Extra Strength Bayer Aspirin Caplets & Tablets 617
Extended-Release Bayer 8-Hour Aspirin 616
Extra Strength Bayer Plus Aspirin Caplets 617
Extra Strength Bayer PM Aspirin Plus Sleep Aid 617
Aspirin Regimen Bayer 81 mg Tablets with Calcium 615
Aspirin Regimen Bayer Adult Low Strength 81 mg Tablets 613
Aspirin Regimen Bayer Children's Chewable Aspirin 616
Aspirin Regimen Bayer Regular Strength 325 mg Caplets 613
Bufferin Analgesic Tablets 636
Arthritis Strength Bufferin Analgesic Caplets 637
Extra Strength Bufferin Analgesic Tablets 637
Cama Arthritis Pain Reliever 748
Darvon Compound-65 Pulvules 1475
Easprin 1971
Ecotrin 2625
Ecotrin Enteric Coated Aspirin Maximum Strength Tablets and Caplets 775
Ecotrin Enteric Coated Aspirin Regular Strength Tablets 2625
Empirin Aspirin Tablets 818
Excedrin Extra-Strength Analgesic Tablets, Caplets, and Geltabs 734
Fiorinal Capsules 2388
Fiorinal with Codeine Capsules 2390
Fiorinal Tablets 2388
Goody's Extra Strength Headache Powders 632
Goody's Extra Strength Pain Relief Tablets 632
Halfprin Tablets 1413
Norgesic 1554
Percodan Tablets 955
Percodan-Demi Tablets 956
Robaxisal Tablets 2246
Soma Compound w/Codeine Tablets 2784
Soma Compound Tablets 2783
St. Joseph Adult Chewable Aspirin (81 mg.) 768
Talwin Compound 2466
Vanquish Analgesic Caplets 627
Bendroflumethiazide (Potential for enhanced hypokalemia; serum potassium levels should be monitored frequently).
No products indexed under this heading.
Bumetanide (Potential for enhanced hypokalemia; serum potassium levels should be monitored frequently). Products include:
Bumex 2260
Butabarbital (Increased metabolic clearance of fludrocortisone acetate because of the induction of hepatic enzymes).
No products indexed under this heading.
Butalbital (Increased metabolic clearance of fludrocortisone acetate because of the induction of hepatic enzymes). Products include:
Axocet Capsules 2469
Esgic-plus Capsules 1012
Esgic-plus Tablets 1012
Fioricet Tablets 2386
Fioricet with Codeine Capsules 2387
Fiorinal Capsules 2388
Fiorinal with Codeine Capsules 2390
Fiorinal Tablets 2388
Phrenilin 790
Sedapap Tablets 50 mg/650 mg .. 1826
Chlorothiazide (Potential for enhanced hypokalemia; serum potassium levels should be monitored frequently). Products include:
Aldoclor Tablets 1638
Diupres Tablets 1691
Diuril Oral 1694
Chlorothiazide Sodium (Potential for enhanced hypokalemia; serum potassium levels should be monitored frequently). Products include:
Diuril Sodium Intravenous 1693
Chlorotrianisene (Increased levels of corticosteroid-binding globulin, thereby increasing the bound (inactive) fraction).
No products indexed under this heading.
Chlorpropamide (Diminished antidiabetic effect; monitor symptoms of hyperglycemia). Products include:
Diabinese Tablets 2002
Deslanoside (Enhanced possibility of arrhythmias or digitalis toxicity associated with hypokalemia).
No products indexed under this heading.
Dicumarol (Decreased prothrombin time response).
No products indexed under this heading.
Dienestrol (Increased levels of corticosteroid-binding globulin, thereby increasing the bound (inactive) fraction). Products include:
Ortho Dienestrol Cream 1922
Diethylstilbestrol (Increased levels of corticosteroid-binding globulin, thereby increasing the bound (inactive) fraction). Products include:
Diethylstilbestrol Tablets 1477
Digitoxin (Enhanced possibility of arrhythmias or digitalis toxicity associated with hypokalemia). Products include:
Crystodigin Tablets 1472
Digoxin (Enhanced possibility of arrhythmias or digitalis toxicity associated with hypokalemia). Products include:
Lanoxicaps 1110
Lanoxin Elixir Pediatric 1113
Lanoxin Injection 1116
Lanoxin Injection Pediatric 1119
Lanoxin Tablets 1121
Estradiol (Increased levels of corticosteroid-binding globulin, thereby increasing the bound (inactive) fraction). Products include:
Climara Transdermal System 640
Estrace Cream and Tablets 751
Estraderm Transdermal System 842
Estring Vaginal Ring 2086
Vivelle Transdermal System 880
Estrogens, Conjugated (Increased levels of corticosteroid-binding globulin, thereby increasing the bound (inactive) fraction). Products include:
PMB 200 and PMB 400 2890
Premarin Intravenous 2893
Premarin Tablets 2896
Premarin Vaginal Cream 2898
Premphase 2900
Prempro 2905
Estrogens, Esterified (Increased levels of corticosteroid-binding globulin, thereby increasing the bound (inactive) fraction). Products include:
ESTRATAB Tablets (0.3, 0.625, 1.25, 2.5 mg) 2715
Estratest 2718
Menest Tablets 2671
Estropipate (Increased levels of corticosteroid-binding globulin, thereby increasing the bound (inactive) fraction). Products include:
Ogen Tablets 2103
Ogen Vaginal Cream 2106
Ortho-Est 1925
Ethacrynic Acid (Potential for enhanced hypokalemia; serum potassium levels should be monitored frequently). Products include:
Edecrin Tablets 1698
Ethinyl Estradiol (Increased levels of corticosteroid-binding globulin, thereby increasing the bound (inactive) fraction). Products include:
Brevicon 2563
Demulen 2580
Desogen Tablets 1867
Levlen/Tri-Levlen 646
Lo/Ovral Tablets 2852
Lo/Ovral-28 Tablets 2857
Modicon 1928
Nordette-21 Tablets 2863
Nordette-28 Tablets 2866
Norinyl 2563
Ortho-Cept 1907
Ortho-Cyclen/Ortho-Tri-Cyclen 1914
Ortho-Novum 1928
Ortho-Cyclen/Ortho Tri-Cyclen 1914
Ovcon 765
Ovral Tablets 2877
Ovral-28 Tablets 2878
Levlen/Tri-Levlen 646
Tri-Norinyl 2607
Triphasil-21 Tablets 2919
Triphasil-28 Tablets 2924
Fluoxymesterone (Enhanced tendency toward edema). Products include:
Halotestin Tablets 2095
Fosphenytoin Sodium (Increased metabolic clearance of fludrocortisone acetate because of the induction of hepatic enzymes). Products include:
Cerebyx Injection 1956
Furosemide (Potential for enhanced hypokalemia; serum potassium levels should be monitored frequently). Products include:
Lasix Injection, Oral Solution and Tablets 1267
Glimepiride (Diminished antidiabetic effect; monitor symptoms of hyperglycemia). Products include:
Amaryl Tablets 1241
Glipizide (Diminished antidiabetic effect; monitor symptoms of hyperglycemia). Products include:
Glucotrol Tablets 2011
Glucotrol XL Extended Release Tablets 2012
Glyburide (Diminished antidiabetic effect; monitor symptoms of hyperglycemia). Products include:
DiaBeta Tablets 1265
Glynase PresTab Tablets 2091
Micronase Tablets 2099

IMPORTANT NOTE: Always consult each drug listing in the patient's regimen for possible interactions.

Hydrochlorothiazide (Potential for enhanced hypokalemia; serum potassium levels should be monitored frequently). Products include:

Aldactazide Tablets ... 2556
Aldoril Tablets ... 1644
Apresazide Capsules ... 824
Capozide Tablets ... 744
Dyazide Capsules ... 2653
Esidrix Tablets ... 839
Esimil Tablets ... 840
HydroDIURIL Tablets ... 1716
Hydropres Tablets ... 1718
Hyzaar Tablets ... 1720
Inderide Tablets ... 2838
Inderide LA Long Acting Capsules .. 2840
Lopressor HCT Tablets ... 850
Lotensin HCT Tablets ... 855
Moduretic Tablets ... 1748
Oretic Tablets ... 450
Prinzide Tablets ... 1780
Ser-Ap-Es Tablets ... 867
Timolide Tablets ... 1791
Vaseretic Tablets ... 1810
Zestoretic Tablets ... 2968
Ziac ... 1459

Hydroflumethiazide (Potential for enhanced hypokalemia; serum potassium levels should be monitored frequently). Products include:

Diucardin Tablets ... 2824

Insulin, Human (Diminished antidiabetic effect; monitor symptoms of hyperglycemia).

No products indexed under this heading.

Insulin, Human Isophane Suspension (Diminished antidiabetic effect; monitor symptoms of hyperglycemia). Products include:

Novolin N Human Insulin 10 ml Vials ... 1846

Insulin, Human NPH (Diminished antidiabetic effect; monitor symptoms of hyperglycemia). Products include:

Humulin N, 100 Units ... 1495
Novolin N PenFill 1.5 ml Cartridges Durable Insulin Delivery System ... 1849
Novolin N Prefilled Syringe Disposable Insulin Delivery System ... 1850

Insulin, Human Regular (Diminished antidiabetic effect; monitor symptoms of hyperglycemia). Products include:

Humulin R, 100 Units ... 1497
Novolin R Human Insulin 10 ml Vials ... 1846
Novolin R PenFill 1.5 ml Cartridges Durable Insulin Delivery System ... 1849
Novolin R Prefilled Syringe Disposable Insulin Delivery System ... 1850
Velosulin BR Human Insulin 10 ml Vials ... 1847

Insulin, Human, Zinc Suspension (Diminished antidiabetic effect; monitor symptoms of hyperglycemia). Products include:

Humulin L, 100 Units ... 1494
Humulin U, 100 Units ... 1498
Novolin L Human Insulin 10 ml Vials ... 1846

Insulin Lispro, Human (Diminished antidiabetic effect; monitor symptoms of hyperglycemia). Products include:

Humalog Injection ... 1488

Insulin, NPH (Diminished antidiabetic effect; monitor symptoms of hyperglycemia). Products include:

NPH, 100 Units ... 1502
Pork NPH, 100 Units ... 1506
Purified Pork NPH Isophane Insulin ... 1852

Insulin, Regular (Diminished antidiabetic effect; monitor symptoms of hyperglycemia). Products include:

Regular, 100 Units ... 1503
Pork Regular, 100 Units ... 1507
Pork Regular (Concentrated), 500 Units ... 1508
Purified Pork Regular Insulin ... 1852

Insulin, Zinc Crystals (Diminished antidiabetic effect; monitor symptoms of hyperglycemia). Products include:

NPH, 100 Units ... 1502

Insulin, Zinc Suspension (Diminished antidiabetic effect; monitor symptoms of hyperglycemia). Products include:

Iletin I ... 1501
Lente, 100 Units ... 1501
Iletin II ... 1504
Pork Lente, 100 Units ... 1504
Purified Pork Lente Insulin ... 1852

Mephobarbital (Increased metabolic clearance of fludrocortisone acetate because of the induction of hepatic enzymes). Products include:

Mebaral Tablets ... 2452

Metformin Hydrochloride (Diminished antidiabetic effect; monitor symptoms of hyperglycemia). Products include:

Glucophage Tablets ... 754

Methandrostinolone (Enhanced tendency toward edema).

Methyclothiazide (Potential for enhanced hypokalemia; serum potassium levels should be monitored frequently). Products include:

Enduron Tablets ... 424

Methyltestosterone (Enhanced tendency toward edema). Products include:

Android Capsules, 10 mg ... 1297
Estratest ... 2718
Testred Capsules, 10 mg ... 1308

Norethandrolone (Enhanced tendency toward edema).

Oxandrolone (Enhanced tendency toward edema). Products include:

Oxandrin ... 783

Oxymetholone (Enhanced tendency toward edema).

No products indexed under this heading.

Pentobarbital Sodium (Increased metabolic clearance of fludrocortisone acetate because of the induction of hepatic enzymes). Products include:

Nembutal Sodium Capsules ... 440
Nembutal Sodium Solution ... 442
Nembutal Sodium Suppositories ... 444

Phenobarbital (Increased metabolic clearance of fludrocortisone acetate because of the induction of hepatic enzymes). Products include:

Arco-Lase Plus Tablets ... 513
Bellergal-S Tablets ... 2375
Donnatal ... 2234
Donnatal Extentabs ... 2234
Donnatal Tablets ... 2234
Phenobarbital Elixir and Tablets ... 1523
Quadrinal Tablets ... 1398

Phenytoin (Increased metabolic clearance of fludrocortisone acetate because of the induction of hepatic enzymes). Products include:

Dilantin Infatabs ... 1967
Dilantin-125 Suspension ... 1969

Phenytoin Sodium (Increased metabolic clearance of fludrocortisone acetate because of the induction of hepatic enzymes). Products include:

Dilantin Kapseals ... 1965

Polyestradiol Phosphate (Increased levels of corticosteroid-binding globulin, thereby increasing the bound (inactive) fraction).

No products indexed under this heading.

Polythiazide (Potential for enhanced hypokalemia; serum potassium levels should be monitored frequently). Products include:

Minizide Capsules ... 2016

Quinestrol (Increased levels of corticosteroid-binding globulin, thereby increasing the bound (inactive) fraction).

No products indexed under this heading.

Rifampin (Increased metabolic clearance of fludrocortisone acetate because of the induction of hepatic enzymes). Products include:

Rifadin ... 1276
Rifamate Capsules ... 1278
Rifater ... 1280
Rimactane Capsules ... 865

Secobarbital Sodium (Increased metabolic clearance of fludrocortisone acetate because of the induction of hepatic enzymes). Products include:

Seconal Sodium Pulvules ... 1529

Stanozolol (Enhanced tendency toward edema). Products include:

Winstrol Tablets ... 2468

Thiamylal Sodium (Increased metabolic clearance of fludrocortisone acetate because of the induction of hepatic enzymes).

No products indexed under this heading.

Tolazamide (Diminished antidiabetic effect; monitor symptoms of hyperglycemia).

No products indexed under this heading.

Tolbutamide (Diminished antidiabetic effect; monitor symptoms of hyperglycemia).

No products indexed under this heading.

Torsemide (Potential for enhanced hypokalemia; serum potassium levels should be monitored frequently). Products include:

Demadex Tablets and Injection ... 691

Warfarin Sodium (Decreased prothrombin time response). Products include:

Coumadin ... 941

FLORONE CREAM 0.05%
(Diflorasone Diacetate) ... 921
None cited in PDR database.

FLORONE E EMOLLIENT CREAM 0.05%
(Diflorasone Diacetate) ... 921
None cited in PDR database.

FLORONE OINTMENT 0.05%
(Diflorasone Diacetate) ... 921
None cited in PDR database.

FLOVENT 44 MCG INHALATION AEROSOL
(Fluticasone Propionate) ... 1089
None cited in PDR database.

FLOVENT 110 MCG INHALATION AEROSOL
(Fluticasone Propionate) ... 1089
None cited in PDR database.

FLOVENT 220 MCG INHALATION AEROSOL
(Fluticasone Propionate) ... 1089
None cited in PDR database.

FLOXIN I.V.
(Ofloxacin) ... 1580
May interact with oral anticoagulants, xanthine bronchodilators, nonsteroidal anti-inflammatory agents, insulin, oral hypoglycemic agents, drugs which undergo biotransformation by cytochrome p-450 mixed function oxidase, and certain other agents. Compounds in these categories include:

Acarbose (Potentiation of hypoglycemic action). Products include:

Precose ... 604

Aminophylline (Increased steady-state theophylline levels; concurrent therapy may prolong the half-life of theophylline, elevate serum theophylline levels, and increase the risk of theophylline-related adverse reactions).

No products indexed under this heading.

Chlorpropamide (Potentiation of hypoglycemic action). Products include:

Diabinese Tablets ... 2002

Cimetidine (May interfere with the elimination of quinolones resulting in significant increase in half-life and AUC of some quinolones; this interaction has not been studied with ofloxacin). Products include:

Tagamet HB Tablets ... ▣ 786
Tagamet Tablets ... 2694

Cimetidine Hydrochloride (May interfere with the elimination of quinolones resulting in significant increase in half-life and AUC of some quinolones; this interaction has not been studied with ofloxacin). Products include:

Tagamet ... 2694

Cyclosporine (Potential for prolonged half-life and elevated serum levels of cyclosporine). Products include:

Neoral ... 2405
Sandimmune ... 2416

Diclofenac Potassium (Increased risk of CNS stimulation and convulsive seizures). Products include:

Cataflam Tablets ... 833

Diclofenac Sodium (Increased risk of CNS stimulation and convulsive seizures). Products include:

Voltaren Ophthalmic Sterile Ophthalmic Solution ... ⊙ 264
Cataflam/Voltaren/Voltaren-XR ... 833

Dicumarol (Potential for enhanced effects of the oral anticoagulant).

No products indexed under this heading.

Drugs which undergo biotransformation by cytochrome P-450 mixed function oxidase (Quinolone antibacterials inhibit cytochrome P450 enzyme activity resulting in prolonged half-life for some drugs that are also metabolized by this system).

Dyphylline (Increased steady-state theophylline levels; concurrent therapy may prolong the half-life of theophylline, elevate serum theophylline levels, and increase the risk of theophylline-related adverse reactions). Products include:

Lufyllin & Lufyllin-400 Tablets ... 2778
Lufyllin-GG Elixir & Tablets ... 2779

Etodolac (Increased risk of CNS stimulation and convulsive seizures). Products include:

Lodine Capsules and Tablets ... 2849

Fenbufen (Increased risk of CNS stimulation convulsive seizures).

Fenoprofen Calcium (Increased risk of CNS stimulation and convulsive seizures). Products include:

Nalfon 200 Pulvules & Nalfon Tablets ... 933

Flurbiprofen (Increased risk of CNS stimulation and convulsive seizures).

No products indexed under this heading.

(▣ Described in PDR For Nonprescription Drugs) (⊙ Described in PDR For Ophthalmology)

Glimepiride (Potentiation of hypoglycemic action). Products include:
Amaryl Tablets 1241

Glipizide (Potentiation of hypoglycemic action). Products include:
Glucotrol Tablets 2011
Glucotrol XL Extended Release Tablets 2012

Glyburide (Potentiation of hypoglycemic action). Products include:
DiaBeta Tablets 1265
Glynase PresTab Tablets 2091
Micronase Tablets 2099

Ibuprofen (Increased risk of CNS stimulation and convulsive seizures). Products include:
Advil Cold and Sinus Caplets and Tablets 837
Advil Ibuprofen Tablets, Caplets and Gel Caplets 836
Children's Motrin Ibuprofen Oral Suspension 1558
IBU Tablets 1389
Ibuprohm 713
Motrin IB Caplets, Tablets, and Gelcaps 802
Motrin Ibuprofen Suspension, Oral Drops, Chewable Tablets, Caplets 1563
Nuprin Ibuprofen/Analgesic Tablets & Caplets 645
Vicks DayQuil SINUS Pressure & PAIN Relief with IBUPROFEN 735

Indomethacin (Increased risk of CNS stimulation and convulsive seizures). Products include:
Indocin 1723

Indomethacin Sodium Trihydrate (Increased risk of CNS stimulation and convulsive seizures). Products include:
Indocin I.V. 1727

Insulin, Human (Potentiation of hypoglycemic action).
No products indexed under this heading.

Insulin, Human Isophane Suspension (Potentiation of hypoglycemic action). Products include:
Novolin N Human Insulin 10 ml Vials 1846

Insulin, Human NPH (Potentiation of hypoglycemic action). Products include:
Humulin N, 100 Units 1495
Novolin N PenFill 1.5 ml Cartridges Durable Insulin Delivery System 1849
Novolin N Prefilled Syringe Disposable Insulin Delivery System 1850

Insulin, Human Regular (Potentiation of hypoglycemic action). Products include:
Humulin R, 100 Units 1497
Novolin R Human Insulin 10 ml Vials 1846
Novolin R PenFill 1.5 ml Cartridges Durable Insulin Delivery System 1849
Novolin R Prefilled Syringe Disposable Insulin Delivery System 1850
Velosulin BR Human Insulin 10 ml Vials 1847

Insulin, Human, Zinc Suspension (Potentiation of hypoglycemic action). Products include:
Humulin L, 100 Units 1494
Humulin U, 100 Units 1498
Novolin L Human Insulin 10 ml Vials 1846

Insulin Lispro, Human (Potentiation of hypoglycemic action). Products include:
Humalog Injection 1488

Insulin, NPH (Potentiation of hypoglycemic action). Products include:
NPH, 100 Units 1502
Pork NPH, 100 Units 1506
Purified Pork NPH Isophane Insulin 1852

Insulin, Regular (Potentiation of hypoglycemic action). Products include:
Regular, 100 Units 1503
Pork Regular, 100 Units 1507
Pork Regular (Concentrated), 500 Units 1508
Purified Pork Regular Insulin 1852

Insulin, Zinc Crystals (Potentiation of hypoglycemic action). Products include:
NPH, 100 Units 1502

Insulin, Zinc Suspension (Potentiation of hypoglycemic action). Products include:
Iletin I 1501
Lente, 100 Units 1501
Iletin II 1504
Pork Lente, 100 Units 1504
Purified Pork Lente Insulin 1852

Ketoprofen (Increased risk of CNS stimulation and convulsive seizures). Products include:
Actron Caplets and Tablets 608
Orudis Capsules 2874
Orudis KT 842
Oruvail Capsules 2874

Ketorolac Tromethamine (Increased risk of CNS stimulation and convulsive seizures). Products include:
Acular Sterile Ophthalmic Solution 470
Toradol 2319

Meclofenamate Sodium (Increased risk of CNS stimulation and convulsive seizures).
No products indexed under this heading.

Mefenamic Acid (Increased risk of CNS stimulation and convulsive seizures). Products include:
Ponstel 1982

Metformin Hydrochloride (Potentiation of hypoglycemic action). Products include:
Glucophage Tablets 754

Nabumetone (Increased risk of CNS stimulation and convulsive seizures). Products include:
Relafen Tablets 2688

Naproxen (Increased risk of CNS stimulation and convulsive seizures). Products include:
Anaprox/Naprosyn 2277

Naproxen Sodium (Increased risk of CNS stimulation and convulsive seizures). Products include:
Aleve 2124
Anaprox/Naprosyn 2277
Naprelan Tablets 2861

Oxaprozin (Increased risk of CNS stimulation and convulsive seizures). Products include:
Daypro Caplets 2578

Phenylbutazone (Increased risk of CNS stimulation and convulsive seizures).
No products indexed under this heading.

Piroxicam (Increased risk of CNS stimulation and convulsive seizures). Products include:
Feldene Capsules 2008

Probenecid (Potential to affect renal tubular secretion; this interaction has not been studied with ofloxacin). Products include:
Benemid Tablets 1651
ColBENEMID Tablets 1662

Sulindac (Increased risk of CNS stimulation and convulsive seizures). Products include:
Clinoril Tablets 1658

Theophylline (Increased steady-state theophylline levels; concurrent therapy may prolong the half-life of theophylline, elevate serum theophylline levels, and increase the risk of theophylline-related adverse reactions). Products include:
Marax Tablets & DF Syrup 2015
Quibron 2227

Theophylline Anhydrous (Increased steady-state theophylline levels; concurrent therapy may prolong the half-life of theophylline, elevate serum theophylline levels, and increase the risk of theophylline-related adverse reactions). Products include:
Aerolate 1003
Primatene Tablets 844
Respbid Tablets 687
Slo-bid Gyrocaps 2201
Theo-24 Extended Release Capsules 2753
Theo-Dur Extended-Release Tablets 1367
Theo-X Extended-Release Tablets .. 793
Uni-Dur Extended-Release Tablets .. 1374
Uniphyl 400 mg and 600 mg Tablets 2157

Theophylline Calcium Salicylate (Increased steady-state theophylline levels; concurrent therapy may prolong the half-life of theophylline, elevate serum theophylline levels, and increase the risk of theophylline-related adverse reactions). Products include:
Quadrinal Tablets 1398

Theophylline Sodium Glycinate (Increased steady-state theophylline levels; concurrent therapy may prolong the half-life of theophylline, elevate serum theophylline levels, and increase the risk of theophylline-related adverse reactions).
No products indexed under this heading.

Tolazamide (Potentiation of hypoglycemic action).
No products indexed under this heading.

Tolbutamide (Potentiation of hypoglycemic action).
No products indexed under this heading.

Tolmetin Sodium (Increased risk of CNS stimulation and convulsive seizures). Products include:
Tolectin (200, 400 and 600 mg) .. 1591

Warfarin Sodium (Potential for enhanced effects of the oral anticoagulant). Products include:
Coumadin 941

FLOXIN TABLETS (200 MG, 300 MG, 400 MG)
(Ofloxacin) 1577
May interact with xanthine bronchodilators, antacids containing aluminium, calcium and magnesium, oral anticoagulants, non-steroidal anti-inflammatory agents, insulin, oral hypoglycemic agents, drugs which undergo biotransformation by cytochrome p-450 mixed function oxidase, and certain other agents. Compounds in these categories include:

Acarbose (Potentiation of hypoglycemic action). Products include:
Precose 604

Aluminum Carbonate (May substantially interfere with the absorption of quinolones). Products include:
Basaljel Capsules 2810
Basaljel Suspension 2810
Basaljel Tablets 2810

Aluminum Hydroxide (May substantially interfere with the absorption of quinolones). Products include:
ALternaGEL Liquid 1358
Maximum Strength Ascriptin 650
Cama Arthritis Pain Reliever 748
Gaviscon Extra Strength Relief Formula Antacid Tablets 778
Gaviscon Extra Strength Relief Formula Liquid Antacid 779
Gaviscon Liquid Antacid 779
Gelusil Antacid-Anti-gas Liquid ... 819
Gelusil Antacid-Anti-gas Tablets .. 819
Maalox Antacid/Anti-Gas Tablets .. 889
Maalox Heartburn Relief Suspension 658
Maalox Antacid Liquid 888
Extra Strength Maalox Antacid/ Anti-Gas Liquid and Tablets 888
Mylanta 1359
Tempo Soft Antacid 799

Aluminum Hydroxide Gel (May substantially interfere with the absorption of quinolones). Products include:
ALternaGEL Liquid 675
Aludrox Oral Suspension 850
Amphojel Suspension 2802
Amphojel Suspension without Flavor 2802
Amphojel Tablets 2802
Ascriptin 650
Gaviscon Antacid Tablets 778
Gaviscon-2 Antacid Tablets 779
Mylanta Liquid 676
Mylanta Double Strength Liquid .. 676
Nephrox Suspension 671

Aminophylline (Increased steady-state theophylline levels; concurrent therapy may prolong the half-life of theophylline, elevate serum theophylline levels, and increase the risk of theophylline-related adverse reactions).
No products indexed under this heading.

Chlorpropamide (Potentiation of hypoglycemic action). Products include:
Diabinese Tablets 2002

Cimetidine (May interfere with the elimination of quinolones resulting in significant increase in half-life and AUC of some quinolones; this interaction has not been studied with ofloxacin). Products include:
Tagamet HB Tablets 786
Tagamet Tablets 2694

Cimetidine Hydrochloride (May interfere with the elimination of quinolones resulting in significant increase in half-life and AUC of some quinolones; this interaction has not been studied with ofloxacin). Products include:
Tagamet 2694

Cyclosporine (Potential for prolonged half-life and elevated serum levels of cyclosporine). Products include:
Neoral 2405
Sandimmune 2416

Diclofenac Potassium (Increased risk of CNS stimulation and convulsive seizures). Products include:
Cataflam Tablets 833

Diclofenac Sodium (Increased risk of CNS stimulation and convulsive seizures). Products include:
Voltaren Ophthalmic Sterile Ophthalmic Solution 264
Cataflam/Voltaren/Voltaren-XR 833

Dicumarol (Potential for enhanced effects of the oral anticoagulant).
No products indexed under this heading.

Drugs which undergo biotransformation by cytochrome P-450 mixed function oxidase (Quinolone antibacterials inhibit cytochrome P450 enzyme activity

IMPORTANT NOTE: Always consult each drug listing in the patient's regimen for possible interactions.

resulting in prolonged half-life for some drugs that are also metabolized by this system).

Dyphylline (Increased steady-state theophylline levels; concurrent therapy may prolong the half-life of theophylline, elevate serum theophylline levels, and increase the risk of theophylline-related adverse reactions). Products include:
- Lufyllin & Lufyllin-400 Tablets 2778
- Lufyllin-GG Elixir & Tablets 2779

Etodolac (Increased risk of CNS stimulation and convulsive seizures). Products include:
- Lodine Capsules and Tablets 2849

Fenoprofen Calcium (Increased risk of CNS stimulation and convulsive seizures). Products include:
- Nalfon 200 Pulvules & Nalfon Tablets 933

Flurbiprofen (Increased risk of CNS stimulation and convulsive seizures).
- No products indexed under this heading.

Glimepiride (Potentiation of hypoglycemic action). Products include:
- Amaryl Tablets 1241

Glipizide (Potentiation of hypoglycemic action). Products include:
- Glucotrol Tablets 2011
- Glucotrol XL Extended Release Tablets 2012

Glyburide (Potentiation of hypoglycemic action). Products include:
- DiaBeta Tablets 1265
- Glynase PresTab Tablets 2091
- Micronase Tablets 2099

Ibuprofen (Increased risk of CNS stimulation and convulsive seizures). Products include:
- Advil Cold and Sinus Caplets and Tablets .... ND 837
- Advil Ibuprofen Tablets, Caplets and Gel Caplets .... ND 836
- Children's Motrin Ibuprofen Oral Suspension 1558
- IBU Tablets 1389
- Ibuprohm .... ND 713
- Motrin IB Caplets, Tablets, and Gelcaps .... ND 802
- Motrin Ibuprofen Suspension, Oral Drops, Chewable Tablets, Caplets 1563
- Nuprin Ibuprofen/Analgesic Tablets & Caplets .... ND 645
- Vicks DayQuil SINUS Pressure & PAIN Relief with IBUPROFEN .... ND 735

Indomethacin (Increased risk of CNS stimulation and convulsive seizures). Products include:
- Indocin 1723

Indomethacin Sodium Trihydrate (Increased risk of CNS stimulation and convulsive seizures). Products include:
- Indocin I.V. 1727

Insulin, Human (Potentiation of hypoglycemic action).
- No products indexed under this heading.

Insulin, Human Isophane Suspension (Potentiation of hypoglycemic action). Products include:
- Novolin N Human Insulin 10 ml Vials 1846

Insulin, Human NPH (Potentiation of hypoglycemic action). Products include:
- Humulin N, 100 Units 1495
- Novolin N PenFill 1.5 ml Cartridges Durable Insulin Delivery System 1849
- Novolin N Prefilled Syringe Disposable Insulin Delivery System 1850

Insulin, Human Regular (Potentiation of hypoglycemic action). Products include:
- Humulin R, 100 Units 1497
- Novolin R Human Insulin 10 ml Vials 1846
- Novolin R PenFill 1.5 ml Cartridges Durable Insulin Delivery System 1849
- Novolin R Prefilled Syringe Disposable Insulin Delivery System 1850
- Velosulin BR Human Insulin 10 ml Vials 1847

Insulin, Human, Zinc Suspension (Potentiation of hypoglycemic action). Products include:
- Humulin L, 100 Units 1494
- Humulin U, 100 Units 1498
- Novolin L Human Insulin 10 ml Vials 1846

Insulin Lispro, Human (Potentiation of hypoglycemic action). Products include:
- Humalog Injection 1488

Insulin, NPH (Potentiation of hypoglycemic action). Products include:
- NPH, 100 Units 1502
- Pork NPH, 100 Units 1506
- Purified Pork NPH Isophane Insulin 1852

Insulin, Regular (Potentiation of hypoglycemic action). Products include:
- Regular, 100 Units 1503
- Pork Regular, 100 Units 1507
- Pork Regular (Concentrated), 500 Units 1508
- Purified Pork Regular Insulin 1852

Insulin, Zinc Crystals (Potentiation of hypoglycemic action). Products include:
- NPH, 100 Units 1502

Insulin, Zinc Suspension (Potentiation of hypoglycemic action). Products include:
- Iletin I 1501
- Lente, 100 Units 1501
- Iletin II 1504
- Pork Lente, 100 Units 1504
- Purified Pork Lente Insulin 1852

Ketoprofen (Increased risk of CNS stimulation and convulsive seizures). Products include:
- Actron Caplets and Tablets .... ND 608
- Orudis Capsules 2874
- Orudis KT .... ND 842
- Oruvail Capsules 2874

Ketorolac Tromethamine (Increased risk of CNS stimulation and convulsive seizures). Products include:
- Acular Sterile Ophthalmic Solution 470
- Toradol 2319

Magaldrate (May substantially interfere with the absorption of quinolones).
- No products indexed under this heading.

Magnesium Hydroxide (May substantially interfere with the absorption of quinolones). Products include:
- Aludrox Oral Suspension .... ND 850
- Ascriptin .... ND 650
- Di-Gel Antacid/Anti-Gas .... ND 762
- Gelusil Antacid-Anti-gas Liquid .... ND 819
- Gelusil Antacid-Anti-gas Tablets .... ND 819
- Maalox Antacid/Anti-Gas Tablets 889
- Maalox Antacid Liquid 888
- Extra Strength Maalox Antacid/Anti-Gas Liquid and Tablets 888
- Mylanta Fast-Acting 1359
- Mylanta Gelcaps Antacid .... ND 678
- Fast-Acting Mylanta Liquid Antacid 1359
- Mylanta Tablets .... ND 677
- Maximum-Strength Fast-Acting Mylanta Liquid Antacid 1359
- Mylanta Double Strength Tablets .. ND 677
- Phillips' Milk of Magnesia Liquid .... ND 627
- Rolaids Antacid Tablets .... ND 807
- Tempo Soft Antacid .... ND 799

Magnesium Oxide (May substantially interfere with the absorption of quinolones). Products include:
- Beelith Tablets 632
- Bufferin Analgesic Tablets .... ND 636
- Arthritis Strength Bufferin Analgesic Caplets .... ND 637
- Extra Strength Bufferin Analgesic Tablets .... ND 637
- Caltrate PLUS .... ND 681
- Cama Arthritis Pain Reliever .... ND 748
- Mag-Ox 400 666
- Uro-Mag 666

Meclofenamate Sodium (Increased risk of CNS stimulation and convulsive seizures).
- No products indexed under this heading.

Mefenamic Acid (Increased risk of CNS stimulation and convulsive seizures). Products include:
- Ponstel 1982

Metformin Hydrochloride (Potentiation of hypoglycemic action). Products include:
- Glucophage Tablets 754

Nabumetone (Increased risk of CNS stimulation and convulsive seizures). Products include:
- Relafen Tablets 2688

Naproxen (Increased risk of CNS stimulation and convulsive seizures). Products include:
- Anaprox/Naprosyn 2277

Naproxen Sodium (Increased risk of CNS stimulation and convulsive seizures). Products include:
- Aleve 2124
- Anaprox/Naprosyn 2277
- Naprelan Tablets 2861

Oxaprozin (Increased risk of CNS stimulation and convulsive seizures). Products include:
- Daypro Caplets 2578

Phenylbutazone (Increased risk of CNS stimulation and convulsive seizures).
- No products indexed under this heading.

Piroxicam (Increased risk of CNS stimulation and convulsive seizures). Products include:
- Feldene Capsules 2008

Probenecid (Potential to affect renal tubular secretion; this interaction has not been studied with ofloxacin). Products include:
- Benemid Tablets 1651
- ColBENEMID Tablets 1662

Sucralfate (May substantially interfere with the absorption of quinolones). Products include:
- Carafate Suspension 1250
- Carafate Tablets 1249

Sulindac (Increased risk of CNS stimulation and convulsive seizures). Products include:
- Clinoril Tablets 1658

Theophylline (Increased steady-state theophylline levels; concurrent therapy may prolong the half-life of theophylline, elevate serum theophylline levels, and increase the risk of theophylline-related adverse reactions). Products include:
- Marax Tablets & DF Syrup 2015
- Quibron 2227

Theophylline Anhydrous (Increased steady-state theophylline levels; concurrent therapy may prolong the half-life of theophylline, elevate serum theophylline levels, and increase the risk of theophylline-related adverse reactions). Products include:
- Aerolate 1003
- Primatene Tablets .... ND 844
- Respbid Tablets 687
- Slo-bid Gyrocaps 2201
- Theo-24 Extended Release Capsules 2753
- Theo-Dur Extended-Release Tablets 1367
- Theo-X Extended-Release Tablets .. 793
- Uni-Dur Extended-Release Tablets .. 1374
- Uniphyl 400 mg and 600 mg Tablets 2157

Theophylline Calcium Salicylate (Increased steady-state theophylline levels; concurrent therapy may prolong the half-life of theophylline, elevate serum theophylline levels, and increase the risk of theophylline-related adverse reactions). Products include:
- Quadrinal Tablets 1398

Theophylline Sodium Glycinate (Increased steady-state theophylline levels; concurrent therapy may prolong the half-life of theophylline, elevate serum theophylline levels, and increase the risk of theophylline-related adverse reactions).
- No products indexed under this heading.

Tolazamide (Potentiation of hypoglycemic action).
- No products indexed under this heading.

Tolbutamide (Potentiation of hypoglycemic action).
- No products indexed under this heading.

Tolmetin Sodium (Increased risk of CNS stimulation and convulsive seizures). Products include:
- Tolectin (200, 400 and 600 mg) .. 1591

Warfarin Sodium (Potential for enhanced effects of the oral anticoagulant). Products include:
- Coumadin 941

Zinc Sulfate (May substantially interfere with the absorption of quinolones). Products include:
- Clear Eyes ACR Astringent/Lubricant Eye Redness Reliever Eye Drops .... ◉ 314
- Visine A.C. Seasonal Relief From Pollen and Dust .... ◉ 301

Food Interactions

Food, unspecified (Food does not affect the C_{max} and AUC_{∞} of the drug, but T_{max} is prolonged).

FLUDARA FOR INJECTION

(Fludarabine Phosphate) 658
May interact with:

Pentostatin (Co-administration may produce severe pulmonary toxicity; the use of Fludara in combination with pentostatin is not recommended). Products include:
- Nipent for Injection 2733

FLUMADINE TABLETS & SYRUP

(Rimantadine Hydrochloride) 1013
May interact with:

Acetaminophen (Coadministration reduces the peak concentration and AUC values for rimantadine). Products include:
- Actifed Cold & Sinus Caplets and Tablets .... ND 808
- Actifed Sinus Daytime/Nighttime Tablets and Caplets .... ND 809
- Alka-Seltzer Fast Relief Caplets .... ND 610
- Alka-Seltzer Plus Liqui-Gels .... ND 612
- Alka-Seltzer Plus Flu & Body Aches Effervescent Tablets .... ND 612
- Alka-Seltzer Plus Flu & Body Aches Liqui-Gels Non-Drowsy Formula .... ND 613
- Alka-Seltzer Plus Night-Time Cold Medicine Liqui-Gels .... ND 612
- Allerest No Drowsiness .... ND 649
- Allerest Sinus Pain Formula .... ND 649
- Axocet Capsules 2469
- Benadryl Allergy/Cold Tablets .... ND 811
- Benadryl Allergy Sinus Headache Caplets .... ND 813
- Children's TYLENOL acetaminophen Chewable Tablets, Elixir,

(ND Described in PDR For Nonprescription Drugs) (◉ Described in PDR For Ophthalmology)

Suspension Liquid, and Suspension Drops ... 1559
Children's TYLENOL Cold Multi-Symptom Chewable Tablets and Liquid ... 1559
Children's TYLENOL Cold Plus Cough Multi Symptom Chewable Tablets and Liquid ... 1560
Children's TYLENOL Flu Suspension Liquid ... 1560
Allergy-Sinus Comtrex Multi-Symptom Allergy-Sinus Formula Tablets and Caplets ... ▣ 639
Comtrex Multi-Symptom ... ▣ 638
Comtrex Non-Drowsy ... ▣ 640
Contac Day Allergy/Sinus Caplets ▣ 771
Contac Day & Night ... ▣ 772
Contac Night Allergy/Sinus Caplets ... ▣ 771
Contac Severe Cold and Flu Formula Caplets ... ▣ 773
Contac Severe Cold & Flu Non-Drowsy ... ▣ 774
Coricidin Cold + Flu Tablets ... ▣ 760
Coricidin 'D' Decongestant Tablets ... ▣ 760
DHCplus Capsules ... 2148
Darvon-N/Darvocet-N ... 1473
Dimetapp Allergy Sinus Caplets ... ▣ 838
Dimetapp Cold & Fever Suspension ... ▣ 839
Drixoral Cold and Flu Extended-Release Tablets ... ▣ 764
Drixoral Cough + Sore Throat Liquid Caps ... ▣ 763
Drixoral Allergy/Sinus Extended Release Tablets ... ▣ 765
Esgic-plus Capsules ... 1012
Esgic-plus Tablets ... 1012
Aspirin Free Excedrin Analgesic Caplets and Geltabs ... 734
Excedrin Extra-Strength Analgesic Tablets, Caplets, and Geltabs ... 734
Excedrin P.M. Analgesic/Sleeping Aid Tablets, Caplets, Liquigels ... 735
Fioricet Tablets ... 2386
Fioricet with Codeine Capsules ... 2387
Goody's Extra Strength Headache Powders ... ▣ 632
Goody's Extra Strength Pain Relief Tablets ... ▣ 632
Hycomine Compound Tablets ... 948
Hydrocet Capsules ... 787
Infants' TYLENOL acetaminophen Suspension Drops ... 1559
Infants' TYLENOL Cold Decongestant & Fever-Reducer Drops ... 1561
Junior Strength TYLENOL acetaminophen Coated Caplets and Chewable Tablets ... 1562
Lorcet 10/650 Tablets ... 1016
Lortab ... 2751
Lurline PMS Tablets ... 1000
Maximum Strength Multi-Symptom Formula Midol ... ▣ 621
PMS Multi-Symptom Formula Midol ... ▣ 622
Maximum Strength Midol Teen Multi-Symptom Formula ... ▣ 621
Midrin Capsules ... 788
Panodol Tablets and Caplets ... ▣ 783
Children's Panadol Chewable Tablets, Liquid, Infant's Drops ... ▣ 783
Percocet Tablets ... 955
Percogesic Analgesic Tablets ... ▣ 727
Phrenilin ... 790
Pyrroxate Caplets ... ▣ 742
Robitussin Cold, Cough & Flu Liqui-Gels ... ▣ 844
Robitussin Night-Time Cold Formula ... ▣ 847
Sedapap Tablets 50 mg/650 mg ... 1826
Sinarest ... ▣ 663
Sine-Aid Maximum Strength Sinus Headache Gelcaps, Caplets and Tablets ... 1570
Sine-Off No Drowsiness Formula Caplets ... ▣ 784
Sine-Off Sinus Medicine ... ▣ 784
Singlet Tablets ... ▣ 785
Sinulin Tablets ... 792
Sinutab Sinus Allergy Medication, Maximum Strength Tablets and Caplets ... ▣ 823
Sinutab Sinus Medication, Maximum Strength Without Drowsiness Formula, Tablets & Caplets ... ▣ 824
Sudafed Cold and Cough Liquid Caps ... ▣ 826
Sudafed Severe Cold Formula Caplets ... ▣ 828
Sudafed Severe Cold Formula Tablets ... ▣ 828
Sudafed Sinus Caplets ... ▣ 829
Sudafed Sinus Tablets ... ▣ 829
Talacen Caplets ... 2464
TheraFlu Flu and Cold Medicine ... ▣ 750
Theraflu Maximum Strength Flu and Cold Medicine For Sore Throat ... ▣ 751
TheraFlu Flu, Cold and Cough Medicine ... ▣ 750
TheraFlu Maximum Strength Nighttime Flu, Cold & Cough Medicine ... ▣ 751
TheraFlu Maximum Strength Non-Drowsy Formula Flu, Cold & Cough Medicine ... ▣ 751
TheraFlu Maximum Strength, Non-Drowsy Formula Flu, Cold and Cough Caplets ... ▣ 752
Theraflu Maximum Strength Sinus Non-Drowsy Formula Caplets ... ▣ 752
Triaminic Sore Throat Formula ... ▣ 755
Triaminicin Tablets ... ▣ 756
TYLENOL acetaminophen Extended Relief Caplets ... 1570
TYLENOL acetaminophen, Extra Strength Adult Liquid Pain Reliever ... 1570
TYLENOL acetaminophen, Extra Strength Gelcaps, Geltabs, Caplets, Tablets ... 1570
TYLENOL acetaminophen, Regular Strength Caplets and Tablets ... 1570
TYLENOL Allergy Sinus, Maximum Strength Caplets and Gelcaps ... 1571
TYLENOL Allergy Sinus NightTime, Maximum Strength Caplets ... 1571
TYLENOL Cold Medication, Multi-Symptom Formula Tablets and Caplets ... 1572
TYLENOL Cold Medication, Multi-Symptom Hot Liquid Packets ... 1572
TYLENOL Cold Medication, No Drowsiness Formula Caplets and Gelcaps ... 1572
TYLENOL Cold Severe Congestion Caplets ... 1573
TYLENOL Cough Medication, Multi Symptom ... 1574
TYLENOL Cough Medication with Decongestant, Multi Symptom ... 1574
TYLENOL Flu No Drowsiness Formula, Maximum Strength Gelcaps ... 1575
TYLENOL Flu NightTime, Maximum Strength Gelcaps ... 1575
TYLENOL Flu NightTime, Maximum Strength Hot Medication Packets ... 1575
TYLENOL Headache Plus Pain Reliever with Antacid, Extra Strength Caplets ... ▣ 705
TYLENOL PM Pain Reliever/Sleep Aid, Extra Strength Gelcaps, Caplets, Geltabs ... 1576
TYLENOL Severe Allergy Medication Caplets ... 1571
TYLENOL Sinus, Maximum Strength Geltabs, Gelcaps, Caplets and Tablets ... 1576
Tylenol with Codeine ... 1592
Tylox Capsules ... 1593
Unisom With Pain Relief-Nighttime Sleep Aid and Pain Reliever ... 1991
Vanquish Analgesic Caplets ... ▣ 627
Vicks 44 LiquiCaps Cough, Cold & Flu Relief ... ▣ 728
Vicks 44M Cough, Cold & Flu Relief ... ▣ 729
Vicks DayQuil LiquiCaps/Liquid Multi-Symptom Cold/Flu Relief ... ▣ 734
Vicks Nyquil Hot Therapy ... ▣ 735
Vicks NyQuil LiquiCaps/Liquid Multi-Symptom Cold/Flu Relief, Original and Cherry Flavors ... ▣ 736
Vicodin Tablets ... 1404
Vicodin ES Tablets ... 1405
Vicodin HP Tablets ... 1403
Wygesic Tablets ... 2930
Zydone Capsules ... 967

Aspirin (Coadministration reduces the peak concentration and AUC values for rimantadine). Products include:
Alka-Seltzer Cherry Effervescent Antacid and Pain Reliever ... ▣ 609
Alka-Seltzer Extra Strength Effervescent Antacid and Pain Reliever ... ▣ 609
Alka-Seltzer Lemon Lime Effervescent Antacid and Pain Reliever ... ▣ 609
Alka-Seltzer Original Effervescent Antacid and Pain Reliever ... ▣ 609
Alka-Seltzer Plus ... ▣ 611
Alka-Seltzer Plus Sinus Medicine ... ▣ 611
Ascriptin ... ▣ 650
Arthritis Strength BC Powder ... ▣ 631
BC Cold Powder Multi-Symptom Formula (Cold-Sinus-Allergy) ... ▣ 631
BC Cold Powder Non-Drowsy Formula (Cold-Sinus) ... ▣ 631
BC Powder ... ▣ 631
Genuine Bayer Aspirin Tablets & Caplets ... ▣ 618
Extra Strength Bayer Arthritis Pain Regimen Formula ... ▣ 615
Extra Strength Bayer Aspirin Caplets & Tablets ... ▣ 617
Extended-Release Bayer 8-Hour Aspirin ... ▣ 616
Extra Strength Bayer Plus Aspirin Caplets ... ▣ 617
Extra Strength Bayer PM Aspirin Plus Sleep Aid ... ▣ 617
Aspirin Regimen Bayer 81 mg Tablets with Calcium ... ▣ 615
Aspirin Regimen Bayer Adult Low Strength 81 mg Tablets ... ▣ 613
Aspirin Regimen Bayer Children's Chewable Aspirin ... ▣ 616
Aspirin Regimen Bayer Regular Strength 325 mg Caplets ... ▣ 613
Bufferin Analgesic Tablets ... ▣ 636
Arthritis Strength Bufferin Analgesic Caplets ... ▣ 637
Extra Strength Bufferin Analgesic Tablets ... ▣ 637
Cama Arthritis Pain Reliever ... ▣ 748
Darvon Compound-65 Pulvules ... 1475
Easprin ... 1971
Ecotrin ... 2625
Ecotrin Enteric Coated Aspirin Maximum Strength Tablets and Caplets ... ▣ 775
Ecotrin Enteric Coated Aspirin Regular Strength Tablets ... 2625
Empirin Aspirin Tablets ... ▣ 818
Excedrin Extra-Strength Analgesic Tablets, Caplets, and Geltabs ... 734
Fiorinal Capsules ... 2388
Fiorinal with Codeine Capsules ... 2390
Fiorinal Tablets ... 2388
Goody's Extra Strength Headache Powders ... ▣ 632
Goody's Extra Strength Pain Relief Tablets ... ▣ 632
Halfprin Tablets ... 1413
Norgesic ... 1554
Percodan Tablets ... 955
Percodan-Demi Tablets ... 956
Robaxisal Tablets ... 2246
Soma Compound w/Codeine Tablets ... 2784
Soma Compound Tablets ... 2783
St. Joseph Adult Chewable Aspirin (81 mg.) ... ▣ 768
Talwin Compound ... 2466
Vanquish Analgesic Caplets ... ▣ 627

Cimetidine (Potential for reduced clearance of total rimantadine). Products include:
Tagamet HB Tablets ... ▣ 786
Tagamet Tablets ... 2694

Cimetidine Hydrochloride (Potential for reduced clearance of total rimantadine). Products include:
Tagamet ... 2694

FLUORACAINE
(Fluorescein Sodium, Proparacaine Hydrochloride) ... ◎ 208
None cited in PDR database.

FLUORESCITE INJECTION
(Fluorescein Sodium) ... ◎ 217
None cited in PDR database.

FLUORESCITE SYRINGE
(Fluorescein Sodium) ... ◎ 217
None cited in PDR database.

FLUORI-METHANE
(Dichlorodifluoromethane, Trichloromonofluoromethane) ... 1040
None cited in PDR database.

FLUOR-I-STRIP
(Fluorescein Sodium) ... ◎ 319
None cited in PDR database.

FLUOR-I-STRIP A.T.
(Fluorescein Sodium) ... ◎ 320
None cited in PDR database.

FLUOROPLEX TOPICAL SOLUTION & CREAM 1%
(Fluorouracil) ... 475
None cited in PDR database.

FLUOROURACIL INJECTION
(Fluorouracil) ... 2282
May interact with alkylating agents and certain other agents. Compounds in these categories include:

Busulfan (Fluorouracil should be used with extreme caution in patients with previous use of alkylating agents). Products include:
Myleran Tablets ... 1209

Carmustine (BCNU) (Fluorouracil should be used with extreme caution in patients with previous use of alkylating agents). Products include:
BiCNU ... 696

Chlorambucil (Fluorouracil should be used with extreme caution in patients with previous use of alkylating agents). Products include:
Leukeran Tablets ... 1205

Cyclophosphamide (Fluorouracil should be used with extreme caution in patients with previous use of alkylating agents). Products include:
Cytoxan ... 700

Dacarbazine (Fluorouracil should be used with extreme caution in patients with previous use of alkylating agents). Products include:
DTIC-Dome ... 593

Leucovorin Calcium (May enhance the toxicity of fluorouracil). Products include:
Leucovorin Calcium for Injection, Wellcovorin Brand ... 1203
Leucovorin Calcium for Injection ... 1313
Leucovorin Calcium Tablets, Wellcovorin Brand ... 1204
Leucovorin Calcium Tablets ... 1315

Lomustine (CCNU) (Fluorouracil should be used with extreme caution in patients with previous use of alkylating agents). Products include:
CeeNU Capsules ... 699

Mechlorethamine Hydrochloride (Fluorouracil should be used with extreme caution in patients with previous use of alkylating agents). Products include:
Mustargen ... 1752

Melphalan (Fluorouracil should be used with extreme caution in patients with previous use of alkylating agents). Products include:
Alkeran Tablets ... 1198

Thiotepa (Fluorouracil should be used with extreme caution in patients with previous use of alkylating agents). Products include:
Thioplex (Thiotepa For Injection) ... 1329

FLUOTHANE
(Halothane) ... 2830
May interact with nondepolarizing neuromuscular blocking agents, ganglionic blocking agents, and cer-

IMPORTANT NOTE: Always consult each drug listing in the patient's regimen for possible interactions.

Fluothane / Interactions Index

tain other agents. Compounds in these categories include:

Atracurium Besylate (Actions augmented by Fluothane). Products include:
- Tracrium Injection 1155

Cisatracurium Besylate (Actions augmented by Fluothane). Products include:
- Nimbex Injection 1131

Epinephrine Hydrochloride (Simultaneous use may induce ventricular tachycardia or fibrillation). Products include:
- Ana-Kit Anaphylaxis Emergency Treatment Kit 611

Guanethidine Monosulfate (Actions augmented by Fluothane). Products include:
- Esimil Tablets 840
- Ismelin Tablets 845

Mecamylamine Hydrochloride (Actions augmented by Fluothane). Products include:
- Inversine Tablets 1729

Metocurine Iodide (Actions augmented by Fluothane). Products include:
- Metubine Iodide Vials 932

Mivacurium Chloride (Actions augmented by Fluothane). Products include:
- Mivacron 1125

Norepinephrine Bitartrate (Simultaneous use may induce ventricular tachycardia or fibrillation). Products include:
- Levophed Bitartrate Injection 2445

Pancuronium Bromide (Actions augmented by Fluothane).
- No products indexed under this heading.

Rocuronium Bromide (Actions augmented by Fluothane). Products include:
- Zemuron Injection 1885

Trimethaphan Camsylate (Actions augmented by Fluothane).
- No products indexed under this heading.

Vecuronium Bromide (Actions augmented by Fluothane). Products include:
- Norcuron for Injection 1875

FLURESS
(Fluorescein Sodium, Benoxinate Hydrochloride) .... ⊚ 208
None cited in PDR database.

FLUVIRIN (INFLUENZA VIRUS VACCINE)
(Influenza Virus Vaccine) 1608
May interact with xanthine bronchodilators, corticosteroids, antineoplastics, cytotoxic drugs, alkylating agents, and certain other agents. Compounds in these categories include:

Altretamine (Potential for reduced antibody response in active immunization procedures). Products include:
- Hexalen Capsules 2760

Aminophylline (Influenza immunization can inhibit the clearance of theophylline).
- No products indexed under this heading.

Anastrozole (Potential for reduced antibody response in active immunization procedures). Products include:
- Arimidex Tablets 2932

Asparaginase (Potential for reduced antibody response in active immunization procedures). Products include:
- Elspar 1700

Betamethasone Acetate (Potential for reduced antibody response in active immunization procedures). Products include:
- Celestone Soluspan Suspension 2484

Betamethasone Sodium Phosphate (Potential for reduced antibody response in active immunization procedures). Products include:
- Celestone Soluspan Suspension 2484

Bicalutamide (Potential for reduced antibody response in active immunization procedures). Products include:
- Casodex Tablets 2934

Bleomycin Sulfate (Potential for reduced antibody response in active immunization procedures). Products include:
- Blenoxane 697

Busulfan (Potential for reduced antibody response in active immunization procedures). Products include:
- Myleran Tablets 1209

Carboplatin (Potential for reduced antibody response in active immunization procedures). Products include:
- Paraplatin for Injection 713

Carmustine (BCNU) (Potential for reduced antibody response in active immunization procedures). Products include:
- BiCNU 696

Chlorambucil (Potential for reduced antibody response in active immunization procedures). Products include:
- Leukeran Tablets 1205

Cisplatin (Potential for reduced antibody response in active immunization procedures). Products include:
- Platinol for Injection 717
- Platinol-AQ Injection 719

Cortisone Acetate (Potential for reduced antibody response in active immunization procedures). Products include:
- Cortone Acetate Sterile Suspension ... 1663
- Cortone Acetate Tablets 1664

Cyclophosphamide (Potential for reduced antibody response in active immunization procedures). Products include:
- Cytoxan 700

Dacarbazine (Potential for reduced antibody response in active immunization procedures). Products include:
- DTIC-Dome 593

Daunorubicin Citrate (Potential for reduced antibody response in active immunization procedures). Products include:
- DaunoXome 1842

Daunorubicin Hydrochloride (Potential for reduced antibody response in active immunization procedures). Products include:
- Cerubidine for Injection 634

Dexamethasone (Potential for reduced antibody response in active immunization procedures). Products include:
- AK-Trol Ointment & Suspension .... ⊚ 205
- Decadron Elixir 1676
- Decadron Tablets 1678
- Decaspray Topical Aerosol 1689
- Maxitrol Ophthalmic Ointment and Suspension .... ⊚ 222

- TobraDex Ophthalmic Suspension and Ointment 469

Dexamethasone Acetate (Potential for reduced antibody response in active immunization procedures). Products include:
- Dalalone D.P. Injectable 1009
- Decadron-LA Sterile Suspension ... 1687

Dexamethasone Sodium Phosphate (Potential for reduced antibody response in active immunization procedures). Products include:
- Decadron Phosphate Injection 1680
- Decadron Phosphate Sterile Ophthalmic Ointment 1684
- Decadron Phosphate Sterile Ophthalmic Solution 1685
- Decadron Phosphate Topical Cream 1686
- Decadron Phosphate with Xylocaine Injection, Sterile 1683
- Dexacort Phosphate in Respihaler ... 1606
- Dexacort Phosphate in Turbinaire ... 1607
- NeoDecadron Sterile Ophthalmic Ointment 1755
- NeoDecadron Sterile Ophthalmic Solution 1756
- NeoDecadron Topical Cream 1757

Docetaxel (Potential for reduced antibody response in active immunization procedures). Products include:
- Taxotere for Injection Concentrate ... 2204

Doxorubicin Hydrochloride (Potential for reduced antibody response in active immunization procedures). Products include:
- Adriamycin PFS 2056
- Adriamycin RDF 2056
- Doxil 2613
- Doxorubicin Astra 531
- Rubex for Injection 721

Dyphylline (Influenza immunization can inhibit the clearance of theophylline). Products include:
- Lufyllin & Lufyllin-400 Tablets 2778
- Lufyllin-GG Elixir & Tablets 2779

Estramustine Phosphate Sodium (Potential for reduced antibody response in active immunization procedures). Products include:
- Emcyt Capsules 2085

Etoposide (Potential for reduced antibody response in active immunization procedures). Products include:
- Etoposide Injection 539
- VePesid Capsules and Injection 727

Floxuridine (Potential for reduced antibody response in active immunization procedures). Products include:
- Sterile FUDR 2284

Fludrocortisone Acetate (Potential for reduced antibody response in active immunization procedures). Products include:
- Florinef Acetate Tablets 506

Fluorouracil (Potential for reduced antibody response in active immunization procedures). Products include:
- Efudex 2280
- Fluoroplex Topical Solution & Cream 1% 475
- Fluorouracil Injection 2282

Flutamide (Potential for reduced antibody response in active immunization procedures). Products include:
- Eulexin Capsules 2498

Gemcitabine (Potential for reduced antibody response in active immunization procedures). Products include:
- Gemzar for Injection 1482

Hydrocortisone (Potential for reduced antibody response in active immunization procedures). Products include:
- Anusol-HC Cream 2.5% 1953

- Aquanil HC Lotion 1989
- Maximum Strength Cortaid Spray ⊡ 800
- CORTENEMA 2713
- Cortisporin Ointment 1074
- Cortisporin Ophthalmic Ointment Sterile 1074
- Cortisporin Ophthalmic Suspension Sterile 1075
- Cortisporin Otic Solution Sterile ... 1076
- Cortisporin Otic Suspension Sterile ... 1077
- Cortizone-5 .... ⊡ 795
- Cortizone-10 .... ⊡ 795
- Hydrocortone Tablets 1715
- Hytone 922
- Hytone Ointment 2 ½% 923
- Massengill Medicated Soft Cloth Towelettes 2628
- Pediotic Suspension Sterile 1140
- Preparation H Hydrocortisone 1% Cream .... ⊡ 843
- ProctoCream-HC 2.5% 2552
- VōSoL HC Otic Solution 2786

Hydrocortisone Acetate (Potential for reduced antibody response in active immunization procedures). Products include:
- Analpram-HC Rectal Cream 1% and 2.5% 993
- Anusol HC-1 Hydrocortisone Anti-Itch Ointment .... ⊡ 810
- Anusol-HC Suppositories 1954
- Caldecort Anti-Itch Hydrocortisone Cream .... ⊡ 651
- Coly-Mycin S Otic w/Neomycin & Hydrocortisone 1965
- Cortaid .... ⊡ 800
- Cortifoam 2540
- Cortisporin Cream 1073
- Epifoam 2543
- Hydrocortone Acetate Sterile Suspension 1712
- Mantadil Cream 1124
- Nupercainal Hydrocortisone 1% Cream .... ⊡ 661
- Pramosone Cream, Lotion & Ointment 995
- ProctoFoam-HC 2552
- Terra-Cortril Ophthalmic Suspension 2033

Hydrocortisone Sodium Phosphate (Potential for reduced antibody response in active immunization procedures). Products include:
- Hydrocortone Phosphate Injection, Sterile 1713

Hydrocortisone Sodium Succinate (Potential for reduced antibody response in active immunization procedures).
- No products indexed under this heading.

Hydroxyurea (Potential for reduced antibody response in active immunization procedures). Products include:
- Hydrea Capsules 705

Idarubicin Hydrochloride (Potential for reduced antibody response in active immunization procedures). Products include:
- Idamycin Injection 2096

Ifosfamide (Potential for reduced antibody response in active immunization procedures). Products include:
- IFEX 706

Interferon alfa-2A, Recombinant (Potential for reduced antibody response in active immunization procedures). Products include:
- Roferon-A Injection 2308

Interferon alfa-2B, Recombinant (Potential for reduced antibody response in active immunization procedures). Products include:
- Intron A for Injection 2506

Irinotecan Hydrochloride (Potential for reduced antibody response in active immunization procedures).
- No products indexed under this heading.

(⊡ Described in PDR For Nonprescription Drugs)   (⊚ Described in PDR For Ophthalmology)

427 **Interactions Index** **Fosamax**

Levamisole Hydrochloride (Potential for reduced antibody response in active immunization procedures). Products include:
Ergamisol Tablets 1340

Lomustine (CCNU) (Potential for reduced antibody response in active immunization procedures). Products include:
CeeNU Capsules 699

Mechlorethamine Hydrochloride (Potential for reduced antibody response in active immunization procedures). Products include:
Mustargen 1752

Megestrol Acetate (Potential for reduced antibody response in active immunization procedures). Products include:
Megace Oral Suspension 708
Megace Tablets 710

Melphalan (Potential for reduced antibody response in active immunization procedures). Products include:
Alkeran Tablets 1198

Mercaptopurine (Potential for reduced antibody response in active immunization procedures). Products include:
Purinethol Tablets 1214

Methotrexate Sodium (Potential for reduced antibody response in active immunization procedures). Products include:
Methotrexate Sodium Tablets, Injection, for Injection and LPF Injection 1322

Methylprednisolone Acetate (Potential for reduced antibody response in active immunization procedures).
No products indexed under this heading.

Methylprednisolone Sodium Succinate (Potential for reduced antibody response in active immunization procedures).
No products indexed under this heading.

Mitomycin (Mitomycin-C) (Potential for reduced antibody response in active immunization procedures). Products include:
Mutamycin for Injection 712

Mitotane (Potential for reduced antibody response in active immunization procedures). Products include:
Lysodren Tablets 707

Mitoxantrone Hydrochloride (Potential for reduced antibody response in active immunization procedures). Products include:
Novantrone for Injection 1327

Paclitaxel (Potential for reduced antibody response in active immunization procedures). Products include:
Taxol Injection 723

Prednisolone Acetate (Potential for reduced antibody response in active immunization procedures). Products include:
AK-CIDE .... ⊙ 203
AK-CIDE Ointment .... ⊙ 203
Blephamide Liquifilm Sterile Ophthalmic Suspension 472
Blephamide Ointment .... ⊙ 234
Econopred & Econopred Plus Ophthalmic Suspensions .... ⊙ 216
Poly-Pred Liquifilm .... ⊙ 246
Pred Forte .... ⊙ 247
Pred Mild .... ⊙ 250
Pred-G Liquifilm Sterile Ophthalmic Suspension .... ⊙ 248
Pred-G S.O.P. Sterile Ophthalmic Ointment .... ⊙ 249

Prednisolone Sodium Phosphate (Potential for reduced antibody response in active immunization procedures). Products include:
AK-PRED .... ⊙ 204
Hydeltrasol Injection, Sterile 1708
Pediapred Oral Solution 1618

Prednisolone Tebutate (Potential for reduced antibody response in active immunization procedures). Products include:
Hydeltra-T.B.A. Sterile Suspension 1710

Prednisone (Potential for reduced antibody response in active immunization procedures).
No products indexed under this heading.

Procarbazine Hydrochloride (Potential for reduced antibody response in active immunization procedures). Products include:
Matulane Capsules 2300

Streptozocin (Potential for reduced antibody response in active immunization procedures). Products include:
Zanosar Sterile Powder 2119

Tamoxifen Citrate (Potential for reduced antibody response in active immunization procedures). Products include:
Nolvadex Tablets 2957

Teniposide (Potential for reduced antibody response in active immunization procedures). Products include:
Vumon for Injection 729

Theophylline (Influenza immunization can inhibit the clearance of theophylline). Products include:
Marax Tablets & DF Syrup 2015
Quibron 2227

Theophylline Anhydrous (Influenza immunization can inhibit the clearance of theophylline). Products include:
Aerolate 1003
Primatene Tablets .... ⊡ 844
Respbid Tablets 687
Slo-bid Gyrocaps 2201
Theo-24 Extended Release Capsules 2753
Theo-Dur Extended-Release Tablets 1367
Theo-X Extended-Release Tablets .. 793
Uni-Dur Extended-Release Tablets .. 1374
Uniphyl 400 mg and 600 mg Tablets 2157

Theophylline Calcium Salicylate (Influenza immunization can inhibit the clearance of theophylline). Products include:
Quadrinal Tablets 1398

Theophylline Sodium Glycinate (Influenza immunization can inhibit the clearance of theophylline).
No products indexed under this heading.

Thioguanine (Potential for reduced antibody response in active immunization procedures). Products include:
Thioguanine Tablets, Tabloid Brand 1225

Thiotepa (Potential for reduced antibody response in active immunization procedures). Products include:
Thioplex (Thiotepa For Injection) 1329

Topotecan Hydrochloride (Potential for reduced antibody response in active immunization procedures). Products include:
Hycamtin for Injection 2665

Triamcinolone (Potential for reduced antibody response in active immunization procedures).
No products indexed under this heading.

Triamcinolone Acetonide (Potential for reduced antibody response in active immunization procedures). Products include:
Azmacort Oral Inhaler 2175
Nasacort AQ Nasal Spray 2191
Nasacort Nasal Inhaler 2189

Triamcinolone Diacetate (Potential for reduced antibody response in active immunization procedures).
No products indexed under this heading.

Triamcinolone Hexacetonide (Potential for reduced antibody response in active immunization procedures).
No products indexed under this heading.

Vincristine Sulfate (Potential for reduced antibody response in active immunization procedures). Products include:
Oncovin Solution Vials & Hyporets 1521

Vinorelbine Tartrate (Potential for reduced antibody response in active immunization procedures). Products include:
Navelbine Injection 1212

Warfarin Sodium (Influenza immunization can inhibit the clearance of warfarin). Products include:
Coumadin 941

FOOD FOR THOUGHT
(Nutritional Beverage) .... ⊡ 833
May interact with:

Aluminum Carbonate (Concomitant use with aluminum-containing antacids should be avoided). Products include:
Basaljel Capsules 2810
Basaljel Suspension 2810
Basaljel Tablets 2810

Aluminum Hydroxide (Concomitant use with aluminum-containing antacids should be avoided). Products include:
ALternaGEL Liquid 1358
Maximum Strength Ascriptin .... ⊡ 650
Cama Arthritis Pain Reliever .... ⊡ 748
Gaviscon Extra Strength Relief Formula Antacid Tablets .... ⊡ 778
Gaviscon Extra Strength Relief Formula Liquid Antacid .... ⊡ 779
Gaviscon Liquid Antacid .... ⊡ 779
Gelusil Antacid-Anti-gas Liquid .... ⊡ 819
Gelusil Antacid-Anti-gas Tablets .... ⊡ 819
Maalox Antacid/Anti-Gas Tablets 889
Maalox Heartburn Relief Suspension .... ⊡ 658
Maalox Antacid Liquid 888
Extra Strength Maalox Antacid/Anti-Gas Liquid and Tablets 888
Mylanta 1359
Tempo Soft Antacid .... ⊡ 799

Aluminum Hydroxide Gel (Concomitant use with aluminum-containing antacids should be avoided). Products include:
ALternaGEL Liquid .... ⊡ 675
Aludrox Oral Suspension .... ⊡ 850
Amphojel Suspension 2802
Amphojel Suspension without Flavor 2802
Amphojel Tablets 2802
Ascriptin .... ⊡ 650
Gaviscon Antacid Tablets .... ⊡ 778
Gaviscon-2 Antacid Tablets .... ⊡ 779
Mylanta Liquid .... ⊡ 676
Mylanta Double Strength Liquid .... ⊡ 676
Nephrox Suspension .... ⊡ 671

FORMULA MAGIC ANTIBACTERIAL POWDER
(Benzethonium Chloride) .... ⊡ 647
None cited in PDR database.

FORTAZ
(Ceftazidime) 1092
May interact with aminoglycosides and certain other agents. Compounds in these categories include:

Amikacin Sulfate (Potential for nephrotoxicity following concomitant administration). Products include:
Amikacin Sulfate Injection, USP 523
Amikacin Sulfate Injection, USP 981
Amikin Injectable 502

Chloramphenicol (Possibility of antagonism *in vivo*, particularly when bactericidal activity is desired; avoid this combination). Products include:
Chloromycetin Ophthalmic Ointment, 1% .... ⊙ 298
Chloromycetin Ophthalmic Solution .... ⊙ 299
Chloroptic S.O.P. .... ⊙ 236
Chloroptic Sterile Ophthalmic Solution .... ⊙ 236

Chloramphenicol Palmitate (Possibility of antagonism *in vivo*, particularly when bactericidal activity is desired; avoid this combination).
No products indexed under this heading.

Chloramphenicol Sodium Succinate (Possibility of antagonism *in vivo*, particularly when bactericidal activity is desired; avoid this combination). Products include:
Chloromycetin Sodium Succinate 1960

Furosemide (Potential for nephrotoxicity following concomitant administration). Products include:
Lasix Injection, Oral Solution and Tablets 1267

Gentamicin Sulfate (Potential for nephrotoxicity following concomitant administration). Products include:
Garamycin Cream 0.1% 2501
Garamycin Injectable 2502
Garamycin Ointment 0.1% 2501
Garamycin Ophthalmic 2501
Genoptic Sterile Ophthalmic Solution .... ⊙ 241
Genoptic Sterile Ophthalmic Ointment .... ⊙ 241
Gentak .... ⊙ 209
Pred-G Liquifilm Sterile Ophthalmic Suspension .... ⊙ 248
Pred-G S.O.P. Sterile Ophthalmic Ointment .... ⊙ 249

Kanamycin Sulfate (Potential for nephrotoxicity following concomitant administration).
No products indexed under this heading.

Streptomycin Sulfate (Potential for nephrotoxicity following concomitant administration). Products include:
Streptomycin Sulfate Injection 2031

Tobramycin (Potential for nephrotoxicity following concomitant administration). Products include:
AKTOB .... ⊙ 207
TobraDex Ophthalmic Suspension and Ointment 469
Tobrex Ophthalmic Ointment and Solution .... ⊙ 226

Tobramycin Sulfate (Potential for nephrotoxicity following concomitant administration). Products include:
Nebcin Vials, Hyporets & ADD-Vantage 1518

FOSAMAX TABLETS
(Alendronate Sodium) 1703
May interact with antacids containing aluminium, calcium and magnesium and certain other agents. Compounds in these categories include:

Aluminum Carbonate (May interfere with the absorption of alendronate). Products include:
Basaljel Capsules 2810
Basaljel Suspension 2810
Basaljel Tablets 2810

IMPORTANT NOTE: Always consult each drug listing in the patient's regimen for possible interactions.

Fosamax Interactions Index 428

Aluminum Hydroxide (May interfere with the absorption of alendronate). Products include:
- ALternaGEL Liquid ... 1358
- Maximum Strength Ascriptin ... ▣ 650
- Cama Arthritis Pain Reliever ... ▣ 748
- Gaviscon Extra Strength Relief Formula Antacid Tablets ... ▣ 778
- Gaviscon Extra Strength Relief Formula Liquid Antacid ... ▣ 779
- Gaviscon Liquid Antacid ... ▣ 779
- Gelusil Antacid-Anti-gas Liquid ... ▣ 819
- Gelusil Antacid-Anti-gas Tablets ... ▣ 819
- Maalox Antacid/Anti-Gas Tablets ... 889
- Maalox Heartburn Relief Suspension ... ▣ 658
- Maalox Antacid Liquid ... 888
- Extra Strength Maalox Antacid/Anti-Gas Liquid and Tablets ... 888
- Mylanta ... 1359
- Tempo Soft Antacid ... ▣ 799

Aluminum Hydroxide Gel (May interfere with the absorption of alendronate). Products include:
- ALternaGEL Liquid ... ▣ 675
- Aludrox Oral Suspension ... ▣ 850
- Amphojel Suspension ... 2802
- Amphojel Suspension without Flavor ... 2802
- Amphojel Tablets ... 2802
- Ascriptin ... ▣ 650
- Gaviscon Antacid Tablets ... ▣ 778
- Gaviscon-2 Antacid Tablets ... ▣ 779
- Mylanta Liquid ... ▣ 676
- Mylanta Double Strength Liquid ... ▣ 676
- Nephrox Suspension ... ▣ 671

Aspirin (Concomitant therapy with doses of Fosamax greater than 10 mg/day and aspirin-containing compounds, the incidence of upper gastrointestinal adverse events may increase). Products include:
- Alka-Seltzer Cherry Effervescent Antacid and Pain Reliever ... ▣ 609
- Alka-Seltzer Extra Strength Effervescent Antacid and Pain Reliever ... ▣ 609
- Alka-Seltzer Lemon Lime Effervescent Antacid and Pain Reliever ... ▣ 609
- Alka-Seltzer Original Effervescent Antacid and Pain Reliever ... ▣ 609
- Alka-Seltzer Plus ... ▣ 611
- Alka-Seltzer Plus Sinus Medicine ... ▣ 611
- Ascriptin ... ▣ 650
- Arthritis Strength BC Powder ... ▣ 631
- BC Cold Powder Multi-Symptom Formula (Cold-Sinus-Allergy) ... ▣ 631
- BC Cold Powder Non-Drowsy Formula (Cold-Sinus) ... ▣ 631
- BC Powder ... ▣ 631
- Genuine Bayer Aspirin Tablets & Caplets ... ▣ 618
- Extra Strength Bayer Arthritis Pain Regimen Formula ... ▣ 615
- Extra Strength Bayer Aspirin Caplets & Tablets ... ▣ 617
- Extended-Release Bayer 8-Hour Aspirin ... ▣ 616
- Extra Strength Bayer Plus Aspirin Caplets ... ▣ 617
- Extra Strength Bayer PM Aspirin Plus Sleep Aid ... ▣ 617
- Aspirin Regimen Bayer 81 mg Tablets with Calcium ... ▣ 615
- Aspirin Regimen Bayer Adult Low Strength 81 mg Tablets ... ▣ 613
- Aspirin Regimen Bayer Children's Chewable Aspirin ... ▣ 616
- Aspirin Regimen Bayer Regular Strength 325 mg Caplets ... ▣ 613
- Bufferin Analgesic Tablets ... ▣ 636
- Arthritis Strength Bufferin Analgesic Caplets ... ▣ 637
- Extra Strength Bufferin Analgesic Tablets ... ▣ 637
- Cama Arthritis Pain Reliever ... ▣ 748
- Darvon Compound-65 Pulvules ... 1475
- Easprin ... 1971
- Ecotrin ... 2625
- Ecotrin Enteric Coated Aspirin Maximum Strength Tablets and Caplets ... ▣ 775
- Ecotrin Enteric Coated Aspirin Regular Strength Tablets ... 2625
- Empirin Aspirin Tablets ... ▣ 818
- Excedrin Extra-Strength Analgesic Tablets, Caplets, and Geltabs ... 734
- Fiorinal Capsules ... 2388
- Fiorinal with Codeine Capsules ... 2390
- Fiorinal Tablets ... 2388
- Goody's Extra Strength Headache Powders ... ▣ 632
- Goody's Extra Strength Pain Relief Tablets ... ▣ 632
- Halfprin Tablets ... 1413
- Norgesic ... 1554
- Percodan Tablets ... 955
- Percodan-Demi Tablets ... 956
- Robaxisal Tablets ... 2246
- Soma Compound w/Codeine Tablets ... 2784
- Soma Compound Tablets ... 2783
- St. Joseph Adult Chewable Aspirin (81 mg.) ... ▣ 768
- Talwin Compound ... 2466
- Vanquish Analgesic Caplets ... ▣ 627

Calcium Citrate (May interfere with the absorption of alendronate). Products include:
- Citracal Tablets ... 1828

Calcium Glubionate (May interfere with the absorption of alendronate).
- No products indexed under this heading.

Magaldrate (May interfere with the absorption of alendronate).
- No products indexed under this heading.

Magnesium Hydroxide (May interfere with the absorption of alendronate). Products include:
- Aludrox Oral Suspension ... ▣ 850
- Ascriptin ... ▣ 650
- Di-Gel Antacid/Anti-Gas ... ▣ 762
- Gelusil Antacid-Anti-gas Liquid ... ▣ 819
- Gelusil Antacid-Anti-gas Tablets ... ▣ 819
- Maalox Antacid/Anti-Gas Tablets ... 889
- Maalox Antacid Liquid ... 888
- Extra Strength Maalox Antacid/Anti-Gas Liquid and Tablets ... 888
- Mylanta Fast-Acting ... 1359
- Mylanta Gelcaps Antacid ... ▣ 678
- Fast-Acting Mylanta Liquid Antacid 1359
- Mylanta Tablets ... ▣ 677
- Maximum-Strength Fast-Acting Mylanta Liquid Antacid ... 1359
- Mylanta Double Strength Tablets ... ▣ 677
- Phillips' Milk of Magnesia Liquid ... ▣ 627
- Rolaids Antacid Tablets ... ▣ 807
- Tempo Soft Antacid ... ▣ 799

Magnesium Oxide (May interfere with the absorption of alendronate). Products include:
- Beelith Tablets ... 632
- Bufferin Analgesic Tablets ... ▣ 636
- Arthritis Strength Bufferin Analgesic Caplets ... ▣ 637
- Extra Strength Bufferin Analgesic Tablets ... ▣ 637
- Caltrate PLUS ... ▣ 681
- Cama Arthritis Pain Reliever ... ▣ 748
- Mag-Ox 400 ... 666
- Uro-Mag ... 666

Ranitidine Hydrochloride (Intravenous ranitidine has shown to double the bioavailability of oral alendronate; clinical significance of this increased bioavailability and whether similar increases will occur with oral ranitidine is unknown). Products include:
- Zantac ... 1182
- Zantac Injection ... 1180
- Zantac Syrup ... 1182

Food Interactions

Beverages, caffeine-containing (Concomitant administration of alendronate with coffee reduces bioavailability by approximately 60%).

Meal, unspecified (Standardized breakfast decreases bioavailability by approximately 40% when alendronate is administered either 0.5 or 1 hour before breakfast).

Orange Juice (Concomitant administration of alendronate with orange juice reduces bioavailability by approximately 60%).

FOSCAVIR INJECTION
(Foscarnet Sodium) ... 541

May interact with aminoglycosides, drugs known to influence serum calcium levels (selected), inhibitors of renal tubular secretion or resorption, and certain other agents. Compounds in these categories include:

Amikacin Sulfate (Concurrent administration should be avoided because of foscarnet's tendency to cause renal impairment). Products include:
- Amikacin Sulfate Injection, USP ... 523
- Amikacin Sulfate Injection, USP ... 981
- Amikin Injectable ... 502

Amphotericin B (Concurrent administration should be avoided because of foscarnet's tendency to cause renal impairment). Products include:
- Abelcet Injection ... 1540
- Fungizone Intravenous ... 507
- Fungizone Oral Suspension ... 704

Carboplatin (Potential for increased hypocalcemia). Products include:
- Paraplatin for Injection ... 713

Cisplatin (Potential for increased hypocalcemia). Products include:
- Platinol for Injection ... 717
- Platinol-AQ Injection ... 719

Gallium Nitrate (Potential for increased hypocalcemia). Products include:
- Ganite ... 2711

Gentamicin Sulfate (Concurrent administration should be avoided because of foscarnet's tendency to cause renal impairment). Products include:
- Garamycin Cream 0.1% ... 2501
- Garamycin Injectable ... 2502
- Garamycin Ointment 0.1% ... 2501
- Garamycin Ophthalmic ... 2501
- Genoptic Sterile Ophthalmic Solution ... ⊙ 241
- Genoptic Sterile Ophthalmic Ointment ... ⊙ 241
- Gentak ... ⊙ 209
- Pred-G Liquifilm Sterile Ophthalmic Suspension ... ⊙ 248
- Pred-G S.O.P. Sterile Ophthalmic Ointment ... ⊙ 249

Kanamycin Sulfate (Concurrent administration should be avoided because of foscarnet's tendency to cause renal impairment).
- No products indexed under this heading.

Pentamidine Isethionate (Concomitant administration with intravenous pentamidine may cause hypocalcemia).
- No products indexed under this heading.

Probenecid (Elimination of foscarnet may be impaired). Products include:
- Benemid Tablets ... 1651
- ColBENEMID Tablets ... 1662

Sodium Polystyrene Sulfonate (Potential for increased hypocalcemia). Products include:
- Kayexalate ... 2444
- Sodium Polystyrene Sulfonate Suspension ... 2367

Streptomycin Sulfate (Concurrent administration should be avoided because of foscarnet's tendency to cause renal impairment). Products include:
- Streptomycin Sulfate Injection ... 2031

Sulfinpyrazone (Elimination of foscarnet may be impaired). Products include:
- Anturane ... 823

Tobramycin (Concurrent administration should be avoided because of foscarnet's tendency to cause renal impairment). Products include:
- AKTOB ... ⊙ 207
- TobraDex Ophthalmic Suspension and Ointment ... 469
- Tobrex Ophthalmic Ointment and Solution ... ⊙ 226

Tobramycin Sulfate (Concurrent administration should be avoided because of foscarnet's tendency to cause renal impairment). Products include:
- Nebcin Vials, Hyporets & ADD-Vantage ... 1518

Zidovudine (Potential for additive effects on anemia). Products include:
- Retrovir Capsules ... 1216
- Retrovir I.V. Infusion ... 1221
- Retrovir Syrup ... 1216

FOTOTAR CREAM
(Coal Tar) ... 1300

None cited in PDR database.

FRAGMIN INJECTION
(Dalteparin Sodium) ... 2088

May interact with oral anticoagulants and platelet inhibitors. Compounds in these categories include:

Aspirin (Potential for increased risk of bleeding). Products include:
- Alka-Seltzer Cherry Effervescent Antacid and Pain Reliever ... ▣ 609
- Alka-Seltzer Extra Strength Effervescent Antacid and Pain Reliever ... ▣ 609
- Alka-Seltzer Lemon Lime Effervescent Antacid and Pain Reliever ... ▣ 609
- Alka-Seltzer Original Effervescent Antacid and Pain Reliever ... ▣ 609
- Alka-Seltzer Plus ... ▣ 611
- Alka-Seltzer Plus Sinus Medicine ... ▣ 611
- Ascriptin ... ▣ 650
- Arthritis Strength BC Powder ... ▣ 631
- BC Cold Powder Multi-Symptom Formula (Cold-Sinus-Allergy) ... ▣ 631
- BC Cold Powder Non-Drowsy Formula (Cold-Sinus) ... ▣ 631
- BC Powder ... ▣ 631
- Genuine Bayer Aspirin Tablets & Caplets ... ▣ 618
- Extra Strength Bayer Arthritis Pain Regimen Formula ... ▣ 615
- Extra Strength Bayer Aspirin Caplets & Tablets ... ▣ 617
- Extended-Release Bayer 8-Hour Aspirin ... ▣ 616
- Extra Strength Bayer Plus Aspirin Caplets ... ▣ 617
- Extra Strength Bayer PM Aspirin Plus Sleep Aid ... ▣ 617
- Aspirin Regimen Bayer 81 mg Tablets with Calcium ... ▣ 615
- Aspirin Regimen Bayer Adult Low Strength 81 mg Tablets ... ▣ 613
- Aspirin Regimen Bayer Children's Chewable Aspirin ... ▣ 616
- Aspirin Regimen Bayer Regular Strength 325 mg Caplets ... ▣ 613
- Bufferin Analgesic Tablets ... ▣ 636
- Arthritis Strength Bufferin Analgesic Caplets ... ▣ 637
- Extra Strength Bufferin Analgesic Tablets ... ▣ 637
- Cama Arthritis Pain Reliever ... ▣ 748
- Darvon Compound-65 Pulvules ... 1475
- Easprin ... 1971
- Ecotrin ... 2625
- Ecotrin Enteric Coated Aspirin Maximum Strength Tablets and Caplets ... ▣ 775
- Ecotrin Enteric Coated Aspirin Regular Strength Tablets ... 2625
- Empirin Aspirin Tablets ... ▣ 818
- Excedrin Extra-Strength Analgesic Tablets, Caplets, and Geltabs ... 734
- Fiorinal Capsules ... 2388
- Fiorinal with Codeine Capsules ... 2390
- Fiorinal Tablets ... 2388
- Goody's Extra Strength Headache Powders ... ▣ 632

(▣ Described in PDR For Nonprescription Drugs) (⊙ Described in PDR For Ophthalmology)

Goody's Extra Strength Pain Relief Tablets	632
Halfprin Tablets	1413
Norgesic	1554
Percodan Tablets	955
Percodan-Demi Tablets	956
Robaxisal Tablets	2246
Soma Compound w/Codeine Tablets	2784
Soma Compound Tablets	2783
St. Joseph Adult Chewable Aspirin (81 mg.)	768
Talwin Compound	2466
Vanquish Analgesic Caplets	627

Azlocillin Sodium (Potential for increased risk of bleeding).
No products indexed under this heading.

Carbenicillin Indanyl Sodium (Potential for increased risk of bleeding). Products include:
Geocillin Tablets	2009

Choline Magnesium Trisalicylate (Potential for increased risk of bleeding). Products include:
Trilisate	2155

Diclofenac Potassium (Potential for increased risk of bleeding). Products include:
Cataflam Tablets	833

Diclofenac Sodium (Potential for increased risk of bleeding). Products include:
Voltaren Ophthalmic Sterile Ophthalmic Solution	264
Cataflam/Voltaren/Voltaren-XR	833

Dicumarol (Potential for increased risk of bleeding).
No products indexed under this heading.

Diflunisal (Potential for increased risk of bleeding). Products include:
Dolobid Tablets	1695

Dipyridamole (Potential for increased risk of bleeding). Products include:
Persantine Tablets	686

Fenoprofen Calcium (Potential for increased risk of bleeding). Products include:
Nalfon 200 Pulvules & Nalfon Tablets	933

Flurbiprofen (Potential for increased risk of bleeding).
No products indexed under this heading.

Ibuprofen (Potential for increased risk of bleeding). Products include:
Advil Cold and Sinus Caplets and Tablets	837
Advil Ibuprofen Tablets, Caplets and Gel Caplets	836
Children's Motrin Ibuprofen Oral Suspension	1558
IBU Tablets	1389
Ibuprohm	713
Motrin IB Caplets, Tablets, and Gelcaps	802
Motrin Ibuprofen Suspension, Oral Drops, Chewable Tablets, Caplets	1563
Nuprin Ibuprofen/Analgesic Tablets & Caplets	645
Vicks DayQuil SINUS Pressure & PAIN Relief with IBUPROFEN	735

Indomethacin (Potential for increased risk of bleeding). Products include:
Indocin	1723

Indomethacin Sodium Trihydrate (Potential for increased risk of bleeding). Products include:
Indocin I.V.	1727

Ketoprofen (Potential for increased risk of bleeding). Products include:
Actron Caplets and Tablets	608
Orudis Capsules	2874
Orudis KT	842
Oruvail Capsules	2874

Magnesium Salicylate (Potential for increased risk of bleeding). Products include:
Backache Caplets	635
Doan's Extra-Strength Analgesic	653
Extra Strength Doan's P.M.	653
Doan's Regular Strength Analgesic	654
Mobigesic Tablets	607

Meclofenamate Sodium (Potential for increased risk of bleeding).
No products indexed under this heading.

Mefenamic Acid (Potential for increased risk of bleeding). Products include:
Ponstel	1982

Mezlocillin Sodium (Potential for increased risk of bleeding). Products include:
Mezlin	594
Mezlin Pharmacy Bulk Package	597

Nafcillin Sodium (Potential for increased risk of bleeding).
No products indexed under this heading.

Naproxen (Potential for increased risk of bleeding). Products include:
Anaprox/Naprosyn	2277

Naproxen Sodium (Potential for increased risk of bleeding). Products include:
Aleve	2124
Anaprox/Naprosyn	2277
Naprelan Tablets	2861

Penicillin G Benzathine (Potential for increased risk of bleeding). Products include:
Bicillin C-R Injection	2810
Bicillin C-R 900/300 Injection	2812
Bicillin L-A Injection	2813

Penicillin G Procaine (Potential for increased risk of bleeding). Products include:
Bicillin C-R Injection	2810
Bicillin C-R 900/300 Injection	2812

Phenylbutazone (Potential for increased risk of bleeding).
No products indexed under this heading.

Piroxicam (Potential for increased risk of bleeding). Products include:
Feldene Capsules	2008

Salsalate (Potential for increased risk of bleeding). Products include:
Disalcid	1549
Mono-Gesic Tablets	810
Salflex Tablets	791

Sulindac (Potential for increased risk of bleeding). Products include:
Clinoril Tablets	1658

Ticarcillin Disodium (Potential for increased risk of bleeding). Products include:
Ticar for Injection	2704
Timentin for Injection	2706

Ticlopidine Hydrochloride (Potential for increased risk of bleeding). Products include:
Ticlid Tablets	2317

Tolmetin Sodium (Potential for increased risk of bleeding). Products include:
Tolectin (200, 400 and 600 mg)	1591

Warfarin Sodium (Potential for increased risk of bleeding). Products include:
Coumadin	941

STERILE FUDR
(Floxuridine) ... 2284

May interact with alkylating agents. Compounds in this category include:

Bone Marrow Depressants, unspecified (Increased toxicity of FUDR).

Busulfan (FUDR should be used with extreme caution in patients with previous use of alkylating agents). Products include:
Myleran Tablets	1209

Carmustine (BCNU) (FUDR should be used with extreme caution in patients with previous use of alkylating agents). Products include:
BiCNU	696

Chlorambucil (FUDR should be used with extreme caution in patients with previous use of alkylating agents). Products include:
Leukeran Tablets	1205

Cyclophosphamide (FUDR should be used with extreme caution in patients with previous use of alkylating agents). Products include:
Cytoxan	700

Dacarbazine (FUDR should be used with extreme caution in patients with previous use of alkylating agents). Products include:
DTIC-Dome	593

Lomustine (CCNU) (FUDR should be used with extreme caution in patients with previous use of alkylating agents). Products include:
CeeNU Capsules	699

Mechlorethamine Hydrochloride (FUDR should be used with extreme caution in patients with previous use of alkylating agents). Products include:
Mustargen	1752

Melphalan (FUDR should be used with extreme caution in patients with previous use of alkylating agents). Products include:
Alkeran Tablets	1198

Thiotepa (FUDR should be used with extreme caution in patients with previous use of alkylating agents). Products include:
Thioplex (Thiotepa For Injection)	1329

FULVICIN P/G TABLETS
(Griseofulvin) ... 2499

May interact with barbiturates, oral anticoagulants, oral contraceptives, and certain other agents. Compounds in these categories include:

Aprobarbital (Depresses griseofulvin activity).
No products indexed under this heading.

Butabarbital (Depresses griseofulvin activity).
No products indexed under this heading.

Butalbital (Depresses griseofulvin activity). Products include:
Axocet Capsules	2469
Esgic-plus Capsules	1012
Esgic-plus Tablets	1012
Fioricet Tablets	2386
Fioricet with Codeine Capsules	2387
Fiorinal Capsules	2388
Fiorinal with Codeine Capsules	2390
Fiorinal Tablets	2388
Phrenilin	790
Sedapap Tablets 50 mg/650 mg	1826

Desogestrel (Decreased contraceptive effects; possible menstrual irregularities). Products include:
Desogen Tablets	1867
Ortho-Cept	1907

Dicumarol (Decreased anticoagulant effects).
No products indexed under this heading.

Ethinyl Estradiol (Decreased contraceptive effects; possible menstrual irregularities). Products include:
Brevicon	2563
Demulen	2580
Desogen Tablets	1867
Levlen/Tri-Levlen	646
Lo/Ovral Tablets	2852
Lo/Ovral-28 Tablets	2857
Modicon	1928
Nordette-21 Tablets	2863
Nordette-28 Tablets	2866
Norinyl	2563
Ortho-Cept	1907
Ortho-Cyclen/Ortho-Tri-Cyclen	1914
Ortho-Novum	1928
Ortho-Cyclen/Ortho Tri-Cyclen	1914
Ovcon	765
Ovral Tablets	2877
Ovral-28 Tablets	2878
Levlen/Tri-Levlen	646
Tri-Norinyl	2607
Triphasil-21 Tablets	2919
Triphasil-28 Tablets	2924

Ethynodiol Diacetate (Decreased contraceptive effects; possible menstrual irregularities). Products include:
Demulen	2580

Levonorgestrel (Decreased contraceptive effects; possible menstrual irregularities). Products include:
Levlen/Tri-Levlen	646
Nordette-21 Tablets	2863
Nordette-28 Tablets	2866
Norplant System	2868
Levlen/Tri-Levlen	646
Triphasil-21 Tablets	2919
Triphasil-28 Tablets	2924

Mephobarbital (Depresses griseofulvin activity). Products include:
Mebaral Tablets	2452

Mestranol (Decreased contraceptive effects; possible menstrual irregularities). Products include:
Norinyl	2563
Ortho-Novum	1928

Norethindrone (Decreased contraceptive effects; possible menstrual irregularities). Products include:
Brevicon	2563
Micronor Tablets	1903
Modicon	1928
Norinyl	2563
Nor-Q D Tablets	2598
Ortho-Novum	1928
Ovcon	765
Tri-Norinyl	2607

Norethynodrel (Decreased contraceptive effects; possible menstrual irregularities).
No products indexed under this heading.

Norgestimate (Decreased contraceptive effects; possible menstrual irregularities). Products include:
Ortho-Cyclen/Ortho-Tri-Cyclen	1914
Ortho-Cyclen/Ortho-Tri-Cyclen	1914

Norgestrel (Decreased contraceptive effects; possible menstrual irregularities). Products include:
Lo/Ovral Tablets	2852
Lo/Ovral-28 Tablets	2857
Ovral Tablets	2877
Ovral-28 Tablets	2878
Ovrette Tablets	2878

Pentobarbital Sodium (Depresses griseofulvin activity). Products include:
Nembutal Sodium Capsules	440
Nembutal Sodium Solution	442
Nembutal Sodium Suppositories	444

Phenobarbital (Depresses griseofulvin activity). Products include:
Arco-Lase Plus Tablets	513
Bellergal-S Tablets	2375
Donnatal	2234
Donnatal Extentabs	2234
Donnatal	2234
Phenobarbital Elixir and Tablets	1523
Quadrinal Tablets	1398

Secobarbital Sodium (Depresses griseofulvin activity). Products include:
Seconal Sodium Pulvules	1529

IMPORTANT NOTE: Always consult each drug listing in the patient's regimen for possible interactions.

Fulvicin P/G — Interactions Index — 430

Thiamylal Sodium (Depresses griseofulvin activity).
No products indexed under this heading.

Warfarin Sodium (Decreased anticoagulant effects). Products include:
Coumadin ... 941

Food Interactions

Alcohol (Potentiation of effects of alcohol).

FULVICIN P/G 165 & 330 TABLETS

(Griseofulvin) ... 2500
May interact with oral anticoagulants, barbiturates, oral contraceptives, and certain other agents. Compounds in these categories include:

Aprobarbital (Depresses griseofulvin activity).
No products indexed under this heading.

Butabarbital (Depresses griseofulvin activity).
No products indexed under this heading.

Butalbital (Depresses griseofulvin activity). Products include:
Axocet Capsules ... 2469
Esgic-plus Capsules ... 1012
Esgic-plus Tablets ... 1012
Fioricet Tablets ... 2386
Fioricet with Codeine Capsules ... 2387
Fiorinal Capsules ... 2388
Fiorinal with Codeine Capsules ... 2390
Fiorinal Tablets ... 2388
Phrenilin ... 790
Sedapap Tablets 50 mg/650 mg ... 1826

Desogestrel (Decreased contraceptive effects; possible menstrual irregularities). Products include:
Desogen Tablets ... 1867
Ortho-Cept ... 1907

Dicumarol (Decreased anticoagulant effect).
No products indexed under this heading.

Ethinyl Estradiol (Decreased contraceptive effects; possible menstrual irregularities). Products include:
Brevicon ... 2563
Demulen ... 2580
Desogen Tablets ... 1867
Levlen/Tri-Levlen ... 646
Lo/Ovral Tablets ... 2852
Lo/Ovral-28 Tablets ... 2857
Modicon ... 1928
Nordette-21 Tablets ... 2863
Nordette-28 Tablets ... 2866
Norinyl ... 2563
Ortho-Cept ... 1907
Ortho-Cyclen/Ortho-Tri-Cyclen ... 1914
Ortho-Novum ... 1928
Ortho-Cyclen/Ortho Tri-Cyclen ... 1914
Ovcon ... 765
Ovral Tablets ... 2877
Ovral-28 Tablets ... 2878
Levlen/Tri-Levlen ... 646
Tri-Norinyl ... 2607
Triphasil-21 Tablets ... 2919
Triphasil-28 Tablets ... 2924

Ethynodiol Diacetate (Decreased contraceptive effects; possible menstrual irregularities). Products include:
Demulen ... 2580

Levonorgestrel (Decreased contraceptive effects; possible menstrual irregularities). Products include:
Levlen/Tri-Levlen ... 646
Nordette-21 Tablets ... 2863
Nordette-28 Tablets ... 2866
Norplant System ... 2868
Levlen/Tri-Levlen ... 646
Triphasil-21 Tablets ... 2919
Triphasil-28 Tablets ... 2924

Mephobarbital (Depresses griseofulvin activity). Products include:
Mebaral Tablets ... 2452

Mestranol (Decreased contraceptive effects; possible menstrual irregularities). Products include:
Norinyl ... 2563
Ortho-Novum ... 1928

Norethindrone (Decreased contraceptive effects; possible menstrual irregularities). Products include:
Brevicon ... 2563
Micronor Tablets ... 1903
Modicon ... 1928
Norinyl ... 2563
Nor-Q D Tablets ... 2598
Ortho-Novum ... 1928
Ovcon ... 765
Tri-Norinyl ... 2607

Norethynodrel (Decreased contraceptive effects; possible menstrual irregularities).
No products indexed under this heading.

Norgestimate (Decreased contraceptive effects; possible menstrual irregularities). Products include:
Ortho-Cyclen/Ortho-Tri-Cyclen ... 1914
Ortho-Cyclen/Ortho Tri-Cyclen ... 1914

Norgestrel (Decreased contraceptive effects; possible menstrual irregularities). Products include:
Lo/Ovral Tablets ... 2852
Lo/Ovral-28 Tablets ... 2857
Ovral Tablets ... 2877
Ovral-28 Tablets ... 2878
Ovrette Tablets ... 2878

Pentobarbital Sodium (Depresses griseofulvin activity). Products include:
Nembutal Sodium Capsules ... 440
Nembutal Sodium Solution ... 442
Nembutal Sodium Suppositories ... 444

Phenobarbital (Depresses griseofulvin activity). Products include:
Arco-Lase Plus Tablets ... 513
Bellergal-S Tablets ... 2375
Donnatal ... 2234
Donnatal Extentabs ... 2234
Donnatal Tablets ... 2234
Phenobarbital Elixir and Tablets ... 1523
Quadrinal Tablets ... 1398

Secobarbital Sodium (Depresses griseofulvin activity). Products include:
Seconal Sodium Pulvules ... 1529

Thiamylal Sodium (Depresses griseofulvin activity).
No products indexed under this heading.

Warfarin Sodium (Decreased anticoagulant effect). Products include:
Coumadin ... 941

Food Interactions

Alcohol (Potentiation of effects of alcohol).

FUNGIZONE INTRAVENOUS

(Amphotericin B) ... 507
May interact with antineoplastics, nitrogen-mustard-type alkylating agents, corticosteroids, cardiac glycosides, aminoglycosides, imidazoles, muscle relaxants, and certain other agents. Compounds in these categories include:

ACTH (May potentiate amphotericin B-induced hypokalemia which may predispose the patient to cardiac dysfunction; avoid concomitant use).
No products indexed under this heading.

Altretamine (May enhance the potential for renal toxicity, bronchospasm and hypotension). Products include:
Hexalen Capsules ... 2760

Amikacin Sulfate (May enhance the potential for drug-induced renal toxicity, and should be used concomitantly only with great caution). Products include:
Amikacin Sulfate Injection, USP ... 523
Amikacin Sulfate Injection, USP ... 981
Amikin Injectable ... 502

Anastrozole (May enhance the potential for renal toxicity, bronchospasm and hypotension). Products include:
Arimidex Tablets ... 2932

Asparaginase (May enhance the potential for renal toxicity, bronchospasm and hypotension). Products include:
Elspar ... 1700

Atracurium Besylate (Amphotericin B-induced hypokalemia may enhance the curariform effect of skeletal muscle relaxants). Products include:
Tracrium Injection ... 1155

Baclofen (Amphotericin B-induced hypokalemia may enhance the curariform effect of skeletal muscle relaxants). Products include:
Lioresal Intrathecal ... 1634
Lioresal Tablets ... 847

Betamethasone Acetate (May potentiate amphotericin B-induced hypokalemia which may predispose the patient to cardiac dysfunction; avoid concomitant use). Products include:
Celestone Soluspan Suspension ... 2484

Betamethasone Sodium Phosphate (May potentiate amphotericin B-induced hypokalemia which may predispose the patient to cardiac dysfunction; avoid concomitant use). Products include:
Celestone Soluspan Suspension ... 2484

Bicalutamide (May enhance the potential for renal toxicity, bronchospasm and hypotension). Products include:
Casodex Tablets ... 2934

Bleomycin Sulfate (May enhance the potential for renal toxicity, bronchospasm and hypotension). Products include:
Blenoxane ... 697

Busulfan (May enhance the potential for renal toxicity, bronchospasm and hypotension). Products include:
Myleran Tablets ... 1209

Carboplatin (May enhance the potential for renal toxicity, bronchospasm and hypotension). Products include:
Paraplatin for Injection ... 713

Carisoprodol (Amphotericin B-induced hypokalemia may enhance the curariform effect of skeletal muscle relaxants). Products include:
Soma Compound w/Codeine Tablets ... 2784
Soma Compound Tablets ... 2783
Soma Tablets ... 2782

Carmustine (BCNU) (May enhance the potential for renal toxicity, bronchospasm and hypotension). Products include:
BiCNU ... 696

Chlorambucil (May enhance the potential for renal toxicity, bronchospasm and hypotension). Products include:
Leukeran Tablets ... 1205

Chlorzoxazone (Amphotericin B-induced hypokalemia may enhance the curariform effect of skeletal muscle relaxants). Products include:
Parafon Forte DSC Caplets ... 1590

Cisatracurium Besylate (Amphotericin B-induced hypokalemia may enhance the curariform effect of skeletal muscle relaxants). Products include:
Nimbex Injection ... 1131

Cisplatin (May enhance the potential for renal toxicity, bronchospasm and hypotension). Products include:
Platinol for Injection ... 717
Platinol-AQ Injection ... 719

Clotrimazole (*In vitro* studies with combination therapy suggest that imidazoles may induce fungal resistance to amphotericin-B). Products include:
Prescription Strength Desenex AF Cream ... [ND] 653
Lotrimin ... 2514
Lotrimin AF Antifungal Cream, Lotion and Solution ... [ND] 766
Lotrisone Cream ... 2515
Mycelex OTC Cream Antifungal ... [ND] 622
Mycelex Troches ... 601
Mycelex-7 Vaginal Cream Antifungal ... [ND] 622
Mycelex-7 Vaginal Antifungal Cream with 7 Disposable Applicators ... [ND] 623
Mycelex-7 Vaginal Inserts Antifungal ... [ND] 623
Mycelex-7 Combination-Pack Vaginal Inserts & External Vulvar Cream ... [ND] 623
Mycelex-G 500 mg Vaginal Tablets 602

Cortisone Acetate (May potentiate amphotericin B-induced hypokalemia which may predispose the patient to cardiac dysfunction; avoid concomitant use). Products include:
Cortone Acetate Sterile Suspension ... 1663
Cortone Acetate Tablets ... 1664

Cyclobenzaprine Hydrochloride (Amphotericin B-induced hypokalemia may enhance the curariform effect of skeletal muscle relaxants). Products include:
Flexeril Tablets ... 1701

Cyclophosphamide (May enhance the potential for renal toxicity, bronchospasm and hypotension). Products include:
Cytoxan ... 700

Cyclosporine (May enhance the potential for drug-induced renal toxicity, and should be used concomitantly only with great caution). Products include:
Neoral ... 2405
Sandimmune ... 2416

Dacarbazine (May enhance the potential for renal toxicity, bronchospasm and hypotension). Products include:
DTIC-Dome ... 593

Dantrolene Sodium (Amphotericin B-induced hypokalemia may enhance the curariform effect of skeletal muscle relaxants). Products include:
Dantrium Capsules ... 2131
Dantrium Intravenous ... 2132

Daunorubicin Citrate (May enhance the potential for renal toxicity, bronchospasm and hypotension). Products include:
DaunoXome ... 1842

Daunorubicin Hydrochloride (May enhance the potential for renal toxicity, bronchospasm and hypotension). Products include:
Cerubidine for Injection ... 634

([ND] Described in PDR For Nonprescription Drugs) (⊚ Described in PDR For Ophthalmology)

431 **Interactions Index** **Fungizone I.V.**

Deslanoside (Amphotericin B-induced hypokalemia may potentiate digitalis toxicity).
No products indexed under this heading.

Dexamethasone (May potentiate amphotericin B-induced hypokalemia which may predispose the patient to cardiac dysfunction; avoid concomitant use). Products include:
AK-Trol Ointment & Suspension .... ◉ 205
Decadron Elixir 1676
Decadron Tablets 1678
Decaspray Topical Aerosol 1689
Maxitrol Ophthalmic Ointment and Suspension .... ◉ 222
TobraDex Ophthalmic Suspension and Ointment 469

Dexamethasone Acetate (May potentiate amphotericin B-induced hypokalemia which may predispose the patient to cardiac dysfunction; avoid concomitant use). Products include:
Dalalone D.P. Injectable 1009
Decadron-LA Sterile Suspension 1687

Dexamethasone Sodium Phosphate (May potentiate amphotericin B-induced hypokalemia which may predispose the patient to cardiac dysfunction; avoid concomitant use). Products include:
Decadron Phosphate Injection 1680
Decadron Phosphate Sterile Ophthalmic Ointment 1684
Decadron Phosphate Sterile Ophthalmic Solution 1685
Decadron Phosphate Topical Cream 1686
Decadron Phosphate with Xylocaine Injection, Sterile 1683
Dexacort Phosphate in Respihaler .. 1606
Dexacort Phosphate in Turbinaire .. 1607
NeoDecadron Sterile Ophthalmic Ointment 1755
NeoDecadron Sterile Ophthalmic Solution 1756
NeoDecadron Topical Cream 1757

Digitoxin (Amphotericin B-induced hypokalemia may potentiate digitalis toxicity). Products include:
Crystodigin Tablets 1472

Digoxin (Amphotericin B-induced hypokalemia may potentiate digitalis toxicity). Products include:
Lanoxicaps 1110
Lanoxin Elixir Pediatric 1113
Lanoxin Injection 1116
Lanoxin Injection Pediatric 1119
Lanoxin Tablets 1121

Docetaxel (May enhance the potential for renal toxicity, bronchospasm and hypotension). Products include:
Taxotere for Injection Concentrate 2204

Doxacurium Chloride (Amphotericin B-induced hypokalemia may enhance the curariform effect of skeletal muscle relaxants). Products include:
Nuromax Injection 1136

Doxorubicin Hydrochloride (May enhance the potential for renal toxicity, bronchospasm and hypotension). Products include:
Adriamycin PFS 2056
Adriamycin RDF 2056
Doxil 2613
Doxorubicin Astra 531
Rubex for Injection 721

Estramustine Phosphate Sodium (May enhance the potential for renal toxicity, bronchospasm and hypotension). Products include:
Emcyt Capsules 2085

Etoposide (May enhance the potential for renal toxicity, bronchospasm and hypotension). Products include:
Etoposide Injection 539
VePesid Capsules and Injection 727

Floxuridine (May enhance the potential for renal toxicity, bronchospasm and hypotension). Products include:
Sterile FUDR 2284

Fluconazole (*In vitro* studies with combination therapy suggest that imidazoles may induce fungal resistance to amphotericin-B). Products include:
Diflucan Tablets, Injection, and Oral Suspension 2003

Flucytosine (Concomitant use may increase the toxicity of flucytosine by possibly increasing its cellular uptake and/or impairing its renal excretion). Products include:
Ancobon Capsules 2254

Fludrocortisone Acetate (May potentiate amphotericin B-induced hypokalemia which may predispose the patient to cardiac dysfunction; avoid concomitant use). Products include:
Florinef Acetate Tablets 506

Fluorouracil (May enhance the potential for renal toxicity, bronchospasm and hypotension). Products include:
Efudex 2280
Fluoroplex Topical Solution & Cream 1% 475
Fluorouracil Injection 2282

Flutamide (May enhance the potential for renal toxicity, bronchospasm and hypotension). Products include:
Eulexin Capsules 2498

Gemcitabine Hydrochloride (May enhance the potential for renal toxicity, bronchospasm and hypotension). Products include:
Gemzar for Injection 1482

Gentamicin Sulfate (May enhance the potential for drug-induced renal toxicity, and should be used concomitantly only with great caution). Products include:
Garamycin Cream 0.1% 2501
Garamycin Injectable 2502
Garamycin Ointment 0.1% 2501
Garamycin Ophthalmic 2501
Genoptic Sterile Ophthalmic Solution .... ◉ 241
Genoptic Sterile Ophthalmic Ointment .... ◉ 241
Gentak .... ◉ 209
Pred-G Liquifilm Sterile Ophthalmic Suspension .... ◉ 248
Pred-G S.O.P. Sterile Ophthalmic Ointment .... ◉ 249

Hydrocortisone (May potentiate amphotericin B-induced hypokalemia which may predispose the patient to cardiac dysfunction; avoid concomitant use). Products include:
Anusol-HC Cream 2.5% 1953
Aquanil HC Lotion 1989
Maximum Strength Cortaid Spray ▣ 800
CORTENEMA 2713
Cortisporin Ointment 1074
Cortisporin Ophthalmic Ointment Sterile 1074
Cortisporin Ophthalmic Suspension Sterile 1075
Cortisporin Otic Solution Sterile 1076
Cortisporin Otic Suspension Sterile 1077
Cortizone-5 .... ▣ 795
Cortizone-10 .... ▣ 795
Hydrocortone Tablets 1715
Hytone 922
Hytone Ointment 2 ½% 923
Massengill Medicated Soft Cloth Towelettes 2628
Pediotic Suspension Sterile 1140
Preparation H Hydrocortisone 1% Cream .... ▣ 843
ProctoCream-HC 2.5% 2552
VōSoL HC Otic Solution 2786

Hydrocortisone Acetate (May potentiate amphotericin B-induced hypokalemia which may predispose the patient to cardiac dysfunction; avoid concomitant use). Products include:
Analpram-HC Rectal Cream 1% and 2.5% 993
Anusol HC-1 Hydrocortisone Anti-Itch Ointment .... ▣ 810
Anusol-HC Suppositories 1954
Caldecort Anti-Itch Hydrocortisone Cream .... ▣ 651
Coly-Mycin S Otic w/Neomycin & Hydrocortisone 1965
Cortaid .... ▣ 800
Cortifoam 2540
Cortisporin Cream 1073
Epifoam 2543
Hydrocortone Acetate Sterile Suspension 1712
Mantadil Cream 1124
Nupercainal Hydrocortisone 1% Cream .... ▣ 661
Pramosone Cream, Lotion & Ointment 995
ProctoFoam-HC 2552
Terra-Cortril Ophthalmic Suspension 2033

Hydrocortisone Sodium Phosphate (May potentiate amphotericin B-induced hypokalemia which may predispose the patient to cardiac dysfunction; avoid concomitant use). Products include:
Hydrocortone Phosphate Injection, Sterile 1713

Hydrocortisone Sodium Succinate (May potentiate amphotericin B-induced hypokalemia which may predispose the patient to cardiac dysfunction; avoid concomitant use).
No products indexed under this heading.

Hydroxyurea (May enhance the potential for renal toxicity, bronchospasm and hypotension). Products include:
Hydrea Capsules 705

Idarubicin Hydrochloride (May enhance the potential for renal toxicity, bronchospasm and hypotension). Products include:
Idamycin Injection 2096

Ifosfamide (May enhance the potential for renal toxicity, bronchospasm and hypotension). Products include:
IFEX 706

Interferon alfa-2A, Recombinant (May enhance the potential for renal toxicity, bronchospasm and hypotension). Products include:
Roferon-A Injection 2308

Interferon alfa-2B, Recombinant (May enhance the potential for renal toxicity, bronchospasm and hypotension). Products include:
Intron A for Injection 2506

Irinotecan Hydrochloride (May enhance the potential for renal toxicity, bronchospasm and hypotension).
No products indexed under this heading.

Kanamycin Sulfate (May enhance the potential for drug-induced renal toxicity, and should be used concomitantly only with great caution).
No products indexed under this heading.

Ketoconazole (*In vitro* studies with combination therapy suggest that imidazoles may induce fungal resistance to amphotericin-B). Products include:
Nizoral 2% Cream 1344
Nizoral 2% Shampoo 1344
Nizoral Tablets 1345

Leukocyte transfusions (Potential for acute pulmonary toxicity with concomitant administration).

Levamisole Hydrochloride (May enhance the potential for renal toxicity, bronchospasm and hypotension). Products include:
Ergamisol Tablets 1340

Lomustine (CCNU) (May enhance the potential for renal toxicity, bronchospasm and hypotension). Products include:
CeeNU Capsules 699

Mechlorethamine Hydrochloride (May enhance the potential for renal toxicity, bronchospasm and hypotension). Products include:
Mustargen 1752

Megestrol Acetate (May enhance the potential for renal toxicity, bronchospasm and hypotension). Products include:
Megace Oral Suspension 708
Megace Tablets 710

Melphalan (May enhance the potential for renal toxicity, bronchospasm and hypotension). Products include:
Alkeran Tablets 1198

Mercaptopurine (May enhance the potential for renal toxicity, bronchospasm and hypotension). Products include:
Purinethol Tablets 1214

Metaxalone (Amphotericin B-induced hypokalemia may enhance the curariform effect of skeletal muscle relaxants). Products include:
Skelaxin Tablets 793

Methocarbamol (Amphotericin B-induced hypokalemia may enhance the curariform effect of skeletal muscle relaxants). Products include:
Robaxin Injectable 2245
Robaxin Tablets 2246
Robaxisal Tablets 2246

Methotrexate Sodium (May enhance the potential for renal toxicity, bronchospasm and hypotension). Products include:
Methotrexate Sodium Tablets, Injection, for Injection and LPF Injection 1322

Methylprednisolone Acetate (May potentiate amphotericin B-induced hypokalemia which may predispose the patient to cardiac dysfunction; avoid concomitant use).
No products indexed under this heading.

Methylprednisolone Sodium Succinate (May potentiate amphotericin B-induced hypokalemia which may predispose the patient to cardiac dysfunction; avoid concomitant use).
No products indexed under this heading.

Metocurine Iodide (Amphotericin B-induced hypokalemia may enhance the curariform effect of skeletal muscle relaxants). Products include:
Metubine Iodide Vials 932

Miconazole (*In vitro* studies with combination therapy suggest that imidazoles may induce fungal resistance to amphotericin-B).
No products indexed under this heading.

Miconazole Nitrate (*In vitro* studies with combination therapy suggest that imidazoles may induce fungal resistance to amphotericin-B). Products include:
Prescription Strength Desenex Spray Powder and Spray Liquid ▣ 653
Lotrimin AF Antifungal Spray Liquid, Spray Powder, Spray Deodorant Powder, Powder and Jock Itch Spray Powder .... ▣ 766
Monistat Dual-Pak 1906
Monistat 3 Vaginal Suppositories 1905

IMPORTANT NOTE: Always consult each drug listing in the patient's regimen for possible interactions.

Fungizone I.V. — Interactions Index

Monistat-Derm (miconazole nitrate 2%) Cream 1944
Ting Antifungal Spray Powder .... ⊞ 666

Mitomycin (Mitomycin-C) (May enhance the potential for renal toxicity, bronchospasm and hypotension). Products include:
Mutamycin for Injection 712

Mitotane (May enhance the potential for renal toxicity, bronchospasm and hypotension). Products include:
Lysodren Tablets 707

Mitoxantrone Hydrochloride (May enhance the potential for renal toxicity, bronchospasm and hypotension). Products include:
Novantrone for Injection 1327

Mivacurium Chloride (Amphotericin B-induced hypokalemia may enhance the curariform effect of skeletal muscle relaxants). Products include:
Mivacron 1125

Orphenadrine Citrate (Amphotericin B-induced hypokalemia may enhance the curariform effect of skeletal muscle relaxants). Products include:
Norflex 1554
Norgesic 1554

Paclitaxel (May enhance the potential for renal toxicity, bronchospasm and hypotension). Products include:
Taxol Injection 723

Pancuronium Bromide (Amphotericin B-induced hypokalemia may enhance the curariform effect of skeletal muscle relaxants).
No products indexed under this heading.

Pentamidine Isethionate (May enhance the potential for drug-induced renal toxicity, and should be used concomitantly only with great caution).
No products indexed under this heading.

Prednisolone Acetate (May potentiate amphotericin B-induced hypokalemia which may predispose the patient to cardiac dysfunction; avoid concomitant use). Products include:
AK-CIDE .... ⊙ 203
AK-CIDE Ointment .... ⊙ 203
Blephamide Liquifilm Sterile Ophthalmic Suspension 472
Blephamide Ointment .... ⊙ 234
Econopred & Econopred Plus Ophthalmic Suspensions .... ⊙ 216
Poly-Pred Liquifilm .... ⊙ 246
Pred Forte .... ⊙ 247
Pred Mild .... ⊙ 250
Pred-G Liquifilm Sterile Ophthalmic Suspension .... ⊙ 248
Pred-G S.O.P. Sterile Ophthalmic Ointment .... ⊙ 249

Prednisolone Sodium Phosphate (May potentiate amphotericin B-induced hypokalemia which may predispose the patient to cardiac dysfunction; avoid concomitant use). Products include:
AK-PRED .... ⊙ 204
Hydeltrasol Injection, Sterile 1708
Pediapred Oral Solution 1618

Prednisolone Tebutate (May potentiate amphotericin B-induced hypokalemia which may predispose the patient to cardiac dysfunction; avoid concomitant use). Products include:
Hydeltra-T.B.A. Sterile Suspension 1710

Prednisone (May potentiate amphotericin B-induced hypokalemia which may predispose the patient to cardiac dysfunction; avoid concomitant use).
No products indexed under this heading.

Procarbazine Hydrochloride (May enhance the potential for renal toxicity, bronchospasm and hypotension). Products include:
Matulane Capsules 2300

Rocuronium Bromide (Amphotericin B-induced hypokalemia may enhance the curariform effect of skeletal muscle relaxants). Products include:
Zemuron Injection 1885

Streptomycin Sulfate (May enhance the potential for drug-induced renal toxicity, and should be used concomitantly only with great caution). Products include:
Streptomycin Sulfate Injection 2031

Streptozocin (May enhance the potential for renal toxicity, bronchospasm and hypotension). Products include:
Zanosar Sterile Powder 2119

Succinylcholine Chloride (Amphotericin B-induced hypokalemia may enhance the curariform effect of skeletal muscle relaxants). Products include:
Anectine 1062

Tamoxifen Citrate (May enhance the potential for renal toxicity, bronchospasm and hypotension). Products include:
Nolvadex Tablets 2957

Teniposide (May enhance the potential for renal toxicity, bronchospasm and hypotension). Products include:
Vumon for Injection 729

Thioguanine (May enhance the potential for renal toxicity, bronchospasm and hypotension). Products include:
Thioguanine Tablets, Tabloid Brand 1225

Thiotepa (May enhance the potential for renal toxicity, bronchospasm and hypotension). Products include:
Thioplex (Thiotepa For Injection) 1329

Tobramycin (May enhance the potential for drug-induced renal toxicity, and should be used concomitantly only with great caution). Products include:
AKTOB .... ⊙ 207
TobraDex Ophthalmic Suspension and Ointment 469
Tobrex Ophthalmic Ointment and Solution .... ⊙ 226

Tobramycin Sulfate (May enhance the potential for drug-induced renal toxicity, and should be used concomitantly only with great caution). Products include:
Nebcin Vials, Hyporets & ADD-Vantage 1518

Topotecan Hydrochloride (May enhance the potential for renal toxicity, bronchospasm and hypotension). Products include:
Hycamtin for Injection 2665

Triamcinolone (May potentiate amphotericin B-induced hypokalemia which may predispose the patient to cardiac dysfunction; avoid concomitant use).
No products indexed under this heading.

Triamcinolone Acetonide (May potentiate amphotericin B-induced hypokalemia which may predispose the patient to cardiac dysfunction; avoid concomitant use). Products include:
Azmacort Oral Inhaler 2175
Nasacort AQ Nasal Spray 2191
Nasacort Nasal Inhaler 2189

Triamcinolone Diacetate (May potentiate amphotericin B-induced hypokalemia which may predispose the patient to cardiac dysfunction; avoid concomitant use).
No products indexed under this heading.

Triamcinolone Hexacetonide (May potentiate amphotericin B-induced hypokalemia which may predispose the patient to cardiac dysfunction; avoid concomitant use).
No products indexed under this heading.

Tubocurarine Chloride (Amphotericin B-induced hypokalemia may enhance the curariform effect of skeletal muscle relaxants).
No products indexed under this heading.

Vecuronium Bromide (Amphotericin B-induced hypokalemia may enhance the curariform effect of skeletal muscle relaxants). Products include:
Norcuron for Injection 1875

Vincristine Sulfate (May enhance the potential for renal toxicity, bronchospasm and hypotension). Products include:
Oncovin Solution Vials & Hyporets 1521

Vinorelbine Tartrate (May enhance the potential for renal toxicity, bronchospasm and hypotension). Products include:
Navelbine Injection 1212

FUNGIZONE ORAL SUSPENSION
(Amphotericin B) 704
May interact with:

Ketoconazole (Antagonism between amphotericin B and imidazole derivative such as ketoconazole has been reported; the clinical significance of this phenomenon is unknown). Products include:
Nizoral 2% Cream 1344
Nizoral 2% Shampoo 1344
Nizoral Tablets 1345

Miconazole (Antagonism between amphotericin B and imidazole derivative such as miconazole has been reported; the clinical significance of this phenomenon is unknown).
No products indexed under this heading.

FURACIN SOLUBLE DRESSING
(Nitrofurazone) 2220
None cited in PDR database.

FURACIN TOPICAL CREAM
(Nitrofurazone) 2220
None cited in PDR database.

FUROXONE LIQUID
(Furazolidone) 2221
May interact with anorexiants, monoamine oxidase inhibitors, antihistamines, hypnotics and sedatives, narcotic analgesics, tranquilizers, indirect-acting sympathomimetic amines, and certain other agents. Compounds in these categories include:

Acrivastine (Predisposition to hypertensive crises; use with caution at reduced dosages). Products include:
Semprex-D Capsules 1620

Alfentanil Hydrochloride (Predisposition to hypertensive crises; use with caution at reduced dosages). Products include:
Alfenta Injection 1334

Alprazolam (Predisposition to hypertensive crises; use with caution at reduced dosages). Products include:
Xanax Tablets 2115

Amphetamine Resins (Predisposition to hypertensive crises; concurrent administration is contraindicated).
No products indexed under this heading.

Astemizole (Predisposition to hypertensive crises; use with caution at reduced dosages). Products include:
Hismanal Tablets 1341

Azatadine Maleate (Predisposition to hypertensive crises; use with caution at reduced dosages). Products include:
Trinalin Repetabs Tablets 1373

Benzphetamine Hydrochloride (Predisposition to hypertensive crises; concurrent administration is contraindicated).
No products indexed under this heading.

Bromodiphenhydramine Hydrochloride (Predisposition to hypertensive crises; use with caution at reduced dosages).
No products indexed under this heading.

Brompheniramine Maleate (Predisposition to hypertensive crises; use with caution at reduced dosages). Products include:
Alka-Seltzer Plus Sinus Medicine .... ⊞ 611
Bromfed Capsules (Extended-Release) 1832
Bromfed Syrup .... ⊞ 712
Bromfed Tablets 1832
Bromfed-DM Cough Syrup 1832
Bromfed-PD Capsules (Extended-Release) 1832
Dimetane-DC Cough Syrup 2232
Dimetane-DX Cough Syrup 2233
Dimetapp Allergy Dye-Free Elixir .... ⊞ 838
Dimetapp Allergy Sinus Caplets .... ⊞ 838
Dimetapp Cold & Allergy Chewable Tablets .... ⊞ 838
Dimetapp Cold & Cough Liqui-Gels .... ⊞ 839
Dimetapp Cold & Fever Suspension .... ⊞ 839
Dimetapp DM Elixir .... ⊞ 840
Dimetapp Elixir .... ⊞ 840
Dimetapp Extentabs .... ⊞ 841
Dimetapp Tablets/Liqui-Gels .... ⊞ 841
Rondec Chewable Tablets 974
Vicks DayQuil Allergy Relief 12-Hour Extended Release Tablets .... ⊞ 733
Vicks DayQuil Allergy Relief 4-Hour Tablets .... ⊞ 733

Buprenorphine (Predisposition to hypertensive crises; use with caution at reduced dosages). Products include:
Buprenex Injectable 2170

Buspirone Hydrochloride (Predisposition to hypertensive crises; use with caution at reduced dosages). Products include:
BuSpar Tablets 738

Cetirizine Hydrochloride (Predisposition to hypertensive crises; use with caution at reduced dosages). Products include:
Zyrtec Tablets 2053

Chlordiazepoxide (Predisposition to hypertensive crises; use with caution at reduced dosages). Products include:
Limbitrol 2333

Chlordiazepoxide Hydrochloride (Predisposition to hypertensive crises; use with caution at reduced dosages). Products include:
Librax Capsules 2330
Librium Capsules 2331
Librium Injectable 2332

(⊞ Described in PDR For Nonprescription Drugs)   (⊙ Described in PDR For Ophthalmology)

Chlorpheniramine Maleate
(Predisposition to hypertensive crises; use with caution at reduced dosages). Products include:
Alka-Seltzer Plus Cold Medicine .... ⚫ 611
Alka-Seltzer Plus Cold Medicine Liqui-Gels .... ⚫ 612
Alka-Seltzer Plus Cold & Cough Medicine .... ⚫ 611
Alka-Seltzer Plus Cold & Cough Medicine Liqui-Gels .... ⚫ 612
Alka-Seltzer Plus Flu & Body Aches Effervescent Tablets.............. ⚫ 612
Allerest Maximum Strength .... ⚫ 649
Allerest Sinus Pain Formula .... ⚫ 649
Ana-Kit Anaphylaxis Emergency Treatment Kit 611
Atrohist Pediatric Capsules 1603
Atrohist Plus Tablets 1605
BC Cold Powder Multi-Symptom Formula (Cold-Sinus-Allergy) .... ⚫ 631
Cerose DM .... ⚫ 853
Cheracol Plus Head Cold/Cough Formula .... ⚫ 741
Children's TYLENOL Cold Multi-Symptom Chewable Tablets and Liquid 1559
Children's TYLENOL Cold Plus Cough Multi Symptom Chewable Tablets and Liquid 1560
Children's TYLENOL Flu Suspension Liquid 1560
Children's Vicks DayQuil Allergy Relief .... ⚫ 730
Children's Vicks NyQuil Cold/Cough Relief .... ⚫ 731
Chlor-Trimeton Allergy Decongestant Tablets .... ⚫ 759
Chlor-Trimeton Allergy Tablets .... ⚫ 758
Allergy-Sinus Comtrex Multi-Symptom Allergy-Sinus Formula Tablets and Caplets .... ⚫ 639
Comtrex Multi-Symptom .... ⚫ 638
Contac Continuous Action Nasal Decongestant/Antihistamine 12 Hour Capsules .... ⚫ 773
Contac Maximum Strength Continuous Action Decongestant/Antihistamine 12 Hour Caplets... ⚫ 772
Contac Severe Cold and Flu Formula Caplets .... ⚫ 773
Coricidin Cold + Flu Tablets............. ⚫ 760
Coricidin Cough + Cold Tablets ...... ⚫ 760
Coricidin 'D' Decongestant Tablets .... ⚫ 760
D.A. II Tablets 972
D.A. Chewable Tablets......................... 970
Dura-Tap/PD Capsules 970
Dura-Vent/DA Tablets 972
Efidac 24 Chlorpheniramine............. 655
Extendryl 1003
Fedahist Gyrocaps................................. 2545
Hycomine Compound Tablets 948
Kronofed-A 994
Nolamine Timed-Release Tablets 790
Novahistine Elixir .... ⚫ 782
Ornade Spansule Capsules 2678
PediaCare Cough-Cold Chewable Tablets and Liquid........................... 1569
PediaCare NightRest Cough-Cold Liquid 1569
Pediatric Vicks 44m Cough & Cold Relief .... ⚫ 737
Pyrroxate Caplets .... ⚫ 742
Ryna .... ⚫ 804
Sinarest .... ⚫ 663
Sine-Off Sinus Medicine .... ⚫ 784
Singlet Tablets .... ⚫ 785
Sinulin Tablets 792
Sinutab Sinus Allergy Medication, Maximum Strength Tablets and Caplets .... ⚫ 823
Sudafed Cold & Allergy Tablets....... ⚫ 826
Teldrin 12 Hour Antihistamine/Nasal Decongestant Allergy Relief Capsules .... ⚫ 786
TheraFlu Flu and Cold Medicine .... ⚫ 750
Theraflu Maximum Strength Flu and Cold Medicine For Sore Throat .... ⚫ 751
TheraFlu Flu, Cold and Cough Medicine .... ⚫ 750
TheraFlu Maximum Strength Nighttime Flu, Cold & Cough Medicine .... ⚫ 751
Triaminic Night Time 754
Triaminic Syrup 755
Triaminic Triaminicol Cold & Cough 756
Triaminicin Tablets 756
Tussend 1830

TYLENOL Allergy Sinus, Maximum Strength Caplets and Gelcaps ... 1571
TYLENOL Cold Medication, Multi-Symptom Formula Tablets and Caplets 1572
TYLENOL Cold Medication, Multi-Symptom Hot Liquid Packets 1572
Vicks 44 LiquiCaps Cough, Cold & Flu Relief .... ⚫ 728
Vicks 44M Cough, Cold & Flu Relief .... ⚫ 729

Chlorpheniramine Polistirex
(Predisposition to hypertensive crises; use with caution at reduced dosages). Products include:
Tussionex Pennkinetic Extended-Release Suspension 1624

Chlorpheniramine Tannate
(Predisposition to hypertensive crises; use with caution at reduced dosages). Products include:
Atrohist Pediatric Suspension 1604
Atrohist Pediatric Suspension Dye-Free 1604
Rynatan 2781
Rynatuss 2782

Chlorpromazine (Predisposition to hypertensive crises; use with caution at reduced dosages). Products include:
Thorazine Suppositories..................... 2701

Chlorprothixene (Predisposition to hypertensive crises; use with caution at reduced dosages).
No products indexed under this heading.

Chlorprothixene Hydrochloride
(Predisposition to hypertensive crises; use with caution at reduced dosages).
No products indexed under this heading.

Clemastine Fumarate (Predisposition to hypertensive crises; use with caution at reduced dosages). Products include:
Tavist Syrup 2426
Tavist Tablets 2427
Tavist-1 12 Hour Relief Tablets .... ⚫ 749
Tavist-D 12 Hour Relief Tablets .... ⚫ 750

Clorazepate Dipotassium (Predisposition to hypertensive crises; use with caution at reduced dosages). Products include:
Tranxene 459

Codeine Phosphate (Predisposition to hypertensive crises; use with caution at reduced dosages). Products include:
Brontex 2130
Dimetane-DC Cough Syrup 2232
Fioricet with Codeine Capsules 2387
Fiorinal with Codeine Capsules 2390
Nucofed 2225
Phenergan with Codeine.................. 2883
Phenergan VC with Codeine 2888
Robitussin A-C Syrup 2248
Robitussin-DAC Syrup 2249
Ryna .... ⚫ 804
Soma Compound w/Codeine Tablets 2784
Tylenol with Codeine 1592

Cyproheptadine Hydrochloride
(Predisposition to hypertensive crises; use with caution at reduced dosages). Products include:
Periactin 1767

Dexchlorpheniramine Maleate
(Predisposition to hypertensive crises; use with caution at reduced dosages).
No products indexed under this heading.

Dextroamphetamine Sulfate
(Predisposition to hypertensive crises; concurrent administration is contraindicated). Products include:
Adderall Tablets 2209
Dexedrine 2648
DextroStat-Dextroamphetamine Sulfate Tablets 2211

Dezocine (Predisposition to hypertensive crises; use with caution at reduced dosages). Products include:
Dalgan Injection 529

Diazepam (Predisposition to hypertensive crises; use with caution at reduced dosages). Products include:
Dizac (diazepam injectable emulsion) CIV 1862
Valium Injectable 2336
Valium Tablets 2335

Diethylpropion Hydrochloride
(Predisposition to hypertensive crises; use with caution at reduced dosages).
No products indexed under this heading.

Diphenhydramine Citrate (Predisposition to hypertensive crises; use with caution at reduced dosages). Products include:
Excedrin P.M. Analgesic/Sleeping Aid Tablets, Caplets, Liquigels ... 735

Diphenhydramine Hydrochloride (Predisposition to hypertensive crises; use with caution at reduced dosages). Products include:
Actifed Allergy Daytime/Nighttime Caplets .... ⚫ 808
Actifed Sinus Daytime/Nighttime Tablets and Caplets .... ⚫ 809
Extra Strength Bayer PM Aspirin Plus Sleep Aid .... ⚫ 617
Benadryl Allergy Chewables .... ⚫ 811
Benadryl Allergy/Cold Tablets .... ⚫ 811
Benadryl Allergy Decongestant Liquid Medication .... ⚫ 812
Benadryl Allergy Decongestant Tablets .... ⚫ 812
Benadryl Allergy Liquid Medication... ⚫ 813
Benadryl Allergy .... ⚫ 811
Benadryl Allergy Sinus Headache Caplets .... ⚫ 813
Benadryl Dye-Free Allergy Liquigel Softgels .... ⚫ 813
Benadryl Dye-Free Allergy Liquid Medication .... ⚫ 814
Benadryl Itch Relief Stick Extra Strength .... ⚫ 814
Benadryl Cream .... ⚫ 814
Benadryl Gel .... ⚫ 815
Benadryl Spray .... ⚫ 815
Benadryl Injection 1955
Contac Day & Night Cold/Flu Night Caplets .... ⚫ 772
Contac Night Allergy/Sinus Caplets .... ⚫ 771
Extra Strength Doan's P.M. .... ⚫ 653
Excedrin P.M. Analgesic/Sleeping Aid Tablets, Caplets, Liquigels... ⚫ 643
Nytol QuickCaps Caplets .... ⚫ 632
Sleepinal Night-time Sleep Aid Capsules and Softgels .... ⚫ 798
TYLENOL Allergy Sinus NightTime, Maximum Strength Caplets 1571
TYLENOL Flu NightTime, Maximum Strength Gelcaps 1575
TYLENOL Flu NightTime, Maximum Strength Hot Medication Packets 1575
TYLENOL PM Pain Reliever/Sleep Aid, Extra Strength Gelcaps, Caplets, Geltabs 1576
TYLENOL Severe Allergy Medication Caplets 1571
Maximum Strength Unisom Sleepgels 1990
Unisom With Pain Relief-Nighttime Sleep Aid and Pain Reliever... 1991

Diphenylpyraline Hydrochloride (Predisposition to hypertensive crises; use with caution at reduced dosages).
No products indexed under this heading.

Droperidol (Predisposition to hypertensive crises; use with caution at reduced dosages). Products include:
Inapsine Injection 462

Ephedrine Hydrochloride (Predisposition to hypertensive crises; concurrent administration is contraindicated). Products include:
Primatene Tablets .... ⚫ 844

Quadrinal Tablets 1398

Ephedrine Sulfate (Predisposition to hypertensive crises; concurrent administration is contraindicated). Products include:
Marax Tablets & DF Syrup............... 2015

Ephedrine Tannate (Predisposition to hypertensive crises; concurrent administration is contraindicated). Products include:
Rynatuss 2782

Estazolam (Predisposition to hypertensive crises; use with caution at reduced dosages). Products include:
ProSom Tablets 457

Ethchlorvynol (Predisposition to hypertensive crises; use with caution at reduced dosages). Products include:
Placidyl Capsules 456

Ethinamate (Predisposition to hypertensive crises; use with caution at reduced dosages).
No products indexed under this heading.

Fenfluramine Hydrochloride
(Predisposition to hypertensive crises; concurrent administration is contraindicated). Products include:
Pondimin Tablets 2239

Fentanyl (Predisposition to hypertensive crises; use with caution at reduced dosages). Products include:
Duragesic Transdermal System..... 1336

Fentanyl Citrate (Predisposition to hypertensive crises; use with caution at reduced dosages). Products include:
Sublimaze Injection 463

Fluphenazine Decanoate (Predisposition to hypertensive crises; use with caution at reduced dosages). Products include:
Prolixin Decanoate 510

Fluphenazine Enanthate (Predisposition to hypertensive crises; use with caution at reduced dosages). Products include:
Prolixin Enanthate 510

Fluphenazine Hydrochloride
(Predisposition to hypertensive crises; use with caution at reduced dosages). Products include:
Prolixin 510

Flurazepam Hydrochloride (Predisposition to hypertensive crises; use with caution at reduced dosages). Products include:
Dalmane Capsules 2329

Glutethimide (Predisposition to hypertensive crises; use with caution at reduced dosages).
No products indexed under this heading.

Haloperidol (Predisposition to hypertensive crises; use with caution at reduced dosages). Products include:
Haldol Injection, Tablets and Concentrate 1585

Haloperidol Decanoate (Predisposition to hypertensive crises; use with caution at reduced dosages). Products include:
Haldol Decanoate 1587

Hydrocodone Bitartrate (Predisposition to hypertensive crises; use with caution at reduced dosages). Products include:
Codiclear DH Syrup 808
Duratuss HD Elixir 2750
Histussin D Liquid 670
Hycodan Tablets and Syrup 946
Hycomine Compound Tablets 948
Hycomine 947
Hycotuss Expectorant Syrup 950
Hydrocet Capsules 787
Lorcet 10/650 Tablets 1016
Lortab 2751

IMPORTANT NOTE: Always consult each drug listing in the patient's regimen for possible interactions.

Furoxone Interactions Index 434

Tussend 1830
Tussend Expectorant 1831
Vicodin Tablets 1404
Vicodin ES Tablets 1405
Vicodin HP Tablets 1403
Vicodin Tuss Expectorant 1406
Zydone Capsules 967

Hydrocodone Polistirex (Predisposition to hypertensive crises; use with caution at reduced dosages). Products include:
Tussionex Pennkinetic Extended-Release Suspension 1624

Hydromorphone Hydrochloride (Predisposition to hypertensive crises; use with caution at reduced dosages). Products include:
Dilaudid Ampules 1382
Dilaudid Cough Syrup 1383
Dilaudid-HP Injection 1384
Dilaudid-HP Lyophilized Powder 250 mg 1384
Dilaudid 1382
Dilaudid Oral Liquid 1386
Dilaudid 1382
Dilaudid Tablets - 8 mg 1386

Hydroxyzine Hydrochloride (Predisposition to hypertensive crises; use with caution at reduced dosages). Products include:
Atarax Tablets & Syrup 1992
Marax Tablets & DF Syrup 2015
Vistaril Intramuscular Solution 2042

Isocarboxazid (Predisposition to hypertensive crises; concurrent administration is contraindicated).
No products indexed under this heading.

Levorphanol Tartrate (Predisposition to hypertensive crises; use with caution at reduced dosages). Products include:
Levo-Dromoran 2297

Loratadine (Predisposition to hypertensive crises; use with caution at reduced dosages). Products include:
Claritin Tablets 2485
Claritin-D Tablets 2487

Lorazepam (Predisposition to hypertensive crises; use with caution at reduced dosages). Products include:
Ativan Injection 2805
Ativan Tablets 2807

Loxapine Hydrochloride (Predisposition to hypertensive crises; use with caution at reduced dosages). Products include:
Loxitane 1426

Loxapine Succinate (Predisposition to hypertensive crises; use with caution at reduced dosages). Products include:
Loxitane Capsules 1426

Mazindol (Predisposition to hypertensive crises; concurrent administration is contraindicated). Products include:
Sanorex Tablets 2423

Meperidine Hydrochloride (Predisposition to hypertensive crises; use with caution at reduced dosages). Products include:
Demerol 2438
Mepergan Injection 2859

Meprobamate (Predisposition to hypertensive crises; use with caution at reduced dosages). Products include:
Miltown Tablets 2780
PMB 200 and PMB 400 2890

Mesoridazine Besylate (Predisposition to hypertensive crises; use with caution at reduced dosages). Products include:
Serentil 689

Methadone Hydrochloride (Predisposition to hypertensive crises; use with caution at reduced dosages). Products include:
Methadone Hydrochloride Oral Concentrate 2356
Methadone Hydrochloride Oral Solution & Tablets 2357

Methamphetamine Hydrochloride (Predisposition to hypertensive crises; concurrent administration is contraindicated). Products include:
Desoxyn Gradumet Tablets 422

Methdilazine Hydrochloride (Predisposition to hypertensive crises; use with caution at reduced dosages).
No products indexed under this heading.

Midazolam Hydrochloride (Predisposition to hypertensive crises; use with caution at reduced dosages). Products include:
Versed Injection 2324

Molindone Hydrochloride (Predisposition to hypertensive crises; use with caution at reduced dosages). Products include:
Moban Tablets and Concentrate 1036

Morphine Sulfate (Predisposition to hypertensive crises; use with caution at reduced dosages). Products include:
Astramorph/PF Injection, USP (Preservative-Free) 526
Duramorph Injection 983
Infumorph 200 and Infumorph 500 Sterile Solutions 985
Kadian Capsules 2948
MS Contin Tablets 2149
MSIR 2152
Oramorph SR (Morphine Sulfate Sustained Release Tablets) 2359
RMS Suppositories CII 2766
Roxanol 2365

Naphazoline Hydrochloride (Predisposition to hypertensive crises; concurrent administration is contraindicated). Products include:
Albalon Solution with Liquifilm ◉ 229
Clear Eyes ACR Astringent/Lubricant Eye Redness Reliever Eye Drops ◉ 314
Clear Eyes Lubricant Eye Redness Reliever ◉ 314
4-Way Fast Acting Nasal Spray (regular & mentholated) ■D 644
Naphcon-A Ophthalmic Solution 469
OcuHist ◉ 300
Privine ■D 663
Vasocon-A ◉ 263

Opium Alkaloids (Predisposition to hypertensive crises; use with caution at reduced dosages).
No products indexed under this heading.

Oxazepam (Predisposition to hypertensive crises; use with caution at reduced dosages). Products include:
Serax Capsules 2916
Serax Tablets 2916

Oxycodone Hydrochloride (Predisposition to hypertensive crises; use with caution at reduced dosages). Products include:
OxyContin Tablets 2163
OxyIR Capsules 2167
Percocet Tablets 955
Percodan Tablets 955
Percodan-Demi Tablets 956
Roxicodone Tablets, Oral Solution & Intensol (Oxycodone) 2366
Tylox Capsules 1593

Oxymetazoline Hydrochloride (Predisposition to hypertensive crises; concurrent administration is contraindicated). Products include:
Afrin ■D 757
Duration 12 Hour Nasal Spray ■D 766
4-Way 12 Hour Nasal Spray ■D 644
Neo-Synephrine Maximum Strength 12 Hour Nasal Spray ■D 624
Neo-Synephrine 12 Hour ■D 624
12 Hour Nöstrilla ■D 660
Vicks Sinex 12-Hour Nasal Decongestant Spray and Ultra Fine Mist ■D 738
Visine L.R. Eye Drops ■D 719
Visine L.R. Eye Drops ◉ 301

Perphenazine (Predisposition to hypertensive crises; use with caution at reduced dosages). Products include:
Etrafon 2495
Triavil Tablets 1800
Trilafon 2532

Phendimetrazine Tartrate (Predisposition to hypertensive crises; concurrent administration is contraindicated). Products include:
Bontril Slow-Release Capsules 786
Prelu-2 Timed Release Capsules 687

Phenelzine Sulfate (Predisposition to hypertensive crises; concurrent administration is contraindicated). Products include:
Nardil 1977

Phenmetrazine Hydrochloride (Predisposition to hypertensive crises; concurrent administration is contraindicated).
No products indexed under this heading.

Phenylephrine Hydrochloride (Predisposition to hypertensive crises; concurrent administration is contraindicated). Products include:
Atrohist Plus Tablets 1605
Cerose DM ■D 853
D.A. II Tablets 972
D.A. Chewable Tablets 970
Dura-Vent/DA Tablets 972
Extendryl 1003
4-Way Fast Acting Nasal Spray (regular & mentholated) ■D 644
Hemorid ■D 797
Hycomine Compound Tablets 948
Neo-Synephrine Hydrochloride 1% Carpuject 2455
Neo-Synephrine Hydrochloride 1% Injection 2455
Neo-Synephrine Hydrochloride (Ophthalmic) 2456
Neo-Synephrine ■D 624
Novahistine Elixir ■D 782
Phenergan VC 2886
Phenergan VC with Codeine 2888
Preparation H ■D 842
Tympagesic Ear Drops 2476
Vicks Sinex Nasal Spray and Ultra Fine Mist ■D 738

Phenylpropanolamine Hydrochloride (Predisposition to hypertensive crises; concurrent administration is contraindicated). Products include:
Acutrim ■D 648
Atrohist Plus Tablets 1605
BC Cold Powder Multi-Symptom Formula (Cold-Sinus-Allergy) ■D 631
BC Cold Powder Non-Drowsy Formula (Cold-Sinus) ■D 631
Cheracol Plus Head Cold/Cough Formula ■D 741
Comtrex Multi-Symptom Cold Reliever Liqui-Gels ■D 638
Comtrex Multi-Symptom Non-Drowsy Liqui-gels ■D 640
Contac Continuous Action Nasal Decongestant/Antihistamine 12 Hour Capsules ■D 773
Contac Maximum Strength Continuous Action Decongestant/Antihistamine 12 Hour Caplets ■D 772
Contac Severe Cold and Flu Formula Caplets ■D 773
Coricidin 'D' Decongestant Tablets ■D 760
Dexatrim ■D 795
Dexatrim Plus Vitamins Caplets ■D 796
Dimetane-DC Cough Syrup 2232
Dimetapp Allergy Sinus Caplets ■D 838
Dimetapp Cold & Allergy Chewable Tablets ■D 838
Dimetapp Cold & Cough Liqui-Gels ■D 839
Dimetapp DM Elixir ■D 840
Dimetapp Elixir ■D 840
Dimetapp Extentabs ■D 841
Dimetapp Tablets/Liqui-Gels ■D 841
Dura-Vent Tablets 971
Entex LA Tablets 972
Exgest LA Tablets 787
Hycomine 947
Nolamine Timed-Release Tablets 790
Ornade Spansule Capsules 2678
Propagest Tablets 791
Pyrroxate Caplets ■D 742
Robitussin-CF ■D 846
Sinulin Tablets 792
Tavist-D 12 Hour Relief Tablets ■D 750
Teldrin 12 Hour Antihistamine/Nasal Decongestant Allergy Relief Capsules ■D 786
Triaminic Expectorant ■D 753
Triaminic Syrup ■D 755
Triaminic Triaminicol Cold & Cough ■D 756
Triaminic DM Syrup ■D 756
Triaminicin Tablets ■D 756
Vicks DayQuil Allergy Relief 12-Hour Extended Release Tablets ■D 733
Vicks DayQuil Allergy Relief 4-Hour Tablets ■D 733
Vicks DayQuil SINUS Pressure & CONGESTION Relief ■D 734

Prazepam (Predisposition to hypertensive crises; use with caution at reduced dosages).
No products indexed under this heading.

Prochlorperazine (Predisposition to hypertensive crises; use with caution at reduced dosages). Products include:
Compazine 2644

Promethazine Hydrochloride (Predisposition to hypertensive crises; use with caution at reduced dosages). Products include:
Mepergan Injection 2859
Phenergan with Codeine 2883
Phenergan with Dextromethorphan 2885
Phenergan Injection 2880
Phenergan Suppositories 2882
Phenergan Syrup 2881
Phenergan Tablets 2882
Phenergan VC 2886
Phenergan VC with Codeine 2888

Propofol (Predisposition to hypertensive crises; use with caution at reduced dosages). Products include:
Diprivan Injectable Emulsion 2939

Propoxyphene Hydrochloride (Predisposition to hypertensive crises; use with caution at reduced dosages). Products include:
Darvon 1475
Wygesic Tablets 2930

Propoxyphene Napsylate (Predisposition to hypertensive crises; use with caution at reduced dosages). Products include:
Darvon-N/Darvocet-N 1473

Pseudoephedrine Hydrochloride (Predisposition to hypertensive crises; concurrent administration is contraindicated). Products include:
Actifed Allergy Daytime/Nighttime Caplets ■D 808
Actifed Cold & Allergy Tablets ■D 807
Actifed Cold & Sinus Caplets and Tablets ■D 808
Actifed Sinus Daytime/Nighttime Tablets and Caplets ■D 809
Advil Cold and Sinus Caplets and Tablets ■D 837
Alka-Seltzer Plus Liqui-Gels ■D 612
Alka-Seltzer Plus Flu & Body Aches Liqui-Gels Non-Drowsy Formula ■D 613
Alka-Seltzer Plus Night-Time Cold Medicine Liqui-Gels ■D 612
Allerest Maximum Strength ■D 649
Allerest No Drowsiness ■D 649
Allerest Sinus Pain Formula ■D 649
Atrohist Pediatric Capsules 1603
Benadryl Allergy/Cold Tablets ■D 811
Benadryl Allergy Decongestant Liquid Medication ■D 812
Benadryl Allergy Decongestant Tablets ■D 812
Benadryl Allergy Sinus Headache Caplets ■D 813
Benylin Multisymptom ■D 816

(■D Described in PDR For Nonprescription Drugs) (◉ Described in PDR For Ophthalmology)

Interactions Index

Bromfed Capsules (Extended-Release) 1832
Bromfed Syrup 712
Bromfed Tablets 1832
Bromfed-DM Cough Syrup 1832
Bromfed-PD Capsules (Extended-Release) 1832
Children's TYLENOL Cold Multi-Symptom Chewable Tablets and Liquid 1559
Children's TYLENOL Cold Plus Cough Multi Symptom Chewable Tablets and Liquid 1560
Children's TYLENOL Flu Suspension Liquid 1560
Children's Vicks DayQuil Allergy Relief 730
Children's Vicks NyQuil Cold/Cough Relief 731
Allergy-Sinus Comtrex Multi-Symptom Allergy-Sinus Formula Tablets and Caplets 639
Comtrex Multi-Symptom 638
Comtrex Multi-Symptom Non-Drowsy Caplets 640
Congess 1003
Contac Day Allergy/Sinus Caplets 771
Contac Day & Night 772
Contac Night Allergy/Sinus Caplets 771
Contac Severe Cold & Flu Non-Drowsy 774
Deconsal II Tablets 1605
Dimetane-DX Cough Syrup 2233
Dimetapp Cold & Fever Suspension 839
Dimetapp Decongestant Pediatric Drops 840
Dorcol Children's Cough Syrup 748
Drixoral Cough + Congestion Liquid Caps 763
Dura-Tap/PD Capsules 970
Duratuss Tablets 2750
Duratuss HD Elixir 2750
Efidac/24 655
Entex PSE Tablets 973
Fedahist Gyrocaps 2545
Guaifed 1833
Guaifed Syrup 712
Guaimax-D Tablets 809
Histussin D Liquid 670
Infants' TYLENOL Cold Decongestant & Fever-Reducer Drops 1561
Kronofed-A 994
Novahistine DMX 782
Nucofed 2225
PediaCare Cough-Cold Chewable Tablets and Liquid 1569
PediaCare Infants' Decongestant Drops 1569
PediaCare Infants' Drops Decongestant Plus Cough 1569
PediaCare NightRest Cough-Cold Liquid 1569
Pediatric Vicks 44d Cough & Head Congestion Relief 736
Pediatric Vicks 44m Cough & Cold Relief 737
Robitussin Cold & Cough Liqui-Gels 844
Robitussin Cold, Cough & Flu Liqui-Gels 844
Robitussin Maximum Strength Cough & Cold 847
Robitussin Night-Time Cold Formula 847
Robitussin Pediatric Cough & Cold Formula 848
Robitussin Pediatric Drops 849
Robitussin Severe Congestion Liqui-Gels 845
Robitussin-DAC Syrup 2249
Robitussin-PE 846
Rondec Oral Drops 974
Rondec Syrup 974
Rondec Tablet 974
Rondec Chewable Tablets 974
Rondec-TR Tablet 974
Ryna 804
Seldane-D Extended-Release Tablets 1286
Semprex-D Capsules 1620
Sinarest 663
Sine-Aid Maximum Strength Sinus Headache Gelcaps, Caplets and Tablets 1570
Sine-Off No Drowsiness Formula Caplets 784
Sine-Off Sinus Medicine 784
Singlet Tablets 785
Sinutab Non-Drying Liquid Caps 823

Sinutab Sinus Allergy Medication, Maximum Strength Tablets and Caplets 823
Sinutab Sinus Medication, Maximum Strength Without Drowsiness Formula, Tablets & Caplets 824
Sudafed Children's Cold & Cough Liquid Medication 825
Sudafed Children's Nasal Decongestant Liquid Medication 826
Sudafed Cold & Allergy Tablets 826
Sudafed Cold and Cough Liquid Caps 826
Sudafed Nasal Decongestant Tablets, 30 mg. 825
Sudafed Nasal Decongestant Tablets, 60 mg. 825
Sudafed Non-Drying Sinus Liquid Caps 827
Sudafed Pediatric Nasal Decongestant Liquid Oral Drops 827
Sudafed Severe Cold Formula Caplets 828
Sudafed Severe Cold Formula Tablets 828
Sudafed Sinus Caplets 829
Sudafed Sinus Tablets 829
Sudafed 12 Hour Caplets 830
Syn-Rx Tablets 1622
Syn-Rx DM Tablets 1623
TheraFlu Flu and Cold Medicine 750
Theraflu Maximum Strength Flu and Cold Medicine For Sore Throat 751
TheraFlu Flu, Cold and Cough Medicine 750
TheraFlu Maximum Strength Nighttime Flu, Cold & Cough Medicine 751
TheraFlu Maximum Strength Non-Drowsy Formula Flu, Cold & Cough Medicine 751
TheraFlu Maximum Strength, Non-Drowsy Formula Flu, Cold and Cough Caplets 752
Theraflu Maximum Strength Sinus Non-Drowsy Formula Caplets 752
Triaminic AM Cough and Decongestant Formula 753
Triaminic AM Decongestant Formula 753
Triaminic Infant Oral Decongestant Drops 754
Triaminic Night Time 754
Triaminic Sore Throat Formula 755
Tussend 1830
Tussend Expectorant 1831
TYLENOL Allergy Sinus, Maximum Strength Caplets and Gelcaps 1571
TYLENOL Allergy Sinus NightTime, Maximum Strength Caplets 1571
TYLENOL Cold Medication, Multi-Symptom Formula Tablets and Caplets 1572
TYLENOL Cold Medication, Multi-Symptom Hot Liquid Packets 1572
TYLENOL Cold Medication, No Drowsiness Formula Caplets and Gelcaps 1572
TYLENOL Cold Severe Congestion Caplets 1573
TYLENOL Cough Medication with Decongestant, Multi Symptom 1574
TYLENOL Flu No Drowsiness Formula, Maximum Strength Gelcaps 1575
TYLENOL Flu NightTime, Maximum Strength Gelcaps 1575
TYLENOL Flu NightTime, Maximum Strength Hot Medication Packets 1575
TYLENOL Sinus, Maximum Strength Geltabs, Gelcaps, Caplets and Tablets 1576
Vicks 44 LiquiCaps Cough, Cold & Flu Relief 728
Vicks 44 LiquiCaps Non-Drowsy Cough & Cold Relief 729
Vicks 44D Cough & Head Congestion Relief 728
Vicks 44M Cough, Cold & Flu Relief 729
Vicks DayQuil LiquiCaps/Liquid Multi-Symptom Cold/Flu Relief 734
Vicks DayQuil SINUS Pressure & PAIN Relief with IBUPROFEN 735
Vicks Nyquil Hot Therapy 735
Vicks NyQuil LiquiCaps/Liquid Multi-Symptom Cold/Flu Relief, Original and Cherry Flavors 736

Pyrilamine Maleate (Predisposition to hypertensive crises; use with caution at reduced dosages). Products include:
4-Way Fast Acting Nasal Spray (regular & mentholated) 644
Maximum Strength Multi-Symptom Formula Midol 621
PMS Multi-Symptom Formula Midol 622

Pyrilamine Tannate (Predisposition to hypertensive crises; use with caution at reduced dosages). Products include:
Atrohist Pediatric Suspension 1604
Atrohist Pediatric Suspension Dye-Free 1604
Rynatan 2781

Quazepam (Predisposition to hypertensive crises; use with caution at reduced dosages). Products include:
Doral Tablets 2773

Secobarbital Sodium (Predisposition to hypertensive crises; use with caution at reduced dosages). Products include:
Seconal Sodium Pulvules 1529

Selegiline Hydrochloride (Predisposition to hypertensive crises; concurrent administration is contraindicated). Products include:
Eldepryl Capsules 2729

Sufentanil Citrate (Predisposition to hypertensive crises; use with caution at reduced dosages). Products include:
Sufenta Injection 1355

Temazepam (Predisposition to hypertensive crises; use with caution at reduced dosages). Products include:
Restoril Capsules 2413

Terfenadine (Predisposition to hypertensive crises; use with caution at reduced dosages). Products include:
Seldane Tablets 1284
Seldane-D Extended-Release Tablets 1286

Tetrahydrozoline Hydrochloride (Predisposition to hypertensive crises; concurrent administration is contraindicated). Products include:
Collyrium Fresh 316
Murine Tears Plus Lubricant Redness Reliever Eye Drops 744
Murine Tears Plus Lubricant Redness Reliever Eye Drops 315
Visine A.C. Seasonal Relief From Pollen and Dust 301
Visine Moisturizing Eye Drops 301
Visine Original Eye Drops 301

Thioridazine Hydrochloride (Predisposition to hypertensive crises; use with caution at reduced dosages). Products include:
Mellaril 2398

Thiothixene (Predisposition to hypertensive crises; use with caution at reduced dosages). Products include:
Navane Capsules and Concentrate 2018
Navane Intramuscular 2019

Tranylcypromine Sulfate (Predisposition to hypertensive crises; concurrent administration is contraindicated). Products include:
Parnate Tablets 2679

Triazolam (Predisposition to hypertensive crises; use with caution at reduced dosages). Products include:
Halcion Tablets 2093

Trifluoperazine Hydrochloride (Predisposition to hypertensive crises; use with caution at reduced dosages). Products include:
Stelazine 2692

Trimeprazine Tartrate (Predisposition to hypertensive crises; use with caution at reduced dosages).
No products indexed under this heading.

Tripelennamine Hydrochloride (Predisposition to hypertensive crises; use with caution at reduced dosages). Products include:
PBZ Tablets 863
PBZ-SR Tablets 862

Triprolidine Hydrochloride (Predisposition to hypertensive crises; use with caution at reduced dosages). Products include:
Actifed Cold & Allergy Tablets 807
Actifed Cold & Sinus Caplets and Tablets 808

Tyramine (Predisposition to hypertensive crises; concurrent administration is contraindicated).

Zolpidem Tartrate (Predisposition to hypertensive crises; use with caution at reduced dosages). Products include:
Ambien Tablets 2559

Food Interactions

Alcohol (Possible disulfiram-like reaction may occur; alcohol intake should be avoided during or within four days after Furoxone therapy).

Beans, broad (Concurrent and/or sequential intake must be avoided).

Beer, unspecified (Concurrent and/or sequential intake must be avoided).

Cheese, strong, unpasteurized (Concurrent and/or sequential intake must be avoided).

Food with high concentration of tyramine (Concurrent and/or sequential intake must be avoided).

Herring, pickled (Concurrent and/or sequential intake must be avoided).

Liver, chicken (Concurrent and/or sequential intake must be avoided).

Wine, unspecified (Concurrent and/or sequential intake must be avoided).

Yeast extract (Concurrent and/or sequential intake must be avoided).

FUROXONE TABLETS
(Furazolidone) 2221
See Furoxone Liquid

GAMIMUNE N, 5% IMMUNE GLOBULIN INTRAVENOUS (HUMAN), 5%
(Globulin, Immune (Human)) 612
May interact with:

Measles, Mumps & Rubella Virus Vaccine Live (Antibodies in Gamimune N, 5% may interfere with the response to live virus vaccine; use of such vaccines should be deferred until approximately 6 months after Gamimune N, 10% administration). Products include:
M-M-R II 1730

GAMIMUNE N, 10% IMMUNE GLOBULIN INTRAVENOUS (HUMAN), 10%
(Globulin, Immune (Human)) 615
May interact with:

Measles, Mumps & Rubella Virus Vaccine Live (Antibodies in Gamimune N, 10% may interfere with the response to live virus vaccine; use of such vaccines should be deferred until approximately 6 months after Gamimune N., 10% administration). Products include:
M-M-R II 1730

IMPORTANT NOTE: Always consult each drug listing in the patient's regimen for possible interactions.

GAMMAGARD S/D, IMMUNE GLOBULIN, INTRAVENOUS (HUMAN)
(Globulin, Immune (Human)) 577
May interact with:

Measles, Mumps & Rubella Virus Vaccine Live (Antibodies in immune globulin may interfere with patient response to vaccine). Products include:
M-M-R II 1730

GAMMAR-P I.V., IMMUNE GLOBULIN INTRAVENOUS (HUMAN)
(Globulin, Immune (Human)) 798
May interact with:

Live Virus Vaccines (Immune globulin preparations may interfere with the response by pediatric patients to live viral vaccines).

Measles Virus Vaccine Live (Immune globulin preparations may interfere with the response by pediatric patients to measles vaccines). Products include:
Attenuvax 1650

Measles, Mumps & Rubella Virus Vaccine Live (Immune globulin preparations may interfere with the response by pediatric patients to MMR vaccines). Products include:
M-M-R II 1730

GANITE
(Gallium Nitrate) 2711
May interact with aminoglycosides and certain other agents. Compounds in these categories include:

Amikacin Sulfate (Concomitant administration increases the risk for developing severe renal insufficiency). Products include:
Amikacin Sulfate Injection, USP 523
Amikacin Sulfate Injection, USP 981
Amikin Injectable 502

Amphotericin B (Concomitant administration increases the risk for developing severe renal insufficiency). Products include:
Abelcet Injection 1540
Fungizone Intravenous 507
Fungizone Oral Suspension 704

Gentamicin Sulfate (Concomitant administration increases the risk for developing severe renal insufficiency). Products include:
Garamycin Cream 0.1% 2501
Garamycin Injectable 2502
Garamycin Ointment 0.1% 2501
Garamycin Ophthalmic 2501
Genoptic Sterile Ophthalmic Solution .... ⊚ 241
Genoptic Sterile Ophthalmic Ointment .... ⊚ 241
Gentak .... ⊚ 209
Pred-G Liquifilm Sterile Ophthalmic Suspension .... ⊚ 248
Pred-G S.O.P. Sterile Ophthalmic Ointment .... ⊚ 249

Kanamycin Sulfate (Concomitant administration increases the risk for developing severe renal insufficiency).
No products indexed under this heading.

Nephrotoxic Drugs (Concomitant administration may increase the risk for development of renal insufficiency).

Streptomycin Sulfate (Concomitant administration increases the risk for developing severe renal insufficiency). Products include:
Streptomycin Sulfate Injection 2031

Tobramycin (Concomitant administration increases the risk for developing severe renal insufficiency). Products include:
AKTOB .... ⊚ 207
TobraDex Ophthalmic Suspension and Ointment 469
Tobrex Ophthalmic Ointment and Solution .... ⊚ 226

Tobramycin Sulfate (Concomitant administration increases the risk for developing severe renal insufficiency). Products include:
Nebcin Vials, Hyporets & ADD-Vantage 1518

GANTANOL TABLETS
(Sulfamethoxazole) 2285
May interact with thiazides, oral anticoagulants, and certain other agents. Compounds in these categories include:

Bendroflumethiazide (Increased incidence of thrombopenia with purpura in elderly).
No products indexed under this heading.

Chlorothiazide (Increased incidence of thrombopenia with purpura in elderly). Products include:
Aldoclor Tablets 1638
Diupres Tablets 1691
Diuril Oral 1694

Chlorothiazide Sodium (Increased incidence of thrombopenia with purpura in elderly). Products include:
Diuril Sodium Intravenous 1693

Dicumarol (Increased prothrombin time).
No products indexed under this heading.

Hydrochlorothiazide (Increased incidence of thrombopenia with purpura in elderly). Products include:
Aldactazide Tablets 2556
Aldoril Tablets 1644
Apresazide Capsules 824
Capozide Tablets 744
Dyazide Capsules 2653
Esidrix Tablets 839
Esimil Tablets 840
HydroDIURIL Tablets 1716
Hydropres Tablets 1718
Hyzaar Tablets 1720
Inderide Tablets 2838
Inderide LA Long Acting Capsules .. 2840
Lopressor HCT Tablets 850
Lotensin HCT Tablets 855
Moduretic Tablets 1748
Oretic Tablets 450
Prinzide Tablets 1780
Ser-Ap-Es Tablets 867
Timolide Tablets 1791
Vaseretic Tablets 1810
Zestoretic Tablets 2968
Ziac 1459

Hydroflumethiazide (Increased incidence of thrombopenia with purpura in elderly). Products include:
Diucardin Tablets 2824

Methotrexate Sodium (May be displaced from protein-binding sites, thus increasing free methotrexate concentrations). Products include:
Methotrexate Sodium Tablets, Injection, for Injection and LPF Injection 1322

Methyclothiazide (Increased incidence of thrombopenia with purpura in elderly). Products include:
Enduron Tablets 424

Phenytoin (May inhibit hepatic metabolism; possible excessive phenytoin effect). Products include:
Dilantin Infatabs 1967
Dilantin-125 Suspension 1969

Phenytoin Sodium (May inhibit hepatic metabolism; possible excessive phenytoin effect). Products include:
Dilantin Kapseals 1965

Polythiazide (Increased incidence of thrombopenia with purpura in elderly). Products include:
Minizide Capsules 2016

Warfarin Sodium (Increased prothrombin time). Products include:
Coumadin 941

GANTRISIN PEDIATRIC SUSPENSION
(Acetyl Sulfisoxazole) 2286
May interact with oral anticoagulants, sulfonylureas, and certain other agents. Compounds in these categories include:

Chlorpropamide (Sulfisoxazole can potentiate the hypoglycemic activity of sulfonylurea). Products include:
Diabinese Tablets 2002

Dicumarol (Prolonged prothrombin time).
No products indexed under this heading.

Glimepiride (Sulfisoxazole can potentiate the hypoglycemic activity of sulfonylurea). Products include:
Amaryl Tablets 1241

Glipizide (Sulfisoxazole can potentiate the hypoglycemic activity of sulfonylurea). Products include:
Glucotrol Tablets 2011
Glucotrol XL Extended Release Tablets 2012

Glyburide (Sulfisoxazole can potentiate the hypoglycemic activity of sulfonylurea). Products include:
DiaBeta Tablets 1265
Glynase PresTab Tablets 2091
Micronase Tablets 2099

Methotrexate Sodium (Displaced from plasma protein-binding sites). Products include:
Methotrexate Sodium Tablets, Injection, for Injection and LPF Injection 1322

Sodium Thiopental (Potential for decrease in the amount of thiopental required for anesthesia and in a shortening of the awakening time when concomitantly administered with I.V. sulfisoxazole).
No products indexed under this heading.

Tolazamide (Sulfisoxazole can potentiate the hypoglycemic activity of sulfonylurea).
No products indexed under this heading.

Tolbutamide (Sulfisoxazole can potentiate the hypoglycemic activity of sulfonylurea).
No products indexed under this heading.

Warfarin Sodium (Prolonged prothrombin time). Products include:
Coumadin 941

GANTRISIN SYRUP
(Acetyl Sulfisoxazole) 2286
See Gantrisin Pediatric Suspension

GANTRISIN TABLETS
(Sulfisoxazole) 2286
See Gantrisin Pediatric Suspension

GARAMYCIN CREAM 0.1%
(Gentamicin Sulfate) 2501
None cited in PDR database.

GARAMYCIN INJECTABLE
(Gentamicin Sulfate) 2502
May interact with aminoglycosides, cephalosporins, anesthetics, neuromuscular blocking agents, and certain other agents. Compounds in these categories include:

Alfentanil Hydrochloride (Increased potential for neuromuscular blockade and respiratory paralysis). Products include:
Alfenta Injection 1334

Amikacin Sulfate (Concurrent and/or sequential use increases the risk of neurotoxicity and/or nephrotoxicity). Products include:
Amikacin Sulfate Injection, USP 523
Amikacin Sulfate Injection, USP 981
Amikin Injectable 502

Atracurium Besylate (Increased potential for neuromuscular blockade and respiratory paralysis). Products include:
Tracrium Injection 1155

Carbenicillin Indanyl Sodium (Potential for reduction in gentamicin serum half-life in patients with severe renal impairment receiving concomitant carbenicillin and gentamicin). Products include:
Geocillin Tablets 2009

Cefaclor (Potential for increased nephrotoxicity). Products include:
Ceclor Pulvules & Suspension 1470

Cefadroxil (Potential for increased nephrotoxicity). Products include:
Duricef Capsules, Tablets, and Oral Suspension 750

Cefamandole Nafate (Potential for increased nephrotoxicity). Products include:
Mandol Vials, Faspak & ADD-Vantage 1516

Cefazolin Sodium (Potential for increased nephrotoxicity). Products include:
Ancef Injection 2632
Kefzol Vials, Faspak & ADD-Vantage 1511

Cefixime (Potential for increased nephrotoxicity). Products include:
Suprax 1443

Cefmetazole Sodium (Potential for increased nephrotoxicity).
No products indexed under this heading.

Cefonicid Sodium (Potential for increased nephrotoxicity). Products include:
Monocid Injection 2674

Cefoperazone Sodium (Potential for increased nephrotoxicity). Products include:
Cefobid Intravenous/Intramuscular 1996
Cefobid Pharmacy Bulk Package - Not for Direct Infusion 1999

Ceforanide (Potential for increased nephrotoxicity).
No products indexed under this heading.

Cefotaxime Sodium (Potential for increased nephrotoxicity). Products include:
Claforan Sterile and Injection 1259

Cefotetan (Potential for increased nephrotoxicity). Products include:
Cefotan 2936

Cefoxitin Sodium (Potential for increased nephrotoxicity). Products include:
Mefoxin 1734
Mefoxin Premixed Intravenous Solution 1737

Cefpodoxime Proxetil (Potential for increased nephrotoxicity). Products include:
Vantin for Oral Suspension and Vantin Tablets 2112

(▣ Described in PDR For Nonprescription Drugs)   (⊚ Described in PDR For Ophthalmology)

Interactions Index

Cefprozil (Potential for increased nephrotoxicity). Products include:
Cefzil Tablets and Oral Suspension ... 747

Ceftazidime (Potential for increased nephrotoxicity). Products include:
Ceptaz ... 1070
Fortaz ... 1092
Tazicef for Injection ... 2697
Tazidime Vials, Faspak & ADD-Vantage ... 1531

Ceftizoxime Sodium (Potential for increased nephrotoxicity). Products include:
Cefizox for Intramuscular or Intravenous Use ... 1025

Ceftriaxone Sodium (Potential for increased nephrotoxicity). Products include:
Rocephin Injectable Vials, ADD-Vantage, Galaxy Container ... 2305

Cefuroxime Axetil (Potential for increased nephrotoxicity). Products include:
Ceftin ... 1067

Cefuroxime Sodium (Potential for increased nephrotoxicity). Products include:
Kefurox Vials, Faspak & ADD-Vantage ... 1509
Zinacef ... 1184

Cephalexin (Potential for increased nephrotoxicity). Products include:
Keflex Pulvules & Oral Suspension ... 930

Cephaloridine (Concurrent and/or sequential use increases the risk of neurotoxicity and/or nephrotoxicity).

Cephalothin Sodium (Potential for increased nephrotoxicity).

Cephapirin Sodium (Potential for increased nephrotoxicity).
No products indexed under this heading.

Cephradine (Potential for increased nephrotoxicity).
No products indexed under this heading.

Cisatracurium Besylate (Increased potential for neuromuscular blockade and respiratory paralysis). Products include:
Nimbex Injection ... 1131

Cisplatin (Concurrent and/or sequential use increases the risk of neurotoxicity and/or nephrotoxicity). Products include:
Platinol for Injection ... 717
Platinol-AQ Injection ... 719

Colistin Sulfate (Concurrent and/or sequential use increases the risk of neurotoxicity and/or nephrotoxicity). Products include:
Coly-Mycin S Otic w/Neomycin & Hydrocortisone ... 1965

Doxacurium Chloride (Increased potential for neuromuscular blockade and respiratory paralysis). Products include:
Nuromax Injection ... 1136

Enflurane (Increased potential for neuromuscular blockade and respiratory paralysis).
No products indexed under this heading.

Ethacrynic Acid (Potential for increased ototoxicity; concurrent use should be avoided). Products include:
Edecrin Tablets ... 1698

Fentanyl Citrate (Increased potential for neuromuscular blockade and respiratory paralysis). Products include:
Sublimaze Injection ... 463

Furosemide (Potential for increased ototoxicity; concurrent use should be avoided). Products include:
Lasix Injection, Oral Solution and Tablets ... 1267

Halothane (Increased potential for neuromuscular blockade and respiratory paralysis). Products include:
Fluothane ... 2830

Isoflurane (Increased potential for neuromuscular blockade and respiratory paralysis).
No products indexed under this heading.

Kanamycin Sulfate (Concurrent and/or sequential use increases the risk of neurotoxicity and/or nephrotoxicity).
No products indexed under this heading.

Ketamine Hydrochloride (Increased potential for neuromuscular blockade and respiratory paralysis).
No products indexed under this heading.

Lithium Carbonate (Increased potential for neuromuscular blockade and respiratory paralysis). Products include:
Eskalith ... 2658
Lithium Carbonate Capsules & Tablets ... 2352
Lithonate/Lithotabs/Lithobid ... 2721

Lithium Citrate (Increased potential for neuromuscular blockade and respiratory paralysis).
No products indexed under this heading.

Loracarbef (Potential for increased nephrotoxicity). Products include:
Lorabid Suspension and Pulvules ... 1513

Methohexital Sodium (Increased potential for neuromuscular blockade and respiratory paralysis).
No products indexed under this heading.

Metocurine Iodide (Increased potential for neuromuscular blockade and respiratory paralysis). Products include:
Metubine Iodide Vials ... 932

Midazolam Hydrochloride (Increased potential for neuromuscular blockade and respiratory paralysis). Products include:
Versed Injection ... 2324

Mivacurium Chloride (Increased potential for neuromuscular blockade and respiratory paralysis). Products include:
Mivacron ... 1125

Neomycin Sulfate (Concurrent and/or sequential use increases the risk of neurotoxicity and/or nephrotoxicity). Products include:
AK-Spore ... 205
AK-Trol Ointment & Suspension ... 205
Coly-Mycin S Otic w/Neomycin & Hydrocortisone ... 1965
Cortisporin Cream ... 1073
Cortisporin Ointment ... 1074
Cortisporin Ophthalmic Ointment Sterile ... 1074
Cortisporin Ophthalmic Suspension Sterile ... 1075
Cortisporin Otic Solution Sterile ... 1076
Cortisporin Otic Suspension Sterile ... 1077
Maxitrol Ophthalmic Ointment and Suspension ... 222
Mycitracin ... 803
NeoDecadron Sterile Ophthalmic Ointment ... 1755
NeoDecadron Sterile Ophthalmic Solution ... 1756
NeoDecadron Topical Cream ... 1757
Neosporin G.U. Irrigant Sterile ... 1130
Neosporin Ointment ... 821
Neosporin Plus Maximum Strength Cream ... 821
Neosporin Plus Maximum Strength Ointment ... 822
Neosporin Ophthalmic Ointment Sterile ... 1130
Neosporin Ophthalmic Solution Sterile ... 1131
Pediotic Suspension Sterile ... 1140
Poly-Pred Liquifilm ... 246

Neomycin, oral (Concurrent and/or sequential use increases the risk of neurotoxicity and/or nephrotoxicity).

Pancuronium Bromide (Increased potential for neuromuscular blockade and respiratory paralysis).
No products indexed under this heading.

Paromomycin Sulfate (Concurrent and/or sequential use increases the risk of neurotoxicity and/or nephrotoxicity).
No products indexed under this heading.

Polymyxin B Sulfate (Concurrent and/or sequential use increases the risk of neurotoxicity and/or nephrotoxicity). Products include:
AK-Spore ... 205
AK-Trol Ointment & Suspension ... 205
Betadine Brand First Aid Antibiotics & Moisturizer Ointment ... 2144
Cortisporin Cream ... 1073
Cortisporin Ointment ... 1074
Cortisporin Ophthalmic Ointment Sterile ... 1074
Cortisporin Ophthalmic Suspension Sterile ... 1075
Cortisporin Otic Solution Sterile ... 1076
Cortisporin Otic Suspension Sterile ... 1077
Maxitrol Ophthalmic Ointment and Suspension ... 222
Mycitracin ... 803
Neosporin G.U. Irrigant Sterile ... 1130
Neosporin Ointment ... 821
Neosporin Plus Maximum Strength Cream ... 821
Neosporin Plus Maximum Strength Ointment ... 822
Neosporin Ophthalmic Ointment Sterile ... 1130
Neosporin Ophthalmic Solution Sterile ... 1131
Pediotic Suspension Sterile ... 1140
Poly-Pred Liquifilm ... 246
Polysporin Ointment ... 822
Polysporin Ophthalmic Ointment Sterile ... 1140
Polysporin Powder ... 823
Polytrim Ophthalmic Solution Sterile ... 479
TERAK Ointment ... 210
Terramycin with Polymyxin B Sulfate Ophthalmic Ointment ... 2035

Propofol (Increased potential for neuromuscular blockade and respiratory paralysis). Products include:
Diprivan Injectable Emulsion ... 2939

Rocuronium Bromide (Increased potential for neuromuscular blockade and respiratory paralysis). Products include:
Zemuron Injection ... 1885

Streptomycin Sulfate (Concurrent and/or sequential use increases the risk of neurotoxicity and/or nephrotoxicity). Products include:
Streptomycin Sulfate Injection ... 2031

Succinylcholine Chloride (Increased potential for neuromuscular blockade and respiratory paralysis). Products include:
Anectine ... 1062

Sufentanil Citrate (Increased potential for neuromuscular blockade and respiratory paralysis). Products include:
Sufenta Injection ... 1355

Thiamylal Sodium (Increased potential for neuromuscular blockade and respiratory paralysis).
No products indexed under this heading.

Tobramycin (Concurrent and/or sequential use increases the risk of neurotoxicity and/or nephrotoxicity). Products include:
AKTOB ... 207
TobraDex Ophthalmic Suspension and Ointment ... 469
Tobrex Ophthalmic Ointment and Solution ... 226

Tobramycin Sulfate (Concurrent and/or sequential use increases the risk of neurotoxicity and/or nephrotoxicity). Products include:
Nebcin Vials, Hyporets & ADD-Vantage ... 1518

Tubocurarine Chloride (Increased potential for neuromuscular blockade and respiratory paralysis).
No products indexed under this heading.

Vancomycin Hydrochloride (Concurrent and/or sequential use increases the risk of neurotoxicity and/or nephrotoxicity). Products include:
Vancocin HCl, Oral Solution & Pulvules ... 1536
Vancocin HCl, Vials & ADD-Vantage ... 1534

Vecuronium Bromide (Increased potential for neuromuscular blockade and respiratory paralysis). Products include:
Norcuron for Injection ... 1875

Viomycin (Concurrent and/or sequential use increases the risk of neurotoxicity and/or nephrotoxicity).

GARAMYCIN OINTMENT 0.1%
(Gentamicin Sulfate) ... 2501
None cited in PDR database.

GARAMYCIN OPHTHALMIC OINTMENT—STERILE
(Gentamicin Sulfate) ... 2501
None cited in PDR database.

GARAMYCIN OPHTHALMIC SOLUTION—STERILE
(Gentamicin Sulfate) ... 2501
None cited in PDR database.

GARLIQUE
(Garlic Extract) ... 791
None cited in PDR database.

GAS-X CHEWABLE TABLETS
(Simethicone) ... 749
None cited in PDR database.

EXTRA STRENGTH GAS-X CHEWABLE TABLETS
(Simethicone) ... 749
None cited in PDR database.

EXTRA STRENGTH GAS-X SOFTGELS
(Simethicone) ... 749
None cited in PDR database.

GASTROCROM CAPSULES
(Cromolyn Sodium) ... 1611
May interact with:

Isoproterenol Hydrochloride (Concurrent use at extremely high doses of both drugs appears to have increased resorptions and malformations in animal studies). Products include:
Isuprel Hydrochloride Solution ... 2443
Isuprel Injection ... 2441
Isuprel Mistometer ... 2442

IMPORTANT NOTE: Always consult each drug listing in the patient's regimen for possible interactions.

GASTROCROM ORAL CONCENTRATE
(Cromolyn Sodium) 1611
May interact with:

Isoproterenol Hydrochloride (Concurrent use at extremely high doses of both drugs appears to have increased resorptions and malformations in animal studies). Products include:
Isuprel Hydrochloride Solution 2443
Isuprel Injection 2441
Isuprel Mistometer 2442

GAVISCON ANTACID TABLETS
(Aluminum Hydroxide Gel, Magnesium Trisilicate) .... ▣ 778
May interact with:

Prescription Drugs, unspecified (Concurrent use with certain unspecified drugs is not recommended; consult your physicians.)

GAVISCON-2 ANTACID TABLETS
(Aluminum Hydroxide Gel, Magnesium Trisilicate) .... ▣ 779
May interact with:

Prescription Drugs, unspecified (Concurrent use with certain unspecified drugs is not recommended; consult your physicians.)

GAVISCON EXTRA STRENGTH RELIEF FORMULA ANTACID TABLETS
(Aluminum Hydroxide, Magnesium Carbonate) .... ▣ 778
May interact with:

Prescription Drugs, unspecified (Concurrent use with certain unspecified drugs is not recommended; consult your physicians.)

GAVISCON EXTRA STRENGTH RELIEF FORMULA LIQUID ANTACID
(Aluminum Hydroxide, Magnesium Carbonate) .... ▣ 779
May interact with:

Prescription Drugs, unspecified (Concurrent use with certain unspecified drugs is not recommended; consult your physicians.)

GAVISCON LIQUID ANTACID
(Aluminum Hydroxide, Magnesium Carbonate) .... ▣ 779
May interact with:

Prescription Drugs, unspecified (Concurrent use with certain unspecified drugs is not recommended; consult your physicians.)

GELUSIL ANTACID-ANTI-GAS LIQUID
(Aluminum Hydroxide, Magnesium Hydroxide, Simethicone) .... ▣ 819
May interact with:

Prescription Drugs, unspecified (Concurrent use is not recommended; consult your doctor.)

GELUSIL ANTACID-ANTI-GAS TABLETS
(Aluminum Hydroxide, Magnesium Hydroxide, Simethicone) .... ▣ 819
May interact with:

Prescription Drugs, unspecified (Concurrent use is not recommended; consult your doctor.)

GEMZAR FOR INJECTION
(Gemcitabine Hydrochloride) 1482
None cited in PDR database.

GENOPTIC STERILE OPHTHALMIC SOLUTION
(Gentamicin Sulfate) .... ⊙ 241
None cited in PDR database.

GENOPTIC STERILE OPHTHALMIC OINTMENT
(Gentamicin Sulfate) .... ⊙ 241
None cited in PDR database.

GENOTROPIN INJECTION
(Somatropin) 2090
May interact with glucocorticoids. Compounds in this category include:

Betamethasone Acetate (Concomitant glucocorticoid therapy may inhibit human growth promoting effect). Products include:
Celestone Soluspan Suspension 2484

Betamethasone Sodium Phosphate (Concomitant glucocorticoid therapy may inhibit human growth promoting effect). Products include:
Celestone Soluspan Suspension 2484

Cortisone Acetate (Concomitant glucocorticoid therapy may inhibit human growth promoting effect). Products include:
Cortone Acetate Sterile Suspension 1663
Cortone Acetate Tablets 1664

Dexamethasone (Concomitant glucocorticoid therapy may inhibit human growth promoting effect). Products include:
AK-Trol Ointment & Suspension .... ⊙ 205
Decadron Elixir 1676
Decadron Tablets 1678
Decaspray Topical Aerosol 1689
Maxitrol Ophthalmic Ointment and Suspension .... ⊙ 222
TobraDex Ophthalmic Suspension and Ointment 469

Dexamethasone Acetate (Concomitant glucocorticoid therapy may inhibit human growth promoting effect). Products include:
Dalalone D.P. Injectable 1009
Decadron-LA Sterile Suspension 1687

Dexamethasone Sodium Phosphate (Concomitant glucocorticoid therapy may inhibit human growth promoting effect). Products include:
Decadron Phosphate Injection 1680
Decadron Phosphate Sterile Ophthalmic Ointment 1684
Decadron Phosphate Sterile Ophthalmic Solution 1685
Decadron Phosphate Topical Cream 1686
Decadron Phosphate with Xylocaine Injection, Sterile 1683
Dexacort Phosphate in Respihaler ... 1606
Dexacort Phosphate in Turbinaire .. 1607
NeoDecadron Sterile Ophthalmic Ointment 1755
NeoDecadron Sterile Ophthalmic Solution 1756
NeoDecadron Topical Cream 1757

Fludrocortisone Acetate (Concomitant glucocorticoid therapy may inhibit human growth promoting effect). Products include:
Florinef Acetate Tablets 506

Hydrocortisone (Concomitant glucocorticoid therapy may inhibit human growth promoting effect). Products include:
Anusol-HC Cream 2.5% 1953
Aquanil HC Lotion 1989
Maximum Strength Cortaid Spray ▣ 800
CORTENEMA 2713
Cortisporin Ointment 1074
Cortisporin Ophthalmic Ointment Sterile 1074
Cortisporin Ophthalmic Suspension Sterile 1075
Cortisporin Otic Solution Sterile ... 1076
Cortisporin Otic Suspension Sterile 1077
Cortizone-5 .... ▣ 795
Cortizone-10 .... ▣ 795
Hydrocortone Tablets 1715
Hytone 922
Hytone Ointment 2 ½% 923
Massengill Medicated Soft Cloth Towelettes 2628
Pediotic Suspension Sterile 1140
Preparation H Hydrocortisone 1% Cream .... ▣ 843
ProctoCream-HC 2.5% 2552
VōSoL HC Otic Solution 2786

Hydrocortisone Acetate (Concomitant glucocorticoid therapy may inhibit human growth promoting effect). Products include:
Analpram-HC Rectal Cream 1% and 2.5% 993
Anusol HC-1 Hydrocortisone Anti-Itch Ointment .... ▣ 810
Anusol-HC Suppositories 1954
Caldecort Anti-Itch Hydrocortisone Cream .... ▣ 651
Coly-Mycin S Otic w/Neomycin & Hydrocortisone 1965
Cortaid .... ▣ 800
Cortifoam 2540
Cortisporin Cream 1073
Epifoam 2543
Hydrocortone Acetate Sterile Suspension 1712
Mantadil Cream 1124
Nupercainal Hydrocortisone 1% Cream .... ▣ 661
Pramosone Cream, Lotion & Ointment 995
ProctoFoam-HC 2552
Terra-Cortril Ophthalmic Suspension 2033

Hydrocortisone Sodium Phosphate (Concomitant glucocorticoid therapy may inhibit human growth promoting effect). Products include:
Hydrocortone Phosphate Injection, Sterile 1713

Hydrocortisone Sodium Succinate (Concomitant glucocorticoid therapy may inhibit human growth promoting effect).
No products indexed under this heading.

Methylprednisolone Acetate (Concomitant glucocorticoid therapy may inhibit human growth promoting effect).
No products indexed under this heading.

Methylprednisolone Sodium Succinate (Concomitant glucocorticoid therapy may inhibit human growth promoting effect).
No products indexed under this heading.

Prednisolone Acetate (Concomitant glucocorticoid therapy may inhibit human growth promoting effect). Products include:
AK-CIDE .... ⊙ 203
AK-CIDE Ointment .... ⊙ 203
Blephamide Liquifilm Sterile Ophthalmic Suspension 472
Blephamide Ointment .... ⊙ 234
Econopred & Econopred Plus Ophthalmic Suspensions .... ⊙ 216
Poly-Pred Liquifilm .... ⊙ 246
Pred Forte .... ⊙ 247
Pred Mild .... ⊙ 250
Pred-G Liquifilm Sterile Ophthalmic Suspension .... ⊙ 248
Pred-G S.O.P. Sterile Ophthalmic Ointment .... ⊙ 249

Prednisolone Sodium Phosphate (Concomitant glucocorticoid therapy may inhibit human growth promoting effect). Products include:
AK-PRED .... ⊙ 204
Hydeltrasol Injection, Sterile 1708
Pediapred Oral Solution 1618

Prednisolone Tebutate (Concomitant glucocorticoid therapy may inhibit human growth promoting effect). Products include:
Hydeltra-T.B.A. Sterile Suspension 1710

Prednisone (Concomitant glucocorticoid therapy may inhibit human growth promoting effect).
No products indexed under this heading.

Triamcinolone (Concomitant glucocorticoid therapy may inhibit human growth promoting effect).
No products indexed under this heading.

Triamcinolone Acetonide (Concomitant glucocorticoid therapy may inhibit human growth promoting effect). Products include:
Azmacort Oral Inhaler 2175
Nasacort AQ Nasal Spray 2191
Nasacort Nasal Inhaler 2189

Triamcinolone Diacetate (Concomitant glucocorticoid therapy may inhibit human growth promoting effect).
No products indexed under this heading.

Triamcinolone Hexacetonide (Concomitant glucocorticoid therapy may inhibit human growth promoting effect).
No products indexed under this heading.

GENTAK
(Gentamicin Sulfate) .... ⊙ 209
None cited in PDR database.

GENTAK OPHTHALMIC OINTMENT
(Gentamicin Sulfate) .... ⊙ 209
None cited in PDR database.

GEOCILLIN TABLETS
(Carbenicillin Indanyl Sodium) 2009
May interact with:

Probenecid (Geocillin blood levels may be increased and prolonged). Products include:
Benemid Tablets 1651
ColBENEMID Tablets 1662

GEREF (SERMORELIN ACETATE FOR INJECTION)
(Sermorelin Acetate) 2995
May interact with drugs directly affecting the pituitary secretion of somatotropin, cyclooxygenase inhibitors, antimuscarinic drugs, antithyroid agents, and certain other agents. Compounds in these categories include:

Aspirin (The Geref test should not be conducted in the presence of this drug). Products include:
Alka-Seltzer Cherry Effervescent Antacid and Pain Reliever ..... ▣ 609
Alka-Seltzer Extra Strength Effervescent Antacid and Pain Reliever .... ▣ 609
Alka-Seltzer Lemon Lime Effervescent Antacid and Pain Reliever .... ▣ 609
Alka-Seltzer Original Effervescent Antacid and Pain Reliever ..... ▣ 609
Alka-Seltzer Plus .... ▣ 611
Alka-Seltzer Plus Sinus Medicine .. ▣ 611
Ascriptin .... ▣ 650
Arthritis Strength BC Powder ...... ▣ 631
BC Cold Powder Multi-Symptom Formula (Cold-Sinus-Allergy) .... ▣ 631

(▣ Described in PDR For Nonprescription Drugs) (⊙ Described in PDR For Ophthalmology)

439 **Interactions Index** **Geref**

- BC Cold Powder Non-Drowsy Formula (Cold-Sinus) ▭ 631
- BC Powder ▭ 631
- Genuine Bayer Aspirin Tablets & Caplets ▭ 618
- Extra Strength Bayer Arthritis Pain Regimen Formula ▭ 615
- Extra Strength Bayer Aspirin Caplets & Tablets ▭ 617
- Extended-Release Bayer 8-Hour Aspirin ▭ 616
- Extra Strength Bayer Plus Aspirin Caplets ▭ 617
- Extra Strength Bayer PM Aspirin Plus Sleep Aid ▭ 617
- Aspirin Regimen Bayer 81 mg Tablets with Calcium ▭ 615
- Aspirin Regimen Bayer Adult Low Strength 81 mg Tablets ▭ 613
- Aspirin Regimen Bayer Children's Chewable Aspirin ▭ 616
- Aspirin Regimen Bayer Regular Strength 325 mg Caplets ▭ 613
- Bufferin Analgesic Tablets ▭ 636
- Arthritis Strength Bufferin Analgesic Caplets ▭ 637
- Extra Strength Bufferin Analgesic Tablets ▭ 637
- Cama Arthritis Pain Reliever ▭ 748
- Darvon Compound-65 Pulvules 1475
- Easprin 1971
- Ecotrin 2625
- Ecotrin Enteric Coated Aspirin Maximum Strength Tablets and Caplets ▭ 775
- Ecotrin Enteric Coated Aspirin Regular Strength Tablets 2625
- Empirin Aspirin Tablets ▭ 818
- Excedrin Extra-Strength Analgesic Tablets, Caplets, and Geltabs 734
- Fiorinal Capsules 2388
- Fiorinal with Codeine Capsules 2390
- Fiorinal Tablets 2388
- Goody's Extra Strength Headache Powders ▭ 632
- Goody's Extra Strength Pain Relief Tablets ▭ 632
- Halfprin Tablets 1413
- Norgesic 1554
- Percodan Tablets 955
- Percodan-Demi Tablets 956
- Robaxisal Tablets 2246
- Soma Compound w/Codeine Tablets 2784
- Soma Compound Tablets 2783
- St. Joseph Adult Chewable Aspirin (81 mg.) ▭ 768
- Talwin Compound 2466
- Vanquish Analgesic Caplets ▭ 627

Atropine Sulfate (Response to Geref may be blunted). Products include:
- Arco-Lase Plus Tablets 513
- Atrohist Plus Tablets 1605
- Donnatal 2234
- Donnatal Extentabs 2234
- Donnatal Tablets 2234
- Lomotil 2591
- Motofen Tablets 789
- Urised Tablets 2123

Belladonna Alkaloids (Response to Geref may be blunted). Products include:
- Bellergal-S Tablets 2375
- Hyland's Bedwetting Tablets ▭ 788
- Hyland's EnurAid Tablets ▭ 789
- Hyland's Headache Tablets ▭ 790
- Hyland's Teething Tablets ▭ 790
- Similasan Eye Drops #1 ▭ 769

Betamethasone Acetate (The Geref test should not be conducted in the presence of this drug). Products include:
- Celestone Soluspan Suspension 2484

Betamethasone Sodium Phosphate (The Geref test should not be conducted in the presence of this drug). Products include:
- Celestone Soluspan Suspension 2484

Clidinium Bromide (Response to Geref may be blunted). Products include:
- Librax Capsules 2330

Cortisone Acetate (The Geref test should not be conducted in the presence of this drug). Products include:
- Cortone Acetate Sterile Suspension 1663
- Cortone Acetate Tablets 1664

Dexamethasone (The Geref test should not be conducted in the presence of this drug). Products include:
- AK-Trol Ointment & Suspension ⊛ 205
- Decadron Elixir 1676
- Decadron Tablets 1678
- Decaspray Topical Aerosol 1689
- Maxitrol Ophthalmic Ointment and Suspension ⊛ 222
- TobraDex Ophthalmic Suspension and Ointment 469

Dexamethasone Acetate (The Geref test should not be conducted in the presence of this drug). Products include:
- Dalalone D.P. Injectable 1009
- Decadron-LA Sterile Suspension 1687

Dexamethasone Sodium Phosphate (The Geref test should not be conducted in the presence of this drug). Products include:
- Decadron Phosphate Injection 1680
- Decadron Phosphate Sterile Ophthalmic Ointment 1684
- Decadron Phosphate Sterile Ophthalmic Solution 1685
- Decadron Phosphate Topical Cream 1686
- Decadron Phosphate with Xylocaine Injection, Sterile 1683
- Dexacort Phosphate in Respihaler 1606
- Dexacort Phosphate in Turbinaire 1607
- NeoDecadron Sterile Ophthalmic Ointment 1755
- NeoDecadron Sterile Ophthalmic Solution 1756
- NeoDecadron Topical Cream 1757

Dicyclomine Hydrochloride (Response to Geref may be blunted). Products include:
- Bentyl 1246

Glycopyrrolate (Response to Geref may be blunted). Products include:
- Robinul Forte Tablets 2247
- Robinul Injectable 2247
- Robinul Tablets 2247

Hydrocortisone (The Geref test should not be conducted in the presence of this drug). Products include:
- Anusol-HC Cream 2.5% 1953
- Aquanil HC Lotion 1989
- Maximum Strength Cortaid Spray ▭ 800
- CORTENEMA 2713
- Cortisporin Ointment 1074
- Cortisporin Ophthalmic Ointment Sterile 1074
- Cortisporin Ophthalmic Suspension Sterile 1075
- Cortisporin Otic Solution Sterile 1076
- Cortisporin Otic Suspension Sterile 1077
- Cortizone-5 ▭ 795
- Cortizone-10 ▭ 795
- Hydrocortone Tablets 1715
- Hytone 922
- Hytone Ointment 2 ½% 923
- Massengill Medicated Soft Cloth Towelettes 2628
- Pediotic Suspension Sterile 1140
- Preparation H Hydrocortisone 1% Cream ▭ 843
- ProctoCream-HC 2.5% 2552
- VōSoL HC Otic Solution 2786

Hydrocortisone Acetate (The Geref test should not be conducted in the presence of this drug). Products include:
- Analpram-HC Rectal Cream 1% and 2.5% 993
- Anusol HC-1 Hydrocortisone Anti-Itch Ointment ▭ 810
- Anusol-HC Suppositories 1954
- Caldecort Anti-Itch Hydrocortisone Cream ▭ 651
- Coly-Mycin S Otic w/Neomycin & Hydrocortisone 1965
- Cortaid ▭ 800
- Cortifoam 2540
- Cortisporin Cream 1073
- Epifoam 2543
- Hydrocortone Acetate Sterile Suspension 1712
- Mantadil Cream 1124
- Nupercainal Hydrocortisone 1% Cream ▭ 661
- Pramosone Cream, Lotion & Ointment 995
- ProctoFoam-HC 2552
- Terra-Cortril Ophthalmic Suspension 2033

Hydrocortisone Sodium Phosphate (The Geref test should not be conducted in the presence of this drug). Products include:
- Hydrocortone Phosphate Injection, Sterile 1713

Hydrocortisone Sodium Succinate (The Geref test should not be conducted in the presence of this drug).
- No products indexed under this heading.

Hyoscyamine (Response to Geref may be blunted). Products include:
- Cystospaz Tablets 2123
- Urised Tablets 2123

Hyoscyamine Sulfate (Response to Geref may be blunted). Products include:
- Arco-Lase Plus Tablets 513
- Atrohist Plus Tablets 1605
- Cystospaz-M Capsules 2123
- Donnatal 2234
- Donnatal Extentabs 2234
- Donnatal Tablets 2234
- Kutrase Capsules 2546
- Levsin/Levsinex/Levbid 2549

Indomethacin (The Geref test should not be conducted in the presence of this drug). Products include:
- Indocin 1723

Indomethacin Sodium Trihydrate (The Geref test should not be conducted in the presence of this drug). Products include:
- Indocin I.V. 1727

Insulin, Human (The Geref test should not be conducted in the presence of this drug).
- No products indexed under this heading.

Insulin, Human Isophane Suspension (The Geref test should not be conducted in the presence of this drug). Products include:
- Novolin N Human Insulin 10 ml Vials 1846

Insulin, Human NPH (The Geref test should not be conducted in the presence of this drug). Products include:
- Humulin N, 100 Units 1495
- Novolin N PenFill 1.5 ml Cartridges Durable Insulin Delivery System 1849
- Novolin N Prefilled Syringe Disposable Insulin Delivery System 1850

Insulin, Human Regular (The Geref test should not be conducted in the presence of this drug). Products include:
- Humulin R, 100 Units 1497
- Novolin R Human Insulin 10 ml Vials 1846
- Novolin R PenFill 1.5 ml Cartridges Durable Insulin Delivery System 1849
- Novolin R Prefilled Syringe Disposable Insulin Delivery System 1850
- Velosulin BR Human Insulin 10 ml Vials 1847

Insulin, Human, Zinc Suspension (The Geref test should not be conducted in the presence of this drug). Products include:
- Humulin L, 100 Units 1494
- Humulin U, 100 Units 1498
- Novolin L Human Insulin 10 ml Vials 1846

Insulin, NPH (The Geref test should not be conducted in the presence of this drug). Products include:
- NPH, 100 Units 1502
- Pork NPH, 100 Units 1506
- Purified Pork NPH Isophane Insulin 1852

Insulin, Regular (The Geref test should not be conducted in the presence of this drug). Products include:
- Regular, 100 Units 1503
- Pork Regular, 100 Units 1507
- Pork Regular (Concentrated), 500 Units 1508
- Purified Pork Regular Insulin 1852

Insulin, Zinc Crystals (The Geref test should not be conducted in the presence of this drug). Products include:
- NPH, 100 Units 1502

Insulin, Zinc Suspension (The Geref test should not be conducted in the presence of this drug). Products include:
- Iletin I 1501
- Lente, 100 Units 1501
- Iletin II 1504
- Pork Lente, 100 Units 1504
- Purified Pork Lente Insulin 1852

Ipratropium Bromide (Response to Geref may be blunted). Products include:
- Atrovent Inhalation Aerosol 674
- Atrovent Inhalation Solution 675
- Atrovent Nasal Spray 0.03% 676
- Atrovent Nasal Spray 0.06% 678

Levodopa (Somatropin levels may be transiently elevated by levodopa). Products include:
- Atamet Tablets 567
- Larodopa Tablets 2296
- Sinemet Tablets 959
- Sinemet CR Tablets 961

Mepenzolate Bromide (Response to Geref may be blunted).
- No products indexed under this heading.

Methimazole (Response to Geref may be blunted). Products include:
- Tapazole Tablets 1361

Methylprednisolone Acetate (The Geref test should not be conducted in the presence of this drug).
- No products indexed under this heading.

Methylprednisolone Sodium Succinate (The Geref test should not be conducted in the presence of this drug).
- No products indexed under this heading.

Oxyphenonium Bromide (Response to Geref may be blunted).

Prednisolone Acetate (The Geref test should not be conducted in the presence of this drug). Products include:
- AK-CIDE ⊛ 203
- AK-CIDE Ointment ⊛ 203
- Blephamide Liquifilm Sterile Ophthalmic Suspension 472
- Blephamide Ointment ⊛ 234
- Econopred & Econopred Plus Ophthalmic Suspensions ⊛ 216
- Poly-Pred Liquifilm ⊛ 246
- Pred Forte ⊛ 247
- Pred Mild ⊛ 250
- Pred-G Liquifilm Sterile Ophthalmic Suspension ⊛ 248
- Pred-G S.O.P. Sterile Ophthalmic Ointment ⊛ 249

Prednisolone Sodium Phosphate (The Geref test should not be conducted in the presence of this drug). Products include:
- AK-PRED ⊛ 204
- Hydeltrasol Injection, Sterile 1708
- Pediapred Oral Solution 1618

IMPORTANT NOTE: Always consult each drug listing in the patient's regimen for possible interactions.

Prednisolone Tebutate (The Geref test should not be conducted in the presence of this drug). Products include:

Hydeltra-T.B.A. Sterile Suspension 1710

Prednisone (The Geref test should not be conducted in the presence of this drug).

No products indexed under this heading.

Propantheline Bromide (Response to Geref may be blunted). Products include:

Pro-Banthine Tablets 2226

Propylthiouracil (Response to Geref may be blunted).

No products indexed under this heading.

Scopolamine (Response to Geref may be blunted). Products include:

Transderm Scōp Transdermal Therapeutic System 890

Scopolamine Hydrobromide (Response to Geref may be blunted). Products include:

Atrohist Plus Tablets 1605
Donnatal 2234
Donnatal Extentabs 2234
Donnatal Tablets 2234

Triamcinolone (The Geref test should not be conducted in the presence of this drug).

No products indexed under this heading.

Triamcinolone Acetonide (The Geref test should not be conducted in the presence of this drug). Products include:

Azmacort Oral Inhaler 2175
Nasacort AQ Nasal Spray 2191
Nasacort Nasal Inhaler 2189

Triamcinolone Diacetate (The Geref test should not be conducted in the presence of this drug).

No products indexed under this heading.

Triamcinolone Hexacetonide (The Geref test should not be conducted in the presence of this drug).

No products indexed under this heading.

Tridihexethyl Chloride (Response to Geref may be blunted).

No products indexed under this heading.

GERIMED TABLETS

(Vitamins with Minerals) 1000
None cited in PDR database.

GINKOBA

(Ginkgo Biloba) ▣ 721
None cited in PDR database.

GINKGO BILOBA PLUS

(Garlic Extract, Ginseng) ▣ 680
None cited in PDR database.

GINSANA

(Ginseng) ▣ 721
None cited in PDR database.

GLAUCTABS 25 MG

(Methazolamide) ◉ 209
May interact with corticosteroids and certain other agents. Compounds in these categories include:

Aspirin (Concomitant use with high-dose aspirin may result in anorexia, tachypnea, lethargy, coma, and death). Products include:

Alka-Seltzer Cherry Effervescent Antacid and Pain Reliever ▣ 609
Alka-Seltzer Extra Strength Effervescent Antacid and Pain Reliever ▣ 609
Alka-Seltzer Lemon Lime Effervescent Antacid and Pain Reliever ▣ 609
Alka-Seltzer Original Effervescent Antacid and Pain Reliever ▣ 609
Alka-Seltzer Plus ▣ 611
Alka-Seltzer Plus Sinus Medicine ▣ 611
Ascriptin ▣ 650
Arthritis Strength BC Powder ▣ 631
BC Cold Powder Multi-Symptom Formula (Cold-Sinus-Allergy) ▣ 631
BC Cold Powder Non-Drowsy Formula (Cold-Sinus) ▣ 631
BC Powder ▣ 631
Genuine Bayer Aspirin Tablets & Caplets ▣ 618
Extra Strength Bayer Arthritis Pain Regimen Formula ▣ 615
Extra Strength Bayer Aspirin Caplets & Tablets ▣ 617
Extended-Release Bayer 8-Hour Aspirin ▣ 616
Extra Strength Bayer Plus Aspirin Caplets ▣ 617
Extra Strength Bayer PM Aspirin Plus Sleep Aid ▣ 617
Aspirin Regimen Bayer 81 mg Tablets with Calcium ▣ 615
Aspirin Regimen Bayer Adult Low Strength 81 mg Tablets ▣ 613
Aspirin Regimen Bayer Children's Chewable Aspirin ▣ 616
Aspirin Regimen Bayer Regular Strength 325 mg Caplets ▣ 613
Bufferin Analgesic Tablets ▣ 636
Arthritis Strength Bufferin Analgesic Caplets ▣ 637
Extra Strength Bufferin Analgesic Tablets ▣ 637
Cama Arthritis Pain Reliever ▣ 748
Darvon Compound-65 Pulvules 1475
Easprin 1971
Ecotrin 2625
Ecotrin Enteric Coated Aspirin Maximum Strength Tablets and Caplets ▣ 775
Ecotrin Enteric Coated Aspirin Regular Strength Tablets 2625
Empirin Aspirin Tablets ▣ 818
Excedrin Extra-Strength Analgesic Tablets, Caplets, and Geltabs 734
Fiorinal Capsules 2388
Fiorinal with Codeine Capsules 2390
Fiorinal Tablets 2388
Goody's Extra Strength Headache Powders ▣ 632
Goody's Extra Strength Pain Relief Tablets ▣ 632
Halfprin Tablets 1413
Norgesic 1554
Percodan Tablets 955
Percodan-Demi Tablets 956
Robaxisal Tablets 2246
Soma Compound w/Codeine Tablets 2784
Soma Compound Tablets 2783
St. Joseph Adult Chewable Aspirin (81 mg.) ▣ 768
Talwin Compound 2466
Vanquish Analgesic Caplets ▣ 627

Betamethasone Acetate (Potential for developing hypokalemia). Products include:

Celestone Soluspan Suspension 2484

Betamethasone Sodium Phosphate (Potential for developing hypokalemia). Products include:

Celestone Soluspan Suspension 2484

Cortisone Acetate (Potential for developing hypokalemia). Products include:

Cortone Acetate Sterile Suspension 1663
Cortone Acetate Tablets 1664

Dexamethasone (Potential for developing hypokalemia). Products include:

AK-Trol Ointment & Suspension ◉ 205
Decadron Elixir 1676
Decadron Tablets 1678
Decaspray Topical Aerosol 1689
Maxitrol Ophthalmic Ointment and Suspension ◉ 222
TobraDex Ophthalmic Suspension and Ointment 469

Dexamethasone Acetate (Potential for developing hypokalemia). Products include:

Dalalone D.P. Injectable 1009
Decadron-LA Sterile Suspension 1687

Dexamethasone Sodium Phosphate (Potential for developing hypokalemia). Products include:

Decadron Phosphate Injection 1680
Decadron Phosphate Sterile Ophthalmic Ointment 1684
Decadron Phosphate Sterile Ophthalmic Solution 1685
Decadron Phosphate Topical Cream 1686
Decadron Phosphate with Xylocaine Injection, Sterile 1683
Dexacort Phosphate in Respihaler 1606
Dexacort Phosphate in Turbinaire 1607
NeoDecadron Sterile Ophthalmic Ointment 1755
NeoDecadron Sterile Ophthalmic Solution 1756
NeoDecadron Topical Cream 1757

Fludrocortisone Acetate (Potential for developing hypokalemia). Products include:

Florinef Acetate Tablets 506

Hydrocortisone (Potential for developing hypokalemia). Products include:

Anusol-HC Cream 2.5% 1953
Aquanil HC Lotion 1989
Maximum Strength Cortaid Spray ▣ 800
CORTENEMA 2713
Cortisporin Ointment 1074
Cortisporin Ophthalmic Ointment Sterile 1074
Cortisporin Ophthalmic Suspension Sterile 1075
Cortisporin Otic Solution Sterile 1076
Cortisporin Otic Suspension Sterile 1077
Cortizone-5 ▣ 795
Cortizone-10 ▣ 795
Hydrocortone Tablets 1715
Hytone 922
Hytone Ointment 2 ½% 923
Massengill Medicated Soft Cloth Towelettes 2628
Pediotic Suspension Sterile 1140
Preparation H Hydrocortisone 1% Cream ▣ 843
ProctoCream-HC 2.5% 2552
VōSoL HC Otic Solution 2786

Hydrocortisone Acetate (Potential for developing hypokalemia). Products include:

Analpram-HC Rectal Cream 1% and 2.5% 993
Anusol HC-1 Hydrocortisone Anti-Itch Ointment ▣ 810
Anusol-HC Suppositories 1954
Caldecort Anti-Itch Hydrocortisone Cream ▣ 651
Coly-Mycin S Otic w/Neomycin & Hydrocortisone 1965
Cortaid ▣ 800
Cortifoam 2540
Cortisporin Cream 1073
Epifoam 2543
Hydrocortone Acetate Sterile Suspension 1712
Mantadil Cream 1124
Nupercainal Hydrocortisone 1% Cream ▣ 661
Pramosone Cream, Lotion & Ointment 995
ProctoFoam-HC 2552
Terra-Cortril Ophthalmic Suspension 2033

Hydrocortisone Sodium Phosphate (Potential for developing hypokalemia). Products include:

Hydrocortone Phosphate Injection, Sterile 1713

Hydrocortisone Sodium Succinate (Potential for developing hypokalemia).

No products indexed under this heading.

Methylprednisolone Acetate (Potential for developing hypokalemia).

No products indexed under this heading.

Methylprednisolone Sodium Succinate (Potential for developing hypokalemia).

No products indexed under this heading.

Prednisolone Acetate (Potential for developing hypokalemia). Products include:

AK-CIDE ◉ 203
AK-CIDE Ointment ◉ 203
Blephamide Liquifilm Sterile Ophthalmic Suspension 472
Blephamide Ointment ◉ 234
Econopred & Econopred Plus Ophthalmic Suspensions ◉ 216
Poly-Pred Liquifilm ◉ 246
Pred Forte ◉ 247
Pred Mild ◉ 250
Pred-G Liquifilm Sterile Ophthalmic Suspension ◉ 248
Pred-G S.O.P. Sterile Ophthalmic Ointment ◉ 249

Prednisolone Sodium Phosphate (Potential for developing hypokalemia). Products include:

AK-PRED ◉ 204
Hydeltrasol Injection, Sterile 1708
Pediapred Oral Solution 1618

Prednisolone Tebutate (Potential for developing hypokalemia). Products include:

Hydeltra-T.B.A. Sterile Suspension 1710

Prednisone (Potential for developing hypokalemia).

No products indexed under this heading.

Triamcinolone (Potential for developing hypokalemia).

No products indexed under this heading.

Triamcinolone Acetonide (Potential for developing hypokalemia). Products include:

Azmacort Oral Inhaler 2175
Nasacort AQ Nasal Spray 2191
Nasacort Nasal Inhaler 2189

Triamcinolone Diacetate (Potential for developing hypokalemia).

No products indexed under this heading.

Triamcinolone Hexacetonide (Potential for developing hypokalemia).

No products indexed under this heading.

GLAUCTABS 50 MG

(Methazolamide) ◉ 209
See **GlaucTabs 25 mg**

GLUCAGON FOR INJECTION VIALS AND EMERGENCY KIT

(Glucagon) 1485
None cited in PDR database.

GLUCERNA SPECIALIZED NUTRITION WITH FIBER FOR PATIENTS WITH ABNORMAL GLUCOSE TOLERANCE

(Nutritional Supplement) 2338
None cited in PDR database.

GLUCOPHAGE TABLETS

(Metformin Hydrochloride) 754
May interact with radiographic iodinated contrast media, cationic drugs that are eliminated by renal tubular secretion, diuretics, corticosteroids, phenothiazines, thyroid preparations, estrogens, oral contraceptives, calcium channel blockers, sympathomimetics, and certain other agents. Compounds in these categories include:

Albuterol (Potential for loss of glycemic control). Products include:

Proventil Inhalation Aerosol 2524
Ventolin Inhalation Aerosol and Refill 1170

Albuterol Sulfate (Potential for loss of glycemic control). Products include:
- Airet Albuterol Sulfate Inhalation Solution ... 1602
- Albuterol Sulfate, USP Solution for Inhalation, Arm-a-Med ... 522
- Proventil Inhalation Solution 0.083% ... 2527
- Proventil Repetabs Tablets ... 2529
- Proventil Solution for Inhalation 0.5% ... 2525
- Proventil Syrup ... 2528
- Proventil Tablets ... 2529
- Ventolin Inhalation Solution ... 1171
- Ventolin Nebules Inhalation Solution ... 1172
- Ventolin Rotacaps for Inhalation ... 1173
- Ventolin Syrup ... 1175
- Ventolin Tablets ... 1176
- Volmax Extended-Release Tablets ... 1835

Amiloride Hydrochloride (Potential for loss of glycemic control; theoretical potential for interaction with metformin by competing for common renal tubular transport system). Products include:
- Midamor Tablets ... 1746
- Moduretic Tablets ... 1748

Amlodipine Besylate (Potential for loss of glycemic control). Products include:
- Lotrel Capsules ... 858
- Norvasc Tablets ... 2020

Bendroflumethiazide (Potential for loss of glycemic control).
- No products indexed under this heading.

Bepridil Hydrochloride (Potential for loss of glycemic control). Products include:
- Vascor Tablets (200 and 300 mg) ... 1597

Betamethasone Acetate (Potential for loss of glycemic control). Products include:
- Celestone Soluspan Suspension ... 2484

Betamethasone Sodium Phosphate (Potential for loss of glycemic control). Products include:
- Celestone Soluspan Suspension ... 2484

Bumetanide (Potential for loss of glycemic control). Products include:
- Bumex ... 2260

Chlorothiazide (Potential for loss of glycemic control). Products include:
- Aldoclor Tablets ... 1638
- Diupres Tablets ... 1691
- Diuril Oral ... 1694

Chlorothiazide Sodium (Potential for loss of glycemic control). Products include:
- Diuril Sodium Intravenous ... 1693

Chlorotrianisene (Potential for loss of glycemic control).
- No products indexed under this heading.

Chlorpromazine (Potential for loss of glycemic control). Products include:
- Thorazine Suppositories ... 2701

Chlorpromazine Hydrochloride (Potential for loss of glycemic control). Products include:
- Thorazine ... 2701

Chlorthalidone (Potential for loss of glycemic control). Products include:
- Combipres Tablets ... 682
- Tenoretic Tablets ... 2963
- Thalitone ... 1293

Cimetidine (Co-administered with oral cimetidine may increase peak metformin plasma and whole blood concentrations by 60% and a 40% increase in plasma and whole blood metformin AUC). Products include:
- Tagamet HB Tablets ... 786
- Tagamet Tablets ... 2694

Cortisone Acetate (Potential for loss of glycemic control). Products include:
- Cortone Acetate Sterile Suspension ... 1663
- Cortone Acetate Tablets ... 1664

Desogestrel (Potential for loss of glycemic control). Products include:
- Desogen Tablets ... 1867
- Ortho-Cept ... 1907

Dexamethasone (Potential for loss of glycemic control). Products include:
- AK-Trol Ointment & Suspension ... 205
- Decadron Elixir ... 1676
- Decadron Tablets ... 1678
- Decaspray Topical Aerosol ... 1689
- Maxitrol Ophthalmic Ointment and Suspension ... 222
- TobraDex Ophthalmic Suspension and Ointment ... 469

Dexamethasone Acetate (Potential for loss of glycemic control). Products include:
- Dalalone D.P. Injectable ... 1009
- Decadron-LA Sterile Suspension ... 1687

Dexamethasone Sodium Phosphate (Potential for loss of glycemic control). Products include:
- Decadron Phosphate Injection ... 1680
- Decadron Phosphate Sterile Ophthalmic Ointment ... 1684
- Decadron Phosphate Sterile Ophthalmic Solution ... 1685
- Decadron Phosphate Topical Cream ... 1686
- Decadron Phosphate with Xylocaine Injection, Sterile ... 1683
- Dexacort Phosphate in Respihaler ... 1606
- Dexacort Phosphate in Turbinaire ... 1607
- NeoDecadron Sterile Ophthalmic Ointment ... 1755
- NeoDecadron Sterile Ophthalmic Solution ... 1756
- NeoDecadron Topical Cream ... 1757

Diatrizoate Meglumine (Potential for acute alteration of renal function; metformin should be temporarily withheld in patients undergoing radiologic studies involving parenteral iodinated contrast material).

Diatrizoate Sodium (Potential for acute alteration of renal function; metformin should be temporarily withheld in patients undergoing radiologic studies involving parenteral iodinated contrast material).

Dienestrol (Potential for loss of glycemic control). Products include:
- Ortho Dienestrol Cream ... 1922

Diethylstilbestrol (Potential for loss of glycemic control). Products include:
- Diethylstilbestrol Tablets ... 1477

Digoxin (Theoretical potential for interaction with metformin by competing for common renal tubular transport system). Products include:
- Lanoxicaps ... 1110
- Lanoxin Elixir Pediatric ... 1113
- Lanoxin Injection ... 1116
- Lanoxin Injection Pediatric ... 1119
- Lanoxin Tablets ... 1121

Diltiazem Hydrochloride (Potential for loss of glycemic control). Products include:
- Cardizem CD Capsules ... 1251
- Cardizem SR Capsules ... 1255
- Cardizem Injectable ... 1253
- Cardizem Tablets ... 1257
- Dilacor XR Extended-release Capsules ... 2183
- Tiazac Capsules ... 1019

Dobutamine Hydrochloride (Potential for loss of glycemic control). Products include:
- Dobutrex Solution Vials ... 1480

Dopamine Hydrochloride (Potential for loss of glycemic control).
- No products indexed under this heading.

Ephedrine Hydrochloride (Potential for loss of glycemic control). Products include:
- Primatene Tablets ... 844
- Quadrinal Tablets ... 1398

Ephedrine Sulfate (Potential for loss of glycemic control). Products include:
- Marax Tablets & DF Syrup ... 2015

Ephedrine Tannate (Potential for loss of glycemic control). Products include:
- Rynatuss ... 2782

Epinephrine (Potential for loss of glycemic control). Products include:
- EPIFRIN ... 237
- EpiPen ... 808
- Marcaine with Epinephrine ... 2446
- Primatene Mist ... 843
- Sensorcaine with Epinephrine Injection ... 554
- Sus-Phrine Injection ... 1017
- Xylocaine with Epinephrine Injections ... 562

Epinephrine Bitartrate (Potential for loss of glycemic control). Products include:
- Sensorcaine-MPF with Epinephrine Injection ... 554

Epinephrine Hydrochloride (Potential for loss of glycemic control). Products include:
- Ana-Kit Anaphylaxis Emergency Treatment Kit ... 611

Estradiol (Potential for loss of glycemic control). Products include:
- Climara Transdermal System ... 640
- Estrace Cream and Tablets ... 751
- Estraderm Transdermal System ... 842
- Estring Vaginal Ring ... 2086
- Vivelle Transdermal System ... 880

Estrogens, Conjugated (Potential for loss of glycemic control). Products include:
- PMB 200 and PMB 400 ... 2890
- Premarin Intravenous ... 2893
- Premarin Tablets ... 2896
- Premarin Vaginal Cream ... 2898
- Premphase ... 2900
- Prempro ... 2905

Estrogens, Esterified (Potential for loss of glycemic control). Products include:
- ESTRATAB Tablets (0.3, 0.625, 1.25, 2.5 mg) ... 2715
- Estratest ... 2718
- Menest Tablets ... 2671

Estropipate (Potential for loss of glycemic control). Products include:
- Ogen Tablets ... 2103
- Ogen Vaginal Cream ... 2106
- Ortho-Est ... 1925

Ethacrynic Acid (Potential for loss of glycemic control). Products include:
- Edecrin Tablets ... 1698

Ethinyl Estradiol (Potential for loss of glycemic control). Products include:
- Brevicon ... 2563
- Demulen ... 2580
- Desogen Tablets ... 1867
- Levlen/Tri-Levlen ... 646
- Lo/Ovral Tablets ... 2852
- Lo/Ovral-28 Tablets ... 2857
- Modicon ... 1928
- Nordette-21 Tablets ... 2863
- Nordette-28 Tablets ... 2866
- Norinyl ... 2563
- Ortho-Cept ... 1907
- Ortho-Cyclen/Ortho-Tri-Cyclen ... 1914
- Ortho-Novum ... 1928
- Ortho-Cyclen/Ortho Tri-Cyclen ... 1914
- Ovcon ... 765
- Ovral Tablets ... 2877
- Ovral-28 Tablets ... 2878
- Levlen/Tri-Levlen ... 646
- Tri-Norinyl ... 2607
- Triphasil-21 Tablets ... 2919
- Triphasil-28 Tablets ... 2924

Ethiodized Oil (Potential for acute alteration of renal function; metformin should be temporarily withheld in patients undergoing radiologic studies involving parenteral iodinated contrast material).
- No products indexed under this heading.

Ethynodiol Diacetate (Potential for loss of glycemic control). Products include:
- Demulen ... 2580

Felodipine (Potential for loss of glycemic control). Products include:
- Plendil Extended-Release Tablets ... 514

Fludrocortisone Acetate (Potential for loss of glycemic control). Products include:
- Florinef Acetate Tablets ... 506

Fluphenazine Decanoate (Potential for loss of glycemic control). Products include:
- Prolixin Decanoate ... 510

Fluphenazine Enanthate (Potential for loss of glycemic control). Products include:
- Prolixin Enanthate ... 510

Fluphenazine Hydrochloride (Potential for loss of glycemic control). Products include:
- Prolixin ... 510

Furosemide (Increases metformin plasma and blood C_{max} by 22% and blood AUC by 15%; the C_{max} and AUC of furosemide were 31% and 12% smaller when co-administered; potential for loss of glycemic control). Products include:
- Lasix Injection, Oral Solution and Tablets ... 1267

Gadopentetate Dimeglumine (Potential for acute alteration of renal function; metformin should be temporarily withheld in patients undergoing radiologic studies involving parenteral iodinated contrast material).
- No products indexed under this heading.

Glyburide (Decrease in glyburide AUC and C_{max} have been observed, but were highly variable). Products include:
- DiaBeta Tablets ... 1265
- Glynase PresTab Tablets ... 2091
- Micronase Tablets ... 2099

Hydrochlorothiazide (Potential for loss of glycemic control). Products include:
- Aldactazide Tablets ... 2556
- Aldoril Tablets ... 1644
- Apresazide Capsules ... 824
- Capozide Tablets ... 744
- Dyazide Capsules ... 2653
- Esidrix Tablets ... 839
- Esimil Tablets ... 840
- HydroDIURIL Tablets ... 1716
- Hydropres Tablets ... 1718
- Hyzaar Tablets ... 1720
- Inderide Tablets ... 2838
- Inderide LA Long Acting Capsules ... 2840
- Lopressor HCT Tablets ... 850
- Lotensin HCT Tablets ... 855
- Moduretic Tablets ... 1748
- Oretic Tablets ... 450
- Prinzide Tablets ... 1780
- Ser-Ap-Es Tablets ... 867
- Timolide Tablets ... 1791
- Vaseretic Tablets ... 1810
- Zestoretic Tablets ... 2968
- Ziac ... 1459

Hydrocortisone (Potential for loss of glycemic control). Products include:
- Anusol-HC Cream 2.5% ... 1953
- Aquanil HC Lotion ... 1989
- Maximum Strength Cortaid Spray ... 800
- CORTENEMA ... 2713
- Cortisporin Ointment ... 1074
- Cortisporin Ophthalmic Ointment Sterile ... 1074

IMPORTANT NOTE: Always consult each drug listing in the patient's regimen for possible interactions.

Glucophage **Interactions Index** **442**

Cortisporin Ophthalmic Suspension Sterile ... 1075
Cortisporin Otic Solution Sterile ... 1076
Cortisporin Otic Suspension Sterile 1077
Cortizone-5 ... 795
Cortizone-10 ... 795
Hydrocortone Tablets ... 1715
Hytone ... 922
Hytone Ointment 2 ½% ... 923
Massengill Medicated Soft Cloth Towelettes ... 2628
Pediotic Suspension Sterile ... 1140
Preparation H Hydrocortisone 1% Cream ... 843
ProctoCream-HC 2.5% ... 2552
VōSoL HC Otic Solution ... 2786

Hydrocortisone Acetate (Potential for loss of glycemic control). Products include:
Analpram-HC Rectal Cream 1% and 2.5% ... 993
Anusol HC-1 Hydrocortisone Anti-Itch Ointment ... 810
Anusol-HC Suppositories ... 1954
Caldecort Anti-Itch Hydrocortisone Cream ... 651
Coly-Mycin S Otic w/Neomycin & Hydrocortisone ... 1965
Cortaid ... 800
Cortifoam ... 2540
Cortisporin Cream ... 1073
Epifoam ... 2543
Hydrocortone Acetate Sterile Suspension ... 1712
Mantadil Cream ... 1124
Nupercainal Hydrocortisone 1% Cream ... 661
Pramosone Cream, Lotion & Ointment ... 995
ProctoFoam-HC ... 2552
Terra-Cortril Ophthalmic Suspension ... 2033

Hydrocortisone Sodium Phosphate (Potential for loss of glycemic control). Products include:
Hydrocortone Phosphate Injection, Sterile ... 1713

Hydrocortisone Sodium Succinate (Potential for loss of glycemic control).
No products indexed under this heading.

Hydroflumethiazide (Potential for loss of glycemic control). Products include:
Diucardin Tablets ... 2824

Indapamide (Potential for loss of glycemic control).
No products indexed under this heading.

Iodamide Meglumine (Potential for acute alteration of renal function; metformin should be temporarily withheld in patients undergoing radiologic studies involving parenteral iodinated contrast material).
No products indexed under this heading.

Iohexol (Potential for acute alteration of renal function; metformin should be temporarily withheld in patients undergoing radiologic studies involving parenteral iodinated contrast material).
No products indexed under this heading.

Iopamidol (Potential for acute alteration of renal function; metformin should be temporarily withheld in patients undergoing radiologic studies involving parenteral iodinated contrast material).
No products indexed under this heading.

Iothalamate Meglumine (Potential for acute alteration of renal function; metformin should be temporarily withheld in patients undergoing radiologic studies involving parenteral iodinated contrast material).
No products indexed under this heading.

Iopanoic Acid (Potential for acute alteration of renal function; metformin should be temporarily withheld in patients undergoing radiologic studies involving parenteral iodinated contrast material).

Ioxaglate Meglumine (Potential for acute alteration of renal function; metformin should be temporarily withheld in patients undergoing radiologic studies involving parenteral iodinated contrast material).
No products indexed under this heading.

Ioxaglate Sodium (Potential for acute alteration of renal function; metformin should be temporarily withheld in patients undergoing radiologic studies involving parenteral iodinated contrast material).
No products indexed under this heading.

Isoniazid (Potential for loss of glycemic control). Products include:
Nydrazid Injection ... 509
Rifamate Capsules ... 1278
Rifater ... 1280

Isoproterenol Hydrochloride (Potential for loss of glycemic control). Products include:
Isuprel Hydrochloride Solution ... 2443
Isuprel Injection ... 2441
Isuprel Mistometer ... 2442

Isoproterenol Sulfate (Potential for loss of glycemic control). Products include:
Norisodrine with Calcium Iodide Syrup ... 446

Isradipine (Potential for loss of glycemic control). Products include:
DynaCirc Capsules ... 2381
DynaCirc CR Tablets ... 2383

Levonorgestrel (Potential for loss of glycemic control). Products include:
Levlen/Tri-Levlen ... 646
Nordette-21 Tablets ... 2863
Nordette-28 Tablets ... 2866
Norplant System ... 2868
Levlen/Tri-Levlen ... 646
Triphasil-21 Tablets ... 2919
Triphasil-28 Tablets ... 2924

Levothyroxine Sodium (Potential for loss of glycemic control). Products include:
Eltroxin Tablets ... 2214
Levothroid Tablets ... 1015
Levothyroxine Sodium, USP for Injection ... 546
Levoxyl Tablets ... 918
Synthroid ... 1410

Liothyronine Sodium (Potential for loss of glycemic control). Products include:
Cytomel Tablets ... 2647
Triostat Injection ... 2708

Liotrix (Potential for loss of glycemic control).
No products indexed under this heading.

Mesoridazine Besylate (Potential for loss of glycemic control). Products include:
Serentil ... 689

Mestranol (Potential for loss of glycemic control). Products include:
Norinyl ... 2563
Ortho-Novum ... 1928

Metaproterenol Sulfate (Potential for loss of glycemic control). Products include:
Alupent ... 672
Metaproterenol Sulfate Inhalation Solution, USP, Arm-a-Med ... 547

Metaraminol Bitartrate (Potential for loss of glycemic control). Products include:
Aramine Injection ... 1649

Methotrimeprazine (Potential for loss of glycemic control). Products include:
Levoprome ... 1321

Methoxamine Hydrochloride (Potential for loss of glycemic control). Products include:
Vasoxyl Injection ... 1169

Methyclothiazide (Potential for loss of glycemic control). Products include:
Enduron Tablets ... 424

Methylprednisolone Acetate (Potential for loss of glycemic control).
No products indexed under this heading.

Methylprednisolone Sodium Succinate (Potential for loss of glycemic control).
No products indexed under this heading.

Metolazone (Potential for loss of glycemic control). Products include:
Mykrox Tablets ... 1617
Zaroxolyn Tablets ... 1625

Morphine Sulfate (Theoretical potential for interaction with metformin by competing for common renal tubular transport system). Products include:
Astramorph/PF Injection, USP (Preservative-Free) ... 526
Duramorph Injection ... 983
Infumorph 200 and Infumorph 500 Sterile Solutions ... 985
Kadian Capsules ... 2948
MS Contin Tablets ... 2149
MSIR ... 2152
Oramorph SR (Morphine Sulfate Sustained Release Tablets) ... 2359
RMS Suppositories CII ... 2766
Roxanol ... 2365

Nicardipine Hydrochloride (Potential for loss of glycemic control). Products include:
Cardene Capsules ... 2261
Cardene I.V. ... 2815
Cardene SR Capsules ... 2264

Nicotinic Acid (Potential for loss of glycemic control).
No products indexed under this heading.

Nifedipine (Enhances the absorption of metformin by increasing plasma metformin C_{max} and AUC; potential for loss of glycemic control). Products include:
Adalat Capsules (10 mg and 20 mg) ... 580
Adalat CC ... 582
Procardia Capsules ... 2024
Procardia XL Extended Release Tablets ... 2026

Nimodipine (Potential for loss of glycemic control). Products include:
Nimotop Capsules ... 603

Nisoldipine (Potential for loss of glycemic control). Products include:
Sular Tablets ... 2961

Norepinephrine Bitartrate (Potential for loss of glycemic control). Products include:
Levophed Bitartrate Injection ... 2445

Norethindrone (Potential for loss of glycemic control). Products include:
Brevicon ... 2563
Micronor Tablets ... 1903
Modicon ... 1928
Norinyl ... 2563
Nor-Q D Tablets ... 2598
Ortho-Novum ... 1928
Ovcon ... 765
Tri-Norinyl ... 2607

Norethynodrel (Potential for loss of glycemic control).
No products indexed under this heading.

Norgestimate (Potential for loss of glycemic control). Products include:
Ortho-Cyclen/Ortho-Tri-Cyclen ... 1914
Ortho-Cyclen/Ortho Tri-Cyclen ... 1914

Norgestrel (Potential for loss of glycemic control). Products include:
Lo/Ovral Tablets ... 2852
Lo/Ovral-28 Tablets ... 2857
Ovral Tablets ... 2877
Ovral-28 Tablets ... 2878
Ovrette Tablets ... 2878

Perphenazine (Potential for loss of glycemic control). Products include:
Etrafon ... 2495
Triavil Tablets ... 1800
Trilafon ... 2532

Phenylephrine Bitartrate (Potential for loss of glycemic control).
No products indexed under this heading.

Phenylephrine Hydrochloride (Potential for loss of glycemic control). Products include:
Atrohist Plus Tablets ... 1605
Cerose DM ... 853
D.A. II Tablets ... 972
D.A. Chewable Tablets ... 970
Dura-Vent/DA Tablets ... 972
Extendryl ... 1003
4-Way Fast Acting Nasal Spray (regular & mentholated) ... 644
Hemorid ... 797
Hycomine Compound Tablets ... 948
Neo-Synephrine Hydrochloride 1% Carpuject ... 2455
Neo-Synephrine Hydrochloride 1% Injection ... 2455
Neo-Synephrine Hydrochloride (Ophthalmic) ... 2456
Neo-Synephrine ... 624
Novahistine Elixir ... 782
Phenergan VC ... 2886
Phenergan VC with Codeine ... 2888
Preparation H ... 842
Tympagesic Ear Drops ... 2476
Vicks Sinex Nasal Spray and Ultra Fine Mist ... 738

Phenylephrine Tannate (Potential for loss of glycemic control). Products include:
Atrohist Pediatric Suspension ... 1604
Atrohist Pediatric Suspension Dye-Free ... 1604
Rynatan ... 2781
Rynatuss ... 2782

Phenylpropanolamine Hydrochloride (Potential for loss of glycemic control). Products include:
Acutrim ... 648
Atrohist Plus Tablets ... 1605
BC Cold Powder Multi-Symptom Formula (Cold-Sinus-Allergy) ... 631
BC Cold Powder Non-Drowsy Formula (Cold-Sinus) ... 631
Cheracol Plus Head Cold/Cough Formula ... 741
Comtrex Multi-Symptom Cold Reliever Liqui-Gels ... 638
Comtrex Multi-Symptom Non-Drowsy Liqui-gels ... 640
Contac Continuous Action Nasal Decongestant/Antihistamine 12 Hour Capsules ... 773
Contac Maximum Strength Continuous Action Decongestant/Antihistamine 12 Hour Caplets ... 772
Contac Severe Cold and Flu Formula Caplets ... 773
Coricidin 'D' Decongestant Tablets ... 760
Dexatrim ... 795
Dexatrim Plus Vitamins Caplets ... 796
Dimetane-DC Cough Syrup ... 2232
Dimetapp Allergy Sinus Caplets ... 838
Dimetapp Cold & Allergy Chewable Tablets ... 838
Dimetapp Cold & Cough Liqui-Gels ... 839
Dimetapp DM Elixir ... 840
Dimetapp Elixir ... 840
Dimetapp Extentabs ... 841
Dimetapp Tablets/Liqui-Gels ... 841
Dura-Vent Tablets ... 971
Entex LA Tablets ... 972
Exgest LA Tablets ... 787

(Described in PDR For Nonprescription Drugs) (⊙ Described in PDR For Ophthalmology)

Interactions Index — Glucophage

Hycomine 947
Nolamine Timed-Release Tablets 790
Ornade Spansule Capsules 2678
Propagest Tablets 791
Pyrroxate Caplets ..... ℞ 742
Robitussin-CF ..... ℞ 846
Sinulin Tablets 792
Tavist-D 12 Hour Relief Tablets .... ℞ 750
Teldrin 12 Hour Antihistamine/Nasal Decongestant Allergy Relief Capsules ..... ℞ 786
Triaminic Expectorant ..... ℞ 753
Triaminic Syrup ..... ℞ 755
Triaminic Triaminicol Cold & Cough ..... ℞ 756
Triaminic DM Syrup ..... ℞ 756
Triaminicin Tablets ..... ℞ 756
Vicks DayQuil Allergy Relief 12-Hour Extended Release Tablets.. ℞ 733
Vicks DayQuil Allergy Relief 4-Hour Tablets ..... ℞ 733
Vicks DayQuil SINUS Pressure & CONGESTION Relief ..... ℞ 734

Phenytoin (Potential for loss of glycemic control). Products include:
Dilantin Infatabs 1967
Dilantin-125 Suspension 1969

Phenytoin Sodium (Potential for loss of glycemic control). Products include:
Dilantin Kapseals 1965

Pirbuterol Acetate (Potential for loss of glycemic control). Products include:
Maxair Autohaler 1550
Maxair Inhaler 1552

Polyestradiol Phosphate (Potential for loss of glycemic control).
No products indexed under this heading.

Polythiazide (Potential for loss of glycemic control). Products include:
Minizide Capsules 2016

Prednisolone Acetate (Potential for loss of glycemic control). Products include:
AK-CIDE ..... ◎ 203
AK-CIDE Ointment ..... ◎ 203
Blephamide Liquifilm Sterile Ophthalmic Suspension 472
Blephamide Ointment ..... ◎ 234
Econopred & Econopred Plus Ophthalmic Suspensions ..... ◎ 216
Poly-Pred Liquifilm ..... ◎ 246
Pred Forte ..... ◎ 247
Pred Mild ..... ◎ 250
Pred-G Liquifilm Sterile Ophthalmic Suspension ..... ◎ 248
Pred-G S.O.P. Sterile Ophthalmic Ointment ..... ◎ 249

Prednisolone Sodium Phosphate (Potential for loss of glycemic control). Products include:
AK-PRED ..... ◎ 204
Hydeltrasol Injection, Sterile 1708
Pediapred Oral Solution 1618

Prednisolone Tebutate (Potential for loss of glycemic control). Products include:
Hydeltra-T.B.A. Sterile Suspension 1710

Prednisone (Potential for loss of glycemic control).
No products indexed under this heading.

Procainamide Hydrochloride (Theoretical potential for interaction with metformin by competing for common renal tubular transport system). Products include:
Procanbid Extended-Release Tablets 1983

Prochlorperazine (Potential for loss of glycemic control). Products include:
Compazine 2644

Promethazine Hydrochloride (Potential for loss of glycemic control). Products include:
Mepergan Injection 2859
Phenergan with Codeine 2883
Phenergan with Dextromethorphan 2885
Phenergan Injection 2880

Phenergan Suppositories 2882
Phenergan Syrup 2881
Phenergan Tablets 2882
Phenergan VC 2886
Phenergan VC with Codeine 2888

Pseudoephedrine Hydrochloride (Potential for loss of glycemic control). Products include:
Actifed Allergy Daytime/Nighttime Caplets ..... ℞ 808
Actifed Cold & Allergy Tablets ..... ℞ 807
Actifed Cold & Sinus Caplets and Tablets ..... ℞ 808
Actifed Sinus Daytime/Nighttime Tablets and Caplets ..... ℞ 809
Advil Cold and Sinus Caplets and Tablets ..... ℞ 837
Alka-Seltzer Plus Liqui-Gels ..... ℞ 612
Alka-Seltzer Plus Flu & Body Aches Liqui-Gels Non-Drowsy Formula ..... ℞ 613
Alka-Seltzer Plus Night-Time Cold Medicine Liqui-Gels ..... ℞ 612
Allerest Maximum Strength ..... ℞ 649
Allerest No Drowsiness ..... ℞ 649
Allerest Sinus Pain Formula ..... ℞ 649
Atrohist Pediatric Capsules 1603
Benadryl Allergy/Cold Tablets ..... ℞ 811
Benadryl Allergy Decongestant Liquid Medication ..... ℞ 812
Benadryl Allergy Decongestant Tablets ..... ℞ 812
Benadryl Allergy Sinus Headache Caplets ..... ℞ 813
Benylin Multisymptom ..... ℞ 816
Bromfed Capsules (Extended-Release) 1832
Bromfed Syrup ..... ℞ 712
Bromfed Tablets 1832
Bromfed-DM Cough Syrup 1832
Bromfed-PD Capsules (Extended-Release) 1832
Children's TYLENOL Cold Multi-Symptom Chewable Tablets and Liquid 1559
Children's TYLENOL Cold Plus Cough Multi Symptom Chewable Tablets and Liquid 1560
Children's TYLENOL Flu Suspension Liquid 1560
Children's Vicks DayQuil Allergy Relief ..... ℞ 730
Children's Vicks NyQuil Cold/Cough Relief ..... ℞ 731
Allergy-Sinus Comtrex Multi-Symptom Allergy-Sinus Formula Tablets and Caplets ..... ℞ 639
Comtrex Multi-Symptom ..... ℞ 638
Comtrex Multi-Symptom Non-Drowsy Caplets ..... ℞ 640
Congess 1003
Contac Day Allergy/Sinus Caplets ℞ 771
Contac Day & Night ..... ℞ 772
Contac Night Allergy/Sinus Caplets ..... ℞ 771
Contac Severe Cold & Flu Non-Drowsy ..... ℞ 774
Deconsal II Tablets 1605
Dimetane-DX Cough Syrup 2233
Dimetapp Cold & Fever Suspension ..... ℞ 839
Dimetapp Decongestant Pediatric Drops ..... ℞ 840
Dorcol Children's Cough Syrup ..... ℞ 748
Drixoral Cough + Congestion Liquid Caps ..... ℞ 763
Dura-Tap/PD Capsules 970
Duratuss Tablets 2750
Duratuss HD Elixir 2750
Efidac/24 655
Entex PSE Tablets 973
Fedahist Gyrocaps 2545
Guaifed 1833
Guaifed Syrup ..... ℞ 712
Guaimax-D Tablets 809
Histussin D Liquid 670
Infants' TYLENOL Cold Decongestant & Fever-Reducer Drops 1561
Kronofed-A 994
Novahistine DMX 782
Nucofed 2225
PediaCare Cough-Cold Chewable Tablets and Liquid 1569
PediaCare Infants' Decongestant Drops 1569
PediaCare Infants' Drops Decongestant Plus Cough 1569
PediaCare NightRest Cough-Cold Liquid 1569

Pediatric Vicks 44d Cough & Head Congestion Relief ..... ℞ 736
Pediatric Vicks 44m Cough & Cold Relief ..... ℞ 737
Robitussin Cold & Cough Liqui-Gels ..... ℞ 844
Robitussin Cold, Cough & Flu Liqui-Gels ..... ℞ 844
Robitussin Maximum Strength Cough & Cold ..... ℞ 847
Robitussin Night-Time Cold Formula ..... ℞ 847
Robitussin Pediatric Cough & Cold Formula ..... ℞ 848
Robitussin Pediatric Drops ..... ℞ 849
Robitussin Severe Congestion Liqui-Gels ..... ℞ 845
Robitussin-DAC Syrup 2249
Robitussin-PE ..... ℞ 846
Rondec Oral Drops 974
Rondec Syrup 974
Rondec Tablet 974
Rondec Chewable Tablets 974
Rondec-TR Tablet 974
Ryna ..... ℞ 804
Seldane-D Extended-Release Tablets 1286
Semprex-D Capsules 1620
Sinarest ..... ℞ 663
Sine-Aid Maximum Strength Sinus Headache Gelcaps, Caplets and Tablets 1570
Sine-Off No Drowsiness Formula Caplets ..... ℞ 784
Sine-Off Sinus Medicine ..... ℞ 784
Singlet Tablets ..... ℞ 785
Sinutab Non-Drying Liquid Caps ..... ℞ 823
Sinutab Sinus Allergy Medication, Maximum Strength Tablets and Caplets ..... ℞ 823
Sinutab Sinus Medication, Maximum Strength Without Drowsiness Formula, Tablets & Caplets ..... ℞ 824
Sudafed Children's Cold & Cough Liquid Medication ..... ℞ 825
Sudafed Children's Nasal Decongestant Liquid Medication ..... ℞ 826
Sudafed Cold & Allergy Tablets ..... ℞ 826
Sudafed Cold and Cough Liquid Caps ..... ℞ 826
Sudafed Nasal Decongestant Tablets, 30 mg ..... ℞ 825
Sudafed Nasal Decongestant Tablets, 60 mg ..... ℞ 825
Sudafed Non-Drying Sinus Liquid Caps ..... ℞ 827
Sudafed Pediatric Nasal Decongestant Liquid Oral Drops ..... ℞ 827
Sudafed Severe Cold Formula Caplets ..... ℞ 828
Sudafed Severe Cold Formula Tablets ..... ℞ 828
Sudafed Sinus Caplets ..... ℞ 829
Sudafed Sinus Tablets ..... ℞ 829
Sudafed 12 Hour Caplets ..... ℞ 824
Syn-Rx Tablets 1622
Syn-Rx DM Tablets 1623
TheraFlu Flu and Cold Medicine ..... ℞ 750
Theraflu Maximum Strength Flu and Cold Medicine For Sore Throat ..... ℞ 751
TheraFlu Flu, Cold and Cough Medicine ..... ℞ 750
TheraFlu Maximum Strength Nighttime Flu, Cold & Cough Medicine ..... ℞ 751
TheraFlu Maximum Strength Non-Drowsy Formula Flu, Cold & Cough Medicine ..... ℞ 751
TheraFlu Maximum Strength, Non-Drowsy Formula Flu, Cold and Cough Caplets ..... ℞ 752
Theraflu Maximum Strength Sinus Non-Drowsy Formula Caplets ..... ℞ 752
Triaminic AM Cough and Decongestant Formula ..... ℞ 753
Triaminic AM Decongestant Formula ..... ℞ 753
Triaminic Infant Oral Decongestant Drops ..... ℞ 754
Triaminic Night Time ..... ℞ 754
Triaminic Sore Throat Formula ..... ℞ 755
Tussend 1830
Tussend Expectorant 1831
TYLENOL Allergy Sinus, Maximum Strength Caplets and Gelcaps 1571
TYLENOL Allergy Sinus NightTime, Maximum Strength Caplets 1571

TYLENOL Cold Medication, Multi-Symptom Formula Tablets and Caplets 1572
TYLENOL Cold Medication, Multi-Symptom Hot Liquid Packets 1572
TYLENOL Cold Medication, No Drowsiness Formula Caplets and Gelcaps 1572
TYLENOL Cold Severe Congestion Caplets 1573
TYLENOL Cough Medication with Decongestant, Multi Symptom 1574
TYLENOL Flu No Drowsiness Formula, Maximum Strength Gelcaps 1575
TYLENOL Flu NightTime, Maximum Strength Gelcaps 1575
TYLENOL Flu NightTime, Maximum Strength Hot Medication Packets 1575
TYLENOL Sinus, Maximum Strength Geltabs, Gelcaps, Caplets and Tablets 1576
Vicks 44 LiquiCaps Cough, Cold & Flu Relief ..... ℞ 728
Vicks 44 LiquiCaps Non-Drowsy Cough & Cold Relief ..... ℞ 729
Vicks 44D Cough & Head Congestion Relief ..... ℞ 728
Vicks 44M Cough, Cold & Flu Relief ..... ℞ 729
Vicks DayQuil LiquiCaps/Liquid Multi-Symptom Cold/Flu Relief .. ℞ 734
Vicks DayQuil SINUS Pressure & PAIN Relief with IBUPROFEN ..... ℞ 735
Vicks Nyquil Hot Therapy ..... ℞ 735
Vicks NyQuil LiquiCaps/Liquid Multi-Symptom Cold/Flu Relief, Original and Cherry Flavors ..... ℞ 736

Pseudoephedrine Sulfate (Potential for loss of glycemic control). Products include:
Chlor-Trimeton Allergy Decongestant Tablets ..... ℞ 759
Claritin-D Tablets 2487
Drixoral Cold and Allergy Sustained-Action Tablets ..... ℞ 763
Drixoral Cold and Flu Extended-Release Tablets ..... ℞ 764
Drixoral Non-Drowsy Formula Extended-Release Tablets ..... ℞ 764
Drixoral Allergy/Sinus Extended Release Tablets ..... ℞ 765
Trinalin Repetabs Tablets 1373

Quinestrol (Potential for loss of glycemic control).
No products indexed under this heading.

Quinidine Gluconate (Theoretical potential for interaction with metformin by competing for common renal tubular transport system). Products include:
Quinaglute Dura-Tabs Tablets 644

Quinidine Polygalacturonate (Theoretical potential for interaction with metformin by competing for common renal tubular transport system). Products include:
Cardioquin Tablets 2146

Quinidine Sulfate (Theoretical potential for interaction with metformin by competing for common renal tubular transport system). Products include:
Quinidex Extentabs 2240

Quinine Sulfate (Theoretical potential for interaction with metformin by competing for common renal tubular transport system).
No products indexed under this heading.

Ranitidine Hydrochloride (Theoretical potential for interaction with metformin by competing for common renal tubular transport system). Products include:
Zantac 1182
Zantac Injection 1180
Zantac Syrup 1182

Salmeterol Xinafoate (Potential for loss of glycemic control). Products include:
Serevent Inhalation Aerosol 1149

IMPORTANT NOTE: Always consult each drug listing in the patient's regimen for possible interactions.

Spironolactone (Potential for loss of glycemic control). Products include:
Aldactazide Tablets 2556
Aldactone Tablets 2558

Terbutaline Sulfate (Potential for loss of glycemic control). Products include:
Brethaire Inhaler 830
Brethine Ampuls 832
Brethine Tablets 831
Bricanyl Subcutaneous Injection 1247
Bricanyl Tablets 1248

Thioridazine Hydrochloride (Potential for loss of glycemic control). Products include:
Mellaril 2398

Thyroglobulin (Potential for loss of glycemic control).
No products indexed under this heading.

Thyroid (Potential for loss of glycemic control).
No products indexed under this heading.

Thyroxine (Potential for loss of glycemic control).
No products indexed under this heading.

Thyroxine Sodium (Potential for loss of glycemic control).
No products indexed under this heading.

Torsemide (Potential for loss of glycemic control). Products include:
Demadex Tablets and Injection 691

Triamcinolone (Potential for loss of glycemic control).
No products indexed under this heading.

Triamcinolone Acetonide (Potential for loss of glycemic control). Products include:
Azmacort Oral Inhaler 2175
Nasacort AQ Nasal Spray 2191
Nasacort Nasal Inhaler 2189

Triamcinolone Diacetate (Potential for loss of glycemic control).
No products indexed under this heading.

Triamcinolone Hexacetonide (Potential for loss of glycemic control).
No products indexed under this heading.

Triamterene (Potential for loss of glycemic control; theoretical potential for interaction with metformin by competing for common renal tubular transport system). Products include:
Dyazide Capsules 2653
Dyrenium Capsules 2655

Trifluoperazine Hydrochloride (Potential for loss of glycemic control). Products include:
Stelazine 2692

Trimethoprim (Theoretical potential for interaction with metformin by competing for common renal tubular transport system). Products include:
Bactrim DS Tablets 2257
Bactrim I.V. Infusion 2255
Bactrim 2257
Proloprim Tablets 1141
Septra 1146
Septra I.V. Infusion 1142
Septra I.V. Infusion ADD-Vantage Vials 1144
Septra 1146
Trimpex Tablets 2323

Trimethoprim Sulfate (Theoretical potential for interaction with metformin by competing for common renal tubular transport system). Products include:
Polytrim Ophthalmic Solution Sterile 479

Tyropanoate Sodium (Potential for acute alteration of renal function; metformin should be temporarily withheld in patients undergoing radiologic studies involving parenteral iodinated contrast material).
No products indexed under this heading.

Vancomycin Hydrochloride (Theoretical potential for interaction with metformin by competing for common renal tubular transport system). Products include:
Vancocin HCl, Oral Solution & Pulvules 1536
Vancocin HCl, Vials & ADD-Vantage 1534

Verapamil Hydrochloride (Potential for loss of glycemic control). Products include:
Calan SR Caplets 2571
Calan Tablets 2568
Covera-HS Tablets 2573
Isoptin Injectable 1391
Isoptin Oral Tablets 1393
Isoptin SR Tablets 1395
Verelan Capsules 1455

Food Interactions

Alcohol (Alcohol potentiates the effect of metfomrin on lactate metabolism; patients should be warned against excessive alcohol intake, acute or chronic).

Food, unspecified (Food decreases the extent and slightly delays the absorption of metformin).

GLUCOTROL TABLETS
(Glipizide) 2011
May interact with highly protein bound drugs (selected), salicylates, non-steroidal anti-inflammatory agents, sulfonamides, oral anticoagulants, monoamine oxidase inhibitors, beta blockers, diuretics, thiazides, corticosteroids, phenothiazines, thyroid preparations, oral contraceptives, estrogens, calcium channel blockers, sympathomimetics, and certain other agents. Compounds in these categories include:

Acebutolol Hydrochloride (Co-administration with beta blockers may result in hypoglycemia). Products include:
Sectral Capsules 2914

Albuterol (Sympathomimetics tend to produce hyperglycemia and concurrent use may lead to loss of control). Products include:
Proventil Inhalation Aerosol 2524
Ventolin Inhalation Aerosol and Refill 1170

Albuterol Sulfate (Sympathomimetics tend to produce hyperglycemia and concurrent use may lead to loss of control). Products include:
Airet Albuterol Sulfate Inhalation Solution 1602
Albuterol Sulfate, USP Solution for Inhalation, Arm-a-Med 522
Proventil Inhalation Solution 0.083% 2527
Proventil Repetabs Tablets 2529
Proventil Solution for Inhalation 0.5% 2525
Proventil Syrup 2528
Proventil Tablets 2529
Ventolin Inhalation Solution 1171
Ventolin Nebules Inhalation Solution 1172
Ventolin Rotacaps for Inhalation 1173
Ventolin Syrup 1175
Ventolin Tablets 1176
Volmax Extended-Release Tablets 1835

Amiloride Hydrochloride (Diuretics tend to produce hyperglycemia and concurrent use may lead to loss of control). Products include:
Midamor Tablets 1746
Moduretic Tablets 1748

Amiodarone Hydrochloride (Co-administration with drugs that are highly protein bound may result in hypoglycemia). Products include:
Cordarone Intravenous 2821
Cordarone Tablets 2818

Amitriptyline Hydrochloride (Co-administration with drugs that are highly protein bound may result in hypoglycemia). Products include:
Elavil 2945
Etrafon 2495
Limbitrol 2333
Triavil Tablets 1800

Amlodipine Besylate (Calcium channel blockers tend to produce hyperglycemia and concurrent use may lead to loss of control). Products include:
Lotrel Capsules 858
Norvasc Tablets 2020

Aspirin (Co-administration with salicylates may result in hypoglycemia). Products include:
Alka-Seltzer Cherry Effervescent Antacid and Pain Reliever ▣ 609
Alka-Seltzer Extra Strength Effervescent Antacid and Pain Reliever ▣ 609
Alka-Seltzer Lemon Lime Effervescent Antacid and Pain Reliever ▣ 609
Alka-Seltzer Original Effervescent Antacid and Pain Reliever ▣ 609
Alka-Seltzer Plus ▣ 611
Alka-Seltzer Plus Sinus Medicine ▣ 611
Ascriptin ▣ 650
Arthritis Strength BC Powder ▣ 631
BC Cold Powder Multi-Symptom Formula (Cold-Sinus-Allergy) ▣ 631
BC Cold Powder Non-Drowsy Formula (Cold-Sinus) ▣ 631
BC Powder ▣ 631
Genuine Bayer Aspirin Tablets & Caplets ▣ 618
Extra Strength Bayer Arthritis Pain Regimen Formula ▣ 615
Extra Strength Bayer Aspirin Caplets & Tablets ▣ 617
Extended-Release Bayer 8-Hour Aspirin ▣ 616
Extra Strength Bayer Plus Aspirin Caplets ▣ 617
Extra Strength Bayer PM Aspirin Plus Sleep Aid ▣ 617
Aspirin Regimen Bayer 81 mg Tablets with Calcium ▣ 615
Aspirin Regimen Bayer Adult Low Strength 81 mg Tablets ▣ 613
Aspirin Regimen Bayer Children's Chewable Aspirin ▣ 616
Aspirin Regimen Bayer Regular Strength 325 mg Caplets ▣ 613
Bufferin Analgesic Tablets ▣ 636
Arthritis Strength Bufferin Analgesic Caplets ▣ 637
Extra Strength Bufferin Analgesic Tablets ▣ 637
Cama Arthritis Pain Reliever ▣ 748
Darvon Compound-65 Pulvules 1475
Easprin 1971
Ecotrin 2625
Ecotrin Enteric Coated Aspirin Maximum Strength Tablets and Caplets ▣ 775
Ecotrin Enteric Coated Aspirin Regular Strength Tablets 2625
Empirin Aspirin Tablets ▣ 818
Excedrin Extra-Strength Analgesic Tablets, Caplets, and Geltabs 734
Fiorinal Capsules 2388
Fiorinal with Codeine Capsules 2390
Fiorinal Tablets 2388
Goody's Extra Strength Headache Powders ▣ 632
Goody's Extra Strength Pain Relief Tablets ▣ 632
Halfprin Tablets 1413
Norgesic 1554
Percodan Tablets 955
Percodan-Demi Tablets 956
Robaxisal Tablets 2246
Soma Compound w/Codeine Tablets 2784
Soma Compound Tablets 2783
St. Joseph Adult Chewable Aspirin (81 mg.) ▣ 768
Talwin Compound 2466
Vanquish Analgesic Caplets ▣ 627

Atenolol (Co-administration with beta blockers may result in hypoglycemia). Products include:
Tenoretic Tablets 2963
Tenormin Tablets and I.V. Injection 2965

Atovaquone (Co-administration with drugs that are highly protein bound may result in hypoglycemia). Products include:
Mepron Suspension 1206

Bendroflumethiazide (Thiazides tend to produce hyperglycemia and concurrent use may lead to loss of control).
No products indexed under this heading.

Bepridil Hydrochloride (Calcium channel blockers tend to produce hyperglycemia and concurrent use may lead to loss of control). Products include:
Vascor Tablets (200 and 300 mg) 1597

Betamethasone Acetate (Corticosteroids tend to produce hyperglycemia and concurrent use may lead to loss of control). Products include:
Celestone Soluspan Suspension 2484

Betamethasone Sodium Phosphate (Corticosteroids tend to produce hyperglycemia and concurrent use may lead to loss of control). Products include:
Celestone Soluspan Suspension 2484

Betaxolol Hydrochloride (Co-administration with beta blockers may result in hypoglycemia). Products include:
Betoptic Ophthalmic Solution 465
Betoptic S Ophthalmic Suspension 467
Kerlone Tablets 2588

Bisoprolol Fumarate (Co-administration with beta blockers may result in hypoglycemia). Products include:
Zebeta Tablets 1457
Ziac 1459

Bumetanide (Diuretics tend to produce hyperglycemia and concurrent use may lead to loss of control). Products include:
Bumex 2260

Carteolol Hydrochloride (Co-administration with beta blockers may result in hypoglycemia). Products include:
Cartrol Tablets 413
Ocupress Ophthalmic Solution, 1% Sterile ⊚ 297

Cefonicid Sodium (Co-administration with drugs that are highly protein bound may result in hypoglycemia). Products include:
Monocid Injection 2674

Chloramphenicol (Co-administration with chloramphenicol may result in hypoglycemia). Products include:
Chloromycetin Ophthalmic Ointment, 1% ⊚ 298
Chloromycetin Ophthalmic Solution ⊚ 299
Chloroptic S.O.P. ⊚ 236
Chloroptic Sterile Ophthalmic Solution ⊚ 236

Chloramphenicol Palmitate (Co-administration with chloramphenicol may result in hypoglycemia).
No products indexed under this heading.

Chloramphenicol Sodium Succinate (Co-administration with chloramphenicol may result in hypoglycemia). Products include:
Chloromycetin Sodium Succinate 1960

(▣ Described in PDR For Nonprescription Drugs) (⊚ Described in PDR For Ophthalmology)

445 **Interactions Index** **Glucotrol**

Chlordiazepoxide (Co-administration with drugs that are highly protein bound may result in hypoglycemia). Products include:

Limbitrol 2333

Chlordiazepoxide Hydrochloride (Co-administration with drugs that are highly protein bound may result in hypoglycemia). Products include:

Librax Capsules 2330
Librium Capsules 2331
Librium Injectable 2332

Chlorothiazide (Thiazides tend to produce hyperglycemia and concurrent use may lead to loss of control). Products include:

Aldoclor Tablets 1638
Diupres Tablets 1691
Diuril Oral 1694

Chlorothiazide Sodium (Thiazides tend to produce hyperglycemia and concurrent use may lead to loss of control). Products include:

Diuril Sodium Intravenous 1693

Chlorotrianisene (Estrogens tend to produce hyperglycemia and concurrent use may lead to loss of control).

No products indexed under this heading.

Chlorpromazine (Phenothiazines tend to produce hyperglycemia and concurrent use may lead to loss of control). Products include:

Thorazine Suppositories 2701

Chlorpromazine Hydrochloride (Phenothiazines tend to produce hyperglycemia and concurrent use may lead to loss of control). Products include:

Thorazine 2701

Chlorpropamide (Co-administration with sulfonamides may result in hypoglycemia). Products include:

Diabinese Tablets 2002

Chlorthalidone (Diuretics tend to produce hyperglycemia and concurrent use may lead to loss of control). Products include:

Combipres Tablets 682
Tenoretic Tablets 2963
Thalitone 1293

Choline Magnesium Trisalicylate (Co-administration with salicylates may result in hypoglycemia). Products include:

Trilisate 2155

Clomipramine Hydrochloride (Co-administration with drugs that are highly protein bound may result in hypoglycemia). Products include:

Anafranil Capsules 819

Clozapine (Co-administration with drugs that are highly protein bound may result in hypoglycemia). Products include:

Clozaril Tablets 2377

Cortisone Acetate (Corticosteroids tend to produce hyperglycemia and concurrent use may lead to loss of control). Products include:

Cortone Acetate Sterile Suspension 1663
Cortone Acetate Tablets 1664

Cyclosporine (Co-administration with drugs that are highly protein bound may result in hypoglycemia). Products include:

Neoral 2405
Sandimmune 2416

Desogestrel (Oral contraceptives tend to produce hyperglycemia and concurrent use may lead to loss of control). Products include:

Desogen Tablets 1867
Ortho-Cept 1907

Dexamethasone (Corticosteroids tend to produce hyperglycemia and concurrent use may lead to loss of control). Products include:

AK-Trol Ointment & Suspension .... ◉ 205
Decadron Elixir 1676
Decadron Tablets 1678
Decaspray Topical Aerosol 1689
Maxitrol Ophthalmic Ointment and Suspension .... ◉ 222
TobraDex Ophthalmic Suspension and Ointment 469

Dexamethasone Acetate (Corticosteroids tend to produce hyperglycemia and concurrent use may lead to loss of control). Products include:

Dalalone D.P. Injectable 1009
Decadron-LA Sterile Suspension 1687

Dexamethasone Sodium Phosphate (Corticosteroids tend to produce hyperglycemia and concurrent use may lead to loss of control). Products include:

Decadron Phosphate Injection 1680
Decadron Phosphate Sterile Ophthalmic Ointment 1684
Decadron Phosphate Sterile Ophthalmic Solution 1685
Decadron Phosphate Topical Cream 1686
Decadron Phosphate with Xylocaine Injection, Sterile 1683
Dexacort Phosphate in Respihaler 1606
Dexacort Phosphate in Turbinaire 1607
NeoDecadron Sterile Ophthalmic Ointment 1755
NeoDecadron Sterile Ophthalmic Solution 1756
NeoDecadron Topical Cream 1757

Diazepam (Co-administration with drugs that are highly protein bound may result in hypoglycemia). Products include:

Dizac (diazepam injectable emulsion) CIV 1862
Valium Injectable 2336
Valium Tablets 2335

Diclofenac Potassium (Co-administration with nonsteroidal anti-inflammatory agents may result in hypoglycemia). Products include:

Cataflam Tablets 833

Diclofenac Sodium (Co-administration with nonsteroidal anti-inflammatory agents may result in hypoglycemia). Products include:

Voltaren Ophthalmic Sterile Ophthalmic Solution .... ◉ 264
Cataflam/Voltaren/Voltaren-XR 833

Dicumarol (Co-administration with coumarins may result in hypoglycemia).

No products indexed under this heading.

Dienestrol (Estrogens tend to produce hyperglycemia and concurrent use may lead to loss of control). Products include:

Ortho Dienestrol Cream 1922

Diethylstilbestrol (Estrogens tend to produce hyperglycemia and concurrent use may lead to loss of control). Products include:

Diethylstilbestrol Tablets 1477

Diflunisal (Co-administration with salicylates may result in hypoglycemia). Products include:

Dolobid Tablets 1695

Diltiazem Hydrochloride (Calcium channel blockers tend to produce hyperglycemia and concurrent use may lead to loss of control). Products include:

Cardizem CD Capsules 1251
Cardizem SR Capsules 1255
Cardizem Injectable 1253
Cardizem Tablets 1257
Dilacor XR Extended-release Capsules 2183
Tiazac Capsules 1019

Dipyridamole (Co-administration with drugs that are highly protein bound may result in hypoglycemia). Products include:

Persantine Tablets 686

Dobutamine Hydrochloride (Sympathomimetics tend to produce hyperglycemia and concurrent use may lead to loss of control). Products include:

Dobutrex Solution Vials 1480

Dopamine Hydrochloride (Sympathomimetics tend to produce hyperglycemia and concurrent use may lead to loss of control).

No products indexed under this heading.

Ephedrine Hydrochloride (Sympathomimetics tend to produce hyperglycemia and concurrent use may lead to loss of control). Products include:

Primatene Tablets .... ▣ 844
Quadrinal Tablets 1398

Ephedrine Sulfate (Sympathomimetics tend to produce hyperglycemia and concurrent use may lead to loss of control). Products include:

Marax Tablets & DF Syrup 2015

Ephedrine Tannate (Sympathomimetics tend to produce hyperglycemia and concurrent use may lead to loss of control). Products include:

Rynatuss 2782

Epinephrine (Sympathomimetics tend to produce hyperglycemia and concurrent use may lead to loss of control). Products include:

EPIFRIN .... ◉ 237
EpiPen 808
Marcaine with Epinephrine 2446
Primatene Mist .... ▣ 843
Sensorcaine with Epinephrine Injection 554
Sus-Phrine Injection 1017
Xylocaine with Epinephrine Injections 562

Epinephrine Bitartrate (Sympathomimetics tend to produce hyperglycemia and concurrent use may lead to loss of control). Products include:

Sensorcaine-MPF with Epinephrine Injection 554

Epinephrine Hydrochloride (Sympathomimetics tend to produce hyperglycemia and concurrent use may lead to loss of control). Products include:

Ana-Kit Anaphylaxis Emergency Treatment Kit 611

Esmolol Hydrochloride (Co-administration with beta blockers may result in hypoglycemia). Products include:

Brevibloc (esmolol HCl) Injection 1860

Estradiol (Estrogens tend to produce hyperglycemia and concurrent use may lead to loss of control). Products include:

Climara Transdermal System 640
Estrace Cream and Tablets 751
Estraderm Transdermal System 842
Estring Vaginal Ring 2086
Vivelle Transdermal System 880

Estrogens, Conjugated (Estrogens tend to produce hyperglycemia and concurrent use may lead to loss of control). Products include:

PMB 200 and PMB 400 2890
Premarin Intravenous 2893
Premarin Tablets 2896
Premarin Vaginal Cream 2898
Premphase 2900
Prempro 2905

Estrogens, Esterified (Estrogens tend to produce hyperglycemia and concurrent use may lead to loss of control). Products include:

ESTRATAB Tablets (0.3, 0.625, 1.25, 2.5 mg) 2715
Estratest 2718
Menest Tablets 2671

Estropipate (Estrogens tend to produce hyperglycemia and concurrent use may lead to loss of control). Products include:

Ogen Tablets 2103
Ogen Vaginal Cream 2106
Ortho-Est 1925

Ethacrynic Acid (Diuretics tend to produce hyperglycemia and concurrent use may lead to loss of control). Products include:

Edecrin Tablets 1698

Ethinyl Estradiol (Estrogens tend to produce hyperglycemia and concurrent use may lead to loss of control). Products include:

Brevicon 2563
Demulen 2580
Desogen Tablets 1867
Levlen/Tri-Levlen 646
Lo/Ovral Tablets 2852
Lo/Ovral-28 Tablets 2857
Modicon 1928
Nordette-21 Tablets 2863
Nordette-28 Tablets 2866
Norinyl 2563
Ortho-Cept 1907
Ortho-Cyclen/Ortho-Tri-Cyclen 1914
Ortho-Novum 1928
Ortho-Cyclen/Ortho Tri-Cyclen 1914
Ovcon 765
Ovral Tablets 2877
Ovral-28 Tablets 2878
Levlen/Tri-Levlen 646
Tri-Norinyl 2607
Triphasil-21 Tablets 2919
Triphasil-28 Tablets 2924

Ethynodiol Diacetate (Oral contraceptives tend to produce hyperglycemia and concurrent use may lead to loss of control). Products include:

Demulen 2580

Etodolac (Co-administration with nonsteroidal anti-inflammatory agents may result in hypoglycemia). Products include:

Lodine Capsules and Tablets 2849

Felodipine (Calcium channel blockers tend to produce hyperglycemia and concurrent use may lead to loss of control). Products include:

Plendil Extended-Release Tablets 514

Fenoprofen Calcium (Co-administration with nonsteroidal anti-inflammatory agents may result in hypoglycemia). Products include:

Nalfon 200 Pulvules & Nalfon Tablets 933

Fluconazole (Co-administration with oral fluconazole has resulted in an increase in Glucotrol AUC by 56.9%). Products include:

Diflucan Tablets, Injection, and Oral Suspension 2003

Fludrocortisone Acetate (Corticosteroids tend to produce hyperglycemia and concurrent use may lead to loss of control). Products include:

Florinef Acetate Tablets 506

Fluphenazine Decanoate (Phenothiazines tend to produce hyperglycemia and concurrent use may lead to loss of control). Products include:

Prolixin Decanoate 510

Fluphenazine Enanthate (Phenothiazines tend to produce hyperglycemia and concurrent use may lead to loss of control). Products include:

Prolixin Enanthate 510

IMPORTANT NOTE: Always consult each drug listing in the patient's regimen for possible interactions.

Glucotrol / Interactions Index

Fluphenazine Hydrochloride (Phenothiazines tend to produce hyperglycemia and concurrent use may lead to loss of control). Products include:
- Prolixin 510

Flurazepam Hydrochloride (Co-administration with drugs that are highly protein bound may result in hypoglycemia). Products include:
- Dalmane Capsules 2329

Flurbiprofen (Co-administration with nonsteroidal anti-inflammatory agents may result in hypoglycemia).
- No products indexed under this heading.

Furazolidone (Co-administration with monamine oxidase inhibitors may result in hypoglycemia). Products include:
- Furoxone 2221

Furosemide (Diuretics tend to produce hyperglycemia and concurrent use may lead to loss of control). Products include:
- Lasix Injection, Oral Solution and Tablets 1267

Glyburide (Co-administration with sulfonamides may result in hypoglycemia). Products include:
- DiaBeta Tablets 1265
- Glynase PresTab Tablets 2091
- Micronase Tablets 2099

Hydrochlorothiazide (Thiazides tend to produce hyperglycemia and concurrent use may lead to loss of control). Products include:
- Aldactazide Tablets 2556
- Aldoril Tablets 1644
- Apresazide Capsules 824
- Capozide Tablets 744
- Dyazide Capsules 2653
- Esidrix Tablets 839
- Esimil Tablets 840
- HydroDIURIL Tablets 1716
- Hydropres Tablets 1718
- Hyzaar Tablets 1720
- Inderide Tablets 2838
- Inderide LA Long Acting Capsules .. 2840
- Lopressor HCT Tablets 850
- Lotensin HCT Tablets 855
- Moduretic Tablets 1748
- Oretic Tablets 450
- Prinzide Tablets 1780
- Ser-Ap-Es Tablets 867
- Timolide Tablets 1791
- Vaseretic Tablets 1810
- Zestoretic Tablets 2968
- Ziac 1459

Hydrocortisone (Corticosteroids tend to produce hyperglycemia and concurrent use may lead to loss of control). Products include:
- Anusol-HC Cream 2.5% 1953
- Aquanil HC Lotion 1989
- Maximum Strength Cortaid Spray ▣ 800
- CORTENEMA 2713
- Cortisporin Ointment 1074
- Cortisporin Ophthalmic Ointment Sterile 1074
- Cortisporin Ophthalmic Suspension Sterile 1075
- Cortisporin Otic Solution Sterile 1076
- Cortisporin Otic Suspension Sterile 1077
- Cortizone-5 .... ▣ 795
- Cortizone-10 .... ▣ 795
- Hydrocortone Tablets 1715
- Hytone 922
- Hytone Ointment 2 ½ % 923
- Massengill Medicated Soft Cloth Towelettes 2628
- Pediotic Suspension Sterile 1140
- Preparation H Hydrocortisone 1% Cream .... ▣ 843
- ProctoCream-HC 2.5% 2552
- VōSoL HC Otic Solution 2786

Hydrocortisone Acetate (Corticosteroids tend to produce hyperglycemia and concurrent use may lead to loss of control). Products include:
- Analpram-HC Rectal Cream 1% and 2.5% 993
- Anusol HC-1 Hydrocortisone Anti-Itch Ointment .... ▣ 810
- Anusol-HC Suppositories 1954
- Caldecort Anti-Itch Hydrocortisone Cream .... ▣ 651
- Coly-Mycin S Otic w/Neomycin & Hydrocortisone 1965
- Cortaid .... ▣ 800
- Cortifoam 2540
- Cortisporin Cream 1073
- Epifoam 2543
- Hydrocortone Acetate Sterile Suspension 1712
- Mantadil Cream 1124
- Nupercainal Hydrocortisone 1% Cream .... ▣ 661
- Pramosone Cream, Lotion & Ointment 995
- ProctoFoam-HC 2552
- Terra-Cortril Ophthalmic Suspension 2033

Hydrocortisone Sodium Phosphate (Corticosteroids tend to produce hyperglycemia and concurrent use may lead to loss of control). Products include:
- Hydrocortone Phosphate Injection, Sterile 1713

Hydrocortisone Sodium Succinate (Corticosteroids tend to produce hyperglycemia and concurrent use may lead to loss of control).
- No products indexed under this heading.

Hydroflumethiazide (Thiazides tend to produce hyperglycemia and concurrent use may lead to loss of control). Products include:
- Diucardin Tablets 2824

Ibuprofen (Co-administration with nonsteroidal anti-inflammatory agents may result in hypoglycemia). Products include:
- Advil Cold and Sinus Caplets and Tablets .... ▣ 837
- Advil Ibuprofen Tablets, Caplets and Gel Caplets .... ▣ 836
- Children's Motrin Ibuprofen Oral Suspension 1558
- IBU Tablets 1389
- Ibuprohm .... ▣ 713
- Motrin IB Caplets, Tablets, and Gelcaps .... ▣ 802
- Motrin Ibuprofen Suspension, Oral Drops, Chewable Tablets, Caplets 1563
- Nuprin Ibuprofen/Analgesic Tablets & Caplets .... ▣ 645
- Vicks DayQuil SINUS Pressure & PAIN Relief with IBUPROFEN ...... ▣ 735

Imipramine Hydrochloride (Co-administration with drugs that are highly protein bound may result in hypoglycemia). Products include:
- Tofranil Ampuls 873
- Tofranil Tablets 875

Imipramine Pamoate (Co-administration with drugs that are highly protein bound may result in hypoglycemia). Products include:
- Tofranil-PM Capsules 876

Indapamide (Diuretics tend to produce hyperglycemia and concurrent use may lead to loss of control).
- No products indexed under this heading.

Indomethacin (Co-administration with nonsteroidal anti-inflammatory agents may result in hypoglycemia). Products include:
- Indocin 1723

Indomethacin Sodium Trihydrate (Co-administration with nonsteroidal anti-inflammatory agents may result in hypoglycemia). Products include:
- Indocin I.V. 1727

Isocarboxazid (Co-administration with monamine oxidase inhibitors may result in hypoglycemia).
- No products indexed under this heading.

Isoniazid (Isoniazid tends to produce hyperglycemia and concurrent use may lead to loss of control). Products include:
- Nydrazid Injection 509
- Rifamate Capsules 1278
- Rifater 1280

Isoproterenol Hydrochloride (Sympathomimetics tend to produce hyperglycemia and concurrent use may lead to loss of control). Products include:
- Isuprel Hydrochloride Solution 2443
- Isuprel Injection 2441
- Isuprel Mistometer 2442

Isoproterenol Sulfate (Sympathomimetics tend to produce hyperglycemia and concurrent use may lead to loss of control). Products include:
- Norisodrine with Calcium Iodide Syrup 446

Isradipine (Calcium channel blockers tend to produce hyperglycemia and concurrent use may lead to loss of control). Products include:
- DynaCirc Capsules 2381
- DynaCirc CR Tablets 2383

Ketoprofen (Co-administration with nonsteroidal anti-inflammatory agents may result in hypoglycemia). Products include:
- Actron Caplets and Tablets .... ▣ 608
- Orudis Capsules 2874
- Orudis KT .... ▣ 842
- Oruvail Capsules 2874

Ketorolac Tromethamine (Co-administration with nonsteroidal anti-inflammatory agents may result in hypoglycemia). Products include:
- Acular Sterile Ophthalmic Solution 470
- Toradol 2319

Labetalol Hydrochloride (Co-administration with beta blockers may result in hypoglycemia). Products include:
- Normodyne Injection 2519
- Normodyne Tablets 2522
- Trandate 1158

Levobunolol Hydrochloride (Co-administration with beta blockers may result in hypoglycemia). Products include:
- Betagan .... ⊙ 230

Levonorgestrel (Oral contraceptives tend to produce hyperglycemia and concurrent use may lead to loss of control). Products include:
- Levlen/Tri-Levlen 646
- Nordette-21 Tablets 2863
- Nordette-28 Tablets 2866
- Norplant System 2868
- Levlen/Tri-Levlen 646
- Triphasil-21 Tablets 2919
- Triphasil-28 Tablets 2924

Levothyroxine Sodium (Thyroid products tend to produce hyperglycemia and concurrent use may lead to loss of control). Products include:
- Eltroxin Tablets 2214
- Levothroid Tablets 1015
- Levothyroxine Sodium, USP for Injection 546
- Levoxyl Tablets 918
- Synthroid 1410

Liothyronine Sodium (Thyroid products tend to produce hyperglycemia and concurrent use may lead to loss of control). Products include:
- Cytomel Tablets 2647
- Triostat Injection 2708

Liotrix (Thyroid products tend to produce hyperglycemia and concurrent use may lead to loss of control).
- No products indexed under this heading.

Magnesium Salicylate (Co-administration with salicylates may result in hypoglycemia). Products include:
- Backache Caplets .... ▣ 635
- Doan's Extra-Strength Analgesic ..... ▣ 653
- Extra Strength Doan's P.M. .... ▣ 653
- Doan's Regular Strength Analgesic .... ▣ 654
- Mobigesic Tablets .... ▣ 607

Meclofenamate Sodium (Co-administration with nonsteroidal anti-inflammatory agents may result in hypoglycemia).
- No products indexed under this heading.

Mefenamic Acid (Co-administration with nonsteroidal anti-inflammatory agents may result in hypoglycemia). Products include:
- Ponstel 1982

Mesoridazine Besylate (Phenothiazines tend to produce hyperglycemia and concurrent use may lead to loss of control). Products include:
- Serentil 689

Mestranol (Oral contraceptives tend to produce hyperglycemia and concurrent use may lead to loss of control). Products include:
- Norinyl 2563
- Ortho-Novum 1928

Metaproterenol Sulfate (Sympathomimetics tend to produce hyperglycemia and concurrent use may lead to loss of control). Products include:
- Alupent 672
- Metaproterenol Sulfate Inhalation Solution, USP, Arm-a-Med 547

Metaraminol Bitartrate (Sympathomimetics tend to produce hyperglycemia and concurrent use may lead to loss of control). Products include:
- Aramine Injection 1649

Methotrimeprazine (Phenothiazines tend to produce hyperglycemia and concurrent use may lead to loss of control). Products include:
- Levoprome 1321

Methoxamine Hydrochloride (Sympathomimetics tend to produce hyperglycemia and concurrent use may lead to loss of control). Products include:
- Vasoxyl Injection 1169

Methyclothiazide (Thiazides tend to produce hyperglycemia and concurrent use may lead to loss of control). Products include:
- Enduron Tablets 424

Methylprednisolone Acetate (Corticosteroids tend to produce hyperglycemia and concurrent use may lead to loss of control).
- No products indexed under this heading.

Methylprednisolone Sodium Succinate (Corticosteroids tend to produce hyperglycemia and concurrent use may lead to loss of control).
- No products indexed under this heading.

Metipranolol Hydrochloride (Co-administration with beta blockers may result in hypoglycemia). Products include:
- OptiPranolol (Metipranolol 0.3%) Sterile Ophthalmic Solution .... ⊙ 256

Metolazone (Diuretics tend to produce hyperglycemia and concurrent use may lead to loss of control). Products include:
- Mykrox Tablets 1617
- Zaroxolyn Tablets 1625

(▣ Described in PDR For Nonprescription Drugs)   (⊙ Described in PDR For Ophthalmology)

447 **Interactions Index** **Glucotrol**

Metoprolol Succinate (Co-administration with beta blockers may result in hypoglycemia). Products include:
- Toprol-XL Tablets ... 560

Metoprolol Tartrate (Co-administration with beta blockers may result in hypoglycemia). Products include:
- Lopressor ... 848
- Lopressor HCT Tablets ... 850

Miconazole (Co-administration with oral miconazole and oral hypoglycemic agents has resulted in severe hypoglycemia).
- No products indexed under this heading.

Midazolam Hydrochloride (Co-administration with drugs that are highly protein bound may result in hypoglycemia). Products include:
- Versed Injection ... 2324

Nabumetone (Co-administration with nonsteroidal anti-inflammatory agents may result in hypoglycemia). Products include:
- Relafen Tablets ... 2688

Nadolol (Co-administration with beta blockers may result in hypoglycemia).
- No products indexed under this heading.

Naproxen (Co-administration with nonsteroidal anti-inflammatory agents may result in hypoglycemia). Products include:
- Anaprox/Naprosyn ... 2277

Naproxen Sodium (Co-administration with nonsteroidal anti-inflammatory agents may result in hypoglycemia). Products include:
- Aleve ... 2124
- Anaprox/Naprosyn ... 2277
- Naprelan Tablets ... 2861

Nicardipine Hydrochloride (Calcium channel blockers tend to produce hyperglycemia and concurrent use may lead to loss of control). Products include:
- Cardene Capsules ... 2261
- Cardene I.V. ... 2815
- Cardene SR Capsules ... 2264

Nicotinic Acid (Nicotinic acid tends to produce hyperglycemia and concurrent use may lead to loss of control).
- No products indexed under this heading.

Nifedipine (Calcium channel blockers tend to produce hyperglycemia and concurrent use may lead to loss of control). Products include:
- Adalat Capsules (10 mg and 20 mg) ... 580
- Adalat CC ... 582
- Procardia Capsules ... 2024
- Procardia XL Extended Release Tablets ... 2026

Nimodipine (Calcium channel blockers tend to produce hyperglycemia and concurrent use may lead to loss of control). Products include:
- Nimotop Capsules ... 603

Nisoldipine (Calcium channel blockers tend to produce hyperglycemia and concurrent use may lead to loss of control). Products include:
- Sular Tablets ... 2961

Norepinephrine Bitartrate (Sympathomimetics tend to produce hyperglycemia and concurrent use may lead to loss of control). Products include:
- Levophed Bitartrate Injection ... 2445

Norethindrone (Oral contraceptives tend to produce hyperglycemia and concurrent use may lead to loss of control). Products include:
- Brevicon ... 2563
- Micronor Tablets ... 1903
- Modicon ... 1928
- Norinyl ... 2563
- Nor-Q D Tablets ... 2598
- Ortho-Novum ... 1928
- Ovcon ... 765
- Tri-Norinyl ... 2607

Norethynodrel (Oral contraceptives tend to produce hyperglycemia and concurrent use may lead to loss of control).
- No products indexed under this heading.

Norgestimate (Oral contraceptives tend to produce hyperglycemia and concurrent use may lead to loss of control). Products include:
- Ortho-Cyclen/Ortho-Tri-Cyclen ... 1914
- Ortho-Cyclen/Ortho Tri-Cyclen ... 1914

Norgestrel (Oral contraceptives tend to produce hyperglycemia and concurrent use may lead to loss of control). Products include:
- Lo/Ovral Tablets ... 2852
- Lo/Ovral-28 Tablets ... 2857
- Ovral Tablets ... 2877
- Ovral-28 Tablets ... 2878
- Ovrette Tablets ... 2878

Nortriptyline Hydrochloride (Co-administration with drugs that are highly protein bound may result in hypoglycemia). Products include:
- Pamelor ... 2409

Oxaprozin (Co-administration with nonsteroidal anti-inflammatory agents may result in hypoglycemia). Products include:
- Daypro Caplets ... 2578

Oxazepam (Co-administration with drugs that are highly protein bound may result in hypoglycemia). Products include:
- Serax Capsules ... 2916
- Serax Tablets ... 2916

Penbutolol Sulfate (Co-administration with beta blockers may result in hypoglycemia). Products include:
- Levatol Tablets ... 2547

Perphenazine (Phenothiazines tend to produce hyperglycemia and concurrent use may lead to loss of control). Products include:
- Etrafon ... 2495
- Triavil Tablets ... 1800
- Trilafon ... 2532

Phenelzine Sulfate (Co-administration with monamine oxidase inhibitors may result in hypoglycemia). Products include:
- Nardil ... 1977

Phenylbutazone (Co-administration with nonsteroidal anti-inflammatory agents may result in hypoglycemia).
- No products indexed under this heading.

Phenylephrine Bitartrate (Sympathomimetics tend to produce hyperglycemia and concurrent use may lead to loss of control).
- No products indexed under this heading.

Phenylephrine Hydrochloride (Sympathomimetics tend to produce hyperglycemia and concurrent use may lead to loss of control). Products include:
- Atrohist Plus Tablets ... 1605
- Cerose DM ... 853
- D.A. II Tablets ... 972
- D.A. Chewable Tablets ... 970
- Dura-Vent/DA Tablets ... 972
- Extendryl ... 1003
- 4-Way Fast Acting Nasal Spray (regular & mentholated) ... 644
- Hemorid ... 797
- Hycomine Compound Tablets ... 948
- Neo-Synephrine Hydrochloride 1% Carpuject ... 2455
- Neo-Synephrine Hydrochloride 1% Injection ... 2455
- Neo-Synephrine Hydrochloride (Ophthalmic) ... 2456
- Neo-Synephrine ... 624
- Novahistine Elixir ... 782
- Phenergan VC ... 2886
- Phenergan VC with Codeine ... 2888
- Preparation H ... 842
- Tympagesic Ear Drops ... 2476
- Vicks Sinex Nasal Spray and Ultra Fine Mist ... 738

Phenylephrine Tannate (Sympathomimetics tend to produce hyperglycemia and concurrent use may lead to loss of control). Products include:
- Atrohist Pediatric Suspension ... 1604
- Atrohist Pediatric Suspension Dye-Free ... 1604
- Rynatan ... 2781
- Rynatuss ... 2782

Phenylpropanolamine Hydrochloride (Sympathomimetics tend to produce hyperglycemia and concurrent use may lead to loss of control). Products include:
- Acutrim ... 648
- Atrohist Plus Tablets ... 1605
- BC Cold Powder Multi-Symptom Formula (Cold-Sinus-Allergy) ... 631
- BC Cold Powder Non-Drowsy Formula (Cold-Sinus) ... 631
- Cheracol Plus Head Cold/Cough Formula ... 741
- Comtrex Multi-Symptom Cold Reliever Liqui-Gels ... 638
- Comtrex Multi-Symptom Non-Drowsy Liqui-gels ... 640
- Contac Continuous Action Nasal Decongestant/Antihistamine 12 Hour Capsules ... 773
- Contac Maximum Strength Continuous Action Decongestant/Antihistamine 12 Hour Caplets ... 772
- Contac Severe Cold and Flu Formula Caplets ... 773
- Coricidin 'D' Decongestant Tablets ... 760
- Dexatrim ... 795
- Dexatrim Plus Vitamins Caplets ... 796
- Dimetane-DC Cough Syrup ... 2232
- Dimetapp Allergy Sinus Caplets ... 838
- Dimetapp Cold & Allergy Chewable Tablets ... 838
- Dimetapp Cold & Cough Liqui-Gels ... 839
- Dimetapp DM Elixir ... 840
- Dimetapp Elixir ... 840
- Dimetapp Extentabs ... 841
- Dimetapp Tablets/Liqui-Gels ... 841
- Dura-Vent Tablets ... 971
- Entex LA Tablets ... 972
- Exgest LA Tablets ... 787
- Hycomine ... 947
- Nolamine Timed-Release Tablets ... 790
- Ornade Spansule Capsules ... 2678
- Propagest Tablets ... 791
- Pyrroxate Caplets ... 742
- Robitussin-CF ... 846
- Sinulin Tablets ... 792
- Tavist-D 12 Hour Relief Tablets ... 750
- Teldrin 12 Hour Antihistaminé/Nasal Decongestant Allergy Relief Capsules ... 786
- Triaminic Expectorant ... 753
- Triaminic Syrup ... 755
- Triaminic Triaminicol Cold & Cough ... 756
- Triaminic DM Syrup ... 756
- Triaminicin Tablets ... 756
- Vicks DayQuil Allergy Relief 12-Hour Extended Release Tablets ... 733
- Vicks DayQuil Allergy Relief 4-Hour Tablets ... 733
- Vicks DayQuil SINUS Pressure & CONGESTION Relief ... 734

Phenytoin (Phenytoin tends to produce hyperglycemia and concurrent use may lead to loss of control). Products include:
- Dilantin Infatabs ... 1967
- Dilantin-125 Suspension ... 1969

Phenytoin Sodium (Phenytoin tends to produce hyperglycemia and concurrent use may lead to loss of control). Products include:
- Dilantin Kapseals ... 1965

Pindolol (Co-administration with beta blockers may result in hypoglycemia). Products include:
- Visken Tablets ... 2428

Pirbuterol Acetate (Sympathomimetics tend to produce hyperglycemia and concurrent use may lead to loss of control). Products include:
- Maxair Autohaler ... 1550
- Maxair Inhaler ... 1552

Piroxicam (Co-administration with nonsteroidal anti-inflammatory agents may result in hypoglycemia). Products include:
- Feldene Capsules ... 2008

Polyestradiol Phosphate (Estrogens tend to produce hyperglycemia and concurrent use may lead to loss of control).
- No products indexed under this heading.

Polythiazide (Thiazides tend to produce hyperglycemia and concurrent use may lead to loss of control). Products include:
- Minizide Capsules ... 2016

Prednisolone Acetate (Corticosteroids tend to produce hyperglycemia and concurrent use may lead to loss of control). Products include:
- AK-CIDE ... ◉ 203
- AK-CIDE Ointment ... ◉ 203
- Blephamide Liquifilm Sterile Ophthalmic Suspension ... 472
- Blephamide Ointment ... ◉ 234
- Econopred & Econopred Plus Ophthalmic Suspensions ... ◉ 216
- Poly-Pred Liquifilm ... ◉ 246
- Pred Forte ... ◉ 247
- Pred Mild ... ◉ 250
- Pred-G Liquifilm Sterile Ophthalmic Suspension ... ◉ 248
- Pred-G S.O.P. Sterile Ophthalmic Ointment ... ◉ 249

Prednisolone Sodium Phosphate (Corticosteroids tend to produce hyperglycemia and concurrent use may lead to loss of control). Products include:
- AK-PRED ... ◉ 204
- Hydeltrasol Injection, Sterile ... 1708
- Pediapred Oral Solution ... 1618

Prednisolone Tebutate (Corticosteroids tend to produce hyperglycemia and concurrent use may lead to loss of control). Products include:
- Hydeltra-T.B.A. Sterile Suspension ... 1710

Prednisone (Corticosteroids tend to produce hyperglycemia and concurrent use may lead to loss of control).
- No products indexed under this heading.

Probenecid (Co-administration with probenecid may result in hypoglycemia). Products include:
- Benemid Tablets ... 1651
- ColBENEMID Tablets ... 1662

Prochlorperazine (Phenothiazines tend to produce hyperglycemia and concurrent use may lead to loss of control). Products include:
- Compazine ... 2644

Promethazine Hydrochloride (Phenothiazines tend to produce hyperglycemia and concurrent use may lead to loss of control). Products include:
- Mepergan Injection ... 2859
- Phenergan with Codeine ... 2883
- Phenergan with Dextromethorphan ... 2885
- Phenergan Injection ... 2880
- Phenergan Suppositories ... 2882
- Phenergan Syrup ... 2881
- Phenergan Tablets ... 2882
- Phenergan VC ... 2886
- Phenergan VC with Codeine ... 2888

IMPORTANT NOTE: Always consult each drug listing in the patient's regimen for possible interactions.

Glucotrol — Interactions Index

Propranolol Hydrochloride (Co-administration with beta blockers may result in hypoglycemia). Products include:
- Inderal ... 2834
- Inderal LA Long Acting Capsules ... 2836
- Inderide Tablets ... 2838
- Inderide LA Long Acting Capsules ... 2840

Pseudoephedrine Hydrochloride (Sympathomimetics tend to produce hyperglycemia and concurrent use may lead to loss of control). Products include:
- Actifed Allergy Daytime/Nighttime Caplets ... 808
- Actifed Cold & Allergy Tablets ... 807
- Actifed Cold & Sinus Caplets and Tablets ... 808
- Actifed Sinus Daytime/Nighttime Tablets and Caplets ... 809
- Advil Cold and Sinus Caplets and Tablets ... 837
- Alka-Seltzer Plus Liqui-Gels ... 612
- Alka-Seltzer Plus Flu & Body Aches Liqui-Gels Non-Drowsy Formula ... 613
- Alka-Seltzer Plus Night-Time Cold Medicine Liqui-Gels ... 612
- Allerest Maximum Strength ... 649
- Allerest No Drowsiness ... 649
- Allerest Sinus Pain Formula ... 649
- Atrohist Pediatric Capsules ... 1603
- Benadryl Allergy/Cold Tablets ... 811
- Benadryl Allergy Decongestant Liquid Medication ... 812
- Benadryl Allergy Decongestant Tablets ... 812
- Benadryl Allergy Sinus Headache Caplets ... 813
- Benylin Multisymptom ... 816
- Bromfed Capsules (Extended-Release) ... 1832
- Bromfed Syrup ... 712
- Bromfed Tablets ... 1832
- Bromfed-DM Cough Syrup ... 1832
- Bromfed-PD Capsules (Extended-Release) ... 1832
- Children's TYLENOL Cold Multi-Symptom Chewable Tablets and Liquid ... 1559
- Children's TYLENOL Cold Plus Cough Multi Symptom Chewable Tablets and Liquid ... 1560
- Children's TYLENOL Flu Suspension Liquid ... 1560
- Children's Vicks DayQuil Allergy Relief ... 730
- Children's Vicks NyQuil Cold/Cough Relief ... 731
- Allergy-Sinus Comtrex Multi-Symptom Allergy-Sinus Formula Tablets and Caplets ... 639
- Comtrex Multi-Symptom ... 638
- Comtrex Multi-Symptom Non-Drowsy Caplets ... 640
- Congess ... 1003
- Contac Day Allergy/Sinus Caplets ... 771
- Contac Day & Night ... 772
- Contac Night Allergy/Sinus Caplets ... 771
- Contac Severe Cold & Flu Non-Drowsy ... 774
- Deconsal II Tablets ... 1605
- Dimetane-DX Cough Syrup ... 2233
- Dimetapp Cold & Fever Suspension ... 839
- Dimetapp Decongestant Pediatric Drops ... 840
- Dorcol Children's Cough Syrup ... 748
- Drixoral Cough + Congestion Liquid Caps ... 763
- Dura-Tap/PD Capsules ... 970
- Duratuss Tablets ... 2750
- Duratuss HD Elixir ... 2750
- Efidac/24 ... 655
- Entex PSE Tablets ... 973
- Fedahist Gyrocaps ... 2545
- Guaifed ... 1833
- Guaifed Syrup ... 712
- Guaimax-D Tablets ... 809
- Histussin D Liquid ... 670
- Infants' TYLENOL Cold Decongestant & Fever-Reducer Drops ... 1561
- Kronofed-A ... 994
- Novahistine DMX ... 782
- Nucofed ... 2225
- PediaCare Cough-Cold Chewable Tablets and Liquid ... 1569
- PediaCare Infants' Decongestant Drops ... 1569
- PediaCare Infants' Drops Decongestant Plus Cough ... 1569
- PediaCare NightRest Cough-Cold Liquid ... 1569
- Pediatric Vicks 44d Cough & Head Congestion Relief ... 736
- Pediatric Vicks 44m Cough & Cold Relief ... 737
- Robitussin Cold & Cough Liqui-Gels ... 844
- Robitussin Cold, Cough & Flu Liqui-Gels ... 844
- Robitussin Maximum Strength Cough & Cold ... 847
- Robitussin Night-Time Cold Formula ... 847
- Robitussin Pediatric Cough & Cold Formula ... 848
- Robitussin Pediatric Drops ... 849
- Robitussin Severe Congestion Liqui-Gels ... 846
- Robitussin-DAC Syrup ... 2249
- Robitussin-PE ... 846
- Rondec Oral Drops ... 974
- Rondec Syrup ... 974
- Rondec Tablet ... 974
- Rondec Chewable Tablets ... 974
- Rondec-TR Tablet ... 974
- Ryna ... 804
- Seldane-D Extended-Release Tablets ... 1286
- Semprex-D Capsules ... 1620
- Sinarest ... 663
- Sine-Aid Maximum Strength Sinus Headache Gelcaps, Caplets and Tablets ... 1570
- Sine-Off No Drowsiness Formula Caplets ... 784
- Sine-Off Sinus Medicine ... 784
- Singlet Tablets ... 785
- Sinutab Non-Drying Liquid Caps ... 823
- Sinutab Sinus Allergy Medication, Maximum Strength Tablets and Caplets ... 823
- Sinutab Sinus Medication, Maximum Strength Without Drowsiness Formula, Tablets & Caplets ... 824
- Sudafed Children's Cold & Cough Liquid Medication ... 825
- Sudafed Children's Nasal Decongestant Liquid Medication ... 826
- Sudafed Cold & Cough Liquid Caps ... 826
- Sudafed Cold and Cough Liquid Caps ... 826
- Sudafed Nasal Decongestant Tablets, 30 mg ... 825
- Sudafed Nasal Decongestant Tablets, 60 mg ... 825
- Sudafed Non-Drying Sinus Liquid Caps ... 827
- Sudafed Pediatric Nasal Decongestant Liquid Oral Drops ... 827
- Sudafed Severe Cold Formula Caplets ... 828
- Sudafed Severe Cold Formula Tablets ... 828
- Sudafed Sinus Caplets ... 829
- Sudafed Sinus Tablets ... 829
- Sudafed 12 Hour Caplets ... 824
- Syn-Rx Tablets ... 1622
- Syn-Rx DM Tablets ... 1623
- TheraFlu Flu and Cold Medicine ... 750
- TheraFlu Maximum Strength Flu and Cold Medicine For Sore Throat ... 751
- TheraFlu Flu, Cold and Cough Medicine ... 750
- TheraFlu Maximum Strength Nighttime Flu, Cold & Cough Medicine ... 751
- TheraFlu Maximum Strength Non-Drowsy Formula Flu, Cold & Cough Medicine ... 751
- TheraFlu Maximum Strength, Non-Drowsy Formula Flu, Cold and Cough Caplets ... 752
- Theraflu Maximum Strength Sinus Non-Drowsy Formula Caplets ... 752
- Triaminic AM Cough and Decongestant Formula ... 753
- Triaminic AM Decongestant Formula ... 753
- Triaminic Infant Oral Decongestant Drops ... 754
- Triaminic Night Time ... 754
- Triaminic Sore Throat Formula ... 755
- Tussend ... 1830
- Tussend Expectorant ... 1831
- TYLENOL Allergy Sinus, Maximum Strength Caplets and Gelcaps ... 1571
- TYLENOL Allergy Sinus NightTime, Maximum Strength Caplets ... 1571
- TYLENOL Cold Medication, Multi-Symptom Formula Tablets and Caplets ... 1572
- TYLENOL Cold Medication, Multi-Symptom Hot Liquid Packets ... 1572
- TYLENOL Cold Medication, No Drowsiness Formula Caplets and Gelcaps ... 1572
- TYLENOL Cold Severe Congestion Caplets ... 1573
- TYLENOL Cough Medication with Decongestant, Multi Symptom ... 1574
- TYLENOL Flu No Drowsiness Formula, Maximum Strength Gelcaps ... 1575
- TYLENOL Flu NightTime, Maximum Strength Gelcaps ... 1575
- TYLENOL Flu NightTime, Maximum Strength Hot Medication Packets ... 1575
- TYLENOL Sinus, Maximum Strength Geltabs, Gelcaps, Caplets and Tablets ... 1576
- Vicks 44 LiquiCaps Cough, Cold & Flu Relief ... 728
- Vicks 44 LiquiCaps Non-Drowsy Cough & Cold Relief ... 729
- Vicks 44D Cough & Head Congestion Relief ... 728
- Vicks 44M Cough, Cold & Flu Relief ... 729
- Vicks DayQuil LiquiCaps/Liquid Multi-Symptom Cold/Flu Relief ... 734
- Vicks DayQuil SINUS Pressure & PAIN Relief with IBUPROFEN ... 735
- Vicks Nyquil Hot Therapy ... 735
- Vicks NyQuil LiquiCaps/Liquid Multi-Symptom Cold/Flu Relief, Original and Cherry Flavors ... 736

Pseudoephedrine Sulfate (Sympathomimetics tend to produce hyperglycemia and concurrent use may lead to loss of control). Products include:
- Chlor-Trimeton Allergy Decongestant Tablets ... 759
- Claritin-D Tablets ... 2487
- Drixoral Cold and Allergy Sustained-Action Tablets ... 763
- Drixoral Cold and Flu Extended-Release Tablets ... 764
- Drixoral Non-Drowsy Formula Extended-Release Tablets ... 764
- Drixoral Allergy/Sinus Extended Release Tablets ... 765
- Trinalin Repetabs Tablets ... 1373

Quinestrol (Estrogens tend to produce hyperglycemia and concurrent use may lead to loss of control).
No products indexed under this heading.

Salmeterol Xinafoate (Sympathomimetics tend to produce hyperglycemia and concurrent use may lead to loss of control). Products include:
- Serevent Inhalation Aerosol ... 1149

Salsalate (Co-administration with salicylates may result in hypoglycemia). Products include:
- Disalcid ... 1549
- Mono-Gesic Tablets ... 810
- Salflex Tablets ... 791

Selegiline Hydrochloride (Co-administration with monamine oxidase inhibitors may result in hypoglycemia). Products include:
- Eldepryl Capsules ... 2729

Sotalol Hydrochloride (Co-administration with beta blockers may result in hypoglycemia). Products include:
- Betapace Tablets ... 637

Spironolactone (Diuretics tend to produce hyperglycemia and concurrent use may lead to loss of control). Products include:
- Aldactazide Tablets ... 2556
- Aldactone Tablets ... 2558

Sulfacytine (Co-administration with sulfonamides may result in hypoglycemia).

Sulfamethizole (Co-administration with sulfonamides may result in hypoglycemia). Products include:
- Urobiotic-250 Capsules ... 2038

Sulfamethoxazole (Co-administration with sulfonamides may result in hypoglycemia). Products include:
- Bactrim DS Tablets ... 2257
- Bactrim I.V. Infusion ... 2255
- Bactrim ... 2257
- Gantanol Tablets ... 2285
- Septra ... 1146
- Septra I.V. Infusion ... 1142
- Septra I.V. Infusion ADD-Vantage Vials ... 1144
- Septra ... 1146

Sulfasalazine (Co-administration with sulfonamides may result in hypoglycemia). Products include:
- Azulfidine ... 2059

Sulfinpyrazone (Co-administration with sulfonamides may result in hypoglycemia). Products include:
- Anturane ... 823

Sulfisoxazole (Co-administration with sulfonamides may result in hypoglycemia). Products include:
- Gantrisin Tablets ... 2286

Sulfisoxazole Diolamine (Co-administration with sulfonamides may result in hypoglycemia).
No products indexed under this heading.

Sulindac (Co-administration with nonsteroidal anti-inflammatory agents may result in hypoglycemia). Products include:
- Clinoril Tablets ... 1658

Temazepam (Co-administration with drugs that are highly protein bound may result in hypoglycemia). Products include:
- Restoril Capsules ... 2413

Terbutaline Sulfate (Sympathomimetics tend to produce hyperglycemia and concurrent use may lead to loss of control). Products include:
- Brethaire Inhaler ... 830
- Brethine Ampuls ... 832
- Brethine Tablets ... 831
- Bricanyl Subcutaneous Injection ... 1247
- Bricanyl Tablets ... 1248

Thioridazine Hydrochloride (Phenothiazines tend to produce hyperglycemia and concurrent use may lead to loss of control). Products include:
- Mellaril ... 2398

Thyroglobulin (Thyroid products tend to produce hyperglycemia and concurrent use may lead to loss of control).
No products indexed under this heading.

Thyroid (Thyroid products tend to produce hyperglycemia and concurrent use may lead to loss of control).
No products indexed under this heading.

Thyroxine (Thyroid products tend to produce hyperglycemia and concurrent use may lead to loss of control).
No products indexed under this heading.

Thyroxine Sodium (Thyroid products tend to produce hyperglycemia and concurrent use may lead to loss of control).
No products indexed under this heading.

Timolol Hemihydrate (Co-administration with beta blockers may result in hypoglycemia). Products include:
- Betimol 0.25%, 0.5% ... 259

(🅡 Described in PDR For Nonprescription Drugs)   (◎ Described in PDR For Ophthalmology)

Timolol Maleate (Co-administration with beta blockers may result in hypoglycemia). Products include:
- Blocadren Tablets ... 1654
- Timolide Tablets ... 1791
- Timoptic in Ocudose ... 1796
- Timoptic Sterile Ophthalmic Solution ... 1794
- Timoptic-XE ... 1798

Tolazamide (Co-administration with sulfonamides may result in hypoglycemia).
- No products indexed under this heading.

Tolbutamide (Co-administration with sulfonamides may result in hypoglycemia).
- No products indexed under this heading.

Tolmetin Sodium (Co-administration with nonsteroidal anti-inflammatory agents may result in hypoglycemia). Products include:
- Tolectin (200, 400 and 600 mg) .. 1591

Torsemide (Diuretics tend to produce hyperglycemia and concurrent use may lead to loss of control). Products include:
- Demadex Tablets and Injection ... 691

Tranylcypromine Sulfate (Co-administration with monamine oxidase inhibitors may result in hypoglycemia). Products include:
- Parnate Tablets ... 2679

Triamcinolone (Corticosteroids tend to produce hyperglycemia and concurrent use may lead to loss of control).
- No products indexed under this heading.

Triamcinolone Acetonide (Corticosteroids tend to produce hyperglycemia and concurrent use may lead to loss of control). Products include:
- Azmacort Oral Inhaler ... 2175
- Nasacort AQ Nasal Spray ... 2191
- Nasacort Nasal Inhaler ... 2189

Triamcinolone Diacetate (Corticosteroids tend to produce hyperglycemia and concurrent use may lead to loss of control).
- No products indexed under this heading.

Triamcinolone Hexacetonide (Corticosteroids tend to produce hyperglycemia and concurrent use may lead to loss of control).
- No products indexed under this heading.

Triamterene (Diuretics tend to produce hyperglycemia and concurrent use may lead to loss of control). Products include:
- Dyazide Capsules ... 2653
- Dyrenium Capsules ... 2655

Trifluoperazine Hydrochloride (Phenothiazines tend to produce hyperglycemia and concurrent use may lead to loss of control). Products include:
- Stelazine ... 2692

Trimipramine Maleate (Co-administration with drugs that are highly protein bound may result in hypoglycemia). Products include:
- Surmontil Capsules ... 2917

Verapamil Hydrochloride (Calcium channel blockers tend to produce hyperglycemia and concurrent use may lead to loss of control). Products include:
- Calan SR Caplets ... 2571
- Calan Tablets ... 2568
- Covera-HS Tablets ... 2573
- Isoptin Injectable ... 1391
- Isoptin Oral Tablets ... 1393
- Isoptin SR Tablets ... 1395
- Verelan Capsules ... 1455

Warfarin Sodium (Co-administration with coumarins may result in hypoglycemia). Products include:
- Coumadin ... 941

Food Interactions

Alcohol (Co-administration with alcohol may result in hypoglycemia).

Food, unspecified (Delays absorption by 40 minutes; administer 30 minutes prior to meals).

GLUCOTROL XL EXTENDED RELEASE TABLETS

(Glipizide) ... 2012

May interact with highly protein bound drugs (selected), salicylates, non-steroidal anti-inflammatory agents, sulfonamides, oral anticoagulants, monoamine oxidase inhibitors, beta blockers, diuretics, thiazides, corticosteroids, phenothiazines, thyroid preparations, oral contraceptives, estrogens, calcium channel blockers, sympathomimetics, and certain other agents. Compounds in these categories include:

Acebutolol Hydrochloride (Co-administration with beta blockers may result in hypoglycemia). Products include:
- Sectral Capsules ... 2914

Albuterol (Sympathomimetics tend to produce hyperglycemia and concurrent use may lead to loss of control). Products include:
- Proventil Inhalation Aerosol ... 2524
- Ventolin Inhalation Aerosol and Refill ... 1170

Albuterol Sulfate (Sympathomimetics tend to produce hyperglycemia and concurrent use may lead to loss of control). Products include:
- Airet Albuterol Sulfate Inhalation Solution ... 1602
- Albuterol Sulfate, USP Solution for Inhalation, Arm-a-Med ... 522
- Proventil Inhalation Solution 0.083% ... 2527
- Proventil Repetabs Tablets ... 2529
- Proventil Solution for Inhalation 0.5% ... 2525
- Proventil Syrup ... 2528
- Proventil Tablets ... 2529
- Ventolin Inhalation Solution ... 1171
- Ventolin Nebules Inhalation Solution ... 1172
- Ventolin Rotacaps for Inhalation ... 1173
- Ventolin Syrup ... 1175
- Ventolin Tablets ... 1176
- Volmax Extended-Release Tablets .. 1835

Amiloride Hydrochloride (Diuretics tend to produce hyperglycemia and concurrent use may lead to loss of control). Products include:
- Midamor Tablets ... 1746
- Moduretic Tablets ... 1748

Amiodarone Hydrochloride (Co-administration with drugs that are highly protein bound may result in hypoglycemia). Products include:
- Cordarone Intravenous ... 2821
- Cordarone Tablets ... 2818

Amitriptyline Hydrochloride (Co-administration with drugs that are highly protein bound may result in hypoglycemia). Products include:
- Elavil ... 2945
- Etrafon ... 2495
- Limbitrol ... 2333
- Triavil Tablets ... 1800

Amlodipine Besylate (Calcium channel blockers tend to produce hyperglycemia and concurrent use may lead to loss of control). Products include:
- Lotrel Capsules ... 858
- Norvasc Tablets ... 2020

Aspirin (Co-administration with salicylates may result in hypoglycemia). Products include:
- Alka-Seltzer Cherry Effervescent Antacid and Pain Reliever ... 609
- Alka-Seltzer Extra Strength Effervescent Antacid and Pain Reliever ... 609
- Alka-Seltzer Lemon Lime Effervescent Antacid and Pain Reliever ... 609
- Alka-Seltzer Original Effervescent Antacid and Pain Reliever ... 609
- Alka-Seltzer Plus ... 611
- Alka-Seltzer Plus Sinus Medicine .. 611
- Ascriptin ... 650
- Arthritis Strength BC Powder ... 631
- BC Cold Powder Multi-Symptom Formula (Cold-Sinus-Allergy) ... 631
- BC Cold Powder Non-Drowsy Formula (Cold-Sinus) ... 631
- BC Powder ... 631
- Genuine Bayer Aspirin Tablets & Caplets ... 618
- Extra Strength Bayer Arthritis Pain Regimen Formula ... 615
- Extra Strength Bayer Aspirin Caplets & Tablets ... 617
- Extended-Release Bayer 8-Hour Aspirin ... 616
- Extra Strength Bayer Plus Aspirin Caplets ... 617
- Extra Strength Bayer PM Aspirin Plus Sleep Aid ... 617
- Aspirin Regimen Bayer 81 mg Tablets with Calcium ... 615
- Aspirin Regimen Bayer Adult Low Strength 81 mg Tablets ... 613
- Aspirin Regimen Bayer Children's Chewable Aspirin ... 616
- Aspirin Regimen Bayer Regular Strength 325 mg Caplets ... 613
- Bufferin Analgesic Tablets ... 636
- Arthritis Strength Bufferin Analgesic Caplets ... 637
- Extra Strength Bufferin Analgesic Tablets ... 637
- Cama Arthritis Pain Reliever ... 748
- Darvon Compound-65 Pulvules ... 1475
- Easprin ... 1971
- Ecotrin ... 2625
- Ecotrin Enteric Coated Aspirin Maximum Strength Tablets and Caplets ... 775
- Ecotrin Enteric Coated Aspirin Regular Strength Tablets ... 2625
- Empirin Aspirin Tablets ... 818
- Excedrin Extra-Strength Analgesic Tablets, Caplets, and Geltabs ... 734
- Fiorinal Capsules ... 2388
- Fiorinal with Codeine Capsules ... 2390
- Fiorinal Tablets ... 2388
- Goody's Extra Strength Headache Powders ... 632
- Goody's Extra Strength Pain Relief Tablets ... 632
- Halfprin Tablets ... 1413
- Norgesic ... 1554
- Percodan Tablets ... 955
- Percodan-Demi Tablets ... 956
- Robaxisal Tablets ... 2246
- Soma Compound w/Codeine Tablets ... 2784
- Soma Compound Tablets ... 2783
- St. Joseph Adult Chewable Aspirin (81 mg.) ... 768
- Talwin Compound ... 2466
- Vanquish Analgesic Caplets ... 627

Atenolol (Co-administration with beta blockers may result in hypoglycemia). Products include:
- Tenoretic Tablets ... 2963
- Tenormin Tablets and I.V. Injection 2965

Atovaquone (Co-administration with drugs that are highly protein bound may result in hypoglycemia). Products include:
- Mepron Suspension ... 1206

Bendroflumethiazide (Thiazides tend to produce hyperglycemia and concurrent use may lead to loss of control).
- No products indexed under this heading.

Bepridil Hydrochloride (Calcium channel blockers tend to produce hyperglycemia and concurrent use may lead to loss of control). Products include:
- Vascor Tablets (200 and 300 mg) 1597

Betamethasone Acetate (Corticosteroids tend to produce hyperglycemia and concurrent use may lead to loss of control). Products include:
- Celestone Soluspan Suspension ... 2484

Betamethasone Sodium Phosphate (Corticosteroids tend to produce hyperglycemia and concurrent use may lead to loss of control). Products include:
- Celestone Soluspan Suspension ... 2484

Betaxolol Hydrochloride (Co-administration with beta blockers may result in hypoglycemia). Products include:
- Betoptic Ophthalmic Solution ... 465
- Betoptic S Ophthalmic Suspension ... 467
- Kerlone Tablets ... 2588

Bisoprolol Fumarate (Co-administration with beta blockers may result in hypoglycemia). Products include:
- Zebeta Tablets ... 1457
- Ziac ... 1459

Bumetanide (Diuretics tend to produce hyperglycemia and concurrent use may lead to loss of control). Products include:
- Bumex ... 2260

Carteolol Hydrochloride (Co-administration with beta blockers may result in hypoglycemia). Products include:
- Cartrol Tablets ... 413
- Ocupress Ophthalmic Solution, 1% Sterile ... ⊙ 297

Cefonicid Sodium (Co-administration with drugs that are highly protein bound may result in hypoglycemia). Products include:
- Monocid Injection ... 2674

Chloramphenicol (Co-administration with chloramphenicol may result in hypoglycemia). Products include:
- Chloromycetin Ophthalmic Ointment, 1% ... ⊙ 298
- Chloromycetin Ophthalmic Solution ... ⊙ 299
- Chloroptic S.O.P. ... ⊙ 236
- Chloroptic Sterile Ophthalmic Solution ... ⊙ 236

Chloramphenicol Palmitate (Co-administration with chloramphenicol may result in hypoglycemia).
- No products indexed under this heading.

Chloramphenicol Sodium Succinate (Co-administration with chloramphenicol may result in hypoglycemia). Products include:
- Chloromycetin Sodium Succinate ... 1960

Chlordiazepoxide (Co-administration with drugs that are highly protein bound may result in hypoglycemia). Products include:
- Limbitrol ... 2333

Chlordiazepoxide Hydrochloride (Co-administration with drugs that are highly protein bound may result in hypoglycemia). Products include:
- Librax Capsules ... 2330
- Librium Capsules ... 2331
- Librium Injectable ... 2332

Chlorothiazide (Thiazides tend to produce hyperglycemia and concurrent use may lead to loss of control). Products include:
- Aldoclor Tablets ... 1638
- Diupres Tablets ... 1691
- Diuril Oral ... 1694

IMPORTANT NOTE: Always consult each drug listing in the patient's regimen for possible interactions.

Glucotrol XL / Interactions Index

Chlorothiazide Sodium (Thiazides tend to produce hyperglycemia and concurrent use may lead to loss of control). Products include:
- Diuril Sodium Intravenous 1693

Chlorotrianisene (Estrogens tend to produce hyperglycemia and concurrent use may lead to loss of control).
- No products indexed under this heading.

Chlorpromazine (Phenothiazines tend to produce hyperglycemia and concurrent use may lead to loss of control). Products include:
- Thorazine Suppositories 2701

Chlorpromazine Hydrochloride (Phenothiazines tend to produce hyperglycemia and concurrent use may lead to loss of control). Products include:
- Thorazine 2701

Chlorpropamide (Co-administration with sulfonamides may result in hypoglycemia). Products include:
- Diabinese Tablets 2002

Chlorthalidone (Diuretics tend to produce hyperglycemia and concurrent use may lead to loss of control). Products include:
- Combipres Tablets 682
- Tenoretic Tablets 2963
- Thalitone 1293

Choline Magnesium Trisalicylate (Co-administration with salicylates may result in hypoglycemia). Products include:
- Trilisate 2155

Clomipramine Hydrochloride (Co-administration with drugs that are highly protein bound may result in hypoglycemia). Products include:
- Anafranil Capsules 819

Clozapine (Co-administration with drugs that are highly protein bound may result in hypoglycemia). Products include:
- Clozaril Tablets 2377

Cortisone Acetate (Corticosteroids tend to produce hyperglycemia and concurrent use may lead to loss of control). Products include:
- Cortone Acetate Sterile Suspension 1663
- Cortone Acetate Tablets 1664

Cyclosporine (Co-administration with drugs that are highly protein bound may result in hypoglycemia). Products include:
- Neoral 2405
- Sandimmune 2416

Desogestrel (Oral contraceptives tend to produce hyperglycemia and concurrent use may lead to loss of control). Products include:
- Desogen Tablets 1867
- Ortho-Cept 1907

Dexamethasone (Corticosteroids tend to produce hyperglycemia and concurrent use may lead to loss of control). Products include:
- AK-Trol Ointment & Suspension 205
- Decadron Elixir 1676
- Decadron Tablets 1678
- Decaspray Topical Aerosol 1689
- Maxitrol Ophthalmic Ointment and Suspension 222
- TobraDex Ophthalmic Suspension and Ointment 469

Dexamethasone Acetate (Corticosteroids tend to produce hyperglycemia and concurrent use may lead to loss of control). Products include:
- Dalalone D.P. Injectable 1009
- Decadron-LA Sterile Suspension 1687

Dexamethasone Sodium Phosphate (Corticosteroids tend to produce hyperglycemia and concurrent use may lead to loss of control). Products include:
- Decadron Phosphate Injection 1680
- Decadron Phosphate Sterile Ophthalmic Ointment 1684
- Decadron Phosphate Sterile Ophthalmic Solution 1685
- Decadron Phosphate Topical Cream 1686
- Decadron Phosphate with Xylocaine Injection, Sterile 1683
- Dexacort Phosphate in Respihaler .. 1606
- Dexacort Phosphate in Turbinaire .. 1607
- NeoDecadron Sterile Ophthalmic Ointment 1755
- NeoDecadron Sterile Ophthalmic Solution 1756
- NeoDecadron Topical Cream 1757

Diazepam (Co-administration with drugs that are highly protein bound may result in hypoglycemia). Products include:
- Dizac (diazepam injectable emulsion) CIV 1862
- Valium Injectable 2336
- Valium Tablets 2335

Diclofenac Potassium (Co-administration with nonsteroidal anti-inflammatory agents may result in hypoglycemia). Products include:
- Cataflam Tablets 833

Diclofenac Sodium (Co-administration with nonsteroidal anti-inflammatory agents may result in hypoglycemia). Products include:
- Voltaren Ophthalmic Sterile Ophthalmic Solution .... ◉ 264
- Cataflam/Voltaren/Voltaren-XR 833

Dicumarol (Co-administration with coumarins may result in hypoglycemia).
- No products indexed under this heading.

Dienestrol (Estrogens tend to produce hyperglycemia and concurrent use may lead to loss of control). Products include:
- Ortho Dienestrol Cream 1922

Diethylstilbestrol (Estrogens tend to produce hyperglycemia and concurrent use may lead to loss of control). Products include:
- Diethylstilbestrol Tablets 1477

Diflunisal (Co-administration with salicylates may result in hypoglycemia). Products include:
- Dolobid Tablets 1695

Diltiazem Hydrochloride (Calcium channel blockers tend to produce hyperglycemia and concurrent use may lead to loss of control). Products include:
- Cardizem CD Capsules 1251
- Cardizem SR Capsules 1255
- Cardizem Injectable 1253
- Cardizem Tablets 1257
- Dilacor XR Extended-release Capsules 2183
- Tiazac Capsules 1019

Dipyridamole (Co-administration with drugs that are highly protein bound may result in hypoglycemia). Products include:
- Persantine Tablets 686

Dobutamine Hydrochloride (Sympathomimetics tend to produce hyperglycemia and concurrent use may lead to loss of control). Products include:
- Dobutrex Solution Vials 1480

Dopamine Hydrochloride (Sympathomimetics tend to produce hyperglycemia and concurrent use may lead to loss of control).
- No products indexed under this heading.

Ephedrine Hydrochloride (Sympathomimetics tend to produce hyperglycemia and concurrent use may lead to loss of control). Products include:
- Primatene Tablets .... ▣ 844
- Quadrinal Tablets 1398

Ephedrine Sulfate (Sympathomimetics tend to produce hyperglycemia and concurrent use may lead to loss of control). Products include:
- Marax Tablets & DF Syrup 2015

Ephedrine Tannate (Sympathomimetics tend to produce hyperglycemia and concurrent use may lead to loss of control). Products include:
- Rynatuss 2782

Epinephrine (Sympathomimetics tend to produce hyperglycemia and concurrent use may lead to loss of control). Products include:
- EPIFRIN .... ◉ 237
- EpiPen 808
- Marcaine with Epinephrine 2446
- Primatene Mist .... ▣ 843
- Sensorcaine with Epinephrine Injection 554
- Sus-Phrine Injection 1017
- Xylocaine with Epinephrine Injections 562

Epinephrine Bitartrate (Sympathomimetics tend to produce hyperglycemia and concurrent use may lead to loss of control). Products include:
- Sensorcaine-MPF with Epinephrine Injection 554

Epinephrine Hydrochloride (Sympathomimetics tend to produce hyperglycemia and concurrent use may lead to loss of control). Products include:
- Ana-Kit Anaphylaxis Emergency Treatment Kit 611

Esmolol Hydrochloride (Co-administration with beta blockers may result in hypoglycemia). Products include:
- Brevibloc (esmolol HCl) Injection 1860

Estradiol (Estrogens tend to produce hyperglycemia and concurrent use may lead to loss of control). Products include:
- Climara Transdermal System 640
- Estrace Cream and Tablets 751
- Estraderm Transdermal System 842
- Estring Vaginal Ring 2086
- Vivelle Transdermal System 880

Estrogens, Conjugated (Estrogens tend to produce hyperglycemia and concurrent use may lead to loss of control). Products include:
- PMB 200 and PMB 400 2890
- Premarin Intravenous 2893
- Premarin Tablets 2896
- Premarin Vaginal Cream 2898
- Premphase 2900
- Prempro 2905

Estrogens, Esterified (Estrogens tend to produce hyperglycemia and concurrent use may lead to loss of control). Products include:
- ESTRATAB Tablets (0.3, 0.625, 1.25, 2.5 mg) 2715
- Estratest 2718
- Menest Tablets 2671

Estropipate (Estrogens tend to produce hyperglycemia and concurrent use may lead to loss of control). Products include:
- Ogen Tablets 2103
- Ogen Vaginal Cream 2106
- Ortho-Est 1925

Ethacrynic Acid (Diuretics tend to produce hyperglycemia and concurrent use may lead to loss of control). Products include:
- Edecrin Tablets 1698

Ethinyl Estradiol (Estrogens tend to produce hyperglycemia and concurrent use may lead to loss of control). Products include:
- Brevicon 2563
- Demulen 2580
- Desogen Tablets 1867
- Levlen/Tri-Levlen 646
- Lo/Ovral Tablets 2852
- Lo/Ovral-28 Tablets 2857
- Modicon 1928
- Nordette-21 Tablets 2863
- Nordette-28 Tablets 2866
- Norinyl 2563
- Ortho-Cept 1907
- Ortho-Cyclen/Ortho-Tri-Cyclen ... 1914
- Ortho-Novum 1928
- Ortho-Cyclen/Ortho-Tri-Cyclen ... 1914
- Ovcon 765
- Ovral Tablets 2877
- Ovral-28 Tablets 2878
- Levlen/Tri-Levlen 646
- Tri-Norinyl 2607
- Triphasil-21 Tablets 2919
- Triphasil-28 Tablets 2924

Ethynodiol Diacetate (Oral contraceptives tend to produce hyperglycemia and concurrent use may lead to loss of control). Products include:
- Demulen 2580

Etodolac (Co-administration with nonsteroidal anti-inflammatory agents may result in hypoglycemia). Products include:
- Lodine Capsules and Tablets 2849

Felodipine (Calcium channel blockers tend to produce hyperglycemia and concurrent use may lead to loss of control). Products include:
- Plendil Extended-Release Tablets 514

Fenoprofen Calcium (Co-administration with nonsteroidal anti-inflammatory agents may result in hypoglycemia). Products include:
- Nalfon 200 Pulvules & Nalfon Tablets 933

Fluconazole (Co-administration with oral fluconazole has resulted in an increase in Glucotrol AUC by 56.9%). Products include:
- Diflucan Tablets, Injection, and Oral Suspension 2003

Fludrocortisone Acetate (Corticosteroids tend to produce hyperglycemia and concurrent use may lead to loss of control). Products include:
- Florinef Acetate Tablets 506

Fluphenazine Decanoate (Phenothiazines tend to produce hyperglycemia and concurrent use may lead to loss of control). Products include:
- Prolixin Decanoate 510

Fluphenazine Enanthate (Phenothiazines tend to produce hyperglycemia and concurrent use may lead to loss of control). Products include:
- Prolixin Enanthate 510

Fluphenazine Hydrochloride (Phenothiazines tend to produce hyperglycemia and concurrent use may lead to loss of control). Products include:
- Prolixin 510

Flurazepam Hydrochloride (Co-administration with drugs that are highly protein bound may result in hypoglycemia). Products include:
- Dalmane Capsules 2329

Flurbiprofen (Co-administration with nonsteroidal anti-inflammatory agents may result in hypoglycemia).
- No products indexed under this heading.

Furazolidone (Co-administration with monamine oxidase inhibitors may result in hypoglycemia). Products include:
- Furoxone 2221

(▣ Described in PDR For Nonprescription Drugs) (◉ Described in PDR For Ophthalmology)

Furosemide (Diuretics tend to produce hyperglycemia and concurrent use may lead to loss of control). Products include:
Lasix Injection, Oral Solution and Tablets ... 1267

Glyburide (Co-administration with sulfonamides may result in hypoglycemia). Products include:
DiaBeta Tablets ... 1265
Glynase PresTab Tablets ... 2091
Micronase Tablets ... 2099

Hydrochlorothiazide (Thiazides tend to produce hyperglycemia and concurrent use may lead to loss of control). Products include:
Aldactazide Tablets ... 2556
Aldoril Tablets ... 1644
Apresazide Capsules ... 824
Capozide Tablets ... 744
Dyazide Capsules ... 2653
Esidrix Tablets ... 839
Esimil Tablets ... 840
HydroDIURIL Tablets ... 1716
Hydropres Tablets ... 1718
Hyzaar Tablets ... 1720
Inderide Tablets ... 2838
Inderide LA Long Acting Capsules .. 2840
Lopressor HCT Tablets ... 850
Lotensin HCT Tablets ... 855
Moduretic Tablets ... 1748
Oretic Tablets ... 450
Prinzide Tablets ... 1780
Ser-Ap-Es Tablets ... 867
Timolide Tablets ... 1791
Vaseretic Tablets ... 1810
Zestoretic Tablets ... 2968
Ziac ... 1459

Hydrocortisone (Corticosteroids tend to produce hyperglycemia and concurrent use may lead to loss of control). Products include:
Anusol-HC Cream 2.5% ... 1953
Aquanil HC Lotion ... 1989
Maximum Strength Cortaid Spray ... 800
CORTENEMA ... 2713
Cortisporin Ointment ... 1074
Cortisporin Ophthalmic Ointment Sterile ... 1074
Cortisporin Ophthalmic Suspension Sterile ... 1075
Cortisporin Otic Solution Sterile ... 1076
Cortisporin Otic Suspension Sterile 1077
Cortizone-5 ... 795
Cortizone-10 ... 795
Hydrocortone Tablets ... 1715
Hytone ... 922
Hytone Ointment 2 ½ % ... 923
Massengill Medicated Soft Cloth Towelettes ... 2628
Pediotic Suspension Sterile ... 1140
Preparation H Hydrocortisone 1% Cream ... 843
ProctoCream-HC 2.5% ... 2552
VōSoL HC Otic Solution ... 2786

Hydrocortisone Acetate (Corticosteroids tend to produce hyperglycemia and concurrent use may lead to loss of control). Products include:
Analpram-HC Rectal Cream 1% and 2.5% ... 993
Anusol HC-1 Hydrocortisone Anti-Itch Ointment ... 810
Anusol-HC Suppositories ... 1954
Caldecort Anti-Itch Hydrocortisone Cream ... 651
Coly-Mycin S Otic w/Neomycin & Hydrocortisone ... 1965
Cortaid ... 800
Cortifoam ... 2540
Cortisporin Cream ... 1073
Epifoam ... 2543
Hydrocortone Acetate Sterile Suspension ... 1712
Mantadil Cream ... 1124
Nupercainal Hydrocortisone 1% Cream ... 661
Pramosone Cream, Lotion & Ointment ... 995
ProctoFoam-HC ... 2552
Terra-Cortril Ophthalmic Suspension ... 2033

Hydrocortisone Sodium Phosphate (Corticosteroids tend to produce hyperglycemia and concurrent use may lead to loss of control). Products include:
Hydrocortone Phosphate Injection, Sterile ... 1713

Hydrocortisone Sodium Succinate (Corticosteroids tend to produce hyperglycemia and concurrent use may lead to loss of control).
No products indexed under this heading.

Hydroflumethiazide (Thiazides tend to produce hyperglycemia and concurrent use may lead to loss of control). Products include:
Diucardin Tablets ... 2824

Ibuprofen (Co-administration with nonsteroidal anti-inflammatory agents may result in hypoglycemia). Products include:
Actron Caplets and Tablets ... 608
Advil Cold and Sinus Caplets and Tablets ... 837
Advil Ibuprofen Tablets, Caplets and Gel Caplets ... 836
Children's Motrin Ibuprofen Oral Suspension ... 1558
IBU Tablets ... 1389
Ibuprohm ... 713
Motrin IB Caplets, Tablets, and Gelcaps ... 802
Motrin Ibuprofen Suspension, Oral Drops, Chewable Tablets, Caplets ... 1563
Nuprin Ibuprofen/Analgesic Tablets & Caplets ... 645
Vicks DayQuil SINUS Pressure & PAIN Relief with IBUPROFEN ... 735

Imipramine Hydrochloride (Co-administration with drugs that are highly protein bound may result in hypoglycemia). Products include:
Tofranil Ampuls ... 873
Tofranil Tablets ... 875

Imipramine Pamoate (Co-administration with drugs that are highly protein bound may result in hypoglycemia). Products include:
Tofranil-PM Capsules ... 876

Indapamide (Diuretics tend to produce hyperglycemia and concurrent use may lead to loss of control).
No products indexed under this heading.

Indomethacin (Co-administration with nonsteroidal anti-inflammatory agents may result in hypoglycemia). Products include:
Indocin ... 1723

Indomethacin Sodium Trihydrate (Co-administration with nonsteroidal anti-inflammatory agents may result in hypoglycemia). Products include:
Indocin I.V. ... 1727

Isocarboxazid (Co-administration with monamine oxidase inhibitors may result in hypoglycemia).
No products indexed under this heading.

Isoniazid (Isoniazid tends to produce hyperglycemia and concurrent use may lead to loss of control). Products include:
Nydrazid Injection ... 509
Rifamate Capsules ... 1278
Rifater ... 1280

Isoproterenol Hydrochloride (Sympathomimetics tend to produce hyperglycemia and concurrent use may lead to loss of control). Products include:
Isuprel Hydrochloride Solution ... 2443
Isuprel Injection ... 2441
Isuprel Mistometer ... 2442

Isoproterenol Sulfate (Sympathomimetics tend to produce hyperglycemia and concurrent use may lead to loss of control). Products include:
Norisodrine with Calcium Iodide Syrup ... 446

Isradipine (Calcium channel blockers tend to produce hyperglycemia and concurrent use may lead to loss of control). Products include:
DynaCirc Capsules ... 2381
DynaCirc CR Tablets ... 2383

Ketoprofen (Co-administration with nonsteroidal anti-inflammatory agents may result in hypoglycemia). Products include:
Actron Caplets and Tablets ... 608
Orudis Capsules ... 2874
Orudis KT ... 842
Oruvail Capsules ... 2874

Ketorolac Tromethamine (Co-administration with nonsteroidal anti-inflammatory agents may result in hypoglycemia). Products include:
Acular Sterile Ophthalmic Solution ... 470
Toradol ... 2319

Labetalol Hydrochloride (Co-administration with beta blockers may result in hypoglycemia). Products include:
Normodyne Injection ... 2519
Normodyne Tablets ... 2522
Trandate ... 1158

Levobunolol Hydrochloride (Co-administration with beta blockers may result in hypoglycemia). Products include:
Betagan ... 230

Levonorgestrel (Oral contraceptives tend to produce hyperglycemia and concurrent use may lead to loss of control). Products include:
Levlen/Tri-Levlen ... 646
Nordette-21 Tablets ... 2863
Nordette-28 Tablets ... 2866
Norplant System ... 2868
Levlen/Tri-Levlen ... 646
Triphasil-21 Tablets ... 2919
Triphasil-28 Tablets ... 2924

Levothyroxine Sodium (Thyroid products tend to produce hyperglycemia and concurrent use may lead to loss of control). Products include:
Eltroxin Tablets ... 2214
Levothroid Tablets ... 1015
Levothyroxine Sodium, USP for Injection ... 546
Levoxyl Tablets ... 918
Synthroid ... 1410

Liothyronine Sodium (Thyroid products tend to produce hyperglycemia and concurrent use may lead to loss of control). Products include:
Cytomel Tablets ... 2647
Triostat Injection ... 2708

Liotrix (Thyroid products tend to produce hyperglycemia and concurrent use may lead to loss of control).
No products indexed under this heading.

Magnesium Salicylate (Co-administration with salicylates may result in hypoglycemia). Products include:
Backache Caplets ... 635
Doan's Extra-Strength Analgesic ... 653
Extra Strength Doan's P.M. ... 653
Doan's Regular Strength Analgesic ... 654
Mobigesic Tablets ... 607

Meclofenamate Sodium (Co-administration with nonsteroidal anti-inflammatory agents may result in hypoglycemia).
No products indexed under this heading.

Mefenamic Acid (Co-administration with nonsteroidal anti-inflammatory agents may result in hypoglycemia). Products include:
Ponstel ... 1982

Mesoridazine Besylate (Phenothiazines tend to produce hyperglycemia and concurrent use may lead to loss of control). Products include:
Serentil ... 689

Mestranol (Oral contraceptives tend to produce hyperglycemia and concurrent use may lead to loss of control). Products include:
Norinyl ... 2563
Ortho-Novum ... 1928

Metaproterenol Sulfate (Sympathomimetics tend to produce hyperglycemia and concurrent use may lead to loss of control). Products include:
Alupent ... 672
Metaproterenol Sulfate Inhalation Solution, USP, Arm-a-Med ... 547

Metaraminol Bitartrate (Sympathomimetics tend to produce hyperglycemia and concurrent use may lead to loss of control). Products include:
Aramine Injection ... 1649

Methotrimeprazine (Phenothiazines tend to produce hyperglycemia and concurrent use may lead to loss of control). Products include:
Levoprome ... 1321

Methoxamine Hydrochloride (Sympathomimetics tend to produce hyperglycemia and concurrent use may lead to loss of control). Products include:
Vasoxyl Injection ... 1169

Methyclothiazide (Thiazides tend to produce hyperglycemia and concurrent use may lead to loss of control). Products include:
Enduron Tablets ... 424

Methylprednisolone Acetate (Corticosteroids tend to produce hyperglycemia and concurrent use may lead to loss of control).
No products indexed under this heading.

Methylprednisolone Sodium Succinate (Corticosteroids tend to produce hyperglycemia and concurrent use may lead to loss of control).
No products indexed under this heading.

Metipranolol Hydrochloride (Co-administration with beta blockers may result in hypoglycemia). Products include:
OptiPranolol (Metipranolol 0.3%) Sterile Ophthalmic Solution ... 256

Metolazone (Diuretics tend to produce hyperglycemia and concurrent use may lead to loss of control). Products include:
Mykrox Tablets ... 1617
Zaroxolyn Tablets ... 1625

Metoprolol Succinate (Co-administration with beta blockers may result in hypoglycemia). Products include:
Toprol-XL Tablets ... 560

Metoprolol Tartrate (Co-administration with beta blockers may result in hypoglycemia). Products include:
Lopressor ... 848
Lopressor HCT Tablets ... 850

Miconazole (Co-administration with oral miconazole and oral hypoglycemic agents has resulted in severe hypoglycemia).
No products indexed under this heading.

IMPORTANT NOTE: Always consult each drug listing in the patient's regimen for possible interactions.

Glucotrol XL — Interactions Index — 452

Midazolam Hydrochloride (Co-administration with drugs that are highly protein bound may result in hypoglycemia). Products include:
Versed Injection ... 2324

Nabumetone (Co-administration with nonsteroidal anti-inflammatory agents may result in hypoglycemia). Products include:
Relafen Tablets ... 2688

Nadolol (Co-administration with beta blockers may result in hypoglycemia).
No products indexed under this heading.

Naproxen (Co-administration with nonsteroidal anti-inflammatory agents may result in hypoglycemia). Products include:
Anaprox/Naprosyn ... 2277

Naproxen Sodium (Co-administration with nonsteroidal anti-inflammatory agents may result in hypoglycemia). Products include:
Aleve ... 2124
Anaprox/Naprosyn ... 2277
Naprelan Tablets ... 2861

Nicardipine Hydrochloride (Calcium channel blockers tend to produce hyperglycemia and concurrent use may lead to loss of control). Products include:
Cardene Capsules ... 2261
Cardene I.V. ... 2815
Cardene SR Capsules ... 2264

Nicotinic Acid (Nicotinic acid tends to produce hyperglycemia and concurrent use may lead to loss of control).
No products indexed under this heading.

Nifedipine (Calcium channel blockers tend to produce hyperglycemia and concurrent use may lead to loss of control). Products include:
Adalat Capsules (10 mg and 20 mg) ... 580
Adalat CC ... 582
Procardia Capsules ... 2024
Procardia XL Extended Release Tablets ... 2026

Nimodipine (Calcium channel blockers tend to produce hyperglycemia and concurrent use may lead to loss of control). Products include:
Nimotop Capsules ... 603

Nisoldipine (Calcium channel blockers tend to produce hyperglycemia and concurrent use may lead to loss of control). Products include:
Sular Tablets ... 2961

Norepinephrine Bitartrate (Sympathomimetics tend to produce hyperglycemia and concurrent use may lead to loss of control). Products include:
Levophed Bitartrate Injection ... 2445

Norethindrone (Oral contraceptives tend to produce hyperglycemia and concurrent use may lead to loss of control). Products include:
Brevicon ... 2563
Micronor Tablets ... 1903
Modicon ... 1928
Norinyl ... 2563
Nor-Q D Tablets ... 2598
Ortho-Novum ... 1928
Ovcon ... 765
Tri-Norinyl ... 2607

Norethynodrel (Oral contraceptives tend to produce hyperglycemia and concurrent use may lead to loss of control).
No products indexed under this heading.

Norgestimate (Oral contraceptives tend to produce hyperglycemia and concurrent use may lead to loss of control). Products include:
Ortho-Cyclen/Ortho-Tri-Cyclen ... 1914
Ortho-Cyclen/Ortho Tri-Cyclen ... 1914

Norgestrel (Oral contraceptives tend to produce hyperglycemia and concurrent use may lead to loss of control). Products include:
Lo/Ovral Tablets ... 2852
Lo/Ovral-28 Tablets ... 2857
Ovral Tablets ... 2877
Ovral-28 Tablets ... 2878
Ovrette Tablets ... 2878

Nortriptyline Hydrochloride (Co-administration with drugs that are highly protein bound may result in hypoglycemia). Products include:
Pamelor ... 2409

Oxaprozin (Co-administration with nonsteroidal anti-inflammatory agents may result in hypoglycemia). Products include:
Daypro Caplets ... 2578

Oxazepam (Co-administration with drugs that are highly protein bound may result in hypoglycemia). Products include:
Serax Capsules ... 2916
Serax Tablets ... 2916

Penbutolol Sulfate (Co-administration with beta blockers may result in hypoglycemia). Products include:
Levatol Tablets ... 2547

Perphenazine (Phenothiazines tend to produce hyperglycemia and concurrent use may lead to loss of control). Products include:
Etrafon ... 2495
Triavil Tablets ... 1800
Trilafon ... 2532

Phenelzine Sulfate (Co-administration with monamine oxidase inhibitors may result in hypoglycemia). Products include:
Nardil ... 1977

Phenylbutazone (Co-administration with nonsteroidal anti-inflammatory agents may result in hypoglycemia).
No products indexed under this heading.

Phenylephrine Bitartrate (Sympathomimetics tend to produce hyperglycemia and concurrent use may lead to loss of control).
No products indexed under this heading.

Phenylephrine Hydrochloride (Sympathomimetics tend to produce hyperglycemia and concurrent use may lead to loss of control). Products include:
Atrohist Plus Tablets ... 1605
Cerose DM ... ◘ 853
D.A. II Tablets ... 972
D.A. Chewable Tablets ... 970
Dura-Vent/DA Tablets ... 972
Extendryl ... 1003
4-Way Fast Acting Nasal Spray (regular & mentholated) ... ◘ 644
Hemorid ... ◘ 797
Hycomine Compound Tablets ... 948
Neo-Synephrine Hydrochloride 1% Carpuject ... 2455
Neo-Synephrine Hydrochloride 1% Injection ... 2455
Neo-Synephrine Hydrochloride (Ophthalmic) ... 2456
Neo-Synephrine ... ◘ 624
Novahistine Elixir ... ◘ 782
Phenergan VC ... 2886
Phenergan VC with Codeine ... 2888
Preparation H ... ◘ 842
Tympagesic Ear Drops ... 2476
Vicks Sinex Nasal Spray and Ultra Fine Mist ... ◘ 738

Phenylephrine Tannate (Sympathomimetics tend to produce hyperglycemia and concurrent use may lead to loss of control). Products include:
Atrohist Pediatric Suspension ... 1604
Atrohist Pediatric Suspension Dye-Free ... 1604
Rynatan ... 2781
Rynatuss ... 2782

Phenylpropanolamine Hydrochloride (Sympathomimetics tend to produce hyperglycemia and concurrent use may lead to loss of control). Products include:
Acutrim ... ◘ 648
Atrohist Plus Tablets ... 1605
BC Cold Powder Multi-Symptom Formula (Cold-Sinus-Allergy) ... ◘ 631
BC Cold Powder Non-Drowsy Formula (Cold-Sinus) ... ◘ 631
Cheracol Plus Head Cold/Cough Formula ... ◘ 741
Comtrex Multi-Symptom Cold Reliever Liqui-Gels ... ◘ 638
Comtrex Multi-Symptom Non-Drowsy Liqui-gels ... ◘ 640
Contac Continuous Action Nasal Decongestant/Antihistamine 12 Hour Capsules ... ◘ 773
Contac Maximum Strength Continuous Action Decongestant/Antihistamine 12 Hour Caplets ... ◘ 772
Contac Severe Cold and Flu Formula Caplets ... ◘ 773
Coricidin 'D' Decongestant Tablets ... ◘ 760
Dexatrim ... ◘ 795
Dexatrim Plus Vitamins Caplets ... ◘ 796
Dimetane-DC Cough Syrup ... 2232
Dimetapp Allergy Sinus Caplets ... ◘ 838
Dimetapp Cold & Allergy Chewable Tablets ... ◘ 838
Dimetapp Cold & Cough Liqui-Gels ... ◘ 839
Dimetapp DM Elixir ... ◘ 840
Dimetapp Elixir ... ◘ 840
Dimetapp Extentabs ... ◘ 841
Dimetapp Tablets/Liqui-Gels ... ◘ 841
Dura-Vent Tablets ... 971
Entex LA Tablets ... 972
Exgest LA Tablets ... 787
Hycomine ... 947
Nolamine Timed-Release Tablets ... 790
Ornade Spansule Capsules ... 2678
Propagest Tablets ... 791
Pyrroxate Caplets ... ◘ 742
Robitussin-CF ... ◘ 846
Sinulin Tablets ... 792
Tavist-D 12 Hour Relief Tablets ... ◘ 750
Teldrin 12 Hour Antihistamine/Nasal Decongestant Allergy Relief Capsules ... ◘ 786
Triaminic Expectorant ... ◘ 753
Triaminic Syrup ... ◘ 755
Triaminic Triaminicol Cold & Cough ... ◘ 756
Triaminic DM Syrup ... ◘ 756
Triaminicin Tablets ... ◘ 756
Vicks DayQuil Allergy Relief 12-Hour Extended Release Tablets ... ◘ 733
Vicks DayQuil Allergy Relief 4-Hour Tablets ... ◘ 733
Vicks DayQuil SINUS Pressure & CONGESTION Relief ... ◘ 734

Phenytoin (Phenytoin tends to produce hyperglycemia and concurrent use may lead to loss of control). Products include:
Dilantin Infatabs ... 1967
Dilantin-125 Suspension ... 1969

Phenytoin Sodium (Phenytoin tends to produce hyperglycemia and concurrent use may lead to loss of control). Products include:
Dilantin Kapseals ... 1965

Pindolol (Co-administration with beta blockers may result in hypoglycemia). Products include:
Visken Tablets ... 2428

Pirbuterol Acetate (Sympathomimetics tend to produce hyperglycemia and concurrent use may lead to loss of control). Products include:
Maxair Autohaler ... 1550
Maxair Inhaler ... 1552

Piroxicam (Co-administration with nonsteroidal anti-inflammatory agents may result in hypoglycemia). Products include:
Feldene Capsules ... 2008

Polyestradiol Phosphate (Estrogens tend to produce hyperglycemia and concurrent use may lead to loss of control).
No products indexed under this heading.

Polythiazide (Thiazides tend to produce hyperglycemia and concurrent use may lead to loss of control). Products include:
Minizide Capsules ... 2016

Prednisolone Acetate (Corticosteroids tend to produce hyperglycemia and concurrent use may lead to loss of control). Products include:
AK-CIDE ... ⊙ 203
AK-CIDE Ointment ... ⊙ 203
Blephamide Liquifilm Sterile Ophthalmic Suspension ... 472
Blephamide Ointment ... ⊙ 234
Econopred & Econopred Plus Ophthalmic Suspensions ... ⊙ 216
Poly-Pred Liquifilm ... ⊙ 246
Pred Forte ... ⊙ 247
Pred Mild ... ⊙ 250
Pred-G Liquifilm Sterile Ophthalmic Suspension ... ⊙ 248
Pred-G S.O.P. Sterile Ophthalmic Ointment ... ⊙ 249

Prednisolone Sodium Phosphate (Corticosteroids tend to produce hyperglycemia and concurrent use may lead to loss of control). Products include:
AK-PRED ... ⊙ 204
Hydeltrasol Injection, Sterile ... 1708
Pediapred Oral Solution ... 1618

Prednisolone Tebutate (Corticosteroids tend to produce hyperglycemia and concurrent use may lead to loss of control). Products include:
Hydeltra-T.B.A. Sterile Suspension ... 1710

Prednisone (Corticosteroids tend to produce hyperglycemia and concurrent use may lead to loss of control).
No products indexed under this heading.

Probenecid (Co-administration with probenecid may result in hypoglycemia). Products include:
Benemid Tablets ... 1651
ColBENEMID Tablets ... 1662

Prochlorperazine (Phenothiazines tend to produce hyperglycemia and concurrent use may lead to loss of control). Products include:
Compazine ... 2644

Promethazine Hydrochloride (Phenothiazines tend to produce hyperglycemia and concurrent use may lead to loss of control). Products include:
Mepergan Injection ... 2859
Phenergan with Codeine ... 2883
Phenergan with Dextromethorphan ... 2885
Phenergan Injection ... 2880
Phenergan Suppositories ... 2882
Phenergan Syrup ... 2881
Phenergan Tablets ... 2882
Phenergan VC ... 2886
Phenergan VC with Codeine ... 2888

Propranolol Hydrochloride (Co-administration with beta blockers may result in hypoglycemia). Products include:
Inderal ... 2834
Inderal LA Long Acting Capsules ... 2836
Inderide Tablets ... 2838
Inderide LA Long Acting Capsules ... 2840

(◘ Described in PDR For Nonprescription Drugs) (⊙ Described in PDR For Ophthalmology)

Pseudoephedrine Hydrochloride (Sympathomimetics tend to produce hyperglycemia and concurrent use may lead to loss of control). Products include:

Actifed Allergy Daytime/Nighttime Caplets	808
Actifed Cold & Allergy Tablets	807
Actifed Cold & Sinus Caplets and Tablets	808
Actifed Sinus Daytime/Nighttime Tablets and Caplets	809
Advil Cold and Sinus Caplets and Tablets	837
Alka-Seltzer Plus Liqui-Gels	612
Alka-Seltzer Plus Flu & Body Aches Liqui-Gels Non-Drowsy Formula	613
Alka-Seltzer Plus Night-Time Cold Medicine Liqui-Gels	612
Allerest Maximum Strength	649
Allerest No Drowsiness	649
Allerest Sinus Pain Formula	649
Atrohist Pediatric Capsules	1603
Benadryl Allergy/Cold Tablets	811
Benadryl Allergy Decongestant Liquid Medication	812
Benadryl Allergy Decongestant Tablets	812
Benadryl Allergy Sinus Headache Caplets	813
Benylin Multisymptom	816
Bromfed Capsules (Extended-Release)	1832
Bromfed Syrup	712
Bromfed Tablets	1832
Bromfed-DM Cough Syrup	1832
Bromfed-PD Capsules (Extended-Release)	1832
Children's TYLENOL Cold Multi-Symptom Chewable Tablets and Liquid	1559
Children's TYLENOL Cold Plus Cough Multi Symptom Chewable Tablets and Liquid	1560
Children's TYLENOL Flu Suspension Liquid	1560
Children's Vicks DayQuil Allergy Relief	730
Children's Vicks NyQuil Cold/Cough Relief	731
Allergy-Sinus Comtrex Multi-Symptom Allergy-Sinus Formula Tablets and Caplets	639
Comtrex Multi-Symptom	638
Comtrex Multi-Symptom Non-Drowsy Caplets	640
Congess	1003
Contac Day Allergy/Sinus Caplets	771
Contac Day & Night	772
Contac Night Allergy/Sinus Caplets	771
Contac Severe Cold & Flu Non-Drowsy	774
Deconsal II Tablets	1605
Dimetane-DX Cough Syrup	2233
Dimetapp Cold & Fever Suspension	839
Dimetapp Decongestant Pediatric Drops	840
Dorcol Children's Cough Syrup	748
Drixoral Cough + Congestion Liquid Caps	763
Dura-Tap/PD Capsules	970
Duratuss Tablets	2750
Duratuss HD Elixir	2750
Efidac/24	655
Entex PSE Tablets	973
Fedahist Gyrocaps	2545
Guaifed	1833
Guaifed Syrup	712
Guaimax-D Tablets	809
Histussin D Liquid	670
Infants' TYLENOL Cold Decongestant & Fever-Reducer Drops	1561
Kronofed-A	994
Novahistine DMX	782
Nucofed	2225
PediaCare Cough-Cold Chewable Tablets and Liquid	1569
PediaCare Infants' Decongestant Drops	1569
PediaCare Infants' Drops Decongestant Plus Cough	1569
PediaCare NightRest Cough-Cold Liquid	1569
Pediatric Vicks 44d Cough & Head Congestion Relief	736
Pediatric Vicks 44m Cough & Cold Relief	737
Robitussin Cold & Cough Liqui-Gels	844
Robitussin Cold, Cough & Flu Liqui-Gels	844
Robitussin Maximum Strength Cough & Cold	847
Robitussin Night-Time Cold Formula	847
Robitussin Pediatric Cough & Cold Formula	848
Robitussin Pediatric Drops	849
Robitussin Severe Congestion Liqui-Gels	845
Robitussin-DAC Syrup	2249
Robitussin-PE	846
Rondec Oral Drops	974
Rondec Syrup	974
Rondec Tablet	974
Rondec Chewable Tablets	974
Rondec-TR Tablet	974
Ryna	804
Seldane-D Extended-Release Tablets	1286
Semprex-D Capsules	1620
Sinarest	663
Sine-Aid Maximum Strength Sinus Headache Gelcaps, Caplets and Tablets	1570
Sine-Off No Drowsiness Formula Caplets	784
Sine-Off Sinus Medicine	784
Singlet Tablets	785
Sinutab Non-Drying Liquid Caps	823
Sinutab Sinus Allergy Medication, Maximum Strength Tablets and Caplets	823
Sinutab Sinus Medication, Maximum Strength Without Drowsiness Formula, Tablets & Caplets	824
Sudafed Children's Cold & Cough Liquid Medication	825
Sudafed Children's Nasal Decongestant Liquid Medication	826
Sudafed Cold & Allergy Tablets	826
Sudafed Cold and Cough Liquid Caps	826
Sudafed Nasal Decongestant Tablets, 30 mg	825
Sudafed Nasal Decongestant Tablets, 60 mg	825
Sudafed Non-Drying Sinus Liquid Caps	827
Sudafed Pediatric Nasal Decongestant Liquid Oral Drops	827
Sudafed Severe Cold Formula Caplets	828
Sudafed Severe Cold Formula Tablets	828
Sudafed Sinus Caplets	829
Sudafed Sinus Tablets	829
Sudafed 12 Hour Caplets	824
Syn-Rx Tablets	1622
Syn-Rx DM Tablets	1623
TheraFlu Flu and Cold Medicine	750
Theraflu Maximum Strength Flu and Cold Medicine For Sore Throat	751
TheraFlu Flu, Cold and Cough Medicine	750
TheraFlu Maximum Strength Nighttime Flu, Cold & Cough Medicine	751
TheraFlu Maximum Strength Non-Drowsy Formula Flu, Cold & Cough Medicine	751
TheraFlu Maximum Strength, Non-Drowsy Formula Flu, Cold and Cough Caplets	752
TheraFlu Maximum Strength Sinus Non-Drowsy Formula Caplets	752
Triaminic AM Cough and Decongestant Formula	753
Triaminic AM Decongestant Formula	753
Triaminic Infant Oral Decongestant Drops	754
Triaminic Night Time	754
Triaminic Sore Throat Formula	755
Tussend	1830
Tussend Expectorant	1831
TYLENOL Allergy Sinus, Maximum Strength Caplets and Gelcaps	1571
TYLENOL Allergy Sinus NightTime, Maximum Strength Caplets	1571
TYLENOL Cold Medication, Multi-Symptom Formula Tablets and Caplets	1572
TYLENOL Cold Medication, Multi-Symptom Hot Liquid Packets	1572
TYLENOL Cold Medication, No Drowsiness Formula Caplets and Gelcaps	1572
TYLENOL Cold Severe Congestion Caplets	1573
TYLENOL Cough Medication with Decongestant, Multi Symptom	1574
TYLENOL Flu No Drowsiness Formula, Maximum Strength Gelcaps	1575
TYLENOL Flu NightTime, Maximum Strength Gelcaps	1575
TYLENOL Flu NightTime, Maximum Strength Hot Medication Packets	1575
TYLENOL Sinus, Maximum Strength Geltabs, Gelcaps, Caplets and Tablets	1576
Vicks 44 LiquiCaps Cough, Cold & Flu Relief	728
Vicks 44 LiquiCaps Non-Drowsy Cough & Cold Relief	729
Vicks 44D Cough & Head Congestion Relief	728
Vicks 44M Cough, Cold & Flu Relief	729
Vicks DayQuil LiquiCaps/Liquid Multi-Symptom Cold/Flu Relief	734
Vicks DayQuil SINUS Pressure & PAIN Relief with IBUPROFEN	735
Vicks Nyquil Hot Therapy	735
Vicks NyQuil LiquiCaps/Liquid Multi-Symptom Cold/Flu Relief, Original and Cherry Flavors	736

Pseudoephedrine Sulfate (Sympathomimetics tend to produce hyperglycemia and concurrent use may lead to loss of control). Products include:

Chlor-Trimeton Allergy Decongestant Tablets	759
Claritin-D Tablets	2487
Drixoral Cold and Allergy Sustained-Action Tablets	763
Drixoral Cold and Flu Extended-Release Tablets	764
Drixoral Non-Drowsy Formula Extended-Release Tablets	764
Drixoral Allergy/Sinus Extended Release Tablets	765
Trinalin Repetabs Tablets	1373

Quinestrol (Estrogens tend to produce hyperglycemia and concurrent use may lead to loss of control).
No products indexed under this heading.

Salmeterol Xinafoate (Sympathomimetics tend to produce hyperglycemia and concurrent use may lead to loss of control). Products include:

Serevent Inhalation Aerosol	1149

Salsalate (Co-administration with salicylates may result in hypoglycemia). Products include:

Disalcid	1549
Mono-Gesic Tablets	810
Salflex Tablets	791

Selegiline Hydrochloride (Co-administration with monamine oxidase inhibitors may result in hypoglycemia). Products include:

Eldepryl Capsules	2729

Sotalol Hydrochloride (Co-administration with beta blockers may result in hypoglycemia). Products include:

Betapace Tablets	637

Spironolactone (Diuretics tend to produce hyperglycemia and concurrent use may lead to loss of control). Products include:

Aldactazide Tablets	2556
Aldactone Tablets	2558

Sulfacytine (Co-administration with sulfonamides may result in hypoglycemia).

Sulfamethizole (Co-administration with sulfonamides may result in hypoglycemia). Products include:

Urobiotic-250 Capsules	2038

Sulfamethoxazole (Co-administration with sulfonamides may result in hypoglycemia). Products include:

Bactrim DS Tablets	2257
Bactrim I.V. Infusion	2255
Bactrim	2257
Gantanol Tablets	2285
Septra	1146
Septra I.V. Infusion	1142
Septra I.V. Infusion ADD-Vantage Vials	1144
Septra	1146

Sulfasalazine (Co-administration with sulfonamides may result in hypoglycemia). Products include:

Azulfidine	2059

Sulfinpyrazone (Co-administration with sulfonamides may result in hypoglycemia). Products include:

Anturane	823

Sulfisoxazole (Co-administration with sulfonamides may result in hypoglycemia). Products include:

Gantrisin Tablets	2286

Sulfisoxazole Diolamine (Co-administration with sulfonamides may result in hypoglycemia).
No products indexed under this heading.

Sulindac (Co-administration with nonsteroidal anti-inflammatory agents may result in hypoglycemia). Products include:

Clinoril Tablets	1658

Temazepam (Co-administration with drugs that are highly protein bound may result in hypoglycemia). Products include:

Restoril Capsules	2413

Terbutaline Sulfate (Sympathomimetics tend to produce hyperglycemia and concurrent use may lead to loss of control). Products include:

Brethaire Inhaler	830
Brethine Ampuls	832
Brethine Tablets	831
Bricanyl Subcutaneous Injection	1247
Bricanyl Tablets	1248

Thioridazine Hydrochloride (Phenothiazines tend to produce hyperglycemia and concurrent use may lead to loss of control). Products include:

Mellaril	2398

Thyroglobulin (Thyroid products tend to produce hyperglycemia and concurrent use may lead to loss of control).
No products indexed under this heading.

Thyroid (Thyroid products tend to produce hyperglycemia and concurrent use may lead to loss of control).
No products indexed under this heading.

Thyroxine (Thyroid products tend to produce hyperglycemia and concurrent use may lead to loss of control).
No products indexed under this heading.

Thyroxine Sodium (Thyroid products tend to produce hyperglycemia and concurrent use may lead to loss of control).
No products indexed under this heading.

Timolol Hemihydrate (Co-administration with beta blockers may result in hypoglycemia). Products include:

Betimol 0.25%, 0.5%	259

Timolol Maleate (Co-administration with beta blockers may result in hypoglycemia). Products include:

Blocadren Tablets	1654
Timolide Tablets	1791
Timoptic in Ocudose	1796
Timoptic Sterile Ophthalmic Solution	1794

IMPORTANT NOTE: Always consult each drug listing in the patient's regimen for possible interactions.

Glucotrol XL — Interactions Index — 454

Timoptic-XE 1798

Tolazamide (Co-administration with sulfonamides may result in hypoglycemia).
 No products indexed under this heading.

Tolbutamide (Co-administration with sulfonamides may result in hypoglycemia).
 No products indexed under this heading.

Tolmetin Sodium (Co-administration with nonsteroidal anti-inflammatory agents may result in hypoglycemia). Products include:
 Tolectin (200, 400 and 600 mg) .. 1591

Torsemide (Diuretics tend to produce hyperglycemia and concurrent use may lead to loss of control). Products include:
 Demadex Tablets and Injection 691

Tranylcypromine Sulfate (Co-administration with monamine oxidase inhibitors may result in hypoglycemia). Products include:
 Parnate Tablets 2679

Triamcinolone (Corticosteroids tend to produce hyperglycemia and concurrent use may lead to loss of control).
 No products indexed under this heading.

Triamcinolone Acetonide (Corticosteroids tend to produce hyperglycemia and concurrent use may lead to loss of control). Products include:
 Azmacort Oral Inhaler 2175
 Nasacort AQ Nasal Spray 2191
 Nasacort Nasal Inhaler 2189

Triamcinolone Diacetate (Corticosteroids tend to produce hyperglycemia and concurrent use may lead to loss of control).
 No products indexed under this heading.

Triamcinolone Hexacetonide (Corticosteroids tend to produce hyperglycemia and concurrent use may lead to loss of control).
 No products indexed under this heading.

Triamterene (Diuretics tend to produce hyperglycemia and concurrent use may lead to loss of control). Products include:
 Dyazide Capsules 2653
 Dyrenium Capsules 2655

Trifluoperazine Hydrochloride (Phenothiazines tend to produce hyperglycemia and concurrent use may lead to loss of control). Products include:
 Stelazine 2692

Trimipramine Maleate (Co-administration with drugs that are highly protein bound may result in hypoglycemia). Products include:
 Surmontil Capsules 2917

Verapamil Hydrochloride (Calcium channel blockers tend to produce hyperglycemia and concurrent use may lead to loss of control). Products include:
 Calan SR Caplets 2571
 Calan Tablets 2568
 Covera-HS Tablets 2573
 Isoptin Injectable 1391
 Isoptin Oral Tablets 1393
 Isoptin SR Tablets 1395
 Verelan Capsules 1455

Warfarin Sodium (Co-administration with coumarins may result in hypoglycemia). Products include:
 Coumadin 941

Food Interactions

Alcohol (Co-administration with alcohol may result in hypoglycemia).

Diet, high-lipid (Administration of Glucotrol XL immediately before a high-fat breakfast resulted in a 40% increase in the glipizide mean Cmax value; the effect on the AUC was not significant).

GLYNASE PRESTAB TABLETS
(Glyburide) 2091
May interact with beta blockers, thiazides, calcium channel blockers, non-steroidal anti-inflammatory agents, salicylates, sulfonamides, oral anticoagulants, monoamine oxidase inhibitors, sympathomimetics, oral contraceptives, diuretics, corticosteroids, phenothiazines, thyroid preparations, estrogens, and certain other agents. Compounds in these categories include:

Acebutolol Hydrochloride (Co-administration with beta blockers may potentiate hypoglycemic action; beta blockers may mask signs and symptoms of hypoglycemia). Products include:
 Sectral Capsules 2914

Albuterol (Co-administration with sympathomimetics tends to produce hyperglycemia and may lead to loss of control). Products include:
 Proventil Inhalation Aerosol 2524
 Ventolin Inhalation Aerosol and Refill 1170

Albuterol Sulfate (Co-administration with sympathomimetics tends to produce hyperglycemia and may lead to loss of control). Products include:
 Airet Albuterol Sulfate Inhalation Solution 1602
 Albuterol Sulfate, USP Solution for Inhalation, Arm-a-Med 522
 Proventil Inhalation Solution 0.083% 2527
 Proventil Repetabs Tablets 2529
 Proventil Solution for Inhalation 0.5% 2525
 Proventil Syrup 2528
 Proventil Tablets 2529
 Ventolin Inhalation Solution 1171
 Ventolin Nebules Inhalation Solution 1172
 Ventolin Rotacaps for Inhalation 1173
 Ventolin Syrup 1175
 Ventolin Tablets 1176
 Volmax Extended-Release Tablets ... 1835

Amiloride Hydrochloride (Co-administration with diuretics tends to produce hyperglycemia and may lead to loss of control). Products include:
 Midamor Tablets 1746
 Moduretic Tablets 1748

Amlodipine Besylate (Co-administration with calcium channel blockers tends to produce hyperglycemia and may lead to loss of control). Products include:
 Lotrel Capsules 858
 Norvasc Tablets 2020

Aspirin (Co-administration with salicylates may potentiate hypoglycemic action). Products include:
 Alka-Seltzer Cherry Effervescent Antacid and Pain Reliever 609
 Alka-Seltzer Extra Strength Effervescent Antacid and Pain Reliever 609
 Alka-Seltzer Lemon Lime Effervescent Antacid and Pain Reliever 609
 Alka-Seltzer Original Effervescent Antacid and Pain Reliever 609
 Alka-Seltzer Plus 611
 Alka-Seltzer Plus Sinus Medicine 611
 Ascriptin 650
 Arthritis Strength BC Powder 631
 BC Cold Powder Multi-Symptom Formula (Cold-Sinus-Allergy) 631
 BC Cold Powder Non-Drowsy Formula (Cold-Sinus) 631
 BC Powder 631
 Genuine Bayer Aspirin Tablets & Caplets 618
 Extra Strength Bayer Arthritis Pain Regimen Formula 615
 Extra Strength Bayer Aspirin Caplets & Tablets 617
 Extended-Release Bayer 8-Hour Aspirin 616
 Extra Strength Bayer Plus Aspirin Caplets 617
 Extra Strength Bayer PM Aspirin Plus Sleep Aid 617
 Aspirin Regimen Bayer 81 mg Tablets with Calcium 615
 Aspirin Regimen Bayer Adult Low Strength 81 mg Tablets 613
 Aspirin Regimen Bayer Children's Chewable Aspirin 616
 Aspirin Regimen Bayer Regular Strength 325 mg Caplets 613
 Bufferin Analgesic Tablets 636
 Arthritis Strength Bufferin Analgesic Caplets 637
 Extra Strength Bufferin Analgesic Tablets 637
 Cama Arthritis Pain Reliever 748
 Darvon Compound-65 Pulvules 1475
 Easprin 1971
 Ecotrin 2625
 Ecotrin Enteric Coated Aspirin Maximum Strength Tablets and Caplets 775
 Ecotrin Enteric Coated Aspirin Regular Strength Tablets 2625
 Empirin Aspirin Tablets 818
 Excedrin Extra-Strength Analgesic Tablets, Caplets, and Geltabs 734
 Fiorinal Capsules 2388
 Fiorinal with Codeine Capsules 2390
 Fiorinal Tablets 2388
 Goody's Extra Strength Headache Powders 632
 Goody's Extra Strength Pain Relief Tablets 632
 Halfprin Tablets 1413
 Norgesic 1554
 Percodan Tablets 955
 Percodan-Demi Tablets 956
 Robaxisal Tablets 2246
 Soma Compound w/Codeine Tablets 2784
 Soma Compound Tablets 2783
 St. Joseph Adult Chewable Aspirin (81 mg.) 768
 Talwin Compound 2466
 Vanquish Analgesic Caplets 627

Atenolol (Co-administration with beta blockers may potentiate hypoglycemic action; beta blockers may mask signs and symptoms of hypoglycemia). Products include:
 Tenoretic Tablets 2963
 Tenormin Tablets and I.V. Injection 2965

Bendroflumethiazide (Co-administration with thiazides tends to produce hyperglycemia and may lead to loss of control).
 No products indexed under this heading.

Bepridil Hydrochloride (Co-administration with calcium channel blockers tends to produce hyperglycemia and may lead to loss of control). Products include:
 Vascor Tablets (200 and 300 mg) 1597

Betamethasone Acetate (Co-administration with corticosteroids tends to produce hyperglycemia and may lead to loss of control). Products include:
 Celestone Soluspan Suspension 2484

Betamethasone Sodium Phosphate (Co-administration with corticosteroids tends to produce hyperglycemia and may lead to loss of control). Products include:
 Celestone Soluspan Suspension 2484

Betaxolol Hydrochloride (Co-administration with beta blockers may potentiate hypoglycemic action; beta blockers may mask signs and symptoms of hypoglycemia). Products include:
 Betoptic Ophthalmic Solution 465
 Betoptic S Ophthalmic Suspension ... 467
 Kerlone Tablets 2588

Bisoprolol Fumarate (Co-administration with beta blockers may potentiate hypoglycemic action; beta blockers may mask signs and symptoms of hypoglycemia). Products include:
 Zebeta Tablets 1457
 Ziac 1459

Bumetanide (Co-administration with diuretics tends to produce hyperglycemia and may lead to loss of control). Products include:
 Bumex 2260

Carteolol Hydrochloride (Co-administration with beta blockers may potentiate hypoglycemic action; beta blockers may mask signs and symptoms of hypoglycemia). Products include:
 Cartrol Tablets 413
 Ocupress Ophthalmic Solution, 1% Sterile 297

Chloramphenicol (Co-administration with chloramphenicol may potentiate hypoglycemic action). Products include:
 Chloromycetin Ophthalmic Ointment, 1% 298
 Chloromycetin Ophthalmic Solution 299
 Chloroptic S.O.P. 236
 Chloroptic Sterile Ophthalmic Solution 236

Chloramphenicol Palmitate (Co-administration with chloramphenicol may potentiate hypoglycemic action).
 No products indexed under this heading.

Chloramphenicol Sodium Succinate (Co-administration with chloramphenicol may potentiate hypoglycemic action). Products include:
 Chloromycetin Sodium Succinate 1960

Chlorothiazide (Co-administration with thiazides tends to produce hyperglycemia and may lead to loss of control). Products include:
 Aldoclor Tablets 1638
 Diupres Tablets 1691
 Diuril Oral 1694

Chlorothiazide Sodium (Co-administration with thiazides tends to produce hyperglycemia and may lead to loss of control). Products include:
 Diuril Sodium Intravenous 1693

Chlorotrianisene (Co-administration with estrogens tends to produce hyperglycemia and may lead to loss of control).
 No products indexed under this heading.

Chlorpromazine (Co-administration with phenothiazines tends to produce hyperglycemia and may lead to loss of control). Products include:
 Thorazine Suppositories 2701

Chlorpromazine Hydrochloride (Co-administration with phenothiazines tends to produce hyperglycemia and may lead to loss of control). Products include:
 Thorazine 2701

Chlorpropamide (Co-administration with sulfonamides may potentiate hypoglycemic action). Products include:
 Diabinese Tablets 2002

Chlorthalidone (Co-administration with diuretics tends to produce hyperglycemia and may lead to loss of control). Products include:
 Combipres Tablets 682
 Tenoretic Tablets 2963
 Thalitone 1293

(▣ Described in PDR For Nonprescription Drugs)   (⊙ Described in PDR For Ophthalmology)

Choline Magnesium Trisalicylate (Co-administration with salicylates may potentiate hypoglycemic action). Products include:

Trilisate 2155

Ciprofloxacin (Co-administration with ciprofloxacin has been reported to result in potentiation of hypoglycemic action). Products include:

Cipro I.V. 587
Cipro I.V. Pharmacy Bulk Package.. 590

Ciprofloxacin Hydrochloride (Co-administration with ciprofloxacin has been reported to result in potentiation of hypoglycemic action). Products include:

Ciloxan Ophthalmic Solution........ 468
Cipro Tablets........ 584

Cortisone Acetate (Co-administration with corticosteroids tends to produce hyperglycemia and may lead to loss of control). Products include:

Cortone Acetate Sterile Suspension 1663
Cortone Acetate Tablets........ 1664

Desogestrel (Co-administration with oral contraceptives tends to produce hyperglycemia and may lead to loss of control). Products include:

Desogen Tablets........ 1867
Ortho-Cept 1907

Dexamethasone (Co-administration with corticosteroids tends to produce hyperglycemia and may lead to loss of control). Products include:

AK-Trol Ointment & Suspension .... ◉ 205
Decadron Elixir 1676
Decadron Tablets........ 1678
Decaspray Topical Aerosol 1689
Maxitrol Ophthalmic Ointment and Suspension .... ◉ 222
TobraDex Ophthalmic Suspension and Ointment........ 469

Dexamethasone Acetate (Co-administration with corticosteroids tends to produce hyperglycemia and may lead to loss of control). Products include:

Dalalone D.P. Injectable 1009
Decadron-LA Sterile Suspension...... 1687

Dexamethasone Sodium Phosphate (Co-administration with corticosteroids tends to produce hyperglycemia and may lead to loss of control). Products include:

Decadron Phosphate Injection 1680
Decadron Phosphate Sterile Ophthalmic Ointment 1684
Decadron Phosphate Sterile Ophthalmic Solution 1685
Decadron Phosphate Topical Cream........ 1686
Decadron Phosphate with Xylocaine Injection, Sterile 1683
Dexacort Phosphate in Respihaler .. 1606
Dexacort Phosphate in Turbinaire .. 1607
NeoDecadron Sterile Ophthalmic Ointment 1755
NeoDecadron Sterile Ophthalmic Solution 1756
NeoDecadron Topical Cream 1757

Diclofenac Potassium (Co-administration with nonsteroidal anti-inflammatory agents may potentiate hypoglycemic action). Products include:

Cataflam Tablets 833

Diclofenac Sodium (Co-administration with nonsteroidal anti-inflammatory agents may potentiate hypoglycemic action). Products include:

Voltaren Ophthalmic Sterile Ophthalmic Solution .... ◉ 264
Cataflam/Voltaren/Voltaren-XR 833

Dicumarol (Co-administration may potentiate or weaken the effects of coumarin derivatives).

No products indexed under this heading.

Dienestrol (Co-administration with estrogens tends to produce hyperglycemia and may lead to loss of control). Products include:

Ortho Dienestrol Cream 1922

Diethylstilbestrol (Co-administration with estrogens tends to produce hyperglycemia and may lead to loss of control). Products include:

Diethylstilbestrol Tablets 1477

Diflunisal (Co-administration with salicylates may potentiate hypoglycemic action). Products include:

Dolobid Tablets........ 1695

Diltiazem Hydrochloride (Co-administration with calcium channel blockers tends to produce hyperglycemia and may lead to loss of control). Products include:

Cardizem CD Capsules 1251
Cardizem SR Capsules 1255
Cardizem Injectable 1253
Cardizem Tablets........ 1257
Dilacor XR Extended-release Capsules 2183
Tiazac Capsules 1019

Dobutamine Hydrochloride (Co-administration with sympathomimetics tends to produce hyperglycemia and may lead to loss of control). Products include:

Dobutrex Solution Vials........ 1480

Dopamine Hydrochloride (Co-administration with sympathomimetics tends to produce hyperglycemia and may lead to loss of control).

No products indexed under this heading.

Ephedrine Hydrochloride (Co-administration with sympathomimetics tends to produce hyperglycemia and may lead to loss of control). Products include:

Primatene Tablets 844
Quadrinal Tablets 1398

Ephedrine Sulfate (Co-administration with sympathomimetics tends to produce hyperglycemia and may lead to loss of control). Products include:

Marax Tablets & DF Syrup........ 2015

Ephedrine Tannate (Co-administration with sympathomimetics tends to produce hyperglycemia and may lead to loss of control). Products include:

Rynatuss 2782

Epinephrine (Co-administration with sympathomimetics tends to produce hyperglycemia and may lead to loss of control). Products include:

EPIFRIN .... ◉ 237
EpiPen 808
Marcaine with Epinephrine 2446
Primatene Mist 843
Sensorcaine with Epinephrine Injection........ 554
Sus-Phrine Injection 1017
Xylocaine with Epinephrine Injections........ 562

Epinephrine Bitartrate (Co-administration with sympathomimetics tends to produce hyperglycemia and may lead to loss of control). Products include:

Sensorcaine-MPF with Epinephrine Injection 554

Epinephrine Hydrochloride (Co-administration with sympathomimetics tends to produce hyperglycemia and may lead to loss of control). Products include:

Ana-Kit Anaphylaxis Emergency Treatment Kit 611

Esmolol Hydrochloride (Co-administration with beta blockers may potentiate hypoglycemic action; beta blockers may mask signs and symptoms of hypoglycemia). Products include:

Brevibloc (esmolol HCl) Injection 1860

Estradiol (Co-administration with estrogens tends to produce hyperglycemia and may lead to loss of control). Products include:

Climara Transdermal System........ 640
Estrace Cream and Tablets........ 751
Estraderm Transdermal System 842
Estring Vaginal Ring........ 2086
Vivelle Transdermal System 880

Estrogens, Conjugated (Co-administration with estrogens tends to produce hyperglycemia and may lead to loss of control). Products include:

PMB 200 and PMB 400 2890
Premarin Intravenous 2893
Premarin Tablets 2896
Premarin Vaginal Cream........ 2898
Premphase 2900
Prempro........ 2905

Estrogens, Esterified (Co-administration with estrogens tends to produce hyperglycemia and may lead to loss of control). Products include:

ESTRATAB Tablets (0.3, 0.625, 1.25, 2.5 mg)........ 2715
Estratest 2718
Menest Tablets 2671

Estropipate (Co-administration with estrogens tends to produce hyperglycemia and may lead to loss of control). Products include:

Ogen Tablets 2103
Ogen Vaginal Cream........ 2106
Ortho-Est........ 1925

Ethacrynic Acid (Co-administration with diuretics tends to produce hyperglycemia and may lead to loss of control). Products include:

Edecrin Tablets........ 1698

Ethinyl Estradiol (Co-administration with estrogens tends to produce hyperglycemia and may lead to loss of control). Products include:

Brevicon........ 2563
Demulen 2580
Desogen Tablets........ 1867
Levlen/Tri-Levlen 646
Lo/Ovral Tablets 2852
Lo/Ovral-28 Tablets........ 2857
Modicon 1928
Nordette-21 Tablets........ 2863
Nordette-28 Tablets........ 2866
Norinyl 2563
Ortho-Cept 1907
Ortho-Cyclen/Ortho-Tri-Cyclen 1914
Ortho-Novum........ 1928
Ortho-Cyclen/Ortho Tri-Cyclen 1914
Ovcon 765
Ovral Tablets 2877
Ovral-28 Tablets 2878
Levlen/Tri-Levlen........ 646
Tri-Norinyl........ 2607
Triphasil-21 Tablets 2919
Triphasil-28 Tablets 2924

Ethynodiol Diacetate (Co-administration with oral contraceptives tends to produce hyperglycemia and may lead to loss of control). Products include:

Demulen 2580

Etodolac (Co-administration with nonsteroidal anti-inflammatory agents may potentiate hypoglycemic action). Products include:

Lodine Capsules and Tablets 2849

Felodipine (Co-administration with calcium channel blockers tends to produce hyperglycemia and may lead to loss of control). Products include:

Plendil Extended-Release Tablets.... 514

Fenoprofen Calcium (Co-administration with nonsteroidal anti-inflammatory agents may potentiate hypoglycemic action). Products include:

Nalfon 200 Pulvules & Nalfon Tablets 933

Fludrocortisone Acetate (Co-administration with corticosteroids tends to produce hyperglycemia and may lead to loss of control). Products include:

Florinef Acetate Tablets 506

Fluphenazine Decanoate (Co-administration with phenothiazines tends to produce hyperglycemia and may lead to loss of control). Products include:

Prolixin Decanoate 510

Fluphenazine Enanthate (Co-administration with phenothiazines tends to produce hyperglycemia and may lead to loss of control). Products include:

Prolixin Enanthate........ 510

Fluphenazine Hydrochloride (Co-administration with phenothiazines tends to produce hyperglycemia and may lead to loss of control). Products include:

Prolixin........ 510

Flurbiprofen (Co-administration with nonsteroidal anti-inflammatory agents may potentiate hypoglycemic action).

No products indexed under this heading.

Fosphenytoin Sodium (Co-administration with phenytoin tends to produce hyperglycemia and may lead to loss of control). Products include:

Cerebyx Injection........ 1956

Furazolidone (Co-administration with monoamine oxidase inhibitors may potentiate hypoglycemic action). Products include:

Furoxone 2221

Furosemide (Co-administration with diuretics tends to produce hyperglycemia and may lead to loss of control). Products include:

Lasix Injection, Oral Solution and Tablets 1267

Glipizide (Co-administration with sulfonamides may potentiate hypoglycemic action). Products include:

Glucotrol Tablets 2011
Glucotrol XL Extended Release Tablets 2012

Hydrochlorothiazide (Co-administration with thiazides tends to produce hyperglycemia and may lead to loss of control). Products include:

Aldactazide Tablets 2556
Aldoril Tablets........ 1644
Apresazide Capsules 824
Capozide Tablets 744
Dyazide Capsules........ 2653
Esidrix Tablets 839
Esimil Tablets 840
HydroDIURIL Tablets 1716
Hydropres Tablets........ 1718
Hyzaar Tablets 1720
Inderide Tablets 2838
Inderide LA Long Acting Capsules .. 2840
Lopressor HCT Tablets 850
Lotensin HCT Tablets 855
Moduretic Tablets 1748
Oretic Tablets 450
Prinzide Tablets 1780
Ser-Ap-Es Tablets 867
Timolide Tablets........ 1791
Vaseretic Tablets 1810
Zestoretic Tablets 2968
Ziac 1459

IMPORTANT NOTE: Always consult each drug listing in the patient's regimen for possible interactions.

Glynase **Interactions Index** 456

Hydrocortisone (Co-administration with corticosteroids tends to produce hyperglycemia and may lead to loss of control). Products include:

Anusol-HC Cream 2.5% 1953
Aquanil HC Lotion 1989
Maximum Strength Cortaid Spray ⊞ 800
CORTENEMA 2713
Cortisporin Ointment 1074
Cortisporin Ophthalmic Ointment Sterile 1074
Cortisporin Ophthalmic Suspension Sterile 1075
Cortisporin Otic Solution Sterile 1076
Cortisporin Otic Suspension Sterile 1077
Cortizone-5 ⊞ 795
Cortizone-10 ⊞ 795
Hydrocortone Tablets 1715
Hytone 922
Hytone Ointment 2 ½% 923
Massengill Medicated Soft Cloth Towelettes 2628
Pediotic Suspension Sterile 1140
Preparation H Hydrocortisone 1% Cream ⊞ 843
ProctoCream-HC 2.5% 2552
VōSoL HC Otic Solution 2786

Hydrocortisone Acetate (Co-administration with corticosteroids tends to produce hyperglycemia and may lead to loss of control). Products include:

Analpram-HC Rectal Cream 1% and 2.5% 993
Anusol HC-1 Hydrocortisone Anti-Itch Ointment ⊞ 810
Anusol-HC Suppositories 1954
Caldecort Anti-Itch Hydrocortisone Cream ⊞ 651
Coly-Mycin S Otic w/Neomycin & Hydrocortisone 1965
Cortaid ⊞ 800
Cortifoam 2540
Cortisporin Cream 1073
Epifoam 2543
Hydrocortone Acetate Sterile Suspension 1712
Mantadil Cream 1124
Nupercainal Hydrocortisone 1% Cream ⊞ 661
Pramosone Cream, Lotion & Ointment 995
ProctoFoam-HC 2552
Terra-Cortril Ophthalmic Suspension 2033

Hydrocortisone Sodium Phosphate (Co-administration with corticosteroids tends to produce hyperglycemia and may lead to loss of control). Products include:

Hydrocortone Phosphate Injection, Sterile 1713

Hydrocortisone Sodium Succinate (Co-administration with corticosteroids tends to produce hyperglycemia and may lead to loss of control).

No products indexed under this heading.

Hydroflumethiazide (Co-administration with thiazides tends to produce hyperglycemia and may lead to loss of control). Products include:

Diucardin Tablets 2824

Ibuprofen (Co-administration with nonsteroidal anti-inflammatory agents may potentiate hypoglycemic action). Products include:

Advil Cold and Sinus Caplets and Tablets ⊞ 837
Advil Ibuprofen Tablets, Caplets and Gel Caplets ⊞ 836
Children's Motrin Ibuprofen Oral Suspension 1558
IBU Tablets 1389
Ibuprohm ⊞ 713
Motrin IB Caplets, Tablets, and Gelcaps ⊞ 802
Motrin Ibuprofen Suspension, Oral Drops, Chewable Tablets, Caplets 1563
Nuprin Ibuprofen/Analgesic Tablets & Caplets ⊞ 645
Vicks DayQuil SINUS Pressure & PAIN Relief with IBUPROFEN ⊞ 735

Indapamide (Co-administration with diuretics tends to produce hyperglycemia and may lead to loss of control).

No products indexed under this heading.

Indomethacin (Co-administration with nonsteroidal anti-inflammatory agents may potentiate hypoglycemic action). Products include:

Indocin 1723

Indomethacin Sodium Trihydrate (Co-administration with nonsteroidal anti-inflammatory agents may potentiate hypoglycemic action). Products include:

Indocin I.V. 1727

Isocarboxazid (Co-administration with monoamine oxidase inhibitors may potentiate hypoglycemic action).

No products indexed under this heading.

Isoniazid (Co-administration with isoniazid tends to produce hyperglycemia and may lead to loss of control). Products include:

Nydrazid Injection 509
Rifamate Capsules 1278
Rifater 1280

Isoproterenol Hydrochloride (Co-administration with sympathomimetics tends to produce hyperglycemia and may lead to loss of control). Products include:

Isuprel Hydrochloride Solution 2443
Isuprel Injection 2441
Isuprel Mistometer 2442

Isoproterenol Sulfate (Co-administration with sympathomimetics tends to produce hyperglycemia and may lead to loss of control). Products include:

Norisodrine with Calcium Iodide Syrup 446

Isradipine (Co-administration with calcium channel blockers tends to produce hyperglycemia and may lead to loss of control). Products include:

DynaCirc Capsules 2381
DynaCirc CR Tablets 2383

Ketoprofen (Co-administration with nonsteroidal anti-inflammatory agents may potentiate hypoglycemic action). Products include:

Actron Caplets and Tablets ⊞ 608
Orudis Capsules 2874
Orudis KT ⊞ 842
Oruvail Capsules 2874

Ketorolac Tromethamine (Co-administration with nonsteroidal anti-inflammatory agents may potentiate hypoglycemic action). Products include:

Acular Sterile Ophthalmic Solution 470
Toradol 2319

Labetalol Hydrochloride (Co-administration with beta blockers may potentiate hypoglycemic action; beta blockers may mask signs and symptoms of hypoglycemia). Products include:

Normodyne Injection 2519
Normodyne Tablets 2522
Trandate 1158

Levobunolol Hydrochloride (Co-administration with beta blockers may potentiate hypoglycemic action; beta blockers may mask signs and symptoms of hypoglycemia). Products include:

Betagan ⊙ 230

Levonorgestrel (Co-administration with oral contraceptives tends to produce hyperglycemia and may lead to loss of control). Products include:

Levlen/Tri-Levlen 646
Nordette-21 Tablets 2863
Nordette-28 Tablets 2866
Norplant System 2868
Levlen/Tri-Levlen 646
Triphasil-21 Tablets 2919
Triphasil-28 Tablets 2924

Levothyroxine Sodium (Co-administration with thyroid preparations tends to produce hyperglycemia and may lead to loss of control). Products include:

Eltroxin Tablets 2214
Levothroid Tablets 1015
Levothyroxine Sodium, USP for Injection 546
Levoxyl Tablets 918
Synthroid 1410

Liothyronine Sodium (Co-administration with thyroid preparations tends to produce hyperglycemia and may lead to loss of control). Products include:

Cytomel Tablets 2647
Triostat Injection 2708

Liotrix (Co-administration with thyroid preparations tends to produce hyperglycemia and may lead to loss of control).

No products indexed under this heading.

Magnesium Salicylate (Co-administration with salicylates may potentiate hypoglycemic action). Products include:

Backache Caplets ⊞ 635
Doan's Extra-Strength Analgesic ⊞ 653
Extra Strength Doan's P.M. ⊞ 653
Doan's Regular Strength Analgesic ⊞ 654
Mobigesic Tablets ⊞ 607

Meclofenamate Sodium (Co-administration with nonsteroidal anti-inflammatory agents may potentiate hypoglycemic action).

No products indexed under this heading.

Mefenamic Acid (Co-administration with nonsteroidal anti-inflammatory agents may potentiate hypoglycemic action). Products include:

Ponstel 1982

Mesoridazine Besylate (Co-administration with phenothiazines tends to produce hyperglycemia and may lead to loss of control). Products include:

Serentil 689

Mestranol (Co-administration with oral contraceptives tends to produce hyperglycemia and may lead to loss of control). Products include:

Norinyl 2563
Ortho-Novum 1928

Metaproterenol Sulfate (Co-administration with sympathomimetics tends to produce hyperglycemia and may lead to loss of control). Products include:

Alupent 672
Metaproterenol Sulfate Inhalation Solution, USP, Arm-a-Med 547

Metaraminol Bitartrate (Co-administration with sympathomimetics tends to produce hyperglycemia and may lead to loss of control). Products include:

Aramine Injection 1649

Metformin Hydrochloride (Co-administration has resulted in highly variable decreases in glyburide AUC and C_{max}). Products include:

Glucophage Tablets 754

Methotrimeprazine (Co-administration with phenothiazines tends to produce hyperglycemia and may lead to loss of control). Products include:

Levoprome 1321

Methoxamine Hydrochloride (Co-administration with sympathomimetics tends to produce hyperglycemia and may lead to loss of control). Products include:

Vasoxyl Injection 1169

Methyclothiazide (Co-administration with thiazides tends to produce hyperglycemia and may lead to loss of control). Products include:

Enduron Tablets 424

Methylprednisolone Acetate (Co-administration with corticosteroids tends to produce hyperglycemia and may lead to loss of control).

No products indexed under this heading.

Methylprednisolone Sodium Succinate (Co-administration with corticosteroids tends to produce hyperglycemia and may lead to loss of control).

No products indexed under this heading.

Metipranolol Hydrochloride (Co-administration with beta blockers may potentiate hypoglycemic action; beta blockers may mask signs and symptoms of hypoglycemia). Products include:

OptiPranolol (Metipranolol 0.3%) Sterile Ophthalmic Solution ⊙ 256

Metolazone (Co-administration with diuretics tend to produce hyperglycemia and may lead to loss of control). Products include:

Mykrox Tablets 1617
Zaroxolyn Tablets 1625

Metoprolol Succinate (Co-administration with beta blockers may potentiate hypoglycemic action; beta blockers may mask signs and symptoms of hypoglycemia). Products include:

Toprol-XL Tablets 560

Metoprolol Tartrate (Co-administration with beta blockers may potentiate hypoglycemic action; beta blockers may mask signs and symptoms of hypoglycemia). Products include:

Lopressor 848
Lopressor HCT Tablets 850

Miconazole (A potential interaction between miconazole and oral hypoglycemic agents leading to severe hypoglycemia has been reported).

No products indexed under this heading.

Nabumetone (Co-administration with nonsteroidal anti-inflammatory agents may potentiate hypoglycemic action). Products include:

Relafen Tablets 2688

Nadolol (Co-administration with beta blockers may potentiate hypoglycemic action; beta blockers may mask signs and symptoms of hypoglycemia).

No products indexed under this heading.

Naproxen (Co-administration with nonsteroidal anti-inflammatory agents may potentiate hypoglycemic action). Products include:

Anaprox/Naprosyn 2277

Naproxen Sodium (Co-administration with nonsteroidal anti-inflammatory agents may potentiate hypoglycemic action). Products include:

Aleve 2124
Anaprox/Naprosyn 2277
Naprelan Tablets 2861

(⊞ Described in PDR For Nonprescription Drugs) (⊙ Described in PDR For Ophthalmology)

Interactions Index

Niacin (Co-administration with nicotinic acid produces hyperglycemia and may lead to loss of control). Products include:
- Kyo-Chrome .... ⓔ 680
- Nicotinex Elixir .... ⓔ 671
- Slo-Niacin Tablets 2767

Nicardipine Hydrochloride (Co-administration with calcium channel blockers tends to produce hyperglycemia and may lead to loss of control). Products include:
- Cardene Capsules 2261
- Cardene I.V. 2815
- Cardene SR Capsules 2264

Nifedipine (Co-administration with calcium channel blockers tends to produce hyperglycemia and may lead to loss of control). Products include:
- Adalat Capsules (10 mg and 20 mg) 580
- Adalat CC 582
- Procardia Capsules 2024
- Procardia XL Extended Release Tablets 2026

Nimodipine (Co-administration with calcium channel blockers tends to produce hyperglycemia and may lead to loss of control). Products include:
- Nimotop Capsules 603

Nisoldipine (Co-administration with calcium channel blockers tends to produce hyperglycemia and may lead to loss of control). Products include:
- Sular Tablets 2961

Norepinephrine Bitartrate (Co-administration with sympathomimetics tends to produce hyperglycemia and may lead to loss of control). Products include:
- Levophed Bitartrate Injection 2445

Norethindrone (Co-administration with oral contraceptives tends to produce hyperglycemia and may lead to loss of control). Products include:
- Brevicon 2563
- Micronor Tablets 1903
- Modicon 1928
- Norinyl 2563
- Nor-Q D Tablets 2598
- Ortho-Novum 1928
- Ovcon 765
- Tri-Norinyl 2607

Norethynodrel (Co-administration with oral contraceptives tends to produce hyperglycemia and may lead to loss of control).
No products indexed under this heading.

Norgestimate (Co-administration with oral contraceptives tends to produce hyperglycemia and may lead to loss of control). Products include:
- Ortho-Cyclen/Ortho-Tri-Cyclen 1914
- Ortho-Cyclen/Ortho Tri-Cyclen 1914

Norgestrel (Co-administration with oral contraceptives tends to produce hyperglycemia and may lead to loss of control). Products include:
- Lo/Ovral Tablets 2852
- Lo/Ovral-28 Tablets 2857
- Ovral Tablets 2877
- Ovral-28 Tablets 2878
- Ovrette Tablets 2878

Oxaprozin (Co-administration with nonsteroidal anti-inflammatory agents may potentiate hypoglycemic action). Products include:
- Daypro Caplets 2578

Penbutolol Sulfate (Co-administration with beta blockers may potentiate hypoglycemic action; beta blockers may mask signs and symptoms of hypoglycemia). Products include:
- Levatol Tablets 2547

Perphenazine (Co-administration with phenothiazines tends to produce hyperglycemia and may lead to loss of control). Products include:
- Etrafon 2495
- Triavil Tablets 1800
- Trilafon 2532

Phenelzine Sulfate (Co-administration with monoamine oxidase inhibitors may potentiate hypoglycemic action). Products include:
- Nardil 1977

Phenylbutazone (Co-administration with nonsteroidal anti-inflammatory agents may potentiate hypoglycemic action).
No products indexed under this heading.

Phenylephrine Bitartrate (Co-administration with sympathomimetics tends to produce hyperglycemia and may lead to loss of control).
No products indexed under this heading.

Phenylephrine Hydrochloride (Co-administration with sympathomimetics tends to produce hyperglycemia and may lead to loss of control). Products include:
- Atrohist Plus Tablets 1605
- Cerose DM .... ⓔ 853
- D.A. II Tablets 972
- D.A. Chewable Tablets 970
- Dura-Vent/DA Tablets 972
- Extendryl 1003
- 4-Way Fast Acting Nasal Spray (regular & mentholated) .... ⓔ 644
- Hemorid 797
- Hycomine Compound Tablets 948
- Neo-Synephrine Hydrochloride 1% Carpuject 2455
- Neo-Synephrine Hydrochloride 1% Injection 2455
- Neo-Synephrine Hydrochloride (Ophthalmic) 2456
- Neo-Synephrine .... ⓔ 624
- Novahistine Elixir 782
- Phenergan VC 2886
- Phenergan VC with Codeine 2888
- Preparation H .... ⓔ 842
- Tympagesic Ear Drops 2476
- Vicks Sinex Nasal Spray and Ultra Fine Mist .... ⓔ 738

Phenylephrine Tannate (Co-administration with sympathomimetics tends to produce hyperglycemia and may lead to loss of control). Products include:
- Atrohist Pediatric Suspension 1604
- Atrohist Pediatric Suspension Dye-Free 1604
- Rynatan 2781
- Rynatuss 2782

Phenylpropanolamine Hydrochloride (Co-administration with sympathomimetics tends to produce hyperglycemia and may lead to loss of control). Products include:
- Acutrim .... ⓔ 648
- Atrohist Plus Tablets 1605
- BC Cold Powder Multi-Symptom Formula (Cold-Sinus-Allergy) ..... ⓔ 631
- BC Cold Powder Non-Drowsy Formula (Cold-Sinus) .... ⓔ 631
- Cheracol Plus Head Cold/Cough Formula .... ⓔ 741
- Comtrex Multi-Symptom Cold Reliever Liqui-Gels .... ⓔ 638
- Comtrex Multi-Symptom Non-Drowsy Liqui-gels .... ⓔ 640
- Contac Continuous Action Nasal Decongestant/Antihistamine 12 Hour Capsules .... ⓔ 773
- Contac Maximum Strength Continuous Action Decongestant/Antihistamine 12 Hour Caplets .. ⓔ 772
- Contac Severe Cold and Flu Formula Caplets .... ⓔ 773
- Coricidin 'D' Decongestant Tablets .... ⓔ 760
- Dexatrim .... ⓔ 795
- Dexatrim Plus Vitamins Caplets ..... ⓔ 796
- Dimetane-DC Cough Syrup 2232
- Dimetapp Allergy Sinus Caplets ..... ⓔ 838
- Dimetapp Cold & Allergy Chewable Tablets .... ⓔ 838
- Dimetapp Cold & Cough Liqui-Gels .... ⓔ 839
- Dimetapp DM Elixir .... ⓔ 840
- Dimetapp Elixir .... ⓔ 840
- Dimetapp Extentabs .... ⓔ 841
- Dimetapp Tablets/Liqui-Gels .... ⓔ 841
- Dura-Vent Tablets 971
- Entex LA Tablets 972
- Exgest LA Tablets 787
- Hycomine 947
- Nolamine Timed-Release Tablets 790
- Ornade Spansule Capsules 2678
- Propagest Tablets 791
- Pyrroxate Caplets .... ⓔ 742
- Robitussin-CF .... ⓔ 846
- Sinulin Tablets 792
- Tavist-D 12 Hour Relief Tablets ..... ⓔ 750
- Teldrin 12 Hour Antihistamine/Nasal Decongestant Allergy Relief Capsules .... ⓔ 786
- Triaminic Expectorant .... ⓔ 753
- Triaminic Syrup .... ⓔ 755
- Triaminic Triaminicol Cold & Cough .... ⓔ 756
- Triaminic DM Syrup .... ⓔ 756
- Triaminicin Tablets .... ⓔ 756
- Vicks DayQuil Allergy Relief 12-Hour Extended Release Tablets.. ⓔ 733
- Vicks DayQuil Allergy Relief 4-Hour Tablets .... ⓔ 733
- Vicks DayQuil SINUS Pressure & CONGESTION Relief .... ⓔ 734

Phenytoin (Co-administration with phenytoin tends to produce hyperglycemia and may lead to loss of control). Products include:
- Dilantin Infatabs 1967
- Dilantin-125 Suspension 1969

Phenytoin Sodium (Co-administration with phenytoin tends to produce hyperglycemia and may lead to loss of control). Products include:
- Dilantin Kapseals 1965

Pindolol (Co-administration with beta blockers may potentiate hypoglycemic action; beta blockers may mask signs and symptoms of hypoglycemia). Products include:
- Visken Tablets 2428

Pirbuterol Acetate (Co-administration with sympathomimetics tends to produce hyperglycemia and may lead to loss of control). Products include:
- Maxair Autohaler 1550
- Maxair Inhaler 1552

Piroxicam (Co-administration with nonsteroidal anti-inflammatory agents may potentiate hypoglycemic action). Products include:
- Feldene Capsules 2008

Polyestradiol Phosphate (Co-administration with estrogens tends to produce hyperglycemia and may lead to loss of control).
No products indexed under this heading.

Polythiazide (Co-administration with thiazides tends to produce hyperglycemia and may lead to loss of control). Products include:
- Minizide Capsules 2016

Prednisolone Acetate (Co-administration with corticosteroids tends to produce hyperglycemia and may lead to loss of control). Products include:
- AK-CIDE .... ⓞ 203
- AK-CIDE Ointment .... ⓞ 203
- Blephamide Liquifilm Sterile Ophthalmic Suspension 472
- Blephamide Ointment .... ⓞ 234
- Econopred & Econopred Plus Ophthalmic Suspensions .... ⓞ 216
- Poly-Pred Liquifilm .... ⓞ 246
- Pred Forte .... ⓞ 247
- Pred Mild .... ⓞ 250
- Pred-G Liquifilm Sterile Ophthalmic Suspension .... ⓞ 248
- Pred-G S.O.P. Sterile Ophthalmic Ointment .... ⓞ 249

Prednisolone Sodium Phosphate (Co-administration with corticosteroids tends to produce hyperglycemia and may lead to loss of control). Products include:
- AK-PRED .... ⓞ 204
- Hydeltrasol Injection, Sterile 1708
- Pediapred Oral Solution 1618

Prednisolone Tebutate (Co-administration with corticosteroids tends to produce hyperglycemia and may lead to loss of control). Products include:
- Hydeltra-T.B.A. Sterile Suspension 1710

Prednisone (Co-administration with corticosteroids tends to produce hyperglycemia and may lead to loss of control).
No products indexed under this heading.

Probenecid (Co-administration with probenecid may potentiate hypoglycemic action). Products include:
- Benemid Tablets 1651
- ColBENEMID Tablets 1662

Prochlorperazine (Co-administration with phenothiazines tends to produce hyperglycemia and may lead to loss of control). Products include:
- Compazine 2644

Promethazine Hydrochloride (Co-administration with phenothiazines tends to produce hyperglycemia and may lead to loss of control). Products include:
- Mepergan Injection 2859
- Phenergan with Codeine 2883
- Phenergan with Dextromethorphan 2885
- Phenergan Injection 2880
- Phenergan Suppositories 2882
- Phenergan Syrup 2881
- Phenergan Tablets 2882
- Phenergan VC 2886
- Phenergan VC with Codeine 2888

Propranolol Hydrochloride (Co-administration with beta blockers may potentiate hypoglycemic action; beta blockers may mask signs and symptoms of hypoglycemia). Products include:
- Inderal 2834
- Inderal LA Long Acting Capsules ... 2836
- Inderide Tablets 2838
- Inderide LA Long Acting Capsules .. 2840

Pseudoephedrine Hydrochloride (Co-administration with sympathomimetics tends to produce hyperglycemia and may lead to loss of control). Products include:
- Actifed Allergy Daytime/Nighttime Caplets .... ⓔ 808
- Actifed Cold & Allergy Tablets .... ⓔ 807
- Actifed Cold & Sinus Caplets and Tablets .... ⓔ 808
- Actifed Sinus Daytime/Nighttime Tablets and Caplets .... ⓔ 809
- Advil Cold and Sinus Caplets and Tablets .... ⓔ 837
- Alka-Seltzer Plus Liqui-Gels .... ⓔ 612
- Alka-Seltzer Plus Flu & Body Aches Liqui-Gels Non-Drowsy Formula .... ⓔ 613
- Alka-Seltzer Plus Night-Time Cold Medicine Liqui-Gels .... ⓔ 612
- Allerest Maximum Strength .... ⓔ 649
- Allerest No Drowsiness .... ⓔ 649
- Allerest Sinus Pain Formula .... ⓔ 649
- Atrohist Pediatric Capsules 1603
- Benadryl Allergy/Cold Tablets .... ⓔ 811
- Benadryl Allergy Decongestant Liquid Medication .... ⓔ 812
- Benadryl Allergy Decongestant Tablets .... ⓔ 812
- Benadryl Allergy Sinus Headache Caplets .... ⓔ 813

IMPORTANT NOTE: Always consult each drug listing in the patient's regimen for possible interactions.

| Benylin Multisymptom ▫ 816
| Bromfed Capsules (Extended-Release) 1832
| Bromfed Syrup ▫ 712
| Bromfed Tablets 1832
| Bromfed-DM Cough Syrup ▫ 1832
| Bromfed-PD Capsules (Extended-Release) 1832
| Children's TYLENOL Cold Multi-Symptom Chewable Tablets and Liquid 1559
| Children's TYLENOL Cold Plus Cough Multi Symptom Chewable Tablets and Liquid 1560
| Children's TYLENOL Flu Suspension Liquid 1560
| Children's Vicks DayQuil Allergy Relief ▫ 730
| Children's Vicks NyQuil Cold/Cough Relief ▫ 731
| Allergy-Sinus Comtrex Multi-Symptom Allergy-Sinus Formula Tablets and Caplets ▫ 639
| Comtrex Multi-Symptom ▫ 638
| Comtrex Multi-Symptom Non-Drowsy Caplets ▫ 640
| Congess 1003
| Contac Day Allergy/Sinus Caplets ▫ 771
| Contac Day & Night ▫ 772
| Contac Night Allergy/Sinus Caplets ▫ 771
| Contac Severe Cold & Flu Non-Drowsy ▫ 774
| Deconsal II Tablets 1605
| Dimetane-DX Cough Syrup 2233
| Dimetapp Cold & Fever Suspension ▫ 839
| Dimetapp Decongestant Pediatric Drops ▫ 840
| Dorcol Children's Cough Syrup ▫ 748
| Drixoral Cough + Congestion Liquid Caps ▫ 763
| Dura-Tap/PD Capsules 970
| Duratuss Tablets 2750
| Duratuss HD Elixir 2750
| Efidac/24 ▫ 655
| Entex PSE Tablets 973
| Fedahist Gyrocaps 2545
| Guaifed 1833
| Guaifed Syrup ▫ 712
| Guaimax-D Tablets 809
| Histussin D Liquid 670
| Infants' TYLENOL Cold Decongestant & Fever-Reducer Drops 1561
| Kronofed-A 994
| Novahistine DMX ▫ 782
| Nucofed 2225
| PediaCare Cough-Cold Chewable Tablets and Liquid 1569
| PediaCare Infants' Decongestant Drops 1569
| PediaCare Infants' Drops Decongestant Plus Cough 1569
| PediaCare NightRest Cough-Cold Liquid 1569
| Pediatric Vicks 44d Cough & Head Congestion Relief ▫ 736
| Pediatric Vicks 44m Cough & Cold Relief ▫ 737
| Robitussin Cold & Cough Liqui-Gels ▫ 844
| Robitussin Cold, Cough & Flu Liqui-Gels ▫ 844
| Robitussin Maximum Strength Cough & Cold ▫ 847
| Robitussin Night-Time Cold Formula ▫ 847
| Robitussin Pediatric Cough & Cold Formula ▫ 848
| Robitussin Pediatric Drops ▫ 849
| Robitussin Severe Congestion Liqui-Gels ▫ 845
| Robitussin-DAC Syrup 2249
| Robitussin-PE ▫ 846
| Rondec Oral Drops 974
| Rondec Syrup 974
| Rondec Tablet 974
| Rondec Chewable Tablets 974
| Rondec-TR Tablet 974
| Ryna ▫ 804
| Seldane-D Extended-Release Tablets 1286
| Semprex-D Capsules 1620
| Sinarest ▫ 663
| Sine-Aid Maximum Strength Sinus Headache Gelcaps, Caplets and Tablets 1570
| Sine-Off No Drowsiness Formula Caplets ▫ 784
| Sine-Off Sinus Medicine ▫ 784
| Singlet Tablets ▫ 785
| Sinutab Non-Drying Liquid Caps ▫ 823
| Sinutab Sinus Allergy Medication, Maximum Strength Tablets and Caplets ▫ 823
| Sinutab Sinus Medication, Maximum Strength Without Drowsiness Formula, Tablets & Caplets ▫ 824
| Sudafed Children's Cold & Cough Liquid Medication ▫ 825
| Sudafed Children's Nasal Decongestant Liquid Medication ▫ 826
| Sudafed Cold & Allergy Tablets ▫ 826
| Sudafed Cold and Cough Liquid Caps ▫ 826
| Sudafed Nasal Decongestant Tablets, 30 mg ▫ 825
| Sudafed Nasal Decongestant Tablets, 60 mg ▫ 825
| Sudafed Non-Drying Sinus Liquid Caps ▫ 827
| Sudafed Pediatric Nasal Decongestant Liquid Oral Drops ▫ 827
| Sudafed Severe Cold Formula Caplets ▫ 828
| Sudafed Severe Cold Formula Tablets ▫ 828
| Sudafed Sinus Caplets ▫ 829
| Sudafed Sinus Tablets ▫ 829
| Sudafed 12 Hour Caplets ▫ 824
| Syn-Rx Tablets 1622
| Syn-Rx DM Tablets 1623
| TheraFlu Flu and Cold Medicine ▫ 750
| Theraflu Maximum Strength Flu and Cold Medicine For Sore Throat ▫ 751
| TheraFlu Flu, Cold and Cough Medicine ▫ 750
| TheraFlu Maximum Strength Nighttime Flu, Cold & Cough Medicine ▫ 751
| TheraFlu Maximum Strength Non-Drowsy Formula Flu, Cold & Cough Medicine ▫ 751
| TheraFlu Maximum Strength, Non-Drowsy Formula Flu, Cold and Cough Caplets ▫ 752
| Theraflu Maximum Strength Sinus Non-Drowsy Formula Caplets ▫ 752
| Triaminic AM Cough and Decongestant Formula ▫ 753
| Triaminic AM Decongestant Formula ▫ 753
| Triaminic Infant Oral Decongestant Drops ▫ 754
| Triaminic Night Time ▫ 754
| Triaminic Sore Throat Formula ▫ 755
| Tussend 1830
| Tussend Expectorant 1831
| TYLENOL Allergy Sinus, Maximum Strength Caplets and Gelcaps 1571
| TYLENOL Allergy Sinus NightTime, Maximum Strength Caplets 1571
| TYLENOL Cold Medication, Multi-Symptom Formula Tablets and Caplets 1572
| TYLENOL Cold Medication, Multi-Symptom Hot Liquid Packets 1572
| TYLENOL Cold Medication, No Drowsiness Formula Caplets and Gelcaps 1572
| TYLENOL Cold Severe Congestion Caplets 1573
| TYLENOL Cough Medication with Decongestant, Multi Symptom 1574
| TYLENOL Flu No Drowsiness Formula, Maximum Strength Gelcaps 1575
| TYLENOL Flu NightTime, Maximum Strength Gelcaps 1575
| TYLENOL Flu NightTime, Maximum Strength Hot Medication Packets 1575
| TYLENOL Sinus, Maximum Strength Geltabs, Gelcaps, Caplets and Tablets 1576
| Vicks 44 LiquiCaps Cough, Cold & Flu Relief ▫ 728
| Vicks 44 LiquiCaps Non-Drowsy Cough & Cold Relief ▫ 729
| Vicks 44D Cough & Head Congestion Relief ▫ 728
| Vicks 44M Cough, Cold & Flu Relief ▫ 729
| Vicks DayQuil LiquiCaps/Liquid Multi-Symptom Cold/Flu Relief ▫ 734
| Vicks DayQuil SINUS Pressure & PAIN Relief with IBUPROFEN ▫ 735
| Vicks Nyquil Hot Therapy ▫ 735
| Vicks NyQuil LiquiCaps/Liquid Multi-Symptom Cold/Flu Relief, Original and Cherry Flavors ▫ 736

Pseudoephedrine Sulfate (Co-administration with sympathomimetics tends to produce hyperglycemia and may lead to loss of control). Products include:
| Chlor-Trimeton Allergy Decongestant Tablets ▫ 759
| Claritin-D Tablets 2487
| Drixoral Cold and Allergy Sustained-Action Tablets ▫ 763
| Drixoral Cold and Flu Extended-Release Tablets ▫ 764
| Drixoral Non-Drowsy Formula Extended-Release Tablets ▫ 764
| Drixoral Allergy/Sinus Extended Release Tablets ▫ 765
| Trinalin Repetabs Tablets 1373

Quinestrol (Co-administration with estrogens tends to produce hyperglycemia and may lead to loss of control).
No products indexed under this heading.

Salmeterol Xinafoate (Co-administration with sympathomimetics tends to produce hyperglycemia and may lead to loss of control). Products include:
| Serevent Inhalation Aerosol 1149

Salsalate (Co-administration with salicylates may potentiate hypoglycemic action). Products include:
| Disalcid 1549
| Mono-Gesic Tablets 810
| Salflex Tablets 791

Selegiline Hydrochloride (Co-administration with monoamine oxidase inhibitors may potentiate hypoglycemic action). Products include:
| Eldepryl Capsules 2729

Sotalol Hydrochloride (Co-administration with beta blockers may potentiate hypoglycemic action; beta blockers may mask signs and symptoms of hypoglycemia). Products include:
| Betapace Tablets 637

Spironolactone (Co-administration with diuretics tends to produce hyperglycemia and may lead to loss of control). Products include:
| Aldactazide Tablets 2556
| Aldactone Tablets 2558

Sulfacytine (Co-administration with sulfonamides may potentiate hypoglycemic action).

Sulfamethizole (Co-administration with sulfonamides may potentiate hypoglycemic action). Products include:
| Urobiotic-250 Capsules 2038

Sulfamethoxazole (Co-administration with sulfonamides may potentiate hypoglycemic action). Products include:
| Bactrim DS Tablets 2257
| Bactrim I.V. Infusion 2255
| Bactrim 2257
| Gantanol Tablets 2285
| Septra 1146
| Septra I.V. Infusion 1142
| Septra I.V. Infusion ADD-Vantage Vials 1144
| Septra 1146

Sulfasalazine (Co-administration with sulfonamides may potentiate hypoglycemic action). Products include:
| Azulfidine 2059

Sulfinpyrazone (Co-administration with sulfonamides may potentiate hypoglycemic action). Products include:
| Anturane 823

Sulfisoxazole (Co-administration with sulfonamides may potentiate hypoglycemic action). Products include:
| Gantrisin Tablets 2286

Sulfisoxazole Diolamine (Co-administration with sulfonamides may potentiate hypoglycemic action).
No products indexed under this heading.

Sulindac (Co-administration with nonsteroidal anti-inflammatory agents may potentiate hypoglycemic action). Products include:
| Clinoril Tablets 1658

Terbutaline Sulfate (Co-administration with sympathomimetics tends to produce hyperglycemia and may lead to loss of control). Products include:
| Brethaire Inhaler 830
| Brethine Ampuls 832
| Brethine Tablets 831
| Bricanyl Subcutaneous Injection 1247
| Bricanyl Tablets 1248

Thioridazine Hydrochloride (Co-administration with phenothiazines tends to produce hyperglycemia and may lead to loss of control). Products include:
| Mellaril 2398

Thyroglobulin (Co-administration with thyroid preparations tends to produce hyperglycemia and may lead to loss of control).
No products indexed under this heading.

Thyroid (Co-administration with thyroid preparations tends to produce hyperglycemia and may lead to loss of control).
No products indexed under this heading.

Thyroxine (Co-administration with thyroid preparations tends to produce hyperglycemia and may lead to loss of control).
No products indexed under this heading.

Thyroxine Sodium (Co-administration with thyroid preparations tends to produce hyperglycemia and may lead to loss of control).
No products indexed under this heading.

Timolol Hemihydrate (Co-administration with beta blockers may potentiate hypoglycemic action; beta blockers may mask signs and symptoms of hypoglycemia). Products include:
| Betimol 0.25%, 0.5% ⊙ 259

Timolol Maleate (Co-administration with beta blockers may potentiate hypoglycemic action; beta blockers may mask signs and symptoms of hypoglycemia). Products include:
| Blocadren Tablets 1654
| Timolide Tablets 1791
| Timoptic in Ocudose 1796
| Timoptic Sterile Ophthalmic Solution 1794
| Timoptic-XE 1798

Tolazamide (Co-administration with sulfonamides may potentiate hypoglycemic action).
No products indexed under this heading.

Tolbutamide (Co-administration with sulfonamides may potentiate hypoglycemic action).
No products indexed under this heading.

Tolmetin Sodium (Co-administration with nonsteroidal anti-inflammatory agents may potentiate hypoglycemic action). Products include:
| Tolectin (200, 400 and 600 mg) 1591

(▫ Described in PDR For Nonprescription Drugs)   (⊙ Described in PDR For Ophthalmology)

459 Interactions Index Gris-Peg

Torsemide (Co-administration with diuretics tends to produce hyperglycemia and may lead to loss of control). Products include:
Demadex Tablets and Injection 691
Tranylcypromine Sulfate (Co-administration with monoamine oxidase inhibitors may potentiate hypoglycemic action). Products include:
Parnate Tablets 2679
Triamcinolone (Co-administration with corticosteroids tends to produce hyperglycemia and may lead to loss of control).
No products indexed under this heading.
Triamcinolone Acetonide (Co-administration with corticosteroids tends to produce hyperglycemia and may lead to loss of control). Products include:
Azmacort Oral Inhaler 2175
Nasacort AQ Nasal Spray 2191
Nasacort Nasal Inhaler 2189
Triamcinolone Diacetate (Co-administration with corticosteroids tends to produce hyperglycemia and may lead to loss of control).
No products indexed under this heading.
Triamcinolone Hexacetonide (Co-administration with corticosteroids tends to produce hyperglycemia and may lead to loss of control).
No products indexed under this heading.
Triamterene (Co-administration with diuretics tends to produce hyperglycemia and may lead to loss of control). Products include:
Dyazide Capsules 2653
Dyrenium Capsules 2655
Trifluoperazine Hydrochloride (Co-administration with phenothiazines tends to produce hyperglycemia and may lead to loss of control). Products include:
Stelazine 2692
Verapamil Hydrochloride (Co-administration with calcium channel blockers tends to produce hyperglycemia and may lead to loss of control). Products include:
Calan SR Caplets 2571
Calan Tablets 2568
Covera-HS Tablets 2573
Isoptin Injectable 1391
Isoptin Oral Tablets 1393
Isoptin SR Tablets 1395
Verelan Capsules 1455
Warfarin Sodium (Co-administration may potentiate or weaken the effects of coumarin derivatives). Products include:
Coumadin 941

GLY-OXIDE LIQUID
(Carbamide Peroxide) 779
None cited in PDR database.

GOLYTELY
(Polyethylene Glycol) 694
May interact with:

Oral Medications, unspecified (Those administered within one hour of GoLYTELY usage may be flushed from the gastrointestinal tract and not absorbed).

Food Interactions
Food, unspecified (For best results, no solid food should be consumed during 3 to 4 hour period before drinking solution).

GOODY'S EXTRA STRENGTH HEADACHE POWDERS
(Aspirin, Acetaminophen, Caffeine) 632
None cited in PDR database.

GOODY'S EXTRA STRENGTH PAIN RELIEF TABLETS
(Aspirin, Acetaminophen, Caffeine) 632
None cited in PDR database.

GRANULEX
(Trypsin, Balsam Peru, Castor Oil) 940
None cited in PDR database.

GRIFULVIN V (GRISEOFULVIN TABLETS) MICROSIZE (GRISEOFULVIN ORAL SUSPENSION) MICROSIZE
(Griseofulvin) 1944
May interact with oral anticoagulants, barbiturates, and oral contraceptives. Compounds in these categories include:
Aprobarbital (Usually depresses griseofulvin activity; may necessitate dosage increase).
No products indexed under this heading.
Butabarbital (Usually depresses griseofulvin activity; may necessitate dosage increase).
No products indexed under this heading.
Butalbital (Usually depresses griseofulvin activity; may necessitate dosage increase). Products include:
Axocet Capsules 2469
Esgic-plus Capsules 1012
Esgic-plus Tablets 1012
Fioricet Tablets 2386
Fioricet with Codeine Capsules 2387
Fiorinal Capsules 2388
Fiorinal with Codeine Capsules 2390
Fiorinal Tablets 2388
Phrenilin 790
Sedapap Tablets 50 mg/650 mg .. 1826
Desogestrel (Reduced contraceptive efficacy; increased incidence of breakthrough bleeding). Products include:
Desogen Tablets 1867
Ortho-Cept 1907
Dicumarol (Dosage adjustment of anticoagulant may be necessary).
No products indexed under this heading.
Ethinyl Estradiol (Reduced contraceptive efficacy; increased incidence of breakthrough bleeding). Products include:
Brevicon 2563
Demulen 2580
Desogen Tablets 1867
Levlen/Tri-Levlen 646
Lo/Ovral Tablets 2852
Lo/Ovral-28 Tablets 2857
Modicon 1928
Nordette-21 Tablets 2863
Nordette-28 Tablets 2866
Norinyl 2563
Ortho-Cept 1907
Ortho-Cyclen/Ortho-Tri-Cyclen 1914
Ortho-Novum 1928
Ortho-Cyclen/Ortho Tri-Cyclen 1914
Ovcon 765
Ovral Tablets 2877
Ovral-28 Tablets 2878
Levlen/Tri-Levlen 646
Tri-Norinyl 2607
Triphasil-21 Tablets 2919
Triphasil-28 Tablets 2924
Ethynodiol Diacetate (Reduced contraceptive efficacy; increased incidence of breakthrough bleeding). Products include:
Demulen 2580
Levonorgestrel (Reduced contraceptive efficacy; increased incidence of breakthrough bleeding). Products include:
Levlen/Tri-Levlen 646
Nordette-21 Tablets 2863
Nordette-28 Tablets 2866
Norplant System 2868
Levlen/Tri-Levlen 646
Triphasil-21 Tablets 2919
Triphasil-28 Tablets 2924
Mephobarbital (Usually depresses griseofulvin activity; may necessitate dosage increase). Products include:
Mebaral Tablets 2452
Mestranol (Reduced contraceptive efficacy; increased incidence of breakthrough bleeding). Products include:
Norinyl 2563
Ortho-Novum 1928
Norethindrone (Reduced contraceptive efficacy; increased incidence of breakthrough bleeding). Products include:
Brevicon 2563
Micronor Tablets 1903
Modicon 1928
Norinyl 2563
Nor-Q D Tablets 2598
Ortho-Novum 1928
Ovcon 765
Tri-Norinyl 2607
Norethynodrel (Reduced contraceptive efficacy; increased incidence of breakthrough bleeding).
No products indexed under this heading.
Norgestimate (Reduced contraceptive efficacy; increased incidence of breakthrough bleeding). Products include:
Ortho-Cyclen/Ortho-Tri-Cyclen 1914
Ortho-Cyclen/Ortho Tri-Cyclen 1914
Norgestrel (Reduced contraceptive efficacy; increased incidence of breakthrough bleeding). Products include:
Lo/Ovral Tablets 2852
Lo/Ovral-28 Tablets 2857
Ovral Tablets 2877
Ovral-28 Tablets 2878
Ovrette Tablets 2878
Pentobarbital Sodium (Usually depresses griseofulvin activity; may necessitate dosage increase). Products include:
Nembutal Sodium Capsules 440
Nembutal Sodium Solution 442
Nembutal Sodium Suppositories 444
Phenobarbital (Usually depresses griseofulvin activity; may necessitate dosage increase). Products include:
Arco-Lase Plus Tablets 513
Bellergal-S Tablets 2375
Donnatal 2234
Donnatal Extentabs 2234
Donnatal Tablets 2234
Phenobarbital Elixir and Tablets 1523
Quadrinal Tablets 1398
Secobarbital Sodium (Usually depresses griseofulvin activity; may necessitate dosage increase). Products include:
Seconal Sodium Pulvules 1529
Thiamylal Sodium (Usually depresses griseofulvin activity; may necessitate dosage increase).
No products indexed under this heading.
Warfarin Sodium (Dosage adjustment of anticoagulant may be necessary). Products include:
Coumadin 941

GRIS-PEG TABLETS, 125 MG & 250 MG
(Griseofulvin) 476
May interact with oral anticoagulants, barbiturates, oral contraceptives, and certain other agents. Compounds in these categories include:
Aprobarbital (Barbiturates usually depress griseofulvin activity and co-administration may require dosage adjustment of the antifungal agent).
No products indexed under this heading.
Butabarbital (Barbiturates usually depress griseofulvin activity and co-administration may require dosage adjustment of the antifungal agent).
No products indexed under this heading.
Butalbital (Barbiturates usually depress griseofulvin activity and co-administration may require dosage adjustment of the antifungal agent). Products include:
Axocet Capsules 2469
Esgic-plus Capsules 1012
Esgic-plus Tablets 1012
Fioricet Tablets 2386
Fioricet with Codeine Capsules 2387
Fiorinal Capsules 2388
Fiorinal with Codeine Capsules 2390
Fiorinal Tablets 2388
Phrenilin 790
Sedapap Tablets 50 mg/650 mg .. 1826
Desogestrel (Co-administration with oral contraceptives has been shown to result in breakthrough bleeding and spotting based on literature reports). Products include:
Desogen Tablets 1867
Ortho-Cept 1907
Dicumarol (Decreased activity of anticoagulants; dosage adjustment may be required).
No products indexed under this heading.
Ethinyl Estradiol (Co-administration with oral contraceptives has been shown to result in breakthrough bleeding and spotting based on literature reports). Products include:
Brevicon 2563
Demulen 2580
Desogen Tablets 1867
Levlen/Tri-Levlen 646
Lo/Ovral Tablets 2852
Lo/Ovral-28 Tablets 2857
Modicon 1928
Nordette-21 Tablets 2863
Nordette-28 Tablets 2866
Norinyl 2563
Ortho-Cept 1907
Ortho-Cyclen/Ortho-Tri-Cyclen 1914
Ortho-Novum 1928
Ortho-Cyclen/Ortho Tri-Cyclen 1914
Ovcon 765
Ovral Tablets 2877
Ovral-28 Tablets 2878
Levlen/Tri-Levlen 646
Tri-Norinyl 2607
Triphasil-21 Tablets 2919
Triphasil-28 Tablets 2924
Ethynodiol Diacetate (Co-administration with oral contraceptives has been shown to result in breakthrough bleeding and spotting based on literature reports). Products include:
Demulen 2580
Levonorgestrel (Co-administration with oral contraceptives has been shown to result in breakthrough bleeding and spotting based on literature reports). Products include:
Levlen/Tri-Levlen 646
Nordette-21 Tablets 2863
Nordette-28 Tablets 2866
Norplant System 2868
Levlen/Tri-Levlen 646
Triphasil-21 Tablets 2919
Triphasil-28 Tablets 2924

Mephobarbital (Barbiturates usually depress griseofulvin activity and co-administration may require dosage adjustment of the antifungal agent). Products include:
- Mebaral Tablets ... 2452

Mestranol (Co-administration with oral contraceptives has been shown to result in breakthrough bleeding and spotting based on literature reports). Products include:
- Norinyl ... 2563
- Ortho-Novum ... 1928

Norethindrone (Co-administration with oral contraceptives has been shown to result in breakthrough bleeding and spotting based on literature reports). Products include:
- Brevicon ... 2563
- Micronor Tablets ... 1903
- Modicon ... 1928
- Norinyl ... 2563
- Nor-Q D Tablets ... 2598
- Ortho-Novum ... 1928
- Ovcon ... 765
- Tri-Norinyl ... 2607

Norethynodrel (Co-administration with oral contraceptives has been shown to result in breakthrough bleeding and spotting based on literature reports).
- No products indexed under this heading.

Norgestimate (Co-administration with oral contraceptives has been shown to result in breakthrough bleeding and spotting based on literature reports). Products include:
- Ortho-Cyclen/Ortho-Tri-Cyclen ... 1914
- Ortho-Cyclen/Ortho Tri-Cyclen ... 1914

Norgestrel (Co-administration with oral contraceptives has been shown to result in breakthrough bleeding and spotting based on literature reports). Products include:
- Lo/Ovral Tablets ... 2852
- Lo/Ovral-28 Tablets ... 2857
- Ovral Tablets ... 2877
- Ovral-28 Tablets ... 2878
- Ovrette Tablets ... 2878

Pentobarbital Sodium (Barbiturates usually depress griseofulvin activity and co-administration may require dosage adjustment of the antifungal agent). Products include:
- Nembutal Sodium Capsules ... 440
- Nembutal Sodium Solution ... 442
- Nembutal Sodium Suppositories ... 444

Phenobarbital (Barbiturates usually depress griseofulvin activity and co-administration may require dosage adjustment of the antifungal agent). Products include:
- Arco-Lase Plus Tablets ... 513
- Bellergal-S Tablets ... 2375
- Donnatal ... 2234
- Donnatal Extentabs ... 2234
- Donnatal Tablets ... 2234
- Phenobarbital Elixir and Tablets ... 1523
- Quadrinal Tablets ... 1398

Secobarbital Sodium (Barbiturates usually depress griseofulvin activity and co-administration may require dosage adjustment of the antifungal agent). Products include:
- Seconal Sodium Pulvules ... 1529

Thiamylal Sodium (Barbiturates usually depress griseofulvin activity and co-administration may require dosage adjustment of the antifungal agent).
- No products indexed under this heading.

Warfarin Sodium (Decreased activity of anticoagulants; dosage adjustment may be required). Products include:
- Coumadin ... 941

Food Interactions

Alcohol (Griseofulvin potentiates the effects of alcohol, producing tachycardia and flushing).

GUAIFED CAPSULES (EXTENDED-RELEASE)

(Guaifenesin, Pseudoephedrine Hydrochloride) ... 1833

May interact with monoamine oxidase inhibitors, beta blockers, veratrum alkaloids, cardiac glycosides, and certain other agents. Compounds in these categories include:

Acebutolol Hydrochloride (Increased effect of sympathomimetic). Products include:
- Sectral Capsules ... 2914

Antidepressant Medications, unspecified (Effect not specified).

Atenolol (Increased effect of sympathomimetic). Products include:
- Tenoretic Tablets ... 2963
- Tenormin Tablets and I.V. Injection 2965

Betaxolol Hydrochloride (Increased effect of sympathomimetic). Products include:
- Betoptic Ophthalmic Solution ... 465
- Betoptic S Ophthalmic Suspension 467
- Kerlone Tablets ... 2588

Bisoprolol Fumarate (Increased effect of sympathomimetic). Products include:
- Zebeta Tablets ... 1457
- Ziac ... 1459

Blood Pressure Medications, unspecified (Effect not specified).
- No products indexed under this heading.

Carteolol Hydrochloride (Increased effect of sympathomimetic). Products include:
- Cartrol Tablets ... 413
- Ocupress Ophthalmic Solution, 1% Sterile ... ⊙ 297

Cryptenamine Preparations (Reduced antihypertensive effects).

Deslanoside (Increased possibility of cardiac arrhythmias).
- No products indexed under this heading.

Digitoxin (Increased possibility of cardiac arrhythmias). Products include:
- Crystodigin Tablets ... 1472

Digoxin (Increased possibility of cardiac arrhythmias). Products include:
- Lanoxicaps ... 1110
- Lanoxin Elixir Pediatric ... 1113
- Lanoxin Injection ... 1116
- Lanoxin Injection Pediatric ... 1119
- Lanoxin Tablets ... 1121

Esmolol Hydrochloride (Increased effect of sympathomimetic). Products include:
- Brevibloc (esmolol HCl) Injection ... 1860

Furazolidone (Increased effect of sympathomimetic; concurrent therapy is contraindicated). Products include:
- Furoxone ... 2221

Isocarboxazid (Increased effect of sympathomimetic; concurrent therapy is contraindicated).
- No products indexed under this heading.

Labetalol Hydrochloride (Increased effect of sympathomimetic). Products include:
- Normodyne Injection ... 2519
- Normodyne Tablets ... 2522
- Trandate ... 1158

Levobunolol Hydrochloride (Increased effect of sympathomimetic). Products include:
- Betagan ... ⊙ 230

Mecamylamine Hydrochloride (Reduced antihypertensive effects). Products include:
- Inversine Tablets ... 1729

Methyldopa (Reduced antihypertensive effects). Products include:
- Aldoclor Tablets ... 1638
- Aldomet Oral ... 1640
- Aldoril Tablets ... 1644

Methyldopate Hydrochloride (Reduced antihypertensive effects). Products include:
- Aldomet Ester HCl Injection ... 1642

Metipranolol Hydrochloride (Increased effect of sympathomimetic). Products include:
- OptiPranolol (Metipranolol 0.3%) Sterile Ophthalmic Solution ... ⊙ 256

Metoprolol Succinate (Increased effect of sympathomimetic). Products include:
- Toprol-XL Tablets ... 560

Metoprolol Tartrate (Increased effect of sympathomimetic). Products include:
- Lopressor ... 848
- Lopressor HCT Tablets ... 850

Nadolol (Increased effect of sympathomimetic).
- No products indexed under this heading.

Penbutolol Sulfate (Increased effect of sympathomimetic). Products include:
- Levatol Tablets ... 2547

Phenelzine Sulfate (Increased effect of sympathomimetic; concurrent therapy is contraindicated). Products include:
- Nardil ... 1977

Pindolol (Increased effect of sympathomimetic). Products include:
- Visken Tablets ... 2428

Propranolol Hydrochloride (Increased effect of sympathomimetic). Products include:
- Inderal ... 2834
- Inderal LA Long Acting Capsules ... 2836
- Inderide Tablets ... 2838
- Inderide LA Long Acting Capsules .. 2840

Reserpine (Reduced antihypertensive effects). Products include:
- Diupres Tablets ... 1691
- Hydropres Tablets ... 1718
- Ser-Ap-Es Tablets ... 867

Selegiline Hydrochloride (Increased effect of sympathomimetic; concurrent therapy is contraindicated). Products include:
- Eldepryl Capsules ... 2729

Sotalol Hydrochloride (Increased effect of sympathomimetic). Products include:
- Betapace Tablets ... 637

Timolol Hemihydrate (Increased effect of sympathomimetic). Products include:
- Betimol 0.25%, 0.5% ... ⊙ 259

Timolol Maleate (Increased effect of sympathomimetic). Products include:
- Blocadren Tablets ... 1654
- Timolide Tablets ... 1791
- Timoptic in Ocudose ... 1796
- Timoptic Sterile Ophthalmic Solution ... 1794
- Timoptic-XE ... 1798

Tranylcypromine Sulfate (Increased effect of sympathomimetic; concurrent therapy is contraindicated). Products include:
- Parnate Tablets ... 2679

GUAIFED-PD CAPSULES (EXTENDED-RELEASE)

(Guaifenesin, Pseudoephedrine Hydrochloride) ... 1833

See **Guaifed Capsules (Extended-Release)**

GUAIFED SYRUP

(Guaifenesin, Pseudoephedrine Hydrochloride) ... ▣ 712

May interact with monoamine oxidase inhibitors. Compounds in this category include:

Furazolidone (Concurrent and/or sequential use is not recommended). Products include:
- Furoxone ... 2221

Isocarboxazid (Concurrent and/or sequential use is not recommended).
- No products indexed under this heading.

Phenelzine Sulfate (Concurrent and/or sequential use is not recommended). Products include:
- Nardil ... 1977

Selegiline Hydrochloride (Concurrent and/or sequential use is not recommended). Products include:
- Eldepryl Capsules ... 2729

Tranylcypromine Sulfate (Concurrent and/or sequential use is not recommended). Products include:
- Parnate Tablets ... 2679

GUAIMAX-D TABLETS

(Pseudoephedrine Hydrochloride, Guaifenesin) ... 809

May interact with monoamine oxidase inhibitors, beta blockers, veratrum alkaloids, catecholamine depleting drugs, and certain other agents. Compounds in these categories include:

Acebutolol Hydrochloride (Increases effects of sympathomimetics). Products include:
- Sectral Capsules ... 2914

Atenolol (Increases effects of sympathomimetics). Products include:
- Tenoretic Tablets ... 2963
- Tenormin Tablets and I.V. Injection 2965

Betaxolol Hydrochloride (Increases effects of sympathomimetics). Products include:
- Betoptic Ophthalmic Solution ... 465
- Betoptic S Ophthalmic Suspension 467
- Kerlone Tablets ... 2588

Bisoprolol Fumarate (Increases effects of sympathomimetics). Products include:
- Zebeta Tablets ... 1457
- Ziac ... 1459

Carteolol Hydrochloride (Increases effects of sympathomimetics). Products include:
- Cartrol Tablets ... 413
- Ocupress Ophthalmic Solution, 1% Sterile ... ⊙ 297

Cryptenamine Preparations (Reduced antihypertensive effects).

Deserpidine (Reduced antihypertensive effects).
- No products indexed under this heading.

Esmolol Hydrochloride (Increases effects of sympathomimetics). Products include:
- Brevibloc (esmolol HCl) Injection ... 1860

Furazolidone (Increases effects of sympathomimetics; concurrent use is contraindicated). Products include:
- Furoxone ... 2221

Guanethidine Monosulfate (Reduced antihypertensive effects). Products include:
- Esimil Tablets ... 840
- Ismelin Tablets ... 845

Isocarboxazid (Increases effects of sympathomimetics; concurrent use is contraindicated).
- No products indexed under this heading.

(▣ Described in PDR For Nonprescription Drugs) (⊙ Described in PDR For Ophthalmology)

461 **Interactions Index** **Habitrol**

Labetalol Hydrochloride (Increases effects of sympathomimetics). Products include:
Normodyne Injection ... 2519
Normodyne Tablets ... 2522
Trandate ... 1158
Levobunolol Hydrochloride (Increases effects of sympathomimetics). Products include:
Betagan ... ◉ 230
Mecamylamine Hydrochloride (Reduced antihypertensive effects). Products include:
Inversine Tablets ... 1729
Methyldopa (Reduced antihypertensive effects). Products include:
Aldoclor Tablets ... 1638
Aldomet Oral ... 1640
Aldoril Tablets ... 1644
Metipranolol Hydrochloride (Increases effects of sympathomimetics). Products include:
OptiPranolol (Metipranolol 0.3%) Sterile Ophthalmic Solution ... ◉ 256
Metoprolol Succinate (Increases effects of sympathomimetics). Products include:
Toprol-XL Tablets ... 560
Metoprolol Tartrate (Increases effects of sympathomimetics). Products include:
Lopressor ... 848
Lopressor HCT Tablets ... 850
Nadolol (Increases effects of sympathomimetics).
No products indexed under this heading.
Penbutolol Sulfate (Increases effects of sympathomimetics). Products include:
Levatol Tablets ... 2547
Phenelzine Sulfate (Increases effects of sympathomimetics; concurrent use is contraindicated). Products include:
Nardil ... 1977
Pindolol (Increases effects of sympathomimetics). Products include:
Visken Tablets ... 2428
Propranolol Hydrochloride (Increases effects of sympathomimetics). Products include:
Inderal ... 2834
Inderal LA Long Acting Capsules ... 2836
Inderide Tablets ... 2838
Inderide LA Long Acting Capsules .. 2840
Rauwolfia Serpentina (Reduced antihypertensive effects).
No products indexed under this heading.
Rescinnamine (Reduced antihypertensive effects).
No products indexed under this heading.
Reserpine (Reduced antihypertensive effects). Products include:
Diupres Tablets ... 1691
Hydropres Tablets ... 1718
Ser-Ap-Es Tablets ... 867
Selegiline Hydrochloride (Increases effects of sympathomimetics; concurrent use is contraindicated). Products include:
Eldepryl Capsules ... 2729
Sotalol Hydrochloride (Increases effects of sympathomimetics). Products include:
Betapace Tablets ... 637
Timolol Hemihydrate (Increases effects of sympathomimetics). Products include:
Betimol 0.25%, 0.5% ... ◉ 259
Timolol Maleate (Increases effects of sympathomimetics). Products include:
Blocadren Tablets ... 1654
Timolide Tablets ... 1791
Timoptic in Ocudose ... 1796
Timoptic Sterile Ophthalmic Solution ... 1794
Timoptic-XE ... 1798
Tranylcypromine Sulfate (Increases effects of sympathomimetics; concurrent use is contraindicated). Products include:
Parnate Tablets ... 2679

HMS LIQUIFILM
(Medrysone) ... ◉ 241
None cited in PDR database.

HABITROL NICOTINE TRANSDERMAL SYSTEM
(Nicotine) ... 884
May interact with insulin and certain other agents. Compounds in these categories include:

Acetaminophen (Deinduction of hepatic enzymes on smoking cessation; may require a decrease in dose at cessation of smoking). Products include:
Actifed Cold & Sinus Caplets and Tablets ... ▣ 808
Actifed Sinus Daytime/Nighttime Tablets and Caplets ... ▣ 809
Alka-Seltzer Fast Relief Caplets ... ▣ 610
Alka-Seltzer Plus Liqui-Gels ... ▣ 612
Alka-Seltzer Plus Flu & Body Aches Effervescent Tablets ... ▣ 612
Alka-Seltzer Plus Flu & Body Aches Liqui-Gels Non-Drowsy Formula ... ▣ 613
Alka-Seltzer Plus Night-Time Cold Medicine Liqui-Gels ... ▣ 612
Allerest No Drowsiness ... ▣ 649
Allerest Sinus Pain Formula ... ▣ 649
Axocet Capsules ... 2469
Benadryl Allergy/Cold Tablets ... ▣ 811
Benadryl Allergy Sinus Headache Caplets ... ▣ 813
Children's TYLENOL acetaminophen Chewable Tablets, Elixir, Suspension Liquid, and Suspension Drops ... 1559
Children's TYLENOL Cold Multi-Symptom Chewable Tablets and Liquid ... 1559
Children's TYLENOL Cold Plus Cough Multi Symptom Chewable Tablets and Liquid ... 1560
Children's TYLENOL Flu Suspension Liquid ... 1560
Allergy-Sinus Comtrex Multi-Symptom Allergy-Sinus Formula Tablets and Caplets ... ▣ 639
Comtrex Multi-Symptom ... ▣ 638
Comtrex Non-Drowsy ... ▣ 640
Contac Day Allergy/Sinus Caplets ▣ 771
Contac Day & Night ... ▣ 772
Contac Night Allergy/Sinus Caplets ... ▣ 771
Contac Severe Cold and Flu Formula Caplets ... ▣ 773
Contac Severe Cold & Flu Non-Drowsy ... ▣ 774
Coricidin Cold + Flu Tablets ... ▣ 760
Coricidin 'D' Decongestant Tablets ... ▣ 760
DHCplus Capsules ... 2148
Darvon-N/Darvocet-N ... 1473
Dimetapp Allergy Sinus Caplets ... ▣ 838
Dimetapp Cold & Fever Suspension ... ▣ 839
Drixoral Cold and Flu Extended-Release Tablets ... ▣ 764
Drixoral Cough + Sore Throat Liquid Caps ... ▣ 763
Drixoral Allergy/Sinus Extended Release Tablets ... ▣ 765
Esgic-plus Capsules ... 1012
Esgic-plus Tablets ... 1012
Aspirin Free Excedrin Analgesic Caplets and Geltabs ... 734
Excedrin Extra-Strength Analgesic Tablets, Caplets, and Geltabs ... 734
Excedrin P.M. Analgesic/Sleeping Aid Tablets, Caplets, Liquigels ... 735
Fioricet Tablets ... 2386
Fioricet with Codeine Capsules ... 2387
Goody's Extra Strength Headache Powders ... ▣ 632
Goody's Extra Strength Pain Relief Tablets ... ▣ 632
Hycomine Compound Tablets ... 948
Hydrocet Capsules ... 787
Infants' TYLENOL acetaminophen Suspension Drops ... 1559
Infants' TYLENOL Cold Decongestant & Fever-Reducer Drops ... 1561
Junior Strength TYLENOL acetaminophen Coated Caplets and Chewable Tablets ... 1562
Lorcet 10/650 Tablets ... 1016
Lortab ... 2751
Lurline PMS Tablets ... 1000
Maximum Strength Multi-Symptom Formula Midol ... ▣ 621
PMS Multi-Symptom Formula Midol ... ▣ 622
Maximum Strength Midol Teen Multi-Symptom Formula ... ▣ 621
Midrin Capsules ... 788
Panodol Tablets and Caplets ... ▣ 783
Children's Panadol Chewable Tablets, Liquid, Infant's Drops ... ▣ 783
Percocet Tablets ... 955
Percogesic Analgesic Tablets ... ▣ 727
Phrenilin ... 790
Pyrroxate Caplets ... ▣ 742
Robitussin Cold, Cough & Flu Liqui-Gels ... ▣ 844
Robitussin Night-Time Cold Formula ... ▣ 847
Sedapap Tablets 50 mg/650 mg .. 1826
Sinarest ... ▣ 663
Sine-Aid Maximum Strength Sinus Headache Gelcaps, Caplets and Tablets ... 1570
Sine-Off No Drowsiness Formula Caplets ... ▣ 784
Sine-Off Sinus Medicine ... ▣ 784
Singlet Tablets ... ▣ 785
Sinulin Tablets ... 792
Sinutab Sinus Allergy Medication, Maximum Strength Tablets and Caplets ... ▣ 823
Sinutab Sinus Medication, Maximum Strength Without Drowsiness Formula, Tablets & Caplets ... ▣ 824
Sudafed Cold and Cough Liquid Caps ... ▣ 826
Sudafed Severe Cold Formula Caplets ... ▣ 828
Sudafed Severe Cold Formula Tablets ... ▣ 828
Sudafed Sinus Caplets ... ▣ 829
Sudafed Sinus Tablets ... ▣ 829
Talacen Caplets ... 2464
TheraFlu Flu and Cold Medicine ... ▣ 750
Theraflu Maximum Strength Flu and Cold Medicine For Sore Throat ... ▣ 751
TheraFlu Flu, Cold and Cough Medicine ... ▣ 750
TheraFlu Maximum Strength Nighttime Flu, Cold & Cough Medicine ... ▣ 751
TheraFlu Maximum Strength Non-Drowsy Formula Flu, Cold & Cough Medicine ... ▣ 751
TheraFlu Maximum Strength, Non-Drowsy Formula Flu, Cold and Cough Caplets ... ▣ 752
Theraflu Maximum Strength Sinus Non-Drowsy Formula Caplets ... ▣ 752
Triaminic Sore Throat Formula ... ▣ 755
Triaminicin Tablets ... ▣ 756
TYLENOL acetaminophen Extended Relief Caplets ... 1570
TYLENOL acetaminophen, Extra Strength Adult Liquid Pain Reliever ... 1570
TYLENOL acetaminophen, Extra Strength Gelcaps, Geltabs, Caplets, Tablets ... 1570
TYLENOL acetaminophen, Regular Strength Caplets and Tablets ... 1570
TYLENOL Allergy Sinus, Maximum Strength Caplets and Gelcaps ... 1571
TYLENOL Allergy Sinus NightTime, Maximum Strength Caplets ... 1571
TYLENOL Cold Medication, Multi-Symptom Formula Tablets and Caplets ... 1572
TYLENOL Cold Medication, Multi-Symptom Hot Liquid Packets ... 1572
TYLENOL Cold Medication, No Drowsiness Formula Caplets and Gelcaps ... 1572
TYLENOL Cold Severe Congestion Caplets ... 1573
TYLENOL Cough Medication, Multi Symptom ... 1574
TYLENOL Cough Medication with Decongestant, Multi Symptom ... 1574
TYLENOL Flu No Drowsiness Formula, Maximum Strength Gelcaps ... 1575
TYLENOL Flu NightTime, Maximum Strength Gelcaps ... 1575
TYLENOL Flu NightTime, Maximum Strength Hot Medication Packets ... 1575
TYLENOL Headache Plus Pain Reliever with Antacid, Extra Strength Caplets ... ▣ 705
TYLENOL PM Pain Reliever/Sleep Aid, Extra Strength Gelcaps, Caplets, Geltabs ... 1576
TYLENOL Severe Allergy Medication Caplets ... 1571
TYLENOL Sinus, Maximum Strength Geltabs, Gelcaps, Caplets and Tablets ... 1576
Tylenol with Codeine ... 1592
Tylox Capsules ... 1593
Unisom With Pain Relief-Nighttime Sleep Aid and Pain Reliever ... 1991
Vanquish Analgesic Caplets ... ▣ 627
Vicks 44 LiquiCaps Cough, Cold & Flu Relief ... ▣ 728
Vicks 44M Cough, Cold & Flu Relief ... ▣ 729
Vicks DayQuil LiquiCaps/Liquid Multi-Symptom Cold/Flu Relief .. ▣ 734
Vicks Nyquil Hot Therapy ... ▣ 735
Vicks NyQuil LiquiCaps/Liquid Multi-Symptom Cold/Flu Relief, Original and Cherry Flavors ... ▣ 736
Vicodin Tablets ... 1404
Vicodin ES Tablets ... 1405
Vicodin HP Tablets ... 1403
Wygesic Tablets ... 2930
Zydone Capsules ... 967
Aminophylline (Deinduction of hepatic enzymes on smoking cessation; may require a decrease in dose at cessation of smoking).
No products indexed under this heading.
Caffeine (Deinduction of hepatic enzymes on smoking cessation; may require a decrease in dose at cessation of smoking). Products include:
Arthritis Strength BC Powder ... ▣ 631
BC Powder ... ▣ 631
Cafergot ... 2376
DHCplus Capsules ... 2148
Darvon Compound-65 Pulvules ... 1475
Esgic-plus Capsules ... 1012
Esgic-plus Tablets ... 1012
Aspirin Free Excedrin Analgesic Caplets and Geltabs ... 734
Excedrin Extra-Strength Analgesic Tablets, Caplets, and Geltabs ... 734
Fioricet Tablets ... 2386
Fioricet with Codeine Capsules ... 2387
Fiorinal Capsules ... 2388
Fiorinal with Codeine Capsules ... 2390
Fiorinal Tablets ... 2388
Goody's Extra Strength Headache Powders ... ▣ 632
Goody's Extra Strength Pain Relief Tablets ... ▣ 632
Maximum Strength Multi-Symptom Formula Midol ... ▣ 621
No Doz Maximum Strength Caplets ... ▣ 644
Norgesic ... 1554
Vanquish Analgesic Caplets ... ▣ 627
Wigraine Tablets ... 1884
Caffeine Anhydrous (Deinduction of hepatic enzymes on smoking cessation; may require a decrease in dose at cessation of smoking).
No products indexed under this heading.
Caffeine Citrate (Deinduction of hepatic enzymes on smoking cessation; may require a decrease in dose at cessation of smoking).
No products indexed under this heading.
Caffeine Sodium Benzoate (Deinduction of hepatic enzymes on smoking cessation; may require a decrease in dose at cessation of smoking).
No products indexed under this heading.

IMPORTANT NOTE: Always consult each drug listing in the patient's regimen for possible interactions.

Habitrol **Interactions Index** **462**

Dyphylline (Deinduction of hepatic enzymes on smoking cessation; may require a decrease in dose at cessation of smoking). Products include:
- Lufyllin & Lufyllin-400 Tablets 2778
- Lufyllin-GG Elixir & Tablets 2779

Imipramine Hydrochloride (Deinduction of hepatic enzymes on smoking cessation; may require a decrease in dose at cessation of smoking). Products include:
- Tofranil Ampuls 873
- Tofranil Tablets 875

Imipramine Pamoate (Deinduction of hepatic enzymes on smoking cessation; may require a decrease in dose at cessation of smoking). Products include:
- Tofranil-PM Capsules 876

Insulin, Human (Increased subcutaneous insulin absorption with smoking cessation).
- No products indexed under this heading.

Insulin, Human Isophane Suspension (Increased subcutaneous insulin absorption with smoking cessation). Products include:
- Novolin N Human Insulin 10 ml Vials 1846

Insulin, Human NPH (Increased subcutaneous insulin absorption with smoking cessation). Products include:
- Humulin N, 100 Units 1495
- Novolin N PenFill 1.5 ml Cartridges Durable Insulin Delivery System 1849
- Novolin N Prefilled Syringe Disposable Insulin Delivery System 1850

Insulin, Human Regular (Increased subcutaneous insulin absorption with smoking cessation). Products include:
- Humulin R, 100 Units 1497
- Novolin R Human Insulin 10 ml Vials 1846
- Novolin R PenFill 1.5 ml Cartridges Durable Insulin Delivery System 1849
- Novolin R Prefilled Syringe Disposable Insulin Delivery System 1850
- Velosulin BR Human Insulin 10 ml Vials 1847

Insulin, Human, Zinc Suspension (Increased subcutaneous insulin absorption with smoking cessation). Products include:
- Humulin L, 100 Units 1494
- Humulin U, 100 Units 1498
- Novolin L Human Insulin 10 ml Vials 1846

Insulin Lispro, Human (Increased subcutaneous insulin absorption with smoking cessation). Products include:
- Humalog Injection 1488

Insulin, NPH (Increased subcutaneous insulin absorption with smoking cessation). Products include:
- NPH, 100 Units 1502
- Pork NPH, 100 Units 1506
- Purified Pork NPH Isophane Insulin 1852

Insulin, Regular (Increased subcutaneous insulin absorption with smoking cessation). Products include:
- Regular, 100 Units 1503
- Pork Regular, 100 Units 1507
- Pork Regular (Concentrated), 500 Units 1508
- Purified Pork Regular Insulin 1852

Insulin, Zinc Crystals (Increased subcutaneous insulin absorption with smoking cessation). Products include:
- NPH, 100 Units 1502

Insulin, Zinc Suspension (Increased subcutaneous insulin absorption with smoking cessation). Products include:
- Iletin I 1501
- Lente, 100 Units 1501
- Iletin II 1504
- Pork Lente, 100 Units 1504
- Purified Pork Lente Insulin 1852

Isoproterenol Hydrochloride (Decrease in circulating catecholamines with smoking cessation). Products include:
- Isuprel Hydrochloride Solution 2443
- Isuprel Injection 2441
- Isuprel Mistometer 2442

Labetalol Hydrochloride (Decrease in circulating catecholamines with smoking cessation). Products include:
- Normodyne Injection 2519
- Normodyne Tablets 2522
- Trandate 1158

Oxazepam (Deinduction of hepatic enzymes on smoking cessation; may require a decrease in dose at cessation of smoking). Products include:
- Serax Capsules 2916
- Serax Tablets 2916

Pentazocine Hydrochloride (Deinduction of hepatic enzymes on smoking cessation; may require a decrease in dose at cessation of smoking). Products include:
- Talacen Caplets 2464
- Talwin Compound 2466
- Talwin Nx Tablets 2467

Pentazocine Lactate (Deinduction of hepatic enzymes on smoking cessation; may require a decrease in dose at cessation of smoking). Products include:
- Talwin Injection 2465

Phenylephrine Hydrochloride (Decrease in circulating catecholamines with smoking cessation). Products include:
- Atrohist Plus Tablets 1605
- Cerose DM .... ▣ 853
- D.A. II Tablets 972
- D.A. Chewable Tablets 970
- Dura-Vent/DA Tablets 972
- Extendryl 1003
- 4-Way Fast Acting Nasal Spray (regular & mentholated) .... ▣ 644
- Hemorid .... ▣ 797
- Hycomine Compound Tablets 948
- Neo-Synephrine Hydrochloride 1% Carpuject 2455
- Neo-Synephrine Hydrochloride 1% Injection 2455
- Neo-Synephrine Hydrochloride (Ophthalmic) 2456
- Neo-Synephrine .... ▣ 624
- Novahistine Elixir .... ▣ 782
- Phenergan VC 2886
- Phenergan VC with Codeine 2888
- Preparation H .... ▣ 842
- Tympagesic Ear Drops 2476
- Vicks Sinex Nasal Spray and Ultra Fine Mist .... ▣ 738

Prazosin Hydrochloride (Decrease in circulating catecholamines with smoking cessation). Products include:
- Minipress Capsules 2015
- Minizide Capsules 2016

Propranolol Hydrochloride (Deinduction of hepatic enzymes on smoking cessation; may require a decrease in dose at cessation of smoking). Products include:
- Inderal 2834
- Inderal LA Long Acting Capsules 2836
- Inderide Tablets 2838
- Inderide LA Long Acting Capsules 2840

Theophylline (Deinduction of hepatic enzymes on smoking cessation; may require a decrease in dose at cessation of smoking). Products include:
- Marax Tablets & DF Syrup 2015
- Quibron 2227

Theophylline Anhydrous (Deinduction of hepatic enzymes on smoking cessation; may require a decrease in dose at cessation of smoking). Products include:
- Aerolate 1003
- Primatene Tablets .... ▣ 844
- Respbid Tablets 687
- Slo-bid Gyrocaps 2201
- Theo-24 Extended Release Capsules 2753
- Theo-Dur Extended-Release Tablets 1367
- Theo-X Extended-Release Tablets 793
- Uni-Dur Extended-Release Tablets 1374
- Uniphyl 400 mg and 600 mg Tablets 2157

Theophylline Calcium Salicylate (Deinduction of hepatic enzymes on smoking cessation; may require a decrease in dose at cessation of smoking). Products include:
- Quadrinal Tablets 1398

Theophylline Sodium Glycinate (Deinduction of hepatic enzymes on smoking cessation; may require a decrease in dose at cessation of smoking).
- No products indexed under this heading.

HALCION TABLETS
(Triazolam) 2093
May interact with benzodiazepines, psychotropics, anticonvulsants, antihistamines, central nervous system depressants, erythromycin, and certain other agents. Compounds in these categories include:

Acrivastine (Additive CNS depressant effects). Products include:
- Semprex-D Capsules 1620

Alfentanil Hydrochloride (Additive CNS depressant effects). Products include:
- Alfenta Injection 1334

Alprazolam (Additive CNS depressant effects). Products include:
- Xanax Tablets 2115

Amitriptyline Hydrochloride (Additive CNS depressant effects). Products include:
- Elavil 2945
- Etrafon 2495
- Limbitrol 2333
- Triavil Tablets 1800

Amoxapine (Additive CNS depressant effects). Products include:
- Asendin Tablets 1419

Aprobarbital (Additive CNS depressant effects).
- No products indexed under this heading.

Astemizole (Additive CNS depressant effects). Products include:
- Hismanal Tablets 1341

Azatadine Maleate (Additive CNS depressant effects). Products include:
- Trinalin Repetabs Tablets 1373

Bromodiphenhydramine Hydrochloride (Additive CNS depressant effects).
- No products indexed under this heading.

Brompheniramine Maleate (Additive CNS depressant effects). Products include:
- Alka-Seltzer Plus Sinus Medicine .... ▣ 611
- Bromfed Capsules (Extended-Release) 1832
- Bromfed Syrup .... ▣ 712
- Bromfed Tablets 1832
- Bromfed-DM Cough Syrup 1832
- Bromfed-PD Capsules (Extended-Release) 1832
- Dimetane-DC Cough Syrup 2232
- Dimetane-DX Cough Syrup 2233
- Dimetapp Allergy Dye-Free Elixir .... ▣ 838
- Dimetapp Allergy Sinus Caplets .... ▣ 838
- Dimetapp Cold & Allergy Chewable Tablets .... ▣ 838
- Dimetapp Cold & Cough Liqui-Gels .... ▣ 839
- Dimetapp Cold & Fever Suspension .... ▣ 839
- Dimetapp DM Elixir .... ▣ 840
- Dimetapp Elixir .... ▣ 840
- Dimetapp Extentabs .... ▣ 841
- Dimetapp Tablets/Liqui-Gels .... ▣ 841
- Rondec Chewable Tablets 974
- Vicks DayQuil Allergy Relief 12-Hour Extended Release Tablets .... ▣ 733
- Vicks DayQuil Allergy Relief 4-Hour Tablets .... ▣ 733

Buprenorphine (Additive CNS depressant effects). Products include:
- Buprenex Injectable 2170

Buspirone Hydrochloride (Additive CNS depressant effects). Products include:
- BuSpar Tablets 738

Butabarbital (Additive CNS depressant effects).
- No products indexed under this heading.

Butalbital (Additive CNS depressant effects). Products include:
- Axocet Capsules 2469
- Esgic-plus Capsules 1012
- Esgic-plus Tablets 1012
- Fioricet Tablets 2386
- Fioricet with Codeine Capsules 2387
- Fiorinal Capsules 2388
- Fiorinal with Codeine Capsules 2390
- Fiorinal Tablets 2388
- Phrenilin 790
- Sedapap Tablets 50 mg/650 mg 1826

Carbamazepine (Additive CNS depressant effects). Products include:
- Atretol Tablets 569
- Tegretol/Tegretol-XR 870

Cetirizine Hydrochloride (Additive CNS depressant effects). Products include:
- Zyrtec Tablets 2053

Chlordiazepoxide (Additive CNS depressant effects). Products include:
- Limbitrol 2333

Chlordiazepoxide Hydrochloride (Additive CNS depressant effects). Products include:
- Librax Capsules 2330
- Librium Capsules 2331
- Librium Injectable 2332

Chlorpheniramine Maleate (Additive CNS depressant effects). Products include:
- Alka-Seltzer Plus Cold Medicine .... ▣ 611
- Alka-Seltzer Plus Cold Medicine Liqui-Gels .... ▣ 612
- Alka-Seltzer Plus Cold & Cough Medicine .... ▣ 611
- Alka-Seltzer Plus Cold & Cough Medicine Liqui-Gels .... ▣ 612
- Alka-Seltzer Plus Flu & Body Aches Effervescent Tablets .... ▣ 612
- Allerest Maximum Strength .... ▣ 649
- Allerest Sinus Pain Formula .... ▣ 649
- Ana-Kit Anaphylaxis Emergency Treatment Kit 611
- Atrohist Pediatric Capsules 1603
- Atrohist Plus Tablets 1605
- BC Cold Powder Multi-Symptom Formula (Cold-Sinus-Allergy) .... ▣ 631
- Cerose DM .... ▣ 853
- Cheracol Plus Head Cold/Cough Formula .... ▣ 741
- Children's TYLENOL Cold Multi-Symptom Chewable Tablets and Liquid 1559
- Children's TYLENOL Cold Plus Cough Multi Symptom Chewable Tablets and Liquid 1560
- Children's TYLENOL Flu Suspension Liquid 1560
- Children's Vicks DayQuil Allergy Relief .... ▣ 730
- Children's Vicks NyQuil Cold/Cough Relief .... ▣ 731
- Chlor-Trimeton Allergy Decongestant Tablets .... ▣ 759

(▣ Described in PDR For Nonprescription Drugs) (⊚ Described in PDR For Ophthalmology)

Interactions Index — Halcion

Chlor-Trimeton Allergy Tablets 758
Allergy-Sinus Comtrex Multi-Symptom Allergy-Sinus Formula Tablets and Caplets 639
Comtrex Multi-Symptom 638
Contac Continuous Action Nasal Decongestant/Antihistamine 12 Hour Capsules 773
Contac Maximum Strength Continuous Action Decongestant/Antihistamine 12 Hour Caplets 772
Contac Severe Cold and Flu Formula Caplets 773
Coricidin Cold + Flu Tablets 760
Coricidin Cough + Cold Tablets 760
Coricidin 'D' Decongestant Tablets 760
D.A. II Tablets 972
D.A. Chewable Tablets 970
Dura-Tap/PD Capsules 970
Dura-Vent/DA Tablets 972
Efidac 24 Chlorpheniramine 655
Extendryl 1003
Fedahist Gyrocaps 2545
Hycomine Compound Tablets 948
Kronofed-A 994
Nolamine Timed-Release Tablets 790
Novahistine Elixir 782
Ornade Spansule Capsules 2678
PediaCare Cough-Cold Chewable Tablets and Liquid 1569
PediaCare NightRest Cough-Cold Liquid 1569
Pediatric Vicks 44m Cough & Cold Relief 737
Pyrroxate Caplets 742
Ryna 804
Sinarest 663
Sine-Off Sinus Medicine 784
Singlet Tablets 785
Sinulin Tablets 792
Sinutab Sinus Allergy Medication, Maximum Strength Tablets and Caplets 823
Sudafed Cold & Allergy Tablets 826
Teldrin 12 Hour Antihistamine/Nasal Decongestant Allergy Relief Capsules 786
TheraFlu Flu and Cold Medicine 750
Theraflu Maximum Strength Flu and Cold Medicine For Sore Throat 751
TheraFlu Flu, Cold and Cough Medicine 750
TheraFlu Maximum Strength Nighttime Flu, Cold & Cough Medicine 751
Triaminic Night Time 754
Triaminic Syrup 755
Triaminic Triaminicol Cold & Cough 756
Triaminicin Tablets 756
Tussend 1830
TYLENOL Allergy Sinus, Maximum Strength Caplets and Gelcaps 1571
TYLENOL Cold Medication, Multi-Symptom Formula Tablets and Caplets 1572
TYLENOL Cold Medication, Multi-Symptom Hot Liquid Packets 1572
Vicks 44 LiquiCaps Cough, Cold & Flu Relief 728
Vicks 44M Cough, Cold & Flu Relief 729

Chlorpheniramine Polistirex (Additive CNS depressant effects). Products include:
Tussionex Pennkinetic Extended-Release Suspension 1624

Chlorpheniramine Tannate (Additive CNS depressant effects). Products include:
Atrohist Pediatric Suspension 1604
Atrohist Pediatric Suspension Dye-Free 1604
Rynatan 2781
Rynatuss 2782

Chlorpromazine (Additive CNS depressant effects). Products include:
Thorazine Suppositories 2701

Chlorpromazine Hydrochloride (Additive CNS depressant effects). Products include:
Thorazine 2701

Chlorprothixene (Additive CNS depressant effects).
No products indexed under this heading.

Chlorprothixene Hydrochloride (Additive CNS depressant effects).
No products indexed under this heading.

Chlorprothixene Lactate (Additive CNS depressant effects).
No products indexed under this heading.

Cimetidine (Co-administration causes an approximate doubling of the elimination half-life and plasma levels of triazolam). Products include:
Tagamet HB Tablets 786
Tagamet Tablets 2694

Cimetidine Hydrochloride (Co-administration causes an approximate doubling of the elimination half-life and plasma levels of triazolam). Products include:
Tagamet 2694

Clemastine Fumarate (Additive CNS depressant effects). Products include:
Tavist Syrup 2426
Tavist Tablets 2427
Tavist-1 12 Hour Relief Tablets 749
Tavist-D 12 Hour Relief Tablets 750

Clonazepam (Additive CNS depressant effects). Products include:
Klonopin Tablets 2294

Clorazepate Dipotassium (Additive CNS depressant effects). Products include:
Tranxene 459

Clozapine (Additive CNS depressant effects). Products include:
Clozaril Tablets 2377

Codeine Phosphate (Additive CNS depressant effects). Products include:
Brontex 2130
Dimetane-DC Cough Syrup 2232
Fioricet with Codeine Capsules 2387
Fiorinal with Codeine Capsules 2390
Nucofed 2225
Phenergan with Codeine 2883
Phenergan VC with Codeine 2888
Robitussin A-C Syrup 2248
Robitussin-DAC Syrup 2249
Ryna 804
Soma Compound w/Codeine Tablets 2784
Tylenol with Codeine 1592

Cyproheptadine Hydrochloride (Additive CNS depressant effects). Products include:
Periactin 1767

Desflurane (Additive CNS depressant effects). Products include:
Suprane (desflurane, USP) 1865

Desipramine Hydrochloride (Additive CNS depressant effects). Products include:
Norpramin Tablets 1273

Dexchlorpheniramine Maleate (Additive CNS depressant effects).
No products indexed under this heading.

Dezocine (Additive CNS depressant effects). Products include:
Dalgan Injection 529

Diazepam (Additive CNS depressant effects). Products include:
Dizac (diazepam injectable emulsion) CIV 1862
Valium Injectable 2336
Valium Tablets 2335

Diphenhydramine Citrate (Additive CNS depressant effects). Products include:
Excedrin P.M. Analgesic/Sleeping Aid Tablets, Caplets, Liquigels 735

Diphenhydramine Hydrochloride (Additive CNS depressant effects). Products include:
Actifed Allergy Daytime/Nighttime Caplets 808
Actifed Sinus Daytime/Nighttime Tablets and Caplets 809
Extra Strength Bayer PM Aspirin Plus Sleep Aid 617
Benadryl Allergy Chewables 811
Benadryl Allergy/Cold Tablets 811
Benadryl Allergy Decongestant Liquid Medication 812
Benadryl Allergy Decongestant Tablets 812
Benadryl Allergy Liquid Medication 813
Benadryl Allergy 811
Benadryl Allergy Sinus Headache Caplets 813
Benadryl Dye-Free Allergy Liquigel Softgels 813
Benadryl Dye-Free Allergy Liquid Medication 814
Benadryl Itch Relief Stick Extra Strength 814
Benadryl Cream 814
Benadryl Gel 815
Benadryl Spray 815
Benadryl Injection 1955
Contac Day & Night Cold/Flu Night Caplets 772
Contac Night Allergy/Sinus Caplets 771
Extra Strength Doan's P.M. 653
Excedrin P.M. Analgesic/Sleeping Aid Tablets, Caplets, Liquigels 643
Nytol QuickCaps Caplets 632
Sleepinal Night-time Sleep Aid Capsules and Softgels 798
TYLENOL Allergy Sinus NightTime, Maximum Strength Caplets 1571
TYLENOL Flu NightTime, Maximum Strength Gelcaps 1575
TYLENOL Flu NightTime, Maximum Strength Hot Medication Packets 1575
TYLENOL PM Pain Reliever/Sleep Aid, Extra Strength Gelcaps, Caplets, Geltabs 1576
TYLENOL Severe Allergy Medication Caplets 1571
Maximum Strength Unisom Sleepgels 1990
Unisom With Pain Relief-Nighttime Sleep Aid and Pain Reliever 1991

Diphenylpyraline Hydrochloride (Additive CNS depressant effects).
No products indexed under this heading.

Divalproex Sodium (Additive CNS depressant effects). Products include:
Depakote Tablets 418

Doxepin Hydrochloride (Additive CNS depressant effects). Products include:
Adapin Capsules 1542
Sinequan 2028
Zonalon Cream 1042

Droperidol (Additive CNS depressant effects). Products include:
Inapsine Injection 462

Enflurane (Additive CNS depressant effects).
No products indexed under this heading.

Erythromycin (Co-administration causes an approximate doubling of the elimination half-life and plasma levels of triazolam). Products include:
A/T/S 2% Acne Topical Gel 1244
A/T/S 2% Acne Topical Solution 1244
Benzamycin Topical Gel 919
E-Mycin Tablets 1388
Emgel 2% Topical Gel 1081
ERYC 1972
Erycette (erythromycin 2%) Topical Solution 1943
Ery-Tab Tablets 426
Erythromycin Base Filmtab 430
Erythromycin Delayed-Release Capsules, USP 431
Ilotycin Ophthalmic Ointment 928
PCE Dispertab Tablets 453
T-Stat 2.0% Topical Solution and Pads 2797
THERAMYCIN Z 2% Solution 1629

Erythromycin Estolate (Co-administration causes an approximate doubling of the elimination half-life and plasma levels of triazolam). Products include:
Ilosone 927

Erythromycin Ethylsuccinate (Co-administration causes an approximate doubling of the elimination half-life and plasma levels of triazolam). Products include:
E.E.S. 427
EryPed 425
Pediazole Suspension 2340

Erythromycin Glucaptate (Co-administration causes an approximate doubling of the elimination half-life and plasma levels of triazolam). Products include:
Ilotycin Glucaptate, IV, Vials 929

Erythromycin Stearate (Co-administration causes an approximate doubling of the elimination half-life and plasma levels of triazolam). Products include:
Erythrocin Stearate Filmtab 429

Estazolam (Additive CNS depressant effects). Products include:
ProSom Tablets 457

Ethchlorvynol (Additive CNS depressant effects). Products include:
Placidyl Capsules 456

Ethinamate (Additive CNS depressant effects).
No products indexed under this heading.

Ethosuximide (Additive CNS depressant effects). Products include:
Zarontin Capsules 1986
Zarontin Syrup 1986

Ethotoin (Additive CNS depressant effects). Products include:
Peganone Tablets 455

Felbamate (Additive CNS depressant effects). Products include:
Felbatol 2774

Fentanyl (Additive CNS depressant effects). Products include:
Duragesic Transdermal System 1336

Fentanyl Citrate (Additive CNS depressant effects). Products include:
Sublimaze Injection 463

Fluphenazine Decanoate (Additive CNS depressant effects). Products include:
Prolixin Decanoate 510

Fluphenazine Enanthate (Additive CNS depressant effects). Products include:
Prolixin Enanthate 510

Fluphenazine Hydrochloride (Additive CNS depressant effects). Products include:
Prolixin 510

Flurazepam Hydrochloride (Additive CNS depressant effects). Products include:
Dalmane Capsules 2329

Fosphenytoin Sodium (Additive CNS depressant effects). Products include:
Cerebyx Injection 1956

Glutethimide (Additive CNS depressant effects).
No products indexed under this heading.

Halazepam (Additive CNS depressant effects).
No products indexed under this heading.

IMPORTANT NOTE: Always consult each drug listing in the patient's regimen for possible interactions.

Interactions Index

Haloperidol (Additive CNS depressant effects). Products include:
- Haldol Injection, Tablets and Concentrate ... 1585

Haloperidol Decanoate (Additive CNS depressant effects). Products include:
- Haldol Decanoate ... 1587

Hydrocodone Bitartrate (Additive CNS depressant effects). Products include:
- Codiclear DH Syrup ... 808
- Duratuss HD Elixir ... 2750
- Histussin D Liquid ... 670
- Hycodan Tablets and Syrup ... 946
- Hycomine Compound Tablets ... 948
- Hycomine ... 947
- Hycotuss Expectorant Syrup ... 950
- Hydrocet Capsules ... 787
- Lorcet 10/650 Tablets ... 1016
- Lortab ... 2751
- Tussend ... 1830
- Tussend Expectorant ... 1831
- Vicodin Tablets ... 1404
- Vicodin ES Tablets ... 1405
- Vicodin HP Tablets ... 1403
- Vicodin Tuss Expectorant ... 1406
- Zydone Capsules ... 967

Hydrocodone Polistirex (Additive CNS depressant effects). Products include:
- Tussionex Pennkinetic Extended-Release Suspension ... 1624

Hydromorphone Hydrochloride (Additive CNS depressant effects). Products include:
- Dilaudid Ampules ... 1382
- Dilaudid Cough Syrup ... 1383
- Dilaudid-HP Injection ... 1384
- Dilaudid-HP Lyophilized Powder 250 mg ... 1384
- Dilaudid ... 1382
- Dilaudid Oral Liquid ... 1386
- Dilaudid ... 1382
- Dilaudid Tablets - 8 mg ... 1386

Hydroxyzine Hydrochloride (Additive CNS depressant effects). Products include:
- Atarax Tablets & Syrup ... 1992
- Marax Tablets & DF Syrup ... 2015
- Vistaril Intramuscular Solution ... 2042

Imipramine Hydrochloride (Additive CNS depressant effects). Products include:
- Tofranil Ampuls ... 873
- Tofranil Tablets ... 875

Imipramine Pamoate (Additive CNS depressant effects). Products include:
- Tofranil-PM Capsules ... 876

Isocarboxazid (Additive CNS depressant effects).
- No products indexed under this heading.

Isoflurane (Additive CNS depressant effects).
- No products indexed under this heading.

Ketamine Hydrochloride (Additive CNS depressant effects).
- No products indexed under this heading.

Lamotrigine (Additive CNS depressant effects). Products include:
- Lamictal Tablets ... 1105

Levomethadyl Acetate Hydrochloride (Additive CNS depressant effects). Products include:
- Orlaam Oral Solution ... 2361

Levorphanol Tartrate (Additive CNS depressant effects). Products include:
- Levo-Dromoran ... 2297

Lithium Carbonate (Additive CNS depressant effects). Products include:
- Eskalith ... 2658
- Lithium Carbonate Capsules & Tablets ... 2352
- Lithonate/Lithotabs/Lithobid ... 2721

Lithium Citrate (Additive CNS depressant effects).
- No products indexed under this heading.

Loratadine (Additive CNS depressant effects). Products include:
- Claritin Tablets ... 2485
- Claritin-D Tablets ... 2487

Lorazepam (Additive CNS depressant effects). Products include:
- Ativan Injection ... 2805
- Ativan Tablets ... 2807

Loxapine Hydrochloride (Additive CNS depressant effects). Products include:
- Loxitane ... 1426

Loxapine Succinate (Additive CNS depressant effects). Products include:
- Loxitane Capsules ... 1426

Maprotiline Hydrochloride (Additive CNS depressant effects). Products include:
- Ludiomil Tablets ... 861

Meperidine Hydrochloride (Additive CNS depressant effects). Products include:
- Demerol ... 2438
- Mepergan Injection ... 2859

Mephenytoin (Additive CNS depressant effects). Products include:
- Mesantoin Tablets ... 2400

Mephobarbital (Additive CNS depressant effects). Products include:
- Mebaral Tablets ... 2452

Meprobamate (Additive CNS depressant effects). Products include:
- Miltown Tablets ... 2780
- PMB 200 and PMB 400 ... 2890

Mesoridazine Besylate (Additive CNS depressant effects). Products include:
- Serentil ... 689

Methadone Hydrochloride (Additive CNS depressant effects). Products include:
- Methadone Hydrochloride Oral Concentrate ... 2356
- Methadone Hydrochloride Oral Solution & Tablets ... 2357

Methdilazine Hydrochloride (Additive CNS depressant effects).
- No products indexed under this heading.

Methohexital Sodium (Additive CNS depressant effects).
- No products indexed under this heading.

Methotrimeprazine (Additive CNS depressant effects). Products include:
- Levoprome ... 1321

Methoxyflurane (Additive CNS depressant effects).
- No products indexed under this heading.

Methsuximide (Additive CNS depressant effects). Products include:
- Celontin Kapseals ... 1955

Midazolam Hydrochloride (Additive CNS depressant effects). Products include:
- Versed Injection ... 2324

Molindone Hydrochloride (Additive CNS depressant effects). Products include:
- Moban Tablets and Concentrate ... 1036

Morphine Sulfate (Additive CNS depressant effects). Products include:
- Astramorph/PF Injection, USP (Preservative-Free) ... 526
- Duramorph Injection ... 983
- Infumorph 200 and Infumorph 500 Sterile Solutions ... 985
- Kadian Capsules ... 2948
- MS Contin Tablets ... 2149
- MSIR ... 2152
- Oramorph SR (Morphine Sulfate Sustained Release Tablets) ... 2359
- RMS Suppositories CII ... 2766
- Roxanol ... 2365

Nortriptyline Hydrochloride (Additive CNS depressant effects). Products include:
- Pamelor ... 2409

Opium Alkaloids (Additive CNS depressant effects).
- No products indexed under this heading.

Oxazepam (Additive CNS depressant effects). Products include:
- Serax Capsules ... 2916
- Serax Tablets ... 2916

Oxycodone Hydrochloride (Additive CNS depressant effects). Products include:
- OxyContin Tablets ... 2163
- OxyIR Capsules ... 2167
- Percocet Tablets ... 955
- Percodan Tablets ... 955
- Percodan-Demi Tablets ... 956
- Roxicodone Tablets, Oral Solution & Intensol (Oxycodone) ... 2366
- Tylox Capsules ... 1593

Paramethadione (Additive CNS depressant effects).
- No products indexed under this heading.

Pentobarbital Sodium (Additive CNS depressant effects). Products include:
- Nembutal Sodium Capsules ... 440
- Nembutal Sodium Solution ... 442
- Nembutal Sodium Suppositories ... 444

Perphenazine (Additive CNS depressant effects). Products include:
- Etrafon ... 2495
- Triavil Tablets ... 1800
- Trilafon ... 2532

Phenacemide (Additive CNS depressant effects). Products include:
- Phenurone Tablets ... 455

Phenelzine Sulfate (Additive CNS depressant effects). Products include:
- Nardil ... 1977

Phenobarbital (Additive CNS depressant effects). Products include:
- Arco-Lase Plus Tablets ... 513
- Bellergal-S Tablets ... 2375
- Donnatal ... 2234
- Donnatal Extentabs ... 2234
- Donnatal Tablets ... 2234
- Phenobarbital Elixir and Tablets ... 1523
- Quadrinal Tablets ... 1398

Phensuximide (Additive CNS depressant effects).
- No products indexed under this heading.

Phenytoin (Additive CNS depressant effects). Products include:
- Dilantin Infatabs ... 1967
- Dilantin-125 Suspension ... 1969

Phenytoin Sodium (Additive CNS depressant effects). Products include:
- Dilantin Kapseals ... 1965

Prazepam (Additive CNS depressant effects).
- No products indexed under this heading.

Primidone (Additive CNS depressant effects). Products include:
- Mysoline ... 2860

Prochlorperazine (Additive CNS depressant effects). Products include:
- Compazine ... 2644

Promethazine Hydrochloride (Additive CNS depressant effects). Products include:
- Mepergan Injection ... 2859
- Phenergan with Codeine ... 2883
- Phenergan with Dextromethorphan ... 2885
- Phenergan Injection ... 2880
- Phenergan Suppositories ... 2882
- Phenergan Syrup ... 2881
- Phenergan Tablets ... 2882
- Phenergan VC ... 2886
- Phenergan VC with Codeine ... 2888

Propofol (Additive CNS depressant effects). Products include:
- Diprivan Injectable Emulsion ... 2939

Propoxyphene Hydrochloride (Additive CNS depressant effects). Products include:
- Darvon ... 1475
- Wygesic Tablets ... 2930

Propoxyphene Napsylate (Additive CNS depressant effects). Products include:
- Darvon-N/Darvocet-N ... 1473

Protriptyline Hydrochloride (Additive CNS depressant effects). Products include:
- Vivactil Tablets ... 1820

Pyrilamine Maleate (Additive CNS depressant effects). Products include:
- 4-Way Fast Acting Nasal Spray (regular & mentholated) ... ⊞ 644
- Maximum Strength Multi-Symptom Formula Midol ... ⊞ 621
- PMS Multi-Symptom Formula Midol ... ⊞ 622

Pyrilamine Tannate (Additive CNS depressant effects). Products include:
- Atrohist Pediatric Suspension ... 1604
- Atrohist Pediatric Suspension Dye-Free ... 1604
- Rynatan ... 2781

Quazepam (Additive CNS depressant effects). Products include:
- Doral Tablets ... 2773

Risperidone (Additive CNS depressant effects). Products include:
- Risperdal Tablets ... 1348

Secobarbital Sodium (Additive CNS depressant effects). Products include:
- Seconal Sodium Pulvules ... 1529

Sevoflurane (Additive CNS depressant effects).
- No products indexed under this heading.

Sufentanil Citrate (Additive CNS depressant effects). Products include:
- Sufenta Injection ... 1355

Temazepam (Additive CNS depressant effects). Products include:
- Restoril Capsules ... 2413

Terfenadine (Additive CNS depressant effects). Products include:
- Seldane Tablets ... 1284
- Seldane-D Extended-Release Tablets ... 1286

Thiamylal Sodium (Additive CNS depressant effects).
- No products indexed under this heading.

Thioridazine Hydrochloride (Additive CNS depressant effects). Products include:
- Mellaril ... 2398

Thiothixene (Additive CNS depressant effects). Products include:
- Navane Capsules and Concentrate ... 2018
- Navane Intramuscular ... 2019

Tranylcypromine Sulfate (Additive CNS depressant effects). Products include:
- Parnate Tablets ... 2679

Trifluoperazine Hydrochloride (Additive CNS depressant effects). Products include:
- Stelazine ... 2692

Trimeprazine Tartrate (Additive CNS depressant effects).
- No products indexed under this heading.

Trimethadione (Additive CNS depressant effects).
- No products indexed under this heading.

(⊞ Described in PDR For Nonprescription Drugs) (⊙ Described in PDR For Ophthalmology)

Trimipramine Maleate (Additive CNS depressant effects). Products include:
Surmontil Capsules 2917
Tripelennamine Hydrochloride (Additive CNS depressant effects). Products include:
PBZ Tablets 863
PBZ-SR Tablets 862
Triprolidine Hydrochloride (Additive CNS depressant effects). Products include:
Actifed Cold & Allergy Tablets .... ⬛ 807
Actifed Cold & Sinus Caplets and Tablets .... ⬛ 808
Valproic Acid (Additive CNS depressant effects). Products include:
Depakene 416
Zolpidem Tartrate (Additive CNS depressant effects). Products include:
Ambien Tablets 2559

Food Interactions
Alcohol (Additive CNS depressant effects).

HALDOL DECANOATE 50 (50 MG/ML) INJECTION
(Haloperidol Decanoate) 1587
May interact with narcotic analgesics, general anesthetics, oral anticoagulants, lithium preparations, central nervous system depressants, anticonvulsants, anticholinergics, anticholinergic-type antiparkinsonism drugs, and certain other agents. Compounds in these categories include:

Alfentanil Hydrochloride (CNS depressant potentiated). Products include:
Alfenta Injection 1334
Alprazolam (CNS depressant potentiated). Products include:
Xanax Tablets 2115
Aprobarbital (CNS depressant potentiated).
No products indexed under this heading.
Atropine Sulfate (Possible increase in intraocular pressure when anticholinergic drugs including antiparkinson agents are administered concomitantly with haloperidol). Products include:
Arco-Lase Plus Tablets 513
Atrohist Plus Tablets 1605
Donnatal 2234
Donnatal Extentabs 2234
Donnatal Tablets 2234
Lomotil 2591
Motofen Tablets 789
Urised Tablets 2123
Belladonna Alkaloids (Possible increase in intraocular pressure when anticholinergic drugs including antiparkinson agents are administered concomitantly with haloperidol). Products include:
Bellergal-S Tablets 2375
Hyland's Bedwetting Tablets .... ⬛ 788
Hyland's EnurAid Tablets .... ⬛ 789
Hyland's Headache Tablets .... ⬛ 790
Hyland's Teething Tablets .... ⬛ 790
Similasan Eye Drops #1 .... ⬛ 769
Benztropine Mesylate (Possible increase in intraocular pressure when antiparkinson agents are administered concomitantly with haloperidol). Products include:
Cogentin 1661
Biperiden Hydrochloride (Possible increase in intraocular pressure when antiparkinson agents are administered concomitantly with haloperidol). Products include:
Akineton 1380

Buprenorphine (CNS depressant potentiated). Products include:
Buprenex Injectable 2170
Buspirone Hydrochloride (CNS depressant potentiated). Products include:
BuSpar Tablets 738
Butabarbital (CNS depressant potentiated).
No products indexed under this heading.
Butalbital (CNS depressant potentiated). Products include:
Axocet Capsules 2469
Esgic-plus Capsules 1012
Esgic-plus Tablets 1012
Fioricet Tablets 2386
Fioricet with Codeine Capsules 2387
Fiorinal Capsules 2388
Fiorinal with Codeine Capsules 2390
Fiorinal Tablets 2388
Phrenilin 790
Sedapap Tablets 50 mg/650 mg .. 1826
Carbamazepine (Haloperidol may lower the convulsive threshold; adequate anticonvulsant therapy should be maintained). Products include:
Atretol Tablets 569
Tegretol/Tegretol-XR 870
Chlordiazepoxide (CNS depressant potentiated). Products include:
Limbitrol 2333
Chlordiazepoxide Hydrochloride (CNS depressant potentiated). Products include:
Librax Capsules 2330
Librium Capsules 2331
Librium Injectable 2332
Chlorpromazine (CNS depressant potentiated). Products include:
Thorazine Suppositories 2701
Chlorprothixene (CNS depressant potentiated).
No products indexed under this heading.
Chlorprothixene Hydrochloride (CNS depressant potentiated).
No products indexed under this heading.
Chlorprothixene Lactate (CNS depressant potentiated).
No products indexed under this heading.
Clidinium Bromide (Possible increase in intraocular pressure when anticholinergic drugs including antiparkinson agents are administered concomitantly with haloperidol). Products include:
Librax Capsules 2330
Clorazepate Dipotassium (CNS depressant potentiated). Products include:
Tranxene 459
Clozapine (CNS depressant potentiated). Products include:
Clozaril Tablets 2377
Codeine Phosphate (CNS depressant potentiated). Products include:
Brontex 2130
Dimetane-DC Cough Syrup 2232
Fioricet with Codeine Capsules 2387
Fiorinal with Codeine Capsules 2390
Nucofed 2225
Phenergan with Codeine 2883
Phenergan VC with Codeine 2888
Robitussin A-C Syrup 2248
Robitussin-DAC Syrup 2249
Ryna .... ⬛ 804
Soma Compound w/Codeine Tablets 2784
Tylenol with Codeine 1592
Desflurane (CNS depressant potentiated). Products include:
Suprane (desflurane, USP) 1865
Dezocine (CNS depressant potentiated). Products include:
Dalgan Injection 529

Diazepam (CNS depressant potentiated). Products include:
Dizac (diazepam injectable emulsion) CIV 1862
Valium Injectable 2336
Valium Tablets 2335
Dicumarol (Co-administration with one anticoagulant has resulted in an isolated instance of interference with the anticoagulant effects).
No products indexed under this heading.
Dicyclomine Hydrochloride (Possible increase in intraocular pressure when anticholinergic drugs including antiparkinson agents are administered concomitantly with haloperidol). Products include:
Bentyl 1246
Diphenhydramine Hydrochloride (Possible increase in intraocular pressure when antiparkinson agents are administered concomitantly with haloperidol). Products include:
Actifed Allergy Daytime/Nighttime Caplets .... ⬛ 808
Actifed Sinus Daytime/Nighttime Tablets and Caplets .... ⬛ 809
Extra Strength Bayer PM Aspirin Plus Sleep Aid .... ⬛ 617
Benadryl Allergy Chewables .... ⬛ 811
Benadryl Allergy/Cold Tablets .... ⬛ 811
Benadryl Allergy Decongestant Liquid Medication .... ⬛ 812
Benadryl Allergy Decongestant Tablets .... ⬛ 812
Benadryl Allergy Liquid Medication .... ⬛ 813
Benadryl Allergy .... ⬛ 811
Benadryl Allergy Sinus Headache Caplets .... ⬛ 813
Benadryl Dye-Free Allergy Liquigel Softgels .... ⬛ 813
Benadryl Dye-Free Allergy Liquid Medication .... ⬛ 814
Benadryl Itch Relief Stick Extra Strength .... ⬛ 814
Benadryl Cream .... ⬛ 814
Benadryl Gel .... ⬛ 815
Benadryl Spray .... ⬛ 815
Benadryl Injection 1955
Contac Day & Night Cold/Flu Night Caplets .... ⬛ 772
Contac Night Allergy/Sinus Caplets .... ⬛ 771
Extra Strength Doan's P.M. .... ⬛ 653
Excedrin P.M. Analgesic/Sleeping Aid Tablets, Caplets, Liquigels .... ⬛ 643
Nytol QuickCaps Caplets .... ⬛ 632
Sleepinal Night-time Sleep Aid Capsules and Softgels .... ⬛ 798
TYLENOL Allergy Sinus NightTime, Maximum Strength Caplets 1571
TYLENOL Flu NightTime, Maximum Strength Gelcaps 1575
TYLENOL Flu NightTime, Maximum Strength Hot Medication Packets 1575
TYLENOL PM Pain Reliever/Sleep Aid, Extra Strength Gelcaps, Caplets, Geltabs 1576
TYLENOL Severe Allergy Medication Caplets 1571
Maximum Strength Unisom Sleepgels 1990
Unisom With Pain Relief-Nighttime Sleep Aid and Pain Reliever. 1991
Divalproex Sodium (Haloperidol may lower the convulsive threshold; adequate anticonvulsant therapy should be maintained). Products include:
Depakote Tablets 418
Droperidol (CNS depressant potentiated). Products include:
Inapsine Injection 462
Enflurane (CNS depressant potentiated).
No products indexed under this heading.

Epinephrine Hydrochloride (Haloperidol may block vasopressor activity of epinephrine ;). Products include:
Ana-Kit Anaphylaxis Emergency Treatment Kit 611
Estazolam (CNS depressant potentiated). Products include:
ProSom Tablets 457
Ethchlorvynol (CNS depressant potentiated). Products include:
Placidyl Capsules 456
Ethinamate (CNS depressant potentiated).
No products indexed under this heading.
Ethosuximide (Haloperidol may lower the convulsive threshold; adequate anticonvulsant therapy should be maintained). Products include:
Zarontin Capsules 1986
Zarontin Syrup 1986
Ethotoin (Haloperidol may lower the convulsive threshold; adequate anticonvulsant therapy should be maintained). Products include:
Peganone Tablets 455
Felbamate (Haloperidol may lower the convulsive threshold; adequate anticonvulsant therapy should be maintained). Products include:
Felbatol 2774
Fentanyl (CNS depressant potentiated). Products include:
Duragesic Transdermal System 1336
Fentanyl Citrate (CNS depressant potentiated). Products include:
Sublimaze Injection 463
Fluphenazine Decanoate (CNS depressant potentiated). Products include:
Prolixin Decanoate 510
Fluphenazine Enanthate (CNS depressant potentiated). Products include:
Prolixin Enanthate 510
Fluphenazine Hydrochloride (CNS depressant potentiated). Products include:
Prolixin 510
Flurazepam Hydrochloride (CNS depressant potentiated). Products include:
Dalmane Capsules 2329
Fosphenytoin Sodium (Haloperidol may lower the convulsive threshold; adequate anticonvulsant therapy should be maintained). Products include:
Cerebyx Injection 1956
Glutethimide (CNS depressant potentiated).
No products indexed under this heading.
Glycopyrrolate (Possible increase in intraocular pressure when anticholinergic drugs including antiparkinson agents are administered concomitantly with haloperidol). Products include:
Robinul Forte Tablets 2247
Robinul Injectable 2247
Robinul Tablets 2247
Haloperidol (CNS depressant potentiated). Products include:
Haldol Injection, Tablets and Concentrate 1585
Hydrocodone Bitartrate (CNS depressant potentiated). Products include:
Codiclear DH Syrup 808
Duratuss HD Elixir 2750
Histussin D Liquid 670
Hycodan Tablets and Syrup 946
Hycomine Compound Tablets 948
Hycomine 947
Hycotuss Expectorant Syrup 950
Hydrocet Capsules 787
Lorcet 10/650 Tablets 1016

IMPORTANT NOTE: Always consult each drug listing in the patient's regimen for possible interactions.

Haldol Decanoate — Interactions Index — 466

Lortab 2751
Tussend 1830
Tussend Expectorant 1831
Vicodin Tablets 1404
Vicodin ES Tablets 1405
Vicodin HP Tablets 1403
Vicodin Tuss Expectorant 1406
Zydone Capsules 967

Hydrocodone Polistirex (CNS depressant potentiated). Products include:
Tussionex Pennkinetic Extended-Release Suspension 1624

Hydromorphone Hydrochloride (CNS depressant potentiated). Products include:
Dilaudid Ampules 1382
Dilaudid Cough Syrup 1383
Dilaudid-HP Injection 1384
Dilaudid-HP Lyophilized Powder 250 mg 1384
Dilaudid 1382
Dilaudid Oral Liquid 1386
Dilaudid 1382
Dilaudid Tablets - 8 mg 1386

Hydroxyzine Hydrochloride (CNS depressant potentiated). Products include:
Atarax Tablets & Syrup 1992
Marax Tablets & DF Syrup 2015
Vistaril Intramuscular Solution 2042

Hyoscyamine (Possible increase in intraocular pressure when anticholinergic drugs including antiparkinson agents are administered concomitantly with haloperidol). Products include:
Cystospaz Tablets 2123
Urised Tablets 2123

Hyoscyamine Sulfate (Possible increase in intraocular pressure when anticholinergic drugs including antiparkinson agents are administered concomitantly with haloperidol). Products include:
Arco-Lase Plus Tablets 513
Atrohist Plus Tablets 1605
Cystospaz-M Capsules 2123
Donnatal 2234
Donnatal Extentabs 2234
Donnatal Tablets 2234
Kutrase Capsules 2546
Levsin/Levsinex/Levbid 2549

Ipratropium Bromide (Possible increase in intraocular pressure when anticholinergic drugs including antiparkinson agents are administered concomitantly with haloperidol). Products include:
Atrovent Inhalation Aerosol 674
Atrovent Inhalation Solution 675
Atrovent Nasal Spray 0.03% 676
Atrovent Nasal Spray 0.06% 678

Isoflurane (CNS depressant potentiated).
No products indexed under this heading.

Ketamine Hydrochloride (CNS depressant potentiated).
No products indexed under this heading.

Lamotrigine (Haloperidol may lower the convulsive threshold; adequate anticonvulsant therapy should be maintained). Products include:
Lamictal Tablets 1105

Levomethadyl Acetate Hydrochloride (CNS depressant potentiated). Products include:
Orlaam Oral Solution 2361

Levorphanol Tartrate (CNS depressant potentiated). Products include:
Levo-Dromoran 2297

Lithium Carbonate (Co-administration in a few patients has resulted in an encephalopathic syndrome characterized by weakness, lethargy, fever, confusion, and leukocytosis followed by irreversible brain damage). Products include:
Eskalith 2658
Lithium Carbonate Capsules & Tablets 2352
Lithonate/Lithotabs/Lithobid 2721

Lithium Citrate (Co-administration in a few patients has resulted in an encephalopathic syndrome characterized by weakness, lethargy, fever, confusion, and leukocytosis followed by irreversible brain damage).
No products indexed under this heading.

Lorazepam (CNS depressant potentiated). Products include:
Ativan Injection 2805
Ativan Tablets 2807

Loxapine Hydrochloride (CNS depressant potentiated). Products include:
Loxitane 1426

Loxapine Succinate (CNS depressant potentiated). Products include:
Loxitane Capsules 1426

Mepenzolate Bromide (Possible increase in intraocular pressure when anticholinergic drugs including antiparkinson agents are administered concomitantly with haloperidol).
No products indexed under this heading.

Meperidine Hydrochloride (CNS depressant potentiated). Products include:
Demerol 2438
Mepergan Injection 2859

Mephenytoin (Haloperidol may lower the convulsive threshold; adequate anticonvulsant therapy should be maintained). Products include:
Mesantoin Tablets 2400

Mephobarbital (CNS depressant potentiated). Products include:
Mebaral Tablets 2452

Meprobamate (CNS depressant potentiated). Products include:
Miltown Tablets 2780
PMB 200 and PMB 400 2890

Mesoridazine Besylate (CNS depressant potentiated). Products include:
Serentil 689

Methadone Hydrochloride (CNS depressant potentiated). Products include:
Methadone Hydrochloride Oral Concentrate 2356
Methadone Hydrochloride Oral Solution & Tablets 2357

Methohexital Sodium (CNS depressant potentiated).
No products indexed under this heading.

Methotrimeprazine (CNS depressant potentiated). Products include:
Levoprome 1321

Methoxyflurane (CNS depressant potentiated).
No products indexed under this heading.

Methsuximide (Haloperidol may lower the convulsive threshold; adequate anticonvulsant therapy should be maintained). Products include:
Celontin Kapseals 1955

Midazolam Hydrochloride (CNS depressant potentiated). Products include:
Versed Injection 2324

Molindone Hydrochloride (CNS depressant potentiated). Products include:
Moban Tablets and Concentrate 1036

Morphine Sulfate (CNS depressant potentiated). Products include:
Astramorph/PF Injection, USP (Preservative-Free) 526
Duramorph Injection 983
Infumorph 200 and Infumorph 500 Sterile Solutions 985
Kadian Capsules 2948
MS Contin Tablets 2149
MSIR 2152
Oramorph SR (Morphine Sulfate Sustained Release Tablets) 2359
RMS Suppositories CII 2766
Roxanol 2365

Opium Alkaloids (CNS depressant potentiated).
No products indexed under this heading.

Oxazepam (CNS depressant potentiated). Products include:
Serax Capsules 2916
Serax Tablets 2916

Oxybutynin Chloride (Possible increase in intraocular pressure when anticholinergic drugs including antiparkinson agents are administered concomitantly with haloperidol). Products include:
Ditropan 1267

Oxycodone Hydrochloride (CNS depressant potentiated). Products include:
OxyContin Tablets 2163
OxyIR Capsules 2167
Percocet Tablets 955
Percodan Tablets 955
Percodan-Demi Tablets 956
Roxicodone Tablets, Oral Solution & Intensol (Oxycodone) 2366
Tylox Capsules 1593

Paramethadione (Haloperidol may lower the convulsive threshold; adequate anticonvulsant therapy should be maintained).
No products indexed under this heading.

Pentobarbital Sodium (CNS depressant potentiated). Products include:
Nembutal Sodium Capsules 440
Nembutal Sodium Solution 442
Nembutal Sodium Suppositories 444

Perphenazine (CNS depressant potentiated). Products include:
Etrafon 2495
Triavil Tablets 1800
Trilafon 2532

Phenacemide (Haloperidol may lower the convulsive threshold; adequate anticonvulsant therapy should be maintained). Products include:
Phenurone Tablets 455

Phenobarbital (Haloperidol may lower the convulsive threshold; adequate anticonvulsant therapy should be maintained; CNS depressant potentiated). Products include:
Arco-Lase Plus Tablets 513
Bellergal-S Tablets 2375
Donnatal 2234
Donnatal Extentabs 2234
Donnatal Tablets 2234
Phenobarbital Elixir and Tablets ... 1523
Quadrinal Tablets 1398

Phensuximide (Haloperidol may lower the convulsive threshold; adequate anticonvulsant therapy should be maintained).
No products indexed under this heading.

Phenytoin (Haloperidol may lower the convulsive threshold; adequate anticonvulsant therapy should be maintained). Products include:
Dilantin Infatabs 1967
Dilantin-125 Suspension 1969

Phenytoin Sodium (Haloperidol may lower the convulsive threshold; adequate anticonvulsant therapy should be maintained). Products include:
Dilantin Kapseals 1965

Prazepam (CNS depressant potentiated).
No products indexed under this heading.

Primidone (Haloperidol may lower the convulsive threshold; adequate anticonvulsant therapy should be maintained). Products include:
Mysoline 2860

Prochlorperazine (CNS depressant potentiated). Products include:
Compazine 2644

Procyclidine Hydrochloride (Possible increase in intraocular pressure when antiparkinson agents are administered concomitantly with haloperidol). Products include:
Kemadrin Tablets 1105

Promethazine Hydrochloride (CNS depressant potentiated). Products include:
Mepergan Injection 2859
Phenergan with Codeine 2883
Phenergan with Dextromethorphan 2885
Phenergan Injection 2880
Phenergan Suppositories 2882
Phenergan Syrup 2881
Phenergan Tablets 2882
Phenergan VC 2886
Phenergan VC with Codeine 2888

Propantheline Bromide (Possible increase in intraocular pressure when anticholinergic drugs including antiparkinson agents are administered concomitantly with haloperidol). Products include:
Pro-Banthine Tablets 2226

Propofol (CNS depressant potentiated). Products include:
Diprivan Injectable Emulsion 2939

Propoxyphene Hydrochloride (CNS depressant potentiated). Products include:
Darvon 1475
Wygesic Tablets 2930

Propoxyphene Napsylate (CNS depressant potentiated). Products include:
Darvon-N/Darvocet-N 1473

Quazepam (CNS depressant potentiated). Products include:
Doral Tablets 2773

Risperidone (CNS depressant potentiated). Products include:
Risperdal Tablets 1348

Scopolamine (Possible increase in intraocular pressure when anticholinergic drugs including antiparkinson agents are administered concomitantly with haloperidol). Products include:
Transderm Scōp Transdermal Therapeutic System 890

Scopolamine Hydrobromide (Possible increase in intraocular pressure when anticholinergic drugs including antiparkinson agents are administered concomitantly with haloperidol). Products include:
Atrohist Plus Tablets 1605
Donnatal 2234
Donnatal Extentabs 2234
Donnatal Tablets 2234

Secobarbital Sodium (CNS depressant potentiated). Products include:
Seconal Sodium Pulvules 1529

Sevoflurane (CNS depressant potentiated).
No products indexed under this heading.

(◨ Described in PDR For Nonprescription Drugs)   (⊚ Described in PDR For Ophthalmology)

Sufentanil Citrate (CNS depressant potentiated). Products include:
Sufenta Injection 1355
Temazepam (CNS depressant potentiated). Products include:
Restoril Capsules 2413
Thiamylal Sodium (CNS depressant potentiated).
No products indexed under this heading.
Thioridazine Hydrochloride (CNS depressant potentiated). Products include:
Mellaril 2398
Thiothixene (CNS depressant potentiated). Products include:
Navane Capsules and Concentrate ... 2018
Navane Intramuscular 2019
Triazolam (CNS depressant potentiated). Products include:
Halcion Tablets 2093
Tridihexethyl Chloride (Possible increase in intraocular pressure when antiparkinson agents are administered concomitantly with haloperidol).
No products indexed under this heading.
Trifluoperazine Hydrochloride (CNS depressant potentiated). Products include:
Stelazine 2692
Trihexyphenidyl Hydrochloride (Possible increase in intraocular pressure when antiparkinson agents are administered concomitantly with haloperidol). Products include:
Artane 1418
Trimethadione (Haloperidol may lower the convulsive threshold; adequate anticonvulsant therapy should be maintained).
No products indexed under this heading.
Valproic Acid (Haloperidol may lower the convulsive threshold; adequate anticonvulsant therapy should be maintained). Products include:
Depakene 416
Warfarin Sodium (Co-administration with one anticoagulant has resulted in an isolated instance of interference with the anticoagulant effects). Products include:
Coumadin 941
Zolpidem Tartrate (CNS depressant potentiated). Products include:
Ambien Tablets 2559

Food Interactions
Alcohol (CNS depressant potentiated).

HALDOL DECANOATE 100 (100 MG/ML) INJECTION
(Haloperidol Decanoate) 1587
See **Haldol Decanoate 50 (50 mg/mL) Injection**

HALDOL INJECTION, TABLETS AND CONCENTRATE
(Haloperidol) 1585
May interact with central nervous system depressants, general anesthetics, narcotic analgesics, oral anticoagulants, anticonvulsants, lithium preparations, anticholinergics, anticholinergic-type antiparkinsonism drugs, and certain other agents. Compounds in these categories include:

Alfentanil Hydrochloride (CNS depressant potentiated). Products include:
Alfenta Injection 1334

Alprazolam (CNS depressant potentiated). Products include:
Xanax Tablets 2115
Aprobarbital (CNS depressant potentiated).
No products indexed under this heading.
Atropine Sulfate (Possible increase in intraocular pressure when anticholinergic drugs including antiparkinson agents are administered concomitantly with haloperidol). Products include:
Arco-Lase Plus Tablets 513
Atrohist Plus Tablets 1605
Donnatal 2234
Donnatal Extentabs 2234
Donnatal Tablets 2234
Lomotil 2591
Motofen Tablets 789
Urised Tablets 2123
Belladonna Alkaloids (Possible increase in intraocular pressure when anticholinergic drugs including antiparkinson agents are administered concomitantly with haloperidol). Products include:
Bellergal-S Tablets 2375
Hyland's Bedwetting Tablets 788
Hyland's EnurAid Tablets 789
Hyland's Headache Tablets 790
Hyland's Teething Tablets 790
Similasan Eye Drops # 1 769
Benztropine Mesylate (Possible increase in intraocular pressure when antiparkinson agents are administered concomitantly with haloperidol). Products include:
Cogentin 1661
Biperiden Hydrochloride (Possible increase in intraocular pressure when antiparkinson agents are administered concomitantly with haloperidol). Products include:
Akineton 1380
Buprenorphine (CNS depressant potentiated). Products include:
Buprenex Injectable 2170
Buspirone Hydrochloride (CNS depressant potentiated). Products include:
BuSpar Tablets 738
Butabarbital (CNS depressant potentiated).
No products indexed under this heading.
Butalbital (CNS depressant potentiated). Products include:
Axocet Capsules 2469
Esgic-plus Capsules 1012
Esgic-plus Tablets 1012
Fioricet Tablets 2386
Fioricet with Codeine Capsules 2387
Fiorinal Capsules 2388
Fiorinal with Codeine Capsules 2390
Fiorinal Tablets 2388
Phrenilin 790
Sedapap Tablets 50 mg/650 mg 1826
Carbamazepine (Haloperidol may lower the convulsive threshold; adequate anticonvulsant therapy should be maintained). Products include:
Atretol Tablets 569
Tegretol/Tegretol-XR 870
Chlordiazepoxide (CNS depressant potentiated). Products include:
Limbitrol 2333
Chlordiazepoxide Hydrochloride (CNS depressant potentiated). Products include:
Librax Capsules 2330
Librium Capsules 2331
Librium Injectable 2332
Chlorpromazine (CNS depressant potentiated). Products include:
Thorazine Suppositories 2701
Chlorpromazine Hydrochloride (CNS depressant potentiated). Products include:
Thorazine 2701

Chlorprothixene (CNS depressant potentiated).
No products indexed under this heading.
Chlorprothixene Hydrochloride (CNS depressant potentiated).
No products indexed under this heading.
Chlorprothixene Lactate (CNS depressant potentiated).
No products indexed under this heading.
Clidinium Bromide (Possible increase in intraocular pressure when anticholinergic drugs including antiparkinson agents are administered concomitantly with haloperidol). Products include:
Librax Capsules 2330
Clorazepate Dipotassium (CNS depressant potentiated). Products include:
Tranxene 459
Clozapine (CNS depressant potentiated). Products include:
Clozaril Tablets 2377
Codeine Phosphate (CNS depressant potentiated). Products include:
Brontex 2130
Dimetane-DC Cough Syrup 2232
Fioricet with Codeine Capsules 2387
Fiorinal with Codeine Capsules 2390
Nucofed 2225
Phenergan with Codeine 2883
Phenergan VC with Codeine 2888
Robitussin A-C Syrup 2248
Robitussin-DAC Syrup 2249
Ryna 804
Soma Compound w/Codeine Tablets 2784
Tylenol with Codeine 1592
Desflurane (CNS depressant potentiated). Products include:
Suprane (desflurane, USP) 1865
Dezocine (CNS depressant potentiated). Products include:
Dalgan Injection 529
Diazepam (CNS depressant potentiated). Products include:
Dizac (diazepam injectable emulsion) CIV 1862
Valium Injectable 2336
Valium Tablets 2335
Dicumarol (Co-administration with one anticoagulant has resulted in an isolated instance of interference with the anticoagulant effects).
No products indexed under this heading.
Dicyclomine Hydrochloride (Possible increase in intraocular pressure when anticholinergic drugs including antiparkinson agents are administered concomitantly with haloperidol). Products include:
Bentyl 1246
Diphenhydramine Hydrochloride (Possible increase in intraocular pressure when antiparkinson agents are administered concomitantly with haloperidol). Products include:
Actifed Allergy Daytime/Nighttime Caplets 808
Actifed Sinus Daytime/Nighttime Tablets and Caplets 809
Extra Strength Bayer PM Aspirin Plus Sleep Aid 617
Benadryl Allergy Chewables 811
Benadryl Allergy/Cold Tablets 811
Benadryl Allergy Decongestant Liquid Medication 812
Benadryl Allergy Decongestant Tablets 812
Benadryl Allergy Liquid Medication 813
Benadryl Allergy 811
Benadryl Allergy Sinus Headache Caplets 813

Benadryl Dye-Free Allergy Liquigel Softgels 813
Benadryl Dye-Free Allergy Liquid Medication 814
Benadryl Itch Relief Stick Extra Strength 814
Benadryl Cream 814
Benadryl Gel 815
Benadryl Spray 815
Benadryl Injection 1955
Contac Day & Night Cold/Flu Night Caplets 772
Contac Night Allergy/Sinus Caplets 771
Extra Strength Doan's P.M. 653
Excedrin P.M. Analgesic/Sleeping Aid Tablets, Caplets, Liquigels ... 643
Nytol QuickCaps Caplets 632
Sleepinal Night-time Sleep Aid Capsules and Softgels 798
TYLENOL Allergy Sinus NightTime, Maximum Strength Caplets 1571
TYLENOL Flu NightTime, Maximum Strength Gelcaps 1575
TYLENOL Flu NightTime, Maximum Strength Hot Medication Packets 1575
TYLENOL PM Pain Reliever/Sleep Aid, Extra Strength Gelcaps, Caplets, Geltabs 1576
TYLENOL Severe Allergy Medication Caplets 1571
Maximum Strength Unisom Sleepgels 1990
Unisom With Pain Relief-Nighttime Sleep Aid and Pain Reliever 1991
Divalproex Sodium (Haloperidol may lower the convulsive threshold; adequate anticonvulsant therapy should be maintained). Products include:
Depakote Tablets 418
Droperidol (CNS depressant potentiated). Products include:
Inapsine Injection 462
Enflurane (CNS depressant potentiated).
No products indexed under this heading.
Epinephrine Hydrochloride (Haloperidol may block vasopressor activity of epinephrine). Products include:
Ana-Kit Anaphylaxis Emergency Treatment Kit 611
Estazolam (CNS depressant potentiated). Products include:
ProSom Tablets 457
Ethchlorvynol (CNS depressant potentiated). Products include:
Placidyl Capsules 456
Ethinamate (CNS depressant potentiated).
No products indexed under this heading.
Ethosuximide (Haloperidol may lower the convulsive threshold; adequate anticonvulsant therapy should be maintained). Products include:
Zarontin Capsules 1986
Zarontin Syrup 1986
Ethotoin (Haloperidol may lower the convulsive threshold; adequate anticonvulsant therapy should be maintained). Products include:
Peganone Tablets 455
Felbamate (Haloperidol may lower the convulsive threshold; adequate anticonvulsant therapy should be maintained). Products include:
Felbatol 2774
Fentanyl (CNS depressant potentiated). Products include:
Duragesic Transdermal System 1336
Fentanyl Citrate (CNS depressant potentiated). Products include:
Sublimaze Injection 463
Fluphenazine Decanoate (CNS depressant potentiated). Products include:
Prolixin Decanoate 510

IMPORTANT NOTE: Always consult each drug listing in the patient's regimen for possible interactions.

Haldol — Interactions Index — 468

Fluphenazine Enanthate (CNS depressant potentiated). Products include:
- Prolixin Enanthate 510

Fluphenazine Hydrochloride (CNS depressant potentiated). Products include:
- Prolixin 510

Flurazepam Hydrochloride (CNS depressant potentiated). Products include:
- Dalmane Capsules 2329

Fosphenytoin Sodium (Haloperidol may lower the convulsive threshold; adequate anticonvulsant therapy should be maintained). Products include:
- Cerebyx Injection 1956

Glutethimide (CNS depressant potentiated).
- No products indexed under this heading.

Glycopyrrolate (Possible increase in intraocular pressure when anticholinergic drugs including antiparkinson agents are administered concomitantly with haloperidol). Products include:
- Robinul Forte Tablets 2247
- Robinul Injectable 2247
- Robinul Tablets 2247

Haloperidol Decanoate (CNS depressant potentiated). Products include:
- Haldol Decanoate 1587

Hydrocodone Bitartrate (CNS depressant potentiated). Products include:
- Codiclear DH Syrup 808
- Duratuss HD Elixir 2750
- Histussin D Liquid 670
- Hycodan Tablets and Syrup 946
- Hycomine Compound Tablets ... 948
- Hycomine 947
- Hycotuss Expectorant Syrup 950
- Hydrocet Capsules 787
- Lorcet 10/650 Tablets 1016
- Lortab 2751
- Tussend 1830
- Tussend Expectorant 1831
- Vicodin Tablets 1404
- Vicodin ES Tablets 1405
- Vicodin HP Tablets 1403
- Vicodin Tuss Expectorant 1406
- Zydone Capsules 967

Hydrocodone Polistirex (CNS depressant potentiated). Products include:
- Tussionex Pennkinetic Extended-Release Suspension 1624

Hydromorphone Hydrochloride (CNS depressant potentiated). Products include:
- Dilaudid Ampules 1382
- Dilaudid Cough Syrup 1383
- Dilaudid-HP Injection 1384
- Dilaudid-HP Lyophilized Powder 250 mg 1384
- Dilaudid 1382
- Dilaudid Oral Liquid 1386
- Dilaudid 1382
- Dilaudid Tablets - 8 mg 1386

Hydroxyzine Hydrochloride (CNS depressant potentiated). Products include:
- Atarax Tablets & Syrup 1992
- Marax Tablets & DF Syrup 2015
- Vistaril Intramuscular Solution .. 2042

Hyoscyamine (Possible increase in intraocular pressure when anticholinergic drugs including antiparkinson agents are administered concomitantly with haloperidol). Products include:
- Cystospaz Tablets 2123
- Urised Tablets 2123

Hyoscyamine Sulfate (Possible increase in intraocular pressure when anticholinergic drugs including antiparkinson agents are administered concomitantly with haloperidol). Products include:
- Arco-Lase Plus Tablets 513
- Atrohist Plus Tablets 1605
- Cystospaz-M Capsules 2123
- Donnatal 2234
- Donnatal Extentabs 2234
- Donnatal Tablets 2234
- Kutrase Capsules 2546
- Levsin/Levsinex/Levbid 2549

Ipratropium Bromide (Possible increase in intraocular pressure when anticholinergic drugs including antiparkinson agents are administered concomitantly with haloperidol). Products include:
- Atrovent Inhalation Aerosol 674
- Atrovent Inhalation Solution ... 675
- Atrovent Nasal Spray 0.03% 676
- Atrovent Nasal Spray 0.06% 678

Isoflurane (CNS depressant potentiated).
- No products indexed under this heading.

Ketamine Hydrochloride (CNS depressant potentiated).
- No products indexed under this heading.

Lamotrigine (Haloperidol may lower the convulsive threshold; adequate anticonvulsant therapy should be maintained). Products include:
- Lamictal Tablets 1105

Levomethadyl Acetate Hydrochloride (CNS depressant potentiated). Products include:
- Orlaam Oral Solution 2361

Levorphanol Tartrate (CNS depressant potentiated). Products include:
- Levo-Dromoran 2297

Lithium Carbonate (Co-administration in a few patients has resulted in an encephalopathic syndrome characterized by weakness, lethargy, fever, confusion, and leukocytosis followed by irreversible brain damage). Products include:
- Eskalith 2658
- Lithium Carbonate Capsules & Tablets 2352
- Lithonate/Lithotabs/Lithobid ... 2721

Lithium Citrate (Co-administration in a few patients has resulted in an encephalopathic syndrome characterized by weakness, lethargy, fever, confusion, and leukocytosis followed by irreversible brain damage).
- No products indexed under this heading.

Lorazepam (CNS depressant potentiated). Products include:
- Ativan Injection 2805
- Ativan Tablets 2807

Loxapine Hydrochloride (CNS depressant potentiated). Products include:
- Loxitane 1426

Loxapine Succinate (CNS depressant potentiated). Products include:
- Loxitane Capsules 1426

Mepenzolate Bromide (Possible increase in intraocular pressure when anticholinergic drugs including antiparkinson agents are administered concomitantly with haloperidol).
- No products indexed under this heading.

Meperidine Hydrochloride (CNS depressant potentiated). Products include:
- Demerol 2438

Mepergan Injection 2859

Mephenytoin (Haloperidol may lower the convulsive threshold; adequate anticonvulsant therapy should be maintained). Products include:
- Mesantoin Tablets 2400

Mephobarbital (CNS depressant potentiated). Products include:
- Mebaral Tablets 2452

Meprobamate (CNS depressant potentiated). Products include:
- Miltown Tablets 2780
- PMB 200 and PMB 400 2890

Mesoridazine Besylate (CNS depressant potentiated). Products include:
- Serentil 689

Methadone Hydrochloride (CNS depressant potentiated). Products include:
- Methadone Hydrochloride Oral Concentrate 2356
- Methadone Hydrochloride Oral Solution & Tablets 2357

Methohexital Sodium (CNS depressant potentiated).
- No products indexed under this heading.

Methotrimeprazine (CNS depressant potentiated). Products include:
- Levoprome 1321

Methoxyflurane (CNS depressant potentiated).
- No products indexed under this heading.

Methsuximide (Haloperidol may lower the convulsive threshold; adequate anticonvulsant therapy should be maintained). Products include:
- Celontin Kapseals 1955

Midazolam Hydrochloride (CNS depressant potentiated). Products include:
- Versed Injection 2324

Molindone Hydrochloride (CNS depressant potentiated). Products include:
- Moban Tablets and Concentrate 1036

Morphine Sulfate (CNS depressant potentiated). Products include:
- Astramorph/PF Injection, USP (Preservative-Free) 526
- Duramorph Injection 983
- Infumorph 200 and Infumorph 500 Sterile Solutions 985
- Kadian Capsules 2948
- MS Contin Tablets 2149
- MSIR 2152
- Oramorph SR (Morphine Sulfate Sustained Release Tablets) .. 2359
- RMS Suppositories CII 2766
- Roxanol 2365

Opium Alkaloids (CNS depressant potentiated).
- No products indexed under this heading.

Oxazepam (CNS depressant potentiated). Products include:
- Serax Capsules 2916
- Serax Tablets 2916

Oxybutynin Chloride (Possible increase in intraocular pressure when anticholinergic drugs including antiparkinson agents are administered concomitantly with haloperidol). Products include:
- Ditropan 1267

Oxycodone Hydrochloride (CNS depressant potentiated). Products include:
- OxyContin Tablets 2163
- OxyIR Capsules 2167
- Percocet Tablets 955
- Percodan Tablets 955
- Percodan-Demi Tablets 956
- Roxicodone Tablets, Oral Solution & Intensol (Oxycodone) 2366
- Tylox Capsules 1593

Paramethadione (Haloperidol may lower the convulsive threshold; adequate anticonvulsant therapy should be maintained).
- No products indexed under this heading.

Pentobarbital Sodium (CNS depressant potentiated). Products include:
- Nembutal Sodium Capsules 440
- Nembutal Sodium Solution 442
- Nembutal Sodium Suppositories 444

Perphenazine (CNS depressant potentiated). Products include:
- Etrafon 2495
- Triavil Tablets 1800
- Trilafon 2532

Phenacemide (Haloperidol may lower the convulsive threshold; adequate anticonvulsant therapy should be maintained). Products include:
- Phenurone Tablets 455

Phenobarbital (Haloperidol may lower the convulsive threshold; adequate anticonvulsant therapy should be maintained; CNS depressant potentiated). Products include:
- Arco-Lase Plus Tablets 513
- Bellergal-S Tablets 2375
- Donnatal 2234
- Donnatal Extentabs 2234
- Donnatal Tablets 2234
- Phenobarbital Elixir and Tablets . 1523
- Quadrinal Tablets 1398

Phensuximide (Haloperidol may lower the convulsive threshold; adequate anticonvulsant therapy should be maintained).
- No products indexed under this heading.

Phenytoin (Haloperidol may lower the convulsive threshold; adequate anticonvulsant therapy should be maintained). Products include:
- Dilantin Infatabs 1967
- Dilantin-125 Suspension 1969

Phenytoin Sodium (Haloperidol may lower the convulsive threshold; adequate anticonvulsant therapy should be maintained). Products include:
- Dilantin Kapseals 1965

Prazepam (CNS depressant potentiated).
- No products indexed under this heading.

Primidone (Haloperidol may lower the convulsive threshold; adequate anticonvulsant therapy should be maintained). Products include:
- Mysoline 2860

Prochlorperazine (CNS depressant potentiated). Products include:
- Compazine 2644

Procyclidine Hydrochloride (Possible increase in intraocular pressure when antiparkinson agents are administered concomitantly with haloperidol). Products include:
- Kemadrin Tablets 1105

Promethazine Hydrochloride (CNS depressant potentiated). Products include:
- Mepergan Injection 2859
- Phenergan with Codeine 2883
- Phenergan with Dextromethorphan .. 2885
- Phenergan Injection 2880
- Phenergan Suppositories 2882
- Phenergan Syrup 2881
- Phenergan Tablets 2882
- Phenergan VC 2886
- Phenergan VC with Codeine ... 2888

Propantheline Bromide (Possible increase in intraocular pressure when anticholinergic drugs including antiparkinson agents are administered concomitantly with haloperidol). Products include:
- Pro-Banthine Tablets 2226

Interactions Index

Propofol (CNS depressant potentiated). Products include:
- Diprivan Injectable Emulsion ... 2939

Propoxyphene Hydrochloride (CNS depressant potentiated). Products include:
- Darvon ... 1475
- Wygesic Tablets ... 2930

Propoxyphene Napsylate (CNS depressant potentiated). Products include:
- Darvon-N/Darvocet-N ... 1473

Quazepam (CNS depressant potentiated). Products include:
- Doral Tablets ... 2773

Risperidone (CNS depressant potentiated). Products include:
- Risperdal Tablets ... 1348

Scopolamine (Possible increase in intraocular pressure when anticholinergic drugs including antiparkinson agents are administered concomitantly with haloperidol). Products include:
- Transderm Scōp Transdermal Therapeutic System ... 890

Scopolamine Hydrobromide (Possible increase in intraocular pressure when anticholinergic drugs including antiparkinson agents are administered concomitantly with haloperidol). Products include:
- Atrohist Plus Tablets ... 1605
- Donnatal ... 2234
- Donnatal Extentabs ... 2234
- Donnatal Tablets ... 2234

Secobarbital Sodium (CNS depressant potentiated). Products include:
- Seconal Sodium Pulvules ... 1529

Sevoflurane (CNS depressant potentiated).
- No products indexed under this heading.

Sufentanil Citrate (CNS depressant potentiated). Products include:
- Sufenta Injection ... 1355

Temazepam (CNS depressant potentiated). Products include:
- Restoril Capsules ... 2413

Thiamylal Sodium (CNS depressant potentiated).
- No products indexed under this heading.

Thioridazine Hydrochloride (CNS depressant potentiated). Products include:
- Mellaril ... 2398

Thiothixene (CNS depressant potentiated). Products include:
- Navane Capsules and Concentrate ... 2018
- Navane Intramuscular ... 2019

Triazolam (CNS depressant potentiated). Products include:
- Halcion Tablets ... 2093

Tridihexethyl Chloride (Possible increase in intraocular pressure when antiparkinson agents are administered concomitantly with haloperidol).
- No products indexed under this heading.

Trifluoperazine Hydrochloride (CNS depressant potentiated). Products include:
- Stelazine ... 2692

Trihexyphenidyl Hydrochloride (Possible increase in intraocular pressure when antiparkinson agents are administered concomitantly with haloperidol). Products include:
- Artane ... 1418

Trimethadione (Haloperidol may lower the convulsive threshold; adequate anticonvulsant therapy should be maintained).
- No products indexed under this heading.

Valproic Acid (Haloperidol may lower the convulsive threshold; adequate anticonvulsant therapy should be maintained). Products include:
- Depakene ... 416

Warfarin Sodium (Co-administration with one anticoagulant has resulted in an isolated instance of interference with the anticoagulant effects). Products include:
- Coumadin ... 941

Zolpidem Tartrate (CNS depressant potentiated). Products include:
- Ambien Tablets ... 2559

Food Interactions

Alcohol (CNS depressant potentiated).

HALFPRIN TABLETS
(Aspirin) ... 1413
None cited in PDR database.

HALLS JUNIORS SUGAR FREE COUGH SUPPRESSANT DROPS
(Menthol) ... 806
None cited in PDR database.

HALLS MENTHO-LYPTUS COUGH SUPPRESSANT DROPS
(Menthol) ... 806
None cited in PDR database.

HALLS PLUS MAXIMUM STRENGTH COUGH SUPPRESSANT DROPS
(Menthol) ... 806
None cited in PDR database.

HALLS SUGAR FREE MENTHO-LYPTUS COUGH SUPPRESSANT DROPS
(Menthol) ... 806
None cited in PDR database.

HALLS VITAMIN C DROPS
(Vitamin C) ... 807
None cited in PDR database.

HALOG CREAM, OINTMENT & SOLUTION 0.1%
(Halcinonide) ... 2795
None cited in PDR database.

HALOG-E CREAM 0.1%
(Halcinonide) ... 2795
None cited in PDR database.

HALOTESTIN TABLETS
(Fluoxymesterone) ... 2095
May interact with oral anticoagulants, insulin, and certain other agents. Compounds in these categories include:

Dicumarol (Androgens may increase sensitivity to oral anticoagulants).
- No products indexed under this heading.

Insulin, Human (The metabolic effects of androgens may decrease blood glucose and, therefore, insulin requirements).
- No products indexed under this heading.

Insulin, Human Isophane Suspension (The metabolic effects of androgens may decrease blood glucose and, therefore, insulin requirements). Products include:
- Novolin N Human Insulin 10 ml Vials ... 1846

Insulin, Human NPH (The metabolic effects of androgens may decrease blood glucose and, therefore, insulin requirements). Products include:
- Humulin N, 100 Units ... 1495
- Novolin N PenFill 1.5 ml Cartridges Durable Insulin Delivery System ... 1849
- Novolin N Prefilled Syringe Disposable Insulin Delivery System ... 1850

Insulin, Human Regular (The metabolic effects of androgens may decrease blood glucose and, therefore, insulin requirements). Products include:
- Humulin R, 100 Units ... 1497
- Novolin R Human Insulin 10 ml Vials ... 1846
- Novolin R PenFill 1.5 ml Cartridges Durable Insulin Delivery System ... 1849
- Novolin R Prefilled Syringe Disposable Insulin Delivery System ... 1850
- Velosulin BR Human Insulin 10 ml Vials ... 1847

Insulin, Human, Zinc Suspension (The metabolic effects of androgens may decrease blood glucose and, therefore, insulin requirements). Products include:
- Humulin L, 100 Units ... 1494
- Humulin U, 100 Units ... 1498
- Novolin L Human Insulin 10 ml Vials ... 1846

Insulin Lispro, Human (The metabolic effects of androgens may decrease blood glucose and, therefore, insulin requirements). Products include:
- Humalog Injection ... 1488

Insulin, NPH (The metabolic effects of androgens may decrease blood glucose and, therefore, insulin requirements). Products include:
- NPH, 100 Units ... 1502
- Pork NPH, 100 Units ... 1506
- Purified Pork NPH Isophane Insulin ... 1852

Insulin, Regular (The metabolic effects of androgens may decrease blood glucose and, therefore, insulin requirements). Products include:
- Regular, 100 Units ... 1503
- Pork Regular, 100 Units ... 1507
- Pork Regular (Concentrated), 500 Units ... 1508
- Purified Pork Regular Insulin ... 1852

Insulin, Zinc Crystals (The metabolic effects of androgens may decrease blood glucose and, therefore, insulin requirements). Products include:
- NPH, 100 Units ... 1502

Insulin, Zinc Suspension (The metabolic effects of androgens may decrease blood glucose and, therefore, insulin requirements). Products include:
- Iletin I ... 1501
- Lente, 100 Units ... 1501
- Iletin II ... 1504
- Pork Lente, 100 Units ... 1504
- Purified Pork Lente Insulin ... 1852

Oxyphenbutazone (Elevated serum levels of oxyphenbutazone).
- No products indexed under this heading.

Warfarin Sodium (Androgens may increase sensitivity to oral anticoagulants). Products include:
- Coumadin ... 941

HAVRIX
(Hepatitis A Vaccine, Inactivated) ... 2663
May interact with anticoagulants. Compounds in this category include:

Dalteparin Sodium (Havrix should be given with caution to individuals on anticoagulant therapy). Products include:
- Fragmin Injection ... 2088

Dicumarol (Havrix should be given with caution to individuals on anticoagulant therapy).
- No products indexed under this heading.

Enoxaparin (Havrix should be given with caution to individuals on anticoagulant therapy). Products include:
- Lovenox Injection ... 2187

Heparin Calcium (Havrix should be given with caution to individuals on anticoagulant therapy).
- No products indexed under this heading.

Heparin Sodium (Havrix should be given with caution to individuals on anticoagulant therapy). Products include:
- Heparin Lock Flush Solution ... 2831
- Heparin Sodium Injection ... 2832
- Heparin Sodium Vials ... 1486

Warfarin Sodium (Havrix should be given with caution to individuals on anticoagulant therapy). Products include:
- Coumadin ... 941

HEAD & SHOULDERS INTENSIVE TREATMENT DANDRUFF AND SEBORRHEIC DERMATITIS SHAMPOO
(Selenium Sulfide) ... 723
None cited in PDR database.

HEALON
(Sodium Hyaluronate) ... 302
None cited in PDR database.

HEALON GV
(Sodium Hyaluronate) ... 303
None cited in PDR database.

HEALTHY HEART
(Vitamins, Multiple) ... 1860
None cited in PDR database.

HELIDAC THERAPY
(Tetracycline Hydrochloride, Bismuth Subsalicylate, Metronidazole) ... 2135
May interact with oral anticoagulants, oral hypoglycemic agents, insulin, antacids containing aluminium, calcium and magnesium, iron containing oral preparations, penicillins, oral contraceptives, lithium preparations, and certain other agents. Compounds in these categories include:

Acarbose (Possible enhanced hypoglycemic effect when given with salicylates). Products include:
- Precose ... 604

Aluminum Carbonate (Impairs absorption of tetracyclines). Products include:
- Basaljel Capsules ... 2810
- Basaljel Suspension ... 2810
- Basaljel Tablets ... 2810

Aluminum Hydroxide (Impairs absorption of tetracyclines). Products include:
- ALternaGEL Liquid ... 1358
- Maximum Strength Ascriptin ... 650
- Cama Arthritis Pain Reliever ... 748
- Gaviscon Extra Strength Relief Formula Antacid Tablets ... 778
- Gaviscon Extra Strength Relief Formula Liquid Antacid ... 779
- Gaviscon Liquid Antacid ... 779
- Gelusil Antacid-Anti-gas Liquid ... 819
- Gelusil Antacid-Anti-gas Tablets ... 819
- Maalox Antacid/Anti-Gas Tablets ... 889
- Maalox Heartburn Relief Suspension ... 658
- Maalox Antacid Liquid ... 888
- Extra Strength Maalox Antacid/Anti-Gas Liquid and Tablets ... 888
- Mylanta ... 1359

IMPORTANT NOTE: Always consult each drug listing in the patient's regimen for possible interactions.

Helidac Therapy — Interactions Index — 470

Tempo Soft Antacid ■ 799

Aluminum Hydroxide Gel (Impairs absorption of tetracyclines). Products include:
- ALternaGEL Liquid ■ 675
- Aludrox Oral Suspension ■ 850
- Amphojel Suspension 2802
- Amphojel Suspension without Flavor 2802
- Amphojel Tablets 2802
- Ascriptin ■ 650
- Gaviscon Antacid Tablets ■ 778
- Gaviscon-2 Antacid Tablets ■ 779
- Mylanta Liquid ■ 676
- Mylanta Double Strength Liquid ■ 676
- Nephrox Suspension ■ 671

Amoxicillin Trihydrate (Tetracycline, a bacteriostatic antibiotic, may interfere with the bactericidal action of penicillin). Products include:
- Amoxil 2631
- Augmentin 2637
- Augmentin Tablets 2640

Ampicillin (Tetracycline, a bacteriostatic antibiotic, may interfere with the bactericidal action of penicillin). Products include:
- Omnipen Capsules 2872
- Omnipen for Oral Suspension 2873

Ampicillin Sodium (Tetracycline, a bacteriostatic antibiotic, may interfere with the bactericidal action of penicillin). Products include:
- Unasyn 2035

Ampicillin Trihydrate (Tetracycline, a bacteriostatic antibiotic, may interfere with the bactericidal action of penicillin).
- No products indexed under this heading.

Aspirin (Caution is recommended if co-administered). Products include:
- Alka-Seltzer Cherry Effervescent Antacid and Pain Reliever ■ 609
- Alka-Seltzer Extra Strength Effervescent Antacid and Pain Reliever ■ 609
- Alka-Seltzer Lemon Lime Effervescent Antacid and Pain Reliever ■ 609
- Alka-Seltzer Original Effervescent Antacid and Pain Reliever ■ 609
- Alka-Seltzer Plus ■ 611
- Alka-Seltzer Plus Sinus Medicine ■ 611
- Ascriptin ■ 650
- Arthritis Strength BC Powder ■ 631
- BC Cold Powder Multi-Symptom Formula (Cold-Sinus-Allergy) ■ 631
- BC Cold Powder Non-Drowsy Formula (Cold-Sinus) ■ 631
- BC Powder ■ 631
- Genuine Bayer Aspirin Tablets & Caplets ■ 618
- Extra Strength Bayer Arthritis Pain Regimen Formula ■ 615
- Extra Strength Bayer Aspirin Caplets & Tablets ■ 617
- Extended-Release Bayer 8-Hour Aspirin ■ 616
- Extra Strength Bayer Plus Aspirin Caplets ■ 617
- Extra Strength Bayer PM Aspirin Plus Sleep Aid ■ 617
- Aspirin Regimen Bayer 81 mg Tablets with Calcium ■ 615
- Aspirin Regimen Bayer Adult Low Strength 81 mg Tablets ■ 613
- Aspirin Regimen Bayer Children's Chewable Aspirin ■ 616
- Aspirin Regimen Bayer Regular Strength 325 mg Caplets ■ 613
- Bufferin Analgesic Tablets ■ 636
- Arthritis Strength Bufferin Analgesic Caplets ■ 637
- Extra Strength Bufferin Analgesic Tablets ■ 637
- Cama Arthritis Pain Reliever ■ 748
- Darvon Compound-65 Pulvules 1475
- Easprin 1971
- Ecotrin 2625
- Ecotrin Enteric Coated Aspirin Maximum Strength Tablets and Caplets ■ 775
- Ecotrin Enteric Coated Aspirin Regular Strength Tablets 2625
- Empirin Aspirin Tablets ■ 818
- Excedrin Extra-Strength Analgesic Tablets, Caplets, and Geltabs 734
- Fiorinal Capsules 2388
- Fiorinal with Codeine Capsules 2390
- Fiorinal Tablets 2388
- Goody's Extra Strength Headache Powders ■ 632
- Goody's Extra Strength Pain Relief Tablets ■ 632
- Halfprin Tablets 1413
- Norgesic 1554
- Percodan Tablets 955
- Percodan-Demi Tablets 956
- Robaxisal Tablets 2246
- Soma Compound w/Codeine Tablets 2784
- Soma Compound Tablets 2783
- St. Joseph Adult Chewable Aspirin (81 mg.) ■ 768
- Talwin Compound 2466
- Vanquish Analgesic Caplets ■ 627

Azlocillin Sodium (Tetracycline, a bacteriostatic antibiotic, may interfere with the bactericidal action of penicillin).
- No products indexed under this heading.

Bacampicillin Hydrochloride (Tetracycline, a bacteriostatic antibiotic, may interfere with the bactericidal action of penicillin). Products include:
- Spectrobid Tablets 2030

Bismuth (There is an anticipated reduction in tetracycline systemic absorption due to an interaction with bismuth and/or calcium carbonate, an excipient of bismuth subsalicylate tablets; the clinical significance is unknown).
- No products indexed under this heading.

Carbenicillin Disodium (Tetracycline, a bacteriostatic antibiotic, may interfere with the bactericidal action of penicillin).
- No products indexed under this heading.

Carbenicillin Indanyl Sodium (Tetracycline, a bacteriostatic antibiotic, may interfere with the bactericidal action of penicillin). Products include:
- Geocillin Tablets 2009

Chlorpropamide (Possible enhanced hypoglycemic effect when given with salicylates). Products include:
- Diabinese Tablets 2002

Cimetidine (Co-administration may prolong the half-life and decrease plasma clearance of metronidazole). Products include:
- Tagamet HB Tablets ■ 786
- Tagamet Tablets 2694

Cimetidine Hydrochloride (Co-administration may prolong the half-life and decrease plasma clearance of metronidazole). Products include:
- Tagamet 2694

Desogestrel (Concurrent use of tetracycline may render oral contraceptives less effective). Products include:
- Desogen Tablets 1867
- Ortho-Cept 1907

Dicloxacillin Sodium (Tetracycline, a bacteriostatic antibiotic, may interfere with the bactericidal action of penicillin).
- No products indexed under this heading.

Dicumarol (Tetracycline depresses plasma prothrombin activity; metronidazole potentiates the anticoagulant resulting in prolongation of prothrombin time; salicylates may cause an increased risk of bleeding when co-administered).
- No products indexed under this heading.

Disulfiram (Psychotic reactions have been reported in alcoholic patients who are using metronidazole and disulfiram concurrently; metronidazole should not be given to patients who have taken disulfiram within the last 2 weeks). Products include:
- Antabuse Tablets 2802

Ethinyl Estradiol (Concurrent use of tetracycline may render oral contraceptives less effective). Products include:
- Brevicon 2563
- Demulen 2580
- Desogen Tablets 1867
- Levlen/Tri-Levlen 646
- Lo/Ovral Tablets 2852
- Lo/Ovral-28 Tablets 2857
- Modicon 1928
- Nordette-21 Tablets 2863
- Nordette-28 Tablets 2866
- Norinyl 2563
- Ortho-Cept 1907
- Ortho-Cyclen/Ortho-Tri-Cyclen 1914
- Ortho-Novum 1928
- Ortho-Cyclen/Ortho Tri-Cyclen 1914
- Ovcon 765
- Ovral Tablets 2877
- Ovral-28 Tablets 2878
- Levlen/Tri-Levlen 646
- Tri-Norinyl 2607
- Triphasil-21 Tablets 2919
- Triphasil-28 Tablets 2924

Ethynodiol Diacetate (Concurrent use of tetracycline may render oral contraceptives less effective). Products include:
- Demulen 2580

Ferrous Fumarate (Impairs absorption of tetracyclines). Products include:
- Chromagen Capsules 2470
- Chromagen FA 2471
- Chromagen Forte 2471
- Ferro-Sequels ■ 684
- Nephro-Fer Tablets 2168
- Nephro-Fer Rx Tablets 2168
- Nephro-Vite + Fe Tablets 2170
- Stresstabs + Iron ■ 685
- Trinsicon Capsules 2759
- Vitron-C Tablets ■ 667

Ferrous Gluconate (Impairs absorption of tetracyclines). Products include:
- Megadose 513

Ferrous Sulfate (Impairs absorption of tetracyclines). Products include:
- Feosol Capsules ■ 777
- Feosol Elixir 2627
- Feosol Tablets 2627
- Fero-Folic-500 Filmtab 433
- Fero-Grad-500 Filmtab 434
- Fero-Gradumet Filmtab 434
- Iberet Tablets 437
- Iberet-500 Liquid 438
- Iberet-Folic-500 Filmtab 433
- Iberet-Liquid 438
- Irospan 1000
- Slow Fe Tablets 889
- Slow Fe with Folic Acid 890

Fosphenytoin Sodium (Co-administration may accelerate the elimination of metronidazole; potential for impaired clearance of phenytoin). Products include:
- Cerebyx Injection 1956

Glimepiride (Possible enhanced hypoglycemic effect when given with salicylates). Products include:
- Amaryl Tablets 1241

Glipizide (Possible enhanced hypoglycemic effect when given with salicylates). Products include:
- Glucotrol Tablets 2011
- Glucotrol XL Extended Release Tablets 2012

Glyburide (Possible enhanced hypoglycemic effect when given with salicylates). Products include:
- DiaBeta Tablets 1265
- Glynase PresTab Tablets 2091
- Micronase Tablets 2099

Insulin, Human (Possible enhanced hypoglycemic effect when given with salicylates).
- No products indexed under this heading.

Insulin, Human Isophane Suspension (Possible enhanced hypoglycemic effect when given with salicylates). Products include:
- Novolin N Human Insulin 10 ml Vials 1846

Insulin, Human NPH (Possible enhanced hypoglycemic effect when given with salicylates). Products include:
- Humulin N, 100 Units 1495
- Novolin N PenFill 1.5 ml Cartridges Durable Insulin Delivery System 1849
- Novolin N Prefilled Syringe Disposable Insulin Delivery System 1850

Insulin, Human Regular (Possible enhanced hypoglycemic effect when given with salicylates). Products include:
- Humulin R, 100 Units 1497
- Novolin R Human Insulin 10 ml Vials 1846
- Novolin R PenFill 1.5 ml Cartridges Durable Insulin Delivery System 1849
- Novolin R Prefilled Syringe Disposable Insulin Delivery System 1850
- Velosulin BR Human Insulin 10 ml Vials 1847

Insulin, Human, Zinc Suspension (Possible enhanced hypoglycemic effect when given with salicylates). Products include:
- Humulin L, 100 Units 1494
- Humulin U, 100 Units 1498
- Novolin L Human Insulin 10 ml Vials 1846

Insulin Lispro, Human (Possible enhanced hypoglycemic effect when given with salicylates). Products include:
- Humalog Injection 1488

Insulin, NPH (Possible enhanced hypoglycemic effect when given with salicylates). Products include:
- NPH, 100 Units 1502
- Pork NPH, 100 Units 1506
- Purified Pork NPH Isophane Insulin 1852

Insulin, Regular (Possible enhanced hypoglycemic effect when given with salicylates). Products include:
- Regular, 100 Units 1503
- Pork Regular, 100 Units 1507
- Pork Regular (Concentrated), 500 Units 1508
- Purified Pork Regular Insulin 1852

Insulin, Zinc Crystals (Possible enhanced hypoglycemic effect when given with salicylates). Products include:
- NPH, 100 Units 1502

Insulin, Zinc Suspension (Possible enhanced hypoglycemic effect when given with salicylates). Products include:
- Iletin I 1501
- Lente, 100 Units 1501
- Iletin II 1504
- Pork Lente, 100 Units 1504
- Purified Pork Lente Insulin 1852

Levonorgestrel (Concurrent use of tetracycline may render oral contraceptives less effective). Products include:
- Levlen/Tri-Levlen 646
- Nordette-21 Tablets 2863
- Nordette-28 Tablets 2866
- Norplant System 2868
- Levlen/Tri-Levlen 646
- Triphasil-21 Tablets 2919
- Triphasil-28 Tablets 2924

(■ Described in PDR For Nonprescription Drugs) (◉ Described in PDR For Ophthalmology)

Lithium Carbonate (In patients stabilized on relatively high doses of lithium, short-term metronidazole therapy may elevate serum lithium levels with possible signs of lithium toxicity). Products include:
- Eskalith ... 2658
- Lithium Carbonate Capsules & Tablets ... 2352
- Lithonate/Lithotabs/Lithobid ... 2721

Lithium Citrate (In patients stabilized on relatively high doses of lithium, short-term metronidazole therapy may elevate serum lithium levels with possible signs of lithium toxicity).
- No products indexed under this heading.

Magaldrate (Impairs absorption of tetracyclines).
- No products indexed under this heading.

Magnesium Hydroxide (Impairs absorption of tetracyclines). Products include:
- Aludrox Oral Suspension ... 850
- Ascriptin ... 650
- Di-Gel Antacid/Anti-Gas ... 762
- Gelusil Antacid-Anti-gas Liquid ... 819
- Gelusil Antacid-Anti-gas Tablets ... 819
- Maalox Antacid/Anti-Gas Tablets ... 889
- Maalox Antacid Liquid ... 888
- Extra Strength Maalox Antacid/Anti-Gas Liquid and Tablets ... 888
- Mylanta Fast-Acting ... 1359
- Mylanta Gelcaps Antacid ... 678
- Fast-Acting Mylanta Liquid Antacid 1359
- Mylanta Tablets ... 677
- Maximum-Strength Fast-Acting Mylanta Liquid Antacid ... 1359
- Mylanta Double Strength Tablets ... 677
- Phillips' Milk of Magnesia Liquid ... 627
- Rolaids Antacid Tablets ... 807
- Tempo Soft Antacid ... 799

Magnesium Oxide (Impairs absorption of tetracyclines). Products include:
- Beelith Tablets ... 632
- Bufferin Analgesic Tablets ... 636
- Arthritis Strength Bufferin Analgesic Caplets ... 637
- Extra Strength Bufferin Analgesic Tablets ... 637
- Caltrate PLUS ... 681
- Cama Arthritis Pain Reliever ... 748
- Mag-Ox 400 ... 666
- Uro-Mag ... 666

Mestranol (Concurrent use of tetracycline may render oral contraceptives less effective). Products include:
- Norinyl ... 2563
- Ortho-Novum ... 1928

Metformin Hydrochloride (Possible enhanced hypoglycemic effect when given with salicylates). Products include:
- Glucophage Tablets ... 754

Methoxyflurane (Co-administration has resulted in fatal renal toxicity).
- No products indexed under this heading.

Mezlocillin Sodium (Tetracycline, a bacteriostatic antibiotic, may interfere with the bactericidal action of penicillin). Products include:
- Mezlin ... 594
- Mezlin Pharmacy Bulk Package ... 597

Nafcillin Sodium (Tetracycline, a bacteriostatic antibiotic, may interfere with the bactericidal action of penicillin).
- No products indexed under this heading.

Norethindrone (Concurrent use of tetracycline may render oral contraceptives less effective). Products include:
- Brevicon ... 2563
- Micronor Tablets ... 1903
- Modicon ... 1928
- Norinyl ... 2563
- Nor-Q D Tablets ... 2598
- Ortho-Novum ... 1928
- Ovcon ... 765
- Tri-Norinyl ... 2607

Norethynodrel (Concurrent use of tetracycline may render oral contraceptives less effective).
- No products indexed under this heading.

Norgestimate (Concurrent use of tetracycline may render oral contraceptives less effective). Products include:
- Ortho-Cyclen/Ortho-Tri-Cyclen ... 1914
- Ortho-Cyclen/Ortho Tri-Cyclen ... 1914

Norgestrel (Concurrent use of tetracycline may render oral contraceptives less effective). Products include:
- Lo/Ovral Tablets ... 2852
- Lo/Ovral-28 Tablets ... 2857
- Ovral Tablets ... 2877
- Ovral-28 Tablets ... 2878
- Ovrette Tablets ... 2878

Penicillin G Benzathine (Tetracycline, a bacteriostatic antibiotic, may interfere with the bactericidal action of penicillin). Products include:
- Bicillin C-R Injection ... 2810
- Bicillin C-R 900/300 Injection ... 2812
- Bicillin L-A Injection ... 2813

Penicillin G Potassium (Tetracycline, a bacteriostatic antibiotic, may interfere with the bactericidal action of penicillin). Products include:
- Pfizerpen for Injection ... 2022

Penicillin G Procaine (Tetracycline, a bacteriostatic antibiotic, may interfere with the bactericidal action of penicillin). Products include:
- Bicillin C-R Injection ... 2810
- Bicillin C-R 900/300 Injection ... 2812

Penicillin G Sodium (Tetracycline, a bacteriostatic antibiotic, may interfere with the bactericidal action of penicillin).
- No products indexed under this heading.

Penicillin V Potassium (Tetracycline, a bacteriostatic antibiotic, may interfere with the bactericidal action of penicillin). Products include:
- Pen•Vee K ... 2879

Phenobarbital (Co-administration may accelerate the elimination of metronidazole). Products include:
- Arco-Lase Plus Tablets ... 513
- Bellergal-S Tablets ... 2375
- Donnatal ... 2234
- Donnatal Extentabs ... 2234
- Donnatal Tablets ... 2234
- Phenobarbital Elixir and Tablets ... 1523
- Quadrinal Tablets ... 1398

Phenytoin (Co-administration may accelerate the elimination of metronidazole; potential for impaired clearance of phenytoin). Products include:
- Dilantin Infatabs ... 1967
- Dilantin-125 Suspension ... 1969

Phenytoin Sodium (Co-administration may accelerate the elimination of metronidazole; potential for impaired clearance of phenytoin). Products include:
- Dilantin Kapseals ... 1965

Polysaccharide-Iron Complex (Impairs absorption of tetracyclines). Products include:
- Niferex-150 Capsules ... 811
- Niferex Elixir ... 811
- Niferex-150 Forte Capsules ... 811
- Niferex ... 811
- Niferex-PN Tablets ... 811
- Nu-Iron 150 Capsules ... 1826
- Nu-Iron Elixir ... 1826

Probenecid (Caution is recommended if co-administered). Products include:
- Benemid Tablets ... 1651
- ColBENEMID Tablets ... 1662

Sodium Bicarbonate (Oral sodium bicarbonate impairs absorption of tetracyclines). Products include:
- Alka-Seltzer Cherry Effervescent Antacid and Pain Reliever ... 609
- Alka-Seltzer Extra Strength Effervescent Antacid and Pain Reliever ... 609
- Alka-Seltzer Gold Effervescent Antacid ... 611
- Alka-Seltzer Lemon Lime Effervescent Antacid and Pain Reliever ... 609
- Alka-Seltzer Original Effervescent Antacid and Pain Reliever ... 609
- Arm & Hammer Pure Baking Soda ... 648
- Colyte and Colyte-flavored ... 2540
- GoLYTELY ... 694
- Massengill Disposable Douches ... 780
- Massengill Liquid Concentrate ... 780
- NuLYTELY ... 694
- Cherry Flavor NuLYTELY ... 694

Sulfinpyrazone (Caution is recommended if co-administered). Products include:
- Anturane ... 823

Ticarcillin Disodium (Tetracycline, a bacteriostatic antibiotic, may interfere with the bactericidal action of penicillin). Products include:
- Ticar for Injection ... 2704
- Timentin for Injection ... 2706

Tolazamide (Possible enhanced hypoglycemic effect when given with salicylates).
- No products indexed under this heading.

Tolbutamide (Possible enhanced hypoglycemic effect when given with salicylates).
- No products indexed under this heading.

Warfarin Sodium (Tetracycline depresses plasma prothrombin activity; metronidazole potentiates the anticoagulant resulting in prolongation of prothrombin time; salicylates may cause an increased risk of bleeding when co-administered). Products include:
- Coumadin ... 941

Zinc Gluconate (Oral zinc preparations impair absorption of tetracyclines). Products include:
- Megadose ... 513

Food Interactions

Alcohol (Concurrent use has resulted in abdominal cramps, nausea, vomiting, headaches, and flushing; avoid alcoholic beverages concurrently and/or at least 1 day afterward).

Dairy products (Impairs absorption of tetracyclines).

HEMORID CREME

(Petrolatum, White, Mineral Oil, Pramoxine Hydrochloride, Phenylephrine Hydrochloride) ... 797

See **Hemorid Ointment**

HEMORID FOR WOMEN CLEANSER

(Cleanser) ... 797

None cited in PDR database.

HEMORID OINTMENT

(Phenylephrine Hydrochloride, Mineral Oil, Petrolatum, White, Pramoxine Hydrochloride) ... 797

May interact with:

Antidepressant Medications, unspecified (Concurrent use is not recommended without first consulting a physician).

Blood Pressure Medications, unspecified (Concurrent use is not recommended without first consulting a physician).
- No products indexed under this heading.

HEMORID SUPPOSITORIES

(Zinc Oxide, Phenylephrine Hydrochloride, Fat, Hard) ... 797

See **Hemorid Ointment**

HEPARIN LOCK FLUSH SOLUTION

(Heparin Sodium) ... 2831

May interact with cardiac glycosides, antihistamines, tetracyclines, non-steroidal anti-inflammatory agents, platelet inhibitors, and certain other agents. Compounds in these categories include:

Acrivastine (Anticoagulant action partially counteracted). Products include:
- Semprex-D Capsules ... 1620

Aspirin (Interferes with platelet-aggregation reactions and may induce bleeding). Products include:
- Alka-Seltzer Cherry Effervescent Antacid and Pain Reliever ... 609
- Alka-Seltzer Extra Strength Effervescent Antacid and Pain Reliever ... 609
- Alka-Seltzer Lemon Lime Effervescent Antacid and Pain Reliever ... 609
- Alka-Seltzer Original Effervescent Antacid and Pain Reliever ... 609
- Alka-Seltzer Plus ... 611
- Alka-Seltzer Plus Sinus Medicine ... 611
- Ascriptin ... 650
- Arthritis Strength BC Powder ... 631
- BC Cold Powder Multi-Symptom Formula (Cold-Sinus-Allergy) ... 631
- BC Cold Powder Non-Drowsy Formula (Cold-Sinus) ... 631
- BC Powder ... 631
- Genuine Bayer Aspirin Tablets & Caplets ... 618
- Extra Strength Bayer Arthritis Pain Regimen Formula ... 615
- Extra Strength Bayer Aspirin Caplets & Tablets ... 617
- Extended-Release Bayer 8-Hour Aspirin ... 616
- Extra Strength Bayer Plus Aspirin Caplets ... 617
- Extra Strength Bayer PM Aspirin Plus Sleep Aid ... 617
- Aspirin Regimen Bayer 81 mg Tablets with Calcium ... 615
- Aspirin Regimen Bayer Adult Low Strength 81 mg Tablets ... 613
- Aspirin Regimen Bayer Children's Chewable Aspirin ... 616
- Aspirin Regimen Bayer Regular Strength 325 mg Caplets ... 613
- Bufferin Analgesic Tablets ... 636
- Arthritis Strength Bufferin Analgesic Caplets ... 637
- Extra Strength Bufferin Analgesic Tablets ... 637
- Cama Arthritis Pain Reliever ... 748
- Darvon Compound-65 Pulvules ... 1475
- Easprin ... 1971
- Ecotrin ... 2625
- Ecotrin Enteric Coated Aspirin Maximum Strength Tablets and Caplets ... 775
- Ecotrin Enteric Coated Aspirin Regular Strength Tablets ... 2625
- Empirin Aspirin Tablets ... 818
- Excedrin Extra-Strength Analgesic Tablets, Caplets, and Geltabs ... 734
- Fiorinal Capsules ... 2388
- Fiorinal with Codeine Capsules ... 2390
- Fiorinal Tablets ... 2388
- Goody's Extra Strength Headache Powders ... 632
- Goody's Extra Strength Pain Relief Tablets ... 632
- Halfprin Tablets ... 1413
- Norgesic ... 1554
- Percodan Tablets ... 955
- Percodan-Demi Tablets ... 956

IMPORTANT NOTE: Always consult each drug listing in the patient's regimen for possible interactions.

Heparin Lock Flush | Interactions Index | 472

Robaxisal Tablets ... 2246
Soma Compound w/Codeine Tablets ... 2784
Soma Compound Tablets ... 2783
St. Joseph Adult Chewable Aspirin (81 mg.) ... ■ 768
Talwin Compound ... 2466
Vanquish Analgesic Caplets ... ■ 627

Astemizole (Anticoagulant action partially counteracted). Products include:
Hismanal Tablets ... 1341

Azatadine Maleate (Anticoagulant action partially counteracted). Products include:
Trinalin Repetabs Tablets ... 1373

Azlocillin Sodium (Interferes with platelet-aggregation reactions and may induce bleeding).
No products indexed under this heading.

Bromodiphenhydramine Hydrochloride (Anticoagulant action partially counteracted).
No products indexed under this heading.

Brompheniramine Maleate (Anticoagulant action partially counteracted). Products include:
Alka-Seltzer Plus Sinus Medicine .. ■ 611
Bromfed Capsules (Extended-Release) ... 1832
Bromfed Syrup ... ■ 712
Bromfed Tablets ... 1832
Bromfed-DM Cough Syrup ... 1832
Bromfed-PD Capsules (Extended-Release) ... 1832
Dimetane-DC Cough Syrup ... 2232
Dimetane-DX Cough Syrup ... 2233
Dimetapp Allergy Dye-Free Elixir ... ■ 838
Dimetapp Allergy Sinus Caplets ... ■ 838
Dimetapp Cold & Allergy Chewable Tablets ... ■ 838
Dimetapp Cold & Cough Liqui-Gels ... ■ 839
Dimetapp Cold & Fever Suspension ... ■ 839
Dimetapp DM Elixir ... ■ 840
Dimetapp Elixir ... ■ 840
Dimetapp Extentabs ... ■ 841
Dimetapp Tablets/Liqui-Gels ... ■ 841
Rondec Chewable Tablets ... 974
Vicks DayQuil Allergy Relief 12-Hour Extended Release Tablets .. ■ 733
Vicks DayQuil Allergy Relief 4-Hour Tablets ... ■ 733

Carbenicillin Indanyl Sodium (Interferes with platelet-aggregation reactions and may induce bleeding). Products include:
Geocillin Tablets ... 2009

Cetirizine Hydrochloride (Anticoagulant action partially counteracted). Products include:
Zyrtec Tablets ... 2053

Chlorpheniramine Maleate (Anticoagulant action partially counteracted). Products include:
Alka-Seltzer Plus Cold Medicine ... ■ 611
Alka-Seltzer Plus Cold Medicine Liqui-Gels ... ■ 612
Alka-Seltzer Plus Cold & Cough Medicine ... ■ 611
Alka-Seltzer Plus Cold & Cough Medicine Liqui-Gels ... ■ 612
Alka-Seltzer Plus Flu & Body Aches Effervescent Tablets ... ■ 612
Allerest Maximum Strength ... ■ 649
Allerest Sinus Pain Formula ... ■ 649
Ana-Kit Anaphylaxis Emergency Treatment Kit ... 611
Atrohist Pediatric Capsules ... 1603
Atrohist Plus Tablets ... 1605
BC Cold Powder Multi-Symptom Formula (Cold-Sinus-Allergy) ... ■ 631
Cerose DM ... ■ 853
Cheracol Plus Head Cold/Cough Formula ... ■ 741
Children's TYLENOL Cold Multi-Symptom Chewable Tablets and Liquid ... 1559
Children's TYLENOL Cold Plus Cough Multi Symptom Chewable Tablets and Liquid ... 1560
Children's TYLENOL Flu Suspension Liquid ... 1560
Children's Vicks DayQuil Allergy Relief ... ■ 730
Children's Vicks NyQuil Cold/Cough Relief ... ■ 731
Chlor-Trimeton Allergy Decongestant Tablets ... ■ 759
Chlor-Trimeton Allergy Tablets ... ■ 758
Allergy-Sinus Comtrex Multi-Symptom Allergy-Sinus Formula Tablets and Caplets ... ■ 639
Comtrex Multi-Symptom ... ■ 638
Contac Continuous Action Nasal Decongestant/Antihistamine 12 Hour Capsules ... ■ 773
Contac Maximum Strength Continuous Action Decongestant/Antihistamine 12 Hour Caplets .. ■ 772
Contac Severe Cold and Flu Formula Caplets ... ■ 773
Coricidin Cold + Flu Tablets ... ■ 760
Coricidin Cough + Cold Tablets ... ■ 760
Coricidin 'D' Decongestant Tablets ... ■ 760
D.A. II Tablets ... 972
D.A. Chewable Tablets ... 970
Dura-Tap/PD Capsules ... 970
Dura-Vent/DA Tablets ... 972
Efidac 24 Chlorpheniramine ... ■ 655
Extendryl ... 1003
Fedahist Gyrocaps ... 2545
Hycomine Compound Tablets ... 948
Kronofed-A ... 994
Nolamine Timed-Release Tablets ... 790
Novahistine Elixir ... ■ 782
Ornade Spansule Capsules ... 2678
PediaCare Cough-Cold Chewable Tablets and Liquid ... 1569
PediaCare NightRest Cough-Cold Liquid ... 1569
Pediatric Vicks 44m Cough & Cold Relief ... ■ 737
Pyrroxate Caplets ... ■ 742
Ryna ... ■ 804
Sinarest ... ■ 663
Sine-Off Sinus Medicine ... ■ 784
Singlet Tablets ... ■ 785
Sinulin Tablets ... 792
Sinutab Sinus Allergy Medication, Maximum Strength Tablets and Caplets ... ■ 823
Sudafed Cold & Allergy Tablets ... ■ 826
Teldrin 12 Hour Antihistamine/Nasal Decongestant Allergy Relief Capsules ... ■ 786
TheraFlu Flu and Cold Medicine ... ■ 750
Theraflu Maximum Strength Flu and Cold Medicine For Sore Throat ... ■ 751
TheraFlu Flu, Cold and Cough Medicine ... ■ 750
TheraFlu Maximum Strength Nighttime Flu, Cold & Cough Medicine ... ■ 751
Triaminic Night Time ... ■ 754
Triaminic Syrup ... ■ 755
Triaminic Triaminicol Cold & Cough ... ■ 756
Triaminicin Tablets ... ■ 756
Tussend ... 1830
TYLENOL Allergy Sinus, Maximum Strength Caplets and Gelcaps ... 1571
TYLENOL Cold Medication, Multi-Symptom Formula Tablets and Caplets ... 1572
TYLENOL Cold Medication, Multi-Symptom Hot Liquid Packets ... 1572
Vicks 44 LiquiCaps Cough, Cold & Flu Relief ... ■ 728
Vicks 44M Cough, Cold & Flu Relief ... ■ 729

Chlorpheniramine Polistirex (Anticoagulant action partially counteracted). Products include:
Tussionex Pennkinetic Extended-Release Suspension ... 1624

Chlorpheniramine Tannate (Anticoagulant action partially counteracted). Products include:
Atrohist Pediatric Suspension ... 1604
Atrohist Pediatric Suspension Dye-Free ... 1604
Rynatan ... 2781
Rynatuss ... 2782

Choline Magnesium Trisalicylate (Interferes with platelet-aggregation reactions and may induce bleeding). Products include:
Trilisate ... 2155

Clemastine Fumarate (Anticoagulant action partially counteracted). Products include:
Tavist Syrup ... 2426
Tavist Tablets ... 2427
Tavist-1 12 Hour Relief Tablets ... ■ 749
Tavist-D 12 Hour Relief Tablets ... ■ 750

Cyproheptadine Hydrochloride (Anticoagulant action partially counteracted). Products include:
Periactin ... 1767

Demeclocycline Hydrochloride (Anticoagulant action partially counteracted). Products include:
Declomycin Tablets ... 1421

Deslanoside (Anticoagulant action partially counteracted).
No products indexed under this heading.

Dexchlorpheniramine Maleate (Anticoagulant action partially counteracted).
No products indexed under this heading.

Dextran 40 (Interferes with platelet-aggregation reactions and may induce bleeding).
No products indexed under this heading.

Diclofenac Potassium (Interferes with platelet-aggregation reactions and may induce bleeding). Products include:
Cataflam Tablets ... 833

Diclofenac Sodium (Interferes with platelet-aggregation reactions and may induce bleeding). Products include:
Voltaren Ophthalmic Sterile Ophthalmic Solution ... ⊙ 264
Cataflam/Voltaren/Voltaren-XR ... 833

Diflunisal (Interferes with platelet-aggregation reactions and may induce bleeding). Products include:
Dolobid Tablets ... 1695

Digitoxin (Anticoagulant action partially counteracted). Products include:
Crystodigin Tablets ... 1472

Digoxin (Anticoagulant action partially counteracted). Products include:
Lanoxicaps ... 1110
Lanoxin Elixir Pediatric ... 1113
Lanoxin Injection ... 1116
Lanoxin Injection Pediatric ... 1119
Lanoxin Tablets ... 1121

Diphenhydramine Citrate (Anticoagulant action partially counteracted). Products include:
Excedrin P.M. Analgesic/Sleeping Aid Tablets, Caplets, Liquigels ... 735

Diphenylpyraline Hydrochloride (Anticoagulant action partially counteracted).
No products indexed under this heading.

Dipyridamole (Interferes with platelet-aggregation reactions and may induce bleeding). Products include:
Persantine Tablets ... 686

Doxycycline Calcium (Anticoagulant action partially counteracted). Products include:
Vibramycin Calcium Oral Suspension Syrup ... 2038

Doxycycline Hyclate (Anticoagulant action partially counteracted). Products include:
Doryx Capsules ... 1970
Vibramycin Hyclate Capsules ... 2038
Vibramycin Hyclate Intravenous ... 2040
Vibra-Tabs Film Coated Tablets ... 2038

Doxycycline Monohydrate (Anticoagulant action partially counteracted). Products include:
Monodox Capsules ... 1858
Vibramycin Monohydrate for Oral Suspension ... 2038

Etodolac (Interferes with platelet-aggregation reactions and may induce bleeding). Products include:
Lodine Capsules and Tablets ... 2849

Fenoprofen Calcium (Interferes with platelet-aggregation ractions and may induce bleeding). Products include:
Nalfon 200 Pulvules & Nalfon Tablets ... 933

Flurbiprofen (Interferes with platelet-aggregation reactions and may induce bleeding).
No products indexed under this heading.

Hydroxychloroquine Sulfate (Interferes with platelet-aggregation reactions and may induce bleeding). Products include:
Plaquenil Sulfate Tablets ... 2459

Ibuprofen (Interferes with platelet-aggregation reactions and may induce bleeding). Products include:
Advil Cold and Sinus Caplets and Tablets ... ■ 837
Advil Ibuprofen Tablets, Caplets and Gel Caplets ... ■ 836
Children's Motrin Ibuprofen Oral Suspension ... 1558
IBU Tablets ... 1389
Ibuprohm ... ■ 713
Motrin IB Caplets, Tablets, and Gelcaps ... ■ 802
Motrin Ibuprofen Suspension, Oral Drops, Chewable Tablets, Caplets ... 1563
Nuprin Ibuprofen/Analgesic Tablets & Caplets ... ■ 645
Vicks DayQuil SINUS Pressure & PAIN Relief with IBUPROFEN ... ■ 735

Indomethacin (Interferes with platelet-aggregation reactions and may induce bleeding). Products include:
Indocin ... 1723

Indomethacin Sodium Trihydrate (Interferes with platelet-aggregation reactions and may induce bleeding). Products include:
Indocin I.V. ... 1727

Ketoprofen (Interferes with platelet-aggregation reactions and may induce bleeding). Products include:
Actron Caplets and Tablets ... ■ 608
Orudis Capsules ... 2874
Orudis KT ... ■ 842
Oruvail Capsules ... 2874

Ketorolac Tromethamine (Interferes with platelet-aggregation reactions and may induce bleeding). Products include:
Acular Sterile Ophthalmic Solution ... 470
Toradol ... 2319

Loratadine (Anticoagulant action partially counteracted). Products include:
Claritin Tablets ... 2485
Claritin-D Tablets ... 2487

Magnesium Salicylate (Interferes with platelet-aggregation reactions and may induce bleeding). Products include:
Backache Caplets ... ■ 635
Doan's Extra-Strength Analgesic ... ■ 653
Extra Strength Doan's P.M. ... ■ 653
Doan's Regular Strength Analgesic ... ■ 654
Mobigesic Tablets ... ■ 607

Meclofenamate Sodium (Interferes with platelet-aggregation reactions and may induce bleeding).
No products indexed under this heading.

Mefenamic Acid (Interferes with platelet-aggregation reactions and may induce bleeding). Products include:
Ponstel ... 1982

(■ Described in PDR For Nonprescription Drugs) (⊙ Described in PDR For Ophthalmology)

Methacycline Hydrochloride (Anticoagulant action partially counteracted).
No products indexed under this heading.

Methdilazine Hydrochloride (Anticoagulant action partially counteracted).
No products indexed under this heading.

Mezlocillin Sodium (Interferes with platelet-aggregation reactions and may induce bleeding). Products include:
Mezlin 594
Mezlin Pharmacy Bulk Package 597

Minocycline Hydrochloride (Anticoagulant action partially counteracted). Products include:
DYNACIN Capsules 1627
Minocin Intravenous 1428
Minocin Oral Suspension 1431
Minocin Pellet-Filled Capsules 1429

Nabumetone (Interferes with platelet-aggregation reactions and may induce bleeding). Products include:
Relafen Tablets 2688

Nafcillin Sodium (Interferes with platelet-aggregation reactions and may induce bleeding).
No products indexed under this heading.

Naproxen (Interferes with platelet-aggregation reactions and may induce bleeding). Products include:
Anaprox/Naprosyn 2277

Naproxen Sodium (Interferes with platelet-aggregation reactions and may induce bleeding). Products include:
Aleve 2124
Anaprox/Naprosyn 2277
Naprelan Tablets 2861

Nicotine Polacrilex (Anticoagulant action partially counteracted).
No products indexed under this heading.

Oxaprozin (Interferes with platelet-aggregation reactions and may induce bleeding). Products include:
Daypro Caplets 2578

Oxytetracycline (Anticoagulant action partially counteracted). Products include:
Terramycin Intramuscular Solution 2034

Oxytetracycline Hydrochloride (Anticoagulant action partially counteracted). Products include:
TERAK Ointment .... © 210
Terra-Cortril Ophthalmic Suspension 2033
Terramycin with Polymyxin B Sulfate Ophthalmic Ointment 2035
Urobiotic-250 Capsules 2038

Penicillin G Benzathine (Interferes with platelet-aggregation reactions and may induce bleeding). Products include:
Bicillin C-R Injection 2810
Bicillin C-R 900/300 Injection 2812
Bicillin L-A Injection 2813

Penicillin G Procaine (Interferes with platelet-aggregation reactions and may induce bleeding). Products include:
Bicillin C-R Injection 2810
Bicillin C-R 900/300 Injection 2812

Phenylbutazone (Interferes with platelet-aggregation reactions and may induce bleeding).
No products indexed under this heading.

Piroxicam (Interferes with platelet-aggregation reactions and may induce bleeding). Products include:
Feldene Capsules 2008

Promethazine Hydrochloride (Anticoagulant action partially counteracted). Products include:
Mepergan Injection 2859
Phenergan with Codeine 2883
Phenergan with Dextromethorphan 2885
Phenergan Injection 2880
Phenergan Suppositories 2882
Phenergan Syrup 2881
Phenergan Tablets 2882
Phenergan VC 2886
Phenergan VC with Codeine 2888

Pyrilamine Maleate (Anticoagulant action partially counteracted). Products include:
4-Way Fast Acting Nasal Spray (regular & mentholated) .... ⊞ 644
Maximum Strength Multi-Symptom Formula Midol .... ⊞ 621
PMS Multi-Symptom Formula Midol .... ⊞ 622

Pyrilamine Tannate (Anticoagulant action partially counteracted). Products include:
Atrohist Pediatric Suspension 1604
Atrohist Pediatric Suspension Dye-Free 1604
Rynatan 2781

Salsalate (Interferes with platelet-aggregation reactions and may induce bleeding). Products include:
Disalcid 1549
Mono-Gesic Tablets 810
Salflex Tablets 791

Sulindac (Interferes with platelet-aggregation reactions and may induce bleeding). Products include:
Clinoril Tablets 1658

Terfenadine (Anticoagulant action partially counteracted). Products include:
Seldane Tablets 1284
Seldane-D Extended-Release Tablets 1286

Tetracycline Hydrochloride (Anticoagulant action partially counteracted). Products include:
Achromycin V Capsules 1417
Helidac Therapy 2135

Ticarcillin Disodium (Interferes with platelet-aggregation reactions and may induce bleeding). Products include:
Ticar for Injection 2704
Timentin for Injection 2706

Ticlopidine Hydrochloride (Interferes with platelet-aggregation reactions and may induce bleeding). Products include:
Ticlid Tablets 2317

Tolmetin Sodium (Interferes with platelet-aggregation reactions and may induce bleeding). Products include:
Tolectin (200, 400 and 600 mg) .. 1591

Trimeprazine Tartrate (Anticoagulant action partially counteracted).
No products indexed under this heading.

Tripelennamine Hydrochloride (Anticoagulant action partially counteracted). Products include:
PBZ Tablets 863
PBZ-SR Tablets 862

Triprolidine Hydrochloride (Anticoagulant action partially counteracted). Products include:
Actifed Cold & Allergy Tablets .... ⊞ 807
Actifed Cold & Sinus Caplets and Tablets .... ⊞ 808

HEPARIN SODIUM INJECTION
(Heparin Sodium) 2832
May interact with cardiac glycosides, antihistamines, oral anticoagulants, tetracyclines, non-steroidal anti-inflammatory agents, platelet inhibitors, and certain other agents. Compounds in these categories include:

Acrivastine (Anticoagulant action partially counteracted). Products include:
Semprex-D Capsules 1620

Aspirin (Interferes with platelet-aggregation reactions and may induce bleeding). Products include:
Alka-Seltzer Cherry Effervescent Antacid and Pain Reliever .... ⊞ 609
Alka-Seltzer Extra Strength Effervescent Antacid and Pain Reliever .... ⊞ 609
Alka-Seltzer Lemon Lime Effervescent Antacid and Pain Reliever .... ⊞ 609
Alka-Seltzer Original Effervescent Antacid and Pain Reliever .... ⊞ 609
Alka-Seltzer Plus .... ⊞ 611
Alka-Seltzer Plus Sinus Medicine .. ⊞ 611
Ascriptin .... ⊞ 650
Arthritis Strength BC Powder .... ⊞ 631
BC Cold Powder Multi-Symptom Formula (Cold-Sinus-Allergy) ..... ⊞ 631
BC Cold Powder Non-Drowsy Formula (Cold-Sinus) .... ⊞ 631
BC Powder .... ⊞ 631
Genuine Bayer Aspirin Tablets & Caplets .... ⊞ 618
Extra Strength Bayer Arthritis Pain Regimen Formula .... ⊞ 615
Extra Strength Bayer Aspirin Caplets & Tablets .... ⊞ 617
Extended-Release Bayer 8-Hour Aspirin .... ⊞ 616
Extra Strength Bayer Plus Aspirin Caplets .... ⊞ 617
Extra Strength Bayer PM Aspirin Plus Sleep Aid .... ⊞ 617
Aspirin Regimen Bayer 81 mg Tablets with Calcium .... ⊞ 615
Aspirin Regimen Bayer Adult Low Strength 81 mg Tablets .... ⊞ 613
Aspirin Regimen Bayer Children's Chewable Aspirin .... ⊞ 616
Aspirin Regimen Bayer Regular Strength 325 mg Caplets .... ⊞ 613
Bufferin Analgesic Tablets .... ⊞ 636
Arthritis Strength Bufferin Analgesic Caplets .... ⊞ 637
Extra Strength Bufferin Analgesic Tablets .... ⊞ 637
Cama Arthritis Pain Reliever .... ⊞ 748
Darvon Compound-65 Pulvules 1475
Easprin 1971
Ecotrin 2625
Ecotrin Enteric Coated Aspirin Maximum Strength Tablets and Caplets 775
Ecotrin Enteric Coated Aspirin Regular Strength Tablets 2625
Empirin Aspirin Tablets .... ⊞ 818
Excedrin Extra-Strength Analgesic Tablets, Caplets, and Geltabs 734
Fiorinal Capsules 2388
Fiorinal with Codeine Capsules 2390
Fiorinal Tablets 2388
Goody's Extra Strength Headache Powders .... ⊞ 632
Goody's Extra Strength Pain Relief Tablets .... ⊞ 632
Halfprin Tablets 1413
Norgesic 1554
Percodan Tablets 955
Percodan-Demi Tablets 956
Robaxisal Tablets 2246
Soma Compound w/Codeine Tablets 2784
Soma Compound Tablets 2783
St. Joseph Adult Chewable Aspirin (81 mg.) .... ⊞ 768
Talwin Compound 2466
Vanquish Analgesic Caplets .... ⊞ 627

Astemizole (Anticoagulant action partially counteracted). Products include:
Hismanal Tablets 1341

Azatadine Maleate (Anticoagulant action partially counteracted). Products include:
Trinalin Repetabs Tablets 1373

Azlocillin Sodium (Interferes with platelet-aggregation reactions and may induce bleeding).
No products indexed under this heading.

Bromodiphenhydramine Hydrochloride (Anticoagulant action partially counteracted).
No products indexed under this heading.

Brompheniramine Maleate (Anticoagulant action partially counteracted). Products include:
Alka-Seltzer Plus Sinus Medicine .. ⊞ 611
Bromfed Capsules (Extended-Release) 1832
Bromfed Syrup .... ⊞ 712
Bromfed Tablets 1832
Bromfed-DM Cough Syrup 1832
Bromfed-PD Capsules (Extended-Release) 1832
Dimetane-DC Cough Syrup 2232
Dimetane-DX Cough Syrup 2233
Dimetapp Allergy Dye-Free Elixir ... ⊞ 838
Dimetapp Allergy Sinus Caplets .... ⊞ 838
Dimetapp Cold & Allergy Chewable Tablets .... ⊞ 838
Dimetapp Cold & Cough Liqui-Gels .... ⊞ 839
Dimetapp Cold & Fever Suspension .... ⊞ 839
Dimetapp DM Elixir .... ⊞ 840
Dimetapp Elixir .... ⊞ 840
Dimetapp Extentabs .... ⊞ 841
Dimetapp Tablets/Liqui-Gels .... ⊞ 841
Rondec Chewable Tablets 974
Vicks DayQuil Allergy Relief 12-Hour Extended Release Tablets . ⊞ 733
Vicks DayQuil Allergy Relief 4-Hour Tablets .... ⊞ 733

Carbenicillin Indanyl Sodium (Interferes with platelet-aggregation reactions and may induce bleeding). Products include:
Geocillin Tablets 2009

Cetirizine Hydrochloride (Anticoagulant action partially counteracted). Products include:
Zyrtec Tablets 2053

Chlorpheniramine Maleate (Anticoagulant action partially counteracted). Products include:
Alka-Seltzer Plus Cold Medicine .... ⊞ 611
Alka-Seltzer Plus Cold Medicine Liqui-Gels .... ⊞ 612
Alka-Seltzer Plus Cold & Cough Medicine .... ⊞ 611
Alka-Seltzer Plus Cold & Cough Medicine Liqui-Gels .... ⊞ 612
Alka-Seltzer Plus Flu & Body Aches Effervescent Tablets .... ⊞ 612
Allerest Maximum Strength .... ⊞ 649
Allerest Sinus Pain Formula .... ⊞ 649
Ana-Kit Anaphylaxis Emergency Treatment Kit 611
Atrohist Pediatric Capsules 1603
Atrohist Plus Tablets 1605
BC Cold Powder Multi-Symptom Formula (Cold-Sinus-Allergy) ..... ⊞ 631
Cerose DM .... ⊞ 853
Cheracol Plus Head Cold/Cough Formula .... ⊞ 741
Children's TYLENOL Cold Multi-Symptom Chewable Tablets and Liquid 1559
Children's TYLENOL Cold Plus Cough Multi Symptom Chewable Tablets and Liquid 1560
Children's TYLENOL Flu Suspension Liquid 1560
Children's Vicks DayQuil Allergy Relief .... ⊞ 730
Children's Vicks NyQuil Cold/Cough Relief .... ⊞ 731
Chlor-Trimeton Allergy Decongestant Tablets .... ⊞ 759
Chlor-Trimeton Allergy Tablets ..... ⊞ 758
Allergy-Sinus Comtrex Multi-Symptom Allergy-Sinus Formula Tablets and Caplets .... ⊞ 639
Comtrex Multi-Symptom .... ⊞ 638
Contac Continuous Action Nasal Decongestant/Antihistamine 12 Hour Capsules .... ⊞ 773
Contac Maximum Strength Continuous Action Decongestant/Antihistamine 12 Hour Caplets .. ⊞ 772
Contac Severe Cold and Flu Formula Caplets .... ⊞ 773
Coricidin Cold + Flu Tablets .... ⊞ 760
Coricidin Cough + Cold Tablets .... ⊞ 760
Coricidin 'D' Decongestant Tablets .... ⊞ 760

IMPORTANT NOTE: Always consult each drug listing in the patient's regimen for possible interactions.

D.A. II Tablets	972
D.A. Chewable Tablets	970
Dura-Tap/PD Capsules	970
Dura-Vent/DA Capsules	972
Efidac 24 Chlorpheniramine	▣ 655
Extendryl	1003
Fedahist Gyrocaps	2545
Hycomine Compound Tablets	948
Kronofed-A	994
Nolamine Timed-Release Tablets	790
Novahistine Elixir	▣ 782
Ornade Spansule Capsules	2678
PediaCare Cough-Cold Chewable Tablets and Liquid	1569
PediaCare NightRest Cough-Cold Liquid	1569
Pediatric Vicks 44m Cough & Cold Relief	▣ 737
Pyrroxate Caplets	▣ 742
Ryna	▣ 804
Sinarest	▣ 663
Sine-Off Sinus Medicine	▣ 784
Singlet Tablets	▣ 785
Sinulin Tablets	792
Sinutab Sinus Allergy Medication, Maximum Strength Tablets and Caplets	▣ 823
Sudafed Cold & Allergy Tablets	▣ 826
Teldrin 12 Hour Antihistamine/Nasal Decongestant Allergy Relief Capsules	▣ 786
TheraFlu Flu and Cold Medicine	▣ 750
Theraflu Maximum Strength Flu and Cold Medicine For Sore Throat	▣ 751
TheraFlu Flu, Cold and Cough Medicine	▣ 750
TheraFlu Maximum Strength Nighttime Flu, Cold & Cough Medicine	▣ 751
Triaminic Night Time	▣ 754
Triaminic Syrup	▣ 755
Triaminic Triaminicol Cold & Cough	▣ 756
Triaminicin Tablets	▣ 756
Tussend	1830
TYLENOL Allergy Sinus, Maximum Strength Caplets and Gelcaps	1571
TYLENOL Cold Medication, Multi-Symptom Formula Tablets and Caplets	1572
TYLENOL Cold Medication, Multi-Symptom Hot Liquid Packets	1572
Vicks 44 LiquiCaps Cough, Cold & Flu Relief	▣ 728
Vicks 44M Cough, Cold & Flu Relief	▣ 729

Chlorpheniramine Polistirex (Anticoagulant action partially counteracted). Products include:
Tussionex Pennkinetic Extended-Release Suspension	1624

Chlorpheniramine Tannate (Anticoagulant action partially counteracted). Products include:
Atrohist Pediatric Suspension	1604
Atrohist Pediatric Suspension Dye-Free	1604
Rynatan	2781
Rynatuss	2782

Choline Magnesium Trisalicylate (Interferes with platelet-aggregation reactions and may induce bleeding). Products include:
Trilisate	2155

Clemastine Fumarate (Anticoagulant action partially counteracted). Products include:
Tavist Syrup	2426
Tavist Tablets	2427
Tavist-1 12 Hour Relief Tablets	▣ 749
Tavist-D 12 Hour Relief Tablets	▣ 750

Cyproheptadine Hydrochloride (Anticoagulant action partially counteracted). Products include:
Periactin	1767

Demeclocycline Hydrochloride (Anticoagulant action partially counteracted). Products include:
Declomycin Tablets	1421

Deslanoside (Anticoagulant action partially counteracted).
No products indexed under this heading.

Dexchlorpheniramine Maleate (Anticoagulant action partially counteracted).
No products indexed under this heading.

Dextran 40 (Interferes with platelet-aggregation reactions and may induce bleeding).
No products indexed under this heading.

Diclofenac Potassium (Interferes with platelet-aggregation reactions and may induce bleeding). Products include:
Cataflam Tablets	833

Diclofenac Sodium (Interferes with platelet-aggregation reactions and may induce bleeding). Products include:
Voltaren Ophthalmic Sterile Ophthalmic Solution	ⓞ 264
Cataflam/Voltaren/Voltaren-XR	833

Dicumarol (Prolonged prothrombin time).
No products indexed under this heading.

Diflunisal (Interferes with platelet-aggregation reactions and may induce bleeding). Products include:
Dolobid Tablets	1695

Digitoxin (Anticoagulant action partially counteracted). Products include:
Crystodigin Tablets	1472

Digoxin (Anticoagulant action partially counteracted). Products include:
Lanoxicaps	1110
Lanoxin Elixir Pediatric	1113
Lanoxin Injection	1116
Lanoxin Injection Pediatric	1119
Lanoxin Tablets	1121

Diphenhydramine Citrate (Anticoagulant action partially counteracted). Products include:
Excedrin P.M. Analgesic/Sleeping Aid Tablets, Caplets, Liquigels	735

Diphenhydramine Hydrochloride (Anticoagulant action partially counteracted). Products include:
Actifed Allergy Daytime/Nighttime Caplets	▣ 808
Actifed Sinus Daytime/Nighttime Tablets and Caplets	▣ 809
Extra Strength Bayer PM Aspirin Plus Sleep Aid	▣ 617
Benadryl Allergy Chewables	▣ 811
Benadryl Allergy/Cold Tablets	▣ 811
Benadryl Allergy Decongestant Liquid Medication	▣ 812
Benadryl Allergy Decongestant Tablets	▣ 812
Benadryl Allergy Liquid Medication	▣ 813
Benadryl Allergy	▣ 811
Benadryl Allergy Sinus Headache Caplets	▣ 813
Benadryl Dye-Free Allergy Liquigel Softgels	▣ 813
Benadryl Dye-Free Allergy Liquid Medication	▣ 814
Benadryl Itch Relief Stick Extra Strength	▣ 814
Benadryl Cream	▣ 814
Benadryl Gel	▣ 815
Benadryl Spray	▣ 815
Benadryl Injection	1955
Contac Day & Night Cold/Flu Night Caplets	▣ 772
Contac Night Allergy/Sinus Caplets	▣ 771
Extra Strength Doan's P.M.	▣ 653
Excedrin P.M. Analgesic/Sleeping Aid Tablets, Caplets, Liquigels	▣ 643
Nytol QuickCaps Caplets	▣ 632
Sleepinal Night-time Sleep Aid Capsules and Softgels	▣ 798
TYLENOL Allergy Sinus NightTime, Maximum Strength Caplets	1571
TYLENOL Flu NightTime, Maximum Strength Gelcaps	1575
TYLENOL Flu NightTime, Maximum Strength Hot Medication Packets	1575
TYLENOL PM Pain Reliever/Sleep Aid, Extra Strength Gelcaps, Caplets, Geltabs	1576
TYLENOL Severe Allergy Medication Caplets	1571
Maximum Strength Unisom Sleepgels	1990
Unisom With Pain Relief-Nighttime Sleep Aid and Pain Reliever	1991

Diphenylpyraline Hydrochloride (Anticoagulant action partially counteracted).
No products indexed under this heading.

Dipyridamole (Interferes with platelet-aggregation reactions and may induce bleeding). Products include:
Persantine Tablets	686

Doxycycline Calcium (Anticoagulant action partially counteracted). Products include:
Vibramycin Calcium Oral Suspension Syrup	2038

Doxycycline Hyclate (Anticoagulant action partially counteracted). Products include:
Doryx Capsules	1970
Vibramycin Hyclate Capsules	2038
Vibramycin Hyclate Intravenous	2040
Vibra-Tabs Film Coated Tablets	2038

Doxycycline Monohydrate (Anticoagulant action partially counteracted). Products include:
Monodox Capsules	1858
Vibramycin Monohydrate for Oral Suspension	2038

Etodolac (Interferes with platelet-aggregation reactions and may induce bleeding). Products include:
Lodine Capsules and Tablets	2849

Fenoprofen Calcium (Interferes with platelet-aggregation reactions and may induce bleeding). Products include:
Nalfon 200 Pulvules & Nalfon Tablets	933

Flurbiprofen (Interferes with platelet-aggregation reactions and may induce bleeding).
No products indexed under this heading.

Hydroxychloroquine Sulfate (Interferes with platelet-aggregation reactions and may induce bleeding). Products include:
Plaquenil Sulfate Tablets	2459

Ibuprofen (Interferes with platelet-aggregation reactions and may induce bleeding). Products include:
Advil Cold and Sinus Caplets and Tablets	▣ 837
Advil Ibuprofen Tablets, Caplets and Gel Caplets	▣ 836
Children's Motrin Ibuprofen Oral Suspension	1558
IBU Tablets	1389
Ibuprohm	▣ 713
Motrin IB Caplets, Tablets, and Gelcaps	▣ 802
Motrin Ibuprofen Suspension, Oral Drops, Chewable Tablets, Caplets	1563
Nuprin Ibuprofen/Analgesic Tablets & Caplets	▣ 645
Vicks DayQuil SINUS Pressure & PAIN Relief with IBUPROFEN	▣ 735

Indomethacin (Interferes with platelet-aggregation reactions and may induce bleeding). Products include:
Indocin	1723

Indomethacin Sodium Trihydrate (Interferes with platelet-aggregation reactions and may induce bleeding). Products include:
Indocin I.V.	1727

Ketoprofen (Interferes with platelet-aggregation reactions and may induce bleeding). Products include:
Actron Caplets and Tablets	▣ 608
Orudis Capsules	2874
Orudis KT	▣ 842
Oruvail Capsules	2874

Ketorolac Tromethamine (Interferes with platelet-aggregation reactions and may induce bleeding). Products include:
Acular Sterile Ophthalmic Solution	470
Toradol	2319

Loratadine (Anticoagulant action partially counteracted). Products include:
Claritin Tablets	2485
Claritin-D Tablets	2487

Magnesium Salicylate (Interferes with platelet-aggregation reactions and may induce bleeding). Products include:
Backache Caplets	▣ 635
Doan's Extra-Strength Analgesic	▣ 653
Extra Strength Doan's P.M.	▣ 653
Doan's Regular Strength Analgesic	▣ 654
Mobigesic Tablets	▣ 607

Meclofenamate Sodium (Interferes with platelet-aggregation reactions and may induce bleeding).
No products indexed under this heading.

Mefenamic Acid (Interferes with platelet-aggregation reactions and may induce bleeding). Products include:
Ponstel	1982

Methacycline Hydrochloride (Anticoagulant action partially counteracted).
No products indexed under this heading.

Methdilazine Hydrochloride (Anticoagulant action partially counteracted).
No products indexed under this heading.

Mezlocillin Sodium (Interferes with platelet-aggregation reactions and may induce bleeding). Products include:
Mezlin	594
Mezlin Pharmacy Bulk Package	597

Minocycline Hydrochloride (Anticoagulant action partially counteracted). Products include:
DYNACIN Capsules	1627
Minocin Intravenous	1428
Minocin Oral Suspension	1431
Minocin Pellet-Filled Capsules	1429

Nabumetone (Interferes with platelet-aggregation reactions and may induce bleeding). Products include:
Relafen Tablets	2688

Nafcillin Sodium (Interferes with platelet-aggregation reactions and may induce bleeding).
No products indexed under this heading.

Naproxen (Interferes with platelet-aggregation reactions and may induce bleeding). Products include:
Anaprox/Naprosyn	2277

Naproxen Sodium (Interferes with platelet-aggregation reactions and may induce bleeding). Products include:
Aleve	2124
Anaprox/Naprosyn	2277
Naprelan Tablets	2861

Nicotine Polacrilex (Anticoagulant action partially counteracted).
No products indexed under this heading.

Oxaprozin (Interferes with platelet-aggregation reactions and may induce bleeding). Products include:
Daypro Caplets	2578

Oxytetracycline (Anticoagulant action partially counteracted). Products include:
Terramycin Intramuscular Solution	2034

(▣ Described in PDR For Nonprescription Drugs)   (ⓞ Described in PDR For Ophthalmology)

Oxytetracycline Hydrochloride (Anticoagulant action partially counteracted). Products include:
TERAK Ointment .... ⊙ 210
Terra-Cortril Ophthalmic Suspension 2033
Terramycin with Polymyxin B Sulfate Ophthalmic Ointment 2035
Urobiotic-250 Capsules 2038

Penicillin G Benzathine (Interferes with platelet-aggregation reactions and may induce bleeding). Products include:
Bicillin C-R Injection 2810
Bicillin C-R 900/300 Injection 2812
Bicillin L-A Injection 2813

Penicillin G Procaine (Interferes with platelet-aggregation reactions and may induce bleeding). Products include:
Bicillin C-R Injection 2810
Bicillin C-R 900/300 Injection 2812

Phenylbutazone (Interferes with platelet-aggregation reactions and may induce bleeding).
No products indexed under this heading.

Piroxicam (Interferes with platelet-aggregation reactions and may induce bleeding). Products include:
Feldene Capsules 2008

Promethazine Hydrochloride (Anticoagulant action partially counteracted). Products include:
Mepergan Injection 2859
Phenergan with Codeine 2883
Phenergan with Dextromethorphan 2885
Phenergan Injection 2880
Phenergan Suppositories 2882
Phenergan Syrup 2881
Phenergan Tablets 2882
Phenergan VC 2886
Phenergan VC with Codeine 2888

Pyrilamine Maleate (Anticoagulant action partially counteracted). Products include:
4-Way Fast Acting Nasal Spray (regular & mentholated) .... ⊙ 644
Maximum Strength Multi-Symptom Formula Midol .... ⊙ 621
PMS Multi-Symptom Formula Midol .... ⊙ 622

Pyrilamine Tannate (Anticoagulant action partially counteracted). Products include:
Atrohist Pediatric Suspension 1604
Atrohist Pediatric Suspension Dye-Free 1604
Rynatan 2781

Salsalate (Interferes with platelet-aggregation reactions and may induce bleeding). Products include:
Disalcid 1549
Mono-Gesic Tablets 810
Salflex Tablets 791

Sulindac (Interferes with platelet-aggregation reactions and may induce bleeding). Products include:
Clinoril Tablets 1658

Terfenadine (Anticoagulant action partially counteracted). Products include:
Seldane Tablets 1284
Seldane-D Extended-Release Tablets 1286

Tetracycline Hydrochloride (Anticoagulant action partially counteracted). Products include:
Achromycin V Capsules 1417
Helidac Therapy 2135

Ticarcillin Disodium (Interferes with platelet-aggregation reactions and may induce bleeding). Products include:
Ticar for Injection 2704
Timentin for Injection 2706

Ticlopidine Hydrochloride (Interferes with platelet-aggregation reactions and may induce bleeding). Products include:
Ticlid Tablets 2317

Tolmetin Sodium (Interferes with platelet-aggregation reactions and may induce bleeding). Products include:
Tolectin (200, 400 and 600 mg) .. 1591

Trimeprazine Tartrate (Anticoagulant action partially counteracted).
No products indexed under this heading.

Tripelennamine Hydrochloride (Anticoagulant action partially counteracted). Products include:
PBZ Tablets 863
PBZ-SR Tablets 862

Triprolidine Hydrochloride (Anticoagulant action partially counteracted). Products include:
Actifed Cold & Allergy Tablets .... ⊙ 807
Actifed Cold & Sinus Caplets and Tablets .... ⊙ 808

Warfarin Sodium (Prolonged prothrombin time). Products include:
Coumadin 941

HEPARIN SODIUM VIALS
(Heparin Sodium) 1486

May interact with oral anticoagulants, non-steroidal anti-inflammatory agents, salicylates, cardiac glycosides, high doses of parenteral penicillins, phenothiazines, tetracyclines, antihistamines, platelet inhibitors, cephalosporins with methylthiotetrazole side chains, macrolide antibiotics, and certain other agents. Compounds in these categories include:

Acrivastine (Antagonizes the antithrombotic activity of heparin). Products include:
Semprex-D Capsules 1620

Aspirin (Coadministration may result in an additive or synergistic activity and can result in an increased risk of bleeding). Products include:
Alka-Seltzer Cherry Effervescent Antacid and Pain Reliever ...... ⊙ 609
Alka-Seltzer Extra Strength Effervescent Antacid and Pain Reliever .... ⊙ 609
Alka-Seltzer Lemon Lime Effervescent Antacid and Pain Reliever .... ⊙ 609
Alka-Seltzer Original Effervescent Antacid and Pain Reliever ...... ⊙ 609
Alka-Seltzer Plus .... ⊙ 611
Alka-Seltzer Plus Sinus Medicine .. ⊙ 611
Ascriptin .... ⊙ 650
Arthritis Strength BC Powder .... ⊙ 631
BC Cold Powder Multi-Symptom Formula (Cold-Sinus-Allergy) ... ⊙ 631
BC Cold Powder Non-Drowsy Formula (Cold-Sinus) .... ⊙ 631
BC Powder .... ⊙ 631
Genuine Bayer Aspirin Tablets & Caplets .... ⊙ 618
Extra Strength Bayer Arthritis Pain Regimen Formula .... ⊙ 615
Extra Strength Bayer Aspirin Caplets & Tablets .... ⊙ 617
Extended-Release Bayer 8-Hour Aspirin .... ⊙ 616
Extra Strength Bayer Plus Aspirin Caplets .... ⊙ 617
Extra Strength Bayer PM Aspirin Plus Sleep Aid .... ⊙ 617
Aspirin Regimen Bayer 81 mg Tablets with Calcium .... ⊙ 615
Aspirin Regimen Bayer Adult Low Strength 81 mg Tablets .... ⊙ 613
Aspirin Regimen Bayer Children's Chewable Aspirin .... ⊙ 616
Aspirin Regimen Bayer Regular Strength 325 mg Caplets .... ⊙ 613
Bufferin Analgesic Tablets .... ⊙ 636
Arthritis Strength Bufferin Analgesic Caplets .... ⊙ 637
Extra Strength Bufferin Analgesic Tablets .... ⊙ 637
Cama Arthritis Pain Reliever .... ⊙ 748
Darvon Compound-65 Pulvules 1475
Easprin 1971
Ecotrin 2625
Ecotrin Enteric Coated Aspirin Maximum Strength Tablets and Caplets .... ⊙ 775
Ecotrin Enteric Coated Aspirin Regular Strength Tablets 2625
Empirin Aspirin Tablets .... ⊙ 818
Excedrin Extra-Strength Analgesic Tablets, Caplets, and Geltabs 734
Fiorinal Capsules 2388
Fiorinal with Codeine Capsules 2390
Fiorinal Tablets 2388
Goody's Extra Strength Headache Powders .... ⊙ 632
Goody's Extra Strength Pain Relief Tablets .... ⊙ 632
Halfprin Tablets 1413
Norgesic 1554
Percodan Tablets 955
Percodan-Demi Tablets 956
Robaxisal Tablets 2246
Soma Compound w/Codeine Tablets 2784
Soma Compound Tablets 2783
St. Joseph Adult Chewable Aspirin (81 mg.) .... ⊙ 768
Talwin Compound 2466
Vanquish Analgesic Caplets .... ⊙ 627

Astemizole (Antagonizes the antithrombotic activity of heparin). Products include:
Hismanal Tablets 1341

Azatadine Maleate (Antagonizes the antithrombotic activity of heparin). Products include:
Trinalin Repetabs Tablets 1373

Azithromycin (Loss of pharmacological activity of either or both drugs). Products include:
Zithromax 2043
Zithromax Tablets 2046

Azlocillin Sodium (Coadministration may result in an additive or synergistic activity and can result in an increased risk of bleeding).
No products indexed under this heading.

Bromodiphenhydramine Hydrochloride (Antagonizes the antithrombotic activity of heparin).
No products indexed under this heading.

Brompheniramine Maleate (Antagonizes the antithrombotic activity of heparin). Products include:
Alka-Seltzer Plus Sinus Medicine .. ⊙ 611
Bromfed Capsules (Extended-Release) 1832
Bromfed Syrup .... ⊙ 712
Bromfed Tablets 1832
Bromfed-DM Cough Syrup 1832
Bromfed-PD Capsules (Extended-Release) 1832
Dimetane-DC Cough Syrup 2232
Dimetane-DX Cough Syrup 2233
Dimetapp Allergy Dye-Free Elixir... ⊙ 838
Dimetapp Allergy Sinus Caplets ... ⊙ 838
Dimetapp Cold & Allergy Chewable Tablets .... ⊙ 838
Dimetapp Cold & Cough Liqui-Gels .... ⊙ 839
Dimetapp Cold & Fever Suspension .... ⊙ 839
Dimetapp DM Elixir .... ⊙ 840
Dimetapp Elixir .... ⊙ 840
Dimetapp Extentabs .... ⊙ 841
Dimetapp Tablets/Liqui-Gels .... ⊙ 841
Rondec Chewable Tablets 974
Vicks DayQuil Allergy Relief 12-Hour Extended Release Tablets.. ⊙ 733
Vicks DayQuil Allergy Relief 4-Hour Tablets .... ⊙ 733

Carbenicillin Indanyl Sodium (Co-administration may result in an additive or synergistic activity and can result in an increased risk of bleeding). Products include:
Geocillin Tablets 2009

Cefamandole Nafate (Co-administration may result in an additive or synergistic activity and can result in an increased risk of bleeding). Products include:
Mandol Vials, Faspak & ADD-Vantage 1516

Cefmetazole Sodium (Co-administration may result in an additive or synergistic activity and can result in an increased risk of bleeding).
No products indexed under this heading.

Cefoperazone Sodium (Co-administration may result in an additive or synergistic activity and can result in an increased risk of bleeding). Products include:
Cefobid Intravenous/Intramuscular 1996
Cefobid Pharmacy Bulk Package - Not for Direct Infusion 1999

Cefotetan (Co-administration may result in additive or synergistic activity and can result in an increased risk of bleeding). Products include:
Cefotan 2936

Cetirizine Hydrochloride (Antagonizes the antithrombotic activity of heparin). Products include:
Zyrtec Tablets 2053

Chlorpheniramine Maleate (Antagonizes the antithrombotic activity of heparin). Products include:
Alka-Seltzer Plus Cold Medicine ... ⊙ 611
Alka-Seltzer Plus Cold Medicine Liqui-Gels .... ⊙ 612
Alka-Seltzer Plus Cold & Cough Medicine .... ⊙ 611
Alka-Seltzer Plus Cold & Cough Medicine Liqui-Gels .... ⊙ 612
Alka-Seltzer Plus Flu & Body Aches Effervescent Tablets ...... ⊙ 612
Allerest Maximum Strength .... ⊙ 649
Allerest Sinus Pain Formula .... ⊙ 649
Ana-Kit Anaphylaxis Emergency Treatment Kit 611
Atrohist Pediatric Capsules 1603
Atrohist Plus Tablets 1605
BC Cold Powder Multi-Symptom Formula (Cold-Sinus-Allergy) ... ⊙ 631
Cerose DM .... ⊙ 853
Cheracol Plus Head Cold/Cough Formula .... ⊙ 741
Children's TYLENOL Cold Multi-Symptom Chewable Tablets and Liquid 1559
Children's TYLENOL Cold Plus Cough Multi Symptom Chewable Tablets and Liquid 1560
Children's TYLENOL Flu Suspension Liquid 1560
Children's Vicks DayQuil Allergy Relief .... ⊙ 730
Children's Vicks NyQuil Cold/Cough Relief .... ⊙ 731
Chlor-Trimeton Allergy Decongestant Tablets .... ⊙ 759
Chlor-Trimeton Allergy Tablets ..... ⊙ 758
Allergy-Sinus Comtrex Multi-Symptom Allergy-Sinus Formula Tablets and Caplets .... ⊙ 639
Comtrex Multi-Symptom .... ⊙ 638
Contac Continuous Action Nasal Decongestant/Antihistamine 12 Hour Capsules .... ⊙ 773
Contac Maximum Strength Continuous Action Decongestant/Antihistamine 12 Hour Caplets .. ⊙ 772
Contac Severe Cold and Flu Formula Caplets .... ⊙ 773
Coricidin Cold + Flu Tablets .... ⊙ 760
Coricidin Cough + Cold Tablets .... ⊙ 760
Coricidin 'D' Decongestant Tablets .... ⊙ 760
D.A. II Tablets 972
D.A. Chewable Tablets 970
Dura-Tap/PD Capsules 970
Dura-Vent/DA Tablets 972
Efidac 24 Chlorpheniramine 655
Extendryl 1003
Fedahist Gyrocaps 2545
Hycomine Compound Tablets 948
Kronofed-A 994
Nolamine Timed-Release Tablets 790
Novahistine Elixir .... ⊙ 782
Ornade Spansule Capsules 2678
PediaCare Cough-Cold Chewable Tablets and Liquid 1569
PediaCare NightRest Cough-Cold Liquid 1569

IMPORTANT NOTE: Always consult each drug listing in the patient's regimen for possible interactions.

Heparin Sodium **Interactions Index** **476**

Pediatric Vicks 44m Cough & Cold Relief ▣ 737
Pyrroxate Caplets ▣ 742
Ryna ▣ 804
Sinarest ▣ 663
Sine-Off Sinus Medicine ▣ 784
Singlet Tablets ▣ 785
Sinulin Tablets 792
Sinutab Sinus Allergy Medication, Maximum Strength Tablets and Caplets ▣ 823
Sudafed Cold & Allergy Tablets ▣ 826
Teldrin 12 Hour Antihistamine/Nasal Decongestant Allergy Relief Capsules ▣ 786
TheraFlu Flu and Cold Medicine ▣ 750
Theraflu Maximum Strength Flu and Cold Medicine For Sore Throat ▣ 751
TheraFlu Flu, Cold and Cough Medicine ▣ 750
TheraFlu Maximum Strength Nighttime Flu, Cold & Cough Medicine ▣ 751
Triaminic Night Time ▣ 754
Triaminic Syrup ▣ 755
Triaminic Triaminicol Cold & Cough ▣ 756
Triaminicin Tablets ▣ 756
Tussend 1830
TYLENOL Allergy Sinus, Maximum Strength Caplets and Gelcaps 1571
TYLENOL Cold Medication, Multi-Symptom Formula Tablets and Caplets 1572
TYLENOL Cold Medication, Multi-Symptom Hot Liquid Packets 1572
Vicks 44 LiquiCaps Cough, Cold & Flu Relief ▣ 728
Vicks 44M Cough, Cold & Flu Relief ▣ 729

Chlorpheniramine Polistirex (Antagonizes the antithrombotic activity of heparin). Products include:
Tussionex Pennkinetic Extended-Release Suspension 1624

Chlorpheniramine Tannate (Antagonizes the antithrombotic activity of heparin). Products include:
Atrohist Pediatric Suspension 1604
Atrohist Pediatric Suspension Dye-Free 1604
Rynatan 2781
Rynatuss 2782

Chlorpromazine (Antagonizes the antithrombotic activity of heparin). Products include:
Thorazine Suppositories 2701

Choline Magnesium Trisalicylate (Co-administration may result in an additive or synergistic activity and can result in an increased risk of bleeding). Products include:
Trilisate 2155

Clarithromycin (Loss of pharmacological activity of either or both drugs). Products include:
Biaxin 406

Clemastine Fumarate (Antagonizes the antithrombotic activity of heparin). Products include:
Tavist Syrup 2426
Tavist Tablets 2427
Tavist-1 12 Hour Relief Tablets ▣ 749
Tavist-D 12 Hour Relief Tablets ▣ 750

Cyproheptadine Hydrochloride (Antagonizes the antithrombotic activity of heparin). Products include:
Periactin 1767

Demeclocycline Hydrochloride (Loss of pharmacological activity of either or both drugs). Products include:
Declomycin Tablets 1421

Deslanoside (Antagonizes the antithrombotic activity of heparin).
No products indexed under this heading.

Dexchlorpheniramine Maleate (Antagonizes the antithrombotic activity of heparin).
No products indexed under this heading.

Dextran 40 (Interferes with platelet aggregation reactions).
No products indexed under this heading.

Dextran 70 (Interferes with platelet aggregation reactions). Products include:
Hyskon Hysteroscopy Fluid 1633
OcuCoat and OcuCoat PF Eye Drops ⊙ 322
Tears Naturale II Lubricant Eye Drops 469
Tears Naturale Free Lubricant Eye Drops 469

Diclofenac Potassium (Co-administration may result in an additive or synergistic activity and can result in an increased risk of bleeding). Products include:
Cataflam Tablets 833

Diclofenac Sodium (Co-administration may result in an additive or synergistic activity and can result in an increased risk of bleeding). Products include:
Voltaren Ophthalmic Sterile Ophthalmic Solution ⊙ 264
Cataflam/Voltaren/Voltaren-XR 833

Dicumarol (One-stage prothrombin time prolonged).
No products indexed under this heading.

Diflunisal (Co-administration may result in an additive or synergistic activity and can result in an increased risk of bleeding). Products include:
Dolobid Tablets 1695

Digitoxin (Antagonizes the antithrombotic activity of heparin). Products include:
Crystodigin Tablets 1472

Digoxin (Antagonizes the antithrombotic activity of heparin). Products include:
Lanoxicaps 1110
Lanoxin Elixir Pediatric 1113
Lanoxin Injection 1116
Lanoxin Injection Pediatric 1119
Lanoxin Tablets 1121

Diphenhydramine Citrate (Antagonizes the antithrombotic activity of heparin). Products include:
Excedrin P.M. Analgesic/Sleeping Aid Tablets, Caplets, Liquigels 735

Diphenhydramine Hydrochloride (Antagonizes the antithrombotic activity of heparin). Products include:
Actifed Allergy Daytime/Nighttime Caplets ▣ 808
Actifed Sinus Daytime/Nighttime Tablets and Caplets ▣ 809
Extra Strength Bayer PM Aspirin Plus Sleep Aid ▣ 617
Benadryl Allergy Chewables ▣ 811
Benadryl Allergy/Cold Tablets ▣ 811
Benadryl Allergy Decongestant Liquid Medication ▣ 812
Benadryl Allergy Decongestant Tablets ▣ 812
Benadryl Allergy Liquid Medication ▣ 813
Benadryl Allergy ▣ 811
Benadryl Allergy Sinus Headache Caplets ▣ 813
Benadryl Dye-Free Allergy Liquigel Softgels ▣ 813
Benadryl Dye-Free Allergy Liquid Medication ▣ 814
Benadryl Itch Relief Stick Extra Strength ▣ 814
Benadryl Cream ▣ 814
Benadryl Gel ▣ 815
Benadryl Spray ▣ 815
Benadryl Injection 1955
Contac Day & Night Cold/Flu Night Caplets ▣ 772
Contac Night Allergy/Sinus Caplets ▣ 771
Extra Strength Doan's P.M. ▣ 653
Excedrin P.M. Analgesic/Sleeping Aid Tablets, Caplets, Liquigels ▣ 643
Nytol QuickCaps Caplets ▣ 632
Sleepinal Night-time Sleep Aid Capsules and Softgels ▣ 798
TYLENOL Allergy Sinus NightTime, Maximum Strength Caplets 1571
TYLENOL Flu NightTime, Maximum Strength Gelcaps 1575
TYLENOL Flu NightTime, Maximum Strength Hot Medication Packets 1575
TYLENOL PM Pain Reliever/Sleep Aid, Extra Strength Gelcaps, Caplets, Geltabs 1576
TYLENOL Severe Allergy Medication Caplets 1571
Maximum Strength Unisom Sleepgels 1990
Unisom With Pain Relief-Nighttime Sleep Aid and Pain Reliever 1991

Diphenylpyraline Hydrochloride (Antagonizes the antithrombotic activity of heparin).
No products indexed under this heading.

Dipyridamole (Co-administration may result in an additive or synergistic activity and can result in an increased risk of bleeding). Products include:
Persantine Tablets 686

Dirithromycin (Loss of pharmacological activity of either or both drugs). Products include:
Dynabac 668

Doxycycline Calcium (Loss of pharmacological activity of either or both drugs). Products include:
Vibramycin Calcium Oral Suspension Syrup 2038

Doxycycline Hyclate (Loss of pharmacological activity of either or both drugs). Products include:
Doryx Capsules 1970
Vibramycin Hyclate Capsules 2038
Vibramycin Hyclate Intravenous 2040
Vibra-Tabs Film Coated Tablets 2038

Doxycycline Monohydrate (Loss of pharmacological activity of either or both drugs). Products include:
Monodox Capsules 1858
Vibramycin Monohydrate for Oral Suspension 2038

Erythromycin (Loss of pharmacological activity of either or both drugs). Products include:
A/T/S 2% Acne Topical Gel 1244
A/T/S 2% Acne Topical Solution 1244
Benzamycin Topical Gel 919
E-Mycin Tablets 1388
Emgel 2% Topical Gel 1081
ERYC 1972
Erycette (erythromycin 2%) Topical Solution 1943
Ery-Tab Tablets 426
Erythromycin Base Filmtab 430
Erythromycin Delayed-Release Capsules, USP 431
Ilotycin Ophthalmic Ointment 928
PCE Dispertab Tablets 453
T-Stat 2.0% Topical Solution and Pads 2797
THERAMYCIN Z 2% Solution 1629

Erythromycin Estolate (Loss of pharmacological activity of either or both drugs). Products include:
Ilosone 927

Erythromycin Ethylsuccinate (Loss of pharmacological activity of either or both drugs). Products include:
E.E.S. 427
EryPed 425
Pediazole Suspension 2340

Erythromycin Gluceptate (Loss of pharmacological activity of either or both drugs). Products include:
Ilotycin Gluceptate, IV, Vials 929

Erythromycin Stearate (Loss of pharmacological activity of either or both drugs). Products include:
Erythrocin Stearate Filmtab 429

Etodolac (Co-administration may result in an additive or synergistic activity and can result in an increased risk of bleeding). Products include:
Lodine Capsules and Tablets 2849

Fenoprofen Calcium (Co-administration may result in an additive or synergistic activity and can result in an increased risk of bleeding). Products include:
Nalfon 200 Pulvules & Nalfon Tablets 933

Fluphenazine Decanoate (Antagonizes the antithrombotic activity of heparin). Products include:
Prolixin Decanoate 510

Fluphenazine Enanthate (Antagonizes the antithrombotic activity of heparin). Products include:
Prolixin Enanthate 510

Fluphenazine Hydrochloride (Antagonizes the antithrombotic activity of heparin). Products include:
Prolixin 510

Flurbiprofen (Co-administration may result in an additive or synergistic activity and can result in an increased risk of bleeding).
No products indexed under this heading.

Gentamicin Sulfate (Loss of pharmacological activity of either or both drugs). Products include:
Garamycin Cream 0.1% 2501
Garamycin Injectable 2502
Garamycin Ointment 0.1% 2501
Garamycin Ophthalmic 2501
Genoptic Sterile Ophthalmic Solution ⊙ 241
Genoptic Sterile Ophthalmic Ointment ⊙ 241
Gentak ⊙ 209
Pred-G Liquifilm Sterile Ophthalmic Suspension ⊙ 248
Pred-G S.O.P. Sterile Ophthalmic Ointment ⊙ 249

Ibuprofen (Co-administration may result in an additive or synergistic activity and can result in an increased risk of bleeding). Products include:
Advil Cold and Sinus Caplets and Tablets ▣ 837
Advil Ibuprofen Tablets, Caplets and Gel Caplets ▣ 836
Children's Motrin Ibuprofen Oral Suspension 1558
IBU Tablets 1389
Ibuprohm ▣ 713
Motrin IB Caplets, Tablets, and Gelcaps ▣ 802
Motrin Ibuprofen Suspension, Oral Drops, Chewable Tablets, Caplets 1563
Nuprin Ibuprofen/Analgesic Tablets & Caplets ▣ 645
Vicks DayQuil SINUS Pressure & PAIN Relief with IBUPROFEN ▣ 735

Indomethacin (Co-administration may result in an additive or synergistic activity and can result in an increased risk of bleeding). Products include:
Indocin 1723

Indomethacin Sodium Trihydrate (Co-administration may result in an additive or synergistic activity and can result in an increased risk of bleeding). Products include:
Indocin I.V. 1727

(▣ Described in PDR For Nonprescription Drugs) (⊙ Described in PDR For Ophthalmology)

477 **Interactions Index** **Hep-B-Gammagee**

Ketoprofen (Co-administration may result in an additive or synergistic activity and can result in an increased risk of bleeding). Products include:
- Actron Caplets and Tablets ◘ 608
- Orudis Capsules 2874
- Orudis KT ◘ 842
- Oruvail Capsules 2874

Ketorolac Tromethamine (Co-administration may result in an additive or synergistic activity and can result in an increased risk of bleeding). Products include:
- Acular Sterile Ophthalmic Solution 470
- Toradol 2319

Loratadine (Antagonizes the antithrombotic activity of heparin). Products include:
- Claritin Tablets 2485
- Claritin-D Tablets 2487

Magnesium Salicylate (Co-administration may result in an additive or synergistic activity and can result in an increased risk of bleeding). Products include:
- Backache Caplets ◘ 635
- Doan's Extra-Strength Analgesic ◘ 653
- Extra Strength Doan's P.M. ◘ 653
- Doan's Regular Strength Analgesic ◘ 654
- Mobigesic Tablets ◘ 607

Meclofenamate Sodium (Co-administration may result in an additive or synergistic activity and can result in an increased risk of bleeding).
- No products indexed under this heading.

Mefenamic Acid (Co-administration may result in an additive or synergistic activity and can result in an increased risk of bleeding). Products include:
- Ponstel 1982

Mesoridazine Besylate (Antagonizes the antithrombotic activity of heparin). Products include:
- Serentil 689

Methacycline Hydrochloride (Loss of pharmacological activity of either or both drugs).
- No products indexed under this heading.

Methdilazine Hydrochloride (Antagonizes the antithrombotic activity of heparin).
- No products indexed under this heading.

Methotrimeprazine (Antagonizes the antithrombotic activity of heparin). Products include:
- Levoprome 1321

Mezlocillin Sodium (Co-administration may result in an additive or synergistic activity and can result in an increased risk of bleeding). Products include:
- Mezlin 594
- Mezlin Pharmacy Bulk Package 597

Minocycline Hydrochloride (Loss of pharmacological activity of either or both drugs). Products include:
- DYNACIN Capsules 1627
- Minocin Intravenous 1428
- Minocin Oral Suspension 1431
- Minocin Pellet-Filled Capsules 1429

Moxalactam Disodium (Co-administration may result in an additive or synergistic activity and can result in an increased risk of bleeding).

Nabumetone (Co-administration may result in an additive or synergistic activity and can result in an increased risk of bleeding). Products include:
- Relafen Tablets 2688

Nafcillin Sodium (Co-administration may result in an additive or synergistic activity and can result in an increased risk of bleeding).
- No products indexed under this heading.

Naproxen (Co-administration may result in an additive or synergistic activity and can result in an increased risk of bleeding). Products include:
- Anaprox/Naprosyn 2277

Naproxen Sodium (Co-administration may result in an additive or synergistic activity and can result in an increased risk of bleeding). Products include:
- Aleve 2124
- Anaprox/Naprosyn 2277
- Naprelan Tablets 2861

Neomycin, oral (Loss of pharmacological activity of either or both drugs).

Nicotine Polacrilex (Antagonizes the antithrombotic activity of heparin).
- No products indexed under this heading.

Nitroglycerin Intravenous (May require higher doses of heparin; close monitoring of the partial thromboplastin time is required).

Oxaprozin (Co-administration may result in an additive or synergistic activity and can result in an increased risk of bleeding). Products include:
- Daypro Caplets 2578

Oxytetracycline Hydrochloride (Loss of pharmacological activity of either or both drugs). Products include:
- TERAK Ointment ◉ 210
- Terra-Cortril Ophthalmic Suspension 2033
- Terramycin with Polymyxin B Sulfate Ophthalmic Ointment 2035
- Urobiotic-250 Capsules 2038

Penicillin G Benzathine (Co-administration may result in an additive or synergistic activity and can result in an increased risk of bleeding). Products include:
- Bicillin C-R Injection 2810
- Bicillin C-R 900/300 Injection 2812
- Bicillin L-A Injection 2813

Penicillin G Procaine (Co-administration may result in an additive or synergistic activity and can result in an increased risk of bleeding). Products include:
- Bicillin C-R Injection 2810
- Bicillin C-R 900/300 Injection 2812

Perphenazine (Antagonizes the antithrombotic activity of heparin). Products include:
- Etrafon 2495
- Triavil Tablets 1800
- Trilafon 2532

Phenylbutazone (Co-administration may result in an additive or synergistic activity and can result in an increased risk of bleeding).
- No products indexed under this heading.

Piroxicam (Co-administration may result in an additive or synergistic activity and can result in an increased risk of bleeding). Products include:
- Feldene Capsules 2008

Polymyxin B Sulfate (Loss of pharmacological activity of either or both drugs). Products include:
- AK-Spore ◉ 205
- AK-Trol Ointment & Suspension ◉ 205
- Betadine Brand First Aid Antibiotics & Moisturizer Ointment 2144
- Cortisporin Cream 1073
- Cortisporin Ointment 1074
- Cortisporin Ophthalmic Ointment Sterile 1074
- Cortisporin Ophthalmic Suspension Sterile 1075
- Cortisporin Otic Solution Sterile 1076
- Cortisporin Otic Suspension Sterile 1077
- Maxitrol Ophthalmic Ointment and Suspension ◉ 222
- Mycitracin ◘ 803
- Neosporin G.U. Irrigant Sterile 1130
- Neosporin Ointment ◘ 821
- Neosporin Plus Maximum Strength Cream ◘ 821
- Neosporin Plus Maximum Strength Ointment ◘ 822
- Neosporin Ophthalmic Ointment Sterile 1130
- Neosporin Ophthalmic Solution Sterile 1131
- Pediotic Suspension Sterile 1140
- Poly-Pred Liquifilm ◉ 246
- Polysporin Ointment ◘ 822
- Polysporin Ophthalmic Ointment Sterile 1140
- Polysporin Powder ◘ 823
- Polytrim Ophthalmic Solution Sterile 479
- TERAK Ointment ◉ 210
- Terramycin with Polymyxin B Sulfate Ophthalmic Ointment 2035

Prochlorperazine (Antagonizes the antithrombotic activity of heparin). Products include:
- Compazine 2644

Promethazine Hydrochloride (Antagonizes the antithrombotic activity of heparin). Products include:
- Mepergan Injection 2859
- Phenergan with Codeine 2883
- Phenergan with Dextromethorphan 2885
- Phenergan Injection 2880
- Phenergan Suppositories 2882
- Phenergan Syrup 2881
- Phenergan Tablets 2882
- Phenergan VC 2886
- Phenergan VC with Codeine 2888

Pyrilamine Maleate (Antagonizes the antithrombotic activity of heparin). Products include:
- 4-Way Fast Acting Nasal Spray (regular & mentholated) ◘ 644
- Maximum Strength Multi-Symptom Formula Midol ◘ 621
- PMS Multi-Symptom Formula Midol ◘ 622

Pyrilamine Tannate (Antagonizes the antithrombotic activity of heparin). Products include:
- Atrohist Pediatric Suspension 1604
- Atrohist Pediatric Suspension Dye-Free 1604
- Rynatan 2781

Salsalate (Co-administration may result in an additive or synergistic activity and can result in an increased risk of bleeding). Products include:
- Disalcid 1549
- Mono-Gesic Tablets 810
- Salflex Tablets 791

Streptomycin Sulfate (Loss of pharmacological activity of either or both drugs). Products include:
- Streptomycin Sulfate Injection 2031

Sulindac (Co-administration may result in an additive or synergistic activity and can result in an increased risk of bleeding). Products include:
- Clinoril Tablets 1658

Terfenadine (Antagonizes the antithrombotic activity of heparin). Products include:
- Seldane Tablets 1284
- Seldane-D Extended-Release Tablets 1286

Tetracycline Hydrochloride (Loss of pharmacological activity of either or both drugs). Products include:
- Achromycin V Capsules 1417
- Helidac Therapy 2135

Thioridazine Hydrochloride (Antagonizes the antithrombotic activity of heparin). Products include:
- Mellaril 2398

Ticarcillin Disodium (Co-administration may result in an additive or synergistic activity and can result in an increased risk of bleeding). Products include:
- Ticar for Injection 2704
- Timentin for Injection 2706

Ticlopidine Hydrochloride (Co-administration may result in an additive or synergistic activity and can result in an increased risk of bleeding). Products include:
- Ticlid Tablets 2317

Tolmetin Sodium (Co-administration may result in an additive or synergistic activity and can result in an increased risk of bleeding). Products include:
- Tolectin (200, 400 and 600 mg) 1591

Trifluoperazine Hydrochloride (Antagonizes the antithrombotic activity of heparin). Products include:
- Stelazine 2692

Trimeprazine Tartrate (Antagonizes the antithrombotic activity of heparin).
- No products indexed under this heading.

Tripelennamine Hydrochloride (Antagonizes the antithrombotic activity of heparin). Products include:
- PBZ Tablets 863
- PBZ-SR Tablets 862

Triprolidine Hydrochloride (Antagonizes the antithrombotic activity of heparin). Products include:
- Actifed Cold & Allergy Tablets ◘ 807
- Actifed Cold & Sinus Caplets and Tablets ◘ 808

Troleandomycin (Loss of pharmacological activity of either or both drugs). Products include:
- Tao Capsules 2033

Vitamin C (Antagonizes the antithrombotic activity of heparin). Products include:
- ACES Antioxidant Soft Gels ◘ 647
- Chromagen Capsules 2470
- Chromagen FA 2471
- Chromagen Forte 2471
- Dexatrim Maximum Strength Plus Vitamin C/Caffeine-Free Caplets ◘ 795
- Ester-C Mineral Ascorbates Powder ◘ 673
- Fero-Folic-500 Filmtab 433
- Fero-Grad-500 Filmtab 434
- Halls Vitamin C Drops ◘ 807
- Irospan 1000
- Materna Tablets 1427
- Niferex w/Vitamin C Tablets 811
- One-A-Day Antioxidant Plus ◘ 625
- Protegra Antioxidant Vitamin & Mineral Supplement ◘ 685
- Sunkist Children's Chewable Multivitamins - Plus Extra C ◘ 665
- Sunkist Vitamin C ◘ 666
- Trinsicon Capsules 2759
- Venolax ◘ 686
- Vitron-C Tablets ◘ 667

Warfarin Sodium (One-stage prothrombin time prolonged). Products include:
- Coumadin 941

HEP-B-GAMMAGEE (Hepatitis B Immune Globulin (Human)) 1706

May interact with:

Measles Virus Vaccine Live (Interference with immune response to live virus vaccines). Products include:
- Attenuvax 1650

IMPORTANT NOTE: Always consult each drug listing in the patient's regimen for possible interactions.

Measles & Rubella Virus Vaccine Live (Interference with immune response to live virus vaccines). Products include:
M-R-VAX II ... 1732

Measles, Mumps & Rubella Virus Vaccine Live (Interference with immune response to live virus vaccines). Products include:
M-M-R II ... 1730

Rubella Virus Vaccine Live (Interference with immune response to live virus vaccines). Products include:
Meruvax II ... 1740

Rubella & Mumps Virus Vaccine Live (Interference with immune response to live virus vaccines). Products include:
Biavax II ... 1653

HEP-FORTE CAPSULES
(Vitamins with Minerals) ... 1558
None cited in PDR database.

HEPLIVE CAPSULES
(Vitamins with Minerals) ... 461
None cited in PDR database.

HERPECIN-L COLD SORE LIP BALM STICK
(Allantoin) ... 812
None cited in PDR database.

HERRICK LACRIMAL PLUGS
(Silicone) ... ⊙ 275
None cited in PDR database.

HESPAN INJECTION
(Hetastarch) ... 945
None cited in PDR database.

HEXALEN CAPSULES
(Altretamine) ... 2760
May interact with monoamine oxidase inhibitors and certain other agents. Compounds in these categories include:

Cimetidine (Increases altretamine's half-life and toxicity in a rat model). Products include:
Tagamet HB Tablets ... ▣ 786
Tagamet Tablets ... 2694

Cimetidine Hydrochloride (Increases altretamine's half-life and toxicity in a rat model). Products include:
Tagamet ... 2694

Furazolidone (Potential for severe orthostatic hypotension). Products include:
Furoxone ... 2221

Isocarboxazid (Potential for severe orthostatic hypotension).
No products indexed under this heading.

Phenelzine Sulfate (Potential for severe orthostatic hypotension). Products include:
Nardil ... 1977

Pyridoxine Hydrochloride (May adversely affect response duration; should not be administered with Hexalen and/or Cisplatin).
No products indexed under this heading.

Selegiline Hydrochloride (Potential for severe orthostatic hypotension). Products include:
Eldepryl Capsules ... 2729

Tranylcypromine Sulfate (Potential for severe orthostatic hypotension). Products include:
Parnate Tablets ... 2679

HELIXATE, ANTIHEMOPHILIC FACTOR (RECOMBINANT)
(Antihemophilic Factor (Recombinant)) ... 799
None cited in PDR database.

HIBICLENS ANTIMICROBIAL SKIN CLEANSER
(Chlorhexidine Gluconate) ... 2947
None cited in PDR database.

HIBISTAT GERMICIDAL HAND RINSE
(Chlorhexidine Gluconate) ... 2948
None cited in PDR database.

HIBISTAT TOWELETTE
(Chlorhexidine Gluconate) ... 2948
None cited in PDR database.

HIBTITER
(Haemophilus B Conjugate Vaccine) .. 1423
May interact with immunosuppressive agents, corticosteroids, cytotoxic drugs, alkylating agents, and anticoagulants. Compounds in these categories include:

Azathioprine (Reduces antibody response to active immunization procedures). Products include:
Azathioprine Tablets ... 2349
Imuran ... 1103

Betamethasone Acetate (Reduces antibody response to active immunization procedures). Products include:
Celestone Soluspan Suspension ... 2484

Betamethasone Sodium Phosphate (Reduces antibody response to active immunization procedures). Products include:
Celestone Soluspan Suspension ... 2484

Bleomycin Sulfate (Reduces antibody response to active immunization procedures). Products include:
Blenoxane ... 697

Busulfan (Reduces antibody response to active immunization procedures). Products include:
Myleran Tablets ... 1209

Carmustine (BCNU) (Reduces antibody response to active immunization procedures). Products include:
BiCNU ... 696

Chlorambucil (Reduces antibody response to active immunization procedures). Products include:
Leukeran Tablets ... 1205

Cortisone Acetate (Reduces antibody response to active immunization procedures). Products include:
Cortone Acetate Sterile Suspension ... 1663
Cortone Acetate Tablets ... 1664

Cyclophosphamide (Reduces antibody response to active immunization procedures). Products include:
Cytoxan ... 700

Cyclosporine (Reduces antibody response to active immunization procedures). Products include:
Neoral ... 2405
Sandimmune ... 2416

Dacarbazine (Reduces antibody response to active immunization procedures). Products include:
DTIC-Dome ... 593

Dalteparin Sodium (HibTITER should be given with caution to children on anticoagulant therapy). Products include:
Fragmin Injection ... 2088

Daunorubicin Hydrochloride (Reduces antibody response to active immunization procedures). Products include:
Cerubidine for Injection ... 634

Dexamethasone (Reduces antibody response to active immunization procedures). Products include:
AK-Trol Ointment & Suspension ... ⊙ 205
Decadron Elixir ... 1676
Decadron Tablets ... 1678
Decaspray Topical Aerosol ... 1689
Maxitrol Ophthalmic Ointment and Suspension ... ⊙ 222
TobraDex Ophthalmic Suspension and Ointment ... 469

Dexamethasone Acetate (Reduces antibody response to active immunization procedures). Products include:
Dalalone D.P. Injectable ... 1009
Decadron-LA Sterile Suspension ... 1687

Dexamethasone Sodium Phosphate (Reduces antibody response to active immunization procedures). Products include:
Decadron Phosphate Injection ... 1680
Decadron Phosphate Sterile Ophthalmic Ointment ... 1684
Decadron Phosphate Sterile Ophthalmic Solution ... 1685
Decadron Phosphate Topical Cream ... 1686
Decadron Phosphate with Xylocaine Injection, Sterile ... 1683
Dexacort Phosphate in Respihaler .. 1606
Dexacort Phosphate in Turbinaire .. 1607
NeoDecadron Sterile Ophthalmic Ointment ... 1755
NeoDecadron Sterile Ophthalmic Solution ... 1756
NeoDecadron Topical Cream ... 1757

Dicumarol (HibTITER should be given with caution to children on anticoagulant therapy).
No products indexed under this heading.

Doxorubicin Hydrochloride (Reduces antibody response to active immunization procedures). Products include:
Adriamycin PFS ... 2056
Adriamycin RDF ... 2056
Doxil ... 2613
Doxorubicin Astra ... 531
Rubex for Injection ... 721

Enoxaparin (HibTITER should be given with caution to children on anticoagulant therapy). Products include:
Lovenox Injection ... 2187

Fludrocortisone Acetate (Reduces antibody response to active immunization procedures). Products include:
Florinef Acetate Tablets ... 506

Fluorouracil (Reduces antibody response to active immunization procedures). Products include:
Efudex ... 2280
Fluoroplex Topical Solution & Cream 1% ... 475
Fluorouracil Injection ... 2282

Heparin Calcium (HibTITER should be given with caution to children on anticoagulant therapy).
No products indexed under this heading.

Heparin Sodium (HibTITER should be given with caution to children on anticoagulant therapy). Products include:
Heparin Lock Flush Solution ... 2831
Heparin Sodium Injection ... 2832
Heparin Sodium Vials ... 1486

Hydrocortisone (Reduces antibody response to active immunization procedures). Products include:
Anusol-HC Cream 2.5% ... 1953
Aquanil HC Lotion ... 1989
Maximum Strength Cortaid Spray ▣ 800
CORTENEMA ... 2713
Cortisporin Ointment ... 1074
Cortisporin Ophthalmic Ointment Sterile ... 1074
Cortisporin Ophthalmic Suspension Sterile ... 1075
Cortisporin Otic Solution Sterile ... 1076
Cortisporin Otic Suspension Sterile 1077
Cortizone-5 ... ▣ 795
Cortizone-10 ... ▣ 795
Hydrocortone Tablets ... 1715
Hytone ... 922
Hytone Ointment 2 ½% ... 923
Massengill Medicated Soft Cloth Towelettes ... 2628
Pediotic Suspension Sterile ... 1140
Preparation H Hydrocortisone 1% Cream ... ▣ 843
ProctoCream-HC 2.5% ... 2552
VōSoL HC Otic Solution ... 2786

Hydrocortisone Acetate (Reduces antibody response to active immunization procedures). Products include:
Analpram-HC Rectal Cream 1% and 2.5% ... 993
Anusol HC-1 Hydrocortisone Anti-Itch Ointment ... ▣ 810
Anusol-HC Suppositories ... 1954
Caldecort Anti-Itch Hydrocortisone Cream ... ▣ 651
Coly-Mycin S Otic w/Neomycin & Hydrocortisone ... 1965
Cortaid ... ▣ 800
Cortifoam ... 2540
Cortisporin Cream ... 1073
Epifoam ... 2543
Hydrocortone Acetate Sterile Suspension ... 1712
Mantadil Cream ... 1124
Nupercainal Hydrocortisone 1% Cream ... ▣ 661
Pramosone Cream, Lotion & Ointment ... 995
ProctoFoam-HC ... 2552
Terra-Cortril Ophthalmic Suspension ... 2033

Hydrocortisone Sodium Phosphate (Reduces antibody response to active immunization procedures). Products include:
Hydrocortone Phosphate Injection, Sterile ... 1713

Hydrocortisone Sodium Succinate (Reduces antibody response to active immunization procedures).
No products indexed under this heading.

Hydroxyurea (Reduces antibody response to active immunization procedures). Products include:
Hydrea Capsules ... 705

Immune Globulin (Human) (Reduces antibody response to active immunization procedures).
No products indexed under this heading.

Immune Globulin Intravenous (Human) (Reduces antibody response to active immunization procedures).

Lomustine (CCNU) (Reduces antibody response to active immunization procedures). Products include:
CeeNU Capsules ... 699

Mechlorethamine Hydrochloride (Reduces antibody response to active immunization procedures). Products include:
Mustargen ... 1752

Melphalan (Reduces antibody response to active immunization procedures). Products include:
Alkeran Tablets ... 1198

Methotrexate Sodium (Reduces antibody response to active immunization procedures). Products include:
Methotrexate Sodium Tablets, Injection, for Injection and LPF Injection ... 1322

(▣ Described in PDR For Nonprescription Drugs) (⊙ Described in PDR For Ophthalmology)

479 **Interactions Index** **Histussin D**

Methylprednisolone Acetate (Reduces antibody response to active immunization procedures).
No products indexed under this heading.

Methylprednisolone Sodium Succinate (Reduces antibody response to active immunization procedures).
No products indexed under this heading.

Mitotane (Reduces antibody response to active immunization procedures). Products include:
- Lysodren Tablets 707

Mitoxantrone Hydrochloride (Reduces antibody response to active immunization procedures). Products include:
- Novantrone for Injection 1327

Muromonab-CD3 (Reduces antibody response to active immunization procedures). Products include:
- Orthoclone OKT3 Sterile Solution .. 1892

Mycophenolate Mofetil (Reduces antibody response to active immunization procedures). Products include:
- CellCept Capsules 2265

Prednisolone Acetate (Reduces antibody response to active immunization procedures). Products include:
- AK-CIDE .... ◉ 203
- AK-CIDE Ointment .... ◉ 203
- Blephamide Liquifilm Sterile Ophthalmic Suspension 472
- Blephamide Ointment .... ◉ 234
- Econopred & Econopred Plus Ophthalmic Suspensions .... ◉ 216
- Poly-Pred Liquifilm .... ◉ 246
- Pred Forte .... ◉ 247
- Pred Mild .... ◉ 250
- Pred-G Liquifilm Sterile Ophthalmic Suspension .... ◉ 248
- Pred-G S.O.P. Sterile Ophthalmic Ointment .... ◉ 249

Prednisolone Sodium Phosphate (Reduces antibody response to active immunization procedures). Products include:
- AK-PRED .... ◉ 204
- Hydeltrasol Injection, Sterile 1708
- Pediapred Oral Solution 1618

Prednisolone Tebutate (Reduces antibody response to active immunization procedures). Products include:
- Hydeltra-T.B.A. Sterile Suspension 1710

Prednisone (Reduces antibody response to active immunization procedures).
No products indexed under this heading.

Procarbazine Hydrochloride (Reduces antibody response to active immunization procedures). Products include:
- Matulane Capsules 2300

Tacrolimus (Reduces antibody response to active immunization procedures). Products include:
- Prograf 1028

Tamoxifen Citrate (Reduces antibody response to active immunization procedures). Products include:
- Nolvadex Tablets 2957

Thiotepa (Reduces antibody response to active immunization procedures). Products include:
- Thioplex (Thiotepa For Injection) 1329

Triamcinolone (Reduces antibody response to active immunization procedures).
No products indexed under this heading.

Triamcinolone Acetonide (Reduces antibody response to active immunization procedures). Products include:
- Azmacort Oral Inhaler 2175
- Nasacort AQ Nasal Spray 2191
- Nasacort Nasal Inhaler 2189

Triamcinolone Diacetate (Reduces antibody response to active immunization procedures).
No products indexed under this heading.

Triamcinolone Hexacetonide (Reduces antibody response to active immunization procedures).
No products indexed under this heading.

Vincristine Sulfate (Reduces antibody response to active immunization procedures). Products include:
- Oncovin Solution Vials & Hyporets 1521

Warfarin Sodium (HibTITER should be given with caution to children on anticoagulant therapy). Products include:
- Coumadin 941

HISMANAL TABLETS
(Astemizole) 1341
May interact with macrolide antibiotics and certain other agents. Compounds in these categories include:

Azithromycin (Concomitant administration is contraindicated; potential for syncope with Torsade de Pointes). Products include:
- Zithromax 2043
- Zithromax Tablets 2046

Clarithromycin (Concomitant administration is contraindicated; potential for syncope with Torsade de Pointes). Products include:
- Biaxin 406

Dirithromycin (Concomitant administration is contraindicated; potential for syncope with Torsade de Pointes). Products include:
- Dynabac 668

Erythromycin (Concomitant administration is contraindicated; potential for syncope with Torsade de Pointes). Products include:
- A/T/S 2% Acne Topical Gel 1244
- A/T/S 2% Acne Topical Solution 1244
- Benzamycin Topical Gel 919
- E-Mycin Tablets 1388
- Emgel 2% Topical Gel 1081
- ERYC 1972
- Erycette (erythromycin 2%) Topical Solution 1943
- Ery-Tab Tablets 426
- Erythromycin Base Filmtab 430
- Erythromycin Delayed-Release Capsules, USP 431
- Ilotycin Ophthalmic Ointment 928
- PCE Dispertab Tablets 453
- T-Stat 2.0% Topical Solution and Pads 2797
- THERAMYCIN Z 2% Solution 1629

Erythromycin Estolate (Concomitant administration is contraindicated; potential for syncope with Torsade de Pointes). Products include:
- Ilosone 927

Erythromycin Ethylsuccinate (Concomitant administration is contraindicated; potential for syncope with Torsade de Pointes). Products include:
- E.E.S. 427
- EryPed 425
- Pediazole Suspension 2340

Erythromycin Gluceptate (Concomitant administration is contraindicated; potential for syncope with Torsade de Pointes). Products include:
- Ilotycin Gluceptate, IV, Vials 929

Erythromycin Stearate (Concomitant administration is contraindicated; potential for syncope with Torsade de Pointes). Products include:
- Erythrocin Stearate Filmtab 429

Fluconazole (Concomitant use with astemizole is not recommended due to chemical similarity of fluconazole to ketoconazole). Products include:
- Diflucan Tablets, Injection, and Oral Suspension 2003

Itraconazole (Concomitant administration with astemizole is contraindicated based on the chemical resemblance of itraconazole and ketoconazole). Products include:
- Sporanox Capsules 1352

Ketoconazole (Concomitant administration with ketoconazole tablets is contraindicated; potential for cardiovascular events including electrographic QT prolongation). Products include:
- Nizoral 2% Cream 1344
- Nizoral 2% Shampoo 1344
- Nizoral Tablets 1345

Metronidazole (Concomitant use with astemizole is not recommended due to chemical similarity of metronidazole to ketoconazole). Products include:
- Flagyl 375 Capsules 2587
- Flagyl I.V. RTU 2373
- Helidac Therapy 2135
- MetroCream 1034
- MetroGel 1034
- MetroGel-Vaginal 917
- Protostat Tablets 1939

Metronidazole Hydrochloride (Concomitant use with astemizole is not recommended due to chemical similarity of metronidazole to ketoconazole). Products include:
- Flagyl I.V. 2373

Miconazole (Concomitant use with astemizole is not recommended due to chemical similarity of intravenous form of miconazole to ketoconazole).
No products indexed under this heading.

Quinine (Co-administration is contraindicated; use of a single dose of 430 mg quinine with astemizole has resulted in elevated plasma levels of astemizole and its metabolite which is accompanied by electrocardiographic QT prolongation).

Troleandomycin (Concomitant administration is contraindicated; potential for syncope with Torsades de Pointes). Products include:
- Tao Capsules 2033

Food Interactions

Meal, unspecified (Reduces the absorption by 60%; patients should be instructed to take Hismanal on an empty stomach, e.g. at least 2 hours after a meal).

Tonic water (May elevate plasma levels of astemizole and desmethyastemizole; potential for insignificant prolongation of the QT interval).

HISTUSSIN D LIQUID
(Hydrocodone Bitartrate, Pseudoephedrine Hydrochloride) 670
May interact with monoamine oxidase inhibitors, narcotic analgesics, general anesthetics, tranquilizers, hypnotics and sedatives, central nervous system depressants, tricyclic antidepressants, beta blockers, and certain other agents. Compounds in these categories include:

Acebutolol Hydrochloride (MAO inhibitors potentiate the sympathomimetic effects of pseudoephedrine). Products include:
- Sectral Capsules 2914

Alfentanil Hydrochloride (Co-administration may produce additive CNS depressant effects). Products include:
- Alfenta Injection 1334

Alprazolam (Co-administration may produce additive CNS depressant effects). Products include:
- Xanax Tablets 2115

Amitriptyline Hydrochloride (Co-administration may produce additive CNS depressant effects). Products include:
- Elavil 2945
- Etrafon 2495
- Limbitrol 2333
- Triavil Tablets 1800

Amoxapine (Co-administration may produce additive CNS depressant effects). Products include:
- Asendin Tablets 1419

Aprobarbital (Co-administration may produce additive CNS depressant effects).
No products indexed under this heading.

Atenolol (MAO inhibitors potentiate the sympathomimetic effects of pseudoephedrine). Products include:
- Tenoretic Tablets 2963
- Tenormin Tablets and I.V. Injection 2965

Betaxolol Hydrochloride (MAO inhibitors potentiate the sympathomimetic effects of pseudoephedrine). Products include:
- Betoptic Ophthalmic Solution 465
- Betoptic S Ophthalmic Suspension 467
- Kerlone Tablets 2588

Bisoprolol Fumarate (MAO inhibitors potentiate the sympathomimetic effects of pseudoephedrine). Products include:
- Zebeta Tablets 1457
- Ziac 1459

Buprenorphine (Co-administration may produce additive CNS depressant effects). Products include:
- Buprenex Injectable 2170

Buspirone Hydrochloride (Co-administration may produce additive CNS depressant effects). Products include:
- BuSpar Tablets 738

Butabarbital (Co-administration may produce additive CNS depressant effects).
No products indexed under this heading.

Butalbital (Co-administration may produce additive CNS depressant effects). Products include:
- Axocet Capsules 2469
- Esgic-plus Capsules 1012
- Esgic-plus Tablets 1012
- Fioricet Tablets 2386
- Fioricet with Codeine Capsules 2387
- Fiorinal Capsules 2388
- Fiorinal with Codeine Capsules 2390
- Fiorinal Tablets 2388
- Phrenilin 790
- Sedapap Tablets 50 mg/650 mg .. 1826

Carteolol Hydrochloride (MAO inhibitors potentiate the sympathomimetic effects of pseudoephedrine). Products include:
- Cartrol Tablets 413
- Ocupress Ophthalmic Solution, 1% Sterile .... ◉ 297

Chlordiazepoxide (Co-administration may produce additive CNS depressant effects). Products include:
- Limbitrol 2333

IMPORTANT NOTE: Always consult each drug listing in the patient's regimen for possible interactions.

Chlordiazepoxide Hydrochloride (Co-administration may produce additive CNS depressant effects). Products include:
- Librax Capsules 2330
- Librium Capsules 2331
- Librium Injectable 2332

Chlorpromazine (Co-administration may produce additive CNS depressant effects). Products include:
- Thorazine Suppositories 2701

Chlorpromazine Hydrochloride (Co-administration may produce additive CNS depressant effects). Products include:
- Thorazine 2701

Chlorprothixene (Co-administration may produce additive CNS depressant effects).
No products indexed under this heading.

Chlorprothixene Hydrochloride (Co-administration may produce additive CNS depressant effects).
No products indexed under this heading.

Chlorprothixene Lactate (Co-administration may produce additive CNS depressant effects).
No products indexed under this heading.

Clomipramine Hydrochloride (Co-administration may produce additive CNS depressant effects). Products include:
- Anafranil Capsules 819

Clorazepate Dipotassium (Co-administration may produce additive CNS depressant effects). Products include:
- Tranxene 459

Clozapine (Co-administration may produce additive CNS depressant effects). Products include:
- Clozaril Tablets 2377

Codeine Phosphate (Co-administration may produce additive CNS depressant effects). Products include:
- Brontex 2130
- Dimetane-DC Cough Syrup ... 2232
- Fioricet with Codeine Capsules ... 2387
- Fiorinal with Codeine Capsules ... 2390
- Nucofed 2225
- Phenergan with Codeine 2883
- Phenergan VC with Codeine ... 2888
- Robitussin A-C Syrup 2248
- Robitussin-DAC Syrup 2249
- Ryna 804
- Soma Compound w/Codeine Tablets 2784
- Tylenol with Codeine 1592

Desflurane (Co-administration may produce additive CNS depressant effects). Products include:
- Suprane (desflurane, USP) ... 1865

Desipramine Hydrochloride (Co-administration may produce additive CNS depressant effects). Products include:
- Norpramin Tablets 1273

Dezocine (Co-administration may produce additive CNS depressant effects). Products include:
- Dalgan Injection 529

Diazepam (Co-administration may produce additive CNS depressant effects). Products include:
- Dizac (diazepam injectable emulsion) CIV 1862
- Valium Injectable 2336
- Valium Tablets 2335

Doxepin Hydrochloride (Co-administration may produce additive CNS depressant effects). Products include:
- Adapin Capsules 1542
- Sinequan 2028
- Zonalon Cream 1042

Droperidol (Co-administration may produce additive CNS depressant effects). Products include:
- Inapsine Injection 462

Enflurane (Co-administration may produce additive CNS depressant effects).
No products indexed under this heading.

Esmolol Hydrochloride (MAO inhibitors potentiate the sympathomimetic effects of pseudoephedrine). Products include:
- Brevibloc (esmolol HCl) Injection ... 1860

Estazolam (Co-administration may produce additive CNS depressant effects). Products include:
- ProSom Tablets 457

Ethchlorvynol (Co-administration may produce additive CNS depressant effects). Products include:
- Placidyl Capsules 456

Ethinamate (Co-administration may produce additive CNS depressant effects).
No products indexed under this heading.

Fentanyl (Co-administration may produce additive CNS depressant effects). Products include:
- Duragesic Transdermal System ... 1336

Fentanyl Citrate (Co-administration may produce additive CNS depressant effects). Products include:
- Sublimaze Injection 463

Fluphenazine Decanoate (Co-administration may produce additive CNS depressant effects). Products include:
- Prolixin Decanoate 510

Fluphenazine Enanthate (Co-administration may produce additive CNS depressant effects). Products include:
- Prolixin Enanthate 510

Fluphenazine Hydrochloride (Co-administration may produce additive CNS depressant effects). Products include:
- Prolixin 510

Flurazepam Hydrochloride (Co-administration may produce additive CNS depressant effects). Products include:
- Dalmane Capsules 2329

Furazolidone (MAO inhibitors potentiate the sympathomimetic effects of pseudoephedrine; concurrent and/or sequential use is contraindicated). Products include:
- Furoxone 2221

Glutethimide (Co-administration may produce additive CNS depressant effects).
No products indexed under this heading.

Haloperidol (Co-administration may produce additive CNS depressant effects). Products include:
- Haldol Injection, Tablets and Concentrate 1585

Haloperidol Decanoate (Co-administration may produce additive CNS depressant effects). Products include:
- Haldol Decanoate 1587

Hydrocodone Polistirex (Co-administration may produce additive CNS depressant effects). Products include:
- Tussionex Pennkinetic Extended-Release Suspension 1624

Hydromorphone Hydrochloride (Co-administration may produce additive CNS depressant effects). Products include:
- Dilaudid Ampules 1382
- Dilaudid Cough Syrup 1383
- Dilaudid-HP Injection 1384
- Dilaudid-HP Lyophilized Powder 250 mg 1384
- Dilaudid 1382
- Dilaudid Oral Liquid 1386
- Dilaudid 1382
- Dilaudid Tablets - 8 mg 1386

Hydroxyzine Hydrochloride (Co-administration may produce additive CNS depressant effects). Products include:
- Atarax Tablets & Syrup 1992
- Marax Tablets & DF Syrup ... 2015
- Vistaril Intramuscular Solution ... 2042

Imipramine Hydrochloride (Co-administration may produce additive CNS depressant effects). Products include:
- Tofranil Ampuls 873
- Tofranil Tablets 875

Imipramine Pamoate (Co-administration may produce additive CNS depressant effects). Products include:
- Tofranil-PM Capsules 876

Isocarboxazid (MAO inhibitors potentiate the sympathomimetic effects of pseudoephedrine; concurrent and/or sequential use is contraindicated).
No products indexed under this heading.

Isoflurane (Co-administration may produce additive CNS depressant effects).
No products indexed under this heading.

Ketamine Hydrochloride (Co-administration may produce additive CNS depressant effects).
No products indexed under this heading.

Labetalol Hydrochloride (MAO inhibitors potentiate the sympathomimetic effects of pseudoephedrine). Products include:
- Normodyne Injection 2519
- Normodyne Tablets 2522
- Trandate 1158

Levobunolol Hydrochloride (MAO inhibitors potentiate the sympathomimetic effects of pseudoephedrine). Products include:
- Betagan .... ⓞ 230

Levomethadyl Acetate Hydrochloride (Co-administration may produce additive CNS depressant effects). Products include:
- Orlaam Oral Solution 2361

Levorphanol Tartrate (Co-administration may produce additive CNS depressant effects). Products include:
- Levo-Dromoran 2297

Lorazepam (Co-administration may produce additive CNS depressant effects). Products include:
- Ativan Injection 2805
- Ativan Tablets 2807

Loxapine Hydrochloride (Co-administration may produce additive CNS depressant effects). Products include:
- Loxitane 1426

Loxapine Succinate (Co-administration may produce additive CNS depressant effects). Products include:
- Loxitane Capsules 1426

Maprotiline Hydrochloride (Co-administration may produce additive CNS depressant effects). Products include:
- Ludiomil Tablets 861

Mecamylamine Hydrochloride (Sympathomimetic amines may reduce the antihypertensive effects of mecamylamine). Products include:
- Inversine Tablets 1729

Meperidine Hydrochloride (Co-administration may produce additive CNS depressant effects). Products include:
- Demerol 2438
- Mepergan Injection 2859

Mephobarbital (Co-administration may produce additive CNS depressant effects). Products include:
- Mebaral Tablets 2452

Meprobamate (Co-administration may produce additive CNS depressant effects). Products include:
- Miltown Tablets 2780
- PMB 200 and PMB 400 2890

Mesoridazine Besylate (Co-administration may produce additive CNS depressant effects). Products include:
- Serentil 689

Methadone Hydrochloride (Co-administration may produce additive CNS depressant effects). Products include:
- Methadone Hydrochloride Oral Concentrate 2356
- Methadone Hydrochloride Oral Solution & Tablets 2357

Methohexital Sodium (Co-administration may produce additive CNS depressant effects).
No products indexed under this heading.

Methotrimeprazine (Co-administration may produce additive CNS depressant effects). Products include:
- Levoprome 1321

Methoxyflurane (Co-administration may produce additive CNS depressant effects).
No products indexed under this heading.

Methyldopa (Sympathomimetic amines may reduce the antihypertensive effects of methyldopa). Products include:
- Aldoclor Tablets 1638
- Aldomet Oral 1640
- Aldoril Tablets 1644

Methyldopate Hydrochloride (Sympathomimetic amines may reduce the antihypertensive effects of methyldopa). Products include:
- Aldomet Ester HCl Injection ... 1642

Metipranolol Hydrochloride (MAO inhibitors potentiate the sympathomimetic effects of pseudoephedrine). Products include:
- OptiPranolol (Metipranolol 0.3%) Sterile Ophthalmic Solution ... ⓞ 256

Metoprolol Succinate (MAO inhibitors potentiate the sympathomimetic effects of pseudoephedrine). Products include:
- Toprol-XL Tablets 560

Metoprolol Tartrate (MAO inhibitors potentiate the sympathomimetic effects of pseudoephedrine). Products include:
- Lopressor 848
- Lopressor HCT Tablets 850

Midazolam Hydrochloride (Co-administration may produce additive CNS depressant effects). Products include:
- Versed Injection 2324

Molindone Hydrochloride (Co-administration may produce additive CNS depressant effects). Products include:
- Moban Tablets and Concentrate ... 1036

(▣ Described in PDR For Nonprescription Drugs)   (ⓞ Described in PDR For Ophthalmology)

481 **Interactions Index** **Hivid**

Morphine Sulfate (Co-administration may produce additive CNS depressant effects). Products include:
- Astramorph/PF Injection, USP (Preservative-Free) 526
- Duramorph Injection 983
- Infumorph 200 and Infumorph 500 Sterile Solutions 985
- Kadian Capsules 2948
- MS Contin Tablets 2149
- MSIR 2152
- Oramorph SR (Morphine Sulfate Sustained Release Tablets) 2359
- RMS Suppositories CII 2766
- Roxanol 2365

Nadolol (MAO inhibitors potentiate the sympathomimetic effects of pseudoephedrine).
- No products indexed under this heading.

Nortriptyline Hydrochloride (Co-administration may produce additive CNS depressant effects). Products include:
- Pamelor 2409

Opium Alkaloids (Co-administration may produce additive CNS depressant effects).
- No products indexed under this heading.

Oxazepam (Co-administration may produce additive CNS depressant effects). Products include:
- Serax Capsules 2916
- Serax Tablets 2916

Oxycodone Hydrochloride (Co-administration may produce additive CNS depressant effects). Products include:
- OxyContin Tablets 2163
- OxyIR Capsules 2167
- Percocet Tablets 955
- Percodan Tablets 955
- Percodan-Demi Tablets 956
- Roxicodone Tablets, Oral Solution & Intensol (Oxycodone) 2366
- Tylox Capsules 1593

Penbutolol Sulfate (MAO inhibitors potentiate the sympathomimetic effects of pseudoephedrine). Products include:
- Levatol Tablets 2547

Pentobarbital Sodium (Co-administration may produce additive CNS depressant effects). Products include:
- Nembutal Sodium Capsules 440
- Nembutal Sodium Solution 442
- Nembutal Sodium Suppositories 444

Perphenazine (Co-administration may produce additive CNS depressant effects). Products include:
- Etrafon 2495
- Triavil Tablets 1800
- Trilafon 2532

Phenelzine Sulfate (MAO inhibitors potentiate the sympathomimetic effects of pseudoephedrine; concurrent and/or sequential use is contraindicated). Products include:
- Nardil 1977

Phenobarbital (Co-administration may produce additive CNS depressant effects). Products include:
- Arco-Lase Plus Tablets 513
- Bellergal-S Tablets 2375
- Donnatal 2234
- Donnatal Extentabs 2234
- Donnatal Tablets 2234
- Phenobarbital Elixir and Tablets 1523
- Quadrinal Tablets 1398

Pindolol (MAO inhibitors potentiate the sympathomimetic effects of pseudoephedrine). Products include:
- Visken Tablets 2428

Prazepam (Co-administration may produce additive CNS depressant effects).
- No products indexed under this heading.

Prochlorperazine (Co-administration may produce additive CNS depressant effects). Products include:
- Compazine 2644

Promethazine Hydrochloride (Co-administration may produce additive CNS depressant effects). Products include:
- Mepergan Injection 2859
- Phenergan with Codeine 2883
- Phenergan with Dextromethorphan 2885
- Phenergan Injection 2880
- Phenergan Suppositories 2882
- Phenergan Syrup 2881
- Phenergan Tablets 2882
- Phenergan VC 2886
- Phenergan VC with Codeine 2888

Propofol (Co-administration may produce additive CNS depressant effects). Products include:
- Diprivan Injectable Emulsion 2939

Propoxyphene Hydrochloride (Co-administration may produce additive CNS depressant effects). Products include:
- Darvon 1475
- Wygesic Tablets 2930

Propoxyphene Napsylate (Co-administration may produce additive CNS depressant effects). Products include:
- Darvon-N/Darvocet-N 1473

Propranolol Hydrochloride (MAO inhibitors potentiate the sympathomimetic effects of pseudoephedrine). Products include:
- Inderal 2834
- Inderal LA Long Acting Capsules 2836
- Inderide Tablets 2838
- Inderide LA Long Acting Capsules .. 2840

Protriptyline Hydrochloride (Co-administration may produce additive CNS depressant effects). Products include:
- Vivactil Tablets 1820

Quazepam (Co-administration may produce additive CNS depressant effects). Products include:
- Doral Tablets 2773

Reserpine (Sympathomimetic amines may reduce the antihypertensive effects of reserpine). Products include:
- Diupres Tablets 1691
- Hydropres Tablets 1718
- Ser-Ap-Es Tablets 867

Risperidone (Co-administration may produce additive CNS depressant effects). Products include:
- Risperdal Tablets 1348

Secobarbital Sodium (Co-administration may produce additive CNS depressant effects). Products include:
- Seconal Sodium Pulvules 1529

Selegiline Hydrochloride (MAO inhibitors potentiate the sympathomimetic effects of pseudoephedrine; concurrent and/or sequential use is contraindicated). Products include:
- Eldepryl Capsules 2729

Sevoflurane (Co-administration may produce additive CNS depressant effects).
- No products indexed under this heading.

Sotalol Hydrochloride (MAO inhibitors potentiate the sympathomimetic effects of pseudoephedrine). Products include:
- Betapace Tablets 637

Sufentanil Citrate (Co-administration may produce additive CNS depressant effects). Products include:
- Sufenta Injection 1355

Temazepam (Co-administration may produce additive CNS depressant effects). Products include:
- Restoril Capsules 2413

Thiamylal Sodium (Co-administration may produce additive CNS depressant effects).
- No products indexed under this heading.

Thioridazine Hydrochloride (Co-administration may produce additive CNS depressant effects). Products include:
- Mellaril 2398

Thiothixene (Co-administration may produce additive CNS depressant effects). Products include:
- Navane Capsules and Concentrate 2018
- Navane Intramuscular 2019

Timolol Hemihydrate (MAO inhibitors potentiate the sympathomimetic effects of pseudoephedrine). Products include:
- Betimol 0.25%, 0.5% .... ◉ 259

Timolol Maleate (MAO inhibitors potentiate the sympathomimetic effects of pseudoephedrine). Products include:
- Blocadren Tablets 1654
- Timolide Tablets 1791
- Timoptic in Ocudose 1796
- Timoptic Sterile Ophthalmic Solution 1794
- Timoptic-XE 1798

Tranylcypromine Sulfate (MAO inhibitors potentiate the sympathomimetic effects of pseudoephedrine; concurrent and/or sequential use is contraindicated). Products include:
- Parnate Tablets 2679

Triazolam (Co-administration may produce additive CNS depressant effects). Products include:
- Halcion Tablets 2093

Trifluoperazine Hydrochloride (Co-administration may produce additive CNS depressant effects). Products include:
- Stelazine 2692

Trimipramine Maleate (Co-administration may produce additive CNS depressant effects). Products include:
- Surmontil Capsules 2917

Zolpidem Tartrate (Co-administration may produce additive CNS depressant effects). Products include:
- Ambien Tablets 2559

Food Interactions

Alcohol (Co-administration may produce additive CNS depressant effects).

HIVID TABLETS

(Zalcitabine) 2287

May interact with aminoglycosides, drugs that are known to cause peripheral neuropathy and pancreatitis (selected), antacids containing aluminium, calcium and magnesium, and certain other agents. Compounds in these categories include:

Altretamine (Potential for increased peripheral neuropathy; concomitant use should be avoided). Products include:
- Hexalen Capsules 2760

Aluminum Carbonate (Absorption of zalcitabine is moderately reduced (approximately 25%) when coadministered with magnesium/aluminum containing antacids). Products include:
- Basaljel Capsules 2810
- Basaljel Suspension 2810
- Basaljel Tablets 2810

Aluminum Hydroxide (Absorption of zalcitabine is moderately reduced (approximately 25%) when coadministered with magnesium/aluminum containing antacids). Products include:
- ALternaGEL Liquid 1358
- Maximum Strength Ascriptin 650
- Cama Arthritis Pain Reliever 748
- Gaviscon Extra Strength Relief Formula Antacid Tablets 778
- Gaviscon Extra Strength Relief Formula Liquid Antacid 779
- Gaviscon Liquid Antacid 779
- Gelusil Antacid-Anti-gas Liquid 819
- Gelusil Antacid-Anti-gas Tablets 819
- Maalox Antacid/Anti-Gas Tablets 889
- Maalox Heartburn Relief Suspension 658
- Maalox Antacid Liquid 888
- Extra Strength Maalox Antacid/Anti-Gas Liquid and Tablets 888
- Mylanta 1359
- Tempo Soft Antacid 799

Aluminum Hydroxide Gel (Absorption of zalcitabine is moderately reduced (approximately 25%) when coadministered with magnesium/aluminum containing antacids). Products include:
- ALternaGEL Liquid 675
- Aludrox Oral Suspension 850
- Amphojel Suspension 2802
- Amphojel Suspension without Flavor 2802
- Amphojel Tablets 2802
- Ascriptin 650
- Gaviscon Antacid Tablets 778
- Gaviscon-2 Antacid Tablets 779
- Mylanta Liquid 676
- Mylanta Double Strength Liquid 676
- Nephrox Suspension 671

Amikacin Sulfate (Increases the risk of developing peripheral neuropathy or other Hivid-associated toxicities by interfering with the renal clearance of zalcitabine). Products include:
- Amikacin Sulfate Injection, USP 523
- Amikacin Sulfate Injection, USP 981
- Amikin Injectable 502

Amphotericin B (Increases the risk of developing peripheral neuropathy or other Hivid-associated toxicities by interfering with the renal clearance of zalcitabine). Products include:
- Abelcet Injection 1540
- Fungizone Intravenous 507
- Fungizone Oral Suspension 704

Auranofin (Potential for increased peripheral neuropathy; concomitant use should be avoided). Products include:
- Ridaura Capsules 2691

Carboplatin (Potential for increased peripheral neuropathy; concomitant use should be avoided). Products include:
- Paraplatin for Injection 713

Chloramphenicol (Potential for increased peripheral neuropathy; concomitant use should be avoided). Products include:
- Chloromycetin Ophthalmic Ointment, 1% .... ◉ 298
- Chloromycetin Ophthalmic Solution .... ◉ 299
- Chloroptic S.O.P. .... ◉ 236
- Chloroptic Sterile Ophthalmic Solution .... ◉ 236

Chloramphenicol Palmitate (Potential for increased peripheral neuropathy; concomitant use should be avoided).
- No products indexed under this heading.

Chloramphenicol Sodium Succinate (Potential for increased peripheral neuropathy; concomitant use should be avoided). Products include:
- Chloromycetin Sodium Succinate 1960

Hivid **Interactions Index** 482

Cimetidine (Concomitant administration decreases the elimination of zalcitabine, most likely by inhibition of renal tubular secretion of zalcitabine). Products include:

Tagamet HB Tablets ▣ 786
Tagamet Tablets 2694

Cimetidine Hydrochloride (Concomitant administration decreases the elimination of zalcitabine, most likely by inhibition of renal tubular secretion of zalcitabine). Products include:

Tagamet 2694

Cisplatin (Potential for increased peripheral neuropathy; concomitant use should be avoided). Products include:

Platinol for Injection 717
Platinol-AQ Injection 719

Dapsone (Potential for increased peripheral neuropathy; concomitant use should be avoided). Products include:

Dapsone Tablets USP 1331

Didanosine (Concomitant use is not recommended). Products include:

Videx Tablets, Powder for Oral Solution, & Pediatric Powder for Oral Solution 2980

Disulfiram (Potential for increased peripheral neuropathy; concomitant use should be avoided). Products include:

Antabuse Tablets 2802

Ethionamide (Potential for increased peripheral neuropathy; concomitant use should be avoided). Products include:

Trecator-SC Tablets 2919

Foscarnet Sodium (Increases the risk of developing peripheral neuropathy or other Hivid-associated toxicities by interfering with the renal clearance of zalcitabine). Products include:

Foscavir Injection 541

Gentamicin Sulfate (Increases the risk of developing peripheral neuropathy or other Hivid-associated toxicities by interfering with the renal clearance of zalcitabine). Products include:

Garamycin Cream 0.1% 2501
Garamycin Injectable 2502
Garamycin Ointment 0.1% 2501
Garamycin Ophthalmic 2501
Genoptic Sterile Ophthalmic Solution ⊙ 241
Genoptic Sterile Ophthalmic Ointment ⊙ 241
Gentak ⊙ 209
Pred-G Liquifilm Sterile Ophthalmic Suspension ⊙ 248
Pred-G S.O.P. Sterile Ophthalmic Ointment ⊙ 249

Glutethimide (Potential for increased peripheral neuropathy; concomitant use should be avoided).

No products indexed under this heading.

Gold Sodium Thiomalate (Potential for increased peripheral neuropathy; concomitant use should be avoided). Products include:

Myochrysine Injection 1754

Hydralazine Hydrochloride (Potential for increased peripheral neuropathy; concomitant use should be avoided). Products include:

Apresazide Capsules 824
Apresoline Hydrochloride Tablets 826
Hydralazine Hydrochloride Injection USP 2712
Ser-Ap-Es Tablets 867

Iodoquinol (Potential for increased peripheral neuropathy; concomitant use should be avoided). Products include:

Yodoxin Tablets 1235

Isoniazid (Potential for increased peripheral neuropathy; concomitant use should be avoided). Products include:

Nydrazid Injection 509
Rifamate Capsules 1278
Rifater 1280

Kanamycin Sulfate (Increases the risk of developing peripheral neuropathy or other Hivid-associated toxicities by interfering with the renal clearance of zalcitabine).

No products indexed under this heading.

Leuprolide Acetate (Potential for increased peripheral neuropathy; concomitant use should be avoided). Products include:

Lupron Depot 3.75 mg 2739
Lupron Depot 7.5 mg 2741
Lupron Depot - 3 Month 22.5 mg 2743
Lupron Depot-PED 7.5 mg, 11.25 mg and 15 mg 2744
Lupron Injection 2736
Lupron Injection Pediatric 2737

Magaldrate (Absorption of zalcitabine is moderately reduced (approximately 25%) when coadministered with magnesium/aluminum containing antacids).

No products indexed under this heading.

Magnesium Hydroxide (Absorption of zalcitabine is moderately reduced (approximately 25%) when co-administered with magnesium/aluminum containing antacids). Products include:

Aludrox Oral Suspension ▣ 850
Ascriptin ▣ 650
Di-Gel Antacid/Anti-Gas ▣ 762
Gelusil Antacid-Anti-gas Liquid ▣ 819
Gelusil Antacid-Anti-gas Tablets ▣ 819
Maalox Antacid/Anti-Gas Tablets 889
Maalox Antacid Liquid 888
Extra Strength Maalox Antacid/Anti-Gas Liquid and Tablets 888
Mylanta Fast-Acting 1359
Mylanta Gelcaps Antacid ▣ 678
Fast-Acting Mylanta Liquid Antacid 1359
Mylanta Tablets ▣ 677
Maximum-Strength Fast-Acting Mylanta Liquid Antacid 1359
Mylanta Double Strength Tablets ▣ 677
Phillips' Milk of Magnesia Liquid ▣ 627
Rolaids Antacid Tablets ▣ 807
Tempo Soft Antacid ▣ 799

Magnesium Oxide (Absorption of zalcitabine is moderately reduced (approximately 25%) when co-administered with magnesium/aluminum containing antacids). Products include:

Beelith Tablets 632
Bufferin Analgesic Tablets ▣ 636
Arthritis Strength Bufferin Analgesic Caplets ▣ 637
Extra Strength Bufferin Analgesic Tablets ▣ 637
Caltrate PLUS ▣ 681
Cama Arthritis Pain Reliever ▣ 748
Mag-Ox 400 666
Uro-Mag 666

Metoclopramide Hydrochloride (Co-administration may reduce bioavailability (approximately 10%)). Products include:

Reglan 2243

Metronidazole (Potential for increased peripheral neuropathy; concomitant use should be avoided). Products include:

Flagyl 375 Capsules 2587
Flagyl I.V. RTU 2373
Helidac Therapy 2135
MetroCream 1034
MetroGel 1034
MetroGel-Vaginal 917
Protostat Tablets 1939

Nitrofurantoin (Potential for increased peripheral neuropathy; concomitant use should be avoided). Products include:

Macrodantin Capsules 2140

Pentamidine Isethionate (Death due to fulminant pancreatitis possibly related to intravenous pentamidine and Hivid has been reported; treatment with Hivid should be interrupted if intravenous pentamidine is required to treat Pneumocystis carinii pneumonia).

No products indexed under this heading.

Phenytoin (Potential for increased peripheral neuropathy; concomitant use should be avoided). Products include:

Dilantin Infatabs 1967
Dilantin-125 Suspension 1969

Phenytoin Sodium (Potential for increased peripheral neuropathy; concomitant use should be avoided). Products include:

Dilantin Kapseals 1965

Probenecid (Concomitant administration decreases the elimination of zalcitabine, most likely by inhibition of renal tubular secretion of zalcitabine). Products include:

Benemid Tablets 1651
ColBENEMID Tablets 1662

Ribavirin (Potential for increased peripheral neuropathy; concomitant use should be avoided). Products include:

Virazole 1310

Streptomycin Sulfate (Increases the risk of developing peripheral neuropathy or other Hivid-associated toxicities by interfering with the renal clearance of zalcitabine). Products include:

Streptomycin Sulfate Injection 2031

Sulfamethoxazole (Potential for increased peripheral neuropathy; concomitant use should be avoided). Products include:

Bactrim DS Tablets 2257
Bactrim I.V. Infusion 2255
Bactrim 2257
Gantanol Tablets 2285
Septra 1146
Septra I.V. Infusion 1142
Septra I.V. Infusion ADD-Vantage Vials 1144
Septra 1146

Tobramycin (Increases the risk of developing peripheral neuropathy or other Hivid-associated toxicities by interfering with the renal clearance of zalcitabine). Products include:

AKTOB ⊙ 207
TobraDex Ophthalmic Suspension and Ointment 469
Tobrex Ophthalmic Ointment and Solution ⊙ 226

Tobramycin Sulfate (Increases the risk of developing peripheral neuropathy or other Hivid-associated toxicities by interfering with the renal clearance of zalcitabine). Products include:

Nebcin Vials, Hyporets & ADD-Vantage 1518

Vincristine Sulfate (Potential for increased peripheral neuropathy; concomitant use should be avoided). Products include:

Oncovin Solution Vials & Hyporets 1521

Food Interactions

Food, unspecified (The absorption rate of a 15 mg oral dose of zalactabine was reduced when administered with food).

HUMALOG INJECTION

(Insulin Lispro, Human) 1488

May interact with corticosteroids, estrogens, oral contraceptives, phenothiazines, thyroid preparations, salicylates, oral hypoglycemic agents, ACE inhibitors, beta blockers, and certain other agents. Compounds in these categories include:

Acarbose (Co-administration with drugs with hypoglycemic activity, such as oral hypoglycemic agents, may result in decreased insulin requirements). Products include:

Precose 604

Acebutolol Hydrochloride (Co-administration with drugs with hypoglycemic activity, such as beta blocker, may result in decreased insulin requirements; beta blockers may mask the symptoms of hypoglycemia in some patients). Products include:

Sectral Capsules 2914

Aspirin (Co-administration with drugs with hypoglycemic activity, such as salicylates, may result in decreased insulin requirements). Products include:

Alka-Seltzer Cherry Effervescent Antacid and Pain Reliever ▣ 609
Alka-Seltzer Extra Strength Effervescent Antacid and Pain Reliever ▣ 609
Alka-Seltzer Lemon Lime Effervescent Antacid and Pain Reliever ▣ 609
Alka-Seltzer Original Effervescent Antacid and Pain Reliever ▣ 609
Alka-Seltzer Plus ▣ 611
Alka-Seltzer Plus Sinus Medicine ▣ 611
Ascriptin ▣ 650
Arthritis Strength BC Powder ▣ 631
BC Cold Powder Multi-Symptom Formula (Cold-Sinus-Allergy) ▣ 631
BC Cold Powder Non-Drowsy Formula (Cold-Sinus) ▣ 631
BC Powder ▣ 631
Genuine Bayer Aspirin Tablets & Caplets ▣ 618
Extra Strength Bayer Arthritis Pain Regimen Formula ▣ 615
Extra Strength Bayer Aspirin Caplets & Tablets ▣ 617
Extended-Release Bayer 8-Hour Aspirin ▣ 616
Extra Strength Bayer Plus Aspirin Caplets ▣ 617
Extra Strength Bayer PM Aspirin Plus Sleep Aid ▣ 617
Aspirin Regimen Bayer 81 mg Tablets with Calcium ▣ 615
Aspirin Regimen Bayer Adult Low Strength 81 mg Tablets ▣ 613
Aspirin Regimen Bayer Children's Chewable Aspirin ▣ 616
Aspirin Regimen Bayer Regular Strength 325 mg Caplets ▣ 613
Bufferin Analgesic Tablets ▣ 636
Arthritis Strength Bufferin Analgesic Caplets ▣ 637
Extra Strength Bufferin Analgesic Tablets ▣ 637
Cama Arthritis Pain Reliever ▣ 748
Darvon Compound-65 Pulvules 1475
Easprin 1971
Ecotrin 2625
Ecotrin Enteric Coated Aspirin Maximum Strength Tablets and Caplets ▣ 775
Ecotrin Enteric Coated Aspirin Regular Strength Tablets 2625
Empirin Aspirin Tablets ▣ 818
Excedrin Extra-Strength Analgesic Tablets, Caplets, and Geltabs 734
Fiorinal Capsules 2388
Fiorinal with Codeine Capsules 2390
Fiorinal Tablets 2388
Goody's Extra Strength Headache Powders ▣ 632
Goody's Extra Strength Pain Relief Tablets ▣ 632
Halfprin Tablets 1413
Norgesic 1554
Percodan Tablets 955
Percodan-Demi Tablets 956
Robaxisal Tablets 2246

(▣ Described in PDR For Nonprescription Drugs) (⊙ Described in PDR For Ophthalmology)

483 **Interactions Index** **Humalog**

Soma Compound w/Codeine Tablets ... 2784
Soma Compound Tablets ... 2783
St. Joseph Adult Chewable Aspirin (81 mg.) ... 768
Talwin Compound ... 2466
Vanquish Analgesic Caplets ... 627

Atenolol (Co-administration with drugs with hypoglycemic activity, such as beta blocker, may result in decreased insulin requirements; beta blockers may mask the symptoms of hypoglycemia in some patients). Products include:
Tenoretic Tablets ... 2963
Tenormin Tablets and I.V. Injection 2965

Benazepril Hydrochloride (Co-administration with drugs with hypoglycemic activity, such as certain ACE inhibitors, may result in decreased insulin requirements). Products include:
Lotensin Tablets ... 852
Lotensin HCT Tablets ... 855
Lotrel Capsules ... 858

Betamethasone Acetate (Co-administration may result in increased insulin requirements). Products include:
Celestone Soluspan Suspension ... 2484

Betamethasone Sodium Phosphate (Co-administration may result in increased insulin requirements). Products include:
Celestone Soluspan Suspension ... 2484

Betaxolol Hydrochloride (Co-administration with drugs with hypoglycemic activity, such as beta blocker, may result in decreased insulin requirements; beta blockers may mask the symptoms of hypoglycemia in some patients). Products include:
Betoptic Ophthalmic Solution ... 465
Betoptic S Ophthalmic Suspension 467
Kerlone Tablets ... 2588

Bisoprolol Fumarate (Co-administration with drugs with hypoglycemic activity, such as beta blocker, may result in decreased insulin requirements; beta blockers may mask the symptoms of hypoglycemia in some patients). Products include:
Zebeta Tablets ... 1457
Ziac ... 1459

Captopril (Co-administration with drugs with hypoglycemic activity, such as certain ACE inhibitors, may result in decreased insulin requirements). Products include:
Capoten Tablets ... 740
Capozide Tablets ... 744

Carteolol Hydrochloride (Co-administration with drugs with hypoglycemic activity, such as beta blocker, may result in decreased insulin requirements; beta blockers may mask the symptoms of hypoglycemia in some patients). Products include:
Cartrol Tablets ... 413
Ocupress Ophthalmic Solution, 1% Sterile ... ◎ 297

Chlorotrianisene (Co-administration may result in increased insulin requirements).
No products indexed under this heading.

Chlorpromazine (Co-administration with phenothiazines may result in increased insulin requirements). Products include:
Thorazine Suppositories ... 2701

Chlorpromazine Hydrochloride (Co-administration with phenothiazines may result in increased insulin requirements). Products include:
Thorazine ... 2701

Chlorpropamide (Co-administration with drugs with hypoglycemic activity, such as oral hypoglycemic agents, may result in decreased insulin requirements). Products include:
Diabinese Tablets ... 2002

Choline Magnesium Trisalicylate (Co-administration with drugs with hypoglycemic activity, such as salicylates, may result in decreased insulin requirements). Products include:
Trilisate ... 2155

Cortisone Acetate (Co-administration may result in increased insulin requirements). Products include:
Cortone Acetate Sterile Suspension ... 1663
Cortone Acetate Tablets ... 1664

Desogestrel (Co-administration with oral contraceptives may result in increased insulin requirements). Products include:
Desogen Tablets ... 1867
Ortho-Cept ... 1907

Dexamethasone (Co-administration may result in increased insulin requirements). Products include:
AK-Trol Ointment & Suspension ... ◎ 205
Decadron Elixir ... 1676
Decadron Tablets ... 1678
Decaspray Topical Aerosol ... 1689
Maxitrol Ophthalmic Ointment and Suspension ... ◎ 222
TobraDex Ophthalmic Suspension and Ointment ... 469

Dexamethasone Acetate (Co-administration may result in increased insulin requirements). Products include:
Dalalone D.P. Injectable ... 1009
Decadron-LA Sterile Suspension ... 1687

Dexamethasone Sodium Phosphate (Co-administration may result in increased insulin requirements). Products include:
Decadron Phosphate Injection ... 1680
Decadron Phosphate Sterile Ophthalmic Ointment ... 1684
Decadron Phosphate Sterile Ophthalmic Solution ... 1685
Decadron Phosphate Topical Cream ... 1686
Decadron Phosphate with Xylocaine Injection, Sterile ... 1683
Dexacort Phosphate in Respihaler .. 1606
Dexacort Phosphate in Turbinaire .. 1607
NeoDecadron Sterile Ophthalmic Ointment ... 1755
NeoDecadron Sterile Ophthalmic Solution ... 1756
NeoDecadron Topical Cream ... 1757

Dienestrol (Co-administration may result in increased insulin requirements). Products include:
Ortho Dienestrol Cream ... 1922

Diethylstilbestrol (Co-administration may result in increased insulin requirements). Products include:
Diethylstilbestrol Tablets ... 1477

Diflunisal (Co-administration with drugs with hypoglycemic activity, such as salicylates, may result in decreased insulin requirements). Products include:
Dolobid Tablets ... 1695

Enalapril Maleate (Co-administration with drugs with hypoglycemic activity, such as certain ACE inhibitors, may result in decreased insulin requirements). Products include:
Vaseretic Tablets ... 1810
Vasotec Tablets ... 1816

Enalaprilat (Co-administration with drugs with hypoglycemic activity, such as certain ACE inhibitors, may result in decreased insulin requirements). Products include:
Vasotec I.V. ... 1814

Esmolol Hydrochloride (Co-administration with drugs with hypoglycemic activity, such as beta blocker, may result in decreased insulin requirements; beta blockers may mask the symptoms of hypoglycemia in some patients). Products include:
Brevibloc (esmolol HCl) Injection ... 1860

Estradiol (Co-administration may result in increased insulin requirements). Products include:
Climara Transdermal System ... 640
Estrace Cream and Tablets ... 751
Estraderm Transdermal System ... 842
Estring Vaginal Ring ... 2086
Vivelle Transdermal System ... 880

Estrogens, Conjugated (Co-administration may result in increased insulin requirements). Products include:
PMB 200 and PMB 400 ... 2890
Premarin Intravenous ... 2893
Premarin Tablets ... 2896
Premarin Vaginal Cream ... 2898
Premphase ... 2900
Prempro ... 2905

Estrogens, Esterified (Co-administration may result in increased insulin requirements). Products include:
ESTRATAB Tablets (0.3, 0.625, 1.25, 2.5 mg) ... 2715
Estratest ... 2718
Menest Tablets ... 2671

Estropipate (Co-administration may result in increased insulin requirements). Products include:
Ogen Tablets ... 2103
Ogen Vaginal Cream ... 2106
Ortho-Est ... 1925

Ethinyl Estradiol (Co-administration with oral contraceptives may result in increased insulin requirements). Products include:
Brevicon ... 2563
Demulen ... 2580
Desogen Tablets ... 1867
Levlen/Tri-Levlen ... 646
Lo/Ovral Tablets ... 2852
Lo/Ovral-28 Tablets ... 2857
Modicon ... 1928
Nordette-21 Tablets ... 2863
Nordette-28 Tablets ... 2866
Norinyl ... 2563
Ortho-Cept ... 1907
Ortho-Cyclen/Ortho-Tri-Cyclen ... 1914
Ortho-Novum ... 1928
Ortho-Cyclen/Ortho Tri-Cyclen ... 1914
Ovcon ... 765
Ovral Tablets ... 2877
Ovral-28 Tablets ... 2878
Levlen/Tri-Levlen ... 646
Tri-Norinyl ... 2607
Triphasil-21 Tablets ... 2919
Triphasil-28 Tablets ... 2924

Ethynodiol Diacetate (Co-administration with oral contraceptives may result in increased insulin requirements). Products include:
Demulen ... 2580

Fludrocortisone Acetate (Co-administration may result in increased insulin requirements). Products include:
Florinef Acetate Tablets ... 506

Fluphenazine Decanoate (Co-administration with phenothiazines may result in increased insulin requirements). Products include:
Prolixin Decanoate ... 510

Fluphenazine Enanthate (Co-administration with phenothiazines may result in increased insulin requirements). Products include:
Prolixin Enanthate ... 510

Fluphenazine Hydrochloride (Co-administration with phenothiazines may result in increased insulin requirements). Products include:
Prolixin ... 510

Fosinopril Sodium (Co-administration with drugs with hypoglycemic activity, such as certain ACE inhibitors, may result in decreased insulin requirements). Products include:
Monopril Tablets ... 762

Glimepiride (Co-administration with drugs with hypoglycemic activity, such as oral hypoglycemic agents, may result in decreased insulin requirements). Products include:
Amaryl Tablets ... 1241

Glipizide (Co-administration with drugs with hypoglycemic activity, such as oral hypoglycemic agents, may result in decreased insulin requirements). Products include:
Glucotrol Tablets ... 2011
Glucotrol XL Extended Release Tablets ... 2012

Glyburide (Co-administration with drugs with hypoglycemic activity, such as oral hypoglycemic agents, may result in decreased insulin requirements). Products include:
DiaBeta Tablets ... 1265
Glynase PresTab Tablets ... 2091
Micronase Tablets ... 2099

Hydrocortisone (Co-administration may result in increased insulin requirements). Products include:
Anusol-HC Cream 2.5% ... 1953
Aquanil HC Lotion ... 1989
Maximum Strength Cortaid Spray ... 800
CORTENEMA ... 2713
Cortisporin Ointment ... 1074
Cortisporin Ophthalmic Ointment Sterile ... 1074
Cortisporin Ophthalmic Suspension Sterile ... 1075
Cortisporin Otic Solution Sterile ... 1076
Cortisporin Otic Suspension Sterile 1077
Cortizone-5 ... 795
Cortizone-10 ... 795
Hydrocortone Tablets ... 1715
Hytone ... 922
Hytone Ointment 2 ½% ... 923
Massengill Medicated Soft Cloth Towelettes ... 2628
Pediotic Suspension Sterile ... 1140
Preparation H Hydrocortisone 1% Cream ... 843
ProctoCream-HC 2.5% ... 2552
VōSoL HC Otic Solution ... 2786

Hydrocortisone Acetate (Co-administration may result in increased insulin requirements). Products include:
Analpram-HC Rectal Cream 1% and 2.5% ... 993
Anusol HC-1 Hydrocortisone Anti-Itch Ointment ... 810
Anusol-HC Suppositories ... 1954
Caldecort Anti-Itch Hydrocortisone Cream ... 651
Coly-Mycin S Otic w/Neomycin & Hydrocortisone ... 1965
Cortaid ... 800
Cortifoam ... 2540
Cortisporin Cream ... 1073
Epifoam ... 2543
Hydrocortone Acetate Sterile Suspension ... 1712
Mantadil Cream ... 1124
Nupercainal Hydrocortisone 1% Cream ... 661
Pramosone Cream, Lotion & Ointment ... 995
ProctoFoam-HC ... 2552
Terra-Cortril Ophthalmic Suspension ... 2033

Hydrocortisone Sodium Phosphate (Co-administration may result in increased insulin requirements). Products include:
Hydrocortone Phosphate Injection, Sterile ... 1713

Hydrocortisone Sodium Succinate (Co-administration may result in increased insulin requirements).
No products indexed under this heading.

IMPORTANT NOTE: Always consult each drug listing in the patient's regimen for possible interactions.

Humalog | **Interactions Index** | **484**

Isoniazid (Co-administration may result in increased insulin requirements). Products include:
- Nydrazid Injection 509
- Rifamate Capsules 1278
- Rifater 1280

Labetalol Hydrochloride (Co-administration with drugs with hypoglycemic activity, such as beta blocker, may result in decreased insulin requirements; beta blockers may mask the symptoms of hypoglycemia in some patients). Products include:
- Normodyne Injection 2519
- Normodyne Tablets 2522
- Trandate 1158

Levobunolol Hydrochloride (Co-administration with drugs with hypoglycemic activity, such as beta blocker, may result in decreased insulin requirements; beta blockers may mask the symptoms of hypoglycemia in some patients). Products include:
- Betagan .... ◉ 230

Levonorgestrel (Co-administration with oral contraceptives may result in increased insulin requirements). Products include:
- Levlen/Tri-Levlen 646
- Nordette-21 Tablets 2863
- Nordette-28 Tablets 2866
- Norplant System 2868
- Levlen/Tri-Levlen 646
- Triphasil-21 Tablets 2919
- Triphasil-28 Tablets 2924

Levothyroxine Sodium (Co-administration with thyroid replacement therapy may result in increased insulin requirements). Products include:
- Eltroxin Tablets 2214
- Levothroid Tablets 1015
- Levothyroxine Sodium, USP for Injection 546
- Levoxyl Tablets 918
- Synthroid 1410

Liothyronine Sodium (Co-administration with thyroid replacement therapy may result in increased insulin requirements). Products include:
- Cytomel Tablets 2647
- Triostat Injection 2708

Liotrix (Co-administration with thyroid replacement therapy may result in increased insulin requirements).
- No products indexed under this heading.

Lisinopril (Co-administration with drugs with hypoglycemic activity, such as certain ACE inhibitors, may result in decreased insulin requirements). Products include:
- Prinivil Tablets 1776
- Prinzide Tablets 1780
- Zestoretic Tablets 2968
- Zestril Tablets 2972

Magnesium Salicylate (Co-administration with drugs with hypoglycemic activity, such as salicylates, may result in decreased insulin requirements). Products include:
- Backache Caplets .... ▣ 635
- Doan's Extra-Strength Analgesic .... ▣ 653
- Extra Strength Doan's P.M. .... ▣ 653
- Doan's Regular Strength Analgesic .... ▣ 654
- Mobigesic Tablets .... ▣ 607

Mesoridazine Besylate (Co-administration with phenothiazines may result in increased insulin requirements). Products include:
- Serentil 689

Mestranol (Co-administration with oral contraceptives may result in increased insulin requirements). Products include:
- Norinyl 2563
- Ortho-Novum 1928

Metformin Hydrochloride (Co-administration with drugs with hypoglycemic activity, such as oral hypoglycemic agents, may result in decreased insulin requirements). Products include:
- Glucophage Tablets 754

Methotrimeprazine (Co-administration with phenothiazines may result in increased insulin requirements). Products include:
- Levoprome 1321

Methylprednisolone Acetate (Co-administration may result in increased insulin requirements).
- No products indexed under this heading.

Methylprednisolone Sodium Succinate (Co-administration may result in increased insulin requirements).
- No products indexed under this heading.

Metipranolol Hydrochloride (Co-administration with drugs with hypoglycemic activity, such as beta blocker, may result in decreased insulin requirements; beta blockers may mask the symptoms of hypoglycemia in some patients). Products include:
- OptiPranolol (Metipranolol 0.3%) Sterile Ophthalmic Solution .... ◉ 256

Metoprolol Succinate (Co-administration with drugs with hypoglycemic activity, such as beta blocker, may result in decreased insulin requirements; beta blockers may mask the symptoms of hypoglycemia in some patients). Products include:
- Toprol-XL Tablets 560

Metoprolol Tartrate (Co-administration with drugs with hypoglycemic activity, such as beta blocker, may result in decreased insulin requirements; beta blockers may mask the symptoms of hypoglycemia in some patients). Products include:
- Lopressor 848
- Lopressor HCT Tablets 850

Moexipril Hydrochloride (Co-administration with drugs with hypoglycemic activity, such as certain ACE inhibitors, may result in decreased insulin requirements). Products include:
- Univasc Tablets 2553

Nadolol (Co-administration with drugs with hypoglycemic activity, such as beta blocker, may result in decreased insulin requirements; beta blockers may mask the symptoms of hypoglycemia in some patients).
- No products indexed under this heading.

Niacin (Co-administration may result in increased insulin requirements). Products include:
- Kyo-Chrome .... ▣ 680
- Nicotinex Elixir .... ▣ 671
- Slo-Niacin Tablets 2767

Norethindrone (Co-administration with oral contraceptives may result in increased insulin requirements). Products include:
- Brevicon 2563
- Micronor Tablets 1903
- Modicon 1928
- Norinyl 2563
- Nor-Q D Tablets 2598
- Ortho-Novum 1928
- Ovcon 765
- Tri-Norinyl 2607

Norethynodrel (Co-administration with oral contraceptives may result in increased insulin requirements).
- No products indexed under this heading.

Norgestimate (Co-administration with oral contraceptives may result in increased insulin requirements). Products include:
- Ortho-Cyclen/Ortho-Tri-Cyclen 1914
- Ortho-Cyclen/Ortho Tri-Cyclen 1914

Norgestrel (Co-administration with oral contraceptives may result in increased insulin requirements). Products include:
- Lo/Ovral Tablets 2852
- Lo/Ovral-28 Tablets 2857
- Ovral Tablets 2877
- Ovral-28 Tablets 2878
- Ovrette Tablets 2878

Octreotide Acetate (Co-administration with drugs with hypoglycemic activity, such as inhibitors of pancreatic function, may result in decreased insulin requirements). Products include:
- Sandostatin Injection 2421

Penbutolol Sulfate (Co-administration with drugs with hypoglycemic activity, such as beta blocker, may result in decreased insulin requirements; beta blockers may mask the symptoms of hypoglycemia in some patients). Products include:
- Levatol Tablets 2547

Perphenazine (Co-administration with phenothiazines may result in increased insulin requirements). Products include:
- Etrafon 2495
- Triavil Tablets 1800
- Trilafon 2532

Phenelzine Sulfate (Co-administration with drugs with hypoglycemic activity, such as certain MAO inhibitor antidepressants, may result in decreased insulin requirements). Products include:
- Nardil 1977

Pindolol (Co-administration with drugs with hypoglycemic activity, such as beta blocker, may result in decreased insulin requirements; beta blockers may mask the symptoms of hypoglycemia in some patients). Products include:
- Visken Tablets 2428

Polyestradiol Phosphate (Co-administration may result in increased insulin requirements).
- No products indexed under this heading.

Prednisolone Acetate (Co-administration may result in increased insulin requirements). Products include:
- AK-CIDE .... ◉ 203
- AK-CIDE Ointment .... ◉ 203
- Blephamide Liquifilm Sterile Ophthalmic Suspension 472
- Blephamide Ointment .... ◉ 234
- Econopred & Econopred Plus Ophthalmic Suspensions .... ◉ 216
- Poly-Pred Liquifilm .... ◉ 246
- Pred Forte .... ◉ 247
- Pred Mild .... ◉ 250
- Pred-G Liquifilm Sterile Ophthalmic Suspension .... ◉ 248
- Pred-G S.O.P. Sterile Ophthalmic Ointment .... ◉ 249

Prednisolone Sodium Phosphate (Co-administration may result in increased insulin requirements). Products include:
- AK-PRED .... ◉ 204
- Hydeltrasol Injection, Sterile 1708
- Pediapred Oral Solution 1618

Prednisolone Tebutate (Co-administration may result in increased insulin requirements). Products include:
- Hydeltra-T.B.A. Sterile Suspension 1710

Prednisone (Co-administration may result in increased insulin requirements).
- No products indexed under this heading.

Prochlorperazine (Co-administration with phenothiazines may result in increased insulin requirements). Products include:
- Compazine 2644

Promethazine Hydrochloride (Co-administration with phenothiazines may result in increased insulin requirements). Products include:
- Mepergan Injection 2859
- Phenergan with Codeine 2883
- Phenergan with Dextromethorphan 2885
- Phenergan Injection 2880
- Phenergan Suppositories 2882
- Phenergan Syrup 2881
- Phenergan Tablets 2882
- Phenergan VC 2886
- Phenergan VC with Codeine 2888

Propranolol Hydrochloride (Co-administration with drugs with hypoglycemic activity, such as beta blocker, may result in decreased insulin requirements; beta blockers may mask the symptoms of hypoglycemia in some patients). Products include:
- Inderal 2834
- Inderal LA Long Acting Capsules 2836
- Inderide Tablets 2838
- Inderide LA Long Acting Capsules .. 2840

Quinapril Hydrochloride (Co-administration with drugs with hypoglycemic activity, such as certain ACE inhibitors, may result in decreased insulin requirements). Products include:
- Accupril Tablets 1950

Quinestrol (Co-administration may result in increased insulin requirements).
- No products indexed under this heading.

Ramipril (Co-administration with drugs with hypoglycemic activity, such as certain ACE inhibitors, may result in decreased insulin requirements). Products include:
- Altace Capsules 1238

Salsalate (Co-administration with drugs with hypoglycemic activity, such as salicylates, may result in decreased insulin requirements). Products include:
- Disalcid 1549
- Mono-Gesic Tablets 810
- Salflex Tablets 791

Sotalol Hydrochloride (Co-administration with drugs with hypoglycemic activity, such as beta blocker, may result in decreased insulin requirements; beta blockers may mask the symptoms of hypoglycemia in some patients). Products include:
- Betapace Tablets 637

Spirapril Hydrochloride (Co-administration with drugs with hypoglycemic activity, such as certain ACE inhibitors, may result in decreased insulin requirements).
- No products indexed under this heading.

Sulfacytine (Co-administration with drugs with hypoglycemic activity, such as sulfa antibiotics, may result in decreased insulin requirements).

Sulfamethizole (Co-administration with drugs with hypoglycemic activity, such as sulfa antibiotics, may result in decreased insulin requirements). Products include:
- Urobiotic-250 Capsules 2038

(▣ Described in PDR For Nonprescription Drugs) (◉ Described in PDR For Ophthalmology)

Sulfamethoxazole (Co-administration with drugs with hypoglycemic activity, such as sulfa antibiotics, may result in decreased insulin requirements). Products include:
Bactrim DS Tablets 2257
Bactrim I.V. Infusion 2255
Bactrim 2257
Gantanol Tablets 2285
Septra 1146
Septra I.V. Infusion 1142
Septra I.V. Infusion ADD-Vantage Vials 1144
Septra 1146

Sulfasalazine (Co-administration with drugs with hypoglycemic activity, such as sulfa antibiotics, may result in decreased insulin requirements). Products include:
Azulfidine 2059

Sulfisoxazole (Co-administration with drugs with hypoglycemic activity, such as sulfa antibiotics, may result in decreased insulin requirements). Products include:
Gantrisin Tablets 2286

Thioridazine Hydrochloride (Co-administration with phenothiazines may result in increased insulin requirements). Products include:
Mellaril 2398

Thyroglobulin (Co-administration with thyroid replacement therapy may result in increased insulin requirements).
No products indexed under this heading.

Thyroid (Co-administration with thyroid replacement therapy may result in increased insulin requirements).
No products indexed under this heading.

Thyroxine (Co-administration with thyroid replacement therapy may result in increased insulin requirements).
No products indexed under this heading.

Thyroxine Sodium (Co-administration with thyroid replacement therapy may result in increased insulin requirements).
No products indexed under this heading.

Timolol Hemihydrate (Co-administration with drugs with hypoglycemic activity, such as beta blocker, may result in decreased insulin requirements; beta blockers may mask the symptoms of hypoglycemia in some patients). Products include:
Betimol 0.25%, 0.5% .... ⓡ 259

Timolol Maleate (Co-administration with drugs with hypoglycemic activity, such as beta blocker, may result in decreased insulin requirements; beta blockers may mask the symptoms of hypoglycemia in some patients). Products include:
Blocadren Tablets 1654
Timolide Tablets 1791
Timoptic in Ocudose 1796
Timoptic Sterile Ophthalmic Solution 1794
Timoptic-XE 1798

Tolazamide (Co-administration with drugs with hypoglycemic activity, such as oral hypoglycemic agents, may result in decreased insulin requirements).
No products indexed under this heading.

Tolbutamide (Co-administration with drugs with hypoglycemic activity, such as oral hypoglycemic agents, may result in decreased insulin requirements).
No products indexed under this heading.

Trandolapril (Co-administration with drugs with hypoglycemic activity, such as certain ACE inhibitors, may result in decreased insulin requirements). Products include:
Mavik Tablets 1407

Tranylcypromine Sulfate (Co-administration with drugs with hypoglycemic activity, such as certain MAO inhibitor antidepressants, may result in decreased insulin requirements). Products include:
Parnate Tablets 2679

Triamcinolone (Co-administration may result in increased insulin requirements).
No products indexed under this heading.

Triamcinolone Acetonide (Co-administration may result in increased insulin requirements). Products include:
Azmacort Oral Inhaler 2175
Nasacort AQ Nasal Spray 2191
Nasacort Nasal Inhaler 2189

Triamcinolone Diacetate (Co-administration may result in increased insulin requirements).
No products indexed under this heading.

Triamcinolone Hexacetonide (Co-administration may result in increased insulin requirements).
No products indexed under this heading.

Trifluoperazine Hydrochloride (Co-administration with phenothiazines may result in increased insulin requirements). Products include:
Stelazine 2692

Food Interactions

Alcohol (Co-administration with drugs with hypoglycemic activity may result in decreased insulin requirements).

HUMATE-P, ANTIHEMOPHILIC FACTOR (HUMAN), DRIED PASTEURIZED
(Antihemophilic Factor (Human)) 801
None cited in PDR database.

HUMATROPE VIALS
(Somatropin) 1490
May interact with glucocorticoids. Compounds in this category include:

Betamethasone Acetate (Excessive glucocorticoid therapy will inhibit the growth promoting effect of somatropin). Products include:
Celestone Soluspan Suspension 2484

Betamethasone Sodium Phosphate (Excessive glucocorticoid therapy will inhibit the growth promoting effect of somatropin). Products include:
Celestone Soluspan Suspension 2484

Cortisone Acetate (Excessive glucocorticoid therapy will inhibit the growth promoting effect of somatropin). Products include:
Cortone Acetate Sterile Suspension 1663
Cortone Acetate Tablets 1664

Dexamethasone (Excessive glucocorticoid therapy will inhibit the growth promoting effect of somatropin). Products include:
AK-Trol Ointment & Suspension .... ⓡ 205
Decadron Elixir 1676
Decadron Tablets 1678
Decaspray Topical Aerosol 1689
Maxitrol Ophthalmic Ointment and Suspension .... ⓡ 222
TobraDex Ophthalmic Suspension and Ointment 469

Dexamethasone Acetate (Excessive glucocorticoid therapy will inhibit the growth promoting effect of somatropin). Products include:
Dalalone D.P. Injectable 1009
Decadron-LA Sterile Suspension 1687

Dexamethasone Sodium Phosphate (Excessive glucocorticoid therapy will inhibit the growth promoting effect of somatropin). Products include:
Decadron Phosphate Injection 1680
Decadron Phosphate Sterile Ophthalmic Ointment 1684
Decadron Phosphate Sterile Ophthalmic Solution 1685
Decadron Phosphate Topical Cream 1686
Decadron Phosphate with Xylocaine Injection, Sterile 1683
Dexacort Phosphate in Respihaler .. 1606
Dexacort Phosphate in Turbinaire .. 1607
NeoDecadron Sterile Ophthalmic Ointment 1755
NeoDecadron Sterile Ophthalmic Solution 1756
NeoDecadron Topical Cream .. 1757

Fludrocortisone Acetate (Excessive glucocorticoid therapy will inhibit the growth promoting effect of somatropin). Products include:
Florinef Acetate Tablets 506

Hydrocortisone (Excessive glucocorticoid therapy will inhibit the growth promoting effect of somatropin). Products include:
Anusol-HC Cream 2.5% 1953
Aquanil HC Lotion 1989
Maximum Strength Cortaid Spray ⓡ 800
CORTENEMA 2713
Cortisporin Ointment 1074
Cortisporin Ophthalmic Ointment Sterile 1074
Cortisporin Ophthalmic Suspension Sterile 1075
Cortisporin Otic Solution Sterile .. 1076
Cortisporin Otic Suspension Sterile 1077
Cortizone-5 .... ⓡ 795
Cortizone-10 .... ⓡ 795
Hydrocortone Tablets 1715
Hytone 922
Hytone Ointment 2 ½% 923
Massengill Medicated Soft Cloth Towelettes 2628
Pediotic Suspension Sterile 1140
Preparation H Hydrocortisone 1% Cream .... ⓡ 843
ProctoCream-HC 2.5% 2552
VōSoL HC Otic Solution........... 2786

Hydrocortisone Acetate (Excessive glucocorticoid therapy will inhibit the growth promoting effect of somatropin). Products include:
Analpram-HC Rectal Cream 1% and .5% 993
Anusol HC-1 Hydrocortisone Anti-Itch Ointment .... ⓡ 810
Anusol-HC Suppositories 1954
Caldecort Anti-Itch Hydrocortisone Cream .... ⓡ 651
Coly-Mycin S Otic w/Neomycin & Hydrocortisone 1965
Cortaid .... ⓡ 800
Cortifoam 2540
Cortisporin Cream 1073
Epifoam 2543
Hydrocortone Acetate Sterile Suspension 1712
Mantadil Cream 1124
Nupercainal Hydrocortisone 1% Cream .... ⓡ 661
Pramosone Cream, Lotion & Ointment 995
ProctoFoam-HC 2552
Terra-Cortril Ophthalmic Suspension 2033

Hydrocortisone Sodium Phosphate (Excessive glucocorticoid therapy will inhibit the growth promoting effect of somatropin). Products include:
Hydrocortone Phosphate Injection, Sterile 1713

Hydrocortisone Sodium Succinate (Excessive glucocorticoid therapy will inhibit the growth promoting effect of somatropin).
No products indexed under this heading.

Methylprednisolone Acetate (Excessive glucocorticoid therapy will inhibit the growth promoting effect of somatropin).
No products indexed under this heading.

Methylprednisolone Sodium Succinate (Excessive glucocorticoid therapy will inhibit the growth promoting effect of somatropin).
No products indexed under this heading.

Prednisolone Acetate (Excessive glucocorticoid therapy will inhibit the growth promoting effect of somatropin). Products include:
AK-CIDE .... ⓡ 203
AK-CIDE Ointment .... ⓡ 203
Blephamide Liquifilm Sterile Ophthalmic Suspension 472
Blephamide Ointment .... ⓡ 234
Econopred & Econopred Plus Ophthalmic Suspensions ... ⓡ 216
Poly-Pred Liquifilm .... ⓡ 246
Pred Forte .... ⓡ 247
Pred Mild .... ⓡ 250
Pred-G Liquifilm Sterile Ophthalmic Suspension .... ⓡ 248
Pred-G S.O.P. Sterile Ophthalmic Ointment .... ⓡ 249

Prednisolone Sodium Phosphate (Excessive glucocorticoid therapy will inhibit the growth promoting effect of somatropin). Products include:
AK-PRED .... ⓡ 204
Hydeltrasol Injection, Sterile .. 1708
Pediapred Oral Solution 1618

Prednisolone Tebutate (Excessive glucocorticoid therapy will inhibit the growth promoting effect of somatropin). Products include:
Hydeltra-T.B.A. Sterile Suspension 1710

Prednisone (Excessive glucocorticoid therapy will inhibit the growth promoting effect of somatropin).
No products indexed under this heading.

Triamcinolone (Excessive glucocorticoid therapy will inhibit the growth promoting effect of somatropin).
No products indexed under this heading.

Triamcinolone Acetonide (Excessive glucocorticoid therapy will inhibit the growth promoting effect of somatropin). Products include:
Azmacort Oral Inhaler 2175
Nasacort AQ Nasal Spray 2191
Nasacort Nasal Inhaler 2189

Triamcinolone Diacetate (Excessive glucocorticoid therapy will inhibit the growth promoting effect of somatropin).
No products indexed under this heading.

Triamcinolone Hexacetonide (Excessive glucocorticoid therapy will inhibit the growth promoting effect of somatropin).
No products indexed under this heading.

HUMEGON FOR INJECTION
(Menotropins) 1873
None cited in PDR database.

HUMIBID DM TABLETS
(Guaifenesin, Dextromethorphan Hydrobromide) 1612

IMPORTANT NOTE: Always consult each drug listing in the patient's regimen for possible interactions.

Humibid — Interactions Index — 486

Humibid
May interact with monoamine oxidase inhibitors. Compounds in this category include:

Furazolidone (Concurrent and/or sequential use is contraindicated). Products include:
- Furoxone ... 2221

Isocarboxazid (Concurrent and/or sequential use is contraindicated).
- No products indexed under this heading.

Phenelzine Sulfate (Concurrent and/or sequential use is contraindicated). Products include:
- Nardil ... 1977

Selegiline Hydrochloride (Concurrent and/or sequential use is contraindicated). Products include:
- Eldepryl Capsules ... 2729

Tranylcypromine Sulfate (Concurrent and/or sequential use is contraindicated). Products include:
- Parnate Tablets ... 2679

HUMIBID L.A. TABLETS
(Guaifenesin) ... 1612
None cited in PDR database.

HUMIBID PEDIATRIC CAPSULES
(Guaifenesin) ... 1612
None cited in PDR database.

HUMORSOL STERILE OPHTHALMIC SOLUTION
(Demecarium Bromide) ... 1707
May interact with cholinergic agents and certain other agents. Compounds in these categories include:

Edrophonium Chloride (Additive adverse effects). Products include:
- Tensilon Injectable ... 1307

Neostigmine Bromide (Additive adverse effects). Products include:
- Prostigmin Tablets ... 1306

Neostigmine Methylsulfate (Additive adverse effects). Products include:
- Prostigmin Injectable ... 1305

Pyridostigmine Bromide (Additive adverse effects). Products include:
- Mestinon Injectable ... 1300
- Mestinon ... 1300

Succinylcholine Chloride (Possible respiratory and cardiovascular collapse). Products include:
- Anectine ... 1062

HUMULIN 50/50, 100 UNITS
(Insulin, Human Isophane Suspension, Insulin, Human) ... 1491
See Pork Regular, 100 Units

HUMULIN 70/30, 100 UNITS
(Insulin, Human Regular and Human NPH Mixture) ... 1492
See Pork Regular, 100 Units

HUMULIN L, 100 UNITS
(Insulin, Human, Zinc Suspension) ... 1494
See Pork Regular, 100 Units

HUMULIN N, 100 UNITS
(Insulin, Human NPH) ... 1495
See Pork Regular, 100 Units

HUMULIN R, 100 UNITS
(Insulin, Human Regular) ... 1497
See Pork Regular, 100 Units

HUMULIN U, 100 UNITS
(Insulin, Human, Zinc Suspension) ... 1498
See Pork Regular, 100 Units

HYCAMTIN FOR INJECTION
(Topotecan Hydrochloride) ... 2665
May interact with:

Cisplatin (Co-administration has resulted in severe myelosuppression; case of neutropenia and fatal neutropenic sepsis has been reported). Products include:
- Platinol for Injection ... 717
- Platinol-AQ Injection ... 719

Filgrastim (Co-administration of G-CSF can prolong the duration of neutropenia, so if G-CSF is to be used, it should not be initiated until day 6 of the course of therapy). Products include:
- Neupogen for Injection ... 495

HYCODAN TABLETS AND SYRUP
(Hydrocodone Bitartrate, Homatropine Methylbromide) ... 946
May interact with central nervous system depressants, narcotic analgesics, antihistamines, antipsychotic agents, tranquilizers, monoamine oxidase inhibitors, tricyclic antidepressants, and certain other agents. Compounds in these categories include:

Acrivastine (Exhibits an additive CNS depression). Products include:
- Semprex-D Capsules ... 1620

Alfentanil Hydrochloride (Exhibits an additive CNS depression). Products include:
- Alfenta Injection ... 1334

Alprazolam (Exhibits an additive CNS depression). Products include:
- Xanax Tablets ... 2115

Amitriptyline Hydrochloride (Increased effect of either the antidepressant or hydrocodone). Products include:
- Elavil ... 2945
- Etrafon ... 2495
- Limbitrol ... 2333
- Triavil Tablets ... 1800

Amoxapine (Increased effect of either the antidepressant or hydrocodone). Products include:
- Asendin Tablets ... 1419

Aprobarbital (Exhibits an additive CNS depression).
- No products indexed under this heading.

Astemizole (Exhibits an additive CNS depression). Products include:
- Hismanal Tablets ... 1341

Azatadine Maleate (Exhibits an additive CNS depression). Products include:
- Trinalin Repetabs Tablets ... 1373

Bromodiphenhydramine Hydrochloride (Exhibits an additive CNS depression).
- No products indexed under this heading.

Brompheniramine Maleate (Exhibits an additive CNS depression). Products include:
- Alka-Seltzer Plus Sinus Medicine ... ■ 611
- Bromfed Capsules (Extended-Release) ... 1832
- Bromfed Syrup ... ■ 712
- Bromfed Tablets ... 1832
- Bromfed-DM Cough Syrup ... 1832
- Bromfed-PD Capsules (Extended-Release) ... 1832
- Dimetane-DC Cough Syrup ... 2232
- Dimetane-DX Cough Syrup ... 2233
- Dimetapp Allergy Dye-Free Elixir ... ■ 838
- Dimetapp Allergy Sinus Caplets ... ■ 838
- Dimetapp Cold & Allergy Chewable Tablets ... ■ 838
- Dimetapp Cold & Cough Liqui-Gels ... ■ 839
- Dimetapp Cold & Fever Suspension ... ■ 839
- Dimetapp DM Elixir ... ■ 840
- Dimetapp Elixir ... ■ 840
- Dimetapp Extentabs ... ■ 841
- Dimetapp Tablets/Liqui-Gels ... ■ 841
- Rondec Chewable Tablets ... 974
- Vicks DayQuil Allergy Relief 12-Hour Extended Release Tablets ... ■ 733
- Vicks DayQuil Allergy Relief 4-Hour Tablets ... ■ 733

Buprenorphine (Exhibits an additive CNS depression). Products include:
- Buprenex Injectable ... 2170

Buspirone Hydrochloride (Exhibits an additive CNS depression). Products include:
- BuSpar Tablets ... 738

Butabarbital (Exhibits an additive CNS depression).
- No products indexed under this heading.

Butalbital (Exhibits an additive CNS depression). Products include:
- Axocet Capsules ... 2469
- Esgic-plus Capsules ... 1012
- Esgic-plus Tablets ... 1012
- Fioricet Tablets ... 2386
- Fioricet with Codeine Capsules ... 2387
- Fiorinal Capsules ... 2388
- Fiorinal with Codeine Capsules ... 2390
- Fiorinal Tablets ... 2388
- Phrenilin ... 790
- Sedapap Tablets 50 mg/650 mg ... 1826

Cetirizine Hydrochloride (Exhibits an additive CNS depression). Products include:
- Zyrtec Tablets ... 2053

Chlordiazepoxide (Exhibits an additive CNS depression). Products include:
- Limbitrol ... 2333

Chlordiazepoxide Hydrochloride (Exhibits an additive CNS depression). Products include:
- Librax Capsules ... 2330
- Librium Capsules ... 2331
- Librium Injectable ... 2332

Chlorpheniramine Maleate (Exhibits an additive CNS depression). Products include:
- Alka-Seltzer Plus Cold Medicine ... ■ 611
- Alka-Seltzer Plus Cold Medicine Liqui-Gels ... ■ 612
- Alka-Seltzer Plus Cold & Cough Medicine ... ■ 611
- Alka-Seltzer Plus Cold & Cough Medicine Liqui-Gels ... ■ 612
- Alka-Seltzer Plus Flu & Body Aches Effervescent Tablets ... ■ 612
- Allerest Maximum Strength ... ■ 649
- Allerest Sinus Pain Formula ... ■ 649
- Ana-Kit Anaphylaxis Emergency Treatment Kit ... 611
- Atrohist Pediatric Capsules ... 1603
- Atrohist Plus Tablets ... 1605
- BC Cold Powder Multi-Symptom Formula (Cold-Sinus-Allergy) ... ■ 631
- Cerose DM ... 853
- Cheracol Plus Head Cold/Cough Formula ... ■ 741
- Children's TYLENOL Cold Multi-Symptom Chewable Tablets and Liquid ... 1559
- Children's TYLENOL Cold Plus Cough Multi Symptom Chewable Tablets and Liquid ... 1560
- Children's TYLENOL Flu Suspension Liquid ... 1560
- Children's Vicks DayQuil Allergy Relief ... ■ 730
- Children's Vicks NyQuil Cold/Cough Relief ... ■ 731
- Chlor-Trimeton Allergy Decongestant Tablets ... 759
- Chlor-Trimeton Allergy Tablets ... 758
- Allergy-Sinus Comtrex Multi-Symptom Allergy-Sinus Formula Tablets and Caplets ... ■ 639
- Comtrex Multi-Symptom ... ■ 638
- Contac Continuous Action Nasal Decongestant/Antihistamine 12 Hour Capsules ... ■ 773
- Contac Maximum Strength Continuous Action Decongestant/Antihistamine 12 Hour Caplets ... ■ 772
- Contac Severe Cold and Flu Formula Caplets ... ■ 773
- Coricidin Cold + Flu Tablets ... ■ 760
- Coricidin Cough + Cold Tablets ... ■ 760
- Coricidin 'D' Decongestant Tablets ... ■ 760
- D.A. II Tablets ... 972
- D.A. Chewable Tablets ... 970
- Dura-Tap/PD Capsules ... 970
- Dura-Vent/DA Tablets ... 972
- Efidac 24 Chlorpheniramine ... ■ 655
- Extendryl ... 1003
- Fedahist Gyrocaps ... 2545
- Hycomine Compound Tablets ... 948
- Kronofed-A ... 994
- Nolamine Timed-Release Tablets ... 790
- Novahistine Elixir ... 782
- Ornade Spansule Capsules ... 2678
- PediaCare Cough-Cold Chewable Tablets and Liquid ... 1569
- PediaCare NightRest Cough-Cold Liquid ... 1569
- Pediatric Vicks 44m Cough & Cold Relief ... ■ 737
- Pyrroxate Caplets ... 742
- Ryna ... 804
- Sinarest ... 663
- Sine-Off Sinus Medicine ... 784
- Singlet Tablets ... 785
- Sinulin Tablets ... 792
- Sinutab Sinus Allergy Medication, Maximum Strength Tablets and Caplets ... ■ 823
- Sudafed Cold & Allergy Tablets ... ■ 826
- Teldrin 12 Hour Antihistamine/Nasal Decongestant Allergy Relief Capsules ... ■ 786
- TheraFlu Flu and Cold Medicine ... ■ 750
- Theraflu Maximum Strength Flu and Cold Medicine For Sore Throat ... ■ 751
- TheraFlu Flu, Cold and Cough Medicine ... ■ 750
- TheraFlu Maximum Strength Nighttime Flu, Cold & Cough Medicine ... ■ 751
- Triaminic Night Time ... ■ 754
- Triaminic Syrup ... ■ 755
- Triaminic Triaminicol Cold & Cough ... ■ 756
- Triaminicin Tablets ... ■ 756
- Tussend ... 1830
- TYLENOL Allergy Sinus, Maximum Strength Caplets and Gelcaps ... 1571
- TYLENOL Cold Medication, Multi-Symptom Formula Tablets and Caplets ... 1572
- TYLENOL Cold Medication, Multi-Symptom Hot Liquid Packets ... 1572
- Vicks 44 LiquiCaps Cough, Cold & Flu Relief ... ■ 728
- Vicks 44M Cough, Cold & Flu Relief ... ■ 729

Chlorpheniramine Polistirex (Exhibits an additive CNS depression). Products include:
- Tussionex Pennkinetic Extended-Release Suspension ... 1624

Chlorpheniramine Tannate (Exhibits an additive CNS depression). Products include:
- Atrohist Pediatric Suspension ... 1604
- Atrohist Pediatric Suspension Dye-Free ... 1604
- Rynatan ... 2781
- Rynatuss ... 2782

Chlorpromazine (Exhibits an additive CNS depression). Products include:
- Thorazine Suppositories ... 2701

Chlorpromazine Hydrochloride (Exhibits an additive CNS depression). Products include:
- Thorazine ... 2701

Chlorprothixene (Exhibits an additive CNS depression).
- No products indexed under this heading.

Chlorprothixene Hydrochloride (Exhibits an additive CNS depression).
- No products indexed under this heading.

Chlorprothixene Lactate (Exhibits an additive CNS depression).
- No products indexed under this heading.

(■ Described in PDR For Nonprescription Drugs)   (● Described in PDR For Ophthalmology)

Clemastine Fumarate (Exhibits an additive CNS depression). Products include:
- Tavist Syrup ... 2426
- Tavist Tablets ... 2427
- Tavist-1 12 Hour Relief Tablets ... 749
- Tavist-D 12 Hour Relief Tablets ... 750

Clomipramine Hydrochloride (Increased effect of either the antidepressant or hydrocodone). Products include:
- Anafranil Capsules ... 819

Clorazepate Dipotassium (Exhibits an additive CNS depression). Products include:
- Tranxene ... 459

Clozapine (Exhibits an additive CNS depression). Products include:
- Clozaril Tablets ... 2377

Codeine Phosphate (Exhibits an additive CNS depression). Products include:
- Brontex ... 2130
- Dimetane-DC Cough Syrup ... 2232
- Fioricet with Codeine Capsules ... 2387
- Fiorinal with Codeine Capsules ... 2390
- Nucofed ... 2225
- Phenergan with Codeine ... 2883
- Phenergan VC with Codeine ... 2888
- Robitussin A-C Syrup ... 2248
- Robitussin-DAC Syrup ... 2249
- Ryna ... 804
- Soma Compound w/Codeine Tablets ... 2784
- Tylenol with Codeine ... 1592

Cyproheptadine Hydrochloride (Exhibits an additive CNS depression). Products include:
- Periactin ... 1767

Desflurane (Exhibits an additive CNS depression). Products include:
- Suprane (desflurane, USP) ... 1865

Desipramine Hydrochloride (Increased effect of either the antidepressant or hydrocodone). Products include:
- Norpramin Tablets ... 1273

Dexchlorpheniramine Maleate (Exhibits an additive CNS depression).
- No products indexed under this heading.

Dezocine (Exhibits an additive CNS depression). Products include:
- Dalgan Injection ... 529

Diazepam (Exhibits an additive CNS depression). Products include:
- Dizac (diazepam injectable emulsion) CIV ... 1862
- Valium Injectable ... 2336
- Valium Tablets ... 2335

Diphenhydramine Citrate (Exhibits an additive CNS depression). Products include:
- Excedrin P.M. Analgesic/Sleeping Aid Tablets, Caplets, Liquigels ... 735

Diphenhydramine Hydrochloride (Exhibits an additive CNS depression). Products include:
- Actifed Allergy Daytime/Nighttime Caplets ... 808
- Actifed Sinus Daytime/Nighttime Tablets and Caplets ... 809
- Extra Strength Bayer PM Aspirin Plus Sleep Aid ... 617
- Benadryl Allergy Chewables ... 811
- Benadryl Allergy/Cold Tablets ... 811
- Benadryl Allergy Decongestant Liquid Medication ... 812
- Benadryl Allergy Decongestant Tablets ... 812
- Benadryl Allergy Liquid Medication ... 813
- Benadryl Allergy ... 811
- Benadryl Allergy Sinus Headache Caplets ... 813
- Benadryl Dye-Free Allergy Liquigel Softgels ... 813
- Benadryl Dye-Free Allergy Liquid Medication ... 814
- Benadryl Itch Relief Stick Extra Strength ... 814
- Benadryl Cream ... 814
- Benadryl Gel ... 815
- Benadryl Spray ... 815
- Benadryl Injection ... 1955
- Contac Day & Night Cold/Flu Night Caplets ... 772
- Contac Night Allergy/Sinus Caplets ... 771
- Extra Strength Doan's P.M. ... 653
- Excedrin P.M. Analgesic/Sleeping Aid Tablets, Caplets, Liquigels ... 643
- Nytol QuickCaps Caplets ... 632
- Sleepinal Night-time Sleep Aid Capsules and Softgels ... 798
- TYLENOL Allergy Sinus NightTime, Maximum Strength Caplets ... 1571
- TYLENOL Flu NightTime, Maximum Strength Gelcaps ... 1575
- TYLENOL Flu NightTime, Maximum Strength Hot Medication Packets ... 1575
- TYLENOL PM Pain Reliever/Sleep Aid, Extra Strength Gelcaps, Caplets, Geltabs ... 1576
- TYLENOL Severe Allergy Medication Caplets ... 1571
- Maximum Strength Unisom Sleepgels ... 1990
- Unisom With Pain Relief-Nighttime Sleep Aid and Pain Reliever ... 1991

Diphenylpyraline Hydrochloride (Exhibits an additive CNS depression).
- No products indexed under this heading.

Doxepin Hydrochloride (Increased effect of either the antidepressant or hydrocodone). Products include:
- Adapin Capsules ... 1542
- Sinequan ... 2028
- Zonalon Cream ... 1042

Droperidol (Exhibits an additive CNS depression). Products include:
- Inapsine Injection ... 462

Enflurane (Exhibits an additive CNS depression).
- No products indexed under this heading.

Estazolam (Exhibits an additive CNS depression). Products include:
- ProSom Tablets ... 457

Ethchlorvynol (Exhibits an additive CNS depression). Products include:
- Placidyl Capsules ... 456

Ethinamate (Exhibits an additive CNS depression).
- No products indexed under this heading.

Fentanyl (Exhibits an additive CNS depression). Products include:
- Duragesic Transdermal System ... 1336

Fentanyl Citrate (Exhibits an additive CNS depression). Products include:
- Sublimaze Injection ... 463

Fluphenazine Decanoate (Exhibits an additive CNS depression). Products include:
- Prolixin Decanoate ... 510

Fluphenazine Enanthate (Exhibits an additive CNS depression). Products include:
- Prolixin Enanthate ... 510

Fluphenazine Hydrochloride (Exhibits an additive CNS depression). Products include:
- Prolixin ... 510

Flurazepam Hydrochloride (Exhibits an additive CNS depression). Products include:
- Dalmane Capsules ... 2329

Furazolidone (May increase the effect of either MAO inhibitor or hydrocodone). Products include:
- Furoxone ... 2221

Glutethimide (Exhibits an additive CNS depression).
- No products indexed under this heading.

Haloperidol (Exhibits an additive CNS depression). Products include:
- Haldol Injection, Tablets and Concentrate ... 1585

Haloperidol Decanoate (Exhibits an additive CNS depression). Products include:
- Haldol Decanoate ... 1587

Hydrocodone Polistirex (Exhibits an additive CNS depression). Products include:
- Tussionex Pennkinetic Extended-Release Suspension ... 1624

Hydromorphone Hydrochloride (Exhibits an additive CNS depression). Products include:
- Dilaudid Ampules ... 1382
- Dilaudid Cough Syrup ... 1383
- Dilaudid-HP Injection ... 1384
- Dilaudid-HP Lyophilized Powder 250 mg ... 1384
- Dilaudid ... 1382
- Dilaudid Oral Liquid ... 1386
- Dilaudid ... 1382
- Dilaudid Tablets - 8 mg ... 1386

Hydroxyzine Hydrochloride (Exhibits an additive CNS depression). Products include:
- Atarax Tablets & Syrup ... 1992
- Marax Tablets & DF Syrup ... 2015
- Vistaril Intramuscular Solution ... 2042

Imipramine Hydrochloride (Increased effect of either the antidepressant or hydrocodone). Products include:
- Tofranil Ampuls ... 873
- Tofranil Tablets ... 875

Imipramine Pamoate (Increased effect of either the antidepressant or hydrocodone). Products include:
- Tofranil-PM Capsules ... 876

Isocarboxazid (May increase the effect of either MAO inhibitor or hydrocodone).
- No products indexed under this heading.

Isoflurane (Exhibits an additive CNS depression).
- No products indexed under this heading.

Ketamine Hydrochloride (Exhibits an additive CNS depression).
- No products indexed under this heading.

Levomethadyl Acetate Hydrochloride (Exhibits an additive CNS depression). Products include:
- Orlaam Oral Solution ... 2361

Levorphanol Tartrate (Exhibits an additive CNS depression). Products include:
- Levo-Dromoran ... 2297

Lithium Carbonate (Exhibits an additive CNS depression). Products include:
- Eskalith ... 2658
- Lithium Carbonate Capsules & Tablets ... 2352
- Lithonate/Lithotabs/Lithobid ... 2721

Lithium Citrate (Exhibits an additive CNS depression).
- No products indexed under this heading.

Loratadine (Exhibits an additive CNS depression). Products include:
- Claritin Tablets ... 2485
- Claritin-D Tablets ... 2487

Lorazepam (Exhibits an additive CNS depression). Products include:
- Ativan Injection ... 2805
- Ativan Tablets ... 2807

Loxapine Hydrochloride (Exhibits an additive CNS depression). Products include:
- Loxitane ... 1426

Loxapine Succinate (Exhibits an additive CNS depression). Products include:
- Loxitane Capsules ... 1426

Maprotiline Hydrochloride (Increased effect of either the antidepressant or hydrocodone). Products include:
- Ludiomil Tablets ... 861

Meperidine Hydrochloride (Exhibits an additive CNS depression). Products include:
- Demerol ... 2438
- Mepergan Injection ... 2859

Mephobarbital (Exhibits an additive CNS depression). Products include:
- Mebaral Tablets ... 2452

Meprobamate (Exhibits an additive CNS depression). Products include:
- Miltown Tablets ... 2780
- PMB 200 and PMB 400 ... 2890

Mesoridazine Besylate (Exhibits an additive CNS depression). Products include:
- Serentil ... 689

Methadone Hydrochloride (Exhibits an additive CNS depression). Products include:
- Methadone Hydrochloride Oral Concentrate ... 2356
- Methadone Hydrochloride Oral Solution & Tablets ... 2357

Methdilazine Hydrochloride (Exhibits an additive CNS depression).
- No products indexed under this heading.

Methohexital Sodium (Exhibits an additive CNS depression).
- No products indexed under this heading.

Methotrimeprazine (Exhibits an additive CNS depression). Products include:
- Levoprome ... 1321

Methoxyflurane (Exhibits an additive CNS depression).
- No products indexed under this heading.

Midazolam Hydrochloride (Exhibits an additive CNS depression). Products include:
- Versed Injection ... 2324

Molindone Hydrochloride (Exhibits an additive CNS depression). Products include:
- Moban Tablets and Concentrate ... 1036

Morphine Sulfate (Exhibits an additive CNS depression). Products include:
- Astramorph/PF Injection, USP (Preservative-Free) ... 526
- Duramorph Injection ... 983
- Infumorph 200 and Infumorph 500 Sterile Solutions ... 985
- Kadian Capsules ... 2948
- MS Contin Tablets ... 2149
- MSIR ... 2152
- Oramorph SR (Morphine Sulfate Sustained Release Tablets) ... 2359
- RMS Suppositories CII ... 2766
- Roxanol ... 2365

Nortriptyline Hydrochloride (Increased effect of either the antidepressant or hydrocodone). Products include:
- Pamelor ... 2409

Opium Alkaloids (Exhibits an additive CNS depression).
- No products indexed under this heading.

Oxazepam (Exhibits an additive CNS depression). Products include:
- Serax Capsules ... 2916
- Serax Tablets ... 2916

Oxycodone Hydrochloride (Exhibits an additive CNS depression). Products include:
- OxyContin Tablets ... 2163
- OxyIR Capsules ... 2167
- Percocet Tablets ... 955
- Percodan Tablets ... 955

IMPORTANT NOTE: Always consult each drug listing in the patient's regimen for possible interactions.

Percodan-Demi Tablets ... 956
Roxicodone Tablets, Oral Solution & Intensol (Oxycodone) ... 2366
Tylox Capsules ... 1593

Pentobarbital Sodium (Exhibits an additive CNS depression). Products include:
Nembutal Sodium Capsules ... 440
Nembutal Sodium Solution ... 442
Nembutal Sodium Suppositories ... 444

Perphenazine (Exhibits an additive CNS depression). Products include:
Etrafon ... 2495
Triavil Tablets ... 1800
Trilafon ... 2532

Phenelzine Sulfate (May increase the effect of either MAO inhibitor or hydrocodone). Products include:
Nardil ... 1977

Phenobarbital (Exhibits an additive CNS depression). Products include:
Arco-Lase Plus Tablets ... 513
Bellergal-S Tablets ... 2375
Donnatal ... 2234
Donnatal Extentabs ... 2234
Donnatal Tablets ... 2234
Phenobarbital Elixir and Tablets ... 1523
Quadrinal Tablets ... 1398

Pimozide (Exhibits an additive CNS depression). Products include:
Orap Tablets ... 1037

Prazepam (Exhibits an additive CNS depression).
No products indexed under this heading.

Prochlorperazine (Exhibits an additive CNS depression). Products include:
Compazine ... 2644

Promethazine Hydrochloride (Exhibits an additive CNS depression). Products include:
Mepergan Injection ... 2859
Phenergan with Codeine ... 2883
Phenergan with Dextromethorphan 2885
Phenergan Injection ... 2880
Phenergan Suppositories ... 2882
Phenergan Syrup ... 2881
Phenergan Tablets ... 2882
Phenergan VC ... 2886
Phenergan VC with Codeine ... 2888

Propofol (Exhibits an additive CNS depression). Products include:
Diprivan Injectable Emulsion ... 2939

Propoxyphene Hydrochloride (Exhibits an additive CNS depression). Products include:
Darvon ... 1475
Wygesic Tablets ... 2930

Propoxyphene Napsylate (Exhibits an additive CNS depression). Products include:
Darvon-N/Darvocet-N ... 1473

Protriptyline Hydrochloride (Increased effect of either the antidepressant or hydrocodone). Products include:
Vivactil Tablets ... 1820

Pyrilamine Maleate (Exhibits an additive CNS depression). Products include:
4-Way Fast Acting Nasal Spray (regular & mentholated) ... ▣ 644
Maximum Strength Multi-Symptom Formula Midol ... ▣ 621
PMS Multi-Symptom Formula Midol ... ▣ 622

Pyrilamine Tannate (Exhibits an additive CNS depression). Products include:
Atrohist Pediatric Suspension ... 1604
Atrohist Pediatric Suspension Dye-Free ... 1604
Rynatan ... 2781

Quazepam (Exhibits an additive CNS depression). Products include:
Doral Tablets ... 2773

Risperidone (Exhibits an additive CNS depression). Products include:
Risperdal Tablets ... 1348

Secobarbital Sodium (Exhibits an additive CNS depression). Products include:
Seconal Sodium Pulvules ... 1529

Selegiline Hydrochloride (May increase the effect of either MAO inhibitor or hydrocodone). Products include:
Eldepryl Capsules ... 2729

Sevoflurane (Exhibits an additive CNS depression).
No products indexed under this heading.

Sufentanil Citrate (Exhibits an additive CNS depression). Products include:
Sufenta Injection ... 1355

Temazepam (Exhibits an additive CNS depression). Products include:
Restoril Capsules ... 2413

Terfenadine (Exhibits an additive CNS depression). Products include:
Seldane Tablets ... 1284
Seldane-D Extended-Release Tablets ... 1286

Thiamylal Sodium (Exhibits an additive CNS depression).
No products indexed under this heading.

Thioridazine Hydrochloride (Exhibits an additive CNS depression). Products include:
Mellaril ... 2398

Thiothixene (Exhibits an additive CNS depression). Products include:
Navane Capsules and Concentrate 2018
Navane Intramuscular ... 2019

Tranylcypromine Sulfate (May increase the effect of either MAO inhibitor or hydrocodone). Products include:
Parnate Tablets ... 2679

Triazolam (Exhibits an additive CNS depression). Products include:
Halcion Tablets ... 2093

Trifluoperazine Hydrochloride (Exhibits an additive CNS depression). Products include:
Stelazine ... 2692

Trimeprazine Tartrate (Exhibits an additive CNS depression).
No products indexed under this heading.

Trimipramine Maleate (Increased effect of either the antidepressant or hydrocodone). Products include:
Surmontil Capsules ... 2917

Tripelennamine Hydrochloride (Exhibits an additive CNS depression). Products include:
PBZ Tablets ... 863
PBZ-SR Tablets ... 862

Triprolidine Hydrochloride (Exhibits an additive CNS depression). Products include:
Actifed Cold & Allergy Tablets ... ▣ 807
Actifed Cold & Sinus Caplets and Tablets ... ▣ 808

Zolpidem Tartrate (Exhibits an additive CNS depression). Products include:
Ambien Tablets ... 2559

Food Interactions

Alcohol (Exhibits an additive CNS depression).

HYCOMINE COMPOUND TABLETS

(Hydrocodone Bitartrate, Chlorpheniramine Maleate, Acetaminophen, Phenylephrine Hydrochloride) ... 948
May interact with monoamine oxidase inhibitors, narcotic analgesics, general anesthetics, central nervous system depressants, phenothiazines, tranquilizers, hypnotics and sedatives, sympathomimetics, beta blockers, and certain other agents. Compounds in these categories include:

Acebutolol Hydrochloride (Potential for hypertensive crises). Products include:
Sectral Capsules ... 2914

Albuterol (Additive elevation of blood pressure). Products include:
Proventil Inhalation Aerosol ... 2524
Ventolin Inhalation Aerosol and Refill ... 1170

Albuterol Sulfate (Additive elevation of blood pressure). Products include:
Airet Albuterol Sulfate Inhalation Solution ... 1602
Albuterol Sulfate, USP Solution for Inhalation, Arm-a-Med ... 522
Proventil Inhalation Solution 0.083% ... 2527
Proventil Repetabs Tablets ... 2529
Proventil Solution for Inhalation 0.5% ... 2525
Proventil Syrup ... 2528
Proventil Tablets ... 2529
Ventolin Inhalation Solution ... 1171
Ventolin Nebules Inhalation Solution ... 1172
Ventolin Rotacaps for Inhalation ... 1173
Ventolin Syrup ... 1175
Ventolin Tablets ... 1176
Volmax Extended-Release Tablets .. 1835

Alfentanil Hydrochloride (Exhibits an additive CNS depression). Products include:
Alfenta Injection ... 1334

Alprazolam (Exhibits an additive CNS depression). Products include:
Xanax Tablets ... 2115

Aprobarbital (Exhibits an additive CNS depression).
No products indexed under this heading.

Atenolol (Potential for hypertensive crises). Products include:
Tenoretic Tablets ... 2963
Tenormin Tablets and I.V. Injection 2965

Betaxolol Hydrochloride (Potential for hypertensive crises). Products include:
Betoptic Ophthalmic Solution ... 465
Betoptic S Ophthalmic Suspension 467
Kerlone Tablets ... 2588

Bisoprolol Fumarate (Potential for hypertensive crises). Products include:
Zebeta Tablets ... 1457
Ziac ... 1459

Buprenorphine (Exhibits an additive CNS depression). Products include:
Buprenex Injectable ... 2170

Buspirone Hydrochloride (Exhibits an additive CNS depression). Products include:
BuSpar Tablets ... 738

Butabarbital (Exhibits an additive CNS depression).
No products indexed under this heading.

Butalbital (Exhibits an additive CNS depression). Products include:
Axocet Capsules ... 2469
Esgic-plus Capsules ... 1012
Esgic-plus Tablets ... 1012
Fioricet Tablets ... 2386
Fioricet with Codeine Capsules ... 2387
Fiorinal Capsules ... 2388
Fiorinal with Codeine Capsules ... 2390
Fiorinal Tablets ... 2388
Phrenilin ... 790
Sedapap Tablets 50 mg/650 mg .. 1826

Carteolol Hydrochloride (Potential for hypertensive crises). Products include:
Cartrol Tablets ... 413
Ocupress Ophthalmic Solution, 1% Sterile ... ◉ 297

Chlordiazepoxide (Exhibits an additive CNS depression). Products include:
Limbitrol ... 2333

Chlordiazepoxide Hydrochloride (Exhibits an additive CNS depression). Products include:
Librax Capsules ... 2330
Librium Capsules ... 2331
Librium Injectable ... 2332

Chlorpromazine (Exhibits an additive CNS depression). Products include:
Thorazine Suppositories ... 2701

Chlorpromazine Hydrochloride (Exhibits an additive CNS depression). Products include:
Thorazine ... 2701

Chlorprothixene (Exhibits an additive CNS depression).
No products indexed under this heading.

Chlorprothixene Hydrochloride (Exhibits an additive CNS depression).
No products indexed under this heading.

Chlorprothixene Lactate (Exhibits an additive CNS depression).
No products indexed under this heading.

Clorazepate Dipotassium (Exhibits an additive CNS depression). Products include:
Tranxene ... 459

Clozapine (Exhibits an additive CNS depression). Products include:
Clozaril Tablets ... 2377

Codeine Phosphate (Exhibits an additive CNS depression). Products include:
Brontex ... 2130
Dimetane-DC Cough Syrup ... 2232
Fioricet with Codeine Capsules ... 2387
Fiorinal with Codeine Capsules ... 2390
Nucofed ... 2225
Phenergan with Codeine ... 2883
Phenergan VC with Codeine ... 2888
Robitussin A-C Syrup ... 2248
Robitussin-DAC Syrup ... 2249
Ryna ... ▣ 804
Soma Compound w/Codeine Tablets ... 2784
Tylenol with Codeine ... 1592

Desflurane (Exhibits an additive CNS depression). Products include:
Suprane (desflurane, USP) ... 1865

Dezocine (Exhibits an additive CNS depression). Products include:
Dalgan Injection ... 529

Diazepam (Exhibits an additive CNS depression). Products include:
Dizac (diazepam injectable emulsion) CIV ... 1862
Valium Injectable ... 2336
Valium Tablets ... 2335

Dobutamine Hydrochloride (Additive elevation of blood pressure). Products include:
Dobutrex Solution Vials ... 1480

Dopamine Hydrochloride (Additive elevation of blood pressure).
No products indexed under this heading.

Droperidol (Exhibits an additive CNS depression). Products include:
Inapsine Injection ... 462

Enflurane (Exhibits an additive CNS depression).
No products indexed under this heading.

Ephedrine Hydrochloride (Additive elevation of blood pressure). Products include:
Primatene Tablets ... ▣ 844
Quadrinal Tablets ... 1398

(▣ Described in PDR For Nonprescription Drugs) (◉ Described in PDR For Ophthalmology)

Ephedrine Sulfate (Additive elevation of blood pressure). Products include:
- Marax Tablets & DF Syrup ... 2015

Ephedrine Tannate (Additive elevation of blood pressure). Products include:
- Rynatuss ... 2782

Epinephrine (Additive elevation of blood pressure). Products include:
- EPIFRIN ... ⊚ 237
- EpiPen ... 808
- Marcaine with Epinephrine ... 2446
- Primatene Mist ... ▣ 843
- Sensorcaine with Epinephrine Injection ... 554
- Sus-Phrine Injection ... 1017
- Xylocaine with Epinephrine Injections ... 562

Epinephrine Bitartrate (Additive elevation of blood pressure). Products include:
- Sensorcaine-MPF with Epinephrine Injection ... 554

Epinephrine Hydrochloride (Additive elevation of blood pressure). Products include:
- Ana-Kit Anaphylaxis Emergency Treatment Kit ... 611

Esmolol Hydrochloride (Potential for hypertensive crises). Products include:
- Brevibloc (esmolol HCl) Injection ... 1860

Estazolam (Exhibits an additive CNS depression). Products include:
- ProSom Tablets ... 457

Ethchlorvynol (Exhibits an additive CNS depression). Products include:
- Placidyl Capsules ... 456

Ethinamate (Exhibits an additive CNS depression).
- No products indexed under this heading.

Fentanyl (Exhibits an additive CNS depression). Products include:
- Duragesic Transdermal System ... 1336

Fentanyl Citrate (Exhibits an additive CNS depression). Products include:
- Sublimaze Injection ... 463

Fluphenazine Decanoate (Exhibits an additive CNS depression). Products include:
- Prolixin Decanoate ... 510

Fluphenazine Enanthate (Exhibits an additive CNS depression). Products include:
- Prolixin Enanthate ... 510

Fluphenazine Hydrochloride (Exhibits an additive CNS depression). Products include:
- Prolixin ... 510

Flurazepam Hydrochloride (Exhibits an additive CNS depression). Products include:
- Dalmane Capsules ... 2329

Furazolidone (Additive elevation of blood pressure; concurrent use is contraindicated; prolongs the anticholinergic effects of antihistamines). Products include:
- Furoxone ... 2221

Glutethimide (Exhibits an additive CNS depression).
- No products indexed under this heading.

Haloperidol (Exhibits an additive CNS depression). Products include:
- Haldol Injection, Tablets and Concentrate ... 1585

Haloperidol Decanoate (Exhibits an additive CNS depression). Products include:
- Haldol Decanoate ... 1587

Hydrocodone Polistirex (Exhibits an additive CNS depression). Products include:
- Tussionex Pennkinetic Extended-Release Suspension ... 1624

Hydromorphone Hydrochloride (Exhibits an additive CNS depression). Products include:
- Dilaudid Ampules ... 1382
- Dilaudid Cough Syrup ... 1383
- Dilaudid-HP Injection ... 1384
- Dilaudid-HP Lyophilized Powder 250 mg ... 1384
- Dilaudid ... 1382
- Dilaudid Oral Liquid ... 1386
- Dilaudid ... 1382
- Dilaudid Tablets - 8 mg ... 1386

Hydroxyzine Hydrochloride (Exhibits an additive CNS depression). Products include:
- Atarax Tablets & Syrup ... 1992
- Marax Tablets & DF Syrup ... 2015
- Vistaril Intramuscular Solution ... 2042

Indomethacin (Potential for hypertensive crises). Products include:
- Indocin ... 1723

Indomethacin Sodium Trihydrate (Potential for hypertensive crises). Products include:
- Indocin I.V. ... 1727

Isocarboxazid (Additive elevation of blood pressure; concurrent use is contraindicated; prolongs the anticholinergic effects of antihistamines).
- No products indexed under this heading.

Isoflurane (Exhibits an additive CNS depression).
- No products indexed under this heading.

Isoproterenol Hydrochloride (Additive elevation of blood pressure). Products include:
- Isuprel Hydrochloride Solution ... 2443
- Isuprel Injection ... 2441
- Isuprel Mistometer ... 2442

Isoproterenol Sulfate (Additive elevation of blood pressure). Products include:
- Norisodrine with Calcium Iodide Syrup ... 446

Ketamine Hydrochloride (Exhibits an additive CNS depression).
- No products indexed under this heading.

Labetalol Hydrochloride (Potential for hypertensive crises). Products include:
- Normodyne Injection ... 2519
- Normodyne Tablets ... 2522
- Trandate ... 1158

Levobunolol Hydrochloride (Potential for hypertensive crises). Products include:
- Betagan ... ⊚ 230

Levomethadyl Acetate Hydrochloride (Exhibits an additive CNS depression). Products include:
- Orlaam Oral Solution ... 2361

Levorphanol Tartrate (Exhibits an additive CNS depression). Products include:
- Levo-Dromoran ... 2297

Lorazepam (Exhibits an additive CNS depression). Products include:
- Ativan Injection ... 2805
- Ativan Tablets ... 2807

Loxapine Hydrochloride (Exhibits an additive CNS depression). Products include:
- Loxitane ... 1426

Loxapine Succinate (Exhibits an additive CNS depression). Products include:
- Loxitane Capsules ... 1426

Meperidine Hydrochloride (Exhibits an additive CNS depression). Products include:
- Demerol ... 2438
- Mepergan Injection ... 2859

Mephobarbital (Exhibits an additive CNS depression). Products include:
- Mebaral Tablets ... 2452

Meprobamate (Exhibits an additive CNS depression). Products include:
- Miltown Tablets ... 2780
- PMB 200 and PMB 400 ... 2890

Mesoridazine Besylate (Exhibits an additive CNS depression). Products include:
- Serentil ... 689

Metaproterenol Sulfate (Additive elevation of blood pressure). Products include:
- Alupent ... 672
- Metaproterenol Sulfate Inhalation Solution, USP, Arm-a-Med ... 547

Metaraminol Bitartrate (Additive elevation of blood pressure). Products include:
- Aramine Injection ... 1649

Methadone Hydrochloride (Exhibits an additive CNS depression). Products include:
- Methadone Hydrochloride Oral Concentrate ... 2356
- Methadone Hydrochloride Oral Solution & Tablets ... 2357

Methohexital Sodium (Exhibits an additive CNS depression).
- No products indexed under this heading.

Methotrimeprazine (Exhibits an additive CNS depression). Products include:
- Levoprome ... 1321

Methoxamine Hydrochloride (Additive elevation of blood pressure). Products include:
- Vasoxyl Injection ... 1169

Methoxyflurane (Exhibits an additive CNS depression).
- No products indexed under this heading.

Methyldopa (Potential for hypertensive crises). Products include:
- Aldoclor Tablets ... 1638
- Aldomet Oral ... 1640
- Aldoril Tablets ... 1644

Metipranolol Hydrochloride (Potential for hypertensive crises). Products include:
- OptiPranolol (Metipranolol 0.3%) Sterile Ophthalmic Solution ... ⊚ 256

Metoprolol Succinate (Potential for hypertensive crises). Products include:
- Toprol-XL Tablets ... 560

Metoprolol Tartrate (Potential for hypertensive crises). Products include:
- Lopressor ... 848
- Lopressor HCT Tablets ... 850

Midazolam Hydrochloride (Exhibits an additive CNS depression). Products include:
- Versed Injection ... 2324

Molindone Hydrochloride (Exhibits an additive CNS depression). Products include:
- Moban Tablets and Concentrate ... 1036

Morphine Sulfate (Exhibits an additive CNS depression). Products include:
- Astramorph/PF Injection, USP (Preservative-Free) ... 526
- Duramorph Injection ... 983
- Infumorph 200 and Infumorph 500 Sterile Solutions ... 985
- Kadian Capsules ... 2948
- MS Contin Tablets ... 2149
- MSIR ... 2152
- Oramorph SR (Morphine Sulfate Sustained Release Tablets) ... 2359
- RMS Suppositories CII ... 2766
- Roxanol ... 2365

Nadolol (Potential for hypertensive crises).
- No products indexed under this heading.

Norepinephrine Bitartrate (Additive elevation of blood pressure). Products include:
- Levophed Bitartrate Injection ... 2445

Opium Alkaloids (Exhibits an additive CNS depression).
- No products indexed under this heading.

Oxazepam (Exhibits an additive CNS depression). Products include:
- Serax Capsules ... 2916
- Serax Tablets ... 2916

Oxycodone Hydrochloride (Exhibits an additive CNS depression). Products include:
- OxyContin Tablets ... 2163
- OxyIR Capsules ... 2167
- Percocet Tablets ... 955
- Percodan Tablets ... 955
- Percodan-Demi Tablets ... 956
- Roxicodone Tablets, Oral Solution & Intensol (Oxycodone) ... 2366
- Tylox Capsules ... 1593

Penbutolol Sulfate (Potential for hypertensive crises). Products include:
- Levatol Tablets ... 2547

Pentobarbital Sodium (Exhibits an additive CNS depression). Products include:
- Nembutal Sodium Capsules ... 440
- Nembutal Sodium Solution ... 442
- Nembutal Sodium Suppositories ... 444

Perphenazine (Exhibits an additive CNS depression). Products include:
- Etrafon ... 2495
- Triavil Tablets ... 1800
- Trilafon ... 2532

Phenelzine Sulfate (Additive elevation of blood pressure; concurrent use is contraindicated; prolongs the anticholinergic effects of antihistamines). Products include:
- Nardil ... 1977

Phenobarbital (Exhibits an additive CNS depression). Products include:
- Arco-Lase Plus Tablets ... 513
- Bellergal-S Tablets ... 2375
- Donnatal ... 2234
- Donnatal Extentabs ... 2234
- Donnatal Tablets ... 2234
- Phenobarbital Elixir and Tablets ... 1523
- Quadrinal Tablets ... 1398

Phenylephrine Bitartrate (Additive elevation of blood pressure).
- No products indexed under this heading.

Phenylephrine Tannate (Additive elevation of blood pressure). Products include:
- Atrohist Pediatric Suspension ... 1604
- Atrohist Pediatric Suspension Dye-Free ... 1604
- Rynatan ... 2781
- Rynatuss ... 2782

Phenylpropanolamine Hydrochloride (Additive elevation of blood pressure). Products include:
- Acutrim ... ▣ 648
- Atrohist Plus Tablets ... 1605
- BC Cold Powder Multi-Symptom Formula (Cold-Sinus-Allergy) ... ▣ 631
- BC Cold Powder Non-Drowsy Formula (Cold-Sinus) ... ▣ 631
- Cheracol Plus Head Cold/Cough Formula ... ▣ 741
- Comtrex Multi-Symptom Cold Reliever Liqui-Gels ... ▣ 638
- Comtrex Multi-Symptom Non-Drowsy Liqui-gels ... ▣ 640

IMPORTANT NOTE: Always consult each drug listing in the patient's regimen for possible interactions.

Hycomine Compound — Interactions Index — 490

Contac Continuous Action Nasal Decongestant/Antihistamine 12 Hour Capsules ▣ 773
Contac Maximum Strength Continuous Action Decongestant/Antihistamine 12 Hour Caplets ▣ 772
Contac Severe Cold and Flu Formula Caplets ▣ 773
Coricidin 'D' Decongestant Tablets ▣ 760
Dexatrim ▣ 795
Dexatrim Plus Vitamins Caplets ▣ 796
Dimetane-DC Cough Syrup 2232
Dimetapp Allergy Sinus Caplets ▣ 838
Dimetapp Cold & Allergy Chewable Tablets ▣ 838
Dimetapp Cold & Cough Liqui-Gels ▣ 839
Dimetapp DM Elixir ▣ 840
Dimetapp Elixir ▣ 840
Dimetapp Extentabs ▣ 841
Dimetapp Tablets/Liqui-Gels ▣ 841
Dura-Vent Tablets 971
Entex LA Tablets 972
Exgest LA Tablets 787
Hycomine 947
Nolamine Timed-Release Tablets 790
Ornade Spansule Capsules 2678
Propagest Tablets 791
Pyrroxate Caplets ▣ 742
Robitussin-CF ▣ 846
Sinulin Tablets 792
Tavist-D 12 Hour Relief Tablets ▣ 750
Teldrin 12 Hour Antihistamine/Nasal Decongestant Allergy Relief Capsules ▣ 786
Triaminic Expectorant ▣ 753
Triaminic Syrup ▣ 755
Triaminic Triaminicol Cold & Cough ▣ 756
Triaminic DM Syrup ▣ 756
Triaminicin Tablets ▣ 756
Vicks DayQuil Allergy Relief 12-Hour Extended Release Tablets ▣ 733
Vicks DayQuil Allergy Relief 4-Hour Tablets ▣ 733
Vicks DayQuil SINUS Pressure & CONGESTION Relief ▣ 734

Pindolol (Potential for hypertensive crises). Products include:
Visken Tablets 2428

Pirbuterol Acetate (Additive elevation of blood pressure). Products include:
Maxair Autohaler 1550
Maxair Inhaler 1552

Prazepam (Exhibits an additive CNS depression).
No products indexed under this heading.

Prochlorperazine (Exhibits an additive CNS depression). Products include:
Compazine 2644

Promethazine Hydrochloride (Exhibits an additive CNS depression). Products include:
Mepergan Injection 2859
Phenergan with Codeine 2883
Phenergan with Dextromethorphan 2885
Phenergan Injection 2880
Phenergan Suppositories 2882
Phenergan Syrup 2881
Phenergan Tablets 2882
Phenergan VC 2886
Phenergan VC with Codeine 2888

Propofol (Exhibits an additive CNS depression). Products include:
Diprivan Injectable Emulsion 2939

Propoxyphene Hydrochloride (Exhibits an additive CNS depression). Products include:
Darvon 1475
Wygesic Tablets 2930

Propoxyphene Napsylate (Exhibits an additive CNS depression). Products include:
Darvon-N/Darvocet-N 1473

Propranolol Hydrochloride (Potential for hypertensive crises). Products include:
Inderal 2834
Inderal LA Long Acting Capsules 2836
Inderide Tablets 2838
Inderide LA Long Acting Capsules 2840

Pseudoephedrine Hydrochloride (Additive elevation of blood pressure). Products include:
Actifed Allergy Daytime/Nighttime Caplets ▣ 808
Actifed Cold & Allergy Tablets ▣ 807
Actifed Cold & Sinus Caplets and Tablets ▣ 808
Actifed Sinus Daytime/Nighttime Tablets and Caplets ▣ 809
Advil Cold and Sinus Caplets and Tablets ▣ 837
Alka-Seltzer Plus Liqui-Gels ▣ 612
Alka-Seltzer Plus Flu & Body Aches Liqui-Gels Non-Drowsy Formula ▣ 613
Alka-Seltzer Plus Night-Time Cold Medicine Liqui-Gels ▣ 612
Allerest Maximum Strength ▣ 649
Allerest No Drowsiness ▣ 649
Allerest Sinus Pain Formula ▣ 649
Atrohist Pediatric Capsules 1603
Benadryl Allergy/Cold Tablets ▣ 811
Benadryl Allergy Decongestant Liquid Medication ▣ 812
Benadryl Allergy Decongestant Tablets ▣ 812
Benadryl Allergy Sinus Headache Caplets ▣ 813
Benylin Multisymptom ▣ 816
Bromfed Capsules (Extended-Release) 1832
Bromfed Syrup ▣ 712
Bromfed Tablets 1832
Bromfed-DM Cough Syrup 1832
Bromfed-PD Capsules (Extended-Release) 1832
Children's TYLENOL Cold Multi-Symptom Chewable Tablets and Liquid 1559
Children's TYLENOL Cold Plus Cough Multi Symptom Chewable Tablets and Liquid 1560
Children's TYLENOL Flu Suspension Liquid 1560
Children's Vicks DayQuil Allergy Relief ▣ 730
Children's Vicks NyQuil Cold/Cough Relief ▣ 731
Allergy-Sinus Comtrex Multi-Symptom Allergy-Sinus Formula Tablets and Caplets ▣ 639
Comtrex Multi-Symptom ▣ 638
Comtrex Multi-Symptom Non-Drowsy Caplets ▣ 640
Congess 1003
Contac Day Allergy/Sinus Caplets ▣ 771
Contac Day & Night ▣ 772
Contac Night Allergy/Sinus Caplets ▣ 771
Contac Severe Cold & Flu Non-Drowsy ▣ 774
Deconsal II Tablets 1605
Dimetane-DX Cough Syrup 2233
Dimetapp Cold & Fever Suspension ▣ 839
Dimetapp Decongestant Pediatric Drops ▣ 840
Dorcol Children's Cough Syrup ▣ 748
Drixoral Cough + Congestion Liquid Caps ▣ 763
Dura-Tap/PD Capsules 970
Duratuss Tablets 2750
Duratuss HD Elixir 2750
Efidac/24 ▣ 655
Entex PSE Tablets 973
Fedahist Gyrocaps 2545
Guaifed 1833
Guaifed Syrup ▣ 712
Guaimax-D Tablets 809
Histussin D Liquid 670
Infants' TYLENOL Cold Decongestant & Fever-Reducer Drops 1561
Kronofed-A 994
Novahistine DMX ▣ 782
Nucofed 2225
PediaCare Cough-Cold Chewable Tablets and Liquid 1569
PediaCare Infants' Decongestant Drops 1569
PediaCare Infants' Drops Decongestant Plus Cough 1569
PediaCare NightRest Cough-Cold Liquid 1569
Pediatric Vicks 44d Cough & Head Congestion Relief ▣ 736
Pediatric Vicks 44m Cough & Cold Relief ▣ 737
Robitussin Cold & Cough Liqui-Gels ▣ 844
Robitussin Cold, Cough & Flu Liqui-Gels ▣ 844
Robitussin Maximum Strength Cough & Cold ▣ 847
Robitussin Night-Time Cold Formula ▣ 847
Robitussin Pediatric Cough & Cold Formula ▣ 848
Robitussin Pediatric Drops ▣ 849
Robitussin Severe Congestion Liqui-Gels ▣ 845
Robitussin-DAC Syrup 2249
Robitussin-PE ▣ 846
Rondec Oral Drops 974
Rondec Syrup 974
Rondec Tablet 974
Rondec Chewable Tablets 974
Rondec-TR Tablet 974
Ryna ▣ 804
Seldane-D Extended-Release Tablets 1286
Semprex-D Capsules 1620
Sinarest ▣ 663
Sine-Aid Maximum Strength Sinus Headache Gelcaps, Caplets and Tablets 1570
Sine-Off No Drowsiness Formula Caplets ▣ 784
Sine-Off Sinus Medicine ▣ 784
Singlet Tablets ▣ 785
Sinutab Non-Drying Liquid Caps ▣ 823
Sinutab Sinus Allergy Medication, Maximum Strength Tablets and Caplets ▣ 823
Sinutab Sinus Medication, Maximum Strength Without Drowsiness Formula, Tablets & Caplets ▣ 824
Sudafed Children's Cold & Cough Liquid Medication ▣ 825
Sudafed Children's Nasal Decongestant Liquid Medication ▣ 826
Sudafed Cold & Allergy Tablets ▣ 826
Sudafed Cold and Cough Liquid Caps ▣ 826
Sudafed Nasal Decongestant Tablets, 30 mg ▣ 825
Sudafed Nasal Decongestant Tablets, 60 mg ▣ 825
Sudafed Non-Drying Sinus Liquid Caps ▣ 827
Sudafed Pediatric Nasal Decongestant Liquid Oral Drops ▣ 827
Sudafed Severe Cold Formula Caplets ▣ 828
Sudafed Severe Cold Formula Tablets ▣ 828
Sudafed Sinus Caplets ▣ 829
Sudafed Sinus Tablets ▣ 829
Sudafed 12 Hour Caplets ▣ 824
Syn-Rx Tablets 1622
Syn-Rx DM Tablets 1623
TheraFlu Flu and Cold Medicine ▣ 750
Theraflu Maximum Strength Flu and Cold Medicine For Sore Throat ▣ 751
TheraFlu Flu, Cold and Cough Medicine ▣ 750
TheraFlu Maximum Strength Nighttime Flu, Cold & Cough Medicine ▣ 751
TheraFlu Maximum Strength Non-Drowsy Formula Flu, Cold & Cough Medicine ▣ 751
TheraFlu Maximum Strength, Non-Drowsy Formula Flu, Cold and Cough Caplets ▣ 752
Theraflu Maximum Strength Sinus Non-Drowsy Formula Caplets ▣ 752
Triaminic AM Cough and Decongestant Formula ▣ 753
Triaminic AM Decongestant Formula ▣ 753
Triaminic Infant Oral Decongestant Drops ▣ 754
Triaminic Night Time ▣ 754
Triaminic Sore Throat Formula ▣ 755
Tussend 1830
Tussend Expectorant 1831
TYLENOL Allergy Sinus, Maximum Strength Caplets and Gelcaps 1571
TYLENOL Allergy Sinus NightTime, Maximum Strength Caplets 1571
TYLENOL Cold Medication, Multi-Symptom Formula Tablets and Caplets 1572
TYLENOL Cold Medication, Multi-Symptom Hot Liquid Packets 1572
TYLENOL Cold Medication, No Drowsiness Formula Caplets and Gelcaps 1572
TYLENOL Cold Severe Congestion Caplets 1573
TYLENOL Cough Medication with Decongestant, Multi Symptom 1574
TYLENOL Flu No Drowsiness Formula, Maximum Strength Gelcaps 1575
TYLENOL Flu NightTime, Maximum Strength Gelcaps 1575
TYLENOL Flu NightTime, Maximum Strength Hot Medication Packets 1575
TYLENOL Sinus, Maximum Strength Geltabs, Gelcaps, Caplets and Tablets 1576
Vicks 44 LiquiCaps Cough, Cold & Flu Relief ▣ 728
Vicks 44 LiquiCaps Non-Drowsy Cough & Cold Relief ▣ 729
Vicks 44D Cough & Head Congestion Relief ▣ 728
Vicks 44M Cough, Cold & Flu Relief ▣ 729
Vicks DayQuil LiquiCaps/Liquid Multi-Symptom Cold/Flu Relief ▣ 734
Vicks DayQuil SINUS Pressure & PAIN Relief with IBUPROFEN ▣ 735
Vicks Nyquil Hot Therapy ▣ 735
Vicks NyQuil LiquiCaps/Liquid Multi-Symptom Cold/Flu Relief, Original and Cherry Flavors ▣ 736

Pseudoephedrine Sulfate (Additive elevation of blood pressure). Products include:
Chlor-Trimeton Allergy Decongestant Tablets ▣ 759
Claritin-D Tablets 2487
Drixoral Cold and Allergy Sustained-Action Tablets ▣ 763
Drixoral Cold and Flu Extended-Release Tablets ▣ 764
Drixoral Non-Drowsy Formula Extended-Release Tablets ▣ 764
Drixoral Allergy/Sinus Extended Release Tablets ▣ 765
Trinalin Repetabs Tablets 1373

Quazepam (Exhibits an additive CNS depression). Products include:
Doral Tablets 2773

Risperidone (Exhibits an additive CNS depression). Products include:
Risperdal Tablets 1348

Salmeterol Xinafoate (Additive elevation of blood pressure). Products include:
Serevent Inhalation Aerosol 1149

Secobarbital Sodium (Exhibits an additive CNS depression). Products include:
Seconal Sodium Pulvules 1529

Selegiline Hydrochloride (Additive elevation of blood pressure; concurrent use is contraindicated; prolongs the anticholinergic effects of antihistamines). Products include:
Eldepryl Capsules 2729

Sevoflurane (Exhibits an additive CNS depression).
No products indexed under this heading.

Sotalol Hydrochloride (Potential for hypertensive crises). Products include:
Betapace Tablets 637

Sufentanil Citrate (Exhibits an additive CNS depression). Products include:
Sufenta Injection 1355

Temazepam (Exhibits an additive CNS depression). Products include:
Restoril Capsules 2413

Terbutaline Sulfate (Additive elevation of blood pressure). Products include:
Brethaire Inhaler 830
Brethine Ampuls 832
Brethine Tablets 831
Bricanyl Subcutaneous Injection 1247
Bricanyl Tablets 1248

Thiamylal Sodium (Exhibits an additive CNS depression).
No products indexed under this heading.

(▣ Described in PDR For Nonprescription Drugs) (◉ Described in PDR For Ophthalmology)

Interactions Index

Thioridazine Hydrochloride (Exhibits an additive CNS depression). Products include:
- Mellaril ... 2398

Thiothixene (Exhibits an additive CNS depression). Products include:
- Navane Capsules and Concentrate ... 2018
- Navane Intramuscular ... 2019

Timolol Hemihydrate (Potential for hypertensive crises). Products include:
- Betimol 0.25%, 0.5% ... ⓔ 259

Timolol Maleate (Potential for hypertensive crises). Products include:
- Blocadren Tablets ... 1654
- Timolide Tablets ... 1791
- Timoptic in Ocudose ... 1796
- Timoptic Sterile Ophthalmic Solution ... 1794
- Timoptic-XE ... 1798

Tranylcypromine Sulfate (Additive elevation of blood pressure; concurrent use is contraindicated; prolongs the anticholinergic effects of antihistamines). Products include:
- Parnate Tablets ... 2679

Triazolam (Exhibits an additive CNS depression). Products include:
- Halcion Tablets ... 2093

Trifluoperazine Hydrochloride (Exhibits an additive CNS depression). Products include:
- Stelazine ... 2692

Zolpidem Tartrate (Exhibits an additive CNS depression). Products include:
- Ambien Tablets ... 2559

Food Interactions

Alcohol (Exhibits an additive CNS depression).

HYCOMINE PEDIATRIC SYRUP
(Hydrocodone Bitartrate, Phenylpropanolamine Hydrochloride) ... 947
May interact with sympathomimetics, monoamine oxidase inhibitors, beta blockers, central nervous system depressants, narcotic analgesics, hypnotics and sedatives, general anesthetics, phenothiazines, tranquilizers, and certain other agents. Compounds in these categories include:

Acebutolol Hydrochloride (Concurrent use may produce additive elevation in blood pressure). Products include:
- Sectral Capsules ... 2914

Albuterol (Concurrent use may produce additive elevation of blood pressure). Products include:
- Proventil Inhalation Aerosol ... 2524
- Ventolin Inhalation Aerosol and Refill ... 1170

Albuterol Sulfate (Concurrent use may produce additive elevation of blood pressure). Products include:
- Airet Albuterol Sulfate Inhalation Solution ... 1602
- Albuterol Sulfate, USP Solution for Inhalation, Arm-a-Med ... 522
- Proventil Inhalation Solution 0.083% ... 2527
- Proventil Repetabs Tablets ... 2529
- Proventil Solution for Inhalation 0.5% ... 2525
- Proventil Syrup ... 2528
- Proventil Tablets ... 2529
- Ventolin Inhalation Solution ... 1171
- Ventolin Nebules Inhalation Solution ... 1172
- Ventolin Rotacaps for Inhalation ... 1173
- Ventolin Syrup ... 1175
- Ventolin Tablets ... 1176
- Volmax Extended-Release Tablets ... 1835

Alfentanil Hydrochloride (Additive CNS depression). Products include:
- Alfenta Injection ... 1334

Alprazolam (Additive CNS depression). Products include:
- Xanax Tablets ... 2115

Aprobarbital (Additive CNS depression).
No products indexed under this heading.

Atenolol (Concurrent use may produce additive elevation in blood pressure). Products include:
- Tenoretic Tablets ... 2963
- Tenormin Tablets and I.V. Injection ... 2965

Betaxolol Hydrochloride (Concurrent use may produce additive elevation in blood pressure). Products include:
- Betoptic Ophthalmic Solution ... 465
- Betoptic S Ophthalmic Suspension ... 467
- Kerlone Tablets ... 2588

Bisoprolol Fumarate (Concurrent use may produce additive elevation in blood pressure). Products include:
- Zebeta Tablets ... 1457
- Ziac ... 1459

Buprenorphine (Additive CNS depression). Products include:
- Buprenex Injectable ... 2170

Buspirone Hydrochloride (Additive CNS depression). Products include:
- BuSpar Tablets ... 738

Butabarbital (Additive CNS depression).
No products indexed under this heading.

Butalbital (Additive CNS depression). Products include:
- Axocet Capsules ... 2469
- Esgic-plus Capsules ... 1012
- Esgic-plus Tablets ... 1012
- Fioricet Tablets ... 2386
- Fioricet with Codeine Capsules ... 2387
- Fiorinal Capsules ... 2388
- Fiorinal with Codeine Capsules ... 2390
- Fiorinal Tablets ... 2388
- Phrenilin ... 790
- Sedapap Tablets 50 mg/650 mg ... 1826

Carteolol Hydrochloride (Concurrent use may produce additive elevation in blood pressure). Products include:
- Cartrol Tablets ... 413
- Ocupress Ophthalmic Solution, 1% Sterile ... ⓔ 297

Chlordiazepoxide (Additive CNS depression). Products include:
- Limbitrol ... 2333

Chlordiazepoxide Hydrochloride (Additive CNS depression). Products include:
- Librax Capsules ... 2330
- Librium Capsules ... 2331
- Librium Injectable ... 2332

Chlorpromazine (Additive CNS depression). Products include:
- Thorazine Suppositories ... 2701

Chlorpromazine Hydrochloride (Additive CNS depression). Products include:
- Thorazine ... 2701

Chlorprothixene (Additive CNS depression).
No products indexed under this heading.

Chlorprothixene Hydrochloride (Additive CNS depression).
No products indexed under this heading.

Chlorprothixene Lactate (Additive CNS depression).
No products indexed under this heading.

Clorazepate Dipotassium (Additive CNS depression). Products include:
- Tranxene ... 459

Clozapine (Additive CNS depression). Products include:
- Clozaril Tablets ... 2377

Codeine Phosphate (Additive CNS depression). Products include:
- Brontex ... 2130
- Dimetane-DC Cough Syrup ... 2232
- Fioricet with Codeine Capsules ... 2387
- Fiorinal with Codeine Capsules ... 2390
- Nucofed ... 2225
- Phenergan with Codeine ... 2883
- Phenergan VC with Codeine ... 2888
- Robitussin A-C Syrup ... 2248
- Robitussin-DAC Syrup ... 2249
- Ryna ... ⓔ 804
- Soma Compound w/Codeine Tablets ... 2784
- Tylenol with Codeine ... 1592

Desflurane (Additive CNS depression). Products include:
- Suprane (desflurane, USP) ... 1865

Dezocine (Additive CNS depression). Products include:
- Dalgan Injection ... 529

Diazepam (Additive CNS depression). Products include:
- Dizac (diazepam injectable emulsion) CIV ... 1862
- Valium Injectable ... 2336
- Valium Tablets ... 2335

Dobutamine Hydrochloride (Concurrent use may produce additive elevation of blood pressure). Products include:
- Dobutrex Solution Vials ... 1480

Dopamine Hydrochloride (Concurrent use may produce additive elevation of blood pressure).
No products indexed under this heading.

Droperidol (Additive CNS depression). Products include:
- Inapsine Injection ... 462

Enflurane (Additive CNS depression).
No products indexed under this heading.

Ephedrine Hydrochloride (Concurrent use may produce additive elevation of blood pressure). Products include:
- Primatene Tablets ... ⓔ 844
- Quadrinal Tablets ... 1398

Ephedrine Sulfate (Concurrent use may produce additive elevation of blood pressure). Products include:
- Marax Tablets & DF Syrup ... 2015

Ephedrine Tannate (Concurrent use may produce additive elevation of blood pressure). Products include:
- Rynatuss ... 2782

Epinephrine (Concurrent use may produce additive elevation of blood pressure). Products include:
- EPIFRIN ... ⓔ 237
- EpiPen ... 808
- Marcaine with Epinephrine ... 2446
- Primatene Mist ... ⓔ 843
- Sensorcaine with Epinephrine Injection ... 554
- Sus-Phrine Injection ... 1017
- Xylocaine with Epinephrine Injections ... 562

Epinephrine Bitartrate (Concurrent use may produce additive elevation of blood pressure). Products include:
- Sensorcaine-MPF with Epinephrine ... 554

Epinephrine Hydrochloride (Concurrent use may produce additive elevation of blood pressure). Products include:
- Ana-Kit Anaphylaxis Emergency Treatment Kit ... 611

Esmolol Hydrochloride (Concurrent use may produce additive elevation in blood pressure). Products include:
- Brevibloc (esmolol HCl) Injection ... 1860

Estazolam (Additive CNS depression). Products include:
- ProSom Tablets ... 457

Ethchlorvynol (Additive CNS depression). Products include:
- Placidyl Capsules ... 456

Ethinamate (Additive CNS depression).
No products indexed under this heading.

Fentanyl (Additive CNS depression). Products include:
- Duragesic Transdermal System ... 1336

Fentanyl Citrate (Additive CNS depression). Products include:
- Sublimaze Injection ... 463

Fluphenazine Decanoate (Additive CNS depression). Products include:
- Prolixin Decanoate ... 510

Fluphenazine Enanthate (Additive CNS depression). Products include:
- Prolixin Enanthate ... 510

Fluphenazine Hydrochloride (Additive CNS depression). Products include:
- Prolixin ... 510

Flurazepam Hydrochloride (Additive CNS depression). Products include:
- Dalmane Capsules ... 2329

Furazolidone (Potential for hypertensive crises; concurrent use is contraindicated). Products include:
- Furoxone ... 2221

Glutethimide (Additive CNS depression).
No products indexed under this heading.

Haloperidol (Additive CNS depression). Products include:
- Haldol Injection, Tablets and Concentrate ... 1585

Haloperidol Decanoate (Additive CNS depression). Products include:
- Haldol Decanoate ... 1587

Hydrocodone Polistirex (Additive CNS depression). Products include:
- Tussionex Pennkinetic Extended-Release Suspension ... 1624

Hydromorphone Hydrochloride (Additive CNS depression). Products include:
- Dilaudid Ampules ... 1382
- Dilaudid Cough Syrup ... 1383
- Dilaudid-HP Injection ... 1384
- Dilaudid-HP Lyophilized Powder 250 mg ... 1384
- Dilaudid ... 1382
- Dilaudid Oral Liquid ... 1386
- Dilaudid ... 1382
- Dilaudid Tablets - 8 mg ... 1386

Hydroxyzine Hydrochloride (Additive CNS depression). Products include:
- Atarax Tablets & Syrup ... 1992
- Marax Tablets & DF Syrup ... 2015
- Vistaril Intramuscular Solution ... 2042

Indomethacin (Hypertensive crisis can occur with concurrent use). Products include:
- Indocin ... 1723

Indomethacin Sodium Trihydrate (Hypertensive crisis can occur with concurrent use). Products include:
- Indocin I.V. ... 1727

IMPORTANT NOTE: Always consult each drug listing in the patient's regimen for possible interactions.

Isocarboxazid (Potential for hypertensive crises; concurrent use is contraindicated).
  No products indexed under this heading.
Isoflurane (Additive CNS depression).
  No products indexed under this heading.
Isoproterenol Hydrochloride (Concurrent use may produce additive elevation of blood pressure). Products include:
  Isuprel Hydrochloride Solution ... 2443
  Isuprel Injection ... 2441
  Isuprel Mistometer ... 2442
Isoproterenol Sulfate (Concurrent use may produce additive elevation of blood pressure). Products include:
  Norisodrine with Calcium Iodide Syrup ... 446
Ketamine Hydrochloride (Additive CNS depression).
  No products indexed under this heading.
Labetalol Hydrochloride (Concurrent use may produce additive elevation in blood pressure). Products include:
  Normodyne Injection ... 2519
  Normodyne Tablets ... 2522
  Trandate ... 1158
Levobunolol Hydrochloride (Concurrent use may produce additive elevation in blood pressure). Products include:
  Betagan ... ⊚ 230
Levomethadyl Acetate Hydrochloride (Additive CNS depression). Products include:
  Orlaam Oral Solution ... 2361
Levorphanol Tartrate (Additive CNS depression). Products include:
  Levo-Dromoran ... 2297
Lorazepam (Additive CNS depression). Products include:
  Ativan Injection ... 2805
  Ativan Tablets ... 2807
Loxapine Hydrochloride (Additive CNS depression). Products include:
  Loxitane ... 1426
Loxapine Succinate (Additive CNS depression). Products include:
  Loxitane Capsules ... 1426
Meperidine Hydrochloride (Additive CNS depression). Products include:
  Demerol ... 2438
  Mepergan Injection ... 2859
Mephobarbital (Additive CNS depression). Products include:
  Mebaral Tablets ... 2452
Meprobamate (Additive CNS depression). Products include:
  Miltown Tablets ... 2780
  PMB 200 and PMB 400 ... 2890
Mesoridazine Besylate (Additive CNS depression). Products include:
  Serentil ... 689
Metaproterenol Sulfate (Concurrent use may produce additive elevation of blood pressure). Products include:
  Alupent ... 672
  Metaproterenol Sulfate Inhalation Solution, USP, Arm-a-Med ... 547
Metaraminol Bitartrate (Concurrent use may produce additive elevation in blood pressure). Products include:
  Aramine Injection ... 1649
Methadone Hydrochloride (Additive CNS depression). Products include:
  Methadone Hydrochloride Oral Concentrate ... 2356

Methadone Hydrochloride Oral Solution & Tablets ... 2357
Methohexital Sodium (Additive CNS depression).
  No products indexed under this heading.
Methotrimeprazine (Additive CNS depression). Products include:
  Levoprome ... 1321
Methoxamine Hydrochloride (Concurrent use may produce additive elevation of blood pressure). Products include:
  Vasoxyl Injection ... 1169
Methoxyflurane (Additive CNS depression).
  No products indexed under this heading.
Methyldopa (Hypertensive crisis can occur with concurrent use). Products include:
  Aldoclor Tablets ... 1638
  Aldomet Oral ... 1640
  Aldoril Tablets ... 1644
Methyldopate Hydrochloride (Hypertensive crisis can occur with concurrent use). Products include:
  Aldomet Ester HCl Injection ... 1642
Metipranolol Hydrochloride (Concurrent use may produce additive elevation in blood pressure). Products include:
  OptiPranolol (Metipranolol 0.3%) Sterile Ophthalmic Solution ... ⊚ 256
Metoprolol Succinate (Concurrent use may produce additive elevation in blood pressure). Products include:
  Toprol-XL Tablets ... 560
Metoprolol Tartrate (Concurrent use may produce additive elevation in blood pressure). Products include:
  Lopressor ... 848
  Lopressor HCT Tablets ... 850
Midazolam Hydrochloride (Additive CNS depression). Products include:
  Versed Injection ... 2324
Molindone Hydrochloride (Additive CNS depression). Products include:
  Moban Tablets and Concentrate ... 1036
Morphine Sulfate (Additive CNS depression). Products include:
  Astramorph/PF Injection, USP (Preservative-Free) ... 526
  Duramorph Injection ... 983
  Infumorph 200 and Infumorph 500 Sterile Solutions ... 985
  Kadian Capsules ... 2948
  MS Contin Tablets ... 2149
  MSIR ... 2152
  Oramorph SR (Morphine Sulfate Sustained Release Tablets) ... 2359
  RMS Suppositories CII ... 2766
  Roxanol ... 2365
Nadolol (Concurrent use may produce additive elevation in blood pressure).
  No products indexed under this heading.
Norepinephrine Bitartrate (Concurrent use may produce additive elevation in blood pressure). Products include:
  Levophed Bitartrate Injection ... 2445
Opium Alkaloids (Additive CNS depression).
  No products indexed under this heading.
Oxazepam (Additive CNS depression). Products include:
  Serax Capsules ... 2916
  Serax Tablets ... 2916
Oxycodone Hydrochloride (Additive CNS depression). Products include:
  OxyContin Tablets ... 2163
  OxyIR Capsules ... 2167

Percocet Tablets ... 955
Percodan Tablets ... 955
Percodan-Demi Tablets ... 956
Roxicodone Tablets, Oral Solution & Intensol (Oxycodone) ... 2366
Tylox Capsules ... 1593
Penbutolol Sulfate (Concurrent use may produce additive elevation in blood pressure). Products include:
  Levatol Tablets ... 2547
Pentobarbital Sodium (Additive CNS depression). Products include:
  Nembutal Sodium Capsules ... 440
  Nembutal Sodium Solution ... 442
  Nembutal Sodium Suppositories ... 444
Perphenazine (Additive CNS depression). Products include:
  Etrafon ... 2495
  Triavil Tablets ... 1800
  Trilafon ... 2532
Phenelzine Sulfate (Potential for hypertensive crises; concurrent use is contraindicated). Products include:
  Nardil ... 1977
Phenobarbital (Additive CNS depression). Products include:
  Arco-Lase Plus Tablets ... 513
  Bellergal-S Tablets ... 2375
  Donnatal ... 2234
  Donnatal Extentabs ... 2234
  Donnatal Tablets ... 2234
  Phenobarbital Elixir and Tablets ... 1523
  Quadrinal Tablets ... 1398
Phenylephrine Bitartrate (Concurrent use may produce additive elevation of blood pressure).
  No products indexed under this heading.
Phenylephrine Hydrochloride (Concurrent use may produce additive elevation of blood pressure). Products include:
  Atrohist Plus Tablets ... 1605
  Cerose DM ... ▣ 853
  D.A. II Tablets ... 972
  D.A. Chewable Tablets ... 970
  Dura-Vent/DA Tablets ... 972
  Extendryl ... 1003
  4-Way Fast Acting Nasal Spray (regular & mentholated) ... ▣ 644
  Hemoril ... ▣ 797
  Hycomine Compound Tablets ... 948
  Neo-Synephrine Hydrochloride 1% Carpuject ... 2455
  Neo-Synephrine Hydrochloride 1% Injection ... 2455
  Neo-Synephrine Hydrochloride (Ophthalmic) ... 2456
  Neo-Synephrine ... ▣ 624
  Novahistine Elixir ... ▣ 782
  Phenergan VC ... 2886
  Phenergan VC with Codeine ... 2888
  Preparation H ... ▣ 842
  Tympagesic Ear Drops ... 2476
  Vicks Sinex Nasal Spray and Ultra Fine Mist ... ▣ 738
Phenylephrine Tannate (Concurrent use may produce additive elevation of blood pressure). Products include:
  Atrohist Pediatric Suspension ... 1604
  Atrohist Pediatric Suspension Dye-Free ... 1604
  Rynatan ... 2781
  Rynatuss ... 2782
Pindolol (Concurrent use may produce additive elevation of blood pressure). Products include:
  Visken Tablets ... 2428
Pirbuterol Acetate (Concurrent use may produce additive elevation of blood pressure). Products include:
  Maxair Autohaler ... 1550
  Maxair Inhaler ... 1552
Prazepam (Additive CNS depression).
  No products indexed under this heading.
Prochlorperazine (Additive CNS depression). Products include:
  Compazine ... 2644

Promethazine Hydrochloride (Additive CNS depression). Products include:
  Mepergan Injection ... 2859
  Phenergan with Codeine ... 2883
  Phenergan with Dextromethorphan ... 2885
  Phenergan Injection ... 2880
  Phenergan Suppositories ... 2882
  Phenergan Syrup ... 2881
  Phenergan Tablets ... 2882
  Phenergan VC ... 2886
  Phenergan VC with Codeine ... 2888
Propofol (Additive CNS depression). Products include:
  Diprivan Injectable Emulsion ... 2939
Propoxyphene Hydrochloride (Additive CNS depression). Products include:
  Darvon ... 1475
  Wygesic Tablets ... 2930
Propoxyphene Napsylate (Additive CNS depression). Products include:
  Darvon-N/Darvocet-N ... 1473
Propranolol Hydrochloride (Concurrent use may produce additive elevation in blood pressure). Products include:
  Inderal ... 2834
  Inderal LA Long Acting Capsules ... 2836
  Inderide Tablets ... 2838
  Inderide LA Long Acting Capsules ... 2840
Pseudoephedrine Hydrochloride (Concurrent use may produce additive elevation in blood pressure). Products include:
  Actifed Allergy Daytime/Nighttime Caplets ... ▣ 808
  Actifed Cold & Allergy Tablets ... ▣ 807
  Actifed Cold & Sinus Caplets and Tablets ... ▣ 808
  Actifed Sinus Daytime/Nighttime Tablets and Caplets ... ▣ 809
  Advil Cold and Sinus Caplets and Tablets ... ▣ 837
  Alka-Seltzer Plus Liqui-Gels ... ▣ 612
  Alka-Seltzer Plus Flu & Body Aches Liqui-Gels Non-Drowsy Formula ... ▣ 613
  Alka-Seltzer Plus Night-Time Cold Medicine Liqui-Gels ... ▣ 612
  Allerest Maximum Strength ... ▣ 649
  Allerest No Drowsiness ... ▣ 649
  Allerest Sinus Pain Formula ... ▣ 649
  Atrohist Pediatric Capsules ... 1603
  Benadryl Allergy/Cold Tablets ... ▣ 811
  Benadryl Allergy Decongestant Liquid Medication ... ▣ 812
  Benadryl Allergy Decongestant Tablets ... ▣ 812
  Benadryl Allergy Sinus Headache Caplets ... ▣ 813
  Benylin Multisymptom ... ▣ 816
  Bromfed Capsules (Extended-Release) ... 1832
  Bromfed Syrup ... ▣ 712
  Bromfed Tablets ... 1832
  Bromfed-DM Cough Syrup ... 1832
  Bromfed-PD Capsules (Extended-Release) ... 1832
  Children's TYLENOL Cold Multi-Symptom Chewable Tablets and Liquid ... 1559
  Children's TYLENOL Cold Plus Cough Multi Symptom Chewable Tablets and Liquid ... 1560
  Children's TYLENOL Flu Suspension Liquid ... 1560
  Children's Vicks DayQuil Allergy Relief ... ▣ 730
  Children's Vicks NyQuil Cold/Cough Relief ... ▣ 731
  Allergy-Sinus Comtrex Multi-Symptom Allergy-Sinus Formula Tablets and Caplets ... ▣ 639
  Comtrex Multi-Symptom ... ▣ 638
  Comtrex Multi-Symptom Non-Drowsy Caplets ... ▣ 640
  Congess ... 1003
  Contac Day Allergy/Sinus Caplets ... ▣ 771
  Contac Day & Night ... ▣ 772
  Contac Night Allergy/Sinus Caplets ... ▣ 771
  Contac Severe Cold & Flu Non-Drowsy ... ▣ 774
  Deconsal II Tablets ... 1605
  Dimetane-DX Cough Syrup ... 2233

(▣ Described in PDR For Nonprescription Drugs)   (⊚ Described in PDR For Ophthalmology)

Dimetapp Cold & Fever Suspension	839
Dimetapp Decongestant Pediatric Drops	840
Dorcol Children's Cough Syrup	748
Drixoral Cough + Congestion Liquid Caps	763
Dura-Tap/PD Capsules	970
Duratuss Tablets	2750
Duratuss HD Elixir	2750
Efidac/24	655
Entex PSE Tablets	973
Fedahist Gyrocaps	2545
Guaifed	1833
Guaifed Syrup	712
Guaimax-D Tablets	809
Histussin D Liquid	670
Infants' TYLENOL Cold Decongestant & Fever-Reducer Drops	1561
Kronofed-A	994
Novahistine DMX	782
Nucofed	2225
PediaCare Cough-Cold Chewable Tablets and Liquid	1569
PediaCare Infants' Decongestant Drops	1569
PediaCare Infants' Drops Decongestant Plus Cough	1569
PediaCare NightRest Cough-Cold Liquid	1569
Pediatric Vicks 44d Cough & Head Congestion Relief	736
Pediatric Vicks 44m Cough & Cold Relief	737
Robitussin Cold & Cough Liqui-Gels	844
Robitussin Cold, Cough & Flu Liqui-Gels	844
Robitussin Maximum Strength Cough & Cold	847
Robitussin Night-Time Cold Formula	847
Robitussin Pediatric Cough & Cold Formula	848
Robitussin Pediatric Drops	849
Robitussin Severe Congestion Liqui-Gels	845
Robitussin-DAC Syrup	2249
Robitussin-PE	846
Rondec Oral Drops	974
Rondec Syrup	974
Rondec Tablet	974
Rondec Chewable Tablets	974
Rondec-TR Tablet	974
Ryna	804
Seldane-D Extended-Release Tablets	1286
Semprex-D Capsules	1620
Sinarest	663
Sine-Aid Maximum Strength Sinus Headache Gelcaps, Caplets and Tablets	1570
Sine-Off No Drowsiness Formula Caplets	784
Sine-Off Sinus Medicine	784
Singlet Tablets	785
Sinutab Non-Drying Liquid Caps	823
Sinutab Sinus Allergy Medication, Maximum Strength Tablets and Caplets	823
Sinutab Sinus Medication, Maximum Strength Without Drowsiness Formula, Tablets & Caplets	824
Sudafed Children's Cold & Cough Liquid Medication	825
Sudafed Children's Nasal Decongestant Liquid Medication	826
Sudafed Cold & Allergy Tablets	826
Sudafed Cold and Cough Liquid Caps	826
Sudafed Nasal Decongestant Tablets, 30 mg	825
Sudafed Nasal Decongestant Tablets, 60 mg	825
Sudafed Non-Drying Sinus Liquid Caps	827
Sudafed Pediatric Nasal Decongestant Liquid Oral Drops	827
Sudafed Severe Cold Formula Caplets	828
Sudafed Severe Cold Formula Tablets	828
Sudafed Sinus Caplets	829
Sudafed Sinus Tablets	829
Sudafed 12 Hour Caplets	824
Syn-Rx Tablets	1622
Syn-Rx DM Tablets	1623
TheraFlu Flu and Cold Medicine	750
Theraflu Maximum Strength Flu and Cold Medicine For Sore Throat	751
TheraFlu Flu, Cold and Cough Medicine	750
TheraFlu Maximum Strength Nighttime Flu, Cold & Cough Medicine	751
TheraFlu Maximum Strength Non-Drowsy Formula Flu, Cold & Cough Medicine	751
TheraFlu Maximum Strength, Non-Drowsy Formula Flu, Cold and Cough Caplets	752
Theraflu Maximum Strength Sinus Non-Drowsy Formula Caplets	752
Triaminic AM Cough and Decongestant Formula	753
Triaminic AM Decongestant Formula	753
Triaminic Infant Oral Decongestant Drops	754
Triaminic Night Time	754
Triaminic Sore Throat Formula	755
Tussend	1830
Tussend Expectorant	1831
TYLENOL Allergy Sinus, Maximum Strength Caplets and Gelcaps	1571
TYLENOL Allergy Sinus NightTime, Maximum Strength Caplets	1571
TYLENOL Cold Medication, Multi-Symptom Formula Tablets and Caplets	1572
TYLENOL Cold Medication, Multi-Symptom Hot Liquid Packets	1572
TYLENOL Cold Medication, No Drowsiness Formula Caplets and Gelcaps	1572
TYLENOL Cold Severe Congestion Caplets	1573
TYLENOL Cough Medication with Decongestant, Multi Symptom	1574
TYLENOL Flu No Drowsiness Formula, Maximum Strength Gelcaps	1575
TYLENOL Flu NightTime, Maximum Strength Gelcaps	1575
TYLENOL Flu NightTime, Maximum Strength Hot Medication Packets	1575
TYLENOL Sinus, Maximum Strength Geltabs, Gelcaps, Caplets and Tablets	1576
Vicks 44 LiquiCaps Cough, Cold & Flu Relief	728
Vicks 44 LiquiCaps Non-Drowsy Cough & Cold Relief	729
Vicks 44D Cough & Head Congestion Relief	728
Vicks 44M Cough, Cold & Flu Relief	729
Vicks DayQuil LiquiCaps/Liquid Multi-Symptom Cold/Flu Relief	734
Vicks DayQuil SINUS Pressure & PAIN Relief with IBUPROFEN	735
Vicks Nyquil Hot Therapy	735
Vicks NyQuil LiquiCaps/Liquid Multi-Symptom Cold/Flu Relief, Original and Cherry Flavors	736

Pseudoephedrine Sulfate (Concurrent use may produce additive elevation of blood pressure). Products include:
Chlor-Trimeton Allergy Decongestant Tablets	759
Claritin-D Tablets	2487
Drixoral Cold and Allergy Sustained-Action Tablets	763
Drixoral Cold and Flu Extended-Release Tablets	764
Drixoral Non-Drowsy Formula Extended-Release Tablets	764
Drixoral Allergy/Sinus Extended Release Tablets	765
Trinalin Repetabs Tablets	1373

Quazepam (Additive CNS depression). Products include:
| Doral Tablets | 2773 |

Risperidone (Additive CNS depression). Products include:
| Risperdal Tablets | 1348 |

Salmeterol Xinafoate (Concurrent use may produce additive elevation of blood pressure). Products include:
| Serevent Inhalation Aerosol | 1149 |

Secobarbital Sodium (Additive CNS depression). Products include:
| Seconal Sodium Pulvules | 1529 |

Selegiline Hydrochloride (Potential for hypertensive crises; concurrent use is contraindicated). Products include:
| Eldepryl Capsules | 2729 |

Sevoflurane (Additive CNS depression).
No products indexed under this heading.

Sotalol Hydrochloride (Concurrent use may produce additive elevation in blood pressure). Products include:
| Betapace Tablets | 637 |

Sufentanil Citrate (Additive CNS depression). Products include:
| Sufenta Injection | 1355 |

Temazepam (Additive CNS depression). Products include:
| Restoril Capsules | 2413 |

Terbutaline Sulfate (Concurrent use may produce additive elevation of blood pressure). Products include:
Brethaire Inhaler	830
Brethine Ampuls	832
Brethine Tablets	831
Bricanyl Subcutaneous Injection	1247
Bricanyl Tablets	1248

Thiamylal Sodium (Additive CNS depression).
No products indexed under this heading.

Thioridazine Hydrochloride (Additive CNS depression). Products include:
| Mellaril | 2398 |

Thiothixene (Additive CNS depression). Products include:
| Navane Capsules and Concentrate | 2018 |
| Navane Intramuscular | 2019 |

Timolol Hemihydrate (Concurrent use may produce additive elevation in blood pressure). Products include:
| Betimol 0.25%, 0.5% | 259 |

Timolol Maleate (Concurrent use may produce additive elevation in blood pressure). Products include:
Blocadren Tablets	1654
Timolide Tablets	1791
Timoptic in Ocudose	1796
Timoptic Sterile Ophthalmic Solution	1794
Timoptic-XE	1798

Tranylcypromine Sulfate (Potential for hypertensive crises; concurrent use is contraindicated). Products include:
| Parnate Tablets | 2679 |

Triazolam (Additive CNS depression). Products include:
| Halcion Tablets | 2093 |

Trifluoperazine Hydrochloride (Additive CNS depression). Products include:
| Stelazine | 2692 |

Zolpidem Tartrate (Additive CNS depression). Products include:
| Ambien Tablets | 2559 |

HYCOMINE SYRUP
(Hydrocodone Bitartrate, Phenylpropanolamine Hydrochloride) 947
See Hycomine Pediatric Syrup

HYCOTUSS EXPECTORANT SYRUP
(Hydrocodone Bitartrate, Guaifenesin) 950
May interact with central nervous system depressants, narcotic analgesics, antipsychotic agents, tranquilizers, and certain other agents. Compounds in these categories include:

Alfentanil Hydrochloride (Exhibits an additive CNS depression). Products include:
| Alfenta Injection | 1334 |

Alprazolam (Exhibits an additive CNS depression). Products include:
| Xanax Tablets | 2115 |

Aprobarbital (Exhibits an additive CNS depression).
No products indexed under this heading.

Buprenorphine (Exhibits an additive CNS depression). Products include:
| Buprenex Injectable | 2170 |

Buspirone Hydrochloride (Exhibits an additive CNS depression). Products include:
| BuSpar Tablets | 738 |

Butabarbital (Exhibits an additive CNS depression).
No products indexed under this heading.

Butalbital (Exhibits an additive CNS depression). Products include:
Axocet Capsules	2469
Esgic-plus Capsules	1012
Esgic-plus Tablets	1012
Fioricet Tablets	2386
Fioricet with Codeine Capsules	2387
Fiorinal Capsules	2388
Fiorinal with Codeine Capsules	2390
Fiorinal Tablets	2388
Phrenilin	790
Sedapap Tablets 50 mg/650 mg	1826

Chlordiazepoxide (Exhibits an additive CNS depression). Products include:
| Limbitrol | 2333 |

Chlordiazepoxide Hydrochloride (Exhibits an additive CNS depression). Products include:
Librax Capsules	2330
Librium Capsules	2331
Librium Injectable	2332

Chlorpromazine (Exhibits an additive CNS depression). Products include:
| Thorazine Suppositories | 2701 |

Chlorpromazine Hydrochloride (Exhibits an additive CNS depression). Products include:
| Thorazine | 2701 |

Chlorprothixene (Exhibits an additive CNS depression).
No products indexed under this heading.

Chlorprothixene Hydrochloride (Exhibits an additive CNS depression).
No products indexed under this heading.

Chlorprothixene Lactate (Exhibits an additive CNS depression).
No products indexed under this heading.

Clorazepate Dipotassium (Exhibits an additive CNS depression). Products include:
| Tranxene | 459 |

Clozapine (Exhibits an additive CNS depression). Products include:
| Clozaril Tablets | 2377 |

Codeine Phosphate (Exhibits an additive CNS depression). Products include:
Brontex	2130
Dimetane-DC Cough Syrup	2232
Fioricet with Codeine Capsules	2387
Fiorinal with Codeine Capsules	2390
Nucofed	2225
Phenergan with Codeine	2883
Phenergan VC with Codeine	2888
Robitussin A-C Syrup	2248
Robitussin-DAC Syrup	2249
Ryna	804
Soma Compound w/Codeine Tablets	2784

IMPORTANT NOTE: Always consult each drug listing in the patient's regimen for possible interactions.

Hycotuss **Interactions Index** 494

Tylenol with Codeine 1592

Desflurane (Exhibits an additive CNS depression). Products include:

Suprane (desflurane, USP) 1865

Dezocine (Exhibits an additive CNS depression). Products include:

Dalgan Injection 529

Diazepam (Exhibits an additive CNS depression). Products include:

Dizac (diazepam injectable emulsion) CIV 1862
Valium Injectable 2336
Valium Tablets 2335

Droperidol (Exhibits an additive CNS depression). Products include:

Inapsine Injection 462

Enflurane (Exhibits an additive CNS depression).

No products indexed under this heading.

Estazolam (Exhibits an additive CNS depression). Products include:

ProSom Tablets 457

Ethchlorvynol (Exhibits an additive CNS depression). Products include:

Placidyl Capsules 456

Ethinamate (Exhibits an additive CNS depression).

No products indexed under this heading.

Fentanyl (Exhibits an additive CNS depression). Products include:

Duragesic Transdermal System 1336

Fentanyl Citrate (Exhibits an additive CNS depression). Products include:

Sublimaze Injection 463

Fluphenazine Decanoate (Exhibits an additive CNS depression). Products include:

Prolixin Decanoate 510

Fluphenazine Enanthate (Exhibits an additive CNS depression). Products include:

Prolixin Enanthate 510

Fluphenazine Hydrochloride (Exhibits an additive CNS depression). Products include:

Prolixin 510

Flurazepam Hydrochloride (Exhibits an additive CNS depression). Products include:

Dalmane Capsules 2329

Glutethimide (Exhibits an additive CNS depression).

No products indexed under this heading.

Haloperidol (Exhibits an additive CNS depression). Products include:

Haldol Injection, Tablets and Concentrate 1585

Haloperidol Decanoate (Exhibits an additive CNS depression). Products include:

Haldol Decanoate 1587

Hydrocodone Polistirex (Exhibits an additive CNS depression). Products include:

Tussionex Pennkinetic Extended-Release Suspension 1624

Hydromorphone Hydrochloride (Exhibits an additive CNS depression). Products include:

Dilaudid Ampules 1382
Dilaudid Cough Syrup 1383
Dilaudid-HP Injection 1384
Dilaudid-HP Lyophilized Powder 250 mg 1384
Dilaudid 1382
Dilaudid Oral Liquid 1386
Dilaudid 1382
Dilaudid Tablets - 8 mg 1386

Hydroxyzine Hydrochloride (Exhibits an additive CNS depression). Products include:

Atarax Tablets & Syrup 1992
Marax Tablets & DF Syrup 2015
Vistaril Intramuscular Solution 2042

Isoflurane (Exhibits an additive CNS depression).

No products indexed under this heading.

Ketamine Hydrochloride (Exhibits an additive CNS depression).

No products indexed under this heading.

Levomethadyl Acetate Hydrochloride (Exhibits an additive CNS depression). Products include:

Orlaam Oral Solution 2361

Levorphanol Tartrate (Exhibits an additive CNS depression). Products include:

Levo-Dromoran 2297

Lithium Carbonate (Exhibits an additive CNS depression). Products include:

Eskalith 2658
Lithium Carbonate Capsules & Tablets 2352
Lithonate/Lithotabs/Lithobid 2721

Lithium Citrate (Exhibits an additive CNS depression).

No products indexed under this heading.

Lorazepam (Exhibits an additive CNS depression). Products include:

Ativan Injection 2805
Ativan Tablets 2807

Loxapine Hydrochloride (Exhibits an additive CNS depression). Products include:

Loxitane 1426

Loxapine Succinate (Exhibits an additive CNS depression). Products include:

Loxitane Capsules 1426

Meperidine Hydrochloride (Exhibits an additive CNS depression). Products include:

Demerol 2438
Mepergan Injection 2859

Mephobarbital (Exhibits an additive CNS depression). Products include:

Mebaral Tablets 2452

Meprobamate (Exhibits an additive CNS depression). Products include:

Miltown Tablets 2780
PMB 200 and PMB 400 2890

Mesoridazine Besylate (Exhibits an additive CNS depression). Products include:

Serentil 689

Methadone Hydrochloride (Exhibits an additive CNS depression). Products include:

Methadone Hydrochloride Oral Concentrate 2356
Methadone Hydrochloride Oral Solution & Tablets 2357

Methohexital Sodium (Exhibits an additive CNS depression).

No products indexed under this heading.

Methotrimeprazine (Exhibits an additive CNS depression). Products include:

Levoprome 1321

Methoxyflurane (Exhibits an additive CNS depression).

No products indexed under this heading.

Midazolam Hydrochloride (Exhibits an additive CNS depression). Products include:

Versed Injection 2324

Molindone Hydrochloride (Exhibits an additive CNS depression). Products include:

Moban Tablets and Concentrate 1036

Morphine Sulfate (Exhibits an additive CNS depression). Products include:

Astramorph/PF Injection, USP (Preservative-Free) 526
Duramorph Injection 983
Infumorph 200 and Infumorph 500 Sterile Solutions 985
Kadian Capsules 2948
MS Contin Tablets 2149
MSIR 2152
Oramorph SR (Morphine Sulfate Sustained Release Tablets) 2359
RMS Suppositories CII 2766
Roxanol 2365

Opium Alkaloids (Exhibits an additive CNS depression).

No products indexed under this heading.

Oxazepam (Exhibits an additive CNS depression). Products include:

Serax Capsules 2916
Serax Tablets 2916

Oxycodone Hydrochloride (Exhibits an additive CNS depression). Products include:

OxyContin Tablets 2163
OxyIR Capsules 2167
Percocet Tablets 955
Percodan Tablets 955
Percodan-Demi Tablets 956
Roxicodone Tablets, Oral Solution & Intensol (Oxycodone) 2366
Tylox Capsules 1593

Pentobarbital Sodium (Exhibits an additive CNS depression). Products include:

Nembutal Sodium Capsules 440
Nembutal Sodium Solution 442
Nembutal Sodium Suppositories 444

Perphenazine (Exhibits an additive CNS depression). Products include:

Etrafon 2495
Triavil Tablets 1800
Trilafon 2532

Phenobarbital (Exhibits an additive CNS depression). Products include:

Arco-Lase Plus Tablets 513
Bellergal-S Tablets 2375
Donnatal 2234
Donnatal Extentabs 2234
Donnatal Tablets 2234
Phenobarbital Elixir and Tablets 1523
Quadrinal Tablets 1398

Pimozide (Exhibits an additive CNS depression). Products include:

Orap Tablets 1037

Prazepam (Exhibits an additive CNS depression).

No products indexed under this heading.

Prochlorperazine (Exhibits an additive CNS depression). Products include:

Compazine 2644

Promethazine Hydrochloride (Exhibits an additive CNS depression). Products include:

Mepergan Injection 2859
Phenergan with Codeine 2883
Phenergan with Dextromethorphan 2885
Phenergan Injection 2880
Phenergan Suppositories 2882
Phenergan Syrup 2881
Phenergan Tablets 2882
Phenergan VC 2886
Phenergan VC with Codeine 2888

Propofol (Exhibits an additive CNS depression). Products include:

Diprivan Injectable Emulsion 2939

Propoxyphene Hydrochloride (Exhibits an additive CNS depression). Products include:

Darvon 1475
Wygesic Tablets 2930

Propoxyphene Napsylate (Exhibits an additive CNS depression). Products include:

Darvon-N/Darvocet-N 1473

Quazepam (Exhibits an additive CNS depression). Products include:

Doral Tablets 2773

Risperidone (Exhibits an additive CNS depression). Products include:

Risperdal Tablets 1348

Secobarbital Sodium (Exhibits an additive CNS depression). Products include:

Seconal Sodium Pulvules 1529

Sevoflurane (Exhibits an additive CNS depression).

No products indexed under this heading.

Sufentanil Citrate (Exhibits an additive CNS depression). Products include:

Sufenta Injection 1355

Temazepam (Exhibits an additive CNS depression). Products include:

Restoril Capsules 2413

Thiamylal Sodium (Exhibits an additive CNS depression).

No products indexed under this heading.

Thioridazine Hydrochloride (Exhibits an additive CNS depression). Products include:

Mellaril 2398

Thiothixene (Exhibits an additive CNS depression). Products include:

Navane Capsules and Concentrate 2018
Navane Intramuscular 2019

Triazolam (Exhibits an additive CNS depression). Products include:

Halcion Tablets 2093

Trifluoperazine Hydrochloride (Exhibits an additive CNS depression). Products include:

Stelazine 2692

Zolpidem Tartrate (Exhibits an additive CNS depression). Products include:

Ambien Tablets 2559

Food Interactions

Alcohol (Exhibits an additive CNS depression).

HYDELTRASOL INJECTION, STERILE
(Prednisolone Sodium Phosphate) 1708
May interact with oral hypoglycemic agents, insulin, oral anticoagulants, potassium-depleting diuretics, and certain other agents. Compounds in these categories include:

Acarbose (Potential for increased requirements of oral hypoglycemic agents). Products include:

Precose 604

Aspirin (Aspirin should be used cautiously in conjunction with corticosteroids in hypoprothrombinemia). Products include:

Alka-Seltzer Cherry Effervescent Antacid and Pain Reliever .... ◙ 609
Alka-Seltzer Extra Strength Effervescent Antacid and Pain Reliever .... ◙ 609
Alka-Seltzer Lemon Lime Effervescent Antacid and Pain Reliever .... ◙ 609
Alka-Seltzer Original Effervescent Antacid and Pain Reliever .... ◙ 609
Alka-Seltzer Plus .... ◙ 611
Alka-Seltzer Plus Sinus Medicine .... ◙ 611
Ascriptin .... ◙ 650
Arthritis Strength BC Powder .... ◙ 631
BC Cold Powder Multi-Symptom Formula (Cold-Sinus-Allergy) .... ◙ 631
BC Cold Powder Non-Drowsy Formula (Cold-Sinus) .... ◙ 631
BC Powder .... ◙ 631
Genuine Bayer Aspirin Tablets & Caplets .... ◙ 618
Extra Strength Bayer Arthritis Pain Regimen Formula .... ◙ 615
Extra Strength Bayer Aspirin Caplets & Tablets .... ◙ 617

(◙ Described in PDR For Nonprescription Drugs) (◎ Described in PDR For Ophthalmology)

495 Interactions Index Hydeltra-T.B.A.

Extended-Release Bayer 8-Hour Aspirin 616
Extra Strength Bayer Plus Aspirin Caplets 617
Extra Strength Bayer PM Aspirin Plus Sleep Aid 617
Aspirin Regimen Bayer 81 mg Tablets with Calcium 615
Aspirin Regimen Bayer Adult Low Strength 81 mg Tablets 613
Aspirin Regimen Bayer Children's Chewable Aspirin 616
Aspirin Regimen Bayer Regular Strength 325 mg Caplets 613
Bufferin Analgesic Tablets 636
Arthritis Strength Bufferin Analgesic Caplets 637
Extra Strength Bufferin Analgesic Tablets 637
Cama Arthritis Pain Reliever 748
Darvon Compound-65 Pulvules 1475
Easprin 1971
Ecotrin 2625
Ecotrin Enteric Coated Aspirin Maximum Strength Tablets and Caplets 775
Ecotrin Enteric Coated Aspirin Regular Strength Tablets 2625
Empirin Aspirin Tablets 818
Excedrin Extra-Strength Analgesic Tablets, Caplets, and Geltabs 734
Fiorinal Capsules 2388
Fiorinal with Codeine Capsules 2390
Fiorinal Tablets 2388
Goody's Extra Strength Headache Powders 632
Goody's Extra Strength Pain Relief Tablets 632
Halfprin Tablets 1413
Norgesic 1554
Percodan Tablets 955
Percodan-Demi Tablets 956
Robaxisal Tablets 2246
Soma Compound w/Codeine Tablets 2784
Soma Compound Tablets 2783
St. Joseph Adult Chewable Aspirin (81 mg.) 768
Talwin Compound 2466
Vanquish Analgesic Caplets 627

Bendroflumethiazide (Co-administration may result in hypokalemia).
No products indexed under this heading.

Chlorothiazide (Co-administration may result in hypokalemia). Products include:
Aldoclor Tablets 1638
Diupres Tablets 1691
Diuril Oral 1694

Chlorothiazide Sodium (Co-administration may result in hypokalemia). Products include:
Diuril Sodium Intravenous 1693

Chlorpropamide (Potential for increased requirements of oral hypoglycemic agents). Products include:
Diabinese Tablets 2002

Dicumarol (Potential for altered response to coumarin anticoagulants).
No products indexed under this heading.

Ephedrine (Enhances metabolic clearance of corticosteroids resulting in decreased blood levels and lessened physiologic activity).

Ephedrine Hydrochloride (Enhances metabolic clearance of corticosteroids resulting in decreased blood levels and lessened physiologic activity). Products include:
Primatene Tablets 844
Quadrinal Tablets 1398

Ephedrine Sulfate (Enhances metabolic clearance of corticosteroids resulting in decreased blood levels and lessened physiologic activity). Products include:
Marax Tablets & DF Syrup 2015

Ephedrine Tannate (Enhances metabolic clearance of corticosteroids resulting in decreased blood levels and lessened physiologic activity). Products include:
Rynatuss 2782

Fosphenytoin Sodium (Enhances metabolic clearance of corticosteroids resulting in decreased blood levels and lessened physiologic activity). Products include:
Cerebyx Injection 1956

Glimepiride (Potential for increased requirements of oral hypoglycemic agents). Products include:
Amaryl Tablets 1241

Glipizide (Potential for increased requirements of oral hypoglycemic agents). Products include:
Glucotrol Tablets 2011
Glucotrol XL Extended Release Tablets 2012

Glyburide (Potential for increased requirements of oral hypoglycemic agents). Products include:
DiaBeta Tablets 1265
Glynase PresTab Tablets 2091
Micronase Tablets 2099

Hydrochlorothiazide (Co-administration may result in hypokalemia). Products include:
Aldactazide Tablets 2556
Aldoril Tablets 1644
Apresazide Capsules 824
Capozide Tablets 744
Dyazide Capsules 2653
Esidrix Tablets 839
Esimil Tablets 840
HydroDIURIL Tablets 1716
Hydropres Tablets 1718
Hyzaar Tablets 1720
Inderide Tablets 2838
Inderide LA Long Acting Capsules 2840
Lopressor HCT Tablets 850
Lotensin HCT Tablets 855
Moduretic Tablets 1748
Oretic Tablets 450
Prinzide Tablets 1780
Ser-Ap-Es Tablets 867
Timolide Tablets 1791
Vaseretic Tablets 1810
Zestoretic Tablets 2968
Ziac 1459

Hydroflumethiazide (Co-administration may result in hypokalemia). Products include:
Diucardin Tablets 2824

Insulin, Human (Potential for increased requirements of insulin).
No products indexed under this heading.

Insulin, Human Isophane Suspension (Potential for increased requirements of insulin). Products include:
Novolin N Human Insulin 10 ml Vials 1846

Insulin, Human NPH (Potential for increased requirements of insulin). Products include:
Humulin N, 100 Units 1495
Novolin N PenFill 1.5 ml Cartridges Durable Insulin Delivery System 1849
Novolin N Prefilled Syringe Disposable Insulin Delivery System 1850

Insulin, Human Regular (Potential for increased requirements of insulin). Products include:
Humulin R, 100 Units 1497
Novolin R Human Insulin 10 ml Vials 1846
Novolin R PenFill 1.5 ml Cartridges Durable Insulin Delivery System 1849
Novolin R Prefilled Syringe Disposable Insulin Delivery System 1850
Velosulin BR Human Insulin 10 ml Vials 1847

Insulin, Human, Zinc Suspension (Potential for increased requirements of insulin). Products include:
Humulin L, 100 Units 1494
Humulin U, 100 Units 1498
Novolin L Human Insulin 10 ml Vials 1846

Insulin Lispro, Human (Potential for increased requirements of insulin). Products include:
Humalog Injection 1488

Insulin, NPH (Potential for increased requirements of insulin). Products include:
NPH, 100 Units 1502
Pork NPH, 100 Units 1506
Purified Pork NPH Isophane Insulin 1852

Insulin, Regular (Potential for increased requirements of insulin). Products include:
Regular, 100 Units 1503
Pork Regular, 100 Units 1507
Pork Regular (Concentrated), 500 Units 1508
Purified Pork Regular Insulin 1852

Insulin, Zinc Crystals (Potential for increased requirements of insulin). Products include:
NPH, 100 Units 1502

Insulin, Zinc Suspension (Potential for increased requirements of insulin). Products include:
Iletin I 1501
Lente, 100 Units 1501
Iletin II 1504
Pork Lente, 100 Units 1504
Purified Pork Lente Insulin 1852

Live Virus Vaccines (Co-administration is contraindicated in patients receiving immunosuppressive doses of corticosteroids).

Metformin Hydrochloride (Potential for increased requirements of oral hypoglycemic agents). Products include:
Glucophage Tablets 754

Methyclothiazide (Co-administration may result in hypokalemia). Products include:
Enduron Tablets 424

Phenobarbital (Enhances metabolic clearance of corticosteroids resulting in decreased blood levels and lessened physiologic activity). Products include:
Arco-Lase Plus Tablets 513
Bellergal-S Tablets 2375
Donnatal 2234
Donnatal Extentabs 2234
Donnatal Tablets 2234
Phenobarbital Elixir and Tablets 1523
Quadrinal Tablets 1398

Phenytoin (Enhances metabolic clearance of corticosteroids resulting in decreased blood levels and lessened physiologic activity). Products include:
Dilantin Infatabs 1967
Dilantin-125 Suspension 1969

Phenytoin Sodium (Enhances metabolic clearance of corticosteroids resulting in decreased blood levels and lessened physiologic activity). Products include:
Dilantin Kapseals 1965

Polythiazide (Co-administration may result in hypokalemia). Products include:
Minizide Capsules 2016

Rifampin (Enhances metabolic clearance of corticosteroids resulting in decreased blood levels and lessened physiologic activity). Products include:
Rifadin 1276
Rifamate Capsules 1278
Rifater 1280
Rimactane Capsules 865

Tolazamide (Potential for increased requirements of oral hypoglycemic agents).
No products indexed under this heading.

Tolbutamide (Potential for increased requirements of oral hypoglycemic agents).
No products indexed under this heading.

Warfarin Sodium (Potential for altered response to coumarin anticoagulants). Products include:
Coumadin 941

HYDELTRA-T.B.A. STERILE SUSPENSION
(Prednisolone Tebutate) 1710
May interact with oral anticoagulants, potassium-depleting diuretics, insulin, oral hypoglycemic agents, and certain other agents. Compounds in these categories include:

Acarbose (Potential for increased requirements of oral hypoglycemic agents). Products include:
Precose 604

Aspirin (Aspirin should be used cautiously in conjunction with corticosteroids in hypoprothrombinemia). Products include:
Alka-Seltzer Cherry Effervescent Antacid and Pain Reliever 609
Alka-Seltzer Extra Strength Effervescent Antacid and Pain Reliever 609
Alka-Seltzer Lemon Lime Effervescent Antacid and Pain Reliever 609
Alka-Seltzer Original Effervescent Antacid and Pain Reliever 609
Alka-Seltzer Plus 611
Alka-Seltzer Plus Sinus Medicine 611
Ascriptin 650
Arthritis Strength BC Powder 631
BC Cold Powder Multi-Symptom Formula (Cold-Sinus-Allergy) 631
BC Cold Powder Non-Drowsy Formula (Cold-Sinus) 631
BC Powder 631
Genuine Bayer Aspirin Tablets & Caplets 618
Extra Strength Bayer Arthritis Pain Regimen Formula 615
Extra Strength Bayer Aspirin Caplets & Tablets 617
Extended-Release Bayer 8-Hour Aspirin 616
Extra Strength Bayer Plus Aspirin Caplets 617
Extra Strength Bayer PM Aspirin Plus Sleep Aid 617
Aspirin Regimen Bayer 81 mg Tablets with Calcium 615
Aspirin Regimen Bayer Adult Low Strength 81 mg Tablets 613
Aspirin Regimen Bayer Children's Chewable Aspirin 616
Aspirin Regimen Bayer Regular Strength 325 mg Caplets 613
Bufferin Analgesic Tablets 636
Arthritis Strength Bufferin Analgesic Caplets 637
Extra Strength Bufferin Analgesic Tablets 637
Cama Arthritis Pain Reliever 748
Darvon Compound-65 Pulvules 1475
Easprin 1971
Ecotrin 2625
Ecotrin Enteric Coated Aspirin Maximum Strength Tablets and Caplets 775
Ecotrin Enteric Coated Aspirin Regular Strength Tablets 2625
Empirin Aspirin Tablets 818
Excedrin Extra-Strength Analgesic Tablets, Caplets, and Geltabs 734
Fiorinal Capsules 2388
Fiorinal with Codeine Capsules 2390
Fiorinal Tablets 2388
Goody's Extra Strength Headache Powders 632
Goody's Extra Strength Pain Relief Tablets 632
Halfprin Tablets 1413
Norgesic 1554

IMPORTANT NOTE: Always consult each drug listing in the patient's regimen for possible interactions.

Percodan Tablets ... 955
Percodan-Demi Tablets ... 956
Robaxisal Tablets ... 2246
Soma Compound w/Codeine Tablets ... 2784
Soma Compound Tablets ... 2783
St. Joseph Adult Chewable Aspirin (81 mg.) ... 768
Talwin Compound ... 2466
Vanquish Analgesic Caplets ... 627

Bendroflumethiazide (Co-administration may result in hypokalemia).
No products indexed under this heading.

Chlorothiazide (Co-administration may result in hypokalemia). Products include:
Aldoclor Tablets ... 1638
Diupres Tablets ... 1691
Diuril Oral ... 1694

Chlorothiazide Sodium (Co-administration may result in hypokalemia). Products include:
Diuril Sodium Intravenous ... 1693

Chlorpropamide (Potential for increased requirements of oral hypoglycemic agents). Products include:
Diabinese Tablets ... 2002

Dicumarol (Potential for altered response to coumarin anticoagulants).
No products indexed under this heading.

Ephedrine (Enhances metabolic clearance of corticosteroids resulting in decreased blood levels and lessened physiologic activity).

Ephedrine Hydrochloride (Enhances metabolic clearance of corticosteroids resulting in decreased blood levels and lessened physiologic activity). Products include:
Primatene Tablets ... 844
Quadrinal Tablets ... 1398

Ephedrine Sulfate (Enhances metabolic clearance of corticosteroids resulting in decreased blood levels and lessened physiologic activity). Products include:
Marax Tablets & DF Syrup ... 2015

Ephedrine Tannate (Enhances metabolic clearance of corticosteroids resulting in decreased blood levels and lessened physiologic activity). Products include:
Rynatuss ... 2782

Glimepiride (Potential for increased requirements of oral hypoglycemic agents). Products include:
Amaryl Tablets ... 1241

Glipizide (Potential for increased requirements of oral hypoglycemic agents). Products include:
Glucotrol Tablets ... 2011
Glucotrol XL Extended Release Tablets ... 2012

Glyburide (Potential for increased requirements of oral hypoglycemic agents). Products include:
DiaBeta Tablets ... 1265
Glynase PresTab Tablets ... 2091
Micronase Tablets ... 2099

Hydrochlorothiazide (Co-administration may result in hypokalemia). Products include:
Aldactazide Tablets ... 2556
Aldoril Tablets ... 1644
Apresazide Capsules ... 824
Capozide Tablets ... 744
Dyazide Capsules ... 2653
Esidrix Tablets ... 839
Esimil Tablets ... 840
HydroDIURIL Tablets ... 1716
Hydropres Tablets ... 1718
Hyzaar Tablets ... 1720
Inderide Tablets ... 2838
Inderide LA Long Acting Capsules ... 2840
Lopressor HCT Tablets ... 850
Lotensin HCT Tablets ... 855
Moduretic Tablets ... 1748
Oretic Tablets ... 450
Prinzide Tablets ... 1780
Ser-Ap-Es Tablets ... 867
Timolide Tablets ... 1791
Vaseretic Tablets ... 1810
Zestoretic Tablets ... 2968
Ziac ... 1459

Hydroflumethiazide (Co-administration may result in hypokalemia). Products include:
Diucardin Tablets ... 2824

Insulin, Human (Potential for increased requirements of insulin).
No products indexed under this heading.

Insulin, Human Isophane Suspension (Potential for increased requirements of insulin). Products include:
Novolin N Human Insulin 10 ml Vials ... 1846

Insulin, Human NPH (Potential for increased requirements of insulin). Products include:
Humulin N, 100 Units ... 1495
Novolin N PenFill 1.5 ml Cartridges Durable Insulin Delivery System ... 1849
Novolin N Prefilled Syringe Disposable Insulin Delivery System ... 1850

Insulin, Human Regular (Potential for increased requirements of insulin). Products include:
Humulin R, 100 Units ... 1497
Novolin R Human Insulin 10 ml Vials ... 1846
Novolin R PenFill 1.5 ml Cartridges Durable Insulin Delivery System ... 1849
Novolin R Prefilled Syringe Disposable Insulin Delivery System ... 1850
Velosulin BR Human Insulin 10 ml Vials ... 1847

Insulin, Human, Zinc Suspension (Potential for increased requirements of insulin). Products include:
Humulin L, 100 Units ... 1494
Humulin U, 100 Units ... 1498
Novolin L Human Insulin 10 ml Vials ... 1846

Insulin Lispro, Human (Potential for increased requirements of insulin). Products include:
Humalog Injection ... 1488

Insulin, NPH (Potential for increased requirements of insulin). Products include:
NPH, 100 Units ... 1502
Pork NPH, 100 Units ... 1506
Purified Pork NPH Isophane Insulin ... 1852

Insulin, Regular (Potential for increased requirements of insulin). Products include:
Regular, 100 Units ... 1503
Pork Regular, 100 Units ... 1507
Pork Regular (Concentrated), 500 Units ... 1508
Purified Pork Regular Insulin ... 1852

Insulin, Zinc Crystals (Potential for increased requirements of insulin). Products include:
NPH, 100 Units ... 1502

Insulin, Zinc Suspension (Potential for increased requirements of insulin). Products include:
Iletin I ... 1501
Lente, 100 Units ... 1501
Iletin II ... 1504
Pork Lente, 100 Units ... 1504
Purified Pork Lente Insulin ... 1852

Live Virus Vaccines (Co-administration is contraindicated in patients receiving immunosuppressive doses of corticosteroids).

Metformin Hydrochloride (Potential for increased requirements of oral hypoglycemic agents). Products include:
Glucophage Tablets ... 754

Methyclothiazide (Co-administration may result in hypokalemia). Products include:
Enduron Tablets ... 424

Phenobarbital (Enhances metabolic clearance of corticosteroids resulting in decreased blood levels and lessened physiologic activity). Products include:
Arco-Lase Plus Tablets ... 513
Bellergal-S Tablets ... 2375
Donnatal ... 2234
Donnatal Extentabs ... 2234
Donnatal Tablets ... 2234
Phenobarbital Elixir and Tablets ... 1523
Quadrinal Tablets ... 1398

Phenytoin (Enhances metabolic clearance of corticosteroids resulting in decreased blood levels and lessened physiologic activity). Products include:
Dilantin Infatabs ... 1967
Dilantin-125 Suspension ... 1969

Phenytoin Sodium (Enhances metabolic clearance of corticosteroids resulting in decreased blood levels and lessened physiologic activity). Products include:
Dilantin Kapseals ... 1965

Polythiazide (Co-administration may result in hypokalemia). Products include:
Minizide Capsules ... 2016

Rifampin (Enhances metabolic clearance of corticosteroids resulting in decreased blood levels and lessened physiologic activity). Products include:
Rifadin ... 1276
Rifamate Capsules ... 1278
Rifater ... 1280
Rimactane Capsules ... 865

Tolazamide (Potential for increased requirements of oral hypoglycemic agents).
No products indexed under this heading.

Tolbutamide (Potential for increased requirements of oral hypoglycemic agents).
No products indexed under this heading.

Warfarin Sodium (Potential for altered response to coumarin anticoagulants). Products include:
Coumadin ... 941

HYDERGINE LC LIQUID CAPSULES
(Ergoloid Mesylates) ... 2392
None cited in PDR database.

HYDERGINE LIQUID
(Ergoloid Mesylates) ... 2392
None cited in PDR database.

HYDERGINE ORAL TABLETS
(Ergoloid Mesylates) ... 2392
None cited in PDR database.

HYDRALAZINE HYDROCHLORIDE INJECTION USP
(Hydralazine Hydrochloride) ... 2712
May interact with monoamine oxidase inhibitors and certain other agents. Compounds in these categories include:

Diazoxide (Profound hypotensive episodes may occur when diazoxide injection and hydralazine are used concomitantly). Products include:
Hyperstat I.V. Injection ... 2504
Proglycem ... 575

Furazolidone (MAO inhibitors should be used with caution in patients receiving hydralazine). Products include:
Furoxone ... 2221

Isocarboxazid (MAO inhibitors should be used with caution in patients receiving hydralazine).
No products indexed under this heading.

Phenelzine Sulfate (MAO inhibitors should be used with caution in patients receiving hydralazine). Products include:
Nardil ... 1977

Selegiline Hydrochloride (MAO inhibitors should be used with caution in patients receiving hydralazine). Products include:
Eldepryl Capsules ... 2729

Tranylcypromine Sulfate (MAO inhibitors should be used with caution in patients receiving hydralazine). Products include:
Parnate Tablets ... 2679

HYDREA CAPSULES
(Hydroxyurea) ... 705
None cited in PDR database.

HYDROCET CAPSULES
(Acetaminophen, Hydrocodone Bitartrate) ... 787
May interact with monoamine oxidase inhibitors, tricyclic antidepressants, central nervous system depressants, antipsychotic agents, narcotic analgesics, antihistamines, and certain other agents. Compounds in these categories include:

Acrivastine (Additive CNS depression). Products include:
Semprex-D Capsules ... 1620

Alfentanil Hydrochloride (Additive CNS depression). Products include:
Alfenta Injection ... 1334

Alprazolam (Additive CNS depression). Products include:
Xanax Tablets ... 2115

Amitriptyline Hydrochloride (Enhanced effect of either/both drugs). Products include:
Elavil ... 2945
Etrafon ... 2495
Limbitrol ... 2333
Triavil Tablets ... 1800

Amoxapine (Enhanced effect of either/both drugs). Products include:
Asendin Tablets ... 1419

Aprobarbital (Additive CNS depression).
No products indexed under this heading.

Astemizole (Additive CNS depression). Products include:
Hismanal Tablets ... 1341

Azatadine Maleate (Additive CNS depression). Products include:
Trinalin Repetabs Tablets ... 1373

Bromodiphenhydramine Hydrochloride (Additive CNS depression).
No products indexed under this heading.

Brompheniramine Maleate (Additive CNS depression). Products include:
Alka-Seltzer Plus Sinus Medicine ... 611
Bromfed Capsules (Extended-Release) ... 1832
Bromfed Syrup ... 712
Bromfed Tablets ... 1832
Bromfed-DM Cough Syrup ... 1832
Bromfed-PD Capsules (Extended-Release) ... 1832
Dimetane-DC Cough Syrup ... 2232
Dimetane-DX Cough Syrup ... 2233

Interactions Index — Hydrocet

Dimetapp Allergy Dye-Free Elixir 838
Dimetapp Allergy Sinus Caplets 838
Dimetapp Cold & Allergy Chewable Tablets 838
Dimetapp Cold & Cough LiquiGels 839
Dimetapp Cold & Fever Suspension 839
Dimetapp DM Elixir 840
Dimetapp Elixir 840
Dimetapp Extentabs 841
Dimetapp Tablets/Liqui-Gels 841
Rondec Chewable Tablets 974
Vicks DayQuil Allergy Relief 12-Hour Extended Release Tablets... 733
Vicks DayQuil Allergy Relief 4-Hour Tablets 733

Buprenorphine (Additive CNS depression). Products include:
Buprenex Injectable 2170

Buspirone Hydrochloride (Additive CNS depression). Products include:
BuSpar Tablets 738

Butabarbital (Additive CNS depression).
No products indexed under this heading.

Butalbital (Additive CNS depression). Products include:
Axocet Capsules 2469
Esgic-plus Capsules 1012
Esgic-plus Tablets 1012
Fioricet Tablets 2386
Fioricet with Codeine Capsules 2387
Fiorinal Capsules 2388
Fiorinal with Codeine Capsules 2390
Fiorinal Tablets 2388
Phrenilin 790
Sedapap Tablets 50 mg/650 mg .. 1826

Cetirizine Hydrochloride (Additive CNS depression). Products include:
Zyrtec Tablets 2053

Chlordiazepoxide (Additive CNS depression). Products include:
Limbitrol 2333

Chlordiazepoxide Hydrochloride (Additive CNS depression). Products include:
Librax Capsules 2330
Librium Capsules 2331
Librium Injectable 2332

Chlorpheniramine Maleate (Additive CNS depression). Products include:
Alka-Seltzer Plus Cold Medicine 611
Alka-Seltzer Plus Cold Medicine Liqui-Gels 612
Alka-Seltzer Plus Cold & Cough Medicine 611
Alka-Seltzer Plus Cold & Cough Medicine Liqui-Gels 612
Alka-Seltzer Plus Flu & Body Aches Effervescent Tablets 612
Allerest Maximum Strength 649
Allerest Sinus Pain Formula 649
Ana-Kit Anaphylaxis Emergency Treatment Kit 611
Atrohist Pediatric Capsules 1603
Atrohist Plus Tablets 1605
BC Cold Powder Multi-Symptom Formula (Cold-Sinus-Allergy) 631
Cerose DM 853
Cheracol Plus Head Cold/Cough Formula 741
Children's TYLENOL Cold Multi-Symptom Chewable Tablets and Liquid 1559
Children's TYLENOL Cold Plus Cough Multi Symptom Chewable Tablets and Liquid 1560
Children's TYLENOL Flu Suspension Liquid 1560
Children's Vicks DayQuil Allergy Relief 730
Children's Vicks NyQuil Cold/Cough Relief 731
Chlor-Trimeton Allergy Decongestant Tablets 759
Chlor-Trimeton Allergy Tablets 758
Allergy-Sinus Comtrex Multi-Symptom Allergy-Sinus Formula Tablets and Caplets 639
Comtrex Multi-Symptom 638

Contac Continuous Action Nasal Decongestant/Antihistamine 12 Hour Capsules 773
Contac Maximum Strength Continuous Action Decongestant/Antihistamine 12 Hour Caplets 772
Contac Severe Cold and Flu Formula Caplets 773
Coricidin Cold + Flu Tablets 760
Coricidin Cough + Cold Tablets 760
Coricidin 'D' Decongestant Tablets 760
D.A. II Tablets 972
D.A. Chewable Tablets 970
Dura-Tap/PD Capsules 970
Dura-Vent/DA Tablets 972
Efidac 24 Chlorpheniramine 655
Extendryl 1003
Fedahist Gyrocaps 2545
Hycomine Compound Tablets 948
Kronofed-A 994
Nolamine Timed-Release Tablets 790
Novahistine Elixir 782
Ornade Spansule Capsules 2678
PediaCare Cough-Cold Chewable Tablets and Liquid 1569
PediaCare NightRest Cough-Cold Liquid 1569
Pediatric Vicks 44m Cough & Cold Relief 737
Pyrroxate Caplets 742
Ryna 804
Sinarest 663
Sine-Off Sinus Medicine 784
Singlet Tablets 785
Sinulin Tablets 792
Sinutab Sinus Allergy Medication, Maximum Strength Tablets and Caplets 823
Sudafed Cold & Allergy Tablets 826
Teldrin 12 Hour Antihistamine/Nasal Decongestant Allergy Relief Capsules 786
TheraFlu Flu and Cold Medicine 750
Theraflu Maximum Strength Flu and Cold Medicine For Sore Throat 751
TheraFlu Flu, Cold and Cough Medicine 750
TheraFlu Maximum Strength Nighttime Flu, Cold & Cough Medicine 751
Triaminic Night Time 754
Triaminic Syrup 755
Triaminic Triaminicol Cold & Cough 756
Triaminicin Tablets 756
Tussend 1830
TYLENOL Allergy Sinus, Maximum Strength Caplets and Gelcaps 1571
TYLENOL Cold Medication, Multi-Symptom Formula Tablets and Caplets 1572
TYLENOL Cold Medication, Multi-Symptom Hot Liquid Packets 1572
Vicks 44 LiquiCaps Cough, Cold & Flu Relief 728
Vicks 44M Cough, Cold & Flu Relief 729

Chlorpheniramine Polistirex (Additive CNS depression). Products include:
Tussionex Pennkinetic Extended-Release Suspension 1624

Chlorpheniramine Tannate (Additive CNS depression). Products include:
Atrohist Pediatric Suspension 1604
Atrohist Pediatric Suspension Dye-Free 1604
Rynatan 2781
Rynatuss 2782

Chlorpromazine (Additive CNS depression). Products include:
Thorazine Suppositories 2701

Chlorpromazine Hydrochloride (Additive CNS depression). Products include:
Thorazine 2701

Chlorprothixene (Additive CNS depression).
No products indexed under this heading.

Chlorprothixene Hydrochloride (Additive CNS depression).
No products indexed under this heading.

Chlorprothixene Lactate (Additive CNS depression).
No products indexed under this heading.

Clemastine Fumarate (Additive CNS depression). Products include:
Tavist Syrup 2426
Tavist Tablets 2427
Tavist-1 12 Hour Relief Tablets 749
Tavist-D 12 Hour Relief Tablets 750

Clomipramine Hydrochloride (Enhanced effect of either/both drugs). Products include:
Anafranil Capsules 819

Clorazepate Dipotassium (Additive CNS depression). Products include:
Tranxene 459

Clozapine (Additive CNS depression). Products include:
Clozaril Tablets 2377

Codeine Phosphate (Additive CNS depression). Products include:
Brontex 2130
Dimetane-DC Cough Syrup 2232
Fioricet with Codeine Capsules 2387
Fiorinal with Codeine Capsules 2390
Nucofed 2225
Phenergan with Codeine 2883
Phenergan VC with Codeine 2888
Robitussin A-C Syrup 2248
Robitussin-DAC Syrup 2249
Ryna 804
Soma Compound w/Codeine Tablets 2784
Tylenol with Codeine 1592

Cyproheptadine Hydrochloride (Additive CNS depression). Products include:
Periactin 1767

Desflurane (Additive CNS depression). Products include:
Suprane (desflurane, USP) 1865

Desipramine Hydrochloride (Enhanced effect of either/both drugs). Products include:
Norpramin Tablets 1273

Dexchlorpheniramine Maleate (Additive CNS depression).
No products indexed under this heading.

Dezocine (Additive CNS depression). Products include:
Dalgan Injection 529

Diazepam (Additive CNS depression). Products include:
Dizac (diazepam injectable emulsion) CIV 1862
Valium Injectable 2336
Valium Tablets 2335

Diphenhydramine Citrate (Additive CNS depression). Products include:
Excedrin P.M. Analgesic/Sleeping Aid Tablets, Caplets, Liquigels 735

Diphenhydramine Hydrochloride (Additive CNS depression). Products include:
Actifed Allergy Daytime/Nighttime Caplets 808
Actifed Sinus Daytime/Nighttime Tablets and Caplets 809
Extra Strength Bayer PM Aspirin Plus Sleep Aid 617
Benadryl Allergy Chewables 811
Benadryl Allergy/Cold Tablets 811
Benadryl Allergy Decongestant Liquid Medication 812
Benadryl Allergy Decongestant Tablets 812
Benadryl Allergy Liquid Medication 813
Benadryl Allergy 811
Benadryl Allergy Sinus Headache Caplets 813
Benadryl Dye-Free Allergy Liquigel Softgels 813
Benadryl Dye-Free Allergy Liquid Medication 814
Benadryl Itch Relief Stick Extra Strength 814
Benadryl Cream 814

Benadryl Gel 815
Benadryl Spray 815
Benadryl Injection 1955
Contac Day & Night Cold/Flu Night Caplets 772
Contac Night Cold/Sinus Caplets 771
Extra Strength Doan's P.M. 653
Excedrin P.M. Analgesic/Sleeping Aid Tablets, Caplets, Liquigels 643
Nytol QuickCaps Caplets 632
Sleepinal Night-time Sleep Aid Capsules and Softgels 798
TYLENOL Allergy Sinus NightTime, Maximum Strength Caplets 1571
TYLENOL Flu NightTime, Maximum Strength Gelcaps 1575
TYLENOL Flu NightTime, Maximum Strength Hot Medication Packets 1575
TYLENOL PM Pain Reliever/Sleep Aid, Extra Strength Gelcaps, Caplets, Geltabs 1576
TYLENOL Severe Allergy Medication Caplets 1571
Maximum Strength Unisom Sleepgels 1990
Unisom With Pain Relief-Nighttime Sleep Aid and Pain Reliever 1991

Diphenylpyraline Hydrochloride (Additive CNS depression).
No products indexed under this heading.

Doxepin Hydrochloride (Enhanced effect of either/both drugs). Products include:
Adapin Capsules 1542
Sinequan 2028
Zonalon Cream 1042

Droperidol (Additive CNS depression). Products include:
Inapsine Injection 462

Enflurane (Additive CNS depression).
No products indexed under this heading.

Estazolam (Additive CNS depression). Products include:
ProSom Tablets 457

Ethchlorvynol (Additive CNS depression). Products include:
Placidyl Capsules 456

Ethinamate (Additive CNS depression).
No products indexed under this heading.

Fentanyl (Additive CNS depression). Products include:
Duragesic Transdermal System 1336

Fentanyl Citrate (Additive CNS depression). Products include:
Sublimaze Injection 463

Fluphenazine Decanoate (Additive CNS depression). Products include:
Prolixin Decanoate 510

Fluphenazine Enanthate (Additive CNS depression). Products include:
Prolixin Enanthate 510

Fluphenazine Hydrochloride (Additive CNS depression). Products include:
Prolixin 510

Flurazepam Hydrochloride (Additive CNS depression). Products include:
Dalmane Capsules 2329

Furazolidone (Enhanced effect of either/both drugs). Products include:
Furoxone 2221

Glutethimide (Additive CNS depression).
No products indexed under this heading.

Haloperidol (Additive CNS depression). Products include:
Haldol Injection, Tablets and Concentrate 1585

IMPORTANT NOTE: Always consult each drug listing in the patient's regimen for possible interactions.

Hydrocet / Interactions Index

Haloperidol Decanoate (Additive CNS depression). Products include:
- Haldol Decanoate 1587

Hydrocodone Polistirex (Additive CNS depression). Products include:
- Tussionex Pennkinetic Extended-Release Suspension 1624

Hydromorphone Hydrochloride (Additive CNS depression). Products include:
- Dilaudid Ampules 1382
- Dilaudid Cough Syrup 1383
- Dilaudid-HP Injection 1384
- Dilaudid-HP Lyophilized Powder 250 mg 1384
- Dilaudid 1382
- Dilaudid Oral Liquid 1386
- Dilaudid 1382
- Dilaudid Tablets - 8 mg 1386

Hydroxyzine Hydrochloride (Additive CNS depression). Products include:
- Atarax Tablets & Syrup 1992
- Marax Tablets & DF Syrup 2015
- Vistaril Intramuscular Solution 2042

Imipramine Hydrochloride (Enhanced effect of either/both drugs). Products include:
- Tofranil Ampuls 873
- Tofranil Tablets 875

Imipramine Pamoate (Enhanced effect of either/both drugs). Products include:
- Tofranil-PM Capsules 876

Isocarboxazid (Enhanced effect of either/both drugs). No products indexed under this heading.

Isoflurane (Additive CNS depression). No products indexed under this heading.

Ketamine Hydrochloride (Additive CNS depression). No products indexed under this heading.

Levomethadyl Acetate Hydrochloride (Additive CNS depression). Products include:
- Orlaam Oral Solution 2361

Levorphanol Tartrate (Additive CNS depression). Products include:
- Levo-Dromoran 2297

Lithium Carbonate (Additive CNS depression). Products include:
- Eskalith 2658
- Lithium Carbonate Capsules & Tablets 2352
- Lithonate/Lithotabs/Lithobid 2721

Lithium Citrate (Additive CNS depression). No products indexed under this heading.

Loratadine (Additive CNS depression). Products include:
- Claritin Tablets 2485
- Claritin-D Tablets 2487

Lorazepam (Additive CNS depression). Products include:
- Ativan Injection 2805
- Ativan Tablets 2807

Loxapine Hydrochloride (Additive CNS depression). Products include:
- Loxitane 1426

Loxapine Succinate (Additive CNS depression). Products include:
- Loxitane Capsules 1426

Maprotiline Hydrochloride (Enhanced effect of either/both drugs). Products include:
- Ludiomil Tablets 861

Meperidine Hydrochloride (Additive CNS depression). Products include:
- Demerol 2438
- Mepergan Injection 2859

Mephobarbital (Additive CNS depression). Products include:
- Mebaral Tablets 2452

Meprobamate (Additive CNS depression). Products include:
- Miltown Tablets 2780
- PMB 200 and PMB 400 2890

Mesoridazine Besylate (Additive CNS depression). Products include:
- Serentil 689

Methadone Hydrochloride (Additive CNS depression). Products include:
- Methadone Hydrochloride Oral Concentrate 2356
- Methadone Hydrochloride Oral Solution & Tablets 2357

Methdilazine Hydrochloride (Additive CNS depression). No products indexed under this heading.

Methohexital Sodium (Additive CNS depression). No products indexed under this heading.

Methotrimeprazine (Additive CNS depression). Products include:
- Levoprome 1321

Methoxyflurane (Additive CNS depression). No products indexed under this heading.

Midazolam Hydrochloride (Additive CNS depression). Products include:
- Versed Injection 2324

Molindone Hydrochloride (Additive CNS depression). Products include:
- Moban Tablets and Concentrate 1036

Morphine Sulfate (Additive CNS depression). Products include:
- Astramorph/PF Injection, USP (Preservative-Free) 526
- Duramorph Injection 983
- Infumorph 200 and Infumorph 500 Sterile Solutions 985
- Kadian Capsules 2948
- MS Contin Tablets 2149
- MSIR 2152
- Oramorph SR (Morphine Sulfate Sustained Release Tablets) 2359
- RMS Suppositories CII 2766
- Roxanol 2365

Nortriptyline Hydrochloride (Enhanced effect of either/both drugs). Products include:
- Pamelor 2409

Opium Alkaloids (Additive CNS depression). No products indexed under this heading.

Oxazepam (Additive CNS depression). Products include:
- Serax Capsules 2916
- Serax Tablets 2916

Oxycodone Hydrochloride (Additive CNS depression). Products include:
- OxyContin Tablets 2163
- OxyIR Capsules 2167
- Percocet Tablets 955
- Percodan Tablets 955
- Percodan-Demi Tablets 956
- Roxicodone Tablets, Oral Solution & Intensol (Oxycodone) 2366
- Tylox Capsules 1593

Pentobarbital Sodium (Additive CNS depression). Products include:
- Nembutal Sodium Capsules 440
- Nembutal Sodium Solution 442
- Nembutal Sodium Suppositories 444

Perphenazine (Additive CNS depression). Products include:
- Etrafon 2495
- Triavil Tablets 1800
- Trilafon 2532

Phenelzine Sulfate (Enhanced effect of either/both drugs). Products include:
- Nardil 1977

Phenobarbital (Additive CNS depression). Products include:
- Arco-Lase Plus Tablets 513
- Bellergal-S Tablets 2375
- Donnatal 2234
- Donnatal Extentabs 2234
- Donnatal Tablets 2234
- Phenobarbital Elixir and Tablets 1523
- Quadrinal Tablets 1398

Pimozide (Additive CNS depression). Products include:
- Orap Tablets 1037

Prazepam (Additive CNS depression). No products indexed under this heading.

Prochlorperazine (Additive CNS depression). Products include:
- Compazine 2644

Promethazine Hydrochloride (Additive CNS depression). Products include:
- Mepergan Injection 2859
- Phenergan with Codeine 2883
- Phenergan with Dextromethorphan 2885
- Phenergan Injection 2880
- Phenergan Suppositories 2882
- Phenergan Syrup 2881
- Phenergan Tablets 2882
- Phenergan VC 2886
- Phenergan VC with Codeine 2888

Propofol (Additive CNS depression). Products include:
- Diprivan Injectable Emulsion 2939

Propoxyphene Hydrochloride (Additive CNS depression). Products include:
- Darvon 1475
- Wygesic Tablets 2930

Propoxyphene Napsylate (Additive CNS depression). Products include:
- Darvon-N/Darvocet-N 1473

Protriptyline Hydrochloride (Enhanced effect of either/both drugs). Products include:
- Vivactil Tablets 1820

Pyrilamine Maleate (Additive CNS depression). Products include:
- 4-Way Fast Acting Nasal Spray (regular & mentholated) 644
- Maximum Strength Multi-Symptom Formula Midol 621
- PMS Multi-Symptom Formula Midol 622

Pyrilamine Tannate (Additive CNS depression). Products include:
- Atrohist Pediatric Suspension 1604
- Atrohist Pediatric Suspension Dye-Free 1604
- Rynatan 2781

Quazepam (Additive CNS depression). Products include:
- Doral Tablets 2773

Risperidone (Additive CNS depression). Products include:
- Risperdal Tablets 1348

Secobarbital Sodium (Additive CNS depression). Products include:
- Seconal Sodium Pulvules 1529

Selegiline Hydrochloride (Enhanced effect of either/both drugs). Products include:
- Eldepryl Capsules 2729

Sevoflurane (Additive CNS depression). No products indexed under this heading.

Sufentanil Citrate (Additive CNS depression). Products include:
- Sufenta Injection 1355

Temazepam (Additive CNS depression). Products include:
- Restoril Capsules 2413

Terfenadine (Additive CNS depression). Products include:
- Seldane Tablets 1284
- Seldane-D Extended-Release Tablets 1286

Thiamylal Sodium (Additive CNS depression). No products indexed under this heading.

Thioridazine Hydrochloride (Additive CNS depression). Products include:
- Mellaril 2398

Thiothixene (Additive CNS depression). Products include:
- Navane Capsules and Concentrate 2018
- Navane Intramuscular 2019

Tranylcypromine Sulfate (Enhanced effect of either/both drugs). Products include:
- Parnate Tablets 2679

Triazolam (Additive CNS depression). Products include:
- Halcion Tablets 2093

Tridihexethyl Chloride (Paralytic ileus). No products indexed under this heading.

Trifluoperazine Hydrochloride (Additive CNS depression). Products include:
- Stelazine 2692

Trihexyphenidyl Hydrochloride (Paralytic ileus). Products include:
- Artane 1418

Trimeprazine Tartrate (Additive CNS depression). No products indexed under this heading.

Trimipramine Maleate (Enhanced effect of either/both drugs). Products include:
- Surmontil Capsules 2917

Tripelennamine Hydrochloride (Additive CNS depression). Products include:
- PBZ Tablets 863
- PBZ-SR Tablets 862

Triprolidine Hydrochloride (Additive CNS depression). Products include:
- Actifed Cold & Allergy Tablets 807
- Actifed Cold & Sinus Caplets and Tablets 808

Zolpidem Tartrate (Additive CNS depression). Products include:
- Ambien Tablets 2559

Food Interactions
Alcohol (Additive CNS depression).

HYDROCORTONE ACETATE STERILE SUSPENSION
(Hydrocortisone Acetate) 1712

May interact with oral anticoagulants, potassium-depleting diuretics, insulin, oral hypoglycemic agents, and certain other agents. Compounds in these categories include:

Acarbose (Potential for increased requirements of oral hypoglycemic agents). Products include:
- Precose 604

Aspirin (Aspirin should be used cautiously in conjunction with corticosteroids in hypoprothrombinemia). Products include:
- Alka-Seltzer Cherry Effervescent Antacid and Pain Reliever 609
- Alka-Seltzer Extra Strength Effervescent Antacid and Pain Reliever 609
- Alka-Seltzer Lemon Lime Effervescent Antacid and Pain Reliever 609
- Alka-Seltzer Original Effervescent Antacid and Pain Reliever 609
- Alka-Seltzer Plus 611
- Alka-Seltzer Plus Sinus Medicine 611
- Ascriptin 650
- Arthritis Strength BC Powder 631
- BC Cold Powder Multi-Symptom Formula (Cold-Sinus-Allergy) 631

(▣ Described in PDR For Nonprescription Drugs)   (◎ Described in PDR For Ophthalmology)

499 Interactions Index Hydrocortone Phosphate

BC Cold Powder Non-Drowsy Formula (Cold-Sinus) 631
BC Powder 631
Genuine Bayer Aspirin Tablets & Caplets 618
Extra Strength Bayer Arthritis Pain Regimen Formula 615
Extra Strength Bayer Aspirin Caplets & Tablets 617
Extended-Release Bayer 8-Hour Aspirin 616
Extra Strength Bayer Plus Aspirin Caplets 617
Extra Strength Bayer PM Aspirin Plus Sleep Aid 617
Aspirin Regimen Bayer 81 mg Tablets with Calcium 615
Aspirin Regimen Bayer Adult Low Strength 81 mg Tablets 613
Aspirin Regimen Bayer Children's Chewable Aspirin 616
Aspirin Regimen Bayer Regular Strength 325 mg Caplets 613
Bufferin Analgesic Tablets 636
Arthritis Strength Bufferin Analgesic Caplets 637
Extra Strength Bufferin Analgesic Tablets 637
Cama Arthritis Pain Reliever 748
Darvon Compound-65 Pulvules 1475
Easprin 1971
Ecotrin 2625
Ecotrin Enteric Coated Aspirin Maximum Strength Tablets and Caplets 775
Ecotrin Enteric Coated Aspirin Regular Strength Tablets 2625
Empirin Aspirin Tablets 818
Excedrin Extra-Strength Analgesic Tablets, Caplets, and Geltabs 734
Fiorinal Capsules 2388
Fiorinal with Codeine Capsules 2390
Fiorinal Tablets 2388
Goody's Extra Strength Headache Powders 632
Goody's Extra Strength Pain Relief Tablets 632
Halfprin Tablets 1413
Norgesic 1554
Percodan Tablets 955
Percodan-Demi Tablets 956
Robaxisal Tablets 2246
Soma Compound w/Codeine Tablets 2784
Soma Compound Tablets 2783
St. Joseph Adult Chewable Aspirin (81 mg.) 768
Talwin Compound 2466
Vanquish Analgesic Caplets 627

Bendroflumethiazide (Co-administration may result in hypokalemia).
No products indexed under this heading.

Chlorothiazide (Co-administration may result in hypokalemia). Products include:
Aldoclor Tablets 1638
Diupres Tablets 1691
Diuril Oral 1694

Chlorothiazide Sodium (Co-administration may result in hypokalemia). Products include:
Diuril Sodium Intravenous 1693

Chlorpropamide (Potential for increased requirements of oral hypoglycemic agents). Products include:
Diabinese Tablets 2002

Dicumarol (Potential for altered response to coumarin anticoagulants).
No products indexed under this heading.

Ephedrine (Enhances metabolic clearance of corticosteroids resulting in decreased blood levels and lessened physiologic activity).

Ephedrine Hydrochloride (Enhances metabolic clearance of corticosteroids resulting in decreased blood levels and lessened physiologic activity). Products include:
Primatene Tablets 844
Quadrinal Tablets 1398

Ephedrine Sulfate (Enhances metabolic clearance of corticosteroids resulting in decreased blood levels and lessened physiologic activity). Products include:
Marax Tablets & DF Syrup 2015

Ephedrine Tannate (Enhances metabolic clearance of corticosteroids resulting in decreased blood levels and lessened physiologic activity). Products include:
Rynatuss 2782

Fosphenytoin Sodium (Enhances metabolic clearance of corticosteroids resulting in decreased blood levels and lessened physiologic activity). Products include:
Cerebyx Injection 1956

Glimepiride (Potential for increased requirements of oral hypoglycemic agents). Products include:
Amaryl Tablets 1241

Glipizide (Potential for increased requirements of oral hypoglycemic agents). Products include:
Glucotrol Tablets 2011
Glucotrol XL Extended Release Tablets 2012

Glyburide (Potential for increased requirements of oral hypoglycemic agents). Products include:
DiaBeta Tablets 1265
Glynase PresTab Tablets 2091
Micronase Tablets 2099

Hydrochlorothiazide (Co-administration may result in hypokalemia). Products include:
Aldactazide Tablets 2556
Aldoril Tablets 1644
Apresazide Capsules 824
Capozide Tablets 744
Dyazide Capsules 2653
Esidrix Tablets 839
Esimil Tablets 840
HydroDIURIL Tablets 1716
Hydropres Tablets 1718
Hyzaar Tablets 1720
Inderide Tablets 2838
Inderide LA Long Acting Capsules 2840
Lopressor HCT Tablets 850
Lotensin HCT Tablets 855
Moduretic Tablets 1748
Oretic Tablets 450
Prinzide Tablets 1780
Ser-Ap-Es Tablets 867
Timolide Tablets 1791
Vaseretic Tablets 1810
Zestoretic Tablets 2968
Ziac 1459

Hydroflumethiazide (Co-administration may result in hypokalemia). Products include:
Diucardin Tablets 2824

Insulin, Human (Potential for increased requirements of insulin).
No products indexed under this heading.

Insulin, Human Isophane Suspension (Potential for increased requirements of insulin). Products include:
Novolin N Human Insulin 10 ml Vials 1846

Insulin, Human NPH (Potential for increased requirements of insulin). Products include:
Humulin N, 100 Units 1495
Novolin N PenFill 1.5 ml Cartridges Durable Insulin Delivery System 1849
Novolin N Prefilled Syringe Disposable Insulin Delivery System 1850

Insulin, Human Regular (Potential for increased requirements of insulin). Products include:
Humulin R, 100 Units 1497
Novolin R Human Insulin 10 ml Vials 1846
Novolin R PenFill 1.5 ml Cartridges Durable Insulin Delivery System 1849
Novolin R Prefilled Syringe Disposable Insulin Delivery System 1850
Velosulin BR Human Insulin 10 ml Vials 1847

Insulin, Human, Zinc Suspension (Potential for increased requirements of insulin). Products include:
Humulin L, 100 Units 1494
Humulin U, 100 Units 1498
Novolin L Human Insulin 10 ml Vials 1846

Insulin Lispro, Human (Potential for increased requirements of insulin). Products include:
Humalog Injection 1488

Insulin, NPH (Potential for increased requirements of insulin). Products include:
NPH, 100 Units 1502
Pork NPH, 100 Units 1506
Purified Pork NPH Isophane Insulin 1852

Insulin, Regular (Potential for increased requirements of insulin). Products include:
Regular, 100 Units 1503
Pork Regular, 100 Units 1507
Pork Regular (Concentrated), 500 Units 1508
Purified Pork Regular Insulin 1852

Insulin, Zinc Crystals (Potential for increased requirements of insulin). Products include:
NPH, 100 Units 1502

Insulin, Zinc Suspension (Potential for increased requirements of insulin). Products include:
Iletin I 1501
Lente, 100 Units 1501
Iletin II 1504
Pork Lente, 100 Units 1504
Purified Pork Lente Insulin 1852

Live Virus Vaccines (Co-administration is contraindicated in patients receiving immunosuppressive doses of corticosteroids).

Metformin Hydrochloride (Potential for increased requirements of oral hypoglycemic agents). Products include:
Glucophage Tablets 754

Methyclothiazide (Co-administration may result in hypokalemia). Products include:
Enduron Tablets 424

Phenobarbital (Enhances metabolic clearance of corticosteroids resulting in decreased blood levels and lessened physiologic activity). Products include:
Arco-Lase Plus Tablets 513
Bellergal-S Tablets 2375
Donnatal 2234
Donnatal Extentabs 2234
Donnatal Tablets 2234
Phenobarbital Elixir and Tablets 1523
Quadrinal Tablets 1398

Phenytoin (Enhances metabolic clearance of corticosteroids resulting in decreased blood levels and lessened physiologic activity). Products include:
Dilantin Infatabs 1967
Dilantin-125 Suspension 1969

Phenytoin Sodium (Enhances metabolic clearance of corticosteroids resulting in decreased blood levels and lessened physiologic activity). Products include:
Dilantin Kapseals 1965

Polythiazide (Co-administration may result in hypokalemia). Products include:
Minizide Capsules 2016

Rifampin (Enhances metabolic clearance of corticosteroids resulting in decreased blood levels and lessened physiologic activity). Products include:
Rifadin 1276
Rifamate Capsules 1278
Rifater 1280
Rimactane Capsules 865

Tolazamide (Potential for increased requirements of oral hypoglycemic agents).
No products indexed under this heading.

Tolbutamide (Potential for increased requirements of oral hypoglycemic agents).
No products indexed under this heading.

Warfarin Sodium (Potential for altered response to coumarin anticoagulants). Products include:
Coumadin 941

HYDROCORTONE PHOSPHATE INJECTION, STERILE
(Hydrocortisone Sodium Phosphate) 1713
May interact with oral anticoagulants, potassium-depleting diuretics, insulin, oral hypoglycemic agents, and certain other agents. Compounds in these categories include:

Acarbose (Potential for increased requirements of oral hypoglycemic agents). Products include:
Precose 604

Aspirin (Aspirin should be used cautiously in conjunction with corticosteroids in hypoprothrombinemia). Products include:
Alka-Seltzer Cherry Effervescent Antacid and Pain Reliever 609
Alka-Seltzer Extra Strength Effervescent Antacid and Pain Reliever 609
Alka-Seltzer Lemon Lime Effervescent Antacid and Pain Reliever 609
Alka-Seltzer Original Effervescent Antacid and Pain Reliever 609
Alka-Seltzer Plus 611
Alka-Seltzer Plus Sinus Medicine 611
Ascriptin 650
Arthritis Strength BC Powder 631
BC Cold Powder Multi-Symptom Formula (Cold-Sinus-Allergy) 631
BC Cold Powder Non-Drowsy Formula (Cold-Sinus) 631
BC Powder 631
Genuine Bayer Aspirin Tablets & Caplets 618
Extra Strength Bayer Arthritis Pain Regimen Formula 615
Extra Strength Bayer Aspirin Caplets & Tablets 617
Extended-Release Bayer 8-Hour Aspirin 616
Extra Strength Bayer Plus Aspirin Caplets 617
Extra Strength Bayer PM Aspirin Plus Sleep Aid 617
Aspirin Regimen Bayer 81 mg Tablets with Calcium 615
Aspirin Regimen Bayer Adult Low Strength 81 mg Tablets 613
Aspirin Regimen Bayer Children's Chewable Aspirin 616
Aspirin Regimen Bayer Regular Strength 325 mg Caplets 613
Bufferin Analgesic Tablets 636
Arthritis Strength Bufferin Analgesic Caplets 637
Extra Strength Bufferin Analgesic Tablets 637
Cama Arthritis Pain Reliever 748
Darvon Compound-65 Pulvules 1475
Easprin 1971
Ecotrin 2625
Ecotrin Enteric Coated Aspirin Maximum Strength Tablets and Caplets 775
Ecotrin Enteric Coated Aspirin Regular Strength Tablets 2625
Empirin Aspirin Tablets 818

IMPORTANT NOTE: Always consult each drug listing in the patient's regimen for possible interactions.

Hydrocortone Phosphate / Interactions Index

Excedrin Extra-Strength Analgesic Tablets, Caplets, and Geltabs 734
Fiorinal Capsules 2388
Fiorinal with Codeine Capsules 2390
Fiorinal Tablets 2388
Goody's Extra Strength Headache Powders ..... ▥ 632
Goody's Extra Strength Pain Relief Tablets ..... ▥ 632
Halfprin Tablets 1413
Norgesic 1554
Percodan Tablets 955
Percodan-Demi Tablets 956
Robaxisal Tablets 2246
Soma Compound w/Codeine Tablets 2784
Soma Compound Tablets 2783
St. Joseph Adult Chewable Aspirin (81 mg.) ..... ▥ 768
Talwin Compound 2466
Vanquish Analgesic Caplets ..... ▥ 627

Bendroflumethiazide (Co-administration may result in hypokalemia).
No products indexed under this heading.

Chlorothiazide (Co-administration may result in hypokalemia). Products include:
Aldoclor Tablets 1638
Diupres Tablets 1691
Diuril Oral 1694

Chlorothiazide Sodium (Co-administration may result in hypokalemia). Products include:
Diuril Sodium Intravenous 1693

Chlorpropamide (Potential for increased requirements of oral hypoglycemic agents). Products include:
Diabinese Tablets 2002

Dicumarol (Potential for altered response to coumarin anticoagulants).
No products indexed under this heading.

Ephedrine (Enhances metabolic clearance of corticosteroids resulting in decreased blood levels and lessened physiologic activity).

Ephedrine Hydrochloride (Enhances metabolic clearance of corticosteroids resulting in decreased blood levels and lessened physiologic activity). Products include:
Primatene Tablets ..... ▥ 844
Quadrinal Tablets 1398

Ephedrine Sulfate (Enhances metabolic clearance of corticosteroids resulting in decreased blood levels and lessened physiologic activity). Products include:
Marax Tablets & DF Syrup 2015

Ephedrine Tannate (Enhances metabolic clearance of corticosteroids resulting in decreased blood levels and lessened physiologic activity). Products include:
Rynatuss 2782

Fosphenytoin Sodium (Enhances metabolic clearance of corticosteroids resulting in decreased physiologic activity). Products include:
Cerebyx Injection 1956

Glimepiride (Potential for increased requirements of oral hypoglycemic agents). Products include:
Amaryl Tablets 1241

Glipizide (Potential for increased requirements of oral hypoglycemic agents). Products include:
Glucotrol Tablets 2011
Glucotrol XL Extended Release Tablets 2012

Glyburide (Potential for increased requirements of oral hypoglycemic agents). Products include:
DiaBeta Tablets 1265
Glynase PresTab Tablets 2091
Micronase Tablets 2099

Hydrochlorothiazide (Co-administration may result in hypokalemia). Products include:
Aldactazide Tablets 2556
Aldoril Tablets 1644
Apresazide Capsules 824
Capozide Tablets 744
Dyazide Capsules 2653
Esidrix Tablets 839
Esimil Tablets 840
HydroDIURIL Tablets 1716
Hydropres Tablets 1718
Hyzaar Tablets 1720
Inderide Tablets 2838
Inderide LA Long Acting Capsules 2840
Lopressor HCT Tablets 850
Lotensin HCT Tablets 855
Moduretic Tablets 1748
Oretic Tablets 450
Prinzide Tablets 1780
Ser-Ap-Es Tablets 867
Timolide Tablets 1791
Vaseretic Tablets 1810
Zestoretic Tablets 2968
Ziac 1459

Hydroflumethiazide (Co-administration may result in hypokalemia). Products include:
Diucardin Tablets 2824

Insulin, Human (Potential for increased requirements of insulin).
No products indexed under this heading.

Insulin, Human Isophane Suspension (Potential for increased requirements of insulin). Products include:
Novolin N Human Insulin 10 ml Vials 1846

Insulin, Human NPH (Potential for increased requirements of insulin). Products include:
Humulin N, 100 Units 1495
Novolin N PenFill 1.5 ml Cartridges Durable Insulin Delivery System 1849
Novolin N Prefilled Syringe Disposable Insulin Delivery System 1850

Insulin, Human Regular (Potential for increased requirements of insulin). Products include:
Humulin R, 100 Units 1497
Novolin R Human Insulin 10 ml Vials 1846
Novolin R PenFill 1.5 ml Cartridges Durable Insulin Delivery System 1849
Novolin R Prefilled Syringe Disposable Insulin Delivery System 1850
Velosulin BR Human Insulin 10 ml Vials 1847

Insulin, Human, Zinc Suspension (Potential for increased requirements of insulin). Products include:
Humulin L, 100 Units 1494
Humulin U, 100 Units 1498
Novolin L Human Insulin 10 ml Vials 1846

Insulin Lispro, Human (Potential for increased requirements of insulin). Products include:
Humalog Injection 1488

Insulin, NPH (Potential for increased requirements of insulin). Products include:
NPH, 100 Units 1502
Pork NPH, 100 Units 1506
Purified Pork NPH Isophane Insulin 1852

Insulin, Regular (Potential for increased requirements of insulin). Products include:
Regular, 100 Units 1503
Pork Regular, 100 Units 1507
Pork Regular (Concentrated), 500 Units 1508
Purified Pork Regular Insulin 1852

Insulin, Zinc Crystals (Potential for increased requirements of insulin). Products include:
NPH, 100 Units 1502

Insulin, Zinc Suspension (Potential for increased requirements of insulin). Products include:
Iletin I 1501
Lente, 100 Units 1501
Iletin II 1504
Pork Lente, 100 Units 1504
Purified Pork Lente Insulin 1852

Live Virus Vaccines (Co-administration is contraindicated in patients receiving immunosuppressive doses of corticosteroids).

Metformin Hydrochloride (Potential for increased requirements of oral hypoglycemic agents). Products include:
Glucophage Tablets 754

Methyclothiazide (Co-administration may result in hypokalemia). Products include:
Enduron Tablets 424

Phenobarbital (Enhances metabolic clearance of corticosteroids resulting in decreased blood levels and lessened physiologic activity). Products include:
Arco-Lase Plus Tablets 513
Bellergal-S Tablets 2375
Donnatal 2234
Donnatal Extentabs 2234
Donnatal Tablets 2234
Phenobarbital Elixir and Tablets 1523
Quadrinal Tablets 1398

Phenytoin (Enhances metabolic clearance of corticosteroids resulting in decreased blood levels and lessened physiologic activity). Products include:
Dilantin Infatabs 1967
Dilantin-125 Suspension 1969

Phenytoin Sodium (Enhances metabolic clearance of corticosteroids resulting in decreased blood levels and lessened physiologic activity). Products include:
Dilantin Kapseals 1965

Polythiazide (Co-administration may result in hypokalemia). Products include:
Minizide Capsules 2016

Rifampin (Enhances metabolic clearance of corticosteroids resulting in decreased blood levels and lessened physiologic activity). Products include:
Rifadin 1276
Rifamate Capsules 1278
Rifater 1280
Rimactane Capsules 865

Tolazamide (Potential for increased requirements of oral hypoglycemic agents).
No products indexed under this heading.

Tolbutamide (Potential for increased requirements of oral hypoglycemic agents).
No products indexed under this heading.

Warfarin Sodium (Potential for altered response to coumarin anticoagulants). Products include:
Coumadin 941

HYDROCORTONE TABLETS
(Hydrocortisone) 1715
May interact with oral anticoagulants, oral hypoglycemic agents, insulin, potassium-depleting diuretics, and certain other agents. Compounds in these categories include:

Acarbose (Potential for increased requirements of oral hypoglycemic agents). Products include:
Precose 604

Aspirin (Aspirin should be used cautiously in conjunction with corticosteroids in hypoprothrombinemia). Products include:
Alka-Seltzer Cherry Effervescent Antacid and Pain Reliever ..... ▥ 609
Alka-Seltzer Extra Strength Effervescent Antacid and Pain Reliever ..... ▥ 609
Alka-Seltzer Lemon Lime Effervescent Antacid and Pain Reliever ..... ▥ 609
Alka-Seltzer Original Effervescent Antacid and Pain Reliever ..... ▥ 609
Alka-Seltzer Plus ..... ▥ 611
Alka-Seltzer Plus Sinus Medicine ..... ▥ 611
Ascriptin ..... ▥ 650
Arthritis Strength BC Powder ..... ▥ 631
BC Cold Powder Multi-Symptom Formula (Cold-Sinus-Allergy) ..... ▥ 631
BC Cold Powder Non-Drowsy Formula (Cold-Sinus) ..... ▥ 631
BC Powder ..... ▥ 631
Genuine Bayer Aspirin Tablets & Caplets ..... ▥ 618
Extra Strength Bayer Arthritis Pain Regimen Formula ..... ▥ 615
Extra Strength Bayer Aspirin Caplets & Tablets ..... ▥ 617
Extended-Release Bayer 8-Hour Aspirin ..... ▥ 616
Extra Strength Bayer Plus Aspirin Caplets ..... ▥ 617
Extra Strength Bayer PM Aspirin Plus Sleep Aid ..... ▥ 617
Aspirin Regimen Bayer 81 mg Tablets with Calcium ..... ▥ 615
Aspirin Regimen Bayer Adult Low Strength 81 mg Tablets ..... ▥ 613
Aspirin Regimen Bayer Children's Chewable Aspirin ..... ▥ 616
Aspirin Regimen Bayer Regular Strength 325 mg Caplets ..... ▥ 613
Bufferin Analgesic Tablets ..... ▥ 636
Arthritis Strength Bufferin Analgesic Caplets ..... ▥ 637
Extra Strength Bufferin Analgesic Tablets ..... ▥ 637
Cama Arthritis Pain Reliever ..... ▥ 748
Darvon Compound-65 Pulvules 1475
Easprin 1971
Ecotrin 2625
Ecotrin Enteric Coated Aspirin Maximum Strength Tablets and Caplets ..... ▥ 775
Ecotrin Enteric Coated Aspirin Regular Strength Tablets 2625
Empirin Aspirin Tablets ..... ▥ 818
Excedrin Extra-Strength Analgesic Tablets, Caplets, and Geltabs 734
Fiorinal Capsules 2388
Fiorinal with Codeine Capsules 2390
Fiorinal Tablets 2388
Goody's Extra Strength Headache Powders ..... ▥ 632
Goody's Extra Strength Pain Relief Tablets ..... ▥ 632
Halfprin Tablets 1413
Norgesic 1554
Percodan Tablets 955
Percodan-Demi Tablets 956
Robaxisal Tablets 2246
Soma Compound w/Codeine Tablets 2784
Soma Compound Tablets 2783
St. Joseph Adult Chewable Aspirin (81 mg.) ..... ▥ 768
Talwin Compound 2466
Vanquish Analgesic Caplets ..... ▥ 627

Bendroflumethiazide (Co-administration may result in hypokalemia).
No products indexed under this heading.

Chlorothiazide (Co-administration may result in hypokalemia). Products include:
Aldoclor Tablets 1638
Diupres Tablets 1691
Diuril Oral 1694

Chlorothiazide Sodium (Co-administration may result in hypokalemia). Products include:
Diuril Sodium Intravenous 1693

Chlorpropamide (Potential for increased requirements of oral hypoglycemic agents). Products include:
Diabinese Tablets 2002

(▥ Described in PDR For Nonprescription Drugs)   (◉ Described in PDR For Ophthalmology)

Dicumarol (Potential for altered response to coumarin anticoagulants).
- No products indexed under this heading.

Ephedrine (Enhances metabolic clearance of corticosteroids resulting in decreased blood levels and lessened physiologic activity).

Ephedrine Hydrochloride (Enhances metabolic clearance of corticosteroids resulting in decreased blood levels and lessened physiologic activity). Products include:
- Primatene Tablets ... OTC 844
- Quadrinal Tablets ... 1398

Ephedrine Sulfate (Enhances metabolic clearance of corticosteroids resulting in decreased blood levels and lessened physiologic activity). Products include:
- Marax Tablets & DF Syrup ... 2015

Ephedrine Tannate (Enhances metabolic clearance of corticosteroids resulting in decreased blood levels and lessened physiologic activity). Products include:
- Rynatuss ... 2782

Fosphenytoin Sodium (Enhances metabolic clearance of corticosteroids resulting in decreased blood levels and lessened physiologic activity). Products include:
- Cerebyx Injection ... 1956

Glimepiride (Potential for increased requirements of oral hypoglycemic agents). Products include:
- Amaryl Tablets ... 1241

Glipizide (Potential for increased requirements of oral hypoglycemic agents). Products include:
- Glucotrol Tablets ... 2011
- Glucotrol XL Extended Release Tablets ... 2012

Glyburide (Potential for increased requirements of oral hypoglycemic agents). Products include:
- DiaBeta Tablets ... 1265
- Glynase PresTab Tablets ... 2091
- Micronase Tablets ... 2099

Hydrochlorothiazide (Co-administration may result in hypokalemia). Products include:
- Aldactazide Tablets ... 2556
- Aldoril Tablets ... 1644
- Apresazide Capsules ... 824
- Capozide Tablets ... 744
- Dyazide Capsules ... 2653
- Esidrix Tablets ... 839
- Esimil Tablets ... 840
- HydroDIURIL Tablets ... 1716
- Hydropres Tablets ... 1718
- Hyzaar Tablets ... 1720
- Inderide Tablets ... 2838
- Inderide LA Long Acting Capsules .. 2840
- Lopressor HCT Tablets ... 850
- Lotensin HCT Tablets ... 855
- Moduretic Tablets ... 1748
- Oretic Tablets ... 450
- Prinzide Tablets ... 1780
- Ser-Ap-Es Tablets ... 867
- Timolide Tablets ... 1791
- Vaseretic Tablets ... 1810
- Zestoretic Tablets ... 2968
- Ziac ... 1459

Hydroflumethiazide (Co-administration may result in hypokalemia). Products include:
- Diucardin Tablets ... 2824

Insulin, Human (Potential for increased requirements of insulin).
- No products indexed under this heading.

Insulin, Human Isophane Suspension (Potential for increased requirements of insulin). Products include:
- Novolin N Human Insulin 10 ml Vials ... 1846

Insulin, Human NPH (Potential for increased requirements of insulin). Products include:
- Humulin N, 100 Units ... 1495
- Novolin N PenFill 1.5 ml Cartridges Durable Insulin Delivery System ... 1849
- Novolin N Prefilled Syringe Disposable Insulin Delivery System ... 1850

Insulin, Human Regular (Potential for increased requirements of insulin). Products include:
- Humulin R, 100 Units ... 1497
- Novolin R Human Insulin 10 ml Vials ... 1846
- Novolin R PenFill 1.5 ml Cartridges Durable Insulin Delivery System ... 1849
- Novolin R Prefilled Syringe Disposable Insulin Delivery System ... 1850
- Velosulin BR Human Insulin 10 ml Vials ... 1847

Insulin, Human, Zinc Suspension (Potential for increased requirements of insulin). Products include:
- Humulin L, 100 Units ... 1494
- Humulin U, 100 Units ... 1498
- Novolin L Human Insulin 10 ml Vials ... 1846

Insulin Lispro, Human (Potential for increased requirements of insulin). Products include:
- Humalog Injection ... 1488

Insulin, NPH (Potential for increased requirements of insulin). Products include:
- NPH, 100 Units ... 1502
- Pork NPH, 100 Units ... 1506
- Purified Pork NPH Isophane Insulin ... 1852

Insulin, Regular (Potential for increased requirements of insulin). Products include:
- Regular, 100 Units ... 1503
- Pork Regular, 100 Units ... 1507
- Pork Regular (Concentrated), 500 Units ... 1508
- Purified Pork Regular Insulin ... 1852

Insulin, Zinc Crystals (Potential for increased requirements of insulin). Products include:
- NPH, 100 Units ... 1502

Insulin, Zinc Suspension (Potential for increased requirements of insulin). Products include:
- Iletin I ... 1501
- Lente, 100 Units ... 1501
- Iletin II ... 1504
- Pork Lente, 100 Units ... 1504
- Purified Pork Lente Insulin ... 1852

Live Virus Vaccines (Co-administration is contraindicated in patients receiving immunosuppressive doses of corticosteroids).

Metformin Hydrochloride (Potential for increased requirements of oral hypoglycemic agents). Products include:
- Glucophage Tablets ... 754

Methyclothiazide (Co-administration may result in hypokalemia). Products include:
- Enduron Tablets ... 424

Phenobarbital (Enhances metabolic clearance of corticosteroids resulting in decreased blood levels and lessened physiologic activity). Products include:
- Arco-Lase Plus Tablets ... 513
- Bellergal-S Tablets ... 2375
- Donnatal ... 2234
- Donnatal Extentabs ... 2234
- Donnatal Tablets ... 2234
- Phenobarbital Elixir and Tablets ... 1523
- Quadrinal Tablets ... 1398

Phenytoin (Enhances metabolic clearance of corticosteroids resulting in decreased blood levels and lessened physiologic activity). Products include:
- Dilantin Infatabs ... 1967
- Dilantin-125 Suspension ... 1969

Phenytoin Sodium (Enhances metabolic clearance of corticosteroids resulting in decreased blood levels and lessened physiologic activity). Products include:
- Dilantin Kapseals ... 1965

Polythiazide (Co-administration may result in hypokalemia). Products include:
- Minizide Capsules ... 2016

Rifampin (Enhances metabolic clearance of corticosteroids resulting in decreased blood levels and lessened physiologic activity). Products include:
- Rifadin ... 1276
- Rifamate Capsules ... 1278
- Rifater ... 1280
- Rimactane Capsules ... 865

Tolazamide (Potential for increased requirements of oral hypoglycemic agents).
- No products indexed under this heading.

Tolbutamide (Potential for increased requirements of oral hypoglycemic agents).
- No products indexed under this heading.

Warfarin Sodium (Potential for altered response to coumarin anticoagulants). Products include:
- Coumadin ... 941

HYDRODIURIL TABLETS

(Hydrochlorothiazide) ... 1716

May interact with antihypertensives, lithium preparations, corticosteroids, cardiac glycosides, insulin, non-steroidal anti-inflammatory agents, barbiturates, narcotic analgesics, oral hypoglycemic agents, bile acid sequestering agents, and certain other agents. Compounds in these categories include:

Acarbose (Hyperglycemia may occur with thiazide diuretics; dosage adjustment of the oral antidiabetic drug may be required). Products include:
- Precose ... 604

Acebutolol Hydrochloride (Potentiation of antihypertensive drugs). Products include:
- Sectral Capsules ... 2914

ACTH (Intensified electrolyte depletion, particularly hypokalemia).
- No products indexed under this heading.

Alfentanil Hydrochloride (Potentiation of orthostatic hypotension). Products include:
- Alfenta Injection ... 1334

Amlodipine Besylate (Potentiation of antihypertensive drugs). Products include:
- Lotrel Capsules ... 858
- Norvasc Tablets ... 2020

Aprobarbital (Potentiation of orthostatic hypotension).
- No products indexed under this heading.

Atenolol (Potentiation of antihypertensive drugs). Products include:
- Tenoretic Tablets ... 2963
- Tenormin Tablets and I.V. Injection 2965

Atracurium Besylate (Possible increased responsiveness to the muscle relaxants). Products include:
- Tracrium Injection ... 1155

Benazepril Hydrochloride (Potentiation of antihypertensive drugs). Products include:
- Lotensin Tablets ... 852
- Lotensin HCT Tablets ... 855
- Lotrel Capsules ... 858

Bendroflumethiazide (Potentiation of antihypertensive drugs).
- No products indexed under this heading.

Betamethasone Acetate (Intensified electrolyte depletion, particularly hypokalemia). Products include:
- Celestone Soluspan Suspension ... 2484

Betamethasone Sodium Phosphate (Intensified electrolyte depletion, particularly hypokalemia). Products include:
- Celestone Soluspan Suspension ... 2484

Betaxolol Hydrochloride (Potentiation of antihypertensive drugs). Products include:
- Betoptic Ophthalmic Solution ... 465
- Betoptic S Ophthalmic Suspension 467
- Kerlone Tablets ... 2588

Bisoprolol Fumarate (Potentiation of antihypertensive drugs). Products include:
- Zebeta Tablets ... 1457
- Ziac ... 1459

Buprenorphine (Potentiation of orthostatic hypotension). Products include:
- Buprenex Injectable ... 2170

Butabarbital (Potentiation of orthostatic hypotension).
- No products indexed under this heading.

Butalbital (Potentiation of orthostatic hypotension). Products include:
- Axocet Capsules ... 2469
- Esgic-plus Capsules ... 1012
- Esgic-plus Tablets ... 1012
- Fioricet Tablets ... 2386
- Fioricet with Codeine Capsules ... 2387
- Fiorinal Capsules ... 2388
- Fiorinal with Codeine Capsules ... 2390
- Fiorinal Tablets ... 2388
- Phrenilin ... 790
- Sedapap Tablets 50 mg/650 mg .. 1826

Captopril (Potentiation of antihypertensive drugs). Products include:
- Capoten Tablets ... 740
- Capozide Tablets ... 744

Carteolol Hydrochloride (Potentiation of antihypertensive drugs). Products include:
- Cartrol Tablets ... 413
- Ocupress Ophthalmic Solution, 1% Sterile ... ⊛ 297

Chlorothiazide (Potentiation of antihypertensive drugs). Products include:
- Aldoclor Tablets ... 1638
- Diupres Tablets ... 1691
- Diuril Oral ... 1694

Chlorothiazide Sodium (Potentiation of antihypertensive drugs). Products include:
- Diuril Sodium Intravenous ... 1693

Chlorpropamide (Hyperglycemia may occur with thiazide diuretics; dosage adjustment of oral hypoglycemic may be neessary). Products include:
- Diabinese Tablets ... 2002

Chlorthalidone (Potentiation of antihypertensive drugs). Products include:
- Combipres Tablets ... 682
- Tenoretic Tablets ... 2963
- Thalitone ... 1293

Cholestyramine (Cholestyramine resin has potential of binding hydrochlorothiazide and reducing its absorption from the GI tract by up to 85%). Products include:
- Questran ... 774

IMPORTANT NOTE: Always consult each drug listing in the patient's regimen for possible interactions.

HydroDIURIL — Interactions Index — 502

Cisatracurium Besylate (Possible increased responsiveness to the muscle relaxants). Products include:
- Nimbex Injection 1131

Clonidine (Potentiation of antihypertensive drugs). Products include:
- Catapres-TTS 680

Clonidine Hydrochloride (Potentiation of antihypertensive drugs). Products include:
- Catapres Tablets 679
- Combipres Tablets 682

Codeine Phosphate (Potentiation of orthostatic hypotension). Products include:
- Brontex 2130
- Dimetane-DC Cough Syrup 2232
- Fioricet with Codeine Capsules 2387
- Fiorinal with Codeine Capsules 2390
- Nucofed 2225
- Phenergan with Codeine 2883
- Phenergan VC with Codeine 2888
- Robitussin A-C Syrup 2248
- Robitussin-DAC Syrup 2249
- Ryna .... ▣ 804
- Soma Compound w/Codeine Tablets 2784
- Tylenol with Codeine 1592

Colestipol Hydrochloride (Colestipol resin has potential of binding hydrochlorothiazide and reducing its absorption from the GI tract by up to 43%). Products include:
- Colestid 2073

Cortisone Acetate (Intensified electrolyte depletion, particularly hypokalemia). Products include:
- Cortone Acetate Sterile Suspension 1663
- Cortone Acetate Tablets 1664

Deserpidine (Potentiation of antihypertensive drugs).
- No products indexed under this heading.

Deslanoside (Resultant hypokalemia may exaggerate cardiac toxicity of digitalis).
- No products indexed under this heading.

Dexamethasone (Intensified electrolyte depletion, particularly hypokalemia). Products include:
- AK-Trol Ointment & Suspension .... ⊙ 205
- Decadron Elixir 1676
- Decadron Tablets 1678
- Decaspray Topical Aerosol 1689
- Maxitrol Ophthalmic Ointment and Suspension .... ⊙ 222
- TobraDex Ophthalmic Suspension and Ointment 469

Dexamethasone Acetate (Intensified electrolyte depletion, particularly hypokalemia). Products include:
- Dalalone D.P. Injectable 1009
- Decadron-LA Sterile Suspension 1687

Dexamethasone Sodium Phosphate (Intensified electrolyte depletion, particularly hypokalemia). Products include:
- Decadron Phosphate Injection 1680
- Decadron Phosphate Sterile Ophthalmic Ointment 1684
- Decadron Phosphate Sterile Ophthalmic Solution 1685
- Decadron Phosphate Topical Cream 1686
- Decadron Phosphate with Xylocaine Injection, Sterile 1683
- Dexacort Phosphate in Respihaler .. 1606
- Dexacort Phosphate in Turbinaire .. 1607
- NeoDecadron Sterile Ophthalmic Ointment 1755
- NeoDecadron Sterile Ophthalmic Solution 1756
- NeoDecadron Topical Cream 1757

Dezocine (Potentiation of orthostatic hypotension). Products include:
- Dalgan Injection 529

Diazoxide (Potentiation of antihypertensive drugs). Products include:
- Hyperstat I.V. Injection 2504
- Proglycem 575

Diclofenac Potassium (Reduced diuretic, natriuretic, and antihypertensive effects). Products include:
- Cataflam Tablets 833

Diclofenac Sodium (Reduced diuretic, natriuretic, and antihypertensive effects). Products include:
- Voltaren Ophthalmic Sterile Ophthalmic Solution .... ⊙ 264
- Cataflam/Voltaren/Voltaren-XR 833

Digitoxin (Resultant hypokalemia may exaggerate cardiac toxicity of digitalis). Products include:
- Crystodigin Tablets 1472

Digoxin (Resultant hypokalemia may exaggerate cardiac toxicity of digitalis). Products include:
- Lanoxicaps 1110
- Lanoxin Elixir Pediatric 1113
- Lanoxin Injection 1116
- Lanoxin Injection Pediatric 1119
- Lanoxin Tablets 1121

Diltiazem Hydrochloride (Potentiation of antihypertensive drugs). Products include:
- Cardizem CD Capsules 1251
- Cardizem SR Capsules 1255
- Cardizem Injectable 1253
- Cardizem Tablets 1257
- Dilacor XR Extended-release Capsules 2183
- Tiazac Capsules 1019

Doxazosin Mesylate (Potentiation of antihypertensive drugs). Products include:
- Cardura Tablets 1993

Enalapril Maleate (Potentiation of antihypertensive drugs). Products include:
- Vaseretic Tablets 1810
- Vasotec Tablets 1816

Enalaprilat (Potentiation of antihypertensive drugs). Products include:
- Vasotec I.V. 1814

Esmolol Hydrochloride (Potentiation of antihypertensive drugs). Products include:
- Brevibloc (esmolol HCl) Injection 1860

Etodolac (Reduced diuretic, natriuretic, and antihypertensive effects). Products include:
- Lodine Capsules and Tablets 2849

Felodipine (Potentiation of antihypertensive drugs). Products include:
- Plendil Extended-Release Tablets 514

Fenoprofen Calcium (Reduced diuretic, natriuretic, and antihypertensive effects). Products include:
- Nalfon 200 Pulvules & Nalfon Tablets 933

Fentanyl (Potentiation of orthostatic hypotension). Products include:
- Duragesic Transdermal System 1336

Fentanyl Citrate (Potentiation of orthostatic hypotension). Products include:
- Sublimaze Injection 463

Fludrocortisone Acetate (Intensified electrolyte depletion, particularly hypokalemia). Products include:
- Florinef Acetate Tablets 506

Flurbiprofen (Reduced diuretic, natriuretic, and antihypertensive effects).
- No products indexed under this heading.

Fosinopril Sodium (Potentiation of antihypertensive drugs). Products include:
- Monopril Tablets 762

Furosemide (Potentiation of antihypertensive drugs). Products include:
- Lasix Injection, Oral Solution and Tablets 1267

Glimepiride (Hyperglycemia may occur with thiazide diuretics; dosage adjustment of the oral antidiabetic drug may be required). Products include:
- Amaryl Tablets 1241

Glipizide (Hyperglycemia may occur with thiazide diuretics; dosage adjustment of the oral antidiabetic drug may be required). Products include:
- Glucotrol Tablets 2011
- Glucotrol XL Extended Release Tablets 2012

Glyburide (Hyperglycemia may occur with thiazide diuretics; dosage adjustment of the oral antidiabetic drug may be required). Products include:
- DiaBeta Tablets 1265
- Glynase PresTab Tablets 2091
- Micronase Tablets 2099

Guanabenz Acetate (Potentiation of antihypertensive drugs).
- No products indexed under this heading.

Guanethidine Monosulfate (Potentiation of antihypertensive drugs). Products include:
- Esimil Tablets 840
- Ismelin Tablets 845

Hydralazine Hydrochloride (Potentiation of antihypertensive drugs). Products include:
- Apresazide Capsules 824
- Apresoline Hydrochloride Tablets .. 826
- Hydralazine Hydrochloride Injection USP 2712
- Ser-Ap-Es Tablets 867

Hydrocodone Bitartrate (Potentiation of orthostatic hypotension). Products include:
- Codiclear DH Syrup 808
- Duratuss HD Elixir 2750
- Histussin D Liquid 670
- Hycodan Tablets and Syrup 946
- Hycomine Compound Tablets 948
- Hycomine 947
- Hycotuss Expectorant Syrup 950
- Hydrocet Capsules 787
- Lorcet 10/650 Tablets 1016
- Lortab 2751
- Tussend 1830
- Tussend Expectorant 1831
- Vicodin Tablets 1404
- Vicodin ES Tablets 1405
- Vicodin HP Tablets 1403
- Vicodin Tuss Expectorant 1406
- Zydone Capsules 967

Hydrocodone Polistirex (Potentiation of orthostatic hypotension). Products include:
- Tussionex Pennkinetic Extended-Release Suspension 1624

Hydrocortisone (Intensified electrolyte depletion, particularly hypokalemia). Products include:
- Anusol-HC Cream 2.5% 1953
- Aquanil HC Lotion 1989
- Maximum Strength Cortaid Spray ▣ 800
- CORTENEMA 2713
- Cortisporin Cream 1074
- Cortisporin Ophthalmic Ointment Sterile 1074
- Cortisporin Ophthalmic Suspension Sterile 1075
- Cortisporin Otic Solution Sterile 1076
- Cortisporin Otic Suspension Sterile 1077
- Cortizone-5 .... ▣ 795
- Cortizone-10 .... ▣ 795
- Hydrocortone Tablets 1715
- Hytone 922
- Hytone Ointment 2 ½% 923
- Massengill Medicated Soft Cloth Towelettes 2628
- Pediotic Suspension Sterile 1140
- Preparation H Hydrocortisone 1% Cream .... ▣ 843
- ProctoCream-HC 2.5% 2552
- VōSoL HC Otic Solution 2786

Hydrocortisone Acetate (Intensified electrolyte depletion, particularly hypokalemia). Products include:
- Analpram-HC Rectal Cream 1% and 2.5% 993
- Anusol HC-1 Hydrocortisone Anti-Itch Ointment .... ▣ 810
- Anusol-HC Suppositories 1954
- Caldecort Anti-Itch Hydrocortisone Cream .... ▣ 651
- Coly-Mycin S Otic w/Neomycin & Hydrocortisone 1965
- Cortaid .... ▣ 800
- Cortifoam 2540
- Cortisporin Cream 1073
- Epifoam 2543
- Hydrocortone Acetate Sterile Suspension 1712
- Mantadil Cream 1124
- Nupercainal Hydrocortisone 1% Cream .... ▣ 661
- Pramosone Cream, Lotion & Ointment 995
- ProctoFoam-HC 2552
- Terra-Cortril Ophthalmic Suspension 2033

Hydrocortisone Sodium Phosphate (Intensified electrolyte depletion, particularly hypokalemia). Products include:
- Hydrocortone Phosphate Injection, Sterile 1713

Hydrocortisone Sodium Succinate (Intensified electrolyte depletion, particularly hypokalemia).
- No products indexed under this heading.

Hydroflumethiazide (Potentiation of antihypertensive drugs). Products include:
- Diucardin Tablets 2824

Hydromorphone Hydrochloride (Potentiation of orthostatic hypotension). Products include:
- Dilaudid Ampules 1382
- Dilaudid Cough Syrup 1383
- Dilaudid-HP Injection 1384
- Dilaudid-HP Lyophilized Powder 250 mg 1384
- Dilaudid 1382
- Dilaudid Oral Liquid 1386
- Dilaudid 1382
- Dilaudid Tablets - 8 mg 1386

Ibuprofen (Reduced diuretic, natriuretic, and antihypertensive effects). Products include:
- Advil Cold and Sinus Caplets and Tablets .... ▣ 837
- Advil Ibuprofen Tablets, Caplets and Gel Caplets .... ▣ 836
- Children's Motrin Ibuprofen Oral Suspension 1558
- IBU Tablets 1389
- Ibuprohm .... ▣ 713
- Motrin IB Caplets, Tablets, and Gelcaps .... ▣ 802
- Motrin Ibuprofen Suspension, Oral Drops, Chewable Tablets, Caplets 1563
- Nuprin Ibuprofen/Analgesic Tablets & Caplets .... ▣ 645
- Vicks DayQuil SINUS Pressure & PAIN Relief with IBUPROFEN .... ▣ 735

Indapamide (Potentiation of antihypertensive drugs).
- No products indexed under this heading.

Indomethacin (Reduced diuretic, natriuretic, and antihypertensive effects). Products include:
- Indocin 1723

Indomethacin Sodium Trihydrate (Reduced diuretic, natriuretic, and antihypertensive effects). Products include:
- Indocin I.V. 1727

Insulin, Human (Hyperglycemia may occur with thiazide diuretics; dosage adjustment of insulin may be required).
- No products indexed under this heading.

(▣ Described in PDR For Nonprescription Drugs)   (⊙ Described in PDR For Ophthalmology)

Insulin, Human Isophane Suspension (Hyperglycemia may occur with thiazide diuretics; dosage adjustment of insulin may be required). Products include:
Novolin N Human Insulin 10 ml Vials 1846

Insulin, Human NPH (Hyperglycemia may occur with thiazide diuretics; dosage adjustment of insulin may be required). Products include:
Humulin N, 100 Units 1495
Novolin N PenFill 1.5 ml Cartridges Durable Insulin Delivery System 1849
Novolin N Prefilled Syringe Disposable Insulin Delivery System 1850

Insulin, Human Regular (Hyperglycemia may occur with thiazide diuretics; dosage adjustment of insulin may be required). Products include:
Humulin R, 100 Units 1497
Novolin R Human Insulin 10 ml Vials 1846
Novolin R PenFill 1.5 ml Cartridges Durable Insulin Delivery System 1849
Novolin R Prefilled Syringe Disposable Insulin Delivery System 1850
Velosulin BR Human Insulin 10 ml Vials 1847

Insulin, Human, Zinc Suspension (Hyperglycemia may occur with thiazide diuretics; dosage adjustment of insulin may be required). Products include:
Humulin L, 100 Units 1494
Humulin U, 100 Units 1498
Novolin L Human Insulin 10 ml Vials 1846

Insulin Lispro, Human (Hyperglycemia may occur with thiazide diuretics; dosage adjustment of insulin may be required). Products include:
Humalog Injection 1488

Insulin, NPH (Hyperglycemia may occur with thiazide diuretics; dosage adjustment of insulin may be required). Products include:
NPH, 100 Units 1502
Pork NPH, 100 Units 1506
Purified Pork NPH Isophane Insulin 1852

Insulin, Regular (Hyperglycemia may occur with thiazide diuretics; dosage adjustment of insulin may be required). Products include:
Regular, 100 Units 1503
Pork Regular, 100 Units 1507
Pork Regular (Concentrated), 500 Units 1508
Purified Pork Regular Insulin 1852

Insulin, Zinc Crystals (Hyperglycemia may occur with thiazide diuretics; dosage adjustment of insulin may be required). Products include:
NPH, 100 Units 1502

Insulin, Zinc Suspension (Hyperglycemia may occur with thiazide diuretics; dosage adjustment of insulin may be required). Products include:
Iletin I 1501
Lente, 100 Units 1501
Iletin II 1504
Pork Lente, 100 Units 1504
Purified Pork Lente Insulin 1852

Isradipine (Potentiation of antihypertensive drugs). Products include:
DynaCirc Capsules 2381
DynaCirc CR Tablets 2383

Ketoprofen (Reduced diuretic, natriuretic, antihypertensive effects). Products include:
Actron Caplets and Tablets 608
Orudis Capsules 2874
Orudis KT 842
Oruvail Capsules 2874

Ketorolac Tromethamine (Reduced diuretic, natriuretic, and antihypertensive effects). Products include:
Acular Sterile Ophthalmic Solution 470
Toradol 2319

Labetalol Hydrochloride (Potentiation of antihypertensive drugs). Products include:
Normodyne Injection 2519
Normodyne Tablets 2522
Trandate 1158

Levorphanol Tartrate (Potentiation of orthostatic hypotension). Products include:
Levo-Dromoran 2297

Lisinopril (Potentiation of antihypertensive drugs). Products include:
Prinivil Tablets 1776
Prinzide Tablets 1780
Zestoretic Tablets 2968
Zestril Tablets 2972

Lithium Carbonate (Diuretics reduce the renal clearance of lithium and add a high risk of lithium toxicity). Products include:
Eskalith 2658
Lithium Carbonate Capsules & Tablets 2352
Lithonate/Lithotabs/Lithobid 2721

Lithium Citrate (Diuretics reduce the renal clearance of lithium and add a high risk of lithium toxicity).
No products indexed under this heading.

Losartan Potassium (Potentiation of antihypertensive drugs). Products include:
Cozaar Tablets 1668
Hyzaar Tablets 1720

Mecamylamine Hydrochloride (Potentiation of antihypertensive drugs). Products include:
Inversine Tablets 1729

Meclofenamate Sodium (Reduced diuretic, natriuretic, and antihypertensive effects).
No products indexed under this heading.

Mefenamic Acid (Reduced diuretic, natriuretic, and antihypertensive effects). Products include:
Ponstel 1982

Meperidine Hydrochloride (Potentiation of orthostatic hypotension). Products include:
Demerol 2438
Mepergan Injection 2859

Mephobarbital (Potentiation of orthostatic hypotension). Products include:
Mebaral Tablets 2452

Metformin Hydrochloride (Hyperglycemia may occur with thiazide diuretics; dosage adjustment of oral hypoglycemic may be necessary). Products include:
Glucophage Tablets 754

Methadone Hydrochloride (Potentiation of orthostatic hypotension). Products include:
Methadone Hydrochloride Oral Concentrate 2356
Methadone Hydrochloride Oral Solution & Tablets 2357

Methyclothiazide (Potentiation of antihypertensive drugs). Products include:
Enduron Tablets 424

Methyldopa (Potentiation of antihypertensive drugs). Products include:
Aldoclor Tablets 1638
Aldomet Oral 1640
Aldoril Tablets 1644

Methyldopate Hydrochloride (Potentiation of antihypertensive drugs). Products include:
Aldomet Ester HCl Injection 1642

Methylprednisolone Acetate (Intensified electrolyte depletion, particularly hypokalemia).
No products indexed under this heading.

Methylprednisolone Sodium Succinate (Intensified electrolyte depletion, particularly hypokalemia).
No products indexed under this heading.

Metocurine Iodide (Possible increased responsiveness to the muscle relaxants). Products include:
Metubine Iodide Vials 932

Metolazone (Potentiation of antihypertensive drugs). Products include:
Mykrox Tablets 1617
Zaroxolyn Tablets 1625

Metoprolol Succinate (Potentiation of antihypertensive drugs). Products include:
Toprol-XL Tablets 560

Metoprolol Tartrate (Potentiation of antihypertensive drugs). Products include:
Lopressor 848
Lopressor HCT Tablets 850

Metyrosine (Potentiation of antihypertensive drugs). Products include:
Demser Capsules 1690

Minoxidil (Potentiation of antihypertensive drugs).
No products indexed under this heading.

Mivacurium Chloride (Possible increased responsiveness to the muscle relaxants). Products include:
Mivacron 1125

Moexipril Hydrochloride (Potentiation of antihypertensive drugs). Products include:
Univasc Tablets 2553

Morphine Sulfate (Potentiation of orthostatic hypotension). Products include:
Astramorph/PF Injection, USP (Preservative-Free) 526
Duramorph Injection 983
Infumorph 200 and Infumorph 500 Sterile Solutions 985
Kadian Capsules 2948
MS Contin Tablets 2149
MSIR 2152
Oramorph SR (Morphine Sulfate Sustained Release Tablets) 2359
RMS Suppositories CII 2766
Roxanol 2365

Nabumetone (Reduced diuretic, natriuretic, and antihypertensive effects). Products include:
Relafen Tablets 2688

Nadolol (Potentiation of antihypertensive drugs).
No products indexed under this heading.

Naproxen (Reduced diuretic, natriuretic, and antihypertensive effects). Products include:
Anaprox/Naprosyn 2277

Naproxen Sodium (Reduced diuretic, natriuretic, and antihypertensive effects). Products include:
Aleve 2124
Anaprox/Naprosyn 2277
Naprelan Tablets 2861

Nicardipine Hydrochloride (Potentiation of ahtihypertensive drugs). Products include:
Cardene Capsules 2261
Cardene I.V. 2815
Cardene SR Capsules 2264

Nifedipine (Potentiation of antihypertensive drugs). Products include:
Adalat Capsules (10 mg and 20 mg) 580
Adalat CC 582
Procardia Capsules 2024
Procardia XL Extended Release Tablets 2026

Nisoldipine (Potentiation of antihypertensive drugs). Products include:
Sular Tablets 2961

Nitroglycerin (Potentiation of antihypertensive drugs). Products include:
Deponit NTG Transdermal Delivery System 2541
Nitro-Bid IV 1270
Nitro-Bid Ointment 1272
Nitro-Dur (nitroglycerin) Transdermal Infusion System 1365
Nitrolingual Spray 2193
Nitrostat Tablets 1981
Transderm-Nitro Transdermal Therapeutic System 878

Norepinephrine Bitartrate (Decreased arterial responsiveness to norepinephrine). Products include:
Levophed Bitartrate Injection 2445

Opium Alkaloids (Potentiation of orthostatic hypotension).
No products indexed under this heading.

Oxaprozin (Reduced diuretic, natriuretic, and antihypertensive effects). Products include:
Daypro Caplets 2578

Oxycodone Hydrochloride (Potentiation of orthostatic hypotension). Products include:
OxyContin Tablets 2163
OxyIR Capsules 2167
Percocet Tablets 955
Percodan Tablets 955
Percodan-Demi Tablets 956
Roxicodone Tablets, Oral Solution & Intensol (Oxycodone) 2366
Tylox Capsules 1593

Pancuronium Bromide (Possible increased responsiveness to the muscle relaxants).
No products indexed under this heading.

Penbutolol Sulfate (Potentiation of antihypertensive drugs). Products include:
Levatol Tablets 2547

Pentobarbital Sodium (Potentiation of orthostatic hypotension). Products include:
Nembutal Sodium Capsules 440
Nembutal Sodium Solution 442
Nembutal Sodium Suppositories ... 444

Phenobarbital (Potentiation of orthostatic hypotension). Products include:
Arco-Lase Plus Tablets 513
Bellergal-S Tablets 2375
Donnatal 2234
Donnatal Extentabs 2234
Donnatal Tablets 2234
Phenobarbital Elixir and Tablets .. 1523
Quadrinal Tablets 1398

Phenoxybenzamine Hydrochloride (Potentiation of antihypertensive drugs). Products include:
Dibenzyline Capsules 2650

Phentolamine Mesylate (Potentiation of antihypertensive drugs). Products include:
Regitine Vials 864

Phenylbutazone (Reduced diuretic, natriuretic, and antihypertensive effects).
No products indexed under this heading.

Pindolol (Potentiation of antihypertensive drugs). Products include:
Visken Tablets 2428

Piroxicam (Reduced diuretic, natriuretic, and antihypertensive effects). Products include:
Feldene Capsules 2008

Polythiazide (Potentiation of antihypertensive drugs). Products include:
Minizide Capsules 2016

IMPORTANT NOTE: Always consult each drug listing in the patient's regimen for possible interactions.

HydroDIURIL — Interactions Index

Prazosin Hydrochloride (Potentiation of antihypertensive drugs). Products include:
- Minipress Capsules 2015
- Minizide Capsules 2016

Prednisolone Acetate (Intensified electrolyte depletion, particularly hypokalemia). Products include:
- AK-CIDE .... ⊙ 203
- AK-CIDE Ointment .... ⊙ 203
- Blephamide Liquifilm Sterile Ophthalmic Suspension 472
- Blephamide Ointment .... ⊙ 234
- Econopred & Econopred Plus Ophthalmic Suspensions .... ⊙ 216
- Poly-Pred Liquifilm .... ⊙ 246
- Pred Forte .... ⊙ 247
- Pred Mild .... ⊙ 250
- Pred-G Liquifilm Sterile Ophthalmic Suspension .... ⊙ 248
- Pred-G S.O.P. Sterile Ophthalmic Ointment .... ⊙ 249

Prednisolone Sodium Phosphate (Intensified electrolyte depletion, particularly hypokalemia). Products include:
- AK-PRED .... ⊙ 204
- Hydeltrasol Injection, Sterile 1708
- Pediapred Oral Solution 1618

Prednisolone Tebutate (Intensified electrolyte depletion, particularly hypokalemia). Products include:
- Hydeltra-T.B.A. Sterile Suspension 1710

Prednisone (Intensified electrolyte depletion, particularly hypokalemia).
No products indexed under this heading.

Propoxyphene Hydrochloride (Potentiation of orthostatic hypotension). Products include:
- Darvon 1475
- Wygesic Tablets 2930

Propoxyphene Napsylate (Potentiation of orthostatic hypotension). Products include:
- Darvon-N/Darvocet-N 1473

Propranolol Hydrochloride (Potentiation of antihypertensive drugs). Products include:
- Inderal 2834
- Inderal LA Long Acting Capsules 2836
- Inderide Tablets 2838
- Inderide LA Long Acting Capsules .. 2840

Quinapril Hydrochloride (Potentiation of antihypertensive drugs). Products include:
- Accupril Tablets 1950

Ramipril (Potentiation of antihypertensive drugs). Products include:
- Altace Capsules 1238

Rauwolfia Serpentina (Potentiation of antihypertensive drugs).
No products indexed under this heading.

Rescinnamine (Potentiation of antihypertensive drugs).
No products indexed under this heading.

Reserpine (Potentiation of antihypertensive drugs). Products include:
- Diupres Tablets 1691
- Hydropres Tablets 1718
- Ser-Ap-Es Tablets 867

Rocuronium Bromide (Possible increased responsiveness to the muscle relaxants). Products include:
- Zemuron Injection 1885

Secobarbital Sodium (Potentiation of orthostatic hypotension). Products include:
- Seconal Sodium Pulvules 1529

Sodium Nitroprusside (Potentiation of antihypertensive drugs).
No products indexed under this heading.

Sotalol Hydrochloride (Potentiation of antihypertensive drugs). Products include:
- Betapace Tablets 637

Spirapril Hydrochloride (Potentiation of antihypertensive drugs).
No products indexed under this heading.

Sufentanil Citrate (Potentiation of orthostatic hypotension). Products include:
- Sufenta Injection 1355

Sulindac (Reduced diuretic, natriuretic, and antihypertensive effects). Products include:
- Clinoril Tablets 1658

Terazosin Hydrochloride (Potentiation of antihypertensive drugs). Products include:
- Hytrin Capsules 434

Thiamylal Sodium (Potentiation of orthostatic hypotension).
No products indexed under this heading.

Timolol Maleate (Potentiation of antihypertensive drugs). Products include:
- Blocadren Tablets 1654
- Timolide Tablets 1791
- Timoptic in Ocudose 1796
- Timoptic Sterile Ophthalmic Solution 1794
- Timoptic-XE 1798

Tolazamide (Hyperglycemia may occur with thiazide diuretics; dosage adjustment of the oral antidiabetic drug may be required).
No products indexed under this heading.

Tolbutamide (Hyperglycemia may occur with thiazide diuretics; dosage adjustment of the oral antidiabetic drug may be required).
No products indexed under this heading.

Tolmetin Sodium (Reduced diuretic, natriuretic, and antihypertensive effects). Products include:
- Tolectin (200, 400 and 600 mg) .. 1591

Torsemide (Potentiation of antihypertensive drugs). Products include:
- Demadex Tablets and Injection 691

Triamcinolone (Intensified electrolyte depletion, particularly hypokalemia).
No products indexed under this heading.

Triamcinolone Acetonide (Intensified electrolyte depletion, particularly hypokalemia). Products include:
- Azmacort Oral Inhaler 2175
- Nasacort AQ Nasal Spray 2191
- Nasacort Nasal Inhaler 2189

Triamcinolone Diacetate (Intensified electrolyte depletion, particularly hypokalemia).
No products indexed under this heading.

Triamcinolone Hexacetonide (Intensified electrolyte depletion, particularly hypokalemia).
No products indexed under this heading.

Trimethaphan Camsylate (Potentiation of antihypertensive drugs).
No products indexed under this heading.

Tubocurarine Chloride (Increased responsiveness to tubocurarine).
No products indexed under this heading.

Vecuronium Bromide (Possible increased responsiveness to the muscle relaxants). Products include:
- Norcuron for Injection 1875

Verapamil Hydrochloride (Potentiation of antihypertensive drugs). Products include:
- Calan SR Caplets 2571
- Calan Tablets 2568
- Covera-HS Tablets 2573
- Isoptin Injectable 1391
- Isoptin Oral Tablets 1393
- Isoptin SR Tablets 1395
- Verelan Capsules 1455

Food Interactions

Alcohol (Potentiation of orthostatic hypotension).

HYDROPRES TABLETS

(Reserpine, Hydrochlorothiazide) 1718
May interact with antihypertensives, lithium preparations, corticosteroids, insulin, non-steroidal anti-inflammatory agents, barbiturates, narcotic analgesics, monoamine oxidase inhibitors, oral hypoglycemic agents, cardiac glycosides, bile acid sequestering agents, and certain other agents. Compounds in these categories include:

Acarbose (Hyperglycemia may occur; dosage adjustment of the antidiabetic drug may be required). Products include:
- Precose 604

Acebutolol Hydrochloride (Potentiation of antihypertensive drugs). Products include:
- Sectral Capsules 2914

ACTH (Potential for intensified electrolyte depletion, particularly hypokalemia).
No products indexed under this heading.

Alfentanil Hydrochloride (Potentiation of orthostatic hypotension; enhanced CNS depressant effects of reserpine). Products include:
- Alfenta Injection 1334

Amlodipine Besylate (Potentiation of antihypertensive drugs). Products include:
- Lotrel Capsules 858
- Norvasc Tablets 2020

Aprobarbital (Potentiation of orthostatic hypotension produced by thiazides; enhances CNS depressant effects of reserpine).
No products indexed under this heading.

Atenolol (Potentiation of antihypertensive drugs). Products include:
- Tenoretic Tablets 2963
- Tenormin Tablets and I.V. Injection 2965

Benazepril Hydrochloride (Potentiation of antihypertensive drugs). Products include:
- Lotensin Tablets 852
- Lotensin HCT Tablets 855
- Lotrel Capsules 858

Bendroflumethiazide (Potentiation of antihypertensive drugs).
No products indexed under this heading.

Betamethasone Acetate (Potential for intensified electrolyte depletion, particularly hypokalemia). Products include:
- Celestone Soluspan Suspension 2484

Betamethasone Sodium Phosphate (Potential for intensified electrolyte depletion, particularly hypokalemia). Products include:
- Celestone Soluspan Suspension 2484

Betaxolol Hydrochloride (Potentiation of antihypertensive drugs). Products include:
- Betoptic Ophthalmic Solution 465
- Betoptic S Ophthalmic Suspension 467
- Kerlone Tablets 2588

Bisoprolol Fumarate (Potentiation of antihypertensive drugs). Products include:
- Zebeta Tablets 1457
- Ziac 1459

Buprenorphine (Potentiation of orthostatic hypotension; enhanced CNS depressant effects of reserpine). Products include:
- Buprenex Injectable 2170

Butabarbital (Potentiation of orthostatic hypotension produced by thiazides; enhances CNS depressant effects of reserpine).
No products indexed under this heading.

Butalbital (Potentiation of orthostatic hypotension produced by thiazides; enhances CNS depressant effects of reserpine). Products include:
- Axocet Capsules 2469
- Esgic-plus Capsules 1012
- Esgic-plus Tablets 1012
- Fioricet Tablets 2386
- Fioricet with Codeine Capsules 2387
- Fiorinal Capsules 2388
- Fiorinal with Codeine Capsules 2390
- Fiorinal Tablets 2388
- Phrenilin 790
- Sedapap Tablets 50 mg/650 mg .. 1826

Captopril (Potentiation of antihypertensive drugs). Products include:
- Capoten Tablets 740
- Capozide Tablets 744

Carteolol Hydrochloride (Potentiation of antihypertensive drugs). Products include:
- Cartrol Tablets 413
- Ocupress Ophthalmic Solution, 1% Sterile .... ⊙ 297

Chlorothiazide (Potentiation of antihypertensive drugs). Products include:
- Aldoclor Tablets 1638
- Diupres Tablets 1691
- Diuril Oral 1694

Chlorothiazide Sodium (Potentiation of antihypertensive drugs). Products include:
- Diuril Sodium Intravenous 1693

Chlorpropamide (Hyperglycemia may occur; dosage adjustment of the antidiabetic drug may be required). Products include:
- Diabinese Tablets 2002

Chlorthalidone (Potentiation of antihypertensive drugs). Products include:
- Combipres Tablets 682
- Tenoretic Tablets 2963
- Thalitone 1293

Cholestyramine (Cholestyramine resin has potential of binding hydrochlorothiazide and reducing its absorption from the GI tract by up to 85%). Products include:
- Questran 774

Clobetasol Propionate (Hypokalemia). Products include:
- Cormax Ointment 1856
- Cormax Scalp Application 1857
- Temovate Cream 1152
- Temovate E Emollient 1154
- Temovate Gel 1153
- Temovate Ointment 1152
- Temovate Scalp Application 1153

Clonidine (Potentiation of antihypertensive drugs). Products include:
- Catapres-TTS 680

Clonidine Hydrochloride (Potentiation of antihypertensive drugs). Products include:
- Catapres Tablets 679
- Combipres Tablets 682

Codeine Phosphate (Potentiation of orthostatic hypotension; enhanced CNS depressant effects of reserpine). Products include:
- Brontex 2130
- Dimetane-DC Cough Syrup 2232
- Fioricet with Codeine Capsules 2387
- Fiorinal with Codeine Capsules 2390
- Nucofed 2225
- Phenergan with Codeine 2883
- Phenergan VC with Codeine 2888

(⊡ Described in PDR For Nonprescription Drugs)   *(⊙ Described in PDR For Ophthalmology)*

Robitussin A-C Syrup 2248
Robitussin-DAC Syrup 2249
Ryna ND 804
Soma Compound w/Codeine Tablets 2784
Tylenol with Codeine 1592

Colestipol Hydrochloride (Colestipol resin has potential of binding hydrochlorothiazide and reducing its absorption from the GI tract by up to 43%). Products include:
Colestid 2073

Cortisone Acetate (Potential for intensified electrolyte depletion, particularly hypokalemia). Products include:
Cortone Acetate Sterile Suspension 1663
Cortone Acetate Tablets 1664

Deserpidine (Potentiation of antihypertensive drugs).
No products indexed under this heading.

Deslanoside (Thiazide-induced hypokalemia may exaggerate or sensitize the response of the heart to toxic effects of digitalis, e.g., increased ventricular irritability; reserpine causes cardiac arrhythmia, use cautiously with digitalis).
No products indexed under this heading.

Dexamethasone (Potential for intensified electrolyte depletion, particularly hypokalemia). Products include:
AK-Trol Ointment & Suspension ◉ 205
Decadron Elixir 1676
Decadron Tablets 1678
Decaspray Topical Aerosol 1689
Maxitrol Ophthalmic Ointment and Suspension ◉ 222
TobraDex Ophthalmic Suspension and Ointment 469

Dexamethasone Acetate (Potential for intensified electrolyte depletion, particularly hypokalemia). Products include:
Dalalone D.P. Injectable 1009
Decadron-LA Sterile Suspension 1687

Dexamethasone Sodium Phosphate (Potential for intensified electrolyte depletion, particularly hypokalemia). Products include:
Decadron Phosphate Injection 1680
Decadron Phosphate Sterile Ophthalmic Ointment 1684
Decadron Phosphate Sterile Ophthalmic Solution 1685
Decadron Phosphate Topical Cream 1686
Decadron Phosphate with Xylocaine Injection, Sterile 1683
Dexacort Phosphate in Respihaler 1606
Dexacort Phosphate in Turbinaire 1607
NeoDecadron Sterile Ophthalmic Ointment 1755
NeoDecadron Sterile Ophthalmic Solution 1756
NeoDecadron Topical Cream 1757

Dezocine (Potentiation of orthostatic hypotension; enhanced CNS depressant effects of reserpine). Products include:
Dalgan Injection 529

Diazoxide (Potentiation of antihypertensive drugs). Products include:
Hyperstat I.V. Injection 2504
Proglycem 575

Diclofenac Potassium (Reduced diuretic, natriuretic, and antihypertensive effects). Products include:
Cataflam Tablets 833

Diclofenac Sodium (Reduced diuretic, natriuretic, and antihypertensive effects). Products include:
Voltaren Ophthalmic Sterile Ophthalmic Solution ◉ 264
Cataflam/Voltaren/Voltaren-XR 833

Digitoxin (Thiazide-induced hypokalemia may exaggerate or sensitize the response of the heart to toxic effects of digitalis, e.g., increased ventricular irritability; reserpine causes cardiac arrhythmia, use cautiously with digitalis). Products include:
Crystodigin Tablets 1472

Digoxin (Thiazide-induced hypokalemia may exaggerate or sensitize the response of the heart to toxic effects of digitalis, e.g., increased ventricular irritability; reserpine causes cardiac arrhythmia, use cautiously with digitalis). Products include:
Lanoxicaps 1110
Lanoxin Elixir Pediatric 1113
Lanoxin Injection 1116
Lanoxin Injection Pediatric 1119
Lanoxin Tablets 1121

Diltiazem Hydrochloride (Potentiation of antihypertensive drugs). Products include:
Cardizem CD Capsules 1251
Cardizem SR Capsules 1255
Cardizem Injectable 1253
Cardizem Tablets 1257
Dilacor XR Extended-release Capsules 2183
Tiazac Capsules 1019

Doxazosin Mesylate (Potentiation of antihypertensive drugs). Products include:
Cardura Tablets 1993

Enalapril Maleate (Potentiation of antihypertensive drugs). Products include:
Vaseretic Tablets 1810
Vasotec Tablets 1816

Enalaprilat (Potentiation of antihypertensive drugs). Products include:
Vasotec I.V. 1814

Esmolol Hydrochloride (Potentiation of antihypertensive drugs). Products include:
Brevibloc (esmolol HCl) Injection 1860

Etodolac (Reduced diuretic, natriuretic, and antihypertensive effects). Products include:
Lodine Capsules and Tablets 2849

Felodipine (Potentiation of antihypertensive drugs). Products include:
Plendil Extended-Release Tablets 514

Fenoprofen Calcium (Reduced diuretic, natriuretic, and antihypertensive effects). Products include:
Nalfon 200 Pulvules & Nalfon Tablets 933

Fentanyl (Potentiation of orthostatic hypotension; enhanced CNS depressant effects of reserpine). Products include:
Duragesic Transdermal System 1336

Fentanyl Citrate (Potentiation of orthostatic hypotension; enhanced CNS depressant effects of reserpine). Products include:
Sublimaze Injection 463

Fludrocortisone Acetate (Potential for intensified electrolyte depletion, particularly hypokalemia). Products include:
Florinef Acetate Tablets 506

Flurbiprofen (Reduced diuretic, natriuretic, and antihypertensive effects).
No products indexed under this heading.

Fosinopril Sodium (Potentiation of antihypertensive drugs). Products include:
Monopril Tablets 762

Furazolidone (Concurrent use is contraindicated). Products include:
Furoxone 2221

Furosemide (Potentiation of antihypertensive drugs). Products include:
Lasix Injection, Oral Solution and Tablets 1267

Glimepiride (Hyperglycemia may occur; dosage adjustment of the antidiabetic drug may be required). Products include:
Amaryl Tablets 1241

Glipizide (Hyperglycemia may occur; dosage adjustment of the antidiabetic drug may be required). Products include:
Glucotrol Tablets 2011
Glucotrol XL Extended Release Tablets 2012

Glyburide (Hyperglycemia may occur; dosage adjustment of the antidiabetic drug may be required). Products include:
DiaBeta Tablets 1265
Glynase PresTab Tablets 2091
Micronase Tablets 2099

Guanabenz Acetate (Potentiation of antihypertensive drugs).
No products indexed under this heading.

Guanethidine Monosulfate (Potentiation of antihypertensive drugs). Products include:
Esimil Tablets 840
Ismelin Tablets 845

Hydralazine Hydrochloride (Potentiation of antihypertensive drugs). Products include:
Apresazide Capsules 824
Apresoline Hydrochloride Tablets 826
Hydralazine Hydrochloride Injection USP 2712
Ser-Ap-Es Tablets 867

Hydrocodone Bitartrate (Potentiation of orthostatic hypotension; enhanced CNS depressant effects of reserpine). Products include:
Codiclear DH Syrup 808
Duratuss HD Elixir 2750
Histussin D Liquid 670
Hycodan Tablets and Syrup 946
Hycomine Compound Tablets 948
Hycomine 947
Hycotuss Expectorant Syrup 950
Hydrocet Capsules 787
Lorcet 10/650 Tablets 1016
Lortab 2751
Tussend 1830
Tussend Expectorant 1831
Vicodin Tablets 1404
Vicodin ES Tablets 1405
Vicodin HP Tablets 1403
Vicodin Tuss Expectorant 1406
Zydone Capsules 967

Hydrocodone Polistirex (Potentiation of orthostatic hypotension; enhanced CNS depressant effects of reserpine). Products include:
Tussionex Pennkinetic Extended-Release Suspension 1624

Hydrocortisone (Potential for intensified electrolyte depletion, particularly hypokalemia). Products include:
Anusol-HC Cream 2.5% 1953
Aquanil HC Lotion 1989
Maximum Strength Cortaid Spray ND 800
CORTENEMA 2713
Cortisporin Ointment 1074
Cortisporin Ophthalmic Ointment Sterile 1074
Cortisporin Ophthalmic Suspension Sterile 1075
Cortisporin Otic Solution Sterile 1076
Cortisporin Otic Suspension Sterile 1077
Cortizone-5 ND 795
Cortizone-10 ND 795
Hydrocortone Tablets 1715
Hytone 922
Hytone Ointment 2 ½% 923
Massengill Medicated Soft Cloth Towelettes 2628
Pediotic Suspension Sterile 1140
Preparation H Hydrocortisone 1% Cream ND 843
ProctoCream-HC 2.5% 2552
VōSoL HC Otic Solution 2786

Hydrocortisone Acetate (Potential for intensified electrolyte depletion, particularly hypokalemia). Products include:
Analpram-HC Rectal Cream 1% and 2.5% 993
Anusol HC-1 Hydrocortisone Anti-Itch Ointment ND 810
Anusol-HC Suppositories 1954
Caldecort Anti-Itch Hydrocortisone Cream ND 651
Coly-Mycin S Otic w/Neomycin & Hydrocortisone 1965
Cortaid ND 800
Cortifoam 2540
Cortisporin Cream 1073
Epifoam 2543
Hydrocortone Acetate Sterile Suspension 1712
Mantadil Cream 1124
Nupercainal Hydrocortisone 1% Cream ND 661
Pramosone Cream, Lotion & Ointment 995
ProctoFoam-HC 2552
Terra-Cortril Ophthalmic Suspension 2033

Hydrocortisone Sodium Phosphate (Potential for intensified electrolyte depletion, particularly hypokalemia). Products include:
Hydrocortone Phosphate Injection, Sterile 1713

Hydrocortisone Sodium Succinate (Potential for intensified electrolyte depletion, particularly hypokalemia).
No products indexed under this heading.

Hydroflumethiazide (Potentiation of antihypertensive drugs). Products include:
Diucardin Tablets 2824

Hydromorphone Hydrochloride (Potentiation of orthostatic hypotension; enhanced CNS depressant effects of reserpine). Products include:
Dilaudid Ampules 1382
Dilaudid Cough Syrup 1383
Dilaudid-HP Injection 1384
Dilaudid-HP Lyophilized Powder 250 mg 1384
Dilaudid 1382
Dilaudid Oral Liquid 1386
Dilaudid 1382
Dilaudid Tablets - 8 mg 1386

Ibuprofen (Reduced diuretic, natriuretic, and antihypertensive effects). Products include:
Advil Cold and Sinus Caplets and Tablets ND 837
Advil Ibuprofen Tablets, Caplets and Gel Caplets ND 836
Children's Motrin Ibuprofen Oral Suspension 1558
IBU Tablets 1389
Ibuprohm ND 713
Motrin IB Caplets, Tablets, and Gelcaps ND 802
Motrin Ibuprofen Suspension, Oral Drops, Chewable Tablets, Caplets 1563
Nuprin Ibuprofen/Analgesic Tablets & Caplets ND 645
Vicks DayQuil SINUS Pressure & PAIN Relief with IBUPROFEN ND 735

Indapamide (Potentiation of antihypertensive drugs).
No products indexed under this heading.

Indomethacin (Reduced diuretic, natriuretic, and antihypertensive effects). Products include:
Indocin 1723

Indomethacin Sodium Trihydrate (Reduced diuretic, natriuretic, and antihypertensive effects). Products include:
Indocin I.V. 1727

IMPORTANT NOTE: Always consult each drug listing in the patient's regimen for possible interactions.

Hydropres — Interactions Index

Insulin, Human (Hyperglycemia may occur; dosage adjustment of insulin may be required).
No products indexed under this heading.

Insulin, Human Isophane Suspension (Hyperglycemia may occur; dosage adjustment of insulin may be required). Products include:
Novolin N Human Insulin 10 ml Vials 1846

Insulin, Human NPH (Hyperglycemia may occur; dosage adjustment of insulin may be required). Products include:
Humulin N, 100 Units 1495
Novolin N PenFill 1.5 ml Cartridges Durable Insulin Delivery System 1849
Novolin N Prefilled Syringe Disposable Insulin Delivery System 1850

Insulin, Human Regular (Hyperglycemia may occur; dosage adjustment of insulin may be required). Products include:
Humulin R, 100 Units 1497
Novolin R Human Insulin 10 ml Vials 1846
Novolin R PenFill 1.5 ml Cartridges Durable Insulin Delivery System 1849
Novolin R Prefilled Syringe Disposable Insulin Delivery System 1850
Velosulin BR Human Insulin 10 ml Vials 1847

Insulin, Human, Zinc Suspension (Hyperglycemia may occur; dosage adjustment of insulin may be required). Products include:
Humulin L, 100 Units 1494
Humulin U, 100 Units 1498
Novolin L Human Insulin 10 ml Vials 1846

Insulin Lispro, Human (Hyperglycemia may occur; dosage adjustment of insulin may be required). Products include:
Humalog Injection 1488

Insulin, NPH (Hyperglycemia may occur; dosage adjustment of insulin may be required). Products include:
NPH, 100 Units 1502
Pork NPH, 100 Units 1506
Purified Pork NPH Isophane Insulin 1852

Insulin, Regular (Hyperglycemia may occur; dosage adjustment of insulin may be required). Products include:
Regular, 100 Units 1503
Pork Regular, 100 Units 1507
Pork Regular (Concentrated), 500 Units 1508
Purified Pork Regular Insulin 1852

Insulin, Zinc Crystals (Hyperglycemia may occur; dosage adjustment of insulin may be required). Products include:
NPH, 100 Units 1502

Insulin, Zinc Suspension (Hyperglycemia may occur; dosage adjustment of insulin may be required). Products include:
Iletin I 1501
Lente, 100 Units 1501
Iletin II 1504
Pork Lente, 100 Units 1504
Purified Pork Lente Insulin 1852

Isocarboxazid (Concurrent use is contraindicated).
No products indexed under this heading.

Isradipine (Potentiation of antihypertensive drugs). Products include:
DynaCirc Capsules 2381
DynaCirc CR Tablets 2383

Ketoprofen (Reduced diuretic, natriuretic, and antihypertensive effects). Products include:
Actron Caplets and Tablets 608
Orudis Capsules 2874

Orudis KT 842
Oruvail Capsules 2874

Ketorolac Tromethamine (Reduced diuretic, natriuretic, and antihypertensive effects). Products include:
Acular Sterile Ophthalmic Solution 470
Toradol 2319

Labetalol Hydrochloride (Potentiation of antihypertensive drugs). Products include:
Normodyne Injection 2519
Normodyne Tablets 2522
Trandate 1158

Levorphanol Tartrate (Potentiation of orthostatic hypotension; enhanced CNS depressant effects of reserpine). Products include:
Levo-Dromoran 2297

Lisinopril (Potentiation of antihypertensive drugs). Products include:
Prinivil Tablets 1776
Prinzide Tablets 1780
Zestoretic Tablets 2968
Zestril Tablets 2972

Lithium Carbonate (Reduced renal clearance of lithium with resultant risk of lithium toxicity). Products include:
Eskalith 2658
Lithium Carbonate Capsules & Tablets 2352
Lithonate/Lithotabs/Lithobid 2721

Lithium Citrate (Reduced renal clearance of lithium with resultant risk of lithium toxicity).
No products indexed under this heading.

Losartan Potassium (Potentiation of antihypertensive drugs). Products include:
Cozaar Tablets 1668
Hyzaar Tablets 1720

Mecamylamine Hydrochloride (Potentiation of antihypertensive drugs). Products include:
Inversine Tablets 1729

Meclofenamate Sodium (Reduced diuretic, natriuretic, and antihypertensive effects).
No products indexed under this heading.

Mefenamic Acid (Reduced diuretic, natriuretic, and antihypertensive effects). Products include:
Ponstel 1982

Meperidine Hydrochloride (Potentiation of orthostatic hypotension; enhanced CNS depressant effects of reserpine). Products include:
Demerol 2438
Mepergan Injection 2859

Mephobarbital (Potentiation of orthostatic hypotension produced by thiazides; enhances CNS depressant effects of reserpine). Products include:
Mebaral Tablets 2452

Metformin Hydrochloride (Hyperglycemia may occur; dosage adjustment of the antidiabetic drug may be required). Products include:
Glucophage Tablets 754

Methadone Hydrochloride (Potentiation of orthostatic hypotension; enhanced CNS depressant effects of reserpine). Products include:
Methadone Hydrochloride Oral Concentrate 2356
Methadone Hydrochloride Oral Solution & Tablets 2357

Methyclothiazide (Potentiation of antihypertensive drugs). Products include:
Enduron Tablets 424

Methyldopa (Potentiation of antihypertensive drugs). Products include:
Aldoclor Tablets 1638

Aldomet Oral 1640
Aldoril Tablets 1644

Methyldopate Hydrochloride (Potentiation of antihypertensive drugs). Products include:
Aldomet Ester HCl Injection 1642

Methylprednisolone Acetate (Potential for intensified electrolyte depletion, particularly hypokalemia).
No products indexed under this heading.

Methylprednisolone Sodium Succinate (Potential for intensified electrolyte depletion, particularly hypokalemia).
No products indexed under this heading.

Metolazone (Potentiation of antihypertensive drugs). Products include:
Mykrox Tablets 1617
Zaroxolyn Tablets 1625

Metoprolol Succinate (Potentiation of antihypertensive drugs). Products include:
Toprol-XL Tablets 560

Metoprolol Tartrate (Potentiation of antihypertensive drugs). Products include:
Lopressor 848
Lopressor HCT Tablets 850

Metyrosine (Potentiation of antihypertensive drugs). Products include:
Demser Capsules 1690

Minoxidil (Potentiation of antihypertensive drugs).
No products indexed under this heading.

Moexipril Hydrochloride (Potentiation of antihypertensive drugs). Products include:
Univasc Tablets 2553

Morphine Sulfate (Potentiation of orthostatic hypotension; enhanced CNS depressant effects of reserpine). Products include:
Astramorph/PF Injection, USP (Preservative-Free) 526
Duramorph Injection 983
Infumorph 200 and Infumorph 500 Sterile Solutions 985
Kadian Capsules 2948
MS Contin Tablets 2149
MSIR 2152
Oramorph SR (Morphine Sulfate Sustained Release Tablets) 2359
RMS Suppositories CII 2766
Roxanol 2365

Nabumetone (Reduced diuretic, natriuretic, and antihypertensive effects). Products include:
Relafen Tablets 2688

Nadolol (Potentiation of antihypertensive drugs).
No products indexed under this heading.

Naproxen (Reduced diuretic, natriuretic, and antihypertensive effects). Products include:
Anaprox/Naprosyn 2277

Naproxen Sodium (Reduced diuretic, natriuretic, and antihypertensive effects). Products include:
Aleve 2124
Anaprox/Naprosyn 2277
Naprelan Tablets 2861

Nicardipine Hydrochloride (Potentiation of antihypertensive drugs). Products include:
Cardene Capsules 2261
Cardene I.V. 2815
Cardene SR Capsules 2264

Nifedipine (Potentiation of antihypertensive drugs). Products include:
Adalat Capsules (10 mg and 20 mg) 580
Adalat CC 582
Procardia Capsules 2024
Procardia XL Extended Release Tablets 2026

Nisoldipine (Potentiation of antihypertensive drugs). Products include:
Sular Tablets 2961

Nitroglycerin (Potentiation of antihypertensive drugs). Products include:
Deponit NTG Transdermal Delivery System 2541
Nitro-Bid IV 1270
Nitro-Bid Ointment 1272
Nitro-Dur (nitroglycerin) Transdermal Infusion System 1365
Nitrolingual Spray 2193
Nitrostat Tablets 1981
Transderm-Nitro Transdermal Therapeutic System 878

Norepinephrine Bitartrate (Decreased arterial responsiveness to norepinephrine). Products include:
Levophed Bitartrate Injection 2445

Opium Alkaloids (Potentiation of orthostatic hypotension; enhanced CNS depressant effects of reserpine).
No products indexed under this heading.

Oxaprozin (Reduced diuretic, natriuretic, and antihypertensive effects). Products include:
Daypro Caplets 2578

Oxycodone Hydrochloride (Potentiation of orthostatic hypotension; enhanced CNS depressant effects of reserpine). Products include:
OxyContin Tablets 2163
OxyIR Capsules 2167
Percocet Tablets 955
Percodan Tablets 955
Percodan-Demi Tablets 956
Roxicodone Tablets, Oral Solution & Intensol (Oxycodone) 2366
Tylox Capsules 1593

Penbutolol Sulfate (Potentiation of antihypertensive drugs). Products include:
Levatol Tablets 2547

Pentobarbital Sodium (Potentiation of orthostatic hypotension produced by thiazides; enhances CNS depressant effects of reserpine). Products include:
Nembutal Sodium Capsules 440
Nembutal Sodium Solution 442
Nembutal Sodium Suppositories 444

Phenelzine Sulfate (Concurrent use is contraindicated). Products include:
Nardil 1977

Phenobarbital (Potentiation of orthostatic hypotension produced by thiazides; enhances CNS depressant effects of reserpine). Products include:
Arco-Lase Plus Tablets 513
Bellergal-S Tablets 2375
Donnatal 2234
Donnatal Extentabs 2234
Donnatal Tablets 2234
Phenobarbital Elixir and Tablets 1523
Quadrinal Tablets 1398

Phenoxybenzamine Hydrochloride (Potentiation of antihypertensive drugs). Products include:
Dibenzyline Capsules 2650

Phentolamine Mesylate (Potentiation of antihypertensive drugs). Products include:
Regitine Vials 864

Phenylbutazone (Reduced diuretic, natriuretic, and antihypertensive effects).
No products indexed under this heading.

Pindolol (Potentiation of antihypertensive drugs). Products include:
Visken Tablets 2428

Piroxicam (Reduced diuretic, natriuretic, and antihypertensive effects). Products include:
Feldene Capsules 2008

(■ Described in PDR For Nonprescription Drugs)   (⊚ Described in PDR For Ophthalmology)

Polythiazide (Potentiation of antihypertensive drugs). Products include:
  Minizide Capsules 2016
Prazosin Hydrochloride (Potentiation of antihypertensive drugs). Products include:
  Minipress Capsules.................. 2015
  Minizide Capsules 2016
Prednisolone Acetate (Potential for intensified electrolyte depletion, particularly hypokalemia). Products include:
  AK-CIDE .... ⓘ 203
  AK-CIDE Ointment .... ⓘ 203
  Blephamide Liquifilm Sterile Ophthalmic Suspension.................. 472
  Blephamide Ointment .... ⓘ 234
  Econopred & Econopred Plus Ophthalmic Suspensions ...... ⓘ 216
  Poly-Pred Liquifilm 246
  Pred Forte................................. 247
  Pred Mild.................................. 250
  Pred-G Liquifilm Sterile Ophthalmic Suspension............... ⓘ 248
  Pred-G S.O.P. Sterile Ophthalmic Ointment................... ⓘ 249
Prednisolone Sodium Phosphate (Potential for intensified electrolyte depletion, particularly hypokalemia). Products include:
  AK-PRED .... ⓘ 204
  Hydeltrasol Injection, Sterile 1708
  Pediapred Oral Solution 1618
Prednisolone Tebutate (Potential for intensified electrolyte depletion, particularly hypokalemia). Products include:
  Hydeltra-T.B.A. Sterile Suspension 1710
Prednisone (Potential for intensified electrolyte depletion, particularly hypokalemia).
  No products indexed under this heading.
Propoxyphene Hydrochloride (Potentiation of orthostatic hypotension; enhanced CNS depressant effects of reserpine). Products include:
  Darvon 1475
  Wygesic Tablets 2930
Propoxyphene Napsylate (Potentiation of orthostatic hypotension; enhanced CNS depressant effects of reserpine). Products include:
  Darvon-N/Darvocet-N 1473
Propranolol Hydrochloride (Potentiation of antihypertensive drugs). Products include:
  Inderal 2834
  Inderal LA Long Acting Capsules 2836
  Inderide Tablets 2838
  Inderide LA Long Acting Capsules ... 2840
Quinapril Hydrochloride (Potentiation of antihypertensive drugs). Products include:
  Accupril Tablets 1950
Quinidine Gluconate (Reserpine causes cardiac arrhythmia, use cautiously with quinidine). Products include:
  Quinaglute Dura-Tabs Tablets 644
Quinidine Polygalacturonate (Reserpine causes cardiac arrhythmia, use cautiously with quinidine). Products include:
  Cardioquin Tablets 2146
Quinidine Sulfate (Reserpine causes cardiac arrhythmia, use cautiously with quinidine). Products include:
  Quinidex Extentabs 2240
Ramipril (Potentiation of antihypertensive drugs). Products include:
  Altace Capsules 1238
Rauwolfia Serpentina (Potentiation of antihypertensive drugs).
  No products indexed under this heading.

Rescinnamine (Potentiation of antihypertensive drugs).
  No products indexed under this heading.
Secobarbital Sodium (Potentiation of orthostatic hypotension produced by thiazides; enhances CNS depressant effects of reserpine). Products include:
  Seconal Sodium Pulvules 1529
Selegiline Hydrochloride (Concurrent use is contraindicated). Products include:
  Eldepryl Capsules 2729
Sodium Nitroprusside (Potentiation of antihypertensive drugs).
  No products indexed under this heading.
Sotalol Hydrochloride (Potentiation of antihypertensive drugs). Products include:
  Betapace Tablets 637
Spirapril Hydrochloride (Potentiation of antihypertensive drugs).
  No products indexed under this heading.
Sufentanil Citrate (Potentiation of orthostatic hypotension; enhanced CNS depressant effects of reserpine). Products include:
  Sufenta Injection 1355
Sulindac (Reduced diuretic, natriuretic, and antihypertensive effects). Products include:
  Clinoril Tablets 1658
Terazosin Hydrochloride (Potentiation of antihypertensive drugs). Products include:
  Hytrin Capsules 434
Thiamylal Sodium (Potentiation of orthostatic hypotension produced by thiazides; enhances CNS depressant effects of reserpine).
  No products indexed under this heading.
Timolol Maleate (Potentiation of antihypertensive drugs). Products include:
  Blocadren Tablets 1654
  Timolide Tablets 1791
  Timoptic in Ocudose 1796
  Timoptic Sterile Ophthalmic Solution.................................. 1794
  Timoptic-XE 1798
Tolazamide (Hyperglycemia may occur; dosage adjustment of the antidiabetic drug may be required).
  No products indexed under this heading.
Tolbutamide (Hyperglycemia may occur; dosage adjustment of the antidiabetic drug may be required).
  No products indexed under this heading.
Tolmetin Sodium (Reduced diuretic, natriuretic, and antihypertensive effects). Products include:
  Tolectin (200, 400 and 600 mg) .. 1591
Torsemide (Potentiation of antihypertensive drugs). Products include:
  Demadex Tablets and Injection 691
Tranylcypromine Sulfate (Concurrent use is contraindicated). Products include:
  Parnate Tablets 2679
Triamcinolone (Potential for intensified electrolyte depletion, particularly hypokalemia).
  No products indexed under this heading.
Triamcinolone Acetonide (Potential for intensified electrolyte depletion, particularly hypokalemia). Products include:
  Azmacort Oral Inhaler 2175
  Nasacort AQ Nasal Spray 2191
  Nasacort Nasal Inhaler 2189

Triamcinolone Diacetate (Potential for intensified electrolyte depletion, particularly hypokalemia).
  No products indexed under this heading.
Triamcinolone Hexacetonide (Potential for intensified electrolyte depletion, particularly hypokalemia).
  No products indexed under this heading.
Trimethaphan Camsylate (Potentiation of antihypertensive drugs).
  No products indexed under this heading.
Tubocurarine Chloride (Increased responsiveness to tubocurarine).
  No products indexed under this heading.
Verapamil Hydrochloride (Potentiation of antihypertensive drugs). Products include:
  Calan SR Caplets 2571
  Calan Tablets 2568
  Covera-HS Tablets 2573
  Isoptin Injectable 1391
  Isoptin Oral Tablets 1393
  Isoptin SR Tablets 1395
  Verelan Capsules 1455

Food Interactions

Alcohol (Potentiation of orthostatic hypotension).

HYLAND'S ARNICAID TABLETS
(Homeopathic Medications) .... ⓘ 788
None cited in PDR database.

HYLAND'S BEDWETTING TABLETS
(Homeopathic Medications) .... ⓘ 788
None cited in PDR database.

HYLAND'S CALMS FORTé TABLETS
(Homeopathic Medications) .... ⓘ 788
None cited in PDR database.

HYLAND'S CLEARAC
(Homeopathic Medications) .... ⓘ 789
None cited in PDR database.

HYLAND'S COLIC TABLETS
(Homeopathic Medications) .... ⓘ 789
None cited in PDR database.

HYLAND'S COUGH SYRUP WITH HONEY
(Ipecac) .... ⓘ 789
None cited in PDR database.

HYLAND'S C-PLUS COLD TABLETS
(Homeopathic Medications) .... ⓘ 789
None cited in PDR database.

HYLAND'S ENURAID TABLETS
(Homeopathic Medications) .... ⓘ 789
None cited in PDR database.

HYLAND'S HEADACHE TABLETS
(Homeopathic Medications, Ipecac, Belladonna Alkaloids).................. ⓘ 790
None cited in PDR database.

HYLAND'S LEG CRAMPS TABLETS
(Homeopathic Medications) .... ⓘ 790
None cited in PDR database.

HYLAND'S TEETHING TABLETS
(Calcium Phosphate, Homeopathic Medications) .... ⓘ 790
None cited in PDR database.

HYLOREL TABLETS
(Guanadrel Sulfate) 1613
May interact with monoamine oxidase inhibitors, phenothiazines, tricyclic antidepressants, vasodilators, sympathomimetic bronchodilators, alpha adrenergic blockers, direct-acting sympathomimetic amines, indirect-acting sympathomimetic amines, beta blockers, catecholamine depleting drugs, and certain other agents. Compounds in these categories include:

Acebutolol Hydrochloride (May cause excessive postural hypotension and bradycardia). Products include:
  Sectral Capsules 2914
Albuterol (May interfere with the hypotensive effect). Products include:
  Proventil Inhalation Aerosol 2524
  Ventolin Inhalation Aerosol and Refill 1170
Albuterol Sulfate (May interfere with the hypotensive effect). Products include:
  Airet Albuterol Sulfate Inhalation Solution 1602
  Albuterol Sulfate, USP Solution for Inhalation, Arm-a-Med 522
  Proventil Inhalation Solution 0.083%............................... 2527
  Proventil Repetabs Tablets 2529
  Proventil Solution for Inhalation 0.5%................................ 2525
  Proventil Syrup 2528
  Proventil Tablets 2529
  Ventolin Inhalation Solution 1171
  Ventolin Nebules Inhalation Solution.................................. 1172
  Ventolin Rotacaps for Inhalation 1173
  Ventolin Syrup 1175
  Ventolin Tablets 1176
  Volmax Extended-Release Tablets .. 1835
Amitriptyline Hydrochloride (Possible reversal of the effects of guanadrel; tricyclic antidepressant, if discontinued abruptly, may enhance effect of guanadrel). Products include:
  Elavil 2945
  Etrafon 2495
  Limbitrol 2333
  Triavil Tablets 1800
Amoxapine (Possible reversal of the effects of guanadrel; tricyclic antidepressant, if discontinued abruptly, may enhance effect of guanadrel). Products include:
  Asendin Tablets 1419
Amphetamine Resins (May reverse the effects of neuronal blocking agents).
  No products indexed under this heading.
Atenolol (May cause excessive postural hypotension and bradycardia). Products include:
  Tenoretic Tablets 2963
  Tenormin Tablets and I.V. Injection 2965
Betaxolol Hydrochloride (May cause excessive postural hypotension and bradycardia). Products include:
  Betoptic Ophthalmic Solution........... 465
  Betoptic S Ophthalmic Suspension 467
  Kerlone Tablets 2588
Bisoprolol Fumarate (May cause excessive postural hypotension and bradycardia). Products include:
  Zebeta Tablets 1457
  Ziac 1459
Bitolterol Mesylate (May interfere with the hypotensive effect). Products include:
  Tornalate Solution for Inhalation, 0.2%.................................. 976
  Tornalate Metered Dose Inhaler 978

IMPORTANT NOTE: Always consult each drug listing in the patient's regimen for possible interactions.

Hylorel / Interactions Index

Carteolol Hydrochloride (May cause excessive postural hypotension and bradycardia). Products include:
- Cartrol Tablets 413
- Ocupress Ophthalmic Solution, 1% Sterile .... ⊚ 297

Chlorpromazine (Possible reversal of the effects of guanadrel). Products include:
- Thorazine Suppositories 2701

Chlorpromazine Hydrochloride (Possible reversal of the effects of guanadrel). Products include:
- Thorazine 2701

Clomipramine Hydrochloride (Possible reversal of the effects of guanadrel; tricyclic antidepressant, if discontinued abruptly, may enhance effect of guanadrel). Products include:
- Anafranil Capsules 819

Deserpidine (May cause excessive postural hypotension and bradycardia).
- No products indexed under this heading.

Desipramine Hydrochloride (Possible reversal of the effects of guanadrel; tricyclic antidepressant, if discontinued abruptly, may enhance effect of guanadrel). Products include:
- Norpramin Tablets 1273

Dextroamphetamine Sulfate (May reverse the effects of neuronal blocking agents). Products include:
- Adderall Tablets 2209
- Dexedrine 2648
- DextroStat-Dextroamphetamine Sulfate Tablets 2211

Diazoxide (Comcomitant use may increase the potential for symptomatic or orthostatic hypotension). Products include:
- Hyperstat I.V. Injection 2504
- Proglycem 575

Doxazosin Mesylate (May cause excessive postural hypotension and bradycardia). Products include:
- Cardura Tablets 1993

Doxepin Hydrochloride (Possible reversal of the effects of guanadrel; tricyclic antidepressant, if discontinued abruptly, may enhance effect of guanadrel). Products include:
- Adapin Capsules 1542
- Sinequan 2028
- Zonalon Cream 1042

Ephedrine Hydrochloride (May interfere with the hypotensive effect; may reverse the effects of neuronal blocking agents). Products include:
- Primatene Tablets .... ▣ 844
- Quadrinal Tablets 1398

Ephedrine Sulfate (May interfere with the hypotensive effect; may reverse the effects of neuronal blocking agents). Products include:
- Marax Tablets & DF Syrup 2015

Ephedrine Tannate (May interfere with the hypotensive effect; may reverse the effects of neuronal blocking agents). Products include:
- Rynatuss 2782

Epinephrine (May interfere with the hypotensive effect). Products include:
- EPIFRIN .... ⊚ 237
- EpiPen 808
- Marcaine with Epinephrine 2446
- Primatene Mist .... ▣ 843
- Sensorcaine with Epinephrine Injection 554
- Sus-Phrine Injection 1017
- Xylocaine with Epinephrine Injections 562

Epinephrine Hydrochloride (May interfere with the hypotensive effect; enhances the activity of direct acting sympathomimetic amines). Products include:
- Ana-Kit Anaphylaxis Emergency Treatment Kit 611

Epoprostenol Sodium (Comcomitant use may increase the potential for symptomatic or orthostatic hypotension). Products include:
- Flolan for Injection 1085

Esmolol Hydrochloride (May cause excessive postural hypotension and bradycardia). Products include:
- Brevibloc (esmolol HCl) Injection .. 1860

Ethylnorepinephrine Hydrochloride (May interfere with the hypotensive effect).
- No products indexed under this heading.

Fluphenazine Decanoate (Possible reversal of the effects of guanadrel). Products include:
- Prolixin Decanoate 510

Fluphenazine Enanthate (Possible reversal of the effects of guanadrel). Products include:
- Prolixin Enanthate 510

Fluphenazine Hydrochloride (Possible reversal of the effects of guanadrel). Products include:
- Prolixin 510

Furazolidone (Concurrent or sequential use with MAO inhibitor is contraindicated). Products include:
- Furoxone 2221

Guanethidine Monosulfate (May cause excessive postural hypotension and bradycardia). Products include:
- Esimil Tablets 840
- Ismelin Tablets 845

Hydralazine Hydrochloride (Comcomitant use may increase the potential for symptomatic or orthostatic hypotension). Products include:
- Apresazide Capsules 824
- Apresoline Hydrochloride Tablets .. 826
- Hydralazine Hydrochloride Injection USP 2712
- Ser-Ap-Es Tablets 867

Imipramine Hydrochloride (Possible reversal of the effects of guanadrel; tricyclic antidepressant, if discontinued abruptly, may enhance effect of guanadrel). Products include:
- Tofranil Ampuls 873
- Tofranil Tablets 875

Imipramine Pamoate (Possible reversal of the effects of guanadrel; tricyclic antidepressant, if discontinued abruptly, may enhance effect of guanadrel). Products include:
- Tofranil-PM Capsules 876

Isocarboxazid (Concurrent or sequential use with MAO inhibitor is contraindicated).
- No products indexed under this heading.

Isoetharine (May interfere with the hypotensive effect). Products include:
- Bronkometer Aerosol 2432
- Bronkosol Solution 2432
- Isoetharine Inhalation Solution, USP, Arm-a-Med 545

Isoproterenol Hydrochloride (May interfere with the hypotensive effect; enhances the activity of direct acting sympathomimetic amines). Products include:
- Isuprel Hydrochloride Solution ... 2443
- Isuprel Injection 2441
- Isuprel Mistometer 2442

Isoproterenol Sulfate (May interfere with the hypotensive effect; enhances the activity of direct acting sympathomimetic amines). Products include:
- Norisodrine with Calcium Iodide Syrup 446

Labetalol Hydrochloride (May cause excessive postural hypotension and bradycardia). Products include:
- Normodyne Injection 2519
- Normodyne Tablets 2522
- Trandate 1158

Levobunolol Hydrochloride (May cause excessive postural hypotension and bradycardia). Products include:
- Betagan .... ⊚ 230

Maprotiline Hydrochloride (Possible reversal of the effects of guanadrel; tricyclic antidepressant, if discontinued abruptly, may enhance effect of guanadrel). Products include:
- Ludiomil Tablets 861

Mesoridazine Besylate (Possible reversal of the effects of guanadrel). Products include:
- Serentil 689

Metaproterenol Sulfate (May interfere with the hypotensive effect). Products include:
- Alupent 672
- Metaproterenol Sulfate Inhalation Solution, USP, Arm-a-Med ... 547

Metaraminol Bitartrate (Enhances the activity of direct acting sympathomimetic amines). Products include:
- Aramine Injection 1649

Methotrimeprazine (Possible reversal of the effects of guanadrel). Products include:
- Levoprome 1321

Metipranolol Hydrochloride (May cause excessive postural hypotension and bradycardia). Products include:
- OptiPranolol (Metipranolol 0.3%) Sterile Ophthalmic Solution .. ⊚ 256

Metoprolol Succinate (May cause excessive postural hypotension and bradycardia). Products include:
- Toprol-XL Tablets 560

Metoprolol Tartrate (May cause excessive postural hypotension and bradycardia). Products include:
- Lopressor 848
- Lopressor HCT Tablets 850

Minoxidil (Comcomitant use may increase the potential for symptomatic or orthostatic hypotension).
- No products indexed under this heading.

Nadolol (May cause excessive postural hypotension and bradycardia).
- No products indexed under this heading.

Norepinephrine Bitartrate (Enhanced effect of norepinephrine). Products include:
- Levophed Bitartrate Injection ... 2445

Norepinephrine Hydrochloride (Enhances the activity of direct acting sympathomimetic amines).

Nortriptyline Hydrochloride (Possible reversal of the effects of guanadrel; tricyclic antidepressant, if discontinued abruptly, may enhance effect of guanadrel). Products include:
- Pamelor 2409

Penbutolol Sulfate (May cause excessive postural hypotension and bradycardia). Products include:
- Levatol Tablets 2547

Perphenazine (Possible reversal of the effects of guanadrel). Products include:
- Etrafon 2495
- Triavil Tablets 1800
- Trilafon 2532

Phenelzine Sulfate (Concurrent or sequential use with MAO inhibitor is contraindicated). Products include:
- Nardil 1977

Phenylephrine Hydrochloride (Enhances the activity of direct acting sympathomimetic amines). Products include:
- Atrohist Plus Tablets 1605
- Cerose DM .... ▣ 853
- D.A. II Tablets 972
- D.A. Chewable Tablets 970
- Dura-Vent/DA Tablets 972
- Extendryl 1003
- 4-Way Fast Acting Nasal Spray (regular & mentholated) ..... ▣ 644
- Hemorid .... ▣ 797
- Hycomine Compound Tablets 948
- Neo-Synephrine Hydrochloride 1% Carpuject 2455
- Neo-Synephrine Hydrochloride 1% Injection 2455
- Neo-Synephrine Hydrochloride (Ophthalmic) 2456
- Neo-Synephrine .... ▣ 624
- Novahistine Elixir .... ▣ 782
- Phenergan VC 2886
- Phenergan VC with Codeine 2888
- Preparation H .... ▣ 842
- Tympagesic Ear Drops 2476
- Vicks Sinex Nasal Spray and Ultra Fine Mist .... ▣ 738

Phenylephrine Tannate (Enhances the activity of direct acting sympathomimetic amines). Products include:
- Atrohist Pediatric Suspension ... 1604
- Atrohist Pediatric Suspension Dye-Free 1604
- Rynatan 2781
- Rynatuss 2782

Phenylpropanolamine Hydrochloride (May reverse the effects of neuronal blocking agents). Products include:
- Acutrim .... ▣ 648
- Atrohist Plus Tablets 1605
- BC Cold Powder Multi-Symptom Formula (Cold-Sinus-Allergy) ... ▣ 631
- BC Cold Powder Non-Drowsy Formula (Cold-Sinus) .... ▣ 631
- Cheracol Plus Head Cold/Cough Formula .... ▣ 741
- Comtrex Multi-Symptom Cold Reliever Liqui-Gels .... ▣ 638
- Comtrex Multi-Symptom Non-Drowsy Liqui-gels .... ▣ 640
- Contac Continuous Action Nasal Decongestant/Antihistamine 12 Hour Capsules .... ▣ 773
- Contac Maximum Strength Continuous Action Decongestant/Antihistamine 12 Hour Caplets ... ▣ 772
- Contac Severe Cold and Flu Formula Caplets .... ▣ 773
- Coricidin 'D' Decongestant Tablets .... ▣ 760
- Dexatrim 795
- Dexatrim Plus Vitamins Caplets ... ▣ 796
- Dimetane-DC Cough Syrup 2232
- Dimetapp Allergy Sinus Caplets ... ▣ 838
- Dimetapp Cold & Allergy Chewable Tablets .... ▣ 838
- Dimetapp Cold & Cough Liqui-Gels .... ▣ 839
- Dimetapp DM Elixir .... ▣ 840
- Dimetapp Elixir .... ▣ 840
- Dimetapp Extentabs .... ▣ 841
- Dimetapp Tablets/Liqui-Gels .. ▣ 841
- Dura-Vent Tablets 971
- Entex LA Tablets 972
- Exgest LA Tablets 787
- Hycomine 947
- Nolamine Timed-Release Tablets ... 790
- Ornade Spansule Capsules 2678
- Propagest Tablets 791
- Pyrroxate Caplets .... ▣ 742
- Robitussin-CF .... ▣ 846
- Sinulin Tablets 792
- Tavist-D 12 Hour Relief Tablets ... ▣ 750

(▣ Described in PDR For Nonprescription Drugs)   (⊚ Described in PDR For Ophthalmology)

508

509 **Interactions Index** **Hyperstat I.V.**

Teldrin 12 Hour Antihistamine/ Nasal Decongestant Allergy Relief Capsules 786
Triaminic Expectorant 753
Triaminic Syrup 755
Triaminic Triaminicol Cold & Cough 756
Triaminic DM Syrup 756
Triaminicin Tablets 756
Vicks DayQuil Allergy Relief 12-Hour Extended Release Tablets.. 733
Vicks DayQuil Allergy Relief 4-Hour Tablets 733
Vicks DayQuil SINUS Pressure & CONGESTION Relief 734

Pindolol (May cause excessive postural hypotension and bradycardia). Products include:
Visken Tablets 2428

Pirbuterol Acetate (May interfere with the hypotensive effect). Products include:
Maxair Autohaler 1550
Maxair Inhaler 1552

Prazosin Hydrochloride (May cause excessive postural hypotension and bradycardia). Products include:
Minipress Capsules 2015
Minizide Capsules 2016

Prochlorperazine (Possible reversal of the effects of guanadrel). Products include:
Compazine 2644

Promethazine Hydrochloride (Possible reversal of the effects of guanadrel). Products include:
Mepergan Injection 2859
Phenergan with Codeine 2883
Phenergan with Dextromethorphan 2885
Phenergan Injection 2880
Phenergan Suppositories 2882
Phenergan Syrup 2881
Phenergan Tablets 2882
Phenergan VC 2886
Phenergan VC with Codeine 2888

Propranolol Hydrochloride (May cause excessive postural hypotension and bradycardia). Products include:
Inderal 2834
Inderal LA Long Acting Capsules ... 2836
Inderide Tablets 2838
Inderide LA Long Acting Capsules .. 2840

Protriptyline Hydrochloride (Possible reversal of the effects of guanadrel; tricyclic antidepressant, if discontinued abruptly, may enhance effect of guanadrel). Products include:
Vivactil Tablets 1820

Rauwolfia Serpentina (May cause excessive postural hypotension and bradycardia).
No products indexed under this heading.

Rescinnamine (May cause excessive postural hypotension and bradycardia).
No products indexed under this heading.

Reserpine (May cause excessive postural hypotension and bradycardia). Products include:
Diupres Tablets 1691
Hydropres Tablets 1718
Ser-Ap-Es Tablets 867

Salmeterol Xinafoate (May interfere with the hypotensive effect). Products include:
Serevent Inhalation Aerosol 1149

Selegiline Hydrochloride (Concurrent or sequential use with MAO inhibitor is contraindicated). Products include:
Eldepryl Capsules 2729

Sotalol Hydrochloride (May cause excessive postural hypotension and bradycardia). Products include:
Betapace Tablets 637

Terazosin Hydrochloride (May cause excessive postural hypotension and bradycardia). Products include:
Hytrin Capsules 434

Terbutaline Sulfate (May interfere with the hypotensive effect). Products include:
Brethaire Inhaler 830
Brethine Ampuls 832
Brethine Tablets 831
Bricanyl Subcutaneous Injection 1247
Bricanyl Tablets 1248

Thioridazine Hydrochloride (Possible reversal of the effects of guanadrel). Products include:
Mellaril 2398

Timolol Hemihydrate (May cause excessive postural hypotension and bradycardia). Products include:
Betimol 0.25%, 0.5% .... ⊛ 259

Timolol Maleate (May cause excessive postural hypotension and bradycardia). Products include:
Blocadren Tablets 1654
Timolide Tablets 1791
Timoptic in Ocudose 1796
Timoptic Sterile Ophthalmic Solution 1794
Timoptic-XE 1798

Tranylcypromine Sulfate (Concurrent or sequential use with MAO inhibitor is contraindicated). Products include:
Parnate Tablets 2679

Trifluoperazine Hydrochloride (Possible reversal of the effects of guanadrel). Products include:
Stelazine 2692

Trimipramine Maleate (Possible reversal of the effects of guanadrel; tricyclic antidepressant, if discontinued abruptly, may enhance effect of guanadrel). Products include:
Surmontil Capsules 2917

Food Interactions

Alcohol (Exaggerates postural hypotension).

HYPERAB RABIES IMMUNE GLOBULIN (HUMAN)
(Rabies Immune Globulin (Human)) .. 618
May interact with:

Measles Virus Vaccine Live (Interference with the response to live viral vaccines). Products include:
Attenuvax 1650

Measles & Rubella Virus Vaccine Live (Interference with the response to live viral vaccines). Products include:
M-R-VAX II 1732

Measles, Mumps & Rubella Virus Vaccine Live (Interference with the response to live viral vaccines). Products include:
M-M-R II 1730

Mumps Virus Vaccine, Live (Interference with the response to live viral vaccines). Products include:
Mumpsvax 1751

Poliovirus Vaccine, Live, Oral, Trivalent, Types 1,2,3 (Sabin) (Interference with the response to live viral vaccines). Products include:
Orimune 1433

Rubella Virus Vaccine Live (Interference with the response to live viral vaccines). Products include:
Meruvax II 1740

Rubella & Mumps Virus Vaccine Live (Interference with the response to live viral vaccines). Products include:
Biavax II 1653

HYPERHEP HEPATITIS B IMMUNE GLOBULIN (HUMAN)
(Hepatitis B Immune Globulin (Human)) 619
May interact with:

Vaccines (Live) (May interfere with response. Use should be deferred for 3 months after administration of HyperHep).

HYPERSTAT I.V. INJECTION
(Diazoxide) 2504
May interact with antihypertensives, oral anticoagulants, beta blockers, diuretics, and certain other agents. Compounds in these categories include:

Acebutolol Hydrochloride (An undesirable hypotension may result when diazoxide is administered to patients who have received other antihypertensive agents within six hours; do not administer within six hours). Products include:
Sectral Capsules 2914

Amiloride Hydrochloride (Potentiates the hyperuricemic and antihypertensive effects of diazoxide). Products include:
Midamor Tablets 1746
Moduretic Tablets 1748

Amlodipine Besylate (An undesirable hypotension may result when diazoxide is administered to patients who have received other antihypertensive agents within six hours). Products include:
Lotrel Capsules 858
Norvasc Tablets 2020

Atenolol (An undesirable hypotension may result when diazoxide is administered to patients who have received other antihypertensive agents within six hours; do not administer within six hours). Products include:
Tenoretic Tablets 2963
Tenormin Tablets and I.V. Injection 2965

Benazepril Hydrochloride (An undesirable hypotension may result when diazoxide is administered to patients who have received other antihypertensive agents within six hours). Products include:
Lotensin Tablets 852
Lotensin HCT Tablets 855
Lotrel Capsules 858

Bendroflumethiazide (Potentiates the hyperuricemic and antihypertensive effects of diazoxide).
No products indexed under this heading.

Betaxolol Hydrochloride (An undesirable hypotension may result when diazoxide is administered to patients who have received other antihypertensive agents within six hours; do not administer within six hours). Products include:
Betoptic Ophthalmic Solution 465
Betoptic S Ophthalmic Suspension 467
Kerlone Tablets 2588

Bisoprolol Fumarate (An undesirable hypotension may result when diazoxide is administered to patients who have received other antihypertensive agents within six hours; do not administer within six hours). Products include:
Zebeta Tablets 1457
Ziac 1459

Bumetanide (Potentiates the hyperuricemic and antihypertensive effects of diazoxide). Products include:
Bumex 2260

Captopril (An undesirable hypotension may result when diazoxide is administered to patients who have received other antihypertensive agents within six hours). Products include:
Capoten Tablets 740
Capozide Tablets 744

Carteolol Hydrochloride (An undesirable hypotension may result when diazoxide is administered to patients who have received other antihypertensive agents within six hours; do not administer within six hours). Products include:
Cartrol Tablets 413
Ocupress Ophthalmic Solution, 1% Sterile .... ⊛ 297

Chlorothiazide (Potentiates the hyperuricemic and antihypertensive effects of diazoxide). Products include:
Aldoclor Tablets 1638
Diupres Tablets 1691
Diuril Oral 1694

Chlorothiazide Sodium (Potentiates the hyperuricemic and antihypertensive effects of diazoxide). Products include:
Diuril Sodium Intravenous 1693

Chlorthalidone (Potentiates the hyperuricemic and antihypertensive effects of diazoxide). Products include:
Combipres Tablets 682
Tenoretic Tablets 2963
Thalitone 1293

Clonidine (An undesirable hypotension may result when diazoxide is administered to patients who have received other antihypertensive agents within six hours). Products include:
Catapres-TTS 680

Clonidine Hydrochloride (An undesirable hypotension may result when diazoxide is administered to patients who have received other antihypertensive agents within six hours). Products include:
Catapres Tablets 679
Combipres Tablets 682

Deserpidine (An undesirable hypotension may result when diazoxide is administered to patients who have received other antihypertensive agents within six hours).
No products indexed under this heading.

Dicumarol (Increased blood levels of coumarin derivatives due to displacement from protein binding sites).
No products indexed under this heading.

Diltiazem Hydrochloride (An undesirable hypotension may result when diazoxide is administered to patients who have received other antihypertensive agents within six hours). Products include:
Cardizem CD Capsules 1251
Cardizem SR Capsules 1255
Cardizem Injectable 1253
Cardizem Tablets 1257
Dilacor XR Extended-release Capsules 2183
Tiazac Capsules 1019

Doxazosin Mesylate (An undesirable hypotension may result when diazoxide is administered to patients who have received other antihypertensive agents within six hours). Products include:
Cardura Tablets 1993

IMPORTANT NOTE: Always consult each drug listing in the patient's regimen for possible interactions.

Hyperstat I.V. Interactions Index 510

Enalapril Maleate (An undesirable hypotension may result when diazoxide is administered to patients who have received other antihypertensive agents within six hours). Products include:
Vaseretic Tablets ... 1810
Vasotec Tablets ... 1816
Enalaprilat (An undesirable hypotension may result when diazoxide is administered to patients who have received other antihypertensive agents within six hours). Products include:
Vasotec I.V. ... 1814
Esmolol Hydrochloride (An undesirable hypotension may result when diazoxide is administered to patients who have received other antihypertensive agents within six hours; do not administer within six hours). Products include:
Brevibloc (esmolol HCl) Injection ... 1860
Ethacrynic Acid (Potentiates the hyperuricemic and antihypertensive effects of diazoxide). Products include:
Edecrin Tablets ... 1698
Felodipine (An undesirable hypotension may result when diazoxide is administered to patients who have received other antihypertensive agents within six hours). Products include:
Plendil Extended-Release Tablets ... 514
Fosinopril Sodium (An undesirable hypotension may result when diazoxide is administered to patients who have received other antihypertensive agents within six hours). Products include:
Monopril Tablets ... 762
Furosemide (Potentiates the hyperuricemic and antihypertensive effects of diazoxide). Products include:
Lasix Injection, Oral Solution and Tablets ... 1267
Guanabenz Acetate (An undesirable hypotension may result when diazoxide is administered to patients who have received other antihypertensive agents within six hours).
No products indexed under this heading.
Guanethidine Monosulfate (An undesirable hypotension may result when diazoxide is administered to patients who have received other antihypertensive agents within six hours). Products include:
Esimil Tablets ... 840
Ismelin Tablets ... 845
Hydralazine Hydrochloride (Co-administration with methyldopa and hydralazine has produced excessive hypotension; do not administer within six hours). Products include:
Apresazide Capsules ... 824
Apresoline Hydrochloride Tablets ... 826
Hydralazine Hydrochloride Injection USP ... 2712
Ser-Ap-Es Tablets ... 867
Hydrochlorothiazide (Potentiates the hyperuricemic and antihypertensive effects of diazoxide). Products include:
Aldactazide Tablets ... 2556
Aldoril Tablets ... 1644
Apresazide Capsules ... 824
Capozide Tablets ... 744
Dyazide Capsules ... 2653
Esidrix Tablets ... 839
Esimil Tablets ... 840
HydroDIURIL Tablets ... 1716
Hydropres Tablets ... 1718
Hyzaar Tablets ... 1720
Inderide Tablets ... 2838
Inderide LA Long Acting Capsules ... 2840
Lopressor HCT Tablets ... 850
Lotensin HCT Tablets ... 855
Moduretic Tablets ... 1748
Oretic Tablets ... 450
Prinzide Tablets ... 1780
Ser-Ap-Es Tablets ... 867
Timolide Tablets ... 1791
Vaseretic Tablets ... 1810
Zestoretic Tablets ... 2968
Ziac ... 1459
Hydroflumethiazide (Potentiates the hyperuricemic and antihypertensive effects of diazoxide). Products include:
Diucardin Tablets ... 2824
Indapamide (Potentiates the hyperuricemic and antihypertensive effects of diazoxide).
No products indexed under this heading.
Isradipine (An undesirable hypotension may result when diazoxide is administered to patients who have received other antihypertensive agents within six hours). Products include:
DynaCirc Capsules ... 2381
DynaCirc CR Tablets ... 2383
Labetalol Hydrochloride (An undesirable hypotension may result when diazoxide is administered to patients who have received other antihypertensive agents within six hours; do not administer within six hours). Products include:
Normodyne Injection ... 2519
Normodyne Tablets ... 2522
Trandate ... 1158
Levobunolol Hydrochloride (An undesirable hypotension may result when diazoxide is administered to patients who have received other antihypertensive agents within six hours; do not administer within six hours). Products include:
Betagan ... ⊙ 230
Lisinopril (An undesirable hypotension may result when diazoxide is administered to patients who have received other antihypertensive agents within six hours). Products include:
Prinivil Tablets ... 1776
Prinzide Tablets ... 1780
Zestoretic Tablets ... 2968
Zestril Tablets ... 2972
Losartan Potassium (An undesirable hypotension may result when diazoxide is administered to patients who have received other antihypertensive agents within six hours). Products include:
Cozaar Tablets ... 1668
Hyzaar Tablets ... 1720
Mecamylamine Hydrochloride (An undesirable hypotension may result when diazoxide is administered to patients who have received other antihypertensive agents within six hours). Products include:
Inversine Tablets ... 1729
Methyclothiazide (Potentiates the hyperuricemic and antihypertensive effects of diazoxide). Products include:
Enduron Tablets ... 424
Methyldopa (Co-administration with methyldopa and hydralazine has produced excessive hypotension; do not administer within six hours). Products include:
Aldoclor Tablets ... 1638
Aldomet Oral ... 1640
Aldoril Tablets ... 1644
Methyldopate Hydrochloride (Co-administration with methyldopa and hydralazine has produced excessive hypotension; do not administer within six hours). Products include:
Aldomet Ester HCl Injection ... 1642
Metipranolol Hydrochloride (An undesirable hypotension may result when diazoxide is administered to patients who have received other antihypertensive agents within six hours; do not administer within six hours). Products include:
OptiPranolol (Metipranolol 0.3%) Sterile Ophthalmic Solution ... ⊙ 256
Metolazone (Potentiates the hyperuricemic and antihypertensive effects of diazoxide). Products include:
Mykrox Tablets ... 1617
Zaroxolyn Tablets ... 1625
Metoprolol Succinate (An undesirable hypotension may result when diazoxide is administered to patients who have received other antihypertensive agents within six hours; do not administer within six hours). Products include:
Toprol-XL Tablets ... 560
Metoprolol Tartrate (An undesirable hypotension may result when diazoxide is administered to patients who have received other antihypertensive agents within six hours; do not administer within six hours). Products include:
Lopressor ... 848
Lopressor HCT Tablets ... 850
Metyrosine (An undesirable hypotension may result when diazoxide is administered to patients who have received other antihypertensive agents within six hours). Products include:
Demser Capsules ... 1690
Minoxidil (An undesirable hypotension may result when diazoxide is administered to patients who have received other antihypertensive agents within six hours; do not administer within six hours).
No products indexed under this heading.
Moexipril Hydrochloride (An undesirable hypotension may result when diazoxide is administered to patients who have received other antihypertensive agents within six hours). Products include:
Univasc Tablets ... 2553
Nadolol (An undesirable hypotension may result when diazoxide is administered to patients who have received other antihypertensive agents within six hours; do not administer within six hours).
No products indexed under this heading.
Nicardipine Hydrochloride (An undesirable hypotension may result when diazoxide is administered to patients who have received other antihypertensive agents within six hours). Products include:
Cardene Capsules ... 2261
Cardene I.V. ... 2815
Cardene SR Capsules ... 2264
Nifedipine (An undesirable hypotension may result when diazoxide is administered to patients who have received other antihypertensive agents within six hours). Products include:
Adalat Capsules (10 mg and 20 mg) ... 580
Adalat CC ... 582
Procardia Capsules ... 2024
Procardia XL Extended Release Tablets ... 2026
Nisoldipine (An undesirable hypotension may result when diazoxide is administered to patients who have received other antihypertensive agents within six hours). Products include:
Sular Tablets ... 2961
Nitroglycerin (An undesirable hypotension may result when diazoxide is administered to patients who have received other antihypertensive agents within six hours; do not administer within six hours). Products include:
Deponit NTG Transdermal Delivery System ... 2541
Nitro-Bid IV ... 1270
Nitro-Bid Ointment ... 1272
Nitro-Dur (nitroglycerin) Transdermal Infusion System ... 1365
Nitrolingual Spray ... 2193
Nitrostat Tablets ... 1981
Transderm-Nitro Transdermal Therapeutic System ... 878
Papaverine Hydrochloride (An undesirable hypotension may result when diazoxide is administered to patients who have received other antihypertensive agents within six hours; do not administer within six hours). Products include:
Papaverine Hydrochloride Vials and Ampoules ... 1523
Penbutolol Sulfate (An undesirable hypotension may result when diazoxide is administered to patients who have received other antihypertensive agents within six hours; do not administer within six hours). Products include:
Levatol Tablets ... 2547
Phenoxybenzamine Hydrochloride (An undesirable hypotension may result when diazoxide is administered to patients who have received other antihypertensive agents within six hours). Products include:
Dibenzyline Capsules ... 2650
Phentolamine Mesylate (An undesirable hypotension may result when diazoxide is administered to patients who have received other antihypertensive agents within six hours). Products include:
Regitine Vials ... 864
Pindolol (An undesirable hypotension may result when diazoxide is administered to patients who have received other antihypertensive agents within six hours; do not administer within six hours). Products include:
Visken Tablets ... 2428
Polythiazide (Potentiates the hyperuricemic and antihypertensive effects of diazoxide). Products include:
Minizide Capsules ... 2016
Prazosin Hydrochloride (An undesirable hypotension may result when diazoxide is administered to patients who have received other antihypertensive agents within six hours; do not administer within six hours). Products include:
Minipress Capsules ... 2015
Minizide Capsules ... 2016
Propranolol Hydrochloride (An undesirable hypotension may result when diazoxide is administered to patients who have received other antihypertensive agents within six hours; do not administer within six hours). Products include:
Inderal ... 2834
Inderal LA Long Acting Capsules ... 2836
Inderide Tablets ... 2838
Inderide LA Long Acting Capsules ... 2840

(▣ Described in PDR For Nonprescription Drugs) (⊙ Described in PDR For Ophthalmology)

Quinapril Hydrochloride (An undesirable hypotension may result when diazoxide is administered to patients who have received other antihypertensive agents within six hours). Products include:
Accupril Tablets 1950

Ramipril (An undesirable hypotension may result when diazoxide is administered to patients who have received other antihypertensive agents within six hours). Products include:
Altace Capsules 1238

Rauwolfia Serpentina (An undesirable hypotension may result when diazoxide is administered to patients who have received other antihypertensive agents within six hours).
No products indexed under this heading.

Rescinnamine (An undesirable hypotension may result when diazoxide is administered to patients who have received other antihypertensive agents within six hours).
No products indexed under this heading.

Reserpine (Co-administration with reserpine and hydralazine has produced maternal hypotension and fetal bradycardia in a patient in labor; do not administer within six hours). Products include:
Diupres Tablets 1691
Hydropres Tablets 1718
Ser-Ap-Es Tablets 867

Sodium Nitroprusside (An undesirable hypotension may result when diazoxide is administered to patients who have received other antihypertensive agents within six hours).
No products indexed under this heading.

Sotalol Hydrochloride (An undesirable hypotension may result when diazoxide is administered to patients who have received other antihypertensive agents within six hours; do not administer within six hours). Products include:
Betapace Tablets 637

Spirapril Hydrochloride (An undesirable hypotension may result when diazoxide is administered to patients who have received other antihypertensive agents within six hours).
No products indexed under this heading.

Spironolactone (Potentiates the hyperuricemic and antihypertensive effects of diazoxide). Products include:
Aldactazide Tablets 2556
Aldactone Tablets 2558

Terazosin Hydrochloride (An undesirable hypotension may result when diazoxide is administered to patients who have received other antihypertensive agents within six hours). Products include:
Hytrin Capsules 434

Timolol Hemihydrate (An undesirable hypotension may result when diazoxide is administered to patients who have received other antihypertensive agents within six hours). Products include:
Betimol 0.25%, 0.5% .... ⓔ 259

Timolol Maleate (An undesirable hypotension may result when diazoxide is administered to patients who have received other antihypertensive agents within six hours; do not administer within six hours). Products include:
Blocadren Tablets 1654
Timolide Tablets 1791
Timoptic in Ocudose 1796
Timoptic Sterile Ophthalmic Solution 1794
Timoptic-XE 1798

Torsemide (Potentiates the hyperuricemic and antihypertensive effects of diazoxide). Products include:
Demadex Tablets and Injection 691

Triamterene (Potentiates the hyperuricemic and antihypertensive effects of diazoxide). Products include:
Dyazide Capsules 2653
Dyrenium Capsules 2655

Trimethaphan Camsylate (An undesirable hypotension may result when diazoxide is administered to patients who have received other antihypertensive agents within six hours).
No products indexed under this heading.

Verapamil Hydrochloride (An undesirable hypotension may result when diazoxide is administered to patients who have received other antihypertensive agents within six hours). Products include:
Calan SR Caplets 2571
Calan Tablets 2568
Covera-HS Tablets 2573
Isoptin Injectable 1391
Isoptin Oral Tablets 1393
Isoptin SR Tablets 1395
Verelan Capsules 1455

Warfarin Sodium (Increased blood levels of coumarin derivatives due to displacement from protein binding sites). Products include:
Coumadin 941

HYPER-TET TETANUS IMMUNE GLOBULIN (HUMAN)
(Tetanus Immune Globulin (Human)) 621
May interact with:

Vaccines (Live) (May interfere with response. Use should be deferred for 3 months).

HYPOTEARS LUBRICANT EYE DROPS
(Polyvinyl Alcohol) .... ⓔ 262
None cited in PDR database.

HYPOTEARS OINTMENT
(Petrolatum, White) .... ⓔ 262
None cited in PDR database.

HYPOTEARS PF LUBRICANT EYE DROPS
(Polyvinyl Alcohol) .... ⓔ 262
None cited in PDR database.

HYPRHO-D FULL DOSE RHO (D) IMMUNE GLOBULIN (HUMAN)
(Immune Globulin (Human)) 623
May interact with:

Measles Virus Vaccine Live (Interference with response to live vaccines). Products include:
Attenuvax 1650

Measles & Rubella Virus Vaccine Live (Interference with response to live vaccines). Products include:
M-R-VAX II 1732

Measles, Mumps & Rubella Virus Vaccine Live (Interference with response to live vaccines). Products include:
M-M-R II 1730

Rubella Virus Vaccine Live (Interference with response to live vaccines). Products include:
Meruvax II 1740

Rubella & Mumps Virus Vaccine Live (Interference with response to live vaccines). Products include:
Biavax II 1653

HYPRHO-D MINI-DOSE RHO (D) IMMUNE GLOBULIN (HUMAN)
(Immune Globulin (Human)) 622
May interact with:

Measles Virus Vaccine Live (Interference with response to live vaccines). Products include:
Attenuvax 1650

Measles & Rubella Virus Vaccine Live (Interference with response to live vaccines). Products include:
M-R-VAX II 1732

Measles, Mumps & Rubella Virus Vaccine Live (Interference with response to live vaccines). Products include:
M-M-R II 1730

Rubella Virus Vaccine Live (Interference with response to live vaccines). Products include:
Meruvax II 1740

Rubella & Mumps Virus Vaccine Live (Interference with response to live vaccines). Products include:
Biavax II 1653

HYSKON HYSTEROSCOPY FLUID
(Dextran 70) 1633
None cited in PDR database.

HYTONE CREAM 2 ½%
(Hydrocortisone) 922
None cited in PDR database.

HYTONE LOTION 2 ½%
(Hydrocortisone) 922
None cited in PDR database.

HYTONE OINTMENT 2 ½%
(Hydrocortisone) 923
None cited in PDR database.

HYTRIN CAPSULES
(Terazosin Hydrochloride) 434
May interact with antihypertensives and certain other agents. Compounds in these categories include:

Acebutolol Hydrochloride (Possibility of significant hypotension; dosage adjustment may be necessary). Products include:
Sectral Capsules 2914

Amlodipine Besylate (Possibility of significant hypotension; dosage adjustment may be necessary). Products include:
Lotrel Capsules 858
Norvasc Tablets 2020

Atenolol (Possibility of significant hypotension; dosage adjustment may be necessary). Products include:
Tenoretic Tablets 2963
Tenormin Tablets and I.V. Injection 2965

Benazepril Hydrochloride (Possibility of significant hypotension; dosage adjustment may be necessary). Products include:
Lotensin Tablets 852
Lotensin HCT Tablets 855
Lotrel Capsules 858

Bendroflumethiazide (Possibility of significant hypotension; dosage adjustment may be necessary).
No products indexed under this heading.

Betaxolol Hydrochloride (Possibility of significant hypotension; dosage adjustment may be necessary). Products include:
Betoptic Ophthalmic Solution 465
Betoptic S Ophthalmic Suspension 467
Kerlone Tablets 2588

Bisoprolol Fumarate (Possibility of significant hypotension; dosage adjustment may be necessary). Products include:
Zebeta Tablets 1457
Ziac 1459

Captopril (Co-administration increases terazosin's maximum plasma concentrations linearly with dose at steady-state after administration of terazosin plus captopril). Products include:
Capoten Tablets 740
Capozide Tablets 744

Carteolol Hydrochloride (Possibility of significant hypotension; dosage adjustment may be necessary). Products include:
Cartrol Tablets 413
Ocupress Ophthalmic Solution, 1% Sterile .... ⓔ 297

Chlorothiazide (Possibility of significant hypotension; dosage adjustment may be necessary). Products include:
Aldoclor Tablets 1638
Diupres Tablets 1691
Diuril Oral 1694

Chlorothiazide Sodium (Possibility of significant hypotension; dosage adjustment may be necessary). Products include:
Diuril Sodium Intravenous 1693

Chlorthalidone (Possibility of significant hypotension; dosage adjustment may be necessary). Products include:
Combipres Tablets 682
Tenoretic Tablets 2963
Thalitone 1293

Clonidine (Possibility of significant hypotension; dosage adjustment may be necessary). Products include:
Catapres-TTS 680

Clonidine Hydrochloride (Possibility of significant hypotension; dosage adjustment may be necessary). Products include:
Catapres Tablets 679
Combipres Tablets 682

Deserpidine (Possibility of significant hypotension; dosage adjustment may be necessary).
No products indexed under this heading.

Diazoxide (Possibility of significant hypotension; dosage adjustment may be necessary). Products include:
Hyperstat I.V. Injection 2504
Proglycem 575

Diltiazem Hydrochloride (Possibility of significant hypotension; dosage adjustment may be necessary). Products include:
Cardizem CD Capsules 1251
Cardizem SR Capsules 1255
Cardizem Injectable 1253
Cardizem Tablets 1257

IMPORTANT NOTE: Always consult each drug listing in the patient's regimen for possible interactions.

Hytrin / Interactions Index

Doxazosin Mesylate (Possibility of significant hypotension; dosage adjustment may be necessary). Products include:
- Dilacor XR Extended-release Capsules 2183
- Tiazac Capsules 1019
- Cardura Tablets 1993

Enalapril Maleate (Possibility of significant hypotension; dosage adjustment may be necessary). Products include:
- Vaseretic Tablets 1810
- Vasotec Tablets 1816

Enalaprilat (Possibility of significant hypotension; dosage adjustment may be necessary). Products include:
- Vasotec I.V. 1814

Esmolol Hydrochloride (Possibility of significant hypotension; dosage adjustment may be necessary). Products include:
- Brevibloc (esmolol HCl) Injection 1860

Felodipine (Possibility of significant hypotension; dosage adjustment may be necessary). Products include:
- Plendil Extended-Release Tablets 514

Fosinopril Sodium (Possibility of significant hypotension; dosage adjustment may be necessary). Products include:
- Monopril Tablets 762

Furosemide (Possibility of significant hypotension; dosage adjustment may be necessary). Products include:
- Lasix Injection, Oral Solution and Tablets 1267

Guanabenz Acetate (Possibility of significant hypotension; dosage adjustment may be necessary).
- No products indexed under this heading.

Guanethidine Monosulfate (Possibility of significant hypotension; dosage adjustment may be necessary). Products include:
- Esimil Tablets 840
- Ismelin Tablets 845

Hydralazine Hydrochloride (Possibility of significant hypotension; dosage adjustment may be necessary). Products include:
- Apresazide Capsules 824
- Apresoline Hydrochloride Tablets .. 826
- Hydralazine Hydrochloride Injection USP 2712
- Ser-Ap-Es Tablets 867

Hydrochlorothiazide (Possibility of significant hypotension; dosage adjustment may be necessary). Products include:
- Aldactazide Tablets 2556
- Aldoril Tablets 1644
- Apresazide Capsules 824
- Capozide Tablets 744
- Dyazide Capsules 2653
- Esidrix Tablets 839
- Esimil Tablets 840
- HydroDIURIL Tablets 1716
- Hydropres Tablets 1718
- Hyzaar Tablets 1720
- Inderide Tablets 2838
- Inderide LA Long Acting Capsules .. 2840
- Lopressor HCT Tablets 850
- Lotensin HCT Tablets 855
- Moduretic Tablets 1748
- Oretic Tablets 450
- Prinzide Tablets 1780
- Ser-Ap-Es Tablets 867
- Timolide Tablets 1791
- Vaseretic Tablets 1810
- Zestoretic Tablets 2968
- Ziac 1459

Hydroflumethiazide (Possibility of significant hypotension; dosage adjustment may be necessary). Products include:
- Diucardin Tablets 2824

Indapamide (Possibility of significant hypotension; dosage adjustment may be necessary).
- No products indexed under this heading.

Isradipine (Possibility of significant hypotension; dosage adjustment may be necessary). Products include:
- DynaCirc Capsules 2381
- DynaCirc CR Tablets 2383

Labetalol Hydrochloride (Possibility of significant hypotension; dosage adjustment may be necessary). Products include:
- Normodyne Injection 2519
- Normodyne Tablets 2522
- Trandate 1158

Lisinopril (Possibility of significant hypotension; dosage adjustment may be necessary). Products include:
- Prinivil Tablets 1776
- Prinzide Tablets 1780
- Zestoretic Tablets 2968
- Zestril Tablets 2972

Losartan Potassium (Possibility of significant hypotension; dosage adjustment may be necessary). Products include:
- Cozaar Tablets 1668
- Hyzaar Tablets 1720

Mecamylamine Hydrochloride (Possibility of significant hypotension; dosage adjustment may be necessary). Products include:
- Inversine Tablets 1729

Methyclothiazide (Possibility of significant hypotension; dosage adjustment may be necessary). Products include:
- Enduron Tablets 424

Methyldopa (Possibility of significant hypotension; dosage adjustment may be necessary). Products include:
- Aldoclor Tablets 1638
- Aldomet Oral 1640
- Aldoril Tablets 1644

Methyldopate Hydrochloride (Possibility of significant hypotension; dosage adjustment may be necessary). Products include:
- Aldomet Ester HCl Injection 1642

Metolazone (Possibility of significant hypotension; dosage adjustment may be necessary). Products include:
- Mykrox Tablets 1617
- Zaroxolyn Tablets 1625

Metoprolol Succinate (Possibility of significant hypotension; dosage adjustment may be necessary). Products include:
- Toprol-XL Tablets 560

Metoprolol Tartrate (Possibility of significant hypotension; dosage adjustment may be necessary). Products include:
- Lopressor 848
- Lopressor HCT Tablets 850

Metyrosine (Possibility of significant hypotension; dosage adjustment may be necessary). Products include:
- Demser Capsules 1690

Minoxidil (Possibility of significant hypotension; dosage adjustment may be necessary).
- No products indexed under this heading.

Moexipril Hydrochloride (Possibility of significant hypotension; dosage adjustment may be necessary). Products include:
- Univasc Tablets 2553

Nadolol (Possibility of significant hypotension; dosage adjustment may be necessary).
- No products indexed under this heading.

Nicardipine Hydrochloride (Possibility of significant hypotension; dosage adjustment may be necessary). Products include:
- Cardene Capsules 2261
- Cardene I.V. 2815
- Cardene SR Capsules 2264

Nifedipine (Possibility of significant hypotension; dosage adjustment may be necessary). Products include:
- Adalat Capsules (10 mg and 20 mg) 580
- Adalat CC 582
- Procardia Capsules 2024
- Procardia XL Extended Release Tablets 2026

Nisoldipine (Possibility of significant hypotension; dosage adjustment may be necessary). Products include:
- Sular Tablets 2961

Nitroglycerin (Possibility of significant hypotension; dosage adjustment may be necessary). Products include:
- Deponit NTG Transdermal Delivery System 2541
- Nitro-Bid IV 1270
- Nitro-Bid Ointment 1272
- Nitro-Dur (nitroglycerin) Transdermal Infusion System 1365
- Nitrolingual Spray 2193
- Nitrostat Tablets 1981
- Transderm-Nitro Transdermal Therapeutic System 878

Penbutolol Sulfate (Possibility of significant hypotension; dosage adjustment may be necessary). Products include:
- Levatol Tablets 2547

Phenoxybenzamine Hydrochloride (Possibility of significant hypotension; dosage adjustment may be necessary). Products include:
- Dibenzyline Capsules 2650

Phentolamine Mesylate (Possibility of significant hypotension; dosage adjustment may be necessary). Products include:
- Regitine Vials 864

Pindolol (Possibility of significant hypotension; dosage adjustment may be necessary). Products include:
- Visken Tablets 2428

Polythiazide (Possibility of significant hypotension; dosage adjustment may be necessary). Products include:
- Minizide Capsules 2016

Prazosin Hydrochloride (Possibility of significant hypotension; dosage adjustment may be necessary). Products include:
- Minipress Capsules 2015
- Minizide Capsules 2016

Propranolol Hydrochloride (Possibility of significant hypotension; dosage adjustment may be necessary). Products include:
- Inderal 2834
- Inderal LA Long Acting Capsules 2836
- Inderide Tablets 2838
- Inderide LA Long Acting Capsules .. 2840

Quinapril Hydrochloride (Possibility of significant hypotension; dosage adjustment may be necessary). Products include:
- Accupril Tablets 1950

Ramipril (Possibility of significant hypotension; dosage adjustment may be necessary). Products include:
- Altace Capsules 1238

Rauwolfia Serpentina (Possibility of significant hypotension; dosage adjustment may be necessary).
- No products indexed under this heading.

Rescinnamine (Possibility of significant hypotension; dosage adjustment may be necessary).
- No products indexed under this heading.

Reserpine (Possibility of significant hypotension; dosage adjustment may be necessary). Products include:
- Diupres Tablets 1691
- Hydropres Tablets 1718
- Ser-Ap-Es Tablets 867

Sodium Nitroprusside (Possibility of significant hypotension; dosage adjustment may be necessary).
- No products indexed under this heading.

Sotalol Hydrochloride (Possibility of significant hypotension; dosage adjustment may be necessary). Products include:
- Betapace Tablets 637

Spirapril Hydrochloride (Possibility of significant hypotension; dosage adjustment may be necessary).
- No products indexed under this heading.

Timolol Maleate (Possibility of significant hypotension; dosage adjustment may be necessary). Products include:
- Blocadren Tablets 1654
- Timolide Tablets 1791
- Timoptic in Ocudose 1796
- Timoptic Sterile Ophthalmic Solution 1794
- Timoptic-XE 1798

Torsemide (Possibility of significant hypotension; dosage adjustment may be necessary). Products include:
- Demadex Tablets and Injection 691

Trimethaphan Camsylate (Possibility of significant hypotension; dosage adjustment may be necessary).
- No products indexed under this heading.

Verapamil Hydrochloride (Co-administration increases terazosin's mean AUC$_{0-24}$ by 11% to 24% with associated increase in C$_{max}$ (25%) and C$_{min}$ (32%)). Products include:
- Calan SR Caplets 2571
- Calan Tablets 2568
- Covera-HS Tablets 2573
- Isoptin Injectable 1391
- Isoptin Oral Tablets 1393
- Isoptin SR Tablets 1395
- Verelan Capsules 1455

Food Interactions

Food, unspecified (Delays the time to peak concentration by about 40 minutes; minimal effect on the extent of absorption).

HYZAAR TABLETS
(Losartan Potassium, Hydrochlorothiazide) 1720

May interact with barbiturates, narcotic analgesics, oral hypoglycemic agents, insulin, antihypertensives, corticosteroids, lithium preparations, non-steroidal anti-inflammatory agents, nondepolarizing neuromuscular blocking agents, and certain other agents. Compounds in these categories include:

Acarbose (Hyperglycemia may occur with thiazide diuretics; dosage adjustment of the antidiabetic drug may be required). Products include:
- Precose 604

(℞ Described in PDR For Nonprescription Drugs)   (⊚ Described in PDR For Ophthalmology)

Acebutolol Hydrochloride (Additive effect or potentiation of other antihypertensives). Products include:
- Sectral Capsules ... 2914

ACTH (Potential for intensified electrolyte depletion particularly hypokalemia).
- No products indexed under this heading.

Alfentanil Hydrochloride (Potentiation of orthostatic hypotension). Products include:
- Alfenta Injection ... 1334

Amlodipine Besylate (Additive effect or potentiation of other antihypertensives). Products include:
- Lotrel Capsules ... 858
- Norvasc Tablets ... 2020

Aprobarbital (Potentiation of orthostatic hypotension).
- No products indexed under this heading.

Atenolol (Additive effect or potentiation of other antihypertensives). Products include:
- Tenoretic Tablets ... 2963
- Tenormin Tablets and I.V. Injection 2965

Atracurium Besylate (Possible increased responsiveness to the muscle relaxant). Products include:
- Tracrium Injection ... 1155

Benazepril Hydrochloride (Additive effect or potentiation of other antihypertensives). Products include:
- Lotensin Tablets ... 852
- Lotensin HCT Tablets ... 855
- Lotrel Capsules ... 858

Bendroflumethiazide (Additive effect or potentiation of other antihypertensives).
- No products indexed under this heading.

Betamethasone Acetate (Potential for intensified electrolyte depletion particularly hypokalemia). Products include:
- Celestone Soluspan Suspension ... 2484

Betamethasone Sodium Phosphate (Potential for intensified electrolyte depletion particularly hypokalemia). Products include:
- Celestone Soluspan Suspension ... 2484

Betaxolol Hydrochloride (Additive effect or potentiation of other antihypertensives). Products include:
- Betoptic Ophthalmic Solution ... 465
- Betoptic S Ophthalmic Suspension 467
- Kerlone Tablets ... 2588

Bisoprolol Fumarate (Additive effect or potentiation of other antihypertensives). Products include:
- Zebeta Tablets ... 1457
- Ziac ... 1459

Buprenorphine (Potentiation of orthostatic hypotension). Products include:
- Buprenex Injectable ... 2170

Butabarbital (Potentiation of orthostatic hypotension).
- No products indexed under this heading.

Butalbital (Potentiation of orthostatic hypotension). Products include:
- Axocet Capsules ... 2469
- Esgic-plus Capsules ... 1012
- Esgic-plus Tablets ... 1012
- Fioricet Tablets ... 2386
- Fioricet with Codeine Capsules ... 2387
- Fiorinal Capsules ... 2388
- Fiorinal with Codeine Capsules ... 2390
- Fiorinal Tablets ... 2388
- Phrenilin ... 790
- Sedapap Tablets 50 mg/650 mg .. 1826

Captopril (Additive effect or potentiation of other antihypertensives). Products include:
- Capoten Tablets ... 740
- Capozide Tablets ... 744

Carteolol Hydrochloride (Additive effect or potentiation of other antihypertensives). Products include:
- Cartrol Tablets ... 413
- Ocupress Ophthalmic Solution, 1% Sterile ... ◉ 297

Chlorothiazide (Additive effect or potentiation of other antihypertensives). Products include:
- Aldoclor Tablets ... 1638
- Diupres Tablets ... 1691
- Diuril Oral ... 1694

Chlorothiazide Sodium (Additive effect or potentiation of other antihypertensives). Products include:
- Diuril Sodium Intravenous ... 1693

Chlorpropamide (Hyperglycemia may occur with thiazide diuretics; dosage adjustment of the antidiabetic drug may be required). Products include:
- Diabinese Tablets ... 2002

Chlorthalidone (Additive effect or potentiation of other antihypertensives). Products include:
- Combipres Tablets ... 682
- Tenoretic Tablets ... 2963
- Thalitone ... 1293

Cholestyramine (Absorption of hydrochlorothiazide is impaired in the presence of anionic exchange resins; cholestyramine binds hydrochlorothiazide and reduces its absorption from GI tract by up to 85%). Products include:
- Questran ... 774

Cimetidine (Co-administration may lead to an increase of about 18% in AUC of losartan but did not affect the pharmacokinetics of its active metabolite). Products include:
- Tagamet HB Tablets ... 786
- Tagamet Tablets ... 2694

Cimetidine Hydrochloride (Co-administration may lead to an increase of about 18% in AUC of losartan but did not affect the pharmacokinetics of its active metabolite). Products include:
- Tagamet ... 2694

Cisatracurium Besylate (Possible increased responsiveness to the muscle relaxant). Products include:
- Nimbex Injection ... 1131

Clonidine (Additive effect or potentiation of other antihypertensives). Products include:
- Catapres-TTS ... 680

Clonidine Hydrochloride (Additive effect or potentiation of other antihypertensives). Products include:
- Catapres Tablets ... 679
- Combipres Tablets ... 682

Codeine Phosphate (Potentiation of orthostatic hypotension). Products include:
- Brontex ... 2130
- Dimetane-DC Cough Syrup ... 2232
- Fioricet with Codeine Capsules ... 2387
- Fiorinal with Codeine Capsules ... 2390
- Nucofed ... 2225
- Phenergan with Codeine ... 2883
- Phenergan VC with Codeine ... 2888
- Robitussin A-C Syrup ... 2248
- Robitussin-DAC Syrup ... 2249
- Ryna ... 804
- Soma Compound w/Codeine Tablets ... 2784
- Tylenol with Codeine ... 1592

Colestipol Hydrochloride (Absorption of hydrochlorothiazide is impaired in the presence of anionic exchange resins; cholestyramine binds hydrochlorothiazide and reduces its absorption from GI tract by up to 85%). Products include:
- Colestid ... 2073

Cortisone Acetate (Potential for intensified electrolyte depletion particularly hypokalemia). Products include:
- Cortone Acetate Sterile Suspension ... 1663
- Cortone Acetate Tablets ... 1664

Deserpidine (Additive effect or potentiation of other antihypertensives).
- No products indexed under this heading.

Dexamethasone (Potential for intensified electrolyte depletion particularly hypokalemia). Products include:
- AK-Trol Ointment & Suspension ... ◉ 205
- Decadron Elixir ... 1676
- Decadron Tablets ... 1678
- Decaspray Topical Aerosol ... 1689
- Maxitrol Ophthalmic Ointment and Suspension ... ◉ 222
- TobraDex Ophthalmic Suspension and Ointment ... 469

Dexamethasone Acetate (Potential for intensified electrolyte depletion particularly hypokalemia). Products include:
- Dalalone D.P. Injectable ... 1009
- Decadron-LA Sterile Suspension ... 1687

Dexamethasone Sodium Phosphate (Potential for intensified electrolyte depletion particularly hypokalemia). Products include:
- Decadron Phosphate Injection ... 1680
- Decadron Phosphate Sterile Ophthalmic Ointment ... 1684
- Decadron Phosphate Sterile Ophthalmic Solution ... 1685
- Decadron Phosphate Topical Cream ... 1686
- Decadron Phosphate with Xylocaine Injection, Sterile ... 1683
- Dexacort Phosphate in Respihaler .. 1606
- Dexacort Phosphate in Turbinaire .. 1607
- NeoDecadron Sterile Ophthalmic Ointment ... 1755
- NeoDecadron Sterile Ophthalmic Solution ... 1756
- NeoDecadron Topical Cream ... 1757

Dezocine (Potentiation of orthostatic hypotension). Products include:
- Dalgan Injection ... 529

Diazoxide (Additive effect or potentiation of other antihypertensives). Products include:
- Hyperstat I.V. Injection ... 2504
- Proglycem ... 575

Diclofenac Potassium (Potential reduced diuretic, natriuretic, and antihypertensive effects). Products include:
- Cataflam Tablets ... 833

Diclofenac Sodium (Potential reduced diuretic, natriuretic, and antihypertensive effects). Products include:
- Voltaren Ophthalmic Sterile Ophthalmic Solution ... ◉ 264
- Cataflam/Voltaren/Voltaren-XR ... 833

Diltiazem Hydrochloride (Additive effect or potentiation of other antihypertensives). Products include:
- Cardizem CD Capsules ... 1251
- Cardizem SR Capsules ... 1255
- Cardizem Injectable ... 1253
- Cardizem Tablets ... 1257
- Dilacor XR Extended-release Capsules ... 2183
- Tiazac Capsules ... 1019

Doxazosin Mesylate (Additive effect or potentiation of other antihypertensives). Products include:
- Cardura Tablets ... 1993

Enalapril Maleate (Additive effect or potentiation of other antihypertensives). Products include:
- Vaseretic Tablets ... 1810
- Vasotec Tablets ... 1816

Enalaprilat (Additive effect or potentiation of other antihypertensives). Products include:
- Vasotec I.V. ... 1814

Esmolol Hydrochloride (Additive effect or potentiation of other antihypertensives). Products include:
- Brevibloc (esmolol HCl) Injection ... 1860

Etodolac (Potential reduced diuretic, natriuretic, and antihypertensive effects). Products include:
- Lodine Capsules and Tablets ... 2849

Felodipine (Additive effect or potentiation of other antihypertensives). Products include:
- Plendil Extended-Release Tablets ... 514

Fenoprofen Calcium (Potential reduced diuretic, natriuretic, and antihypertensive effects). Products include:
- Nalfon 200 Pulvules & Nalfon Tablets ... 933

Fentanyl (Potentiation of orthostatic hypotension). Products include:
- Duragesic Transdermal System ... 1336

Fentanyl Citrate (Potentiation of orthostatic hypotension). Products include:
- Sublimaze Injection ... 463

Fludrocortisone Acetate (Potential for intensified electrolyte depletion particularly hypokalemia). Products include:
- Florinef Acetate Tablets ... 506

Flurbiprofen (Potential reduced diuretic, natriuretic, and antihypertensive effects).
- No products indexed under this heading.

Fosinopril Sodium (Additive effect or potentiation of other antihypertensives). Products include:
- Monopril Tablets ... 762

Furosemide (Additive effect or potentiation of other antihypertensives). Products include:
- Lasix Injection, Oral Solution and Tablets ... 1267

Gestodene (*In Vitro* studies show significant inhibition of the formation of the active metabolite by inhibitors of P450 3A4 such as gestodene; pharmacodynamic consequences of concomitant use is undefined).
- No products indexed under this heading.

Glimepiride (Hyperglycemia may occur with thiazide diuretics; dosage adjustment of the antidiabetic drug may be required). Products include:
- Amaryl Tablets ... 1241

Glipizide (Hyperglycemia may occur with thiazide diuretics; dosage adjustment of the antidiabetic drug may be required). Products include:
- Glucotrol Tablets ... 2011
- Glucotrol XL Extended Release Tablets ... 2012

Glyburide (Hyperglycemia may occur with thiazide diuretics; dosage adjustment of the antidiabetic drug may be required). Products include:
- DiaBeta Tablets ... 1265
- Glynase PresTab Tablets ... 2091
- Micronase Tablets ... 2099

Guanabenz Acetate (Additive effect or potentiation of other antihypertensives).
- No products indexed under this heading.

Guanethidine Monosulfate (Additive effect or potentiation of other antihypertensives). Products include:
- Esimil Tablets ... 840
- Ismelin Tablets ... 845

IMPORTANT NOTE: Always consult each drug listing in the patient's regimen for possible interactions.

Hyzaar **Interactions Index** 514

Hydralazine Hydrochloride (Additive effect or potentiation of other antihypertensives). Products include:
- Apresazide Capsules 824
- Apresoline Hydrochloride Tablets .. 826
- Hydralazine Hydrochloride Injection USP 2712
- Ser-Ap-Es Tablets 867

Hydrocodone Bitartrate (Potentiation of orthostatic hypotension). Products include:
- Codiclear DH Syrup 808
- Duratuss HD Elixir 2750
- Histussin D Liquid 670
- Hycodan Tablets and Syrup 946
- Hycomine Compound Tablets 948
- Hycomine 947
- Hycotuss Expectorant Syrup 950
- Hydrocet Capsules 787
- Lorcet 10/650 Tablets 1016
- Lortab 2751
- Tussend 1830
- Tussend Expectorant 1831
- Vicodin Tablets 1404
- Vicodin ES Tablets 1405
- Vicodin HP Tablets 1403
- Vicodin Tuss Expectorant 1406
- Zydone Capsules 967

Hydrocodone Polistirex (Potentiation of orthostatic hypotension). Products include:
- Tussionex Pennkinetic Extended-Release Suspension 1624

Hydrocortisone (Potential for intensified electrolyte depletion particularly hypokalemia). Products include:
- Anusol-HC Cream 2.5% 1953
- Aquanil HC Lotion 1989
- Maximum Strength Cortaid Spray ⊞ 800
- CORTENEMA 2713
- Cortisporin Ointment 1074
- Cortisporin Ophthalmic Ointment Sterile 1074
- Cortisporin Ophthalmic Suspension Sterile 1075
- Cortisporin Otic Solution Sterile 1076
- Cortisporin Otic Suspension Sterile 1077
- Cortizone-5 .... ⊞ 795
- Cortizone-10 .... ⊞ 795
- Hydrocortone Tablets 1715
- Hytone 922
- Hytone Ointment 2 ½% 923
- Massengill Medicated Soft Cloth Towelettes 2628
- Pediotic Suspension Sterile 1140
- Preparation H Hydrocortisone 1% Cream .... ⊞ 843
- ProctoCream-HC 2.5% 2552
- VōSoL HC Otic Solution 2786

Hydrocortisone Acetate (Potential for intensified electrolyte depletion particularly hypokalemia). Products include:
- Analpram-HC Rectal Cream 1% and 2.5% 993
- Anusol HC-1 Hydrocortisone Anti-Itch Ointment .... ⊞ 810
- Anusol-HC Suppositories 1954
- Caldecort Anti-Itch Hydrocortisone Cream .... ⊞ 651
- Coly-Mycin S Otic w/Neomycin & Hydrocortisone 1965
- Cortaid .... ⊞ 800
- Cortifoam 2540
- Cortisporin Cream 1073
- Epifoam 2543
- Hydrocortone Acetate Sterile Suspension 1712
- Mantadil Cream 1124
- Nupercainal Hydrocortisone 1% Cream .... ⊞ 661
- Pramosone Cream, Lotion & Ointment 995
- ProctoFoam-HC 2552
- Terra-Cortril Ophthalmic Suspension 2033

Hydrocortisone Sodium Phosphate (Potential for intensified electrolyte depletion particularly hypokalemia). Products include:
- Hydrocortone Phosphate Injection, Sterile 1713

Hydrocortisone Sodium Succinate (Potential for intensified electrolyte depletion particularly hypokalemia).
- No products indexed under this heading.

Hydroflumethiazide (Additive effect or potentiation of other antihypertensives). Products include:
- Diucardin Tablets 2824

Hydromorphone Hydrochloride (Potentiation of orthostatic hypotension). Products include:
- Dilaudid Ampules 1382
- Dilaudid Cough Syrup 1383
- Dilaudid-HP Injection 1384
- Dilaudid-HP Lyophilized Powder 250 mg 1384
- Dilaudid 1382
- Dilaudid Oral Liquid 1386
- Dilaudid 1382
- Dilaudid Tablets - 8 mg 1386

Ibuprofen (Potential reduced diuretic, natriuretic, and antihypertensive effects). Products include:
- Advil Cold and Sinus Caplets and Tablets .... ⊞ 837
- Advil Ibuprofen Tablets, Caplets and Gel Caplets .... ⊞ 836
- Children's Motrin Ibuprofen Oral Suspension 1558
- IBU Tablets 1389
- Ibuprohm .... ⊞ 713
- Motrin IB Caplets, Tablets, and Gelcaps .... ⊞ 802
- Motrin Ibuprofen Suspension, Oral Drops, Chewable Tablets, Caplets 1563
- Nuprin Ibuprofen/Analgesic Tablets & Caplets .... ⊞ 645
- Vicks DayQuil SINUS Pressure & PAIN Relief with IBUPROFEN .... ⊞ 735

Indapamide (Additive effect or potentiation of other antihypertensives).
- No products indexed under this heading.

Indomethacin (Potential reduced diuretic, natriuretic, and antihypertensive effects). Products include:
- Indocin 1723

Indomethacin Sodium Trihydrate (Potential reduced diuretic, natriuretic, and antihypertensive effects). Products include:
- Indocin I.V. 1727

Insulin, Human (Hyperglycemia may occur with thiazide diuretics; dosage adjustment of the antidiabetic drug may be required).
- No products indexed under this heading.

Insulin, Human Isophane Suspension (Hyperglycemia may occur with thiazide diuretics; dosage adjustment of the antidiabetic drug may be required). Products include:
- Novolin N Human Insulin 10 ml Vials 1846

Insulin, Human NPH (Hyperglycemia may occur with thiazide diuretics; dosage adjustment of the antidiabetic drug may be required). Products include:
- Humulin N, 100 Units 1495
- Novolin N PenFill 1.5 ml Cartridges Durable Insulin Delivery System 1849
- Novolin N Prefilled Syringe Disposable Insulin Delivery System 1850

Insulin, Human Regular (Hyperglycemia may occur with thiazide diuretics; dosage adjustment of the antidiabetic drug may be required). Products include:
- Humulin R, 100 Units 1497
- Novolin R Human Insulin 10 ml Vials 1846
- Novolin R PenFill 1.5 ml Cartridges Durable Insulin Delivery System 1849
- Novolin R Prefilled Syringe Disposable Insulin Delivery System 1850
- Velosulin BR Human Insulin 10 ml Vials 1847

Insulin, Human, Zinc Suspension (Hyperglycemia may occur with thiazide diuretics; dosage adjustment of the antidiabetic drug may be required). Products include:
- Humulin L, 100 Units 1494
- Humulin U, 100 Units 1498
- Novolin L Human Insulin 10 ml Vials 1846

Insulin Lispro, Human (Hyperglycemia may occur with thiazide diuretics; dosage adjustment of the antidiabetic drug may be required). Products include:
- Humalog Injection 1488

Insulin, NPH (Hyperglycemia may occur with thiazide diuretics; dosage adjustment of the antidiabetic drug may be required). Products include:
- NPH, 100 Units 1502
- Pork NPH, 100 Units 1506
- Purified Pork NPH Isophane Insulin 1852

Insulin, Regular (Hyperglycemia may occur with thiazide diuretics; dosage adjustment of the antidiabetic drug may be required). Products include:
- Regular, 100 Units 1503
- Pork Regular, 100 Units 1507
- Pork Regular (Concentrated), 500 Units 1508
- Purified Pork Regular Insulin 1852

Insulin, Zinc Crystals (Hyperglycemia may occur with thiazide diuretics; dosage adjustment of the antidiabetic drug may be required). Products include:
- NPH, 100 Units 1502

Insulin, Zinc Suspension (Hyperglycemia may occur with thiazide diuretics; dosage adjustment of the antidiabetic drug may be required). Products include:
- Iletin I 1501
- Lente, 100 Units 1501
- Iletin II 1504
- Pork Lente, 100 Units 1504
- Purified Pork Lente Insulin 1852

Isradipine (Additive effect or potentiation of other antihypertensives). Products include:
- DynaCirc Capsules 2381
- DynaCirc CR Tablets 2383

Ketoconazole (*In Vitro* studies show significant inhibition of the formation of the active metabolite by inhibitors of P450 3A4 such as ketoconazole or complete inhibition by the combination of ketoconazole and sulfaphenazole; pharmacodynamic consequences of concomitant use is undefined). Products include:
- Nizoral 2% Cream 1344
- Nizoral 2% Shampoo 1344
- Nizoral Tablets 1345

Ketoprofen (Potential reduced diuretic, natriuretic, and antihypertensive effects). Products include:
- Actron Caplets and Tablets .... ⊞ 608
- Orudis Capsules 2874
- Orudis KT .... ⊞ 842
- Oruvail Capsules 2874

Ketorolac Tromethamine (Potential reduced diuretic, natriuretic, and antihypertensive effects). Products include:
- Acular Sterile Ophthalmic Solution 470
- Toradol 2319

Labetalol Hydrochloride (Additive effect or potentiation of other antihypertensives). Products include:
- Normodyne Injection 2519
- Normodyne Tablets 2522
- Trandate 1158

Levorphanol Tartrate (Potentiation of orthostatic hypotension). Products include:
- Levo-Dromoran 2297

Lisinopril (Additive effect or potentiation of other antihypertensives). Products include:
- Prinivil Tablets 1776
- Prinzide Tablets 1780
- Zestoretic Tablets 2968
- Zestril Tablets 2972

Lithium Carbonate (Diuretics reduce the renal clearance of lithium and add a high risk of lithium toxicity; concurrent use should be avoided). Products include:
- Eskalith 2658
- Lithium Carbonate Capsules & Tablets 2352
- Lithonate/Lithotabs/Lithobid 2721

Lithium Citrate (Diuretics reduce the renal clearance of lithium and add a high risk of lithium toxicity; concurrent use should be avoided).
- No products indexed under this heading.

Mecamylamine Hydrochloride (Additive effect or potentiation of other antihypertensives). Products include:
- Inversine Tablets 1729

Meclofenamate Sodium (Potential reduced diuretic, natriuretic, and antihypertensive effects).
- No products indexed under this heading.

Mefenamic Acid (Potential reduced diuretic, natriuretic, and antihypertensive effects). Products include:
- Ponstel 1982

Meperidine Hydrochloride (Potentiation of orthostatic hypotension). Products include:
- Demerol 2438
- Mepergan Injection 2859

Mephobarbital (Potentiation of orthostatic hypotension). Products include:
- Mebaral Tablets 2452

Metformin Hydrochloride (Hyperglycemia may occur with thiazide diuretics; dosage adjustment of the antidiabetic drug may be required). Products include:
- Glucophage Tablets 754

Methadone Hydrochloride (Potentiation of orthostatic hypotension). Products include:
- Methadone Hydrochloride Oral Concentrate 2356
- Methadone Hydrochloride Oral Solution & Tablets 2357

Methyclothiazide (Additive effect or potentiation of other antihypertensives). Products include:
- Enduron Tablets 424

Methyldopa (Additive effect or potentiation of other antihypertensives). Products include:
- Aldoclor Tablets 1638
- Aldomet Oral 1640
- Aldoril Tablets 1644

Methyldopate Hydrochloride (Additive effect or potentiation of other antihypertensives). Products include:
- Aldomet Ester HCl Injection 1642

Methylprednisolone Acetate (Potential for intensified electrolyte depletion particularly hypokalemia).
- No products indexed under this heading.

Methylprednisolone Sodium Succinate (Potential for intensified electrolyte depletion particularly hypokalemia).
- No products indexed under this heading.

(⊞ Described in PDR For Nonprescription Drugs) (⊚ Described in PDR For Ophthalmology)

Metocurine Iodide (Possible increased responsiveness to the muscle relaxant). Products include:
- Metubine Iodide Vials 932

Metolazone (Additive effect or potentiation of other antihypertensives). Products include:
- Mykrox Tablets 1617
- Zaroxolyn Tablets 1625

Metoprolol Succinate (Additive effect or potentiation of other antihypertensives). Products include:
- Toprol-XL Tablets 560

Metoprolol Tartrate (Additive effect or potentiation of other antihypertensives). Products include:
- Lopressor 848
- Lopressor HCT Tablets 850

Metyrosine (Additive effect or potentiation of other antihypertensives). Products include:
- Demser Capsules 1690

Minoxidil (Additive effect or potentiation of other antihypertensives).
No products indexed under this heading.

Mivacurium Chloride (Possible increased responsiveness to the muscle relaxant). Products include:
- Mivacron 1125

Moexipril Hydrochloride (Additive effect or potentiation of other antihypertensives). Products include:
- Univasc Tablets 2553

Morphine Sulfate (Potentiation of orthostatic hypotension). Products include:
- Astramorph/PF Injection, USP (Preservative-Free) 526
- Duramorph Injection 983
- Infumorph 200 and Infumorph 500 Sterile Solutions 985
- Kadian Capsules 2948
- MS Contin Tablets 2149
- MSIR 2152
- Oramorph SR (Morphine Sulfate Sustained Release Tablets) 2359
- RMS Suppositories CII 2766
- Roxanol 2365

Nabumetone (Potential reduced diuretic, natriuretic, and antihypertensive effects). Products include:
- Relafen Tablets 2688

Nadolol (Additive effect or potentiation of other antihypertensives).
No products indexed under this heading.

Naproxen (Potential reduced diuretic, natriuretic, and antihypertensive effects). Products include:
- Anaprox/Naprosyn 2277

Naproxen Sodium (Potential reduced diuretic, natriuretic, and antihypertensive effects). Products include:
- Aleve 2124
- Anaprox/Naprosyn 2277
- Naprelan Tablets 2861

Nicardipine Hydrochloride (Additive effect or potentiation of other antihypertensives). Products include:
- Cardene Capsules 2261
- Cardene I.V. 2815
- Cardene SR Capsules 2264

Nifedipine (Additive effect or potentiation of other antihypertensives). Products include:
- Adalat Capsules (10 mg and 20 mg) 580
- Adalat CC 582
- Procardia Capsules 2024
- Procardia XL Extended Release Tablets 2026

Nisoldipine (Additive effect or potentiation of other antihypertensives). Products include:
- Sular Tablets 2961

Nitroglycerin (Additive effect or potentiation of other antihypertensives). Products include:
- Deponit NTG Transdermal Delivery System 2541
- Nitro-Bid IV 1270
- Nitro-Bid Ointment 1272
- Nitro-Dur (nitroglycerin) Transdermal Infusion System 1365
- Nitrolingual Spray 2193
- Nitrostat Tablets 1981
- Transderm-Nitro Transdermal Therapeutic System 878

Norepinephrine Bitartrate (Possible decreased response to pressor amines). Products include:
- Levophed Bitartrate Injection 2445

Opium Alkaloids (Potentiation of orthostatic hypotension).
No products indexed under this heading.

Oxaprozin (Potential reduced diuretic, natriuretic, and antihypertensive effects). Products include:
- Daypro Caplets 2578

Oxycodone Hydrochloride (Potentiation of orthostatic hypotension). Products include:
- OxyContin Tablets 2163
- OxyIR Capsules 2167
- Percocet Tablets 955
- Percodan Tablets 955
- Percodan-Demi Tablets 956
- Roxicodone Tablets, Oral Solution & Intensol (Oxycodone) 2366
- Tylox Capsules 1593

Pancuronium Bromide (Possible increased responsiveness to the muscle relaxant).
No products indexed under this heading.

Penbutolol Sulfate (Additive effect or potentiation of other antihypertensives). Products include:
- Levatol Tablets 2547

Pentobarbital Sodium (Potentiation of orthostatic hypotension). Products include:
- Nembutal Sodium Capsules 440
- Nembutal Sodium Solution 442
- Nembutal Sodium Suppositories 444

Phenobarbital (Co-administration may lead to a reduction of about 20% in AUC of losartan and its active metabolite; potentiation of orthostatic hypotension). Products include:
- Arco-Lase Plus Tablets 513
- Bellergal-S Tablets 2375
- Donnatal 2234
- Donnatal Extentabs 2234
- Donnatal Tablets 2234
- Phenobarbital Elixir and Tablets 1523
- Quadrinal Tablets 1398

Phenoxybenzamine Hydrochloride (Additive effect or potentiation of other antihypertensives). Products include:
- Dibenzyline Capsules 2650

Phentolamine Mesylate (Additive effect or potentiation of other antihypertensives). Products include:
- Regitine Vials 864

Phenylbutazone (Potential reduced diuretic, natriuretic, and antihypertensive effects).
No products indexed under this heading.

Pindolol (Additive effect or potentiation of other antihypertensives). Products include:
- Visken Tablets 2428

Piroxicam (Potential reduced diuretic, natriuretic, and antihypertensive effects). Products include:
- Feldene Capsules 2008

Polythiazide (Additive effect or potentiation of other antihypertensives). Products include:
- Minizide Capsules 2016

Prazosin Hydrochloride (Additive effect or potentiation of other antihypertensives). Products include:
- Minipress Capsules 2015
- Minizide Capsules 2016

Prednisolone Acetate (Potential for intensified electrolyte depletion particularly hypokalemia). Products include:
- AK-CIDE .... ⊚ 203
- AK-CIDE Ointment .... ⊚ 203
- Blephamide Liquifilm Sterile Ophthalmic Suspension 472
- Blephamide Ointment .... ⊚ 234
- Econopred & Econopred Plus Ophthalmic Suspensions .... ⊚ 216
- Poly-Pred Liquifilm .... ⊚ 246
- Pred Forte .... ⊚ 247
- Pred Mild .... ⊚ 250
- Pred-G Liquifilm Sterile Ophthalmic Suspension .... ⊚ 248
- Pred-G S.O.P. Sterile Ophthalmic Ointment .... ⊚ 249

Prednisolone Sodium Phosphate (Potential for intensified electrolyte depletion particularly hypokalemia). Products include:
- AK-PRED .... ⊚ 204
- Hydeltrasol Injection, Sterile 1708
- Pediapred Oral Solution 1618

Prednisolone Tebutate (Potential for intensified electrolyte depletion particularly hypokalemia). Products include:
- Hydeltra-T.B.A. Sterile Suspension 1710

Prednisone (Potential for intensified electrolyte depletion particularly hypokalemia).
No products indexed under this heading.

Propoxyphene Hydrochloride (Potentiation of orthostatic hypotension). Products include:
- Darvon 1475
- Wygesic Tablets 2930

Propoxyphene Napsylate (Potentiation of orthostatic hypotension). Products include:
- Darvon-N/Darvocet-N 1473

Propranolol Hydrochloride (Additive effect or potentiation of other antihypertensives). Products include:
- Inderal 2834
- Inderal LA Long Acting Capsules 2836
- Inderide Tablets 2838
- Inderide LA Long Acting Capsules 2840

Quinapril Hydrochloride (Additive effect or potentiation of other antihypertensives). Products include:
- Accupril Tablets 1950

Ramipril (Additive effect or potentiation of other antihypertensives). Products include:
- Altace Capsules 1238

Rauwolfia Serpentina (Additive effect or potentiation of other antihypertensives).
No products indexed under this heading.

Rescinnamine (Additive effect or potentiation of other antihypertensives).
No products indexed under this heading.

Reserpine (Additive effect or potentiation of other antihypertensives). Products include:
- Diupres Tablets 1691
- Hydropres Tablets 1718
- Ser-Ap-Es Tablets 867

Rocuronium Bromide (Possible increased responsiveness to the muscle relaxant). Products include:
- Zemuron Injection 1885

Secobarbital Sodium (Potentiation of orthostatic hypotension). Products include:
- Seconal Sodium Pulvules 1529

Sodium Nitroprusside (Additive effect or potentiation of other antihypertensives).
No products indexed under this heading.

Sotalol Hydrochloride (Additive effect or potentiation of other antihypertensives). Products include:
- Betapace Tablets 637

Spirapril Hydrochloride (Additive effect or potentiation of other antihypertensives).
No products indexed under this heading.

Sufentanil Citrate (Potentiation of orthostatic hypotension). Products include:
- Sufenta Injection 1355

Sulfaphenazole (*In Vitro* studies show significant inhibition of the formation of the active metabolite by inhibitors of P450 3A4 such as sulfaphenazole; pharmacodynamic consequences of concomitant use is undefined).
No products indexed under this heading.

Sulindac (Potential reduced diuretic, natriuretic, and antihypertensive effects). Products include:
- Clinoril Tablets 1658

Terazosin Hydrochloride (Additive effect or potentiation of other antihypertensives). Products include:
- Hytrin Capsules 434

Thiamylal Sodium (Potentiation of orthostatic hypotension).
No products indexed under this heading.

Timolol Maleate (Additive effect or potentiation of other antihypertensives). Products include:
- Blocadren Tablets 1654
- Timolide Tablets 1791
- Timoptic in Ocudose 1796
- Timoptic Sterile Ophthalmic Solution 1794
- Timoptic-XE 1798

Tolazamide (Hyperglycemia may occur with thiazide diuretics; dosage adjustment of the antidiabetic drug may be required).
No products indexed under this heading.

Tolbutamide (Hyperglycemia may occur with thiazide diuretics; dosage adjustment of the antidiabetic drug may be required).
No products indexed under this heading.

Tolmetin Sodium (Potential reduced diuretic, natriuretic, and antihypertensive effects). Products include:
- Tolectin (200, 400 and 600 mg) 1591

Torsemide (Additive effect or potentiation of other antihypertensives). Products include:
- Demadex Tablets and Injection 691

Triamcinolone (Potential for intensified electrolyte depletion particularly hypokalemia).
No products indexed under this heading.

Triamcinolone Acetonide (Potential for intensified electrolyte depletion particularly hypokalemia). Products include:
- Azmacort Oral Inhaler 2175
- Nasacort AQ Nasal Spray 2191
- Nasacort Nasal Inhaler 2189

Triamcinolone Diacetate (Potential for intensified electrolyte depletion particularly hypokalemia).
No products indexed under this heading.

IMPORTANT NOTE: Always consult each drug listing in the patient's regimen for possible interactions.

Triamcinolone Hexacetonide (Potential for intensified electrolyte depletion particularly hypokalemia).
No products indexed under this heading.

Trimethaphan Camsylate (Additive effect or potentiation of other antihypertensives).
No products indexed under this heading.

Troleandomycin (*In Vitro* studies show significant inhibition of the formation of the active metabolite by inhibitors of P450 3A4 such as troleandomycin; pharmacodynamic consequences of concomitant use is undefined). Products include:
Tao Capsules ... 2033

Vecuronium Bromide (Possible increased responsiveness to the muscle relaxant). Products include:
Norcuron for Injection ... 1875

Verapamil Hydrochloride (Additive effect or potentiation of other antihypertensives). Products include:
Calan SR Caplets ... 2571
Calan Tablets ... 2568
Covera-HS Tablets ... 2573
Isoptin Injectable ... 1391
Isoptin Oral Tablets ... 1393
Isoptin SR Tablets ... 1395
Verelan Capsules ... 1455

Food Interactions

Alcohol (Potentiation of orthostatic hypotension).

Meal, unspecified (Meal slows absorption and decreases C_{max} but has minor effects on losartan AUC or on the AUC of the metabolite).

IBU TABLETS
(Ibuprofen) ... 1389
May interact with oral anticoagulants, thiazides, lithium preparations, and certain other agents. Compounds in these categories include:

Aspirin (Yields a net decrease in anti-inflammatory activity with lowered blood levels of non-aspirin drug in animal studies). Products include:
Alka-Seltzer Cherry Effervescent Antacid and Pain Reliever ... ▣ 609
Alka-Seltzer Extra Strength Effervescent Antacid and Pain Reliever ... ▣ 609
Alka-Seltzer Lemon Lime Effervescent Antacid and Pain Reliever ... ▣ 609
Alka-Seltzer Original Effervescent Antacid and Pain Reliever ... ▣ 609
Alka-Seltzer Plus ... ▣ 611
Alka-Seltzer Plus Sinus Medicine ... ▣ 611
Ascriptin ... ▣ 650
Arthritis Strength BC Powder ... ▣ 631
BC Cold Powder Multi-Symptom Formula (Cold-Sinus-Allergy) ... ▣ 631
BC Cold Powder Non-Drowsy Formula (Cold-Sinus) ... ▣ 631
BC Powder ... ▣ 631
Genuine Bayer Aspirin Tablets & Caplets ... ▣ 618
Extra Strength Bayer Arthritis Pain Regimen Formula ... ▣ 615
Extra Strength Bayer Aspirin Caplets & Tablets ... ▣ 617
Extended-Release Bayer 8-Hour Aspirin ... ▣ 616
Extra Strength Bayer Plus Aspirin Caplets ... ▣ 617
Extra Strength Bayer PM Aspirin Plus Sleep Aid ... ▣ 617
Aspirin Regimen Bayer 81 mg Tablets with Calcium ... ▣ 615
Aspirin Regimen Bayer Adult Low Strength 81 mg Tablets ... ▣ 613
Aspirin Regimen Bayer Children's Chewable Aspirin ... ▣ 616
Aspirin Regimen Bayer Regular Strength 325 mg Caplets ... ▣ 613
Bufferin Analgesic Tablets ... ▣ 636
Arthritis Strength Bufferin Analgesic Caplets ... ▣ 637
Extra Strength Bufferin Analgesic Tablets ... ▣ 637
Cama Arthritis Pain Reliever ... ▣ 748
Darvon Compound-65 Pulvules ... 1475
Easprin ... 1971
Ecotrin ... 2625
Ecotrin Enteric Coated Aspirin Maximum Strength Tablets and Caplets ... ▣ 775
Ecotrin Enteric Coated Aspirin Regular Strength Tablets ... 2625
Empirin Aspirin Tablets ... ▣ 818
Excedrin Extra-Strength Analgesic Tablets, Caplets, and Geltabs ... 734
Fiorinal Capsules ... 2388
Fiorinal with Codeine Capsules ... 2390
Fiorinal Tablets ... 2388
Goody's Extra Strength Headache Powders ... ▣ 632
Goody's Extra Strength Pain Relief Tablets ... ▣ 632
Halfprin Tablets ... 1413
Norgesic ... 1554
Percodan Tablets ... 955
Percodan-Demi Tablets ... 956
Robaxisal Tablets ... 2246
Soma Compound w/Codeine Tablets ... 2784
Soma Compound Tablets ... 2783
St. Joseph Adult Chewable Aspirin (81 mg.) ... ▣ 768
Talwin Compound ... 2466
Vanquish Analgesic Caplets ... ▣ 627

Bendroflumethiazide (Ibuprofen can reduce the natriuretic effect of thiazide diuretics in some patients).
No products indexed under this heading.

Chlorothiazide (Ibuprofen can reduce the natriuretic effect of thiazide diuretics in some patients). Products include:
Aldoclor Tablets ... 1638
Diupres Tablets ... 1691
Diuril Oral ... 1694

Chlorothiazide Sodium (Ibuprofen can reduce the natriuretic effect of thiazide diuretics in some patients). Products include:
Diuril Sodium Intravenous ... 1693

Dicumarol (Concurrent use may result in bleeding).
No products indexed under this heading.

Furosemide (Ibuprofen can reduce the natriurectic effect furosemide). Products include:
Lasix Injection, Oral Solution and Tablets ... 1267

Hydrochlorothiazide (Ibuprofen can reduce the natriuretic effect of thiazide diuretics in some patients). Products include:
Aldactazide Tablets ... 2556
Aldoril Tablets ... 1644
Apresazide Capsules ... 824
Capozide Tablets ... 744
Dyazide Capsules ... 2653
Esidrix Tablets ... 839
Esimil Tablets ... 840
HydroDIURIL Tablets ... 1716
Hydropres Tablets ... 1718
Hyzaar Tablets ... 1720
Inderide Tablets ... 2838
Inderide LA Long Acting Capsules ... 2840
Lopressor HCT Tablets ... 850
Lotensin HCT Tablets ... 855
Moduretic Tablets ... 1748
Oretic Tablets ... 450
Prinzide Tablets ... 1780
Ser-Ap-Es Tablets ... 867
Timolide Tablets ... 1791
Vaseretic Tablets ... 1810
Zestoretic Tablets ... 2968
Ziac ... 1459

Hydroflumethiazide (Ibuprofen can reduce the natriuretic effect of thiazide diuretics in some patients). Products include:
Diucardin Tablets ... 2824

Lithium Carbonate (Ibuprofen can produce an elevation of plasma lithium levels and a reduction in renal lithium clearance). Products include:
Eskalith ... 2658
Lithium Carbonate Capsules & Tablets ... 2352
Lithonate/Lithotabs/Lithobid ... 2721

Lithium Citrate (Ibuprofen can produce an elevation of plasma lithium levels and a reduction in renal lithium clearance).
No products indexed under this heading.

Methotrexate Sodium (Potential for enhanced methotrexate toxicity possibly resulting from competitively inhibiting methotrexate accumulation). Products include:
Methotrexate Sodium Tablets, Injection, for Injection and LPF Injection ... 1322

Methyclothiazide (Ibuprofen can reduce the natriuretic effect of thiazide diuretics in some patients). Products include:
Enduron Tablets ... 424

Polythiazide (Ibuprofen can reduce the natriuretic effect of thiazide diuretics in some patients). Products include:
Minizide Capsules ... 2016

Warfarin Sodium (Concurrent use may result in bleeding). Products include:
Coumadin ... 941

Food Interactions

Food, unspecified (Food affects the rate but not the extent of absorption).

IBERET FILMTAB
(Vitamin B Complex With Vitamin C, Ferrous Sulfate) ... 437
None cited in PDR database.

IBERET-500 FILMTAB
(Vitamin B Complex With Vitamin C, Ferrous Sulfate) ... 437
None cited in PDR database.

IBERET-500 LIQUID
(Vitamin B Complex With Vitamin C, Ferrous Sulfate) ... 438
None cited in PDR database.

IBERET-FOLIC-500 FILMTAB
(Vitamin B Complex With Vitamin C, Ferrous Sulfate) ... 433
See **Fero-Folic-500 Filmtab**

IBERET-LIQUID
(Vitamin B Complex With Vitamin C, Ferrous Sulfate) ... 438
None cited in PDR database.

IBUPROHM (IBUPROFEN) CAPLETS, 200 MG
(Ibuprofen) ... ▣ 713
May interact with aspirin and acetaminophen containing products. Compounds in this category include:

Acetaminophen (Concurrent use not recommended). Products include:
Actifed Cold & Sinus Caplets and Tablets ... ▣ 808
Actifed Sinus Daytime/Nighttime Tablets and Caplets ... ▣ 809
Alka-Seltzer Fast Relief Caplets ... ▣ 610
Alka-Seltzer Plus Liqui-Gels ... ▣ 612
Alka-Seltzer Plus Flu & Body Aches Effervescent Tablets ... ▣ 612
Alka-Seltzer Plus Flu & Body Aches Liqui-Gels Non-Drowsy Formula ... ▣ 613
Alka-Seltzer Plus Night-Time Cold Medicine Liqui-Gels ... ▣ 612
Allerest No Drowsiness ... ▣ 649
Allerest Sinus Pain Formula ... ▣ 649
Axocet Capsules ... 2469
Benadryl Allergy/Cold Tablets ... ▣ 811
Benadryl Allergy Sinus Headache Caplets ... ▣ 813
Children's TYLENOL acetaminophen Chewable Tablets, Elixir, Suspension Liquid, and Suspension Drops ... 1559
Children's TYLENOL Cold Multi-Symptom Chewable Tablets and Liquid ... 1559
Children's TYLENOL Cold Plus Cough Multi Symptom Chewable Tablets and Liquid ... 1560
Children's TYLENOL Flu Suspension Liquid ... 1560
Allergy-Sinus Comtrex Multi-Symptom Allergy-Sinus Formula Tablets and Caplets ... ▣ 639
Comtrex Multi-Symptom ... ▣ 638
Comtrex Non-Drowsy ... ▣ 640
Contac Day Allergy/Sinus Caplets ▣ 771
Contac Day & Night ... ▣ 772
Contac Night Allergy/Sinus Caplets ... ▣ 771
Contac Severe Cold and Flu Formula Caplets ... ▣ 773
Contac Severe Cold & Flu Non-Drowsy ... ▣ 774
Coricidin Cold + Flu Tablets ... ▣ 760
Coricidin 'D' Decongestant Tablets ... ▣ 760
DHCplus Capsules ... 2148
Darvon-N/Darvocet-N ... 1473
Dimetapp Allergy Sinus Caplets ... ▣ 838
Dimetapp Cold & Fever Suspension ... ▣ 839
Drixoral Cold and Flu Extended-Release Tablets ... ▣ 764
Drixoral Cough + Sore Throat Liquid Caps ... ▣ 763
Drixoral Allergy/Sinus Extended Release Tablets ... ▣ 765
Esgic-plus Capsules ... 1012
Esgic-plus Tablets ... 1012
Aspirin Free Excedrin Analgesic Caplets and Geltabs ... 734
Excedrin Extra-Strength Analgesic Tablets, Caplets, and Geltabs ... 734
Excedrin P.M. Analgesic/Sleeping Aid Tablets, Caplets, Liquigels ... 735
Fioricet Tablets ... 2386
Fioricet with Codeine Capsules ... 2387
Goody's Extra Strength Headache Powders ... ▣ 632
Goody's Extra Strength Pain Relief Tablets ... ▣ 632
Hycomine Compound Tablets ... 948
Hydrocet Capsules ... 787
Infants' TYLENOL acetaminophen Suspension Drops ... 1559
Infants' TYLENOL Cold Decongestant & Fever-Reducer Drops ... 1561
Junior Strength TYLENOL acetaminophen Coated Caplets and Chewable Tablets ... 1562
Lorcet 10/650 Tablets ... 1016
Lortab ... 2751
Lurline PMS Tablets ... 1000
Maximum Strength Multi-Symptom Formula Midol ... ▣ 621
PMS Multi-Symptom Formula Midol ... ▣ 622
Maximum Strength Midol Teen Multi-Symptom Formula ... ▣ 621
Midrin Capsules ... 788
Panodol Tablets and Caplets ... ▣ 783
Children's Panadol Chewable Tablets, Liquid, Infant's Drops ... ▣ 783
Percocet Tablets ... 955
Percogesic Analgesic Tablets ... ▣ 727
Phrenilin ... 790
Pyrroxate Caplets ... ▣ 742
Robitussin Cold, Cough & Flu Liqui-Gels ... ▣ 844
Robitussin Night-Time Cold Formula ... ▣ 847
Sedapap Tablets 50 mg/650 mg ... 1826
Sinarest ... ▣ 663
Sine-Aid Maximum Strength Sinus Headache Gelcaps, Caplets and Tablets ... 1570
Sine-Off No Drowsiness Formula Caplets ... ▣ 784
Sine-Off Sinus Medicine ... ▣ 784
Singlet Tablets ... ▣ 785
Sinulin Tablets ... 792

517 **Interactions Index** **Pork Regular, 100 Units**

Sinutab Sinus Allergy Medication, Maximum Strength Tablets and Caplets ... 823
Sinutab Sinus Medication, Maximum Strength Without Drowsiness Formula, Tablets & Caplets ... 824
Sudafed Cold and Cough Liquid Caps ... 826
Sudafed Severe Cold Formula Caplets ... 828
Sudafed Severe Cold Formula Tablets ... 828
Sudafed Sinus Caplets ... 829
Sudafed Sinus Tablets ... 829
Talacen Caplets ... 2464
TheraFlu Flu and Cold Medicine ... 750
Theraflu Maximum Strength Flu and Cold Medicine For Sore Throat ... 751
TheraFlu Flu, Cold and Cough Medicine ... 750
TheraFlu Maximum Strength Nighttime Flu, Cold & Cough Medicine ... 751
TheraFlu Maximum Strength Non-Drowsy Formula Flu, Cold & Cough Medicine ... 751
TheraFlu Maximum Strength, Non-Drowsy Formula Flu, Cold and Cough Caplets ... 752
Theraflu Maximum Strength Sinus Non-Drowsy Formula Caplets ... 752
Triaminic Sore Throat Formula ... 755
Triaminicin Tablets ... 756
TYLENOL acetaminophen Extended Relief Caplets ... 1570
TYLENOL acetaminophen, Extra Strength Adult Liquid Pain Reliever ... 1570
TYLENOL acetaminophen, Extra Strength Gelcaps, Geltabs, Caplets, Tablets ... 1570
TYLENOL acetaminophen, Regular Strength Caplets and Tablets ... 1570
TYLENOL Allergy Sinus, Maximum Strength Caplets and Gelcaps ... 1571
TYLENOL Allergy Sinus NightTime, Maximum Strength Caplets ... 1571
TYLENOL Cold Medication, Multi-Symptom Formula Tablets and Caplets ... 1572
TYLENOL Cold Medication, Multi-Symptom Hot Liquid Packets ... 1572
TYLENOL Cold Medication, No Drowsiness Formula Caplets and Gelcaps ... 1572
TYLENOL Cold Severe Congestion Caplets ... 1573
TYLENOL Cough Medication, Multi Symptom ... 1574
TYLENOL Cough Medication with Decongestant, Multi Symptom ... 1574
TYLENOL Flu No Drowsiness Formula, Maximum Strength Gelcaps ... 1575
TYLENOL Flu NightTime, Maximum Strength Gelcaps ... 1575
TYLENOL Flu NightTime, Maximum Strength Hot Medication Packets ... 1575
TYLENOL Headache Plus Pain Reliever with Antacid, Extra Strength Caplets ... 705
TYLENOL PM Pain Reliever/Sleep Aid, Extra Strength Gelcaps, Caplets, Geltabs ... 1576
TYLENOL Severe Allergy Medication Caplets ... 1571
TYLENOL Sinus, Maximum Strength Geltabs, Gelcaps, Caplets and Tablets ... 1576
Tylenol with Codeine ... 1592
Tylox Capsules ... 1593
Unisom With Pain Relief-Nighttime Sleep Aid and Pain Reliever ... 1991
Vanquish Analgesic Caplets ... 627
Vicks 44 LiquiCaps Cough, Cold & Flu Relief ... 728
Vicks 44M Cough, Cold & Flu Relief ... 729
Vicks DayQuil LiquiCaps/Liquid Multi-Symptom Cold/Flu Relief ... 734
Vicks Nyquil Hot Therapy ... 735
Vicks NyQuil LiquiCaps/Liquid Multi-Symptom Cold/Flu Relief, Original and Cherry Flavors ... 736
Vicodin Tablets ... 1404
Vicodin ES Tablets ... 1405
Vicodin HP Tablets ... 1403
Wygesic Tablets ... 2930
Zydone Capsules ... 967

Aspirin (Concurrent use not recommended). Products include:
Alka-Seltzer Cherry Effervescent Antacid and Pain Reliever ... 609
Alka-Seltzer Extra Strength Effervescent Antacid and Pain Reliever ... 609
Alka-Seltzer Lemon Lime Effervescent Antacid and Pain Reliever ... 609
Alka-Seltzer Original Effervescent Antacid and Pain Reliever ... 609
Alka-Seltzer Plus ... 611
Alka-Seltzer Plus Sinus Medicine ... 611
Ascriptin ... 650
Arthritis Strength BC Powder ... 631
BC Cold Powder Multi-Symptom Formula (Cold-Sinus-Allergy) ... 631
BC Cold Powder Non-Drowsy Formula (Cold-Sinus) ... 631
BC Powder ... 631
Genuine Bayer Aspirin Tablets & Caplets ... 618
Extra Strength Bayer Arthritis Pain Regimen Formula ... 615
Extra Strength Bayer Aspirin Caplets & Tablets ... 617
Extended-Release Bayer 8-Hour Aspirin ... 616
Extra Strength Bayer Plus Aspirin Caplets ... 617
Extra Strength Bayer PM Aspirin Plus Sleep Aid ... 617
Aspirin Regimen Bayer 81 mg Tablets with Calcium ... 615
Aspirin Regimen Bayer Adult Low Strength 81 mg Tablets ... 613
Aspirin Regimen Bayer Children's Chewable Aspirin ... 616
Aspirin Regimen Bayer Regular Strength 325 mg Caplets ... 613
Bufferin Analgesic Tablets ... 636
Arthritis Strength Bufferin Analgesic Caplets ... 637
Extra Strength Bufferin Analgesic Tablets ... 637
Cama Arthritis Pain Reliever ... 748
Darvon Compound-65 Pulvules ... 1475
Easprin ... 1971
Ecotrin ... 2625
Ecotrin Enteric Coated Aspirin Maximum Strength Tablets and Caplets ... 775
Ecotrin Enteric Coated Aspirin Regular Strength Tablets ... 2625
Empirin Aspirin Tablets ... 818
Excedrin Extra-Strength Analgesic Tablets, Caplets, and Geltabs ... 734
Fiorinal Capsules ... 2388
Fiorinal with Codeine Capsules ... 2390
Fiorinal Tablets ... 2388
Goody's Extra Strength Headache Powders ... 632
Goody's Extra Strength Pain Relief Tablets ... 632
Halfprin Tablets ... 1413
Norgesic ... 1554
Percodan Tablets ... 955
Percodan-Demi Tablets ... 956
Robaxisal Tablets ... 2246
Soma Compound w/Codeine Tablets ... 2784
Soma Compound Tablets ... 2783
St. Joseph Adult Chewable Aspirin (81 mg.) ... 768
Talwin Compound ... 2466
Vanquish Analgesic Caplets ... 627

IBUPROHM (IBUPROFEN) TABLETS, 200 MG
(Ibuprofen) ... 713
See **Ibuprohm (Ibuprofen) Caplets, 200 mg**

IDAMYCIN INJECTION
(Idarubicin Hydrochloride) ... 2096
May interact with anthracyclines. Compounds in this category include:

Daunorubicin Citrate (Previous therapy with anthracyclines is co-factor for increased cardiac toxicity). Products include:
DaunoXome ... 1842

Daunorubicin Hydrochloride (Previous therapy with anthracyclines is co-factor for increased cardiac toxicity). Products include:
Cerubidine for Injection ... 634

Doxorubicin Hydrochloride (Previous therapy with anthracyclines is co-factor for increased cardiac toxicity). Products include:
Adriamycin PFS ... 2056
Adriamycin RDF ... 2056
Doxil ... 2613
Doxorubicin Astra ... 531
Rubex for Injection ... 721

IFEX
(Ifosfamide) ... 706
May interact with:

Bone Marrow Depressants, unspecified (Adjustments in dosing may be necessary).

ILETIN I
(Insulin, Zinc Suspension) ... 1501
See **Pork Regular, 100 Units**

LENTE, 100 UNITS
(Insulin, Zinc Suspension) ... 1501
See **Pork Regular, 100 Units**

NPH, 100 UNITS
(Insulin, NPH) ... 1502
See **Pork Regular, 100 Units**

REGULAR, 100 UNITS
(Insulin, Regular) ... 1503
See **Pork Regular, 100 Units**

ILETIN II
(Insulin, Zinc Suspension) ... 1504
See **Pork Regular, 100 Units**

PORK LENTE, 100 UNITS
(Insulin, Zinc Suspension) ... 1504
See **Pork Regular, 100 Units**

PORK NPH, 100 UNITS
(Insulin, NPH) ... 1506
See **Pork Regular, 100 Units**

PORK REGULAR, 100 UNITS
(Insulin, Regular) ... 1507
May interact with corticosteroids, oral contraceptives, thyroid preparations, salicylates, oral hypoglycemic agents, and certain other agents. Compounds in these categories include:

Acarbose (Co-administration with drugs with hypoglycemic activity, such as oral hypoglycemic agents, may result in decreased insulin requirements). Products include:
Precose ... 604

Aspirin (Co-administration with drugs with hypoglycemic activity, such as salicylates, may result in decreased insulin requirements). Products include:
Alka-Seltzer Cherry Effervescent Antacid and Pain Reliever ... 609
Alka-Seltzer Extra Strength Effervescent Antacid and Pain Reliever ... 609
Alka-Seltzer Lemon Lime Effervescent Antacid and Pain Reliever ... 609
Alka-Seltzer Original Effervescent Antacid and Pain Reliever ... 609
Alka-Seltzer Plus ... 611
Alka-Seltzer Plus Sinus Medicine ... 611
Ascriptin ... 650
Arthritis Strength BC Powder ... 631
BC Cold Powder Multi-Symptom Formula (Cold-Sinus-Allergy) ... 631
BC Cold Powder Non-Drowsy Formula (Cold-Sinus) ... 631
BC Powder ... 631
Genuine Bayer Aspirin Tablets & Caplets ... 618
Extra Strength Bayer Arthritis Pain Regimen Formula ... 615
Extra Strength Bayer Aspirin Caplets & Tablets ... 617
Extended-Release Bayer 8-Hour Aspirin ... 616
Extra Strength Bayer Plus Aspirin Caplets ... 617
Extra Strength Bayer PM Aspirin Plus Sleep Aid ... 617
Aspirin Regimen Bayer 81 mg Tablets with Calcium ... 615
Aspirin Regimen Bayer Adult Low Strength 81 mg Tablets ... 613
Aspirin Regimen Bayer Children's Chewable Aspirin ... 616
Aspirin Regimen Bayer Regular Strength 325 mg Caplets ... 613
Bufferin Analgesic Tablets ... 636
Arthritis Strength Bufferin Analgesic Caplets ... 637
Extra Strength Bufferin Analgesic Tablets ... 637
Cama Arthritis Pain Reliever ... 748
Darvon Compound-65 Pulvules ... 1475
Easprin ... 1971
Ecotrin ... 2625
Ecotrin Enteric Coated Aspirin Maximum Strength Tablets and Caplets ... 775
Ecotrin Enteric Coated Aspirin Regular Strength Tablets ... 2625
Empirin Aspirin Tablets ... 818
Excedrin Extra-Strength Analgesic Tablets, Caplets, and Geltabs ... 734
Fiorinal Capsules ... 2388
Fiorinal with Codeine Capsules ... 2390
Fiorinal Tablets ... 2388
Goody's Extra Strength Headache Powders ... 632
Goody's Extra Strength Pain Relief Tablets ... 632
Halfprin Tablets ... 1413
Norgesic ... 1554
Percodan Tablets ... 955
Percodan-Demi Tablets ... 956
Robaxisal Tablets ... 2246
Soma Compound w/Codeine Tablets ... 2784
Soma Compound Tablets ... 2783
St. Joseph Adult Chewable Aspirin (81 mg.) ... 768
Talwin Compound ... 2466
Vanquish Analgesic Caplets ... 627

Betamethasone Acetate (Co-administration may result in increased insulin requirements). Products include:
Celestone Soluspan Suspension ... 2484

Betamethasone Sodium Phosphate (Co-administration may result in increased insulin requirements). Products include:
Celestone Soluspan Suspension ... 2484

Chlorpropamide (Co-administration with drugs with hypoglycemic activity, such as oral hypoglycemic agents, may result in decreased insulin requirements). Products include:
Diabinese Tablets ... 2002

Choline Magnesium Trisalicylate (Co-administration with drugs with hypoglycemic activity, such as salicylates, may result in decreased insulin requirements). Products include:
Trilisate ... 2155

Cortisone Acetate (Co-administration may result in increased insulin requirements). Products include:
Cortone Acetate Sterile Suspension ... 1663
Cortone Acetate Tablets ... 1664

Desogestrel (Co-administration with oral contraceptives may result in increased insulin requirements). Products include:
Desogen Tablets ... 1867
Ortho-Cept ... 1907

Dexamethasone (Co-administration may result in increased insulin requirements). Products include:
AK-Trol Ointment & Suspension ... ◉ 205
Decadron Elixir ... 1676

IMPORTANT NOTE: Always consult each drug listing in the patient's regimen for possible interactions.

Dexamethasone Acetate (Co-administration may result in increased insulin requirements). Products include:
Dalalone D.P. Injectable	1009
Decadron-LA Sterile Suspension	1687

Dexamethasone Sodium Phosphate (Co-administration may result in increased insulin requirements). Products include:
Decadron Phosphate Injection	1680
Decadron Phosphate Sterile Ophthalmic Ointment	1684
Decadron Phosphate Sterile Ophthalmic Solution	1685
Decadron Phosphate Topical Cream	1686
Decadron Phosphate with Xylocaine Injection, Sterile	1683
Dexacort Phosphate in Respihaler	1606
Dexacort Phosphate in Turbinaire	1607
NeoDecadron Sterile Ophthalmic Ointment	1755
NeoDecadron Sterile Ophthalmic Solution	1756
NeoDecadron Topical Cream	1757

Diflunisal (Co-administration with drugs with hypoglycemic activity, such as salicylates, may result in decreased insulin requirements). Products include:
Dolobid Tablets	1695

Ethinyl Estradiol (Co-administration with oral contraceptives may result in increased insulin requirements). Products include:
Brevicon	2563
Demulen	2580
Desogen Tablets	1867
Levlen/Tri-Levlen	646
Lo/Ovral Tablets	2852
Lo/Ovral-28 Tablets	2857
Modicon	1928
Nordette-21 Tablets	2863
Nordette-28 Tablets	2866
Norinyl	2563
Ortho-Cept	1907
Ortho-Cyclen/Ortho-Tri-Cyclen	1914
Ortho-Novum	1928
Ortho-Cyclen/Ortho Tri-Cyclen	1914
Ovcon	765
Ovral Tablets	2877
Ovral-28 Tablets	2878
Levlen/Tri-Levlen	646
Tri-Norinyl	2607
Triphasil-21 Tablets	2919
Triphasil-28 Tablets	2924

Ethynodiol Diacetate (Co-administration with oral contraceptives may result in increased insulin requirements). Products include:
Demulen	2580

Fludrocortisone Acetate (Co-administration may result in increased insulin requirements). Products include:
Florinef Acetate Tablets	506

Glimepiride (Co-administration with drugs with hypoglycemic activity, such as oral hypoglycemic agents, may result in decreased insulin requirements). Products include:
Amaryl Tablets	1241

Glipizide (Co-administration with drugs with hypoglycemic activity, such as oral hypoglycemic agents, may result in decreased insulin requirements). Products include:
Glucotrol Tablets	2011
Glucotrol XL Extended Release Tablets	2012

Glyburide (Co-administration with drugs with hypoglycemic activity, such as oral hypoglycemic agents, may result in decreased insulin requirements). Products include:
DiaBeta Tablets	1265
Glynase PresTab Tablets	2091
Micronase Tablets	2099

Hydrocortisone (Co-administration may result in increased insulin requirements). Products include:
Anusol-HC Cream 2.5%	1953
Aquanil HC Lotion	1989
Maximum Strength Cortaid Spray	800
CORTENEMA	2713
Cortisporin Ointment	1074
Cortisporin Ophthalmic Ointment Sterile	1074
Cortisporin Ophthalmic Suspension Sterile	1075
Cortisporin Otic Solution Sterile	1076
Cortisporin Otic Suspension Sterile	1077
Cortizone-5	795
Cortizone-10	795
Hydrocortone Tablets	1715
Hytone	922
Hytone Ointment 2 ½%	923
Massengill Medicated Soft Cloth Towelettes	2628
Pediotic Suspension Sterile	1140
Preparation H Hydrocortisone 1% Cream	843
ProctoCream-HC 2.5%	2552
VōSoL HC Otic Solution	2786

Hydrocortisone Acetate (Co-administration may result in increased insulin requirements). Products include:
Analpram-HC Rectal Cream 1% and 2.5%	993
Anusol HC-1 Hydrocortisone Anti-Itch Ointment	810
Anusol-HC Suppositories	1954
Caldecort Anti-Itch Hydrocortisone Cream	651
Coly-Mycin S Otic w/Neomycin & Hydrocortisone	1965
Cortaid	800
Cortifoam	2540
Cortisporin Cream	1073
Epifoam	2543
Hydrocortone Acetate Sterile Suspension	1712
Mantadil Cream	1124
Nupercainal Hydrocortisone 1% Cream	661
Pramosone Cream, Lotion & Ointment	995
ProctoFoam-HC	2552
Terra-Cortril Ophthalmic Suspension	2033

Hydrocortisone Sodium Phosphate (Co-administration may result in increased insulin requirements). Products include:
Hydrocortone Phosphate Injection, Sterile	1713

Hydrocortisone Sodium Succinate (Co-administration may result in increased insulin requirements).
No products indexed under this heading.

Levonorgestrel (Co-administration with oral contraceptives may result in increased insulin requirements). Products include:
Levlen/Tri-Levlen	646
Nordette-21 Tablets	2863
Nordette-28 Tablets	2866
Norplant System	2868
Levlen/Tri-Levlen	646
Triphasil-21 Tablets	2919
Triphasil-28 Tablets	2924

Levothyroxine Sodium (Co-administration with thyroid replacement therapy may result in increased insulin requirements). Products include:
Eltroxin Tablets	2214
Levothroid Tablets	1015
Levothyroxine Sodium, USP for Injection	546
Levoxyl Tablets	918
Synthroid	1410

Liothyronine Sodium (Co-administration with thyroid replacement therapy may result in increased insulin requirements). Products include:
Cytomel Tablets	2647
Triostat Injection	2708

Liotrix (Co-administration with thyroid replacement therapy may result in increased insulin requirements).
No products indexed under this heading.

Magnesium Salicylate (Co-administration with drugs with hypoglycemic activity, such as salicylates, may result in decreased insulin requirements). Products include:
Backache Caplets	635
Doan's Extra-Strength Analgesic	653
Extra Strength Doan's P.M.	653
Doan's Regular Strength Analgesic	654
Mobigesic Tablets	607

Mestranol (Co-administration with oral contraceptives may result in increased insulin requirements). Products include:
Norinyl	2563
Ortho-Novum	1928

Metformin Hydrochloride (Co-administration with drugs with hypoglycemic activity, such as oral hypoglycemic agents, may result in decreased insulin requirements). Products include:
Glucophage Tablets	754

Methylprednisolone Acetate (Co-administration may result in increased insulin requirements).
No products indexed under this heading.

Methylprednisolone Sodium Succinate (Co-administration may result in increased insulin requirements).
No products indexed under this heading.

Norethindrone (Co-administration with oral contraceptives may result in increased insulin requirements). Products include:
Brevicon	2563
Micronor Tablets	1903
Modicon	1928
Norinyl	2563
Nor-Q D Tablets	2598
Ortho-Novum	1928
Ovcon	765
Tri-Norinyl	2607

Norethynodrel (Co-administration with oral contraceptives may result in increased insulin requirements).
No products indexed under this heading.

Norgestimate (Co-administration with oral contraceptives may result in increased insulin requirements). Products include:
Ortho-Cyclen/Ortho-Tri-Cyclen	1914
Ortho-Cyclen/Ortho Tri-Cyclen	1914

Norgestrel (Co-administration with oral contraceptives may result in increased insulin requirements). Products include:
Lo/Ovral Tablets	2852
Lo/Ovral-28 Tablets	2857
Ovral Tablets	2877
Ovral-28 Tablets	2878
Ovrette Tablets	2878

Phenelzine Sulfate (Co-administration with drugs with hypoglycemic activity, such as certain MAO inhibitor antidepressants, may result in decreased insulin requirements). Products include:
Nardil	1977

Prednisolone Acetate (Co-administration may result in increased insulin requirements). Products include:
AK-CIDE	203
AK-CIDE Ointment	203
Blephamide Liquifilm Sterile Ophthalmic Suspension	472
Blephamide Ointment	234
Econopred & Econopred Plus Ophthalmic Suspensions	216
Poly-Pred Liquifilm	246
Pred Forte	247
Pred Mild	250
Pred-G Liquifilm Sterile Ophthalmic Suspension	248
Pred-G S.O.P. Sterile Ophthalmic Ointment	249

Prednisolone Sodium Phosphate (Co-administration may result in increased insulin requirements). Products include:
AK-PRED	204
Hydeltrasol Injection, Sterile	1708
Pediapred Oral Solution	1618

Prednisolone Tebutate (Co-administration may result in increased insulin requirements). Products include:
Hydeltra-T.B.A. Sterile Suspension	1710

Prednisone (Co-administration may result in increased insulin requirements).
No products indexed under this heading.

Salsalate (Co-administration with drugs with hypoglycemic activity, such as salicylates, may result in decreased insulin requirements). Products include:
Disalcid	1549
Mono-Gesic Tablets	810
Salflex Tablets	791

Sulfacytine (Co-administration with drugs with hypoglycemic activity, such as sulfa antibiotics, may result in decreased insulin requirements).

Sulfamethizole (Co-administration with drugs with hypoglycemic activity, such as sulfa antibiotics, may result in decreased insulin requirements). Products include:
Urobiotic-250 Capsules	2038

Sulfamethoxazole (Co-administration with drugs with hypoglycemic activity, such as sulfa antibiotics, may result in decreased insulin requirements). Products include:
Bactrim DS Tablets	2257
Bactrim I.V. Infusion	2255
Bactrim	2257
Gantanol Tablets	2285
Septra	1146
Septra I.V. Infusion	1142
Septra I.V. Infusion ADD-Vantage Vials	1144
Septra	1146

Sulfasalazine (Co-administration with drugs with hypoglycemic activity, such as sulfa antibiotics, may result in decreased insulin requirements). Products include:
Azulfidine	2059

Sulfisoxazole (Co-administration with drugs with hypoglycemic activity, such as sulfa antibiotics, may result in devreased insulin requirements). Products include:
Gantrisin Tablets	2286

Thyroglobulin (Co-administration with thyroid replacement therapy may result in increased insulin requirements).
No products indexed under this heading.

(▣ Described in PDR For Nonprescription Drugs)   (⊚ Described in PDR For Ophthalmology)

Thyroid (Co-administration with thyroid replacement therapy may result in increased insulin requirements).
  No products indexed under this heading.

Thyroxine (Co-administration with thyroid replacement therapy may result in increased insulin requirements).
  No products indexed under this heading.

Thyroxine Sodium (Co-administration with thyroid replacement therapy may result in increased insulin requirements).
  No products indexed under this heading.

Tolazamide (Co-administration with drugs with hypoglycemic activity, such as oral hypoglycemic agents, may result in decreased insulin requirements).
  No products indexed under this heading.

Tolbutamide (Co-administration with drugs with hypoglycemic activity, such as oral hypoglycemic agents, may result in decreased insulin requirements).
  No products indexed under this heading.

Tranylcypromine Sulfate (Co-administration with drugs with hypoglycemic activity, such as certain MAO inhibitor antidepressants, may result in decreased insulin requirements). Products include:
  Parnate Tablets 2679

Triamcinolone (Co-administration may result in increased insulin requirements).
  No products indexed under this heading.

Triamcinolone Acetonide (Co-administration may result in increased insulin requirements). Products include:
  Azmacort Oral Inhaler 2175
  Nasacort AQ Nasal Spray 2191
  Nasacort Nasal Inhaler 2189

Triamcinolone Diacetate (Co-administration may result in increased insulin requirements).
  No products indexed under this heading.

Triamcinolone Hexacetonide (Co-administration may result in increased insulin requirements).
  No products indexed under this heading.

PORK REGULAR (CONCENTRATED), 500 UNITS
(Insulin, Regular) 1508
  See   Pork Regular, 100 Units

ILOSONE LIQUID, ORAL SUSPENSIONS
(Erythromycin Estolate) 927
  See Ilosone Pulvules & Tablets

ILOSONE PULVULES & TABLETS
(Erythromycin Estolate) 927
May interact with drugs which undergo biotransformation by cytochrome p-450 mixed function oxidase, oral anticoagulants, xanthine bronchodilators, and certain other agents. Compounds in these categories include:

Alfentanil Hydrochloride (Concurrent use may be associated with elevation in serum level of alfentanil; monitor serum levels closely). Products include:
  Alfenta Injection 1334

Aminophylline (Co-administration with high doses of theophylline may be associated with increased serum theophylline levels and potential theophylline toxicity).
  No products indexed under this heading.

Astemizole (Concomitant use may significantly alter the metabolism of astemizole; rare cases of serious cardiovascular adverse events, including electrocardiographic QT/QTc interval prolongation, death, cardiac arrest, torsades de pointes and other ventricular arrhythmias have been reported; concurrent use is contraindicated). Products include:
  Hismanal Tablets 1341

Bromocriptine Mesylate (Concurrent use may be associated with elevation in serum level of bromocriptine; monitor serum levels closely). Products include:
  Parlodel 2411

Carbamazepine (Concurrent use may be associated with elevation in serum level of carbamazepine; monitor serum levels closely). Products include:
  Atretol Tablets 569
  Tegretol/Tegretol-XR 870

Clindamycin Hydrochloride (Antagonistic under some conditions).
  No products indexed under this heading.

Clindamycin Palmitate Hydrochloride (Antagonistic under some conditions).
  No products indexed under this heading.

Cyclosporine (Concurrent use may be associated with elevation in serum level of cyclosporine; monitor serum levels closely). Products include:
  Neoral 2405
  Sandimmune 2416

Dicumarol (Concomitant therapy may result in increased anticoagulant effects).
  No products indexed under this heading.

Digoxin (Co-administration may result in elevated digoxin serum levels). Products include:
  Lanoxicaps 1110
  Lanoxin Elixir Pediatric 1113
  Lanoxin Injection 1116
  Lanoxin Injection Pediatric............. 1119
  Lanoxin Tablets 1121

Dihydroergotamine Mesylate (Concurrent use has been associated with acute ergot toxicity characterized by severe peripheral vasospasm and dysesthesia). Products include:
  D.H.E. 45 Injection 2381

Disopyramide Phosphate (Concurrent use may be associated with elevation in serum level of disopyramide; monitor serum levels closely). Products include:
  Norpace 2596

Divalproex Sodium (Concurrent use may be associated with elevation in serum level of valproate; monitor serum levels closely). Products include:
  Depakote Tablets 418

Drugs which undergo biotransformation by cytochrome P-450 mixed function oxidase (Concurrent use may be associated with elevation in serum level of drugs metabolized by the cytochrome P-450 system).

Dyphylline (Co-administration with high doses of theophylline may be associated with increased serum theophylline levels and potential theophylline toxicity). Products include:
  Lufyllin & Lufyllin-400 Tablets 2778
  Lufyllin-GG Elixir & Tablets 2779

Ergotamine Tartrate (Concurrent use has been associated with acute ergot toxicity characterized by severe peripheral vasospasm and dysesthesia). Products include:
  Bellergal-S Tablets 2375
  Cafergot 2376
  Ergomar Tablets 1543
  Wigraine Tablets 1884

Hexobarbital (Concurrent use may be associated with elevation in serum level of hexobarbital; monitor serum levels closely).

Lincomycin Hydrochloride Monohydrate (Antagonistic under some conditions).
  No products indexed under this heading.

Lovastatin (Potential for rhabdomyolysis with or without renal impairment in seriously ill patients; concurrent use may be associated with elevation in serum level of lovastatin; monitor serum levels closely). Products include:
  Mevacor Tablets 1742

Midazolam Hydrochloride (Decreased clearance of midazolam; potential for increased pharmacologic effect of midazolam). Products include:
  Versed Injection 2324

Phenytoin (Concurrent use may be associated with elevation in serum level of phenytoin; monitor serum levels closely). Products include:
  Dilantin Infatabs 1967
  Dilantin-125 Suspension 1969

Phenytoin Sodium (Concurrent use may be associated with elevation in serum level of phenytoin; monitor serum levels closely). Products include:
  Dilantin Kapseals 1965

Probenecid (Inhibits tubular reabsorption of erythromycin). Products include:
  Benemid Tablets 1651
  ColBENEMID Tablets 1662

Terfenadine (Concomitant use may significantly alter the metabolism of terfenadine; rare cases of serious cardiovascular adverse events, including electrocardiographic QT/QTc interval prolongation, death, cardiac arrest, torsades de pointes and other ventricular arrhythmias have been reported; concurrent use is contraindicated). Products include:
  Seldane Tablets 1284
  Seldane-D Extended-Release Tablets 1286

Theophylline (Co-administration with high doses of theophylline may be associated with increased serum theophylline levels and potential theophylline toxicity). Products include:
  Marax Tablets & DF Syrup 2015
  Quibron 2227

Theophylline Anhydrous (Co-administration with high doses of theophylline may be associated with increased serum theophylline levels and potential theophylline toxicity). Products include:
  Aerolate 1003
  Primatene Tablets 844
  Respbid Tablets 687
  Slo-bid Gyrocaps 2201
  Theo-24 Extended Release Capsules 2753
  Theo-Dur Extended-Release Tablets 1367
  Theo-X Extended-Release Tablets .. 793
  Uni-Dur Extended-Release Tablets .. 1374
  Uniphyl 400 mg and 600 mg Tablets 2157

Theophylline Calcium Salicylate (Co-administration with high doses of theophylline may be associated with increased serum theophylline levels and potential theophylline toxicity). Products include:
  Quadrinal Tablets 1398

Theophylline Sodium Glycinate (Co-administration with high doses of theophylline may be associated with increased serum theophylline levels and potential theophylline toxicity).
  No products indexed under this heading.

Triazolam (Decreased clearance of triazolam; potential for increased pharmacologic effect of triazolam). Products include:
  Halcion Tablets 2093

Valproic Acid (Concurrent use may be associated with elevation in serum level of valproate; monitor serum levels closely). Products include:
  Depakene 416

Warfarin Sodium (Concomitant therapy may result in increased anticoagulant effects). Products include:
  Coumadin 941

ILOTYCIN GLUCEPTATE, IV, VIALS
(Erythromycin Glucoptate) 929
May interact with oral anticoagulants, drugs which undergo biotransformation by cytochrome p-450 mixed function oxidase, xanthine bronchodilators, and certain other agents. Compounds in these categories include:

Alfentanil Hydrochloride (Concurrent use may be associated with elevation in serum level of alfentanil; monitor serum levels closely). Products include:
  Alfenta Injection 1334

Aminophylline (Co-administration with high doses of theophylline may be associated with increased serum theophylline levels and potential theophylline toxicity).
  No products indexed under this heading.

Astemizole (Concomitant use may significantly alter the metabolism of astemizole; rare cases of serious cardiovascular adverse events, including electrocardiographic QT/QTc interval prolongation, death, cardiac arrest, torsades de pointes and other ventricular arrhythmias have been reported; concurrent use is contraindicated). Products include:
  Hismanal Tablets 1341

Bromocriptine Mesylate (Concurrent use may be associated with elevation in serum level of bromocriptine; monitor serum levels closely). Products include:
  Parlodel 2411

Carbamazepine (Concurrent use may be associated with elevation in serum level of carbamazepine; monitor serum levels closely). Products include:
  Atretol Tablets 569
  Tegretol/Tegretol-XR 870

IMPORTANT NOTE: Always consult each drug listing in the patient's regimen for possible interactions.

Ilotycin Gluceptate, IV — Interactions Index

Cyclosporine (Concurrent use may be associated with elevation in serum level of cyclosporine; monitor serum levels closely). Products include:
- Neoral 2405
- Sandimmune 2416

Dicumarol (Concomitant therapy may result in increased anticoagulant effects).
- No products indexed under this heading.

Digoxin (Co-administration may result in elevated digoxin serum levels). Products include:
- Lanoxicaps 1110
- Lanoxin Elixir Pediatric 1113
- Lanoxin Injection 1116
- Lanoxin Injection Pediatric 1119
- Lanoxin Tablets 1121

Dihydroergotamine Mesylate (Concurrent use has been associated with acute ergot toxicity characterized by severe peripheral vasospasm and dysesthesia). Products include:
- D.H.E. 45 Injection 2381

Disopyramide Phosphate (Concurrent use may be associated with elevation in serum level of disopyramide; monitor serum levels closely). Products include:
- Norpace 2596

Drugs which undergo biotransformation by cytochrome P-450 mixed function oxidase (Concurrent use may be associated with elevation in serum level of drugs metabolized by the cytochrome P-450 system).

Dyphylline (Co-administration with high doses of theophylline may be associated with increased serum theophylline levels and potential theophylline toxicity). Products include:
- Lufyllin & Lufyllin-400 Tablets 2778
- Lufyllin-GG Elixir & Tablets 2779

Ergotamine Tartrate (Concurrent use has been associated with acute ergot toxicity characterized by severe peripheral vasospasm and dysesthesia). Products include:
- Bellergal-S Tablets 2375
- Cafergot 2376
- Ergomar Tablets 1543
- Wigraine Tablets 1884

Hexobarbital (Concurrent use may be associated with elevation in serum level of hexobarbital; monitor serum levels closely).

Lovastatin (Potential for rhabdomyolysis with or without renal impairment in seriously ill patients; concurrent use may be associated with elevation in serum level of lovastatin; monitor serum levels closely). Products include:
- Mevacor Tablets 1742

Midazolam Hydrochloride (Decreased clearance of midazolam; potential for increased pharmacologic effect of midazolam). Products include:
- Versed Injection 2324

Phenytoin (Concurrent use may be associated with elevation in serum level of phenytoin; monitor serum levels closely). Products include:
- Dilantin Infatabs 1967
- Dilantin-125 Suspension 1969

Phenytoin Sodium (Concurrent use may be associated with elevation in serum level of phenytoin; monitor serum levels closely). Products include:
- Dilantin Kapseals 1965

Terfenadine (Concomitant use may significantly alter the metabolism of terfenadine; rare cases of serious cardiovascular adverse events, including electrocardiographic QT/QTc interval prolongation, death, cardiac arrest, torsades de pointes and other ventricular arrhythmias have been reported; concurrent use is contraindicated). Products include:
- Seldane Tablets 1284
- Seldane-D Extended-Release Tablets 1286

Theophylline (Co-administration with high doses of theophylline may be associated with increased serum theophylline levels and potential theophylline toxicity). Products include:
- Marax Tablets & DF Syrup 2015
- Quibron 2227

Theophylline Anhydrous (Co-administration with high doses of theophylline may be associated with increased serum theophylline levels and potential theophylline toxicity). Products include:
- Aerolate 1003
- Primatene Tablets .... ⊞ 844
- Respbid Tablets 687
- Slo-bid Gyrocaps 2201
- Theo-24 Extended Release Capsules 2753
- Theo-Dur Extended- Release Tablets 1367
- Theo-X Extended-Release Tablets 793
- Uni-Dur Extended-Release Tablets 1374
- Uniphyl 400 mg and 600 mg Tablets 2157

Theophylline Calcium Salicylate (Co-administration with high doses of theophylline may be associated with increased serum theophylline levels and potential theophylline toxicity). Products include:
- Quadrinal Tablets 1398

Theophylline Sodium Glycinate (Co-administration with high doses of theophylline may be associated with increased serum theophylline levels and potential theophylline toxicity).
- No products indexed under this heading.

Triazolam (Decreased clearance of triazolam; potential for increased pharmacologic effect of triazolam). Products include:
- Halcion Tablets 2093

Warfarin Sodium (Concomitant therapy may result in increased anticoagulant effects). Products include:
- Coumadin 941

ILOTYCIN OPHTHALMIC OINTMENT
(Erythromycin) 928
None cited in PDR database.

IMDUR
(Isosorbide Mononitrate) 1362
May interact with calcium channel blockers, vasodilators, and certain other agents. Compounds in these categories include:

Amlodipine Besylate (Potential for marked symptomatic orthostatic hypotension; dosage adjustments may be necessary). Products include:
- Lotrel Capsules 858
- Norvasc Tablets 2020

Bepridil Hydrochloride (Potential for marked symptomatic orthostatic hypotension; dosage adjustments may be necessary). Products include:
- Vascor Tablets (200 and 300 mg) 1597

Diazoxide (Additive vasodilating effects). Products include:
- Hyperstat I.V. Injection 2504
- Proglycem 575

Diltiazem Hydrochloride (Potential for marked symptomatic orthostatic hypotension; dosage adjustments may be necessary). Products include:
- Cardizem CD Capsules 1251
- Cardizem SR Capsules 1255
- Cardizem Injectable 1253
- Cardizem Tablets 1257
- Dilacor XR Extended-release Capsules 2183
- Tiazac Capsules 1019

Epoprostenol Sodium (Additive vasodilating effects). Products include:
- Flolan for Injection 1085

Felodipine (Potential for marked symptomatic orthostatic hypotension; dosage adjustments may be necessary). Products include:
- Plendil Extended-Release Tablets 514

Hydralazine Hydrochloride (Additive vasodilating effects). Products include:
- Apresazide Capsules 824
- Apresoline Hydrochloride Tablets 826
- Hydralazine Hydrochloride Injection USP 2712
- Ser-Ap-Es Tablets 867

Isradipine (Potential for marked symptomatic orthostatic hypotension; dosage adjustments may be necessary). Products include:
- DynaCirc Capsules 2381
- DynaCirc CR Tablets 2383

Minoxidil (Additive vasodilating effects).
- No products indexed under this heading.

Nicardipine Hydrochloride (Potential for marked symptomatic orthostatic hypotension; dosage adjustments may be necessary). Products include:
- Cardene Capsules 2261
- Cardene I.V. 2815
- Cardene SR Capsules 2264

Nifedipine (Potential for marked symptomatic orthostatic hypotension; dosage adjustments may be necessary). Products include:
- Adalat Capsules (10 mg and 20 mg) 580
- Adalat CC 582
- Procardia Capsules 2024
- Procardia XL Extended Release Tablets 2026

Nimodipine (Potential for marked symptomatic orthostatic hypotension; dosage adjustments may be necessary). Products include:
- Nimotop Capsules 603

Nisoldipine (Potential for marked symptomatic orthostatic hypotension; dosage adjustments may be necessary). Products include:
- Sular Tablets 2961

Verapamil Hydrochloride (Potential for marked symptomatic orthostatic hypotension; dosage adjustments may be necessary). Products include:
- Calan SR Caplets 2571
- Calan Tablets 2568
- Covera-HS Tablets 2573
- Isoptin Injectable 1391
- Isoptin Oral Tablets 1393
- Isoptin SR Tablets 1395
- Verelan Capsules 1455

Food Interactions
Alcohol (Additive vasodilating effects).
Food, unspecified (May decrease the rate (increase in T_{max}) but not the extent (AUC) of absorption).

IMITREX INJECTION
(Sumatriptan Succinate) 1095
May interact with ergot-containing drugs, monoamine oxidase inhibitors, and certain other agents. Compounds in these categories include:

Dihydroergotamine Mesylate (Co-administration has resulted in prolonged vasospastic reactions due to theoretical basis of additive effects; use of these agents concurrently or within 24 hours is contraindicated). Products include:
- D.H.E. 45 Injection 2381

Ergotamine Tartrate (Co-administration has resulted in prolonged vasospastic reactions due to theoretical basis of additive effects; use of these agents concurrently or within 24 hours is contraindicated). Products include:
- Bellergal-S Tablets 2375
- Cafergot 2376
- Ergomar Tablets 1543
- Wigraine Tablets 1884

Fluoxetine Hydrochloride (Co-administration with a selective serotonin reuptake inhibitor has resulted in rare reports of weakness, hyperreflexia, and incoordination). Products include:
- Prozac Pulvules & Liquid, Oral Solution 935

Fluvoxamine Maleate (Co-administration with a selective serotonin reuptake inhibitor has resulted in rare reports of weakness, hyperreflexia, and incoordination). Products include:
- LUVOX Tablets 2723

Furazolidone (Co-administration with an MAO-A inhibitor reduces sumatriptan clearance with a significant increase in systemic exposure; concurrent use with MAO-A inhibitor is not ordinarily recommended). Products include:
- Furoxone 2221

Isocarboxazid (Co-administration with an MAO-A inhibitor reduces sumatriptan clearance with a significant increase in systemic exposure; concurrent use with MAO-A inhibitor is not ordinarily recommended).
- No products indexed under this heading.

Methylergonovine Maleate (Co-administration has resulted in prolonged vasospastic reactions due to theoretical basis of additive effects; use of these agents concurrently or within 24 hours is contraindicated). Products include:
- Methergine 2401

Methysergide Maleate (Co-administration has resulted in prolonged vasospastic reactions due to theoretical basis of additive effects; use of these agents concurrently or within 24 hours is contraindicated). Products include:
- Sansert Tablets 2424

Paroxetine Hydrochloride (Co-administration with a selective serotonin reuptake inhibitor has resulted in rare reports of weakness, hyperreflexia, and incoordination). Products include:
- Paxil Tablets 2681

Phenelzine Sulfate (Co-administration with an MAO-A inhibitor reduces sumatriptan clearance with a significant increase in systemic exposure; concurrent use with MAO-A inhibitor is not ordinarily recommended). Products include:
- Nardil 1977

(⊞ Described in PDR For Nonprescription Drugs) (⊙ Described in PDR For Ophthalmology)

Selegiline Hydrochloride (Sumatriptan is metabolized by MAO-A isoenzyme; co-administration with an MAO-A inhibitor reduces sumatriptan clearance with a significant increase in systemic exposure; no significant effect was seen with an MAO-B inhibitor. Products include:
Eldepryl Capsules 2729

Sertraline Hydrochloride (Co-administration with a selective serotonin reuptake inhibitor has resulted in rare reports of weakness, hyperreflexia, and incoordination). Products include:
Zoloft Tablets 2051

Tranylcypromine Sulfate (Co-administration with an MAO-A inhibitor reduces sumatriptan clearance with a significant increase in systemic exposure; concurrent use with MAO-A inhibitor is not ordinarily recommended). Products include:
Parnate Tablets 2679

IMITREX TABLETS
(Sumatriptan Succinate) 1099
May interact with monoamine oxidase inhibitors, ergot-containing drugs, and certain other agents. Compounds in these categories include:

Dihydroergotamine Mesylate (Ergot-containing drugs have been reported to cause prolonged vasospastic reactions which may result in additive effects; concurrent use within 24 hours of each other should be avoided). Products include:
D.H.E. 45 Injection 2381

Ergotamine Tartrate (Ergot-containing drugs have been reported to cause prolonged vasospastic reactions which may result in additive effects; concurrent use within 24 hours of each other should be avoided). Products include:
Bellergal-S Tablets 2375
Cafergot 2376
Ergomar Tablets 1543
Wigraine Tablets 1884

Furazolidone (Concurrent and/or sequential use is contraindicated; MAOI can markedly increase sumatriptan systemic exposure; potential for marked increase in sumatriptan AUC and half-life and decrease in Cl$_p$/F). Products include:
Furoxone 2221

Isocarboxazid (Concurrent and/or sequential use is contraindicated; MAOI can markedly increase sumatriptan systemic exposure; potential for marked increase in sumatriptan AUC and half-life and marked decrease in Cl$_p$/F).
No products indexed under this heading.

Methylergonovine Maleate (Ergot-containing drugs have been reported to cause prolonged vasospastic reactions which may result in additive effects; concurrent use within 24 hours of each other should be avoided). Products include:
Methergine 2401

Methysergide Maleate (Ergot-containing drugs have been reported to cause prolonged vasospastic reactions which may result in additive effects; concurrent use within 24 hours of each other should be avoided). Products include:
Sansert Tablets 2424

Phenelzine Sulfate (Concurrent and/or sequential use is contraindicated; MAOI can markedly increase sumatriptan systemic exposure; potential for marked increase in sumatriptan AUC and half-life and marked decrease in Cl$_p$/F). Products include:
Nardil 1977

Selegiline Hydrochloride (Concurrent and/or sequential use is contraindicated; MAOI can markedly increase sumatriptan systemic exposure; potential for marked increase in sumatriptan AUC and half-life and marked decrease in Cl$_p$/F). Products include:
Eldepryl Capsules 2729

Tranylcypromine Sulfate (Concurrent and/or sequential use is contraindicated; MAOI can markedly increase sumatriptan systemic exposure; potential for marked increase in sumatriptan AUC and half-life and marked decrease in Cl$_p$/F). Products include:
Parnate Tablets 2679

Food Interactions
Food, unspecified (Delays the T$_{max}$ slightly by about 0.5 hour with no significant effect on the bioavailability).

IMODIUM A-D CAPLETS AND LIQUID
(Loperamide Hydrochloride) 1561
None cited in PDR database.

IMODIUM CAPSULES
(Loperamide Hydrochloride) 1343
None cited in PDR database.

IMOGAM RABIES IMMUNE GLOBULIN (HUMAN)
(Rabies Immune Globulin (Human)) .. 897
May interact with:

Measles Virus Vaccine Live (Antibodies may interfere with the immune response to the vaccine). Products include:
Attenuvax 1650

IMOVAX RABIES VACCINE
(Rabies Vaccine) 899
May interact with corticosteroids and immunosuppressive agents. Compounds in these categories include:

Azathioprine (Can interfere with the development of active immunity and predispose the patient to develop rabies). Products include:
Azathioprine Tablets 2349
Imuran 1103

Betamethasone Acetate (Can interfere with the development of active immunity and predispose the patient to develop rabies). Products include:
Celestone Soluspan Suspension .. 2484

Betamethasone Sodium Phosphate (Can interfere with the development of active immunity and predispose the patient to develop rabies). Products include:
Celestone Soluspan Suspension .. 2484

Cortisone Acetate (Can interfere with the development of active immunity and predispose the patient to develop rabies). Products include:
Cortone Acetate Sterile Suspension .. 1663
Cortone Acetate Tablets 1664

Cyclosporine (Can interfere with the development of active immunity and predispose the patient to develop rabies). Products include:
Neoral 2405

Sandimmune 2416

Dexamethasone (Can interfere with the development of active immunity and predispose the patient to develop rabies). Products include:
AK-Trol Ointment & Suspension ... 205
Decadron Elixir 1676
Decadron Tablets 1678
Decaspray Topical Aerosol 1689
Maxitrol Ophthalmic Ointment and Suspension 222
TobraDex Ophthalmic Suspension and Ointment 469

Dexamethasone Acetate (Can interfere with the development of active immunity and predispose the patient to develop rabies). Products include:
Dalalone D.P. Injectable 1009
Decadron-LA Sterile Suspension 1687

Dexamethasone Sodium Phosphate (Can interfere with the development of active immunity and predispose the patient to develop rabies). Products include:
Decadron Phosphate Injection 1680
Decadron Phosphate Sterile Ophthalmic Ointment 1684
Decadron Phosphate Sterile Ophthalmic Solution 1685
Decadron Phosphate Topical Cream 1686
Decadron Phosphate with Xylocaine Injection, Sterile 1683
Dexacort Phosphate in Respihaler .. 1606
Dexacort Phosphate in Turbinaire .. 1607
NeoDecadron Sterile Ophthalmic Ointment 1755
NeoDecadron Sterile Ophthalmic Solution 1756
NeoDecadron Topical Cream ... 1757

Fludrocortisone Acetate (Can interfere with the development of active immunity and predispose the patient to develop rabies). Products include:
Florinef Acetate Tablets 506

Hydrocortisone (Can interfere with the development of active immunity and predispose the patient to develop rabies). Products include:
Anusol-HC Cream 2.5% 1953
Aquanil HC Lotion 1989
Maximum Strength Cortaid Spray .. 800
CORTENEMA 2713
Cortisporin Ointment 1074
Cortisporin Ophthalmic Ointment Sterile 1074
Cortisporin Ophthalmic Suspension Sterile 1075
Cortisporin Otic Solution Sterile ... 1076
Cortisporin Otic Suspension Sterile ... 1077
Cortizone-5 795
Cortizone-10 795
Hydrocortone Tablets 1715
Hytone 922
Hytone Ointment 2 ½% 923
Massengill Medicated Soft Cloth Towelettes 2628
Pediotic Suspension Sterile ... 1140
Preparation H Hydrocortisone 1% Cream 843
ProctoCream-HC 2.5% 2552
VōSol HC Otic Solution 2786

Hydrocortisone Acetate (Can interfere with the development of active immunity and predispose the patient to develop rabies). Products include:
Analpram-HC Rectal Cream 1% and 2.5% 993
Anusol HC-1 Hydrocortisone Anti-Itch Ointment 810
Anusol-HC Suppositories 1954
Caldecort Anti-Itch Hydrocortisone Cream 651
Coly-Mycin S Otic w/Neomycin & Hydrocortisone 1965
Cortaid 800
Cortifoam 2540
Cortisporin Cream 1073
Epifoam 2543
Hydrocortone Acetate Sterile Suspension 1712

Mantadil Cream 1124
Nupercainal Hydrocortisone 1% Cream 661
Pramosone Cream, Lotion & Ointment 995
ProctoFoam-HC 2552
Terra-Cortril Ophthalmic Suspension 2033

Hydrocortisone Sodium Phosphate (Can interfere with the development of active immunity and predispose the patient to develop rabies). Products include:
Hydrocortone Phosphate Injection, Sterile 1713

Hydrocortisone Sodium Succinate (Can interfere with the development of active immunity and predispose the patient to develop rabies).
No products indexed under this heading.

Immune Globulin (Human) (Can interfere with the development of active immunity and predispose the patient to develop rabies).
No products indexed under this heading.

Immune Globulin Intravenous (Human) (Can interfere with the development of active immunity and predispose the patient to develop rabies).

Methylprednisolone Acetate (Can interfere with the development of active immunity and predispose the patient to develop rabies).
No products indexed under this heading.

Methylprednisolone Sodium Succinate (Can interfere with the development of active immunity and predispose the patient to develop rabies).
No products indexed under this heading.

Muromonab-CD3 (Can interfere with the development of active immunity and predispose the patient to develop rabies). Products include:
Orthoclone OKT3 Sterile Solution .. 1892

Mycophenolate Mofetil (Can interfere with the development of active immunity and predispose the patient to develop rabies). Products include:
CellCept Capsules 2265

Prednisolone Acetate (Can interfere with the development of active immunity and predispose the patient to develop rabies). Products include:
AK-CIDE 203
AK-CIDE Ointment 203
Blephamide Liquifilm Sterile Ophthalmic Suspension 472
Blephamide Ointment 234
Econopred & Econopred Plus Ophthalmic Suspensions ... 216
Poly-Pred Liquifilm 246
Pred Forte 247
Pred Mild 250
Pred-G Liquifilm Sterile Ophthalmic Suspension 248
Pred-G S.O.P. Sterile Ophthalmic Ointment 249

Prednisolone Sodium Phosphate (Can interfere with the development of active immunity and predispose the patient to develop rabies). Products include:
AK-PRED 204
Hydeltrasol Injection, Sterile .. 1708
Pediapred Oral Solution 1618

Prednisolone Tebutate (Can interfere with the development of active immunity and predispose the patient to develop rabies). Products include:
Hydeltra-T.B.A. Sterile Suspension .. 1710

IMPORTANT NOTE: Always consult each drug listing in the patient's regimen for possible interactions.

Imovax | **Interactions Index** | **522**

Prednisone (Can interfere with the development of active immunity and predispose the patient to develop rabies).
No products indexed under this heading.

Tacrolimus (Can interfere with the development of active immunity and predispose the patient to develop rabies). Products include:
- Prograf ... 1028

Triamcinolone (Can interfere with the development of active immunity and predispose the patient to develop rabies).
No products indexed under this heading.

Triamcinolone Acetonide (Can interfere with the development of active immunity and predispose the patient to develop rabies). Products include:
- Azmacort Oral Inhaler ... 2175
- Nasacort AQ Nasal Spray ... 2191
- Nasacort Nasal Inhaler ... 2189

Triamcinolone Diacetate (Can interfere with the development of active immunity and predispose the patient to develop rabies).
No products indexed under this heading.

Triamcinolone Hexacetonide (Can interfere with the development of active immunity and predispose the patient to develop rabies).
No products indexed under this heading.

IMPREGON CONCENTRATE
(Tetrachlorosalicylanilide) ... 1003
None cited in PDR database.

IMURAN INJECTION
(Azathioprine) ... 1103
See **Imuran Tablets**

IMURAN TABLETS
(Azathioprine) ... 1103
May interact with ACE inhibitors and certain other agents. Compounds in these categories include:

Allopurinol (Inhibits the principal pathway for detoxification of azathioprine; reduce azathioprine dosage by 1/3 to 1/4 the usual dose). Products include:
- Zyloprim Tablets ... 1194

Benazepril Hydrochloride (Co-administration has been reported to induce anemia and severe leukopenia). Products include:
- Lotensin Tablets ... 852
- Lotensin HCT Tablets ... 855
- Lotrel Capsules ... 858

Captopril (Co-administration has been reported to induce anemia and severe leukopenia). Products include:
- Capoten Tablets ... 740
- Capozide Tablets ... 744

Enalapril Maleate (Co-administration has been reported to induce anemia and severe leukopenia). Products include:
- Vaseretic Tablets ... 1810
- Vasotec Tablets ... 1816

Enalaprilat (Co-administration has been reported to induce anemia and severe leukopenia). Products include:
- Vasotec I.V. ... 1814

Fosinopril Sodium (Co-administration has been reported to induce anemia and severe leukopenia). Products include:
- Monopril Tablets ... 762

Lisinopril (Co-administration has been reported to induce anemia and severe leukopenia). Products include:
- Prinivil Tablets ... 1776
- Prinzide Tablets ... 1780
- Zestoretic Tablets ... 2968
- Zestril Tablets ... 2972

Moexipril Hydrochloride (Co-administration has been reported to induce anemia and severe leukopenia). Products include:
- Univasc Tablets ... 2553

Quinapril Hydrochloride (Co-administration has been reported to induce anemia and severe leukopenia). Products include:
- Accupril Tablets ... 1950

Ramipril (Co-administration has been reported to induce anemia and severe leukopenia). Products include:
- Altace Capsules ... 1238

Spirapril Hydrochloride (Co-administration has been reported to induce anemia and severe leukopenia).
No products indexed under this heading.

Sulfamethoxazole (Co-administration with sulfamethoxazole/trimethoprim may lead to exaggerated leukopenia, especially in renal transplant recipients). Products include:
- Bactrim DS Tablets ... 2257
- Bactrim I.V. Infusion ... 2255
- Bactrim ... 2257
- Gantanol Tablets ... 2285
- Septra ... 1146
- Septra I.V. Infusion ... 1142
- Septra I.V. Infusion ADD-Vantage Vials ... 1144
- Septra ... 1146

Trandolapril (Co-administration has been reported to induce anemia and severe leukopenia). Products include:
- Mavik Tablets ... 1407

Trimethoprim (Co-administration with sulfamethoxazole/trimethoprim may lead to exaggerated leukopenia, especially in renal transplant recipients). Products include:
- Bactrim DS Tablets ... 2257
- Bactrim I.V. Infusion ... 2255
- Bactrim ... 2257
- Proloprim Tablets ... 1141
- Septra ... 1146
- Septra I.V. Infusion ... 1142
- Septra I.V. Infusion ADD-Vantage Vials ... 1144
- Septra ... 1146
- Trimpex Tablets ... 2323

Warfarin Sodium (Azathioprine may inhibit the anticoagulant effect of warfarin). Products include:
- Coumadin ... 941

INAPSINE INJECTION
(Droperidol) ... 462
May interact with central nervous system depressants, barbiturates, tranquilizers, narcotic analgesics, general anesthetics, and certain other agents. Compounds in these categories include:

Alfentanil Hydrochloride (Additive or potentiating effects). Products include:
- Alfenta Injection ... 1334

Alprazolam (Additive or potentiating effects). Products include:
- Xanax Tablets ... 2115

Aprobarbital (Additive or potentiating effects).
No products indexed under this heading.

Buprenorphine (Additive or potentiating effects). Products include:
- Buprenex Injectable ... 2170

Buspirone Hydrochloride (Additive or potentiating effects). Products include:
- BuSpar Tablets ... 738

Butabarbital (Additive or potentiating effects).
No products indexed under this heading.

Butalbital (Additive or potentiating effects). Products include:
- Axocet Capsules ... 2469
- Esgic-plus Capsules ... 1012
- Esgic-plus Tablets ... 1012
- Fioricet Tablets ... 2386
- Fioricet with Codeine Capsules ... 2387
- Fiorinal Capsules ... 2388
- Fiorinal with Codeine Capsules ... 2390
- Fiorinal Tablets ... 2388
- Phrenilin ... 790
- Sedapap Tablets 50 mg/650 mg .. 1826

Chlordiazepoxide (Additive or potentiating effects). Products include:
- Limbitrol ... 2333

Chlordiazepoxide Hydrochloride (Additive or potentiating effects). Products include:
- Librax Capsules ... 2330
- Librium Capsules ... 2331
- Librium Injectable ... 2332

Chlorpromazine (Additive or potentiating effects). Products include:
- Thorazine Suppositories ... 2701

Chlorpromazine Hydrochloride (Additive or potentiating effects). Products include:
- Thorazine ... 2701

Chlorprothixene (Additive or potentiating effects).
No products indexed under this heading.

Chlorprothixene Hydrochloride (Additive or potentiating effects).
No products indexed under this heading.

Chlorprothixene Lactate (Additive or potentiating effects).
No products indexed under this heading.

Clorazepate Dipotassium (Additive or potentiating effects). Products include:
- Tranxene ... 459

Clozapine (Additive or potentiating effects). Products include:
- Clozaril Tablets ... 2377

Codeine Phosphate (Additive or potentiating effects). Products include:
- Brontex ... 2130
- Dimetane-DC Cough Syrup ... 2232
- Fioricet with Codeine Capsules ... 2387
- Fiorinal with Codeine Capsules ... 2390
- Nucofed ... 2225
- Phenergan with Codeine ... 2883
- Phenergan VC with Codeine ... 2888
- Robitussin A-C Syrup ... 2248
- Robitussin-DAC Syrup ... 2249
- Ryna ... ◘ 804
- Soma Compound w/Codeine Tablets ... 2784
- Tylenol with Codeine ... 1592

Desflurane (Additive or potentiating effects). Products include:
- Suprane (desflurane, USP) ... 1865

Dezocine (Additive or potentiating effects). Products include:
- Dalgan Injection ... 529

Diazepam (Additive or potentiating effects). Products include:
- Dizac (diazepam injectable emulsion) CIV ... 1862
- Valium Injectable ... 2336
- Valium Tablets ... 2335

Enflurane (Additive or potentiating effects).
No products indexed under this heading.

Epinephrine (Epinephrine may cause paradoxical hypotension due to alpha blockade produced by Inapsine). Products include:
- EPIFRIN ... ◉ 237
- EpiPen ... 808
- Marcaine with Epinephrine ... 2446
- Primatene Mist ... ◘ 843
- Sensorcaine with Epinephrine Injection ... 554
- Sus-Phrine Injection ... 1017
- Xylocaine with Epinephrine Injections ... 562

Estazolam (Additive or potentiating effects). Products include:
- ProSom Tablets ... 457

Ethchlorvynol (Additive or potentiating effects). Products include:
- Placidyl Capsules ... 456

Ethinamate (Additive or potentiating effects).
No products indexed under this heading.

Fentanyl (Additive or potentiating effects). Products include:
- Duragesic Transdermal System ... 1336

Fentanyl Citrate (Additive or potentiating effects). Products include:
- Sublimaze Injection ... 463

Fluphenazine Decanoate (Additive or potentiating effects). Products include:
- Prolixin Decanoate ... 510

Fluphenazine Enanthate (Additive or potentiating effects). Products include:
- Prolixin Enanthate ... 510

Fluphenazine Hydrochloride (Additive or potentiating effects). Products include:
- Prolixin ... 510

Flurazepam Hydrochloride (Additive or potentiating effects). Products include:
- Dalmane Capsules ... 2329

Glutethimide (Additive or potentiating effects).
No products indexed under this heading.

Haloperidol (Additive or potentiating effects). Products include:
- Haldol Injection, Tablets and Concentrate ... 1585

Haloperidol Decanoate (Additive or potentiating effects). Products include:
- Haldol Decanoate ... 1587

Hydrocodone Bitartrate (Additive or potentiating effects). Products include:
- Codiclear DH Syrup ... 808
- Duratuss HD Elixir ... 2750
- Histussin D Liquid ... 670
- Hycodan Tablets and Syrup ... 946
- Hycomine Compound Tablets ... 948
- Hycomine ... 947
- Hycotuss Expectorant Syrup ... 950
- Hydrocet Capsules ... 787
- Lorcet 10/650 Tablets ... 1016
- Lortab ... 2751
- Tussend ... 1830
- Tussend Expectorant ... 1831
- Vicodin Tablets ... 1404
- Vicodin ES Tablets ... 1405
- Vicodin HP Tablets ... 1403
- Vicodin Tuss Expectorant ... 1406
- Zydone Capsules ... 967

Hydrocodone Polistirex (Additive or potentiating effects). Products include:
- Tussionex Pennkinetic Extended-Release Suspension ... 1624

Hydromorphone Hydrochloride (Additive or potentiating effects). Products include:
- Dilaudid Ampules ... 1382
- Dilaudid Cough Syrup ... 1383
- Dilaudid-HP Injection ... 1384
- Dilaudid-HP Lyophilized Powder 250 mg ... 1384
- Dilaudid ... 1382

(◘ Described in PDR For Nonprescription Drugs) (◉ Described in PDR For Ophthalmology)

523 **Interactions Index** **Inderal**

Dilaudid Oral Liquid 1386
Dilaudid 1382
Dilaudid Tablets - 8 mg 1386

Hydroxyzine Hydrochloride (Additive or potentiating effects). Products include:
Atarax Tablets & Syrup 1992
Marax Tablets & DF Syrup 2015
Vistaril Intramuscular Solution 2042

Isoflurane (Additive or potentiating effects).
No products indexed under this heading.

Ketamine Hydrochloride (Additive or potentiating effects).
No products indexed under this heading.

Levomethadyl Acetate Hydrochloride (Additive or potentiating effects). Products include:
Orlaam Oral Solution 2361

Levorphanol Tartrate (Additive or potentiating effects). Products include:
Levo-Dromoran 2297

Lorazepam (Additive or potentiating effects). Products include:
Ativan Injection 2805
Ativan Tablets 2807

Loxapine Hydrochloride (Additive or potentiating effects). Products include:
Loxitane 1426

Loxapine Succinate (Additive or potentiating effects). Products include:
Loxitane Capsules 1426

Meperidine Hydrochloride (Additive or potentiating effects). Products include:
Demerol 2438
Mepergan Injection 2859

Mephobarbital (Additive or potentiating effects). Products include:
Mebaral Tablets 2452

Meprobamate (Additive or potentiating effects). Products include:
Miltown Tablets 2780
PMB 200 and PMB 400 2890

Mesoridazine Besylate (Additive or potentiating effects). Products include:
Serentil 689

Methadone Hydrochloride (Additive or potentiating effects). Products include:
Methadone Hydrochloride Oral Concentrate 2356
Methadone Hydrochloride Oral Solution & Tablets 2357

Methohexital Sodium (Additive or potentiating effects).
No products indexed under this heading.

Methotrimeprazine (Additive or potentiating effects). Products include:
Levoprome 1321

Methoxyflurane (Additive or potentiating effects).
No products indexed under this heading.

Midazolam Hydrochloride (Additive or potentiating effects). Products include:
Versed Injection 2324

Molindone Hydrochloride (Additive or potentiating effects). Products include:
Moban Tablets and Concentrate 1036

Morphine Sulfate (Additive or potentiating effects). Products include:
Astramorph/PF Injection, USP (Preservative-Free) 526
Duramorph Injection 983
Infumorph 200 and Infumorph 500 Sterile Solutions 985
Kadian Capsules 2948
MS Contin Tablets 2149
MSIR 2152
Oramorph SR (Morphine Sulfate Sustained Release Tablets) 2359
RMS Suppositories CII 2766
Roxanol 2365

Opium Alkaloids (Additive or potentiating effects).
No products indexed under this heading.

Oxazepam (Additive or potentiating effects). Products include:
Serax Capsules 2916
Serax Tablets 2916

Oxycodone Hydrochloride (Additive or potentiating effects). Products include:
OxyContin Tablets 2163
OxyIR Capsules 2167
Percocet Tablets 955
Percodan Tablets 955
Percodan-Demi Tablets 956
Roxicodone Tablets, Oral Solution & Intensol (Oxycodone) 2366
Tylox Capsules 1593

Pentobarbital Sodium (Additive or potentiating effects). Products include:
Nembutal Sodium Capsules 440
Nembutal Sodium Solution 442
Nembutal Sodium Suppositories 444

Perphenazine (Additive or potentiating effects). Products include:
Etrafon 2495
Triavil Tablets 1800
Trilafon 2532

Phenobarbital (Additive or potentiating effects). Products include:
Arco-Lase Plus Tablets 513
Bellergal-S Tablets 2375
Donnatal 2234
Donnatal Extentabs 2234
Donnatal Tablets 2234
Phenobarbital Elixir and Tablets 1523
Quadrinal Tablets 1398

Prazepam (Additive or potentiating effects).
No products indexed under this heading.

Prochlorperazine (Additive or potentiating effects). Products include:
Compazine 2644

Promethazine Hydrochloride (Additive or potentiating effects). Products include:
Mepergan Injection 2859
Phenergan with Codeine 2883
Phenergan with Dextromethorphan 2885
Phenergan Injection 2880
Phenergan Suppositories 2882
Phenergan Syrup 2881
Phenergan Tablets 2882
Phenergan VC 2886
Phenergan VC with Codeine 2888

Propofol (Additive or potentiating effects). Products include:
Diprivan Injectable Emulsion 2939

Propoxyphene Hydrochloride (Additive or potentiating effects). Products include:
Darvon 1475
Wygesic Tablets 2930

Propoxyphene Napsylate (Additive or potentiating effects). Products include:
Darvon-N/Darvocet-N 1473

Quazepam (Additive or potentiating effects). Products include:
Doral Tablets 2773

Risperidone (Additive or potentiating effects). Products include:
Risperdal Tablets 1348

Secobarbital Sodium (Additive or potentiating effects). Products include:
Seconal Sodium Pulvules 1529

Sevoflurane (Additive or potentiating effects).
No products indexed under this heading.

Sufentanil Citrate (Additive or potentiating effects). Products include:
Sufenta Injection 1355

Temazepam (Additive or potentiating effects). Products include:
Restoril Capsules 2413

Thiamylal Sodium (Additive or potentiating effects).
No products indexed under this heading.

Thioridazine Hydrochloride (Additive or potentiating effects). Products include:
Mellaril 2398

Thiothixene (Additive or potentiating effects). Products include:
Navane Capsules and Concentrate 2018
Navane Intramuscular 2019

Triazolam (Additive or potentiating effects). Products include:
Halcion Tablets 2093

Trifluoperazine Hydrochloride (Additive or potentiating effects). Products include:
Stelazine 2692

Zolpidem Tartrate (Additive or potentiating effects). Products include:
Ambien Tablets 2559

INDERAL INJECTABLE
(Propranolol Hydrochloride) **2834**
May interact with insulin, catecholamine depleting drugs, calcium channel blockers, non-steroidal anti-inflammatory agents, beta-adrenergic stimulating agents, oral hypoglycemic agents, and certain other agents. Compounds in these categories include:

Acarbose (Delay in the recovery of blood glucose to normal levels following insulin-induced hypoglycemia). Products include:
Precose 604

Albuterol (Propranolol may block bronchodilation produced by exogenous catecholamine stimulation of beta receptors). Products include:
Proventil Inhalation Aerosol 2524
Ventolin Inhalation Aerosol and Refill 1170

Albuterol Sulfate (Propranolol may block bronchodilation produced by exogenous catecholamine stimulation of beta receptors). Products include:
Airet Albuterol Sulfate Inhalation Solution 1602
Albuterol Sulfate, USP Solution for Inhalation, Arm-a-Med 522
Proventil Inhalation Solution 0.083% 2527
Proventil Repetabs Tablets 2529
Proventil Solution for Inhalation 0.5% 2525
Proventil Syrup 2528
Proventil Tablets 2529
Ventolin Inhalation Solution 1171
Ventolin Nebules Inhalation Solution 1172
Ventolin Rotacaps for Inhalation 1173
Ventolin Syrup 1175
Ventolin Tablets 1176
Volmax Extended-Release Tablets .. 1835

Aluminum Hydroxide (Greatly reduces intestinal absorption of propranolol). Products include:
ALternaGEL Liquid 1358
Maximum Strength Ascriptin 650
Cama Arthritis Pain Reliever 748
Gaviscon Extra Strength Relief Formula Antacid Tablets 778
Gaviscon Extra Strength Relief Formula Liquid Antacid 779
Gaviscon Liquid Antacid 779
Gelusil Antacid-Anti-gas Liquid 819
Gelusil Antacid-Anti-gas Tablets 819
Maalox Antacid/Anti-Gas Tablets 889
Maalox Heartburn Relief Suspension 658
Maalox Antacid Liquid 888
Extra Strength Maalox Antacid/Anti-Gas Liquid and Tablets 888
Mylanta 1359
Tempo Soft Antacid 799

Aluminum Hydroxide Gel (Greatly reduces intestinal absorption of propranolol). Products include:
ALternaGEL Liquid 675
Aludrox Oral Suspension 850
Amphojel Suspension 2802
Amphojel Suspension without Flavor 2802
Amphojel Tablets 2802
Ascriptin 650
Gaviscon Antacid Tablets 778
Gaviscon-2 Antacid Tablets 779
Mylanta Liquid 676
Mylanta Double Strength Liquid 676
Nephrox Suspension 671

Aminophylline (Reduced theophylline clearance).
No products indexed under this heading.

Amlodipine Besylate (Both agents may depress myocardial contractility or AV conduction resulting in increased adverse reactions). Products include:
Lotrel Capsules 858
Norvasc Tablets 2020

Antipyrine (Reduced clearance of antipyrine). Products include:
Auralgan Otic Solution 2810
Tympagesic Ear Drops 2476

Bepridil Hydrochloride (Both agents may depress myocardial contractility or AV conduction resulting in increased adverse reactions). Products include:
Vascor Tablets (200 and 300 mg) 1597

Bitolterol Mesylate (Propranolol may block bronchodilation produced by exogenous catecholamine stimulation of beta receptors). Products include:
Tornalate Solution for Inhalation, 0.2% 976
Tornalate Metered Dose Inhaler 978

Chlorpromazine (Increased plasma levels of both drugs). Products include:
Thorazine Suppositories 2701

Chlorpromazine Hydrochloride (Increased plasma levels of both drugs). Products include:
Thorazine 2701

Chlorpropamide (Delay in the recovery of blood glucose to normal levels following insulin-induced hypoglycemia). Products include:
Diabinese Tablets 2002

Cimetidine (Decreases hepatic metabolism of propranolol resulting in increased blood levels). Products include:
Tagamet HB Tablets 786
Tagamet Tablets 2694

Cimetidine Hydrochloride (Decreases hepatic metabolism of propranolol resulting in increased blood levels). Products include:
Tagamet 2694

Deserpidine (May produce an excessive hypotension with bradycardia and orthostatic effects).
No products indexed under this heading.

Diclofenac Potassium (Blunts antihypertensive effect of beta blocker). Products include:
Cataflam Tablets 833

Diclofenac Sodium (Blunts antihypertensive effect of beta blocker). Products include:
Voltaren Ophthalmic Sterile Ophthalmic Solution .... ⊙ 264
Cataflam/Voltaren/Voltaren-XR 833

IMPORTANT NOTE: Always consult each drug listing in the patient's regimen for possible interactions.

Inderal Interactions Index 524

Diltiazem Hydrochloride (Both agents may depress myocardial contractility or AV conduction resulting in increased adverse reactions). Products include:
- Cardizem CD Capsules ... 1251
- Cardizem SR Capsules ... 1255
- Cardizem Injectable ... 1253
- Cardizem Tablets ... 1257
- Dilacor XR Extended-release Capsules ... 2183
- Tiazac Capsules ... 1019

Dobutamine Hydrochloride (Reversed effects of propranolol). Products include:
- Dobutrex Solution Vials ... 1480

Dyphylline (Reduced theophylline clearance). Products include:
- Lufyllin & Lufyllin-400 Tablets ... 2778
- Lufyllin-GG Elixir & Tablets ... 2779

Ephedrine Hydrochloride (Propranolol may block bronchodilation produced by exogenous catecholamine stimulation of beta receptors). Products include:
- Primatene Tablets ... ⊡ 844
- Quadrinal Tablets ... 1398

Ephedrine Sulfate (Propranolol may block bronchodilation produced by exogenous catecholamine stimulation of beta receptors). Products include:
- Marax Tablets & DF Syrup ... 2015

Ephedrine Tannate (Propranolol may block bronchodilation produced by exogenous catecholamine stimulation of beta receptors). Products include:
- Rynatuss ... 2782

Epinephrine (Propranolol may block bronchodilation produced by exogenous catecholamine stimulation of beta receptors). Products include:
- EPIFRIN ... ⊙ 237
- EpiPen ... 808
- Marcaine with Epinephrine ... 2446
- Primatene Mist ... ⊡ 843
- Sensorcaine with Epinephrine Injection ... 554
- Sus-Phrine Injection ... 1017
- Xylocaine with Epinephrine Injections ... 562

Epinephrine Hydrochloride (Propranolol may block bronchodilation produced by exogenous catecholamine stimulation of beta receptors). Products include:
- Ana-Kit Anaphylaxis Emergency Treatment Kit ... 611

Ethylnorepinephrine Hydrochloride (Propranolol may block bronchodilation produced by exogenous catecholamine stimulation of beta receptors).
- No products indexed under this heading.

Etodolac (Blunts antihypertensive effect of beta blocker). Products include:
- Lodine Capsules and Tablets ... 2849

Felodipine (Both agents may depress myocardial contractility or AV conduction resulting in increased adverse reactions). Products include:
- Plendil Extended-Release Tablets ... 514

Fenoprofen Calcium (Blunts antihypertensive effect of beta blocker). Products include:
- Nalfon 200 Pulvules & Nalfon Tablets ... 933

Flurbiprofen (Blunts antihypertensive effect of beta blocker).
- No products indexed under this heading.

Glimepiride (Delay in the recovery of blood glucose to normal levels following insulin-induced hypoglycemia). Products include:
- Amaryl Tablets ... 1241

Glipizide (Delay in the recovery of blood glucose to normal levels following insulin-induced hypoglycemia). Products include:
- Glucotrol Tablets ... 2011
- Glucotrol XL Extended Release Tablets ... 2012

Glyburide (Delay in the recovery of blood glucose to normal levels following insulin-induced hypoglycemia). Products include:
- DiaBeta Tablets ... 1265
- Glynase PresTab Tablets ... 2091
- Micronase Tablets ... 2099

Guanethidine Monosulfate (May produce an excessive hypotension with bradycardia and orthostatic effects). Products include:
- Esimil Tablets ... 840
- Ismelin Tablets ... 845

Haloperidol (Hypotension and cardiac arrest have been reported with the concomitant use of propranolol and haloperidol). Products include:
- Haldol Injection, Tablets and Concentrate ... 1585

Haloperidol Decanoate (Hypotension and cardiac arrest have been reported with the concomitant use of propranolol and haloperidol). Products include:
- Haldol Decanoate ... 1587

Ibuprofen (Blunts antihypertensive effect of beta blocker). Products include:
- Advil Cold and Sinus Caplets and Tablets ... ⊡ 837
- Advil Ibuprofen Tablets, Caplets and Gel Caplets ... ⊡ 836
- Children's Motrin Ibuprofen Oral Suspension ... 1558
- IBU Tablets ... 1389
- Ibuprohm ... ⊡ 713
- Motrin IB Caplets, Tablets, and Gelcaps ... ⊡ 802
- Motrin Ibuprofen Suspension, Oral Drops, Chewable Tablets, Caplets ... 1563
- Nuprin Ibuprofen/Analgesic Tablets & Caplets ... ⊡ 645
- Vicks DayQuil SINUS Pressure & PAIN Relief with IBUPROFEN ... ⊡ 735

Indomethacin (Blunts antihypertensive effect of beta blocker). Products include:
- Indocin ... 1723

Indomethacin Sodium Trihydrate (Blunts antihypertensive effect of beta blocker). Products include:
- Indocin I.V. ... 1727

Insulin, Human (Delayed recovery of blood glucose to normal levels following insulin-induced hypoglycemia).
- No products indexed under this heading.

Insulin, Human Isophane Suspension (Delayed recovery of blood glucose to normal levels following insulin-induced hypoglycemia). Products include:
- Novolin N Human Insulin 10 ml Vials ... 1846

Insulin, Human NPH (Delayed recovery of blood glucose to normal levels following insulin-induced hypoglycemia). Products include:
- Humulin N, 100 Units ... 1495
- Novolin N PenFill 1.5 ml Cartridges Durable Insulin Delivery System ... 1849
- Novolin N Prefilled Syringe Disposable Insulin Delivery System ... 1850

Insulin, Human Regular (Delayed recovery of blood glucose to normal levels following insulin-induced hypoglycemia). Products include:
- Humulin R, 100 Units ... 1497
- Novolin R Human Insulin 10 ml Vials ... 1846
- Novolin R PenFill 1.5 ml Cartridges Durable Insulin Delivery System ... 1849
- Novolin R Prefilled Syringe Disposable Insulin Delivery System ... 1850
- Velosulin BR Human Insulin 10 ml Vials ... 1847

Insulin, Human, Zinc Suspension (Delayed recovery of blood glucose to normal levels following insulin-induced hypoglycemia). Products include:
- Humulin L, 100 Units ... 1494
- Humulin U, 100 Units ... 1498
- Novolin L Human Insulin 10 ml Vials ... 1846

Insulin Lispro, Human (Delayed recovery of blood glucose to normal levels following insulin-induced hypoglycemia). Products include:
- Humalog Injection ... 1488

Insulin, NPH (Delayed recovery of blood glucose to normal levels following insulin-induced hypoglycemia). Products include:
- NPH, 100 Units ... 1502
- Pork NPH, 100 Units ... 1506
- Purified Pork NPH Isophane Insulin ... 1852

Insulin, Regular (Delayed recovery of blood glucose to normal levels following insulin-induced hypoglycemia). Products include:
- Regular, 100 Units ... 1503
- Pork Regular, 100 Units ... 1507
- Pork Regular (Concentrated), 500 Units ... 1508
- Purified Pork Regular Insulin ... 1852

Insulin, Zinc Crystals (Delayed recovery of blood glucose to normal levels following insulin-induced hypoglycemia). Products include:
- NPH, 100 Units ... 1502

Insulin, Zinc Suspension (Delayed recovery of blood glucose to normal levels following insulin-induced hypoglycemia). Products include:
- Iletin I ... 1501
- Lente, 100 Units ... 1501
- Iletin II ... 1504
- Pork Lente, 100 Units ... 1504
- Purified Pork Lente Insulin ... 1852

Isoetharine (Propranolol may block bronchodilation produced by exogenous catecholamine stimulation of beta receptors). Products include:
- Bronkometer Aerosol ... 2432
- Bronkosol Solution ... 2432
- Isoetharine Inhalation Solution, USP, Arm-a-Med ... 545

Isoproterenol Hydrochloride (Propranolol may block bronchodilation produced by exogenous catecholamine stimulation of beta receptors). Products include:
- Isuprel Hydrochloride Solution ... 2443
- Isuprel Injection ... 2441
- Isuprel Mistometer ... 2442

Isoproterenol Sulfate (Propranolol may block bronchodilation produced by exogenous catecholamine stimulation of beta receptors). Products include:
- Norisodrine with Calcium Iodide Syrup ... 446

Isradipine (Both agents may depress myocardial contractility or AV conduction resulting in increased adverse reactions). Products include:
- DynaCirc Capsules ... 2381
- DynaCirc CR Tablets ... 2383

Ketoprofen (Blunts antihypertensive effect of beta blocker). Products include:
- Actron Caplets and Tablets ... ⊡ 608
- Orudis Capsules ... 2874
- Orudis KT ... ⊡ 842
- Oruvail Capsules ... 2874

Ketorolac Tromethamine (Blunts antihypertensive effect of beta blocker). Products include:
- Acular Sterile Ophthalmic Solution ... 470
- Toradol ... 2319

Levothyroxine Sodium (Concurrent use may result in lower than expected T_3 concentration). Products include:
- Eltroxin Tablets ... 2214
- Levothroid Tablets ... 1015
- Levothyroxine Sodium, USP for Injection ... 546
- Levoxyl Tablets ... 918
- Synthroid ... 1410

Lidocaine Hydrochloride (Reduced clearance of lidocaine). Products include:
- Decadron Phosphate with Xylocaine Injection, Sterile ... 1683
- Unguentine Plus ... ⊡ 712
- Xylocaine Injections ... 562

Meclofenamate Sodium (Blunts antihypertensive effect of beta blocker).
- No products indexed under this heading.

Mefenamic Acid (Blunts antihypertensive effect of beta blocker). Products include:
- Ponstel ... 1982

Metaproterenol Sulfate (Propranolol may block bronchodilation produced by exogenous catecholamine stimulation of beta receptors). Products include:
- Alupent ... 672
- Metaproterenol Sulfate Inhalation Solution, USP, Arm-a-Med ... 547

Metformin Hydrochloride (Delay in the recovery of blood glucose to normal levels following insulin-induced hypoglycemia). Products include:
- Glucophage Tablets ... 754

Nabumetone (Blunts antihypertensive effect of beta blocker). Products include:
- Relafen Tablets ... 2688

Naproxen (Blunts antihypertensive effect of beta blocker). Products include:
- Anaprox/Naprosyn ... 2277

Naproxen Sodium (Blunts antihypertensive effect of beta blocker). Products include:
- Aleve ... 2124
- Anaprox/Naprosyn ... 2277
- Naprelan Tablets ... 2861

Nicardipine Hydrochloride (Both agents may depress myocardial contractility or AV conduction resulting in increased adverse reactions). Products include:
- Cardene Capsules ... 2261
- Cardene I.V. ... 2815
- Cardene SR Capsules ... 2264

Nifedipine (Both agents may depress myocardial contractility or AV conduction resulting in increased adverse reactions). Products include:
- Adalat Capsules (10 mg and 20 mg) ... 580
- Adalat CC ... 582
- Procardia Capsules ... 2024
- Procardia XL Extended Release Tablets ... 2026

Nimodipine (Both agents may depress myocardial contractility or AV conduction resulting in increased adverse reactions). Products include:
- Nimotop Capsules ... 603

Nisoldipine (Both agents may depress myocardial contractility or AV conduction resulting in increased adverse reactions). Products include:
- Sular Tablets ... 2961

(⊡ Described in PDR For Nonprescription Drugs) (⊙ Described in PDR For Ophthalmology)

525 **Interactions Index** **Inderal LA**

Oxaprozin (Blunts antihypertensive effect of beta blocker). Products include:

Daypro Caplets 2578

Phenobarbital (Accelerates propranolol clearance). Products include:

Arco-Lase Plus Tablets 513
Bellergal-S Tablets 2375
Donnatal 2234
Donnatal Extentabs 2234
Donnatal Tablets 2234
Phenobarbital Elixir and Tablets 1523
Quadrinal Tablets 1398

Phenylbutazone (Blunts antihypertensive effect of beta blocker).

No products indexed under this heading.

Phenytoin (Accelerates propranolol clearance). Products include:

Dilantin Infatabs 1967
Dilantin-125 Suspension 1969

Phenytoin Sodium (Accelerates propranolol clearance). Products include:

Dilantin Kapseals 1965

Pirbuterol Acetate (Propranolol may block bronchodilation produced by exogenous catecholamine stimulation of beta receptors). Products include:

Maxair Autohaler 1550
Maxair Inhaler 1552

Piroxicam (Blunts antihypertensive effect of beta blocker). Products include:

Feldene Capsules 2008

Rauwolfia Serpentina (May produce an excessive hypotension with bradycardia and orthostatic effects).

No products indexed under this heading.

Rescinnamine (May produce an excessive hypotension with bradycardia and orthostatic effects).

No products indexed under this heading.

Reserpine (May produce an excessive hypotension with bradycardia and orthostatic effects). Products include:

Diupres Tablets 1691
Hydropres Tablets 1718
Ser-Ap-Es Tablets 867

Rifampin (Accelerates propranolol clearance). Products include:

Rifadin 1276
Rifamate Capsules 1278
Rifater 1280
Rimactane Capsules 865

Salmeterol Xinafoate (Propranolol may block bronchodilation produced by exogenous catecholamine stimulation of beta receptors). Products include:

Serevent Inhalation Aerosol 1149

Sulindac (Blunts antihypertensive effect of beta blocker). Products include:

Clinoril Tablets 1658

Terbutaline Sulfate (Propranolol may block bronchodilation produced by exogenous catecholamine stimulation of beta receptors). Products include:

Brethaire Inhaler 830
Brethine Ampuls 832
Brethine Tablets 831
Bricanyl Subcutaneous Injection 1247
Bricanyl Tablets 1248

Theophylline (Reduced theophylline clearance). Products include:

Marax Tablets & DF Syrup 2015
Quibron 2227

Theophylline Anhydrous (Reduced theophylline clearance). Products include:

Aerolate 1003
Primatene Tablets .... ⊡ 844
Respbid Tablets 687
Slo-bid Gyrocaps 2201
Theo-24 Extended Release Capsules 2753
Theo-Dur Extended-Release Tablets 1367
Theo-X Extended-Release Tablets 793
Uni-Dur Extended-Release Tablets 1374
Uniphyl 400 mg and 600 mg Tablets 2157

Theophylline Calcium Salicylate (Reduced theophylline clearance). Products include:

Quadrinal Tablets 1398

Theophylline Sodium Glycinate (Reduced theophylline clearance).

No products indexed under this heading.

Tolazamide (Delay in the recovery of blood glucose to normal levels following insulin-induced hypoglycemia).

No products indexed under this heading.

Tolbutamide (Delay in the recovery of blood glucose to normal levels following insulin-induced hypoglycemia).

No products indexed under this heading.

Tolmetin Sodium (Blunts antihypertensive effect of beta blocker). Products include:

Tolectin (200, 400 and 600 mg) 1591

Verapamil Hydrochloride (Both agents may depress myocardial contractility or AV conduction resulting in increased adverse reactions). Products include:

Calan SR Caplets 2571
Calan Tablets 2568
Covera-HS Tablets 2573
Isoptin Injectable 1391
Isoptin Oral Tablets 1393
Isoptin SR Tablets 1395
Verelan Capsules 1455

Food Interactions

Alcohol (Slows the rate of absorption of propranolol).

INDERAL TABLETS

(Propranolol Hydrochloride) 2834
See **Inderal Injectable**

INDERAL LA LONG ACTING CAPSULES

(Propranolol Hydrochloride) 2836
May interact with catecholamine depleting drugs, calcium channel blockers, insulin, beta-adrenergic stimulating agents, oral hypoglycemic agents, non-steroidal anti-inflammatory agents, and certain other agents. Compounds in these categories include:

Acarbose (Delay in the recovery of blood glucose to normal levels following insulin-induced hypoglycemia). Products include:

Precose 604

Albuterol (Propranolol may block bronchodilation produced by exogenous catecholamine stimulation of beta receptors). Products include:

Proventil Inhalation Aerosol 2524
Ventolin Inhalation Aerosol and Refill 1170

Albuterol Sulfate (Propranolol may block bronchodilation produced by exogenous catecholamine stimulation of beta receptors). Products include:

Airet Albuterol Sulfate Inhalation Solution 1602
Albuterol Sulfate, USP Solution for Inhalation, Arm-a-Med 522
Proventil Inhalation Solution 0.083% 2527
Proventil Repetabs Tablets 2529
Proventil Solution for Inhalation 0.5% 2525
Proventil Syrup 2528
Proventil Tablets 2529
Ventolin Inhalation Solution 1171
Ventolin Nebules Inhalation Solution 1172
Ventolin Rotacaps for Inhalation 1173
Ventolin Syrup 1175
Ventolin Tablets 1176
Volmax Extended-Release Tablets 1835

Aluminum Hydroxide Gel (Intestinal absorption of propranolol greatly reduced). Products include:

ALternaGEL Liquid .... ⊡ 675
Aludrox Oral Suspension .... ⊡ 850
Amphojel Suspension 2802
Amphojel Suspension without Flavor 2802
Amphojel Tablets 2802
Ascriptin .... ⊡ 650
Gaviscon Antacid Tablets .... ⊡ 778
Gaviscon-2 Antacid Tablets .... ⊡ 779
Mylanta Liquid .... ⊡ 676
Mylanta Double Strength Liquid .... ⊡ 676
Nephrox Suspension .... ⊡ 671

Amlodipine Besylate (Caution should be exercised when administered concomitantly). Products include:

Lotrel Capsules 858
Norvasc Tablets 2020

Antipyrine (Reduced clearance of antipyrine). Products include:

Auralgan Otic Solution 2810
Tympagesic Ear Drops 2476

Bepridil Hydrochloride (Caution should be exercised when administered concomitantly). Products include:

Vascor Tablets (200 and 300 mg) 1597

Bitolterol Mesylate (Propranolol may block bronchodilation produced by exogenous catecholamine stimulation of beta receptors). Products include:

Tornalate Solution for Inhalation, 0.2% 976
Tornalate Metered Dose Inhaler 978

Chlorpromazine (Increased plasma levels of both drugs). Products include:

Thorazine Suppositories 2701

Chlorpromazine Hydrochloride (Increased plasma levels of both drugs). Products include:

Thorazine 2701

Chlorpropamide (Delay in the recovery of blood glucose to normal levels following insulin-induced hypoglycemia). Products include:

Diabinese Tablets 2002

Cimetidine (Delayed elimination and increased blood levels of propranolol). Products include:

Tagamet HB Tablets .... ⊡ 786
Tagamet Tablets 2694

Cimetidine Hydrochloride (Delayed elimination and increased blood levels of propranolol). Products include:

Tagamet 2694

Deserpidine (May produce excessive hypotension with bradycardia and orthostatic effects).

No products indexed under this heading.

Diclofenac Potassium (Blunts antihypertensive effect of beta blocker). Products include:

Cataflam Tablets 833

Diclofenac Sodium (Blunts antihypertensive effect of beta blocker). Products include:

Voltaren Ophthalmic Sterile Ophthalmic Solution .... ◉ 264
Cataflam/Voltaren/Voltaren-XR 833

Diltiazem Hydrochloride (Caution should be exercised when administered concomitantly). Products include:

Cardizem CD Capsules 1251
Cardizem SR Capsules 1255
Cardizem Injectable 1253
Cardizem Tablets 1257
Dilacor XR Extended-release Capsules 2183
Tiazac Capsules 1019

Ephedrine Hydrochloride (Propranolol may block bronchodilation produced by exogenous catecholamine stimulation of beta receptors). Products include:

Primatene Tablets .... ⊡ 844
Quadrinal Tablets 1398

Ephedrine Sulfate (Propranolol may block bronchodilation produced by exogenous catecholamine stimulation of beta receptors). Products include:

Marax Tablets & DF Syrup 2015

Ephedrine Tannate (Propranolol may block bronchodilation produced by exogenous catecholamine stimulation of beta receptors). Products include:

Rynatuss 2782

Epinephrine (Propranolol may block bronchodilation produced by exogenous catecholamine stimulation of beta receptors). Products include:

EPIFRIN .... ◉ 237
EpiPen 808
Marcaine with Epinephrine 2446
Primatene Mist .... ⊡ 843
Sensorcaine with Epinephrine Injection 554
Sus-Phrine Injection 1017
Xylocaine with Epinephrine Injections 562

Epinephrine Hydrochloride (Propranolol may block bronchodilation produced by exogenous catecholamine stimulation of beta receptors). Products include:

Ana-Kit Anaphylaxis Emergency Treatment Kit 611

Ethylnorepinephrine Hydrochloride (Propranolol may block bronchodilation produced by exogenous catecholamine stimulation of beta receptors).

No products indexed under this heading.

Etodolac (Blunts antihypertensive effect of beta blocker). Products include:

Lodine Capsules and Tablets 2849

Felodipine (Caution should be exercised when administered concomitantly). Products include:

Plendil Extended-Release Tablets 514

Fenoprofen Calcium (Blunts antihypertensive effect of beta blocker). Products include:

Nalfon 200 Pulvules & Nalfon Tablets 933

Flurbiprofen (Blunts antihypertensive effect of beta blocker).

No products indexed under this heading.

Glimepiride (Delay in the recovery of blood glucose to normal levels following insulin-induced hypoglycemia). Products include:

Amaryl Tablets 1241

Glipizide (Delay in the recovery of blood glucose to normal levels following insulin-induced hypoglycemia). Products include:

Glucotrol Tablets 2011
Glucotrol XL Extended Release Tablets 2012

Glyburide (Delay in the recovery of blood glucose to normal levels following insulin-induced hypoglycemia). Products include:

DiaBeta Tablets 1265
Glynase PresTab Tablets 2091
Micronase Tablets 2099

IMPORTANT NOTE: Always consult each drug listing in the patient's regimen for possible interactions.

Guanethidine Monosulfate (May produce excessive hypotension with bradycardia and orthostatic effects). Products include:
- Esimil Tablets 840
- Ismelin Tablets 845

Haloperidol (Hypotension and cardiac arrest have been reported with the concomitant use of propranolol and haloperidol). Products include:
- Haldol Injection, Tablets and Concentrate 1585

Haloperidol Decanoate (Hypotension and cardiac arrest have been reported with the concomitant use of propranolol and haloperidol). Products include:
- Haldol Decanoate 1587

Ibuprofen (Blunts antihypertensive effect of beta blocker). Products include:
- Advil Cold and Sinus Caplets and Tablets .... ◘◘ 837
- Advil Ibuprofen Tablets, Caplets and Gel Caplets .... ◘◘ 836
- Children's Motrin Ibuprofen Oral Suspension 1558
- IBU Tablets 1389
- Ibuprohm .... ◘◘ 713
- Motrin IB Caplets, Tablets, and Gelcaps .... ◘◘ 802
- Motrin Ibuprofen Suspension, Oral Drops, Chewable Tablets, Caplets 1563
- Nuprin Ibuprofen/Analgesic Tablets & Caplets .... ◘◘ 645
- Vicks DayQuil SINUS Pressure & PAIN Relief with IBUPROFEN ..... ◘◘ 735

Indomethacin (Blunts antihypertensive effect of beta blocker). Products include:
- Indocin 1723

Indomethacin Sodium Trihydrate (Blunts antihypertensive effect of beta blocker). Products include:
- Indocin I.V. 1727

Insulin, Human (Delayed recovery of blood glucose to normal levels following insulin-induced hypoglycemia).
- No products indexed under this heading.

Insulin, Human Isophane Suspension (Delayed recovery of blood glucose to normal levels following insulin-induced hypoglycemia). Products include:
- Novolin N Human Insulin 10 ml Vials 1846

Insulin, Human NPH (Delayed recovery of blood glucose to normal levels following insulin-induced hypoglycemia). Products include:
- Humulin N, 100 Units 1495
- Novolin N PenFill 1.5 ml Cartridges Durable Insulin Delivery System 1849
- Novolin N Prefilled Syringe Disposable Insulin Delivery System 1850

Insulin, Human Regular (Delayed recovery of blood glucose to normal levels following insulin-induced hypoglycemia). Products include:
- Humulin R, 100 Units 1497
- Novolin R Human Insulin 10 ml Vials 1846
- Novolin R PenFill 1.5 ml Cartridges Durable Insulin Delivery System 1849
- Novolin R Prefilled Syringe Disposable Insulin Delivery System 1850
- Velosulin BR Human Insulin 10 ml Vials 1847

Insulin, Human, Zinc Suspension (Delayed recovery of blood glucose to normal levels following insulin-induced hypoglycemia). Products include:
- Humulin L, 100 Units 1494

- Humulin U, 100 Units 1498
- Novolin L Human Insulin 10 ml Vials 1846

Insulin Lispro, Human (Delayed recovery of blood glucose to normal levels following insulin-induced hypoglycemia). Products include:
- Humalog Injection 1488

Insulin, NPH (Delayed recovery of blood glucose to normal levels following insulin-induced hypoglycemia). Products include:
- NPH, 100 Units 1502
- Pork NPH, 100 Units 1506
- Purified Pork NPH Isophane Insulin 1852

Insulin, Regular (Delayed recovery of blood glucose to normal levels following insulin-induced hypoglycemia). Products include:
- Regular, 100 Units 1503
- Pork Regular, 100 Units 1507
- Pork Regular (Concentrated), 500 Units 1508
- Purified Pork Regular Insulin 1852

Insulin, Zinc Crystals (Delayed recovery of blood glucose to normal levels following insulin-induced hypoglycemia). Products include:
- NPH, 100 Units 1502

Insulin, Zinc Suspension (Delayed recovery of blood glucose to normal levels following insulin-induced hypoglycemia). Products include:
- Iletin I 1501
- Lente, 100 Units 1501
- Iletin II 1504
- Pork Lente, 100 Units 1504
- Purified Pork Lente Insulin 1852

Isoetharine (Propranolol may block bronchodilation produced by exogenous catecholamine stimulation of beta receptors). Products include:
- Bronkometer Aerosol 2432
- Bronkosol Solution 2432
- Isoetharine Inhalation Solution, USP, Arm-a-Med 545

Isoproterenol Hydrochloride (Propranolol may block bronchodilation produced by exogenous catecholamine stimulation of beta receptors). Products include:
- Isuprel Hydrochloride Solution 2443
- Isuprel Injection 2441
- Isuprel Mistometer 2442

Isoproterenol Sulfate (Propranolol may block bronchodilation produced by exogenous catecholamine stimulation of beta receptors). Products include:
- Norisodrine with Calcium Iodide Syrup 446

Isradipine (Caution should be exercised when administered concomitantly). Products include:
- DynaCirc Capsules 2381
- DynaCirc CR Tablets 2383

Ketoprofen (Blunts antihypertensive effect of beta blocker). Products include:
- Actron Caplets and Tablets .... ◘◘ 608
- Orudis Capsules 2874
- Orudis KT .... ◘◘ 842
- Oruvail Capsules 2874

Ketorolac Tromethamine (Blunts antihypertensive effect of beta blocker). Products include:
- Acular Sterile Ophthalmic Solution 470
- Toradol 2319

Levothyroxine Sodium (Concurrent use may result in lower than expected T_3 concentration). Products include:
- Eltroxin Tablets 2214
- Levothroid Tablets 1015
- Levothyroxine Sodium, USP for Injection 546

- Levoxyl Tablets 918
- Synthroid 1410

Lidocaine Hydrochloride (Reduced clearance of lidocaine). Products include:
- Decadron Phosphate with Xylocaine Injection, Sterile 1683
- Unguentine Plus .... ◘◘ 712
- Xylocaine Injections 562

Meclofenamate Sodium (Blunts antihypertensive effect of beta blocker).
- No products indexed under this heading.

Mefenamic Acid (Blunts antihypertensive effect of beta blocker). Products include:
- Ponstel 1982

Metaproterenol Sulfate (Propranolol may block bronchodilation produced by exogenous catecholamine stimulation of beta receptors). Products include:
- Alupent 672
- Metaproterenol Sulfate Inhalation Solution, USP, Arm-a-Med 547

Metformin Hydrochloride (Delay in the recovery of blood glucose to normal levels following insulin-induced hypoglycemia). Products include:
- Glucophage Tablets 754

Nabumetone (Blunts antihypertensive effect of beta blocker). Products include:
- Relafen Tablets 2688

Naproxen (Blunts antihypertensive effect of beta blocker). Products include:
- Anaprox/Naprosyn 2277

Naproxen Sodium (Blunts antihypertensive effect of beta blocker). Products include:
- Aleve 2124
- Anaprox/Naprosyn 2277
- Naprelan Tablets 2861

Nicardipine Hydrochloride (Caution should be exercised when administered concomitantly). Products include:
- Cardene Capsules 2261
- Cardene I.V. 2815
- Cardene SR Capsules 2264

Nifedipine (Caution should be exercised when administered concomitantly). Products include:
- Adalat Capsules (10 mg and 20 mg) 580
- Adalat CC 582
- Procardia Capsules 2024
- Procardia XL Extended Release Tablets 2026

Nimodipine (Caution should be exercised when administered concomitantly). Products include:
- Nimotop Capsules 603

Nisoldipine (Caution should be exercised when administered concomitantly). Products include:
- Sular Tablets 2961

Oxaprozin (Blunts antihypertensive effect of beta blocker). Products include:
- Daypro Caplets 2578

Phenobarbital (Propranolol clearance accelerated). Products include:
- Arco-Lase Plus Tablets 513
- Bellergal-S Tablets 2375
- Donnatal 2234
- Donnatal Extentabs 2234
- Donnatal Tablets 2234
- Phenobarbital Elixir and Tablets ... 1523
- Quadrinal Tablets 1398

Phenylbutazone (Blunts antihypertensive effect of beta blocker).
- No products indexed under this heading.

Phenytoin (Propranolol clearance accelerated). Products include:
- Dilantin Infatabs 1967
- Dilantin-125 Suspension 1969

Phenytoin Sodium (Propranolol clearance accelerated). Products include:
- Dilantin Kapseals 1965

Pirbuterol Acetate (Propranolol may block bronchodilation produced by exogenous catecholamine stimulation of beta receptors). Products include:
- Maxair Autohaler 1550
- Maxair Inhaler 1552

Piroxicam (Blunts antihypertensive effect of beta blocker). Products include:
- Feldene Capsules 2008

Rauwolfia Serpentina (May produce excessive hypotension with bradycardia and orthostatic effects).
- No products indexed under this heading.

Rescinnamine (May produce excessive hypotension with bradycardia and orthostatic effects).
- No products indexed under this heading.

Reserpine (May produce excessive hypotension with bradycardia and orthostatic effects). Products include:
- Diupres Tablets 1691
- Hydropres Tablets 1718
- Ser-Ap-Es Tablets 867

Rifampin (Propranolol clearance accelerated). Products include:
- Rifadin 1276
- Rifamate Capsules 1278
- Rifater 1280
- Rimactane Capsules 865

Salmeterol Xinafoate (Propranolol may block bronchodilation produced by exogenous catecholamine stimulation of beta receptors). Products include:
- Serevent Inhalation Aerosol 1149

Sulindac (Blunts antihypertensive effect of beta blocker). Products include:
- Clinoril Tablets 1658

Terbutaline Sulfate (Propranolol may block bronchodilation produced by exogenous catecholamine stimulation of beta receptors). Products include:
- Brethaire Inhaler 830
- Brethine Ampuls 832
- Brethine Tablets 831
- Bricanyl Subcutaneous Injection ... 1247
- Bricanyl Tablets 1248

Theophylline (Reduced theophylline clearance). Products include:
- Marax Tablets & DF Syrup 2015
- Quibron 2227

Theophylline Anhydrous (Reduced theophylline clearance). Products include:
- Aerolate 1003
- Primatene Tablets .... ◘◘ 844
- Respbid Tablets 687
- Slo-bid Gyrocaps 2201
- Theo-24 Extended Release Capsules 2753
- Theo-Dur Extended-Release Tablets 1367
- Theo-X Extended-Release Tablets 793
- Uni-Dur Extended-Release Tablets .. 1374
- Uniphyl 400 mg and 600 mg Tablets 2157

Theophylline Calcium Salicylate (Reduced theophylline clearance). Products include:
- Quadrinal Tablets 1398

Theophylline Sodium Glycinate (Reduced theophylline clearance).
- No products indexed under this heading.

527 **Interactions Index** **Inderide**

Tolazamide (Delay in the recovery of blood glucose to normal levels following insulin-induced hypoglycemia).
No products indexed under this heading.
Tolbutamide (Delay in the recovery of blood glucose to normal levels following insulin-induced hypoglycemia).
No products indexed under this heading.
Tolmetin Sodium (Blunts antihypertensive effect of beta blocker). Products include:
Tolectin (200, 400 and 600 mg) .. 1591
Verapamil Hydrochloride (Intravenous use of beta blocker and verapamil has resulted in serious adverse reactions in patients with severe cardiomyopathy, CHF or recent MI). Products include:
Calan SR Caplets ... 2571
Calan Tablets ... 2568
Covera-HS Tablets ... 2573
Isoptin Injectable ... 1391
Isoptin Oral Tablets ... 1393
Isoptin SR Tablets ... 1395
Verelan Capsules ... 1455

Food Interactions

Alcohol (Absorption rate of propranolol slowed).

INDERIDE TABLETS
(Propranolol Hydrochloride, Hydrochlorothiazide) ... 2838
May interact with antihypertensives, catecholamine depleting drugs, cardiac glycosides, corticosteroids, calcium channel blockers, ganglionic blocking agents, insulin, non-steroidal anti-inflammatory agents, barbiturates, narcotic analgesics, xanthine bronchodilators, and certain other agents. Compounds in these categories include:

Acebutolol Hydrochloride (Potentiated or additive action). Products include:
Sectral Capsules ... 2914
ACTH (Hypokalemia may develop with concomitant use).
No products indexed under this heading.
Alfentanil Hydrochloride (Aggravates orthostatic hypotension). Products include:
Alfenta Injection ... 1334
Aluminum Hydroxide (Greatly reduces intestinal absorption of propranolol). Products include:
ALternaGEL Liquid ... 1358
Maximum Strength Ascriptin ... ⊞ 650
Cama Arthritis Pain Reliever ... ⊞ 748
Gaviscon Extra Strength Relief Formula Antacid Tablets ... ⊞ 778
Gaviscon Extra Strength Relief Formula Liquid Antacid ... ⊞ 779
Gaviscon Liquid Antacid ... ⊞ 779
Gelusil Antacid-Anti-gas Liquid ... ⊞ 819
Gelusil Antacid-Anti-gas Tablets ... ⊞ 819
Maalox Antacid/Anti-Gas Tablets ... 889
Maalox Heartburn Relief Suspension ... ⊞ 658
Maalox Antacid Liquid ... 888
Extra Strength Maalox Antacid/Anti-Gas Liquid and Tablets ... 888
Mylanta ... 1359
Tempo Soft Antacid ... ⊞ 799
Aluminum Hydroxide Gel (Greatly reduces intestinal absorption of propranolol). Products include:
ALternaGEL Liquid ... ⊞ 675
Aludrox Oral Suspension ... ⊞ 850
Amphojel Suspension ... 2802
Amphojel Suspension without Flavor ... 2802
Amphojel Tablets ... 2802
Ascriptin ... ⊞ 650
Gaviscon Antacid Tablets ... ⊞ 778
Gaviscon-2 Antacid Tablets ... ⊞ 779
Mylanta Liquid ... ⊞ 676
Mylanta Double Strength Liquid ... ⊞ 676
Nephrox Suspension ... ⊞ 671
Aminophylline (Reduced theophylline clearance).
No products indexed under this heading.
Amlodipine Besylate (Both agents may depress myocardial contractility or AV conduction resulting in increased adverse reactions). Products include:
Lotrel Capsules ... 858
Norvasc Tablets ... 2020
Antipyrine (Reduced clearance of antipyrine). Products include:
Auralgan Otic Solution ... 2810
Tympagesic Ear Drops ... 2476
Aprobarbital (Aggravates orthostatic hypotension).
No products indexed under this heading.
Atenolol (Potentiated or additive action). Products include:
Tenoretic Tablets ... 2963
Tenormin Tablets and I.V. Injection 2965
Benazepril Hydrochloride (Potentiated or additive action). Products include:
Lotensin Tablets ... 852
Lotensin HCT Tablets ... 855
Lotrel Capsules ... 858
Bendroflumethiazide (Potentiated or additive action).
No products indexed under this heading.
Bepridil Hydrochloride (Both agents may depress myocardial contractility or AV conduction resulting in increased adverse reactions). Products include:
Vascor Tablets (200 and 300 mg) 1597
Betamethasone Acetate (Hypokalemia may develop with concomitant use). Products include:
Celestone Soluspan Suspension ... 2484
Betamethasone Sodium Phosphate (Hypokalemia may develop with concomitant use). Products include:
Celestone Soluspan Suspension ... 2484
Betaxolol Hydrochloride (Potentiated or additive action). Products include:
Betoptic Ophthalmic Solution ... 465
Betoptic S Ophthalmic Suspension 467
Kerlone Tablets ... 2588
Bisoprolol Fumarate (Potentiated or additive action). Products include:
Zebeta Tablets ... 1457
Ziac ... 1459
Buprenorphine (Aggravates orthostatic hypotension). Products include:
Buprenex Injectable ... 2170
Butabarbital (Aggravates orthostatic hypotension).
No products indexed under this heading.
Butalbital (Aggravates orthostatic hypotension). Products include:
Axocet Capsules ... 2469
Esgic-plus Capsules ... 1012
Esgic-plus Tablets ... 1012
Fioricet Tablets ... 2386
Fioricet with Codeine Capsules ... 2387
Fiorinal Capsules ... 2388
Fiorinal with Codeine Capsules ... 2390
Fiorinal Tablets ... 2388
Phrenilin ... 790
Sedapap Tablets 50 mg/650 mg .. 1826
Captopril (Potentiated or additive action). Products include:
Capoten Tablets ... 740
Capozide Tablets ... 744
Carteolol Hydrochloride (Potentiated or additive action). Products include:
Cartrol Tablets ... 413
Ocupress Ophthalmic Solution, 1% Sterile ... ◉ 297
Chlorothiazide (Potentiated or additive action). Products include:
Aldoclor Tablets ... 1638
Diupres Tablets ... 1691
Diuril Oral ... 1694
Chlorothiazide Sodium (Potentiated or additive action). Products include:
Diuril Sodium Intravenous ... 1693
Chlorpromazine (Increased plasma levels of both drugs). Products include:
Thorazine Suppositories ... 2701
Chlorthalidone (Potentiated or additive action). Products include:
Combipres Tablets ... 682
Tenoretic Tablets ... 2963
Thalitone ... 1293
Cimetidine (Decreases hepatic metabolism of propranolol resulting in increased blood levels). Products include:
Tagamet HB Tablets ... ⊞ 786
Tagamet Tablets ... 2694
Cimetidine Hydrochloride (Decreases hepatic metabolism of propranolol resulting in increased blood levels). Products include:
Tagamet ... 2694
Clonidine (Potentiated or additive action). Products include:
Catapres-TTS ... 680
Clonidine Hydrochloride (Potentiated or additive action). Products include:
Catapres Tablets ... 679
Combipres Tablets ... 682
Codeine Phosphate (Aggravates orthostatic hypotension). Products include:
Brontex ... 2130
Dimetane-DC Cough Syrup ... 2232
Fioricet with Codeine Capsules ... 2387
Fiorinal with Codeine Capsules ... 2390
Nucofed ... 2225
Phenergan with Codeine ... 2883
Phenergan VC with Codeine ... 2888
Robitussin A-C Syrup ... 2248
Robitussin-DAC Syrup ... 2249
Ryna ... ⊞ 804
Soma Compound w/Codeine Tablets ... 2784
Tylenol with Codeine ... 1592
Cortisone Acetate (Hypokalemia may develop with concomitant use). Products include:
Cortone Acetate Sterile Suspension ... 1663
Cortone Acetate Tablets ... 1664
Deserpidine (May produce an excessive hypotension with bradycardia and orthostatic effects).
No products indexed under this heading.
Deslanoside (Hypokalemia can sensitize or exaggerate the response of the heart to digitalis toxicity).
No products indexed under this heading.
Dexamethasone (Hypokalemia may develop with concomitant use). Products include:
AK-Trol Ointment & Suspension ... ◉ 205
Decadron Elixir ... 1676
Decadron Tablets ... 1678
Decaspray Topical Aerosol ... 1689
Maxitrol Ophthalmic Ointment and Suspension ... ◉ 222
TobraDex Ophthalmic Suspension and Ointment ... 469
Dexamethasone Acetate (Hypokalemia may develop with concomitant use). Products include:
Dalalone D.P. Injectable ... 1009
Decadron-LA Sterile Suspension ... 1687
Dexamethasone Sodium Phosphate (Hypokalemia may develop with concomitant use). Products include:
Decadron Phosphate Injection ... 1680
Decadron Phosphate Sterile Ophthalmic Ointment ... 1684
Decadron Phosphate Sterile Ophthalmic Solution ... 1685
Decadron Phosphate Topical Cream ... 1686
Decadron Phosphate with Xylocaine Injection, Sterile ... 1683
Dexacort Phosphate in Respihaler .. 1606
Dexacort Phosphate in Turbinaire .. 1607
NeoDecadron Sterile Ophthalmic Ointment ... 1755
NeoDecadron Sterile Ophthalmic Solution ... 1756
NeoDecadron Topical Cream ... 1757
Dezocine (Aggravates orthostatic hypotension). Products include:
Dalgan Injection ... 529
Diazoxide (Potentiated or additive action). Products include:
Hyperstat I.V. Injection ... 2504
Proglycem ... 575
Diclofenac Potassium (Blunting of the antihypertensive effect). Products include:
Cataflam Tablets ... 833
Diclofenac Sodium (Blunting of the antihypertensive effect). Products include:
Voltaren Ophthalmic Sterile Ophthalmic Solution ... ◉ 264
Cataflam/Voltaren/Voltaren-XR ... 833
Digitoxin (Hypokalemia can sensitize or exaggerate the response of the heart to digitalis toxicity). Products include:
Crystodigin Tablets ... 1472
Digoxin (Hypokalemia can sensitize or exaggerate the response of the heart to digitalis toxicity). Products include:
Lanoxicaps ... 1110
Lanoxin Elixir Pediatric ... 1113
Lanoxin Injection ... 1116
Lanoxin Injection Pediatric ... 1119
Lanoxin Tablets ... 1121
Diltiazem Hydrochloride (Both agents may depress myocardial contractility or AV conduction resulting in increased adverse reactions). Products include:
Cardizem CD Capsules ... 1251
Cardizem SR Capsules ... 1255
Cardizem Injectable ... 1253
Cardizem Tablets ... 1257
Dilacor XR Extended-release Capsules ... 2183
Tiazac Capsules ... 1019
Doxazosin Mesylate (Potentiated or additive action). Products include:
Cardura Tablets ... 1993
Dyphylline (Reduced theophylline clearance). Products include:
Lufyllin & Lufyllin-400 Tablets ... 2778
Lufyllin-GG Elixir & Tablets ... 2779
Enalapril Maleate (Potentiated or additive action). Products include:
Vaseretic Tablets ... 1810
Vasotec Tablets ... 1816
Enalaprilat (Potentiated or additive action). Products include:
Vasotec I.V. ... 1814
Esmolol Hydrochloride (Potentiated or additive action). Products include:
Brevibloc (esmolol HCl) Injection ... 1860
Etodolac (Blunting of the antihypertensive effect). Products include:
Lodine Capsules and Tablets ... 2849
Felodipine (Both agents may depress myocardial contractility or AV conduction resulting in increased adverse reactions). Products include:
Plendil Extended-Release Tablets ... 514

IMPORTANT NOTE: Always consult each drug listing in the patient's regimen for possible interactions.

Interactions Index

Fenoprofen Calcium (Blunting of the antihypertensive effect). Products include:
- Nalfon 200 Pulvules & Nalfon Tablets ... 933

Fentanyl (Aggravates orthostatic hypotension). Products include:
- Duragesic Transdermal System ... 1336

Fentanyl Citrate (Aggravates orthostatic hypotension). Products include:
- Sublimaze Injection ... 463

Fludrocortisone Acetate (Hypokalemia may develop with concomitant use). Products include:
- Florinef Acetate Tablets ... 506

Flurbiprofen (Blunting of the antihypertensive effect).
- No products indexed under this heading.

Fosinopril Sodium (Potentiated or additive action). Products include:
- Monopril Tablets ... 762

Furosemide (Potentiated or additive action). Products include:
- Lasix Injection, Oral Solution and Tablets ... 1267

Guanabenz Acetate (Potentiated or additive action).
- No products indexed under this heading.

Guanethidine Monosulfate (May produce an excessive hypotension with bradycardia and orthostatic effects). Products include:
- Esimil Tablets ... 840
- Ismelin Tablets ... 845

Haloperidol (Concomitant use may result in hypotension and coronary arrest). Products include:
- Haldol Injection, Tablets and Concentrate ... 1585

Haloperidol Decanoate (Concomitant use may result in hypotension and coronary arrest). Products include:
- Haldol Decanoate ... 1587

Hydralazine Hydrochloride (Potentiated or additive action). Products include:
- Apresazide Capsules ... 824
- Apresoline Hydrochloride Tablets ... 826
- Hydralazine Hydrochloride Injection USP ... 2712
- Ser-Ap-Es Tablets ... 867

Hydrocodone Bitartrate (Aggravates orthostatic hypotension). Products include:
- Codiclear DH Syrup ... 808
- Duratuss HD Elixir ... 2750
- Histussin D Liquid ... 670
- Hycodan Tablets and Syrup ... 946
- Hycomine Compound Tablets ... 948
- Hycomine ... 947
- Hycotuss Expectorant Syrup ... 950
- Hydrocet Capsules ... 787
- Lorcet 10/650 Tablets ... 1016
- Lortab ... 2751
- Tussend ... 1830
- Tussend Expectorant ... 1831
- Vicodin Tablets ... 1404
- Vicodin ES Tablets ... 1405
- Vicodin HP Tablets ... 1403
- Vicodin Tuss Expectorant ... 1406
- Zydone Capsules ... 967

Hydrocodone Polistirex (Aggravates orthostatic hypotension). Products include:
- Tussionex Pennkinetic Extended-Release Suspension ... 1624

Hydrocortisone (Hypokalemia may develop with concomitant use). Products include:
- Anusol-HC Cream 2.5% ... 1953
- Aquanil HC Lotion ... 1989
- Maximum Strength Cortaid Spray ... 800
- CORTENEMA ... 2713
- Cortisporin Ointment ... 1074
- Cortisporin Ophthalmic Ointment Sterile ... 1074
- Cortisporin Ophthalmic Suspension Sterile ... 1075
- Cortisporin Otic Solution Sterile ... 1076
- Cortisporin Otic Suspension Sterile ... 1077
- Cortizone-5 ... 795
- Cortizone-10 ... 795
- Hydrocortone Tablets ... 1715
- Hytone ... 922
- Hytone Ointment 2 ½% ... 923
- Massengill Medicated Soft Cloth Towelettes ... 2628
- Pediotic Suspension Sterile ... 1140
- Preparation H Hydrocortisone 1% Cream ... 843
- ProctoCream-HC 2.5% ... 2552
- VōSoL HC Otic Solution ... 2786

Hydrocortisone Acetate (Hypokalemia may develop with concomitant use). Products include:
- Analpram-HC Rectal Cream 1% and 2.5% ... 993
- Anusol HC-1 Hydrocortisone Anti-Itch Ointment ... 810
- Anusol-HC Suppositories ... 1954
- Caldecort Anti-Itch Hydrocortisone Cream ... 651
- Coly-Mycin S Otic w/Neomycin & Hydrocortisone ... 1965
- Cortaid ... 800
- Cortifoam ... 2540
- Cortisporin Cream ... 1073
- Epifoam ... 2543
- Hydrocortone Acetate Sterile Suspension ... 1712
- Mantadil Cream ... 1124
- Nupercainal Hydrocortisone 1% Cream ... 661
- Pramosone Cream, Lotion & Ointment ... 995
- ProctoFoam-HC ... 2552
- Terra-Cortril Ophthalmic Suspension ... 2033

Hydrocortisone Sodium Phosphate (Hypokalemia may develop with concomitant use). Products include:
- Hydrocortone Phosphate Injection, Sterile ... 1713

Hydrocortisone Sodium Succinate (Hypokalemia may develop with concomitant use).
- No products indexed under this heading.

Hydroflumethiazide (Potentiated or additive action). Products include:
- Diucardin Tablets ... 2824

Hydromorphone Hydrochloride (Aggravates orthostatic hypotension). Products include:
- Dilaudid Ampules ... 1382
- Dilaudid Cough Syrup ... 1383
- Dilaudid-HP Injection ... 1384
- Dilaudid-HP Lyophilized Powder 250 mg ... 1384
- Dilaudid ... 1382
- Dilaudid Oral Liquid ... 1386
- Dilaudid ... 1382
- Dilaudid Tablets - 8 mg ... 1386

Ibuprofen (Blunting of the antihypertensive effect). Products include:
- Advil Cold and Sinus Caplets and Tablets ... 837
- Advil Ibuprofen Tablets, Caplets and Gel Caplets ... 836
- Children's Motrin Ibuprofen Oral Suspension ... 1558
- IBU Tablets ... 1389
- Ibuprohm ... 713
- Motrin IB Caplets, Tablets, and Gelcaps ... 802
- Motrin Ibuprofen Suspension, Oral Drops, Chewable Tablets, Caplets ... 1563
- Nuprin Ibuprofen/Analgesic Tablets & Caplets ... 645
- Vicks DayQuil SINUS Pressure & PAIN Relief with IBUPROFEN ... 735

Indapamide (Potentiated or additive action).
- No products indexed under this heading.

Indomethacin (Blunting of the antihypertensive effect). Products include:
- Indocin ... 1723

Indomethacin Sodium Trihydrate (Blunting of the antihypertensive effect). Products include:
- Indocin I.V. ... 1727

Insulin, Human (Insulin requirements may be altered).
- No products indexed under this heading.

Insulin, Human Isophane Suspension (Insulin requirements may be altered). Products include:
- Novolin N Human Insulin 10 ml Vials ... 1846

Insulin, Human NPH (Insulin requirements may be altered). Products include:
- Humulin N, 100 Units ... 1495
- Novolin N PenFill 1.5 ml Cartridges Durable Insulin Delivery System ... 1849
- Novolin N Prefilled Syringe Disposable Insulin Delivery System ... 1850

Insulin, Human Regular (Insulin requirements may be altered). Products include:
- Humulin R, 100 Units ... 1497
- Novolin R Human Insulin 10 ml Vials ... 1846
- Novolin R PenFill 1.5 ml Cartridges Durable Insulin Delivery System ... 1849
- Novolin R Prefilled Syringe Disposable Insulin Delivery System ... 1850
- Velosulin BR Human Insulin 10 ml Vials ... 1847

Insulin, Human, Zinc Suspension (Insulin requirements may be altered). Products include:
- Humulin L, 100 Units ... 1494
- Humulin U, 100 Units ... 1498
- Novolin L Human Insulin 10 ml Vials ... 1846

Insulin Lispro, Human (Insulin requirements may be altered). Products include:
- Humalog Injection ... 1488

Insulin, NPH (Insulin requirements may be altered). Products include:
- NPH, 100 Units ... 1502
- Pork NPH, 100 Units ... 1506
- Purified Pork NPH Isophane Insulin ... 1852

Insulin, Regular (Insulin requirements may be altered). Products include:
- Regular, 100 Units ... 1503
- Pork Regular, 100 Units ... 1507
- Pork Regular (Concentrated), 500 Units ... 1508
- Purified Pork Regular Insulin ... 1852

Insulin, Zinc Crystals (Insulin requirements may be altered). Products include:
- NPH, 100 Units ... 1502

Insulin, Zinc Suspension (Insulin requirements may be altered). Products include:
- Iletin I ... 1501
- Lente, 100 Units ... 1501
- Iletin II ... 1504
- Pork Lente, 100 Units ... 1504
- Purified Pork Lente Insulin ... 1852

Isradipine (Both agents may depress myocardial contractility or AV conduction resulting in increased adverse reactions). Products include:
- DynaCirc Capsules ... 2381
- DynaCirc CR Tablets ... 2383

Ketoprofen (Blunting of the antihypertensive effect). Products include:
- Actron Caplets and Tablets ... 608
- Orudis Capsules ... 2874
- Orudis KT ... 842
- Oruvail Capsules ... 2874

Ketorolac Tromethamine (Blunting of the antihypertensive effect). Products include:
- Acular Sterile Ophthalmic Solution ... 470
- Toradol ... 2319

Labetalol Hydrochloride (Potentiated or additive action). Products include:
- Normodyne Injection ... 2519
- Normodyne Tablets ... 2522
- Trandate ... 1158

Levorphanol Tartrate (Aggravates orthostatic hypotension). Products include:
- Levo-Dromoran ... 2297

Lidocaine Hydrochloride (Reduced clearance of lidocaine). Products include:
- Decadron Phosphate with Xylocaine Injection, Sterile ... 1683
- Unguentine Plus ... 712
- Xylocaine Injections ... 562

Lisinopril (Potentiated or additive action). Products include:
- Prinivil Tablets ... 1776
- Prinzide Tablets ... 1780
- Zestoretic Tablets ... 2968
- Zestril Tablets ... 2972

Losartan Potassium (Potentiated or additive action). Products include:
- Cozaar Tablets ... 1668
- Hyzaar Tablets ... 1720

Mecamylamine Hydrochloride (Potentiated or additive action). Products include:
- Inversine Tablets ... 1729

Meclofenamate Sodium (Blunting of the antihypertensive effect).
- No products indexed under this heading.

Mefenamic Acid (Blunting of the antihypertensive effect). Products include:
- Ponstel ... 1982

Meperidine Hydrochloride (Aggravates orthostatic hypotension). Products include:
- Demerol ... 2438
- Mepergan Injection ... 2859

Mephobarbital (Aggravates orthostatic hypotension). Products include:
- Mebaral Tablets ... 2452

Methadone Hydrochloride (Aggravates orthostatic hypotension). Products include:
- Methadone Hydrochloride Oral Concentrate ... 2356
- Methadone Hydrochloride Oral Solution & Tablets ... 2357

Methyclothiazide (Potentiated or additive action). Products include:
- Enduron Tablets ... 424

Methyldopa (Potentiated or additive action). Products include:
- Aldoclor Tablets ... 1638
- Aldomet Oral ... 1640
- Aldoril Tablets ... 1644

Methyldopate Hydrochloride (Potentiated or additive action). Products include:
- Aldomet Ester HCl Injection ... 1642

Methylprednisolone Acetate (Hypokalemia may develop with concomitant use).
- No products indexed under this heading.

Methylprednisolone Sodium Succinate (Hypokalemia may develop with concomitant use).
- No products indexed under this heading.

Metolazone (Potentiated or additive action). Products include:
- Mykrox Tablets ... 1617
- Zaroxolyn Tablets ... 1625

Metoprolol Succinate (Potentiated or additive action). Products include:
- Toprol-XL Tablets ... 560

Metoprolol Tartrate (Potentiated or additive action). Products include:
- Lopressor ... 848
- Lopressor HCT Tablets ... 850

(■ Described in PDR For Nonprescription Drugs) (● Described in PDR For Ophthalmology)

Metyrosine (Potentiated or additive action). Products include:
- Demser Capsules 1690

Minoxidil (Potentiated or additive action).
- No products indexed under this heading.

Moexipril Hydrochloride (Potentiated or additive action). Products include:
- Univasc Tablets 2553

Morphine Sulfate (Aggravates orthostatic hypotension). Products include:
- Astramorph/PF Injection, USP (Preservative-Free) 526
- Duramorph Injection 983
- Infumorph 200 and Infumorph 500 Sterile Solutions 985
- Kadian Capsules 2948
- MS Contin Tablets 2149
- MSIR 2152
- Oramorph SR (Morphine Sulfate Sustained Release Tablets) 2359
- RMS Suppositories CII 2766
- Roxanol 2365

Nabumetone (Blunting of the antihypertensive effect). Products include:
- Relafen Tablets 2688

Nadolol (Potentiated or additive action).
- No products indexed under this heading.

Naproxen (Blunting of the antihypertensive effect). Products include:
- Anaprox/Naprosyn 2277

Naproxen Sodium (Blunting of the antihypertensive effect). Products include:
- Aleve 2124
- Anaprox/Naprosyn 2277
- Naprelan Tablets 2861

Nicardipine Hydrochloride (Both agents may depress myocardial contractility or AV conduction resulting in increased adverse reactions). Products include:
- Cardene Capsules 2261
- Cardene I.V. 2815
- Cardene SR Capsules 2264

Nifedipine (Both agents may depress myocardial contractility or AV conduction resulting in increased adverse reactions). Products include:
- Adalat Capsules (10 mg and 20 mg) 580
- Adalat CC 582
- Procardia Capsules 2024
- Procardia XL Extended Release Tablets 2026

Nimodipine (Both agents may depress myocardial contractility or AV conduction resulting in increased adverse reactions). Products include:
- Nimotop Capsules 603

Nisoldipine (Both agents may depress myocardial contractility or AV conduction resulting in increased adverse reactions). Products include:
- Sular Tablets 2961

Nitroglycerin (Potentiated or additive action). Products include:
- Deponit NTG Transdermal Delivery System 2541
- Nitro-Bid IV 1270
- Nitro-Bid Ointment 1272
- Nitro-Dur (nitroglycerin) Transdermal Infusion System 1365
- Nitrolingual Spray 2193
- Nitrostat Tablets 1981
- Transderm-Nitro Transdermal Therapeutic System 878

Norepinephrine Bitartrate (Decreased arterial responsiveness to norepinephrine). Products include:
- Levophed Bitartrate Injection 2445

Opium Alkaloids (Aggravates orthostatic hypotension).
- No products indexed under this heading.

Oxaprozin (Blunting of the antihypertensive effect). Products include:
- Daypro Caplets 2578

Oxycodone Hydrochloride (Aggravates orthostatic hypotension). Products include:
- OxyContin Tablets 2163
- OxyIR Capsules 2167
- Percocet Tablets 955
- Percodan Tablets 955
- Percodan-Demi Tablets 956
- Roxicodone Tablets, Oral Solution & Intensol (Oxycodone) 2366
- Tylox Capsules 1593

Penbutolol Sulfate (Potentiated or additive action). Products include:
- Levatol Tablets 2547

Pentobarbital Sodium (Aggravates orthostatic hypotension). Products include:
- Nembutal Sodium Capsules 440
- Nembutal Sodium Solution 442
- Nembutal Sodium Suppositories 444

Phenobarbital (Accelerates propranolol clearance). Products include:
- Arco-Lase Plus Tablets 513
- Bellergal-S Tablets 2375
- Donnatal 2234
- Donnatal Extentabs 2234
- Donnatal Tablets 2234
- Phenobarbital Elixir and Tablets 1523
- Quadrinal Tablets 1398

Phenoxybenzamine Hydrochloride (Potentiated or additive action). Products include:
- Dibenzyline Capsules 2650

Phentolamine Mesylate (Potentiated or additive action). Products include:
- Regitine Vials 864

Phenylbutazone (Blunting of the antihypertensive effect).
- No products indexed under this heading.

Phenytoin (Accelerates propranolol clearance). Products include:
- Dilantin Infatabs 1967
- Dilantin-125 Suspension 1969

Phenytoin Sodium (Accelerates propranolol clearance). Products include:
- Dilantin Kapseals 1965

Pindolol (Potentiated or additive action). Products include:
- Visken Tablets 2428

Piroxicam (Blunting of the antihypertensive effect). Products include:
- Feldene Capsules 2008

Polythiazide (Potentiated or additive action). Products include:
- Minizide Capsules 2016

Prazosin Hydrochloride (Potentiated or additive action). Products include:
- Minipress Capsules 2015
- Minizide Capsules 2016

Prednisolone Acetate (Hypokalemia may develop with concomitant use). Products include:
- AK-CIDE ..... ◉ 203
- AK-CIDE Ointment ..... ◉ 203
- Blephamide Liquifilm Sterile Ophthalmic Suspension 472
- Blephamide Ointment ..... ◉ 234
- Econopred & Econopred Plus Ophthalmic Suspensions ..... ◉ 216
- Poly-Pred Liquifilm ..... ◉ 246
- Pred Forte ..... ◉ 247
- Pred Mild ..... ◉ 250
- Pred-G Liquifilm Sterile Ophthalmic Suspension ..... ◉ 248
- Pred-G S.O.P. Sterile Ophthalmic Ointment ..... ◉ 249

Prednisolone Sodium Phosphate (Hypokalemia may develop with concomitant use). Products include:
- AK-PRED ..... ◉ 204
- Hydeltrasol Injection, Sterile 1708
- Pediapred Oral Solution 1618

Prednisolone Tebutate (Hypokalemia may develop with concomitant use). Products include:
- Hydeltra-T.B.A. Sterile Suspension 1710

Prednisone (Hypokalemia may develop with concomitant use).
- No products indexed under this heading.

Propoxyphene Hydrochloride (Aggravates orthostatic hypotension). Products include:
- Darvon 1475
- Wygesic Tablets 2930

Propoxyphene Napsylate (Aggravates orthostatic hypotension). Products include:
- Darvon-N/Darvocet-N 1473

Quinapril Hydrochloride (Potentiated or additive action). Products include:
- Accupril Tablets 1950

Ramipril (Potentiated or additive action). Products include:
- Altace Capsules 1238

Rauwolfia Serpentina (May produce an excessive hypotension with bradycardia and orthostatic effects).
- No products indexed under this heading.

Rescinnamine (May produce an excessive hypotension with bradycardia and orthostatic effects).
- No products indexed under this heading.

Reserpine (May produce an excessive hypotension with bradycardia and orthostatic effects). Products include:
- Diupres Tablets 1691
- Hydropres Tablets 1718
- Ser-Ap-Es Tablets 867

Rifampin (Accelerates propranolol clearance). Products include:
- Rifadin 1276
- Rifamate Capsules 1278
- Rifater 1280
- Rimactane Capsules 865

Secobarbital Sodium (Aggravates orthostatic hypotension). Products include:
- Seconal Sodium Pulvules 1529

Sodium Nitroprusside (Potentiated or additive action).
- No products indexed under this heading.

Sotalol Hydrochloride (Potentiated or additive action). Products include:
- Betapace Tablets 637

Spirapril Hydrochloride (Potentiated or additive action).
- No products indexed under this heading.

Sufentanil Citrate (Aggravates orthostatic hypotension). Products include:
- Sufenta Injection 1355

Sulindac (Blunting of the antihypertensive effect). Products include:
- Clinoril Tablets 1658

Terazosin Hydrochloride (Potentiated or additive action). Products include:
- Hytrin Capsules 434

Theophylline (Reduced theophylline clearance). Products include:
- Marax Tablets & DF Syrup 2015
- Quibron 2227

Theophylline Anhydrous (Reduced theophylline clearance). Products include:
- Aerolate 1003
- Primatene Tablets 844
- Respbid Tablets 687
- Slo-bid Gyrocaps 2201
- Theo-24 Extended Release Capsules 2753
- Theo-Dur Extended-Release Tablets 1367
- Theo-X Extended-Release Tablets .. 793
- Uni-Dur Extended-Release Tablets .. 1374
- Uniphyl 400 mg and 600 mg Tablets 2157

Theophylline Calcium Salicylate (Reduced theophylline clearance). Products include:
- Quadrinal Tablets 1398

Theophylline Sodium Glycinate (Reduced theophylline clearance).
- No products indexed under this heading.

Thiamylal Sodium (Aggravates orthostatic hypotension).
- No products indexed under this heading.

Thyroxine (Lower than expected T3 concentration).
- No products indexed under this heading.

Thyroxine Sodium (Lower than expected T3 concentration).
- No products indexed under this heading.

Timolol Maleate (Potentiated or additive action). Products include:
- Blocadren Tablets 1654
- Timolide Tablets 1791
- Timoptic in Ocudose 1796
- Timoptic Sterile Ophthalmic Solution 1794
- Timoptic-XE 1798

Tolmetin Sodium (Blunting of the antihypertensive effect). Products include:
- Tolectin (200, 400 and 600 mg) .. 1591

Torsemide (Potentiated or additive action). Products include:
- Demadex Tablets and Injection 691

Triamcinolone (Hypokalemia may develop with concomitant use).
- No products indexed under this heading.

Triamcinolone Acetonide (Hypokalemia may develop with concomitant use). Products include:
- Azmacort Oral Inhaler 2175
- Nasacort AQ Nasal Spray 2191
- Nasacort Nasal Inhaler 2189

Triamcinolone Diacetate (Hypokalemia may develop with concomitant use).
- No products indexed under this heading.

Triamcinolone Hexacetonide (Hypokalemia may develop with concomitant use).
- No products indexed under this heading.

Trimethaphan Camsylate (Potentiated or additive action).
- No products indexed under this heading.

Tubocurarine Chloride (Increased responsiveness to tubocurarine).
- No products indexed under this heading.

Verapamil Hydrochloride (Both agents may depress myocardial contractility or AV conduction resulting in increased adverse reactions; on rare occasions, the concomitant use with intravenous forms has resulted in serious adverse reactions). Products include:
- Calan SR Caplets 2571
- Calan Tablets 2568
- Covera-HS Tablets 2573
- Isoptin Injectable 1391
- Isoptin Oral Tablets 1393
- Isoptin SR Tablets 1395
- Verelan Capsules 1455

Food Interactions

Alcohol (Slows the rate of absorption of propranolol).

IMPORTANT NOTE: Always consult each drug listing in the patient's regimen for possible interactions.

Inderide LA | Interactions Index | 530

INDERIDE LA LONG ACTING CAPSULES
(Propranolol Hydrochloride, Hydrochlorothiazide) 2840
May interact with antihypertensives, catecholamine depleting drugs, cardiac glycosides, calcium channel blockers, corticosteroids, insulin, barbiturates, non-steroidal anti-inflammatory agents, narcotic analgesics, and certain other agents. Compounds in these categories include:

Acebutolol Hydrochloride (Potentiated or additive action). Products include:
Sectral Capsules 2914

ACTH (Hypokalemia may develop with concomitant use).
No products indexed under this heading.

Alfentanil Hydrochloride (May aggravate orthostatic hypotension). Products include:
Alfenta Injection 1334

Amlodipine Besylate (Both agents may depress myocardial contractility or AV conduction resulting in increased adverse reactions). Products include:
Lotrel Capsules 858
Norvasc Tablets 2020

Aprobarbital (May aggravate orthostatic hypotension).
No products indexed under this heading.

Atenolol (Potentiated or additive action). Products include:
Tenoretic Tablets 2963
Tenormin Tablets and I.V. Injection 2965

Benazepril Hydrochloride (Potentiated or additive action). Products include:
Lotensin Tablets 852
Lotensin HCT Tablets 855
Lotrel Capsules 858

Bendroflumethiazide (Potentiated or additive action).
No products indexed under this heading.

Bepridil Hydrochloride (Both agents may depress myocardial contractility or AV conduction resulting in increased adverse reactions). Products include:
Vascor Tablets (200 and 300 mg) 1597

Betamethasone Acetate (Hypokalemia may develop with concomitant use). Products include:
Celestone Soluspan Suspension 2484

Betamethasone Sodium Phosphate (Hypokalemia may develop with concomitant use). Products include:
Celestone Soluspan Suspension 2484

Betaxolol Hydrochloride (Potentiated or additive action). Products include:
Betoptic Ophthalmic Solution........ 465
Betoptic S Ophthalmic Suspension 467
Kerlone Tablets 2588

Bisoprolol Fumarate (Potentiated or additive action). Products include:
Zebeta Tablets 1457
Ziac 1459

Buprenorphine (May aggravate orthostatic hypotension). Products include:
Buprenex Injectable 2170

Butabarbital (May aggravate orthostatic hypotension).
No products indexed under this heading.

Butalbital (May aggravate orthostatic hypotension). Products include:
Axocet Capsules 2469
Esgic-plus Capsules 1012
Esgic-plus Tablets 1012
Fioricet Tablets 2386
Fioricet with Codeine Capsules 2387
Fiorinal Capsules 2388
Fiorinal with Codeine Capsules 2390
Fiorinal Tablets 2388
Phrenilin 790
Sedapap Tablets 50 mg/650 mg .. 1826

Captopril (Potentiated or additive action). Products include:
Capoten Tablets 740
Capozide Tablets 744

Carteolol Hydrochloride (Potentiated or additive action). Products include:
Cartrol Tablets 413
Ocupress Ophthalmic Solution, 1% Sterile........ ⊙ 297

Chlorothiazide (Potentiated or additive action). Products include:
Aldoclor Tablets 1638
Diupres Tablets 1691
Diuril Oral 1694

Chlorothiazide Sodium (Potentiated or additive action). Products include:
Diuril Sodium Intravenous 1693

Chlorthalidone (Potentiated or additive action). Products include:
Combipres Tablets 682
Tenoretic Tablets 2963
Thalitone 1293

Clonidine (Potentiated or additive action). Products include:
Catapres-TTS 680

Clonidine Hydrochloride (Potentiated or additive action). Products include:
Catapres Tablets 679
Combipres Tablets 682

Codeine Phosphate (May aggravate orthostatic hypotension). Products include:
Brontex 2130
Dimetane-DC Cough Syrup 2232
Fioricet with Codeine Capsules 2387
Fiorinal with Codeine Capsules 2390
Nucofed 2225
Phenergan with Codeine 2883
Phenergan VC with Codeine 2888
Robitussin A-C Syrup 2248
Robitussin-DAC Syrup 2249
Ryna .... ▣ 804
Soma Compound w/Codeine Tablets 2784
Tylenol with Codeine 1592

Cortisone Acetate (Hypokalemia may develop with concomitant use). Products include:
Cortone Acetate Sterile Suspension 1663
Cortone Acetate Tablets 1664

Deserpidine (May produce an excessive hypotension with bradycardia and orthostatic effects).
No products indexed under this heading.

Deslanoside (Hypokalemia produced by thiazides can exaggerate cardiotoxicity of digitalis).
No products indexed under this heading.

Dexamethasone (Hypokalemia may develop with concomitant use). Products include:
AK-Trol Ointment & Suspension .... ⊙ 205
Decadron Elixir 1676
Decadron Tablets 1678
Decaspray Topical Aerosol 1689
Maxitrol Ophthalmic Ointment and Suspension .... ⊙ 222
TobraDex Ophthalmic Suspension and Ointment 469

Dexamethasone Acetate (Hypokalemia may develop with concomitant use). Products include:
Dalalone D.P. Injectable 1009
Decadron-LA Sterile Suspension 1687

Dexamethasone Sodium Phosphate (Hypokalemia may develop with concomitant use). Products include:
Decadron Phosphate Injection 1680
Decadron Phosphate Sterile Ophthalmic Ointment 1684
Decadron Phosphate Sterile Ophthalmic Solution 1685
Decadron Phosphate Topical Cream 1686
Decadron Phosphate with Xylocaine Injection, Sterile 1683
Dexacort Phosphate in Respihaler .. 1606
Dexacort Phosphate in Turbinaire .. 1607
NeoDecadron Sterile Ophthalmic Ointment 1755
NeoDecadron Sterile Ophthalmic Solution 1756
NeoDecadron Topical Cream 1757

Dezocine (May aggravate orthostatic hypotension). Products include:
Dalgan Injection 529

Diazoxide (Potentiated or additive action). Products include:
Hyperstat I.V. Injection 2504
Proglycem 575

Diclofenac Potassium (Blunts antihypertensive effect of beta blocker). Products include:
Cataflam Tablets 833

Diclofenac Sodium (Blunts antihypertensive effect of beta blocker). Products include:
Voltaren Ophthalmic Sterile Ophthalmic Solution .... ⊙ 264
Cataflam/Voltaren/Voltaren-XR 833

Digitoxin (Hypokalemia produced by thiazides can exaggerate cardiotoxicity of digitalis). Products include:
Crystodigin Tablets 1472

Digoxin (Hypokalemia produced by thiazides can exaggerate cardiotoxicity of digitalis). Products include:
Lanoxicaps 1110
Lanoxin Elixir Pediatric 1113
Lanoxin Injection 1116
Lanoxin Injection Pediatric 1119
Lanoxin Tablets 1121

Diltiazem Hydrochloride (Both agents may depress myocardial contractility or AV conduction resulting in increased adverse reactions). Products include:
Cardizem CD Capsules 1251
Cardizem SR Capsules 1255
Cardizem Injectable 1253
Cardizem Tablets 1257
Dilacor XR Extended-release Capsules 2183
Tiazac Capsules 1019

Doxazosin Mesylate (Potentiated or additive action). Products include:
Cardura Tablets 1993

Enalapril Maleate (Potentiated or additive action). Products include:
Vaseretic Tablets 1810
Vasotec Tablets 1816

Enalaprilat (Potentiated or additive action). Products include:
Vasotec I.V. 1814

Esmolol Hydrochloride (Potentiated or additive action). Products include:
Brevibloc (esmolol HCl) Injection 1860

Etodolac (Blunts antihypertensive effect of beta blocker). Products include:
Lodine Capsules and Tablets 2849

Felodipine (Both agents may depress myocardial contractility or AV conduction resulting in increased adverse reactions). Products include:
Plendil Extended-Release Tablets 514

Fenoprofen Calcium (Blunts antihypertensive effect of beta blocker). Products include:
Nalfon 200 Pulvules & Nalfon Tablets 933

Fentanyl (May aggravate orthostatic hypotension). Products include:
Duragesic Transdermal System........ 1336

Fentanyl Citrate (May aggravate orthostatic hypotension). Products include:
Sublimaze Injection 463

Fludrocortisone Acetate (Hypokalemia may develop with concomitant use). Products include:
Florinef Acetate Tablets 506

Flurbiprofen (Blunts antihypertensive effect of beta blocker).
No products indexed under this heading.

Fosinopril Sodium (Potentiated or additive action). Products include:
Monopril Tablets 762

Furosemide (Potentiated or additive action). Products include:
Lasix Injection, Oral Solution and Tablets 1267

Guanabenz Acetate (Potentiated or additive action).
No products indexed under this heading.

Guanethidine Monosulfate (May produce an excessive hypotension with bradycardia and orthostatic effects). Products include:
Esimil Tablets 840
Ismelin Tablets 845

Haloperidol (Hypotension and cardiac arrest have been reported with the concomitant use of propranolol and haloperidol). Products include:
Haldol Injection, Tablets and Concentrate 1585

Haloperidol Decanoate (Hypotension and cardiac arrest have been reported with the concomitant use of propranolol and haloperidol). Products include:
Haldol Decanoate 1587

Hydralazine Hydrochloride (Potentiated or additive action). Products include:
Apresazide Capsules 824
Apresoline Hydrochloride Tablets .. 826
Hydralazine Hydrochloride Injection USP 2712
Ser-Ap-Es Tablets 867

Hydrocodone Bitartrate (May aggravate orthostatic hypotension). Products include:
Codiclear DH Syrup 808
Duratuss HD Elixir 2750
Histussin D Liquid 670
Hycodan Tablets and Syrup 946
Hycomine Compound Tablets 948
Hycomine 947
Hycotuss Expectorant Syrup 950
Hydrocet Capsules 787
Lorcet 10/650 Tablets 1016
Lortab 2751
Tussend 1830
Tussend Expectorant 1831
Vicodin Tablets 1404
Vicodin ES Tablets 1405
Vicodin HP Tablets 1403
Vicodin Tuss Expectorant 1406
Zydone Capsules 967

Hydrocodone Polistirex (May aggravate orthostatic hypotension). Products include:
Tussionex Pennkinetic Extended-Release Suspension 1624

Hydrocortisone (Hypokalemia may develop with concomitant use). Products include:
Anusol-HC Cream 2.5% 1953
Aquanil HC Lotion 1989
Maximum Strength Cortaid Spray ▣ 800
CORTENEMA 2713
Cortisporin Ointment 1074
Cortisporin Ophthalmic Ointment Sterile 1074
Cortisporin Ophthalmic Suspension Sterile 1075
Cortisporin Otic Solution Sterile 1076
Cortisporin Otic Suspension Sterile 1077
Cortizone-5 .... ▣ 795
Cortizone-10 .... ▣ 795
Hydrocortone Tablets 1715

(▣ Described in PDR For Nonprescription Drugs) (⊙ Described in PDR For Ophthalmology)

Hytone ... 922
Hytone Ointment 2 ½% ... 923
Massengill Medicated Soft Cloth Towelettes ... 2628
Pediotic Suspension Sterile ... 1140
Preparation H Hydrocortisone 1% Cream ... 843
ProctoCream-HC 2.5% ... 2552
VōSoL HC Otic Solution ... 2786

Hydrocortisone Acetate (Hypokalemia may develop with concomitant use). Products include:
Analpram-HC Rectal Cream 1% and 2.5% ... 993
Anusol HC-1 Hydrocortisone Anti-Itch Ointment ... 810
Anusol-HC Suppositories ... 1954
Caldecort Anti-Itch Hydrocortisone Cream ... 651
Coly-Mycin S Otic w/Neomycin & Hydrocortisone ... 1965
Cortaid ... 800
Cortifoam ... 2540
Cortisporin Cream ... 1073
Epifoam ... 2543
Hydrocortone Acetate Sterile Suspension ... 1712
Mantadil Cream ... 1124
Nupercainal Hydrocortisone 1% Cream ... 661
Pramosone Cream, Lotion & Ointment ... 995
ProctoFoam-HC ... 2552
Terra-Cortril Ophthalmic Suspension ... 2033

Hydrocortisone Sodium Phosphate (Hypokalemia may develop with concomitant use). Products include:
Hydrocortone Phosphate Injection, Sterile ... 1713

Hydrocortisone Sodium Succinate (Hypokalemia may develop with concomitant use).
No products indexed under this heading.

Hydroflumethiazide (Potentiated or additive action). Products include:
Diucardin Tablets ... 2824

Hydromorphone Hydrochloride (May aggravate orthostatic hypotension). Products include:
Dilaudid Ampules ... 1382
Dilaudid Cough Syrup ... 1383
Dilaudid-HP Injection ... 1384
Dilaudid-HP Lyophilized Powder 250 mg ... 1384
Dilaudid ... 1382
Dilaudid Oral Liquid ... 1386
Dilaudid ... 1382
Dilaudid Tablets - 8 mg ... 1386

Ibuprofen (Blunts antihypertensive effect of beta blocker). Products include:
Advil Cold and Sinus Caplets and Tablets ... 837
Advil Ibuprofen Tablets, Caplets and Gel Caplets ... 836
Children's Motrin Ibuprofen Oral Suspension ... 1558
IBU Tablets ... 1389
Ibuprohm ... 713
Motrin IB Caplets, Tablets, and Gelcaps ... 802
Motrin Ibuprofen Suspension, Oral Drops, Chewable Tablets, Caplets ... 1563
Nuprin Ibuprofen/Analgesic Tablets & Caplets ... 645
Vicks DayQuil SINUS Pressure & PAIN Relief with IBUPROFEN ... 735

Indapamide (Potentiated or additive action).
No products indexed under this heading.

Indomethacin (Blunts antihypertensive effect of beta blocker). Products include:
Indocin ... 1723

Indomethacin Sodium Trihydrate (Blunts antihypertensive effect of beta blocker). Products include:
Indocin I.V. ... 1727

Insulin, Human (Insulin requirements may be increased, decreased, or unchanged).
No products indexed under this heading.

Insulin, Human Isophane Suspension (Insulin requirements may be increased, decreased, or unchanged). Products include:
Novolin N Human Insulin 10 ml Vials ... 1846

Insulin, Human NPH (Insulin requirements may be increased, decreased, or unchanged). Products include:
Humulin N, 100 Units ... 1495
Novolin N PenFill 1.5 ml Cartridges Durable Insulin Delivery System ... 1849
Novolin N Prefilled Syringe Disposable Insulin Delivery System ... 1850

Insulin, Human Regular (Insulin requirements may be increased, decreased, or unchanged). Products include:
Humulin R, 100 Units ... 1497
Novolin R Human Insulin 10 ml Vials ... 1846
Novolin R PenFill 1.5 ml Cartridges Durable Insulin Delivery System ... 1849
Novolin R Prefilled Syringe Disposable Insulin Delivery System ... 1850
Velosulin BR Human Insulin 10 ml Vials ... 1847

Insulin, Human, Zinc Suspension (Insulin requirements may be increased, decreased, or unchanged). Products include:
Humulin L, 100 Units ... 1494
Humulin U, 100 Units ... 1498
Novolin L Human Insulin 10 ml Vials ... 1846

Insulin Lispro, Human (Insulin requirements may be increased, decreased, or unchanged). Products include:
Humalog Injection ... 1488

Insulin, NPH (Insulin requirements may be increased, decreased, or unchanged). Products include:
NPH, 100 Units ... 1502
Pork NPH, 100 Units ... 1506
Purified Pork NPH Isophane Insulin ... 1852

Insulin, Regular (Insulin requirements may be increased, decreased, or unchanged). Products include:
Regular, 100 Units ... 1503
Pork Regular, 100 Units ... 1507
Pork Regular (Concentrated), 500 Units ... 1508
Purified Pork Regular Insulin ... 1852

Insulin, Zinc Crystals (Insulin requirements may be increased, decreased, or unchanged). Products include:
NPH, 100 Units ... 1502

Insulin, Zinc Suspension (Insulin requirements may be increased, decreased, or unchanged). Products include:
Iletin I ... 1501
Lente, 100 Units ... 1501
Iletin II ... 1504
Pork Lente, 100 Units ... 1504
Purified Pork Lente Insulin ... 1852

Isradipine (Both agents may depress myocardial contractility or AV conduction resulting in increased adverse reactions). Products include:
DynaCirc Capsules ... 2381
DynaCirc CR Tablets ... 2383

Ketoprofen (Blunts antihypertensive effect of beta blocker). Products include:
Actron Caplets and Tablets ... 608
Orudis Capsules ... 2874
Orudis KT ... 842
Oruvail Capsules ... 2874

Ketorolac Tromethamine (Blunts antihypertensive effect of beta blocker). Products include:
Acular Sterile Ophthalmic Solution ... 470
Toradol ... 2319

Labetalol Hydrochloride (Potentiated or additive action). Products include:
Normodyne Injection ... 2519
Normodyne Tablets ... 2522
Trandate ... 1158

Levorphanol Tartrate (May aggravate orthostatic hypotension). Products include:
Levo-Dromoran ... 2297

Lisinopril (Potentiated or additive action). Products include:
Prinivil Tablets ... 1776
Prinzide Tablets ... 1780
Zestoretic Tablets ... 2968
Zestril Tablets ... 2972

Losartan Potassium (Potentiated or additive action). Products include:
Cozaar Tablets ... 1668
Hyzaar Tablets ... 1720

Mecamylamine Hydrochloride (Potentiated or additive action). Products include:
Inversine Tablets ... 1729

Meclofenamate Sodium (Blunts antihypertensive effect of beta blocker).
No products indexed under this heading.

Mefenamic Acid (Blunts antihypertensive effect of beta blocker). Products include:
Ponstel ... 1982

Meperidine Hydrochloride (May aggravate orthostatic hypotension). Products include:
Demerol ... 2438
Mepergan Injection ... 2859

Mephobarbital (May aggravate orthostatic hypotension). Products include:
Mebaral Tablets ... 2452

Methadone Hydrochloride (May aggravate orthostatic hypotension). Products include:
Methadone Hydrochloride Oral Concentrate ... 2356
Methadone Hydrochloride Oral Solution & Tablets ... 2357

Methyclothiazide (Potentiated or additive action). Products include:
Enduron Tablets ... 424

Methyldopa (Potentiated or additive action). Products include:
Aldoclor Tablets ... 1638
Aldomet Oral ... 1640
Aldoril Tablets ... 1644

Methyldopate Hydrochloride (Potentiated or additive action). Products include:
Aldomet Ester HCl Injection ... 1642

Methylprednisolone Acetate (Hypokalemia may develop with concomitant use).
No products indexed under this heading.

Methylprednisolone Sodium Succinate (Hypokalemia may develop with concomitant use).
No products indexed under this heading.

Metolazone (Potentiated or additive action). Products include:
Mykrox Tablets ... 1617
Zaroxolyn Tablets ... 1625

Metoprolol Succinate (Potentiated or additive action). Products include:
Toprol-XL Tablets ... 560

Metoprolol Tartrate (Potentiated or additive action). Products include:
Lopressor ... 848
Lopressor HCT Tablets ... 850

Metyrosine (Potentiated or additive action). Products include:
Demser Capsules ... 1690

Minoxidil (Potentiated or additive action).
No products indexed under this heading.

Moexipril Hydrochloride (Potentiated or additive action). Products include:
Univasc Tablets ... 2553

Morphine Sulfate (May aggravate orthostatic hypotension). Products include:
Astramorph/PF Injection, USP (Preservative-Free) ... 526
Duramorph Injection ... 983
Infumorph 200 and Infumorph 500 Sterile Solutions ... 985
Kadian Capsules ... 2948
MS Contin Tablets ... 2149
MSIR ... 2152
Oramorph SR (Morphine Sulfate Sustained Release Tablets) ... 2359
RMS Suppositories CII ... 2766
Roxanol ... 2365

Nabumetone (Blunts antihypertensive effect of beta blocker). Products include:
Relafen Tablets ... 2688

Nadolol (Potentiated or additive action).
No products indexed under this heading.

Naproxen (Blunts antihypertensive effect of beta blocker). Products include:
Anaprox/Naprosyn ... 2277

Naproxen Sodium (Blunts antihypertensive effect of beta blocker). Products include:
Aleve ... 2124
Anaprox/Naprosyn ... 2277
Naprelan Tablets ... 2861

Nicardipine Hydrochloride (Both agents may depress myocardial contractility or AV conduction resulting in increased adverse reactions). Products include:
Cardene Capsules ... 2261
Cardene I.V. ... 2815
Cardene SR Capsules ... 2264

Nifedipine (Both agents may depress myocardial contractility or AV conduction resulting in increased adverse reactions). Products include:
Adalat Capsules (10 mg and 20 mg) ... 580
Adalat CC ... 582
Procardia Capsules ... 2024
Procardia XL Extended Release Tablets ... 2026

Nimodipine (Both agents may depress myocardial contractility or AV conduction resulting in increased adverse reactions). Products include:
Nimotop Capsules ... 603

Nisoldipine (Both agents may depress myocardial contractility or AV conduction resulting in increased adverse reactions). Products include:
Sular Tablets ... 2961

Nitroglycerin (Potentiated or additive action). Products include:
Deponit NTG Transdermal Delivery System ... 2541
Nitro-Bid IV ... 1270
Nitro-Bid Ointment ... 1272
Nitro-Dur (nitroglycerin) Transdermal Infusion System ... 1365
Nitrolingual Spray ... 2193
Nitrostat Tablets ... 1981
Transderm-Nitro Transdermal Therapeutic System ... 878

Norepinephrine Bitartrate (Decreased arterial responsiveness to norepinephrine). Products include:
Levophed Bitartrate Injection ... 2445

IMPORTANT NOTE: Always consult each drug listing in the patient's regimen for possible interactions.

Inderide LA | Interactions Index | 532

Opium Alkaloids (May aggravate orthostatic hypotension).
No products indexed under this heading.

Oxaprozin (Blunts antihypertensive effect of beta blocker). Products include:
Daypro Caplets ... 2578

Oxycodone Hydrochloride (May aggravate orthostatic hypotension). Products include:
OxyContin Tablets ... 2163
OxyIR Capsules ... 2167
Percocet Tablets ... 955
Percodan Tablets ... 955
Percodan-Demi Tablets ... 956
Roxicodone Tablets, Oral Solution & Intensol (Oxycodone) ... 2366
Tylox Capsules ... 1593

Penbutolol Sulfate (Potentiated or additive action). Products include:
Levatol Tablets ... 2547

Pentobarbital Sodium (May aggravate orthostatic hypotension). Products include:
Nembutal Sodium Capsules ... 440
Nembutal Sodium Solution ... 442
Nembutal Sodium Suppositories ... 444

Phenobarbital (May aggravate orthostatic hypotension). Products include:
Arco-Lase Plus Tablets ... 513
Bellergal-S Tablets ... 2375
Donnatal ... 2234
Donnatal Extentabs ... 2234
Donnatal Tablets ... 2234
Phenobarbital Elixir and Tablets ... 1523
Quadrinal Tablets ... 1398

Phenoxybenzamine Hydrochloride (Potentiated or additive action). Products include:
Dibenzyline Capsules ... 2650

Phentolamine Mesylate (Potentiated or additive action). Products include:
Regitine Vials ... 864

Phenylbutazone (Blunts antihypertensive effect of beta blocker).
No products indexed under this heading.

Pindolol (Potentiated or additive action). Products include:
Visken Tablets ... 2428

Piroxicam (Blunts antihypertensive effect of beta blocker). Products include:
Feldene Capsules ... 2008

Polythiazide (Potentiated or additive action). Products include:
Minizide Capsules ... 2016

Prazosin Hydrochloride (Potentiated). Products include:
Minipress Capsules ... 2015
Minizide Capsules ... 2016

Prednisolone Acetate (Hypokalemia may develop with concomitant use). Products include:
AK-CIDE ... ⊚ 203
AK-CIDE Ointment ... ⊚ 203
Blephamide Liquifilm Sterile Ophthalmic Suspension ... 472
Blephamide Ointment ... ⊚ 234
Econopred & Econopred Plus Ophthalmic Suspensions ... ⊚ 216
Poly-Pred Liquifilm ... ⊚ 246
Pred Forte ... ⊚ 247
Pred Mild ... ⊚ 250
Pred-G Liquifilm Sterile Ophthalmic Suspension ... ⊚ 248
Pred-G S.O.P. Sterile Ophthalmic Ointment ... ⊚ 249

Prednisolone Sodium Phosphate (Hypokalemia may develop with concomitant use). Products include:
AK-PRED ... ⊚ 204
Hydeltrasol Injection, Sterile ... 1708
Pediapred Oral Solution ... 1618

Prednisolone Tebutate (Hypokalemia may develop with concomitant use). Products include:
Hydeltra-T.B.A. Sterile Suspension 1710

Prednisone (Hypokalemia may develop with concomitant use).
No products indexed under this heading.

Propoxyphene Hydrochloride (May aggravate orthostatic hypotension). Products include:
Darvon ... 1475
Wygesic Tablets ... 2930

Propoxyphene Napsylate (May aggravate orthostatic hypotension). Products include:
Darvon-N/Darvocet-N ... 1473

Quinapril Hydrochloride (Potentiated or additive action). Products include:
Accupril Tablets ... 1950

Ramipril (Potentiated or additive action). Products include:
Altace Capsules ... 1238

Rauwolfia Serpentina (May produce an excessive hypotension with bradycardia and orthostatic effects).
No products indexed under this heading.

Rescinnamine (May produce an excessive hypotension with bradycardia and orthostatic effects).
No products indexed under this heading.

Reserpine (May produce an excessive hypotension with bradycardia and orthostatic effects). Products include:
Diupres Tablets ... 1691
Hydropres Tablets ... 1718
Ser-Ap-Es Tablets ... 867

Secobarbital Sodium (May aggravate orthostatic hypotension). Products include:
Seconal Sodium Pulvules ... 1529

Sodium Nitroprusside (Potentiated or additive action).
No products indexed under this heading.

Sotalol Hydrochloride (Potentiated or additive action). Products include:
Betapace Tablets ... 637

Spirapril Hydrochloride (Potentiated or additive action).
No products indexed under this heading.

Sufentanil Citrate (May aggravate orthostatic hypotension). Products include:
Sufenta Injection ... 1355

Sulindac (Blunts antihypertensive effect of beta blocker). Products include:
Clinoril Tablets ... 1658

Terazosin Hydrochloride (Potentiated or additive action). Products include:
Hytrin Capsules ... 434

Thiamylal Sodium (May aggravate orthostatic hypotension).
No products indexed under this heading.

Timolol Maleate (Potentiated or additive action). Products include:
Blocadren Tablets ... 1654
Timolide Tablets ... 1791
Timoptic in Ocudose ... 1796
Timoptic Sterile Ophthalmic Solution ... 1794
Timoptic-XE ... 1798

Tolmetin Sodium (Blunts antihypertensive effect of beta blocker). Products include:
Tolectin (200, 400 and 600 mg) .. 1591

Torsemide (Potentiated or additive action). Products include:
Demadex Tablets and Injection ... 691

Triamcinolone (Hypokalemia may develop with concomitant use).
No products indexed under this heading.

Triamcinolone Acetonide (Hypokalemia may develop with concomitant use). Products include:
Azmacort Oral Inhaler ... 2175
Nasacort AQ Nasal Spray ... 2191
Nasacort Nasal Inhaler ... 2189

Triamcinolone Diacetate (Hypokalemia may develop with concomitant use).
No products indexed under this heading.

Triamcinolone Hexacetonide (Hypokalemia may develop with concomitant use).
No products indexed under this heading.

Trimethaphan Camsylate (Potentiated).
No products indexed under this heading.

Tubocurarine Chloride (Increased responsiveness to tubocurarine).
No products indexed under this heading.

Verapamil Hydrochloride (Both agents may depress myocardial contractility or AV conduction resulting in increased adverse reactions; on rare occasions, the concomitant use with intravenous forms has resulted in serious adverse reactions). Products include:
Calan SR Caplets ... 2571
Calan Tablets ... 2568
Covera-HS Tablets ... 2573
Isoptin Injectable ... 1391
Isoptin Oral Tablets ... 1393
Isoptin SR Tablets ... 1395
Verelan Capsules ... 1455

Food Interactions

Alcohol (May aggravate orthostatic hypotension).

INDOCIN CAPSULES
(Indomethacin) ... 1723
May interact with loop diuretics, oral anticoagulants, thiazides, potassium sparing diuretics, beta blockers, non-steroidal anti-inflammatory agents, and certain other agents. Compounds in these categories include:

Acebutolol Hydrochloride (Blunting of antihypertensive effect of beta blockers). Products include:
Sectral Capsules ... 2914

Amiloride Hydrochloride (Reduced diuretic, natriuretic, and antihypertensive effects and increased serum potassium levels). Products include:
Midamor Tablets ... 1746
Moduretic Tablets ... 1748

Aspirin (Decreases indomethacin blood levels). Products include:
Alka-Seltzer Cherry Effervescent Antacid and Pain Reliever ... ▣ 609
Alka-Seltzer Extra Strength Effervescent Antacid and Pain Reliever ... ▣ 609
Alka-Seltzer Lemon Lime Effervescent Antacid and Pain Reliever ... ▣ 609
Alka-Seltzer Original Effervescent Antacid and Pain Reliever ... ▣ 609
Alka-Seltzer Plus ... ▣ 611
Alka-Seltzer Plus Sinus Medicine .. ▣ 611
Ascriptin ... ▣ 650
Arthritis Strength BC Powder ... ▣ 631
BC Cold Powder Multi-Symptom Formula (Cold-Sinus-Allergy) ... ▣ 631
BC Cold Powder Non-Drowsy Formula (Cold-Sinus) ... ▣ 631
BC Powder ... ▣ 631
Genuine Bayer Aspirin Tablets & Caplets ... ▣ 618
Extra Strength Bayer Arthritis Pain Regimen Formula ... ▣ 615
Extra Strength Bayer Aspirin Caplets & Tablets ... ▣ 617
Extended-Release Bayer 8-Hour Aspirin ... ▣ 616
Extra Strength Bayer Plus Aspirin Caplets ... ▣ 617
Extra Strength Bayer PM Aspirin Plus Sleep Aid ... ▣ 617
Aspirin Regimen Bayer 81 mg Tablets with Calcium ... ▣ 615
Aspirin Regimen Bayer Adult Low Strength 81 mg Tablets ... ▣ 613
Aspirin Regimen Bayer Children's Chewable Aspirin ... ▣ 616
Aspirin Regimen Bayer Regular Strength 325 mg Caplets ... ▣ 613
Bufferin Analgesic Tablets ... ▣ 636
Arthritis Strength Bufferin Analgesic Caplets ... ▣ 637
Extra Strength Bufferin Analgesic Tablets ... ▣ 637
Cama Arthritis Pain Reliever ... ▣ 748
Darvon Compound-65 Pulvules ... 1475
Easprin ... 1971
Ecotrin ... 2625
Ecotrin Enteric Coated Aspirin Maximum Strength Tablets and Caplets ... ▣ 775
Ecotrin Enteric Coated Aspirin Regular Strength Tablets ... 2625
Empirin Aspirin Tablets ... ▣ 818
Excedrin Extra-Strength Analgesic Tablets, Caplets, and Geltabs ... 734
Fiorinal Capsules ... 2388
Fiorinal with Codeine Capsules ... 2390
Fiorinal Tablets ... 2388
Goody's Extra Strength Headache Powders ... ▣ 632
Goody's Extra Strength Pain Relief Tablets ... ▣ 632
Halfprin Tablets ... 1413
Norgesic ... 1554
Percodan Tablets ... 955
Percodan-Demi Tablets ... 956
Robaxisal Tablets ... 2246
Soma Compound w/Codeine Tablets ... 2784
Soma Compound Tablets ... 2783
St. Joseph Adult Chewable Aspirin (81 mg.) ... ▣ 768
Talwin Compound ... 2466
Vanquish Analgesic Caplets ... ▣ 627

Atenolol (Blunting of antihypertensive effect of beta blockers). Products include:
Tenoretic Tablets ... 2963
Tenormin Tablets and I.V. Injection 2965

Bendroflumethiazide (Reduced diuretic, natriuretic, and antihypertensive effects of thiazide diuretics).
No products indexed under this heading.

Betaxolol Hydrochloride (Blunting of antihypertensive effect of beta blockers). Products include:
Betoptic Ophthalmic Solution ... 465
Betoptic S Ophthalmic Suspension 467
Kerlone Tablets ... 2588

Bisoprolol Fumarate (Blunting of antihypertensive effect of beta blockers). Products include:
Zebeta Tablets ... 1457
Ziac ... 1459

Bumetanide (Reduced diuretic, natriuretic, and antihypertensive effects of loop diuretics). Products include:
Bumex ... 2260

Captopril (Reduced antihypertensive effect of captopril). Products include:
Capoten Tablets ... 740
Capozide Tablets ... 744

Carteolol Hydrochloride (Blunting of antihypertensive effect of beta blockers). Products include:
Cartrol Tablets ... 413
Ocupress Ophthalmic Solution, 1% Sterile ... ⊚ 297

(▣ Described in PDR For Nonprescription Drugs) (⊚ Described in PDR For Ophthalmology)

533 **Interactions Index** **Indocin**

Chlorothiazide (Reduced diuretic, natriuretic, and antihypertensive effects of thiazide diuretics). Products include:

- Aldoclor Tablets 1638
- Diupres Tablets 1691
- Diuril Oral 1694

Chlorothiazide Sodium (Reduced diuretic, natriuretic, and antihypertensive effects of thiazide diuretics). Products include:

- Diuril Sodium Intravenous 1693

Cyclosporine (Increase in cyclosporine-induced toxicity). Products include:

- Neoral 2405
- Sandimmune 2416

Dexamethasone (False-negative results in dexamethasone suppression test). Products include:

- AK-Trol Ointment & Suspension .... ◉ 205
- Decadron Elixir 1676
- Decadron Tablets 1678
- Decaspray Topical Aerosol 1689
- Maxitrol Ophthalmic Ointment and Suspension .... ◉ 222
- TobraDex Ophthalmic Suspension and Ointment 469

Dexamethasone Acetate (False-negative results in dexamethasone suppression test). Products include:

- Dalalone D.P. Injectable 1009
- Decadron-LA Sterile Suspension 1687

Dexamethasone Sodium Phosphate (False-negative results in dexamethasone suppression test). Products include:

- Decadron Phosphate Injection 1680
- Decadron Phosphate Sterile Ophthalmic Ointment 1684
- Decadron Phosphate Sterile Ophthalmic Solution 1685
- Decadron Phosphate Topical Cream 1686
- Decadron Phosphate with Xylocaine Injection, Sterile 1683
- Dexacort Phosphate in Respihaler .. 1606
- Dexacort Phosphate in Turbinaire .. 1607
- NeoDecadron Sterile Ophthalmic Ointment 1755
- NeoDecadron Sterile Ophthalmic Solution 1756
- NeoDecadron Topical Cream 1757

Diclofenac Potassium (Concomitant use is not recommended due to the increased possibility of gastrointestinal toxicity, with little or no increase in efficacy). Products include:

- Cataflam Tablets 833

Diclofenac Sodium (Concomitant use is not recommended due to the increased possibility of gastrointestinal toxicity, with little or no increase in efficacy). Products include:

- Voltaren Ophthalmic Sterile Ophthalmic Solution .... ◉ 264
- Cataflam/Voltaren/Voltaren-XR 833

Dicumarol (Possible alterations of the prothrombin time; clinical studies have shown that indomethacin does not influence the hypoprothrombinemia).

No products indexed under this heading.

Diflunisal (Co-administration results in decreased renal clearance and significant increase in the plasma levels of indomethacin; in some patients combined therapy has been associated with fatal gastrointestinal hemorrhage; concurrent use is not recommended). Products include:

- Dolobid Tablets 1695

Digoxin (Increased serum digoxin concentration and prolonged half-life). Products include:

- Lanoxicaps 1110
- Lanoxin Elixir Pediatric 1113
- Lanoxin Injection 1116
- Lanoxin Injection Pediatric 1119
- Lanoxin Tablets 1121

Esmolol Hydrochloride (Blunting of antihypertensive effect of beta blockers). Products include:

- Brevibloc (esmolol HCl) Injection 1860

Ethacrynic Acid (Reduced diuretic, natriuretic, and antihypertensive effects of loop diuretics). Products include:

- Edecrin Tablets 1698

Etodolac (Concomitant use is not recommended due to the increased possibility of gastrointestinal toxicity, with little or no increase in efficacy). Products include:

- Lodine Capsules and Tablets 2849

Fenoprofen Calcium (Concomitant use is not recommended due to the increased possibility of gastrointestinal toxicity, with little or no increase in efficacy). Products include:

- Nalfon 200 Pulvules & Nalfon Tablets 933

Flurbiprofen (Concomitant use is not recommended due to the increased possibility of gastrointestinal toxicity, with little or no increase in efficacy).

No products indexed under this heading.

Furosemide (Indomethacin reduces basal plasma renin activity (PRA) induced by furosemide; reduced diuretic, natriuretic, and antihypertensive effects of loop diuretics). Products include:

- Lasix Injection, Oral Solution and Tablets 1267

Hydrochlorothiazide (Reduced diuretic, natriuretic, and antihypertensive effects of thiazide diuretics). Products include:

- Aldactazide Tablets 2556
- Aldoril Tablets 1644
- Apresazide Capsules 824
- Capozide Tablets 744
- Dyazide Capsules 2653
- Esidrix Tablets 839
- Esimil Tablets 840
- HydroDIURIL Tablets 1716
- Hydropres Tablets 1718
- Hyzaar Tablets 1720
- Inderide Tablets 2838
- Inderide LA Long Acting Capsules .. 2840
- Lopressor HCT Tablets 850
- Lotensin HCT Tablets 855
- Moduretic Tablets 1748
- Oretic Tablets 450
- Prinzide Tablets 1780
- Ser-Ap-Es Tablets 867
- Timolide Tablets 1791
- Vaseretic Tablets 1810
- Zestoretic Tablets 2968
- Ziac 1459

Hydroflumethiazide (Reduced diuretic, natriuretic, and antihypertensive effects of thiazide diuretics). Products include:

- Diucardin Tablets 2824

Ibuprofen (Concomitant use is not recommended due to the increased possibility of gastrointestinal toxicity, with little or no increase in efficacy). Products include:

- Advil Cold and Sinus Caplets and Tablets .... ᴮᴰ 837
- Advil Ibuprofen Tablets, Caplets and Gel Caplets .... ᴮᴰ 836
- Children's Motrin Ibuprofen Oral Suspension 1558
- IBU Tablets 1389
- Ibuprohm .... ᴮᴰ 713
- Motrin IB Caplets, Tablets, and Gelcaps .... ᴮᴰ 802
- Motrin Ibuprofen Suspension, Oral Drops, Chewable Tablets, Caplets 1563
- Nuprin Ibuprofen/Analgesic Tablets & Caplets .... ᴮᴰ 645
- Vicks DayQuil SINUS Pressure & PAIN Relief with IBUPROFEN ...... ᴮᴰ 735

Ketoprofen (Concomitant use is not recommended due to the increased possibility of gastrointestinal toxicity, with little or no increase in efficacy). Products include:

- Actron Caplets and Tablets .... ᴮᴰ 608
- Orudis Capsules 2874
- Orudis KT .... ᴮᴰ 842
- Oruvail Capsules 2874

Ketorolac Tromethamine (Concomitant use is not recommended due to the increased possibility of gastrointestinal toxicity, with little or no increase in efficacy). Products include:

- Acular Sterile Ophthalmic Solution 470
- Toradol 2319

Labetalol Hydrochloride (Blunting of antihypertensive effect of beta blockers). Products include:

- Normodyne Injection 2519
- Normodyne Tablets 2522
- Trandate 1158

Levobunolol Hydrochloride (Blunting of antihypertensive effect of beta blockers). Products include:

- Betagan .... ◉ 230

Lithium Carbonate (Co-administration produces a clinically relevant elevation of plasma lithium and reduction in renal lithium clearance with a potential for lithium toxicity). Products include:

- Eskalith 2658
- Lithium Carbonate Capsules & Tablets 2352
- Lithonate/Lithotabs/Lithobid 2721

Lithium Citrate (Co-administration produces a clinically relevant elevation of plasma lithium and reduction in renal lithium clearance with a potential for lithium toxicity).

No products indexed under this heading.

Meclofenamate Sodium (Concomitant use is not recommended due to the increased possibility of gastrointestinal toxicity, with little or no increase in efficacy).

No products indexed under this heading.

Mefenamic Acid (Concomitant use is not recommended due to the increased possibility of gastrointestinal toxicity, with little or no increase in efficacy). Products include:

- Ponstel 1982

Methotrexate Sodium (Potentiation of methotrexate toxicity). Products include:

- Methotrexate Sodium Tablets, Injection, for Injection and LPF Injection 1322

Methyclothiazide (Reduced diuretic, natriuretic, and antihypertensive effects of thiazide diuretics). Products include:

- Enduron Tablets 424

Metipranolol Hydrochloride (Blunting of antihypertensive effect of beta blockers). Products include:

- OptiPranolol (Metipranolol 0.3%) Sterile Ophthalmic Solution .... ◉ 256

Metoprolol Succinate (Blunting of antihypertensive effect of beta blockers). Products include:

- Toprol-XL Tablets 560

Metoprolol Tartrate (Blunting of antihypertensive effect of beta blockers). Products include:

- Lopressor 848
- Lopressor HCT Tablets 850

Nabumetone (Concomitant use is not recommended due to the increased possibility of gastrointestinal toxicity, with little or no increase in efficacy). Products include:

- Relafen Tablets 2688

Nadolol (Blunting of antihypertensive effect of beta blockers).

No products indexed under this heading.

Naproxen (Concomitant use is not recommended due to the increased possibility of gastrointestinal toxicity, with little or no increase in efficacy). Products include:

- Anaprox/Naprosyn 2277

Naproxen Sodium (Concomitant use is not recommended due to the increased possibility of gastrointestinal toxicity, with little or no increase in efficacy). Products include:

- Aleve 2124
- Anaprox/Naprosyn 2277
- Naprelan Tablets 2861

Nephrotoxic Drugs (Overt renal decompensation).

Oxaprozin (Concomitant use is not recommended due to the increased possibility of gastrointestinal toxicity, with little or no increase in efficacy). Products include:

- Daypro Caplets 2578

Penbutolol Sulfate (Blunting of antihypertensive effect of beta blockers). Products include:

- Levatol Tablets 2547

Phenylbutazone (Concomitant use is not recommended due to the increased possibility of gastrointestinal toxicity, with little or no increase in efficacy).

No products indexed under this heading.

Pindolol (Blunting of antihypertensive effect of beta blockers). Products include:

- Visken Tablets 2428

Piroxicam (Concomitant use is not recommended due to the increased possibility of gastrointestinal toxicity, with little or no increase in efficacy). Products include:

- Feldene Capsules 2008

Polythiazide (Reduced diuretic, natriuretic, and antihypertensive effects of thiazide diuretics). Products include:

- Minizide Capsules 2016

Probenecid (Increased plasma levels of indomethacin). Products include:

- Benemid Tablets 1651
- ColBENEMID Tablets 1662

Propranolol Hydrochloride (Blunting of antihypertensive effect of beta blockers). Products include:

- Inderal 2834
- Inderal LA Long Acting Capsules 2836
- Inderide Tablets 2838
- Inderide LA Long Acting Capsules .. 2840

Sotalol Hydrochloride (Blunting of antihypertensive effect of beta blockers). Products include:

- Betapace Tablets 637

Spironolactone (Reduced diuretic, natriuretic, and antihypertensive effects and increased serum potassium levels). Products include:

- Aldactazide Tablets 2556
- Aldactone Tablets 2558

Sulindac (Concomitant use is not recommended due to the increased possibility of gastrointestinal toxicity, with little or no increase in efficacy). Products include:

- Clinoril Tablets 1658

Timolol Hemihydrate (Blunting of antihypertensive effect of beta blockers). Products include:

- Betimol 0.25%, 0.5% .... ◉ 259

Timolol Maleate (Blunting of antihypertensive effect of beta blockers). Products include:

- Blocadren Tablets 1654

IMPORTANT NOTE: Always consult each drug listing in the patient's regimen for possible interactions.

Indocin / Interactions Index

Indocin

Drug	Page
Timolide Tablets	1791
Timoptic in Ocudose	1796
Timoptic Sterile Ophthalmic Solution	1794
Timoptic-XE	1798

Tolmetin Sodium (Concomitant use is not recommended due to the increased possibility of gastrointestinal toxicity, with little or no increase in efficacy). Products include:
- Tolectin (200, 400 and 600 mg) .. 1591

Torsemide (Reduced diuretic, natriuretic, and antihypertensive effects of loop diuretics). Products include:
- Demadex Tablets and Injection 691

Triamterene (The addition of triamterene to maintenance schedule of indomethacin has resulted in reversible acute renal failure; potential for increased hyperkalemia; concurrent therapy should be avoided). Products include:
- Dyazide Capsules 2653
- Dyrenium Capsules 2655

Warfarin Sodium (Possible alterations of the prothrombin time; clinical studies have shown that indomethacin does not influence the hypoprothrombinemia). Products include:
- Coumadin 941

INDOCIN I.V.
(Indomethacin Sodium Trihydrate) 1727
May interact with cardiac glycosides and certain other agents. Compounds in these categories include:

Amikacin Sulfate (Serum levels of amikacin significantly elevated). Products include:
- Amikacin Sulfate Injection, USP .. 523
- Amikacin Sulfate Injection, USP 981
- Amikin Injectable 502

Deslanoside (Half-life of digitalis may be prolonged when given concomitantly).
- No products indexed under this heading.

Digitoxin (Half-life of digitalis may be prolonged when given concomitantly). Products include:
- Crystodigin Tablets 1472

Digoxin (Half-life of digitalis may be prolonged when given concomitantly). Products include:
- Lanoxicaps 1110
- Lanoxin Elixir Pediatric 1113
- Lanoxin Injection 1116
- Lanoxin Injection Pediatric 1119
- Lanoxin Tablets 1121

Furosemide (Blunted natriuretic effect of furosemide). Products include:
- Lasix Injection, Oral Solution and Tablets 1267

Gentamicin Sulfate (Serum levels of gentamicin significantly elevated). Products include:
- Garamycin Cream 0.1 % 2501
- Garamycin Injectable 2502
- Garamycin Ointment 0.1 % 2501
- Garamycin Ophthalmic 2501
- Genoptic Sterile Ophthalmic Solution .... ⊚ 241
- Genoptic Sterile Ophthalmic Ointment .... ⊚ 241
- Gentak .... ⊚ 209
- Pred-G Liquifilm Sterile Ophthalmic Suspension .... ⊚ 248
- Pred-G S.O.P. Sterile Ophthalmic Ointment .... ⊚ 249

INDOCIN ORAL SUSPENSION
(Indomethacin) 1723
See Indocin Capsules

INDOCIN SR CAPSULES
(Indomethacin) 1723
See Indocin Capsules

INDOCIN SUPPOSITORIES
(Indomethacin) 1723
See Indocin Capsules

INFANTS' TYLENOL ACETAMINOPHEN SUSPENSION DROPS
(Acetaminophen) 1559
None cited in PDR database.

INFANTS' TYLENOL COLD DECONGESTANT & FEVER-REDUCER DROPS
(Acetaminophen, Pseudoephedrine Hydrochloride) 1561
May interact with monoamine oxidase inhibitors. Compounds in this category include:

Furazolidone (Concurrent and/or sequential use is not recommended). Products include:
- Furoxone 2221

Isocarboxazid (Concurrent and/or sequential use is not recommended).
- No products indexed under this heading.

Phenelzine Sulfate (Concurrent and/or sequential use is not recommended). Products include:
- Nardil 1977

Selegiline Hydrochloride (Concurrent and/or sequential use is not recommended). Products include:
- Eldepryl Capsules 2729

Tranylcypromine Sulfate (Concurrent and/or sequential use is not recommended). Products include:
- Parnate Tablets 2679

INFED (IRON DEXTRAN INJECTION, USP)
(Iron Dextran) 2478
None cited in PDR database.

INFLUENZA VIRUS VACCINE, TRIVALENT, TYPES A AND B (CHROMATOGRAPH- AND FILTER-PURIFIED SUBVIRON ANTIGEN) FLUSHIELD, 1996-1997 FORMULA
(Influenza Virus Vaccine) 2842
May interact with corticosteroids, alkylating agents, cytotoxic drugs, xanthine bronchodilators, and certain other agents. Compounds in these categories include:

Aminophylline (Potential for elevated theophylline serum concentrations resulting in possible enhanced effects or toxicity).
- No products indexed under this heading.

Betamethasone Acetate (Individual receiving large amount of corticosteroids as immunosuppressive agents may not respond optimally to active immunization procedures). Products include:
- Celestone Soluspan Suspension 2484

Betamethasone Sodium Phosphate (Individual receiving large amount of corticosteroids as immunosuppressive agents may not respond optimally to active immunization procedures). Products include:
- Celestone Soluspan Suspension 2484

Bleomycin Sulfate (Individual receiving large amount of cytotoxic agents may not respond optimally to active immunization procedures). Products include:
- Blenoxane 697

Busulfan (Individual receiving large amount of alkylating agents may not respond optimally to active immunization procedures). Products include:
- Myleran Tablets 1209

Carmustine (BCNU) (Individual receiving large amount of alkylating agents may not respond optimally to active immunization procedures). Products include:
- BiCNU 696

Chlorambucil (Individual receiving large amount of alkylating agents may not respond optimally to active immunization procedures). Products include:
- Leukeran Tablets 1205

Cortisone Acetate (Individual receiving large amount of corticosteroids as immunosuppressive agents may not respond optimally to active immunization procedures). Products include:
- Cortone Acetate Sterile Suspension 1663
- Cortone Acetate Tablets 1664

Cyclophosphamide (Individual receiving large amount of alkylating agents may not respond optimally to active immunization procedures). Products include:
- Cytoxan 700

Dacarbazine (Individual receiving large amount of alkylating agents may not respond optimally to active immunization procedures). Products include:
- DTIC-Dome 593

Daunorubicin Hydrochloride (Individual receiving large amount of cytotoxic agents may not respond optimally to active immunization procedures). Products include:
- Cerubidine for Injection 634

Dexamethasone (Individual receiving large amount of corticosteroids as immunosuppressive agents may not respond optimally to active immunization procedures). Products include:
- AK-Trol Ointment & Suspension .... ⊚ 205
- Decadron Elixir 1676
- Decadron Tablets 1678
- Decaspray Topical Aerosol 1689
- Maxitrol Ophthalmic Ointment and Suspension .... ⊚ 222
- TobraDex Ophthalmic Suspension and Ointment 469

Dexamethasone Acetate (Individual receiving large amount of corticosteroids as immunosuppressive agents may not respond optimally to active immunization procedures). Products include:
- Dalalone D.P. Injectable 1009
- Decadron-LA Sterile Suspension .. 1687

Dexamethasone Sodium Phosphate (Individual receiving large amount of corticosteroids as immunosuppressive agents may not respond optimally to active immunization procedures). Products include:
- Decadron Phosphate Injection 1680
- Decadron Phosphate Sterile Ophthalmic Ointment 1684
- Decadron Phosphate Sterile Ophthalmic Solution 1685
- Decadron Phosphate Topical Cream 1686
- Decadron Phosphate with Xylocaine Injection, Sterile 1683
- Dexacort Phosphate in Respihaler 1606
- Dexacort Phosphate in Turbinaire .. 1607

- NeoDecadron Sterile Ophthalmic Ointment 1755
- NeoDecadron Sterile Ophthalmic Solution 1756
- NeoDecadron Topical Cream 1757

Doxorubicin Hydrochloride (Individual receiving large amount of cytotoxic agents may not respond optimally to active immunization procedures). Products include:
- Adriamycin PFS 2056
- Adriamycin RDF 2056
- Doxil 2613
- Doxorubicin Astra 531
- Rubex for Injection 721

Dyphylline (Potential for elevated theophylline serum concentrations resulting in possible enhanced effects or toxicity). Products include:
- Lufyllin & Lufyllin-400 Tablets 2778
- Lufyllin-GG Elixir & Tablets 2779

Fludrocortisone Acetate (Individual receiving large amount of corticosteroids as immunosuppressive agents may not respond optimally to active immunization procedures). Products include:
- Florinef Acetate Tablets 506

Fluorouracil (Individual receiving large amount of cytotoxic agents may not respond optimally to active immunization procedures). Products include:
- Efudex 2280
- Fluoroplex Topical Solution & Cream 1 % 475
- Fluorouracil Injection 2282

Hydrocortisone (Individual receiving large amount of corticosteroids as immunosuppressive agents may not respond optimally to active immunization procedures). Products include:
- Anusol-HC Cream 2.5 % 1953
- Aquanil HC Lotion 1989
- Maximum Strength Cortaid Spray ⊞ 800
- CORTENEMA 2713
- Cortisporin Ointment 1074
- Cortisporin Ophthalmic Ointment Sterile 1074
- Cortisporin Ophthalmic Suspension Sterile 1075
- Cortisporin Otic Solution Sterile ... 1076
- Cortisporin Otic Suspension Sterile 1077
- Cortizone-5 .... ⊞ 795
- Cortizone-10 .... ⊞ 795
- Hydrocortone Tablets 1715
- Hytone 922
- Hytone Ointment 2 ½ % 923
- Massengill Medicated Soft Cloth Towelettes 2628
- Pediotic Suspension Sterile 1140
- Preparation H Hydrocortisone 1 % Cream .... ⊞ 843
- ProctoCream-HC 2.5 % 2552
- VōSoL HC Otic Solution 2786

Hydrocortisone Acetate (Individual receiving large amount of corticosteroids as immunosuppressive agents may not respond optimally to active immunization procedures). Products include:
- Analpram-HC Rectal Cream 1 % and 2.5 % 993
- Anusol HC-1 Hydrocortisone Anti-Itch Ointment .... ⊞ 810
- Anusol-HC Suppositories 1954
- Caldecort Anti-Itch Hydrocortisone Cream .... ⊞ 651
- Coly-Mycin S Otic w/Neomycin & Hydrocortisone 1965
- Cortaid .... ⊞ 800
- Cortifoam 2540
- Cortisporin Cream 1073
- Epifoam 2543
- Hydrocortone Acetate Sterile Suspension 1712
- Mantadil Cream 1124
- Nupercainal Hydrocortisone 1 % Cream .... ⊞ 661
- Pramosone Cream, Lotion & Ointment 995
- ProctoFoam-HC 2552
- Terra-Cortril Ophthalmic Suspension 2033

(⊞ Described in PDR For Nonprescription Drugs) (⊚ Described in PDR For Ophthalmology)

Hydrocortisone Sodium Phosphate (Individual receiving large amount of corticosteroids as immunosuppressive agents may not respond optimally to active immunization procedures). Products include:
   Hydrocortone Phosphate Injection, Sterile 1713

Hydrocortisone Sodium Succinate (Individual receiving large amount of corticosteroids as immunosuppressive agents may not respond optimally to active immunization procedures).
   No products indexed under this heading.

Hydroxyurea (Individual receiving large amount of cytotoxic agents may not respond optimally to active immunization procedures). Products include:
   Hydrea Capsules 705

Lomustine (CCNU) (Individual receiving large amount of alkylating agents may not respond optimally to active immunization procedures). Products include:
   CeeNU Capsules 699

Mechlorethamine Hydrochloride (Individual receiving large amount of alkylating agents may not respond optimally to active immunization procedures). Products include:
   Mustargen................................... 1752

Melphalan (Individual receiving large amount of alkylating agents may not respond optimally to active immunization procedures). Products include:
   Alkeran Tablets 1198

Methotrexate Sodium (Individual receiving large amount of cytotoxic agents may not respond optimally to active immunization procedures). Products include:
   Methotrexate Sodium Tablets, Injection, for Injection and LPF Injection 1322

Methylprednisolone Acetate (Individual receiving large amount of corticosteroids as immunosuppressive agents may not respond optimally to active immunization procedures).
   No products indexed under this heading.

Methylprednisolone Sodium Succinate (Individual receiving large amount of corticosteroids as immunosuppressive agents may not respond optimally to active immunization procedures).
   No products indexed under this heading.

Mitotane (Individual receiving large amount of cytotoxic agents may not respond optimally to active immunization procedures). Products include:
   Lysodren Tablets 707

Mitoxantrone Hydrochloride (Individual receiving large amount of cytotoxic agents may not respond optimally to active immunization procedures). Products include:
   Novantrone for Injection............. 1327

Prednisolone Acetate (Individual receiving large amount of corticosteroids as immunosuppressive agents may not respond optimally to active immunization procedures). Products include:
   AK-CIDE .... ⊙ 203
   AK-CIDE Ointment .... ⊙ 203
   Blephamide Liquifilm Sterile Ophthalmic Suspension 472
   Blephamide Ointment .... ⊙ 234
   Econopred & Econopred Plus Ophthalmic Suspensions .... ⊙ 216
   Poly-Pred Liquifilm .... ⊙ 246
   Pred Forte .... ⊙ 247
   Pred Mild .... ⊙ 250
   Pred-G Liquifilm Sterile Ophthalmic Suspension .... ⊙ 248
   Pred-G S.O.P. Sterile Ophthalmic Ointment .... ⊙ 249

Prednisolone Sodium Phosphate (Individual receiving large amount of corticosteroids as immunosuppressive agents may not respond optimally to active immunization procedures). Products include:
   AK-PRED .... ⊙ 204
   Hydeltrasol Injection, Sterile 1708
   Pediapred Oral Solution 1618

Prednisolone Tebutate (Individual receiving large amount of corticosteroids as immunosuppressive agents may not respond optimally to active immunization procedures). Products include:
   Hydeltra-T.B.A. Sterile Suspension 1710

Prednisone (Individual receiving large amount of corticosteroids as immunosuppressive agents may not respond optimally to active immunization procedures).
   No products indexed under this heading.

Procarbazine Hydrochloride (Individual receiving large amount of cytotoxic agents may not respond optimally to active immunization procedures). Products include:
   Matulane Capsules 2300

Tamoxifen Citrate (Individual receiving large amount of cytotoxic agents may not respond optimally to active immunization procedures). Products include:
   Nolvadex Tablets 2957

Theophylline (Potential for elevated theophylline serum concentrations resulting in possible enhanced effects or toxicity). Products include:
   Marax Tablets & DF Syrup......... 2015
   Quibron 2227

Theophylline Anhydrous (Potential for elevated theophylline serum concentrations resulting in possible enhanced effects or toxicity). Products include:
   Aerolate 1003
   Primatene Tablets .... ⊙ 844
   Respbid Tablets 687
   Slo-bid Gyrocaps 2201
   Theo-24 Extended Release Capsules 2753
   Theo-Dur Extended-Release Tablets 1367
   Theo-X Extended-Release Tablets .. 793
   Uni-Dur Extended-Release Tablets. 1374
   Uniphyl 400 mg and 600 mg Tablets 2157

Theophylline Calcium Salicylate (Potential for elevated theophylline serum concentrations resulting in possible enhanced effects or toxicity). Products include:
   Quadrinal Tablets 1398

Theophylline Sodium Glycinate (Potential for elevated theophylline serum concentrations resulting in possible enhanced effects or toxicity).
   No products indexed under this heading.

Thiotepa (Individual receiving large amount of alkylating agents may not respond optimally to active immunization procedures). Products include:
   Thioplex (Thiotepa For Injection) 1329

Triamcinolone (Individual receiving large amount of corticosteroids as immunosuppressive agents may not respond optimally to active immunization procedures).
   No products indexed under this heading.

Triamcinolone Acetonide (Individual receiving large amount of corticosteroids as immunosuppressive agents may not respond optimally to active immunization procedures). Products include:
   Azmacort Oral Inhaler 2175
   Nasacort AQ Nasal Spray 2191
   Nasacort Nasal Inhaler 2189

Triamcinolone Diacetate (Individual receiving large amount of corticosteroids as immunosuppressive agents may not respond optimally to active immunization procedures).
   No products indexed under this heading.

Triamcinolone Hexacetonide (Individual receiving large amount of corticosteroids as immunosuppressive agents may not respond optimally to active immunization procedures).
   No products indexed under this heading.

Vincristine Sulfate (Individual receiving large amount of cytotoxic agents may not respond optimally to active immunization procedures). Products include:
   Oncovin Solution Vials & Hyporets 1521

Warfarin Sodium (Potential for hypoprothrombinemia resulting in possible enhanced effects or toxicity). Products include:
   Coumadin 941

INFUMORPH 200 AND INFUMORPH 500 STERILE SOLUTIONS

(Morphine Sulfate) 985
May interact with central nervous system depressants, antihistamines, antipsychotic agents, and certain other agents. Compounds in these categories include:

Acrivastine (Potentiates CNS depressant effects). Products include:
   Semprex-D Capsules 1620

Alfentanil Hydrochloride (Potentiates CNS depressant effects). Products include:
   Alfenta Injection 1334

Alprazolam (Potentiates CNS depressant effects). Products include:
   Xanax Tablets 2115

Aprobarbital (Potentiates CNS depressant effects).
   No products indexed under this heading.

Astemizole (Potentiates CNS depressant effects). Products include:
   Hismanal Tablets 1341

Azatadine Maleate (Potentiates CNS depressant effects). Products include:
   Trinalin Repetabs Tablets 1373

Bromodiphenhydramine Hydrochloride (Potentiates CNS depressant effects).
   No products indexed under this heading.

Brompheniramine Maleate (Potentiates CNS depressant effects). Products include:
   Alka-Seltzer Plus Sinus Medicine .. ⊙ 611
   Bromfed Capsules (Extended-Release) 1832
   Bromfed Syrup .... ⊙ 712
   Bromfed Tablets 1832
   Bromfed-DM Cough Syrup......... 1832
   Bromfed-PD Capsules (Extended-Release) 1832
   Dimetane-DC Cough Syrup 2232
   Dimetane-DX Cough Syrup 2233
   Dimetapp Allergy Dye-Free Elixir.. ⊙ 838
   Dimetapp Allergy Sinus Caplets .. ⊙ 838
   Dimetapp Cold & Allergy Chewable Tablets .... ⊙ 838
   Dimetapp Cold & Cough Liqui-Gels .... ⊙ 839
   Dimetapp Cold & Fever Suspension .... ⊙ 839
   Dimetapp DM Elixir .... ⊙ 840
   Dimetapp Elixir .... ⊙ 840
   Dimetapp Extentabs .... ⊙ 841
   Dimetapp Tablets/Liqui-Gels ..... ⊙ 841
   Rondec Chewable Tablets 974
   Vicks DayQuil Allergy Relief 12-Hour Extended Release Tablets.. 733
   Vicks DayQuil Allergy Relief 4-Hour Tablets 733

Buprenorphine (Potentiates CNS depressant effects). Products include:
   Buprenex Injectable 2170

Buspirone Hydrochloride (Potentiates CNS depressant effects). Products include:
   BuSpar Tablets 738

Butabarbital (Potentiates CNS depressant effects).
   No products indexed under this heading.

Butalbital (Potentiates CNS depressant effects). Products include:
   Axocet Capsules........................ 2469
   Esgic-plus Capsules 1012
   Esgic-plus Tablets 1012
   Fioricet Tablets 2386
   Fioricet with Codeine Capsules .. 2387
   Fiorinal Capsules 2388
   Fiorinal with Codeine Capsules .. 2390
   Fiorinal Tablets 2388
   Phrenilin 790
   Sedapap Tablets 50 mg/650 mg .. 1826

Cetirizine Hydrochloride (Potentiates CNS depressant effects). Products include:
   Zyrtec Tablets 2053

Chlordiazepoxide (Potentiates CNS depressant effects). Products include:
   Limbitrol 2333

Chlordiazepoxide Hydrochloride (Potentiates CNS depressant effects). Products include:
   Librax Capsules 2330
   Librium Capsules 2331
   Librium Injectable 2332

Chlorpheniramine Maleate (Potentiates CNS depressant effects). Products include:
   Alka-Seltzer Plus Cold Medicine 611
   Alka-Seltzer Plus Cold Medicine Liqui-Gels .... ⊙ 612
   Alka-Seltzer Plus Cold & Cough Medicine .... ⊙ 611
   Alka-Seltzer Plus Cold & Cough Medicine Liqui-Gels.................. ⊙ 612
   Alka-Seltzer Plus Flu & Body Aches Effervescent Tablets ...... ⊙ 612
   Allerest Maximum Strength........... ⊙ 649
   Allerest Sinus Pain Formula ...... ⊙ 649
   Ana-Kit Anaphylaxis Emergency Treatment Kit 611
   Atrohist Pediatric Capsules 1603
   Atrohist Plus Tablets 1605
   BC Cold Powder Multi-Symptom Formula (Cold-Sinus-Allergy) .... ⊙ 631
   Cerose DM .... ⊙ 853
   Cheracol Plus Head Cold/Cough Formula 741
   Children's TYLENOL Cold Multi-Symptom Chewable Tablets and Liquid 1559
   Children's TYLENOL Cold Plus Cough Multi Symptom Chewable Tablets and Liquid 1560
   Children's TYLENOL Flu Suspension Liquid 1560
   Children's Vicks DayQuil Allergy Relief....................................... ⊙ 730
   Children's Vicks NyQuil Cold/Cough Relief............................ ⊙ 731
   Chlor-Trimeton Allergy Decongestant Tablets .... ⊙ 759

IMPORTANT NOTE: Always consult each drug listing in the patient's regimen for possible interactions.

Infumorph | Interactions Index | 536

Chlor-Trimeton Allergy Tablets ▣ 758
Allergy-Sinus Comtrex Multi-Symptom Allergy-Sinus Formula Tablets and Caplets ▣ 639
Comtrex Multi-Symptom ▣ 638
Contac Continuous Action Nasal Decongestant/Antihistamine 12 Hour Capsules ▣ 773
Contac Maximum Strength Continuous Action Decongestant/Antihistamine 12 Hour Caplets ▣ 772
Contac Severe Cold and Flu Formula Caplets ▣ 773
Coricidin Cold + Flu Tablets ▣ 760
Coricidin Cough + Cold Tablets ▣ 760
Coricidin 'D' Decongestant Tablets ▣ 760
D.A. II Tablets 972
D.A. Chewable Tablets 970
Dura-Tap/PD Capsules 970
Dura-Vent/DA Tablets 972
Efidac 24 Chlorpheniramine ▣ 655
Extendryl 1003
Fedahist Gyrocaps 2545
Hycomine Compound Tablets 948
Kronofed-A 994
Nolamine Timed-Release Tablets 790
Novahistine Elixir ▣ 782
Ornade Spansule Capsules 2678
PediaCare Cough-Cold Chewable Tablets and Liquid 1569
PediaCare NightRest Cough-Cold Liquid 1569
Pediatric Vicks 44m Cough & Cold Relief ▣ 737
Pyrroxate Caplets ▣ 742
Ryna ▣ 804
Sinarest ▣ 663
Sine-Off Sinus Medicine ▣ 784
Singlet Tablets ▣ 785
Sinulin Tablets 792
Sinutab Sinus Allergy Medication, Maximum Strength Tablets and Caplets ▣ 823
Sudafed Cold & Allergy Tablets ▣ 826
Teldrin 12 Hour Antihistamine/Nasal Decongestant Allergy Relief Capsules ▣ 786
TheraFlu Flu and Cold Medicine ▣ 750
Theraflu Maximum Strength Flu and Cold Medicine For Sore Throat ▣ 751
TheraFlu Flu, Cold and Cough Medicine ▣ 750
TheraFlu Maximum Strength Nighttime Flu, Cold & Cough Medicine ▣ 751
Triaminic Night Time ▣ 754
Triaminic Syrup ▣ 755
Triaminic Triaminicol Cold & Cough ▣ 756
Triaminicin Tablets ▣ 756
Tussend 1830
TYLENOL Allergy Sinus, Maximum Strength Caplets and Gelcaps 1571
TYLENOL Cold Medication, Multi-Symptom Formula Tablets and Caplets 1572
TYLENOL Cold Medication, Multi-Symptom Hot Liquid Packets 1572
Vicks 44 LiquiCaps Cough, Cold & Flu Relief ▣ 728
Vicks 44M Cough, Cold & Flu Relief ▣ 729

Chlorpheniramine Polistirex (Potentiates CNS depressant effects). Products include:
Tussionex Pennkinetic Extended-Release Suspension 1624

Chlorpheniramine Tannate (Potentiates CNS depressant effects). Products include:
Atrohist Pediatric Suspension 1604
Atrohist Pediatric Suspension Dye-Free 1604
Rynatan 2781
Rynatuss 2782

Chlorpromazine (Potentiates CNS depressant effects; increases the risk of respiratory depression). Products include:
Thorazine Suppositories 2701

Chlorprothixene (Potentiates CNS depressant effects; increases the risk of respiratory depression).
No products indexed under this heading.

Chlorprothixene Hydrochloride (Potentiates CNS depressant effects; increases the risk of respiratory depression).
No products indexed under this heading.

Chlorprothixene Lactate (Potentiates CNS depressant effects).
No products indexed under this heading.

Clemastine Fumarate (Potentiates CNS depressant effects). Products include:
Tavist Syrup 2426
Tavist Tablets 2427
Tavist-1 12 Hour Relief Tablets ▣ 749
Tavist-D 12 Hour Relief Tablets ▣ 750

Clorazepate Dipotassium (Potentiates CNS depressant effects). Products include:
Tranxene 459

Clozapine (Potentiates CNS depressant effects; increases the risk of respiratory depression). Products include:
Clozaril Tablets 2377

Codeine Phosphate (Potentiates CNS depressant effects). Products include:
Brontex 2130
Dimetane-DC Cough Syrup 2232
Fioricet with Codeine Capsules 2387
Fiorinal with Codeine Capsules 2390
Nucofed 2225
Phenergan with Codeine 2883
Phenergan VC with Codeine 2888
Robitussin A-C Syrup 2248
Robitussin-DAC Syrup 2249
Ryna ▣ 804
Soma Compound w/Codeine Tablets 2784
Tylenol with Codeine 1592

Cyproheptadine Hydrochloride (Potentiates CNS depressant effects). Products include:
Periactin 1767

Desflurane (Potentiates CNS depressant effects). Products include:
Suprane (desflurane, USP) 1865

Dexchlorpheniramine Maleate (Potentiates CNS depressant effects).
No products indexed under this heading.

Dezocine (Potentiates CNS depressant effects). Products include:
Dalgan Injection 529

Diazepam (Potentiates CNS depressant effects). Products include:
Dizac (diazepam injectable emulsion) CIV 1862
Valium Injectable 2336
Valium Tablets 2335

Diphenhydramine Citrate (Potentiates CNS depressant effects). Products include:
Excedrin P.M. Analgesic/Sleeping Aid Tablets, Caplets, Liquigels 735

Diphenhydramine Hydrochloride (Potentiates CNS depressant effects). Products include:
Actifed Allergy Daytime/Nighttime Caplets ▣ 808
Actifed Sinus Daytime/Nighttime Tablets and Caplets ▣ 809
Extra Strength Bayer PM Aspirin Plus Sleep Aid ▣ 617
Benadryl Allergy Chewables ▣ 811
Benadryl Allergy/Cold Tablets ▣ 811
Benadryl Allergy Decongestant Liquid Medication ▣ 812
Benadryl Allergy Decongestant Tablets ▣ 812
Benadryl Allergy Liquid Medication ▣ 813
Benadryl Allergy ▣ 811
Benadryl Allergy Sinus Headache Caplets ▣ 813
Benadryl Dye-Free Allergy Liqui-gel Softgels ▣ 813
Benadryl Dye-Free Allergy Liquid Medication ▣ 814
Benadryl Itch Relief Stick Extra Strength ▣ 814
Benadryl Cream ▣ 814
Benadryl Gel ▣ 815
Benadryl Spray ▣ 815
Benadryl Injection 1955
Contac Day & Night Cold/Flu Night Caplets ▣ 772
Contac Night Allergy/Sinus Caplets ▣ 771
Extra Strength Doan's P.M. ▣ 653
Excedrin P.M. Analgesic/Sleeping Aid Tablets, Caplets, Liquigels ▣ 643
Nytol QuickCaps Caplets ▣ 632
Sleepinal Night-time Sleep Aid Capsules and Softgels ▣ 798
TYLENOL Allergy Sinus NightTime, Maximum Strength Caplets 1571
TYLENOL Flu NightTime, Maximum Strength Gelcaps 1575
TYLENOL Flu NightTime, Maximum Strength Hot Medication Packets 1575
TYLENOL PM Pain Reliever/Sleep Aid, Extra Strength Gelcaps, Caplets, Geltabs 1576
TYLENOL Severe Allergy Medication Caplets 1571
Maximum Strength Unisom Sleepgels 1990
Unisom With Pain Relief-Nighttime Sleep Aid and Pain Reliever 1991

Diphenylpyraline Hydrochloride (Potentiates CNS depressant effects).
No products indexed under this heading.

Droperidol (Potentiates CNS depressant effects). Products include:
Inapsine Injection 462

Enflurane (Potentiates CNS depressant effects).
No products indexed under this heading.

Estazolam (Potentiates CNS depressant effects). Products include:
ProSom Tablets 457

Ethchlorvynol (Potentiates CNS depressant effects). Products include:
Placidyl Capsules 456

Ethinamate (Potentiates CNS depressant effects).
No products indexed under this heading.

Fentanyl (Potentiates CNS depressant effects). Products include:
Duragesic Transdermal System 1336

Fentanyl Citrate (Potentiates CNS depressant effects). Products include:
Sublimaze Injection 463

Fluphenazine Decanoate (Potentiates CNS depressant effects; increases the risk of respiratory depression). Products include:
Prolixin Decanoate 510

Fluphenazine Enanthate (Potentiates CNS depressant effects; increases the risk of respiratory depression). Products include:
Prolixin Enanthate 510

Fluphenazine Hydrochloride (Potentiates CNS depressant effects; increases the risk of respiratory depression). Products include:
Prolixin 510

Flurazepam Hydrochloride (Potentiates CNS depressant effects). Products include:
Dalmane Capsules 2329

Glutethimide (Potentiates CNS depressant effects).
No products indexed under this heading.

Haloperidol (Potentiates CNS depressant effects; increases the risk of respiratory depression). Products include:
Haldol Injection, Tablets and Concentrate 1585

Haloperidol Decanoate (Potentiates CNS depressant effects; increases the risk of respiratory depression). Products include:
Haldol Decanoate 1587

Hydrocodone Bitartrate (Potentiates CNS depressant effects). Products include:
Codiclear DH Syrup 808
Duratuss HD Elixir 2750
Histussin D Liquid 670
Hycodan Tablets and Syrup 946
Hycomine Compound Tablets 948
Hycomine 947
Hycotuss Expectorant Syrup 950
Hydrocet Capsules 787
Lorcet 10/650 Tablets 1016
Lortab 2751
Tussend 1830
Tussend Expectorant 1831
Vicodin Tablets 1404
Vicodin ES Tablets 1405
Vicodin HP Tablets 1403
Vicodin Tuss Expectorant 1406
Zydone Capsules 967

Hydrocodone Polistirex (Potentiates CNS depressant effects). Products include:
Tussionex Pennkinetic Extended-Release Suspension 1624

Hydroxyzine Hydrochloride (Potentiates CNS depressant effects). Products include:
Atarax Tablets & Syrup 1992
Marax Tablets & DF Syrup 2015
Vistaril Intramuscular Solution 2042

Isoflurane (Potentiates CNS depressant effects).
No products indexed under this heading.

Ketamine Hydrochloride (Potentiates CNS depressant effects).
No products indexed under this heading.

Levomethadyl Acetate Hydrochloride (Potentiates CNS depressant effects). Products include:
Orlaam Oral Solution 2361

Levorphanol Tartrate (Potentiates CNS depressant effects). Products include:
Levo-Dromoran 2297

Lithium Carbonate (Potentiates CNS depressant effects; increases the risk of respiratory depression). Products include:
Eskalith 2658
Lithium Carbonate Capsules & Tablets 2352
Lithonate/Lithotabs/Lithobid 2721

Lithium Citrate (Potentiates CNS depressant effects; increases the risk of respiratory depression).
No products indexed under this heading.

Loratadine (Potentiates CNS depressant effects). Products include:
Claritin Tablets 2485
Claritin-D Tablets 2487

Lorazepam (Potentiates CNS depressant effects). Products include:
Ativan Injection 2805
Ativan Tablets 2807

Loxapine Hydrochloride (Potentiates CNS depressant effects; increases the risk of respiratory depression). Products include:
Loxitane 1426

Loxapine Succinate (Potentiates CNS depressant effects; increases the risk of respiratory depression). Products include:
Loxitane Capsules 1426

Meperidine Hydrochloride (Potentiates CNS depressant effects). Products include:
Demerol 2438
Mepergan Injection 2859

(▣ Described in PDR For Nonprescription Drugs) (⊙ Described in PDR For Ophthalmology)

537 **Interactions Index** **Inversine**

Mephobarbital (Potentiates CNS depressant effects). Products include:
- Mebaral Tablets 2452

Meprobamate (Potentiates CNS depressant effects). Products include:
- Miltown Tablets 2780
- PMB 200 and PMB 400 2890

Mesoridazine Besylate (Potentiates CNS depressant effects; increases the risk of respiratory depression). Products include:
- Serentil 689

Methadone Hydrochloride (Potentiates CNS depressant effects). Products include:
- Methadone Hydrochloride Oral Concentrate 2356
- Methadone Hydrochloride Oral Solution & Tablets 2357

Methdilazine Hydrochloride (Potentiates CNS depressant effects).
- No products indexed under this heading.

Methohexital Sodium (Potentiates CNS depressant effects).
- No products indexed under this heading.

Methotrimeprazine (Potentiates CNS depressant effects; increases the risk of respiratory depression). Products include:
- Levoprome 1321

Methoxyflurane (Potentiates CNS depressant effects).
- No products indexed under this heading.

Midazolam Hydrochloride (Potentiates CNS depressant effects). Products include:
- Versed Injection 2324

Molindone Hydrochloride (Potentiates CNS depressant effects; increases the risk of respiratory depression). Products include:
- Moban Tablets and Concentrate 1036

Opium Alkaloids (Potentiates CNS depressant effects).
- No products indexed under this heading.

Oxazepam (Potentiates CNS depressant effects). Products include:
- Serax Capsules 2916
- Serax Tablets 2916

Oxycodone Hydrochloride (Potentiates CNS depressant effects). Products include:
- OxyContin Tablets 2163
- OxyIR Capsules 2167
- Percocet Tablets 955
- Percodan Tablets 955
- Percodan-Demi Tablets 956
- Roxicodone Tablets, Oral Solution & Intensol (Oxycodone) 2366
- Tylox Capsules 1593

Pentobarbital Sodium (Potentiates CNS depressant effects). Products include:
- Nembutal Sodium Capsules 440
- Nembutal Sodium Solution 442
- Nembutal Sodium Suppositories 444

Perphenazine (Potentiates CNS depressant effects; increases the risk of respiratory depression). Products include:
- Etrafon 2495
- Triavil Tablets 1800
- Trilafon 2532

Phenobarbital (Potentiates CNS depressant effects). Products include:
- Arco-Lase Plus Tablets 513
- Bellergal-S Tablets 2375
- Donnatal 2234
- Donnatal Extentabs 2234
- Donnatal Tablets 2234
- Phenobarbital Elixir and Tablets 1523
- Quadrinal Tablets 1398

Pimozide (Potentiates CNS depressant effects; increases the risk of respiratory depression). Products include:
- Orap Tablets 1037

Prazepam (Potentiates CNS depressant effects).
- No products indexed under this heading.

Prochlorperazine (Potentiates CNS depressant effects; increases the risk of respiratory depression). Products include:
- Compazine 2644

Promethazine Hydrochloride (Potentiates CNS depressant effects; increases the risk of respiratory depression). Products include:
- Mepergan Injection 2859
- Phenergan with Codeine 2883
- Phenergan with Dextromethorphan 2885
- Phenergan Injection 2880
- Phenergan Suppositories 2882
- Phenergan Syrup 2881
- Phenergan Tablets 2882
- Phenergan VC 2886
- Phenergan VC with Codeine 2888

Propofol (Potentiates CNS depressant effects). Products include:
- Diprivan Injectable Emulsion 2939

Propoxyphene Hydrochloride (Potentiates CNS depressant effects). Products include:
- Darvon 1475
- Wygesic Tablets 2930

Propoxyphene Napsylate (Potentiates CNS depressant effects). Products include:
- Darvon-N/Darvocet-N 1473

Pyrilamine Maleate (Potentiates CNS depressant effects). Products include:
- 4-Way Fast Acting Nasal Spray (regular & mentholated) .... ⊞ 644
- Maximum Strength Multi-Symptom Formula Midol .... ⊞ 621
- PMS Multi-Symptom Formula Midol .... ⊞ 622

Pyrilamine Tannate (Potentiates CNS depressant effects). Products include:
- Atrohist Pediatric Suspension 1604
- Atrohist Pediatric Suspension Dye-Free 1604
- Rynatan 2781

Quazepam (Potentiates CNS depressant effects). Products include:
- Doral Tablets 2773

Risperidone (Potentiates CNS depressant effects; increases the risk of respiratory depression). Products include:
- Risperdal Tablets 1348

Secobarbital Sodium (Potentiates CNS depressant effects). Products include:
- Seconal Sodium Pulvules 1529

Sevoflurane (Potentiates CNS depressant effects).
- No products indexed under this heading.

Sufentanil Citrate (Potentiates CNS depressant effects). Products include:
- Sufenta Injection 1355

Temazepam (Potentiates CNS depressant effects). Products include:
- Restoril Capsules 2413

Terfenadine (Potentiates CNS depressant effects). Products include:
- Seldane Tablets 1284
- Seldane-D Extended-Release Tablets 1286

Thiamylal Sodium (Potentiates CNS depressant effects).
- No products indexed under this heading.

Thioridazine Hydrochloride (Potentiates CNS depressant effects; increases the risk of respiratory depression). Products include:
- Mellaril 2398

Thiothixene (Potentiates CNS depressant effects; increases the risk of respiratory depression). Products include:
- Navane Capsules and Concentrate 2018
- Navane Intramuscular 2019

Triazolam (Potentiates CNS depressant effects). Products include:
- Halcion Tablets 2093

Trifluoperazine Hydrochloride (Potentiates CNS depressant effects; increases the risk of respiratory depression). Products include:
- Stelazine 2692

Trimeprazine Tartrate (Potentiates CNS depressant effects).
- No products indexed under this heading.

Tripelennamine Hydrochloride (Potentiates CNS depressant effects). Products include:
- PBZ Tablets 863
- PBZ-SR Tablets 862

Triprolidine Hydrochloride (Potentiates CNS depressant effects). Products include:
- Actifed Cold & Allergy Tablets .... ⊞ 807
- Actifed Cold & Sinus Caplets and Tablets .... ⊞ 808

Zolpidem Tartrate (Potentiates CNS depressant effects). Products include:
- Ambien Tablets 2559

Food Interactions

Alcohol (Potentiates CNS depressant effects).

INNOGEL PLUS
(Pyrethrum Extract, Piperonyl Butoxide) .... ⊞ 673
None cited in PDR database.

INOCOR LACTATE INJECTION
(Amrinone Lactate) 2439
May interact with:

Disopyramide Phosphate (Co-administration has produced excessive hypotension in one case; concurrent administration should be undertaken with caution). Products include:
- Norpace 2596

INTAL INHALER
(Cromolyn Sodium) 2185
May interact with:

Isoproterenol Hydrochloride (The addition of cromolyn sodium increases incidence of both resorptions and malformations in animal studies). Products include:
- Isuprel Hydrochloride Solution 2443
- Isuprel Injection 2441
- Isuprel Mistometer 2442

INTAL NEBULIZER SOLUTION
(Cromolyn Sodium) 2186
May interact with:

Isoproterenol Hydrochloride (The addition of cromolyn sodium increases the incidence of both resorption and malformations in animal studies). Products include:
- Isuprel Hydrochloride Solution 2443
- Isuprel Injection 2441
- Isuprel Mistometer 2442

INTRON A FOR INJECTION
(Interferon alfa-2B, Recombinant) 2506
May interact with xanthine bronchodilators and certain other agents. Compounds in these categories include:

Aminophylline (Co-administration results in decreased theophylline clearance resulting in a 100% increase in serum theophylline levels).
- No products indexed under this heading.

Bone Marrow Depressants, unspecified (Careful monitoring of the WBC count is indicated).

Dyphylline (Co-administration results in decreased theophylline clearance resulting in a 100% increase in serum theophylline levels). Products include:
- Lufyllin & Lufyllin-400 Tablets 2778
- Lufyllin-GG Elixir & Tablets 2779

Theophylline (Co-administration results in decreased theophylline clearance resulting in a 100% increase in serum theophylline levels). Products include:
- Marax Tablets & DF Syrup 2015
- Quibron 2227

Theophylline Anhydrous (Co-administration results in decreased theophylline clearance resulting in a 100% increase in serum theophylline levels). Products include:
- Aerolate 1003
- Primatene Tablets .... ⊞ 844
- Respbid Tablets 687
- Slo-bid Gyrocaps 2201
- Theo-24 Extended Release Capsules 2753
- Theo-Dur Extended-Release Tablets 1367
- Theo-X Extended-Release Tablets .. 793
- Uni-Dur Extended-Release Tablets .. 1374
- Uniphyl 400 mg and 600 mg Tablets 2157

Theophylline Calcium Salicylate (Co-administration results in decreased theophylline clearance resulting in a 100% increase in serum theophylline levels). Products include:
- Quadrinal Tablets 1398

Theophylline Sodium Glycinate (Co-administration results in decreased theophylline clearance resulting in a 100% increase in serum theophylline levels).
- No products indexed under this heading.

Zidovudine (Concomitant administration may result in a higher incidence of neutropenia). Products include:
- Retrovir Capsules 1216
- Retrovir I.V. Infusion 1221
- Retrovir Syrup 1216

INVERSINE TABLETS
(Mecamylamine Hydrochloride) 1729
May interact with sulfonamides, general anesthetics, antihypertensives, and certain other agents. Compounds in these categories include:

Acebutolol Hydrochloride (Potentiation of Inversine). Products include:
- Sectral Capsules 2914

Amlodipine Besylate (Potentiation of Inversine). Products include:
- Lotrel Capsules 858
- Norvasc Tablets 2020

Antibiotics, unspecified (Patients receiving antibiotics generally should not be treated with ganglionic blockers).

Atenolol (Potentiation of Inversine). Products include:
- Tenoretic Tablets 2963

IMPORTANT NOTE: Always consult each drug listing in the patient's regimen for possible interactions.

Inversine — Interactions Index

Inversine
Tenormin Tablets and I.V. Injection ... 2965

Benazepril Hydrochloride (Potentiation of Inversine). Products include:
- Lotensin Tablets ... 852
- Lotensin HCT Tablets ... 855
- Lotrel Capsules ... 858

Bendroflumethiazide (Potentiation of Inversine; patients receiving sulfonamides generally should not be treated with ganglion blockers).
No products indexed under this heading.

Betaxolol Hydrochloride (Potentiation of Inversine). Products include:
- Betoptic Ophthalmic Solution ... 465
- Betoptic S Ophthalmic Suspension ... 467
- Kerlone Tablets ... 2588

Bisoprolol Fumarate (Potentiation of Inversine). Products include:
- Zebeta Tablets ... 1457
- Ziac ... 1459

Captopril (Potentiation of Inversine). Products include:
- Capoten Tablets ... 740
- Capozide Tablets ... 744

Carteolol Hydrochloride (Potentiation of Inversine). Products include:
- Cartrol Tablets ... 413
- Ocupress Ophthalmic Solution, 1% Sterile ... ⊚ 297

Chlorothiazide (Potentiation of Inversine; patients receiving sulfonamides generally should not be treated with ganglion blockers). Products include:
- Aldoclor Tablets ... 1638
- Diupres Tablets ... 1691
- Diuril Oral ... 1694

Chlorothiazide Sodium (Potentiation of Inversine; patients receiving sulfonamides generally should not be treated with ganglion blockers). Products include:
- Diuril Sodium Intravenous ... 1693

Chlorpropamide (Patients receiving sulfonamides generally should not be treated with ganglionic blockers). Products include:
- Diabinese Tablets ... 2002

Chlorthalidone (Potentiation of Inversine). Products include:
- Combipres Tablets ... 682
- Tenoretic Tablets ... 2963
- Thalitone ... 1293

Clonidine (Potentiation of Inversine). Products include:
- Catapres-TTS ... 680

Clonidine Hydrochloride (Potentiation of Inversine). Products include:
- Catapres Tablets ... 679
- Combipres Tablets ... 682

Deserpidine (Potentiation of Inversine).
No products indexed under this heading.

Diazoxide (Potentiation of Inversine). Products include:
- Hyperstat I.V. Injection ... 2504
- Proglycem ... 575

Diltiazem Hydrochloride (Potentiation of Inversine). Products include:
- Cardizem CD Capsules ... 1251
- Cardizem SR Capsules ... 1255
- Cardizem Injectable ... 1253
- Cardizem Tablets ... 1257
- Dilacor XR Extended-release Capsules ... 2183
- Tiazac Capsules ... 1019

Doxazosin Mesylate (Potentiation of Inversine). Products include:
- Cardura Tablets ... 1993

Enalapril Maleate (Potentiation of Inversine). Products include:
- Vaseretic Tablets ... 1810

Vasotec Tablets ... 1816

Enalaprilat (Potentiation of Inversine). Products include:
- Vasotec I.V. ... 1814

Enflurane (Potentiation of Inversine).
No products indexed under this heading.

Esmolol Hydrochloride (Potentiation of Inversine). Products include:
- Brevibloc (esmolol HCl) Injection ... 1860

Felodipine (Potentiation of Inversine). Products include:
- Plendil Extended-Release Tablets ... 514

Fosinopril Sodium (Potentiation of Inversine). Products include:
- Monopril Tablets ... 762

Furosemide (Potentiation of Inversine). Products include:
- Lasix Injection, Oral Solution and Tablets ... 1267

Glipizide (Patients receiving sulfonamides generally should not be treated with ganglionic blockers). Products include:
- Glucotrol Tablets ... 2011
- Glucotrol XL Extended Release Tablets ... 2012

Glyburide (Patients receiving sulfonamides generally should not be treated with ganglion blockers). Products include:
- DiaBeta Tablets ... 1265
- Glynase PresTab Tablets ... 2091
- Micronase Tablets ... 2099

Guanabenz Acetate (Potentiation of Inversine).
No products indexed under this heading.

Guanethidine Monosulfate (Potentiation of Inversine). Products include:
- Esimil Tablets ... 840
- Ismelin Tablets ... 845

Hydralazine Hydrochloride (Potentiation of Inversine). Products include:
- Apresazide Capsules ... 824
- Apresoline Hydrochloride Tablets ... 826
- Hydralazine Hydrochloride Injection USP ... 2712
- Ser-Ap-Es Tablets ... 867

Hydrochlorothiazide (Potentiation of Inversine; patients receiving sulfonamides generally should not receive ganglion blockers). Products include:
- Aldactazide Tablets ... 2556
- Aldoril Tablets ... 1644
- Apresazide Capsules ... 824
- Capozide Tablets ... 744
- Dyazide Capsules ... 2653
- Esidrix Tablets ... 839
- Esimil Tablets ... 840
- HydroDIURIL Tablets ... 1716
- Hydropres Tablets ... 1718
- Hyzaar Tablets ... 1720
- Inderide Tablets ... 2838
- Inderide LA Long Acting Capsules ... 2840
- Lopressor HCT Tablets ... 850
- Lotensin HCT Tablets ... 855
- Moduretic Tablets ... 1748
- Oretic Tablets ... 450
- Prinzide Tablets ... 1780
- Ser-Ap-Es Tablets ... 867
- Timolide Tablets ... 1791
- Vaseretic Tablets ... 1810
- Zestoretic Tablets ... 2968
- Ziac ... 1459

Hydroflumethiazide (Potentiation of Inversine; patients receiving sulfonamides generally should not be treated with ganglion blockers). Products include:
- Diucardin Tablets ... 2824

Indapamide (Potentiation of Inversine).
No products indexed under this heading.

Isoflurane (Potentiation of Inversine).
No products indexed under this heading.

Isradipine (Potentiation of Inversine). Products include:
- DynaCirc Capsules ... 2381
- DynaCirc CR Tablets ... 2383

Labetalol Hydrochloride (Potentiation of Inversine). Products include:
- Normodyne Injection ... 2519
- Normodyne Tablets ... 2522
- Trandate ... 1158

Lisinopril (Potentiation of Inversine). Products include:
- Prinivil Tablets ... 1776
- Prinzide Tablets ... 1780
- Zestoretic Tablets ... 2968
- Zestril Tablets ... 2972

Losartan Potassium (Potentiation of Inversine). Products include:
- Cozaar Tablets ... 1668
- Hyzaar Tablets ... 1720

Methohexital Sodium (Potentiation of Inversine).
No products indexed under this heading.

Methoxyflurane (Potentiation of Inversine).
No products indexed under this heading.

Methyclothiazide (Potentiation of Inversine; patients receiving sulfonamides generally should not be treated with ganglion blockers). Products include:
- Enduron Tablets ... 424

Methyldopa (Potentiation of Inversine). Products include:
- Aldoclor Tablets ... 1638
- Aldomet Oral ... 1640
- Aldoril Tablets ... 1644

Methyldopate Hydrochloride (Potentiation of Inversine). Products include:
- Aldomet Ester HCl Injection ... 1642

Metolazone (Potentiation of Inversine). Products include:
- Mykrox Tablets ... 1617
- Zaroxolyn Tablets ... 1625

Metoprolol Succinate (Potentiation of Inversine). Products include:
- Toprol-XL Tablets ... 560

Metoprolol Tartrate (Potentiation of Inversine). Products include:
- Lopressor ... 848
- Lopressor HCT Tablets ... 850

Metyrosine (Potentiation of Inversine). Products include:
- Demser Capsules ... 1690

Minoxidil (Potentiation of Inversine).
No products indexed under this heading.

Moexipril Hydrochloride (Potentiation of Inversine). Products include:
- Univasc Tablets ... 2553

Nadolol (Potentiation of Inversine).
No products indexed under this heading.

Nicardipine Hydrochloride (Potentiation of Inversine). Products include:
- Cardene Capsules ... 2261
- Cardene I.V. ... 2815
- Cardene SR Capsules ... 2264

Nifedipine (Potentiation of Inversine). Products include:
- Adalat Capsules (10 mg and 20 mg) ... 580
- Adalat CC ... 582
- Procardia Capsules ... 2024
- Procardia XL Extended Release Tablets ... 2026

Nisoldipine (Potentiation of Inversine). Products include:
- Sular Tablets ... 2961

Nitroglycerin (Potentiation of Inversine). Products include:
- Deponit NTG Transdermal Delivery System ... 2541
- Nitro-Bid IV ... 1270
- Nitro-Bid Ointment ... 1272
- Nitro-Dur (nitroglycerin) Transdermal Infusion System ... 1365
- Nitrolingual Spray ... 2193
- Nitrostat Tablets ... 1981
- Transderm-Nitro Transdermal Therapeutic System ... 878

Penbutolol Sulfate (Potentiation of Inversine). Products include:
- Levatol Tablets ... 2547

Phenoxybenzamine Hydrochloride (Potentiation of Inversine). Products include:
- Dibenzyline Capsules ... 2650

Phentolamine Mesylate (Potentiation of Inversine). Products include:
- Regitine Vials ... 864

Pindolol (Potentiation of Inversine). Products include:
- Visken Tablets ... 2428

Polythiazide (Potentiation of Inversine; patients receiving sulfonamides generally should not be treated with ganglion blockers). Products include:
- Minizide Capsules ... 2016

Prazosin Hydrochloride (Potentiation of Inversine). Products include:
- Minipress Capsules ... 2015
- Minizide Capsules ... 2016

Propofol (Potentiation of Inversine). Products include:
- Diprivan Injectable Emulsion ... 2939

Propranolol Hydrochloride (Potentiation of Inversine). Products include:
- Inderal ... 2834
- Inderal LA Long Acting Capsules ... 2836
- Inderide Tablets ... 2838
- Inderide LA Long Acting Capsules ... 2840

Quinapril Hydrochloride (Potentiation of Inversine). Products include:
- Accupril Tablets ... 1950

Ramipril (Potentiation of Inversine). Products include:
- Altace Capsules ... 1238

Rauwolfia Serpentina (Potentiation of Inversine).
No products indexed under this heading.

Rescinnamine (Potentiation of Inversine).
No products indexed under this heading.

Reserpine (Potentiation of Inversine). Products include:
- Diupres Tablets ... 1691
- Hydropres Tablets ... 1718
- Ser-Ap-Es Tablets ... 867

Sevoflurane (Potentiation of Inversine).
No products indexed under this heading.

Sodium Nitroprusside (Potentiation of Inversine).
No products indexed under this heading.

Sotalol Hydrochloride (Potentiation of Inversine). Products include:
- Betapace Tablets ... 637

Spirapril Hydrochloride (Potentiation of Inversine).
No products indexed under this heading.

Sulfamethizole (Patients receiving sulfonamides generally should not be treated with ganglionic blockers). Products include:
- Urobiotic-250 Capsules ... 2038

(▣ Described in PDR For Nonprescription Drugs)   (⊚ Described in PDR For Ophthalmology)

Sulfamethoxazole (Patients receiving sulfonamides generally should not be treated with ganglionic blockers). Products include:

- Bactrim DS Tablets 2257
- Bactrim I.V. Infusion 2255
- Bactrim 2257
- Gantanol Tablets 2285
- Septra 1146
- Septra I.V. Infusion 1142
- Septra I.V. Infusion ADD-Vantage Vials 1144
- Septra 1146

Sulfasalazine (Patients receiving sulfonamides generally should not be treated with ganglionic blockers). Products include:

- Azulfidine 2059

Sulfinpyrazone (Patients receiving sulfonamides generally should not be treated with ganglionic blockers). Products include:

- Anturane 823

Sulfisoxazole (Patients receiving sulfonamides generally should not be treated with ganglionic blockers). Products include:

- Gantrisin Tablets 2286

Sulfisoxazole Diolamine (Patients receiving sulfonamides generally should not be treated with ganglionic blockers).

No products indexed under this heading.

Terazosin Hydrochloride (Potentiation of Inversine). Products include:

- Hytrin Capsules 434

Timolol Maleate (Potentiation of Inversine). Products include:

- Blocadren Tablets 1654
- Timolide Tablets 1791
- Timoptic in Ocudose 1796
- Timoptic Sterile Ophthalmic Solution 1794
- Timoptic-XE 1798

Tolazamide (Patients receiving sulfonamides generally should not be treated with ganglionic blockers).

No products indexed under this heading.

Tolbutamide (Patients receiving sulfonamides generally should not be treated with ganglionic blockers).

No products indexed under this heading.

Torsemide (Potentiation of Inversine). Products include:

- Demadex Tablets and Injection 691

Trimethaphan Camsylate (Potentiation of Inversine).

No products indexed under this heading.

Verapamil Hydrochloride (Potentiation of Inversine). Products include:

- Calan SR Caplets 2571
- Calan Tablets 2568
- Covera-HS Tablets 2573
- Isoptin Injectable 1391
- Isoptin Oral Tablets 1393
- Isoptin SR Tablets 1395
- Verelan Capsules 1455

Food Interactions

Alcohol (Potentiation of Inversine).

INVIRASE CAPSULES

(Saquinavir Mesylate) 2291

May interact with calcium channel blockers and certain other agents. Compounds in these categories include:

Amlodipine Besylate (Potential for elevated plasma concentrations of compounds that are substrate of CYP3A4, such as calcium channel blockers). Products include:

- Lotrel Capsules 858
- Norvasc Tablets 2020

Astemizole (Potential for elevated astemizole plasma levels, which may in turn prolong QT intervals leading to rare cases of serious cardiovascular adverse events due to inhibition of cytochrome P4503A). Products include:

- Hismanal Tablets 1341

Bepridil Hydrochloride (Potential for elevated plasma concentrations of compounds that are substrate of CYP3A4, such as calcium channel blockers). Products include:

- Vascor Tablets (200 and 300 mg) 1597

Carbamazepine (Co-administration may reduce saquinavir plasma concentrations through CYP3A4 induction). Products include:

- Atretol Tablets 569
- Tegretol/Tegretol-XR 870

Cisapride (Potential for elevated cisapride plasma levels, which in turn prolong QT intervals leading to rare cases of serious cardiovascular adverse events due to inhibition of cytochrome P4503A4). Products include:

- Propulsid 1346

Clindamycin Hydrochloride (Potential for elevated plasma concentrations of compounds that are substrate of CYP3A4, such as clindamycin).

No products indexed under this heading.

Clindamycin Palmitate Hydrochloride (Potential for elevated plasma concentrations of compounds that are substrate of CYP3A4, such as clindamycin).

No products indexed under this heading.

Clindamycin Phosphate (Potential for elevated plasma concentrations of compounds that are substrate of CYP3A4, such as clindamycin). Products include:

- Cleocin Phosphate Injection 2068
- Cleocin T Topical 2072
- Cleocin Vaginal Cream 2070

Dapsone (Potential for elevated plasma concentrations of compounds that are substrate of CYP3A4, such as dapsone). Products include:

- Dapsone Tablets USP 1331

Dexamethasone (Co-administration may reduce saquinavir plasma concentrations through CYP3A4 induction). Products include:

- AK-Trol Ointment & Suspension ..... ◉ 205
- Decadron Elixir 1676
- Decadron Tablets 1678
- Decaspray Topical Aerosol 1689
- Maxitrol Ophthalmic Ointment and Suspension ..... ◉ 222
- TobraDex Ophthalmic Suspension and Ointment 469

Dexamethasone Acetate (Co-administration may reduce saquinavir plasma concentrations through CYP3A4 induction). Products include:

- Dalalone D.P. Injectable 1009
- Decadron-LA Sterile Suspension 1687

Dexamethasone Sodium Phosphate (Co-administration may reduce saquinavir plasma concentrations through CYP3A4 induction). Products include:

- Decadron Phosphate Injection 1680
- Decadron Phosphate Sterile Ophthalmic Ointment 1684
- Decadron Phosphate Sterile Ophthalmic Solution 1685
- Decadron Phosphate Topical Cream 1686
- Decadron Phosphate with Xylocaine Injection, Sterile 1683
- Dexacort Phosphate in Respihaler 1606
- Dexacort Phosphate in Turbinaire 1607
- NeoDecadron Sterile Ophthalmic Ointment 1755
- NeoDecadron Sterile Ophthalmic Solution 1756
- NeoDecadron Topical Cream 1757

Diltiazem Hydrochloride (Potential for elevated plasma concentrations of compounds that are substrate of CYP3A4, such as calcium channel blockers). Products include:

- Cardizem CD Capsules 1251
- Cardizem SR Capsules 1255
- Cardizem Injectable 1253
- Cardizem Tablets 1257
- Dilacor XR Extended-release Capsules 2183
- Tiazac Capsules 1019

Felodipine (Potential for elevated plasma concentrations of compounds that are substrate of CYP3A4, such as calcium channel blockers). Products include:

- Plendil Extended-Release Tablets 514

Isradipine (Potential for elevated plasma concentrations of compounds that are substrate of CYP3A4, such as calcium channel blockers). Products include:

- DynaCirc Capsules 2381
- DynaCirc CR Tablets 2383

Ketoconazole (Co-administration results in steady-state saquinavir AUC Cmax values that are three times those seen with saquinavir alone; no dosage adjustments are required). Products include:

- Nizoral 2% Cream 1344
- Nizoral 2% Shampoo 1344
- Nizoral Tablets 1345

Nicardipine Hydrochloride (Potential for elevated plasma concentrations of compounds that are substrate of CYP3A4, such as calcium channel blockers). Products include:

- Cardene Capsules 2261
- Cardene I.V. 2815
- Cardene SR Capsules 2264

Nifedipine (Potential for elevated plasma concentrations of compounds that are substrate of CYP3A4, such as calcium channel blockers). Products include:

- Adalat Capsules (10 mg and 20 mg) 580
- Adalat CC 582
- Procardia Capsules 2024
- Procardia XL Extended Release Tablets 2026

Nimodipine (Potential for elevated plasma concentrations of compounds that are substrate of CYP3A4, such as calcium channel blockers). Products include:

- Nimotop Capsules 603

Nisoldipine (Potential for elevated plasma concentrations of compounds that are substrate of CYP3A4, such as calcium channel blockers). Products include:

- Sular Tablets 2961

Phenobarbital (Co-administration may reduce saquinavir plasma concentrations through CYP3A4 induction). Products include:

- Arco-Lase Plus Tablets 513
- Bellergal-S Tablets 2375
- Donnatal 2234
- Donnatal Extentabs 2234
- Donnatal Tablets 2234
- Phenobarbital Elixir and Tablets 1523
- Quadrinal Tablets 1398

Phenytoin (Co-administration may reduce saquinavir plasma concentrations through CYP3A4 induction). Products include:

- Dilantin Infatabs 1967
- Dilantin-125 Suspension 1969

Phenytoin Sodium (Co-administration may reduce saquinavir plasma concentrations through CYP3A4 induction). Products include:

- Dilantin Kapseals 1965

Quinidine Gluconate (Potential for elevated plasma concentrations of compounds that are substrate of CYP3A4, such as quinidine). Products include:

- Quinaglute Dura-Tabs Tablets 644

Quinidine Polygalacturonate (Potential for elevated plasma concentrations of compounds that are substrate of CYP3A4, such as quinidine). Products include:

- Cardioquin Tablets 2146

Quinidine Sulfate (Potential for elevated plasma concentrations of compounds that are substrate of CYP3A4, such as quinidine). Products include:

- Quinidex Extentabs 2240

Rifabutin (Preliminary data indicates that rifabutin decreases steady-state AUC of saquinavir by 40%). Products include:

- Mycobutin Capsules 2101

Rifampin (Co-administration results in a decreased steady-state AUC and Cmax of saquinavir by approximately 80%; concomitant use is not recommended). Products include:

- Rifadin 1276
- Rifamate Capsules 1278
- Rifater 1280
- Rimactane Capsules 865

Terfenadine (Potential for elevated terfenadine plasma levels, which may in turn prolong QT intervals leading to rare cases of serious cardiovascular adverse events due to inhibition of cytochrome P4503A). Products include:

- Seldane Tablets 1284
- Seldane-D Extended-Release Tablets 1286

Triazolam (Potential for elevated plasma concentrations of compounds that are substrate of CYP3A4, such as triazolam). Products include:

- Halcion Tablets 2093

Verapamil Hydrochloride (Potential for elevated plasma concentrations of compounds that are substrate of CYP3A4, such as calcium channel blockers). Products include:

- Calan SR Caplets 2571
- Calan Tablets 2568
- Covera-HS Tablets 2573
- Isoptin Injectable 1391
- Isoptin Oral Tablets 1393
- Isoptin SR Tablets 1395
- Verelan Capsules 1455

Food Interactions

Food, unspecified (Saquinavir 24-AUC and Cmax following a high-caloric meal is on average two times higher than a lower calorie, lower fat meal; patients should be advised to take saquinavir within 2 hours after a full meal).

IONAMIN CAPSULES

(Phentermine Resin) 1615

May interact with monoamine oxidase inhibitors, insulin, and certain other agents. Compounds in these categories include:

Furazolidone (Concurrent use is contraindicated). Products include:

- Furoxone 2221

Guanethidine Monosulfate (Decreased hypotensive effect of guanethidine). Products include:

- Esimil Tablets 840

IMPORTANT NOTE: Always consult each drug listing in the patient's regimen for possible interactions.

Interactions Index

Ismelin Tablets 845
Insulin, Human (Insulin requirement may be altered in diabetics).
 No products indexed under this heading.
Insulin, Human Isophane Suspension (Insulin requirement may be altered in diabetics). Products include:
 Novolin N Human Insulin 10 ml Vials 1846
Insulin, Human NPH (Insulin requirement may be altered in diabetics). Products include:
 Humulin N, 100 Units 1495
 Novolin N PenFill 1.5 ml Cartridges Durable Insulin Delivery System 1849
 Novolin N Prefilled Syringe Disposable Insulin Delivery System 1850
Insulin, Human Regular (Insulin requirement may be altered in diabetics). Products include:
 Humulin R, 100 Units 1497
 Novolin R Human Insulin 10 ml Vials 1846
 Novolin R PenFill 1.5 ml Cartridges Durable Insulin Delivery System 1849
 Novolin R Prefilled Syringe Disposable Insulin Delivery System 1850
 Velosulin BR Human Insulin 10 ml Vials 1847
Insulin, Human, Zinc Suspension (Insulin requirement may be altered in diabetics). Products include:
 Humulin L, 100 Units 1494
 Humulin U, 100 Units 1498
 Novolin L Human Insulin 10 ml Vials 1846
Insulin Lispro, Human (Insulin requirement may be altered in diabetics). Products include:
 Humalog Injection 1488
Insulin, NPH (Insulin requirement may be altered in diabetics). Products include:
 NPH, 100 Units 1502
 Pork NPH, 100 Units 1506
 Purified Pork NPH Isophane Insulin 1852
Insulin, Regular (Insulin requirement may be altered in diabetics). Products include:
 Regular, 100 Units 1503
 Pork Regular, 100 Units 1507
 Pork Regular (Concentrated), 500 Units 1508
 Purified Pork Regular Insulin 1852
Insulin, Zinc Crystals (Insulin requirement may be altered in diabetics). Products include:
 NPH, 100 Units 1502
Insulin, Zinc Suspension (Insulin requirement may be altered in diabetics). Products include:
 Iletin I 1501
 Lente, 100 Units 1501
 Iletin II 1504
 Pork Lente, 100 Units 1504
 Purified Pork Lente Insulin 1852
Isocarboxazid (Concurrent use is contraindicated).
 No products indexed under this heading.
Phenelzine Sulfate (Concurrent use is contraindicated). Products include:
 Nardil 1977
Selegiline Hydrochloride (Concurrent use is contraindicated). Products include:
 Eldepryl Capsules 2729
Tranylcypromine Sulfate (Concurrent use is contraindicated). Products include:
 Parnate Tablets 2679

Food Interactions

Alcohol (Possibility of adverse interactions).

IOPIDINE STERILE OPHTHALMIC SOLUTION
(Apraclonidine Hydrochloride) .... ⊚ 218
May interact with monoamine oxidase inhibitors. Compounds in this category include:

Furazolidone (Concurrent therapy is contraindicated). Products include:
 Furoxone 2221
Isocarboxazid (Concurrent therapy is contraindicated).
 No products indexed under this heading.
Phenelzine Sulfate (Concurrent therapy is contraindicated). Products include:
 Nardil 1977
Selegiline Hydrochloride (Concurrent therapy is contraindicated). Products include:
 Eldepryl Capsules 2729
Tranylcypromine Sulfate (Concurrent therapy is contraindicated). Products include:
 Parnate Tablets 2679

IOPIDINE 0.5%
(Apraclonidine Hydrochloride) .... ⊚ 219
May interact with monoamine oxidase inhibitors, central nervous system depressants, barbiturates, narcotic analgesics, general anesthetics, hypnotics and sedatives, tricyclic antidepressants, antipsychotic agents, insulin, beta blockers, antihypertensives, and cardiac glycosides. Compounds in these categories include:

Acebutolol Hydrochloride (Apraclonidine reduces pulse and blood pressure, caution is advised when used concurrently). Products include:
 Sectral Capsules 2914
Alfentanil Hydrochloride (Possible additive or potentiating effect with CNS depressant). Products include:
 Alfenta Injection 1334
Alprazolam (Possible additive or potentiating effect with CNS depressant). Products include:
 Xanax Tablets 2115
Amitriptyline Hydrochloride (Tricyclic antidepressants have been reported to blunt the hypotensive effect of clonidine; it is not known whether the concurrent use with apraclonidine can lead to reduction in IOP lowering effect). Products include:
 Elavil 2945
 Etrafon 2495
 Limbitrol 2333
 Triavil Tablets 1800
Amlodipine Besylate (Apraclonidine reduces pulse and blood pressure, caution is advised when used concurrently). Products include:
 Lotrel Capsules 858
 Norvasc Tablets 2020
Amoxapine (Tricyclic antidepressants have been reported to blunt the hypotensive effect of clonidine; it is not known whether the concurrent use with apraclonidine can lead to reduction in IOP lowering effect). Products include:
 Asendin Tablets 1419

Aprobarbital (Possible additive or potentiating effect with CNS depressant).
 No products indexed under this heading.
Atenolol (Apraclonidine reduces pulse and blood pressure, caution is advised when used concurrently). Products include:
 Tenoretic Tablets 2963
 Tenormin Tablets and I.V. Injection 2965
Benazepril Hydrochloride (Apraclonidine reduces pulse and blood pressure, caution is advised when used concurrently). Products include:
 Lotensin Tablets 852
 Lotensin HCT Tablets 855
 Lotrel Capsules 858
Bendroflumethiazide (Apraclonidine reduces pulse and blood pressure, caution is advised when used concurrently).
 No products indexed under this heading.
Betaxolol Hydrochloride (Apraclonidine reduces pulse and blood pressure, caution is advised when used concurrently). Products include:
 Betoptic Ophthalmic Solution 465
 Betoptic S Ophthalmic Suspension 467
 Kerlone Tablets 2588
Bisoprolol Fumarate (Apraclonidine reduces pulse and blood pressure, caution is advised when used concurrently). Products include:
 Zebeta Tablets 1457
 Ziac 1459
Buprenorphine (Possible additive or potentiating effect with CNS depressant). Products include:
 Buprenex Injectable 2170
Buspirone Hydrochloride (Possible additive or potentiating effect with CNS depressant). Products include:
 BuSpar Tablets 738
Butabarbital (Possible additive or potentiating effect with CNS depressant).
 No products indexed under this heading.
Butalbital (Possible additive or potentiating effect with CNS depressant). Products include:
 Axocet Capsules 2469
 Esgic-plus Capsules 1012
 Esgic-plus Tablets 1012
 Fioricet Tablets 2386
 Fioricet with Codeine Capsules 2387
 Fiorinal Capsules 2388
 Fiorinal with Codeine Capsules 2390
 Fiorinal Tablets 2388
 Phrenilin 790
 Sedapap Tablets 50 mg/650 mg .. 1826
Captopril (Apraclonidine reduces pulse and blood pressure, caution is advised when used concurrently). Products include:
 Capoten Tablets 740
 Capozide Tablets 744
Carteolol Hydrochloride (Apraclonidine reduces pulse and blood pressure, caution is advised when used concurrently). Products include:
 Cartrol Tablets 413
 Ocupress Ophthalmic Solution, 1% Sterile .... ⊚ 297
Chlordiazepoxide (Possible additive or potentiating effect with CNS depressant). Products include:
 Limbitrol 2333
Chlordiazepoxide Hydrochloride (Possible additive or potentiating effect with CNS depressant). Products include:
 Librax Capsules 2330

 Librium Capsules 2331
 Librium Injectable 2332
Chlorothiazide (Apraclonidine reduces pulse and blood pressure, caution is advised when used concurrently). Products include:
 Aldoclor Tablets 1638
 Diupres Tablets 1691
 Diuril Oral 1694
Chlorothiazide Sodium (Apraclonidine reduces pulse and blood pressure, caution is advised when used concurrently). Products include:
 Diuril Sodium Intravenous 1693
Chlorpromazine (An additive hypotensive effect has been reported with the combination of systemic clonidine and neuroleptic therapy; possible additive or potentiating effect with CNS depressant). Products include:
 Thorazine Suppositories 2701
Chlorpromazine Hydrochloride (An additive hypotensive effect has been reported with the combination of systemic clonidine and neuroleptic therapy; possible additive or potentiating effect with CNS depressant). Products include:
 Thorazine 2701
Chlorprothixene (An additive hypotensive effect has been reported with the combination of systemic clonidine and neuroleptic therapy; possible additive or potentiating effect with CNS depressant).
 No products indexed under this heading.
Chlorprothixene Hydrochloride (An additive hypotensive effect has been reported with the combination of systemic clonidine and neuroleptic therapy; possible additive or potentiating effect with CNS depressant).
 No products indexed under this heading.
Chlorprothixene Lactate (Possible additive or potentiating effect with CNS depressant).
 No products indexed under this heading.
Chlorthalidone (Apraclonidine reduces pulse and blood pressure, caution is advised when used concurrently). Products include:
 Combipres Tablets 682
 Tenoretic Tablets 2963
 Thalitone 1293
Clomipramine Hydrochloride (Tricyclic antidepressants have been reported to blunt the hypotensive effect of clonidine; it is not known whether the concurrent use with apraclonidine can lead to reduction in IOP lowering effect). Products include:
 Anafranil Capsules 819
Clonidine (Apraclonidine reduces pulse and blood pressure, caution is advised when used concurrently). Products include:
 Catapres-TTS 680
Clonidine Hydrochloride (Apraclonidine reduces pulse and blood pressure, caution is advised when used concurrently). Products include:
 Catapres Tablets 679
 Combipres Tablets 682
Clorazepate Dipotassium (Possible additive or potentiating effect with CNS depressant). Products include:
 Tranxene 459

(⊞ Described in PDR For Nonprescription Drugs)   (⊚ Described in PDR For Ophthalmology)

541 **Interactions Index** **Iopidine**

Clozapine (An additive hypotensive effect has been reported with the combination of systemic clonidine and neuroleptic therapy; possible additive or potentiating effect with CNS depressant). Products include:

Clozaril Tablets ... 2377

Codeine Phosphate (Possible additive or potentiating effect with CNS depressant). Products include:

Brontex ... 2130
Dimetane-DC Cough Syrup ... 2232
Fioricet with Codeine Capsules ... 2387
Fiorinal with Codeine Capsules ... 2390
Nucofed ... 2225
Phenergan with Codeine ... 2883
Phenergan VC with Codeine ... 2888
Robitussin A-C Syrup ... 2248
Robitussin-DAC Syrup ... 2249
Ryna ... 804
Soma Compound w/Codeine Tablets ... 2784
Tylenol with Codeine ... 1592

Deserpidine (Apraclonidine reduces pulse and blood pressure, caution is advised when used concurrently).

No products indexed under this heading.

Desflurane (Possible additive or potentiating effect with CNS depressant). Products include:

Suprane (desflurane, USP) ... 1865

Desipramine Hydrochloride (Tricyclic antidepressants have been reported to blunt the hypotensive effect of clonidine; it is not known whether the concurrent use with apraclonidine can lead to reduction in IOP lowering effect). Products include:

Norpramin Tablets ... 1273

Deslanoside (Apraclonidine reduces pulse and blood pressure, caution is advised when used concurrently).

No products indexed under this heading.

Dezocine (Possible additive or potentiating effect with CNS depressant). Products include:

Dalgan Injection ... 529

Diazepam (Possible additive or potentiating effect with CNS depressant). Products include:

Dizac (diazepam injectable emulsion) CIV ... 1862
Valium Injectable ... 2336
Valium Tablets ... 2335

Diazoxide (Apraclonidine reduces pulse and blood pressure, caution is advised when used concurrently). Products include:

Hyperstat I.V. Injection ... 2504
Proglycem ... 575

Digitoxin (Apraclonidine reduces pulse and blood pressure, caution is advised when used concurrently). Products include:

Crystodigin Tablets ... 1472

Digoxin (Apraclonidine reduces pulse and blood pressure, caution is advised when used concurrently). Products include:

Lanoxicaps ... 1110
Lanoxin Elixir Pediatric ... 1113
Lanoxin Injection ... 1116
Lanoxin Injection Pediatric ... 1119
Lanoxin Tablets ... 1121

Diltiazem Hydrochloride (Apraclonidine reduces pulse and blood pressure, caution is advised when used concurrently). Products include:

Cardizem CD Capsules ... 1251
Cardizem SR Capsules ... 1255
Cardizem Injectable ... 1253
Cardizem Tablets ... 1257
Dilacor XR Extended-release Capsules ... 2183
Tiazac Capsules ... 1019

Doxazosin Mesylate (Apraclonidine reduces pulse and blood pressure, caution is advised when used concurrently). Products include:

Cardura Tablets ... 1993

Doxepin Hydrochloride (Tricyclic antidepressants have been reported to blunt the hypotensive effect of clonidine; it is not known whether the concurrent use with apraclonidine can lead to reduction in IOP lowering effect). Products include:

Adapin Capsules ... 1542
Sinequan ... 2028
Zonalon Cream ... 1042

Droperidol (Possible additive or potentiating effect with CNS depressant). Products include:

Inapsine Injection ... 462

Enalapril Maleate (Apraclonidine reduces pulse and blood pressure, caution is advised when used concurrently). Products include:

Vaseretic Tablets ... 1810
Vasotec Tablets ... 1816

Enalaprilat (Apraclonidine reduces pulse and blood pressure, caution is advised when used concurrently). Products include:

Vasotec I.V. ... 1814

Enflurane (Possible additive or potentiating effect with CNS depressant).

No products indexed under this heading.

Esmolol Hydrochloride (Apraclonidine reduces pulse and blood pressure, caution is advised when used concurrently). Products include:

Brevibloc (esmolol HCl) Injection ... 1860

Estazolam (Possible additive or potentiating effect with CNS depressant). Products include:

ProSom Tablets ... 457

Ethchlorvynol (Possible additive or potentiating effect with CNS depressant). Products include:

Placidyl Capsules ... 456

Ethinamate (Possible additive or potentiating effect with CNS depressant).

No products indexed under this heading.

Felodipine (Apraclonidine reduces pulse and blood pressure, caution is advised when used concurrently). Products include:

Plendil Extended-Release Tablets ... 514

Fentanyl (Possible additive or potentiating effect with CNS depressant). Products include:

Duragesic Transdermal System ... 1336

Fentanyl Citrate (Possible additive or potentiating effect with CNS depressant). Products include:

Sublimaze Injection ... 463

Fluphenazine Decanoate (An additive hypotensive effect has been reported with the combination of systemic clonidine and neuroleptic therapy; possible additive or potentiating effect with CNS depressant). Products include:

Prolixin Decanoate ... 510

Fluphenazine Enanthate (An additive hypotensive effect has been reported with the combination of systemic clonidine and neuroleptic therapy; possible additive or potentiating effect with CNS depressant). Products include:

Prolixin Enanthate ... 510

Fluphenazine Hydrochloride (An additive hypotensive effect has been reported with the combination of systemic clonidine and neuroleptic therapy; possible additive or potentiating effect with CNS depressant). Products include:

Prolixin ... 510

Flurazepam Hydrochloride (Possible additive or potentiating effect with CNS depressant). Products include:

Dalmane Capsules ... 2329

Fosinopril Sodium (Apraclonidine reduces pulse and blood pressure, caution is advised when used concurrently). Products include:

Monopril Tablets ... 762

Furazolidone (Concurrent use is contraindicated). Products include:

Furoxone ... 2221

Furosemide (Apraclonidine reduces pulse and blood pressure, caution is advised when used concurrently). Products include:

Lasix Injection, Oral Solution and Tablets ... 1267

Glutethimide (Possible additive or potentiating effect with CNS depressant).

No products indexed under this heading.

Guanabenz Acetate (Apraclonidine reduces pulse and blood pressure, caution is advised when used concurrently).

No products indexed under this heading.

Guanethidine Monosulfate (Apraclonidine reduces pulse and blood pressure, caution is advised when used concurrently). Products include:

Esimil Tablets ... 840
Ismelin Tablets ... 845

Haloperidol (An additive hypotensive effect has been reported with the combination of systemic clonidine and neuroleptic therapy; possible additive or potentiating effect with CNS depressant). Products include:

Haldol Injection, Tablets and Concentrate ... 1585

Haloperidol Decanoate (An additive hypotensive effect has been reported with the combination of systemic clonidine and neuroleptic therapy; possible additive or potentiating effect with CNS depressant). Products include:

Haldol Decanoate ... 1587

Hydralazine Hydrochloride (Apraclonidine reduces pulse and blood pressure, caution is advised when used concurrently). Products include:

Apresazide Capsules ... 824
Apresoline Hydrochloride Tablets ... 826
Hydralazine Hydrochloride Injection USP ... 2712
Ser-Ap-Es Tablets ... 867

Hydrochlorothiazide (Apraclonidine reduces pulse and blood pressure, caution is advised when used concurrently). Products include:

Aldactazide Tablets ... 2556
Aldoril Tablets ... 1644
Apresazide Capsules ... 824
Capozide Tablets ... 744
Dyazide Capsules ... 2653
Esidrix Tablets ... 839
Esimil Tablets ... 840
HydroDIURIL Tablets ... 1716
Hydropres Tablets ... 1718
Hyzaar Tablets ... 1720
Inderide Tablets ... 2838
Inderide LA Long Acting Capsules ... 2840
Lopressor HCT Tablets ... 850
Lotensin HCT Tablets ... 855
Moduretic Tablets ... 1748
Oretic Tablets ... 450
Prinzide Tablets ... 1780
Ser-Ap-Es Tablets ... 867
Timolide Tablets ... 1791
Vaseretic Tablets ... 1810
Zestoretic Tablets ... 2968
Ziac ... 1459

Hydrocodone Bitartrate (Possible additive or potentiating effect with CNS depressant). Products include:

Codiclear DH Syrup ... 808
Duratuss HD Elixir ... 2750
Histussin D Liquid ... 670
Hycodan Tablets and Syrup ... 946
Hycomine Compound Tablets ... 948
Hycomine ... 947
Hycotuss Expectorant Syrup ... 950
Hydrocet Capsules ... 787
Lorcet 10/650 Tablets ... 1016
Lortab ... 2751
Tussend ... 1830
Tussend Expectorant ... 1831
Vicodin Tablets ... 1404
Vicodin ES Tablets ... 1405
Vicodin HP Tablets ... 1403
Vicodin Tuss Expectorant ... 1406
Zydone Capsules ... 967

Hydrocodone Polistirex (Possible additive or potentiating effect with CNS depressant). Products include:

Tussionex Pennkinetic Extended-Release Suspension ... 1624

Hydroflumethiazide (Apraclonidine reduces pulse and blood pressure, caution is advised when used concurrently). Products include:

Diucardin Tablets ... 2824

Hydromorphone Hydrochloride (Possible additive or potentiating effect with CNS depressant). Products include:

Dilaudid Ampules ... 1382
Dilaudid Cough Syrup ... 1383
Dilaudid-HP Injection ... 1384
Dilaudid-HP Lyophilized Powder 250 mg ... 1384
Dilaudid ... 1382
Dilaudid Oral Liquid ... 1386
Dilaudid ... 1382
Dilaudid Tablets - 8 mg ... 1386

Hydroxyzine Hydrochloride (Possible additive or potentiating effect with CNS depressant). Products include:

Atarax Tablets & Syrup ... 1992
Marax Tablets & DF Syrup ... 2015
Vistaril Intramuscular Solution ... 2042

Imipramine Hydrochloride (Tricyclic antidepressants have been reported to blunt the hypotensive effect of clonidine; it is not known whether the concurrent use with apraclonidine can lead to reduction in IOP lowering effect). Products include:

Tofranil Ampuls ... 873
Tofranil Tablets ... 875

Imipramine Pamoate (Tricyclic antidepressants have been reported to blunt the hypotensive effect of clonidine; it is not known whether the concurrent use with apraclonidine can lead to reduction in IOP lowering effect). Products include:

Tofranil-PM Capsules ... 876

Indapamide (Apraclonidine reduces pulse and blood pressure, caution is advised when used concurrently).

No products indexed under this heading.

Insulin, Human (Systemic clonidine may inhibit the production of catecholamines in response to insulin-induced hypoglycemia and mask the signs and symptoms of hypoglycemia).

No products indexed under this heading.

IMPORTANT NOTE: Always consult each drug listing in the patient's regimen for possible interactions.

Iopidine Interactions Index 542

Insulin, Human Isophane Suspension (Systemic clonidine may inhibit the production of catecholamines in response to insulin-induced hypoglycemia and mask the signs and symptoms of hypoglycemia). Products include:
- Novolin N Human Insulin 10 ml Vials ... 1846

Insulin, Human NPH (Systemic clonidine may inhibit the production of catecholamines in response to insulin-induced hypoglycemia and mask the signs and symptoms of hypoglycemia). Products include:
- Humulin N, 100 Units ... 1495
- Novolin N PenFill 1.5 ml Cartridges Durable Insulin Delivery System ... 1849
- Novolin N Prefilled Syringe Disposable Insulin Delivery System ... 1850

Insulin, Human Regular (Systemic clonidine may inhibit the production of catecholamines in response to insulin-induced hypoglycemia and mask the signs and symptoms of hypoglycemia). Products include:
- Humulin R, 100 Units ... 1497
- Novolin R Human Insulin 10 ml Vials ... 1846
- Novolin R PenFill 1.5 ml Cartridges Durable Insulin Delivery System ... 1849
- Novolin R Prefilled Syringe Disposable Insulin Delivery System ... 1850
- Velosulin BR Human Insulin 10 ml Vials ... 1847

Insulin, Human, Zinc Suspension (Systemic clonidine may inhibit the production of catecholamines in response to insulin-induced hypoglycemia and mask the signs and symptoms of hypoglycemia). Products include:
- Humulin L, 100 Units ... 1494
- Humulin U, 100 Units ... 1498
- Novolin L Human Insulin 10 ml Vials ... 1846

Insulin Lispro, Human (Systemic clonidine may inhibit the production of catecholamines in response to insulin-induced hypoglycemia and mask the signs and symptoms of hypoglycemia). Products include:
- Humalog Injection ... 1488

Insulin, NPH (Systemic clonidine may inhibit the production of catecholamines in response to insulin-induced hypoglycemia and mask the signs and symptoms of hypoglycemia). Products include:
- NPH, 100 Units ... 1502
- Pork NPH, 100 Units ... 1506
- Purified Pork NPH Isophane Insulin ... 1852

Insulin, Regular (Systemic clonidine may inhibit the production of catecholamines in response to insulin-induced hypoglycemia and mask the signs and symptoms of hypoglycemia). Products include:
- Regular, 100 Units ... 1503
- Pork Regular, 100 Units ... 1507
- Pork Regular (Concentrated), 500 Units ... 1508
- Purified Pork Regular Insulin ... 1852

Insulin, Zinc Crystals (Systemic clonidine may inhibit the production of catecholamines in response to insulin-induced hypoglycemia and mask the signs and symptoms of hypoglycemia). Products include:
- NPH, 100 Units ... 1502

Insulin, Zinc Suspension (Systemic clonidine may inhibit the production of catecholamines in response to insulin-induced hypoglycemia and mask the signs and symptoms of hypoglycemia). Products include:
- Iletin I ... 1501
- Lente, 100 Units ... 1501
- Iletin II ... 1504
- Pork Lente, 100 Units ... 1504
- Purified Pork Lente Insulin ... 1852

Isocarboxazid (Concurrent use is contraindicated).
- No products indexed under this heading.

Isoflurane (Possible additive or potentiating effect with CNS depressant).
- No products indexed under this heading.

Isradipine (Apraclonidine reduces pulse and blood pressure, caution is advised when used concurrently). Products include:
- DynaCirc Capsules ... 2381
- DynaCirc CR Tablets ... 2383

Ketamine Hydrochloride (Possible additive or potentiating effect with CNS depressant).
- No products indexed under this heading.

Labetalol Hydrochloride (Apraclonidine reduces pulse and blood pressure, caution is advised when used concurrently). Products include:
- Normodyne Injection ... 2519
- Normodyne Tablets ... 2522
- Trandate ... 1158

Levobunolol Hydrochloride (Apraclonidine reduces pulse and blood pressure, caution is advised when used concurrently). Products include:
- Betagan ... ◉ 230

Levomethadyl Acetate Hydrochloride (Possible additive or potentiating effect with CNS depressant). Products include:
- Orlaam Oral Solution ... 2361

Levorphanol Tartrate (Possible additive or potentiating effect with CNS depressant). Products include:
- Levo-Dromoran ... 2297

Lisinopril (Apraclonidine reduces pulse and blood pressure, caution is advised when used concurrently). Products include:
- Prinivil Tablets ... 1776
- Prinzide Tablets ... 1780
- Zestoretic Tablets ... 2968
- Zestril Tablets ... 2972

Lithium Carbonate (An additive hypotensive effect has been reported with the combination of systemic clonidine and neuroleptic therapy). Products include:
- Eskalith ... 2658
- Lithium Carbonate Capsules & Tablets ... 2352
- Lithonate/Lithotabs/Lithobid ... 2721

Lithium Citrate (An additive hypotensive effect has been reported with the combination of systemic clonidine and neuroleptic therapy).
- No products indexed under this heading.

Lorazepam (Possible additive or potentiating effect with CNS depressant). Products include:
- Ativan Injection ... 2805
- Ativan Tablets ... 2807

Losartan Potassium (Apraclonidine reduces pulse and blood pressure, caution is advised when used concurrently). Products include:
- Cozaar Tablets ... 1668
- Hyzaar Tablets ... 1720

Loxapine Hydrochloride (An additive hypotensive effect has been reported with the combination of systemic clonidine and neuroleptic therapy; possible additive or potentiating effect with CNS depressant). Products include:
- Loxitane ... 1426

Loxapine Succinate (An additive hypotensive effect has been reported with the combination of systemic clonidine and neuroleptic therapy; possible additive or potentiating effect with CNS depressant). Products include:
- Loxitane Capsules ... 1426

Maprotiline Hydrochloride (Tricyclic antidepressants have been reported to blunt the hypotensive effect of clonidine; it is not known whether the concurrent use with apraclonidine can lead to reduction in IOP lowering effect). Products include:
- Ludiomil Tablets ... 861

Mecamylamine Hydrochloride (Apraclonidine reduces pulse and blood pressure, caution is advised when used concurrently). Products include:
- Inversine Tablets ... 1729

Meperidine Hydrochloride (Possible additive or potentiating effect with CNS depressant). Products include:
- Demerol ... 2438
- Mepergan Injection ... 2859

Mephobarbital (Possible additive or potentiating effect with CNS depressant). Products include:
- Mebaral Tablets ... 2452

Meprobamate (Possible additive or potentiating effect with CNS depressant). Products include:
- Miltown Tablets ... 2780
- PMB 200 and PMB 400 ... 2890

Mesoridazine Besylate (An additive hypotensive effect has been reported with the combination of systemic clonidine and neuroleptic therapy; possible additive or potentiating effect with cns depressant). Products include:
- Serentil ... 689

Methadone Hydrochloride (Possible additive or potentiating effect with CNS depressant). Products include:
- Methadone Hydrochloride Oral Concentrate ... 2356
- Methadone Hydrochloride Oral Solution & Tablets ... 2357

Methohexital Sodium (Possible additive or potentiating effect with CNS depressant).
- No products indexed under this heading.

Methotrimeprazine (An additive hypotensive effect has been reported with the combination of systemic clonidine and neuroleptic therapy; possible additive or potentiating effect with CNS depressant). Products include:
- Levoprome ... 1321

Methoxyflurane (Possible additive or potentiating effect with CNS depressant).
- No products indexed under this heading.

Methyclothiazide (Apraclonidine reduces pulse and blood pressure, caution is advised when used concurrently). Products include:
- Enduron Tablets ... 424

Methyldopa (Apraclonidine reduces pulse and blood pressure, caution is advised when used concurrently). Products include:
- Aldoclor Tablets ... 1638
- Aldomet Oral ... 1640
- Aldoril Tablets ... 1644

Methyldopate Hydrochloride (Apraclonidine reduces pulse and blood pressure, caution is advised when used concurrently). Products include:
- Aldomet Ester HCl Injection ... 1642

Metipranolol Hydrochloride (Apraclonidine reduces pulse and blood pressure, caution is advised when used concurrently). Products include:
- OptiPranolol (Metipranolol 0.3%) Sterile Ophthalmic Solution ... ◉ 256

Metolazone (Apraclonidine reduces pulse and blood pressure, caution is advised when used concurrently). Products include:
- Mykrox Tablets ... 1617
- Zaroxolyn Tablets ... 1625

Metoprolol Succinate (Apraclonidine reduces pulse and blood pressure, caution is advised when used concurrently). Products include:
- Toprol-XL Tablets ... 560

Metoprolol Tartrate (Apraclonidine reduces pulse and blood pressure, caution is advised when used concurrently). Products include:
- Lopressor ... 848
- Lopressor HCT Tablets ... 850

Metyrosine (Apraclonidine reduces pulse and blood pressure, caution is advised when used concurrently). Products include:
- Demser Capsules ... 1690

Midazolam Hydrochloride (Possible additive or potentiating effect with CNS depressant). Products include:
- Versed Injection ... 2324

Minoxidil (Apraclonidine reduces pulse and blood pressure, caution is advised when used concurrently).
- No products indexed under this heading.

Moexipril Hydrochloride (Apraclonidine reduces pulse and blood pressure, caution is advised when used concurrently). Products include:
- Univasc Tablets ... 2553

Molindone Hydrochloride (An additive hypotensive effect has been reported with the combination of systemic clonidine and neuroleptic therapy; possible additive or potentiating effect with CNS depressant). Products include:
- Moban Tablets and Concentrate ... 1036

Morphine Sulfate (Possible additive or potentiating effect with CNS depressant). Products include:
- Astramorph/PF Injection, USP (Preservative-Free) ... 526
- Duramorph Injection ... 983
- Infumorph 200 and Infumorph 500 Sterile Solutions ... 985
- Kadian Capsules ... 2948
- MS Contin Tablets ... 2149
- MSIR ... 2152
- Oramorph SR (Morphine Sulfate Sustained Release Tablets) ... 2359
- RMS Suppositories CII ... 2766
- Roxanol ... 2365

Nadolol (Apraclonidine reduces pulse and blood pressure, caution is advised when used concurrently).
- No products indexed under this heading.

(Described in PDR For Nonprescription Drugs) (◉ Described in PDR For Ophthalmology)

Nicardipine Hydrochloride (Apraclonidine reduces pulse and blood pressure, caution is advised when used concurrently). Products include:
Cardene Capsules 2261
Cardene I.V. 2815
Cardene SR Capsules 2264

Nifedipine (Apraclonidine reduces pulse and blood pressure, caution is advised when used concurrently). Products include:
Adalat Capsules (10 mg and 20 mg) 580
Adalat CC 582
Procardia Capsules 2024
Procardia XL Extended Release Tablets 2026

Nisoldipine (Apraclonidine reduces pulse and blood pressure, caution is advised when used concurrently). Products include:
Sular Tablets 2961

Nitroglycerin (Apraclonidine reduces pulse and blood pressure, caution is advised when used concurrently). Products include:
Deponit NTG Transdermal Delivery System 2541
Nitro-Bid IV 1270
Nitro-Bid Ointment 1272
Nitro-Dur (nitroglycerin) Transdermal Infusion System 1365
Nitrolingual Spray 2193
Nitrostat Tablets 1981
Transderm-Nitro Transdermal Therapeutic System 878

Nortriptyline Hydrochloride (Tricyclic antidepressants have been reported to blunt the hypotensive effect of clonidine; it is not known whether the concurrent use with apraclonidine can lead to reduction in IOP lowering effect). Products include:
Pamelor 2409

Opium Alkaloids (Possible additive or potentiating effect with CNS depressant).
No products indexed under this heading.

Oxazepam (Possible additive or potentiating effect with CNS depressant). Products include:
Serax Capsules 2916
Serax Tablets 2916

Oxycodone Hydrochloride (Possible additive or potentiating effect with CNS depressant). Products include:
OxyContin Tablets 2163
OxyIR Capsules 2167
Percocet Tablets 955
Percodan Tablets 955
Percodan-Demi Tablets 956
Roxicodone Tablets, Oral Solution & Intensol (Oxycodone) 2366
Tylox Capsules 1593

Penbutolol Sulfate (Apraclonidine reduces pulse and blood pressure, caution is advised when used concurrently). Products include:
Levatol Tablets 2547

Pentobarbital Sodium (Possible additive or potentiating effect with CNS depressant). Products include:
Nembutal Sodium Capsules 440
Nembutal Sodium Solution 442
Nembutal Sodium Suppositories 444

Perphenazine (An additive hypotensive effect has been reported with the combination of systemic clonidine and neuroleptic therapy; possible additive or potentiating effect with CNS depressant). Products include:
Etrafon 2495
Triavil Tablets 1800
Trilafon 2532

Phenelzine Sulfate (Concurrent use is contraindicated). Products include:
Nardil 1977

Phenobarbital (Possible additive or potentiating effect with CNS depressant). Products include:
Arco-Lase Plus Tablets 513
Bellergal-S Tablets 2375
Donnatal 2234
Donnatal Extentabs 2234
Donnatal Tablets 2234
Phenobarbital Elixir and Tablets 1523
Quadrinal Tablets 1398

Phenoxybenzamine Hydrochloride (Apraclonidine reduces pulse and blood pressure, caution is advised when used concurrently). Products include:
Dibenzyline Capsules 2650

Phentolamine Mesylate (Apraclonidine reduces pulse and blood pressure, caution is advised when used concurrently). Products include:
Regitine Vials 864

Pimozide (An additive hypotensive effect has been reported with the combination of systemic clonidine and neuroleptic therapy). Products include:
Orap Tablets 1037

Pindolol (Apraclonidine reduces pulse and blood pressure, caution is advised when used concurrently). Products include:
Visken Tablets 2428

Polythiazide (Apraclonidine reduces pulse and blood pressure, caution is advised when used concurrently). Products include:
Minizide Capsules 2016

Prazepam (Possible additive or potentiating effect with CNS depressant).
No products indexed under this heading.

Prazosin Hydrochloride (Apraclonidine reduces pulse and blood pressure, caution is advised when used concurrently). Products include:
Minipress Capsules 2015
Minizide Capsules 2016

Prochlorperazine (An additive hypotensive effect has been reported with the combination of systemic clonidine and neuroleptic therapy; possible additive or potentiating effect with CNS depressant). Products include:
Compazine 2644

Promethazine Hydrochloride (An additive hypotensive effect has been reported with the combination of systemic clonidine and neuroleptic therapy; possible additive or potentiating effect with CNS depressant). Products include:
Mepergan Injection 2859
Phenergan with Codeine 2883
Phenergan with Dextromethorphan 2885
Phenergan Injection 2880
Phenergan Suppositories 2882
Phenergan Syrup 2881
Phenergan Tablets 2882
Phenergan VC 2886
Phenergan VC with Codeine 2888

Propofol (Possible additive or potentiating effect with CNS depressant). Products include:
Diprivan Injectable Emulsion 2939

Propoxyphene Hydrochloride (Possible additive or potentiating effect with CNS depressant). Products include:
Darvon 1475
Wygesic Tablets 2930

Propoxyphene Napsylate (Possible additive or potentiating effect with CNS depressant). Products include:
Darvon-N/Darvocet-N 1473

Propranolol Hydrochloride (Apraclonidine reduces pulse and blood pressure, caution is advised when used concurrently). Products include:
Inderal 2834
Inderal LA Long Acting Capsules 2836
Inderide Tablets 2838
Inderide LA Long Acting Capsules 2840

Protriptyline Hydrochloride (Tricyclic antidepressants have been reported to blunt the hypotensive effect of clonidine; it is not known whether the concurrent use with apraclonidine can lead to reduction in IOP lowering effect). Products include:
Vivactil Tablets 1820

Quazepam (Possible additive or potentiating effect with CNS depressant). Products include:
Doral Tablets 2773

Quinapril Hydrochloride (Apraclonidine reduces pulse and blood pressure, caution is advised when used concurrently). Products include:
Accupril Tablets 1950

Ramipril (Apraclonidine reduces pulse and blood pressure, caution is advised when used concurrently). Products include:
Altace Capsules 1238

Rauwolfia Serpentina (Apraclonidine reduces pulse and blood pressure, caution is advised when used concurrently).
No products indexed under this heading.

Rescinnamine (Apraclonidine reduces pulse and blood pressure, caution is advised when used concurrently).
No products indexed under this heading.

Reserpine (Apraclonidine reduces pulse and blood pressure, caution is advised when used concurrently). Products include:
Diupres Tablets 1691
Hydropres Tablets 1718
Ser-Ap-Es Tablets 867

Risperidone (An additive hypotensive effect has been reported with the combination of systemic clonidine and neuroleptic therapy; possible additive or potentiating effect with CNS depressant). Products include:
Risperdal Tablets 1348

Secobarbital Sodium (Possible additive or potentiating effect with CNS depressant). Products include:
Seconal Sodium Pulvules 1529

Selegiline Hydrochloride (Concurrent use is contraindicated). Products include:
Eldepryl Capsules 2729

Sevoflurane (Possible additive or potentiating effect with CNS depressant).
No products indexed under this heading.

Sodium Nitroprusside (Apraclonidine reduces pulse and blood pressure, caution is advised when used concurrently).
No products indexed under this heading.

Sotalol Hydrochloride (Apraclonidine reduces pulse and blood pressure, caution is advised when used concurrently). Products include:
Betapace Tablets 637

Spirapril Hydrochloride (Apraclonidine reduces pulse and blood pressure, caution is advised when used concurrently).
No products indexed under this heading.

Sufentanil Citrate (Possible additive or potentiating effect with CNS depressant). Products include:
Sufenta Injection 1355

Temazepam (Possible additive or potentiating effect with CNS depressant). Products include:
Restoril Capsules 2413

Terazosin Hydrochloride (Apraclonidine reduces pulse and blood pressure, caution is advised when used concurrently). Products include:
Hytrin Capsules 434

Thiamylal Sodium (Possible additive or potentiating effect with CNS depressant).
No products indexed under this heading.

Thioridazine Hydrochloride (An additive hypotensive effect has been reported with the combination of systemic clonidine and neuroleptic therapy; possible additive or potentiating effect with CNS depressant). Products include:
Mellaril 2398

Thiothixene (An additive hypotensive effect has been reported with the combination of systemic clonidine and neuroleptic therapy; possible additive or potentiating effect with CNS depressant). Products include:
Navane Capsules and Concentrate 2018
Navane Intramuscular 2019

Timolol Hemihydrate (Apraclonidine reduces pulse and blood pressure, caution is advised when used concurrently). Products include:
Betimol 0.25%, 0.5% .... ◉ 259

Timolol Maleate (Apraclonidine reduces pulse and blood pressure, caution is advised when used concurrently). Products include:
Blocadren Tablets 1654
Timolide Tablets 1791
Timoptic in Ocudose 1796
Timoptic Sterile Ophthalmic Solution 1794
Timoptic-XE 1798

Torsemide (Apraclonidine reduces pulse and blood pressure, caution is advised when used concurrently). Products include:
Demadex Tablets and Injection 691

Tranylcypromine Sulfate (Concurrent use is contraindicated). Products include:
Parnate Tablets 2679

Triazolam (Possible additive or potentiating effect with CNS depressant). Products include:
Halcion Tablets 2093

Trifluoperazine Hydrochloride (An additive hypotensive effect has been reported with the combination of systemic clonidine and neuroleptic therapy; possible additive or potentiating effect with CNS depressant). Products include:
Stelazine 2692

IMPORTANT NOTE: Always consult each drug listing in the patient's regimen for possible interactions.

Iopidine — Interactions Index

Trimethaphan Camsylate (Apraclonidine reduces pulse and blood pressure, caution is advised when used concurrently).
No products indexed under this heading.

Trimipramine Maleate (Tricyclic antidepressants have been reported to blunt the hypotensive effect of clonidine; it is not known whether the concurrent use with apraclonidine can lead to reduction in IOP lowering effect). Products include:
- Surmontil Capsules 2917

Verapamil Hydrochloride (Apraclonidine reduces pulse and blood pressure, caution is advised when used concurrently). Products include:
- Calan SR Caplets 2571
- Calan Tablets 2568
- Covera-HS Tablets 2573
- Isoptin Injectable 1391
- Isoptin Oral Tablets 1393
- Isoptin SR Tablets 1395
- Verelan Capsules 1455

Zolpidem Tartrate (Possible additive or potentiating effect with CNS depressant). Products include:
- Ambien Tablets 2559

IPOL POLIOVIRUS VACCINE INACTIVATED
(Poliovirus Vaccine Inactivated, Trivalent Types 1,2,3) 903
None cited in PDR database.

IROSPAN CAPSULES
(Ferrous Sulfate, Vitamin C) 1000
None cited in PDR database.

IROSPAN TABLETS
(Ferrous Sulfate, Vitamin C) 1000
None cited in PDR database.

ISMELIN TABLETS
(Guanethidine Monosulfate) 845
May interact with monoamine oxidase inhibitors, tricyclic antidepressants, phenothiazines, estrogens, thiazides, oral contraceptives, cardiac glycosides, and certain other agents. Compounds in these categories include:

Amitriptyline Hydrochloride (Reduces hypotensive effect). Products include:
- Elavil 2945
- Etrafon 2495
- Limbitrol 2333
- Triavil Tablets 1800

Amoxapine (Reduces hypotensive effect). Products include:
- Asendin Tablets 1419

Bendroflumethiazide (Enhances antihypertensive action of Ismelin).
No products indexed under this heading.

Chlorothiazide (Enhances antihypertensive action of Ismelin). Products include:
- Aldoclor Tablets 1638
- Diupres Tablets 1691
- Diuril Oral 1694

Chlorothiazide Sodium (Enhances antihypertensive action of Ismelin). Products include:
- Diuril Sodium Intravenous 1693

Chlorotrianisene (Reduces hypotensive effect).
No products indexed under this heading.

Chlorpromazine (Reduces hypotensive effect). Products include:
- Thorazine Suppositories 2701

Clomipramine Hydrochloride (Reduces hypotensive effect). Products include:
- Anafranil Capsules 819

Deserpidine (May result in excessive postural hypotension, bradycardia, and mental depression).
No products indexed under this heading.

Desipramine Hydrochloride (Reduces hypotensive effect). Products include:
- Norpramin Tablets 1273

Deslanoside (Slow heart rate).
No products indexed under this heading.

Desogestrel (Reduces hypotensive effect). Products include:
- Desogen Tablets 1867
- Ortho-Cept 1907

Dienestrol (Reduces hypotensive effect). Products include:
- Ortho Dienestrol Cream 1922

Diethylstilbestrol (Reduces hypotensive effect). Products include:
- Diethylstilbestrol Tablets 1477

Digitoxin (Slow heart rate). Products include:
- Crystodigin Tablets 1472

Digoxin (Slow heart rate). Products include:
- Lanoxicaps 1110
- Lanoxin Elixir Pediatric 1113
- Lanoxin Injection 1116
- Lanoxin Injection Pediatric 1119
- Lanoxin Tablets 1121

Doxepin Hydrochloride (Reduces hypotensive effect). Products include:
- Adapin Capsules 1542
- Sinequan 2028
- Zonalon Cream 1042

Ephedrine Hydrochloride (Reduces hypotensive effect). Products include:
- Primatene Tablets 844
- Quadrinal Tablets 1398

Ephedrine Sulfate (Reduces hypotensive effect). Products include:
- Marax Tablets & DF Syrup 2015

Ephedrine Tannate (Reduces hypotensive effect). Products include:
- Rynatuss 2782

Estradiol (Reduces hypotensive effect). Products include:
- Climara Transdermal System 640
- Estrace Cream and Tablets 751
- Estraderm Transdermal System 842
- Estring Vaginal Ring 2086
- Vivelle Transdermal System 880

Estrogens, Conjugated (Reduces hypotensive effect). Products include:
- PMB 200 and PMB 400 2890
- Premarin Intravenous 2893
- Premarin Tablets 2896
- Premarin Vaginal Cream 2898
- Premphase 2900
- Prempro 2905

Estrogens, Esterified (Reduces hypotensive effect). Products include:
- ESTRATAB Tablets (0.3, 0.625, 1.25, 2.5 mg) 2715
- Estratest 2718
- Menest Tablets 2671

Estropipate (Reduces hypotensive effect). Products include:
- Ogen Tablets 2103
- Ogen Vaginal Cream 2106
- Ortho-Est 1925

Ethinyl Estradiol (Reduces hypotensive effect). Products include:
- Brevicon 2563
- Demulen 2580
- Desogen Tablets 1867
- Levlen/Tri-Levlen 646
- Lo/Ovral Tablets 2852
- Lo/Ovral-28 Tablets 2857
- Modicon 1928
- Nordette-21 Tablets 2863
- Nordette-28 Tablets 2866
- Norinyl 2563
- Ortho-Cept 1907
- Ortho-Cyclen/Ortho Tri-Cyclen 1914
- Ortho-Novum 1928
- Ortho-Cyclen/Ortho Tri-Cyclen 1914
- Ovcon 765
- Ovral Tablets 2877
- Ovral-28 Tablets 2878
- Levlen/Tri-Levlen 646
- Tri-Norinyl 2607
- Triphasil-21 Tablets 2919
- Triphasil-28 Tablets 2924

Ethynodiol Diacetate (Reduces hypotensive effect). Products include:
- Demulen 2580

Fluphenazine Decanoate (Reduces hypotensive effect). Products include:
- Prolixin Decanoate 510

Fluphenazine Enanthate (Reduces hypotensive effect). Products include:
- Prolixin Enanthate 510

Fluphenazine Hydrochloride (Reduces hypotensive effect). Products include:
- Prolixin 510

Furazolidone (Concurrent use contraindicated). Products include:
- Furoxone 2221

Hydrochlorothiazide (Enhances antihypertensive action of Ismelin). Products include:
- Aldactazide Tablets 2556
- Aldoril Tablets 1644
- Apresazide Capsules 824
- Capozide Tablets 744
- Dyazide Capsules 2653
- Esidrix Tablets 839
- Esimil Tablets 840
- HydroDIURIL Tablets 1716
- Hydropres Tablets 1718
- Hyzaar Tablets 1720
- Inderide Tablets 2838
- Inderide LA Long Acting Capsules 2840
- Lopressor HCT Tablets 850
- Lotensin HCT Tablets 855
- Moduretic Tablets 1748
- Oretic Tablets 450
- Prinzide Tablets 1780
- Ser-Ap-Es Tablets 867
- Timolide Tablets 1791
- Vaseretic Tablets 1810
- Zestoretic Tablets 2968
- Ziac 1459

Hydroflumethiazide (Enhances antihypertensive action of Ismelin). Products include:
- Diucardin Tablets 2824

Imipramine Hydrochloride (Reduces hypotensive effect). Products include:
- Tofranil Ampuls 873
- Tofranil Tablets 875

Imipramine Pamoate (Reduces hypotensive effect). Products include:
- Tofranil-PM Capsules 876

Isocarboxazid (Concurrent use contraindicated).
No products indexed under this heading.

Levonorgestrel (Reduces hypotensive effect). Products include:
- Levlen/Tri-Levlen 646
- Nordette-21 Tablets 2863
- Nordette-28 Tablets 2866
- Norplant System 2868
- Levlen/Tri-Levlen 646
- Triphasil-21 Tablets 2919
- Triphasil-28 Tablets 2924

Maprotiline Hydrochloride (Reduces hypotensive effect). Products include:
- Ludiomil Tablets 861

Mesoridazine Besylate (Reduces hypotensive effect). Products include:
- Serentil 689

Mestranol (Reduces hypotensive effect). Products include:
- Norinyl 2563
- Ortho-Novum 1928

Methotrimeprazine (Reduces hypotensive effect). Products include:
- Levoprome 1321

Methyclothiazide (Reduces hypotensive effect). Products include:
- Enduron Tablets 424

Methylphenidate Hydrochloride (Reduces hypotensive effect). Products include:
- Ritalin 866

Norethindrone (Reduces hypotensive effect). Products include:
- Brevicon 2563
- Micronor Tablets 1903
- Modicon 1928
- Norinyl 2563
- Nor-Q D Tablets 2598
- Ortho-Novum 1928
- Ovcon 765
- Tri-Norinyl 2607

Norethynodrel (Reduces hypotensive effect).
No products indexed under this heading.

Norgestimate (Reduces hypotensive effect). Products include:
- Ortho-Cyclen/Ortho Tri-Cyclen 1914
- Ortho-Cyclen/Ortho Tri-Cyclen 1914

Norgestrel (Reduces hypotensive effect). Products include:
- Lo/Ovral Tablets 2852
- Lo/Ovral-28 Tablets 2857
- Ovral Tablets 2877
- Ovral-28 Tablets 2878
- Ovrette Tablets 2878

Nortriptyline Hydrochloride (Reduces hypotensive effect). Products include:
- Pamelor 2409

Perphenazine (Reduces hypotensive effect). Products include:
- Etrafon 2495
- Triavil Tablets 1800
- Trilafon 2532

Phenelzine Sulfate (Concurrent use contraindicated). Products include:
- Nardil 1977

Polyestradiol Phosphate (Reduces hypotensive effect).
No products indexed under this heading.

Polythiazide (Enhances antihypertensive action of Ismelin). Products include:
- Minizide Capsules 2016

Prochlorperazine (Reduces hypotensive effect). Products include:
- Compazine 2644

Promethazine Hydrochloride (Reduces hypotensive effect). Products include:
- Mepergan Injection 2859
- Phenergan with Codeine 2883
- Phenergan with Dextromethorphan 2885
- Phenergan Injection 2880
- Phenergan Suppositories 2882
- Phenergan Syrup 2881
- Phenergan Tablets 2882
- Phenergan VC 2886
- Phenergan VC with Codeine 2888

Protriptyline Hydrochloride (Reduces hypotensive effect). Products include:
- Vivactil Tablets 1820

Quinestrol (Reduces hypotensive effect).
No products indexed under this heading.

Rauwolfia Serpentina (May result in excessive postural hypotension, bradycardia, and mental depression).
No products indexed under this heading.

(⊞ Described in PDR For Nonprescription Drugs) (⊙ Described in PDR For Ophthalmology)

545 **Interactions Index** **Isoetharine Arm-A-Med**

Rescinnamine (May result in excessive postural hypotension, bradycardia, and mental depression).
No products indexed under this heading.
Reserpine (May result in excessive postural hypotension, bradycardia, and mental depression). Products include:
Diupres Tablets ... 1691
Hydropres Tablets ... 1718
Ser-Ap-Es Tablets ... 867
Selegiline Hydrochloride (Concurrent use contraindicated). Products include:
Eldepryl Capsules ... 2729
Thioridazine Hydrochloride (Reduces hypotensive effect). Products include:
Mellaril ... 2398
Tranylcypromine Sulfate (Concurrent use contraindicated). Products include:
Parnate Tablets ... 2679
Trifluoperazine Hydrochloride (Reduces hypotensive effect). Products include:
Stelazine ... 2692
Trimipramine Maleate (Reduces hypotensive effect). Products include:
Surmontil Capsules ... 2917

Food Interactions

Alcohol (Aggravates orthostatic hypotensive effects).

ISMO TABLETS
(Isosorbide Mononitrate) ... **2844**
May interact with vasodilators, calcium channel blockers, and certain other agents. Compounds in these categories include:

Amlodipine Besylate (Potential for marked symptomatic orthostatic hypotension). Products include:
Lotrel Capsules ... 858
Norvasc Tablets ... 2020
Bepridil Hydrochloride (Potential for marked symptomatic orthostatic hypotension). Products include:
Vascor Tablets (200 and 300 mg) 1597
Diazoxide (Additive vasodilating effects). Products include:
Hyperstat I.V. Injection ... 2504
Proglycem ... 575
Diltiazem Hydrochloride (Potential for marked symptomatic orthostatic hypotension). Products include:
Cardizem CD Capsules ... 1251
Cardizem SR Capsules ... 1255
Cardizem Injectable ... 1253
Cardizem Tablets ... 1257
Dilacor XR Extended-release Capsules ... 2183
Tiazac Capsules ... 1019
Epoprostenol Sodium (Additive vasodilating effects). Products include:
Flolan for Injection ... 1085
Felodipine (Potential for marked symptomatic orthostatic hypotension). Products include:
Plendil Extended-Release Tablets ... 514
Hydralazine Hydrochloride (Additive vasodilating effects). Products include:
Apresazide Capsules ... 824
Apresoline Hydrochloride Tablets ... 826
Hydralazine Hydrochloride Injection USP ... 2712
Ser-Ap-Es Tablets ... 867
Isradipine (Potential for marked symptomatic orthostatic hypotension). Products include:
DynaCirc Capsules ... 2381
DynaCirc CR Tablets ... 2383
Minoxidil (Additive vasodilating effects).
No products indexed under this heading.
Nicardipine Hydrochloride (Potential for marked symptomatic orthostatic hypotension). Products include:
Cardene Capsules ... 2261
Cardene I.V. ... 2815
Cardene SR Capsules ... 2264
Nifedipine (Potential for marked symptomatic orthostatic hypotension). Products include:
Adalat Capsules (10 mg and 20 mg) ... 580
Adalat CC ... 582
Procardia Capsules ... 2024
Procardia XL Extended Release Tablets ... 2026
Nimodipine (Potential for marked symptomatic orthostatic hypotension). Products include:
Nimotop Capsules ... 603
Nisoldipine (Potential for marked symptomatic orthostatic hypotension). Products include:
Sular Tablets ... 2961
Verapamil Hydrochloride (Potential for marked symptomatic orthostatic hypotension). Products include:
Calan SR Caplets ... 2571
Calan Tablets ... 2568
Covera-HS Tablets ... 2573
Isoptin Injectable ... 1391
Isoptin Oral Tablets ... 1393
Isoptin SR Tablets ... 1395
Verelan Capsules ... 1455

Food Interactions

Alcohol (Additive vasodilating effects).

ISMOTIC 45% W/V SOLUTION
(Isosorbide) ... ◉ 221
None cited in PDR database.

ISOETHARINE INHALATION SOLUTION, USP, ARM-A-MED
(Isoetharine) ... 545
May interact with sympathomimetics. Compounds in this category include:

Albuterol (May cause excessive tachycardia). Products include:
Proventil Inhalation Aerosol ... 2524
Ventolin Inhalation Aerosol and Refill ... 1170
Albuterol Sulfate (May cause excessive tachycardia). Products include:
Airet Albuterol Sulfate Inhalation Solution ... 1602
Albuterol Sulfate, USP Solution for Inhalation, Arm-a-Med ... 522
Proventil Inhalation Solution 0.083% ... 2527
Proventil Repetabs Tablets ... 2529
Proventil Solution for Inhalation 0.5% ... 2525
Proventil Syrup ... 2528
Proventil Tablets ... 2529
Ventolin Inhalation Solution ... 1171
Ventolin Nebules Inhalation Solution ... 1172
Ventolin Rotacaps for Inhalation ... 1173
Ventolin Syrup ... 1175
Ventolin Tablets ... 1176
Volmax Extended-Release Tablets .. 1835
Dobutamine Hydrochloride (May cause excessive tachycardia). Products include:
Dobutrex Solution Vials ... 1480
Dopamine Hydrochloride (May cause excessive tachycardia).
No products indexed under this heading.
Ephedrine Hydrochloride (May cause excessive tachycardia). Products include:
Primatene Tablets ... ▣ 844
Quadrinal Tablets ... 1398
Ephedrine Sulfate (May cause excessive tachycardia). Products include:
Marax Tablets & DF Syrup ... 2015
Ephedrine Tannate (May cause excessive tachycardia). Products include:
Rynatuss ... 2782
Epinephrine (May cause excessive tachycardia). Products include:
EPIFRIN ... ◉ 237
EpiPen ... 808
Marcaine with Epinephrine ... 2446
Primatene Mist ... ▣ 843
Sensorcaine with Epinephrine Injection ... 554
Sus-Phrine Injection ... 1017
Xylocaine with Epinephrine Injections ... 562
Epinephrine Bitartrate (May cause excessive tachycardia). Products include:
Sensorcaine-MPF with Epinephrine Injection ... 554
Epinephrine Hydrochloride (May cause excessive tachycardia). Products include:
Ana-Kit Anaphylaxis Emergency Treatment Kit ... 611
Isoproterenol Hydrochloride (May cause excessive tachycardia). Products include:
Isuprel Hydrochloride Solution ... 2443
Isuprel Injection ... 2441
Isuprel Mistometer ... 2442
Isoproterenol Sulfate (May cause excessive tachycardia). Products include:
Norisodrine with Calcium Iodide Syrup ... 446
Metaproterenol Sulfate (May cause excessive tachycardia). Products include:
Alupent ... 672
Metaproterenol Sulfate Inhalation Solution, USP, Arm-a-Med ... 547
Metaraminol Bitartrate (May cause excessive tachycardia). Products include:
Aramine Injection ... 1649
Methoxamine Hydrochloride (May cause excessive tachycardia). Products include:
Vasoxyl Injection ... 1169
Norepinephrine Bitartrate (May cause excessive tachycardia). Products include:
Levophed Bitartrate Injection ... 2445
Phenylephrine Bitartrate (May cause excessive tachycardia).
No products indexed under this heading.
Phenylephrine Hydrochloride (May cause excessive tachycardia). Products include:
Atrohist Plus Tablets ... 1605
Cerose DM ... ▣ 853
D.A. II Tablets ... 972
D.A. Chewable Tablets ... 970
Dura-Vent/DA Tablets ... 972
Extendryl ... 1003
4-Way Fast Acting Nasal Spray (regular & mentholated) ... ▣ 644
Hemorid ... ▣ 797
Hycomine Compound Tablets ... 948
Neo-Synephrine Hydrochloride 1% Carpuject ... 2455
Neo-Synephrine Hydrochloride 1% Injection ... 2455
Neo-Synephrine Hydrochloride (Ophthalmic) ... 2456
Neo-Synephrine ... ▣ 624
Novahistine Elixir ... ▣ 782
Phenergan VC ... 2886
Phenergan VC with Codeine ... 2888
Preparation H ... ▣ 842
Tympagesic Ear Drops ... 2476
Vicks Sinex Nasal Spray and Ultra Fine Mist ... ▣ 738
Phenylephrine Tannate (May cause excessive tachycardia). Products include:
Atrohist Pediatric Suspension ... 1604
Atrohist Pediatric Suspension Dye-Free ... 1604
Rynatan ... 2781
Rynatuss ... 2782
Phenylpropanolamine Hydrochloride (May cause excessive tachycardia). Products include:
Acutrim ... ▣ 648
Atrohist Plus Tablets ... 1605
BC Cold Powder Multi-Symptom Formula (Cold-Sinus-Allergy) ... ▣ 631
BC Cold Powder Non-Drowsy Formula (Cold-Sinus) ... ▣ 631
Cheracol Plus Head Cold/Cough Formula ... ▣ 741
Comtrex Multi-Symptom Cold Reliever Liqui-Gels ... ▣ 638
Comtrex Multi-Symptom Non-Drowsy Liqui-gels ... ▣ 640
Contac Continuous Action Nasal Decongestant/Antihistamine 12 Hour Capsules ... ▣ 773
Contac Maximum Strength Continuous Action Decongestant/Antihistamine 12 Hour Caplets .. ▣ 772
Contac Severe Cold and Flu Formula Caplets ... ▣ 773
Coricidin 'D' Decongestant Tablets ... ▣ 760
Dexatrim ... ▣ 795
Dexatrim Plus Vitamins Caplets ... ▣ 796
Dimetane-DC Cough Syrup ... 2232
Dimetapp Allergy Sinus Caplets ... ▣ 838
Dimetapp Cold & Allergy Chewable Tablets ... ▣ 838
Dimetapp Cold & Cough Liqui-Gels ... ▣ 839
Dimetapp DM Elixir ... ▣ 840
Dimetapp Elixir ... ▣ 840
Dimetapp Extentabs ... ▣ 841
Dimetapp Tablets/Liqui-Gels ... ▣ 841
Dura-Vent Tablets ... 971
Entex LA Tablets ... 972
Exgest LA Tablets ... 787
Hycomine ... 947
Nolamine Timed-Release Tablets ... 790
Ornade Spansule Capsules ... 2678
Propagest Tablets ... 791
Pyrroxate Caplets ... ▣ 742
Robitussin-CF ... ▣ 846
Sinulin Tablets ... 792
Tavist-D 12 Hour Relief Tablets ... ▣ 750
Teldrin 12 Hour Antihistamine/Nasal Decongestant Allergy Relief Capsules ... ▣ 786
Triaminic Expectorant ... ▣ 753
Triaminic Syrup ... ▣ 755
Triaminic Triaminicol Cold & Cough ... ▣ 756
Triaminic DM Syrup ... ▣ 756
Triaminicin Tablets ... ▣ 756
Vicks DayQuil Allergy Relief 12-Hour Extended Release Tablets.. ▣ 733
Vicks DayQuil Allergy Relief 4-Hour Tablets ... ▣ 733
Vicks DayQuil SINUS Pressure & CONGESTION Relief ... ▣ 734
Pirbuterol Acetate (May cause excessive tachycardia). Products include:
Maxair Autohaler ... 1550
Maxair Inhaler ... 1552
Pseudoephedrine Hydrochloride (May cause excessive tachycardia). Products include:
Actifed Allergy Daytime/Nighttime Caplets ... ▣ 808
Actifed Cold & Allergy Tablets ... ▣ 807
Actifed Cold & Sinus Caplets and Tablets ... ▣ 808
Actifed Sinus Daytime/Nighttime Tablets and Caplets ... ▣ 809
Advil Cold and Sinus Caplets and Tablets ... ▣ 837
Alka-Seltzer Plus Liqui-Gels ... ▣ 612
Alka-Seltzer Plus Flu & Body Aches Liqui-Gels Non-Drowsy Formula ... ▣ 613
Alka-Seltzer Plus Night-Time Cold Medicine Liqui-Gels ... ▣ 612
Allerest Maximum Strength ... ▣ 649
Allerest No Drowsiness ... ▣ 649
Allerest Sinus Pain Formula ... ▣ 649

IMPORTANT NOTE: Always consult each drug listing in the patient's regimen for possible interactions.

Isoetharine Arm-A-Med / Interactions Index

Product	Page
Atrohist Pediatric Capsules	1603
Benadryl Allergy/Cold Tablets	▣ 811
Benadryl Allergy Decongestant Liquid Medication	▣ 812
Benadryl Allergy Decongestant Tablets	▣ 812
Benadryl Allergy Sinus Headache Caplets	▣ 813
Benylin Multisymptom	▣ 816
Bromfed Capsules (Extended-Release)	1832
Bromfed Syrup	▣ 712
Bromfed Tablets	1832
Bromfed-DM Cough Syrup	1832
Bromfed-PD Capsules (Extended-Release)	1832
Children's TYLENOL Cold Multi-Symptom Chewable Tablets and Liquid	1559
Children's TYLENOL Cold Plus Cough Multi Symptom Chewable Tablets and Liquid	1560
Children's TYLENOL Flu Suspension Liquid	1560
Children's Vicks DayQuil Allergy Relief	▣ 730
Children's Vicks NyQuil Cold/Cough Relief	▣ 731
Allergy-Sinus Comtrex Multi-Symptom Allergy-Sinus Formula Tablets and Caplets	▣ 639
Comtrex Multi-Symptom	▣ 638
Comtrex Multi-Symptom Non-Drowsy Caplets	▣ 640
Congess	1003
Contac Day Allergy/Sinus Caplets	▣ 771
Contac Day & Night	▣ 772
Contac Night Allergy/Sinus Caplets	▣ 771
Contac Severe Cold & Flu Non-Drowsy	▣ 774
Deconsal II Tablets	1605
Dimetane-DX Cough Syrup	2233
Dimetapp Cold & Fever Suspension	▣ 839
Dimetapp Decongestant Pediatric Drops	▣ 840
Dorcol Children's Cough Syrup	▣ 748
Drixoral Cough + Congestion Liquid Caps	▣ 763
Dura-Tap/PD Capsules	970
Duratuss Tablets	2750
Duratuss HD Elixir	2750
Efidac/24	▣ 655
Entex PSE Tablets	973
Fedahist Gyrocaps	2545
Guaifed	1833
Guaifed Syrup	▣ 712
Guaimax-D Tablets	809
Histussin D Liquid	670
Infants' TYLENOL Cold Decongestant & Fever-Reducer Drops	1561
Kronofed-A	994
Novahistine DMX	▣ 782
Nucofed	2225
PediaCare Cough-Cold Chewable Tablets and Liquid	1569
PediaCare Infants' Decongestant Drops	1569
PediaCare Infants' Drops Decongestant Plus Cough	1569
PediaCare NightRest Cough-Cold Liquid	1569
Pediatric Vicks 44d Cough & Head Congestion Relief	▣ 736
Pediatric Vicks 44m Cough & Cold Relief	▣ 737
Robitussin Cold & Cough Liqui-Gels	▣ 844
Robitussin Cold, Cough & Flu Liqui-Gels	▣ 844
Robitussin Maximum Strength Cough & Cold	▣ 847
Robitussin Night-Time Cold Formula	▣ 847
Robitussin Pediatric Cough & Cold Formula	▣ 848
Robitussin Pediatric Drops	▣ 849
Robitussin Severe Congestion Liqui-Gels	▣ 845
Robitussin-DAC Syrup	2249
Robitussin-PE	▣ 846
Rondec Oral Drops	974
Rondec Syrup	974
Rondec Tablet	974
Rondec Chewable Tablets	974
Rondec-TR Tablet	974
Ryna	▣ 804
Seldane-D Extended-Release Tablets	1286
Semprex-D Capsules	1620
Sinarest	▣ 663
Sine-Aid Maximum Strength Sinus Headache Gelcaps, Caplets and Tablets	1570
Sine-Off No Drowsiness Formula Caplets	▣ 784
Sine-Off Sinus Medicine	▣ 784
Singlet Tablets	▣ 785
Sinutab Non-Drying Liquid Caps	▣ 823
Sinutab Sinus Allergy Medication, Maximum Strength Tablets and Caplets	▣ 823
Sinutab Sinus Medication, Maximum Strength Without Drowsiness Formula, Tablets & Caplets	▣ 824
Sudafed Children's Cold & Cough Liquid Medication	▣ 825
Sudafed Children's Nasal Decongestant Liquid Medication	▣ 826
Sudafed Cold & Allergy Tablets	▣ 826
Sudafed Cold and Cough Liquid Caps	▣ 826
Sudafed Nasal Decongestant Tablets, 30 mg	▣ 825
Sudafed Nasal Decongestant Tablets, 60 mg	▣ 825
Sudafed Non-Drying Sinus Liquid Caps	▣ 827
Sudafed Pediatric Nasal Decongestant Liquid Oral Drops	▣ 827
Sudafed Severe Cold Formula Caplets	▣ 828
Sudafed Severe Cold Formula Tablets	▣ 828
Sudafed Sinus Caplets	▣ 829
Sudafed Sinus Tablets	▣ 829
Sudafed 12 Hour Caplets	▣ 824
Syn-Rx Tablets	1622
Syn-Rx DM Tablets	1623
TheraFlu and Cold Medicine	▣ 750
TheraFlu Maximum Strength Flu and Cold Medicine For Sore Throat	▣ 751
TheraFlu Flu, Cold and Cough Medicine	▣ 750
TheraFlu Maximum Strength Nighttime Flu, Cold & Cough Medicine	▣ 751
TheraFlu Maximum Strength Non-Drowsy Formula Flu, Cold & Cough Medicine	▣ 751
TheraFlu Maximum Strength, Non-Drowsy Formula Flu, Cold and Cough Caplets	▣ 752
Theraflu Maximum Strength Sinus Non-Drowsy Formula Caplets	▣ 752
Triaminic AM Cough and Decongestant Formula	▣ 753
Triaminic AM Decongestant Formula	▣ 753
Triaminic Infant Oral Decongestant Drops	▣ 754
Triaminic Night Time	▣ 754
Triaminic Sore Throat Formula	▣ 755
Tussend	1830
Tussend Expectorant	1831
TYLENOL Allergy Sinus, Maximum Strength Caplets and Gelcaps	1571
TYLENOL Allergy Sinus NightTime, Maximum Strength Caplets	1571
TYLENOL Cold Medication, Multi-Symptom Formula Tablets and Caplets	1572
TYLENOL Cold Medication, Multi-Symptom Hot Liquid Packets	1572
TYLENOL Cold Medication, No Drowsiness Formula Caplets and Gelcaps	1572
TYLENOL Cold Severe Congestion Caplets	1573
TYLENOL Cough Medication with Decongestant, Multi Symptom	1574
TYLENOL Flu No Drowsiness Formula, Maximum Strength Gelcaps	1575
TYLENOL Flu NightTime, Maximum Strength Gelcaps	1575
TYLENOL Flu NightTime, Maximum Strength Hot Medication Packets	1575
TYLENOL Sinus, Maximum Strength Geltabs, Gelcaps, Caplets and Tablets	1576
Vicks 44 LiquiCaps Cough, Cold & Flu Relief	▣ 728
Vicks 44 LiquiCaps Non-Drowsy Cough & Cold Relief	▣ 729
Vicks 44D Cough & Head Congestion Relief	▣ 728
Vicks 44M Cough, Cold & Flu Relief	▣ 729
Vicks DayQuil LiquiCaps/Liquid Multi-Symptom Cold/Flu Relief	▣ 734
Vicks DayQuil SINUS Pressure & PAIN Relief with IBUPROFEN	▣ 735
Vicks Nyquil Hot Therapy	▣ 735
Vicks NyQuil LiquiCaps/Liquid Multi-Symptom Cold/Flu Relief, Original and Cherry Flavors	▣ 736

Pseudoephedrine Sulfate (May cause excessive tachycardia). Products include:

Chlor-Trimeton Allergy Decongestant Tablets	▣ 759
Claritin-D Tablets	2487
Drixoral Cold and Allergy Sustained-Action Tablets	▣ 763
Drixoral Cold and Flu Extended-Release Tablets	▣ 764
Drixoral Non-Drowsy Formula Extended-Release Tablets	▣ 764
Drixoral Allergy/Sinus Extended Release Tablets	▣ 765
Trinalin Repetabs Tablets	1373

Salmeterol Xinafoate (May cause excessive tachycardia). Products include:

Serevent Inhalation Aerosol	1149

Terbutaline Sulfate (May cause excessive tachycardia). Products include:

Brethaire Inhaler	830
Brethine Ampuls	832
Brethine Tablets	831
Bricanyl Subcutaneous Injection	1247
Bricanyl Tablets	1248

ISOPTIN AMPULES 5MG/2ML

(Verapamil Hydrochloride) 1391
May interact with beta blockers, alpha adrenergic blockers, inhalant anesthetics, nondepolarizing neuromuscular blocking agents, cardiac glycosides, lithium preparations, highly protein bound drugs (selected), and certain other agents. Compounds in these categories include:

Acebutolol Hydrochloride (Concomitant intravenous beta blocker therapy results in serious toxicity in patients with CHF, recent MI or severe cardiomyopathy). Products include:

Sectral Capsules	2914

Amiodarone Hydrochloride (Administer with caution to patients receiving other highly protein bound drugs). Products include:

Cordarone Intravenous	2821
Cordarone Tablets	2818

Amitriptyline Hydrochloride (Administer with caution to patients receiving other highly protein bound drugs). Products include:

Elavil	2945
Etrafon	2495
Limbitrol	2333
Triavil Tablets	1800

Atenolol (Concomitant intravenous beta blocker therapy results in serious toxicity in patients with CHF, recent MI or severe cardiomyopathy). Products include:

Tenoretic Tablets	2963
Tenormin Tablets and I.V. Injection	2965

Atovaquone (Administer with caution to patients receiving other highly protein bound drugs). Products include:

Mepron Suspension	1206

Atracurium Besylate (Verapamil may potentiate the activity of neuromuscular blocking agents). Products include:

Tracrium Injection	1155

Betaxolol Hydrochloride (Concomitant intravenous beta blocker therapy results in serious toxicity in patients with CHF, recent MI or severe cardiomyopathy). Products include:

Betoptic Ophthalmic Solution	465
Betoptic S Ophthalmic Suspension	467
Kerlone Tablets	2588

Bisoprolol Fumarate (Concomitant intravenous beta blocker therapy results in serious toxicity in patients with CHF, recent MI or severe cardiomyopathy). Products include:

Zebeta Tablets	1457
Ziac	1459

Carbamazepine (Increased carbamazepine concentrations resulting in increased side effects of carbamazepine). Products include:

Atretol Tablets	569
Tegretol/Tegretol-XR	870

Carteolol Hydrochloride (Concomitant intravenous beta blocker therapy results in serious toxicity in patients with CHF, recent MI or severe cardiomyopathy). Products include:

Cartrol Tablets	413
Ocupress Ophthalmic Solution, 1% Sterile	⊙ 297

Cefonicid Sodium (Administer with caution to patients receiving other highly protein bound drugs). Products include:

Monocid Injection	2674

Chlordiazepoxide (Administer with caution to patients receiving other highly protein bound drugs). Products include:

Limbitrol	2333

Chlordiazepoxide Hydrochloride (Administer with caution to patients receiving other highly protein bound drugs). Products include:

Librax Capsules	2330
Librium Capsules	2331
Librium Injectable	2332

Chlorpromazine (Administer with caution to patients receiving other highly protein bound drugs). Products include:

Thorazine Suppositories	2701

Chlorpromazine Hydrochloride (Administer with caution to patients receiving other highly protein bound drugs). Products include:

Thorazine	2701

Cimetidine (Variable results on verapamil clearance). Products include:

Tagamet HB Tablets	▣ 786
Tagamet Tablets	2694

Cimetidine Hydrochloride (Variable results on verapamil clearance). Products include:

Tagamet	2694

Cisatracurium Besylate (Verapamil may potentiate the activity of neuromuscular blocking agents). Products include:

Nimbex Injection	1131

Clomipramine Hydrochloride (Administer with caution to patients receiving other highly protein bound drugs). Products include:

Anafranil Capsules	819

Clozapine (Administer with caution to patients receiving other highly protein bound drugs). Products include:

Clozaril Tablets	2377

Cyclosporine (Increased serum levels of cyclosporin; administer with caution to patients receiving other highly protein bound drugs). Products include:

Neoral	2405

(▣ Described in PDR For Nonprescription Drugs)   (⊙ Described in PDR For Ophthalmology)

Interactions Index — Isoptin Injectable

Sandimmune 2416

Dantrolene Sodium (Concomitant use of both drugs by intravenous route may result in cardiovascular collapse). Products include:
- Dantrium Capsules 2131
- Dantrium Intravenous 2132

Desflurane (Excessive cardiovascular depression). Products include:
- Suprane (desflurane, USP) 1865

Deslanoside (Both drugs slow AV conduction resulting in possible AV block or excessive bradycardia).
No products indexed under this heading.

Diazepam (Administer with caution to patients receiving other highly protein bound drugs). Products include:
- Dizac (diazepam injectable emulsion) CIV 1862
- Valium Injectable 2336
- Valium Tablets 2335

Diclofenac Potassium (Administer with caution to patients receiving other highly protein bound drugs). Products include:
- Cataflam Tablets 833

Diclofenac Sodium (Administer with caution to patients receiving other highly protein bound drugs). Products include:
- Voltaren Ophthalmic Sterile Ophthalmic Solution .... ⓒ 264
- Cataflam/Voltaren/Voltaren-XR 833

Digitoxin (Both drugs slow AV conduction resulting in possible AV block or excessive bradycardia). Products include:
- Crystodigin Tablets 1472

Digoxin (Both drugs slow AV conduction resulting in possible AV block or excessive bradycardia). Products include:
- Lanoxicaps 1110
- Lanoxin Elixir Pediatric 1113
- Lanoxin Injection 1116
- Lanoxin Injection Pediatric 1119
- Lanoxin Tablets 1121

Dipyridamole (Administer with caution to patients receiving other highly protein bound drugs). Products include:
- Persantine Tablets 686

Disopyramide Phosphate (Do not administer within 48 hours before or 24 hours after verapamil). Products include:
- Norpace 2596

Doxazosin Mesylate (Exaggerated hypotensive response). Products include:
- Cardura Tablets 1993

Enflurane (Excessive cardiovascular depression).
No products indexed under this heading.

Esmolol Hydrochloride (Concomitant intravenous beta blocker therapy results in serious toxicity in patients with CHF, recent MI or severe cardiomyopathy). Products include:
- Brevibloc (esmolol HCl) Injection 1860

Fenoprofen Calcium (Administer with caution to patients receiving other highly protein bound drugs). Products include:
- Nalfon 200 Pulvules & Nalfon Tablets 933

Flecainide Acetate (Additive effects on myocardial contractility, AV conduction, and repolarization). Products include:
- Tambocor Tablets 1555

Flurazepam Hydrochloride (Administer with caution to patients receiving other highly protein bound drugs). Products include:
- Dalmane Capsules 2329

Flurbiprofen (Administer with caution to patients receiving other highly protein bound drugs).
No products indexed under this heading.

Glipizide (Administer with caution to patients receiving other highly protein bound drugs). Products include:
- Glucotrol Tablets 2011
- Glucotrol XL Extended Release Tablets 2012

Halothane (Excessive cardiovascular depression). Products include:
- Fluothane 2830

Ibuprofen (Administer with caution to patients receiving other highly protein bound drugs). Products include:
- Advil Cold and Sinus Caplets and Tablets .... ⓒ 837
- Advil Ibuprofen Tablets, Caplets and Gel Caplets .... ⓒ 836
- Children's Motrin Ibuprofen Oral Suspension 1558
- IBU Tablets 1389
- Ibuprohm .... ⓒ 713
- Motrin IB Caplets, Tablets, and Gelcaps .... ⓒ 802
- Motrin Ibuprofen Suspension, Oral Drops, Chewable Tablets, Caplets 1563
- Nuprin Ibuprofen/Analgesic Tablets & Caplets .... ⓒ 645
- Vicks DayQuil SINUS Pressure & PAIN Relief with IBUPROFEN .. ⓒ 735

Imipramine Hydrochloride (Administer with caution to patients receiving other highly protein bound drugs). Products include:
- Tofranil Ampuls 873
- Tofranil Tablets 875

Imipramine Pamoate (Administer with caution to patients receiving other highly protein bound drugs). Products include:
- Tofranil-PM Capsules 876

Indomethacin (Administer with caution to patients receiving other highly protein bound drugs). Products include:
- Indocin 1723

Indomethacin Sodium Trihydrate (Administer with caution to patients receiving other highly protein bound drugs). Products include:
- Indocin I.V. 1727

Isoflurane (Excessive cardiovascular depression).
No products indexed under this heading.

Ketoprofen (Administer with caution to patients receiving other highly protein bound drugs). Products include:
- Actron Caplets and Tablets .... ⓒ 608
- Orudis Capsules 2874
- Orudis KT .... ⓒ 842
- Oruvail Capsules 2874

Ketorolac Tromethamine (Administer with caution to patients receiving other highly protein bound drugs). Products include:
- Acular Sterile Ophthalmic Solution .. 470
- Toradol 2319

Labetalol Hydrochloride (Concomitant intravenous beta blocker therapy results in serious toxicity in patients with CHF, recent MI or severe cardiomyopathy). Products include:
- Normodyne Injection 2519
- Normodyne Tablets 2522
- Trandate 1158

Levobunolol Hydrochloride (Concomitant intravenous beta blocker therapy results in serious toxicity in patients with CHF, recent MI or severe cardiomyopathy). Products include:
- Betagan .... ⓒ 230

Lithium Carbonate (Increased sensitivity to effects of lithium). Products include:
- Eskalith 2658
- Lithium Carbonate Capsules & Tablets 2352
- Lithonate/Lithotabs/Lithobid 2721

Lithium Citrate (Increased sensitivity to effects of lithium).
No products indexed under this heading.

Meclofenamate Sodium (Administer with caution to patients receiving other highly protein bound drugs).
No products indexed under this heading.

Mefenamic Acid (Administer with caution to patients receiving other highly protein bound drugs). Products include:
- Ponstel 1982

Methoxyflurane (Excessive cardiovascular depression).
No products indexed under this heading.

Metipranolol Hydrochloride (Concomitant intravenous beta blocker therapy results in serious toxicity in patients with CHF, recent MI or severe cardiomyopathy). Products include:
- OptiPranolol (Metipranolol 0.3%) Sterile Ophthalmic Solution ...... ⓒ 256

Metocurine Iodide (Verapamil may potentiate the activity of neuromuscular blocking agents). Products include:
- Metubine Iodide Vials 932

Metoprolol Succinate (Concomitant intravenous beta blocker therapy results in serious toxicity in patients with CHF, recent MI or severe cardiomyopathy). Products include:
- Toprol-XL Tablets 560

Metoprolol Tartrate (Concomitant intravenous beta blocker therapy results in serious toxicity in patients with CHF, recent MI or severe cardiomyopathy). Products include:
- Lopressor 848
- Lopressor HCT Tablets 850

Midazolam Hydrochloride (Administer with caution to patients receiving other highly protein bound drugs). Products include:
- Versed Injection 2324

Mivacurium Chloride (Verapamil may potentiate the activity of neuromuscular blocking agents). Products include:
- Mivacron 1125

Nadolol (Concomitant intravenous beta blocker therapy results in serious toxicity in patients with CHF, recent MI or severe cardiomyopathy).
No products indexed under this heading.

Naproxen (Administer with caution to patients receiving other highly protein bound drugs). Products include:
- Anaprox/Naprosyn 2277

Naproxen Sodium (Administer with caution to patients receiving other highly protein bound drugs). Products include:
- Aleve 2124

- Anaprox/Naprosyn 2277
- Naprelan Tablets 2861

Nortriptyline Hydrochloride (Administer with caution to patients receiving other highly protein bound drugs). Products include:
- Pamelor 2409

Oxaprozin (Administer with caution to patients receiving other highly protein bound drugs). Products include:
- Daypro Caplets 2578

Oxazepam (Administer with caution to patients receiving other highly protein bound drugs). Products include:
- Serax Capsules 2916
- Serax Tablets 2916

Pancuronium Bromide (Verapamil may potentiate the activity of neuromuscular blocking agents).
No products indexed under this heading.

Penbutolol Sulfate (Concomitant intravenous beta blocker therapy results in serious toxicity in patients with CHF, recent MI or severe cardiomyopathy). Products include:
- Levatol Tablets 2547

Phenobarbital (Increases verapamil serum levels). Products include:
- Arco-Lase Plus Tablets 513
- Bellergal-S Tablets 2375
- Donnatal 2234
- Donnatal Extentabs 2234
- Donnatal 2234
- Phenobarbital Elixir and Tablets .. 1523
- Quadrinal Tablets 1398

Phenylbutazone (Administer with caution to patients receiving other highly protein bound drugs).
No products indexed under this heading.

Pindolol (Concomitant intravenous beta blocker therapy results in serious toxicity in patients with CHF, recent MI or severe cardiomyopathy). Products include:
- Visken Tablets 2428

Piroxicam (Administer with caution to patients receiving other highly protein bound drugs). Products include:
- Feldene Capsules 2008

Prazosin Hydrochloride (Exaggerated hypotensive response). Products include:
- Minipress Capsules 2015
- Minizide Capsules 2016

Propranolol Hydrochloride (Concomitant intravenous beta blocker therapy results in serious toxicity in patients with CHF, recent MI or severe cardiomyopathy). Products include:
- Inderal 2834
- Inderal LA Long Acting Capsules .. 2836
- Inderide Tablets 2838
- Inderide LA Long Acting Capsules .. 2840

Quinidine Gluconate (Exaggerated hypotensive response). Products include:
- Quinaglute Dura-Tabs Tablets 644

Quinidine Polygalacturonate (Exaggerated hypotensive response). Products include:
- Cardioquin Tablets 2146

Quinidine Sulfate (Exaggerated hypotensive response). Products include:
- Quinidex Extentabs 2240

Rifampin (Markedly reduces oral verapamil bioavailability). Products include:
- Rifadin 1276
- Rifamate Capsules 1278
- Rifater 1280
- Rimactane Capsules 865

IMPORTANT NOTE: Always consult each drug listing in the patient's regimen for possible interactions.

Isoptin Injectable | **Interactions Index** | **548**

Rocuronium Bromide (Verapamil may potentiate the activity of neuromuscular blocking agents). Products include:
- Zemuron Injection 1885

Sotalol Hydrochloride (Concomitant intravenous beta blocker therapy results in serious toxicity in patients with CHF, recent MI or severe cardiomyopathy). Products include:
- Betapace Tablets 637

Sulindac (Administer with caution to patients receiving other highly protein bound drugs). Products include:
- Clinoril Tablets 1658

Temazepam (Administer with caution to patients receiving other highly protein bound drugs). Products include:
- Restoril Capsules 2413

Terazosin Hydrochloride (Exaggerated hypotensive response). Products include:
- Hytrin Capsules 434

Timolol Hemihydrate (Concomitant intravenous beta blocker therapy results in serious toxicity in patients with CHF, recent MI or severe cardiomyopathy). Products include:
- Betimol 0.25%, 0.5% .... ◉ 259

Timolol Maleate (Concomitant intravenous beta blocker therapy results in serious toxicity in patients with CHF, recent MI or severe cardiomyopathy). Products include:
- Blocadren Tablets 1654
- Timolide Tablets 1791
- Timoptic in Ocudose 1796
- Timoptic Sterile Ophthalmic Solution 1794
- Timoptic-XE 1798

Tolbutamide (Administer with caution to patients receiving other highly protein bound drugs).
- No products indexed under this heading.

Tolmetin Sodium (Administer with caution to patients receiving other highly protein bound drugs). Products include:
- Tolectin (200, 400 and 600 mg) .. 1591

Trimipramine Maleate (Administer with caution to patients receiving other highly protein bound drugs). Products include:
- Surmontil Capsules 2917

Vecuronium Bromide (Verapamil may potentiate the activity of neuromuscular blocking agents). Products include:
- Norcuron for Injection 1875

Warfarin Sodium (Administer with caution to patients receiving other highly protein bound drugs). Products include:
- Coumadin 941

ISOPTIN FOR INTRAVENOUS INJECTION 5MG/2ML
(Verapamil Hydrochloride) 1391
See **Isoptin Ampules 5mg/2mL**

ISOPTIN ORAL TABLETS
(Verapamil Hydrochloride) 1393
May interact with antihypertensives, ACE inhibitors, beta blockers, cardiac glycosides, quinidine, lithium preparations, inhalant anesthetics, neuromuscular blocking agents, and certain other agents. Compounds in these categories include:

Acebutolol Hydrochloride (Concomitant therapy may result in additive negative effects on heart rate, AV conduction, and/or cardiac contractility; excessive bradycardia and AV block has been reported with concurrent use in hypertensive patients; possible additive effect on blood pressure). Products include:
- Sectral Capsules 2914

Amlodipine Besylate (Co-administration with oral antihypertensive agents will usually have an additive effect on lowering blood pressure). Products include:
- Lotrel Capsules 858
- Norvasc Tablets 2020

Atenolol (Concomitant therapy may result in additive negative effects on heart rate, AV conduction, and/or cardiac contractility; excessive bradycardia and AV block has been reported with concurrent use in hypertensive patients; possible additive effect on blood pressure). Products include:
- Tenoretic Tablets 2963
- Tenormin Tablets and I.V. Injection 2965

Atracurium Besylate (Verapamil may potentiate the activity of neuromuscular blocking drugs). Products include:
- Tracrium Injection 1155

Benazepril Hydrochloride (Co-administration with oral antihypertensive agents will usually have an additive effect on lowering blood pressure). Products include:
- Lotensin Tablets 852
- Lotensin HCT Tablets 855
- Lotrel Capsules 858

Bendroflumethiazide (Co-administration with oral antihypertensive agents will usually have an additive effect on lowering blood pressure).
- No products indexed under this heading.

Betaxolol Hydrochloride (Concomitant therapy may result in additive negative effects on heart rate, AV conduction, and/or cardiac contractility; excessive bradycardia and AV block has been reported with concurrent use in hypertensive patients; possible additive effect on blood pressure). Products include:
- Betoptic Ophthalmic Solution 465
- Betoptic S Ophthalmic Suspension 467
- Kerlone Tablets 2588

Bisoprolol Fumarate (Concomitant therapy may result in additive negative effects on heart rate, AV conduction, and/or cardiac contractility; excessive bradycardia and AV block has been reported with concurrent use in hypertensive patients; possible additive effect on blood pressure). Products include:
- Zebeta Tablets 1457
- Ziac 1459

Captopril (Co-administration with oral antihypertensive agents will usually have an additive effect on lowering blood pressure). Products include:
- Capoten Tablets 740
- Capozide Tablets 744

Carbamazepine (Verapamil therapy may increase carbamazepine concentrations during combined therapy resulting in side effects such as diplopia, headache, ataxia, or dizziness). Products include:
- Atretol Tablets 569
- Tegretol/Tegretol-XR 870

Carteolol Hydrochloride (Concomitant therapy may result in additive negative effects on heart rate, AV conduction, and/or cardiac contractility; excessive bradycardia and AV block has been reported with concurrent use in hypertensive patients; possible additive effect on blood pressure). Products include:
- Cartrol Tablets 413
- Ocupress Ophthalmic Solution, 1% Sterile .... ◉ 297

Chlorothiazide (Co-administration with oral antihypertensive agents will usually have an additive effect on lowering blood pressure). Products include:
- Aldoclor Tablets 1638
- Diupres Tablets 1691
- Diuril Oral 1694

Chlorothiazide Sodium (Co-administration with oral antihypertensive agents will usually have an additive effect on lowering blood pressure). Products include:
- Diuril Sodium Intravenous 1693

Chlorthalidone (Co-administration with oral antihypertensive agents will usually have an additive effect on lowering blood pressure). Products include:
- Combipres Tablets 682
- Tenoretic Tablets 2963
- Thalitone 1293

Cimetidine (Variable results on verapamil clearance acute studies, either reduced or unchanged). Products include:
- Tagamet HB Tablets .... ▣ 786
- Tagamet Tablets 2694

Cimetidine Hydrochloride (Variable results on verapamil clearance acute studies, either reduced or unchanged). Products include:
- Tagamet 2694

Cisatracurium Besylate (Verapamil may potentiate the activity of neuromuscular blocking drugs). Products include:
- Nimbex Injection 1131

Clonidine (Co-administration with oral antihypertensive agents will usually have an additive effect on lowering blood pressure). Products include:
- Catapres-TTS 680

Clonidine Hydrochloride (Co-administration with oral antihypertensive agents will usually have an additive effect on lowering blood pressure). Products include:
- Catapres Tablets 679
- Combipres Tablets 682

Cyclosporine (Verapamil therapy may increase serum levels of cyclosporine). Products include:
- Neoral 2405
- Sandimmune 2416

Deserpidine (Co-administration with oral antihypertensive agents will usually have an additive effect on lowering blood pressure).
- No products indexed under this heading.

Desflurane (Potential for excessive cardiovascular depression based on animal studies). Products include:
- Suprane (desflurane, USP) 1865

Deslanoside (Chronic verapamil treatment can increase serum digoxin levels by 50% to 70% resulting in digitalis toxicity; influence on digoxin kinetics is magnified in hepatic cirrhosis patients).
- No products indexed under this heading.

Diazoxide (Co-administration with oral antihypertensive agents will usually have an additive effect on lowering blood pressure). Products include:
- Hyperstat I.V. Injection 2504
- Proglycem 575

Digitoxin (Chronic verapamil treatment can increase serum digoxin levels by 50% to 70% resulting in digitalis toxicity; influence on digoxin kinetics is magnified in hepatic cirrhosis patients). Products include:
- Crystodigin Tablets 1472

Digoxin (Chronic verapamil treatment can increase serum digoxin levels by 50% to 70% resulting in digitalis toxicity; influence on digoxin kinetics is magnified in hepatic cirrhosis patients). Products include:
- Lanoxicaps 1110
- Lanoxin Elixir Pediatric 1113
- Lanoxin Injection 1116
- Lanoxin Injection Pediatric 1119
- Lanoxin Tablets 1121

Diltiazem Hydrochloride (Co-administration with oral antihypertensive agents will usually have an additive effect on lowering blood pressure). Products include:
- Cardizem CD Capsules 1251
- Cardizem SR Capsules 1255
- Cardizem Injectable 1253
- Cardizem Tablets 1257
- Dilacor XR Extended-release Capsules 2183
- Tiazac Capsules 1019

Disopyramide Phosphate (Disopyramide should not be administered within 48 hours before or 24 hours after verapamil administration). Products include:
- Norpace 2596

Doxacurium Chloride (Verapamil may potentiate the activity of neuromuscular blocking drugs). Products include:
- Nuromax Injection 1136

Doxazosin Mesylate (Concomitant use of agents that attenuate alpha-adrenergic function, such as doxazosin, may result in excessive reduction in blood pressure). Products include:
- Cardura Tablets 1993

Enalapril Maleate (Co-administration with oral antihypertensive agents will usually have an additive effect on lowering blood pressure). Products include:
- Vaseretic Tablets 1810
- Vasotec Tablets 1816

Enalaprilat (Co-administration with oral antihypertensive agents will usually have an additive effect on lowering blood pressure). Products include:
- Vasotec I.V. 1814

Enflurane (Potential for excessive cardiovascular depression based on animal studies).
- No products indexed under this heading.

Esmolol Hydrochloride (Concomitant therapy may result in additive negative effects on heart rate, AV conduction, and/or cardiac contractility; excessive bradycardia and AV block has been reported with concurrent use in hypertensive patients; possible additive effect on blood pressure). Products include:
- Brevibloc (esmolol HCl) Injection 1860

Felodipine (Co-administration with oral antihypertensive agents will usually have an additive effect on lowering blood pressure). Products include:
- Plendil Extended-Release Tablets 514

(▣ Described in PDR For Nonprescription Drugs) (◉ Described in PDR For Ophthalmology)

Flecainide Acetate (Co-administration may have additive effects on myocardial contractility, AV conduction, and repolarization). Products include:
  Tambocor Tablets 1555

Fosinopril Sodium (Co-administration with oral antihypertensive agents will usually have an additive effect on lowering blood pressure). Products include:
  Monopril Tablets 762

Furosemide (Co-administration with oral antihypertensive agents will usually have an additive effect on lowering blood pressure). Products include:
  Lasix Injection, Oral Solution and Tablets 1267

Guanabenz Acetate (Co-administration with oral antihypertensive agents will usually have an additive effect on lowering blood pressure).
  No products indexed under this heading.

Guanethidine Monosulfate (Co-administration with oral antihypertensive agents will usually have an additive effect on lowering blood pressure). Products include:
  Esimil Tablets 840
  Ismelin Tablets 845

Halothane (Potential for excessive cardiovascular depression based on animal studies). Products include:
  Fluothane 2830

Hydralazine Hydrochloride (Co-administration with oral antihypertensive agents will usually have an additive effect on lowering blood pressure). Products include:
  Apresazide Capsules 824
  Apresoline Hydrochloride Tablets .. 826
  Hydralazine Hydrochloride Injection USP 2712
  Ser-Ap-Es Tablets 867

Hydrochlorothiazide (Co-administration with oral antihypertensive agents will usually have an additive effect on lowering blood pressure). Products include:
  Aldactazide Tablets 2556
  Aldoril Tablets 1644
  Apresazide Capsules 824
  Capozide Tablets 744
  Dyazide Capsules 2653
  Esidrix Tablets 839
  Esimil Tablets 840
  HydroDIURIL Tablets 1716
  Hydropres Tablets 1718
  Hyzaar Tablets 1720
  Inderide Tablets 2838
  Inderide LA Long Acting Capsules .. 2840
  Lopressor HCT Tablets 850
  Lotensin HCT Tablets 855
  Moduretic Tablets 1748
  Oretic Tablets 450
  Prinzide Tablets 1780
  Ser-Ap-Es Tablets 867
  Timolide Tablets 1791
  Vaseretic Tablets 1810
  Zestoretic Tablets 2968
  Ziac 1459

Hydroflumethiazide (Co-administration with oral antihypertensive agents will usually have an additive effect on lowering blood pressure). Products include:
  Diucardin Tablets 2824

Indapamide (Co-administration with oral antihypertensive agents will usually have an additive effect on lowering blood pressure).
  No products indexed under this heading.

Isoflurane (Potential for excessive cardiovascular depression based on animal studies).
  No products indexed under this heading.

Isradipine (Co-administration with oral antihypertensive agents will usually have an additive effect on lowering blood pressure). Products include:
  DynaCirc Capsules 2381
  DynaCirc CR Tablets 2383

Labetalol Hydrochloride (Concomitant therapy may result in additive negative effects on heart rate, AV conduction, and/or cardiac contractility; excessive bradycardia and AV block has been reported with concurrent use in hypertensive patients; possible additive effect on blood pressure). Products include:
  Normodyne Injection 2519
  Normodyne Tablets 2522
  Trandate 1158

Levobunolol Hydrochloride (Concomitant therapy may result in additive negative effects on heart rate, AV conduction, and/or cardiac contractility; excessive bradycardia and AV block has been reported with concurrent use in hypertensive patients; possible additive effect on blood pressure). Products include:
  Betagan .... ⊙ 230

Lisinopril (Co-administration with oral antihypertensive agents will usually have an additive effect on lowering blood pressure). Products include:
  Prinivil Tablets 1776
  Prinzide Tablets 1780
  Zestoretic Tablets 2968
  Zestril Tablets 2972

Lithium Carbonate (Combined therapy of oral verapamil and lithium may result in a lowering of serum lithium levels in patients on receiving chronic stable oral lithium; potential for increased sensitivity to the effect of lithium). Products include:
  Eskalith 2658
  Lithium Carbonate Capsules & Tablets 2352
  Lithonate/Lithotabs/Lithobid ... 2721

Lithium Citrate (Combined therapy of oral verapamil and lithium may result in a lowering of serum lithium levels in patients on receiving chronic stable oral lithium; potential for increased sensitivity to the effect of lithium).
  No products indexed under this heading.

Losartan Potassium (Co-administration with oral antihypertensive agents will usually have an additive effect on lowering blood pressure). Products include:
  Cozaar Tablets 1668
  Hyzaar Tablets 1720

Mecamylamine Hydrochloride (Co-administration with oral antihypertensive agents will usually have an additive effect on lowering blood pressure). Products include:
  Inversine Tablets 1729

Methoxyflurane (Potential for excessive cardiovascular depression based on animal studies).
  No products indexed under this heading.

Methyclothiazide (Co-administration with oral antihypertensive agents will usually have an additive effect on lowering blood pressure). Products include:
  Enduron Tablets 424

Methyldopa (Co-administration with oral antihypertensive agents will usually have an additive effect on lowering blood pressure). Products include:
  Aldoclor Tablets 1638
  Aldomet Oral 1640
  Aldoril Tablets 1644

Methyldopate Hydrochloride (Co-administration with oral antihypertensive agents will usually have an additive effect on lowering blood pressure). Products include:
  Aldomet Ester HCl Injection ... 1642

Metipranolol Hydrochloride (Concomitant therapy may result in additive negative effects on heart rate, AV conduction, and/or cardiac contractility; excessive bradycardia and AV block has been reported with concurrent use in hypertensive patients; possible additive effect on blood pressure). Products include:
  OptiPranolol (Metipranolol 0.3%) Sterile Ophthalmic Solution ..... ⊙ 256

Metocurine Iodide (Verapamil may potentiate the activity of neuromuscular blocking drugs). Products include:
  Metubine Iodide Vials 932

Metolazone (Co-administration with oral antihypertensive agents will usually have an additive effect on lowering blood pressure). Products include:
  Mykrox Tablets 1617
  Zaroxolyn Tablets 1625

Metoprolol Succinate (Co-administration has resulted in a decrease in metoprolol clearance; concomitant therapy may result in additive negative effects on heart rate, AV conduction, and/or cardiac contractility; excessive bradycardia and AV block has been reported with concurrent use in hypertensive patients). Products include:
  Toprol-XL Tablets 560

Metoprolol Tartrate (Co-administration has resulted in a decrease in metoprolol clearance; concomitant therapy may result in additive negative effects on heart rate, AV conduction, and/or cardiac contractility; excessive bradycardia and AV block has been reported with concurrent use in hypertensive patients). Products include:
  Lopressor 848
  Lopressor HCT Tablets 850

Metyrosine (Co-administration with oral antihypertensive agents will usually have an additive effect on lowering blood pressure). Products include:
  Demser Capsules 1690

Minoxidil (Co-administration with oral antihypertensive agents will usually have an additive effect on lowering blood pressure).
  No products indexed under this heading.

Mivacurium Chloride (Verapamil may potentiate the activity of neuromuscular blocking drugs). Products include:
  Mivacron 1125

Moexipril Hydrochloride (Co-administration with oral antihypertensive agents will usually have an additive effect on lowering blood pressure). Products include:
  Univasc Tablets 2553

Nadolol (Concomitant therapy may result in additive negative effects on heart rate, AV conduction, and/or cardiac contractility; excessive bradycardia and AV block has been reported with concurrent use in hypertensive patients; possible additive effect on blood pressure).
  No products indexed under this heading.

Nicardipine Hydrochloride (Co-administration with oral antihypertensive agents will usually have an additive effect on lowering blood pressure). Products include:
  Cardene Capsules 2261
  Cardene I.V. 2815
  Cardene SR Capsules 2264

Nifedipine (Co-administration with oral antihypertensive agents will usually have an additive effect on lowering blood pressure). Products include:
  Adalat Capsules (10 mg and 20 mg) 580
  Adalat CC 582
  Procardia Capsules 2024
  Procardia XL Extended Release Tablets 2026

Nisoldipine (Co-administration with oral antihypertensive agents will usually have an additive effect on lowering blood pressure). Products include:
  Sular Tablets 2961

Nitroglycerin (Co-administration with oral antihypertensive agents will usually have an additive effect on lowering blood pressure). Products include:
  Deponit NTG Transdermal Delivery System 2541
  Nitro-Bid IV 1270
  Nitro-Bid Ointment 1272
  Nitro-Dur (nitroglycerin) Transdermal Infusion System 1365
  Nitrolingual Spray 2193
  Nitrostat Tablets 1981
  Transderm-Nitro Transdermal Therapeutic System 878

Pancuronium Bromide (Verapamil may potentiate the activity of neuromuscular blocking drugs).
  No products indexed under this heading.

Penbutolol Sulfate (Concomitant therapy may result in additive negative effects on heart rate, AV conduction, and/or cardiac contractility; excessive bradycardia and AV block has been reported with concurrent use in hypertensive patients; possible additive effect on blood pressure). Products include:
  Levatol Tablets 2547

Phenobarbital (Combined therapy with phenobarbital may increase verapamil clearance). Products include:
  Arco-Lase Plus Tablets 513
  Bellergal-S Tablets 2375
  Donnatal 2234
  Donnatal Extentabs 2234
  Donnatal Tablets 2234
  Phenobarbital Elixir and Tablets .. 1523
  Quadrinal Tablets 1398

Phenoxybenzamine Hydrochloride (Co-administration with oral antihypertensive agents will usually have an additive effect on lowering blood pressure). Products include:
  Dibenzyline Capsules 2650

Phentolamine Mesylate (Co-administration with oral antihypertensive agents will usually have an additive effect on lowering blood pressure). Products include:
  Regitine Vials 864

Pindolol (Concomitant therapy may result in additive negative effects on heart rate, AV conduction, and/or cardiac contractility; excessive bradycardia and AV block has been reported with concurrent use in hypertensive patients; possible additive effect on blood pressure). Products include:
  Visken Tablets 2428

IMPORTANT NOTE: Always consult each drug listing in the patient's regimen for possible interactions.

Isoptin Oral

Polythiazide (Co-administration with oral antihypertensive agents will usually have an additive effect on lowering blood pressure). Products include:
- Minizide Capsules 2016

Prazosin Hydrochloride (Concomitant use of agents that attenuate alpha-adrenergic function, such as prazosin, has resulted in excessive reduction in blood pressure). Products include:
- Minipress Capsules 2015
- Minizide Capsules 2016

Propranolol Hydrochloride (Concomitant therapy may result in additive negative effects on heart rate, AV conduction, and/or cardiac contractility; excessive bradycardia and AV block has been reported with concurrent use in hypertensive patients; possible additive effect on blood pressure). Products include:
- Inderal 2834
- Inderal LA Long Acting Capsules 2836
- Inderide Tablets 2838
- Inderide LA Long Acting Capsules .. 2840

Quinapril Hydrochloride (Co-administration with oral antihypertensive agents will usually have an additive effect on lowering blood pressure). Products include:
- Accupril Tablets 1950

Quinidine Gluconate (In a small number of patients with hypertrophic cardiomyopathy, co-administration has resulted in significant hypotension; combined use in these patients should probably be avoided). Products include:
- Quinaglute Dura-Tabs Tablets 644

Quinidine Polygalacturonate (In a small number of patients with hypertrophic cardiomyopathy, co-administration has resulted in significant hypotension; combined use in these patients should probably be avoided). Products include:
- Cardioquin Tablets 2146

Quinidine Sulfate (In a small number of patients with hypertrophic cardiomyopathy, co-administration has resulted in significant hypotension; combined use in these patients should probably be avoided). Products include:
- Quinidex Extentabs 2240

Ramipril (Co-administration with oral antihypertensive agents will usually have an additive effect on lowering blood pressure). Products include:
- Altace Capsules 1238

Rauwolfia Serpentina (Co-administration with oral antihypertensive agents will usually have an additive effect on lowering blood pressure).
- No products indexed under this heading.

Rescinnamine (Co-administration with oral antihypertensive agents will usually have an additive effect on lowering blood pressure).
- No products indexed under this heading.

Reserpine (Co-administration with oral antihypertensive agents will usually have an additive effect on lowering blood pressure). Products include:
- Diupres Tablets 1691
- Hydropres Tablets 1718
- Ser-Ap-Es Tablets 867

Rifampin (Combined therapy with rifampin may markedly reduce oral verapamil bioavailability). Products include:
- Rifadin 1276
- Rifamate Capsules 1278
- Rifater 1280
- Rimactane Capsules 865

Rocuronium Bromide (Verapamil may potentiate the activity of neuromuscular blocking drugs). Products include:
- Zemuron Injection 1885

Sodium Nitroprusside (Co-administration with oral antihypertensive agents will usually have an additive effect on lowering blood pressure).
- No products indexed under this heading.

Sotalol Hydrochloride (Concomitant therapy may result in additive negative effects on heart rate, AV conduction, and/or cardiac contractility; excessive bradycardia and AV block has been reported with concurrent use in hypertensive patients; possible additive effect on blood pressure). Products include:
- Betapace Tablets 637

Spirapril Hydrochloride (Co-administration with oral antihypertensive agents will usually have an additive effect on lowering blood pressure).
- No products indexed under this heading.

Succinylcholine Chloride (Verapamil may potentiate the activity of neuromuscular blocking drugs). Products include:
- Anectine 1062

Terazosin Hydrochloride (Concomitant use of agents that attenuate alpha-adrenergic function, such as terazosin, may result in excessive reduction in blood pressure). Products include:
- Hytrin Capsules 434

Timolol Hemihydrate (Co-administration of oral verapamil and timolol eye drops has resulted in asymptomatic bradycardia with a wandering atrial pacemaker). Products include:
- Betimol 0.25%, 0.5% .... ⊚ 259

Timolol Maleate (Co-administration of oral verapamil and timolol eye drops has resulted in asymptomatic bradycardia with a wandering atrial pacemaker; concomitant therapy may result in additive negative effects on heart rate, AV conduction, and/or cardiac contractility; excessive bradycardia and AV block has been reported with concurrent use in hypertensive patients). Products include:
- Blocadren Tablets 1654
- Timolide Tablets 1791
- Timoptic in Ocudose 1796
- Timoptic Sterile Ophthalmic Solution 1794
- Timoptic-XE 1798

Torsemide (Co-administration with oral antihypertensive agents will usually have an additive effect on lowering blood pressure). Products include:
- Demadex Tablets and Injection 691

Trandolapril (Co-administration with oral antihypertensive agents will usually have an additive effect on lowering blood pressure). Products include:
- Mavik Tablets 1407

Trimethaphan Camsylate (Co-administration with oral antihypertensive agents will usually have an additive effect on lowering blood pressure).
- No products indexed under this heading.

Tubocurarine Chloride (Verapamil may potentiate the activity of neuromuscular blocking drugs).
- No products indexed under this heading.

Vecuronium Bromide (Verapamil may potentiate the activity of neuromuscular blocking drugs). Products include:
- Norcuron for Injection 1875

ISOPTIN SR TABLETS
(Verapamil Hydrochloride) 1395

May interact with antihypertensives, beta blockers, diuretics, inhalant anesthetics, neuromuscular blocking agents, vasodilators, ACE inhibitors, xanthine bronchodilators, lithium preparations, alpha adrenergic blockers, cardiac glycosides, and certain other agents. Compounds in these categories include:

Acebutolol Hydrochloride (Additive negative effects on heart rate, AV conduction and/or cardiac contractility; additive effect on lowering blood pressure). Products include:
- Sectral Capsules 2914

Amiloride Hydrochloride (Additive effect on lowering blood pressure). Products include:
- Midamor Tablets 1746
- Moduretic Tablets 1748

Aminophylline (Inhibition of theophylline clearance and increased plasma levels of theophylline).
- No products indexed under this heading.

Amlodipine Besylate (Additive effect on lowering blood pressure). Products include:
- Lotrel Capsules 858
- Norvasc Tablets 2020

Atenolol (Additive negative effects on heart rate, AV conduction and/or cardiac contractility; potential for a variable effect on atenolol clearance; additive effect on lowering blood pressure). Products include:
- Tenoretic Tablets 2963
- Tenormin Tablets and I.V. Injection 2965

Atracurium Besylate (Verapamil may potentiate the activity of neuromuscular blocking agents). Products include:
- Tracrium Injection 1155

Benazepril Hydrochloride (Additive effect on lowering blood pressure). Products include:
- Lotensin Tablets 852
- Lotensin HCT Tablets 855
- Lotrel Capsules 858

Bendroflumethiazide (Additive effect on lowering blood pressure).
- No products indexed under this heading.

Betaxolol Hydrochloride (Additive effect on lowering blood pressure). Products include:
- Betoptic Ophthalmic Solution 465
- Betoptic S Ophthalmic Suspension 467
- Kerlone Tablets 2588

Bisoprolol Fumarate (Additive negative effects on heart rate, AV conduction and/or cardiac contractility; additive effect on lowering blood pressure). Products include:
- Zebeta Tablets 1457
- Ziac 1459

Bumetanide (Additive effect on lowering blood pressure). Products include:
- Bumex 2260

Captopril (Additive effect on lowering blood pressure). Products include:
- Capoten Tablets 740
- Capozide Tablets 744

Carbamazepine (Increased carbamazepine concentrations; potential for diplopia, headache, ataxia, or dizziness). Products include:
- Atretol Tablets 569
- Tegretol/Tegretol-XR 870

Carteolol Hydrochloride (Additive negative effects on heart rate, AV conduction and/or cardiac contractility; additive effect on lowering blood pressure). Products include:
- Cartrol Tablets 413
- Ocupress Ophthalmic Solution, 1% Sterile .... ⊚ 297

Chlorothiazide (Additive effect on lowering blood pressure). Products include:
- Aldoclor Tablets 1638
- Diupres Tablets 1691
- Diuril Oral 1694

Chlorothiazide Sodium (Additive effect on lowering blood pressure). Products include:
- Diuril Sodium Intravenous 1693

Chlorthalidone (Additive effect on lowering blood pressure). Products include:
- Combipres Tablets 682
- Tenoretic Tablets 2963
- Thalitone 1293

Cimetidine (Possible reduced verapamil clearance). Products include:
- Tagamet HB Tablets .... ⊞ 786
- Tagamet Tablets 2694

Cimetidine Hydrochloride (Possible reduced verapamil clearance). Products include:
- Tagamet 2694

Cisatracurium Besylate (Verapamil may potentiate the activity of neuromuscular blocking agents). Products include:
- Nimbex Injection 1131

Clonidine (Additive effect on lowering blood pressure). Products include:
- Catapres-TTS 680

Clonidine Hydrochloride (Adverse effects on cardiac function). Products include:
- Catapres Tablets 679
- Combipres Tablets 682

Cyclosporine (Increased serum levels of cyclosporin). Products include:
- Neoral 2405
- Sandimmune 2416

Deserpidine (Additive effect on lowering blood pressure).
- No products indexed under this heading.

Desflurane (Potential for excessive cardiovascular depression). Products include:
- Suprane (desflurane, USP) 1865

Deslanoside (Chronic verapamil treatment can increase serum digoxin levels and this can result in digitalis toxicity).
- No products indexed under this heading.

Diazoxide (Additive effect on lowering blood pressure). Products include:
- Hyperstat I.V. Injection 2504
- Proglycem 575

Digitoxin (Chronic verapamil treatment can increase serum digoxin levels and this can result in digitalis toxicity). Products include:
- Crystodigin Tablets 1472

Digoxin (Chronic verapamil treatment can increase serum digoxin levels and this can result in digitalis toxicity). Products include:
- Lanoxicaps 1110
- Lanoxin Elixir Pediatric 1113

(⊞ Described in PDR For Nonprescription Drugs) (⊚ Described in PDR For Ophthalmology)

Interactions Index — Isoptin SR

Lanoxin Injection 1116
Lanoxin Injection Pediatric........ 1119
Lanoxin Tablets 1121

Diltiazem Hydrochloride (Additive effect on lowering blood pressure). Products include:
  Cardizem CD Capsules 1251
  Cardizem SR Capsules 1255
  Cardizem Injectable 1253
  Cardizem Tablets 1257
  Dilacor XR Extended-release Capsules 2183
  Tiazac Capsules 1019

Disopyramide Phosphate (Should not be administered within 48 hours before or 24 hours after verapamil administration). Products include:
  Norpace 2596

Doxacurium Chloride (Verapamil may potentiate the activity of neuromuscular blocking agents). Products include:
  Nuromax Injection 1136

Doxazosin Mesylate (May result in a reduction in blood pressure that is excessive in some patients). Products include:
  Cardura Tablets 1993

Dyphylline (Inhibition of theophylline clearance and increased plasma levels of theophylline). Products include:
  Lufyllin & Lufyllin-400 Tablets ... 2778
  Lufyllin-GG Elixir & Tablets 2779

Enalapril Maleate (Additive effect on lowering blood pressure). Products include:
  Vaseretic Tablets 1810
  Vasotec Tablets 1816

Enalaprilat (Additive effect on lowering blood pressure). Products include:
  Vasotec I.V. 1814

Enflurane (Potential for excessive cardiovascular depression).
  No products indexed under this heading.

Epoprostenol Sodium (Additive effect on lowering blood pressure). Products include:
  Flolan for Injection 1085

Esmolol Hydrochloride (Additive negative effects on heart rate, AV conduction and/or cardiac contractility; additive effect on lowering blood pressure cardiac contractility; additive effect on lowering blood pressure). Products include:
  Brevibloc (esmolol HCl) Injection 1860

Ethacrynic Acid (Additive effect on lowering blood pressure). Products include:
  Edecrin Tablets 1698

Felodipine (Additive effect on lowering blood pressure). Products include:
  Plendil Extended-Release Tablets... 514

Flecainide Acetate (Additive effects on myocardial contractility, AV conduction, and repolarization; additive negative inotropic effect). Products include:
  Tambocor Tablets 1555

Fosinopril Sodium (Additive effect on lowering blood pressure). Products include:
  Monopril Tablets 762

Furosemide (Additive effect on lowering blood pressure). Products include:
  Lasix Injection, Oral Solution and Tablets 1267

Guanabenz Acetate (Additive effect on lowering blood pressure).
  No products indexed under this heading.

Guanethidine Monosulfate (Additive effect on lowering blood pressure). Products include:
  Esimil Tablets 840
  Ismelin Tablets 845

Halothane (Potential for excessive cardiovascular depression). Products include:
  Fluothane 2830

Hydralazine Hydrochloride (Additive effect on lowering blood pressure). Products include:
  Apresazide Capsules 824
  Apresoline Hydrochloride Tablets .. 826
  Hydralazine Hydrochloride Injection USP 2712
  Ser-Ap-Es Tablets 867

Hydrochlorothiazide (Additive effect on lowering blood pressure). Products include:
  Aldactazide Tablets 2556
  Aldoril Tablets 1644
  Apresazide Capsules 824
  Capozide Tablets 744
  Dyazide Capsules 2653
  Esidrix Tablets 839
  Esimil Tablets 840
  HydroDIURIL Tablets 1716
  Hydropres Tablets 1718
  Hyzaar Tablets 1720
  Inderide Tablets 2838
  Inderide LA Long Acting Capsules .. 2840
  Lopressor HCT Tablets 850
  Lotensin HCT Tablets 855
  Moduretic Tablets 1748
  Oretic Tablets 450
  Prinzide Tablets 1780
  Ser-Ap-Es Tablets 867
  Timolide Tablets 1791
  Vaseretic Tablets 1810
  Zestoretic Tablets 2968
  Ziac 1459

Hydroflumethiazide (Additive effect on lowering blood pressure). Products include:
  Diucardin Tablets 2824

Indapamide (Additive effect on lowering blood pressure).
  No products indexed under this heading.

Isoflurane (Potential for excessive cardiovascular depression).
  No products indexed under this heading.

Isradipine (Additive effect on lowering blood pressure). Products include:
  DynaCirc Capsules 2381
  DynaCirc CR Tablets 2383

Labetalol Hydrochloride (Additive negative effects on heart rate, AV conduction and/or cardiac contractility; additive effect on lowering blood pressure). Products include:
  Normodyne Injection 2519
  Normodyne Tablets 2522
  Trandate 1158

Levobunolol Hydrochloride (Additive negative effects on heart rate, AV conduction and/or cardiac contractility; additive effect on lowering blood pressure). Products include:
  Betagan ....© 230

Lisinopril (Additive effect on lowering blood pressure). Products include:
  Prinivil Tablets 1776
  Prinzide Tablets 1780
  Zestoretic Tablets 2968
  Zestril Tablets 2972

Lithium Carbonate (May result in lowering of serum lithium levels and increased sensitivity to the effects of lithium). Products include:
  Eskalith 2658
  Lithium Carbonate Capsules & Tablets 2352
  Lithonate/Lithotabs/Lithobid 2721

Lithium Citrate (May result in lowering of serum lithium levels and increased sensitivity to the effects of lithium).
  No products indexed under this heading.

Losartan Potassium (Additive effect on lowering blood pressure). Products include:
  Cozaar Tablets 1668
  Hyzaar Tablets 1720

Mecamylamine Hydrochloride (Additive effect on lowering blood pressure). Products include:
  Inversine Tablets 1729

Methoxyflurane (Potential for excessive cardiovascular depression).
  No products indexed under this heading.

Methyclothiazide (Additive effect on lowering blood pressure). Products include:
  Enduron Tablets 424

Methyldopa (Additive effect on lowering blood pressure). Products include:
  Aldoclor Tablets 1638
  Aldomet Oral 1640
  Aldoril Tablets 1644

Methyldopate Hydrochloride (Additive effect on lowering blood pressure). Products include:
  Aldomet Ester HCl Injection 1642

Metipranolol Hydrochloride (Additive negative effects on heart rate, AV conduction and/or cardiac contractility; additive effect on lowering blood pressure). Products include:
  OptiPranolol (Metipranolol 0.3%) Sterile Ophthalmic Solution.....© 256

Metocurine Iodide (Verapamil may potentiate the activity of neuromuscular blocking agents). Products include:
  Metubine Iodide Vials 932

Metolazone (Additive effect on lowering blood pressure). Products include:
  Mykrox Tablets 1617
  Zaroxolyn Tablets 1625

Metoprolol Succinate (Additive negative effects on heart rate, AV conduction and/or cardiac contractility; a decrease in metoprolol clearance; additive effect on lowering blood pressure). Products include:
  Toprol-XL Tablets 560

Metoprolol Tartrate (Additive negative effects on heart rate, AV conduction and/or cardiac contractility; a decrease in metoprolol clearance; additive effect on lowering blood pressure). Products include:
  Lopressor 848
  Lopressor HCT Tablets 850

Metyrosine (Additive effect on lowering blood pressure). Products include:
  Demser Capsules 1690

Minoxidil (Additive effect on lowering blood pressure).
  No products indexed under this heading.

Mivacurium Chloride (Verapamil may potentiate the activity of neuromuscular blocking agents). Products include:
  Mivacron 1125

Moexipril Hydrochloride (Additive effect on lowering blood pressure). Products include:
  Univasc Tablets 2553

Nadolol (Additive negative effects on heart rate, AV conduction and/or cardiac contractility; additive effect on lowering blood pressure).
  No products indexed under this heading.

Nicardipine Hydrochloride (Additive effect on lowering blood pressure). Products include:
  Cardene Capsules 2261
  Cardene I.V. 2815
  Cardene SR Capsules 2264

Nifedipine (Additive effect on lowering blood pressure). Products include:
  Adalat Capsules (10 mg and 20 mg) 580
  Adalat CC 582
  Procardia Capsules 2024
  Procardia XL Extended Release Tablets 2026

Nisoldipine (Additive effect on lowering blood pressure). Products include:
  Sular Tablets 2961

Nitroglycerin (Additive effect on lowering blood pressure). Products include:
  Deponit NTG Transdermal Delivery System 2541
  Nitro-Bid IV 1270
  Nitro-Bid Ointment 1272
  Nitro-Dur (nitroglycerin) Transdermal Infusion System 1365
  Nitrolingual Spray 2193
  Nitrostat Tablets 1981
  Transderm-Nitro Transdermal Therapeutic System 878

Pancuronium Bromide (Verapamil may potentiate the activity of neuromuscular blocking agents).
  No products indexed under this heading.

Penbutolol Sulfate (Additive negative effects on heart rate, AV conduction and/or cardiac contractility; additive effect on lowering blood pressure). Products include:
  Levatol Tablets 2547

Phenobarbital (Increases verapamil clearance). Products include:
  Arco-Lase Plus Tablets 513
  Bellergal-S Tablets 2375
  Donnatal 2234
  Donnatal Extentabs 2234
  Donnatal Tablets 2234
  Phenobarbital Elixir and Tablets .. 1523
  Quadrinal Tablets 1398

Phenoxybenzamine Hydrochloride (Additive effect on lowering blood pressure). Products include:
  Dibenzyline Capsules 2650

Phentolamine Mesylate (Additive effect on lowering blood pressure). Products include:
  Regitine Vials 864

Pindolol (Additive negative effects on heart rate, AV conduction and/or cardiac contractility; additive effect on lowering blood pressure). Products include:
  Visken Tablets 2428

Polythiazide (Additive effect on lowering blood pressure). Products include:
  Minizide Capsules 2016

Prazosin Hydrochloride (May result in a reduction in blood pressure that is excessive in some patients). Products include:
  Minipress Capsules 2015
  Minizide Capsules 2016

Propranolol Hydrochloride (Additive negative effects on heart rate, AV conduction and/or cardiac contractility; potential for a decrease in propranolol clearance; additive effect on lowering blood pressure). Products include:
  Inderal 2834

IMPORTANT NOTE: Always consult each drug listing in the patient's regimen for possible interactions.

Isoptin SR — Inderal LA Long Acting Capsules ... 2836
Inderide Tablets ... 2838
Inderide LA Long Acting Capsules .. 2840

Quinapril Hydrochloride (Additive effect on lowering blood pressure). Products include:
Accupril Tablets ... 1950

Quinidine Gluconate (Hypotension (in patients with hypertrophic cardiomyopathy); increased quinidine levels). Products include:
Quinaglute Dura-Tabs Tablets ... 644

Quinidine Polygalacturonate (Hypotension (in patients with hypertrophic cardiomyopathy); increased quinidine levels). Products include:
Cardioquin Tablets ... 2146

Quinidine Sulfate (Hypotension (in patients with hypertrophic cardiomyopathy); increased quinidine levels). Products include:
Quinidex Extentabs ... 2240

Ramipril (Additive effect on lowering blood pressure). Products include:
Altace Capsules ... 1238

Rauwolfia Serpentina (Additive effect on lowering blood pressure).
No products indexed under this heading.

Rescinnamine (Additive effect on lowering blood pressure).
No products indexed under this heading.

Reserpine (Additive effect on lowering blood pressure). Products include:
Diupres Tablets ... 1691
Hydropres Tablets ... 1718
Ser-Ap-Es Tablets ... 867

Rifampin (Reduces oral verapamil bioavailability). Products include:
Rifadin ... 1276
Rifamate Capsules ... 1278
Rifater ... 1280
Rimactane Capsules ... 865

Rocuronium Bromide (Verapamil may potentiate the activity of neuromuscular blocking agents). Products include:
Zemuron Injection ... 1885

Sodium Nitroprusside (Additive effect on lowering blood pressure).
No products indexed under this heading.

Sotalol Hydrochloride (Additive negative effects on heart rate, AV conduction and/or cardiac contractility). Products include:
Betapace Tablets ... 637

Spirapril Hydrochloride (Additive effect on lowering blood pressure).
No products indexed under this heading.

Spironolactone (Additive effect on lowering blood pressure). Products include:
Aldactazide Tablets ... 2556
Aldactone Tablets ... 2558

Succinylcholine Chloride (Verapamil may potentiate the activity of neuromuscular blocking agents). Products include:
Anectine ... 1062

Terazosin Hydrochloride (May result in a reduction in blood pressure that is excessive in some patients). Products include:
Hytrin Capsules ... 434

Theophylline (Inhibition of theophylline clearance and increased plasma levels of theophylline). Products include:
Marax Tablets & DF Syrup ... 2015
Quibron ... 2227

Theophylline Anhydrous (Inhibition of theophylline clearance and increased plasma levels of theophylline). Products include:
Aerolate ... 1003
Primatene Tablets ... ⊞ 844
Respbid Tablets ... 687
Slo-bid Gyrocaps ... 2201
Theo-24 Extended Release Capsules ... 2753
Theo-Dur Extended-Release Tablets ... 1367
Theo-X Extended-Release Tablets .. 793
Uni-Dur Extended-Release Tablets .. 1374
Uniphyl 400 mg and 600 mg Tablets ... 2157

Theophylline Calcium Salicylate (Inhibition of theophylline clearance and increased plasma levels of theophylline). Products include:
Quadrinal Tablets ... 1398

Theophylline Sodium Glycinate (Inhibition of theophylline clearance and increased plasma levels of theophylline). Products include:
No products indexed under this heading.

Timolol Hemihydrate (Asymptomatic bradycardia with wandering atrial pacemaker has been observed with ophthalmic timolol and oral verapamil). Products include:
Betimol 0.25%, 0.5% ... ⊚ 259

Timolol Maleate (Asymptomatic bradycardia with wandering atrial pacemaker has been observed with ophthalmic timolol and oral verapamil; additive negative effects on heart rate, AV conduction and/or cardiac contractility). Products include:
Blocadren Tablets ... 1654
Timolide Tablets ... 1791
Timoptic in Ocudose ... 1796
Timoptic Sterile Ophthalmic Solution ... 1794
Timoptic-XE ... 1798

Torsemide (Additive effect on lowering blood pressure). Products include:
Demadex Tablets and Injection ... 691

Trandolapril (Additive effect on lowering blood pressure). Products include:
Mavik Tablets ... 1407

Triamterene (Additive effect on lowering blood pressure). Products include:
Dyazide Capsules ... 2653
Dyrenium Capsules ... 2655

Trimethaphan Camsylate (Additive effect on lowering blood pressure).
No products indexed under this heading.

Tubocurarine Chloride (Verapamil may potentiate the activity of neuromuscular blocking agents).
No products indexed under this heading.

Vecuronium Bromide (Verapamil prolongs recovery from the neuromuscular blockade; may potentiate the activity of neuromuscular blocking agents). Products include:
Norcuron for Injection ... 1875

Food Interactions
Food, unspecified (Produces decreased bioavailability (AUC) but a narrower peak to trough ratio).

ISOPTO CARBACHOL OPHTHALMIC SOLUTION
(Carbachol) ... ⊚ 221
None cited in PDR database.

ISOPTO CARPINE OPHTHALMIC SOLUTION
(Pilocarpine Hydrochloride) ... ⊚ 221
None cited in PDR database.

ISORDIL SUBLINGUAL TABLETS
(Isosorbide Dinitrate) ... 2845
May interact with vasodilators and certain other agents. Compounds in these categories include:

Diazoxide (The vasodilating effects of isosorbide dinitrate may be additive with those of other vasodilators). Products include:
Hyperstat I.V. Injection ... 2504
Proglycem ... 575

Epoprostenol Sodium (The vasodilating effects of isosorbide dinitrate may be additive with those of other vasodilators). Products include:
Flolan for Injection ... 1085

Hydralazine Hydrochloride (The vasodilating effects of isosorbide dinitrate may be additive with those of other vasodilators). Products include:
Apresazide Capsules ... 824
Apresoline Hydrochloride Tablets .. 826
Hydralazine Hydrochloride Injection USP ... 2712
Ser-Ap-Es Tablets ... 867

Minoxidil (The vasodilating effects of isosorbide dinitrate may be additive with those of other vasodilators).
No products indexed under this heading.

Food Interactions
Alcohol (Alcohol exhibits additive vasodilating effects).

ISORDIL TEMBIDS CAPSULES
(Isosorbide Dinitrate) ... 2847
May interact with vasodilators and certain other agents. Compounds in these categories include:

Diazoxide (The vasodilating effects of isosorbide dinitrate may be additive with those of other vasodilators). Products include:
Hyperstat I.V. Injection ... 2504
Proglycem ... 575

Epoprostenol Sodium (The vasodilating effects of isosorbide dinitrate may be additive with those of other vasodilators). Products include:
Flolan for Injection ... 1085

Hydralazine Hydrochloride (The vasodilating effects of isosorbide dinitrate may be additive with those of other vasodilators). Products include:
Apresazide Capsules ... 824
Apresoline Hydrochloride Tablets .. 826
Hydralazine Hydrochloride Injection USP ... 2712
Ser-Ap-Es Tablets ... 867

Minoxidil (The vasodilating effects of isosorbide dinitrate may be additive with those of other vasodilators).
No products indexed under this heading.

Food Interactions
Alcohol (Alcohol exhibits additive vasodilating effects).

ISORDIL TEMBIDS CONTROLLED-RELEASE TABLETS
(Isosorbide Dinitrate) ... 2847
See **Isordil Tembids Capsules**

ISORDIL TITRADOSE TABLETS
(Isosorbide Dinitrate) ... 2848
May interact with vasodilators and certain other agents. Compounds in these categories include:

Diazoxide (The vasodilating effects of isosorbide dinitrate may be additive with those of other vasodilators). Products include:
Hyperstat I.V. Injection ... 2504
Proglycem ... 575

Epoprostenol Sodium (The vasodilating effects of isosorbide dinitrate may be additive with those of other vasodilators). Products include:
Flolan for Injection ... 1085

Hydralazine Hydrochloride (The vasodilating effects of isosorbide dinitrate may be additive with those of other vasodilators). Products include:
Apresazide Capsules ... 824
Apresoline Hydrochloride Tablets .. 826
Hydralazine Hydrochloride Injection USP ... 2712
Ser-Ap-Es Tablets ... 867

Minoxidil (The vasodilating effects of isosorbide dinitrate may be additive with those of other vasodilators).
No products indexed under this heading.

Food Interactions
Alcohol (Alcohol exhibits additive vasodilating effects).

ISPAN PERFLUOROPROPANE
(Perfluoropropane) ... ⊚ 267
None cited in PDR database.

ISPAN SULFUR HEXAFLUORIDE
(Sulfur Hexafluoride) ... ⊚ 266
None cited in PDR database.

ISUPREL HYDROCHLORIDE SOLUTION
(Isoproterenol Hydrochloride) ... 2443
May interact with beta blockers, monoamine oxidase inhibitors, tricyclic antidepressants, sympathomimetic bronchodilators, and sympathomimetic aerosol bronchodilators. Compounds in these categories include:

Acebutolol Hydrochloride (Inhibition of the effects of each other). Products include:
Sectral Capsules ... 2914

Albuterol (Potential for deleterious cardiovascular effects; should not be used concomitantly). Products include:
Proventil Inhalation Aerosol ... 2524
Ventolin Inhalation Aerosol and Refill ... 1170

Albuterol Sulfate (Potential for deleterious cardiovascular effects). Products include:
Airet Albuterol Sulfate Inhalation Solution ... 1602
Albuterol Sulfate, USP Solution for Inhalation, Arm-a-Med ... 522
Proventil Inhalation Solution 0.083% ... 2527
Proventil Repetabs Tablets ... 2529
Proventil Solution for Inhalation 0.5% ... 2525
Proventil Syrup ... 2528
Proventil Tablets ... 2529
Ventolin Inhalation Solution ... 1171
Ventolin Nebules Inhalation Solution ... 1172
Ventolin Rotacaps for Inhalation ... 1173
Ventolin Syrup ... 1175
Ventolin Tablets ... 1176
Volmax Extended-Release Tablets . 1835

(⊞ Described in PDR For Nonprescription Drugs)   (⊚ Described in PDR For Ophthalmology)

553 **Interactions Index** **K-Dur**

Amitriptyline Hydrochloride (The action of beta adrenergic agonists on the vascular system may be potentiated). Products include:
- Elavil 2945
- Etrafon 2495
- Limbitrol 2333
- Triavil Tablets 1800

Amoxapine (The action of beta adrenergic agonists on the vascular system may be potentiated). Products include:
- Asendin Tablets 1419

Atenolol (Inhibition of the effects of each other). Products include:
- Tenoretic Tablets 2963
- Tenormin Tablets and I.V. Injection 2965

Betaxolol Hydrochloride (Inhibition of the effects of each other). Products include:
- Betoptic Ophthalmic Solution 465
- Betoptic S Ophthalmic Suspension 467
- Kerlone Tablets 2588

Bisoprolol Fumarate (Inhibition of the effects of each other). Products include:
- Zebeta Tablets 1457
- Ziac 1459

Bitolterol Mesylate (Potential for deleterious cardiovascular effects; should not be used concomitantly). Products include:
- Tornalate Solution for Inhalation, 0.2% 976
- Tornalate Metered Dose Inhaler 978

Carteolol Hydrochloride (Inhibition of the effects of each other). Products include:
- Cartrol Tablets 413
- Ocupress Ophthalmic Solution, 1% Sterile .... ◉ 297

Clomipramine Hydrochloride (The action of beta adrenergic agonists on the vascular system may be potentiated). Products include:
- Anafranil Capsules 819

Desipramine Hydrochloride (The action of beta adrenergic agonists on the vascular system may be potentiated). Products include:
- Norpramin Tablets 1273

Doxepin Hydrochloride (The action of beta adrenergic agonists on the vascular system may be potentiated). Products include:
- Adapin Capsules 1542
- Sinequan 2028
- Zonalon Cream 1042

Ephedrine Hydrochloride (Potential for deleterious cardiovascular effects). Products include:
- Primatene Tablets .... ▣ 844
- Quadrinal Tablets 1398

Ephedrine Sulfate (Potential for deleterious cardiovascular effects). Products include:
- Marax Tablets & DF Syrup 2015

Ephedrine Tannate (Potential for deleterious cardiovascular effects). Products include:
- Rynatuss 2782

Epinephrine (Potential for deleterious cardiovascular effects). Products include:
- EPIFRIN .... ◉ 237
- EpiPen 808
- Marcaine with Epinephrine 2446
- Primatene Mist .... ▣ 843
- Sensorcaine with Epinephrine Injection 554
- Sus-Phrine Injection 1017
- Xylocaine with Epinephrine Injections 562

Epinephrine Hydrochloride (Potential for deleterious cardiovascular effects). Products include:
- Ana-Kit Anaphylaxis Emergency Treatment Kit 611

Esmolol Hydrochloride (Inhibition of the effects of each other). Products include:
- Brevibloc (esmolol HCl) Injection 1860

Ethylnorepinephrine Hydrochloride (Potential for deleterious cardiovascular effects).
- No products indexed under this heading.

Furazolidone (The action of beta adrenergic agonists on the vascular system may be potentiated). Products include:
- Furoxone 2221

Imipramine Hydrochloride (The action of beta adrenergic agonists on the vascular system may be potentiated). Products include:
- Tofranil Ampuls 873
- Tofranil Tablets 875

Imipramine Pamoate (The action of beta adrenergic agonists on the vascular system may be potentiated). Products include:
- Tofranil-PM Capsules 876

Isocarboxazid (The action of beta adrenergic agonists on the vascular system may be potentiated).
- No products indexed under this heading.

Isoetharine (Potential for deleterious cardiovascular effects; should not be used concomitantly). Products include:
- Bronkometer Aerosol 2432
- Bronkosol Solution 2432
- Isoetharine Inhalation Solution, USP, Arm-a-Med 545

Isoproterenol Sulfate (Potential for deleterious cardiovascular effects; should not be used concomitantly). Products include:
- Norisodrine with Calcium Iodide Syrup 446

Labetalol Hydrochloride (Inhibition of the effects of each other). Products include:
- Normodyne Injection 2519
- Normodyne Tablets 2522
- Trandate 1158

Levobunolol Hydrochloride (Inhibition of the effects of each other). Products include:
- Betagan .... ◉ 230

Maprotiline Hydrochloride (The action of beta adrenergic agonists on the vascular system may be potentiated). Products include:
- Ludiomil Tablets 861

Metaproterenol Sulfate (Potential for deleterious cardiovascular effects; should not be used concomitantly). Products include:
- Alupent 672
- Metaproterenol Sulfate Inhalation Solution, USP, Arm-a-Med 547

Metipranolol Hydrochloride (Inhibition of the effects of each other). Products include:
- OptiPranolol (Metipranolol 0.3%) Sterile Ophthalmic Solution .... ◉ 256

Metoprolol Succinate (Inhibition of the effects of each other). Products include:
- Toprol-XL Tablets 560

Metoprolol Tartrate (Inhibition of the effects of each other). Products include:
- Lopressor 848
- Lopressor HCT Tablets 850

Nadolol (Inhibition of the effects of each other).
- No products indexed under this heading.

Nortriptyline Hydrochloride (The action of beta adrenergic agonists on the vascular system may be potentiated). Products include:
- Pamelor 2409

Penbutolol Sulfate (Inhibition of the effects of each other). Products include:
- Levatol Tablets 2547

Phenelzine Sulfate (The action of beta adrenergic agonists on the vascular system may be potentiated). Products include:
- Nardil 1977

Pindolol (Inhibition of the effects of each other). Products include:
- Visken Tablets 2428

Pirbuterol Acetate (Potential for deleterious cardiovascular effects; should not be used concomitantly). Products include:
- Maxair Autohaler 1550
- Maxair Inhaler 1552

Propranolol Hydrochloride (Inhibition of the effects of each other). Products include:
- Inderal 2834
- Inderal LA Long Acting Capsules 2836
- Inderide Tablets 2838
- Inderide LA Long Acting Capsules .. 2840

Protriptyline Hydrochloride (The action of beta adrenergic agonists on the vascular system may be potentiated). Products include:
- Vivactil Tablets 1820

Salmeterol Xinafoate (Potential for deleterious cardiovascular effects; should not be used concomitantly). Products include:
- Serevent Inhalation Aerosol 1149

Selegiline Hydrochloride (The action of beta adrenergic agonists on the vascular system may be potentiated). Products include:
- Eldepryl Capsules 2729

Sotalol Hydrochloride (Inhibition of the effects of each other). Products include:
- Betapace Tablets 637

Terbutaline Sulfate (Potential for deleterious cardiovascular effects; should not be used concomitantly). Products include:
- Brethaire Inhaler 830
- Brethine Ampuls 832
- Brethine Tablets 831
- Bricanyl Subcutaneous Injection 1247
- Bricanyl Tablets 1248

Timolol Hemihydrate (Inhibition of the effects of each other). Products include:
- Betimol 0.25%, 0.5% .... ◉ 259

Timolol Maleate (Inhibition of the effects of each other). Products include:
- Blocadren Tablets 1654
- Timolide Tablets 1791
- Timoptic in Ocudose 1796
- Timoptic Sterile Ophthalmic Solution 1794
- Timoptic-XE 1798

Tranylcypromine Sulfate (The action of beta adrenergic agonists on the vascular system may be potentiated). Products include:
- Parnate Tablets 2679

Trimipramine Maleate (The action of beta adrenergic agonists on the vascular system may be potentiated). Products include:
- Surmontil Capsules 2917

ISUPREL INJECTION
(Isoproterenol Hydrochloride) 2441
May interact with inhalant anesthetics and certain other agents. Compounds in these categories include:

Desflurane (Myocardium sensitized to sympathomimetic amines). Products include:
- Suprane (desflurane, USP) 1865

Enflurane (Myocardium sensitized to sympathomimetic amines).
- No products indexed under this heading.

Epinephrine Hydrochloride (May induce serious arrhythmias). Products include:
- Ana-Kit Anaphylaxis Emergency Treatment Kit 611

Halothane (Myocardium sensitized to sympathomimetic amines). Products include:
- Fluothane 2830

Isoflurane (Myocardium sensitized to sympathomimetic amines).
- No products indexed under this heading.

Methoxyflurane (Myocardium sensitized to sympathomimetic amines).
- No products indexed under this heading.

ISUPREL MISTOMETER
(Isoproterenol Hydrochloride) 2442
May interact with:

Epinephrine Hydrochloride (May induce serious arrhythmias). Products include:
- Ana-Kit Anaphylaxis Emergency Treatment Kit 611

ITCH-X GEL
(Pramoxine Hydrochloride, Benzyl Alcohol) .... ▣ 607
None cited in PDR database.

ITCH-X SPRAY
(Pramoxine Hydrochloride, Benzyl Alcohol) .... ▣ 607
None cited in PDR database.

JE-VAX
(Japanese Encephalitis Vaccine Inactivated) 904
None cited in PDR database.

JEVITY ISOTONIC LIQUID NUTRITION WITH FIBER
(Nutritional Supplement) 2339
None cited in PDR database.

JEVITY PLUS 1.2 CAL/ML, HIGH-NITROGEN LIQUID NUTRITION WITH PATENTED FIBER BLEND
(Nutritional Supplement) 2339
None cited in PDR database.

JUNIOR STRENGTH TYLENOL ACETAMINOPHEN COATED CAPLETS AND CHEWABLE TABLETS
(Acetaminophen) 1562
None cited in PDR database.

K-DUR MICROBURST RELEASE SYSTEM (POTASSIUM CHLORIDE, USP) E.R. TABLETS
(Potassium Chloride) 1364
May interact with potassium sparing diuretics, ACE inhibitors, and anticholinergics. Compounds in these categories include:

Amiloride Hydrochloride (Coadministration of these agents can produce severe hyperkalemia; concurrent use is not recommended). Products include:
- Midamor Tablets 1746
- Moduretic Tablets 1748

IMPORTANT NOTE: Always consult each drug listing in the patient's regimen for possible interactions.

K-Dur / Interactions Index

Atropine Sulfate
(Concurrent use with anticholinergic drugs or other agents with anticholinergic properties at sufficient doses to exert anticholinergic effects is contraindicated). Products include:
- Arco-Lase Plus Tablets ... 513
- Atrohist Plus Tablets ... 1605
- Donnatal ... 2234
- Donnatal Extentabs ... 2234
- Donnatal Tablets ... 2234
- Lomotil ... 2591
- Motofen Tablets ... 789
- Urised Tablets ... 2123

Belladonna Alkaloids
(Concurrent use with anticholinergic drugs or other agents with anticholinergic properties at sufficient doses to exert anticholinergic effects is contraindicated). Products include:
- Bellergal-S Tablets ... 2375
- Hyland's Bedwetting Tablets ... 788
- Hyland's EnurAid Tablets ... 789
- Hyland's Headache Tablets ... 790
- Hyland's Teething Tablets ... 790
- Similasan Eye Drops #1 ... 769

Benazepril Hydrochloride
(Potential for increased potassium retention). Products include:
- Lotensin Tablets ... 852
- Lotensin HCT Tablets ... 855
- Lotrel Capsules ... 858

Benztropine Mesylate
(Concurrent use with anticholinergic drugs or other agents with anticholinergic properties at sufficient doses to exert anticholinergic effects is contraindicated). Products include:
- Cogentin ... 1661

Biperiden Hydrochloride
(Concurrent use with anticholinergic drugs or other agents with anticholinergic properties at sufficient doses to exert anticholinergic effects is contraindicated). Products include:
- Akineton ... 1380

Captopril
(Potential for increased potassium retention). Products include:
- Capoten Tablets ... 740
- Capozide Tablets ... 744

Clidinium Bromide
(Concurrent use with anticholinergic drugs or other agents with anticholinergic properties at sufficient doses to exert anticholinergic effects is contraindicated). Products include:
- Librax Capsules ... 2330

Dicyclomine Hydrochloride
(Concurrent use with anticholinergic drugs or other agents with anticholinergic properties at sufficient doses to exert anticholinergic effects is contraindicated). Products include:
- Bentyl ... 1246

Enalapril Maleate
(Potential for increased potassium retention). Products include:
- Vaseretic Tablets ... 1810
- Vasotec Tablets ... 1816

Enalaprilat
(Potential for increased potassium retention). Products include:
- Vasotec I.V. ... 1814

Fosinopril Sodium
(Potential for increased potassium retention). Products include:
- Monopril Tablets ... 762

Glycopyrrolate
(Concurrent use with anticholinergic drugs or other agents with anticholinergic properties at sufficient doses to exert anticholinergic effects is contraindicated). Products include:
- Robinul Forte Tablets ... 2247
- Robinul Injectable ... 2247
- Robinul Tablets ... 2247

Hyoscyamine
(Concurrent use with anticholinergic drugs or other agents with anticholinergic properties at sufficient doses to exert anticholinergic effects is contraindicated). Products include:
- Cystospaz Tablets ... 2123
- Urised Tablets ... 2123

Hyoscyamine Sulfate
(Concurrent use with anticholinergic drugs or other agents with anticholinergic properties at sufficient doses to exert anticholinergic effects is contraindicated). Products include:
- Arco-Lase Plus Tablets ... 513
- Atrohist Plus Tablets ... 1605
- Cystospaz-M Capsules ... 2123
- Donnatal ... 2234
- Donnatal Extentabs ... 2234
- Donnatal Tablets ... 2234
- Kutrase Capsules ... 2546
- Levsin/Levsinex/Levbid ... 2549

Ipratropium Bromide
(Concurrent use with anticholinergic drugs or other agents with anticholinergic properties at sufficient doses to exert anticholinergic effects is contraindicated). Products include:
- Atrovent Inhalation Aerosol ... 674
- Atrovent Inhalation Solution ... 675
- Atrovent Nasal Spray 0.03% ... 676
- Atrovent Nasal Spray 0.06% ... 678

Lisinopril
(Potential for increased potassium retention). Products include:
- Prinivil Tablets ... 1776
- Prinzide Tablets ... 1780
- Zestoretic Tablets ... 2968
- Zestril Tablets ... 2972

Mepenzolate Bromide
(Concurrent use with anticholinergic drugs or other agents with anticholinergic properties at sufficient doses to exert anticholinergic effects is contraindicated).
No products indexed under this heading.

Moexipril Hydrochloride
(Potential for increased potassium retention). Products include:
- Univasc Tablets ... 2553

Oxybutynin Chloride
(Concurrent use with anticholinergic drugs or other agents with anticholinergic properties at sufficient doses to exert anticholinergic effects is contraindicated). Products include:
- Ditropan ... 1267

Procyclidine Hydrochloride
(Concurrent use with anticholinergic drugs or other agents with anticholinergic properties at sufficient doses to exert anticholinergic effects is contraindicated). Products include:
- Kemadrin Tablets ... 1105

Propantheline Bromide
(Concurrent use with anticholinergic drugs or other agents with anticholinergic properties at sufficient doses to exert anticholinergic effects is contraindicated). Products include:
- Pro-Banthine Tablets ... 2226

Quinapril Hydrochloride
(Potential for increased potassium retention). Products include:
- Accupril Tablets ... 1950

Ramipril
(Potential for increased potassium retention). Products include:
- Altace Capsules ... 1238

Scopolamine
(Concurrent use with anticholinergic drugs or other agents with anticholinergic properties at sufficient doses to exert anticholinergic effects is contraindicated). Products include:
- Transderm Scōp Transdermal Therapeutic System ... 890

Scopolamine Hydrobromide
(Concurrent use with anticholinergic drugs or other agents with anticholinergic properties at sufficient doses to exert anticholinergic effects is contraindicated). Products include:
- Atrohist Plus Tablets ... 1605
- Donnatal ... 2234
- Donnatal Extentabs ... 2234
- Donnatal Tablets ... 2234

Spirapril Hydrochloride
(Potential for increased potassium retention).
No products indexed under this heading.

Spironolactone
(Co-administration of these agents can produce severe hyperkalemia; concurrent use is not recommended). Products include:
- Aldactazide Tablets ... 2556
- Aldactone Tablets ... 2558

Trandolapril
(Potential for increased potassium retention). Products include:
- Mavik Tablets ... 1407

Triamterene
(Co-administration of these agents can produce severe hyperkalemia; concurrent use is not recommended). Products include:
- Dyazide Capsules ... 2653
- Dyrenium Capsules ... 2655

Tridihexethyl Chloride
(Concurrent use with anticholinergic drugs or other agents with anticholinergic properties at sufficient doses to exert anticholinergic effects is contraindicated).
No products indexed under this heading.

Trihexyphenidyl Hydrochloride
(Concurrent use with anticholinergic drugs or other agents with anticholinergic properties at sufficient doses to exert anticholinergic effects is contraindicated). Products include:
- Artane ... 1418

K-LOR POWDER PACKETS
(Potassium Chloride) ... 438
May interact with potassium sparing diuretics and ACE inhibitors. Compounds in these categories include:

Amiloride Hydrochloride
(Co-administration of these agents can produce severe hyperkalemia; concurrent use is not recommended). Products include:
- Midamor Tablets ... 1746
- Moduretic Tablets ... 1748

Benazepril Hydrochloride
(Potential for hyperkalemia). Products include:
- Lotensin Tablets ... 852
- Lotensin HCT Tablets ... 855
- Lotrel Capsules ... 858

Captopril
(Potential for hyperkalemia). Products include:
- Capoten Tablets ... 740
- Capozide Tablets ... 744

Enalapril Maleate
(Potential for hyperkalemia). Products include:
- Vaseretic Tablets ... 1810
- Vasotec Tablets ... 1816

Enalaprilat
(Potential for hyperkalemia). Products include:
- Vasotec I.V. ... 1814

Fosinopril Sodium
(Potential for hyperkalemia). Products include:
- Monopril Tablets ... 762

Lisinopril
(Potential for hyperkalemia). Products include:
- Prinivil Tablets ... 1776
- Prinzide Tablets ... 1780
- Zestoretic Tablets ... 2968
- Zestril Tablets ... 2972

Moexipril Hydrochloride
(Potential for hyperkalemia). Products include:
- Univasc Tablets ... 2553

Quinapril Hydrochloride
(Potential for hyperkalemia). Products include:
- Accupril Tablets ... 1950

Ramipril
(Potential for hyperkalemia). Products include:
- Altace Capsules ... 1238

Spirapril Hydrochloride
(Potential for hyperkalemia).
No products indexed under this heading.

Spironolactone
(Co-administration of these agents can produce severe hyperkalemia; concurrent use is not recommended). Products include:
- Aldactazide Tablets ... 2556
- Aldactone Tablets ... 2558

Trandolapril
(Potential for hyperkalemia). Products include:
- Mavik Tablets ... 1407

Triamterene
(Co-administration of these agents can produce severe hyperkalemia; concurrent use is not recommended). Products include:
- Dyazide Capsules ... 2653
- Dyrenium Capsules ... 2655

K-NORM CAPSULES
(Potassium Chloride) ... 1615
May interact with potassium sparing diuretics, ACE inhibitors, and anticholinergics. Compounds in these categories include:

Amiloride Hydrochloride
(Concurrent administration can produce severe hyperkalemia). Products include:
- Midamor Tablets ... 1746
- Moduretic Tablets ... 1748

Atropine Sulfate
(Anticholinergic drugs can be cause for delay or arrest in tablet passage through the gastrointestinal tract; concomitant administration of drugs capable of decreasing GI motility should be avoided). Products include:
- Arco-Lase Plus Tablets ... 513
- Atrohist Plus Tablets ... 1605
- Donnatal ... 2234
- Donnatal Extentabs ... 2234
- Donnatal Tablets ... 2234
- Lomotil ... 2591
- Motofen Tablets ... 789
- Urised Tablets ... 2123

Belladonna Alkaloids
(Anticholinergic drugs can be cause for delay or arrest in tablet passage through the gastrointestinal tract; concomitant administration of drugs capable of decreasing GI motility should be avoided). Products include:
- Bellergal-S Tablets ... 2375
- Hyland's Bedwetting Tablets ... 788
- Hyland's EnurAid Tablets ... 789
- Hyland's Headache Tablets ... 790
- Hyland's Teething Tablets ... 790
- Similasan Eye Drops #1 ... 769

Benazepril Hydrochloride
(Potential for severe hyperkalemia). Products include:
- Lotensin Tablets ... 852
- Lotensin HCT Tablets ... 855
- Lotrel Capsules ... 858

Benztropine Mesylate
(Anticholinergic drugs can be cause for delay or arrest in tablet passage through the gastrointestinal tract; concomitant administration of drugs capable of decreasing GI motility should be avoided). Products include:
- Cogentin ... 1661

(⊡ Described in PDR For Nonprescription Drugs) (⊚ Described in PDR For Ophthalmology)

Biperiden Hydrochloride (Anticholinergic drugs can be cause for delay or arrest in tablet passage through the gastrointestinal tract; concomitant administration of drugs capable of decreasing GI motility should be avoided). Products include:
- Akineton ... 1380

Captopril (Potential for severe hyperkalemia). Products include:
- Capoten Tablets ... 740
- Capozide Tablets ... 744

Clidinium Bromide (Anticholinergic drugs can be cause for delay or arrest in tablet passage through the gastrointestinal tract; concomitant administration of drugs capable of decreasing GI motility should be avoided). Products include:
- Librax Capsules ... 2330

Dicyclomine Hydrochloride (Anticholinergic drugs can be cause for delay or arrest in tablet passage through the gastrointestinal tract; concomitant administration of drugs capable of decreasing GI motility should be avoided). Products include:
- Bentyl ... 1246

Enalapril Maleate (Potential for severe hyperkalemia). Products include:
- Vaseretic Tablets ... 1810
- Vasotec Tablets ... 1816

Enalaprilat (Potential for severe hyperkalemia). Products include:
- Vasotec I.V. ... 1814

Fosinopril Sodium (Potential for severe hyperkalemia). Products include:
- Monopril Tablets ... 762

Glycopyrrolate (Anticholinergic drugs can be cause for delay or arrest in tablet passage through the gastrointestinal tract; concomitant administration of drugs capable of decreasing GI motility should be avoided). Products include:
- Robinul Forte Tablets ... 2247
- Robinul Injectable ... 2247
- Robinul Tablets ... 2247

Hyoscyamine (Anticholinergic drugs can be cause for delay or arrest in tablet passage through the gastrointestinal tract; concomitant administration of drugs capable of decreasing GI motility should be avoided). Products include:
- Cystospaz Tablets ... 2123
- Urised Tablets ... 2123

Hyoscyamine Sulfate (Anticholinergic drugs can be cause for delay or arrest in tablet passage through the gastrointestinal tract; concomitant administration of drugs capable of decreasing GI motility should be avoided). Products include:
- Arco-Lase Plus Tablets ... 513
- Atrohist Plus Tablets ... 1605
- Cystospaz-M Capsules ... 2123
- Donnatal ... 2234
- Donnatal Extentabs ... 2234
- Donnatal Tablets ... 2234
- Kutrase Capsules ... 2546
- Levsin/Levsinex/Levbid ... 2549

Ipratropium Bromide (Anticholinergic drugs can be cause for delay or arrest in tablet passage through the gastrointestinal tract; concomitant administration of drugs capable of decreasing GI motility should be avoided). Products include:
- Atrovent Inhalation Aerosol ... 674
- Atrovent Inhalation Solution ... 675
- Atrovent Nasal Spray 0.03% ... 676
- Atrovent Nasal Spray 0.06% ... 678

Lisinopril (Potential for severe hyperkalemia). Products include:
- Prinivil Tablets ... 1776
- Prinzide Tablets ... 1780
- Zestoretic Tablets ... 2968
- Zestril Tablets ... 2972

Mepenzolate Bromide (Anticholinergic drugs can be cause for delay or arrest in tablet passage through the gastrointestinal tract; concomitant administration of drugs capable of decreasing GI motility should be avoided).

No products indexed under this heading.

Moexipril Hydrochloride (Potential for severe hyperkalemia). Products include:
- Univasc Tablets ... 2553

Oxybutynin Chloride (Anticholinergic drugs can be cause for delay or arrest in tablet passage through the gastrointestinal tract; concomitant administration of drugs capable of decreasing GI motility should be avoided). Products include:
- Ditropan ... 1267

Procyclidine Hydrochloride (Anticholinergic drugs can be cause for delay or arrest in tablet passage through the gastrointestinal tract; concomitant administration of drugs capable of decreasing GI motility should be avoided). Products include:
- Kemadrin Tablets ... 1105

Propantheline Bromide (Anticholinergic drugs can be cause for delay or arrest in tablet passage through the gastrointestinal tract; concomitant administration of drugs capable of decreasing GI motility should be avoided). Products include:
- Pro-Banthine Tablets ... 2226

Quinapril Hydrochloride (Potential for severe hyperkalemia). Products include:
- Accupril Tablets ... 1950

Ramipril (Potential for severe hyperkalemia). Products include:
- Altace Capsules ... 1238

Scopolamine (Anticholinergic drugs can be cause for delay or arrest in tablet passage through the gastrointestinal tract; concomitant administration of drugs capable of decreasing GI motility should be avoided). Products include:
- Transderm Scōp Transdermal Therapeutic System ... 890

Scopolamine Hydrobromide (Anticholinergic drugs can be cause for delay or arrest in tablet passage through the gastrointestinal tract; concomitant administration of drugs capable of decreasing GI motility should be avoided). Products include:
- Atrohist Plus Tablets ... 1605
- Donnatal ... 2234
- Donnatal Extentabs ... 2234
- Donnatal Tablets ... 2234

Spirapril Hydrochloride (Potential for severe hyperkalemia).

No products indexed under this heading.

Spironolactone (Concurrent administration can produce severe hyperkalemia). Products include:
- Aldactazide Tablets ... 2556
- Aldactone Tablets ... 2558

Trandolapril (Potential for severe hyperkalemia). Products include:
- Mavik Tablets ... 1407

Triamterene (Concurrent administration can produce severe hyperkalemia). Products include:
- Dyazide Capsules ... 2653
- Dyrenium Capsules ... 2655

Tridihexethyl Chloride (Anticholinergic drugs can be cause for delay or arrest in tablet passage through the gastrointestinal tract; concomitant administration of drugs capable of decreasing GI motility should be avoided).

No products indexed under this heading.

Trihexyphenidyl Hydrochloride (Anticholinergic drugs can be cause for delay or arrest in tablet passage through the gastrointestinal tract; concomitant administration of drugs capable of decreasing GI motility should be avoided). Products include:
- Artane ... 1418

K-PHOS NEUTRAL TABLETS

(Potassium Phosphate, Monobasic, Sodium Phosphate, Monobasic, Sodium Phosphate, Dibasic) ... 633

May interact with antacids containing aluminium, calcium and magnesium, calcium preparations, potassium preparations, potassium sparing diuretics, and certain other agents. Compounds in these categories include:

ACTH (Concurrent use with corticotropin may result in hypernatremia).

No products indexed under this heading.

Aluminum Carbonate (Co-administration with antacids may bind the phosphate and prevent its absorption). Products include:
- Basaljel Capsules ... 2810
- Basaljel Suspension ... 2810
- Basaljel Tablets ... 2810

Aluminum Hydroxide (Co-administration with antacids may bind the phosphate and prevent its absorption). Products include:
- ALternaGEL Liquid ... 1358
- Maximum Strength Ascriptin ... PD 650
- Cama Arthritis Pain Reliever ... PD 748
- Gaviscon Extra Strength Relief Formula Antacid Tablets ... PD 778
- Gaviscon Extra Strength Relief Formula Liquid Antacid ... PD 779
- Gaviscon Liquid Antacid ... PD 779
- Gelusil Antacid-Anti-gas Liquid ... PD 819
- Gelusil Antacid-Anti-gas Tablets ... PD 819
- Maalox Antacid/Anti-Gas Tablets ... 889
- Maalox Heartburn Relief Suspension ... PD 658
- Maalox Antacid Liquid ... 888
- Extra Strength Maalox Antacid/Anti-Gas Liquid and Tablets ... 888
- Mylanta ... 1359
- Tempo Soft Antacid ... PD 799

Aluminum Hydroxide Gel (Co-administration with antacids may bind the phosphate and prevent its absorption). Products include:
- ALternaGEL Liquid ... PD 675
- Aludrox Oral Suspension ... PD 850
- Amphojel Suspension ... 2802
- Amphojel Suspension without Flavor ... 2802
- Amphojel Tablets ... 2802
- Ascriptin ... PD 650
- Gaviscon Antacid Tablets ... PD 778
- Gaviscon-2 Antacid Tablets ... PD 779
- Mylanta Liquid ... PD 676
- Mylanta Double Strength Liquid ... PD 676
- Nephrox Suspension ... PD 671

Amiloride Hydrochloride (Concurrent use with potassium-sparing diuretics may cause hyperkalemia). Products include:
- Midamor Tablets ... 1746
- Moduretic Tablets ... 1748

Calcium Carbonate (Concurrent use with calcium-containing preparations may antagonize the effects of phosphates in the treatment of hypercalcemia). Products include:
- Alka-Mints Chewable Antacid ... PD 609
- Alka-Seltzer Fast Relief Caplets ... PD 610
- Ascriptin ... PD 650
- Extra Strength Bayer Plus Aspirin Caplets ... PD 617
- Aspirin Regimen Bayer 81 mg Tablets with Calcium ... PD 615
- Bufferin Analgesic Tablets ... PD 636
- Arthritis Strength Bufferin Analgesic Caplets ... PD 637
- Extra Strength Bufferin Analgesic Tablets ... PD 637
- Calci-Chew Tablets ... 2168
- Calci-Mix Capsules ... 2168
- Caltrate 600 ... PD 681
- Caltrate PLUS ... PD 681
- Caltrate 600 + D ... PD 681
- Cotazym Capsules ... 1866
- Di-Gel Antacid/Anti-Gas ... PD 762
- Florical Capsules and Tablets ... 1825
- Gerimed Tablets ... 1000
- Maalox Antacid Caplets ... PD 657
- Marblen ... PD 671
- Materna Tablets ... 1427
- Monocal Tablets ... 1825
- Mylanta Fast-Acting ... 1359
- Mylanta Gelcaps Antacid ... PD 678
- Mylanta Soothing Lozenges ... 1360
- Mylanta Tablets ... PD 677
- Mylanta Double Strength Tablets ... PD 677
- Nephro-Calci Tablets ... 2168
- One-A-Day Calcium Plus ... PD 625
- Rolaids Antacid Tablets ... PD 807
- Rolaids Antacid Calcium Rich/Sodium Free Tablets ... PD 807
- Tempo Soft Antacid ... PD 799
- Titralac ... PD 686
- Titralac Plus ... PD 687
- Tums Antacid/Calcium Supplement Tablets ... PD 787
- Tums Anti-gas/Antacid Formula Tablets, Assorted Fruit ... PD 788
- Tums E-X Antacid/Calcium Supplement Tablets ... PD 787
- Tums 500 Calcium Supplement ... PD 788
- Tums ULTRA Antacid/Calcium Supplement Tablets ... PD 787
- TYLENOL Headache Plus Pain Reliever with Antacid, Extra Strength Caplets ... PD 705

Calcium Chloride (Concurrent use with calcium-containing preparations may antagonize the effects of phosphates in the treatment of hypercalcemia).

No products indexed under this heading.

Calcium Citrate (Concurrent use with calcium-containing preparations may antagonize the effects of phosphates in the treatment of hypercalcemia). Products include:
- Citracal Tablets ... 1828

Calcium Glubionate (Concurrent use with calcium-containing preparations may antagonize the effects of phosphates in the treatment of hypercalcemia).

No products indexed under this heading.

Deserpidine (Concurrent use with antihypertensives, such as rauwolfia alkaloids, may result in hypernatremia).

No products indexed under this heading.

Diazoxide (Concurrent use with antihypertensives, such as diazoxide, may result in hypernatremia). Products include:
- Hyperstat I.V. Injection ... 2504
- Proglycem ... 575

Fludrocortisone Acetate (Concurrent use with mineralocorticoids may result in hypernatremia). Products include:
- Florinef Acetate Tablets ... 506

IMPORTANT NOTE: Always consult each drug listing in the patient's regimen for possible interactions.

K-Phos Neutral / Interactions Index

Guanethidine Monosulfate (Concurrent use with antihypertensives, such as guanethidine, may result in hypernatremia). Products include:
- Esimil Tablets ... 840
- Ismelin Tablets ... 845

Hydralazine Hydrochloride (Concurrent use with antihypertensives, such as hydralazine, may result in hypernatremia). Products include:
- Apresazide Capsules ... 824
- Apresoline Hydrochloride Tablets ... 826
- Hydralazine Hydrochloride Injection USP ... 2712
- Ser-Ap-Es Tablets ... 867

Magaldrate (Co-administration with antacids may bind the phosphate and prevent its absorption).
No products indexed under this heading.

Magnesium Hydroxide (Co-administration with antacids may bind the phosphate and prevent its absorption). Products include:
- Aludrox Oral Suspension ... 850
- Ascriptin ... 650
- Di-Gel Antacid/Anti-Gas ... 762
- Gelusil Antacid-Anti-gas Liquid ... 819
- Gelusil Antacid-Anti-gas Tablets ... 819
- Maalox Antacid/Anti-Gas Tablets ... 889
- Maalox Antacid Liquid ... 888
- Extra Strength Maalox Antacid/Anti-Gas Liquid and Tablets ... 888
- Mylanta Fast-Acting ... 1359
- Mylanta Gelcaps Antacid ... 678
- Fast-Acting Mylanta Liquid Antacid ... 1359
- Mylanta Tablets ... 677
- Maximum-Strength Fast-Acting Mylanta Liquid Antacid ... 1359
- Mylanta Double Strength Tablets ... 677
- Phillips' Milk of Magnesia Liquid ... 627
- Rolaids Antacid Tablets ... 807
- Tempo Soft Antacid ... 799

Magnesium Oxide (Co-administration with antacids may bind the phosphate and prevent its absorption). Products include:
- Beelith Tablets ... 632
- Bufferin Analgesic Tablets ... 636
- Arthritis Strength Bufferin Analgesic Caplets ... 637
- Extra Strength Bufferin Analgesic Tablets ... 637
- Caltrate PLUS ... 681
- Cama Arthritis Pain Reliever ... 748
- Mag-Ox 400 ... 666
- Uro-Mag ... 666

Methyldopa (Concurrent use with antihypertensives, such as methyldopa, may result in hypernatremia). Products include:
- Aldoclor Tablets ... 1638
- Aldomet Oral ... 1640
- Aldoril Tablets ... 1644

Potassium Acid Phosphate (Concurrent use with potassium-containing medications may cause hyperkalemia). Products include:
- K-Phos Original Formula 'Sodium Free' Tablets ... 633

Potassium Bicarbonate (Concurrent use with potassium-containing medications may cause hyperkalemia). Products include:
- Alka-Seltzer Gold Effervescent Antacid ... 611

Potassium Chloride (Concurrent use with potassium-containing medications may cause hyperkalemia). Products include:
- Chlor-3 Condiment ... 1003
- Colyte and Colyte-flavored ... 2540
- GoLYTELY ... 694
- K-Dur Microburst Release System (potassium chloride, USP) E.R. Tablets ... 1364
- K-Lor Powder Packets ... 438
- K-Norm Capsules ... 1615
- K-Tab Filmtab ... 439
- Micro-K ... 2237
- Micro-K LS Packets ... 2238
- NuLYTELY ... 694
- Cherry Flavor NuLYTELY ... 694
- Rum-K Syrup ... 1004
- Slow-K Extended-Release Tablets ... 869

Potassium Citrate (Concurrent use with potassium-containing medications may cause hyperkalemia). Products include:
- Polycitra Syrup ... 574
- Polycitra-K Crystals ... 574
- Polycitra-K Oral Solution ... 575
- Polycitra-LC ... 574
- Urocit-K Tablets ... 1828

Potassium Gluconate (Concurrent use with potassium-containing medications may cause hyperkalemia).
No products indexed under this heading.

Potassium Phosphate, Dibasic (Concurrent use with potassium-containing medications may cause hyperkalemia).
No products indexed under this heading.

Rauwolfia Serpentina (Concurrent use with antihypertensives, such as rauwolfia alkaloids, may result in hypernatremia).
No products indexed under this heading.

Rescinnamine (Concurrent use with antihypertensives, such as rauwolfia alkaloids, may result in hypernatremia).
No products indexed under this heading.

Reserpine (Concurrent use with antihypertensives, such as rauwolfia alkaloids, may result in hypernatremia). Products include:
- Diupres Tablets ... 1691
- Hydropres Tablets ... 1718
- Ser-Ap-Es Tablets ... 867

Spironolactone (Concurrent use with potassium-sparing diuretics may cause hyperkalemia). Products include:
- Aldactazide Tablets ... 2556
- Aldactone Tablets ... 2558

Triamterene (Concurrent use with potassium-sparing diuretics may cause hyperkalemia). Products include:
- Dyazide Capsules ... 2653
- Dyrenium Capsules ... 2655

Vitamin D (Concurrent use with vitamin D may antagonize the effects of phosphates in the treatment of hypercalcemia). Products include:
- Caltrate PLUS ... 681
- Caltrate 600 + D ... 681
- Dical-D Tablets & Wafers ... 424
- Materna Tablets ... 1427
- Megadose ... 513
- One-A-Day Calcium Plus ... 625

K-PHOS ORIGINAL FORMULA 'SODIUM FREE' TABLETS

(Potassium Acid Phosphate) ... 633
May interact with antacids, potassium sparing diuretics, salicylates, potassium preparations, and certain other agents. Compounds in these categories include:

Aluminum Carbonate (May bind phosphate and prevent its absorption). Products include:
- Basaljel Capsules ... 2810
- Basaljel Suspension ... 2810
- Basaljel Tablets ... 2810

Aluminum Hydroxide (May bind phosphate and prevent its absorption). Products include:
- ALternaGEL Liquid ... 1358
- Maximum Strength Ascriptin ... 650
- Cama Arthritis Pain Reliever ... 748
- Gaviscon Extra Strength Relief Formula Antacid Tablets ... 778
- Gaviscon Extra Strength Relief Formula Liquid Antacid ... 779
- Gaviscon Liquid Antacid ... 779
- Gelusil Antacid-Anti-gas Liquid ... 819
- Gelusil Antacid-Anti-gas Tablets ... 819
- Maalox Antacid/Anti-Gas Tablets ... 889
- Maalox Heartburn Relief Suspension ... 658
- Maalox Antacid Liquid ... 888
- Extra Strength Maalox Antacid/Anti-Gas Liquid and Tablets ... 888
- Mylanta ... 1359
- Tempo Soft Antacid ... 799

Aluminum Hydroxide Gel (May bind phosphate and prevent its absorption). Products include:
- ALternaGEL Liquid ... 675
- Aludrox Oral Suspension ... 850
- Amphojel Suspension ... 2802
- Amphojel Suspension without Flavor ... 2802
- Amphojel Tablets ... 2802
- Ascriptin ... 650
- Gaviscon Antacid Tablets ... 778
- Gaviscon-2 Antacid Tablets ... 779
- Mylanta Liquid ... 676
- Mylanta Double Strength Liquid ... 676
- Nephrox Suspension ... 671

Amiloride Hydrochloride (Hyperkalemia). Products include:
- Midamor Tablets ... 1746
- Moduretic Tablets ... 1748

Aspirin (Increased serum salicylate levels; possible toxicity). Products include:
- Alka-Seltzer Cherry Effervescent Antacid and Pain Reliever ... 609
- Alka-Seltzer Extra Strength Effervescent Antacid and Pain Reliever ... 609
- Alka-Seltzer Lemon Lime Effervescent Antacid and Pain Reliever ... 609
- Alka-Seltzer Original Effervescent Antacid and Pain Reliever ... 609
- Alka-Seltzer Plus ... 611
- Alka-Seltzer Plus Sinus Medicine ... 611
- Ascriptin ... 650
- Arthritis Strength BC Powder ... 631
- BC Cold Powder Multi-Symptom Formula (Cold-Sinus-Allergy) ... 631
- BC Cold Powder Non-Drowsy Formula (Cold-Sinus) ... 631
- BC Powder ... 631
- Genuine Bayer Aspirin Tablets & Caplets ... 618
- Extra Strength Bayer Arthritis Pain Regimen Formula ... 615
- Extra Strength Bayer Aspirin Caplets & Tablets ... 617
- Extended-Release Bayer 8-Hour Aspirin ... 616
- Extra Strength Bayer Plus Aspirin Caplets ... 617
- Extra Strength Bayer PM Aspirin Plus Sleep Aid ... 617
- Aspirin Regimen Bayer 81 mg Tablets with Calcium ... 615
- Aspirin Regimen Bayer Adult Low Strength 81 mg Tablets ... 613
- Aspirin Regimen Bayer Children's Chewable Aspirin ... 616
- Aspirin Regimen Bayer Regular Strength 325 mg Caplets ... 613
- Bufferin Analgesic Tablets ... 636
- Arthritis Strength Bufferin Analgesic Caplets ... 637
- Extra Strength Bufferin Analgesic Tablets ... 637
- Cama Arthritis Pain Reliever ... 748
- Darvon Compound-65 Pulvules ... 1475
- Easprin ... 1971
- Ecotrin ... 2625
- Ecotrin Enteric Coated Aspirin Maximum Strength Tablets and Caplets ... 775
- Ecotrin Enteric Coated Aspirin Regular Strength Tablets ... 2625
- Empirin Aspirin Tablets ... 818
- Excedrin Extra-Strength Analgesic Tablets, Caplets, and Geltabs ... 734
- Fiorinal Capsules ... 2388
- Fiorinal with Codeine Capsules ... 2390
- Fiorinal Tablets ... 2388
- Goody's Extra Strength Headache Powders ... 632
- Goody's Extra Strength Pain Relief Tablets ... 632
- Halfprin Tablets ... 1413
- Norgesic ... 1554
- Percodan Tablets ... 955
- Percodan-Demi Tablets ... 956
- Robaxisal Tablets ... 2246
- Soma Compound w/Codeine Tablets ... 2784
- Soma Compound Tablets ... 2783
- St. Joseph Adult Chewable Aspirin (81 mg.) ... 768
- Talwin Compound ... 2466
- Vanquish Analgesic Caplets ... 627

Choline Magnesium Trisalicylate (Increased serum salicylate levels; possible toxicity). Products include:
- Trilisate ... 2155

Diflunisal (Increased serum salicylate levels; possible toxicity). Products include:
- Dolobid Tablets ... 1695

Magaldrate (May bind phosphate and prevent its absorption).
No products indexed under this heading.

Magnesium Hydroxide (May bind phosphate and prevent its absorption). Products include:
- Aludrox Oral Suspension ... 850
- Ascriptin ... 650
- Di-Gel Antacid/Anti-Gas ... 762
- Gelusil Antacid-Anti-gas Liquid ... 819
- Gelusil Antacid-Anti-gas Tablets ... 819
- Maalox Antacid/Anti-Gas Tablets ... 889
- Maalox Antacid Liquid ... 888
- Extra Strength Maalox Antacid/Anti-Gas Liquid and Tablets ... 888
- Mylanta Fast-Acting ... 1359
- Mylanta Gelcaps Antacid ... 678
- Fast-Acting Mylanta Liquid Antacid ... 1359
- Mylanta Tablets ... 677
- Maximum-Strength Fast-Acting Mylanta Liquid Antacid ... 1359
- Mylanta Double Strength Tablets ... 677
- Phillips' Milk of Magnesia Liquid ... 627
- Rolaids Antacid Tablets ... 807
- Tempo Soft Antacid ... 799

Magnesium Oxide (May bind phosphate and prevent its absorption). Products include:
- Beelith Tablets ... 632
- Bufferin Analgesic Tablets ... 636
- Arthritis Strength Bufferin Analgesic Caplets ... 637
- Extra Strength Bufferin Analgesic Tablets ... 637
- Caltrate PLUS ... 681
- Cama Arthritis Pain Reliever ... 748
- Mag-Ox 400 ... 666
- Uro-Mag ... 666

Magnesium Salicylate (Increased serum salicylate levels; possible toxicity). Products include:
- Backache Caplets ... 635
- Doan's Extra-Strength Analgesic ... 653
- Extra Strength Doan's P.M. ... 653
- Doan's Regular Strength Analgesic ... 654
- Mobigesic Tablets ... 607

Potassium Bicarbonate (Potential for hyperkalemia). Products include:
- Alka-Seltzer Gold Effervescent Antacid ... 611

Potassium Chloride (Potential for hyperkalemia). Products include:
- Chlor-3 Condiment ... 1003
- Colyte and Colyte-flavored ... 2540
- GoLYTELY ... 694
- K-Dur Microburst Release System (potassium chloride, USP) E.R. Tablets ... 1364
- K-Lor Powder Packets ... 438
- K-Norm Capsules ... 1615
- K-Tab Filmtab ... 439
- Micro-K ... 2237
- Micro-K LS Packets ... 2238
- NuLYTELY ... 694
- Cherry Flavor NuLYTELY ... 694
- Rum-K Syrup ... 1004
- Slow-K Extended-Release Tablets ... 869

Potassium Citrate (Potential for hyperkalemia). Products include:
- Polycitra Syrup ... 574
- Polycitra-K Crystals ... 574
- Polycitra-K Oral Solution ... 575
- Polycitra-LC ... 574
- Urocit-K Tablets ... 1828

(▣ Described in PDR For Nonprescription Drugs) (Ⓞ Described in PDR For Ophthalmology)

Potassium Gluconate (Potential for hyperkalemia).
No products indexed under this heading.

Potassium Phosphate, Dibasic (Potential for hyperkalemia).
No products indexed under this heading.

Potassium Phosphate, Monobasic (Potential for hyperkalemia). Products include:
K-Phos Neutral Tablets 633
K-Phos Original Formula 'Sodium Free' Tablets 633

Salsalate (Increased serum salicylate levels; possible toxicity). Products include:
Disalcid 1549
Mono-Gesic Tablets 810
Salflex Tablets 791

Spironolactone (Hyperkalemia). Products include:
Aldactazide Tablets 2556
Aldactone Tablets 2558

Triamterene (Hyperkalemia). Products include:
Dyazide Capsules 2653
Dyrenium Capsules 2655

K-TAB FILMTAB
(Potassium Chloride) 439
May interact with potassium sparing diuretics, ACE inhibitors, and anticholinergics. Compounds in these categories include:

Amiloride Hydrochloride (Potential for severe hyperkalemia). Products include:
Midamor Tablets 1746
Moduretic Tablets 1748

Atropine Sulfate (Anticholinergic drugs can be cause for delay or arrest in tablet passage through the gastrointestinal tract; concomitant administration of drugs capable of decreasing GI motility should be avoided). Products include:
Arco-Lase Plus Tablets 513
Atrohist Plus Tablets 1605
Donnatal 2234
Donnatal Extentabs 2234
Donnatal Tablets 2234
Lomotil 2591
Motofen Tablets 789
Urised Tablets 2123

Belladonna Alkaloids (Anticholinergic drugs can be cause for delay or arrest in tablet passage through the gastrointestinal tract; concomitant administration of drugs capable of decreasing GI motility should be avoided). Products include:
Bellergal-S Tablets 2375
Hyland's Bedwetting Tablets 788
Hyland's EnurAid Tablets 789
Hyland's Headache Tablets 790
Hyland's Teething Tablets 790
Similasan Eye Drops #1 769

Benazepril Hydrochloride (Concomitant therapy may result in hyperkalemia; close monitoring is advised). Products include:
Lotensin Tablets 852
Lotensin HCT Tablets 855
Lotrel Capsules 858

Benztropine Mesylate (Anticholinergic drugs can be cause for delay or arrest in tablet passage through the gastrointestinal tract; concomitant administration of drugs capable of decreasing GI motility should be avoided). Products include:
Cogentin 1661

Biperiden Hydrochloride (Anticholinergic drugs can be cause for delay or arrest in tablet passage through the gastrointestinal tract; concomitant administration of drugs capable of decreasing GI motility should be avoided). Products include:
Akineton 1380

Captopril (Concomitant therapy may result in hyperkalemia; close monitoring is advised). Products include:
Capoten Tablets 740
Capozide Tablets 744

Clidinium Bromide (Anticholinergic drugs can be cause for delay or arrest in tablet passage through the gastrointestinal tract; concomitant administration of drugs capable of decreasing GI motility should be avoided). Products include:
Librax Capsules 2330

Dicyclomine Hydrochloride (Anticholinergic drugs can be cause for delay or arrest in tablet passage through the gastrointestinal tract; concomitant administration of drugs capable of decreasing GI motility should be avoided). Products include:
Bentyl 1246

Enalapril Maleate (Concomitant therapy may result in hyperkalemia; close monitoring is advised). Products include:
Vaseretic Tablets 1810
Vasotec Tablets 1816

Enalaprilat (Concomitant therapy may result in hyperkalemia; close monitoring is advised). Products include:
Vasotec I.V. 1814

Fosinopril Sodium (Concomitant therapy may result in hyperkalemia; close monitoring is advised). Products include:
Monopril Tablets 762

Glycopyrrolate (Anticholinergic drugs can be cause for delay or arrest in tablet passage through the gastrointestinal tract; concomitant administration of drugs capable of decreasing GI motility should be avoided). Products include:
Robinul Forte Tablets 2247
Robinul Injectable 2247
Robinul Tablets 2247

Hyoscyamine (Anticholinergic drugs can be cause for delay or arrest in tablet passage through the gastrointestinal tract; concomitant administration of drugs capable of decreasing GI motility should be avoided). Products include:
Cystospaz Tablets 2123
Urised Tablets 2123

Hyoscyamine Sulfate (Anticholinergic drugs can be cause for delay or arrest in tablet passage through the gastrointestinal tract; concomitant administration of drugs capable of decreasing GI motility should be avoided). Products include:
Arco-Lase Plus Tablets 513
Atrohist Plus Tablets 1605
Cystospaz-M Capsules 2123
Donnatal 2234
Donnatal Extentabs 2234
Donnatal Tablets 2234
Kutrase Capsules 2546
Levsin/Levsinex/Levbid 2549

Ipratropium Bromide (Anticholinergic drugs can be cause for delay or arrest in tablet passage through the gastrointestinal tract; concomitant administration of drugs capable of decreasing GI motility should be avoided). Products include:
Atrovent Inhalation Aerosol 674
Atrovent Inhalation Solution 675
Atrovent Nasal Spray 0.03% 676
Atrovent Nasal Spray 0.06% 678

Lisinopril (Concomitant therapy may result in hyperkalemia; close monitoring is advised). Products include:
Prinivil Tablets 1776
Prinzide Tablets 1780
Zestoretic Tablets 2968
Zestril Tablets 2972

Mepenzolate Bromide (Anticholinergic drugs can be cause for delay or arrest in tablet passage through the gastrointestinal tract; concomitant administration of drugs capable of decreasing GI motility should be avoided).
No products indexed under this heading.

Moexipril Hydrochloride (Concomitant therapy may result in hyperkalemia; close monitoring is advised). Products include:
Univasc Tablets 2553

Oxybutynin Chloride (Anticholinergic drugs can be cause for delay or arrest in tablet passage through the gastrointestinal tract; concomitant administration of drugs capable of decreasing GI motility should be avoided). Products include:
Ditropan 1267

Procyclidine Hydrochloride (Anticholinergic drugs can be cause for delay or arrest in tablet passage through the gastrointestinal tract; concomitant administration of drugs capable of decreasing GI motility should be avoided). Products include:
Kemadrin Tablets 1105

Propantheline Bromide (Anticholinergic drugs can be cause for delay or arrest in tablet passage through the gastrointestinal tract; concomitant administration of drugs capable of decreasing GI motility should be avoided). Products include:
Pro-Banthine Tablets 2226

Quinapril Hydrochloride (Concomitant therapy may result in hyperkalemia; close monitoring is advised). Products include:
Accupril Tablets 1950

Ramipril (Concomitant therapy may result in hyperkalemia; close monitoring is advised). Products include:
Altace Capsules 1238

Scopolamine (Anticholinergic drugs can be cause for delay or arrest in tablet passage through the gastrointestinal tract; concomitant administration of drugs capable of decreasing GI motility should be avoided). Products include:
Transderm Scōp Transdermal Therapeutic System 890

Scopolamine Hydrobromide (Anticholinergic drugs can be cause for delay or arrest in tablet passage through the gastrointestinal tract; concomitant administration of drugs capable of decreasing GI motility should be avoided). Products include:
Atrohist Plus Tablets 1605
Donnatal 2234

Donnatal Extentabs 2234
Donnatal Tablets 2234

Spirapril Hydrochloride (Concomitant therapy may result in hyperkalemia; close monitoring is advised).
No products indexed under this heading.

Spironolactone (Potential for severe hyperkalemia). Products include:
Aldactazide Tablets 2556
Aldactone Tablets 2558

Trandolapril (Concomitant therapy may result in hyperkalemia; close monitoring is advised). Products include:
Mavik Tablets 1407

Triamterene (Potential for severe hyperkalemia). Products include:
Dyazide Capsules 2653
Dyrenium Capsules 2655

Tridihexethyl Chloride (Anticholinergic drugs can be cause for delay or arrest in tablet passage through the gastrointestinal tract; concomitant administration of drugs capable of decreasing GI motility should be avoided).
No products indexed under this heading.

Trihexyphenidyl Hydrochloride (Anticholinergic drugs can be cause for delay or arrest in tablet passage through the gastrointestinal tract; concomitant administration of drugs capable of decreasing GI motility should be avoided). Products include:
Artane 1418

KADIAN CAPSULES
(Morphine Sulfate) 2948
May interact with central nervous system depressants, hypnotics and sedatives, general anesthetics, phenothiazines, tranquilizers, neuromuscular blocking agents, mixed agonist/antagonist opioid analgesics, monoamine oxidase inhibitors, diuretics, and certain other agents. Compounds in these categories include:

Alfentanil Hydrochloride (Co-administration may increase the risk of respiratory depression, hypotension and profound sedation and coma; when such combined therapy is contemplated, the initial dose of one or both agents should be reduced by at least 50%). Products include:
Alfenta Injection 1334

Alprazolam (Co-administration may increase the risk of respiratory depression, hypotension and profound sedation and coma; when such combined therapy is contemplated, the initial dose of one or both agents should be reduced by at least 50%). Products include:
Xanax Tablets 2115

Amiloride Hydrochloride (Morphine can reduce the efficacy of diuretics by inducing the release of antidiuretic hormone and by causing spasm of the sphincter of the bladder leading to acute retention of urine). Products include:
Midamor Tablets 1746
Moduretic Tablets 1748

Aprobarbital (Co-administration may increase the risk of respiratory depression, hypotension and profound sedation and coma; when such combined therapy is contemplated, the initial dose of one or both agents should be reduced by at least 50%).
No products indexed under this heading.

IMPORTANT NOTE: Always consult each drug listing in the patient's regimen for possible interactions.

Atracurium Besylate (Morphine may enhance the neuromuscular blocking action of skeletal relaxants and produce an increased degree of respiratory depression). Products include:
- Tracrium Injection 1155

Bendroflumethiazide (Morphine can reduce the efficacy of diuretics by inducing the release of antidiuretic hormone and by causing spasm of the sphincter of the bladder leading to acute retention of urine).
- No products indexed under this heading.

Bumetanide (Morphine can reduce the efficacy of diuretics by inducing the release of antidiuretic hormone and by causing spasm of the sphincter of the bladder leading to acute retention of urine). Products include:
- Bumex 2260

Buprenorphine (May reduce the analgesic effect and/or precipitate withdrawal symptoms). Products include:
- Buprenex Injectable 2170

Buspirone Hydrochloride (Co-administration may increase the risk of respiratory depression, hypotension and profound sedation and coma; when such combined therapy is contemplated, the initial dose of one or both agents should be reduced by at least 50%). Products include:
- BuSpar Tablets 738

Butabarbital (Co-administration may increase the risk of respiratory depression, hypotension and profound sedation and coma; when such combined therapy is contemplated, the initial dose of one or both agents should be reduced by at least 50%).
- No products indexed under this heading.

Butalbital (Co-administration may increase the risk of respiratory depression, hypotension and profound sedation and coma; when such combined therapy is contemplated, the initial dose of one or both agents should be reduced by at least 50%). Products include:
- Axocet Capsules 2469
- Esgic-plus Capsules 1012
- Esgic-plus Tablets 1012
- Fioricet Tablets 2386
- Fioricet with Codeine Capsules ... 2387
- Fiorinal Capsules 2388
- Fiorinal with Codeine Capsules ... 2390
- Fiorinal Tablets 2388
- Phrenilin 790
- Sedapap Tablets 50 mg/650 mg .. 1826

Butorphanol Tartrate (May reduce the analgesic effect and/or precipitate withdrawal symptoms). Products include:
- Stadol 779

Chlordiazepoxide (Co-administration may increase the risk of respiratory depression, hypotension and profound sedation and coma; when such combined therapy is contemplated, the initial dose of one or both agents should be reduced by at least 50%). Products include:
- Limbitrol 2333

Chlordiazepoxide Hydrochloride (Co-administration may increase the risk of respiratory depression, hypotension and profound sedation and coma; when such combined therapy is contemplated, the initial dose of one or both agents should be reduced by at least 50%). Products include:
- Librax Capsules 2330
- Librium Capsules 2331
- Librium Injectable 2332

Chlorothiazide (Morphine can reduce the efficacy of diuretics by inducing the release of antidiuretic hormone and by causing spasm of the sphincter of the bladder leading to acute retention of urine). Products include:
- Aldoclor Tablets 1638
- Diupres Tablets 1691
- Diuril Oral 1694

Chlorothiazide Sodium (Morphine can reduce the efficacy of diuretics by inducing the release of antidiuretic hormone and by causing spasm of the sphincter of the bladder leading to acute retention of urine). Products include:
- Diuril Sodium Intravenous 1693

Chlorpromazine (Co-administration may increase the risk of respiratory depression, hypotension and profound sedation and coma; when such combined therapy is contemplated, the initial dose of one or both agents should be reduced by at least 50%). Products include:
- Thorazine Suppositories 2701

Chlorpromazine Hydrochloride (Co-administration may increase the risk of respiratory depression, hypotension and profound sedation and coma; when such combined therapy is contemplated, the initial dose of one or both agents should be reduced by at least 50%). Products include:
- Thorazine 2701

Chlorprothixene (Co-administration may increase the risk of respiratory depression, hypotension and profound sedation and coma; when such combined therapy is contemplated, the initial dose of one or both agents should be reduced by at least 50%).
- No products indexed under this heading.

Chlorprothixene Hydrochloride (Co-administration may increase the risk of respiratory depression, hypotension and profound sedation and coma; when such combined therapy is contemplated, the initial dose of one or both agents should be reduced by at least 50%).
- No products indexed under this heading.

Chlorprothixene Lactate (Co-administration may increase the risk of respiratory depression, hypotension and profound sedation and coma; when such combined therapy is contemplated, the initial dose of one or both agents should be reduced by at least 50%).
- No products indexed under this heading.

Chlorthalidone (Morphine can reduce the efficacy of diuretics by inducing the release of antidiuretic hormone and by causing spasm of the sphincter of the bladder leading to acute retention of urine). Products include:
- Combipres Tablets 682
- Tenoretic Tablets 2963
- Thalitone 1293

Cimetidine (Co-administration has resulted in an isolated report of confusion and severe respiratory depression). Products include:
- Tagamet HB Tablets 786
- Tagamet Tablets 2694

Cimetidine Hydrochloride (Co-administration has resulted in an isolated report of confusion and severe respiratory depression). Products include:
- Tagamet 2694

Cisatracurium Besylate (Morphine may enhance the neuromuscular blocking action of skeletal relaxants and produce an increased degree of respiratory depression). Products include:
- Nimbex Injection 1131

Clorazepate Dipotassium (Co-administration may increase the risk of respiratory depression, hypotension and profound sedation and coma; when such combined therapy is contemplated, the initial dose of one or both agents should be reduced by at least 50%). Products include:
- Tranxene 459

Clozapine (Co-administration may increase the risk of respiratory depression, hypotension and profound sedation and coma; when such combined therapy is contemplated, the initial dose of one or both agents should be reduced by at least 50%). Products include:
- Clozaril Tablets 2377

Codeine Phosphate (Co-administration may increase the risk of respiratory depression, hypotension and profound sedation and coma; when such combined therapy is contemplated, the initial dose of one or both agents should be reduced by at least 50%). Products include:
- Brontex 2130
- Dimetane-DC Cough Syrup 2232
- Fioricet with Codeine Capsules ... 2387
- Fiorinal with Codeine Capsules ... 2390
- Nucofed 2225
- Phenergan with Codeine 2883
- Phenergan VC with Codeine 2888
- Robitussin A-C Syrup 2248
- Robitussin-DAC Syrup 2249
- Ryna 804
- Soma Compound w/Codeine Tablets 2784
- Tylenol with Codeine 1592

Desflurane (Co-administration may increase the risk of respiratory depression, hypotension and profound sedation and coma; when such combined therapy is contemplated, the initial dose of one or both agents should be reduced by at least 50%). Products include:
- Suprane (desflurane, USP) 1865

Dezocine (Co-administration may increase the risk of respiratory depression, hypotension and profound sedation and coma; when such combined therapy is contemplated, the initial dose of one or both agents should be reduced by at least 50%). Products include:
- Dalgan Injection 529

Diazepam (Co-administration may increase the risk of respiratory depression, hypotension and profound sedation and coma; when such combined therapy is contemplated, the initial dose of one or both agents should be reduced by at least 50%). Products include:
- Dizac (diazepam injectable emulsion) CIV 1862
- Valium Injectable 2336
- Valium Tablets 2335

Doxacurium Chloride (Morphine may enhance the neuromuscular blocking action of skeletal relaxants and produce an increased degree of respiratory depression). Products include:
- Nuromax Injection 1136

Droperidol (Co-administration may increase the risk of respiratory depression, hypotension and profound sedation and coma; when such combined therapy is contemplated, the initial dose of one or both agents should be reduced by at least 50%). Products include:
- Inapsine Injection 462

Enflurane (Co-administration may increase the risk of respiratory depression, hypotension and profound sedation and coma; when such combined therapy is contemplated, the initial dose of one or both agents should be reduced by at least 50%).
- No products indexed under this heading.

Estazolam (Co-administration may increase the risk of respiratory depression, hypotension and profound sedation and coma; when such combined therapy is contemplated, the initial dose of one or both agents should be reduced by at least 50%). Products include:
- ProSom Tablets 457

Ethacrynic Acid (Morphine can reduce the efficacy of diuretics by inducing the release of antidiuretic hormone and by causing spasm of the sphincter of the bladder leading to acute retention of urine). Products include:
- Edecrin Tablets 1698

Ethchlorvynol (Co-administration may increase the risk of respiratory depression, hypotension and profound sedation and coma; when such combined therapy is contemplated, the initial dose of one or both agents should be reduced by at least 50%). Products include:
- Placidyl Capsules 456

Ethinamate (Co-administration may increase the risk of respiratory depression, hypotension and profound sedation and coma; when such combined therapy is contemplated, the initial dose of one or both agents should be reduced by at least 50%).
- No products indexed under this heading.

Fentanyl (Co-administration may increase the risk of respiratory depression, hypotension and profound sedation and coma; when such combined therapy is contemplated, the initial dose of one or both agents should be reduced by at least 50%). Products include:
- Duragesic Transdermal System .. 1336

Fentanyl Citrate (Co-administration may increase the risk of respiratory depression, hypotension and profound sedation and coma; when such combined therapy is contemplated, the initial dose of one or both agents should be reduced by at least 50%). Products include:
- Sublimaze Injection 463

Fluphenazine Decanoate (Co-administration may increase the risk of respiratory depression, hypotension and profound sedation and coma; when such combined therapy is contemplated, the initial dose of one or both agents should be reduced by at least 50%). Products include:
- Prolixin Decanoate 510

(▣ Described in PDR For Nonprescription Drugs)   (⊙ Described in PDR For Ophthalmology)

Fluphenazine Enanthate (Co-administration may increase the risk of respiratory depression, hypotension and profound sedation and coma; when such combined therapy is contemplated, the initial dose of one or both agents should be reduced by at least 50%). Products include:
   Prolixin Enanthate 510

Fluphenazine Hydrochloride (Co-administration may increase the risk of respiratory depression, hypotension and profound sedation and coma; when such combined therapy is contemplated, the initial dose of one or both agents should be reduced by at least 50%). Products include:
   Prolixin 510

Flurazepam Hydrochloride (Co-administration may increase the risk of respiratory depression, hypotension and profound sedation and coma; when such combined therapy is contemplated, the initial dose of one or both agents should be reduced by at least 50%). Products include:
   Dalmane Capsules 2329

Furazolidone (MAO inhibitors have been reported to intensify the effects of opioids causing anxiety, confusion and significant depression of respiration or coma; concurrent and/or sequential use is not recommended). Products include:
   Furoxone 2221

Furosemide (Morphine can reduce the efficacy of diuretics by inducing the release of antidiuretic hormone and by causing spasm of the sphincter of the bladder leading to acute retention of urine). Products include:
   Lasix Injection, Oral Solution and Tablets 1267

Glutethimide (Co-administration may increase the risk of respiratory depression, hypotension and profound sedation and coma; when such combined therapy is contemplated, the initial dose of one or both agents should be reduced by at least 50%).
   No products indexed under this heading.

Haloperidol (Co-administration may increase the risk of respiratory depression, hypotension and profound sedation and coma; when such combined therapy is contemplated, the initial dose of one or both agents should be reduced by at least 50%). Products include:
   Haldol Injection, Tablets and Concentrate 1585

Haloperidol Decanoate (Co-administration may increase the risk of respiratory depression, hypotension and profound sedation and coma; when such combined therapy is contemplated, the initial dose of one or both agents should be reduced by at least 50%). Products include:
   Haldol Decanoate 1587

Hydrochlorothiazide (Morphine can reduce the efficacy of diuretics by inducing the release of antidiuretic hormone and by causing spasm of the sphincter of the bladder leading to acute retention of urine). Products include:
   Aldactazide Tablets 2556
   Aldoril Tablets 1644
   Apresazide Capsules 824
   Capozide Tablets 744
   Dyazide Capsules 2653
   Esidrix Tablets 839
   Esimil Tablets 840
   HydroDIURIL Tablets 1716
   Hydropres Tablets 1718
   Hyzaar Tablets 1720
   Inderide Tablets 2838
   Inderide LA Long Acting Capsules .. 2840
   Lopressor HCT Tablets 850
   Lotensin HCT Tablets 855
   Moduretic Tablets 1748
   Oretic Tablets 450
   Prinzide Tablets 1780
   Ser-Ap-Es Tablets 867
   Timolide Tablets 1791
   Vaseretic Tablets 1810
   Zestoretic Tablets 2968
   Ziac 1459

Hydrocodone Bitartrate (Co-administration may increase the risk of respiratory depression, hypotension and profound sedation and coma; when such combined therapy is contemplated, the initial dose of one or both agents should be reduced by at least 50%). Products include:
   Codiclear DH Syrup 808
   Duratuss HD Elixir 2750
   Histussin D Liquid 670
   Hycodan Tablets and Syrup 946
   Hycomine Compound Tablets 948
   Hycomine 947
   Hycotuss Expectorant Syrup 950
   Hydrocet Capsules 787
   Lorcet 10/650 Tablets 1016
   Lortab 2751
   Tussend 1830
   Tussend Expectorant 1831
   Vicodin Tablets 1404
   Vicodin ES Tablets 1405
   Vicodin HP Tablets 1403
   Vicodin Tuss Expectorant 1406
   Zydone Capsules 967

Hydrocodone Polistirex (Co-administration may increase the risk of respiratory depression, hypotension and profound sedation and coma; when such combined therapy is contemplated, the initial dose of one or both agents should be reduced by at least 50%). Products include:
   Tussionex Pennkinetic Extended-Release Suspension 1624

Hydroflumethiazide (Morphine can reduce the efficacy of diuretics by inducing the release of antidiuretic hormone and by causing spasm of the sphincter of the bladder leading to acute retention of urine). Products include:
   Diucardin Tablets 2824

Hydroxyzine Hydrochloride (Co-administration may increase the risk of respiratory depression, hypotension and profound sedation and coma; when such combined therapy is contemplated, the initial dose of one or both agents should be reduced by at least 50%). Products include:
   Atarax Tablets & Syrup 1992
   Marax Tablets & DF Syrup 2015
   Vistaril Intramuscular Solution 2042

Indapamide (Morphine can reduce the efficacy of diuretics by inducing the release of antidiuretic hormone and by causing spasm of the sphincter of the bladder leading to acute retention of urine).
   No products indexed under this heading.

Isocarboxazid (MAO inhibitors have been reported to intensify the effects of opioids causing anxiety, confusion and significant depression of respiration or coma; concurrent and/or sequential use is not recommended).
   No products indexed under this heading.

Isoflurane (Co-administration may increase the risk of respiratory depression, hypotension and profound sedation and coma; when such combined therapy is contemplated, the initial dose of one or both agents should be reduced by at least 50%).
   No products indexed under this heading.

Ketamine Hydrochloride (Co-administration may increase the risk of respiratory depression, hypotension and profound sedation and coma; when such combined therapy is contemplated, the initial dose of one or both agents should be reduced by at least 50%).
   No products indexed under this heading.

Levomethadyl Acetate Hydrochloride (Co-administration may increase the risk of respiratory depression, hypotension and profound sedation and coma; when such combined therapy is contemplated, the initial dose of one or both agents should be reduced by at least 50%). Products include:
   Orlaam Oral Solution 2361

Levorphanol Tartrate (Co-administration may increase the risk of respiratory depression, hypotension and profound sedation and coma; when such combined therapy is contemplated, the initial dose of one or both agents should be reduced by at least 50%). Products include:
   Levo-Dromoran 2297

Lorazepam (Co-administration may increase the risk of respiratory depression, hypotension and profound sedation and coma; when such combined therapy is contemplated, the initial dose of one or both agents should be reduced by at least 50%). Products include:
   Ativan Injection 2805
   Ativan Tablets 2807

Loxapine Hydrochloride (Co-administration may increase the risk of respiratory depression, hypotension and profound sedation and coma; when such combined therapy is contemplated, the initial dose of one or both agents should be reduced by at least 50%). Products include:
   Loxitane 1426

Loxapine Succinate (Co-administration may increase the risk of respiratory depression, hypotension and profound sedation and coma; when such combined therapy is contemplated, the initial dose of one or both agents should be reduced by at least 50%). Products include:
   Loxitane Capsules 1426

Meperidine Hydrochloride (Co-administration may increase the risk of respiratory depression, hypotension and profound sedation and coma; when such combined therapy is contemplated, the initial dose of one or both agents should be reduced by at least 50%). Products include:
   Demerol 2438
   Mepergan Injection 2859

Mephobarbital (Co-administration may increase the risk of respiratory depression, hypotension and profound sedation and coma; when such combined therapy is contemplated, the initial dose of one or both agents should be reduced by at least 50%). Products include:
   Mebaral Tablets 2452

Meprobamate (Co-administration may increase the risk of respiratory depression, hypotension and profound sedation and coma; when such combined therapy is contemplated, the initial dose of one or both agents should be reduced by at least 50%). Products include:
   Miltown Tablets 2780
   PMB 200 and PMB 400 2890

Mesoridazine Besylate (Co-administration may increase the risk of respiratory depression, hypotension and profound sedation and coma; when such combined therapy is contemplated, the initial dose of one or both agents should be reduced by at least 50%). Products include:
   Serentil 689

Methadone Hydrochloride (Co-administration may increase the risk of respiratory depression, hypotension and profound sedation and coma; when such combined therapy is contemplated, the initial dose of one or both agents should be reduced by at least 50%). Products include:
   Methadone Hydrochloride Oral Concentrate 2356
   Methadone Hydrochloride Oral Solution & Tablets 2357

Methohexital Sodium (Co-administration may increase the risk of respiratory depression, hypotension and profound sedation and coma; when such combined therapy is contemplated, the initial dose of one or both agents should be reduced by at least 50%).
   No products indexed under this heading.

Methotrimeprazine (Co-administration may increase the risk of respiratory depression, hypotension and profound sedation and coma; when such combined therapy is contemplated, the initial dose of one or both agents should be reduced by at least 50%). Products include:
   Levoprome 1321

Methoxyflurane (Co-administration may increase the risk of respiratory depression, hypotension and profound sedation and coma; when such combined therapy is contemplated, the initial dose of one or both agents should be reduced by at least 50%).
   No products indexed under this heading.

Methyclothiazide (Morphine can reduce the efficacy of diuretics by inducing the release of antidiuretic hormone and by causing spasm of the sphincter of the bladder leading to acute retention of urine). Products include:
   Enduron Tablets 424

Metocurine Iodide (Morphine may enhance the neuromuscular blocking action of skeletal relaxants and produce an increased degree of respiratory depression). Products include:
   Metubine Iodide Vials 932

Metolazone (Morphine can reduce the efficacy of diuretics by inducing the release of antidiuretic hormone and by causing spasm of the sphincter of the bladder leading to acute retention of urine). Products include:
   Mykrox Tablets 1617
   Zaroxolyn Tablets 1625

IMPORTANT NOTE: Always consult each drug listing in the patient's regimen for possible interactions.

Kadian / Interactions Index

Midazolam Hydrochloride (Co-administration may increase the risk of respiratory depression, hypotension and profound sedation and coma; when such combined therapy is contemplated, the initial dose of one or both agents should be reduced by at least 50%). Products include:
- Versed Injection 2324

Mivacurium Chloride (Morphine may enhance the neuromuscular blocking action of skeletal relaxants and produce an increased degree of respiratory depression). Products include:
- Mivacron 1125

Molindone Hydrochloride (Co-administration may increase the risk of respiratory depression, hypotension and profound sedation and coma; when such combined therapy is contemplated, the initial dose of one or both agents should be reduced by at least 50%). Products include:
- Moban Tablets and Concentrate 1036

Nalbuphine Hydrochloride (May reduce the analgesic effect and/or precipitate withdrawal symptoms). Products include:
- Nubain Injection 952

Opium Alkaloids (Co-administration may increase the risk of respiratory depression, hypotension and profound sedation and coma; when such combined therapy is contemplated, the initial dose of one or both agents should be reduced by at least 50%).
- No products indexed under this heading.

Oxazepam (Co-administration may increase the risk of respiratory depression, hypotension and profound sedation and coma; when such combined therapy is contemplated, the initial dose of one or both agents should be reduced by at least 50%). Products include:
- Serax Capsules 2916
- Serax Tablets 2916

Oxycodone Hydrochloride (Co-administration may increase the risk of respiratory depression, hypotension and profound sedation and coma; when such combined therapy is contemplated, the initial dose of one or both agents should be reduced by at least 50%). Products include:
- OxyContin Tablets 2163
- OxyIR Capsules 2167
- Percocet Tablets 955
- Percodan Tablets 955
- Percodan-Demi Tablets 956
- Roxicodone Tablets, Oral Solution & Intensol (Oxycodone) 2366
- Tylox Capsules 1593

Pancuronium Bromide (Morphine may enhance the neuromuscular blocking action of skeletal relaxants and produce an increased degree of respiratory depression).
- No products indexed under this heading.

Pentazocine Hydrochloride (May reduce the analgesic effect and/or precipitate withdrawal symptoms). Products include:
- Talacen Caplets 2464
- Talwin Compound 2466
- Talwin Nx Tablets 2467

Pentazocine Lactate (May reduce the analgesic effect and/or precipitate withdrawal symptoms). Products include:
- Talwin Injection 2465

Pentobarbital Sodium (Co-administration may increase the risk of respiratory depression, hypotension and profound sedation and coma; when such combined therapy is contemplated, the initial dose of one or both agents should be reduced by at least 50%). Products include:
- Nembutal Sodium Capsules 440
- Nembutal Sodium Solution 442
- Nembutal Sodium Suppositories 444

Perphenazine (Co-administration may increase the risk of respiratory depression, hypotension and profound sedation and coma; when such combined therapy is contemplated, the initial dose of one or both agents should be reduced by at least 50%). Products include:
- Etrafon 2495
- Triavil Tablets 1800
- Trilafon 2532

Phenelzine Sulfate (MAO inhibitors have been reported to intensify the effects of opioids causing anxiety, confusion and significant depression of respiration or coma; concurrent and/or sequential use is not recommended). Products include:
- Nardil 1977

Phenobarbital (Co-administration may increase the risk of respiratory depression, hypotension and profound sedation and coma; when such combined therapy is contemplated, the initial dose of one or both agents should be reduced by at least 50%). Products include:
- Arco-Lase Plus Tablets 513
- Bellergal-S Tablets 2375
- Donnatal 2234
- Donnatal Extentabs 2234
- Donnatal Tablets 2234
- Phenobarbital Elixir and Tablets ... 1523
- Quadrinal Tablets 1398

Polythiazide (Morphine can reduce the efficacy of diuretics by inducing the release of antidiuretic hormone and by causing spasm of the sphincter of the bladder leading to acute retention of urine). Products include:
- Minizide Capsules 2016

Prazepam (Co-administration may increase the risk of respiratory depression, hypotension and profound sedation and coma; when such combined therapy is contemplated, the initial dose of one or both agents should be reduced by at least 50%).
- No products indexed under this heading.

Prochlorperazine (Co-administration may increase the risk of respiratory depression, hypotension and profound sedation and coma; when such combined therapy is contemplated, the initial dose of one or both agents should be reduced by at least 50%). Products include:
- Compazine 2644

Promethazine Hydrochloride (Co-administration may increase the risk of respiratory depression, hypotension and profound sedation and coma; when such combined therapy is contemplated, the initial dose of one or both agents should be reduced by at least 50%). Products include:
- Meperigan Injection 2859
- Phenergan with Codeine 2883
- Phenergan with Dextromethorphan ... 2885
- Phenergan Injection 2880
- Phenergan Suppositories 2882
- Phenergan Syrup 2881
- Phenergan Tablets 2882
- Phenergan VC 2886
- Phenergan VC with Codeine 2888

Propofol (Co-administration may increase the risk of respiratory depression, hypotension and profound sedation and coma; when such combined therapy is contemplated, the initial dose of one or both agents should be reduced by at least 50%). Products include:
- Diprivan Injectable Emulsion 2939

Propoxyphene Hydrochloride (Co-administration may increase the risk of respiratory depression, hypotension and profound sedation and coma; when such combined therapy is contemplated, the initial dose of one or both agents should be reduced by at least 50%). Products include:
- Darvon 1475
- Wygesic Tablets 2930

Propoxyphene Napsylate (Co-administration may increase the risk of respiratory depression, hypotension and profound sedation and coma; when such combined therapy is contemplated, the initial dose of one or both agents should be reduced by at least 50%). Products include:
- Darvon-N/Darvocet-N 1473

Quazepam (Co-administration may increase the risk of respiratory depression, hypotension and profound sedation and coma; when such combined therapy is contemplated, the initial dose of one or both agents should be reduced by at least 50%). Products include:
- Doral Tablets 2773

Risperidone (Co-administration may increase the risk of respiratory depression, hypotension and profound sedation and coma; when such combined therapy is contemplated, the initial dose of one or both agents should be reduced by at least 50%). Products include:
- Risperdal Tablets 1348

Rocuronium Bromide (Morphine may enhance the neuromuscular blocking action of skeletal relaxants and produce an increased degree of respiratory depression). Products include:
- Zemuron Injection 1885

Secobarbital Sodium (Co-administration may increase the risk of respiratory depression, hypotension and profound sedation and coma; when such combined therapy is contemplated, the initial dose of one or both agents should be reduced by at least 50%). Products include:
- Seconal Sodium Pulvules 1529

Selegiline Hydrochloride (MAO inhibitors have been reported to intensify the effects of opioids causing anxiety, confusion and significant depression of respiration or coma; concurrent and/or sequential use is not recommended). Products include:
- Eldepryl Capsules 2729

Sevoflurane (Co-administration may increase the risk of respiratory depression, hypotension and profound sedation and coma; when such combined therapy is contemplated, the initial dose of one or both agents should be reduced by at least 50%).
- No products indexed under this heading.

Spironolactone (Morphine can reduce the efficacy of diuretics by inducing the release of antidiuretic hormone and by causing spasm of the sphincter of the bladder leading to acute retention of urine). Products include:
- Aldactazide Tablets 2556
- Aldactone Tablets 2558

Succinylcholine Chloride (Morphine may enhance the neuromuscular blocking action of skeletal relaxants and produce an increased degree of respiratory depression). Products include:
- Anectine 1062

Sufentanil Citrate (Co-administration may increase the risk of respiratory depression, hypotension and profound sedation and coma; when such combined therapy is contemplated, the initial dose of one or both agents should be reduced by at least 50%). Products include:
- Sufenta Injection 1355

Temazepam (Co-administration may increase the risk of respiratory depression, hypotension and profound sedation and coma; when such combined therapy is contemplated, the initial dose of one or both agents should be reduced by at least 50%). Products include:
- Restoril Capsules 2413

Thiamylal Sodium (Co-administration may increase the risk of respiratory depression, hypotension and profound sedation and coma; when such combined therapy is contemplated, the initial dose of one or both agents should be reduced by at least 50%).
- No products indexed under this heading.

Thioridazine Hydrochloride (Co-administration may increase the risk of respiratory depression, hypotension and profound sedation and coma; when such combined therapy is contemplated, the initial dose of one or both agents should be reduced by at least 50%). Products include:
- Mellaril 2398

Thiothixene (Co-administration may increase the risk of respiratory depression, hypotension and profound sedation and coma; when such combined therapy is contemplated, the initial dose of one or both agents should be reduced by at least 50%). Products include:
- Navane Capsules and Concentrate ... 2018
- Navane Intramuscular 2019

Torsemide (Morphine can reduce the efficacy of diuretics by inducing the release of antidiuretic hormone and by causing spasm of the sphincter of the bladder leading to acute retention of urine). Products include:
- Demadex Tablets and Injection 691

Tranylcypromine Sulfate (MAO inhibitors have been reported to intensify the effects of opioids causing anxiety, confusion and significant depression of respiration or coma; concurrent and/or sequential use is not recommended). Products include:
- Parnate Tablets 2679

Triamterene (Morphine can reduce the efficacy of diuretics by inducing the release of antidiuretic hormone and by causing spasm of the sphincter of the bladder leading to acute retention of urine). Products include:
- Dyazide Capsules 2653

(■ Described in PDR For Nonprescription Drugs) (◉ Described in PDR For Ophthalmology)

Dyrenium Capsules 2655

Triazolam (Co-administration may increase the risk of respiratory depression, hypotension and profound sedation and coma; when such combined therapy is contemplated, the initial dose of one or both agents should be reduced by at least 50%). Products include:
Halcion Tablets 2093

Trifluoperazine Hydrochloride (Co-administration may increase the risk of respiratory depression, hypotension and profound sedation and coma; when such combined therapy is contemplated, the initial dose of one or both agents should be reduced by at least 50%). Products include:
Stelazine 2692

Vecuronium Bromide (Morphine may enhance the neuromuscular blocking action of skeletal relaxants and produce an increased degree of respiratory depression). Products include:
Norcuron for Injection 1875

Zolpidem Tartrate (Co-administration may increase the risk of respiratory depression, hypotension and profound sedation and coma; when such combined therapy is contemplated, the initial dose of one or both agents should be reduced by at least 50%). Products include:
Ambien Tablets 2559

Food Interactions

Alcohol (Co-administration may increase the risk of respiratory depression, hypotension and profound sedation and coma).

Food, unspecified (Concurrent administration of food slows the rate of absorption; the extent of absorption is not affected).

KAO LECTROLYTE
(Electrolyte Supplement) 2099
None cited in PDR database.

KAOPECTATE CONCENTRATED ANTI-DIARRHEAL, PEPPERMINT FLAVOR
(Attapulgite) 802
None cited in PDR database.

KAOPECTATE CONCENTRATED ANTI-DIARRHEAL, REGULAR FLAVOR
(Attapulgite) 802
None cited in PDR database.

KAOPECTATE CHILDREN'S LIQUID
(Attapulgite) 802
None cited in PDR database.

KAOPECTATE MAXIMUM STRENGTH CAPLETS
(Attapulgite) 802
None cited in PDR database.

KAYEXALATE
(Sodium Polystyrene Sulfonate) 2444
May interact with antacids, cardiac glycosides, and certain other agents. Compounds in these categories include:

Aluminum Carbonate (May reduce potassium exchange capability). Products include:
Basaljel Capsules 2810
Basaljel Suspension 2810
Basaljel Tablets 2810

Aluminum Hydroxide (May reduce potassium exchange capability; potential for intestinal obstruction). Products include:
ALternaGEL Liquid 1358
Maximum Strength Ascriptin 650
Cama Arthritis Pain Reliever 748
Gaviscon Extra Strength Relief Formula Antacid Tablets 778
Gaviscon Extra Strength Relief Formula Liquid Antacid 779
Gaviscon Liquid Antacid 779
Gelusil Antacid-Anti-gas Liquid .. 819
Gelusil Antacid-Anti-gas Tablets .. 819
Maalox Antacid/Anti-Gas Tablets .. 889
Maalox Heartburn Relief Suspension 658
Maalox Antacid Liquid 888
Extra Strength Maalox Antacid/ Anti-Gas Liquid and Tablets .. 888
Mylanta 1359
Tempo Soft Antacid 799

Aluminum Hydroxide Gel (May reduce potassium exchange capability; potential for intestinal obstruction). Products include:
ALternaGEL Liquid 675
Aludrox Oral Suspension 850
Amphojel Suspension 2802
Amphojel Suspension without Flavor 2802
Amphojel Tablets 2802
Ascriptin 650
Gaviscon Antacid Tablets 778
Gaviscon-2 Antacid Tablets 779
Mylanta 676
Mylanta Double Strength Liquid .. 676
Nephrox Suspension 671

Deslanoside (Cardiac toxicity of digitalis may be exaggerated).
No products indexed under this heading.

Digitoxin (Cardiac toxicity of digitalis may be exaggerated). Products include:
Crystodigin Tablets 1472

Digoxin (Cardiac toxicity of digitalis may be exaggerated). Products include:
Lanoxicaps 1110
Lanoxin Elixir Pediatric 1113
Lanoxin Injection 1116
Lanoxin Injection Pediatric 1119
Lanoxin Tablets 1121

Magaldrate (May reduce potassium exchange capability).
No products indexed under this heading.

Magnesium Hydroxide (May reduce potassium exchange capability; potential for grand mal seizure). Products include:
Aludrox Oral Suspension 850
Ascriptin 650
Di-Gel Antacid/Anti-Gas 762
Gelusil Antacid-Anti-gas Liquid .. 819
Gelusil Antacid-Anti-gas Tablets .. 819
Maalox Antacid/Anti-Gas Tablets .. 889
Maalox Antacid Liquid 888
Extra Strength Maalox Antacid/ Anti-Gas Liquid and Tablets .. 888
Mylanta Fast-Acting
Mylanta Gelcaps Antacid 678
Fast-Acting Mylanta Liquid Antacid .. 1359
Mylanta Tablets 677
Maximum-Strength Fast-Acting Mylanta Liquid Antacid 1359
Mylanta Double Strength Tablets .. 677
Phillips' Milk of Magnesia Liquid .. 627
Rolaids Antacid Tablets 807
Tempo Soft Antacid 799

Magnesium Oxide (May reduce potassium exchange capability). Products include:
Beelith Tablets 632
Bufferin Analgesic Tablets 636
Arthritis Strength Bufferin Analgesic Caplets 637
Extra Strength Bufferin Analgesic Tablets 637
Caltrate PLUS 681
Cama Arthritis Pain Reliever .. 748
Mag-Ox 400 666
Uro-Mag 666

KEFLEX PULVULES & ORAL SUSPENSION
(Cephalexin) 930
None cited in PDR database.

KEFTAB TABLETS
(Cephalexin Hydrochloride) 931
None cited in PDR database.

KEFUROX VIALS, FASPAK & ADD-VANTAGE
(Cefuroxime Sodium) 1509
May interact with aminoglycosides and diuretics. Compounds in these categories include:

Amikacin Sulfate (Nephrotoxicity). Products include:
Amikacin Sulfate Injection, USP .. 523
Amikacin Sulfate Injection, USP .. 981
Amikin Injectable 502

Amiloride Hydrochloride (Possible adverse effects on renal function). Products include:
Midamor Tablets 1746
Moduretic Tablets 1748

Bendroflumethiazide (Possible adverse effects on renal function).
No products indexed under this heading.

Bumetanide (Possible adverse effects on renal function). Products include:
Bumex 2260

Chlorothiazide (Possible adverse effects on renal function). Products include:
Aldoclor Tablets 1638
Diupres Tablets 1691
Diuril Oral 1694

Chlorothiazide Sodium (Possible adverse effects on renal function). Products include:
Diuril Sodium Intravenous 1693

Chlorthalidone (Possible adverse effects on renal function). Products include:
Combipres Tablets 682
Tenoretic Tablets 2963
Thalitone 1293

Ethacrynic Acid (Possible adverse effects on renal function). Products include:
Edecrin Tablets 1698

Furosemide (Possible adverse effects on renal function). Products include:
Lasix Injection, Oral Solution and Tablets 1267

Gentamicin Sulfate (Nephrotoxicity). Products include:
Garamycin Cream 0.1% 2501
Garamycin Injectable 2502
Garamycin Ointment 0.1% 2501
Garamycin Ophthalmic 2501
Genoptic Sterile Ophthalmic Solution 241
Genoptic Sterile Ophthalmic Ointment 241
Gentak 209
Pred-G Liquifilm Sterile Ophthalmic Suspension 248
Pred-G S.O.P. Sterile Ophthalmic Ointment 249

Hydrochlorothiazide (Possible adverse effects on renal function). Products include:
Aldactazide Tablets 2556
Aldoril Tablets 1644
Apresazide Capsules 824
Capozide Tablets 744
Dyazide Capsules 2653
Esidrix Tablets 839
Esimil Tablets 840
HydroDIURIL Tablets 1716
Hydropres Tablets 1718
Hyzaar Tablets 1720
Inderide Tablets 2838
Inderide LA Long Acting Capsules .. 2840
Lopressor HCT Tablets 850
Lotensin HCT Tablets 855
Moduretic Tablets 1748
Oretic Tablets 450
Prinzide Tablets 1780
Ser-Ap-Es Tablets 867
Timolide Tablets 1791
Vaseretic Tablets 1810
Zestoretic Tablets 2968
Ziac 1459

Hydroflumethiazide (Possible adverse effects on renal function). Products include:
Diucardin Tablets 2824

Indapamide (Possible adverse effects on renal function).
No products indexed under this heading.

Kanamycin Sulfate (Nephrotoxicity).
No products indexed under this heading.

Methyclothiazide (Possible adverse effects on renal function). Products include:
Enduron Tablets 424

Metolazone (Possible adverse effects on renal function). Products include:
Mykrox Tablets 1617
Zaroxolyn Tablets 1625

Polythiazide (Possible adverse effects on renal function). Products include:
Minizide Capsules 2016

Spironolactone (Possible adverse effects on renal function). Products include:
Aldactazide Tablets 2556
Aldactone Tablets 2558

Streptomycin Sulfate (Nephrotoxicity). Products include:
Streptomycin Sulfate Injection .. 2031

Tobramycin (Nephrotoxicity). Products include:
AKTOB 207
TobraDex Ophthalmic Suspension and Ointment 469
Tobrex Ophthalmic Ointment and Solution 226

Tobramycin Sulfate (Nephrotoxicity). Products include:
Nebcin Vials, Hyporets & ADD-Vantage 1518

Torsemide (Possible adverse effects on renal function). Products include:
Demadex Tablets and Injection .. 691

Triamterene (Possible adverse effects on renal function). Products include:
Dyazide Capsules 2653
Dyrenium Capsules 2655

KEFZOL VIALS, FASPAK & ADD-VANTAGE
(Cefazolin Sodium) 1511
May interact with:

Probenecid (Increases and prolongs cephalosporin blood levels). Products include:
Benemid Tablets 1651
ColBENEMID Tablets 1662

KEMADRIN TABLETS
(Procyclidine Hydrochloride) 1105
None cited in PDR database.

KERI LOTION - ORIGINAL FORMULA
(Mineral Oil) 644
None cited in PDR database.

KERI LOTION - SILKY SMOOTH
(Petrolatum) 644
None cited in PDR database.

KERI LOTION - SENSITIVE SKIN
(Petrolatum) 644
None cited in PDR database.

IMPORTANT NOTE: Always consult each drug listing in the patient's regimen for possible interactions.

Kerlone Interactions Index 562

KERLONE TABLETS
(Betaxolol Hydrochloride) 2588
May interact with catecholamine depleting drugs, calcium channel blockers, and certain other agents. Compounds in these categories include:

Amlodipine Besylate (Potential for hypotension, AV conduction disturbances, and LVF in patients with impaired cardiac function). Products include:
Lotrel Capsules 858
Norvasc Tablets 2020

Bepridil Hydrochloride (Potential for hypotension, AV conduction disturbances, and LVF in patients with impaired cardiac function). Products include:
Vascor Tablets (200 and 300 mg) 1597

Clonidine (Potential for withdrawal reactions). Products include:
Catapres-TTS 680

Clonidine Hydrochloride (Potential for withdrawal). Products include:
Catapres Tablets 679
Combipres Tablets 682

Deserpidine (Additive effect resulting in marked bradycardia, vertigo, syncope or postural hypotension).
No products indexed under this heading.

Diltiazem Hydrochloride (Potential for hypotension, AV conduction disturbances, and LVF in patients with impaired cardiac function). Products include:
Cardizem CD Capsules 1251
Cardizem SR Capsules 1255
Cardizem Injectable 1253
Cardizem Tablets 1257
Dilacor XR Extended-release Capsules 2183
Tiazac Capsules 1019

Felodipine (Potential for hypotension, AV conduction disturbances, and LVF in patients with impaired cardiac function). Products include:
Plendil Extended-Release Tablets 514

Guanethidine Monosulfate (Additive effect resulting in marked bradycardia, vertigo, syncope or postural hypotension). Products include:
Esimil Tablets 840
Ismelin Tablets 845

Isradipine (Potential for hypotension, AV conduction disturbances, and LVF in patients with impaired cardiac function). Products include:
DynaCirc Capsules 2381
DynaCirc CR Tablets 2383

Nicardipine Hydrochloride (Potential for hypotension, AV conduction disturbances, and LVF in patients with impaired cardiac function). Products include:
Cardene Capsules 2261
Cardene I.V. 2815
Cardene SR Capsules 2264

Nifedipine (Potential for hypotension, AV conduction disturbances, and LVF in patients with impaired cardiac function). Products include:
Adalat Capsules (10 mg and 20 mg) 580
Adalat CC 582
Procardia Capsules 2024
Procardia XL Extended Release Tablets 2026

Nimodipine (Potential for hypotension, AV conduction disturbances, and LVF in patients with impaired cardiac function). Products include:
Nimotop Capsules 603

Nisoldipine (Potential for hypotension, AV conduction disturbances, and LVF in patients with impaired cardiac function). Products include:
Sular Tablets 2961

Rauwolfia Serpentina (Additive effect resulting in marked bradycardia, vertigo, syncope or postural hypotension).
No products indexed under this heading.

Rescinnamine (Additive effect resulting in marked bradycardia, vertigo, syncope or postural hypotension).
No products indexed under this heading.

Reserpine (Additive effect resulting in marked bradycardia, vertigo, syncope or postural hypotension). Products include:
Diupres Tablets 1691
Hydropres Tablets 1718
Ser-Ap-Es Tablets 867

Verapamil Hydrochloride (Potential for hypotension, AV conduction disturbances, and LVF in patients with impaired cardiac function). Products include:
Calan SR Caplets 2571
Calan Tablets 2568
Covera-HS Tablets 2573
Isoptin Injectable 1391
Isoptin Oral Tablets 1393
Isoptin SR Tablets 1395
Verelan Capsules 1455

KLONOPIN TABLETS
(Clonazepam) 2294
May interact with narcotic analgesics, barbiturates, hypnotics and sedatives, tranquilizers, phenothiazines, monoamine oxidase inhibitors, tricyclic antidepressants, anticonvulsants, and certain other agents. Compounds in these categories include:

Alfentanil Hydrochloride (Potentiates CNS-depressant action). Products include:
Alfenta Injection 1334

Alprazolam (Potentiates CNS-depressant action). Products include:
Xanax Tablets 2115

Amitriptyline Hydrochloride (Potentiates CNS-depressant action). Products include:
Elavil 2945
Etrafon 2495
Limbitrol 2333
Triavil Tablets 1800

Amoxapine (Potentiates CNS-depressant action). Products include:
Asendin Tablets 1419

Aprobarbital (Potentiates CNS-depressant action).
No products indexed under this heading.

Buprenorphine (Potentiates CNS-depressant action). Products include:
Buprenex Injectable 2170

Buspirone Hydrochloride (Potentiates CNS-depressant action). Products include:
BuSpar Tablets 738

Butabarbital (Potentiates CNS-depressant action).
No products indexed under this heading.

Butalbital (Potentiates CNS-depressant action). Products include:
Axocet Capsules 2469
Esgic-plus Capsules 1012
Esgic-plus Tablets 1012
Fioricet Tablets 2386
Fioricet with Codeine Capsules 2387
Fiorinal Capsules 2388
Fiorinal with Codeine Capsules 2390
Fiorinal Tablets 2388
Phrenilin 790
Sedapap Tablets 50 mg/650 mg 1826

Carbamazepine (Potentiates CNS-depressant action). Products include:
Atretol Tablets 569
Tegretol/Tegretol-XR 870

Chlordiazepoxide (Potentiates CNS-depressant action). Products include:
Limbitrol 2333

Chlordiazepoxide Hydrochloride (Potentiates CNS-depressant action). Products include:
Librax Capsules 2330
Librium Capsules 2331
Librium Injectable 2332

Chlorpromazine (Potentiates CNS-depressant action). Products include:
Thorazine Suppositories 2701

Chlorprothixene (Potentiates CNS-depressant action).
No products indexed under this heading.

Chlorprothixene Hydrochloride (Potentiates CNS-depressant action).
No products indexed under this heading.

Clomipramine Hydrochloride (Potentiates CNS-depressant action). Products include:
Anafranil Capsules 819

Clorazepate Dipotassium (Potentiates CNS-depressant action). Products include:
Tranxene 459

Codeine Phosphate (Potentiates CNS-depressant action). Products include:
Brontex 2130
Dimetane-DC Cough Syrup 2232
Fioricet with Codeine Capsules 2387
Fiorinal with Codeine Capsules 2390
Nucofed 2225
Phenergan with Codeine 2883
Phenergan VC with Codeine 2888
Robitussin A-C Syrup 2248
Robitussin-DAC Syrup 2249
Ryna ▣ 804
Soma Compound w/Codeine Tablets 2784
Tylenol with Codeine 1592

Desipramine Hydrochloride (Potentiates CNS-depressant action). Products include:
Norpramin Tablets 1273

Dezocine (Potentiates CNS-depressant action). Products include:
Dalgan Injection 529

Diazepam (Potentiates CNS-depressant action). Products include:
Dizac (diazepam injectable emulsion) CIV 1862
Valium Injectable 2336
Valium Tablets 2335

Divalproex Sodium (Potentiates CNS-depressant action). Products include:
Depakote Tablets 418

Doxepin Hydrochloride (Potentiates CNS-depressant action). Products include:
Adapin Capsules 1542
Sinequan 2028
Zonalon Cream 1042

Droperidol (Potentiates CNS-depressant action). Products include:
Inapsine Injection 462

Estazolam (Potentiates CNS-depressant action). Products include:
ProSom Tablets 457

Ethchlorvynol (Potentiates CNS-depressant action). Products include:
Placidyl Capsules 456

Ethinamate (Potentiates CNS-depressant action).
No products indexed under this heading.

Ethosuximide (Potentiates CNS-depressant action). Products include:
Zarontin Capsules 1986
Zarontin Syrup 1986

Ethotoin (Potentiates CNS-depressant action). Products include:
Peganone Tablets 455

Felbamate (Potentiates CNS-depressant action). Products include:
Felbatol 2774

Fentanyl (Potentiates CNS-depressant action). Products include:
Duragesic Transdermal System 1336

Fentanyl Citrate (Potentiates CNS-depressant action). Products include:
Sublimaze Injection 463

Fluphenazine Decanoate (Potentiates CNS-depressant action). Products include:
Prolixin Decanoate 510

Fluphenazine Enanthate (Potentiates CNS-depressant action). Products include:
Prolixin Enanthate 510

Fluphenazine Hydrochloride (Potentiates CNS-depressant action). Products include:
Prolixin 510

Flurazepam Hydrochloride (Potentiates CNS-depressant action). Products include:
Dalmane Capsules 2329

Furazolidone (Potentiates CNS-depressant action). Products include:
Furoxone 2221

Glutethimide (Potentiates CNS-depressant action).
No products indexed under this heading.

Haloperidol (Potentiates CNS-depressant action). Products include:
Haldol Injection, Tablets and Concentrate 1585

Haloperidol Decanoate (Potentiates CNS-depressant action). Products include:
Haldol Decanoate 1587

Hydrocodone Bitartrate (Potentiates CNS-depressant action). Products include:
Codiclear DH Syrup 808
Duratuss HD Elixir 2750
Histussin D Liquid 670
Hycodan Tablets and Syrup 946
Hycomine Compound Tablets 948
Hycomine 947
Hycotuss Expectorant Syrup 950
Hydrocet Capsules 787
Lorcet 10/650 Tablets 1016
Lortab 2751
Tussend 1830
Tussend Expectorant 1831
Vicodin Tablets 1404
Vicodin ES Tablets 1405
Vicodin HP Tablets 1403
Vicodin Tuss Expectorant 1406
Zydone Capsules 967

Hydrocodone Polistirex (Potentiates CNS-depressant action). Products include:
Tussionex Pennkinetic Extended-Release Suspension 1624

Hydromorphone Hydrochloride (Potentiates CNS-depressant action). Products include:
Dilaudid Ampules 1382
Dilaudid Cough Syrup 1383
Dilaudid-HP Injection 1384
Dilaudid-HP Lyophilized Powder 250 mg 1384
Dilaudid 1382
Dilaudid Oral Liquid 1386
Dilaudid 1382
Dilaudid Tablets - 8 mg 1386

Hydroxyzine Hydrochloride (Potentiates CNS-depressant action). Products include:
Atarax Tablets & Syrup 1992
Marax Tablets & DF Syrup 2015

(▣ Described in PDR For Nonprescription Drugs) (◉ Described in PDR For Ophthalmology)

Interactions Index

Vistaril Intramuscular Solution......... 2042

Imipramine Hydrochloride (Potentiates CNS-depressant action). Products include:
- Tofranil Ampuls 873
- Tofranil Tablets 875

Imipramine Pamoate (Potentiates CNS-depressant action). Products include:
- Tofranil-PM Capsules 876

Isocarboxazid (Potentiates CNS-depressant action).
No products indexed under this heading.

Lamotrigine (Potentiates CNS-depressant action). Products include:
- Lamictal Tablets 1105

Levorphanol Tartrate (Potentiates CNS-depressant action). Products include:
- Levo-Dromoran 2297

Lorazepam (Potentiates CNS-depressant action). Products include:
- Ativan Injection 2805
- Ativan Tablets 2807

Loxapine Hydrochloride (Potentiates CNS-depressant action). Products include:
- Loxitane 1426

Maprotiline Hydrochloride (Potentiates CNS-depressant action). Products include:
- Ludiomil Tablets 861

Meperidine Hydrochloride (Potentiates CNS-depressant action). Products include:
- Demerol 2438
- Mepergan Injection 2859

Mephenytoin (Potentiates CNS-depressant action). Products include:
- Mesantoin Tablets 2400

Mephobarbital (Potentiates CNS-depressant action). Products include:
- Mebaral Tablets 2452

Meprobamate (Potentiates CNS-depressant action). Products include:
- Miltown Tablets 2780
- PMB 200 and PMB 400 2890

Mesoridazine Besylate (Potentiates CNS-depressant action). Products include:
- Serentil 689

Methadone Hydrochloride (Potentiates CNS-depressant action). Products include:
- Methadone Hydrochloride Oral Concentrate 2356
- Methadone Hydrochloride Oral Solution & Tablets 2357

Methotrimeprazine (Potentiates CNS-depressant action). Products include:
- Levoprome 1321

Methsuximide (Potentiates CNS-depressant action). Products include:
- Celontin Kapseals 1955

Midazolam Hydrochloride (Potentiates CNS-depressant action). Products include:
- Versed Injection 2324

Molindone Hydrochloride (Potentiates CNS-depressant action). Products include:
- Moban Tablets and Concentrate 1036

Morphine Sulfate (Potentiates CNS-depressant action). Products include:
- Astramorph/PF Injection, USP (Preservative-Free) 526
- Duramorph Injection 983
- Infumorph 200 and Infumorph 500 Sterile Solutions 985
- Kadian Capsules 2948
- MS Contin Tablets 2149
- MSIR 2152
- Oramorph SR (Morphine Sulfate Sustained Release Tablets) 2359
- RMS Suppositories CII 2766
- Roxanol 2365

Nortriptyline Hydrochloride (Potentiates CNS-depressant action). Products include:
- Pamelor 2409

Opium Alkaloids (Potentiates CNS-depressant action).
No products indexed under this heading.

Oxazepam (Potentiates CNS-depressant action). Products include:
- Serax Capsules 2916
- Serax Tablets 2916

Oxycodone Hydrochloride (Potentiates CNS-depressant action). Products include:
- OxyContin Tablets 2163
- OxyIR Capsules 2167
- Percocet Tablets 955
- Percodan Tablets 955
- Percodan-Demi Tablets 956
- Roxicodone Tablets, Oral Solution & Intensol (Oxycodone) 2366
- Tylox Capsules 1593

Paramethadione (Potentiates CNS-depressant action).
No products indexed under this heading.

Pentobarbital Sodium (Potentiates CNS-depressant action). Products include:
- Nembutal Sodium Capsules 440
- Nembutal Sodium Solution 442
- Nembutal Sodium Suppositories 444

Perphenazine (Potentiates CNS-depressant action). Products include:
- Etrafon 2495
- Triavil Tablets 1800
- Trilafon 2532

Phenacemide (Potentiates CNS-depressant action). Products include:
- Phenurone Tablets 455

Phenelzine Sulfate (Potentiates CNS-depressant action). Products include:
- Nardil 1977

Phenobarbital (Potentiates CNS-depressant action). Products include:
- Arco-Lase Plus Tablets 513
- Bellergal-S Tablets 2375
- Donnatal 2234
- Donnatal Extentabs 2234
- Donnatal Tablets 2234
- Phenobarbital Elixir and Tablets 1523
- Quadrinal Tablets 1398

Phenothiazine Derivatives (Potentiates CNS-depressant action).

Phensuximide (Potentiates CNS-depressant action).
No products indexed under this heading.

Phenytoin (Potentiates CNS-depressant action). Products include:
- Dilantin Infatabs 1967
- Dilantin-125 Suspension 1969

Phenytoin Sodium (Potentiates CNS-depressant action). Products include:
- Dilantin Kapseals 1965

Prazepam (Potentiates CNS-depressant action).
No products indexed under this heading.

Primidone (Potentiates CNS-depressant action). Products include:
- Mysoline 2860

Prochlorperazine (Potentiates CNS-depressant action). Products include:
- Compazine 2644

Promethazine Hydrochloride (Potentiates CNS-depressant action). Products include:
- Mepergan Injection 2859
- Phenergan with Codeine 2883
- Phenergan with Dextromethorphan 2885
- Phenergan Injection 2880
- Phenergan Suppositories 2882
- Phenergan Syrup 2881
- Phenergan Tablets 2882
- Phenergan VC 2886
- Phenergan VC with Codeine 2888

Propofol (Potentiates CNS-depressant action). Products include:
- Diprivan Injectable Emulsion 2939

Propoxyphene Hydrochloride (Potentiates CNS-depressant action). Products include:
- Darvon 1475
- Wygesic Tablets 2930

Propoxyphene Napsylate (Potentiates CNS-depressant action). Products include:
- Darvon-N/Darvocet-N 1473

Protriptyline Hydrochloride (Potentiates CNS-depressant action). Products include:
- Vivactil Tablets 1820

Quazepam (Potentiates CNS-depressant action). Products include:
- Doral Tablets 2773

Secobarbital Sodium (Potentiates CNS-depressant action). Products include:
- Seconal Sodium Pulvules 1529

Selegiline Hydrochloride (Potentiates CNS-depressant action). Products include:
- Eldepryl Capsules 2729

Sufentanil Citrate (Potentiates CNS-depressant action). Products include:
- Sufenta Injection 1355

Temazepam (Potentiates CNS-depressant action). Products include:
- Restoril Capsules 2413

Thiamylal Sodium (Potentiates CNS-depressant action).
No products indexed under this heading.

Thioridazine Hydrochloride (Potentiates CNS-depressant action). Products include:
- Mellaril 2398

Thiothixene (Potentiates CNS-depressant action). Products include:
- Navane Capsules and Concentrate 2018
- Navane Intramuscular 2019

Tranylcypromine Sulfate (Potentiates CNS-depressant action). Products include:
- Parnate Tablets 2679

Triazolam (Potentiates CNS-depressant action). Products include:
- Halcion Tablets 2093

Trifluoperazine Hydrochloride (Potentiates CNS-depressant action). Products include:
- Stelazine 2692

Trimethadione (Potentiates CNS-depressant action).
No products indexed under this heading.

Trimipramine Maleate (Potentiates CNS-depressant action). Products include:
- Surmontil Capsules 2917

Valproic Acid (Potentiates CNS-depressant action). Products include:
- Depakene 416

Zolpidem Tartrate (Potentiates CNS-depressant action). Products include:
- Ambien Tablets 2559

Food Interactions

Alcohol (Potentiates CNS-depressant action).

Konsyl

KOāTE-HP ANTIHEMOPHILIC FACTOR (HUMAN)
(Antihemophilic Factor (Human)) 624
None cited in PDR database.

KOGENATE ANTIHEMOPHILIC FACTOR (RECOMBINANT)
(Antihemophilic Factor (Recombinant)) 626
None cited in PDR database.

KONDREMUL
(Mineral Oil) 656
May interact with stool softener laxatives. Compounds in this category include:

Docusate Calcium (Concurrent use is not recommended). Products include:
- Doxidan Liqui-Gels 801
- Surfak Liqui-Gels 803

Docusate Potassium (Concurrent use is not recommended).
No products indexed under this heading.

Docusate Sodium (Concurrent use is not recommended). Products include:
- Colace Capsules, Syrup, Liquid 2212
- Colace Microenema 2213
- Colace-T 50 mg Tablets 2213
- Colace-T 100 mg Tablets 2213
- Correctol Extra Gentle Stool Softener 762
- Dialose Tablets 1358
- Dialose Plus Tablets 1358
- Extra Gentle Ex-Lax Laxative Pills 749
- Fleet Sof-Lax 1003
- Fleet Sof-Lax Overnight 1003
- Peri-Colace Capsules and Syrup 2226
- Phillips' Gelcaps 627
- Senokot-S Tablets 2154

KONSYL FIBER TABLETS
(Calcium Polycarbophil) 679
May interact with tetracyclines. Compounds in this category include:

Demeclocycline Hydrochloride (Take KONSYL at least one hour before or two hours after taking the antibiotic). Products include:
- Declomycin Tablets 1421

Doxycycline Calcium (Take KONSYL at least one hour before or two hours after taking the antibiotic). Products include:
- Vibramycin Calcium Oral Suspension Syrup 2038

Doxycycline Hyclate (Take KONSYL at least one hour before or two hours after taking the antibiotic). Products include:
- Doryx Capsules 1970
- Vibramycin Hyclate Capsules 2038
- Vibramycin Hyclate Intravenous 2040
- Vibra-Tabs Film Coated Tablets 2038

Doxycycline Monohydrate (Take KONSYL at least one hour before or two hours after taking the antibiotic). Products include:
- Monodox Capsules 1858
- Vibramycin Monohydrate for Oral Suspension 2038

Methacycline Hydrochloride (Take KONSYL at least one hour before or two hours after taking the antibiotic).
No products indexed under this heading.

Minocycline Hydrochloride (Take KONSYL at least one hour before or two hours after taking the antibiotic). Products include:
- DYNACIN Capsules 1627
- Minocin Intravenous 1428
- Minocin Oral Suspension 1431
- Minocin Pellet-Filled Capsules 1429

IMPORTANT NOTE: Always consult each drug listing in the patient's regimen for possible interactions.

Konsyl — Interactions Index

Oxytetracycline Hydrochloride (Take KONSYL at least one hour before or two hours after taking the antibiotic). Products include:
- TERAK Ointment ... ⓞ 210
- Terra-Cortril Ophthalmic Suspension ... 2033
- Terramycin with Polymyxin B Sulfate Ophthalmic Ointment ... 2035
- Urobiotic-250 Capsules ... 2038

Tetracycline Hydrochloride (Take KONSYL at least one hour before or two hours after taking the antibiotic). Products include:
- Achromycin V Capsules ... 1417
- Helidac Therapy ... 2135

KONSYL POWDER SUGAR FREE UNFLAVORED
(Psyllium Preparations) ... ▣ 680
None cited in PDR database.

KONINE 80 FACTOR IX COMPLEX
(Factor IX Complex) ... 627
None cited in PDR database.

KRONOFED-A KRONOCAPS
(Chlorpheniramine Maleate, Pseudoephedrine Hydrochloride) ... 994
None cited in PDR database.

KRONOFED-A-JR. KRONOCAPS
(Pseudoephedrine Hydrochloride, Chlorpheniramine Maleate) ... 994
None cited in PDR database.

KUTRASE CAPSULES
(Hyoscyamine Sulfate, Phenyltoloxamine Citrate, Amylase, Cellulase, Lipase, Protease) ... 2546
None cited in PDR database.

KU-ZYME CAPSULES
(Amylase, Lipase, Cellulase, Protease) ... 2546
None cited in PDR database.

KU-ZYME HP CAPSULES
(Pancrelipase) ... 2547
May interact with:

Ferrous Fumarate (Decreased serum response to oral iron). Products include:
- Chromagen Capsules ... 2470
- Chromagen FA ... 2471
- Chromagen Forte ... 2471
- Ferro-Sequels ... ▣ 684
- Nephro-Fer Tablets ... 2168
- Nephro-Fer Rx Tablets ... 2168
- Nephro-Vite + Fe Tablets ... 2170
- Stresstabs + Iron ... ▣ 685
- Trinsicon Capsules ... 2759
- Vitron-C Tablets ... 667

Ferrous Gluconate (Decreased serum response to oral iron). Products include:
- Megadose ... 513

Ferrous Sulfate (Decreased serum response to oral iron). Products include:
- Feosol Capsules ... ▣ 777
- Feosol Elixir ... 2627
- Feosol Tablets ... 2627
- Fero-Folic-500 Filmtab ... 433
- Fero-Grad-500 Filmtab ... 434
- Fero-Gradumet Filmtab ... 434
- Iberet Tablets ... 437
- Iberet-500 Liquid ... 438
- Iberet-Folic-500 Filmtab ... 433
- Iberet-Liquid ... 438
- Irospan ... 1000
- Slow Fe Tablets ... 889
- Slow Fe with Folic Acid ... 890

KWELL CREAM & LOTION
(Lindane) ... 2172
May interact with:

Oil Based Products (May enhance absorption; avoid concomitant use).

KWELL SHAMPOO
(Lindane) ... 2173
May interact with:

Oil Based Products (Oils may enhance absorption; avoid using immediately before or after using Kwell Shampoo).

Oils, unspecified (Oils may enhance absorption; avoid using immediately before or after using Kwell Shampoo).

KYO-CHROME
(Chromium Picolinate, Garlic Extract, Niacin) ... ▣ 680
None cited in PDR database.

KYOLIC AGED GARLIC EXTRACT CAPLETS
(Garlic Extract) ... ▣ 680
None cited in PDR database.

KYTRIL INJECTION
(Granisetron Hydrochloride) ... 2667
May interact with drugs affecting hepatic drug metabolizing enzyme systems and certain other agents. Compounds in these categories include:

Carbamazepine (May change the clearance and hence, the half-life of granisetron). Products include:
- Atretol Tablets ... 569
- Tegretol/Tegretol-XR ... 870

Cimetidine (May change the clearance and hence the half-life of granisetron). Products include:
- Tagamet HB Tablets ... ▣ 786
- Tagamet Tablets ... 2694

Cimetidine Hydrochloride (May change the clearance and hence, the half-life of granisetron). Products include:
- Tagamet ... 2694

Phenobarbital (May change the clearance and hence the half-life of granisetron). Products include:
- Arco-Lase Plus Tablets ... 513
- Bellergal-S Tablets ... 2375
- Donnatal ... 2234
- Donnatal Extentabs ... 2234
- Donnatal Tablets ... 2234
- Phenobarbital Elixir and Tablets ... 1523
- Quadrinal Tablets ... 1398

Phenytoin (May change the clearance and hence, the half-life of granisetron). Products include:
- Dilantin Infatabs ... 1967
- Dilantin-125 Suspension ... 1969

Phenytoin Sodium (May change the clearance and hence, the half-life of granisetron). Products include:
- Dilantin Kapseals ... 1965

Rifampin (May change the clearance and hence, the half-life of granisetron). Products include:
- Rifadin ... 1276
- Rifamate Capsules ... 1278
- Rifater ... 1280
- Rimactane Capsules ... 865

KYTRIL TABLETS
(Granisetron Hydrochloride) ... 2669
May interact with drugs affecting hepatic drug metabolizing enzyme systems. Compounds in this category include:

Carbamazepine (May change the clearance and, hence the half-life of granisetron). Products include:
- Atretol Tablets ... 569
- Tegretol/Tegretol-XR ... 870

Cimetidine (May change the clearance and, hence the half-life of granisetron). Products include:
- Tagamet HB Tablets ... ▣ 786
- Tagamet Tablets ... 2694

Cimetidine Hydrochloride (May change the clearance and, hence the half-life of granisetron). Products include:
- Tagamet ... 2694

Phenobarbital (May change the clearance and, hence the half-life of granisetron). Products include:
- Arco-Lase Plus Tablets ... 513
- Bellergal-S Tablets ... 2375
- Donnatal ... 2234
- Donnatal Extentabs ... 2234
- Donnatal Tablets ... 2234
- Phenobarbital Elixir and Tablets ... 1523
- Quadrinal Tablets ... 1398

Phenytoin (May change the clearance and, hence the half-life of granisetron). Products include:
- Dilantin Infatabs ... 1967
- Dilantin-125 Suspension ... 1969

Phenytoin Sodium (May change the clearance and, hence the half-life of granisetron). Products include:
- Dilantin Kapseals ... 1965

Food Interactions
Food, unspecified (When oral granisetron was administered with food, AUC was decreased by 5% and C_{max} increased by 30% in non-fasted individuals).

LAC-HYDRIN 12% LOTION
(Ammonium Lactate) ... 2796
None cited in PDR database.

LACRISERT STERILE OPHTHALMIC INSERT
(Hydroxypropyl Cellulose) ... 1730
None cited in PDR database.

LACTAID DROPS
(Lactase (beta-d-Galactosidase)) ... 1562
None cited in PDR database.

LACTAID EXTRA STRENGTH CAPLETS
(Lactase (beta-d-Galactosidase)) ... 1562
None cited in PDR database.

LACTAID ORIGINAL STRENGTH CAPLETS
(Lactase (beta-d-Galactosidase)) ... 1562
None cited in PDR database.

LAMICTAL TABLETS
(Lamotrigine) ... 1105
May interact with dihydrofolate reductase inhibitors and certain other agents. Compounds in these categories include:

Carbamazepine (Potential for higher incidence of dizziness, diplopia, ataxia, and blurred vision; decreases lamotrigine steady-state concentrations by approximately 40%). Products include:
- Atretol Tablets ... 569
- Tegretol/Tegretol-XR ... 870

Divalproex Sodium (Decreases the clearance of lamotrigine, i.e., more than doubles the elimination $t_{1/2}$ of lamotrigine, whether given with or without hepatic enzyme inducing antiepileptic drugs; the steady-state valproic acid concentrations in plasma may be decreased by an average of 25%). Products include:
- Depakote Tablets ... 418

Methotrexate Sodium (Lamotrigine is an inhibitor of dihydrofolate reductase; prescribers should be aware of this action when used concurrently with agents which inhibit folate metabolism). Products include:
- Methotrexate Sodium Tablets, Injection, for Injection and LPF Injection ... 1322

Phenobarbital (Decreases lamotrigine steady-state concentrations by approximately 40%). Products include:
- Arco-Lase Plus Tablets ... 513
- Bellergal-S Tablets ... 2375
- Donnatal ... 2234
- Donnatal Extentabs ... 2234
- Donnatal Tablets ... 2234
- Phenobarbital Elixir and Tablets ... 1523
- Quadrinal Tablets ... 1398

Phenytoin (Decreases lamotrigine steady-state concentrations by approximately 45% to 54%). Products include:
- Dilantin Infatabs ... 1967
- Dilantin-125 Suspension ... 1969

Phenytoin Sodium (Decreases lamotrigine steady-state concentrations by approximately 45% to 54%). Products include:
- Dilantin Kapseals ... 1965

Primidone (Decreases lamotrigine steady-state concentrations by approximately 40%). Products include:
- Mysoline ... 2860

Sodium Valproate (Decreases the clearance of lamotrigine, i.e., more than doubles the elimination $t_{1/2}$ of lamotrigine, whether given with or without hepatic enzyme-inducing antiepileptic drugs; the steady-state valproic acid concentrations in plasma may be decreased by an average of 25%).

Trimethoprim (Lamotrigine is an inhibitor of dihydrofolate reductase; prescribers should be aware of this action when used concurrently with agents which inhibit folate metabolism). Products include:
- Bactrim DS Tablets ... 2257
- Bactrim I.V. Infusion ... 2255
- Bactrim ... 2257
- Proloprim Tablets ... 1141
- Septra ... 1146
- Septra I.V. Infusion ... 1142
- Septra I.V. Infusion ADD-Vantage Vials ... 1144
- Septra ... 1146
- Trimpex Tablets ... 2323

Trimetrexate Glucuronate (Lamotrigine is an inhibitor of dihydrofolate reductase; prescribers should be aware of this action when used concurrently with agents which inhibit folate metabolism). Products include:
- Neutrexin for Injection ... 2761

Valproic Acid (Decreases the clearance of lamotrigine, i.e., more than doubles the elimination $t_{1/2}$ of lamotrigine, whether given with or without hepatic enzyme-inducing antiepileptic drugs; the steady-state valproic acid concentrations in plasma may be decreased by an average of 25%). Products include:
- Depakene ... 416

(▣ Described in PDR For Nonprescription Drugs)   (ⓞ Described in PDR For Ophthalmology)

LAMISIL CREAM 1%
(Terbinafine Hydrochloride)................2393
None cited in PDR database.

LAMISIL TABLETS
(Terbinafine Hydrochloride)................2394
May interact with:

Caffeine Citrate (Terbinafine decreases the clearance of intravenously administered caffeine by 19%).
No products indexed under this heading.

Cimetidine (Terbinafine clearance is decreased 33% by cimetidine, a CYP450 enzyme inhibitor). Products include:
Tagamet HB Tablets............................ 786
Tagamet Tablets 2694

Cyclosporine (Terbinafine increases the clearance of cyclosporine by 15%; terbinafine clearance is unaffected by cyclosporine). Products include:
Neoral 2405
Sandimmune 2416

Rifampin (Terbinafine clearance is increased 100% by rifampin, a CYP450 enzyme inducer). Products include:
Rifadin 1276
Rifamate Capsules 1278
Rifater 1280
Rimactane Capsules 865

Terfenadine (Terbinafine clearance is decreased 16% by terfenadine). Products include:
Seldane Tablets 1284
Seldane-D Extended-Release Tablets 1286

Food Interactions
Food, unspecified (Co-administration has resulted in an increase in the AUC of terbinafine of less than 20%).

LAMPRENE CAPSULES
(Clofazimine) 846
None cited in PDR database.

LANOXICAPS
(Digoxin) 1110
May interact with potassium-depleting corticosteroids, potassium-depleting diuretics, antacids, sympathomimetics, beta blockers, calcium channel blockers, thyroid preparations, tetracyclines, macrolide antibiotics, erythromycin, and certain other agents. Compounds in these categories include:

Acebutolol Hydrochloride (Additive effects on AV node conduction). Products include:
Sectral Capsules 2914

Albuterol (Both agents enhance ectopic pacemaker activity; concomitant use increases the risk of cardiac arrhythmias). Products include:
Proventil Inhalation Aerosol 2524
Ventolin Inhalation Aerosol and Refill 1170

Albuterol Sulfate (Both agents enhance ectopic pacemaker activity; concomitant use increases the risk of cardiac arrhythmias). Products include:
Airet Albuterol Sulfate Inhalation Solution 1602
Albuterol Sulfate, USP Solution for Inhalation, Arm-a-Med 522
Proventil Inhalation Solution 0.083%... 2527
Proventil Repetabs Tablets 2529
Proventil Solution for Inhalation 0.5% 2525
Proventil Syrup 2528
Proventil Tablets 2529
Ventolin Inhalation Solution............... 1171
Ventolin Nebules Inhalation Solution.. 1172
Ventolin Rotacaps for Inhalation 1173
Ventolin Syrup 1175
Ventolin Tablets 1176
Volmax Extended-Release Tablets .. 1835

Alprazolam (Causes a rise in serum digoxin concentration, with the implication that digitalis intoxication may result). Products include:
Xanax Tablets 2115

Aluminum Carbonate (Interferes with intestinal digoxin absorption). Products include:
Basaljel Capsules 2810
Basaljel Suspension 2810
Basaljel Tablets 2810

Aluminum Hydroxide (Interferes with intestinal digoxin absorption). Products include:
ALternaGEL Liquid 1358
Maximum Strength Ascriptin 650
Cama Arthritis Pain Reliever 748
Gaviscon Extra Strength Relief Formula Antacid Tablets................. 778
Gaviscon Extra Strength Relief Formula Liquid Antacid 779
Gaviscon Liquid Antacid 779
Gelusil Antacid-Anti-gas Liquid 819
Gelusil Antacid-Anti-gas Tablets 819
Maalox Antacid/Anti-Gas Tablets 889
Maalox Heartburn Relief Suspension 658
Maalox Antacid Liquid 888
Extra Strength Maalox Antacid/ Anti-Gas Liquid and Tablets 888
Mylanta 1359
Tempo Soft Antacid 799

Aluminum Hydroxide Gel (Interferes with intestinal digoxin absorption). Products include:
ALternaGEL Liquid 675
Aludrox Oral Suspension 850
Amphojel Suspension 2802
Amphojel Suspension without Flavor 2802
Amphojel Tablets 2802
Ascriptin 650
Gaviscon Antacid Tablets.................. 778
Gaviscon-2 Antacid Tablets 779
Mylanta Liquid 676
Mylanta Double Strength Liquid 676
Nephrox Suspension 671

Amiodarone Hydrochloride (Causes a rise in serum digoxin concentration, with the implication that digitalis intoxication may result). Products include:
Cordarone Intravenous 2821
Cordarone Tablets............................. 2818

Amlodipine Besylate (Additive effects on AV node conduction). Products include:
Lotrel Capsules 858
Norvasc Tablets 2020

Amphotericin B (Amphotericin B-induced hypokalemia sensitizes the myocardium to digitalis resulting in possible digitalis toxicity). Products include:
Abelcet Injection................................ 1540
Fungizone Intravenous 507
Fungizone Oral Suspension 704

Anticancer Drugs, unspecified (Interferes with intestinal digoxin absorption).

Atenolol (Additive effects on AV node conduction). Products include:
Tenoretic Tablets............................... 2963
Tenormin Tablets and I.V. Injection 2965

Azithromycin (Co-administration results in increased digoxin absorption and serum levels). Products include:
Zithromax 2043
Zithromax Tablets 2046

Bendroflumethiazide (Diuretic-induced hypokalemia sensitizes the myocardium to digitalis resulting in possible digitalis toxicity).
No products indexed under this heading.

Bepridil Hydrochloride (Additive effects on AV node conduction). Products include:
Vascor Tablets (200 and 300 mg) 1597

Betamethasone Acetate (Corticosteroid-induced hypokalemia sensitizes the myocardium to digitalis resulting in possible digitalis toxicity). Products include:
Celestone Soluspan Suspension 2484

Betamethasone Sodium Phosphate (Corticosteroid-induced hypokalemia sensitizes the myocardium to digitalis resulting in possible digitalis toxicity). Products include:
Celestone Soluspan Suspension 2484

Betaxolol Hydrochloride (Additive effects on AV node conduction). Products include:
Betoptic Ophthalmic Solution 465
Betoptic S Ophthalmic Suspension 467
Kerlone Tablets 2588

Bisoprolol Fumarate (Additive effects on AV node conduction). Products include:
Zebeta Tablets 1457
Ziac 1459

Calcium, intravenous (May produce serious arrhythmias in digitalized patients).
No products indexed under this heading.

Carteolol Hydrochloride (Additive effects on Av node conduction). Products include:
Cartrol Tablets 413
Ocupress Ophthalmic Solution, 1% Sterile.. 297

Chlorothiazide (Diuretic-induced hypokalemia sensitizes the myocardium to digitalis resulting in possible digitalis toxicity). Products include:
Aldoclor Tablets 1638
Diupres Tablets 1691
Diuril Oral 1694

Chlorothiazide Sodium (Diuretic-induced hypokalemia sensitizes the myocardium to digitalis resulting in possible digitalis toxicity). Products include:
Diuril Sodium Intravenous 1693

Chlorthalidone (Diuretic-induced hypokalemia sensitizes the myocardium to digitalis resulting in possible digitalis toxicity). Products include:
Combipres Tablets 682
Tenoretic Tablets............................... 2963
Thalitone 1293

Cholestyramine (Interferes with intestinal digoxin absorption). Products include:
Questran 774

Clarithromycin (Co-administration results in increased digoxin absorption and serum levels). Products include:
Biaxin 406

Cortisone Acetate (Corticosteroid-induced hypokalemia sensitizes the myocardium to digitalis resulting in possible digitalis toxicity). Products include:
Cortone Acetate Sterile Suspension 1663
Cortone Acetate Tablets................... 1664

Demeclocycline Hydrochloride (May increase digoxin absorption in patients who convert digoxin to inactive metabolites in the gut resulting in increased serum levels of digoxin). Products include:
Declomycin Tablets 1421

Desoxycorticosterone Acetate (Contributing factor to digitalis toxicity).

Dexamethasone (Corticosteroid-induced hypokalemia sensitizes the myocardium to digitalis resulting in possible digitalis toxicity). Products include:
AK-Trol Ointment & Suspension 205
Decadron Elixir 1676
Decadron Tablets 1678
Decaspray Topical Aerosol 1689
Maxitrol Ophthalmic Ointment and Suspension 222
TobraDex Ophthalmic Suspension and Ointment................................... 469

Dexamethasone Acetate (Corticosteroid-induced hypokalemia sensitizes the myocardium to digitalis resulting in possible digitalis toxicity). Products include:
Dalalone D.P. Injectable 1009
Decadron-LA Sterile Suspension..... 1687

Dexamethasone Sodium Phosphate (Corticosteroid-induced hypokalemia sensitizes the myocardium to digitalis resulting in possible digitalis toxicity). Products include:
Decadron Phosphate Injection 1680
Decadron Phosphate Sterile Ophthalmic Ointment 1684
Decadron Phosphate Sterile Ophthalmic Solution 1685
Decadron Phosphate Topical Cream... 1686
Decadron Phosphate with Xylocaine Injection, Sterile...................... 1683
Dexacort Phosphate in Respihaler .. 1606
Dexacort Phosphate in Turbinaire .. 1607
NeoDecadron Sterile Ophthalmic Ointment... 1755
NeoDecadron Sterile Ophthalmic Solution 1756
NeoDecadron Topical Cream 1757

Diltiazem Hydrochloride (Additive effects on AV node conduction). Products include:
Cardizem CD Capsules 1251
Cardizem SR Capsules 1255
Cardizem Injectable 1253
Cardizem Tablets............................... 1257
Dilacor XR Extended-release Capsules 2183
Tiazac Capsules 1019

Diphenoxylate Hydrochloride (Increases digoxin absorption). Products include:
Lomotil 2591

Dirithromycin (Co-administration results in increased digoxin absorption and serum levels). Products include:
Dynabac 668

Dobutamine Hydrochloride (Both agents enhance ectopic pacemaker activity; concomitant use increases the risk of cardiac arrhythmias). Products include:
Dobutrex Solution Vials..................... 1480

Dopamine Hydrochloride (Both agents enhance ectopic pacemaker activity; concomitant use increases the risk of cardiac arrhythmias).
No products indexed under this heading.

Doxycycline Hyclate (May increase digoxin absorption in patients who convert digoxin to inactive metabolites in the gut resulting in increased serum levels of digoxin). Products include:
Doryx Capsules.................................. 1970
Vibramycin Hyclate Capsules 2038
Vibramycin Hyclate Intravenous 2040
Vibra-Tabs Film Coated Tablets 2038

Doxycycline Monohydrate (May increase digoxin absorption in patients who convert digoxin to inactive metabolites in the gut resulting in increased serum levels of digoxin). Products include:
Monodox Capsules 1858
Vibramycin Monohydrate for Oral Suspension 2038

IMPORTANT NOTE: Always consult each drug listing in the patient's regimen for possible interactions.

Interactions Index

Lanoxicaps

Ephedrine Hydrochloride (Both agents enhance ectopic pacemaker activity; concomitant use increases the risk of cardiac arrhythmias). Products include:
- Primatene Tablets .... ⊞ 844
- Quadrinal Tablets 1398

Ephedrine Sulfate (Both agents enhance ectopic pacemaker activity; concomitant use increases the risk of cardiac arrhythmias). Products include:
- Marax Tablets & DF Syrup 2015

Ephedrine Tannate (Both agents enhance ectopic pacemaker activity; concomitant use increases the risk of cardiac arrhythmias). Products include:
- Rynatuss 2782

Epinephrine (Both agents enhance ectopic pacemaker activity; concomitant use increases the risk of cardiac arrhythmias). Products include:
- EPIFRIN .... ⊙ 237
- EpiPen 808
- Marcaine with Epinephrine 2446
- Primatene Mist .... ⊞ 843
- Sensorcaine with Epinephrine Injection ... 554
- Sus-Phrine Injection 1017
- Xylocaine with Epinephrine Injections 562

Epinephrine Bitartrate (Both agents enhance ectopic pacemaker activity; concomitant use increases the risk of cardiac arrhythmias). Products include:
- Sensorcaine-MPF with Epinephrine Injection ... 554

Epinephrine Hydrochloride (Both agents enhance ectopic pacemaker activity; concomitant use increases the risk of cardiac arrhythmias). Products include:
- Ana-Kit Anaphylaxis Emergency Treatment Kit ... 611

Erythromycin (Co-administration results in increased digoxin absorption and serum levels). Products include:
- A/T/S 2% Acne Topical Gel 1244
- A/T/S 2% Acne Topical Solution 1244
- Benzamycin Topical Gel 919
- E-Mycin Tablets 1388
- Emgel 2% Topical Gel 1081
- ERYC 1972
- Erycette (erythromycin 2%) Topical Solution ... 1943
- Ery-Tab Tablets 426
- Erythromycin Base Filmtab 430
- Erythromycin Delayed-Release Capsules, USP ... 431
- Ilotycin Ophthalmic Ointment 928
- PCE Dispertab Tablets 453
- T-Stat 2.0% Topical Solution and Pads 2797
- THERAMYCIN Z 2% Solution 1629

Erythromycin Estolate (Co-administration results in increased digoxin absorption and serum levels). Products include:
- Ilosone 927

Erythromycin Ethylsuccinate (Co-administration results in increased digoxin absorption and serum levels). Products include:
- E.E.S. 427
- EryPed 425
- Pediazole Suspension 2340

Erythromycin Gluceptate (Co-administration results in increased digoxin absorption and serum levels). Products include:
- Ilotycin Gluceptate, IV, Vials 929

Erythromycin Stearate (Co-administration results in increased digoxin absorption and serum levels). Products include:
- Erythrocin Stearate Filmtab 429

Esmolol Hydrochloride (Additive effects on AV node conduction). Products include:
- Brevibloc (esmolol HCl) Injection 1860

Felodipine (Additive effects on AV node conduction). Products include:
- Plendil Extended-Release Tablets 514

Furosemide (Diuretic-induced hypokalemia sensitizes the myocardium to digitalis resulting in possible digitalis toxicity). Products include:
- Lasix Injection, Oral Solution and Tablets ... 1267

Hydrochlorothiazide (Diuretic-induced hypokalemia sensitizes the myocardium to digitalis resulting in possible digitalis toxicity). Products include:
- Aldactazide Tablets 2556
- Aldoril Tablets 1644
- Apresazide Capsules 824
- Capozide Tablets 744
- Dyazide Capsules 2653
- Esidrix Tablets 839
- Esimil Tablets 840
- HydroDIURIL Tablets 1716
- Hydropres Tablets 1718
- Hyzaar Tablets 1720
- Inderide Tablets 2838
- Inderide LA Long Acting Capsules 2840
- Lopressor HCT Tablets 850
- Lotensin HCT Tablets 855
- Moduretic Tablets 1748
- Oretic Tablets 450
- Prinzide Tablets 1780
- Ser-Ap-Es Tablets 867
- Timolide Tablets 1791
- Vaseretic Tablets 1810
- Zestoretic Tablets 2968
- Ziac 1459

Hydrocortisone (Corticosteroid-induced hypokalemia sensitizes the myocardium to digitalis resulting in possible digitalis toxicity). Products include:
- Anusol-HC Cream 2.5% 1953
- Aquanil HC Lotion 1989
- Maximum Strength Cortaid Spray .... ⊞ 800
- CORTENEMA 2713
- Cortisporin Ointment 1074
- Cortisporin Ophthalmic Ointment Sterile .. 1074
- Cortisporin Ophthalmic Suspension Sterile ... 1075
- Cortisporin Otic Solution Sterile 1076
- Cortisporin Otic Suspension Sterile 1077
- Cortizone-5 .... ⊞ 795
- Cortizone-10 .... ⊞ 795
- Hydrocortone Tablets 1715
- Hytone 922
- Hytone Ointment 2 ½% 923
- Massengill Medicated Soft Cloth Towelettes ... 2628
- Pediotic Suspension Sterile 1140
- Preparation H Hydrocortisone 1% Cream .... ⊞ 843
- ProctoCream-HC 2.5% 2552
- VōSoL HC Otic Solution 2786

Hydrocortisone Acetate (Corticosteroid-induced hypokalemia sensitizes the myocardium to digitalis resulting in possible digitalis toxicity). Products include:
- Analpram-HC Rectal Cream 1% and 2.5% 993
- Anusol HC-1 Hydrocortisone Anti-Itch Ointment ... ⊞ 810
- Anusol-HC Suppositories 1954
- Caldecort Anti-Itch Hydrocortisone Cream ... ⊞ 651
- Coly-Mycin S Otic w/Neomycin & Hydrocortisone ... 1965
- Cortaid .... ⊞ 800
- Cortifoam 2540
- Cortisporin Cream 1073
- Epifoam 2543
- Hydrocortone Acetate Sterile Suspension ... 1712
- Mantadil Cream 1124
- Nupercainal Hydrocortisone 1% Cream ...... ⊞ 661
- Pramosone Cream, Lotion & Ointment 995
- ProctoFoam-HC 2552
- Terra-Cortril Ophthalmic Suspension 2033

Hydrocortisone Sodium Phosphate (Corticosteroid-induced hypokalemia sensitizes the myocardium to digitalis resulting in possible digitalis toxicity). Products include:
- Hydrocortone Phosphate Injection, Sterile ... 1713

Hydrocortisone Sodium Succinate (Corticosteroid-induced hypokalemia sensitizes the myocardium to digitalis resulting in possible digitalis toxicity).
No products indexed under this heading.

Hydroflumethiazide (Diuretic-induced hypokalemia sensitizes the myocardium to digitalis resulting in possible digitalis toxicity). Products include:
- Diucardin Tablets 2824

Indapamide (Diuretic-induced hypokalemia sensitizes the myocardium to digitalis resulting in possible digitalis toxicity).
No products indexed under this heading.

Indomethacin (Causes a rise in serum digoxin concentration, with the implication that digitalis intoxication may result). Products include:
- Indocin 1723

Indomethacin Sodium Trihydrate (Causes a rise in serum digoxin concentration, with the implication that digitalis intoxication may result). Products include:
- Indocin I.V. 1727

Isoproterenol Hydrochloride (Both agents enhance ectopic pacemaker activity; concomitant use increases the risk of cardiac arrhythmias). Products include:
- Isuprel Hydrochloride Solution 2443
- Isuprel Injection 2441
- Isuprel Mistometer 2442

Isoproterenol Sulfate (Both agents enhance ectopic pacemaker activity; concomitant use increases the risk of cardiac arrhythmias). Products include:
- Norisodrine with Calcium Iodide Syrup 446

Isradipine (Additive effects on AV node conduction). Products include:
- DynaCirc Capsules 2381
- DynaCirc CR Tablets 2383

Itraconazole (Causes a rise in serum digoxin concentration, with the implication that digitalis intoxication may result). Products include:
- Sporanox Capsules 1352

Kaolin (Interferes with intestinal digoxin absorption).
No products indexed under this heading.

Labetalol Hydrochloride (Additive effects on AV node conduction). Products include:
- Normodyne Injection 2519
- Normodyne Tablets 2522
- Trandate 1158

Levobunolol Hydrochloride (Additive effects on AV node conduction). Products include:
- Betagan .... ⊙ 230

Liothyronine Sodium (Hypothyroid patients may require increased digoxin dose). Products include:
- Cytomel Tablets 2647
- Triostat Injection 2708

Magaldrate (Interferes with intestinal digoxin absorption).
No products indexed under this heading.

Magnesium Hydroxide (Interferes with intestinal digoxin absorption). Products include:
- Aludrox Oral Suspension .... ⊞ 850
- Ascriptin .... ⊞ 650
- Di-Gel Antacid/Anti-Gas .... ⊞ 762
- Gelusil Antacid-Anti-gas Liquid .... ⊞ 819
- Gelusil Antacid-Anti-Gas Tablets .... ⊞ 819
- Maalox Antacid/Anti-Gas Tablets 889
- Maalox Antacid Liquid 888
- Extra Strength Maalox Antacid/Anti-Gas Liquid and Tablets ... 888
- Mylanta Fast-Acting 1359
- Mylanta Gelcaps Antacid .... ⊞ 678
- Fast-Acting Mylanta Liquid Antacid 1359
- Mylanta Tablets .... ⊞ 677
- Maximum-Strength Fast-Acting Mylanta Tablets ... 1359
- Mylanta Double Strength Tablets .... ⊞ 677
- Phillips' Milk of Magnesia Liquid .... ⊞ 627
- Rolaids Antacid Tablets .... ⊞ 807
- Tempo Soft Antacid .... ⊞ 799

Magnesium Oxide (Interferes with intestinal digoxin absorption). Products include:
- Beelith Tablets 632
- Bufferin Analgesic Tablets .... ⊞ 636
- Arthritis Strength Bufferin Analgesic Caplets ... ⊞ 637
- Extra Strength Bufferin Analgesic Tablets ... ⊞ 637
- Caltrate PLUS .... ⊞ 681
- Cama Arthritis Pain Reliever .... ⊞ 748
- Mag-Ox 400 666
- Uro-Mag 666

Metaproterenol Sulfate (Both agents enhance ectopic pacemaker activity; concomitant use increases the risk of cardiac arrhythmias). Products include:
- Alupent 672
- Metaproterenol Sulfate Inhalation Solution, USP, Arm-a-Med ... 547

Metaraminol Bitartrate (Both agents enhance ectopic pacemaker activity; concomitant use increases the risk of cardiac arrhythmias). Products include:
- Aramine Injection 1649

Methoxamine Hydrochloride (Both agents enhance ectopic pacemaker activity; concomitant use increases the risk of cardiac arrhythmias). Products include:
- Vasoxyl Injection 1169

Methyclothiazide (Diuretic-induced hypokalemia sensitizes the myocardium to digitalis resulting in possible digitalis toxicity). Products include:
- Enduron Tablets 424

Methylprednisolone Acetate (Corticosteroid-induced hypokalemia sensitizes the myocardium to digitalis resulting in possible digitalis toxicity).
No products indexed under this heading.

Methylprednisolone Sodium Succinate (Corticosteroid-induced hypokalemia sensitizes the myocardium to digitalis resulting in possible digitalis toxicity).
No products indexed under this heading.

Metipranolol Hydrochloride (Additive effects on AV node conduction). Products include:
- OptiPranolol (Metipranolol 0.3%) Sterile Ophthalmic Solution ... ⊙ 256

Metolazone (Diuretic-induced hypokalemia sensitizes the myocardium to digitalis resulting in possible digitalis toxicity). Products include:
- Mykrox Tablets 1617
- Zaroxolyn Tablets 1625

Metoprolol Succinate (Additive effects on AV node conduction). Products include:
- Toprol-XL Tablets 560

Metoprolol Tartrate (Additive effects on AV node conduction). Products include:
- Lopressor 848
- Lopressor HCT Tablets 850

(⊞ Described in PDR For Nonprescription Drugs)   (⊙ Described in PDR For Ophthalmology)

Minocycline Hydrochloride (May increase digoxin absorption in patients who convert digoxin to inactive metabolites in the gut resulting in increased serum levels of digoxin). Products include:

- DYNACIN Capsules ... 1627
- Minocin Intravenous ... 1428
- Minocin Oral Suspension ... 1431
- Minocin Pellet-Filled Capsules ... 1429

Nadolol (Additive effects on AV node conduction).

- No products indexed under this heading.

Neomycin, oral (Interferes with intestinal digoxin absorption).

Nephrotoxic Drugs (May impair the excretion of digoxin).

Nicardipine Hydrochloride (Additive effects on AV node conduction). Products include:

- Cardene Capsules ... 2261
- Cardene I.V. ... 2815
- Cardene SR Capsules ... 2264

Nifedipine (Additive effects on AV node conduction). Products include:

- Adalat Capsules (10 mg and 20 mg) ... 580
- Adalat CC ... 582
- Procardia Capsules ... 2024
- Procardia XL Extended Release Tablets ... 2026

Nimodipine (Additive effects on AV node conduction). Products include:

- Nimotop Capsules ... 603

Nisoldipine (Additive effects on AV node conduction). Products include:

- Sular Tablets ... 2961

Norepinephrine Bitartrate (Both agents enhance ectopic pacemaker activity; concomitant use increases the risk of cardiac arrhythmias). Products include:

- Levophed Bitartrate Injection ... 2445

Oxytetracycline Hydrochloride (May increase digoxin absorption in patients who convert digoxin to inactive metabolites in the gut resulting in increased serum levels of digoxin). Products include:

- TERAK Ointment ... ⊙ 210
- Terra-Cortril Ophthalmic Suspension ... 2033
- Terramycin with Polymyxin B Sulfate Ophthalmic Ointment ... 2035
- Urobiotic-250 Capsules ... 2038

Pectin (Interferes with intestinal digoxin absorption). Products include:

- Celestial Seasonings Soothers Herbal Throat Drops ... ▣ 805

Penbutolol Sulfate (Additive effects on AV node conduction). Products include:

- Levatol Tablets ... 2547

Phenylephrine Bitartrate (Both agents enhance ectopic pacemaker activity; concomitant use increases the risk of cardiac arrhythmias).

- No products indexed under this heading.

Phenylephrine Hydrochloride (Both agents enhance ectopic pacemaker activity; concomitant use increases the risk of cardiac arrhythmias). Products include:

- Atrohist Plus Tablets ... 1605
- Cerose DM ... ▣ 853
- D.A. II Tablets ... 972
- D.A. Chewable Tablets ... 970
- Dura-Vent/DA Tablets ... 972
- Extendryl ... 1003
- 4-Way Fast Acting Nasal Spray (regular & mentholated) ... ▣ 644
- Hemorid ... ▣ 797
- Hycomine Compound Tablets ... 948
- Neo-Synephrine Hydrochloride 1% Carpuject ... 2455
- Neo-Synephrine Hydrochloride 1% Injection ... 2455
- Neo-Synephrine Hydrochloride (Ophthalmic) ... 2456
- Neo-Synephrine ... ▣ 624
- Novahistine Elixir ... ▣ 782
- Phenergan VC ... 2886
- Phenergan VC with Codeine ... 2888
- Preparation H ... ▣ 842
- Tympagesic Ear Drops ... 2476
- Vicks Sinex Nasal Spray and Ultra Fine Mist ... ▣ 738

Phenylephrine Tannate (Both agents enhance ectopic pacemaker activity; concomitant use increases the risk of cardiac arrhythmias). Products include:

- Atrohist Pediatric Suspension ... 1604
- Atrohist Pediatric Suspension Dye-Free ... 1604
- Rynatan ... 2781
- Rynatuss ... 2782

Phenylpropanolamine Hydrochloride (Both agents enhance ectopic pacemaker activity; concomitant use increases the risk of cardiac arrhythmias). Products include:

- Acutrim ... ▣ 648
- Atrohist Plus Tablets ... 1605
- BC Cold Powder Multi-Symptom Formula (Cold-Sinus-Allergy) ... ▣ 631
- BC Cold Powder Non-Drowsy Formula (Cold-Sinus) ... ▣ 631
- Cheracol Plus Head Cold/Cough Formula ... ▣ 741
- Comtrex Multi-Symptom Cold Reliever Liqui-Gels ... ▣ 638
- Comtrex Multi-Symptom Non-Drowsy Liqui-gels ... ▣ 640
- Contac Continuous Action Nasal Decongestant/Antihistamine 12 Hour Capsules ... ▣ 773
- Contac Maximum Strength Continuous Action Decongestant/Antihistamine 12 Hour Caplets ... ▣ 772
- Contac Severe Cold and Flu Formula Caplets ... ▣ 773
- Coricidin 'D' Decongestant Tablets ... ▣ 760
- Dexatrim ... ▣ 795
- Dexatrim Plus Vitamins Caplets ... ▣ 796
- Dimetane-DC Cough Syrup ... 2232
- Dimetapp Allergy Sinus Caplets ... ▣ 838
- Dimetapp Cold & Allergy Chewable Tablets ... ▣ 838
- Dimetapp Cold & Cough Liqui-Gels ... ▣ 839
- Dimetapp DM Elixir ... ▣ 840
- Dimetapp Elixir ... ▣ 840
- Dimetapp Extentabs ... ▣ 841
- Dimetapp Tablets/Liqui-Gels ... ▣ 841
- Dura-Vent Tablets ... 971
- Entex LA Tablets ... 972
- Exgest LA Tablets ... 787
- Hycomine ... 947
- Nolamine Timed-Release Tablets ... 790
- Ornade Spansule Capsules ... 2678
- Propagest Tablets ... 791
- Pyrroxate Caplets ... ▣ 742
- Robitussin-CF ... ▣ 846
- Sinulin Tablets ... 792
- Tavist-D 12 Hour Relief Tablets ... ▣ 750
- Teldrin 12 Hour Antihistamine/Nasal Decongestant Allergy Relief Capsules ... ▣ 786
- Triaminic Expectorant ... ▣ 753
- Triaminic Syrup ... ▣ 755
- Triaminic Triaminicol Cold & Cough ... ▣ 756
- Triaminic DM Syrup ... ▣ 756
- Triaminicin Tablets ... ▣ 756
- Vicks DayQuil Allergy Relief 12-Hour Extended Release Tablets ... ▣ 733
- Vicks DayQuil Allergy Relief 4-Hour Tablets ... ▣ 733
- Vicks DayQuil SINUS Pressure & CONGESTION Relief ... ▣ 734

Pindolol (Additive effects on AV node conduction). Products include:

- Visken Tablets ... 2428

Pirbuterol Acetate (Both agents enhance ectopic pacemaker activity; concomitant use increases the risk of cardiac arrhythmias). Products include:

- Maxair Autohaler ... 1550
- Maxair Inhaler ... 1552

Polythiazide (Diuretic-induced hypokalemia sensitizes the myocardium to digitalis resulting in possible digitalis toxicity). Products include:

- Minizide Capsules ... 2016

Prednisolone Acetate (Corticosteroid-induced hypokalemia sensitizes the myocardium to digitalis resulting in possible digitalis toxicity). Products include:

- AK-CIDE ... ⊙ 203
- AK-CIDE Ointment ... ⊙ 203
- Blephamide Liquifilm Sterile Ophthalmic Suspension ... 472
- Blephamide Ointment ... ⊙ 234
- Econopred & Econopred Plus Ophthalmic Suspensions ... ⊙ 216
- Poly-Pred Liquifilm ... ⊙ 246
- Pred Forte ... ⊙ 247
- Pred Mild ... ⊙ 250
- Pred-G Liquifilm Sterile Ophthalmic Suspension ... ⊙ 248
- Pred-G S.O.P. Sterile Ophthalmic Ointment ... ⊙ 249

Prednisolone Sodium Phosphate (Corticosteroid-induced hypokalemia sensitizes the myocardium to digitalis resulting in possible digitalis toxicity). Products include:

- AK-PRED ... ⊙ 204
- Hydeltrasol Injection, Sterile ... 1708
- Pediapred Oral Solution ... 1618

Prednisolone Tebutate (Corticosteroid-induced hypokalemia sensitizes the myocardium to digitalis resulting in possible digitalis toxicity). Products include:

- Hydeltra-T.B.A. Sterile Suspension 1710

Prednisone (Corticosteroid-induced hypokalemia sensitizes the myocardium to digitalis resulting in possible digitalis toxicity).

- No products indexed under this heading.

Propafenone Hydrochloride (Causes a rise in serum digoxin concentration, with the implication that digitalis intoxication may result). Products include:

- Rythmol Tablets–150mg, 225mg, 300mg ... 1399

Propantheline Bromide (Increases digoxin absorption). Products include:

- Pro-Banthine Tablets ... 2226

Propranolol Hydrochloride (Additive effects on AV node conduction). Products include:

- Inderal ... 2834
- Inderal LA Long Acting Capsules ... 2836
- Inderide Tablets ... 2838
- Inderide LA Long Acting Capsules .. 2840

Pseudoephedrine Hydrochloride (Both agents enhance ectopic pacemaker activity; concomitant use increases the risk of cardiac arrhythmias). Products include:

- Actifed Allergy Daytime/Nighttime Caplets ... ▣ 808
- Actifed Cold & Allergy Tablets ... ▣ 807
- Actifed Cold & Sinus Caplets and Tablets ... ▣ 808
- Actifed Sinus Daytime/Nighttime Tablets and Caplets ... ▣ 809
- Advil Cold and Sinus Caplets and Tablets ... ▣ 837
- Alka-Seltzer Plus Liqui-Gels ... ▣ 612
- Alka-Seltzer Plus Flu & Body Aches Liqui-Gels Non-Drowsy Formula ... ▣ 613
- Alka-Seltzer Plus Night-Time Cold Medicine Liqui-Gels ... ▣ 612
- Allerest Maximum Strength ... ▣ 649
- Allerest No Drowsiness ... ▣ 649
- Allerest Sinus Pain Formula ... ▣ 649
- Atrohist Pediatric Capsules ... 1603
- Benadryl Allergy/Cold Tablets ... ▣ 811
- Benadryl Allergy Decongestant Liquid Medication ... ▣ 812
- Benadryl Allergy Decongestant Tablets ... ▣ 812
- Benadryl Allergy Sinus Headache Caplets ... ▣ 813
- Benylin Multisymptom ... ▣ 816
- Bromfed Capsules (Extended-Release) ... 1832
- Bromfed Syrup ... ▣ 712
- Bromfed Tablets ... 1832
- Bromfed-DM Cough Syrup ... 1832
- Bromfed-PD Capsules (Extended-Release) ... 1832
- Children's TYLENOL Cold Multi-Symptom Chewable Tablets and Liquid ... 1559
- Children's TYLENOL Cold Plus Cough Multi Symptom Chewable Tablets and Liquid ... 1560
- Children's TYLENOL Flu Suspension Liquid ... 1560
- Children's Vicks DayQuil Allergy Relief ... ▣ 730
- Children's Vicks NyQuil Cold/Cough Relief ... ▣ 731
- Allergy-Sinus Comtrex Multi-Symptom Allergy-Sinus Formula Tablets and Caplets ... ▣ 639
- Comtrex Multi-Symptom ... ▣ 638
- Comtrex Multi-Symptom Non-Drowsy Caplets ... ▣ 640
- Congess ... 1003
- Contac Day Allergy/Sinus Caplets ▣ 771
- Contac Day & Night ... ▣ 772
- Contac Night Allergy/Sinus Caplets ... ▣ 771
- Contac Severe Cold & Flu Non-Drowsy ... ▣ 774
- Deconsal II Tablets ... 1605
- Dimetane-DX Cough Syrup ... 2233
- Dimetapp Cold & Fever Suspension ... ▣ 839
- Dimetapp Decongestant Pediatric Drops ... ▣ 840
- Dorcol Children's Cough Syrup ... ▣ 748
- Drixoral Cough + Congestion Liquid Caps ... ▣ 763
- Dura-Tap/PD Capsules ... 970
- Duratuss Tablets ... 2750
- Duratuss HD Elixir ... 2750
- Efidac/24 ... ▣ 655
- Entex PSE Tablets ... 973
- Fedahist Gyrocaps ... 2545
- Guaifed ... 1833
- Guaifed Syrup ... ▣ 712
- Guaimax-D Tablets ... 809
- Histussin D Liquid ... 670
- Infants' TYLENOL Cold Decongestant & Fever-Reducer Drops ... 1561
- Kronofed-A ... 994
- Novahistine DMX ... ▣ 782
- Nucofed ... 2225
- PediaCare Cough-Cold Chewable Tablets and Liquid ... 1569
- PediaCare Infants' Decongestant Drops ... 1569
- PediaCare Infants' Drops Decongestant Plus Cough ... 1569
- PediaCare NightRest Cough-Cold Liquid ... 1569
- Pediatric Vicks 44d Cough & Head Congestion Relief ... ▣ 736
- Pediatric Vicks 44m Cough & Cold Relief ... ▣ 737
- Robitussin Cold & Cough Liqui-Gels ... ▣ 844
- Robitussin Cold, Cough & Flu Liqui-Gels ... ▣ 844
- Robitussin Maximum Strength Cough & Cold ... ▣ 847
- Robitussin Night-Time Cold Formula ... ▣ 847
- Robitussin Pediatric Cough & Cold Formula ... ▣ 848
- Robitussin Pediatric Drops ... ▣ 849
- Robitussin Severe Congestion Liqui-Gels ... ▣ 845
- Robitussin-DAC Syrup ... 2249
- Robitussin-PE ... ▣ 846
- Rondec Oral Drops ... 974
- Rondec Syrup ... 974
- Rondec Tablet ... 974
- Rondec Chewable Tablets ... 974
- Rondec-TR Tablet ... 974
- Ryna ... ▣ 804
- Seldane-D Extended-Release Tablets ... 1286
- Semprex-D Capsules ... 1620
- Sinarest ... ▣ 663
- Sine-Aid Maximum Strength Sinus Headache Gelcaps, Caplets and Tablets ... 1570
- Sine-Off No Drowsiness Formula Caplets ... ▣ 784
- Sine-Off Sinus Medicine ... ▣ 784
- Singlet Tablets ... ▣ 785
- Sinutab Non-Drying Liquid Caps ... ▣ 823

IMPORTANT NOTE: Always consult each drug listing in the patient's regimen for possible interactions.

Lanoxicaps **Interactions Index** **568**

Sinutab Sinus Allergy Medication, Maximum Strength Tablets and Caplets ▣ 823
Sinutab Sinus Medication, Maximum Strength Without Drowsiness Formula, Tablets & Caplets ▣ 824
Sudafed Children's Cold & Cough Liquid Medication ▣ 825
Sudafed Children's Nasal Decongestant Liquid Medication ▣ 826
Sudafed Cold & Allergy Tablets ▣ 826
Sudafed Cold and Cough Liquid Caps ▣ 826
Sudafed Nasal Decongestant Tablets, 30 mg ▣ 825
Sudafed Nasal Decongestant Tablets, 60 mg ▣ 825
Sudafed Non-Drying Sinus Liquid Caps ▣ 827
Sudafed Pediatric Nasal Decongestant Liquid Oral Drops ▣ 827
Sudafed Severe Cold Formula Caplets ▣ 828
Sudafed Severe Cold Formula Tablets ▣ 828
Sudafed Sinus Caplets ▣ 829
Sudafed Sinus Tablets ▣ 829
Sudafed 12 Hour Caplets ▣ 824
Syn-Rx Tablets 1622
Syn-Rx DM Tablets 1623
TheraFlu Flu and Cold Medicine ▣ 750
Theraflu Maximum Strength Flu and Cold Medicine For Sore Throat ▣ 751
TheraFlu Flu, Cold and Cough Medicine ▣ 750
TheraFlu Maximum Strength Nighttime Flu, Cold & Cough Medicine ▣ 751
TheraFlu Maximum Strength Non-Drowsy Formula Flu, Cold & Cough Medicine ▣ 751
TheraFlu Maximum Strength, Non-Drowsy Formula Flu, Cold and Cough Caplets ▣ 752
Theraflu Maximum Strength Sinus Non-Drowsy Formula Caplets ▣ 752
Triaminic AM Cough and Decongestant Formula ▣ 753
Triaminic AM Decongestant Formula ▣ 753
Triaminic Infant Oral Decongestant Drops ▣ 754
Triaminic Night Time ▣ 754
Triaminic Sore Throat Formula ▣ 755
Tussend 1830
Tussend Expectorant 1831
TYLENOL Allergy Sinus, Maximum Strength Caplets and Gelcaps 1571
TYLENOL Allergy Sinus NightTime, Maximum Strength Caplets 1571
TYLENOL Cold Medication, Multi-Symptom Formula Tablets and Caplets 1572
TYLENOL Cold Medication, Multi-Symptom Hot Liquid Packets 1572
TYLENOL Cold Medication, No Drowsiness Formula Caplets and Gelcaps 1572
TYLENOL Cold Severe Congestion Caplets 1573
TYLENOL Cough Medication with Decongestant, Multi Symptom 1574
TYLENOL Flu No Drowsiness Formula, Maximum Strength Gelcaps 1575
TYLENOL Flu NightTime, Maximum Strength Gelcaps 1575
TYLENOL Flu NightTime, Maximum Strength Hot Medication Packets 1575
TYLENOL Sinus, Maximum Strength Geltabs, Gelcaps, Caplets and Tablets 1576
Vicks 44 LiquiCaps Cough, Cold & Flu Relief ▣ 728
Vicks 44 LiquiCaps Non-Drowsy Cough & Cold Relief ▣ 729
Vicks 44D Cough & Head Congestion Relief ▣ 728
Vicks 44M Cough, Cold & Flu Relief ▣ 729
Vicks DayQuil LiquiCaps/Liquid Multi-Symptom Cold/Flu Relief ▣ 734
Vicks DayQuil SINUS Pressure & PAIN Relief with IBUPROFEN ▣ 735
Vicks Nyquil Hot Therapy ▣ 735
Vicks NyQuil LiquiCaps/Liquid Multi-Symptom Cold/Flu Relief, Original and Cherry Flavors ▣ 736

Pseudoephedrine Sulfate (Both agents enhance ectopic pacemaker activity; concomitant use increases the risk of cardiac arrhythmias). Products include:
Chlor-Trimeton Allergy Decongestant Tablets ▣ 759
Claritin-D Tablets 2487
Drixoral Cold and Allergy Sustained-Action Tablets ▣ 763
Drixoral Cold and Flu Extended-Release Tablets ▣ 764
Drixoral Non-Drowsy Formula Extended-Release Tablets ▣ 764
Drixoral Allergy/Sinus Extended Release Tablets ▣ 765
Trinalin Repetabs Tablets 1373

Quinidine Gluconate (Causes a rise in serum digoxin concentration, with the implication that digitalis intoxication may result). Products include:
Quinaglute Dura-Tabs Tablets 644

Quinidine Polygalacturonate (Causes a rise in serum digoxin concentration, with the implication that digitalis intoxication may result). Products include:
Cardioquin Tablets 2146

Quinidine Sulfate (Causes a rise in serum digoxin concentration, with the implication that digitalis intoxication may result). Products include:
Quinidex Extentabs 2240

Salmeterol Xinafoate (Both agents enhance ectopic pacemaker activity; concomitant use increases the risk of cardiac arrhythmias). Products include:
Serevent Inhalation Aerosol 1149

Sotalol Hydrochloride (Additive effects on AV node conduction). Products include:
Betapace Tablets 637

Succinylcholine Chloride (May cause arrhythmias). Products include:
Anectine 1062

Sulfasalazine (Interferes with intestinal digoxin absorption). Products include:
Azulfidine 2059

Terbutaline Sulfate (Both agents enhance ectopic pacemaker activity; concomitant use increases the risk of cardiac arrhythmias). Products include:
Brethaire Inhaler 830
Brethine Ampuls 832
Brethine Tablets 831
Bricanyl Subcutaneous Injection 1247
Bricanyl Tablets 1248

Tetracycline Hydrochloride (Co-administration results in increased digoxin absorption and serum levels). Products include:
Achromycin V Capsules 1417
Helidac Therapy 2135

Thyroid (Hypothyroid patients may require increased digoxin dose).
No products indexed under this heading.

Thyroxine (Hypothyroid patients may require increased digoxin dose).
No products indexed under this heading.

Timolol Hemihydrate (Additive effects on AV node conduction). Products include:
Betimol 0.25%, 0.5% ◉ 259

Timolol Maleate (Additive effects on AV node conduction). Products include:
Blocadren Tablets 1654
Timolide Tablets 1791
Timoptic in Ocudose 1796
Timoptic Sterile Ophthalmic Solution 1794
Timoptic-XE 1798

Torsemide (Diuretic-induced hypokalemia sensitizes the myocardium to digitalis resulting in possible digitalis toxicity). Products include:
Demadex Tablets and Injection 691

Triamcinolone (Corticosteroid-induced hypokalemia sensitizes the myocardium to digitalis resulting in possible digitalis toxicity).
No products indexed under this heading.

Triamcinolone Acetonide (Corticosteroid-induced hypokalemia sensitizes the myocardium to digitalis resulting in possible digitalis toxicity). Products include:
Azmacort Oral Inhaler 2175
Nasacort AQ Nasal Spray 2191
Nasacort Nasal Inhaler 2189

Triamcinolone Diacetate (Corticosteroid-induced hypokalemia sensitizes the myocardium to digitalis resulting in possible digitalis toxicity).
No products indexed under this heading.

Triamcinolone Hexacetonide (Corticosteroid-induced hypokalemia sensitizes the myocardium to digitalis resulting in possible digitalis toxicity).
No products indexed under this heading.

Troleandomycin (Co-administration results in increased digoxin absorption and serum levels). Products include:
Tao Capsules 2033

Verapamil Hydrochloride (Causes a rise in serum digoxin concentration, with the implication that digitalis intoxication may result). Products include:
Calan SR Caplets 2571
Calan Tablets 2568
Covera-HS Tablets 2573
Isoptin Injectable 1391
Isoptin Oral Tablets 1393
Isoptin SR Tablets 1395
Verelan Capsules 1455

Food Interactions

Meal, high in bran fiber (Reduces the amount of digoxin from an oral dose).

Meal, unspecified (The rate of absorption is slowed).

LANOXIN ELIXIR PEDIATRIC
(Digoxin) 1113
May interact with potassium-depleting corticosteroids, potassium-depleting diuretics, antacids, sympathomimetics, beta blockers, calcium channel blockers, thyroid preparations, tetracyclines, macrolide antibiotics, erythromycin, and certain other agents. Compounds in these categories include:

Acebutolol Hydrochloride (Additive effects on AV node conduction). Products include:
Sectral Capsules 2914

Albuterol (Both agents enhance ectopic pacemaker activity; concomitant use increases the risk of cardiac arrhythmias). Products include:
Proventil Inhalation Aerosol 2524
Ventolin Inhalation Aerosol and Refill 1170

Albuterol Sulfate (Both agents enhance ectopic pacemaker activity; concomitant use increases the risk of cardiac arrhythmias). Products include:
Airet Albuterol Sulfate Inhalation Solution 1602
Albuterol Sulfate, USP Solution for Inhalation, Arm-a-Med 522
Proventil Inhalation Solution 0.083% 2527
Proventil Repetabs Tablets 2529
Proventil Solution for Inhalation 0.5% 2525
Proventil Syrup 2528
Proventil Tablets 2529
Ventolin Inhalation Solution 1171
Ventolin Nebules Inhalation Solution 1172
Ventolin Rotacaps for Inhalation 1173
Ventolin Syrup 1175
Ventolin Tablets 1176
Volmax Extended-Release Tablets 1835

Alprazolam (Causes a rise in serum digoxin concentration, with the implication that digitalis intoxication may result). Products include:
Xanax Tablets 2115

Aluminum Carbonate (Interferes with intestinal digoxin absorption). Products include:
Basaljel Capsules 2810
Basaljel Suspension 2810
Basaljel Tablets 2810

Aluminum Hydroxide (Interferes with intestinal digoxin absorption). Products include:
ALternaGEL Liquid 1358
Maximum Strength Ascriptin ▣ 650
Cama Arthritis Pain Reliever ▣ 748
Gaviscon Extra Strength Relief Formula Antacid Tablets ▣ 778
Gaviscon Extra Strength Relief Formula Liquid Antacid ▣ 779
Gaviscon Liquid Antacid ▣ 779
Gelusil Antacid-Anti-gas Liquid ▣ 819
Gelusil Antacid-Anti-gas Tablets ▣ 819
Maalox Antacid/Anti-Gas Tablets 889
Maalox Heartburn Relief Suspension ▣ 658
Maalox Antacid Liquid 888
Extra Strength Maalox Antacid/Anti-Gas Liquid and Tablets 888
Mylanta 1359
Tempo Soft Antacid ▣ 799

Aluminum Hydroxide Gel (Interferes with intestinal digoxin absorption). Products include:
ALternaGEL Liquid ▣ 675
Aludrox Oral Suspension ▣ 850
Amphojel Suspension 2802
Amphojel Suspension without Flavor 2802
Amphojel Tablets 2802
Ascriptin ▣ 650
Gaviscon Antacid Tablets ▣ 778
Gaviscon-2 Antacid Tablets ▣ 779
Mylanta Liquid ▣ 676
Mylanta Double Strength Liquid ▣ 676
Nephrox Suspension ▣ 671

Amiodarone Hydrochloride (Causes a rise in serum digoxin concentration, with the implication that digitalis intoxication may result). Products include:
Cordarone Intravenous 2821
Cordarone Tablets 2818

Amlodipine Besylate (Additive effects on AV node conduction). Products include:
Lotrel Capsules 858
Norvasc Tablets 2020

Amphotericin B (Amphotericin B-induced hypokalemia sensitizes the myocardium to digitalis resulting in possible digitalis toxicity). Products include:
Abelcet Injection 1540
Fungizone Intravenous 507
Fungizone Oral Suspension 704

Anticancer Drugs, unspecified (Interferes with intestinal digoxin absorption).

Atenolol (Additive effects on AV node conduction). Products include:
Tenoretic Tablets 2963
Tenormin Tablets and I.V. Injection 2965

Azithromycin (Co-administration results in increased digoxin absorption and serum levels). Products include:
Zithromax 2043
Zithromax Tablets 2046

(▣ Described in PDR For Nonprescription Drugs) (◉ Described in PDR For Ophthalmology)

Bendroflumethiazide (Diuretic-induced hypokalemia sensitizes the myocardium to digitalis resulting in possible digitalis toxicity).

No products indexed under this heading.

Bepridil Hydrochloride (Additive effects on AV node conduction). Products include:

Vascor Tablets (200 and 300 mg) 1597

Betamethasone Acetate (Corticosteroid-induced hypokalemia sensitizes the myocardium to digitalis resulting in possible digitalis toxicity). Products include:

Celestone Soluspan Suspension 2484

Betamethasone Sodium Phosphate (Corticosteroid-induced hypokalemia sensitizes the myocardium to digitalis resulting in possible digitalis toxicity). Products include:

Celestone Soluspan Suspension 2484

Betaxolol Hydrochloride (Additive effects on AV node conduction). Products include:

Betoptic Ophthalmic Solution........... 465
Betoptic S Ophthalmic Suspension 467
Kerlone Tablets.................................... 2588

Bisoprolol Fumarate (Additive effects on AV node conduction). Products include:

Zebeta Tablets 1457
Ziac 1459

Calcium, intravenous (May produce serious arrhythmias in digitalized patients).

No products indexed under this heading.

Carteolol Hydrochloride (Additive effects on AV node conduction). Products include:

Cartrol Tablets 413
Ocupress Ophthalmic Solution, 1% Sterile....................................... ◉ 297

Chlorothiazide (Diuretic-induced hypokalemia sensitizes the myocardium to digitalis resulting in possible digitalis toxicity). Products include:

Aldoclor Tablets 1638
Diupres Tablets 1691
Diuril Oral 1694

Chlorothiazide Sodium (Diuretic-induced hypokalemia sensitizes the myocardium to digitalis resulting in possible digitalis toxicity). Products include:

Diuril Sodium Intravenous 1693

Chlorthalidone (Diuretic-induced hypokalemia sensitizes the myocardium to digitalis resulting in possible digitalis toxicity). Products include:

Combipres Tablets 682
Tenoretic Tablets.................................. 2963
Thalitone 1293

Cholestyramine (Interferes with intestinal digoxin absorption). Products include:

Questran 774

Clarithromycin (Co-administration results in increased digoxin absorption and serum levels). Products include:

Biaxin 406

Cortisone Acetate (Corticosteroid-induced hypokalemia sensitizes the myocardium to digitalis resulting in possible digitalis toxicity). Products include:

Cortone Acetate Sterile Suspension 1663
Cortone Acetate Tablets...................... 1664

Demeclocycline Hydrochloride (May increase digoxin absorption in patients who convert digoxin to inactive metabolites in the gut resulting in increased serum levels of digoxin). Products include:

Declomycin Tablets.............................. 1421

Dexamethasone (Corticosteroid-induced hypokalemia sensitizes the myocardium to digitalis resulting in possible digitalis toxicity). Products include:

AK-Trol Ointment & Suspension .... ◉ 205
Decadron Elixir 1676
Decadron Tablets.................................. 1678
Decaspray Topical Aerosol 1689
Maxitrol Ophthalmic Ointment and Suspension .... ◉ 222
TobraDex Ophthalmic Suspension and Ointment...................................... 469

Dexamethasone Acetate (Corticosteroid-induced hypokalemia sensitizes the myocardium to digitalis resulting in possible digitalis toxicity). Products include:

Dalalone D.P. Injectable 1009
Decadron-LA Sterile Suspension...... 1687

Dexamethasone Sodium Phosphate (Corticosteroid-induced hypokalemia sensitizes the myocardium to digitalis resulting in possible digitalis toxicity). Products include:

Decadron Phosphate Injection 1680
Decadron Phosphate Sterile Ophthalmic Ointment.............................. 1684
Decadron Phosphate Sterile Ophthalmic Solution 1685
Decadron Phosphate Topical Cream 1686
Decadron Phosphate with Xylocaine Injection, Sterile 1683
Dexacort Phosphate in Respihaler .. 1606
Dexacort Phosphate in Turbinaire .. 1607
NeoDecadron Sterile Ophthalmic Ointment 1755
NeoDecadron Sterile Ophthalmic Solution 1756
NeoDecadron Topical Cream 1757

Diltiazem Hydrochloride (Additive effects on AV node conduction). Products include:

Cardizem CD Capsules 1251
Cardizem SR Capsules 1255
Cardizem Injectable 1253
Cardizem Tablets.................................. 1257
Dilacor XR Extended-release Capsules 2183
Tiazac Capsules 1019

Diphenoxylate Hydrochloride (Increases digoxin absorption). Products include:

Lomotil 2591

Dirithromycin (Co-administration results in increased digoxin absorption and serum levels). Products include:

Dynabac... 668

Dobutamine Hydrochloride (Both agents enhance ectopic pacemaker activity; concomitant use increases the risk of cardiac arrhythmias). Products include:

Dobutrex Solution Vials....................... 1480

Dopamine Hydrochloride (Both agents enhance ectopic pacemaker activity; concomitant use increases the risk of cardiac arrhythmias).

No products indexed under this heading.

Doxycycline Hyclate (May increase digoxin absorption in patients who convert digoxin to inactive metabolites in the gut resulting in increased serum levels of digoxin). Products include:

Doryx Capsules...................................... 1970
Vibramycin Hyclate Capsules............ 2038
Vibramycin Hyclate Intravenous 2040
Vibra-Tabs Film Coated Tablets 2038

Doxycycline Monohydrate (May increase digoxin absorption in patients who convert digoxin to inactive metabolites in the gut resulting in increased serum levels of digoxin). Products include:

Monodox Capsules 1858
Vibramycin Monohydrate for Oral Suspension 2038

Ephedrine Hydrochloride (Both agents enhance ectopic pacemaker activity; concomitant use increases the risk of cardiac arrhythmias). Products include:

Primatene Tablets .... ■D 844
Quadrinal Tablets 1398

Ephedrine Sulfate (Both agents enhance ectopic pacemaker activity; concomitant use increases the risk of cardiac arrhythmias). Products include:

Marax Tablets & DF Syrup.................. 2015

Ephedrine Tannate (Both agents enhance ectopic pacemaker activity; concomitant use increases the risk of cardiac arrhythmias). Products include:

Rynatuss 2782

Epinephrine (Both agents enhance ectopic pacemaker activity; concomitant use increases the risk of cardiac arrhythmias). Products include:

EPIFRIN .... ◉ 237
EpiPen 808
Marcaine with Epinephrine 2446
Primatene Mist .... ■D 843
Sensorcaine with Epinephrine Injection 554
Sus-Phrine Injection 1017
Xylocaine with Epinephrine Injections.. 562

Epinephrine Bitartrate (Both agents enhance ectopic pacemaker activity; concomitant use increases the risk of cardiac arrhythmias). Products include:

Sensorcaine-MPF with Epinephrine Injection 554

Epinephrine Hydrochloride (Both agents enhance ectopic pacemaker activity; concomitant use increases the risk of cardiac arrhythmias). Products include:

Ana-Kit Anaphylaxis Emergency Treatment Kit 611

Erythromycin (Co-administration results in increased digoxin absorption and serum levels). Products include:

A/T/S 2% Acne Topical Gel.............. 1244
A/T/S 2% Acne Topical Solution.... 1244
Benzamycin Topical Gel 919
E-Mycin Tablets 1388
Emgel 2% Topical Gel......................... 1081
ERYC.. 1972
Erycette (erythromycin 2%) Topical Solution... 1943
Ery-Tab Tablets 426
Erythromycin Base Filmtab 430
Erythromycin Delayed-Release Capsules, USP..................................... 431
Ilotycin Ophthalmic Ointment........... 928
PCE Dispertab Tablets 453
T-Stat 2.0% Topical Solution and Pads 2797
THERAMYCIN Z 2% Solution........... 1629

Erythromycin Estolate (Co-administration results in increased digoxin absorption and serum levels). Products include:

Ilosone 927

Erythromycin Ethylsuccinate (Co-administration results in increased digoxin absorption and serum levels). Products include:

E.E.S. 427
EryPed 425
Pediazole Suspension 2340

Erythromycin Gluceptate (Co-administration results in increased digoxin absorption and serum levels). Products include:

Ilotycin Gluceptate, IV, Vials 929

Erythromycin Stearate (Co-administration results in increased digoxin absorption and serum levels). Products include:

Erythrocin Stearate Filmtab 429

Esmolol Hydrochloride (Additive effects on AV node conduction). Products include:

Brevibloc (esmolol HCl) Injection 1860

Felodipine (Additive effects on AV node conduction). Products include:

Plendil Extended-Release Tablets.... 514

Furosemide (Diuretic-induced hypokalemia sensitizes the myocardium to digitalis resulting in possible digitalis toxicity). Products include:

Lasix Injection, Oral Solution and Tablets 1267

Hydrochlorothiazide (Diuretic-induced hypokalemia sensitizes the myocardium to digitalis resulting in possible digitalis toxicity). Products include:

Aldactazide Tablets 2556
Aldoril Tablets....................................... 1644
Apresazide Capsules 824
Capozide Tablets 744
Dyazide Capsules................................. 2653
Esidrix Tablets 839
Esimil Tablets 840
HydroDIURIL Tablets 1716
Hydropres Tablets................................ 1718
Hyzaar Tablets 1720
Inderide Tablets 2838
Inderide LA Long Acting Capsules .. 2840
Lopressor HCT Tablets 850
Lotensin HCT Tablets 855
Moduretic Tablets 1748
Oretic Tablets 450
Prinzide Tablets 1780
Ser-Ap-Es Tablets 867
Timolide Tablets................................... 1791
Vaseretic Tablets 1810
Zestoretic Tablets 2968
Ziac 1459

Hydrocortisone (Corticosteroid-induced hypokalemia sensitizes the myocardium to digitalis resulting in possible digitalis toxicity). Products include:

Anusol-HC Cream 2.5% 1953
Aquanil HC Lotion 1989
Maximum Strength Cortaid Spray ■D 800
CORTENEMA.. 2713
Cortisporin Ointment........................... 1074
Cortisporin Ophthalmic Ointment Sterile 1074
Cortisporin Ophthalmic Suspension Sterile 1075
Cortisporin Otic Solution Sterile 1076
Cortisporin Otic Suspension Sterile 1077
Cortizone-5 .... ■D 795
Cortizone-10 .... ■D 795
Hydrocortone Tablets 1715
Hytone 922
Hytone Ointment 2 ½% 923
Massengill Medicated Soft Cloth Towelettes.. 2628
Pediotic Suspension Sterile............... 1140
Preparation H Hydrocortisone 1% Cream .... ■D 843
ProctoCream-HC 2.5%....................... 2552
VōSoL HC Otic Solution...................... 2786

Hydrocortisone Acetate (Corticosteroid-induced hypokalemia sensitizes the myocardium to digitalis resulting in possible digitalis toxicity). Products include:

Analpram-HC Rectal Cream 1% and 2.5% 993
Anusol HC-1 Hydrocortisone Anti-Itch Ointment .... ■D 810
Anusol-HC Suppositories 1954
Caldecort Anti-Itch Hydrocortisone Cream .... ■D 651
Coly-Mycin S Otic w/Neomycin & Hydrocortisone 1965
Cortaid .... ■D 800
Cortifoam 2540
Cortisporin Cream................................ 1073
Epifoam 2543
Hydrocortone Acetate Sterile Suspension 1712
Mantadil Cream 1124
Nupercainal Hydrocortisone 1% Cream .... ■D 661
Pramosone Cream, Lotion & Ointment 995
ProctoFoam-HC 2552
Terra-Cortril Ophthalmic Suspension 2033

IMPORTANT NOTE: Always consult each drug listing in the patient's regimen for possible interactions.

Hydrocortisone Sodium Phosphate (Corticosteroid-induced hypokalemia sensitizes the myocardium to digitalis resulting in possible digitalis toxicity). Products include:
Hydrocortone Phosphate Injection, Sterile ... 1713

Hydrocortisone Sodium Succinate (Corticosteroid-induced hypokalemia sensitizes the myocardium to digitalis resulting in possible digitalis toxicity).
No products indexed under this heading.

Hydroflumethiazide (Diuretic-induced hypokalemia sensitizes the myocardium to digitalis resulting in possible digitalis toxicity). Products include:
Diucardin Tablets ... 2824

Indapamide (Diuretic-induced hypokalemia sensitizes the myocardium to digitalis resulting in possible digitalis toxicity).
No products indexed under this heading.

Indomethacin (Causes a rise in serum digoxin concentration, with the implication that digitalis intoxication may result). Products include:
Indocin ... 1723

Indomethacin Sodium Trihydrate (Causes a rise in serum digoxin concentration, with the implication that digitalis intoxication may result). Products include:
Indocin I.V. ... 1727

Isoproterenol Hydrochloride (Both agents enhance ectopic pacemaker activity; concomitant use increases the risk of cardiac arrhythmias). Products include:
Isuprel Hydrochloride Solution ... 2443
Isuprel Injection ... 2441
Isuprel Mistometer ... 2442

Isoproterenol Sulfate (Both agents enhance ectopic pacemaker activity; concomitant use increases the risk of cardiac arrhythmias). Products include:
Norisodrine with Calcium Iodide Syrup ... 446

Isradipine (Additive effects on AV node conduction). Products include:
DynaCirc Capsules ... 2381
DynaCirc CR Tablets ... 2383

Itraconazole (Causes a rise in serum digoxin concentration, with the implication that digitalis intoxication may result). Products include:
Sporanox Capsules ... 1352

Labetalol Hydrochloride (Additive effects on AV node conduction). Products include:
Normodyne Injection ... 2519
Normodyne Tablets ... 2522
Trandate ... 1158

Levobunolol Hydrochloride (Additive effects on AV node conduction). Products include:
Betagan ... Ⓞ 230

Levothyroxine Sodium (Hypothyroid patients may require increased digoxin dose). Products include:
Eltroxin Tablets ... 2214
Levothroid Tablets ... 1015
Levothyroxine Sodium, USP for Injection ... 546
Levoxyl Tablets ... 918
Synthroid ... 1410

Liothyronine Sodium (Hypothyroid patients may require increased digoxin dose). Products include:
Cytomel Tablets ... 2647
Triostat Injection ... 2708

Liotrix (Hypothyroid patients may require increased digoxin dose).
No products indexed under this heading.

Magaldrate (Interferes with intestinal digoxin absorption).
No products indexed under this heading.

Magnesium Hydroxide (Interferes with intestinal digoxin absorption). Products include:
Aludrox Oral Suspension ... ND 850
Ascriptin ... ND 650
Di-Gel Antacid/Anti-Gas ... ND 762
Gelusil Antacid-Anti-gas Liquid ... ND 819
Gelusil Antacid-Anti-gas Tablets ... ND 819
Maalox Antacid/Anti-Gas Tablets ... 889
Maalox Antacid Liquid ... 888
Extra Strength Maalox Antacid/Anti-Gas Liquid and Tablets ... 888
Mylanta Fast-Acting ... 1359
Mylanta Gelcaps Antacid ... 678
Fast-Acting Mylanta Liquid Antacid 1359
Mylanta Tablets ... ND 677
Maximum-Strength Fast-Acting Mylanta Liquid Antacid ... 1359
Mylanta Double Strength Tablets ... ND 677
Phillips' Milk of Magnesia Liquid ... ND 627
Rolaids Antacid Tablets ... ND 807
Tempo Soft Antacid ... ND 799

Magnesium Oxide (Interferes with intestinal digoxin absorption). Products include:
Beelith Tablets ... 632
Bufferin Analgesic Tablets ... ND 636
Arthritis Strength Bufferin Analgesic Caplets ... ND 637
Extra Strength Bufferin Analgesic Tablets ... ND 637
Caltrate PLUS ... ND 681
Cama Arthritis Pain Reliever ... ND 748
Mag-Ox 400 ... 666
Uro-Mag ... 666

Metaproterenol Sulfate (Both agents enhance ectopic pacemaker activity; concomitant use increases the risk of cardiac arrhythmias). Products include:
Alupent ... 672
Metaproterenol Sulfate Inhalation Solution, USP, Arm-a-Med ... 547

Metaraminol Bitartrate (Both agents enhance ectopic pacemaker activity; concomitant use increases the risk of cardiac arrhythmias). Products include:
Aramine Injection ... 1649

Methoxamine Hydrochloride (Both agents enhance ectopic pacemaker activity; concomitant use increases the risk of cardiac arrhythmias). Products include:
Vasoxyl Injection ... 1169

Methyclothiazide (Diuretic-induced hypokalemia sensitizes the myocardium to digitalis resulting in possible digitalis toxicity). Products include:
Enduron Tablets ... 424

Methylprednisolone Acetate (Corticosteroid-induced hypokalemia sensitizes the myocardium to digitalis resulting in possible digitalis toxicity).
No products indexed under this heading.

Methylprednisolone Sodium Succinate (Corticosteroid-induced hypokalemia sensitizes the myocardium to digitalis resulting in possible digitalis toxicity).
No products indexed under this heading.

Metipranolol Hydrochloride (Additive effects on AV node conduction). Products include:
OptiPranolol (Metipranolol 0.3%) Sterile Ophthalmic Solution ... Ⓞ 256

Metolazone (Diuretic-induced hypokalemia sensitizes the myocardium to digitalis resulting in possible digitalis toxicity). Products include:
Mykrox Tablets ... 1617
Zaroxolyn Tablets ... 1625

Metoprolol Succinate (Additive effects on AV node conduction). Products include:
Toprol-XL Tablets ... 560

Metoprolol Tartrate (Additive effects on AV node conduction). Products include:
Lopressor ... 848
Lopressor HCT Tablets ... 850

Minocycline Hydrochloride (May increase digoxin absorption in patients who convert digoxin to inactive metabolites in the gut resulting in increased serum levels of digoxin). Products include:
DYNACIN Capsules ... 1627
Minocin Intravenous ... 1428
Minocin Oral Suspension ... 1431
Minocin Pellet-Filled Capsules ... 1429

Nadolol (Additive effects on AV node conduction).
No products indexed under this heading.

Neomycin, oral (Interferes with intestinal digoxin absorption).

Nephrotoxic Drugs (May impair the excretion of digoxin).

Nicardipine Hydrochloride (Additive effects on AV node conduction). Products include:
Cardene Capsules ... 2261
Cardene I.V. ... 2815
Cardene SR Capsules ... 2264

Nifedipine (Additive effects on AV node conduction). Products include:
Adalat Capsules (10 mg and 20 mg) ... 580
Adalat CC ... 582
Procardia Capsules ... 2024
Procardia XL Extended Release Tablets ... 2026

Nimodipine (Additive effects on AV node conduction). Products include:
Nimotop Capsules ... 603

Nisoldipine (Additive effects on AV node conduction). Products include:
Sular Tablets ... 2961

Norepinephrine Bitartrate (Both agents enhance ectopic pacemaker activity; concomitant use increases the risk of cardiac arrhythmias). Products include:
Levophed Bitartrate Injection ... 2445

Oxytetracycline Hydrochloride (May increase digoxin absorption in patients who convert digoxin to inactive metabolites in the gut resulting in increased serum levels of digoxin). Products include:
TERAK Ointment ... Ⓞ 210
Terra-Cortril Ophthalmic Suspension ... 2033
Terramycin with Polymyxin B Sulfate Ophthalmic Ointment ... 2035
Urobiotic-250 Capsules ... 2038

Pectin (Low digoxin serum concentration; interferes with intestinal digoxin absorption). Products include:
Celestial Seasonings Soothers Herbal Throat Drops ... ND 805

Penbutolol Sulfate (Additive effects on AV node conduction). Products include:
Levatol Tablets ... 2547

Phenylephrine Bitartrate (Both agents enhance ectopic pacemaker activity; concomitant use increases the risk of cardiac arrhythmias).
No products indexed under this heading.

Phenylephrine Hydrochloride (Both agents enhance ectopic pacemaker activity; concomitant use increases the risk of cardiac arrhythmias). Products include:
Atrohist Plus Tablets ... 1605

Cerose DM ... ND 853
D.A. II Tablets ... 972
D.A. Chewable Tablets ... 970
Dura-Vent/DA Tablets ... 972
Extendryl ... 1003
4-Way Fast Acting Nasal Spray (regular & mentholated) ... ND 644
Hemorid ... ND 797
Hycomine Compound Tablets ... 948
Neo-Synephrine Hydrochloride 1% Carpuject ... 2455
Neo-Synephrine Hydrochloride 1% Injection ... 2455
Neo-Synephrine Hydrochloride (Ophthalmic) ... 2456
Neo-Synephrine ... ND 624
Novahistine Elixir ... ND 782
Phenergan VC ... 2886
Phenergan VC with Codeine ... 2888
Preparation H ... ND 842
Tympagesic Ear Drops ... 2476
Vicks Sinex Nasal Spray and Ultra Fine Mist ... ND 738

Phenylephrine Tannate (Both agents enhance ectopic pacemaker activity; concomitant use increases the risk of cardiac arrhythmias). Products include:
Atrohist Pediatric Suspension ... 1604
Atrohist Pediatric Suspension Dye-Free ... 1604
Rynatan ... 2781
Rynatuss ... 2782

Phenylpropanolamine Hydrochloride (Both agents enhance ectopic pacemaker activity; concomitant use increases the risk of cardiac arrhythmias). Products include:
Acutrim ... ND 648
Atrohist Plus Tablets ... 1605
BC Cold Powder Multi-Symptom Formula (Cold-Sinus-Allergy) ... ND 631
BC Cold Powder Non-Drowsy Formula (Cold-Sinus) ... ND 631
Cheracol Plus Head Cold/Cough Formula ... ND 741
Comtrex Multi-Symptom Cold Reliever Liqui-Gels ... ND 638
Comtrex Multi-Symptom Non-Drowsy Liqui-gels ... ND 640
Contac Continuous Action Nasal Decongestant/Antihistamine 12 Hour Capsules ... ND 773
Contac Maximum Strength Continuous Action Decongestant/Antihistamine 12 Hour Caplets ... ND 772
Contac Severe Cold and Flu Formula Caplets ... ND 773
Coricidin 'D' Decongestant Tablets ... ND 760
Dexatrim ... ND 795
Dexatrim Plus Vitamins Caplets ... ND 796
Dimetane-DC Cough Syrup ... 2232
Dimetapp Allergy Sinus Caplets ... ND 838
Dimetapp Cold & Allergy Chewable Tablets ... ND 838
Dimetapp Cold & Cough Liqui-Gels ... ND 839
Dimetapp DM Elixir ... ND 840
Dimetapp Elixir ... ND 840
Dimetapp Extentabs ... ND 841
Dimetapp Tablets/Liqui-Gels ... ND 841
Dura-Vent Tablets ... 971
Entex LA Tablets ... 972
Exgest LA Tablets ... 787
Hycomine ... 947
Nolamine Timed-Release Tablets ... 790
Ornade Spansule Capsules ... 2678
Propagest Tablets ... 791
Pyrroxate Caplets ... ND 742
Robitussin-CF ... ND 846
Sinulin Tablets ... 792
Tavist-D 12 Hour Relief Tablets ... ND 750
Teldrin 12 Hour Antihistamine/Nasal Decongestant Allergy Relief Capsules ... ND 786
Triaminic Expectorant ... ND 753
Triaminic Syrup ... ND 755
Triaminic Triaminicol Cold & Cough ... ND 756
Triaminic DM Syrup ... ND 756
Triaminicin Tablets ... ND 756
Vicks DayQuil Allergy Relief 12-Hour Extended Release Tablets ... ND 733
Vicks DayQuil Allergy Relief 4-Hour Tablets ... ND 733
Vicks DayQuil SINUS Pressure & CONGESTION Relief ... ND 734

(ND Described in PDR For Nonprescription Drugs)   (Ⓞ Described in PDR For Ophthalmology)

571 **Interactions Index** **Lanoxin Elixir**

Pindolol (Additive effects on AV node conduction). Products include:

Visken Tablets ... 2428

Pirbuterol Acetate (Both agents enhance ectopic pacemaker activity; concomitant use increases the risk of cardiac arrhythmias). Products include:

Maxair Autohaler ... 1550
Maxair Inhaler ... 1552

Polythiazide (Diuretic-induced hypokalemia sensitizes the myocardium to digitalis resulting in possible digitalis toxicity). Products include:

Minizide Capsules ... 2016

Prednisolone Acetate (Corticosteroid-induced hypokalemia sensitizes the myocardium to digitalis resulting in possible digitalis toxicity). Products include:

AK-CIDE ... ◉ 203
AK-CIDE Ointment ... ◉ 203
Blephamide Liquifilm Sterile Ophthalmic Suspension ... 472
Blephamide Ointment ... ◉ 234
Econopred & Econopred Plus Ophthalmic Suspensions ... ◉ 216
Poly-Pred Liquifilm ... ◉ 246
Pred Forte ... ◉ 247
Pred Mild ... ◉ 250
Pred-G Liquifilm Sterile Ophthalmic Suspension ... ◉ 248
Pred-G S.O.P. Sterile Ophthalmic Ointment ... ◉ 249

Prednisolone Sodium Phosphate (Corticosteroid-induced hypokalemia sensitizes the myocardium to digitalis resulting in possible digitalis toxicity). Products include:

AK-PRED ... ◉ 204
Hydeltrasol Injection, Sterile ... 1708
Pediapred Oral Solution ... 1618

Prednisolone Tebutate (Corticosteroid-induced hypokalemia sensitizes the myocardium to digitalis resulting in possible digitalis toxicity). Products include:

Hydeltra-T.B.A. Sterile Suspension 1710

Prednisone (Corticosteroid-induced hypokalemia sensitizes the myocardium to digitalis resulting in possible digitalis toxicity).

No products indexed under this heading.

Propafenone Hydrochloride (Causes a rise in serum digoxin concentration, with the implication that digitalis intoxication may result). Products include:

Rythmol Tablets–150mg, 225mg, 300mg ... 1399

Propantheline Bromide (Increases digoxin absorption). Products include:

Pro-Banthine Tablets ... 2226

Propranolol Hydrochloride (Additive effects on AV node conduction). Products include:

Inderal ... 2834
Inderal LA Long Acting Capsules ... 2836
Inderide Tablets ... 2838
Inderide LA Long Acting Capsules .. 2840

Pseudoephedrine Hydrochloride (Both agents enhance ectopic pacemaker activity; concomitant use increases the risk of cardiac arrhythmias). Products include:

Actifed Allergy Daytime/Nighttime Caplets ... ED 808
Actifed Cold & Allergy Tablets ... ED 807
Actifed Cold & Sinus Caplets and Tablets ... ED 808
Actifed Sinus Daytime/Nighttime Tablets and Caplets ... ED 809
Advil Cold and Sinus Caplets and Tablets ... ED 837
Alka-Seltzer Plus Liqui-Gels ... ED 612
Alka-Seltzer Plus Flu & Body Aches Liqui-Gels Non-Drowsy Formula ... ED 613
Alka-Seltzer Plus Night-Time Cold Medicine Liqui-Gels ... ED 612
Allerest Maximum Strength ... ED 649
Allerest No Drowsiness ... ED 649
Allerest Sinus Pain Formula ... ED 649
Atrohist Pediatric Capsules ... 1603
Benadryl Allergy/Cold Tablets ... ED 811
Benadryl Allergy Decongestant Liquid Medication ... ED 812
Benadryl Allergy Decongestant Tablets ... ED 812
Benadryl Allergy Sinus Headache Caplets ... ED 813
Benylin Multisymptom ... ED 816
Bromfed Capsules (Extended-Release) ... 1832
Bromfed Syrup ... ED 712
Bromfed Tablets ... 1832
Bromfed-DM Cough Syrup ... 1832
Bromfed-PD Capsules (Extended-Release) ... 1832
Children's TYLENOL Cold Multi-Symptom Chewable Tablets and Liquid ... 1559
Children's TYLENOL Cold Plus Cough Multi Symptom Chewable Tablets and Liquid ... 1560
Children's TYLENOL Flu Suspension Liquid ... 1560
Children's Vicks DayQuil Allergy Relief ... ED 730
Children's Vicks NyQuil Cold/Cough Relief ... ED 731
Allergy-Sinus Comtrex Multi-Symptom Allergy-Sinus Formula Tablets and Caplets ... ED 639
Comtrex Multi-Symptom ... ED 638
Comtrex Multi-Symptom Non-Drowsy Caplets ... ED 640
Congess ... 1003
Contac Day Allergy/Sinus Caplets ED 771
Contac Day & Night ... ED 772
Contac Night Allergy/Sinus Caplets ... ED 771
Contac Severe Cold & Flu Non-Drowsy ... ED 774
Deconsal II Tablets ... 1605
Dimetane-DX Cough Syrup ... 2233
Dimetapp Cold & Fever Suspension ... ED 839
Dimetapp Decongestant Pediatric Drops ... ED 840
Dorcol Children's Cough Syrup ... ED 748
Drixoral Cough + Congestion Liquid Caps ... ED 763
Dura-Tap/PD Capsules ... 970
Duratuss Tablets ... 2750
Duratuss HD Elixir ... 2750
Efidac/24 ... ED 655
Entex PSE Tablets ... 973
Fedahist Gyrocaps ... 2545
Guaifed ... 1833
Guaifed Syrup ... ED 712
Guaimax-D Tablets ... 809
Histussin D Liquid ... 670
Infants' TYLENOL Cold Decongestant & Fever-Reducer Drops ... 1561
Kronofed-A ... 994
Novahistine DMX ... ED 782
Nucofed ... 2225
PediaCare Cough-Cold Chewable Tablets and Liquid ... 1569
PediaCare Infants' Decongestant Drops ... 1569
PediaCare Infants' Drops Decongestant Plus Cough ... 1569
PediaCare NightRest Cough-Cold Liquid ... 1569
Pediatric Vicks 44d Cough & Head Congestion Relief ... ED 736
Pediatric Vicks 44m Cough & Cold Relief ... ED 737
Robitussin Cold & Cough Liqui-Gels ... ED 844
Robitussin Cold, Cough & Flu Liqui-Gels ... ED 844
Robitussin Maximum Strength Cough & Cold ... ED 847
Robitussin Night-Time Cold Formula ... ED 847
Robitussin Pediatric Cough & Cold Formula ... ED 848
Robitussin Pediatric Drops ... ED 849
Robitussin Severe Congestion Liqui-Gels ... ED 845
Robitussin-DAC Syrup ... 2249
Robitussin-PE ... ED 846
Rondec Oral Drops ... 974
Rondec Syrup ... 974
Rondec Tablet ... 974
Rondec Chewable Tablets ... 974
Rondec-TR Tablet ... 974
Ryna ... ED 804
Seldane-D Extended-Release Tablets ... 1286
Semprex-D Capsules ... 1620
Sinarest ... ED 663
Sine-Aid Maximum Strength Sinus Headache Gelcaps, Caplets and Tablets ... 1570
Sine-Off No Drowsiness Formula Caplets ... ED 784
Sine-Off Sinus Medicine ... ED 784
Singlet Tablets ... ED 785
Sinutab Non-Drying Liquid Caps ... ED 823
Sinutab Sinus Allergy Medication, Maximum Strength Tablets and Caplets ... ED 823
Sinutab Sinus Medication, Maximum Strength Without Drowsiness Formula, Tablets & Caplets ... ED 824
Sudafed Children's Cold & Cough Liquid Medication ... ED 825
Sudafed Children's Nasal Decongestant Liquid Medication ... ED 826
Sudafed Cold & Allergy Tablets ... ED 826
Sudafed Cold and Cough Liquid Caps ... ED 826
Sudafed Nasal Decongestant Tablets, 30 mg ... ED 825
Sudafed Nasal Decongestant Tablets, 60 mg ... ED 825
Sudafed Non-Drying Sinus Liquid Caps ... ED 827
Sudafed Pediatric Nasal Decongestant Liquid Oral Drops ... ED 827
Sudafed Severe Cold Formula Caplets ... ED 828
Sudafed Severe Cold Formula Tablets ... ED 828
Sudafed Sinus Caplets ... ED 829
Sudafed Sinus Tablets ... ED 829
Sudafed 12 Hour Caplets ... ED 824
Syn-Rx Tablets ... 1622
Syn-Rx DM Tablets ... 1623
TheraFlu Flu and Cold Medicine ... ED 750
Theraflu Maximum Strength Flu and Cold Medicine For Sore Throat ... ED 751
TheraFlu Flu, Cold and Cough Medicine ... ED 750
TheraFlu Maximum Strength Nighttime Flu, Cold & Cough Medicine ... ED 751
TheraFlu Maximum Strength Non-Drowsy Formula Flu, Cold & Cough Medicine ... ED 751
TheraFlu Maximum Strength, Non-Drowsy Formula Flu, Cold and Cough Caplets ... ED 752
Theraflu Maximum Strength Sinus Non-Drowsy Formula Caplets ... ED 752
Triaminic AM Cough and Decongestant Formula ... ED 753
Triaminic AM Decongestant Formula ... ED 753
Triaminic Infant Oral Decongestant Drops ... ED 754
Triaminic Night Time ... ED 754
Triaminic Sore Throat Formula ... ED 755
Tussend ... 1830
Tussend Expectorant ... 1831
TYLENOL Allergy Sinus, Maximum Strength Caplets and Gelcaps ... 1571
TYLENOL Allergy Sinus NightTime, Maximum Strength Caplets ... 1571
TYLENOL Cold Medication, Multi-Symptom Formula Tablets and Caplets ... 1572
TYLENOL Cold Medication, Multi-Symptom Hot Liquid Packets ... 1572
TYLENOL Cold Medication, No Drowsiness Formula Caplets and Gelcaps ... 1572
TYLENOL Cold Severe Congestion Caplets ... 1573
TYLENOL Cough Medication with Decongestant, Multi Symptom ... 1574
TYLENOL Flu No Drowsiness Formula, Maximum Strength Gelcaps ... 1575
TYLENOL Flu NightTime, Maximum Strength Gelcaps ... 1575
TYLENOL Flu NightTime, Maximum Strength Hot Medication Packets ... 1575
TYLENOL Sinus, Maximum Strength Geltabs, Gelcaps, Caplets and Tablets ... 1576
Vicks 44 LiquiCaps Cough, Cold & Flu Relief ... ED 728
Vicks 44 LiquiCaps Non-Drowsy Cough & Cold Relief ... ED 729
Vicks 44D Cough & Head Congestion Relief ... ED 728
Vicks 44M Cough, Cold & Flu Relief ... ED 729
Vicks DayQuil LiquiCaps/Liquid Multi-Symptom Cold/Flu Relief .. ED 734
Vicks DayQuil SINUS Pressure & PAIN Relief with IBUPROFEN ... ED 735
Vicks Nyquil Hot Therapy ... ED 735
Vicks NyQuil LiquiCaps/Liquid Multi-Symptom Cold/Flu Relief, Original and Cherry Flavors ... ED 736

Pseudoephedrine Sulfate (Both agents enhance ectopic pacemaker activity; concomitant use increases the risk of cardiac arrhythmias). Products include:

Chlor-Trimeton Allergy Decongestant Tablets ... ED 759
Claritin-D Tablets ... 2487
Drixoral Cold and Allergy Sustained-Action Tablets ... ED 763
Drixoral Cold and Flu Extended-Release Tablets ... ED 764
Drixoral Non-Drowsy Formula Extended-Release Tablets ... ED 764
Drixoral Allergy/Sinus Extended Release Tablets ... ED 765
Trinalin Repetabs Tablets ... 1373

Quinidine Gluconate (Causes a rise in serum digoxin concentration, with the implication that digitalis intoxication may result). Products include:

Quinaglute Dura-Tabs Tablets ... 644

Quinidine Polygalacturonate (Causes a rise in serum digoxin concentration, with the implication that digitalis intoxication may result). Products include:

Cardioquin Tablets ... 2146

Quinidine Sulfate (Causes a rise in serum digoxin concentration, with the implication that digitalis intoxication may result). Products include:

Quinidex Extentabs ... 2240

Salmeterol Xinafoate (Both agents enhance ectopic pacemaker activity; concomitant use increases the risk of cardiac arrhythmias). Products include:

Serevent Inhalation Aerosol ... 1149

Sodium Bicarbonate (Interferes with intestinal digoxin absorption). Products include:

Alka-Seltzer Cherry Effervescent Antacid and Pain Reliever ... ED 609
Alka-Seltzer Extra Strength Effervescent Antacid and Pain Reliever ... ED 609
Alka-Seltzer Gold Effervescent Antacid ... ED 611
Alka-Seltzer Lemon Lime Effervescent Antacid and Pain Reliever ... ED 609
Alka-Seltzer Original Effervescent Antacid and Pain Reliever ... ED 609
Arm & Hammer Pure Baking Soda ... ED 648
Colyte and Colyte-flavored ... 2540
GoLYTELY ... 694
Massengill Disposable Douches ... ED 780
Massengill Liquid Concentrate ... ED 780
NuLYTELY ... 694
Cherry Flavor NuLYTELY ... 694

Sotalol Hydrochloride (Additive effects on AV node conduction). Products include:

Betapace Tablets ... 637

Succinylcholine Chloride (May cause arrhythmias). Products include:

Anectine ... 1062

Sulfasalazine (Low digoxin serum concentration; interferes with intestinal digoxin absorption). Products include:

Azulfidine ... 2059

IMPORTANT NOTE: Always consult each drug listing in the patient's regimen for possible interactions.

Lanoxin Elixir

Terbutaline Sulfate (Both agents enhance ectopic pacemaker activity; concomitant use increases the risk of cardiac arrhythmias). Products include:
- Brethaire Inhaler 830
- Brethine Ampuls 832
- Brethine Tablets 831
- Bricanyl Subcutaneous Injection 1247
- Bricanyl Tablets 1248

Tetracycline Hydrochloride (Co-administration results in increased digoxin absorption and serum levels). Products include:
- Achromycin V Capsules 1417
- Helidac Therapy 2135

Thyroglobulin (Hypothyroid patients may require increased digoxin dose).
- No products indexed under this heading.

Thyroid (Hypothyroid patients may require increased digoxin dose).
- No products indexed under this heading.

Thyroxine (Hypothyroid patients may require increased digoxin dose).
- No products indexed under this heading.

Thyroxine Sodium (Hypothyroid patients may require increased digoxin dose).
- No products indexed under this heading.

Timolol Hemihydrate (Additive effects on AV node conduction). Products include:
- Betimol 0.25%, 0.5% .... ⊚ 259

Timolol Maleate (Additive effects on AV node conduction). Products include:
- Blocadren Tablets 1654
- Timolide Tablets 1791
- Timoptic in Ocudose 1796
- Timoptic Sterile Ophthalmic Solution 1794
- Timoptic-XE 1798

Triamcinolone (Corticosteroid-induced hypokalemia sensitizes the myocardium to digitalis resulting in possible digitalis toxicity).
- No products indexed under this heading.

Triamcinolone Acetonide (Corticosteroid-induced hypokalemia sensitizes the myocardium to digitalis resulting in possible digitalis toxicity). Products include:
- Azmacort Oral Inhaler 2175
- Nasacort AQ Nasal Spray 2191
- Nasacort Nasal Inhaler 2189

Triamcinolone Diacetate (Corticosteroid-induced hypokalemia sensitizes the myocardium to digitalis resulting in possible digitalis toxicity).
- No products indexed under this heading.

Triamcinolone Hexacetonide (Corticosteroid-induced hypokalemia sensitizes the myocardium to digitalis resulting in possible digitalis toxicity).
- No products indexed under this heading.

Troleandomycin (Co-administration results in increased digoxin absorption and serum levels). Products include:
- Tao Capsules 2033

Verapamil Hydrochloride (Causes a rise in serum digoxin concentration, with the implication that digitalis intoxication may result). Products include:
- Calan SR Caplets 2571
- Calan Tablets 2568
- Covera-HS Tablets 2573
- Isoptin Injectable 1391
- Isoptin Oral Tablets 1393
- Isoptin SR Tablets 1395
- Verelan Capsules 1455

Food Interactions

Meal, high in bran fiber (The amount of digoxin from an oral dose may be reduced).

Meal, unspecified (Slows the rate of absorption).

LANOXIN INJECTION
(Digoxin) 1116
May interact with potassium-depleting corticosteroids, potassium-depleting diuretics, antacids, sympathomimetics, beta blockers, calcium channel blockers, thyroid preparations, tetracyclines, macrolide antibiotics, erythromycin, and certain other agents. Compounds in these categories include:

Acebutolol Hydrochloride (Additive effects on AV node conduction). Products include:
- Sectral Capsules 2914

Albuterol (Both agents enhance ectopic pacemaker activity; concomitant use increases the risk of cardiac arrhythmias). Products include:
- Proventil Inhalation Aerosol 2524
- Ventolin Inhalation Aerosol and Refill 1170

Albuterol Sulfate (Both agents enhance ectopic pacemaker activity; concomitant use increases the risk of cardiac arrhythmias). Products include:
- Airet Albuterol Sulfate Inhalation Solution 1602
- Albuterol Sulfate, USP Solution for Inhalation, Arm-a-Med 522
- Proventil Inhalation Solution 0.083% 2527
- Proventil Repetabs Tablets 2529
- Proventil Solution for Inhalation 0.5% 2525
- Proventil Syrup 2528
- Proventil Tablets 2529
- Ventolin Inhalation Solution 1171
- Ventolin Nebules Inhalation Solution 1172
- Ventolin Rotacaps for Inhalation 1173
- Ventolin Syrup 1175
- Ventolin Tablets 1176
- Volmax Extended-Release Tablets 1835

Alprazolam (Causes a rise in serum digoxin concentration, with the implication that digitalis intoxication may result). Products include:
- Xanax Tablets 2115

Aluminum Carbonate (Interferes with intestinal digoxin absorption). Products include:
- Basaljel Capsules 2810
- Basaljel Suspension 2810
- Basaljel Tablets 2810

Aluminum Hydroxide (Interferes with intestinal digoxin absorption). Products include:
- ALternaGEL Liquid 1358
- Maximum Strength Ascriptin .... ⊡ 650
- Cama Arthritis Pain Reliever .... ⊡ 748
- Gaviscon Extra Strength Relief Formula Antacid Tablets .... ⊡ 778
- Gaviscon Extra Strength Relief Formula Liquid Antacid .... ⊡ 779
- Gaviscon Liquid Antacid .... ⊡ 779
- Gelusil Antacid-Anti-gas Liquid .... ⊡ 819
- Gelusil Antacid-Anti-gas Tablets .... ⊡ 819
- Maalox Antacid/Anti-Gas Tablets 889
- Maalox Heartburn Relief Suspension 658
- Maalox Antacid Liquid 888
- Extra Strength Maalox Antacid/Anti-Gas Liquid and Tablets 888
- Mylanta 1359
- Tempo Soft Antacid .... ⊡ 799

Aluminum Hydroxide Gel (Interferes with intestinal digoxin absorption). Products include:
- ALternaGEL Liquid .... ⊡ 675
- Aludrox Oral Suspension .... ⊡ 850
- Amphojel Suspension 2802
- Amphojel Suspension without Flavor 2802
- Amphojel Tablets 2802
- Ascriptin .... ⊡ 650
- Gaviscon Antacid Tablets .... ⊡ 778
- Gaviscon-2 Antacid Tablets .... ⊡ 779
- Mylanta Liquid .... ⊡ 676
- Mylanta Double Strength Liquid .... ⊡ 676
- Nephrox Suspension .... ⊡ 671

Amiodarone Hydrochloride (Causes a rise in serum digoxin concentration, with the implication that digitalis intoxication may result). Products include:
- Cordarone Intravenous 2821
- Cordarone Tablets 2818

Amlodipine Besylate (Additive effects on AV node conduction). Products include:
- Lotrel Capsules 858
- Norvasc Tablets 2020

Amphotericin B (Amphotericin B-induced hypokalemia sensitizes the myocardium to digitalis resulting in possible digitalis toxicity). Products include:
- Abelcet Injection 1540
- Fungizone Intravenous 507
- Fungizone Oral Suspension 704

Antibiotics, unspecified (Increases digoxin absorption in patients who inactivate digoxin by bacterial metabolism).

Anticancer Drugs, unspecified (Interferes with intestinal digoxin absorption).

Atenolol (Additive effects on AV node conduction). Products include:
- Tenoretic Tablets 2963
- Tenormin Tablets and I.V. Injection 2965

Azithromycin (Co-administration results in increased digoxin serum levels). Products include:
- Zithromax 2043
- Zithromax Tablets 2046

Bendroflumethiazide (Diuretic-induced hypokalemia sensitizes the myocardium to digitalis resulting in possible digitalis toxicity).
- No products indexed under this heading.

Bepridil Hydrochloride (Additive effects on AV node conduction). Products include:
- Vascor Tablets (200 and 300 mg) 1597

Betamethasone Acetate (Corticosteroid-induced hypokalemia sensitizes the myocardium to digitalis resulting in possible digitalis toxicity). Products include:
- Celestone Soluspan Suspension 2484

Betamethasone Sodium Phosphate (Corticosteroid-induced hypokalemia sensitizes the myocardium to digitalis resulting in possible digitalis toxicity). Products include:
- Celestone Soluspan Suspension 2484

Betaxolol Hydrochloride (Additive effects on AV node conduction). Products include:
- Betoptic Ophthalmic Solution 465
- Betoptic S Ophthalmic Suspension 467
- Kerlone Tablets 2588

Bisoprolol Fumarate (Additive effects on AV node conduction). Products include:
- Zebeta Tablets 1457
- Ziac 1459

Calcium, intravenous (May produce serious arrhythmias in digitalized patients).
- No products indexed under this heading.

Carteolol Hydrochloride (Additive effects on AV node conduction). Products include:
- Cartrol Tablets 413
- Ocupress Ophthalmic Solution, 1% Sterile .... ⊚ 297

Chlorothiazide (Diuretic-induced hypokalemia sensitizes the myocardium to digitalis resulting in possible digitalis toxicity). Products include:
- Aldoclor Tablets 1638
- Diupres Tablets 1691
- Diuril Oral 1694

Chlorothiazide Sodium (Diuretic-induced hypokalemia sensitizes the myocardium to digitalis resulting in possible digitalis toxicity). Products include:
- Diuril Sodium Intravenous 1693

Chlorthalidone (Diuretic-induced hypokalemia sensitizes the myocardium to digitalis resulting in possible digitalis toxicity). Products include:
- Combipres Tablets 682
- Tenoretic Tablets 2963
- Thalitone 1293

Cholestyramine (Interferes with intestinal digoxin absorption). Products include:
- Questran 774

Clarithromycin (Co-administration results in increased digoxin serum levels). Products include:
- Biaxin 406

Cortisone Acetate (Corticosteroid-induced hypokalemia sensitizes the myocardium to digitalis resulting in possible digitalis toxicity). Products include:
- Cortone Acetate Sterile Suspension 1663
- Cortone Acetate Tablets 1664

Demeclocycline Hydrochloride (May increase digoxin absorption in patients who convert digoxin to inactive metabolites in the gut resulting in increased serum levels of digoxin). Products include:
- Declomycin Tablets 1421

Dexamethasone (Corticosteroid-induced hypokalemia sensitizes the myocardium to digitalis resulting in possible digitalis toxicity). Products include:
- AK-Trol Ointment & Suspension .... ⊚ 205
- Decadron Elixir 1676
- Decadron Tablets 1678
- Decaspray Topical Aerosol 1689
- Maxitrol Ophthalmic Ointment and Suspension .... ⊚ 222
- TobraDex Ophthalmic Suspension and Ointment 469

Dexamethasone Acetate (Corticosteroid-induced hypokalemia sensitizes the myocardium to digitalis resulting in possible digitalis toxicity). Products include:
- Dalalone D.P. Injectable 1009
- Decadron-LA Sterile Suspension 1687

Dexamethasone Sodium Phosphate (Corticosteroid-induced hypokalemia sensitizes the myocardium to digitalis resulting in possible digitalis toxicity). Products include:
- Decadron Phosphate Injection 1680
- Decadron Phosphate Sterile Ophthalmic Ointment 1684
- Decadron Phosphate Sterile Ophthalmic Solution 1685
- Decadron Phosphate Topical Cream 1686
- Decadron Phosphate with Xylocaine Injection, Sterile 1683
- Dexacort Phosphate in Respihaler 1606
- Dexacort Phosphate in Turbinaire 1607
- NeoDecadron Sterile Ophthalmic Ointment 1755
- NeoDecadron Sterile Ophthalmic Solution 1756
- NeoDecadron Topical Cream 1757

Diltiazem Hydrochloride (Additive effects on AV node conduction). Products include:
- Cardizem CD Capsules 1251
- Cardizem SR Capsules 1255
- Cardizem Injectable 1253
- Cardizem Tablets 1257

(⊡ Described in PDR For Nonprescription Drugs)   (⊚ Described in PDR For Ophthalmology)

Interactions Index — Lanoxin Injection

Dilacor XR Extended-release Capsules ... 2183
Tiazac Capsules ... 1019

Diphenoxylate Hydrochloride (Increases digoxin absorption). Products include:
Lomotil ... 2591

Dirithromycin (Co-administration results in increased digoxin serum levels). Products include:
Dynabac ... 668

Dobutamine Hydrochloride (Both agents enhance ectopic pacemaker activity; concomitant use increases the risk of cardiac arrhythmias). Products include:
Dobutrex Solution Vials ... 1480

Dopamine Hydrochloride (Both agents enhance ectopic pacemaker activity; concomitant use increases the risk of cardiac arrhythmias). Products include:
No products indexed under this heading.

Doxycycline Hyclate (May increase digoxin absorption in patients who convert digoxin to inactive metabolites in the gut resulting in increased serum levels of digoxin). Products include:
Doryx Capsules ... 1970
Vibramycin Hyclate Capsules ... 2038
Vibramycin Hyclate Intravenous ... 2040
Vibra-Tabs Film Coated Tablets ... 2038

Doxycycline Monohydrate (May increase digoxin absorption in patients who convert digoxin to inactive metabolites in the gut resulting in increased serum levels of digoxin). Products include:
Monodox Capsules ... 1858
Vibramycin Monohydrate for Oral Suspension ... 2038

Ephedrine Hydrochloride (Both agents enhance ectopic pacemaker activity; concomitant use increases the risk of cardiac arrhythmias). Products include:
Primatene Tablets ... 844
Quadrinal Tablets ... 1398

Ephedrine Sulfate (Both agents enhance ectopic pacemaker activity; concomitant use increases the risk of cardiac arrhythmias). Products include:
Marax Tablets & DF Syrup ... 2015

Ephedrine Tannate (Both agents enhance ectopic pacemaker activity; concomitant use increases the risk of cardiac arrhythmias). Products include:
Rynatuss ... 2782

Epinephrine (Both agents enhance ectopic pacemaker activity; concomitant use increases the risk of cardiac arrhythmias). Products include:
EPIFRIN ... 237
EpiPen ... 808
Marcaine with Epinephrine ... 2446
Primatene Mist ... 843
Sensorcaine with Epinephrine Injection ... 554
Sus-Phrine Injection ... 1017
Xylocaine with Epinephrine Injections ... 562

Epinephrine Bitartrate (Both agents enhance ectopic pacemaker activity; concomitant use increases the risk of cardiac arrhythmias). Products include:
Sensorcaine-MPF with Epinephrine Injection ... 554

Epinephrine Hydrochloride (Both agents enhance ectopic pacemaker activity; concomitant use increases the risk of cardiac arrhythmias). Products include:
Ana-Kit Anaphylaxis Emergency Treatment Kit ... 611

Erythromycin (Co-administration results in increased digoxin serum levels). Products include:
A/T/S 2% Acne Topical Gel ... 1244
A/T/S 2% Acne Topical Solution ... 1244
Benzamycin Topical Gel ... 919
E-Mycin Tablets ... 1388
Emgel 2% Topical Gel ... 1081
ERYC ... 1972
Erycette (erythromycin 2%) Topical Solution ... 1943
Ery-Tab Tablets ... 426
Erythromycin Base Filmtab ... 430
Erythromycin Delayed-Release Capsules, USP ... 431
Ilotycin Ophthalmic Ointment ... 928
PCE Dispertab Tablets ... 453
T-Stat 2.0% Topical Solution and Pads ... 2797
THERAMYCIN Z 2% Solution ... 1629

Erythromycin Estolate (Co-administration results in increased digoxin serum levels). Products include:
Ilosone ... 927

Erythromycin Ethylsuccinate (Co-administration results in increased digoxin serum levels). Products include:
E.E.S. ... 427
EryPed ... 425
Pediazole Suspension ... 2340

Erythromycin Gluceptate (Co-administration results in increased digoxin serum levels). Products include:
Ilotycin Gluceptate, IV, Vials ... 929

Erythromycin Stearate (Co-administration results in increased digoxin serum levels). Products include:
Erythrocin Stearate Filmtab ... 429

Esmolol Hydrochloride (Additive effects on AV node conduction). Products include:
Brevibloc (esmolol HCl) Injection ... 1860

Felodipine (Additive effects on AV node conduction). Products include:
Plendil Extended-Release Tablets ... 514

Furosemide (Diuretic-induced hypokalemia sensitizes the myocardium to digitalis resulting in possible digitalis toxicity). Products include:
Lasix Injection, Oral Solution and Tablets ... 1267

Hydrochlorothiazide (Diuretic-induced hypokalemia sensitizes the myocardium to digitalis resulting in possible digitalis toxicity). Products include:
Aldactazide Tablets ... 2556
Aldoril Tablets ... 1644
Apresazide Capsules ... 824
Capozide Tablets ... 744
Dyazide Capsules ... 2653
Esidrix Tablets ... 839
Esimil Tablets ... 840
HydroDIURIL Tablets ... 1716
Hydropres Tablets ... 1718
Hyzaar Tablets ... 1720
Inderide Tablets ... 2838
Inderide LA Long Acting Capsules ... 2840
Lopressor HCT Tablets ... 850
Lotensin HCT Tablets ... 855
Moduretic Tablets ... 1748
Oretic Tablets ... 450
Prinzide Tablets ... 1780
Ser-Ap-Es Tablets ... 867
Timolide Tablets ... 1791
Vaseretic Tablets ... 1810
Zestoretic Tablets ... 2968
Ziac ... 1459

Hydrocortisone (Corticosteroid-induced hypokalemia sensitizes the myocardium to digitalis resulting in possible digitalis toxicity). Products include:
Anusol-HC Cream 2.5% ... 1953
Aquanil HC Lotion ... 1989
Maximum Strength Cortaid Spray ... 800
CORTENEMA ... 2713

Cortisporin Ointment ... 1074
Cortisporin Ophthalmic Ointment Sterile ... 1074
Cortisporin Ophthalmic Suspension Sterile ... 1075
Cortisporin Otic Solution Sterile ... 1076
Cortisporin Otic Suspension Sterile ... 1077
Cortizone-5 ... 795
Cortizone-10 ... 795
Hydrocortone Tablets ... 1715
Hytone ... 922
Hytone Ointment 2 ½% ... 923
Massengill Medicated Soft Cloth Towelettes ... 2628
Pediotic Suspension Sterile ... 1140
Preparation H Hydrocortisone 1% Cream ... 843
ProctoCream-HC 2.5% ... 2552
VōSol HC Otic Solution ... 2786

Hydrocortisone Acetate (Corticosteroid-induced hypokalemia sensitizes the myocardium to digitalis resulting in possible digitalis toxicity). Products include:
Analpram-HC Rectal Cream 1% and 2.5% ... 993
Anusol HC-1 Hydrocortisone Anti-Itch Ointment ... 810
Anusol-HC Suppositories ... 1954
Caldecort Anti-Itch Hydrocortisone Cream ... 651
Coly-Mycin S Otic w/Neomycin & Hydrocortisone ... 1965
Cortaid ... 800
Cortifoam ... 2540
Cortisporin Cream ... 1073
Epifoam ... 2543
Hydrocortone Acetate Sterile Suspension ... 1712
Mantadil Cream ... 1124
Nupercainal Hydrocortisone 1% Cream ... 661
Pramosone Cream, Lotion & Ointment ... 995
ProctoFoam-HC ... 2552
Terra-Cortril Ophthalmic Suspension ... 2033

Hydrocortisone Sodium Phosphate (Corticosteroid-induced hypokalemia sensitizes the myocardium to digitalis resulting in possible digitalis toxicity). Products include:
Hydrocortone Phosphate Injection, Sterile ... 1713

Hydrocortisone Sodium Succinate (Corticosteroid-induced hypokalemia sensitizes the myocardium to digitalis resulting in possible digitalis toxicity).
No products indexed under this heading.

Hydroflumethiazide (Diuretic-induced hypokalemia sensitizes the myocardium to digitalis resulting in possible digitalis toxicity). Products include:
Diucardin Tablets ... 2824

Indapamide (Diuretic-induced hypokalemia sensitizes the myocardium to digitalis resulting in possible digitalis toxicity).
No products indexed under this heading.

Indomethacin (Causes a rise in serum digoxin concentration, with the implication that digitalis intoxication may result). Products include:
Indocin ... 1723

Indomethacin Sodium Trihydrate (Causes a rise in serum digoxin concentration, with the implication that digitalis intoxication may result). Products include:
Indocin I.V. ... 1727

Isoproterenol Hydrochloride (Both agents enhance ectopic pacemaker activity; concomitant use increases the risk of cardiac arrhythmias). Products include:
Isuprel Hydrochloride Solution ... 2443
Isuprel Injection ... 2441
Isuprel Mistometer ... 2442

Isoproterenol Sulfate (Both agents enhance ectopic pacemaker activity; concomitant use increases the risk of cardiac arrhythmias). Products include:
Norisodrine with Calcium Iodide Syrup ... 446

Isradipine (Additive effects on AV node conduction). Products include:
DynaCirc Capsules ... 2381
DynaCirc CR Tablets ... 2383

Itraconazole (Causes a rise in serum digoxin concentration, with the implication that digitalis intoxication may result). Products include:
Sporanox Capsules ... 1352

Labetalol Hydrochloride (Additive effects on AV node conduction). Products include:
Normodyne Injection ... 2519
Normodyne Tablets ... 2522
Trandate ... 1158

Levobunolol Hydrochloride (Additive effects on AV node conduction). Products include:
Betagan ... 230

Levothyroxine Sodium (Hypothyroid patients may require increased digoxin dose). Products include:
Eltroxin Tablets ... 2214
Levothroid Tablets ... 1015
Levothyroxine Sodium, USP for Injection ... 546
Levoxyl Tablets ... 918
Synthroid ... 1410

Liothyronine Sodium (Hypothyroid patients may require increased digoxin dose). Products include:
Cytomel Tablets ... 2647
Triostat Injection ... 2708

Liotrix (Hypothyroid patients may require increased digoxin dose).
No products indexed under this heading.

Magaldrate (Interferes with intestinal digoxin absorption).
No products indexed under this heading.

Magnesium Hydroxide (Interferes with intestinal digoxin absorption). Products include:
Aludrox Oral Suspension ... 850
Ascriptin ... 650
Di-Gel Antacid/Anti-Gas ... 762
Gelusil Antacid-Anti-gas Liquid ... 819
Gelusil Antacid-Anti-gas Tablets ... 819
Maalox Antacid/Anti-Gas Tablets ... 889
Maalox Antacid Liquid ... 888
Extra Strength Maalox Antacid/Anti-Gas Liquid and Tablets ... 888
Mylanta Fast-Acting ... 1359
Mylanta Gelcaps Antacid ... 678
Fast-Acting Mylanta Liquid Antacid ... 1359
Mylanta Tablets ... 677
Maximum-Strength Fast-Acting Mylanta Liquid Antacid ... 1359
Mylanta Double Strength Tablets ... 677
Phillips' Milk of Magnesia Liquid ... 807
Rolaids Antacid Tablets ... 807
Tempo Soft Antacid ... 799

Magnesium Oxide (Interferes with intestinal digoxin absorption). Products include:
Beelith Tablets ... 632
Bufferin Analgesic Tablets ... 636
Arthritis Strength Bufferin Analgesic Caplets ... 637
Extra Strength Bufferin Analgesic Tablets ... 637
Caltrate PLUS ... 681
Cama Arthritis Pain Reliever ... 748
Mag-Ox 400 ... 666
Uro-Mag ... 666

Metaproterenol Sulfate (Both agents enhance ectopic pacemaker activity; concomitant use increases the risk of cardiac arrhythmias). Products include:
Alupent ... 672
Metaproterenol Sulfate Inhalation Solution, USP, Arm-a-Med ... 547

IMPORTANT NOTE: Always consult each drug listing in the patient's regimen for possible interactions.

Metaraminol Bitartrate (Both agents enhance ectopic pacemaker activity; concomitant use increases the risk of cardiac arrhythmias). Products include:
  Aramine Injection 1649

Methoxamine Hydrochloride (Both agents enhance ectopic pacemaker activity; concomitant use increases the risk of cardiac arrhythmias). Products include:
  Vasoxyl Injection 1169

Methyclothiazide (Diuretic-induced hypokalemia sensitizes the myocardium to digitalis resulting in possible digitalis toxicity). Products include:
  Enduron Tablets 424

Methylprednisolone Acetate (Corticosteroid-induced hypokalemia sensitizes the myocardium to digitalis resulting in possible digitalis toxicity).
  No products indexed under this heading.

Methylprednisolone Sodium Succinate (Corticosteroid-induced hypokalemia sensitizes the myocardium to digitalis resulting in possible digitalis toxicity).
  No products indexed under this heading.

Metipranolol Hydrochloride (Additive effects on AV node conduction). Products include:
  OptiPranolol (Metipranolol 0.3%) Sterile Ophthalmic Solution .... ⊙ 256

Metolazone (Diuretic-induced hypokalemia sensitizes the myocardium to digitalis resulting in possible digitalis toxicity). Products include:
  Mykrox Tablets 1617
  Zaroxolyn Tablets 1625

Metoprolol Succinate (Additive effects on AV node conduction). Products include:
  Toprol-XL Tablets 560

Metoprolol Tartrate (Additive effects on AV node conduction). Products include:
  Lopressor 848
  Lopressor HCT Tablets 850

Minocycline Hydrochloride (May increase digoxin absorption in patients who convert digoxin to inactive metabolites in the gut resulting in increased serum levels of digoxin). Products include:
  DYNACIN Capsules 1627
  Minocin Intravenous 1428
  Minocin Oral Suspension 1431
  Minocin Pellet-Filled Capsules 1429

Nadolol (Additive effects on AV node conduction).
  No products indexed under this heading.

Neomycin, oral (Interferes with intestinal digoxin absorption).

Nephrotoxic Drugs (May impair the excretion of digoxin).

Nicardipine Hydrochloride (Additive effects on AV node conduction). Products include:
  Cardene Capsules 2261
  Cardene I.V. 2815
  Cardene SR Capsules 2264

Nifedipine (Additive effects on AV node conduction). Products include:
  Adalat Capsules (10 mg and 20 mg) 580
  Adalat CC 582
  Procardia Capsules 2024
  Procardia XL Extended Release Tablets 2026

Nimodipine (Additive effects on AV node conduction). Products include:
  Nimotop Capsules 603

Nisoldipine (Additive effects on AV node conduction). Products include:
  Sular Tablets 2961

Norepinephrine Bitartrate (Both agents enhance ectopic pacemaker activity, concomitant use increases the risk of cardiac arrhythmias). Products include:
  Levophed Bitartrate Injection 2445

Oxytetracycline Hydrochloride (May increase digoxin absorption in patients who convert digoxin to inactive metabolites in the gut resulting in increased serum levels of digoxin). Products include:
  TERAK Ointment .... ⊙ 210
  Terra-Cortril Ophthalmic Suspension 2033
  Terramycin with Polymyxin B Sulfate Ophthalmic Ointment 2035
  Urobiotic-250 Capsules 2038

Pectin (Low digoxin serum concentration; interferes with intestinal digoxin absorption). Products include:
  Celestial Seasonings Soothers Herbal Throat Drops .... ᴾ 805

Penbutolol Sulfate (Additive effects on AV node conduction). Products include:
  Levatol Tablets 2547

Phenylephrine Bitartrate (Both agents enhance ectopic pacemaker activity, concomitant use increases the risk of cardiac arrhythmias).
  No products indexed under this heading.

Phenylephrine Hydrochloride (Both agents enhance ectopic pacemaker activity, concomitant use increases the risk of cardiac arrhythmias). Products include:
  Atrohist Plus Tablets 1605
  Cerose DM .... ᴾ 853
  D.A. II Tablets 972
  D.A. Chewable Tablets 970
  Dura-Vent/DA Tablets 972
  Extendryl 1003
  4-Way Fast Acting Nasal Spray (regular & mentholated) .... ᴾ 644
  Hemorid .... ᴾ 797
  Hycomine Compound Tablets 948
  Neo-Synephrine Hydrochloride 1% Carpuject 2455
  Neo-Synephrine Hydrochloride 1% Injection 2455
  Neo-Synephrine Hydrochloride (Ophthalmic) 2456
  Neo-Synephrine .... ᴾ 624
  Novahistine Elixir .... ᴾ 782
  Phenergan VC 2886
  Phenergan VC with Codeine 2888
  Preparation H .... ᴾ 842
  Tympagesic Ear Drops 2476
  Vicks Sinex Nasal Spray and Ultra Fine Mist .... ᴾ 738

Phenylephrine Tannate (Both agents enhance ectopic pacemaker activity, concomitant use increases the risk of cardiac arrhythmias). Products include:
  Atrohist Pediatric Suspension 1604
  Atrohist Pediatric Suspension Dye-Free 1604
  Rynatan 2781
  Rynatuss 2782

Phenylpropanolamine Hydrochloride (Both agents enhance ectopic pacemaker activity, concomitant use increases the risk of cardiac arrhythmias). Products include:
  Acutrim .... ᴾ 648
  Atrohist Plus Tablets 1605
  BC Cold Powder Multi-Symptom Formula (Cold-Sinus-Allergy) .... ᴾ 631
  BC Cold Powder Non-Drowsy Formula (Cold-Sinus) .... ᴾ 631
  Cheracol Plus Head Cold/Cough Formula .... ᴾ 741
  Comtrex Multi-Symptom Cold Reliever Liqui-Gels .... ᴾ 638
  Comtrex Multi-Symptom Non-Drowsy Liqui-gels .... ᴾ 640
  Contac Continuous Action Nasal Decongestant/Antihistamine 12 Hour Capsules .... ᴾ 773
  Contac Maximum Strength Continuous Action Decongestant/Antihistamine 12 Hour Caplets .... ᴾ 772
  Contac Severe Cold and Flu Formula Caplets .... ᴾ 773
  Coricidin 'D' Decongestant Tablets .... ᴾ 760
  Dexatrim .... ᴾ 795
  Dexatrim Plus Vitamins Caplets .... ᴾ 796
  Dimetane-DC Cough Syrup 2232
  Dimetapp Allergy Sinus Caplets .... ᴾ 838
  Dimetapp Cold & Allergy Chewable Tablets .... ᴾ 838
  Dimetapp Cold & Cough Liqui-Gels .... ᴾ 839
  Dimetapp DM Elixir .... ᴾ 840
  Dimetapp Elixir .... ᴾ 840
  Dimetapp Extentabs .... ᴾ 841
  Dimetapp Tablets/Liqui-Gels .... ᴾ 841
  Dura-Vent Tablets 971
  Entex LA Tablets 972
  Exgest LA Tablets 787
  Hycomine 947
  Nolamine Timed-Release Tablets 790
  Ornade Spansule Capsules 2678
  Propagest Tablets 791
  Pyrroxate Caplets .... ᴾ 742
  Robitussin-CF 846
  Sinulin Tablets 792
  Tavist-D 12 Hour Relief Tablets .... ᴾ 750
  Teldrin 12 Hour Antihistamine/Nasal Decongestant Allergy Relief Capsules .... ᴾ 786
  Triaminic Expectorant .... ᴾ 753
  Triaminic Syrup .... ᴾ 755
  Triaminic Triaminicol Cold & Cough .... ᴾ 756
  Triaminic DM Syrup .... ᴾ 756
  Triaminicin Tablets .... ᴾ 756
  Vicks DayQuil Allergy Relief 12-Hour Extended Release Tablets .... ᴾ 733
  Vicks DayQuil Allergy Relief 4-Hour Tablets .... ᴾ 733
  Vicks DayQuil SINUS Pressure & CONGESTION Relief .... ᴾ 734

Pindolol (Additive effects on AV node conduction). Products include:
  Visken Tablets 2428

Pirbuterol Acetate (Both agents enhance ectopic pacemaker activity, concomitant use increases the risk of cardiac arrhythmias). Products include:
  Maxair Autohaler 1550
  Maxair Inhaler 1552

Polythiazide (Diuretic-induced hypokalemia sensitizes the myocardium to digitalis resulting in possible digitalis toxicity). Products include:
  Minizide Capsules 2016

Prednisolone Acetate (Corticosteroid-induced hypokalemia sensitizes the myocardium to digitalis resulting in possible digitalis toxicity). Products include:
  AK-CIDE .... ⊙ 203
  AK-CIDE Ointment .... ⊙ 203
  Blephamide Liquifilm Sterile Ophthalmic Suspension 472
  Blephamide Ointment .... ⊙ 234
  Econopred & Econopred Plus Ophthalmic Suspensions .... ⊙ 216
  Poly-Pred Liquifilm .... ⊙ 246
  Pred Forte .... ⊙ 247
  Pred Mild .... ⊙ 250
  Pred-G Liquifilm Sterile Ophthalmic Suspension .... ⊙ 248
  Pred-G S.O.P. Sterile Ophthalmic Ointment .... ⊙ 249

Prednisolone Sodium Phosphate (Corticosteroid-induced hypokalemia sensitizes the myocardium to digitalis resulting in possible digitalis toxicity). Products include:
  AK-PRED .... ⊙ 204
  Hydeltrasol Injection, Sterile 1708
  Pediapred Oral Solution 1618

Prednisolone Tebutate (Corticosteroid-induced hypokalemia sensitizes the myocardium to digitalis resulting in possible digitalis toxicity). Products include:
  Hydeltra-T.B.A. Sterile Suspension 1710

Prednisone (Corticosteroid-induced hypokalemia sensitizes the myocardium to digitalis resulting in possible digitalis toxicity).
  No products indexed under this heading.

Propafenone Hydrochloride (Causes a rise in serum digoxin concentration, with the implication that digitalis intoxication may result). Products include:
  Rythmol Tablets–150mg, 225mg, 300mg 1399

Propantheline Bromide (Increases digoxin absorption). Products include:
  Pro-Banthine Tablets 2226

Propranolol Hydrochloride (Additive effects on AV node conduction). Products include:
  Inderal 2834
  Inderal LA Long Acting Capsules 2836
  Inderide Tablets 2838
  Inderide LA Long Acting Capsules 2840

Pseudoephedrine Hydrochloride (Both agents enhance ectopic pacemaker activity, concomitant use increases the risk of cardiac arrhythmias). Products include:
  Actifed Allergy Daytime/Nighttime Caplets .... ᴾ 808
  Actifed Cold & Allergy Tablets .... ᴾ 807
  Actifed Cold & Sinus Caplets and Tablets .... ᴾ 808
  Actifed Sinus Daytime/Nighttime Tablets and Caplets .... ᴾ 809
  Advil Cold and Sinus Caplets and Tablets .... ᴾ 837
  Alka-Seltzer Plus Liqui-Gels .... ᴾ 612
  Alka-Seltzer Plus Flu & Body Aches Liqui-Gels Non-Drowsy Formula .... ᴾ 613
  Alka-Seltzer Plus Night-Time Cold Medicine Liqui-Gels .... ᴾ 612
  Allerest Maximum Strength .... ᴾ 649
  Allerest No Drowsiness .... ᴾ 649
  Allerest Sinus Pain Formula .... ᴾ 649
  Atrohist Pediatric Capsules 1603
  Benadryl Allergy/Cold Tablets .... ᴾ 811
  Benadryl Allergy Decongestant Liquid Medication .... ᴾ 812
  Benadryl Allergy Decongestant Tablets .... ᴾ 812
  Benadryl Allergy Sinus Headache Caplets .... ᴾ 813
  Benylin Multisymptom .... ᴾ 816
  Bromfed Capsules (Extended-Release) 1832
  Bromfed Syrup .... ᴾ 712
  Bromfed Tablets 1832
  Bromfed-DM Cough Syrup 1832
  Bromfed-PD Capsules (Extended-Release) 1832
  Children's TYLENOL Cold Multi-Symptom Chewable Tablets and Liquid 1559
  Children's TYLENOL Cold Plus Cough Multi Symptom Chewable Tablets and Liquid 1560
  Children's TYLENOL Flu Suspension Liquid 1560
  Children's Vicks DayQuil Allergy Relief .... ᴾ 730
  Children's Vicks NyQuil Cold/Cough Relief .... ᴾ 731
  Allergy-Sinus Comtrex Multi-Symptom Allergy-Sinus Formula Tablets and Caplets .... ᴾ 639
  Comtrex Multi-Symptom .... ᴾ 638
  Comtrex Multi-Symptom Non-Drowsy Caplets .... ᴾ 640
  Congess 1003
  Contac Day Allergy/Sinus Caplets .... ᴾ 771
  Contac Day & Night .... ᴾ 772
  Contac Night Allergy/Sinus Caplets .... ᴾ 771
  Contac Severe Cold & Flu Non-Drowsy .... ᴾ 774
  Deconsal II Tablets 1605
  Dimetane-DX Cough Syrup 2233

(ᴾ Described in PDR For Nonprescription Drugs)   (⊙ Described in PDR For Ophthalmology)

Dimetapp Cold & Fever Suspension ... 839
Dimetapp Decongestant Pediatric Drops ... 840
Dorcol Children's Cough Syrup ... 748
Drixoral Cough + Congestion Liquid Caps ... 763
Dura-Tap/PD Capsules ... 970
Duratuss Tablets ... 2750
Duratuss HD Elixir ... 2750
Efidac/24 ... 655
Entex PSE Tablets ... 973
Fedahist Gyrocaps ... 2545
Guaifed ... 1833
Guaifed Syrup ... 712
Guaimax-D Tablets ... 809
Histussin D Liquid ... 670
Infants' TYLENOL Cold Decongestant & Fever-Reducer Drops ... 1561
Kronofed-A ... 994
Novahistine DMX ... 782
Nucofed ... 2225
PediaCare Cough-Cold Chewable Tablets and Liquid ... 1569
PediaCare Infants' Decongestant Drops ... 1569
PediaCare Infants' Drops Decongestant Plus Cough ... 1569
PediaCare NightRest Cough-Cold Liquid ... 1569
Pediatric Vicks 44d Cough & Head Congestion Relief ... 736
Pediatric Vicks 44m Cough & Cold Relief ... 737
Robitussin Cold & Cough Liqui-Gels ... 844
Robitussin Cold, Cough & Flu Liqui-Gels ... 844
Robitussin Maximum Strength Cough & Cold ... 847
Robitussin Night-Time Cold Formula ... 847
Robitussin Pediatric Cough & Cold Formula ... 848
Robitussin Pediatric Drops ... 849
Robitussin Severe Congestion Liqui-Gels ... 845
Robitussin-DAC Syrup ... 2249
Robitussin-PE ... 846
Rondec Oral Drops ... 974
Rondec Syrup ... 974
Rondec Tablet ... 974
Rondec Chewable Tablets ... 974
Rondec-TR Tablet ... 974
Ryna ... 804
Seldane-D Extended-Release Tablets ... 1286
Semprex-D Capsules ... 1620
Sinarest ... 663
Sine-Aid Maximum Strength Sinus Headache Gelcaps, Caplets and Tablets ... 1570
Sine-Off No Drowsiness Formula Caplets ... 784
Sine-Off Sinus Medicine ... 784
Singlet Tablets ... 785
Sinutab Non-Drying Liquid Caps ... 823
Sinutab Sinus Allergy Medication, Maximum Strength Tablets and Caplets ... 823
Sinutab Sinus Medication, Maximum Strength Without Drowsiness Formula, Tablets & Caplets ... 824
Sudafed Children's Cold & Cough Liquid Medication ... 825
Sudafed Children's Nasal Decongestant Liquid Medication ... 826
Sudafed Cold & Allergy Tablets ... 826
Sudafed Cold and Cough Liquid Caps ... 826
Sudafed Nasal Decongestant Tablets, 30 mg ... 825
Sudafed Nasal Decongestant Tablets, 60 mg ... 825
Sudafed Non-Drying Sinus Liquid Caps ... 827
Sudafed Pediatric Nasal Decongestant Liquid Oral Drops ... 827
Sudafed Severe Cold Formula Caplets ... 828
Sudafed Severe Cold Formula Tablets ... 828
Sudafed Sinus Caplets ... 829
Sudafed Sinus Tablets ... 829
Sudafed 12 Hour Caplets ... 824
Syn-Rx Tablets ... 1622
Syn-Rx DM Tablets ... 1623
TheraFlu Flu and Cold Medicine ... 750
Theraflu Maximum Strength Flu and Cold Medicine For Sore Throat ... 751
TheraFlu Flu, Cold and Cough Medicine ... 750
TheraFlu Maximum Strength Nighttime Flu, Cold & Cough Medicine ... 751
TheraFlu Maximum Strength Non-Drowsy Formula Flu, Cold & Cough Medicine ... 751
TheraFlu Maximum Strength, Non-Drowsy Formula Flu, Cold and Cough Caplets ... 752
Theraflu Maximum Strength Sinus Non-Drowsy Formula Caplets ... 752
Triaminic AM Cough and Decongestant Formula ... 753
Triaminic AM Decongestant Formula ... 753
Triaminic Infant Oral Decongestant Drops ... 754
Triaminic Night Time ... 754
Triaminic Sore Throat Formula ... 755
Tussend ... 1830
Tussend Expectorant ... 1831
TYLENOL Allergy Sinus, Maximum Strength Caplets and Gelcaps ... 1571
TYLENOL Allergy Sinus NightTime, Maximum Strength Caplets ... 1571
TYLENOL Cold Medication, Multi-Symptom Formula Tablets and Caplets ... 1572
TYLENOL Cold Medication, Multi-Symptom Hot Liquid Packets ... 1572
TYLENOL Cold Medication, No Drowsiness Formula Caplets and Gelcaps ... 1572
TYLENOL Cold Severe Congestion Caplets ... 1573
TYLENOL Cough Medication with Decongestant, Multi Symptom ... 1574
TYLENOL Flu No Drowsiness Formula, Maximum Strength Gelcaps ... 1575
TYLENOL Flu NightTime, Maximum Strength Gelcaps ... 1575
TYLENOL Flu NightTime, Maximum Strength Hot Medication Packets ... 1575
TYLENOL Sinus, Maximum Strength Geltabs, Gelcaps, Caplets and Tablets ... 1576
Vicks 44 LiquiCaps Cough, Cold & Flu Relief ... 728
Vicks 44 LiquiCaps Non-Drowsy Cough & Cold Relief ... 729
Vicks 44D Cough & Head Congestion Relief ... 728
Vicks 44M Cough, Cold & Flu Relief ... 729
Vicks DayQuil LiquiCaps/Liquid Multi-Symptom Cold/Flu Relief ... 734
Vicks DayQuil SINUS Pressure & PAIN Relief with IBUPROFEN ... 735
Vicks Nyquil Hot Therapy ... 735
Vicks NyQuil LiquiCaps/Liquid Multi-Symptom Cold/Flu Relief, Original and Cherry Flavors ... 736

Pseudoephedrine Sulfate (Both agents enhance ectopic pacemaker activity; concomitant use increases the risk of cardiac arrhythmias). Products include:

Chlor-Trimeton Allergy Decongestant Tablets ... 759
Claritin-D Tablets ... 2487
Drixoral Cold and Allergy Sustained-Action Tablets ... 763
Drixoral Cold and Flu Extended-Release Tablets ... 764
Drixoral Non-Drowsy Formula Extended-Release Tablets ... 764
Drixoral Allergy/Sinus Extended Release Tablets ... 765
Trinalin Repetabs Tablets ... 1373

Quinidine Gluconate (Causes a rise in serum digoxin concentration, with the implication that digitalis intoxication may result). Products include:

Quinaglute Dura-Tabs Tablets ... 644

Quinidine Polygalacturonate (Causes a rise in serum digoxin concentration, with the implication that digitalis intoxication may result). Products include:

Cardioquin Tablets ... 2146

Quinidine Sulfate (Causes a rise in serum digoxin concentration, with the implication that digitalis intoxication may result). Products include:

Quinidex Extentabs ... 2240

Salmeterol Xinafoate (Both agents enhance ectopic pacemaker activity; concomitant use increases the risk of cardiac arrhythmias). Products include:

Serevent Inhalation Aerosol ... 1149

Sodium Bicarbonate (Interferes with intestinal digoxin absorption). Products include:

Alka-Seltzer Cherry Effervescent Antacid and Pain Reliever ... 609
Alka-Seltzer Extra Strength Effervescent Antacid and Pain Reliever ... 609
Alka-Seltzer Gold Effervescent Antacid ... 611
Alka-Seltzer Lemon Lime Effervescent Antacid and Pain Reliever ... 609
Alka-Seltzer Original Effervescent Antacid and Pain Reliever ... 609
Arm & Hammer Pure Baking Soda ... 648
Colyte and Colyte-flavored ... 2540
GoLYTELY ... 694
Massengill Disposable Douches ... 780
Massengill Liquid Concentrate ... 780
NuLYTELY ... 694
Cherry Flavor NuLYTELY ... 694

Sotalol Hydrochloride (Additive effects on AV node conduction). Products include:

Betapace Tablets ... 637

Succinylcholine Chloride (May cause arrhythmias). Products include:

Anectine ... 1062

Sulfasalazine (Low digoxin serum concentration; interferes with intestinal digoxin absorption). Products include:

Azulfidine ... 2059

Terbutaline Sulfate (Both agents enhance ectopic pacemaker activity, concomitant use increases the risk of cardiac arrhythmias). Products include:

Brethaire Inhaler ... 830
Brethine Ampuls ... 832
Brethine Tablets ... 831
Bricanyl Subcutaneous Injection ... 1247
Bricanyl Tablets ... 1248

Tetracycline Hydrochloride (Co-administration results in increased digoxin serum levels). Products include:

Achromycin V Capsules ... 1417
Helidac Therapy ... 2135

Thyroglobulin (Hypothyroid patients may require increased digoxin dose).

No products indexed under this heading.

Thyroid (Hypothyroid patients may require increased digoxin dose).

No products indexed under this heading.

Thyroxine (Hypothyroid patients may require increased digoxin dose).

No products indexed under this heading.

Thyroxine Sodium (Hypothyroid patients may require increased digoxin dose).

No products indexed under this heading.

Timolol Hemihydrate (Additive effects on AV node conduction). Products include:

Betimol 0.25%, 0.5% ... ◉ 259

Timolol Maleate (Additive effects on AV node conduction). Products include:

Blocadren Tablets ... 1654
Timolide Tablets ... 1791
Timoptic in Ocudose ... 1796
Timoptic Sterile Ophthalmic Solution ... 1794
Timoptic-XE ... 1798

Triamcinolone (Corticosteroid-induced hypokalemia sensitizes the myocardium to digitalis resulting in possible digitalis toxicity).

No products indexed under this heading.

Triamcinolone Acetonide (Corticosteroid-induced hypokalemia sensitizes the myocardium to digitalis resulting in possible digitalis toxicity). Products include:

Azmacort Oral Inhaler ... 2175
Nasacort AQ Nasal Spray ... 2191
Nasacort Nasal Inhaler ... 2189

Triamcinolone Diacetate (Corticosteroid-induced hypokalemia sensitizes the myocardium to digitalis resulting in possible digitalis toxicity).

No products indexed under this heading.

Triamcinolone Hexacetonide (Corticosteroid-induced hypokalemia sensitizes the myocardium to digitalis resulting in possible digitalis toxicity).

No products indexed under this heading.

Troleandomycin (Co-administration results in increased digoxin serum levels). Products include:

Tao Capsules ... 2033

Verapamil Hydrochloride (Causes a rise in serum digoxin concentration, with the implication that digitalis intoxication may result). Products include:

Calan SR Caplets ... 2571
Calan Tablets ... 2568
Covera-HS Tablets ... 2573
Isoptin Injectable ... 1391
Isoptin Oral Tablets ... 1393
Isoptin SR Tablets ... 1395
Verelan Capsules ... 1455

LANOXIN INJECTION PEDIATRIC

(Digoxin) ... 1119

May interact with potassium-depleting corticosteroids, potassium-depleting diuretics, antacids, sympathomimetics, beta blockers, calcium channel blockers, thyroid preparations, tetracyclines, macrolide antibiotics, erythromycin, and certain other agents. Compounds in these categories include:

Acebutolol Hydrochloride (Additive effects on AV node conduction). Products include:

Sectral Capsules ... 2914

Albuterol (Both agents enhance ectopic pacemaker activity; concomitant use increases the risk of cardiac arrhythmias). Products include:

Proventil Inhalation Aerosol ... 2524
Ventolin Inhalation Aerosol and Refill ... 1170

Albuterol Sulfate (Both agents enhance ectopic pacemaker activity; concomitant use increases the risk of cardiac arrhythmias). Products include:

Airet Albuterol Sulfate Inhalation Solution ... 1602
Albuterol Sulfate, USP Solution for Inhalation, Arm-a-Med ... 522
Proventil Inhalation Solution 0.083% ... 2527
Proventil Repetabs Tablets ... 2529
Proventil Solution for Inhalation 0.5% ... 2525
Proventil Syrup ... 2528
Proventil Tablets ... 2529
Ventolin Inhalation Solution ... 1171
Ventolin Nebules Inhalation Solution ... 1172
Ventolin Rotacaps for Inhalation ... 1173
Ventolin Syrup ... 1175

IMPORTANT NOTE: Always consult each drug listing in the patient's regimen for possible interactions.

Lanoxin Injection Pediatric — **Interactions Index** — **576**

- Ventolin Tablets 1176
- Volmax Extended-Release Tablets 1835

Alprazolam (Causes a rise in serum digoxin concentration, with the implication that digitalis intoxication may result). Products include:

- Xanax Tablets 2115

Aluminum Carbonate (Interferes with intestinal digoxin absorption). Products include:

- Basaljel Capsules 2810
- Basaljel Suspension 2810
- Basaljel Tablets 2810

Aluminum Hydroxide (Interferes with intestinal digoxin absorption). Products include:

- ALternaGEL Liquid 1358
- Maximum Strength Ascriptin ▣ 650
- Cama Arthritis Pain Reliever ▣ 748
- Gaviscon Extra Strength Relief Formula Antacid Tablets ▣ 778
- Gaviscon Extra Strength Relief Formula Liquid Antacid ▣ 779
- Gaviscon Liquid Antacid ▣ 779
- Gelusil Antacid-Anti-gas Liquid ▣ 819
- Gelusil Antacid-Anti-gas Tablets ▣ 819
- Maalox Antacid/Anti-Gas Tablets 889
- Maalox Heartburn Relief Suspension ▣ 658
- Maalox Antacid Liquid 888
- Extra Strength Maalox Antacid/Anti-Gas Liquid and Tablets 888
- Mylanta 1359
- Tempo Soft Antacid ▣ 799

Aluminum Hydroxide Gel (Interferes with intestinal digoxin absorption). Products include:

- ALternaGEL Liquid ▣ 675
- Aludrox Oral Suspension ▣ 850
- Amphojel Suspension 2802
- Amphojel Suspension without Flavor 2802
- Amphojel Tablets 2802
- Ascriptin ▣ 650
- Gaviscon Antacid Tablets ▣ 778
- Gaviscon-2 Antacid Tablets ▣ 779
- Mylanta Liquid ▣ 676
- Mylanta Double Strength Liquid ▣ 676
- Nephrox Suspension ▣ 671

Amiodarone Hydrochloride (Causes a rise in serum digoxin concentration, with the implication that digitalis intoxication may result). Products include:

- Cordarone Intravenous 2821
- Cordarone Tablets 2818

Amlodipine Besylate (Additive effects on AV node conduction). Products include:

- Lotrel Capsules 858
- Norvasc Tablets 2020

Amphotericin B (Amphotericin B-induced hypokalemia sensitizes the myocardium to digitalis resulting in possible digitalis toxicity). Products include:

- Abelcet Injection 1540
- Fungizone Intravenous 507
- Fungizone Oral Suspension 704

Anticancer Drugs, unspecified (Interferes with intestinal digoxin absorption).

Atenolol (Additive effects on AV node conduction). Products include:

- Tenoretic Tablets 2963
- Tenormin Tablets and I.V. Injection 2965

Azithromycin (Co-administration results in increased digoxin). Products include:

- Zithromax 2043
- Zithromax Tablets 2046

Bendroflumethiazide (Diuretic-induced hypokalemia sensitizes the myocardium to digitalis resulting in possible digitalis toxicity).

- No products indexed under this heading.

Bepridil Hydrochloride (Additive effects on AV node conduction). Products include:

- Vascor Tablets (200 and 300 mg) 1597

Betamethasone Acetate (Corticosteroid-induced hypokalemia sensitizes the myocardium to digitalis resulting in possible digitalis toxicity). Products include:

- Celestone Soluspan Suspension 2484

Betamethasone Sodium Phosphate (Corticosteroid-induced hypokalemia sensitizes the myocardium to digitalis resulting in possible digitalis toxicity). Products include:

- Celestone Soluspan Suspension 2484

Betaxolol Hydrochloride (Additive effects on AV node conduction). Products include:

- Betoptic Ophthalmic Solution 465
- Betoptic S Ophthalmic Suspension 467
- Kerlone Tablets 2588

Bisoprolol Fumarate (Additive effects on AV node conduction). Products include:

- Zebeta Tablets 1457
- Ziac 1459

Calcium, intravenous (May produce serious arrhythmias in digitalized patients).

- No products indexed under this heading.

Carteolol Hydrochloride (Additive effects on AV node conduction). Products include:

- Cartrol Tablets 413
- Ocupress Ophthalmic Solution, 1% Sterile ⊙ 297

Chlorothiazide (Diuretic-induced hypokalemia sensitizes the myocardium to digitalis resulting in possible digitalis toxicity). Products include:

- Aldoclor Tablets 1638
- Diupres Tablets 1691
- Diuril Oral 1694

Chlorothiazide Sodium (Diuretic-induced hypokalemia sensitizes the myocardium to digitalis resulting in possible digitalis toxicity). Products include:

- Diuril Sodium Intravenous 1693

Chlorthalidone (Diuretic-induced hypokalemia sensitizes the myocardium to digitalis resulting in possible digitalis toxicity). Products include:

- Combipres Tablets 682
- Tenoretic Tablets 2963
- Thalitone 1293

Cholestyramine (Interferes with intestinal digoxin absorption). Products include:

- Questran 774

Clarithromycin (Co-administration results in increased digoxin). Products include:

- Biaxin 406

Cortisone Acetate (Corticosteroid-induced hypokalemia sensitizes the myocardium to digitalis resulting in possible digitalis toxicity). Products include:

- Cortone Acetate Sterile Suspension 1663
- Cortone Acetate Tablets 1664

Demeclocycline Hydrochloride (May increase digoxin absorption in patients who convert digoxin to inactive metabolites in the gut resulting in increased serum levels of digoxin). Products include:

- Declomycin Tablets 1421

Dexamethasone (Corticosteroid-induced hypokalemia sensitizes the myocardium to digitalis resulting in possible digitalis toxicity). Products include:

- AK-Trol Ointment & Suspension ⊙ 205
- Decadron Elixir 1676
- Decadron Tablets 1678
- Decaspray Topical Aerosol 1689
- Maxitrol Ophthalmic Ointment and Suspension ⊙ 222
- TobraDex Ophthalmic Suspension and Ointment 469

Dexamethasone Acetate (Corticosteroid-induced hypokalemia sensitizes the myocardium to digitalis resulting in possible digitalis toxicity). Products include:

- Dalalone D.P. Injectable 1009
- Decadron-LA Sterile Suspension 1687

Dexamethasone Sodium Phosphate (Corticosteroid-induced hypokalemia sensitizes the myocardium to digitalis resulting in possible digitalis toxicity). Products include:

- Decadron Phosphate Injection 1680
- Decadron Phosphate Sterile Ophthalmic Ointment 1684
- Decadron Phosphate Sterile Ophthalmic Solution 1685
- Decadron Phosphate Topical Cream 1686
- Decadron Phosphate with Xylocaine Injection, Sterile 1683
- Dexacort Phosphate in Respihaler 1606
- Dexacort Phosphate in Turbinaire 1607
- NeoDecadron Sterile Ophthalmic Ointment 1755
- NeoDecadron Sterile Ophthalmic Solution 1756
- NeoDecadron Topical Cream 1757

Diltiazem Hydrochloride (Additive effects on AV node conduction). Products include:

- Cardizem CD Capsules 1251
- Cardizem SR Capsules 1255
- Cardizem Injectable 1253
- Cardizem Tablets 1257
- Dilacor XR Extended-release Capsules 2183
- Tiazac Capsules 1019

Diphenoxylate Hydrochloride (Increases digoxin absorption). Products include:

- Lomotil 2591

Dirithromycin (Co-administration results in increased digoxin). Products include:

- Dynabac 668

Dobutamine Hydrochloride (Both agents enhance ectopic pacemaker activity; concomitant use increases the risk of cardiac arrhythmias). Products include:

- Dobutrex Solution Vials 1480

Dopamine Hydrochloride (Both agents enhance ectopic pacemaker activity; concomitant use increases the risk of cardiac arrhythmias).

- No products indexed under this heading.

Doxycycline Hyclate (May increase digoxin absorption in patients who convert digoxin to inactive metabolites in the gut resulting in increased serum levels of digoxin). Products include:

- Doryx Capsules 1970
- Vibramycin Hyclate Capsules 2038
- Vibramycin Hyclate Intravenous 2040
- Vibra-Tabs Film Coated Tablets 2038

Doxycycline Monohydrate (May increase digoxin absorption in patients who convert digoxin to inactive metabolites in the gut resulting in increased serum levels of digoxin). Products include:

- Monodox Capsules 1858
- Vibramycin Monohydrate for Oral Suspension 2038

Ephedrine Hydrochloride (Both agents enhance ectopic pacemaker activity; concomitant use increases the risk of cardiac arrhythmias). Products include:

- Primatene Tablets ▣ 844
- Quadrinal Tablets 1398

Ephedrine Sulfate (Both agents enhance ectopic pacemaker activity; concomitant use increases the risk of cardiac arrhythmias). Products include:

- Marax Tablets & DF Syrup 2015

Ephedrine Tannate (Both agents enhance ectopic pacemaker activity; concomitant use increases the risk of cardiac arrhythmias). Products include:

- Rynatuss 2782

Epinephrine (Both agents enhance ectopic pacemaker activity; concomitant use increases the risk of cardiac arrhythmias). Products include:

- EPIFRIN ⊙ 237
- EpiPen 808
- Marcaine with Epinephrine 2446
- Primatene Mist ▣ 843
- Sensorcaine with Epinephrine Injection 554
- Sus-Phrine Injection 1017
- Xylocaine with Epinephrine Injections 562

Epinephrine Bitartrate (Both agents enhance ectopic pacemaker activity; concomitant use increases the risk of cardiac arrhythmias). Products include:

- Sensorcaine-MPF with Epinephrine Injection 554

Epinephrine Hydrochloride (Both agents enhance ectopic pacemaker activity; concomitant use increases the risk of cardiac arrhythmias). Products include:

- Ana-Kit Anaphylaxis Emergency Treatment Kit 611

Erythromycin (Co-administration results in increased digoxin serum levels). Products include:

- A/T/S 2% Acne Topical Gel 1244
- A/T/S 2% Acne Topical Solution 1244
- Benzamycin Topical Gel 919
- E-Mycin Tablets 1388
- Emgel 2% Topical Gel 1081
- ERYC 1972
- Erycette (erythromycin 2%) Topical Solution 1943
- Ery-Tab Tablets 426
- Erythromycin Base Filmtab 430
- Erythromycin Delayed-Release Capsules, USP 431
- Ilotycin Ophthalmic Ointment 928
- PCE Dispertab Tablets 453
- T-Stat 2.0% Topical Solution and Pads 2797
- THERAMYCIN Z 2% Solution 1629

Erythromycin Estolate (Co-administration results in increased digoxin). Products include:

- Ilosone 927

Erythromycin Ethylsuccinate (Co-administration results in increased digoxin). Products include:

- E.E.S. 427
- EryPed 425
- Pediazole Suspension 2340

Erythromycin Gluceptate (Co-administration results in increased digoxin). Products include:

- Ilotycin Gluceptate, IV, Vials 929

Erythromycin Stearate (Co-administration results in increased digoxin). Products include:

- Erythrocin Stearate Filmtab 429

Esmolol Hydrochloride (Additive effects on AV node conduction). Products include:

- Brevibloc (esmolol HCl) Injection 1860

Felodipine (Additive effects on AV node conduction). Products include:

- Plendil Extended-Release Tablets 514

Furosemide (Diuretic-induced hypokalemia sensitizes the myocardium to digitalis resulting in possible digitalis toxicity). Products include:

- Lasix Injection, Oral Solution and Tablets 1267

(▣ Described in PDR For Nonprescription Drugs) (⊙ Described in PDR For Ophthalmology)

Hydrochlorothiazide (Diuretic-induced hypokalemia sensitizes the myocardium to digitalis resulting in possible digitalis toxicity). Products include:
Aldactazide Tablets	2556
Aldoril Tablets	1644
Apresazide Capsules	824
Capozide Tablets	744
Dyazide Capsules	2653
Esidrix Tablets	839
Esimil Tablets	840
HydroDIURIL Tablets	1716
Hydropres Tablets	1718
Hyzaar Tablets	1720
Inderide Tablets	2838
Inderide LA Long Acting Capsules	2840
Lopressor HCT Tablets	850
Lotensin HCT Tablets	855
Moduretic Tablets	1748
Oretic Tablets	450
Prinzide Tablets	1780
Ser-Ap-Es Tablets	867
Timolide Tablets	1791
Vaseretic Tablets	1810
Zestoretic Tablets	2968
Ziac	1459

Hydrocortisone (Corticosteroid-induced hypokalemia sensitizes the myocardium to digitalis resulting in possible digitalis toxicity). Products include:
Anusol-HC Cream 2.5%	1953
Aquanil HC Lotion	1989
Maximum Strength Cortaid Spray	800
CORTENEMA	2713
Cortisporin Ointment	1074
Cortisporin Ophthalmic Ointment Sterile	1074
Cortisporin Ophthalmic Suspension Sterile	1075
Cortisporin Otic Solution Sterile	1076
Cortisporin Otic Suspension Sterile	1077
Cortizone-5	795
Cortizone-10	795
Hydrocortone Tablets	1715
Hytone	922
Hytone Ointment 2 ½%	923
Massengill Medicated Soft Cloth Towelettes	2628
Pediotic Suspension Sterile	1140
Preparation H Hydrocortisone 1% Cream	843
ProctoCream-HC 2.5%	2552
VōSoL HC Otic Solution	2786

Hydrocortisone Acetate (Corticosteroid-induced hypokalemia sensitizes the myocardium to digitalis resulting in possible digitalis toxicity). Products include:
Analpram-HC Rectal Cream 1% and 2.5%	993
Anusol HC-1 Hydrocortisone Anti-Itch Ointment	810
Anusol-HC Suppositories	1954
Caldecort Anti-Itch Hydrocortisone Cream	651
Coly-Mycin S Otic w/Neomycin & Hydrocortisone	1965
Cortaid	800
Cortifoam	2540
Cortisporin Cream	1073
Epifoam	2543
Hydrocortone Acetate Sterile Suspension	1712
Mantadil Cream	1124
Nupercainal Hydrocortisone 1% Cream	661
Pramosone Cream, Lotion & Ointment	995
ProctoFoam-HC	2552
Terra-Cortril Ophthalmic Suspension	2033

Hydrocortisone Sodium Phosphate (Corticosteroid-induced hypokalemia sensitizes the myocardium to digitalis resulting in possible digitalis toxicity). Products include:
Hydrocortone Phosphate Injection, Sterile	1713

Hydrocortisone Sodium Succinate (Corticosteroid-induced hypokalemia sensitizes the myocardium to digitalis resulting in possible digitalis toxicity).
No products indexed under this heading.

Hydroflumethiazide (Diuretic-induced hypokalemia sensitizes the myocardium to digitalis resulting in possible digitalis toxicity). Products include:
Diucardin Tablets	2824

Indapamide (Diuretic-induced hypokalemia sensitizes the myocardium to digitalis resulting in possible digitalis toxicity).
No products indexed under this heading.

Indomethacin (Causes a rise in serum digoxin concentration, with the implication that digitalis intoxication may result). Products include:
Indocin	1723

Indomethacin Sodium Trihydrate (Causes a rise in serum digoxin concentration, with the implication that digitalis intoxication may result). Products include:
Indocin I.V.	1727

Isoproterenol Hydrochloride (Both agents enhance ectopic pacemaker activity; concomitant use increases the risk of cardiac arrhythmias). Products include:
Isuprel Hydrochloride Solution	2443
Isuprel Injection	2441
Isuprel Mistometer	2442

Isoproterenol Sulfate (Both agents enhance ectopic pacemaker activity; concomitant use increases the risk of cardiac arrhythmias). Products include:
Norisodrine with Calcium Iodide Syrup	446

Isradipine (Additive effects on AV node conduction). Products include:
DynaCirc Capsules	2381
DynaCirc CR Tablets	2383

Itraconazole (Causes a rise in serum digoxin concentration, with the implication that digitalis intoxication may result). Products include:
Sporanox Capsules	1352

Labetalol Hydrochloride (Additive effects on AV node conduction). Products include:
Normodyne Injection	2519
Normodyne Tablets	2522
Trandate	1158

Levobunolol Hydrochloride (Additive effects on AV node conduction). Products include:
Betagan	230

Levothyroxine Sodium (Hypothyroid patients may require increased digoxin dose). Products include:
Eltroxin Tablets	2214
Levothroid Tablets	1015
Levothyroxine Sodium, USP for Injection	546
Levoxyl Tablets	918
Synthroid	1410

Liothyronine Sodium (Hypothyroid patients may require increased digoxin dose). Products include:
Cytomel Tablets	2647
Triostat Injection	2708

Liotrix (Hypothyroid patients may require increased digoxin dose).
No products indexed under this heading.

Magaldrate (Interferes with intestinal digoxin absorption).
No products indexed under this heading.

Magnesium Hydroxide (Interferes with intestinal digoxin absorption). Products include:
Aludrox Oral Suspension	850
Ascriptin	650
Di-Gel Antacid/Anti-Gas	762
Gelusil Antacid-Anti-Gas Liquid	819
Gelusil Antacid-Anti-gas Tablets	819
Maalox Antacid/Anti-Gas Tablets	889
Maalox Antacid Liquid	888
Extra Strength Maalox Antacid/Anti-Gas Liquid and Tablets	888
Mylanta Fast-Acting	1359
Mylanta Gelcaps Antacid	678
Fast-Acting Mylanta Liquid Antacid	1359
Mylanta Tablets	677
Maximum-Strength Fast-Acting Mylanta Liquid Antacid	1359
Mylanta Double Strength Tablets	677
Phillips' Milk of Magnesia Liquid	627
Rolaids Antacid Tablets	807
Tempo Soft Antacid	799

Magnesium Oxide (Interferes with intestinal digoxin absorption). Products include:
Beelith Tablets	632
Bufferin Analgesic Tablets	636
Arthritis Strength Bufferin Analgesic Caplets	637
Extra Strength Bufferin Analgesic Tablets	637
Caltrate PLUS	681
Cama Arthritis Pain Reliever	748
Mag-Ox 400	666
Uro-Mag	666

Metaproterenol Sulfate (Both agents enhance ectopic pacemaker activity; concomitant use increases the risk of cardiac arrhythmias). Products include:
Alupent	672
Metaproterenol Sulfate Inhalation Solution, USP, Arm-a-Med	547

Metaraminol Bitartrate (Both agents enhance ectopic pacemaker activity; concomitant use increases the risk of cardiac arrhythmias). Products include:
Aramine Injection	1649

Methoxamine Hydrochloride (Both agents enhance ectopic pacemaker activity; concomitant use increases the risk of cardiac arrhythmias). Products include:
Vasoxyl Injection	1169

Methyclothiazide (Diuretic-induced hypokalemia sensitizes the myocardium to digitalis resulting in possible digitalis toxicity). Products include:
Enduron Tablets	424

Methylprednisolone Acetate (Corticosteroid-induced hypokalemia sensitizes the myocardium to digitalis resulting in possible digitalis toxicity).
No products indexed under this heading.

Methylprednisolone Sodium Succinate (Corticosteroid-induced hypokalemia sensitizes the myocardium to digitalis resulting in possible digitalis toxicity).
No products indexed under this heading.

Metipranolol Hydrochloride (Additive effects on AV node conduction). Products include:
OptiPranolol (Metipranolol 0.3%) Sterile Ophthalmic Solution	256

Metolazone (Diuretic-induced hypokalemia sensitizes the myocardium to digitalis resulting in possible digitalis toxicity). Products include:
Mykrox Tablets	1617
Zaroxolyn Tablets	1625

Metoprolol Succinate (Additive effects on AV node conduction). Products include:
Toprol-XL Tablets	560

Metoprolol Tartrate (Additive effects on AV node conduction). Products include:
Lopressor	848
Lopressor HCT Tablets	850

Minocycline Hydrochloride (May increase digoxin absorption in patients who convert digoxin to inactive metabolites in the gut resulting in increased serum levels of digoxin). Products include:
DYNACIN Capsules	1627
Minocin Intravenous	1428
Minocin Oral Suspension	1431
Minocin Pellet-Filled Capsules	1429

Nadolol (Additive effects on AV node conduction).
No products indexed under this heading.

Neomycin, oral (Interferes with intestinal digoxin absorption).

Nephrotoxic Drugs (May impair the excretion of digoxin).

Nicardipine Hydrochloride (Additive effects on AV node conduction). Products include:
Cardene Capsules	2261
Cardene I.V.	2815
Cardene SR Capsules	2264

Nifedipine (Additive effects on AV node conduction). Products include:
Adalat Capsules (10 mg and 20 mg)	580
Adalat CC	582
Procardia Capsules	2024
Procardia XL Extended Release Tablets	2026

Nimodipine (Additive effects on AV node conduction). Products include:
Nimotop Capsules	603

Nisoldipine (Additive effects on AV node conduction). Products include:
Sular Tablets	2961

Norepinephrine Bitartrate (Both agents enhance ectopic pacemaker activity; concomitant use increases the risk of cardiac arrhythmias). Products include:
Levophed Bitartrate Injection	2445

Oxytetracycline Hydrochloride (May increase digoxin absorption in patients who convert digoxin to inactive metabolites in the gut resulting in increased serum levels of digoxin). Products include:
TERAK Ointment	210
Terra-Cortril Ophthalmic Suspension	2033
Terramycin with Polymyxin B Sulfate Ophthalmic Ointment	2035
Urobiotic-250 Capsules	2038

Pectin (Low digoxin serum concentration; interferes with intestinal digoxin absorption). Products include:
Celestial Seasonings Soothers Herbal Throat Drops	805

Penbutolol Sulfate (Additive effects on AV node conduction). Products include:
Levatol Tablets	2547

Phenylephrine Bitartrate (Both agents enhance ectopic pacemaker activity; concomitant use increases the risk of cardiac arrhythmias).
No products indexed under this heading.

Phenylephrine Hydrochloride (Both agents enhance ectopic pacemaker activity; concomitant use increases the risk of cardiac arrhythmias). Products include:
Atrohist Plus Tablets	1605
Cerose DM	853
D.A. II Tablets	972
D.A. Chewable Tablets	970
Dura-Vent/DA Tablets	972
Extendryl	1003

IMPORTANT NOTE: Always consult each drug listing in the patient's regimen for possible interactions.

Lanoxin Injection Pediatric | Interactions Index | 578

4-Way Fast Acting Nasal Spray (regular & mentholated) ▣ 644
Hemorid ▣ 797
Hycomine Compound Tablets 948
Neo-Synephrine Hydrochloride 1% Carpuject 2455
Neo-Synephrine Hydrochloride 1% Injection 2455
Neo-Synephrine Hydrochloride (Ophthalmic) 2456
Neo-Synephrine ▣ 624
Novahistine Elixir ▣ 782
Phenergan VC 2886
Phenergan VC with Codeine 2888
Preparation H ▣ 842
Tympagesic Ear Drops 2476
Vicks Sinex Nasal Spray and Ultra Fine Mist ▣ 738

Phenylephrine Tannate (Both agents enhance ectopic pacemaker activity; concomitant use increases the risk of cardiac arrhythmias). Products include:
Atrohist Pediatric Suspension 1604
Atrohist Pediatric Suspension Dye-Free 1604
Rynatan 2781
Rynatuss 2782

Phenylpropanolamine Hydrochloride (Both agents enhance ectopic pacemaker activity; concomitant use increases the risk of cardiac arrhythmias). Products include:
Acutrim ▣ 648
Atrohist Plus Tablets 1605
BC Cold Powder Multi-Symptom Formula (Cold-Sinus-Allergy) ▣ 631
BC Cold Powder Non-Drowsy Formula (Cold-Sinus) ▣ 631
Cheracol Plus Head Cold/Cough Formula ▣ 741
Comtrex Multi-Symptom Cold Reliever Liqui-Gels ▣ 638
Comtrex Multi-Symptom Non-Drowsy Liqui-gels ▣ 640
Contac Continuous Action Nasal Decongestant/Antihistamine 12 Hour Capsules ▣ 773
Contac Maximum Strength Continuous Action Decongestant/Antihistamine 12 Hour Caplets ▣ 772
Contac Severe Cold and Flu Formula Caplets ▣ 773
Coricidin 'D' Decongestant Tablets ▣ 760
Dexatrim ▣ 795
Dexatrim Plus Vitamins Caplets ▣ 796
Dimetane-DC Cough Syrup 2232
Dimetapp Allergy Sinus Caplets ▣ 838
Dimetapp Cold & Allergy Chewable Tablets ▣ 838
Dimetapp Cold & Cough Liqui-Gels ▣ 839
Dimetapp DM Elixir ▣ 840
Dimetapp Elixir ▣ 840
Dimetapp Extentabs ▣ 841
Dimetapp Tablets/Liqui-Gels ▣ 841
Dura-Vent Tablets 971
Entex LA Tablets 972
Exgest LA Tablets 787
Hycomine 947
Nolamine Timed-Release Tablets 790
Ornade Spansule Capsules 2678
Propagest Tablets 791
Pyrroxate Caplets ▣ 742
Robitussin-CF ▣ 846
Sinulin Tablets 792
Tavist-D 12 Hour Relief Tablets ▣ 750
Teldrin 12 Hour Antihistamine/Nasal Decongestant Allergy Relief Capsules ▣ 786
Triaminic Expectorant ▣ 753
Triaminic Syrup ▣ 755
Triaminic Triaminicol Cold & Cough ▣ 756
Triaminic DM Syrup ▣ 756
Triaminicin Tablets ▣ 756
Vicks DayQuil Allergy Relief 12-Hour Extended Release Tablets ▣ 733
Vicks DayQuil Allergy Relief 4-Hour Tablets ▣ 733
Vicks DayQuil SINUS Pressure & CONGESTION Relief ▣ 734

Pindolol (Additive effects on AV node conduction). Products include:
Visken Tablets 2428

Pirbuterol Acetate (Both agents enhance ectopic pacemaker activity; concomitant use increases the risk of cardiac arrhythmias). Products include:
Maxair Autohaler 1550
Maxair Inhaler 1552

Polythiazide (Diuretic-induced hypokalemia sensitizes the myocardium to digitalis resulting in possible digitalis toxicity). Products include:
Minizide Capsules 2016

Prednisolone Acetate (Corticosteroid-induced hypokalemia sensitizes the myocardium to digitalis resulting in possible digitalis toxicity). Products include:
AK-CIDE ⊙ 203
AK-CIDE Ointment ⊙ 203
Blephamide Liquifilm Sterile Ophthalmic Suspension 472
Blephamide Ointment ⊙ 234
Econopred & Econopred Plus Ophthalmic Suspensions ⊙ 216
Poly-Pred Liquifilm ⊙ 246
Pred Forte ⊙ 247
Pred Mild ⊙ 250
Pred-G Liquifilm Sterile Ophthalmic Suspension ⊙ 248
Pred-G S.O.P. Sterile Ophthalmic Ointment ⊙ 249

Prednisolone Sodium Phosphate (Corticosteroid-induced hypokalemia sensitizes the myocardium to digitalis resulting in possible digitalis toxicity). Products include:
AK-PRED ⊙ 204
Hydeltrasol Injection, Sterile 1708
Pediapred Oral Solution 1618

Prednisolone Tebutate (Corticosteroid-induced hypokalemia sensitizes the myocardium to digitalis resulting in possible digitalis toxicity). Products include:
Hydeltra-T.B.A. Sterile Suspension 1710

Prednisone (Corticosteroid-induced hypokalemia sensitizes the myocardium to digitalis resulting in possible digitalis toxicity).
No products indexed under this heading.

Propafenone Hydrochloride (Causes a rise in serum digoxin concentration, with the implication that digitalis intoxication may result). Products include:
Rythmol Tablets–150mg, 225mg, 300mg 1399

Propantheline Bromide (Increases digoxin absorption). Products include:
Pro-Banthine Tablets 2226

Propranolol Hydrochloride (Additive effects on AV node conduction). Products include:
Inderal 2834
Inderal LA Long Acting Capsules 2836
Inderide Tablets 2838
Inderide LA Long Acting Capsules 2840

Pseudoephedrine Hydrochloride (Both agents enhance ectopic pacemaker activity; concomitant use increases the risk of cardiac arrhythmias). Products include:
Actifed Allergy Daytime/Nighttime Caplets ▣ 808
Actifed Cold & Allergy Tablets ▣ 807
Actifed Cold & Sinus Caplets and Tablets ▣ 808
Actifed Sinus Daytime/Nighttime Tablets and Caplets ▣ 809
Advil Cold and Sinus Caplets and Tablets ▣ 837
Alka-Seltzer Plus Liqui-Gels ▣ 612
Alka-Seltzer Plus Flu & Body Aches Liqui-Gels Non-Drowsy Formula ▣ 613
Alka-Seltzer Plus Night-Time Cold Medicine Liqui-Gels ▣ 612
Allerest Maximum Strength ▣ 649
Allerest No Drowsiness ▣ 649
Allerest Sinus Pain Formula ▣ 649
Atrohist Pediatric Capsules 1603
Benadryl Allergy/Cold Tablets ▣ 811
Benadryl Allergy Decongestant Liquid Medication ▣ 812
Benadryl Allergy Decongestant Tablets ▣ 812
Benadryl Allergy Sinus Headache Caplets ▣ 813
Benylin Multisymptom ▣ 816
Bromfed Capsules (Extended-Release) 1832
Bromfed Syrup ▣ 712
Bromfed Tablets 1832
Bromfed-DM Cough Syrup 1832
Bromfed-PD Capsules (Extended-Release) 1832
Children's TYLENOL Cold Multi-Symptom Chewable Tablets and Liquid 1559
Children's TYLENOL Cold Plus Cough Multi Symptom Chewable Tablets and Liquid 1560
Children's TYLENOL Flu Suspension Liquid 1560
Children's Vicks DayQuil Allergy Relief ▣ 730
Children's Vicks NyQuil Cold/Cough Relief ▣ 731
Allergy-Sinus Comtrex Multi-Symptom Allergy-Sinus Formula Tablets and Caplets ▣ 639
Comtrex Multi-Symptom ▣ 638
Comtrex Multi-Symptom Non-Drowsy Caplets ▣ 640
Congess 1003
Contac Day Allergy/Sinus Caplets ▣ 771
Contac Day & Night ▣ 772
Contac Night Allergy/Sinus Caplets ▣ 771
Contac Severe Cold & Flu Non-Drowsy ▣ 774
Deconsal II Tablets 1605
Dimetane-DX Cough Syrup 2233
Dimetapp Cold & Fever Suspension ▣ 839
Dimetapp Decongestant Pediatric Drops ▣ 840
Dorcol Children's Cough Syrup ▣ 748
Drixoral Cough + Congestion Liquid Caps ▣ 763
Dura-Tap/PD Capsules 970
Duratuss Tablets 2750
Duratuss HD Elixir 2750
Efidac/24 ▣ 655
Entex PSE Tablets 973
Fedahist Gyrocaps 2545
Guaifed 1833
Guaifed Syrup ▣ 712
Guaimax-D Tablets 809
Histussin D Liquid 670
Infants' TYLENOL Cold Decongestant & Fever-Reducer Drops 1561
Kronofed-A 994
Novahistine DMX ▣ 782
Nucofed 2225
PediaCare Cough-Cold Chewable Tablets and Liquid 1569
PediaCare Infants' Decongestant Drops 1569
PediaCare Infants' Drops Decongestant Plus Cough 1569
PediaCare NightRest Cough-Cold Liquid 1569
Pediatric Vicks 44d Cough & Head Congestion Relief ▣ 736
Pediatric Vicks 44m Cough & Cold Relief ▣ 737
Robitussin Cold & Cough Liqui-Gels ▣ 844
Robitussin Cold, Cough & Flu Liqui-Gels ▣ 844
Robitussin Maximum Strength Cough & Cold ▣ 847
Robitussin Night-Time Cold Formula ▣ 847
Robitussin Pediatric Cough & Cold Formula ▣ 848
Robitussin Pediatric Drops ▣ 849
Robitussin Severe Congestion Liqui-Gels ▣ 845
Robitussin-DAC Syrup 2249
Robitussin-PE ▣ 846
Rondec Oral Drops 974
Rondec Syrup 974
Rondec Tablet 974
Rondec Chewable Tablets 974
Rondec-TR Tablet 974
Ryna ▣ 804
Seldane-D Extended-Release Tablets 1286
Semprex-D Capsules 1620
Sinarest ▣ 663
Sine-Aid Maximum Strength Sinus Headache Gelcaps, Caplets and Tablets 1570
Sine-Off No Drowsiness Formula Caplets ▣ 784
Sine-Off Sinus Medicine ▣ 784
Singlet Tablets ▣ 785
Sinutab Non-Drying Liquid Caps ▣ 823
Sinutab Sinus Allergy Medication, Maximum Strength Tablets and Caplets ▣ 823
Sinutab Sinus Medication, Maximum Strength Without Drowsiness Formula, Tablets & Caplets ▣ 824
Sudafed Children's Cold & Cough Liquid Medication ▣ 825
Sudafed Children's Nasal Decongestant Liquid Medication ▣ 826
Sudafed Cold & Allergy Tablets ▣ 826
Sudafed Cold and Cough Liquid Caps ▣ 826
Sudafed Nasal Decongestant Tablets, 30 mg ▣ 825
Sudafed Nasal Decongestant Tablets, 60 mg ▣ 825
Sudafed Non-Drying Sinus Liquid Caps ▣ 827
Sudafed Pediatric Nasal Decongestant Liquid Oral Drops ▣ 827
Sudafed Severe Cold Formula Caplets ▣ 828
Sudafed Severe Cold Formula Tablets ▣ 828
Sudafed Sinus Caplets ▣ 829
Sudafed Sinus Tablets ▣ 829
Sudafed 12 Hour Caplets ▣ 824
Syn-Rx Tablets 1622
Syn-Rx DM Tablets 1623
TheraFlu Flu and Cold Medicine ▣ 750
Theraflu Maximum Strength Flu and Cold Medicine For Sore Throat ▣ 751
TheraFlu Flu, Cold and Cough Medicine ▣ 750
TheraFlu Maximum Strength Nighttime Flu, Cold & Cough Medicine ▣ 751
TheraFlu Maximum Strength Non-Drowsy Formula Flu, Cold & Cough Medicine ▣ 751
TheraFlu Maximum Strength, Non-Drowsy Formula Flu, Cold and Cough Caplets ▣ 752
Theraflu Maximum Strength Sinus Non-Drowsy Formula Caplets ▣ 752
Triaminic AM Cough and Decongestant Formula ▣ 753
Triaminic AM Decongestant Formula ▣ 753
Triaminic Infant Oral Decongestant Drops ▣ 754
Triaminic Night Time ▣ 754
Triaminic Sore Throat Formula ▣ 755
Tussend 1830
Tussend Expectorant 1831
TYLENOL Allergy Sinus, Maximum Strength Caplets and Gelcaps 1571
TYLENOL Allergy Sinus NightTime, Maximum Strength Caplets 1571
TYLENOL Cold Medication, Multi-Symptom Formula Tablets and Caplets 1572
TYLENOL Cold Medication, Multi-Symptom Hot Liquid Packets 1572
TYLENOL Cold Medication, No Drowsiness Formula Caplets and Gelcaps 1572
TYLENOL Cold Severe Congestion Caplets 1573
TYLENOL Cough Medication with Decongestant, Multi Symptom 1574
TYLENOL Flu No Drowsiness Formula, Maximum Strength Gelcaps 1575
TYLENOL Flu NightTime, Maximum Strength Gelcaps 1575
TYLENOL Flu NightTime, Maximum Strength Hot Medication Packets 1575
TYLENOL Sinus, Maximum Strength Geltabs, Gelcaps, Caplets and Tablets 1576
Vicks 44 LiquiCaps Cough, Cold & Flu Relief ▣ 728
Vicks 44 LiquiCaps Non-Drowsy Cough & Cold Relief ▣ 729
Vicks 44D Cough & Head Congestion Relief ▣ 728
Vicks 44M Cough, Cold & Flu Relief ▣ 729

(▣ Described in PDR For Nonprescription Drugs) (⊙ Described in PDR For Ophthalmology)

Vicks DayQuil LiquiCaps/Liquid Multi-Symptom Cold/Flu Relief .. 734
Vicks DayQuil SINUS Pressure & PAIN Relief with IBUPROFEN 735
Vicks Nyquil Hot Therapy 735
Vicks NyQuil LiquiCaps/Liquid Multi-Symptom Cold/Flu Relief, Original and Cherry Flavors....... 736

Pseudoephedrine Sulfate (Both agents enhance ectopic pacemaker activity; concomitant use increases the risk of cardiac arrhythmias). Products include:
Chlor-Trimeton Allergy Decongestant Tablets 759
Claritin-D Tablets 2487
Drixoral Cold and Allergy Sustained-Action Tablets 763
Drixoral Cold and Flu Extended-Release Tablets 764
Drixoral Non-Drowsy Formula Extended-Release Tablets 764
Drixoral Allergy/Sinus Extended Release Tablets 765
Trinalin Repetabs Tablets 1373

Quinidine Gluconate (Causes a rise in serum digoxin concentration, with the implication that digitalis intoxication may result). Products include:
Quinaglute Dura-Tabs Tablets 644

Quinidine Polygalacturonate (Causes a rise in serum digoxin concentration, with the implication that digitalis intoxication may result). Products include:
Cardioquin Tablets 2146

Quinidine Sulfate (Causes a rise in serum digoxin concentration, with the implication that digitalis intoxication may result). Products include:
Quinidex Extentabs 2240

Salmeterol Xinafoate (Both agents enhance ectopic pacemaker activity; concomitant use increases the risk of cardiac arrhythmias). Products include:
Serevent Inhalation Aerosol.............. 1149

Sodium Bicarbonate (Interferes with intestinal digoxin absorption). Products include:
Alka-Seltzer Cherry Effervescent Antacid and Pain Reliever 609
Alka-Seltzer Extra Strength Effervescent Antacid and Pain Reliever 609
Alka-Seltzer Gold Effervescent Antacid 611
Alka-Seltzer Lemon Lime Effervescent Antacid and Pain Reliever 609
Alka-Seltzer Original Effervescent Antacid and Pain Reliever 609
Arm & Hammer Pure Baking Soda 648
Colyte and Colyte-flavored................ 2540
GoLYTELY.. 694
Massengill Disposable Douches...... 780
Massengill Liquid Concentrate 780
NuLYTELY... 694
Cherry Flavor NuLYTELY 694

Sotalol Hydrochloride (Additive effects on AV node conduction). Products include:
Betapace Tablets 637

Succinylcholine Chloride (May cause arrhythmias). Products include:
Anectine 1062

Sulfasalazine (Low digoxin serum concentration; interferes with intestinal digoxin absorption). Products include:
Azulfidine 2059

Terbutaline Sulfate (Both agents enhance ectopic pacemaker activity; concomitant use increases the risk of cardiac arrhythmias). Products include:
Brethaire Inhaler 830
Brethine Ampuls 832
Brethine Tablets 831
Bricanyl Subcutaneous Injection 1247
Bricanyl Tablets 1248

Tetracycline Hydrochloride (Co-administration results in increased digoxin serum levels). Products include:
Achromycin V Capsules 1417
Helidac Therapy 2135

Thyroglobulin (Hypothyroid patients may require increased digoxin dose).
No products indexed under this heading.

Thyroid (Hypothyroid patients may require increased digoxin dose).
No products indexed under this heading.

Thyroxine (Hypothyroid patients may require increased digoxin dose).
No products indexed under this heading.

Thyroxine Sodium (Hypothyroid patients may require increased digoxin dose).
No products indexed under this heading.

Timolol Hemihydrate (Additive effects on AV node conduction). Products include:
Betimol 0.25%, 0.5% 259

Timolol Maleate (Additive effects on AV node conduction). Products include:
Blocadren Tablets 1654
Timolide Tablets 1791
Timoptic in Ocudose 1796
Timoptic Sterile Ophthalmic Solution 1794
Timoptic-XE 1798

Triamcinolone (Corticosteroid-induced hypokalemia sensitizes the myocardium to digitalis resulting in possible digitalis toxicity).
No products indexed under this heading.

Triamcinolone Acetonide (Corticosteroid-induced hypokalemia sensitizes the myocardium to digitalis resulting in possible digitalis toxicity). Products include:
Azmacort Oral Inhaler 2175
Nasacort AQ Nasal Spray 2191
Nasacort Nasal Inhaler 2189

Triamcinolone Diacetate (Corticosteroid-induced hypokalemia sensitizes the myocardium to digitalis resulting in possible digitalis toxicity).
No products indexed under this heading.

Triamcinolone Hexacetonide (Corticosteroid-induced hypokalemia sensitizes the myocardium to digitalis resulting in possible digitalis toxicity).
No products indexed under this heading.

Troleandomycin (Co-administration results in increased digoxin). Products include:
Tao Capsules 2033

Verapamil Hydrochloride (Causes a rise in serum digoxin concentration, with the implication that digitalis intoxication may result). Products include:
Calan SR Caplets 2571
Calan Tablets 2568
Covera-HS Tablets 2573
Isoptin Injectable 1391
Isoptin Oral Tablets 1393
Isoptin SR Tablets 1395
Verelan Capsules 1455

LANOXIN TABLETS
(Digoxin) 1121
May interact with potassium-depleting corticosteroids, potassium-depleting diuretics, antacids, sympathomimetics, beta blockers, calcium channel blockers, thyroid preparations, tetracyclines, macrolide antibiotics, erythromycin, and certain other agents. Compounds in these categories include:

Acebutolol Hydrochloride (Additive effects on AV node conduction). Products include:
Sectral Capsules 2914

Albuterol (Both agents enhance ectopic pacemaker activity; concomitant use increases the risk of cardiac arrhythmias). Products include:
Proventil Inhalation Aerosol 2524
Ventolin Inhalation Aerosol and Refill 1170

Albuterol Sulfate (Both agents enhance ectopic pacemaker activity; concomitant use increases the risk of cardiac arrhythmias). Products include:
Airet Albuterol Sulfate Inhalation Solution 1602
Albuterol Sulfate, USP Solution for Inhalation, Arm-a-Med 522
Proventil Inhalation Solution 0.083% 2527
Proventil Repetabs Tablets 2529
Proventil Solution for Inhalation 0.5% 2525
Proventil Syrup 2528
Proventil Tablets 2529
Ventolin Inhalation Solution 1171
Ventolin Nebules Inhalation Solution 1172
Ventolin Rotacaps for Inhalation ... 1173
Ventolin Syrup 1175
Ventolin Tablets 1176
Volmax Extended-Release Tablets .. 1835

Alprazolam (Causes a rise in serum digoxin concentration, with the implication that digitalis intoxication may result). Products include:
Xanax Tablets 2115

Aluminum Carbonate (Interferes with intestinal digoxin absorption). Products include:
Basaljel Capsules 2810
Basaljel Suspension 2810
Basaljel Tablets 2810

Aluminum Hydroxide (Interferes with intestinal digoxin absorption). Products include:
ALternaGEL Liquid 1358
Maximum Strength Ascriptin 650
Cama Arthritis Pain Reliever........... 748
Gaviscon Extra Strength Relief Formula Antacid Tablets 778
Gaviscon Extra Strength Relief Formula Liquid Antacid 779
Gaviscon Liquid Antacid 779
Gelusil Antacid-Anti-gas Liquid 819
Gelusil Antacid-Anti-gas Tablets 819
Maalox Antacid/Anti-Gas Tablets ... 889
Maalox Heartburn Relief Suspension 658
Maalox Antacid Liquid 888
Extra Strength Maalox Antacid/ Anti-Gas Liquid and Tablets 888
Mylanta 1359
Tempo Soft Antacid 799

Aluminum Hydroxide Gel (Interferes with intestinal digoxin absorption). Products include:
ALternaGEL Liquid 675
Aludrox Oral Suspension 850
Amphojel Suspension 2802
Amphojel Suspension without Flavor 2802
Amphojel Tablets 2802
Ascriptin 650
Gaviscon Antacid Tablets................ 778
Gaviscon-2 Antacid Tablets 779
Mylanta Liquid 676
Mylanta Double Strength Liquid 676
Nephrox Suspension 671

Amiodarone Hydrochloride (Causes a rise in serum digoxin concentration, with the implication that digitalis intoxication may result). Products include:
Cordarone Intravenous 2821
Cordarone Tablets 2818

Amlodipine Besylate (Additive effects on AV node conduction). Products include:
Lotrel Capsules 858
Norvasc Tablets 2020

Amphotericin B (Amphotericin B-induced hypokalemia sensitizes the myocardium to digitalis resulting in possible digitalis toxicity). Products include:
Abelcet Injection.............................. 1540
Fungizone Intravenous 507
Fungizone Oral Suspension 704

Anticancer Drugs, unspecified (Interferes with intestinal digoxin absorption).

Atenolol (Additive effects on AV node conduction). Products include:
Tenoretic Tablets 2963
Tenormin Tablets and I.V. Injection 2965

Azithromycin (Co-administration results in increased digoxin absorption and serum levels). Products include:
Zithromax 2043
Zithromax Tablets 2046

Bendroflumethiazide (Diuretic-induced hypokalemia sensitizes the myocardium to digitalis resulting in possible digitalis toxicity).
No products indexed under this heading.

Bepridil Hydrochloride (Additive effects on AV node conduction). Products include:
Vascor Tablets (200 and 300 mg) 1597

Betamethasone Acetate (Corticosteroid-induced hypokalemia sensitizes the myocardium to digitalis resulting in possible digitalis toxicity). Products include:
Celestone Soluspan Suspension 2484

Betamethasone Sodium Phosphate (Corticosteroid-induced hypokalemia sensitizes the myocardium to digitalis resulting in possible digitalis toxicity). Products include:
Celestone Soluspan Suspension 2484

Betaxolol Hydrochloride (Additive effects on AV node conduction). Products include:
Betoptic Ophthalmic Solution 465
Betoptic S Ophthalmic Suspension 467
Kerlone Tablets 2588

Bisoprolol Fumarate (Additive effects on AV node conduction). Products include:
Zebeta Tablets 1457
Ziac 1459

Calcium, intravenous (May produce serious arrhythmias in digitalized patients).
No products indexed under this heading.

Carteolol Hydrochloride (Additive effects on AV node conduction). Products include:
Cartrol Tablets 413
Ocupress Ophthalmic Solution, 1% Sterile 297

Chlorothiazide (Diuretic-induced hypokalemia sensitizes the myocardium to digitalis resulting in possible digitalis toxicity). Products include:
Aldoclor Tablets 1638
Diupres Tablets 1691
Diuril Oral 1694

Chlorothiazide Sodium (Diuretic-induced hypokalemia sensitizes the myocardium to digitalis resulting in possible digitalis toxicity). Products include:
Diuril Sodium Intravenous 1693

Chlorthalidone (Diuretic-induced hypokalemia sensitizes the myocardium to digitalis resulting in possible digitalis toxicity). Products include:
Combipres Tablets 682
Tenoretic Tablets 2963

IMPORTANT NOTE: Always consult each drug listing in the patient's regimen for possible interactions.

Lanoxin Tablets — Interactions Index — 580

Thalitone 1293

Cholestyramine (Interferes with intestinal digoxin absorption). Products include:
Questran 774

Clarithromycin (Co-administration results in increased digoxin absorption and serum levels). Products include:
Biaxin 406

Cortisone Acetate (Corticosteroid-induced hypokalemia sensitizes the myocardium to digitalis resulting in possible digitalis toxicity). Products include:
Cortone Acetate Sterile Suspension 1663
Cortone Acetate Tablets 1664

Demeclocycline Hydrochloride (May increase digoxin absorption in patients who convert digoxin to inactive metabolites in the gut resulting in increased serum levels of digoxin). Products include:
Declomycin Tablets 1421

Dexamethasone (Corticosteroid-induced hypokalemia sensitizes the myocardium to digitalis resulting in possible digitalis toxicity). Products include:
AK-Trol Ointment & Suspension .... ⊙ 205
Decadron Elixir 1676
Decadron Tablets 1678
Decaspray Topical Aerosol 1689
Maxitrol Ophthalmic Ointment and Suspension .... ⊙ 222
TobraDex Ophthalmic Suspension and Ointment 469

Dexamethasone Acetate (Corticosteroid-induced hypokalemia sensitizes the myocardium to digitalis resulting in possible digitalis toxicity). Products include:
Dalalone D.P. Injectable 1009
Decadron-LA Sterile Suspension 1687

Dexamethasone Sodium Phosphate (Corticosteroid-induced hypokalemia sensitizes the myocardium to digitalis resulting in possible digitalis toxicity). Products include:
Decadron Phosphate Injection 1680
Decadron Phosphate Sterile Ophthalmic Ointment 1684
Decadron Phosphate Sterile Ophthalmic Solution 1685
Decadron Phosphate Topical Cream 1686
Decadron Phosphate with Xylocaine Injection, Sterile 1683
Dexacort Phosphate in Respihaler 1606
Dexacort Phosphate in Turbinaire 1607
NeoDecadron Sterile Ophthalmic Ointment 1755
NeoDecadron Sterile Ophthalmic Solution 1756
NeoDecadron Topical Cream 1757

Diltiazem Hydrochloride (Additive effects on AV node conduction). Products include:
Cardizem CD Capsules 1251
Cardizem SR Capsules 1255
Cardizem Injectable 1253
Cardizem Tablets 1257
Dilacor XR Extended-release Capsules 2183
Tiazac Capsules 1019

Diphenoxylate Hydrochloride (Increases digoxin absorption). Products include:
Lomotil 2591

Dirithromycin (Co-administration results in increased digoxin absorption and serum levels). Products include:
Dynabac 668

Dobutamine Hydrochloride (Both agents enhance ectopic pacemaker activity; concomitant use increases the risk of cardiac arrhythmias). Products include:
Dobutrex Solution Vials 1480

Dopamine Hydrochloride (Both agents enhance ectopic pacemaker activity; concomitant use increases the risk of cardiac arrhythmias).
No products indexed under this heading.

Doxycycline Hyclate (May increase digoxin absorption in patients who convert digoxin to inactive metabolites in the gut resulting in increased serum levels of digoxin). Products include:
Doryx Capsules 1970
Vibramycin Hyclate Capsules 2038
Vibramycin Hyclate Intravenous 2040
Vibra-Tabs Film Coated Tablets 2038

Doxycycline Monohydrate (May increase digoxin absorption in patients who convert digoxin to inactive metabolites in the gut resulting in increased serum levels of digoxin). Products include:
Monodox Capsules 1858
Vibramycin Monohydrate for Oral Suspension 2038

Ephedrine Hydrochloride (Both agents enhance ectopic pacemaker activity; concomitant use increases the risk of cardiac arrhythmias). Products include:
Primatene Tablets .... ⊡ 844
Quadrinal Tablets 1398

Ephedrine Sulfate (Both agents enhance ectopic pacemaker activity; concomitant use increases the risk of cardiac arrhythmias). Products include:
Marax Tablets & DF Syrup 2015

Ephedrine Tannate (Both agents enhance ectopic pacemaker activity; concomitant use increases the risk of cardiac arrhythmias). Products include:
Rynatuss 2782

Epinephrine (Both agents enhance ectopic pacemaker activity; concomitant use increases the risk of cardiac arrhythmias). Products include:
EPIFRIN .... ⊙ 237
EpiPen 808
Marcaine with Epinephrine 2446
Primatene Mist .... ⊡ 843
Sensorcaine with Epinephrine Injection 554
Sus-Phrine Injection 1017
Xylocaine with Epinephrine Injections 562

Epinephrine Bitartrate (Both agents enhance ectopic pacemaker activity; concomitant use increases the risk of cardiac arrhythmias). Products include:
Sensorcaine-MPF with Epinephrine Injection 554

Epinephrine Hydrochloride (Both agents enhance ectopic pacemaker activity; concomitant use increases the risk of cardiac arrhythmias). Products include:
Ana-Kit Anaphylaxis Emergency Treatment Kit 611

Erythromycin (Co-administration results in increased digoxin absorption and serum levels). Products include:
A/T/S 2% Acne Topical Gel 1244
A/T/S 2% Acne Topical Solution 1244
Benzamycin Topical Gel 919
E-Mycin Tablets 1388
Emgel 2% Topical Gel 1081
ERYC 1972
Erycette (erythromycin 2%) Topical Solution 1943
Ery-Tab Tablets 426
Erythromycin Base Filmtab 430
Erythromycin Delayed-Release Capsules, USP 431
Ilotycin Ophthalmic Ointment 928
PCE Dispertab Tablets 453
T-Stat 2.0% Topical Solution and Pads 2797
THERAMYCIN Z 2% Solution 1629

Erythromycin Estolate (Co-administration results in increased digoxin absorption and serum levels). Products include:
Ilosone 927

Erythromycin Ethylsuccinate (Co-administration results in increased digoxin absorption and serum levels). Products include:
E.E.S. 427
EryPed 425
Pediazole Suspension 2340

Erythromycin Gluceptate (Co-administration results in increased digoxin absorption and serum levels). Products include:
Ilotycin Gluceptate, IV, Vials 929

Erythromycin Stearate (Co-administration results in increased digoxin absorption and serum levels). Products include:
Erythrocin Stearate Filmtab 429

Esmolol Hydrochloride (Additive effects on AV node conduction). Products include:
Brevibloc (esmolol HCl) Injection 1860

Felodipine (Additive effects on AV node conduction). Products include:
Plendil Extended-Release Tablets 514

Furosemide (Diuretic-induced hypokalemia sensitizes the myocardium to digitalis resulting in possible digitalis toxicity). Products include:
Lasix Injection, Oral Solution and Tablets 1267

Hydrochlorothiazide (Diuretic-induced hypokalemia sensitizes the myocardium to digitalis resulting in possible digitalis toxicity). Products include:
Aldactazide Tablets 2556
Aldoril Tablets 1644
Apresazide Capsules 824
Capozide Tablets 744
Dyazide Capsules 2653
Esidrix Tablets 839
Esimil Tablets 840
HydroDIURIL Tablets 1716
Hydropres Tablets 1718
Hyzaar Tablets 1720
Inderide Tablets 2838
Inderide LA Long Acting Capsules 2840
Lopressor HCT Tablets 850
Lotensin HCT Tablets 855
Moduretic Tablets 1748
Oretic Tablets 450
Prinzide Tablets 1780
Ser-Ap-Es Tablets 867
Timolide Tablets 1791
Vaseretic Tablets 1810
Zestoretic Tablets 2968
Ziac 1459

Hydrocortisone (Corticosteroid-induced hypokalemia sensitizes the myocardium to digitalis resulting in possible digitalis toxicity). Products include:
Anusol-HC Cream 2.5% 1953
Aquanil HC Lotion 1989
Maximum Strength Cortaid Spray .... ⊡ 800
CORTENEMA 2713
Cortisporin Ointment 1074
Cortisporin Ophthalmic Ointment Sterile 1074
Cortisporin Ophthalmic Suspension Sterile 1075
Cortisporin Otic Solution Sterile 1076
Cortisporin Otic Suspension Sterile 1077
Cortizone-5 .... ⊡ 795
Cortizone-10 .... ⊡ 795
Hydrocortone Tablets 1715
Hytone 922
Hytone Ointment 2 ½% 923
Massengill Medicated Soft Cloth Towelettes 2628
Pediotic Suspension Sterile 1140
Preparation H Hydrocortisone 1% Cream .... ⊡ 843
ProctoCream-HC 2.5% 2552
VōSoL HC Otic Solution 2786

Hydrocortisone Acetate (Corticosteroid-induced hypokalemia sensitizes the myocardium to digitalis resulting in possible digitalis toxicity). Products include:
Analpram-HC Rectal Cream 1% and 2.5% 993
Anusol HC-1 Hydrocortisone Anti-Itch Ointment .... ⊡ 810
Anusol-HC Suppositories 1954
Caldecort Anti-Itch Hydrocortisone Cream .... ⊡ 651
Coly-Mycin S Otic w/Neomycin & Hydrocortisone 1965
Cortaid .... ⊡ 800
Cortifoam 2540
Cortisporin Cream 1073
Epifoam 2543
Hydrocortone Acetate Sterile Suspension 1712
Mantadil Cream 1124
Nupercainal Hydrocortisone 1% Cream .... ⊡ 661
Pramosone Cream, Lotion & Ointment 995
ProctoFoam-HC 2552
Terra-Cortril Ophthalmic Suspension 2033

Hydrocortisone Sodium Phosphate (Corticosteroid-induced hypokalemia sensitizes the myocardium to digitalis resulting in possible digitalis toxicity). Products include:
Hydrocortone Phosphate Injection, Sterile 1713

Hydrocortisone Sodium Succinate (Corticosteroid-induced hypokalemia sensitizes the myocardium to digitalis resulting in possible digitalis toxicity).
No products indexed under this heading.

Hydroflumethiazide (Diuretic-induced hypokalemia sensitizes the myocardium to digitalis resulting in possible digitalis toxicity). Products include:
Diucardin Tablets 2824

Indapamide (Diuretic-induced hypokalemia sensitizes the myocardium to digitalis resulting in possible digitalis toxicity).
No products indexed under this heading.

Indomethacin (Causes a rise in serum digoxin concentration, with the implication that digitalis intoxication may result). Products include:
Indocin 1723

Indomethacin Sodium Trihydrate (Causes a rise in serum digoxin concentration, with the implication that digitalis intoxication may result). Products include:
Indocin I.V. 1727

Isoproterenol Hydrochloride (Both agents enhance ectopic pacemaker activity; concomitant use increases the risk of cardiac arrhythmias). Products include:
Isuprel Hydrochloride Solution 2443
Isuprel Injection 2441
Isuprel Mistometer 2442

Isoproterenol Sulfate (Both agents enhance ectopic pacemaker activity; concomitant use increases the risk of cardiac arrhythmias). Products include:
Norisodrine with Calcium Iodide Syrup 446

Isradipine (Additive effects on AV node conduction). Products include:
DynaCirc Capsules 2381
DynaCirc CR Tablets 2383

Itraconazole (Causes a rise in serum digoxin concentration, with the implication that digitalis intoxication may result). Products include:
Sporanox Capsules 1352

(⊡ Described in PDR For Nonprescription Drugs) (⊙ Described in PDR For Ophthalmology)

Kaolin (Low digoxin serum concentration; interferes with intestinal digoxin absorption).
No products indexed under this heading.

Labetalol Hydrochloride (Additive effects on AV node conduction). Products include:
Normodyne Injection 2519
Normodyne Tablets 2522
Trandate 1158

Levobunolol Hydrochloride (Additive effects on AV node conduction). Products include:
Betagan .... ◉ 230

Liothyronine Sodium (Hypothyroid patients may require increased digoxin dose). Products include:
Cytomel Tablets 2647
Triostat Injection 2708

Magaldrate (Interferes with intestinal digoxin absorption).
No products indexed under this heading.

Magnesium Hydroxide (Interferes with intestinal digoxin absorption). Products include:
Aludrox Oral Suspension .... ▣ 850
Ascriptin .... ▣ 650
Di-Gel Antacid/Anti-Gas .... ▣ 762
Gelusil Antacid-Anti-gas Liquid .... ▣ 819
Gelusil Antacid-Anti-gas Tablets .... ▣ 819
Maalox Antacid/Anti-Gas Tablets 889
Maalox Antacid Liquid 888
Extra Strength Maalox Antacid/Anti-Gas Liquid and Tablets 888
Mylanta Fast-Acting 1359
Mylanta Gelcaps Antacid .... ▣ 678
Fast-Acting Mylanta Liquid Antacid 1359
Mylanta Tablets .... ▣ 677
Maximum-Strength Fast-Acting Mylanta Liquid Antacid 1359
Mylanta Double Strength Tablets .... ▣ 677
Phillips' Milk of Magnesia Liquid .... ▣ 627
Rolaids Antacid Tablets .... ▣ 807
Tempo Soft Antacid .... ▣ 799

Magnesium Oxide (Interferes with intestinal digoxin absorption). Products include:
Beelith Tablets 632
Bufferin Analgesic Tablets .... ▣ 636
Arthritis Strength Bufferin Analgesic Caplets .... ▣ 637
Extra Strength Bufferin Analgesic Tablets .... ▣ 637
Caltrate PLUS .... ▣ 681
Cama Arthritis Pain Reliever .... ▣ 748
Mag-Ox 400 666
Uro-Mag 666

Metaproterenol Sulfate (Both agents enhance ectopic pacemaker activity; concomitant use increases the risk of cardiac arrhythmias). Products include:
Alupent 672
Metaproterenol Sulfate Inhalation Solution, USP, Arm-a-Med 547

Metaraminol Bitartrate (Both agents enhance ectopic pacemaker activity; concomitant use increases the risk of cardiac arrhythmias). Products include:
Aramine Injection 1649

Methoxamine Hydrochloride (Both agents enhance ectopic pacemaker activity; concomitant use increases the risk of cardiac arrhythmias). Products include:
Vasoxyl Injection 1169

Methyclothiazide (Diuretic-induced hypokalemia sensitizes the myocardium to digitalis resulting in possible digitalis toxicity). Products include:
Enduron Tablets 424

Methylprednisolone Acetate (Corticosteroid-induced hypokalemia sensitizes the myocardium to digitalis resulting in possible digitalis toxicity).
No products indexed under this heading.

Methylprednisolone Sodium Succinate (Corticosteroid-induced hypokalemia sensitizes the myocardium to digitalis resulting in possible digitalis toxicity).
No products indexed under this heading.

Metipranolol Hydrochloride (Additive effects on AV node conduction). Products include:
OptiPranolol (Metipranolol 0.3%) Sterile Ophthalmic Solution .... ◉ 256

Metoclopramide Hydrochloride (Reduces intestinal digoxin absorption, resulting in unexpectedly low serum concentration). Products include:
Reglan 2243

Metolazone (Diuretic-induced hypokalemia sensitizes the myocardium to digitalis resulting in possible digitalis toxicity). Products include:
Mykrox Tablets 1617
Zaroxolyn Tablets 1625

Metoprolol Succinate (Additive effects on AV node conduction). Products include:
Toprol-XL Tablets 560

Metoprolol Tartrate (Additive effects on AV node conduction). Products include:
Lopressor 848
Lopressor HCT Tablets 850

Minocycline Hydrochloride (May increase digoxin absorption in patients who convert digoxin to inactive metabolites in the gut resulting in increased serum levels of digoxin). Products include:
DYNACIN Capsules 1627
Minocin Intravenous 1428
Minocin Oral Suspension 1431
Minocin Pellet-Filled Capsules 1429

Nadolol (Additive effects on AV node conduction).
No products indexed under this heading.

Neomycin, oral (Interferes with intestinal digoxin absorption).

Nephrotoxic Drugs (May impair the excretion of digoxin).

Nicardipine Hydrochloride (Additive effects on AV node conduction). Products include:
Cardene Capsules 2261
Cardene I.V. 2815
Cardene SR Capsules 2264

Nifedipine (Additive effects on AV node conduction). Products include:
Adalat Capsules (10 mg and 20 mg) 580
Adalat CC 582
Procardia Capsules 2024
Procardia XL Extended Release Tablets 2026

Nimodipine (Additive effects on AV node conduction). Products include:
Nimotop Capsules 603

Nisoldipine (Additive effects on AV node conduction). Products include:
Sular Tablets 2961

Norepinephrine Bitartrate (Both agents enhance ectopic pacemaker activity; concomitant use increases the risk of cardiac arrhythmias). Products include:
Levophed Bitartrate Injection 2445

Oxytetracycline Hydrochloride (May increase digoxin absorption in patients who convert digoxin to inactive metabolites in the gut resulting in increased serum levels of digoxin). Products include:
TERAK Ointment .... ◉ 210
Terra-Cortril Ophthalmic Suspension 2033
Terramycin with Polymyxin B Sulfate Ophthalmic Ointment 2035
Urobiotic-250 Capsules 2038

Pectin (Low digoxin serum concentration; interferes with intestinal digoxin absorption). Products include:
Celestial Seasonings Soothers Herbal Throat Drops .... ▣ 805

Penbutolol Sulfate (Additive effects on AV node conduction). Products include:
Levatol Tablets 2547

Phenylephrine Bitartrate (Both agents enhance ectopic pacemaker activity; concomitant use increases the risk of cardiac arrhythmias).
No products indexed under this heading.

Phenylephrine Hydrochloride (Both agents enhance ectopic pacemaker activity; concomitant use increases the risk of cardiac arrhythmias). Products include:
Atrohist Plus Tablets 1605
Cerose DM .... ▣ 853
D.A. II Tablets 972
D.A. Chewable Tablets 970
Dura-Vent/DA Tablets 972
Extendryl 1003
4-Way Fast Acting Nasal Spray (regular & mentholated) .... ▣ 644
Hemorid .... ▣ 797
Hycomine Compound Tablets 948
Neo-Synephrine Hydrochloride 1% Carpuject 2455
Neo-Synephrine Hydrochloride 1% Injection 2455
Neo-Synephrine Hydrochloride (Ophthalmic) 2456
Neo-Synephrine .... ▣ 624
Novahistine Elixir .... ▣ 782
Phenergan VC 2886
Phenergan VC with Codeine 2888
Preparation H .... ▣ 842
Tympagesic Ear Drops 2476
Vicks Sinex Nasal Spray and Ultra Fine Mist .... ▣ 738

Phenylephrine Tannate (Both agents enhance ectopic pacemaker activity; concomitant use increases the risk of cardiac arrhythmias). Products include:
Atrohist Pediatric Suspension 1604
Atrohist Pediatric Suspension Dye-Free 1604
Rynatan 2781
Rynatuss 2782

Phenylpropanolamine Hydrochloride (Both agents enhance ectopic pacemaker activity; concomitant use increases the risk of cardiac arrhythmias). Products include:
Acutrim .... ▣ 648
Atrohist Plus Tablets 1605
BC Cold Powder Multi-Symptom Formula (Cold-Sinus-Allergy) .... ▣ 631
BC Cold Powder Non-Drowsy Formula (Cold-Sinus) .... ▣ 631
Cheracol Plus Head Cold/Cough Formula .... ▣ 741
Comtrex Multi-Symptom Cold Reliever Liqui-Gels .... ▣ 638
Comtrex Multi-Symptom Non-Drowsy Liqui-gels .... ▣ 640
Contac Continuous Action Nasal Decongestant/Antihistamine 12 Hour Capsules .... ▣ 773
Contac Maximum Strength Continuous Action Decongestant/Antihistamine 12 Hour Caplets .... ▣ 772
Contac Severe Cold and Flu Formula Caplets .... ▣ 773
Coricidin 'D' Decongestant Tablets .... ▣ 760
Dexatrim .... ▣ 795
Dexatrim Plus Vitamins Caplets .... ▣ 796
Dimetane-DC Cough Syrup 2232
Dimetapp Allergy Sinus Caplets .... ▣ 838
Dimetapp Cold & Allergy Chewable Tablets .... ▣ 838
Dimetapp Cold & Cough Liqui-Gels .... ▣ 839
Dimetapp DM Elixir .... ▣ 840
Dimetapp Elixir .... ▣ 840
Dimetapp Extentabs .... ▣ 841
Dimetapp Tablets/Liqui-Gels .... ▣ 841
Dura-Vent Tablets 971
Entex LA Tablets 972
Exgest LA Tablets 787
Hycomine 947
Nolamine Timed-Release Tablets 790
Ornade Spansule Capsules 2678
Propagest Tablets 791
Pyrroxate Caplets .... ▣ 742
Robitussin-CF .... ▣ 846
Sinulin Tablets 792
Tavist-D 12 Hour Relief Tablets .... ▣ 750
Teldrin 12 Hour Antihistamine/Nasal Decongestant Allergy Relief Capsules .... ▣ 786
Triaminic Expectorant .... ▣ 753
Triaminic Syrup .... ▣ 755
Triaminic Triaminicol Cold & Cough .... ▣ 756
Triaminic DM Syrup .... ▣ 756
Triaminicin Tablets .... ▣ 756
Vicks DayQuil Allergy Relief 12-Hour Extended Release Tablets .... ▣ 733
Vicks DayQuil Allergy Relief 4-Hour Tablets .... ▣ 733
Vicks DayQuil SINUS Pressure & CONGESTION Relief .... ▣ 734

Pindolol (Additive effects on AV node conduction). Products include:
Visken Tablets 2428

Pirbuterol Acetate (Both agents enhance ectopic pacemaker activity; concomitant use increases the risk of cardiac arrhythmias). Products include:
Maxair Autohaler 1550
Maxair Inhaler 1552

Polythiazide (Diuretic-induced hypokalemia sensitizes the myocardium to digitalis resulting in possible digitalis toxicity). Products include:
Minizide Capsules 2016

Prednisolone Acetate (Corticosteroid-induced hypokalemia sensitizes the myocardium to digitalis resulting in possible digitalis toxicity). Products include:
AK-CIDE .... ◉ 203
AK-CIDE Ointment .... ◉ 203
Blephamide Liquifilm Sterile Ophthalmic Suspension 472
Blephamide Ointment .... ◉ 234
Econopred & Econopred Plus Ophthalmic Suspensions .... ◉ 216
Poly-Pred Liquifilm .... ◉ 246
Pred Forte .... ◉ 247
Pred Mild .... ◉ 250
Pred-G Liquifilm Sterile Ophthalmic Suspension .... ◉ 248
Pred-G S.O.P. Sterile Ophthalmic Ointment .... ◉ 249

Prednisolone Sodium Phosphate (Corticosteroid-induced hypokalemia sensitizes the myocardium to digitalis resulting in possible digitalis toxicity). Products include:
AK-PRED .... ◉ 204
Hydeltrasol Injection, Sterile 1708
Pediapred Oral Solution 1618

Prednisolone Tebutate (Corticosteroid-induced hypokalemia sensitizes the myocardium to digitalis resulting in possible digitalis toxicity). Products include:
Hydeltra-T.B.A. Sterile Suspension 1710

Prednisone (Corticosteroid-induced hypokalemia sensitizes the myocardium to digitalis resulting in possible digitalis toxicity).
No products indexed under this heading.

Propafenone Hydrochloride (Causes a rise in serum digoxin concentration, with the implication that digitalis intoxication may result). Products include:
Rythmol Tablets–150mg, 225mg, 300mg 1399

Propantheline Bromide (Increases digoxin absorption). Products include:
Pro-Banthine Tablets 2226

IMPORTANT NOTE: Always consult each drug listing in the patient's regimen for possible interactions.

Lanoxin Tablets | Interactions Index | 582

Propranolol Hydrochloride (Additive effects on AV node conduction). Products include:

Inderal	2834
Inderal LA Long Acting Capsules	2836
Inderide Tablets	2838
Inderide LA Long Acting Capsules	2840

Pseudoephedrine Hydrochloride (Both agents enhance ectopic pacemaker activity; concomitant use increases the risk of cardiac arrhythmias). Products include:

Actifed Allergy Daytime/Nighttime Caplets	808
Actifed Cold & Allergy Tablets	807
Actifed Cold & Sinus Caplets and Tablets	808
Actifed Sinus Daytime/Nighttime Tablets and Caplets	809
Advil Cold and Sinus Caplets and Tablets	837
Alka-Seltzer Plus Liqui-Gels	612
Alka-Seltzer Plus Flu & Body Aches Liqui-Gels Non-Drowsy Formula	613
Alka-Seltzer Plus Night-Time Cold Medicine Liqui-Gels	612
Allerest Maximum Strength	649
Allerest No Drowsiness	649
Allerest Sinus Pain Formula	649
Atrohist Pediatric Capsules	1603
Benadryl Allergy/Cold Tablets	811
Benadryl Allergy Decongestant Liquid Medication	812
Benadryl Allergy Decongestant Tablets	812
Benadryl Allergy Sinus Headache Caplets	813
Benylin Multisymptom	816
Bromfed Capsules (Extended-Release)	1832
Bromfed Syrup	712
Bromfed Tablets	1832
Bromfed-DM Cough Syrup	1832
Bromfed-PD Capsules (Extended-Release)	1832
Children's TYLENOL Cold Multi-Symptom Chewable Tablets and Liquid	1559
Children's TYLENOL Cold Plus Cough Multi Symptom Chewable Tablets and Liquid	1560
Children's TYLENOL Flu Suspension Liquid	1560
Children's Vicks DayQuil Allergy Relief	730
Children's Vicks NyQuil Cold/Cough Relief	731
Allergy-Sinus Comtrex Multi-Symptom Allergy-Sinus Formula Tablets and Caplets	639
Comtrex Multi-Symptom	638
Comtrex Multi-Symptom Non-Drowsy Caplets	640
Congess	1003
Contac Day Allergy/Sinus Caplets	771
Contac Day & Night	772
Contac Night Allergy/Sinus Caplets	771
Contac Severe Cold & Flu Non-Drowsy	774
Deconsal II Tablets	1605
Dimetane-DX Cough Syrup	2233
Dimetapp Cold & Fever Suspension	839
Dimetapp Decongestant Pediatric Drops	840
Dorcol Children's Cough Syrup	748
Drixoral Cough + Congestion Liquid Caps	763
Dura-Tap/PD Capsules	970
Duratuss Tablets	2750
Duratuss HD Elixir	2750
Efidac/24	655
Entex PSE Tablets	973
Fedahist Gyrocaps	2545
Guaifed	1833
Guaifed Syrup	712
Guaimax-D Tablets	809
Histussin D Liquid	670
Infants' TYLENOL Cold Decongestant & Fever-Reducer Drops	1561
Kronofed-A	994
Novahistine DMX	782
Nucofed	2225
PediaCare Cough-Cold Chewable Tablets and Liquid	1569
PediaCare Infants' Decongestant Drops	1569
PediaCare Infants' Drops Decongestant Plus Cough	1569
PediaCare NightRest Cough-Cold Liquid	1569
Pediatric Vicks 44d Cough & Head Congestion Relief	736
Pediatric Vicks 44m Cough & Cold Relief	737
Robitussin Cold & Cough Liqui-Gels	844
Robitussin Cold, Cough & Flu Liqui-Gels	844
Robitussin Maximum Strength Cough & Cold	847
Robitussin Night-Time Cold Formula	847
Robitussin Pediatric Cough & Cold Formula	848
Robitussin Pediatric Drops	849
Robitussin Severe Congestion Liqui-Gels	845
Robitussin-DAC Syrup	2249
Robitussin-PE	846
Rondec Oral Drops	974
Rondec Syrup	974
Rondec Tablet	974
Rondec Chewable Tablets	974
Rondec-TR Tablet	974
Ryna	804
Seldane-D Extended-Release Tablets	1286
Semprex-D Capsules	1620
Sinarest	663
Sine-Aid Maximum Strength Sinus Headache Gelcaps, Caplets and Tablets	1570
Sine-Off No Drowsiness Formula Caplets	784
Sine-Off Sinus Medicine	784
Singlet Tablets	785
Sinutab Non-Drying Liquid Caps	823
Sinutab Sinus Allergy Medication, Maximum Strength Tablets and Caplets	823
Sinutab Sinus Medication, Maximum Strength Without Drowsiness Formula, Tablets & Caplets	824
Sudafed Children's Cold & Cough Liquid Medication	825
Sudafed Children's Nasal Decongestant Liquid Medication	826
Sudafed Cold & Allergy Tablets	826
Sudafed Cold and Cough Liquid Caps	826
Sudafed Nasal Decongestant Tablets, 30 mg	825
Sudafed Nasal Decongestant Tablets, 60 mg	825
Sudafed Non-Drying Sinus Liquid Caps	827
Sudafed Pediatric Nasal Decongestant Liquid Oral Drops	827
Sudafed Severe Cold Formula Caplets	828
Sudafed Severe Cold Formula Tablets	828
Sudafed Sinus Caplets	829
Sudafed Sinus Tablets	829
Sudafed 12 Hour Caplets	824
Syn-Rx Tablets	1622
Syn-Rx DM Tablets	1623
TheraFlu Flu and Cold Medicine	750
TheraFlu Maximum Strength Flu and Cold Medicine For Sore Throat	751
TheraFlu Flu, Cold and Cough Medicine	750
TheraFlu Maximum Strength Nighttime Flu, Cold & Cough Medicine	751
TheraFlu Maximum Strength Non-Drowsy Formula Flu, Cold & Cough Medicine	751
TheraFlu Maximum Strength, Non-Drowsy Formula Flu, Cold and Cough Caplets	752
Theraflu Maximum Strength Sinus Non-Drowsy Formula Caplets	752
Triaminic AM Cough and Decongestant Formula	753
Triaminic AM Decongestant Formula	753
Triaminic Infant Oral Decongestant Drops	754
Triaminic Night Time	754
Triaminic Sore Throat Formula	755
Tussend	1830
Tussend Expectorant	1831
TYLENOL Allergy Sinus, Maximum Strength Caplets and Gelcaps	1571
TYLENOL Allergy Sinus NightTime, Maximum Strength Caplets	1571
TYLENOL Cold Medication, Multi-Symptom Formula Tablets and Caplets	1572
TYLENOL Cold Medication, Multi-Symptom Hot Liquid Packets	1572
TYLENOL Cold Medication, No Drowsiness Formula Caplets and Gelcaps	1572
TYLENOL Cold Severe Congestion Caplets	1573
TYLENOL Cough Medication with Decongestant, Multi Symptom	1574
TYLENOL Flu No Drowsiness Formula, Maximum Strength Gelcaps	1575
TYLENOL Flu NightTime, Maximum Strength Gelcaps	1575
TYLENOL Flu NightTime, Maximum Strength Hot Medication Packets	1575
TYLENOL Sinus, Maximum Strength Geltabs, Gelcaps, Caplets and Tablets	1576
Vicks 44 LiquiCaps Cough, Cold & Flu Relief	728
Vicks 44 LiquiCaps Non-Drowsy Cough & Cold Relief	729
Vicks 44D Cough & Head Congestion Relief	728
Vicks 44M Cough, Cold & Flu Relief	729
Vicks DayQuil LiquiCaps/Liquid Multi-Symptom Cold/Flu Relief	734
Vicks DayQuil SINUS Pressure & PAIN Relief with IBUPROFEN	735
Vicks Nyquil Hot Therapy	735
Vicks NyQuil LiquiCaps/Liquid Multi-Symptom Cold/Flu Relief, Original and Cherry Flavors	736

Pseudoephedrine Sulfate (Both agents enhance ectopic pacemaker activity; concomitant use increases the risk of cardiac arrhythmias). Products include:

Chlor-Trimeton Allergy Decongestant Tablets	759
Claritin-D Tablets	2487
Drixoral Cold and Allergy Sustained-Action Tablets	763
Drixoral Cold and Flu Extended-Release Tablets	764
Drixoral Non-Drowsy Formula Extended-Release Tablets	764
Drixoral Allergy/Sinus Extended Release Tablets	765
Trinalin Repetabs Tablets	1373

Quinidine Gluconate (Causes a rise in serum digoxin concentration, with the implication that digitalis intoxication may result). Products include:

Quinaglute Dura-Tabs Tablets	644

Quinidine Polygalacturonate (Causes a rise in serum digoxin concentration, with the implication that digitalis intoxication may result). Products include:

Cardioquin Tablets	2146

Quinidine Sulfate (Causes a rise in serum digoxin concentration, with the implication that digitalis intoxication may result). Products include:

Quinidex Extentabs	2240

Salmeterol Xinafoate (Both agents enhance ectopic pacemaker activity; concomitant use increases the risk of cardiac arrhythmias). Products include:

Serevent Inhalation Aerosol	1149

Sotalol Hydrochloride (Additive effects on AV node conduction). Products include:

Betapace Tablets	637

Succinylcholine Chloride (May cause arrhythmias). Products include:

Anectine	1062

Sulfasalazine (Low serum digoxin; interferes with intestinal digoxin absorption). Products include:

Azulfidine	2059

Terbutaline Sulfate (Both agents enhance ectopic pacemaker activity; concomitant use increases the risk of cardiac arrhythmias). Products include:

Brethaire Inhaler	830
Brethine Ampuls	832
Brethine Tablets	831
Bricanyl Subcutaneous Injection	1247
Bricanyl Tablets	1248

Tetracycline Hydrochloride (Co-administration results in increased digoxin absorption and serum levels). Products include:

Achromycin V Capsules	1417
Helidac Therapy	2135

Thyroid (Hypothyroid patients may require increased digoxin dose).
No products indexed under this heading.

Thyroxine (Hypothyroid patients may require increased digoxin dose).
No products indexed under this heading.

Timolol Hemihydrate (Additive effects on AV node conduction). Products include:

Betimol 0.25%, 0.5%	259

Timolol Maleate (Additive effects on AV node conduction). Products include:

Blocadren Tablets	1654
Timolide Tablets	1791
Timoptic in Ocudose	1796
Timoptic Sterile Ophthalmic Solution	1794
Timoptic-XE	1798

Triamcinolone (Corticosteroid-induced hypokalemia sensitizes the myocardium to digitalis resulting in possible digitalis toxicity).
No products indexed under this heading.

Triamcinolone Acetonide (Corticosteroid-induced hypokalemia sensitizes the myocardium to digitalis resulting in possible digitalis toxicity). Products include:

Azmacort Oral Inhaler	2175
Nasacort AQ Nasal Spray	2191
Nasacort Nasal Inhaler	2189

Triamcinolone Diacetate (Corticosteroid-induced hypokalemia sensitizes the myocardium to digitalis resulting in possible digitalis toxicity).
No products indexed under this heading.

Triamcinolone Hexacetonide (Corticosteroid-induced hypokalemia sensitizes the myocardium to digitalis resulting in possible digitalis toxicity).
No products indexed under this heading.

Troleandomycin (Co-administration results in increased digoxin absorption and serum levels). Products include:

Tao Capsules	2033

Verapamil Hydrochloride (Causes a rise in serum digoxin concentration, with the implication that digitalis intoxication may result). Products include:

Calan SR Caplets	2571
Calan Tablets	2568
Covera-HS Tablets	2573
Isoptin Injectable	1391
Isoptin Oral Tablets	1393
Isoptin SR Tablets	1395
Verelan Capsules	1455

Food Interactions

Meal, high in bran fiber (The amount of digoxin from an oral dose may be reduced).

Meal, unspecified (Slows the rate of absorption).

(▣ Described in PDR For Nonprescription Drugs) (⊙ Described in PDR For Ophthalmology)

LARIAM TABLETS
(Mefloquine Hydrochloride) 2295
May interact with beta blockers, anticonvulsants, and certain other agents. Compounds in these categories include:

Acebutolol Hydrochloride (May produce electrocardiographic abnormalities or cardiac arrest). Products include:
Sectral Capsules 2914

Atenolol (May produce electrocardiographic abnormalities or cardiac arrest). Products include:
Tenoretic Tablets 2963
Tenormin Tablets and I.V. Injection 2965

Betaxolol Hydrochloride (May produce electrocardiographic abnormalities or cardiac arrest). Products include:
Betoptic Ophthalmic Solution 465
Betoptic S Ophthalmic Suspension 467
Kerlone Tablets 2588

Bisoprolol Fumarate (May produce electrocardiographic abnormalities or cardiac arrest). Products include:
Zebeta Tablets 1457
Ziac 1459

Carbamazepine (Potential for loss of seizure control and lower than expected serum levels). Products include:
Atretol Tablets 569
Tegretol/Tegretol-XR 870

Carteolol Hydrochloride (May produce electrocardiographic abnormalities or cardiac arrest). Products include:
Cartrol Tablets 413
Ocupress Ophthalmic Solution, 1% Sterile .... ⊙ 297

Chloroquine Hydrochloride (Increased risk of convulsions). Products include:
Aralen Hydrochloride Injection 2430

Chloroquine Phosphate (Increased risk of convulsions). Products include:
Aralen Phosphate Tablets 2431

Divalproex Sodium (Potential for loss of seizure control and lower than expected serum levels). Products include:
Depakote Tablets 418

Esmolol Hydrochloride (May produce electrocardiographic abnormalities or cardiac arrest). Products include:
Brevibloc (esmolol HCl) Injection 1860

Ethosuximide (Potential for loss of seizure control and lower than expected serum levels). Products include:
Zarontin Capsules 1986
Zarontin Syrup 1986

Ethotoin (Potential for loss of seizure control and lower than expected serum levels). Products include:
Peganone Tablets 455

Felbamate (Potential for loss of seizure control and lower than expected serum levels). Products include:
Felbatol 2774

Halofantrine (Concurrent use may result in potentially fatal prolongation of Qtc interval; concurrent and/or sequential use is not recommended).
No products indexed under this heading.

Labetalol Hydrochloride (May produce electrocardiographic abnormalities or cardiac arrest). Products include:
Normodyne Injection 2519
Normodyne Tablets 2522

Trandate 1158

Lamotrigine (Potential for loss of seizure control and lower than expected serum levels). Products include:
Lamictal Tablets 1105

Levobunolol Hydrochloride (May produce electrocardiographic abnormalities or cardiac arrest). Products include:
Betagan .... ⊙ 230

Mephenytoin (Potential for loss of seizure control and lower than expected serum levels). Products include:
Mesantoin Tablets 2400

Methsuximide (Potential for loss of seizure control and lower than expected serum levels). Products include:
Celontin Kapseals 1955

Metipranolol Hydrochloride (May produce electrocardiographic abnormalities or cardiac arrest). Products include:
OptiPranolol (Metipranolol 0.3%) Sterile Ophthalmic Solution.......... ⊙ 256

Metoprolol Succinate (May produce electrocardiographic abnormalities or cardiac arrest). Products include:
Toprol-XL Tablets 560

Metoprolol Tartrate (May produce electrocardiographic abnormalities or cardiac arrest). Products include:
Lopressor 848
Lopressor HCT Tablets 850

Nadolol (May produce electrocardiographic abnormalities or cardiac arrest).
No products indexed under this heading.

Paramethadione (Potential for loss of seizure control and lower than expected serum levels).
No products indexed under this heading.

Penbutolol Sulfate (May produce electrocardiographic abnormalities or cardiac arrest). Products include:
Levatol Tablets 2547

Phenacemide (Potential for loss of seizure control and lower than expected serum levels). Products include:
Phenurone Tablets 455

Phenobarbital (Potential for loss of seizure control and lower than expected serum levels). Products include:
Arco-Lase Plus Tablets 513
Bellergal-S Tablets 2375
Donnatal 2234
Donnatal Extentabs 2234
Donnatal Tablets 2234
Phenobarbital Elixir and Tablets 1523
Quadrinal Tablets 1398

Phensuximide (Potential for loss of seizure control and lower than expected serum levels).
No products indexed under this heading.

Phenytoin (Potential for loss of seizure control and lower than expected serum levels). Products include:
Dilantin Infatabs 1967
Dilantin-125 Suspension 1969

Phenytoin Sodium (Potential for loss of seizure control and lower than expected serum levels). Products include:
Dilantin Kapseals 1965

Pindolol (May produce electrocardiographic abnormalities or cardiac arrest). Products include:
Visken Tablets 2428

Primidone (Potential for loss of seizure control and lower than expected serum levels). Products include:
Mysoline 2860

Propranolol Hydrochloride (May produce electrocardiographic abnormalities or cardiac arrest). Products include:
Inderal 2834
Inderal LA Long Acting Capsules 2836
Inderide Tablets 2838
Inderide LA Long Acting Capsules .. 2840

Quinidine Gluconate (May produce electrocardiographic abnormalities or cardiac arrest). Products include:
Quinaglute Dura-Tabs Tablets 644

Quinidine Polygalacturonate (May produce electrocardiographic abnormalities or cardiac arrest). Products include:
Cardioquin Tablets 2146

Quinidine Sulfate (May produce electrocardiographic abnormalities or cardiac arrest). Products include:
Quinidex Extentabs 2240

Quinine Sulfate (Increased risk of convulsions; potential for electrocardiographic abnormalities or cardiac arrest).
No products indexed under this heading.

Sotalol Hydrochloride (May produce electrocardiographic abnormalities or cardiac arrest). Products include:
Betapace Tablets 637

Timolol Hemihydrate (May produce electrocardiographic abnormalities or cardiac arrest). Products include:
Betimol 0.25%, 0.5% .... ⊙ 259

Timolol Maleate (May produce electrocardiographic abnormalities or cardiac arrest). Products include:
Blocadren Tablets 1654
Timolide Tablets 1791
Timoptic in Ocudose 1796
Timoptic Sterile Ophthalmic Solution 1794
Timoptic-XE 1798

Trimethadione (Potential for loss of seizure control and lower than expected serum levels).
No products indexed under this heading.

Valproic Acid (Potential for loss of seizure control and lower than expected serum levels). Products include:
Depakene 416

LARODOPA TABLETS
(Levodopa) 2296
May interact with monoamine oxidase inhibitors and antihypertensives. Compounds in these categories include:

Acebutolol Hydrochloride (Postural hypotensive episodes have been reported). Products include:
Sectral Capsules 2914

Amlodipine Besylate (Postural hypotensive episodes have been reported). Products include:
Lotrel Capsules 858
Norvasc Tablets 2020

Atenolol (Postural hypotensive episodes have been reported). Products include:
Tenoretic Tablets 2963
Tenormin Tablets and I.V. Injection 2965

Benazepril Hydrochloride (Postural hypotensive episodes have been reported). Products include:
Lotensin Tablets 852
Lotensin HCT Tablets 855

Lotrel Capsules 858

Bendroflumethiazide (Postural hypotensive episodes have been reported).
No products indexed under this heading.

Betaxolol Hydrochloride (Postural hypotensive episodes have been reported). Products include:
Betoptic Ophthalmic Solution 465
Betoptic S Ophthalmic Suspension 467
Kerlone Tablets 2588

Bisoprolol Fumarate (Postural hypotensive episodes have been reported). Products include:
Zebeta Tablets 1457
Ziac 1459

Captopril (Postural hypotensive episodes have been reported). Products include:
Capoten Tablets 740
Capozide Tablets 744

Carteolol Hydrochloride (Postural hypotensive episodes have been reported). Products include:
Cartrol Tablets 413
Ocupress Ophthalmic Solution, 1% Sterile .... ⊙ 297

Chlorothiazide (Postural hypotensive episodes have been reported). Products include:
Aldoclor Tablets 1638
Diupres Tablets 1691
Diuril Oral 1694

Chlorothiazide Sodium (Postural hypotensive episodes have been reported). Products include:
Diuril Sodium Intravenous 1693

Chlorthalidone (Postural hypotensive episodes have been reported). Products include:
Combipres Tablets 682
Tenoretic Tablets 2963
Thalitone 1293

Clonidine (Postural hypotensive episodes have been reported). Products include:
Catapres-TTS 680

Clonidine Hydrochloride (Postural hypotensive episodes have been reported). Products include:
Catapres Tablets 679
Combipres Tablets 682

Deserpidine (Postural hypotensive episodes have been reported).
No products indexed under this heading.

Diazoxide (Postural hypotensive episodes have been reported). Products include:
Hyperstat I.V. Injection 2504
Proglycem 575

Diltiazem Hydrochloride (Postural hypotensive episodes have been reported). Products include:
Cardizem CD Capsules 1251
Cardizem SR Capsules 1255
Cardizem Injectable 1253
Cardizem Tablets 1257
Dilacor XR Extended-release Capsules 2183
Tiazac Capsules 1019

Doxazosin Mesylate (Postural hypotensive episodes have been reported). Products include:
Cardura Tablets 1993

Enalapril Maleate (Postural hypotensive episodes have been reported). Products include:
Vaseretic Tablets 1810
Vasotec Tablets 1816

Enalaprilat (Postural hypotensive episodes have been reported). Products include:
Vasotec I.V. 1814

Esmolol Hydrochloride (Postural hypotensive episodes have been reported). Products include:
Brevibloc (esmolol HCl) Injection 1860

IMPORTANT NOTE: Always consult each drug listing in the patient's regimen for possible interactions.

Felodipine (Postural hypotensive episodes have been reported). Products include:

- Plendil Extended-Release Tablets 514

Fosinopril Sodium (Postural hypotensive episodes have been reported). Products include:

- Monopril Tablets 762

Furazolidone (Concurrent administration is contraindicated). Products include:

- Furoxone 2221

Furosemide (Postural hypotensive episodes have been reported). Products include:

- Lasix Injection, Oral Solution and Tablets 1267

Guanabenz Acetate (Postural hypotensive episodes have been reported).

- No products indexed under this heading.

Guanethidine Monosulfate (Postural hypotensive episodes have been reported). Products include:

- Esimil Tablets 840
- Ismelin Tablets 845

Hydralazine Hydrochloride (Postural hypotensive episodes have been reported). Products include:

- Apresazide Capsules 824
- Apresoline Hydrochloride Tablets .. 826
- Hydralazine Hydrochloride Injection USP 2712
- Ser-Ap-Es Tablets 867

Hydrochlorothiazide (Postural hypotensive episodes have been reported). Products include:

- Aldactazide Tablets 2556
- Aldoril Tablets 1644
- Apresazide Capsules 824
- Capozide Tablets 744
- Dyazide Capsules 2653
- Esidrix Tablets 839
- Esimil Tablets 840
- HydroDIURIL Tablets 1716
- Hydropres Tablets 1718
- Hyzaar Tablets 1720
- Inderide Tablets 2838
- Inderide LA Long Acting Capsules .. 2840
- Lopressor HCT Tablets 850
- Lotensin HCT Tablets 855
- Moduretic Tablets 1748
- Oretic Tablets 450
- Prinzide Tablets 1780
- Ser-Ap-Es Tablets 867
- Timolide Tablets 1791
- Vaseretic Tablets 1810
- Zestoretic Tablets 2968
- Ziac 1459

Hydroflumethiazide (Postural hypotensive episodes have been reported). Products include:

- Diucardin Tablets 2824

Indapamide (Postural hypotensive episodes have been reported).

- No products indexed under this heading.

Isocarboxazid (Concurrent administration is contraindicated).

- No products indexed under this heading.

Isradipine (Postural hypotensive episodes have been reported). Products include:

- DynaCirc Capsules 2381
- DynaCirc CR Tablets 2383

Labetalol Hydrochloride (Postural hypotensive episodes have been reported). Products include:

- Normodyne Injection 2519
- Normodyne Tablets 2522
- Trandate 1158

Lisinopril (Postural hypotensive episodes have been reported). Products include:

- Prinivil Tablets 1776
- Prinzide Tablets 1780
- Zestoretic Tablets 2968
- Zestril Tablets 2972

Losartan Potassium (Postural hypotensive episodes have been reported). Products include:

- Cozaar Tablets 1668
- Hyzaar Tablets 1720

Mecamylamine Hydrochloride (Postural hypotensive episodes have been reported). Products include:

- Inversine Tablets 1729

Methyclothiazide (Postural hypotensive episodes have been reported). Products include:

- Enduron Tablets 424

Methyldopa (Postural hypotensive episodes have been reported). Products include:

- Aldoclor Tablets 1638
- Aldomet Oral 1640
- Aldoril Tablets 1644

Methyldopate Hydrochloride (Postural hypotensive episodes have been reported). Products include:

- Aldomet Ester HCl Injection 1642

Metolazone (Postural hypotensive episodes have been reported). Products include:

- Mykrox Tablets 1617
- Zaroxolyn Tablets 1625

Metoprolol Succinate (Postural hypotensive episodes have been reported). Products include:

- Toprol-XL Tablets 560

Metoprolol Tartrate (Postural hypotensive episodes have been reported). Products include:

- Lopressor 848
- Lopressor HCT Tablets 850

Metyrosine (Postural hypotensive episodes have been reported). Products include:

- Demser Capsules 1690

Minoxidil (Postural hypotensive episodes have been reported).

- No products indexed under this heading.

Moexipril Hydrochloride (Postural hypotensive episodes have been reported). Products include:

- Univasc Tablets 2553

Nadolol (Postural hypotensive episodes have been reported).

- No products indexed under this heading.

Nicardipine Hydrochloride (Postural hypotensive episodes have been reported). Products include:

- Cardene Capsules 2261
- Cardene I.V. 2815
- Cardene SR Capsules 2264

Nifedipine (Postural hypotensive episodes have been reported). Products include:

- Adalat Capsules (10 mg and 20 mg) 580
- Adalat CC 582
- Procardia Capsules 2024
- Procardia XL Extended Release Tablets 2026

Nisoldipine (Postural hypotensive episodes have been reported). Products include:

- Sular Tablets 2961

Nitroglycerin (Postural hypotensive episodes have been reported). Products include:

- Deponit NTG Transdermal Delivery System 2541
- Nitro-Bid IV 1270
- Nitro-Bid Ointment 1272
- Nitro-Dur (nitroglycerin) Transdermal Infusion System 1365
- Nitrolingual Spray 2193
- Nitrostat Tablets 1981
- Transderm-Nitro Transdermal Therapeutic System 878

Penbutolol Sulfate (Postural hypotensive episodes have been reported). Products include:

- Levatol Tablets 2547

Phenelzine Sulfate (Concurrent administration is contraindicated). Products include:

- Nardil 1977

Phenoxybenzamine Hydrochloride (Postural hypotensive episodes have been reported). Products include:

- Dibenzyline Capsules 2650

Phentolamine Mesylate (Postural hypotensive episodes have been reported). Products include:

- Regitine Vials 864

Pindolol (Postural hypotensive episodes have been reported). Products include:

- Visken Tablets 2428

Polythiazide (Postural hypotensive episodes have been reported). Products include:

- Minizide Capsules 2016

Prazosin Hydrochloride (Postural hypotensive episodes have been reported). Products include:

- Minipress Capsules 2015
- Minizide Capsules 2016

Propranolol Hydrochloride (Postural hypotensive episodes have been reported). Products include:

- Inderal 2834
- Inderal LA Long Acting Capsules 2836
- Inderide Tablets 2838
- Inderide LA Long Acting Capsules .. 2840

Quinapril Hydrochloride (Postural hypotensive episodes have been reported). Products include:

- Accupril Tablets 1950

Ramipril (Postural hypotensive episodes have been reported). Products include:

- Altace Capsules 1238

Rauwolfia Serpentina (Postural hypotensive episodes have been reported).

- No products indexed under this heading.

Rescinnamine (Postural hypotensive episodes have been reported).

- No products indexed under this heading.

Reserpine (Postural hypotensive episodes have been reported). Products include:

- Diupres Tablets 1691
- Hydropres Tablets 1718
- Ser-Ap-Es Tablets 867

Selegiline Hydrochloride (Concurrent administration is contraindicated). Products include:

- Eldepryl Capsules 2729

Sodium Nitroprusside (Postural hypotensive episodes have been reported).

- No products indexed under this heading.

Sotalol Hydrochloride (Postural hypotensive episodes have been reported). Products include:

- Betapace Tablets 637

Spirapril Hydrochloride (Postural hypotensive episodes have been reported).

- No products indexed under this heading.

Terazosin Hydrochloride (Postural hypotensive episodes have been reported). Products include:

- Hytrin Capsules 434

Timolol Maleate (Postural hypotensive episodes have been reported). Products include:

- Blocadren Tablets 1654
- Timolide Tablets 1791
- Timoptic in Ocudose 1796
- Timoptic Sterile Ophthalmic Solution 1794
- Timoptic-XE 1798

Torsemide (Postural hypotensive episodes have been reported). Products include:

- Demadex Tablets and Injection 691

Tranylcypromine Sulfate (Concurrent administration is contraindicated). Products include:

- Parnate Tablets 2679

Trimethaphan Camsylate (Postural hypotensive episodes have been reported).

- No products indexed under this heading.

Verapamil Hydrochloride (Postural hypotensive episodes have been reported). Products include:

- Calan SR Caplets 2571
- Calan Tablets 2568
- Covera-HS Tablets 2573
- Isoptin Injectable 1391
- Isoptin Oral Tablets 1393
- Isoptin SR Tablets 1395
- Verelan Capsules 1455

LASIX INJECTION, ORAL SOLUTION AND TABLETS

(Furosemide) 1267

May interact with aminoglycosides, salicylates, lithium preparations, antihypertensives, cardiac glycosides, corticosteroids, barbiturates, narcotic analgesics, and certain other agents. Compounds in these categories include:

Acebutolol Hydrochloride (Co-administration may add to or potentiate the therapeutic effect of other antihypertensive drugs). Products include:

- Sectral Capsules 2914

ACTH (Co-administration may increase the risk of hypokalemia).

- No products indexed under this heading.

Alfentanil Hydrochloride (Orthostatic hypotension may be aggravated by narcotics). Products include:

- Alfenta Injection 1334

Amikacin Sulfate (Co-administration may increase the ototoxic potential of aminoglycoside antibiotics). Products include:

- Amikacin Sulfate Injection, USP 523
- Amikacin Sulfate Injection, USP 981
- Amikin Injectable 502

Amlodipine Besylate (Co-administration may add to or potentiate the therapeutic effect of other antihypertensive drugs). Products include:

- Lotrel Capsules 858
- Norvasc Tablets 2020

Aprobarbital (Orthostatic hypotension may be aggravated by barbiturates).

- No products indexed under this heading.

Aspirin (Co-administration may temporarily reduce creatinine clearance in patients with chronic renal insufficiency). Products include:

- Alka-Seltzer Cherry Effervescent Antacid and Pain Reliever .... ▣ 609
- Alka-Seltzer Extra Strength Effervescent Antacid and Pain Reliever .... ▣ 609
- Alka-Seltzer Lemon Lime Effervescent Antacid and Pain Reliever .... ▣ 609
- Alka-Seltzer Original Effervescent Antacid and Pain Reliever .... ▣ 609
- Alka-Seltzer Plus .... ▣ 611
- Alka-Seltzer Plus Sinus Medicine .. ▣ 611
- Ascriptin .... ▣ 650
- Arthritis Strength BC Powder .... ▣ 631
- BC Cold Powder Multi-Symptom Formula (Cold-Sinus-Allergy) .... ▣ 631
- BC Cold Powder Non-Drowsy Formula (Cold-Sinus) .... ▣ 631
- BC Powder .... ▣ 631

(▣ Described in PDR For Nonprescription Drugs) (⊚ Described in PDR For Ophthalmology)

Interactions Index

Genuine Bayer Aspirin Tablets & Caplets ... 618
Extra Strength Bayer Arthritis Pain Regimen Formula ... 615
Extra Strength Bayer Aspirin Caplets & Tablets ... 617
Extended-Release Bayer 8-Hour Aspirin ... 616
Extra Strength Bayer Plus Aspirin Caplets ... 617
Extra Strength Bayer PM Aspirin Plus Sleep Aid ... 617
Aspirin Regimen Bayer 81 mg Tablets with Calcium ... 615
Aspirin Regimen Bayer Adult Low Strength 81 mg Tablets ... 613
Aspirin Regimen Bayer Children's Chewable Aspirin ... 616
Aspirin Regimen Bayer Regular Strength 325 mg Caplets ... 613
Bufferin Analgesic Tablets ... 636
Arthritis Strength Bufferin Analgesic Caplets ... 637
Extra Strength Bufferin Analgesic Tablets ... 637
Cama Arthritis Pain Reliever ... 748
Darvon Compound-65 Pulvules ... 1475
Easprin ... 1971
Ecotrin ... 2625
Ecotrin Enteric Coated Aspirin Maximum Strength Tablets and Caplets ... 775
Ecotrin Enteric Coated Aspirin Regular Strength Tablets ... 2625
Empirin Aspirin Tablets ... 818
Excedrin Extra-Strength Analgesic Tablets, Caplets, and Geltabs ... 734
Fiorinal Capsules ... 2388
Fiorinal with Codeine Capsules ... 2390
Fiorinal Tablets ... 2388
Goody's Extra Strength Headache Powders ... 632
Goody's Extra Strength Pain Relief Tablets ... 632
Halfprin Tablets ... 1413
Norgesic ... 1554
Percodan Tablets ... 955
Percodan-Demi Tablets ... 956
Robaxisal Tablets ... 2246
Soma Compound w/Codeine Tablets ... 2784
Soma Compound Tablets ... 2783
St. Joseph Adult Chewable Aspirin (81 mg.) ... 768
Talwin Compound ... 2466
Vanquish Analgesic Caplets ... 627

Atenolol (Co-administration may add to or potentiate the therapeutic effect of other antihypertensive drugs). Products include:
Tenoretic Tablets ... 2963
Tenormin Tablets and I.V. Injection 2965

Benazepril Hydrochloride (Co-administration may add to or potentiate the therapeutic effect of other antihypertensive drugs). Products include:
Lotensin Tablets ... 852
Lotensin HCT Tablets ... 855
Lotrel Capsules ... 858

Bendroflumethiazide (Co-administration may add to or potentiate the therapeutic effect of other antihypertensive drugs).
No products indexed under this heading.

Betamethasone Acetate (Co-administration may increase the risk of hypokalemia). Products include:
Celestone Soluspan Suspension ... 2484

Betamethasone Sodium Phosphate (Co-administration may increase the risk of hypokalemia). Products include:
Celestone Soluspan Suspension ... 2484

Betaxolol Hydrochloride (Co-administration may add to or potentiate the therapeutic effect of other antihypertensive drugs). Products include:
Betoptic Ophthalmic Solution ... 465
Betoptic S Ophthalmic Suspension ... 467
Kerlone Tablets ... 2588

Bisoprolol Fumarate (Co-administration may add to or potentiate the therapeutic effect of other antihypertensive drugs). Products include:
Zebeta Tablets ... 1457
Ziac ... 1459

Buprenorphine (Orthostatic hypotension may be aggravated by narcotics). Products include:
Buprenex Injectable ... 2170

Butabarbital (Orthostatic hypotension may be aggravated by barbiturates).
No products indexed under this heading.

Butalbital (Orthostatic hypotension may be aggravated by barbiturates). Products include:
Axocet Capsules ... 2469
Esgic-plus Capsules ... 1012
Esgic-plus Tablets ... 1012
Fioricet Tablets ... 2386
Fioricet with Codeine Capsules ... 2387
Fiorinal Capsules ... 2388
Fiorinal with Codeine Capsules ... 2390
Fiorinal Tablets ... 2388
Phrenilin ... 790
Sedapap Tablets 50 mg/650 mg .. 1826

Captopril (Co-administration may add to or potentiate the therapeutic effect of other antihypertensive drugs). Products include:
Capoten Tablets ... 740
Capozide Tablets ... 744

Carteolol Hydrochloride (Co-administration may add to or potentiate the therapeutic effect of other antihypertensive drugs). Products include:
Cartrol Tablets ... 413
Ocupress Ophthalmic Solution, 1% Sterile ... 297

Chlorothiazide (Co-administration may add to or potentiate the therapeutic effect of other antihypertensive drugs). Products include:
Aldoclor Tablets ... 1638
Diupres Tablets ... 1691
Diuril Oral ... 1694

Chlorothiazide Sodium (Co-administration may add to or potentiate the therapeutic effect of other antihypertensive drugs). Products include:
Diuril Sodium Intravenous ... 1693

Chlorthalidone (Co-administration may add to or potentiate the therapeutic effect of other antihypertensive drugs). Products include:
Combipres Tablets ... 682
Tenoretic Tablets ... 2963
Thalitone ... 1293

Choline Magnesium Trisalicylate (Patients receiving high doses of salicylates concomitantly may experience salicylate toxicity at lower doses because of competitive renal excretory sites). Products include:
Trilisate ... 2155

Clonidine (Co-administration may add to or potentiate the therapeutic effect of other antihypertensive drugs). Products include:
Catapres-TTS ... 680

Clonidine Hydrochloride (Co-administration may add to or potentiate the therapeutic effect of other antihypertensive drugs). Products include:
Catapres Tablets ... 679
Combipres Tablets ... 682

Codeine Phosphate (Orthostatic hypotension may be aggravated by narcotics). Products include:
Brontex ... 2130

Dimetane-DC Cough Syrup ... 2232
Fioricet with Codeine Capsules ... 2387
Fiorinal with Codeine Capsules ... 2390
Nucofed ... 2225
Phenergan with Codeine ... 2883
Phenergan VC with Codeine ... 2888
Robitussin A-C Syrup ... 2248
Robitussin-DAC Syrup ... 2249
Ryna ... 804
Soma Compound w/Codeine Tablets ... 2784
Tylenol with Codeine ... 1592

Cortisone Acetate (Co-administration may increase the risk of hypokalemia). Products include:
Cortone Acetate Sterile Suspension ... 1663
Cortone Acetate Tablets ... 1664

Deserpidine (Co-administration may add to or potentiate the therapeutic effect of other antihypertensive drugs).
No products indexed under this heading.

Deslanoside (Digitalis therapy may exaggerate metabolic effects of hypokalemia, especially myocardial effects).
No products indexed under this heading.

Dexamethasone (Co-administration may increase the risk of hypokalemia). Products include:
AK-Trol Ointment & Suspension ... 205
Decadron Elixir ... 1676
Decadron Tablets ... 1678
Decaspray Topical Aerosol ... 1689
Maxitrol Ophthalmic Ointment and Suspension ... 222
TobraDex Ophthalmic Suspension and Ointment ... 469

Dexamethasone Acetate (Co-administration may increase the risk of hypokalemia). Products include:
Dalalone D.P. Injectable ... 1009
Decadron-LA Sterile Suspension ... 1687

Dexamethasone Sodium Phosphate (Co-administration may increase the risk of hypokalemia). Products include:
Decadron Phosphate Injection ... 1680
Decadron Phosphate Sterile Ophthalmic Ointment ... 1684
Decadron Phosphate Sterile Ophthalmic Solution ... 1685
Decadron Phosphate Topical Cream ... 1686
Decadron Phosphate with Xylocaine Injection, Sterile ... 1683
Dexacort Phosphate in Respihaler ... 1606
Dexacort Phosphate in Turbinaire ... 1607
NeoDecadron Sterile Ophthalmic Ointment ... 1755
NeoDecadron Sterile Ophthalmic Solution ... 1756
NeoDecadron Topical Cream ... 1757

Dezocine (Orthostatic hypotension may be aggravated by narcotics). Products include:
Dalgan Injection ... 529

Diazoxide (Co-administration may add to or potentiate the therapeutic effect of other antihypertensive drugs). Products include:
Hyperstat I.V. Injection ... 2504
Proglycem ... 575

Diclofenac Potassium (Co-administration has resulted in increased BUN, serum creatinine, and serum potassium levels, and weight gain). Products include:
Cataflam Tablets ... 833

Diclofenac Sodium (Co-administration has resulted in increased BUN, serum creatinine, and serum potassium levels, and weight gain). Products include:
Voltaren Ophthalmic Sterile Ophthalmic Solution ... 264
Cataflam/Voltaren/Voltaren-XR ... 833

Diflunisal (Patients receiving high doses of salicylates concomitantly may experience salicylate toxicity at lower doses because of competitive renal excretory sites). Products include:
Dolobid Tablets ... 1695

Digitoxin (Digitalis therapy may exaggerate metabolic effects of hypokalemia, especially myocardial effects). Products include:
Crystodigin Tablets ... 1472

Digoxin (Digitalis therapy may exaggerate metabolic effects of hypokalemia, especially myocardial effects). Products include:
Lanoxicaps ... 1110
Lanoxin Elixir Pediatric ... 1113
Lanoxin Injection ... 1116
Lanoxin Injection Pediatric ... 1119
Lanoxin Tablets ... 1121

Diltiazem Hydrochloride (Co-administration may add to or potentiate the therapeutic effect of other antihypertensive drugs). Products include:
Cardizem CD Capsules ... 1251
Cardizem SR Capsules ... 1255
Cardizem Injectable ... 1253
Cardizem Tablets ... 1257
Dilacor XR Extended-release Capsules ... 2183
Tiazac Capsules ... 1019

Doxazosin Mesylate (Co-administration may add to or potentiate the therapeutic effect of other antihypertensive drugs). Products include:
Cardura Tablets ... 1993

Enalapril Maleate (Co-administration may add to or potentiate the therapeutic effect of other antihypertensive drugs). Products include:
Vaseretic Tablets ... 1810
Vasotec Tablets ... 1816

Enalaprilat (Co-administration may add to or potentiate the therapeutic effect of other antihypertensive drugs). Products include:
Vasotec I.V. ... 1814

Esmolol Hydrochloride (Co-administration may add to or potentiate the therapeutic effect of other antihypertensive drugs). Products include:
Brevibloc (esmolol HCl) Injection ... 1860

Ethacrynic Acid (Increased risk of ototoxic potential). Products include:
Edecrin Tablets ... 1698

Etodolac (Co-administration has resulted in increased BUN, serum creatinine, and serum potassium levels, and weight gain). Products include:
Lodine Capsules and Tablets ... 2849

Felodipine (Co-administration may add to or potentiate the therapeutic effect of other antihypertensive drugs). Products include:
Plendil Extended-Release Tablets ... 514

Fenoprofen Calcium (Co-administration has resulted in increased BUN, serum creatinine, and potassium levels, and weight gain). Products include:
Nalfon 200 Pulvules & Nalfon Tablets ... 933

Fentanyl (Orthostatic hypotension may be aggravated by narcotics). Products include:
Duragesic Transdermal System ... 1336

Fentanyl Citrate (Orthostatic hypotension may be aggravated by narcotics). Products include:
Sublimaze Injection ... 463

IMPORTANT NOTE: Always consult each drug listing in the patient's regimen for possible interactions.

Lasix   Interactions Index   586

Fludrocortisone Acetate (Co-administration may increase the risk of hypokalemia). Products include:
- Florinef Acetate Tablets 506

Flurbiprofen (Co-administration has resulted in increased BUN, serum creatinine, and serum potassium levels, and weight gain).
- No products indexed under this heading.

Fosinopril Sodium (Co-administration may add to or potentiate the therapeutic effect of other antihypertensive drugs). Products include:
- Monopril Tablets 762

Gentamicin Sulfate (Co-administration may increase the ototoxic potential of aminoglycoside antibiotics). Products include:
- Garamycin Cream 0.1% 2501
- Garamycin Injectable 2502
- Garamycin Ointment 0.1% 2501
- Garamycin Ophthalmic 2501
- Genoptic Sterile Ophthalmic Solution ...... ⊙ 241
- Genoptic Sterile Ophthalmic Ointment ...... ⊙ 241
- Gentak ...... ⊙ 209
- Pred-G Liquifilm Sterile Ophthalmic Suspension ...... ⊙ 248
- Pred-G S.O.P. Sterile Ophthalmic Ointment ...... ⊙ 249

Guanabenz Acetate (Co-administration may add to or potentiate the therapeutic effect of other antihypertensive drugs).
- No products indexed under this heading.

Guanethidine Monosulfate (Co-administration may add to or potentiate the therapeutic effect of other antihypertensive drugs). Products include:
- Esimil Tablets 840
- Ismelin Tablets 845

Hydralazine Hydrochloride (Co-administration may add to or potentiate the therapeutic effect of other antihypertensive drugs). Products include:
- Apresazide Capsules 824
- Apresoline Hydrochloride Tablets 826
- Hydralazine Hydrochloride Injection USP 2712
- Ser-Ap-Es Tablets 867

Hydrochlorothiazide (Co-administration may add to or potentiate the therapeutic effect of other antihypertensive drugs). Products include:
- Aldactazide Tablets 2556
- Aldoril Tablets 1644
- Apresazide Capsules 824
- Capozide Tablets 744
- Dyazide Capsules 2653
- Esidrix Tablets 839
- Esimil Tablets 840
- HydroDIURIL Tablets 1716
- Hydropres Tablets 1718
- Hyzaar Tablets 1720
- Inderide Tablets 2838
- Inderide LA Long Acting Capsules 2840
- Lopressor HCT Tablets 850
- Lotensin HCT Tablets 855
- Moduretic Tablets 1748
- Oretic Tablets 450
- Prinzide Tablets 1780
- Ser-Ap-Es Tablets 867
- Timolide Tablets 1791
- Vaseretic Tablets 1810
- Zestoretic Tablets 2968
- Ziac 1459

Hydrocodone Bitartrate (Orthostatic hypotension may be aggravated by narcotics). Products include:
- Codiclear DH Syrup 808
- Duratuss HD Elixir 2750
- Histussin D Liquid 670
- Hycodan Tablets and Syrup 946
- Hycomine Compound Tablets 948
- Hycomine 947
- Hycotuss Expectorant Syrup 950
- Hydrocet Capsules 787
- Lorcet 10/650 Tablets 1016
- Lortab 2751
- Tussend 1830
- Tussend Expectorant 1831
- Vicodin Tablets 1404
- Vicodin ES Tablets 1405
- Vicodin HP Tablets 1403
- Vicodin Tuss Expectorant 1406
- Zydone Tablets 967

Hydrocodone Polistirex (Orthostatic hypotension may be aggravated by narcotics). Products include:
- Tussionex Pennkinetic Extended-Release Suspension 1624

Hydrocortisone (Co-administration may increase the risk of hypokalemia). Products include:
- Anusol-HC Cream 2.5% 1953
- Aquanil HC Lotion 1989
- Maximum Strength Cortaid Spray ...... ⊞ 800
- CORTENEMA 2713
- Cortisporin Ointment 1074
- Cortisporin Ophthalmic Ointment Sterile 1074
- Cortisporin Ophthalmic Suspension Sterile 1075
- Cortisporin Otic Solution Sterile 1076
- Cortisporin Otic Suspension Sterile 1077
- Cortizone-5 ...... ⊞ 795
- Cortizone-10 ...... ⊞ 795
- Hydrocortone Tablets 1715
- Hytone 922
- Hytone Ointment 2 ½% 923
- Massengill Medicated Soft Cloth Towelettes 2628
- Pediotic Suspension Sterile 1140
- Preparation H Hydrocortisone 1% Cream ...... ⊞ 843
- ProctoCream-HC 2.5% 2552
- VōSoL HC Otic Solution 2786

Hydrocortisone Acetate (Co-administration may increase the risk of hypokalemia). Products include:
- Analpram-HC Rectal Cream 1% and 2.5% 993
- Anusol HC-1 Hydrocortisone Anti-Itch Ointment ...... ⊞ 810
- Anusol-HC Suppositories 1954
- Caldecort Anti-Itch Hydrocortisone Cream ...... ⊞ 651
- Coly-Mycin S Otic w/Neomycin & Hydrocortisone 1965
- Cortaid ...... ⊞ 800
- Cortifoam 2540
- Cortisporin Cream 1073
- Epifoam 2543
- Hydrocortone Acetate Sterile Suspension 1712
- Mantadil Cream 1124
- Nupercainal Hydrocortisone 1% Cream ...... ⊞ 661
- Pramosone Cream, Lotion & Ointment 995
- ProctoFoam-HC 2552
- Terra-Cortril Ophthalmic Suspension 2033

Hydrocortisone Sodium Phosphate (Co-administration may increase the risk of hypokalemia). Products include:
- Hydrocortone Phosphate Injection, Sterile 1713

Hydrocortisone Sodium Succinate (Co-administration may increase the risk of hypokalemia).
- No products indexed under this heading.

Hydroflumethiazide (Co-administration may add to or potentiate the therapeutic effect of other antihypertensive drugs). Products include:
- Diucardin Tablets 2824

Hydromorphone Hydrochloride (Orthostatic hypotension may be aggravated by narcotics). Products include:
- Dilaudid Ampules 1382
- Dilaudid Cough Syrup 1383
- Dilaudid-HP Injection 1384
- Dilaudid-HP Lyophilized Powder 250 mg 1384
- Dilaudid 1382
- Dilaudid Oral Liquid 1386
- Dilaudid 1382
- Dilaudid Tablets - 8 mg 1386

Ibuprofen (Co-administration has resulted in increased BUN, serum creatinine, and serum potassium levels, and weight gain). Products include:
- Advil Cold and Sinus Caplets and Tablets ...... ⊞ 837
- Advil Ibuprofen Tablets, Caplets and Gel Caplets ...... ⊞ 836
- Children's Motrin Ibuprofen Oral Suspension 1558
- IBU Tablets 1389
- Ibuprohm ...... ⊞ 713
- Motrin IB Caplets, Tablets, and Gelcaps ...... ⊞ 802
- Motrin Ibuprofen Suspension, Oral Drops, Chewable Tablets, Caplets 1563
- Nuprin Ibuprofen/Analgesic Tablets & Caplets ...... ⊞ 645
- Vicks DayQuil SINUS Pressure & PAIN Relief with IBUPROFEN ...... ⊞ 735

Indapamide (Co-administration may add to or potentiate the therapeutic effect of other antihypertensive drugs).
- No products indexed under this heading.

Indomethacin (Co-administration may reduce the natriuretic and antihypertensive effects). Products include:
- Indocin 1723

Indomethacin Sodium Trihydrate (Co-administration may reduce the natriuretic and antihypertensive effects). Products include:
- Indocin I.V. 1727

Isradipine (Co-administration may add to or potentiate the therapeutic effect of other antihypertensive drugs). Products include:
- DynaCirc Capsules 2381
- DynaCirc CR Tablets 2383

Kanamycin Sulfate (Co-administration may increase the ototoxic potential of aminoglycoside antibiotics).
- No products indexed under this heading.

Ketoprofen (Co-administration has resulted in increased BUN, serum creatinine, and serum potassium levels, and weight gain). Products include:
- Actron Caplets and Tablets ...... ⊞ 608
- Orudis Capsules 2874
- Orudis KT ...... ⊞ 842
- Oruvail Capsules 2874

Ketorolac Tromethamine (Co-administration has resulted in increased BUN, serum creatinine, and serum potassium levels, and weight gain). Products include:
- Acular Sterile Ophthalmic Solution 470
- Toradol 2319

Labetalol Hydrochloride (Co-administration may add to or potentiate the therapeutic effect of other antihypertensive drugs). Products include:
- Normodyne Injection 2519
- Normodyne Tablets 2522
- Trandate 1158

Levorphanol Tartrate (Orthostatic hypotension may be aggravated by narcotics). Products include:
- Levo-Dromoran 2297

Lisinopril (Co-administration may add to or potentiate the therapeutic effect of other antihypertensive drugs). Products include:
- Prinivil Tablets 1776
- Prinzide Tablets 1780
- Zestoretic Tablets 2968
- Zestril Tablets 2972

Lithium Carbonate (Co-administration may reduce lithium renal clearance and add a high risk of lithium toxicity). Products include:
- Eskalith 2658
- Lithium Carbonate Capsules & Tablets 2352
- Lithonate/Lithotabs/Lithobid 2721

Lithium Citrate (Co-administration may reduce lithium renal clearance and add a high risk of lithium toxicity).
- No products indexed under this heading.

Losartan Potassium (Co-administration may add to or potentiate the therapeutic effect of other antihypertensive drugs). Products include:
- Cozaar Tablets 1668
- Hyzaar Tablets 1720

Magnesium Salicylate (Patients receiving high doses of salicylates concomitantly may experience salicylate toxicity at lower doses because of competitive renal excretory sites). Products include:
- Backache Caplets ...... ⊞ 635
- Doan's Extra-Strength Analgesic ...... ⊞ 653
- Extra Strength Doan's P.M. ...... ⊞ 653
- Doan's Regular Strength Analgesic ...... ⊞ 654
- Mobigesic Tablets ...... ⊞ 607

Mecamylamine Hydrochloride (Co-administration may add to or potentiate the therapeutic effect of other antihypertensive drugs). Products include:
- Inversine Tablets 1729

Meclofenamate Sodium (Co-administration has resulted in increased BUN, serum creatinine, and serum potassium levels, and weight gain).
- No products indexed under this heading.

Mefenamic Acid (Co-administration has resulted in increased BUN, serum creatinine, and serum potassium levels, and weight gain). Products include:
- Ponstel 1982

Meperidine Hydrochloride (Orthostatic hypotension may be aggravated by narcotics). Products include:
- Demerol 2438
- Mepergan Injection 2859

Mephobarbital (Orthostatic hypotension may be aggravated by barbiturates). Products include:
- Mebaral Tablets 2452

Methadone Hydrochloride (Orthostatic hypotension may be aggravated by narcotics). Products include:
- Methadone Hydrochloride Oral Concentrate 2356
- Methadone Hydrochloride Oral Solution & Tablets 2357

Methyclothiazide (Co-administration may add to or potentiate the therapeutic effect of other antihypertensive drugs). Products include:
- Enduron Tablets 424

Methyldopa (Co-administration may add to or potentiate the therapeutic effect of other antihypertensive drugs). Products include:
- Aldoclor Tablets 1638
- Aldomet Oral 1640
- Aldoril Tablets 1644

Methyldopate Hydrochloride (Co-administration may add to or potentiate the therapeutic effect of other antihypertensive drugs). Products include:
- Aldomet Ester HCl Injection 1642

(⊞ Described in PDR For Nonprescription Drugs)   (⊙ Described in PDR For Ophthalmology)

Methylprednisolone Acetate (Co-administration may increase the risk of hypokalemia).
No products indexed under this heading.

Methylprednisolone Sodium Succinate (Co-administration may increase the risk of hypokalemia).
No products indexed under this heading.

Metolazone (Co-administration may add to or potentiate the therapeutic effect of other antihypertensive drugs). Products include:
Mykrox Tablets 1617
Zaroxolyn Tablets 1625

Metoprolol Succinate (Co-administration may add to or potentiate the therapeutic effect of other antihypertensive drugs). Products include:
Toprol-XL Tablets 560

Metoprolol Tartrate (Co-administration may add to or potentiate the therapeutic effect of other antihypertensive drugs). Products include:
Lopressor 848
Lopressor HCT Tablets 850

Metyrosine (Co-administration may add to or potentiate the therapeutic effect of other antihypertensive drugs). Products include:
Demser Capsules 1690

Minoxidil (Co-administration may add to or potentiate the therapeutic effect of other antihypertensive drugs).
No products indexed under this heading.

Moexipril Hydrochloride (Co-administration may add to or potentiate the therapeutic effect of other antihypertensive drugs). Products include:
Univasc Tablets 2553

Morphine Sulfate (Orthostatic hypotension may be aggravated by narcotics). Products include:
Astramorph/PF Injection, USP (Preservative-Free) 526
Duramorph Injection 983
Infumorph 200 and Infumorph 500 Sterile Solutions 985
Kadian Capsules 2948
MS Contin Tablets 2149
MSIR 2152
Oramorph SR (Morphine Sulfate Sustained Release Tablets) 2359
RMS Suppositories CII 2766
Roxanol 2365

Nabumetone (Co-administration has resulted in increased BUN, serum creatinine, and serum potassium levels, and weight gain). Products include:
Relafen Tablets 2688

Nadolol (Co-administration may add to or potentiate the therapeutic effect of other antihypertensive drugs).
No products indexed under this heading.

Naproxen (Co-administration has resulted in increased BUN, serum creatinine, and serum potassium levels, and weight gain). Products include:
Anaprox/Naprosyn 2277

Naproxen Sodium (Co-administration has resulted in increased BUN, serum creatinine, and serum potassium levels, and weight gain). Products include:
Aleve 2124
Anaprox/Naprosyn 2277
Naprelan Tablets 2861

Nicardipine Hydrochloride (Co-administration may add to or potentiate the therapeutic effect of other antihypertensive drugs). Products include:
Cardene Capsules 2261
Cardene I.V. 2815
Cardene SR Capsules 2264

Nifedipine (Co-administration may add to or potentiate the therapeutic effect of other antihypertensive drugs). Products include:
Adalat Capsules (10 mg and 20 mg) 580
Adalat CC 582
Procardia Capsules 2024
Procardia XL Extended Release Tablets 2026

Nisoldipine (Co-administration may add to or potentiate the therapeutic effect of other antihypertensive drugs). Products include:
Sular Tablets 2961

Nitroglycerin (Co-administration may add to or potentiate the therapeutic effect of other antihypertensive drugs). Products include:
Deponit NTG Transdermal Delivery System 2541
Nitro-Bid IV 1270
Nitro-Bid Ointment 1272
Nitro-Dur (nitroglycerin) Transdermal Infusion System 1365
Nitrolingual Spray 2193
Nitrostat Tablets 1981
Transderm-Nitro Transdermal Therapeutic System 878

Norepinephrine Bitartrate (Furosemide may decrease arterial responsiveness to norepinephrine). Products include:
Levophed Bitartrate Injection 2445

Opium Alkaloids (Orthostatic hypotension may be aggravated by narcotics).
No products indexed under this heading.

Oxaprozin (Co-administration has resulted in increased BUN, serum creatinine, and serum potassium levels, and weight gain). Products include:
Daypro Caplets 2578

Oxycodone Hydrochloride (Orthostatic hypotension may be aggravated by narcotics). Products include:
OxyContin Tablets 2163
OxyIR Capsules 2167
Percocet Tablets 955
Percodan Tablets 955
Percodan-Demi Tablets 956
Roxicodone Tablets, Oral Solution & Intensol (Oxycodone) 2366
Tylox Capsules 1593

Penbutolol Sulfate (Co-administration may add to or potentiate the therapeutic effect of other antihypertensive drugs). Products include:
Levatol Tablets 2547

Pentobarbital Sodium (Orthostatic hypotension may be aggravated by barbiturates). Products include:
Nembutal Sodium Capsules 440
Nembutal Sodium Solution 442
Nembutal Sodium Suppositories ... 444

Phenobarbital (Orthostatic hypotension may be aggravated by barbiturates). Products include:
Arco-Lase Plus Tablets 513
Bellergal-S Tablets 2375
Donnatal 2234
Donnatal Extentabs 2234
Donnatal Tablets 2234
Phenobarbital Elixir and Tablets ... 1523
Quadrinal Tablets 1398

Phenoxybenzamine Hydrochloride (Co-administration may add to or potentiate the therapeutic effect of other antihypertensive drugs). Products include:
Dibenzyline Capsules 2650

Phentolamine Mesylate (Co-administration may add to or potentiate the therapeutic effect of other antihypertensive drugs). Products include:
Regitine Vials 864

Phenylbutazone (Co-administration has resulted in increased BUN, serum creatinine, and serum potassium levels, and weight gain).
No products indexed under this heading.

Pindolol (Co-administration may add to or potentiate the therapeutic effect of other antihypertensive drugs). Products include:
Visken Tablets 2428

Piroxicam (Co-administration has resulted in increased BUN, serum creatinine, and serum potassium levels, and weight gain). Products include:
Feldene Capsules 2008

Polythiazide (Co-administration may add to or potentiate the therapeutic effect of other antihypertensive drugs). Products include:
Minizide Capsules 2016

Prazosin Hydrochloride (Co-administration may add to or potentiate the therapeutic effect of other antihypertensive drugs). Products include:
Minipress Capsules 2015
Minizide Capsules 2016

Prednisolone Acetate (Co-administration may increase the risk of hypokalemia). Products include:
AK-CIDE .... ⊚ 203
AK-CIDE Ointment .... ⊚ 203
Blephamide Liquifilm Sterile Ophthalmic Suspension 472
Blephamide Ointment .... ⊚ 234
Econopred & Econopred Plus Ophthalmic Suspensions .... ⊚ 216
Poly-Pred Liquifilm .... ⊚ 246
Pred Forte .... ⊚ 247
Pred Mild .... ⊚ 250
Pred-G Liquifilm Sterile Ophthalmic Suspension .... ⊚ 248
Pred-G S.O.P. Sterile Ophthalmic Ointment .... ⊚ 249

Prednisolone Sodium Phosphate (Co-administration may increase the risk of hypokalemia). Products include:
AK-PRED .... ⊚ 204
Hydeltrasol Injection, Sterile 1708
Pediapred Oral Solution 1618

Prednisolone Tebutate (Co-administration may increase the risk of hypokalemia). Products include:
Hydeltra-T.B.A. Sterile Suspension ... 1710

Prednisone (Co-administration may increase the risk of hypokalemia).
No products indexed under this heading.

Propoxyphene Hydrochloride (Orthostatic hypotension may be aggravated by narcotics). Products include:
Darvon 1475
Wygesic Tablets 2930

Propoxyphene Napsylate (Orthostatic hypotension may be aggravated by narcotics). Products include:
Darvon-N/Darvocet-N 1473

Propranolol Hydrochloride (Co-administration may add to or potentiate the therapeutic effect of other antihypertensive drugs). Products include:
Inderal 2834
Inderal LA Long Acting Capsules 2836
Inderide Tablets 2838
Inderide LA Long Acting Capsules .. 2840

Quinapril Hydrochloride ().
Products include:
Accupril Tablets 1950

Ramipril (Co-administration may add to or potentiate the therapeutic effect of other antihypertensive drugs). Products include:
Altace Capsules 1238

Rauwolfia Serpentina (Co-administration may add to or potentiate the therapeutic effect of other antihypertensive drugs).
No products indexed under this heading.

Rescinnamine (Co-administration may add to or potentiate the therapeutic effect of other antihypertensive drugs).
No products indexed under this heading.

Reserpine (Co-administration may add to or potentiate the therapeutic effect of other antihypertensive drugs). Products include:
Diupres Tablets 1691
Hydropres Tablets 1718
Ser-Ap-Es Tablets 867

Salsalate (Patients receiving high doses of salicylates concomitantly may experience salicylate toxicity at lower doses because of competitive renal excretory sites). Products include:
Disalcid 1549
Mono-Gesic Tablets 810
Salflex Tablets 791

Secobarbital Sodium (Orthostatic hypotension may be aggravated by barbiturates). Products include:
Seconal Sodium Pulvules 1529

Sodium Nitroprusside (Co-administration may add to or potentiate the therapeutic effect of other antihypertensive drugs).
No products indexed under this heading.

Sotalol Hydrochloride (Co-administration may add to or potentiate the therapeutic effect of other antihypertensive drugs). Products include:
Betapace Tablets 637

Spirapril Hydrochloride (Co-administration may add to or potentiate the therapeutic effect of other antihypertensive drugs).
No products indexed under this heading.

Streptomycin Sulfate (Co-administration may increase the ototoxic potential of aminoglycoside antibiotics). Products include:
Streptomycin Sulfate Injection 2031

Succinylcholine Chloride (Furosemide may potentiate the action of succinylcholine). Products include:
Anectine 1062

Sufentanil Citrate (Orthostatic hypotension may be aggravated by narcotics). Products include:
Sufenta Injection 1355

Sulindac (Co-administration has resulted in increased BUN, serum creatinine, and serum potassium levels, and weight gain). Products include:
Clinoril Tablets 1658

IMPORTANT NOTE: Always consult each drug listing in the patient's regimen for possible interactions.

Terazosin Hydrochloride (Co-administration may add to or potentiate the therapeutic effect of other antihypertensive drugs). Products include:

Hytrin Capsules 434

Thiamylal Sodium (Orthostatic hypotension may be aggravated by barbiturates).

No products indexed under this heading.

Timolol Maleate (Co-administration may add to or potentiate the therapeutic effect of other antihypertensive drugs). Products include:

Blocadren Tablets 1654
Timolide Tablets 1791
Timoptic in Ocudose 1796
Timoptic Sterile Ophthalmic Solution 1794
Timoptic-XE 1798

Tobramycin (Co-administration may increase the ototoxic potential of aminoglycoside antibiotics). Products include:

AKTOB .... ◉ 207
TobraDex Ophthalmic Suspension and Ointment 469
Tobrex Ophthalmic Ointment and Solution .... ◉ 226

Tobramycin Sulfate (Co-administration may increase the ototoxic potential of aminoglycoside antibiotics). Products include:

Nebcin Vials, Hyporets & ADD-Vantage 1518

Tolmetin Sodium (Co-administration has resulted in increased BUN, serum creatinine, and serum potassium levels, and weight gain). Products include:

Tolectin (200, 400 and 600 mg) .. 1591

Torsemide (Co-administration may add to or potentiate the therapeutic effect of other antihypertensive drugs). Products include:

Demadex Tablets and Injection 691

Triamcinolone (Co-administration may increase the risk of hypokalemia).

No products indexed under this heading.

Triamcinolone Acetonide (Co-administration may increase the risk of hypokalemia). Products include:

Azmacort Oral Inhaler 2175
Nasacort AQ Nasal Spray 2191
Nasacort Nasal Inhaler 2189

Triamcinolone Diacetate (Co-administration may increase the risk of hypokalemia).

No products indexed under this heading.

Triamcinolone Hexacetonide (Co-administration may increase the risk of hypokalemia).

No products indexed under this heading.

Trimethaphan Camsylate (Co-administration may add to or potentiate the therapeutic effect of other antihypertensive drugs).

No products indexed under this heading.

Tubocurarine Chloride (Furosemide has a tendency to antagonize the skeletal muscle relaxing effect of tubocurarine).

No products indexed under this heading.

Verapamil Hydrochloride (Co-administration may add to or potentiate the therapeutic effect of other antihypertensive drugs). Products include:

Calan SR Caplets 2571
Calan Tablets 2568
Covera-HS Tablets 2573
Isoptin Injectable 1391
Isoptin Oral Tablets 1393
Isoptin SR Tablets 1395
Verelan Capsules 1455

Food Interactions

Alcohol (Orthostatic hypotension may be aggravated by alcohol).

LAVOPTIK EYE WASH

(Isotonic Solution) .... ▣ 681
None cited in PDR database.

LESCOL CAPSULES

(Fluvastatin Sodium) 2395
May interact with fibrates, erythromycin, and certain other agents. Compounds in these categories include:

Cholestyramine (Administration of fluvastatin with, or up to 4 hours after cholestyramine results in significant reductions in AUC and C_{max} of fluvastatin, however, use of fluvastatin 4 hours after resin results in clinically significant additive effect). Products include:

Questran 774

Cimetidine (Co-administration results in a significant increase in the fluvastatin C_{max} and AUC and a decrease in plasma clearance). Products include:

Tagamet HB Tablets .... ▣ 786
Tagamet Tablets 2694

Cimetidine Hydrochloride (Co-administration results in a significant increase in the fluvastatin C_{max} and AUC and a decrease in plasma clearance). Products include:

Tagamet 2694

Clofibrate (Myopathy has occasionally been associated with fibrates; combined use should generally be avoided). Products include:

Atromid-S Capsules 2808

Cyclosporine (The risk of myopathy and/or rhabdomyolysis during treatment with HMG-CoA reductase inhibitor has been reported to be increased with concurrent cyclosporine; caution should be exercised). Products include:

Neoral 2405
Sandimmune 2416

Digoxin (Co-administration in patients on chronic digoxin may result in a small increase in digoxin C_{max} (11%) and urinary clearance). Products include:

Lanoxicaps 1110
Lanoxin Elixir Pediatric 1113
Lanoxin Injection 1116
Lanoxin Injection Pediatric 1119
Lanoxin Tablets 1121

Erythromycin (The risk of myopathy and/or rhabdomyolysis during treatment with HMG-CoA reductase inhibitor has been reported to be increased with concurrent erythromycin; caution should be exercised). Products include:

A/T/S 2% Acne Topical Gel 1244
A/T/S 2% Acne Topical Solution 1244
Benzamycin Topical Gel 919
E-Mycin Tablets 1388
Emgel 2% Topical Gel 1081
ERYC 1972
Erycette (erythromycin 2%) Topical Solution 1943
Ery-Tab Tablets 426
Erythromycin Base Filmtab 430
Erythromycin Delayed-Release Capsules, USP 431
Ilotycin Ophthalmic Ointment 928
PCE Dispertab Tablets 453
T-Stat 2.0% Topical Solution and Pads 2797
THERAMYCIN Z 2% Solution 1629

Erythromycin Estolate (The risk of myopathy and/or rhabdomyolysis during treatment with HMG-CoA reductase inhibitor has been reported to be increased with concurrent erythromycin; caution should be exercised). Products include:

Ilosone 927

Erythromycin Ethylsuccinate (The risk of myopathy and/or rhabdomyolysis during treatment with HMG-CoA reductase inhibitor has been reported to be increased with concurrent erythromycin; caution should be exercised). Products include:

E.E.S. 427
EryPed 425
Pediazole Suspension 2340

Erythromycin Gluceptate (The risk of myopathy and/or rhabdomyolysis during treatment with HMG-CoA reductase inhibitor has been reported to be increased with concurrent erythromycin; caution should be exercised). Products include:

Ilotycin Gluceptate, IV, Vials 929

Erythromycin Stearate (The risk of myopathy and/or rhabdomyolysis during treatment with HMG-CoA reductase inhibitor has been reported to be increased with concurrent erythromycin; caution should be exercised). Products include:

Erythrocin Stearate Filmtab 429

Gemfibrozil (The risk of myopathy and/or rhabdomyolysis during treatment with HMG-CoA reductase inhibitor has been reported to be increased with concurrent gemfibrozil; combined use should generally be avoided). Products include:

Lopid Tablets 1974

Ketoconazole (Caution should be exercised if used concurrently with drugs that may decrease the levels of endogenous steroid hormones; increase potential for endocrine dysfunction). Products include:

Nizoral 2% Cream 1344
Nizoral 2% Shampoo 1344
Nizoral Tablets 1345

Nicotinic Acid (The risk of myopathy and/or rhabdomyolysis during treatment with HMG-CoA reductase inhibitor has been reported to be increased with concurrent niacin; caution should be exercised).

No products indexed under this heading.

Omeprazole (Co-administration results in a significant increase in the fluvastatin C_{max} and AUC and a decrease in plasma clearance). Products include:

Prilosec Delayed-Release Capsules 516

Ranitidine Hydrochloride (Co-administration results in a significant increase in the fluvastatin C_{max} and AUC and a decrease in plasma clearance). Products include:

Zantac 1182
Zantac Injection 1180
Zantac Syrup 1182

Rifampin (Co-administration in patients pretreated with rifampin results in significant reduction in C_{max} (59%) and AUC (51%) with a large increase (95%) in plasma clearance). Products include:

Rifadin 1276
Rifamate Capsules 1278
Rifater 1280
Rimactane Capsules 865

Spironolactone (Caution should be exercised if used concurrently with drugs that may decrease the levels of endogenous steroid hormones; increase potential for endocrine dysfunction). Products include:

Aldactazide Tablets 2556
Aldactone Tablets 2558

Warfarin Sodium (Bleeding and/or increased prothrombin time has been reported with other HMG-CoA reductase inhibitors when used concurrently; no interactions at therapeutic concentrations have been demonstrated with fluvastatin and warfarin). Products include:

Coumadin 941

Food Interactions

Meal, unspecified (Administration of fluvastatin with the evening meal results in a two-fold decrease in C_{max} and more than two-fold increase in t_{max} as compared to patients receiving the drug 4 hours after evening meal).

LEUCOVORIN CALCIUM FOR INJECTION, WELLCOVORIN BRAND

(Leucovorin Calcium) 1203
May interact with:

Fluorouracil (Co-administration has resulted in rare reports of seizures and/or syncope with high doses of leucovorin and fluorouracil for the treatment of malignancies in patients with prior history of seizures or CNS abnormalities). Products include:

Efudex 2280
Fluoroplex Topical Solution & Cream 1% 475
Fluorouracil Injection 2282

Fosphenytoin Sodium (Co-administration with folic acid or its derivatives in large amounts may counteract antiepileptic effects). Products include:

Cerebyx Injection 1956

Phenobarbital (Co-administration with folic acid or its derivatives in large amounts may counteract antiepileptic effects). Products include:

Arco-Lase Plus Tablets 513
Bellergal-S Tablets 2375
Donnatal 2234
Donnatal Extentabs 2234
Donnatal Tablets 2234
Phenobarbital Elixir and Tablets 1523
Quadrinal Tablets 1398

Phenytoin (Co-administration with folic acid or its derivatives in large amounts may counteract antiepileptic effects). Products include:

Dilantin Infatabs 1967
Dilantin-125 Suspension 1969

Phenytoin Sodium (Co-administration with folic acid or its derivatives in large amounts may counteract antiepileptic effects). Products include:

Dilantin Kapseals 1965

Primidone (Co-administration with folic acid or its derivatives in large amounts may counteract antiepileptic effects). Products include:

Mysoline 2860

Sulfamethoxazole (Concomitant use of leucovorin with trimethoprim-sulfamethoxazole for the acute treatment of *Pneumocystis carinii* pneumonia in patients with HIV infection is associated with increased rates of treatment failure and morbidity). Products include:

Bactrim DS Tablets 2257
Bactrim I.V. Infusion 2255
Bactrim 2257
Gantanol Tablets 2285

(▣ Described in PDR For Nonprescription Drugs) (◉ Described in PDR For Ophthalmology)

Septra ... 1146
Septra I.V. Infusion ... 1142
Septra I.V. Infusion ADD-Vantage Vials ... 1144
Septra ... 1146

Trimethoprim (Concomitant use of leucovorin with trimethprim-sulfamethoxazole for the acute treatment of *Pneumocystis carinii* pneumonia in patients with HIV infection is associated with increased rates of treatment failure and morbidity). Products include:

Bactrim DS Tablets ... 2257
Bactrim I.V. Infusion ... 2255
Bactrim ... 2257
Proloprim Tablets ... 1141
Septra ... 1146
Septra I.V. Infusion ... 1142
Septra I.V. Infusion ADD-Vantage Vials ... 1144
Septra ... 1146
Trimpex Tablets ... 2323

LEUCOVORIN CALCIUM FOR INJECTION

(Leucovorin Calcium) ... 1313
May interact with:

Fluorouracil (Enhanced toxicity of fluorouracil). Products include:

Efudex ... 2280
Fluoroplex Topical Solution & Cream 1% ... 475
Fluorouracil Injection ... 2282

Fosphenytoin Sodium (Folic acid in large amounts may counteract antiepileptic effects and increase frequency of seizures in susceptible children). Products include:

Cerebyx Injection ... 1956

Methotrexate Sodium (High doses of leucovorin may reduce the efficacy of intrathecally administered methotrexate). Products include:

Methotrexate Sodium Tablets, Injection, for Injection and LPF Injection ... 1322

Phenobarbital (Folic acid in large amounts may counteract antiepileptic effects and increase frequency of seizures in susceptible children). Products include:

Arco-Lase Plus Tablets ... 513
Bellergal-S Tablets ... 2375
Donnatal ... 2234
Donnatal Extentabs ... 2234
Donnatal Tablets ... 2234
Phenobarbital Elixir and Tablets ... 1523
Quadrinal Tablets ... 1398

Phenytoin (Folic acid in large amounts may counteract antiepileptic effects and increase frequency of seizures in susceptible children). Products include:

Dilantin Infatabs ... 1967
Dilantin-125 Suspension ... 1969

Phenytoin Sodium (Folic acid in large amounts may counteract antiepileptic effects and increase frequency of seizures in susceptible children). Products include:

Dilantin Kapseals ... 1965

Primidone (Folic acid in large amounts may counteract antiepileptic effects and increase frequency of seizures in susceptible children). Products include:

Mysoline ... 2860

LEUCOVORIN CALCIUM TABLETS, WELLCOVORIN BRAND

(Leucovorin Calcium) ... 1204
May interact with:

Fluorouracil (Concomitant administration results in enhanced toxicity of fluorouracil). Products include:

Efudex ... 2280
Fluoroplex Topical Solution & Cream 1% ... 475
Fluorouracil Injection ... 2282

Fosphenytoin Sodium (Folic acid in large amounts may counteract antiepileptic effects and increase frequency of seizures in susceptible children). Products include:

Cerebyx Injection ... 1956

Phenobarbital (Folic acid in large amounts may counteract antiepileptic effects and increase frequency of seizures in susceptible children). Products include:

Arco-Lase Plus Tablets ... 513
Bellergal-S Tablets ... 2375
Donnatal ... 2234
Donnatal Extentabs ... 2234
Donnatal Tablets ... 2234
Phenobarbital Elixir and Tablets ... 1523
Quadrinal Tablets ... 1398

Phenytoin (Folic acid in large amounts may counteract antiepileptic effects and increase frequency of seizures in susceptible children). Products include:

Dilantin Infatabs ... 1967
Dilantin-125 Suspension ... 1969

Phenytoin Sodium (Folic acid in large amounts may counteract antiepileptic effects and increase frequency of seizures in susceptible children). Products include:

Dilantin Kapseals ... 1965

Primidone (Folic acid in large amounts may counteract antiepileptic effects and increase frequency of seizures in susceptible children). Products include:

Mysoline ... 2860

Sulfamethoxazole (Concomitant use of leucovorin with trimethoprim-sulfamethoxazole for the acute treatment of *Pneumocystis carinii* pneumonia in patients with HIV infection is associated with increased rates of treatment failure and morbidity). Products include:

Bactrim DS Tablets ... 2257
Bactrim I.V. Infusion ... 2255
Bactrim ... 2257
Gantanol Tablets ... 2285
Septra ... 1146
Septra I.V. Infusion ... 1142
Septra I.V. Infusion ADD-Vantage Vials ... 1144
Septra ... 1146

Trimethoprim (Concomitant use of leucovorin with trimethoprim-sulfamethoxazole for the acute treatment of *Pneumocystis carinii* pneumonia in patients with HIV infection is associated with increased rates of treatment failure and morbidity). Products include:

Bactrim DS Tablets ... 2257
Bactrim I.V. Infusion ... 2255
Bactrim ... 2257
Proloprim Tablets ... 1141
Septra ... 1146
Septra I.V. Infusion ... 1142
Septra I.V. Infusion ADD-Vantage Vials ... 1144
Septra ... 1146
Trimpex Tablets ... 2323

LEUCOVORIN CALCIUM TABLETS

(Leucovorin Calcium) ... 1315
May interact with:

Fluorouracil (Enhanced toxicity of fluorouracil). Products include:

Efudex ... 2280
Fluoroplex Topical Solution & Cream 1% ... 475
Fluorouracil Injection ... 2282

Fosphenytoin Sodium (Folic acid in large amounts may counteract antiepileptic effects and increase frequency of seizures in susceptible children). Products include:

Cerebyx Injection ... 1956

Methotrexate Sodium (High doses of leucovorin may reduce the efficacy of intrathecally administered methotrexate). Products include:

Methotrexate Sodium Tablets, Injection, for Injection and LPF Injection ... 1322

Phenobarbital (Folic acid in large amounts may counteract antiepileptic effects and increase frequency of seizures in susceptible children). Products include:

Arco-Lase Plus Tablets ... 513
Bellergal-S Tablets ... 2375
Donnatal ... 2234
Donnatal Extentabs ... 2234
Donnatal Tablets ... 2234
Phenobarbital Elixir and Tablets ... 1523
Quadrinal Tablets ... 1398

Phenytoin (Folic acid in large amounts may counteract antiepileptic effects and increase frequency of seizures in susceptible children). Products include:

Dilantin Infatabs ... 1967
Dilantin-125 Suspension ... 1969

Phenytoin Sodium (Folic acid in large amounts may counteract antiepileptic effects and increase frequency of seizures in susceptible children). Products include:

Dilantin Kapseals ... 1965

Primidone (Folic acid in large amounts may counteract antiepileptic effects and increase frequency of seizures in susceptible children). Products include:

Mysoline ... 2860

LEUKERAN TABLETS

(Chlorambucil) ... 1205
None cited in PDR database.

LEUKINE

(Sargramostim) ... 1317
May interact with drugs with myelproliferative effects and cytotoxic drugs. Compounds in these categories include:

Betamethasone Acetate (May potentiate the myeloproliferative effect). Products include:

Celestone Soluspan Suspension ... 2484

Betamethasone Sodium Phosphate (May potentiate the myeloproliferative effect). Products include:

Celestone Soluspan Suspension ... 2484

Bleomycin Sulfate (Coadministration within 24 hours preceding or following chemotherapy is not recommended because of potential sensitivity of rapidly dividing hematopoietic progenitor cells to cytotoxic therapy). Products include:

Blenoxane ... 697

Cortisone Acetate (May potentiate the myeloproliferative effect). Products include:

Cortone Acetate Sterile Suspension ... 1663
Cortone Acetate Tablets ... 1664

Daunorubicin Hydrochloride (Coadministration within 24 hours preceding or following chemotherapy is not recommended because of potential sensitivity of rapidly dividing hematopoietic progenitor cells to cytotoxic therapy). Products include:

Cerubidine for Injection ... 634

Dexamethasone (May potentiate the myeloproliferative effect). Products include:

AK-Trol Ointment & Suspension ... ◉ 205
Decadron Elixir ... 1676
Decadron Tablets ... 1678
Decaspray Topical Aerosol ... 1689
Maxitrol Ophthalmic Ointment and Suspension ... ◉ 222
TobraDex Ophthalmic Suspension and Ointment ... 469

Dexamethasone Acetate (May potentiate the myeloproliferative effect). Products include:

Dalalone D.P. Injectable ... 1009
Decadron-LA Sterile Suspension ... 1687

Dexamethasone Sodium Phosphate (May potentiate the myeloproliferative effect). Products include:

Decadron Phosphate Injection ... 1680
Decadron Phosphate Sterile Ophthalmic Ointment ... 1684
Decadron Phosphate Sterile Ophthalmic Solution ... 1685
Decadron Phosphate Topical Cream ... 1686
Decadron Phosphate with Xylocaine Injection, Sterile ... 1683
Dexacort Phosphate in Respihaler .. 1606
Dexacort Phosphate in Turbinaire .. 1607
NeoDecadron Sterile Ophthalmic Ointment ... 1755
NeoDecadron Sterile Ophthalmic Solution ... 1756
NeoDecadron Topical Cream ... 1757

Doxorubicin Hydrochloride (Coadministration within 24 hours preceding or following chemotherapy is not recommended because of potential sensitivity of rapidly dividing hematopoietic progenitor cells to cytotoxic therapy). Products include:

Adriamycin PFS ... 2056
Adriamycin RDF ... 2056
Doxil ... 2613
Doxorubicin Astra ... 531
Rubex for Injection ... 721

Fluorouracil (Coadministration within 24 hours preceding or following chemotherapy is not recommended because of potential sensitivity of rapidly dividing hematopoietic progenitor cells to cytotoxic therapy). Products include:

Efudex ... 2280
Fluoroplex Topical Solution & Cream 1% ... 475
Fluorouracil Injection ... 2282

Hydrocortisone (May potentiate the myeloproliferative effect). Products include:

Anusol-HC Cream 2.5% ... 1953
Aquanil HC Lotion ... 1989
Maximum Strength Cortaid Spray ... 800
CORTENEMA ... 2713
Cortisporin Ointment ... 1074
Cortisporin Ophthalmic Ointment Sterile ... 1074
Cortisporin Ophthalmic Suspension Sterile ... 1075
Cortisporin Otic Solution Sterile ... 1076
Cortisporin Otic Suspension Sterile 1077
Cortizone-5 ... 795
Cortizone-10 ... 795
Hydrocortone Tablets ... 1715
Hytone ... 922
Hytone Ointment 2 ½% ... 923
Massengill Medicated Soft Cloth Towelettes ... 2628
Pediotic Suspension Sterile ... 1140
Preparation H Hydrocortisone 1% Cream ... 843
ProctoCream-HC 2.5% ... 2552
VōSoL HC Otic Solution ... 2786

Hydrocortisone Acetate (May potentiate the myeloproliferative effect). Products include:

Analpram-HC Rectal Cream 1% and 2.5% ... 993
Anusol HC-1 Hydrocortisone Anti-Itch Ointment ... 810
Anusol-HC Suppositories ... 1954
Caldecort Anti-Itch Hydrocortisone Cream ... 651

IMPORTANT NOTE: Always consult each drug listing in the patient's regimen for possible interactions.

Leukine **Interactions Index** 590

Coly-Mycin S Otic w/Neomycin & Hydrocortisone ... 1965
Cortaid ... ▣ 800
Cortifoam ... 2540
Cortisporin Cream ... 1073
Epifoam ... 2543
Hydrocortone Acetate Sterile Suspension ... 1712
Mantadil Cream ... 1124
Nupercainal Hydrocortisone 1% Cream ... ▣ 661
Pramosone Cream, Lotion & Ointment ... 995
ProctoFoam-HC ... 2552
Terra-Cortril Ophthalmic Suspension ... 2033

Hydrocortisone Sodium Phosphate (May potentiate the myeloproliferative effect). Products include:
Hydrocortone Phosphate Injection, Sterile ... 1713

Hydrocortisone Sodium Succinate (May potentiate the myeloproliferative effect).
No products indexed under this heading.

Hydroxyurea (Coadministration within 24 hours preceding or following chemotherapy is not recommended because of potential sensitivity of rapidly dividing hematopoietic progenitor cells to cytotoxic therapy). Products include:
Hydrea Capsules ... 705

Lithium Carbonate (May potentiate the myeloproliferative effect). Products include:
Eskalith ... 2658
Lithium Carbonate Capsules & Tablets ... 2352
Lithonate/Lithotabs/Lithobid ... 2721

Lithium Citrate (May potentiate the myeloproliferative effect).
No products indexed under this heading.

Methotrexate Sodium (Coadministration within 24 hours preceding or following chemotherapy is not recommended because of potential sensitivity of rapidly dividing hematopoietic progenitor cells to cytotoxic therapy). Products include:
Methotrexate Sodium Tablets, Injection, for Injection and LPF Injection ... 1322

Methylprednisolone Acetate (May potentiate the myeloproliferative effect).
No products indexed under this heading.

Methylprednisolone Sodium Succinate (May potentiate the myeloproliferative effect).
No products indexed under this heading.

Mitotane (Coadministration within 24 hours preceding or following chemotherapy is not recommended because of potential sensitivity of rapidly dividing hematopoietic progenitor cells to cytotoxic therapy). Products include:
Lysodren Tablets ... 707

Mitoxantrone Hydrochloride (Coadministration within 24 hours preceding or following chemotherapy is not recommended because of potential sensitivity of rapidly dividing hematopoietic progenitor cells to cytotoxic therapy). Products include:
Novantrone for Injection ... 1327

Prednisolone Acetate (May potentiate the myeloproliferative effect). Products include:
AK-CIDE ... ⊙ 203
AK-CIDE Ointment ... ⊙ 203
Blephamide Liquifilm Sterile Ophthalmic Suspension ... 472
Blephamide Ointment ... ⊙ 234
Econopred & Econopred Plus Ophthalmic Suspensions ... ⊙ 216
Poly-Pred Liquifilm ... ⊙ 246
Pred Forte ... ⊙ 247
Pred Mild ... ⊙ 250
Pred-G Liquifilm Sterile Ophthalmic Suspension ... ⊙ 248
Pred-G S.O.P. Sterile Ophthalmic Ointment ... ⊙ 249

Prednisolone Sodium Phosphate (May potentiate the myeloproliferative effect). Products include:
AK-PRED ... ⊙ 204
Hydeltrasol Injection, Sterile ... 1708
Pediapred Oral Solution ... 1618

Prednisolone Tebutate (May potentiate the myeloproliferative effect). Products include:
Hydeltra-T.B.A. Sterile Suspension 1710

Prednisone (May potentiate the myeloproliferative effect).
No products indexed under this heading.

Procarbazine Hydrochloride (Coadministration within 24 hours preceding or following chemotherapy is not recommended because of potential sensitivity of rapidly dividing hematopoietic progenitor cells to cytotoxic therapy). Products include:
Matulane Capsules ... 2300

Tamoxifen Citrate (Coadministration within 24 hours preceding or following chemotherapy is not recommended because of potential sensitivity of rapidly dividing hematopoietic progenitor cells to cytotoxic therapy). Products include:
Nolvadex Tablets ... 2957

Triamcinolone (May potentiate the myeloproliferative effect).
No products indexed under this heading.

Triamcinolone Acetonide (May potentiate the myeloproliferative effect). Products include:
Azmacort Oral Inhaler ... 2175
Nasacort AQ Nasal Spray ... 2191
Nasacort Nasal Inhaler ... 2189

Triamcinolone Diacetate (May potentiate the myeloproliferative effect).
No products indexed under this heading.

Triamcinolone Hexacetonide (May potentiate the myeloproliferative effect).
No products indexed under this heading.

Vincristine Sulfate (Coadministration within 24 hours preceding or following chemotherapy is not recommended because of potential sensitivity of rapidly dividing hematopoietic progenitor cells to cytotoxic therapy). Products include:
Oncovin Solution Vials & Hyporets 1521

LEUSTATIN
(Cladribine) ... 1889
May interact with:

Bone Marrow Depressants, unspecified (Caution should be exercised if co-administered with other drugs known to cause myelosuppression).

LEVATOL TABLETS
(Penbutolol Sulfate) ... 2547
May interact with calcium channel blockers, catecholamine depleting drugs, insulin, and certain other agents. Compounds in these categories include:

Amlodipine Besylate (Synergistic hypotensive effects, bradycardia, and arrhythmias have been reported in some patients on beta blockers when an oral calcium antagonist was added to the treatment regimen). Products include:
Lotrel Capsules ... 858
Norvasc Tablets ... 2020

Bepridil Hydrochloride (Synergistic hypotensive effects, bradycardia, and arrhythmias have been reported in some patients on beta blockers when an oral calcium antagonist was added to the treatment regimen). Products include:
Vascor Tablets (200 and 300 mg) 1597

Deserpidine (Concurrent use with catecholamine-depleting drugs should be avoided).
No products indexed under this heading.

Diltiazem Hydrochloride (Synergistic hypotensive effects, bradycardia, and arrhythmias have been reported in some patients on beta blockers when an oral calcium antagonist was added to the treatment regimen). Products include:
Cardizem CD Capsules ... 1251
Cardizem SR Capsules ... 1255
Cardizem Injectable ... 1253
Cardizem Tablets ... 1257
Dilacor XR Extended-release Capsules ... 2183
Tiazac Capsules ... 1019

Epinephrine (Patients with a history of anaphylactic reaction may be unresponsive to the usual dose of epinephrine). Products include:
EPIFRIN ... ⊙ 237
EpiPen ... 808
Marcaine with Epinephrine ... 2446
Primatene Mist ... ▣ 843
Sensorcaine with Epinephrine Injection ... 554
Sus-Phrine Injection ... 1017
Xylocaine with Epinephrine Injections ... 562

Epinephrine Hydrochloride (Patients with a history of anaphylactic reaction may be unresponsive to the usual dose of epinephrine). Products include:
Ana-Kit Anaphylaxis Emergency Treatment Kit ... 611

Felodipine (Synergistic hypotensive effects, bradycardia, and arrhythmias have been reported in some patients on beta blockers when an oral calcium antagonist was added to the treatment regimen). Products include:
Plendil Extended-Release Tablets ... 514

Guanethidine Monosulfate (Concurrent use with catecholamine-depleting drugs should be avoided). Products include:
Esimil Tablets ... 840
Ismelin Tablets ... 845

Insulin, Human (Beta blockade may prevent the appearance of signs and symptoms of acute hypoglycemia; beta blockade also reduces the release of insulin in response to hyperglycemia).
No products indexed under this heading.

Insulin, Human Isophane Suspension (Beta blockade may prevent the appearance of signs and symptoms of acute hypoglycemia; beta blockade also reduces the release of insulin in response to hyperglycemia). Products include:
Novolin N Human Insulin 10 ml Vials ... 1846

Insulin, Human NPH (Beta blockade may prevent the appearance of signs and symptoms of acute hypoglycemia; beta blockade also reduces the release of insulin in response to hyperglycemia). Products include:
Humulin N, 100 Units ... 1495
Novolin N PenFill 1.5 ml Cartridges Durable Insulin Delivery System ... 1849
Novolin N Prefilled Syringe Disposable Insulin Delivery System ... 1850

Insulin, Human Regular (Beta blockade may prevent the appearance of signs and symptoms of acute hypoglycemia; beta blockade also reduces the release of insulin in response to hyperglycemia). Products include:
Humulin R, 100 Units ... 1497
Novolin R Human Insulin 10 ml Vials ... 1846
Novolin R PenFill 1.5 ml Cartridges Durable Insulin Delivery System ... 1849
Novolin R Prefilled Syringe Disposable Insulin Delivery System ... 1850
Velosulin BR Human Insulin 10 ml Vials ... 1847

Insulin, Human, Zinc Suspension (Beta blockade may prevent the appearance of signs and symptoms of acute hypoglycemia; beta blockade also reduces the release of insulin in response to hyperglycemia). Products include:
Humulin L, 100 Units ... 1494
Humulin U, 100 Units ... 1498
Novolin L Human Insulin 10 ml Vials ... 1846

Insulin Lispro, Human (Beta blockade may prevent the appearance of signs and symptoms of acute hypoglycemia; beta blockade also reduces the release of insulin in response to hyperglycemia). Products include:
Humalog Injection ... 1488

Insulin, NPH (Beta blockade may prevent the appearance of signs and symptoms of acute hypoglycemia; beta blockade also reduces the release of insulin in response to hyperglycemia). Products include:
NPH, 100 Units ... 1502
Pork NPH, 100 Units ... 1506
Purified Pork NPH Isophane Insulin ... 1852

Insulin, Regular (Beta blockade may prevent the appearance of signs and symptoms of acute hypoglycemia; beta blockade also reduces the release of insulin in response to hyperglycemia). Products include:
Regular, 100 Units ... 1503
Pork Regular, 100 Units ... 1507
Pork Regular (Concentrated), 500 Units ... 1508
Purified Pork Regular Insulin ... 1852

Insulin, Zinc Crystals (Beta blockade may prevent the appearance of signs and symptoms of acute hypoglycemia; beta blockade also reduces the release of insulin in response to hyperglycemia). Products include:
NPH, 100 Units ... 1502

Insulin, Zinc Suspension (Beta blockade may prevent the appearance of signs and symptoms of acute hypoglycemia; beta blockade also reduces the release of insulin in response to hyperglycemia). Products include:
Iletin I ... 1501
Lente, 100 Units ... 1501
Iletin II ... 1504
Pork Lente, 100 Units ... 1504
Purified Pork Lente Insulin ... 1852

(▣ Described in PDR For Nonprescription Drugs) (⊙ Described in PDR For Ophthalmology)

591 Interactions Index Levo-Dromoran

Isradipine (Synergistic hypotensive effects, bradycardia, and arrhythmias have been reported in some patients on beta blockers when an oral calcium antagonist was added to the treatment regimen). Products include:
DynaCirc Capsules 2381
DynaCirc CR Tablets 2383

Lidocaine Hydrochloride (Penbutolol increases the volume of distribution of lidocaine; this could result in a requirement for higher loading doses of lidocaine). Products include:
Decadron Phosphate with Xylocaine Injection, Sterile 1683
Unguentine Plus .... ⊞ 712
Xylocaine Injections 562

Nicardipine Hydrochloride (Synergistic hypotensive effects, bradycardia, and arrhythmias have been reported in some patients on beta blockers when an oral calcium antagonist was added to the treatment regimen). Products include:
Cardene Capsules 2261
Cardene I.V. 2815
Cardene SR Capsules 2264

Nifedipine (Synergistic hypotensive effects, bradycardia, and arrhythmias have been reported in some patients on beta blockers when an oral calcium antagonist was added to the treatment regimen). Products include:
Adalat Capsules (10 mg and 20 mg) 580
Adalat CC 582
Procardia Capsules 2024
Procardia XL Extended Release Tablets 2026

Nimodipine (Synergistic hypotensive effects, bradycardia, and arrhythmias have been reported in some patients on beta blockers when an oral calcium antagonist was added to the treatment regimen). Products include:
Nimotop Capsules 603

Nisoldipine (Synergistic hypotensive effects, bradycardia, and arrhythmias have been reported in some patients on beta blockers when an oral calcium antagonist was added to the treatment regimen). Products include:
Sular Tablets 2961

Rauwolfia Serpentina (Concurrent use with catecholamine-depleting drugs should be avoided).
No products indexed under this heading.

Rescinnamine (Concurrent use with catecholamine-depleting drugs should be avoided).
No products indexed under this heading.

Reserpine (Concurrent use with catecholamine-depleting drugs should be avoided). Products include:
Diupres Tablets 1691
Hydropres Tablets 1718
Ser-Ap-Es Tablets 867

Verapamil Hydrochloride (Synergistic hypotensive effects, bradycardia, and arrhythmias have been reported in some patients on beta blockers when an oral calcium antagonist was added to the treatment regimen). Products include:
Calan SR Caplets 2571
Calan Tablets 2568
Covera-HS Tablets 2573
Isoptin Injectable 1391
Isoptin Oral Tablets 1393
Isoptin SR Tablets 1395
Verelan Capsules 1455

Food Interactions

Alcohol (Concurrent use increases the number of errors in the eye-hand psychomotor function test).

LEVBID EXTENDED-RELEASE TABLETS
(Hyoscyamine Sulfate) 2549
See **Levsin Drops**

LEVER 2000 ANTIBACTERIAL BAR AND LIQUID
(Triclosan) .... ⊞ 686
None cited in PDR database.

LEVLEN 21 TABLETS
(Levonorgestrel, Ethinyl Estradiol) 646
May interact with barbiturates, tetracyclines, and certain other agents. Compounds in these categories include:

Ampicillin (Potential for reduced efficacy and increased incidence of breakthrough bleeding and menstrual irregularities with concomitant use). Products include:
Omnipen Capsules 2872
Omnipen for Oral Suspension 2873

Ampicillin Sodium (Potential for reduced efficacy and increased incidence of breakthrough bleeding and menstrual irregularities with concomitant use). Products include:
Unasyn 2035

Aprobarbital (Potential for reduced efficacy and increased incidence of breakthrough bleeding and menstrual irregularities with concomitant use).
No products indexed under this heading.

Butabarbital (Potential for reduced efficacy and increased incidence of breakthrough bleeding and menstrual irregularities with concomitant use).
No products indexed under this heading.

Butalbital (Potential for reduced efficacy and increased incidence of breakthrough bleeding and menstrual irregularities with concomitant use). Products include:
Axocet Capsules 2469
Esgic-plus Capsules 1012
Esgic-plus Tablets 1012
Fioricet Tablets 2386
Fioricet with Codeine Capsules 2387
Fiorinal Capsules 2388
Fiorinal with Codeine Capsules 2390
Fiorinal Tablets 2388
Phrenilin 790
Sedapap Tablets 50 mg/650 mg .. 1826

Demeclocycline Hydrochloride (Potential for reduced efficacy and increased incidence of breakthrough bleeding and menstrual irregularities with concomitant use). Products include:
Declomycin Tablets 1421

Doxycycline Calcium (Potential for reduced efficacy and increased incidence of breakthrough bleeding and menstrual irregularities with concomitant use). Products include:
Vibramycin Calcium Oral Suspension Syrup 2038

Doxycycline Hyclate (Potential for reduced efficacy and increased incidence of breakthrough bleeding and menstrual irregularities with concomitant use). Products include:
Doryx Capsules 1970
Vibramycin Hyclate Capsules 2038
Vibramycin Hyclate Intravenous 2040
Vibra-Tabs Film Coated Tablets 2038

Doxycycline Monohydrate (Potential for reduced efficacy and increased incidence of breakthrough bleeding and menstrual irregularities with concomitant use). Products include:
Monodox Capsules 1858
Vibramycin Monohydrate for Oral Suspension 2038

Fosphenytoin Sodium (Potential for reduced efficacy and increased incidence of breakthrough bleeding and menstrual irregularities with concomitant use). Products include:
Cerebyx Injection 1956

Griseofulvin (Potential for reduced efficacy and increased incidence of breakthrough bleeding and menstrual irregularities with concomitant use). Products include:
Fulvicin P/G Tablets 2499
Fulvicin P/G 165 & 330 Tablets 2500
Grifulvin V (griseofulvin tablets) Microsize (griseofulvin oral suspension) Microsize 1944
Gris-PEG Tablets, 125 mg & 250 mg 476

Mephobarbital (Potential for reduced efficacy and increased incidence of breakthrough bleeding and menstrual irregularities with concomitant use). Products include:
Mebaral Tablets 2452

Methacycline Hydrochloride (Potential for reduced efficacy and increased incidence of breakthrough bleeding and menstrual irregularities with concomitant use).
No products indexed under this heading.

Minocycline Hydrochloride (Potential for reduced efficacy and increased incidence of breakthrough bleeding and menstrual irregularities with concomitant use). Products include:
DYNACIN Capsules 1627
Minocin Intravenous 1428
Minocin Oral Suspension 1431
Minocin Pellet-Filled Capsules 1429

Oxytetracycline Hydrochloride (Potential for reduced efficacy and increased incidence of breakthrough bleeding and menstrual irregularities with concomitant use). Products include:
TERAK Ointment .... ⊚ 210
Terra-Cortril Ophthalmic Suspension 2033
Terramycin with Polymyxin B Sulfate Ophthalmic Ointment 2035
Urobiotic-250 Capsules 2038

Pentobarbital Sodium (Potential for reduced efficacy and increased incidence of breakthrough bleeding and menstrual irregularities with concomitant use). Products include:
Nembutal Sodium Capsules 440
Nembutal Sodium Solution 442
Nembutal Sodium Suppositories 444

Phenobarbital (Potential for reduced efficacy and increased incidence of breakthrough bleeding and menstrual irregularities with concomitant use). Products include:
Arco-Lase Plus Tablets 513
Bellergal-S Tablets 2375
Donnatal 2234
Donnatal Extentabs 2234
Donnatal Tablets 2234
Phenobarbital Elixir and Tablets 1523
Quadrinal Tablets 1398

Phenylbutazone (Potential for reduced efficacy and increased incidence of breakthrough bleeding and menstrual irregularities with concomitant use).
No products indexed under this heading.

Phenytoin (Potential for reduced efficacy and increased incidence of breakthrough bleeding and menstrual irregularities with concomitant use). Products include:
Dilantin Infatabs 1967
Dilantin-125 Suspension 1969

Phenytoin Sodium (Potential for reduced efficacy and increased incidence of breakthrough bleeding and menstrual irregularities with concomitant use). Products include:
Dilantin Kapseals 1965

Rifampin (Co-administration has been associated with reduced efficacy and increased incidence of breakthrough bleeding and menstrual irregularities). Products include:
Rifadin 1276
Rifamate Capsules 1278
Rifater 1280
Rimactane Capsules 865

Secobarbital Sodium (Potential for reduced efficacy and increased incidence of breakthrough bleeding and menstrual irregularities with concomitant use). Products include:
Seconal Sodium Pulvules 1529

Tetracycline Hydrochloride (Potential for reduced efficacy and increased incidence of breakthrough bleeding and menstrual irregularities with concomitant use). Products include:
Achromycin V Capsules 1417
Helidac Therapy 2135

Thiamylal Sodium (Potential for reduced efficacy and increased incidence of breakthrough bleeding and menstrual irregularities with concomitant use).
No products indexed under this heading.

LEVLEN 28 TABLETS
(Levonorgestrel, Ethinyl Estradiol) 646
See **Levlen 21 Tablets**

LEVO-DROMORAN INJECTABLE
(Levorphanol Tartrate) 2297
May interact with central nervous system depressants, hypnotics and sedatives, narcotic analgesics, general anesthetics, barbiturates, tricyclic antidepressants, phenothiazines, tranquilizers, antihistamines, mixed agonist/antagonist opioid analgesics, monoamine oxidase inhibitors, skeletal muscle relaxants, and certain other agents. Compounds in these categories include:

Acrivastine (Concurrent use may result in additive central nervous system depressant effects, including respiratory depression, hypotension, profound sedation and coma). Products include:
Semprex-D Capsules 1620

Alfentanil Hydrochloride (Concurrent use may result in additive central nervous system depressant effects, including respiratory depression, hypotension, profound sedation and coma). Products include:
Alfenta Injection 1334

Alprazolam (Concurrent use may result in additive central nervous system depressant effects, including respiratory depression, hypotension, profound sedation and coma). Products include:
Xanax Tablets 2115

IMPORTANT NOTE: Always consult each drug listing in the patient's regimen for possible interactions.

Levo-Dromoran | Interactions Index | 592

Amitriptyline Hydrochloride (Concurrent use may result in additive central nervous system depressant effects, including respiratory depression, hypotension, profound sedation and coma). Products include:

Elavil	2945
Etrafon	2495
Limbitrol	2333
Triavil Tablets	1800

Amoxapine (Concurrent use may result in additive central nervous system depressant effects, including respiratory depression, hypotension, profound sedation and coma). Products include:

Asendin Tablets	1419

Aprobarbital (Concurrent use may result in additive central nervous system depressant effects, including respiratory depression, hypotension, profound sedation and coma).
No products indexed under this heading.

Astemizole (Concurrent use may result in additive central nervous system depressant effects, including respiratory depression, hypotension, profound sedation and coma). Products include:

Hismanal Tablets	1341

Azatadine Maleate (Concurrent use may result in additive central nervous system depressant effects, including respiratory depression, hypotension, profound sedation and coma). Products include:

Trinalin Repetabs Tablets	1373

Baclofen (Concurrent use may result in additive central nervous system depressant effects, including respiratory depression, hypotension, profound sedation and coma). Products include:

Lioresal Intrathecal	1634
Lioresal Tablets	847

Bromodiphenhydramine Hydrochloride (Concurrent use may result in additive central nervous system depressant effects, including respiratory depression, hypotension, profound sedation and coma).
No products indexed under this heading.

Brompheniramine Maleate (Concurrent use may result in additive central nervous system depressant effects, including respiratory depression, hypotension, profound sedation and coma). Products include:

Alka-Seltzer Plus Sinus Medicine	▣ 611
Bromfed Capsules (Extended-Release)	1832
Bromfed Syrup	▣ 712
Bromfed Tablets	1832
Bromfed-DM Cough Syrup	1832
Bromfed-PD Capsules (Extended-Release)	1832
Dimetane-DC Cough Syrup	2232
Dimetane-DX Cough Syrup	2233
Dimetapp Allergy Dye-Free Elixir	▣ 838
Dimetapp Allergy Sinus Caplets	▣ 838
Dimetapp Cold & Allergy Chewable Tablets	▣ 838
Dimetapp Cold & Cough Liqui-Gels	▣ 839
Dimetapp Cold & Fever Suspension	▣ 839
Dimetapp DM Elixir	▣ 840
Dimetapp Elixir	▣ 840
Dimetapp Extentabs	▣ 841
Dimetapp Tablets/Liqui-Gels	▣ 841
Rondec Chewable Tablets	974
Vicks DayQuil Allergy Relief 12-Hour Extended Release Tablets	▣ 733
Vicks DayQuil Allergy Relief 4-Hour Tablets	▣ 733

Buprenorphine (In patients on pure opioid agonist therapy, mixed agonist/antagonist analgesics may precipitate withdrawal symptoms). Products include:

Buprenex Injectable	2170

Buspirone Hydrochloride (Concurrent use may result in additive central nervous system depressant effects, including respiratory depression, hypotension, profound sedation and coma). Products include:

BuSpar Tablets	738

Butabarbital (Concurrent use may result in additive central nervous system depressant effects, including respiratory depression, hypotension, profound sedation and coma).
No products indexed under this heading.

Butalbital (Concurrent use may result in additive central nervous system depressant effects, including respiratory depression, hypotension, profound sedation and coma). Products include:

Axocet Capsules	2469
Esgic-plus Capsules	1012
Esgic-plus Tablets	1012
Fioricet Tablets	2386
Fioricet with Codeine Capsules	2387
Fiorinal Capsules	2388
Fiorinal with Codeine Capsules	2390
Fiorinal Tablets	2388
Phrenilin	790
Sedapap Tablets 50 mg/650 mg	1826

Butorphanol Tartrate (In patients on pure opioid agonist therapy, mixed agonist/antagonist analgesics may precipitate withdrawal symptoms). Products include:

Stadol	779

Carisoprodol (Concurrent use may result in additive central nervous system depressant effects, including respiratory depression, hypotension, profound sedation and coma). Products include:

Soma Compound w/Codeine Tablets	2784
Soma Compound Tablets	2783
Soma Tablets	2782

Cetirizine Hydrochloride (Concurrent use may result in additive central nervous system depressant effects, including respiratory depression, hypotension, profound sedation and coma). Products include:

Zyrtec Tablets	2053

Chlordiazepoxide (Concurrent use may result in additive central nervous system depressant effects, including respiratory depression, hypotension, profound sedation and coma). Products include:

Limbitrol	2333

Chlordiazepoxide Hydrochloride (Concurrent use may result in additive central nervous system depressant effects, including respiratory depression, hypotension, profound sedation and coma). Products include:

Librax Capsules	2330
Librium Capsules	2331
Librium Injectable	2332

Chlorpheniramine Maleate (Concurrent use may result in additive central nervous system depressant effects, including respiratory depression, hypotension, profound sedation and coma). Products include:

Alka-Seltzer Plus Cold Medicine	▣ 611
Alka-Seltzer Plus Cold Medicine Liqui-Gels	▣ 612
Alka-Seltzer Plus Cold & Cough Medicine	▣ 611
Alka-Seltzer Plus Cold & Cough Medicine Liqui-Gels	▣ 612
Alka-Seltzer Plus Flu & Body Aches Effervescent Tablets	▣ 612
Allerest Maximum Strength	▣ 649
Allerest Sinus Pain Formula	▣ 649
Ana-Kit Anaphylaxis Emergency Treatment Kit	611
Atrohist Pediatric Capsules	1603
Atrohist Plus Tablets	1605
BC Cold Powder Multi-Symptom Formula (Cold-Sinus-Allergy)	▣ 631
Cerose DM	853
Cheracol Plus Head Cold/Cough Formula	▣ 741
Children's TYLENOL Cold Multi-Symptom Chewable Tablets and Liquid	1559
Children's TYLENOL Cold Plus Cough Multi Symptom Chewable Tablets and Liquid	1560
Children's TYLENOL Flu Suspension Liquid	1560
Children's Vicks DayQuil Allergy Relief	▣ 730
Children's Vicks NyQuil Cold/Cough Relief	▣ 731
Chlor-Trimeton Allergy Decongestant Tablets	▣ 759
Chlor-Trimeton Allergy Tablets	▣ 758
Allergy-Sinus Comtrex Multi-Symptom Allergy-Sinus Formula Tablets and Caplets	▣ 639
Comtrex Multi-Symptom	▣ 638
Contac Continuous Action Nasal Decongestant/Antihistamine 12 Hour Capsules	▣ 773
Contac Maximum Strength Continuous Action Decongestant/Antihistamine 12 Hour Caplets	▣ 772
Contac Severe Cold and Flu Formula Caplets	▣ 773
Coricidin Cold + Flu Tablets	▣ 760
Coricidin Cough + Cold Tablets	▣ 760
Coricidin 'D' Decongestant Tablets	▣ 760
D.A. II Tablets	972
D.A. Chewable Tablets	970
Dura-Tap/PD Capsules	970
Dura-Vent/DA Tablets	972
Efidac 24 Chlorpheniramine	▣ 655
Extendryl	1003
Fedahist Gyrocaps	2545
Hycomine Compound Tablets	948
Kronofed-A	994
Nolamine Timed-Release Tablets	790
Novahistine Elixir	▣ 782
Ornade Spansule Capsules	2678
PediaCare Cough-Cold Chewable Tablets and Liquid	1569
PediaCare NightRest Cough-Cold Liquid	1569
Pediatric Vicks 44m Cough & Cold Relief	▣ 737
Pyrroxate Caplets	▣ 742
Ryna	▣ 804
Sinarest	▣ 663
Sine-Off Sinus Medicine	▣ 784
Singlet Tablets	▣ 785
Sinulin Tablets	792
Sinutab Sinus Allergy Medication, Maximum Strength Tablets and Caplets	▣ 823
Sudafed Cold & Allergy Tablets	▣ 826
Teldrin 12 Hour Antihistamine/Nasal Decongestant Allergy Relief Capsules	▣ 786
TheraFlu Flu and Cold Medicine	▣ 750
Theraflu Maximum Strength Flu and Cold Medicine For Sore Throat	▣ 751
TheraFlu Flu, Cold and Cough Medicine	▣ 750
TheraFlu Maximum Strength Nighttime Flu, Cold & Cough Medicine	▣ 751
Triaminic Night Time	▣ 754
Triaminic Syrup	▣ 755
Triaminic Triaminicol Cold & Cough	▣ 756
Triaminicin Tablets	▣ 756
Tussend	1830
TYLENOL Allergy Sinus, Maximum Strength Caplets and Gelcaps	1571
TYLENOL Cold Medication, Multi-Symptom Formula Tablets and Caplets	1572
TYLENOL Cold Medication, Multi-Symptom Hot Liquid Packets	1572
Vicks 44 LiquiCaps Cough, Cold & Flu Relief	▣ 728
Vicks 44M Cough, Cold & Flu Relief	▣ 729

Chlorpheniramine Polistirex (Concurrent use may result in additive central nervous system depressant effects, including respiratory depression, hypotension, profound sedation and coma). Products include:

Tussionex Pennkinetic Extended-Release Suspension	1624

Chlorpheniramine Tannate (Concurrent use may result in additive central nervous system depressant effects, including respiratory depression, hypotension, profound sedation and coma). Products include:

Atrohist Pediatric Suspension	1604
Atrohist Pediatric Suspension Dye-Free	1604
Rynatan	2781
Rynatuss	2782

Chlorpromazine (Concurrent use may result in additive central nervous system depressant effects, including respiratory depression, hypotension, profound sedation and coma). Products include:

Thorazine Suppositories	2701

Chlorpromazine Hydrochloride (Concurrent use may result in additive central nervous system depressant effects, including respiratory depression, hypotension, profound sedation and coma). Products include:

Thorazine	2701

Chlorprothixene (Concurrent use may result in additive central nervous system depressant effects, including respiratory depression, hypotension, profound sedation and coma).
No products indexed under this heading.

Chlorprothixene Hydrochloride (Concurrent use may result in additive central nervous system depressant effects, including respiratory depression, hypotension, profound sedation and coma).
No products indexed under this heading.

Chlorprothixene Lactate (Concurrent use may result in additive central nervous system depressant effects, including respiratory depression, hypotension, profound sedation and coma).
No products indexed under this heading.

Chlorzoxazone (Concurrent use may result in additive central nervous system depressant effects, including respiratory depression, hypotension, profound sedation and coma). Products include:

Parafon Forte DSC Caplets	1590

Clemastine Fumarate (Concurrent use may result in additive central nervous system depressant effects, including respiratory depression, hypotension, profound sedation and coma). Products include:

Tavist Syrup	2426
Tavist Tablets	2427
Tavist-1 12 Hour Relief Tablets	▣ 749
Tavist-D 12 Hour Relief Tablets	▣ 750

Clomipramine Hydrochloride (Concurrent use may result in additive central nervous system depressant effects, including respiratory depression, hypotension, profound sedation and coma). Products include:

Anafranil Capsules	819

(▣ Described in PDR For Nonprescription Drugs)   (◉ Described in PDR For Ophthalmology)

Interactions Index

Clorazepate Dipotassium (Concurrent use may result in additive central nervous system depressant effects, including respiratory depression, hypotension, profound sedation and coma). Products include:
Tranxene 459

Clozapine (Concurrent use may result in additive central nervous system depressant effects, including respiratory depression, hypotension, profound sedation and coma). Products include:
Clozaril Tablets 2377

Codeine Phosphate (Concurrent use may result in additive central nervous system depressant effects, including respiratory depression, hypotension, profound sedation and coma). Products include:
Brontex 2130
Dimetane-DC Cough Syrup 2232
Fioricet with Codeine Capsules 2387
Fiorinal with Codeine Capsules 2390
Nucofed 2225
Phenergan with Codeine 2883
Phenergan VC with Codeine 2888
Robitussin A-C Syrup 2248
Robitussin-DAC Syrup 2249
Ryna 804
Soma Compound w/Codeine Tablets 2784
Tylenol with Codeine 1592

Cyclobenzaprine Hydrochloride (Concurrent use may result in additive central nervous system depressant effects, including respiratory depression, hypotension, profound sedation and coma). Products include:
Flexeril Tablets 1701

Cyproheptadine Hydrochloride (Concurrent use may result in additive central nervous system depressant effects, including respiratory depression, hypotension, profound sedation and coma). Products include:
Periactin 1767

Dantrolene Sodium (Concurrent use may result in additive central nervous system depressant effects, including respiratory depression, hypotension, profound sedation and coma). Products include:
Dantrium Capsules 2131
Dantrium Intravenous 2132

Desflurane (Concurrent use may result in additive central nervous system depressant effects, including respiratory depression, hypotension, profound sedation and coma). Products include:
Suprane (desflurane, USP) 1865

Desipramine Hydrochloride (Concurrent use may result in additive central nervous system depressant effects, including respiratory depression, hypotension, profound sedation and coma). Products include:
Norpramin Tablets 1273

Dexchlorpheniramine Maleate (Concurrent use may result in additive central nervous system depressant effects, including respiratory depression, hypotension, profound sedation and coma).
No products indexed under this heading.

Dezocine (In patients on pure opioid agonist therapy, mixed agonist/antagonist analgesics may precipitate withdrawal symptoms). Products include:
Dalgan Injection 529

Diazepam (Concurrent use may result in additive central nervous system depressant effects, including respiratory depression, hypotension, profound sedation and coma). Products include:
Dizac (diazepam injectable emulsion) CIV 1862
Valium Injectable 2336
Valium Tablets 2335

Diphenhydramine Citrate (Concurrent use may result in additive central nervous system depressant effects, including respiratory depression, hypotension, profound sedation and coma). Products include:
Excedrin P.M. Analgesic/Sleeping Aid Tablets, Caplets, Liquigels 735

Diphenhydramine Hydrochloride (Concurrent use may result in additive central nervous system depressant effects, including respiratory depression, hypotension, profound sedation and coma). Products include:
Actifed Allergy Daytime/Nighttime Caplets 808
Actifed Sinus Daytime/Nighttime Tablets and Caplets 809
Extra Strength Bayer PM Aspirin Plus Sleep Aid 617
Benadryl Allergy Chewables 811
Benadryl Allergy/Cold Tablets 811
Benadryl Allergy Decongestant Liquid Medication 812
Benadryl Allergy Decongestant Tablets 812
Benadryl Allergy Liquid Medication 813
Benadryl Allergy 811
Benadryl Allergy Sinus Headache Caplets 813
Benadryl Dye-Free Allergy Liquigel Softgels 813
Benadryl Dye-Free Allergy Liquid Medication 814
Benadryl Itch Relief Stick Extra Strength 814
Benadryl Cream 814
Benadryl Gel 815
Benadryl Spray 815
Benadryl Injection 1955
Contac Day & Night Cold/Flu Night Caplets 772
Contac Night Allergy/Sinus Caplets 771
Extra Strength Doan's P.M. 653
Excedrin P.M. Analgesic/Sleeping Aid Tablets, Caplets, Liquigels 643
Nytol QuickCaps Caplets 632
Sleepinal Night-time Sleep Aid Capsules and Softgels 798
TYLENOL Allergy Sinus NightTime, Maximum Strength Caplets 1571
TYLENOL Flu NightTime, Maximum Strength Gelcaps 1575
TYLENOL Flu NightTime, Maximum Strength Hot Medication Packets 1575
TYLENOL PM Pain Reliever/Sleep Aid, Extra Strength Gelcaps, Caplets, Geltabs 1576
TYLENOL Severe Allergy Medication Caplets 1571
Maximum Strength Unisom Sleepgels 1990
Unisom With Pain Relief-Nighttime Sleep Aid and Pain Reliever 1991

Diphenylpyraline Hydrochloride (Concurrent use may result in additive central nervous system depressant effects, including respiratory depression, hypotension, profound sedation and coma).
No products indexed under this heading.

Doxepin Hydrochloride (Concurrent use may result in additive central nervous system depressant effects, including respiratory depression, hypotension, profound sedation and coma). Products include:
Adapin Capsules 1542
Sinequan 2028
Zonalon Cream 1042

Droperidol (Concurrent use may result in additive central nervous system depressant effects, including respiratory depression, hypotension, profound sedation and coma). Products include:
Inapsine Injection 462

Enflurane (Concurrent use may result in additive central nervous system depressant effects, including respiratory depression, hypotension, profound sedation and coma).
No products indexed under this heading.

Estazolam (Concurrent use may result in additive central nervous system depressant effects, including respiratory depression, hypotension, profound sedation and coma). Products include:
ProSom Tablets 457

Ethchlorvynol (Concurrent use may result in additive central nervous system depressant effects, including respiratory depression, hypotension, profound sedation and coma). Products include:
Placidyl Capsules 456

Ethinamate (Concurrent use may result in additive central nervous system depressant effects, including respiratory depression, hypotension, profound sedation and coma).
No products indexed under this heading.

Fentanyl (Concurrent use may result in additive central nervous system depressant effects, including respiratory depression, hypotension, profound sedation and coma). Products include:
Duragesic Transdermal System 1336

Fentanyl Citrate (Concurrent use may result in additive central nervous system depressant effects, including respiratory depression, hypotension, profound sedation and coma). Products include:
Sublimaze Injection 463

Fluphenazine Decanoate (Concurrent use may result in additive central nervous system depressant effects, including respiratory depression, hypotension, profound sedation and coma). Products include:
Prolixin Decanoate 510

Fluphenazine Enanthate (Concurrent use may result in additive central nervous system depressant effects, including respiratory depression, hypotension, profound sedation and coma). Products include:
Prolixin Enanthate 510

Fluphenazine Hydrochloride (Concurrent use may result in additive central nervous system depressant effects, including respiratory depression, hypotension, profound sedation and coma). Products include:
Prolixin 510

Flurazepam Hydrochloride (Concurrent use may result in additive central nervous system depressant effects, including respiratory depression, hypotension, profound sedation and coma). Products include:
Dalmane Capsules 2329

Furazolidone (Although no interaction between MAO inhibitors and levorphanol has been observed, concurrent use is not recommended). Products include:
Furoxone 2221

Glutethimide (Concurrent use may result in additive central nervous system depressant effects, including respiratory depression, hypotension, profound sedation and coma).
No products indexed under this heading.

Haloperidol (Concurrent use may result in additive central nervous system depressant effects, including respiratory depression, hypotension, profound sedation and coma). Products include:
Haldol Injection, Tablets and Concentrate 1585

Haloperidol Decanoate (Concurrent use may result in additive central nervous system depressant effects, including respiratory depression, hypotension, profound sedation and coma). Products include:
Haldol Decanoate 1587

Hydrocodone Bitartrate (Concurrent use may result in additive central nervous system depressant effects, including respiratory depression, hypotension, profound sedation and coma). Products include:
Codiclear DH Syrup 808
Duratuss HD Elixir 2750
Histussin D Liquid 670
Hycodan Tablets and Syrup 946
Hycomine Compound Tablets 948
Hycomine 947
Hycotuss Expectorant Syrup 950
Hydrocet Capsules 787
Lorcet 10/650 Tablets 1016
Lortab 2751
Tussend 1830
Tussend Expectorant 1831
Vicodin Tablets 1404
Vicodin ES Tablets 1405
Vicodin HP Tablets 1403
Vicodin Tuss Expectorant 1406
Zydone Capsules 967

Hydrocodone Polistirex (Concurrent use may result in additive central nervous system depressant effects, including respiratory depression, hypotension, profound sedation and coma). Products include:
Tussionex Pennkinetic Extended-Release Suspension 1624

Hydromorphone Hydrochloride (Concurrent use may result in additive central nervous system depressant effects, including respiratory depression, hypotension, profound sedation and coma). Products include:
Dilaudid Ampules 1382
Dilaudid Cough Syrup 1383
Dilaudid-HP Injection 1384
Dilaudid-HP Lyophilized Powder 250 mg 1384
Dilaudid 1382
Dilaudid Oral Liquid 1386
Dilaudid 1382
Dilaudid Tablets - 8 mg. 1386

Hydroxyzine Hydrochloride (Concurrent use may result in additive central nervous system depressant effects, including respiratory depression, hypotension, profound sedation and coma). Products include:
Atarax Tablets & Syrup 1992
Marax Tablets & DF Syrup 2015
Vistaril Intramuscular Solution 2042

Imipramine Hydrochloride (Concurrent use may result in additive central nervous system depressant effects, including respiratory depression, hypotension, profound sedation and coma). Products include:
Tofranil Ampuls 873
Tofranil Tablets 875

IMPORTANT NOTE: Always consult each drug listing in the patient's regimen for possible interactions.

Levo-Dromoran Interactions Index 594

Imipramine Pamoate (Concurrent use may result in additive central nervous system depressant effects, including respiratory depression, hypotension, profound sedation and coma). Products include:
Tofranil-PM Capsules ... 876

Isocarboxazid (Although no interaction between MAO inhibitors and levorphanol has been observed, concurrent use is not recommended).
No products indexed under this heading.

Isoflurane (Concurrent use may result in additive central nervous system depressant effects, including respiratory depression, hypotension, profound sedation and coma).
No products indexed under this heading.

Ketamine Hydrochloride (Concurrent use may result in additive central nervous system depressant effects, including respiratory depression, hypotension, profound sedation and coma).
No products indexed under this heading.

Levomethadyl Acetate Hydrochloride (Concurrent use may result in additive central nervous system depressant effects, including respiratory depression, hypotension, profound sedation and coma). Products include:
Orlaam Oral Solution ... 2361

Loratadine (Concurrent use may result in additive central nervous system depressant effects, including respiratory depression, hypotension, profound sedation and coma). Products include:
Claritin Tablets ... 2485
Claritin-D Tablets ... 2487

Lorazepam (Concurrent use may result in additive central nervous system depressant effects, including respiratory depression, hypotension, profound sedation and coma). Products include:
Ativan Injection ... 2805
Ativan Tablets ... 2807

Loxapine Hydrochloride (Concurrent use may result in additive central nervous system depressant effects, including respiratory depression, hypotension, profound sedation and coma). Products include:
Loxitane ... 1426

Loxapine Succinate (Concurrent use may result in additive central nervous system depressant effects, including respiratory depression, hypotension, profound sedation and coma). Products include:
Loxitane Capsules ... 1426

Maprotiline Hydrochloride (Concurrent use may result in additive central nervous system depressant effects, including respiratory depression, hypotension, profound sedation and coma). Products include:
Ludiomil Tablets ... 861

Meperidine Hydrochloride (Concurrent use may result in additive central nervous system depressant effects, including respiratory depression, hypotension, profound sedation and coma). Products include:
Demerol ... 2438
Mepergan Injection ... 2859

Mephobarbital (Concurrent use may result in additive central nervous system depressant effects, including respiratory depression, hypotension, profound sedation and coma). Products include:
Mebaral Tablets ... 2452

Meprobamate (Concurrent use may result in additive central nervous system depressant effects, including respiratory depression, hypotension, profound sedation and coma). Products include:
Miltown Tablets ... 2780
PMB 200 and PMB 400 ... 2890

Mesoridazine Besylate (Concurrent use may result in additive central nervous system depressant effects, including respiratory depression, hypotension, profound sedation and coma). Products include:
Serentil ... 689

Metaxalone (Concurrent use may result in additive central nervous system depressant effects, including respiratory depression, hypotension, profound sedation and coma). Products include:
Skelaxin Tablets ... 793

Methadone Hydrochloride (Concurrent use may result in additive central nervous system depressant effects, including respiratory depression, hypotension, profound sedation and coma). Products include:
Methadone Hydrochloride Oral Concentrate ... 2356
Methadone Hydrochloride Oral Solution & Tablets ... 2357

Methdilazine Hydrochloride (Concurrent use may result in additive central nervous system depressant effects, including respiratory depression, hypotension, profound sedation and coma).
No products indexed under this heading.

Methocarbamol (Concurrent use may result in additive central nervous system depressant effects, including respiratory depression, hypotension, profound sedation and coma). Products include:
Robaxin Injectable ... 2245
Robaxin Tablets ... 2246
Robaxisal Tablets ... 2246

Methohexital Sodium (Concurrent use may result in additive central nervous system depressant effects, including respiratory depression, hypotension, profound sedation and coma).
No products indexed under this heading.

Methotrimeprazine (Concurrent use may result in additive central nervous system depressant effects, including respiratory depression, hypotension, profound sedation and coma). Products include:
Levoprome ... 1321

Methoxyflurane (Concurrent use may result in additive central nervous system depressant effects, including respiratory depression, hypotension, profound sedation and coma).
No products indexed under this heading.

Midazolam Hydrochloride (Concurrent use may result in additive central nervous system depressant effects, including respiratory depression, hypotension, profound sedation and coma). Products include:
Versed Injection ... 2324

Molindone Hydrochloride (Concurrent use may result in additive central nervous system depressant effects, including respiratory depression, hypotension, profound sedation and coma). Products include:
Moban Tablets and Concentrate ... 1036

Morphine Sulfate (Concurrent use may result in additive central nervous system depressant effects, including respiratory depression, hypotension, profound sedation and coma). Products include:
Astramorph/PF Injection, USP (Preservative-Free) ... 526
Duramorph Injection ... 983
Infumorph 200 and Infumorph 500 Sterile Solutions ... 985
Kadian Capsules ... 2948
MS Contin Tablets ... 2149
MSIR ... 2152
Oramorph SR (Morphine Sulfate Sustained Release Tablets) ... 2359
RMS Suppositories CII ... 2766
Roxanol ... 2365

Nalbuphine Hydrochloride (In patients on pure opioid agonist therapy, mixed agonist/antagonist analgesics may precipitate withdrawal symptoms). Products include:
Nubain Injection ... 952

Nortriptyline Hydrochloride (Concurrent use may result in additive central nervous system depressant effects, including respiratory depression, hypotension, profound sedation and coma). Products include:
Pamelor ... 2409

Opium Alkaloids (Concurrent use may result in additive central nervous system depressant effects, including respiratory depression, hypotension, profound sedation and coma).
No products indexed under this heading.

Orphenadrine Citrate (Concurrent use may result in additive central nervous system depressant effects, including respiratory depression, hypotension, profound sedation and coma). Products include:
Norflex ... 1554
Norgesic ... 1554

Oxazepam (Concurrent use may result in additive central nervous system depressant effects, including respiratory depression, hypotension, profound sedation and coma). Products include:
Serax Capsules ... 2916
Serax Tablets ... 2916

Oxycodone Hydrochloride (Concurrent use may result in additive central nervous system depressant effects, including respiratory depression, hypotension, profound sedation and coma). Products include:
OxyContin Tablets ... 2163
OxyIR Capsules ... 2167
Percocet Tablets ... 955
Percodan Tablets ... 955
Percodan-Demi Tablets ... 956
Roxicodone Tablets, Oral Solution & Intensol (Oxycodone) ... 2366
Tylox Capsules ... 1593

Pentazocine Hydrochloride (In patients on pure opioid agonist therapy, mixed agonist/antagonist analgesics may precipitate withdrawal symptoms). Products include:
Talacen Caplets ... 2464
Talwin Compound ... 2466
Talwin Nx Tablets ... 2467

Pentazocine Lactate (In patients on pure opioid agonist therapy, mixed agonist/antagonist analgesics may precipitate withdrawal symptoms). Products include:
Talwin Injection ... 2465

Pentobarbital Sodium (Concurrent use may result in additive central nervous system depressant effects, including respiratory depression, hypotension, profound sedation and coma). Products include:
Nembutal Sodium Capsules ... 440
Nembutal Sodium Solution ... 442
Nembutal Sodium Suppositories ... 444

Perphenazine (Concurrent use may result in additive central nervous system depressant effects, including respiratory depression, hypotension, profound sedation and coma). Products include:
Etrafon ... 2495
Triavil Tablets ... 1800
Trilafon ... 2532

Phenelzine Sulfate (Although no interaction between MAO inhibitors and levorphanol has been observed, concurrent use is not recommended). Products include:
Nardil ... 1977

Phenobarbital (Concurrent use may result in additive central nervous system depressant effects, including respiratory depression, hypotension, profound sedation and coma). Products include:
Arco-Lase Plus Tablets ... 513
Bellergal-S Tablets ... 2375
Donnatal ... 2234
Donnatal Extentabs ... 2234
Donnatal Tablets ... 2234
Phenobarbital Elixir and Tablets ... 1523
Quadrinal Tablets ... 1398

Prazepam (Concurrent use may result in additive central nervous system depressant effects, including respiratory depression, hypotension, profound sedation and coma).
No products indexed under this heading.

Prochlorperazine (Concurrent use may result in additive central nervous system depressant effects, including respiratory depression, hypotension, profound sedation and coma). Products include:
Compazine ... 2644

Promethazine Hydrochloride (Concurrent use may result in additive central nervous system depressant effects, including respiratory depression, hypotension, profound sedation and coma). Products include:
Mepergan Injection ... 2859
Phenergan with Codeine ... 2883
Phenergan with Dextromethorphan ... 2885
Phenergan Injection ... 2880
Phenergan Suppositories ... 2882
Phenergan Syrup ... 2881
Phenergan Tablets ... 2882
Phenergan VC ... 2886
Phenergan VC with Codeine ... 2888

Propofol (Concurrent use may result in additive central nervous system depressant effects, including respiratory depression, hypotension, profound sedation and coma). Products include:
Diprivan Injectable Emulsion ... 2939

Propoxyphene Hydrochloride (Concurrent use may result in additive central nervous system depressant effects, including respiratory depression, hypotension, profound sedation and coma). Products include:
Darvon ... 1475
Wygesic Tablets ... 2930

(Described in PDR For Nonprescription Drugs) (◉ Described in PDR For Ophthalmology)

Propoxyphene Napsylate (Concurrent use may result in additive central nervous system depressant effects, including respiratory depression, hypotension, profound sedation and coma). Products include:
Darvon-N/Darvocet-N 1473

Protriptyline Hydrochloride (Concurrent use may result in additive central nervous system depressant effects, including respiratory depression, hypotension, profound sedation and coma). Products include:
Vivactil Tablets 1820

Pyrilamine Maleate (Concurrent use may result in additive central nervous system depressant effects, including respiratory depression, hypotension, profound sedation and coma). Products include:
4-Way Fast Acting Nasal Spray (regular & mentholated) 644
Maximum Strength Multi-Symptom Formula Midol 621
PMS Multi-Symptom Formula Midol 622

Pyrilamine Tannate (Concurrent use may result in additive central nervous system depressant effects, including respiratory depression, hypotension, profound sedation and coma). Products include:
Atrohist Pediatric Suspension 1604
Atrohist Pediatric Suspension Dye-Free 1604
Rynatan 2781

Quazepam (Concurrent use may result in additive central nervous system depressant effects, including respiratory depression, hypotension, profound sedation and coma). Products include:
Doral Tablets 2773

Risperidone (Concurrent use may result in additive central nervous system depressant effects, including respiratory depression, hypotension, profound sedation and coma). Products include:
Risperdal Tablets 1348

Secobarbital Sodium (Concurrent use may result in additive central nervous system depressant effects, including respiratory depression, hypotension, profound sedation and coma). Products include:
Seconal Sodium Pulvules 1529

Selegiline Hydrochloride (Although no interaction between MAO inhibitors and levorphanol has been observed, concurrent use is not recommended). Products include:
Eldepryl Capsules 2729

Sevoflurane (Concurrent use may result in additive central nervous system depressant effects, including respiratory depression, hypotension, profound sedation and coma). No products indexed under this heading.

Sufentanil Citrate (Concurrent use may result in additive central nervous system depressant effects, including respiratory depression, hypotension, profound sedation and coma). Products include:
Sufenta Injection 1355

Temazepam (Concurrent use may result in additive central nervous system depressant effects, including respiratory depression, hypotension, profound sedation and coma). Products include:
Restoril Capsules 2413

Terfenadine (Concurrent use may result in additive central nervous system depressant effects, including respiratory depression, hypotension, profound sedation and coma). Products include:
Seldane Tablets 1284
Seldane-D Extended-Release Tablets 1286

Thiamylal Sodium (Concurrent use may result in additive central nervous system depressant effects, including respiratory depression, hypotension, profound sedation and coma). No products indexed under this heading.

Thioridazine Hydrochloride (Concurrent use may result in additive central nervous system depressant effects, including respiratory depression, hypotension, profound sedation and coma). Products include:
Mellaril 2398

Thiothixene (Concurrent use may result in additive central nervous system depressant effects, including respiratory depression, hypotension, profound sedation and coma). Products include:
Navane Capsules and Concentrate ... 2018
Navane Intramuscular 2019

Tranylcypromine Sulfate (Although no interaction between MAO inhibitors and levorphanol has been observed, concurrent use is not recommended). Products include:
Parnate Tablets 2679

Triazolam (Concurrent use may result in additive central nervous system depressant effects, including respiratory depression, hypotension, profound sedation and coma). Products include:
Halcion Tablets 2093

Trifluoperazine Hydrochloride (Concurrent use may result in additive central nervous system depressant effects, including respiratory depression, hypotension, profound sedation and coma). Products include:
Stelazine 2692

Trimeprazine Tartrate (Concurrent use may result in additive central nervous system depressant effects, including respiratory depression, hypotension, profound sedation and coma). No products indexed under this heading.

Trimipramine Maleate (Concurrent use may result in additive central nervous system depressant effects, including respiratory depression, hypotension, profound sedation and coma). Products include:
Surmontil Capsules 2917

Tripelennamine Hydrochloride (Concurrent use may result in additive central nervous system depressant effects, including respiratory depression, hypotension, profound sedation and coma). Products include:
PBZ Tablets 863
PBZ-SR Tablets 862

Triprolidine Hydrochloride (Concurrent use may result in additive central nervous system depressant effects, including respiratory depression, hypotension, profound sedation and coma). Products include:
Actifed Cold & Allergy Tablets 807

Actifed Cold & Sinus Caplets and Tablets 808

Zolpidem Tartrate (Concurrent use may result in additive central nervous system depressant effects, including respiratory depression, hypotension, profound sedation and coma). Products include:
Ambien Tablets 2559

Food Interactions

Alcohol (Concurrent use may result in additive central nervous system depressant effects, including respiratory depression, hypotension, profound sedation and coma).

LEVO-DROMORAN TABLETS
(Levorphanol Tartrate) 2297
See Levo-Dromoran Injectable

LEVOPHED BITARTRATE INJECTION
(Norepinephrine Bitartrate) 2445
May interact with monoamine oxidase inhibitors, tricyclic antidepressants, and certain other agents. Compounds in these categories include:

Amitriptyline Hydrochloride (Severe prolonged hypertension). Products include:
Elavil 2945
Etrafon 2495
Limbitrol 2333
Triavil Tablets 1800

Amoxapine (Severe prolonged hypertension). Products include:
Asendin Tablets 1419

Clomipramine Hydrochloride (Severe prolonged hypertension). Products include:
Anafranil Capsules 819

Cyclopropane (Increases cardiac autonomic irritability).

Desipramine Hydrochloride (Severe prolonged hypertension). Products include:
Norpramin Tablets 1273

Doxepin Hydrochloride (Severe prolonged hypertension). Products include:
Adapin Capsules 1542
Sinequan 2028
Zonalon Cream 1042

Furazolidone (Severe prolonged hypertension). Products include:
Furoxone 2221

Halothane (Increases cardiac autonomic irritability). Products include:
Fluothane 2830

Imipramine Hydrochloride (Severe prolonged hypertension). Products include:
Tofranil Ampuls 873
Tofranil Tablets 875

Imipramine Pamoate (Severe prolonged hypertension). Products include:
Tofranil-PM Capsules 876

Isocarboxazid (Severe prolonged hypertension). No products indexed under this heading.

Maprotiline Hydrochloride (Severe prolonged hypertension). Products include:
Ludiomil Tablets 861

Nortriptyline Hydrochloride (Severe prolonged hypertension). Products include:
Pamelor 2409

Phenelzine Sulfate (Severe prolonged hypertension). Products include:
Nardil 1977

Protriptyline Hydrochloride (Severe prolonged hypertension). Products include:
Vivactil Tablets 1820

Selegiline Hydrochloride (Severe prolonged hypertension). Products include:
Eldepryl Capsules 2729

Tranylcypromine Sulfate (Severe prolonged hypertension). Products include:
Parnate Tablets 2679

Trimipramine Maleate (Severe prolonged hypertension). Products include:
Surmontil Capsules 2917

LEVOPROME
(Methotrimeprazine) 1321
May interact with monoamine oxidase inhibitors, antihypertensives, central nervous system depressants, narcotic analgesics, barbiturates, general anesthetics, antihistamines, and certain other agents. Compounds in these categories include:

Acebutolol Hydrochloride (Concurrent use is contraindicated). Products include:
Sectral Capsules 2914

Acrivastine (Potentiation of CNS depression). Products include:
Semprex-D Capsules 1620

Alfentanil Hydrochloride (Potential for additive effects; the dosage of either drug should be reduced and critically adjusted when used concomitantly or in sequence). Products include:
Alfenta Injection 1334

Alprazolam (Potential for additive effects; the dosage of either drug should be reduced and critically adjusted when used concomitantly or in sequence). Products include:
Xanax Tablets 2115

Amlodipine Besylate (Concurrent use is contraindicated). Products include:
Lotrel Capsules 858
Norvasc Tablets 2020

Analgesics, unspecified (Potentiation of CNS depression).

Aprobarbital (Potential for additive effects; the dosage of either drug should be reduced and critically adjusted when used concomitantly or in sequence). No products indexed under this heading.

Aspirin (Potential for additive effects; the dosage of either drug should be reduced and critically adjusted when used concomitantly or in sequence). Products include:
Alka-Seltzer Cherry Effervescent Antacid and Pain Reliever 609
Alka-Seltzer Extra Strength Effervescent Antacid and Pain Reliever 609
Alka-Seltzer Lemon Lime Effervescent Antacid and Pain Reliever 609
Alka-Seltzer Original Effervescent Antacid and Pain Reliever 609
Alka-Seltzer Plus 611
Alka-Seltzer Plus Sinus Medicine ... 611
Ascriptin 631
Arthritis Strength BC Powder 631
BC Cold Powder Multi-Symptom Formula (Cold-Sinus-Allergy) 631
BC Cold Powder Non-Drowsy Formula (Cold-Sinus) 631
BC Powder 631
Genuine Bayer Aspirin Tablets & Caplets 618
Extra Strength Bayer Arthritis Pain Regimen Formula 615
Extra Strength Bayer Aspirin Caplets & Tablets 617

IMPORTANT NOTE: Always consult each drug listing in the patient's regimen for possible interactions.

Levoprome **Interactions Index** 596

Extended-Release Bayer 8-Hour Aspirin ND 616
Extra Strength Bayer Plus Aspirin Caplets ND 617
Extra Strength Bayer PM Aspirin Plus Sleep Aid ND 617
Aspirin Regimen Bayer 81 mg Tablets with Calcium ND 615
Aspirin Regimen Bayer Adult Low Strength 81 mg Tablets ND 613
Aspirin Regimen Bayer Children's Chewable Aspirin ND 616
Aspirin Regimen Bayer Regular Strength 325 mg Caplets ND 613
Bufferin Analgesic Tablets ND 636
Arthritis Strength Bufferin Analgesic Caplets ND 637
Extra Strength Bufferin Analgesic Tablets ND 637
Cama Arthritis Pain Reliever ND 748
Darvon Compound-65 Pulvules 1475
Easprin 1971
Ecotrin 2625
Ecotrin Enteric Coated Aspirin Maximum Strength Tablets and Caplets ND 775
Ecotrin Enteric Coated Aspirin Regular Strength Tablets 2625
Empirin Aspirin Tablets ND 818
Excedrin Extra-Strength Analgesic Tablets, Caplets, and Geltabs 734
Fiorinal Capsules 2388
Fiorinal with Codeine Capsules 2390
Fiorinal Tablets 2388
Goody's Extra Strength Headache Powders ND 632
Goody's Extra Strength Pain Relief Tablets ND 632
Halfprin Tablets 1413
Norgesic 1554
Percodan Tablets 955
Percodan-Demi Tablets 956
Robaxisal Tablets 2246
Soma Compound w/Codeine Tablets 2784
Soma Compound Tablets 2783
St. Joseph Adult Chewable Aspirin (81 mg.) ND 768
Talwin Compound 2466
Vanquish Analgesic Caplets ND 627

Astemizole (Potentiation of CNS depression). Products include:
Hismanal Tablets 1341

Atenolol (Concurrent use is contraindicated). Products include:
Tenoretic Tablets 2963
Tenormin Tablets and I.V. Injection 2965

Atropine Sulfate (Potential for tachycardia, hypotension, undesirable CNS effects such as stimulation, delirium, and extrapyramidal symptoms may be aggravated). Products include:
Arco-Lase Plus Tablets 513
Atrohist Plus Tablets 1605
Donnatal 2234
Donnatal Extentabs 2234
Donnatal Tablets 2234
Lomotil 2591
Motofen Tablets 789
Urised Tablets 2123

Azatadine Maleate (Potentiation of CNS depression). Products include:
Trinalin Repetabs Tablets 1373

Benazepril Hydrochloride (Concurrent use is contraindicated). Products include:
Lotensin Tablets 852
Lotensin HCT Tablets 855
Lotrel Capsules 858

Bendroflumethiazide (Concurrent use is contraindicated).
No products indexed under this heading.

Betaxolol Hydrochloride (Concurrent use is contraindicated). Products include:
Betoptic Ophthalmic Solution 465
Betoptic S Ophthalmic Suspension 467
Kerlone Tablets 2588

Bisoprolol Fumarate (Concurrent use is contraindicated). Products include:
Zebeta Tablets 1457
Ziac 1459

Bromodiphenhydramine Hydrochloride (Potentiation of CNS depression).
No products indexed under this heading.

Brompheniramine Maleate (Potentiation of CNS depression). Products include:
Alka-Seltzer Plus Sinus Medicine ND 611
Bromfed Capsules (Extended-Release) 1832
Bromfed Syrup ND 712
Bromfed Tablets 1832
Bromfed-DM Cough Syrup 1832
Bromfed-PD Capsules (Extended-Release) 1832
Dimetane-DC Cough Syrup 2232
Dimetane-DX Cough Syrup 2233
Dimetapp Allergy Dye-Free Elixir ND 838
Dimetapp Allergy Sinus Caplets ND 838
Dimetapp Cold & Allergy Chewable Tablets ND 838
Dimetapp Cold & Cough Liqui-Gels ND 839
Dimetapp Cold & Fever Suspension ND 839
Dimetapp DM Elixir ND 840
Dimetapp Elixir ND 840
Dimetapp Extentabs ND 841
Dimetapp Tablets/Liqui-Gels ND 841
Rondec Chewable Tablets 974
Vicks DayQuil Allergy Relief 12-Hour Extended Release Tablets ND 733
Vicks DayQuil Allergy Relief 4-Hour Tablets ND 733

Buprenorphine (Potential for additive effects; the dosage of either drug should be reduced and critically adjusted when used concomitantly or in sequence). Products include:
Buprenex Injectable 2170

Buspirone Hydrochloride (Potential for additive effects; the dosage of either drug should be reduced and critically adjusted when used concomitantly or in sequence). Products include:
BuSpar Tablets 738

Butabarbital (Potential for additive effects; the dosage of either drug should be reduced and critically adjusted when used concomitantly or in sequence).
No products indexed under this heading.

Butalbital (Potential for additive effects; the dosage of either drug should be reduced and critically adjusted when used concomitantly or in sequence). Products include:
Axocet Capsules 2469
Esgic-plus Capsules 1012
Esgic-plus Tablets 1012
Fioricet Tablets 2386
Fioricet with Codeine Capsules 2387
Fiorinal Capsules 2388
Fiorinal with Codeine Capsules 2390
Fiorinal Tablets 2388
Phrenilin 790
Sedapap Tablets 50 mg/650 mg 1826

Captopril (Concurrent use is contraindicated). Products include:
Capoten Tablets 740
Capozide Tablets 744

Carteolol Hydrochloride (Concurrent use is contraindicated). Products include:
Cartrol Tablets 413
Ocupress Ophthalmic Solution, 1% Sterile ⊙ 297

Cetirizine Hydrochloride (Potentiation of CNS depression). Products include:
Zyrtec Tablets 2053

Chlordiazepoxide (Potential for additive effects; the dosage of either drug should be reduced and critically adjusted when used concomitantly or in sequence). Products include:
Limbitrol 2333

Chlordiazepoxide Hydrochloride (Potential for additive effects; the dosage of either drug should be reduced and critically adjusted when used concomitantly or in sequence). Products include:
Librax Capsules 2330
Librium Capsules 2331
Librium Injectable 2332

Chlorothiazide (Concurrent use is contraindicated). Products include:
Aldoclor Tablets 1638
Diupres Tablets 1691
Diuril Oral 1694

Chlorothiazide Sodium (Concurrent use is contraindicated). Products include:
Diuril Sodium Intravenous 1693

Chlorpheniramine Maleate (Potentiation of CNS depression). Products include:
Alka-Seltzer Plus Cold Medicine ND 611
Alka-Seltzer Plus Cold Medicine Liqui-Gels ND 612
Alka-Seltzer Plus Cold & Cough Medicine ND 611
Alka-Seltzer Plus Cold & Cough Medicine Liqui-Gels ND 612
Alka-Seltzer Plus Flu & Body Aches Effervescent Tablets ND 612
Allerest Maximum Strength ND 649
Allerest Sinus Pain Formula ND 649
Ana-Kit Anaphylaxis Emergency Treatment Kit 611
Atrohist Pediatric Capsules 1603
Atrohist Plus Tablets 1605
BC Cold Powder Multi-Symptom Formula (Cold-Sinus-Allergy) ND 631
Cerose DM ND 853
Cheracol Plus Head Cold/Cough Formula ND 741
Children's TYLENOL Cold Multi-Symptom Chewable Tablets and Liquid 1559
Children's TYLENOL Cold Plus Cough Multi Symptom Chewable Tablets and Liquid 1560
Children's TYLENOL Flu Suspension Liquid 1560
Children's Vicks DayQuil Allergy Relief ND 730
Children's Vicks NyQuil Cold/Cough Relief ND 731
Chlor-Trimeton Allergy Decongestant Tablets ND 759
Chlor-Trimeton Allergy Tablets ND 758
Allergy-Sinus Comtrex Multi-Symptom Allergy-Sinus Formula Tablets and Caplets ND 639
Comtrex Multi-Symptom ND 638
Contac Continuous Action Nasal Decongestant/Antihistamine 12 Hour Capsules ND 773
Contac Maximum Strength Continuous Action Decongestant/Antihistamine 12 Hour Caplets ND 772
Contac Severe Cold and Flu Formula Caplets ND 773
Coricidin Cold + Flu Tablets ND 760
Coricidin Cough + Cold Tablets ND 760
Coricidin 'D' Decongestant Tablets ND 760
D.A. II Tablets 972
D.A. Chewable Tablets 970
Dura-Tap/PD Capsules 970
Dura-Vent/DA Tablets 972
Efidac 24 Chlorpheniramine ND 655
Extendryl 1003
Fedahist Gyrocaps 2545
Hycomine Compound Tablets 948
Kronofed-A 994
Nolamine Timed-Release Tablets 790
Novahistine Elixir ND 782
Ornade Spansule Capsules 2678
PediaCare Cough-Cold Chewable Tablets and Liquid 1569
PediaCare NightRest Cough-Cold Liquid 1569
Pediatric Vicks 44m Cough & Cold Relief ND 737
Pyrroxate Caplets ND 742
Ryna ND 804
Sinarest ND 663
Sine-Off Sinus Medicine ND 784
Singlet Tablets ND 785
Sinulin Tablets 792
Sinutab Sinus Allergy Medication, Maximum Strength Tablets and Caplets ND 823
Sudafed Cold & Allergy Tablets ND 826
Teldrin 12 Hour Antihistamine/Nasal Decongestant Allergy Relief Capsules ND 786
TheraFlu Flu and Cold Medicine ND 750
Theraflu Maximum Strength Flu and Cold Medicine For Sore Throat ND 751
TheraFlu Flu, Cold and Cough Medicine ND 750
TheraFlu Maximum Strength Nighttime Flu, Cold & Cough Medicine ND 751
Triaminic Night Time ND 754
Triaminic Syrup ND 755
Triaminic Triaminicol Cold & Cough ND 756
Triaminicin Tablets ND 756
Tussend 1830
TYLENOL Allergy Sinus, Maximum Strength Caplets and Gelcaps 1571
TYLENOL Cold Medication, Multi-Symptom Formula Tablets and Caplets 1572
TYLENOL Cold Medication, Multi-Symptom Hot Liquid Packets 1572
Vicks 44 LiquiCaps Cough, Cold & Flu Relief ND 728
Vicks 44M Cough, Cold & Flu Relief ND 729

Chlorpheniramine Polistirex (Potentiation of CNS depression). Products include:
Tussionex Pennkinetic Extended-Release Suspension 1624

Chlorpheniramine Tannate (Potentiation of CNS depression). Products include:
Atrohist Pediatric Suspension 1604
Atrohist Pediatric Suspension Dye-Free 1604
Rynatan 2781
Rynatuss 2782

Chlorpromazine (Potential for additive effects; the dosage of either drug should be reduced and critically adjusted when used concomitantly or in sequence). Products include:
Thorazine Suppositories 2701

Chlorpromazine Hydrochloride (Potential for additive effects; the dosage of either drug should be reduced and critically adjusted when used concomitantly or in sequence). Products include:
Thorazine 2701

Chlorprothixene (Potential for additive effects; the dosage of either drug should be reduced and critically adjusted when used concomitantly or in sequence).
No products indexed under this heading.

Chlorprothixene Hydrochloride (Potential for additive effects; the dosage of either drug should be reduced and critically adjusted when used concomitantly or in sequence).
No products indexed under this heading.

Chlorprothixene Lactate (Potential for additive effects; the dosage of either drug should be reduced and critically adjusted when used concomitantly or in sequence).
No products indexed under this heading.

Chlorthalidone (Concurrent use is contraindicated). Products include:
Combipres Tablets 682
Tenoretic Tablets 2963
Thalitone 1293

Clemastine Fumarate (Potentiation of CNS depression). Products include:
Tavist Syrup 2426
Tavist Tablets 2427
Tavist-1 12 Hour Relief Tablets ND 749
Tavist-D 12 Hour Relief Tablets ND 750

(ND Described in PDR For Nonprescription Drugs) (⊙ Described in PDR For Ophthalmology)

Interactions Index

Clonidine (Concurrent use is contraindicated). Products include:
- Catapres-TTS 680

Clonidine Hydrochloride (Concurrent use is contraindicated). Products include:
- Catapres Tablets 679
- Combipres Tablets 682

Clorazepate Dipotassium (Potential for additive effects; the dosage of either drug should be reduced and critically adjusted when used concomitantly or in sequence). Products include:
- Tranxene 459

Clozapine (Potential for additive effects; the dosage of either drug should be reduced and critically adjusted when used concomitantly or in sequence). Products include:
- Clozaril Tablets 2377

Codeine Phosphate (Potential for additive effects; the dosage of either drug should be reduced and critically adjusted when used concomitantly or in sequence). Products include:
- Brontex 2130
- Dimetane-DC Cough Syrup 2232
- Fioricet with Codeine Capsules 2387
- Fiorinal with Codeine Capsules 2390
- Nucofed 2225
- Phenergan with Codeine 2883
- Phenergan VC with Codeine 2888
- Robitussin A-C Syrup 2248
- Robitussin-DAC Syrup 2249
- Ryna 804
- Soma Compound w/Codeine Tablets 2784
- Tylenol with Codeine 1592

Cyproheptadine Hydrochloride (Potentiation of CNS depression). Products include:
- Periactin 1767

Deserpidine (Concurrent use is contraindicated).
- No products indexed under this heading.

Desflurane (Potential for additive effects; the dosage of either drug should be reduced and critically adjusted when used concomitantly or in sequence). Products include:
- Suprane (desflurane, USP) 1865

Dexchlorpheniramine Maleate (Potentiation of CNS depression).
- No products indexed under this heading.

Dezocine (Potential for additive effects; the dosage of either drug should be reduced and critically adjusted when used concomitantly or in sequence). Products include:
- Dalgan Injection 529

Diazepam (Potential for additive effects; the dosage of either drug should be reduced and critically adjusted when used concomitantly or in sequence). Products include:
- Dizac (diazepam injectable emulsion) CIV 1862
- Valium Injectable 2336
- Valium Tablets 2335

Diazoxide (Concurrent use is contraindicated). Products include:
- Hyperstat I.V. Injection 2504
- Proglycem 575

Diltiazem Hydrochloride (Concurrent use is contraindicated). Products include:
- Cardizem CD Capsules 1251
- Cardizem SR Capsules 1255
- Cardizem Injectable 1253
- Cardizem Tablets 1257
- Dilacor XR Extended-release Capsules 2183
- Tiazac Capsules 1019

Diphenhydramine Citrate (Potentiation of CNS depression). Products include:
- Excedrin P.M. Analgesic/Sleeping Aid Tablets, Caplets, Liquigels 735

Diphenhydramine Hydrochloride (Potentiation of CNS depression). Products include:
- Actifed Allergy Daytime/Nighttime Caplets 808
- Actifed Sinus Daytime/Nighttime Tablets and Caplets 809
- Extra Strength Bayer PM Aspirin Plus Sleep Aid 617
- Benadryl Allergy Chewables 811
- Benadryl Allergy/Cold Tablets 811
- Benadryl Allergy Decongestant Liquid Medication 812
- Benadryl Allergy Decongestant Tablets 812
- Benadryl Allergy Liquid Medication 813
- Benadryl Allergy 811
- Benadryl Allergy Sinus Headache Caplets 813
- Benadryl Dye-Free Allergy Liquigel Softgels 813
- Benadryl Dye-Free Allergy Liquid Medication 814
- Benadryl Itch Relief Stick Extra Strength 814
- Benadryl Cream 814
- Benadryl Gel 815
- Benadryl Spray 815
- Benadryl Injection 1955
- Contac Day & Night Cold/Flu Night Caplets 772
- Contac Night Allergy/Sinus Caplets 771
- Extra Strength Doan's P.M. 653
- Excedrin P.M. Analgesic/Sleeping Aid Tablets, Caplets, Liquigels 643
- Nytol QuickCaps Caplets 632
- Sleepinal Night-time Sleep Aid Capsules and Softgels 798
- TYLENOL Allergy Sinus NightTime, Maximum Strength Caplets 1571
- TYLENOL Flu NightTime, Maximum Strength Gelcaps 1575
- TYLENOL Flu NightTime, Maximum Strength Hot Medication Packets 1575
- TYLENOL PM Pain Reliever/Sleep Aid, Extra Strength Gelcaps, Caplets, Geltabs 1576
- TYLENOL Severe Allergy Medication Caplets 1571
- Maximum Strength Unisom Sleepgels 1990
- Unisom With Pain Relief-Nighttime Sleep Aid and Pain Reliever 1991

Diphenylpyraline Hydrochloride (Potentiation of CNS depression).
- No products indexed under this heading.

Doxazosin Mesylate (Concurrent use is contraindicated). Products include:
- Cardura Tablets 1993

Droperidol (Potential for additive effects; the dosage of either drug should be reduced and critically adjusted when used concomitantly or in sequence). Products include:
- Inapsine Injection 462

Enalapril Maleate (Concurrent use is contraindicated). Products include:
- Vaseretic Tablets 1810
- Vasotec Tablets 1816

Enalaprilat (Concurrent use is contraindicated). Products include:
- Vasotec I.V. 1814

Enflurane (Potential for additive effects; the dosage of either drug should be reduced and critically adjusted when used concomitantly or in sequence).
- No products indexed under this heading.

Epinephrine Hydrochloride (Potential for paradoxical decrease in blood pressure). Products include:
- Ana-Kit Anaphylaxis Emergency Treatment Kit 611

Esmolol Hydrochloride (Concurrent use is contraindicated). Products include:
- Brevibloc (esmolol HCl) Injection 1860

Estazolam (Potential for additive effects; the dosage of either drug should be reduced and critically adjusted when used concomitantly or in sequence). Products include:
- ProSom Tablets 457

Ethchlorvynol (Potential for additive effects; the dosage of either drug should be reduced and critically adjusted when used concomitantly or in sequence). Products include:
- Placidyl Capsules 456

Ethinamate (Potential for additive effects; the dosage of either drug should be reduced and critically adjusted when used concomitantly or in sequence).
- No products indexed under this heading.

Felodipine (Concurrent use is contraindicated). Products include:
- Plendil Extended-Release Tablets 514

Fentanyl (Potential for additive effects; the dosage of either drug should be reduced and critically adjusted when used concomitantly or in sequence). Products include:
- Duragesic Transdermal System 1336

Fentanyl Citrate (Potential for additive effects; the dosage of either drug should be reduced and critically adjusted when used concomitantly or in sequence). Products include:
- Sublimaze Injection 463

Fluphenazine Decanoate (Potential for additive effects; the dosage of either drug should be reduced and critically adjusted when used concomitantly or in sequence). Products include:
- Prolixin Decanoate 510

Fluphenazine Enanthate (Potential for additive effects; the dosage of either drug should be reduced and critically adjusted when used concomitantly or in sequence). Products include:
- Prolixin Enanthate 510

Fluphenazine Hydrochloride (Potential for additive effects; the dosage of either drug should be reduced and critically adjusted when used concomitantly or in sequence). Products include:
- Prolixin 510

Flurazepam Hydrochloride (Potential for additive effects; the dosage of either drug should be reduced and critically adjusted when used concomitantly or in sequence). Products include:
- Dalmane Capsules 2329

Fosinopril Sodium (Concurrent use is contraindicated). Products include:
- Monopril Tablets 762

Furazolidone (Concurrent use is contraindicated). Products include:
- Furoxone 2221

Furosemide (Concurrent use is contraindicated). Products include:
- Lasix Injection, Oral Solution and Tablets 1267

Glutethimide (Potential for additive effects; the dosage of either drug should be reduced and critically adjusted when used concomitantly or in sequence).
- No products indexed under this heading.

Guanabenz Acetate (Concurrent use is contraindicated).
- No products indexed under this heading.

Guanethidine Monosulfate (Concurrent use is contraindicated). Products include:
- Esimil Tablets 840
- Ismelin Tablets 845

Haloperidol (Potential for additive effects; the dosage of either drug should be reduced and critically adjusted when used concomitantly or in sequence). Products include:
- Haldol Injection, Tablets and Concentrate 1585

Haloperidol Decanoate (Potential for additive effects; the dosage of either drug should be reduced and critically adjusted when used concomitantly or in sequence). Products include:
- Haldol Decanoate 1587

Hydralazine Hydrochloride (Concurrent use is contraindicated). Products include:
- Apresazide Capsules 824
- Apresoline Hydrochloride Tablets 826
- Hydralazine Hydrochloride Injection USP 2712
- Ser-Ap-Es Tablets 867

Hydrochlorothiazide (Concurrent use is contraindicated). Products include:
- Aldactazide Tablets 2556
- Aldoril Tablets 1644
- Apresazide Capsules 824
- Capozide Tablets 744
- Dyazide Capsules 2653
- Esidrix Tablets 839
- Esimil Tablets 840
- HydroDIURIL Tablets 1716
- Hydropres Tablets 1718
- Hyzaar Tablets 1720
- Inderide Tablets 2838
- Inderide LA Long Acting Capsules 2840
- Lopressor HCT Tablets 850
- Lotensin HCT Tablets 855
- Moduretic Tablets 1748
- Oretic Tablets 450
- Prinzide Tablets 1780
- Ser-Ap-Es Tablets 867
- Timolide Tablets 1791
- Vaseretic Tablets 1810
- Zestoretic Tablets 2968
- Ziac 1459

Hydrocodone Bitartrate (Potential for additive effects; the dosage of either drug should be reduced and critically adjusted when used concomitantly or in sequence). Products include:
- Codiclear DH Syrup 808
- Duratuss HD Elixir 2750
- Histussin D Liquid 670
- Hycodan Tablets and Syrup 946
- Hycomine Compound Tablets 948
- Hycomine 947
- Hycotuss Expectorant Syrup 950
- Hydrocet Capsules 787
- Lorcet 10/650 Tablets 1016
- Lortab 2751
- Tussend 1830
- Tussend Expectorant 1831
- Vicodin Tablets 1404
- Vicodin ES Tablets 1405
- Vicodin HP Tablets 1403
- Vicodin Tuss Expectorant 1406
- Zydone Capsules 967

Hydrocodone Polistirex (Potential for additive effects; the dosage of either drug should be reduced and critically adjusted when used concomitantly or in sequence). Products include:
- Tussionex Pennkinetic Extended-Release Suspension 1624

IMPORTANT NOTE: Always consult each drug listing in the patient's regimen for possible interactions.

Levoprome / Interactions Index

Hydroflumethiazide (Concurrent use is contraindicated). Products include:
- Diucardin Tablets 2824

Hydromorphone Hydrochloride (Potential for additive effects; the dosage of either drug should be reduced and critically adjusted when used concomitantly or in sequence. Products include:
- Dilaudid Ampules 1382
- Dilaudid Cough Syrup 1383
- Dilaudid-HP Injection 1384
- Dilaudid-HP Lyophilized Powder 250 mg 1384
- Dilaudid 1382
- Dilaudid Oral Liquid 1386
- Dilaudid 1382
- Dilaudid Tablets - 8 mg. 1386

Hydroxyzine Hydrochloride (Potential for additive effects; the dosage of either drug should be reduced and critically adjusted when used concomitantly or in sequence). Products include:
- Atarax Tablets & Syrup 1992
- Marax Tablets & DF Syrup 2015
- Vistaril Intramuscular Solution 2042

Indapamide (Concurrent use is contraindicated).
- No products indexed under this heading.

Isocarboxazid (Concurrent use is contraindicated).
- No products indexed under this heading.

Isoflurane (Potential for additive effects; the dosage of either drug should be reduced and critically adjusted when used concomitantly or in sequence).
- No products indexed under this heading.

Isradipine (Concurrent use is contraindicated). Products include:
- DynaCirc Capsules 2381
- DynaCirc CR Tablets 2383

Ketamine Hydrochloride (Potential for additive effects; the dosage of either drug should be reduced and critically adjusted when used concomitantly or in sequence).
- No products indexed under this heading.

Labetalol Hydrochloride (Concurrent use is contraindicated). Products include:
- Normodyne Injection 2519
- Normodyne Tablets 2522
- Trandate 1158

Levomethadyl Acetate Hydrochloride (Potential for additive effects; the dosage of either drug should be reduced and critically adjusted when used concomitantly or in sequence). Products include:
- Orlaam Oral Solution 2361

Levorphanol Tartrate (Potential for additive effects; the dosage of either drug should be reduced and critically adjusted when used concomitantly or in sequence). Products include:
- Levo-Dromoran 2297

Lisinopril (Concurrent use is contraindicated). Products include:
- Prinivil Tablets 1776
- Prinzide Tablets 1780
- Zestoretic Tablets 2968
- Zestril Tablets 2972

Loratadine (Potentiation of CNS depression). Products include:
- Claritin Tablets 2485
- Claritin-D Tablets 2487

Lorazepam (Potential for additive effects; the dosage of either drug should be reduced and critically adjusted when used concomitantly or in sequence). Products include:
- Ativan Injection 2805
- Ativan Tablets 2807

Losartan Potassium (Concurrent use is contraindicated). Products include:
- Cozaar Tablets 1668
- Hyzaar Tablets 1720

Loxapine Hydrochloride (Potential for additive effects; the dosage of either drug should be reduced and critically adjusted when used concomitantly or in sequence). Products include:
- Loxitane 1426

Loxapine Succinate (Potential for additive effects; the dosage of either drug should be reduced and critically adjusted when used concomitantly or in sequence). Products include:
- Loxitane Capsules 1426

Mecamylamine Hydrochloride (Concurrent use is contraindicated). Products include:
- Inversine Tablets 1729

Meperidine Hydrochloride (Potential for additive effects; the dosage of either drug should be reduced and critically adjusted when used concomitantly or in sequence). Products include:
- Demerol 2438
- Mepergan Injection 2859

Mephobarbital (Potential for additive effects; the dosage of either drug should be reduced and critically adjusted when used concomitantly or in sequence). Products include:
- Mebaral Tablets 2452

Meprobamate (Potential for additive effects; the dosage of either drug should be reduced and critically adjusted when used concomitantly or in sequence). Products include:
- Miltown Tablets 2780
- PMB 200 and PMB 400 2890

Mesoridazine Besylate (Potential for additive effects; the dosage of either drug should be reduced and critically adjusted when used concomitantly or in sequence). Products include:
- Serentil 689

Methadone Hydrochloride (Potential for additive effects; the dosage of either drug should be reduced and critically adjusted when used concomitantly or in sequence). Products include:
- Methadone Hydrochloride Oral Concentrate 2356
- Methadone Hydrochloride Oral Solution & Tablets 2357

Methdilazine Hydrochloride (Potentiation of CNS depression).
- No products indexed under this heading.

Methohexital Sodium (Potential for additive effects; the dosage of either drug should be reduced and critically adjusted when used concomitantly or in sequence).
- No products indexed under this heading.

Methoxyflurane (Potential for additive effects; the dosage of either drug should be reduced and critically adjusted when used concomitantly or in sequence).
- No products indexed under this heading.

Methyclothiazide (Concurrent use is contraindicated). Products include:
- Enduron Tablets 424

Methyldopa (Concurrent use is contraindicated). Products include:
- Aldoclor Tablets 1638
- Aldomet Oral 1640
- Aldoril Tablets 1644

Methyldopate Hydrochloride (Concurrent use is contraindicated). Products include:
- Aldomet Ester HCl Injection 1642

Metolazone (Concurrent use is contraindicated). Products include:
- Mykrox Tablets 1617
- Zaroxolyn Tablets 1625

Metoprolol Succinate (Concurrent use is contraindicated). Products include:
- Toprol-XL Tablets 560

Metoprolol Tartrate (Concurrent use is contraindicated). Products include:
- Lopressor 848
- Lopressor HCT Tablets 850

Metyrosine (Concurrent use is contraindicated). Products include:
- Demser Capsules 1690

Midazolam Hydrochloride (Potential for additive effects; the dosage of either drug should be reduced and critically adjusted when used concomitantly or in sequence). Products include:
- Versed Injection 2324

Minoxidil (Concurrent use is contraindicated).
- No products indexed under this heading.

Moexipril Hydrochloride (Concurrent use is contraindicated). Products include:
- Univasc Tablets 2553

Molindone Hydrochloride (Potential for additive effects; the dosage of either drug should be reduced and critically adjusted when used concomitantly or in sequence). Products include:
- Moban Tablets and Concentrate 1036

Morphine Sulfate (Potential for additive effects; the dosage of either drug should be reduced and critically adjusted when used concomitantly or in sequence). Products include:
- Astramorph/PF Injection, USP (Preservative-Free) 526
- Duramorph Injection 983
- Infumorph 200 and Infumorph 500 Sterile Solutions 985
- Kadian Capsules 2948
- MS Contin Tablets 2149
- MSIR 2152
- Oramorph SR (Morphine Sulfate Sustained Release Tablets) 2359
- RMS Suppositories CII 2766
- Roxanol 2365

Nadolol (Concurrent use is contraindicated).
- No products indexed under this heading.

Nicardipine Hydrochloride (Concurrent use is contraindicated). Products include:
- Cardene Capsules 2261
- Cardene I.V. 2815
- Cardene SR Capsules 2264

Nifedipine (Concurrent use is contraindicated). Products include:
- Adalat Capsules (10 mg and 20 mg) 580
- Adalat CC 582
- Procardia Capsules 2024
- Procardia XL Extended Release Tablets 2026

Nisoldipine (Concurrent use is contraindicated). Products include:
- Sular Tablets 2961

Nitroglycerin (Concurrent use is contraindicated). Products include:
- Deponit NTG Transdermal Delivery System 2541
- Nitro-Bid IV 1270
- Nitro-Bid Ointment 1272
- Nitro-Dur (nitroglycerin) Transdermal Infusion System 1365
- Nitrolingual Spray 2193
- Nitrostat Tablets 1981
- Transderm-Nitro Transdermal Therapeutic System 878

Opium Alkaloids (Potential for additive effects; the dosage of either drug should be reduced and critically adjusted when used concomitantly or in sequence).
- No products indexed under this heading.

Oxazepam (Potential for additive effects; the dosage of either drug should be reduced and critically adjusted when used concomitantly or in sequence). Products include:
- Serax Capsules 2916
- Serax Tablets 2916

Oxycodone Hydrochloride (Potential for additive effects; the dosage of either drug should be reduced and critically adjusted when used concomitantly or in sequence). Products include:
- OxyContin Tablets 2163
- OxyIR Capsules 2167
- Percocet Tablets 955
- Percodan Tablets 955
- Percodan-Demi Tablets 956
- Roxicodone Tablets, Oral Solution & Intensol (Oxycodone) 2366
- Tylox Capsules 1593

Penbutolol Sulfate (Concurrent use is contraindicated). Products include:
- Levatol Tablets 2547

Pentobarbital Sodium (Potential for additive effects; the dosage of either drug should be reduced and critically adjusted when used concomitantly or in sequence). Products include:
- Nembutal Sodium Capsules 440
- Nembutal Sodium Solution 442
- Nembutal Sodium Suppositories 444

Perphenazine (Potential for additive effects; the dosage of either drug should be reduced and critically adjusted when used concomitantly or in sequence). Products include:
- Etrafon 2495
- Triavil Tablets 1800
- Trilafon 2532

Phenelzine Sulfate (Concurrent use is contraindicated). Products include:
- Nardil 1977

Phenobarbital (Potential for additive effects; the dosage of either drug should be reduced and critically adjusted when used concomitantly or in sequence). Products include:
- Arco-Lase Plus Tablets 513
- Bellergal-S Tablets 2375
- Donnatal 2234
- Donnatal Extentabs 2234
- Donnatal Tablets 2234
- Phenobarbital Elixir and Tablets 1523
- Quadrinal Tablets 1398

Phenoxybenzamine Hydrochloride (Concurrent use is contraindicated). Products include:
- Dibenzyline Capsules 2650

Phentolamine Mesylate (Concurrent use is contraindicated). Products include:
- Regitine Vials 864

Pindolol (Concurrent use is contraindicated). Products include:
- Visken Tablets 2428

Polythiazide (Concurrent use is contraindicated). Products include:
- Minizide Capsules 2016

Prazepam (Potential for additive effects; the dosage of either drug should be reduced and critically adjusted when used concomitantly or in sequence).
- No products indexed under this heading.

(▣ Described in PDR For Nonprescription Drugs)   (◉ Described in PDR For Ophthalmology)

599 **Interactions Index** **Levothroid Tablets**

Prazosin Hydrochloride (Concurrent use is contraindicated). Products include:
- Minipress Capsules ... 2015
- Minizide Capsules ... 2016

Prochlorperazine (Potential for additive effects; the dosage of either drug should be reduced and critically adjusted when used concomitantly or in sequence). Products include:
- Compazine ... 2644

Promethazine Hydrochloride (Potential for additive effects; the dosage of either drug should be reduced and critically adjusted when used concomitantly or in sequence; potentiation of CNS depression). Products include:
- Mepergan Injection ... 2859
- Phenergan with Codeine ... 2883
- Phenergan with Dextromethorphan 2885
- Phenergan Injection ... 2880
- Phenergan Suppositories ... 2882
- Phenergan Syrup ... 2881
- Phenergan Tablets ... 2882
- Phenergan VC ... 2886
- Phenergan VC with Codeine ... 2888

Propofol (Potential for additive effects; the dosage of either drug should be reduced and critically adjusted when used concomitantly or in sequence). Products include:
- Diprivan Injectable Emulsion ... 2939

Propoxyphene Hydrochloride (Potential for additive effects; the dosage of either drug should be reduced and critically adjusted when used concomitantly or in sequence). Products include:
- Darvon ... 1475
- Wygesic Tablets ... 2930

Propoxyphene Napsylate (Potential for additive effects; the dosage of either drug should be reduced and critically adjusted when used concomitantly or in sequence). Products include:
- Darvon-N/Darvocet-N ... 1473

Propranolol Hydrochloride (Concurrent use is contraindicated). Products include:
- Inderal ... 2834
- Inderal LA Long Acting Capsules ... 2836
- Inderide Tablets ... 2838
- Inderide LA Long Acting Capsules .. 2840

Pyrilamine Maleate (Potentiation of CNS depression). Products include:
- 4-Way Fast Acting Nasal Spray (regular & mentholated) ... 644
- Maximum Strength Multi-Symptom Formula Midol ... 621
- PMS Multi-Symptom Formula Midol ... 622

Pyrilamine Tannate (Potentiation of CNS depression). Products include:
- Atrohist Pediatric Suspension ... 1604
- Atrohist Pediatric Suspension Dye-Free ... 1604
- Rynatan ... 2781

Quazepam (Potential for additive effects; the dosage of either drug should be reduced and critically adjusted when used concomitantly or in sequence). Products include:
- Doral Tablets ... 2773

Quinapril Hydrochloride (Concurrent use is contraindicated). Products include:
- Accupril Tablets ... 1950

Ramipril (Concurrent use is contraindicated). Products include:
- Altace Capsules ... 1238

Rauwolfia Serpentina (Concurrent use is contraindicated).
- No products indexed under this heading.

Rescinnamine (Concurrent use is contraindicated).
- No products indexed under this heading.

Reserpine (Potential for additive effects; the dosage of either drug should be reduced and critically adjusted when used concomitantly or in sequence; concurrent use is contraindicated). Products include:
- Diupres Tablets ... 1691
- Hydropres Tablets ... 1718
- Ser-Ap-Es Tablets ... 867

Risperidone (Potential for additive effects; the dosage of either drug should be reduced and critically adjusted when used concomitantly or in sequence). Products include:
- Risperdal Tablets ... 1348

Scopolamine (Potential for tachycardia, hypotension, undesirable CNS effects such as stimulation, delirium, and extrapyramidal symptoms may be aggravated). Products include:
- Transderm Scōp Transdermal Therapeutic System ... 890

Scopolamine Hydrobromide (Potential for tachycardia, hypotension, undesirable CNS effects such as stimulation, delirium, and extrapyramidal symptoms may be aggravated). Products include:
- Atrohist Plus Tablets ... 1605
- Donnatal ... 2234
- Donnatal Extentabs ... 2234
- Donnatal Tablets ... 2234

Secobarbital Sodium (Potential for additive effects; the dosage of either drug should be reduced and critically adjusted when used concomitantly or in sequence). Products include:
- Seconal Sodium Pulvules ... 1529

Selegiline Hydrochloride (Concurrent use is contraindicated). Products include:
- Eldepryl Capsules ... 2729

Sevoflurane (Potential for additive effects; the dosage of either drug should be reduced and critically adjusted when used concomitantly or in sequence).
- No products indexed under this heading.

Sodium Nitroprusside (Concurrent use is contraindicated).
- No products indexed under this heading.

Sotalol Hydrochloride (Concurrent use is contraindicated). Products include:
- Betapace Tablets ... 637

Spirapril Hydrochloride (Concurrent use is contraindicated).
- No products indexed under this heading.

Succinylcholine Chloride (Potential for tachycardia, hypotension, undesirable CNS effects such as stimulation, delirium, and extrapyramidal symptoms may be aggravated). Products include:
- Anectine ... 1062

Sufentanil Citrate (Potential for additive effects; the dosage of either drug should be reduced and critically adjusted when used concomitantly or in sequence). Products include:
- Sufenta Injection ... 1355

Temazepam (Potential for additive effects; the dosage of either drug should be reduced and critically adjusted when used concomitantly or in sequence). Products include:
- Restoril Capsules ... 2413

Terazosin Hydrochloride (Concurrent use is contraindicated). Products include:
- Hytrin Capsules ... 434

Terfenadine (Potentiation of CNS depression). Products include:
- Seldane Tablets ... 1284
- Seldane-D Extended-Release Tablets ... 1286

Thiamylal Sodium (Potential for additive effects; the dosage of either drug should be reduced and critically adjusted when used concomitantly or in sequence).
- No products indexed under this heading.

Thioridazine Hydrochloride (Potential for additive effects; the dosage of either drug should be reduced and critically adjusted when used concomitantly or in sequence). Products include:
- Mellaril ... 2398

Thiothixene (Potential for additive effects; the dosage of either drug should be reduced and critically adjusted when used concomitantly or in sequence). Products include:
- Navane Capsules and Concentrate 2018
- Navane Intramuscular ... 2019

Timolol Maleate (Concurrent use is contraindicated). Products include:
- Blocadren Tablets ... 1654
- Timolide Tablets ... 1791
- Timoptic in Ocudose ... 1796
- Timoptic Sterile Ophthalmic Solution ... 1794
- Timoptic-XE ... 1798

Torsemide (Concurrent use is contraindicated). Products include:
- Demadex Tablets and Injection ... 691

Tranylcypromine Sulfate (Concurrent use is contraindicated). Products include:
- Parnate Tablets ... 2679

Triazolam (Potential for additive effects; the dosage of either drug should be reduced and critically adjusted when used concomitantly or in sequence). Products include:
- Halcion Tablets ... 2093

Trifluoperazine Hydrochloride (Potential for additive effects; the dosage of either drug should be reduced and critically adjusted when used concomitantly or in sequence). Products include:
- Stelazine ... 2692

Trimeprazine Tartrate (Potentiation of CNS depression).
- No products indexed under this heading.

Trimethaphan Camsylate (Concurrent use is contraindicated).
- No products indexed under this heading.

Tripelennamine Hydrochloride (Potentiation of CNS depression). Products include:
- PBZ Tablets ... 863
- PBZ-SR Tablets ... 862

Triprolidine Hydrochloride (Potentiation of CNS depression). Products include:
- Actifed Cold & Allergy Tablets ... 807
- Actifed Cold & Sinus Caplets and Tablets ... 808

Verapamil Hydrochloride (Concurrent use is contraindicated). Products include:
- Calan SR Caplets ... 2571
- Calan Tablets ... 2568
- Covera-HS Tablets ... 2573
- Isoptin Injectable ... 1391
- Isoptin Oral Tablets ... 1393
- Isoptin SR Tablets ... 1395
- Verelan Capsules ... 1455

Zolpidem Tartrate (Potential for additive effects; the dosage of either drug should be reduced and critically adjusted when used concomitantly or in sequence). Products include:
- Ambien Tablets ... 2559

Food Interactions

Alcohol (Potentiation of CNS depression).

LEVOTHROID TABLETS
(Levothyroxine Sodium) ... 1015
May interact with oral hypoglycemic agents, insulin, oral anticoagulants, oral contraceptives, estrogens, and certain other agents. Compounds in these categories include:

Acarbose (Dosage of hypoglycemic agent may need to be adjusted). Products include:
- Precose ... 604

Chlorotrianisene (Estrogens tend to increase serum thyroxine-binding globulin; patients with non-functioning thyroid may need to adjust thyroid dosage).
- No products indexed under this heading.

Chlorpropamide (Dosage of hypoglycemic agent may need to be adjusted). Products include:
- Diabinese Tablets ... 2002

Cholestyramine (Binds both T_4 and T_3 in the intestine, thus impairing absorption of thyroid hormone; four to five hours should elapse between administration of cholestyramine and thyroid hormone). Products include:
- Questran ... 774

Colestipol Hydrochloride (Binds both T_4 and T_3 in the intestine, thus impairing absorption of thyroid hormone; four to five hours should elapse between administration of cholestyramine and thyroid hormone). Products include:
- Colestid ... 2073

Desogestrel (Estrogens tend to increase serum thyroxine-binding globulin; patients with non-functioning thyroid may need to adjust thyroid dosage). Products include:
- Desogen Tablets ... 1867
- Ortho-Cept ... 1907

Dicumarol (Anticoagulant effects may be potentiated; dosage adjustment should be made).
- No products indexed under this heading.

Dienestrol (Estrogens tend to increase serum thyroxine-binding globulin; patients with non-functioning thyroid may need to adjust thyroid dosage). Products include:
- Ortho Dienestrol Cream ... 1922

Diethylstilbestrol (Estrogens tend to increase serum thyroxine-binding globulin; patients with non-functioning thyroid may need to adjust thyroid dosage). Products include:
- Diethylstilbestrol Tablets ... 1477

Epinephrine Hydrochloride (Enhanced coronary insufficiency). Products include:
- Ana-Kit Anaphylaxis Emergency Treatment Kit ... 611

Estradiol (Estrogens tend to increase serum thyroxine-binding globulin; patients with non-functioning thyroid may need to adjust thyroid dosage). Products include:
- Climara Transdermal System ... 640
- Estrace Cream and Tablets ... 751
- Estraderm Transdermal System ... 842
- Estring Vaginal Ring ... 2086
- Vivelle Transdermal System ... 880

IMPORTANT NOTE: Always consult each drug listing in the patient's regimen for possible interactions.

Levothroid Tablets — Interactions Index

Estrogens, Conjugated (Estrogens tend to increase serum thyroxine-binding globulin; patients with non-functioning thyroid may need to adjust thyroid dosage). Products include:

PMB 200 and PMB 400	2890
Premarin Intravenous	2893
Premarin Tablets	2896
Premarin Vaginal Cream	2898
Premphase	2900
Prempro	2905

Estrogens, Esterified (Estrogens tend to increase serum thyroxine-binding globulin; patients with non-functioning thyroid may need to adjust thyroid dosage). Products include:

ESTRATAB Tablets (0.3, 0.625, 1.25, 2.5 mg)	2715
Estratest	2718
Menest Tablets	2671

Estropipate (Estrogens tend to increase serum thyroxine-binding globulin; patients with non-functioning thyroid may need to adjust thyroid dosage). Products include:

Ogen Tablets	2103
Ogen Vaginal Cream	2106
Ortho-Est	1925

Ethinyl Estradiol (Estrogens tend to increase serum thyroxine-binding globulin; patients with non-functioning thyroid may need to adjust thyroid dosage). Products include:

Brevicon	2563
Demulen	2580
Desogen Tablets	1867
Levlen/Tri-Levlen	646
Lo/Ovral Tablets	2852
Lo/Ovral-28 Tablets	2857
Modicon	1928
Nordette-21 Tablets	2863
Nordette-28 Tablets	2866
Norinyl	2563
Ortho-Cept	1907
Ortho-Cyclen/Ortho-Tri-Cyclen	1914
Ortho-Novum	1928
Ortho-Cyclen/Ortho Tri-Cyclen	1914
Ovcon	765
Ovral Tablets	2877
Ovral-28 Tablets	2878
Levlen/Tri-Levlen	646
Tri-Norinyl	2607
Triphasil-21 Tablets	2919
Triphasil-28 Tablets	2924

Ethynodiol Diacetate (Estrogens tend to increase serum thyroxine-binding globulin; patients with non-functioning thyroid may need to adjust thyroid dosage). Products include:

Demulen	2580

Glimepiride (Dosage of hypoglycemic agent may need to be adjusted). Products include:

Amaryl Tablets	1241

Glipizide (Dosage of hypoglycemic agent may need to be adjusted). Products include:

Glucotrol Tablets	2011
Glucotrol XL Extended Release Tablets	2012

Glyburide (Dosage of hypoglycemic agent may need to be adjusted). Products include:

DiaBeta Tablets	1265
Glynase PresTab Tablets	2091
Micronase Tablets	2099

Insulin, Human (Dosage of insulin may need to be adjusted).
No products indexed under this heading.

Insulin, Human Isophane Suspension (Dosage of insulin may need to be adjusted). Products include:

Novolin N Human Insulin 10 ml Vials	1846

Insulin, Human NPH (Dosage of insulin may need to be adjusted). Products include:

Humulin N, 100 Units	1495
Novolin N PenFill 1.5 ml Cartridges Durable Insulin Delivery System	1849
Novolin N Prefilled Syringe Disposable Insulin Delivery System	1850

Insulin, Human Regular (Dosage of insulin may need to be adjusted). Products include:

Humulin R, 100 Units	1497
Novolin R Human Insulin 10 ml Vials	1846
Novolin R PenFill 1.5 ml Cartridges Durable Insulin Delivery System	1849
Novolin R Prefilled Syringe Disposable Insulin Delivery System	1850
Velosulin BR Human Insulin 10 ml Vials	1847

Insulin, Human, Zinc Suspension (Dosage of insulin may need to be adjusted). Products include:

Humulin L, 100 Units	1494
Humulin U, 100 Units	1498
Novolin L Human Insulin 10 ml Vials	1846

Insulin Lispro, Human (Dosage of insulin may need to be adjusted). Products include:

Humalog Injection	1488

Insulin, NPH (Dosage of insulin may need to be adjusted). Products include:

NPH, 100 Units	1502
Pork NPH, 100 Units	1506
Purified Pork NPH Isophane Insulin	1852

Insulin, Regular (Dosage of insulin may need to be adjusted). Products include:

Regular, 100 Units	1503
Pork Regular, 100 Units	1507
Pork Regular (Concentrated), 500 Units	1508
Purified Pork Regular Insulin	1852

Insulin, Zinc Crystals (Dosage of insulin may need to be adjusted). Products include:

NPH, 100 Units	1502

Insulin, Zinc Suspension (Dosage of insulin may need to be adjusted). Products include:

Iletin I	1501
Lente, 100 Units	1501
Iletin II	1504
Pork Lente, 100 Units	1504
Purified Pork Lente Insulin	1852

Levonorgestrel (Estrogens tend to increase serum thyroxine-binding globulin; patients with non-functioning thyroid may need to adjust thyroid dosage). Products include:

Levlen/Tri-Levlen	646
Nordette-21 Tablets	2863
Nordette-28 Tablets	2866
Norplant System	2868
Levlen/Tri-Levlen	646
Triphasil-21 Tablets	2919
Triphasil-28 Tablets	2924

Mestranol (Estrogens tend to increase serum thyroxine-binding globulin; patients with non-functioning thyroid may need to adjust thyroid dosage). Products include:

Norinyl	2563
Ortho-Novum	1928

Metformin Hydrochloride (Dosage of hypoglycemic agent may need to be adjusted). Products include:

Glucophage Tablets	754

Norethindrone (Estrogens tend to increase serum thyroxine-binding globulin; patients with non-functioning thyroid may need to adjust thyroid dosage). Products include:

Brevicon	2563
Micronor Tablets	1903
Modicon	1928
Norinyl	2563
Nor-Q D Tablets	2598
Ortho-Novum	1928
Ovcon	765
Tri-Norinyl	2607

Norethynodrel (Estrogens tend to increase serum thyroxine-binding globulin; patients with non-functioning thyroid may need to adjust thyroid dosage).
No products indexed under this heading.

Norgestimate (Estrogens tend to increase serum thyroxine-binding globulin; patients with non-functioning thyroid may need to adjust thyroid dosage). Products include:

Ortho-Cyclen/Ortho Tri-Cyclen	1914
Ortho-Cyclen/Ortho Tri-Cyclen	1914

Norgestrel (Estrogens tend to increase serum thyroxine-binding globulin; patients with non-functioning thyroid may need to adjust thyroid dosage). Products include:

Lo/Ovral Tablets	2852
Lo/Ovral-28 Tablets	2857
Ovral Tablets	2877
Ovral-28 Tablets	2878
Ovrette Tablets	2878

Polyestradiol Phosphate (Estrogens tend to increase serum thyroxine-binding globulin; patients with non-functioning thyroid may need to adjust thyroid dosage).
No products indexed under this heading.

Quinestrol (Estrogens tend to increase serum thyroxine-binding globulin; patients with non-functioning thyroid may need to adjust thyroid dosage).
No products indexed under this heading.

Tolazamide (Dosage of hypoglycemic agent may need to be adjusted).
No products indexed under this heading.

Tolbutamide (Dosage of hypoglycemic agent may need to be adjusted).
No products indexed under this heading.

Warfarin Sodium (Anticoagulant effects may be potentiated; dosage adjustment should be made). Products include:

Coumadin	941

LEVOTHYROXINE SODIUM, USP FOR INJECTION

(Levothyroxine Sodium) 546
May interact with oral anticoagulants, estrogens, insulin, and oral hypoglycemic agents. Compounds in these categories include:

Acarbose (Initiating thyroid replacement therapy may cause increases in hypoglycemic requirements). Products include:

Precose	604

Chlorotrianisene (Estrogens or estrogen-containing oral contraceptives tend to increase serum thyroxine-binding globulin (TBG); increase in thyroid requirements in patients with nonfunctioning thyroid gland on combined therapy).
No products indexed under this heading.

Chlorpropamide (Initiating thyroid replacement therapy may cause increases in hypoglycemic requirements). Products include:

Diabinese Tablets	2002

Dicumarol (Thyroid hormones appear to increase catabolism of vitamin K-dependent clotting factor; concurrent therapy may result in impairment of compensatory increases in clotting factor synthesis; anticoagulant dosage adjustment may be required).
No products indexed under this heading.

Dienestrol (Estrogens or estrogen-containing oral contraceptives tend to increase serum thyroxine-binding globulin (TBG); increase in thyroid requirements in patients with non-functioning thyroid gland on combined therapy). Products include:

Ortho Dienestrol Cream	1922

Diethylstilbestrol (Estrogens or estrogen-containing oral contraceptives tend to increase serum thyroxine-binding globulin (TBG); increase in thyroid requirements in patients with nonfunctioning thyroid gland on combined therapy). Products include:

Diethylstilbestrol Tablets	1477

Estradiol (Estrogens or estrogen-containing oral contraceptives tend to increase serum thyroxine-binding globulin (TBG); increase in thyroid requirements in patients with non-functioning thyroid gland on combined therapy). Products include:

Climara Transdermal System	640
Estrace Cream and Tablets	751
Estraderm Transdermal System	842
Estring Vaginal Ring	2086
Vivelle Transdermal System	880

Estrogens, Conjugated (Estrogens or estrogen-containing oral contraceptives tend to increase serum thyroxine-binding globulin (TBG); increase in thyroid requirements in patients with nonfunctioning thyroid gland on combined therapy). Products include:

PMB 200 and PMB 400	2890
Premarin Intravenous	2893
Premarin Tablets	2896
Premarin Vaginal Cream	2898
Premphase	2900
Prempro	2905

Estrogens, Esterified (Estrogens or estrogen-containing oral contraceptives tend to increase serum thyroxine-binding globulin (TBG); increase in thyroid requirements in patients with nonfunctioning thyroid gland on combined therapy). Products include:

ESTRATAB Tablets (0.3, 0.625, 1.25, 2.5 mg)	2715
Estratest	2718
Menest Tablets	2671

Estropipate (Estrogens or estrogen-containing oral contraceptives tend to increase serum thyroxine-binding globulin (TBG); increase in thyroid requirements in patients with nonfunctioning thyroid gland on combined therapy). Products include:

Ogen Tablets	2103
Ogen Vaginal Cream	2106
Ortho-Est	1925

Ethinyl Estradiol (Estrogens or estrogen-containing oral contraceptives tend to increase serum thyroxine-binding globulin (TBG); increase in thyroid requirements in patients with nonfunctioning thyroid gland on combined therapy). Products include:

Brevicon	2563
Demulen	2580
Desogen Tablets	1867
Levlen/Tri-Levlen	646
Lo/Ovral Tablets	2852
Lo/Ovral-28 Tablets	2857

(⊞ Described in PDR For Nonprescription Drugs)   (⊚ Described in PDR For Ophthalmology)

Modicon	1928
Nordette-21 Tablets	2863
Nordette-28 Tablets	2866
Norinyl	2563
Ortho-Cept	1907
Ortho-Cyclen/Ortho-Tri-Cyclen	1914
Ortho-Novum	1928
Ortho-Cyclen/Ortho Tri-Cyclen	1914
Ovcon	765
Ovral Tablets	2877
Ovral-28 Tablets	2878
Levlen/Tri-Levlen	646
Tri-Norinyl	2607
Triphasil-21 Tablets	2919
Triphasil-28 Tablets	2924

Glimepiride (Initiating thyroid replacement therapy may cause increases in hypoglycemic requirements). Products include:

Amaryl Tablets	1241

Glipizide (Initiating thyroid replacement therapy may cause increases in hypoglycemic requirements). Products include:

Glucotrol Tablets	2011
Glucotrol XL Extended Release Tablets	2012

Glyburide (Initiating thyroid replacement therapy may cause increases in hypoglycemic requirements). Products include:

DiaBeta Tablets	1265
Glynase PresTab Tablets	2091
Micronase Tablets	2099

Insulin, Human (Initiating thyroid replacement therapy may cause increases in insulin requirements).
No products indexed under this heading.

Insulin, Human Isophane Suspension (Initiating thyroid replacement therapy may cause increases in insulin requirements). Products include:

Novolin N Human Insulin 10 ml Vials	1846

Insulin, Human NPH (Initiating thyroid replacement therapy may cause increases in insulin requirements). Products include:

Humulin N, 100 Units	1495
Novolin N PenFill 1.5 ml Cartridges Durable Insulin Delivery System	1849
Novolin N Prefilled Syringe Disposable Insulin Delivery System	1850

Insulin, Human Regular (Initiating thyroid replacement therapy may cause increases in insulin requirements). Products include:

Humulin R, 100 Units	1497
Novolin R Human Insulin 10 ml Vials	1846
Novolin R PenFill 1.5 ml Cartridges Durable Insulin Delivery System	1849
Novolin R Prefilled Syringe Disposable Insulin Delivery System	1850
Velosulin BR Human Insulin 10 ml Vials	1847

Insulin, Human, Zinc Suspension (Initiating thyroid replacement therapy may cause increases in insulin requirements). Products include:

Humulin L, 100 Units	1494
Humulin U, 100 Units	1498
Novolin L Human Insulin 10 ml Vials	1846

Insulin Lispro, Human (Initiating thyroid replacement therapy may cause increases in insulin requirements). Products include:

Humalog Injection	1488

Insulin, NPH (Initiating thyroid replacement therapy may cause increases in insulin requirements). Products include:

NPH, 100 Units	1502
Pork NPH, 100 Units	1506
Purified Pork NPH Isophane Insulin	1852

Insulin, Regular (Initiating thyroid replacement therapy may cause increases in insulin requirements). Products include:

Regular, 100 Units	1503
Pork Regular, 100 Units	1507
Pork Regular (Concentrated), 500 Units	1508
Purified Pork Regular Insulin	1852

Insulin, Zinc Crystals (Initiating thyroid replacement therapy may cause increases in insulin requirements). Products include:

NPH, 100 Units	1502

Insulin, Zinc Suspension (Initiating thyroid replacement therapy may cause increases in insulin requirements). Products include:

Iletin I	1501
Lente, 100 Units	1501
Iletin II	1504
Pork Lente, 100 Units	1504
Purified Pork Lente Insulin	1852

Metformin Hydrochloride (Initiating thyroid replacement therapy may cause increases in hypoglycemic requirements). Products include:

Glucophage Tablets	754

Polyestradiol Phosphate (Estrogens or estrogen-containing oral contraceptives tend to increase serum thyroxine-binding globulin (TBG); increase in thyroid requirements in patients with nonfunctioning thyroid gland on combined therapy).
No products indexed under this heading.

Quinestrol (Estrogens or estrogen-containing oral contraceptives tend to increase serum thyroxine-binding globulin (TBG); increase in thyroid requirements in patients with non-functioning thyroid gland on combined therapy).
No products indexed under this heading.

Tolazamide (Initiating thyroid replacement therapy may cause increases in hypoglycemic requirements).
No products indexed under this heading.

Tolbutamide (Initiating thyroid replacement therapy may cause increases in hypoglycemic requirements).
No products indexed under this heading.

Warfarin Sodium (Thyroid hormones appear to increase catabolism of vitamin K-dependent clotting factor; concurrent therapy may result in impairment of compensatory increases in clotting factor synthesis; anticoagulant dosage adjustment may be required). Products include:

Coumadin	941

LEVOXYL TABLETS

(Levothyroxine Sodium) 918
May interact with insulin, oral hypoglycemic agents, oral anticoagulants, estrogens, and certain other agents. Compounds in these categories include:

Acarbose (May cause an increase in the required dosage of oral hypoglycemics). Products include:

Precose	604

Chlorotrianisene (Increases serum thyroxine-binding globulin (TBG) in patients with a non-functioning thyroid gland who are receiving thyroid replacement therapy thus decreasing thyroxine and increasing thyroid requirements in patients who are on estrogens or estrogen containing oral contraceptives).
No products indexed under this heading.

Chlorpropamide (May cause an increase in the required dosage of oral hypoglycemics). Products include:

Diabinese Tablets	2002

Cholestyramine (Impairs absorption; 4 to 5 hours should elapse between administration of cholestyramine and thyroid hormones). Products include:

Questran	774

Dicumarol (Close supervision is advised; possible reduction in anticoagulant dosage).
No products indexed under this heading.

Dienestrol (Increases serum thyroxine-binding globulin (TBG) in patients with a non-functioning thyroid gland who are receiving thyroid replacement therapy thus decreasing thyroxine and increasing thyroid requirements in patients who are on estrogens or estrogen containing oral contraceptives). Products include:

Ortho Dienestrol Cream	1922

Diethylstilbestrol (Increases serum thyroxine-binding globulin (TBG) in patients with a non-functioning thyroid gland who are receiving thyroid replacement therapy thus decreasing thyroxine and increasing thyroid requirements in patients who are on estrogens or estrogen containing oral contraceptives). Products include:

Diethylstilbestrol Tablets	1477

Estradiol (Increases serum thyroxine-binding globulin (TBG) in patients with a non-functioning thyroid gland who are receiving thyroid replacement therapy thus decreasing thyroxine and increasing thyroid requirements in patients who are on estrogens or estrogen containing oral contraceptives). Products include:

Climara Transdermal System	640
Estrace Cream and Tablets	751
Estraderm Transdermal System	842
Estring Vaginal Ring	2086
Vivelle Transdermal System	880

Estrogens, Conjugated (Increases serum thyroxine-binding globulin (TBG) in patients with a non-functioning thyroid gland who are receiving thyroid replacement therapy thus decreasing thyroxine and increasing thyroid requirements in patients who are on estrogens or estrogen containing oral contraceptives). Products include:

PMB 200 and PMB 400	2890
Premarin Intravenous	2893
Premarin Tablets	2896
Premarin Vaginal Cream	2898
Premphase	2900
Prempro	2905

Estrogens, Esterified (Increases serum thyroxine-binding globulin (TBG) in patients with a non-functioning thyroid gland who are receiving thyroid replacement therapy thus decreasing thyroxine and increasing thyroid requirements in patients who are on estrogens or estrogen containing oral contraceptives). Products include:

ESTRATAB Tablets (0.3, 0.625, 1.25, 2.5 mg)	2715
Estratest	2718
Menest Tablets	2671

Estropipate (Increases serum thyroxine-binding globulin (TBG) in patients with a non-functioning thyroid gland who are receiving thyroid replacement therapy thus decreasing thyroxine and increasing thyroid requirements in patients who are on estrogens or estrogen containing oral contraceptives). Products include:

Ogen Tablets	2103
Ogen Vaginal Cream	2106
Ortho-Est	1925

Ethinyl Estradiol (Increases serum thyroxine-binding globulin (TBG) in patients with a non-functioning thyroid gland who are receiving thyroid replacement therapy thus decreasing thyroxine and increasing thyroid requirements in patients who are on estrogens or estrogen containing oral contraceptives). Products include:

Brevicon	2563
Demulen	2580
Desogen Tablets	1867
Levlen/Tri-Levlen	646
Lo/Ovral Tablets	2852
Lo/Ovral-28 Tablets	2857
Modicon	1928
Nordette-21 Tablets	2863
Nordette-28 Tablets	2866
Norinyl	2563
Ortho-Cept	1907
Ortho-Cyclen/Ortho-Tri-Cyclen	1914
Ortho-Novum	1928
Ortho-Cyclen/Ortho Tri-Cyclen	1914
Ovcon	765
Ovral Tablets	2877
Ovral-28 Tablets	2878
Levlen/Tri-Levlen	646
Tri-Norinyl	2607
Triphasil-21 Tablets	2919
Triphasil-28 Tablets	2924

Glimepiride (May cause an increase in the required dosage of oral hypoglycemics). Products include:

Amaryl Tablets	1241

Glipizide (May cause an increase in the required dosage of oral hypoglycemics). Products include:

Glucotrol Tablets	2011
Glucotrol XL Extended Release Tablets	2012

Glyburide (May cause an increase in the required dosage of oral hypoglycemics). Products include:

DiaBeta Tablets	1265
Glynase PresTab Tablets	2091
Micronase Tablets	2099

Insulin, Human (May cause an increase in the required dosage of insulin).
No products indexed under this heading.

Insulin, Human Isophane Suspension (May cause an increase in the required dosage of insulin). Products include:

Novolin N Human Insulin 10 ml Vials	1846

Insulin, Human NPH (May cause an increase in the required dosage of insulin). Products include:

Humulin N, 100 Units	1495
Novolin N PenFill 1.5 ml Cartridges Durable Insulin Delivery System	1849

IMPORTANT NOTE: Always consult each drug listing in the patient's regimen for possible interactions.

Levoxyl | Interactions Index | 602

Novolin N Prefilled Syringe Disposable Insulin Delivery System 1850

Insulin, Human Regular (May cause an increase in the required dosage of insulin). Products include:
- Humulin R, 100 Units 1497
- Novolin R Human Insulin 10 ml Vials 1846
- Novolin R PenFill 1.5 ml Cartridges Durable Insulin Delivery System 1849
- Novolin R Prefilled Syringe Disposable Insulin Delivery System 1850
- Velosulin BR Human Insulin 10 ml Vials 1847

Insulin, Human, Zinc Suspension (May cause an increase in the required dosage of insulin). Products include:
- Humulin L, 100 Units 1494
- Humulin U, 100 Units 1498
- Novolin L Human Insulin 10 ml Vials 1846

Insulin Lispro, Human (May cause an increase in the required dosage of insulin). Products include:
- Humalog Injection 1488

Insulin, NPH (May cause an increase in the required dosage of insulin). Products include:
- NPH, 100 Units 1502
- Pork NPH, 100 Units 1506
- Purified Pork NPH Isophane Insulin 1852

Insulin, Regular (May cause an increase in the required dosage of insulin). Products include:
- Regular, 100 Units 1503
- Pork Regular, 100 Units 1507
- Pork Regular (Concentrated), 500 Units 1508
- Purified Pork Regular Insulin 1852

Insulin, Zinc Crystals (May cause an increase in the required dosage of insulin). Products include:
- NPH, 100 Units 1502

Insulin, Zinc Suspension (May cause an increase in the required dosage of insulin). Products include:
- Iletin I 1501
- Lente, 100 Units 1501
- Iletin II 1504
- Pork Lente, 100 Units 1504
- Purified Pork Lente Insulin 1852

Metformin Hydrochloride (May cause an increase in the required dosage of oral hypoglycemics). Products include:
- Glucophage Tablets 754

Polyestradiol Phosphate (Increases serum thyroxine-binding globulin (TBG) in patients with a non-functioning thyroid gland who are receiving thyroid replacement therapy thus decreasing thyroxine and increasing thyroid requirements in patients who are on estrogens or estrogen containing oral contraceptives).
- No products indexed under this heading.

Quinestrol (Increases serum thyroxine-binding globulin (TBG) in patients with a non-functioning thyroid gland who are receiving thyroid replacement therapy thus decreasing thyroxine and increasing thyroid requirements in patients who are on estrogens or estrogen containing oral contraceptives).
- No products indexed under this heading.

Tolazamide (May cause an increase in the required dosage of oral hypoglycemics).
- No products indexed under this heading.

Tolbutamide (May cause an increase in the required dosage of oral hypoglycemics).
- No products indexed under this heading.

Warfarin Sodium (Close supervision is advised; possible reduction in anticoagulant dosage). Products include:
- Coumadin 941

LEVSIN DROPS
(Hyoscyamine Sulfate) 2549

May interact with antimuscarinic drugs, phenothiazines, monoamine oxidase inhibitors, tricyclic antidepressants, antihistamines, antacids, and certain other agents. Compounds in these categories include:

Acrivastine (Additive adverse effects). Products include:
- Semprex-D Capsules 1620

Aluminum Carbonate (Interferes with absorption of Levsin). Products include:
- Basaljel Capsules 2810
- Basaljel Suspension 2810
- Basaljel Tablets 2810

Aluminum Hydroxide (Interferes with absorption of Levsin). Products include:
- ALternaGEL Liquid 1358
- Maximum Strength Ascriptin .... ▣ 650
- Cama Arthritis Pain Reliever .... ▣ 748
- Gaviscon Extra Strength Relief Formula Antacid Tablets .... ▣ 778
- Gaviscon Extra Strength Relief Formula Liquid Antacid .... ▣ 779
- Gaviscon Liquid Antacid .... ▣ 779
- Gelusil Antacid-Anti-gas Liquid .... ▣ 819
- Gelusil Antacid-Anti-gas Tablets .... ▣ 819
- Maalox Antacid/Anti-Gas Tablets 889
- Maalox Heartburn Relief Suspension .... ▣ 658
- Maalox Antacid Liquid 888
- Extra Strength Maalox Antacid/Anti-Gas Liquid and Tablets 888
- Mylanta 1359
- Tempo Soft Antacid .... ▣ 799

Aluminum Hydroxide Gel (Interferes with absorption of Levsin). Products include:
- ALternaGEL Liquid .... ▣ 675
- Aludrox Oral Suspension .... ▣ 850
- Amphojel Suspension 2802
- Amphojel Suspension without Flavor 2802
- Amphojel Tablets 2802
- Ascriptin .... ▣ 650
- Gaviscon Antacid Tablets .... ▣ 778
- Gaviscon-2 Antacid Tablets .... ▣ 779
- Mylanta Liquid .... ▣ 676
- Mylanta Double Strength Liquid .... ▣ 676
- Nephrox Suspension .... ▣ 671

Amantadine Hydrochloride (Additive adverse effects). Products include:
- Symmetrel Capsules 965
- Symmetrel Syrup 963

Amitriptyline Hydrochloride (Additive adverse effects). Products include:
- Elavil 2945
- Etrafon 2495
- Limbitrol 2333
- Triavil Tablets 1800

Amoxapine (Additive adverse effects). Products include:
- Asendin Tablets 1419

Astemizole (Additive adverse effects). Products include:
- Hismanal Tablets 1341

Atropine Sulfate (Additive adverse effects). Products include:
- Arco-Lase Plus Tablets 513
- Atrohist Plus Tablets 1605
- Donnatal 2234
- Donnatal Extentabs 2234
- Donnatal Tablets 2234
- Lomotil 2591
- Motofen Tablets 789
- Urised Tablets 2123

Azatadine Maleate (Additive adverse effects). Products include:
- Trinalin Repetabs Tablets 1373

Belladonna Alkaloids (Additive adverse effects). Products include:
- Bellergal-S Tablets 2375
- Hyland's Bedwetting Tablets .... ▣ 788
- Hyland's EnurAid Tablets .... ▣ 789
- Hyland's Headache Tablets .... ▣ 790
- Hyland's Teething Tablets .... ▣ 790
- Similasan Eye Drops #1 .... ▣ 769

Bromodiphenhydramine Hydrochloride (Additive adverse effects).
- No products indexed under this heading.

Brompheniramine Maleate (Additive adverse effects). Products include:
- Alka-Seltzer Plus Sinus Medicine .... ▣ 611
- Bromfed Capsules (Extended-Release) 1832
- Bromfed Syrup .... ▣ 712
- Bromfed Tablets 1832
- Bromfed-DM Cough Syrup 1832
- Bromfed-PD Capsules (Extended-Release) 1832
- Dimetane-DC Cough Syrup 2232
- Dimetane-DX Cough Syrup 2233
- Dimetapp Allergy Dye-Free Elixir .... ▣ 838
- Dimetapp Allergy Sinus Caplets .... ▣ 838
- Dimetapp Cold & Allergy Chewable Tablets .... ▣ 838
- Dimetapp Cold & Cough Liqui-Gels .... ▣ 839
- Dimetapp Cold & Fever Suspension .... ▣ 839
- Dimetapp DM Elixir .... ▣ 840
- Dimetapp Elixir .... ▣ 840
- Dimetapp Extentabs .... ▣ 841
- Dimetapp Tablets/Liqui-Gels .... ▣ 841
- Rondec Chewable Tablets 974
- Vicks DayQuil Allergy Relief 12-Hour Extended Release Tablets .... ▣ 733
- Vicks DayQuil Allergy Relief 4-Hour Tablets .... ▣ 733

Cetirizine Hydrochloride (Additive adverse effects). Products include:
- Zyrtec Tablets 2053

Chlorpheniramine Maleate (Additive adverse effects). Products include:
- Alka-Seltzer Plus Cold Medicine .... ▣ 611
- Alka-Seltzer Plus Cold Medicine Liqui-Gels .... ▣ 612
- Alka-Seltzer Plus Cold & Cough Medicine .... ▣ 611
- Alka-Seltzer Plus Cold & Cough Medicine Liqui-Gels .... ▣ 612
- Alka-Seltzer Plus Flu & Body Aches Effervescent Tablets .... ▣ 612
- Allerest Maximum Strength .... ▣ 649
- Allerest Sinus Pain Formula .... ▣ 649
- Ana-Kit Anaphylaxis Emergency Treatment Kit 611
- Atrohist Pediatric Capsules 1603
- Atrohist Plus Tablets 1605
- BC Cold Powder Multi-Symptom Formula (Cold-Sinus-Allergy) .... ▣ 631
- Cerose DM .... ▣ 853
- Cheracol Plus Head Cold/Cough Formula .... ▣ 741
- Children's TYLENOL Cold Multi-Symptom Chewable Tablets and Liquid 1559
- Children's TYLENOL Cold Plus Cough Multi Symptom Chewable Tablets and Liquid 1560
- Children's TYLENOL Flu Suspension Liquid 1560
- Children's Vicks DayQuil Allergy Relief .... ▣ 730
- Children's Vicks NyQuil Cold/Cough Relief .... ▣ 731
- Chlor-Trimeton Allergy Decongestant Tablets .... ▣ 759
- Chlor-Trimeton Allergy Tablets .... ▣ 758
- Allergy-Sinus Comtrex Multi-Symptom Allergy-Sinus Formula Tablets and Caplets .... ▣ 639
- Comtrex Multi-Symptom .... ▣ 638
- Contac Continuous Action Nasal Decongestant/Antihistamine 12 Hour Capsules .... ▣ 773
- Contac Maximum Strength Continuous Action Decongestant/Antihistamine 12 Hour Caplets .... ▣ 772
- Contac Severe Cold and Flu Formula Caplets .... ▣ 773
- Coricidin Cold + Flu Tablets .... ▣ 760
- Coricidin Cough + Cold Tablets .... ▣ 760
- Coricidin 'D' Decongestant Tablets .... ▣ 760
- D.A. II Tablets 972
- D.A. Chewable Tablets 970
- Dura-Tap/PD Capsules 970
- Dura-Vent/DA Tablets 972
- Efidac 24 Chlorpheniramine .... ▣ 655
- Extendryl 1003
- Fedahist Gyrocaps 2545
- Hycomine Compound Tablets 948
- Kronofed-A 994
- Nolamine Timed-Release Tablets 790
- Novahistine Elixir .... ▣ 782
- Ornade Spansule Capsules 2678
- PediaCare Cough-Cold Chewable Tablets and Liquid 1569
- PediaCare NightRest Cough-Cold Liquid 1569
- Pediatric Vicks 44m Cough & Cold Relief .... ▣ 737
- Pyrroxate Caplets .... ▣ 742
- Ryna .... ▣ 804
- Sinarest .... ▣ 663
- Sine-Off Sinus Medicine .... ▣ 784
- Singlet Tablets .... ▣ 785
- Sinulin Tablets 792
- Sinutab Sinus Allergy Medication, Maximum Strength Tablets and Caplets .... ▣ 823
- Sudafed Cold & Allergy Tablets .... ▣ 826
- Teldrin 12 Hour Antihistamine/Nasal Decongestant Allergy Relief Capsules .... ▣ 786
- TheraFlu Flu and Cold Medicine .... ▣ 750
- Theraflu Maximum Strength Flu and Cold Medicine For Sore Throat .... ▣ 751
- TheraFlu Flu, Cold and Cough Medicine .... ▣ 750
- TheraFlu Maximum Strength Nighttime Flu, Cold & Cough Medicine .... ▣ 751
- Triaminic Night Time .... ▣ 754
- Triaminic Syrup .... ▣ 755
- Triaminic Triaminicol Cold & Cough .... ▣ 756
- Triaminicin Tablets .... ▣ 756
- Tussend 1830
- TYLENOL Allergy Sinus, Maximum Strength Caplets and Gelcaps 1571
- TYLENOL Cold Medication, Multi-Symptom Formula Tablets and Caplets 1572
- TYLENOL Cold Medication, Multi-Symptom Hot Liquid Packets 1572
- Vicks 44 LiquiCaps Cough, Cold & Flu Relief .... ▣ 728
- Vicks 44M Cough, Cold & Flu Relief .... ▣ 729

Chlorpheniramine Polistirex (Additive adverse effects). Products include:
- Tussionex Pennkinetic Extended-Release Suspension 1624

Chlorpheniramine Tannate (Additive adverse effects). Products include:
- Atrohist Pediatric Suspension 1604
- Atrohist Pediatric Suspension Dye-Free 1604
- Rynatan 2781
- Rynatuss 2782

Chlorpromazine (Additive adverse effects). Products include:
- Thorazine Suppositories 2701

Chlorpromazine Hydrochloride (Additive adverse effects). Products include:
- Thorazine 2701

Clemastine Fumarate (Additive adverse effects). Products include:
- Tavist Syrup 2426
- Tavist Tablets 2427
- Tavist-1 12 Hour Relief Tablets .... ▣ 749
- Tavist-D 12 Hour Relief Tablets .... ▣ 750

Clidinium Bromide (Additive adverse effects). Products include:
- Librax Capsules 2330

Clomipramine Hydrochloride (Additive adverse effects). Products include:
- Anafranil Capsules 819

(▣ Described in PDR For Nonprescription Drugs) (◉ Described in PDR For Ophthalmology)

Cyproheptadine Hydrochloride (Additive adverse effects). Products include:
Periactin 1767

Desipramine Hydrochloride (Additive adverse effects). Products include:
Norpramin Tablets 1273

Dexchlorpheniramine Maleate (Additive adverse effects).
No products indexed under this heading.

Dicyclomine Hydrochloride (Additive adverse effects). Products include:
Bentyl 1246

Diphenhydramine Citrate (Additive adverse effects). Products include:
Excedrin P.M. Analgesic/Sleeping Aid Tablets, Caplets, Liquigels 735

Diphenhydramine Hydrochloride (Additive adverse effects). Products include:
Actifed Allergy Daytime/Nighttime Caplets 808
Actifed Sinus Daytime/Nighttime Tablets and Caplets 809
Extra Strength Bayer PM Aspirin Plus Sleep Aid 617
Benadryl Allergy Chewables 811
Benadryl Allergy/Cold Tablets 811
Benadryl Allergy Decongestant Liquid Medication 812
Benadryl Allergy Decongestant Tablets 812
Benadryl Allergy Liquid Medication 813
Benadryl Allergy 811
Benadryl Allergy Sinus Headache Caplets 813
Benadryl Dye-Free Allergy Liquigel Softgels 813
Benadryl Dye-Free Allergy Liquid Medication 814
Benadryl Itch Relief Stick Extra Strength 814
Benadryl Cream 814
Benadryl Gel 815
Benadryl Spray 815
Benadryl Injection 1955
Contac Day & Night Cold/Flu Night Caplets 772
Contac Night Allergy/Sinus Caplets 771
Extra Strength Doan's P.M. 653
Excedrin P.M. Analgesic/Sleeping Aid Tablets, Caplets, Liquigels 643
Nytol QuickCaps Caplets 632
Sleepinal Night-time Sleep Aid Capsules and Softgels 798
TYLENOL Allergy Sinus NightTime, Maximum Strength Caplets 1571
TYLENOL Flu NightTime, Maximum Strength Gelcaps 1575
TYLENOL Flu NightTime, Maximum Strength Hot Medication Packets 1575
TYLENOL PM Pain Reliever/Sleep Aid, Extra Strength Gelcaps, Caplets, Geltabs 1576
TYLENOL Severe Allergy Medication Caplets 1571
Maximum Strength Unisom Sleepgels 1990
Unisom With Pain Relief-Nighttime Sleep Aid and Pain Reliever 1991

Diphenylpyraline Hydrochloride (Additive adverse effects).
No products indexed under this heading.

Doxepin Hydrochloride (Additive adverse effects). Products include:
Adapin Capsules 1542
Sinequan 2028
Zonalon Cream 1042

Fluphenazine Decanoate (Additive adverse effects). Products include:
Prolixin Decanoate 510

Fluphenazine Enanthate (Additive adverse effects). Products include:
Prolixin Enanthate 510

Fluphenazine Hydrochloride (Additive adverse effects). Products include:
Prolixin 510

Furazolidone (Additive adverse effects). Products include:
Furoxone 2221

Glycopyrrolate (Additive adverse effects). Products include:
Robinul Forte Tablets 2247
Robinul Injectable 2247
Robinul Tablets 2247

Haloperidol (Additive adverse effects). Products include:
Haldol Injection, Tablets and Concentrate 1585

Haloperidol Decanoate (Additive adverse effects). Products include:
Haldol Decanoate 1587

Hyoscyamine (Additive adverse effects). Products include:
Cystospaz Tablets 2123
Urised Tablets 2123

Imipramine Hydrochloride (Additive adverse effects). Products include:
Tofranil Ampuls 873
Tofranil Tablets 875

Imipramine Pamoate (Additive adverse effects). Products include:
Tofranil-PM Capsules 876

Ipratropium Bromide (Additive adverse effects). Products include:
Atrovent Inhalation Aerosol 674
Atrovent Inhalation Solution 675
Atrovent Nasal Spray 0.03% 676
Atrovent Nasal Spray 0.06% 678

Isocarboxazid (Additive adverse effects).
No products indexed under this heading.

Loratadine (Additive adverse effects). Products include:
Claritin Tablets 2485
Claritin-D Tablets 2487

Magaldrate (Interferes with absorption of Levsin).
No products indexed under this heading.

Magnesium Hydroxide (Interferes with absorption of Levsin). Products include:
Aludrox Oral Suspension 850
Ascriptin 650
Di-Gel Antacid/Anti-Gas 762
Gelusil Antacid-Anti-gas Liquid 819
Gelusil Antacid-Anti-gas Tablets 819
Maalox Antacid/Anti-Gas Tablets 889
Maalox Antacid Liquid 888
Extra Strength Maalox Antacid/Anti-Gas Liquid and Tablets ... 888
Mylanta Fast-Acting 1359
Mylanta Gelcaps Antacid 678
Fast-Acting Mylanta Liquid Antacid 1359
Mylanta Tablets 677
Maximum Strength Fast-Acting Mylanta Liquid Antacid 1359
Mylanta Double Strength Plus ... 678
Phillips' Milk of Magnesia Liquid 627
Rolaids Antacid Tablets 807
Tempo Soft Antacid 799

Magnesium Oxide (Interferes with absorption of Levsin). Products include:
Beelith Tablets 632
Bufferin Analgesic Tablets 636
Arthritis Strength Bufferin Analgesic Caplets 637
Extra Strength Bufferin Analgesic Tablets 637
Caltrate PLUS 681
Cama Arthritis Pain Reliever 748
Mag-Ox 400 666
Uro-Mag 666

Maprotiline Hydrochloride (Additive adverse effects). Products include:
Ludiomil Tablets 861

Mepenzolate Bromide (Additive adverse effects).
No products indexed under this heading.

Mesoridazine Besylate (Additive adverse effects). Products include:
Serentil 689

Methdilazine Hydrochloride (Additive adverse effects).
No products indexed under this heading.

Methotrimeprazine (Additive adverse effects). Products include:
Levoprome 1321

Nortriptyline Hydrochloride (Additive adverse effects). Products include:
Pamelor 2409

Oxyphenonium Bromide (Additive adverse effects).

Perphenazine (Additive adverse effects). Products include:
Etrafon 2495
Triavil Tablets 1800
Trilafon 2532

Phenelzine Sulfate (Additive adverse effects). Products include:
Nardil 1977

Prochlorperazine (Additive adverse effect). Products include:
Compazine 2644

Promethazine Hydrochloride (Additive adverse effects). Products include:
Mepergan Injection 2859
Phenergan with Codeine 2883
Phenergan with Dextromethorphan 2885
Phenergan Injection 2880
Phenergan Suppositories 2882
Phenergan Syrup 2881
Phenergan Tablets 2882
Phenergan VC 2886
Phenergan VC with Codeine 2888

Propantheline Bromide (Additive adverse effects). Products include:
Pro-Banthine Tablets 2226

Protriptyline Hydrochloride (Additive adverse effects). Products include:
Vivactil Tablets 1820

Pyrilamine Maleate (Additive adverse effects). Products include:
4-Way Fast Acting Nasal Spray (regular & mentholated) 644
Maximum Strength Multi-Symptom Formula Midol 621
PMS Multi-Symptom Formula Midol 622

Pyrilamine Tannate (Additive adverse effects). Products include:
Atrohist Pediatric Suspension 1604
Atrohist Pediatric Suspension Dye-Free 1604
Rynatan 2781

Scopolamine (Additive adverse effects). Products include:
Transderm Scōp Transdermal Therapeutic System 890

Scopolamine Hydrobromide (Additive adverse effects). Products include:
Atrohist Plus Tablets 1605
Donnatal 2234
Donnatal Extentabs 2234
Donnatal Tablets 2234

Selegiline Hydrochloride (Additive adverse effects). Products include:
Eldepryl Capsules 2729

Terfenadine (Additive adverse effects). Products include:
Seldane Tablets 1284
Seldane-D Extended-Release Tablets 1286

Thioridazine Hydrochloride (Additive adverse effects). Products include:
Mellaril 2398

Tranylcypromine Sulfate (Additive adverse effects). Products include:
Parnate Tablets 2679

Tridihexethyl Chloride (Additive adverse effects).
No products indexed under this heading.

Trifluoperazine Hydrochloride (Additive adverse effects). Products include:
Stelazine 2692

Trimeprazine Tartrate (Additive adverse effects).
No products indexed under this heading.

Trimipramine Maleate (Additive adverse effects). Products include:
Surmontil Capsules 2917

Tripelennamine Hydrochloride (Additive adverse effects). Products include:
PBZ Tablets 863
PBZ-SR Tablets 862

Triprolidine Hydrochloride (Additive adverse effects). Products include:
Actifed Cold & Allergy Tablets 807
Actifed Cold & Sinus Caplets and Tablets 808

LEVSIN ELIXIR
(Hyoscyamine Sulfate) 2549
See **Levsin Drops**

LEVSIN INJECTION
(Hyoscyamine Sulfate) 2549
See **Levsin Drops**

LEVSIN TABLETS
(Hyoscyamine Sulfate) 2549
See **Levsin Drops**

LEVSIN/SL TABLETS
(Hyoscyamine Sulfate) 2549
See **Levsin Drops**

LEVSINEX TIMECAPS
(Hyoscyamine Sulfate) 2549
See **Levsin Drops**

LIBRAX CAPSULES
(Chlordiazepoxide Hydrochloride, Clidinium Bromide) 2330
May interact with monoamine oxidase inhibitors, phenothiazines, central nervous system depressants, oral anticoagulants, and certain other agents. Compounds in these categories include:

Alfentanil Hydrochloride (Co-administration may produce additive CNS depressant effects). Products include:
Alfenta Injection 1334

Alprazolam (Co-administration may produce additive CNS depressant effects). Products include:
Xanax Tablets 2115

Aprobarbital (Co-administration may produce additive CNS depressant effects).
No products indexed under this heading.

Buprenorphine (Co-administration may produce additive CNS depressant effects). Products include:
Buprenex Injectable 2170

Buspirone Hydrochloride (Co-administration may produce additive CNS depressant effects). Products include:
BuSpar Tablets 738

Butabarbital (Co-administration may produce additive CNS depressant effects).
No products indexed under this heading.

Butalbital (Co-administration may produce additive CNS depressant effects). Products include:
Axocet Capsules 2469
Esgic-plus Capsules 1012

IMPORTANT NOTE: Always consult each drug listing in the patient's regimen for possible interactions.

Librax — Interactions Index

Esgic-plus Tablets 1012
Fioricet Tablets 2386
Fioricet with Codeine Capsules ... 2387
Fiorinal Capsules 2388
Fiorinal with Codeine Capsules ... 2390
Fiorinal Tablets 2388
Phrenilin 790
Sedapap Tablets 50 mg/650 mg .. 1826

Chlordiazepoxide (Co-administration may produce additive CNS depressant effects). Products include:
Limbitrol 2333

Chlorpromazine (Phenothiazines may have potentiating effects). Products include:
Thorazine Suppositories 2701

Chlorpromazine Hydrochloride (Phenothiazines may have potentiating effects). Products include:
Thorazine 2701

Chlorprothixene (Co-administration may produce additive CNS depressant effects).
No products indexed under this heading.

Chlorprothixene Hydrochloride (Co-administration may produce additive CNS depressant effects).
No products indexed under this heading.

Chlorprothixene Lactate (Co-administration may produce additive CNS depressant effects).
No products indexed under this heading.

Clorazepate Dipotassium (Co-administration may produce additive CNS depressant effects). Products include:
Tranxene 459

Clozapine (Co-administration may produce additive CNS depressant effects). Products include:
Clozaril Tablets 2377

Codeine Phosphate (Co-administration may produce additive CNS depressant effects). Products include:
Brontex 2130
Dimetane-DC Cough Syrup 2232
Fioricet with Codeine Capsules ... 2387
Fiorinal with Codeine Capsules ... 2390
Nucofed 2225
Phenergan with Codeine 2883
Phenergan VC with Codeine ... 2888
Robitussin A-C Syrup 2248
Robitussin-DAC Syrup 2249
Ryna .... ▣ 804
Soma Compound w/Codeine Tablets 2784
Tylenol with Codeine 1592

Desflurane (Co-administration may produce additive CNS depressant effects). Products include:
Suprane (desflurane, USP) 1865

Dezocine (Co-administration may produce additive CNS depressant effects). Products include:
Dalgan Injection 529

Diazepam (Co-administration may produce additive CNS depressant effects). Products include:
Dizac (diazepam injectable emulsion) CIV 1862
Valium Injectable 2336
Valium Tablets 2335

Dicumarol (Co-administration of chlordiazepoxide and oral anticoagulants has produced variable effects on blood coagulation).
No products indexed under this heading.

Droperidol (Co-administration may produce additive CNS depressant effects). Products include:
Inapsine Injection 462

Enflurane (Co-administration may produce additive CNS depressant effects).
No products indexed under this heading.

Estazolam (Co-administration may produce additive CNS depressant effects). Products include:
ProSom Tablets 457

Ethchlorvynol (Co-administration may produce additive CNS depressant effects). Products include:
Placidyl Capsules 456

Ethinamate (Co-administration may produce additive CNS depressant effects).
No products indexed under this heading.

Fentanyl (Co-administration may produce additive CNS depressant effects). Products include:
Duragesic Transdermal System 1336

Fentanyl Citrate (Co-administration may produce additive CNS depressant effects). Products include:
Sublimaze Injection 463

Fluphenazine Decanoate (Phenothiazines may have potentiating effects). Products include:
Prolixin Decanoate 510

Fluphenazine Enanthate (Phenothiazines may have potentiating effects). Products include:
Prolixin Enanthate 510

Fluphenazine Hydrochloride (Phenothiazines may have potentiating effects). Products include:
Prolixin 510

Flurazepam Hydrochloride (Co-administration may produce additive CNS depressant effects). Products include:
Dalmane Capsules 2329

Furazolidone (MAO inhibitors may have potentiating effects). Products include:
Furoxone 2221

Glutethimide (Co-administration may produce additive CNS depressant effects).
No products indexed under this heading.

Haloperidol (Co-administration may produce additive CNS depressant effects). Products include:
Haldol Injection, Tablets and Concentrate 1585

Haloperidol Decanoate (Co-administration may produce additive CNS depressant effects). Products include:
Haldol Decanoate 1587

Hydrocodone Bitartrate (Co-administration may produce additive CNS depressant effects). Products include:
Codiclear DH Syrup 808
Duratuss HD Elixir 2750
Histussin D Liquid 670
Hycodan Tablets and Syrup 946
Hycomine Compound Tablets 948
Hycomine 947
Hycotuss Expectorant Syrup 950
Hydrocet Capsules 787
Lorcet 10/650 Tablets 1016
Lortab 2751
Tussend 1830
Tussend Expectorant 1831
Vicodin Tablets 1404
Vicodin ES Tablets 1405
Vicodin HP Tablets 1403
Vicodin Tuss Expectorant 1406
Zydone Tablets 967

Hydrocodone Polistirex (Co-administration may produce additive CNS depressant effects). Products include:
Tussionex Pennkinetic Extended-Release Suspension 1624

Hydromorphone Hydrochloride (Co-administration may produce additive CNS depressant effects). Products include:
Dilaudid Ampules 1382
Dilaudid Cough Syrup 1383
Dilaudid-HP Injection 1384
Dilaudid-HP Lyophilized Powder 250 mg 1384
Dilaudid 1382
Dilaudid Oral Liquid 1386
Dilaudid 1382
Dilaudid Tablets - 8 mg 1386

Hydroxyzine Hydrochloride (Co-administration may produce additive CNS depressant effects). Products include:
Atarax Tablets & Syrup 1992
Marax Tablets & DF Syrup 2015
Vistaril Intramuscular Solution 2042

Isocarboxazid (MAO inhibitors may have potentiating effects).
No products indexed under this heading.

Isoflurane (Co-administration may produce additive CNS depressant effects).
No products indexed under this heading.

Ketamine Hydrochloride (Co-administration may produce additive CNS depressant effects).
No products indexed under this heading.

Levomethadyl Acetate Hydrochloride (Co-administration may produce additive CNS depressant effects). Products include:
Orlaam Oral Solution 2361

Levorphanol Tartrate (Co-administration may produce additive CNS depressant effects). Products include:
Levo-Dromoran 2297

Lorazepam (Co-administration may produce additive CNS depressant effects). Products include:
Ativan Injection 2805
Ativan Tablets 2807

Loxapine Hydrochloride (Co-administration may produce additive CNS depressant effects). Products include:
Loxitane 1426

Loxapine Succinate (Co-administration may produce additive CNS depressant effects). Products include:
Loxitane Capsules 1426

Meperidine Hydrochloride (Co-administration may produce additive CNS depressant effects). Products include:
Demerol 2438
Mepergan Injection 2859

Mephobarbital (Co-administration may produce additive CNS depressant effects). Products include:
Mebaral Tablets 2452

Meprobamate (Co-administration may produce additive CNS depressant effects). Products include:
Miltown Tablets 2780
PMB 200 and PMB 400 2890

Mesoridazine Besylate (Phenothiazines may have potentiating effects). Products include:
Serentil 689

Methadone Hydrochloride (Co-administration may produce additive CNS depressant effects). Products include:
Methadone Hydrochloride Oral Concentrate 2356
Methadone Hydrochloride Oral Solution & Tablets 2357

Methohexital Sodium (Co-administration may produce additive CNS depressant effects).
No products indexed under this heading.

Methotrimeprazine (Phenothiazines may have potentiating effects). Products include:
Levoprome 1321

Methoxyflurane (Co-administration may produce additive CNS depressant effects).
No products indexed under this heading.

Midazolam Hydrochloride (Co-administration may produce additive CNS depressant effects). Products include:
Versed Injection 2324

Molindone Hydrochloride (Co-administration may produce additive CNS depressant effects). Products include:
Moban Tablets and Concentrate ... 1036

Morphine Sulfate (Co-administration may produce additive CNS depressant effects). Products include:
Astramorph/PF Injection, USP (Preservative-Free) 526
Duramorph Injection 983
Infumorph 200 and Infumorph 500 Sterile Solutions 985
Kadian Capsules 2948
MS Contin Tablets 2149
MSIR 2152
Oramorph SR (Morphine Sulfate Sustained Release Tablets) 2359
RMS Suppositories CII 2766
Roxanol 2365

Opium Alkaloids (Co-administration may produce additive CNS depressant effects).
No products indexed under this heading.

Oxazepam (Co-administration may produce additive CNS depressant effects). Products include:
Serax Capsules 2916
Serax Tablets 2916

Oxycodone Hydrochloride (Co-administration may produce additive CNS depressant effects). Products include:
OxyContin Tablets 2163
OxyIR Capsules 2167
Percocet Tablets 955
Percodan Tablets 955
Percodan-Demi Tablets 956
Roxicodone Tablets, Oral Solution & Intensol (Oxycodone) 2366
Tylox Capsules 1593

Pentobarbital Sodium (Co-administration may produce additive CNS depressant effects). Products include:
Nembutal Sodium Capsules 440
Nembutal Sodium Solution 442
Nembutal Sodium Suppositories 444

Perphenazine (Phenothiazines may have potentiating effects). Products include:
Etrafon 2495
Triavil Tablets 1800
Trilafon 2532

Phenelzine Sulfate (MAO inhibitors may have potentiating effects). Products include:
Nardil 1977

Phenobarbital (Co-administration may produce additive CNS depressant effects). Products include:
Arco-Lase Plus Tablets 513
Bellergal-S Tablets 2375
Donnatal 2234
Donnatal Extentabs 2234
Donnatal Tablets 2234
Phenobarbital Elixir and Tablets 1523
Quadrinal Tablets 1398

Prazepam (Co-administration may produce additive CNS depressant effects).
No products indexed under this heading.

Prochlorperazine (Phenothiazines may have potentiating effects). Products include:
Compazine 2644

(▣ Described in PDR For Nonprescription Drugs)   (⊚ Described in PDR For Ophthalmology)

Interactions Index — Librium

Promethazine Hydrochloride (Phenothiazines may have potentiating effects). Products include:
- Mepergan Injection ... 2859
- Phenergan with Codeine ... 2883
- Phenergan with Dextromethorphan ... 2885
- Phenergan Injection ... 2880
- Phenergan Suppositories ... 2882
- Phenergan Syrup ... 2881
- Phenergan Tablets ... 2882
- Phenergan VC ... 2886
- Phenergan VC with Codeine ... 2888

Propofol (Co-administration may produce additive CNS depressant effects). Products include:
- Diprivan Injectable Emulsion ... 2939

Propoxyphene Hydrochloride (Co-administration may produce additive CNS depressant effects). Products include:
- Darvon ... 1475
- Wygesic Tablets ... 2930

Propoxyphene Napsylate (Co-administration may produce additive CNS depressant effects). Products include:
- Darvon-N/Darvocet-N ... 1473

Quazepam (Co-administration may produce additive CNS depressant effects). Products include:
- Doral Tablets ... 2773

Risperidone (Co-administration may produce additive CNS depressant effects). Products include:
- Risperdal Tablets ... 1348

Secobarbital Sodium (Co-administration may produce additive CNS depressant effects). Products include:
- Seconal Sodium Pulvules ... 1529

Selegiline Hydrochloride (MAO inhibitors may have potentiating effects). Products include:
- Eldepryl Capsules ... 2729

Sevoflurane (Co-administration may produce additive CNS depressant effects).
- No products indexed under this heading.

Sufentanil Citrate (Co-administration may produce additive CNS depressant effects). Products include:
- Sufenta Injection ... 1355

Temazepam (Co-administration may produce additive CNS depressant effects). Products include:
- Restoril Capsules ... 2413

Thiamylal Sodium (Co-administration may produce additive CNS depressant effects).
- No products indexed under this heading.

Thioridazine Hydrochloride (Phenothiazines may have potentiating effects). Products include:
- Mellaril ... 2398

Thiothixene (Co-administration may produce additive CNS depressant effects). Products include:
- Navane Capsules and Concentrate ... 2018
- Navane Intramuscular ... 2019

Tranylcypromine Sulfate (MAO inhibitors may have potentiating effects). Products include:
- Parnate Tablets ... 2679

Triazolam (Co-administration may produce additive CNS depressant effects). Products include:
- Halcion Tablets ... 2093

Trifluoperazine Hydrochloride (Phenothiazines may have potentiating effects). Products include:
- Stelazine ... 2692

Warfarin Sodium (Co-administration of chlordiazepoxide and oral anticoagulants has produced variable effects on blood coagulation). Products include:
- Coumadin ... 941

Zolpidem Tartrate (Co-administration may produce additive CNS depressant effects). Products include:
- Ambien Tablets ... 2559

Food Interactions

Alcohol (Co-administration may produce additive CNS depressant effects).

LIBRIUM CAPSULES

(Chlordiazepoxide Hydrochloride) ... 2331
May interact with monoamine oxidase inhibitors, phenothiazines, oral anticoagulants, central nervous system depressants, and certain other agents. Compounds in these categories include:

Alfentanil Hydrochloride (Potential for additive effects). Products include:
- Alfenta Injection ... 1334

Alprazolam (Potential for additive effects). Products include:
- Xanax Tablets ... 2115

Aprobarbital (Potential for additive effects).
- No products indexed under this heading.

Buprenorphine (Potential for additive effects). Products include:
- Buprenex Injectable ... 2170

Buspirone Hydrochloride (Potential for additive effects). Products include:
- BuSpar Tablets ... 738

Butabarbital (Potential for additive effects).
- No products indexed under this heading.

Butalbital (Potential for additive effects). Products include:
- Axocet Capsules ... 2469
- Esgic-plus Capsules ... 1012
- Esgic-plus Tablets ... 1012
- Fioricet Tablets ... 2386
- Fioricet with Codeine Capsules ... 2387
- Fiorinal Capsules ... 2388
- Fiorinal with Codeine Capsules ... 2390
- Fiorinal Tablets ... 2388
- Phrenilin ... 790
- Sedapap Tablets 50 mg/650 mg ... 1826

Chlordiazepoxide (Potential for additive effects). Products include:
- Limbitrol ... 2333

Chlorpromazine (Concomitant use should be avoided due to the possibility of potentiation). Products include:
- Thorazine Suppositories ... 2701

Chlorpromazine Hydrochloride (Concomitant use should be avoided due to the possibility of potentiation). Products include:
- Thorazine ... 2701

Chlorprothixene (Potential for additive effects).
- No products indexed under this heading.

Chlorprothixene Hydrochloride (Potential for additive effects).
- No products indexed under this heading.

Chlorprothixene Lactate (Potential for additive effects).
- No products indexed under this heading.

Clorazepate Dipotassium (Potential for additive effects). Products include:
- Tranxene ... 459

Clozapine (Potential for additive effects). Products include:
- Clozaril Tablets ... 2377

Codeine Phosphate (Potential for additive effects). Products include:
- Brontex ... 2130
- Dimetane-DC Cough Syrup ... 2232
- Fioricet with Codeine Capsules ... 2387
- Fiorinal with Codeine Capsules ... 2390
- Nucofed ... 2225
- Phenergan with Codeine ... 2883
- Phenergan VC with Codeine ... 2888
- Robitussin A-C Syrup ... 2248
- Robitussin-DAC Syrup ... 2249
- Ryna ... 804
- Soma Compound w/Codeine Tablets ... 2784
- Tylenol with Codeine ... 1592

Desflurane (Potential for additive effects). Products include:
- Suprane (desflurane, USP) ... 1865

Dezocine (Potential for additive effects). Products include:
- Dalgan Injection ... 529

Diazepam (Potential for additive effects). Products include:
- Dizac (diazepam injectable emulsion) CIV ... 1862
- Valium Injection ... 2336
- Valium Tablets ... 2335

Dicumarol (Variable effects on blood coagulation have been reported very rarely with concomitant use).
- No products indexed under this heading.

Droperidol (Potential for additive effects). Products include:
- Inapsine Injection ... 462

Enflurane (Potential for additive effects).
- No products indexed under this heading.

Estazolam (Potential for additive effects). Products include:
- ProSom Tablets ... 457

Ethchlorvynol (Potential for additive effects). Products include:
- Placidyl Capsules ... 456

Ethinamate (Potential for additive effects).
- No products indexed under this heading.

Fentanyl (Potential for additive effects). Products include:
- Duragesic Transdermal System ... 1336

Fentanyl Citrate (Potential for additive effects). Products include:
- Sublimaze Injection ... 463

Fluphenazine Decanoate (Concomitant use should be avoided due to the possibility of potentiation). Products include:
- Prolixin Decanoate ... 510

Fluphenazine Enanthate (Concomitant use should be avoided due to the possibility of potentiation). Products include:
- Prolixin Enanthate ... 510

Fluphenazine Hydrochloride (Concomitant use should be avoided due to the possibility of potentiation). Products include:
- Prolixin ... 510

Flurazepam Hydrochloride (Potential for additive effects). Products include:
- Dalmane Capsules ... 2329

Furazolidone (Concomitant use should be avoided due to the possibility of potentiation). Products include:
- Furoxone ... 2221

Glutethimide (Potential for additive effects).
- No products indexed under this heading.

Haloperidol (Potential for additive effects). Products include:
- Haldol Injection, Tablets and Concentrate ... 1585

Haloperidol Decanoate (Potential for additive effects). Products include:
- Haldol Decanoate ... 1587

Hydrocodone Bitartrate (Potential for additive effects). Products include:
- Codiclear DH Syrup ... 808
- Duratuss HD Elixir ... 2750
- Histussin D Liquid ... 670
- Hycodan Tablets and Syrup ... 946
- Hycomine Compound Tablets ... 948
- Hycomine ... 947
- Hycotuss Expectorant Syrup ... 950
- Hydrocet Capsules ... 787
- Lorcet 10/650 Tablets ... 1016
- Lortab ... 2751
- Tussend ... 1830
- Tussend Expectorant ... 1831
- Vicodin Tablets ... 1404
- Vicodin ES Tablets ... 1405
- Vicodin HP Tablets ... 1403
- Vicodin Tuss Expectorant ... 1406
- Zydone Capsules ... 967

Hydrocodone Polistirex (Potential for additive effects). Products include:
- Tussionex Pennkinetic Extended-Release Suspension ... 1624

Hydroxyzine Hydrochloride (Potential for additive effects). Products include:
- Atarax Tablets & Syrup ... 1992
- Marax Tablets & DF Syrup ... 2015
- Vistaril Intramuscular Solution ... 2042

Isocarboxazid (Concomitant use should be avoided due to the possibility of potentiation).
- No products indexed under this heading.

Isoflurane (Potential for additive effects).
- No products indexed under this heading.

Ketamine Hydrochloride (Potential for additive effects).
- No products indexed under this heading.

Levomethadyl Acetate Hydrochloride (Potential for additive effects). Products include:
- Orlaam Oral Solution ... 2361

Levorphanol Tartrate (Potential for additive effects). Products include:
- Levo-Dromoran ... 2297

Lorazepam (Potential for additive effects). Products include:
- Ativan Injection ... 2805
- Ativan Tablets ... 2807

Loxapine Hydrochloride (Potential for additive effects). Products include:
- Loxitane ... 1426

Loxapine Succinate (Potential for additive effects). Products include:
- Loxitane Capsules ... 1426

Meperidine Hydrochloride (Potential for additive effects). Products include:
- Demerol ... 2438
- Mepergan Injection ... 2859

Mephobarbital (Potential for additive effects). Products include:
- Mebaral Tablets ... 2452

Meprobamate (Potential for additive effects). Products include:
- Miltown Tablets ... 2780
- PMB 200 and PMB 400 ... 2890

Mesoridazine Besylate (Concomitant use should be avoided due to the possibility of potentiation). Products include:
- Serentil ... 689

IMPORTANT NOTE: Always consult each drug listing in the patient's regimen for possible interactions.

Librium — Interactions Index

Methadone Hydrochloride (Potential for additive effects). Products include:
- Methadone Hydrochloride Oral Concentrate 2356
- Methadone Hydrochloride Oral Solution & Tablets 2357

Methohexital Sodium (Potential for additive effects).
- No products indexed under this heading.

Methotrimeprazine (Concomitant use should be avoided due to the possibility of potentiation). Products include:
- Levoprome 1321

Methoxyflurane (Potential for additive effects).
- No products indexed under this heading.

Midazolam Hydrochloride (Potential for additive effects). Products include:
- Versed Injection 2324

Molindone Hydrochloride (Potential for additive effects). Products include:
- Moban Tablets and Concentrate 1036

Morphine Sulfate (Potential for additive effects). Products include:
- Astramorph/PF Injection, USP (Preservative-Free) 526
- Duramorph Injection 983
- Infumorph 200 and Infumorph 500 Sterile Solutions 985
- Kadian Capsules 2948
- MS Contin Tablets 2149
- MSIR 2152
- Oramorph SR (Morphine Sulfate Sustained Release Tablets) 2359
- RMS Suppositories CII 2766
- Roxanol 2365

Opium Alkaloids (Potential for additive effects).
- No products indexed under this heading.

Oxazepam (Potential for additive effects). Products include:
- Serax Capsules 2916
- Serax Tablets 2916

Oxycodone Hydrochloride (Potential for additive effects). Products include:
- OxyContin Tablets 2163
- OxyIR Capsules 2167
- Percocet Tablets 955
- Percodan Tablets 955
- Percodan-Demi Tablets 956
- Roxicodone Tablets, Oral Solution & Intensol (Oxycodone) 2366
- Tylox Capsules 1593

Pentobarbital Sodium (Potential for additive effects). Products include:
- Nembutal Sodium Capsules 440
- Nembutal Sodium Solution 442
- Nembutal Sodium Suppositories...... 444

Perphenazine (Concomitant use should be avoided due to the possibility of potentiation). Products include:
- Etrafon 2495
- Triavil Tablets 1800
- Trilafon 2532

Phenelzine Sulfate (Concomitant use should be avoided due to the possibility of potentiation). Products include:
- Nardil 1977

Phenobarbital (Potential for additive effects). Products include:
- Arco-Lase Plus Tablets 513
- Bellergal-S Tablets 2375
- Donnatal 2234
- Donnatal Extentabs 2234
- Donnatal Tablets 2234
- Phenobarbital Elixir and Tablets ... 1523
- Quadrinal Tablets 1398

Prazepam (Potential for additive effects).
- No products indexed under this heading.

Prochlorperazine (Concomitant use should be avoided due to the possibility of potentiation). Products include:
- Compazine 2644

Promethazine Hydrochloride (Concomitant use should be avoided due to the possibility of potentiation). Products include:
- Mepergan Injection 2859
- Phenergan with Codeine 2883
- Phenergan with Dextromethorphan ... 2885
- Phenergan Injection 2880
- Phenergan Suppositories 2882
- Phenergan Syrup 2881
- Phenergan Tablets 2882
- Phenergan VC 2886
- Phenergan VC with Codeine 2888

Propofol (Potential for additive effects). Products include:
- Diprivan Injectable Emulsion 2939

Propoxyphene Hydrochloride (Potential for additive effects). Products include:
- Darvon 1475
- Wygesic Tablets 2930

Propoxyphene Napsylate (Potential for additive effects). Products include:
- Darvon-N/Darvocet-N 1473

Quazepam (Potential for additive effects). Products include:
- Doral Tablets 2773

Risperidone (Potential for additive effects). Products include:
- Risperdal Tablets 1348

Secobarbital Sodium (Potential for additive effects). Products include:
- Seconal Sodium Pulvules 1529

Selegiline Hydrochloride (Concomitant use should be avoided due to the possibility of potentiation). Products include:
- Eldepryl Capsules 2729

Sevoflurane (Potential for additive effects).
- No products indexed under this heading.

Sufentanil Citrate (Potential for additive effects). Products include:
- Sufenta Injection 1355

Temazepam (Potential for additive effects). Products include:
- Restoril Capsules 2413

Thiamylal Sodium (Potential for additive effects).
- No products indexed under this heading.

Thioridazine Hydrochloride (Concomitant use should be avoided due to the possibility of potentiation). Products include:
- Mellaril 2398

Thiothixene (Potential for additive effects). Products include:
- Navane Capsules and Concentrate ... 2018
- Navane Intramuscular 2019

Tranylcypromine Sulfate (Concomitant use should be avoided due to the possibility of potentiation). Products include:
- Parnate Tablets 2679

Triazolam (Potential for additive effects). Products include:
- Halcion Tablets 2093

Trifluoperazine Hydrochloride (Concomitant use should be avoided due to the possibility of potentiation). Products include:
- Stelazine 2692

Warfarin Sodium (Variable effects on blood coagulation have been reported very rarely with concomitant use). Products include:
- Coumadin 941

Zolpidem Tartrate (Potential for additive effects). Products include:
- Ambien Tablets 2559

Food Interactions

Alcohol (Potential for additive effects).

LIBRIUM INJECTABLE

(Chlordiazepoxide Hydrochloride).......2332
May interact with central nervous system depressants, monoamine oxidase inhibitors, phenothiazines, and certain other agents. Compounds in these categories include:

Alfentanil Hydrochloride (Additive effect). Products include:
- Alfenta Injection 1334

Alprazolam (Additive effect). Products include:
- Xanax Tablets 2115

Aprobarbital (Additive effect).
- No products indexed under this heading.

Buprenorphine (Additive effect). Products include:
- Buprenex Injectable 2170

Buspirone Hydrochloride (Additive effect). Products include:
- BuSpar Tablets 738

Butabarbital (Additive effect).
- No products indexed under this heading.

Butalbital (Additive effect). Products include:
- Axocet Capsules 2469
- Esgic-plus Capsules 1012
- Esgic-plus Tablets 1012
- Fioricet Tablets 2386
- Fioricet with Codeine Capsules 2387
- Fiorinal Capsules 2388
- Fiorinal with Codeine Capsules 2390
- Fiorinal Tablets 2388
- Phrenilin 790
- Sedapap Tablets 50 mg/650 mg .. 1826

Chlordiazepoxide (Additive effect). Products include:
- Limbitrol 2333

Chlorpromazine (Additive effect; potentiates Librium). Products include:
- Thorazine Suppositories 2701

Chlorprothixene (Additive effect).
- No products indexed under this heading.

Chlorprothixene Hydrochloride (Additive effect).
- No products indexed under this heading.

Chlorprothixene Lactate (Additive effect).
- No products indexed under this heading.

Clorazepate Dipotassium (Additive effect). Products include:
- Tranxene 459

Clozapine (Additive effect). Products include:
- Clozaril Tablets 2377

Codeine Phosphate (Additive effect). Products include:
- Brontex 2130
- Dimetane-DC Cough Syrup 2232
- Fioricet with Codeine Capsules 2387
- Fiorinal with Codeine Capsules 2390
- Nucofed 2225
- Phenergan with Codeine 2883
- Phenergan VC with Codeine 2888
- Robitussin A-C Syrup 2248
- Robitussin-DAC Syrup 2249
- Ryna .... ⊡ 804
- Soma Compound w/Codeine Tablets 2784
- Tylenol with Codeine 1592

Desflurane (Additive effect). Products include:
- Suprane (desflurane, USP) 1865

Dezocine (Additive effect). Products include:
- Dalgan Injection 529

Diazepam (Additive effect). Products include:
- Dizac (diazepam injectable emulsion) CIV 1862
- Valium Injectable 2336
- Valium Tablets 2335

Droperidol (Additive effect). Products include:
- Inapsine Injection 462

Enflurane (Additive effect).
- No products indexed under this heading.

Estazolam (Additive effect). Products include:
- ProSom Tablets 457

Ethchlorvynol (Additive effect). Products include:
- Placidyl Capsules 456

Ethinamate (Additive effect).
- No products indexed under this heading.

Fentanyl (Additive effect). Products include:
- Duragesic Transdermal System 1336

Fentanyl Citrate (Additive effect). Products include:
- Sublimaze Injection 463

Fluphenazine Decanoate (Additive effect; potentiates Librium). Products include:
- Prolixin Decanoate 510

Fluphenazine Enanthate (Additive effect; potentiates Librium). Products include:
- Prolixin Enanthate 510

Fluphenazine Hydrochloride (Additive effect; potentiates Librium). Products include:
- Prolixin 510

Flurazepam Hydrochloride (Additive effect). Products include:
- Dalmane Capsules 2329

Furazolidone (Potentiates Librium). Products include:
- Furoxone 2221

Glutethimide (Additive effect).
- No products indexed under this heading.

Haloperidol (Additive effect). Products include:
- Haldol Injection, Tablets and Concentrate 1585

Haloperidol Decanoate (Additive effect). Products include:
- Haldol Decanoate 1587

Hydrocodone Bitartrate (Additive effect). Products include:
- Codiclear DH Syrup 808
- Duratuss HD Elixir 2750
- Histussin D Liquid 670
- Hycodan Tablets and Syrup 946
- Hycomine Compound Tablets 948
- Hycomine 947
- Hycotuss Expectorant Syrup 950
- Hydrocet Capsules 787
- Lorcet 10/650 Tablets 1016
- Lortab 2751
- Tussend 1830
- Tussend Expectorant 1831
- Vicodin Tablets 1404
- Vicodin ES Tablets 1405
- Vicodin HP Tablets 1403
- Vicodin Tuss Expectorant 1406
- Zydone Capsules 967

Hydrocodone Polistirex (Additive effect). Products include:
- Tussionex Pennkinetic Extended-Release Suspension 1624

Hydroxyzine Hydrochloride (Additive effect). Products include:
- Atarax Tablets & Syrup 1992
- Marax Tablets & DF Syrup 2015
- Vistaril Intramuscular Solution 2042

(⊡ Described in PDR For Nonprescription Drugs)   (◎ Described in PDR For Ophthalmology)

Isocarboxazid (Potentiates Librium).
No products indexed under this heading.

Isoflurane (Additive effect).
No products indexed under this heading.

Ketamine Hydrochloride (Additive effect).
No products indexed under this heading.

Levomethadyl Acetate Hydrochloride (Additive effect). Products include:
Orlaam Oral Solution 2361

Levorphanol Tartrate (Additive effect). Products include:
Levo-Dromoran 2297

Lorazepam (Additive effect). Products include:
Ativan Injection 2805
Ativan Tablets 2807

Loxapine Hydrochloride (Additive effect). Products include:
Loxitane 1426

Loxapine Succinate (Additive effect). Products include:
Loxitane Capsules 1426

Meperidine Hydrochloride (Additive effect). Products include:
Demerol 2438
Mepergan Injection 2859

Mephobarbital (Additive effect). Products include:
Mebaral Tablets 2452

Meprobamate (Additive effect). Products include:
Miltown Tablets 2780
PMB 200 and PMB 400 2890

Mesoridazine Besylate (Additive effect; potentiates Librium). Products include:
Serentil 689

Methadone Hydrochloride (Additive effect). Products include:
Methadone Hydrochloride Oral Concentrate 2356
Methadone Hydrochloride Oral Solution & Tablets 2357

Methohexital Sodium (Additive effect).
No products indexed under this heading.

Methotrimeprazine (Additive effect). Products include:
Levoprome 1321

Methoxyflurane (Additive effect).
No products indexed under this heading.

Midazolam Hydrochloride (Additive effect). Products include:
Versed Injection 2324

Molindone Hydrochloride (Additive effect). Products include:
Moban Tablets and Concentrate 1036

Morphine Sulfate (Additive effect). Products include:
Astramorph/PF Injection, USP (Preservative-Free) 526
Duramorph Injection 983
Infumorph 200 and Infumorph 500 Sterile Solutions 985
Kadian Capsules 2948
MS Contin Tablets 2149
MSIR 2152
Oramorph SR (Morphine Sulfate Sustained Release Tablets) 2359
RMS Suppositories CII 2766
Roxanol 2365

Opium Alkaloids (Additive effect).
No products indexed under this heading.

Oxazepam (Additive effect). Products include:
Serax Capsules 2916
Serax Tablets 2916

Oxycodone Hydrochloride (Additive effect). Products include:
OxyContin Tablets 2163

OxyIR Capsules 2167
Percocet Tablets 955
Percodan Tablets 955
Percodan-Demi Tablets 956
Roxicodone Tablets, Oral Solution & Intensol (Oxycodone) 2366
Tylox Capsules 1593

Pentobarbital Sodium (Additive effect). Products include:
Nembutal Sodium Capsules 440
Nembutal Sodium Solution 442
Nembutal Sodium Suppositories 444

Perphenazine (Additive effect; potentiates Librium). Products include:
Etrafon 2495
Triavil Tablets 1800
Trilafon 2532

Phenelzine Sulfate (Potentiates Librium). Products include:
Nardil 1977

Phenobarbital (Additive effect). Products include:
Arco-Lase Plus Tablets 513
Bellergal-S Tablets 2375
Donnatal 2234
Donnatal Extentabs 2234
Donnatal Tablets 2234
Phenobarbital Elixir and Tablets 1523
Quadrinal Tablets 1398

Prazepam (Additive effect).
No products indexed under this heading.

Prochlorperazine (Additive effect; potentiates Librium). Products include:
Compazine 2644

Promethazine Hydrochloride (Additive effect; potentiates Librium). Products include:
Mepergan Injection 2859
Phenergan with Codeine 2883
Phenergan with Dextromethorphan .. 2885
Phenergan Injection 2880
Phenergan Suppositories 2882
Phenergan Syrup 2881
Phenergan Tablets 2882
Phenergan VC 2886
Phenergan VC with Codeine 2888

Propofol (Additive effect). Products include:
Diprivan Injectable Emulsion 2939

Propoxyphene Hydrochloride (Additive effect). Products include:
Darvon 1475
Wygesic Tablets 2930

Propoxyphene Napsylate (Additive effect). Products include:
Darvon-N/Darvocet-N 1473

Quazepam (Additive effect). Products include:
Doral Tablets 2773

Risperidone (Additive effect). Products include:
Risperdal Tablets 1348

Secobarbital Sodium (Additive effect). Products include:
Seconal Sodium Pulvules 1529

Selegiline Hydrochloride (Potentiates Librium). Products include:
Eldepryl Capsules 2729

Sevoflurane (Additive effect).
No products indexed under this heading.

Sufentanil Citrate (Additive effect). Products include:
Sufenta Injection 1355

Temazepam (Additive effect). Products include:
Restoril Capsules 2413

Thiamylal Sodium (Additive effect).
No products indexed under this heading.

Thioridazine Hydrochloride (Additive effect; potentiates Librium). Products include:
Mellaril 2398

Thiothixene (Additive effect). Products include:
Navane Capsules and Concentrate .. 2018
Navane Intramuscular 2019

Tranylcypromine Sulfate (Potentiates Librium). Products include:
Parnate Tablets 2679

Triazolam (Additive effect). Products include:
Halcion Tablets 2093

Trifluoperazine Hydrochloride (Additive effect). Products include:
Stelazine 2692

Zolpidem Tartrate (Additive effect). Products include:
Ambien Tablets 2559

Food Interactions

Alcohol (Additive effect).

LID WIPES-SPF
(Peg-200 Glyceryl Monotallowate) .. 210
None cited in PDR database.

LIDEX CREAM 0.05%
(Fluocinonide) 2299
None cited in PDR database.

LIDEX GEL 0.05%
(Fluocinonide) 2299
None cited in PDR database.

LIDEX OINTMENT 0.05%
(Fluocinonide) 2299
None cited in PDR database.

LIDEX TOPICAL SOLUTION 0.05%
(Fluocinonide) 2299
None cited in PDR database.

LIDEX-E CREAM 0.05%
(Fluocinonide) 2299
None cited in PDR database.

LIMBITROL DS TABLETS
(Chlordiazepoxide, Amitriptyline Hydrochloride) 2333
See **Limbitrol Tablets**

LIMBITROL TABLETS
(Chlordiazepoxide, Amitriptyline Hydrochloride) 2333
May interact with monoamine oxidase inhibitors, anticholinergics, central nervous system depressants, antidepressant drugs, phenothiazines, thyroid preparations, quinidine, and certain other agents. Compounds in these categories include:

Alfentanil Hydrochloride (Co-administration may produce additive effects resulting in harmful level of sedation and CNS depression). Products include:
Alfenta Injection 1334

Alprazolam (Co-administration may produce additive effects resulting in harmful level of sedation and CNS depression). Products include:
Xanax Tablets 2115

Amoxapine (May inhibit the activity of cytochrome P450 2D6 isoenzyme and are substrates for P450 2D6 and may make normal metabolizers resemble poor metabolizers resulting in higher than expected plasma levels of tricyclic antidepressants). Products include:
Asendin Tablets 1419

Aprobarbital (Co-administration may produce additive effects resulting in harmful level of sedation and CNS depression).
No products indexed under this heading.

Atropine Sulfate (Severe constipation may result with concurrent use of tricyclic antidepressants and anticholinergic drugs). Products include:
Arco-Lase Plus Tablets 513
Atrohist Plus Tablets 1605
Donnatal 2234
Donnatal Extentabs 2234
Donnatal Tablets 2234
Lomotil 2591
Motofen Tablets 789
Urised Tablets 2123

Belladonna Alkaloids (Severe constipation may result with concurrent use of tricyclic antidepressants and anticholinergic drugs). Products include:
Bellergal-S Tablets 2375
Hyland's Bedwetting Tablets 788
Hyland's EnurAid Tablets 789
Hyland's Headache Tablets 790
Hyland's Teething Tablets 790
Similasan Eye Drops #1 769

Benztropine Mesylate (Severe constipation may result with concurrent use of tricyclic antidepressants and anticholinergic drugs). Products include:
Cogentin 1661

Biperiden Hydrochloride (Severe constipation may result with concurrent use of tricyclic antidepressants and anticholinergic drugs). Products include:
Akineton 1380

Buprenorphine (Co-administration may produce additive effects resulting in harmful level of sedation and CNS depression). Products include:
Buprenex Injectable 2170

Bupropion Hydrochloride (May inhibit the activity of cytochrome P450 2D6 isoenzyme and are substrates for P450 2D6 and may make normal metabolizers resemble poor metabolizers resulting in higher than expected plasma levels of tricyclic antidepressants). Products include:
Wellbutrin Tablets 1177

Buspirone Hydrochloride (Co-administration may produce additive effects resulting in harmful level of sedation and CNS depression). Products include:
BuSpar Tablets 738

Butabarbital (Co-administration may produce additive effects resulting in harmful level of sedation and CNS depression).
No products indexed under this heading.

Butalbital (Co-administration may produce additive effects resulting in harmful level of sedation and CNS depression). Products include:
Axocet Capsules 2469
Esgic-plus Capsules 1012
Esgic-plus Tablets 1012
Fioricet Tablets 2386
Fioricet with Codeine Capsules 2387
Fiorinal Capsules 2388
Fiorinal with Codeine Capsules 2390
Fiorinal Tablets 2388
Phrenilin 790
Sedapap Tablets 50 mg/650 mg .. 1826

Chlordiazepoxide Hydrochloride (Co-administration may produce additive effects resulting in harmful level of sedation and CNS depression). Products include:
Librax Capsules 2330
Librium Capsules 2331
Librium Injectable 2332

IMPORTANT NOTE: Always consult each drug listing in the patient's regimen for possible interactions.

Chlorpromazine (May inhibit the activity of cytochrome P450 2D6 isoenzyme and are substrates for P450 2D6 and may make normal metabolizers resemble poor metabolizers resulting in higher than expected plasma levels of tricyclic antidepressants; co-administration may produce additive effects resulting in harmful level of sedation and CNS depression). Products include:
   Thorazine Suppositories 2701

Chlorpromazine Hydrochloride (May inhibit the activity of cytochrome P450 2D6 isoenzyme and are substrates for P450 2D6 and may make normal metabolizers resemble poor metabolizers resulting in higher than expected plasma levels of tricyclic antidepressants; co-administration may produce additive effects resulting in harmful level of sedation and CNS depression). Products include:
   Thorazine 2701

Chlorprothixene (Co-administration may produce additive effects resulting in harmful level of sedation and CNS depression).
   No products indexed under this heading.

Chlorprothixene Hydrochloride (Co-administration may produce additive effects resulting in harmful level of sedation and CNS depression).
   No products indexed under this heading.

Chlorprothixene Lactate (Co-administration may produce additive effects resulting in harmful level of sedation and CNS depression).
   No products indexed under this heading.

Cimetidine (Cimetidine is reported to reduce hepatic metabolism of certain tricyclic antidepressants and benzodiazepines, thereby delaying elimination and increasing steady-state concentrations of these drugs). Products include:
   Tagamet HB Tablets .... ▣ 786
   Tagamet Tablets 2694

Cimetidine Hydrochloride (Cimetidine is reported to reduce hepatic metabolism of certain tricyclic antidepressants and benzodiazepines, thereby delaying elimination and increasing steady-state concentrations of these drugs). Products include:
   Tagamet 2694

Clidinium Bromide (Severe constipation may result with concurrent use of tricyclic antidepressants and anticholinergic drugs). Products include:
   Librax Capsules 2330

Clonidine (Amitriptyline may block the antihypertensive effects). Products include:
   Catapres-TTS 680

Clonidine Hydrochloride (Amitriptyline may block the antihypertensive effects). Products include:
   Catapres Tablets 679
   Combipres Tablets 682

Clorazepate Dipotassium (Co-administration may produce additive effects resulting in harmful level of sedation and CNS depression). Products include:
   Tranxene 459

Clozapine (Co-administration may produce additive effects resulting in harmful level of sedation and CNS depression). Products include:
   Clozaril Tablets 2377

Codeine Phosphate (Co-administration may produce additive effects resulting in harmful level of sedation and CNS depression). Products include:
   Brontex 2130
   Dimetane-DC Cough Syrup 2232
   Fioricet with Codeine Capsules .. 2387
   Fiorinal with Codeine Capsules .. 2390
   Nucofed 2225
   Phenergan with Codeine 2883
   Phenergan VC with Codeine 2888
   Robitussin A-C Syrup 2248
   Robitussin-DAC Syrup 2249
   Ryna .... ▣ 804
   Soma Compound w/Codeine Tablets 2784
   Tylenol with Codeine 1592

Desflurane (Co-administration may produce additive effects resulting in harmful level of sedation and CNS depression). Products include:
   Suprane (desflurane, USP) 1865

Desipramine Hydrochloride (May inhibit the activity of cytochrome P450 2D6 isoenzyme and are substrates for P450 2D6 and may make normal metabolizers resemble poor metabolizers resulting in higher than expected plasma levels of tricyclic antidepressants). Products include:
   Norpramin Tablets 1273

Dezocine (Co-administration may produce additive effects resulting in harmful level of sedation and CNS depression). Products include:
   Dalgan Injection 529

Diazepam (Co-administration may produce additive effects resulting in harmful level of sedation and CNS depression). Products include:
   Dizac (diazepam injectable emulsion) CIV 1862
   Valium Injectable 2336
   Valium Tablets 2335

Dicyclomine Hydrochloride (Severe constipation may result with concurrent use of tricyclic antidepressants and anticholinergic drugs). Products include:
   Bentyl 1246

Doxepin Hydrochloride (May inhibit the activity of cytochrome P450 2D6 isoenzyme and are substrates for P450 2D6 and may make normal metabolizers resemble poor metabolizers resulting in higher than expected plasma levels of tricyclic antidepressants). Products include:
   Adapin Capsules 1542
   Sinequan 2028
   Zonalon Cream 1042

Droperidol (Co-administration may produce additive effects resulting in harmful level of sedation and CNS depression). Products include:
   Inapsine Injection 462

Enflurane (Co-administration may produce additive effects resulting in harmful level of sedation and CNS depression).
   No products indexed under this heading.

Estazolam (Co-administration may produce additive effects resulting in harmful level of sedation and CNS depression). Products include:
   ProSom Tablets 457

Ethchlorvynol (Co-administration may produce additive effects resulting in harmful level of sedation and CNS depression). Products include:
   Placidyl Capsules 456

Ethinamate (Co-administration may produce additive effects resulting in harmful level of sedation and CNS depression).
   No products indexed under this heading.

Fentanyl (Co-administration may produce additive effects resulting in harmful level of sedation and CNS depression). Products include:
   Duragesic Transdermal System .. 1336

Fentanyl Citrate (Co-administration may produce additive effects resulting in harmful level of sedation and CNS depression). Products include:
   Sublimaze Injection 463

Flecainide Acetate (May inhibit the activity of cytochrome P450 2D6 isoenzyme and are substrates for P450 2D6 and may make normal metabolizers resemble poor metabolizers resulting in higher than expected plasma levels of tricyclic antidepressants). Products include:
   Tambocor Tablets 1555

Fluoxetine Hydrochloride (Selective serotonin reuptake inhibitors, such as fluoxetine, may have variable extent of inhibition of P450 2D6; potential for higher than expected plasma levels of tricyclic antidepressants; due to long half-life of fluoxetine, at least 5 weeks should elapse before initiating TCA treatment in a patient being withdrawn from fluoxetine). Products include:
   Prozac Pulvules & Liquid, Oral Solution 935

Fluphenazine Decanoate (May inhibit the activity of cytochrome P450 2D6 isoenzyme and are substrates for P450 2D6 and may make normal metabolizers resemble poor metabolizers resulting in higher than expected plasma levels of tricyclic antidepressants; co-administration may produce additive effects resulting in harmful level of sedation and CNS depression). Products include:
   Prolixin Decanoate 510

Fluphenazine Enanthate (May inhibit the activity of cytochrome P450 2D6 isoenzyme and are substrates for P450 2D6 and may make normal metabolizers resemble poor metabolizers resulting in higher than expected plasma levels of tricyclic antidepressants; co-administration may produce additive effects resulting in harmful level of sedation and CNS depression). Products include:
   Prolixin Enanthate 510

Fluphenazine Hydrochloride (May inhibit the activity of cytochrome P450 2D6 isoenzyme and are substrates for P450 2D6 and may make normal metabolizers resemble poor metabolizers resulting in higher than expected plasma levels of tricyclic antidepressants; co-administration may produce additive effects resulting in harmful level of sedation and CNS depression). Products include:
   Prolixin 510

Flurazepam Hydrochloride (Co-administration may produce additive effects resulting in harmful level of sedation and CNS depression). Products include:
   Dalmane Capsules 2329

Furazolidone (Co-administration of tricyclic antidepressants and MAO inhibitor has produced hyperpyretic crises, severe convulsions, and deaths; concurrent and/or sequential use is contraindicated). Products include:
   Furoxone 2221

Glutethimide (Co-administration may produce additive effects resulting in harmful level of sedation and CNS depression).
   No products indexed under this heading.

Glycopyrrolate (Severe constipation may result with concurrent use of tricyclic antidepressants and anticholinergic drugs). Products include:
   Robinul Forte Tablets 2247
   Robinul Injectable 2247
   Robinul Tablets 2247

Guanadrel Sulfate (Amitriptyline may block the antihypertensive effects). Products include:
   Hylorel Tablets 1613

Guanethidine Monosulfate (Amitriptyline may block the antihypertensive effects). Products include:
   Esimil Tablets 840
   Ismelin Tablets 845

Haloperidol (Co-administration may produce additive effects resulting in harmful level of sedation and CNS depression). Products include:
   Haldol Injection, Tablets and Concentrate 1585

Haloperidol Decanoate (Co-administration may produce additive effects resulting in harmful level of sedation and CNS depression). Products include:
   Haldol Decanoate 1587

Hydrocodone Bitartrate (Co-administration may produce additive effects resulting in harmful level of sedation and CNS depression). Products include:
   Codiclear DH Syrup 808
   Duratuss HD Elixir 2750
   Histussin D Liquid 670
   Hycodan Tablets and Syrup 946
   Hycomine Compound Tablets .. 948
   Hycomine 947
   Hycotuss Expectorant Syrup 950
   Hydrocet Capsules 787
   Lorcet 10/650 Tablets 1016
   Lortab 2751
   Tussend 1830
   Tussend Expectorant 1831
   Vicodin Tablets 1404
   Vicodin ES Tablets 1405
   Vicodin HP Tablets 1403
   Vicodin Tuss Expectorant 1406
   Zydone Capsules 967

Hydrocodone Polistirex (Co-administration may produce additive effects resulting in harmful level of sedation and CNS depression). Products include:
   Tussionex Pennkinetic Extended-Release Suspension 1624

Hydromorphone Hydrochloride (Co-administration may produce additive effects resulting in harmful level of sedation and CNS depression). Products include:
   Dilaudid Ampules 1382
   Dilaudid Cough Syrup 1383
   Dilaudid-HP Injection 1384
   Dilaudid-HP Lyophilized Powder 250 mg 1384
   Dilaudid 1382
   Dilaudid Oral Liquid 1386
   Dilaudid 1382
   Dilaudid Tablets - 8 mg. 1386

Hydroxyzine Hydrochloride (Co-administration may produce additive effects resulting in harmful level of sedation and CNS depression). Products include:
   Atarax Tablets & Syrup 1992

(▣ Described in PDR For Nonprescription Drugs)   (⊙ Described in PDR For Ophthalmology)

609 **Interactions Index** **Limbitrol**

Marax Tablets & DF Syrup.................. 2015
Vistaril Intramuscular Solution.......... 2042

Hyoscyamine (Severe constipation may result with concurrent use of tricyclic antidepressants and anticholinergic drugs). Products include:
Cystospaz Tablets.................................. 2123
Urised Tablets.. 2123

Hyoscyamine Sulfate (Severe constipation may result with concurrent use of tricyclic antidepressants and anticholinergic drugs). Products include:
Arco-Lase Plus Tablets 513
Atrohist Plus Tablets 1605
Cystospaz-M Capsules 2123
Donnatal 2234
Donnatal Extentabs................................ 2234
Donnatal Tablets 2234
Kutrase Capsules.................................... 2546
Levsin/Levsinex/Levbid 2549

Imipramine Hydrochloride (May inhibit the activity of cytochrome P450 2D6 isoenzyme and are substrates for P450 2D6 and may make normal metabolizers resemble poor metabolizers resulting in higher than expected plasma levels of tricyclic antidepressants). Products include:
Tofranil Ampuls 873
Tofranil Tablets 875

Imipramine Pamoate (May inhibit the activity of cytochrome P450 2D6 isoenzyme and are substrates for P450 2D6 and may make normal metabolizers resemble poor metabolizers resulting in higher than expected plasma levels of tricyclic antidepressants). Products include:
Tofranil-PM Capsules............................ 876

Ipratropium Bromide (Severe constipation may result with concurrent use of tricyclic antidepressants and anticholinergic drugs). Products include:
Atrovent Inhalation Aerosol................ 674
Atrovent Inhalation Solution 675
Atrovent Nasal Spray 0.03%............ 676
Atrovent Nasal Spray 0.06%............ 678

Isocarboxazid (Co-administration of tricyclic antidepressants and MAO inhibitor has produced hyperpyretic crises, severe convulsions, and deaths; concurrent and/or sequential use is contraindicated).
No products indexed under this heading.

Isoflurane (Co-administration may produce additive effects resulting in harmful level of sedation and CNS depression).
No products indexed under this heading.

Ketamine Hydrochloride (Co-administration may produce additive effects resulting in harmful level of sedation and CNS depression).
No products indexed under this heading.

Levomethadyl Acetate Hydrochloride (Co-administration may produce additive effects resulting in harmful level of sedation and CNS depression). Products include:
Orlaam Oral Solution 2361

Levorphanol Tartrate (Co-administration may produce additive effects resulting in harmful level of sedation and CNS depression). Products include:
Levo-Dromoran....................................... 2297

Levothyroxine Sodium (Close supervision is required when Limbitrol is given to patients on thyroid medications). Products include:
Eltroxin Tablets...................................... 2214
Levothroid Tablets 1015
Levothyroxine Sodium, USP for Injection 546
Levoxyl Tablets....................................... 918
Synthroid.. 1410

Liothyronine Sodium (Close supervision is required when Limbitrol is given to patients on thyroid medications). Products include:
Cytomel Tablets 2647
Triostat Injection 2708

Liotrix (Close supervision is required when Limbitrol is given to patients on thyroid medications).
No products indexed under this heading.

Lorazepam (Co-administration may produce additive effects resulting in harmful level of sedation and CNS depression). Products include:
Ativan Injection....................................... 2805
Ativan Tablets... 2807

Loxapine Hydrochloride (Co-administration may produce additive effects resulting in harmful level of sedation and CNS depression). Products include:
Loxitane 1426

Loxapine Succinate (Co-administration may produce additive effects resulting in harmful level of sedation and CNS depression). Products include:
Loxitane Capsules 1426

Maprotiline Hydrochloride (May inhibit the activity of cytochrome P450 2D6 isoenzyme and are substrates for P450 2D6 and may make normal metabolizers resemble poor metabolizers resulting in higher than expected plasma levels of tricyclic antidepressants). Products include:
Ludiomil Tablets..................................... 861

Mepenzolate Bromide (Severe constipation may result with concurrent use of tricyclic antidepressants and anticholinergic drugs).
No products indexed under this heading.

Meperidine Hydrochloride (Co-administration may produce additive effects resulting in harmful level of sedation and CNS depression). Products include:
Demerol 2438
Mepergan Injection 2859

Mephobarbital (Co-administration may produce additive effects resulting in harmful level of sedation and CNS depression). Products include:
Mebaral Tablets 2452

Meprobamate (Co-administration may produce additive effects resulting in harmful level of sedation and CNS depression). Products include:
Miltown Tablets 2780
PMB 200 and PMB 400 2890

Mesoridazine Besylate (May inhibit the activity of cytochrome P450 2D6 isoenzyme and are substrates for P450 2D6 and may make normal metabolizers resemble poor metabolizers resulting in higher than expected plasma levels of tricyclic antidepressants; co-administration may produce additive effects resulting in harmful level of sedation and CNS depression). Products include:
Serentil.. 689

Methadone Hydrochloride (Co-administration may produce additive effects resulting in harmful level of sedation and CNS depression). Products include:
Methadone Hydrochloride Oral Concentrate 2356
Methadone Hydrochloride Oral Solution & Tablets.............................. 2357

Methohexital Sodium (Co-administration may produce additive effects resulting in harmful level of sedation and CNS depression).
No products indexed under this heading.

Methotrimeprazine (May inhibit the activity of cytochrome P450 2D6 isoenzyme and are substrates for P450 2D6 and may make normal metabolizers resemble poor metabolizers resulting in higher than expected plasma levels of tricyclic antidepressants; co-administration may produce adcditive effects resulting in harmful level of sedation and CNS depression). Products include:
Levoprome 1321

Methoxyflurane (Co-administration may produce additive effects resulting in harmful level of sedation and CNS depression).
No products indexed under this heading.

Midazolam Hydrochloride (Co-administration may produce additive effects resulting in harmful level of sedation and CNS depression). Products include:
Versed Injection 2324

Mirtazapine (May inhibit the activity of cytochrome P450 2D6 isoenzyme and are substrates for P450 2D6 and may make normal metabolizers resemble poor metabolizers resulting in higher than expected plasma levels of tricyclic antidepressants). Products include:
Remeron Tablets 1878

Molindone Hydrochloride (Co-administration may produce additive effects resulting in harmful level of sedation and CNS depression). Products include:
Moban Tablets and Concentrate...... 1036

Morphine Sulfate (Co-administration may produce additive effects resulting in harmful level of sedation and CNS depression). Products include:
Astramorph/PF Injection, USP (Preservative-Free) 526
Duramorph Injection 983
Infumorph 200 and Infumorph 500 Sterile Solutions....................... 985
Kadian Capsules..................................... 2948
MS Contin Tablets.................................. 2149
MSIR 2152
Oramorph SR (Morphine Sulfate Sustained Release Tablets)........... 2359
RMS Suppositories CII........................ 2766
Roxanol 2365

Nefazodone Hydrochloride (May inhibit the activity of cytochrome P450 2D6 isoenzyme and are substrates for P450 2D6 and may make normal metabolizers resemble poor metabolizers resulting in higher than expected plasma levels of tricyclic antidepressants). Products include:
Serzone Tablets 776

Nortriptyline Hydrochloride (May inhibit the activity of cytochrome P450 2D6 isoenzyme and are substrates for P450 2D6 and may make normal metabolizers resemble poor metabolizers resulting in higher than expected plasma levels of tricyclic antidepressants). Products include:
Pamelor 2409

Opium Alkaloids (Co-administration may produce additive effects resulting in harmful level of sedation and CNS depression).
No products indexed under this heading.

Oxazepam (Co-administration may produce additive effects resulting in harmful level of sedation and CNS depression). Products include:
Serax Capsules 2916
Serax Tablets... 2916

Oxybutynin Chloride (Severe constipation may result with concurrent use of tricyclic antidepressants and anticholinergic drugs). Products include:
Ditropan.. 1267

Oxycodone Hydrochloride (Co-administration may produce additive effects resulting in harmful level of sedation and CNS depression). Products include:
OxyContin Tablets.................................. 2163
OxyIR Capsules....................................... 2167
Percocet Tablets 955
Percodan Tablets..................................... 955
Percodan-Demi Tablets........................ 956
Roxicodone Tablets, Oral Solution & Intensol (Oxycodone) 2366
Tylox Capsules 1593

Paroxetine Hydrochloride (Selective serotonin reuptake inhibitors, such as sertraline, may have variable extent of inhibition of P450 2D6; potential for higher than expected plasma levels of tricyclic antidepressants). Products include:
Paxil Tablets 2681

Pentobarbital Sodium (Co-administration may produce additive effects resulting in harmful level of sedation and CNS depression). Products include:
Nembutal Sodium Capsules 440
Nembutal Sodium Solution 442
Nembutal Sodium Suppositories...... 444

Perphenazine (May inhibit the activity of cytochrome P450 2D6 isoenzyme and are substrates for P450 2D6 and may make normal metabolizers resemble poor metabolizers resulting in higher than expected plasma levels of tricyclic antidepressants; co-administration may produce additive effects resulting in harmful level of sedation and CNS depression). Products include:
Etrafon 2495
Triavil Tablets 1800
Trilafon... 2532

Phenelzine Sulfate (Co-administration of tricyclic antidepressants and MAO inhibitor has produced hyperpyretic crises, severe convulsions, and deaths; concurrent and/or sequential use is contraindicated). Products include:
Nardil 1977

Phenobarbital (Co-administration may produce additive effects resulting in harmful level of sedation and CNS depression). Products include:
Arco-Lase Plus Tablets 513
Bellergal-S Tablets 2375
Donnatal 2234
Donnatal Extentabs................................ 2234
Donnatal Tablets 2234
Phenobarbital Elixir and Tablets...... 1523
Quadrinal Tablets 1398

Prazepam (Co-administration may produce additive effects resulting in harmful level of sedation and CNS depression).
No products indexed under this heading.

IMPORTANT NOTE: Always consult each drug listing in the patient's regimen for possible interactions.

Limbitrol — Interactions Index

Prochlorperazine (May inhibit the activity of cytochrome P450 2D6 isoenzyme and are substrates for P450 2D6 and may make normal metabolizers resemble poor metabolizers resulting in higher than expected plasma levels of tricyclic antidepressants; co-administration may produce additive effects resulting in harmful level of sedation and CNS depression). Products include:
- Compazine 2644

Procyclidine Hydrochloride (Severe constipation may result with concurrent use of tricyclic antidepressants and anticholinergic drugs). Products include:
- Kemadrin Tablets 1105

Promethazine Hydrochloride (May inhibit the activity of cytochrome P450 2D6 isoenzyme and are substrates for P450 2D6 and may make normal metabolizers resemble poor metabolizers resulting in higher than expected plasma levels of tricyclic antidepressants; co-administration may produce additive effects resulting in harmful level of sedation and CNS depression). Products include:
- Mepergan Injection 2859
- Phenergan with Codeine 2883
- Phenergan with Dextromethorphan 2885
- Phenergan Injection 2880
- Phenergan Suppositories 2882
- Phenergan Syrup 2881
- Phenergan Tablets 2882
- Phenergan VC 2886
- Phenergan VC with Codeine 2888

Propafenone Hydrochloride (May inhibit the activity of cytochrome P450 2D6 isoenzyme and are substrates for P450 2D6 and may make normal metabolizers resemble poor metabolizers resulting in higher than expected plasma levels of tricyclic antidepressants). Products include:
- Rythmol Tablets–150mg, 225mg, 300mg 1399

Propantheline Bromide (Severe constipation may result with concurrent use of tricyclic antidepressants and anticholinergic drugs). Products include:
- Pro-Banthine Tablets 2226

Propofol (Co-administration may produce additive effects resulting in harmful level of sedation and CNS depression). Products include:
- Diprivan Injectable Emulsion 2939

Propoxyphene Hydrochloride (Co-administration may produce additive effects resulting in harmful level of sedation and CNS depression). Products include:
- Darvon 1475
- Wygesic Tablets 2930

Propoxyphene Napsylate (Co-administration may produce additive effects resulting in harmful level of sedation and CNS depression). Products include:
- Darvon-N/Darvocet-N 1473

Protriptyline Hydrochloride (May inhibit the activity of cytochrome P450 2D6 isoenzyme and are substrates for P450 2D6 and may make normal metabolizers resemble poor metabolizers resulting in higher than expected plasma levels of tricyclic antidepressants). Products include:
- Vivactil Tablets 1820

Quazepam (Co-administration may produce additive effects resulting in harmful level of sedation and CNS depression). Products include:
- Doral Tablets 2773

Quinidine Gluconate (May inhibit the activity of cytochrome P450 2D6 isoenzyme and may make normal metabolizers resemble poor metabolizers resulting in higher than expected plasma levels of tricyclic antidepressants). Products include:
- Quinaglute Dura-Tabs Tablets 644

Quinidine Polygalacturonate (May inhibit the activity of cytochrome P450 2D6 isoenzyme and may make normal metabolizers resemble poor metabolizers resulting in higher than expected plasma levels of tricyclic antidepressants). Products include:
- Cardioquin Tablets 2146

Quinidine Sulfate (May inhibit the activity of cytochrome P450 2D6 isoenzyme and may make normal metabolizers resemble poor metabolizers resulting in higher than expected plasma levels of tricyclic antidepressants). Products include:
- Quinidex Extentabs 2240

Risperidone (Co-administration may produce additive effects resulting in harmful level of sedation and CNS depression). Products include:
- Risperdal Tablets 1348

Scopolamine (Severe constipation may result with concurrent use of tricyclic antidepressants and anticholinergic drugs). Products include:
- Transderm Scōp Transdermal Therapeutic System 890

Scopolamine Hydrobromide (Severe constipation may result with concurrent use of tricyclic antidepressants and anticholinergic drugs). Products include:
- Atrohist Plus Tablets 1605
- Donnatal 2234
- Donnatal Extentabs 2234
- Donnatal Tablets 2234

Secobarbital Sodium (Co-administration may produce additive effects resulting in harmful level of sedation and CNS depression). Products include:
- Seconal Sodium Pulvules 1529

Selegiline Hydrochloride (Co-administration of tricyclic antidepressants and MAO inhibitor has produced hyperpyretic crises, severe convulsions, and deaths; concurrent and/or sequential use is contraindicated). Products include:
- Eldepryl Capsules 2729

Sertraline Hydrochloride (Selective serotonin reuptake inhibitors, such as sertraline, may have variable extent of inhibition of P450 2D6; potential for higher than expected plasma levels of tricyclic antidepressants). Products include:
- Zoloft Tablets 2051

Sevoflurane (Co-administration may produce additive effects resulting in harmful level of sedation and CNS depression).
  No products indexed under this heading.

Sufentanil Citrate (Co-administration may produce additive effects resulting in harmful level of sedation and CNS depression). Products include:
- Sufenta Injection 1355

Temazepam (Co-administration may produce additive effects resulting in harmful level of sedation and CNS depression). Products include:
- Restoril Capsules 2413

Thiamylal Sodium (Co-administration may produce additive effects resulting in harmful level of sedation and CNS depression).
  No products indexed under this heading.

Thioridazine Hydrochloride (May inhibit the activity of cytochrome P450 2D6 isoenzyme and are substrates for P450 2D6 and may make normal metabolizers resemble poor metabolizers resulting in higher than expected plasma levels of tricyclic antidepressants; co-administration may produce additive effects resulting in harmful level of sedation and CNS depression). Products include:
- Mellaril 2398

Thiothixene (Co-administration may produce additive effects resulting in harmful level of sedation and CNS depression). Products include:
- Navane Capsules and Concentrate 2018
- Navane Intramuscular 2019

Thyroglobulin (Close supervision is required when Limbitrol is given to patients on thyroid medications).
  No products indexed under this heading.

Thyroid (Close supervision is required when Limbitrol is given to patients on thyroid medications).
  No products indexed under this heading.

Thyroxine (Close supervision is required when Limbitrol is given to patients on thyroid medications).
  No products indexed under this heading.

Thyroxine Sodium (Close supervision is required when Limbitrol is given to patients on thyroid medications).
  No products indexed under this heading.

Tranylcypromine Sulfate (Co-administration of tricyclic antidepressants and MAO inhibitor has produced hyperpyretic crises, severe convulsions, and deaths; concurrent and/or sequential use is contraindicated). Products include:
- Parnate Tablets 2679

Trazodone Hydrochloride (May inhibit the activity of cytochrome P450 2D6 isoenzyme and are substrates for P450 2D6 and may make normal metabolizers resemble poor metabolizers resulting in higher than expected plasma levels of tricyclic antidepressants). Products include:
- Desyrel and Desyrel Dividose 504

Triazolam (Co-administration may produce additive effects resulting in harmful level of sedation and CNS depression). Products include:
- Halcion Tablets 2093

Tridihexethyl Chloride (Severe constipation may result with concurrent use of tricyclic antidepressants and anticholinergic drugs).
  No products indexed under this heading.

Trifluoperazine Hydrochloride (May inhibit the activity of cytochrome P450 2D6 isoenzyme and are substrates for P450 2D6 and may make normal metabolizers resemble poor metabolizers resulting in higher than expected plasma levels of tricyclic antidepressants; co-administration may produce additive effects resulting in harmful level of sedation and CNS depression). Products include:
- Stelazine 2692

Trihexyphenidyl Hydrochloride (Severe constipation may result with concurrent use of tricyclic antidepressants and anticholinergic drugs). Products include:
- Artane 1418

Trimipramine Maleate (May inhibit the activity of cytochrome P450 2D6 isoenzyme and are substrates for P450 2D6 and may make normal metabolizers resemble poor metabolizers resulting in higher than expected plasma levels of tricyclic antidepressants). Products include:
- Surmontil Capsules 2917

Venlafaxine Hydrochloride (May inhibit the activity of cytochrome P450 2D6 isoenzyme and are substrates for P450 2D6 and may make normal metabolizers resemble poor metabolizers resulting in higher than expected plasma levels of tricyclic antidepressants). Products include:
- Effexor 2825

Zolpidem Tartrate (Co-administration may produce additive effects resulting in harmful level of sedation and CNS depression). Products include:
- Ambien Tablets 2559

Food Interactions

Alcohol (Concurrent use may produce additive effects resulting in harmful level of sedation and CNS depression).

LINDANE LOTION USP 1%
(Lindane) 481
May interact with:

Oils, unspecified (May enhance absorption; avoid concurrent use).

LINDANE SHAMPOO USP 1%
(Lindane) 483
May interact with:

Oils, unspecified (May enhance absorption; avoid concurrent use).

LIORESAL INTRATHECAL
(Baclofen) 1634
May interact with central nervous system depressants and certain other agents. Compounds in these categories include:

Alfentanil Hydrochloride (CNS depressant effect of Lioresal Intrathecal may be additive to those of other CNS depressants). Products include:
- Alfenta Injection 1334

Alprazolam (CNS depressant effect of Lioresal Intrathecal may be additive to those of other CNS depressants). Products include:
- Xanax Tablets 2115

Aprobarbital (CNS depressant effect of Lioresal Intrathecal may be additive to those of other CNS depressants).
  No products indexed under this heading.

Buprenorphine (CNS depressant effect of Lioresal Intrathecal may be additive to those of other CNS depressants). Products include:
- Buprenex Injectable 2170

Buspirone Hydrochloride (CNS depressant effect of Lioresal Intrathecal may be additive to those of other CNS depressants). Products include:
- BuSpar Tablets 738

(▣ Described in PDR For Nonprescription Drugs)   (⊙ Described in PDR For Ophthalmology)

611 **Interactions Index** **Lioresal Intrathecal**

Butabarbital (CNS depressant effect of Lioresal Intrathecal may be additive to those of other CNS depressants).
No products indexed under this heading.

Butalbital (CNS depressant effect of Lioresal Intrathecal may be additive to those of other CNS depressants). Products include:
Axocet Capsules 2469
Esgic-plus Capsules 1012
Esgic-plus Tablets 1012
Fioricet Tablets 2386
Fioricet with Codeine Capsules 2387
Fiorinal Capsules 2388
Fiorinal with Codeine Capsules 2390
Fiorinal Tablets 2388
Phrenilin 790
Sedapap Tablets 50 mg/650 mg .. 1826

Chlordiazepoxide (CNS depressant effect of Lioresal Intrathecal may be additive to those of other CNS depressants). Products include:
Limbitrol 2333

Chlordiazepoxide Hydrochloride (CNS depressant effect of Lioresal Intrathecal may be additive to those of other CNS depressants). Products include:
Librax Capsules 2330
Librium Capsules 2331
Librium Injectable 2332

Chlorpromazine (CNS depressant effect of Lioresal Intrathecal may be additive to those of other CNS depressants). Products include:
Thorazine Suppositories 2701

Chlorpromazine Hydrochloride (CNS depressant effect of Lioresal Intrathecal may be additive to those of other CNS depressants). Products include:
Thorazine 2701

Chlorprothixene (CNS depressant effect of Lioresal Intrathecal may be additive to those of other CNS depressants).
No products indexed under this heading.

Chlorprothixene Hydrochloride (CNS depressant effect of Lioresal Intrathecal may be additive to those of other CNS depressants).
No products indexed under this heading.

Chlorprothixene Lactate (CNS depressant effect of Lioresal Intrathecal may be additive to those of other CNS depressants).
No products indexed under this heading.

Clorazepate Dipotassium (CNS depressant effect of Lioresal Intrathecal may be additive to those of other CNS depressants). Products include:
Tranxene 459

Clozapine (CNS depressant effect of Lioresal Intrathecal may be additive to those of other CNS depressants). Products include:
Clozaril Tablets 2377

Codeine Phosphate (CNS depressant effect of Lioresal Intrathecal may be additive to those of other CNS depressants). Products include:
Brontex 2130
Dimetane-DC Cough Syrup 2232
Fioricet with Codeine Capsules 2387
Fiorinal with Codeine Capsules 2390
Nucofed 2225
Phenergan with Codeine 2883
Phenergan VC with Codeine 2888
Robitussin A-C Syrup 2248
Robitussin-DAC Syrup 2249
Ryna 804
Soma Compound w/Codeine Tablets 2784
Tylenol with Codeine 1592

Desflurane (CNS depressant effect of Lioresal Intrathecal may be additive to those of other CNS depressants). Products include:
Suprane (desflurane, USP) 1865

Dezocine (CNS depressant effect of Lioresal Intrathecal may be additive to those of other CNS depressants). Products include:
Dalgan Injection 529

Diazepam (CNS depressant effect of Lioresal Intrathecal may be additive to those of other CNS depressants). Products include:
Dizac (diazepam injectable emulsion) CIV 1862
Valium Injectable 2336
Valium Tablets 2335

Droperidol (CNS depressant effect of Lioresal Intrathecal may be additive to those of other CNS depressants). Products include:
Inapsine Injection 462

Enflurane (CNS depressant effect of Lioresal Intrathecal may be additive to those of other CNS depressants).
No products indexed under this heading.

Estazolam (CNS depressant effect of Lioresal Intrathecal may be additive to those of other CNS depressants). Products include:
ProSom Tablets 457

Ethchlorvynol (CNS depressant effect of Lioresal Intrathecal may be additive to those of other CNS depressants). Products include:
Placidyl Capsules 456

Ethinamate (CNS depressant effect of Lioresal Intrathecal may be additive to those of other CNS depressants).
No products indexed under this heading.

Fentanyl (CNS depressant effect of Lioresal Intrathecal may be additive to those of other CNS depressants). Products include:
Duragesic Transdermal System 1336

Fentanyl Citrate (CNS depressant effect of Lioresal Intrathecal may be additive to those of other CNS depressants). Products include:
Sublimaze Injection 463

Fluphenazine Decanoate (CNS depressant effect of Lioresal Intrathecal may be additive to those of other CNS depressants). Products include:
Prolixin Decanoate 510

Fluphenazine Enanthate (CNS depressant effect of Lioresal Intrathecal may be additive to those of other CNS depressants). Products include:
Prolixin Enanthate 510

Fluphenazine Hydrochloride (CNS depressant effect of Lioresal Intrathecal may be additive to those of other CNS depressants). Products include:
Prolixin 510

Flurazepam Hydrochloride (CNS depressant effect of Lioresal Intrathecal may be additive to those of other CNS depressants). Products include:
Dalmane Capsules 2329

Glutethimide (CNS depressant effect of Lioresal Intrathecal may be additive to those of other CNS depressants).
No products indexed under this heading.

Haloperidol (CNS depressant effect of Lioresal Intrathecal may be additive to those of other CNS depressants). Products include:
Haldol Injection, Tablets and Concentrate 1585

Haloperidol Decanoate (CNS depressant effect of Lioresal Intrathecal may be additive to those of other CNS depressants). Products include:
Haldol Decanoate 1587

Hydrocodone Bitartrate (CNS depressant effect of Lioresal Intrathecal may be additive to those of other CNS depressants). Products include:
Codiclear DH Syrup 808
Duratuss HD Elixir 2750
Histussin D Liquid 670
Hycodan Tablets and Syrup 946
Hycomine Compound Tablets 948
Hycomine 947
Hycotuss Expectorant Syrup 950
Hydrocet Capsules 787
Lorcet 10/650 Tablets 1016
Lortab 2751
Tussend 1830
Tussend Expectorant 1831
Vicodin Tablets 1404
Vicodin ES Tablets 1405
Vicodin HP Tablets 1403
Vicodin Tuss Expectorant 1406
Zydone Capsules 967

Hydrocodone Polistirex (CNS depressant effect of Lioresal Intrathecal may be additive to those of other CNS depressants). Products include:
Tussionex Pennkinetic Extended-Release Suspension 1624

Hydroxyzine Hydrochloride (CNS depressant effect of Lioresal Intrathecal may be additive to those of other CNS depressants). Products include:
Atarax Tablets & Syrup 1992
Marax Tablets & DF Syrup 2015
Vistaril Intramuscular Solution 2042

Isoflurane (CNS depressant effect of Lioresal Intrathecal may be additive to those of other CNS depressants).
No products indexed under this heading.

Ketamine Hydrochloride (CNS depressant effect of Lioresal Intrathecal may be additive to those of other CNS depressants).
No products indexed under this heading.

Levomethadyl Acetate Hydrochloride (CNS depressant effect of Lioresal Intrathecal may be additive to those of other CNS depressants). Products include:
Orlaam Oral Solution 2361

Levorphanol Tartrate (CNS depressant effect of Lioresal Intrathecal may be additive to those of other CNS depressants). Products include:
Levo-Dromoran 2297

Lorazepam (CNS depressant effect of Lioresal Intrathecal may be additive to those of other CNS depressants). Products include:
Ativan Injection 2805
Ativan Tablets 2807

Loxapine Hydrochloride (CNS depressant effect of Lioresal Intrathecal may be additive to those of other CNS depressants). Products include:
Loxitane 1426

Loxapine Succinate (CNS depressant effect of Lioresal Intrathecal may be additive to those of other CNS depressants). Products include:
Loxitane Capsules 1426

Meperidine Hydrochloride (CNS depressant effect of Lioresal Intrathecal may be additive to those of other CNS depressants). Products include:
Demerol 2438
Mepergan Injection 2859

Mephobarbital (CNS depressant effect of Lioresal Intrathecal may be additive to those of other CNS depressants). Products include:
Mebaral Tablets 2452

Meprobamate (CNS depressant effect of Lioresal Intrathecal may be additive to those of other CNS depressants). Products include:
Miltown Tablets 2780
PMB 200 and PMB 400 2890

Mesoridazine Besylate (CNS depressant effect of Lioresal Intrathecal may be additive to those of other CNS depressants). Products include:
Serentil 689

Methadone Hydrochloride (CNS depressant effect of Lioresal Intrathecal may be additive to those of other CNS depressants). Products include:
Methadone Hydrochloride Oral Concentrate 2356
Methadone Hydrochloride Oral Solution & Tablets 2357

Methohexital Sodium (CNS depressant effect of Lioresal Intrathecal may be additive to those of other CNS depressants).
No products indexed under this heading.

Methotrimeprazine (CNS depressant effect of Lioresal Intrathecal may be additive to those of other CNS depressants). Products include:
Levoprome 1321

Methoxyflurane (CNS depressant effect of Lioresal Intrathecal may be additive to those of other CNS depressants).
No products indexed under this heading.

Midazolam Hydrochloride (CNS depressant effect of Lioresal Intrathecal may be additive to those of other CNS depressants). Products include:
Versed Injection 2324

Molindone Hydrochloride (CNS depressant effect of Lioresal Intrathecal may be additive to those of other CNS depressants). Products include:
Moban Tablets and Concentrate 1036

Morphine Sulfate (CNS depressant effect of Lioresal Intrathecal may be additive to those of other CNS depressants; potential for hypotension and dyspnea with concurrent administration of Lioresal Intrathecal and epidural morphine). Products include:
Astramorph/PF Injection, USP (Preservative-Free) 526
Duramorph Injection 983
Infumorph 200 and Infumorph 500 Sterile Solutions 985
Kadian Capsules 2948
MS Contin Tablets 2149
MSIR 2152
Oramorph SR (Morphine Sulfate Sustained Release Tablets) 2359
RMS Suppositories CII 2766
Roxanol 2365

Opium Alkaloids (CNS depressant effect of Lioresal Intrathecal may be additive to those of other CNS depressants).
No products indexed under this heading.

IMPORTANT NOTE: Always consult each drug listing in the patient's regimen for possible interactions.

Lioresal Intrathecal / Interactions Index

Oxazepam (CNS depressant effect of Lioresal Intrathecal may be additive to those of other CNS depressants). Products include:
- Serax Capsules 2916
- Serax Tablets 2916

Oxycodone Hydrochloride (CNS depressant effect of Lioresal Intrathecal may be additive to those of other CNS depressants). Products include:
- OxyContin Tablets 2163
- OxyIR Capsules 2167
- Percocet Tablets 955
- Percodan Tablets 955
- Percodan-Demi Tablets 956
- Roxicodone Tablets, Oral Solution & Intensol (Oxycodone) 2366
- Tylox Capsules 1593

Pentobarbital Sodium (CNS depressant effect of Lioresal Intrathecal may be additive to those of other CNS depressants). Products include:
- Nembutal Sodium Capsules 440
- Nembutal Sodium Solution 442
- Nembutal Sodium Suppositories 444

Perphenazine (CNS depressant effect of Lioresal Intrathecal may be additive to those of other CNS depressants). Products include:
- Etrafon 2495
- Triavil Tablets 1800
- Trilafon 2532

Phenobarbital (CNS depressant effect of Lioresal Intrathecal may be additive to those of other CNS depressants). Products include:
- Arco-Lase Plus Tablets 513
- Bellergal-S Tablets 2375
- Donnatal 2234
- Donnatal Extentabs 2234
- Donnatal Tablets 2234
- Phenobarbital Elixir and Tablets 1523
- Quadrinal Tablets 1398

Prazepam (CNS depressant effect of Lioresal Intrathecal may be additive to those of other CNS depressants).
No products indexed under this heading.

Prochlorperazine (CNS depressant effect of Lioresal Intrathecal may be additive to those of other CNS depressants). Products include:
- Compazine 2644

Promethazine Hydrochloride (CNS depressant effect of Lioresal Intrathecal may be additive to those of other CNS depressants). Products include:
- Mepergan Injection 2859
- Phenergan with Codeine 2883
- Phenergan with Dextromethorphan 2885
- Phenergan Injection 2880
- Phenergan Suppositories 2882
- Phenergan Syrup 2881
- Phenergan Tablets 2882
- Phenergan VC 2886
- Phenergan VC with Codeine 2888

Propofol (CNS depressant effect of Lioresal Intrathecal may be additive to those of other CNS depressants). Products include:
- Diprivan Injectable Emulsion 2939

Propoxyphene Hydrochloride (CNS depressant effect of Lioresal Intrathecal may be additive to those of other CNS depressants). Products include:
- Darvon 1475
- Wygesic Tablets 2930

Propoxyphene Napsylate (CNS depressant effect of Lioresal Intrathecal may be additive to those of other CNS depressants). Products include:
- Darvon-N/Darvocet-N 1473

Quazepam (CNS depressant effect of Lioresal Intrathecal may be additive to those of other CNS depressants). Products include:
- Doral Tablets 2773

Risperidone (CNS depressant effect of Lioresal Intrathecal may be additive to those of other CNS depressants). Products include:
- Risperdal Tablets 1348

Secobarbital Sodium (CNS depressant effect of Lioresal Intrathecal may be additive to those of other CNS depressants). Products include:
- Seconal Sodium Pulvules 1529

Sevoflurane (CNS depressant effect of Lioresal Intrathecal may be additive to those of other CNS depressants).
No products indexed under this heading.

Sufentanil Citrate (CNS depressant effect of Lioresal Intrathecal may be additive to those of other CNS depressants). Products include:
- Sufenta Injection 1355

Temazepam (CNS depressant effect of Lioresal Intrathecal may be additive to those of other CNS depressants). Products include:
- Restoril Capsules 2413

Thiamylal Sodium (CNS depressant effect of Lioresal Intrathecal may be additive to those of other CNS depressants).
No products indexed under this heading.

Thioridazine Hydrochloride (CNS depressant effect of Lioresal Intrathecal may be additive to those of other CNS depressants). Products include:
- Mellaril 2398

Thiothixene (CNS depressant effect of Lioresal Intrathecal may be additive to those of other CNS depressants). Products include:
- Navane Capsules and Concentrate 2018
- Navane Intramuscular 2019

Triazolam (CNS depressant effect of Lioresal Intrathecal may be additive to those of other CNS depressants). Products include:
- Halcion Tablets 2093

Trifluoperazine Hydrochloride (CNS depressant effect of Lioresal Intrathecal may be additive to those of other CNS depressants). Products include:
- Stelazine 2692

Zolpidem Tartrate (CNS depressant effect of Lioresal Intrathecal may be additive to those of other CNS depressants). Products include:
- Ambien Tablets 2559

Food Interactions

Alcohol (CNS depressant effect of Lioresal Intrathecal may be additive to those of alcohol).

LIORESAL TABLETS
(Baclofen) 847

May interact with central nervous system depressants and certain other agents. Compounds in these categories include:

Alfentanil Hydrochloride (Additive depressant effect). Products include:
- Alfenta Injection 1334

Alprazolam (Additive depressant effect). Products include:
- Xanax Tablets 2115

Aprobarbital (Additive depressant effect).
No products indexed under this heading.

Buprenorphine (Additive depressant effect). Products include:
- Buprenex Injectable 2170

Buspirone Hydrochloride (Additive depressant effect). Products include:
- BuSpar Tablets 738

Butabarbital (Additive depressant effect).
No products indexed under this heading.

Butalbital (Additive depressant effect). Products include:
- Axocet Capsules 2469
- Esgic-plus Capsules 1012
- Esgic-plus Tablets 1012
- Fioricet Tablets 2386
- Fioricet with Codeine Capsules 2387
- Fiorinal Capsules 2388
- Fiorinal with Codeine Capsules 2390
- Fiorinal Tablets 2388
- Phrenilin 790
- Sedapap Tablets 50 mg/650 mg 1826

Chlordiazepoxide (Additive depressant effect). Products include:
- Limbitrol 2333

Chlordiazepoxide Hydrochloride (Additive depressant effect). Products include:
- Librax Capsules 2330
- Librium Capsules 2331
- Librium Injectable 2332

Chlorpromazine (Additive depressant effect). Products include:
- Thorazine Suppositories 2701

Chlorprothixene (Additive depressant effect).
No products indexed under this heading.

Chlorprothixene Hydrochloride (Additive depressant effect). Products include:
No products indexed under this heading.

Chlorprothixene Lactate (Additive depressant effect).
No products indexed under this heading.

Clorazepate Dipotassium (Additive depressant effect). Products include:
- Tranxene 459

Clozapine (Additive depressant effect). Products include:
- Clozaril Tablets 2377

Codeine Phosphate (Additive depressant effect). Products include:
- Brontex 2130
- Dimetane-DC Cough Syrup 2232
- Fioricet with Codeine Capsules 2387
- Fiorinal with Codeine Capsules 2390
- Nucofed 2225
- Phenergan with Codeine 2883
- Phenergan VC with Codeine 2888
- Robitussin A-C Syrup 2248
- Robitussin-DAC Syrup 2249
- Ryna .... ▩ 804
- Soma Compound w/Codeine Tablets 2784
- Tylenol with Codeine 1592

Desflurane (Additive depressant effect). Products include:
- Suprane (desflurane, USP) 1865

Dezocine (Additive depressant effect). Products include:
- Dalgan Injection 529

Diazepam (Additive depressant effect). Products include:
- Dizac (diazepam injectable emulsion) CIV 1862
- Valium Injectable 2336
- Valium Tablets 2335

Droperidol (Additive depressant effect). Products include:
- Inapsine Injection 462

Enflurane (Additive depressant effect).
No products indexed under this heading.

Estazolam (Additive depressant effect). Products include:
- ProSom Tablets 457

Ethchlorvynol (Additive depressant effect). Products include:
- Placidyl Capsules 456

Ethinamate (Additive depressant effect).
No products indexed under this heading.

Fentanyl (Additive depressant effect). Products include:
- Duragesic Transdermal System 1336

Fentanyl Citrate (Additive depressant effect). Products include:
- Sublimaze Injection 463

Fluphenazine Decanoate (Additive depressant effect). Products include:
- Prolixin Decanoate 510

Fluphenazine Enanthate (Additive depressant effect). Products include:
- Prolixin Enanthate 510

Fluphenazine Hydrochloride (Additive depressant effect). Products include:
- Prolixin 510

Flurazepam Hydrochloride (Additive depressant effect). Products include:
- Dalmane Capsules 2329

Glutethimide (Additive depressant effect).
No products indexed under this heading.

Haloperidol (Additive depressant effect). Products include:
- Haldol Injection, Tablets and Concentrate 1585

Haloperidol Decanoate (Additive depressant effect). Products include:
- Haldol Decanoate 1587

Hydrocodone Bitartrate (Additive depressant effect). Products include:
- Codiclear DH Syrup 808
- Duratuss HD Elixir 2750
- Histussin D Liquid 670
- Hycodan Tablets and Syrup 946
- Hycomine Compound Tablets 948
- Hycomine 947
- Hycotuss Expectorant Syrup 950
- Hydrocet Capsules 787
- Lorcet 10/650 Tablets 1016
- Lortab 2751
- Tussend 1830
- Tussend Expectorant 1831
- Vicodin Tablets 1404
- Vicodin ES Tablets 1405
- Vicodin HP Tablets 1403
- Vicodin Tuss Expectorant 1406
- Zydone Capsules 967

Hydrocodone Polistirex (Additive depressant effect). Products include:
- Tussionex Pennkinetic Extended-Release Suspension 1624

Hydromorphone Hydrochloride (Additive depressant effect). Products include:
- Dilaudid Ampules 1382
- Dilaudid Cough Syrup 1383
- Dilaudid-HP Injection 1384
- Dilaudid-HP Lyophilized Powder 250 mg 1384
- Dilaudid 1382
- Dilaudid Oral Liquid 1386
- Dilaudid 1382
- Dilaudid Tablets - 8 mg 1386

Hydroxyzine Hydrochloride (Additive depressant effect). Products include:
- Atarax Tablets & Syrup 1992
- Marax Tablets & DF Syrup 2015
- Vistaril Intramuscular Solution 2042

(▩ Described in PDR For Nonprescription Drugs)   (⊙ Described in PDR For Ophthalmology)

Interactions Index — Lithium Carbonate

Isoflurane (Additive depressant effect).
No products indexed under this heading.

Ketamine Hydrochloride (Additive depressant effect).
No products indexed under this heading.

Levomethadyl Acetate Hydrochloride (Additive depressant effect). Products include:
Orlaam Oral Solution 2361

Levorphanol Tartrate (Additive depressant effect). Products include:
Levo-Dromoran 2297

Lorazepam (Additive depressant effect). Products include:
Ativan Injection 2805
Ativan Tablets 2807

Loxapine Hydrochloride (Additive depressant effect). Products include:
Loxitane 1426

Loxapine Succinate (Additive depressant effect). Products include:
Loxitane Capsules 1426

Meperidine Hydrochloride (Additive depressant effect). Products include:
Demerol 2438
Mepergan Injection 2859

Mephobarbital (Additive depressant effect). Products include:
Mebaral Tablets 2452

Meprobamate (Additive depressant effect). Products include:
Miltown Tablets 2780
PMB 200 and PMB 400 2890

Mesoridazine Besylate (Additive depressant effect). Products include:
Serentil 689

Methadone Hydrochloride (Additive depressant effect). Products include:
Methadone Hydrochloride Oral Concentrate 2356
Methadone Hydrochloride Oral Solution & Tablets 2357

Methohexital Sodium (Additive depressant effect).
No products indexed under this heading.

Methotrimeprazine (Additive depressant effect). Products include:
Levoprome 1321

Methoxyflurane (Additive depressant effect).
No products indexed under this heading.

Midazolam Hydrochloride (Additive depressant effect). Products include:
Versed Injection 2324

Molindone Hydrochloride (Additive depressant effect). Products include:
Moban Tablets and Concentrate 1036

Morphine Sulfate (Additive depressant effect). Products include:
Astramorph/PF Injection, USP (Preservative-Free) 526
Duramorph Injection 983
Infumorph 200 and Infumorph 500 Sterile Solutions 985
Kadian Capsules 2948
MS Contin Tablets 2149
MSIR 2152
Oramorph SR (Morphine Sulfate Sustained Release Tablets) 2359
RMS Suppositories CII 2766
Roxanol 2365

Opium Alkaloids (Additive depressant effect).
No products indexed under this heading.

Oxazepam (Additive depressant effect). Products include:
Serax Capsules 2916
Serax Tablets 2916

Oxycodone Hydrochloride (Additive depressant effect). Products include:
OxyContin Tablets 2163
OxyIR Capsules 2167
Percocet Tablets 955
Percodan Tablets 955
Percodan-Demi Tablets 956
Roxicodone Tablets, Oral Solution & Intensol (Oxycodone) 2366
Tylox Capsules 1593

Pentobarbital Sodium (Additive depressant effects). Products include:
Nembutal Sodium Capsules 440
Nembutal Sodium Solution 442
Nembutal Sodium Suppositories 444

Perphenazine (Additive depressant effect). Products include:
Etrafon 2495
Triavil Tablets 1800
Trilafon 2532

Phenobarbital (Additive depressant effect). Products include:
Arco-Lase Plus Tablets 513
Bellergal-S Tablets 2375
Donnatal 2234
Donnatal Extentabs 2234
Donnatal Tablets 2234
Phenobarbital Elixir and Tablets 1523
Quadrinal Tablets 1398

Prazepam (Additive depressant effect).
No products indexed under this heading.

Prochlorperazine (Additive depressant effect). Products include:
Compazine 2644

Promethazine Hydrochloride (Additive depressant effect). Products include:
Mepergan Injection 2859
Phenergan with Codeine 2883
Phenergan with Dextromethorphan 2885
Phenergan Injection 2880
Phenergan Suppositories 2882
Phenergan Syrup 2881
Phenergan Tablets 2882
Phenergan VC 2886
Phenergan VC with Codeine 2888

Propofol (Additive depressant effect). Products include:
Diprivan Injectable Emulsion 2939

Propoxyphene Hydrochloride (Additive depressant effect). Products include:
Darvon 1475
Wygesic Tablets 2930

Propoxyphene Napsylate (Additive depressant effect). Products include:
Darvon-N/Darvocet-N 1473

Quazepam (Additive depressant effect). Products include:
Doral Tablets 2773

Risperidone (Additive depressant effect). Products include:
Risperdal Tablets 1348

Secobarbital Sodium (Additive depressant effect). Products include:
Seconal Sodium Pulvules 1529

Sevoflurane (Additive depressant effect).
No products indexed under this heading.

Sufentanil Citrate (Additive depressant effect). Products include:
Sufenta Injection 1355

Temazepam (Additive depressant effect). Products include:
Restoril Capsules 2413

Thiamylal Sodium (Additive depressant effect).
No products indexed under this heading.

Thioridazine Hydrochloride (Additive depressant effect). Products include:
Mellaril 2398

Thiothixene (Additive depressant effect). Products include:
Navane Capsules and Concentrate 2018
Navane Intramuscular 2019

Triazolam (Additive depressant effect). Products include:
Halcion Tablets 2093

Trifluoperazine Hydrochloride (Additive depressant effect). Products include:
Stelazine 2692

Zolpidem Tartrate (Additive depressant effect). Products include:
Ambien Tablets 2559

Food Interactions

Alcohol (Additive depressant effect).

LISTERINE ANTISEPTIC (Eucalyptol, Menthol, Methyl Salicylate) 820
None cited in PDR database.

COOL MINT LISTERINE (Thymol, Eucalyptol, Methyl Salicylate, Menthol) 820
None cited in PDR database.

FRESHBURST LISTERINE (Thymol, Eucalyptol, Methyl Salicylate, Menthol) 820
None cited in PDR database.

LISTERMINT (Sodium Lauryl Sulfate, Sodium Benzoate, Zinc Chloride) 820
None cited in PDR database.

LITHIUM CARBONATE CAPSULES & TABLETS
(Lithium Carbonate) 2352
May interact with antipsychotic agents, nondepolarizing neuromuscular blocking agents, non-steroidal anti-inflammatory agents, diuretics, ACE inhibitors, and certain other agents. Compounds in these categories include:

Amiloride Hydrochloride (High risk of lithium toxicity). Products include:
Midamor Tablets 1746
Moduretic Tablets 1748

Atracurium Besylate (Prolonged effects of neuromuscular blockers). Products include:
Tracrium Injection 1155

Benazepril Hydrochloride (Reduces lithium clearance and increases serum lithium levels resulting in risk of lithium toxicity). Products include:
Lotensin Tablets 852
Lotensin HCT Tablets 855
Lotrel Capsules 858

Bendroflumethiazide (High risk of lithium toxicity).
No products indexed under this heading.

Bumetanide (High risk of lithium toxicity). Products include:
Bumex 2260

Captopril (Reduces lithium clearance and increases serum lithium levels resulting in risk of lithium toxicity). Products include:
Capoten Tablets 740
Capozide Tablets 744

Chlorothiazide (High risk of lithium toxicity). Products include:
Aldoclor Tablets 1638
Diupres Tablets 1691
Diuril Oral 1694

Chlorothiazide Sodium (High risk of lithium toxicity). Products include:
Diuril Sodium Intravenous 1693

Chlorpromazine (Neurological toxicity has occurred; encephalopathic syndrome followed by irreversible brain damage). Products include:
Thorazine Suppositories 2701

Chlorprothixene (Neurological toxicity has occurred; encephalopathic syndrome followed by irreversible brain damage).
No products indexed under this heading.

Chlorprothixene Hydrochloride (Neurological toxicity has occurred; encephalopathic syndrome followed by irreversible brain damage).
No products indexed under this heading.

Chlorthalidone (High risk of lithium toxicity). Products include:
Combipres Tablets 682
Tenoretic Tablets 2963
Thalitone 1293

Cisatracurium Besylate (Prolonged effects of neuromuscular blockers). Products include:
Nimbex Injection 1131

Clozapine (Neurological toxicity has occurred; encephalopathic syndrome followed by irreversible brain damage). Products include:
Clozaril Tablets 2377

Diclofenac Potassium (Significant increase in steady state plasma lithium levels; possible lithium toxicity). Products include:
Cataflam Tablets 833

Diclofenac Sodium (Significant increase in steady state plasma lithium levels; possible lithium toxicity). Products include:
Voltaren Ophthalmic Sterile Ophthalmic Solution 264
Cataflam/Voltaren/Voltaren-XR 833

Enalapril Maleate (Reduces lithium clearance and increases serum lithium levels resulting in risk of lithium toxicity). Products include:
Vaseretic Tablets 1810
Vasotec Tablets 1816

Enalaprilat (Reduces lithium clearance and increases serum lithium levels resulting in risk of lithium toxicity). Products include:
Vasotec I.V. 1814

Ethacrynic Acid (High risk of lithium toxicity). Products include:
Edecrin Tablets 1698

Etodolac (Significant increase in steady state plasma lithium levels; possible lithium toxicity). Products include:
Lodine Capsules and Tablets 2849

Fenoprofen Calcium (Significant increase in steady state plasma lithium levels; possible lithium toxicity). Products include:
Nalfon 200 Pulvules & Nalfon Tablets 933

Fluphenazine Decanoate (Neurological toxicity has occurred; encephalopathic syndrome followed by irreversible brain damage). Products include:
Prolixin Decanoate 510

Fluphenazine Enanthate (Neurological toxicity has occurred; encephalopathic syndrome followed by irreversible brain damage). Products include:
Prolixin Enanthate 510

Fluphenazine Hydrochloride (Neurological toxicity has occurred; encephalopathic syndrome followed by irreversible brain damage). Products include:
Prolixin 510

IMPORTANT NOTE: Always consult each drug listing in the patient's regimen for possible interactions.

Flurbiprofen (Significant increase in steady state plasma lithium levels; possible lithium toxicity).
- No products indexed under this heading.

Fosinopril Sodium (Reduces lithium clearance and increases serum lithium levels resulting in risk of lithium toxicity). Products include:
- Monopril Tablets ... 762

Furosemide (High risk of lithium toxicity). Products include:
- Lasix Injection, Oral Solution and Tablets ... 1267

Haloperidol (Neurological toxicity has occurred; encephalopathic syndrome followed by irreversible brain damage). Products include:
- Haldol Injection, Tablets and Concentrate ... 1585

Haloperidol Decanoate (Neurological toxicity has occurred; encephalopathic syndrome followed by irreversible brain damage). Products include:
- Haldol Decanoate ... 1587

Hydrochlorothiazide (High risk of lithium toxicity). Products include:
- Aldactazide Tablets ... 2556
- Aldoril Tablets ... 1644
- Apresazide Capsules ... 824
- Capozide Tablets ... 744
- Dyazide Capsules ... 2653
- Esidrix Tablets ... 839
- Esimil Tablets ... 840
- HydroDIURIL Tablets ... 1716
- Hydropres Tablets ... 1718
- Hyzaar Tablets ... 1720
- Inderide Tablets ... 2838
- Inderide LA Long Acting Capsules .. 2840
- Lopressor HCT Tablets ... 850
- Lotensin HCT Tablets ... 855
- Moduretic Tablets ... 1748
- Oretic Tablets ... 450
- Prinzide Tablets ... 1780
- Ser-Ap-Es Tablets ... 867
- Timolide Tablets ... 1791
- Vaseretic Tablets ... 1810
- Zestoretic Tablets ... 2968
- Ziac ... 1459

Hydroflumethiazide (High risk of lithium toxicity). Products include:
- Diucardin Tablets ... 2824

Ibuprofen (Significant increase in steady state plasma lithium levels; possible lithium toxicity). Products include:
- Advil Cold and Sinus Caplets and Tablets ... ▣ 837
- Advil Ibuprofen Tablets, Caplets and Gel Caplets ... ▣ 836
- Children's Motrin Ibuprofen Oral Suspension ... 1558
- IBU Tablets ... 1389
- Ibuprohm ... ▣ 713
- Motrin IB Caplets, Tablets, and Gelcaps ... ▣ 802
- Motrin Ibuprofen Suspension, Oral Drops, Chewable Tablets, Caplets ... 1563
- Nuprin Ibuprofen/Analgesic Tablets & Caplets ... ▣ 645
- Vicks DayQuil SINUS Pressure & PAIN Relief with IBUPROFEN ... ▣ 735

Indapamide (High risk of lithium toxicity).
- No products indexed under this heading.

Indomethacin (Significant increase in steady state plasma lithium levels; possible lithium toxicity). Products include:
- Indocin ... 1723

Indomethacin Sodium Trihydrate (Significant increase in steady state plasma lithium levels; possible lithium toxicity). Products include:
- Indocin I.V. ... 1727

Ketoprofen (Significant increase in steady state plasma lithium levels; possible lithium toxicity). Products include:
- Actron Caplets and Tablets ... ▣ 608
- Orudis Capsules ... 2874
- Orudis KT ... ▣ 842
- Oruvail Capsules ... 2874

Ketorolac Tromethamine (Significant increase in steady state plasma lithium levels; possible lithium toxicity). Products include:
- Acular Sterile Ophthalmic Solution 470
- Toradol ... 2319

Lisinopril (Reduces lithium clearance and increases serum lithium levels resulting in risk of lithium toxicity). Products include:
- Prinivil Tablets ... 1776
- Prinzide Tablets ... 1780
- Zestoretic Tablets ... 2968
- Zestril Tablets ... 2972

Loxapine Hydrochloride (Neurological toxicity has occurred; encephalopathic syndrome followed by irreversible brain damage). Products include:
- Loxitane ... 1426

Meclofenamate Sodium (Significant increase in steady state plasma lithium levels; possible lithium toxicity).
- No products indexed under this heading.

Mefenamic Acid (Significant increase in steady state plasma lithium levels; possible lithium toxicity). Products include:
- Ponstel ... 1982

Mesoridazine Besylate (Neurological toxicity has occurred; encephalopathic syndrome followed by irreversible brain damage). Products include:
- Serentil ... 689

Methyclothiazide (High risk of lithium toxicity). Products include:
- Enduron Tablets ... 424

Metocurine Iodide (Prolonged effects of neuromuscular blockers). Products include:
- Metubine Iodide Vials ... 932

Metolazone (High risk of lithium toxicity). Products include:
- Mykrox Tablets ... 1617
- Zaroxolyn Tablets ... 1625

Mivacurium Chloride (Prolonged effects of neuromuscular blockers). Products include:
- Mivacron ... 1125

Moexipril Hydrochloride (Reduces lithium clearance and increases serum lithium levels resulting in risk of lithium toxicity). Products include:
- Univasc Tablets ... 2553

Molindone Hydrochloride (Neurological toxicity has occurred; encephalopathic syndrome followed by irreversible brain damage). Products include:
- Moban Tablets and Concentrate ... 1036

Nabumetone (Significant increase in steady state plasma lithium levels; possible lithium toxicity). Products include:
- Relafen Tablets ... 2688

Naproxen (Significant increase in steady state plasma lithium levels; possible lithium toxicity). Products include:
- Anaprox/Naprosyn ... 2277

Naproxen Sodium (Significant increase in steady state plasma lithium levels; possible lithium toxicity). Products include:
- Aleve ... 2124
- Anaprox/Naprosyn ... 2277
- Naprelan Tablets ... 2861

Oxaprozin (Significant increase in steady state plasma lithium levels; possible lithium toxicity). Products include:
- Daypro Caplets ... 2578

Pancuronium Bromide (Prolonged effects of neuromuscular blockers).
- No products indexed under this heading.

Perphenazine (Neurological toxicity has occurred; encephalopathic syndrome followed by irreversible brain damage). Products include:
- Etrafon ... 2495
- Triavil Tablets ... 1800
- Trilafon ... 2532

Phenylbutazone (Significant increase in steady state plasma lithium levels; possible lithium toxicity).
- No products indexed under this heading.

Pimozide (Neurological toxicity has occurred; encephalopathic syndrome followed by irreversible brain damage). Products include:
- Orap Tablets ... 1037

Piroxicam (Significant increase in steady state plasma lithium levels; possible lithium toxicity). Products include:
- Feldene Capsules ... 2008

Polythiazide (High risk of lithium toxicity). Products include:
- Minizide Capsules ... 2016

Prochlorperazine (Neurological toxicity has occurred; encephalopathic syndrome followed by irreversible brain damage). Products include:
- Compazine ... 2644

Promethazine Hydrochloride (Neurological toxicity has occurred; encephalopathic syndrome followed by irreversible brain damage). Products include:
- Mepergan Injection ... 2859
- Phenergan with Codeine ... 2883
- Phenergan with Dextromethorphan 2885
- Phenergan Injection ... 2880
- Phenergan Suppositories ... 2882
- Phenergan Syrup ... 2881
- Phenergan Tablets ... 2882
- Phenergan VC ... 2886
- Phenergan VC with Codeine ... 2888

Quinapril Hydrochloride (Reduces lithium clearance and increases serum lithium levels resulting in risk of lithium toxicity). Products include:
- Accupril Tablets ... 1950

Ramipril (Reduces lithium clearance and increases serum lithium levels resulting in risk of lithium toxicity). Products include:
- Altace Capsules ... 1238

Risperidone (Neurological toxicity has occurred; encephalopathic syndrome followed by irreversible brain damage). Products include:
- Risperdal Tablets ... 1348

Rocuronium Bromide (Prolonged effects of neuromuscular blockers). Products include:
- Zemuron Injection ... 1885

Spirapril Hydrochloride (Reduces lithium clearance and increases serum lithium levels resulting in risk of lithium toxicity).
- No products indexed under this heading.

Spironolactone (High risk of lithium toxicity). Products include:
- Aldactazide Tablets ... 2556
- Aldactone Tablets ... 2558

Sulindac (Significant increase in steady state plasma lithium levels; possible lithium toxicity). Products include:
- Clinoril Tablets ... 1658

Thioridazine Hydrochloride (Neurological toxicity has occurred; encephalopathic syndrome followed by irreversible brain damage). Products include:
- Mellaril ... 2398

Thiothixene (Neurological toxicity has occurred; encephalopathic syndrome followed by irreversible brain damage). Products include:
- Navane Capsules and Concentrate 2018
- Navane Intramuscular ... 2019

Tolmetin Sodium (Significant increase in steady state plasma lithium levels; possible lithium toxicity). Products include:
- Tolectin (200, 400 and 600 mg) .. 1591

Torsemide (High risk of lithium toxicity). Products include:
- Demadex Tablets and Injection ... 691

Trandolapril (Reduces lithium clearance and increases serum lithium levels resulting in risk of lithium toxicity). Products include:
- Mavik Tablets ... 1407

Triamterene (High risk of lithium toxicity). Products include:
- Dyazide Capsules ... 2653
- Dyrenium Capsules ... 2655

Trifluoperazine Hydrochloride (Neurological toxicity has occurred; encephalopathic syndrome followed by irreversible brain damage). Products include:
- Stelazine ... 2692

Vecuronium Bromide (Prolonged effects of neuromuscular blockers). Products include:
- Norcuron for Injection ... 1875

LITHOBID SLOW-RELEASE TABLETS

(Lithium Carbonate) ... 2721

See **LITHONATE Capsules**

LITHONATE CAPSULES

(Lithium Carbonate) ... 2721

May interact with ACE inhibitors, diuretics, calcium channel blockers, antipsychotic agents, thiazides, neuromuscular blocking agents, xanthine bronchodilators, non-steroidal anti-inflammatory agents, and certain other agents. Compounds in these categories include:

Acetazolamide (Lowers serum lithium concentrations by increasing urinary lithium excretions). Products include:
- Diamox Sequels (Sustained Release) ... ⊙ 318
- Diamox Tablets ... ⊙ 317

Amiloride Hydrochloride (Concomitant use should be avoided; potential for lithium toxicity). Products include:
- Midamor Tablets ... 1746
- Moduretic Tablets ... 1748

Aminophylline (Lowers serum lithium concentrations by increasing urinary lithium excretions).
- No products indexed under this heading.

Amlodipine Besylate (Concurrent use may increase the risk of neurotoxicity in the form of ataxia, tremors, nausea, vomiting, diarrhea, and/or tinnitus). Products include:
- Lotrel Capsules ... 858
- Norvasc Tablets ... 2020

(▣ Described in PDR For Nonprescription Drugs) (⊙ Described in PDR For Ophthalmology)

Atracurium Besylate (Prolonged effects of neuromuscular blocking agents). Products include:
- Tracrium Injection ... 1155

Benazepril Hydrochloride (Concomitant use should be avoided; potential for lithium toxicity). Products include:
- Lotensin Tablets ... 852
- Lotensin HCT Tablets ... 855
- Lotrel Capsules ... 858

Bendroflumethiazide (Concomitant use should be avoided; potential for lithium toxicity).
- No products indexed under this heading.

Bepridil Hydrochloride (Concurrent use may increase the risk of neurotoxicity in the form of ataxia, tremors, nausea, vomiting, diarrhea, and/or tinnitus). Products include:
- Vascor Tablets (200 and 300 mg) 1597

Bumetanide (Concomitant use should be avoided; potential for lithium toxicity). Products include:
- Bumex ... 2260

Captopril (Concomitant use should be avoided; potential for lithium toxicity). Products include:
- Capoten Tablets ... 740
- Capozide Tablets ... 744

Carbamazepine (Increased risk of neurotoxic side effects). Products include:
- Atretol Tablets ... 569
- Tegretol/Tegretol-XR ... 870

Chlorothiazide (Concomitant use should be avoided; potential for lithium toxicity). Products include:
- Aldoclor Tablets ... 1638
- Diupres Tablets ... 1691
- Diuril Oral ... 1694

Chlorothiazide Sodium (Concomitant use should be avoided; potential for lithium toxicity). Products include:
- Diuril Sodium Intravenous ... 1693

Chlorpromazine (Possible haloperidol-type interaction has been extended to other antipsychotics). Products include:
- Thorazine Suppositories ... 2701

Chlorprothixene (Possible haloperidol-type interaction has been extended to other antipsychotics).
- No products indexed under this heading.

Chlorprothixene Hydrochloride (Possible haloperidol-type interaction has been extended to other antipsychotics).
- No products indexed under this heading.

Chlorthalidone (Concomitant use should be avoided; potential for lithium toxicity). Products include:
- Combipres Tablets ... 682
- Tenoretic Tablets ... 2963
- Thalitone ... 1293

Cisatracurium Besylate (Prolonged effects of neuromuscular blocking agents). Products include:
- Nimbex Injection ... 1131

Clozapine (Possible haloperidol-type interaction has been extended to other antipsychotics). Products include:
- Clozaril Tablets ... 2377

Decamethonium (Prolonged effects of neuromuscular blocking agents).

Diclofenac Potassium (Potential for increased steady-state plasma lithium levels resulting in lithium toxicity). Products include:
- Cataflam Tablets ... 833

Diclofenac Sodium (Potential for increased steady-state plasma lithium levels resulting in lithium toxicity). Products include:
- Voltaren Ophthalmic Sterile Ophthalmic Solution ... ◉ 264
- Cataflam/Voltaren/Voltaren-XR ... 833

Diltiazem Hydrochloride (Concurrent use may increase the risk of neurotoxicity in the form of ataxia, tremors, nausea, vomiting, diarrhea, and/or tinnitus). Products include:
- Cardizem CD Capsules ... 1251
- Cardizem SR Capsules ... 1255
- Cardizem Injectable ... 1253
- Cardizem Tablets ... 1257
- Dilacor XR Extended-release Capsules ... 2183
- Tiazac Capsules ... 1019

Doxacurium Chloride (Prolonged effects of neuromuscular blocking agents). Products include:
- Nuromax Injection ... 1136

Dyphylline (Lowers serum lithium concentrations by increasing urinary lithium excretions). Products include:
- Lufyllin & Lufyllin-400 Tablets ... 2778
- Lufyllin-GG Elixir & Tablets ... 2779

Enalapril Maleate (Concomitant use should be avoided; potential for lithium toxicity). Products include:
- Vaseretic Tablets ... 1810
- Vasotec Tablets ... 1816

Enalaprilat (Concomitant use should be avoided; potential for lithium toxicity). Products include:
- Vasotec I.V. ... 1814

Ethacrynic Acid (Concomitant use should be avoided; potential for lithium toxicity). Products include:
- Edecrin Tablets ... 1698

Etodolac (Potential for increased steady-state plasma lithium levels resulting in lithium toxicity). Products include:
- Lodine Capsules and Tablets ... 2849

Felodipine (Concurrent use may increase the risk of neurotoxicity in the form of ataxia, tremors, nausea, vomiting, diarrhea, and/or tinnitus). Products include:
- Plendil Extended-Release Tablets ... 514

Fenoprofen Calcium (Potential for increased steady-state plasma lithium levels resulting in lithium toxicity). Products include:
- Nalfon 200 Pulvules & Nalfon Tablets ... 933

Fluoxetine Hydrochloride (Concurrent use has resulted in both increased and decreased lithium levels). Products include:
- Prozac Pulvules & Liquid, Oral Solution ... 935

Fluphenazine Decanoate (Possible haloperidol-type interaction has been extended to other antipsychotics). Products include:
- Prolixin Decanoate ... 510

Fluphenazine Enanthate (Possible haloperidol-type interaction has been extended to other antipsychotics). Products include:
- Prolixin Enanthate ... 510

Fluphenazine Hydrochloride (Possible haloperidol-type interaction has been extended to other antipsychotics). Products include:
- Prolixin ... 510

Flurbiprofen (Potential for increased steady-state plasma lithium levels resulting in lithium toxicity).
- No products indexed under this heading.

Fosinopril Sodium (Concomitant use should be avoided; potential for lithium toxicity). Products include:
- Monopril Tablets ... 762

Furosemide (Concomitant use should be avoided; potential for lithium toxicity). Products include:
- Lasix Injection, Oral Solution and Tablets ... 1267

Haloperidol (Concomitant use may lead to encephalopathic syndrome followed by irreversible brain damage). Products include:
- Haldol Injection, Tablets and Concentrate ... 1585

Haloperidol Decanoate (Concomitant use may lead to encephalopathic syndrome followed by irreversible brain damage). Products include:
- Haldol Decanoate ... 1587

Hydrochlorothiazide (Concomitant use should be avoided; potential for lithium toxicity). Products include:
- Aldactazide Tablets ... 2556
- Aldoril Tablets ... 1644
- Apresazide Capsules ... 824
- Capozide Tablets ... 744
- Dyazide Capsules ... 2653
- Esidrix Tablets ... 839
- Esimil Tablets ... 840
- HydroDIURIL Tablets ... 1716
- Hydropres Tablets ... 1718
- Hyzaar Tablets ... 1720
- Inderide Tablets ... 2838
- Inderide LA Long Acting Capsules .. 2840
- Lopressor HCT Tablets ... 850
- Lotensin HCT Tablets ... 855
- Moduretic Tablets ... 1748
- Oretic Tablets ... 450
- Prinzide Tablets ... 1780
- Ser-Ap-Es Tablets ... 867
- Timolide Tablets ... 1791
- Vaseretic Tablets ... 1810
- Zestoretic Tablets ... 2968
- Ziac ... 1459

Hydroflumethiazide (Concomitant use should be avoided; potential for lithium toxicity). Products include:
- Diucardin Tablets ... 2824

Ibuprofen (Potential for increased steady-state plasma lithium levels resulting in lithium toxicity). Products include:
- Advil Cold and Sinus Caplets and Tablets ... 837
- Advil Ibuprofen Tablets, Caplets and Gel Caplets ... 836
- Children's Motrin Ibuprofen Oral Suspension ... 1558
- IBU Tablets ... 1389
- Ibuprohm ... 713
- Motrin IB Caplets, Tablets, and Gelcaps ... 802
- Motrin Ibuprofen Suspension, Oral Drops, Chewable Tablets, Caplets ... 1563
- Nuprin Ibuprofen/Analgesic Tablets & Caplets ... 645
- Vicks DayQuil SINUS Pressure & PAIN Relief with IBUPROFEN ... 735

Indapamide (Concomitant use should be avoided; potential for lithium toxicity).
- No products indexed under this heading.

Indomethacin (Potential for increased steady-state plasma lithium levels resulting in lithium toxicity). Products include:
- Indocin ... 1723

Indomethacin Sodium Trihydrate (Potential for increased steady-state plasma lithium levels resulting in lithium toxicity). Products include:
- Indocin I.V. ... 1727

Isradipine (Concurrent use may increase the risk of neurotoxicity in the form of ataxia, tremors, nausea, vomiting, diarrhea, and/or tinnitus). Products include:
- DynaCirc Capsules ... 2381
- DynaCirc CR Tablets ... 2383

Ketoprofen (Potential for increased steady-state plasma lithium levels resulting in lithium toxicity). Products include:
- Actron Caplets and Tablets ... 608
- Orudis Capsules ... 2874
- Orudis KT ... 842
- Oruvail Capsules ... 2874

Ketorolac Tromethamine (Potential for increased steady-state plasma lithium levels resulting in lithium toxicity). Products include:
- Acular Sterile Ophthalmic Solution 470
- Toradol ... 2319

Lisinopril (Concomitant use should be avoided; potential for lithium toxicity). Products include:
- Prinivil Tablets ... 1776
- Prinzide Tablets ... 1780
- Zestoretic Tablets ... 2968
- Zestril Tablets ... 2972

Loxapine Hydrochloride (Possible haloperidol-type interaction has been extended to other antipsychotics). Products include:
- Loxitane ... 1426

Loxapine Succinate (Possible haloperidol-type interaction has been extended to other antipsychotics). Products include:
- Loxitane Capsules ... 1426

Meclofenamate Sodium (Potential for increased steady-state plasma lithium levels resulting in lithium toxicity).
- No products indexed under this heading.

Mefenamic Acid (Potential for increased steady-state plasma lithium levels resulting in lithium toxicity). Products include:
- Ponstel ... 1982

Mesoridazine Besylate (Possible haloperidol-type interaction has been extended to other antipsychotics). Products include:
- Serentil ... 689

Methyclothiazide (Concomitant use should be avoided; potential for lithium toxicity). Products include:
- Enduron Tablets ... 424

Metocurine Iodide (Prolonged effects of neuromuscular blocking agents). Products include:
- Metubine Iodide Vials ... 932

Metolazone (Concomitant use should be avoided; potential for lithium toxicity). Products include:
- Mykrox Tablets ... 1617
- Zaroxolyn Tablets ... 1625

Metronidazole (Concurrent use may provoke lithium toxicity due to reduced renal clearance). Products include:
- Flagyl 375 Capsules ... 2587
- Flagyl I.V. RTU ... 2373
- Helidac Therapy ... 2135
- MetroCream ... 1034
- MetroGel ... 1034
- MetroGel-Vaginal ... 917
- Protostat Tablets ... 1939

Mivacurium Chloride (Prolonged effects of neuromuscular blocking agents). Products include:
- Mivacron ... 1125

Moexipril Hydrochloride (Concomitant use should be avoided; potential for lithium toxicity). Products include:
- Univasc Tablets ... 2553

IMPORTANT NOTE: Always consult each drug listing in the patient's regimen for possible interactions.

Lithonate/Lithotabs/Lithobid — Interactions Index

Molindone Hydrochloride (Possible haloperidol-type interaction has been extended to other antipsychotics). Products include:
- Moban Tablets and Concentrate 1036

Nabumetone (Potential for increased steady-state plasma lithium levels resulting in lithium toxicity). Products include:
- Relafen Tablets 2688

Naproxen (Potential for increased steady-state plasma lithium levels resulting in lithium toxicity). Products include:
- Anaprox/Naprosyn 2277

Naproxen Sodium (Potential for increased steady-state plasma lithium levels resulting in lithium toxicity). Products include:
- Aleve 2124
- Anaprox/Naprosyn 2277
- Naprelan Tablets 2861

Nicardipine Hydrochloride (Concurrent use may increase the risk of neurotoxicity in the form of ataxia, tremors, nausea, vomiting, diarrhea, and/or tinnitus). Products include:
- Cardene Capsules 2261
- Cardene I.V. 2815
- Cardene SR Capsules 2264

Nifedipine (Concurrent use may increase the risk of neurotoxicity in the form of ataxia, tremors, nausea, vomiting, diarrhea, and/or tinnitus). Products include:
- Adalat Capsules (10 mg and 20 mg) 580
- Adalat CC 582
- Procardia Capsules 2024
- Procardia XL Extended Release Tablets 2026

Nimodipine (Concurrent use may increase the risk of neurotoxicity in the form of ataxia, tremors, nausea, vomiting, diarrhea, and/or tinnitus). Products include:
- Nimotop Capsules 603

Nisoldipine (Concurrent use may increase the risk of neurotoxicity in the form of ataxia, tremors, nausea, vomiting, diarrhea, and/or tinnitus). Products include:
- Sular Tablets 2961

Oxaprozin (Potential for increased steady-state plasma lithium levels resulting in lithium toxicity). Products include:
- Daypro Caplets 2578

Pancuronium Bromide (Prolonged effects of neuromuscular blocking agents).
- No products indexed under this heading.

Perphenazine (Possible haloperidol-type interaction has been extended to other antipsychotics). Products include:
- Etrafon 2495
- Triavil Tablets 1800
- Trilafon 2532

Phenylbutazone (Potential for increased steady-state plasma lithium levels resulting in lithium toxicity).
- No products indexed under this heading.

Pimozide (Possible haloperidol-type interaction has been extended to other antipsychotics). Products include:
- Orap Tablets 1037

Piroxicam (Potential for increased steady-state plasma lithium levels resulting in lithium toxicity). Products include:
- Feldene Capsules 2008

Polythiazide (Concomitant use should be avoided; potential for lithium toxicity). Products include:
- Minizide Capsules 2016

Potassium Iodide (Concomitant extended use of iodide preparation may produce hypothyroidism). Products include:
- Hyland's C-Plus Cold Tablets 789
- Pima Syrup 1004
- Quadrinal Tablets 1398
- SSKI Solution 2767
- Thyro-Block Tablets 2785

Prochlorperazine (Possible haloperidol-type interaction has been extended to other antipsychotics). Products include:
- Compazine 2644

Promethazine Hydrochloride (Possible haloperidol-type interaction has been extended to other antipsychotics). Products include:
- Mepergan Injection 2859
- Phenergan with Codeine 2883
- Phenergan with Dextromethorphan 2885
- Phenergan Injection 2880
- Phenergan Suppositories 2882
- Phenergan Syrup 2881
- Phenergan Tablets 2882
- Phenergan VC 2886
- Phenergan VC with Codeine 2888

Quinapril Hydrochloride (Concomitant use should be avoided; potential for lithium toxicity). Products include:
- Accupril Tablets 1950

Ramipril (Concomitant use should be avoided; potential for lithium toxicity). Products include:
- Altace Capsules 1238

Risperidone (Possible haloperidol-type interaction has been extended to other antipsychotics). Products include:
- Risperdal Tablets 1348

Rocuronium Bromide (Prolonged effects of neuromuscular blocking agents). Products include:
- Zemuron Injection 1885

Sodium Bicarbonate (Lowers serum lithium concentrations by increasing urinary lithium excretions). Products include:
- Alka-Seltzer Cherry Effervescent Antacid and Pain Reliever 609
- Alka-Seltzer Extra Strength Effervescent Antacid and Pain Reliever 609
- Alka-Seltzer Gold Effervescent Antacid 611
- Alka-Seltzer Lemon Lime Effervescent Antacid and Pain Reliever 609
- Alka-Seltzer Original Effervescent Antacid and Pain Reliever 609
- Arm & Hammer Pure Baking Soda 648
- Colyte and Colyte-flavored 2540
- GoLYTELY 694
- Massengill Disposable Douches 780
- Massengill Liquid Concentrate 780
- NuLYTELY 694
- Cherry Flavor NuLYTELY 694

Spirapril Hydrochloride (Concomitant use should be avoided; potential for lithium toxicity).
- No products indexed under this heading.

Spironolactone (Concomitant use should be avoided; potential for lithium toxicity). Products include:
- Aldactazide Tablets 2556
- Aldactone Tablets 2558

Succinylcholine Chloride (Prolonged effects of neuromuscular blocking agents). Products include:
- Anectine 1062

Sulindac (Potential for increased steady-state plasma lithium levels resulting in lithium toxicity). Products include:
- Clinoril Tablets 1658

Theophylline (Lowers serum lithium concentrations by increasing urinary lithium excretions). Products include:
- Marax Tablets & DF Syrup 2015
- Quibron 2227

Theophylline Anhydrous (Lowers serum lithium concentrations by increasing urinary lithium excretions). Products include:
- Aerolate 1003
- Primatene Tablets 844
- Respbid Tablets 687
- Slo-bid Gyrocaps 2201
- Theo-24 Extended Release Capsules 2753
- Theo-Dur Extended-Release Tablets 1367
- Theo-X Extended-Release Tablets .. 793
- Uni-Dur Extended-Release Tablets .. 1374
- Uniphyl 400 mg and 600 mg Tablets 2157

Theophylline Calcium Salicylate (Lowers serum lithium concentrations by increasing urinary lithium excretions). Products include:
- Quadrinal Tablets 1398

Theophylline Sodium Glycinate (Lowers serum lithium concentrations by increasing urinary lithium excretions).
- No products indexed under this heading.

Thioridazine Hydrochloride (Possible haloperidol-type interaction has been extended to other antipsychotics). Products include:
- Mellaril 2398

Thiothixene (Possible haloperidol-type interaction has been extended to other antipsychotics). Products include:
- Navane Capsules and Concentrate 2018
- Navane Intramuscular 2019

Tolmetin Sodium (Potential for increased steady-state plasma lithium levels resulting in lithium toxicity). Products include:
- Tolectin (200, 400 and 600 mg) .. 1591

Torsemide (Concomitant use should be avoided; potential for lithium toxicity). Products include:
- Demadex Tablets and Injection 691

Trandolapril (Concomitant use should be avoided; potential for lithium toxicity). Products include:
- Mavik Tablets 1407

Triamterene (Concomitant use should be avoided; potential for lithium toxicity). Products include:
- Dyazide Capsules 2653
- Dyrenium Capsules 2655

Trifluoperazine Hydrochloride (Possible haloperidol-type interaction has been extended to other antipsychotics). Products include:
- Stelazine 2692

Vecuronium Bromide (Prolonged effects of neuromuscular blocking agents). Products include:
- Norcuron for Injection 1875

Verapamil Hydrochloride (Concurrent use may increase the risk of neurotoxicity in the form of ataxia, tremors, nausea, vomiting, diarrhea, and/or tinnitus). Products include:
- Calan SR Caplets 2571
- Calan Tablets 2568
- Covera-HS Tablets 2573
- Isoptin Injectable 1391
- Isoptin Oral Tablets 1393
- Isoptin SR Tablets 1395
- Verelan Capsules 1455

LITHOTABS TABLETS
(Lithium Carbonate) 2721
See LITHONATE Capsules

LIVOSTIN
(Levocabastine Hydrochloride) 262
None cited in PDR database.

LOCOID CREAM, OINTMENT AND TOPICAL SOLUTION
(Hydrocortisone Butyrate) 994
None cited in PDR database.

LODINE CAPSULES AND TABLETS
(Etodolac) 2849
May interact with lithium preparations and certain other agents. Compounds in these categories include:

Aluminum Carbonate (Co-administration with antacids has no apparent effect on the extent of absorption, however, antacids can decrease the peak concentration reached by 15% to 20%). Products include:
- Basaljel Capsules 2810
- Basaljel Suspension 2810
- Basaljel Tablets 2810

Aluminum Hydroxide (Co-administration with antacids has no apparent effect on the extent of absorption, however, antacids can decrease the peak concentration reached by 15% to 20%). Products include:
- ALternaGEL Liquid 1358
- Maximum Strength Ascriptin 650
- Cama Arthritis Pain Reliever 748
- Gaviscon Extra Strength Relief Formula Antacid Tablets 778
- Gaviscon Extra Strength Relief Formula Liquid Antacid 779
- Gaviscon Liquid Antacid 779
- Gelusil Antacid-Anti-gas Liquid 819
- Gelusil Antacid-Anti-gas Tablets 819
- Maalox Antacid/Anti-Gas Tablets 889
- Maalox Heartburn Relief Suspension 658
- Maalox Antacid Liquid 888
- Extra Strength Maalox Antacid/Anti-Gas Liquid and Tablets 888
- Mylanta 1359
- Tempo Soft Antacid 799

Aluminum Hydroxide Gel (Co-administration with antacids has no apparent effect on the extent of absorption, however, antacids can decrease the peak concentration reached by 15% to 20%). Products include:
- ALternaGEL Liquid 675
- Aludrox Oral Suspension 850
- Amphojel Suspension 2802
- Amphojel Suspension without Flavor 2802
- Amphojel Tablets 2802
- Ascriptin 650
- Gaviscon Antacid Tablets 778
- Gaviscon-2 Antacid Tablets 779
- Mylanta Liquid 676
- Mylanta Double Strength Liquid 676
- Nephrox Suspension 671

Aspirin (Co-administration reduces protein binding, although the clearance of free Etodolac is not altered; concurrent use is not recommended because of potential for increased adverse effects). Products include:
- Alka-Seltzer Cherry Effervescent Antacid and Pain Reliever 609
- Alka-Seltzer Extra Strength Effervescent Antacid and Pain Reliever 609
- Alka-Seltzer Lemon Lime Effervescent Antacid and Pain Reliever 609
- Alka-Seltzer Original Effervescent Antacid and Pain Reliever 609
- Alka-Seltzer Plus 611
- Alka-Seltzer Plus Sinus Medicine .. 611
- Ascriptin 650
- Arthritis Strength BC Powder 631

(■ Described in PDR For Nonprescription Drugs)   (◉ Described in PDR For Ophthalmology)

BC Cold Powder Multi-Symptom Formula (Cold-Sinus-Allergy) 631
BC Cold Powder Non-Drowsy Formula (Cold-Sinus) 631
BC Powder 631
Genuine Bayer Aspirin Tablets & Caplets 618
Extra Strength Bayer Arthritis Pain Regimen Formula 615
Extra Strength Bayer Aspirin Caplets & Tablets 617
Extended-Release Bayer 8-Hour Aspirin 616
Extra Strength Bayer Plus Aspirin Caplets 617
Extra Strength Bayer PM Aspirin Plus Sleep Aid 617
Aspirin Regimen Bayer 81 mg Tablets with Calcium 615
Aspirin Regimen Bayer Adult Low Strength 81 mg Tablets 613
Aspirin Regimen Bayer Children's Chewable Aspirin 616
Aspirin Regimen Bayer Regular Strength 325 mg Caplets 613
Bufferin Analgesic Tablets 636
Arthritis Strength Bufferin Analgesic Caplets 637
Extra Strength Bufferin Analgesic Tablets 637
Cama Arthritis Pain Reliever 748
Darvon Compound-65 Pulvules 1475
Easprin 1971
Ecotrin 2625
Ecotrin Enteric Coated Aspirin Maximum Strength Tablets and Caplets 775
Ecotrin Enteric Coated Aspirin Regular Strength Tablets 2625
Empirin Aspirin Tablets 818
Excedrin Extra-Strength Analgesic Tablets, Caplets, and Geltabs 734
Fiorinal Capsules 2388
Fiorinal with Codeine Capsules 2390
Fiorinal Tablets 2388
Goody's Extra Strength Headache Powders 632
Goody's Extra Strength Pain Relief Tablets 632
Halfprin Tablets 1413
Norgesic 1554
Percodan Tablets 955
Percodan-Demi Tablets 956
Robaxisal Tablets 2246
Soma Compound w/Codeine Tablets 2784
Soma Compound Tablets 2783
St. Joseph Adult Chewable Aspirin (81 mg.) 768
Talwin Compound 2466
Vanquish Analgesic Caplets 627

Cyclosporine (Etodolac, like other NSAIDs, may cause changes in the elimination of cyclosporine; nephrotoxicity associated with cyclosporine may also be enhanced). Products include:
Neoral 2405
Sandimmune 2416

Digoxin (Etodolac, like other NSAIDs, may cause changes in the elimination of digoxin through its effects on renal prostaglandins, leading to elevated serum levels of digoxin and increased toxicity). Products include:
Lanoxicaps 1110
Lanoxin Elixir Pediatric 1113
Lanoxin Injection 1116
Lanoxin Injection Pediatric 1119
Lanoxin Tablets 1121

Lithium Carbonate (Etodolac, like other NSAIDs, may cause changes in the elimination of lithium through its effects on renal prostaglandins, leading to elevated serum levels of lithium and increased toxicity). Products include:
Eskalith 2658
Lithium Carbonate Capsules & Tablets 2352
Lithonate/Lithotabs/Lithobid 2721

Lithium Citrate (Etodolac, like other NSAIDs, may cause changes in the elimination of lithium through its effects on renal prostaglandins, leading to elevated serum levels of lithium and increased toxicity).
No products indexed under this heading.

Magnesium Hydroxide (Co-administration with antacids has no apparent effect on the extent of absorption, however, antacids can decrease the peak concentration reached by 15% to 20%). Products include:
Aludrox Oral Suspension 850
Ascriptin 650
Di-Gel Antacid/Anti-Gas 762
Gelusil Antacid-Anti-gas Liquid 819
Gelusil Antacid-Anti-gas Tablets 819
Maalox Antacid/Anti-Gas Tablets 889
Maalox Antacid Liquid 888
Extra Strength Maalox Antacid/Anti-Gas Liquid and Tablets 888
Mylanta Fast-Acting 1359
Mylanta Gelcaps Antacid 678
Fast-Acting Mylanta Liquid Antacid 1359
Mylanta Tablets 677
Maximum-Strength Fast-Acting Mylanta Liquid Antacid 1359
Mylanta Double Strength Tablets 677
Phillips' Milk of Magnesia Liquid 627
Rolaids Antacid Tablets 807
Tempo Soft Antacid 799

Magnesium Oxide (Co-administration with antacids has no apparent effect on the extent of absorption, however, antacids can decrease the peak concentration reached by 15% to 20%). Products include:
Beelith Tablets 632
Bufferin Analgesic Tablets 636
Arthritis Strength Bufferin Analgesic Caplets 637
Extra Strength Bufferin Analgesic Tablets 637
Caltrate PLUS 681
Cama Arthritis Pain Reliever 748
Mag-Ox 400 666
Uro-Mag 666

Methotrexate Sodium (Etodolac, like other NSAIDs, may cause changes in the elimination of methotrexate through its effects on renal prostaglandins, leading to elevated serum levels of methotrexate and increased toxicity). Products include:
Methotrexate Sodium Tablets, Injection, for Injection and LPF Injection 1322

Phenylbutazone (Co-administration causes an increase (by about 80%) in the free fraction of etodolac; concomitant use is not recommended).
No products indexed under this heading.

Warfarin Sodium (Co-administration results in reduced protein binding of warfarin with a few spontaneous reports of prolonged prothrombin times; caution should be exercised). Products include:
Coumadin 941

Food Interactions

Food, unspecified (Reduces the peak concentration reached by approximately one-half and increases the time-to-peak concentration by 1.4 to 3.8 hours).

LOMOTIL LIQUID

(Diphenoxylate Hydrochloride, Atropine Sulfate) 2591
May interact with monoamine oxidase inhibitors, barbiturates, tranquilizers, and certain other agents. Compounds in these categories include:

Alprazolam (Potentiation of tranquilizers). Products include:
Xanax Tablets 2115

Aprobarbital (Potentiation of barbiturates).
No products indexed under this heading.

Buspirone Hydrochloride (Potentiation of tranquilizers). Products include:
BuSpar Tablets 738

Butabarbital (Potentiation of barbiturates).
No products indexed under this heading.

Butalbital (Potentiation of barbiturates). Products include:
Axocet Capsules 2469
Esgic-plus Capsules 1012
Esgic-plus Tablets 1012
Fioricet Tablets 2386
Fioricet with Codeine Capsules 2387
Fiorinal Capsules 2388
Fiorinal with Codeine Capsules 2390
Fiorinal Tablets 2388
Phrenilin 790
Sedapap Tablets 50 mg/650 mg 1826

Chlordiazepoxide (Potentiation of tranquilizers). Products include:
Limbitrol 2333

Chlordiazepoxide Hydrochloride (Potentiation of tranquilizers). Products include:
Librax Capsules 2330
Librium Capsules 2331
Librium Injectable 2332

Chlorpromazine (Potentiation of tranquilizers). Products include:
Thorazine Suppositories 2701

Chlorprothixene (Potentiation of tranquilizers).
No products indexed under this heading.

Chlorprothixene Lactate (Potentiation of tranquilizers).
No products indexed under this heading.

Clorazepate Dipotassium (Potentiation of tranquilizers). Products include:
Tranxene 459

Diazepam (Potentiation of tranquilizers). Products include:
Dizac (diazepam injectable emulsion) CIV 1862
Valium Injectable 2336
Valium Tablets 2335

Droperidol (Potentiation of tranquilizers). Products include:
Inapsine Injection 462

Fluphenazine Decanoate (Potentiation of tranquilizers). Products include:
Prolixin Decanoate 510

Fluphenazine Enanthate (Potentiation of tranquilizers). Products include:
Prolixin Enanthate 510

Fluphenazine Hydrochloride (Potentiation of tranquilizers). Products include:
Prolixin 510

Furazolidone (Hypertensive crisis). Products include:
Furoxone 2221

Haloperidol (Potentiation of tranquilizers). Products include:
Haldol Injection, Tablets and Concentrate 1585

Haloperidol Decanoate (Potentiation of tranquilizers). Products include:
Haldol Decanoate 1587

Hydroxyzine Hydrochloride (Potentiation of tranquilizers). Products include:
Atarax Tablets & Syrup 1992
Marax Tablets & DF Syrup 2015
Vistaril Intramuscular Solution 2042

Isocarboxazid (Hypertensive crisis).
No products indexed under this heading.

Lorazepam (Potentiation of tranquilizers). Products include:
Ativan Injection 2805
Ativan Tablets 2807

Loxapine Hydrochloride (Potentiation of tranquilizers). Products include:
Loxitane 1426

Mephobarbital (Potentiation of barbiturates). Products include:
Mebaral Tablets 2452

Meprobamate (Potentiation of tranquilizers). Products include:
Miltown Tablets 2780
PMB 200 and PMB 400 2890

Mesoridazine Besylate (Potentiation of tranquilizers). Products include:
Serentil 689

Molindone Hydrochloride (Potentiation of tranquilizers). Products include:
Moban Tablets and Concentrate 1036

Oxazepam (Potentiation of tranquilizers). Products include:
Serax Capsules 2916
Serax Tablets 2916

Pentobarbital Sodium (Potentiation of barbiturates). Products include:
Nembutal Sodium Capsules 440
Nembutal Sodium Solution 442
Nembutal Sodium Suppositories 444

Perphenazine (Potentiation of tranquilizers). Products include:
Etrafon 2495
Triavil Tablets 1800
Trilafon 2532

Phenelzine Sulfate (Hypertensive crisis). Products include:
Nardil 1977

Phenobarbital (Potentiation of barbiturates). Products include:
Arco-Lase Plus Tablets 513
Bellergal-S Tablets 2375
Donnatal 2234
Donnatal Extentabs 2234
Donnatal Tablets 2234
Phenobarbital Elixir and Tablets 1523
Quadrinal Tablets 1398

Prazepam (Potentiation of tranquilizers).
No products indexed under this heading.

Prochlorperazine (Potentiation of tranquilizers). Products include:
Compazine 2644

Promethazine Hydrochloride (Potentiation of tranquilizers). Products include:
Mepergan Injection 2859
Phenergan with Codeine 2883
Phenergan with Dextromethorphan 2885
Phenergan Injection 2880
Phenergan Suppositories 2882
Phenergan Syrup 2881
Phenergan Tablets 2882
Phenergan VC 2886
Phenergan VC with Codeine 2888

Secobarbital Sodium (Potentiation of barbiturates). Products include:
Seconal Sodium Pulvules 1529

Selegiline Hydrochloride (Hypertensive crisis). Products include:
Eldepryl Capsules 2729

Thiamylal Sodium (Potentiation of barbiturates).
No products indexed under this heading.

Thioridazine Hydrochloride (Potentiation of tranquilizers). Products include:
Mellaril 2398

IMPORTANT NOTE: Always consult each drug listing in the patient's regimen for possible interactions.

Lomotil — Interactions Index

Thiothixene (Potentiation of tranquilizers). Products include:
- Navane Capsules and Concentrate ... 2018
- Navane Intramuscular ... 2019

Tranylcypromine Sulfate (Hypertensive crisis). Products include:
- Parnate Tablets ... 2679

Trifluoperazine Hydrochloride (Potentiation of tranquilizers). Products include:
- Stelazine ... 2692

Food Interactions
Alcohol (Potentiation of alcohol).

LOMOTIL TABLETS
(Diphenoxylate Hydrochloride, Atropine Sulfate) ... 2591
See **Lomotil Liquid**

LO/OVRAL TABLETS
(Norgestrel, Ethinyl Estradiol) ... 2852
May interact with barbiturates and certain other agents. Compounds in these categories include:

Ampicillin Sodium (Reduced efficacy; increased incidence of breakthrough bleeding). Products include:
- Unasyn ... 2035

Aprobarbital (Reduced efficacy; increased incidence of breakthrough bleeding).
- No products indexed under this heading.

Butabarbital (Reduced efficacy; increased incidence of breakthrough bleeding).
- No products indexed under this heading.

Butalbital (Reduced efficacy; increased incidence of breakthrough bleeding). Products include:
- Axocet Capsules ... 2469
- Esgic-plus Capsules ... 1012
- Esgic-plus Tablets ... 1012
- Fioricet Tablets ... 2386
- Fioricet with Codeine Capsules ... 2387
- Fiorinal Capsules ... 2388
- Fiorinal with Codeine Capsules ... 2390
- Fiorinal Tablets ... 2388
- Phrenilin ... 790
- Sedapap Tablets 50 mg/650 mg .. 1826

Mephobarbital (Reduced efficacy; increased incidence of breakthrough bleeding). Products include:
- Mebaral Tablets ... 2452

Oxytetracycline (Reduced efficacy; increased incidence of breakthrough bleeding). Products include:
- Terramycin Intramuscular Solution 2034

Oxytetracycline Hydrochloride (Reduced efficacy; increased incidence of breakthrough bleeding). Products include:
- TERAK Ointment ... ⊙ 210
- Terra-Cortril Ophthalmic Suspension ... 2033
- Terramycin with Polymyxin B Sulfate Ophthalmic Ointment ... 2035
- Urobiotic-250 Capsules ... 2038

Pentobarbital Sodium (Reduced efficacy; increased incidence of breakthrough bleeding). Products include:
- Nembutal Sodium Capsules ... 440
- Nembutal Sodium Solution ... 442
- Nembutal Sodium Suppositories ... 444

Phenobarbital (Reduced efficacy; increased incidence of breakthrough bleeding). Products include:
- Arco-Lase Plus Tablets ... 513
- Bellergal-S Tablets ... 2375
- Donnatal ... 2234
- Donnatal Extentabs ... 2234
- Donnatal Tablets ... 2234
- Phenobarbital Elixir and Tablets ... 1523
- Quadrinal Tablets ... 1398

Phenylbutazone (Reduced efficacy; increased incidence of breakthrough bleeding).
- No products indexed under this heading.

Phenytoin Sodium (Reduced efficacy; increased incidence of breakthrough bleeding). Products include:
- Dilantin Kapseals ... 1965

Rifampin (Reduced efficacy; increased incidence of breakthrough bleeding). Products include:
- Rifadin ... 1276
- Rifamate Capsules ... 1278
- Rifater ... 1280
- Rimactane Capsules ... 865

Secobarbital Sodium (Reduced efficacy; increased incidence of breakthrough bleeding). Products include:
- Seconal Sodium Pulvules ... 1529

Tetracycline Hydrochloride (Reduced efficacy; increased incidence of breakthrough bleeding). Products include:
- Achromycin V Capsules ... 1417
- Helidac Therapy ... 2135

Thiamylal Sodium (Reduced efficacy; increased incidence of breakthrough bleeding).
- No products indexed under this heading.

LO/OVRAL-28 TABLETS
(Norgestrel, Ethinyl Estradiol) ... 2857
See **Lo/Ovral Tablets**

LOPID TABLETS
(Gemfibrozil) ... 1974
May interact with anticoagulants, hmg-coa reductase inhibitors, and certain other agents. Compounds in these categories include:

Dalteparin Sodium (May affect prothrombin time resulting in bleeding complication). Products include:
- Fragmin Injection ... 2088

Dicumarol (May affect prothrombin time resulting in bleeding complication).
- No products indexed under this heading.

Enoxaparin (May affect prothrombin time resulting in bleeding complication). Products include:
- Lovenox Injection ... 2187

Fluvastatin Sodium (Potential for severe myopathy, rhabdomyolysis, and acute renal failure). Products include:
- Lescol Capsules ... 2395

Heparin Calcium (May affect prothrombin time resulting in bleeding complication).
- No products indexed under this heading.

Heparin Sodium (May affect prothrombin time resulting in bleeding complication). Products include:
- Heparin Lock Flush Solution ... 2831
- Heparin Sodium Injection ... 2832
- Heparin Sodium Vials ... 1486

Lovastatin (Potential for severe myopathy, rhabdomyolysis, and acute renal failure). Products include:
- Mevacor Tablets ... 1742

Pravastatin Sodium (Potential for severe myopathy, rhabdomyolysis, and acute renal failure). Products include:
- Pravachol Tablets ... 770

Simvastatin (Potential for severe myopathy, rhabdomyolysis, and acute renal failure). Products include:
- Zocor Tablets ... 1821

Warfarin Sodium (May affect prothrombin time resulting in bleeding complication). Products include:
- Coumadin ... 941

LOPRESSOR INJECTION
(Metoprolol Tartrate) ... 848
May interact with catecholamine depleting drugs and certain other agents. Compounds in these categories include:

Deserpidine (Potential for additive effect).
- No products indexed under this heading.

Epinephrine Hydrochloride (Potential for unresponsiveness to epinephrine to treat allergic reactions in certain patients). Products include:
- Ana-Kit Anaphylaxis Emergency Treatment Kit ... 611

Guanethidine Monosulfate (Potential for additive effect). Products include:
- Esimil Tablets ... 840
- Ismelin Tablets ... 845

Rauwolfia Serpentina (Potential for additive effect).
- No products indexed under this heading.

Rescinnamine (Potential for additive effect).
- No products indexed under this heading.

Reserpine (Potential for additive effect). Products include:
- Diupres Tablets ... 1691
- Hydropres Tablets ... 1718
- Ser-Ap-Es Tablets ... 867

LOPRESSOR TABLETS
(Metoprolol Tartrate) ... 848
See **Lopressor Injection**

LOPRESSOR HCT TABLETS
(Metoprolol Tartrate, Hydrochlorothiazide) ... 850
May interact with catecholamine depleting drugs, cardiac glycosides, corticosteroids, peripheral adrenergic blockers, ganglionic blocking agents, antihypertensives, non-steroidal anti-inflammatory agents, barbiturates, narcotic analgesics, and certain other agents. Compounds in these categories include:

Acebutolol Hydrochloride (Potentiation of antihypertensive action). Products include:
- Sectral Capsules ... 2914

ACTH (Hypokalemia may develop during concomitant use).
- No products indexed under this heading.

Alfentanil Hydrochloride (Orthostatic hypotension may be potentiated). Products include:
- Alfenta Injection ... 1334

Amlodipine Besylate (Potentiation of antihypertensive action). Products include:
- Lotrel Capsules ... 858
- Norvasc Tablets ... 2020

Aprobarbital (Orthostatic hypotension may be potentiated).
- No products indexed under this heading.

Atenolol (Potentiation of antihypertensive action). Products include:
- Tenoretic Tablets ... 2963
- Tenormin Tablets and I.V. Injection 2965

Benazepril Hydrochloride (Potentiation of antihypertensive action). Products include:
- Lotensin Tablets ... 852
- Lotensin HCT Tablets ... 855
- Lotrel Capsules ... 858

Bendroflumethiazide (Potentiation of antihypertensive action).
- No products indexed under this heading.

Betamethasone Acetate (Hypokalemia may develop during concomitant use). Products include:
- Celestone Soluspan Suspension ... 2484

Betamethasone Sodium Phosphate (Hypokalemia may develop during concomitant use). Products include:
- Celestone Soluspan Suspension ... 2484

Betaxolol Hydrochloride (Potentiation of antihypertensive action). Products include:
- Betoptic Ophthalmic Solution ... 465
- Betoptic S Ophthalmic Suspension ... 467
- Kerlone Tablets ... 2588

Bisoprolol Fumarate (Potentiation of antihypertensive action). Products include:
- Zebeta Tablets ... 1457
- Ziac ... 1459

Buprenorphine (Orthostatic hypotension may be potentiated). Products include:
- Buprenex Injectable ... 2170

Butabarbital (Orthostatic hypotension may be potentiated).
- No products indexed under this heading.

Butalbital (Orthostatic hypotension may be potentiated). Products include:
- Axocet Capsules ... 2469
- Esgic-plus Capsules ... 1012
- Esgic-plus Tablets ... 1012
- Fioricet Tablets ... 2386
- Fioricet with Codeine Capsules ... 2387
- Fiorinal Capsules ... 2388
- Fiorinal with Codeine Capsules ... 2390
- Fiorinal Tablets ... 2388
- Phrenilin ... 790
- Sedapap Tablets 50 mg/650 mg .. 1826

Captopril (Potentiation of antihypertensive action). Products include:
- Capoten Tablets ... 740
- Capozide Tablets ... 744

Carteolol Hydrochloride (Potentiation of antihypertensive action). Products include:
- Cartrol Tablets ... 413
- Ocupress Ophthalmic Solution, 1% Sterile ... ⊙ 297

Chlorothiazide (Potentiation of antihypertensive action). Products include:
- Aldoclor Tablets ... 1638
- Diupres Tablets ... 1691
- Diuril Oral ... 1694

Chlorothiazide Sodium (Potentiation of antihypertensive action). Products include:
- Diuril Sodium Intravenous ... 1693

Chlorthalidone (Potentiation of antihypertensive action). Products include:
- Combipres Tablets ... 682
- Tenoretic Tablets ... 2963
- Thalitone ... 1293

Cholestyramine (Impairs the oral absorption of hydrochlorothiazide from gastrointestinal tract by up to 85%). Products include:
- Questran ... 774

Clonidine (Potentiation of antihypertensive action). Products include:
- Catapres-TTS ... 680

Clonidine Hydrochloride (Potentiation of antihypertensive action). Products include:
- Catapres Tablets ... 679
- Combipres Tablets ... 682

Codeine Phosphate (Orthostatic hypotension may be potentiated). Products include:
- Brontex ... 2130
- Dimetane-DC Cough Syrup ... 2232
- Fioricet with Codeine Capsules ... 2387

Fiorinal with Codeine Capsules 2390
Nucofed 2225
Phenergan with Codeine 2883
Phenergan VC with Codeine 2888
Robitussin A-C Syrup 2248
Robitussin-DAC Syrup 2249
Ryna 804
Soma Compound w/Codeine Tablets 2784
Tylenol with Codeine 1592

Colestipol Hydrochloride (Impairs the oral absorption of hydrochlorothiazide from gastrointestinal tract by up to 43%). Products include:
Colestid 2073

Cortisone Acetate (Hypokalemia may develop during concomitant use). Products include:
Cortone Acetate Sterile Suspension 1663
Cortone Acetate Tablets 1664

Deserpidine (Potentiation of antihypertensive action; potential for additive effects).
No products indexed under this heading.

Deslanoside (Potential for toxic effects of deslanoside on heart).
No products indexed under this heading.

Dexamethasone (Hypokalemia may develop during concomitant use). Products include:
AK-Trol Ointment & Suspension .... ◉ 205
Decadron Elixir 1676
Decadron Tablets 1678
Decaspray Topical Aerosol 1689
Maxitrol Ophthalmic Ointment and Suspension .... ◉ 222
TobraDex Ophthalmic Suspension and Ointment 469

Dexamethasone Acetate (Hypokalemia may develop during concomitant use). Products include:
Dalalone D.P. Injectable 1009
Decadron-LA Sterile Suspension 1687

Dexamethasone Sodium Phosphate (Hypokalemia may develop during concomitant use). Products include:
Decadron Phosphate Injection 1680
Decadron Phosphate Sterile Ophthalmic Ointment 1684
Decadron Phosphate Sterile Ophthalmic Solution 1685
Decadron Phosphate Topical Cream 1686
Decadron Phosphate with Xylocaine Injection, Sterile 1683
Dexacort Phosphate in Respihaler 1606
Dexacort Phosphate in Turbinaire 1607
NeoDecadron Sterile Ophthalmic Ointment 1755
NeoDecadron Sterile Ophthalmic Solution 1756
NeoDecadron Topical Cream 1757

Dezocine (Orthostatic hypotension may be potentiated). Products include:
Dalgan Injection 529

Diazoxide (Potentiation of antihypertensive action). Products include:
Hyperstat I.V. Injection 2504
Proglycem 575

Diclofenac Potassium (Reduces diuretic, natriuretic and antihypertensive effects of thiazides). Products include:
Cataflam Tablets 833

Diclofenac Sodium (Reduces diuretic, natriuretic and antihypertensive effects of thiazides). Products include:
Voltaren Ophthalmic Sterile Ophthalmic Solution .... ◉ 264
Cataflam/Voltaren/Voltaren-XR 833

Digitoxin (Potential for toxic effects of digitalis on heart). Products include:
Crystodigin Tablets 1472

Digoxin (Potential for toxic effects of digitalis on heart). Products include:
Lanoxicaps 1110
Lanoxin Elixir Pediatric 1113
Lanoxin Injection 1116
Lanoxin Injection Pediatric 1119
Lanoxin Tablets 1121

Diltiazem Hydrochloride (Potentiation of antihypertensive action). Products include:
Cardizem CD Capsules 1251
Cardizem SR Capsules 1255
Cardizem Injectable 1253
Cardizem Tablets 1257
Dilacor XR Extended-release Capsules 2183
Tiazac Capsules 1019

Doxazosin Mesylate (Potentiation of antihypertensive action). Products include:
Cardura Tablets 1993

Enalapril Maleate (Potentiation of antihypertensive action). Products include:
Vaseretic Tablets 1810
Vasotec Tablets 1816

Enalaprilat (Potentiation of antihypertensive effects). Products include:
Vasotec I.V. 1814

Epinephrine Hydrochloride (Potential for unresponsiveness to epinephrine to treat allergic reactions in certain patients). Products include:
Ana-Kit Anaphylaxis Emergency Treatment Kit 611

Esmolol Hydrochloride (Potentiation of antihypertensive action). Products include:
Brevibloc (esmolol HCl) Injection 1860

Etodolac (Reduces diuretic, natriuretic and antihypertensive effects of thiazides). Products include:
Lodine Capsules and Tablets 2849

Felodipine (Potentiation of antihypertensive action). Products include:
Plendil Extended-Release Tablets 514

Fenoprofen Calcium (Reduces diuretic, natriuretic and antihypertensive effects of thiazides). Products include:
Nalfon 200 Pulvules & Nalfon Tablets 933

Fentanyl (Orthostatic hypotension may be potentiated). Products include:
Duragesic Transdermal System 1336

Fentanyl Citrate (Orthostatic hypotension may be potentiated). Products include:
Sublimaze Injection 463

Fludrocortisone Acetate (Hypokalemia may develop during concomitant use). Products include:
Florinef Acetate Tablets 506

Flurbiprofen (Reduces diuretic, natriuretic and antihypertensive effects of thiazides).
No products indexed under this heading.

Fosinopril Sodium (Potentiation of antihypertensive action). Products include:
Monopril Tablets 762

Furosemide (Potentiation of antihypertensive action). Products include:
Lasix Injection, Oral Solution and Tablets 1267

Guanabenz Acetate (Potentiation of antihypertensive action).
No products indexed under this heading.

Guanethidine Monosulfate (Potentiation of antihypertensive action). Products include:
Esimil Tablets 840
Ismelin Tablets 845

Hydralazine Hydrochloride (Potentiation of antihypertensive action). Products include:
Apresazide Capsules 824
Apresoline Hydrochloride Tablets 826
Hydralazine Hydrochloride Injection USP 2712
Ser-Ap-Es Tablets 867

Hydrocodone Bitartrate (Orthostatic hypotension may be potentiated). Products include:
Codiclear DH Syrup 808
Duratuss HD Elixir 2750
Histussin D Liquid 670
Hycodan Tablets and Syrup 946
Hycomine Compound Tablets 948
Hycomine 947
Hycotuss Expectorant Syrup 950
Hydrocet Capsules 787
Lorcet 10/650 Tablets 1016
Lortab 2751
Tussend 1830
Tussend Expectorant 1831
Vicodin Tablets 1404
Vicodin ES Tablets 1405
Vicodin HP Tablets 1403
Vicodin Tuss Expectorant 1406
Zydone Capsules 967

Hydrocodone Polistirex (Orthostatic hypotension may be potentiated). Products include:
Tussionex Pennkinetic Extended-Release Suspension 1624

Hydrocortisone (Hypokalemia may develop during concomitant use). Products include:
Anusol-HC Cream 2.5% 1953
Aquanil HC Lotion 1989
Maximum Strength Cortaid Spray 800
CORTENEMA 2713
Cortisporin Ointment 1074
Cortisporin Ophthalmic Ointment Sterile 1074
Cortisporin Ophthalmic Suspension Sterile 1075
Cortisporin Otic Solution Sterile 1076
Cortisporin Otic Suspension Sterile 1077
Cortizone-5 795
Cortizone-10 795
Hydrocortone Tablets 1715
Hytone 922
Hytone Ointment 2 ½% 923
Massengill Medicated Soft Cloth Towelettes 2628
Pediotic Suspension Sterile 1140
Preparation H Hydrocortisone 1% Cream 843
ProctoCream-HC 2.5% 2552
VōSoL HC Otic Solution 2786

Hydrocortisone Acetate (Hypokalemia may develop during concomitant use). Products include:
Analpram-HC Rectal Cream 1% and 2.5% 993
Anusol HC-1 Hydrocortisone Anti-Itch Ointment 810
Anusol-HC Suppositories 1954
Caldecort Anti-Itch Hydrocortisone Cream 651
Coly-Mycin S Otic w/Neomycin & Hydrocortisone 1965
Cortaid 800
Cortifoam 2540
Cortisporin Cream 1073
Epifoam 2543
Hydrocortone Acetate Sterile Suspension 1712
Mantadil Cream 1124
Nupercainal Hydrocortisone 1% Cream 661
Pramosone Cream, Lotion & Ointment 995
ProctoFoam-HC 2552
Terra-Cortril Ophthalmic Suspension 2033

Hydrocortisone Sodium Phosphate (Hypokalemia may develop during concomitant use). Products include:
Hydrocortone Phosphate Injection, Sterile 1713

Hydrocortisone Sodium Succinate (Hypokalemia may develop during concomitant use).
No products indexed under this heading.

Hydroflumethiazide (Potentiation of antihypertensive action). Products include:
Diucardin Tablets 2824

Hydromorphone Hydrochloride (Orthostatic hypotension may be potentiated). Products include:
Dilaudid Ampules 1382
Dilaudid Cough Syrup 1383
Dilaudid-HP Injection 1384
Dilaudid-HP Lyophilized Powder 250 mg 1384
Dilaudid 1382
Dilaudid Oral Liquid 1386
Dilaudid 1382
Dilaudid Tablets - 8 mg 1386

Ibuprofen (Reduces diuretic, natriuretic and antihypertensive effects of thiazides). Products include:
Advil Cold and Sinus Caplets and Tablets 837
Advil Ibuprofen Tablets, Caplets and Gel Caplets 836
Children's Motrin Ibuprofen Oral Suspension 1558
IBU Tablets 1389
Ibuprohm 713
Motrin IB Caplets, Tablets, and Gelcaps 802
Motrin Ibuprofen Suspension, Oral Drops, Chewable Tablets, Caplets 1563
Nuprin Ibuprofen/Analgesic Tablets & Caplets 645
Vicks DayQuil SINUS Pressure & PAIN Relief with IBUPROFEN 735

Indapamide (Potentiation of antihypertensive action).
No products indexed under this heading.

Indomethacin (Reduces diuretic, natriuretic and antihypertensive effects of thiazides). Products include:
Indocin 1723

Indomethacin Sodium Trihydrate (Reduces diuretic, natriuretic and antihypertensive effects of thiazides). Products include:
Indocin I.V. 1727

Isradipine (Potentiation of antihypertensive action). Products include:
DynaCirc Capsules 2381
DynaCirc CR Tablets 2383

Ketoprofen (Reduces diuretic, natriuretic and antihypertensive effects of thiazides). Products include:
Actron Caplets and Tablets 608
Orudis Capsules 2874
Orudis KT 842
Oruvail Capsules 2874

Ketorolac Tromethamine (Reduces diuretic, natriuretic and antihypertensive effects of thiazides). Products include:
Acular Sterile Ophthalmic Solution 470
Toradol 2319

Labetalol Hydrochloride (Potentiation of antihypertensive action). Products include:
Normodyne Injection 2519
Normodyne Tablets 2522
Trandate 1158

Levorphanol Tartrate (Orthostatic hypotension may be potentiated). Products include:
Levo-Dromoran 2297

Lisinopril (Potentiation of antihypertensive effects). Products include:
Prinivil Tablets 1776
Prinzide Tablets 1780
Zestoretic Tablets 2968
Zestril Tablets 2972

IMPORTANT NOTE: Always consult each drug listing in the patient's regimen for possible interactions.

Lopressor HCT — Interactions Index — 620

Lithium Carbonate (Lithium renal clearance is reduced, increasing risk of lithium toxicity). Products include:
- Eskalith 2658
- Lithium Carbonate Capsules & Tablets 2352
- Lithonate/Lithotabs/Lithobid 2721

Lithium Citrate (Lithium renal clearance is reduced, increasing risk of lithium toxicity).
- No products indexed under this heading.

Losartan Potassium (Potentiation of antihypertensive action). Products include:
- Cozaar Tablets 1668
- Hyzaar Tablets 1720

Mecamylamine Hydrochloride (Potentiation of antihypertensive action). Products include:
- Inversine Tablets 1729

Meclofenamate Sodium (Reduces diuretic, natriuretic and antihypertensive effects of thiazides).
- No products indexed under this heading.

Mefenamic Acid (Reduces diuretic, natriuretic and antihypertensive effects of thiazides). Products include:
- Ponstel 1982

Meperidine Hydrochloride (Orthostatic hypotension may be potentiated). Products include:
- Demerol 2438
- Mepergan Injection 2859

Mephobarbital (Orthostatic hypotension may be potentiated). Products include:
- Mebaral Tablets 2452

Methadone Hydrochloride (Orthostatic hypotension may be potentiated). Products include:
- Methadone Hydrochloride Oral Concentrate 2356
- Methadone Hydrochloride Oral Solution & Tablets 2357

Methyclothiazide (Potentiation of antihypertensive action). Products include:
- Enduron Tablets 424

Methyldopa (Potentiation of antihypertensive action; hemolytic anemia). Products include:
- Aldoclor Tablets 1638
- Aldomet Oral 1640
- Aldoril Tablets 1644

Methyldopate Hydrochloride (Potentiation of antihypertensive action; hemolytic anemia). Products include:
- Aldomet Ester HCl Injection 1642

Methylprednisolone Acetate (Hypokalemia may develop during concomitant use).
- No products indexed under this heading.

Methylprednisolone Sodium Succinate (Hypokalemia may develop during concomitant use).
- No products indexed under this heading.

Metolazone (Potentiation of antihypertensive action). Products include:
- Mykrox Tablets 1617
- Zaroxolyn Tablets 1625

Metoprolol Succinate (Potentiation of antihypertensive action). Products include:
- Toprol-XL Tablets 560

Metyrosine (Potentiation of antihypertensive action). Products include:
- Demser Capsules 1690

Minoxidil (Potentiation of antihypertensive action).
- No products indexed under this heading.

Moexipril Hydrochloride (Potentiation of antihypertensive action). Products include:
- Univasc Tablets 2553

Morphine Sulfate (Orthostatic hypotension may be potentiated). Products include:
- Astramorph/PF Injection, USP (Preservative-Free) 526
- Duramorph Injection 983
- Infumorph 200 and Infumorph 500 Sterile Solutions 985
- Kadian Capsules 2948
- MS Contin Tablets 2149
- MSIR 2152
- Oramorph SR (Morphine Sulfate Sustained Release Tablets) 2359
- RMS Suppositories CII 2766
- Roxanol 2365

Nabumetone (Reduces diuretic, natriuretic and antihypertensive effects of thiazides). Products include:
- Relafen Tablets 2688

Nadolol (Potentiation of antihypertensive action).
- No products indexed under this heading.

Naproxen (Reduces diuretic, natriuretic and antihypertensive effects of thiazides). Products include:
- Anaprox/Naprosyn 2277

Naproxen Sodium (Reduces diuretic, natriuretic and antihypertensive effects of thiazides). Products include:
- Aleve 2124
- Anaprox/Naprosyn 2277
- Naprelan Tablets 2861

Nicardipine Hydrochloride (Potentiation of antihypertensive action). Products include:
- Cardene Capsules 2261
- Cardene I.V. 2815
- Cardene SR Capsules 2264

Nifedipine (Potentiation of antihypertensive action). Products include:
- Adalat Capsules (10 mg and 20 mg) 580
- Adalat CC 582
- Procardia Capsules 2024
- Procardia XL Extended Release Tablets 2026

Nisoldipine (Potentiation of antihypertensive action). Products include:
- Sular Tablets 2961

Nitroglycerin (Potentiation of antihypertensive action). Products include:
- Deponit NTG Transdermal Delivery System 2541
- Nitro-Bid IV 1270
- Nitro-Bid Ointment 1272
- Nitro-Dur (nitroglycerin) Transdermal Infusion System 1365
- Nitrolingual Spray 2193
- Nitrostat Tablets 1981
- Transderm-Nitro Transdermal Therapeutic System 878

Norepinephrine Bitartrate (Arterial responsiveness may be decreased, but not enough to preclude effectiveness of pressor agent). Products include:
- Levophed Bitartrate Injection ... 2445

Opium Alkaloids (Orthostatic hypotension may be potentiated).
- No products indexed under this heading.

Oxaprozin (Reduces diuretic, natriuretic and antihypertensive effects of thiazides). Products include:
- Daypro Caplets 2578

Oxycodone Hydrochloride (Orthostatic hypotension may be potentiated). Products include:
- OxyContin Tablets 2163
- OxyIR Capsules 2167
- Percocet Tablets 955
- Percodan Tablets 955
- Percodan-Demi Tablets 956
- Roxicodone Tablets, Oral Solution & Intensol (Oxycodone) 2366
- Tylox Capsules 1593

Penbutolol Sulfate (Potentiation of antihypertensive action). Products include:
- Levatol Tablets 2547

Pentobarbital Sodium (Orthostatic hypotension may be potentiated). Products include:
- Nembutal Sodium Capsules 440
- Nembutal Sodium Solution 442
- Nembutal Sodium Suppositories .. 444

Phenobarbital (Orthostatic hypotension may be potentiated). Products include:
- Arco-Lase Plus Tablets 513
- Bellergal-S Tablets 2375
- Donnatal 2234
- Donnatal Extentabs 2234
- Donnatal Tablets 2234
- Phenobarbital Elixir and Tablets .. 1523
- Quadrinal Tablets 1398

Phenoxybenzamine Hydrochloride (Potentiation of antihypertensive action). Products include:
- Dibenzyline Capsules 2650

Phentolamine Mesylate (Potentiation of antihypertensive action). Products include:
- Regitine Vials 864

Phenylbutazone (Reduces diuretic, natriuretic and antihypertensive effects of thiazides).
- No products indexed under this heading.

Pindolol (Potentiation of antihypertensive action). Products include:
- Visken Tablets 2428

Piroxicam (Reduces diuretic, natriuretic and antihypertensive effects of thiazides). Products include:
- Feldene Capsules 2008

Polythiazide (Potentiation of antihypertensive action). Products include:
- Minizide Capsules 2016

Prazosin Hydrochloride (Potentiation of antihypertensive action). Products include:
- Minipress Capsules 2015
- Minizide Capsules 2016

Prednisolone Acetate (Hypokalemia may develop during concomitant use). Products include:
- AK-CIDE .... ⊚ 203
- AK-CIDE Ointment .... ⊚ 203
- Blephamide Liquifilm Sterile Ophthalmic Suspension 472
- Blephamide Ointment .... ⊚ 234
- Econopred & Econopred Plus Ophthalmic Suspensions ..... ⊚ 216
- Poly-Pred Liquifilm .... ⊚ 246
- Pred Forte .... ⊚ 247
- Pred Mild .... ⊚ 250
- Pred-G Liquifilm Sterile Ophthalmic Suspension .... ⊚ 248
- Pred-G S.O.P. Sterile Ophthalmic Ointment .... ⊚ 249

Prednisolone Sodium Phosphate (Hypokalemia may develop during concomitant use). Products include:
- AK-PRED .... ⊚ 204
- Hydeltrasol Injection, Sterile 1708
- Pediapred Oral Solution 1618

Prednisolone Tebutate (Hypokalemia may develop during concomitant use). Products include:
- Hydeltra-T.B.A. Sterile Suspension 1710

Prednisone (Hypokalemia may develop during concomitant use).
- No products indexed under this heading.

Propoxyphene Hydrochloride (Orthostatic hypotension may be potentiated). Products include:
- Darvon 1475
- Wygesic Tablets 2930

Propoxyphene Napsylate (Orthostatic hypotension may be potentiated). Products include:
- Darvon-N/Darvocet-N 1473

Propranolol Hydrochloride (Potentiation of antihypertensive action). Products include:
- Inderal 2834
- Inderal LA Long Acting Capsules 2836
- Inderide Tablets 2838
- Inderide LA Long Acting Capsules .. 2840

Quinapril Hydrochloride (Potentiation of antihypertensive action). Products include:
- Accupril Tablets 1950

Ramipril (Potentiation of antihypertensive action). Products include:
- Altace Capsules 1238

Rauwolfia Serpentina (Potentiation of antihypertensive action; potential for additive effects).
- No products indexed under this heading.

Rescinnamine (Potentiation of antihypertensive action; potential for additive effects).
- No products indexed under this heading.

Reserpine (Potentiation of antihypertensive action; potential for additive effects). Products include:
- Diupres Tablets 1691
- Hydropres Tablets 1718
- Ser-Ap-Es Tablets 867

Secobarbital Sodium (Orthostatic hypotension may be potentiated). Products include:
- Seconal Sodium Pulvules 1529

Sodium Nitroprusside (Potentiation of antihypertensive action).
- No products indexed under this heading.

Sotalol Hydrochloride (Potentiation of antihypertensive action). Products include:
- Betapace Tablets 637

Spirapril Hydrochloride (Potentiation of antihypertensive action).
- No products indexed under this heading.

Sufentanil Citrate (Orthostatic hypotension may be potentiated). Products include:
- Sufenta Injection 1355

Sulindac (Reduces diuretic, natriuretic and antihypertensive effects of thiazides). Products include:
- Clinoril Tablets 1658

Terazosin Hydrochloride (Potentiation of antihypertensive action). Products include:
- Hytrin Capsules 434

Thiamylal Sodium (Orthostatic hypotension may be potentiated).
- No products indexed under this heading.

Timolol Maleate (Potentiation of antihypertensive action). Products include:
- Blocadren Tablets 1654
- Timolide Tablets 1791
- Timoptic in Ocudose 1796
- Timoptic Sterile Ophthalmic Solution 1794
- Timoptic-XE 1798

Tolmetin Sodium (Reduces diuretic, natriuretic and antihypertensive effects of thiazides). Products include:
- Tolectin (200, 400 and 600 mg) .. 1591

Torsemide (Potentiation of antihypertensive action). Products include:
- Demadex Tablets and Injection .. 691

Triamcinolone (Hypokalemia may develop during concomitant use).
- No products indexed under this heading.

(▣ Described in PDR For Nonprescription Drugs) (⊚ Described in PDR For Ophthalmology)

Triamcinolone Acetonide (Hypokalemia may develop during concomitant use). Products include:
   Azmacort Oral Inhaler 2175
   Nasacort AQ Nasal Spray........... 2191
   Nasacort Nasal Inhaler 2189

Triamcinolone Diacetate (Hypokalemia may develop during concomitant use).
   No products indexed under this heading.

Triamcinolone Hexacetonide (Hypokalemia may develop during concomitant use).
   No products indexed under this heading.

Trimethaphan Camsylate (Potentiation of antihypertensive action).
   No products indexed under this heading.

Tubocurarine Chloride (Increase responsiveness to tubocurarine).
   No products indexed under this heading.

Verapamil Hydrochloride (Potentiation of antihypertensive action). Products include:
   Calan SR Caplets 2571
   Calan Tablets 2568
   Covera-HS Tablets 2573
   Isoptin Injectable 1391
   Isoptin Oral Tablets 1393
   Isoptin SR Tablets 1395
   Verelan Capsules 1455

Food Interactions
Alcohol (Orthostatic hypotension may be potentiated).

LOPROX 1% CREAM AND LOTION
(Ciclopirox Olamine) 1269
None cited in PDR database.

LORABID SUSPENSION AND PULVULES
(Loracarbef) 1513
May interact with:

Probenecid (Inhibits renal excretion resulting in an approximately 80% increase in the AUC for loracarbef). Products include:
   Benemid Tablets 1651
   ColBENEMID Tablets 1662

Food Interactions
Food, unspecified (Delays the peak plasma concentration with no change in the total absorption).

LORCET 10/650 TABLETS
(Hydrocodone Bitartrate, Acetaminophen).............................1016
May interact with narcotic analgesics, tricyclic antidepressants, monoamine oxidase inhibitors, tranquilizers, central nervous system depressants, anticholinergics, and certain other agents. Compounds in these categories include:

Alfentanil Hydrochloride (Potential for additive CNS depression). Products include:
   Alfenta Injection 1334

Alprazolam (Potential for additive CNS depression). Products include:
   Xanax Tablets 2115

Amitriptyline Hydrochloride (Increased effect of either the antidepressant or hydrocodone). Products include:
   Elavil 2945
   Etrafon 2495
   Limbitrol 2333
   Triavil Tablets 1800

Amoxapine (Increased effect of either the antidepressant or hydrocodone). Products include:
   Asendin Tablets 1419

Aprobarbital (Potential for additive CNS depression).
   No products indexed under this heading.

Atropine Sulfate (Concurrent use may produce paralytic ileus). Products include:
   Arco-Lase Plus Tablets 513
   Atrohist Plus Tablets 1605
   Donnatal 2234
   Donnatal Extentabs 2234
   Donnatal Tablets 2234
   Lomotil 2591
   Motofen Tablets 789
   Urised Tablets 2123

Belladonna Alkaloids (Concurrent use may produce paralytic ileus). Products include:
   Bellergal-S Tablets 2375
   Hyland's Bedwetting Tablets ... 788
   Hyland's EnurAid Tablets 789
   Hyland's Headache Tablets 790
   Hyland's Teething Tablets 790
   Similasan Eye Drops #1 769

Benztropine Mesylate (Concurrent use may produce paralytic ileus). Products include:
   Cogentin 1661

Biperiden Hydrochloride (Concurrent use may produce paralytic ileus). Products include:
   Akineton 1380

Buprenorphine (Potential for additive CNS depression). Products include:
   Buprenex Injectable 2170

Buspirone Hydrochloride (Potential for additive CNS depression). Products include:
   BuSpar Tablets 738

Butabarbital (Potential for additive CNS depression).
   No products indexed under this heading.

Butalbital (Potential for additive CNS depression). Products include:
   Axocet Capsules 2469
   Esgic-plus Capsules 1012
   Esgic-plus Tablets 1012
   Fioricet Tablets 2386
   Fioricet with Codeine Capsules .. 2387
   Fiorinal Capsules 2388
   Fiorinal with Codeine Capsules .. 2390
   Fiorinal Tablets 2388
   Phrenilin 790
   Sedapap Tablets 50 mg/650 mg .. 1826

Chlordiazepoxide (Potential for additive CNS depression). Products include:
   Limbitrol 2333

Chlordiazepoxide Hydrochloride (Potential for additive CNS depression). Products include:
   Librax Capsules 2330
   Librium Capsules 2331
   Librium Injectable 2332

Chlorpromazine (Potential for additive CNS depression). Products include:
   Thorazine Suppositories 2701

Chlorpromazine Hydrochloride (Potential for additive CNS depression). Products include:
   Thorazine 2701

Chlorprothixene (Potential for additive CNS depression).
   No products indexed under this heading.

Chlorprothixene Hydrochloride (Potential for additive CNS depression).
   No products indexed under this heading.

Chlorprothixene Lactate (Potential for additive CNS depression).
   No products indexed under this heading.

Clidinium Bromide (Concurrent use may produce paralytic ileus). Products include:
   Librax Capsules 2330

Clomipramine Hydrochloride (Increased effect of either the antidepressant or hydrocodone). Products include:
   Anafranil Capsules 819

Clorazepate Dipotassium (Potential for additive CNS depression). Products include:
   Tranxene 459

Clozapine (Potential for additive CNS depression). Products include:
   Clozaril Tablets 2377

Codeine Phosphate (Potential for additive CNS depression). Products include:
   Brontex 2130
   Dimetane-DC Cough Syrup 2232
   Fioricet with Codeine Capsules .. 2387
   Fiorinal with Codeine Capsules .. 2390
   Nucofed 2225
   Phenergan with Codeine 2883
   Phenergan VC with Codeine 2888
   Robitussin A-C Syrup 2248
   Robitussin-DAC Syrup 2249
   Ryna 804
   Soma Compound w/Codeine Tablets 2784
   Tylenol with Codeine 1592

Desflurane (Potential for additive CNS depression). Products include:
   Suprane (desflurane, USP) 1865

Desipramine Hydrochloride (Increased effect of either the antidepressant or hydrocodone). Products include:
   Norpramin Tablets 1273

Dezocine (Potential for additive CNS depression). Products include:
   Dalgan Injection 529

Diazepam (Potential for additive CNS depression). Products include:
   Dizac (diazepam injectable emulsion) CIV 1862
   Valium Injectable 2336
   Valium Tablets 2335

Dicyclomine Hydrochloride (Concurrent use may produce paralytic ileus). Products include:
   Bentyl 1246

Doxepin Hydrochloride (Increased effect of either the antidepressant or hydrocodone). Products include:
   Adapin Capsules 1542
   Sinequan 2028
   Zonalon Cream 1042

Droperidol (Potential for additive CNS depression). Products include:
   Inapsine Injection 462

Enflurane (Potential for additive CNS depression).
   No products indexed under this heading.

Estazolam (Potential for additive CNS depression). Products include:
   ProSom Tablets 457

Ethchlorvynol (Potential for additive CNS depression). Products include:
   Placidyl Capsules 456

Ethinamate (Potential for additive CNS depression).
   No products indexed under this heading.

Fentanyl (Potential for additive CNS depression). Products include:
   Duragesic Transdermal System .. 1336

Fentanyl Citrate (Potential for additive CNS depression). Products include:
   Sublimaze Injection 463

Fluphenazine Decanoate (Potential for additive CNS depression). Products include:
   Prolixin Decanoate 510

Fluphenazine Enanthate (Potential for additive CNS depression). Products include:
   Prolixin Enanthate 510

Fluphenazine Hydrochloride (Potential for additive CNS depression). Products include:
   Prolixin 510

Flurazepam Hydrochloride (Potential for additive CNS depression). Products include:
   Dalmane Capsules 2329

Furazolidone (Increased effect of either the antidepressant or hydrocodone). Products include:
   Furoxone 2221

Glutethimide (Potential for additive CNS depression).
   No products indexed under this heading.

Glycopyrrolate (Concurrent use may produce paralytic ileus). Products include:
   Robinul Forte Tablets 2247
   Robinul Injectable 2247
   Robinul Tablets 2247

Haloperidol (Potential for additive CNS depression). Products include:
   Haldol Injection, Tablets and Concentrate 1585

Haloperidol Decanoate (Potential for additive CNS depression). Products include:
   Haldol Decanoate 1587

Hydrocodone Polistirex (Potential for additive CNS depression). Products include:
   Tussionex Pennkinetic Extended-Release Suspension 1624

Hydromorphone Hydrochloride (Potential for additive CNS depression). Products include:
   Dilaudid Ampules 1382
   Dilaudid Cough Syrup 1383
   Dilaudid-HP Injection 1384
   Dilaudid-HP Lyophilized Powder 250 mg 1384
   Dilaudid 1382
   Dilaudid Oral Liquid 1386
   Dilaudid 1382
   Dilaudid Tablets - 8 mg. 1386

Hydroxyzine Hydrochloride (Potential for additive CNS depression). Products include:
   Atarax Tablets & Syrup 1992
   Marax Tablets & DF Syrup 2015
   Vistaril Intramuscular Solution .. 2042

Hyoscyamine (Concurrent use may produce paralytic ileus). Products include:
   Cystospaz Tablets 2123
   Urised Tablets 2123

Hyoscyamine Sulfate (Concurrent use may produce paralytic ileus). Products include:
   Arco-Lase Plus Tablets 513
   Atrohist Plus Tablets 1605
   Cystospaz-M Capsules 2123
   Donnatal 2234
   Donnatal Extentabs 2234
   Donnatal Tablets 2234
   Kutrase Capsules 2546
   Levsin/Levsinex/Levbid 2549

Imipramine Hydrochloride (Increased effect of either the antidepressant or hydrocodone). Products include:
   Tofranil Ampuls 873
   Tofranil Tablets 875

Imipramine Pamoate (Increased effect of either the antidepressant or hydrocodone). Products include:
   Tofranil-PM Capsules 876

IMPORTANT NOTE: Always consult each drug listing in the patient's regimen for possible interactions.

Lorcet 10/650 — Interactions Index

Ipratropium Bromide (Concurrent use may produce paralytic ileus). Products include:
- Atrovent Inhalation Aerosol 674
- Atrovent Inhalation Solution 675
- Atrovent Nasal Spray 0.03% 676
- Atrovent Nasal Spray 0.06% 678

Isocarboxazid (Increased effect of either the antidepressant or hydrocodone).
- No products indexed under this heading.

Isoflurane (Potential for additive CNS depression).
- No products indexed under this heading.

Ketamine Hydrochloride (Potential for additive CNS depression).
- No products indexed under this heading.

Levomethadyl Acetate Hydrochloride (Potential for additive CNS depression). Products include:
- Orlaam Oral Solution 2361

Levorphanol Tartrate (Potential for additive CNS depression). Products include:
- Levo-Dromoran 2297

Lorazepam (Potential for additive CNS depression). Products include:
- Ativan Injection 2805
- Ativan Tablets 2807

Loxapine Hydrochloride (Potential for additive CNS depression). Products include:
- Loxitane 1426

Loxapine Succinate (Potential for additive CNS depression). Products include:
- Loxitane Capsules 1426

Maprotiline Hydrochloride (Increased effect of either the antidepressant or hydrocodone). Products include:
- Ludiomil Tablets 861

Mepenzolate Bromide (Concurrent use may produce paralytic ileus).
- No products indexed under this heading.

Meperidine Hydrochloride (Potential for additive CNS depression). Products include:
- Demerol 2438
- Mepergan Injection 2859

Mephobarbital (Potential for additive CNS depression). Products include:
- Mebaral Tablets 2452

Meprobamate (Potential for additive CNS depression). Products include:
- Miltown Tablets 2780
- PMB 200 and PMB 400 2890

Mesoridazine Besylate (Potential for additive CNS depression). Products include:
- Serentil 689

Methadone Hydrochloride (Potential for additive CNS depression). Products include:
- Methadone Hydrochloride Oral Concentrate 2356
- Methadone Hydrochloride Oral Solution & Tablets 2357

Methohexital Sodium (Potential for additive CNS depression).
- No products indexed under this heading.

Methotrimeprazine (Potential for additive CNS depression). Products include:
- Levoprome 1321

Methoxyflurane (Potential for additive CNS depression).
- No products indexed under this heading.

Midazolam Hydrochloride (Potential for additive CNS depression). Products include:
- Versed Injection 2324

Molindone Hydrochloride (Potential for additive CNS depression). Products include:
- Moban Tablets and Concentrate 1036

Morphine Sulfate (Potential for additive CNS depression). Products include:
- Astramorph/PF Injection, USP (Preservative-Free) 526
- Duramorph Injection 983
- Infumorph 200 and Infumorph 500 Sterile Solutions 985
- Kadian Capsules 2948
- MS Contin Tablets 2149
- MSIR 2152
- Oramorph SR (Morphine Sulfate Sustained Release Tablets) 2359
- RMS Suppositories CII 2766
- Roxanol 2365

Nortriptyline Hydrochloride (Increased effect of either the antidepressant or hydrocodone). Products include:
- Pamelor 2409

Opium Alkaloids (Potential for additive CNS depression).
- No products indexed under this heading.

Oxazepam (Potential for additive CNS depression). Products include:
- Serax Capsules 2916
- Serax Tablets 2916

Oxybutynin Chloride (Concurrent use may produce paralytic ileus). Products include:
- Ditropan 1267

Oxycodone Hydrochloride (Potential for additive CNS depression). Products include:
- OxyContin Tablets 2163
- OxyIR Capsules 2167
- Percocet Tablets 955
- Percodan Tablets 955
- Percodan-Demi Tablets 956
- Roxicodone Tablets, Oral Solution & Intensol (Oxycodone) 2366
- Tylox Capsules 1593

Pentobarbital Sodium (Potential for additive CNS depression). Products include:
- Nembutal Sodium Capsules 440
- Nembutal Sodium Solution 442
- Nembutal Sodium Suppositories 444

Perphenazine (Potential for additive CNS depression). Products include:
- Etrafon 2495
- Triavil Tablets 1800
- Trilafon 2532

Phenelzine Sulfate (Increased effect of either the antidepressant or hydrocodone). Products include:
- Nardil 1977

Phenobarbital (Potential for additive CNS depression). Products include:
- Arco-Lase Plus Tablets 513
- Bellergal-S Tablets 2375
- Donnatal 2234
- Donnatal Extentabs 2234
- Donnatal Tablets 2234
- Phenobarbital Elixir and Tablets 1523
- Quadrinal Tablets 1398

Prazepam (Potential for additive CNS depression).
- No products indexed under this heading.

Prochlorperazine (Potential for additive CNS depression). Products include:
- Compazine 2644

Procyclidine Hydrochloride (Concurrent use may produce paralytic ileus). Products include:
- Kemadrin Tablets 1105

Promethazine Hydrochloride (Potential for additive CNS depression). Products include:
- Mepergan Injection 2859
- Phenergan with Codeine 2883
- Phenergan with Dextromethorphan 2885
- Phenergan Injection 2880
- Phenergan Suppositories 2882
- Phenergan Syrup 2881
- Phenergan Tablets 2882
- Phenergan VC 2886
- Phenergan VC with Codeine 2888

Propantheline Bromide (Concurrent use may produce paralytic ileus). Products include:
- Pro-Banthine Tablets 2226

Propofol (Potential for additive CNS depression). Products include:
- Diprivan Injectable Emulsion 2939

Propoxyphene Hydrochloride (Potential for additive CNS depression). Products include:
- Darvon 1475
- Wygesic Tablets 2930

Propoxyphene Napsylate (Potential for additive CNS depression). Products include:
- Darvon-N/Darvocet-N 1473

Protriptyline Hydrochloride (Increased effect of either the antidepressant or hydrocodone). Products include:
- Vivactil Tablets 1820

Quazepam (Potential for additive CNS depression). Products include:
- Doral Tablets 2773

Risperidone (Potential for additive CNS depression). Products include:
- Risperdal Tablets 1348

Scopolamine (Concurrent use may produce paralytic ileus). Products include:
- Transderm Scōp Transdermal Therapeutic System 890

Scopolamine Hydrobromide (Concurrent use may produce paralytic ileus). Products include:
- Atrohist Plus Tablets 1605
- Donnatal 2234
- Donnatal Extentabs 2234
- Donnatal Tablets 2234

Secobarbital Sodium (Potential for additive CNS depression). Products include:
- Seconal Sodium Pulvules 1529

Selegiline Hydrochloride (Increased effect of either the antidepressant or hydrocodone). Products include:
- Eldepryl Capsules 2729

Sevoflurane (Potential for additive CNS depression).
- No products indexed under this heading.

Sufentanil Citrate (Potential for additive CNS depression). Products include:
- Sufenta Injection 1355

Temazepam (Potential for additive CNS depression). Products include:
- Restoril Capsules 2413

Thiamylal Sodium (Potential for additive CNS depression).
- No products indexed under this heading.

Thioridazine Hydrochloride (Potential for additive CNS depression). Products include:
- Mellaril 2398

Thiothixene (Potential for additive CNS depression). Products include:
- Navane Capsules and Concentrate 2018
- Navane Intramuscular 2019

Tranylcypromine Sulfate (Increased effect of either the antidepressant or hydrocodone). Products include:
- Parnate Tablets 2679

Triazolam (Potential for additive CNS depression). Products include:
- Halcion Tablets 2093

Tridihexethyl Chloride (Concurrent use may produce paralytic ileus).
- No products indexed under this heading.

Trifluoperazine Hydrochloride (Potential for additive CNS depression). Products include:
- Stelazine 2692

Trihexyphenidyl Hydrochloride (Concurrent use may produce paralytic ileus). Products include:
- Artane 1418

Trimipramine Maleate (Increased effect of either the antidepressant or hydrocodone). Products include:
- Surmontil Capsules 2917

Zolpidem Tartrate (Potential for additive CNS depression). Products include:
- Ambien Tablets 2559

Food Interactions

Alcohol (Potential for additive CNS depression).

LORTAB 2.5/500 TABLETS
(Hydrocodone Bitartrate, Acetaminophen) 2751
See **Lortab 10/500 Tablets**

LORTAB 5/500 TABLETS
(Hydrocodone Bitartrate, Acetaminophen) 2751
See **Lortab 10/500 Tablets**

LORTAB 7.5/500 TABLETS
(Hydrocodone Bitartrate, Acetaminophen) 2751
See **Lortab 10/500 Tablets**

LORTAB 10/500 TABLETS
(Acetaminophen, Hydrocodone Bitartrate) 2751

May interact with central nervous system depressants, antihistamines, narcotic analgesics, tranquilizers, monoamine oxidase inhibitors, tricyclic antidepressants, and certain other agents. Compounds in these categories include:

Acrivastine (Co-administration may exhibit additive CNS depression). Products include:
- Semprex-D Capsules 1620

Alfentanil Hydrochloride (Co-administration may exhibit additive CNS depression). Products include:
- Alfenta Injection 1334

Alprazolam (Co-administration may exhibit additive CNS depression). Products include:
- Xanax Tablets 2115

Amitriptyline Hydrochloride (Co-administration may increase the effect of either the antidepressant or hydrocodone). Products include:
- Elavil 2945
- Etrafon 2495
- Limbitrol 2333
- Triavil Tablets 1800

Amoxapine (Co-administration may increase the effect of either the antidepressant or hydrocodone). Products include:
- Asendin Tablets 1419

Aprobarbital (Co-administration may exhibit additive CNS depression).
- No products indexed under this heading.

(▣ Described in PDR For Nonprescription Drugs)   (⊚ Described in PDR For Ophthalmology)

Astemizole (Co-administration may exhibit additive CNS depression). Products include:
- Hismanal Tablets ... 1341

Azatadine Maleate (Co-administration may exhibit additive CNS depression). Products include:
- Trinalin Repetabs Tablets ... 1373

Bromodiphenhydramine Hydrochloride (Co-administration may exhibit additive CNS depression).
- No products indexed under this heading.

Brompheniramine Maleate (Co-administration may exhibit additive CNS depression). Products include:
- Alka-Seltzer Plus Sinus Medicine ... 611
- Bromfed Capsules (Extended-Release) ... 1832
- Bromfed Syrup ... 712
- Bromfed Tablets ... 1832
- Bromfed-DM Cough Syrup ... 1832
- Bromfed-PD Capsules (Extended-Release) ... 1832
- Dimetane-DC Cough Syrup ... 2232
- Dimetane-DX Cough Syrup ... 2233
- Dimetapp Allergy Dye-Free Elixir ... 838
- Dimetapp Allergy Sinus Caplets ... 838
- Dimetapp Cold & Allergy Chewable Tablets ... 838
- Dimetapp Cold & Cough Liqui-Gels ... 839
- Dimetapp Cold & Fever Suspension ... 839
- Dimetapp DM Elixir ... 840
- Dimetapp Elixir ... 840
- Dimetapp Extentabs ... 841
- Dimetapp Tablets/Liqui-Gels ... 841
- Rondec Chewable Tablets ... 974
- Vicks DayQuil Allergy Relief 12-Hour Extended Release Tablets ... 733
- Vicks DayQuil Allergy Relief 4-Hour Tablets ... 733

Buprenorphine (Co-administration may exhibit additive CNS depression). Products include:
- Buprenex Injectable ... 2170

Buspirone Hydrochloride (Co-administration may exhibit additive CNS depression). Products include:
- BuSpar Tablets ... 738

Butabarbital (Co-administration may exhibit additive CNS depression).
- No products indexed under this heading.

Butalbital (Co-administration may exhibit additive CNS depression). Products include:
- Axocet Capsules ... 2469
- Esgic-plus Capsules ... 1012
- Esgic-plus Tablets ... 1012
- Fioricet Tablets ... 2386
- Fioricet with Codeine Capsules ... 2387
- Fiorinal Capsules ... 2388
- Fiorinal with Codeine Capsules ... 2390
- Fiorinal Tablets ... 2388
- Phrenilin ... 790
- Sedapap Tablets 50 mg/650 mg ... 1826

Cetirizine Hydrochloride (Co-administration may exhibit additive CNS depression). Products include:
- Zyrtec Tablets ... 2053

Chlordiazepoxide (Co-administration may exhibit additive CNS depression). Products include:
- Limbitrol ... 2333

Chlordiazepoxide Hydrochloride (Co-administration may exhibit additive CNS depression). Products include:
- Librax Capsules ... 2330
- Librium Capsules ... 2331
- Librium Injectable ... 2332

Chlorpheniramine Maleate (Co-administration may exhibit additive CNS depression). Products include:
- Alka-Seltzer Plus Cold Medicine ... 611
- Alka-Seltzer Plus Cold Medicine Liqui-Gels ... 612
- Alka-Seltzer Plus Cold & Cough Medicine ... 611
- Alka-Seltzer Plus Cold & Cough Medicine Liqui-Gels ... 612
- Alka-Seltzer Plus Flu & Body Aches Effervescent Tablets ... 612
- Allerest Maximum Strength ... 649
- Allerest Sinus Pain Formula ... 649
- Ana-Kit Anaphylaxis Emergency Treatment Kit ... 611
- Atrohist Pediatric Capsules ... 1603
- Atrohist Plus Tablets ... 1605
- BC Cold Powder Multi-Symptom Formula (Cold-Sinus-Allergy) ... 631
- Cerose DM ... 853
- Cheracol Plus Head Cold/Cough Formula ... 741
- Children's TYLENOL Cold Multi-Symptom Chewable Tablets and Liquid ... 1559
- Children's TYLENOL Cold Plus Cough Multi Symptom Chewable Tablets and Liquid ... 1560
- Children's TYLENOL Flu Suspension Liquid ... 1560
- Children's Vicks DayQuil Allergy Relief ... 730
- Children's Vicks NyQuil Cold/Cough Relief ... 731
- Chlor-Trimeton Allergy Decongestant Tablets ... 759
- Chlor-Trimeton Allergy Tablets ... 758
- Allergy-Sinus Comtrex Multi-Symptom Allergy-Sinus Formula Tablets and Caplets ... 639
- Comtrex Multi-Symptom ... 638
- Contac Continuous Action Nasal Decongestant/Antihistamine 12 Hour Capsules ... 773
- Contac Maximum Strength Continuous Action Decongestant/Antihistamine 12 Hour Caplets ... 772
- Contac Severe Cold and Flu Formula Caplets ... 773
- Coricidin Cold + Flu Tablets ... 760
- Coricidin Cough + Cold Tablets ... 760
- Coricidin 'D' Decongestant Tablets ... 760
- D.A. II Tablets ... 972
- D.A. Chewable Tablets ... 970
- Dura-Tap/PD Capsules ... 970
- Dura-Vent/DA Tablets ... 972
- Efidac 24 Chlorpheniramine ... 655
- Extendryl ... 1003
- Fedahist Gyrocaps ... 2545
- Hycomine Compound Tablets ... 948
- Kronofed-A ... 994
- Nolamine Timed-Release Tablets ... 790
- Novahistine Elixir ... 782
- Ornade Spansule Capsules ... 2678
- PediaCare Cough-Cold Chewable Tablets and Liquid ... 1569
- PediaCare NightRest Cough-Cold Liquid ... 1569
- Pediatric Vicks 44m Cough & Cold Relief ... 737
- Pyrroxate Caplets ... 742
- Ryna ... 804
- Sinarest ... 663
- Sine-Off Sinus Medicine ... 784
- Singlet Tablets ... 785
- Sinulin Tablets ... 792
- Sinutab Sinus Allergy Medication, Maximum Strength Tablets and Caplets ... 823
- Sudafed Cold & Allergy Tablets ... 826
- Teldrin 12 Hour Antihistamine/Nasal Decongestant Allergy Relief Capsules ... 786
- TheraFlu Flu and Cold Medicine ... 750
- Theraflu Maximum Strength Flu and Cold Medicine For Sore Throat ... 751
- TheraFlu Flu, Cold and Cough Medicine ... 750
- TheraFlu Maximum Strength Nighttime Flu, Cold & Cough Medicine ... 751
- Triaminic Night Time ... 754
- Triaminic Syrup ... 755
- Triaminic Triaminicol Cold & Cough ... 756
- Triaminicin Tablets ... 756
- Tussend ... 1830
- TYLENOL Allergy Sinus, Maximum Strength Caplets and Gelcaps ... 1571
- TYLENOL Cold Medication, Multi-Symptom Formula Tablets and Caplets ... 1572
- TYLENOL Cold Medication, Multi-Symptom Hot Liquid Packets ... 1572
- Vicks 44 LiquiCaps Cough, Cold & Flu Relief ... 728
- Vicks 44M Cough, Cold & Flu Relief ... 729

Chlorpheniramine Polistirex (Co-administration may exhibit additive CNS depression). Products include:
- Tussionex Pennkinetic Extended-Release Suspension ... 1624

Chlorpheniramine Tannate (Co-administration may exhibit additive CNS depression). Products include:
- Atrohist Pediatric Suspension ... 1604
- Atrohist Pediatric Suspension Dye-Free ... 1604
- Rynatan ... 2781
- Rynatuss ... 2782

Chlorpromazine (Co-administration may exhibit additive CNS depression). Products include:
- Thorazine Suppositories ... 2701

Chlorpromazine Hydrochloride (Co-administration may exhibit additive CNS depression). Products include:
- Thorazine ... 2701

Chlorprothixene (Co-administration may exhibit additive CNS depression).
- No products indexed under this heading.

Chlorprothixene Hydrochloride (Co-administration may exhibit additive CNS depression).
- No products indexed under this heading.

Chlorprothixene Lactate (Co-administration may exhibit additive CNS depression).
- No products indexed under this heading.

Clemastine Fumarate (Co-administration may exhibit additive CNS depression). Products include:
- Tavist Syrup ... 2426
- Tavist Tablets ... 2427
- Tavist-1 12 Hour Relief Tablets ... 749
- Tavist-D 12 Hour Relief Tablets ... 750

Clomipramine Hydrochloride (Co-administration may increase the effect of either the antidepressant or hydrocodone). Products include:
- Anafranil Capsules ... 819

Clorazepate Dipotassium (Co-administration may exhibit additive CNS depression). Products include:
- Tranxene ... 459

Clozapine (Co-administration may exhibit additive CNS depression). Products include:
- Clozaril Tablets ... 2377

Codeine Phosphate (Co-administration may exhibit additive CNS depression). Products include:
- Brontex ... 2130
- Dimetane-DC Cough Syrup ... 2232
- Fioricet with Codeine Capsules ... 2387
- Fiorinal with Codeine Capsules ... 2390
- Nucofed ... 2225
- Phenergan with Codeine ... 2883
- Phenergan VC with Codeine ... 2888
- Robitussin A-C Syrup ... 2248
- Robitussin-DAC Syrup ... 2249
- Ryna ... 804
- Soma Compound w/Codeine Tablets ... 2784
- Tylenol with Codeine ... 1592

Cyproheptadine Hydrochloride (Co-administration may exhibit additive CNS depression). Products include:
- Periactin ... 1767

Desflurane (Co-administration may exhibit additive CNS depression). Products include:
- Suprane (desflurane, USP) ... 1865

Desipramine Hydrochloride (Co-administration may increase the effect of either the antidepressant or hydrocodone). Products include:
- Norpramin Tablets ... 1273

Dexchlorpheniramine Maleate (Co-administration may exhibit additive CNS depression).
- No products indexed under this heading.

Dezocine (Co-administration may exhibit additive CNS depression). Products include:
- Dalgan Injection ... 529

Diazepam (Co-administration may exhibit additive CNS depression). Products include:
- Dizac (diazepam injectable emulsion) CIV ... 1862
- Valium Injectable ... 2336
- Valium Tablets ... 2335

Diphenhydramine Citrate (Co-administration may exhibit additive CNS depression). Products include:
- Excedrin P.M. Analgesic/Sleeping Aid Tablets, Caplets, Liquigels ... 735

Diphenhydramine Hydrochloride (Co-administration may exhibit additive CNS depression). Products include:
- Actifed Allergy Daytime/Nighttime Caplets ... 808
- Actifed Sinus Daytime/Nighttime Tablets and Caplets ... 809
- Extra Strength Bayer PM Aspirin Plus Sleep Aid ... 617
- Benadryl Allergy Chewables ... 811
- Benadryl Allergy/Cold Tablets ... 811
- Benadryl Allergy Decongestant Liquid Medication ... 812
- Benadryl Allergy Decongestant Tablets ... 812
- Benadryl Allergy Liquid Medication ... 813
- Benadryl Allergy ... 811
- Benadryl Allergy Sinus Headache Caplets ... 813
- Benadryl Dye-Free Allergy Liquigel Softgels ... 813
- Benadryl Dye-Free Allergy Liquid Medication ... 814
- Benadryl Itch Relief Stick Extra Strength ... 814
- Benadryl Cream ... 814
- Benadryl Gel ... 815
- Benadryl Spray ... 815
- Benadryl Injection ... 1955
- Contac Day & Night Cold/Flu Night Caplets ... 772
- Contac Night Allergy/Sinus Caplets ... 771
- Extra Strength Doan's P.M. ... 653
- Excedrin P.M. Analgesic/Sleeping Aid Tablets, Caplets, Liquigels ... 643
- Nytol QuickCaps Caplets ... 632
- Sleepinal Night-time Sleep Aid Capsules and Softgels ... 798
- TYLENOL Allergy Sinus NightTime, Maximum Strength Caplets ... 1571
- TYLENOL Flu NightTime, Maximum Strength Gelcaps ... 1575
- TYLENOL Flu NightTime, Maximum Strength Hot Medication Packets ... 1575
- TYLENOL PM Pain Reliever/Sleep Aid, Extra Strength Gelcaps, Caplets, Geltabs ... 1576
- TYLENOL Severe Allergy Medication Caplets ... 1571
- Maximum Strength Unisom Sleepgels ... 1990
- Unisom With Pain Relief-Nighttime Sleep Aid and Pain Reliever ... 1991

Diphenylpyraline Hydrochloride (Co-administration may exhibit additive CNS depression).
- No products indexed under this heading.

Doxepin Hydrochloride (Co-administration may increase the effect of either the antidepressant or hydrocodone). Products include:
- Adapin Capsules ... 1542
- Sinequan ... 2028
- Zonalon Cream ... 1042

IMPORTANT NOTE: Always consult each drug listing in the patient's regimen for possible interactions.

Lortab | Interactions Index | 624

Droperidol (Co-administration may exhibit additive CNS depression). Products include:
Inapsine Injection ... 462

Enflurane (Co-administration may exhibit additive CNS depression).
No products indexed under this heading.

Estazolam (Co-administration may exhibit additive CNS depression). Products include:
ProSom Tablets ... 457

Ethchlorvynol (Co-administration may exhibit additive CNS depression). Products include:
Placidyl Capsules ... 456

Ethinamate (Co-administration may exhibit additive CNS depression).
No products indexed under this heading.

Fentanyl (Co-administration may exhibit additive CNS depression). Products include:
Duragesic Transdermal System ... 1336

Fentanyl Citrate (Co-administration may exhibit additive CNS depression). Products include:
Sublimaze Injection ... 463

Fluphenazine Decanoate (Co-administration may exhibit additive CNS depression). Products include:
Prolixin Decanoate ... 510

Fluphenazine Enanthate (Co-administration may exhibit additive CNS depression). Products include:
Prolixin Enanthate ... 510

Fluphenazine Hydrochloride (Co-administration may exhibit additive CNS depression). Products include:
Prolixin ... 510

Flurazepam Hydrochloride (Co-administration may exhibit additive CNS depression). Products include:
Dalmane Capsules ... 2329

Furazolidone (Co-administration may increase the effect of either the MAO inhibitor or hydrocodone). Products include:
Furoxone ... 2221

Glutethimide (Co-administration may exhibit additive CNS depression).
No products indexed under this heading.

Haloperidol (Co-administration may exhibit additive CNS depression). Products include:
Haldol Injection, Tablets and Concentrate ... 1585

Haloperidol Decanoate (Co-administration may exhibit additive CNS depression). Products include:
Haldol Decanoate ... 1587

Hydrocodone Polistirex (Co-administration may exhibit additive CNS depression). Products include:
Tussionex Pennkinetic Extended-Release Suspension ... 1624

Hydromorphone Hydrochloride (Co-administration may exhibit additive CNS depression). Products include:
Dilaudid Ampules ... 1382
Dilaudid Cough Syrup ... 1383
Dilaudid-HP Injection ... 1384
Dilaudid-HP Lyophilized Powder 250 mg ... 1384
Dilaudid ... 1382
Dilaudid Oral Liquid ... 1386
Dilaudid ... 1382
Dilaudid Tablets - 8 mg ... 1386

Hydroxyzine Hydrochloride (Co-administration may exhibit additive CNS depression). Products include:
Atarax Tablets & Syrup ... 1992
Marax Tablets & DF Syrup ... 2015
Vistaril Intramuscular Solution ... 2042

Imipramine Hydrochloride (Co-administration may increase the effect of either the antidepressant or hydrocodone). Products include:
Tofranil Ampuls ... 873
Tofranil Tablets ... 875

Imipramine Pamoate (Co-administration may increase the effect of either the antidepressant or hydrocodone). Products include:
Tofranil-PM Capsules ... 876

Isocarboxazid (Co-administration may increase the effect of either the MAO inhibitor or hydrocodone).
No products indexed under this heading.

Isoflurane (Co-administration may exhibit additive CNS depression).
No products indexed under this heading.

Ketamine Hydrochloride (Co-administration may exhibit additive CNS depression).
No products indexed under this heading.

Levomethadyl Acetate Hydrochloride (Co-administration may exhibit additive CNS depression). Products include:
Orlaam Oral Solution ... 2361

Levorphanol Tartrate (Co-administration may exhibit additive CNS depression). Products include:
Levo-Dromoran ... 2297

Loratadine (Co-administration may exhibit additive CNS depression). Products include:
Claritin Tablets ... 2485
Claritin-D Tablets ... 2487

Lorazepam (Co-administration may exhibit additive CNS depression). Products include:
Ativan Injection ... 2805
Ativan Tablets ... 2807

Loxapine Hydrochloride (Co-administration may exhibit additive CNS depression). Products include:
Loxitane ... 1426

Loxapine Succinate (Co-administration may exhibit additive CNS depression). Products include:
Loxitane Capsules ... 1426

Maprotiline Hydrochloride (Co-administration may increase the effect of either the antidepressant or hydrocodone). Products include:
Ludiomil Tablets ... 861

Meperidine Hydrochloride (Co-administration may exhibit additive CNS depression). Products include:
Demerol ... 2438
Mepergan Injection ... 2859

Mephobarbital (Co-administration may exhibit additive CNS depression). Products include:
Mebaral Tablets ... 2452

Meprobamate (Co-administration may exhibit additive CNS depression). Products include:
Miltown Tablets ... 2780
PMB 200 and PMB 400 ... 2890

Mesoridazine Besylate (Co-administration may exhibit additive CNS depression). Products include:
Serentil ... 689

Methadone Hydrochloride (Co-administration may exhibit additive CNS depression). Products include:
Methadone Hydrochloride Oral Concentrate ... 2356
Methadone Hydrochloride Oral Solution & Tablets ... 2357

Methdilazine Hydrochloride (Co-administration may exhibit additive CNS depression).
No products indexed under this heading.

Methohexital Sodium (Co-administration may exhibit additive CNS depression).
No products indexed under this heading.

Methotrimeprazine (Co-administration may exhibit additive CNS depression). Products include:
Levoprome ... 1321

Methoxyflurane (Co-administration may exhibit additive CNS depression).
No products indexed under this heading.

Midazolam Hydrochloride (Co-administration may exhibit additive CNS depression). Products include:
Versed Injection ... 2324

Molindone Hydrochloride (Co-administration may exhibit additive CNS depression). Products include:
Moban Tablets and Concentrate ... 1036

Morphine Sulfate (Co-administration may exhibit additive CNS depression). Products include:
Astramorph/PF Injection, USP (Preservative-Free) ... 526
Duramorph Injection ... 983
Infumorph 200 and Infumorph 500 Sterile Solutions ... 985
Kadian Capsules ... 2948
MS Contin Tablets ... 2149
MSIR ... 2152
Oramorph SR (Morphine Sulfate Sustained Release Tablets) ... 2359
RMS Suppositories CII ... 2766
Roxanol ... 2365

Nortriptyline Hydrochloride (Co-administration may increase the effect of either the antidepressant or hydrocodone). Products include:
Pamelor ... 2409

Opium Alkaloids (Co-administration may exhibit additive CNS depression).
No products indexed under this heading.

Oxazepam (Co-administration may exhibit additive CNS depression). Products include:
Serax Capsules ... 2916
Serax Tablets ... 2916

Oxycodone Hydrochloride (Co-administration may exhibit additive CNS depression). Products include:
OxyContin Tablets ... 2163
OxyIR Capsules ... 2167
Percocet Tablets ... 955
Percodan Tablets ... 955
Percodan-Demi Tablets ... 956
Roxicodone Tablets, Oral Solution & Intensol (Oxycodone) ... 2366
Tylox Capsules ... 1593

Pentobarbital Sodium (Co-administration may exhibit additive CNS depression). Products include:
Nembutal Sodium Capsules ... 440
Nembutal Sodium Solution ... 442
Nembutal Sodium Suppositories ... 444

Perphenazine (Co-administration may exhibit additive CNS depression). Products include:
Etrafon ... 2495
Triavil Tablets ... 1800
Trilafon ... 2532

Phenelzine Sulfate (Co-administration may increase the effect of either the MAO inhibitor or hydrocodone). Products include:
Nardil ... 1977

Phenobarbital (Co-administration may exhibit additive CNS depression). Products include:
Arco-Lase Plus Tablets ... 513
Bellergal-S Tablets ... 2375
Donnatal ... 2234
Donnatal Extentabs ... 2234
Donnatal Tablets ... 2234
Phenobarbital Elixir and Tablets ... 1523
Quadrinal Tablets ... 1398

Prazepam (Co-administration may exhibit additive CNS depression).
No products indexed under this heading.

Prochlorperazine (Co-administration may exhibit additive CNS depression). Products include:
Compazine ... 2644

Promethazine Hydrochloride (Co-administration may exhibit additive CNS depression). Products include:
Mepergan Injection ... 2859
Phenergan with Codeine ... 2883
Phenergan with Dextromethorphan ... 2885
Phenergan Injection ... 2880
Phenergan Suppositories ... 2882
Phenergan Syrup ... 2881
Phenergan Tablets ... 2882
Phenergan VC ... 2886
Phenergan VC with Codeine ... 2888

Propofol (Co-administration may exhibit additive CNS depression). Products include:
Diprivan Injectable Emulsion ... 2939

Propoxyphene Hydrochloride (Co-administration may exhibit additive CNS depression). Products include:
Darvon ... 1475
Wygesic Tablets ... 2930

Propoxyphene Napsylate (Co-administration may exhibit additive CNS depression). Products include:
Darvon-N/Darvocet-N ... 1473

Protriptyline Hydrochloride (Co-administration may increase the effect of either the antidepressant or hydrocodone). Products include:
Vivactil Tablets ... 1820

Pyrilamine Maleate (Co-administration may exhibit additive CNS depression). Products include:
4-Way Fast Acting Nasal Spray (regular & mentholated) ... ◼ 644
Maximum Strength Multi-Symptom Formula Midol ... ◼ 621
PMS Multi-Symptom Formula Midol ... ◼ 622

Pyrilamine Tannate (Co-administration may exhibit additive CNS depression). Products include:
Atrohist Pediatric Suspension ... 1604
Atrohist Pediatric Suspension Dye-Free ... 1604
Rynatan ... 2781

Quazepam (Co-administration may exhibit additive CNS depression). Products include:
Doral Tablets ... 2773

Risperidone (Co-administration may exhibit additive CNS depression). Products include:
Risperdal Tablets ... 1348

Secobarbital Sodium (Co-administration may exhibit additive CNS depression). Products include:
Seconal Sodium Pulvules ... 1529

Selegiline Hydrochloride (Co-administration may increase the effect of either the MAO inhibitor or hydrocodone). Products include:
Eldepryl Capsules ... 2729

Sevoflurane (Co-administration may exhibit additive CNS depression).
No products indexed under this heading.

Sufentanil Citrate (Co-administration may exhibit additive CNS depression). Products include:
Sufenta Injection ... 1355

Temazepam (Co-administration may exhibit additive CNS depression). Products include:
Restoril Capsules ... 2413

(◼ Described in PDR For Nonprescription Drugs) (◉ Described in PDR For Ophthalmology)

625 **Interactions Index** **Lotensin HCT**

Terfenadine (Co-administration may exhibit additive CNS depression). Products include:
- Seldane Tablets 1284
- Seldane-D Extended-Release Tablets 1286

Thiamylal Sodium (Co-administration may exhibit additive CNS depression).
- No products indexed under this heading.

Thioridazine Hydrochloride (Co-administration may exhibit additive CNS depression). Products include:
- Mellaril 2398

Thiothixene (Co-administration may exhibit additive CNS depression). Products include:
- Navane Capsules and Concentrate 2018
- Navane Intramuscular 2019

Tranylcypromine Sulfate (Co-administration may increase the effect of either the MAO inhibitor or hydrocodone). Products include:
- Parnate Tablets 2679

Triazolam (Co-administration may exhibit additive CNS depression). Products include:
- Halcion Tablets 2093

Trifluoperazine Hydrochloride (Co-administration may exhibit additive CNS depression). Products include:
- Stelazine 2692

Trimeprazine Tartrate (Co-administration may exhibit additive CNS depression).
- No products indexed under this heading.

Trimipramine Maleate (Co-administration may increase the effect of either the antidepressant or hydrocodone). Products include:
- Surmontil Capsules 2917

Tripelennamine Hydrochloride (Co-administration may exhibit additive CNS depression). Products include:
- PBZ Tablets 863
- PBZ-SR Tablets 862

Triprolidine Hydrochloride (Co-administration may exhibit additive CNS depression). Products include:
- Actifed Cold & Allergy Tablets 807
- Actifed Cold & Sinus Caplets and Tablets 808

Zolpidem Tartrate (Co-administration may exhibit additive CNS depression). Products include:
- Ambien Tablets 2559

Food Interactions

Alcohol (Co-administration may exhibit additive CNS depression; concurrent use should be avoided).

LORTAB ELIXIR
(Hydrocodone Bitartrate, Acetaminophen) 2751
See **Lortab 10/500 Tablets**

LOTENSIN TABLETS
(Benazepril Hydrochloride) 852
May interact with diuretics, thiazides, potassium sparing diuretics, potassium preparations, lithium preparations, and certain other agents. Compounds in these categories include:

Amiloride Hydrochloride (Co-administration can increase the risk of hyperkalemia; potential for excessive reduction in blood pressure, especially in those whom diuretic therapy was recently instituted). Products include:
- Midamor Tablets 1746
- Moduretic Tablets 1748

Bendroflumethiazide (Benazepril can attenuate potassium loss caused by thiazide diuretics; co-administration may result in excessive reduction in blood pressure, especially in those whom diuretic therapy was recently instituted).
- No products indexed under this heading.

Bumetanide (Co-administration may result in excessive reduction in blood pressure, especially in those whom diuretic therapy was recently instituted). Products include:
- Bumex 2260

Chlorothiazide (Benazepril can attenuate potassium loss caused by thiazide diuretics; co-administration may result in excessive reduction in blood pressure, especially in those whom diuretic therapy was recently instituted). Products include:
- Aldoclor Tablets 1638
- Diupres Tablets 1691
- Diuril Oral 1694

Chlorothiazide Sodium (Benazepril can attenuate potassium loss caused by thiazide diuretics; co-administration may result in excessive reduction in blood pressure, especially in those whom diuretic therapy was recently instituted). Products include:
- Diuril Sodium Intravenous 1693

Chlorthalidone (Co-administration may result in excessive reduction in blood pressure, especially in those whom diuretic therapy was recently instituted). Products include:
- Combipres Tablets 682
- Tenoretic Tablets 2963
- Thalitone 1293

Ethacrynic Acid (Co-administration may result in excessive reduction in blood pressure, especially in those whom diuretic therapy was recently instituted). Products include:
- Edecrin Tablets 1698

Furosemide (Co-administration may result in excessive reduction in blood pressure, especially in those whom diuretic therapy was recently instituted). Products include:
- Lasix Injection, Oral Solution and Tablets 1267

Hydrochlorothiazide (Benazepril can attenuate potassium loss caused by thiazide diuretics; co-administration may result in excessive reduction in blood pressure, especially in those whom diuretic therapy was recently instituted). Products include:
- Aldactazide Tablets 2556
- Aldoril Tablets 1644
- Apresazide Capsules 824
- Capozide Tablets 744
- Dyazide Capsules 2653
- Esidrix Tablets 839
- Esimil Tablets 840
- HydroDIURIL Tablets 1716
- Hydropres Tablets 1718
- Hyzaar Tablets 1720
- Inderide Tablets 2838
- Inderide LA Long Acting Capsules .. 2840
- Lopressor HCT Tablets 850
- Lotensin HCT Tablets 855
- Moduretic Tablets 1748
- Oretic Tablets 450
- Prinzide Tablets 1780
- Ser-Ap-Es Tablets 867
- Timolide Tablets 1791
- Vaseretic Tablets 1810
- Zestoretic Tablets 2968
- Ziac 1459

Hydroflumethiazide (Benazepril can attenuate potassium loss caused by thiazide diuretics; co-administration may result in excessive reduction in blood pressure, especially in those whom diuretic therapy was recently instituted). Products include:
- Diucardin Tablets 2824

Indapamide (Co-administration may result in excessive reduction in blood pressure, especially in those whom diuretic therapy was recently instituted).
- No products indexed under this heading.

Lithium Carbonate (Co-administration has resulted in increased serum lithium levels and symptoms of lithium toxicity). Products include:
- Eskalith 2658
- Lithium Carbonate Capsules & Tablets 2352
- Lithonate/Lithotabs/Lithobid 2721

Lithium Citrate (Co-administration has resulted in increased serum lithium levels and symptoms of lithium toxicity).
- No products indexed under this heading.

Methyclothiazide (Benazepril can attenuate potassium loss caused by thiazide diuretics; co-administration may result in excessive reduction in blood pressure, especially in those whom diuretic therapy was recently instituted). Products include:
- Enduron Tablets 424

Metolazone (Co-administration may result in excessive reduction in blood pressure, especially in those whom diuretic therapy was recently instituted). Products include:
- Mykrox Tablets 1617
- Zaroxolyn Tablets 1625

Polythiazide (Benazepril can attenuate potassium loss caused by thiazide diuretics; co-administration may result in excessive reduction in blood pressure, especially in those whom diuretic therapy was recently instituted). Products include:
- Minizide Capsules 2016

Potassium Acid Phosphate (Co-administration can increase the risk of hyperkalemia). Products include:
- K-Phos Original Formula 'Sodium Free' Tablets 633

Potassium Bicarbonate (Co-administration can increase the risk of hyperkalemia). Products include:
- Alka-Seltzer Gold Effervescent Antacid 611

Potassium Chloride (Co-administration can increase the risk of hyperkalemia). Products include:
- Chlor-3 Condiment 1003
- Colyte and Colyte-flavored 2540
- GoLYTELY 694
- K-Dur Microburst Release System (potassium chloride, USP) E.R. Tablets 1364
- K-Lor Powder Packets 438
- K-Norm Capsules 1615
- K-Tab Filmtab 439
- Micro-K 2237
- Micro-K LS Packets 2238
- NuLYTELY 694
- Cherry Flavor NuLYTELY 694
- Rum-K Syrup 1004
- Slow-K Extended-Release Tablets 869

Potassium Citrate (Co-administration can increase the risk of hyperkalemia). Products include:
- Polycitra Syrup 574
- Polycitra-K Crystals 574
- Polycitra-K Oral Solution 575
- Polycitra-LC 574
- Urocit-K Tablets 1828

Potassium Gluconate (Co-administration can increase the risk of hyperkalemia).
- No products indexed under this heading.

Potassium Phosphate, Dibasic (Co-administration can increase the risk of hyperkalemia).
- No products indexed under this heading.

Potassium Phosphate, Monobasic (Co-administration can increase the risk of hyperkalemia). Products include:
- K-Phos Neutral Tablets 633
- K-Phos Original Formula 'Sodium Free' Tablets 633

Spironolactone (Co-administration can increase the risk of hyperkalemia; potential for excessive reduction in blood pressure, especially in those whom diuretic therapy was recently instituted). Products include:
- Aldactazide Tablets 2556
- Aldactone Tablets 2558

Torsemide (Co-administration may result in excessive reduction in blood pressure, especially in those whom diuretic therapy was recently instituted). Products include:
- Demadex Tablets and Injection 691

Triamterene (Co-administration can increase the risk of hyperkalemia; potential for excessive reduction in blood pressure, especially in those whom diuretic therapy was recently instituted). Products include:
- Dyazide Capsules 2653
- Dyrenium Capsules 2655

LOTENSIN HCT TABLETS
(Benazepril Hydrochloride, Hydrochlorothiazide) 855
May interact with potassium sparing diuretics, potassium preparations, lithium preparations, insulin, non-steroidal anti-inflammatory agents, barbiturates, narcotic analgesics, and certain other agents. Compounds in these categories include:

Alfentanil Hydrochloride (Thiazide-induced orthostatic hypotension potentiated by narcotics). Products include:
- Alfenta Injection 1334

Amiloride Hydrochloride (Increases the risk of hyperkalemia). Products include:
- Midamor Tablets 1746
- Moduretic Tablets 1748

Aprobarbital (Thiazide-induced orthostatic hypotension potentiated by barbiturates).
- No products indexed under this heading.

Buprenorphine (Thiazide-induced orthostatic hypotension potentiated by narcotics). Products include:
- Buprenex Injectable 2170

Butabarbital (Thiazide-induced orthostatic hypotension potentiated by barbiturates).
- No products indexed under this heading.

Butalbital (Thiazide-induced orthostatic hypotension potentiated by barbiturates). Products include:
- Axocet Capsules 2469
- Esgic-plus Capsules 1012
- Esgic-plus Tablets 1012
- Fioricet Tablets 2386
- Fioricet with Codeine Capsules 2387
- Fiorinal Capsules 2388
- Fiorinal with Codeine Capsules 2390
- Fiorinal Tablets 2388
- Phrenilin 790
- Sedapap Tablets 50 mg/650 mg .. 1826

IMPORTANT NOTE: Always consult each drug listing in the patient's regimen for possible interactions.

Lotensin HCT **Interactions Index** **626**

Cholestyramine (Cholestyramine resin has potential of binding hydrochlorothiazide and reducing its absorption from the GI tract by up to 85%). Products include:
- Questran ... 774

Codeine Phosphate (Thiazide-induced orthostatic hypotension potentiated by narcotics). Products include:
- Brontex ... 2130
- Dimetane-DC Cough Syrup ... 2232
- Fioricet with Codeine Capsules ... 2387
- Fiorinal with Codeine Capsules ... 2390
- Nucofed ... 2225
- Phenergan with Codeine ... 2883
- Phenergan VC with Codeine ... 2888
- Robitussin A-C Syrup ... 2248
- Robitussin-DAC Syrup ... 2249
- Ryna ... ▣ 804
- Soma Compound w/Codeine Tablets ... 2784
- Tylenol with Codeine ... 1592

Colestipol Hydrochloride (Colestipol resin has potential of binding hydrochlorothiazide and reducing its absorption from the GI tract by up to 43%). Products include:
- Colestid ... 2073

Dezocine (Thiazide-induced orthostatic hypotension potentiated by narcotics). Products include:
- Dalgan Injection ... 529

Diclofenac Potassium (Reduces diuretic, natriuretic, and antihypertensive effects). Products include:
- Cataflam Tablets ... 833

Diclofenac Sodium (Reduces diuretic, natriuretic, and antihypertensive effects). Products include:
- Voltaren Ophthalmic Sterile Ophthalmic Solution ... ⊙ 264
- Cataflam/Voltaren/Voltaren-XR ... 833

Etodolac (Reduces diuretic, natriuretic, and antihypertensive effects). Products include:
- Lodine Capsules and Tablets ... 2849

Fenoprofen Calcium (Reduces diuretic, natriuretic, and antihypertensive effects). Products include:
- Nalfon 200 Pulvules & Nalfon Tablets ... 933

Fentanyl (Thiazide-induced orthostatic hypotension potentiated by narcotics). Products include:
- Duragesic Transdermal System ... 1336

Fentanyl Citrate (Thiazide-induced orthostatic hypotension potentiated by narcotics). Products include:
- Sublimaze Injection ... 463

Flurbiprofen (Reduces diuretic, natriuretic, and antihypertensive effects).
- No products indexed under this heading.

Hydrocodone Bitartrate (Thiazide-induced orthostatic hypotension potentiated by narcotics). Products include:
- Codiclear DH Syrup ... 808
- Duratuss HD Elixir ... 2750
- Histussin D Liquid ... 670
- Hycodan Tablets and Syrup ... 946
- Hycomine Compound Tablets ... 948
- Hycomine ... 947
- Hycotuss Expectorant Syrup ... 950
- Hydrocet Capsules ... 787
- Lorcet 10/650 Tablets ... 1016
- Lortab ... 2751
- Tussend ... 1830
- Tussend Expectorant ... 1831
- Vicodin Tablets ... 1404
- Vicodin ES Tablets ... 1405
- Vicodin HP Tablets ... 1403
- Vicodin Tuss Expectorant ... 1406
- Zydone Capsules ... 967

Hydrocodone Polistirex (Thiazide-induced orthostatic hypotension potentiated by narcotics). Products include:
- Tussionex Pennkinetic Extended-Release Suspension ... 1624

Hydromorphone Hydrochloride (Thiazide-induced orthostatic hypotension potentiated by narcotics). Products include:
- Dilaudid Ampules ... 1382
- Dilaudid Cough Syrup ... 1383
- Dilaudid-HP Injection ... 1384
- Dilaudid-HP Lyophilized Powder 250 mg ... 1384
- Dilaudid ... 1382
- Dilaudid Oral Liquid ... 1386
- Dilaudid ... 1382
- Dilaudid Tablets - 8 mg ... 1386

Ibuprofen (Reduces diuretic, natriuretic, and antihypertensive effects). Products include:
- Advil Cold and Sinus Caplets and Tablets ... ▣ 837
- Advil Ibuprofen Tablets, Caplets and Gel Caplets ... ▣ 836
- Children's Motrin Ibuprofen Oral Suspension ... 1558
- IBU Tablets ... 1389
- Ibuprohm ... ▣ 713
- Motrin IB Caplets, Tablets, and Gelcaps ... ▣ 802
- Motrin Ibuprofen Suspension, Oral Drops, Chewable Tablets, Caplets ... 1563
- Nuprin Ibuprofen/Analgesic Tablets & Caplets ... ▣ 645
- Vicks DayQuil SINUS Pressure & PAIN Relief with IBUPROFEN ... ▣ 735

Indomethacin (Reduces diuretic, natriuretic, and antihypertensive effects). Products include:
- Indocin ... 1723

Indomethacin Sodium Trihydrate (Reduces diuretic, natriuretic, and antihypertensive effects). Products include:
- Indocin I.V. ... 1727

Insulin, Human (Insulin requirements may be increased, decreased, or unchanged).
- No products indexed under this heading.

Insulin, Human Isophane Suspension (Insulin requirements may be increased, decreased, or unchanged). Products include:
- Novolin N Human Insulin 10 ml Vials ... 1846

Insulin, Human NPH (Insulin requirements may be increased, decreased, or unchanged). Products include:
- Humulin N, 100 Units ... 1495
- Novolin N PenFill 1.5 ml Cartridges Durable Insulin Delivery System ... 1849
- Novolin N Prefilled Syringe Disposable Insulin Delivery System ... 1850

Insulin, Human Regular (Insulin requirements may be increased, decreased, or unchanged). Products include:
- Humulin R, 100 Units ... 1497
- Novolin R Human Insulin 10 ml Vials ... 1846
- Novolin R PenFill 1.5 ml Cartridges Durable Insulin Delivery System ... 1849
- Novolin R Prefilled Syringe Disposable Insulin Delivery System ... 1850
- Velosulin BR Human Insulin 10 ml Vials ... 1847

Insulin, Human, Zinc Suspension (Insulin requirements may be increased, decreased, or unchanged). Products include:
- Humulin L, 100 Units ... 1494
- Humulin U, 100 Units ... 1498
- Novolin L Human Insulin 10 ml Vials ... 1846

Insulin Lispro, Human (Insulin requirements may be increased, decreased, or unchanged). Products include:
- Humalog Injection ... 1488

Insulin, NPH (Insulin requirements may be increased, decreased, or unchanged). Products include:
- NPH, 100 Units ... 1502
- Pork NPH, 100 Units ... 1506
- Purified Pork NPH Isophane Insulin ... 1852

Insulin, Regular (Insulin requirements may be increased, decreased, or unchanged). Products include:
- Regular, 100 Units ... 1503
- Pork Regular, 100 Units ... 1507
- Pork Regular (Concentrated), 500 Units ... 1508
- Purified Pork Regular Insulin ... 1852

Insulin, Zinc Crystals (Insulin requirements may be increased, decreased, or unchanged). Products include:
- NPH, 100 Units ... 1502

Insulin, Zinc Suspension (Insulin requirements may be increased, decreased, or unchanged). Products include:
- Iletin I ... 1501
- Lente, 100 Units ... 1501
- Iletin II ... 1504
- Pork Lente, 100 Units ... 1504
- Purified Pork Lente Insulin ... 1852

Ketoprofen (Reduces diuretic, natriuretic, and antihypertensive effects). Products include:
- Actron Caplets and Tablets ... ▣ 608
- Orudis Capsules ... 2874
- Orudis KT ... ▣ 842
- Oruvail Capsules ... 2874

Ketorolac Tromethamine (Reduces diuretic, natriuretic, and antihypertensive effects). Products include:
- Acular Sterile Ophthalmic Solution 470
- Toradol ... 2319

Levorphanol Tartrate (Thiazide-induced orthostatic hypotension potentiated by narcotics). Products include:
- Levo-Dromoran ... 2297

Lithium Carbonate (Increased serum lithium levels and symptoms of lithium toxicity; potential for reduced lithium renal clearance). Products include:
- Eskalith ... 2658
- Lithium Carbonate Capsules & Tablets ... 2352
- Lithonate/Lithotabs/Lithobid ... 2721

Lithium Citrate (Increased serum lithium levels and symptoms of lithium toxicity; potential for reduced lithium renal clearance).
- No products indexed under this heading.

Meclofenamate Sodium (Reduces diuretic, natriuretic, and antihypertensive effects).
- No products indexed under this heading.

Mefenamic Acid (Reduces diuretic, natriuretic, and antihypertensive effects). Products include:
- Ponstel ... 1982

Meperidine Hydrochloride (Thiazide-induced orthostatic hypotension potentiated by narcotics). Products include:
- Demerol ... 2438
- Mepergan Injection ... 2859

Mephobarbital (Thiazide-induced orthostatic hypotension potentiated by barbiturates). Products include:
- Mebaral Tablets ... 2452

Methadone Hydrochloride (Thiazide-induced orthostatic hypotension potentiated by narcotics). Products include:
- Methadone Hydrochloride Oral Concentrate ... 2356
- Methadone Hydrochloride Oral Solution & Tablets ... 2357

Morphine Sulfate (Thiazide-induced orthostatic hypotension potentiated by narcotics). Products include:
- Astramorph/PF Injection, USP (Preservative-Free) ... 526
- Duramorph Injection ... 983
- Infumorph 200 and Infumorph 500 Sterile Solutions ... 985
- Kadian Capsules ... 2948
- MS Contin Tablets ... 2149
- MSIR ... 2152
- Oramorph SR (Morphine Sulfate Sustained Release Tablets) ... 2359
- RMS Suppositories CII ... 2766
- Roxanol ... 2365

Nabumetone (Reduces diuretic, natriuretic, and antihypertensive effects). Products include:
- Relafen Tablets ... 2688

Naproxen (Reduces diuretic, natriuretic, and antihypertensive effects). Products include:
- Anaprox/Naprosyn ... 2277

Naproxen Sodium (Reduces diuretic, natriuretic, and antihypertensive effects). Products include:
- Aleve ... 2124
- Anaprox/Naprosyn ... 2277
- Naprelan Tablets ... 2861

Norepinephrine Bitartrate (Thiazides may decrease arterial responsiveness to norepinephrine). Products include:
- Levophed Bitartrate Injection ... 2445

Opium Alkaloids (Thiazide-induced orthostatic hypotension potentiated by narcotics).
- No products indexed under this heading.

Oxaprozin (Reduces diuretic, natriuretic, and antihypertensive effects). Products include:
- Daypro Caplets ... 2578

Oxycodone Hydrochloride (Thiazide-induced orthostatic hypotension potentiated by narcotics). Products include:
- OxyContin Tablets ... 2163
- OxyIR Capsules ... 2167
- Percocet Tablets ... 955
- Percodan Tablets ... 955
- Percodan-Demi Tablets ... 956
- Roxicodone Tablets, Oral Solution & Intensol (Oxycodone) ... 2366
- Tylox Capsules ... 1593

Pentobarbital Sodium (Thiazide-induced orthostatic hypotension potentiated by barbiturates). Products include:
- Nembutal Sodium Capsules ... 440
- Nembutal Sodium Solution ... 442
- Nembutal Sodium Suppositories ... 444

Phenobarbital (Thiazide-induced orthostatic hypotension potentiated by barbiturates). Products include:
- Arco-Lase Plus Tablets ... 513
- Bellergal-S Tablets ... 2375
- Donnatal ... 2234
- Donnatal Extentabs ... 2234
- Donnatal Tablets ... 2234
- Phenobarbital Elixir and Tablets ... 1523
- Quadrinal Tablets ... 1398

Phenylbutazone (Reduces diuretic, natriuretic, and antihypertensive effects).
- No products indexed under this heading.

Piroxicam (Reduces diuretic, natriuretic, and antihypertensive effects). Products include:
- Feldene Capsules ... 2008

(▣ Described in PDR For Nonprescription Drugs) (⊙ Described in PDR For Ophthalmology)

Potassium Acid Phosphate (Increases the risk of hyperkalemia). Products include:
- K-Phos Original Formula 'Sodium Free' Tablets ... 633

Potassium Bicarbonate (Increases the risk of hyperkalemia). Products include:
- Alka-Seltzer Gold Effervescent Antacid ... 611

Potassium Chloride (Increases the risk of hyperkalemia). Products include:
- Chlor-3 Condiment ... 1003
- Colyte and Colyte-flavored ... 2540
- GoLYTELY ... 694
- K-Dur Microburst Release System (potassium chloride, USP) E.R. Tablets ... 1364
- K-Lor Powder Packets ... 438
- K-Norm Capsules ... 1615
- K-Tab Filmtab ... 439
- Micro-K ... 2237
- Micro-K LS Packets ... 2238
- NuLYTELY ... 694
- Cherry Flavor NuLYTELY ... 694
- Rum-K Syrup ... 1004
- Slow-K Extended-Release Tablets ... 869

Potassium Citrate (Increases the risk of hyperkalemia). Products include:
- Polycitra Syrup ... 574
- Polycitra-K Crystals ... 574
- Polycitra-K Oral Solution ... 575
- Polycitra-LC ... 574
- Urocit-K Tablets ... 1828

Potassium Gluconate (Increases the risk of hyperkalemia).
No products indexed under this heading.

Potassium Phosphate, Dibasic (Increases the risk of hyperkalemia).
No products indexed under this heading.

Potassium Phosphate, Monobasic (Increases the risk of hyperkalemia). Products include:
- K-Phos Neutral Tablets ... 633
- K-Phos Original Formula 'Sodium Free' Tablets ... 633

Propoxyphene Hydrochloride (Thiazide-induced orthostatic hypotension potentiated by narcotics). Products include:
- Darvon ... 1475
- Wygesic Tablets ... 2930

Propoxyphene Napsylate (Thiazide-induced orthostatic hypotension potentiated by narcotics). Products include:
- Darvon-N/Darvocet-N ... 1473

Secobarbital Sodium (Thiazide-induced orthostatic hypotension potentiated by barbiturates). Products include:
- Seconal Sodium Pulvules ... 1529

Spironolactone (Increases the risk of hyperkalemia). Products include:
- Aldactazide Tablets ... 2556
- Aldactone Tablets ... 2558

Sufentanil Citrate (Thiazide-induced orthostatic hypotension potentiated by narcotics). Products include:
- Sufenta Injection ... 1355

Sulindac (Reduces diuretic, natriuretic, and antihypertensive effects). Products include:
- Clinoril Tablets ... 1658

Thiamylal Sodium (Thiazide-induced orthostatic hypotension potentiated by barbiturates).
No products indexed under this heading.

Tolmetin Sodium (Reduces diuretic, natriuretic, and antihypertensive effects). Products include:
- Tolectin (200, 400 and 600 mg) ... 1591

Triamterene (Increases the risk of hyperkalemia). Products include:
- Dyazide Capsules ... 2653
- Dyrenium Capsules ... 2655

Tubocurarine Chloride (Thiazides may increase the responsiveness to tubocurarine).
No products indexed under this heading.

Food Interactions

Alcohol (Thiazide-induced orthostatic hypotension potentiated by alcohol).

LOTREL CAPSULES
(Amlodipine Besylate, Benazepril Hydrochloride) ... 858
May interact with potassium sparing diuretics, potassium preparations, lithium preparations, and diuretics. Compounds in these categories include:

Amiloride Hydrochloride (Potential for the increased risk of hyperkalemia; patients on diuretics, especially those in whom diuretic therapy was recently instituted, may experience an excessive reduction in blood pressure). Products include:
- Midamor Tablets ... 1746
- Moduretic Tablets ... 1748

Bendroflumethiazide (Patients on diuretics, especially those in whom diuretic therapy was recently instituted, may experience an excessive reduction in blood pressure).
No products indexed under this heading.

Bumetanide (Patients on diuretics, especially those in whom diuretic therapy was recently instituted, may experience an excessive reduction in blood pressure). Products include:
- Bumex ... 2260

Chlorothiazide (Patients on diuretics, especially those in whom diuretic therapy was recently instituted, may experience an excessive reduction in blood pressure). Products include:
- Aldoclor Tablets ... 1638
- Diupres Tablets ... 1691
- Diuril Oral ... 1694

Chlorothiazide Sodium (Patients on diuretics, especially those in whom diuretic therapy was recently instituted, may experience an excessive reduction in blood pressure). Products include:
- Diuril Sodium Intravenous ... 1693

Chlorthalidone (Patients on diuretics, especially those in whom diuretic therapy was recently instituted, may experience an excessive reduction in blood pressure). Products include:
- Combipres Tablets ... 682
- Tenoretic Tablets ... 2963
- Thalitone ... 1293

Ethacrynic Acid (Patients on diuretics, especially those in whom diuretic therapy was recently instituted, may experience an excessive reduction in blood pressure). Products include:
- Edecrin Tablets ... 1698

Furosemide (Patients on diuretics, especially those in whom diuretic therapy was recently instituted, may experience an excessive reduction in blood pressure). Products include:
- Lasix Injection, Oral Solution and Tablets ... 1267

Hydrochlorothiazide (Patients on diuretics, especially those in whom diuretic therapy was recently instituted, may experience an excessive reduction in blood pressure). Products include:
- Aldactazide Tablets ... 2556
- Aldoril Tablets ... 1644
- Apresazide Capsules ... 824
- Capozide Tablets ... 744
- Dyazide Capsules ... 2653
- Esidrix Tablets ... 839
- Esimil Tablets ... 840
- HydroDIURIL Tablets ... 1716
- Hydropres Tablets ... 1718
- Hyzaar Tablets ... 1720
- Inderide Tablets ... 2838
- Inderide LA Long Acting Capsules ... 2840
- Lopressor HCT Tablets ... 850
- Lotensin HCT Tablets ... 855
- Moduretic Tablets ... 1748
- Oretic Tablets ... 450
- Prinzide Tablets ... 1780
- Ser-Ap-Es Tablets ... 867
- Timolide Tablets ... 1791
- Vaseretic Tablets ... 1810
- Zestoretic Tablets ... 2968
- Ziac ... 1459

Hydroflumethiazide (Patients on diuretics, especially those in whom diuretic therapy was recently instituted, may experience an excessive reduction in blood pressure). Products include:
- Diucardin Tablets ... 2824

Indapamide (Patients on diuretics, especially those in whom diuretic therapy was recently instituted, may experience an excessive reduction in blood pressure).
No products indexed under this heading.

Lithium Carbonate (Potential for increased serum lithium levels and symptoms of lithium toxicity). Products include:
- Eskalith ... 2658
- Lithium Carbonate Capsules & Tablets ... 2352
- Lithonate/Lithotabs/Lithobid ... 2721

Lithium Citrate (Potential for increased serum lithium levels and symptoms of lithium toxicity).
No products indexed under this heading.

Methyclothiazide (Patients on diuretics, especially those in whom diuretic therapy was recently instituted, may experience an excessive reduction in blood pressure). Products include:
- Enduron Tablets ... 424

Metolazone (Patients on diuretics, especially those in whom diuretic therapy was recently instituted, may experience an excessive reduction in blood pressure). Products include:
- Mykrox Tablets ... 1617
- Zaroxolyn Tablets ... 1625

Polythiazide (Patients on diuretics, especially those in whom diuretic therapy was recently instituted, may experience an excessive reduction in blood pressure). Products include:
- Minizide Capsules ... 2016

Potassium Acid Phosphate (Potential for the increased risk of hyperkalemia). Products include:
- K-Phos Original Formula 'Sodium Free' Tablets ... 633

Potassium Bicarbonate (Potential for the increased risk of hyperkalemia). Products include:
- Alka-Seltzer Gold Effervescent Antacid ... 611

Potassium Chloride (Potential for the increased risk of hyperkalemia). Products include:
- Chlor-3 Condiment ... 1003
- Colyte and Colyte-flavored ... 2540
- GoLYTELY ... 694
- K-Dur Microburst Release System (potassium chloride, USP) E.R. Tablets ... 1364
- K-Lor Powder Packets ... 438
- K-Norm Capsules ... 1615
- K-Tab Filmtab ... 439
- Micro-K ... 2237
- Micro-K LS Packets ... 2238
- NuLYTELY ... 694
- Cherry Flavor NuLYTELY ... 694
- Rum-K Syrup ... 1004
- Slow-K Extended-Release Tablets ... 869

Potassium Citrate (Potential for the increased risk of hyperkalemia). Products include:
- Polycitra Syrup ... 574
- Polycitra-K Crystals ... 574
- Polycitra-K Oral Solution ... 575
- Polycitra-LC ... 574
- Urocit-K Tablets ... 1828

Potassium Gluconate (Potential for the increased risk of hyperkalemia).
No products indexed under this heading.

Potassium Phosphate, Dibasic (Potential for the increased risk of hyperkalemia).
No products indexed under this heading.

Potassium Phosphate, Monobasic (Potential for the increased risk of hyperkalemia). Products include:
- K-Phos Neutral Tablets ... 633
- K-Phos Original Formula 'Sodium Free' Tablets ... 633

Spironolactone (Potential for the increased risk of hyperkalemia; patients on diuretics, especially those in whom diuretic therapy was recently instituted, may experience an excessive reduction in blood pressure). Products include:
- Aldactazide Tablets ... 2556
- Aldactone Tablets ... 2558

Torsemide (Patients on diuretics, especially those in whom diuretic therapy was recently instituted, may experience an excessive reduction in blood pressure). Products include:
- Demadex Tablets and Injection ... 691

Triamterene (Potential for the increased risk of hyperkalemia; patients on diuretics, especially those in whom diuretic therapy was recently instituted, may experience an excessive reduction in blood pressure). Products include:
- Dyazide Capsules ... 2653
- Dyrenium Capsules ... 2655

LOTRIMIN CREAM 1%
(Clotrimazole) ... 2514
None cited in PDR database.

LOTRIMIN LOTION 1%
(Clotrimazole) ... 2514
None cited in PDR database.

LOTRIMIN SOLUTION 1%
(Clotrimazole) ... 2514
None cited in PDR database.

LOTRIMIN AF ANTIFUNGAL CREAM, LOTION AND SOLUTION
(Clotrimazole) ... 766
None cited in PDR database.

LOTRIMIN AF ANTIFUNGAL SPRAY LIQUID, SPRAY POWDER, SPRAY DEODORANT POWDER, POWDER AND JOCK ITCH SPRAY POWDER
(Miconazole Nitrate) ... 766
None cited in PDR database.

IMPORTANT NOTE: Always consult each drug listing in the patient's regimen for possible interactions.

LOTRISONE CREAM
(Clotrimazole, Betamethasone Dipropionate) 2515
None cited in PDR database.

LOVENOX INJECTION
(Enoxaparin) 2187
May interact with oral anticoagulants, platelet inhibitors, non-steroidal anti-inflammatory agents, salicylates, and certain other agents. Compounds in these categories include:

Aspirin (May enhance the risk of hemorrhage). Products include:
- Alka-Seltzer Cherry Effervescent Antacid and Pain Reliever .... ▣ 609
- Alka-Seltzer Extra Strength Effervescent Antacid and Pain Reliever .... ▣ 609
- Alka-Seltzer Lemon Lime Effervescent Antacid and Pain Reliever .... ▣ 609
- Alka-Seltzer Original Effervescent Antacid and Pain Reliever .... ▣ 609
- Alka-Seltzer Plus .... ▣ 611
- Alka-Seltzer Plus Sinus Medicine .. ▣ 611
- Ascriptin .... ▣ 650
- Arthritis Strength BC Powder....... ▣ 631
- BC Cold Powder Multi-Symptom Formula (Cold-Sinus-Allergy) .... ▣ 631
- BC Cold Powder Non-Drowsy Formula (Cold-Sinus) .... ▣ 631
- BC Powder .... ▣ 631
- Genuine Bayer Aspirin Tablets & Caplets .... ▣ 618
- Extra Strength Bayer Arthritis Pain Regimen Formula .... ▣ 615
- Extra Strength Bayer Aspirin Caplets & Tablets .... ▣ 617
- Extended-Release Bayer 8-Hour Aspirin .... ▣ 616
- Extra Strength Bayer Plus Aspirin Caplets .... ▣ 617
- Extra Strength Bayer PM Aspirin Plus Sleep Aid .... ▣ 617
- Aspirin Regimen Bayer 81 mg Tablets with Calcium .... ▣ 615
- Aspirin Regimen Bayer Adult Low Strength 81 mg Tablets .... ▣ 613
- Aspirin Regimen Bayer Children's Chewable Aspirin .... ▣ 616
- Aspirin Regimen Bayer Regular Strength 325 mg Caplets .... ▣ 613
- Bufferin Analgesic Tablets....... ▣ 636
- Arthritis Strength Bufferin Analgesic Caplets .... ▣ 637
- Extra Strength Bufferin Analgesic Tablets .... ▣ 637
- Cama Arthritis Pain Reliever....... ▣ 748
- Darvon Compound-65 Pulvules 1475
- Easprin 1971
- Ecotrin 2625
- Ecotrin Enteric Coated Aspirin Maximum Strength Tablets and Caplets .... ▣ 775
- Ecotrin Enteric Coated Aspirin Regular Strength Tablets 2625
- Empirin Aspirin Tablets .... ▣ 818
- Excedrin Extra-Strength Analgesic Tablets, Caplets, and Geltabs....... 734
- Fiorinal Capsules 2388
- Fiorinal with Codeine Capsules 2390
- Fiorinal Tablets....... 2388
- Goody's Extra Strength Headache Powders .... ▣ 632
- Goody's Extra Strength Pain Relief Tablets .... ▣ 632
- Halfprin Tablets 1413
- Norgesic....... 1554
- Percodan Tablets....... 955
- Percodan-Demi Tablets....... 956
- Robaxisal Tablets....... 2246
- Soma Compound w/Codeine Tablets....... 2784
- Soma Compound Tablets....... 2783
- St. Joseph Adult Chewable Aspirin (81 mg.) .... ▣ 768
- Talwin Compound 2466
- Vanquish Analgesic Caplets .... ▣ 627

Azlocillin Sodium (May enhance the risk of hemorrhage).
- No products indexed under this heading.

Carbenicillin Indanyl Sodium (May enhance the risk of hemorrhage). Products include:
- Geocillin Tablets....... 2009

Choline Magnesium Trisalicylate (May enhance the risk of hemorrhage). Products include:
- Trilisate 2155

Diclofenac Potassium (May enhance the risk of hemorrhage). Products include:
- Cataflam Tablets 833

Diclofenac Sodium (May enhance the risk of hemorrhage). Products include:
- Voltaren Ophthalmic Sterile Ophthalmic Solution .... ◉ 264
- Cataflam/Voltaren/Voltaren-XR 833

Dicumarol (May enhance the risk of hemorrhage).
- No products indexed under this heading.

Diflunisal (May enhance the risk of hemorrhage). Products include:
- Dolobid Tablets....... 1695

Dipyridamole (May enhance the risk of hemorrhage). Products include:
- Persantine Tablets 686

Etodolac (May enhance the risk of hemorrhage). Products include:
- Lodine Capsules and Tablets 2849

Fenoprofen Calcium (May enhance the risk of hemorrhage). Products include:
- Nalfon 200 Pulvules & Nalfon Tablets 933

Flurbiprofen (May enhance the risk of hemorrhage).
- No products indexed under this heading.

Ibuprofen (May enhance the risk of hemorrhage). Products include:
- Advil Cold and Sinus Caplets and Tablets .... ▣ 837
- Advil Ibuprofen Tablets, Caplets and Gel Caplets .... ▣ 836
- Children's Motrin Ibuprofen Oral Suspension 1558
- IBU Tablets....... 1389
- Ibuprohm....... ▣ 713
- Motrin IB Caplets, Tablets, and Gelcaps .... ▣ 802
- Motrin Ibuprofen Suspension, Oral Drops, Chewable Tablets, Caplets 1563
- Nuprin Ibuprofen/Analgesic Tablets & Caplets .... ▣ 645
- Vicks DayQuil SINUS Pressure & PAIN Relief with IBUPROFEN .... ▣ 735

Indomethacin (May enhance the risk of hemorrhage). Products include:
- Indocin 1723

Indomethacin Sodium Trihydrate (May enhance the risk of hemorrhage). Products include:
- Indocin I.V. 1727

Ketoprofen (May enhance the risk of hemorrhage). Products include:
- Actron Caplets and Tablets....... ▣ 608
- Orudis Capsules....... 2874
- Orudis KT .... ▣ 842
- Oruvail Capsules 2874

Ketorolac Tromethamine (May enhance the risk of hemorrhage). Products include:
- Acular Sterile Ophthalmic Solution 470
- Toradol....... 2319

Magnesium Salicylate (May enhance the risk of hemorrhage). Products include:
- Backache Caplets .... ▣ 635
- Doan's Extra-Strength Analgesic....... ▣ 653
- Extra Strength Doan's P.M....... ▣ 653
- Doan's Regular Strength Analgesic .... ▣ 654
- Mobigesic Tablets .... ▣ 607

Meclofenamate Sodium (May enhance the risk of hemorrhage).
- No products indexed under this heading.

Mefenamic Acid (May enhance the risk of hemorrhage). Products include:
- Ponstel 1982

Mezlocillin Sodium (May enhance the risk of hemorrhage). Products include:
- Mezlin 594
- Mezlin Pharmacy Bulk Package....... 597

Nabumetone (May enhance the risk of hemorrhage). Products include:
- Relafen Tablets....... 2688

Nafcillin Sodium (May enhance the risk of hemorrhage).
- No products indexed under this heading.

Naproxen (May enhance the risk of hemorrhage). Products include:
- Anaprox/Naprosyn 2277

Naproxen Sodium (May enhance the risk of hemorrhage). Products include:
- Aleve 2124
- Anaprox/Naprosyn 2277
- Naprelan Tablets 2861

Oxaprozin (May enhance the risk of hemorrhage). Products include:
- Daypro Caplets 2578

Penicillin G Benzathine (May enhance the risk of hemorrhage). Products include:
- Bicillin C-R Injection 2810
- Bicillin C-R 900/300 Injection 2812
- Bicillin L-A Injection 2813

Penicillin G Procaine (May enhance the risk of hemorrhage). Products include:
- Bicillin C-R Injection 2810
- Bicillin C-R 900/300 Injection 2812

Phenylbutazone (May enhance the risk of hemorrhage).
- No products indexed under this heading.

Piroxicam (May enhance the risk of hemorrhage). Products include:
- Feldene Capsules....... 2008

Salsalate (May enhance the risk of hemorrhage). Products include:
- Disalcid 1549
- Mono-Gesic Tablets 810
- Salflex Tablets....... 791

Sulfinpyrazone (May enhance the risk of hemorrhage). Products include:
- Anturane 823

Sulindac (May enhance the risk of hemorrhage). Products include:
- Clinoril Tablets 1658

Ticarcillin Disodium (May enhance the risk of hemorrhage). Products include:
- Ticar for Injection 2704
- Timentin for Injection....... 2706

Ticlopidine Hydrochloride (May enhance the risk of hemorrhage). Products include:
- Ticlid Tablets 2317

Tolmetin Sodium (May enhance the risk of hemorrhage). Products include:
- Tolectin (200, 400 and 600 mg) .. 1591

Warfarin Sodium (May enhance the risk of hemorrhage). Products include:
- Coumadin 941

LOXITANE C ORAL CONCENTRATE
(Loxapine Hydrochloride) 1426
See **Loxitane Capsules**

LOXITANE CAPSULES
(Loxapine Succinate).......1426
May interact with anticholinergic-type antiparkinsonism drugs, barbiturates, narcotic analgesics, general anesthetics, and certain other agents. Compounds in these categories include:

Alfentanil Hydrochloride (Loxitane is contraindicated in severe narcotic-induced depressed state). Products include:
- Alfenta Injection 1334

Aprobarbital (Loxitane is contraindicated in severe barbiturate-induced depressed state).
- No products indexed under this heading.

Benztropine Mesylate (Use Loxitane cautiously). Products include:
- Cogentin 1661

Biperiden Hydrochloride (Use Loxitane cautiously). Products include:
- Akineton 1380

Buprenorphine (Loxitane is contraindicated in severe narcotic-induced depressed state). Products include:
- Buprenex Injectable 2170

Butabarbital (Loxitane is contraindicated in severe barbiturate-induced depressed state).
- No products indexed under this heading.

Butalbital (Loxitane is contraindicated in severe barbiturate-induced depressed state). Products include:
- Axocet Capsules....... 2469
- Esgic-plus Capsules 1012
- Esgic-plus Tablets 1012
- Fioricet Tablets....... 2386
- Fioricet with Codeine Capsules 2387
- Fiorinal Capsules 2388
- Fiorinal with Codeine Capsules 2390
- Fiorinal Tablets....... 2388
- Phrenilin 790
- Sedapap Tablets 50 mg/650 mg .. 1826

Codeine Phosphate (Loxitane is contraindicated in severe narcotic-induced depressed state). Products include:
- Brontex 2130
- Dimetane-DC Cough Syrup 2232
- Fioricet with Codeine Capsules 2387
- Fiorinal with Codeine Capsules 2390
- Nucofed 2225
- Phenergan with Codeine....... 2883
- Phenergan VC with Codeine 2888
- Robitussin A-C Syrup....... 2248
- Robitussin-DAC Syrup....... 2249
- Ryna .... ▣ 804
- Soma Compound w/Codeine Tablets 2784
- Tylenol with Codeine 1592

Dezocine (Loxitane is contraindicated in severe narcotic-induced depressed state). Products include:
- Dalgan Injection 529

Diphenhydramine Hydrochloride (Use Loxitane cautiously). Products include:
- Actifed Allergy Daytime/Nighttime Caplets....... ▣ 808
- Actifed Sinus Daytime/Nighttime Tablets and Caplets .... ▣ 809
- Extra Strength Bayer PM Aspirin Plus Sleep Aid .... ▣ 617
- Benadryl Allergy Chewables .... ▣ 811
- Benadryl Allergy/Cold Tablets....... ▣ 811
- Benadryl Allergy Decongestant Liquid Medication .... ▣ 812
- Benadryl Allergy Decongestant Tablets .... ▣ 812
- Benadryl Allergy Liquid Medication....... ▣ 813
- Benadryl Allergy....... ▣ 811
- Benadryl Allergy Sinus Headache Caplets .... ▣ 813
- Benadryl Dye-Free Allergy Liqui-gel Softgels....... ▣ 813
- Benadryl Dye-Free Allergy Liquid Medication .... ▣ 814
- Benadryl Itch Relief Stick Extra Strength....... ▣ 814
- Benadryl Cream .... ▣ 814
- Benadryl Gel .... ▣ 815
- Benadryl Spray .... ▣ 815
- Benadryl Injection 1955

(▣ Described in PDR For Nonprescription Drugs) (◉ Described in PDR For Ophthalmology)

Interactions Index

Contac Day & Night Cold/Flu Night Caplets ... ⓐⓓ 772
Contac Night Allergy/Sinus Caplets ... ⓐⓓ 771
Extra Strength Doan's P.M. ... ⓐⓓ 653
Excedrin P.M. Analgesic/Sleeping Aid Tablets, Caplets, Liquigels ... ⓐⓓ 643
Nytol QuickCaps Caplets ... ⓐⓓ 632
Sleepinal Night-time Sleep Aid Capsules and Softgels ... ⓐⓓ 798
TYLENOL Allergy Sinus NightTime, Maximum Strength Caplets ... 1571
TYLENOL Flu NightTime, Maximum Strength Gelcaps ... 1575
TYLENOL Flu NightTime, Maximum Strength Hot Medication Packets ... 1575
TYLENOL PM Pain Reliever/Sleep Aid, Extra Strength Gelcaps, Caplets, Geltabs ... 1576
TYLENOL Severe Allergy Medication Caplets ... 1571
Maximum Strength Unisom Sleepgels ... 1990
Unisom With Pain Relief-Nighttime Sleep Aid and Pain Reliever ... 1991

Enflurane (Loxitane is contraindicated in severe anesthetic-induced depressed state).
No products indexed under this heading.

Epinephrine (Inhibition of vasopressor effect by Loxitane). Products include:
EPIFRIN ... ⓐ 237
EpiPen ... 808
Marcaine with Epinephrine ... 2446
Primatene Mist ... ⓐⓓ 843
Sensorcaine with Epinephrine Injection ... 554
Sus-Phrine Injection ... 1017
Xylocaine with Epinephrine Injections ... 562

Fentanyl (Loxitane is contraindicated in severe narcotic-induced depressed state). Products include:
Duragesic Transdermal System ... 1336

Fentanyl Citrate (Loxitane is contraindicated in severe narcotic-induced depressed state). Products include:
Sublimaze Injection ... 463

Hydrocodone Bitartrate (Loxitane is contraindicated in severe narcotic-induced depressed state). Products include:
Codiclear DH Syrup ... 808
Duratuss HD Elixir ... 2750
Histussin D Liquid ... 670
Hycodan Tablets and Syrup ... 946
Hycomine Compound Tablets ... 948
Hycomine ... 947
Hycotuss Expectorant Syrup ... 950
Hydrocet Capsules ... 787
Lorcet 10/650 Tablets ... 1016
Lortab ... 2751
Tussend ... 1830
Tussend Expectorant ... 1831
Vicodin Tablets ... 1404
Vicodin ES Tablets ... 1405
Vicodin HP Tablets ... 1403
Vicodin Tuss Expectorant ... 1406
Zydone Capsules ... 967

Hydrocodone Polistirex (Loxitane is contraindicated in severe narcotic-induced depressed state). Products include:
Tussionex Pennkinetic Extended-Release Suspension ... 1624

Hydromorphone Hydrochloride (Loxitane is contraindicated in severe narcotic-induced depressed state). Products include:
Dilaudid Ampules ... 1382
Dilaudid Cough Syrup ... 1383
Dilaudid-HP Injection ... 1384
Dilaudid-HP Lyophilized Powder 250 mg ... 1384
Dilaudid ... 1382
Dilaudid Oral Liquid ... 1386
Dilaudid ... 1382
Dilaudid Tablets - 8 mg ... 1386

Isoflurane (Loxitane is contraindicated in severe anesthetic-induced depressed state).
No products indexed under this heading.

Ketamine Hydrochloride (Loxitane is contraindicated in severe anesthetic-induced depressed state).
No products indexed under this heading.

Levorphanol Tartrate (Loxitane is contraindicated in severe narcotic-induced depressed state). Products include:
Levo-Dromoran ... 2297

Meperidine Hydrochloride (Loxitane is contraindicated in severe narcotic-induced depressed state). Products include:
Demerol ... 2438
Mepergan Injection ... 2859

Mephobarbital (Loxitane is contraindicated in severe barbiturate-induced depressed state). Products include:
Mebaral Tablets ... 2452

Methadone Hydrochloride (Loxitane is contraindicated in severe narcotic-induced depressed state). Products include:
Methadone Hydrochloride Oral Concentrate ... 2356
Methadone Hydrochloride Oral Solution & Tablets ... 2357

Methohexital Sodium (Loxitane is contraindicated in severe anesthetic-induced depressed state).
No products indexed under this heading.

Methoxyflurane (Loxitane is contraindicated in severe anesthetic-induced depressed state).
No products indexed under this heading.

Morphine Sulfate (Loxitane is contraindicated in severe narcotic-induced depressed state). Products include:
Astramorph/PF Injection, USP (Preservative-Free) ... 526
Duramorph Injection ... 983
Infumorph 200 and Infumorph 500 Sterile Solutions ... 985
Kadian Capsules ... 2948
MS Contin Tablets ... 2149
MSIR ... 2152
Oramorph SR (Morphine Sulfate Sustained Release Tablets) ... 2359
RMS Suppositories CII ... 2766
Roxanol ... 2365

Opium Alkaloids (Loxitane is contraindicated in severe narcotic-induced depressed state).
No products indexed under this heading.

Oxycodone Hydrochloride (Loxitane is contraindicated in severe narcotic-induced depressed state). Products include:
OxyContin Tablets ... 2163
OxyIR Capsules ... 2167
Percocet Tablets ... 955
Percodan Tablets ... 955
Percodan-Demi Tablets ... 956
Roxicodone Tablets, Oral Solution & Intensol (Oxycodone) ... 2366
Tylox Capsules ... 1593

Pentobarbital Sodium (Loxitane is contraindicated in severe barbiturate-induced depressed state). Products include:
Nembutal Sodium Capsules ... 440
Nembutal Sodium Solution ... 442
Nembutal Sodium Suppositories ... 444

Phenobarbital (Loxitane is contraindicated in severe barbiturate-induced depressed state). Products include:
Arco-Lase Plus Tablets ... 513
Bellergal-S Tablets ... 2375
Donnatal ... 2234
Donnatal Extentabs ... 2234
Donnatal Tablets ... 2234
Phenobarbital Elixir and Tablets ... 1523
Quadrinal Tablets ... 1398

Procyclidine Hydrochloride (Use Loxitane cautiously). Products include:
Kemadrin Tablets ... 1105

Propofol (Loxitane is contraindicated in severe anesthetic-induced depressed state). Products include:
Diprivan Injectable Emulsion ... 2939

Propoxyphene Hydrochloride (Loxitane is contraindicated in severe narcotic-induced depressed state). Products include:
Darvon ... 1475
Wygesic Tablets ... 2930

Propoxyphene Napsylate (Loxitane is contraindicated in severe narcotic-induced depressed state). Products include:
Darvon-N/Darvocet-N ... 1473

Secobarbital Sodium (Loxitane is contraindicated in severe barbiturate-induced depressed state). Products include:
Seconal Sodium Pulvules ... 1529

Sevoflurane (Loxitane is contraindicated in severe anesthetic-induced depressed state).
No products indexed under this heading.

Sufentanil Citrate (Loxitane is contraindicated in severe narcotic-induced depressed state). Products include:
Sufenta Injection ... 1355

Thiamylal Sodium (Loxitane is contraindicated in severe barbiturate-induced depressed state).
No products indexed under this heading.

Tridihexethyl Chloride (Use Loxitane cautiously).
No products indexed under this heading.

Trihexyphenidyl Hydrochloride (Use Loxitane cautiously). Products include:
Artane ... 1418

LOXITANE IM
(Loxapine Hydrochloride) ... 1426
See **Loxitane Capsules**

LUBRIDERM BATH AND SHOWER OIL
(Emollient, Mineral Oil) ... ⓐⓓ 821
None cited in PDR database.

LUBRIDERM DRY SKIN CARE LOTION
(Emollient) ... ⓐⓓ 820
None cited in PDR database.

LUBRIDERM MOISTURE RECOVERY ALPHA HYDROXY CREAM AND LOTION
(Moisturizing formula) ... ⓐⓓ 821
None cited in PDR database.

LUBRIDERM MOISTURE RECOVERY GELCREME
(Cetyl Alcohol, Glycerin, Mineral Oil) ... ⓐⓓ 821
None cited in PDR database.

LUBRIDERM SERIOUSLY SENSITIVE LOTION
(Glycerin, Mineral Oil, Petrolatum) ... ⓐⓓ 821
None cited in PDR database.

LUDIOMIL TABLETS
(Maprotiline Hydrochloride) ... 861
May interact with monoamine oxidase inhibitors, benzodiazepines, phenothiazines, barbiturates, anticholinergics, sympathomimetics, thyroid preparations, central nervous system depressants, and certain other agents. Compounds in these categories include:

Albuterol (Co-administration with sympathomimetics may result in possible additive atropine-like effects). Products include:
Proventil Inhalation Aerosol ... 2524
Ventolin Inhalation Aerosol and Refill ... 1170

Albuterol Sulfate (Co-administration with sympathomimetics may result in possible additive atropine-like effects). Products include:
Airet Albuterol Sulfate Inhalation Solution ... 1602
Albuterol Sulfate, USP Solution for Inhalation, Arm-a-Med ... 522
Proventil Inhalation Solution 0.083% ... 2527
Proventil Repetabs Tablets ... 2529
Proventil Solution for Inhalation 0.5% ... 2525
Proventil Syrup ... 2528
Proventil Tablets ... 2529
Ventolin Inhalation Solution ... 1171
Ventolin Nebules Inhalation Solution ... 1172
Ventolin Rotacaps for Inhalation ... 1173
Ventolin Syrup ... 1175
Ventolin Tablets ... 1176
Volmax Extended-Release Tablets ... 1835

Alfentanil Hydrochloride (Enhanced response to central nervous system depressants). Products include:
Alfenta Injection ... 1334

Alprazolam (Co-administration with benzodiazepines may increase the risk of seizures, especially when the dosage of benzodiazepines is rapidly tapered; enhanced response to central nervous system depressants). Products include:
Xanax Tablets ... 2115

Aprobarbital (Co-administration with certain barbiturates, hepatic enzyme inducers, may decrease the plasma levels of maprotiline; enhanced response to central nervous system depressants).
No products indexed under this heading.

Atropine Sulfate (Co-administration with anticholinergics may result in possible additive atropine-like effects). Products include:
Arco-Lase Plus Tablets ... 513
Atrohist Plus Tablets ... 1605
Donnatal ... 2234
Donnatal Extentabs ... 2234
Donnatal Tablets ... 2234
Lomotil ... 2591
Motofen Tablets ... 789
Urised Tablets ... 2123

Belladonna Alkaloids (Co-administration with anticholinergics may result in possible additive atropine-like effects). Products include:
Bellergal-S Tablets ... 2375
Hyland's Bedwetting Tablets ... ⓐⓓ 788
Hyland's EnurAid Tablets ... ⓐⓓ 789
Hyland's Headache Tablets ... ⓐⓓ 790
Hyland's Teething Tablets ... ⓐⓓ 790
Similasan Eye Drops #1 ... ⓐⓓ 769

Benztropine Mesylate (Co-administration with anticholinergics may result in possible additive atropine-like effects). Products include:
Cogentin ... 1661

Biperiden Hydrochloride (Co-administration with anticholinergics may result in possible additive atropine-like effects). Products include:
Akineton ... 1380

IMPORTANT NOTE: Always consult each drug listing in the patient's regimen for possible interactions.

Ludiomil | Interactions Index | 630

Buprenorphine (Enhanced response to central nervous system depressants). Products include:
- Buprenex Injectable ... 2170

Buspirone Hydrochloride (Enhanced response to central nervous system depressants). Products include:
- BuSpar Tablets ... 738

Butabarbital (Co-administration with certain barbiturates, hepatic enzyme inducers, may decrease the plasma levels of maprotiline; enhanced response to central nervous system depressants).
- No products indexed under this heading.

Butalbital (Co-administration with certain barbiturates, hepatic enzyme inducers, may decrease the plasma levels of maprotiline; enhanced response to central nervous system depressants). Products include:
- Axocet Capsules ... 2469
- Esgic-plus Capsules ... 1012
- Esgic-plus Tablets ... 1012
- Fioricet Tablets ... 2386
- Fioricet with Codeine Capsules ... 2387
- Fiorinal Capsules ... 2388
- Fiorinal with Codeine Capsules ... 2390
- Fiorinal Tablets ... 2388
- Phrenilin ... 790
- Sedapap Tablets 50 mg/650 mg .. 1826

Chlordiazepoxide (Co-administration with benzodiazepines may increase the risk of seizures, especially when the dosage of benzodiazepines is rapidly tapered; enhanced response to central nervous system depressants). Products include:
- Limbitrol ... 2333

Chlordiazepoxide Hydrochloride (Co-administration with benzodiazepines may increase the risk of seizures, especially when the dosage of benzodiazepines is rapidly tapered; enhanced response to central nervous system depressants). Products include:
- Librax Capsules ... 2330
- Librium Capsules ... 2331
- Librium Injectable ... 2332

Chlorpromazine (Co-administration with phenothiazines may increase the risk of seizures; enhanced response to central nervous system depressants). Products include:
- Thorazine Suppositories ... 2701

Chlorpromazine Hydrochloride (Co-administration with phenothiazines may increase the risk of seizures; enhanced response to central nervous system depressants). Products include:
- Thorazine ... 2701

Chlorprothixene (Enhanced response to central nervous system depressants).
- No products indexed under this heading.

Chlorprothixene Hydrochloride (Enhanced response to central nervous system depressants).
- No products indexed under this heading.

Chlorprothixene Lactate (Enhanced response to central nervous system depressants).
- No products indexed under this heading.

Cimetidine (Co-administration with hepatic enzyme inhibitors, such as cimetidine, may increase the plasma levels of maprotiline). Products include:
- Tagamet HB Tablets ... [ND] 786
- Tagamet Tablets ... 2694

Cimetidine Hydrochloride (Co-administration with hepatic enzyme inhibitors, such as cimetidine, may increase the plasma levels of maprotiline). Products include:
- Tagamet ... 2694

Clidinium Bromide (Co-administration with anticholinergics may result in possible additive atropine-like effects). Products include:
- Librax Capsules ... 2330

Clonazepam (Co-administration with benzodiazepines may increase the risk of seizures, especially when the dosage of benzodiazepines is rapidly tapered; enhanced response to central nervous system depressants). Products include:
- Klonopin Tablets ... 2294

Clorazepate Dipotassium (Co-administration with benzodiazepines may increase the risk of seizures, especially when the dosage of benzodiazepines is rapidly tapered; enhanced response to central nervous system depressants). Products include:
- Tranxene ... 459

Clozapine (Enhanced response to central nervous system depressants). Products include:
- Clozaril Tablets ... 2377

Codeine Phosphate (Enhanced response to central nervous system depressants). Products include:
- Brontex ... 2130
- Dimetane-DC Cough Syrup ... 2232
- Fioricet with Codeine Capsules ... 2387
- Fiorinal with Codeine Capsules ... 2390
- Nucofed ... 2225
- Phenergan with Codeine ... 2883
- Phenergan VC with Codeine ... 2888
- Robitussin A-C Syrup ... 2248
- Robitussin-DAC Syrup ... 2249
- Ryna ... [ND] 804
- Soma Compound w/Codeine Tablets ... 2784
- Tylenol with Codeine ... 1592

Desflurane (Enhanced response to central nervous system depressants). Products include:
- Suprane (desflurane, USP) ... 1865

Dezocine (Enhanced response to central nervous system depressants). Products include:
- Dalgan Injection ... 529

Diazepam (Co-administration with benzodiazepines may increase the risk of seizures, especially when the dosage of benzodiazepines is rapidly tapered; enhanced response to central nervous system depressants). Products include:
- Dizac (diazepam injectable emulsion) CIV ... 1862
- Valium Injectable ... 2336
- Valium Tablets ... 2335

Dicyclomine Hydrochloride (Co-administration with anticholinergics may result in possible additive atropine-like effects). Products include:
- Bentyl ... 1246

Dobutamine Hydrochloride (Co-administration with sympathomimetics may result in possible additive atropine-like effects). Products include:
- Dobutrex Solution Vials ... 1480

Dopamine Hydrochloride (Co-administration with sympathomimetics may result in possible additive atropine-like effects).
- No products indexed under this heading.

Droperidol (Enhanced response to central nervous system depressants). Products include:
- Inapsine Injection ... 462

Enflurane (Enhanced response to central nervous system depressants).
- No products indexed under this heading.

Ephedrine Hydrochloride (Co-administration with sympathomimetics may result in possible additive atropine-like effects). Products include:
- Primatene Tablets ... [ND] 844
- Quadrinal Tablets ... 1398

Ephedrine Sulfate (Co-administration with sympathomimetics may result in possible additive atropine-like effects). Products include:
- Marax Tablets & DF Syrup ... 2015

Ephedrine Tannate (Co-administration with sympathomimetics may result in possible additive atropine-like effects). Products include:
- Rynatuss ... 2782

Epinephrine (Co-administration with sympathomimetics may result in possible additive atropine-like effects). Products include:
- EPIFRIN ... ◉ 237
- EpiPen ... 808
- Marcaine with Epinephrine ... 2446
- Primatene Mist ... [ND] 843
- Sensorcaine with Epinephrine Injection ... 554
- Sus-Phrine Injection ... 1017
- Xylocaine with Epinephrine Injections ... 562

Epinephrine Bitartrate (Co-administration with sympathomimetics may result in possible additive atropine-like effects). Products include:
- Sensorcaine-MPF with Epinephrine Injection ... 554

Epinephrine Hydrochloride (Co-administration with sympathomimetics may result in possible additive atropine-like effects). Products include:
- Ana-Kit Anaphylaxis Emergency Treatment Kit ... 611

Estazolam (Co-administration with benzodiazepines may increase the risk of seizures, especially when the dosage of benzodiazepines is rapidly tapered; enhanced response to central nervous system depressants). Products include:
- ProSom Tablets ... 457

Ethchlorvynol (Enhanced response to central nervous system depressants). Products include:
- Placidyl Capsules ... 456

Ethinamate (Enhanced response to central nervous system depressants).
- No products indexed under this heading.

Fentanyl (Enhanced response to central nervous system depressants). Products include:
- Duragesic Transdermal System ... 1336

Fentanyl Citrate (Enhanced response to central nervous system depressants). Products include:
- Sublimaze Injection ... 463

Fluoxetine Hydrochloride (Co-administration with hepatic enzyme inhibitors, such as fluoxetine, may increase the plasma levels of maprotiline). Products include:
- Prozac Pulvules & Liquid, Oral Solution ... 935

Fluphenazine Decanoate (Co-administration with phenothiazines may increase the risk of seizures; enhanced response to central nervous system depressants). Products include:
- Prolixin Decanoate ... 510

Fluphenazine Enanthate (Co-administration with phenothiazines may increase the risk of seizures; enhanced response to central nervous system depressants). Products include:
- Prolixin Enanthate ... 510

Fluphenazine Hydrochloride (Co-administration with phenothiazines may increase the risk of seizures; enhanced response to central nervous system depressants). Products include:
- Prolixin ... 510

Flurazepam Hydrochloride (Co-administration with benzodiazepines may increase the risk of seizures, especially when the dosage of benzodiazepines is rapidly tapered; enhanced response to central nervous system depressants). Products include:
- Dalmane Capsules ... 2329

Furazolidone (Concurrent and/or sequential use with MAO inhibitors is contraindicated). Products include:
- Furoxone ... 2221

Glutethimide (Enhanced response to central nervous system depressants).
- No products indexed under this heading.

Glycopyrrolate (Co-administration with anticholinergics may result in possible additive atropine-like effects). Products include:
- Robinul Forte Tablets ... 2247
- Robinul Injectable ... 2247
- Robinul Tablets ... 2247

Guanethidine Monosulfate (Maprotiline may block the pharmacological effects of guanethidine or similar agents). Products include:
- Esimil Tablets ... 840
- Ismelin Tablets ... 845

Halazepam (Co-administration with benzodiazepines may increase the risk of seizures, especially when the dosage of benzodiazepines is rapidly tapered; enhanced response to central nervous system depressants).
- No products indexed under this heading.

Haloperidol (Enhanced response to central nervous system depressants). Products include:
- Haldol Injection, Tablets and Concentrate ... 1585

Haloperidol Decanoate (Enhanced response to central nervous system depressants). Products include:
- Haldol Decanoate ... 1587

Hydrocodone Bitartrate (Enhanced response to central nervous system depressants). Products include:
- Codiclear DH Syrup ... 808
- Duratuss HD Elixir ... 2750
- Histussin D Liquid ... 670
- Hycodan Tablets and Syrup ... 946
- Hycomine Compound Tablets ... 948
- Hycomine ... 947
- Hycotuss Expectorant Syrup ... 950
- Hydrocet Capsules ... 787
- Lorcet 10/650 Tablets ... 1016
- Lortab ... 2751
- Tussend ... 1830
- Tussend Expectorant ... 1831
- Vicodin Tablets ... 1404
- Vicodin ES Tablets ... 1405
- Vicodin HP Tablets ... 1403
- Vicodin Tuss Expectorant ... 1406
- Zydone Capsules ... 967

([ND] Described in PDR For Nonprescription Drugs) (◉ Described in PDR For Ophthalmology)

Hydrocodone Polistirex (Enhanced response to central nervous system depressants). Products include:
   Tussionex Pennkinetic Extended-Release Suspension 1624

Hydromorphone Hydrochloride (Enhanced response to central nervous system depressants). Products include:
   Dilaudid Ampules 1382
   Dilaudid Cough Syrup 1383
   Dilaudid-HP Injection 1384
   Dilaudid-HP Lyophilized Powder 250 mg 1384
   Dilaudid 1382
   Dilaudid Oral Liquid 1386
   Dilaudid 1382
   Dilaudid Tablets - 8 mg. 1386

Hydroxyzine Hydrochloride (Enhanced response to central nervous system depressants). Products include:
   Atarax Tablets & Syrup 1992
   Marax Tablets & DF Syrup 2015
   Vistaril Intramuscular Solution 2042

Hyoscyamine (Co-administration with anticholinergics may result in possible additive atropine-like effects). Products include:
   Cystospaz Tablets 2123
   Urised Tablets 2123

Hyoscyamine Sulfate (Co-administration with anticholinergics may result in possible additive atropine-like effects). Products include:
   Arco-Lase Plus Tablets 513
   Atrohist Plus Tablets 1605
   Cystospaz-M Capsules 2123
   Donnatal 2234
   Donnatal Extentabs 2234
   Donnatal Tablets 2234
   Kutrase Capsules 2546
   Levsin/Levsinex/Levbid 2549

Ipratropium Bromide (Co-administration with anticholinergics may result in possible additive atropine-like effects). Products include:
   Atrovent Inhalation Aerosol 674
   Atrovent Inhalation Solution 675
   Atrovent Nasal Spray 0.03% 676
   Atrovent Nasal Spray 0.06% 678

Isocarboxazid (Concurrent and/or sequential use with MAO inhibitors is contraindicated).
   No products indexed under this heading.

Isoflurane (Enhanced response to central nervous system depressants).
   No products indexed under this heading.

Isoproterenol Hydrochloride (Co-administration with sympathomimetics may result in possible additive atropine-like effects). Products include:
   Isuprel Hydrochloride Solution 2443
   Isuprel Injection 2441
   Isuprel Mistometer 2442

Isoproterenol Sulfate (Co-administration with sympathomimetics may result in possible additive atropine-like effects). Products include:
   Norisodrine with Calcium Iodide Syrup 446

Ketamine Hydrochloride (Enhanced response to central nervous system depressants).
   No products indexed under this heading.

Levomethadyl Acetate Hydrochloride (Enhanced response to central nervous system depressants). Products include:
   Orlaam Oral Solution 2361

Levorphanol Tartrate (Enhanced response to central nervous system depressants). Products include:
   Levo-Dromoran 2297

Levothyroxine Sodium (Co-administration in patients with hyperthyroidism or those on thyroid drugs may result in possibility of enhanced cardiovascular toxicity of maprotiline). Products include:
   Eltroxin Tablets 2214
   Levothroid Tablets 1015
   Levothyroxine Sodium, USP for Injection 546
   Levoxyl Tablets 918
   Synthroid 1410

Liothyronine Sodium (Co-administration in patients with hyperthyroidism or those on thyroid drugs may result in possibility of enhanced cardiovascular toxicity of maprotiline). Products include:
   Cytomel Tablets 2647
   Triostat Injection 2708

Liotrix (Co-administration in patients with hyperthyroidism or those on thyroid drugs may result in possibility of enhanced cardiovascular toxicity of maprotiline).
   No products indexed under this heading.

Lorazepam (Co-administration with benzodiazepines may increase the risk of seizures, especially when the dosage of benzodiazepines is rapidly tapered; enhanced response to central nervous system depressants). Products include:
   Ativan Injection 2805
   Ativan Tablets 2807

Loxapine Hydrochloride (Enhanced response to central nervous system depressants). Products include:
   Loxitane 1426

Loxapine Succinate (Enhanced response to central nervous system depressants). Products include:
   Loxitane Capsules 1426

Mepenzolate Bromide (Co-administration with anticholinergics may result in possible additive atropine-like effects).
   No products indexed under this heading.

Meperidine Hydrochloride (Enhanced response to central nervous system depressants). Products include:
   Demerol 2438
   Mepergan Injection 2859

Mephobarbital (Co-administration with certain barbiturates, hepatic enzyme inducers, may decrease the plasma levels of maprotiline; enhanced response to central nervous system depressants). Products include:
   Mebaral Tablets 2452

Meprobamate (Enhanced response to central nervous system depressants). Products include:
   Miltown Tablets 2780
   PMB 200 and PMB 400 2890

Mesoridazine Besylate (Co-administration with phenothiazines may increase the risk of seizures; enhanced response to central nervous system depressants). Products include:
   Serentil 689

Metaproterenol Sulfate (Co-administration with sympathomimetics may result in possible additive atropine-like effects). Products include:
   Alupent 672
   Metaproterenol Sulfate Inhalation Solution, USP, Arm-a-Med 547

Metaraminol Bitartrate (Co-administration with sympathomimetics may result in possible additive atropine-like effects). Products include:
   Aramine Injection 1649

Methadone Hydrochloride (Enhanced response to central nervous system depressants). Products include:
   Methadone Hydrochloride Oral Concentrate 2356
   Methadone Hydrochloride Oral Solution & Tablets 2357

Methohexital Sodium (Enhanced response to central nervous system depressants).
   No products indexed under this heading.

Methotrimeprazine (Co-administration with phenothiazines may increase the risk of seizures; enhanced response to central nervous system depressants). Products include:
   Levoprome 1321

Methoxamine Hydrochloride (Co-administration with sympathomimetics may result in possible additive atropine-like effects). Products include:
   Vasoxyl Injection 1169

Methoxyflurane (Enhanced response to central nervous system depressants).
   No products indexed under this heading.

Midazolam Hydrochloride (Co-administration with benzodiazepines may increase the risk of seizures, especially when the dosage of benzodiazepines is rapidly tapered; enhanced response to central nervous system depressants). Products include:
   Versed Injection 2324

Molindone Hydrochloride (Enhanced response to central nervous system depressants). Products include:
   Moban Tablets and Concentrate 1036

Morphine Sulfate (Enhanced response to central nervous system depressants). Products include:
   Astramorph/PF Injection, USP (Preservative-Free) 526
   Duramorph Injection 983
   Infumorph 200 and Infumorph 500 Sterile Solutions 985
   Kadian Capsules 2948
   MS Contin Tablets 2149
   MSIR 2152
   Oramorph SR (Morphine Sulfate Sustained Release Tablets) 2359
   RMS Suppositories CII 2766
   Roxanol 2365

Norepinephrine Bitartrate (Co-administration with sympathomimetics may result in possible additive atropine-like effects). Products include:
   Levophed Bitartrate Injection 2445

Opium Alkaloids (Enhanced response to central nervous system depressants).
   No products indexed under this heading.

Oxazepam (Co-administration with benzodiazepines may increase the risk of seizures, especially when the dosage of benzodiazepines is rapidly tapered; enhanced response to central nervous system depressants). Products include:
   Serax Capsules 2916
   Serax Tablets 2916

Oxybutynin Chloride (Co-administration with anticholinergics may result in possible additive atropine-like effects). Products include:
   Ditropan 1267

Oxycodone Hydrochloride (Enhanced response to central nervous system depressants). Products include:
   OxyContin Tablets 2163
   OxyIR Capsules 2167
   Percocet Tablets 955
   Percodan Tablets 955
   Percodan-Demi Tablets 956
   Roxicodone Tablets, Oral Solution & Intensol (Oxycodone) 2366
   Tylox Capsules 1593

Pentobarbital Sodium (Co-administration with certain barbiturates, hepatic enzyme inducers, may decrease the plasma levels of maprotiline; enhanced response to central nervous system depressants). Products include:
   Nembutal Sodium Capsules 440
   Nembutal Sodium Solution 442
   Nembutal Sodium Suppositories 444

Perphenazine (Co-administration with phenothiazines may increase the risk of seizures; enhanced response to central nervous system depressants). Products include:
   Etrafon 2495
   Triavil Tablets 1800
   Trilafon 2532

Phenelzine Sulfate (Concurrent and/or sequential use with MAO inhibitors is contraindicated). Products include:
   Nardil 1977

Phenobarbital (Co-administration with certain barbiturates, hepatic enzyme inducers, may decrease the plasma levels of maprotiline; enhanced response to central nervous system depressants). Products include:
   Arco-Lase Plus Tablets 513
   Bellergal-S Tablets 2375
   Donnatal 2234
   Donnatal Extentabs 2234
   Donnatal Tablets 2234
   Phenobarbital Elixir and Tablets 1523
   Quadrinal Tablets 1398

Phenylephrine Bitartrate (Co-administration with sympathomimetics may result in possible additive atropine-like effects).
   No products indexed under this heading.

Phenylephrine Hydrochloride (Co-administration with sympathomimetics may result in possible additive atropine-like effects). Products include:
   Atrohist Plus Tablets 1605
   Cerose DM 853
   D.A. II Tablets 972
   D.A. Chewable Tablets 970
   Dura-Vent/DA Tablets 972
   Extendryl 1003
   4-Way Fast Acting Nasal Spray (regular & mentholated) 644
   Hemorid 797
   Hycomine Compound Tablets 948
   Neo-Synephrine Hydrochloride 1% Carpuject 2455
   Neo-Synephrine Hydrochloride 1% Injection 2455
   Neo-Synephrine Hydrochloride (Ophthalmic) 2456
   Neo-Synephrine 624
   Novahistine Elixir 782
   Phenergan VC 2886
   Phenergan VC with Codeine 2888
   Preparation H 842
   Tympagesic Ear Drops 2476
   Vicks Sinex Nasal Spray and Ultra Fine Mist 738

Phenylephrine Tannate (Co-administration with sympathomimetics may result in possible additive atropine-like effects). Products include:
   Atrohist Pediatric Suspension 1604
   Atrohist Pediatric Suspension Dye-Free 1604
   Rynatan 2781
   Rynatuss 2782

IMPORTANT NOTE: Always consult each drug listing in the patient's regimen for possible interactions.

Phenylpropanolamine Hydrochloride (Co-administration with sympathomimetics may result in possible additive atropine-like effects). Products include:

Acutrim	▣ 648
Atrohist Plus Tablets	1605
BC Cold Powder Multi-Symptom Formula (Cold-Sinus-Allergy)	▣ 631
BC Cold Powder Non-Drowsy Formula (Cold-Sinus)	▣ 631
Cheracol Plus Head Cold/Cough Formula	▣ 741
Comtrex Multi-Symptom Cold Reliever Liqui-Gels	▣ 638
Comtrex Multi-Symptom Non-Drowsy Liqui-gels	▣ 640
Contac Continuous Action Nasal Decongestant/Antihistamine 12 Hour Capsules	▣ 773
Contac Maximum Strength Continuous Action Decongestant/Antihistamine 12 Hour Caplets	▣ 772
Contac Severe Cold and Flu Formula Caplets	▣ 773
Coricidin 'D' Decongestant Tablets	▣ 760
Dexatrim	795
Dexatrim Plus Vitamins Caplets	796
Dimetane-DC Cough Syrup	2232
Dimetapp Allergy Sinus Caplets	▣ 838
Dimetapp Cold & Allergy Chewable Tablets	▣ 838
Dimetapp Cold & Cough Liqui-Gels	▣ 839
Dimetapp DM Elixir	▣ 840
Dimetapp Elixir	▣ 840
Dimetapp Extentabs	▣ 841
Dimetapp Tablets/Liqui-Gels	▣ 841
Dura-Vent Tablets	971
Entex LA Tablets	972
Exgest LA Tablets	787
Hycomine	947
Nolamine Timed-Release Tablets	790
Ornade Spansule Capsules	2678
Propagest Tablets	791
Pyrroxate Caplets	742
Robitussin-CF	▣ 846
Sinulin Tablets	792
Tavist-D 12 Hour Relief Tablets	▣ 750
Teldrin 12 Hour Antihistamine/Nasal Decongestant Allergy Relief Capsules	▣ 786
Triaminic Expectorant	▣ 753
Triaminic Syrup	▣ 755
Triaminic Triaminicol Cold & Cough	▣ 756
Triaminic DM Syrup	▣ 756
Triaminicin Tablets	▣ 756
Vicks DayQuil Allergy Relief 12-Hour Extended Release Tablets	▣ 733
Vicks DayQuil Allergy Relief 4-Hour Tablets	▣ 733
Vicks DayQuil SINUS Pressure & CONGESTION Relief	▣ 734

Phenytoin (Co-administration with hepatic enzyme inhibitors, such as phenytoin, may decrease the plasma levels of maprotiline). Products include:

Dilantin Infatabs	1967
Dilantin-125 Suspension	1969

Phenytoin Sodium (Co-administration with hepatic enzyme inhibitors, such as phenytoin, may decrease the plasma levels of maprotiline). Products include:

Dilantin Kapseals	1965

Pirbuterol Acetate (Co-administration with sympathomimetics may result in possible additive atropine-like effects). Products include:

Maxair Autohaler	1550
Maxair Inhaler	1552

Prazepam (Co-administration with benzodiazepines may increase the risk of seizures, especially when the dosage of benzodiazepines is rapidly tapered; enhanced response to central nervous system depressants). No products indexed under this heading.

Prochlorperazine (Co-administration with phenothiazines may increase the risk of seizures; enhanced response to central nervous system depressants). Products include:

Compazine	2644

Procyclidine Hydrochloride (Co-administration with anticholinergics may result in possible additive atropine-like effects). Products include:

Kemadrin Tablets	1105

Promethazine Hydrochloride (Co-administration with phenothiazines may increase the risk of seizures; enhanced response to central nervous system depressants). Products include:

Mepergan Injection	2859
Phenergan with Codeine	2859
Phenergan with Dextromethorphan	2885
Phenergan Injection	2880
Phenergan Suppositories	2882
Phenergan Syrup	2881
Phenergan Tablets	2882
Phenergan VC	2886
Phenergan VC with Codeine	2888

Propantheline Bromide (Co-administration with anticholinergics may result in possible additive atropine-like effects). Products include:

Pro-Banthine Tablets	2226

Propofol (Enhanced response to central nervous system depressants). Products include:

Diprivan Injectable Emulsion	2939

Propoxyphene Hydrochloride (Enhanced response to central nervous system depressants). Products include:

Darvon	1475
Wygesic Tablets	2930

Propoxyphene Napsylate (Enhanced response to central nervous system depressants). Products include:

Darvon-N/Darvocet-N	1473

Pseudoephedrine Hydrochloride (Co-administration with sympathomimetics may result in possible additive atropine-like effects). Products include:

Actifed Allergy Daytime/Nighttime Caplets	▣ 808
Actifed Cold & Allergy Tablets	▣ 807
Actifed Cold & Sinus Caplets and Tablets	▣ 808
Actifed Sinus Daytime/Nighttime Tablets and Caplets	▣ 809
Advil Cold and Sinus Caplets and Tablets	▣ 837
Alka-Seltzer Plus Liqui-Gels	▣ 612
Alka-Seltzer Plus Flu & Body Aches Liqui-Gels Non-Drowsy Formula	▣ 613
Alka-Seltzer Plus Night-Time Cold Medicine Liqui-Gels	▣ 612
Allerest Maximum Strength	▣ 649
Allerest No Drowsiness	▣ 649
Allerest Sinus Pain Formula	▣ 649
Atrohist Pediatric Suspension	1603
Benadryl Allergy/Cold Tablets	▣ 811
Benadryl Allergy Decongestant Liquid Medication	▣ 812
Benadryl Allergy Decongestant Tablets	▣ 812
Benadryl Allergy Sinus Headache Caplets	▣ 813
Benylin Multisymptom	▣ 816
Bromfed Capsules (Extended-Release)	1832
Bromfed Syrup	▣ 712
Bromfed Tablets	1832
Bromfed-DM Cough Syrup	1832
Bromfed-PD Capsules (Extended-Release)	1832
Children's TYLENOL Cold Multi-Symptom Chewable Tablets and Liquid	1559
Children's TYLENOL Cold Plus Cough Multi Symptom Chewable Tablets and Liquid	1560
Children's TYLENOL Flu Suspension Liquid	1560
Children's Vicks DayQuil Allergy Relief	▣ 730
Children's Vicks NyQuil Cold/Cough Relief	▣ 731
Allergy-Sinus Comtrex Multi-Symptom Allergy-Sinus Formula Tablets and Caplets	▣ 639
Comtrex Multi-Symptom	▣ 638
Comtrex Multi-Symptom Non-Drowsy Caplets	▣ 640
Congess	1003
Contac Day Allergy/Sinus Caplets	▣ 771
Contac Day & Night	▣ 772
Contac Night Allergy/Sinus Caplets	▣ 771
Contac Severe Cold & Flu Non-Drowsy	▣ 774
Deconsal II Tablets	1605
Dimetane-DX Cough Syrup	2233
Dimetapp Cold & Fever Suspension	▣ 839
Dimetapp Decongestant Pediatric Drops	▣ 840
Dorcol Children's Cough Syrup	▣ 748
Drixoral Cough + Congestion Liquid Caps	▣ 763
Dura-Tap/PD Capsules	970
Duratuss Tablets	2750
Duratuss HD Elixir	2750
Efidac/24	655
Entex PSE Tablets	973
Fedahist Gyrocaps	2545
Guaifed	1833
Guaifed Syrup	▣ 712
Guaimax-D Tablets	809
Histussin D Liquid	670
Infants' TYLENOL Cold Decongestant & Fever-Reducer Drops	1561
Kronofed-A	994
Novahistine DMX	▣ 782
Nucofed	2225
PediaCare Cough-Cold Chewable Tablets and Liquid	1569
PediaCare Infants' Decongestant Drops	1569
PediaCare Infants' Drops Decongestant Plus Cough	1569
PediaCare NightRest Cough-Cold Liquid	1569
Pediatric Vicks 44d Cough & Head Congestion Relief	▣ 736
Pediatric Vicks 44m Cough & Cold Relief	▣ 737
Robitussin Cold & Cough Liqui-Gels	▣ 844
Robitussin Cold, Cough & Flu Liqui-Gels	▣ 844
Robitussin Maximum Strength Cough & Cold	▣ 847
Robitussin Night-Time Cold Formula	▣ 847
Robitussin Pediatric Cough & Cold Formula	▣ 848
Robitussin Pediatric Drops	▣ 849
Robitussin Severe Congestion Liqui-Gels	▣ 845
Robitussin-DAC Syrup	2249
Robitussin-PE	▣ 846
Rondec Oral Drops	974
Rondec Syrup	974
Rondec Tablet	974
Rondec Chewable Tablets	974
Rondec-TR Tablet	974
Ryna	804
Seldane-D Extended-Release Tablets	1286
Semprex-D Capsules	1620
Sinarest	663
Sine-Aid Maximum Strength Sinus Headache Gelcaps, Caplets and Tablets	1570
Sine-Off No Drowsiness Formula Caplets	784
Sine-Off Sinus Medicine	784
Singlet Tablets	785
Sinutab Non-Drying Liquid Caps	823
Sinutab Sinus Allergy Medication, Maximum Strength Tablets and Caplets	823
Sinutab Sinus Medication, Maximum Strength Without Drowsiness Formula, Tablets & Caplets	824
Sudafed Children's Cold & Cough Liquid Medication	825
Sudafed Children's Nasal Decongestant Liquid Medication	826
Sudafed Cold & Allergy Tablets	▣ 826
Sudafed Cold and Cough Liquid Caps	▣ 826
Sudafed Nasal Decongestant Tablets, 30 mg	▣ 825
Sudafed Nasal Decongestant Tablets, 60 mg	▣ 825
Sudafed Non-Drying Sinus Liquid Caps	▣ 827
Sudafed Pediatric Nasal Decongestant Liquid Oral Drops	▣ 827
Sudafed Severe Cold Formula Caplets	▣ 828
Sudafed Severe Cold Formula Tablets	▣ 828
Sudafed Sinus Caplets	▣ 829
Sudafed Sinus Tablets	▣ 829
Sudafed 12 Hour Caplets	▣ 824
Syn-Rx Tablets	1622
Syn-Rx DM Tablets	1623
TheraFlu Flu and Cold Medicine	▣ 750
TheraFlu Maximum Strength Flu and Cold Medicine For Sore Throat	▣ 751
TheraFlu Flu, Cold and Cough Medicine	▣ 750
TheraFlu Maximum Strength Nighttime Flu, Cold & Cough Medicine	▣ 751
TheraFlu Maximum Strength Non-Drowsy Formula Flu, Cold & Cough Medicine	▣ 751
TheraFlu Maximum Strength, Non-Drowsy Formula Flu, Cold and Cough Caplets	▣ 752
Theraflu Maximum Strength Sinus Non-Drowsy Formula Caplets	▣ 752
Triaminic AM Cough and Decongestant Formula	▣ 753
Triaminic AM Decongestant Formula	▣ 753
Triaminic Infant Oral Decongestant Drops	▣ 754
Triaminic Night Time	▣ 754
Triaminic Sore Throat Formula	▣ 755
Tussend	1830
Tussend Expectorant	1831
TYLENOL Allergy Sinus, Maximum Strength Caplets and Gelcaps	1571
TYLENOL Allergy Sinus NightTime, Maximum Strength Caplets	1571
TYLENOL Cold Medication, Multi-Symptom Formula Tablets and Caplets	1572
TYLENOL Cold Medication, Multi-Symptom Hot Liquid Packets	1572
TYLENOL Cold Medication, No Drowsiness Formula Caplets and Gelcaps	1572
TYLENOL Cold Severe Congestion Caplets	1573
TYLENOL Cough Medication with Decongestant, Multi Symptom	1574
TYLENOL Flu No Drowsiness Formula, Maximum Strength Gelcaps	1575
TYLENOL Flu NightTime, Maximum Strength Gelcaps	1575
TYLENOL Flu NightTime, Maximum Strength Hot Medication Packets	1575
TYLENOL Sinus, Maximum Strength Geltabs, Gelcaps, Caplets and Tablets	1576
Vicks 44 LiquiCaps Cough, Cold & Flu Relief	▣ 728
Vicks 44 LiquiCaps Non-Drowsy Cough & Cold Relief	▣ 729
Vicks 44D Cough & Head Congestion Relief	▣ 728
Vicks 44M Cough, Cold & Flu Relief	▣ 729
Vicks DayQuil LiquiCaps/Liquid Multi-Symptom Cold/Flu Relief	▣ 734
Vicks DayQuil SINUS Pressure & PAIN Relief with IBUPROFEN	▣ 735
Vicks Nyquil Hot Therapy	▣ 735
Vicks NyQuil LiquiCaps/Liquid Multi-Symptom Cold/Flu Relief, Original and Cherry Flavors	▣ 736

Pseudoephedrine Sulfate (Co-administration with sympathomimetics may result in possible additive atropine-like effects). Products include:

Chlor-Trimeton Allergy Decongestant Tablets	▣ 759
Claritin-D Tablets	2487
Drixoral Cold and Allergy Sustained-Action Tablets	▣ 763
Drixoral Cold and Flu Extended-Release Tablets	▣ 764

(▣ Described in PDR For Nonprescription Drugs)   (⊚ Described in PDR For Ophthalmology)

Drixoral Non-Drowsy Formula Extended-Release Tablets 764
Drixoral Allergy/Sinus Extended Release Tablets 765
Trinalin Repetabs Tablets 1373

Quazepam (Co-administration with benzodiazepines may increase the risk of seizures, especially when the dosage of benzodiazepines is rapidly tapered; enhanced response to central nervous system depressants). Products include:
Doral Tablets 2773

Risperidone (Enhanced response to central nervous system depressants). Products include:
Risperdal Tablets 1348

Salmeterol Xinafoate (Co-administration with sympathomimetics may result in possible additive atropine-like effects). Products include:
Serevent Inhalation Aerosol 1149

Scopolamine (Co-administration with anticholinergics may result in possible additive atropine-like effects). Products include:
Transderm Scōp Transdermal Therapeutic System 890

Scopolamine Hydrobromide (Co-administration with anticholinergics may result in possible additive atropine-like effects). Products include:
Atrohist Plus Tablets 1605
Donnatal 2234
Donnatal Extentabs 2234
Donnatal Tablets 2234

Secobarbital Sodium (Co-administration with certain barbiturates, hepatic enzyme inducers, may decrease the plasma levels of maprotiline; enhanced response to central nervous system depressants). Products include:
Seconal Sodium Pulvules 1529

Selegiline Hydrochloride (Concurrent and/or sequential use with MAO inhibitors is contraindicated). Products include:
Eldepryl Capsules 2729

Sevoflurane (Enhanced response to central nervous system depressants).
No products indexed under this heading.

Sufentanil Citrate (Enhanced response to central nervous system depressants). Products include:
Sufenta Injection 1355

Temazepam (Co-administration with benzodiazepines may increase the risk of seizures, especially when the dosage of benzodiazepines is rapidly tapered; enhanced response to central nervous system depressants). Products include:
Restoril Capsules 2413

Terbutaline Sulfate (Co-administration with sympathomimetics may result in possible additive atropine-like effects). Products include:
Brethaire Inhaler 830
Brethine Ampuls 832
Brethine Tablets 831
Bricanyl Subcutaneous Injection 1247
Bricanyl Tablets 1248

Thiamylal Sodium (Co-administration with certain barbiturates, hepatic enzyme inducers, may decrease the plasma levels of maprotiline; enhanced response to central nervous system depressants).
No products indexed under this heading.

Thioridazine Hydrochloride (Co-administration with phenothiazines may increase the risk of seizures; enhanced response to central nervous system depressants). Products include:
Mellaril 2398

Thiothixene (Enhanced response to central nervous system depressants). Products include:
Navane Capsules and Concentrate 2018
Navane Intramuscular 2019

Thyroglobulin (Co-administration in patients with hyperthyroidism or those on thyroid drugs may result in possibility of enhanced cardiovascular toxicity of maprotiline).
No products indexed under this heading.

Thyroid (Co-administration in patients with hyperthyroidism or those on thyroid drugs may result in possibility of enhanced cardiovascular toxicity of maprotiline).
No products indexed under this heading.

Thyroxine (Co-administration in patients with hyperthyroidism or those on thyroid drugs may result in possibility of enhanced cardiovascular toxicity of maprotiline).
No products indexed under this heading.

Thyroxine Sodium (Co-administration in patients with hyperthyroidism or those on thyroid drugs may result in possibility of enhanced cardiovascular toxicity of maprotiline).
No products indexed under this heading.

Tranylcypromine Sulfate (Concurrent and/or sequential use with MAO inhibitors is contraindicated). Products include:
Parnate Tablets 2679

Triazolam (Co-administration with benzodiazepines may increase the risk of seizures, especially when the dosage of benzodiazepines is rapidly tapered; enhanced response to central nervous system depressants). Products include:
Halcion Tablets 2093

Tridihexethyl Chloride (Co-administration with anticholinergics may result in possible additive atropine-like effects).
No products indexed under this heading.

Trifluoperazine Hydrochloride (Co-administration with phenothiazines may increase the risk of seizures; enhanced response to central nervous system depressants). Products include:
Stelazine 2692

Trihexyphenidyl Hydrochloride (Co-administration with anticholinergics may result in possible additive atropine-like effects). Products include:
Artane 1418

Zolpidem Tartrate (Enhanced response to central nervous system depressants). Products include:
Ambien Tablets 2559

Food Interactions

Alcohol (Enhanced response to central nervous system depressants).

LUFYLLIN & LUFYLLIN-400 TABLETS
(Dyphylline) 2778
May interact with sympathomimetic bronchodilators and certain other agents. Compounds in these categories include:

Albuterol (Co-administration with sympathomimetic bronchodilators has been reported to produce synergism). Products include:
Proventil Inhalation Aerosol 2524
Ventolin Inhalation Aerosol and Refill 1170

Albuterol Sulfate (Co-administration with sympathomimetic bronchodilators has been reported to produce synergism). Products include:
Airet Albuterol Sulfate Inhalation Solution 1602
Albuterol Sulfate, USP Solution for Inhalation, Arm-a-Med 522
Proventil Inhalation Solution 0.083% 2527
Proventil Repetabs Tablets 2529
Proventil Solution for Inhalation 0.5% 2525
Proventil Syrup 2528
Proventil Tablets 2529
Ventolin Inhalation Solution 1171
Ventolin Nebules Inhalation Solution 1172
Ventolin Rotacaps for Inhalation 1173
Ventolin Syrup 1175
Ventolin Tablets 1176
Volmax Extended-Release Tablets .. 1835

Bitolterol Mesylate (Co-administration with sympathomimetic bronchodilators has been reported to produce synergism). Products include:
Tornalate Solution for Inhalation, 0.2% 976
Tornalate Metered Dose Inhaler 978

Ephedrine Hydrochloride (Co-administration with sympathomimetic bronchodilators has been reported to produce synergism). Products include:
Primatene Tablets 844
Quadrinal Tablets 1398

Ephedrine Sulfate (Co-administration with sympathomimetic bronchodilators has been reported to produce synergism). Products include:
Marax Tablets & DF Syrup 2015

Ephedrine Tannate (Co-administration with sympathomimetic bronchodilators has been reported to produce synergism). Products include:
Rynatuss 2782

Epinephrine (Co-administration with sympathomimetic bronchodilators has been reported to produce synergism). Products include:
EPIFRIN 237
EpiPen 808
Marcaine with Epinephrine 2446
Primatene Mist 843
Sensorcaine with Epinephrine Injection 554
Sus-Phrine Injection 1017
Xylocaine with Epinephrine Injections 562

Epinephrine Hydrochloride (Co-administration with sympathomimetic bronchodilators has been reported to produce synergism). Products include:
Ana-Kit Anaphylaxis Emergency Treatment Kit 611

Ethylnorepinephrine Hydrochloride (Co-administration with sympathomimetic bronchodilators has been reported to produce synergism).
No products indexed under this heading.

Isoetharine (Co-administration with sympathomimetic bronchodilators has been reported to produce synergism). Products include:
Bronkometer Aerosol 2432
Bronkosol Solution 2432

Isoetharine Inhalation Solution, USP, Arm-a-Med 545

Isoproterenol Hydrochloride (Co-administration with sympathomimetic bronchodilators has been reported to produce synergism). Products include:
Isuprel Hydrochloride Solution 2443
Isuprel Injection 2441
Isuprel Mistometer 2442

Isoproterenol Sulfate (Co-administration with sympathomimetic bronchodilators has been reported to produce synergism). Products include:
Norisodrine with Calcium Iodide Syrup 446

Metaproterenol Sulfate (Co-administration with sympathomimetic bronchodilators has been reported to produce synergism). Products include:
Alupent 672
Metaproterenol Sulfate Inhalation Solution, USP, Arm-a-Med 547

Pirbuterol Acetate (Co-administration with sympathomimetic bronchodilators has been reported to produce synergism). Products include:
Maxair Autohaler 1550
Maxair Inhaler 1552

Probenecid (Concurrent use with probenecid, which competes for tubular secretion, has shown to increase plasma half-life of dyphylline). Products include:
Benemid Tablets 1651
ColBENEMID Tablets 1662

Salmeterol Xinafoate (Co-administration with sympathomimetic bronchodilators has been reported to produce synergism). Products include:
Serevent Inhalation Aerosol 1149

Terbutaline Sulfate (Co-administration with sympathomimetic bronchodilators has been reported to produce synergism). Products include:
Brethaire Inhaler 830
Brethine Ampuls 832
Brethine Tablets 831
Bricanyl Subcutaneous Injection 1247
Bricanyl Tablets 1248

LUFYLLIN-GG ELIXIR & TABLETS
(Dyphylline, Guaifenesin) 2779
May interact with sympathomimetic bronchodilators and certain other agents. Compounds in these categories include:

Albuterol (Co-administration with sympathomimetic bronchodilators has been reported to produce synergism). Products include:
Proventil Inhalation Aerosol 2524
Ventolin Inhalation Aerosol and Refill 1170

Albuterol Sulfate (Co-administration with sympathomimetic bronchodilators has been reported to produce synergism). Products include:
Airet Albuterol Sulfate Inhalation Solution 1602
Albuterol Sulfate, USP Solution for Inhalation, Arm-a-Med 522
Proventil Inhalation Solution 0.083% 2527
Proventil Repetabs Tablets 2529
Proventil Solution for Inhalation 0.5% 2525
Proventil Syrup 2528
Proventil Tablets 2529
Ventolin Inhalation Solution 1171
Ventolin Nebules Inhalation Solution 1172
Ventolin Rotacaps for Inhalation 1173
Ventolin Syrup 1175
Ventolin Tablets 1176

IMPORTANT NOTE: Always consult each drug listing in the patient's regimen for possible interactions.

Lufyllin-GG / Interactions Index

Volmax Extended-Release Tablets .. 1835

Bitolterol Mesylate (Co-administration with sympathomimetic bronchodilators has been reported to produce synergism). Products include:
- Tornalate Solution for Inhalation, 0.2% 976
- Tornalate Metered Dose Inhaler 978

Ephedrine Hydrochloride (Co-administration with sympathomimetic bronchodilators has been reported to produce synergism). Products include:
- Primatene Tablets 844
- Quadrinal Tablets 1398

Ephedrine Sulfate (Co-administration with sympathomimetic bronchodilators has been reported to produce synergism). Products include:
- Marax Tablets & DF Syrup 2015

Ephedrine Tannate (Co-administration with sympathomimetic bronchodilators has been reported to produce synergism). Products include:
- Rynatuss 2782

Epinephrine (Co-administration with sympathomimetic bronchodilators has been reported to produce synergism). Products include:
- EPIFRIN 237
- EpiPen 808
- Marcaine with Epinephrine 2446
- Primatene Mist 843
- Sensorcaine with Epinephrine Injection 554
- Sus-Phrine Injection 1017
- Xylocaine with Epinephrine Injections 562

Epinephrine Hydrochloride (Co-administration with sympathomimetic bronchodilators has been reported to produce synergism). Products include:
- Ana-Kit Anaphylaxis Emergency Treatment Kit 611

Ethylnorepinephrine Hydrochloride (Co-administration with sympathomimetic bronchodilators has been reported to produce synergism).
No products indexed under this heading.

Isoetharine (Co-administration with sympathomimetic bronchodilators has been reported to produce synergism). Products include:
- Bronkometer Aerosol 2432
- Bronkosol Solution 2432
- Isoetharine Inhalation Solution, USP, Arm-a-Med 545

Isoproterenol Hydrochloride (Co-administration with sympathomimetic bronchodilators has been reported to produce synergism). Products include:
- Isuprel Hydrochloride Solution 2443
- Isuprel Injection 2441
- Isuprel Mistometer 2442

Isoproterenol Sulfate (Co-administration with sympathomimetic bronchodilators has been reported to produce synergism). Products include:
- Norisodrine with Calcium Iodide Syrup 446

Metaproterenol Sulfate (Co-administration with sympathomimetic bronchodilators has been reported to produce synergism). Products include:
- Alupent 672
- Metaproterenol Sulfate Inhalation Solution, USP, Arm-a-Med 547

Pirbuterol Acetate (Co-administration with sympathomimetic bronchodilators has been reported to produce synergism). Products include:
- Maxair Autohaler 1550
- Maxair Inhaler 1552

Probenecid (Concurrent use with probenecid, which competes for tubular secretion, has shown to increase plasma half-life of dyphylline). Products include:
- Benemid Tablets 1651
- ColBENEMID Tablets 1662

Salmeterol Xinafoate (Co-administration with sympathomimetic bronchodilators has been reported to produce synergism). Products include:
- Serevent Inhalation Aerosol 1149

Terbutaline Sulfate (Co-administration with sympathomimetic bronchodilators has been reported to produce synergism). Products include:
- Brethaire Inhaler 830
- Brethine Ampuls 832
- Brethine Tablets 831
- Bricanyl Subcutaneous Injection 1247
- Bricanyl Tablets 1248

LUMITENE
(Beta Carotene) 799
May interact with:

Vitamin A (Concurrent use with Vitamin A is not recommended). Products include:
- Aquasol A Vitamin A Capsules, USP 525
- Aquasol A Parenteral 526
- Breath + Plus 603
- Materna Tablets 1427
- Megadose 513
- One-A-Day Antioxidant Plus 625

LUPRON DEPOT 3.75 MG
(Leuprolide Acetate) 2739
None cited in PDR database.

LUPRON DEPOT 7.5 MG
(Leuprolide Acetate) 2741
None cited in PDR database.

LUPRON DEPOT - 3 MONTH 22.5 MG
(Leuprolide Acetate) 2743
None cited in PDR database.

LUPRON DEPOT-PED 7.5 MG, 11.25 MG AND 15 MG
(Leuprolide Acetate) 2744
None cited in PDR database.

LUPRON INJECTION
(Leuprolide Acetate) 2736
None cited in PDR database.

LUPRON INJECTION PEDIATRIC
(Leuprolide Acetate) 2737
None cited in PDR database.

LURIDE DROPS 50 ML
(Sodium Fluoride) 891

Food Interactions
Dairy products (Incompatibility of fluoride with dairy).

LURIDE LOZI-TABS TABLETS
(Sodium Fluoride) 892

Food Interactions
Dairy products (Incompatibility of fluoride with dairy foods results in the formation of poorly absorbed calcium fluoride).

LURLINE PMS TABLETS
(Acetaminophen, Pamabrom) 1000
None cited in PDR database.

LUTREPULSE FOR INJECTION
(Gonadorelin Acetate) 998
May interact with ovulation stimulators. Compounds in this category include:

Chorionic Gonadotropin (Lutrepulse should not be used concomitantly with other ovulation stimulators). Products include:
- Pregnyl for Injection 1878
- Profasi (chorionic gonadotropin for injection, USP) 2620

Clomiphene Citrate (Lutrepulse should not be used concomitantly with other ovulation stimulators). Products include:
- Clomid 1262
- Serophene (clomiphene citrate tablets, USP) 2621

Menotropins (Lutrepulse should not be used concomitantly with other ovulation stimulators). Products include:
- Humegon for Injection 1873
- Pergonal (menotropins for injection, USP) 2618

Urofollitropin (Lutrepulse should not be used concomitantly with other ovulation stimulators). Products include:
- Metrodin (urofollitropin for injection) 2616

LUVOX TABLETS
(Fluvoxamine Maleate) 2723
May interact with monoamine oxidase inhibitors, benzodiazepines metabolized by hepatic oxidation, benzodiazepines metabolized by glucuronidation, xanthine bronchodilators, lithium preparations, tricyclic antidepressants, and certain other agents. Compounds in these categories include:

Alprazolam (Co-administration may result in reduced alprazolam clearance, pharmacokinetic parameters (AUC, C_{max}, $T_{½}$) and steady state plasma concentrations of alprazolam are twice those observed when alprazolam was used alone). Products include:
- Xanax Tablets 2115

Aminophylline (Decreased clearance of theophylline by approximately 3-fold; dose of theophylline should be reduced to one-third of the usual daily dose).
No products indexed under this heading.

Amitriptyline Hydrochloride (Potential for increased plasma tricyclic antidepressants levels). Products include:
- Elavil 2945
- Etrafon 2495
- Limbitrol 2333
- Triavil Tablets 1800

Amoxapine (Potential for increased plasma tricyclic antidepressants levels). Products include:
- Asendin Tablets 1419

Astemizole (Fluvoxamine may be a potent inhibitor of P450IIIA4, co-administration may lead to the potential for QT prolongation and torsade de pointes-type ventricular tachycardia; concurrent use is contraindicated). Products include:
- Hismanal Tablets 1341

Carbamazepine (Elevated plasma carbamazepine levels and symptoms of toxicity). Products include:
- Atretol Tablets 569
- Tegretol/Tegretol-XR 870

Chlordiazepoxide (Potential for reduced clearance of benzodiazepines metabolized by hepatic oxidation). Products include:
- Limbitrol 2333

Chlordiazepoxide Hydrochloride (Potential for reduced clearance of benzodiazepines metabolized by hepatic oxidation). Products include:
- Librax Capsules 2330
- Librium Capsules 2331
- Librium Injectable 2332

Cisapride (Fluvoxamine may be a potent inhibitor of P450IIIA4, co-administration may lead to the potential for QT prolongation and torsade de pointes-type ventricular tachycardia; concurrent use is contraindicated). Products include:
- Propulsid 1346

Clomipramine Hydrochloride (Potential for increased plasma tricyclic antidepressants levels). Products include:
- Anafranil Capsules 819

Clozapine (Elevated serum levels of clozapine). Products include:
- Clozaril Tablets 2377

Desipramine Hydrochloride (Potential for increased plasma tricyclic antidepressants levels). Products include:
- Norpramin Tablets 1273

Diazepam (Reduced clearance of both diazepam and its active metabolite; co-administration is not advisable). Products include:
- Dizac (diazepam injectable emulsion) CIV 1862
- Valium Injectable 2336
- Valium Tablets 2335

Diltiazem Hydrochloride (Co-administration may produce bradycardia). Products include:
- Cardizem CD Capsules 1251
- Cardizem SR Capsules 1255
- Cardizem Injectable 1253
- Cardizem Tablets 1257
- Dilacor XR Extended-release Capsules 2183
- Tiazac Capsules 1019

Doxepin Hydrochloride (Potential for increased plasma tricyclic antidepressants levels). Products include:
- Adapin Capsules 1542
- Sinequan 2028
- Zonalon Cream 1042

Dyphylline (Decreased clearance of theophylline by approximately 3-fold; dose of theophylline should be reduced to one-third of the usual daily dose). Products include:
- Lufyllin & Lufyllin-400 Tablets 2778
- Lufyllin-GG Elixir & Tablets 2779

Estazolam (Potential for reduced clearance of benzodiazepines metabolized by hepatic oxidation). Products include:
- ProSom Tablets 457

Flurazepam Hydrochloride (Potential for reduced clearance of benzodiazepines metabolized by hepatic oxidation). Products include:
- Dalmane Capsules 2329

Furazolidone (Co-administration of another serotonin reuptake inhibitor and MAO inhibitors has resulted in serious, sometimes fatal, reactions including hyperthermia, rigidity, extreme agitation, delirium, and coma; concurrent and/or sequential use of Luvox and an MAOI is not recommended). Products include:
- Furoxone 2221

(▣ Described in PDR For Nonprescription Drugs) (◉ Described in PDR For Ophthalmology)

Halazepam (Potential for reduced clearance of benzodiazepines metabolized by hepatic oxidation).
   No products indexed under this heading.

Imipramine Hydrochloride (Potential for increased plasma tricyclic antidepressants levels). Products include:
   Tofranil Ampuls 873
   Tofranil Tablets 875

Imipramine Pamoate (Potential for increased plasma tricyclic antidepressants levels). Products include:
   Tofranil-PM Capsules 876

Isocarboxazid (Co-administration of another serotonin reuptake inhibitor and MAO inhibitors has resulted in serious, sometimes fatal, reactions including hyperthermia, rigidity, extreme agitation, delirium, and coma; concurrent and/or sequential use of Luvox and an MAOI is not recommended).
   No products indexed under this heading.

Ketoconazole (Caution is advised if used concurrently with inhibitor of P450IIIA4, such as ketoconazole). Products include:
   Nizoral 2% Cream 1344
   Nizoral 2% Shampoo 1344
   Nizoral Tablets 1345

Lithium Carbonate (Co-administration has resulted in seizures; lithium may enhance the serotonergic effects of fluvoxamine). Products include:
   Eskalith 2658
   Lithium Carbonate Capsules & Tablets 2352
   Lithonate/Lithotabs/Lithobid 2721

Lithium Citrate (Co-administration has resulted in seizures; lithium may enhance the serotonergic effects of fluvoxamine).
   No products indexed under this heading.

Lorazepam (Possible substantial decrements in cognitive functioning; the clearance of benzodiazepines metabolized by glucuronidation is unlikely to be affected). Products include:
   Ativan Injection 2805
   Ativan Tablets 2807

Maprotiline Hydrochloride (Potential for increased plasma tricyclic antidepressants levels). Products include:
   Ludiomil Tablets 861

Methadone Hydrochloride (Significantly increased methadone (plasma level:dose) ratios). Products include:
   Methadone Hydrochloride Oral Concentrate 2356
   Methadone Hydrochloride Oral Solution & Tablets 2357

Metoprolol Succinate (Potential for bradycardia, hypotension and orthostatic hypotension). Products include:
   Toprol-XL Tablets 560

Metoprolol Tartrate (Potential for bradycardia, hypotension and orthostatic hypotension). Products include:
   Lopressor 848
   Lopressor HCT Tablets 850

Midazolam Hydrochloride (Potential for reduced clearance of benzodiazepines metabolized by hepatic oxidation). Products include:
   Versed Injection 2324

Nortriptyline Hydrochloride (Potential for increased plasma tricyclic antidepressants levels). Products include:
   Pamelor 2409

Oxazepam (The clearance of benzodiazepines metabolized by glucuronidation is unlikely to be affected). Products include:
   Serax Capsules 2916
   Serax Tablets 2916

Phenelzine Sulfate (Co-administration of another serotonin reuptake inhibitor and MAO inhibitors has resulted in serious, sometimes fatal, reactions including hyperthermia, rigidity, extreme agitation, delirium, and coma; concurrent and/or sequential use of Luvox and an MAOI is not recommended). Products include:
   Nardil 1977

Propranolol Hydrochloride (Potential for five-fold increase in minimum propranolol plasma concentrations; slight potentiation of the propranolol-induced reduction in heart rate and reduction in the exercise diastolic pressure). Products include:
   Inderal 2834
   Inderal LA Long Acting Capsules ... 2836
   Inderide Tablets 2838
   Inderide LA Long Acting Capsules .. 2840

Protriptyline Hydrochloride (Potential for increased plasma tricyclic antidepressants levels). Products include:
   Vivactil Tablets 1820

Quazepam (Potential for reduced clearance of benzodiazepines metabolized by hepatic oxidation). Products include:
   Doral Tablets 2773

Quinidine Gluconate (Fluvoxamine is metabolized, at least in part, by P450IID6 isoenzyme; caution is indicated in patients receiving known inhibitor, such as quinidine, of this isoenzyme). Products include:
   Quinaglute Dura-Tabs Tablets 644

Quinidine Polygalacturonate (Fluvoxamine is metabolized, at least in part, by P450IID6 isoenzyme; caution is indicated in patients receiving known inhibitor, such as quinidine, of this isoenzyme). Products include:
   Cardioquin Tablets 2146

Quinidine Sulfate (Fluvoxamine is metabolized, at least in part, by P450IID6 isoenzyme; caution is indicated in patients receiving known inhibitor, such as quinidine, of this isoenzyme). Products include:
   Quinidex Extentabs 2240

Selegiline Hydrochloride (Co-administration of another serotonin reuptake inhibitor and MAO inhibitors has resulted in serious, sometimes fatal, reactions including hyperthermia, rigidity, extreme agitation, delirium, and coma; concurrent and/or sequential use of Luvox and an MAOI is not recommended). Products include:
   Eldepryl Capsules 2729

Temazepam (The clearance of benzodiazepines metabolized by glucuronidation is unlikely to be affected). Products include:
   Restoril Capsules 2413

Terfenadine (Fluvoxamine may be a potent inhibitor of P450IIIA4, co-administration may lead to the potential for QT prolongation and torsade de pointes-type ventricular tachycardia; concurrent use is contraindicated). Products include:
   Seldane Tablets 1284
   Seldane-D Extended-Release Tablets 1286

Theophylline (Decreased clearance of theophylline by approximately 3-fold; dose of theophylline should be reduced to one-third of the usual daily dose). Products include:
   Marax Tablets & DF Syrup 2015
   Quibron 2227

Theophylline Anhydrous (Decreased clearance of theophylline by approximately 3-fold; dose of theophylline should be reduced to one-third of the usual daily dose). Products include:
   Aerolate 1003
   Primatene Tablets 844
   Respbid Tablets 687
   Slo-bid Gyrocaps 2201
   Theo-24 Extended Release Capsules 2753
   Theo-Dur Extended-Release Tablets 1367
   Theo-X Extended-Release Tablets .. 793
   Uni-Dur Extended-Release Tablets.. 1374
   Uniphyl 400 mg and 600 mg Tablets 2157

Theophylline Calcium Salicylate (Decreased clearance of theophylline by approximately 3-fold; dose of theophylline should be reduced to one-third of the usual daily dose). Products include:
   Quadrinal Tablets 1398

Theophylline Sodium Glycinate (Decreased clearance of theophylline by approximately 3-fold; dose of theophylline should be reduced to one-third of the usual daily dose).
   No products indexed under this heading.

Tranylcypromine Sulfate (Co-administration of another serotonin reuptake inhibitor and MAO inhibitors has resulted in serious, sometimes fatal, reactions including hyperthermia, rigidity, extreme agitation, delirium, and coma; concurrent and/or sequential use of Luvox and an MAOI is not recommended). Products include:
   Parnate Tablets 2679

Triazolam (The clearance of benzodiazepines metabolized by glucuronidation is unlikely to be affected). Products include:
   Halcion Tablets 2093

Trimipramine Maleate (Potential for increased plasma tricyclic antidepressants levels). Products include:
   Surmontil Capsules 2917

L-Tryptophan (Enhances serotogenic effects; potential for severe vomiting).
   No products indexed under this heading.

Warfarin Sodium (Potential for increased plasma concentrations of warfarin and prolonged prothrombin time). Products include:
   Coumadin 941

Food Interactions
Alcohol (Concurrent use should be avoided).

LYSODREN TABLETS
(Mitotane) 707
May interact with oral anticoagulants. Compounds in this category include:

Dicumarol (Potential for accelerated metabolism of coumarin-type anticoagulants).
   No products indexed under this heading.

Warfarin Sodium (Mitotane has been reported to accelerate the metabolism of warfarin by enzyme induction, leading to an increase in dosage requirements for warfarin). Products include:
   Coumadin 941

MDR FITNESS TABS FOR MEN AND WOMEN
(Vitamins with Minerals) 1544
None cited in PDR database.

MICRHOGAM RH₀(D) IMMUNE GLOBULIN (HUMAN)
(Immune Globulin (Human)) 1902
None cited in PDR database.

M-M-R II
(Measles, Mumps & Rubella Virus Vaccine Live) 1730
May interact with immunosuppressive agents. Compounds in this category include:

Azathioprine (Concurrent administration is containdicated). Products include:
   Azathioprine Tablets 2349
   Imuran 1103

Cyclosporine (Concurrent administration is containdicated). Products include:
   Neoral 2405
   Sandimmune 2416

Immune Globulin (Human) (Concurrent administration is containdicated).
   No products indexed under this heading.

Immune Globulin Intravenous (Human) (Concurrent administration is containdicated).

Muromonab-CD3 (Concurrent administration is containdicated). Products include:
   Orthoclone OKT3 Sterile Solution .. 1892

Mycophenolate Mofetil (Concurrent administration is containdicated). Products include:
   CellCept Capsules 2265

Tacrolimus (Concurrent administration is containdicated). Products include:
   Prograf 1028

M-R-VAX II
(Measles & Rubella Virus Vaccine Live) 1732
May interact with immunosuppressive agents. Compounds in this category include:

Azathioprine (Concurrent administration is containdicated). Products include:
   Azathioprine Tablets 2349
   Imuran 1103

Cyclosporine (Concurrent administration is containdicated). Products include:
   Neoral 2405
   Sandimmune 2416

Immune Globulin (Human) (Concurrent administration is containdicated).
   No products indexed under this heading.

Immune Globulin Intravenous (Human) (Concurrent administration is containdicated).

IMPORTANT NOTE: Always consult each drug listing in the patient's regimen for possible interactions.

Muromonab-CD3 (Concurrent administration is contraindicated). Products include:
   Orthoclone OKT3 Sterile Solution .. 1892

Mycophenolate Mofetil (Concurrent administration is contraindicated). Products include:
   CellCept Capsules 2265

Tacrolimus (Concurrent administration is contraindicated). Products include:
   Prograf 1028

MS CONTIN TABLETS
(Morphine Sulfate) 2149
May interact with phenothiazines, general anesthetics, hypnotics and sedatives, tranquilizers, neuromuscular blocking agents, mixed agonist/antagonist opioid analgesics, central nervous system depressants, and certain other agents. Compounds in these categories include:

Alfentanil Hydrochloride (Profound sedation; coma; severe hypotension; respiratory depression). Products include:
   Alfenta Injection 1334

Alprazolam (Profound sedation; coma; severe hypotension; respiratory depression). Products include:
   Xanax Tablets 2115

Aprobarbital (Profound sedation; coma; severe hypotension; respiratory depression).
   No products indexed under this heading.

Atracurium Besylate (Increased respiratory depression). Products include:
   Tracrium Injection 1155

Buprenorphine (Mixed agonist/antagonist analgesics may reduce the analgesic effect or may precipitate withdrawal symptoms). Products include:
   Buprenex Injectable 2170

Buspirone Hydrochloride (Profound sedation; coma; severe hypotension; respiratory depression). Products include:
   BuSpar Tablets 738

Butabarbital (Profound sedation; coma; severe hypotension; respiratory depression).
   No products indexed under this heading.

Butalbital (Profound sedation; coma; severe hypotension; respiratory depression). Products include:
   Axocet Capsules 2469
   Esgic-plus Capsules 1012
   Esgic-plus Tablets 1012
   Fioricet Tablets 2386
   Fioricet with Codeine Capsules 2387
   Fiorinal Capsules 2388
   Fiorinal with Codeine Capsules 2390
   Fiorinal Tablets 2388
   Phrenilin 790
   Sedapap Tablets 50 mg/650 mg .. 1826

Butorphanol Tartrate (Mixed agonist/antagonist analgesics may reduce the analgesic effect or may precipitate withdrawal symptoms). Products include:
   Stadol 779

Chlordiazepoxide (Profound sedation; coma; severe hypotension; respiratory depression). Products include:
   Limbitrol 2333

Chlordiazepoxide Hydrochloride (Profound sedation; coma; severe hypotension; respiratory depression). Products include:
   Librax Capsules 2330
   Librium Capsules 2331
   Librium Injectable 2332

Chlorpromazine (Profound sedation; coma; severe hypotension; respiratory depression). Products include:
   Thorazine Suppositories 2701

Chlorpromazine Hydrochloride (Profound sedation; coma; severe hypotension; respiratory depression). Products include:
   Thorazine 2701

Chlorprothixene (Profound sedation; coma; severe hypotension; respiratory depression).
   No products indexed under this heading.

Chlorprothixene Hydrochloride (Profound sedation; coma; severe hypotension; respiratory depression).
   No products indexed under this heading.

Chlorprothixene Lactate (Profound sedation; coma; severe hypotension; respiratory depression).
   No products indexed under this heading.

Cisatracurium Besylate (Increased respiratory depression). Products include:
   Nimbex Injection 1131

Clorazepate Dipotassium (Profound sedation; coma; severe hypotension; respiratory depression). Products include:
   Tranxene 459

Clozapine (Profound sedation; coma; severe hypotension; respiratory depression). Products include:
   Clozaril Tablets 2377

Codeine Phosphate (Profound sedation; coma; severe hypotension; respiratory depression). Products include:
   Brontex 2130
   Dimetane-DC Cough Syrup 2232
   Fioricet with Codeine Capsules 2387
   Fiorinal with Codeine Capsules 2390
   Nucofed 2225
   Phenergan with Codeine 2883
   Phenergan VC with Codeine .. 2888
   Robitussin A-C Syrup 2248
   Robitussin-DAC Syrup 2249
   Ryna 804
   Soma Compound w/Codeine Tablets 2784
   Tylenol with Codeine 1592

Desflurane (Profound sedation; coma; severe hypotension; respiratory depression). Products include:
   Suprane (desflurane, USP) 1865

Dezocine (Profound sedation; coma; severe hypotension; respiratory depression). Products include:
   Dalgan Injection 529

Diazepam (Profound sedation; coma; severe hypotension; respiratory depression). Products include:
   Dizac (diazepam injectable emulsion) CIV 1862
   Valium Injectable 2336
   Valium Tablets 2335

Doxacurium Chloride (Increased respiratory depression). Products include:
   Nuromax Injection 1136

Droperidol (Profound sedation; coma; severe hypotension; respiratory depression). Products include:
   Inapsine Injection 462

Enflurane (Profound sedation; coma; severe hypotension; respiratory depression).
   No products indexed under this heading.

Estazolam (Profound sedation; coma; severe hypotension; respiratory depression). Products include:
   ProSom Tablets 457

Etchlorvynol (Profound sedation; coma; severe hypotension; respiratory depression). Products include:
   Placidyl Capsules 456

Ethinamate (Profound sedation; coma; severe hypotension; respiratory depression).
   No products indexed under this heading.

Fentanyl (Profound sedation; coma; severe hypotension; respiratory depression). Products include:
   Duragesic Transdermal System 1336

Fentanyl Citrate (Profound sedation; coma; severe hypotension; respiratory depression). Products include:
   Sublimaze Injection 463

Fluphenazine Decanoate (Profound sedation; coma; severe hypotension; respiratory depression). Products include:
   Prolixin Decanoate 510

Fluphenazine Enanthate (Profound sedation; coma; severe hypotension; respiratory depression). Products include:
   Prolixin Enanthate 510

Fluphenazine Hydrochloride (Profound sedation; coma; severe hypotension; respiratory depression). Products include:
   Prolixin 510

Flurazepam Hydrochloride (Profound sedation; coma; severe hypotension; respiratory depression). Products include:
   Dalmane Capsules 2329

Glutethimide (Profound sedation; coma; severe hypotension; respiratory depression).
   No products indexed under this heading.

Haloperidol (Profound sedation; coma; severe hypotension; respiratory depression). Products include:
   Haldol Injection, Tablets and Concentrate 1585

Haloperidol Decanoate (Profound sedation; coma; severe hypotension; respiratory depression). Products include:
   Haldol Decanoate 1587

Hydrocodone Bitartrate (Profound sedation; coma; severe hypotension; respiratory depression). Products include:
   Codiclear DH Syrup 808
   Duratuss HD Elixir 2750
   Histussin D Liquid 670
   Hycodan Tablets and Syrup ... 946
   Hycomine Compound Tablets 948
   Hycomine 947
   Hycotuss Expectorant Syrup 950
   Hydrocet Capsules 787
   Lorcet 10/650 Tablets 1016
   Lortab 2751
   Tussend 1830
   Tussend Expectorant 1831
   Vicodin Tablets 1404
   Vicodin ES Tablets 1405
   Vicodin HP Tablets 1403
   Vicodin Tuss Expectorant 1406
   Zydone Capsules 967

Hydrocodone Polistirex (Profound sedation; coma; severe hypotension; respiratory depression). Products include:
   Tussionex Pennkinetic Extended-Release Suspension 1624

Hydroxyzine Hydrochloride (Profound sedation; coma; severe hypotension; respiratory depression). Products include:
   Atarax Tablets & Syrup 1992
   Marax Tablets & DF Syrup 2015

   Vistaril Intramuscular Solution 2042

Isoflurane (Profound sedation; coma; severe hypotension; respiratory depression).
   No products indexed under this heading.

Ketamine Hydrochloride (Profound sedation; coma; severe hypotension; respiratory depression).
   No products indexed under this heading.

Levomethadyl Acetate Hydrochloride (Profound sedation; coma; severe hypotension; respiratory depression). Products include:
   Orlaam Oral Solution 2361

Levorphanol Tartrate (Profound sedation; coma; severe hypotension; respiratory depression). Products include:
   Levo-Dromoran 2297

Lorazepam (Profound sedation; coma; severe hypotension; respiratory depression). Products include:
   Ativan Injection 2805
   Ativan Tablets 2807

Loxapine Hydrochloride (Profound sedation; coma; severe hypotension; respiratory depression). Products include:
   Loxitane 1426

Loxapine Succinate (Profound sedation; coma; severe hypotension; respiratory depression). Products include:
   Loxitane Capsules 1426

Meperidine Hydrochloride (Profound sedation; coma; severe hypotension; respiratory depression). Products include:
   Demerol 2438
   Mepergan Injection 2859

Mephobarbital (Profound sedation; coma; severe hypotension; respiratory depression). Products include:
   Mebaral Tablets 2452

Meprobamate (Profound sedation; coma; severe hypotension; respiratory depression). Products include:
   Miltown Tablets 2780
   PMB 200 and PMB 400 2890

Mesoridazine Besylate (Profound sedation; coma; severe hypotension; respiratory depression). Products include:
   Serentil 689

Methadone Hydrochloride (Profound sedation; coma; severe hypotension; respiratory depression). Products include:
   Methadone Hydrochloride Oral Concentrate 2356
   Methadone Hydrochloride Oral Solution & Tablets 2357

Methohexital Sodium (Profound sedation; coma; severe hypotension; respiratory depression).
   No products indexed under this heading.

Methotrimeprazine (Profound sedation; coma; severe hypotension; respiratory depression). Products include:
   Levoprome 1321

Methoxyflurane (Profound sedation; coma; severe hypotension; respiratory depression).
   No products indexed under this heading.

Metocurine Iodide (Increased respiratory depression). Products include:
   Metubine Iodide Vials 932

(▣ Described in PDR For Nonprescription Drugs)   (⊚ Described in PDR For Ophthalmology)

Midazolam Hydrochloride (Profound sedation; coma; severe hypotension; respiratory depression). Products include:
Versed Injection 2324

Mivacurium Chloride (Increased respiratory depression). Products include:
Mivacron 1125

Molindone Hydrochloride (Profound sedation; coma; severe hypotension; respiratory depression). Products include:
Moban Tablets and Concentrate 1036

Nalbuphine Hydrochloride (Mixed agonist/antagonist analgesics may reduce the analgesic effect or may precipitate withdrawal symptoms). Products include:
Nubain Injection 952

Opium Alkaloids (Profound sedation; coma; severe hypotension; respiratory depression).
No products indexed under this heading.

Oxazepam (Profound sedation; coma; severe hypotension; respiratory depression). Products include:
Serax Capsules 2916
Serax Tablets 2916

Oxycodone Hydrochloride (Profound sedation; coma; severe hypotension; respiratory depression). Products include:
OxyContin Tablets 2163
OxyIR Capsules 2167
Percocet Tablets 955
Percodan Tablets 955
Percodan-Demi Tablets 956
Roxicodone Tablets, Oral Solution & Intensol (Oxycodone) 2366
Tylox Capsules 1593

Pancuronium Bromide (Increased respiratory depression).
No products indexed under this heading.

Pentazocine Hydrochloride (Mixed agonist/antagonist analgesics may reduce the analgesic effect or may precipitate withdrawal symptoms). Products include:
Talacen Caplets 2464
Talwin Compound 2466
Talwin Nx Tablets 2467

Pentazocine Lactate (Mixed agonist/antagonist analgesics may reduce the analgesic effect or may precipitate withdrawal symptoms). Products include:
Talwin Injection 2465

Pentobarbital Sodium (Profound sedation; coma; severe hypotension; respiratory depression). Products include:
Nembutal Sodium Capsules 440
Nembutal Sodium Solution 442
Nembutal Sodium Suppositories 444

Perphenazine (Profound sedation; coma; severe hypotension; respiratory depression). Products include:
Etrafon 2495
Triavil Tablets 1800
Trilafon 2532

Phenobarbital (Profound sedation; coma; severe hypotension; respiratory depression). Products include:
Arco-Lase Plus Tablets 513
Bellergal-S Tablets 2375
Donnatal 2234
Donnatal Extentabs 2234
Donnatal Tablets 2234
Phenobarbital Elixir and Tablets 1523
Quadrinal Tablets 1398

Prazepam (Profound sedation; coma; severe hypotension; respiratory depression).
No products indexed under this heading.

Prochlorperazine (Profound sedation; coma; severe hypotension; respiratory depression). Products include:
Compazine 2644

Promethazine Hydrochloride (Profound sedation; coma; severe hypotension; respiratory depression). Products include:
Mepergan Injection 2859
Phenergan with Codeine 2883
Phenergan with Dextromethorphan 2885
Phenergan Injection 2880
Phenergan Suppositories 2882
Phenergan Syrup 2881
Phenergan Tablets 2882
Phenergan VC 2886
Phenergan VC with Codeine 2888

Propofol (Profound sedation; coma; severe hypotension; respiratory depression). Products include:
Diprivan Injectable Emulsion 2939

Propoxyphene Hydrochloride (Profound sedation; coma; severe hypotension; respiratory depression). Products include:
Darvon 1475
Wygesic Tablets 2930

Propoxyphene Napsylate (Profound sedation; coma; severe hypotension; respiratory depression). Products include:
Darvon-N/Darvocet-N 1473

Quazepam (Profound sedation; coma; severe hypotension; respiratory depression). Products include:
Doral Tablets 2773

Risperidone (Profound sedation; coma; severe hypotension; respiratory depression). Products include:
Risperdal Tablets 1348

Rocuronium Bromide (Increased respiratory depression). Products include:
Zemuron Injection 1885

Secobarbital Sodium (Profound sedation; coma; severe hypotension; respiratory depression). Products include:
Seconal Sodium Pulvules 1529

Sevoflurane (Profound sedation; coma; severe hypotension; respiratory depression).
No products indexed under this heading.

Succinylcholine Chloride (Increased respiratory depression). Products include:
Anectine 1062

Sufentanil Citrate (Profound sedation; coma; severe hypotension; respiratory depression). Products include:
Sufenta Injection 1355

Temazepam (Profound sedation; coma; severe hypotension; respiratory depression). Products include:
Restoril Capsules 2413

Thiamylal Sodium (Profound sedation; coma; severe hypotension; respiratory depression).
No products indexed under this heading.

Thioridazine Hydrochloride (Profound sedation; coma; severe hypotension; respiratory depression). Products include:
Mellaril 2398

Thiothixene (Profound sedation; coma; severe hypotension; respiratory depression). Products include:
Navane Capsules and Concentrate 2018
Navane Intramuscular 2019

Triazolam (Profound sedation; coma; severe hypotension; respiratory depression). Products include:
Halcion Tablets 2093

Trifluoperazine Hydrochloride (Profound sedation; coma; severe hypotension; respiratory depression). Products include:
Stelazine 2692

Vecuronium Bromide (Increased respiratory depression). Products include:
Norcuron for Injection 1875

Zolpidem Tartrate (Profound sedation; coma; severe hypotension; respiratory depression). Products include:
Ambien Tablets 2559

Food Interactions

Alcohol (Respiratory depression, hypotension and profound sedation or coma may result).

MSIR ORAL CAPSULES
(Morphine Sulfate)..................2152
See **MSIR Oral Solution**

MSIR ORAL SOLUTION
(Morphine Sulfate)..................2152
May interact with hypnotics and sedatives, general anesthetics, phenothiazines, tranquilizers, muscle relaxants, central nervous system depressants, and certain other agents. Compounds in these categories include:

Alfentanil Hydrochloride (Additive depressant effects; potential for respiratory depression, hypotension and profound sedation or coma; the dose of one or both agents should be reduced). Products include:
Alfenta Injection 1334

Alprazolam (Additive depressant effects; potential for respiratory depression, hypotension and profound sedation or coma; the dose of one or both agents should be reduced). Products include:
Xanax Tablets 2115

Aprobarbital (Additive depressant effects; potential for respiratory depression, hypotension and profound sedation or coma; the dose of one or both agents should be reduced).
No products indexed under this heading.

Atracurium Besylate (Increased respiratory depression). Products include:
Tracrium Injection 1155

Baclofen (Increased respiratory depression). Products include:
Lioresal Intrathecal 1634
Lioresal 847

Buprenorphine (Additive depressant effects; potential for respiratory depression, hypotension and profound sedation or coma; the dose of one or both agents should be reduced). Products include:
Buprenex Injectable 2170

Buspirone Hydrochloride (Additive depressant effects; potential for respiratory depression, hypotension and profound sedation or coma; the dose of one or both agents should be reduced). Products include:
BuSpar Tablets 738

Butabarbital (Additive depressant effects; potential for respiratory depression, hypotension and profound sedation or coma; the dose of one or both agents should be reduced).
No products indexed under this heading.

Butalbital (Additive depressant effects; potential for respiratory depression, hypotension and profound sedation or coma; the dose of one or both agents should be reduced). Products include:
Axocet Capsules 2469
Esgic-plus Capsules 1012
Esgic-plus Tablets 1012
Fioricet Tablets 2386
Fioricet with Codeine Capsules 2387
Fiorinal Capsules 2388
Fiorinal with Codeine Capsules 2390
Fiorinal Tablets 2388
Phrenilin 790
Sedapap Tablets 50 mg/650 mg 1826

Carisoprodol (Increased respiratory depression). Products include:
Soma Compound w/Codeine Tablets 2784
Soma Compound Tablets 2783
Soma Tablets 2782

Chlordiazepoxide (Additive depressant effects; potential for respiratory depression, hypotension and profound sedation or coma; the dose of one or both agents should be reduced). Products include:
Limbitrol 2333

Chlordiazepoxide Hydrochloride (Additive depressant effects; potential for respiratory depression, hypotension and profound sedation or coma; the dose of one or both agents should be reduced). Products include:
Librax Capsules 2330
Librium Capsules 2331
Librium Injectable 2332

Chlorpromazine (Additive depressant effects; potential for respiratory depression, hypotension and profound sedation or coma; the dose of one or both agents should be reduced). Products include:
Thorazine Suppositories 2701

Chlorpromazine Hydrochloride (Additive depressant effects; potential for respiratory depression, hypotension and profound sedation or coma; the dose of one or both agents should be reduced). Products include:
Thorazine 2701

Chlorprothixene (Additive depressant effects; potential for respiratory depression, hypotension and profound sedation or coma; the dose of one or both agents should be reduced).
No products indexed under this heading.

Chlorprothixene Hydrochloride (Additive depressant effects; potential for respiratory depression, hypotension and profound sedation or coma; the dose of one or both agents should be reduced).
No products indexed under this heading.

Chlorprothixene Lactate (Additive depressant effects; potential for respiratory depression, hypotension and profound sedation or coma; the dose of one or both agents should be reduced).
No products indexed under this heading.

Chlorzoxazone (Increased respiratory depression). Products include:
Parafon Forte DSC Caplets 1590

Cisatracurium Besylate (Increased respiratory depression). Products include:
Nimbex Injection 1131

IMPORTANT NOTE: Always consult each drug listing in the patient's regimen for possible interactions.

MSIR **Interactions Index** 638

Clorazepate Dipotassium (Additive depressant effects; potential for respiratory depression, hypotension and profound sedation or coma; the dose of one or both agents should be reduced). Products include:
- Tranxene 459

Clozapine (Additive depressant effects; potential for respiratory depression, hypotension and profound sedation or coma; the dose of one or both agents should be reduced). Products include:
- Clozaril Tablets 2377

Codeine Phosphate (Additive depressant effects; potential for respiratory depression, hypotension and profound sedation or coma; the dose of one or both agents should be reduced). Products include:
- Brontex 2130
- Dimetane-DC Cough Syrup 2232
- Fioricet with Codeine Capsules 2387
- Fiorinal with Codeine Capsules 2390
- Nucofed 2225
- Phenergan with Codeine 2883
- Phenergan VC with Codeine 2888
- Robitussin A-C Syrup 2248
- Robitussin-DAC Syrup 2249
- Ryna ⊞ 804
- Soma Compound w/Codeine Tablets 2784
- Tylenol with Codeine 1592

Cyclobenzaprine Hydrochloride (Increased respiratory depression). Products include:
- Flexeril Tablets 1701

Dantrolene Sodium (Increased respiratory depression). Products include:
- Dantrium Capsules 2131
- Dantrium Intravenous 2132

Desflurane (Additive depressant effects; potential for respiratory depression, hypotension and profound sedation or coma; the dose of one or both agents should be reduced). Products include:
- Suprane (desflurane, USP) 1865

Dezocine (Additive depressant effects; potential for respiratory depression, hypotension and profound sedation or coma; the dose of one or both agents should be reduced). Products include:
- Dalgan Injection 529

Diazepam (Additive depressant effects; potential for respiratory depression, hypotension and profound sedation or coma; the dose of one or both agents should be reduced). Products include:
- Dizac (diazepam injectable emulsion) CIV 1862
- Valium Injectable 2336
- Valium Tablets 2335

Doxacurium Chloride (Increased respiratory depression). Products include:
- Nuromax Injection 1136

Droperidol (Additive depressant effects; potential for respiratory depression, hypotension and profound sedation or coma; the dose of one or both agents should be reduced). Products include:
- Inapsine Injection 462

Enflurane (Additive depressant effects; potential for respiratory depression, hypotension and profound sedation or coma; the dose of one or both agents should be reduced).
- No products indexed under this heading.

Estazolam (Additive depressant effects; potential for respiratory depression, hypotension and profound sedation or coma; the dose of one or both agents should be reduced). Products include:
- ProSom Tablets 457

Ethchlorvynol (Additive depressant effects; potential for respiratory depression, hypotension and profound sedation or coma; the dose of one or both agents should be reduced). Products include:
- Placidyl Capsules 456

Ethinamate (Additive depressant effects; potential for respiratory depression, hypotension and profound sedation or coma; the dose of one or both agents should be reduced).
- No products indexed under this heading.

Fentanyl (Additive depressant effects; potential for respiratory depression, hypotension and profound sedation or coma; the dose of one or both agents should be reduced). Products include:
- Duragesic Transdermal System 1336

Fentanyl Citrate (Additive depressant effects; potential for respiratory depression, hypotension and profound sedation or coma; the dose of one or both agents should be reduced). Products include:
- Sublimaze Injection 463

Fluphenazine Decanoate (Additive depressant effects; potential for respiratory depression, hypotension and profound sedation or coma; the dose of one or both agents should be reduced). Products include:
- Prolixin Decanoate 510

Fluphenazine Enanthate (Additive depressant effects; potential for respiratory depression, hypotension and profound sedation or coma; the dose of one or both agents should be reduced). Products include:
- Prolixin Enanthate 510

Fluphenazine Hydrochloride (Additive depressant effects; potential for respiratory depression, hypotension and profound sedation or coma; the dose of one or both agents should be reduced). Products include:
- Prolixin 510

Flurazepam Hydrochloride (Additive depressant effects; potential for respiratory depression, hypotension and profound sedation or coma; the dose of one or both agents should be reduced). Products include:
- Dalmane Capsules 2329

Glutethimide (Additive depressant effects; potential for respiratory depression, hypotension and profound sedation or coma; the dose of one or both agents should be reduced).
- No products indexed under this heading.

Haloperidol (Additive depressant effects; potential for respiratory depression, hypotension and profound sedation or coma; the dose of one or both agents should be reduced). Products include:
- Haldol Injection, Tablets and Concentrate 1585

Haloperidol Decanoate (Additive depressant effects; potential for respiratory depression, hypotension and profound sedation or coma; the dose of one or both agents should be reduced). Products include:
- Haldol Decanoate 1587

Hydrocodone Bitartrate (Additive depressant effects; potential for respiratory depression, hypotension and profound sedation or coma; the dose of one or both agents should be reduced). Products include:
- Codiclear DH Syrup 808
- Duratuss HD Elixir 2750
- Histussin D Liquid 670
- Hycodan Tablets and Syrup 946
- Hycomine Compound Tablets 948
- Hycomine 947
- Hycotuss Expectorant Syrup 950
- Hydrocet Capsules 787
- Lorcet 10/650 Tablets 1016
- Lortab 2751
- Tussend 1830
- Tussend Expectorant 1831
- Vicodin Tablets 1404
- Vicodin ES Tablets 1405
- Vicodin HP Tablets 1403
- Vicodin Tuss Expectorant 1406
- Zydone Capsules 967

Hydrocodone Polistirex (Additive depressant effects; potential for respiratory depression, hypotension and profound sedation or coma; the dose of one or both agents should be reduced). Products include:
- Tussionex Pennkinetic Extended-Release Suspension 1624

Hydroxyzine Hydrochloride (Additive depressant effects; potential for respiratory depression, hypotension and profound sedation or coma; the dose of one or both agents should be reduced). Products include:
- Atarax Tablets & Syrup 1992
- Marax Tablets & DF Syrup 2015
- Vistaril Intramuscular Solution 2042

Isoflurane (Additive depressant effects; potential for respiratory depression, hypotension and profound sedation or coma; the dose of one or both agents should be reduced).
- No products indexed under this heading.

Ketamine Hydrochloride (Additive depressant effects; potential for respiratory depression, hypotension and profound sedation or coma; the dose of one or both agents should be reduced).
- No products indexed under this heading.

Levomethadyl Acetate Hydrochloride (Additive depressant effects; potential for respiratory depression, hypotension and profound sedation or coma; the dose of one or both agents should be reduced). Products include:
- Orlaam Oral Solution 2361

Levorphanol Tartrate (Additive depressant effects; potential for respiratory depression, hypotension and profound sedation or coma; the dose of one or both agents should be reduced). Products include:
- Levo-Dromoran 2297

Lorazepam (Additive depressant effects; potential for respiratory depression, hypotension and profound sedation or coma; the dose of one or both agents should be reduced). Products include:
- Ativan Injection 2805
- Ativan Tablets 2807

Loxapine Hydrochloride (Additive depressant effects; potential for respiratory depression, hypotension and profound sedation or coma; the dose of one or both agents should be reduced). Products include:
- Loxitane 1426

Loxapine Succinate (Additive depressant effects; potential for respiratory depression, hypotension and profound sedation or coma; the dose of one or both agents should be reduced). Products include:
- Loxitane Capsules 1426

Meperidine Hydrochloride (Additive depressant effects; potential for respiratory depression, hypotension and profound sedation or coma; the dose of one or both agents should be reduced). Products include:
- Demerol 2438
- Mepergan Injection 2859

Mephobarbital (Additive depressant effects; potential for respiratory depression, hypotension and profound sedation or coma; the dose of one or both agents should be reduced). Products include:
- Mebaral Tablets 2452

Meprobamate (Additive depressant effects; potential for respiratory depression, hypotension and profound sedation or coma; the dose of one or both agents should be reduced). Products include:
- Miltown Tablets 2780
- PMB 200 and PMB 400 2890

Mesoridazine Besylate (Additive depressant effects; potential for respiratory depression, hypotension and profound sedation or coma; the dose of one or both agents should be reduced). Products include:
- Serentil 689

Metaxalone (Increased respiratory depression). Products include:
- Skelaxin Tablets 793

Methadone Hydrochloride (Additive depressant effects; potential for respiratory depression, hypotension and profound sedation or coma; the dose of one or both agents should be reduced). Products include:
- Methadone Hydrochloride Oral Concentrate 2356
- Methadone Hydrochloride Oral Solution & Tablets 2357

Methocarbamol (Increased respiratory depression). Products include:
- Robaxin Injectable 2245
- Robaxin Tablets 2246
- Robaxisal Tablets 2246

Methohexital Sodium (Additive depressant effects; potential for respiratory depression, hypotension and profound sedation or coma; the dose of one or both agents should be reduced).
- No products indexed under this heading.

Methotrimeprazine (Additive depressant effects; potential for respiratory depression, hypotension and profound sedation or coma; the dose of one or both agents should be reduced). Products include:
- Levoprome 1321

Methoxyflurane (Additive depressant effects; potential for respiratory depression, hypotension and profound sedation or coma; the dose of one or both agents should be reduced).
- No products indexed under this heading.

(⊞ Described in PDR For Nonprescription Drugs) (⊙ Described in PDR For Ophthalmology)

Metocurine Iodide (Increased respiratory depression). Products include:
- Metubine Iodide Vials 932

Midazolam Hydrochloride (Additive depressant effects; potential for respiratory depression, hypotension and profound sedation or coma; the dose of one or both agents should be reduced). Products include:
- Versed Injection 2324

Mivacurium Chloride (Increased respiratory depression). Products include:
- Mivacron 1125

Molindone Hydrochloride (Additive depressant effects; potential for respiratory depression, hypotension and profound sedation or coma; the dose of one or both agents should be reduced). Products include:
- Moban Tablets and Concentrate 1036

Opium Alkaloids (Additive depressant effects; potential for respiratory depression, hypotension and profound sedation or coma; the dose of one or both agents should be reduced).
- No products indexed under this heading.

Orphenadrine Citrate (Increased respiratory depression). Products include:
- Norflex 1554
- Norgesic 1554

Oxazepam (Additive depressant effects; potential for respiratory depression, hypotension and profound sedation or coma; the dose of one or both agents should be reduced). Products include:
- Serax Capsules 2916
- Serax Tablets 2916

Oxycodone Hydrochloride (Additive depressant effects; potential for respiratory depression, hypotension and profound sedation or coma; the dose of one or both agents should be reduced). Products include:
- OxyContin Tablets 2163
- OxyIR Capsules 2167
- Percocet Tablets 955
- Percodan Tablets 955
- Percodan-Demi Tablets 956
- Roxicodone Tablets, Oral Solution & Intensol (Oxycodone) 2366
- Tylox Capsules 1593

Pancuronium Bromide (Increased respiratory depression).
- No products indexed under this heading.

Pentazocine Hydrochloride (Reduced analgesic effect; precipitation of withdrawal). Products include:
- Talacen Caplets 2464
- Talwin Compound 2466
- Talwin Nx Tablets 2467

Pentazocine Lactate (Reduced analgesic effect; precipitation of withdrawal). Products include:
- Talwin Injection 2465

Pentobarbital Sodium (Additive depressant effects; potential for respiratory depression, hypotension and profound sedation or coma; the dose of one or both agents should be reduced). Products include:
- Nembutal Sodium Capsules 440
- Nembutal Sodium Solution 442
- Nembutal Sodium Suppositories 444

Perphenazine (Additive depressant effects; potential for respiratory depression, hypotension and profound sedation or coma; the dose of one or both agents should be reduced). Products include:
- Etrafon 2495
- Triavil Tablets 1800
- Trilafon 2532

Phenobarbital (Additive depressant effects; potential for respiratory depression, hypotension and profound sedation or coma; the dose of one or both agents should be reduced). Products include:
- Arco-Lase Plus Tablets 513
- Bellergal-S Tablets 2375
- Donnatal 2234
- Donnatal Extentabs 2234
- Donnatal Tablets 2234
- Phenobarbital Elixir and Tablets 1523
- Quadrinal Tablets 1398

Prazepam (Additive depressant effects; potential for respiratory depression, hypotension and profound sedation or coma; the dose of one or both agents should be reduced).
- No products indexed under this heading.

Prochlorperazine (Additive depressant effects; potential for respiratory depression, hypotension and profound sedation or coma; the dose of one or both agents should be reduced). Products include:
- Compazine 2644

Promethazine Hydrochloride (Additive depressant effects; potential for respiratory depression, hypotension and profound sedation or coma; the dose of one or both agents should be reduced). Products include:
- Mepergan Injection 2859
- Phenergan with Codeine 2880
- Phenergan with Dextromethorphan .. 2885
- Phenergan Injection 2880
- Phenergan Suppositories 2882
- Phenergan Syrup 2881
- Phenergan Tablets 2882
- Phenergan VC 2886
- Phenergan VC with Codeine 2888

Propofol (Additive depressant effects; potential for respiratory depression, hypotension and profound sedation or coma; the dose of one or both agents should be reduced). Products include:
- Diprivan Injectable Emulsion 2939

Propoxyphene Hydrochloride (Additive depressant effects; potential for respiratory depression, hypotension and profound sedation or coma; the dose of one or both agents should be reduced). Products include:
- Darvon 1475
- Wygesic Tablets 2930

Propoxyphene Napsylate (Additive depressant effects; potential for respiratory depression, hypotension and profound sedation or coma; the dose of one or both agents should be reduced). Products include:
- Darvon-N/Darvocet-N 1473

Quazepam (Additive depressant effects; potential for respiratory depression, hypotension and profound sedation or coma; the dose of one or both agents should be reduced). Products include:
- Doral Tablets 2773

Risperidone (Additive depressant effects; potential for respiratory depression, hypotension and profound sedation or coma; the dose of one or both agents should be reduced). Products include:
- Risperdal Tablets 1348

Rocuronium Bromide (Increased respiratory depression). Products include:
- Zemuron Injection 1885

Secobarbital Sodium (Additive depressant effects; potential for respiratory depression, hypotension and profound sedation or coma; the dose of one or both agents should be reduced). Products include:
- Seconal Sodium Pulvules 1529

Sevoflurane (Additive depressant effects; potential for respiratory depression, hypotension and profound sedation or coma; the dose of one or both agents should be reduced).
- No products indexed under this heading.

Succinylcholine Chloride (Increased respiratory depression). Products include:
- Anectine 1062

Sufentanil Citrate (Additive depressant effects; potential for respiratory depression, hypotension and profound sedation or coma; the dose of one or both agents should be reduced). Products include:
- Sufenta Injection 1355

Temazepam (Additive depressant effects; potential for respiratory depression, hypotension and profound sedation or coma; the dose of one or both agents should be reduced). Products include:
- Restoril Capsules 2413

Thiamylal Sodium (Additive depressant effects; potential for respiratory depression, hypotension and profound sedation or coma; the dose of one or both agents should be reduced).
- No products indexed under this heading.

Thioridazine Hydrochloride (Additive depressant effects; potential for respiratory depression, hypotension and profound sedation or coma; the dose of one or both agents should be reduced). Products include:
- Mellaril 2398

Thiothixene (Additive depressant effects; potential for respiratory depression, hypotension and profound sedation or coma; the dose of one or both agents should be reduced). Products include:
- Navane Capsules and Concentrate .. 2018
- Navane Intramuscular 2019

Triazolam (Additive depressant effects; potential for respiratory depression, hypotension and profound sedation or coma; the dose of one or both agents should be reduced). Products include:
- Halcion Tablets 2093

Trifluoperazine Hydrochloride (Additive depressant effects; potential for respiratory depression, hypotension and profound sedation or coma; the dose of one or both agents should be reduced). Products include:
- Stelazine 2692

Vecuronium Bromide (Increased respiratory depression). Products include:
- Norcuron for Injection 1875

Zolpidem Tartrate (Additive depressant effects; potential for respiratory depression, hypotension and profound sedation or coma; the dose of one or both agents should be reduced). Products include:
- Ambien Tablets 2559

Food Interactions

Alcohol (Additive depressant effects; potential for respiratory depression, hypotension and profound sedation or coma).

MSIR ORAL SOLUTION CONCENTRATE
(Morphine Sulfate) 2152
See **MSIR Oral Solution**

MSIR TABLETS
(Morphine Sulfate) 2152
See **MSIR Oral Solution**

MAALOX ANTACID CAPLETS
(Calcium Carbonate, Magnesium Carbonate) 657
May interact with:

Prescription Drugs, unspecified (Antacids may interact with certain unspecified prescription drugs).

MAALOX ANTACID/ANTI-GAS TABLETS
(Aluminum Hydroxide, Magnesium Hydroxide, Simethicone) 889
May interact with:

Prescription Drugs, unspecified (Antacids may interfere with certain unspecified prescription drugs; resulting effect not specified).

MAALOX ANTI-DIARRHEAL CAPLETS
(Loperamide Hydrochloride) 658
May interact with:

Antibiotics, unspecified (Effect not specified; consult your doctor).

MAALOX ANTI-GAS TABLETS, REGULAR STRENGTH
(Simethicone) 658
None cited in PDR database.

MAALOX ANTI-GAS TABLETS, EXTRA STRENGTH
(Simethicone) 658
None cited in PDR database.

MAALOX HEARTBURN RELIEF SUSPENSION
(Aluminum Hydroxide, Magnesium Carbonate) 658
May interact with:

Prescription Drugs, unspecified (Effect of concurrent use with unspecified prescription drugs not cited).

MAALOX ANTACID LIQUID
(Magnesium Hydroxide, Aluminum Hydroxide) 888
May interact with:

Prescription Drugs, unspecified (Antacids may interact with certain unspecified prescription drugs).

EXTRA STRENGTH MAALOX ANTACID/ANTI-GAS LIQUID AND TABLETS
(Aluminum Hydroxide, Magnesium Hydroxide, Simethicone) 888
May interact with:

Prescription Drugs, unspecified (Antacids may interfere with

IMPORTANT NOTE: Always consult each drug listing in the patient's regimen for possible interactions.

certain unspecified prescription drugs; resulting effect not specified).

MACROBID CAPSULES
(Nitrofurantoin Monohydrate) ...2138
May interact with:

Magnesium Trisilicate (Co-administration with antacids containing magnesium trisilicate reduces both the rate and extent of absorption). Products include:
- Gaviscon Antacid Tablets ... ▣ 778
- Gaviscon-2 Antacid Tablets ... ▣ 779

Probenecid (Inhibition of renal tubular secretion of nitrofurantoin; increases toxicity and could lessen its efficacy as a urinary tract antibacterial). Products include:
- Benemid Tablets ... 1651
- ColBENEMID Tablets ... 1662

Sulfinpyrazone (Inhibition of renal tubular secretion of nitrofurantoin; increases toxicity and could lessen its efficacy as a urinary tract antibacterial). Products include:
- Anturane ... 823

Food Interactions

Food, unspecified (Increases bioavailability by approximately 40%).

MACRODANTIN CAPSULES
(Nitrofurantoin) ...2140
May interact with:

Magnesium Trisilicate (Co-administration with antacids containing magnesium trisilicate reduces both the rate and extent of absorption). Products include:
- Gaviscon Antacid Tablets ... ▣ 778
- Gaviscon-2 Antacid Tablets ... ▣ 779

Probenecid (Inhibition of renal tubular secretion of nitrofurantoin; increases toxicity and could lessen its efficacy as a urinary tract antibacterial). Products include:
- Benemid Tablets ... 1651
- ColBENEMID Tablets ... 1662

Sulfinpyrazone (Inhibition of renal tubular secretion of nitrofurantoin; increases toxicity and could lessen its efficacy as a urinary tract antibacterial). Products include:
- Anturane ... 823

Food Interactions

Food, unspecified (Increases bioavailability of Macrodantin).

MAG-CARB CAPSULES
(Magnesium Carbonate) ...2168
None cited in PDR database.

MAGONATE TABLETS AND LIQUID
(Magnesium Gluconate) ...1003
None cited in PDR database.

MAG-OX 400
(Magnesium Oxide) ... 666
None cited in PDR database.

MAGTAB SR CAPLETS
(Magnesium Lactate) ...1844
None cited in PDR database.

MALTSUPEX LIQUID, POWDER & TABLETS
(Malt Soup Extract) ... ▣ 803
None cited in PDR database.

MANDOL VIALS, FASPAK & ADD-VANTAGE
(Cefamandole Nafate) ...1516
May interact with aminoglycosides and certain other agents. Compounds in these categories include:

Amikacin Sulfate (Nephrotoxicity). Products include:
- Amikacin Sulfate Injection, USP ... 523
- Amikacin Sulfate Injection, USP ... 981
- Amikin Injectable ... 502

Gentamicin Sulfate (Nephrotoxicity). Products include:
- Garamycin Cream 0.1% ... 2501
- Garamycin Injectable ... 2502
- Garamycin Ointment 0.1% ... 2501
- Garamycin Ophthalmic ... 2501
- Genoptic Sterile Ophthalmic Solution ... ◉ 241
- Genoptic Sterile Ophthalmic Ointment ... ◉ 241
- Gentak ... ◉ 209
- Pred-G Liquifilm Sterile Ophthalmic Suspension ... ◉ 248
- Pred-G S.O.P. Sterile Ophthalmic Ointment ... ◉ 249

Kanamycin Sulfate (Nephrotoxicity).
No products indexed under this heading.

Probenecid (Slows tubular excretion and doubles the peak serum levels). Products include:
- Benemid Tablets ... 1651
- ColBENEMID Tablets ... 1662

Streptomycin Sulfate (Nephrotoxicity). Products include:
- Streptomycin Sulfate Injection ... 2031

Tobramycin Sulfate (Nephrotoxicity). Products include:
- Nebcin Vials, Hyporets & ADD-Vantage ... 1518

Food Interactions

Alcohol (Concurrent ingestion of ethanol may result in nausea, vomiting, vasomotor instability with hypotension and peripheral vasodilation).

MANTADIL CREAM
(Chlorcyclizine Hydrochloride) ...1124
None cited in PDR database.

MARAX TABLETS & DF SYRUP
(Ephedrine Sulfate, Theophylline, Hydroxyzine Hydrochloride) ...2015
May interact with central nervous system depressants and certain other agents. Compounds in these categories include:

Alfentanil Hydrochloride (Potentiated). Products include:
- Alfenta Injection ... 1334

Alprazolam (Potentiated). Products include:
- Xanax Tablets ... 2115

Aprobarbital (Potentiated).
No products indexed under this heading.

Buprenorphine (Potentiated). Products include:
- Buprenex Injectable ... 2170

Buspirone Hydrochloride (Potentiated). Products include:
- BuSpar Tablets ... 738

Butabarbital (Potentiated).
No products indexed under this heading.

Butalbital (Potentiated). Products include:
- Axocet Capsules ... 2469
- Esgic-plus Capsules ... 1012
- Esgic-plus Tablets ... 1012
- Fioricet Tablets ... 2386
- Fioricet with Codeine Capsules ... 2387
- Fiorinal Capsules ... 2388
- Fiorinal with Codeine Capsules ... 2390
- Fiorinal Tablets ... 2388
- Phrenilin ... 790
- Sedapap Tablets 50 mg/650 mg ... 1826

Chlordiazepoxide (Potentiated). Products include:
- Limbitrol ... 2333

Chlordiazepoxide Hydrochloride (Potentiated). Products include:
- Librax Capsules ... 2330
- Librium Capsules ... 2331
- Librium Injectable ... 2332

Chlorpromazine (Potentiated). Products include:
- Thorazine Suppositories ... 2701

Chlorprothixene (Potentiated).
No products indexed under this heading.

Chlorprothixene Hydrochloride (Potentiated).
No products indexed under this heading.

Chlorprothixene Lactate (Potentiated).
No products indexed under this heading.

Clorazepate Dipotassium (Potentiated). Products include:
- Tranxene ... 459

Clozapine (Potentiated). Products include:
- Clozaril Tablets ... 2377

Codeine Phosphate (Potentiated). Products include:
- Brontex ... 2130
- Dimetane-DC Cough Syrup ... 2232
- Fioricet with Codeine Capsules ... 2387
- Fiorinal with Codeine Capsules ... 2390
- Nucofed ... 2225
- Phenergan with Codeine ... 2883
- Phenergan VC with Codeine ... 2888
- Robitussin A-C Syrup ... 2248
- Robitussin-DAC Syrup ... 2249
- Ryna ... ▣ 804
- Soma Compound w/Codeine Tablets ... 2784
- Tylenol with Codeine ... 1592

Desflurane (Potentiated). Products include:
- Suprane (desflurane, USP) ... 1865

Dezocine (Potentiated). Products include:
- Dalgan Injection ... 529

Diazepam (Potentiated). Products include:
- Dizac (diazepam injectable emulsion) CIV ... 1862
- Valium Injectable ... 2336
- Valium Tablets ... 2335

Droperidol (Potentiated). Products include:
- Inapsine Injection ... 462

Enflurane (Potentiated).
No products indexed under this heading.

Estazolam (Potentiated). Products include:
- ProSom Tablets ... 457

Ethchlorvynol (Potentiated). Products include:
- Placidyl Capsules ... 456

Ethinamate (Potentiated).
No products indexed under this heading.

Fentanyl (Potentiated). Products include:
- Duragesic Transdermal System ... 1336

Fentanyl Citrate (Potentiated). Products include:
- Sublimaze Injection ... 463

Fluphenazine Decanoate (Potentiated). Products include:
- Prolixin Decanoate ... 510

Fluphenazine Enanthate (Potentiated). Products include:
- Prolixin Enanthate ... 510

Fluphenazine Hydrochloride (Potentiated). Products include:
- Prolixin ... 510

Flurazepam Hydrochloride (Potentiated). Products include:
- Dalmane Capsules ... 2329

Glutethimide (Potentiated).
No products indexed under this heading.

Haloperidol (Potentiated). Products include:
- Haldol Injection, Tablets and Concentrate ... 1585

Haloperidol Decanoate (Potentiated). Products include:
- Haldol Decanoate ... 1587

Hydrocodone Bitartrate (Potentiated). Products include:
- Codiclear DH Syrup ... 808
- Duratuss HD Elixir ... 2750
- Histussin D Liquid ... 670
- Hycodan Tablets and Syrup ... 946
- Hycomine Compound Tablets ... 948
- Hycomine ... 947
- Hycotuss Expectorant Syrup ... 950
- Hydrocet Capsules ... 787
- Lorcet 10/650 Tablets ... 1016
- Lortab ... 2751
- Tussend ... 1830
- Tussend Expectorant ... 1831
- Vicodin Tablets ... 1404
- Vicodin ES Tablets ... 1405
- Vicodin HP Tablets ... 1403
- Vicodin Tuss Expectorant ... 1406
- Zydone Capsules ... 967

Hydrocodone Polistirex (Potentiated). Products include:
- Tussionex Pennkinetic Extended-Release Suspension ... 1624

Isoflurane (Potentiated).
No products indexed under this heading.

Ketamine Hydrochloride (Potentiated).
No products indexed under this heading.

Levomethadyl Acetate Hydrochloride (Potentiated). Products include:
- Orlaam Oral Solution ... 2361

Levorphanol Tartrate (Potentiated). Products include:
- Levo-Dromoran ... 2297

Lorazepam (Potentiated). Products include:
- Ativan Injection ... 2805
- Ativan Tablets ... 2807

Loxapine Hydrochloride (Potentiated). Products include:
- Loxitane ... 1426

Loxapine Succinate (Potentiated). Products include:
- Loxitane Capsules ... 1426

Meperidine Hydrochloride (Potentiated). Products include:
- Demerol ... 2438
- Mepergan Injection ... 2859

Mephobarbital (Potentiated). Products include:
- Mebaral Tablets ... 2452

Meprobamate (Potentiated). Products include:
- Miltown Tablets ... 2780
- PMB 200 and PMB 400 ... 2890

Mesoridazine Besylate (Potentiated). Products include:
- Serentil ... 689

Methadone Hydrochloride (Potentiated). Products include:
- Methadone Hydrochloride Oral Concentrate ... 2356
- Methadone Hydrochloride Oral Solution & Tablets ... 2357

Methohexital Sodium (Potentiated).
No products indexed under this heading.

Methotrimeprazine (Potentiated). Products include:
- Levoprome ... 1321

Methoxyflurane (Potentiated).
No products indexed under this heading.

Midazolam Hydrochloride (Potentiated). Products include:
- Versed Injection ... 2324

641 Interactions Index Marcaine

Molindone Hydrochloride (Potentiated). Products include:
Moban Tablets and Concentrate 1036
Morphine Sulfate (Potentiated). Products include:
Astramorph/PF Injection, USP (Preservative-Free) 526
Duramorph Injection 983
Infumorph 200 and Infumorph 500 Sterile Solutions 985
Kadian Capsules 2948
MS Contin Tablets 2149
MSIR 2152
Oramorph SR (Morphine Sulfate Sustained Release Tablets) 2359
RMS Suppositories CII 2766
Roxanol 2365
Opium Alkaloids (Potentiated).
No products indexed under this heading.
Oxazepam (Potentiated). Products include:
Serax Capsules 2916
Serax Tablets 2916
Oxycodone Hydrochloride (Potentiated). Products include:
OxyContin Tablets 2163
OxyIR Capsules 2167
Percocet Tablets 955
Percodan Tablets 955
Percodan-Demi Tablets 956
Roxicodone Tablets, Oral Solution & Intensol (Oxycodone) 2366
Tylox Capsules 1593
Pentobarbital Sodium (Potentiated). Products include:
Nembutal Sodium Capsules 440
Nembutal Sodium Solution 442
Nembutal Sodium Suppositories 444
Perphenazine (Potentiated). Products include:
Etrafon 2495
Triavil Tablets 1800
Trilafon 2532
Phenobarbital (Potentiated). Products include:
Arco-Lase Plus Tablets 513
Bellergal-S Tablets 2375
Donnatal 2234
Donnatal Extentabs 2234
Donnatal Tablets 2234
Phenobarbital Elixir and Tablets 1523
Quadrinal Tablets 1398
Prazepam (Potentiated).
No products indexed under this heading.
Prochlorperazine (Potentiated). Products include:
Compazine 2644
Promethazine Hydrochloride (Potentiated). Products include:
Mepergan Injection 2859
Phenergan with Codeine 2883
Phenergan with Dextromethorphan 2885
Phenergan Injection 2880
Phenergan Suppositories 2882
Phenergan Syrup 2881
Phenergan Tablets 2882
Phenergan VC 2886
Phenergan VC with Codeine 2888
Propofol (Potentiated). Products include:
Diprivan Injectable Emulsion 2939
Propoxyphene Hydrochloride (Potentiated). Products include:
Darvon 1475
Wygesic Tablets 2930
Propoxyphene Napsylate (Potentiated). Products include:
Darvon-N/Darvocet-N 1473
Quazepam (Potentiated). Products include:
Doral Tablets 2773
Risperidone (Potentiated). Products include:
Risperdal Tablets 1348
Secobarbital Sodium (Potentiated). Products include:
Seconal Sodium Pulvules 1529
Sevoflurane (Potentiated).
No products indexed under this heading.
Sufentanil Citrate (Potentiated). Products include:
Sufenta Injection 1355
Temazepam (Potentiated). Products include:
Restoril Capsules 2413
Thiamylal Sodium (Potentiated).
No products indexed under this heading.
Thioridazine Hydrochloride (Potentiated). Products include:
Mellaril 2398
Thiothixene (Potentiated). Products include:
Navane Capsules and Concentrate 2018
Navane Intramuscular 2019
Triazolam (Potentiated). Products include:
Halcion Tablets 2093
Trifluoperazine Hydrochloride (Potentiated). Products include:
Stelazine 2692
Zolpidem Tartrate (Potentiated). Products include:
Ambien Tablets 2559

Food Interactions
Alcohol (Potentiated).

MARBLEN SUSPENSION PEACH/APRICOT
(Calcium Carbonate, Magnesium Carbonate) 671
None cited in PDR database.

MARBLEN TABLETS
(Calcium Carbonate, Magnesium Carbonate) 671
None cited in PDR database.

MARCAINE WITH EPINEPHRINE
(Bupivacaine Hydrochloride, Epinephrine) 2446
May interact with monoamine oxidase inhibitors, tricyclic antidepressants, ergot-type oxytocic drugs, phenothiazines, and certain other agents. Compounds in these categories include:

Amitriptyline Hydrochloride (Co-administration of local anesthetic solution containing epinephrine to patients receiving tricyclic antidepressants may produce severe prolonged hypertension). Products include:
Elavil 2945
Etrafon 2495
Limbitrol 2333
Triavil Tablets 1800
Amoxapine (Co-administration of local anesthetic solution containing epinephrine to patients receiving tricyclic antidepressants may produce severe prolonged hypertension). Products include:
Asendin Tablets 1419
Chlorpromazine (Phenothiazines may reduce or reverse the pressor effect of epinephrine). Products include:
Thorazine Suppositories 2701
Chlorpromazine Hydrochloride (Phenothiazines may reduce or reverse the pressor effect of epinephrine). Products include:
Thorazine 2701
Clomipramine Hydrochloride (Co-administration of local anesthetic solution containing epinephrine to patients receiving tricyclic antidepressants may produce severe prolonged hypertension). Products include:
Anafranil Capsules 819
Desipramine Hydrochloride (Co-administration of local anesthetic solution containing epinephrine to patients receiving tricyclic antidepressants may produce severe prolonged hypertension). Products include:
Norpramin Tablets 1273
Doxepin Hydrochloride (Co-administration of local anesthetic solution containing epinephrine to patients receiving tricyclic antidepressants may produce severe prolonged hypertension). Products include:
Adapin Capsules 1542
Sinequan 2028
Zonalon Cream 1042
Fluphenazine Decanoate (Phenothiazines may reduce or reverse the pressor effect of epinephrine). Products include:
Prolixin Decanoate 510
Fluphenazine Enanthate (Phenothiazines may reduce or reverse the pressor effect of epinephrine). Products include:
Prolixin Enanthate 510
Fluphenazine Hydrochloride (Phenothiazines may reduce or reverse the pressor effect of epinephrine). Products include:
Prolixin 510
Furazolidone (Co-administration of local anesthetic solution containing epinephrine to patients receiving MAO inhibitors may produce severe prolonged hypertension). Products include:
Furoxone 2221
Haloperidol (Butyrophenones may reduce or reverse the pressor effect of epinephrine). Products include:
Haldol Injection, Tablets and Concentrate 1585
Haloperidol Decanoate (Butyrophenones may reduce or reverse the pressor effect of epinephrine). Products include:
Haldol Decanoate 1587
Imipramine Hydrochloride (Co-administration of local anesthetic solution containing epinephrine to patients receiving tricyclic antidepressants may produce severe prolonged hypertension). Products include:
Tofranil Ampuls 873
Tofranil Tablets 875
Imipramine Pamoate (Co-administration of local anesthetic solution containing epinephrine to patients receiving tricyclic antidepressants may produce severe prolonged hypertension). Products include:
Tofranil-PM Capsules 876
Isocarboxazid (Co-administration of local anesthetic solution containing epinephrine to patients receiving MAO inhibitors may produce severe prolonged hypertension).
No products indexed under this heading.
Maprotiline Hydrochloride (Co-administration of local anesthetic solution containing epinephrine to patients receiving tricyclic antidepressants may produce severe prolonged hypertension). Products include:
Ludiomil Tablets 861
Mesoridazine Besylate (Phenothiazines may reduce or reverse the pressor effect of epinephrine). Products include:
Serentil 689
Methotrimeprazine (Phenothiazines may reduce or reverse the pressor effect of epinephrine). Products include:
Levoprome 1321
Methylergonovine Maleate (Co-administration of local anesthetic solution containing vasopressor to patients receiving ergot-type oxytocic drugs may cause severe persistent hypertension or cerebrovascular accidents). Products include:
Methergine 2401
Nortriptyline Hydrochloride (Co-administration of local anesthetic solution containing epinephrine to patients receiving tricyclic antidepressants may produce severe prolonged hypertension). Products include:
Pamelor 2409
Perphenazine (Phenothiazines may reduce or reverse the pressor effect of epinephrine). Products include:
Etrafon 2495
Triavil Tablets 1800
Trilafon 2532
Phenelzine Sulfate (Co-administration of local anesthetic solution containing epinephrine to patients receiving MAO inhibitors may produce severe prolonged hypertension). Products include:
Nardil 1977
Prochlorperazine (Phenothiazines may reduce or reverse the pressor effect of epinephrine). Products include:
Compazine 2644
Promethazine Hydrochloride (Phenothiazines may reduce or reverse the pressor effect of epinephrine). Products include:
Mepergan Injection 2859
Phenergan with Codeine 2883
Phenergan with Dextromethorphan 2885
Phenergan Injection 2880
Phenergan Suppositories 2882
Phenergan Syrup 2881
Phenergan Tablets 2882
Phenergan VC 2886
Phenergan VC with Codeine 2888
Protriptyline Hydrochloride (Co-administration of local anesthetic solution containing epinephrine to patients receiving tricyclic antidepressants may produce severe prolonged hypertension). Products include:
Vivactil Tablets 1820
Selegiline Hydrochloride (Co-administration of local anesthetic solution containing epinephrine to patients receiving MAO inhibitors may produce severe prolonged hypertension). Products include:
Eldepryl Capsules 2729
Thioridazine Hydrochloride (Phenothiazines may reduce or reverse the pressor effect of epinephrine). Products include:
Mellaril 2398
Tranylcypromine Sulfate (Co-administration of local anesthetic solution containing epinephrine to patients receiving MAO inhibitors may produce severe prolonged hypertension). Products include:
Parnate Tablets 2679
Trifluoperazine Hydrochloride (Phenothiazines may reduce or reverse the pressor effect of epinephrine). Products include:
Stelazine 2692

IMPORTANT NOTE: Always consult each drug listing in the patient's regimen for possible interactions.

Marcaine — Interactions Index — 642

Trimipramine Maleate (Co-administration of local anesthetic solution containing epinephrine to patients receiving tricyclic antidepressants may produce severe prolonged hypertension). Products include:
- Surmontil Capsules 2917

MARCAINE INJECTION
(Bupivacaine Hydrochloride) 2446
See Marcaine with Epinephrine

MARCAINE SPINAL
(Bupivacaine Hydrochloride) 2449
May interact with monoamine oxidase inhibitors, tricyclic antidepressants, vasopressors, and certain other agents. Compounds in these categories include:

Amitriptyline Hydrochloride (Severe, persistent hypertension). Products include:
- Elavil 2945
- Etrafon 2495
- Limbitrol 2333
- Triavil Tablets 1800

Amoxapine (Severe, persistent hypertension). Products include:
- Asendin Tablets 1419

Clomipramine Hydrochloride (Severe, persistent hypertension). Products include:
- Anafranil Capsules 819

Desipramine Hydrochloride (Severe, persistent hypertension). Products include:
- Norpramin Tablets 1273

Dopamine Hydrochloride (Severe, persistent hypertension).
No products indexed under this heading.

Doxepin Hydrochloride (Severe, persistent hypertension). Products include:
- Adapin Capsules 1542
- Sinequan 2028
- Zonalon Cream 1042

Epinephrine Hydrochloride (Severe, persistent hypertension). Products include:
- Ana-Kit Anaphylaxis Emergency Treatment Kit 611

Furazolidone (Severe, persistent hypertension). Products include:
- Furoxone 2221

Imipramine Hydrochloride (Severe, persistent hypertension). Products include:
- Tofranil Ampuls 873
- Tofranil Tablets 875

Imipramine Pamoate (Severe, persistent hypertension). Products include:
- Tofranil-PM Capsules 876

Isocarboxazid (Severe, persistent hypertension).
No products indexed under this heading.

Maprotiline Hydrochloride (Severe, persistent hypertension). Products include:
- Ludiomil Tablets 861

Metaraminol Bitartrate (Severe, persistent hypertension). Products include:
- Aramine Injection 1649

Methoxamine Hydrochloride (Severe, persistent hypertension). Products include:
- Vasoxyl Injection 1169

Norepinephrine Bitartrate (Severe, persistent hypertension). Products include:
- Levophed Bitartrate Injection 2445

Nortriptyline Hydrochloride (Severe, persistent hypertension). Products include:
- Pamelor 2409

Oxytocin (Severe, persistent hypertension). Products include:
- Syntocinon Injection 2425

Oxytocin (Nasal Spray) (Severe, persistent hypertension).

Phenelzine Sulfate (Severe, persistent hypertension). Products include:
- Nardil 1977

Phenylephrine Hydrochloride (Severe, persistent hypertension). Products include:
- Atrohist Plus Tablets 1605
- Cerose DM 853
- D.A. II Tablets 972
- D.A. Chewable Tablets 970
- Dura-Vent/DA Tablets 972
- Extendryl 1003
- 4-Way Fast Acting Nasal Spray (regular & mentholated) 644
- Hemorid 797
- Hycomine Compound Tablets 948
- Neo-Synephrine Hydrochloride 1% Carpuject 2455
- Neo-Synephrine Hydrochloride 1% Injection 2455
- Neo-Synephrine Hydrochloride (Ophthalmic) 2456
- Neo-Synephrine 624
- Novahistine Elixir 782
- Phenergan VC 2886
- Phenergan VC with Codeine 2888
- Preparation H 842
- Tympagesic Ear Drops 2476
- Vicks Sinex Nasal Spray and Ultra Fine Mist 738

Protriptyline Hydrochloride (Severe, persistent hypertension). Products include:
- Vivactil Tablets 1820

Selegiline Hydrochloride (Severe, persistent hypertension). Products include:
- Eldepryl Capsules 2729

Tranylcypromine Sulfate (Severe, persistent hypertension). Products include:
- Parnate Tablets 2679

Trimipramine Maleate (Severe, persistent hypertension). Products include:
- Surmontil Capsules 2917

MARINOL (DRONABINOL) CAPSULES
(Dronabinol) 2353
May interact with central nervous system depressants, benzodiazepines, barbiturates, sympathomimetics, antihistamines, anticholinergics, tricyclic antidepressants, lithium preparations, narcotic analgesics, xanthine bronchodilators, and certain other agents. Compounds in these categories include:

Acrivastine (Co-administration results in additive CNS depression or super-additive tachycardia and drowsiness). Products include:
- Semprex-D Capsules 1620

Albuterol (Co-administration with sympathomimetics may result in additive hypertension, tachycardia, and possibly cardiotoxicity). Products include:
- Proventil Inhalation Aerosol 2524
- Ventolin Inhalation Aerosol and Refill 1170

Albuterol Sulfate (Co-administration with sympathomimetics may result in additive hypertension, tachycardia, and possibly cardiotoxicity). Products include:
- Airet Albuterol Sulfate Inhalation Solution 1602
- Albuterol Sulfate, USP Solution for Inhalation, Arm-a-Med 522
- Proventil Inhalation Solution 0.083% 2527
- Proventil Repetabs Tablets 2529
- Proventil Solution for Inhalation 0.5% 2525
- Proventil Syrup 2528
- Proventil Tablets 2529
- Ventolin Inhalation Solution 1171
- Ventolin Nebules Inhalation Solution 1172
- Ventolin Rotacaps for Inhalation 1173
- Ventolin Syrup 1175
- Ventolin Tablets 1176
- Volmax Extended-Release Tablets 1835

Alfentanil Hydrochloride (Co-administration results in additive drowsiness and CNS depression). Products include:
- Alfenta Injection 1334

Alprazolam (Co-administration results in additive drowsiness and CNS depression). Products include:
- Xanax Tablets 2115

Aminophylline (Increased theophylline metabolism has resulted with smoking marijuana).
No products indexed under this heading.

Amitriptyline Hydrochloride (Co-administration results in additive tachycardia, hypertension, drowsiness). Products include:
- Elavil 2945
- Etrafon 2495
- Limbitrol 2333
- Triavil Tablets 1800

Amoxapine (Co-administration results in additive tachycardia, hypertension, drowsiness). Products include:
- Asendin Tablets 1419

Amphetamine Sulfate (Co-administration with amphetamine may result in additive hypertension, tachycardia, and possibly cardiotoxicity). Products include:
- Adderall Tablets 2209

Aprobarbital (Co-administration results in decreased clearance of barbiturates via competitive inhibition of metabolism; additive drowsiness and CNS depression).
No products indexed under this heading.

Astemizole (Co-administration results in additive CNS depression or super-additive tachycardia and drowsiness). Products include:
- Hismanal Tablets 1341

Atropine Sulfate (Co-administration with anticholinergic agents may result in additive or super-additive tachycardia and drowsiness). Products include:
- Arco-Lase Plus Tablets 513
- Atrohist Plus Tablets 1605
- Donnatal 2234
- Donnatal Extentabs 2234
- Donnatal Tablets 2234
- Lomotil 2591
- Motofen Tablets 789
- Urised Tablets 2123

Azatadine Maleate (Co-administration results in additive CNS depression or super-additive tachycardia and drowsiness). Products include:
- Trinalin Repetabs Tablets 1373

Belladonna Alkaloids (Co-administration with anticholinergic agents may result in additive or super-additive tachycardia and drowsiness). Products include:
- Bellergal-S Tablets 2375
- Hyland's Bedwetting Tablets 788
- Hyland's EnurAid Tablets 789
- Hyland's Headache Tablets 790
- Hyland's Teething Tablets 790
- Similasan Eye Drops #1 769

Benztropine Mesylate (Co-administration with anticholinergic agents may result in additive or super-additive tachycardia and drowsiness). Products include:
- Cogentin 1661

Biperiden Hydrochloride (Co-administration with anticholinergic agents may result in additive or super-additive tachycardia and drowsiness). Products include:
- Akineton 1380

Bromodiphenhydramine Hydrochloride (Co-administration results in additive CNS depression or super-additive tachycardia and drowsiness).
No products indexed under this heading.

Brompheniramine Maleate (Co-administration results in additive CNS depression or super-additive tachycardia and drowsiness). Products include:
- Alka-Seltzer Plus Sinus Medicine 611
- Bromfed Capsules (Extended-Release) 1832
- Bromfed Syrup 712
- Bromfed Tablets 1832
- Bromfed-DM Cough Syrup 1832
- Bromfed-PD Capsules (Extended-Release) 1832
- Dimetane-DC Cough Syrup 2232
- Dimetane-DX Cough Syrup 2233
- Dimetapp Allergy Dye-Free Elixir 838
- Dimetapp Allergy Sinus Caplets 838
- Dimetapp Cold & Allergy Chewable Tablets 838
- Dimetapp Cold & Cough Liqui-Gels 839
- Dimetapp Cold & Fever Suspension 839
- Dimetapp DM Elixir 840
- Dimetapp Elixir 840
- Dimetapp Extentabs 841
- Dimetapp Tablets/Liqui-Gels 841
- Rondec Chewable Tablets 974
- Vicks DayQuil Allergy Relief 12-Hour Extended Release Tablets 733
- Vicks DayQuil Allergy Relief 4-Hour Tablets 733

Buprenorphine (Co-administration results in additive drowsiness and CNS depression). Products include:
- Buprenex Injectable 2170

Buspirone Hydrochloride (Co-administration results in additive drowsiness and CNS depression). Products include:
- BuSpar Tablets 738

Butabarbital (Co-administration results in decreased clearance of barbiturates via competitive inhibition of metabolism; additive drowsiness and CNS depression).
No products indexed under this heading.

Butalbital (Co-administration results in decreased clearance of barbiturates via competitive inhibition of metabolism; additive drowsiness and CNS depression). Products include:
- Axocet Capsules 2469
- Esgic-plus Capsules 1012
- Esgic-plus Tablets 1012
- Fioricet Tablets 2386
- Fioricet with Codeine Capsules 2387
- Fiorinal Capsules 2388
- Fiorinal with Codeine Capsules 2390
- Fiorinal Tablets 2388
- Phrenilin 790
- Sedapap Tablets 50 mg/650 mg 1826

Carisoprodol (Co-administration with muscle relaxants may result in additive drowsiness and CNS depression). Products include:
- Soma Compound w/Codeine Tablets 2784
- Soma Compound Tablets 2783
- Soma Tablets 2782

(Described in PDR For Nonprescription Drugs)   (Described in PDR For Ophthalmology)

Interactions Index

Cetirizine Hydrochloride (Co-administration results in additive CNS depression or super-additive tachycardia and drowsiness). Products include:
- Zyrtec Tablets 2053

Chlordiazepoxide (Co-administration results in additive drowsiness and CNS depression). Products include:
- Limbitrol 2333

Chlordiazepoxide Hydrochloride (Co-administration results in additive drowsiness and CNS depression). Products include:
- Librax Capsules 2330
- Librium Capsules 2331
- Librium Injectable 2332

Chlorpheniramine Maleate (Co-administration results in additive CNS depression or super-additive tachycardia and drowsiness). Products include:
- Alka-Seltzer Plus Cold Medicine 611
- Alka-Seltzer Plus Cold Medicine Liqui-Gels 612
- Alka-Seltzer Plus Cold & Cough Medicine 611
- Alka-Seltzer Plus Cold & Cough Medicine Liqui-Gels 612
- Alka-Seltzer Plus Flu & Body Aches Effervescent Tablets 612
- Allerest Maximum Strength 649
- Allerest Sinus Pain Formula 649
- Ana-Kit Anaphylaxis Emergency Treatment Kit 611
- Atrohist Pediatric Capsules 1603
- Atrohist Plus Tablets 1605
- BC Cold Powder Multi-Symptom Formula (Cold-Sinus-Allergy) 631
- Cerose DM 853
- Cheracol Plus Head Cold/Cough Formula 741
- Children's TYLENOL Cold-Symptom Chewable Tablets and Liquid 1559
- Children's TYLENOL Cold Plus Cough Multi Symptom Chewable Tablets and Liquid 1560
- Children's TYLENOL Flu Suspension Liquid 1560
- Children's Vicks DayQuil Allergy Relief 730
- Children's Vicks NyQuil Cold/Cough Relief 731
- Chlor-Trimeton Allergy Decongestant Tablets 759
- Chlor-Trimeton Allergy Tablets 758
- Allergy-Sinus Comtrex Multi-Symptom Allergy-Sinus Formula Tablets and Caplets 639
- Comtrex Multi-Symptom 638
- Contac Continuous Action Nasal Decongestant/Antihistamine 12 Hour Capsules 773
- Contac Maximum Strength Continuous Action Decongestant/Antihistamine 12 Hour Caplets 772
- Contac Severe Cold and Flu Formula Caplets 773
- Coricidin Cold + Flu Tablets 760
- Coricidin Cough + Cold Tablets 760
- Coricidin 'D' Decongestant Tablets 760
- D.A. II Tablets 972
- D.A. Chewable Tablets 970
- Dura-Tap/PD Capsules 970
- Dura-Vent/DA Tablets 972
- Efidac 24 Chlorpheniramine 655
- Extendryl 1003
- Fedahist Gyrocaps 2545
- Hycomine Compound Tablets 948
- Kronofed-A 994
- Nolamine Timed-Release Tablets 790
- Novahistine Elixir 782
- Ornade Spansule Capsules 2678
- PediaCare Cough-Cold Chewable Tablets and Liquid 1569
- PediaCare NightRest Cough-Cold Liquid 1569
- Pediatric Vicks 44m Cough & Cold Relief 737
- Pyrroxate Caplets 742
- Ryna 804
- Sinarest 663
- Sine-Off Sinus Medicine 784
- Singlet Tablets 785
- Sinulin Tablets 792
- Sinutab Sinus Allergy Medication, Maximum Strength Tablets and Caplets 823
- Sudafed Cold & Allergy Tablets 826
- Teldrin 12 Hour Antihistamine/Nasal Decongestant Allergy Relief Capsules 786
- TheraFlu Flu and Cold Medicine 750
- Theraflu Maximum Strength Flu and Cold Medicine For Sore Throat 751
- TheraFlu Flu, Cold and Cough Medicine 750
- TheraFlu Maximum Strength Nighttime Flu, Cold & Cough Medicine 751
- Triaminic Night Time 754
- Triaminic Syrup 755
- Triaminic Triaminicol Cold & Cough 756
- Triaminicin Tablets 756
- Tussend 1830
- TYLENOL Allergy Sinus, Maximum Strength Caplets and Gelcaps 1571
- TYLENOL Cold Medication, Multi-Symptom Formula Tablets and Caplets 1572
- TYLENOL Cold Medication, Multi-Symptom Hot Liquid Packets 1572
- Vicks 44 LiquiCaps Cough, Cold & Flu Relief 728
- Vicks 44M Cough, Cold & Flu Relief 729

Chlorpheniramine Polistirex (Co-administration results in additive CNS depression or super-additive tachycardia and drowsiness). Products include:
- Tussionex Pennkinetic Extended-Release Suspension 1624

Chlorpheniramine Tannate (Co-administration results in additive CNS depression or super-additive tachycardia and drowsiness). Products include:
- Atrohist Pediatric Suspension 1604
- Atrohist Pediatric Suspension Dye-Free 1604
- Rynatan 2781
- Rynatuss 2782

Chlorpromazine (Co-administration results in additive drowsiness and CNS depression). Products include:
- Thorazine Suppositories 2701

Chlorpromazine Hydrochloride (Co-administration results in additive drowsiness and CNS depression). Products include:
- Thorazine 2701

Chlorprothixene (Co-administration results in additive drowsiness and CNS depression).
No products indexed under this heading.

Chlorprothixene Hydrochloride (Co-administration results in additive drowsiness and CNS depression).
No products indexed under this heading.

Chlorprothixene Lactate (Co-administration results in additive drowsiness and CNS depression).
No products indexed under this heading.

Chlorzoxazone (Co-administration with muscle relaxants may result in additive drowsiness and CNS depression). Products include:
- Parafon Forte DSC Caplets 1590

Clemastine Fumarate (Co-administration results in additive CNS depression or super-additive tachycardia and drowsiness). Products include:
- Tavist Syrup 2426
- Tavist Tablets 2427
- Tavist-1 12 Hour Relief Tablets 749
- Tavist-D 12 Hour Relief Tablets 750

Clidinium Bromide (Co-administration with anticholinergic agents may result in additive or super-additive tachycardia and drowsiness). Products include:
- Librax Capsules 2330

Clomipramine Hydrochloride (Co-administration results in additive tachycardia, hypertension, drowsiness). Products include:
- Anafranil Capsules 819

Clorazepate Dipotassium (Co-administration results in additive drowsiness and CNS depression). Products include:
- Tranxene 459

Clozapine (Co-administration results in additive drowsiness and CNS depression). Products include:
- Clozaril Tablets 2377

Cocaine Hydrochloride (Co-administration with cocaine may result in additive hypertension, tachycardia, and possibly cardiotoxicity). Products include:
- Cocaine Hydrochloride Topical Solutions 529

Codeine Phosphate (Co-administration results in additive drowsiness and CNS depression). Products include:
- Brontex 2130
- Dimetane-DC Cough Syrup 2232
- Fioricet with Codeine Capsules 2387
- Fiorinal with Codeine Capsules 2390
- Nucofed 2225
- Phenergan with Codeine 2883
- Phenergan VC with Codeine 2888
- Robitussin A-C Syrup 2248
- Robitussin-DAC Syrup 2249
- Ryna 804
- Soma Compound w/Codeine Tablets 2784
- Tylenol with Codeine 1592

Cyclobenzaprine Hydrochloride (Co-administration with muscle relaxants may result in additive drowsiness and CNS depression). Products include:
- Flexeril Tablets 1701

Cyproheptadine Hydrochloride (Co-administration results in additive CNS depression or super-additive tachycardia and drowsiness). Products include:
- Periactin 1767

Desflurane (Co-administration results in additive drowsiness and CNS depression). Products include:
- Suprane (desflurane, USP) 1865

Desipramine Hydrochloride (Co-administration results in additive tachycardia, hypertension, drowsiness). Products include:
- Norpramin Tablets 1273

Dexchlorpheniramine Maleate (Co-administration results in additive CNS depression or super-additive tachycardia and drowsiness).
No products indexed under this heading.

Dextroamphetamine Sulfate (Co-administration with amphetamine may result in additive hypertension, tachycardia, and possibly cardiotoxicity). Products include:
- Adderall Tablets 2209
- Dexedrine 2648
- DextroStat-Dextroamphetamine Sulfate Tablets 2211

Dezocine (Co-administration results in additive drowsiness and CNS depression). Products include:
- Dalgan Injection 529

Diazepam (Co-administration results in additive drowsiness and CNS depression). Products include:
- Dizac (diazepam injectable emulsion) CIV 1862
- Valium Injectable 2336
- Valium Tablets 2335

Dicyclomine Hydrochloride (Co-administration with anticholinergic agents may result in additive or super-additive tachycardia and drowsiness). Products include:
- Bentyl 1246

Diphenhydramine Citrate (Co-administration results in additive CNS depression or super-additive tachycardia and drowsiness). Products include:
- Excedrin P.M. Analgesic/Sleeping Aid Tablets, Caplets, Liquigels 735

Diphenhydramine Hydrochloride (Co-administration results in additive CNS depression or super-additive tachycardia and drowsiness). Products include:
- Actifed Allergy Daytime/Nighttime Caplets 808
- Actifed Sinus Daytime/Nighttime Tablets and Caplets 809
- Extra Strength Bayer PM Aspirin Plus Sleep Aid 617
- Benadryl Allergy Chewables 811
- Benadryl Allergy/Cold Tablets 811
- Benadryl Allergy Decongestant Liquid Medication 812
- Benadryl Allergy Decongestant Tablets 812
- Benadryl Allergy Liquid Medication 813
- Benadryl Allergy 811
- Benadryl Allergy Sinus Headache Caplets 813
- Benadryl Dye-Free Allergy Liquigel Softgels 813
- Benadryl Dye-Free Allergy Liquid Medication 814
- Benadryl Itch Relief Stick Extra Strength 814
- Benadryl Cream 814
- Benadryl Gel 815
- Benadryl Spray 815
- Benadryl Injection 1955
- Contac Day & Night Cold/Flu Night Caplets 772
- Contac Night Allergy/Sinus Caplets 771
- Extra Strength Doan's P.M. 653
- Excedrin P.M. Analgesic/Sleeping Aid Tablets, Caplets, Liquigels 643
- Nytol QuickCaps Caplets 632
- Sleepinal Night-time Sleep Aid Capsules and Softgels 798
- TYLENOL Allergy Sinus NightTime, Maximum Strength Caplets 1571
- TYLENOL Flu NightTime, Maximum Strength Gelcaps 1575
- TYLENOL Flu NightTime, Maximum Strength Hot Medication Packets 1575
- TYLENOL PM Pain Reliever/Sleep Aid, Extra Strength Gelcaps, Caplets, Geltabs 1576
- TYLENOL Severe Allergy Medication Caplets 1571
- Maximum Strength Unisom Sleepgels 1990
- Unisom With Pain Relief-Nighttime Sleep Aid and Pain Reliever 1991

Diphenylpyraline Hydrochloride (Co-administration results in additive CNS depression or super-additive tachycardia and drowsiness).
No products indexed under this heading.

Disulfiram (Co-administration of disulfiram in a patient who smoked marijuana has resulted in a reversible hypomanic reaction). Products include:
- Antabuse Tablets 2802

Dobutamine Hydrochloride (Co-administration with sympathomimetics may result in additive hypertension, tachycardia, and possibly cardiotoxicity). Products include:
- Dobutrex Solution Vials 1480

IMPORTANT NOTE: Always consult each drug listing in the patient's regimen for possible interactions.

Marinol — Interactions Index — 644

Dopamine Hydrochloride (Co-administration with sympathomimetics may result in additive hypertension, tachycardia, and possibly cardiotoxicity).

No products indexed under this heading.

Doxepin Hydrochloride (Co-administration results in additive tachycardia, hypertension, drowsiness). Products include:
- Adapin Capsules 1542
- Sinequan 2028
- Zonalon Cream 1042

Droperidol (Co-administration results in additive drowsiness and CNS depression). Products include:
- Inapsine Injection 462

Dyphylline (Increased theophylline metabolism has resulted with smoking marijuana). Products include:
- Lufyllin & Lufyllin-400 Tablets 2778
- Lufyllin-GG Elixir & Tablets 2779

Enflurane (Co-administration results in additive drowsiness and CNS depression).

No products indexed under this heading.

Ephedrine Hydrochloride (Co-administration with sympathomimetics may result in additive hypertension, tachycardia, and possibly cardiotoxicity). Products include:
- Primatene Tablets .... ▣ 844
- Quadrinal Tablets 1398

Ephedrine Sulfate (Co-administration with sympathomimetics may result in additive hypertension, tachycardia, and possibly cardiotoxicity). Products include:
- Marax Tablets & DF Syrup 2015

Ephedrine Tannate (Co-administration with sympathomimetics may result in additive hypertension, tachycardia, and possibly cardiotoxicity). Products include:
- Rynatuss 2782

Epinephrine (Co-administration with sympathomimetics may result in additive hypertension, tachycardia, and possibly cardiotoxicity). Products include:
- EPIFRIN .... ⊚ 237
- EpiPen 808
- Marcaine with Epinephrine 2446
- Primatene Mist .... ▣ 843
- Sensorcaine with Epinephrine Injection 554
- Sus-Phrine Injection 1017
- Xylocaine with Epinephrine Injections 562

Epinephrine Bitartrate (Co-administration with sympathomimetics may result in additive hypertension, tachycardia, and possibly cardiotoxicity). Products include:
- Sensorcaine-MPF with Epinephrine Injection 554

Epinephrine Hydrochloride (Co-administration with sympathomimetics may result in additive hypertension, tachycardia, and possibly cardiotoxicity). Products include:
- Ana-Kit Anaphylaxis Emergency Treatment Kit 611

Estazolam (Co-administration results in additive drowsiness and CNS depression). Products include:
- ProSom Tablets 457

Ethchlorvynol (Co-administration results in additive drowsiness and CNS depression). Products include:
- Placidyl Capsules 456

Ethinamate (Co-administration results in additive drowsiness and CNS depression).

No products indexed under this heading.

Fentanyl (Co-administration results in additive drowsiness and CNS depression). Products include:
- Duragesic Transdermal System 1336

Fentanyl Citrate (Co-administration results in additive drowsiness and CNS depression). Products include:
- Sublimaze Injection 463

Fluoxetine Hydrochloride (Co-administration of fluoxetine in a patient who smoked marijuana has resulted in a hypomanic reaction). Products include:
- Prozac Pulvules & Liquid, Oral Solution 935

Fluphenazine Decanoate (Co-administration results in additive drowsiness and CNS depression). Products include:
- Prolixin Decanoate 510

Fluphenazine Enanthate (Co-administration results in additive drowsiness and CNS depression). Products include:
- Prolixin Enanthate 510

Fluphenazine Hydrochloride (Co-administration results in additive drowsiness and CNS depression). Products include:
- Prolixin 510

Flurazepam Hydrochloride (Co-administration results in additive drowsiness and CNS depression). Products include:
- Dalmane Capsules 2329

Glutethimide (Co-administration results in additive drowsiness and CNS depression).

No products indexed under this heading.

Glycopyrrolate (Co-administration with anticholinergic agents may result in additive or super-additive tachycardia and drowsiness). Products include:
- Robinul Forte Tablets 2247
- Robinul Injectable 2247
- Robinul Tablets 2247

Halazepam (Co-administration results in additive drowsiness and CNS depression).

No products indexed under this heading.

Haloperidol (Co-administration results in additive drowsiness and CNS depression). Products include:
- Haldol Injection, Tablets and Concentrate 1585

Haloperidol Decanoate (Co-administration results in additive drowsiness and CNS depression). Products include:
- Haldol Decanoate 1587

Hydrocodone Bitartrate (Co-administration results in additive drowsiness and CNS depression). Products include:
- Codiclear DH Syrup 808
- Duratuss HD Elixir 2750
- Histussin D Liquid 670
- Hycodan Tablets and Syrup 946
- Hycomine Compound Tablets 948
- Hycomine 947
- Hycotuss Expectorant Syrup 950
- Hydrocet Capsules 787
- Lorcet 10/650 Tablets 1016
- Lortab 2751
- Tussend 1830
- Tussend Expectorant 1831
- Vicodin Tablets 1404
- Vicodin ES Tablets 1405
- Vicodin HP Tablets 1403
- Vicodin Tuss Expectorant 1406
- Zydone Capsules 967

Hydrocodone Polistirex (Co-administration results in additive drowsiness and CNS depression). Products include:
- Tussionex Pennkinetic Extended-Release Suspension 1624

Hydromorphone Hydrochloride (Co-administration results in additive drowsiness and CNS depression). Products include:
- Dilaudid Ampules 1382
- Dilaudid Cough Syrup 1383
- Dilaudid-HP Injection 1384
- Dilaudid-HP Lyophilized Powder 250 mg 1384
- Dilaudid 1382
- Dilaudid Oral Liquid 1386
- Dilaudid 1382
- Dilaudid Tablets - 8 mg 1386

Hydroxyzine Hydrochloride (Co-administration results in additive drowsiness and CNS depression). Products include:
- Atarax Tablets & Syrup 1992
- Marax Tablets & DF Syrup 2015
- Vistaril Intramuscular Solution 2042

Hyoscyamine (Co-administration with anticholinergic agents may result in additive or super-additive tachycardia and drowsiness). Products include:
- Cystospaz Tablets 2123
- Urised Tablets 2123

Hyoscyamine Sulfate (Co-administration with anticholinergic agents may result in additive or super-additive tachycardia and drowsiness). Products include:
- Arco-Lase Plus Tablets 513
- Atrohist Plus Tablets 1605
- Cystospaz-M Capsules 2123
- Donnatal 2234
- Donnatal Extentabs 2234
- Donnatal Tablets 2234
- Kutrase Capsules 2546
- Levsin/Levsinex/Levbid 2549

Imipramine Hydrochloride (Co-administration results in additive tachycardia, hypertension, drowsiness). Products include:
- Tofranil Ampuls 873
- Tofranil Tablets 875

Imipramine Pamoate (Co-administration results in additive tachycardia, hypertension, drowsiness). Products include:
- Tofranil-PM Capsules 876

Ipratropium Bromide (Co-administration with anticholinergic agents may result in additive or super-additive tachycardia and drowsiness). Products include:
- Atrovent Inhalation Aerosol 674
- Atrovent Inhalation Solution 675
- Atrovent Nasal Spray 0.03% 676
- Atrovent Nasal Spray 0.06% 678

Isoflurane (Co-administration results in additive drowsiness and CNS depression).

No products indexed under this heading.

Isoproterenol Hydrochloride (Co-administration with sympathomimetics may result in additive hypertension, tachycardia, and possibly cardiotoxicity). Products include:
- Isuprel Hydrochloride Solution 2443
- Isuprel Injection 2441
- Isuprel Mistometer 2442

Isoproterenol Sulfate (Co-administration with sympathomimetics may result in additive hypertension, tachycardia, and possibly cardiotoxicity). Products include:
- Norisodrine with Calcium Iodide Syrup 446

Ketamine Hydrochloride (Co-administration results in additive drowsiness and CNS depression).

No products indexed under this heading.

Levomethadyl Acetate Hydrochloride (Co-administration results in additive drowsiness and CNS depression). Products include:
- Orlaam Oral Solution 2361

Levorphanol Tartrate (Co-administration results in additive drowsiness and CNS depression). Products include:
- Levo-Dromoran 2297

Lithium Carbonate (Co-administration results in additive drowsiness and CNS depression). Products include:
- Eskalith 2658
- Lithium Carbonate Capsules & Tablets 2352
- Lithonate/Lithotabs/Lithobid 2721

Lithium Citrate (Co-administration results in additive drowsiness and CNS depression).

No products indexed under this heading.

Loratadine (Co-administration results in additive CNS depression or super-additive tachycardia and drowsiness). Products include:
- Claritin Tablets 2485
- Claritin-D Tablets 2487

Lorazepam (Co-administration results in additive drowsiness and CNS depression). Products include:
- Ativan Injection 2805
- Ativan Tablets 2807

Loxapine Hydrochloride (Co-administration results in additive drowsiness and CNS depression). Products include:
- Loxitane 1426

Loxapine Succinate (Co-administration results in additive drowsiness and CNS depression). Products include:
- Loxitane Capsules 1426

Maprotiline Hydrochloride (Co-administration results in additive tachycardia, hypertension, drowsiness). Products include:
- Ludiomil Tablets 861

Mepenzolate Bromide (Co-administration with anticholinergic agents may result in additive or super-additive tachycardia and drowsiness).

No products indexed under this heading.

Meperidine Hydrochloride (Co-administration results in additive drowsiness and CNS depression). Products include:
- Demerol 2438
- Mepergan Injection 2859

Mephobarbital (Co-administration results in decreased clearance of barbiturates via competitive inhibition of metabolism; additive drowsiness and CNS depression). Products include:
- Mebaral Tablets 2452

Meprobamate (Co-administration results in additive drowsiness and CNS depression). Products include:
- Miltown Tablets 2780
- PMB 200 and PMB 400 2890

Mesoridazine Besylate (Co-administration results in additive drowsiness and CNS depression). Products include:
- Serentil 689

Metaproterenol Sulfate (Co-administration with sympathomimetics may result in additive hypertension, tachycardia, and possibly cardiotoxicity). Products include:
- Alupent 672
- Metaproterenol Sulfate Inhalation Solution, USP, Arm-a-Med 547

(▣ Described in PDR For Nonprescription Drugs)   (⊚ Described in PDR For Ophthalmology)

645 **Interactions Index** Marinol

Metaraminol Bitartrate (Co-administration with sympathomimetics may result in additive hypertension, tachycardia, and possibly cardiotoxicity). Products include:
- Aramine Injection 1649

Methadone Hydrochloride (Co-administration results in additive drowsiness and CNS depression). Products include:
- Methadone Hydrochloride Oral Concentrate 2356
- Methadone Hydrochloride Oral Solution & Tablets 2357

Methamphetamine Hydrochloride (Co-administration with amphetamine may result in additive hypertension, tachycardia, and possibly cardiotoxicity). Products include:
- Desoxyn Gradumet Tablets 422

Methdilazine Hydrochloride (Co-administration results in additive CNS depression or super-additive tachycardia and drowsiness).
- No products indexed under this heading.

Methocarbamol (Co-administration with muscle relaxants may result in additive drowsiness and CNS depression). Products include:
- Robaxin Injectable 2245
- Robaxin Tablets 2246
- Robaxisal Tablets 2246

Methohexital Sodium (Co-administration results in additive drowsiness and CNS depression).
- No products indexed under this heading.

Methotrimeprazine (Co-administration results in additive drowsiness and CNS depression). Products include:
- Levoprome 1321

Methoxamine Hydrochloride (Co-administration with sympathomimetics may result in additive hypertension, tachycardia, and possibly cardiotoxicity). Products include:
- Vasoxyl Injection 1169

Methoxyflurane (Co-administration results in additive drowsiness and CNS depression).
- No products indexed under this heading.

Midazolam Hydrochloride (Co-administration results in additive drowsiness and CNS depression). Products include:
- Versed Injection 2324

Molindone Hydrochloride (Co-administration results in additive drowsiness and CNS depression). Products include:
- Moban Tablets and Concentrate 1036

Morphine Sulfate (Co-administration results in additive drowsiness and CNS depression). Products include:
- Astramorph/PF Injection, USP (Preservative-Free) 526
- Duramorph Injection 983
- Infumorph 200 and Infumorph 500 Sterile Solutions 985
- Kadian Capsules 2948
- MS Contin Tablets 2149
- MSIR 2152
- Oramorph SR (Morphine Sulfate Sustained Release Tablets) 2359
- RMS Suppositories CII 2766
- Roxanol 2365

Norepinephrine Bitartrate (Co-administration with sympathomimetics may result in additive hypertension, tachycardia, and possibly cardiotoxicity). Products include:
- Levophed Bitartrate Injection 2445

Nortriptyline Hydrochloride (Co-administration results in additive tachycardia, hypertension, drowsiness). Products include:
- Pamelor 2409

Opium Alkaloids (Co-administration results in additive drowsiness and CNS depression).
- No products indexed under this heading.

Orphenadrine Citrate (Co-administration with muscle relaxants may result in additive drowsiness and CNS depression). Products include:
- Norflex 1554
- Norgesic 1554

Oxazepam (Co-administration results in additive drowsiness and CNS depression). Products include:
- Serax Capsules 2916
- Serax Tablets 2916

Oxybutynin Chloride (Co-administration with anticholinergic agents may result in additive or super-additive tachycardia and drowsiness). Products include:
- Ditropan 1267

Oxycodone Hydrochloride (Co-administration results in additive drowsiness and CNS depression). Products include:
- OxyContin Tablets 2163
- OxyIR Capsules 2167
- Percocet Tablets 955
- Percodan Tablets 955
- Percodan-Demi Tablets 956
- Roxicodone Tablets, Oral Solution & Intensol (Oxycodone) 2366
- Tylox Capsules 1593

Pentobarbital Sodium (Co-administration results in decreased clearance of barbiturates via competitive inhibition of metabolism; additive drowsiness and CNS depression). Products include:
- Nembutal Sodium Capsules 440
- Nembutal Sodium Solution 442
- Nembutal Sodium Suppositories 444

Perphenazine (Co-administration results in additive drowsiness and CNS depression). Products include:
- Etrafon 2495
- Triavil Tablets 1800
- Trilafon 2532

Phenobarbital (Co-administration results in decreased clearance of barbiturates via competitive inhibition of metabolism; additive drowsiness and CNS depression). Products include:
- Arco-Lase Plus Tablets 513
- Bellergal-S Tablets 2375
- Donnatal 2234
- Donnatal Extentabs 2234
- Donnatal Tablets 2234
- Phenobarbital Elixir and Tablets 1523
- Quadrinal Tablets 1398

Phenylephrine Bitartrate (Co-administration with sympathomimetics may result in additive hypertension, tachycardia, and possibly cardiotoxicity).
- No products indexed under this heading.

Phenylephrine Hydrochloride (Co-administration with sympathomimetics may result in additive hypertension, tachycardia, and possibly cardiotoxicity). Products include:
- Atrohist Plus Tablets 1605
- Cerose DM 853
- D.A. II Tablets 972
- D.A. Chewable Tablets 970
- Dura-Vent/DA Tablets 972
- Extendryl 1003
- 4-Way Fast Acting Nasal Spray (regular & mentholated) 644
- Hemorid 797
- Hycomine Compound Tablets 948
- Neo-Synephrine Hydrochloride 1% Carpuject 2455
- Neo-Synephrine Hydrochloride 1% Injection 2455
- Neo-Synephrine Hydrochloride (Ophthalmic) 2456
- Neo-Synephrine 624
- Novahistine Elixir 782
- Phenergan VC 2886
- Phenergan VC with Codeine 2888
- Preparation H 842
- Tympagesic Ear Drops 2476
- Vicks Sinex Nasal Spray and Ultra Fine Mist 738

Phenylephrine Tannate (Co-administration with sympathomimetics may result in additive hypertension, tachycardia, and possibly cardiotoxicity). Products include:
- Atrohist Pediatric Suspension 1604
- Atrohist Pediatric Suspension Dye-Free 1604
- Rynatan 2781
- Rynatuss 2782

Phenylpropanolamine Hydrochloride (Co-administration with sympathomimetics may result in additive hypertension, tachycardia, and possibly cardiotoxicity). Products include:
- Acutrim 648
- Atrohist Plus Tablets 1605
- BC Cold Powder Multi-Symptom Formula (Cold-Sinus-Allergy) 631
- BC Cold Powder Non-Drowsy Formula (Cold-Sinus) 631
- Cheracol Plus Head Cold/Cough Formula 741
- Comtrex Multi-Symptom Cold Reliever Liqui-Gels 638
- Comtrex Multi-Symptom Non-Drowsy Liqui-gels 640
- Contac Continuous Action Nasal Decongestant/Antihistamine 12 Hour Capsules 773
- Contac Maximum Strength Continuous Action Decongestant/Antihistamine 12 Hour Caplets 772
- Contac Severe Cold and Flu Formula Caplets 773
- Coricidin 'D' Decongestant Tablets 760
- Dexatrim 795
- Dexatrim Plus Vitamins Caplets 796
- Dimetane-DC Cough Syrup 2232
- Dimetapp Allergy Sinus Caplets 838
- Dimetapp Cold & Allergy Chewable Tablets 838
- Dimetapp Cold & Cough Liqui-Gels 839
- Dimetapp DM Elixir 840
- Dimetapp Elixir 840
- Dimetapp Extentabs 841
- Dimetapp Tablets/Liqui-Gels 841
- Dura-Vent Tablets 971
- Entex LA Tablets 972
- Exgest LA Tablets 787
- Hycomine 947
- Nolamine Timed-Release Tablets 790
- Ornade Spansule Capsules 2678
- Propagest Tablets 791
- Pyrroxate Caplets 742
- Robitussin-CF 846
- Sinulin Tablets 792
- Tavist-D 12 Hour Relief Tablets 750
- Teldrin 12 Hour Antihistamine/Nasal Decongestant Allergy Relief Capsules 786
- Triaminic Expectorant 753
- Triaminic Syrup 755
- Triaminic Triaminicol Cold & Cough 756
- Triaminic DM Syrup 756
- Triaminicin Tablets 756
- Vicks DayQuil Allergy Relief 12-Hour Extended Release Tablets 733
- Vicks DayQuil Allergy Relief 4-Hour Tablets 733
- Vicks DayQuil SINUS Pressure & CONGESTION Relief 734

Pirbuterol Acetate (Co-administration with sympathomimetics may result in additive hypertension, tachycardia, and possibly cardiotoxicity). Products include:
- Maxair Autohaler 1550
- Maxair Inhaler 1552

Prazepam (Co-administration results in additive drowsiness and CNS depression).
- No products indexed under this heading.

Prochlorperazine (Co-administration results in additive drowsiness and CNS depression). Products include:
- Compazine 2644

Procyclidine Hydrochloride (Co-administration with anticholinergic agents may result in additive or super-additive tachycardia and drowsiness). Products include:
- Kemadrin Tablets 1105

Promethazine Hydrochloride (Co-administration results in additive drowsiness and CNS depression). Products include:
- Mepergan Injection 2859
- Phenergan with Codeine 2883
- Phenergan with Dextromethorphan 2885
- Phenergan Injection 2880
- Phenergan Suppositories 2882
- Phenergan Syrup 2881
- Phenergan Tablets 2882
- Phenergan VC 2886
- Phenergan VC with Codeine 2888

Propantheline Bromide (Co-administration with anticholinergic agents may result in additive or super-additive tachycardia and drowsiness). Products include:
- Pro-Banthine Tablets 2226

Propofol (Co-administration results in additive drowsiness and CNS depression). Products include:
- Diprivan Injectable Emulsion 2939

Propoxyphene Hydrochloride (Co-administration results in additive drowsiness and CNS depression). Products include:
- Darvon 1475
- Wygesic Tablets 2930

Propoxyphene Napsylate (Co-administration results in additive drowsiness and CNS depression). Products include:
- Darvon-N/Darvocet-N 1473

Protriptyline Hydrochloride (Co-administration results in additive tachycardia, hypertension, drowsiness). Products include:
- Vivactil Tablets 1820

Pseudoephedrine Hydrochloride (Co-administration with sympathomimetics may result in additive hypertension, tachycardia, and possibly cardiotoxicity). Products include:
- Actifed Allergy Daytime/Nighttime Caplets 808
- Actifed Cold & Allergy Tablets 807
- Actifed Cold & Sinus Caplets and Tablets 808
- Actifed Sinus Daytime/Nighttime Tablets and Caplets 809
- Advil Cold and Sinus Caplets and Tablets 837
- Alka-Seltzer Plus Liqui-Gels 612
- Alka-Seltzer Plus Flu & Body Aches Liqui-Gels Non-Drowsy Formula 613
- Alka-Seltzer Plus Night-Time Cold Medicine Liqui-Gels 612
- Allerest Maximum Strength 649
- Allerest No Drowsiness 649
- Allerest Sinus Pain Formula 649
- Atrohist Pediatric Capsules 1603
- Benadryl Allergy/Cold Tablets 811
- Benadryl Allergy Decongestant Liquid Medication 812
- Benadryl Allergy Decongestant Tablets 812
- Benadryl Allergy Sinus Headache Caplets 813
- Benylin Multisymptom 816
- Bromfed Capsules (Extended-Release) 1832
- Bromfed Syrup 712
- Bromfed Tablets 1832
- Bromfed-DM Cough Syrup 1832

IMPORTANT NOTE: Always consult each drug listing in the patient's regimen for possible interactions.

Bromfed-PD Capsules (Extended-Release) 1832	Sinutab Sinus Medication, Maximum Strength Without Drowsiness Formula, Tablets & Caplets 824	**Pseudoephedrine Sulfate** (Co-administration with sympathomimetics may result in additive hypertension, tachycardia, and possibly cardiotoxicity). Products include:	**Terbutaline Sulfate** (Co-administration with sympathomimetics may result in additive hypertension, tachycardia, and possibly cardiotoxicity). Products include:
Children's TYLENOL Cold Multi-Symptom Chewable Tablets and Liquid 1559	Sudafed Children's Cold & Cough Liquid Medication 825	Chlor-Trimeton Allergy Decongestant Tablets 759	Brethaire Inhaler 830
Children's TYLENOL Cold Plus Cough Multi Symptom Chewable Tablets and Liquid............ 1560	Sudafed Children's Nasal Decongestant Liquid Medication 826	Claritin-D Tablets............ 2487	Brethine Ampuls 832
Children's TYLENOL Flu Suspension Liquid 1560	Sudafed Cold & Allergy Tablets...... 826	Drixoral Cold and Allergy Sustained-Action Tablets............ 763	Brethine Tablets............ 831
Children's Vicks DayQuil Allergy Relief............ 730	Sudafed Cold and Cough Liquid Caps 826	Drixoral Cold and Flu Extended-Release Tablets............ 764	Bricanyl Subcutaneous Injection 1247
Children's Vicks NyQuil Cold/Cough Relief............ 731	Sudafed Nasal Decongestant Tablets, 30 mg............ 825	Drixoral Non-Drowsy Formula Extended-Release Tablets 764	Bricanyl Tablets............ 1248
Allergy-Sinus Comtrex Multi-Symptom Allergy-Sinus Formula Tablets and Caplets 639	Sudafed Nasal Decongestant Tablets, 60 mg............ 825	Drixoral Allergy/Sinus Extended Release Tablets............ 765	**Terfenadine** (Co-administration results in additive CNS depression or super-additive tachycardia and drowsiness). Products include:
Comtrex Multi-Symptom............ 638	Sudafed Non-Drying Sinus Liquid Caps 827	Trinalin Repetabs Tablets 1373	Seldane Tablets 1284
Comtrex Multi-Symptom Non-Drowsy Caplets 640	Sudafed Pediatric Nasal Decongestant Liquid Oral Drops 827	**Pyrilamine Maleate** (Co-administration results in additive CNS depression or super-additive tachycardia and drowsiness). Products include:	Seldane-D Extended-Release Tablets 1286
Congess 1003	Sudafed Severe Cold Formula Caplets............ 828	4-Way Fast Acting Nasal Spray (regular & mentholated) 644	**Theophylline** (Increased theophylline metabolism has resulted with smoking marijuana). Products include:
Contac Day Allergy/Sinus Caplets 771	Sudafed Severe Cold Formula Tablets 828	Maximum Strength Multi-Symptom Formula Midol 621	Marax Tablets & DF Syrup............ 2015
Contac Day & Night 772	Sudafed Sinus Caplets 829	PMS Multi-Symptom Formula Midol 622	Quibron 2227
Contac Night Allergy/Sinus Caplets 771	Sudafed Sinus Tablets 829	**Pyrilamine Tannate** (Co-administration results in additive CNS depression or super-additive tachycardia and drowsiness). Products include:	**Theophylline Anhydrous** (Increased theophylline metabolism has resulted with smoking marijuana). Products include:
Contac Severe Cold & Flu Non-Drowsy............ 774	Sudafed 12 Hour Caplets 824	Atrohist Pediatric Suspension 1604	Aerolate 1003
Deconsal II Tablets 1605	Syn-Rx Tablets 1622	Atrohist Pediatric Suspension Dye-Free 1604	Primatene Tablets 844
Dimetane-DX Cough Syrup 2233	Syn-Rx DM Tablets 1623	Rynatan 2781	Respbid Tablets 687
Dimetapp Cold & Fever Suspension 839	TheraFlu Flu and Cold Medicine 750	**Quazepam** (Co-administration results in additive drowsiness and CNS depression). Products include:	Slo-bid Gyrocaps 2201
Dimetapp Decongestant Pediatric Drops 840	Theraflu Maximum Strength Flu and Cold Medicine For Sore Throat 751	Doral Tablets 2773	Theo-24 Extended Release Capsules 2753
Dorcol Children's Cough Syrup 748	TheraFlu Flu, Cold and Cough Medicine 750	**Risperidone** (Co-administration results in additive drowsiness and CNS depression). Products include:	Theo-Dur Extended-Release Tablets 1367
Drixoral Cough + Congestion Liquid Caps 763	TheraFlu Maximum Strength Nighttime Flu, Cold & Cough Medicine 751	Risperdal Tablets 1348	Theo-X Extended-Release Tablets 793
Dura-Tap/PD Capsules 970	TheraFlu Maximum Strength Non-Drowsy Formula Flu, Cold & Cough Medicine 751	**Salmeterol Xinafoate** (Co-administration with sympathomimetics may result in additive hypertension, tachycardia, and possibly cardiotoxicity). Products include:	Uni-Dur Extended-Release Tablets 1374
Duratuss Tablets 2750	TheraFlu Maximum Strength, Non-Drowsy Formula Flu, Cold and Cough Caplets 752	Serevent Inhalation Aerosol 1149	Uniphyl 400 mg and 600 mg Tablets 2157
Duratuss HD Elixir 2750	Theraflu Maximum Strength Sinus Non-Drowsy Formula Caplets 752	**Scopolamine** (Co-administration with anticholinergic agents may result in additive or super-additive tachycardia and drowsiness). Products include:	**Theophylline Calcium Salicylate** (Increased theophylline metabolism has resulted with smoking marijuana). Products include:
Efidac/24 655	Triaminic AM Cough and Decongestant Formula 753	Transderm Scōp Transdermal Therapeutic System 890	Quadrinal Tablets 1398
Entex PSE Tablets 973	Triaminic AM Decongestant Formula 753	**Scopolamine Hydrobromide** (Co-administration with anticholinergic agents may result in additive or super-additive tachycardia and drowsiness). Products include:	**Theophylline Sodium Glycinate** (Increased theophylline metabolism has resulted with smoking marijuana).
Fedahist Gyrocaps 2545	Triaminic Infant Oral Decongestant Drops 754	Atrohist Plus Tablets 1605	No products indexed under this heading.
Guaifed 1833	Triaminic Night Time 754	Donnatal 2234	**Thiamylal Sodium** (Co-administration results in decreased clearance of barbiturates via competitive inhibition of metabolism; additive drowsiness and CNS depression).
Guaifed Syrup 712	Triaminic Sore Throat Formula 755	Donnatal Extentabs 2234	No products indexed under this heading.
Guaimax-D Tablets 809	Tussend 1830	Donnatal Tablets 2234	**Thioridazine Hydrochloride** (Co-administration results in additive drowsiness and CNS depression). Products include:
Histussin D Liquid 670	Tussend Expectorant 1831	**Secobarbital Sodium** (Co-administration results in decreased clearance of barbiturates via competitive inhibition of metabolism; additive drowsiness and CNS depression). Products include:	Mellaril 2398
Infants' TYLENOL Cold Decongestant & Fever-Reducer Drops 1561	TYLENOL Allergy Sinus, Maximum Strength Caplets and Gelcaps 1571	Seconal Sodium Pulvules 1529	**Thiothixene** (Co-administration results in additive drowsiness and CNS depression). Products include:
Kronofed-A 994	TYLENOL Allergy Sinus NightTime, Maximum Strength Caplets 1571	**Sevoflurane** (Co-administration results in additive drowsiness and CNS depression).	Navane Capsules and Concentrate 2018
Novahistine DMX 782	TYLENOL Cold Medication, Multi-Symptom Formula Tablets and Caplets 1572	No products indexed under this heading.	Navane Intramuscular 2019
Nucofed 2225	TYLENOL Cold Medication, Multi-Symptom Hot Liquid Packets 1572	**Sufentanil Citrate** (Co-administration results in additive drowsiness and CNS depression). Products include:	**Triazolam** (Co-administration results in additive drowsiness and CNS depression). Products include:
PediaCare Cough-Cold Chewable Tablets and Liquid............ 1569	TYLENOL Cold Medication, No Drowsiness Formula Caplets and Gelcaps 1572	Sufenta Injection 1355	Halcion Tablets 2093
PediaCare Infants' Decongestant Drops 1569	TYLENOL Cold Severe Congestion Caplets 1573	**Temazepam** (Co-administration results in additive drowsiness and CNS depression). Products include:	**Tridihexethyl Chloride** (Co-administration with anticholinergic agents may result in additive or super-additive tachycardia and drowsiness).
PediaCare Infants' Drops Decongestant Plus Cough............ 1569	TYLENOL Cough Medication with Decongestant, Multi Symptom 1574	Restoril Capsules 2413	No products indexed under this heading.
PediaCare NightRest Cough-Cold Liquid 1569	TYLENOL Flu No Drowsiness Formula, Maximum Strength Gelcaps 1575		**Trifluoperazine Hydrochloride** (Co-administration results in additive drowsiness and CNS depression). Products include:
Pediatric Vicks 44d Cough & Head Congestion Relief 736	TYLENOL Flu NightTime, Maximum Strength Gelcaps 1575		Stelazine 2692
Pediatric Vicks 44m Cough & Cold Relief 737	TYLENOL Flu NightTime, Maximum Strength Hot Medication Packets 1575		**Trihexyphenidyl Hydrochloride** (Co-administration with anticholinergic agents may result in additive or super-additive tachycardia and drowsiness). Products include:
Robitussin Cold & Cough Liqui-Gels 844	TYLENOL Sinus, Maximum Strength Geltabs, Gelcaps, Caplets and Tablets 1576		Artane 1418
Robitussin Cold, Cough & Flu Liqui-Gels 844	Vicks 44 LiquiCaps Cough, Cold & Flu Relief 728		
Robitussin Maximum Strength Cough & Cold 847	Vicks 44 LiquiCaps Non-Drowsy Cough & Cold Relief 729		
Robitussin Night-Time Cold Formula 847	Vicks 44D Cough & Head Congestion Relief 728		
Robitussin Pediatric Cough & Cold Formula 848	Vicks 44M Cough, Cold & Flu Relief 729		
Robitussin Pediatric Drops 849	Vicks DayQuil LiquiCaps/Liquid Multi-Symptom Cold/Flu Relief 734		
Robitussin Severe Congestion Liqui-Gels 845	Vicks DayQuil SINUS Pressure & PAIN Relief with IBUPROFEN 735		
Robitussin-DAC Syrup 2249	Vicks Nyquil Hot Therapy 735		
Robitussin-PE 846	Vicks NyQuil LiquiCaps/Liquid Multi-Symptom Cold/Flu Relief, Original and Cherry Flavors 736		
Rondec Oral Drops 974			
Rondec Syrup 974			
Rondec Tablet 974			
Rondec Chewable Tablets 974			
Rondec-TR Tablet 974			
Ryna 804			
Seldane-D Extended-Release Tablets 1286			
Semprex-D Capsules 1620			
Sinarest 663			
Sine-Aid Maximum Strength Sinus Headache Gelcaps, Caplets and Tablets 1570			
Sine-Off No Drowsiness Formula Caplets 784			
Sine-Off Sinus Medicine 784			
Singlet Tablets 785			
Sinutab Non-Drying Liquid Caps 823			
Sinutab Sinus Allergy Medication, Maximum Strength Tablets and Caplets 823			

(■ Described in PDR For Nonprescription Drugs)   (© Described in PDR For Ophthalmology)

Trimeprazine Tartrate (Co-administration results in additive CNS depression or super-additive tachycardia and drowsiness).
- No products indexed under this heading.

Trimipramine Maleate (Co-administration results in additive tachycardia, hypertension, drowsiness). Products include:
- Surmontil Capsules ... 2917

Tripelennamine Hydrochloride (Co-administration results in additive CNS depression or super-additive tachycardia and drowsiness). Products include:
- PBZ Tablets ... 863
- PBZ-SR Tablets ... 862

Triprolidine Hydrochloride (Co-administration results in additive CNS depression or super-additive tachycardia and drowsiness). Products include:
- Actifed Cold & Allergy Tablets ... ◘ 807
- Actifed Cold & Sinus Caplets and Tablets ... ◘ 808

Zolpidem Tartrate (Co-administration results in additive drowsiness and CNS depression). Products include:
- Ambien Tablets ... 2559

Food Interactions

Alcohol (Co-administration results in additive drowsiness and CNS depression).

MARLYN FORMULA 50 CAPSULES
(Amino Acid Preparations, Vitamin B_6) ... 1558
None cited in PDR database.

MASSENGILL DISPOSABLE DOUCHE
(Vinegar) ... 2627
None cited in PDR database.

MASSENGILL FEMININE CLEANSING WASH
(Cleanser) ... 2628
None cited in PDR database.

MASSENGILL FRAGRANCE-FREE SOFT CLOTH TOWELETTE & BABY POWDER SCENT
(Lactic Acid, Potassium Sorbate, Sodium Lactate) ... 2628
None cited in PDR database.

MASSENGILL LIQUID CONCENTRATE
(Povidone Iodine) ... 2627
None cited in PDR database.

MASSENGILL MEDICATED DISPOSABLE DOUCHE
(Povidone Iodine) ... 2628
None cited in PDR database.

MASSENGILL MEDICATED SOFT CLOTH TOWELETTES
(Hydrocortisone) ... 2628
None cited in PDR database.

MASSENGILL POWDER
(Ammonium Alum, Sodium Chloride) 2627
None cited in PDR database.

MATERNA TABLETS
(Vitamins, Prenatal) ... 1427
None cited in PDR database.

MATRIX MICROCLYSMIC GEL
(Propylene Glycol, Glycerin) ... ◘ 647
None cited in PDR database.

MATULANE CAPSULES
(Procarbazine Hydrochloride) ... 2300
May interact with barbiturates, antihistamines, narcotic analgesics, phenothiazines, antihypertensives, sympathomimetics, tricyclic antidepressants, and certain other agents. Compounds in these categories include:

Acebutolol Hydrochloride (Possible potentiation). Products include:
- Sectral Capsules ... 2914

Acrivastine (Possible potentiation; exercise caution to minimize CNS depression). Products include:
- Semprex-D Capsules ... 1620

Albuterol (Procarbazine exhibits some monoamine oxidase inhibitory activity; concurrent use should be avoided). Products include:
- Proventil Inhalation Aerosol ... 2524
- Ventolin Inhalation Aerosol and Refill ... 1170

Albuterol Sulfate (Procarbazine exhibits some monoamine oxidase inhibitory activity; concurrent use should be avoided). Products include:
- Airet Albuterol Sulfate Inhalation Solution ... 1602
- Albuterol Sulfate, USP Solution for Inhalation, Arm-a-Med ... 522
- Proventil Inhalation Solution 0.083% ... 2527
- Proventil Repetabs Tablets ... 2529
- Proventil Solution for Inhalation 0.5% ... 2525
- Proventil Syrup ... 2528
- Proventil Tablets ... 2529
- Ventolin Inhalation Solution ... 1171
- Ventolin Nebules Inhalation Solution ... 1172
- Ventolin Rotacaps for Inhalation ... 1173
- Ventolin Syrup ... 1175
- Ventolin Tablets ... 1176
- Volmax Extended-Release Tablets .. 1835

Alfentanil Hydrochloride (Possible potentiation; exercise caution to minimize CNS depression). Products include:
- Alfenta Injection ... 1334

Amitriptyline Hydrochloride (Procarbazine exhibits some monoamine oxidase inhibitory activity; concurrent use should be avoided). Products include:
- Elavil ... 2945
- Etrafon ... 2495
- Limbitrol ... 2333
- Triavil Tablets ... 1800

Amlodipine Besylate (Possible potentiation). Products include:
- Lotrel Capsules ... 858
- Norvasc Tablets ... 2020

Amoxapine (Procarbazine exhibits some monoamine oxidase inhibitory activity; concurrent use should be avoided). Products include:
- Asendin Tablets ... 1419

Aprobarbital (Possible potentiation; exercise caution to minimize CNS depression).
- No products indexed under this heading.

Astemizole (Possible potentiation; exercise caution to minimize CNS depression). Products include:
- Hismanal Tablets ... 1341

Atenolol (Possible potentiation). Products include:
- Tenoretic Tablets ... 2963
- Tenormin Tablets and I.V. Injection 2965

Azatadine Maleate (Possible potentiation; exercise caution to minimize CNS depression). Products include:
- Trinalin Repetabs Tablets ... 1373

Benazepril Hydrochloride (Possible potentiation). Products include:
- Lotensin Tablets ... 852
- Lotensin HCT Tablets ... 855
- Lotrel Capsules ... 858

Bendroflumethiazide (Possible potentiation).
- No products indexed under this heading.

Betaxolol Hydrochloride (Possible potentiation). Products include:
- Betoptic Ophthalmic Solution ... 465
- Betoptic S Ophthalmic Suspension 467
- Kerlone Tablets ... 2588

Bisoprolol Fumarate (Possible potentiation). Products include:
- Zebeta Tablets ... 1457
- Ziac ... 1459

Bromodiphenhydramine Hydrochloride (Possible potentiation; exercise caution to minimize CNS depression).
- No products indexed under this heading.

Brompheniramine Maleate (Possible potentiation; exercise caution to minimize CNS depression). Products include:
- Alka-Seltzer Plus Sinus Medicine .. ◘ 611
- Bromfed Capsules (Extended-Release) ... 1832
- Bromfed Syrup ... ◘ 712
- Bromfed Tablets ... 1832
- Bromfed-DM Cough Syrup ... 1832
- Bromfed-PD Capsules (Extended-Release) ... 1832
- Dimetane-DC Cough Syrup ... 2232
- Dimetane-DX Cough Syrup ... 2233
- Dimetapp Allergy Dye-Free Elixir ... ◘ 838
- Dimetapp Allergy Sinus Caplets ... ◘ 838
- Dimetapp Cold & Allergy Chewable Tablets ... ◘ 838
- Dimetapp Cold & Cough Liqui-Gels ... ◘ 839
- Dimetapp Cold & Fever Suspension ... ◘ 839
- Dimetapp DM Elixir ... ◘ 840
- Dimetapp Elixir ... ◘ 840
- Dimetapp Extentabs ... ◘ 841
- Dimetapp Tablets/Liqui-Gels ... ◘ 841
- Rondec Chewable Tablets ... 974
- Vicks DayQuil Allergy Relief 12-Hour Extended Release Tablets.. ◘ 733
- Vicks DayQuil Allergy Relief 4-Hour Tablets ... ◘ 733

Buprenorphine (Possible potentiation; exercise caution to minimize CNS depression). Products include:
- Buprenex Injectable ... 2170

Butabarbital (Possible potentiation; exercise caution to minimize CNS depression).
- No products indexed under this heading.

Butalbital (Possible potentiation; exercise caution to minimize CNS depression). Products include:
- Axocet Capsules ... 2469
- Esgic-plus Capsules ... 1012
- Esgic-plus Tablets ... 1012
- Fioricet Tablets ... 2386
- Fioricet with Codeine Capsules ... 2387
- Fiorinal Capsules ... 2388
- Fiorinal with Codeine Capsules ... 2390
- Fiorinal Tablets ... 2388
- Phrenilin ... 790
- Sedapap Tablets 50 mg/650 mg .. 1826

Captopril (Possible potentiation). Products include:
- Capoten Tablets ... 740
- Capozide Tablets ... 744

Carteolol Hydrochloride (Possible potentiation). Products include:
- Cartrol Tablets ... 413
- Ocupress Ophthalmic Solution, 1% Sterile ... ⊙ 297

Cetirizine Hydrochloride (Possible potentiation; exercise caution to minimize CNS depression). Products include:
- Zyrtec Tablets ... 2053

Chlorothiazide (Possible potentiation). Products include:
- Aldoclor Tablets ... 1638
- Diupres Tablets ... 1691
- Diuril Oral ... 1694

Chlorothiazide Sodium (Possible potentiation). Products include:
- Diuril Sodium Intravenous ... 1693

Chlorpheniramine Maleate (Possible potentiation; exercise caution to minimize CNS depression). Products include:
- Alka-Seltzer Plus Cold Medicine ... ◘ 611
- Alka-Seltzer Plus Cold Medicine Liqui-Gels ... ◘ 612
- Alka-Seltzer Plus Cold & Cough Medicine ... ◘ 611
- Alka-Seltzer Plus Cold & Cough Medicine Liqui-Gels ... ◘ 612
- Alka-Seltzer Plus Flu & Body Aches Effervescent Tablets ... ◘ 612
- Allerest Maximum Strength ... ◘ 649
- Allerest Sinus Pain Formula ... ◘ 649
- Ana-Kit Anaphylaxis Emergency Treatment Kit ... 611
- Atrohist Pediatric Capsules ... 1603
- Atrohist Plus Tablets ... 1605
- BC Cold Powder Multi-Symptom Formula (Cold-Sinus-Allergy) ... ◘ 631
- Cerose DM ... ◘ 853
- Cheracol Plus Head Cold/Cough Formula ... ◘ 741
- Children's TYLENOL Cold Multi-Symptom Chewable Tablets and Liquid ... 1559
- Children's TYLENOL Cold Plus Cough Multi Symptom Chewable Tablets and Liquid ... 1560
- Children's TYLENOL Flu Suspension Liquid ... 1560
- Children's Vicks DayQuil Allergy Relief ... ◘ 730
- Children's Vicks NyQuil Cold/Cough Relief ... ◘ 731
- Chlor-Trimeton Allergy Decongestant Tablets ... ◘ 759
- Chlor-Trimeton Allergy Tablets ... ◘ 758
- Allergy-Sinus Comtrex Multi-Symptom Allergy-Sinus Formula Tablets and Caplets ... ◘ 639
- Comtrex Multi-Symptom ... ◘ 638
- Contac Continuous Action Nasal Decongestant/Antihistamine 12 Hour Capsules ... ◘ 773
- Contac Maximum Strength Continuous Action Decongestant/Antihistamine 12 Hour Caplets.. ◘ 772
- Contac Severe Cold and Flu Formula Caplets ... ◘ 773
- Coricidin Cold + Flu Tablets ... ◘ 760
- Coricidin Cough + Cold Tablets ... ◘ 760
- Coricidin 'D' Decongestant Tablets ... ◘ 760
- D.A. II Tablets ... 972
- D.A. Chewable Tablets ... 970
- Dura-Tap/PD Capsules ... 970
- Dura-Vent/DA Tablets ... 972
- Efidac 24 Chlorpheniramine ... ◘ 655
- Extendryl ... 1003
- Fedahist Gyrocaps ... 2545
- Hycomine Compound Tablets ... 948
- Kronofed-A ... 994
- Nolamine Timed-Release Tablets ... 790
- Novahistine Elixir ... ◘ 782
- Ornade Spansule Capsules ... 2678
- PediaCare Cough-Cold Chewable Tablets and Liquid ... 1569
- PediaCare NightRest Cough-Cold Liquid ... 1569
- Pediatric Vicks 44m Cough & Cold Relief ... ◘ 737
- Pyrroxate Caplets ... ◘ 742
- Ryna ... ◘ 804
- Sinarest ... ◘ 663
- Sine-Off Sinus Medicine ... ◘ 784
- Singlet Tablets ... ◘ 785
- Sinulin Tablets ... 792
- Sinutab Sinus Allergy Medication, Maximum Strength Tablets and Caplets ... ◘ 823
- Sudafed Cold & Allergy Tablets ... ◘ 826
- Teldrin 12 Hour Antihistamine/Nasal Decongestant Allergy Relief Capsules ... ◘ 786
- TheraFlu Flu and Cold Medicine ... ◘ 750
- Theraflu Maximum Strength Flu and Cold Medicine For Sore Throat ... ◘ 751
- TheraFlu Flu, Cold and Cough Medicine ... ◘ 750
- TheraFlu Maximum Strength Nighttime Flu, Cold & Cough Medicine ... ◘ 751
- Triaminic Night Time ... ◘ 754
- Triaminic Syrup ... ◘ 755

IMPORTANT NOTE: Always consult each drug listing in the patient's regimen for possible interactions.

Matulane — Interactions Index

Triaminic Triaminicol Cold & Cough ... ▣ 756
Triaminicin Tablets ... ▣ 756
Tussend ... 1830
TYLENOL Allergy Sinus, Maximum Strength Caplets and Gelcaps ... 1571
TYLENOL Cold Medication, Multi-Symptom Formula Tablets and Caplets ... 1572
TYLENOL Cold Medication, Multi-Symptom Hot Liquid Packets ... 1572
Vicks 44 LiquiCaps Cough, Cold & Flu Relief ... ▣ 728
Vicks 44M Cough, Cold & Flu Relief ... ▣ 729

Chlorpheniramine Polistirex (Possible potentiation; exercise caution to minimize CNS depression). Products include:
Tussionex Pennkinetic Extended-Release Suspension ... 1624

Chlorpheniramine Tannate (Possible potentiation; exercise caution to minimize CNS depression). Products include:
Atrohist Pediatric Suspension ... 1604
Atrohist Pediatric Suspension Dye-Free ... 1604
Rynatan ... 2781
Rynatuss ... 2782

Chlorpromazine (Possible potentiation; exercise caution to minimize CNS depression). Products include:
Thorazine Suppositories ... 2701

Chlorpromazine Hydrochloride (Possible potentiation; exercise caution to minimize CNS depression). Products include:
Thorazine ... 2701

Chlorthalidone (Possible potentiation). Products include:
Combipres Tablets ... 682
Tenoretic Tablets ... 2963
Thalitone ... 1293

Clemastine Fumarate (Possible potentiation; exercise caution to minimize CNS depression). Products include:
Tavist Syrup ... 2426
Tavist Tablets ... 2427
Tavist-1 12 Hour Relief Tablets ... ▣ 749
Tavist-D 12 Hour Relief Tablets ... ▣ 750

Clomipramine Hydrochloride (Procarbazine exhibits some monoamine oxidase inhibitory activity; concurrent use should be avoided). Products include:
Anafranil Capsules ... 819

Clonidine (Possible potentiation). Products include:
Catapres-TTS ... 680

Clonidine Hydrochloride (Possible potentiation). Products include:
Catapres Tablets ... 679
Combipres Tablets ... 682

Codeine Phosphate (Possible potentiation; exercise caution to minimize CNS depression). Products include:
Brontex ... 2130
Dimetane-DC Cough Syrup ... 2232
Fioricet with Codeine Capsules ... 2387
Fiorinal with Codeine Capsules ... 2390
Nucofed ... 2225
Phenergan with Codeine ... 2883
Phenergan VC with Codeine ... 2888
Robitussin A-C Syrup ... 2248
Robitussin-DAC Syrup ... 2249
Ryna ... 804
Soma Compound w/Codeine Tablets ... 2784
Tylenol with Codeine ... 1592

Cyproheptadine Hydrochloride (Possible potentiation; exercise caution to minimize CNS depression). Products include:
Periactin ... 1767

Deserpidine (Possible potentiation).
No products indexed under this heading.

Desipramine Hydrochloride (Procarbazine exhibits some monoamine oxidase inhibitory activity; concurrent use should be avoided). Products include:
Norpramin Tablets ... 1273

Dexchlorpheniramine Maleate (Possible potentiation; exercise caution to minimize CNS depression).
No products indexed under this heading.

Dezocine (Possible potentiation; exercise caution to minimize CNS depression). Products include:
Dalgan Injection ... 529

Diazoxide (Possible potentiation). Products include:
Hyperstat I.V. Injection ... 2504
Proglycem ... 575

Diltiazem Hydrochloride (Possible potentiation). Products include:
Cardizem CD Capsules ... 1251
Cardizem SR Capsules ... 1255
Cardizem Injectable ... 1253
Cardizem Tablets ... 1257
Dilacor XR Extended-release Capsules ... 2183
Tiazac Capsules ... 1019

Diphenhydramine Citrate (Possible potentiation; exercise caution to minimize CNS depression). Products include:
Excedrin P.M. Analgesic/Sleeping Aid Tablets, Caplets, Liquigels ... 735

Diphenhydramine Hydrochloride (Possible potentiation; exercise caution to minimize CNS depression). Products include:
Actifed Allergy Daytime/Nighttime Caplets ... ▣ 808
Actifed Sinus Daytime/Nighttime Tablets and Caplets ... ▣ 809
Extra Strength Bayer PM Aspirin Plus Sleep Aid ... 617
Benadryl Allergy Chewables ... ▣ 811
Benadryl Allergy/Cold Tablets ... ▣ 811
Benadryl Allergy Decongestant Liquid Medication ... ▣ 812
Benadryl Allergy Decongestant Tablets ... ▣ 812
Benadryl Allergy Liquid Medication ... ▣ 813
Benadryl Allergy ... ▣ 811
Benadryl Allergy Sinus Headache Caplets ... ▣ 813
Benadryl Dye-Free Allergy Liquigel Softgels ... ▣ 813
Benadryl Dye-Free Allergy Liquid Medication ... ▣ 814
Benadryl Itch Relief Stick Extra Strength ... ▣ 814
Benadryl Cream ... ▣ 814
Benadryl Gel ... ▣ 815
Benadryl Spray ... ▣ 815
Benadryl Injection ... 1955
Contac Day & Night Cold/Flu Night Caplets ... ▣ 772
Contac Night Allergy/Sinus Caplets ... ▣ 771
Extra Strength Doan's P.M. ... ▣ 653
Excedrin P.M. Analgesic/Sleeping Aid Tablets, Caplets, Liquigels ... ▣ 643
Nytol QuickCaps Caplets ... ▣ 632
Sleepinal Night-time Sleep Aid Capsules and Softgels ... ▣ 798
TYLENOL Allergy Sinus NightTime, Maximum Strength Caplets ... 1571
TYLENOL Flu NightTime, Maximum Strength Gelcaps ... 1575
TYLENOL Flu NightTime, Maximum Strength Hot Medication Packets ... 1575
TYLENOL PM Pain Reliever/Sleep Aid, Extra Strength Gelcaps, Caplets, Geltabs ... 1576
TYLENOL Severe Allergy Medication Caplets ... 1571
Maximum Strength Unisom Sleepgels ... 1990
Unisom With Pain Relief-Nighttime Sleep Aid and Pain Reliever ... 1991

Diphenylpyraline Hydrochloride (Possible potentiation; exercise caution to minimize CNS depression).
No products indexed under this heading.

Dobutamine Hydrochloride (Procarbazine exhibits some monoamine oxidase inhibitory activity; concurrent use should be avoided). Products include:
Dobutrex Solution Vials ... 1480

Dopamine Hydrochloride (Procarbazine exhibits some monoamine oxidase inhibitory activity; concurrent use should be avoided).
No products indexed under this heading.

Doxazosin Mesylate (Possible potentiation). Products include:
Cardura Tablets ... 1993

Doxepin Hydrochloride (Procarbazine exhibits some monoamine oxidase inhibitory activity; concurrent use should be avoided). Products include:
Adapin Capsules ... 1542
Sinequan ... 2028
Zonalon Cream ... 1042

Enalapril Maleate (Possible potentiation). Products include:
Vaseretic Tablets ... 1810
Vasotec Tablets ... 1816

Enalaprilat (Possible potentiation). Products include:
Vasotec I.V. ... 1814

Ephedrine Hydrochloride (Procarbazine exhibits some monoamine oxidase inhibitory activity; concurrent use should be avoided). Products include:
Primatene Tablets ... ▣ 844
Quadrinal Tablets ... 1398

Ephedrine Sulfate (Procarbazine exhibits some monoamine oxidase inhibitory activity; concurrent use should be avoided). Products include:
Marax Tablets & DF Syrup ... 2015

Ephedrine Tannate (Procarbazine exhibits some monoamine oxidase inhibitory activity; concurrent use should be avoided). Products include:
Rynatuss ... 2782

Epinephrine (Procarbazine exhibits some monoamine oxidase inhibitory activity; concurrent use should be avoided). Products include:
EPIFRIN ... ⓞ 237
EpiPen ... 808
Marcaine with Epinephrine ... 2446
Primatene Mist ... ▣ 843
Sensorcaine with Epinephrine Injection ... 554
Sus-Phrine Injection ... 1017
Xylocaine with Epinephrine Injections ... 562

Epinephrine Bitartrate (Procarbazine exhibits some monoamine oxidase inhibitory activity; concurrent use should be avoided). Products include:
Sensorcaine-MPF with Epinephrine Injection ... 554

Epinephrine Hydrochloride (Procarbazine exhibits some monoamine oxidase inhibitory activity; concurrent use should be avoided). Products include:
Ana-Kit Anaphylaxis Emergency Treatment Kit ... 611

Esmolol Hydrochloride (Possible potentiation). Products include:
Brevibloc (esmolol HCl) Injection ... 1860

Felodipine (Possible potentiation). Products include:
Plendil Extended-Release Tablets ... 514

Fentanyl (Possible potentiation; exercise caution to minimize CNS depression). Products include:
Duragesic Transdermal System ... 1336

Fentanyl Citrate (Possible potentiation; exercise caution to minimize CNS depression). Products include:
Sublimaze Injection ... 463

Fluphenazine Decanoate (Possible potentiation; exercise caution to minimize CNS depression). Products include:
Prolixin Decanoate ... 510

Fluphenazine Enanthate (Possible potentiation; exercise caution to minimize CNS depression). Products include:
Prolixin Enanthate ... 510

Fluphenazine Hydrochloride (Possible potentiation; exercise caution to minimize CNS depression). Products include:
Prolixin ... 510

Fosinopril Sodium (Possible potentiation). Products include:
Monopril Tablets ... 762

Furosemide (Possible potentiation). Products include:
Lasix Injection, Oral Solution and Tablets ... 1267

Guanabenz Acetate (Possible potentiation).
No products indexed under this heading.

Guanethidine Monosulfate (Possible potentiation). Products include:
Esimil Tablets ... 840
Ismelin Tablets ... 845

Hydralazine Hydrochloride (Possible potentiation). Products include:
Apresazide Capsules ... 824
Apresoline Hydrochloride Tablets ... 826
Hydralazine Hydrochloride Injection USP ... 2712
Ser-Ap-Es Tablets ... 867

Hydrochlorothiazide (Possible potentiation). Products include:
Aldactazide Tablets ... 2556
Aldoril Tablets ... 1644
Apresazide Capsules ... 824
Capozide Tablets ... 744
Dyazide Capsules ... 2653
Esidrix Tablets ... 839
Esimil Tablets ... 840
HydroDIURIL Tablets ... 1716
Hydropres Tablets ... 1718
Hyzaar Tablets ... 1720
Inderide Tablets ... 2838
Inderide LA Long Acting Capsules ... 2840
Lopressor HCT Tablets ... 850
Lotensin HCT Tablets ... 855
Moduretic Tablets ... 1748
Oretic Tablets ... 450
Prinzide Tablets ... 1780
Ser-Ap-Es Tablets ... 867
Timolide Tablets ... 1791
Vaseretic Tablets ... 1810
Zestoretic Tablets ... 2968
Ziac ... 1459

Hydrocodone Bitartrate (Possible potentiation; exercise caution to minimize CNS depression). Products include:
Codiclear DH Syrup ... 808
Duratuss HD Elixir ... 2750
Histussin D Liquid ... 670
Hycodan Tablets and Syrup ... 946
Hycomine Compound Tablets ... 948
Hycomine ... 947
Hycotuss Expectorant Syrup ... 950
Hydrocet Capsules ... 787
Lorcet 10/650 Tablets ... 1016
Lortab ... 2751
Tussend ... 1830
Tussend Expectorant ... 1831
Vicodin Tablets ... 1404
Vicodin ES Tablets ... 1405
Vicodin HP Tablets ... 1403
Vicodin Tuss Expectorant ... 1406
Zydone Capsules ... 967

(▣ Described in PDR For Nonprescription Drugs)   (ⓞ Described in PDR For Ophthalmology)

Hydrocodone Polistirex (Possible potentiation; exercise caution to minimize CNS depression). Products include:
Tussionex Pennkinetic Extended-Release Suspension ... 1624

Hydroflumethiazide (Possible potentiation). Products include:
Diucardin Tablets ... 2824

Hydromorphone Hydrochloride (Possible potentiation; exercise caution to minimize CNS depression). Products include:
Dilaudid Ampules ... 1382
Dilaudid Cough Syrup ... 1383
Dilaudid-HP Injection ... 1384
Dilaudid-HP Lyophilized Powder 250 mg ... 1384
Dilaudid ... 1382
Dilaudid Oral Liquid ... 1386
Dilaudid ... 1382
Dilaudid Tablets - 8 mg ... 1386

Imipramine Hydrochloride (Procarbazine exhibits some monoamine oxidase inhibitory activity; concurrent use should be avoided). Products include:
Tofranil Ampuls ... 873
Tofranil Tablets ... 875

Imipramine Pamoate (Procarbazine exhibits some monoamine oxidase inhibitory activity; concurrent use should be avoided). Products include:
Tofranil-PM Capsules ... 876

Indapamide (Possible potentiation).
No products indexed under this heading.

Isoproterenol Hydrochloride (Procarbazine exhibits some monoamine oxidase inhibitory activity; concurrent use should be avoided). Products include:
Isuprel Hydrochloride Solution ... 2443
Isuprel Injection ... 2441
Isuprel Mistometer ... 2442

Isoproterenol Sulfate (Procarbazine exhibits some monoamine oxidase inhibitory activity; concurrent use should be avoided). Products include:
Norisodrine with Calcium Iodide Syrup ... 446

Isradipine (Possible potentiation). Products include:
DynaCirc Capsules ... 2381
DynaCirc CR Tablets ... 2383

Labetalol Hydrochloride (Possible potentiation). Products include:
Normodyne Injection ... 2519
Normodyne Tablets ... 2522
Trandate ... 1158

Levorphanol Tartrate (Possible potentiation; exercise caution to minimize CNS depression). Products include:
Levo-Dromoran ... 2297

Lisinopril (Possible potentiation). Products include:
Prinivil Tablets ... 1776
Prinzide Tablets ... 1780
Zestoretic Tablets ... 2968
Zestril Tablets ... 2972

Loratadine (Possible potentiation; exercise caution to minimize CNS depression). Products include:
Claritin Tablets ... 2485
Claritin-D Tablets ... 2487

Losartan Potassium (Possible potentiation). Products include:
Cozaar Tablets ... 1668
Hyzaar Tablets ... 1720

Maprotiline Hydrochloride (Procarbazine exhibits some monoamine oxidase inhibitory activity; concurrent use should be avoided). Products include:
Ludiomil Tablets ... 861

Mecamylamine Hydrochloride (Possible potentiation). Products include:
Inversine Tablets ... 1729

Meperidine Hydrochloride (Possible potentiation; exercise caution to minimize CNS depression). Products include:
Demerol ... 2438
Mepergan Injection ... 2859

Mephobarbital (Possible potentiation; exercise caution to minimize CNS depression). Products include:
Mebaral Tablets ... 2452

Mesoridazine Besylate (Possible potentiation; exercise caution to minimize CNS depression). Products include:
Serentil ... 689

Metaproterenol Sulfate (Procarbazine exhibits some monoamine oxidase inhibitory activity; concurrent use should be avoided). Products include:
Alupent ... 672
Metaproterenol Sulfate Inhalation Solution, USP, Arm-a-Med ... 547

Metaraminol Bitartrate (Procarbazine exhibits some monoamine oxidase inhibitory activity; concurrent use should be avoided). Products include:
Aramine Injection ... 1649

Methadone Hydrochloride (Possible potentiation; exercise caution to minimize CNS depression). Products include:
Methadone Hydrochloride Oral Concentrate ... 2356
Methadone Hydrochloride Oral Solution & Tablets ... 2357

Methdilazine Hydrochloride (Possible potentiation; exercise caution to minimize CNS depression).
No products indexed under this heading.

Methotrimeprazine (Possible potentiation; exercise caution to minimize CNS depression). Products include:
Levoprome ... 1321

Methoxamine Hydrochloride (Procarbazine exhibits some monoamine oxidase inhibitory activity; concurrent use should be avoided). Products include:
Vasoxyl Injection ... 1169

Methyclothiazide (Possible potentiation). Products include:
Enduron Tablets ... 424

Methyldopa (Possible potentiation). Products include:
Aldoclor Tablets ... 1638
Aldomet Oral ... 1640
Aldoril Tablets ... 1644

Methyldopate Hydrochloride (Possible potentiation). Products include:
Aldomet Ester HCl Injection ... 1642

Metolazone (Possible potentiation). Products include:
Mykrox Tablets ... 1617
Zaroxolyn Tablets ... 1625

Metoprolol Succinate (Possible potentiation). Products include:
Toprol-XL Tablets ... 560

Metoprolol Tartrate (Possible potentiation). Products include:
Lopressor ... 848
Lopressor HCT Tablets ... 850

Metyrosine (Possible potentiation). Products include:
Demser Capsules ... 1690

Minoxidil (Possible potentiation).
No products indexed under this heading.

Moexipril Hydrochloride (Possible potentiation). Products include:
Univasc Tablets ... 2553

Morphine Sulfate (Possible potentiation; exercise caution to minimize CNS depression). Products include:
Astramorph/PF Injection, USP (Preservative-Free) ... 526
Duramorph Injection ... 983
Infumorph 200 and Infumorph 500 Sterile Solutions ... 985
Kadian Capsules ... 2948
MS Contin Tablets ... 2149
MSIR ... 2152
Oramorph SR (Morphine Sulfate Sustained Release Tablets) ... 2359
RMS Suppositories CII ... 2766
Roxanol ... 2365

Nadolol (Possible potentiation).
No products indexed under this heading.

Nicardipine Hydrochloride (Possible potentiation). Products include:
Cardene Capsules ... 2261
Cardene I.V. ... 2815
Cardene SR Capsules ... 2264

Nifedipine (Possible potentiation). Products include:
Adalat Capsules (10 mg and 20 mg) ... 580
Adalat CC ... 582
Procardia Capsules ... 2024
Procardia XL Extended Release Tablets ... 2026

Nisoldipine (Possible potentiation). Products include:
Sular Tablets ... 2961

Nitroglycerin (Possible potentiation). Products include:
Deponit NTG Transdermal Delivery System ... 2541
Nitro-Bid IV ... 1270
Nitro-Bid Ointment ... 1272
Nitro-Dur (nitroglycerin) Transdermal Infusion System ... 1365
Nitrolingual Spray ... 2193
Nitrostat Tablets ... 1981
Transderm-Nitro Transdermal Therapeutic System ... 878

Norepinephrine Bitartrate (Procarbazine exhibits some monoamine oxidase inhibitory activity; concurrent use should be avoided). Products include:
Levophed Bitartrate Injection ... 2445

Nortriptyline Hydrochloride (Procarbazine exhibits some monoamine oxidase inhibitory activity; concurrent use should be avoided). Products include:
Pamelor ... 2409

Opium Alkaloids (Possible potentiation; exercise caution to minimize CNS depression).
No products indexed under this heading.

Oxycodone Hydrochloride (Possible potentiation; exercise caution to minimize CNS depression). Products include:
OxyContin Tablets ... 2163
OxyIR Capsules ... 2167
Percocet Tablets ... 955
Percodan Tablets ... 955
Percodan-Demi Tablets ... 956
Roxicodone Tablets, Oral Solution & Intensol (Oxycodone) ... 2366
Tylox Capsules ... 1593

Penbutolol Sulfate (Possible potentiation). Products include:
Levatol Tablets ... 2547

Pentobarbital Sodium (Possible potentiation; exercise caution to minimize CNS depression). Products include:
Nembutal Sodium Capsules ... 440
Nembutal Sodium Solution ... 442
Nembutal Sodium Suppositories ... 444

Perphenazine (Possible potentiation; exercise caution to minimize CNS depression). Products include:
Etrafon ... 2495
Triavil Tablets ... 1800
Trilafon ... 2532

Phenobarbital (Possible potentiation; exercise caution to minimize CNS depression). Products include:
Arco-Lase Plus Tablets ... 513
Bellergal-S Tablets ... 2375
Donnatal ... 2234
Donnatal Extentabs ... 2234
Donnatal Tablets ... 2234
Phenobarbital Elixir and Tablets ... 1523
Quadrinal Tablets ... 1398

Phenoxybenzamine Hydrochloride (Possible potentiation). Products include:
Dibenzyline Capsules ... 2650

Phentolamine Mesylate (Possible potentiation). Products include:
Regitine Vials ... 864

Phenylephrine Bitartrate (Procarbazine exhibits some monoamine oxidase inhibitory activity; concurrent use should be avoided).
No products indexed under this heading.

Phenylephrine Hydrochloride (Procarbazine exhibits some monoamine oxidase inhibitory activity; concurrent use should be avoided). Products include:
Atrohist Plus Tablets ... 1605
Cerose DM ... 853
D.A. II Tablets ... 972
D.A. Chewable Tablets ... 970
Dura-Vent/DA Tablets ... 972
Extendryl ... 1003
4-Way Fast Acting Nasal Spray (regular & mentholated) ... 644
Hemorid ... 797
Hycomine Compound Tablets ... 948
Neo-Synephrine Hydrochloride 1% Carpuject ... 2455
Neo-Synephrine Hydrochloride 1% Injection ... 2455
Neo-Synephrine Hydrochloride (Ophthalmic) ... 2456
Neo-Synephrine ... 624
Novahistine Elixir ... 782
Phenergan VC ... 2886
Phenergan VC with Codeine ... 2888
Preparation H ... 842
Tympagesic Ear Drops ... 2476
Vicks Sinex Nasal Spray and Ultra Fine Mist ... 738

Phenylephrine Tannate (Procarbazine exhibits some monoamine oxidase inhibitory activity; concurrent use should be avoided). Products include:
Atrohist Pediatric Suspension ... 1604
Atrohist Pediatric Suspension Dye-Free ... 1604
Rynatan ... 2781
Rynatuss ... 2782

Phenylpropanolamine Hydrochloride (Procarbazine exhibits some monoamine oxidase inhibitory activity; concurrent use should be avoided). Products include:
Acutrim ... 648
Atrohist Plus Tablets ... 1605
BC Cold Powder Multi-Symptom Formula (Cold-Sinus-Allergy) ... 631
BC Cold Powder Non-Drowsy Formula (Cold-Sinus) ... 631
Cheracol Plus Head Cold/Cough Formula ... 741
Comtrex Multi-Symptom Cold Reliever Liqui-Gels ... 638
Comtrex Multi-Symptom Non-Drowsy Liqui-gels ... 640
Contac Continuous Action Nasal Decongestant/Antihistamine 12 Hour Capsules ... 773
Contac Maximum Strength Continuous Action Decongestant/Antihistamine 12 Hour Caplets ... 772
Contac Severe Cold and Flu Formula Caplets ... 773
Coricidin 'D' Decongestant Tablets ... 760

IMPORTANT NOTE: Always consult each drug listing in the patient's regimen for possible interactions.

Matulane — Interactions Index — 650

Dexatrim ... 795
Dexatrim Plus Vitamins Caplets ... 796
Dimetane-DC Cough Syrup ... 2232
Dimetapp Allergy Sinus Caplets ... 838
Dimetapp Cold & Allergy Chewable Tablets ... 838
Dimetapp Cold & Cough Liqui-Gels ... 839
Dimetapp DM Elixir ... 840
Dimetapp Elixir ... 840
Dimetapp Extentabs ... 841
Dimetapp Tablets/Liqui-Gels ... 841
Dura-Vent Tablets ... 971
Entex LA Tablets ... 972
Exgest LA Tablets ... 787
Hycomine ... 947
Nolamine Timed-Release Tablets ... 790
Ornade Spansule Capsules ... 2678
Propagest Tablets ... 791
Pyrroxate Caplets ... 742
Robitussin-CF ... 846
Sinulin Tablets ... 792
Tavist-D 12 Hour Relief Tablets ... 750
Teldrin 12 Hour Antihistamine/Nasal Decongestant Allergy Relief Capsules ... 786
Triaminic Expectorant ... 753
Triaminic Syrup ... 755
Triaminic Triaminicol Cold & Cough ... 756
Triaminic DM Syrup ... 756
Triaminicin Tablets ... 756
Vicks DayQuil Allergy Relief 12-Hour Extended Release Tablets ... 733
Vicks DayQuil Allergy Relief 4-Hour Tablets ... 733
Vicks DayQuil SINUS Pressure & CONGESTION Relief ... 734

Pindolol (Possible potentiation). Products include:
Visken Tablets ... 2428

Pirbuterol Acetate (Procarbazine exhibits some monoamine oxidase inhibitory activity; concurrent use should be avoided). Products include:
Maxair Autohaler ... 1550
Maxair Inhaler ... 1552

Polythiazide (Possible potentiation). Products include:
Minizide Capsules ... 2016

Prazosin Hydrochloride (Possible potentiation). Products include:
Minipress Capsules ... 2015
Minizide Capsules ... 2016

Prochlorperazine (Possible potentiation; exercise caution to minimize CNS depression. Products include:
Compazine ... 2644

Promethazine Hydrochloride (Possible potentiation; exercise caution to minimize CNS depression). Products include:
Meperigan Injection ... 2859
Phenergan with Codeine ... 2883
Phenergan with Dextromethorphan ... 2880
Phenergan Injection ... 2882
Phenergan Suppositories ... 2882
Phenergan Syrup ... 2881
Phenergan Tablets ... 2882
Phenergan VC ... 2886
Phenergan VC with Codeine ... 2888

Propoxyphene Hydrochloride (Possible potentiation; exercise caution to minimize CNS depression). Products include:
Darvon ... 1475
Wygesic Tablets ... 2930

Propoxyphene Napsylate (Possible potentiation; exercise caution to minimize CNS depression). Products include:
Darvon-N/Darvocet-N ... 1473

Propranolol Hydrochloride (Possible potentiation). Products include:
Inderal ... 2834
Inderal LA Long Acting Capsules ... 2836
Inderide Tablets ... 2838
Inderide LA Long Acting Capsules ... 2840

Protriptyline Hydrochloride (Procarbazine exhibits some monoamine oxidase inhibitory activity; concurrent use should be avoided). Products include:
Vivactil Tablets ... 1820

Pseudoephedrine Hydrochloride (Procarbazine exhibits some monoamine oxidase inhibitory activity; concurrent use should be avoided). Products include:
Actifed Allergy Daytime/Nighttime Caplets ... 808
Actifed Cold & Allergy Tablets ... 807
Actifed Cold & Sinus Caplets and Tablets ... 808
Actifed Sinus Daytime/Nighttime Tablets and Caplets ... 809
Advil Cold and Sinus Caplets and Tablets ... 837
Alka-Seltzer Plus Liqui-Gels ... 612
Alka-Seltzer Plus Flu & Body Aches Liqui-Gels Non-Drowsy Formula ... 613
Alka-Seltzer Plus Night-Time Cold Medicine Liqui-Gels ... 612
Allerest Maximum Strength ... 649
Allerest No Drowsiness ... 649
Allerest Sinus Pain Formula ... 649
Atrohist Pediatric Capsules ... 1603
Benadryl Allergy/Cold Tablets ... 811
Benadryl Allergy Decongestant Liquid Medication ... 812
Benadryl Allergy Decongestant Tablets ... 812
Benadryl Allergy Sinus Headache Caplets ... 813
Benylin Multisymptom ... 816
Bromfed Capsules (Extended-Release) ... 1832
Bromfed Syrup ... 712
Bromfed Tablets ... 1832
Bromfed-DM Cough Syrup ... 1832
Bromfed-PD Capsules (Extended-Release) ... 1832
Children's TYLENOL Cold Multi-Symptom Chewable Tablets and Liquid ... 1559
Children's TYLENOL Cold Plus Cough Multi Symptom Chewable Tablets and Liquid ... 1560
Children's TYLENOL Flu Suspension Liquid ... 1560
Children's Vicks DayQuil Allergy Relief ... 730
Children's Vicks NyQuil Cold/Cough Relief ... 731
Allergy-Sinus Comtrex Multi-Symptom Allergy-Sinus Formula Tablets and Caplets ... 639
Comtrex Multi-Symptom ... 638
Comtrex Multi-Symptom Non-Drowsy Caplets ... 640
Congess ... 1003
Contac Day Allergy/Sinus Caplets ... 771
Contac Day & Night ... 772
Contac Night Allergy/Sinus Caplets ... 771
Contac Severe Cold & Flu Non-Drowsy ... 774
Deconsal II Tablets ... 1605
Dimetane-DX Cough Syrup ... 2233
Dimetapp Cold & Fever Suspension ... 839
Dimetapp Decongestant Pediatric Drops ... 840
Dorcol Children's Cough Syrup ... 748
Drixoral Cough + Congestion Liquid Caps ... 763
Dura-Tap/PD Capsules ... 970
Duratuss Tablets ... 2750
Duratuss HD Elixir ... 2750
Efidac/24 ... 655
Entex PSE Tablets ... 973
Fedahist Gyrocaps ... 2545
Guaifed ... 1833
Guaifed Syrup ... 712
Guaimax-D Tablets ... 809
Histussin D Liquid ... 670
Infants' TYLENOL Cold Decongestant & Fever-Reducer Drops ... 1561
Kronofed-A ... 994
Novahistine DMX ... 782
Nucofed ... 2225
PediaCare Cough-Cold Chewable Tablets and Liquid ... 1569
PediaCare Infants' Decongestant Drops ... 1569
PediaCare Infants' Drops Decongestant Plus Cough ... 1569
PediaCare NightRest Cough-Cold Liquid ... 1569
Pediatric Vicks 44d Cough & Head Congestion Relief ... 736
Pediatric Vicks 44m Cough & Cold Relief ... 737
Robitussin Cold & Cough Liqui-Gels ... 844
Robitussin Cold, Cough & Flu Liqui-Gels ... 844
Robitussin Maximum Strength Cough & Cold ... 847
Robitussin Night-Time Cold Formula ... 847
Robitussin Pediatric Cough & Cold Formula ... 848
Robitussin Pediatric Drops ... 849
Robitussin Severe Congestion Liqui-Gels ... 845
Robitussin-DAC Syrup ... 2249
Robitussin-PE ... 846
Rondec Oral Drops ... 974
Rondec Syrup ... 974
Rondec Tablet ... 974
Rondec Chewable Tablets ... 974
Rondec-TR Tablet ... 974
Ryna ... 804
Seldane-D Extended-Release Tablets ... 1286
Semprex-D Capsules ... 1620
Sinarest ... 663
Sine-Aid Maximum Strength Sinus Headache Gelcaps, Caplets and Tablets ... 1570
Sine-Off No Drowsiness Formula Caplets ... 784
Sine-Off Sinus Medicine ... 784
Singlet Tablets ... 785
Sinutab Non-Drying Liquid Caps ... 823
Sinutab Sinus Allergy Medication, Maximum Strength Tablets and Caplets ... 823
Sinutab Sinus Medication, Maximum Strength Without Drowsiness Formula, Tablets & Caplets ... 824
Sudafed Children's Cold & Cough Liquid Medication ... 825
Sudafed Children's Nasal Decongestant Liquid Medication ... 826
Sudafed Cold & Allergy Tablets ... 826
Sudafed Cold and Cough Liquid Caps ... 826
Sudafed Nasal Decongestant Tablets, 30 mg ... 825
Sudafed Nasal Decongestant Tablets, 60 mg ... 825
Sudafed Non-Drying Sinus Liquid Caps ... 827
Sudafed Pediatric Nasal Decongestant Liquid Oral Drops ... 827
Sudafed Severe Cold Formula Caplets ... 828
Sudafed Severe Cold Formula Tablets ... 828
Sudafed Sinus Caplets ... 829
Sudafed Sinus Tablets ... 829
Sudafed 12 Hour Caplets ... 824
Syn-Rx Tablets ... 1622
Syn-Rx DM Tablets ... 1623
TheraFlu Flu and Cold Medicine ... 750
Theraflu Maximum Strength Flu and Cold Medicine For Sore Throat ... 751
TheraFlu, Flu, Cold and Cough Medicine ... 750
TheraFlu Maximum Strength Nighttime Flu, Cold & Cough Medicine ... 751
TheraFlu Maximum Strength Non-Drowsy Formula Flu, Cold & Cough Medicine ... 751
TheraFlu Maximum Strength, Non-Drowsy Formula Flu, Cold and Cough Caplets ... 752
Theraflu Maximum Strength Sinus Non-Drowsy Formula Caplets ... 752
Triaminic AM Cough and Decongestant Formula ... 753
Triaminic AM Decongestant Formula ... 753
Triaminic Infant Oral Decongestant Drops ... 754
Triaminic Night Time ... 754
Triaminic Sore Throat Formula ... 755
Tussend ... 1830
Tussend Expectorant ... 1831
TYLENOL Allergy Sinus, Maximum Strength Caplets and Gelcaps ... 1571
TYLENOL Allergy Sinus NightTime, Maximum Strength Caplets ... 1571
TYLENOL Cold Medication, Multi-Symptom Formula Tablets and Caplets ... 1572
TYLENOL Cold Medication, Multi-Symptom Hot Liquid Packets ... 1572
TYLENOL Cold Medication, No Drowsiness Formula Caplets and Gelcaps ... 1572
TYLENOL Cold Severe Congestion Caplets ... 1573
TYLENOL Cough Medication with Decongestant, Multi Symptom ... 1574
TYLENOL Flu No Drowsiness Formula, Maximum Strength Gelcaps ... 1575
TYLENOL Flu NightTime, Maximum Strength Gelcaps ... 1575
TYLENOL Flu NightTime, Maximum Strength Hot Medication Packets ... 1575
TYLENOL Sinus, Maximum Strength Geltabs, Gelcaps, Caplets and Tablets ... 1576
Vicks 44 LiquiCaps Cough, Cold & Flu Relief ... 728
Vicks 44 LiquiCaps Non-Drowsy Cough & Cold Relief ... 729
Vicks 44D Cough & Head Congestion Relief ... 728
Vicks 44M Cough, Cold & Flu Relief ... 729
Vicks DayQuil LiquiCaps/Liquid Multi-Symptom Cold/Flu Relief ... 734
Vicks DayQuil SINUS Pressure & PAIN Relief with IBUPROFEN ... 735
Vicks Nyquil Hot Therapy ... 735
Vicks NyQuil LiquiCaps/Liquid Multi-Symptom Cold/Flu Relief, Original and Cherry Flavors ... 736

Pseudoephedrine Sulfate (Procarbazine exhibits some monoamine oxidase inhibitory activity; concurrent use should be avoided). Products include:
Chlor-Trimeton Allergy Decongestant Tablets ... 759
Claritin-D Tablets ... 2487
Drixoral Cold and Allergy Sustained-Action Tablets ... 763
Drixoral Cold and Flu Extended-Release Tablets ... 764
Drixoral Non-Drowsy Formula Extended-Release Tablets ... 764
Drixoral Allergy/Sinus Extended Release Tablets ... 765
Trinalin Repetabs Tablets ... 1373

Pyrilamine Maleate (Possible potentiation; exercise caution to minimize CNS depression). Products include:
4-Way Fast Acting Nasal Spray (regular & mentholated) ... 644
Maximum Strength Multi-Symptom Formula Midol ... 621
PMS Multi-Symptom Formula Midol ... 622

Pyrilamine Tannate (Possible potentiation; exercise caution to minimize CNS depression). Products include:
Atrohist Pediatric Suspension ... 1604
Atrohist Pediatric Suspension Dye-Free ... 1604
Rynatan ... 2781

Quinapril Hydrochloride (Possible potentiation). Products include:
Accupril Tablets ... 1950

Ramipril (Possible potentiation). Products include:
Altace Capsules ... 1238

Rauwolfia Serpentina (Possible potentiation).
No products indexed under this heading.

Rescinnamine (Possible potentiation).
No products indexed under this heading.

Reserpine (Possible potentiation). Products include:
Diupres Tablets ... 1691
Hydropres Tablets ... 1718
Ser-Ap-Es Tablets ... 867

(■ Described in PDR For Nonprescription Drugs)   (● Described in PDR For Ophthalmology)

651 **Interactions Index** **Mavik**

Salmeterol Xinafoate (Procarbazine exhibits some monoamine oxidase inhibitory activity; concurrent use should be avoided). Products include:

Serevent Inhalation Aerosol 1149

Secobarbital Sodium (Possible potentiation; exercise caution to minimize CNS depression). Products include:

Seconal Sodium Pulvules 1529

Sodium Nitroprusside (Possible potentiation).

No products indexed under this heading.

Sotalol Hydrochloride (Possible potentiation). Products include:

Betapace Tablets 637

Spirapril Hydrochloride (Possible potentiation).

No products indexed under this heading.

Sufentanil Citrate (Possible potentiation; exercise caution to minimize CNS depression). Products include:

Sufenta Injection 1355

Terazosin Hydrochloride (Possible potentiation). Products include:

Hytrin Capsules 434

Terbutaline Sulfate (Procarbazine exhibits some monoamine oxidase inhibitory activity; concurrent use should be avoided). Products include:

Brethaire Inhaler 830
Brethine Ampuls 832
Brethine Tablets 831
Bricanyl Subcutaneous Injection 1247
Bricanyl Tablets 1248

Terfenadine (Possible potentiation; exercise caution to minimize CNS depression). Products include:

Seldane Tablets 1284
Seldane-D Extended-Release Tablets 1286

Thiamylal Sodium (Possible potentiation; exercise caution to minimize CNS depression).

No products indexed under this heading.

Thioridazine Hydrochloride (Possible potentiation; exercise caution to minimize CNS depression). Products include:

Mellaril 2398

Timolol Maleate (Possible potentiation). Products include:

Blocadren Tablets 1654
Timolide Tablets 1791
Timoptic in Ocudose 1796
Timoptic Sterile Ophthalmic Solution 1794
Timoptic-XE 1798

Torsemide (Possible potentiation). Products include:

Demadex Tablets and Injection 691

Trifluoperazine Hydrochloride (Possible potentiation; exercise caution to minimize CNS depression). Products include:

Stelazine 2692

Trimeprazine Tartrate (Possible potentiation; exercise caution to minimize CNS depression).

No products indexed under this heading.

Trimethaphan Camsylate (Possible potentiation).

No products indexed under this heading.

Trimipramine Maleate (Procarbazine exhibits some monoamine oxidase inhibitory activity; concurrent use should be avoided). Products include:

Surmontil Capsules 2917

Tripelennamine Hydrochloride (Possible potentiation; exercise caution to minimize CNS depression). Products include:

PBZ Tablets 863
PBZ-SR Tablets 862

Triprolidine Hydrochloride (Possible potentiation; exercise caution to minimize CNS depression). Products include:

Actifed Cold & Allergy Tablets 807
Actifed Cold & Sinus Caplets and Tablets 808

Verapamil Hydrochloride (Possible potentiation). Products include:

Calan SR Caplets 2571
Calan Tablets 2568
Covera-HS Tablets 2573
Isoptin Injectable 1391
Isoptin Oral Tablets 1393
Isoptin SR Tablets 1395
Verelan Capsules 1455

Food Interactions

Alcohol (Concurrent use may result in disulfiram-like reaction).

Bananas (Procarbazine exhibits some monoamine oxidase inhibitory activity; concurrent use should be avoided).

Cheese, aged (Procarbazine exhibits some monoamine oxidase inhibitory activity; concurrent use should be avoided).

Food with high concentration of tyramine (Procarbazine exhibits some monoamine oxidase inhibitory activity; concurrent use should be avoided).

Wine, unspecified (Procarbazine exhibits some monoamine oxidase inhibitory activity; concurrent use should be avoided).

Yogurt (Procarbazine exhibits some monoamine oxidase inhibitory activity; concurrent use should be avoided).

MAVIK TABLETS

(Trandolapril) 1407

May interact with lithium preparations, diuretics, potassium sparing diuretics, potassium preparations, and certain other agents. Compounds in these categories include:

Amiloride Hydrochloride (Co-administration increases the risk of hyperkalemia; patients on diuretics, especially those on recently instituted diuretic therapy, may experience an excessive reduction in blood pressure after initiation of therapy with trandolapril). Products include:

Midamor Tablets 1746
Moduretic Tablets 1748

Bendroflumethiazide (Patients on diuretics, especially those on recently instituted diuretic therapy, may experience an excessive reduction in blood pressure after initiation of therapy with trandolapril).

No products indexed under this heading.

Bumetanide (Patients on diuretics, especially those on recently instituted diuretic therapy, may experience an excessive reduction in blood pressure after initiation of therapy with trandolapril). Products include:

Bumex 2260

Chlorothiazide (Patients on diuretics, especially those on recently instituted diuretic therapy, may experience an excessive reduction in blood pressure after initiation of therapy with trandolapril). Products include:

Aldoclor Tablets 1638
Diupres Tablets 1691
Diuril Oral 1694

Chlorothiazide Sodium (Patients on diuretics, especially those on recently instituted diuretic therapy, may experience an excessive reduction in blood pressure after initiation of therapy with trandolapril). Products include:

Diuril Sodium Intravenous 1693

Chlorthalidone (Patients on diuretics, especially those on recently instituted diuretic therapy, may experience an excessive reduction in blood pressure after initiation of therapy with trandolapril). Products include:

Combipres Tablets 682
Tenoretic Tablets 2963
Thalitone 1293

Cimetidine (Co-administration has led to an increase of about 44% in C_{max} for trandolapril with no effect on ACE inhibition). Products include:

Tagamet HB Tablets 786
Tagamet Tablets 2694

Cimetidine Hydrochloride (Co-administration has led to an increase of about 44% in C_{max} for trandolapril with no effect on ACE inhibition). Products include:

Tagamet 2694

Ethacrynic Acid (Patients on diuretics, especially those on recently instituted diuretic therapy, may experience an excessive reduction in blood pressure after initiation of therapy with trandolapril). Products include:

Edecrin Tablets 1698

Furosemide (Co-administration has led to an increase of about 25% in the renal clearance of trandolaprilat with no effect on ACE inhibition; patients on diuretics, especially those on recently instituted diuretic therapy, may experience an excessive reduction in blood pressure after initiation of therapy with trandolapril). Products include:

Lasix Injection, Oral Solution and Tablets 1267

Hydrochlorothiazide (Patients on diuretics, especially those on recently instituted diuretic therapy, may experience an excessive reduction in blood pressure after initiation of therapy with trandolapril). Products include:

Aldactazide Tablets 2556
Aldoril Tablets 1644
Apresazide Capsules 824
Capozide Tablets 744
Dyazide Capsules 2653
Esidrix Tablets 839
Esimil Tablets 840
HydroDIURIL Tablets 1716
Hydropres Tablets 1718
Hyzaar Tablets 1720
Inderide Tablets 2838
Inderide LA Long Acting Capsules 2840
Lopressor HCT Tablets 850
Lotensin HCT Tablets 855
Moduretic Tablets 1748
Oretic Tablets 450
Prinzide Tablets 1780
Ser-Ap-Es Tablets 867
Timolide Tablets 1791
Vaseretic Tablets 1810
Zestoretic Tablets 2968
Ziac 1459

Hydroflumethiazide (Patients on diuretics, especially those on recently instituted diuretic therapy, may experience an excessive reduction in blood pressure after initiation of therapy with trandolapril). Products include:

Diucardin Tablets 2824

Indapamide (Patients on diuretics, especially those on recently instituted diuretic therapy, may experience an excessive reduction in blood pressure after initiation of therapy with trandolapril).

No products indexed under this heading.

Lithium Carbonate (Co-administration of ACE inhibitors and lithium has resulted in increased serum lithium levels and symptoms of lithium toxicity). Products include:

Eskalith 2658
Lithium Carbonate Capsules & Tablets 2352
Lithonate/Lithotabs/Lithobid 2721

Lithium Citrate (Co-administration of ACE inhibitors and lithium has resulted in increased serum lithium levels and symptoms of lithium toxicity).

No products indexed under this heading.

Methyclothiazide (Patients on diuretics, especially those on recently instituted diuretic therapy, may experience an excessive reduction in blood pressure after initiation of therapy with trandolapril). Products include:

Enduron Tablets 424

Metolazone (Patients on diuretics, especially those on recently instituted diuretic therapy, may experience an excessive reduction in blood pressure after initiation of therapy with trandolapril). Products include:

Mykrox Tablets 1617
Zaroxolyn Tablets 1625

Polythiazide (Patients on diuretics, especially those on recently instituted diuretic therapy, may experience an excessive reduction in blood pressure after initiation of therapy with trandolapril). Products include:

Minizide Capsules 2016

Potassium Acid Phosphate (Co-administration increases the risk of hyperkalemia). Products include:

K-Phos Original Formula 'Sodium Free' Tablets 633

Potassium Bicarbonate (Co-administration increases the risk of hyperkalemia). Products include:

Alka-Seltzer Gold Effervescent Antacid 611

Potassium Chloride (Co-administration increases the risk of hyperkalemia). Products include:

Chlor-3 Condiment 1003
Colyte and Colyte-flavored 2540
GoLYTELY 694
K-Dur Microburst Release System (potassium chloride, USP) E.R. Tablets 1364
K-Lor Powder Packets 438
K-Norm Capsules 1615
K-Tab Filmtab 439
Micro-K 2237
Micro-K LS Packets 2238
NuLYTELY 694
Cherry Flavor NuLYTELY 694
Rum-K Syrup 1004
Slow-K Extended-Release Tablets 869

Potassium Citrate (Co-administration increases the risk of hyperkalemia). Products include:

Polycitra Syrup 574
Polycitra-K Crystals 574
Polycitra-K Oral Solution 575
Polycitra-LC 574
Urocit-K Tablets 1828

Potassium Gluconate (Co-administration increases the risk of hyperkalemia).

No products indexed under this heading.

IMPORTANT NOTE: Always consult each drug listing in the patient's regimen for possible interactions.

Mavik — Interactions Index

Potassium Phosphate, Dibasic (Co-administration increases the risk of hyperkalemia).
   No products indexed under this heading.

Potassium Phosphate, Monobasic (Co-administration increases the risk of hyperkalemia). Products include:
K-Phos Neutral Tablets	633
K-Phos Original Formula 'Sodium Free' Tablets	633

Spironolactone (Co-administration increases the risk of hyperkalemia; patients on diuretics, especially those on recently instituted diuretic therapy, may experience an excessive reduction in blood pressure after initiation of therapy with trandolapril). Products include:
Aldactazide Tablets	2556
Aldactone Tablets	2558

Torsemide (Patients on diuretics, especially those on recently instituted diuretic therapy, may experience an excessive reduction in blood pressure after initiation of therapy with trandolapril). Products include:
Demadex Tablets and Injection	691

Triamterene (Co-administration increases the risk of hyperkalemia; patients on diuretics, especially those on recently instituted diuretic therapy, may experience an excessive reduction in blood pressure after initiation of therapy with trandolapril). Products include:
Dyazide Capsules	2653
Dyrenium Capsules	2655

Food Interactions

Food, unspecified (Slows absorption of trandolapril but does not affect AUC or C_{max}).

MAXAIR AUTOHALER
(Pirbuterol Acetate) 1550
May interact with sympathomimetic aerosol bronchodilators, monoamine oxidase inhibitors, and tricyclic antidepressants. Compounds in these categories include:

Albuterol (Potential for additive effects). Products include:
Proventil Inhalation Aerosol	2524
Ventolin Inhalation Aerosol and Refill	1170

Amitriptyline Hydrochloride (Potentiates the action of beta adrenergic agonists on the vascular system). Products include:
Elavil	2945
Etrafon	2495
Limbitrol	2333
Triavil Tablets	1800

Amoxapine (Potentiates the action of beta adrenergic agonists on the vascular system). Products include:
Asendin Tablets	1419

Bitolterol Mesylate (Potential for additive effects). Products include:
Tornalate Solution for Inhalation, 0.2%	976
Tornalate Metered Dose Inhaler	978

Clomipramine Hydrochloride (Potentiates the action of beta adrenergic agonists on the vascular system). Products include:
Anafranil Capsules	819

Desipramine Hydrochloride (Potentiates the action of beta adrenergic agonists on the vascular system). Products include:
Norpramin Tablets	1273

Doxepin Hydrochloride (Potentiates the action of beta adrenergic agonists on the vascular system). Products include:
Adapin Capsules	1542
Sinequan	2028
Zonalon Cream	1042

Furazolidone (Potentiates the action of beta adrenergic agonists on the vascular system). Products include:
Furoxone	2221

Imipramine Hydrochloride (Potentiates the action of beta adrenergic agonists on the vascular system). Products include:
Tofranil Ampuls	873
Tofranil Tablets	875

Imipramine Pamoate (Potentiates the action of beta adrenergic agonists on the vascular system). Products include:
Tofranil-PM Capsules	876

Isocarboxazid (Potentiates the action of beta adrenergic agonists on the vascular system).
   No products indexed under this heading.

Isoetharine (Potential for additive effects). Products include:
Bronkometer Aerosol	2432
Bronkosol Solution	2432
Isoetharine Inhalation Solution, USP, Arm-a-Med	545

Isoproterenol Hydrochloride (Potential for additive effects). Products include:
Isuprel Hydrochloride Solution	2443
Isuprel Injection	2441
Isuprel Mistometer	2442

Maprotiline Hydrochloride (Potentiates the action of beta adrenergic agonists on the vascular system). Products include:
Ludiomil Tablets	861

Metaproterenol Sulfate (Potential for additive effects). Products include:
Alupent	672
Metaproterenol Sulfate Inhalation Solution, USP, Arm-a-Med	547

Nortriptyline Hydrochloride (Potentiates the action of beta adrenergic agonists on the vascular system). Products include:
Pamelor	2409

Phenelzine Sulfate (Potentiates the action of beta adrenergic agonists on the vascular system). Products include:
Nardil	1977

Protriptyline Hydrochloride (Potentiates the action of beta adrenergic agonists on the vascular system). Products include:
Vivactil Tablets	1820

Salmeterol Xinafoate (Potential for additive effects). Products include:
Serevent Inhalation Aerosol	1149

Selegiline Hydrochloride (Potentiates the action of beta adrenergic agonists on the vascular system). Products include:
Eldepryl Capsules	2729

Terbutaline Sulfate (Potential for additive effects). Products include:
Brethaire Inhaler	830
Brethine Ampuls	832
Brethine Tablets	831
Bricanyl Subcutaneous Injection	1247
Bricanyl Tablets	1248

Tranylcypromine Sulfate (Potentiates the action of beta adrenergic agonists on the vascular system). Products include:
Parnate Tablets	2679

Trimipramine Maleate (Potentiates the action of beta adrenergic agonists on the vascular system). Products include:
Surmontil Capsules	2917

MAXAIR INHALER
(Pirbuterol Acetate) 1552
May interact with monoamine oxidase inhibitors, tricyclic antidepressants, and sympathomimetic aerosol bronchodilators. Compounds in these categories include:

Albuterol (Potential for additive effects). Products include:
Proventil Inhalation Aerosol	2524
Ventolin Inhalation Aerosol and Refill	1170

Amitriptyline Hydrochloride (Action of pirbuterol on vascular system may be potentiated). Products include:
Elavil	2945
Etrafon	2495
Limbitrol	2333
Triavil Tablets	1800

Amoxapine (Action of pirbuterol on vascular system may be potentiated). Products include:
Asendin Tablets	1419

Bitolterol Mesylate (Potential for additive effects). Products include:
Tornalate Solution for Inhalation, 0.2%	976
Tornalate Metered Dose Inhaler	978

Clomipramine Hydrochloride (Action of pirbuterol on vascular system may be potentiated). Products include:
Anafranil Capsules	819

Desipramine Hydrochloride (Action of pirbuterol on vascular system may be potentiated). Products include:
Norpramin Tablets	1273

Doxepin Hydrochloride (Action of pirbuterol on vascular system may be potentiated). Products include:
Adapin Capsules	1542
Sinequan	2028
Zonalon Cream	1042

Furazolidone (Action of pirbuterol on vascular system may be potentiated). Products include:
Furoxone	2221

Imipramine Hydrochloride (Action of pirbuterol on vascular system may be potentiated). Products include:
Tofranil Ampuls	873
Tofranil Tablets	875

Imipramine Pamoate (Action of pirbuterol on vascular system may be potentiated). Products include:
Tofranil-PM Capsules	876

Isocarboxazid (Action of pirbuterol on vascular system may be potentiated).
   No products indexed under this heading.

Isoetharine (Potential for additive effects). Products include:
Bronkometer Aerosol	2432
Bronkosol Solution	2432
Isoetharine Inhalation Solution, USP, Arm-a-Med	545

Isoproterenol Hydrochloride (Potential for additive effects). Products include:
Isuprel Hydrochloride Solution	2443
Isuprel Injection	2441
Isuprel Mistometer	2442

Maprotiline Hydrochloride (Action of pirbuterol on vascular system may be potentiated). Products include:
Ludiomil Tablets	861

Metaproterenol Sulfate (Potential for additive effects). Products include:
Alupent	672
Metaproterenol Sulfate Inhalation Solution, USP, Arm-a-Med	547

Nortriptyline Hydrochloride (Action of pirbuterol on vascular system may be potentiated). Products include:
Pamelor	2409

Phenelzine Sulfate (Action of pirbuterol on vascular system may be potentiated). Products include:
Nardil	1977

Protriptyline Hydrochloride (Action of pirbuterol on vascular system may be potentiated). Products include:
Vivactil Tablets	1820

Salmeterol Xinafoate (Potential for additive effects). Products include:
Serevent Inhalation Aerosol	1149

Selegiline Hydrochloride (Action of pirbuterol on vascular system may be potentiated). Products include:
Eldepryl Capsules	2729

Terbutaline Sulfate (Potential for additive effects). Products include:
Brethaire Inhaler	830
Brethine Ampuls	832
Brethine Tablets	831
Bricanyl Subcutaneous Injection	1247
Bricanyl Tablets	1248

Tranylcypromine Sulfate (Action of pirbuterol on vascular system may be potentiated). Products include:
Parnate Tablets	2679

Trimipramine Maleate (Action of pirbuterol on vascular system may be potentiated). Products include:
Surmontil Capsules	2917

MAXAQUIN TABLETS
(Lomefloxacin Hydrochloride) 2593
May interact with xanthine bronchodilators, antacids containing aluminium, calcium and magnesium, oral anticoagulants, and certain other agents. Compounds in these categories include:

Aluminum Carbonate (Interferes with the bioavailability of lomefloxacin). Products include:
Basaljel Capsules	2810
Basaljel Suspension	2810
Basaljel Tablets	2810

Aluminum Hydroxide (Interferes with the bioavailability of lomefloxacin). Products include:
ALternaGEL Liquid	1358
Maximum Strength Ascriptin	⊠ 650
Cama Arthritis Pain Reliever	⊠ 748
Gaviscon Extra Strength Relief Formula Antacid Tablets	⊠ 778
Gaviscon Extra Strength Relief Formula Liquid Antacid	⊠ 779
Gaviscon Liquid Antacid	⊠ 779
Gelusil Antacid-Anti-gas Liquid	⊠ 819
Gelusil Antacid-Anti-gas Tablets	⊠ 819
Maalox Antacid/Anti-Gas Tablets	889
Maalox Heartburn Relief Suspension	⊠ 658
Maalox Antacid Liquid	888
Extra Strength Maalox Antacid/Anti-Gas Liquid and Tablets	888
Mylanta	1359
Tempo Soft Antacid	⊠ 799

Aluminum Hydroxide Gel (Interferes with the bioavailability of lomefloxacin). Products include:
ALternaGEL Liquid	⊠ 675
Aludrox Oral Suspension	⊠ 850
Amphojel Suspension	2802
Amphojel Suspension without Flavor	2802
Amphojel Tablets	2802
Ascriptin	⊠ 650
Gaviscon Antacid Tablets	⊠ 778
Gaviscon-2 Antacid Tablets	⊠ 779
Mylanta Liquid	⊠ 676
Mylanta Double Strength Liquid	⊠ 676
Nephrox Suspension	⊠ 671

(⊠ Described in PDR For Nonprescription Drugs)   (⊚ Described in PDR For Ophthalmology)

Aminophylline (Individual theophylline levels may fluctuate with no clinically significant symptoms of drug interactions).
    No products indexed under this heading.

Caffeine-containing medications (May result in drug-induced central nervous system-related adverse effects in certain patient population at higher levels of caffeine).

Cimetidine (May interfere with the elimination of quinolones). Products include:
    Tagamet HB Tablets 786
    Tagamet Tablets 2694

Cimetidine Hydrochloride (May interfere with the elimination of quinolones). Products include:
    Tagamet 2694

Cyclosporine (Elevated serum levels of cyclosporin have been reported with concomitant use of cyclosporin and quinolones). Products include:
    Neoral 2405
    Sandimmune 2416

Dicumarol (Quinolones may enhance the effects of oral anticoagulants).
    No products indexed under this heading.

Dyphylline (Individual theophylline levels may fluctuate with no clinically significant symptoms of drug interactions). Products include:
    Lufyllin & Lufyllin-400 Tablets 2778
    Lufyllin-GG Elixir & Tablets 2779

Fenbufen (Potential for increased risk of CNS stimulation and convulsive seizures).

Magaldrate (Interferes with the bioavailability of lomefloxacin).
    No products indexed under this heading.

Magnesium Hydroxide (Interferes with the bioavailability of lomefloxacin). Products include:
    Aludrox Oral Suspension 850
    Ascriptin 650
    Di-Gel Antacid/Anti-Gas 762
    Gelusil Antacid-Anti-gas Liquid 819
    Gelusil Antacid-Anti-gas Tablets .. 819
    Maalox Antacid/Anti-Gas Tablets 889
    Maalox Antacid Liquid 888
    Extra Strength Maalox Antacid/Anti-Gas Liquid and Tablets 888
    Mylanta Fast-Acting 1359
    Mylanta Gelcaps Antacid 678
    Fast-Acting Mylanta Liquid Antacid 1359
    Mylanta Tablets 677
    Maximum-Strength Fast-Acting Mylanta Liquid Antacid 1359
    Mylanta Double Strength Tablets .. 677
    Phillips' Milk of Magnesia Liquid ... 627
    Rolaids Antacid Tablets 807
    Tempo Soft Antacid 799

Magnesium Oxide (Interferes with the bioavailability of lomefloxacin). Products include:
    Beelith Tablets 632
    Bufferin Analgesic Tablets 636
    Arthritis Strength Bufferin Analgesic Caplets 637
    Extra Strength Bufferin Analgesic Tablets 637
    Caltrate PLUS 681
    Cama Arthritis Pain Reliever 748
    Mag-Ox 400 666
    Uro-Mag 666

Probenecid (Slows the renal eliminaton of lomefloxacin). Products include:
    Benemid Tablets 1651
    ColBENEMID Tablets 1662

Sucralfate (Interferes with the bioavailability of lomefloxacin). Products include:
    Carafate Suspension 1250
    Carafate Tablets 1249

Theophylline (Individual theophylline levels may fluctuate with no clinically significant symptoms of drug interactions). Products include:
    Marax Tablets & DF Syrup 2015
    Quibron 2227

Theophylline Anhydrous (Individual theophylline levels may fluctuate with no clinically significant symptoms of drug interactions). Products include:
    Aerolate 1003
    Primatene Tablets 844
    Respbid Tablets 687
    Slo-bid Gyrocaps 2201
    Theo-24 Extended Release Capsules 2753
    Theo-Dur Extended-Release Tablets 1367
    Theo-X Extended-Release Tablets ... 793
    Uni-Dur Extended-Release Tablets . 1374
    Uniphyl 400 mg and 600 mg Tablets 2157

Theophylline Calcium Salicylate (Individual theophylline levels may fluctuate with no clinically significant symptoms of drug interactions). Products include:
    Quadrinal Tablets 1398

Theophylline Sodium Glycinate (Individual theophylline levels may fluctuate with no clinically significant symptoms of drug interactions).
    No products indexed under this heading.

Warfarin Sodium (Quinolones may enhance the effects of oral anticoagulants). Products include:
    Coumadin 941

Food Interactions

Food, unspecified (The rate of drug absorption may be delayed by 41%, however, the drug can be taken without regard to meal).

MAXIPIME FOR INJECTION
(Cefepime Hydrochloride) 758
May interact with aminoglycosides and certain other agents. Compounds in these categories include:

Amikacin Sulfate (Co-administration increases the potential for nephrotoxicity and ototoxicity of aminoglycoside antibiotics). Products include:
    Amikacin Sulfate Injection, USP ... 523
    Amikacin Sulfate Injection, USP ... 981
    Amikin Injectable 502

Furosemide (Co-administration with furosemide and other cephalosporins has resulted in nephrotoxicity). Products include:
    Lasix Injection, Oral Solution and Tablets 1267

Gentamicin Sulfate (Co-administration increases the potential for nephrotoxicity and ototoxicity of aminoglycoside antibiotics). Products include:
    Garamycin Cream 0.1% 2501
    Garamycin Injectable 2502
    Garamycin Ointment 0.1% 2501
    Garamycin Ophthalmic 2501
    Genoptic Sterile Ophthalmic Solution 241
    Genoptic Sterile Ophthalmic Ointment 241
    Gentak 209
    Pred-G Liquifilm Sterile Ophthalmic Suspension 248
    Pred-G S.O.P. Sterile Ophthalmic Ointment 249

Kanamycin Sulfate (Co-administration increases the potential for nephrotoxicity and ototoxicity of aminoglycoside antibiotics).
    No products indexed under this heading.

Streptomycin Sulfate (Co-administration increases the potential for nephrotoxicity and ototoxicity of aminoglycoside antibiotics). Products include:
    Streptomycin Sulfate Injection 2031

Tobramycin (Co-administration increases the potential for nephrotoxicity and ototoxicity of aminoglycoside antibiotics). Products include:
    AKTOB 207
    TobraDex Ophthalmic Suspension and Ointment 469
    Tobrex Ophthalmic Ointment and Solution 226

Tobramycin Sulfate (Co-administration increases the potential for nephrotoxicity and ototoxicity of aminoglycoside antibiotics). Products include:
    Nebcin Vials, Hyporets & ADD-Vantage 1518

MAXITROL OPHTHALMIC OINTMENT AND SUSPENSION
(Dexamethasone, Neomycin Sulfate, Polymyxin B Sulfate) 222
None cited in PDR database.

MAY-VITA ELIXIR
(Vitamins with Minerals) 1826
None cited in PDR database.

MEBARAL TABLETS
(Mephobarbital) 2452
May interact with corticosteroids, monoamine oxidase inhibitors, central nervous system depressants, oral anticoagulants, oral contraceptives, and certain other agents. Compounds in these categories include:

Alfentanil Hydrochloride (Additive depressant effects). Products include:
    Alfenta Injection 1334

Alprazolam (Additive depressant effects). Products include:
    Xanax Tablets 2115

Aprobarbital (Additive depressant effects).
    No products indexed under this heading.

Betamethasone Acetate (Enhanced metabolism of exogenous corticosteroids). Products include:
    Celestone Soluspan Suspension .. 2484

Betamethasone Sodium Phosphate (Enhanced metabolism of exogenous corticosteroids). Products include:
    Celestone Soluspan Suspension 2484

Buprenorphine (Additive depressant effects). Products include:
    Buprenex Injectable 2170

Buspirone Hydrochloride (Additive depressant effects). Products include:
    BuSpar Tablets 738

Butabarbital (Additive depressant effects).
    No products indexed under this heading.

Butalbital (Additive depressant effects). Products include:
    Axocet Capsules 2469
    Esgic-plus Capsules 1012
    Esgic-plus Tablets 1012
    Fioricet Tablets 2386
    Fioricet with Codeine Capsules 2387
    Fiorinal Capsules 2388
    Fiorinal with Codeine Capsules 2390
    Fiorinal Tablets 2388
    Phrenilin 790
    Sedapap Tablets 50 mg/650 mg ... 1826

Chlordiazepoxide (Additive depressant effects). Products include:
    Limbitrol 2333

Chlordiazepoxide Hydrochloride (Additive depressant effects). Products include:
    Librax Capsules 2330
    Librium Capsules 2331
    Librium Injectable 2332

Chlorpromazine (Additive depressant effects). Products include:
    Thorazine Suppositories 2701

Chlorprothixene (Additive depressant effects).
    No products indexed under this heading.

Chlorprothixene Hydrochloride (Additive depressant effects).
    No products indexed under this heading.

Chlorprothixene Lactate (Additive depressant effects).
    No products indexed under this heading.

Clorazepate Dipotassium (Additive depressant effects). Products include:
    Tranxene 459

Clozapine (Additive depressant effects). Products include:
    Clozaril Tablets 2377

Codeine Phosphate (Additive depressant effects). Products include:
    Brontex 2130
    Dimetane-DC Cough Syrup 2232
    Fioricet with Codeine Capsules 2387
    Fiorinal with Codeine Capsules 2390
    Nucofed 2225
    Phenergan with Codeine 2883
    Phenergan VC with Codeine 2888
    Robitussin A-C Syrup 2248
    Robitussin-DAC Syrup 2249
    Ryna 804
    Soma Compound w/Codeine Tablets 2784
    Tylenol with Codeine 1592

Cortisone Acetate (Enhanced metabolism of exogenous corticosteroids). Products include:
    Cortone Acetate Sterile Suspension 1663
    Cortone Acetate Tablets 1664

Desflurane (Additive depressant effects). Products include:
    Suprane (desflurane, USP) 1865

Desogestrel (Decreased contraceptive effect). Products include:
    Desogen Tablets 1867
    Ortho-Cept 1907

Dexamethasone (Enhanced metabolism of exogenous corticosteroids). Products include:
    AK-Trol Ointment & Suspension 205
    Decadron Elixir 1676
    Decadron Tablets 1678
    Decaspray Topical Aerosol 1689
    Maxitrol Ophthalmic Ointment and Suspension 222
    TobraDex Ophthalmic Suspension and Ointment 469

Dexamethasone Acetate (Enhanced metabolism of exogenous corticosteroids). Products include:
    Dalalone D.P. Injectable 1009
    Decadron-LA Sterile Suspension ... 1687

Dexamethasone Sodium Phosphate (Enhanced metabolism of exogenous corticosteroids). Products include:
    Decadron Phosphate Injection ... 1680
    Decadron Phosphate Sterile Ophthalmic Ointment 1684
    Decadron Phosphate Sterile Ophthalmic Solution 1685
    Decadron Phosphate Topical Cream 1686
    Decadron Phosphate with Xylocaine Injection, Sterile 1683
    Dexacort Phosphate in Respihaler .. 1606
    Dexacort Phosphate in Turbinaire .. 1607
    NeoDecadron Sterile Ophthalmic Ointment 1755
    NeoDecadron Sterile Ophthalmic Solution 1756

IMPORTANT NOTE: Always consult each drug listing in the patient's regimen for possible interactions.

Mebaral Tablets — Interactions Index — 654

NeoDecadron Topical Cream 1757

Dezocine (Additive depressant effects). Products include:
- Dalgan Injection 529

Diazepam (Additive depressant effects). Products include:
- Dizac (diazepam injectable emulsion) CIV 1862
- Valium Injectable 2336
- Valium Tablets 2335

Dicumarol (Decreased anticoagulant response).
- No products indexed under this heading.

Doxycycline Calcium (Half-life of doxycycline shortened). Products include:
- Vibramycin Calcium Oral Suspension Syrup 2038

Doxycycline Hyclate (Half-life of doxycycline shortened). Products include:
- Doryx Capsules 1970
- Vibramycin Hyclate Capsules 2038
- Vibramycin Hyclate Intravenous 2040
- Vibra-Tabs Film Coated Tablets 2038

Doxycycline Monohydrate (Half-life of doxycycline shortened). Products include:
- Monodox Capsules 1858
- Vibramycin Monohydrate for Oral Suspension 2038

Droperidol (Additive depressant effects). Products include:
- Inapsine Injection 462

Enflurane (Additive depressant effects).
- No products indexed under this heading.

Estazolam (Additive depressant effects). Products include:
- ProSom Tablets 457

Estradiol (Decreased effect of estradiol). Products include:
- Climara Transdermal System 640
- Estrace Cream and Tablets 751
- Estraderm Transdermal System 842
- Estring Vaginal Ring 2086
- Vivelle Transdermal System 880

Estrone (Decreased effect of estrone).
- No products indexed under this heading.

Ethchlorvynol (Additive depressant effects). Products include:
- Placidyl Capsules 456

Ethinamate (Additive depressant effects).
- No products indexed under this heading.

Ethinyl Estradiol (Decreased contraceptive effect). Products include:
- Brevicon 2563
- Demulen 2580
- Desogen Tablets 1867
- Levlen/Tri-Levlen 646
- Lo/Ovral Tablets 2852
- Lo/Ovral-28 Tablets 2857
- Modicon 1928
- Nordette-21 Tablets 2863
- Nordette-28 Tablets 2866
- Norinyl 2563
- Ortho-Cept 1907
- Ortho-Cyclen/Ortho-Tri-Cyclen 1914
- Ortho-Novum 1928
- Ortho-Cyclen/Ortho Tri-Cyclen 1914
- Ovcon 765
- Ovral Tablets 2877
- Ovral-28 Tablets 2878
- Levlen/Tri-Levlen 646
- Tri-Norinyl 2607
- Triphasil-21 Tablets 2919
- Triphasil-28 Tablets 2924

Ethynodiol Diacetate (Decreased contraceptive effect). Products include:
- Demulen 2580

Fentanyl (Additive depressant effects). Products include:
- Duragesic Transdermal System 1336

Fentanyl Citrate (Additive depressant effects). Products include:
- Sublimaze Injection 463

Fludrocortisone Acetate (Enhanced metabolism of exogenous corticosteroids). Products include:
- Florinef Acetate Tablets 506

Fluphenazine Decanoate (Additive depressant effects). Products include:
- Prolixin Decanoate 510

Fluphenazine Enanthate (Additive depressant effects). Products include:
- Prolixin Enanthate 510

Fluphenazine Hydrochloride (Additive depressant effects). Products include:
- Prolixin 510

Flurazepam Hydrochloride (Additive depressant effects). Products include:
- Dalmane Capsules 2329

Furazolidone (Prolongs effects of barbiturates). Products include:
- Furoxone 2221

Glutethimide (Additive depressant effects).
- No products indexed under this heading.

Griseofulvin (Decreased blood levels of griseofulvin). Products include:
- Fulvicin P/G Tablets 2499
- Fulvicin P/G 165 & 330 Tablets 2500
- Grifulvin V (griseofulvin tablets) Microsize (griseofulvin oral suspension) Microsize 1944
- Gris-PEG Tablets, 125 mg & 250 mg 476

Haloperidol (Additive depressant effects). Products include:
- Haldol Injection, Tablets and Concentrate 1585

Haloperidol Decanoate (Additive depressant effects). Products include:
- Haldol Decanoate 1587

Hydrocodone Bitartrate (Additive depressant effects). Products include:
- Codiclear DH Syrup 808
- Duratuss HD Elixir 2750
- Histussin D Liquid 670
- Hycodan Tablets and Syrup 946
- Hycomine Compound Tablets 948
- Hycomine 947
- Hycotuss Expectorant Syrup 950
- Hydrocet Capsules 787
- Lorcet 10/650 Tablets 1016
- Lortab 2751
- Tussend 1830
- Tussend Expectorant 1831
- Vicodin Tablets 1404
- Vicodin ES Tablets 1405
- Vicodin HP Tablets 1403
- Vicodin Tuss Expectorant 1406
- Zydone Capsules 967

Hydrocodone Polistirex (Additive depressant effects). Products include:
- Tussionex Pennkinetic Extended-Release Suspension 1624

Hydrocortisone (Enhanced metabolism of exogenous corticosteroids). Products include:
- Anusol-HC Cream 2.5% 1953
- Aquanil HC Lotion 1989
- Maximum Strength Cortaid Spray ⊞ 800
- CORTENEMA 2713
- Cortisporin Ointment 1074
- Cortisporin Ophthalmic Ointment Sterile 1074
- Cortisporin Ophthalmic Suspension Sterile 1075
- Cortisporin Otic Solution Sterile 1076
- Cortisporin Otic Suspension Sterile 1077
- Cortizone-5 .... ⊞ 795
- Cortizone-10 .... ⊞ 795
- Hydrocortone Tablets 1715
- Hytone 922
- Hytone Ointment 2 ½% 923
- Massengill Medicated Soft Cloth Towelettes 2628
- Pediotic Suspension Sterile 1140
- Preparation H Hydrocortisone 1% Cream .... ⊞ 843
- ProctoCream-HC 2.5% 2552
- VoSoL HC Otic Solution 2786

Hydrocortisone Acetate (Enhanced metabolism of exogenous corticosteroids). Products include:
- Analpram-HC Rectal Cream 1% and 2.5% 993
- Anusol HC-1 Hydrocortisone Anti-Itch Ointment .... ⊞ 810
- Anusol-HC Suppositories 1954
- Caldecort Anti-Itch Hydrocortisone Cream .... ⊞ 651
- Coly-Mycin S Otic w/Neomycin & Hydrocortisone 1965
- Cortaid .... ⊞ 800
- Cortifoam 2540
- Cortisporin Cream 1073
- Epifoam 2543
- Hydrocortone Acetate Sterile Suspension 1712
- Mantadil Cream 1124
- Nupercainal Hydrocortisone 1% Cream .... ⊞ 661
- Pramosone Cream, Lotion & Ointment 995
- ProctoFoam-HC 2552
- Terra-Cortril Ophthalmic Suspension 2033

Hydrocortisone Sodium Phosphate (Enhanced metabolism of exogenous corticosteroids). Products include:
- Hydrocortone Phosphate Injection, Sterile 1713

Hydrocortisone Sodium Succinate (Enhanced metabolism of exogenous corticosteroids).
- No products indexed under this heading.

Hydroxyzine Hydrochloride (Additive depressant effects). Products include:
- Atarax Tablets & Syrup 1992
- Marax Tablets & DF Syrup 2015
- Vistaril Intramuscular Solution 2042

Isocarboxazid (Prolongs effects of barbiturates).
- No products indexed under this heading.

Isoflurane (Additive depressant effects).
- No products indexed under this heading.

Ketamine Hydrochloride (Additive depressant effects).
- No products indexed under this heading.

Levomethadyl Acetate Hydrochloride (Additive depressant effects). Products include:
- Orlaam Oral Solution 2361

Levonorgestrel (Decreased contraceptive effect). Products include:
- Levlen/Tri-Levlen 646
- Nordette-21 Tablets 2863
- Nordette-28 Tablets 2866
- Norplant System 2868
- Levlen/Tri-Levlen 646
- Triphasil-21 Tablets 2919
- Triphasil-28 Tablets 2924

Levorphanol Tartrate (Additive depressant effects). Products include:
- Levo-Dromoran 2297

Lorazepam (Additive depressant effects). Products include:
- Ativan Injection 2805
- Ativan Tablets 2807

Loxapine Hydrochloride (Additive depressant effects). Products include:
- Loxitane 1426

Loxapine Succinate (Additive depressant effects). Products include:
- Loxitane Capsules 1426

Meperidine Hydrochloride (Additive depressant effects). Products include:
- Demerol 2438
- Mepergan Injection 2859

Meprobamate (Additive depressant effects). Products include:
- Miltown Tablets 2780
- PMB 200 and PMB 400 2890

Mesoridazine Besylate (Additive depressant effects). Products include:
- Serentil 689

Mestranol (Decreased contraceptive effect). Products include:
- Norinyl 2563
- Ortho-Novum 1928

Methadone Hydrochloride (Additive depressant effects). Products include:
- Methadone Hydrochloride Oral Concentrate 2356
- Methadone Hydrochloride Oral Solution & Tablets 2357

Methohexital Sodium (Additive depressant effects).
- No products indexed under this heading.

Methotrimeprazine (Additive depressant effects). Products include:
- Levoprome 1321

Methoxyflurane (Additive depressant effects).
- No products indexed under this heading.

Methylprednisolone Acetate (Enhanced metabolism of exogenous corticosteroids).
- No products indexed under this heading.

Methylprednisolone Sodium Succinate (Enhanced metabolism of exogenous corticosteroids).
- No products indexed under this heading.

Midazolam Hydrochloride (Additive depressant effects). Products include:
- Versed Injection 2324

Molindone Hydrochloride (Additive depressant effects). Products include:
- Moban Tablets and Concentrate 1036

Morphine Sulfate (Additive depressant effects). Products include:
- Astramorph/PF Injection, USP (Preservative-Free) 526
- Duramorph Injection 983
- Infumorph 200 and Infumorph 500 Sterile Solutions 985
- Kadian Capsules 2948
- MS Contin Tablets 2149
- MSIR 2152
- Oramorph SR (Morphine Sulfate Sustained Release Tablets) 2359
- RMS Suppositories CII 2766
- Roxanol 2365

Norethindrone (Decreased contraceptive effect). Products include:
- Brevicon 2563
- Micronor Tablets 1903
- Modicon 1928
- Norinyl 2563
- Nor-Q D Tablets 2598
- Ortho-Novum 1928
- Ovcon 765
- Tri-Norinyl 2607

Norethynodrel (Decreased contraceptive effect).
- No products indexed under this heading.

Norgestimate (Decreased contraceptive effect). Products include:
- Ortho-Cyclen/Ortho-Tri-Cyclen 1914
- Ortho-Cyclen/Ortho Tri-Cyclen 1914

Norgestrel (Decreased contraceptive effect). Products include:
- Lo/Ovral Tablets 2852
- Lo/Ovral-28 Tablets 2857
- Ovral Tablets 2877

(⊞ Described in PDR For Nonprescription Drugs) (⊙ Described in PDR For Ophthalmology)

Interactions Index

Ovral-28 Tablets 2878
Ovrette Tablets 2878

Opium Alkaloids (Additive depressant effects).
No products indexed under this heading.

Oxazepam (Additive depressant effects). Products include:
Serax Capsules 2916
Serax Tablets 2916

Oxycodone Hydrochloride (Additive depressant effects). Products include:
OxyContin Tablets 2163
OxyIR Capsules 2167
Percocet Tablets 955
Percodan Tablets 955
Percodan-Demi Tablets 956
Roxicodone Tablets, Oral Solution & Intensol (Oxycodone) 2366
Tylox Capsules 1593

Pentobarbital Sodium (Additive depressant effects). Products include:
Nembutal Sodium Capsules 440
Nembutal Sodium Solution 442
Nembutal Sodium Suppositories ... 444

Perphenazine (Additive depressant effects). Products include:
Etrafon 2495
Triavil Tablets 1800
Trilafon 2532

Phenelzine Sulfate (Prolongs effects of barbiturates). Products include:
Nardil 1977

Phenobarbital (Additive depressant effects). Products include:
Arco-Lase Plus Tablets 513
Bellergal-S Tablets 2375
Donnatal 2234
Donnatal Extentabs 2234
Donnatal Tablets 2234
Phenobarbital Elixir and Tablets ... 1523
Quadrinal Tablets 1398

Phenytoin (Unpredictable effects). Products include:
Dilantin Infatabs 1967
Dilantin-125 Suspension 1969

Phenytoin Sodium (Unpredictable effects). Products include:
Dilantin Kapseals 1965

Prazepam (Additive depressant effects).
No products indexed under this heading.

Prednisolone Acetate (Enhanced metabolism of exogenous corticosteroids). Products include:
AK-CIDE .... ⊙ 203
AK-CIDE Ointment .... ⊙ 203
Blephamide Liquifilm Sterile Ophthalmic Suspension 472
Blephamide Ointment .... ⊙ 234
Econopred & Econopred Plus Ophthalmic Suspensions ... ⊙ 216
Poly-Pred Liquifilm .... ⊙ 246
Pred Forte .... ⊙ 247
Pred Mild .... ⊙ 250
Pred-G Liquifilm Sterile Ophthalmic Suspension .... ⊙ 248
Pred-G S.O.P. Sterile Ophthalmic Ointment .... ⊙ 249

Prednisolone Sodium Phosphate (Enhanced metabolism of exogenous corticosteroids). Products include:
AK-PRED .... ⊙ 204
Hydeltrasol Injection, Sterile ... 1708
Pediapred Oral Solution 1618

Prednisolone Tebutate (Enhanced metabolism of exogenous corticosteroids). Products include:
Hydeltra-T.B.A. Sterile Suspension ... 1710

Prednisone (Enhanced metabolism of exogenous corticosteroids).
No products indexed under this heading.

Prochlorperazine (Additive depressant effects). Products include:
Compazine 2644

Progesterone (Decreased effect of progesterone).
No products indexed under this heading.

Promethazine Hydrochloride (Additive depressant effects). Products include:
Mepergan Injection 2859
Phenergan with Codeine 2883
Phenergan with Dextromethorphan ... 2885
Phenergan Injection 2880
Phenergan Suppositories 2882
Phenergan Syrup 2881
Phenergan Tablets 2882
Phenergan VC 2886
Phenergan VC with Codeine ... 2888

Propofol (Additive depressant effects). Products include:
Diprivan Injectable Emulsion ... 2939

Propoxyphene Hydrochloride (Additive depressant effects). Products include:
Darvon 1475
Wygesic Tablets 2930

Propoxyphene Napsylate (Additive depressant effects). Products include:
Darvon-N/Darvocet-N 1473

Quazepam (Additive depressant effects). Products include:
Doral Tablets 2773

Risperidone (Additive depressant effects). Products include:
Risperdal Tablets 1348

Secobarbital Sodium (Additive depressant effects). Products include:
Seconal Sodium Pulvules 1529

Selegiline Hydrochloride (Prolongs effects of barbiturates). Products include:
Eldepryl Capsules 2729

Sevoflurane (Additive depressant effects).
No products indexed under this heading.

Sodium Valproate (Barbiturate metabolism decreased).

Sufentanil Citrate (Additive depressant effects). Products include:
Sufenta Injection 1355

Temazepam (Additive depressant effects). Products include:
Restoril Capsules 2413

Thiamylal Sodium (Additive depressant effects).
No products indexed under this heading.

Thioridazine Hydrochloride (Additive depressant effects). Products include:
Mellaril 2398

Thiothixene (Additive depressant effects). Products include:
Navane Capsules and Concentrate ... 2018
Navane Intramuscular 2019

Tranylcypromine Sulfate (Prolongs effects of barbiturates). Products include:
Parnate Tablets 2679

Triamcinolone (Enhanced metabolism of exogenous corticosteroids).
No products indexed under this heading.

Triamcinolone Acetonide (Enhanced metabolism of exogenous corticosteroids). Products include:
Azmacort Oral Inhaler 2175
Nasacort AQ Nasal Spray 2191
Nasacort Nasal Inhaler 2189

Triamcinolone Diacetate (Enhanced metabolism of exogenous corticosteroids).
No products indexed under this heading.

Triamcinolone Hexacetonide (Enhanced metabolism of exogenous corticosteroids).
No products indexed under this heading.

Triazolam (Additive depressant effects). Products include:
Halcion Tablets 2093

Trifluoperazine Hydrochloride (Additive depressant effects). Products include:
Stelazine 2692

Valproic Acid (Decreased barbiturate metabolism). Products include:
Depakene 416

Warfarin Sodium (Decreased anticoagulant response). Products include:
Coumadin 941

Zolpidem Tartrate (Additive depressant effects). Products include:
Ambien Tablets 2559

MEDI-QUIK
(Benzalkonium Chloride, Lidocaine) ⊙ 710
None cited in PDR database.

MEFOXIN
(Cefoxitin Sodium) 1734
May interact with aminoglycosides and certain other agents. Compounds in these categories include:

Amikacin Sulfate (Increased nephrotoxicity). Products include:
Amikacin Sulfate Injection, USP ... 523
Amikacin Sulfate Injection, USP ... 981
Amikin Injectable 502

Gentamicin Sulfate (Increased nephrotoxicity). Products include:
Garamycin Cream 0.1% 2501
Garamycin Injectable 2502
Garamycin Ointment 0.1% 2501
Garamycin Ophthalmic 2501
Genoptic Sterile Ophthalmic Solution .... ⊙ 241
Genoptic Sterile Ophthalmic Ointment .... ⊙ 241
Gentak .... ⊙ 209
Pred-G Liquifilm Sterile Ophthalmic Suspension .... ⊙ 248
Pred-G S.O.P. Sterile Ophthalmic Ointment .... ⊙ 249

Kanamycin Sulfate (Increased nephrotoxicity).
No products indexed under this heading.

Probenecid (Slows tubular excretion and produces higher serum levels of cefoxitin). Products include:
Benemid Tablets 1651
ColBENEMID Tablets 1662

Streptomycin Sulfate (Increased nephrotoxicity). Products include:
Streptomycin Sulfate Injection ... 2031

Tobramycin (Increased nephrotoxicity). Products include:
AKTOB .... ⊙ 207
TobraDex Ophthalmic Suspension and Ointment 469
Tobrex Ophthalmic Ointment and Solution .... ⊙ 226

Tobramycin Sulfate (Increased nephrotoxicity). Products include:
Nebcin Vials, Hyporets & ADD-Vantage 1518

MEFOXIN PREMIXED INTRAVENOUS SOLUTION
(Cefoxitin Sodium) 1737
May interact with aminoglycosides and certain other agents. Compounds in these categories include:

Amikacin Sulfate (Increased nephrotoxicity). Products include:
Amikacin Sulfate Injection, USP ... 523
Amikacin Sulfate Injection, USP ... 981
Amikin Injectable 502

Gentamicin Sulfate (Increased nephrotoxicity). Products include:
Garamycin Cream 0.1% 2501
Garamycin Injectable 2502
Garamycin Ointment 0.1% 2501
Garamycin Ophthalmic 2501
Genoptic Sterile Ophthalmic Solution .... ⊙ 241
Genoptic Sterile Ophthalmic Ointment .... ⊙ 241
Gentak .... ⊙ 209
Pred-G Liquifilm Sterile Ophthalmic Suspension .... ⊙ 248
Pred-G S.O.P. Sterile Ophthalmic Ointment .... ⊙ 249

Kanamycin Sulfate (Increased nephrotoxicity).
No products indexed under this heading.

Probenecid (Higher serum levels of cefoxitin). Products include:
Benemid Tablets 1651
ColBENEMID Tablets 1662

Streptomycin Sulfate (Increased nephrotoxicity). Products include:
Streptomycin Sulfate Injection ... 2031

Tobramycin Sulfate (Increased nephrotoxicity). Products include:
Nebcin Vials, Hyporets & ADD-Vantage 1518

MEGA-B
(Vitamin B Complex) 513
None cited in PDR database.

MEGACE ORAL SUSPENSION
(Megestrol Acetate) 708
None cited in PDR database.

MEGACE TABLETS
(Megestrol Acetate) 710
None cited in PDR database.

MEGADOSE
(Vitamins with Minerals) 513
None cited in PDR database.

MELANEX TOPICAL SOLUTION
(Hydroquinone) 1842
May interact with:

Hydrogen Peroxide (May result in transient dark staining of skin areas so treated).
No products indexed under this heading.

MELATONEX
(Melatonin, Vitamin B_6) .... ⊙ 791
None cited in PDR database.

MELATONIN TABLETS
(Melatonin) 461
None cited in PDR database.

MELLARIL CONCENTRATE
(Thioridazine Hydrochloride) 2398
May interact with anesthetics, psychotropics, central nervous system depressants, narcotic analgesics, barbiturates, and certain other agents. Compounds in these categories include:

Alfentanil Hydrochloride (Co-administration results in the potentiation of CNS depression). Products include:
Alfenta Injection 1334

Alprazolam (Co-administration results in the potentiation of CNS depression). Products include:
Xanax Tablets 2115

Amitriptyline Hydrochloride (Co-administration results in the potentiation of CNS depression). Products include:
Elavil 2945
Etrafon 2495

IMPORTANT NOTE: Always consult each drug listing in the patient's regimen for possible interactions.

Mellaril Interactions Index 656

Limbitrol ... 2333
Triavil Tablets ... 1800

Amoxapine (Co-administration results in the potentiation of CNS depression). Products include:
Asendin Tablets ... 1419

Aprobarbital (Co-administration of a barbiturate and a phenothiazine has resulted in a severe respiratory depression and respiratory arrest; co-administration results in the potentiation of CNS depression).
No products indexed under this heading.

Buprenorphine (Co-administration results in the potentiation of CNS depression). Products include:
Buprenex Injectable ... 2170

Buspirone Hydrochloride (Co-administration results in the potentiation of CNS depression). Products include:
BuSpar Tablets ... 738

Butabarbital (Co-administration of a barbiturate and a phenothiazine has resulted in a severe respiratory depression and respiratory arrest; co-administration results in the potentiation of CNS depression).
No products indexed under this heading.

Butalbital (Co-administration of a barbiturate and a phenothiazine has resulted in a severe respiratory depression and respiratory arrest; co-administration results in the potentiation of CNS depression). Products include:
Axocet Capsules ... 2469
Esgic-plus Capsules ... 1012
Esgic-plus Tablets ... 1012
Fioricet Tablets ... 2386
Fioricet with Codeine Capsules ... 2387
Fiorinal Capsules ... 2388
Fiorinal with Codeine Capsules ... 2390
Fiorinal Tablets ... 2388
Phrenilin ... 790
Sedapap Tablets 50 mg/650 mg .. 1826

Chlordiazepoxide (Co-administration results in the potentiation of CNS depression). Products include:
Limbitrol ... 2333

Chlordiazepoxide Hydrochloride (Co-administration results in the potentiation of CNS depression). Products include:
Librax Capsules ... 2330
Librium Capsules ... 2331
Librium Injectable ... 2332

Chlorpromazine (Co-administration results in the potentiation of CNS depression). Products include:
Thorazine Suppositories ... 2701

Chlorpromazine Hydrochloride (Co-administration results in the potentiation of CNS depression). Products include:
Thorazine ... 2701

Chlorprothixene (Co-administration results in the potentiation of CNS depression).
No products indexed under this heading.

Chlorprothixene Hydrochloride (Co-administration results in the potentiation of CNS depression).
No products indexed under this heading.

Chlorprothixene Lactate (Co-administration results in the potentiation of CNS depression).
No products indexed under this heading.

Clorazepate Dipotassium (Co-administration results in the potentiation of CNS depression). Products include:
Tranxene ... 459

Clozapine (Co-administration results in the potentiation of CNS depression). Products include:
Clozaril Tablets ... 2377

Codeine Phosphate (Co-administration results in the potentiation of CNS depression). Products include:
Brontex ... 2130
Dimetane-DC Cough Syrup ... 2232
Fioricet with Codeine Capsules ... 2387
Fiorinal with Codeine Capsules ... 2390
Nucofed ... 2225
Phenergan with Codeine ... 2883
Phenergan VC with Codeine ... 2888
Robitussin A-C Syrup ... 2248
Robitussin-DAC Syrup ... 2249
Ryna ... ▣ 804
Soma Compound w/Codeine Tablets ... 2784
Tylenol with Codeine ... 1592

Desflurane (Co-administration results in the potentiation of CNS depression). Products include:
Suprane (desflurane, USP) ... 1865

Desipramine Hydrochloride (Co-administration results in the potentiation of CNS depression). Products include:
Norpramin Tablets ... 1273

Dezocine (Co-administration results in the potentiation of CNS depression). Products include:
Dalgan Injection ... 529

Diazepam (Co-administration results in the potentiation of CNS depression). Products include:
Dizac (diazepam injectable emulsion) CIV ... 1862
Valium Injectable ... 2336
Valium Tablets ... 2335

Doxepin Hydrochloride (Co-administration results in the potentiation of CNS depression). Products include:
Adapin Capsules ... 1542
Sinequan ... 2028
Zonalon Cream ... 1042

Droperidol (Co-administration results in the potentiation of CNS depression). Products include:
Inapsine Injection ... 462

Enflurane (Co-administration results in the potentiation of CNS depression).
No products indexed under this heading.

Estazolam (Co-administration results in the potentiation of CNS depression). Products include:
ProSom Tablets ... 457

Ethchlorvynol (Co-administration results in the potentiation of CNS depression). Products include:
Placidyl Capsules ... 456

Ethinamate (Co-administration results in the potentiation of CNS depression).
No products indexed under this heading.

Fentanyl (Co-administration results in the potentiation of CNS depression). Products include:
Duragesic Transdermal System ... 1336

Fentanyl Citrate (Co-administration results in the potentiation of CNS depression). Products include:
Sublimaze Injection ... 463

Fluphenazine Decanoate (Co-administration results in the potentiation of CNS depression). Products include:
Prolixin Decanoate ... 510

Fluphenazine Enanthate (Co-administration results in the potentiation of CNS depression). Products include:
Prolixin Enanthate ... 510

Fluphenazine Hydrochloride (Co-administration results in the potentiation of CNS depression). Products include:
Prolixin ... 510

Flurazepam Hydrochloride (Co-administration results in the potentiation of CNS depression). Products include:
Dalmane Capsules ... 2329

Glutethimide (Co-administration results in the potentiation of CNS depression).
No products indexed under this heading.

Haloperidol (Co-administration results in the potentiation of CNS depression). Products include:
Haldol Injection, Tablets and Concentrate ... 1585

Haloperidol Decanoate (Co-administration results in the potentiation of CNS depression). Products include:
Haldol Decanoate ... 1587

Halothane (Co-administration results in the potentiation of CNS depression). Products include:
Fluothane ... 2830

Hydrocodone Bitartrate (Co-administration results in the potentiation of CNS depression). Products include:
Codiclear DH Syrup ... 808
Duratuss HD Elixir ... 2750
Histussin D Liquid ... 670
Hycodan Tablets and Syrup ... 946
Hycomine Compound Tablets ... 948
Hycomine ... 947
Hycotuss Expectorant Syrup ... 950
Hydrocet Capsules ... 787
Lorcet 10/650 Tablets ... 1016
Lortab ... 2751
Tussend ... 1830
Tussend Expectorant ... 1831
Vicodin Tablets ... 1404
Vicodin ES Tablets ... 1405
Vicodin HP Tablets ... 1403
Vicodin Tuss Expectorant ... 1406
Zydone Capsules ... 967

Hydrocodone Polistirex (Co-administration results in the potentiation of CNS depression). Products include:
Tussionex Pennkinetic Extended-Release Suspension ... 1624

Hydromorphone Hydrochloride (Co-administration results in the potentiation of CNS depression). Products include:
Dilaudid Ampules ... 1382
Dilaudid Cough Syrup ... 1383
Dilaudid-HP Injection ... 1384
Dilaudid-HP Lyophilized Powder 250 mg ... 1384
Dilaudid ... 1382
Dilaudid Oral Liquid ... 1386
Dilaudid ... 1382
Dilaudid Tablets - 8 mg ... 1386

Hydroxyzine Hydrochloride (Co-administration results in the potentiation of CNS depression). Products include:
Atarax Tablets & Syrup ... 1992
Marax Tablets & DF Syrup ... 2015
Vistaril Intramuscular Solution ... 2042

Imipramine Hydrochloride (Co-administration results in the potentiation of CNS depression). Products include:
Tofranil Ampuls ... 873
Tofranil Tablets ... 875

Imipramine Pamoate (Co-administration results in the potentiation of CNS depression). Products include:
Tofranil-PM Capsules ... 876

Isocarboxazid (Co-administration results in the potentiation of CNS depression).
No products indexed under this heading.

Isoflurane (Co-administration results in the potentiation of CNS depression).
No products indexed under this heading.

Ketamine Hydrochloride (Co-administration results in the potentiation of CNS depression).
No products indexed under this heading.

Levomethadyl Acetate Hydrochloride (Co-administration results in the potentiation of CNS depression). Products include:
Orlaam Oral Solution ... 2361

Levorphanol Tartrate (Co-administration results in the potentiation of CNS depression). Products include:
Levo-Dromoran ... 2297

Lithium Carbonate (Co-administration results in the potentiation of CNS depression). Products include:
Eskalith ... 2658
Lithium Carbonate Capsules & Tablets ... 2352
Lithonate/Lithotabs/Lithobid ... 2721

Lithium Citrate (Co-administration results in the potentiation of CNS depression).
No products indexed under this heading.

Lorazepam (Co-administration results in the potentiation of CNS depression). Products include:
Ativan Injection ... 2805
Ativan Tablets ... 2807

Loxapine Hydrochloride (Co-administration results in the potentiation of CNS depression). Products include:
Loxitane ... 1426

Loxapine Succinate (Co-administration results in the potentiation of CNS depression). Products include:
Loxitane Capsules ... 1426

Maprotiline Hydrochloride (Co-administration results in the potentiation of CNS depression). Products include:
Ludiomil Tablets ... 861

Meperidine Hydrochloride (Co-administration results in the potentiation of CNS depression). Products include:
Demerol ... 2438
Mepergan Injection ... 2859

Mephobarbital (Co-administration of a barbiturate and a phenothiazine has resulted in a severe respiratory depression and respiratory arrest; co-administration results in the potentiation of CNS depression). Products include:
Mebaral Tablets ... 2452

Meprobamate (Co-administration results in the potentiation of CNS depression). Products include:
Miltown Tablets ... 2780
PMB 200 and PMB 400 ... 2890

Mesoridazine Besylate (Co-administration results in the potentiation of CNS depression). Products include:
Serentil ... 689

Methadone Hydrochloride (Co-administration results in the potentiation of CNS depression). Products include:
Methadone Hydrochloride Oral Concentrate ... 2356
Methadone Hydrochloride Oral Solution & Tablets ... 2357

Methohexital Sodium (Co-administration results in the potentiation of CNS depression).
No products indexed under this heading.

(▣ Described in PDR For Nonprescription Drugs) (◉ Described in PDR For Ophthalmology)

Methotrimeprazine (Co-administration results in the potentiation of CNS depression). Products include:
Levoprome 1321
Methoxyflurane (Co-administration results in the potentiation of CNS depression).
No products indexed under this heading.
Midazolam Hydrochloride (Co-administration results in the potentiation of CNS depression). Products include:
Versed Injection 2324
Molindone Hydrochloride (Co-administration results in the potentiation of CNS depression). Products include:
Moban Tablets and Concentrate 1036
Morphine Sulfate (Co-administration results in the potentiation of CNS depression). Products include:
Astramorph/PF Injection, USP (Preservative-Free) 526
Duramorph Injection 983
Infumorph 200 and Infumorph 500 Sterile Solutions 985
Kadian Capsules 2948
MS Contin Tablets 2149
MSIR 2152
Oramorph SR (Morphine Sulfate Sustained Release Tablets) 2359
RMS Suppositories CII 2766
Roxanol 2365
Nortriptyline Hydrochloride (Co-administration results in the potentiation of CNS depression). Products include:
Pamelor 2409
Opium Alkaloids (Co-administration results in the potentiation of CNS depression).
No products indexed under this heading.
Oxazepam (Co-administration results in the potentiation of CNS depression). Products include:
Serax Capsules 2916
Serax Tablets 2916
Oxycodone Hydrochloride (Co-administration results in the potentiation of CNS depression). Products include:
OxyContin Tablets 2163
OxyIR Capsules 2167
Percocet Tablets 955
Percodan Tablets 955
Percodan-Demi Tablets 956
Roxicodone Tablets, Oral Solution & Intensol (Oxycodone) 2366
Tylox Capsules 1593
Pentobarbital Sodium (Co-administration of a barbiturate and a phenothiazine has resulted in a severe respiratory depression and respiratory arrest; co-administration results in the potentiation of CNS depression). Products include:
Nembutal Sodium Capsules 440
Nembutal Sodium Solution 442
Nembutal Sodium Suppositories 444
Perphenazine (Co-administration results in the potentiation of CNS depression). Products include:
Etrafon 2495
Triavil Tablets 1800
Trilafon 2532
Phenelzine Sulfate (Co-administration results in the potentiation of CNS depression). Products include:
Nardil 1977
Phenobarbital (Co-administration of a barbiturate and a phenothiazine has resulted in a severe respiratory depression and respiratory arrest; co-administration results in the potentiation of CNS depression). Products include:
Arco-Lase Plus Tablets 513
Bellergal-S Tablets 2375

Donnatal 2234
Donnatal Extentabs 2234
Donnatal Tablets 2234
Phenobarbital Elixir and Tablets 1523
Quadrinal Tablets 1398
Pindolol (Co-administration results in a moderate, dose-related increase in the serum levels of thioridazine and two of its metabolites, as well as higher than expected serum pindolol levels). Products include:
Visken Tablets 2428
Prazepam (Co-administration results in the potentiation of CNS depression).
No products indexed under this heading.
Prochlorperazine (Co-administration results in the potentiation of CNS depression). Products include:
Compazine 2644
Promethazine Hydrochloride (Co-administration results in the potentiation of CNS depression). Products include:
Mepergan Injection 2859
Phenergan with Codeine 2883
Phenergan with Dextromethorphan ... 2885
Phenergan Injection 2880
Phenergan Suppositories 2882
Phenergan Syrup 2881
Phenergan Tablets 2882
Phenergan VC 2886
Phenergan VC with Codeine 2888
Propofol (Co-administration results in the potentiation of CNS depression). Products include:
Diprivan Injectable Emulsion 2939
Propoxyphene Hydrochloride (Co-administration results in the potentiation of CNS depression). Products include:
Darvon 1475
Wygesic Tablets 2930
Propoxyphene Napsylate (Co-administration results in the potentiation of CNS depression). Products include:
Darvon-N/Darvocet-N 1473
Propranolol Hydrochloride (Co-administration has been reported to produce increases in plasma levels of thioridazine and its metabolites). Products include:
Inderal 2834
Inderal LA Long Acting Capsules ... 2836
Inderide Tablets 2838
Inderide LA Long Acting Capsules ... 2840
Protriptyline Hydrochloride (Co-administration results in the potentiation of CNS depression). Products include:
Vivactil Tablets 1820
Quazepam (Co-administration results in the potentiation of CNS depression). Products include:
Doral Tablets 2773
Risperidone (Co-administration results in the potentiation of CNS depression). Products include:
Risperdal Tablets 1348
Secobarbital Sodium (Co-administration of a barbiturate and a phenothiazine has resulted in a severe respiratory depression and respiratory arrest; co-administration results in the potentiation of CNS depression). Products include:
Seconal Sodium Pulvules 1529
Sevoflurane (Co-administration results in the potentiation of CNS depression).
No products indexed under this heading.
Sufentanil Citrate (Co-administration results in the potentiation of CNS depression). Products include:
Sufenta Injection 1355

Temazepam (Co-administration results in the potentiation of CNS depression). Products include:
Restoril Capsules 2413
Thiamylal Sodium (Co-administration of a barbiturate and a phenothiazine has resulted in a severe respiratory depression and respiratory arrest; co-administration results in the potentiation of CNS depression).
No products indexed under this heading.
Thiothixene (Co-administration results in the potentiation of CNS depression). Products include:
Navane Capsules and Concentrate ... 2018
Navane Intramuscular 2019
Tranylcypromine Sulfate (Co-administration results in the potentiation of CNS depression). Products include:
Parnate Tablets 2679
Triazolam (Co-administration results in the potentiation of CNS depression). Products include:
Halcion Tablets 2093
Trifluoperazine Hydrochloride (Co-administration results in the potentiation of CNS depression). Products include:
Stelazine 2692
Trimipramine Maleate (Co-administration results in the potentiation of CNS depression). Products include:
Surmontil Capsules 2917
Zolpidem Tartrate (Co-administration results in the potentiation of CNS depression). Products include:
Ambien Tablets 2559

Food Interactions
Alcohol (Concurrent use results in the potentiation of CNS depression).

MELLARIL TABLETS
(Thioridazine Hydrochloride) 2398
See **Mellaril Concentrate**

MELLARIL-S SUSPENSION
(Thioridazine) 2398
See **Mellaril Concentrate**

MENEST TABLETS
(Estrogens, Esterified) 2671
None cited in PDR database.

MENOMUNE-A/C/Y/W-135-
(Meningococcal Polysaccharide Vaccine) 906
May interact with immunosuppressive agents. Compounds in this category include:
Azathioprine (The expected immune response may not be obtained). Products include:
Azathioprine Tablets 2349
Imuran 1103
Cyclosporine (The expected immune response may not be obtained). Products include:
Neoral 2405
Sandimmune 2416
Immune Globulin (Human) (The expected immune response may not be obtained).
No products indexed under this heading.
Immune Globulin Intravenous (Human) (The expected immune response may not be obtained).
Muromonab-CD3 (The expected immune response may not be obtained). Products include:
Orthoclone OKT3 Sterile Solution .. 1892

Mycophenolate Mofetil (The expected immune response may not be obtained). Products include:
CellCept Capsules 2265
Tacrolimus (The expected immune response may not be obtained). Products include:
Prograf 1028

MENTHOLATUM CHERRY CHEST RUB FOR KIDS
(Camphor, Eucalyptus, Oil of, Menthol) 710
None cited in PDR database.

MENTHOLATUM DEEP HEATING EXTRA STRENGTH FORMULA RUB
(Menthol, Methyl Salicylate) 710
None cited in PDR database.

MENTHOLATUM MENTHACIN
(Capsaicin, Menthol) 711
None cited in PDR database.

MENTHOLATUM OINTMENT
(Camphor, Menthol) 711
None cited in PDR database.

MEPERGAN INJECTION
(Meperidine Hydrochloride, Promethazine Hydrochloride) 2859
May interact with narcotic analgesics, general anesthetics, phenothiazines, tranquilizers, hypnotics and sedatives, tricyclic antidepressants, barbiturates, central nervous system depressants, monoamine oxidase inhibitors, and certain other agents. Compounds in these categories include:
Alfentanil Hydrochloride (Respiratory depression, hypotension, profound sedation or coma). Products include:
Alfenta Injection 1334
Alprazolam (Respiratory depression, hypotension, profound sedation or coma). Products include:
Xanax Tablets 2115
Amitriptyline Hydrochloride (Respiratory depression, hypotension, profound sedation or coma). Products include:
Elavil 2945
Etrafon 2495
Limbitrol 2333
Triavil Tablets 1800
Amoxapine (Respiratory depression, hypotension, profound sedation or coma). Products include:
Asendin Tablets 1419
Aprobarbital (Respiratory depression, hypotension, profound sedation or coma).
No products indexed under this heading.
Buprenorphine (Respiratory depression, hypotension, profound sedation or coma). Products include:
Buprenex Injectable 2170
Buspirone Hydrochloride (Respiratory depression, hypotension, profound sedation or coma). Products include:
BuSpar Tablets 738
Butabarbital (Respiratory depression, hypotension, profound sedation or coma).
No products indexed under this heading.
Butalbital (Respiratory depression, hypotension, profound sedation or coma). Products include:
Axocet Capsules 2469
Esgic-plus Capsules 1012

IMPORTANT NOTE: Always consult each drug listing in the patient's regimen for possible interactions.

Mepergan — Interactions Index — 658

Esgic-plus Tablets 1012
Fioricet Tablets 2386
Fioricet with Codeine Capsules ... 2387
Fiorinal Capsules 2388
Fiorinal with Codeine Capsules ... 2390
Fiorinal Tablets 2388
Phrenilin 790
Sedapap Tablets 50 mg/650 mg .. 1826

Chlordiazepoxide (Respiratory depression, hypotension, profound sedation or coma). Products include:
Limbitrol 2333

Chlordiazepoxide Hydrochloride (Respiratory depression, hypotension, profound sedation or coma). Products include:
Librax Capsules 2330
Librium Capsules 2331
Librium Injectable 2332

Chlorpromazine (Respiratory depression, hypotension, profound sedation or coma). Products include:
Thorazine Suppositories 2701

Chlorprothixene (Respiratory depression, hypotension, profound sedation or coma).
No products indexed under this heading.

Chlorprothixene Hydrochloride (Respiratory depression, hypotension, profound sedation or coma).
No products indexed under this heading.

Chlorprothixene Lactate (Respiratory depression, hypotension, profound sedation or coma).
No products indexed under this heading.

Clomipramine Hydrochloride (Respiratory depression, hypotension, profound sedation or coma). Products include:
Anafranil Capsules 819

Clorazepate Dipotassium (Respiratory depression, hypotension, profound sedation or coma). Products include:
Tranxene 459

Clozapine (Respiratory depression, hypotension, profound sedation or coma). Products include:
Clozaril Tablets 2377

Codeine Phosphate (Respiratory depression, hypotension, profound sedation or coma). Products include:
Brontex 2130
Dimetane-DC Cough Syrup 2232
Fioricet with Codeine Capsules .. 2387
Fiorinal with Codeine Capsules .. 2390
Nucofed 2225
Phenergan with Codeine 2883
Phenergan VC with Codeine 2888
Robitussin A-C Syrup 2248
Robitussin-DAC Syrup 2249
Ryna .... ▣ 804
Soma Compound w/Codeine Tablets 2784
Tylenol with Codeine 1592

Desflurane (Respiratory depression, hypotension, profound sedation or coma). Products include:
Suprane (desflurane, USP) 1865

Desipramine Hydrochloride (Respiratory depression, hypotension, profound sedation or coma). Products include:
Norpramin Tablets 1273

Dezocine (Respiratory depression, hypotension, profound sedation or coma). Products include:
Dalgan Injection 529

Diazepam (Respiratory depression, hypotension, profound sedation or coma). Products include:
Dizac (diazepam injectable emulsion) CIV 1862
Valium Injectable 2336
Valium Tablets 2335

Doxepin Hydrochloride (Respiratory depression, hypotension, profound sedation or coma). Products include:
Adapin Capsules 1542
Sinequan 2028
Zonalon Cream 1042

Droperidol (Respiratory depression, hypotension, profound sedation or coma). Products include:
Inapsine Injection 462

Enflurane (Respiratory depression, hypotension, profound sedation or coma).
No products indexed under this heading.

Estazolam (Respiratory depression, hypotension, profound sedation or coma). Products include:
ProSom Tablets 457

Ethchlorvynol (Respiratory depression, hypotension, profound sedation or coma). Products include:
Placidyl Capsules 456

Ethinamate (Respiratory depression, hypotension, profound sedation or coma).
No products indexed under this heading.

Fentanyl (Respiratory depression, hypotension, profound sedation or coma). Products include:
Duragesic Transdermal System .. 1336

Fentanyl Citrate (Respiratory depression, hypotension, profound sedation or coma). Products include:
Sublimaze Injection 463

Fluphenazine Decanoate (Respiratory depression, hypotension, profound sedation or coma). Products include:
Prolixin Decanoate 510

Fluphenazine Enanthate (Respiratory depression, hypotension, profound sedation or coma). Products include:
Prolixin Enanthate 510

Fluphenazine Hydrochloride (Respiratory depression, hypotension, profound sedation or coma). Products include:
Prolixin 510

Flurazepam Hydrochloride (Respiratory depression, hypotension, profound sedation or coma). Products include:
Dalmane Capsules 2329

Furazolidone (Concurrent administration is contraindicated). Products include:
Furoxone 2221

Glutethimide (Respiratory depression, hypotension, profound sedation or coma).
No products indexed under this heading.

Haloperidol (Respiratory depression, hypotension, profound sedation or coma). Products include:
Haldol Injection, Tablets and Concentrate 1585

Haloperidol Decanoate (Respiratory depression, hypotension, profound sedation or coma). Products include:
Haldol Decanoate 1587

Hydrocodone Bitartrate (Respiratory depression, hypotension, profound sedation or coma). Products include:
Codiclear DH Syrup 808
Duratuss HD Elixir 2750
Histussin D Liquid 670
Hycodan Tablets and Syrup 946
Hycomine Compound Tablets ... 948
Hycomine 947
Hycotuss Expectorant Syrup 950
Hydrocet Capsules 787

Lorcet 10/650 Tablets 1016
Lortab 2751
Tussend 1830
Tussend Expectorant 1831
Vicodin Tablets 1404
Vicodin ES Tablets 1405
Vicodin HP Tablets 1403
Vicodin Tuss Expectorant 1406
Zydone Tablets 967

Hydrocodone Polistirex (Respiratory depression, hypotension, profound sedation or coma). Products include:
Tussionex Pennkinetic Extended-Release Suspension 1624

Hydromorphone Hydrochloride (Respiratory depression, hypotension, profound sedation or coma). Products include:
Dilaudid Ampules 1382
Dilaudid Cough Syrup 1383
Dilaudid-HP Injection 1384
Dilaudid-HP Lyophilized Powder 250 mg 1384
Dilaudid 1382
Dilaudid Oral Liquid 1386
Dilaudid 1382
Dilaudid Tablets - 8 mg 1386

Hydroxyzine Hydrochloride (Respiratory depression, hypotension, profound sedation or coma). Products include:
Atarax Tablets & Syrup 1992
Marax Tablets & DF Syrup 2015
Vistaril Intramuscular Solution .. 2042

Imipramine Hydrochloride (Respiratory depression, hypotension, profound sedation or coma). Products include:
Tofranil Ampuls 873
Tofranil Tablets 875

Imipramine Pamoate (Respiratory depression, hypotension, profound sedation or coma). Products include:
Tofranil-PM Capsules 876

Isocarboxazid (Concurrent administration is contraindicated).
No products indexed under this heading.

Isoflurane (Respiratory depression, hypotension, profound sedation or coma).
No products indexed under this heading.

Ketamine Hydrochloride (Respiratory depression, hypotension, profound sedation or coma).
No products indexed under this heading.

Levomethadyl Acetate Hydrochloride (Respiratory depression, hypotension, profound sedation or coma). Products include:
Orlaam Oral Solution 2361

Levorphanol Tartrate (Respiratory depression, hypotension, profound sedation or coma). Products include:
Levo-Dromoran 2297

Lorazepam (Respiratory depression, hypotension, profound sedation or coma). Products include:
Ativan Injection 2805
Ativan Tablets 2807

Loxapine Hydrochloride (Respiratory depression, hypotension, profound sedation or coma). Products include:
Loxitane 1426

Loxapine Succinate (Respiratory depression, hypotension, profound sedation or coma). Products include:
Loxitane Capsules 1426

Maprotiline Hydrochloride (Respiratory depression, hypotension, profound sedation or coma). Products include:
Ludiomil Tablets 861

Mephobarbital (Respiratory depression, hypotension, profound sedation or coma). Products include:
Mebaral Tablets 2452

Meprobamate (Respiratory depression, hypotension, profound sedation or coma). Products include:
Miltown Tablets 2780
PMB 200 and PMB 400 2890

Mesoridazine Besylate (Respiratory depression, hypotension, profound sedation or coma). Products include:
Serentil 689

Methadone Hydrochloride (Respiratory depression, hypotension, profound sedation or coma). Products include:
Methadone Hydrochloride Oral Concentrate 2356
Methadone Hydrochloride Oral Solution & Tablets 2357

Methohexital Sodium (Respiratory depression, hypotension, profound sedation or coma).
No products indexed under this heading.

Methotrimeprazine (Respiratory depression, hypotension, profound sedation or coma). Products include:
Levoprome 1321

Methoxyflurane (Respiratory depression, hypotension, profound sedation or coma).
No products indexed under this heading.

Midazolam Hydrochloride (Respiratory depression, hypotension, profound sedation or coma). Products include:
Versed Injection 2324

Molindone Hydrochloride (Respiratory depression, hypotension, profound sedation or coma). Products include:
Moban Tablets and Concentrate .. 1036

Morphine Sulfate (Respiratory depression, hypotension, profound sedation or coma). Products include:
Astramorph/PF Injection, USP (Preservative-Free) 526
Duramorph Injection 983
Infumorph 200 and Infumorph 500 Sterile Solutions 985
Kadian Capsules 2948
MS Contin Tablets 2149
MSIR 2152
Oramorph SR (Morphine Sulfate Sustained Release Tablets) ... 2359
RMS Suppositories CII 2766
Roxanol 2365

Nortriptyline Hydrochloride (Respiratory depression, hypotension, profound sedation or coma). Products include:
Pamelor 2409

Opium Alkaloids (Respiratory depression, hypotension, profound sedation or coma).
No products indexed under this heading.

Oxazepam (Respiratory depression, hypotension, profound sedation or coma). Products include:
Serax Capsules 2916
Serax Tablets 2916

Oxycodone Hydrochloride (Respiratory depression, hypotension, profound sedation or coma). Products include:
OxyContin Tablets 2163
OxyIR Capsules 2167
Percocet Tablets 955
Percodan Tablets 955
Percodan-Demi Tablets 956
Roxicodone Tablets, Oral Solution & Intensol (Oxycodone) 2366
Tylox Capsules 1593

(▣ Described in PDR For Nonprescription Drugs)   (◉ Described in PDR For Ophthalmology)

Interactions Index

Pentobarbital Sodium (Respiratory depression, hypotension, profound sedation or coma). Products include:
- Nembutal Sodium Capsules 440
- Nembutal Sodium Solution 442
- Nembutal Sodium Suppositories 444

Perphenazine (Respiratory depression, hypotension, profound sedation or coma). Products include:
- Etrafon 2495
- Triavil Tablets 1800
- Trilafon 2532

Phenelzine Sulfate (Concurrent administration is contraindicated). Products include:
- Nardil 1977

Phenobarbital (Respiratory depression, hypotension, profound sedation or coma). Products include:
- Arco-Lase Plus Tablets 513
- Bellergal-S Tablets 2375
- Donnatal 2234
- Donnatal Extentabs 2234
- Donnatal Tablets 2234
- Phenobarbital Elixir and Tablets 1523
- Quadrinal Tablets 1398

Prazepam (Respiratory depression, hypotension, profound sedation or coma).
No products indexed under this heading.

Prochlorperazine (Respiratory depression, hypotension, profound sedation or coma). Products include:
- Compazine 2644

Propofol (Respiratory depression, hypotension, profound sedation or coma). Products include:
- Diprivan Injectable Emulsion 2939

Propoxyphene Hydrochloride (Respiratory depression, hypotension, profound sedation or coma). Products include:
- Darvon 1475
- Wygesic Tablets 2930

Propoxyphene Napsylate (Respiratory depression, hypotension, profound sedation or coma). Products include:
- Darvon-N/Darvocet-N 1473

Protriptyline Hydrochloride (Respiratory depression, hypotension, profound sedation or coma). Products include:
- Vivactil Tablets 1820

Quazepam (Respiratory depression, hypotension, profound sedation or coma). Products include:
- Doral Tablets 2773

Risperidone (Respiratory depression, hypotension, profound sedation or coma). Products include:
- Risperdal Tablets 1348

Secobarbital Sodium (Respiratory depression, hypotension, profound sedation or coma). Products include:
- Seconal Sodium Pulvules 1529

Selegiline Hydrochloride (Concurrent administration is contraindicated). Products include:
- Eldepryl Capsules 2729

Sevoflurane (Respiratory depression, hypotension, profound sedation or coma).
No products indexed under this heading.

Sufentanil Citrate (Respiratory depression, hypotension, profound sedation or coma). Products include:
- Sufenta Injection 1355

Temazepam (Respiratory depression, hypotension, profound sedation or coma). Products include:
- Restoril Capsules 2413

Thiamylal Sodium (Respiratory depression, hypotension, profound sedation or coma).
No products indexed under this heading.

Thioridazine Hydrochloride (Respiratory depression, hypotension, profound sedation or coma). Products include:
- Mellaril 2398

Thiothixene (Respiratory depression, hypotension, profound sedation or coma). Products include:
- Navane Capsules and Concentrate 2018
- Navane Intramuscular 2019

Tranylcypromine Sulfate (Concurrent administration is contraindicated). Products include:
- Parnate Tablets 2679

Triazolam (Respiratory depression, hypotension, profound sedation or coma). Products include:
- Halcion Tablets 2093

Trifluoperazine Hydrochloride (Respiratory depression, hypotension, profound sedation or coma). Products include:
- Stelazine 2692

Trimipramine Maleate (Respiratory depression, hypotension, profound sedation or coma). Products include:
- Surmontil Capsules 2917

Zolpidem Tartrate (Respiratory depression, hypotension, profound sedation or coma). Products include:
- Ambien Tablets 2559

Food Interactions

Alcohol (Respiratory depression, hypotension, profound sedation or coma).

MEPHYTON TABLETS
(Phytonadione) 1739
None cited in PDR database.

MEPRON SUSPENSION
(Atovaquone) 1206
May interact with highly protein bound drugs (selected) and certain other agents. Compounds in these categories include:

Amiodarone Hydrochloride (Atovaquone is highly bound to plasma protein (greater than 99.9%); caution is advised when co-administered with other highly protein bound drugs with narrow therapeutic indices). Products include:
- Cordarone Intravenous 2821
- Cordarone Tablets 2818

Amitriptyline Hydrochloride (Atovaquone is highly bound to plasma protein (greater than 99.9%); caution is advised when co-administered with other highly protein bound drugs with narrow therapeutic indices). Products include:
- Elavil 2945
- Etrafon 2495
- Limbitrol 2333
- Triavil Tablets 1800

Cefonicid Sodium (Atovaquone is highly bound to plasma protein (greater than 99.9%); caution is advised when co-administered with other highly protein bound drugs with narrow therapeutic indices). Products include:
- Monocid Injection 2674

Chlordiazepoxide (Atovaquone is highly bound to plasma protein (greater than 99.9%); caution is advised when co-administered with other highly protein bound drugs with narrow therapeutic indices). Products include:
- Limbitrol 2333

Chlordiazepoxide Hydrochloride (Atovaquone is highly bound to plasma protein (greater than 99.9%); caution is advised when co-administered with other highly protein bound drugs with narrow therapeutic indices). Products include:
- Librax Capsules 2330
- Librium Capsules 2331
- Librium Injectable 2332

Chlorpromazine (Atovaquone is highly bound to plasma protein (greater than 99.9%); caution is advised when co-administered with other highly protein bound drugs with narrow therapeutic indices). Products include:
- Thorazine Suppositories 2701

Chlorpromazine Hydrochloride (Atovaquone is highly bound to plasma protein (greater than 99.9%); caution is advised when co-administered with other highly protein bound drugs with narrow therapeutic indices). Products include:
- Thorazine 2701

Clomipramine Hydrochloride (Atovaquone is highly bound to plasma protein (greater than 99.9%); caution is advised when co-administered with other highly protein bound drugs with narrow therapeutic indices). Products include:
- Anafranil Capsules 819

Clozapine (Atovaquone is highly bound to plasma protein (greater than 99.9%); caution is advised when co-administered with other highly protein bound drugs with narrow therapeutic indices). Products include:
- Clozaril Tablets 2377

Cyclosporine (Atovaquone is highly bound to plasma protein (greater than 99.9%); caution is advised when co-administered with other highly protein bound drugs with narrow therapeutic indices). Products include:
- Neoral 2405
- Sandimmune 2416

Diazepam (Atovaquone is highly bound to plasma protein (greater than 99.9%); caution is advised when co-administered with other highly protein bound drugs with narrow therapeutic indices). Products include:
- Dizac (diazepam injectable emulsion) CIV 1862
- Valium Injectable 2336
- Valium Tablets 2335

Diclofenac Potassium (Atovaquone is highly bound to plasma protein (greater than 99.9%); caution is advised when co-administered with other highly protein bound drugs with narrow therapeutic indices). Products include:
- Cataflam Tablets 833

Diclofenac Sodium (Atovaquone is highly bound to plasma protein (greater than 99.9%); caution is advised when co-administered with other highly protein bound drugs with narrow therapeutic indices). Products include:
- Voltaren Ophthalmic Sterile Ophthalmic Solution .... ⓪ 264
- Cataflam/Voltaren/Voltaren-XR 833

Dipyridamole (Atovaquone is highly bound to plasma protein (greater than 99.9%); caution is advised when co-administered with other highly protein bound drugs with narrow therapeutic indices). Products include:
- Persantine Tablets 686

Fenoprofen Calcium (Atovaquone is highly bound to plasma protein (greater than 99.9%); caution is advised when co-administered with other highly protein bound drugs with narrow therapeutic indices). Products include:
- Nalfon 200 Pulvules & Nalfon Tablets 933

Flurazepam Hydrochloride (Atovaquone is highly bound to plasma protein (greater than 99.9%); caution is advised when co-administered with other highly protein bound drugs with narrow therapeutic indices). Products include:
- Dalmane Capsules 2329

Flurbiprofen (Atovaquone is highly bound to plasma protein (greater than 99.9%); caution is advised when co-administered with other highly protein bound drugs with narrow therapeutic indices).
No products indexed under this heading.

Glipizide (Atovaquone is highly bound to plasma protein (greater than 99.9%); caution is advised when co-administered with other highly protein bound drugs with narrow therapeutic indices). Products include:
- Glucotrol Tablets 2011
- Glucotrol XL Extended Release Tablets 2012

Ibuprofen (Atovaquone is highly bound to plasma protein (greater than 99.9%); caution is advised when co-administered with other highly protein bound drugs with narrow therapeutic indices). Products include:
- Advil Cold and Sinus Caplets and Tablets 837
- Advil Ibuprofen Tablets, Caplets and Gel Caplets 836
- Children's Motrin Ibuprofen Oral Suspension 1558
- IBU Tablets 1389
- Ibuprohm 713
- Motrin IB Caplets, Tablets, and Gelcaps 802
- Motrin Ibuprofen Suspension, Oral Drops, Chewable Tablets, Caplets 1563
- Nuprin Ibuprofen/Analgesic Tablets & Caplets 645
- Vicks DayQuil SINUS Pressure & PAIN Relief with IBUPROFEN 735

Imipramine Hydrochloride (Atovaquone is highly bound to plasma protein (greater than 99.9%); caution is advised when co-administered with other highly protein bound drugs with narrow therapeutic indices). Products include:
- Tofranil Ampuls 873
- Tofranil Tablets 875

IMPORTANT NOTE: Always consult each drug listing in the patient's regimen for possible interactions.

Mepron Suspension / Interactions Index

Imipramine Pamoate (Atovaquone is highly bound to plasma protein (greater than 99.9%); caution is advised when co-administered with other highly protein bound drugs with narrow therapeutic indices). Products include:
- Tofranil-PM Capsules 876

Indomethacin (Atovaquone is highly bound to plasma protein (greater than 99.9%); caution is advised when co-administered with other highly protein bound drugs with narrow therapeutic indices). Products include:
- Indocin 1723

Indomethacin Sodium Trihydrate (Atovaquone is highly bound to plasma protein (greater than 99.9%); caution is advised when co-administered with other highly protein bound drugs with narrow therapeutic indices). Products include:
- Indocin I.V. 1727

Ketoprofen (Atovaquone is highly bound to plasma protein (greater than 99.9%); caution is advised when co-administered with other highly protein bound drugs with narrow therapeutic indices). Products include:
- Actron Caplets and Tablets 608
- Orudis Capsules 2874
- Orudis KT 842
- Oruvail Capsules 2874

Ketorolac Tromethamine (Atovaquone is highly bound to plasma protein (greater than 99.9%); caution is advised when co-administered with other highly protein bound drugs with narrow therapeutic indices). Products include:
- Acular Sterile Ophthalmic Solution . 470
- Toradol 2319

Meclofenamate Sodium (Atovaquone is highly bound to plasma protein (greater than 99.9%); caution is advised when co-administered with other highly protein bound drugs with narrow therapeutic indices).
- No products indexed under this heading.

Mefenamic Acid (Atovaquone is highly bound to plasma protein (greater than 99.9%); caution is advised when co-administered with other highly protein bound drugs with narrow therapeutic indices). Products include:
- Ponstel 1982

Midazolam Hydrochloride (Atovaquone is highly bound to plasma protein (greater than 99.9%); caution is advised when co-administered with other highly protein bound drugs with narrow therapeutic indices). Products include:
- Versed Injection 2324

Naproxen (Atovaquone is highly bound to plasma protein (greater than 99.9%); caution is advised when co-administered with other highly protein bound drugs with narrow therapeutic indices). Products include:
- Anaprox/Naprosyn 2277

Naproxen Sodium (Atovaquone is highly bound to plasma protein (greater than 99.9%); caution is advised when co-administered with other highly protein bound drugs with narrow therapeutic indices). Products include:
- Aleve 2124

- Anaprox/Naprosyn 2277
- Naprelan Tablets 2861

Nortriptyline Hydrochloride (Atovaquone is highly bound to plasma protein (greater than 99.9%); caution is advised when co-administered with other highly protein bound drugs with narrow therapeutic indices). Products include:
- Pamelor 2409

Oxaprozin (Atovaquone is highly bound to plasma protein (greater than 99.9%); caution is advised when co-administered with other highly protein bound drugs with narrow therapeutic indices). Products include:
- Daypro Caplets 2578

Oxazepam (Atovaquone is highly bound to plasma protein (greater than 99.9%); caution is advised when co-administered with other highly protein bound drugs with narrow therapeutic indices). Products include:
- Serax Capsules 2916
- Serax Tablets 2916

Phenylbutazone (Atovaquone is highly bound to plasma protein (greater than 99.9%); caution is advised when co-administered with other highly protein bound drugs with narrow therapeutic indices).
- No products indexed under this heading.

Piroxicam (Atovaquone is highly bound to plasma protein (greater than 99.9%); caution is advised when co-administered with other highly protein bound drugs with narrow therapeutic indices). Products include:
- Feldene Capsules 2008

Propranolol Hydrochloride (Atovaquone is highly bound to plasma protein (greater than 99.9%); caution is advised when co-administered with other highly protein bound drugs with narrow therapeutic indices). Products include:
- Inderal 2834
- Inderal LA Long Acting Capsules ... 2836
- Inderide Tablets 2838
- Inderide LA Long Acting Capsules .. 2840

Rifabutin (Due to structural similarity to rifampin, rifabutin may decrease average steady-state plasma atovaquone concentration). Products include:
- Mycobutin Capsules 2101

Rifampin (Co-administration with oral rifampin in HIV-infected individuals may result in a 52% +/- 13% decrease in the average steady-state plasma atovaquone concentration and a 37% 42% increase in the average steady-state plasma rifampin concentration). Products include:
- Rifadin 1276
- Rifamate Capsules 1278
- Rifater 1280
- Rimactane Capsules 865

Sulfamethoxazole (Co-administration with TMP-SMX may result in slight decrease in average steady-state concentrations of TMP-SMX; this effect is minor and would not expect to produce clinically significant events). Products include:
- Bactrim DS Tablets 2257
- Bactrim I.V. Infusion 2255
- Bactrim 2257
- Gantanol Tablets 2285
- Septra 1146

- Septra I.V. Infusion 1142
- Septra I.V. Infusion ADD-Vantage Vials 1144
- Septra 1146

Sulindac (Atovaquone is highly bound to plasma protein (greater than 99.9%); caution is advised when co-administered with other highly protein bound drugs with narrow therapeutic indices). Products include:
- Clinoril Tablets 1658

Temazepam (Atovaquone is highly bound to plasma protein (greater than 99.9%); caution is advised when co-administered with other highly protein bound drugs with narrow therapeutic indices). Products include:
- Restoril Capsules 2413

Tolbutamide (Atovaquone is highly bound to plasma protein (greater than 99.9%); caution is advised when co-administered with other highly protein bound drugs with narrow therapeutic indices).
- No products indexed under this heading.

Tolmetin Sodium (Atovaquone is highly bound to plasma protein (greater than 99.9%); caution is advised when co-administered with other highly protein bound drugs with narrow therapeutic indices). Products include:
- Tolectin (200, 400 and 600 mg) ... 1591

Trimethoprim (Co-administration with TMP-SMX may result in slight decrease in average steady-state concentrations of TMP-SMX; this effect is minor and would not expect to produce clinically significant events). Products include:
- Bactrim DS Tablets 2257
- Bactrim I.V. Infusion 2255
- Bactrim 2257
- Proloprim Tablets 1141
- Septra 1146
- Septra I.V. Infusion 1142
- Septra I.V. Infusion ADD-Vantage Vials 1144
- Septra 1146
- Trimpex Tablets 2323

Trimipramine Maleate (Atovaquone is highly bound to plasma protein (greater than 99.9%); caution is advised when co-administered with other highly protein bound drugs with narrow therapeutic indices). Products include:
- Surmontil Capsules 2917

Warfarin Sodium (Atovaquone is highly bound to plasma protein (greater than 99.9%); caution is advised when co-administered with other highly protein bound drugs with narrow therapeutic indices). Products include:
- Coumadin 941

Zidovudine (Atovaquone tablets have shown to decrease zidovudine apparent oral clearance leading to an increase in plasma zidovudine AUC; this effect is minor and would not expect to produce clinically significant events). Products include:
- Retrovir Capsules 1216
- Retrovir I.V. Infusion 1221
- Retrovir Syrup 1216

Food Interactions

Food, unspecified (Food enhances absorption by approximately two-fold).

MERREM I.V.
(Meropenem) 2952
May interact with:

Probenecid (Competes with meropenem for active tubular secretion and thus inhibits the renal excretion of meropenem; statistically significant increases in the elimination half-life and the extent of systemic exposure has been reported; co-administration is not recommended). Products include:
- Benemid Tablets 1651
- ColBENEMID Tablets 1662

MERUVAX II
(Rubella Virus Vaccine Live) 1740
May interact with immunosuppressive agents. Compounds in this category include:

Azathioprine (Concurrent administration is contraindicated). Products include:
- Azathioprine Tablets 2349
- Imuran 1103

Cyclosporine (Concurrent administration is contraindicated). Products include:
- Neoral 2405
- Sandimmune 2416

Immune Globulin (Human) (Concurrent administration is contraindicated).
- No products indexed under this heading.

Immune Globulin Intravenous (Human) (Concurrent administration is contraindicated).

Muromonab-CD3 (Concurrent administration is contraindicated). Products include:
- Orthoclone OKT3 Sterile Solution .. 1892

Mycophenolate Mofetil (Concurrent administration is contraindicated). Products include:
- CellCept Capsules 2265

Tacrolimus (Concurrent administration is contraindicated). Products include:
- Prograf 1028

MESANTOIN TABLETS
(Mephenytoin) 2400
May interact with central nervous system depressants and certain other agents. Compounds in these categories include:

Alfentanil Hydrochloride (Co-administration may result in possible additive effects). Products include:
- Alfenta Injection 1334

Alprazolam (Co-administration may result in possible additive effects). Products include:
- Xanax Tablets 2115

Aprobarbital (Co-administration may result in possible additive effects).
- No products indexed under this heading.

Buprenorphine (Co-administration may result in possible additive effects). Products include:
- Buprenex Injectable 2170

Buspirone Hydrochloride (Co-administration may result in possible additive effects). Products include:
- BuSpar Tablets 738

Butabarbital (Co-administration may result in possible additive effects).
- No products indexed under this heading.

(◨ Described in PDR For Nonprescription Drugs)   (◉ Described in PDR For Ophthalmology)

Butalbital (Co-administration may result in possible additive effects). Products include:
- Axocet Capsules ... 2469
- Esgic-plus Capsules ... 1012
- Esgic-plus Tablets ... 1012
- Fioricet Tablets ... 2386
- Fioricet with Codeine Capsules ... 2387
- Fiorinal Capsules ... 2388
- Fiorinal with Codeine Capsules ... 2390
- Fiorinal Tablets ... 2388
- Phrenilin ... 790
- Sedapap Tablets 50 mg/650 mg .. 1826

Chlordiazepoxide (Co-administration may result in possible additive effects). Products include:
- Limbitrol ... 2333

Chlordiazepoxide Hydrochloride (Co-administration may result in possible additive effects). Products include:
- Librax Capsules ... 2330
- Librium Capsules ... 2331
- Librium Injectable ... 2332

Chlorpromazine (Co-administration may result in possible additive effects). Products include:
- Thorazine Suppositories ... 2701

Chlorpromazine Hydrochloride (Co-administration may result in possible additive effects). Products include:
- Thorazine ... 2701

Chlorprothixene (Co-administration may result in possible additive effects).
- No products indexed under this heading.

Chlorprothixene Hydrochloride (Co-administration may result in possible additive effects).
- No products indexed under this heading.

Chlorprothixene Lactate (Co-administration may result in possible additive effects).
- No products indexed under this heading.

Clonazepam (Co-administration may result in possible additive effects). Products include:
- Klonopin Tablets ... 2294

Clorazepate Dipotassium (Co-administration may result in possible additive effects). Products include:
- Tranxene ... 459

Clozapine (Co-administration may result in possible additive effects). Products include:
- Clozaril Tablets ... 2377

Codeine Phosphate (Co-administration may result in possible additive effects). Products include:
- Brontex ... 2130
- Dimetane-DC Cough Syrup ... 2232
- Fioricet with Codeine Capsules ... 2387
- Fiorinal with Codeine Capsules ... 2390
- Nucofed ... 2225
- Phenergan with Codeine ... 2883
- Phenergan VC with Codeine ... 2888
- Robitussin A-C Syrup ... 2248
- Robitussin-DAC Syrup ... 2249
- Ryna ... 804
- Soma Compound w/Codeine Tablets ... 2784
- Tylenol with Codeine ... 1592

Desflurane (Co-administration may result in possible additive effects). Products include:
- Suprane (desflurane, USP) ... 1865

Dezocine (Co-administration may result in possible additive effects). Products include:
- Dalgan Injection ... 529

Diazepam (Co-administration may result in possible additive effects). Products include:
- Dizac (diazepam injectable emulsion) CIV ... 1862
- Valium Injectable ... 2336
- Valium Tablets ... 2335

Droperidol (Co-administration may result in possible additive effects). Products include:
- Inapsine Injection ... 462

Enflurane (Co-administration may result in possible additive effects).
- No products indexed under this heading.

Estazolam (Co-administration may result in possible additive effects). Products include:
- ProSom Tablets ... 457

Ethchlorvynol (Co-administration may result in possible additive effects). Products include:
- Placidyl Capsules ... 456

Ethinamate (Co-administration may result in possible additive effects).
- No products indexed under this heading.

Fentanyl (Co-administration may result in possible additive effects). Products include:
- Duragesic Transdermal System ... 1336

Fentanyl Citrate (Co-administration may result in possible additive effects). Products include:
- Sublimaze Injection ... 463

Fluphenazine Decanoate (Co-administration may result in possible additive effects). Products include:
- Prolixin Decanoate ... 510

Fluphenazine Enanthate (Co-administration may result in possible additive effects). Products include:
- Prolixin Enanthate ... 510

Fluphenazine Hydrochloride (Co-administration may result in possible additive effects). Products include:
- Prolixin ... 510

Flurazepam Hydrochloride (Co-administration may result in possible additive effects). Products include:
- Dalmane Capsules ... 2329

Glutethimide (Co-administration may result in possible additive effects).
- No products indexed under this heading.

Haloperidol (Co-administration may result in possible additive effects). Products include:
- Haldol Injection, Tablets and Concentrate ... 1585

Haloperidol Decanoate (Co-administration may result in possible additive effects). Products include:
- Haldol Decanoate ... 1587

Hydrocodone Bitartrate (Co-administration may result in possible additive effects). Products include:
- Codiclear DH Syrup ... 808
- Duratuss HD Elixir ... 2750
- Histussin D Liquid ... 670
- Hycodan Tablets and Syrup ... 946
- Hycomine Compound Tablets ... 948
- Hycomine ... 947
- Hycotuss Expectorant Syrup ... 950
- Hydrocet Capsules ... 787
- Lorcet 10/650 Tablets ... 1016
- Lortab ... 2751
- Tussend ... 1830
- Tussend Expectorant ... 1831
- Vicodin Tablets ... 1404
- Vicodin ES Tablets ... 1405
- Vicodin HP Tablets ... 1403
- Vicodin Tuss Expectorant ... 1406
- Zydone Capsules ... 967

Hydrocodone Polistirex (Co-administration may result in possible additive effects). Products include:
- Tussionex Pennkinetic Extended-Release Suspension ... 1624

Hydromorphone Hydrochloride (Co-administration may result in possible additive effects). Products include:
- Dilaudid Ampules ... 1382
- Dilaudid Cough Syrup ... 1383
- Dilaudid-HP Injection ... 1384
- Dilaudid-HP Lyophilized Powder 250 mg ... 1384
- Dilaudid ... 1382
- Dilaudid Oral Liquid ... 1386
- Dilaudid ... 1382
- Dilaudid Tablets - 8 mg ... 1386

Hydroxyzine Hydrochloride (Co-administration may result in possible additive effects). Products include:
- Atarax Tablets & Syrup ... 1992
- Marax Tablets & DF Syrup ... 2015
- Vistaril Intramuscular Solution ... 2042

Isoflurane (Co-administration may result in possible additive effects).
- No products indexed under this heading.

Ketamine Hydrochloride (Co-administration may result in possible additive effects).
- No products indexed under this heading.

Levomethadyl Acetate Hydrochloride (Co-administration may result in possible additive effects). Products include:
- Orlaam Oral Solution ... 2361

Levorphanol Tartrate (Co-administration may result in possible additive effects). Products include:
- Levo-Dromoran ... 2297

Lorazepam (Co-administration may result in possible additive effects). Products include:
- Ativan Injection ... 2805
- Ativan Tablets ... 2807

Loxapine Hydrochloride (Co-administration may result in possible additive effects). Products include:
- Loxitane ... 1426

Loxapine Succinate (Co-administration may result in possible additive effects). Products include:
- Loxitane Capsules ... 1426

Meperidine Hydrochloride (Co-administration may result in possible additive effects). Products include:
- Demerol ... 2438
- Mepergan Injection ... 2859

Mephobarbital (Co-administration may result in possible additive effects). Products include:
- Mebaral Tablets ... 2452

Meprobamate (Co-administration may result in possible additive effects). Products include:
- Miltown Tablets ... 2780
- PMB 200 and PMB 400 ... 2890

Mesoridazine Besylate (Co-administration may result in possible additive effects). Products include:
- Serentil ... 689

Methadone Hydrochloride (Co-administration may result in possible additive effects). Products include:
- Methadone Hydrochloride Oral Concentrate ... 2356
- Methadone Hydrochloride Oral Solution & Tablets ... 2357

Methohexital Sodium (Co-administration may result in possible additive effects).
- No products indexed under this heading.

Methotrimeprazine (Co-administration may result in possible additive effects). Products include:
- Levoprome ... 1321

Methoxyflurane (Co-administration may result in possible additive effects).
- No products indexed under this heading.

Midazolam Hydrochloride (Co-administration may result in possible additive effects). Products include:
- Versed Injection ... 2324

Molindone Hydrochloride (Co-administration may result in possible additive effects). Products include:
- Moban Tablets and Concentrate ... 1036

Morphine Sulfate (Co-administration may result in possible additive effects). Products include:
- Astramorph/PF Injection, USP (Preservative-Free) ... 526
- Duramorph Injection ... 983
- Infumorph 200 and Infumorph 500 Sterile Solutions ... 985
- Kadian Capsules ... 2948
- MS Contin Tablets ... 2149
- MSIR ... 2152
- Oramorph SR (Morphine Sulfate Sustained Release Tablets) ... 2359
- RMS Suppositories CII ... 2766
- Roxanol ... 2365

Opium Alkaloids (Co-administration may result in possible additive effects).
- No products indexed under this heading.

Oxazepam (Co-administration may result in possible additive effects). Products include:
- Serax Capsules ... 2916
- Serax Tablets ... 2916

Oxycodone Hydrochloride (Co-administration may result in possible additive effects). Products include:
- OxyContin Tablets ... 2163
- OxyIR Capsules ... 2167
- Percocet Tablets ... 955
- Percodan Tablets ... 955
- Percodan-Demi Tablets ... 956
- Roxicodone Tablets, Oral Solution & Intensol (Oxycodone) ... 2366
- Tylox Capsules ... 1593

Pentobarbital Sodium (Co-administration may result in possible additive effects). Products include:
- Nembutal Sodium Capsules ... 440
- Nembutal Sodium Solution ... 442
- Nembutal Sodium Suppositories ... 444

Perphenazine (Co-administration may result in possible additive effects). Products include:
- Etrafon ... 2495
- Triavil Tablets ... 1800
- Trilafon ... 2532

Phenobarbital (Co-administration may result in possible additive effects). Products include:
- Arco-Lase Plus Tablets ... 513
- Bellergal-S Tablets ... 2375
- Donnatal ... 2234
- Donnatal Extentabs ... 2234
- Donnatal Tablets ... 2234
- Phenobarbital Elixir and Tablets ... 1523
- Quadrinal Tablets ... 1398

Prazepam (Co-administration may result in possible additive effects).
- No products indexed under this heading.

Prochlorperazine (Co-administration may result in possible additive effects). Products include:
- Compazine ... 2644

Promethazine Hydrochloride (Co-administration may result in possible additive effects). Products include:
- Mepergan Injection ... 2859
- Phenergan with Codeine ... 2883
- Phenergan with Dextromethorphan ... 2885
- Phenergan Injection ... 2880
- Phenergan Suppositories ... 2882
- Phenergan Syrup ... 2881
- Phenergan Tablets ... 2882
- Phenergan VC ... 2886
- Phenergan VC with Codeine ... 2888

IMPORTANT NOTE: Always consult each drug listing in the patient's regimen for possible interactions.

Mesantoin — Interactions Index

Propofol (Co-administration may result in possible additive effects). Products include:
- Diprivan Injectable Emulsion 2939

Propoxyphene Hydrochloride (Co-administration may result in possible additive effects). Products include:
- Darvon 1475
- Wygesic Tablets 2930

Propoxyphene Napsylate (Co-administration may result in possible additive effects). Products include:
- Darvon-N/Darvocet-N 1473

Quazepam (Co-administration may result in possible additive effects). Products include:
- Doral Tablets 2773

Risperidone (Co-administration may result in possible additive effects). Products include:
- Risperdal Tablets 1348

Secobarbital Sodium (Co-administration may result in possible additive effects). Products include:
- Seconal Sodium Pulvules 1529

Sevoflurane (Co-administration may result in possible additive effects).
- No products indexed under this heading.

Sufentanil Citrate (Co-administration may result in possible additive effects). Products include:
- Sufenta Injection 1355

Temazepam (Co-administration may result in possible additive effects). Products include:
- Restoril Capsules 2413

Thiamylal Sodium (Co-administration may result in possible additive effects).
- No products indexed under this heading.

Thioridazine Hydrochloride (Co-administration may result in possible additive effects). Products include:
- Mellaril 2398

Thiothixene (Co-administration may result in possible additive effects). Products include:
- Navane Capsules and Concentrate 2018
- Navane Intramuscular 2019

Triazolam (Co-administration may result in possible additive effects). Products include:
- Halcion Tablets 2093

Trifluoperazine Hydrochloride (Co-administration may result in possible additive effects). Products include:
- Stelazine 2692

Zolpidem Tartrate (Co-administration may result in possible additive effects). Products include:
- Ambien Tablets 2559

Food Interactions

Alcohol (Co-administration may result in possible additive effects; acute alcohol intoxication may increase the anticonvulsant effect; chronic alcohol abuse may decrease anticonvulsant effect).

MESNEX INJECTION
(Mesna). 711
None cited in PDR database.

MESTINON INJECTABLE
(Pyridostigmine Bromide) 1300
None cited in PDR database.

MESTINON SYRUP
(Pyridostigmine Bromide) 1300
None cited in PDR database.

MESTINON TABLETS
(Pyridostigmine Bromide) 1300
None cited in PDR database.

MESTINON TIMESPAN TABLETS
(Pyridostigmine Bromide) 1300
None cited in PDR database.

METAMUCIL POWDER, ORANGE FLAVOR
(Psyllium Preparations) 2125
None cited in PDR database.

METAMUCIL ORIGINAL TEXTURE POWDER, REGULAR FLAVOR
(Psyllium Preparations) 2125
None cited in PDR database.

METAMUCIL SMOOTH TEXTURE POWDER, ORANGE FLAVOR
(Psyllium Preparations) 2125
None cited in PDR database.

METAMUCIL SMOOTH TEXTURE POWDER, SUGAR-FREE, ORANGE FLAVOR
(Psyllium Preparations) 2125
None cited in PDR database.

METAMUCIL SMOOTH TEXTURE, SUGAR-FREE, REGULAR FLAVOR
(Psyllium Preparations) 2125
None cited in PDR database.

METAMUCIL WAFERS, APPLE CRISP AND CINNAMON SPICE FLAVORS
(Psyllium Preparations) 2125
None cited in PDR database.

METAPROTERENOL SULFATE INHALATION SOLUTION, USP, ARM-A-MED
(Metaproterenol Sulfate) 547
May interact with sympathomimetics. Compounds in this category include:

Albuterol (Effect not specified). Products include:
- Proventil Inhalation Aerosol 2524
- Ventolin Inhalation Aerosol and Refill 1170

Albuterol Sulfate (Effect not specified). Products include:
- Airet Albuterol Sulfate Inhalation Solution 1602
- Albuterol Sulfate, USP Solution for Inhalation, Arm-a-Med 522
- Proventil Inhalation Solution 0.083% 2527
- Proventil Repetabs Tablets 2529
- Proventil Solution for Inhalation 0.5% 2525
- Proventil Syrup 2528
- Proventil Tablets 2529
- Ventolin Inhalation Solution 1171
- Ventolin Nebules Inhalation Solution 1172
- Ventolin Rotacaps for Inhalation 1173
- Ventolin Syrup 1175
- Ventolin Tablets 1176
- Volmax Extended-Release Tablets 1835

Dobutamine Hydrochloride (Effect not specified). Products include:
- Dobutrex Solution Vials 1480

Dopamine Hydrochloride (Effect not specified).
- No products indexed under this heading.

Ephedrine Hydrochloride (Effect not specified). Products include:
- Primatene Tablets 844
- Quadrinal Tablets 1398

Ephedrine Sulfate (Effect not specified). Products include:
- Marax Tablets & DF Syrup 2015

Ephedrine Tannate (Effect not specified). Products include:
- Rynatuss 2782

Epinephrine (Effect not specified). Products include:
- EPIFRIN 237
- EpiPen 808
- Marcaine with Epinephrine 2446
- Primatene Mist 843
- Sensorcaine with Epinephrine Injection 554
- Sus-Phrine Injection 1017
- Xylocaine with Epinephrine Injections 562

Epinephrine Bitartrate (Effect not specified). Products include:
- Sensorcaine-MPF with Epinephrine Injection 554

Epinephrine Hydrochloride (Effect not specified). Products include:
- Ana-Kit Anaphylaxis Emergency Treatment Kit 611

Isoproterenol Hydrochloride (Effect not specified). Products include:
- Isuprel Hydrochloride Solution 2443
- Isuprel Injection 2441
- Isuprel Mistometer 2442

Isoproterenol Sulfate (Effect not specified). Products include:
- Norisodrine with Calcium Iodide Syrup 446

Metaraminol Bitartrate (Effect not specified). Products include:
- Aramine Injection 1649

Methoxamine Hydrochloride (Effect not specified). Products include:
- Vasoxyl Injection 1169

Norepinephrine Bitartrate (Effect not specified). Products include:
- Levophed Bitartrate Injection 2445

Phenylephrine Bitartrate (Effect not specified).
- No products indexed under this heading.

Phenylephrine Hydrochloride (Effect not specified). Products include:
- Atrohist Plus Tablets 1605
- Cerose DM 853
- D.A. II Tablets 972
- D.A. Chewable Tablets 970
- Dura-Vent/DA Tablets 972
- Extendryl 1003
- 4-Way Fast Acting Nasal Spray (regular & mentholated) 644
- Hemorid 797
- Hycomine Compound Tablets 948
- Neo-Synephrine Hydrochloride 1% Carpuject 2455
- Neo-Synephrine Hydrochloride 1% Injection 2455
- Neo-Synephrine Hydrochloride (Ophthalmic) 2456
- Neo-Synephrine Elixir 624
- Novahistine Elixir 782
- Phenergan VC 2886
- Phenergan VC with Codeine 2888
- Preparation H 842
- Tympagesic Ear Drops 2476
- Vicks Sinex Nasal Spray and Ultra Fine Mist 738

Phenylephrine Tannate (Effect not specified). Products include:
- Atrohist Pediatric Suspension 1604
- Atrohist Pediatric Suspension Dye-Free 1604
- Rynatan 2781
- Rynatuss 2782

Phenylpropanolamine Hydrochloride (Effect not specified). Products include:
- Acutrim 648
- Atrohist Plus Tablets 1605
- BC Cold Powder Multi-Symptom Formula (Cold-Sinus-Allergy) 631
- BC Cold Powder Non-Drowsy Formula (Cold-Sinus) 631
- Cheracol Plus Head Cold/Cough Formula 741
- Comtrex Multi-Symptom Cold Reliever Liqui-Gels 638
- Comtrex Multi-Symptom Non-Drowsy Liqui-gels 640
- Contac Continuous Action Nasal Decongestant/Antihistamine 12 Hour Capsules 773
- Contac Maximum Strength Continuous Action Decongestant/Antihistamine 12 Hour Caplets 772
- Contac Severe Cold and Flu Formula Caplets 773
- Coricidin 'D' Decongestant Tablets 760
- Dexatrim 795
- Dexatrim Plus Vitamins Caplets 796
- Dimetane-DC Cough Syrup 2232
- Dimetapp Allergy Sinus Caplets 838
- Dimetapp Cold & Allergy Chewable Tablets 838
- Dimetapp Cold & Cough Liqui-Gels 839
- Dimetapp DM Elixir 840
- Dimetapp Elixir 840
- Dimetapp Extentabs 841
- Dimetapp Tablets/Liqui-Gels 841
- Dura-Vent Tablets 971
- Entex LA Tablets 972
- Exgest LA Tablets 787
- Hycomine 947
- Nolamine Timed-Release Tablets 790
- Ornade Spansule Capsules 2678
- Propagest Tablets 791
- Pyrroxate Caplets 742
- Robitussin-CF 846
- Sinulin Tablets 792
- Tavist-D 12 Hour Relief Tablets 750
- Teldrin 12 Hour Antihistamine/Nasal Decongestant Allergy Relief Capsules 786
- Triaminic Expectorant 753
- Triaminic Syrup 755
- Triaminic Triaminicol Cold & Cough 756
- Triaminic DM Syrup 756
- Triaminicin Tablets 756
- Vicks DayQuil Allergy Relief 12-Hour Extended Release Tablets 733
- Vicks DayQuil Allergy Relief 4-Hour Tablets 733
- Vicks DayQuil SINUS Pressure & CONGESTION Relief 734

Pirbuterol Acetate (Effect not specified). Products include:
- Maxair Autohaler 1550
- Maxair Inhaler 1552

Pseudoephedrine Hydrochloride (Effect not specified). Products include:
- Actifed Allergy Daytime/Nighttime Caplets 808
- Actifed Cold & Allergy Tablets 807
- Actifed Cold & Sinus Caplets and Tablets 808
- Actifed Sinus Daytime/Nighttime Tablets and Caplets 809
- Advil Cold and Sinus Caplets and Tablets 837
- Alka-Seltzer Plus Liqui-Gels 612
- Alka-Seltzer Plus Flu & Body Aches Liqui-Gels Non-Drowsy Formula 613
- Alka-Seltzer Plus Night-Time Cold Medicine Liqui-Gels 612
- Allerest Maximum Strength 649
- Allerest No Drowsiness 649
- Allerest Sinus Pain Formula 649
- Atrohist Pediatric Capsules 1603
- Benadryl Allergy/Cold Tablets 811
- Benadryl Allergy Decongestant Liquid Medication 812
- Benadryl Allergy Decongestant Tablets 812
- Benadryl Allergy Sinus Headache Caplets 813
- Benylin Multisymptom 816
- Bromfed Capsules (Extended-Release) 1832
- Bromfed Syrup 712
- Bromfed Tablets 1832
- Bromfed-DM Cough Syrup 1832
- Bromfed-PD Capsules (Extended-Release) 1832

(■ Described in PDR For Nonprescription Drugs)   (● Described in PDR For Ophthalmology)

Children's TYLENOL Cold Multi-Symptom Chewable Tablets and Liquid ... 1559
Children's TYLENOL Cold Plus Cough Multi Symptom Chewable Tablets and Liquid ... 1560
Children's TYLENOL Flu Suspension Liquid ... 1560
Children's Vicks DayQuil Allergy Relief ... 730
Children's Vicks NyQuil Cold/Cough Relief ... 731
Allergy-Sinus Comtrex Multi-Symptom Allergy-Sinus Formula Tablets and Caplets ... 639
Comtrex Multi-Symptom ... 638
Comtrex Multi-Symptom Non-Drowsy Caplets ... 640
Congess ... 1003
Contac Day Allergy/Sinus Caplets ... 771
Contac Day & Night ... 772
Contac Night Allergy/Sinus Caplets ... 771
Contac Severe Cold & Flu Non-Drowsy ... 774
Deconsal II Tablets ... 1605
Dimetane-DX Cough Syrup ... 2233
Dimetapp Cold & Fever Suspension ... 839
Dimetapp Decongestant Pediatric Drops ... 840
Dorcol Children's Cough Syrup ... 748
Drixoral Cough + Congestion Liquid Caps ... 763
Dura-Tap/PD Capsules ... 970
Duratuss Tablets ... 2750
Duratuss HD Elixir ... 2750
Efidac/24 ... 655
Entex PSE Tablets ... 973
Fedahist Gyrocaps ... 2545
Guaifed ... 1833
Guaifed Syrup ... 712
Guaimax-D Tablets ... 809
Histussin D Liquid ... 670
Infants' TYLENOL Cold Decongestant & Fever-Reducer Drops ... 1561
Kronofed-A ... 994
Novahistine DMX ... 782
Nucofed ... 2225
PediaCare Cough-Cold Chewable Tablets and Liquid ... 1569
PediaCare Infants' Decongestant Drops ... 1569
PediaCare Infants' Drops Decongestant Plus Cough ... 1569
PediaCare NightRest Cough-Cold Liquid ... 1569
Pediatric Vicks 44d Cough & Head Congestion Relief ... 736
Pediatric Vicks 44m Cough & Cold Relief ... 737
Robitussin Cold & Cough Liqui-Gels ... 844
Robitussin Cold, Cough & Flu Liqui-Gels ... 844
Robitussin Maximum Strength Cough & Cold ... 847
Robitussin Night-Time Cold Formula ... 847
Robitussin Pediatric Cough & Cold Formula ... 848
Robitussin Pediatric Drops ... 849
Robitussin Severe Congestion Liqui-Gels ... 845
Robitussin-DAC Syrup ... 2249
Robitussin-PE ... 846
Rondec Oral Drops ... 974
Rondec Syrup ... 974
Rondec Tablet ... 974
Rondec Chewable Tablets ... 974
Rondec-TR Tablet ... 974
Ryna ... 804
Seldane-D Extended-Release Tablets ... 1286
Semprex-D Capsules ... 1620
Sinarest ... 663
Sine-Aid Maximum Strength Sinus Headache Gelcaps, Caplets and Tablets ... 1570
Sine-Off No Drowsiness Formula Caplets ... 784
Sine-Off Sinus Medicine ... 784
Singlet Tablets ... 785
Sinutab Non-Drying Liquid Caps ... 823
Sinutab Sinus Allergy Medication, Maximum Strength Tablets and Caplets ...
Sinutab Sinus Medication, Maximum Strength Without Drowsiness Formula, Tablets & Caplets ... 824
Sudafed Children's Cold & Cough Liquid Medication ... 825
Sudafed Children's Nasal Decongestant Liquid Medication ... 826
Sudafed Cold & Allergy Tablets ... 826
Sudafed Cold and Cough Liquid Caps ... 826
Sudafed Nasal Decongestant Tablets, 30 mg ... 825
Sudafed Nasal Decongestant Tablets, 60 mg ... 825
Sudafed Non-Drying Sinus Liquid Caps ... 827
Sudafed Pediatric Nasal Decongestant Liquid Oral Drops ... 827
Sudafed Severe Cold Formula Caplets ... 828
Sudafed Severe Cold Formula Tablets ... 828
Sudafed Sinus Caplets ... 829
Sudafed Sinus Tablets ... 829
Sudafed 12 Hour Caplets ... 824
Syn-Rx Tablets ... 1622
Syn-Rx DM Tablets ... 1623
TheraFlu Flu and Cold Medicine ... 750
TheraFlu Maximum Strength Flu and Cold Medicine For Sore Throat ... 751
TheraFlu Flu, Cold and Cough Medicine ... 750
TheraFlu Maximum Strength Nighttime Flu, Cold & Cough Medicine ... 751
TheraFlu Maximum Strength Non-Drowsy Formula Flu, Cold & Cough Medicine ... 751
TheraFlu Maximum Strength, Non-Drowsy Formula Flu, Cold and Cough Caplets ... 752
Theraflu Maximum Strength Sinus Non-Drowsy Formula Caplets ... 752
Triaminic AM Cough and Decongestant Formula ... 753
Triaminic AM Decongestant Formula ... 753
Triaminic Infant Oral Decongestant Drops ... 754
Triaminic Night Time ... 754
Triaminic Sore Throat Formula ... 755
Tussend ... 1830
Tussend Expectorant ... 1831
TYLENOL Allergy Sinus, Maximum Strength Caplets and Gelcaps ... 1571
TYLENOL Allergy Sinus NightTime, Maximum Strength Caplets ... 1571
TYLENOL Cold Medication, Multi-Symptom Formula Tablets and Caplets ... 1572
TYLENOL Cold Medication, Multi-Symptom Hot Liquid Packets ... 1572
TYLENOL Cold Medication, No Drowsiness Formula Caplets and Gelcaps ... 1572
TYLENOL Cold Severe Congestion Caplets ... 1573
TYLENOL Cough Medication with Decongestant, Multi Symptom ... 1574
TYLENOL Flu No Drowsiness Formula, Maximum Strength Gelcaps ... 1575
TYLENOL Flu NightTime, Maximum Strength Gelcaps ... 1575
TYLENOL Flu NightTime, Maximum Strength Hot Medication Packets ... 1575
TYLENOL Sinus, Maximum Strength Geltabs, Gelcaps, Caplets and Tablets ... 1576
Vicks 44 LiquiCaps Cough, Cold & Flu Relief ... 728
Vicks 44 LiquiCaps Non-Drowsy Cough & Cold Relief ... 729
Vicks 44D Cough & Head Congestion Relief ... 728
Vicks 44M Cough, Cold & Flu Relief ... 729
Vicks DayQuil LiquiCaps/Liquid Multi-Symptom Cold/Flu Relief ... 734
Vicks DayQuil SINUS Pressure & PAIN Relief with IBUPROFEN ... 735
Vicks Nyquil Hot Therapy ... 735
Vicks NyQuil LiquiCaps/Liquid Multi-Symptom Cold/Flu Relief, Original and Cherry Flavors ... 736

Pseudoephedrine Sulfate (Effect not specified). Products include:
Chlor-Trimeton Allergy Decongestant Tablets ... 759
Claritin-D Tablets ... 2487
Drixoral Cold and Allergy Sustained-Action Tablets ... 763
Drixoral Cold and Flu Extended-Release Tablets ... 764
Drixoral Non-Drowsy Formula Extended-Release Tablets ... 764
Drixoral Allergy/Sinus Extended Release Tablets ... 765
Trinalin Repetabs Tablets ... 1373

Salmeterol Xinafoate (Effect not specified). Products include:
Serevent Inhalation Aerosol ... 1149

Terbutaline Sulfate (Effect not specified). Products include:
Brethaire Inhaler ... 830
Brethine Ampuls ... 832
Brethine Tablets ... 831
Bricanyl Subcutaneous Injection ... 1247
Bricanyl Tablets ... 1248

METHADONE HYDROCHLORIDE ORAL CONCENTRATE

(Methadone Hydrochloride) ... 2356
May interact with central nervous system depressants, narcotic analgesics, general anesthetics, phenothiazines, tranquilizers, hypnotics and sedatives, tricyclic antidepressants, monoamine oxidase inhibitors, and certain other agents. Compounds in these categories include:

Alfentanil Hydrochloride (Potential for respiratory depression, hypotension, and profound sedation or coma; use caution and reduced dosage in patients who are concurrently receiving these drugs). Products include:
Alfenta Injection ... 1334

Alprazolam (Potential for respiratory depression, hypotension, and profound sedation or coma; use caution and reduced dosage in patients who are concurrently receiving these drugs). Products include:
Xanax Tablets ... 2115

Amitriptyline Hydrochloride (Potential for respiratory depression, hypotension, and profound sedation or coma; use caution and reduced dosage in patients who are concurrently receiving these drugs). Products include:
Elavil ... 2945
Etrafon ... 2495
Limbitrol ... 2333
Triavil Tablets ... 1800

Amoxapine (Potential for respiratory depression, hypotension, and profound sedation or coma; use caution and reduced dosage in patients who are concurrently receiving these drugs). Products include:
Asendin Tablets ... 1419

Aprobarbital (Potential for respiratory depression, hypotension, and profound sedation or coma; use caution and reduced dosage in patients who are concurrently receiving these drugs).
No products indexed under this heading.

Buprenorphine (Potential for respiratory depression, hypotension, and profound sedation or coma; use caution and reduced dosage in patients who are concurrently receiving these drugs). Products include:
Buprenex Injectable ... 2170

Buspirone Hydrochloride (Potential for respiratory depression, hypotension, and profound sedation or coma; use caution and reduced dosage in patients who are concurrently receiving these drugs). Products include:
BuSpar Tablets ... 738

Butabarbital (Potential for respiratory depression, hypotension, and profound sedation or coma; use caution and reduced dosage in patients who are concurrently receiving these drugs).
No products indexed under this heading.

Butalbital (Potential for respiratory depression, hypotension, and profound sedation or coma; use caution and reduced dosage in patients who are concurrently receiving these drugs). Products include:
Axocet Capsules ... 2469
Esgic-plus Capsules ... 1012
Esgic-plus Tablets ... 1012
Fioricet Tablets ... 2386
Fioricet with Codeine Capsules ... 2387
Fiorinal Capsules ... 2388
Fiorinal with Codeine Capsules ... 2390
Fiorinal Tablets ... 2388
Phrenilin ... 790
Sedapap Tablets 50 mg/650 mg ... 1826

Chlordiazepoxide (Potential for respiratory depression, hypotension, and profound sedation or coma; use caution and reduced dosage in patients who are concurrently receiving these drugs). Products include:
Limbitrol ... 2333

Chlordiazepoxide Hydrochloride (Potential for respiratory depression, hypotension, and profound sedation or coma; use caution and reduced dosage in patients who are concurrently receiving these drugs). Products include:
Librax Capsules ... 2330
Librium Capsules ... 2331
Librium Injectable ... 2332

Chlorpromazine (Potential for respiratory depression, hypotension, and profound sedation or coma; use caution and reduced dosage in patients who are concurrently receiving these drugs). Products include:
Thorazine Suppositories ... 2701

Chlorpromazine Hydrochloride (Potential for respiratory depression, hypotension, and profound sedation or coma; use caution and reduced dosage in patients who are concurrently receiving these drugs). Products include:
Thorazine ... 2701

Chlorprothixene (Potential for respiratory depression, hypotension, and profound sedation or coma; use caution and reduced dosage in patients who are concurrently receiving these drugs).
No products indexed under this heading.

Chlorprothixene Hydrochloride (Potential for respiratory depression, hypotension, and profound sedation or coma; use caution and reduced dosage in patients who are concurrently receiving these drugs).
No products indexed under this heading.

Chlorprothixene Lactate (Potential for respiratory depression, hypotension, and profound sedation or coma; use caution and reduced dosage in patients who are concurrently receiving these drugs).
No products indexed under this heading.

Clomipramine Hydrochloride (Potential for respiratory depression, hypotension, and profound sedation or coma; use caution and reduced dosage in patients who are concurrently receiving these drugs). Products include:
Anafranil Capsules ... 819

IMPORTANT NOTE: Always consult each drug listing in the patient's regimen for possible interactions.

Methadone Concentrate — Interactions Index — 664

Clorazepate Dipotassium (Potential for respiratory depression, hypotension, and profound sedation or coma; use caution and reduced dosage in patients who are concurrently receiving these drugs). Products include:
- Tranxene 459

Clozapine (Potential for respiratory depression, hypotension, and profound sedation or coma; use caution and reduced dosage in patients who are concurrently receiving these drugs). Products include:
- Clozaril Tablets 2377

Codeine Phosphate (Potential for respiratory depression, hypotension, and profound sedation or coma; use caution and reduced dosage in patients who are concurrently receiving these drugs). Products include:
- Brontex 2130
- Dimetane-DC Cough Syrup 2232
- Fioricet with Codeine Capsules ... 2387
- Fiorinal with Codeine Capsules ... 2390
- Nucofed 2225
- Phenergan with Codeine 2883
- Phenergan VC with Codeine 2888
- Robitussin A-C Syrup 2248
- Robitussin-DAC Syrup 2249
- Ryna ⊞ 804
- Soma Compound w/Codeine Tablets 2784
- Tylenol with Codeine 1592

Desflurane (Potential for respiratory depression, hypotension, and profound sedation or coma; use caution and reduced dosage in patients who are concurrently receiving these drugs). Products include:
- Suprane (desflurane, USP) 1865

Desipramine Hydrochloride (Potential for respiratory depression, hypotension, and profound sedation or coma; use caution and reduced dosage in patients who are concurrently receiving these drugs). Products include:
- Norpramin Tablets 1273

Dezocine (Potential for respiratory depression, hypotension, and profound sedation or coma; use caution and reduced dosage in patients who are concurrently receiving these drugs). Products include:
- Dalgan Injection 529

Diazepam (Potential for respiratory depression, hypotension, and profound sedation or coma; use caution and reduced dosage in patients who are concurrently receiving these drugs). Products include:
- Dizac (diazepam injectable emulsion) CIV 1862
- Valium Injectable 2336
- Valium Tablets 2335

Doxepin Hydrochloride (Potential for respiratory depression, hypotension, and profound sedation or coma; use caution and reduced dosage in patients who are concurrently receiving these drugs). Products include:
- Adapin Capsules 1542
- Sinequan 2028
- Zonalon Cream 1042

Droperidol (Potential for respiratory depression, hypotension, and profound sedation or coma; use caution and reduced dosage in patients who are concurrently receiving these drugs). Products include:
- Inapsine Injection 462

Enflurane (Potential for respiratory depression, hypotension, and profound sedation or coma; use caution and reduced dosage in patients who are concurrently receiving these drugs).
- No products indexed under this heading.

Estazolam (Potential for respiratory depression, hypotension, and profound sedation or coma; use caution and reduced dosage in patients who are concurrently receiving these drugs). Products include:
- ProSom Tablets 457

Ethchlorvynol (Potential for respiratory depression, hypotension, and profound sedation or coma; use caution and reduced dosage in patients who are concurrently receiving these drugs). Products include:
- Placidyl Capsules 456

Ethinamate (Potential for respiratory depression, hypotension, and profound sedation or coma; use caution and reduced dosage in patients who are concurrently receiving these drugs).
- No products indexed under this heading.

Fentanyl (Potential for respiratory depression, hypotension, and profound sedation or coma; use caution and reduced dosage in patients who are concurrently receiving these drugs). Products include:
- Duragesic Transdermal System ... 1336

Fentanyl Citrate (Potential for respiratory depression, hypotension, and profound sedation or coma; use caution and reduced dosage in patients who are concurrently receiving these drugs). Products include:
- Sublimaze Injection 463

Fluphenazine Decanoate (Potential for respiratory depression, hypotension, and profound sedation or coma; use caution and reduced dosage in patients who are concurrently receiving these drugs). Products include:
- Prolixin Decanoate 510

Fluphenazine Enanthate (Potential for respiratory depression, hypotension, and profound sedation or coma; use caution and reduced dosage in patients who are concurrently receiving these drugs). Products include:
- Prolixin Enanthate 510

Fluphenazine Hydrochloride (Potential for respiratory depression, hypotension, and profound sedation or coma; use caution and reduced dosage in patients who are concurrently receiving these drugs). Products include:
- Prolixin 510

Flurazepam Hydrochloride (Potential for respiratory depression, hypotension, and profound sedation or coma; use caution and reduced dosage in patients who are concurrently receiving these drugs). Products include:
- Dalmane Capsules 2329

Furazolidone (Potential for meperidine/MAOI-type reaction; sensitivity test should be performed). Products include:
- Furoxone 2221

Glutethimide (Potential for respiratory depression, hypotension, and profound sedation or coma; use caution and reduced dosage in patients who are concurrently receiving these drugs).
- No products indexed under this heading.

Haloperidol (Potential for respiratory depression, hypotension, and profound sedation or coma; use caution and reduced dosage in patients who are concurrently receiving these drugs). Products include:
- Haldol Injection, Tablets and Concentrate 1585

Haloperidol Decanoate (Potential for respiratory depression, hypotension, and profound sedation or coma; use caution and reduced dosage in patients who are concurrently receiving these drugs). Products include:
- Haldol Decanoate 1587

Hydrocodone Bitartrate (Potential for respiratory depression, hypotension, and profound sedation or coma; use caution and reduced dosage in patients who are concurrently receiving these drugs). Products include:
- Codiclear DH Syrup 808
- Duratuss HD Elixir 2750
- Histussin D Liquid 670
- Hycodan Tablets and Syrup 946
- Hycomine Compound Tablets ... 948
- Hycomine 947
- Hycotuss Expectorant Syrup 950
- Hydrocet Capsules 787
- Lorcet 10/650 Tablets 1016
- Lortab 2751
- Tussend 1830
- Tussend Expectorant 1831
- Vicodin Tablets 1404
- Vicodin ES Tablets 1405
- Vicodin HP Tablets 1403
- Vicodin Tuss Expectorant 1406
- Zydone Capsules 967

Hydrocodone Polistirex (Potential for respiratory depression, hypotension, and profound sedation or coma; use caution and reduced dosage in patients who are concurrently receiving these drugs). Products include:
- Tussionex Pennkinetic Extended-Release Suspension 1624

Hydromorphone Hydrochloride (Potential for respiratory depression, hypotension, and profound sedation or coma; use caution and reduced dosage in patients who are concurrently receiving these drugs). Products include:
- Dilaudid Ampules 1382
- Dilaudid Cough Syrup 1383
- Dilaudid-HP Injection 1384
- Dilaudid-HP Lyophilized Powder 250 mg 1384
- Dilaudid 1382
- Dilaudid Oral Liquid 1386
- Dilaudid 1382
- Dilaudid Tablets - 8 mg. 1386

Hydroxyzine Hydrochloride (Potential for respiratory depression, hypotension, and profound sedation or coma; use caution and reduced dosage in patients who are concurrently receiving these drugs). Products include:
- Atarax Tablets & Syrup 1992
- Marax Tablets & DF Syrup 2015
- Vistaril Intramuscular Solution ... 2042

Imipramine Hydrochloride (Potential for respiratory depression, hypotension, and profound sedation or coma; use caution and reduced dosage in patients who are concurrently receiving these drugs). Products include:
- Tofranil Ampuls 873

- Tofranil Tablets 875

Imipramine Pamoate (Potential for respiratory depression, hypotension, and profound sedation or coma; use caution and reduced dosage in patients who are concurrently receiving these drugs). Products include:
- Tofranil-PM Capsules 876

Isocarboxazid (Potential for meperidine/MAOI-type reaction; sensitivity test should be performed).
- No products indexed under this heading.

Isoflurane (Potential for respiratory depression, hypotension, and profound sedation or coma; use caution and reduced dosage in patients who are concurrently receiving these drugs).
- No products indexed under this heading.

Ketamine Hydrochloride (Potential for respiratory depression, hypotension, and profound sedation or coma; use caution and reduced dosage in patients who are concurrently receiving these drugs).
- No products indexed under this heading.

Levomethadyl Acetate Hydrochloride (Potential for respiratory depression, hypotension, and profound sedation or coma; use caution and reduced dosage in patients who are concurrently receiving these drugs). Products include:
- Orlaam Oral Solution 2361

Levorphanol Tartrate (Potential for respiratory depression, hypotension, and profound sedation or coma; use caution and reduced dosage in patients who are concurrently receiving these drugs). Products include:
- Levo-Dromoran 2297

Lorazepam (Potential for respiratory depression, hypotension, and profound sedation or coma; use caution and reduced dosage in patients who are concurrently receiving these drugs). Products include:
- Ativan Injection 2805
- Ativan Tablets 2807

Loxapine Hydrochloride (Potential for respiratory depression, hypotension, and profound sedation or coma; use caution and reduced dosage in patients who are concurrently receiving these drugs). Products include:
- Loxitane 1426

Loxapine Succinate (Potential for respiratory depression, hypotension, and profound sedation or coma; use caution and reduced dosage in patients who are concurrently receiving these drugs). Products include:
- Loxitane Capsules 1426

Maprotiline Hydrochloride (Potential for respiratory depression, hypotension, and profound sedation or coma; use caution and reduced dosage in patients who are concurrently receiving these drugs). Products include:
- Ludiomil Tablets 861

Meperidine Hydrochloride (Potential for respiratory depression, hypotension, and profound sedation or coma; use caution and reduced dosage in patients who are concurrently receiving these drugs). Products include:
- Demerol 2438
- Mepergan Injection 2859

(⊞ Described in PDR For Nonprescription Drugs) (⊚ Described in PDR For Ophthalmology)

665 Interactions Index Methadone Concentrate

Mephobarbital (Potential for respiratory depression, hypotension, and profound sedation or coma; use caution and reduced dosage in patients who are concurrently receiving these drugs). Products include:
Mebaral Tablets 2452
Meprobamate (Potential for respiratory depression, hypotension, and profound sedation or coma; use caution and reduced dosage in patients who are concurrently receiving these drugs). Products include:
Miltown Tablets 2780
PMB 200 and PMB 400 2890
Mesoridazine Besylate (Potential for respiratory depression, hypotension, and profound sedation or coma; use caution and reduced dosage in patients who are concurrently receiving these drugs). Products include:
Serentil 689
Methohexital Sodium (Potential for respiratory depression, hypotension, and profound sedation or coma; use caution and reduced dosage in patients who are concurrently receiving these drugs).
No products indexed under this heading.
Methotrimeprazine (Potential for respiratory depression, hypotension, and profound sedation or coma; use caution and reduced dosage in patients who are concurrently receiving these drugs). Products include:
Levoprome 1321
Methoxyflurane (Potential for respiratory depression, hypotension, and profound sedation or coma; use caution and reduced dosage in patients who are concurrently receiving these drugs).
No products indexed under this heading.
Midazolam Hydrochloride (Potential for respiratory depression, hypotension, and profound sedation or coma; use caution and reduced dosage in patients who are concurrently receiving these drugs). Products include:
Versed Injection 2324
Molindone Hydrochloride (Potential for respiratory depression, hypotension, and profound sedation or coma; use caution and reduced dosage in patients who are concurrently receiving these drugs). Products include:
Moban Tablets and Concentrate 1036
Morphine Sulfate (Potential for respiratory depression, hypotension, and profound sedation or coma; use caution and reduced dosage in patients who are concurrently receiving these drugs). Products include:
Astramorph/PF Injection, USP (Preservative-Free) 526
Duramorph Injection 983
Infumorph 200 and Infumorph 500 Sterile Solutions 985
Kadian Capsules 2948
MS Contin Tablets 2149
MSIR 2152
Oramorph SR (Morphine Sulfate Sustained Release Tablets) 2359
RMS Suppositories CII 2766
Roxanol 2365
Nortriptyline Hydrochloride (Potential for respiratory depression, hypotension, and profound sedation or coma; use caution and reduced dosage in patients who are concurrently receiving these drugs). Products include:
Pamelor 2409
Opium Alkaloids (Potential for respiratory depression, hypotension, and profound sedation or coma; use caution and reduced dosage in patients who are concurrently receiving these drugs).
No products indexed under this heading.
Oxazepam (Potential for respiratory depression, hypotension, and profound sedation or coma; use caution and reduced dosage in patients who are concurrently receiving these drugs). Products include:
Serax Capsules 2916
Serax Tablets 2916
Oxycodone Hydrochloride (Potential for respiratory depression, hypotension, and profound sedation or coma; use caution and reduced dosage in patients who are concurrently receiving these drugs). Products include:
OxyContin Tablets 2163
OxyIR Capsules 2167
Percocet Tablets 955
Percodan Tablets 955
Percodan-Demi Tablets 956
Roxicodone Tablets, Oral Solution & Intensol (Oxycodone) 2366
Tylox Capsules 1593
Pentazocine Hydrochloride (Potential for withdrawal symptoms in patients who are on the methadone maintenance program when given pentazocine). Products include:
Talacen Caplets 2464
Talwin Compound 2466
Talwin Nx Tablets 2467
Pentazocine Lactate (Potential for withdrawal symptoms in patients who are on the methadone maintenance program when given pentazocine). Products include:
Talwin Injection 2465
Pentobarbital Sodium (Potential for respiratory depression, hypotension, and profound sedation or coma; use caution and reduced dosage in patients who are concurrently receiving these drugs). Products include:
Nembutal Sodium Capsules 440
Nembutal Sodium Solution 442
Nembutal Sodium Suppositories 444
Perphenazine (Potential for respiratory depression, hypotension, and profound sedation or coma; use caution and reduced dosage in patients who are concurrently receiving these drugs). Products include:
Etrafon 2495
Triavil Tablets 1800
Trilafon 2532
Phenelzine Sulfate (Potential for meperidine/MAOI-type reaction; sensitivity test should be performed). Products include:
Nardil 1977
Phenobarbital (Potential for respiratory depression, hypotension, and profound sedation or coma; use caution and reduced dosage in patients who are concurrently receiving these drugs). Products include:
Arco-Lase Plus Tablets 513
Bellergal-S Tablets 2375
Donnatal 2234
Donnatal Extentabs 2234
Donnatal Tablets 2234
Phenobarbital Elixir and Tablets 1523
Quadrinal Tablets 1398
Prazepam (Potential for respiratory depression, hypotension, and profound sedation or coma; use caution and reduced dosage in patients who are concurrently receiving these drugs).
No products indexed under this heading.
Prochlorperazine (Potential for respiratory depression, hypotension, and profound sedation or coma; use caution and reduced dosage in patients who are concurrently receiving these drugs). Products include:
Compazine 2644
Promethazine Hydrochloride (Potential for respiratory depression, hypotension, and profound sedation or coma; use caution and reduced dosage in patients who are concurrently receiving these drugs). Products include:
Mepergan Injection 2859
Phenergan with Codeine 2883
Phenergan with Dextromethorphan 2885
Phenergan Injection 2880
Phenergan Suppositories 2882
Phenergan Syrup 2881
Phenergan Tablets 2882
Phenergan VC 2886
Phenergan VC with Codeine 2888
Propofol (Potential for respiratory depression, hypotension, and profound sedation or coma; use caution and reduced dosage in patients who are concurrently receiving these drugs). Products include:
Diprivan Injectable Emulsion 2939
Propoxyphene Hydrochloride (Potential for respiratory depression, hypotension, and profound sedation or coma; use caution and reduced dosage in patients who are concurrently receiving these drugs). Products include:
Darvon 1475
Wygesic Tablets 2930
Propoxyphene Napsylate (Potential for respiratory depression, hypotension, and profound sedation or coma; use caution and reduced dosage in patients who are concurrently receiving these drugs). Products include:
Darvon-N/Darvocet-N 1473
Protriptyline Hydrochloride (Potential for respiratory depression, hypotension, and profound sedation or coma; use caution and reduced dosage in patients who are concurrently receiving these drugs). Products include:
Vivactil Tablets 1820
Quazepam (Potential for respiratory depression, hypotension, and profound sedation or coma; use caution and reduced dosage in patients who are concurrently receiving these drugs). Products include:
Doral Tablets 2773
Rifampin (Concurrent administration may reduce the blood concentration of methadone to a degree sufficient to produce withdrawal symptoms). Products include:
Rifadin 1276
Rifamate Capsules 1278
Rifater 1280
Rimactane Capsules 865
Risperidone (Potential for respiratory depression, hypotension, and profound sedation or coma; use caution and reduced dosage in patients who are concurrently receiving these drugs). Products include:
Risperdal Tablets 1348
Secobarbital Sodium (Potential for respiratory depression, hypotension, and profound sedation or coma; use caution and reduced dosage in patients who are concurrently receiving these drugs). Products include:
Seconal Sodium Pulvules 1529
Selegiline Hydrochloride (Potential for meperidine/MAOI-type reaction; sensitivity test should be performed). Products include:
Eldepryl Capsules 2729
Sevoflurane (Potential for respiratory depression, hypotension, and profound sedation or coma; use caution and reduced dosage in patients who are concurrently receiving these drugs).
No products indexed under this heading.
Sufentanil Citrate (Potential for respiratory depression, hypotension, and profound sedation or coma; use caution and reduced dosage in patients who are concurrently receiving these drugs). Products include:
Sufenta Injection 1355
Temazepam (Potential for respiratory depression, hypotension, and profound sedation or coma; use caution and reduced dosage in patients who are concurrently receiving these drugs). Products include:
Restoril Capsules 2413
Thiamylal Sodium (Potential for respiratory depression, hypotension, and profound sedation or coma; use caution and reduced dosage in patients who are concurrently receiving these drugs).
No products indexed under this heading.
Thioridazine Hydrochloride (Potential for respiratory depression, hypotension, and profound sedation or coma; use caution and reduced dosage in patients who are concurrently receiving these drugs). Products include:
Mellaril 2398
Thiothixene (Potential for respiratory depression, hypotension, and profound sedation or coma; use caution and reduced dosage in patients who are concurrently receiving these drugs). Products include:
Navane Capsules and Concentrate 2018
Navane Intramuscular 2019
Tranylcypromine Sulfate (Potential for meperidine/MAOI-type reaction; sensitivity test should be performed). Products include:
Parnate Tablets 2679
Triazolam (Potential for respiratory depression, hypotension, and profound sedation or coma; use caution and reduced dosage in patients who are concurrently receiving these drugs). Products include:
Halcion Tablets 2093
Trifluoperazine Hydrochloride (Potential for respiratory depression, hypotension, and profound sedation or coma; use caution and reduced dosage in patients who are concurrently receiving these drugs). Products include:
Stelazine 2692
Trimipramine Maleate (Potential for respiratory depression, hypotension, and profound sedation or coma; use caution and reduced dosage in patients who are concurrently receiving these drugs). Products include:
Surmontil Capsules 2917

IMPORTANT NOTE: Always consult each drug listing in the patient's regimen for possible interactions.

Methadone Concentrate | Interactions Index | 666

Zolpidem Tartrate (Potential for respiratory depression, hypotension, and profound sedation or coma; use caution and reduced dosage in patients who are concurrently receiving these drugs). Products include:
- Ambien Tablets ... 2559

Food Interactions

Alcohol (Potential for respiratory depression, hypotension, and profound sedation or coma; use caution and reduced dosage in patients who are concurrently receiving these drugs).

METHADONE HYDROCHLORIDE ORAL SOLUTION & TABLETS

(Methadone Hydrochloride) ... 2357
May interact with tricyclic antidepressants, central nervous system depressants, monoamine oxidase inhibitors, and certain other agents. Compounds in these categories include:

Alfentanil Hydrochloride (Respiratory depression, hypotension, and profound sedation or coma may result). Products include:
- Alfenta Injection ... 1334

Alprazolam (Respiratory depression, hypotension, and profound sedation or coma may result). Products include:
- Xanax Tablets ... 2115

Amitriptyline Hydrochloride (Respiratory depression, hypotension, and profound sedation or coma may result). Products include:
- Elavil ... 2945
- Etrafon ... 2495
- Limbitrol ... 2333
- Triavil Tablets ... 1800

Amoxapine (Respiratory depression, hypotension, and profound sedation or coma may result). Products include:
- Asendin Tablets ... 1419

Aprobarbital (Respiratory depression, hypotension, and profound sedation or coma may result).
- No products indexed under this heading.

Buprenorphine (Respiratory depression, hypotension, and profound sedation or coma may result). Products include:
- Buprenex Injectable ... 2170

Buspirone Hydrochloride (Respiratory depression, hypotension, and profound sedation or coma may result). Products include:
- BuSpar Tablets ... 738

Butabarbital (Respiratory depression, hypotension, and profound sedation or coma may result).
- No products indexed under this heading.

Butalbital (Respiratory depression, hypotension, and profound sedation or coma may result). Products include:
- Axocet Capsules ... 2469
- Esgic-plus Capsules ... 1012
- Esgic-plus Tablets ... 1012
- Fioricet Tablets ... 2386
- Fioricet with Codeine Capsules ... 2387
- Fiorinal Capsules ... 2388
- Fiorinal with Codeine Capsules ... 2390
- Fiorinal Tablets ... 2388
- Phrenilin ... 790
- Sedapap Tablets 50 mg/650 mg ... 1826

Chlordiazepoxide (Respiratory depression, hypotension, and profound sedation or coma may result). Products include:
- Limbitrol ... 2333

Chlordiazepoxide Hydrochloride (Respiratory depression, hypotension, and profound sedation or coma may result). Products include:
- Librax Capsules ... 2330
- Librium Capsules ... 2331
- Librium Injectable ... 2332

Chlorpromazine (Respiratory depression, hypotension, and profound sedation or coma may result). Products include:
- Thorazine Suppositories ... 2701

Chlorprothixene (Respiratory depression, hypotension, and profound sedation or coma may result).
- No products indexed under this heading.

Chlorprothixene Hydrochloride (Respiratory depression, hypotension, and profound sedation or coma may result).
- No products indexed under this heading.

Chlorprothixene Lactate (Respiratory depression, hypotension, and profound sedation or coma may result).
- No products indexed under this heading.

Clomipramine Hydrochloride (Respiratory depression, hypotension, and profound sedation or coma may result). Products include:
- Anafranil Capsules ... 819

Clorazepate Dipotassium (Respiratory depression, hypotension, and profound sedation or coma may result). Products include:
- Tranxene ... 459

Clozapine (Respiratory depression, hypotension, and profound sedation or coma may result). Products include:
- Clozaril Tablets ... 2377

Codeine Phosphate (Respiratory depression, hypotension, and profound sedation or coma may result). Products include:
- Brontex ... 2130
- Dimetane-DC Cough Syrup ... 2232
- Fioricet with Codeine Capsules ... 2387
- Fiorinal with Codeine Capsules ... 2390
- Nucofed ... 2225
- Phenergan with Codeine ... 2883
- Phenergan VC with Codeine ... 2888
- Robitussin A-C Syrup ... 2248
- Robitussin-DAC Syrup ... 2249
- Ryna ... ⊞ 804
- Soma Compound w/Codeine Tablets ... 2784
- Tylenol with Codeine ... 1592

Desflurane (Respiratory depression, hypotension, and profound sedation or coma may result). Products include:
- Suprane (desflurane, USP) ... 1865

Desipramine Hydrochloride (Respiratory depression, hypotension, and profound sedation or coma may result). Products include:
- Norpramin Tablets ... 1273

Dezocine (Respiratory depression, hypotension, and profound sedation or coma may result). Products include:
- Dalgan Injection ... 529

Diazepam (Respiratory depression, hypotension, and profound sedation or coma may result). Products include:
- Dizac (diazepam injectable emulsion) CIV ... 1862
- Valium Injectable ... 2336
- Valium Tablets ... 2335

Doxepin Hydrochloride (Respiratory depression, hypotension, and profound sedation or coma may result). Products include:
- Adapin Capsules ... 1542
- Sinequan ... 2028
- Zonalon Cream ... 1042

Droperidol (Respiratory depression, hypotension, and profound sedation or coma may result). Products include:
- Inapsine Injection ... 462

Enflurane (Respiratory depression, hypotension, and profound sedation or coma may result).
- No products indexed under this heading.

Estazolam (Respiratory depression, hypotension, and profound sedation or coma may result). Products include:
- ProSom Tablets ... 457

Ethchlorvynol (Respiratory depression, hypotension, and profound sedation or coma may result). Products include:
- Placidyl Capsules ... 456

Ethinamate (Respiratory depression, hypotension, and profound sedation or coma may result).
- No products indexed under this heading.

Fentanyl (Respiratory depression, hypotension, and profound sedation or coma may result). Products include:
- Duragesic Transdermal System ... 1336

Fentanyl Citrate (Respiratory depression, hypotension, and profound sedation or coma may result). Products include:
- Sublimaze Injection ... 463

Fluphenazine Decanoate (Respiratory depression, hypotension, and profound sedation or coma may result). Products include:
- Prolixin Decanoate ... 510

Fluphenazine Enanthate (Respiratory depression, hypotension, and profound sedation or coma may result). Products include:
- Prolixin Enanthate ... 510

Fluphenazine Hydrochloride (Respiratory depression, hypotension, and profound sedation or coma may result). Products include:
- Prolixin ... 510

Flurazepam Hydrochloride (Respiratory depression, hypotension, and profound sedation or coma may result). Products include:
- Dalmane Capsules ... 2329

Furazolidone (Severe reactions not reported, but a sensitivity test is advised). Products include:
- Furoxone ... 2221

Glutethimide (Respiratory depression, hypotension, and profound sedation or coma may result).
- No products indexed under this heading.

Haloperidol (Respiratory depression, hypotension, and profound sedation or coma may result). Products include:
- Haldol Injection, Tablets and Concentrate ... 1585

Haloperidol Decanoate (Respiratory depression, hypotension, and profound sedation or coma may result). Products include:
- Haldol Decanoate ... 1587

Hydrocodone Bitartrate (Respiratory depression, hypotension, and profound sedation or coma may result). Products include:
- Codiclear DH Syrup ... 808
- Duratuss HD Elixir ... 2750
- Histussin D Liquid ... 670
- Hycodan Tablets and Syrup ... 946
- Hycomine Compound Tablets ... 948
- Hycomine ... 947
- Hycotuss Expectorant Syrup ... 950
- Hydrocet Capsules ... 787
- Lorcet 10/650 Tablets ... 1016
- Lortab ... 2751
- Tussend ... 1830
- Tussend Expectorant ... 1831
- Vicodin Tablets ... 1404
- Vicodin ES Tablets ... 1405
- Vicodin HP Tablets ... 1403
- Vicodin Tuss Expectorant ... 1406
- Zydone Capsules ... 967

Hydrocodone Polistirex (Respiratory depression, hypotension, and profound sedation or coma may result). Products include:
- Tussionex Pennkinetic Extended-Release Suspension ... 1624

Hydroxyzine Hydrochloride (Respiratory depression, hypotension, and profound sedation or coma may result). Products include:
- Atarax Tablets & Syrup ... 1992
- Marax Tablets & DF Syrup ... 2015
- Vistaril Intramuscular Solution ... 2042

Imipramine Hydrochloride (Respiratory depression, hypotension, and profound sedation or coma may result). Products include:
- Tofranil Ampuls ... 873
- Tofranil Tablets ... 875

Imipramine Pamoate (Respiratory depression, hypotension, and profound sedation or coma may result). Products include:
- Tofranil-PM Capsules ... 876

Isocarboxazid (Severe reactions not reported, but a sensitivity test is advised).
- No products indexed under this heading.

Isoflurane (Respiratory depression, hypotension, and profound sedation or coma may result).
- No products indexed under this heading.

Ketamine Hydrochloride (Respiratory depression, hypotension, and profound sedation or coma may result).
- No products indexed under this heading.

Levomethadyl Acetate Hydrochloride (Respiratory depression, hypotension, and profound sedation or coma may result). Products include:
- Orlaam Oral Solution ... 2361

Levorphanol Tartrate (Respiratory depression, hypotension, and profound sedation or coma may result). Products include:
- Levo-Dromoran ... 2297

Lorazepam (Respiratory depression, hypotension, and profound sedation or coma may result). Products include:
- Ativan Injection ... 2805
- Ativan Tablets ... 2807

Loxapine Hydrochloride (Respiratory depression, hypotension, and profound sedation or coma may result). Products include:
- Loxitane ... 1426

Loxapine Succinate (Respiratory depression, hypotension, and profound sedation or coma may result). Products include:
- Loxitane Capsules ... 1426

Maprotiline Hydrochloride (Respiratory depression, hypotension, and profound sedation or coma may result). Products include:
- Ludiomil Tablets ... 861

Meperidine Hydrochloride (Respiratory depression, hypotension, and profound sedation or coma may result). Products include:
- Demerol ... 2438
- Mepergan Injection ... 2859

(⊞ Described in PDR For Nonprescription Drugs) (⊙ Described in PDR For Ophthalmology)

667 **Interactions Index** **Methergine**

Mephobarbital (Respiratory depression, hypotension, and profound sedation or coma may result). Products include:
- Mebaral Tablets ... 2452

Meprobamate (Respiratory depression, hypotension, and profound sedation or coma may result). Products include:
- Miltown Tablets ... 2780
- PMB 200 and PMB 400 ... 2890

Mesoridazine Besylate (Respiratory depression, hypotension, and profound sedation or coma may result). Products include:
- Serentil ... 689

Methohexital Sodium (Respiratory depression, hypotension, and profound sedation or coma may result).
- No products indexed under this heading.

Methotrimeprazine (Respiratory depression, hypotension, and profound sedation or coma may result). Products include:
- Levoprome ... 1321

Methoxyflurane (Respiratory depression, hypotension, and profound sedation or coma may result).
- No products indexed under this heading.

Methyldopate Hydrochloride (Respiratory depression, hypotension, and profound sedation or coma may result). Products include:
- Aldomet Ester HCl Injection ... 1642

Midazolam Hydrochloride (Respiratory depression, hypotension, and profound sedation or coma may result). Products include:
- Versed Injection ... 2324

Molindone Hydrochloride (Respiratory depression, hypotension, and profound sedation or coma may result). Products include:
- Moban Tablets and Concentrate ... 1036

Morphine Sulfate (Respiratory depression, hypotension, and profound sedation or coma may result). Products include:
- Astramorph/PF Injection, USP (Preservative-Free) ... 526
- Duramorph Injection ... 983
- Infumorph 200 and Infumorph 500 Sterile Solutions ... 985
- Kadian Capsules ... 2948
- MS Contin Tablets ... 2149
- MSIR ... 2152
- Oramorph SR (Morphine Sulfate Sustained Release Tablets) ... 2359
- RMS Suppositories CII ... 2766
- Roxanol ... 2365

Nortriptyline Hydrochloride (Respiratory depression, hypotension, and profound sedation or coma may result). Products include:
- Pamelor ... 2409

Opium Alkaloids (Respiratory depression, hypotension, and profound sedation or coma may result).
- No products indexed under this heading.

Oxazepam (Respiratory depression, hypotension, and profound sedation or coma may result). Products include:
- Serax Capsules ... 2916
- Serax Tablets ... 2916

Oxycodone Hydrochloride (Respiratory depression, hypotension, and profound sedation or coma may result). Products include:
- OxyContin Tablets ... 2163
- OxyIR Capsules ... 2167
- Percocet Tablets ... 955
- Percodan Tablets ... 955
- Percodan-Demi Tablets ... 956
- Roxicodone Tablets, Oral Solution & Intensol (Oxycodone) ... 2366
- Tylox Capsules ... 1593

Pentazocine Hydrochloride (Possible withdrawal symptoms). Products include:
- Talacen Caplets ... 2464
- Talwin Compound ... 2466
- Talwin Nx Tablets ... 2467

Pentazocine Lactate (Possible withdrawal symptoms). Products include:
- Talwin Injection ... 2465

Pentobarbital Sodium (Respiratory depression, hypotension, and profound sedation or coma may result). Products include:
- Nembutal Sodium Capsules ... 440
- Nembutal Sodium Solution ... 442
- Nembutal Sodium Suppositories ... 444

Perphenazine (Respiratory depression, hypotension, and profound sedation or coma may result). Products include:
- Etrafon ... 2495
- Triavil Tablets ... 1800
- Trilafon ... 2532

Phenelzine Sulfate (Severe reactions not reported, but a sensitivity test is advised). Products include:
- Nardil ... 1977

Phenobarbital (Respiratory depression, hypotension, and profound sedation or coma may result). Products include:
- Arco-Lase Plus Tablets ... 513
- Bellergal-S Tablets ... 2375
- Donnatal ... 2234
- Donnatal Extentabs ... 2234
- Donnatal Tablets ... 2234
- Phenobarbital Elixir and Tablets ... 1523
- Quadrinal Tablets ... 1398

Prazepam (Respiratory depression, hypotension, and profound sedation or coma may result).
- No products indexed under this heading.

Prochlorperazine (Respiratory depression, hypotension, and profound sedation or coma may result). Products include:
- Compazine ... 2644

Promethazine Hydrochloride (Respiratory depression, hypotension, and profound sedation or coma may result). Products include:
- Mepergan Injection ... 2859
- Phenergan with Codeine ... 2883
- Phenergan with Dextromethorphan ... 2885
- Phenergan Injection ... 2880
- Phenergan Suppositories ... 2882
- Phenergan Syrup ... 2881
- Phenergan Tablets ... 2882
- Phenergan VC ... 2886
- Phenergan VC with Codeine ... 2888

Propofol (Respiratory depression, hypotension, and profound sedation or coma may result). Products include:
- Diprivan Injectable Emulsion ... 2939

Propoxyphene Hydrochloride (Respiratory depression, hypotension, and profound sedation or coma may result). Products include:
- Darvon ... 1475
- Wygesic Tablets ... 2930

Propoxyphene Napsylate (Respiratory depression, hypotension, and profound sedation or coma may result). Products include:
- Darvon-N/Darvocet-N ... 1473

Protriptyline Hydrochloride (Respiratory depression, hypotension, and profound sedation or coma may result). Products include:
- Vivactil Tablets ... 1820

Quazepam (Respiratory depression, hypotension, and profound sedation or coma may result). Products include:
- Doral Tablets ... 2773

Rifampin (Reduced blood concentration of methadone). Products include:
- Rifadin ... 1276
- Rifamate Capsules ... 1278
- Rifater ... 1280
- Rimactane Capsules ... 865

Risperidone (Respiratory depression, hypotension, and profound sedation or coma may result). Products include:
- Risperdal Tablets ... 1348

Secobarbital Sodium (Respiratory depression, hypotension, and profound sedation or coma may result). Products include:
- Seconal Sodium Pulvules ... 1529

Selegiline Hydrochloride (Severe reactions not reported, but a sensitivity test is advised). Products include:
- Eldepryl Capsules ... 2729

Sevoflurane (Respiratory depression, hypotension, and profound sedation or coma may result).
- No products indexed under this heading.

Sufentanil Citrate (Respiratory depression, hypotension, and profound sedation or coma may result). Products include:
- Sufenta Injection ... 1355

Temazepam (Respiratory depression, hypotension, and profound sedation or coma may result). Products include:
- Restoril Capsules ... 2413

Thiamylal Sodium (Respiratory depression, hypotension, and profound sedation or coma may result).
- No products indexed under this heading.

Thioridazine Hydrochloride (Respiratory depression, hypotension, and profound sedation or coma may result). Products include:
- Mellaril ... 2398

Thiothixene (Respiratory depression, hypotension, and profound sedation or coma may result). Products include:
- Navane Capsules and Concentrate ... 2018
- Navane Intramuscular ... 2019

Tranylcypromine Sulfate (Severe reactions not reported, but a sensitivity test is advised). Products include:
- Parnate Tablets ... 2679

Triazolam (Respiratory depression, hypotension, and profound sedation or coma may result). Products include:
- Halcion Tablets ... 2093

Trifluoperazine Hydrochloride (Respiratory depression, hypotension, and profound sedation or coma may result). Products include:
- Stelazine ... 2692

Trimipramine Maleate (Respiratory depression, hypotension, and profound sedation or coma may result). Products include:
- Surmontil Capsules ... 2917

Zolpidem Tartrate (Respiratory depression, hypotension, and profound sedation or coma may result). Products include:
- Ambien Tablets ... 2559

Food Interactions

Alcohol (Respiratory depression, hypotension, and profound sedation or coma may result).

METHERGINE INJECTION

(Methylergonovine Maleate) ... 2401
May interact with vasopressors, ergot-containing drugs, and certain other agents. Compounds in these categories include:

Dihydroergotamine Mesylate (The most common adverse reaction of methylergonovine is hypertension; exercise caution if used concurrently with other ergot alkaloids). Products include:
- D.H.E. 45 Injection ... 2381

Dopamine Hydrochloride (The most common adverse reaction of methylergonovine is hypertension; exercise caution if used concurrently with other vasoconstrictors).
- No products indexed under this heading.

Epinephrine Bitartrate (The most common adverse reaction of methylergonovine is hypertension; exercise caution if used concurrently with other vasoconstrictors). Products include:
- Sensorcaine-MPF with Epinephrine Injection ... 554

Epinephrine Hydrochloride (The most common adverse reaction of methylergonovine is hypertension; exercise caution if used concurrently with other vasoconstrictors). Products include:
- Ana-Kit Anaphylaxis Emergency Treatment Kit ... 611

Ergonovine Maleate (The most common adverse reaction of methylergonovine is hypertension; exercise caution if used concurrently with other ergot alkaloids).
- No products indexed under this heading.

Ergotamine Tartrate (The most common adverse reaction of methylergonovine is hypertension; exercise caution if used concurrently with other ergot alkaloids). Products include:
- Bellergal-S Tablets ... 2375
- Cafergot ... 2376
- Ergomar Tablets ... 1543
- Wigraine Tablets ... 1884

Metaraminol Bitartrate (The most common adverse reaction of methylergonovine is hypertension; exercise caution if used concurrently with other vasoconstrictors). Products include:
- Aramine Injection ... 1649

Methoxamine Hydrochloride (The most common adverse reaction of methylergonovine is hypertension; exercise caution if used concurrently with other vasoconstrictors). Products include:
- Vasoxyl Injection ... 1169

Methysergide Maleate (The most common adverse reaction of methylergonovine is hypertension; exercise caution if used concurrently with other ergot alkaloids). Products include:
- Sansert Tablets ... 2424

Norepinephrine Bitartrate (The most common adverse reaction of methylergonovine is hypertension; exercise caution if used concurrently with other vasoconstrictors). Products include:
- Levophed Bitartrate Injection ... 2445

Phenylephrine Hydrochloride (The most common adverse reaction of methylergonovine is hypertension; exercise caution if used concurrently with other vasoconstrictors). Products include:
- Atrohist Plus Tablets ... 1605
- Cerose DM ... OTC 853
- D.A. II Tablets ... 972
- D.A. Chewable Tablets ... 970
- Dura-Vent/DA Tablets ... 972
- Extendryl ... 1003

IMPORTANT NOTE: Always consult each drug listing in the patient's regimen for possible interactions.

4-Way Fast Acting Nasal Spray (regular & mentholated) ▣ 644
Hemorid ▣ 797
Hycomine Compound Tablets 948
Neo-Synephrine Hydrochloride 1% Carpuject 2455
Neo-Synephrine Hydrochloride 1% Injection 2455
Neo-Synephrine Hydrochloride (Ophthalmic) 2456
Neo-Synephrine ▣ 624
Novahistine Elixir ▣ 782
Phenergan VC 2886
Phenergan VC with Codeine 2888
Preparation H ▣ 842
Tympagesic Ear Drops 2476
Vicks Sinex Nasal Spray and Ultra Fine Mist ▣ 738

METHERGINE TABLETS
(Methylergonovine Maleate) 2401
See **Methergine Injection**

METHOTREXATE SODIUM TABLETS, INJECTION, FOR INJECTION AND LPF INJECTION
(Methotrexate Sodium) 1322
May interact with salicylates, sulfonamides, tetracyclines, non-steroidal anti-inflammatory agents, penicillins, xanthine bronchodilators, and certain other agents. Compounds in these categories include:

Aminophylline (Methotrexate may decrease the clearance of theophylline).
No products indexed under this heading.

Amoxicillin Trihydrate (Penicillins may reduce the renal clearance of methotrexate; concurrent use has resulted in increased serum concentrations of methotrexate with concomitant hematologic and gastrointestinal toxicity). Products include:
Amoxil 2631
Augmentin 2637
Augmentin Tablets 2640

Ampicillin (Penicillins may reduce the renal clearance of methotrexate; concurrent use has resulted in increased serum concentrations of methotrexate with concomitant hematologic and gastrointestinal toxicity). Products include:
Omnipen Capsules 2872
Omnipen for Oral Suspension 2873

Ampicillin Sodium (Penicillins may reduce the renal clearance of methotrexate; concurrent use has resulted in increased serum concentrations of methotrexate with concomitant hematologic and gastrointestinal toxicity). Products include:
Unasyn 2035

Ampicillin Trihydrate (Penicillins may reduce the renal clearance of methotrexate; concurrent use has resulted in increased serum concentrations of methotrexate with concomitant hematologic and gastrointestinal toxicity).
No products indexed under this heading.

Aspirin (Co-administration has been reported to reduce the tubular secretion of methotrexate in an animal model and may enhance its toxicity; salicylates may displace methotrexate from protein binding sites). Products include:
Alka-Seltzer Cherry Effervescent Antacid and Pain Reliever ▣ 609
Alka-Seltzer Extra Strength Effervescent Antacid and Pain Reliever ▣ 609
Alka-Seltzer Lemon Lime Effervescent Antacid and Pain Reliever ▣ 609
Alka-Seltzer Original Effervescent Antacid and Pain Reliever ▣ 609
Alka-Seltzer Plus ▣ 611
Alka-Seltzer Plus Sinus Medicine ▣ 611
Ascriptin ▣ 650
Arthritis Strength BC Powder ▣ 631
BC Cold Powder Multi-Symptom Formula (Cold-Sinus-Allergy) ▣ 631
BC Cold Powder Non-Drowsy Formula (Cold-Sinus) ▣ 631
BC Powder ▣ 631
Genuine Bayer Aspirin Tablets & Caplets ▣ 618
Extra Strength Bayer Arthritis Pain Regimen Formula ▣ 615
Extra Strength Bayer Aspirin Caplets & Tablets ▣ 617
Extended-Release Bayer 8-Hour Aspirin ▣ 616
Extra Strength Bayer Plus Aspirin Caplets ▣ 617
Extra Strength Bayer PM Aspirin Plus Sleep Aid ▣ 617
Aspirin Regimen Bayer 81 mg Tablets with Calcium ▣ 615
Aspirin Regimen Bayer Adult Low Strength 81 mg Tablets ▣ 613
Aspirin Regimen Bayer Children's Chewable Aspirin ▣ 616
Aspirin Regimen Bayer Regular Strength 325 mg Caplets ▣ 613
Bufferin Analgesic Tablets ▣ 636
Arthritis Strength Bufferin Analgesic Caplets ▣ 637
Extra Strength Bufferin Analgesic Tablets ▣ 637
Cama Arthritis Pain Reliever ▣ 748
Darvon Compound-65 Pulvules 1475
Easprin 1971
Ecotrin 2625
Ecotrin Enteric Coated Aspirin Maximum Strength Tablets and Caplets ▣ 775
Ecotrin Enteric Coated Aspirin Regular Strength Tablets 2625
Empirin Aspirin Tablets ▣ 818
Excedrin Extra-Strength Analgesic Tablets, Caplets, and Geltabs 734
Fiorinal Capsules 2388
Fiorinal with Codeine Capsules 2390
Fiorinal Tablets 2388
Goody's Extra Strength Headache Powders ▣ 632
Goody's Extra Strength Pain Relief Tablets ▣ 632
Halfprin Tablets 1413
Norgesic 1554
Percodan Tablets 955
Percodan-Demi Tablets 956
Robaxisal Tablets 2246
Soma Compound w/Codeine Tablets 2784
Soma Compound Tablets 2783
St. Joseph Adult Chewable Aspirin (81 mg.) ▣ 768
Talwin Compound 2466
Vanquish Analgesic Caplets ▣ 627

Azlocillin Sodium (Penicillins may reduce the renal clearance of methotrexate; concurrent use has resulted in increased serum concentrations of methotrexate with concomitant hematologic and gastrointestinal toxicity).
No products indexed under this heading.

Bacampicillin Hydrochloride (Penicillins may reduce the renal clearance of methotrexate; concurrent use has resulted in increased serum concentrations of methotrexate with concomitant hematologic and gastrointestinal toxicity). Products include:
Spectrobid Tablets 2030

Bendroflumethiazide (Co-administration with sulfonamides may displace methotrexate from protein binding sites with potential increase in toxicity).
No products indexed under this heading.

Carbenicillin Disodium (Penicillins may reduce the renal clearance of methotrexate; concurrent use has resulted in increased serum concentrations of methotrexate with concomitant hematologic and gastrointestinal toxicity).
No products indexed under this heading.

Carbenicillin Indanyl Sodium (Penicillins may reduce the renal clearance of methotrexate; concurrent use has resulted in increased serum concentrations of methotrexate with concomitant hematologic and gastrointestinal toxicity). Products include:
Geocillin Tablets 2009

Chloramphenicol Palmitate (Co-administration with oral chloramphenicol may decrease intestinal absorption of methotrexate or interfere with the enterohepatic circulation by inhibiting bowel flora and suppressing metabolism of the drug by bacteria).
No products indexed under this heading.

Chlorothiazide (Co-administration with sulfonamides may displace methotrexate from protein binding sites with potential increase in toxicity). Products include:
Aldoclor Tablets 1638
Diupres Tablets 1691
Diuril Oral 1694

Chlorothiazide Sodium (Co-administration with sulfonamides may displace methotrexate from protein binding sites with potential increase in toxicity). Products include:
Diuril Sodium Intravenous 1693

Chlorpropamide (Co-administration with sulfonamides may displace methotrexate from protein binding sites with potential increase in toxicity). Products include:
Diabinese Tablets 2002

Choline Magnesium Trisalicylate (Co-administration has been reported to reduce the tubular secretion of methotrexate in an animal model and may enhance its toxicity; salicylates may displace methotrexate from protein binding sites). Products include:
Trilisate 2155

Cisplatin (Caution should be exercised if high-dose methotrexate is administered to patients with osteosarcoma in combination with a potentially nephrotoxic chemotherapeutic agent, such as cisplatin). Products include:
Platinol for Injection 717
Platinol-AQ Injection 719

Demeclocycline Hydrochloride (Co-administration with oral tetracycline may decrease intestinal absorption of methotrexate or interfere with the enterohepatic circulation by inhibiting bowel flora and suppressing metabolism of the drug by bacteria). Products include:
Declomycin Tablets 1421

Diclofenac Potassium (Co-administration with high doses of methotrexate therapy has been reported to elevate and prolong serum methotrexate levels in unexpectedly severe, sometimes fatal, bone marrow suppression and gastrointestinal toxicity). Products include:
Cataflam Tablets 833

Diclofenac Sodium (Co-administration with high doses of methotrexate therapy has been reported to elevate and prolong serum methotrexate levels in unexpectedly severe, sometimes fatal, bone marrow suppression and gastrointestinal toxicity). Products include:
Voltaren Ophthalmic Sterile Ophthalmic Solution ◉ 264
Cataflam/Voltaren/Voltaren-XR 833

Dicloxacillin Sodium (Penicillins may reduce the renal clearance of methotrexate; concurrent use has resulted in increased serum concentrations of methotrexate with concomitant hematologic and gastrointestinal toxicity).
No products indexed under this heading.

Diflunisal (Co-administration has been reported to reduce the tubular secretion of methotrexate in an animal model and may enhance its toxicity; salicylates may displace methotrexate from protein binding sites). Products include:
Dolobid Tablets 1695

Doxycycline Calcium (Co-administration with oral tetracycline may decrease intestinal absorption of methotrexate or interfere with the enterohepatic circulation by inhibiting bowel flora and suppressing metabolism of the drug by bacteria). Products include:
Vibramycin Calcium Oral Suspension Syrup 2038

Doxycycline Hyclate (Co-administration with oral tetracycline may decrease intestinal absorption of methotrexate or interfere with the enterohepatic circulation by inhibiting bowel flora and suppressing metabolism of the drug by bacteria). Products include:
Doryx Capsules 1970
Vibramycin Hyclate Capsules 2038
Vibramycin Hyclate Intravenous 2040
Vibra-Tabs Film Coated Tablets 2038

Doxycycline Monohydrate (Co-administration with oral tetracycline may decrease intestinal absorption of methotrexate or interfere with the enterohepatic circulation by inhibiting bowel flora and suppressing metabolism of the drug by bacteria). Products include:
Monodox Capsules 1858
Vibramycin Monohydrate for Oral Suspension 2038

Dyphylline (Methotrexate may decrease the clearance of theophylline). Products include:
Lufyllin & Lufyllin-400 Tablets 2778
Lufyllin-GG Elixir & Tablets 2779

Etodolac (Co-administration with high doses of methotrexate therapy has been reported to elevate and prolong serum methotrexate levels in unexpectedly severe, sometimes fatal, bone marrow suppression and gastrointestinal toxicity). Products include:
Lodine Capsules and Tablets 2849

Etretinate (Co-administration with retinoids may increase the possible risk of hepatotoxicity). Products include:
Tegison Capsules 2314

(▣ Described in PDR For Nonprescription Drugs) (◉ Described in PDR For Ophthalmology)

Fenoprofen Calcium (Co-administration with high doses of methotrexate therapy has been reported to elevate and prolong serum methotrexate levels in unexpectedly severe, sometimes fatal, bone marrow suppression and gastrointestinal toxicity). Products include:

- Nalfon 200 Pulvules & Nalfon Tablets 933

Flurbiprofen (Co-administration with high doses of methotrexate therapy has been reported to elevate and prolong serum methotrexate levels in unexpectedly severe, sometimes fatal, bone marrow suppression and gastrointestinal toxicity).

- No products indexed under this heading.

Folic Acid (Vitamin preparations containing folic acid or its derivatives may decrease response to systemically administered methotrexate). Products include:

- Cefol Filmtab 415
- Chromagen FA 2471
- Chromagen Forte 2471
- Fero-Folic-500 Filmtab 433
- Iberet-Folic-500 Filmtab 433
- Materna Tablets 1427
- Mega-B 513
- Megadose 513
- Nephro-Fer Rx Tablets 2168
- Nephro-Vite + Fe Tablets 2170
- Nephro-Vite Rx Tablets 2170
- Niferex-150 Forte Capsules 811
- Slow Fe with Folic Acid 890
- Trinsicon Capsules 2759

Fosphenytoin Sodium (May displace methotrexate from protein binding sites with potential increase in toxicity). Products include:

- Cerebyx Injection 1956

Glipizide (Co-administration with sulfonamides may displace methotrexate from protein binding sites with potential increase in toxicity). Products include:

- Glucotrol Tablets 2011
- Glucotrol XL Extended Release Tablets 2012

Glyburide (Co-administration with sulfonamides may displace methotrexate from protein binding sites with potential increase in toxicity). Products include:

- DiaBeta Tablets 1265
- Glynase PresTab Tablets 2091
- Micronase Tablets 2099

Hydrochlorothiazide (Co-administration with sulfonamides may displace methotrexate from protein binding sites with potential increase in toxicity). Products include:

- Aldactazide Tablets 2556
- Aldoril Tablets 1644
- Apresazide Capsules 824
- Capozide Tablets 744
- Dyazide Capsules 2653
- Esidrix Tablets 839
- Esimil Tablets 840
- HydroDIURIL Tablets 1716
- Hydropres Tablets 1718
- Hyzaar Tablets 1720
- Inderide Tablets 2838
- Inderide LA Long Acting Capsules .. 2840
- Lopressor HCT Tablets 850
- Lotensin HCT Tablets 855
- Moduretic Tablets 1748
- Oretic Tablets 450
- Prinzide Tablets 1780
- Ser-Ap-Es Tablets 867
- Timolide Tablets 1791
- Vaseretic Tablets 1810
- Zestoretic Tablets 2968
- Ziac 1459

Hydroflumethiazide (Co-administration with sulfonamides may displace methotrexate from protein binding sites with potential increase in toxicity). Products include:

- Diucardin Tablets 2824

Ibuprofen (Co-administration with high doses of methotrexate therapy has been reported to elevate and prolong serum methotrexate levels in unexpectedly severe, sometimes fatal, bone marrow suppression and gastrointestinal toxicity). Products include:

- Advil Cold and Sinus Caplets and Tablets .... ⊞ 837
- Advil Ibuprofen Tablets, Caplets and Gel Caplets .... ⊞ 836
- Children's Motrin Ibuprofen Oral Suspension 1558
- IBU Tablets 1389
- Ibuprohm .... ⊞ 713
- Motrin IB Caplets, Tablets, and Gelcaps .... ⊞ 802
- Motrin Ibuprofen Suspension, Oral Drops, Chewable Tablets, Caplets 1563
- Nuprin Ibuprofen/Analgesic Tablets & Caplets .... ⊞ 645
- Vicks DayQuil SINUS Pressure & PAIN Relief with IBUPROFEN .... ⊞ 735

Indomethacin (Co-administration with high doses of methotrexate therapy has been reported to elevate and prolong serum methotrexate levels in unexpectedly severe, sometimes fatal, bone marrow suppression and gastrointestinal toxicity). Products include:

- Indocin 1723

Indomethacin Sodium Trihydrate (Co-administration with high doses of methotrexate therapy has been reported to elevate and prolong serum methotrexate levels in unexpectedly severe, sometimes fatal, bone marrow suppression and gastrointestinal toxicity). Products include:

- Indocin I.V. 1727

Isotretinoin (Co-administration with retinoids may increase the possible risk of hepatotoxicity). Products include:

- Accutane Capsules 2252

Kanamycin Sulfate (Co-administration with nonabsorbable broad spectrum oral antibiotics, such as kanamycin, may decrease intestinal absorption of methotrexate or interfere with the enterohepatic circulation by inhibiting bowel flora and suppressing metabolism of the drug by bacteria).

- No products indexed under this heading.

Ketoprofen (Co-administration with high doses of methotrexate therapy has been reported to elevate and prolong serum methotrexate levels in unexpectedly severe, sometimes fatal, bone marrow suppression and gastrointestinal toxicity). Products include:

- Actron Caplets and Tablets .... ⊞ 608
- Orudis Capsules 2874
- Orudis KT .... ⊞ 842
- Oruvail Capsules 2874

Ketorolac Tromethamine (Co-administration with high doses of methotrexate therapy has been reported to elevate and prolong serum methotrexate levels in unexpectedly severe, sometimes fatal, bone marrow suppression and gastrointestinal toxicity). Products include:

- Acular Sterile Ophthalmic Solution 470
- Toradol 2319

Magnesium Salicylate (Co-administration has been reported to reduce the tubular secretion of methotrexate in an animal model and may enhance its toxicity; salicylates may displace methotrexate from protein binding sites). Products include:

- Backache Caplets .... ⊞ 635
- Doan's Extra-Strength Analgesic.... ⊞ 653
- Extra Strength Doan's P.M. .... ⊞ 653
- Doan's Regular Strength Analgesic .... ⊞ 654
- Mobigesic Tablets .... ⊞ 607

Meclofenamate Sodium (Co-administration with high doses of methotrexate therapy has been reported to elevate and prolong serum methotrexate levels in unexpectedly severe, sometimes fatal, bone marrow suppression and gastrointestinal toxicity).

- No products indexed under this heading.

Mefenamic Acid (Co-administration with high doses of methotrexate therapy has been reported to elevate and prolong serum methotrexate levels in unexpectedly severe, sometimes fatal, bone marrow suppression and gastrointestinal toxicity). Products include:

- Ponstel 1982

Methacycline Hydrochloride (Co-administration with oral tetracycline may decrease intestinal absorption of methotrexate or interfere with the enterohepatic circulation by inhibiting bowel flora and suppressing metabolism of the drug by bacteria).

- No products indexed under this heading.

Methyclothiazide (Co-administration with sulfonamides may displace methotrexate from protein binding sites with potential increase in toxicity). Products include:

- Enduron Tablets 424

Mezlocillin Sodium (Penicillins may reduce the renal clearance of methotrexate; concurrent use has resulted in increased serum concentrations of methotrexate with concomitant hematologic and gastrointestinal toxicity). Products include:

- Mezlin 594
- Mezlin Pharmacy Bulk Package........ 597

Minocycline Hydrochloride (Co-administration with oral tetracycline may decrease intestinal absorption of methotrexate or interfere with the enterohepatic circulation by inhibiting bowel flora and suppressing metabolism of the drug by bacteria). Products include:

- DYNACIN Capsules 1627
- Minocin Intravenous 1428
- Minocin Oral Suspension 1431
- Minocin Pellet-Filled Capsules 1429

Nabumetone (Co-administration with high doses of methotrexate therapy has been reported to elevate and prolong serum methotrexate levels in unexpectedly severe, sometimes fatal, bone marrow suppression and gastrointestinal toxicity). Products include:

- Relafen Tablets 2688

Nafcillin Sodium (Penicillins may reduce the renal clearance of methotrexate; concurrent use has resulted in increased serum concentrations of methotrexate with concomitant hematologic and gastrointestinal toxicity).

- No products indexed under this heading.

Naproxen (Co-administration with high doses of methotrexate therapy has been reported to elevate and prolong serum methotrexate levels in unexpectedly severe, sometimes fatal, bone marrow suppression and gastrointestinal toxicity). Products include:

- Anaprox/Naprosyn 2277

Naproxen Sodium (Co-administration with high doses of methotrexate therapy has been reported to elevate and prolong serum methotrexate levels in unexpectedly severe, sometimes fatal, bone marrow suppression and gastrointestinal toxicity). Products include:

- Aleve 2124
- Anaprox/Naprosyn 2277
- Naprelan Tablets 2861

Neomycin, oral (Co-administration with nonabsorbable broad spectrum oral antibiotics, such as neomycin, may decrease intestinal absorption of methotrexate or interfere with the enterohepatic circulation by inhibiting bowel flora and suppressing metabolism of the drug by bacteria).

Oxaprozin (Co-administration with high doses of methotrexate therapy has been reported to elevate and prolong serum methotrexate levels in unexpectedly severe, sometimes fatal, bone marrow suppression and gastrointestinal toxicity). Products include:

- Daypro Caplets 2578

Oxytetracycline Hydrochloride (Co-administration with oral tetracycline may decrease intestinal absorption of methotrexate or interfere with the enterohepatic circulation by inhibiting bowel flora and suppressing metabolism of the drug by bacteria). Products include:

- TERAK Ointment .... ⊙ 210
- Terra-Cortril Ophthalmic Suspension 2033
- Terramycin with Polymyxin B Sulfate Ophthalmic Ointment 2035
- Urobiotic-250 Capsules 2038

Penicillin G Benzathine (Penicillins may reduce the renal clearance of methotrexate; concurrent use has resulted in increased serum concentrations of methotrexate with concomitant hematologic and gastrointestinal toxicity). Products include:

- Bicillin C-R Injection 2810
- Bicillin C-R 900/300 Injection 2812
- Bicillin L-A Injection 2813

Penicillin G Potassium (Penicillins may reduce the renal clearance of methotrexate; concurrent use has resulted in increased serum concentrations of methotrexate with concomitant hematologic and gastrointestinal toxicity). Products include:

- Pfizerpen for Injection 2022

Penicillin G Procaine (Penicillins may reduce the renal clearance of methotrexate; concurrent use has resulted in increased serum concentrations of methotrexate with concomitant hematologic and gastrointestinal toxicity). Products include:

- Bicillin C-R Injection 2810
- Bicillin C-R 900/300 Injection 2812

Penicillin G Sodium (Penicillins may reduce the renal clearance of methotrexate; concurrent use has resulted in increased serum concentrations of methotrexate with concomitant hematologic and gastrointestinal toxicity).

- No products indexed under this heading.

IMPORTANT NOTE: Always consult each drug listing in the patient's regimen for possible interactions.

Methotrexate/Rheumatrex — Interactions Index

Penicillin V Potassium (Penicillins may reduce the renal clearance of methotrexate; concurrent use has resulted in increased serum concentrations of methotrexate with concomitant hematologic and gastrointestinal toxicity). Products include:
Pen•Vee K 2879

Phenylbutazone (Co-administration with high doses of methotrexate therapy has been reported to elevate and prolong serum methotrexate levels in unexpectedly severe, sometimes fatal, bone marrow suppression and gastrointestinal toxicity; phenylbutazone may displace methotrexate from protein binding sites).
No products indexed under this heading.

Phenytoin (May displace methotrexate from protein binding sites with potential increase in toxicity). Products include:
Dilantin Infatabs 1967
Dilantin-125 Suspension 1969

Phenytoin Sodium (May displace methotrexate from protein binding sites with potential increase in toxicity). Products include:
Dilantin Kapseals 1965

Piroxicam (Co-administration with high doses of methotrexate therapy has been reported to elevate and prolong serum methotrexate levels in unexpectedly severe, sometimes fatal, bone marrow suppression and gastrointestinal toxicity). Products include:
Feldene Capsules 2008

Polythiazide (Co-administration with sulfonamides may displace methotrexate from protein binding sites with potential increase in toxicity). Products include:
Minizide Capsules 2016

Probenecid (Diminishes renal tubular transport). Products include:
Benemid Tablets 1651
ColBENEMID Tablets 1662

Salsalate (Co-administration has been reported to reduce the tubular secretion of methotrexate in an animal model and may enhance its toxicity; salicylates may displace methotrexate from protein binding sites). Products include:
Disalcid 1549
Mono-Gesic Tablets 810
Salflex Tablets 791

Sulfacytine (Co-administration with sulfonamides may displace methotrexate from protein binding sites with potential increase in toxicity).

Sulfamethizole (Co-administration with sulfonamides may displace methotrexate from protein binding sites with potential increase in toxicity). Products include:
Urobiotic-250 Capsules 2038

Sulfamethoxazole (Trimethoprim/sulfamethoxazole has been reported rarely to increase bone marrow suppression in patients receiving methotrexate, probably by an additive antifolate effect). Products include:
Bactrim DS Tablets 2257
Bactrim I.V. Infusion 2255
Bactrim 2257
Gantanol Tablets 2285
Septra 1146
Septra I.V. Infusion 1142
Septra I.V. Infusion ADD-Vantage Vials 1144
Septra 1146

Sulfasalazine (Co-administration with sulfonamides may displace methotrexate from protein binding sites with potential increase in toxicity). Products include:
Azulfidine 2059

Sulfinpyrazone (Co-administration with sulfonamides may displace methotrexate from protein binding sites with potential increase in toxicity). Products include:
Anturane 823

Sulfisoxazole (Co-administration with sulfonamides may displace methotrexate from protein binding sites with potential increase in toxicity). Products include:
Gantrisin Tablets 2286

Sulfisoxazole Diolamine (Co-administration with sulfonamides may displace methotrexate from protein binding sites with potential increase in toxicity).
No products indexed under this heading.

Sulindac (Co-administration with high doses of methotrexate therapy has been reported to elevate and prolong serum methotrexate levels in unexpectedly severe, sometimes fatal, bone marrow suppression and gastrointestinal toxicity). Products include:
Clinoril Tablets 1658

Tetracycline Hydrochloride (Co-administration with oral tetracycline may decrease intestinal absorption of methotrexate or interfere with the enterohepatic circulation by inhibiting bowel flora and suppressing metabolism of the drug by bacteria). Products include:
Achromycin V Capsules 1417
Helidac Therapy 2135

Theophylline (Methotrexate may decrease the clearance of theophylline). Products include:
Marax Tablets & DF Syrup 2015
Quibron 2227

Theophylline Anhydrous (Methotrexate may decrease the clearance of theophylline). Products include:
Aerolate 1003
Primatene Tablets 844
Respbid Tablets 687
Slo-bid Gyrocaps 2201
Theo-24 Extended Release Capsules 2753
Theo-Dur Extended-Release Tablets 1367
Theo-X Extended-Release Tablets .. 793
Uni-Dur Extended-Release Tablets.. 1374
Uniphyl 400 mg and 600 mg Tablets 2157

Theophylline Calcium Salicylate (Methotrexate may decrease the clearance of theophylline). Products include:
Quadrinal Tablets 1398

Theophylline Sodium Glycinate (Methotrexate may decrease the clearance of theophylline).
No products indexed under this heading.

Ticarcillin Disodium (Penicillins may reduce the renal clearance of methotrexate; concurrent use has resulted in increased serum concentrations of methotrexate with concomitant hematologic and gastrointestinal toxicity). Products include:
Ticar for Injection 2704
Timentin for Injection 2706

Tolazamide (Co-administration with sulfonamides may displace methotrexate from protein binding sites with potential increase in toxicity).
No products indexed under this heading.

Tolbutamide (Co-administration with sulfonamides may displace methotrexate from protein binding sites with potential increase in toxicity).
No products indexed under this heading.

Tolmetin Sodium (Co-administration with high doses of methotrexate therapy has been reported to elevate and prolong serum methotrexate levels in unexpectedly severe, sometimes fatal, bone marrow suppression and gastrointestinal toxicity). Products include:
Tolectin (200, 400 and 600 mg) .. 1591

Tretinoin (Co-administration with retinoids may increase the possible risk of hepatotoxicity). Products include:
Renova (tretinoin emollient cream) 0.05% 1945
Retin-A (tretinoin) Cream/Gel/Liquid 1947
Vesanoid Capsules 2327

Trimethoprim (Trimethoprim/sulfamethoxazole has been reported rarely to increase bone marrow suppression in patients receiving methotrexate, probably by an additive antifolate effect). Products include:
Bactrim DS Tablets 2257
Bactrim I.V. Infusion 2255
Bactrim 2257
Proloprim Tablets 1141
Septra 1146
Septra I.V. Infusion 1142
Septra I.V. Infusion ADD-Vantage Vials 1144
Septra 1146
Trimpex Tablets 2323

Food Interactions

Food, unspecified (Delays absorption and reduces peak concentration).

METROCREAM
(Metronidazole) 1034
May interact with oral anticoagulants. Compounds in this category include:

Dicumarol (Oral metronidazole potentiates the anticoagulant effect resulting in a prolongation of prothrombin time; the effect of topical metronidazole on prothrombin time is not known).
No products indexed under this heading.

Warfarin Sodium (Oral metronidazole potentiates the anticoagulant effect resulting in a prolongation of prothrombin time; the effect of topical metronidazole on prothrombin time is not known). Products include:
Coumadin 941

METRODIN (UROFOLLITROPIN FOR INJECTION)
(Urofollitropin) 2616
None cited in PDR database.

METROGEL
(Metronidazole) 1034
May interact with oral anticoagulants. Compounds in this category include:

Dicumarol (Prolonged prothrombin time and potentiation of oral anticoagulant with systemic metronidazole; the effect of topical metronidazole on prothrombin is unknown).
No products indexed under this heading.

Warfarin Sodium (Prolonged prothrombin time and potentiation of oral anticoagulant with systemic metronidazole; the effect of topical metronidazole on prothrombin is unknown). Products include:
Coumadin 941

METROGEL-VAGINAL
(Metronidazole) 917
May interact with oral anticoagulants and certain other agents. Compounds in these categories include:

Dicumarol (Oral metronidazole potentiates the anticoagulant effect of warfarin).
No products indexed under this heading.

Disulfiram (Psychotic reactions to oral metronidazole have been reported in alcoholics who are using metronidazole and disulfiram concurrently). Products include:
Antabuse Tablets 2802

Warfarin Sodium (Oral metronidazole potentiates the anticoagulant effect of warfarin). Products include:
Coumadin 941

Food Interactions
Alcohol (Possibility of a disulfiram-like reaction).

METUBINE IODIDE VIALS
(Metocurine Iodide) 932
May interact with parenteral tetracyclines, quinidine, and certain other agents. Compounds in these categories include:

Bacitracin (Parenteral administration of high dose of bacitracin may intensify or resemble the neuroblocking action of muscle relaxant).
No products indexed under this heading.

Colistimethate Sodium (Parenteral administration of high dose of sodium colistimethate may intensify or resemble the neuroblocking action of muscle relaxant).
No products indexed under this heading.

Colistin Sulfate (Parenteral administration of high dose of colistin may intensify or resemble the neuroblocking action of muscle relaxant). Products include:
Coly-Mycin S Otic w/Neomycin & Hydrocortisone 1965

Diazepam (Potential for unexpected drug response or prolongation of action; monitor patients carefully). Products include:
Dizac (diazepam injectable emulsion) CIV 1862
Valium Injectable 2336
Valium Tablets 2335

Diethyl Ether (May potentiate neuromuscular blocking action).

Doxycycline Hyclate (Parenteral administration of high dose of tetracyclines may intensify or resemble the neuroblocking action of muscle relaxant). Products include:
Doryx Capsules 1970
Vibramycin Hyclate Capsules 2038
Vibramycin Hyclate Intravenous . 2040
Vibra-Tabs Film Coated Tablets .. 2038

Gentamicin Sulfate (Parenteral administration of high dose of gentamicin may intensify or resemble the neuroblocking action of muscle relaxant). Products include:
Garamycin Cream 0.1% 2501
Garamycin Injectable 2502
Garamycin Ointment 0.1% 2501
Garamycin Ophthalmic 2501
Genoptic Sterile Ophthalmic Solution 241

(▣ Described in PDR For Nonprescription Drugs)　　　　(◉ Described in PDR For Ophthalmology)

671 **Interactions Index** **Mexitil**

Genoptic Sterile Ophthalmic Ointment ⊙ 241
Gentak ⊙ 209
Pred-G Liquifilm Sterile Ophthalmic Suspension ⊙ 248
Pred-G S.O.P. Sterile Ophthalmic Ointment ⊙ 249

Halothane (May potentiate neuromuscular blocking action). Products include:
Fluothane 2830

Isoflurane (May potentiate neuromuscular blocking action).
No products indexed under this heading.

Kanamycin Sulfate (Parenteral administration of high dose of kanamycin may intensify or resemble the neuroblocking action of muscle relaxant).
No products indexed under this heading.

Magnesium Sulfate (The use of magnesium sulfate in preeclamptic patients potentiates both depolarizing and nondepolarizing muscle relaxants).
No products indexed under this heading.

Minocycline Hydrochloride (Parenteral administration of high dose of tetracyclines may intensify or resemble the neuroblocking action of muscle relaxant). Products include:
DYNACIN Capsules 1627
Minocin Intravenous 1428
Minocin Oral Suspension 1431
Minocin Pellet-Filled Capsules 1429

Neomycin Sulfate (Parenteral administration of high dose of neomycin may intensify or resemble the neuroblocking action of muscle relaxant). Products include:
AK-Spore ⊙ 205
AK-Trol Ointment & Suspension ⊙ 205
Coly-Mycin S Otic w/Neomycin & Hydrocortisone 1965
Cortisporin Cream 1073
Cortisporin Ointment 1074
Cortisporin Ophthalmic Ointment Sterile 1074
Cortisporin Ophthalmic Suspension Sterile 1075
Cortisporin Otic Solution Sterile 1076
Cortisporin Otic Suspension Sterile 1077
Maxitrol Ophthalmic Ointment and Suspension ⊙ 222
Mycitracin RD 803
NeoDecadron Sterile Ophthalmic Ointment 1755
NeoDecadron Sterile Ophthalmic Solution 1756
NeoDecadron Topical Cream 1757
Neosporin G.U. Irrigant Sterile 1130
Neosporin Ointment RD 821
Neosporin Plus Maximum Strength Cream RD 821
Neosporin Plus Maximum Strength Ointment RD 822
Neosporin Ophthalmic Ointment Sterile 1130
Neosporin Ophthalmic Solution Sterile 1131
Pediotic Suspension Sterile 1140
Poly-Pred Liquifilm ⊙ 246

Oxytetracycline (Parenteral administration of high dose of tetracyclines may intensify or resemble the neuroblocking action of muscle relaxant). Products include:
Terramycin Intramuscular Solution 2034

Polymyxin B Sulfate (Parenteral administration of high dose of polymyxin B may intensify or resemble the neuroblocking action of muscle relaxant). Products include:
AK-Spore ⊙ 205
AK-Trol Ointment & Suspension ⊙ 205
Betadine Brand First Aid Antibiotics & Moisturizer Ointment 2144
Cortisporin Cream 1073
Cortisporin Ointment 1074
Cortisporin Ophthalmic Ointment Sterile 1074
Cortisporin Ophthalmic Suspension Sterile 1075
Cortisporin Otic Solution Sterile 1076
Cortisporin Otic Suspension Sterile 1077
Maxitrol Ophthalmic Ointment and Suspension ⊙ 222
Mycitracin RD 803
Neosporin G.U. Irrigant Sterile 1130
Neosporin Ointment RD 821
Neosporin Plus Maximum Strength Cream RD 821
Neosporin Plus Maximum Strength Ointment RD 822
Neosporin Ophthalmic Ointment Sterile 1130
Neosporin Ophthalmic Solution Sterile 1131
Pediotic Suspension Sterile 1140
Poly-Pred Liquifilm ⊙ 246
Polysporin Ointment RD 822
Polysporin Ophthalmic Ointment Sterile 1140
Polysporin Powder RD 823
Polytrim Ophthalmic Solution Sterile 479
TERAK Ointment ⊙ 210
Terramycin with Polymyxin B Sulfate Ophthalmic Ointment 2035

Quinidine Gluconate (Administration of quinidine shortly after recovery may produce recurrent paralysis). Products include:
Quinaglute Dura-Tabs Tablets 644

Quinidine Polygalacturonate (Administration of quinidine shortly after recovery may produce recurrent paralysis). Products include:
Cardioquin Tablets 2146

Quinidine Sulfate (Administration of quinidine shortly after recovery may produce recurrent paralysis). Products include:
Quinidex Extentabs 2240

Streptomycin Sulfate (Parenteral administration of high dose of streptomycin may intensify or resemble the neuroblocking action of muscle relaxant). Products include:
Streptomycin Sulfate Injection 2031

Succinylcholine Chloride (Synergistic or antagonistic effects may result when depolarizing and nondepolarizing muscle relaxants are used simultaneously or sequentially). Products include:
Anectine 1062

MEVACOR TABLETS
(Lovastatin) 1742
May interact with erythromycin, fibrates, oral anticoagulants, and certain other agents. Compounds in these categories include:

Clofibrate (Myopathy and rhabdomyolysis have occasionally been associated with fibrates; combined use should generally be avoided). Products include:
Atromid-S Capsules 2808

Cyclosporine (Rhabdomyolysis with renal failure has been reported in a renal transplant patient receiving cyclosporine and lovastatin shortly after a dose increase in the systemic itraconazole). Products include:
Neoral 2405
Sandimmune 2416

Dicumarol (Co-administration has resulted in bleeding and/or prothrombin time in few patients).
No products indexed under this heading.

Erythromycin (Rhabdomyolysis with or without renal impairment has been reported in seriously ill patients receiving erythromycin and lovastatin). Products include:
A/T/S 2% Acne Topical Gel 1244
A/T/S 2% Acne Topical Solution 1244
Benzamycin Topical Gel 919
E-Mycin Tablets 1388
Emgel 2% Topical Gel 1081
ERYC 1972
Erycette (erythromycin 2%) Topical Solution 1943
Ery-Tab Tablets 426
Erythromycin Base Filmtab 430
Erythromycin Delayed-Release Capsules, USP 431
Ilotycin Ophthalmic Ointment 928
PCE Dispertab Tablets 453
T-Stat 2.0% Topical Solution and Pads 2797
THERAMYCIN Z 2% Solution 1629

Erythromycin Estolate (Rhabdomyolysis with or without renal impairment has been reported in seriously ill patients receiving erythromycin and lovastatin). Products include:
Ilosone 927

Erythromycin Ethylsuccinate (Rhabdomyolysis with or without renal impairment has been reported in seriously ill patients receiving erythromycin and lovastatin). Products include:
E.E.S. 427
EryPed 425
Pediazole Suspension 2340

Erythromycin Gluceptate (Rhabdomyolysis with or without renal impairment has been reported in seriously ill patients receiving erythromycin and lovastatin). Products include:
Ilotycin Gluceptate, IV, Vials 929

Erythromycin Stearate (Rhabdomyolysis with or without renal impairment has been reported in seriously ill patients receiving erythromycin and lovastatin). Products include:
Erythrocin Stearate Filmtab 429

Gemfibrozil (Combined therapy has resulted in fulminant rhabdomyolysis; possible risk of severe myopathy, rhabdomyolysis, and acute renal failure; combined use should generally be avoided). Products include:
Lopid Tablets 1974

Itraconazole (Rhabdomyolysis with renal failure has been reported in a renal transplant patient receiving cyclosporine and lovastatin shortly after a dose increase in the systemic itraconazole). Products include:
Sporanox Capsules 1352

Niacin (Combined therapy with lipid lowering doses of niacin may produce muscle weakness, pain, or tenderness; periodic CPK determinations are recommended). Products include:
Kyo-Chrome RD 680
Nicotinex Elixir RD 671
Slo-Niacin Tablets 2767

Warfarin Sodium (Co-administration has resulted in bleeding and/or prothrombin time in few patients). Products include:
Coumadin 941

Food Interactions

Alcohol (Lovastatin should be used with caution in patients who have consumed a substantial quantity of alcohol and have a past history of liver disease; active liver disease and unexplained elevation in transaminase are contraindications to the use of lovastatin).

Meal, unspecified (When lovastatin was given under fasting conditions, plasma concentrations of total inhibitors were on average about two-thirds those found when lovastatin was administered immediately after a standard meal).

MEXITIL CAPSULES
(Mexiletine Hydrochloride) 684
May interact with narcotic analgesics, xanthine bronchodilators, and certain other agents. Compounds in these categories include:

Alfentanil Hydrochloride (Narcotics have been reported to slow the absorption of mexiletine). Products include:
Alfenta Injection 1334

Aluminum Hydroxide (Magnesium-aluminum hydroxide has been reported to slow the absorption of mexiletine). Products include:
ALternaGEL Liquid 1358
Maximum Strength Ascriptin RD 650
Cama Arthritis Pain Reliever RD 748
Gaviscon Extra Strength Relief Formula Antacid Tablets RD 778
Gaviscon Extra Strength Relief Formula Liquid Antacid RD 779
Gaviscon Liquid Antacid RD 779
Gelusil Antacid-Anti-gas Liquid RD 819
Gelusil Antacid-Anti-gas Tablets RD 819
Maalox Antacid/Anti-Gas Tablets 889
Maalox Heartburn Relief Suspension RD 658
Maalox Antacid Liquid 888
Extra Strength Maalox Antacid/Anti-Gas Liquid and Tablets 888
Mylanta 1359
Tempo Soft Antacid RD 799

Aminophylline (Co-administration may lead to increased plasma theophylline levels).
No products indexed under this heading.

Atropine Sulfate (Atropine has been reported to slow the absorption of mexiletine). Products include:
Arco-Lase Plus Tablets 513
Atrohist Plus Tablets 1605
Donnatal 2234
Donnatal Extentabs 2234
Donnatal Tablets 2234
Lomotil 2591
Motofen Tablets 789
Urised Tablets 2123

Buprenorphine (Narcotics have been reported to slow the absorption of mexiletine). Products include:
Buprenex Injectable 2170

Caffeine (Co-administration leads to a decrease in caffeine clearance). Products include:
Arthritis Strength BC Powder RD 631
BC Powder RD 631
Cafergot 2376
DHCplus Capsules 2148
Darvon Compound-65 Pulvules 1475
Esgic-plus Capsules 1012
Esgic-plus Tablets 1012
Aspirin Free Excedrin Analgesic Caplets and Geltabs 734
Excedrin Extra-Strength Analgesic Tablets, Caplets, and Geltabs 734
Fioricet Tablets 2386
Fioricet with Codeine Capsules 2387
Fiorinal Capsules 2388
Fiorinal with Codeine Capsules 2390
Fiorinal Tablets 2388
Goody's Extra Strength Headache Powders RD 632
Goody's Extra Strength Pain Relief Tablets RD 632
Maximum Strength Multi-Symptom Formula Midol RD 621
No Doz Maximum Strength Caplets RD 644
Norgesic 1554
Vanquish Analgesic Caplets RD 627
Wigraine Tablets 1884

Cimetidine (Co-administration has been reported to increase, decrease, or leave unchanged mexiletine plasma levels). Products include:
Tagamet HB Tablets RD 786
Tagamet Tablets 2694

IMPORTANT NOTE: Always consult each drug listing in the patient's regimen for possible interactions.

Mexitil | **Interactions Index** | **672**

Cimetidine Hydrochloride (Co-administration has been reported to increase, decrease, or leave unchanged mexiletine plasma levels). Products include:
Tagamet 2694

Codeine Phosphate (Narcotics have been reported to slow the absorption of mexiletine). Products include:
Brontex 2130
Dimetane-DC Cough Syrup 2232
Fioricet with Codeine Capsules 2387
Fiorinal with Codeine Capsules 2390
Nucofed 2225
Phenergan with Codeine 2883
Phenergan VC with Codeine 2888
Robitussin A-C Syrup 2248
Robitussin-DAC Syrup 2249
Ryna .... ▣ 804
Soma Compound w/Codeine Tablets 2784
Tylenol with Codeine 1592

Dezocine (Narcotics have been reported to slow the absorption of mexiletine). Products include:
Dalgan Injection 529

Digoxin (Mexiletine does not alter serum digoxin levels, but magnesium-aluminum hydroxide, when used to treat gastrointestinal symptoms due to mexiletine, has been reported to lower serum digoxin levels). Products include:
Lanoxicaps 1110
Lanoxin Elixir Pediatric 1113
Lanoxin Injection 1116
Lanoxin Injection Pediatric 1119
Lanoxin Tablets 1121

Dyphylline (Co-administration may lead to increased plasma theophylline levels). Products include:
Lufyllin & Lufyllin-400 Tablets 2778
Lufyllin-GG Elixir & Tablets 2779

Fentanyl (Narcotics have been reported to slow the absorption of mexiletine). Products include:
Duragesic Transdermal System 1336

Fentanyl Citrate (Narcotics have been reported to slow the absorption of mexiletine). Products include:
Sublimaze Injection 463

Hydrocodone Bitartrate (Narcotics have been reported to slow the absorption of mexiletine). Products include:
Codiclear DH Syrup 808
Duratuss HD Elixir 2750
Histussin D Liquid 670
Hycodan Tablets and Syrup 946
Hycomine Compound Tablets 948
Hycomine 947
Hycotuss Expectorant Syrup 950
Hydrocet Capsules 787
Lorcet 10/650 Tablets 1016
Lortab 2751
Tussend 1830
Tussend Expectorant 1831
Vicodin Tablets 1404
Vicodin ES Tablets 1405
Vicodin HP Tablets 1403
Vicodin Tuss Expectorant 1406
Zydone Capsules 967

Hydrocodone Polistirex (Narcotics have been reported to slow the absorption of mexiletine). Products include:
Tussionex Pennkinetic Extended-Release Suspension 1624

Hydromorphone Hydrochloride (Narcotics have been reported to slow the absorption of mexiletine). Products include:
Dilaudid Ampules 1382
Dilaudid Cough Syrup 1383
Dilaudid-HP Injection 1384
Dilaudid-HP Lyophilized Powder 250 mg 1384
Dilaudid 1382
Dilaudid Oral Liquid 1386
Dilaudid 1382
Dilaudid Tablets - 8 mg 1386

Levorphanol Tartrate (Narcotics have been reported to slow the absorption of mexiletine). Products include:
Levo-Dromoran 2297

Magnesium Hydroxide (Magnesium-aluminum hydroxide has been reported to slow the absorption of mexiletine). Products include:
Aludrox Oral Suspension .... ▣ 850
Ascriptin .... ▣ 650
Di-Gel Antacid/Anti-Gas .... ▣ 762
Gelusil Antacid-Anti-gas Liquid .... ▣ 819
Gelusil Antacid-Anti-gas Tablets .... ▣ 819
Maalox Antacid/Anti-Gas Tablets 889
Maalox Antacid Liquid 888
Extra Strength Maalox Antacid/Anti-Gas Liquid and Tablets 888
Mylanta Fast-Acting 1359
Mylanta Gelcaps Antacid .... ▣ 678
Fast-Acting Mylanta Liquid Antacid 1359
Mylanta Tablets .... ▣ 677
Maximum-Strength Fast-Acting Mylanta Liquid Antacid 1359
Mylanta Double Strength Tablets .. ▣ 677
Phillips' Milk of Magnesia Liquid .... ▣ 627
Rolaids Antacid Tablets .... ▣ 807
Tempo Soft Antacid .... ▣ 799

Meperidine Hydrochloride (Narcotics have been reported to slow the absorption of mexiletine). Products include:
Demerol 2438
Mepergan Injection 2859

Methadone Hydrochloride (Narcotics have been reported to slow the absorption of mexiletine). Products include:
Methadone Hydrochloride Oral Concentrate 2356
Methadone Hydrochloride Oral Solution & Tablets 2357

Morphine Sulfate (Narcotics have been reported to slow the absorption of mexiletine). Products include:
Astramorph/PF Injection, USP (Preservative-Free) 526
Duramorph Injection 983
Infumorph 200 and Infumorph 500 Sterile Solutions 985
Kadian Capsules 2948
MS Contin Tablets 2149
MSIR 2152
Oramorph SR (Morphine Sulfate Sustained Release Tablets) 2359
RMS Suppositories CII 2766
Roxanol 2365

Opium Alkaloids (Narcotics have been reported to slow the absorption of mexiletine).
No products indexed under this heading.

Oxycodone Hydrochloride (Narcotics have been reported to slow the absorption of mexiletine). Products include:
OxyContin Tablets 2163
OxyIR Capsules 2167
Percocet Tablets 955
Percodan Tablets 955
Percodan-Demi Tablets 956
Roxicodone Tablets, Oral Solution & Intensol (Oxycodone) 2366
Tylox Capsules 1593

Phenobarbital (Co-administration with hepatic enzyme inducers, such as phenobarbital, results in lowered mexiletine). Products include:
Arco-Lase Plus Tablets 513
Bellergal-S Tablets 2375
Donnatal 2234
Donnatal Extentabs 2234
Donnatal Tablets 2234
Phenobarbital Elixir and Tablets 1523
Quadrinal Tablets 1398

Phenytoin (Co-administration with hepatic enzyme inducers, such as phenytoin, results in lowered mexiletine). Products include:
Dilantin Infatabs 1967
Dilantin-125 Suspension 1969

Phenytoin Sodium (Co-administration with hepatic enzyme inducers, such as phenytoin, results in lowered mexiletine). Products include:
Dilantin Kapseals 1965

Propoxyphene Hydrochloride (Narcotics have been reported to slow the absorption of mexiletine). Products include:
Darvon 1475
Wygesic Tablets 2930

Propoxyphene Napsylate (Narcotics have been reported to slow the absorption of mexiletine). Products include:
Darvon-N/Darvocet-N 1473

Rifampin (Co-administration with hepatic enzyme inducers, such as rifampin, results in lowered mexiletine). Products include:
Rifadin 1276
Rifamate Capsules 1278
Rifater 1280
Rimactane Capsules 865

Sufentanil Citrate (Narcotics have been reported to slow the absorption of mexiletine). Products include:
Sufenta Injection 1355

Theophylline (Co-administration may lead to increased plasma theophylline levels). Products include:
Marax Tablets & DF Syrup 2015
Quibron 2227

Theophylline Anhydrous (Co-administration may lead to increased plasma theophylline levels). Products include:
Aerolate 1003
Primatene Tablets .... ▣ 844
Respbid Tablets 687
Slo-bid Gyrocaps 2201
Theo-24 Extended Release Capsules 2753
Theo-Dur Extended-Release Tablets 1367
Theo-X Extended-Release Tablets .. 793
Uni-Dur Extended-Release Tablets .. 1374
Uniphyl 400 mg and 600 mg Tablets 2157

Theophylline Calcium Salicylate (Co-administration may lead to increased plasma theophylline levels). Products include:
Quadrinal Tablets 1398

Theophylline Sodium Glycinate (Co-administration may lead to increased plasma theophylline levels).
No products indexed under this heading.

MEZLIN
(Mezlocillin Sodium) 594
May interact with aminoglycosides and certain other agents. Compounds in these categories include:

Amikacin Sulfate (Physical incompatibility resulting in substantial inactivation of the aminoglycoside). Products include:
Amikacin Sulfate Injection, USP 523
Amikacin Sulfate Injection, USP 981
Amikin Injectable 502

Gentamicin Sulfate (Physical incompatibility resulting in substantial inactivation of the aminoglycoside). Products include:
Garamycin Cream 0.1% 2501
Garamycin Injectable 2502
Garamycin Ointment 0.1% 2501
Garamycin Ophthalmic 2501
Genoptic Sterile Ophthalmic Solution .... ◎ 241
Genoptic Sterile Ophthalmic Ointment .... ◎ 241
Gentak .... ◎ 209
Pred-G Liquifilm Sterile Ophthalmic Suspension .... ◎ 248
Pred-G S.O.P. Sterile Ophthalmic Ointment .... ◎ 249

Kanamycin Sulfate (Physical incompatibility resulting in substantial inactivation of the aminoglycoside).
No products indexed under this heading.

Probenecid (Increased serum concentrations and prolonged serum half-life of mezlocillin). Products include:
Benemid Tablets 1651
ColBENEMID Tablets 1662

Streptomycin Sulfate (Physical incompatibility resulting in substantial inactivation of the aminoglycoside). Products include:
Streptomycin Sulfate Injection 2031

Tobramycin Sulfate (Physical incompatibility resulting in substantial inactivation of the aminoglycoside). Products include:
Nebcin Vials, Hyporets & ADD-Vantage 1518

MEZLIN PHARMACY BULK PACKAGE
(Mezlocillin Sodium) 597
May interact with:

Probenecid (Prolongs serum half-life of antibiotic). Products include:
Benemid Tablets 1651
ColBENEMID Tablets 1662

MG 217 MEDICATED TAR SHAMPOO
(Coal Tar) .... ▣ 800
None cited in PDR database.

MG 217 MEDICATED TAR-FREE SHAMPOO
(Sulfur, Salicylic Acid) .... ▣ 800
None cited in PDR database.

MG 217 PSORIASIS OINTMENT AND LOTION
(Coal Tar) .... ▣ 800
None cited in PDR database.

MG 217 SAL-ACID OINTMENT
(Salicylic Acid) .... ▣ 800
None cited in PDR database.

MIACALCIN INJECTION
(Calcitonin, Synthetic) 2402
None cited in PDR database.

MIACALCIN NASAL SPRAY
(Calcitonin-Salmon) 2403
May interact with:

Etidronate Disodium (Diphosphonate) (Prior diphosphonate use may reduce the anti-resorptive response to calcitonin-salmon nasal spray).

Pamidronate Disodium (Prior diphosphonate use may reduce the anti-resorptive response to calcitonin-salmon nasal spray). Products include:
Aredia for Injection 827

MICRO-K EXTENCAPS
(Potassium Chloride) 2237
May interact with potassium sparing diuretics, ACE inhibitors, and anticholinergics. Compounds in these categories include:

Amiloride Hydrochloride (Simultaneous administration can produce severe hyperkalemia). Products include:
Midamor Tablets 1746
Moduretic Tablets 1748

(▣ Described in PDR For Nonprescription Drugs) (◎ Described in PDR For Ophthalmology)

Atropine Sulfate (Anticholinergic drugs can be cause for delay or arrest in tablet passage through the gastrointestinal tract; concomitant administration of drugs capable of decreasing GI motility should be avoided). Products include:
Arco-Lase Plus Tablets 513
Atrohist Plus Tablets 1605
Donnatal 2234
Donnatal Extentabs 2234
Donnatal Tablets 2234
Lomotil 2591
Motofen Tablets 789
Urised Tablets 2123

Belladonna Alkaloids (Anticholinergic drugs can be cause for delay or arrest in tablet passage through the gastrointestinal tract; concomitant administration of drugs capable of decreasing GI motility should be avoided). Products include:
Bellergal-S Tablets 2375
Hyland's Bedwetting Tablets 788
Hyland's EnurAid Tablets 789
Hyland's Headache Tablets 790
Hyland's Teething Tablets 790
Similasan Eye Drops #1 769

Benazepril Hydrochloride (Potential for hyperkalemia). Products include:
Lotensin Tablets 852
Lotensin HCT Tablets 855
Lotrel Capsules 858

Benztropine Mesylate (Anticholinergic drugs can be cause for delay or arrest in tablet passage through the gastrointestinal tract; concomitant administration of drugs capable of decreasing GI motility should be avoided). Products include:
Cogentin 1661

Biperiden Hydrochloride (Anticholinergic drugs can be cause for delay or arrest in tablet passage through the gastrointestinal tract; concomitant administration of drugs capable of decreasing GI motility should be avoided). Products include:
Akineton 1380

Captopril (Potential for hyperkalemia). Products include:
Capoten Tablets 740
Capozide Tablets 744

Clidinium Bromide (Anticholinergic drugs can be cause for delay or arrest in tablet passage through the gastrointestinal tract; concomitant administration of drugs capable of decreasing GI motility should be avoided). Products include:
Librax Capsules 2330

Dicyclomine Hydrochloride (Anticholinergic drugs can be cause for delay or arrest in tablet passage through the gastrointestinal tract; concomitant administration of drugs capable of decreasing GI motility should be avoided). Products include:
Bentyl 1246

Enalapril Maleate (Potential for hyperkalemia). Products include:
Vaseretic Tablets 1810
Vasotec Tablets 1816

Enalaprilat (Potential for hyperkalemia). Products include:
Vasotec I.V. 1814

Fosinopril Sodium (Potential for hyperkalemia). Products include:
Monopril Tablets 762

Glycopyrrolate (Anticholinergic drugs can be cause for delay or arrest in tablet passage through the gastrointestinal tract; concomitant administration of drugs capable of decreasing GI motility should be avoided). Products include:
Robinul Forte Tablets 2247
Robinul Injectable 2247
Robinul Tablets 2247

Hyoscyamine (Anticholinergic drugs can be cause for delay or arrest in tablet passage through the gastrointestinal tract; concomitant administration of drugs capable of decreasing GI motility should be avoided). Products include:
Cystospaz Tablets 2123
Urised Tablets 2123

Hyoscyamine Sulfate (Anticholinergic drugs can be cause for delay or arrest in tablet passage through the gastrointestinal tract; concomitant administration of drugs capable of decreasing GI motility should be avoided). Products include:
Arco-Lase Plus Tablets 513
Atrohist Plus Tablets 1605
Cystospaz-M Capsules 2123
Donnatal 2234
Donnatal Extentabs 2234
Donnatal Tablets 2234
Kutrase Capsules 2546
Levsin/Levsinex/Levbid 2549

Ipratropium Bromide (Anticholinergic drugs can be cause for delay or arrest in tablet passage through the gastrointestinal tract; concomitant administration of drugs capable of decreasing GI motility should be avoided). Products include:
Atrovent Inhalation Aerosol 674
Atrovent Inhalation Solution 675
Atrovent Nasal Spray 0.03% 676
Atrovent Nasal Spray 0.06% 678

Lisinopril (Potential for hyperkalemia). Products include:
Prinivil Tablets 1776
Prinzide Tablets 1780
Zestoretic Tablets 2968
Zestril Tablets 2972

Mepenzolate Bromide (Anticholinergic drugs can be cause for delay or arrest in tablet passage through the gastrointestinal tract; concomitant administration of drugs capable of decreasing GI motility should be avoided).
No products indexed under this heading.

Moexipril Hydrochloride (Potential for hyperkalemia). Products include:
Univasc Tablets 2553

Oxybutynin Chloride (Anticholinergic drugs can be cause for delay or arrest in tablet passage through the gastrointestinal tract; concomitant administration of drugs capable of decreasing GI motility should be avoided). Products include:
Ditropan 1267

Procyclidine Hydrochloride (Anticholinergic drugs can be cause for delay or arrest in tablet passage through the gastrointestinal tract; concomitant administration of drugs capable of decreasing GI motility should be avoided). Products include:
Kemadrin Tablets 1105

Propantheline Bromide (Anticholinergic drugs can be cause for delay or arrest in tablet passage through the gastrointestinal tract; concomitant administration of drugs capable of decreasing GI motility should be avoided). Products include:
Pro-Banthine Tablets 2226

Quinapril Hydrochloride (Potential for hyperkalemia). Products include:
Accupril Tablets 1950

Ramipril (Potential for hyperkalemia). Products include:
Altace Capsules 1238

Scopolamine (Anticholinergic drugs can be cause for delay or arrest in tablet passage through the gastrointestinal tract; concomitant administration of drugs capable of decreasing GI motility should be avoided). Products include:
Transderm Scōp Transdermal Therapeutic System 890

Scopolamine Hydrobromide (Anticholinergic drugs can be cause for delay or arrest in tablet passage through the gastrointestinal tract; concomitant administration of drugs capable of decreasing GI motility should be avoided). Products include:
Atrohist Plus Tablets 1605
Donnatal 2234
Donnatal Extentabs 2234
Donnatal Tablets 2234

Spirapril Hydrochloride (Potential for hyperkalemia).
No products indexed under this heading.

Spironolactone (Simultaneous administration can produce severe hyperkalemia). Products include:
Aldactazide Tablets 2556
Aldactone Tablets 2558

Trandolapril (Potential for hyperkalemia). Products include:
Mavik Tablets 1407

Triamterene (Simultaneous administration can produce severe hyperkalemia). Products include:
Dyazide Capsules 2653
Dyrenium Capsules 2655

Tridihexethyl Chloride (Anticholinergic drugs can be cause for delay or arrest in tablet passage through the gastrointestinal tract; concomitant administration of drugs capable of decreasing GI motility should be avoided).
No products indexed under this heading.

Trihexyphenidyl Hydrochloride (Anticholinergic drugs can be cause for delay or arrest in tablet passage through the gastrointestinal tract; concomitant administration of drugs capable of decreasing GI motility should be avoided). Products include:
Artane 1418

MICRO-K 10 EXTENCAPS
(Potassium Chloride) 2237
See Micro-K Extencaps

MICRO-K LS PACKETS
(Potassium Chloride) 2238
May interact with potassium sparing diuretics, anticholinergics, and ACE inhibitors. Compounds in these categories include:

Amiloride Hydrochloride (Co-administration of these agents can produce severe hyperkalemia; concurrent use is not recommended). Products include:
Midamor Tablets 1746
Moduretic Tablets 1748

Atropine Sulfate (Concurrent use with anticholinergic drugs or other agents with anticholinergic properties at sufficient doses to exert anticholinergic effects is contraindicated). Products include:
Arco-Lase Plus Tablets 513

Atrohist Plus Tablets 1605
Donnatal 2234
Donnatal Extentabs 2234
Donnatal Tablets 2234
Lomotil 2591
Motofen Tablets 789
Urised Tablets 2123

Belladonna Alkaloids (Concurrent use with anticholinergic drugs or other agents with anticholinergic properties at sufficient doses to exert anticholinergic effects is contraindicated). Products include:
Bellergal-S Tablets 2375
Hyland's Bedwetting Tablets 788
Hyland's EnurAid Tablets 789
Hyland's Headache Tablets 790
Hyland's Teething Tablets 790
Similasan Eye Drops #1 769

Benazepril Hydrochloride (Potential for hyperkalemia). Products include:
Lotensin Tablets 852
Lotensin HCT Tablets 855
Lotrel Capsules 858

Benztropine Mesylate (Concurrent use with anticholinergic drugs or other agents with anticholinergic properties at sufficient doses to exert anticholinergic effects is contraindicated). Products include:
Cogentin 1661

Biperiden Hydrochloride (Concurrent use with anticholinergic drugs or other agents with anticholinergic properties at sufficient doses to exert anticholinergic effects is contraindicated). Products include:
Akineton 1380

Captopril (Potential for hyperkalemia). Products include:
Capoten Tablets 740
Capozide Tablets 744

Clidinium Bromide (Concurrent use with anticholinergic drugs or other agents with anticholinergic properties at sufficient doses to exert anticholinergic effects is contraindicated). Products include:
Librax Capsules 2330

Dicyclomine Hydrochloride (Concurrent use with anticholinergic drugs or other agents with anticholinergic properties at sufficient doses to exert anticholinergic effects is contraindicated). Products include:
Bentyl 1246

Enalapril Maleate (Potential for hyperkalemia). Products include:
Vaseretic Tablets 1810
Vasotec Tablets 1816

Enalaprilat (Potential for hyperkalemia). Products include:
Vasotec I.V. 1814

Fosinopril Sodium (Potential for hyperkalemia). Products include:
Monopril Tablets 762

Glycopyrrolate (Concurrent use with anticholinergic drugs or other agents with anticholinergic properties at sufficient doses to exert anticholinergic effects is contraindicated). Products include:
Robinul Forte Tablets 2247
Robinul Injectable 2247
Robinul Tablets 2247

Hyoscyamine (Concurrent use with anticholinergic drugs or other agents with anticholinergic properties at sufficient doses to exert anticholinergic effects is contraindicated). Products include:
Cystospaz Tablets 2123
Urised Tablets 2123

IMPORTANT NOTE: Always consult each drug listing in the patient's regimen for possible interactions.

Interactions Index

Hyoscyamine Sulfate (Concurrent use with anticholinergic drugs or other agents with anticholinergic properties at sufficient doses to exert anticholinergic effects is contraindicated). Products include:

Arco-Lase Plus Tablets	513
Atrohist Plus Tablets	1605
Cystospaz-M Capsules	2123
Donnatal	2234
Donnatal Extentabs	2234
Donnatal Tablets	2234
Kutrase Capsules	2546
Levsin/Levsinex/Levbid	2549

Ipratropium Bromide (Concurrent use with anticholinergic drugs or other agents with anticholinergic properties at sufficient doses to exert anticholinergic effects is contraindicated). Products include:

Atrovent Inhalation Aerosol	674
Atrovent Inhalation Solution	675
Atrovent Nasal Spray 0.03%	676
Atrovent Nasal Spray 0.06%	678

Lisinopril (Potential for hyperkalemia). Products include:

Prinivil Tablets	1776
Prinzide Tablets	1780
Zestoretic Tablets	2968
Zestril Tablets	2972

Mepenzolate Bromide (Concurrent use with anticholinergic drugs or other agents with anticholinergic properties at sufficient doses to exert anticholinergic effects is contraindicated).

No products indexed under this heading.

Moexipril Hydrochloride (Potential for hyperkalemia). Products include:

Univasc Tablets	2553

Oxybutynin Chloride (Concurrent use with anticholinergic drugs or other agents with anticholinergic properties at sufficient doses to exert anticholinergic effects is contraindicated). Products include:

Ditropan	1267

Procyclidine Hydrochloride (Concurrent use with anticholinergic drugs or other agents with anticholinergic properties at sufficient doses to exert anticholinergic effects is contraindicated). Products include:

Kemadrin Tablets	1105

Propantheline Bromide (Concurrent use with anticholinergic drugs or other agents with anticholinergic properties at sufficient doses to exert anticholinergic effects is contraindicated). Products include:

Pro-Banthine Tablets	2226

Quinapril Hydrochloride (Potential for hyperkalemia). Products include:

Accupril Tablets	1950

Ramipril (Potential for hyperkalemia). Products include:

Altace Capsules	1238

Scopolamine (Concurrent use with anticholinergic drugs or other agents with anticholinergic properties at sufficient doses to exert anticholinergic effects is contraindicated). Products include:

Transderm Scōp Transdermal Therapeutic System	890

Scopolamine Hydrobromide (Concurrent use with anticholinergic drugs or other agents with anticholinergic properties at sufficient doses to exert anticholinergic effects is contraindicated). Products include:

Atrohist Plus Tablets	1605
Donnatal	2234
Donnatal Extentabs	2234
Donnatal Tablets	2234

Spirapril Hydrochloride (Potential for hyperkalemia).

No products indexed under this heading.

Spironolactone (Co-administration of these agents can produce severe hyperkalemia; concurrent use is not recommended). Products include:

Aldactazide Tablets	2556
Aldactone Tablets	2558

Trandolapril (Potential for hyperkalemia). Products include:

Mavik Tablets	1407

Triamterene (Co-administration of these agents can produce severe hyperkalemia; concurrent use is not recommended). Products include:

Dyazide Capsules	2653
Dyrenium Capsules	2655

Tridihexethyl Chloride (Concurrent use with anticholinergic drugs or other agents with anticholinergic properties at sufficient doses to exert anticholinergic effects is contraindicated).

No products indexed under this heading.

Trihexyphenidyl Hydrochloride (Concurrent use with anticholinergic drugs or other agents with anticholinergic properties at sufficient doses to exert anticholinergic effects is contraindicated). Products include:

Artane	1418

MICRONASE TABLETS
(Glyburide) 2099

May interact with beta blockers, salicylates, non-steroidal anti-inflammatory agents, sulfonamides, oral anticoagulants, monoamine oxidase inhibitors, diuretics, thiazides, corticosteroids, phenothiazines, thyroid preparations, oral contraceptives, estrogens, calcium channel blockers, sympathomimetics, highly protein bound drugs (selected), and certain other agents. Compounds in these categories include:

Acebutolol Hydrochloride (Co-administration with beta blockers may result in hypoglycemia). Products include:

Sectral Capsules	2914

Albuterol (Sympathomimetics tend to produce hyperglycemia and concurrent use may lead to loss of control). Products include:

Proventil Inhalation Aerosol	2524
Ventolin Inhalation Aerosol and Refill	1170

Albuterol Sulfate (Sympathomimetics tend to produce hyperglycemia and concurrent use may lead to loss of control). Products include:

Airet Albuterol Sulfate Inhalation Solution	1602
Albuterol Sulfate, USP Solution for Inhalation, Arm-a-Med	522
Proventil Inhalation Solution 0.083%	2527
Proventil Repetabs Tablets	2529
Proventil Solution for Inhalation 0.5%	2525
Proventil Syrup	2528
Proventil Tablets	2529
Ventolin Inhalation Solution	1171
Ventolin Nebules Inhalation Solution	1172
Ventolin Rotacaps for Inhalation	1173
Ventolin Syrup	1175
Ventolin Tablets	1176
Volmax Extended-Release Tablets	1835

Amiloride Hydrochloride (Diuretics tend to produce hyperglycemia and concurrent use may lead to loss of control). Products include:

Midamor Tablets	1746
Moduretic Tablets	1748

Amiodarone Hydrochloride (Co-administration with drugs that are highly protein bound may result in hypoglycemia). Products include:

Cordarone Intravenous	2821
Cordarone Tablets	2818

Amitriptyline Hydrochloride (Co-administration with drugs that are highly protein bound may result in hypoglycemia). Products include:

Elavil	2945
Etrafon	2495
Limbitrol	2333
Triavil Tablets	1800

Amlodipine Besylate (Calcium channel blockers tend to produce hyperglycemia and concurrent use may lead to loss of control). Products include:

Lotrel Capsules	858
Norvasc Tablets	2020

Aspirin (Co-administration with salicylates may result in hypoglycemia). Products include:

Alka-Seltzer Cherry Effervescent Antacid and Pain Reliever	■□ 609
Alka-Seltzer Extra Strength Effervescent Antacid and Pain Reliever	■□ 609
Alka-Seltzer Lemon Lime Effervescent Antacid and Pain Reliever	■□ 609
Alka-Seltzer Original Effervescent Antacid and Pain Reliever	■□ 609
Alka-Seltzer Plus	■□ 611
Alka-Seltzer Plus Sinus Medicine	■□ 611
Ascriptin	■□ 650
Arthritis Strength BC Powder	■□ 631
BC Cold Powder Multi-Symptom Formula (Cold-Sinus-Allergy)	■□ 631
BC Cold Powder Non-Drowsy Formula (Cold-Sinus)	■□ 631
BC Powder	■□ 631
Genuine Bayer Aspirin Tablets & Caplets	■□ 618
Extra Strength Bayer Arthritis Pain Regimen Formula	■□ 615
Extra Strength Bayer Aspirin Caplets & Tablets	■□ 617
Extended-Release Bayer 8-Hour Aspirin	■□ 616
Extra Strength Bayer Plus Aspirin Caplets	■□ 617
Extra Strength Bayer PM Aspirin Plus Sleep Aid	■□ 617
Aspirin Regimen Bayer 81 mg Tablets with Calcium	■□ 615
Aspirin Regimen Bayer Adult Low Strength 81 mg Tablets	■□ 613
Aspirin Regimen Bayer Children's Chewable Aspirin	■□ 616
Aspirin Regimen Bayer Regular Strength 325 mg Caplets	■□ 613
Bufferin Analgesic Tablets	■□ 636
Arthritis Strength Bufferin Analgesic Caplets	■□ 637
Extra Strength Bufferin Analgesic Tablets	■□ 637
Cama Arthritis Pain Reliever	■□ 748
Darvon Compound-65 Pulvules	1475
Easprin	1971
Ecotrin	2625
Ecotrin Enteric Coated Aspirin Maximum Strength Tablets and Caplets	■□ 775
Ecotrin Enteric Coated Aspirin Regular Strength Tablets	2625
Empirin Aspirin Tablets	■□ 818
Excedrin Extra-Strength Analgesic Tablets, Caplets, and Geltabs	734
Fiorinal Capsules	2388
Fiorinal with Codeine Capsules	2390
Fiorinal Tablets	2388
Goody's Extra Strength Headache Powders	■□ 632
Goody's Extra Strength Pain Relief Tablets	■□ 632
Halfprin Tablets	1413
Norgesic	1554
Percodan Tablets	955
Percodan-Demi Tablets	956
Robaxisal Tablets	2246
Soma Compound w/Codeine Tablets	2784
Soma Compound Tablets	2783
St. Joseph Adult Chewable Aspirin (81 mg.)	■□ 768
Talwin Compound	2466
Vanquish Analgesic Caplets	■□ 627

Atenolol (Co-administration with beta blockers may result in hypoglycemia). Products include:

Tenoretic Tablets	2963
Tenormin Tablets and I.V. Injection	2965

Atovaquone (Co-administration with drugs that are highly protein bound may result in hypoglycemia). Products include:

Mepron Suspension	1206

Bendroflumethiazide (Thiazides tend to produce hyperglycemia and concurrent use may lead to loss of control).

No products indexed under this heading.

Bepridil Hydrochloride (Calcium channel blockers tend to produce hyperglycemia and concurrent use may lead to loss of control). Products include:

Vascor Tablets (200 and 300 mg)	1597

Betamethasone Acetate (Corticosteroids tend to produce hyperglycemia and concurrent use may lead to loss of control). Products include:

Celestone Soluspan Suspension	2484

Betamethasone Sodium Phosphate (Corticosteroids tend to produce hyperglycemia and concurrent use may lead to loss of control). Products include:

Celestone Soluspan Suspension	2484

Betaxolol Hydrochloride (Co-administration with beta blockers may result in hypoglycemia). Products include:

Betoptic Ophthalmic Solution	465
Betoptic S Ophthalmic Suspension	467
Kerlone Tablets	2588

Bisoprolol Fumarate (Co-administration with beta blockers may result in hypoglycemia). Products include:

Zebeta Tablets	1457
Ziac	1459

Bumetanide (Diuretics tend to produce hyperglycemia and concurrent use may lead to loss of control). Products include:

Bumex	2260

Carteolol Hydrochloride (Co-administration with beta blockers may result in hypoglycemia). Products include:

Cartrol Tablets	413
Ocupress Ophthalmic Solution, 1% Sterile	◉ 297

Cefonicid Sodium (Co-administration with drugs that are highly protein bound may result in hypoglycemia). Products include:

Monocid Injection	2674

Chloramphenicol Palmitate (Co-administration with chloramphenicol may result in hypoglycemia).

No products indexed under this heading.

Chloramphenicol Sodium Succinate (Co-administration with chloramphenicol may result in hypoglycemia). Products include:

Chloromycetin Sodium Succinate	1960

Chlordiazepoxide (Co-administration with drugs that are highly protein bound may result in hypoglycemia). Products include:

Limbitrol	2333

Chlordiazepoxide Hydrochloride (Co-administration with drugs that are highly protein bound may result in hypoglycemia). Products include:

Librax Capsules	2330
Librium Capsules	2331
Librium Injectable	2332

(■□ Described in PDR For Nonprescription Drugs)   (◉ Described in PDR For Ophthalmology)

675 **Interactions Index** **Micronase**

Chlorothiazide (Thiazides tend to produce hyperglycemia and concurrent use may lead to loss of control). Products include:
Aldoclor Tablets ... 1638
Diupres Tablets ... 1691
Diuril Oral ... 1694

Chlorothiazide Sodium (Thiazides tend to produce hyperglycemia and concurrent use may lead to loss of control). Products include:
Diuril Sodium Intravenous ... 1693

Chlorotrianisene (Estrogens tend to produce hyperglycemia and concurrent use may lead to loss of control).
No products indexed under this heading.

Chlorpromazine (Phenothiazines tend to produce hyperglycemia and concurrent use may lead to loss of control). Products include:
Thorazine Suppositories ... 2701

Chlorpromazine Hydrochloride (Phenothiazines tend to produce hyperglycemia and concurrent use may lead to loss of control). Products include:
Thorazine ... 2701

Chlorpropamide (Co-administration with sulfonamides may result in hypoglycemia). Products include:
Diabinese Tablets ... 2002

Chlorthalidone (Diuretics tend to produce hyperglycemia and concurrent use may lead to loss of control). Products include:
Combipres Tablets ... 682
Tenoretic Tablets ... 2963
Thalitone ... 1293

Choline Magnesium Trisalicylate (Co-administration with salicylates may result in hypoglycemia). Products include:
Trilisate ... 2155

Ciprofloxacin (Co-administration has resulted in a potentiation of the hypoglycemic action of glyburide). Products include:
Cipro I.V. ... 587
Cipro I.V. Pharmacy Bulk Package ... 590

Ciprofloxacin Hydrochloride (Co-administration has resulted in a potentiation of the hypoglycemic action of glyburide). Products include:
Ciloxan Ophthalmic Solution ... 468
Cipro Tablets ... 584

Clomipramine Hydrochloride (Co-administration with drugs that are highly protein bound may result in hypoglycemia). Products include:
Anafranil Capsules ... 819

Clozapine (Co-administration with drugs that are highly protein bound may result in hypoglycemia). Products include:
Clozaril Tablets ... 2377

Cortisone Acetate (Corticosteroids tend to produce hyperglycemia and concurrent use may lead to loss of control). Products include:
Cortone Acetate Sterile Suspension ... 1663
Cortone Acetate Tablets ... 1664

Cyclosporine (Co-administration with drugs that are highly protein bound may result in hypoglycemia). Products include:
Neoral ... 2405
Sandimmune ... 2416

Desogestrel (Oral contraceptives tend to produce hyperglycemia and concurrent use may lead to loss of control). Products include:
Desogen Tablets ... 1867
Ortho-Cept ... 1907

Dexamethasone (Corticosteroids tend to produce hyperglycemia and concurrent use may lead to loss of control). Products include:
AK-Trol Ointment & Suspension ... ⊛ 205
Decadron Elixir ... 1676
Decadron Tablets ... 1678
Decaspray Topical Aerosol ... 1689
Maxitrol Ophthalmic Ointment and Suspension ... ⊛ 222
TobraDex Ophthalmic Suspension and Ointment ... 469

Dexamethasone Acetate (Corticosteroids tend to produce hyperglycemia and concurrent use may lead to loss of control). Products include:
Dalalone D.P. Injectable ... 1009
Decadron-LA Sterile Suspension ... 1687

Dexamethasone Sodium Phosphate (Corticosteroids tend to produce hyperglycemia and concurrent use may lead to loss of control). Products include:
Decadron Phosphate Injection ... 1680
Decadron Phosphate Sterile Ophthalmic Ointment ... 1684
Decadron Phosphate Sterile Ophthalmic Solution ... 1685
Decadron Phosphate Topical Cream ... 1686
Decadron Phosphate with Xylocaine Injection, Sterile ... 1683
Dexacort Phosphate in Respihaler .. 1606
Dexacort Phosphate in Turbinaire .. 1607
NeoDecadron Sterile Ophthalmic Ointment ... 1755
NeoDecadron Sterile Ophthalmic Solution ... 1756
NeoDecadron Topical Cream ... 1757

Diazepam (Co-administration with drugs that are highly protein bound may result in hypoglycemia). Products include:
Dizac (diazepam injectable emulsion) CIV ... 1862
Valium Injectable ... 2336
Valium Tablets ... 2335

Diclofenac Potassium (Co-administration with nonsteroidal anti-inflammatory agents may result in hypoglycemia). Products include:
Cataflam Tablets ... 833

Diclofenac Sodium (Co-administration with nonsteroidal anti-inflammatory agents may result in hypoglycemia). Products include:
Voltaren Ophthalmic Sterile Ophthalmic Solution ... ⊛ 264
Cataflam/Voltaren/Voltaren-XR ... 833

Dicumarol (Co-administration with coumarins may result in hypoglycemia).
No products indexed under this heading.

Dienestrol (Estrogens tend to produce hyperglycemia and concurrent use may lead to loss of control). Products include:
Ortho Dienestrol Cream ... 1922

Diethylstilbestrol (Estrogens tend to produce hyperglycemia and concurrent use may lead to loss of control). Products include:
Diethylstilbestrol Tablets ... 1477

Diflunisal (Co-administration with salicylates may result in hypoglycemia). Products include:
Dolobid Tablets ... 1695

Diltiazem Hydrochloride (Calcium channel blockers tend to produce hyperglycemia and concurrent use may lead to loss of control). Products include:
Cardizem CD Capsules ... 1251
Cardizem SR Capsules ... 1255
Cardizem Injectable ... 1253
Cardizem Tablets ... 1257
Dilacor XR Extended-release Capsules ... 2183
Tiazac Capsules ... 1019

Dipyridamole (Co-administration with drugs that are highly protein bound may result in hypoglycemia). Products include:
Persantine Tablets ... 686

Dobutamine Hydrochloride (Sympathomimetics tend to produce hyperglycemia and concurrent use may lead to loss of control). Products include:
Dobutrex Solution Vials ... 1480

Dopamine Hydrochloride (Sympathomimetics tend to produce hyperglycemia and concurrent use may lead to loss of control).
No products indexed under this heading.

Ephedrine Hydrochloride (Sympathomimetics tend to produce hyperglycemia and concurrent use may lead to loss of control). Products include:
Primatene Tablets ... [PD] 844
Quadrinal Tablets ... 1398

Ephedrine Sulfate (Sympathomimetics tend to produce hyperglycemia and concurrent use may lead to loss of control). Products include:
Marax Tablets & DF Syrup ... 2015

Ephedrine Tannate (Sympathomimetics tend to produce hyperglycemia and concurrent use may lead to loss of control). Products include:
Rynatuss ... 2782

Epinephrine (Sympathomimetics tend to produce hyperglycemia and concurrent use may lead to loss of control). Products include:
EPIFRIN ... ⊛ 237
EpiPen ... 808
Marcaine with Epinephrine ... 2446
Primatene Mist ... [PD] 843
Sensorcaine with Epinephrine Injection ... 554
Sus-Phrine Injection ... 1017
Xylocaine with Epinephrine Injections ... 562

Epinephrine Bitartrate (Sympathomimetics tend to produce hyperglycemia and concurrent use may lead to loss of control). Products include:
Sensorcaine-MPF with Epinephrine Injection ... 554

Epinephrine Hydrochloride (Sympathomimetics tend to produce hyperglycemia and concurrent use may lead to loss of control). Products include:
Ana-Kit Anaphylaxis Emergency Treatment Kit ... 611

Esmolol Hydrochloride (Co-administration with beta blockers may result in hypoglycemia). Products include:
Brevibloc (esmolol HCl) Injection ... 1860

Estradiol (Estrogens tend to produce hyperglycemia and concurrent use may lead to loss of control). Products include:
Climara Transdermal System ... 640
Estrace Cream and Tablets ... 751
Estraderm Transdermal System ... 842
Estring Vaginal Ring ... 2086
Vivelle Transdermal System ... 880

Estrogens, Conjugated (Estrogens tend to produce hyperglycemia and concurrent use may lead to loss of control). Products include:
PMB 200 and PMB 400 ... 2890
Premarin Intravenous ... 2893
Premarin Tablets ... 2896
Premarin Vaginal Cream ... 2898
Premphase ... 2900
Prempro ... 2905

Estrogens, Esterified (Estrogens tend to produce hyperglycemia and concurrent use may lead to loss of control). Products include:
ESTRATAB Tablets (0.3, 0.625, 1.25, 2.5 mg) ... 2715
Estratest ... 2718
Menest Tablets ... 2671

Estropipate (Estrogens tend to produce hyperglycemia and concurrent use may lead to loss of control). Products include:
Ogen Tablets ... 2103
Ogen Vaginal Cream ... 2106
Ortho-Est ... 1925

Ethacrynic Acid (Diuretics tend to produce hyperglycemia and concurrent use may lead to loss of control). Products include:
Edecrin Tablets ... 1698

Ethinyl Estradiol (Estrogens tend to produce hyperglycemia and concurrent use may lead to loss of control). Products include:
Brevicon ... 2563
Demulen ... 2580
Desogen Tablets ... 1867
Levlen/Tri-Levlen ... 646
Lo/Ovral Tablets ... 2852
Lo/Ovral-28 Tablets ... 2857
Modicon ... 1928
Nordette-21 Tablets ... 2863
Nordette-28 Tablets ... 2866
Norinyl ... 2563
Ortho-Cept ... 1907
Ortho-Cyclen/Ortho-Tri-Cyclen ... 1914
Ortho-Novum ... 1928
Ortho-Cyclen/Ortho Tri-Cyclen ... 1914
Ovcon ... 765
Ovral Tablets ... 2877
Ovral-28 Tablets ... 2878
Levlen/Tri-Levlen ... 646
Tri-Norinyl ... 2607
Triphasil-21 Tablets ... 2919
Triphasil-28 Tablets ... 2924

Ethynodiol Diacetate (Oral contraceptives tend to produce hyperglycemia and concurrent use may lead to loss of control). Products include:
Demulen ... 2580

Etodolac (Co-administration with nonsteroidal anti-inflammatory agents may result in hypoglycemia). Products include:
Lodine Capsules and Tablets ... 2849

Felodipine (Calcium channel blockers tend to produce hyperglycemia and concurrent use may lead to loss of control). Products include:
Plendil Extended-Release Tablets ... 514

Fenoprofen Calcium (Co-administration with nonsteroidal anti-inflammatory agents may result in hypoglycemia). Products include:
Nalfon 200 Pulvules & Nalfon Tablets ... 933

Fludrocortisone Acetate (Corticosteroids tend to produce hyperglycemia and concurrent use may lead to loss of control). Products include:
Florinef Acetate Tablets ... 506

Fluphenazine Decanoate (Phenothiazines tend to produce hyperglycemia and concurrent use may lead to loss of control). Products include:
Prolixin Decanoate ... 510

Fluphenazine Enanthate (Phenothiazines tend to produce hyperglycemia and concurrent use may lead to loss of control). Products include:
Prolixin Enanthate ... 510

Fluphenazine Hydrochloride (Phenothiazines tend to produce hyperglycemia and concurrent use may lead to loss of control). Products include:
Prolixin ... 510

IMPORTANT NOTE: Always consult each drug listing in the patient's regimen for possible interactions.

Micronase **Interactions Index** **676**

Flurazepam Hydrochloride (Co-administration with drugs that are highly protein bound may result in hypoglycemia). Products include:
Dalmane Capsules ... 2329
Flurbiprofen (Co-administration with nonsteroidal anti-inflammatory agents may result in hypoglycemia).
No products indexed under this heading.
Fosphenytoin Sodium (Phenytoin tends to produce hyperglycemia and concurrent use may lead to loss of control). Products include:
Cerebyx Injection ... 1956
Furazolidone (Co-administration with monamine oxidase inhibitors may result in hypoglycemia). Products include:
Furoxone ... 2221
Furosemide (Diuretics tend to produce hyperglycemia and concurrent use may lead to loss of control). Products include:
Lasix Injection, Oral Solution and Tablets ... 1267
Glipizide (Co-administration with sulfonamides may result in hypoglycemia). Products include:
Glucotrol Tablets ... 2011
Glucotrol XL Extended Release Tablets ... 2012
Hydrochlorothiazide (Thiazides tend to produce hyperglycemia and concurrent use may lead to loss of control). Products include:
Aldactazide Tablets ... 2556
Aldoril Tablets ... 1644
Apresazide Capsules ... 824
Capozide Tablets ... 744
Dyazide Capsules ... 2653
Esidrix Tablets ... 839
Esimil Tablets ... 840
HydroDIURIL Tablets ... 1716
Hydropres Tablets ... 1718
Hyzaar Tablets ... 1720
Inderide Tablets ... 2838
Inderide LA Long Acting Capsules .. 2840
Lopressor HCT Tablets ... 850
Lotensin HCT Tablets ... 855
Moduretic Tablets ... 1748
Oretic Tablets ... 450
Prinzide Tablets ... 1780
Ser-Ap-Es Tablets ... 867
Timolide Tablets ... 1791
Vaseretic Tablets ... 1810
Zestoretic Tablets ... 2968
Ziac ... 1459
Hydrocortisone (Corticosteroids tend to produce hyperglycemia and concurrent use may lead to loss of control). Products include:
Anusol-HC Cream 2.5% ... 1953
Aquanil HC Lotion ... 1989
Maximum Strength Cortaid Spray ▣ 800
CORTENEMA ... 2713
Cortisporin Ointment ... 1074
Cortisporin Ophthalmic Ointment Sterile ... 1074
Cortisporin Ophthalmic Suspension Sterile ... 1075
Cortisporin Otic Solution Sterile ... 1076
Cortisporin Otic Suspension Sterile 1077
Cortizone-5 ... ▣ 795
Cortizone-10 ... ▣ 795
Hydrocortone Tablets ... 1715
Hytone ... 922
Hytone Ointment 2 ½% ... 923
Massengill Medicated Soft Cloth Towelettes ... 2628
Pediotic Suspension Sterile ... 1140
Preparation H Hydrocortisone 1% Cream ... ▣ 843
ProctoCream-HC 2.5% ... 2552
VōSoL HC Otic Solution ... 2786
Hydrocortisone Acetate (Corticosteroids tend to produce hyperglycemia and concurrent use may lead to loss of control). Products include:
Analpram-HC Rectal Cream 1% and 2.5% ... 993
Anusol HC-1 Hydrocortisone Anti-Itch Ointment ... ▣ 810
Anusol-HC Suppositories ... 1954
Caldecort Anti-Itch Hydrocortisone Cream ... ▣ 651
Coly-Mycin S Otic w/Neomycin & Hydrocortisone ... 1965
Cortaid ... ▣ 800
Cortifoam ... 2540
Cortisporin Cream ... 1073
Epifoam ... 2543
Hydrocortone Acetate Sterile Suspension ... 1712
Mantadil Cream ... 1124
Nupercainal Hydrocortisone 1% Cream ... ▣ 661
Pramosone Cream, Lotion & Ointment ... 995
ProctoFoam-HC ... 2552
Terra-Cortril Ophthalmic Suspension ... 2033
Hydrocortisone Sodium Phosphate (Corticosteroids tend to produce hyperglycemia and concurrent use may lead to loss of control). Products include:
Hydrocortone Phosphate Injection, Sterile ... 1713
Hydrocortisone Sodium Succinate (Corticosteroids tend to produce hyperglycemia and concurrent use may lead to loss of control).
No products indexed under this heading.
Hydroflumethiazide (Thiazides tend to produce hyperglycemia and concurrent use may lead to loss of control). Products include:
Diucardin Tablets ... 2824
Ibuprofen (Co-administration with nonsteroidal anti-inflammatory agents may result in hypoglycemia). Products include:
Advil Cold and Sinus Caplets and Tablets ... ▣ 837
Advil Ibuprofen Tablets, Caplets and Gel Caplets ... ▣ 836
Children's Motrin Ibuprofen Oral Suspension ... 1558
IBU Tablets ... 1389
Ibuprohm ... ▣ 713
Motrin IB Caplets, Tablets, and Gelcaps ... ▣ 802
Motrin Ibuprofen Suspension, Oral Drops, Chewable Tablets, Caplets ... 1563
Nuprin Ibuprofen/Analgesic Tablets & Caplets ... ▣ 645
Vicks DayQuil SINUS Pressure & PAIN Relief with IBUPROFEN ... ▣ 735
Imipramine Hydrochloride (Co-administration with drugs that are highly protein bound may result in hypoglycemia). Products include:
Tofranil Ampuls ... 873
Tofranil Tablets ... 875
Imipramine Pamoate (Co-administration with drugs that are highly protein bound may result in hypoglycemia). Products include:
Tofranil-PM Capsules ... 876
Indapamide (Diuretics tend to produce hyperglycemia and concurrent use may lead to loss of control).
No products indexed under this heading.
Indomethacin (Co-administration with nonsteroidal anti-inflammatory agents may result in hypoglycemia). Products include:
Indocin ... 1723
Indomethacin Sodium Trihydrate (Co-administration with nonsteroidal anti-inflammatory agents may result in hypoglycemia). Products include:
Indocin I.V. ... 1727
Isocarboxazid (Co-administration with monamine oxidase inhibitors may result in hypoglycemia).
No products indexed under this heading.
Isoniazid (Isoniazid tends to produce hyperglycemia and concurrent use may lead to loss of control). Products include:
Nydrazid Injection ... 509
Rifamate Capsules ... 1278
Rifater ... 1280
Isoproterenol Hydrochloride (Sympathomimetics tend to produce hyperglycemia and concurrent use may lead to loss of control). Products include:
Isuprel Hydrochloride Solution ... 2443
Isuprel Injection ... 2441
Isuprel Mistometer ... 2442
Isoproterenol Sulfate (Sympathomimetics tend to produce hyperglycemia and concurrent use may lead to loss of control). Products include:
Norisodrine with Calcium Iodide Syrup ... 446
Isradipine (Calcium channel blockers tend to produce hyperglycemia and concurrent use may lead to loss of control). Products include:
DynaCirc Capsules ... 2381
DynaCirc CR Tablets ... 2383
Ketoprofen (Co-administration with nonsteroidal anti-inflammatory agents may result in hypoglycemia). Products include:
Actron Caplets and Tablets ... ▣ 608
Orudis Capsules ... 2874
Orudis KT ... ▣ 842
Oruvail Capsules ... 2874
Ketorolac Tromethamine (Co-administration with nonsteroidal anti-inflammatory agents may result in hypoglycemia). Products include:
Acular Sterile Ophthalmic Solution 470
Toradol ... 2319
Labetalol Hydrochloride (Co-administration with beta blockers may result in hypoglycemia). Products include:
Normodyne Injection ... 2519
Normodyne Tablets ... 2522
Trandate ... 1158
Levobunolol Hydrochloride (Co-administration with beta blockers may result in hypoglycemia). Products include:
Betagan ... ◉ 230
Levonorgestrel (Oral contraceptives tend to produce hyperglycemia and concurrent use may lead to loss of control). Products include:
Levlen/Tri-Levlen ... 646
Nordette-21 Tablets ... 2863
Nordette-28 Tablets ... 2866
Norplant System ... 2868
Levlen/Tri-Levlen ... 646
Triphasil-21 Tablets ... 2919
Triphasil-28 Tablets ... 2924
Levothyroxine Sodium (Thyroid products tend to produce hyperglycemia and concurrent use may lead to loss of control). Products include:
Eltroxin Tablets ... 2214
Levothroid Tablets ... 1015
Levothyroxine Sodium, USP for Injection ... 546
Levoxyl Tablets ... 918
Synthroid ... 1410
Liothyronine Sodium (Thyroid products tend to produce hyperglycemia and concurrent use may lead to loss of control). Products include:
Cytomel Tablets ... 2647
Triostat Injection ... 2708
Liotrix (Thyroid products tend to produce hyperglycemia and concurrent use may lead to loss of control).
No products indexed under this heading.
Magnesium Salicylate (Co-administration with salicylates may result in hypoglycemia). Products include:
Backache Caplets ... ▣ 635
Doan's Extra-Strength Analgesic ... ▣ 653
Extra Strength Doan's P.M. ... ▣ 653
Doan's Regular Strength Analgesic ... ▣ 654
Mobigesic Tablets ... ▣ 607
Meclofenamate Sodium (Co-administration with nonsteroidal anti-inflammatory agents may result in hypoglycemia).
No products indexed under this heading.
Mefenamic Acid (Co-administration with nonsteroidal anti-inflammatory agents may result in hypoglycemia). Products include:
Ponstel ... 1982
Mesoridazine Besylate (Phenothiazines tend to produce hyperglycemia and concurrent use may lead to loss of control). Products include:
Serentil ... 689
Mestranol (Oral contraceptives tend to produce hyperglycemia and concurrent use may lead to loss of control). Products include:
Norinyl ... 2563
Ortho-Novum ... 1928
Metaproterenol Sulfate (Sympathomimetics tend to produce hyperglycemia and concurrent use may lead to loss of control). Products include:
Alupent ... 672
Metaproterenol Sulfate Inhalation Solution, USP, Arm-a-Med ... 547
Metaraminol Bitartrate (Sympathomimetics tend to produce hyperglycemia and concurrent use may lead to loss of control). Products include:
Aramine Injection ... 1649
Metformin Hydrochloride (Co-administration in a single-dose study has resulted in a decrease in glyburide AUC and C_{max}, however, these decreases were highly variable; clinical significance of this interaction is uncertain). Products include:
Glucophage Tablets ... 754
Methotrimeprazine (Phenothiazines tend to produce hyperglycemia and concurrent use may lead to loss of control). Products include:
Levoprome ... 1321
Methoxamine Hydrochloride (Sympathomimetics tend to produce hyperglycemia and concurrent use may lead to loss of control). Products include:
Vasoxyl Injection ... 1169
Methyclothiazide (Thiazides tend to produce hyperglycemia and concurrent use may lead to loss of control). Products include:
Enduron Tablets ... 424
Methylprednisolone Acetate (Corticosteroids tend to produce hyperglycemia and concurrent use may lead to loss of control).
No products indexed under this heading.
Methylprednisolone Sodium Succinate (Corticosteroids tend to produce hyperglycemia and concurrent use may lead to loss of control).
No products indexed under this heading.
Metipranolol Hydrochloride (Co-administration with beta blockers may result in hypoglycemia). Products include:
OptiPranolol (Metipranolol 0.3%) Sterile Ophthalmic Solution ... ◉ 256

(▣ Described in PDR For Nonprescription Drugs) (◉ Described in PDR For Ophthalmology)

677 **Interactions Index** **Micronase**

Metolazone (Diuretics tend to produce hyperglycemia and concurrent use may lead to loss of control). Products include:
- Mykrox Tablets ... 1617
- Zaroxolyn Tablets ... 1625

Metoprolol Succinate (Co-administration with beta blockers may result in hypoglycemia). Products include:
- Toprol-XL Tablets ... 560

Metoprolol Tartrate (Co-administration with beta blockers may result in hypoglycemia). Products include:
- Lopressor ... 848
- Lopressor HCT Tablets ... 850

Miconazole (Co-administration with oral miconazole and oral hypoglycemic agents has resulted in severe hypoglycemia).
- No products indexed under this heading.

Midazolam Hydrochloride (Co-administration with drugs that are highly protein bound may result in hypoglycemia). Products include:
- Versed Injection ... 2324

Nabumetone (Co-administration with nonsteroidal anti-inflammatory agents may result in hypoglycemia). Products include:
- Relafen Tablets ... 2688

Nadolol (Co-administration with beta blockers may result in hypoglycemia).
- No products indexed under this heading.

Naproxen (Co-administration with nonsteroidal anti-inflammatory agents may result in hypoglycemia). Products include:
- Anaprox/Naprosyn ... 2277

Naproxen Sodium (Co-administration with nonsteroidal anti-inflammatory agents may result in hypoglycemia). Products include:
- Aleve ... 2124
- Anaprox/Naprosyn ... 2277
- Naprelan Tablets ... 2861

Nicardipine Hydrochloride (Calcium channel blockers tend to produce hyperglycemia and concurrent use may lead to loss of control). Products include:
- Cardene Capsules ... 2261
- Cardene I.V. ... 2815
- Cardene SR Capsules ... 2264

Nicotinic Acid (Nicotinic acid tends to produce hyperglycemia and concurrent use may lead to loss of control).
- No products indexed under this heading.

Nifedipine (Calcium channel blockers tend to produce hyperglycemia and concurrent use may lead to loss of control). Products include:
- Adalat Capsules (10 mg and 20 mg) ... 580
- Adalat CC ... 582
- Procardia Capsules ... 2024
- Procardia XL Extended Release Tablets ... 2026

Nimodipine (Calcium channel blockers tend to produce hyperglycemia and concurrent use may lead to loss of control). Products include:
- Nimotop Capsules ... 603

Nisoldipine (Calcium channel blockers tend to produce hyperglycemia and concurrent use may lead to loss of control). Products include:
- Sular Tablets ... 2961

Norepinephrine Bitartrate (Sympathomimetics tend to produce hyperglycemia and concurrent use may lead to loss of control). Products include:
- Levophed Bitartrate Injection ... 2445

Norethindrone (Oral contraceptives tend to produce hyperglycemia and concurrent use may lead to loss of control). Products include:
- Brevicon ... 2563
- Micronor Tablets ... 1903
- Modicon ... 1928
- Norinyl ... 2563
- Nor-Q D Tablets ... 2598
- Ortho-Novum ... 1928
- Ovcon ... 765
- Tri-Norinyl ... 2607

Norethynodrel (Oral contraceptives tend to produce hyperglycemia and concurrent use may lead to loss of control).
- No products indexed under this heading.

Norgestimate (Oral contraceptives tend to produce hyperglycemia and concurrent use may lead to loss of control). Products include:
- Ortho-Cyclen/Ortho-Tri-Cyclen ... 1914
- Ortho-Cyclen/Ortho Tri-Cyclen ... 1914

Norgestrel (Oral contraceptives tend to produce hyperglycemia and concurrent use may lead to loss of control). Products include:
- Lo/Ovral Tablets ... 2852
- Lo/Ovral-28 Tablets ... 2857
- Ovral Tablets ... 2877
- Ovral-28 Tablets ... 2878
- Ovrette Tablets ... 2878

Nortriptyline Hydrochloride (Co-administration with drugs that are highly protein bound may result in hypoglycemia). Products include:
- Pamelor ... 2409

Oxaprozin (Co-administration with nonsteroidal anti-inflammatory agents may result in hypoglycemia). Products include:
- Daypro Caplets ... 2578

Oxazepam (Co-administration with drugs that are highly protein bound may result in hypoglycemia). Products include:
- Serax Capsules ... 2916
- Serax Tablets ... 2916

Penbutolol Sulfate (Co-administration with beta blockers may result in hypoglycemia). Products include:
- Levatol Tablets ... 2547

Perphenazine (Phenothiazines tend to produce hyperglycemia and concurrent use may lead to loss of control). Products include:
- Etrafon ... 2495
- Triavil Tablets ... 1800
- Trilafon ... 2532

Phenelzine Sulfate (Co-administration with monamine oxidase inhibitors may result in hypoglycemia). Products include:
- Nardil ... 1977

Phenylbutazone (Co-administration with nonsteroidal anti-inflammatory agents may result in hypoglycemia).
- No products indexed under this heading.

Phenylephrine Bitartrate (Sympathomimetics tend to produce hyperglycemia and concurrent use may lead to loss of control).
- No products indexed under this heading.

Phenylephrine Hydrochloride (Sympathomimetics tend to produce hyperglycemia and concurrent use may lead to loss of control). Products include:
- Atrohist Plus Tablets ... 1605
- Cerose DM ... ▣ 853
- D.A. II Tablets ... 972
- D.A. Chewable Tablets ... 970
- Dura-Vent/DA Tablets ... 972
- Extendryl ... 1003
- 4-Way Fast Acting Nasal Spray (regular & mentholated) ... ▣ 644
- Hemorid ... ▣ 797
- Hycomine Compound Tablets ... 948
- Neo-Synephrine Hydrochloride 1% Carpuject ... 2455
- Neo-Synephrine Hydrochloride 1% Injection ... 2455
- Neo-Synephrine Hydrochloride (Ophthalmic) ... 2456
- Neo-Synephrine ... ▣ 624
- Novahistine Elixir ... ▣ 782
- Phenergan VC ... 2886
- Phenergan VC with Codeine ... 2888
- Preparation H ... ▣ 842
- Tympagesic Ear Drops ... 2476
- Vicks Sinex Nasal Spray and Ultra Fine Mist ... ▣ 738

Phenylephrine Tannate (Sympathomimetics tend to produce hyperglycemia and concurrent use may lead to loss of control). Products include:
- Atrohist Pediatric Suspension ... 1604
- Atrohist Pediatric Suspension Dye-Free ... 1604
- Rynatan ... 2781
- Rynatuss ... 2782

Phenylpropanolamine Hydrochloride (Sympathomimetics tend to produce hyperglycemia and concurrent use may lead to loss of control). Products include:
- Acutrim ... ▣ 648
- Atrohist Plus Tablets ... 1605
- BC Cold Powder Multi-Symptom Formula (Cold-Sinus-Allergy) ... ▣ 631
- BC Cold Powder Non-Drowsy Formula (Cold-Sinus) ... ▣ 631
- Cheracol Plus Head Cold/Cough Formula ... ▣ 741
- Comtrex Multi-Symptom Cold Reliever Liqui-Gels ... ▣ 638
- Comtrex Multi-Symptom Non-Drowsy Liqui-gels ... ▣ 640
- Contac Continuous Action Nasal Decongestant/Antihistamine 12 Hour Capsules ... ▣ 773
- Contac Maximum Strength Continuous Action Decongestant/Antihistamine 12 Hour Caplets ... ▣ 772
- Contac Severe Cold and Flu Formula Caplets ... ▣ 773
- Coricidin 'D' Decongestant Tablets ... ▣ 760
- Dexatrim ... ▣ 795
- Dexatrim Plus Vitamins Caplets ... ▣ 796
- Dimetane-DC Cough Syrup ... 2232
- Dimetapp Allergy Sinus Caplets ... ▣ 838
- Dimetapp Cold & Allergy Chewable Tablets ... ▣ 838
- Dimetapp Cold & Cough Liqui-Gels ... ▣ 839
- Dimetapp DM Elixir ... ▣ 840
- Dimetapp Elixir ... ▣ 840
- Dimetapp Extentabs ... ▣ 841
- Dimetapp Tablets/Liqui-Gels ... ▣ 841
- Dura-Vent Tablets ... 971
- Entex LA Tablets ... 972
- Exgest LA Tablets ... 787
- Hycomine ... 947
- Nolamine Timed-Release Tablets ... 790
- Ornade Spansule Capsules ... 2678
- Propagest Tablets ... 791
- Pyrroxate Caplets ... ▣ 742
- Robitussin-CF ... ▣ 846
- Sinulin Tablets ... 792
- Tavist-D 12 Hour Relief Tablets ... ▣ 750
- Teldrin 12 Hour Antihistamine/Nasal Decongestant Allergy Relief Capsules ... ▣ 786
- Triaminic Expectorant ... ▣ 753
- Triaminic Syrup ... ▣ 755
- Triaminic Triaminicol Cold & Cough ... ▣ 756
- Triaminic DM Syrup ... ▣ 756
- Triaminicin Tablets ... ▣ 756
- Vicks DayQuil Allergy Relief 12-Hour Extended Release Tablets ... ▣ 733
- Vicks DayQuil Allergy Relief 4-Hour Tablets ... ▣ 733
- Vicks DayQuil SINUS Pressure & CONGESTION Relief ... ▣ 734

Phenytoin (Phenytoin tends to produce hyperglycemia and concurrent use may lead to loss of control). Products include:
- Dilantin Infatabs ... 1967
- Dilantin-125 Suspension ... 1969

Phenytoin Sodium (Phenytoin tends to produce hyperglycemia and concurrent use may lead to loss of control). Products include:
- Dilantin Kapseals ... 1965

Pindolol (Co-administration with beta blockers may result in hypoglycemia). Products include:
- Visken Tablets ... 2428

Pirbuterol Acetate (Sympathomimetics tend to produce hyperglycemia and concurrent use may lead to loss of control). Products include:
- Maxair Autohaler ... 1550
- Maxair Inhaler ... 1552

Piroxicam (Co-administration with nonsteroidal anti-inflammatory agents may result in hypoglycemia). Products include:
- Feldene Capsules ... 2008

Polyestradiol Phosphate (Estrogens tend to produce hyperglycemia and concurrent use may lead to loss of control).
- No products indexed under this heading.

Polythiazide (Thiazides tend to produce hyperglycemia and concurrent use may lead to loss of control). Products include:
- Minizide Capsules ... 2016

Prednisolone Acetate (Corticosteroids tend to produce hyperglycemia and concurrent use may lead to loss of control). Products include:
- AK-CIDE ... ◉ 203
- AK-CIDE Ointment ... ◉ 203
- Blephamide Liquifilm Sterile Ophthalmic Suspension ... 472
- Blephamide Ointment ... ◉ 234
- Econopred & Econopred Plus Ophthalmic Suspensions ... ◉ 216
- Poly-Pred Liquifilm ... ◉ 246
- Pred Forte ... ◉ 247
- Pred Mild ... ◉ 250
- Pred-G Liquifilm Sterile Ophthalmic Suspension ... ◉ 248
- Pred-G S.O.P. Sterile Ophthalmic Ointment ... ◉ 249

Prednisolone Sodium Phosphate (Corticosteroids tend to produce hyperglycemia and concurrent use may lead to loss of control). Products include:
- AK-PRED ... ◉ 204
- Hydeltrasol Injection, Sterile ... 1708
- Pediapred Oral Solution ... 1618

Prednisolone Tebutate (Corticosteroids tend to produce hyperglycemia and concurrent use may lead to loss of control). Products include:
- Hydeltra-T.B.A. Sterile Suspension 1710

Prednisone (Corticosteroids tend to produce hyperglycemia and concurrent use may lead to loss of control).
- No products indexed under this heading.

Probenecid (Co-administration with probenecid may result in hypoglycemia). Products include:
- Benemid Tablets ... 1651
- ColBENEMID Tablets ... 1662

Prochlorperazine (Phenothiazines tend to produce hyperglycemia and concurrent use may lead to loss of control). Products include:
- Compazine ... 2644

Promethazine Hydrochloride (Phenothiazines tend to produce hyperglycemia and concurrent use may lead to loss of control). Products include:
- Mepergan Injection ... 2859
- Phenergan with Codeine ... 2883
- Phenergan with Dextromethorphan 2885
- Phenergan Injection ... 2880
- Phenergan Suppositories ... 2882
- Phenergan Syrup ... 2881
- Phenergan Tablets ... 2882

IMPORTANT NOTE: Always consult each drug listing in the patient's regimen for possible interactions.

Phenergan VC ... 2886
Phenergan VC with Codeine ... 2888

Propranolol Hydrochloride (Co-administration with beta blockers may result in hypoglycemia). Products include:

Inderal ... 2834
Inderal LA Long Acting Capsules ... 2836
Inderide Tablets ... 2838
Inderide LA Long Acting Capsules .. 2840

Pseudoephedrine Hydrochloride (Sympathomimetics tend to produce hyperglycemia and concurrent use may lead to loss of control). Products include:

Actifed Allergy Daytime/Nighttime Caplets ... ◘ 808
Actifed Cold & Allergy Tablets ... ◘ 807
Actifed Cold & Sinus Caplets and Tablets ... ◘ 808
Actifed Sinus Daytime/Nighttime Tablets and Caplets ... ◘ 809
Advil Cold and Sinus Caplets and Tablets ... ◘ 837
Alka-Seltzer Plus Liqui-Gels ... ◘ 612
Alka-Seltzer Plus Flu & Body Aches Liqui-Gels Non-Drowsy Formula ... ◘ 613
Alka-Seltzer Plus Night-Time Cold Medicine Liqui-Gels ... ◘ 612
Allerest Maximum Strength ... ◘ 649
Allerest No Drowsiness ... ◘ 649
Allerest Sinus Pain Formula ... ◘ 649
Atrohist Pediatric Capsules ... 1603
Benadryl Allergy/Cold Tablets ... ◘ 811
Benadryl Allergy Decongestant Liquid Medication ... ◘ 812
Benadryl Allergy Decongestant Tablets ... ◘ 812
Benadryl Allergy Sinus Headache Caplets ... ◘ 813
Benylin Multisymptom ... ◘ 816
Bromfed Capsules (Extended-Release) ... 1832
Bromfed Syrup ... ◘ 712
Bromfed Tablets ... 1832
Bromfed-DM Cough Syrup ... 1832
Bromfed-PD Capsules (Extended-Release) ... 1832
Children's TYLENOL Cold Multi-Symptom Chewable Tablets and Liquid ... 1559
Children's TYLENOL Cold Plus Cough Multi Symptom Chewable Tablets and Liquid ... 1560
Children's TYLENOL Flu Suspension Liquid ... 1560
Children's Vicks DayQuil Allergy Relief ... ◘ 730
Children's Vicks NyQuil Cold/Cough Relief ... ◘ 731
Allergy-Sinus Comtrex Multi-Symptom Allergy-Sinus Formula Tablets and Caplets ... ◘ 639
Comtrex Multi-Symptom ... ◘ 638
Comtrex Multi-Symptom Non-Drowsy Caplets ... ◘ 640
Congess ... 1003
Contac Day Allergy/Sinus Caplets ◘ 771
Contac Day & Night ... ◘ 772
Contac Night Allergy/Sinus Caplets ... ◘ 771
Contac Severe Cold & Flu Non-Drowsy ... ◘ 774
Deconsal II Tablets ... 1605
Dimetane-DX Cough Syrup ... 2233
Dimetapp Cold & Fever Suspension ... ◘ 839
Dimetapp Decongestant Pediatric Drops ... ◘ 840
Dorcol Children's Cough Syrup ... ◘ 748
Drixoral Cough + Congestion Liquid Caps ... ◘ 763
Dura-Tap/PD Capsules ... 970
Duratuss Tablets ... 2750
Duratuss HD Elixir ... 2750
Efidac/24 ... ◘ 655
Entex PSE Tablets ... 973
Fedahist Gyrocaps ... 2545
Guaifed ... 1833
Guaifed Syrup ... ◘ 712
Guaimax-D Tablets ... 809
Histussin D Liquid ... 670
Infants' TYLENOL Cold Decongestant & Fever-Reducer Drops ... 1561
Kronofed-A ... 994
Novahistine DMX ... ◘ 782
Nucofed ... 2225
PediaCare Cough-Cold Chewable Tablets and Liquid ... 1569
PediaCare Infants' Decongestant Drops ... 1569
PediaCare Infants' Drops Decongestant Plus Cough ... 1569
PediaCare NightRest Cough-Cold Liquid ... 1569
Pediatric Vicks 44d Cough & Head Congestion Relief ... ◘ 736
Pediatric Vicks 44m Cough & Cold Relief ... ◘ 737
Robitussin Cold & Cough Liqui-Gels ... ◘ 844
Robitussin Cold, Cough & Flu Liqui-Gels ... ◘ 844
Robitussin Maximum Strength Cough & Cold ... ◘ 847
Robitussin Night-Time Cold Formula ... ◘ 847
Robitussin Pediatric Cough & Cold Formula ... ◘ 848
Robitussin Pediatric Drops ... ◘ 849
Robitussin Severe Congestion Liqui-Gels ... ◘ 845
Robitussin-DAC Syrup ... 2249
Robitussin-PE ... ◘ 846
Rondec Oral Drops ... 974
Rondec Syrup ... 974
Rondec Tablet ... 974
Rondec Chewable Tablets ... 974
Rondec-TR Tablet ... 974
Ryna ... ◘ 804
Seldane-D Extended-Release Tablets ... 1286
Semprex-D Capsules ... 1620
Sinarest ... ◘ 663
Sine-Aid Maximum Strength Sinus Headache Gelcaps, Caplets and Tablets ... 1570
Sine-Off No Drowsiness Formula Caplets ... ◘ 784
Sine-Off Sinus Medicine ... ◘ 784
Singlet Tablets ... ◘ 785
Sinutab Non-Drying Liquid Caps ... ◘ 823
Sinutab Sinus Allergy Medication, Maximum Strength Tablets and Caplets ... ◘ 823
Sinutab Sinus Medication, Maximum Strength Without Drowsiness Formula, Tablets & Caplets ... ◘ 824
Sudafed Children's Cold & Cough Liquid Medication ... ◘ 825
Sudafed Children's Nasal Decongestant Liquid Medication ... ◘ 826
Sudafed Cold & Allergy Tablets ... ◘ 826
Sudafed Cold and Cough Liquid Caps ... ◘ 826
Sudafed Nasal Decongestant Tablets, 30 mg ... ◘ 825
Sudafed Nasal Decongestant Tablets, 60 mg ... ◘ 825
Sudafed Non-Drying Sinus Liquid Caps ... ◘ 827
Sudafed Pediatric Nasal Decongestant Liquid Oral Drops ... ◘ 827
Sudafed Severe Cold Formula Caplets ... ◘ 828
Sudafed Severe Cold Formula Tablets ... ◘ 828
Sudafed Sinus Caplets ... ◘ 829
Sudafed Sinus Tablets ... ◘ 829
Sudafed 12 Hour Caplets ... ◘ 824
Syn-Rx Tablets ... 1622
Syn-Rx DM Tablets ... 1623
TheraFlu Flu and Cold Medicine ... ◘ 750
Theraflu Maximum Strength Flu and Cold Medicine For Sore Throat ... ◘ 751
TheraFlu Flu, Cold and Cough Medicine ... ◘ 750
TheraFlu Maximum Strength Nighttime Flu, Cold & Cough Medicine ... ◘ 751
TheraFlu Maximum Strength Non-Drowsy Formula Flu, Cold & Cough Medicine ... ◘ 751
TheraFlu Maximum Strength, Non-Drowsy Formula Flu, Cold and Cough Caplets ... ◘ 752
Theraflu Maximum Strength Sinus Non-Drowsy Formula Caplets ... ◘ 752
Triaminic AM Cough and Decongestant Formula ... ◘ 753
Triaminic AM Decongestant Formula ... ◘ 753
Triaminic Infant Oral Decongestant Drops ... ◘ 754
Triaminic Night Time ... ◘ 754
Triaminic Sore Throat Formula ... ◘ 755
Tussend ... 1830
Tussend Expectorant ... 1831
TYLENOL Allergy Sinus, Maximum Strength Caplets and Gelcaps ... 1571
TYLENOL Allergy Sinus NightTime, Maximum Strength Caplets ... 1571
TYLENOL Cold Medication, Multi-Symptom Formula Tablets and Caplets ... 1572
TYLENOL Cold Medication, Multi-Symptom Hot Liquid Packets ... 1572
TYLENOL Cold Medication, No Drowsiness Formula Caplets and Gelcaps ... 1572
TYLENOL Cold Severe Congestion Caplets ... 1573
TYLENOL Cough Medication with Decongestant, Multi Symptom ... 1574
TYLENOL Flu No Drowsiness Formula, Maximum Strength Gelcaps ... 1575
TYLENOL Flu NightTime, Maximum Strength Gelcaps ... 1575
TYLENOL Flu NightTime, Maximum Strength Hot Medication Packets ... 1575
TYLENOL Sinus, Maximum Strength Geltabs, Gelcaps, Caplets and Tablets ... 1576
Vicks 44 LiquiCaps Cough, Cold & Flu Relief ... ◘ 728
Vicks 44 LiquiCaps Non-Drowsy Cough & Cold Relief ... ◘ 729
Vicks 44D Cough & Head Congestion Relief ... ◘ 728
Vicks 44M Cough, Cold & Flu Relief ... ◘ 729
Vicks DayQuil LiquiCaps/Liquid Multi-Symptom Cold/Flu Relief .. ◘ 734
Vicks DayQuil SINUS Pressure & PAIN Relief with IBUPROFEN ... ◘ 735
Vicks Nyquil Hot Therapy ... ◘ 735
Vicks NyQuil LiquiCaps/Liquid Multi-Symptom Cold/Flu Relief, Original and Cherry Flavors ... ◘ 736

Pseudoephedrine Sulfate (Sympathomimetics tend to produce hyperglycemia and concurrent use may lead to loss of control). Products include:

Chlor-Trimeton Allergy Decongestant Tablets ... ◘ 759
Claritin-D Tablets ... 2487
Drixoral Cold and Allergy Sustained-Action Tablets ... ◘ 763
Drixoral Cold and Flu Extended-Release Tablets ... ◘ 764
Drixoral Non-Drowsy Formula Extended-Release Tablets ... ◘ 764
Drixoral Allergy/Sinus Extended Release Tablets ... ◘ 765
Trinalin Repetabs Tablets ... 1373

Quinestrol (Estrogens tend to produce hyperglycemia and concurrent use may lead to loss of control).

No products indexed under this heading.

Salmeterol Xinafoate (Sympathomimetics tend to produce hyperglycemia and concurrent use may lead to loss of control). Products include:

Serevent Inhalation Aerosol ... 1149

Salsalate (Co-administration with salicylates may result in hypoglycemia). Products include:

Disalcid ... 1549
Mono-Gesic Tablets ... 810
Salflex Tablets ... 791

Selegiline Hydrochloride (Co-administration with monamine oxidase inhibitors may result in hypoglycemia). Products include:

Eldepryl Capsules ... 2729

Sotalol Hydrochloride (Co-administration with beta blockers may result in hypoglycemia). Products include:

Betapace Tablets ... 637

Spironolactone (Diuretics tend to produce hyperglycemia and concurrent use may lead to loss of control). Products include:

Aldactazide Tablets ... 2556
Aldactone Tablets ... 2558

Sulfacytine (Co-administration with sulfonamides may result in hypoglycemia).

Sulfamethizole (Co-administration with sulfonamides may result in hypoglycemia). Products include:

Urobiotic-250 Capsules ... 2038

Sulfamethoxazole (Co-administration with sulfonamides may result in hypoglycemia). Products include:

Bactrim DS Tablets ... 2257
Bactrim I.V. Infusion ... 2255
Bactrim ... 2257
Gantanol Tablets ... 2285
Septra ... 1146
Septra I.V. Infusion ... 1142
Septra I.V. Infusion ADD-Vantage Vials ... 1144
Septra ... 1146

Sulfasalazine (Co-administration with sulfonamides may result in hypoglycemia). Products include:

Azulfidine ... 2059

Sulfinpyrazone (Co-administration with sulfonamides may result in hypoglycemia). Products include:

Anturane ... 823

Sulfisoxazole (Co-administration with sulfonamides may result in hypoglycemia). Products include:

Gantrisin Tablets ... 2286

Sulfisoxazole Diolamine (Co-administration with sulfonamides may result in hypoglycemia).

No products indexed under this heading.

Sulindac (Co-administration with nonsteroidal anti-inflammatory agents may result in hypoglycemia). Products include:

Clinoril Tablets ... 1658

Temazepam (Co-administration with drugs that are highly protein bound may result in hypoglycemia). Products include:

Restoril Capsules ... 2413

Terbutaline Sulfate (Sympathomimetics tend to produce hyperglycemia and concurrent use may lead to loss of control). Products include:

Brethaire Inhaler ... 830
Brethine Ampuls ... 832
Brethine Tablets ... 831
Bricanyl Subcutaneous Injection ... 1247
Bricanyl Tablets ... 1248

Thioridazine Hydrochloride (Phenothiazines tend to produce hyperglycemia and concurrent use may lead to loss of control). Products include:

Mellaril ... 2398

Thyroglobulin (Thyroid products tend to produce hyperglycemia and concurrent use may lead to loss of control).

No products indexed under this heading.

Thyroid (Thyroid products tend to produce hyperglycemia and concurrent use may lead to loss of control).

No products indexed under this heading.

Thyroxine (Thyroid products tend to produce hyperglycemia and concurrent use may lead to loss of control).

No products indexed under this heading.

Thyroxine Sodium (Thyroid products tend to produce hyperglycemia and concurrent use may lead to loss of control).

No products indexed under this heading.

Timolol Hemihydrate (Co-administration with beta blockers may result in hypoglycemia). Products include:

Betimol 0.25%, 0.5% ... ⊙ 259

(◘ Described in PDR For Nonprescription Drugs) (⊙ Described in PDR For Ophthalmology)

679 **Interactions Index** **Midamor**

Timolol Maleate (Co-administration with beta blockers may result in hypoglycemia). Products include:
- Blocadren Tablets 1654
- Timolide Tablets 1791
- Timoptic in Ocudose 1796
- Timoptic Sterile Ophthalmic Solution 1794
- Timoptic-XE 1798

Tolazamide (Co-administration with sulfonamides may result in hypoglycemia).
- No products indexed under this heading.

Tolbutamide (Co-administration with sulfonamides may result in hypoglycemia).
- No products indexed under this heading.

Tolmetin Sodium (Co-administration with nonsteroidal anti-inflammatory agents may result in hypoglycemia). Products include:
- Tolectin (200, 400 and 600 mg) 1591

Torsemide (Diuretics tend to produce hyperglycemia and concurrent use may lead to loss of control). Products include:
- Demadex Tablets and Injection 691

Tranylcypromine Sulfate (Co-administration with monamine oxidase inhibitors may result in hypoglycemia). Products include:
- Parnate Tablets 2679

Triamcinolone (Corticosteroids tend to produce hyperglycemia and concurrent use may lead to loss of control).
- No products indexed under this heading.

Triamcinolone Acetonide (Corticosteroids tend to produce hyperglycemia and concurrent use may lead to loss of control). Products include:
- Azmacort Oral Inhaler 2175
- Nasacort AQ Nasal Spray 2191
- Nasacort Nasal Inhaler 2189

Triamcinolone Diacetate (Corticosteroids tend to produce hyperglycemia and concurrent use may lead to loss of control).
- No products indexed under this heading.

Triamcinolone Hexacetonide (Corticosteroids tend to produce hyperglycemia and concurrent use may lead to loss of control).
- No products indexed under this heading.

Triamterene (Diuretics tend to produce hyperglycemia and concurrent use may lead to loss of control). Products include:
- Dyazide Capsules 2653
- Dyrenium Capsules 2655

Trifluoperazine Hydrochloride (Phenothiazines tend to produce hyperglycemia and concurrent use may lead to loss of control). Products include:
- Stelazine 2692

Trimipramine Maleate (Co-administration with drugs that are highly protein bound may result in hypoglycemia). Products include:
- Surmontil Capsules 2917

Verapamil Hydrochloride (Calcium channel blockers tend to produce hyperglycemia and concurrent use may lead to loss of control). Products include:
- Calan SR Caplets 2571
- Calan Tablets 2568
- Covera-HS Tablets 2573
- Isoptin Injectable 1391
- Isoptin Oral Tablets 1393
- Isoptin SR Tablets 1395
- Verelan Capsules 1455

Warfarin Sodium (Co-administration with coumarins may result in hypoglycemia). Products include:
- Coumadin 941

MICRONOR TABLETS
(Norethindrone) 1903

May interact with barbiturates and certain other agents. Compounds in these categories include:

Aprobarbital (The effectiveness of progestin-only oral contraceptives is reduced by hepatic enzyme-inducing agents such as barbiturates).
- No products indexed under this heading.

Butabarbital (The effectiveness of progestin-only oral contraceptives is reduced by hepatic enzyme-inducing agents such as barbiturates).
- No products indexed under this heading.

Butalbital (The effectiveness of progestin-only oral contraceptives is reduced by hepatic enzyme-inducing agents such as barbiturates). Products include:
- Axocet Capsules 2469
- Esgic-plus Capsules 1012
- Esgic-plus Tablets 1012
- Fioricet Tablets 2386
- Fioricet with Codeine Capsules 2387
- Fiorinal Capsules 2388
- Fiorinal with Codeine Capsules 2390
- Fiorinal Tablets 2388
- Phrenilin 790
- Sedapap Tablets 50 mg/650 mg 1826

Carbamazepine (The effectiveness of progestin-only oral contraceptives is reduced by hepatic enzyme-inducing agents such as carbamazepine). Products include:
- Atretol Tablets 569
- Tegretol/Tegretol-XR 870

Fosphenytoin Sodium (The effectiveness of progestin-only oral contraceptives is reduced by hepatic enzyme-inducing agents such as phenytoin). Products include:
- Cerebyx Injection 1956

Mephobarbital (The effectiveness of progestin-only oral contraceptives is reduced by hepatic enzyme-inducing agents such as barbiturates). Products include:
- Mebaral Tablets 2452

Pentobarbital Sodium (The effectiveness of progestin-only oral contraceptives is reduced by hepatic enzyme-inducing agents such as barbiturates). Products include:
- Nembutal Sodium Capsules 440
- Nembutal Sodium Solution 442
- Nembutal Sodium Suppositories 444

Phenobarbital (The effectiveness of progestin-only oral contraceptives is reduced by hepatic enzyme-inducing agents such as barbiturates). Products include:
- Arco-Lase Plus Tablets 513
- Bellergal-S Tablets 2375
- Donnatal 2234
- Donnatal Extentabs 2234
- Donnatal Tablets 2234
- Phenobarbital Elixir and Tablets 1523
- Quadrinal Tablets 1398

Phenytoin (The effectiveness of progestin-only oral contraceptives is reduced by hepatic enzyme-inducing agents such as phenytoin). Products include:
- Dilantin Infatabs 1967
- Dilantin-125 Suspension 1969

Phenytoin Sodium (The effectiveness of progestin-only oral contraceptives is reduced by hepatic enzyme-inducing agents such as phenytoin). Products include:
- Dilantin Kapseals 1965

Rifampin (The effectiveness of progestin-only oral contraceptives is reduced by hepatic enzyme-inducing agents such as rifampin). Products include:
- Rifadin 1276
- Rifamate Capsules 1278
- Rifater 1280
- Rimactane Capsules 865

Secobarbital Sodium (The effectiveness of progestin-only oral contraceptives is reduced by hepatic enzyme-inducing agents such as barbiturates). Products include:
- Seconal Sodium Pulvules 1529

Thiamylal Sodium (The effectiveness of progestin-only oral contraceptives is reduced by hepatic enzyme-inducing agents such as barbiturates).
- No products indexed under this heading.

MIDAMOR TABLETS
(Amiloride Hydrochloride) 1746

May interact with diuretics, potassium sparing diuretics, lithium preparations, non-steroidal anti-inflammatory agents, potassium preparations, ACE inhibitors, and certain other agents. Compounds in these categories include:

Benazepril Hydrochloride (Increased risk of hyperkalemia). Products include:
- Lotensin Tablets 852
- Lotensin HCT Tablets 855
- Lotrel Capsules 858

Bendroflumethiazide (Hyponatremia; hypochloremia; increases in BUN levels).
- No products indexed under this heading.

Bumetanide (Hyponatremia; hypochloremia; increases in BUN levels). Products include:
- Bumex 2260

Captopril (Increased risk of hyperkalemia). Products include:
- Capoten Tablets 740
- Capozide Tablets 744

Chlorothiazide (Hyponatremia; hypochloremia; increases in BUN levels). Products include:
- Aldoclor Tablets 1638
- Diupres Tablets 1691
- Diuril Oral 1694

Chlorothiazide Sodium (Hyponatremia; hypochloremia; increases in BUN levels). Products include:
- Diuril Sodium Intravenous 1693

Chlorthalidone (Hyponatremia; hypochloremia; increases in BUN levels). Products include:
- Combipres Tablets 682
- Tenoretic Tablets 2963
- Thalitone 1293

Diclofenac Potassium (Reduced diuretic, natriuretic, and antihypertensive effects of Midamor). Products include:
- Cataflam Tablets 833

Diclofenac Sodium (Reduced diuretic, natriuretic, and antihypertensive effects of Midamor). Products include:
- Voltaren Ophthalmic Sterile Ophthalmic Solution ⊙ 264
- Cataflam/Voltaren/Voltaren-XR 833

Enalapril Maleate (Increased risk of hyperkalemia). Products include:
- Vaseretic Tablets 1810
- Vasotec Tablets 1816

Enalaprilat (Increased risk of hyperkalemia). Products include:
- Vasotec I.V. 1814

Ethacrynic Acid (Hyponatremia; hypochloremia; increases in BUN levels). Products include:
- Edecrin Tablets 1698

Etodolac (Reduced diuretic, natriuretic, and antihypertensive effects of Midamor). Products include:
- Lodine Capsules and Tablets 2849

Fenoprofen Calcium (Reduced diuretic, natriuretic, and antihypertensive effects of Midamor). Products include:
- Nalfon 200 Pulvules & Nalfon Tablets 933

Flurbiprofen (Reduced diuretic, natriuretic, and antihypertensive effects of Midamor).
- No products indexed under this heading.

Fosinopril Sodium (Increased risk of hyperkalemia). Products include:
- Monopril Tablets 762

Furosemide (Hyponatremia; hypochloremia; increases in BUN levels). Products include:
- Lasix Injection, Oral Solution and Tablets 1267

Hydrochlorothiazide (Hyponatremia; hypochloremia; increases in BUN levels). Products include:
- Aldactazide Tablets 2556
- Aldoril Tablets 1644
- Apresazide Capsules 824
- Capozide Tablets 744
- Dyazide Capsules 2653
- Esidrix Tablets 839
- Esimil Tablets 840
- HydroDIURIL Tablets 1716
- Hydropres Tablets 1718
- Hyzaar Tablets 1720
- Inderide Tablets 2838
- Inderide LA Long Acting Capsules 2840
- Lopressor HCT Tablets 850
- Lotensin HCT Tablets 855
- Moduretic Tablets 1748
- Oretic Tablets 450
- Prinzide Tablets 1780
- Ser-Ap-Es Tablets 867
- Timolide Tablets 1791
- Vaseretic Tablets 1810
- Zestoretic Tablets 2968
- Ziac 1459

Hydroflumethiazide (Hyponatremia; hypochloremia; increases in BUN levels). Products include:
- Diucardin Tablets 2824

Ibuprofen (Reduced diuretic, natriuretic, and antihypertensive effects of Midamor). Products include:
- Advil Cold and Sinus Caplets and Tablets 837
- Advil Ibuprofen Tablets, Caplets and Gel Caplets 836
- Children's Motrin Ibuprofen Oral Suspension 1558
- IBU Tablets 1389
- Ibuprohm 713
- Motrin IB Caplets, Tablets, and Gelcaps 802
- Motrin Ibuprofen Suspension, Oral Drops, Chewable Tablets, Caplets 1563
- Nuprin Ibuprofen/Analgesic Tablets & Caplets 645
- Vicks DayQuil SINUS Pressure & PAIN Relief with IBUPROFEN 735

Indapamide (Hyponatremia; hypochloremia; increases in BUN levels).
- No products indexed under this heading.

Indomethacin (Reduced diuretic, natriuretic, and antihypertensive effects of Midamor; increased serum potassium levels of both drugs). Products include:
- Indocin 1723

IMPORTANT NOTE: Always consult each drug listing in the patient's regimen for possible interactions.

Midamor Interactions Index 680

Indomethacin Sodium Trihydrate (Reduced diuretic, natriuretic, and antihypertensive effects of Midamor; increased serum potassium levels of both drugs). Products include:
- Indocin I.V. 1727

Ketoprofen (Reduced diuretic, natriuretic, and antihypertensive effects of Midamor). Products include:
- Actron Caplets and Tablets .... ◘ 608
- Orudis Capsules 2874
- Orudis KT .... ◘ 842
- Oruvail Capsules 2874

Ketorolac Tromethamine (Reduced diuretic, natriuretic, and antihypertensive effects of Midamor). Products include:
- Acular Sterile Ophthalmic Solution 470
- Toradol 2319

Lisinopril (Increased risk of hyperkalemia). Products include:
- Prinivil Tablets 1776
- Prinzide Tablets 1780
- Zestoretic Tablets 2968
- Zestril Tablets 2972

Lithium Carbonate (High risk of lithium toxicity). Products include:
- Eskalith 2658
- Lithium Carbonate Capsules & Tablets 2352
- Lithonate/Lithotabs/Lithobid 2721

Lithium Citrate (High risk of lithium toxicity).
- No products indexed under this heading.

Meclofenamate Sodium (Reduced diuretic, natiuretic, and antihypertensive effects of Midamor).
- No products indexed under this heading.

Mefenamic Acid (Reduced diuretic, natriuretic, and antihypertensive effects of Midamor). Products include:
- Ponstel 1982

Methyclothiazide (Hyponatremia; hypochloremia; increases in BUN levels). Products include:
- Enduron Tablets 424

Metolazone (Hyponatremia; hypochloremia; increases in BUN levels). Products include:
- Mykrox Tablets 1617
- Zaroxolyn Tablets 1625

Moexipril Hydrochloride (Increased risk of hyperkalemia). Products include:
- Univasc Tablets 2553

Nabumetone (Reduced diuretic, natriuretic, and antihypertensive effects of Midamor). Products include:
- Relafen Tablets 2688

Naproxen (Reduced diuretic, natriuretic, and antihypertensive effects of Midamor). Products include:
- Anaprox/Naprosyn 2277

Naproxen Sodium (Reduced diuretic, natriuretic, and antihypertensive effects of Midamor). Products include:
- Aleve 2124
- Anaprox/Naprosyn 2277
- Naprelan Tablets 2861

Oxaprozin (Reduced diuretic, natriuretic, and antihypertensive effects of Midamor). Products include:
- Daypro Caplets 2578

Phenylbutazone (Reduced diuretic, natriuretic, and antihypertensive effects of Midamor).
- No products indexed under this heading.

Piroxicam (Reduced diuretic, natriuretic, and antihypertensive effects of Midamor). Products include:
- Feldene Capsules 2008

Polythiazide (Hyponatremia; hypochloremia; increases in BUN levels). Products include:
- Minizide Capsules 2016

Potassium Acid Phosphate (Concomitant therapy is contraindicated). Products include:
- K-Phos Original Formula 'Sodium Free' Tablets 633

Potassium Bicarbonate (Concomitant therapy is contraindicated). Products include:
- Alka-Seltzer Gold Effervescent Antacid .... ◘ 611

Potassium Chloride (Concomitant therapy is contraindicated). Products include:
- Chlor-3 Condiment 1003
- Colyte and Colyte-flavored 2540
- GoLYTELY 694
- K-Dur Microburst Release System (potassium chloride, USP) E.R. Tablets 1364
- K-Lor Powder Packets 438
- K-Norm Capsules 1615
- K-Tab Filmtab 439
- Micro-K 2237
- Micro-K LS Packets 2238
- NuLYTELY 694
- Cherry Flavor NuLYTELY 694
- Rum-K Syrup 1004
- Slow-K Extended-Release Tablets 869

Potassium Citrate (Concomitant therapy is contraindicated). Products include:
- Polycitra Syrup 574
- Polycitra-K Crystals 574
- Polycitra-K Oral Solution 575
- Polycitra-LC 574
- Urocit-K Tablets 1828

Potassium Gluconate (Concomitant therapy is contraindicated).
- No products indexed under this heading.

Potassium Phosphate, Dibasic (Concomitant therapy is contraindicated).
- No products indexed under this heading.

Potassium Phosphate, Monobasic (Concomitant therapy is contraindicated). Products include:
- K-Phos Neutral Tablets 633
- K-Phos Original Formula 'Sodium Free' Tablets 633

Quinapril Hydrochloride (Increased risk of hyperkalemia). Products include:
- Accupril Tablets 1950

Ramipril (Increased risk of hyperkalemia). Products include:
- Altace Capsules 1238

Spirapril Hydrochloride (Increased risk of hyperkalemia).
- No products indexed under this heading.

Spironolactone (Do not administer concomitantly; rapid increases in serum potassium). Products include:
- Aldactazide Tablets 2556
- Aldactone Tablets 2558

Sulindac (Reduced diuretic, natriuretic, and antihypertensive effects of Midamor). Products include:
- Clinoril Tablets 1658

Tolmetin Sodium (Reduced diuretic, natriuretic, and antihypertensive effects of Midamor). Products include:
- Tolectin (200, 400 and 600 mg) .. 1591

Torsemide (Hyponatremia; hypochloremia; increases in BUN levels). Products include:
- Demadex Tablets and Injection 691

Trandolapril (Increased risk of hyperkalemia). Products include:
- Mavik Tablets 1407

Triamterene (Do not administer concomitantly; rapid increases in serum potassium). Products include:
- Dyazide Capsules 2653
- Dyrenium Capsules 2655

Food Interactions

Diet, potassium-rich (Potential for rapid increases in serum potassium levels).

MAXIMUM STRENGTH MULTI-SYMPTOM FORMULA MIDOL

(Acetaminophen, Caffeine, Pyrilamine Maleate) .... ◘ 621

May interact with hypnotics and sedatives, tranquilizers, and certain other agents. Compounds in these categories include:

Alprazolam (May increase drowsiness). Products include:
- Xanax Tablets 2115

Buspirone Hydrochloride (May increase drowsiness). Products include:
- BuSpar Tablets 738

Caffeine-containing medications (Concomitant use may cause nervousness, irritability, sleeplessness, and occasionally, rapid heartbeat).

Chlordiazepoxide (May increase drowsiness). Products include:
- Limbitrol 2333

Chlordiazepoxide Hydrochloride (May increase drowsiness). Products include:
- Librax Capsules 2330
- Librium Capsules 2331
- Librium Injectable 2332

Chlorpromazine (May increase drowsiness). Products include:
- Thorazine Suppositories 2701

Chlorprothixene (May increase drowsiness).
- No products indexed under this heading.

Chlorprothixene Hydrochloride (May increase drowsiness).
- No products indexed under this heading.

Clorazepate Dipotassium (May increase drowsiness). Products include:
- Tranxene 459

Diazepam (May increase drowsiness). Products include:
- Dizac (diazepam injectable emulsion) CIV 1862
- Valium Injectable 2336
- Valium Tablets 2335

Droperidol (May increase drowsiness). Products include:
- Inapsine Injection 462

Estazolam (May increase drowsiness). Products include:
- ProSom Tablets 457

Ethchlorvynol (May increase drowsiness). Products include:
- Placidyl Capsules 456

Ethinamate (May increase drowsiness).
- No products indexed under this heading.

Fluphenazine Decanoate (May increase drowsiness). Products include:
- Prolixin Decanoate 510

Fluphenazine Enanthate (May increase drowsiness). Products include:
- Prolixin Enanthate 510

Fluphenazine Hydrochloride (May increase drowsiness). Products include:
- Prolixin 510

Flurazepam Hydrochloride (May increase drowsiness). Products include:
- Dalmane Capsules 2329

Glutethimide (May increase drowsiness).
- No products indexed under this heading.

Haloperidol (May increase drowsiness). Products include:
- Haldol Injection, Tablets and Concentrate 1585

Haloperidol Decanoate (May increase drowsiness). Products include:
- Haldol Decanoate 1587

Hydroxyzine Hydrochloride (May increase drowsiness). Products include:
- Atarax Tablets & Syrup 1992
- Marax Tablets & DF Syrup 2015
- Vistaril Intramuscular Solution 2042

Lorazepam (May increase drowsiness). Products include:
- Ativan Injection 2805
- Ativan Tablets 2807

Loxapine Hydrochloride (May increase drowsiness). Products include:
- Loxitane 1426

Loxapine Succinate (May increase drowsiness). Products include:
- Loxitane Capsules 1426

Meprobamate (May increase drowsiness). Products include:
- Miltown Tablets 2780
- PMB 200 and PMB 400 2890

Mesoridazine Besylate (May increase drowsiness). Products include:
- Serentil 689

Midazolam Hydrochloride (May increase drowsiness). Products include:
- Versed Injection 2324

Molindone Hydrochloride (May increase drowsiness). Products include:
- Moban Tablets and Concentrate 1036

Oxazepam (May increase drowsiness). Products include:
- Serax Capsules 2916
- Serax Tablets 2916

Perphenazine (May increase drowsiness). Products include:
- Etrafon 2495
- Triavil Tablets 1800
- Trilafon 2532

Prazepam (May increase drowsiness).
- No products indexed under this heading.

Prochlorperazine (May increase drowsiness). Products include:
- Compazine 2644

Promethazine Hydrochloride (May increase drowsiness). Products include:
- Mepergan Injection 2859
- Phenergan with Codeine 2883
- Phenergan with Dextromethorphan 2885
- Phenergan Injection 2880
- Phenergan Suppositories 2882
- Phenergan Syrup 2881
- Phenergan Tablets 2882
- Phenergan VC 2886
- Phenergan VC with Codeine 2888

Propofol (May increase drowsiness). Products include:
- Diprivan Injectable Emulsion 2939

Quazepam (May increase drowsiness). Products include:
- Doral Tablets 2773

Secobarbital Sodium (May increase drowsiness). Products include:
- Seconal Sodium Pulvules 1529

(◘ Described in PDR For Nonprescription Drugs) (◉ Described in PDR For Ophthalmology)

681 **Interactions Index** Miltown

Temazepam (May increase drowsiness). Products include:
- Restoril Capsules ... 2413

Thioridazine Hydrochloride (May increase drowsiness). Products include:
- Mellaril ... 2398

Thiothixene (May increase drowsiness). Products include:
- Navane Capsules and Concentrate 2018
- Navane Intramuscular ... 2019

Triazolam (May increase drowsiness). Products include:
- Halcion Tablets ... 2093

Trifluoperazine Hydrochloride (May increase drowsiness). Products include:
- Stelazine ... 2692

Zolpidem Tartrate (May increase drowsiness). Products include:
- Ambien Tablets ... 2559

Food Interactions

Alcohol (May increase drowsiness).

Beverages, caffeine-containing (Concomitant use may cause nervousness, irritability, sleeplessness, and occasionally, rapid heartbeat).

Food, caffeine containing (Concomitant use may cause nervousness, irritability, sleeplessness, and occasionally, rapid heartbeat).

PMS MULTI-SYMPTOM FORMULA MIDOL
(Acetaminophen, Pamabrom, Pyrilamine Maleate) ... 622
May interact with hypnotics and sedatives, tranquilizers, and certain other agents. Compounds in these categories include:

Alprazolam (May increase drowsiness). Products include:
- Xanax Tablets ... 2115

Buspirone Hydrochloride (May increase drowsiness). Products include:
- BuSpar Tablets ... 738

Chlordiazepoxide (May increase drowsiness). Products include:
- Limbitrol ... 2333

Chlordiazepoxide Hydrochloride (May increase drowsiness). Products include:
- Librax Capsules ... 2330
- Librium Capsules ... 2331
- Librium Injectable ... 2332

Chlorpromazine (May increase drowsiness). Products include:
- Thorazine Suppositories ... 2701

Chlorprothixene (May increase drowsiness).
- No products indexed under this heading.

Chlorprothixene Hydrochloride (May increase drowsiness).
- No products indexed under this heading.

Clorazepate Dipotassium (May increase drowsiness). Products include:
- Tranxene ... 459

Diazepam (May increase drowsiness). Products include:
- Dizac (diazepam injectable emulsion) CIV ... 1862
- Valium Injectable ... 2336
- Valium Tablets ... 2335

Droperidol (May increase drowsiness). Products include:
- Inapsine Injection ... 462

Estazolam (May increase drowsiness). Products include:
- ProSom Tablets ... 457

Ethchlorvynol (May increase drowsiness). Products include:
- Placidyl Capsules ... 456

Ethinamate (May increase drowsiness).
- No products indexed under this heading.

Fluphenazine Decanoate (May increase drowsiness). Products include:
- Prolixin Decanoate ... 510

Fluphenazine Enanthate (May increase drowsiness). Products include:
- Prolixin Enanthate ... 510

Fluphenazine Hydrochloride (May increase drowsiness). Products include:
- Prolixin ... 510

Flurazepam Hydrochloride (May increase drowsiness). Products include:
- Dalmane Capsules ... 2329

Glutethimide (May increase drowsiness).
- No products indexed under this heading.

Haloperidol (May increase drowsiness). Products include:
- Haldol Injection, Tablets and Concentrate ... 1585

Haloperidol Decanoate (May increase drowsiness). Products include:
- Haldol Decanoate ... 1587

Hydroxyzine Hydrochloride (May increase drowsiness). Products include:
- Atarax Tablets & Syrup ... 1992
- Marax Tablets & DF Syrup ... 2015
- Vistaril Intramuscular Solution ... 2042

Lorazepam (May increase drowsiness). Products include:
- Ativan Injection ... 2805
- Ativan Tablets ... 2807

Loxapine Hydrochloride (May increase drowsiness). Products include:
- Loxitane ... 1426

Loxapine Succinate (May increase drowsiness). Products include:
- Loxitane Capsules ... 1426

Meprobamate (May increase drowsiness). Products include:
- Miltown Tablets ... 2780
- PMB 200 and PMB 400 ... 2890

Mesoridazine Besylate (May increase drowsiness). Products include:
- Serentil ... 689

Midazolam Hydrochloride (May increase drowsiness). Products include:
- Versed Injection ... 2324

Molindone Hydrochloride (May increase drowsiness). Products include:
- Moban Tablets and Concentrate ... 1036

Oxazepam (May increase drowsiness). Products include:
- Serax Capsules ... 2916
- Serax Tablets ... 2916

Perphenazine (May increase drowsiness). Products include:
- Etrafon ... 2495
- Triavil Tablets ... 1800
- Trilafon ... 2532

Prazepam (May increase drowsiness).
- No products indexed under this heading.

Prochlorperazine (May increase drowsiness). Products include:
- Compazine ... 2644

Promethazine Hydrochloride (May increase drowsiness). Products include:
- Mepergan Injection ... 2859
- Phenergan with Codeine ... 2883
- Phenergan with Dextromethorphan 2885
- Phenergan Injection ... 2880
- Phenergan Suppositories ... 2882
- Phenergan Syrup ... 2881
- Phenergan Tablets ... 2882
- Phenergan VC ... 2886
- Phenergan VC with Codeine ... 2888

Propofol (May increase drowsiness). Products include:
- Diprivan Injectable Emulsion ... 2939

Quazepam (May increase drowsiness). Products include:
- Doral Tablets ... 2773

Secobarbital Sodium (May increase drowsiness). Products include:
- Seconal Sodium Pulvules ... 1529

Temazepam (May increase drowsiness). Products include:
- Restoril Capsules ... 2413

Thioridazine Hydrochloride (May increase drowsiness). Products include:
- Mellaril ... 2398

Thiothixene (May increase drowsiness). Products include:
- Navane Capsules and Concentrate 2018
- Navane Intramuscular ... 2019

Triazolam (May increase drowsiness). Products include:
- Halcion Tablets ... 2093

Trifluoperazine Hydrochloride (May increase drowsiness). Products include:
- Stelazine ... 2692

Zolpidem Tartrate (May increase drowsiness). Products include:
- Ambien Tablets ... 2559

Food Interactions

Alcohol (May increase drowsiness).

MAXIMUM STRENGTH MIDOL TEEN MULTI-SYMPTOM FORMULA
(Acetaminophen, Pamabrom) ... 621
None cited in PDR database.

MIDRIN CAPSULES
(Isometheptene Mucate, Dichloralphenazone, Acetaminophen) ... 788
May interact with monoamine oxidase inhibitors. Compounds in this category include:

Furazolidone (Concurrent therapy contraindicated). Products include:
- Furoxone ... 2221

Isocarboxazid (Concurrent therapy contraindicated).
- No products indexed under this heading.

Phenelzine Sulfate (Concurrent therapy contraindicated). Products include:
- Nardil ... 1977

Selegiline Hydrochloride (Concurrent therapy contraindicated). Products include:
- Eldepryl Capsules ... 2729

Tranylcypromine Sulfate (Concurrent therapy contraindicated). Products include:
- Parnate Tablets ... 2679

MILTOWN TABLETS
(Meprobamate) ... 2780
May interact with central nervous system depressants, psychotropics, and certain other agents. Compounds in these categories include:

Alfentanil Hydrochloride (Additive effects). Products include:
- Alfenta Injection ... 1334

Alprazolam (Additive effects). Products include:
- Xanax Tablets ... 2115

Amitriptyline Hydrochloride (Additive effects). Products include:
- Elavil ... 2945
- Etrafon ... 2495
- Limbitrol ... 2333
- Triavil Tablets ... 1800

Amoxapine (Additive effects). Products include:
- Asendin Tablets ... 1419

Aprobarbital (Additive effects).
- No products indexed under this heading.

Buprenorphine (Additive effects). Products include:
- Buprenex Injectable ... 2170

Buspirone Hydrochloride (Additive effects). Products include:
- BuSpar Tablets ... 738

Butabarbital (Additive effects).
- No products indexed under this heading.

Butalbital (Additive effects). Products include:
- Axocet Capsules ... 2469
- Esgic-plus Capsules ... 1012
- Esgic-plus Tablets ... 1012
- Fioricet Tablets ... 2386
- Fioricet with Codeine Capsules ... 2387
- Fiorinal Capsules ... 2388
- Fiorinal with Codeine Capsules ... 2390
- Fiorinal Tablets ... 2388
- Phrenilin ... 790
- Sedapap Tablets 50 mg/650 mg .. 1826

Chlordiazepoxide (Additive effects). Products include:
- Limbitrol ... 2333

Chlordiazepoxide Hydrochloride (Additive effects). Products include:
- Librax Capsules ... 2330
- Librium Capsules ... 2331
- Librium Injectable ... 2332

Chlorpromazine (Additive effects). Products include:
- Thorazine Suppositories ... 2701

Chlorpromazine Hydrochloride (Additive effects). Products include:
- Thorazine ... 2701

Chlorprothixene (Additive effects).
- No products indexed under this heading.

Chlorprothixene Hydrochloride (Additive effects).
- No products indexed under this heading.

Chlorprothixene Lactate (Additive effects).
- No products indexed under this heading.

Clorazepate Dipotassium (Additive effects). Products include:
- Tranxene ... 459

Clozapine (Additive effects). Products include:
- Clozaril Tablets ... 2377

Codeine Phosphate (Additive effects). Products include:
- Brontex ... 2130
- Dimetane-DC Cough Syrup ... 2232
- Fioricet with Codeine Capsules ... 2387
- Fiorinal with Codeine Capsules ... 2390
- Nucofed ... 2225
- Phenergan with Codeine ... 2883
- Phenergan VC with Codeine ... 2888
- Robitussin A-C Syrup ... 2248
- Robitussin-DAC Syrup ... 2249
- Ryna ... 804
- Soma Compound w/Codeine Tablets ... 2784
- Tylenol with Codeine ... 1592

Desflurane (Additive effects). Products include:
- Suprane (desflurane, USP) ... 1865

Desipramine Hydrochloride (Additive effects). Products include:
- Norpramin Tablets ... 1273

Dezocine (Additive effects). Products include:
- Dalgan Injection ... 529

IMPORTANT NOTE: Always consult each drug listing in the patient's regimen for possible interactions.

Miltown — **Interactions Index** — 682

Diazepam (Additive effects). Products include:
- Dizac (diazepam injectable emulsion) CIV 1862
- Valium Injectable 2336
- Valium Tablets 2335

Doxepin Hydrochloride (Additive effects). Products include:
- Adapin Capsules 1542
- Sinequan 2028
- Zonalon Cream 1042

Droperidol (Additive effects). Products include:
- Inapsine Injection 462

Enflurane (Additive effects).
No products indexed under this heading.

Estazolam (Additive effects). Products include:
- ProSom Tablets 457

Ethchlorvynol (Additive effects). Products include:
- Placidyl Capsules 456

Ethinamate (Additive effects).
No products indexed under this heading.

Fentanyl (Additive effects). Products include:
- Duragesic Transdermal System 1336

Fentanyl Citrate (Additive effects). Products include:
- Sublimaze Injection 463

Fluphenazine Decanoate (Additive effects). Products include:
- Prolixin Decanoate 510

Fluphenazine Enanthate (Additive effects). Products include:
- Prolixin Enanthate 510

Fluphenazine Hydrochloride (Additive effects). Products include:
- Prolixin 510

Flurazepam Hydrochloride (Additive effects). Products include:
- Dalmane Capsules 2329

Glutethimide (Additive effects).
No products indexed under this heading.

Haloperidol (Additive effects). Products include:
- Haldol Injection, Tablets and Concentrate 1585

Haloperidol Decanoate (Additive effects). Products include:
- Haldol Decanoate 1587

Hydrocodone Bitartrate (Additive effects). Products include:
- Codiclear DH Syrup 808
- Duratuss HD Elixir 2750
- Histussin D Liquid 670
- Hycodan Tablets and Syrup 946
- Hycomine Compound Tablets 948
- Hycomine 947
- Hycotuss Expectorant Syrup 950
- Hydrocet Capsules 787
- Lorcet 10/650 Tablets 1016
- Lortab 2751
- Tussend 1830
- Tussend Expectorant 1831
- Vicodin Tablets 1404
- Vicodin ES Tablets 1405
- Vicodin HP Tablets 1403
- Vicodin Tuss Expectorant 1406
- Zydone Capsules 967

Hydrocodone Polistirex (Additive effects). Products include:
- Tussionex Pennkinetic Extended-Release Suspension 1624

Hydroxyzine Hydrochloride (Additive effects). Products include:
- Atarax Tablets & Syrup 1992
- Marax Tablets & DF Syrup 2015
- Vistaril Intramuscular Solution 2042

Imipramine Hydrochloride (Additive effects). Products include:
- Tofranil Ampuls 873
- Tofranil Tablets 875

Imipramine Pamoate (Additive effects). Products include:
- Tofranil-PM Capsules 876

Isocarboxazid (Additive effects).
No products indexed under this heading.

Isoflurane (Additive effects).
No products indexed under this heading.

Ketamine Hydrochloride (Additive effects).
No products indexed under this heading.

Levomethadyl Acetate Hydrochloride (Additive effects). Products include:
- Orlaam Oral Solution 2361

Levorphanol Tartrate (Additive effects). Products include:
- Levo-Dromoran 2297

Lithium Carbonate (Additive effects). Products include:
- Eskalith 2658
- Lithium Carbonate Capsules & Tablets 2352
- Lithonate/Lithotabs/Lithobid 2721

Lithium Citrate (Additive effects).
No products indexed under this heading.

Lorazepam (Additive effects). Products include:
- Ativan Injection 2805
- Ativan Tablets 2807

Loxapine Hydrochloride (Additive effects). Products include:
- Loxitane 1426

Loxapine Succinate (Additive effects). Products include:
- Loxitane Capsules 1426

Maprotiline Hydrochloride (Additive effects). Products include:
- Ludiomil Tablets 861

Meperidine Hydrochloride (Additive effects). Products include:
- Demerol 2438
- Mepergan Injection 2859

Mephobarbital (Additive effects). Products include:
- Mebaral Tablets 2452

Mesoridazine Besylate (Additive effects). Products include:
- Serentil 689

Methadone Hydrochloride (Additive effects). Products include:
- Methadone Hydrochloride Oral Concentrate 2356
- Methadone Hydrochloride Oral Solution & Tablets 2357

Methohexital Sodium (Additive effects).
No products indexed under this heading.

Methotrimeprazine (Additive effects). Products include:
- Levoprome 1321

Methoxyflurane (Additive effects).
No products indexed under this heading.

Midazolam Hydrochloride (Additive effects). Products include:
- Versed Injection 2324

Molindone Hydrochloride (Additive effects). Products include:
- Moban Tablets and Concentrate 1036

Morphine Sulfate (Additive effects). Products include:
- Astramorph/PF Injection, USP (Preservative-Free) 526
- Duramorph Injection 983
- Infumorph 200 and Infumorph 500 Sterile Solutions 985
- Kadian Capsules 2948
- MS Contin Tablets 2149
- MSIR 2152
- Oramorph SR (Morphine Sulfate Sustained Release Tablets) 2359
- RMS Suppositories CII 2766
- Roxanol 2365

Nortriptyline Hydrochloride (Additive effects). Products include:
- Pamelor 2409

Opium Alkaloids (Additive effects).
No products indexed under this heading.

Oxazepam (Additive effects). Products include:
- Serax Capsules 2916
- Serax Tablets 2916

Oxycodone Hydrochloride (Additive effects). Products include:
- OxyContin Tablets 2163
- OxyIR Capsules 2167
- Percocet Tablets 955
- Percodan Tablets 955
- Percodan-Demi Tablets 956
- Roxicodone Tablets, Oral Solution & Intensol (Oxycodone) 2366
- Tylox Capsules 1593

Pentobarbital Sodium (Additive effects). Products include:
- Nembutal Sodium Capsules 440
- Nembutal Sodium Solution 442
- Nembutal Sodium Suppositories 444

Perphenazine (Additive effects). Products include:
- Etrafon 2495
- Triavil Tablets 1800
- Trilafon Tablets 2532

Phenelzine Sulfate (Additive effects). Products include:
- Nardil 1977

Phenobarbital (Additive effects). Products include:
- Arco-Lase Plus Tablets 513
- Bellergal-S Tablets 2375
- Donnatal 2234
- Donnatal Extentabs 2234
- Donnatal Tablets 2234
- Phenobarbital Elixir and Tablets 1523
- Quadrinal Tablets 1398

Prazepam (Additive effects).
No products indexed under this heading.

Prochlorperazine (Additive effects). Products include:
- Compazine 2644

Promethazine Hydrochloride (Additive effects). Products include:
- Mepergan Injection 2859
- Phenergan with Codeine 2883
- Phenergan with Dextromethorphan 2885
- Phenergan Injection 2880
- Phenergan Suppositories 2882
- Phenergan Syrup 2881
- Phenergan Tablets 2882
- Phenergan VC 2886
- Phenergan VC with Codeine 2888

Propofol (Additive effects). Products include:
- Diprivan Injectable Emulsion 2939

Propoxyphene Hydrochloride (Additive effects). Products include:
- Darvon 1475
- Wygesic Tablets 2930

Propoxyphene Napsylate (Additive effects). Products include:
- Darvon-N/Darvocet-N 1473

Protriptyline Hydrochloride (Additive effects). Products include:
- Vivactil Tablets 1820

Quazepam (Additive effects). Products include:
- Doral Tablets 2773

Risperidone (Additive effects). Products include:
- Risperdal Tablets 1348

Secobarbital Sodium (Additive effects). Products include:
- Seconal Sodium Pulvules 1529

Sevoflurane (Additive effects).
No products indexed under this heading.

Sufentanil Citrate (Additive effects). Products include:
- Sufenta Injection 1355

Temazepam (Additive effects). Products include:
- Restoril Capsules 2413

Thiamylal Sodium (Additive effects).
No products indexed under this heading.

Thioridazine Hydrochloride (Additive effects). Products include:
- Mellaril 2398

Thiothixene (Additive effects). Products include:
- Navane Capsules and Concentrate 2018
- Navane Intramuscular 2019

Tranylcypromine Sulfate (Additive effects). Products include:
- Parnate Tablets 2679

Triazolam (Additive effects). Products include:
- Halcion Tablets 2093

Trifluoperazine Hydrochloride (Additive effects). Products include:
- Stelazine 2692

Trimipramine Maleate (Additive effects). Products include:
- Surmontil Capsules 2917

Zolpidem Tartrate (Additive effects). Products include:
- Ambien Tablets 2559

Food Interactions
Alcohol (Additive effects).

MINIPRESS CAPSULES
(Prazosin Hydrochloride) 2015
May interact with beta blockers, diuretics, antihypertensives, and certain other agents. Compounds in these categories include:

Acebutolol Hydrochloride (Additive hypotensive effect; dosage retitration may be required). Products include:
- Sectral Capsules 2914

Amiloride Hydrochloride (Additive hypotensive effect). Products include:
- Midamor Tablets 1746
- Moduretic Tablets 1748

Amlodipine Besylate (Additive hypotensive effect; dosage retitration may be required). Products include:
- Lotrel Capsules 858
- Norvasc Tablets 2020

Atenolol (Additive hypotensive effect; dosage retitration may be required). Products include:
- Tenoretic Tablets 2963
- Tenormin Tablets and I.V. Injection 2965

Benazepril Hydrochloride (Additive hypotensive effect; dosage retitration may be required). Products include:
- Lotensin Tablets 852
- Lotensin HCT Tablets 855
- Lotrel Capsules 858

Bendroflumethiazide (Additive hypotensive effect; dosage retitration may be required).
No products indexed under this heading.

Betaxolol Hydrochloride (Additive hypotensive effect; dosage retitration may be required). Products include:
- Betoptic Ophthalmic Solution 465
- Betoptic S Ophthalmic Suspension 467
- Kerlone Tablets 2588

Bisoprolol Fumarate (Additive hypotensive effect; dosage retitration may be required). Products include:
- Zebeta Tablets 1457
- Ziac 1459

Bumetanide (Additive hypotensive effect). Products include:
- Bumex 2260

Interactions Index — Minipress

Captopril (Additive hypotensive effect; dosage retitration may be required). Products include:
- Capoten Tablets 740
- Capozide Tablets 744

Carteolol Hydrochloride (Additive hypotensive effect; dosage retitration may be required). Products include:
- Cartrol Tablets 413
- Ocupress Ophthalmic Solution, 1% Sterile .... ⦿ 297

Chlorothiazide (Additive hypotensive effect; dosage retitration may be required). Products include:
- Aldoclor Tablets 1638
- Diupres Tablets 1691
- Diuril Oral 1694

Chlorothiazide Sodium (Additive hypotensive effect; dosage retitration may be required). Products include:
- Diuril Sodium Intravenous 1693

Chlorthalidone (Additive hypotensive effect; dosage retitration may be required). Products include:
- Combipres Tablets 682
- Tenoretic Tablets 2963
- Thalitone 1293

Clonidine (Additive hypotensive effect; dosage retitration may be required). Products include:
- Catapres-TTS 680

Clonidine Hydrochloride (Additive hypotensive effect; dosage retitration may be required). Products include:
- Catapres Tablets 679
- Combipres Tablets 682

Deserpidine (Additive hypotensive effect; dosage retitration may be required).
No products indexed under this heading.

Diazoxide (Additive hypotensive effect; dosage retitration may be required). Products include:
- Hyperstat I.V. Injection 2504
- Proglycem 575

Diltiazem Hydrochloride (Additive hypotensive effect; dosage retitration may be required). Products include:
- Cardizem CD Capsules 1251
- Cardizem SR Capsules 1255
- Cardizem Injectable 1253
- Cardizem Tablets 1257
- Dilacor XR Extended-release Capsules 2183
- Tiazac Capsules 1019

Doxazosin Mesylate (Additive hypotensive effect; dosage retitration may be required). Products include:
- Cardura Tablets 1993

Enalapril Maleate (Additive hypotensive effect; dosage retitration may be required). Products include:
- Vaseretic Tablets 1810
- Vasotec Tablets 1816

Enalaprilat (Additive hypotensive effect; dosage retitration may be required). Products include:
- Vasotec I.V. 1814

Esmolol Hydrochloride (Additive hypotensive effect; dosage retitration may be required). Products include:
- Brevibloc (esmolol HCl) Injection 1860

Ethacrynic Acid (Additive hypotensive effect). Products include:
- Edecrin Tablets 1698

Felodipine (Additive hypotensive effect; dosage retitration may be required). Products include:
- Plendil Extended-Release Tablets 514

Fosinopril Sodium (Additive hypotensive effect; dosage retitration may be required). Products include:
- Monopril Tablets 762

Furosemide (Additive hypotensive effect; dosage retitration may be required). Products include:
- Lasix Injection, Oral Solution and Tablets 1267

Guanabenz Acetate (Additive hypotensive effect; dosage retitration may be required).
No products indexed under this heading.

Guanethidine Monosulfate (Additive hypotensive effect; dosage retitration may be required). Products include:
- Esimil Tablets 840
- Ismelin Tablets 845

Hydralazine Hydrochloride (Additive hypotensive effect; dosage retitration may be required). Products include:
- Apresazide Capsules 824
- Apresoline Hydrochloride Tablets .. 826
- Hydralazine Hydrochloride Injection USP 2712
- Ser-Ap-Es Tablets 867

Hydrochlorothiazide (Additive hypotensive effect; dosage retitration may be required). Products include:
- Aldactazide Tablets 2556
- Aldoril Tablets 1644
- Apresazide Capsules 824
- Capozide Tablets 744
- Dyazide Capsules 2653
- Esidrix Tablets 839
- Esimil Tablets 840
- HydroDIURIL Tablets 1716
- Hydropres Tablets 1718
- Hyzaar Tablets 1720
- Inderide Tablets 2838
- Inderide LA Long Acting Capsules .. 2840
- Lopressor HCT Tablets 850
- Lotensin HCT Tablets 855
- Moduretic Tablets 1748
- Oretic Tablets 450
- Prinzide Tablets 1780
- Ser-Ap-Es Tablets 867
- Timolide Tablets 1791
- Vaseretic Tablets 1810
- Zestoretic Tablets 2968
- Ziac 1459

Hydroflumethiazide (Additive hypotensive effect; dosage retitration may be required). Products include:
- Diucardin Tablets 2824

Indapamide (Additive hypotensive effect; dosage retitration may be required).
No products indexed under this heading.

Isradipine (Additive hypotensive effect; dosage retitration may be required). Products include:
- DynaCirc Capsules 2381
- DynaCirc CR Tablets 2383

Labetalol Hydrochloride (Additive hypotensive effect; dosage retitration may be required). Products include:
- Normodyne Injection 2519
- Normodyne Tablets 2522
- Trandate 1158

Levobunolol Hydrochloride (Additive hypotensive effect; dosage retitration may be required). Products include:
- Betagan .... ⦿ 230

Lisinopril (Additive hypotensive effect; dosage retitration may be required). Products include:
- Prinivil Tablets 1776
- Prinzide Tablets 1780
- Zestoretic Tablets 2968
- Zestril Tablets 2972

Losartan Potassium (Additive hypotensive effect; dosage retitration may be required). Products include:
- Cozaar Tablets 1668
- Hyzaar Tablets 1720

Mecamylamine Hydrochloride (Additive hypotensive effect; dosage retitration may be required). Products include:
- Inversine Tablets 1729

Methyclothiazide (Additive hypotensive effect; dosage retitration may be required). Products include:
- Enduron Tablets 424

Methyldopa (Additive hypotensive effect; dosage retitration may be required). Products include:
- Aldoclor Tablets 1638
- Aldomet Oral 1640
- Aldoril Tablets 1644

Methyldopate Hydrochloride (Additive hypotensive effect; dosage retitration may be required). Products include:
- Aldomet Ester HCl Injection 1642

Metipranolol Hydrochloride (Additive hypotensive effect; dosage retitration may be required). Products include:
- OptiPranolol (Metipranolol 0.3%) Sterile Ophthalmic Solution ...... ⦿ 256

Metolazone (Additive hypotensive effect; dosage retitration may be required). Products include:
- Mykrox Tablets 1617
- Zaroxolyn Tablets 1625

Metoprolol Succinate (Additive hypotensive effect; dosage retitration may be required). Products include:
- Toprol-XL Tablets 560

Metoprolol Tartrate (Additive hypotensive effect; dosage retitration may be required). Products include:
- Lopressor 848
- Lopressor HCT Tablets 850

Metyrosine (Additive hypotensive effect; dosage retitration may be required). Products include:
- Demser Capsules 1690

Minoxidil (Additive hypotensive effect; dosage retitration may be required).
No products indexed under this heading.

Moexipril Hydrochloride (Additive hypotensive effect; dosage retitration may be required). Products include:
- Univasc Tablets 2553

Nadolol (Additive hypotensive effect; dosage retitration may be required).
No products indexed under this heading.

Nicardipine Hydrochloride (Additive hypotensive effect; dosage retitration may be required). Products include:
- Cardene Capsules 2261
- Cardene I.V. 2815
- Cardene SR Capsules 2264

Nifedipine (Additive hypotensive effect; dosage retitration may be required). Products include:
- Adalat Capsules (10 mg and 20 mg) 580
- Adalat CC 582
- Procardia Capsules 2024
- Procardia XL Extended Release Tablets 2026

Nisoldipine (Additive hypotensive effect; dosage retitration may be required). Products include:
- Sular Tablets 2961

Nitroglycerin (Additive hypotensive effect; dosage retitration may be required). Products include:
- Deponit NTG Transdermal Delivery System 2541
- Nitro-Bid IV 1270
- Nitro-Bid Ointment 1272
- Nitro-Dur (nitroglycerin) Transdermal Infusion System 1365
- Nitrolingual Spray 2193
- Nitrostat Tablets 1981
- Transderm-Nitro Transdermal Therapeutic System 878

Penbutolol Sulfate (Additive hypotensive effect; dosage retitration may be required). Products include:
- Levatol Tablets 2547

Phenoxybenzamine Hydrochloride (Additive hypotensive effect; dosage retitration may be required). Products include:
- Dibenzyline Capsules 2650

Phentolamine Mesylate (Additive hypotensive effect; dosage retitration may be required). Products include:
- Regitine Vials 864

Pindolol (Additive hypotensive effect; dosage retitration may be required). Products include:
- Visken Tablets 2428

Polythiazide (Additive hypotensive effect; dosage retitration may be required). Products include:
- Minizide Capsules 2016

Propranolol Hydrochloride (Additive hypotensive effect; dosage retitration may be required). Products include:
- Inderal 2834
- Inderal LA Long Acting Capsules ... 2836
- Inderide Tablets 2838
- Inderide LA Long Acting Capsules .. 2840

Quinapril Hydrochloride (Additive hypotensive effect; dosage retitration may be required). Products include:
- Accupril Tablets 1950

Ramipril (Additive hypotensive effect; dosage retitration may be required). Products include:
- Altace Capsules 1238

Rauwolfia Serpentina (Additive hypotensive effect; dosage retitration may be required).
No products indexed under this heading.

Rescinnamine (Additive hypotensive effect; dosage retitration may be required).
No products indexed under this heading.

Reserpine (Additive hypotensive effect; dosage retitration may be required). Products include:
- Diupres Tablets 1691
- Hydropres Tablets 1718
- Ser-Ap-Es Tablets 867

Sodium Nitroprusside (Additive hypotensive effect; dosage retitration may be required).
No products indexed under this heading.

Sotalol Hydrochloride (Additive hypotensive effect; dosage retitration may be required). Products include:
- Betapace Tablets 637

Spirapril Hydrochloride (Additive hypotensive effect; dosage retitration may be required).
No products indexed under this heading.

Spironolactone (Additive hypotensive effect). Products include:
- Aldactazide Tablets 2556
- Aldactone Tablets 2558

IMPORTANT NOTE: Always consult each drug listing in the patient's regimen for possible interactions.

Terazosin Hydrochloride (Additive hypotensive effect; dosage retitration may be required). Products include:

- Hytrin Capsules ... 434

Timolol Hemihydrate (Additive hypotensive effect; dosage retitration may be required). Products include:

- Betimol 0.25%, 0.5% ... ◉ 259

Timolol Maleate (Additive hypotensive effect; dosage retitration may be required). Products include:

- Blocadren Tablets ... 1654
- Timolide Tablets ... 1791
- Timoptic in Ocudose ... 1796
- Timoptic Sterile Ophthalmic Solution ... 1794
- Timoptic-XE ... 1798

Torsemide (Additive hypotensive effect; dosage retitration may be required). Products include:

- Demadex Tablets and Injection ... 691

Triamterene (Additive hypotensive effect). Products include:

- Dyazide Capsules ... 2653
- Dyrenium Capsules ... 2655

Trimethaphan Camsylate (Additive hypotensive effect; dosage retitration may be required).

No products indexed under this heading.

Verapamil Hydrochloride (Additive hypotensive effect; dosage retitration may be required). Products include:

- Calan SR Caplets ... 2571
- Calan Tablets ... 2568
- Covera-HS Tablets ... 2573
- Isoptin Injectable ... 1391
- Isoptin Oral Tablets ... 1393
- Isoptin SR Tablets ... 1395
- Verelan Capsules ... 1455

MINIZIDE CAPSULES

(Prazosin Hydrochloride, Polythiazide) ... 2016

May interact with narcotic analgesics, barbiturates, antihypertensives, cardiac glycosides, corticosteroids, insulin, and certain other agents. Compounds in these categories include:

Acebutolol Hydrochloride (Co-administration may result in additive or potentiative action of other antihypertensives). Products include:

- Sectral Capsules ... 2914

ACTH (Concomitant use with ACTH may increase the risk of developing hypokalemia).

No products indexed under this heading.

Alfentanil Hydrochloride (Co-administration may aggravate orthostatic hypotension). Products include:

- Alfenta Injection ... 1334

Amlodipine Besylate (Co-administration may result in additive or potentiative action of other antihypertensives). Products include:

- Lotrel Capsules ... 858
- Norvasc Tablets ... 2020

Aprobarbital (Co-administration may aggravate orthostatic hypotension).

No products indexed under this heading.

Atenolol (Co-administration may result in additive or potentiative action of other antihypertensives). Products include:

- Tenoretic Tablets ... 2963
- Tenormin Tablets and I.V. Injection 2965

Benazepril Hydrochloride (Co-administration may result in additive or potentiative action of other antihypertensives). Products include:

- Lotensin Tablets ... 852
- Lotensin HCT Tablets ... 855
- Lotrel Capsules ... 858

Bendroflumethiazide (Co-administration may result in additive or potentiative action of other antihypertensives).

No products indexed under this heading.

Betamethasone Acetate (Concomitant use with corticosteroids may increase the risk of developing hypokalemia). Products include:

- Celestone Soluspan Suspension ... 2484

Betamethasone Sodium Phosphate (Concomitant use with corticosteroids may increase the risk of developing hypokalemia). Products include:

- Celestone Soluspan Suspension ... 2484

Betaxolol Hydrochloride (Co-administration may result in additive or potentiative action of other antihypertensives). Products include:

- Betoptic Ophthalmic Solution ... 465
- Betoptic S Ophthalmic Suspension 467
- Kerlone Tablets ... 2588

Bisoprolol Fumarate (Co-administration may result in additive or potentiative action of other antihypertensives). Products include:

- Zebeta Tablets ... 1457
- Ziac ... 1459

Buprenorphine (Co-administration may aggravate orthostatic hypotension). Products include:

- Buprenex Injectable ... 2170

Butabarbital (Co-administration may aggravate orthostatic hypotension).

No products indexed under this heading.

Butalbital (Co-administration may aggravate orthostatic hypotension). Products include:

- Axocet Capsules ... 2469
- Esgic-plus Capsules ... 1012
- Esgic-plus Tablets ... 1012
- Fioricet Tablets ... 2386
- Fioricet with Codeine Capsules ... 2387
- Fiorinal Capsules ... 2388
- Fiorinal with Codeine Capsules ... 2390
- Fiorinal Tablets ... 2388
- Phrenilin ... 790
- Sedapap Tablets 50 mg/650 mg .. 1826

Captopril (Co-administration may result in additive or potentiative action of other antihypertensives). Products include:

- Capoten Tablets ... 740
- Capozide Tablets ... 744

Carteolol Hydrochloride (Co-administration may result in additive or potentiative action of other antihypertensives). Products include:

- Cartrol Tablets ... 413
- Ocupress Ophthalmic Solution, 1% Sterile ... ◉ 297

Chlorothiazide (Co-administration may result in additive or potentiative action of other antihypertensives). Products include:

- Aldoclor Tablets ... 1638
- Diupres Tablets ... 1691
- Diuril Oral ... 1694

Chlorothiazide Sodium (Co-administration may result in additive or potentiative action of other antihypertensives). Products include:

- Diuril Sodium Intravenous ... 1693

Chlorthalidone (Co-administration may result in additive or potentiative action of other antihypertensives). Products include:

- Combipres Tablets ... 682
- Tenoretic Tablets ... 2963
- Thalitone ... 1293

Clonidine (Co-administration may result in additive or potentiative action of other antihypertensives). Products include:

- Catapres-TTS ... 680

Clonidine Hydrochloride (Co-administration may result in additive or potentiative action of other antihypertensives). Products include:

- Catapres Tablets ... 679
- Combipres Tablets ... 682

Codeine Phosphate (Co-administration may aggravate orthostatic hypotension). Products include:

- Brontex ... 2130
- Dimetane-DC Cough Syrup ... 2232
- Fioricet with Codeine Capsules ... 2387
- Fiorinal with Codeine Capsules ... 2390
- Nucofed ... 2225
- Phenergan with Codeine ... 2883
- Phenergan VC with Codeine ... 2888
- Robitussin A-C Syrup ... 2248
- Robitussin-DAC Syrup ... 2249
- Ryna ... ▣ 804
- Soma Compound w/Codeine Tablets ... 2784
- Tylenol with Codeine ... 1592

Cortisone Acetate (Concomitant use with corticosteroids may increase the risk of developing hypokalemia). Products include:

- Cortone Acetate Sterile Suspension ... 1663
- Cortone Acetate Tablets ... 1664

Deserpidine (Co-administration may result in additive or potentiative action of other antihypertensives).

No products indexed under this heading.

Deslanoside (Co-administration with digitalis may exaggerate the metabolic effects of hypokalemia, especially with reference to myocardial activity).

No products indexed under this heading.

Dexamethasone (Concomitant use with corticosteroids may increase the risk of developing hypokalemia). Products include:

- AK-Trol Ointment & Suspension ... ◉ 205
- Decadron Elixir ... 1676
- Decadron Tablets ... 1678
- Decaspray Topical Aerosol ... 1689
- Maxitrol Ophthalmic Ointment and Suspension ... ◉ 222
- TobraDex Ophthalmic Suspension and Ointment ... 469

Dexamethasone Acetate (Concomitant use with corticosteroids may increase the risk of developing hypokalemia). Products include:

- Dalalone D.P. Injectable ... 1009
- Decadron-LA Sterile Suspension ... 1687

Dexamethasone Sodium Phosphate (Concomitant use with corticosteroids may increase the risk of developing hypokalemia). Products include:

- Decadron Phosphate Injection ... 1680
- Decadron Phosphate Sterile Ophthalmic Ointment ... 1684
- Decadron Phosphate Sterile Ophthalmic Solution ... 1685
- Decadron Phosphate Topical Cream ... 1686
- Decadron Phosphate with Xylocaine Injection, Sterile ... 1683
- Dexacort Phosphate in Respihaler .. 1606
- Dexacort Phosphate in Turbinaire .. 1607
- NeoDecadron Sterile Ophthalmic Ointment ... 1755
- NeoDecadron Sterile Ophthalmic Solution ... 1756
- NeoDecadron Topical Cream ... 1757

Dezocine (Co-administration may aggravate orthostatic hypotension). Products include:

- Dalgan Injection ... 529

Diazoxide (Co-administration may result in additive or potentiative action of other antihypertensives). Products include:

- Hyperstat I.V. Injection ... 2504
- Proglycem ... 575

Digitoxin (Co-administration with digitalis may exaggerate the metabolic effects of hypokalemia, especially with reference to myocardial activity). Products include:

- Crystodigin Tablets ... 1472

Digoxin (Co-administration with digitalis may exaggerate the metabolic effects of hypokalemia, especially with reference to myocardial activity). Products include:

- Lanoxicaps ... 1110
- Lanoxin Elixir Pediatric ... 1113
- Lanoxin Injection ... 1116
- Lanoxin Injection Pediatric ... 1119
- Lanoxin Tablets ... 1121

Diltiazem Hydrochloride (Co-administration may result in additive or potentiative action of other antihypertensives). Products include:

- Cardizem CD Capsules ... 1251
- Cardizem SR Capsules ... 1255
- Cardizem Injectable ... 1253
- Cardizem Tablets ... 1257
- Dilacor XR Extended-release Capsules ... 2183
- Tiazac Capsules ... 1019

Doxazosin Mesylate (Co-administration may result in additive or potentiative action of other antihypertensives). Products include:

- Cardura Tablets ... 1993

Enalapril Maleate (Co-administration may result in additive or potentiative action of other antihypertensives). Products include:

- Vaseretic Tablets ... 1810
- Vasotec Tablets ... 1816

Enalaprilat (Co-administration may result in additive or potentiative action of other antihypertensives). Products include:

- Vasotec I.V. ... 1814

Esmolol Hydrochloride (Co-administration may result in additive or potentiative action of other antihypertensives). Products include:

- Brevibloc (esmolol HCl) Injection ... 1860

Felodipine (Co-administration may result in additive or potentiative action of other antihypertensives). Products include:

- Plendil Extended-Release Tablets ... 514

Fentanyl (Co-administration may aggravate orthostatic hypotension). Products include:

- Duragesic Transdermal System ... 1336

Fentanyl Citrate (Co-administration may aggravate orthostatic hypotension). Products include:

- Sublimaze Injection ... 463

Fludrocortisone Acetate (Concomitant use with corticosteroids may increase the risk of developing hypokalemia). Products include:

- Florinef Acetate Tablets ... 506

Fosinopril Sodium (Co-administration may result in additive or potentiative action of other antihypertensives). Products include:

- Monopril Tablets ... 762

Furosemide (Co-administration may result in additive or potentiative action of other antihypertensives). Products include:

- Lasix Injection, Oral Solution and Tablets ... 1267

Guanabenz Acetate (Co-administration may result in additive or potentiative action of other antihypertensives).

No products indexed under this heading.

(▣ Described in PDR For Nonprescription Drugs) (◉ Described in PDR For Ophthalmology)

Guanethidine Monosulfate (Co-administration may result in additive or potentiative action of other antihypertensives). Products include:
Esimil Tablets ... 840
Ismelin Tablets ... 845

Hydralazine Hydrochloride (Co-administration may result in additive or potentiative action of other antihypertensives). Products include:
Apresazide Capsules ... 824
Apresoline Hydrochloride Tablets .. 826
Hydralazine Hydrochloride Injection USP ... 2712
Ser-Ap-Es Tablets ... 867

Hydrochlorothiazide (Co-administration may result in additive or potentiative action of other antihypertensives). Products include:
Aldactazide Tablets ... 2556
Aldoril Tablets ... 1644
Apresazide Capsules ... 824
Capozide Tablets ... 744
Dyazide Capsules ... 2653
Esidrix Tablets ... 839
Esimil Tablets ... 840
HydroDIURIL Tablets ... 1716
Hydropres Tablets ... 1718
Hyzaar Tablets ... 1720
Inderide Tablets ... 2838
Inderide LA Long Acting Capsules .. 2840
Lopressor HCT Tablets ... 850
Lotensin HCT Tablets ... 855
Moduretic Tablets ... 1748
Oretic Tablets ... 450
Prinzide Tablets ... 1780
Ser-Ap-Es Tablets ... 867
Timolide Tablets ... 1791
Vaseretic Tablets ... 1810
Zestoretic Tablets ... 2968
Ziac ... 1459

Hydrocodone Bitartrate (Co-administration may aggravate orthostatic hypotension). Products include:
Codiclear DH Syrup ... 808
Duratuss HD Elixir ... 2750
Histussin D Liquid ... 670
Hycodan Tablets and Syrup ... 946
Hycomine Compound Tablets ... 948
Hycomine ... 947
Hycotuss Expectorant Syrup ... 950
Hydrocet Capsules ... 787
Lorcet 10/650 Tablets ... 1016
Lortab ... 2751
Tussend ... 1830
Tussend Expectorant ... 1831
Vicodin Tablets ... 1404
Vicodin ES Tablets ... 1405
Vicodin HP Tablets ... 1403
Vicodin Tuss Expectorant ... 1406
Zydone Capsules ... 967

Hydrocodone Polistirex (Co-administration may aggravate orthostatic hypotension). Products include:
Tussionex Pennkinetic Extended-Release Suspension ... 1624

Hydrocortisone (Concomitant use with corticosteroids may increase the risk of developing hypokalemia). Products include:
Anusol-HC Cream 2.5% ... 1953
Aquanil HC Lotion ... 1989
Maximum Strength Cortaid Spray ... 800
CORTENEMA ... 2713
Cortisporin Ointment ... 1074
Cortisporin Ophthalmic Ointment Sterile ... 1074
Cortisporin Ophthalmic Suspension Sterile ... 1075
Cortisporin Otic Solution Sterile ... 1076
Cortisporin Otic Suspension Sterile 1077
Cortizone-5 ... 795
Cortizone-10 ... 795
Hydrocortone Tablets ... 1715
Hytone ... 922
Hytone Ointment 2 ½% ... 923
Massengill Medicated Soft Cloth Towelettes ... 2628
Pediotic Suspension Sterile ... 1140
Preparation H Hydrocortisone 1% Cream ... 843
ProctoCream-HC 2.5% ... 2552
VōSoL HC Otic Solution ... 2786

Hydrocortisone Acetate (Concomitant use with corticosteroids may increase the risk of developing hypokalemia). Products include:
Analpram-HC Rectal Cream 1% and 2.5% ... 993
Anusol HC-1 Hydrocortisone Anti-Itch Ointment ... 810
Anusol-HC Suppositories ... 1954
Caldecort Anti-Itch Hydrocortisone Cream ... 651
Coly-Mycin S Otic w/Neomycin & Hydrocortisone ... 1965
Cortaid ... 800
Cortifoam ... 2540
Cortisporin Cream ... 1073
Epifoam ... 2543
Hydrocortone Acetate Sterile Suspension ... 1712
Mantadil Cream ... 1124
Nupercainal Hydrocortisone 1% Cream ... 661
Pramosone Cream, Lotion & Ointment ... 995
ProctoFoam-HC ... 2552
Terra-Cortril Ophthalmic Suspension ... 2033

Hydrocortisone Sodium Phosphate (Concomitant use with corticosteroids may increase the risk of developing hypokalemia). Products include:
Hydrocortone Phosphate Injection, Sterile ... 1713

Hydrocortisone Sodium Succinate (Concomitant use with corticosteroids may increase the risk of developing hypokalemia).
No products indexed under this heading.

Hydroflumethiazide (Co-administration may result in additive or potentiative action of other antihypertensives). Products include:
Diucardin Tablets ... 2824

Hydromorphone Hydrochloride (Co-administration may aggravate orthostatic hypotension). Products include:
Dilaudid Ampules ... 1382
Dilaudid Cough Syrup ... 1383
Dilaudid-HP Injection ... 1384
Dilaudid-HP Lyophilized Powder 250 mg ... 1384
Dilaudid ... 1382
Dilaudid Oral Liquid ... 1386
Dilaudid ... 1382
Dilaudid Tablets - 8 mg ... 1386

Indapamide (Co-administration may result in additive or potentiative action of other antihypertensives).
No products indexed under this heading.

Insulin, Human (Hyperglycemia is a side effect of thiazides, insulin dosage may need to be altered).
No products indexed under this heading.

Insulin, Human Isophane Suspension (Hyperglycemia is a side effect of thiazides, insulin dosage may need to be altered). Products include:
Novolin N Human Insulin 10 ml Vials ... 1846

Insulin, Human NPH (Hyperglycemia is a side effect of thiazides, insulin dosage may need to be altered). Products include:
Humulin N, 100 Units ... 1495
Novolin N PenFill 1.5 ml Cartridges Durable Insulin Delivery System ... 1849
Novolin N Prefilled Syringe Disposable Insulin Delivery System ... 1850

Insulin, Human Regular (Hyperglycemia is a side effect of thiazides, insulin dosage may need to be altered). Products include:
Humulin R, 100 Units ... 1497
Novolin R Human Insulin 10 ml Vials ... 1846
Novolin R PenFill 1.5 ml Cartridges Durable Insulin Delivery System ... 1849
Novolin R Prefilled Syringe Disposable Insulin Delivery System ... 1850
Velosulin BR Human Insulin 10 ml Vials ... 1847

Insulin, Human, Zinc Suspension (Hyperglycemia is a side effect of thiazides, insulin dosage may need to be altered). Products include:
Humulin L, 100 Units ... 1494
Humulin U, 100 Units ... 1498
Novolin L Human Insulin 10 ml Vials ... 1846

Insulin Lispro, Human (Hyperglycemia is a side effect of thiazides, insulin dosage may need to be altered). Products include:
Humalog Injection ... 1488

Insulin, NPH (Hyperglycemia is a side effect of thiazides, insulin dosage may need to be altered). Products include:
NPH, 100 Units ... 1502
Pork NPH, 100 Units ... 1506
Purified Pork NPH Isophane Insulin ... 1852

Insulin, Regular (Hyperglycemia is a side effect of thiazides, insulin dosage may need to be altered). Products include:
Regular, 100 Units ... 1503
Pork Regular, 100 Units ... 1507
Pork Regular (Concentrated), 500 Units ... 1508
Purified Pork Regular Insulin ... 1852

Insulin, Zinc Crystals (Hyperglycemia is a side effect of thiazides, insulin dosage may need to be altered). Products include:
NPH, 100 Units ... 1502

Insulin, Zinc Suspension (Hyperglycemia is a side effect of thiazides, insulin dosage may need to be altered). Products include:
Iletin I ... 1501
Lente, 100 Units ... 1501
Iletin II ... 1504
Pork Lente, 100 Units ... 1504
Purified Pork Lente Insulin ... 1852

Isradipine (Co-administration may result in additive or potentiative action of other antihypertensives). Products include:
DynaCirc Capsules ... 2381
DynaCirc CR Tablets ... 2383

Labetalol Hydrochloride (Co-administration may result in additive or potentiative action of other antihypertensives). Products include:
Normodyne Injection ... 2519
Normodyne Tablets ... 2522
Trandate ... 1158

Levorphanol Tartrate (Co-administration may aggravate orthostatic hypotension). Products include:
Levo-Dromoran ... 2297

Lisinopril (Co-administration may result in additive or potentiative action of other antihypertensives). Products include:
Prinivil Tablets ... 1776
Prinzide Tablets ... 1780
Zestoretic Tablets ... 2968
Zestril Tablets ... 2972

Losartan Potassium (Co-administration may result in additive or potentiative action of other antihypertensives). Products include:
Cozaar Tablets ... 1668
Hyzaar Tablets ... 1720

Mecamylamine Hydrochloride (Co-administration may result in additive or potentiative action of other antihypertensives). Products include:
Inversine Tablets ... 1729

Meperidine Hydrochloride (Co-administration may aggravate orthostatic hypotension). Products include:
Demerol ... 2438
Mepergan Injection ... 2859

Mephobarbital (Co-administration may aggravate orthostatic hypotension). Products include:
Mebaral Tablets ... 2452

Methadone Hydrochloride (Co-administration may aggravate orthostatic hypotension). Products include:
Methadone Hydrochloride Oral Concentrate ... 2356
Methadone Hydrochloride Oral Solution & Tablets ... 2357

Methyclothiazide (Co-administration may result in additive or potentiative action of other antihypertensives). Products include:
Enduron Tablets ... 424

Methyldopa (Co-administration may result in additive or potentiative action of other antihypertensives). Products include:
Aldoclor Tablets ... 1638
Aldomet Oral ... 1640
Aldoril Tablets ... 1644

Methyldopate Hydrochloride (Co-administration may result in additive or potentiative action of other antihypertensives). Products include:
Aldomet Ester HCl Injection ... 1642

Methylprednisolone Acetate (Concomitant use with corticosteroids may increase the risk of developing hypokalemia).
No products indexed under this heading.

Methylprednisolone Sodium Succinate (Concomitant use with corticosteroids may increase the risk of developing hypokalemia).
No products indexed under this heading.

Metolazone (Co-administration may result in additive or potentiative action of other antihypertensives). Products include:
Mykrox Tablets ... 1617
Zaroxolyn Tablets ... 1625

Metoprolol Succinate (Co-administration may result in additive or potentiative action of other antihypertensives). Products include:
Toprol-XL Tablets ... 560

Metoprolol Tartrate (Co-administration may result in additive or potentiative action of other antihypertensives). Products include:
Lopressor ... 848
Lopressor HCT Tablets ... 850

Metyrosine (Co-administration may result in additive or potentiative action of other antihypertensives). Products include:
Demser Capsules ... 1690

Minoxidil (Co-administration may result in additive or potentiative action of other antihypertensives).
No products indexed under this heading.

Moexipril Hydrochloride (Co-administration may result in additive or potentiative action of other antihypertensives). Products include:
Univasc Tablets ... 2553

Morphine Sulfate (Co-administration may aggravate orthostatic hypotension). Products include:
Astramorph/PF Injection, USP (Preservative-Free) ... 526
Duramorph Injection ... 983
Infumorph 200 and Infumorph 500 Sterile Solutions ... 985
Kadian Capsules ... 2948

IMPORTANT NOTE: Always consult each drug listing in the patient's regimen for possible interactions.

Minizide / Interactions Index

MS Contin Tablets 2149
MSIR 2152
Oramorph SR (Morphine Sulfate Sustained Release Tablets) 2359
RMS Suppositories CII 2766
Roxanol 2365

Nadolol (Co-administration may result in additive or potentiative action of other antihypertensives).
No products indexed under this heading.

Nicardipine Hydrochloride (Co-administration may result in additive or potentiative action of other antihypertensives). Products include:
Cardene Capsules 2261
Cardene I.V. 2815
Cardene SR Capsules 2264

Nifedipine (Co-administration may result in additive or potentiative action of other antihypertensives). Products include:
Adalat Capsules (10 mg and 20 mg) 580
Adalat CC 582
Procardia Capsules 2024
Procardia XL Extended Release Tablets 2026

Nisoldipine (Co-administration may result in additive or potentiative action of other antihypertensives). Products include:
Sular Tablets 2961

Nitroglycerin (Co-administration may result in additive or potentiative action of other antihypertensives). Products include:
Deponit NTG Transdermal Delivery System 2541
Nitro-Bid IV 1270
Nitro-Bid Ointment 1272
Nitro-Dur (nitroglycerin) Transdermal Infusion System 1365
Nitrolingual Spray 2193
Nitrostat Tablets 1981
Transderm-Nitro Transdermal Therapeutic System 878

Norepinephrine Bitartrate (Thiazides may decrease the arterial responsiveness to norepinephrine). Products include:
Levophed Bitartrate Injection 2445

Opium Alkaloids (Co-administration may aggravate orthostatic hypotension).
No products indexed under this heading.

Oxycodone Hydrochloride (Co-administration may aggravate orthostatic hypotension). Products include:
OxyContin Tablets 2163
OxyIR Capsules 2167
Percocet Tablets 955
Percodan Tablets 955
Percodan-Demi Tablets 956
Roxicodone Tablets, Oral Solution & Intensol (Oxycodone) 2366
Tylox Capsules 1593

Penbutolol Sulfate (Co-administration may result in additive or potentiative action of other antihypertensives). Products include:
Levatol Tablets 2547

Pentobarbital Sodium (Co-administration may aggravate orthostatic hypotension). Products include:
Nembutal Sodium Capsules 440
Nembutal Sodium Solution 442
Nembutal Sodium Suppositories 444

Phenobarbital (Co-administration may aggravate orthostatic hypotension). Products include:
Arco-Lase Plus Tablets 513
Bellergal-S Tablets 2375
Donnatal 2234
Donnatal Extentabs 2234
Donnatal 2234
Phenobarbital Elixir and Tablets 1523
Quadrinal Tablets 1398

Phenoxybenzamine Hydrochloride (Co-administration may result in additive or potentiative action of other antihypertensives). Products include:
Dibenzyline Capsules 2650

Phentolamine Mesylate (Co-administration may result in additive or potentiative action of other antihypertensives). Products include:
Regitine Vials 864

Pindolol (Co-administration may result in additive or potentiative action of other antihypertensives). Products include:
Visken Tablets 2428

Prednisolone Acetate (Concomitant use with corticosteroids may increase the risk of developing hypokalemia). Products include:
AK-CIDE ..... ⊙ 203
AK-CIDE Ointment ..... ⊙ 203
Blephamide Liquifilm Sterile Ophthalmic Suspension 472
Blephamide Ointment ..... ⊙ 234
Econopred & Econopred Plus Ophthalmic Suspensions ..... ⊙ 216
Poly-Pred Liquifilm ..... ⊙ 246
Pred Forte ..... ⊙ 248
Pred Mild ..... ⊙ 250
Pred-G Liquifilm Sterile Ophthalmic Suspension ..... ⊙ 248
Pred-G S.O.P. Sterile Ophthalmic Ointment ..... ⊙ 249

Prednisolone Sodium Phosphate (Concomitant use with corticosteroids may increase the risk of developing hypokalemia). Products include:
AK-PRED ..... ⊙ 204
Hydeltrasol Injection, Sterile 1708
Pediapred Oral Solution 1618

Prednisolone Tebutate (Concomitant use with corticosteroids may increase the risk of developing hypokalemia). Products include:
Hydeltra-T.B.A. Sterile Suspension 1710

Prednisone (Concomitant use with corticosteroids may increase the risk of developing hypokalemia).
No products indexed under this heading.

Propoxyphene Hydrochloride (Co-administration may aggravate orthostatic hypotension). Products include:
Darvon 1475
Wygesic Tablets 2930

Propoxyphene Napsylate (Co-administration may aggravate orthostatic hypotension). Products include:
Darvon-N/Darvocet-N 1473

Propranolol Hydrochloride (Co-administration may result in additive or potentiative action of other antihypertensives). Products include:
Inderal 2834
Inderal LA Long Acting Capsules 2836
Inderide Tablets 2838
Inderide LA Long Acting Capsules 2840

Quinapril Hydrochloride (Co-administration may result in additive or potentiative action of other antihypertensives). Products include:
Accupril Tablets 1950

Ramipril (Co-administration may result in additive or potentiative action of other antihypertensives). Products include:
Altace Capsules 1238

Rauwolfia Serpentina (Co-administration may result in additive or potentiative action of other antihypertensives).
No products indexed under this heading.

Rescinnamine (Co-administration may result in additive or potentiative action of other antihypertensives).
No products indexed under this heading.

Reserpine (Co-administration may result in additive or potentiative action of other antihypertensives). Products include:
Diupres Tablets 1691
Hydropres Tablets 1718
Ser-Ap-Es Tablets 867

Secobarbital Sodium (Co-administration may aggravate orthostatic hypotension). Products include:
Seconal Sodium Pulvules 1529

Sodium Nitroprusside (Co-administration may result in additive or potentiative action of other antihypertensives).
No products indexed under this heading.

Sotalol Hydrochloride (Co-administration may result in additive or potentiative action of other antihypertensives). Products include:
Betapace Tablets 637

Spirapril Hydrochloride (Co-administration may result in additive or potentiative action of other antihypertensives).
No products indexed under this heading.

Sufentanil Citrate (Co-administration may aggravate orthostatic hypotension). Products include:
Sufenta Injection 1355

Terazosin Hydrochloride (Co-administration may result in additive or potentiative action of other antihypertensives). Products include:
Hytrin Capsules 434

Thiamylal Sodium (Co-administration may aggravate orthostatic hypotension).
No products indexed under this heading.

Timolol Maleate (Co-administration may result in additive or potentiative action of other antihypertensives). Products include:
Blocadren Tablets 1654
Timolide Tablets 1791
Timoptic in Ocudose 1796
Timoptic Sterile Ophthalmic Solution 1794
Timoptic-XE 1798

Torsemide (Co-administration may result in additive or potentiative action of other antihypertensives). Products include:
Demadex Tablets and Injection 691

Trandolapril (Co-administration may result in additive or potentiative action of other antihypertensives). Products include:
Mavik Tablets 1407

Triamcinolone (Concomitant use with corticosteroids may increase the risk of developing hypokalemia).
No products indexed under this heading.

Triamcinolone Acetonide (Concomitant use with corticosteroids may increase the risk of developing hypokalemia). Products include:
Azmacort Oral Inhaler 2175
Nasacort AQ Nasal Spray 2191
Nasacort Nasal Inhaler 2189

Triamcinolone Diacetate (Concomitant use with corticosteroids may increase the risk of developing hypokalemia).
No products indexed under this heading.

Triamcinolone Hexacetonide (Concomitant use with corticosteroids may increase the risk of developing hypokalemia).
No products indexed under this heading.

Trimethaphan Camsylate (Co-administration may result in additive or potentiative action of other antihypertensives).
No products indexed under this heading.

Tubocurarine Chloride (Thiazides may increase the responsiveness to tubocurarine).
No products indexed under this heading.

Verapamil Hydrochloride (Co-administration may result in additive or potentiative action of other antihypertensives). Products include:
Calan SR Caplets 2571
Calan Tablets 2568
Covera-HS Tablets 2573
Isoptin Injectable 1391
Isoptin Oral Tablets 1393
Isoptin SR Tablets 1395
Verelan Capsules 1455

Food Interactions

Alcohol (Concurrent use may aggravate orthostatic hypotension).

MINOCIN INTRAVENOUS
(Minocycline Hydrochloride) 1428
May interact with penicillins, anticoagulants, oral contraceptives, and certain other agents. Compounds in these categories include:

Amoxicillin Trihydrate (Interference with bactericidal action of penicillins; avoid concurrent use). Products include:
Amoxil 2631
Augmentin 2637
Augmentin Tablets 2640

Ampicillin (Interference with bactericidal action of penicillins; avoid concurrent use). Products include:
Omnipen Capsules 2872
Omnipen for Oral Suspension 2873

Ampicillin Sodium (Interference with bactericidal action of penicillins; avoid concurrent use). Products include:
Unasyn 2035

Ampicillin Trihydrate (Interference with bactericidal action of penicillins; avoid concurrent use).
No products indexed under this heading.

Azlocillin Sodium (Interference with bactericidal action of penicillins; avoid concurrent use).
No products indexed under this heading.

Bacampicillin Hydrochloride (Interference with bactericidal action of penicillins; avoid concurrent use). Products include:
Spectrobid Tablets 2030

Carbenicillin Disodium (Interference with bactericidal action of penicillins; avoid concurrent use).
No products indexed under this heading.

Carbenicillin Indanyl Sodium (Interference with bactericidal action of penicillins; avoid concurrent use). Products include:
Geocillin Tablets 2009

Dalteparin Sodium (Depressed plasma prothrombin activity). Products include:
Fragmin Injection 2088

Desogestrel (Reduced efficacy and increased incidence of breakthrough bleeding). Products include:
Desogen Tablets 1867

(▣ Described in PDR For Nonprescription Drugs)   (⊙ Described in PDR For Ophthalmology)

687 **Interactions Index** **Minocin Oral Suspension**

Ortho-Cept ... 1907

Dicloxacillin Sodium (Interference with bactericidal action of penicillins; avoid concurrent use).
No products indexed under this heading.

Dicumarol (Depressed plasma prothrombin activity).
No products indexed under this heading.

Enoxaparin (Depressed plasma prothrombin activity). Products include:
Lovenox Injection ... 2187

Ethinyl Estradiol (Reduced efficacy and increased incidence of breakthrough bleeding). Products include:
Brevicon ... 2563
Demulen ... 2580
Desogen Tablets ... 1867
Levlen/Tri-Levlen ... 646
Lo/Ovral Tablets ... 2852
Lo/Ovral-28 Tablets ... 2857
Modicon ... 1928
Nordette-21 Tablets ... 2863
Nordette-28 Tablets ... 2866
Norinyl ... 2563
Ortho-Cept ... 1907
Ortho-Cyclen/Ortho-Tri-Cyclen ... 1914
Ortho-Novum ... 1928
Ortho-Cyclen/Ortho Tri-Cyclen ... 1914
Ovcon ... 765
Ovral Tablets ... 2877
Ovral-28 Tablets ... 2878
Levlen/Tri-Levlen ... 646
Tri-Norinyl ... 2607
Triphasil-21 Tablets ... 2919
Triphasil-28 Tablets ... 2924

Ethynodiol Diacetate (Reduced efficacy and increased incidence of breakthrough bleeding). Products include:
Demulen ... 2580

Heparin Calcium (Depressed plasma prothrombin activity).
No products indexed under this heading.

Heparin Sodium (Depressed plasma prothrombin activity). Products include:
Heparin Lock Flush Solution ... 2831
Heparin Sodium Injection ... 2832
Heparin Sodium Vials ... 1486

Levonorgestrel (Reduced efficacy and increased incidence of breakthrough bleeding). Products include:
Levlen/Tri-Levlen ... 646
Nordette-21 Tablets ... 2863
Nordette-28 Tablets ... 2866
Norplant System ... 2868
Levlen/Tri-Levlen ... 646
Triphasil-21 Tablets ... 2919
Triphasil-28 Tablets ... 2924

Mestranol (Reduced efficacy and increased incidence of breakthrough bleeding). Products include:
Norinyl ... 2563
Ortho-Novum ... 1928

Mezlocillin Sodium (Interference with bactericidal action of penicillins; avoid concurrent use). Products include:
Mezlin ... 594
Mezlin Pharmacy Bulk Package ... 597

Nafcillin Sodium (Interference with bactericidal action of penicillins; avoid concurrent use).
No products indexed under this heading.

Norethindrone (Reduced efficacy and increased incidence of breakthrough bleeding). Products include:
Brevicon ... 2563
Micronor Tablets ... 1903
Modicon ... 1928
Norinyl ... 2563
Nor-Q D Tablets ... 2598
Ortho-Novum ... 1928
Ovcon ... 765
Tri-Norinyl ... 2607

Norethynodrel (Reduced efficacy and increased incidence of breakthrough bleeding).
No products indexed under this heading.

Norgestimate (Reduced efficacy and increased incidence of breakthrough bleeding). Products include:
Ortho-Cyclen/Ortho-Tri-Cyclen ... 1914
Ortho-Cyclen/Ortho Tri-Cyclen ... 1914

Norgestrel (Reduced efficacy and increased incidence of breakthrough bleeding). Products include:
Lo/Ovral Tablets ... 2852
Lo/Ovral-28 Tablets ... 2857
Ovral Tablets ... 2877
Ovral-28 Tablets ... 2878
Ovrette Tablets ... 2878

Penicillin G Benzathine (Interference with bactericidal action of penicillins; avoid concurrent use). Products include:
Bicillin C-R Injection ... 2810
Bicillin C-R 900/300 Injection ... 2812
Bicillin L-A Injection ... 2813

Penicillin G Potassium (Interference with bactericidal action of penicillins; avoid concurrent use). Products include:
Pfizerpen for Injection ... 2022

Penicillin G Procaine (Interference with bactericidal action of penicillins; avoid concurrent use). Products include:
Bicillin C-R Injection ... 2810
Bicillin C-R 900/300 Injection ... 2812

Penicillin G Sodium (Interference with bactericidal action of penicillins; avoid concurrent use).
No products indexed under this heading.

Penicillin V Potassium (Interference with bactericidal action of penicillins; avoid concurrent use). Products include:
Pen•Vee K ... 2879

Ticarcillin Disodium (Interference with bactericidal action of penicillins; avoid concurrent use). Products include:
Ticar for Injection ... 2704
Timentin for Injection ... 2706

Warfarin Sodium (Depressed plasma prothrombin activity). Products include:
Coumadin ... 941

MINOCIN ORAL SUSPENSION
(Minocycline Hydrochloride) ... 1431
May interact with anticoagulants, oral contraceptives, penicillins, antacids containing aluminium, calcium and magnesium, and certain other agents. Compounds in these categories include:

Aluminum Carbonate (Absorption of tetracyclines is impaired). Products include:
Basaljel Capsules ... 2810
Basaljel Suspension ... 2810
Basaljel Tablets ... 2810

Aluminum Hydroxide (Absorption of tetracyclines is impaired). Products include:
ALternaGEL Liquid ... 1358
Maximum Strength Ascriptin ... 650
Cama Arthritis Pain Reliever ... 748
Gaviscon Extra Strength Relief Formula Antacid Tablets ... 778
Gaviscon Extra Strength Relief Formula Liquid Antacid ... 779
Gaviscon Liquid Antacid ... 779
Gelusil Antacid-Anti-gas Liquid ... 819
Gelusil Antacid-Anti-gas Tablets ... 819
Maalox Antacid/Anti-Gas Tablets ... 889
Maalox Heartburn Relief Suspension ... 658
Maalox Antacid Liquid ... 888
Extra Strength Maalox Antacid/Anti-Gas Liquid and Tablets ... 888
Mylanta ... 1359
Tempo Soft Antacid ... 799

Aluminum Hydroxide Gel (Absorption of tetracyclines is impaired). Products include:
ALternaGEL Liquid ... 675
Aludrox Oral Suspension ... 850
Amphojel Suspension ... 2802
Amphojel Suspension without Flavor ... 2802
Amphojel Tablets ... 2802
Ascriptin ... 650
Gaviscon Antacid Tablets ... 778
Gaviscon-2 Antacid Tablets ... 779
Mylanta Liquid ... 676
Mylanta Double Strength Liquid ... 676
Nephrox Suspension ... 671

Amoxicillin Trihydrate (Interference with bactericidal action of penicillin; avoid concurrent use). Products include:
Amoxil ... 2631
Augmentin ... 2637
Augmentin Tablets ... 2640

Ampicillin (Interference with bactericidal action of penicillin; avoid concurrent use). Products include:
Omnipen Capsules ... 2872
Omnipen for Oral Suspension ... 2873

Ampicillin Sodium (Interference with bactericidal action of penicillin; avoid concurrent use). Products include:
Unasyn ... 2035

Ampicillin Trihydrate (Interference with bactericidal action of penicillin; avoid concurrent use).
No products indexed under this heading.

Azlocillin Sodium (Interference with bactericidal action of penicillin; avoid concurrent use).
No products indexed under this heading.

Bacampicillin Hydrochloride (Interference with bactericidal action of penicillin; avoid concurrent use). Products include:
Spectrobid Tablets ... 2030

Carbenicillin Disodium (Interference with bactericidal action of penicillin; avoid concurrent use).
No products indexed under this heading.

Carbenicillin Indanyl Sodium (Interference with bactericidal action of penicillin; avoid concurrent use). Products include:
Geocillin Tablets ... 2009

Dalteparin Sodium (Depressed plasma prothrombin activity; may require downward adjustment of the anticoagulant dosage). Products include:
Fragmin Injection ... 2088

Desogestrel (Concurrent use may render oral contraceptives less effective; potential for breakthrough bleeding). Products include:
Desogen Tablets ... 1867
Ortho-Cept ... 1907

Dicloxacillin Sodium (Interference with bactericidal action of penicillin; avoid concurrent use).
No products indexed under this heading.

Dicumarol (Depressed plasma prothrombin activity; may require downward adjustment of the anticoagulant dosage).
No products indexed under this heading.

Enoxaparin (Depressed plasma prothrombin activity; may require downward adjustment of the anticoagulant dosage). Products include:
Lovenox Injection ... 2187

Ethinyl Estradiol (Concurrent use may render oral contraceptives less effective; potential for breakthrough bleeding). Products include:
Brevicon ... 2563
Demulen ... 2580
Desogen Tablets ... 1867
Levlen/Tri-Levlen ... 646
Lo/Ovral Tablets ... 2852
Lo/Ovral-28 Tablets ... 2857
Modicon ... 1928
Nordette-21 Tablets ... 2863
Nordette-28 Tablets ... 2866
Norinyl ... 2563
Ortho-Cept ... 1907
Ortho-Cyclen/Ortho-Tri-Cyclen ... 1914
Ortho-Novum ... 1928
Ortho-Cyclen/Ortho Tri-Cyclen ... 1914
Ovcon ... 765
Ovral Tablets ... 2877
Ovral-28 Tablets ... 2878
Levlen/Tri-Levlen ... 646
Tri-Norinyl ... 2607
Triphasil-21 Tablets ... 2919
Triphasil-28 Tablets ... 2924

Ethynodiol Diacetate (Concurrent use may render oral contraceptives less effective; potential for breakthrough bleeding). Products include:
Demulen ... 2580

Ferrous Fumarate (Absorption of tetracyclines is impaired). Products include:
Chromagen Capsules ... 2470
Chromagen FA ... 2471
Chromagen Forte ... 2471
Ferro-Sequels ... 684
Nephro-Fer Tablets ... 2168
Nephro-Fer Rx Tablets ... 2168
Nephro-Vite + Fe Tablets ... 2170
Stresstabs + Iron ... 685
Trinsicon Capsules ... 2759
Vitron-C Tablets ... 667

Ferrous Gluconate (Absorption of tetracyclines is impaired). Products include:
Megadose ... 513

Ferrous Sulfate (Absorption of tetracyclines is impaired). Products include:
Feosol Capsules ... 777
Feosol Elixir ... 2627
Feosol Tablets ... 2627
Fero-Folic-500 Filmtab ... 433
Fero-Grad-500 Filmtab ... 434
Fero-Gradumet Filmtab ... 434
Iberet Tablets ... 437
Iberet-500 Liquid ... 438
Iberet-Folic-500 Filmtab ... 433
Iberet-Liquid ... 438
Irospan ... 1000
Slow Fe Tablets ... 889
Slow Fe with Folic Acid ... 890

Heparin Calcium (Depressed plasma prothrombin activity; may require downward adjustment of the anticoagulant dosage).
No products indexed under this heading.

Heparin Sodium (Depressed plasma prothrombin activity; may require downward adjustment of the anticoagulant dosage). Products include:
Heparin Lock Flush Solution ... 2831
Heparin Sodium Injection ... 2832
Heparin Sodium Vials ... 1486

Levonorgestrel (Concurrent use may render oral contraceptives less effective; potential for breakthrough bleeding). Products include:
Levlen/Tri-Levlen ... 646
Nordette-21 Tablets ... 2863
Nordette-28 Tablets ... 2866
Norplant System ... 2868
Levlen/Tri-Levlen ... 646
Triphasil-21 Tablets ... 2919
Triphasil-28 Tablets ... 2924

Magaldrate (Absorption of tetracyclines is impaired).
No products indexed under this heading.

IMPORTANT NOTE: Always consult each drug listing in the patient's regimen for possible interactions.

Minocin Oral Suspension — Interactions Index — 688

Magnesium Hydroxide (Absorption of tetracyclines is impaired). Products include:
Aludrox Oral Suspension ▣ 850
Ascriptin ▣ 650
Di-Gel Antacid/Anti-Gas ▣ 762
Gelusil Antacid-Anti-gas Liquid ▣ 819
Gelusil Antacid-Anti-gas Tablets ▣ 819
Maalox Antacid/Anti-Gas Tablets 889
Maalox Antacid Liquid 888
Extra Strength Maalox Antacid/Anti-Gas Liquid and Tablets 888
Mylanta Fast-Acting 1359
Mylanta Gelcaps Antacid ▣ 678
Fast-Acting Mylanta Liquid Antacid 1359
Mylanta Tablets ▣ 677
Maximum-Strength Fast-Acting Mylanta Liquid Antacid 1359
Mylanta Double Strength Tablets ▣ 677
Phillips' Milk of Magnesia Liquid ▣ 627
Rolaids Antacid Tablets ▣ 807
Tempo Soft Antacid ▣ 799

Magnesium Oxide (Absorption of tetracyclines is impaired). Products include:
Beelith Tablets 632
Bufferin Analgesic Tablets ▣ 636
Arthritis Strength Bufferin Analgesic Caplets ▣ 637
Extra Strength Bufferin Analgesic Tablets ▣ 637
Caltrate PLUS ▣ 681
Cama Arthritis Pain Reliever ▣ 748
Mag-Ox 400 666
Uro-Mag 666

Mestranol (Concurrent use may render oral contraceptives less effective; potential for breakthrough bleeding). Products include:
Norinyl 2563
Ortho-Novum 1928

Mezlocillin Sodium (Interference with bactericidal action of penicillin; avoid concurrent use). Products include:
Mezlin 594
Mezlin Pharmacy Bulk Package 597

Nafcillin Sodium (Interference with bactericidal action of penicillin; avoid concurrent use).
No products indexed under this heading.

Norethindrone (Concurrent use may render oral contraceptives less effective; potential for breakthrough bleeding). Products include:
Brevicon 2563
Micronor Tablets 1903
Modicon 1928
Norinyl 2563
Nor-Q D Tablets 2598
Ortho-Novum 1928
Ovcon 765
Tri-Norinyl 2607

Norethynodrel (Concurrent use may render oral contraceptives less effective; potential for breakthrough bleeding).
No products indexed under this heading.

Norgestimate (Concurrent use may render oral contraceptives less effective; potential for breakthrough bleeding). Products include:
Ortho-Cyclen/Ortho-Tri-Cyclen 1914
Ortho-Cyclen/Ortho Tri-Cyclen 1914

Norgestrel (Concurrent use may render oral contraceptives less effective; potential for breakthrough bleeding). Products include:
Lo/Ovral Tablets 2852
Lo/Ovral-28 Tablets 2857
Ovral Tablets 2877
Ovral-28 Tablets 2878
Ovrette Tablets 2878

Penicillin G Benzathine (Interference with bactericidal action of penicillin; avoid concurrent use). Products include:
Bicillin C-R Injection 2810
Bicillin C-R 900/300 Injection 2812
Bicillin L-A Injection 2813

Penicillin G Potassium (Interference with bactericidal action of penicillin; avoid concurrent use). Products include:
Pfizerpen for Injection 2022

Penicillin G Procaine (Interference with bactericidal action of penicillin; avoid concurrent use). Products include:
Bicillin C-R Injection 2810
Bicillin C-R 900/300 Injection 2812

Penicillin G Sodium (Interference with bactericidal action of penicillin; avoid concurrent use).
No products indexed under this heading.

Penicillin V Potassium (Interference with bactericidal action of penicillin; avoid concurrent use). Products include:
Pen•Vee K 2879

Ticarcillin Disodium (Interference with bactericidal action of penicillin; avoid concurrent use). Products include:
Ticar for Injection 2704
Timentin for Injection 2706

Warfarin Sodium (Depressed plasma prothrombin activity; may require downward adjustment of the anticoagulant dosage). Products include:
Coumadin 941

MINOCIN PELLET-FILLED CAPSULES
(Minocycline Hydrochloride) 1429
May interact with anticoagulants, oral contraceptives, penicillins, antacids containing aluminium, calcium and magnesium, iron containing oral preparations, and certain other agents. Compounds in these categories include:

Aluminum Carbonate (Absorption of tetracyclines is impaired). Products include:
Basaljel Capsules 2810
Basaljel Suspension 2810
Basaljel Tablets 2810

Aluminum Hydroxide (Absorption of tetracyclines is impaired). Products include:
ALternaGEL Liquid 1358
Maximum Strength Ascriptin ▣ 650
Cama Arthritis Pain Reliever ▣ 748
Gaviscon Extra Strength Relief Formula Antacid Tablets ▣ 778
Gaviscon Extra Strength Relief Formula Liquid Antacid ▣ 779
Gaviscon Liquid Antacid ▣ 779
Gelusil Antacid-Anti-gas Liquid ▣ 819
Gelusil Antacid-Anti-gas Tablets ▣ 819
Maalox Antacid/Anti-Gas Tablets 889
Maalox Heartburn Relief Suspension ▣ 658
Maalox Antacid Liquid 888
Extra Strength Maalox Antacid/Anti-Gas Liquid and Tablets 888
Mylanta 1359
Tempo Soft Antacid ▣ 799

Aluminum Hydroxide Gel (Absorption of tetracyclines is impaired). Products include:
ALternaGEL Liquid ▣ 675
Aludrox Oral Suspension ▣ 850
Amphojel Suspension 2802
Amphojel Suspension without Flavor 2802
Amphojel Tablets 2802
Ascriptin ▣ 650
Gaviscon Antacid Tablets ▣ 778
Gaviscon-2 Antacid Tablets ▣ 779
Mylanta Liquid ▣ 676
Mylanta Double Strength Liquid ▣ 676
Nephrox Suspension ▣ 671

Amoxicillin Trihydrate (Interference with bactericidal action of penicillin; avoid concurrent use). Products include:
Amoxil 2631
Augmentin 2637
Augmentin Tablets 2640

Ampicillin (Interference with bactericidal action of penicllin; avoid concurrent use). Products include:
Omnipen Capsules 2872
Omnipen for Oral Suspension 2873

Ampicillin Sodium (Interference with bactericidal action of penicillin; avoid concurrent use). Products include:
Unasyn 2035

Ampicillin Trihydrate (Interference with bactericidal action of penicillin; avoid concurrent use).
No products indexed under this heading.

Azlocillin Sodium (Interference with bactericidal action of penicillin; avoid concurrent use).
No products indexed under this heading.

Bacampicillin Hydrochloride (Interference with bactericidal action of penicillin; avoid concurrent use). Products include:
Spectrobid Tablets 2030

Carbenicillin Disodium (Interference with bactericidal action of penicillin; avoid concurrent use).
No products indexed under this heading.

Carbenicillin Indanyl Sodium (Interference with bactericidal action of penicillin; avoid concurrent use). Products include:
Geocillin Tablets 2009

Dalteparin Sodium (Depressed plasma prothrombin activity; may require downward adjustment of the anticoagulant dosage). Products include:
Fragmin Injection 2088

Desogestrel (Concurrent use may render oral contraceptives less effective; potential for breakthrough bleeding). Products include:
Desogen Tablets 1867
Ortho-Cept 1907

Dicloxacillin Sodium (Interference with bactericidal action of penicillin; avoid concurrent use).
No products indexed under this heading.

Dicumarol (Depressed plasma prothrombin activity; may require downward adjustment of the anticoagulant dosage).
No products indexed under this heading.

Enoxaparin (Depressed plasma prothrombin activity; may require downward adjustment of the anticoagulant dosage). Products include:
Lovenox Injection 2187

Ethinyl Estradiol (Concurrent use may render oral contraceptives less effective; potential for breakthrough bleeding). Products include:
Brevicon 2563
Demulen 2580
Desogen Tablets 1867
Levlen/Tri-Levlen 646
Lo/Ovral Tablets 2852
Lo/Ovral-28 Tablets 2857
Modicon 1928
Nordette-21 Tablets 2863
Nordette-28 Tablets 2866
Norinyl 2563
Ortho-Cept 1907
Ortho-Cyclen/Ortho-Tri-Cyclen 1914
Ortho-Novum 1928
Ortho-Cyclen/Ortho Tri-Cyclen 1914
Ovcon 765
Ovral Tablets 2877
Ovral-28 Tablets 2878
Levlen/Tri-Levlen 646
Tri-Norinyl 2607
Triphasil-21 Tablets 2919
Triphasil-28 Tablets 2924

Ethynodiol Diacetate (Concurrent use may render oral contraceptives less effective; potential for breakthrough bleeding). Products include:
Demulen 2580

Ferrous Fumarate (Absorption of tetracyclines is impaired). Products include:
Chromagen Capsules 2470
Chromagen FA 2471
Chromagen Forte 2471
Ferro-Sequels ▣ 684
Nephro-Fer Tablets 2168
Nephro-Fer Rx Tablets 2168
Nephro-Vite + Fe Tablets 2170
Stresstabs + Iron ▣ 685
Trinsicon Capsules 2759
Vitron-C Tablets ▣ 667

Ferrous Gluconate (Absorption of tetracyclines is impaired). Products include:
Megadose 513

Ferrous Sulfate (Absorption of tetracyclines is impaired). Products include:
Feosol Capsules ▣ 777
Feosol Elixir 2627
Feosol Tablets 2627
Fero-Folic-500 Filmtab 433
Fero-Grad-500 Filmtab 434
Fero-Gradumet Filmtab 434
Iberet Tablets 437
Iberet-500 Liquid 438
Iberet-Folic-500 Filmtab 433
Iberet-Liquid 438
Irospan 1000
Slow Fe Tablets 889
Slow Fe with Folic Acid 890

Heparin Calcium (Depressed plasma prothrombin activity; may require downward adjustment of the anticoagulant dosage).
No products indexed under this heading.

Heparin Sodium (Depressed plasma prothrombin activity; may require downward adjustment of the anticoagulant dosage). Products include:
Heparin Lock Flush Solution 2831
Heparin Sodium Injection 2832
Heparin Sodium Vials 1486

Levonorgestrel (Concurrent use may render oral contraceptives less effective; potential for breakthrough bleeding). Products include:
Levlen/Tri-Levlen 646
Nordette-21 Tablets 2863
Nordette-28 Tablets 2866
Norplant System 2868
Levlen/Tri-Levlen 646
Triphasil-21 Tablets 2919
Triphasil-28 Tablets 2924

Magaldrate (Absorption of tetracyclines is impaired).
No products indexed under this heading.

Magnesium Hydroxide (Absorption of tetracyclines is impaired). Products include:
Aludrox Oral Suspension ▣ 850
Ascriptin ▣ 650
Di-Gel Antacid/Anti-Gas ▣ 762
Gelusil Antacid-Anti-gas Liquid ▣ 819
Gelusil Antacid-Anti-gas Tablets ▣ 819
Maalox Antacid/Anti-Gas Tablets 889
Maalox Antacid Liquid 888
Extra Strength Maalox Antacid/Anti-Gas Liquid and Tablets 888
Mylanta Fast-Acting 1359
Mylanta Gelcaps Antacid ▣ 678
Fast-Acting Mylanta Liquid Antacid 1359
Mylanta Tablets ▣ 677
Maximum-Strength Fast-Acting Mylanta Liquid Antacid 1359
Mylanta Double Strength Tablets ▣ 677
Phillips' Milk of Magnesia Liquid ▣ 627
Rolaids Antacid Tablets ▣ 807
Tempo Soft Antacid ▣ 799

Magnesium Oxide (Absorption of tetracyclines is impaired). Products include:
Beelith Tablets 632

(▣ Described in PDR For Nonprescription Drugs) (⊙ Described in PDR For Ophthalmology)

Bufferin Analgesic Tablets	◆ 636
Arthritis Strength Bufferin Analgesic Caplets	◆ 637
Extra Strength Bufferin Analgesic Tablets	◆ 637
Caltrate PLUS	◆ 681
Cama Arthritis Pain Reliever	◆ 748
Mag-Ox 400	666
Uro-Mag	666

Mestranol (Concurrent use may render oral contraceptives less effective; potential for breakthrough bleeding). Products include:

Norinyl	2563
Ortho-Novum	1928

Methoxyflurane (Potential for fatal renal toxicity).
No products indexed under this heading.

Mezlocillin Sodium (Interference with bactericidal action of penicillin; avoid concurrent use). Products include:

Mezlin	594
Mezlin Pharmacy Bulk Package	597

Nafcillin Sodium (Interference with bactericidal action of penicillin).
No products indexed under this heading.

Norethindrone (Concurrent use may render oral contraceptives less effective; potential for breakthrough bleeding). Products include:

Brevicon	2563
Micronor Tablets	1903
Modicon	1928
Norinyl	2563
Nor-Q D Tablets	2598
Ortho-Novum	1928
Ovcon	765
Tri-Norinyl	2607

Norethynodrel (Concurrent use may render oral contraceptives less effective; potential for breakthrough bleeding).
No products indexed under this heading.

Norgestimate (Concurrent use may render oral contraceptives less effective; potential for breakthrough bleeding). Products include:

Ortho-Cyclen/Ortho-Tri-Cyclen	1914
Ortho-Cyclen/Ortho-Tri-Cyclen	1914

Norgestrel (Concurrent use may render oral contraceptives less effective; potential for breakthrough bleeding). Products include:

Lo/Ovral Tablets	2852
Lo/Ovral-28 Tablets	2857
Ovral Tablets	2877
Ovral-28 Tablets	2878
Ovrette Tablets	2878

Penicillin G Benzathine (Interference with bactericidal action of penicillin; avoid concurrent use). Products include:

Bicillin C-R Injection	2810
Bicillin C-R 900/300 Injection	2812
Bicillin L-A Injection	2813

Penicillin G Potassium (Interference with bactericidal action of penicillin; avoid concurrent use). Products include:

Pfizerpen for Injection	2022

Penicillin G Procaine (Interference with bactericidal action of penicillin; avoid concurrent use). Products include:

Bicillin C-R Injection	2810
Bicillin C-R 900/300 Injection	2812

Penicillin G Sodium (Interference with bactericidal action of penicillin; avoid concurrent use).
No products indexed under this heading.

Penicillin V Potassium (Interference with bactericidal action of penicillin; avoid concurrent use). Products include:

Pen•Vee K	2879

Polysaccharide-Iron Complex (Absorption of tetracyclines is impaired). Products include:

Niferex-150 Capsules	811
Niferex Elixir	811
Niferex-150 Forte Capsules	811
Niferex	811
Niferex-PN Tablets	811
Nu-Iron 150 Capsules	1826
Nu-Iron Elixir	1826

Ticarcillin Disodium (Interference with bactericidal action of penicillin; avoid concurrent use). Products include:

Ticar for Injection	2704
Timentin for Injection	2706

Warfarin Sodium (Depressed plasma prothrombin activity; may require downward adjustment of the anticoagulant dosage). Products include:

Coumadin	941

Food Interactions

Dairy products (The peak plasma concentrations were slightly decreased (11.2%) and delayed by 1 hour).

Meal with dairy products (The peak plasma concentrations were slightly decreased (11.2%) and delayed by 1 hour).

MINTEZOL CHEWABLE TABLETS
(Thiabendazole) 1747
May interact with xanthine bronchodilators. Compounds in this category include:

Aminophylline (Xanthine toxicity).
No products indexed under this heading.

Dyphylline (Xanthine toxicity). Products include:

Lufyllin & Lufyllin-400 Tablets	2778
Lufyllin-GG Elixir & Tablets	2779

Theophylline (Xanthine toxicity). Products include:

Marax Tablets & DF Syrup	2015
Quibron	2227

Theophylline Anhydrous (Xanthine toxicity). Products include:

Aerolate	1003
Primatene Tablets	◆ 844
Respbid Tablets	687
Slo-bid Gyrocaps	2201
Theo-24 Extended Release Capsules	2753
Theo-Dur Extended-Release Tablets	1367
Theo-X Extended-Release Tablets	793
Uni-Dur Extended-Release Tablets	1374
Uniphyl 400 mg and 600 mg Tablets	2157

Theophylline Calcium Salicylate (Xanthine toxicity). Products include:

Quadrinal Tablets	1398

Theophylline Sodium Glycinate (Xanthine toxicity).
No products indexed under this heading.

Xanthine Preparations (Xanthine toxicity).

MINTEZOL SUSPENSION
(Thiabendazole) 1747
See Mintezol Chewable Tablets

MIOCHOL-E WITH IOCARE STERI-TAGS AND MIOCHOL-E SYSTEM PAK
(Acetylcholine Chloride) .... ◆ 263
May interact with topical nonsteroidal anti-inflammatory agents. Compounds in this category include:

Diclofenac Sodium (Acetylcholine and carbachol have been ineffective when used in patients with topical nonsteroidal anti-inflammatory agents). Products include:

Voltaren Ophthalmic Sterile Ophthalmic Solution	◆ 264
Cataflam/Voltaren/Voltaren-XR	833

Flurbiprofen Sodium (Acetylcholine and carbachol have been ineffective when used in patients with topical nonsteroidal anti-inflammatory agents). Products include:

Ocufen	◆ 242

Suprofen (Acetylcholine and carbachol have been ineffective when used in patients with topical nonsteroidal anti-inflammatory agents).
No products indexed under this heading.

MIOSTAT INTRAOCULAR SOLUTION
(Carbachol) .... ◆ 222
None cited in PDR database.

MITHRACIN
(Plicamycin) 599
None cited in PDR database.

MIVACRON INJECTION
(Mivacurium Chloride) 1125
May interact with aminoglycosides, tetracyclines, lithium preparations, local anesthetics, oral contraceptives, monoamine oxidase inhibitors, glucocorticoids, antineoplastics, and certain other agents. Compounds in these categories include:

Altretamine (Irreversible inhibition of plasma cholinesterase by certain unspecified antineoplastic drugs resulting in possible prolonged neuromuscular block). Products include:

Hexalen Capsules	2760

Amikacin Sulfate (Enhances the neuromuscular blocking action). Products include:

Amikacin Sulfate Injection, USP	523
Amikacin Sulfate Injection, USP	981
Amikin Injectable	502

Anastrozole (Irreversible inhibition of plasma cholinesterase by certain unspecified antineoplastic drugs resulting in possible prolonged neuromuscular block). Products include:

Arimidex Tablets	2932

Asparaginase (Irreversible inhibition of plasma cholinesterase by certain unspecified antineoplastic drugs resulting in possible prolonged neuromuscular block). Products include:

Elspar	1700

Bacitracin (Enhances neuromuscular blocking action).
No products indexed under this heading.

Betamethasone Acetate (Enhances the neuromuscular blocking effects by a reduction in plasma cholinesterase activity induced by chronic administration of glucocorticoids). Products include:

Celestone Soluspan Suspension	2484

Betamethasone Sodium Phosphate (Enhances the neuromuscular blocking effects by a reduction in plasma cholinesterase activity induced by chronic administration of glucocorticoids). Products include:

Celestone Soluspan Suspension	2484

Bicalutamide (Irreversible inhibition of plasma cholinesterase by certain unspecified antineoplastic drugs resulting in possible prolonged neuromuscular block). Products include:

Casodex Tablets	2934

Bleomycin Sulfate (Irreversible inhibition of plasma cholinesterase by certain unspecified antineoplastic drugs resulting in possible prolonged neuromuscular block). Products include:

Blenoxane	697

Bupivacaine Hydrochloride (Enhances neuromuscular blocking action). Products include:

Marcaine	2446
Marcaine Spinal	2449
Sensorcaine	554

Busulfan (Irreversible inhibition of plasma cholinesterase by certain unspecified antineoplastic drugs resulting in possible prolonged neuromuscular block). Products include:

Myleran Tablets	1209

Carbamazepine (Potential for resistance to the neuromuscular blocking action in patients on chronic carbamazepine therapy). Products include:

Atretol Tablets	569
Tegretol/Tegretol-XR	870

Carboplatin (Irreversible inhibition of plasma cholinesterase by certain unspecified antineoplastic drugs resulting in possible prolonged neuromuscular block). Products include:

Paraplatin for Injection	713

Carmustine (BCNU) (Irreversible inhibition of plasma cholinesterase by certain unspecified antineoplastic drugs resulting in possible prolonged neuromuscular block). Products include:

BiCNU	696

Chlorambucil (Irreversible inhibition of plasma cholinesterase by certain unspecified antineoplastic drugs resulting in possible prolonged neuromuscular block). Products include:

Leukeran Tablets	1205

Chloroprocaine Hydrochloride (Enhances neuromuscular blocking action). Products include:

Nescaine/Nescaine MPF	549

Cisplatin (Irreversible inhibition of plasma cholinesterase by certain unspecified antineoplastic drugs resulting in possible prolonged neuromuscular block). Products include:

Platinol for Injection	717
Platinol-AQ Injection	719

Clindamycin Hydrochloride (Enhances neuromuscular blocking action).
No products indexed under this heading.

Clindamycin Palmitate Hydrochloride (Enhances neuromuscular blocking action).
No products indexed under this heading.

Clindamycin Phosphate (Enhances neuromuscular blocking action). Products include:

Cleocin Phosphate Injection	2068
Cleocin T Topical	2072
Cleocin Vaginal Cream	2070

Colistimethate Sodium (Enhances neuromuscular blocking action).
No products indexed under this heading.

IMPORTANT NOTE: Always consult each drug listing in the patient's regimen for possible interactions.

Mivacron Interactions Index 690

Colistin Sulfate (Enhances neuromuscular blocking action). Products include:

Coly-Mycin S Otic w/Neomycin & Hydrocortisone ... 1965

Cortisone Acetate (Enhances the neuromuscular blocking effects by a reduction in plasma cholinesterase activity induced by chronic administration of glucocorticoids). Products include:

Cortone Acetate Sterile Suspension ... 1663
Cortone Acetate Tablets ... 1664

Cyclophosphamide (Irreversible inhibition of plasma cholinesterase by certain unspecified antineoplastic drugs resulting in possible prolonged neuromuscular block). Products include:

Cytoxan ... 700

Dacarbazine (Irreversible inhibition of plasma cholinesterase by certain unspecified antineoplastic drugs resulting in possible prolonged neuromuscular block). Products include:

DTIC-Dome ... 593

Daunorubicin Citrate (Irreversible inhibition of plasma cholinesterase by certain unspecified antineoplastic drugs resulting in possible prolonged neuromuscular block). Products include:

DaunoXome ... 1842

Daunorubicin Hydrochloride (Irreversible inhibition of plasma cholinesterase by certain unspecified antineoplastic drugs resulting in possible prolonged neuromuscular block). Products include:

Cerubidine for Injection ... 634

Demeclocycline Hydrochloride (Enhances neuromuscular blocking action). Products include:

Declomycin Tablets ... 1421

Desogestrel (Enhances the neuromuscular blocking effects by a reduction in plasma cholinesterase activity induced by chronic administration of oral contraceptives). Products include:

Desogen Tablets ... 1867
Ortho-Cept ... 1907

Dexamethasone (Enhances the neuromuscular blocking effects by a reduction in plasma cholinesterase activity induced by chronic administration of glucocorticoids). Products include:

AK-Trol Ointment & Suspension ... ◉ 205
Decadron Elixir ... 1676
Decadron Tablets ... 1678
Decaspray Topical Aerosol ... 1689
Maxitrol Ophthalmic Ointment and Suspension ... ◉ 222
TobraDex Ophthalmic Suspension and Ointment ... 469

Dexamethasone Acetate (Enhances the neuromuscular blocking effects by a reduction in plasma cholinesterase activity induced by chronic administration of glucocorticoids). Products include:

Dalalone D.P. Injectable ... 1009
Decadron-LA Sterile Suspension ... 1687

Dexamethasone Sodium Phosphate (Enhances the neuromuscular blocking effects by a reduction in plasma cholinesterase activity induced by chronic administration of glucocorticoids). Products include:

Decadron Phosphate Injection ... 1680
Decadron Phosphate Sterile Ophthalmic Ointment ... 1684
Decadron Phosphate Sterile Ophthalmic Solution ... 1685
Decadron Phosphate Topical Cream ... 1686
Decadron Phosphate with Xylocaine Injection, Sterile ... 1683
Dexacort Phosphate in Respihaler .. 1606
Dexacort Phosphate in Turbinaire .. 1607
NeoDecadron Sterile Ophthalmic Ointment ... 1755
NeoDecadron Sterile Ophthalmic Solution ... 1756
NeoDecadron Topical Cream ... 1757

Docetaxel (Irreversible inhibition of plasma cholinesterase by certain unspecified antineoplastic drugs resulting in possible prolonged neuromuscular block). Products include:

Taxotere for Injection Concentrate 2204

Doxorubicin Hydrochloride (Irreversible inhibition of plasma cholinesterase by certain unspecified antineoplastic drugs resulting in possible prolonged neuromuscular block). Products include:

Adriamycin PFS ... 2056
Adriamycin RDF ... 2056
Doxil ... 2613
Doxorubicin Astra ... 531
Rubex for Injection ... 721

Doxycycline Calcium (Enhances neuromuscular blocking action). Products include:

Vibramycin Calcium Oral Suspension Syrup ... 2038

Doxycycline Hyclate (Enhances neuromuscular blocking action). Products include:

Doryx Capsules ... 1970
Vibramycin Hyclate Capsules ... 2038
Vibramycin Hyclate Intravenous ... 2040
Vibra-Tabs Film Coated Tablets ... 2038

Doxycycline Monohydrate (Enhances neuromuscular blocking action). Products include:

Monodox Capsules ... 1858
Vibramycin Monohydrate for Oral Suspension ... 2038

Echothiophate Iodide (Irreversible inhibition of plasma cholinesterase by echothiophate resulting in possible prolonged neuromuscular block). Products include:

Phospholine Iodide ... ◉ 323

Enflurane (Decreases ED_{50} of Mivacron by as much as 35% to 40%; prolongs the clinically effective duration of action).

No products indexed under this heading.

Estramustine Phosphate Sodium (Irreversible inhibition of plasma cholinesterase by certain unspecified antineoplastic drugs resulting in possible prolonged neuromuscular block). Products include:

Emcyt Capsules ... 2085

Ethinyl Estradiol (Enhances the neuromuscular blocking effects by a reduction in plasma cholinesterase activity induced by chronic administration of oral contraceptives). Products include:

Brevicon ... 2563
Demulen ... 2580
Desogen Tablets ... 1867
Levlen/Tri-Levlen ... 646
Lo/Ovral Tablets ... 2852
Lo/Ovral-28 Tablets ... 2857
Modicon ... 1928
Nordette-21 Tablets ... 2863
Nordette-28 Tablets ... 2866
Norinyl ... 2563
Ortho-Cept ... 1907
Ortho-Cyclen/Ortho-Tri-Cyclen ... 1914
Ortho-Novum ... 1928
Ortho-Cyclen/Ortho Tri-Cyclen ... 1914
Ovcon ... 765
Ovral Tablets ... 2877
Ovral-28 Tablets ... 2878
Levlen/Tri-Levlen ... 646
Tri-Norinyl ... 2607
Triphasil-21 Tablets ... 2919
Triphasil-28 Tablets ... 2924

Ethynodiol Diacetate (Enhances the neuromuscular blocking effects by a reduction in plasma cholinesterase activity induced by chronic administration of oral contraceptives). Products include:

Demulen ... 2580

Etidocaine Hydrochloride (Enhances neuromuscular blocking action). Products include:

Duranest Injections ... 533

Etoposide (Irreversible inhibition of plasma cholinesterase by certain unspecified antineoplastic drugs resulting in possible prolonged neuromuscular block). Products include:

Etoposide Injection ... 539
VePesid Capsules and Injection ... 727

Floxuridine (Irreversible inhibition of plasma cholinesterase by certain unspecified antineoplastic drugs resulting in possible prolonged neuromuscular block). Products include:

Sterile FUDR ... 2284

Fludrocortisone Acetate (Enhances the neuromuscular blocking effects by a reduction in plasma cholinesterase activity induced by chronic administration of glucocorticoids). Products include:

Florinef Acetate Tablets ... 506

Fluorouracil (Irreversible inhibition of plasma cholinesterase by certain unspecified antineoplastic drugs resulting in possible prolonged neuromuscular block). Products include:

Efudex ... 2280
Fluoroplex Topical Solution & Cream 1% ... 475
Fluorouracil Injection ... 2282

Flutamide (Irreversible inhibition of plasma cholinesterase by certain unspecified antineoplastic drugs resulting in possible prolonged neuromuscular block). Products include:

Eulexin Capsules ... 2498

Fosphenytoin Sodium (Potential for resistance to the neuromuscular blocking action in patients on chronic phenytoin therapy). Products include:

Cerebyx Injection ... 1956

Furazolidone (Enhances the neuromuscular blocking effects by a reduction in plasma cholinesterase activity induced by chronic administration of certain unspecified monoamine oxidase inhibitors). Products include:

Furoxone ... 2221

Gemcitabine Hydrochloride (Irreversible inhibition of plasma cholinesterase by certain unspecified antineoplastic drugs resulting in possible prolonged neuromuscular block). Products include:

Gemzar for Injection ... 1482

Gentamicin Sulfate (Enhances the neuromuscular blocking action). Products include:

Garamycin Cream 0.1% ... 2501
Garamycin Injectable ... 2502
Garamycin Ointment 0.1% ... 2501
Garamycin Ophthalmic ... 2501
Genoptic Sterile Ophthalmic Solution ... ◉ 241
Genoptic Sterile Ophthalmic Ointment ... ◉ 241
Gentak ... ◉ 209
Pred-G Liquifilm Sterile Ophthalmic Suspension ... ◉ 248
Pred-G S.O.P. Sterile Ophthalmic Ointment ... ◉ 249

Halothane (Prolongs the duration of action). Products include:

Fluothane ... 2830

Hydrocortisone (Enhances the neuromuscular blocking effects by a reduction in plasma cholinesterase activity induced by chronic administration of glucocorticoids). Products include:

Anusol-HC Cream 2.5% ... 1953
Aquanil HC Lotion ... 1989
Maximum Strength Cortaid Spray ▣ 800
CORTENEMA ... 2713
Cortisporin Ointment ... 1074
Cortisporin Ophthalmic Ointment Sterile ... 1074
Cortisporin Ophthalmic Suspension Sterile ... 1075
Cortisporin Otic Solution Sterile ... 1076
Cortisporin Otic Suspension Sterile 1077
Cortizone-5 ... ▣ 795
Cortizone-10 ... ▣ 795
Hydrocortone Tablets ... 1715
Hytone ... 922
Hytone Ointment 2 ½% ... 923
Massengill Medicated Soft Cloth Towelettes ... 2628
Pediotic Suspension Sterile ... 1140
Preparation H Hydrocortisone 1% Cream ... ▣ 843
ProctoCream-HC 2.5% ... 2552
VōSoL HC Otic Solution ... 2786

Hydrocortisone Acetate (Enhances the neuromuscular blocking effects by a reduction in plasma cholinesterase activity induced by chronic administration of glucocorticoids). Products include:

Analpram-HC Rectal Cream 1% and 2.5% ... 993
Anusol HC-1 Hydrocortisone Anti-Itch Ointment ... ▣ 810
Anusol-HC Suppositories ... 1954
Caldecort Anti-Itch Hydrocortisone Cream ... ▣ 651
Coly-Mycin S Otic w/Neomycin & Hydrocortisone ... 1965
Cortaid ... ▣ 800
Cortifoam ... 2540
Cortisporin Cream ... 1073
Epifoam ... 2543
Hydrocortone Acetate Sterile Suspension ... 1712
Mantadil Cream ... 1124
Nupercainal Hydrocortisone 1% Cream ... ▣ 661
Pramosone Cream, Lotion & Ointment ... 995
ProctoFoam-HC ... 2552
Terra-Cortril Ophthalmic Suspension ... 2033

Hydrocortisone Sodium Phosphate (Enhances the neuromuscular blocking effects by a reduction in plasma cholinesterase activity induced by chronic administration of glucocorticoids). Products include:

Hydrocortone Phosphate Injection, Sterile ... 1713

Hydrocortisone Sodium Succinate (Enhances the neuromuscular blocking effects by a reduction in plasma cholinesterase activity induced by chronic administration of glucocorticoids).

No products indexed under this heading.

Hydroxyurea (Irreversible inhibition of plasma cholinesterase by certain unspecified antineoplastic drugs resulting in possible prolonged neuromuscular block). Products include:

Hydrea Capsules ... 705

Idarubicin Hydrochloride (Irreversible inhibition of plasma cholinesterase by certain unspecified antineoplastic drugs resulting in possible prolonged neuromuscular block). Products include:

Idamycin Injection ... 2096

Ifosfamide (Irreversible inhibition of plasma cholinesterase by certain unspecified antineoplastic drugs resulting in possible prolonged neuromuscular block). Products include:

IFEX ... 706

(▣ Described in PDR For Nonprescription Drugs) (◉ Described in PDR For Ophthalmology)

Interferon alfa-2A, Recombinant (Irreversible inhibition of plasma cholinesterase by certain unspecified antineoplastic drugs resulting in possible prolonged neuromuscular block). Products include:
- Roferon-A Injection ... 2308

Interferon alfa-2B, Recombinant (Irreversible inhibition of plasma cholinesterase by certain unspecified antineoplastic drugs resulting in possible prolonged neuromuscular block). Products include:
- Intron A for Injection ... 2506

Irinotecan Hydrochloride (Irreversible inhibition of plasma cholinesterase by certain unspecified antineoplastic drugs resulting in possible prolonged neuromuscular block).
- No products indexed under this heading.

Isocarboxazid (Enhances the neuromuscular blocking effects by a reduction in plasma cholinesterase activity induced by chronic administration of certain unspecified monoamine oxidase inhibitors).
- No products indexed under this heading.

Isoflurane (Decreases ED_{50} of Mivacron by as much as 35% to 40%; prolongs the clinically effective duration of action).
- No products indexed under this heading.

Kanamycin Sulfate (Enhances the neuromuscular blocking action).
- No products indexed under this heading.

Levamisole Hydrochloride (Irreversible inhibition of plasma cholinesterase by certain unspecified antineoplastic drugs resulting in possible prolonged neuromuscular block). Products include:
- Ergamisol Tablets ... 1340

Levonorgestrel (Enhances the neuromuscular blocking effects by a reduction in plasma cholinesterase activity induced by chronic administration of oral contraceptives). Products include:
- Levlen/Tri-Levlen ... 646
- Nordette-21 Tablets ... 2863
- Nordette-28 Tablets ... 2866
- Norplant System ... 2868
- Levlen/Tri-Levlen ... 646
- Triphasil-21 Tablets ... 2919
- Triphasil-28 Tablets ... 2924

Lidocaine Hydrochloride (Enhances neuromuscular blocking action). Products include:
- Decadron Phosphate with Xylocaine Injection, Sterile ... 1683
- Unguentine Plus ... [book icon] 712
- Xylocaine Injections ... 562

Lincomycin Hydrochloride (Enhances neuromuscular blocking action).
- No products indexed under this heading.

Lithium Carbonate (Enhances neuromuscular blocking action). Products include:
- Eskalith ... 2658
- Lithium Carbonate Capsules & Tablets ... 2352
- Lithonate/Lithotabs/Lithobid ... 2721

Lithium Citrate (Enhances neuromuscular blocking action).
- No products indexed under this heading.

Lomustine (CCNU) (Irreversible inhibition of plasma cholinesterase by certain unspecified antineoplastic drugs resulting in possible prolonged neuromuscular block). Products include:
- CeeNU Capsules ... 699

Magnesium Salts (Enhances neuromuscular blocking action).

Mechlorethamine Hydrochloride (Irreversible inhibition of plasma cholinesterase by certain unspecified antineoplastic drugs resulting in possible prolonged neuromuscular block). Products include:
- Mustargen ... 1752

Megestrol Acetate (Irreversible inhibition of plasma cholinesterase by certain unspecified antineoplastic drugs resulting in possible prolonged neuromuscular block). Products include:
- Megace Oral Suspension ... 708
- Megace Tablets ... 710

Melphalan (Irreversible inhibition of plasma cholinesterase by certain unspecified antineoplastic drugs resulting in possible prolonged neuromuscular block). Products include:
- Alkeran Tablets ... 1198

Mepivacaine Hydrochloride Injection (Enhances neuromuscular blocking action). Products include:
- Carbocaine Injection ... 2432

Mercaptopurine (Irreversible inhibition of plasma cholinesterase by certain unspecified antineoplastic drugs resulting in possible prolonged neuromuscular block). Products include:
- Purinethol Tablets ... 1214

Mestranol (Enhances the neuromuscular blocking effects by a reduction in plasma cholinesterase activity induced by chronic administration of oral contraceptives). Products include:
- Norinyl ... 2563
- Ortho-Novum ... 1928

Methacycline Hydrochloride (Enhances neuromuscular blocking action).
- No products indexed under this heading.

Methotrexate Sodium (Irreversible inhibition of plasma cholinesterase by certain unspecified antineoplastic drugs resulting in possible prolonged neuromuscular block). Products include:
- Methotrexate Sodium Tablets, Injection, for Injection and LPF Injection ... 1322

Methylprednisolone Acetate (Enhances the neuromuscular blocking effects by a reduction in plasma cholinesterase activity induced by chronic administration of glucocorticoids).
- No products indexed under this heading.

Methylprednisolone Sodium Succinate (Enhances the neuromuscular blocking effects by a reduction in plasma cholinesterase activity induced by chronic administration of glucocorticoids).
- No products indexed under this heading.

Minocycline Hydrochloride (Enhances neuromuscular blocking action). Products include:
- DYNACIN Capsules ... 1627
- Minocin Intravenous ... 1428
- Minocin Oral Suspension ... 1431
- Minocin Pellet-Filled Capsules ... 1429

Mitomycin (Mitomycin-C) (Irreversible inhibition of plasma cholinesterase by certain unspecified antineoplastic drugs resulting in possible prolonged neuromuscular block). Products include:
- Mutamycin for Injection ... 712

Mitotane (Irreversible inhibition of plasma cholinesterase by certain unspecified antineoplastic drugs resulting in possible prolonged neuromuscular block). Products include:
- Lysodren Tablets ... 707

Mitoxantrone Hydrochloride (Irreversible inhibition of plasma cholinesterase by certain unspecified antineoplastic drugs resulting in possible prolonged neuromuscular block). Products include:
- Novantrone for Injection ... 1327

Norethindrone (Enhances the neuromuscular blocking effects by a reduction in plasma cholinesterase activity induced by chronic administration of oral contraceptives). Products include:
- Brevicon ... 2563
- Micronor Tablets ... 1903
- Modicon ... 1928
- Norinyl ... 2563
- Nor-Q D Tablets ... 2598
- Ortho-Novum ... 1928
- Ovcon ... 765
- Tri-Norinyl ... 2607

Norethynodrel (Enhances the neuromuscular blocking effects by a reduction in plasma cholinesterase activity induced by chronic administration of oral contraceptives).
- No products indexed under this heading.

Norgestimate (Enhances the neuromuscular blocking effects by a reduction in plasma cholinesterase activity induced by chronic administration of oral contraceptives). Products include:
- Ortho-Cyclen/Ortho-Tri-Cyclen ... 1914
- Ortho-Cyclen/Ortho Tri-Cyclen ... 1914

Norgestrel (Enhances the neuromuscular blocking effects by a reduction in plasma cholinesterase activity induced by chronic administration of oral contraceptives). Products include:
- Lo/Ovral Tablets ... 2852
- Lo/Ovral-28 Tablets ... 2857
- Ovral Tablets ... 2877
- Ovral-28 Tablets ... 2878
- Ovrette Tablets ... 2878

Oxytetracycline Hydrochloride (Enhances neuromuscular blocking action). Products include:
- TERAK Ointment ... ◉ 210
- Terra-Cortril Ophthalmic Suspension ... 2033
- Terramycin with Polymyxin B Sulfate Ophthalmic Ointment ... 2035
- Urobiotic-250 Capsules ... 2038

Paclitaxel (Irreversible inhibition of plasma cholinesterase by certain unspecified antineoplastic drugs resulting in possible prolonged neuromuscular block). Products include:
- Taxol Injection ... 723

Phenelzine Sulfate (Enhances the neuromuscular blocking effects by a reduction in plasma cholinesterase activity induced by chronic administration of certain unspecified monoamine oxidase inhibitors). Products include:
- Nardil ... 1977

Phenytoin (Potential for resistance to the neuromuscular blocking action in patients on chronic phenytoin therapy). Products include:
- Dilantin Infatabs ... 1967
- Dilantin-125 Suspension ... 1969

Phenytoin Sodium (Potential for resistance to the neuromuscular blocking action in patients on chronic phenytoin therapy). Products include:
- Dilantin Kapseals ... 1965

Polymyxin Preparations (Enhances neuromuscular blocking action).

Prednisolone Acetate (Enhances the neuromuscular blocking effects by a reduction in plasma cholinesterase activity induced by chronic administration of glucocorticoids). Products include:
- AK-CIDE ... ◉ 203
- AK-CIDE Ointment ... ◉ 203
- Blephamide Liquifilm Sterile Ophthalmic Suspension ... 472
- Blephamide Ointment ... ◉ 234
- Econopred & Econopred Plus Ophthalmic Suspensions ... ◉ 216
- Poly-Pred Liquifilm ... ◉ 246
- Pred Forte ... ◉ 247
- Pred Mild ... ◉ 250
- Pred-G Liquifilm Sterile Ophthalmic Suspension ... ◉ 248
- Pred-G S.O.P. Sterile Ophthalmic Ointment ... ◉ 249

Prednisolone Sodium Phosphate (Enhances the neuromuscular blocking effects by a reduction in plasma cholinesterase activity induced by chronic administration of glucocorticoids). Products include:
- AK-PRED ... ◉ 204
- Hydeltrasol Injection, Sterile ... 1708
- Pediapred Oral Solution ... 1618

Prednisolone Tebutate (Enhances the neuromuscular blocking effects by a reduction in plasma cholinesterase activity induced by chronic administration of glucocorticoids). Products include:
- Hydeltra-T.B.A. Sterile Suspension 1710

Prednisone (Enhances the neuromuscular blocking effects by a reduction in plasma cholinesterase activity induced by chronic administration of glucocorticoids).
- No products indexed under this heading.

Procainamide Hydrochloride (Enhances neuromuscular blocking action). Products include:
- Procanbid Extended-Release Tablets ... 1983

Procaine Hydrochloride (Enhances neuromuscular blocking action). Products include:
- Novocain Hydrochloride for Spinal Anesthesia ... 2457

Procarbazine Hydrochloride (Irreversible inhibition of plasma cholinesterase by certain unspecified antineoplastic drugs resulting in possible prolonged neuromuscular block). Products include:
- Matulane Capsules ... 2300

Quinidine Gluconate (Enhances neuromuscular blocking action). Products include:
- Quinaglute Dura-Tabs Tablets ... 644

Quinidine Polygalacturonate (Enhances neuromuscular blocking action). Products include:
- Cardioquin Tablets ... 2146

Quinidine Sulfate (Enhances neuromuscular blocking action). Products include:
- Quinidex Extentabs ... 2240

Selegiline Hydrochloride (Enhances the neuromuscular blocking effects by a reduction in plasma cholinesterase activity induced by chronic administration of certain unspecified monoamine oxidase inhibitors). Products include:
- Eldepryl Capsules ... 2729

Streptomycin Sulfate (Enhances the neuromuscular blocking action). Products include:
- Streptomycin Sulfate Injection ... 2031

IMPORTANT NOTE: Always consult each drug listing in the patient's regimen for possible interactions.

Streptozocin (Irreversible inhibition of plasma cholinesterase by certain unspecified antineoplastic drugs resulting in possible prolonged neuromuscular block). Products include:
Zanosar Sterile Powder 2119

Succinylcholine Chloride (Prior administration of succinylcholine can potentiate neuromuscular blockade). Products include:
Anectine 1062

Tamoxifen Citrate (Irreversible inhibition of plasma cholinesterase by certain unspecified antineoplastic drugs resulting in possible prolonged neuromuscular block). Products include:
Nolvadex Tablets 2957

Teniposide (Irreversible inhibition of plasma cholinesterase by certain unspecified antineoplastic drugs resulting in possible prolonged neuromuscular block). Products include:
Vumon for Injection 729

Tetracaine Hydrochloride (Enhances neuromuscular blocking action). Products include:
Cetacaine Topical Anesthetic 812
Pontocaine Hydrochloride for Spinal Anesthesia 2460

Tetracycline Hydrochloride (Enhances neuromuscular blocking action). Products include:
Achromycin V Capsules 1417
Helidac Therapy 2135

Thioguanine (Irreversible inhibition of plasma cholinesterase by certain unspecified antineoplastic drugs resulting in possible prolonged neuromuscular block). Products include:
Thioguanine Tablets, Tabloid Brand 1225

Thiotepa (Irreversible inhibition of plasma cholinesterase by certain unspecified antineoplastic drugs resulting in possible prolonged neuromuscular block). Products include:
Thioplex (Thiotepa For Injection) 1329

Tobramycin (Enhances the neuromuscular blocking action). Products include:
AKTOB .... ⊡ 207
TobraDex Ophthalmic Suspension and Ointment 469
Tobrex Ophthalmic Ointment and Solution .... ⊡ 226

Tobramycin Sulfate (Enhances the neuromuscular blocking action). Products include:
Nebcin Vials, Hyporets & ADD-Vantage 1518

Topotecan Hydrochloride (Irreversible inhibition of plasma cholinesterase by certain unspecified antineoplastic drugs resulting in possible prolonged neuromuscular block). Products include:
Hycamtin for Injection 2665

Tranylcypromine Sulfate (Enhances the neuromuscular blocking effects by a reduction in plasma cholinesterase activity induced by chronic administration of certain unspecified monoamine oxidase inhibitors). Products include:
Parnate Tablets 2679

Triamcinolone (Enhances the neuromuscular blocking effects by a reduction in plasma cholinesterase activity induced by chronic administration of glucocorticoids). Products include:
No products indexed under this heading.

Triamcinolone Acetonide (Enhances the neuromuscular blocking effects by a reduction in plasma cholinesterase activity induced by chronic administration of glucocorticoids). Products include:
Azmacort Oral Inhaler 2175
Nasacort AQ Nasal Spray 2191
Nasacort Nasal Inhaler 2189

Triamcinolone Diacetate (Enhances the neuromuscular blocking effects by a reduction in plasma cholinesterase activity induced by chronic administration of glucocorticoids).
No products indexed under this heading.

Triamcinolone Hexacetonide (Enhances the neuromuscular blocking effects by a reduction in plasma cholinesterase activity induced by chronic administration of glucocorticoids).
No products indexed under this heading.

Vincristine Sulfate (Irreversible inhibition of plasma cholinesterase by certain unspecified antineoplastic drugs resulting in possible prolonged neuromuscular block). Products include:
Oncovin Solution Vials & Hyporets 1521

Vinorelbine Tartrate (Irreversible inhibition of plasma cholinesterase by certain unspecified antineoplastic drugs resulting in possible prolonged neuromuscular block). Products include:
Navelbine Injection 1212

MIVACRON PREMIXED INFUSION
(Mivacurium Chloride) 1125
See **Mivacron Injection**

MOBAN TABLETS AND CONCENTRATE
(Molindone Hydrochloride) 1036
May interact with tetracyclines and certain other agents. Compounds in these categories include:

Demeclocycline Hydrochloride (Calcium sulfate present as an excipient may interfere with the absorption of oral tetracyclines). Products include:
Declomycin Tablets 1421

Doxycycline Calcium (Calcium sulfate present as an excipient may interfere with the absorption of oral tetracyclines). Products include:
Vibramycin Calcium Oral Suspension Syrup 2038

Doxycycline Hyclate (Calcium sulfate present as an excipient may interfere with the absorption of oral tetracyclines). Products include:
Doryx Capsules 1970
Vibramycin Hyclate Capsules 2038
Vibramycin Hyclate Intravenous 2040
Vibra-Tabs Film Coated Tablets 2038

Doxycycline Monohydrate (Calcium sulfate present as an excipient may interfere with the absorption of oral tetracyclines). Products include:
Monodox Capsules 1858
Vibramycin Monohydrate for Oral Suspension 2038

Methacycline Hydrochloride (Calcium sulfate present as an excipient may interfere with the absorption of oral tetracyclines).
No products indexed under this heading.

Minocycline Hydrochloride (Calcium sulfate present as an excipient may interfere with the absorption of oral tetracyclines). Products include:
DYNACIN Capsules 1627
Minocin Intravenous 1428
Minocin Oral Suspension 1431
Minocin Pellet-Filled Capsules 1429

Oxytetracycline Hydrochloride (Calcium sulfate present as an excipient may interfere with the absorption of oral tetracyclines). Products include:
TERAK Ointment .... ⊙ 210
Terra-Cortril Ophthalmic Suspension 2033
Terramycin with Polymyxin B Sulfate Ophthalmic Ointment 2035
Urobiotic-250 Capsules 2038

Phenytoin Sodium (Calcium sulfate present as an excipient may interfere with the absorption of oral phenytoin sodium). Products include:
Dilantin Kapseals 1965

Tetracycline Hydrochloride (Calcium sulfate present as an excipient may interfere with the absorption of oral tetracyclines). Products include:
Achromycin V Capsules 1417
Helidac Therapy 2135

MOBIGESIC TABLETS
(Magnesium Salicylate, Phenyltoloxamine Citrate) .... ⊡ 607
May interact with hypnotics and sedatives, tranquilizers, and certain other agents. Compounds in these categories include:

Alprazolam (Concurrent use not recommended; consult your doctor). Products include:
Xanax Tablets 2115

Buspirone Hydrochloride (Concurrent use not recommended; consult your doctor). Products include:
BuSpar Tablets 738

Chlordiazepoxide (Concurrent use not recommended; consult your doctor). Products include:
Limbitrol 2333

Chlordiazepoxide Hydrochloride (Concurrent use not recommended; consult your doctor). Products include:
Librax Capsules 2330
Librium Capsules 2331
Librium Injectable 2332

Chlorpromazine (Concurrent use not recommended; consult your doctor). Products include:
Thorazine Suppositories 2701

Chlorpromazine Hydrochloride (Concurrent use not recommended; consult your doctor). Products include:
Thorazine 2701

Chlorprothixene (Concurrent use not recommended; consult your doctor).
No products indexed under this heading.

Chlorprothixene Hydrochloride (Concurrent use not recommended; consult your doctor).
No products indexed under this heading.

Clorazepate Dipotassium (Concurrent use not recommended; consult your doctor). Products include:
Tranxene 459

Diazepam (Concurrent use not recommended; consult your doctor). Products include:
Dizac (diazepam injectable emulsion) CIV 1862

Valium Injectable 2336
Valium Tablets 2335

Droperidol (Concurrent use not recommended; consult your doctor). Products include:
Inapsine Injection 462

Estazolam (Concurrent use not recommended; consult your doctor). Products include:
ProSom Tablets 457

Ethchlorvynol (Concurrent use not recommended; consult your doctor). Products include:
Placidyl Capsules 456

Ethinamate (Concurrent use not recommended; consult your doctor).
No products indexed under this heading.

Fluphenazine Decanoate (Concurrent use not recommended; consult your doctor). Products include:
Prolixin Decanoate 510

Fluphenazine Enanthate (Concurrent use not recommended; consult your doctor). Products include:
Prolixin Enanthate 510

Fluphenazine Hydrochloride (Concurrent use not recommended; consult your doctor). Products include:
Prolixin 510

Flurazepam Hydrochloride (Concurrent use not recommended; consult your doctor). Products include:
Dalmane Capsules 2329

Glutethimide (Concurrent use not recommended; consult your doctor).
No products indexed under this heading.

Haloperidol (Concurrent use not recommended; consult your doctor). Products include:
Haldol Injection, Tablets and Concentrate 1585

Haloperidol Decanoate (Concurrent use not recommended; consult your doctor). Products include:
Haldol Decanoate 1587

Hydroxyzine Hydrochloride (Concurrent use not recommended; consult your doctor). Products include:
Atarax Tablets & Syrup 1992
Marax Tablets & DF Syrup 2015
Vistaril Intramuscular Solution 2042

Lorazepam (Concurrent use not recommended; consult your doctor). Products include:
Ativan Injection 2805
Ativan Tablets 2807

Loxapine Hydrochloride (Concurrent use not recommended; consult your doctor). Products include:
Loxitane 1426

Loxapine Succinate (Concurrent use not recommended; consult your doctor). Products include:
Loxitane Capsules 1426

Meprobamate (Concurrent use not recommended; consult your doctor). Products include:
Miltown Tablets 2780
PMB 200 and PMB 400 2890

Mesoridazine Besylate (Concurrent use not recommended; consult your doctor). Products include:
Serentil 689

Midazolam Hydrochloride (Concurrent use not recommended; consult your doctor). Products include:
Versed Injection 2324

Molindone Hydrochloride (Concurrent use not recommended; consult your doctor). Products include:
Moban Tablets and Concentrate .. 1036

(⊡ Described in PDR For Nonprescription Drugs)   (⊙ Described in PDR For Ophthalmology)

Interactions Index

Oxazepam (Concurrent use not recommended; consult your doctor). Products include:
Serax Capsules 2916
Serax Tablets 2916

Perphenazine (Concurrent use not recommended; consult your doctor). Products include:
Etrafon 2495
Triavil Tablets 1800
Trilafon 2532

Prazepam (Concurrent use not recommended; consult your doctor).
No products indexed under this heading.

Prochlorperazine (Concurrent use not recommended; consult your doctor). Products include:
Compazine 2644

Promethazine Hydrochloride (Concurrent use not recommended; consult your doctor). Products include:
Mepergan Injection 2859
Phenergan with Codeine ... 2883
Phenergan with Dextromethorphan 2885
Phenergan Injection 2880
Phenergan Suppositories .. 2882
Phenergan Syrup 2881
Phenergan Tablets 2882
Phenergan VC 2886
Phenergan VC with Codeine 2888

Propofol (Concurrent use not recommended; consult your doctor). Products include:
Diprivan Injectable Emulsion 2939

Quazepam (Concurrent use not recommended; consult your doctor). Products include:
Doral Tablets 2773

Secobarbital Sodium (Concurrent use not recommended; consult your doctor). Products include:
Seconal Sodium Pulvules .. 1529

Temazepam (Concurrent use not recommended; consult your doctor). Products include:
Restoril Capsules 2413

Thioridazine Hydrochloride (Concurrent use not recommended; consult your doctor). Products include:
Mellaril 2398

Thiothixene (Concurrent use not recommended; consult your doctor). Products include:
Navane Capsules and Concentrate 2018
Navane Intramuscular 2019

Triazolam (Concurrent use not recommended; consult your doctor). Products include:
Halcion Tablets 2093

Trifluoperazine Hydrochloride (Concurrent use not recommended; consult your doctor). Products include:
Stelazine 2692

Zolpidem Tartrate (Concurrent use not recommended; consult your doctor). Products include:
Ambien Tablets 2559

Food Interactions
Alcohol (Avoid concurrent use; may cause drowsiness).

MOBISYL ANALGESIC CREME
(Trolamine Salicylate) 607
None cited in PDR database.

MODICON 21 TABLETS
(Norethindrone, Ethinyl Estradiol) 1928
See Ortho-Novum 7/7/7 □21 Tablets

MODICON 28 TABLETS
(Norethindrone, Ethinyl Estradiol) 1928
See Ortho-Novum 7/7/7 □21 Tablets

MODURETIC TABLETS
(Amiloride Hydrochloride, Hydrochlorothiazide) 1748
May interact with antihypertensives, lithium preparations, non-steroidal anti-inflammatory agents, insulin, cardiac glycosides, corticosteroids, potassium preparations, ACE inhibitors, oral hypoglycemic agents, barbiturates, narcotic analgesics, bile acid sequestering agents, and certain other agents. Compounds in these categories include:

Acarbose (Dosage adjustment of the antidiabetic drug may be required). Products include:
Precose 604

Acebutolol Hydrochloride (Potentiated or additive action). Products include:
Sectral Capsules 2914

ACTH (Hypokalemia).
No products indexed under this heading.

Alfentanil Hydrochloride (Potentiation of orthostatic hypotension). Products include:
Alfenta Injection 1334

Amlodipine Besylate (Potentiated or additive action). Products include:
Lotrel Capsules 858
Norvasc Tablets 2020

Aprobarbital (Potentiation of orthostatic hypotension).
No products indexed under this heading.

Atenolol (Potentiated or additive action). Products include:
Tenoretic Tablets 2963
Tenormin Tablets and I.V. Injection 2965

Benazepril Hydrochloride (Potentiated or additive action; increased risk of hyperkalemia). Products include:
Lotensin Tablets 852
Lotensin HCT Tablets 855
Lotrel Capsules 858

Bendroflumethiazide (Potentiated or additive action).
No products indexed under this heading.

Betamethasone Acetate (Hypokalemia). Products include:
Celestone Soluspan Suspension 2484

Betamethasone Sodium Phosphate (Hypokalemia). Products include:
Celestone Soluspan Suspension 2484

Betaxolol Hydrochloride (Potentiated or additive action). Products include:
Betoptic Ophthalmic Solution 465
Betoptic S Ophthalmic Suspension 467
Kerlone Tablets 2588

Bisoprolol Fumarate (Potentiated or additive action). Products include:
Zebeta Tablets 1457
Ziac 1459

Buprenorphine (Potentiation of orthostatic hypotension). Products include:
Buprenex Injectable 2170

Butabarbital (Potentiation of orthostatic hypotension).
No products indexed under this heading.

Butalbital (Potentiation of orthostatic hypotension). Products include:
Axocet Capsules 2469
Esgic-plus Capsules 1012
Esgic-plus Tablets 1012
Fioricet Tablets 2386
Fioricet with Codeine Capsules .. 2387
Fiorinal Capsules 2388
Fiorinal with Codeine Capsules .. 2390
Fiorinal Tablets 2388
Phrenilin 790
Sedapap Tablets 50 mg/650 mg .. 1826

Captopril (Potentiated or additive action; increased risk of hyperkalemia). Products include:
Capoten Tablets 740
Capozide Tablets 744

Carteolol Hydrochloride (Potentiated or additive action). Products include:
Cartrol Tablets 413
Ocupress Ophthalmic Solution, 1% Sterile 297

Chlorothiazide (Potentiated or additive action). Products include:
Aldoclor Tablets 1638
Diupres Tablets 1691
Diuril Oral 1694

Chlorothiazide Sodium (Potentiated or additive action). Products include:
Diuril Sodium Intravenous ... 1693

Chlorpropamide (Dosage adjustment of the antidiabetic drug may be required). Products include:
Diabinese Tablets 2002

Chlorthalidone (Potentiated or additive effects). Products include:
Combipres Tablets 682
Tenoretic Tablets 2963
Thalitone 1293

Cholestyramine (Cholestyramine resin has potential of binding hydrochlorothiazide and reducing its absorption from the GI tract by up to 85%). Products include:
Questran 774

Clonidine (Potentiated or additive action). Products include:
Catapres-TTS 680

Clonidine Hydrochloride (Potentiated or additive action). Products include:
Catapres Tablets 679
Combipres Tablets 682

Codeine Phosphate (Potentiation of orthostatic hypotension). Products include:
Brontex 2130
Dimetane-DC Cough Syrup .. 2232
Fioricet with Codeine Capsules .. 2387
Fiorinal with Codeine Capsules .. 2390
Nucofed 2225
Phenergan with Codeine ... 2883
Phenergan VC with Codeine 2888
Robitussin A-C Syrup 2248
Robitussin-DAC Syrup 2249
Ryna 804
Soma Compound w/Codeine Tablets 2784
Tylenol with Codeine 1592

Colestipol Hydrochloride (Colestipol resin has potential of binding hydrochlorothiazide and reducing its absorption from the GI tract by up to 43%). Products include:
Colestid 2073

Cortisone Acetate (Hypokalemia). Products include:
Cortone Acetate Sterile Suspension 1663
Cortone Acetate Tablets ... 1664

Deserpidine (Potentiated or additive action).
No products indexed under this heading.

Deslanoside (Potential for exaggerated response of the heart to the toxic effects of digitalis).
No products indexed under this heading.

Dexamethasone (Hypokalemia). Products include:
AK-Trol Ointment & Suspension 205
Decadron Elixir 1676
Decadron Tablets 1678
Decaspray Topical Aerosol 1689
Maxitrol Ophthalmic Ointment and Suspension 222
TobraDex Ophthalmic Suspension and Ointment 469

Dexamethasone Acetate (Hypokalemia). Products include:
Dalalone D.P. Injectable ... 1009
Decadron-LA Sterile Suspension 1687

Dexamethasone Sodium Phosphate (Hypokalemia). Products include:
Decadron Phosphate Injection .. 1680
Decadron Phosphate Sterile Ophthalmic Ointment 1684
Decadron Phosphate Sterile Ophthalmic Solution 1685
Decadron Phosphate Topical Cream 1686
Decadron Phosphate with Xylocaine Injection, Sterile 1683
Dexacort Phosphate in Respihaler .. 1606
Dexacort Phosphate in Turbinaire .. 1607
NeoDecadron Sterile Ophthalmic Ointment 1755
NeoDecadron Sterile Ophthalmic Solution 1756
NeoDecadron Topical Cream 1757

Dezocine (Potentiation of orthostatic hypotension). Products include:
Dalgan Injection 529

Diazoxide (Potentiated or additive action). Products include:
Hyperstat I.V. Injection 2504
Proglycem 575

Diclofenac Potassium (Reduced diuretic, natriuretic, and antihypertensive effects of Moduretic). Products include:
Cataflam Tablets 833

Diclofenac Sodium (Reduced diuretic, natriuretic, and antihypertensive effects of Moduretic). Products include:
Voltaren Ophthalmic Sterile Ophthalmic Solution 264
Cataflam/Voltaren/Voltaren-XR 833

Digitoxin (Potential for exaggerated response of the heart to the toxic effects of digitalis). Products include:
Crystodigin Tablets 1472

Digoxin (Potential for exaggerated response of the heart to the toxic effects of digitalis). Products include:
Lanoxicaps 1110
Lanoxin Elixir Pediatric 1113
Lanoxin Injection 1116
Lanoxin Injection Pediatric ... 1119
Lanoxin Tablets 1121

Diltiazem Hydrochloride (Potentiated or additive action). Products include:
Cardizem CD Capsules 1251
Cardizem SR Capsules 1255
Cardizem Injectable 1253
Cardizem Tablets 1257
Dilacor XR Extended-release Capsules 2183
Tiazac Capsules 1019

Doxazosin Mesylate (Potentiated or additive action). Products include:
Cardura Tablets 1993

Enalapril Maleate (Potentiated or additive action; increased risk of hyperkalemia). Products include:
Vaseretic Tablets 1810
Vasotec Tablets 1816

Enalaprilat (Potentiated or additive action; increased risk of hyperkalemia). Products include:
Vasotec I.V. 1814

Etodolac (Reduced diuretic, natriuretic, and antihypertensive effects of Moduretic). Products include:
Lodine Capsules and Tablets .. 2849

IMPORTANT NOTE: Always consult each drug listing in the patient's regimen for possible interactions.

Moduretic — Interactions Index — 694

Felodipine (Potentiated or additive action). Products include:
- Plendil Extended-Release Tablets 514

Fenoprofen Calcium (Reduced diuretic, natriuretic, and antihypertensive effects of Moduretic). Products include:
- Nalfon 200 Pulvules & Nalfon Tablets 933

Fentanyl (Potentiation of orthostatic hypotension). Products include:
- Duragesic Transdermal System 1336

Fentanyl Citrate (Potentiation of orthostatic hypotension). Products include:
- Sublimaze Injection 463

Fludrocortisone Acetate (Hypokalemia). Products include:
- Florinef Acetate Tablets 506

Flurbiprofen (Reduced diuretic, natriuretic, and antihypertensive effects of Moduretic).
- No products indexed under this heading.

Fosinopril Sodium (Potentiated or additive action; increased risk of hyperkalemia). Products include:
- Monopril Tablets 762

Furosemide (Potentiated or additive action). Products include:
- Lasix Injection, Oral Solution and Tablets 1267

Glimepiride (Dosage adjustment of the antidiabetic drug may be required). Products include:
- Amaryl Tablets 1241

Glipizide (Dosage adjustment of the antidiabetic drug may be required). Products include:
- Glucotrol Tablets 2011
- Glucotrol XL Extended Release Tablets 2012

Glyburide (Dosage adjustment of the antidiabetic drug may be required). Products include:
- DiaBeta Tablets 1265
- Glynase PresTab Tablets 2091
- Micronase Tablets 2099

Guanabenz Acetate (Potentiated or additive action).
- No products indexed under this heading.

Guanethidine Monosulfate (Potentiated or additive action). Products include:
- Esimil Tablets 840
- Ismelin Tablets 845

Hydralazine Hydrochloride (Potentiated or additive effects). Products include:
- Apresazide Capsules 824
- Apresoline Hydrochloride Tablets .. 826
- Hydralazine Hydrochloride Injection USP 2712
- Ser-Ap-Es Tablets 867

Hydrocodone Bitartrate (Potentiation of orthostatic hypotension). Products include:
- Codiclear DH Syrup 808
- Duratuss HD Elixir 2750
- Histussin D Liquid 670
- Hycodan Tablets and Syrup 946
- Hycomine Compound Tablets 948
- Hycomine 947
- Hycotuss Expectorant Syrup 950
- Hydrocet Capsules 787
- Lorcet 10/650 Tablets 1016
- Lortab 2751
- Tussend 1830
- Tussend Expectorant 1831
- Vicodin Tablets 1404
- Vicodin ES Tablets 1405
- Vicodin HP Tablets 1403
- Vicodin Tuss Expectorant 1406
- Zydone Capsules 967

Hydrocodone Polistirex (Potentiation of orthostatic hypotension). Products include:
- Tussionex Pennkinetic Extended-Release Suspension 1624

Hydrocortisone (Hypokalemia). Products include:
- Anusol-HC Cream 2.5% 1953
- Aquanil HC Lotion 1989
- Maximum Strength Cortaid Spray ▣ 800
- CORTENEMA 2713
- Cortisporin Ointment 1074
- Cortisporin Ophthalmic Ointment Sterile 1074
- Cortisporin Ophthalmic Suspension Sterile 1075
- Cortisporin Otic Solution Sterile 1076
- Cortisporin Otic Suspension Sterile . 1077
- Cortizone-5 795
- Cortizone-10 .... ▣ 795
- Hydrocortone Tablets 1715
- Hytone 922
- Hytone Ointment 2 ½% 923
- Massengill Medicated Soft Cloth Towelettes 2628
- Pediotic Suspension Sterile 1140
- Preparation H Hydrocortisone 1% Cream .... ▣ 843
- ProctoCream-HC 2.5% 2552
- VōSoL HC Otic Solution 2786

Hydrocortisone Acetate (Hypokalemia). Products include:
- Analpram-HC Rectal Cream 1% and 2.5% 993
- Anusol HC-1 Hydrocortisone Anti-Itch Ointment .... ▣ 810
- Anusol-HC Suppositories 1954
- Caldecort Anti-Itch Hydrocortisone Cream .... ▣ 651
- Coly-Mycin S Otic w/Neomycin & Hydrocortisone 1965
- Cortaid .... ▣ 800
- Cortifoam 2540
- Cortisporin Cream 1073
- Epifoam 2543
- Hydrocortone Acetate Sterile Suspension 1712
- Mantadil Cream 1124
- Nupercainal Hydrocortisone 1% Cream .... ▣ 661
- Pramosone Cream, Lotion & Ointment 995
- ProctoFoam-HC 2552
- Terra-Cortril Ophthalmic Suspension 2033

Hydrocortisone Sodium Phosphate (Hypokalemia). Products include:
- Hydrocortone Phosphate Injection, Sterile 1713

Hydrocortisone Sodium Succinate (Hypokalemia).
- No products indexed under this heading.

Hydroflumethiazide (Potentiated or additive action). Products include:
- Diucardin Tablets 2824

Hydromorphone Hydrochloride (Potentiation of orthostatic hypotension). Products include:
- Dilaudid Ampules 1382
- Dilaudid Cough Syrup 1383
- Dilaudid-HP Injection 1384
- Dilaudid-HP Lyophilized Powder 250 mg 1384
- Dilaudid 1382
- Dilaudid Oral Liquid 1386
- Dilaudid 1382
- Dilaudid Tablets - 8 mg 1386

Ibuprofen (Reduced diuretic, natriuretic, and antihypertensive effects of Moduretic). Products include:
- Advil Cold and Sinus Caplets and Tablets .... ▣ 837
- Advil Ibuprofen Tablets, Caplets and Gel Caplets ..... ▣ 836
- Children's Motrin Ibuprofen Oral Suspension 1558
- IBU Tablets 1389
- Ibuprohm .... ▣ 713
- Motrin IB Caplets, Tablets, and Gelcaps .... ▣ 802
- Motrin Ibuprofen Suspension, Oral Drops, Chewable Tablets, Caplets 1563
- Nuprin Ibuprofen/Analgesic Tablets & Caplets ..... ▣ 645
- Vicks DayQuil SINUS Pressure & PAIN Relief with IBUPROFEN ...... ▣ 735

Indapamide (Potentiated or additive action).
- No products indexed under this heading.

Indomethacin (Reduced diuretic, natriuretic, and antihypertensive effects of Moduretic; increased serum potassium levels of both drugs). Products include:
- Indocin 1723

Indomethacin Sodium Trihydrate (Reduced diuretic, natriuretic, and antihypertensive effects of Moduretic; increased serum potassium levels of both drugs). Products include:
- Indocin I.V. 1727

Insulin, Human (Altered insulin requirements).
- No products indexed under this heading.

Insulin, Human Isophane Suspension (Altered insulin requirements). Products include:
- Novolin N Human Insulin 10 ml Vials 1846

Insulin, Human NPH (Altered insulin requirements). Products include:
- Humulin N, 100 Units 1495
- Novolin N PenFill 1.5 ml Cartridges Durable Insulin Delivery System 1849
- Novolin N Prefilled Syringe Disposable Insulin Delivery System .. 1850

Insulin, Human Regular (Altered insulin requirements). Products include:
- Humulin R, 100 Units 1497
- Novolin R Human Insulin 10 ml Vials 1846
- Novolin R PenFill 1.5 ml Cartridges Durable Insulin Delivery System 1849
- Novolin R Prefilled Syringe Disposable Insulin Delivery System .. 1850
- Velosulin BR Human Insulin 10 ml Vials 1847

Insulin, Human, Zinc Suspension (Altered insulin requirements). Products include:
- Humulin L, 100 Units 1494
- Humulin U, 100 Units 1498
- Novolin L Human Insulin 10 ml Vials 1846

Insulin Lispro, Human (Altered insulin requirements). Products include:
- Humalog Injection 1488

Insulin, NPH (Altered insulin requirements). Products include:
- NPH, 100 Units 1502
- Pork NPH, 100 Units 1506
- Purified Pork NPH Isophane Insulin 1852

Insulin, Regular (Altered insulin requirements). Products include:
- Regular, 100 Units 1503
- Pork Regular, 100 Units 1507
- Pork Regular (Concentrated), 500 Units 1508
- Purified Pork Regular Insulin 1852

Insulin, Zinc Crystals (Altered insulin requirements). Products include:
- NPH, 100 Units 1502

Insulin, Zinc Suspension (Altered insulin requirements). Products include:
- Iletin I 1501
- Lente, 100 Units 1501
- Iletin II 1504
- Pork Lente, 100 Units 1504
- Purified Pork Lente Insulin 1852

Isradipine (Potentiated or additive action). Products include:
- DynaCirc Capsules 2381
- DynaCirc CR Tablets 2383

Ketoprofen (Reduced diuretic, natriuretic, and antihypertensive effects of Moduretic). Products include:
- Actron Caplets and Tablets .... ▣ 608
- Orudis Capsules 2874
- Orudis KT .... ▣ 842
- Oruvail Capsules 2874

Ketorolac Tromethamine (Reduced diuretic, natriuretic, and antihypertensive effects of Moduretic). Products include:
- Acular Sterile Ophthalmic Solution 470
- Toradol 2319

Labetalol Hydrochloride (Potentiated or additive action). Products include:
- Normodyne Injection 2519
- Normodyne Tablets 2522
- Trandate 1158

Levorphanol Tartrate (Potentiation of orthostatic hypotension). Products include:
- Levo-Dromoran 2297

Lisinopril (Potentiated or additive action; increased risk of hyperkalemia). Products include:
- Prinivil Tablets 1776
- Prinzide Tablets 1780
- Zestoretic Tablets 2968
- Zestril Tablets 2972

Lithium Carbonate (High risk of lithium toxicity). Products include:
- Eskalith 2658
- Lithium Carbonate Capsules & Tablets 2352
- Lithonate/Lithotabs/Lithobid 2721

Lithium Citrate (High risk of lithium toxicity).
- No products indexed under this heading.

Losartan Potassium (Potentiated or additive action). Products include:
- Cozaar Tablets 1668
- Hyzaar Tablets 1720

Mecamylamine Hydrochloride (Potentiated or additive action). Products include:
- Inversine Tablets 1729

Meclofenamate Sodium (Reduced diuretic, natriuretic, and antihypertensive effects of Moduretic).
- No products indexed under this heading.

Mefenamic Acid (Reduced diuretic, natriuretic, and antihypertensive effects of Moduretic). Products include:
- Ponstel 1982

Meperidine Hydrochloride (Potentiation of orthostatic hypotension). Products include:
- Demerol 2438
- Mepergan Injection 2859

Mephobarbital (Potentiation of orthostatic hypotension). Products include:
- Mebaral Tablets 2452

Metformin Hydrochloride (Dosage adjustment of the antidiabetic drug may be required). Products include:
- Glucophage Tablets 754

Methadone Hydrochloride (Potentiation of orthostatic hypotension). Products include:
- Methadone Hydrochloride Oral Concentrate 2356
- Methadone Hydrochloride Oral Solution & Tablets ... 2357

Methyclothiazide (Potentiated or additive action). Products include:
- Enduron Tablets 424

Methyldopa (Potentiated or additive action). Products include:
- Aldoclor Tablets 1638
- Aldomet Oral 1640
- Aldoril Tablets 1644

(▣ Described in PDR For Nonprescription Drugs)   (◉ Described in PDR For Ophthalmology)

Interactions Index — Moduretic

Methyldopate Hydrochloride (Potentiated or additive action). Products include:
- Aldomet Ester HCl Injection 1642

Methylprednisolone Acetate (Hypokalemia).
No products indexed under this heading.

Methylprednisolone Sodium Succinate (Hypokalemia).
No products indexed under this heading.

Metolazone (Potentiated or additive action). Products include:
- Mykrox Tablets 1617
- Zaroxolyn Tablets 1625

Metoprolol Succinate (Potentiated or additive action). Products include:
- Toprol-XL Tablets 560

Metoprolol Tartrate (Potentiated or additive action). Products include:
- Lopressor 848
- Lopressor HCT Tablets 850

Metyrosine (Potentiated or additive action). Products include:
- Demser Capsules 1690

Minoxidil (Potentiated or additive action).
No products indexed under this heading.

Moexipril Hydrochloride (Potentiated or additive action; increased risk of hyperkalemia). Products include:
- Univasc Tablets 2553

Morphine Sulfate (Potentiation of orthostatic hypotension). Products include:
- Astramorph/PF Injection, USP (Preservative-Free) 526
- Duramorph Injection 983
- Infumorph 200 and Infumorph 500 Sterile Solutions 985
- Kadian Capsules 2948
- MS Contin Tablets 2149
- MSIR 2152
- Oramorph SR (Morphine Sulfate Sustained Release Tablets) 2359
- RMS Suppositories CII 2766
- Roxanol 2365

Nabumetone (Reduced diuretic, natriuretic, and antihypertensive effects of Moduretic). Products include:
- Relafen Tablets 2688

Nadolol (Potentiated or additive action).
No products indexed under this heading.

Naproxen (Reduced diuretic, natriuretic, and antihypertensive effects of Moduretic). Products include:
- Anaprox/Naprosyn 2277

Naproxen Sodium (Reduced diuretic, natriuretic, and antihypertensive effects of Moduretic). Products include:
- Aleve 2124
- Anaprox/Naprosyn 2277
- Naprelan Tablets 2861

Nicardipine Hydrochloride (Potentiated or additive action). Products include:
- Cardene Capsules 2261
- Cardene I.V. 2815
- Cardene SR Capsules 2264

Nifedipine (Potentiated or additive action). Products include:
- Adalat Capsules (10 mg and 20 mg) 580
- Adalat CC 582
- Procardia Capsules 2024
- Procardia XL Extended Release Tablets 2026

Nisoldipine (Potentiated or additive action). Products include:
- Sular Tablets 2961

Nitroglycerin (Potentiated or additive action). Products include:
- Deponit NTG Transdermal Delivery System 2541
- Nitro-Bid IV 1270
- Nitro-Bid Ointment 1272
- Nitro-Dur (nitroglycerin) Transdermal Infusion System 1365
- Nitrolingual Spray 2193
- Nitrostat Tablets 1981
- Transderm-Nitro Transdermal Therapeutic System 878

Norepinephrine Bitartrate (Possible decreased response to pressor amines). Products include:
- Levophed Bitartrate Injection 2445

Opium Alkaloids (Potentiation of orthostatic hypotension).
No products indexed under this heading.

Oxaprozin (Reduced diuretic, natriuretic, and antihypertensive effects of Moduretic). Products include:
- Daypro Caplets 2578

Oxycodone Hydrochloride (Potentiation of orthostatic hypotension). Products include:
- OxyContin Tablets 2163
- OxyIR Capsules 2167
- Percocet Tablets 955
- Percodan Tablets 955
- Percodan-Demi Tablets 956
- Roxicodone Tablets, Oral Solution & Intensol (Oxycodone) 2366
- Tylox Capsules 1593

Penbutolol Sulfate (Potentiated or additive action). Products include:
- Levatol Tablets 2547

Pentobarbital Sodium (Potentiation of orthostatic hypotension). Products include:
- Nembutal Sodium Capsules 440
- Nembutal Sodium Solution 442
- Nembutal Sodium Suppositories 444

Phenobarbital (Potentiation of orthostatic hypotension). Products include:
- Arco-Lase Plus Tablets 513
- Bellergal-S Tablets 2375
- Donnatal 2234
- Donnatal Extentabs 2234
- Donnatal Tablets 2234
- Phenobarbital Elixir and Tablets 1523
- Quadrinal Tablets 1398

Phenoxybenzamine Hydrochloride (Potentiated or additive action). Products include:
- Dibenzyline Capsules 2650

Phentolamine Mesylate (Potentiated or additive action). Products include:
- Regitine Vials 864

Phenylbutazone (Reduced diuretic, natriuretic, and antihypertensive effects of Moduretic).
No products indexed under this heading.

Pindolol (Potentiated or additive action). Products include:
- Visken Tablets 2428

Piroxicam (Reduced diuretic, natriuretic, and antihypertensive effects of Moduretic). Products include:
- Feldene Capsules 2008

Polythiazide (Potentiated or additive action). Products include:
- Minizide Capsules 2016

Potassium Acid Phosphate (Potential for rapid increase in serum potassium levels). Products include:
- K-Phos Original Formula 'Sodium Free' Tablets 633

Potassium Bicarbonate (Potential for rapid increase in serum potassium levels). Products include:
- Alka-Seltzer Gold Effervescent Antacid 611

Potassium Chloride (Potential for rapid increase in serum potassium levels). Products include:
- Chlor-3 Condiment 1003
- Colyte and Colyte-flavored 2540
- GoLYTELY 694
- K-Dur Microburst Release System (potassium chloride, USP) E.R. Tablets 1364
- K-Lor Powder Packets 438
- K-Norm Capsules 1615
- K-Tab Filmtab 439
- Micro-K 2237
- Micro-K LS Packets 2238
- NuLYTELY 694
- Cherry Flavor NuLYTELY 694
- Rum-K Syrup 1004
- Slow-K Extended-Release Tablets 869

Potassium Citrate (Potential for rapid increase in serum potassium levels). Products include:
- Polycitra Syrup 574
- Polycitra-K Crystals 574
- Polycitra-K Oral Solution 575
- Polycitra-LC 574
- Urocit-K Tablets 1828

Potassium Gluconate (Potential for rapid increase in serum potassium levels).
No products indexed under this heading.

Potassium Phosphate, Dibasic (Potential for rapid increase in serum potassium levels).
No products indexed under this heading.

Potassium Phosphate, Monobasic (Potential for rapid increase in serum potassium levels). Products include:
- K-Phos Neutral Tablets 633
- K-Phos Original Formula 'Sodium Free' Tablets 633

Prazosin Hydrochloride (Potentiated or additive action). Products include:
- Minipress Capsules 2015
- Minizide Capsules 2016

Prednisolone Acetate (Hypokalemia). Products include:
- AK-CIDE .... ⓢ 203
- AK-CIDE Ointment .... ⓢ 203
- Blephamide Liquifilm Sterile Ophthalmic Suspension 472
- Blephamide Ointment .... ⓢ 234
- Econopred & Econopred Plus Ophthalmic Suspensions .... ⓢ 216
- Poly-Pred Liquifilm .... ⓢ 246
- Pred Forte .... ⓢ 247
- Pred Mild .... ⓢ 250
- Pred-G Liquifilm Sterile Ophthalmic Suspension .... ⓢ 248
- Pred-G S.O.P. Sterile Ophthalmic Ointment .... ⓢ 249

Prednisolone Sodium Phosphate (Hypokalemia). Products include:
- AK-PRED .... ⓢ 204
- Hydeltrasol Injection, Sterile 1708
- Pediapred Oral Solution 1618

Prednisolone Tebutate (Hypokalemia). Products include:
- Hydeltra-T.B.A. Sterile Suspension 1710

Prednisone (Hypokalemia).
No products indexed under this heading.

Propoxyphene Hydrochloride (Potentiation of orthostatic hypotension). Products include:
- Darvon 1475
- Wygesic Tablets 2930

Propoxyphene Napsylate (Potentiation of orthostatic hypotension). Products include:
- Darvon-N/Darvocet-N 1473

Propranolol Hydrochloride (Potentiated or additive action). Products include:
- Inderal 2834
- Inderal LA Long Acting Capsules 2836
- Inderide Tablets 2838
- Inderide LA Long Acting Capsules 2840

Quinapril Hydrochloride (Potentiated or additive action; increased risk of hyperkalemia). Products include:
- Accupril Tablets 1950

Ramipril (Potentiated or additive action; increased risk of hyperkalemia). Products include:
- Altace Capsules 1238

Rauwolfia Serpentina (Potentiated or additive action).
No products indexed under this heading.

Rescinnamine (Potentiated or additive action).
No products indexed under this heading.

Reserpine (Potentiated or additive action). Products include:
- Diupres Tablets 1691
- Hydropres Tablets 1718
- Ser-Ap-Es Tablets 867

Secobarbital Sodium (Potentiation of orthostatic hypotension). Products include:
- Seconal Sodium Pulvules 1529

Sodium Nitroprusside (Potentiated or additive action).
No products indexed under this heading.

Sotalol Hydrochloride (Potentiated or additive action). Products include:
- Betapace Tablets 637

Spirapril Hydrochloride (Potentiated or additive action; increased risk of hyperkalemia).
No products indexed under this heading.

Spironolactone (Potential for rapid increase in serum potassium levels). Products include:
- Aldactazide Tablets 2556
- Aldactone Tablets 2558

Sufentanil Citrate (Potentiation of orthostatic hypotension). Products include:
- Sufenta Injection 1355

Sulindac (Reduced diuretic, natriuretic, and antihypertensive effects of Moduretic). Products include:
- Clinoril Tablets 1658

Terazosin Hydrochloride (Potentiated or additive action). Products include:
- Hytrin Capsules 434

Thiamylal Sodium (Potentiation of orthostatic hypotension).
No products indexed under this heading.

Timolol Maleate (Potentiated or additive action). Products include:
- Blocadren Tablets 1654
- Timolide Tablets 1791
- Timoptic in Ocudose 1796
- Timoptic Sterile Ophthalmic Solution 1794
- Timoptic-XE 1798

Tolazamide (Dosage adjustment of the antidiabetic drug may be required).
No products indexed under this heading.

Tolbutamide (Dosage adjustment of the antidiabetic drug may be required).
No products indexed under this heading.

Tolmetin Sodium (Reduced diuretic, natriuretic, and antihypertensive effects of Moduretic). Products include:
- Tolectin (200, 400 and 600 mg) 1591

Torsemide (Potentiated or additive action; increased risk of hyperkalemia). Products include:
- Demadex Tablets and Injection 691

IMPORTANT NOTE: Always consult each drug listing in the patient's regimen for possible interactions.

Trandolapril (Potentiated or additive action; increased risk of hyperkalemia). Products include:
- Mavik Tablets ... 1407

Triamcinolone (Hypokalemia).
- No products indexed under this heading.

Triamcinolone Acetonide (Hypokalemia). Products include:
- Azmacort Oral Inhaler ... 2175
- Nasacort AQ Nasal Spray ... 2191
- Nasacort Nasal Inhaler ... 2189

Triamcinolone Diacetate (Hypokalemia).
- No products indexed under this heading.

Triamcinolone Hexacetonide (Hypokalemia).
- No products indexed under this heading.

Triamterene (Potential for rapid increase in serum potassium levels). Products include:
- Dyazide Capsules ... 2653
- Dyrenium Capsules ... 2655

Trimethaphan Camsylate (Potentiated or additive action).
- No products indexed under this heading.

Tubocurarine Chloride (Increased responsiveness to tubocurarine).
- No products indexed under this heading.

Verapamil Hydrochloride (Potentiated or additive action). Products include:
- Calan SR Caplets ... 2571
- Calan Tablets ... 2568
- Covera-HS Tablets ... 2573
- Isoptin Injectable ... 1391
- Isoptin Oral Tablets ... 1393
- Isoptin SR Tablets ... 1395
- Verelan Capsules ... 1455

Food Interactions

Alcohol (Potentiation of orthostatic hypotension).

Diet, potassium-rich (Potential for rapid increases in serum potassium levels).

MOISTUREL CREAM
(Dimethicone, Petrolatum) ... 2796
None cited in PDR database.

MOISTUREL LOTION
(Dimethicone) ... 2797
None cited in PDR database.

MONOCAL TABLETS
(Calcium Carbonate, Sodium Monofluorophosphate) ... 1825
None cited in PDR database.

8-MOP CAPSULES
(Methoxsalen) ... 1294
May interact with phenothiazines, tetracyclines, thiazides, sulfonamides, and certain other agents. Compounds in these categories include:

Anthralin (Concomitant therapy, either topically or systemically, with photosensitizing agents requires special care). Products include:
- Drithocreme 0.1%, 0.25%, 0.5%, 1.0% (HP) ... 920
- Dritho-Scalp 0.25%, 0.5% ... 921

Bendroflumethiazide (Concomitant therapy, either topically or systemically, with photosensitizing agents requires special care).
- No products indexed under this heading.

Chlorothiazide (Concomitant therapy, either topically or systemically, with photosensitizing agents requires special care). Products include:
- Aldoclor Tablets ... 1638
- Diupres Tablets ... 1691
- Diuril Oral ... 1694

Chlorothiazide Sodium (Concomitant therapy, either topically or systemically, with photosensitizing agents requires special care). Products include:
- Diuril Sodium Intravenous ... 1693

Chlorpromazine (Concomitant therapy, either topically or systemically, with photosensitizing agents requires special care). Products include:
- Thorazine Suppositories ... 2701

Chlorpromazine Hydrochloride (Concomitant therapy, either topically or systemically, with photosensitizing agents requires special care). Products include:
- Thorazine ... 2701

Chlorpropamide (Concomitant therapy, either topically or systemically, with photosensitizing agents requires special care). Products include:
- Diabinese Tablets ... 2002

Coal Tar (Concomitant therapy, either topically or systemically, with photosensitizing agents requires special care). Products include:
- DHS ... 1989
- Fototar Cream ... 1300
- MG 217 ... ▣ 800
- Pentrax Shampoo ... 1042
- Tegrin Dandruff Shampoo ... ▣ 634
- Tegrin Skin Cream & Tegrin Medicated Soap ... ▣ 634

Demeclocycline Hydrochloride (Concomitant therapy, either topically or systemically, with photosensitizing agents requires special care). Products include:
- Declomycin Tablets ... 1421

Doxycycline Calcium (Concomitant therapy, either topically or systemically, with photosensitizing agents requires special care). Products include:
- Vibramycin Calcium Oral Suspension Syrup ... 2038

Doxycycline Hyclate (Concomitant therapy, either topically or systemically, with photosensitizing agents requires special care). Products include:
- Doryx Capsules ... 1970
- Vibramycin Hyclate Capsules ... 2038
- Vibramycin Hyclate Intravenous ... 2040
- Vibra-Tabs Film Coated Tablets ... 2038

Doxycycline Monohydrate (Concomitant therapy, either topically or systemically, with photosensitizing agents requires special care). Products include:
- Monodox Capsules ... 1858
- Vibramycin Monohydrate for Oral Suspension ... 2038

Fluphenazine Decanoate (Concomitant therapy, either topically or systemically, with photosensitizing agents requires special care). Products include:
- Prolixin Decanoate ... 510

Fluphenazine Enanthate (Concomitant therapy, either topically or systemically, with photosensitizing agents requires special care). Products include:
- Prolixin Enanthate ... 510

Fluphenazine Hydrochloride (Concomitant therapy, either topically or systemically, with photosensitizing agents requires special care). Products include:
- Prolixin ... 510

Glipizide (Concomitant therapy, either topically or systemically, with photosensitizing agents requires special care). Products include:
- Glucotrol Tablets ... 2011
- Glucotrol XL Extended Release Tablets ... 2012

Glyburide (Concomitant therapy, either topically or systemically, with photosensitizing agents requires special care). Products include:
- DiaBeta Tablets ... 1265
- Glynase PresTab Tablets ... 2091
- Micronase Tablets ... 2099

Griseofulvin (Concomitant therapy, either topically or systemically, with photosensitizing agents requires special care). Products include:
- Fulvicin P/G Tablets ... 2499
- Fulvicin P/G 165 & 330 Tablets ... 2500
- Grifulvin V (griseofulvin tablets) Microsize (griseofulvin oral suspension) Microsize ... 1944
- Gris-PEG Tablets, 125 mg & 250 mg ... 476

Hydrochlorothiazide (Concomitant therapy, either topically or systemically, with photosensitizing agents requires special care). Products include:
- Aldactazide Tablets ... 2556
- Aldoril Tablets ... 1644
- Apresazide Capsules ... 824
- Capozide Tablets ... 744
- Dyazide Capsules ... 2653
- Esidrix Tablets ... 839
- Esimil Tablets ... 840
- HydroDIURIL Tablets ... 1716
- Hydropres Tablets ... 1718
- Hyzaar Tablets ... 1720
- Inderide Tablets ... 2838
- Inderide LA Long Acting Capsules ... 2840
- Lopressor HCT Tablets ... 850
- Lotensin HCT Tablets ... 855
- Moduretic Tablets ... 1748
- Oretic Tablets ... 450
- Prinzide Tablets ... 1780
- Ser-Ap-Es Tablets ... 867
- Timolide Tablets ... 1791
- Vaseretic Tablets ... 1810
- Zestoretic Tablets ... 2968
- Ziac ... 1459

Hydroflumethiazide (Concomitant therapy, either topically or systemically, with photosensitizing agents requires special care). Products include:
- Diucardin Tablets ... 2824

Mesoridazine Besylate (Concomitant therapy, either topically or systemically, with photosensitizing agents requires special care). Products include:
- Serentil ... 689

Methacycline Hydrochloride (Concomitant therapy, either topically or systemically, with photosensitizing agents requires special care).
- No products indexed under this heading.

Methotrimeprazine (Concomitant therapy, either topically or systemically, with photosensitizing agents requires special care). Products include:
- Levoprome ... 1321

Methyclothiazide (Concomitant therapy, either topically or systemically, with photosensitizing agents requires special care). Products include:
- Enduron Tablets ... 424

Methylene Blue (Concomitant therapy, either topically or systemically, with photosensitizing agents requires special care). Products include:
- Urised Tablets ... 2123

Minocycline Hydrochloride (Concomitant therapy, either topically or systemically, with photosensitizing agents requires special care). Products include:
- DYNACIN Capsules ... 1627
- Minocin Intravenous ... 1428
- Minocin Oral Suspension ... 1431
- Minocin Pellet-Filled Capsules ... 1429

Nalidixic Acid (Concomitant therapy, either topically or systemically, with photosensitizing agents requires special care). Products include:
- NegGram ... 2453

Oxytetracycline Hydrochloride (Concomitant therapy, either topically or systemically, with photosensitizing agents requires special care). Products include:
- TERAK Ointment ... ⊚ 210
- Terra-Cortril Ophthalmic Suspension ... 2033
- Terramycin with Polymyxin B Sulfate Ophthalmic Ointment ... 2035
- Urobiotic-250 Capsules ... 2038

Perphenazine (Concomitant therapy, either topically or systemically, with photosensitizing agents requires special care). Products include:
- Etrafon ... 2495
- Triavil Tablets ... 1800
- Trilafon ... 2532

Polythiazide (Concomitant therapy, either topically or systemically, with photosensitizing agents requires special care). Products include:
- Minizide Capsules ... 2016

Prochlorperazine (Concomitant therapy, either topically or systemically, with photosensitizing agents requires special care). Products include:
- Compazine ... 2644

Promethazine Hydrochloride (Concomitant therapy, either topically or systemically, with photosensitizing agents requires special care). Products include:
- Mepergan Injection ... 2859
- Phenergan with Codeine ... 2883
- Phenergan with Dextromethorphan ... 2885
- Phenergan Injection ... 2880
- Phenergan Suppositories ... 2882
- Phenergan Syrup ... 2881
- Phenergan Tablets ... 2882
- Phenergan VC ... 2886
- Phenergan VC with Codeine ... 2888

Rose Bengal (Concomitant therapy, either topically or systemically, with photosensitizing agents requires special care).
- No products indexed under this heading.

Sulfacytine (Concomitant therapy, either topically or systemically, with photosensitizing agents requires special care).

Sulfamethizole (Concomitant therapy, either topically or systemically, with photosensitizing agents requires special care). Products include:
- Urobiotic-250 Capsules ... 2038

Sulfamethoxazole (Concomitant therapy, either topically or systemically, with photosensitizing agents requires special care). Products include:
- Bactrim DS Tablets ... 2257
- Bactrim I.V. Infusion ... 2255
- Bactrim ... 2257
- Gantanol Tablets ... 2285
- Septra ... 1146
- Septra I.V. Infusion ... 1142

(▣ Described in PDR For Nonprescription Drugs) (⊚ Described in PDR For Ophthalmology)

697 **Interactions Index** **Monodox**

Septra I.V. Infusion ADD-Vantage Vials 1144
Septra 1146

Sulfasalazine (Concomitant therapy, either topically or systemically, with photosensitizing agents requires special care). Products include:
Azulfidine 2059

Sulfinpyrazone (Concomitant therapy, either topically or systemically, with photosensitizing agents requires special care). Products include:
Anturane 823

Sulfisoxazole (Concomitant therapy, either topically or systemically, with photosensitizing agents requires special care). Products include:
Gantrisin Tablets 2286

Sulfisoxazole Diolamine (Concomitant therapy, either topically or systemically, with photosensitizing agents requires special care).
No products indexed under this heading.

Tetracycline Hydrochloride (Concomitant therapy, either topically or systemically, with photosensitizing agents requires special care). Products include:
Achromycin V Capsules 1417
Helidac Therapy 2135

Thioridazine Hydrochloride (Concomitant therapy, either topically or systemically, with photosensitizing agents requires special care). Products include:
Mellaril 2398

Tolazamide (Concomitant therapy, either topically or systemically, with photosensitizing agents requires special care).
No products indexed under this heading.

Tolbutamide (Concomitant therapy, either topically or systemically, with photosensitizing agents requires special care).
No products indexed under this heading.

Trifluoperazine Hydrochloride (Concomitant therapy, either topically or systemically, with photosensitizing agents requires special care). Products include:
Stelazine 2692

MONISTAT DUAL-PAK
(Miconazole Nitrate) 1906
None cited in PDR database.

MONISTAT 3 VAGINAL SUPPOSITORIES
(Miconazole Nitrate) 1905
None cited in PDR database.

MONISTAT-DERM (MICONAZOLE NITRATE 2%) CREAM
(Miconazole Nitrate) 1944
None cited in PDR database.

MONOCID INJECTION
(Cefonicid Sodium) 2674
May interact with aminoglycosides and certain other agents. Compounds in these categories include:

Amikacin Sulfate (Concomitant administration may result in nephrotoxicity). Products include:
Amikacin Sulfate Injection, USP 523
Amikacin Sulfate Injection, USP 981
Amikin Injectable 502

Gentamicin Sulfate (Concomitant administration may result in nephrotoxicity). Products include:
Garamycin Cream 0.1% 2501
Garamycin Injectable 2502
Garamycin Ointment 0.1% 2501
Garamycin Ophthalmic 2501
Genoptic Sterile Ophthalmic Solution .... ◎ 241
Genoptic Sterile Ophthalmic Ointment .... ◎ 241
Gentak .... ◎ 209
Pred-G Liquifilm Sterile Ophthalmic Suspension .... ◎ 248
Pred-G S.O.P. Sterile Ophthalmic Ointment .... ◎ 249

Kanamycin Sulfate (Concomitant administration may result in nephrotoxicity).
No products indexed under this heading.

Probenecid (Produces higher peak serum levels). Products include:
Benemid Tablets 1651
ColBENEMID Tablets 1662

Streptomycin Sulfate (Concomitant administration may result in nephrotoxicity). Products include:
Streptomycin Sulfate Injection 2031

Tobramycin Sulfate (Concomitant administration may result in nephrotoxicity). Products include:
Nebcin Vials, Hyporets & ADD-Vantage 1518

MONOCLATE-P, FACTOR VIII:C PASTEURIZED, MONOCLONAL ANTIBODY PURIFIED ANTIHEMOPHILIC FACTOR (HUMAN)
(Antihemophilic Factor (Human)) 802
None cited in PDR database.

MONODOX CAPSULES
(Doxycycline Monohydrate) 1858
May interact with barbiturates, oral contraceptives, penicillins, antacids containing aluminium, calcium and magnesium, oral anticoagulants, and certain other agents. Compounds in these categories include:

Aluminum Carbonate (Absorption of tetracyclines is impaired). Products include:
Basaljel Capsules 2810
Basaljel Suspension 2810
Basaljel Tablets 2810

Aluminum Hydroxide (Absorption of tetracyclines is impaired). Products include:
ALternaGEL Liquid 1358
Maximum Strength Ascriptin .... ▣ 650
Cama Arthritis Pain Reliever .... ▣ 748
Gaviscon Extra Strength Relief Formula Antacid Tablets .... ▣ 778
Gaviscon Extra Strength Relief Formula Liquid Antacid .... ▣ 779
Gaviscon Liquid Antacid .... ▣ 779
Gelusil Antacid-Anti-gas Liquid .... ▣ 819
Gelusil Antacid-Anti-gas Tablets .... ▣ 819
Maalox Antacid/Anti-Gas Tablets 889
Maalox Heartburn Relief Suspension .... ▣ 658
Maalox Antacid Liquid 888
Extra Strength Maalox Antacid/Anti-Gas Liquid and Tablets 888
Mylanta 1359
Tempo Soft Antacid .... ▣ 799

Aluminum Hydroxide Gel (Absorption of tetracyclines is impaired). Products include:
ALternaGEL Liquid .... ▣ 675
Aludrox Oral Suspension .... ▣ 850
Amphojel Suspension 2802
Amphojel Suspension without Flavor 2802
Amphojel Tablets 2802
Ascriptin .... ▣ 650
Gaviscon Antacid Tablets .... ▣ 778
Gaviscon-2 Antacid Tablets .... ▣ 779
Mylanta Liquid .... ▣ 676
Mylanta Double Strength Liquid .... ▣ 676
Nephrox Suspension .... ▣ 671

Amoxicillin Trihydrate (Interference with penicillins' bactericidal action). Products include:
Amoxil 2631
Augmentin 2637
Augmentin Tablets 2640

Ampicillin (Interference with penicillins' bactericidal action). Products include:
Omnipen Capsules 2872
Omnipen for Oral Suspension 2873

Ampicillin Sodium (Interference with penicillins' bactericidal action). Products include:
Unasyn 2035

Aprobarbital (Decreases the half-life of doxycycline).
No products indexed under this heading.

Azlocillin Sodium (Interference with penicillins' bactericidal action).
No products indexed under this heading.

Bacampicillin Hydrochloride (Interference with penicillins' bactericidal action). Products include:
Spectrobid Tablets 2030

Butabarbital (Decreases the half-life of doxycycline).
No products indexed under this heading.

Butalbital (Decreases the half-life of doxycycline). Products include:
Axocet Capsules 2469
Esgic-plus Capsules 1012
Esgic-plus Tablets 1012
Fioricet Tablets 2386
Fioricet with Codeine Capsules 2387
Fiorinal Capsules 2388
Fiorinal with Codeine Capsules 2390
Fiorinal Tablets 2388
Phrenilin 790
Sedapap Tablets 50 mg/650 mg 1826

Carbamazepine (Decreases the half-life of doxycycline). Products include:
Atretol Tablets 569
Tegretol/Tegretol-XR 870

Carbenicillin Disodium (Interference with penicillins' bactericidal action).
No products indexed under this heading.

Carbenicillin Indanyl Sodium (Interference with penicillins' bactericidal action). Products include:
Geocillin Tablets 2009

Desogestrel (Concurrent use may render oral contraceptives less effective). Products include:
Desogen Tablets 1867
Ortho-Cept 1907

Dicloxacillin Sodium (Interference with penicillins' bactericidal action).
No products indexed under this heading.

Dicumarol (Depressed plasma prothrombin activity).
No products indexed under this heading.

Ethinyl Estradiol (Concurrent use may render oral contraceptives less effective). Products include:
Brevicon 2563
Demulen 2580
Desogen Tablets 1867
Levlen/Tri-Levlen 646
Lo/Ovral Tablets 2852
Lo/Ovral-28 Tablets 2857
Modicon 1928
Nordette-21 Tablets 2863
Nordette-28 Tablets 2866
Norinyl 2563
Ortho-Cept 1907
Ortho-Cyclen/Ortho-Tri-Cyclen 1914
Ortho-Novum 1928
Ortho-Cyclen/Ortho Tri-Cyclen 1914
Ovcon 765
Ovral Tablets 2877
Ovral-28 Tablets 2878
Levlen/Tri-Levlen 646
Tri-Norinyl 2607
Triphasil-21 Tablets 2919
Triphasil-28 Tablets 2924

Ethynodiol Diacetate (Concurrent use may render oral contraceptives less effective). Products include:
Demulen 2580

Levonorgestrel (Concurrent use may render oral contraceptives less effective). Products include:
Levlen/Tri-Levlen 646
Nordette-21 Tablets 2863
Nordette-28 Tablets 2866
Norplant System 2868
Levlen/Tri-Levlen 646
Triphasil-21 Tablets 2919
Triphasil-28 Tablets 2924

Magaldrate (Absorption of tetracyclines is impaired).
No products indexed under this heading.

Magnesium Hydroxide (Absorption of tetracyclines is impaired). Products include:
Aludrox Oral Suspension .... ▣ 850
Ascriptin .... ▣ 650
Di-Gel Antacid/Anti-Gas .... ▣ 762
Gelusil Antacid-Anti-gas Liquid .... ▣ 819
Gelusil Antacid-Anti-gas Tablets .... ▣ 819
Maalox Antacid/Anti-Gas Tablets 889
Maalox Antacid Liquid 888
Extra Strength Maalox Antacid/Anti-Gas Liquid and Tablets 888
Mylanta Fast-Acting 1359
Mylanta Gelcaps Antacid .... ▣ 678
Fast-Acting Mylanta Liquid Antacid 1359
Mylanta Tablets .... ▣ 677
Maximum-Strength Fast-Acting Mylanta Liquid Antacid 1359
Mylanta Double Strength Tablets .... ▣ 677
Phillips' Milk of Magnesia Liquid .... ▣ 627
Rolaids Antacid Tablets .... ▣ 807
Tempo Soft Antacid .... ▣ 799

Magnesium Oxide (Absorption of tetracyclines is impaired). Products include:
Beelith Tablets 632
Bufferin Analgesic Tablets .... ▣ 636
Arthritis Strength Bufferin Analgesic Caplets .... ▣ 637
Extra Strength Bufferin Analgesic Tablets .... ▣ 637
Caltrate PLUS .... ▣ 681
Cama Arthritis Pain Reliever .... ▣ 748
Mag-Ox 400 666
Uro-Mag 666

Mephobarbital (Decreases the half-life of doxycycline). Products include:
Mebaral Tablets 2452

Mestranol (Concurrent use may render oral contraceptives less effective). Products include:
Norinyl 2563
Ortho-Novum 1928

Methoxyflurane (Potential for fatal renal toxicity).
No products indexed under this heading.

Mezlocillin Sodium (Interference with penicillins' bactericidal action). Products include:
Mezlin 594
Mezlin Pharmacy Bulk Package 597

Nafcillin Sodium (Interference with penicillins' bactericidal action).
No products indexed under this heading.

Norethindrone (Concurrent use may render oral contraceptives less effective). Products include:
Brevicon 2563
Micronor Tablets 1903
Modicon 1928
Norinyl 2563
Nor-Q D Tablets 2598
Ortho-Novum 1928
Ovcon 765
Tri-Norinyl 2607

Norethynodrel (Concurrent use may render oral contraceptives less effective).
No products indexed under this heading.

IMPORTANT NOTE: Always consult each drug listing in the patient's regimen for possible interactions.

Monodox / Interactions Index ... 698

Norgestimate (Concurrent use may render oral contraceptives less effective). Products include:
- Ortho-Cyclen/Ortho-Tri-Cyclen ... 1914
- Ortho-Cyclen/Ortho-Tri-Cyclen ... 1914

Norgestrel (Concurrent use may render oral contraceptives less effective). Products include:
- Lo/Ovral Tablets ... 2852
- Lo/Ovral-28 Tablets ... 2857
- Ovral Tablets ... 2877
- Ovral-28 Tablets ... 2878
- Ovrette Tablets ... 2878

Penicillin G Benzathine (Interference with penicillins' bactericidal action). Products include:
- Bicillin C-R Injection ... 2810
- Bicillin C-R 900/300 Injection ... 2812
- Bicillin L-A Injection ... 2813

Penicillin G Potassium (Interference with penicillins' bactericidal action). Products include:
- Pfizerpen for Injection ... 2022

Penicillin G Procaine (Interference with penicillins' bactericidal action). Products include:
- Bicillin C-R Injection ... 2810
- Bicillin C-R 900/300 Injection ... 2812

Penicillin G Sodium (Interference with penicillins' bactericidal action).
- No products indexed under this heading.

Penicillin V Potassium (Interference with penicillins' bactericidal action). Products include:
- Pen•Vee K ... 2879

Pentobarbital Sodium (Decreases the half-life of doxycycline). Products include:
- Nembutal Sodium Capsules ... 440
- Nembutal Sodium Solution ... 442
- Nembutal Sodium Suppositories ... 444

Phenobarbital (Decreases the half-life of doxycycline). Products include:
- Arco-Lase Plus Tablets ... 513
- Bellergal-S Tablets ... 2375
- Donnatal ... 2234
- Donnatal Extentabs ... 2234
- Donnatal Tablets ... 2234
- Phenobarbital Elixir and Tablets ... 1523
- Quadrinal Tablets ... 1398

Phenytoin (Decreases the half-life of doxycycline). Products include:
- Dilantin Infatabs ... 1967
- Dilantin-125 Suspension ... 1969

Phenytoin Sodium (Decreases the half-life of doxycycline). Products include:
- Dilantin Kapseals ... 1965

Secobarbital Sodium (Decreases the half-life of doxycycline). Products include:
- Seconal Sodium Pulvules ... 1529

Thiamylal Sodium (Decreases the half-life of doxycycline).
- No products indexed under this heading.

Ticarcillin Disodium (Interference with penicillins' bactericidal action). Products include:
- Ticar for Injection ... 2704
- Timentin for Injection ... 2706

Warfarin Sodium (Depressed plasma prothrombin activity). Products include:
- Coumadin ... 941

MONO-GESIC TABLETS
(Salsalate) ... 810
May interact with thyroid preparations, salicylates, antigout agents, anticoagulants, oral hypoglycemic agents, corticosteroids, and penicillins. Compounds in these categories include:

Acarbose (Hypoglycemic effect enhanced). Products include:
- Precose ... 604

Allopurinol (Uricosuric action of gout drugs antagonized). Products include:
- Zyloprim Tablets ... 1194

Amoxicillin Trihydrate (Competition for protein-binding sites). Products include:
- Amoxil ... 2631
- Augmentin ... 2637
- Augmentin Tablets ... 2640

Ampicillin Sodium (Competition for protein-binding sites). Products include:
- Unasyn ... 2035

Aspirin (Potential toxicity). Products include:
- Alka-Seltzer Cherry Effervescent Antacid and Pain Reliever ... 609
- Alka-Seltzer Extra Strength Effervescent Antacid and Pain Reliever ... 609
- Alka-Seltzer Lemon Lime Effervescent Antacid and Pain Reliever ... 609
- Alka-Seltzer Original Effervescent Antacid and Pain Reliever ... 609
- Alka-Seltzer Plus ... 611
- Alka-Seltzer Plus Sinus Medicine ... 611
- Ascriptin ... 650
- Arthritis Strength BC Powder ... 631
- BC Cold Powder Multi-Symptom Formula (Cold-Sinus-Allergy) ... 631
- BC Cold Powder Non-Drowsy Formula (Cold-Sinus) ... 631
- BC Powder ... 631
- Genuine Bayer Aspirin Tablets & Caplets ... 618
- Extra Strength Bayer Arthritis Pain Regimen Formula ... 615
- Extra Strength Bayer Aspirin Caplets & Tablets ... 617
- Extended-Release Bayer 8-Hour Aspirin ... 616
- Extra Strength Bayer Plus Aspirin Caplets ... 617
- Extra Strength Bayer PM Aspirin Plus Sleep Aid ... 617
- Aspirin Regimen Bayer 81 mg Tablets with Calcium ... 615
- Aspirin Regimen Bayer Adult Low Strength 81 mg Tablets ... 613
- Aspirin Regimen Bayer Children's Chewable Aspirin ... 616
- Aspirin Regimen Bayer Regular Strength 325 mg Caplets ... 613
- Bufferin Analgesic Tablets ... 636
- Arthritis Strength Bufferin Analgesic Caplets ... 637
- Extra Strength Bufferin Analgesic Tablets ... 637
- Cama Arthritis Pain Reliever ... 748
- Darvon Compound-65 Pulvules ... 1475
- Easprin ... 1971
- Ecotrin ... 2625
- Ecotrin Enteric Coated Aspirin Maximum Strength Tablets and Caplets ... 775
- Ecotrin Enteric Coated Aspirin Regular Strength Tablets ... 2625
- Empirin Aspirin Tablets ... 818
- Excedrin Extra-Strength Analgesic Tablets, Caplets, and Geltabs ... 734
- Fiorinal Capsules ... 2388
- Fiorinal with Codeine Capsules ... 2390
- Fiorinal Tablets ... 2388
- Goody's Extra Strength Headache Powders ... 632
- Goody's Extra Strength Pain Relief Tablets ... 632
- Halfprin Tablets ... 1413
- Norgesic ... 1554
- Percodan Tablets ... 955
- Percodan-Demi Tablets ... 956
- Robaxisal Tablets ... 2246
- Soma Compound w/Codeine Tablets ... 2784
- Soma Compound Tablets ... 2783
- St. Joseph Adult Chewable Aspirin (81 mg.) ... 768
- Talwin Compound ... 2466
- Vanquish Analgesic Caplets ... 627

Azlocillin Sodium (Competition for protein-binding sites).
- No products indexed under this heading.

Bacampicillin Hydrochloride (Competition for protein-binding sites). Products include:
- Spectrobid Tablets ... 2030

Betamethasone Acetate (Competition for protein-binding sites). Products include:
- Celestone Soluspan Suspension ... 2484

Betamethasone Sodium Phosphate (Competition for protein-binding sites). Products include:
- Celestone Soluspan Suspension ... 2484

Carbenicillin Disodium (Competition for protein-binding sites).
- No products indexed under this heading.

Carbenicillin Indanyl Sodium (Competition for protein-binding sites). Products include:
- Geocillin Tablets ... 2009

Chlorpropamide (Hypoglycemic effect enhanced). Products include:
- Diabinese Tablets ... 2002

Choline Magnesium Trisalicylate (Potential toxicity). Products include:
- Trilisate ... 2155

Cortisone Acetate (Competition for protein-binding sites). Products include:
- Cortone Acetate Sterile Suspension ... 1663
- Cortone Acetate Tablets ... 1664

Dalteparin Sodium (Competition for protein binding predisposes to systemic bleeding). Products include:
- Fragmin Injection ... 2088

Dexamethasone (Competition for protein-binding sites). Products include:
- AK-Trol Ointment & Suspension ... 205
- Decadron Elixir ... 1676
- Decadron Tablets ... 1678
- Decaspray Topical Aerosol ... 1689
- Maxitrol Ophthalmic Ointment and Suspension ... 222
- TobraDex Ophthalmic Suspension and Ointment ... 469

Dexamethasone Acetate (Competition for protein-binding sites). Products include:
- Dalalone D.P. Injectable ... 1009
- Decadron-LA Sterile Suspension ... 1687

Dexamethasone Sodium Phosphate (Competition for protein-binding sites). Products include:
- Decadron Phosphate Injection ... 1680
- Decadron Phosphate Sterile Ophthalmic Ointment ... 1684
- Decadron Phosphate Sterile Ophthalmic Solution ... 1685
- Decadron Phosphate Topical Cream ... 1686
- Decadron Phosphate with Xylocaine Injection, Sterile ... 1683
- Dexacort Phosphate in Respihaler ... 1606
- Dexacort Phosphate in Turbinaire ... 1607
- NeoDecadron Sterile Ophthalmic Ointment ... 1755
- NeoDecadron Sterile Ophthalmic Solution ... 1756
- NeoDecadron Topical Cream ... 1757

Dicloxacillin Sodium (Competition for protein-binding sites).
- No products indexed under this heading.

Dicumarol (Competition for protein binding predisposes to systemic bleeding).
- No products indexed under this heading.

Diflunisal (Potential toxicity). Products include:
- Dolobid Tablets ... 1695

Enoxaparin (Competition for protein binding predisposes to systemic bleeding). Products include:
- Lovenox Injection ... 2187

Fludrocortisone Acetate (Competition for protein-binding sites). Products include:
- Florinef Acetate Tablets ... 506

Glimepiride (Hypoglycemic effect enhanced). Products include:
- Amaryl Tablets ... 1241

Glipizide (Hypoglycemic effect enhanced). Products include:
- Glucotrol Tablets ... 2011
- Glucotrol XL Extended Release Tablets ... 2012

Glyburide (Hypoglycemic effect enhanced). Products include:
- DiaBeta Tablets ... 1265
- Glynase PresTab Tablets ... 2091
- Micronase Tablets ... 2099

Heparin Calcium (Competition for protein binding predisposes to systemic bleeding).
- No products indexed under this heading.

Heparin Sodium (Competition for protein binding predisposes to systemic bleeding). Products include:
- Heparin Lock Flush Solution ... 2831
- Heparin Sodium Injection ... 2832
- Heparin Sodium Vials ... 1486

Hydrocortisone (Competition for protein-binding sites). Products include:
- Anusol-HC Cream 2.5% ... 1953
- Aquanil HC Lotion ... 1989
- Maximum Strength Cortaid Spray ... 800
- CORTENEMA ... 2713
- Cortisporin Ointment ... 1074
- Cortisporin Ophthalmic Ointment Sterile ... 1074
- Cortisporin Ophthalmic Suspension Sterile ... 1075
- Cortisporin Otic Solution Sterile ... 1076
- Cortisporin Otic Suspension Sterile ... 1077
- Cortizone-5 ... 795
- Cortizone-10 ... 795
- Hydrocortone Tablets ... 1715
- Hytone ... 922
- Hytone Ointment 2 ½% ... 923
- Massengill Medicated Soft Cloth Towelettes ... 2628
- Pediotic Suspension Sterile ... 1140
- Preparation H Hydrocortisone 1% Cream ... 843
- ProctoCream-HC 2.5% ... 2552
- VōSoL HC Otic Solution ... 2786

Hydrocortisone Acetate (Competition for protein-binding sites). Products include:
- Analpram-HC Rectal Cream 1% and 2.5% ... 993
- Anusol HC-1 Hydrocortisone Anti-Itch Ointment ... 810
- Anusol-HC Suppositories ... 1954
- Caldecort Anti-Itch Hydrocortisone Cream ... 651
- Coly-Mycin S Otic w/Neomycin & Hydrocortisone ... 1965
- Cortaid ... 800
- Cortifoam ... 2540
- Cortisporin Cream ... 1073
- Epifoam ... 2543
- Hydrocortone Acetate Sterile Suspension ... 1712
- Mantadil Cream ... 1124
- Nupercainal Hydrocortisone 1% Cream ... 661
- Pramosone Cream, Lotion & Ointment ... 995
- ProctoFoam-HC ... 2552
- Terra-Cortril Ophthalmic Suspension ... 2033

Hydrocortisone Sodium Phosphate (Competition for protein-binding sites). Products include:
- Hydrocortone Phosphate Injection, Sterile ... 1713

Hydrocortisone Sodium Succinate (Competition for protein-binding sites).
- No products indexed under this heading.

Levothyroxine Sodium (Depressed plasma T4 value). Products include:
- Eltroxin Tablets ... 2214

(⊞ Described in PDR For Nonprescription Drugs)   (⊚ Described in PDR For Ophthalmology)

Interactions Index — Monopril

Levothroid Tablets 1015
Levothyroxine Sodium, USP for Injection 546
Levoxyl Tablets 918
Synthroid 1410

Liothyronine Sodium (Depressed plasma T4 value). Products include:
Cytomel Tablets 2647
Triostat Injection 2708

Magnesium Salicylate (Potential toxicity). Products include:
Backache Caplets .... ⊞◻ 635
Doan's Extra-Strength Analgesic.... ⊞◻ 653
Extra Strength Doan's P.M. .... ⊞◻ 653
Doan's Regular Strength Analgesic .... ⊞◻ 654
Mobigesic Tablets .... ⊞◻ 607

Metformin Hydrochloride (Hypoglycemic effect enhanced). Products include:
Glucophage Tablets 754

Methotrexate Sodium (Competition for protein-binding sites). Products include:
Methotrexate Sodium Tablets, Injection, for Injection and LPF Injection 1322

Methylprednisolone Acetate (Competition for protein-binding sites).
No products indexed under this heading.

Methylprednisolone Sodium Succinate (Competition for protein-binding sites).
No products indexed under this heading.

Mezlocillin Sodium (Competition for protein-binding sites). Products include:
Mezlin 594
Mezlin Pharmacy Bulk Package...... 597

Nafcillin Sodium (Competition for protein-binding sites).
No products indexed under this heading.

Naproxen (Competition for protein-binding sites). Products include:
Anaprox/Naprosyn 2277

Naproxen Sodium (Competition for protein-binding sites). Products include:
Aleve 2124
Anaprox/Naprosyn 2277
Naprelan Tablets 2861

Penicillin G Benzathine (Competition for protein-binding sites). Products include:
Bicillin C-R Injection 2810
Bicillin C-R 900/300 Injection 2812
Bicillin L-A Injection 2813

Penicillin G Potassium (Competition for protein-binding sites). Products include:
Pfizerpen for Injection 2022

Penicillin G Procaine (Competition for protein-binding sites). Products include:
Bicillin C-R Injection 2810
Bicillin C-R 900/300 Injection 2812

Penicillin G Sodium (Competition for protein-binding sites).
No products indexed under this heading.

Penicillin V Potassium (Competition for protein-binding sites). Products include:
Pen•Vee K 2879

Phenytoin (Competition for protein-binding sites). Products include:
Dilantin Infatabs 1967
Dilantin-125 Suspension 1969

Phenytoin Sodium (Competition for protein-binding sites). Products include:
Dilantin Kapseals 1965

Prednisolone Acetate (Competition for protein-binding sites). Products include:
AK-CIDE .... ◎ 203

AK-CIDE Ointment................. ◎ 203
Blephamide Liquifilm Sterile Ophthalmic Suspension 472
Blephamide Ointment .... ◎ 234
Econopred & Econopred Plus Ophthalmic Suspensions .... ◎ 216
Poly-Pred Liquifilm .... ◎ 246
Pred Forte .... ◎ 247
Pred Mild .... ◎ 250
Pred-G Liquifilm Sterile Ophthalmic Suspension .... ◎ 248
Pred-G S.O.P. Sterile Ophthalmic Ointment .... ◎ 249

Prednisolone Sodium Phosphate (Competition for protein-binding sites). Products include:
AK-PRED .... ◎ 204
Hydeltrasol Injection, Sterile 1708
Pediapred Oral Solution 1618

Prednisolone Tebutate (Competition for protein-binding sites). Products include:
Hydeltra-T.B.A. Sterile Suspension 1710

Prednisone (Competition for protein-binding sites).
No products indexed under this heading.

Probenecid (Uricosuric action of gout drugs antagonized). Products include:
Benemid Tablets 1651
ColBENEMID Tablets 1662

Sulfinpyrazone (Uricosuric action of gout drugs antagonized). Products include:
Anturane 823

Thyroxine (Depressed plasma T4 value; competition for protein-binding sites).
No products indexed under this heading.

Thyroxine Sodium (Depressed plasma T4 value).
No products indexed under this heading.

Ticarcillin Disodium (Competition for protein-binding sites). Products include:
Ticar for Injection 2704
Timentin for Injection 2706

Tolazamide (Hypoglycemic effect enhanced).
No products indexed under this heading.

Tolbutamide (Hypoglycemic effect enhanced).
No products indexed under this heading.

Triamcinolone (Competition for protein-binding sites).
No products indexed under this heading.

Triamcinolone Acetonide (Competition for protein-binding sites). Products include:
Azmacort Oral Inhaler 2175
Nasacort AQ Nasal Spray 2191
Nasacort Nasal Inhaler 2189

Triamcinolone Diacetate (Competition for protein-binding sites).
No products indexed under this heading.

Triamcinolone Hexacetonide (Competition for protein-binding sites).
No products indexed under this heading.

l-Triiodothyronine (Competition for protein-binding sites).

Warfarin Sodium (Competition for protein binding predisposes to systemic bleeding). Products include:
Coumadin 941

Food Interactions

Food that lowers urinary pH (Decreases urinary excretion and increases plasma levels).

Food that raises urinary pH (Increases renal clearance and urinary excretion of salicylic acid).

MONOKET TABLETS
(Isosorbide Mononitrate) 2550
May interact with vasodilators, calcium channel blockers, and certain other agents. Compounds in these categories include:

Amlodipine Besylate (Combination therapy produces marked symptomatic orthostatic hypotension). Products include:
Lotrel Capsules 858
Norvasc Tablets 2020

Bepridil Hydrochloride (Combination therapy produces marked symptomatic orthostatic hypotension). Products include:
Vascor Tablets (200 and 300 mg) 1597

Diazoxide (Additive vasodilating effects). Products include:
Hyperstat I.V. Injection 2504
Proglycem 575

Diltiazem Hydrochloride (Combination therapy produces marked symptomatic orthostatic hypotension). Products include:
Cardizem CD Capsules 1251
Cardizem SR Capsules 1255
Cardizem Injectable 1253
Cardizem Tablets..................... 1257
Dilacor XR Extended-release Capsules 2183
Tiazac Capsules 1019

Epoprostenol Sodium (Additive vasodilating effects). Products include:
Flolan for Injection 1085

Felodipine (Combination therapy produces marked symptomatic orthostatic hypotension). Products include:
Plendil Extended-Release Tablets.... 514

Hydralazine Hydrochloride (Additive vasodilating effects). Products include:
Apresazide Capsules 824
Apresoline Hydrochloride Tablets .. 826
Hydralazine Hydrochloride Injection USP............................... 2712
Ser-Ap-Es Tablets 867

Isradipine (Combination therapy produces marked symptomatic orthostatic hypotension). Products include:
DynaCirc Capsules 2381
DynaCirc CR Tablets 2383

Minoxidil (Additive vasodilating effects).
No products indexed under this heading.

Nicardipine Hydrochloride (Combination therapy produces marked symptomatic orthostatic hypotension). Products include:
Cardene Capsules 2261
Cardene I.V. 2815
Cardene SR Capsules............... 2264

Nifedipine (Combination therapy produces marked symptomatic orthostatic hypotension). Products include:
Adalat Capsules (10 mg and 20 mg) 580
Adalat CC 582
Procardia Capsules................... 2024
Procardia XL Extended Release Tablets 2026

Nimodipine (Combination therapy produces marked symptomatic orthostatic hypotension). Products include:
Nimotop Capsules 603

Nisoldipine (Combination therapy produces marked symptomatic orthostatic hypotension). Products include:
Sular Tablets 2961

Verapamil Hydrochloride (Combination therapy produces marked symptomatic orthostatic hypotension). Products include:
Calan SR Caplets 2571
Calan Tablets 2568
Covera-HS Tablets 2573
Isoptin Injectable 1391
Isoptin Oral Tablets 1393
Isoptin SR Tablets 1395
Verelan Capsules 1455

Food Interactions
Alcohol (Additive vasodilating effects).

MONONINE, COAGULATION FACTOR IX (HUMAN), MONOCLONAL ANTIBODY PURIFIED
(Factor IX (Human)) 804
None cited in PDR database.

MONOPRIL TABLETS
(Fosinopril Sodium) 762
May interact with diuretics, potassium sparing diuretics, potassium preparations, lithium preparations, and certain other agents. Compounds in these categories include:

Aluminum Hydroxide (Co-administration with an antacid containing aluminum hydroxide, magnesium hydroxide, and simethicone has resulted in reduced serum levels and urinary excretion of fosinoprilat; dosing should be separated by two hours). Products include:
ALternaGEL Liquid 1358
Maximum Strength Ascriptin .... ⊞◻ 650
Cama Arthritis Pain Reliever...... ⊞◻ 748
Gaviscon Extra Strength Relief Formula Antacid Tablets ...... ⊞◻ 778
Gaviscon Extra Strength Relief Formula Liquid Antacid........ ⊞◻ 779
Gaviscon Liquid Antacid .... ⊞◻ 779
Gelusil Antacid-Anti-gas Liquid .. ⊞◻ 819
Gelusil Antacid-Anti-gas Tablets .... ⊞◻ 819
Maalox Antacid/Anti-Gas Tablets 889
Maalox Heartburn Relief Suspension .... ⊞◻ 658
Maalox Antacid Liquid 888
Extra Strength Maalox Antacid/ Anti-Gas Liquid and Tablets ... 888
Mylanta 1359
Tempo Soft Antacid .... ⊞◻ 799

Aluminum Hydroxide Gel (Co-administration with an antacid containing aluminum hydroxide, magnesium hydroxide, and simethicone has resulted in reduced serum levels and urinary excretion of fosinoprilat; dosing should be separated by two hours). Products include:
ALternaGEL Liquid .... ⊞◻ 675
Aludrox Oral Suspension .... ⊞◻ 850
Amphojel Suspension 2802
Amphojel Suspension without Flavor 2802
Amphojel Tablets 2802
Ascriptin .... ⊞◻ 650
Gaviscon Antacid Tablets.......... ⊞◻ 778
Gaviscon-2 Antacid Tablets ...... ⊞◻ 779
Mylanta Liquid .... ⊞◻ 676
Mylanta Double Strength Liquid ... ⊞◻ 676
Nephrox Suspension .... ⊞◻ 671

Amiloride Hydrochloride (Potential for hyperkalemia; potential for excessive reduction in blood pressure after initiation of Monopril therapy). Products include:
Midamor Tablets 1746
Moduretic Tablets 1748

Bendroflumethiazide (Potential for excessive reduction in blood pressure after initiation of Monopril therapy).
No products indexed under this heading.

IMPORTANT NOTE: Always consult each drug listing in the patient's regimen for possible interactions.

Monopril — **Interactions Index** — **700**

Bumetanide (Potential for excessive reduction in blood pressure after initiation of Monopril therapy). Products include:
- Bumex 2260

Chlorothiazide (Potential for excessive reduction in blood pressure after initiation of Monopril therapy). Products include:
- Aldoclor Tablets 1638
- Diupres Tablets 1691
- Diuril Oral 1694

Chlorothiazide Sodium (Potential for excessive reduction in blood pressure after initiation of Monopril therapy). Products include:
- Diuril Sodium Intravenous 1693

Chlorthalidone (Potential for excessive reduction in blood pressure after initiation of Monopril therapy). Products include:
- Combipres Tablets 682
- Tenoretic Tablets 2963
- Thalitone 1293

Ethacrynic Acid (Potential for excessive reduction in blood pressure after initiation of Monopril therapy). Products include:
- Edecrin Tablets 1698

Furosemide (Potential for excessive reduction in blood pressure after initiation of Monopril therapy). Products include:
- Lasix Injection, Oral Solution and Tablets 1267

Hydrochlorothiazide (Potential for excessive reduction in blood pressure after initiation of Monopril therapy). Products include:
- Aldactazide Tablets 2556
- Aldoril Tablets 1644
- Apresazide Capsules 824
- Capozide Tablets 744
- Dyazide Capsules 2653
- Esidrix Tablets 839
- Esimil Tablets 840
- HydroDIURIL Tablets 1716
- Hydropres Tablets 1718
- Hyzaar Tablets 1720
- Inderide Tablets 2838
- Inderide LA Long Acting Capsules .. 2840
- Lopressor HCT Tablets 850
- Lotensin HCT Tablets 855
- Moduretic Tablets 1748
- Oretic Tablets 450
- Prinzide Tablets 1780
- Ser-Ap-Es Tablets 867
- Timolide Tablets 1791
- Vaseretic Tablets 1810
- Zestoretic Tablets 2968
- Ziac 1459

Hydroflumethiazide (Potential for excessive reduction in blood pressure after initiation of Monopril therapy). Products include:
- Diucardin Tablets 2824

Indapamide (Potential for excessive reduction in blood pressure after initiation of Monopril therapy).
- No products indexed under this heading.

Lithium Carbonate (Potential for increased lithium levels and symptoms of lithium toxicity). Products include:
- Eskalith 2658
- Lithium Carbonate Capsules & Tablets 2352
- Lithonate/Lithotabs/Lithobid 2721

Lithium Citrate (Potential for increased lithium levels and symptoms of lithium toxicity).
- No products indexed under this heading.

Magnesium Hydroxide (Co-administration with an antacid containing aluminum hydroxide, magnesium hydroxide, and simethicone has resulted in reduced serum levels and urinary excretion of fosinoprilat; dosing should be separated by two hours). Products include:
- Aludrox Oral Suspension .... ⊞ 850
- Ascriptin .... ⊞ 650
- Di-Gel Antacid/Anti-Gas .... ⊞ 762
- Gelusil Antacid-Anti-gas Liquid .... ⊞ 819
- Gelusil Antacid-Anti-gas Tablets .... ⊞ 819
- Maalox Antacid/Anti-Gas Tablets 889
- Maalox Antacid Liquid 888
- Extra Strength Maalox Antacid/Anti-Gas Liquid and Tablets 888
- Mylanta Fast-Acting 1359
- Mylanta Gelcaps Antacid .... ⊞ 678
- Fast-Acting Mylanta Liquid Antacid 1359
- Mylanta Tablets .... ⊞ 677
- Maximum-Strength Fast-Acting Mylanta Liquid Antacid 1359
- Mylanta Double Strength Tablets .. ⊞ 677
- Phillips' Milk of Magnesia Liquid .... ⊞ 627
- Rolaids Antacid Tablets .... ⊞ 807
- Tempo Soft Antacid .... ⊞ 799

Methyclothiazide (Potential for excessive reduction in blood pressure after initiation of Monopril therapy). Products include:
- Enduron Tablets 424

Metolazone (Potential for excessive reduction in blood pressure after initiation of Monopril therapy). Products include:
- Mykrox Tablets 1617
- Zaroxolyn Tablets 1625

Polythiazide (Potential for excessive reduction in blood pressure after initiation of Monopril therapy). Products include:
- Minizide Capsules 2016

Potassium Acid Phosphate (Potential for hyperkalemia). Products include:
- K-Phos Original Formula 'Sodium Free' Tablets 633

Potassium Bicarbonate (Potential for hyperkalemia). Products include:
- Alka-Seltzer Gold Effervescent Antacid .... ⊞ 611

Potassium Chloride (Potential for hyperkalemia). Products include:
- Chlor-3 Condiment 1003
- Colyte and Colyte-flavored 2540
- GoLYTELY 694
- K-Dur Microburst Release System (potassium chloride, USP) E.R. Tablets 1364
- K-Lor Powder Packets 438
- K-Norm Capsules 1615
- K-Tab Filmtab 439
- Micro-K 2237
- Micro-K LS Packets 2238
- NuLYTELY 694
- Cherry Flavor NuLYTELY 694
- Rum-K Syrup 1004
- Slow-K Extended-Release Tablets 869

Potassium Citrate (Potential for hyperkalemia). Products include:
- Polycitra Syrup 574
- Polycitra-K Crystals 574
- Polycitra-K Oral Solution 575
- Polycitra-LC 574
- Urocit-K Tablets 1828

Potassium Gluconate (Potential for hyperkalemia).
- No products indexed under this heading.

Potassium Phosphate, Dibasic (Potential for hyperkalemia).
- No products indexed under this heading.

Potassium Phosphate, Monobasic (Potential for hyperkalemia). Products include:
- K-Phos Neutral Tablets 633
- K-Phos Original Formula 'Sodium Free' Tablets 633

Spironolactone (Potential for hyperkalemia; potential for excessive reduction in blood pressure after initiation of Monopril therapy). Products include:
- Aldactazide Tablets 2556
- Aldactone Tablets 2558

Torsemide (Potential for excessive reduction in blood pressure after initiation of Monopril therapy). Products include:
- Demadex Tablets and Injection 691

Triamterene (Potential for hyperkalemia; potential for excessive reduction in blood pressure after initiation of Monopril therapy). Products include:
- Dyazide Capsules 2653
- Dyrenium Capsules 2655

Food Interactions

Food, unspecified (Rate of absorption may be slowed by the presence of food in the GI tract; the extent of absorption is not affected).

MOTOFEN TABLETS
(Atropine Sulfate, Difenoxin Hydrochloride) 789

May interact with monoamine oxidase inhibitors, barbiturates, tranquilizers, narcotic analgesics, and certain other agents. Compounds in these categories include:

Alfentanil Hydrochloride (Effects potentiated). Products include:
- Alfenta Injection 1334

Alprazolam (Effects potentiated). Products include:
- Xanax Tablets 2115

Aprobarbital (Effects potentiated).
- No products indexed under this heading.

Buprenorphine (Effects potentiated). Products include:
- Buprenex Injectable 2170

Buspirone Hydrochloride (Effects potentiated). Products include:
- BuSpar Tablets 738

Butabarbital (Effects potentiated).
- No products indexed under this heading.

Butalbital (Effects potentiated). Products include:
- Axocet Capsules 2469
- Esgic-plus Capsules 1012
- Esgic-plus Tablets 1012
- Fioricet Tablets 2386
- Fioricet with Codeine Capsules 2387
- Fiorinal Capsules 2388
- Fiorinal with Codeine Capsules 2390
- Fiorinal Tablets 2388
- Phrenilin 790
- Sedapap Tablets 50 mg/650 mg .. 1826

Chlordiazepoxide (Effects potentiated). Products include:
- Limbitrol 2333

Chlordiazepoxide Hydrochloride (Effects potentiated). Products include:
- Librax Capsules 2330
- Librium Capsules 2331
- Librium Injectable 2332

Chlorpromazine (Effects potentiated). Products include:
- Thorazine Suppositories 2701

Chlorprothixene (Effects potentiated).
- No products indexed under this heading.

Chlorprothixene Hydrochloride (Effects potentiated).
- No products indexed under this heading.

Clorazepate Dipotassium (Effects potentiated). Products include:
- Tranxene 459

Codeine Phosphate (Effects potentiated). Products include:
- Brontex 2130
- Dimetane-DC Cough Syrup 2232
- Fioricet with Codeine Capsules 2387
- Fiorinal with Codeine Capsules 2390
- Nucofed 2225
- Phenergan with Codeine 2883
- Phenergan VC with Codeine 2888
- Robitussin A-C Syrup 2248
- Robitussin-DAC Syrup 2249
- Ryna .... ⊞ 804
- Soma Compound w/Codeine Tablets 2784
- Tylenol with Codeine 1592

Dezocine (Effects potentiated). Products include:
- Dalgan Injection 529

Diazepam (Effects potentiated). Products include:
- Dizac (diazepam injectable emulsion) CIV 1862
- Valium Injectable 2336
- Valium Tablets 2335

Droperidol (Effects potentiated). Products include:
- Inapsine Injection 462

Fentanyl (Effects potentiated). Products include:
- Duragesic Transdermal System 1336

Fentanyl Citrate (Effects potentiated). Products include:
- Sublimaze Injection 463

Fluphenazine Decanoate (Effects potentiated). Products include:
- Prolixin Decanoate 510

Fluphenazine Enanthate (Effects potentiated). Products include:
- Prolixin Enanthate 510

Fluphenazine Hydrochloride (Effects potentiated). Products include:
- Prolixin 510

Furazolidone (Concurrent use may precipitate hypertensive crisis). Products include:
- Furoxone 2221

Haloperidol (Effects potentiated). Products include:
- Haldol Injection, Tablets and Concentrate 1585

Haloperidol Decanoate (Effects potentiated). Products include:
- Haldol Decanoate 1587

Hydrocodone Bitartrate (Effects potentiated). Products include:
- Codiclear DH Syrup 808
- Duratuss HD Elixir 2750
- Histussin D Liquid 670
- Hycodan Tablets and Syrup 946
- Hycomine Compound Tablets 948
- Hycomine 947
- Hycotuss Expectorant Syrup 950
- Hydrocet Capsules 787
- Lorcet 10/650 Tablets 1016
- Lortab 2751
- Tussend 1830
- Tussend Expectorant 1831
- Vicodin Tablets 1404
- Vicodin ES Tablets 1405
- Vicodin HP Tablets 1403
- Vicodin Tuss Expectorant 1406
- Zydone Capsules 967

Hydrocodone Polistirex (Effects potentiated). Products include:
- Tussionex Pennkinetic Extended-Release Suspension 1624

Hydromorphone Hydrochloride (Effects potentiated). Products include:
- Dilaudid Ampules 1382
- Dilaudid Cough Syrup 1383
- Dilaudid-HP Injection 1384
- Dilaudid-HP Lyophilized Powder 250 mg 1384
- Dilaudid 1382
- Dilaudid Oral Liquid 1386
- Dilaudid 1382
- Dilaudid Tablets - 8 mg 1386

(⊞ Described in PDR For Nonprescription Drugs) (◉ Described in PDR For Ophthalmology)

Hydroxyzine Hydrochloride (Effects potentiated). Products include:
- Atarax Tablets & Syrup ... 1992
- Marax Tablets & DF Syrup ... 2015
- Vistaril Intramuscular Solution ... 2042

Isocarboxazid (Concurrent use may precipitate hypertensive crisis).
- No products indexed under this heading.

Levorphanol Tartrate (Effects potentiated). Products include:
- Levo-Dromoran ... 2297

Lorazepam (Effects potentiated). Products include:
- Ativan Injection ... 2805
- Ativan Tablets ... 2807

Loxapine Hydrochloride (Effects potentiated). Products include:
- Loxitane ... 1426

Loxapine Succinate (Effects potentiated). Products include:
- Loxitane Capsules ... 1426

Meperidine Hydrochloride (Effects potentiated). Products include:
- Demerol ... 2438
- Mepergan Injection ... 2859

Mephobarbital (Effects potentiated). Products include:
- Mebaral Tablets ... 2452

Meprobamate (Effects potentiated). Products include:
- Miltown Tablets ... 2780
- PMB 200 and PMB 400 ... 2890

Mesoridazine Besylate (Effects potentiated). Products include:
- Serentil ... 689

Methadone Hydrochloride (Effects potentiated). Products include:
- Methadone Hydrochloride Oral Concentrate ... 2356
- Methadone Hydrochloride Oral Solution & Tablets ... 2357

Molindone Hydrochloride (Effects potentiated). Products include:
- Moban Tablets and Concentrate ... 1036

Morphine Sulfate (Effects potentiated). Products include:
- Astramorph/PF Injection, USP (Preservative-Free) ... 526
- Duramorph Injection ... 983
- Infumorph 200 and Infumorph 500 Sterile Solutions ... 985
- Kadian Capsules ... 2948
- MS Contin Tablets ... 2149
- MSIR ... 2152
- Oramorph SR (Morphine Sulfate Sustained Release Tablets) ... 2359
- RMS Suppositories CII ... 2766
- Roxanol ... 2365

Opium Alkaloids (Effects potentiated).
- No products indexed under this heading.

Oxazepam (Effects potentiated). Products include:
- Serax Capsules ... 2916
- Serax Tablets ... 2916

Oxycodone Hydrochloride (Effects potentiated). Products include:
- OxyContin Tablets ... 2163
- OxyIR Capsules ... 2167
- Percocet Tablets ... 955
- Percodan Tablets ... 955
- Percodan-Demi Tablets ... 956
- Roxicodone Tablets, Oral Solution & Intensol (Oxycodone) ... 2366
- Tylox Capsules ... 1593

Pentobarbital Sodium (Effects potentiated). Products include:
- Nembutal Sodium Capsules ... 440
- Nembutal Sodium Solution ... 442
- Nembutal Sodium Suppositories ... 444

Perphenazine (Effects potentiated). Products include:
- Etrafon ... 2495
- Triavil Tablets ... 1800
- Trilafon ... 2532

Phenelzine Sulfate (Concurrent use may precipitate hypertensive crisis). Products include:
- Nardil ... 1977

Phenobarbital (Effects potentiated). Products include:
- Arco-Lase Plus Tablets ... 513
- Bellergal-S Tablets ... 2375
- Donnatal ... 2234
- Donnatal Extentabs ... 2234
- Donnatal Tablets ... 2234
- Phenobarbital Elixir and Tablets ... 1523
- Quadrinal Tablets ... 1398

Prazepam (Effects potentiated).
- No products indexed under this heading.

Prochlorperazine (Effects potentiated). Products include:
- Compazine ... 2644

Promethazine Hydrochloride (Effects potentiated). Products include:
- Mepergan Injection ... 2859
- Phenergan with Codeine ... 2883
- Phenergan with Dextromethorphan ... 2885
- Phenergan Injection ... 2880
- Phenergan Suppositories ... 2882
- Phenergan Syrup ... 2881
- Phenergan Tablets ... 2882
- Phenergan VC ... 2886
- Phenergan VC with Codeine ... 2888

Propoxyphene Hydrochloride (Effects potentiated). Products include:
- Darvon ... 1475
- Wygesic Tablets ... 2930

Propoxyphene Napsylate (Effects potentiated). Products include:
- Darvon-N/Darvocet-N ... 1473

Secobarbital Sodium (Effects potentiated). Products include:
- Seconal Sodium Pulvules ... 1529

Selegiline Hydrochloride (Concurrent use may precipitate hypertensive crisis). Products include:
- Eldepryl Capsules ... 2729

Sufentanil Citrate (Effects potentiated). Products include:
- Sufenta Injection ... 1355

Thiamylal Sodium (Effects potentiated).
- No products indexed under this heading.

Thioridazine Hydrochloride (Effects potentiated). Products include:
- Mellaril ... 2398

Thiothixene (Effects potentiated). Products include:
- Navane Capsules and Concentrate ... 2018
- Navane Intramuscular ... 2019

Tranylcypromine Sulfate (Concurrent use may precipitate hypertensive crisis). Products include:
- Parnate Tablets ... 2679

Trifluoperazine Hydrochloride (Effects potentiated). Products include:
- Stelazine ... 2692

Food Interactions

Alcohol (Effects potentiated).

MOTRIN IB CAPLETS, TABLETS, AND GELCAPS

(Ibuprofen) ... 802

May interact with aspirin and acetaminophen containing products. Compounds in this category include:

Acetaminophen (Concurrent use is not recommended except under a doctor's direction). Products include:
- Actifed Cold & Sinus Caplets and Tablets ... 808
- Actifed Sinus Daytime/Nighttime Tablets and Caplets ... 809
- Alka-Seltzer Fast Relief Caplets ... 610
- Alka-Seltzer Plus Liqui-Gels ... 612
- Alka-Seltzer Plus Flu & Body Aches Effervescent Tablets ... 612
- Alka-Seltzer Plus Flu & Body Aches Liqui-Gels Non-Drowsy Formula ... 613
- Alka-Seltzer Plus Night-Time Cold Medicine Liqui-Gels ... 612
- Allerest No Drowsiness ... 649
- Allerest Sinus Pain Formula ... 649
- Axocet Capsules ... 2469
- Benadryl Allergy/Cold Tablets ... 811
- Benadryl Allergy Sinus Headache Caplets ... 813
- Children's TYLENOL acetaminophen Chewable Tablets, Elixir, Suspension Liquid, and Suspension Drops ... 1559
- Children's TYLENOL Cold Multi-Symptom Chewable Tablets and Liquid ... 1559
- Children's TYLENOL Cold Plus Cough Multi Symptom Chewable Tablets and Liquid ... 1560
- Children's TYLENOL Flu Suspension Liquid ... 1560
- Allergy-Sinus Comtrex Multi-Symptom Allergy-Sinus Formula Tablets and Caplets ... 639
- Comtrex Multi-Symptom ... 638
- Comtrex Non-Drowsy ... 640
- Contac Day Allergy/Sinus Caplets ... 771
- Contac Day & Night ... 772
- Contac Night Allergy/Sinus Caplets ... 771
- Contac Severe Cold and Flu Formula Caplets ... 773
- Contac Severe Cold & Flu Non-Drowsy ... 774
- Coricidin Cold + Flu Tablets ... 760
- Coricidin 'D' Decongestant Tablets ... 760
- DHCplus Capsules ... 2148
- Darvon-N/Darvocet-N ... 1473
- Dimetapp Allergy Sinus Caplets ... 838
- Dimetapp Cold & Fever Suspension ... 839
- Drixoral Cold and Flu Extended-Release Tablets ... 764
- Drixoral Cough + Sore Throat Liquid Caps ... 763
- Drixoral Allergy/Sinus Extended Release Tablets ... 765
- Esgic-plus Capsules ... 1012
- Esgic-plus Tablets ... 1012
- Aspirin Free Excedrin Analgesic Caplets and Geltabs ... 734
- Excedrin Extra-Strength Analgesic Tablets, Caplets, and Geltabs ... 734
- Excedrin P.M. Analgesic/Sleeping Aid Tablets, Caplets, Liquigels ... 735
- Fioricet Tablets ... 2386
- Fioricet with Codeine Capsules ... 2387
- Goody's Extra Strength Headache Powders ... 632
- Goody's Extra Strength Pain Relief Tablets ... 632
- Hycomine Compound Tablets ... 948
- Hydrocet Capsules ... 787
- Infants' TYLENOL acetaminophen Suspension Drops ... 1559
- Infants' TYLENOL Cold Decongestant & Fever-Reducer Drops ... 1561
- Junior Strength TYLENOL acetaminophen Coated Caplets and Chewable Tablets ... 1562
- Lorcet 10/650 Tablets ... 1016
- Lortab ... 2751
- Lurline PMS Tablets ... 1000
- Maximum Strength Multi-Symptom Formula Midol ... 621
- PMS Multi-Symptom Formula Midol ... 622
- Maximum Strength Midol Teen Multi-Symptom Formula ... 621
- Midrin Capsules ... 788
- Panodol Tablets and Caplets ... 783
- Children's Panadol Chewable Tablets, Liquid, Infant's Drops ... 783
- Percocet Tablets ... 955
- Percogesic Analgesic Tablets ... 727
- Phrenilin ... 790
- Pyrroxate Caplets ... 742
- Robitussin Cold, Cough & Flu Liqui-Gels ... 844
- Robitussin Night-Time Cold Formula ... 847
- Sedapap Tablets 50 mg/650 mg ... 1826
- Sinarest ... 663
- Sine-Aid Maximum Strength Sinus Headache Gelcaps, Caplets and Tablets ... 1570
- Sine-Off No Drowsiness Formula Caplets ... 784
- Sine-Off Sinus Medicine ... 784
- Singlet Tablets ... 785
- Sinulin Tablets ... 792
- Sinutab Sinus Allergy Medication, Maximum Strength Tablets and Caplets ... 823
- Sinutab Sinus Medication, Maximum Strength Without Drowsiness Formula, Tablets & Caplets ... 824
- Sudafed Cold and Cough Liquid Caps ... 826
- Sudafed Severe Cold Formula Caplets ... 828
- Sudafed Severe Cold Formula Tablets ... 828
- Sudafed Sinus Caplets ... 829
- Sudafed Sinus Tablets ... 829
- Talacen Caplets ... 2464
- TheraFlu Flu and Cold Medicine ... 750
- Theraflu Maximum Strength Flu and Cold Medicine For Sore Throat ... 751
- TheraFlu Flu, Cold and Cough Medicine ... 750
- TheraFlu Maximum Strength Nighttime Flu, Cold & Cough Medicine ... 751
- TheraFlu Maximum Strength Non-Drowsy Formula Flu, Cold & Cough Medicine ... 751
- TheraFlu Maximum Strength, Non-Drowsy Formula Flu, Cold and Cough Caplets ... 752
- Theraflu Maximum Strength Sinus Non-Drowsy Formula Caplets ... 752
- Triaminic Sore Throat Formula ... 755
- Triaminicin Tablets ... 756
- TYLENOL acetaminophen Extended Relief Caplets ... 1570
- TYLENOL acetaminophen, Extra Strength Adult Liquid Pain Reliever ... 1570
- TYLENOL acetaminophen, Extra Strength Gelcaps, Geltabs, Caplets, Tablets ... 1570
- TYLENOL acetaminophen, Regular Strength Caplets and Tablets ... 1570
- TYLENOL Allergy Sinus, Maximum Strength Caplets and Gelcaps ... 1571
- TYLENOL Allergy Sinus NightTime, Maximum Strength Caplets ... 1571
- TYLENOL Cold Medication, Multi-Symptom Formula Tablets and Caplets ... 1572
- TYLENOL Cold Medication, Multi-Symptom Hot Liquid Packets ... 1572
- TYLENOL Cold Medication, No Drowsiness Formula Caplets and Gelcaps ... 1572
- TYLENOL Cold Severe Congestion Caplets ... 1573
- TYLENOL Cough Medication, Multi Symptom ... 1574
- TYLENOL Cough Medication with Decongestant, Multi Symptom ... 1574
- TYLENOL Flu No Drowsiness Formula, Maximum Strength Gelcaps ... 1575
- TYLENOL Flu NightTime, Maximum Strength Gelcaps ... 1575
- TYLENOL Flu NightTime, Maximum Strength Hot Medication Packets ... 1575
- TYLENOL Headache Plus Pain Reliever with Antacid, Extra Strength Caplets ... 705
- TYLENOL PM Pain Reliever/Sleep Aid, Extra Strength Gelcaps, Caplets, Geltabs ... 1576
- TYLENOL Severe Allergy Medication Caplets ... 1571
- TYLENOL Sinus, Maximum Strength Geltabs, Gelcaps, Caplets and Tablets ... 1576
- Tylenol with Codeine ... 1592
- Tylox Capsules ... 1593
- Unisom With Pain Relief-Nighttime Sleep Aid and Pain Reliever ... 1991
- Vanquish Analgesic Caplets ... 627
- Vicks 44 LiquiCaps Cough, Cold & Flu Relief ... 728
- Vicks 44M Cough, Cold & Flu Relief ... 729
- Vicks DayQuil LiquiCaps/Liquid Multi-Symptom Cold/Flu Relief ... 734
- Vicks Nyquil Hot Therapy ... 735
- Vicks NyQuil LiquiCaps/Liquid Multi-Symptom Cold/Flu Relief, Original and Cherry Flavors ... 736
- Vicodin Tablets ... 1404

IMPORTANT NOTE: Always consult each drug listing in the patient's regimen for possible interactions.

Motrin IB — Interactions Index

Vicodin ES Tablets 1405
Vicodin HP Tablets 1403
Wygesic Tablets 2930
Zydone Capsules 967

Aspirin (Concurrent use is not recommended except under a doctor's direction). Products include:
Alka-Seltzer Cherry Effervescent Antacid and Pain Reliever .... ⊡ 609
Alka-Seltzer Extra Strength Effervescent Antacid and Pain Reliever .... ⊡ 609
Alka-Seltzer Lemon Lime Effervescent Antacid and Pain Reliever .... ⊡ 609
Alka-Seltzer Original Effervescent Antacid and Pain Reliever .... ⊡ 609
Alka-Seltzer Plus .... ⊡ 611
Alka-Seltzer Plus Sinus Medicine .. ⊡ 611
Ascriptin .... ⊡ 650
Arthritis Strength BC Powder ..... ⊡ 631
BC Cold Powder Multi-Symptom Formula (Cold-Sinus-Allergy) .... ⊡ 631
BC Cold Powder Non-Drowsy Formula (Cold-Sinus) .... ⊡ 631
BC Powder .... ⊡ 631
Genuine Bayer Aspirin Tablets & Caplets .... ⊡ 618
Extra Strength Bayer Arthritis Pain Regimen Formula .... ⊡ 615
Extra Strength Bayer Aspirin Caplets & Tablets .... ⊡ 617
Extended-Release Bayer 8-Hour Aspirin .... ⊡ 616
Extra Strength Bayer Plus Aspirin Caplets .... ⊡ 617
Extra Strength Bayer PM Aspirin Plus Sleep Aid .... ⊡ 617
Aspirin Regimen Bayer 81 mg Tablets with Calcium .... ⊡ 615
Aspirin Regimen Bayer Adult Low Strength 81 mg Tablets .... ⊡ 613
Aspirin Regimen Bayer Children's Chewable Aspirin .... ⊡ 616
Aspirin Regimen Bayer Regular Strength 325 mg Caplets .... ⊡ 613
Bufferin Analgesic Tablets .... ⊡ 636
Arthritis Strength Bufferin Analgesic Caplets .... ⊡ 637
Extra Strength Bufferin Analgesic Tablets .... ⊡ 637
Cama Arthritis Pain Reliever ..... ⊡ 748
Darvon Compound-65 Pulvules 1475
Easprin 1971
Ecotrin 2625
Ecotrin Enteric Coated Aspirin Maximum Strength Tablets and Caplets .... ⊡ 775
Ecotrin Enteric Coated Aspirin Regular Strength Tablets 2625
Empirin Aspirin Tablets .... ⊡ 818
Excedrin Extra-Strength Analgesic Tablets, Caplets, and Geltabs 734
Fiorinal Capsules 2388
Fiorinal with Codeine Capsules 2390
Fiorinal Tablets 2388
Goody's Extra Strength Headache Powders .... ⊡ 632
Goody's Extra Strength Pain Relief Tablets .... ⊡ 632
Halfprin Tablets 1413
Norgesic 1554
Percodan Tablets 955
Percodan-Demi Tablets 956
Robaxisal Tablets 2246
Soma Compound w/Codeine Tablets 2784
Soma Compound Tablets 2783
St. Joseph Adult Chewable Aspirin (81 mg.) .... ⊡ 768
Talwin Compound 2466
Vanquish Analgesic Caplets .... ⊡ 627

MOTRIN IBUPROFEN SUSPENSION, ORAL DROPS, CHEWABLE TABLETS, CAPLETS
(Ibuprofen) 1563
May interact with oral anticoagulants, ACE inhibitors, thiazides, lithium preparations, and certain other agents. Compounds in these categories include:

Aspirin (Yields a net decrease in anti-inflammatory activity with lowered blood levels of non-aspirin drug in animal studies). Products include:
Alka-Seltzer Cherry Effervescent Antacid and Pain Reliever .... ⊡ 609
Alka-Seltzer Extra Strength Effervescent Antacid and Pain Reliever .... ⊡ 609
Alka-Seltzer Lemon Lime Effervescent Antacid and Pain Reliever .... ⊡ 609
Alka-Seltzer Original Effervescent Antacid and Pain Reliever .... ⊡ 609
Alka-Seltzer Plus .... ⊡ 611
Alka-Seltzer Plus Sinus Medicine .. ⊡ 611
Ascriptin .... ⊡ 650
Arthritis Strength BC Powder ..... ⊡ 631
BC Cold Powder Multi-Symptom Formula (Cold-Sinus-Allergy) .... ⊡ 631
BC Cold Powder Non-Drowsy Formula (Cold-Sinus) .... ⊡ 631
BC Powder .... ⊡ 631
Genuine Bayer Aspirin Tablets & Caplets .... ⊡ 618
Extra Strength Bayer Arthritis Pain Regimen Formula .... ⊡ 615
Extra Strength Bayer Aspirin Caplets & Tablets .... ⊡ 617
Extended-Release Bayer 8-Hour Aspirin .... ⊡ 616
Extra Strength Bayer Plus Aspirin Caplets .... ⊡ 617
Extra Strength Bayer PM Aspirin Plus Sleep Aid .... ⊡ 617
Aspirin Regimen Bayer 81 mg Tablets with Calcium .... ⊡ 615
Aspirin Regimen Bayer Adult Low Strength 81 mg Tablets .... ⊡ 613
Aspirin Regimen Bayer Children's Chewable Aspirin .... ⊡ 616
Aspirin Regimen Bayer Regular Strength 325 mg Caplets .... ⊡ 613
Bufferin Analgesic Tablets .... ⊡ 636
Arthritis Strength Bufferin Analgesic Caplets .... ⊡ 637
Extra Strength Bufferin Analgesic Tablets .... ⊡ 637
Cama Arthritis Pain Reliever ..... ⊡ 748
Darvon Compound-65 Pulvules 1475
Easprin 1971
Ecotrin 2625
Ecotrin Enteric Coated Aspirin Maximum Strength Tablets and Caplets .... ⊡ 775
Ecotrin Enteric Coated Aspirin Regular Strength Tablets 2625
Empirin Aspirin Tablets .... ⊡ 818
Excedrin Extra-Strength Analgesic Tablets, Caplets, and Geltabs 734
Fiorinal Capsules 2388
Fiorinal with Codeine Capsules 2390
Fiorinal Tablets 2388
Goody's Extra Strength Headache Powders .... ⊡ 632
Goody's Extra Strength Pain Relief Tablets .... ⊡ 632
Halfprin Tablets 1413
Norgesic 1554
Percodan Tablets 955
Percodan-Demi Tablets 956
Robaxisal Tablets 2246
Soma Compound w/Codeine Tablets 2784
Soma Compound Tablets 2783
St. Joseph Adult Chewable Aspirin (81 mg.) .... ⊡ 768
Talwin Compound 2466
Vanquish Analgesic Caplets .... ⊡ 627

Benazepril Hydrochloride (Ibuprofen may diminish the antihypertensive effect). Products include:
Lotensin Tablets 852
Lotensin HCT Tablets 855
Lotrel Capsules 858

Bendroflumethiazide (Ibuprofen can reduce the natriuretic effect of thiazide diuretics in some patients).
No products indexed under this heading.

Captopril (Ibuprofen may diminish the antihypertensive effect). Products include:
Capoten Tablets 740
Capozide Tablets 744

Chlorothiazide (Ibuprofen can reduce the natriuretic effect of thiazide diuretics in some patients). Products include:
Aldoclor Tablets 1638
Diupres Tablets 1691
Diuril Oral 1694

Chlorothiazide Sodium (Ibuprofen can reduce the natriuretic effect of thiazide diuretics in some patients). Products include:
Diuril Sodium Intravenous 1693

Dicumarol (Concurrent use may result in bleeding).
No products indexed under this heading.

Enalapril Maleate (Ibuprofen may diminish the antihypertensive effect). Products include:
Vaseretic Tablets 1810
Vasotec Tablets 1816

Enalaprilat (Ibuprofen may diminish the antihypertensive effect). Products include:
Vasotec I.V. 1814

Fosinopril Sodium (Ibuprofen may diminish the antihypertensive effect). Products include:
Monopril Tablets 762

Furosemide (Ibuprofen can reduce the natriuretic effect furosemide). Products include:
Lasix Injection, Oral Solution and Tablets 1267

Hydrochlorothiazide (Ibuprofen can reduce the natriuretic effect of thiazide diuretics in some patients). Products include:
Aldactazide Tablets 2556
Aldoril Tablets 1644
Apresazide Capsules 824
Capozide Tablets 744
Dyazide Capsules 2653
Esidrix Tablets 839
Esimil Tablets 840
HydroDIURIL Tablets 1716
Hydropres Tablets 1718
Hyzaar Tablets 1720
Inderide Tablets 2838
Inderide LA Long Acting Capsules .. 2840
Lopressor HCT Tablets 850
Lotensin HCT Tablets 855
Moduretic Tablets 1748
Oretic Tablets 450
Prinzide Tablets 1780
Ser-Ap-Es Tablets 867
Timolide Tablets 1791
Vaseretic Tablets 1810
Zestoretic Tablets 2968
Ziac 1459

Hydroflumethiazide (Ibuprofen can reduce the natriuretic effect of thiazide diuretics in some patients). Products include:
Diucardin Tablets 2824

Lisinopril (Ibuprofen may diminish the antihypertensive effect). Products include:
Prinivil Tablets 1776
Prinzide Tablets 1780
Zestoretic Tablets 2968
Zestril Tablets 2972

Lithium Carbonate (Ibuprofen can produce an elevation of plasma lithium levels and a reduction in renal lithium clearance). Products include:
Eskalith 2658
Lithium Carbonate Capsules & Tablets 2352
Lithonate/Lithotabs/Lithobid 2721

Lithium Citrate (Ibuprofen can produce an elevation of plasma lithium levels and a reduction in renal lithium clearance).
No products indexed under this heading.

Methotrexate Sodium (Potential for enhanced methotrexate toxicity possibly resulting from competitively inhibiting methotrexate accumulation). Products include:
Methotrexate Sodium Tablets, Injection, for Injection and LPF Injection 1322

Methyclothiazide (Ibuprofen can reduce the natriuretic effect of thiazide diuretics in some patients). Products include:
Enduron Tablets 424

Moexipril Hydrochloride (Ibuprofen may diminish the antihypertensive effect). Products include:
Univasc Tablets 2553

Polythiazide (Ibuprofen can reduce the natriuretic effect of thiazide diuretics in some patients). Products include:
Minizide Capsules 2016

Quinapril Hydrochloride (Ibuprofen may diminish the antihypertensive effect). Products include:
Accupril Tablets 1950

Ramipril (Ibuprofen may diminish the antihypertensive effect). Products include:
Altace Capsules 1238

Spirapril Hydrochloride (Ibuprofen may diminish the antihypertensive effect).
No products indexed under this heading.

Trandolapril (Ibuprofen may diminish the antihypertensive effect). Products include:
Mavik Tablets 1407

Warfarin Sodium (Concurrent use may result in bleeding). Products include:
Coumadin 941

Food Interactions

Food, unspecified (Food affects the rate but not the extent of absorption; T_{max} is delayed by approximately 30 to 60 minutes and peak levels are reduced by approximately 30 to 50%).

MSTA MUMPS SKIN TEST ANTIGEN
(Mumps Skin Test Antigen) 2988
None cited in PDR database.

MUMPSVAX
(Mumps Virus Vaccine, Live) 1751
May interact with immunosuppressive agents. Compounds in this category include:

Azathioprine (Concurrent administration is contraindicated). Products include:
Azathioprine Tablets 2349
Imuran 1103

Cyclosporine (Concurrent administration is contraindicated). Products include:
Neoral 2405
Sandimmune 2416

Immune Globulin (Human) (Concurrent administration is contraindicated).
No products indexed under this heading.

Immune Globulin Intravenous (Human) (Concurrent administration is contraindicated).

Muromonab-CD3 (Concurrent administration is contraindicated). Products include:
Orthoclone OKT3 Sterile Solution .. 1892

Mycophenolate Mofetil (Concurrent administration is contraindicated). Products include:
CellCept Capsules 2265

(⊡ Described in PDR For Nonprescription Drugs)   (⊙ Described in PDR For Ophthalmology)

Interactions Index — Mustargen

Tacrolimus (Concurrent administration is contraindicated). Products include:
  Prograf 1028

MURINE EAR DROPS
(Carbamide Peroxide) 743
None cited in PDR database.

MURINE EAR WAX REMOVAL SYSTEM
(Carbamide Peroxide) 743
None cited in PDR database.

MURINE TEARS LUBRICANT EYE DROPS
(Polyvinyl Alcohol, Povidone) 315
None cited in PDR database.

MURINE TEARS PLUS LUBRICANT REDNESS RELIEVER EYE DROPS
(Polyvinyl Alcohol, Povidone, Tetrahydrozoline Hydrochloride) 315
None cited in PDR database.

MURO 128 OPHTHALMIC OINTMENT
(Sodium Chloride) 256
None cited in PDR database.

MURO 128 SOLUTION 2% AND 5%
(Sodium Chloride) 255
None cited in PDR database.

MUSTARGEN
(Mechlorethamine Hydrochloride) 1752
May interact with antineoplastics. Compounds in this category include:

Altretamine (Hematopoiesis may be further compromised in patients who have been previously treated with chemotherapeutic agents). Products include:
  Hexalen Capsules 2760

Anastrozole (Hematopoiesis may be further compromised in patients who have been previously treated with chemotherapeutic agents). Products include:
  Arimidex Tablets 2932

Asparaginase (Hematopoiesis may be further compromised in patients who have been previously treated with chemotherapeutic agents). Products include:
  Elspar 1700

Bicalutamide (Hematopoiesis may be further compromised in patients who have been previously treated with chemotherapeutic agents). Products include:
  Casodex Tablets 2934

Bleomycin Sulfate (Hematopoiesis may be further compromised in patients who have been previously treated with chemotherapeutic agents). Products include:
  Blenoxane 697

Busulfan (Hematopoiesis may be further compromised in patients who have been previously treated with chemotherapeutic agents). Products include:
  Myleran Tablets 1209

Carboplatin (Hematopoiesis may be further compromised in patients who have been previously treated with chemotherapeutic agents). Products include:
  Paraplatin for Injection 713

Carmustine (BCNU) (Hematopoiesis may be further compromised in patients who have been previously treated with chemotherapeutic agents). Products include:
  BiCNU 696

Chlorambucil (Hematopoiesis may be further compromised in patients who have been previously treated with chemotherapeutic agents). Products include:
  Leukeran Tablets 1205

Cisplatin (Hematopoiesis may be further compromised in patients who have been previously treated with chemotherapeutic agents). Products include:
  Platinol for Injection 717
  Platinol-AQ Injection 719

Cyclophosphamide (Hematopoiesis may be further compromised in patients who have been previously treated with chemotherapeutic agents). Products include:
  Cytoxan 700

Dacarbazine (Hematopoiesis may be further compromised in patients who have been previously treated with chemotherapeutic agents). Products include:
  DTIC-Dome 593

Daunorubicin Citrate (Hematopoiesis may be further compromised in patients who have been previously treated with chemotherapeutic agents). Products include:
  DaunoXome 1842

Daunorubicin Hydrochloride (Hematopoiesis may be further compromised in patients who have been previously treated with chemotherapeutic agents). Products include:
  Cerubidine for Injection 634

Docetaxel (Hematopoiesis may be further compromised in patients who have been previously treated with chemotherapeutic agents). Products include:
  Taxotere for Injection Concentrate 2204

Doxorubicin Hydrochloride (Hematopoiesis may be further compromised in patients who have been previously treated with chemotherapeutic agents). Products include:
  Adriamycin PFS 2056
  Adriamycin RDF 2056
  Doxil 2613
  Doxorubicin Astra 531
  Rubex for Injection 721

Estramustine Phosphate Sodium (Hematopoiesis may be further compromised in patients who have been previously treated with chemotherapeutic agents). Products include:
  Emcyt Capsules 2085

Etoposide (Hematopoiesis may be further compromised in patients who have been previously treated with chemotherapeutic agents). Products include:
  Etoposide Injection 539
  VePesid Capsules and Injection 727

Floxuridine (Hematopoiesis may be further compromised in patients who have been previously treated with chemotherapeutic agents). Products include:
  Sterile FUDR 2284

Fluorouracil (Hematopoiesis may be further compromised in patients who have been previously treated with chemotherapeutic agents). Products include:
  Efudex 2280
  Fluoroplex Topical Solution & Cream 1% 475
  Fluorouracil Injection 2282

Flutamide (Hematopoiesis may be further compromised in patients who have been previously treated with chemotherapeutic agents). Products include:
  Eulexin Capsules 2498

Gemcitabine Hydrochloride (Hematopoiesis may be further compromised in patients who have been previously treated with chemotherapeutic agents). Products include:
  Gemzar for Injection 1482

Hydroxyurea (Hematopoiesis may be further compromised in patients who have been previously treated with chemotherapeutic agents). Products include:
  Hydrea Capsules 705

Idarubicin Hydrochloride (Hematopoiesis may be further compromised in patients who have been previously treated with chemotherapeutic agents). Products include:
  Idamycin Injection 2096

Ifosfamide (Hematopoiesis may be further compromised in patients who have been previously treated with chemotherapeutic agents). Products include:
  IFEX 706

Interferon alfa-2A, Recombinant (Hematopoiesis may be further compromised in patients who have been previously treated with chemotherapeutic agents). Products include:
  Roferon-A Injection 2308

Interferon alfa-2B, Recombinant (Hematopoiesis may be further compromised in patients who have been previously treated with chemotherapeutic agents). Products include:
  Intron A for Injection 2506

Irinotecan Hydrochloride (Hematopoiesis may be further compromised in patients who have been previously treated with chemotherapeutic agents).
  No products indexed under this heading.

Levamisole Hydrochloride (Hematopoiesis may be further compromised in patients who have been previously treated with chemotherapeutic agents). Products include:
  Ergamisol Tablets 1340

Lomustine (CCNU) (Hematopoiesis may be further compromised in patients who have been previously treated with chemotherapeutic agents). Products include:
  CeeNU Capsules 699

Megestrol Acetate (Hematopoiesis may be further compromised in patients who have been previously treated with chemotherapeutic agents). Products include:
  Megace Oral Suspension ... 708
  Megace Tablets 710

Melphalan (Hematopoiesis may be further compromised in patients who have been previously treated with chemotherapeutic agents). Products include:
  Alkeran Tablets 1198

Mercaptopurine (Hematopoiesis may be further compromised in patients who have been previously treated with chemotherapeutic agents). Products include:
  Purinethol Tablets 1214

Methotrexate Sodium (Hematopoiesis may be further compromised in patients who have been previously treated with chemotherapeutic agents). Products include:
  Methotrexate Sodium Tablets, Injection, for Injection and LPF Injection 1322

Mitomycin (Mitomycin-C) (Hematopoiesis may be further compromised in patients who have been previously treated with chemotherapeutic agents). Products include:
  Mutamycin for Injection 712

Mitotane (Hematopoiesis may be further compromised in patients who have been previously treated with chemotherapeutic agents). Products include:
  Lysodren Tablets 707

Mitoxantrone Hydrochloride (Hematopoiesis may be further compromised in patients who have been previously treated with chemotherapeutic agents). Products include:
  Novantrone for Injection 1327

Paclitaxel (Hematopoiesis may be further compromised in patients who have been previously treated with chemotherapeutic agents). Products include:
  Taxol Injection 723

Procarbazine Hydrochloride (Hematopoiesis may be further compromised in patients who have been previously treated with chemotherapeutic agents). Products include:
  Matulane Capsules 2300

Streptozocin (Hematopoiesis may be further compromised in patients who have been previously treated with chemotherapeutic agents). Products include:
  Zanosar Sterile Powder 2119

Tamoxifen Citrate (Hematopoiesis may be further compromised in patients who have been previously treated with chemotherapeutic agents). Products include:
  Nolvadex Tablets 2957

Teniposide (Hematopoiesis may be further compromised in patients who have been previously treated with chemotherapeutic agents). Products include:
  Vumon for Injection 729

Thioguanine (Hematopoiesis may be further compromised in patients who have been previously treated with chemotherapeutic agents). Products include:
  Thioguanine Tablets, Tabloid Brand 1225

Thiotepa (Hematopoiesis may be further compromised in patients who have been previously treated with chemotherapeutic agents). Products include:
  Thioplex (Thiotepa For Injection) 1329

Topotecan Hydrochloride (Hematopoiesis may be further compromised in patients who have been previously treated with chemotherapeutic agents). Products include:
  Hycamtin for Injection 2665

Vincristine Sulfate (Hematopoiesis may be further compromised in patients who have been previously treated with chemotherapeutic agents). Products include:
  Oncovin Solution Vials & Hyporets 1521

Vinorelbine Tartrate (Hematopoiesis may be further compromised in patients who have been previously treated with chemotherapeutic agents). Products include:
  Navelbine Injection 1212

IMPORTANT NOTE: Always consult each drug listing in the patient's regimen for possible interactions.

MUTAMYCIN FOR INJECTION
(Mitomycin (Mitomycin-C)).................. 712
May interact with antineoplastics, cytotoxic drugs, nitrogen-mustard-type alkylating agents, and certain other agents. Compounds in these categories include:

Altretamine (Adult respiratory distress syndrome). Products include:
- Hexalen Capsules 2760

Anastrozole (Adult respiratory distress syndrome). Products include:
- Arimidex Tablets 2932

Asparaginase (Adult respiratory distress syndrome). Products include:
- Elspar 1700

Bicalutamide (Adult respiratory distress syndrome). Products include:
- Casodex Tablets 2934

Bleomycin Sulfate (Hemolytic uremic syndrome; adult respiratory distress syndrome). Products include:
- Blenoxane 697

Busulfan (Adult respiratory distress syndrome). Products include:
- Myleran Tablets 1209

Carboplatin (Adult respiratory distress syndrome). Products include:
- Paraplatin for Injection 713

Carmustine (BCNU) (Adult respiratory distress syndrome). Products include:
- BiCNU 696

Chlorambucil (Adult respiratory distress syndrome). Products include:
- Leukeran Tablets 1205

Cisplatin (Adult respiratory distress syndrome). Products include:
- Platinol for Injection 717
- Platinol-AQ Injection 719

Cyclophosphamide (Adult respiratory distress syndrome). Products include:
- Cytoxan 700

Dacarbazine (Hemolytic uremic syndrome; adult respiratory distress syndrome). Products include:
- DTIC-Dome 593

Daunorubicin Citrate (Adult respiratory distress syndrome). Products include:
- DaunoXome 1842

Daunorubicin Hydrochloride (Hemolytic uremic syndrome; adult respiratory distress syndrome). Products include:
- Cerubidine for Injection 634

Docetaxel (Adult respiratory distress syndrome). Products include:
- Taxotere for Injection Concentrate 2204

Doxorubicin Hydrochloride (Hemolytic uremic syndrome; adult respiratory distress syndrome). Products include:
- Adriamycin PFS 2056
- Adriamycin RDF 2056
- Doxil 2613
- Doxorubicin Astra 531
- Rubex for Injection 721

Estramustine Phosphate Sodium (Adult respiratory distress syndrome). Products include:
- Emcyt Capsules 2085

Etoposide (Adult respiratory distress syndrome). Products include:
- Etoposide Injection 539
- VePesid Capsules and Injection 727

Floxuridine (Adult respiratory distress syndrome). Products include:
- Sterile FUDR 2284

Fluorouracil (Hemolytic uremic syndrome; adult respiratory distress syndrome). Products include:
- Efudex 2280
- Fluoroplex Topical Solution & Cream 1% 475
- Fluorouracil Injection 2282

Flutamide (Adult respiratory distress syndrome). Products include:
- Eulexin Capsules 2498

Gemcitabine Hydrochloride (Adult respiratory distress syndrome). Products include:
- Gemzar for Injection 1482

Hydroxyurea (Hemolytic uremic syndrome; adult respiratory distress syndrome). Products include:
- Hydrea Capsules 705

Idarubicin Hydrochloride (Adult respiratory distress syndrome). Products include:
- Idamycin Injection 2096

Ifosfamide (Adult respiratory distress syndrome). Products include:
- IFEX 706

Interferon alfa-2A, Recombinant (Adult respiratory distress syndrome). Products include:
- Roferon-A Injection 2308

Interferon alfa-2B, Recombinant (Adult respiratory distress syndrome). Products include:
- Intron A for Injection 2506

Irinotecan Hydrochloride (Adult respiratory distress syndrome).
- No products indexed under this heading.

Levamisole Hydrochloride (Adult respiratory distress syndrome). Products include:
- Ergamisol Tablets 1340

Lomustine (CCNU) (Adult respiratory distress syndrome). Products include:
- CeeNU Capsules 699

Mechlorethamine Hydrochloride (Adult respiratory distress syndrome). Products include:
- Mustargen 1752

Megestrol Acetate (Adult respiratory distress syndrome). Products include:
- Megace Oral Suspension 708
- Megace Tablets 710

Melphalan (Adult respiratory distress syndrome). Products include:
- Alkeran Tablets 1198

Mercaptopurine (Adult respiratory distress syndrome). Products include:
- Purinethol Tablets 1214

Methotrexate Sodium (Hemolytic uremic syndrome; adult respiratory distress syndrome). Products include:
- Methotrexate Sodium Tablets, Injection, for Injection and LPF Injection 1322

Mitotane (Hemolytic uremic syndrome; adult respiratory distress syndrome). Products include:
- Lysodren Tablets 707

Mitoxantrone Hydrochloride (Hemolytic uremic syndrome; adult respiratory distress syndrome). Products include:
- Novantrone for Injection 1327

Paclitaxel (Adult respiratory distress syndrome). Products include:
- Taxol Injection 723

Procarbazine Hydrochloride (Hemolytic uremic syndrome; adult respiratory distress syndrome). Products include:
- Matulane Capsules 2300

Streptozocin (Adult respiratory distress syndrome). Products include:
- Zanosar Sterile Powder 2119

Tamoxifen Citrate (Hemolytic uremic syndrome; adult respiratory distress syndrome). Products include:
- Nolvadex Tablets 2957

Teniposide (Adult respiratory distress syndrome). Products include:
- Vumon for Injection 729

Thioguanine (Adult respiratory distress syndrome). Products include:
- Thioguanine Tablets, Tabloid Brand 1225

Thiotepa (Adult respiratory distress syndrome). Products include:
- Thioplex (Thiotepa For Injection) 1329

Topotecan Hydrochloride (Adult respiratory distress syndrome). Products include:
- Hycamtin for Injection 2665

Vinblastine Sulfate (Acute shortness of breath; severe bronchospasm). Products include:
- Velban Vials 1537

Vincristine Sulfate (Hemolytic uremic syndrome; adult respiratory distress syndrome). Products include:
- Oncovin Solution Vials & Hyporets 1521

Vinorelbine Tartrate (Adult respiratory distress syndrome). Products include:
- Navelbine Injection 1212

MYAMBUTOL TABLETS
(Ethambutol Hydrochloride) 1432
None cited in PDR database.

MYCELEX OTC CREAM ANTIFUNGAL
(Clotrimazole) .... ⊡ 622
None cited in PDR database.

MYCELEX TROCHES
(Clotrimazole) 601
None cited in PDR database.

MYCELEX-7 VAGINAL CREAM ANTIFUNGAL
(Clotrimazole) .... ⊡ 622
None cited in PDR database.

MYCELEX-7 VAGINAL ANTIFUNGAL CREAM WITH 7 DISPOSABLE APPLICATORS
(Clotrimazole) .... ⊡ 623
None cited in PDR database.

MYCELEX-7 VAGINAL INSERTS ANTIFUNGAL
(Clotrimazole) .... ⊡ 623
None cited in PDR database.

MYCELEX-7 COMBINATION-PACK VAGINAL INSERTS & EXTERNAL VULVAR CREAM
(Clotrimazole) .... ⊡ 623
None cited in PDR database.

MYCELEX-G 500 MG VAGINAL TABLETS
(Clotrimazole) 602
None cited in PDR database.

MYCITRACIN PLUS PAIN RELIEVER
(Bacitracin Zinc, Neomycin Sulfate, Lidocaine, Polymyxin B Sulfate) .... ⊡ 803
None cited in PDR database.

MAXIMUM STRENGTH MYCITRACIN TRIPLE ANTIBIOTIC FIRST AID OINTMENT
(Bacitracin Zinc, Neomycin Sulfate, Polymyxin B Sulfate) .... ⊡ 803
None cited in PDR database.

MYCOBUTIN CAPSULES
(Rifabutin) 2101
May interact with narcotic analgesics, oral anticoagulants, corticosteroids, oral contraceptives, oral hypoglycemic agents, cardiac glycosides, barbiturates, beta blockers, progestins, xanthine bronchodilators, anticonvulsants, macrolide antibiotics, and certain other agents. Compounds in these categories include:

Acarbose (Potential for reduced activity of oral hypoglycemic agents through liver enzyme-inducing properties). Products include:
- Precose 604

Acebutolol Hydrochloride (Potential for decreased effects of concurrently administered beta-adrenergic blockers). Products include:
- Sectral Capsules 2914

Alfentanil Hydrochloride (Potential for reduced activity of narcotics through liver enzyme-inducing properties). Products include:
- Alfenta Injection 1334

Aminophylline (Potential for decreased effects of concurrently administered theophylline).
- No products indexed under this heading.

Analgesics, unspecified (Potential for reduced activity of analgesics through liver enzyme-inducing properties).
- No products indexed under this heading.

Aprobarbital (Potential for decreased effects of concurrently administered barbiturates).
- No products indexed under this heading.

Atenolol (Potential for decreased effects of concurrently administered beta-adrenergic blockers). Products include:
- Tenoretic Tablets 2963
- Tenormin Tablets and I.V. Injection 2965

Azithromycin (Concomitant administration with higher doses of rifabutin results in higher incidence of uveitis). Products include:
- Zithromax 2043
- Zithromax Tablets 2046

Betamethasone Acetate (Potential for reduced activity of corticosteroids through liver enzyme-inducing properties). Products include:
- Celestone Soluspan Suspension 2484

Betamethasone Sodium Phosphate (Potential for reduced activity of corticosteroids through liver enzyme-inducing properties). Products include:
- Celestone Soluspan Suspension 2484

Betaxolol Hydrochloride (Potential for decreased effects of concurrently administered beta-adrenergic blockers). Products include:
- Betoptic Ophthalmic Solution 465
- Betoptic S Ophthalmic Suspension 467
- Kerlone Tablets 2588

(⊡ Described in PDR For Nonprescription Drugs)　　　　　(⊚ Described in PDR For Ophthalmology)

Bisoprolol Fumarate (Potential for decreased effects of concurrently administered beta-adrenergic blockers). Products include:
- Zebeta Tablets 1457
- Ziac 1459

Buprenorphine (Potential for reduced activity of narcotics through liver enzyme-inducing properties). Products include:
- Buprenex Injectable 2170

Butabarbital (Potential for decreased effects of concurrently administered barbiturates).
No products indexed under this heading.

Butalbital (Potential for decreased effects of concurrently administered barbiturates). Products include:
- Axocet Capsules 2469
- Esgic-plus Capsules 1012
- Esgic-plus Tablets 1012
- Fioricet Tablets 2386
- Fioricet with Codeine Capsules .. 2387
- Fiorinal Capsules 2388
- Fiorinal with Codeine Capsules . 2390
- Fiorinal Tablets 2388
- Phrenilin 790
- Sedapap Tablets 50 mg/650 mg .. 1826

Carbamazepine (Potential for decreased effects of concurrently administered anticonvulsants). Products include:
- Atretol Tablets 569
- Tegretol/Tegretol-XR 870

Carteolol Hydrochloride (Potential for decreased effects of concurrently administered beta-adrenergic blockers). Products include:
- Cartrol Tablets 413
- Ocupress Ophthalmic Solution, 1% Sterile 297

Chloramphenicol (Potential for decreased effects of concurrently administered chloramphenicol). Products include:
- Chloromycetin Ophthalmic Ointment, 1% 298
- Chloromycetin Ophthalmic Solution 299
- Chloroptic S.O.P. 236
- Chloroptic Sterile Ophthalmic Solution 236

Chloramphenicol Palmitate (Potential for decreased effects of concurrently administered chloramphenicol).
No products indexed under this heading.

Chloramphenicol Sodium Succinate (Potential for decreased effects of concurrently administered chloramphenicol). Products include:
- Chloromycetin Sodium Succinate 1960

Chlorpropamide (Potential for reduced activity of oral sulfonylureas through liver enzyme-inducing properties). Products include:
- Diabinese Tablets 2002

Clarithromycin (Concomitant administration with higher doses of rifabutin results in higher incidence of uveitis). Products include:
- Biaxin 406

Clofibrate (Potential for decreased effects of concurrently administered clofibrate). Products include:
- Atromid-S Capsules 2808

Clonazepam (Potential for decreased effects of concurrently administered anticonvulsants). Products include:
- Klonopin Tablets 2294

Codeine Phosphate (Potential for reduced activity of narcotics through liver enzyme-inducing properties). Products include:
- Brontex 2130

- Dimetane-DC Cough Syrup 2232
- Fioricet with Codeine Capsules 2387
- Fiorinal with Codeine Capsules ... 2390
- Nucofed 2225
- Phenergan with Codeine 2883
- Phenergan VC with Codeine 2888
- Robitussin A-C Syrup 2248
- Robitussin-DAC Syrup 2249
- Ryna 804
- Soma Compound w/Codeine Tablets 2784
- Tylenol with Codeine 1592

Cortisone Acetate (Potential for reduced activity of corticosteroids through liver enzyme-inducing properties). Products include:
- Cortone Acetate Sterile Suspension 1663
- Cortone Acetate Tablets 1664

Cyclosporine (Potential for reduced activity of cyclosporine through liver enzyme-inducing properties). Products include:
- Neoral 2405
- Sandimmune 2416

Dapsone (Potential for reduced activity of dapsone through liver enzyme-inducing properties). Products include:
- Dapsone Tablets USP 1331

Deslanoside (Potential for reduced activity of cardiac glycoside agents through liver enzyme-inducing properties).
No products indexed under this heading.

Desogestrel (Potential for reduced activity of oral contraceptives through liver enzyme-inducing properties). Products include:
- Desogen Tablets 1867
- Ortho-Cept 1907

Dexamethasone (Potential for reduced activity of corticosteroids through liver enzyme-inducing properties). Products include:
- AK-Trol Ointment & Suspension 205
- Decadron Elixir 1676
- Decadron Tablets 1678
- Decaspray Topical Aerosol 1689
- Maxitrol Ophthalmic Ointment and Suspension 222
- TobraDex Ophthalmic Suspension and Ointment 469

Dexamethasone Acetate (Potential for reduced activity of corticosteroids through liver enzyme-inducing properties). Products include:
- Dalalone D.P. Injectable 1009
- Decadron-LA Sterile Suspension ... 1687

Dexamethasone Sodium Phosphate (Potential for reduced activity of corticosteroids through liver enzyme-inducing properties). Products include:
- Decadron Phosphate Injection 1680
- Decadron Phosphate Sterile Ophthalmic Ointment 1684
- Decadron Phosphate Sterile Ophthalmic Solution 1685
- Decadron Phosphate Topical Cream 1686
- Decadron Phosphate with Xylocaine Injection, Sterile 1683
- Dexacort Phosphate in Respihaler .. 1606
- Dexacort Phosphate in Turbinaire .. 1607
- NeoDecadron Sterile Ophthalmic Ointment 1755
- NeoDecadron Sterile Ophthalmic Solution 1756
- NeoDecadron Topical Cream 1757

Dezocine (Potential for reduced activity of narcotics through liver enzyme-inducing properties). Products include:
- Dalgan Injection 529

Diazepam (Potential for decreased effects of concurrently administered diazepam). Products include:
- Dizac (diazepam injectable emulsion) CIV 1862

- Valium Injectable 2336
- Valium Tablets 2335

Dicumarol (Potential for reduced activity of anticoagulants through liver enzyme-inducing properties).
No products indexed under this heading.

Digitoxin (Potential for reduced activity of cardiac glycoside agents through liver enzyme-inducing properties). Products include:
- Crystodigin Tablets 1472

Digoxin (Potential for reduced activity of cardiac glycoside agents through liver enzyme-inducing properties). Products include:
- Lanoxicaps 1110
- Lanoxin Elixir Pediatric 1113
- Lanoxin Injection 1116
- Lanoxin Injection Pediatric 1119
- Lanoxin Tablets 1121

Dirithromycin (Concomitant administration with higher doses of rifabutin results in higher incidence of uveitis). Products include:
- Dynabac 668

Disopyramide Phosphate (Potential for decreased effects of concurrently administered mexiletine). Products include:
- Norpace 2596

Divalproex Sodium (Potential for decreased effects of concurrently administered anticonvulsants). Products include:
- Depakote Tablets 418

Dyphylline (Potential for decreased effects of concurrently administered theophylline). Products include:
- Lufyllin & Lufyllin-400 Tablets 2778
- Lufyllin-GG Elixir & Tablets 2779

Erythromycin (Concomitant administration with higher doses of rifabutin results in higher incidence of uveitis). Products include:
- A/T/S 2% Acne Topical Gel 1244
- A/T/S 2% Acne Topical Solution ... 1244
- Benzamycin Topical Gel 919
- E-Mycin Tablets 1388
- Emgel 2% Topical Gel 1081
- ERYC 1972
- Erycette (erythromycin 2%) Topical Solution 1943
- Ery-Tab Tablets 426
- Erythromycin Base Filmtab 430
- Erythromycin Delayed-Release Capsules, USP 431
- Ilotycin Ophthalmic Ointment ... 928
- PCE Dispertab Tablets 453
- T-Stat 2.0% Topical Solution and Pads 2797
- THERAMYCIN Z 2% Solution ... 1629

Erythromycin Estolate (Concomitant administration with higher doses of rifabutin results in higher incidence of uveitis). Products include:
- Ilosone 927

Erythromycin Ethylsuccinate (Concomitant administration with higher doses of rifabutin results in higher incidence of uveitis). Products include:
- E.E.S. 427
- EryPed 425
- Pediazole Suspension 2340

Erythromycin Gluceptate (Concomitant administration with higher doses of rifabutin results in higher incidence of uveitis). Products include:
- Ilotycin Gluceptate, IV, Vials 929

Erythromycin Stearate (Concomitant administration with higher doses of rifabutin results in higher incidence of uveitis). Products include:
- Erythrocin Stearate Filmtab 429

Esmolol Hydrochloride (Potential for decreased effects of concurrently administered beta-adrenergic blockers). Products include:
- Brevibloc (esmolol HCl) Injection 1860

Ethinyl Estradiol (Potential for reduced activity of oral contraceptives through liver enzyme-inducing properties). Products include:
- Brevicon 2563
- Demulen 2580
- Desogen Tablets 1867
- Levlen/Tri-Levlen 646
- Lo/Ovral Tablets 2852
- Lo/Ovral-28 Tablets 2857
- Modicon 1928
- Nordette-21 Tablets 2863
- Nordette-28 Tablets 2866
- Norinyl 2563
- Ortho-Cept 1907
- Ortho-Cyclen/Ortho-Tri-Cyclen ... 1914
- Ortho-Novum 1928
- Ortho-Cyclen/Ortho-Tri-Cyclen ... 1914
- Ovcon 765
- Ovral Tablets 2877
- Ovral-28 Tablets 2878
- Levlen/Tri-Levlen 646
- Tri-Norinyl 2607
- Triphasil-21 Tablets 2919
- Triphasil-28 Tablets 2924

Ethosuximide (Potential for decreased effects of concurrently administered anticonvulsants). Products include:
- Zarontin Capsules 1986
- Zarontin Syrup 1986

Ethotoin (Potential for decreased effects of concurrently administered anticonvulsants). Products include:
- Peganone Tablets 455

Ethynodiol Diacetate (Potential for reduced activity of oral contraceptives through liver enzyme-inducing properties). Products include:
- Demulen 2580

Felbamate (Potential for decreased effects of concurrently administered anticonvulsants). Products include:
- Felbatol 2774

Fentanyl (Potential for reduced activity of narcotics through liver enzyme-inducing properties). Products include:
- Duragesic Transdermal System 1336

Fentanyl Citrate (Potential for reduced activity of narcotics through liver enzyme-inducing properties). Products include:
- Sublimaze Injection 463

Fluconazole (Concomitant administration with higher doses of rifabutin results in higher incidence of uveitis). Products include:
- Diflucan Tablets, Injection, and Oral Suspension 2003

Fludrocortisone Acetate (Potential for reduced activity of corticosteroids through liver enzyme-inducing properties). Products include:
- Florinef Acetate Tablets 506

Fosphenytoin Sodium (Potential for decreased effects of concurrently administered anticonvulsants). Products include:
- Cerebyx Injection 1956

Glimepiride (Potential for reduced activity of oral sulfonylureas through liver enzyme-inducing properties). Products include:
- Amaryl Tablets 1241

Glipizide (Potential for reduced activity of oral sulfonylureas through liver enzyme-inducing properties). Products include:
- Glucotrol Tablets 2011
- Glucotrol XL Extended Release Tablets 2012

IMPORTANT NOTE: Always consult each drug listing in the patient's regimen for possible interactions.

Glyburide (Potential for reduced activity of oral sulfonylureas through liver enzyme-inducing properties). Products include:
- DiaBeta Tablets 1265
- Glynase PresTab Tablets 2091
- Micronase Tablets 2099

Hydrocodone Bitartrate (Potential for reduced activity of narcotics through liver enzyme-inducing properties). Products include:
- Codiclear DH Syrup 808
- Duratuss HD Elixir 2750
- Histussin D Liquid 670
- Hycodan Tablets and Syrup ... 946
- Hycomine Compound Tablets 948
- Hycomine 947
- Hycotuss Expectorant Syrup 950
- Hydrocet Capsules 787
- Lorcet 10/650 Tablets 1016
- Lortab 2751
- Tussend 1830
- Tussend Expectorant 1831
- Vicodin Tablets 1404
- Vicodin ES Tablets 1405
- Vicodin HP Tablets 1403
- Vicodin Tuss Expectorant 1406
- Zydone Capsules 967

Hydrocodone Polistirex (Potential for reduced activity of narcotics through liver enzyme-inducing properties). Products include:
- Tussionex Pennkinetic Extended-Release Suspension 1624

Hydrocortisone (Potential for reduced activity of corticosteroids through liver enzyme-inducing properties). Products include:
- Anusol-HC Cream 2.5% 1953
- Aquanil HC Lotion 1989
- Maximum Strength Cortaid Spray ⊞ 800
- CORTENEMA 2713
- Cortisporin Ointment 1074
- Cortisporin Ophthalmic Ointment Sterile 1074
- Cortisporin Ophthalmic Suspension Sterile 1075
- Cortisporin Otic Solution Sterile 1076
- Cortisporin Otic Suspension Sterile 1077
- Cortizone-5 .... ⊞ 795
- Cortizone-10 .... ⊞ 795
- Hydrocortone Tablets 1715
- Hytone 922
- Hytone Ointment 2 ½% 923
- Massengill Medicated Soft Cloth Towelettes 2628
- Pediotic Suspension Sterile .. 1140
- Preparation H Hydrocortisone 1% Cream .... ⊞ 843
- ProctoCream-HC 2.5% 2552
- VōSoL HC Otic Solution 2786

Hydrocortisone Acetate (Potential for reduced activity of corticosteroids through liver enzyme-inducing properties). Products include:
- Analpram-HC Rectal Cream 1% and 2.5% 993
- Anusol HC-1 Hydrocortisone Anti-Itch Ointment .... ⊞ 810
- Anusol-HC Suppositories ... 1954
- Caldecort Anti-Itch Hydrocortisone Cream .... ⊞ 651
- Coly-Mycin S Otic w/Neomycin & Hydrocortisone 1965
- Cortaid .... ⊞ 800
- Cortifoam 2540
- Cortisporin Cream 1073
- Epifoam 2543
- Hydrocortone Acetate Sterile Suspension 1712
- Mantadil Cream 1124
- Nupercainal Hydrocortisone 1% Cream .... ⊞ 661
- Pramosone Cream, Lotion & Ointment 995
- ProctoFoam-HC 2552
- Terra-Cortril Ophthalmic Suspension 2033

Hydrocortisone Sodium Phosphate (Potential for reduced activity of corticosteroids through liver enzyme-inducing properties). Products include:
- Hydrocortone Phosphate Injection, Sterile 1713

Hydrocortisone Sodium Succinate (Potential for reduced activity of corticosteroids through liver enzyme-inducing properties).
No products indexed under this heading.

Hydromorphone Hydrochloride (Potential for reduced activity of narcotics through liver enzyme-inducing properties). Products include:
- Dilaudid Ampules 1382
- Dilaudid Cough Syrup 1383
- Dilaudid-HP Injection 1384
- Dilaudid-HP Lyophilized Powder 250 mg 1384
- Dilaudid 1382
- Dilaudid Oral Liquid 1386
- Dilaudid 1382
- Dilaudid Tablets - 8 mg 1386

Ketoconazole (Potential for decreased effects of concurrently administered ketoconazole). Products include:
- Nizoral 2% Cream 1344
- Nizoral 2% Shampoo 1344
- Nizoral Tablets 1345

Labetalol Hydrochloride (Potential for decreased effects of concurrently administered beta-adrenergic blockers). Products include:
- Normodyne Injection 2519
- Normodyne Tablets 2522
- Trandate 1158

Lamotrigine (Potential for decreased effects of concurrently administered anticonvulsants). Products include:
- Lamictal Tablets 1105

Levobunolol Hydrochloride (Potential for decreased effects of concurrently administered beta-adrenergic blockers). Products include:
- Betagan .... ⊚ 230

Levonorgestrel (Potential for reduced activity of oral contraceptives through liver enzyme-inducing properties). Products include:
- Levlen/Tri-Levlen 646
- Nordette-21 Tablets 2863
- Nordette-28 Tablets 2866
- Norplant System 2868
- Levlen/Tri-Levlen 646
- Triphasil-21 Tablets 2919
- Triphasil-28 Tablets 2924

Levorphanol Tartrate (Potential for reduced activity of narcotics through liver enzyme-inducing properties). Products include:
- Levo-Dromoran 2297

Medroxyprogesterone Acetate (Potential for decreased effects of concurrently administered progestins). Products include:
- Amen Tablets 785
- Cycrin Tablets 991
- Depo-Provera Contraceptive Injection 2079
- Depo-Provera Sterile Aqueous Suspension 2083
- Premphase 2900
- Prempro 2905
- Provera Tablets 2110

Megestrol Acetate (Potential for decreased effects of concurrently administered progestins). Products include:
- Megace Oral Suspension ... 708
- Megace Tablets 710

Meperidine Hydrochloride (Potential for reduced activity of narcotics through liver enzyme-inducing properties). Products include:
- Demerol 2438
- Mepergan Injection 2859

Mephenytoin (Potential for decreased effects of concurrently administered anticonvulsants). Products include:
- Mesantoin Tablets 2400

Mephobarbital (Potential for decreased effects of concurrently administered barbiturates). Products include:
- Mebaral Tablets 2452

Mestranol (Potential for reduced activity of oral contraceptives through liver enzyme-inducing properties). Products include:
- Norinyl 2563
- Ortho-Novum 1928

Metformin Hydrochloride (Potential for reduced activity of oral hypoglycemic agents through liver enzyme-inducing properties). Products include:
- Glucophage Tablets 754

Methadone Hydrochloride (Potential for reduced activity of methadone—and narcotics—through liver enzyme-inducing properties). Products include:
- Methadone Hydrochloride Oral Concentrate 2356
- Methadone Hydrochloride Oral Solution & Tablets 2357

Methsuximide (Potential for decreased effects of concurrently administered anticonvulsants). Products include:
- Celontin Kapseals 1955

Methylprednisolone Acetate (Potential for reduced activity of corticosteroids through liver enzyme-inducing properties).
No products indexed under this heading.

Methylprednisolone Sodium Succinate (Potential for reduced activity of corticosteroids through liver enzyme-inducing properties).
No products indexed under this heading.

Metipranolol Hydrochloride (Potential for decreased effects of concurrently administered beta-adrenergic blockers). Products include:
- OptiPranolol (Metipranolol 0.3%) Sterile Ophthalmic Solution .... ⊚ 256

Metoprolol Succinate (Potential for decreased effects of concurrently administered beta-adrenergic blockers). Products include:
- Toprol-XL Tablets 560

Metoprolol Tartrate (Potential for decreased effects of concurrently administered beta-adrenergic blockers). Products include:
- Lopressor 848
- Lopressor HCT Tablets 850

Morphine Sulfate (Potential for reduced activity of narcotics through liver enzyme-inducing properties). Products include:
- Astramorph/PF Injection, USP (Preservative-Free) 526
- Duramorph Injection 983
- Infumorph 200 and Infumorph 500 Sterile Solutions 985
- Kadian Capsules 2948
- MS Contin Tablets 2149
- MSIR 2152
- Oramorph SR (Morphine Sulfate Sustained Release Tablets) 2359
- RMS Suppositories CII 2766
- Roxanol 2365

Nadolol (Potential for decreased effects of concurrently administered beta-adrenergic blockers).
No products indexed under this heading.

Norethindrone (Potential for reduced activity of oral contraceptives through liver enzyme-inducing properties). Products include:
- Brevicon 2563
- Micronor Tablets 1903
- Modicon 1928
- Norinyl 2563
- Nor-Q D Tablets 2598
- Ortho-Novum 1928
- Ovcon 765
- Tri-Norinyl 2607

Norethynodrel (Potential for reduced activity of oral contraceptives through liver enzyme-inducing properties).
No products indexed under this heading.

Norgestimate (Potential for reduced activity of oral contraceptives through liver enzyme-inducing properties). Products include:
- Ortho-Cyclen/Ortho Tri-Cyclen .. 1914
- Ortho-Cyclen/Ortho Tri-Cyclen .. 1914

Norgestrel (Potential for reduced activity of oral contraceptives through liver enzyme-inducing properties). Products include:
- Lo/Ovral Tablets 2852
- Lo/Ovral-28 Tablets 2857
- Ovral Tablets 2877
- Ovral-28 Tablets 2878
- Ovrette Tablets 2878

Opium Alkaloids (Potential for reduced activity of narcotics through liver enzyme-inducing properties).
No products indexed under this heading.

Oxycodone Hydrochloride (Potential for reduced activity of narcotics through liver enzyme-inducing properties). Products include:
- OxyContin Tablets 2163
- OxyIR Capsules 2167
- Percocet Tablets 955
- Percodan Tablets 955
- Percodan-Demi Tablets 956
- Roxicodone Tablets, Oral Solution & Intensol (Oxycodone) 2366
- Tylox Capsules 1593

Paramethadione (Potential for decreased effects of concurrently administered anticonvulsants).
No products indexed under this heading.

Penbutolol Sulfate (Potential for decreased effects of concurrently administered beta-adrenergic blockers). Products include:
- Levatol Tablets 2547

Pentobarbital Sodium (Potential for decreased effects of concurrently administered barbiturates). Products include:
- Nembutal Sodium Capsules .. 440
- Nembutal Sodium Solution .. 442
- Nembutal Sodium Suppositories .. 444

Phenacemide (Potential for decreased effects of concurrently administered anticonvulsants). Products include:
- Phenurone Tablets 455

Phenobarbital (Potential for decreased effects of concurrently administered anticonvulsants and barbiturates). Products include:
- Arco-Lase Plus Tablets 513
- Bellergal-S Tablets 2375
- Donnatal 2234
- Donnatal Extentabs 2234
- Donnatal Tablets 2234
- Phenobarbital Elixir and Tablets .. 1523
- Quadrinal Tablets 1398

Phensuximide (Potential for decreased effects of concurrently administered anticonvulsants).
No products indexed under this heading.

Phenytoin (Potential for decreased effects of concurrently administered anticonvulsants). Products include:
- Dilantin Infatabs 1967
- Dilantin-125 Suspension ... 1969

Phenytoin Sodium (Potential for decreased effects of concurrently administered anticonvulsants). Products include:
- Dilantin Kapseals 1965

Pindolol (Potential for decreased effects of concurrently administered beta-adrenergic blockers). Products include:
- Visken Tablets 2428

Prednisolone Acetate (Potential for reduced activity of corticosteroids through liver enzyme-inducing properties). Products include:
- AK-CIDE .... ⓢ 203
- AK-CIDE Ointment .... ⓢ 203
- Blephamide Liquifilm Sterile Ophthalmic Suspension 472
- Blephamide Ointment .... ⓢ 234
- Econopred & Econopred Plus Ophthalmic Suspensions .... ⓢ 216
- Poly-Pred Liquifilm .... ⓢ 246
- Pred Forte .... ⓢ 247
- Pred Mild .... ⓢ 250
- Pred-G Liquifilm Sterile Ophthalmic Suspension .... ⓢ 248
- Pred-G S.O.P. Sterile Ophthalmic Ointment .... ⓢ 249

Prednisolone Sodium Phosphate (Potential for reduced activity of corticosteroids through liver enzyme-inducing properties). Products include:
- AK-PRED .... ⓢ 204
- Hydeltrasol Injection, Sterile 1708
- Pediapred Oral Solution 1618

Prednisolone Tebutate (Potential for reduced activity of corticosteroids through liver enzyme-inducing properties). Products include:
- Hydeltra-T.B.A. Sterile Suspension 1710

Prednisone (Potential for reduced activity of corticosteroids through liver enzyme-inducing properties).
No products indexed under this heading.

Primidone (Potential for decreased effects of concurrently administered anticonvulsants). Products include:
- Mysoline 2860

Propoxyphene Hydrochloride (Potential for reduced activity of narcotics through liver enzyme-inducing properties). Products include:
- Darvon 1475
- Wygesic Tablets 2930

Propoxyphene Napsylate (Potential for reduced activity of narcotics through liver enzyme-inducing properties). Products include:
- Darvon-N/Darvocet-N 1473

Propranolol Hydrochloride (Potential for decreased effects of concurrently administered beta-adrenergic blockers). Products include:
- Inderal 2834
- Inderal LA Long Acting Capsules 2836
- Inderide Tablets 2838
- Inderide LA Long Acting Capsules 2840

Quinidine Gluconate (Potential for reduced activity of quinidine through liver enzyme-inducing properties). Products include:
- Quinaglute Dura-Tabs Tablets 644

Quinidine Polygalacturonate (Potential for reduced activity of quinidine through liver enzyme-inducing properties). Products include:
- Cardioquin Tablets 2146

Quinidine Sulfate (Potential for reduced activity of quinidine through liver enzyme-inducing properties). Products include:
- Quinidex Extentabs 2240

Secobarbital Sodium (Potential for decreased effects of concurrently administered barbiturates). Products include:
- Seconal Sodium Pulvules 1529

Sotalol Hydrochloride (Potential for decreased effects of concurrently administered beta-adrenergic blockers). Products include:
- Betapace Tablets 637

Sufentanil Citrate (Potential for reduced activity of narcotics through liver enzyme-inducing properties). Products include:
- Sufenta Injection 1355

Theophylline (Potential for decreased effects of concurrently administered theophylline). Products include:
- Marax Tablets & DF Syrup 2015
- Quibron 2227

Theophylline Anhydrous (Potential for decreased effects of concurrently administered theophylline). Products include:
- Aerolate 1003
- Primatene Tablets .... ⓢ 844
- Respbid Tablets 687
- Slo-bid Gyrocaps 2201
- Theo-24 Extended Release Capsules 2753
- Theo-Dur Extended-Release Tablets 1367
- Theo-X Extended-Release Tablets 793
- Uni-Dur Extended-Release Tablets 1374
- Uniphyl 400 mg and 600 mg Tablets 2157

Theophylline Calcium Salicylate (Potential for decreased effects of concurrently administered theophylline). Products include:
- Quadrinal Tablets 1398

Theophylline Sodium Glycinate (Potential for decreased effects of concurrently administered theophylline).
No products indexed under this heading.

Thiamylal Sodium (Potential for decreased effects of concurrently administered barbiturates).
No products indexed under this heading.

Timolol Hemihydrate (Potential for decreased effects of concurrently administered beta-adrenergic blockers). Products include:
- Betimol 0.25%, 0.5% .... ⓢ 259

Timolol Maleate (Potential for decreased effects of concurrently administered beta-adrenergic blockers). Products include:
- Blocadren Tablets 1654
- Timolide Tablets 1791
- Timoptic in Ocudose 1796
- Timoptic Sterile Ophthalmic Solution 1794
- Timoptic-XE 1798

Tolazamide (Potential for reduced activity of oral sulfonylureas through liver enzyme-inducing properties).
No products indexed under this heading.

Tolbutamide (Potential for reduced activity of oral sulfonylureas through liver enzyme-inducing properties).
No products indexed under this heading.

Triamcinolone (Potential for reduced activity of corticosteroids through liver enzyme-inducing properties).
No products indexed under this heading.

Triamcinolone Acetonide (Potential for reduced activity of corticosteroids through liver enzyme-inducing properties). Products include:
- Azmacort Oral Inhaler 2175
- Nasacort AQ Nasal Spray 2191
- Nasacort Nasal Inhaler 2189

Triamcinolone Diacetate (Potential for reduced activity of corticosteroids through liver enzyme-inducing properties).
No products indexed under this heading.

Triamcinolone Hexacetonide (Potential for reduced activity of corticosteroids through liver enzyme-inducing properties).
No products indexed under this heading.

Trimethadione (Potential for decreased effects of concurrently administered anticonvulsants).
No products indexed under this heading.

Troleandomycin (Concomitant administration with higher doses of rifabutin results in higher incidence of uveitis). Products include:
- Tao Capsules 2033

Valproic Acid (Potential for decreased effects of concurrently administered anticonvulsants). Products include:
- Depakene 416

Verapamil Hydrochloride (Potential for decreased effects of concurrently administered verapamil). Products include:
- Calan SR Caplets 2571
- Calan Tablets 2568
- Covera-HS Tablets 2573
- Isoptin Injectable 1391
- Isoptin Oral Tablets 1393
- Isoptin SR Tablets 1395
- Verelan Capsules 1455

Warfarin Sodium (Potential for reduced activity of anticoagulants through liver enzyme-inducing properties). Products include:
- Coumadin 941

Zidovudine (Reduced steady-state plasma levels of zidovudine after repeated Mycobutin dosing). Products include:
- Retrovir Capsules 1216
- Retrovir I.V. Infusion 1221
- Retrovir Syrup 1216

Food Interactions

Diet, high-lipid (High-fat meals slow the rate without influencing the extent of absorption from the capsule dosage form).

MYCOSTATIN CREAM & TOPICAL POWDER
(Nystatin) 2797
None cited in PDR database.

MYCOSTATIN PASTILLES
(Nystatin) 713
None cited in PDR database.

MYKROX TABLETS
(Metolazone) 1617
May interact with lithium preparations, antihypertensives, insulin, barbiturates, narcotic analgesics, loop diuretics, cardiac glycosides, corticosteroids, salicylates, non-steroidal anti-inflammatory agents, oral hypoglycemic agents, and certain other agents. Compounds in these categories include:

Acarbose (Blood glucose concentrations may be raised by metolazone in diabetics). Products include:
- Precose 604

Acebutolol Hydrochloride (Orthostatic hypotension may occur with concurrent therapy). Products include:
- Sectral Capsules 2914

ACTH (Potential for increased hypokalemia).
No products indexed under this heading.

Alfentanil Hydrochloride (Potentiates orthostatic hypotensive effects). Products include:
- Alfenta Injection 1334

Amlodipine Besylate (Orthostatic hypotension may occur with concurrent therapy). Products include:
- Lotrel Capsules 858
- Norvasc Tablets 2020

Aprobarbital (Potentiates orthostatic hypotensive effects).
No products indexed under this heading.

Aspirin (Antihypertensive effects of Mykrox may be decreased). Products include:
- Alka-Seltzer Cherry Effervescent Antacid and Pain Reliever .... ⓢ 609
- Alka-Seltzer Extra Strength Effervescent Antacid and Pain Reliever .... ⓢ 609
- Alka-Seltzer Lemon Lime Effervescent Antacid and Pain Reliever .... ⓢ 609
- Alka-Seltzer Original Effervescent Antacid and Pain Reliever .... ⓢ 609
- Alka-Seltzer Plus .... ⓢ 611
- Alka-Seltzer Plus Sinus Medicine .... ⓢ 611
- Ascriptin 650
- Arthritis Strength BC Powder .... ⓢ 631
- BC Cold Powder Multi-Symptom Formula (Cold-Sinus-Allergy) ..... ⓢ 631
- BC Cold Powder Non-Drowsy Formula (Cold-Sinus) .... ⓢ 631
- BC Powder .... ⓢ 631
- Genuine Bayer Aspirin Tablets & Caplets .... ⓢ 618
- Extra Strength Bayer Arthritis Pain Regimen Formula .... ⓢ 615
- Extra Strength Bayer Aspirin Caplets & Tablets .... ⓢ 617
- Extended-Release Bayer 8-Hour Aspirin .... ⓢ 616
- Extra Strength Bayer Plus Aspirin Caplets .... ⓢ 617
- Extra Strength Bayer PM Aspirin Plus Sleep Aid .... ⓢ 617
- Aspirin Regimen Bayer 81 mg Tablets with Calcium .... ⓢ 615
- Aspirin Regimen Bayer Adult Low Strength 81 mg Tablets .... ⓢ 613
- Aspirin Regimen Bayer Children's Chewable Aspirin .... ⓢ 616
- Aspirin Regimen Bayer Regular Strength 325 mg Caplets .... ⓢ 613
- Bufferin Analgesic Tablets .... ⓢ 636
- Arthritis Strength Bufferin Analgesic Caplets .... ⓢ 637
- Extra Strength Bufferin Analgesic Tablets .... ⓢ 637
- Cama Arthritis Pain Reliever 748
- Darvon Compound-65 Pulvules 1475
- Easprin 1971
- Ecotrin 2625
- Ecotrin Enteric Coated Aspirin Maximum Strength Tablets and Caplets .... ⓢ 775
- Ecotrin Enteric Coated Aspirin Regular Strength Tablets 2625
- Empirin Aspirin Tablets .... ⓢ 818
- Excedrin Extra-Strength Analgesic Tablets, Caplets, and Geltabs 734
- Fiorinal Capsules 2388
- Fiorinal with Codeine Capsules 2390
- Fiorinal Tablets 2388
- Goody's Extra Strength Headache Powders .... ⓢ 632
- Goody's Extra Strength Pain Relief Tablets .... ⓢ 632
- Halfprin Tablets 1413
- Norgesic 1554
- Percodan Tablets 955
- Percodan-Demi Tablets 956
- Robaxisal Tablets 2246
- Soma Compound w/Codeine Tablets 2784
- Soma Compound Tablets 2783
- St. Joseph Adult Chewable Aspirin (81 mg.) .... ⓢ 768
- Talwin Compound 2466
- Vanquish Analgesic Caplets .... ⓢ 627

Atenolol (Orthostatic hypotension may occur with concurrent therapy). Products include:
- Tenoretic Tablets 2963
- Tenormin Tablets and I.V. Injection 2965

Benazepril Hydrochloride (Orthostatic hypotension may occur with concurrent therapy). Products include:
- Lotensin Tablets 852

IMPORTANT NOTE: Always consult each drug listing in the patient's regimen for possible interactions.

Mykrox **Interactions Index** **708**

Lotensin HCT Tablets 855
Lotrel Capsules 858

Bendroflumethiazide (Orthostatic hypotension may occur with concurrent therapy).
No products indexed under this heading.

Betamethasone Acetate (Potential for increased hypokalemia). Products include:
Celestone Soluspan Suspension 2484

Betamethasone Sodium Phosphate (Potential for increased hypokalemia). Products include:
Celestone Soluspan Suspension 2484

Betaxolol Hydrochloride (Orthostatic hypotension may occur with concurrent therapy). Products include:
Betoptic Ophthalmic Solution........ 465
Betoptic S Ophthalmic Suspension 467
Kerlone Tablets........ 2588

Bisoprolol Fumarate (Orthostatic hypotension may occur with concurrent therapy). Products include:
Zebeta Tablets 1457
Ziac 1459

Bumetanide (Large or prolonged losses of fluids and electrolytes may result). Products include:
Bumex 2260

Buprenorphine (Potentiates orthostatic hypotensive effects). Products include:
Buprenex Injectable 2170

Butabarbital (Potentiates orthostatic hypotensive effects).
No products indexed under this heading.

Butalbital (Potentiates orthostatic hypotensive effects). Products include:
Axocet Capsules........ 2469
Esgic-plus Capsules 1012
Esgic-plus Tablets 1012
Fioricet Tablets........ 2386
Fioricet with Codeine Capsules 2387
Fiorinal Capsules 2388
Fiorinal with Codeine Capsules 2390
Fiorinal Tablets........ 2388
Phrenilin 790
Sedapap Tablets 50 mg/650 mg .. 1826

Captopril (Orthostatic hypotension may occur with concurrent therapy). Products include:
Capoten Tablets 740
Capozide Tablets 744

Carteolol Hydrochloride (Orthostatic hypotension may occur with concurrent therapy). Products include:
Cartrol Tablets 413
Ocupress Ophthalmic Solution, 1% Sterile........ ⊚ 297

Chlorothiazide (Orthostatic hypotension may occur with concurrent therapy). Products include:
Aldoclor Tablets 1638
Diupres Tablets 1691
Diuril Oral 1694

Chlorothiazide Sodium (Orthostatic hypotension may occur with concurrent therapy). Products include:
Diuril Sodium Intravenous 1693

Chlorpropamide (Blood glucose concentrations may be raised by metolazone in diabetics). Products include:
Diabinese Tablets 2002

Chlorthalidone (Orthostatic hypotension may occur with concurrent therapy). Products include:
Combipres Tablets 682
Tenoretic Tablets........ 2963
Thalitone 1293

Choline Magnesium Trisalicylate (Antihypertensive effects of Mykrox may be decreased). Products include:
Trilisate 2155

Clonidine (Orthostatic hypotension may occur with concurrent therapy). Products include:
Catapres-TTS........ 680

Clonidine Hydrochloride (Orthostatic hypotension may occur with concurrent therapy). Products include:
Catapres Tablets 679
Combipres Tablets 682

Codeine Phosphate (Potentiates orthostatic hypotensive effects). Products include:
Brontex 2130
Dimetane-DC Cough Syrup 2232
Fioricet with Codeine Capsules 2387
Fiorinal with Codeine Capsules 2390
Nucofed 2225
Phenergan with Codeine........ 2883
Phenergan VC with Codeine 2888
Robitussin A-C Syrup........ 2248
Robitussin-DAC Syrup........ 2249
Ryna .... ▣ 804
Soma Compound w/Codeine Tablets 2784
Tylenol with Codeine 1592

Cortisone Acetate (Potential for increased hypokalemia). Products include:
Cortone Acetate Sterile Suspension 1663
Cortone Acetate Tablets........ 1664

Deserpidine (Orthostatic hypotension may occur with concurrent therapy).
No products indexed under this heading.

Deslanoside (Hypokalemia increases sensitivity of the myocardium to digitalis toxicity).
No products indexed under this heading.

Dexamethasone (Potential for increased hypokalemia). Products include:
AK-Trol Ointment & Suspension .... ⊚ 205
Decadron Elixir 1676
Decadron Tablets........ 1678
Decaspray Topical Aerosol 1689
Maxitrol Ophthalmic Ointment and Suspension .... ⊚ 222
TobraDex Ophthalmic Suspension and Ointment........ 469

Dexamethasone Acetate (Potential for increased hypokalemia). Products include:
Dalalone D.P. Injectable 1009
Decadron-LA Sterile Suspension...... 1687

Dexamethasone Sodium Phosphate (Potential for increased hypokalemia). Products include:
Decadron Phosphate Injection 1680
Decadron Phosphate Sterile Ophthalmic Ointment........ 1684
Decadron Phosphate Sterile Ophthalmic Solution 1685
Decadron Phosphate Topical Cream........ 1686
Decadron Phosphate with Xylocaine Injection, Sterile 1683
Dexacort Phosphate in Respihaler .. 1606
Dexacort Phosphate in Turbinaire .. 1607
NeoDecadron Sterile Ophthalmic Ointment 1755
NeoDecadron Sterile Ophthalmic Solution 1756
NeoDecadron Topical Cream 1757

Dezocine (Potentiates orthostatic hypotensive effects). Products include:
Dalgan Injection 529

Diazoxide (Orthostatic hypotension may occur with concurrent therapy). Products include:
Hyperstat I.V. Injection 2504
Proglycem........ 575

Diclofenac Potassium (Antihypertensive effects of Mykrox may be decreased). Products include:
Cataflam Tablets 833

Diclofenac Sodium (Antihypertensive effects of Mykrox may be decreased). Products include:
Voltaren Ophthalmic Sterile Ophthalmic Solution .... ⊚ 264
Cataflam/Voltaren/Voltaren-XR 833

Dicumarol (May affect the hypoprothrombinemic response to anticoagulants; dosage adjustments may be necessary).
No products indexed under this heading.

Diflunisal (Antihypertensive effects of Mykrox may be decreased). Products include:
Dolobid Tablets........ 1695

Digitoxin (Hypokalemia increases sensitivity of the myocardium to digitalis toxicity). Products include:
Crystodigin Tablets........ 1472

Digoxin (Hypokalemia increases sensitivity of the myocardium to digitalis toxicity). Products include:
Lanoxicaps 1110
Lanoxin Elixir Pediatric 1113
Lanoxin Injection 1116
Lanoxin Injection Pediatric........ 1119
Lanoxin Tablets 1121

Diltiazem Hydrochloride (Orthostatic hypotension may occur with concurrent therapy). Products include:
Cardizem CD Capsules 1251
Cardizem SR Capsules 1255
Cardizem Injectable 1253
Cardizem Tablets........ 1257
Dilacor XR Extended-release Capsules 2183
Tiazac Capsules 1019

Doxazosin Mesylate (Orthostatic hypotension may occur with concurrent therapy). Products include:
Cardura Tablets 1993

Enalapril Maleate (Orthostatic hypotension may occur with concurrent therapy). Products include:
Vaseretic Tablets 1810
Vasotec Tablets 1816

Enalaprilat (Orthostatic hypotension may occur with concurrent therapy). Products include:
Vasotec I.V........ 1814

Esmolol Hydrochloride (Orthostatic hypotension may occur with concurrent therapy). Products include:
Brevibloc (esmolol HCl) Injection 1860

Ethacrynic Acid (Large or prolonged losses of fluids and electrolytes may result). Products include:
Edecrin Tablets........ 1698

Etodolac (Antihypertensive effects of Mykrox may be decreased). Products include:
Lodine Capsules and Tablets 2849

Felodipine (Orthostatic hypotension may occur with concurrent therapy). Products include:
Plendil Extended-Release Tablets.... 514

Fenoprofen Calcium (Antihypertensive effects of Mykrox may be decreased). Products include:
Nalfon 200 Pulvules & Nalfon Tablets 933

Fentanyl (Potentiates orthostatic hypotensive effects). Products include:
Duragesic Transdermal System........ 1336

Fentanyl Citrate (Potentiates orthostatic hypotensive effects). Products include:
Sublimaze Injection........ 463

Fludrocortisone Acetate (Potential for increased hypokalemia). Products include:
Florinef Acetate Tablets 506

Flurbiprofen (Antihypertensive effects of Mykrox may be decreased).
No products indexed under this heading.

Fosinopril Sodium (Orthostatic hypotension may occur with concurrent therapy). Products include:
Monopril Tablets 762

Furosemide (Large or prolonged losses of fluids and electrolytes may result; orthostatic hypotension may occur with concurrent therapy). Products include:
Lasix Injection, Oral Solution and Tablets 1267

Glimepiride (Blood glucose concentrations may be raised by metolazone in diabetics). Products include:
Amaryl Tablets 1241

Glipizide (Blood glucose concentrations may be raised by metolazone in diabetics). Products include:
Glucotrol Tablets 2011
Glucotrol XL Extended Release Tablets 2012

Glyburide (Blood glucose concentrations may be raised by metolazone in diabetics). Products include:
DiaBeta Tablets 1265
Glynase PresTab Tablets 2091
Micronase Tablets........ 2099

Guanabenz Acetate (Orthostatic hypotension may occur with concurrent therapy).
No products indexed under this heading.

Guanethidine Monosulfate (Orthostatic hypotension may occur with concurrent therapy). Products include:
Esimil Tablets 840
Ismelin Tablets 845

Hydralazine Hydrochloride (Orthostatic hypotension may occur with concurrent therapy). Products include:
Apresazide Capsules 824
Apresoline Hydrochloride Tablets .. 826
Hydralazine Hydrochloride Injection USP........ 2712
Ser-Ap-Es Tablets 867

Hydrochlorothiazide (Orthostatic hypotension may occur with concurrent therapy). Products include:
Aldactazide Tablets 2556
Aldoril Tablets........ 1644
Apresazide Capsules 824
Capozide Tablets 744
Dyazide Capsules........ 2653
Esidrix Tablets 839
Esimil Tablets 840
HydroDIURIL Tablets 1716
Hydropres Tablets........ 1718
Hyzaar Tablets 1720
Inderide Tablets 2838
Inderide LA Long Acting Capsules .. 2840
Lopressor HCT Tablets 850
Lotensin HCT Tablets 855
Moduretic Tablets 1748
Oretic Tablets 450
Prinzide Tablets 1780
Ser-Ap-Es Tablets 867
Timolide Tablets........ 1791
Vaseretic Tablets 1810
Zestoretic Tablets 2968
Ziac 1459

Hydrocodone Bitartrate (Potentiates orthostatic hypotensive effects). Products include:
Codiclear DH Syrup 808
Duratuss HD Elixir........ 2750
Histussin D Liquid 670
Hycodan Tablets and Syrup 946
Hycomine Compound Tablets 948
Hycomine 947
Hycotuss Expectorant Syrup 950
Hydrocet Capsules 787

(▣ Described in PDR For Nonprescription Drugs) (⊚ Described in PDR For Ophthalmology)

Lorcet 10/650 Tablets	1016		
Lortab	2751		
Tussend	1830		
Tussend Expectorant	1831		
Vicodin Tablets	1404		
Vicodin ES Tablets	1405		
Vicodin HP Tablets	1403		
Vicodin Tuss Expectorant	1406		
Zydone Capsules	967		

Hydrocodone Polistirex (Potentiates orthostatic hypotensive effects). Products include:

Tussionex Pennkinetic Extended-Release Suspension	1624

Hydrocortisone (Potential for increased hypokalemia). Products include:

Anusol-HC Cream 2.5%	1953
Aquanil HC Lotion	1989
Maximum Strength Cortaid Spray	800
CORTENEMA	2713
Cortisporin Ointment	1074
Cortisporin Ophthalmic Ointment Sterile	1074
Cortisporin Ophthalmic Suspension Sterile	1075
Cortisporin Otic Solution Sterile	1076
Cortisporin Otic Suspension Sterile	1077
Cortizone-5	795
Cortizone-10	795
Hydrocortone Tablets	1715
Hytone	922
Hytone Ointment 2 ½ %	923
Massengill Medicated Soft Cloth Towelettes	2628
Pediotic Suspension Sterile	1140
Preparation H Hydrocortisone 1% Cream	843
ProctoCream-HC 2.5%	2552
VōSoL HC Otic Solution	2786

Hydrocortisone Acetate (Potential for increased hypokalemia). Products include:

Analpram-HC Rectal Cream 1% and 2.5%	993
Anusol HC-1 Hydrocortisone Anti-Itch Ointment	810
Anusol-HC Suppositories	1954
Caldecort Anti-Itch Hydrocortisone Cream	651
Coly-Mycin S Otic w/Neomycin & Hydrocortisone	1965
Cortaid	800
Cortifoam	2540
Cortisporin Cream	1073
Epifoam	2543
Hydrocortone Acetate Sterile Suspension	1712
Mantadil Cream	1124
Nupercainal Hydrocortisone 1% Cream	661
Pramosone Cream, Lotion & Ointment	995
ProctoFoam-HC	2552
Terra-Cortril Ophthalmic Suspension	2033

Hydrocortisone Sodium Phosphate (Potential for increased hypokalemia). Products include:

Hydrocortone Phosphate Injection, Sterile	1713

Hydrocortisone Sodium Succinate (Potential for increased hypokalemia).

No products indexed under this heading.

Hydroflumethiazide (Orthostatic hypotension may occur with concurrent therapy). Products include:

Diucardin Tablets	2824

Hydromorphone Hydrochloride (Potentiates orthostatic hypotensive effects). Products include:

Dilaudid Ampules	1382
Dilaudid Cough Syrup	1383
Dilaudid-HP Injection	1384
Dilaudid-HP Lyophilized Powder 250 mg	1384
Dilaudid	1382
Dilaudid Oral Liquid	1386
Dilaudid	1382
Dilaudid Tablets - 8 mg	1386

Ibuprofen (Antihypertensive effects of Mykrox may be decreased). Products include:

Advil Cold and Sinus Caplets and Tablets	837
Advil Ibuprofen Tablets, Caplets and Gel Caplets	836
Children's Motrin Ibuprofen Oral Suspension	1558
IBU Tablets	1389
Ibuprohm	713
Motrin IB Caplets, Tablets, and Gelcaps	802
Motrin Ibuprofen Suspension, Oral Drops, Chewable Tablets, Caplets	1563
Nuprin Ibuprofen/Analgesic Tablets & Caplets	645
Vicks DayQuil SINUS Pressure & PAIN Relief with IBUPROFEN	735

Indapamide (Orthostatic hypotension may occur with concurrent therapy).

No products indexed under this heading.

Indomethacin (Antihypertensive effects of Mykrox may be decreased). Products include:

Indocin	1723

Indomethacin Sodium Trihydrate (Antihypertensive effects of Mykrox may be decreased). Products include:

Indocin I.V.	1727

Insulin, Human (Blood glucose concentrations may be raised by metolazone in diabetics).

No products indexed under this heading.

Insulin, Human Isophane Suspension (Blood glucose concentrations may be raised by metolazone in diabetics). Products include:

Novolin N Human Insulin 10 ml Vials	1846

Insulin, Human NPH (Blood glucose concentrations may be raised by metolazone in diabetics). Products include:

Humulin N, 100 Units	1495
Novolin N PenFill 1.5 ml Cartridges Durable Insulin Delivery System	1849
Novolin N Prefilled Syringe Disposable Insulin Delivery System	1850

Insulin, Human Regular (Blood glucose concentrations may be raised by metolazone in diabetics). Products include:

Humulin R, 100 Units	1497
Novolin R Human Insulin 10 ml Vials	1846
Novolin R PenFill 1.5 ml Cartridges Durable Insulin Delivery System	1849
Novolin R Prefilled Syringe Disposable Insulin Delivery System	1850
Velosulin BR Human Insulin 10 ml Vials	1847

Insulin, Human, Zinc Suspension (Blood glucose concentrations may be raised by metolazone in diabetics). Products include:

Humulin L, 100 Units	1494
Humulin U, 100 Units	1498
Novolin L Human Insulin 10 ml Vials	1846

Insulin Lispro, Human (Blood glucose concentrations may be raised by metolazone in diabetics). Products include:

Humalog Injection	1488

Insulin, NPH (Blood glucose concentrations may be raised by metolazone in diabetics). Products include:

NPH, 100 Units	1502
Pork NPH, 100 Units	1506
Purified Pork NPH Isophane Insulin	1852

Insulin, Regular (Blood glucose concentrations may be raised by metolazone in diabetics). Products include:

Regular, 100 Units	1503
Pork Regular, 100 Units	1507
Pork Regular (Concentrated), 500 Units	1508
Purified Pork Regular Insulin	1852

Insulin, Zinc Crystals (Blood glucose concentrations may be raised by metolazone in diabetics). Products include:

NPH, 100 Units	1502

Insulin, Zinc Suspension (Blood glucose concentrations may be raised by metolazone in diabetics). Products include:

Iletin I	1501
Lente, 100 Units	1501
Iletin II	1504
Pork Lente, 100 Units	1504
Purified Pork Lente Insulin	1852

Isradipine (Orthostatic hypotension may occur with concurrent therapy). Products include:

DynaCirc Capsules	2381
DynaCirc CR Tablets	2383

Ketoprofen (Antihypertensive effects of Mykrox may be decreased). Products include:

Actron Caplets and Tablets	608
Orudis Capsules	2874
Orudis KT	842
Oruvail Capsules	2874

Ketorolac Tromethamine (Antihypertensive effects of Mykrox may be decreased). Products include:

Acular Sterile Ophthalmic Solution	470
Toradol	2319

Labetalol Hydrochloride (Orthostatic hypotension may occur with concurrent therapy). Products include:

Normodyne Injection	2519
Normodyne Tablets	2522
Trandate	1158

Levorphanol Tartrate (Potentiates orthostatic hypotensive effects). Products include:

Levo-Dromoran	2297

Lisinopril (Orthostatic hypotension may occur with concurrent therapy). Products include:

Prinivil Tablets	1776
Prinzide Tablets	1780
Zestoretic Tablets	2968
Zestril Tablets	2972

Lithium Carbonate (Reduced renal clearance of lithium; high risk of lithium toxicity). Products include:

Eskalith	2658
Lithium Carbonate Capsules & Tablets	2352
Lithonate/Lithotabs/Lithobid	2721

Lithium Citrate (Reduced renal clearance of lithium; high risk of lithium toxicity).

No products indexed under this heading.

Losartan Potassium (Orthostatic hypotension may occur with concurrent therapy). Products include:

Cozaar Tablets	1668
Hyzaar Tablets	1720

Magnesium Salicylate (Antihypertensive effects of Mykrox may be decreased). Products include:

Backache Caplets	635
Doan's Extra-Strength Analgesic	653
Extra Strength Doan's P.M.	653
Doan's Regular Strength Analgesic	654
Mobigesic Tablets	607

Mecamylamine Hydrochloride (Orthostatic hypotension may occur with concurrent therapy). Products include:

Inversine Tablets	1729

Meclofenamate Sodium (Antihypertensive effects of Mykrox may be decreased).

No products indexed under this heading.

Mefenamic Acid (Antihypertensive effects of Mykrox may be decreased). Products include:

Ponstel	1982

Meperidine Hydrochloride (Potentiates orthostatic hypotensive effects). Products include:

Demerol	2438
Mepergan Injection	2859

Mephobarbital (Potentiates orthostatic hypotensive effects). Products include:

Mebaral Tablets	2452

Metformin Hydrochloride (Blood glucose concentrations may be raised by metolazone in diabetics). Products include:

Glucophage Tablets	754

Methadone Hydrochloride (Potentiates orthostatic hypotensive effects). Products include:

Methadone Hydrochloride Oral Concentrate	2356
Methadone Hydrochloride Oral Solution & Tablets	2357

Methenamine (Efficacy of methenamine may be decreased). Products include:

Urised Tablets	2123

Methenamine Hippurate (Efficacy of methenamine may be decreased).

No products indexed under this heading.

Methenamine Mandelate (Efficacy of methenamine may be decreased). Products include:

Uroqid-Acid No. 2 Tablets	633

Methyclothiazide (Orthostatic hypotension may occur with concurrent therapy). Products include:

Enduron Tablets	424

Methyldopa (Orthostatic hypotension may occur with concurrent therapy). Products include:

Aldoclor Tablets	1638
Aldomet Oral	1640
Aldoril Tablets	1644

Methyldopate Hydrochloride (Orthostatic hypotension may occur with concurrent therapy). Products include:

Aldomet Ester HCl Injection	1642

Methylprednisolone Acetate (Potential for increased hypokalemia).

No products indexed under this heading.

Methylprednisolone Sodium Succinate (Potential for increased hypokalemia).

No products indexed under this heading.

Metoprolol Succinate (Orthostatic hypotension may occur with concurrent therapy). Products include:

Toprol-XL Tablets	560

Metoprolol Tartrate (Orthostatic hypotension may occur with concurrent therapy). Products include:

Lopressor	848
Lopressor HCT Tablets	850

Metyrosine (Orthostatic hypotension may occur with concurrent therapy). Products include:

Demser Capsules	1690

Minoxidil (Orthostatic hypotension may occur with concurrent therapy).

No products indexed under this heading.

IMPORTANT NOTE: Always consult each drug listing in the patient's regimen for possible interactions.

Mykrox / Interactions Index

Moexipril Hydrochloride (Orthostatic hypotension may occur with concurrent therapy). Products include:
- Univasc Tablets 2553

Morphine Sulfate (Potentiates orthostatic hypotensive effects). Products include:
- Astramorph/PF Injection, USP (Preservative-Free) 526
- Duramorph Injection 983
- Infumorph 200 and Infumorph 500 Sterile Solutions 985
- Kadian Capsules 2948
- MS Contin Tablets 2149
- MSIR 2152
- Oramorph SR (Morphine Sulfate Sustained Release Tablets) ... 2359
- RMS Suppositories CII 2766
- Roxanol 2365

Nabumetone (Antihypertensive effects of Mykrox may be decreased). Products include:
- Relafen Tablets 2688

Nadolol (Orthostatic hypotension may occur with concurrent therapy).
No products indexed under this heading.

Naproxen (Antihypertensive effects of Mykrox may be decreased). Products include:
- Anaprox/Naprosyn 2277

Naproxen Sodium (Antihypertensive effects of Mykrox may be decreased). Products include:
- Aleve 2124
- Anaprox/Naprosyn 2277
- Naprelan Tablets 2861

Nicardipine Hydrochloride (Orthostatic hypotension may occur with concurrent therapy). Products include:
- Cardene Capsules 2261
- Cardene I.V. 2815
- Cardene SR Capsules 2264

Nifedipine (Orthostatic hypotension may occur with concurrent therapy). Products include:
- Adalat Capsules (10 mg and 20 mg) 580
- Adalat CC 582
- Procardia Capsules 2024
- Procardia XL Extended Release Tablets 2026

Nisoldipine (Orthostatic hypotension may occur with concurrent therapy). Products include:
- Sular Tablets 2961

Nitroglycerin (Orthostatic hypotension may occur with concurrent therapy). Products include:
- Deponit NTG Transdermal Delivery System 2541
- Nitro-Bid IV 1270
- Nitro-Bid Ointment 1272
- Nitro-Dur (nitroglycerin) Transdermal Infusion System 1365
- Nitrolingual Spray 2193
- Nitrostat Tablets 1981
- Transderm-Nitro Transdermal Therapeutic System 878

Norepinephrine Bitartrate (Arterial responsiveness to norepinephrine may be decreased). Products include:
- Levophed Bitartrate Injection 2445

Opium Alkaloids (Potentiates orthostatic hypotensive effects).
No products indexed under this heading.

Oxaprozin (Antihypertensive effects of Mykrox may be decreased). Products include:
- Daypro Caplets 2578

Oxycodone Hydrochloride (Potentiates orthostatic hypotensive effects). Products include:
- OxyContin Tablets 2163
- OxyIR Capsules 2167
- Percocet Tablets 955
- Percodan Tablets 955
- Percodan-Demi Tablets 956
- Roxicodone Tablets, Oral Solution & Intensol (Oxycodone) 2366
- Tylox Capsules 1593

Penbutolol Sulfate (Orthostatic hypotension may occur with concurrent therapy). Products include:
- Levatol Tablets 2547

Pentobarbital Sodium (Potentiates orthostatic hypotensive effects). Products include:
- Nembutal Sodium Capsules 440
- Nembutal Sodium Tablets 442
- Nembutal Sodium Suppositories 444

Phenobarbital (Potentiates orthostatic hypotensive effects). Products include:
- Arco-Lase Plus Tablets 513
- Bellergal-S Tablets 2375
- Donnatal 2234
- Donnatal Extentabs 2234
- Donnatal Tablets 2234
- Phenobarbital Elixir and Tablets . 1523
- Quadrinal Tablets 1398

Phenoxybenzamine Hydrochloride (Orthostatic hypotension may occur with concurrent therapy). Products include:
- Dibenzyline Capsules 2650

Phentolamine Mesylate (Orthostatic hypotension may occur with concurrent therapy). Products include:
- Regitine Vials 864

Phenylbutazone (Antihypertensive effects of Mykrox may be decreased).
No products indexed under this heading.

Pindolol (Orthostatic hypotension may occur with concurrent therapy). Products include:
- Visken Tablets 2428

Piroxicam (Antihypertensive effects of Mykrox may be decreased). Products include:
- Feldene Capsules 2008

Polythiazide (Orthostatic hypotension may occur with concurrent therapy). Products include:
- Minizide Capsules 2016

Prazosin Hydrochloride (Orthostatic hypotension may occur with concurrent therapy). Products include:
- Minipress Capsules 2015
- Minizide Capsules 2016

Prednisolone Acetate (Potential for increased hypokalemia). Products include:
- AK-CIDE .... ⊚ 203
- AK-CIDE Ointment .... ⊚ 203
- Blephamide Liquifilm Sterile Ophthalmic Suspension 472
- Blephamide Ointment .... ⊚ 234
- Econopred & Econopred Plus Ophthalmic Suspensions .... ⊚ 216
- Poly-Pred Liquifilm .... ⊚ 246
- Pred Forte .... ⊚ 247
- Pred Mild .... ⊚ 250
- Pred-G Liquifilm Sterile Ophthalmic Suspension .... ⊚ 248
- Pred-G S.O.P. Sterile Ophthalmic Ointment .... ⊚ 249

Prednisolone Sodium Phosphate (Potential for increased hypokalemia). Products include:
- AK-PRED .... ⊚ 204
- Hydeltrasol Injection, Sterile ... 1708
- Pediapred Oral Solution 1618

Prednisolone Tebutate (Potential for increased hypokalemia). Products include:
- Hydeltra-T.B.A. Sterile Suspension 1710

Prednisone (Potential for increased hypokalemia).
No products indexed under this heading.

Propoxyphene Hydrochloride (Potentiates orthostatic hypotensive effects). Products include:
- Darvon 1475
- Wygesic Tablets 2930

Propoxyphene Napsylate (Potentiates orthostatic hypotensive effects). Products include:
- Darvon-N/Darvocet-N 1473

Propranolol Hydrochloride (Orthostatic hypotension may occur with concurrent therapy). Products include:
- Inderal 2834
- Inderal LA Long Acting Capsules .. 2836
- Inderide Tablets 2838
- Inderide LA Long Acting Capsules . 2840

Quinapril Hydrochloride (Orthostatic hypotension may occur with concurrent therapy). Products include:
- Accupril Tablets 1950

Ramipril (Orthostatic hypotension may occur with concurrent therapy). Products include:
- Altace Capsules 1238

Rauwolfia Serpentina (Orthostatic hypotension may occur with concurrent therapy).
No products indexed under this heading.

Rescinnamine (Orthostatic hypotension may occur with concurrent therapy).
No products indexed under this heading.

Reserpine (Orthostatic hypotension may occur with concurrent therapy). Products include:
- Diupres Tablets 1691
- Hydropres Tablets 1718
- Ser-Ap-Es Tablets 867

Salsalate (Antihypertensive effects of Mykrox may be decreased). Products include:
- Disalcid 1549
- Mono-Gesic Tablets 810
- Salflex Tablets 791

Secobarbital Sodium (Potentiates orthostatic hypotensive effects). Products include:
- Seconal Sodium Pulvules 1529

Sodium Nitroprusside (Orthostatic hypotension may occur with concurrent therapy).
No products indexed under this heading.

Sotalol Hydrochloride (Orthostatic hypotension may occur with concurrent therapy). Products include:
- Betapace Tablets 637

Spirapril Hydrochloride (Orthostatic hypotension may occur with concurrent therapy).
No products indexed under this heading.

Sufentanil Citrate (Potentiates orthostatic hypotensive effects). Products include:
- Sufenta Injection 1355

Sulindac (Antihypertensive effects of Mykrox may be decreased). Products include:
- Clinoril Tablets 1658

Terazosin Hydrochloride (Orthostatic hypotension may occur with concurrent therapy). Products include:
- Hytrin Capsules 434

Thiamylal Sodium (Potentiates orthostatic hypotensive effects).
No products indexed under this heading.

Timolol Maleate (Orthostatic hypotension may occur with concurrent therapy). Products include:
- Blocadren Tablets 1654
- Timolide Tablets 1791
- Timoptic in Ocudose 1796
- Timoptic Sterile Ophthalmic Solution 1794
- Timoptic-XE 1798

Tolazamide (Blood glucose concentrations may be raised by metolazone in diabetics).
No products indexed under this heading.

Tolbutamide (Blood glucose concentrations may be raised by metolazone in diabetics).
No products indexed under this heading.

Tolmetin Sodium (Antihypertensive effects of Mykrox may be decreased). Products include:
- Tolectin (200, 400 and 600 mg) .. 1591

Torsemide (Orthostatic hypotension may occur with concurrent therapy). Products include:
- Demadex Tablets and Injection 691

Triamcinolone (Potential for increased hypokalemia).
No products indexed under this heading.

Triamcinolone Acetonide (Potential for increased hypokalemia). Products include:
- Azmacort Oral Inhaler 2175
- Nasacort AQ Nasal Spray 2191
- Nasacort Nasal Inhaler 2189

Triamcinolone Diacetate (Potential for increased hypokalemia).
No products indexed under this heading.

Triamcinolone Hexacetonide (Potential for increased hypokalemia).
No products indexed under this heading.

Trimethaphan Camsylate (Orthostatic hypotension may occur with concurrent therapy).
No products indexed under this heading.

Tubocurarine Chloride (Neuromuscular blocking effects of curariform drugs may be enhanced).
No products indexed under this heading.

Verapamil Hydrochloride (Orthostatic hypotension may occur with concurrent therapy). Products include:
- Calan SR Caplets 2571
- Calan Tablets 2568
- Covera-HS Tablets 2573
- Isoptin Injectable 1391
- Isoptin Oral Tablets 1393
- Isoptin SR Tablets 1395
- Verelan Capsules 1455

Warfarin Sodium (May affect the hypoprothrombinemic response to anticoagulants; dosage adjustments may be necessary). Products include:
- Coumadin 941

Food Interactions

Alcohol (Potentiates orthostatic hypotensive effects).

FAST-ACTING MYLANTA ANTACID TABLETS
(Calcium Carbonate, Magnesium Hydroxide) 1359
May interact with:

Prescription Drugs, unspecified (Resultant effects of concurrent use not specified).

MYLANTA GAS RELIEF GELCAPS
(Simethicone) 1360
None cited in PDR database.

(⊠ Described in PDR For Nonprescription Drugs)   (⊚ Described in PDR For Ophthalmology)

711 Interactions Index Myochrysine

MYLANTA GAS RELIEF TABLETS-80 MG
(Simethicone)....................................1360
None cited in PDR database.

MAXIMUM STRENGTH FAST-ACTING MYLANTA ANTACID TABLETS
(Calcium Carbonate, Magnesium Hydroxide)..1359
See **Fast-Acting Mylanta Antacid Tablets**

MAXIMUM STRENGTH MYLANTA GAS RELIEF TABLETS-125 MG
(Simethicone)....................................1360
None cited in PDR database.

MYLANTA GELCAPS ANTACID
(Calcium Carbonate, Magnesium Hydroxide)..678
May interact with:

Prescription Drugs, unspecified (Antacids may interact with certain unspecified prescription drugs).

FAST-ACTING MYLANTA LIQUID ANTACID
(Aluminum Hydroxide, Magnesium Hydroxide, Simethicone)....................1359
May interact with:

Prescription Drugs, unspecified (Antacids interact with certain prescription drugs; physician's consultation is required if used concurrently).

MYLANTA SOOTHING LOZENGES
(Calcium Carbonate)............................1360
May interact with:

Prescription Drugs, unspecified (Concurrent use not recommended; consult your doctor).

MAXIMUM-STRENGTH FAST-ACTING MYLANTA LIQUID ANTACID
(Aluminum Hydroxide, Magnesium Hydroxide, Simethicone)....................1359
See **Fast-Acting Mylanta Liquid Antacid**

MYLERAN TABLETS
(Busulfan)..1209
May interact with antineoplastics and certain other agents. Compounds in these categories include:

Altretamine (Potential for rare life-threatening hepatic veno-occlusive disease). Products include:
Hexalen Capsules 2760

Anastrozole (Potential for rare life-threatening hepatic veno-occlusive disease). Products include:
Arimidex Tablets 2932

Asparaginase (Potential for rare life-threatening hepatic veno-occlusive disease). Products include:
Elspar 1700

Bicalutamide (Potential for rare life-threatening hepatic veno-occlusive disease). Products include:
Casodex Tablets................................. 2934

Bleomycin Sulfate (Potential for rare life-threatening hepatic veno-occlusive disease). Products include:
Blenoxane 697

Bone Marrow Depressants, unspecified (Additive myelosuppression).

Carboplatin (Potential for rare life-threatening hepatic veno-occlusive disease). Products include:
Paraplatin for Injection 713

Carmustine (BCNU) (Potential for rare life-threatening hepatic veno-occlusive disease). Products include:
BiCNU.. 696

Chlorambucil (Potential for rare life-threatening hepatic veno-occlusive disease). Products include:
Leukeran Tablets 1205

Cisplatin (Potential for rare life-threatening hepatic veno-occlusive disease). Products include:
Platinol for Injection 717
Platinol-AQ Injection........................... 719

Cyclophosphamide (Potential for rare life-threatening hepatic veno-occlusive disease; potential for cardiac temponade). Products include:
Cytoxan 700

Dacarbazine (Potential for rare life-threatening hepatic veno-occlusive disease). Products include:
DTIC-Dome.. 593

Daunorubicin Citrate (Potential for rare life-threatening hepatic veno-occlusive disease). Products include:
DaunoXome 1842

Daunorubicin Hydrochloride (Potential for rare life-threatening hepatic veno-occlusive disease). Products include:
Cerubidine for Injection 634

Docetaxel (Potential for rare life-threatening hepatic veno-occlusive disease). Products include:
Taxotere for Injection Concentrate 2204

Doxorubicin Hydrochloride (Potential for rare life-threatening hepatic veno-occlusive disease). Products include:
Adriamycin PFS 2056
Adriamycin RDF 2056
Doxil 2613
Doxorubicin Astra 531
Rubex for Injection 721

Estramustine Phosphate Sodium (Potential for rare life-threatening hepatic veno-occlusive disease). Products include:
Emcyt Capsules 2085

Etoposide (Potential for rare life-threatening hepatic veno-occlusive disease). Products include:
Etoposide Injection 539
VePesid Capsules and Injection........ 727

Floxuridine (Potential for rare life-threatening hepatic veno-occlusive disease). Products include:
Sterile FUDR 2284

Fluorouracil (Potential for rare life-threatening hepatic veno-occlusive disease). Products include:
Efudex 2280
Fluoroplex Topical Solution & Cream 1% 475
Fluorouracil Injection 2282

Flutamide (Potential for rare life-threatening hepatic veno-occlusive disease). Products include:
Eulexin Capsules 2498

Gemcitabine Hydrochloride (Potential for rare life-threatening hepatic veno-occlusive disease). Products include:
Gemzar for Injection........................... 1482

Hydroxyurea (Potential for rare life-threatening hepatic veno-occlusive disease). Products include:
Hydrea Capsules 705

Idarubicin Hydrochloride (Potential for rare life-threatening hepatic veno-occlusive disease). Products include:
Idamycin Injection 2096

Ifosfamide (Potential for rare life-threatening hepatic veno-occlusive disease). Products include:
IFEX 706

Interferon alfa-2A, Recombinant (Potential for rare life-threatening hepatic veno-occlusive disease). Products include:
Roferon-A Injection 2308

Interferon alfa-2B, Recombinant (Potential for rare life-threatening hepatic veno-occlusive disease). Products include:
Intron A for Injection 2506

Irinotecan Hydrochloride (Potential for rare life-threatening hepatic veno-occlusive disease).
No products indexed under this heading.

Levamisole Hydrochloride (Potential for rare life-threatening hepatic veno-occlusive disease). Products include:
Ergamisol Tablets 1340

Lomustine (CCNU) (Potential for rare life-threatening hepatic veno-occlusive disease). Products include:
CeeNU Capsules.................................... 699

Mechlorethamine Hydrochloride (Potential for rare life-threatening hepatic veno-occlusive disease). Products include:
Mustargen... 1752

Megestrol Acetate (Potential for rare life-threatening hepatic veno-occlusive disease). Products include:
Megace Oral Suspension 708
Megace Tablets 710

Melphalan (Potential for rare life-threatening hepatic veno-occlusive disease). Products include:
Alkeran Tablets..................................... 1198

Mercaptopurine (Potential for rare life-threatening hepatic veno-occlusive disease). Products include:
Purinethol Tablets 1214

Methotrexate Sodium (Potential for rare life-threatening hepatic veno-occlusive disease). Products include:
Methotrexate Sodium Tablets, Injection, for Injection and LPF Injection 1322

Mitomycin (Mitomycin-C) (Potential for rare life-threatening hepatic veno-occlusive disease). Products include:
Mutamycin for Injection 712

Mitotane (Potential for rare life-threatening hepatic veno-occlusive disease). Products include:
Lysodren Tablets 707

Mitoxantrone Hydrochloride (Potential for rare life-threatening hepatic veno-occlusive disease). Products include:
Novantrone for Injection..................... 1327

Paclitaxel (Potential for rare life-threatening hepatic veno-occlusive disease). Products include:
Taxol Injection...................................... 723

Procarbazine Hydrochloride (Potential for rare life-threatening hepatic veno-occlusive disease). Products include:
Matulane Capsules 2300

Streptozocin (Potential for rare life-threatening hepatic veno-occlusive disease). Products include:
Zanosar Sterile Powder...................... 2119

Tamoxifen Citrate (Potential for rare life-threatening hepatic veno-occlusive disease). Products include:
Nolvadex Tablets 2957

Teniposide (Potential for rare life-threatening hepatic veno-occlusive disease). Products include:
Vumon for Injection 729

Thioguanine (Potential for esophageal varices associated with abnormal liver function tests; potential for rare life-threatening hepatic veno-occulsive disease). Products include:
Thioguanine Tablets, Tabloid Brand 1225

Thiotepa (Potential for rare life-threatening hepatic veno-occlusive disease). Products include:
Thioplex (Thiotepa For Injection) 1329

Topotecan Hydrochloride (Potential for rare life-threatening hepatic veno-occlusive disease). Products include:
Hycamtin for Injection.......................... 2665

Vincristine Sulfate (Potential for rare life-threatening hepatic veno-occlusive disease). Products include:
Oncovin Solution Vials & Hyporets 1521

Vinorelbine Tartrate (Potential for rare life-threatening hepatic veno-occlusive disease). Products include:
Navelbine Injection 1212

MYLICON INFANTS' DROPS
(Simethicone).......................................1358
None cited in PDR database.

MYOCHRYSINE INJECTION
(Gold Sodium Thiomalate) 1754
May interact with cytotoxic drugs and certain other agents. Compounds in these categories include:

Bleomycin Sulfate (Safety of coadministration has NOT been established). Products include:
Blenoxane 697

Daunorubicin Hydrochloride (Safety of coadministration has NOT been established). Products include:
Cerubidine for Injection 634

Doxorubicin Hydrochloride (Safety of coadministration has NOT been established). Products include:
Adriamycin PFS 2056
Adriamycin RDF 2056
Doxil 2613
Doxorubicin Astra 531
Rubex for Injection 721

Fluorouracil (Safety of coadministration has NOT been established). Products include:
Efudex 2280
Fluoroplex Topical Solution & Cream 1% 475
Fluorouracil Injection 2282

Hydroxyurea (Safety of coadministration has NOT been established). Products include:
Hydrea Capsules 705

Methotrexate Sodium (Safety of coadministration has NOT been established). Products include:
Methotrexate Sodium Tablets, Injection, for Injection and LPF Injection 1322

Mitotane (Safety of coadministration has NOT been established). Products include:
Lysodren Tablets 707

Mitoxantrone Hydrochloride (Safety of coadministration has NOT been established). Products include:
Novantrone for Injection..................... 1327

Penicillamine (Do not use concomitantly). Products include:
Cuprimine Capsules 1673
Depen Titratable Tablets 2770

IMPORTANT NOTE: Always consult each drug listing in the patient's regimen for possible interactions.

Myochrysine | **Interactions Index** | **712**

Procarbazine Hydrochloride (Safety of coadministration has NOT been established). Products include:
Matulane Capsules 2300

Tamoxifen Citrate (Safety of coadministration has NOT been established). Products include:
Nolvadex Tablets 2957

Vincristine Sulfate (Safety of coadministration has NOT been established). Products include:
Oncovin Solution Vials & Hyporets 1521

MYOFLEX EXTERNAL ANALGESIC CREME (Trolamine Salicylate) 660
None cited in PDR database.

MYSOLINE SUSPENSION (Primidone) 2860
None cited in PDR database.

MYSOLINE TABLETS (Primidone) 2860
None cited in PDR database.

NAFTIN CREAM 1% (Naftifine Hydrochloride) 477
None cited in PDR database.

NAFTIN GEL 1% (Naftifine Hydrochloride) 477
None cited in PDR database.

NALFON 200 PULVULES & NALFON TABLETS (Fenoprofen Calcium) 933
May interact with oral anticoagulants, loop diuretics, hydantoin anticonvulsants, sulfonylureas, corticosteroids, and certain other agents. Compounds in these categories include:

Aspirin (Co-administration decreases biological half-life of fenoprofen because of an increase in metabolic clearance; concurrent use is not recommended). Products include:
Alka-Seltzer Cherry Effervescent Antacid and Pain Reliever 609
Alka-Seltzer Extra Strength Effervescent Antacid and Pain Reliever 609
Alka-Seltzer Lemon Lime Effervescent Antacid and Pain Reliever 609
Alka-Seltzer Original Effervescent Antacid and Pain Reliever 609
Alka-Seltzer Plus 611
Alka-Seltzer Plus Sinus Medicine .. 611
Ascriptin 650
Arthritis Strength BC Powder 631
BC Cold Powder Multi-Symptom Formula (Cold-Sinus-Allergy) 631
BC Cold Powder Non-Drowsy Formula (Cold-Sinus) 631
BC Powder 631
Genuine Bayer Aspirin Tablets & Caplets 618
Extra Strength Bayer Arthritis Pain Regimen Formula 615
Extra Strength Bayer Aspirin Caplets & Tablets 617
Extended-Release Bayer 8-Hour Aspirin 616
Extra Strength Bayer Plus Aspirin Caplets 617
Extra Strength Bayer PM Aspirin Plus Sleep Aid 617
Aspirin Regimen Bayer 81 mg Tablets with Calcium 615
Aspirin Regimen Bayer Adult Low Strength 81 mg Tablets 613
Aspirin Regimen Bayer Children's Chewable Aspirin 616
Aspirin Regimen Bayer Regular Strength 325 mg Caplets 613
Bufferin Analgesic Tablets 636
Arthritis Strength Bufferin Analgesic Caplets 637
Extra Strength Bufferin Analgesic Tablets 637
Cama Arthritis Pain Reliever 748
Darvon Compound-65 Pulvules 1475
Easprin 1971
Ecotrin 2625
Ecotrin Enteric Coated Aspirin Maximum Strength Tablets and Caplets 775
Ecotrin Enteric Coated Aspirin Regular Strength Tablets 2625
Empirin Aspirin Tablets 818
Excedrin Extra-Strength Analgesic Tablets, Caplets, and Geltabs... 734
Fiorinal Capsules 2388
Fiorinal with Codeine Capsules 2390
Fiorinal Tablets 2388
Goody's Extra Strength Headache Powders 632
Goody's Extra Strength Pain Relief Tablets 632
Halfprin Tablets 1413
Norgesic 1554
Percodan Tablets 955
Percodan-Demi Tablets 956
Robaxisal Tablets 2246
Soma Compound w/Codeine Tablets 2784
Soma Compound Tablets 2783
St. Joseph Adult Chewable Aspirin (81 mg.) 768
Talwin Compound 2466
Vanquish Analgesic Caplets 627

Betamethasone Acetate (Any reduction in steroid dosage, when used concurrently, should be done gradually in order to avoid possible complications of sudden steroid withdrawal). Products include:
Celestone Soluspan Suspension 2484

Betamethasone Sodium Phosphate (Any reduction in steroid dosage, when used concurrently, should be done gradually in order to avoid possible complications of sudden steroid withdrawal). Products include:
Celestone Soluspan Suspension 2484

Bumetanide (Patients treated with loop diuretics may be resistant to the effects of loop diuretics). Products include:
Bumex 2260

Chlorpropamide (Theoretical possibility of displacement from the protein binding sites with resultant increase in activities and toxicity of sulfonylureas). Products include:
Diabinese Tablets 2002

Cortisone Acetate (Any reduction in steroid dosage, when used concurrently, should be done gradually in order to avoid possible complications of sudden steroid withdrawal). Products include:
Cortone Acetate Sterile Suspension 1663
Cortone Acetate Tablets 1664

Dexamethasone (Any reduction in steroid dosage, when used concurrently, should be done gradually in order to avoid possible complications of sudden steroid withdrawal). Products include:
AK-Trol Ointment & Suspension .. 205
Decadron Elixir 1676
Decadron Tablets 1678
Decaspray Topical Aerosol 1689
Maxitrol Ophthalmic Ointment and Suspension 222
TobraDex Ophthalmic Suspension and Ointment 469

Dexamethasone Acetate (Any reduction in steroid dosage, when used concurrently, should be done gradually in order to avoid possible complications of sudden steroid withdrawal). Products include:
Dalalone D.P. Injectable 1009
Decadron-LA Sterile Suspension 1687

Dexamethasone Sodium Phosphate (Any reduction in steroid dosage, when used concurrently, should be done gradually in order to avoid possible complications of sudden steroid withdrawal). Products include:
Decadron Phosphate Injection 1680
Decadron Phosphate Sterile Ophthalmic Ointment 1684
Decadron Phosphate Sterile Ophthalmic Solution 1685
Decadron Phosphate Topical Cream 1686
Decadron Phosphate with Xylocaine Injection, Sterile 1683
Dexacort Phosphate in Respihaler .. 1606
Dexacort Phosphate in Turbinaire .. 1607
NeoDecadron Sterile Ophthalmic Ointment 1755
NeoDecadron Sterile Ophthalmic Solution 1756
NeoDecadron Topical Cream 1757

Dicumarol (Potential for prolonged prothrombin time).
No products indexed under this heading.

Ethacrynic Acid (Patients treated with loop diuretics may be resistant to the effects of loop diuretics). Products include:
Edecrin Tablets 1698

Ethotoin (Theoretical possibility of displacement from the protein binding sites with resultant increase in activities and toxicity of hydantoins). Products include:
Peganone Tablets 455

Fludrocortisone Acetate (Any reduction in steroid dosage, when used concurrently, should be done gradually in order to avoid possible complications of sudden steroid withdrawal). Products include:
Florinef Acetate Tablets 506

Fosphenytoin Sodium (Theoretical possibility of displacement from the protein binding sites with resultant increase in activities and toxicity of hydantoins). Products include:
Cerebyx Injection 1956

Furosemide (Patients treated with loop diuretics may be resistant to the effects of loop diuretics). Products include:
Lasix Injection, Oral Solution and Tablets 1267

Glimepiride (Theoretical possibility of displacement from the protein binding sites with resultant increase in activities and toxicity of sulfonylureas). Products include:
Amaryl Tablets 1241

Glipizide (Theoretical possibility of displacement from the protein binding sites with resultant increase in activities and toxicity of sulfonylureas). Products include:
Glucotrol Tablets 2011
Glucotrol XL Extended Release Tablets 2012

Glyburide (Theoretical possibility of displacement from the protein binding sites with resultant increase in activities and toxicity of sulfonylureas). Products include:
DiaBeta Tablets 1265
Glynase PresTab Tablets 2091
Micronase Tablets 2099

Hydrocortisone (Any reduction in steroid dosage, when used concurrently, should be done gradually in order to avoid possible complications of sudden steroid withdrawal): Products include:
Anusol-HC Cream 2.5% 1953
Aquanil HC Lotion 1989
Maximum Strength Cortaid Spray 800
CORTENEMA 2713
Cortisporin Ointment 1074
Cortisporin Ophthalmic Ointment Sterile 1074
Cortisporin Ophthalmic Suspension Sterile 1075
Cortisporin Otic Solution Sterile 1076
Cortisporin Otic Suspension Sterile 1077
Cortizone-5 795
Cortizone-10 795
Hydrocortone Tablets 1715
Hytone 922
Hytone Ointment 2 ½% 923
Massengill Medicated Soft Cloth Towelettes 2628
Pediotic Suspension Sterile 1140
Preparation H Hydrocortisone 1% Cream 843
ProctoCream-HC 2.5% 2552
VōSoL HC Otic Solution 2786

Hydrocortisone Acetate (Any reduction in steroid dosage, when used concurrently, should be done gradually in order to avoid possible complications of sudden steroid withdrawal). Products include:
Analpram-HC Rectal Cream 1% and 2.5% 993
Anusol HC-1 Hydrocortisone Anti-Itch Ointment 810
Anusol-HC Suppositories 1954
Caldecort Anti-Itch Hydrocortisone Cream 651
Coly-Mycin S Otic w/Neomycin & Hydrocortisone 1965
Cortaid 800
Cortifoam 2540
Cortisporin Cream 1073
Epifoam 2543
Hydrocortone Acetate Sterile Suspension 1712
Mantadil Cream 1124
Nupercainal Hydrocortisone 1% Cream 661
Pramosone Cream, Lotion & Ointment 995
ProctoFoam-HC 2552
Terra-Cortril Ophthalmic Suspension 2033

Hydrocortisone Sodium Phosphate (Any reduction in steroid dosage, when used concurrently, should be done gradually in order to avoid possible complications of sudden steroid withdrawal). Products include:
Hydrocortone Phosphate Injection, Sterile 1713

Hydrocortisone Sodium Succinate (Any reduction in steroid dosage, when used concurrently, should be done gradually in order to avoid possible complications of sudden steroid withdrawal).
No products indexed under this heading.

Mephenytoin (Theoretical possibility of displacement from the protein binding sites with resultant increase in activities and toxicity of hydantoins). Products include:
Mesantoin Tablets 2400

Methylprednisolone Acetate (Any reduction in steroid dosage, when used concurrently, should be done gradually in order to avoid possible complications of sudden steroid withdrawal).
No products indexed under this heading.

Methylprednisolone Sodium Succinate (Any reduction in steroid dosage, when used concurrently, should be done gradually in order to avoid possible complications of sudden steroid withdrawal).
No products indexed under this heading.

Phenobarbital (Chronic administration of phenobarbital may be associated with a decrease in the plasma half-life of fenoprofen). Products include:
Arco-Lase Plus Tablets 513
Bellergal-S Tablets 2375
Donnatal 2234

(Described in PDR For Nonprescription Drugs) (Described in PDR For Ophthalmology)

Donnatal Extentabs 2234
Donnatal Tablets 2234
Phenobarbital Elixir and Tablets 1523
Quadrinal Tablets 1398

Phenytoin (Theoretical possibility of displacement from the protein binding sites with resultant increase in activities and toxicity of hydantoins). Products include:
Dilantin Infatabs 1967
Dilantin-125 Suspension 1969

Phenytoin Sodium (Theoretical possibility of displacement from the protein binding sites with resultant increase in activities and toxicity of hydantoins). Products include:
Dilantin Kapseals 1965

Prednisolone Acetate (Any reduction in steroid dosage, when used concurrently, should be done gradually in order to avoid possible complications of sudden steroid withdrawal). Products include:
AK-CIDE .... ◉ 203
AK-CIDE Ointment .... ◉ 203
Blephamide Liquifilm Sterile Ophthalmic Suspension 472
Blephamide Ointment .... ◉ 234
Econopred & Econopred Plus Ophthalmic Suspensions .... ◉ 216
Poly-Pred Liquifilm .... ◉ 246
Pred Forte .... ◉ 247
Pred Mild .... ◉ 250
Pred-G Liquifilm Sterile Ophthalmic Suspension .... ◉ 248
Pred-G S.O.P. Sterile Ophthalmic Ointment .... ◉ 249

Prednisolone Sodium Phosphate (Any reduction in steroid dosage, when used concurrently, should be done gradually in order to avoid possible complications of sudden steroid withdrawal). Products include:
AK-PRED .... ◉ 204
Hydeltrasol Injection, Sterile 1708
Pediapred Oral Solution 1618

Prednisolone Tebutate (Any reduction in steroid dosage, when used concurrently, should be done gradually in order to avoid possible complications of sudden steroid withdrawal). Products include:
Hydeltra-T.B.A. Sterile Suspension 1710

Prednisone (Any reduction in steroid dosage, when used concurrently, should be done gradually in order to avoid possible complications of sudden steroid withdrawal).
No products indexed under this heading.

Sulfacytine (Theoretical possibility of displacement from the protein binding sites with resultant increase in activities and toxicity of sulfonamides).

Sulfamethizole (Theoretical possibility of displacement from the protein binding sites with resultant increase in activities and toxicity of sulfonamides). Products include:
Urobiotic-250 Capsules 2038

Sulfamethoxazole (Theoretical possibility of displacement from the protein binding sites with resultant increase in activities and toxicity of sulfonamides). Products include:
Bactrim DS Tablets 2257
Bactrim I.V. Infusion 2255
Bactrim 2257
Gantanol Tablets 2285
Septra 1146
Septra I.V. Infusion 1142
Septra I.V. Infusion ADD-Vantage Vials 1144
Septra 1146

Sulfasalazine (Theoretical possibility of displacement from the protein binding sites with resultant increase in activities and toxicity of sulfonamides). Products include:
Azulfidine 2059

Sulfinpyrazone (Theoretical possibility of displacement from the protein binding sites with resultant increase in activities and toxicity of sulfonamides). Products include:
Anturane 823

Sulfisoxazole (Theoretical possibility of displacement from the protein binding sites with resultant increase in activities and toxicity of sulfonamides). Products include:
Gantrisin Tablets 2286

Tolazamide (Theoretical possibility of displacement from the protein binding sites with resultant increase in activities and toxicity of sulfonylureas).
No products indexed under this heading.

Tolbutamide (Theoretical possibility of displacement from the protein binding sites with resultant increase in activities and toxicity of sulfonylureas).
No products indexed under this heading.

Torsemide (Patients treated with loop diuretics may be resistant to the effects of loop diuretics). Products include:
Demadex Tablets and Injection 691

Triamcinolone (Any reduction in steroid dosage, when used concurrently, should be done gradually in order to avoid possible complications of sudden steroid withdrawal).
No products indexed under this heading.

Triamcinolone Acetonide (Any reduction in steroid dosage, when used concurrently, should be done gradually in order to avoid possible complications of sudden steroid withdrawal). Products include:
Azmacort Oral Inhaler 2175
Nasacort AQ Nasal Spray 2191
Nasacort Nasal Inhaler 2189

Triamcinolone Diacetate (Any reduction in steroid dosage, when used concurrently, should be done gradually in order to avoid possible complications of sudden steroid withdrawal).
No products indexed under this heading.

Triamcinolone Hexacetonide (Any reduction in steroid dosage, when used concurrently, should be done gradually in order to avoid possible complications of sudden steroid withdrawal).
No products indexed under this heading.

Warfarin Sodium (Potential for prolonged prothrombin time). Products include:
Coumadin 941

Food Interactions

Dairy products (Peak blood levels are delayed and diminished).

Meal, unspecified (Peak blood levels are delayed and diminished).

NAPHCON-A OPHTHALMIC SOLUTION

(Naphazoline Hydrochloride, Pheniramine Maleate) 469
None cited in PDR database.

NAPRELAN TABLETS

(Naproxen Sodium) 2861
May interact with ACE inhibitors, hydantoin anticonvulsants, sulfonamides, sulfonylureas, lithium preparations, beta blockers, oral anticoagulants, and certain other agents. Compounds in these categories include:

Acebutolol Hydrochloride (Reduced antihypertensive effect of beta blockers). Products include:
Sectral Capsules 2914

Aspirin (Naproxen is displaced from its binding sites during concomitant use of aspirin resulting in lower plasma concentrations and peak plasma levels). Products include:
Alka-Seltzer Cherry Effervescent Antacid and Pain Reliever 609
Alka-Seltzer Extra Strength Effervescent Antacid and Pain Reliever 609
Alka-Seltzer Lemon Lime Effervescent Antacid and Pain Reliever 609
Alka-Seltzer Original Effervescent Antacid and Pain Reliever 609
Alka-Seltzer Plus 611
Alka-Seltzer Plus Sinus Medicine 611
Ascriptin 650
Arthritis Strength BC Powder 631
BC Cold Powder Multi-Symptom Formula (Cold-Sinus-Allergy) 631
BC Cold Powder Non-Drowsy Formula (Cold-Sinus) 631
BC Powder 631
Genuine Bayer Aspirin Tablets & Caplets 618
Extra Strength Bayer Arthritis Pain Regimen Formula 615
Extra Strength Bayer Aspirin Caplets & Tablets 617
Extended-Release Bayer 8-Hour Aspirin 616
Extra Strength Bayer Plus Aspirin Caplets 617
Extra Strength Bayer PM Aspirin Plus Sleep Aid 617
Aspirin Regimen Bayer 81 mg Tablets with Calcium 615
Aspirin Regimen Bayer Adult Low Strength 81 mg Tablets 613
Aspirin Regimen Bayer Children's Chewable Aspirin 616
Aspirin Regimen Bayer Regular Strength 325 mg Caplets 613
Bufferin Analgesic Tablets 636
Arthritis Strength Bufferin Analgesic Caplets 637
Extra Strength Bufferin Analgesic Tablets 637
Cama Arthritis Pain Reliever 748
Darvon Compound-65 Pulvules 1475
Easprin 1971
Ecotrin 2625
Ecotrin Enteric Coated Aspirin Maximum Strength Tablets and Caplets 775
Ecotrin Enteric Coated Aspirin Regular Strength Tablets 2625
Empirin Aspirin Tablets 818
Excedrin Extra-Strength Analgesic Tablets, Caplets, and Geltabs 734
Fiorinal Capsules 2388
Fiorinal with Codeine Capsules 2390
Fiorinal Tablets 2388
Goody's Extra Strength Headache Powders 632
Goody's Extra Strength Pain Relief Tablets 632
Halfprin Tablets 1413
Norgesic 1554
Percodan Tablets 955
Percodan-Demi Tablets 956
Robaxisal Tablets 2246
Soma Compound w/Codeine Tablets 2784
Soma Compound Tablets 2783
St. Joseph Adult Chewable Aspirin (81 mg.) 768
Talwin Compound 2466
Vanquish Analgesic Caplets 627

Atenolol (Reduced antihypertensive effect of beta blockers). Products include:
Tenoretic Tablets 2963
Tenormin Tablets and I.V. Injection 2965

Benazepril Hydrochloride (Co-administration may potentiate renal disease states). Products include:
Lotensin Tablets 852
Lotensin HCT Tablets 855
Lotrel Capsules 858

Bendroflumethiazide (Potential for sulfonamide toxicity).
No products indexed under this heading.

Betaxolol Hydrochloride (Reduced antihypertensive effect of beta blockers). Products include:
Betoptic Ophthalmic Solution 465
Betoptic S Ophthalmic Suspension 467
Kerlone Tablets 2588

Bisoprolol Fumarate (Reduced antihypertensive effect of beta blockers). Products include:
Zebeta Tablets 1457
Ziac 1459

Captopril (Co-administration may potentiate renal disease states). Products include:
Capoten Tablets 740
Capozide Tablets 744

Carteolol Hydrochloride (Reduced antihypertensive effect of beta blockers). Products include:
Cartrol Tablets 413
Ocupress Ophthalmic Solution, 1% Sterile .... ◉ 297

Chlorothiazide (Potential for sulfonamide toxicity). Products include:
Aldoclor Tablets 1638
Diupres Tablets 1691
Diuril Oral 1694

Chlorothiazide Sodium (Potential for sulfonamide toxicity). Products include:
Diuril Sodium Intravenous 1693

Chlorpropamide (Potential for sulfonylurea toxicity). Products include:
Diabinese Tablets 2002

Dicumarol (Naproxen may decrease platelet aggregation and prolong bleeding time; caution is advised if co-administered).
No products indexed under this heading.

Enalapril Maleate (Co-administration may potentiate renal disease states). Products include:
Vaseretic Tablets 1810
Vasotec Tablets 1816

Enalaprilat (Co-administration may potentiate renal disease states). Products include:
Vasotec I.V. 1814

Esmolol Hydrochloride (Reduced antihypertensive effect of beta blockers). Products include:
Brevibloc (esmolol HCl) Injection 1860

Ethotoin (Potential for hydantoin toxicity). Products include:
Peganone Tablets 455

Fosinopril Sodium (Co-administration may potentiate renal disease states). Products include:
Monopril Tablets 762

Furosemide (Potential for inhibition of natriuretic effect of furosemide). Products include:
Lasix Injection, Oral Solution and Tablets 1267

Glimepiride (Potential for sulfonylurea toxicity). Products include:
Amaryl Tablets 1241

Glipizide (Potential for sulfonylurea toxicity). Products include:
Glucotrol Tablets 2011
Glucotrol XL Extended Release Tablets 2012

Glyburide (Potential for sulfonylurea toxicity). Products include:
DiaBeta Tablets 1265
Glynase PresTab Tablets 2091
Micronase Tablets 2099

IMPORTANT NOTE: Always consult each drug listing in the patient's regimen for possible interactions.

Hydrochlorothiazide (Potential for sulfonamide toxicity). Products include:
- Aldactazide Tablets ... 2556
- Aldoril Tablets ... 1644
- Apresazide Capsules ... 824
- Capozide Tablets ... 744
- Dyazide Capsules ... 2653
- Esidrix Tablets ... 839
- Esimil Tablets ... 840
- HydroDIURIL Tablets ... 1716
- Hydropres Tablets ... 1718
- Hyzaar Tablets ... 1720
- Inderide Tablets ... 2838
- Inderide LA Long Acting Capsules ... 2840
- Lopressor HCT Tablets ... 850
- Lotensin HCT Tablets ... 855
- Moduretic Tablets ... 1748
- Oretic Tablets ... 450
- Prinzide Tablets ... 1780
- Ser-Ap-Es Tablets ... 867
- Timolide Tablets ... 1791
- Vaseretic Tablets ... 1810
- Zestoretic Tablets ... 2968
- Ziac ... 1459

Hydroflumethiazide (Potential for sulfonamide toxicity). Products include:
- Diucardin Tablets ... 2824

Labetalol Hydrochloride (Reduced antihypertensive effect of beta blockers). Products include:
- Normodyne Injection ... 2519
- Normodyne Tablets ... 2522
- Trandate ... 1158

Levobunolol Hydrochloride (Reduced antihypertensive effect of beta blockers). Products include:
- Betagan ... ⊚ 230

Lisinopril (Co-administration may potentiate renal disease states). Products include:
- Prinivil Tablets ... 1776
- Prinzide Tablets ... 1780
- Zestoretic Tablets ... 2968
- Zestril Tablets ... 2972

Lithium Carbonate (Inhibition of lithium renal clearance leading to increase in plasma lithium concentrations). Products include:
- Eskalith ... 2658
- Lithium Carbonate Capsules & Tablets ... 2352
- Lithonate/Lithotabs/Lithobid ... 2721

Lithium Citrate (Inhibition of lithium renal clearance leading to increase in plasma lithium concentrations).
- No products indexed under this heading.

Mephenytoin (Potential for hydantoin toxicity). Products include:
- Mesantoin Tablets ... 2400

Methotrexate Sodium (Potential for reduced tubular secretion of methotrexate and possible increased methotrexate toxicity as shown in animal model; caution is recommended). Products include:
- Methotrexate Sodium Tablets, Injection, for Injection and LPF Injection ... 1322

Methyclothiazide (Potential for sulfonamide toxicity). Products include:
- Enduron Tablets ... 424

Metipranolol Hydrochloride (Reduced antihypertensive effect of beta blockers). Products include:
- OptiPranolol (Metipranolol 0.3%) Sterile Ophthalmic Solution ... ⊚ 256

Metoprolol Succinate (Reduced antihypertensive effect of beta blockers). Products include:
- Toprol-XL Tablets ... 560

Metoprolol Tartrate (Reduced antihypertensive effect of beta blockers). Products include:
- ⸺ssor Tablets ... 848
- ⸺ssor HCT Tablets ... 850

Moexipril Hydrochloride (Co-administration may potentiate renal disease states). Products include:
- Univasc Tablets ... 2553

Nadolol (Reduced antihypertensive effect of beta blockers).
- No products indexed under this heading.

Naproxen (Concurrent use of Naprelan with other naproxen products should be avoided since they all circulate in the plasma as the naproxen anion). Products include:
- Anaprox/Naprosyn ... 2277

Penbutolol Sulfate (Reduced antihypertensive effect of beta blockers). Products include:
- Levatol Tablets ... 2547

Phenytoin (Potential for hydantoin toxicity). Products include:
- Dilantin Infatabs ... 1967
- Dilantin-125 Suspension ... 1969

Phenytoin Sodium (Potential for hydantoin toxicity). Products include:
- Dilantin Kapseals ... 1965

Pindolol (Reduced antihypertensive effect of beta blockers). Products include:
- Visken Tablets ... 2428

Polythiazide (Potential for sulfonamide toxicity). Products include:
- Minizide Capsules ... 2016

Probenecid (Probenecid given concurrently increases naproxen anion plasma levels and extends its plasma half-life significantly). Products include:
- Benemid Tablets ... 1651
- ColBENEMID Tablets ... 1662

Propranolol Hydrochloride (Reduced antihypertensive effect of beta blockers). Products include:
- Inderal ... 2834
- Inderal LA Long Acting Capsules ... 2836
- Inderide Tablets ... 2838
- Inderide LA Long Acting Capsules ... 2840

Quinapril Hydrochloride (Co-administration may potentiate renal disease states). Products include:
- Accupril Tablets ... 1950

Ramipril (Co-administration may potentiate renal disease states). Products include:
- Altace Tablets ... 1238

Sotalol Hydrochloride (Reduced antihypertensive effect of beta blockers). Products include:
- Betapace Tablets ... 637

Spirapril Hydrochloride (Co-administration may potentiate renal disease states).
- No products indexed under this heading.

Sulfacytine (Potential for sulfonamide toxicity).

Sulfamethizole (Potential for sulfonamide toxicity). Products include:
- Urobiotic-250 Capsules ... 2038

Sulfamethoxazole (Potential for sulfonamide toxicity). Products include:
- Bactrim DS Tablets ... 2257
- Bactrim I.V. Infusion ... 2255
- Bactrim ... 2257
- Gantanol Tablets ... 2285
- Septra ... 1146
- Septra I.V. Infusion ... 1142
- Septra I.V. Infusion ADD-Vantage Vials ... 1144
- Septra ... 1146

Sulfasalazine (Potential for sulfonamide toxicity). Products include:
- Azulfidine ... 2059

Sulfinpyrazone (Potential for sulfonamide toxicity). Products include:
- Anturane ... 823

Sulfisoxazole (Potential for sulfonamide toxicity). Products include:
- Gantrisin Tablets ... 2286

Sulfisoxazole Diolamine (Potential for sulfonamide toxicity).
- No products indexed under this heading.

Timolol Hemihydrate (Reduced antihypertensive effect of beta blockers). Products include:
- Betimol 0.25%, 0.5% ... ⊚ 259

Timolol Maleate (Reduced antihypertensive effect of beta blockers). Products include:
- Blocadren Tablets ... 1654
- Timolide Tablets ... 1791
- Timoptic in Ocudose ... 1796
- Timoptic Sterile Ophthalmic Solution ... 1794
- Timoptic-XE ... 1798

Tolazamide (Potential for sulfonylurea toxicity).
- No products indexed under this heading.

Tolbutamide (Potential for sulfonylurea toxicity).
- No products indexed under this heading.

Trandolapril (Co-administration may potentiate renal disease states). Products include:
- Mavik Tablets ... 1407

Warfarin Sodium (Naproxen may decrease platelet aggregation and prolong bleeding time; caution is advised if co-administered). Products include:
- Coumadin ... 941

Food Interactions
Food, unspecified (Food causes a slight decrease in the rate of naproxen absorption following Naprelan administration).

NAPROSYN SUSPENSION
(Naproxen) ... 2277
See EC-Naprosyn Delayed-Release Tablets

NAPROSYN TABLETS
(Naproxen) ... 2277
See EC-Naprosyn Delayed-Release Tablets

NARCAN INJECTION
(Naloxone Hydrochloride) ... 950
May interact with:

Cardiotoxic drugs, unspecified (Narcan should be used with caution in patients who have received potentially cardiotoxic drugs).

NARDIL
(Phenelzine Sulfate) ... 1977
May interact with monoamine oxidase inhibitors, antihypertensives, sympathomimetics, dibenzazepines, tricyclic antidepressants, phenylpropanolamine containing anorectics, alpha adrenergic stimulants, antidepressant drugs, anorexiants, beta blockers, thiazides, narcotic analgesics, barbiturates, catecholamine depleting drugs, and certain other agents. Compounds in these categories include:

Acebutolol Hydrochloride (Exaggerated hypotensive effects). Products include:
- Sectral Capsules ... 2914

Albuterol (Potentiation of sympathomimetic agents and related compounds resulting in hypertensive crises; concurrent use is contraindicated). Products include:
- Proventil Inhalation Aerosol ... 2524
- Ventolin Inhalation Aerosol and Refill ... 1170

Albuterol Sulfate (Potentiation of sympathomimetic agents and related compounds resulting in hypertensive crises; concurrent use is contraindicated). Products include:
- Airet Albuterol Sulfate Inhalation Solution ... 1602
- Albuterol Sulfate, USP Solution for Inhalation, Arm-a-Med ... 522
- Proventil Inhalation Solution 0.083% ... 2527
- Proventil Repetabs Tablets ... 2529
- Proventil Solution for Inhalation 0.5% ... 2525
- Proventil Syrup ... 2525
- Proventil Tablets ... 2529
- Ventolin Inhalation Solution ... 1171
- Ventolin Nebules Inhalation Solution ... 1172
- Ventolin Rotacaps for Inhalation ... 1173
- Ventolin Syrup ... 1175
- Ventolin Tablets ... 1176
- Volmax Extended-Release Tablets ... 1835

Alfentanil Hydrochloride (Contraindication warning for meperidine is extended to other narcotics). Products include:
- Alfenta Injection ... 1334

Amitriptyline Hydrochloride (Concurrent or in rapid succession administration is contraindicated). Products include:
- Elavil ... 2945
- Etrafon ... 2495
- Limbitrol ... 2333
- Triavil Tablets ... 1800

Amlodipine Besylate (Exaggerated hypotensive effects). Products include:
- Lotrel Capsules ... 858
- Norvasc Tablets ... 2020

Amoxapine (Concurrent or in rapid succession administration is contraindicated). Products include:
- Asendin Tablets ... 1419

Amphetamine Resins (Potentiation of sympathomimetic agents and related compounds resulting in hypertensive crises; concurrent use is contraindicated).
- No products indexed under this heading.

Amphetamine Sulfate (Potentiation of sympathomimetic agents and related compounds resulting in hypertensive crises; concurrent use is contraindicated). Products include:
- Adderall Tablets ... 2209

Aprobarbital (Potential for increased hypnosis).
- No products indexed under this heading.

Atenolol (Exaggerated hypotensive effects). Products include:
- Tenoretic Tablets ... 2963
- Tenormin Tablets and I.V. Injection ... 2965

Benazepril Hydrochloride (Exaggerated hypotensive effects). Products include:
- Lotensin Tablets ... 852
- Lotensin HCT Tablets ... 855
- Lotrel Capsules ... 858

Bendroflumethiazide (Exaggerated hypotensive effects).
- No products indexed under this heading.

Benzphetamine Hydrochloride (Concurrent administration is not recommended).
- No products indexed under this heading.

Betaxolol Hydrochloride (Exaggerated hypotensive effects). Products include:
- Betoptic Ophthalmic Solution ... 465
- Betoptic S Ophthalmic Suspension ... 467
- Kerlone Tablets ... 2588

Bisoprolol Fumarate (Exaggerated hypotensive effects). Products include:
- Zebeta Tablets ... 1457

◧ Described in PDR For Nonprescription Drugs   (⊚ Described in PDR For Ophthalmology)

Ziac ... 1459

Buprenorphine (Contraindication warning for meperidine is extended to other narcotics). Products include:
Buprenex Injectable ... 2170

Bupropion Hydrochloride (Concurrent administration is contraindicated; at least 14 days should elapse between discontinuation of an MAOI inhibitor and initiation of treatment with bupropion hydrochloride). Products include:
Wellbutrin Tablets ... 1177

Buspirone Hydrochloride (Elevated blood pressure; concurrent therapy is contraindicated). Products include:
BuSpar Tablets ... 738

Butabarbital (Potential for increased hypnosis).
No products indexed under this heading.

Butalbital (Potential for increased hypnosis). Products include:
Axocet Capsules ... 2469
Esgic-plus Capsules ... 1012
Esgic-plus Tablets ... 1012
Fioricet Tablets ... 2386
Fioricet with Codeine Capsules ... 2387
Fiorinal Capsules ... 2388
Fiorinal with Codeine Capsules ... 2390
Fiorinal Tablets ... 2388
Phrenilin ... 790
Sedapap Tablets 50 mg/650 mg ... 1826

Caffeine-containing medications (Concurrent use with excessive caffeine intake should be avoided).

Captopril (Exaggerated hypotensive effects). Products include:
Capoten Tablets ... 740
Capozide Tablets ... 744

Carbamazepine (Concurrent or in rapid succession administration is contraindicated). Products include:
Atretol Tablets ... 569
Tegretol/Tegretol-XR ... 870

Carteolol Hydrochloride (Exaggerated hypotensive effects). Products include:
Cartrol Tablets ... 413
Ocupress Ophthalmic Solution, 1% Sterile ... ◉ 297

Chlorothiazide (Exaggerated hypotensive effects). Products include:
Aldoclor Tablets ... 1638
Diupres Tablets ... 1691
Diuril Oral ... 1694

Chlorothiazide Sodium (Exaggerated hypotensive effects). Products include:
Diuril Sodium Intravenous ... 1693

Chlorthalidone (Exaggerated hypotensive effects). Products include:
Combipres Tablets ... 682
Tenoretic Tablets ... 2963
Thalitone ... 1293

Clomipramine Hydrochloride (Concurrent or in rapid succession administration is contraindicated). Products include:
Anafranil Capsules ... 819

Clonidine (Exaggerated hypotensive effects). Products include:
Catapres-TTS ... 680

Clonidine Hydrochloride (Exaggerated hypotensive effects). Products include:
Catapres Tablets ... 679
Combipres Tablets ... 682

Clozapine (Concurrent or in rapid succession administration is contraindicated). Products include:
Clozaril Tablets ... 2377

Cocaine Hydrochloride (Potentiation of sympathomimetic agents and related compounds resulting in hypertensive crises; concurrent use is contraindicated). Products include:
Cocaine Hydrochloride Topical Solutions ... 529

Codeine Phosphate (Contraindication warning for meperidine is extended to other narcotics). Products include:
Brontex ... 2130
Dimetane-DC Cough Syrup ... 2232
Fioricet with Codeine Capsules ... 2387
Fiorinal with Codeine Capsules ... 2390
Nucofed ... 2225
Phenergan with Codeine ... 2883
Phenergan VC with Codeine ... 2888
Robitussin A-C Syrup ... 2248
Robitussin-DAC Syrup ... 2249
Ryna ... ND 804
Soma Compound w/Codeine Tablets ... 2784
Tylenol with Codeine ... 1592

Cyclobenzaprine Hydrochloride (Possibility of unspecified adverse drug interaction; concurrent or in rapid succession administration should be avoided). Products include:
Flexeril Tablets ... 1701

Deserpidine (Exaggerated hypotensive effects; exercise caution).
No products indexed under this heading.

Desipramine Hydrochloride (Concurrent or in rapid succession administration is contraindicated). Products include:
Norpramin Tablets ... 1273

Dextroamphetamine (Hypertensive crises; concurrent administration is not recommended).
No products indexed under this heading.

Dextroamphetamine Sulfate (Hypertensive crises; concurrent administration is not recommended). Products include:
Adderall Tablets ... 2209
Dexedrine ... 2648
DextroStat-Dextroamphetamine Sulfate Tablets ... 2211

Dextromethorphan Hydrobromide (Concurrent administration is not recommended; may cause drowsiness and bizarre behavior). Products include:
Alka-Seltzer Plus Cold & Cough Medicine ... ND 611
Alka-Seltzer Plus Cold & Cough Medicine Liqui-Gels ... ND 612
Alka-Seltzer Plus Flu & Body Aches Effervescent Tablets ... ND 612
Alka-Seltzer Plus Flu & Body Aches Liqui-Gels Non-Drowsy Formula ... ND 613
Alka-Seltzer Plus Night-Time Cold Medicine ... ND 611
Alka-Seltzer Plus Night-Time Cold Medicine Liqui-Gels ... ND 612
Benylin Adult Formula Cough Suppressant ... ND 817
Benylin Expectorant ... ND 816
Benylin Multisymptom ... ND 816
Benylin Pediatric Cough Suppressant ... ND 817
Bromfed-DM Cough Syrup ... 1832
Cerose DM ... ND 853
Cheracol D Cough Formula ... ND 740
Cheracol Plus Head Cold/Cough Formula ... ND 741
Children's TYLENOL Cold Plus Cough Multi Symptom Chewable Tablets and Liquid ... 1560
Children's TYLENOL Flu Suspension Liquid ... 1560
Children's Vicks NyQuil Cold/Cough Relief ... ND 731
Comtrex Multi-Symptom ... ND 638
Comtrex Non-Drowsy ... ND 640
Contac Day & Night Cold/Flu Caplets ... ND 772
Contac Severe Cold and Flu Formula Caplets ... ND 773
Contac Severe Cold & Flu Non-Drowsy ... ND 774
Coricidin Cough + Cold Tablets ... ND 760
Cough-X Lozenges ... ND 606
Diabe-Tuss DM Syrup ... 1948
Dimetane-DX Cough Syrup ... 2233
Dimetapp Cold & Cough Liqui-Gels ... ND 839
Dimetapp DM Elixir ... ND 840
Dorcol Children's Cough Syrup ... ND 748
Drixoral Cough Liquid Caps ... ND 762
Drixoral Cough + Congestion Liquid Caps ... ND 763
Drixoral Cough + Sore Throat Liquid Caps ... ND 763
Humibid DM Tablets ... 1612
Novahistine DMX ... ND 782
PediaCare Cough-Cold Chewable Tablets and Liquid ... 1569
PediaCare Infants' Drops Decongestant Plus Cough ... 1569
PediaCare NightRest Cough-Cold Liquid ... 1569
Pediatric Vicks 44d Cough & Head Congestion Relief ... ND 736
Pediatric Vicks 44e Cough & Chest Congestion Relief ... ND 737
Pediatric Vicks 44m Cough & Cold Relief ... ND 737
Pertussin Adult Extra Strength ... ND 630
Pertussin Children's Strength ... ND 630
Phenergan with Dextromethorphan 2885
Robitussin Cold & Cough Liqui-Gels ... ND 844
Robitussin Cold, Cough & Flu Liqui-Gels ... ND 844
Robitussin Maximum Strength Cough Suppressant ... ND 847
Robitussin Maximum Strength Cough & Cold ... ND 847
Robitussin Night-Time Cold Formula ... ND 847
Robitussin Pediatric Cough & Cold Formula ... ND 848
Robitussin Pediatric Cough Suppressant ... ND 848
Robitussin Pediatric Drops ... ND 849
Robitussin-CF ... ND 846
Robitussin-DM ... ND 846
Safe Tussin 30 Liquid ... 1413
Sucrets 4-Hour Cough Suppressant ... ND 785
Sudafed Children's Cold & Cough Liquid Medication ... ND 825
Sudafed Cold and Cough Liquid Caps ... ND 826
Sudafed Severe Cold Formula Caplets ... ND 828
Sudafed Severe Cold Formula Tablets ... ND 828
Syn-Rx DM Tablets ... 1623
TheraFlu Flu, Cold and Cough Medicine ... ND 750
TheraFlu Maximum Strength Nighttime Flu, Cold & Cough Medicine ... ND 751
TheraFlu Maximum Strength Non-Drowsy Formula Flu, Cold & Cough Medicine ... ND 751
TheraFlu Maximum Strength, Non-Drowsy Formula Flu, Cold and Cough Caplets ... ND 752
Triaminic AM Cough and Decongestant Formula ... ND 753
Triaminic Night Time ... ND 754
Triaminic Sore Throat Formula ... ND 755
Triaminic Triaminicol Cold & Cough ... ND 756
Triaminic DM Syrup ... ND 756
Tussi-Organidin DM NR Liquid and DM-S NR Liquid ... 2786
TYLENOL Cold Medication, Multi-Symptom Formula Tablets and Caplets ... 1572
TYLENOL Cold Medication, Multi-Symptom Hot Liquid Packets ... 1572
TYLENOL Cold Medication, No Drowsiness Formula Caplets and Gelcaps ... 1572
TYLENOL Cold Severe Congestion Caplets ... 1573
TYLENOL Cough Medication, Multi Symptom ... 1574
TYLENOL Cough Medication with Decongestant, Multi Symptom ... 1574
TYLENOL Flu No Drowsiness Formula, Maximum Strength Gelcaps ... 1575
Vicks 44 Cough Relief ... ND 728
Vicks 44 LiquiCaps Cough, Cold & Flu Relief ... ND 728
Vicks 44 LiquiCaps Non-Drowsy Cough & Cold Relief ... ND 729
Vicks 44D Cough & Head Congestion Relief ... ND 728
Vicks 44E Cough & Chest Congestion Relief ... ND 729
Vicks 44M Cough, Cold & Flu Relief ... ND 729
Vicks DayQuil LiquiCaps/Liquid Multi-Symptom Cold/Flu Relief ... ND 734
Vicks Nyquil Hot Therapy ... ND 735
Vicks NyQuil LiquiCaps/Liquid Multi-Symptom Cold/Flu Relief, Original and Cherry Flavors ... ND 736

Dextromethorphan Polistirex (Concurrent administration is not recommended; may cause drowsiness and bizarre behavior). Products include:
Delsym Extended-Release Suspension ... ND 670

Dezocine (Contraindication warning for meperidine is extended to other narcotics). Products include:
Dalgan Injection ... 529

Diazoxide (Exaggerated hypotensive effects). Products include:
Hyperstat I.V. Injection ... 2504
Proglycem ... 575

Diethylpropion Hydrochloride (Concurrent administration is not recommended).
No products indexed under this heading.

Diltiazem Hydrochloride (Exaggerated hypotensive effects). Products include:
Cardizem CD Capsules ... 1251
Cardizem SR Capsules ... 1255
Cardizem Injectable ... 1253
Cardizem Tablets ... 1257
Dilacor XR Extended-release Capsules ... 2183
Tiazac Capsules ... 1019

Dobutamine Hydrochloride (Potentiation of sympathomimetic agents and related compounds resulting in hypertensive crises; concurrent use is contraindicated). Products include:
Dobutrex Solution Vials ... 1480

Dopamine Hydrochloride (Potentiation of sympathomimetic agents and related compounds resulting in hypertensive crises; concurrent use is contraindicated).
No products indexed under this heading.

Doxazosin Mesylate (Exaggerated hypotensive effects). Products include:
Cardura Tablets ... 1993

Doxepin Hydrochloride (Concurrent or in rapid succession administration is contraindicated). Products include:
Adapin Capsules ... 1542
Sinequan ... 2028
Zonalon Cream ... 1042

Enalapril Maleate (Exaggerated hypotensive effects). Products include:
Vaseretic Tablets ... 1810
Vasotec Tablets ... 1816

Enalaprilat (Exaggerated hypotensive effects). Products include:
Vasotec I.V. ... 1814

Ephedrine Hydrochloride (Potentiation of sympathomimetic agents and related compounds resulting in hypertensive crises; concurrent use is contraindicated). Products include:
Primatene Tablets ... ND 844
Quadrinal Tablets ... 1398

IMPORTANT NOTE: Always consult each drug listing in the patient's regimen for possible interactions.

Nardil — Interactions Index

Ephedrine Sulfate (Potentiation of sympathomimetic agents and related compounds resulting in hypertensive crises; concurrent use is contraindicated). Products include:
- Marax Tablets & DF Syrup 2015

Ephedrine Tannate (Potentiation of sympathomimetic agents and related compounds resulting in hypertensive crises; concurrent use is contraindicated). Products include:
- Rynatuss 2782

Epinephrine (Potentiation of sympathomimetic agents and related compounds resulting in hypertensive crises; concurrent use is contraindicated). Products include:
- EPIFRIN .... ⊚ 237
- EpiPen 808
- Marcaine with Epinephrine 2446
- Primatene Mist .... ▣ 843
- Sensorcaine with Epinephrine Injection 554
- Sus-Phrine Injection 1017
- Xylocaine with Epinephrine Injections 562

Epinephrine Bitartrate (Potentiation of sympathomimetic agents and related compounds resulting in hypertensive crises; concurrent use is contraindicated). Products include:
- Sensorcaine-MPF with Epinephrine Injection 554

Epinephrine Hydrochloride (Potentiation of sympathomimetic agents and related compounds resulting in hypertensive crises; concurrent use is contraindicated). Products include:
- Ana-Kit Anaphylaxis Emergency Treatment Kit 611

Esmolol Hydrochloride (Exaggerated hypotensive effects). Products include:
- Brevibloc (esmolol HCl) Injection 1860

Felodipine (Exaggerated hypotensive effects). Products include:
- Plendil Extended-Release Tablets 514

Fenfluramine Hydrochloride (Concurrent administration is not recommended). Products include:
- Pondimin Tablets 2239

Fentanyl (Contraindication warning for meperidine is extended to other narcotics). Products include:
- Duragesic Transdermal System 1336

Fentanyl Citrate (Contraindication warning for meperidine is extended to other narcotics). Products include:
- Sublimaze Injection 463

Fluoxetine Hydrochloride (Concurrent or in rapid succession administration is contraindicated; serious reactions including hyperthermia, rigidity, myoclonic movements and death have been reported). Products include:
- Prozac Pulvules & Liquid, Oral Solution 935

Fosinopril Sodium (Exaggerated hypotensive effects). Products include:
- Monopril Tablets 762

Furazolidone (Hypertensive crises; at least 10 days should elapse between discontinuation of Nardil and institution of another MAOI). Products include:
- Furoxone 2221

Furosemide (Exaggerated hypotensive effects). Products include:
- Lasix Injection, Oral Solution and Tablets 1267

Guanabenz Acetate (Exaggerated hypotensive effects).
No products indexed under this heading.

Guanethidine Monosulfate (Exaggerated hypotensive effects; contraindication). Products include:
- Esimil Tablets 840
- Ismelin Tablets 845

Hexobarbital (Potential for increased hypnosis).

Hydralazine Hydrochloride (Exaggerated hypotensive effects). Products include:
- Apresazide Capsules 824
- Apresoline Hydrochloride Tablets 826
- Hydralazine Hydrochloride Injection USP 2712
- Ser-Ap-Es Tablets 867

Hydrochlorothiazide (Exaggerated hypotensive effects). Products include:
- Aldactazide Tablets 2556
- Aldoril Tablets 1644
- Apresazide Capsules 824
- Capozide Tablets 744
- Dyazide Capsules 2653
- Esidrix Tablets 839
- Esimil Tablets 840
- HydroDIURIL Tablets 1716
- Hydropres Tablets 1718
- Hyzaar Tablets 1720
- Inderide Tablets 2838
- Inderide LA Long Acting Capsules 2840
- Lopressor HCT Tablets 850
- Lotensin HCT Tablets 855
- Moduretic Tablets 1748
- Oretic Tablets 450
- Prinzide Tablets 1780
- Ser-Ap-Es Tablets 867
- Timolide Tablets 1791
- Vaseretic Tablets 1810
- Zestoretic Tablets 2968
- Ziac 1459

Hydrocodone Bitartrate (Contraindication warning for meperidine is extended to other narcotics). Products include:
- Codiclear DH Syrup 808
- Duratuss HD Elixir 2750
- Histussin D Liquid 670
- Hycodan Tablets and Syrup 946
- Hycomine Compound Tablets 948
- Hycomine 947
- Hycotuss Expectorant Syrup 950
- Hydrocet Capsules 787
- Lorcet 10/650 Tablets 1016
- Lortab 2751
- Tussend 1830
- Tussend Expectorant 1831
- Vicodin Tablets 1404
- Vicodin ES Tablets 1405
- Vicodin HP Tablets 1403
- Vicodin Tuss Expectorant 1406
- Zydone Capsules 967

Hydrocodone Polistirex (Contraindication warning for meperidine is extended to other narcotics). Products include:
- Tussionex Pennkinetic Extended-Release Suspension 1624

Hydroflumethiazide (Exaggerated hypotensive effects). Products include:
- Diucardin Tablets 2824

Hydromorphone Hydrochloride (Contraindication warning for meperidine is extended to other narcotics). Products include:
- Dilaudid Ampules 1382
- Dilaudid Cough Syrup 1383
- Dilaudid-HP Injection 1384
- Dilaudid-HP Lyophilized Powder 250 mg 1384
- Dilaudid 1382
- Dilaudid Oral Liquid 1386
- Dilaudid 1382
- Dilaudid Tablets - 8 mg 1386

Imipramine Hydrochloride (Concurrent or in rapid succession administration is contraindicated). Products include:
- Tofranil Ampuls 873
- Tofranil Tablets 875

Imipramine Pamoate (Concurrent or in rapid succession administration is contraindicated). Products include:
- Tofranil-PM Capsules 876

Indapamide (Exaggerated hypotensive effects).
No products indexed under this heading.

Isocarboxazid (Hypertensive crises; at least 10 days should elapse between discontinuation of Nardil and institution of another MAOI).
No products indexed under this heading.

Isoproterenol Hydrochloride (Potentiation of sympathomimetic agents and related compounds resulting in hypertensive crises; concurrent use is contraindicated). Products include:
- Isuprel Hydrochloride Solution 2443
- Isuprel Injection 2441
- Isuprel Mistometer 2442

Isoproterenol Sulfate (Potentiation of sympathomimetic agents and related compounds resulting in hypertensive crises; concurrent use is contraindicated). Products include:
- Norisodrine with Calcium Iodide Syrup 446

Isradipine (Exaggerated hypotensive effects). Products include:
- DynaCirc Capsules 2381
- DynaCirc CR Tablets 2383

Labetalol Hydrochloride (Exaggerated hypotensive effects). Products include:
- Normodyne Injection 2519
- Normodyne Tablets 2522
- Trandate 1158

Levobunolol Hydrochloride (Exaggerated hypotensive effects). Products include:
- Betagan .... ⊚ 230

Levodopa (Potentiation of sympathomimetic agents and related compounds, including levodopa, resulting in hypertensive crises; concurrent use is contraindicated). Products include:
- Atamet Tablets 567
- Larodopa Tablets 2296
- Sinemet Tablets 959
- Sinemet CR Tablets 961

Levorphanol Tartrate (Contraindication warning for meperidine is extended to other narcotics). Products include:
- Levo-Dromoran 2297

Lisinopril (Exaggerated hypotensive effects). Products include:
- Prinivil Tablets 1776
- Prinzide Tablets 1780
- Zestoretic Tablets 2968
- Zestril Tablets 2972

Losartan Potassium (Exaggerated hypotensive effects). Products include:
- Cozaar Tablets 1668
- Hyzaar Tablets 1720

Maprotiline Hydrochloride (Concurrent or in rapid succession administration is contraindicated). Products include:
- Ludiomil Tablets 861

Mazindol (Concurrent administration is not recommended). Products include:
- Sanorex Tablets 2423

Mecamylamine Hydrochloride (Exaggerated hypotensive effects). Products include:
- Inversine Tablets 1729

Meperidine Hydrochloride (Co-administration with a single dose of meperidine has resulted in excitation, seizures, delirium, hyperpyrexia, circulatory collapse, coma, and death; concurrent use is contraindicated). Products include:
- Demerol 2438
- Mepergan Injection 2859

Mephobarbital (Potential for increased hypnosis). Products include:
- Mebaral Tablets 2452

Metaproterenol Sulfate (Potentiation of sympathomimetic agents and related compounds resulting in hypertensive crises; concurrent use is contraindicated). Products include:
- Alupent 672
- Metaproterenol Sulfate Inhalation Solution, USP, Arm-a-Med 547

Metaraminol Bitartrate (Potentiation of sympathomimetic agents and related compounds resulting in hypertensive crises; concurrent use is contraindicated). Products include:
- Aramine Injection 1649

Methadone Hydrochloride (Contraindication warning for meperidine is extended to other narcotics). Products include:
- Methadone Hydrochloride Oral Concentrate 2356
- Methadone Hydrochloride Oral Solution & Tablets 2357

Methamphetamine Hydrochloride (Concurrent administration is not recommended). Products include:
- Desoxyn Gradumet Tablets 422

Methoxamine Hydrochloride (Potentiation of sympathomimetic agents and related compounds resulting in hypertensive crises; concurrent use is contraindicated). Products include:
- Vasoxyl Injection 1169

Methyclothiazide (Exaggerated hypotensive effects). Products include:
- Enduron Tablets 424

Methyldopa (Potentiation of sympathomimetic agents and related compounds, including methyldopa, resulting in hypertensive crises; concurrent use is contraindicated). Products include:
- Aldoclor Tablets 1638
- Aldomet Oral 1640
- Aldoril Tablets 1644

Methyldopate Hydrochloride (Potentiation of sympathomimetic agents and related compounds, including methyldopa, resulting in hypertensive crises; concurrent use is contraindicated). Products include:
- Aldomet Ester HCl Injection 1642

Methylphenidate Hydrochloride (Potentiation of sympathomimetic agents and related compounds resulting in hypertensive crises; concurrent use is contraindicated). Products include:
- Ritalin 866

Metipranolol Hydrochloride (Exaggerated hypotensive effects). Products include:
- OptiPranolol (Metipranolol 0.3%) Sterile Ophthalmic Solution .... ⊚ 256

Metolazone (Exaggerated hypotensive effects). Products include:
- Mykrox Tablets 1617
- Zaroxolyn Tablets 1625

Metoprolol Succinate (Exaggerated hypotensive effects). Products include:
- Toprol-XL Tablets 560

(▣ Described in PDR For Nonprescription Drugs)   (⊚ Described in PDR For Ophthalmology)

Interactions Index

Metoprolol Tartrate (Exaggerated hypotensive effects). Products include:
- Lopressor ... 848
- Lopressor HCT Tablets ... 850

Metyrosine (Exaggerated hypotensive effects). Products include:
- Demser Capsules ... 1690

Minoxidil (Exaggerated hypotensive effects).
No products indexed under this heading.

Moexipril Hydrochloride (Exaggerated hypotensive effects). Products include:
- Univasc Tablets ... 2553

Morphine Sulfate (Contraindication warning for meperidine is extended to other narcotics). Products include:
- Astramorph/PF Injection, USP (Preservative-Free) ... 526
- Duramorph Injection ... 983
- Infumorph 200 and Infumorph 500 Sterile Solutions ... 985
- Kadian Capsules ... 2948
- MS Contin Tablets ... 2149
- MSIR ... 2152
- Oramorph SR (Morphine Sulfate Sustained Release Tablets) ... 2359
- RMS Suppositories CII ... 2766
- Roxanol ... 2365

Nadolol (Exaggerated hypotensive effects).
No products indexed under this heading.

Naphazoline Hydrochloride (Contraindicated). Products include:
- Albalon Solution with Liquifilm ... ⓔ 229
- Clear Eyes ACR Astringent/Lubricant Eye Redness Reliever Eye Drops ... ⓔ 314
- Clear Eyes Lubricant Eye Redness Reliever ... ⓔ 314
- 4-Way Fast Acting Nasal Spray (regular & mentholated) ... ⓔⓓ 644
- Naphcon-A Ophthalmic Solution ... 469
- OcuHist ... ⓔ 300
- Privine ... ⓔⓓ 663
- Vasocon-A ... ⓔ 263

Nefazodone Hydrochloride (Concurrent or in rapid succession administration is contraindicated). Products include:
- Serzone Tablets ... 776

Nicardipine Hydrochloride (Exaggerated hypotensive effects). Products include:
- Cardene Capsules ... 2261
- Cardene I.V. ... 2815
- Cardene SR Capsules ... 2264

Nifedipine (Exaggerated hypotensive effects). Products include:
- Adalat Capsules (10 mg and 20 mg) ... 580
- Adalat CC ... 582
- Procardia Capsules ... 2024
- Procardia XL Extended Release Tablets ... 2026

Nisoldipine (Exaggerated hypotensive effects). Products include:
- Sular Tablets ... 2961

Nitroglycerin (Exaggerated hypotensive effects). Products include:
- Deponit NTG Transdermal Delivery System ... 2541
- Nitro-Bid IV ... 1270
- Nitro-Bid Ointment ... 1272
- Nitro-Dur (nitroglycerin) Transdermal Infusion System ... 1365
- Nitrolingual Spray ... 2193
- Nitrostat Tablets ... 1981
- Transderm-Nitro Transdermal Therapeutic System ... 878

Norepinephrine Bitartrate (Potentiation of sympathomimetic agents and related compounds resulting in hypertensive crises; concurrent use is contraindicated). Products include:
- Levophed Bitartrate Injection ... 2445

Nortriptyline Hydrochloride (Hypertensive crises; concurrent or in rapid succession administration is contraindicated). Products include:
- Pamelor ... 2409

Opium Alkaloids (Contraindication warning for meperidine is extended to other narcotics).
No products indexed under this heading.

Oxycodone Hydrochloride (Contraindication warning for meperidine is extended to other narcotics). Products include:
- OxyContin Tablets ... 2163
- OxyIR Capsules ... 2167
- Percocet Tablets ... 955
- Percodan Tablets ... 955
- Percodan-Demi Tablets ... 956
- Roxicodone Tablets, Oral Solution & Intensol (Oxycodone) ... 2366
- Tylox Capsules ... 1593

Oxymetazoline Hydrochloride (Contraindicated). Products include:
- Afrin ... ⓔⓓ 757
- Duration 12 Hour Nasal Spray ... ⓔⓓ 766
- 4-Way 12 Hour Nasal Spray ... ⓔⓓ 644
- Neo-Synephrine Maximum Strength 12 Hour Nasal Spray ... ⓔⓓ 624
- Neo-Synephrine 12 Hour ... ⓔⓓ 624
- 12 Hour Nostrilla ... ⓔⓓ 660
- Vicks Sinex 12-Hour Nasal Decongestant Spray and Ultra Fine Mist ... ⓔⓓ 738
- Visine L.R. Eye Drops ... ⓔⓓ 719
- Visine L.R. Eye Drops ... ⓔ 301

Paroxetine Hydrochloride (Concurrent or in rapid succession administration is contraindicated). Products include:
- Paxil Tablets ... 2681

Penbutolol Sulfate (Exaggerated hypotensive effects). Products include:
- Levatol Tablets ... 2547

Pentobarbital Sodium (Potential for increased hypnosis). Products include:
- Nembutal Sodium Capsules ... 440
- Nembutal Sodium Solution ... 442
- Nembutal Sodium Suppositories ... 444

Phendimetrazine Tartrate (Concurrent administration is not recommended). Products include:
- Bontril Slow-Release Capsules ... 786
- Prelu-2 Timed Release Capsules ... 687

Phenmetrazine Hydrochloride (Concurrent administration is not recommended).
No products indexed under this heading.

Phenobarbital (Potential for increased hypnosis). Products include:
- Arco-Lase Plus Tablets ... 513
- Bellergal-S Tablets ... 2375
- Donnatal ... 2234
- Donnatal Extentabs ... 2234
- Donnatal Tablets ... 2234
- Phenobarbital Elixir and Tablets ... 1523
- Quadrinal Tablets ... 1398

Phenoxybenzamine Hydrochloride (Exaggerated hypotensive effects). Products include:
- Dibenzyline Capsules ... 2650

Phentolamine Mesylate (Exaggerated hypotensive effects). Products include:
- Regitine Vials ... 864

d-Phenylalanine (Potentiation of sympathomimetic agents and related compounds resulting in hypertensive crises; concurrent use is contraindicated).

L-Phenylalanine (Potentiation of sympathomimetic agents and related compounds resulting in hypertensive crises; concurrent use is contraindicated).

Phenylephrine Bitartrate (Potentiation of sympathomimetic agents and related compounds resulting in hypertensive crises; concurrent use is contraindicated).
No products indexed under this heading.

Phenylephrine Hydrochloride (Potentiation of sympathomimetic agents and related compounds resulting in hypertensive crises; concurrent use is contraindicated). Products include:
- Atrohist Plus Tablets ... 1605
- Cerose DM ... ⓔⓓ 853
- D.A. II Tablets ... 972
- D.A. Chewable Tablets ... 970
- Dura-Vent/DA Tablets ... 972
- Extendryl ... 1003
- 4-Way Fast Acting Nasal Spray (regular & mentholated) ... ⓔⓓ 644
- Hemoril ... ⓔⓓ 797
- Hycomine Compound Tablets ... 948
- Neo-Synephrine Hydrochloride 1% Carpuject ... 2455
- Neo-Synephrine Hydrochloride 1% Injection ... 2455
- Neo-Synephrine Hydrochloride (Ophthalmic) ... 2456
- Neo-Synephrine ... ⓔⓓ 624
- Novahistine Elixir ... ⓔⓓ 782
- Phenergan VC ... 2886
- Phenergan VC with Codeine ... 2888
- Preparation H ... ⓔⓓ 842
- Tympagesic Ear Drops ... 2476
- Vicks Sinex Nasal Spray and Ultra Fine Mist ... ⓔⓓ 738

Phenylephrine Tannate (Potentiation of sympathomimetic agents and related compounds resulting in hypertensive crises; concurrent use is contraindicated). Products include:
- Atrohist Pediatric Suspension ... 1604
- Atrohist Pediatric Suspension Dye-Free ... 1604
- Rynatan ... 2781
- Rynatuss ... 2782

Phenylpropanolamine Containing Anorectics (Concurrent administration is not recommended).

Phenylpropanolamine Hydrochloride (Potentiation of sympathomimetic agents and related compounds resulting in hypertensive crises; concurrent use is contraindicated). Products include:
- Acutrim ... ⓔⓓ 648
- Atrohist Plus Tablets ... 1605
- BC Cold Powder Multi-Symptom Formula (Cold-Sinus-Allergy) ... ⓔⓓ 631
- BC Cold Powder Non-Drowsy Formula (Cold-Sinus) ... ⓔⓓ 631
- Cheracol Plus Head Cold/Cough Formula ... ⓔⓓ 741
- Comtrex Multi-Symptom Cold Reliever Liqui-Gels ... ⓔⓓ 638
- Comtrex Multi-Symptom Non-Drowsy Liqui-gels ... ⓔⓓ 640
- Contac Continuous Action Nasal Decongestant/Antihistamine 12 Hour Capsules ... ⓔⓓ 773
- Contac Maximum Strength Continuous Action Decongestant/Antihistamine 12 Hour Caplets ... ⓔⓓ 772
- Contac Severe Cold and Flu Formula Caplets ... ⓔⓓ 773
- Coricidin 'D' Decongestant Tablets ... ⓔⓓ 760
- Dexatrim ... ⓔⓓ 795
- Dexatrim Plus Vitamins Caplets ... ⓔⓓ 796
- Dimetane-DC Cough Syrup ... 2232
- Dimetapp Allergy Sinus Caplets ... ⓔⓓ 838
- Dimetapp Cold & Allergy Chewable Tablets ... ⓔⓓ 838
- Dimetapp Cold & Cough Liqui-Gels ... ⓔⓓ 839
- Dimetapp DM Elixir ... ⓔⓓ 840
- Dimetapp Elixir ... ⓔⓓ 840
- Dimetapp Extentabs ... ⓔⓓ 841
- Dimetapp Tablets/Liqui-Gels ... ⓔⓓ 841
- Dura-Vent Tablets ... 971
- Entex LA Tablets ... 972
- Exgest LA Tablets ... 787
- Hycomine ... 947
- Nolamine Timed-Release Tablets ... 790

Nardil

- Ornade Spansule Capsules ... 2678
- Propagest Tablets ... 791
- Pyrroxate Tablets ... ⓔⓓ 742
- Robitussin-CF ... ⓔⓓ 846
- Sinulin Tablets ... 792
- Tavist-D 12 Hour Relief Tablets ... ⓔⓓ 750
- Teldrin 12 Hour Antihistamine/Nasal Decongestant Allergy Relief Capsules ... ⓔⓓ 786
- Triaminic Expectorant ... ⓔⓓ 753
- Triaminic Syrup ... ⓔⓓ 755
- Triaminic Triaminicol Cold & Cough ... ⓔⓓ 756
- Triaminic DM Syrup ... ⓔⓓ 756
- Triaminicin Tablets ... ⓔⓓ 756
- Vicks DayQuil Allergy Relief 12-Hour Extended Release Tablets ... ⓔⓓ 733
- Vicks DayQuil Allergy Relief 4-Hour Tablets ... ⓔⓓ 733
- Vicks DayQuil SINUS Pressure & CONGESTION Relief ... ⓔⓓ 734

Pindolol (Exaggerated hypotensive effects). Products include:
- Visken Tablets ... 2428

Pirbuterol Acetate (Potentiation of sympathomimetic agents and related compounds resulting in hypertensive crises; concurrent use is contraindicated). Products include:
- Maxair Autohaler ... 1550
- Maxair Inhaler ... 1552

Polythiazide (Exaggerated hypotensive effects). Products include:
- Minizide Capsules ... 2016

Prazosin Hydrochloride (Exaggerated hypotensive effects). Products include:
- Minipress Capsules ... 2015
- Minizide Capsules ... 2016

Propoxyphene Hydrochloride (Contraindication warning for meperidine is extended to other narcotics). Products include:
- Darvon ... 1475
- Wygesic Tablets ... 2930

Propoxyphene Napsylate (Contraindication warning for meperidine is extended to other narcotics). Products include:
- Darvon-N/Darvocet-N ... 1473

Propranolol Hydrochloride (Exaggerated hypotensive effects). Products include:
- Inderal ... 2834
- Inderal LA Long Acting Capsules ... 2836
- Inderide Tablets ... 2838
- Inderide LA Long Acting Capsules ... 2840

Protriptyline Hydrochloride (Concurrent or in rapid succession administration is contraindicated). Products include:
- Vivactil Tablets ... 1820

Pseudoephedrine Hydrochloride (Potentiation of sympathomimetic agents and related compounds resulting in hypertensive crises; concurrent use is contraindicated). Products include:
- Actifed Allergy Daytime/Nighttime Caplets ... ⓔⓓ 808
- Actifed Cold & Allergy Tablets ... ⓔⓓ 807
- Actifed Cold & Sinus Caplets and Tablets ... ⓔⓓ 808
- Actifed Sinus Daytime/Nighttime Tablets and Caplets ... ⓔⓓ 809
- Advil Cold and Sinus Caplets and Tablets ... ⓔⓓ 837
- Alka-Seltzer Plus Liqui-Gels ... ⓔⓓ 612
- Alka-Seltzer Plus Flu & Body Aches Liqui-Gels Non-Drowsy Formula ... ⓔⓓ 613
- Alka-Seltzer Plus Night-Time Cold Medicine Liqui-Gels ... ⓔⓓ 612
- Allerest Maximum Strength ... ⓔⓓ 649
- Allerest No Drowsiness ... ⓔⓓ 649
- Allerest Sinus Pain Formula ... ⓔⓓ 649
- Atrohist Pediatric Capsules ... 1603
- Benadryl Allergy/Cold Tablets ... ⓔⓓ 811
- Benadryl Allergy Decongestant Liquid Medication ... ⓔⓓ 812
- Benadryl Allergy Decongestant Tablets ... ⓔⓓ 812
- Benadryl Allergy Sinus Headache Caplets ... ⓔⓓ 813
- Benylin Multisymptom ... ⓔⓓ 816

IMPORTANT NOTE: Always consult each drug listing in the patient's regimen for possible interactions.

Nardil — Interactions Index

Bromfed Capsules (Extended-Release)	1832
Bromfed Syrup	◐ 712
Bromfed Tablets	1832
Bromfed-DM Cough Syrup	1832
Bromfed-PD Capsules (Extended-Release)	1832
Children's TYLENOL Cold Multi-Symptom Chewable Tablets and Liquid	1559
Children's TYLENOL Cold Plus Cough Multi Symptom Chewable Tablets and Liquid	1560
Children's TYLENOL Flu Suspension Liquid	1560
Children's Vicks DayQuil Allergy Relief	◐ 730
Children's Vicks NyQuil Cold/Cough Relief	◐ 731
Allergy-Sinus Comtrex Multi-Symptom Allergy-Sinus Formula Tablets and Caplets	◐ 639
Comtrex Multi-Symptom	◐ 638
Comtrex Multi-Symptom Non-Drowsy Caplets	◐ 640
Congess	1003
Contac Day Allergy/Sinus Caplets	◐ 771
Contac Day & Night	◐ 772
Contac Night Allergy/Sinus Caplets	◐ 771
Contac Severe Cold & Flu Non-Drowsy	◐ 774
Deconsal II Tablets	1605
Dimetane-DX Cough Syrup	2233
Dimetapp Cold & Fever Suspension	◐ 839
Dimetapp Decongestant Pediatric Drops	◐ 840
Dorcol Children's Cough Syrup	◐ 748
Drixoral Cough + Congestion Liquid Caps	◐ 763
Dura-Tap/PD Capsules	970
Duratuss Tablets	2750
Duratuss HD Elixir	2750
Efidac/24	◐ 655
Entex PSE Tablets	973
Fedahist Gyrocaps	2545
Guaifed	1833
Guaifed Syrup	◐ 712
Guaimax-D Tablets	809
Histussin D Liquid	670
Infants' TYLENOL Cold Decongestant & Fever-Reducer Drops	1561
Kronofed-A	994
Novahistine DMX	◐ 782
Nucofed	2225
PediaCare Cough-Cold Chewable Tablets and Liquid	1569
PediaCare Infants' Decongestant Drops	1569
PediaCare Infants' Drops Decongestant Plus Cough	1569
PediaCare NightRest Cough-Cold Liquid	1569
Pediatric Vicks 44d Cough & Head Congestion Relief	◐ 736
Pediatric Vicks 44m Cough & Cold Relief	◐ 737
Robitussin Cold & Cough Liqui-Gels	◐ 844
Robitussin Cold, Cough & Flu Liqui-Geis	◐ 844
Robitussin Maximum Strength Cough & Cold	◐ 847
Robitussin Night-Time Cold Formula	◐ 847
Robitussin Pediatric Cough & Cold Formula	◐ 848
Robitussin Pediatric Drops	◐ 849
Robitussin Severe Congestion Liqui-Gels	◐ 845
Robitussin-DAC Syrup	2249
Robitussin-PE	◐ 846
Rondec Oral Drops	974
Rondec Syrup	974
Rondec Tablet	974
Rondec Chewable Tablets	974
Rondec-TR Tablet	974
Ryna	◐ 804
Seldane-D Extended-Release Tablets	1286
Semprex-D Capsules	1620
Sinarest	◐ 663
Sine-Aid Maximum Strength Sinus Headache Gelcaps, Caplets and Tablets	1570
Sine-Off No Drowsiness Formula Caplets	◐ 784
Sine-Off Sinus Medicine	◐ 784
[...]	◐ 785
Non-Drying Liquid Caps	◐ 823
Sinutab Sinus Allergy Medication, Maximum Strength Tablets and Caplets	◐ 823
Sinutab Sinus Medication, Maximum Strength Without Drowsiness Formula, Tablets & Caplets	◐ 824
Sudafed Children's Cold & Cough Liquid Medication	◐ 825
Sudafed Children's Nasal Decongestant Liquid Medication	◐ 826
Sudafed Cold & Allergy Tablets	◐ 826
Sudafed Cold and Cough Liquid Caps	◐ 826
Sudafed Nasal Decongestant Tablets, 30 mg	◐ 825
Sudafed Nasal Decongestant Tablets, 60 mg	◐ 825
Sudafed Non-Drying Sinus Liquid Caps	◐ 827
Sudafed Pediatric Nasal Decongestant Liquid Oral Drops	◐ 827
Sudafed Severe Cold Formula Caplets	◐ 828
Sudafed Severe Cold Formula Tablets	◐ 828
Sudafed Sinus Caplets	◐ 829
Sudafed Sinus Tablets	◐ 829
Sudafed 12 Hour Caplets	◐ 824
Syn-Rx Tablets	1622
Syn-Rx DM Tablets	1623
TheraFlu Flu and Cold Medicine	◐ 750
Theraflu Maximum Strength Flu and Cold Medicine For Sore Throat	◐ 751
TheraFlu Flu, Cold and Cough Medicine	◐ 750
TheraFlu Maximum Strength Nighttime Flu, Cold & Cough Medicine	◐ 751
TheraFlu Maximum Strength Non-Drowsy Formula Flu, Cold & Cough Medicine	◐ 751
TheraFlu Maximum Strength, Non-Drowsy Formula Flu, Cold and Cough Caplets	◐ 752
Theraflu Maximum Strength Sinus Non-Drowsy Formula Caplets	◐ 752
Triaminic AM Cough and Decongestant Formula	◐ 753
Triaminic AM Decongestant Formula	◐ 753
Triaminic Infant Oral Decongestant Drops	◐ 754
Triaminic Night Time	◐ 754
Triaminic Sore Throat Formula	◐ 755
Tussend	1830
Tussend Expectorant	1831
TYLENOL Allergy Sinus, Maximum Strength Caplets and Gelcaps	1571
TYLENOL Allergy Sinus NightTime, Maximum Strength Caplets	1571
TYLENOL Cold Medication, Multi-Symptom Formula Tablets and Caplets	1572
TYLENOL Cold Medication, Multi-Symptom Hot Liquid Packets	1572
TYLENOL Cold Medication, No Drowsiness Formula Caplets and Gelcaps	1572
TYLENOL Cold Severe Congestion Caplets	1573
TYLENOL Cough Medication with Decongestant, Multi Symptom	1574
TYLENOL Flu No Drowsiness Formula, Maximum Strength Gelcaps	1575
TYLENOL Flu NightTime, Maximum Strength Gelcaps	1575
TYLENOL Flu NightTime, Maximum Strength Hot Medication Packets	1575
TYLENOL Sinus, Maximum Strength Geltabs, Gelcaps, Caplets and Tablets	1576
Vicks 44 LiquiCaps Cough, Cold & Flu Relief	◐ 728
Vicks 44 LiquiCaps Non-Drowsy Cough & Cold Relief	◐ 729
Vicks 44D Cough & Head Congestion Relief	◐ 728
Vicks 44M Cough, Cold & Flu Relief	◐ 729
Vicks DayQuil LiquiCaps/Liquid Multi-Symptom Cold/Flu Relief	◐ 734
Vicks DayQuil SINUS Pressure & PAIN Relief with IBUPROFEN	◐ 735
Vicks Nyquil Hot Therapy	◐ 735
Vicks NyQuil LiquiCaps/Liquid Multi-Symptom Cold/Flu Relief, Original and Cherry Flavors	◐ 736

Pseudoephedrine Sulfate (Potentiation of sympathomimetic agents and related compounds resulting in hypertensive crises; concurrent use is contraindicated). Products include:

Chlor-Trimeton Allergy Decongestant Tablets	◐ 759
Claritin-D Tablets	2487
Drixoral Cold and Allergy Sustained-Action Tablets	◐ 763
Drixoral Cold and Flu Extended-Release Tablets	◐ 764
Drixoral Non-Drowsy Formula Extended-Release Tablets	◐ 764
Drixoral Allergy/Sinus Extended Release Tablets	◐ 765
Trinalin Repetabs Tablets	1373

Quinapril Hydrochloride (Exaggerated hypotensive effects). Products include:

| Accupril Tablets | 1950 |

Ramipril (Exaggerated hypotensive effects). Products include:

| Altace Capsules | 1238 |

Rauwolfia Serpentina (Exaggerated hypotensive effects; exercise caution).
No products indexed under this heading.

Rescinnamine (Exaggerated hypotensive effects; exercise caution).
No products indexed under this heading.

Reserpine (Exaggerated hypotensive effects; exercise caution). Products include:

Diupres Tablets	1691
Hydropres Tablets	1718
Ser-Ap-Es Tablets	867

Salmeterol Xinafoate (Potentiation of sympathomimetic agents and related compounds resulting in hypertensive crises; concurrent use is contraindicated). Products include:

| Serevent Inhalation Aerosol | 1149 |

Secobarbital Sodium (Potential for increased hypnosis). Products include:

| Seconal Sodium Pulvules | 1529 |

Selegiline Hydrochloride (Hypertensive crises; at least 10 days should elapse between discontinuation of Nardil and institution of another MAOI). Products include:

| Eldepryl Capsules | 2729 |

Sertraline Hydrochloride (Concurrent or in rapid succession administration is contraindicated). Products include:

| Zoloft Tablets | 2051 |

Sodium Nitroprusside (Exaggerated hypotensive effects).
No products indexed under this heading.

Sotalol Hydrochloride (Exaggerated hypotensive effects). Products include:

| Betapace Tablets | 637 |

Spirapril Hydrochloride (Exaggerated hypotensive effects).
No products indexed under this heading.

Sufentanil Citrate (Contraindication warning for meperidine is extended to other narcotics). Products include:

| Sufenta Injection | 1355 |

Terazosin Hydrochloride (Exaggerated hypotensive effects). Products include:

| Hytrin Capsules | 434 |

Terbutaline Sulfate (Potentiation of sympathomimetic agents and related compounds resulting in hypertensive crises; concurrent use is contraindicated). Products include:

Brethaire Inhaler	830
Brethine Ampuls	832
Brethine Tablets	831
Bricanyl Subcutaneous Injection	1247
Bricanyl Tablets	1248

Tetrahydrozoline Hydrochloride (Contraindicated). Products include:

Collyrium Fresh	◉ 316
Murine Tears Plus Lubricant Redness Reliever Eye Drops	◐ 744
Murine Tears Plus Lubricant Redness Reliever Eye Drops	◉ 315
Visine A.C. Seasonal Relief From Pollen and Dust	◉ 301
Visine Moisturizing Eye Drops	◉ 301
Visine Original Eye Drops	◉ 301

Thiamylal Sodium (Potential for increased hypnosis).
No products indexed under this heading.

Timolol Hemihydrate (Exaggerated hypotensive effects). Products include:

| Betimol 0.25%, 0.5% | ◉ 259 |

Timolol Maleate (Exaggerated hypotensive effects). Products include:

Blocadren Tablets	1654
Timolide Tablets	1791
Timoptic in Ocudose	1796
Timoptic Sterile Ophthalmic Solution	1794
Timoptic-XE	1798

Torsemide (Exaggerated hypotensive effects). Products include:

| Demadex Tablets and Injection | 691 |

Tranylcypromine Sulfate (Hypertensive crises; at least 10 days should elapse between discontinuation of Nardil and institution of another MAOI). Products include:

| Parnate Tablets | 2679 |

Trimethaphan Camsylate (Exaggerated hypotensive effects).
No products indexed under this heading.

Trimipramine Maleate (Concurrent or in rapid succession administration is contraindicated). Products include:

| Surmontil Capsules | 2917 |

L-Tryptophan (Potentiation of sympathomimetic agents and related compounds, including tryptophan, resulting in hypertensive crises; concurrent use is contraindicated).
No products indexed under this heading.

Tyramine (Concurrent use should be avoided).

L-Tyrosine (Potentiation of sympathomimetic agents and related compounds, including tyrosine, resulting in hypertensive crises; concurrent use is contraindicated). Products include:

| Catemine Enteric Tablets (Tyrosine) | 2750 |

Venlafaxine Hydrochloride (Concurrent or in rapid succession administration is contraindicated). Products include:

| Effexor | 2825 |

Verapamil Hydrochloride (Exaggerated hypotensive effects). Products include:

Calan SR Caplets	2571
Calan Tablets	2568
Covera-HS Tablets	2573
Isoptin Injectable	1391
Isoptin Oral Tablets	1393
Isoptin SR Tablets	1395
Verelan Capsules	1455

Food Interactions

Alcohol (Concurrent use should be avoided).

Beans, broad (Concurrent and/or sequential intake must be avoided).

Beans, Fava (Concurrent and/or sequential intake must be avoided).

(◐ Described in PDR For Nonprescription Drugs)   *(◉ Described in PDR For Ophthalmology)*

Interactions Index

Beer, alcohol-free (Concurrent and/or sequential intake must be avoided).
Beer, reduced-alcohol (Concurrent and/or sequential intake must be avoided).
Beer, unspecified (Concurrent and/or sequential intake must be avoided).
Beverages, caffeine-containing (Excessive caffeine intake should be avoided).
Bologna, Lebanon (Concurrent and/or sequential intake must be avoided).
Cheese, aged (Concurrent and/or sequential intake must be avoided).
Cheese, unspecified (Concurrent and/or sequential intake must be avoided).
Chocolate (Concurrent and/or sequential intake must be avoided).
Fish, smoked (Concurrent and/or sequential intake must be avoided).
Food with high concentration of dopamine (Concurrent and/or sequential intake must be avoided).
Food with high concentration of tyramine (Concurrent and/or sequential intake must be avoided).
Herring, pickled (Concurrent and/or sequential intake must be avoided).
Liver (Concurrent and/or sequential intake must be avoided).
Meat extracts (Concurrent and/or sequential intake must be avoided).
Meat, unspecified (Concurrent and/or sequential intake must be avoided).
Pepperoni (Concurrent and/or sequential intake must be avoided).
Salami, hard (Concurrent and/or sequential intake must be avoided).
Salami, Genoa (Concurrent and/or sequential intake must be avoided).
Sauerkraut (Concurrent and/or sequential intake must be avoided).
Sausage, dry (Concurrent and/or sequential intake must be avoided).
Wine products (Concurrent and/or sequential intake must be avoided).
Wine, unspecified (Concurrent and/or sequential intake must be avoided).
Yeast extract (Concurrent and/or sequential intake must be avoided).
Yeast, brewer's (Concurrent and/or sequential intake must be avoided).
Yogurt (Concurrent and/or sequential intake must be avoided).

NASACORT AQ NASAL SPRAY
(Triamcinolone Acetonide) 2191
May interact with:

Prednisone (Co-administration with alternate day systemic prednisone could increase the likelihood of hypothalamic-pituitary-adrenal suppression).
No products indexed under this heading.

NASACORT NASAL INHALER
(Triamcinolone Acetonide) 2189
May interact with:

Prednisone (Concomitant use with alternate-day systemic prednisone could increase the likelihood of hypothalamic-pituitary-adrenal (HPA) suppression).
No products indexed under this heading.

NASAL MOIST
(Sodium Chloride) 630
None cited in PDR database.

NASALCROM NASAL SOLUTION
(Cromolyn Sodium) 2192
None cited in PDR database.

NASALIDE NASAL SOLUTION 0.025%
(Flunisolide) 2301
None cited in PDR database.

NASAREL NASAL SOLUTION
(Flunisolide) 2302
None cited in PDR database.

NATACYN ANTIFUNGAL OPHTHALMIC SUSPENSION
(Natamycin) 223
None cited in PDR database.

NATALINS RX TABLETS
(Vitamins, Prenatal) 1599
None cited in PDR database.

NAVANE CAPSULES AND CONCENTRATE
(Thiothixene) 2018
May interact with central nervous system depressants, barbiturates, anticholinergics, and certain other agents. Compounds in these categories include:

Alfentanil Hydrochloride (Possible additive effects which may include hypotension). Products include:
Alfenta Injection 1334

Alprazolam (Possible additive effects which may include hypotension). Products include:
Xanax Tablets 2115

Aprobarbital (Thiothixene potentiates the action of barbiturates).
No products indexed under this heading.

Atropine Sulfate (Thiothixene possesses weak anticholinergic properties; concurrent use requires caution because of increased atropine-like effect). Products include:
Arco-Lase Plus Tablets 513
Atrohist Plus Tablets 1605
Donnatal 2234
Donnatal Extentabs 2234
Donnatal Tablets 2234
Lomotil 2591
Motofen Tablets 789
Urised Tablets 2123

Belladonna Alkaloids (Thiothixene possesses weak anticholinergic properties; concurrent use requires caution because of increased atropine-like effect). Products include:
Bellergal-S Tablets 2375
Hyland's Bedwetting Tablets 788
Hyland's EnurAid Tablets 789
Hyland's Headache Tablets 790
Hyland's Teething Tablets 790
Similasan Eye Drops # 1 769

Benztropine Mesylate (Thiothixene possesses weak anticholinergic properties; concurrent use requires caution because of increased atropine-like effect). Products include:
Cogentin 1661

Biperiden Hydrochloride (Thiothixene possesses weak anticholinergic properties; concurrent use requires caution because of increased atropine-like effect). Products include:
Akineton 1380

Buprenorphine (Possible additive effects which may include hypotension). Products include:
Buprenex Injectable 2170

Buspirone Hydrochloride (Possible additive effects which may include hypotension). Products include:
BuSpar Tablets 738

Butabarbital (Thiothixene potentiates the action of barbiturates).
No products indexed under this heading.

Butalbital (Thiothixene potentiates the action of barbiturates). Products include:
Axocet Capsules 2469
Esgic-plus Capsules 1012
Esgic-plus Tablets 1012
Fioricet Tablets 2386
Fioricet with Codeine Capsules 2387
Fiorinal Capsules 2388
Fiorinal with Codeine Capsules 2390
Fiorinal Tablets 2388
Phrenilin 790
Sedapap Tablets 50 mg/650 mg 1826

Chlordiazepoxide (Possible additive effects which may include hypotension). Products include:
Limbitrol 2333

Chlordiazepoxide Hydrochloride (Possible additive effects which may include hypotension). Products include:
Librax Capsules 2330
Librium Capsules 2331
Librium Injectable 2332

Chlorpromazine (Possible additive effects which may include hypotension). Products include:
Thorazine Suppositories 2701

Chlorpromazine Hydrochloride (Possible additive effects which may include hypotension). Products include:
Thorazine 2701

Chlorprothixene (Possible additive effects which may include hypotension).
No products indexed under this heading.

Chlorprothixene Hydrochloride (Possible additive effects which may include hypotension).
No products indexed under this heading.

Chlorprothixene Lactate (Possible additive effects which may include hypotension).
No products indexed under this heading.

Clidinium Bromide (Thiothixene possesses weak anticholinergic properties; concurrent use requires caution because of increased atropine-like effect). Products include:
Librax Capsules 2330

Clorazepate Dipotassium (Possible additive effects which may include hypotension). Products include:
Tranxene 459

Clozapine (Possible additive effects which may include hypotension). Products include:
Clozaril Tablets 2377

Codeine Phosphate (Possible additive effects which may include hypotension). Products include:
Brontex 2130
Dimetane-DC Cough Syrup 2232
Fioricet with Codeine Capsules 2387
Fiorinal with Codeine Capsules 2390
Nucofed 2225
Phenergan with Codeine 2883
Phenergan VC with Codeine 2888
Robitussin A-C Syrup 2248
Robitussin-DAC Syrup 2249
Ryna 804

Navane Oral

Soma Compound w/Codeine Tablets 2784
Tylenol with Codeine 1592

Desflurane (Possible additive effects which may include hypotension). Products include:
Suprane (desflurane, USP) 1865

Dezocine (Possible additive effects which may include hypotension). Products include:
Dalgan Injection 529

Diazepam (Possible additive effects which may include hypotension). Products include:
Dizac (diazepam injectable emulsion) CIV 1862
Valium Injectable 2336
Valium Tablets 2335

Dicyclomine Hydrochloride (Thiothixene possesses weak anticholinergic properties; concurrent use requires caution because of increased atropine-like effect). Products include:
Bentyl 1246

Droperidol (Possible additive effects which may include hypotension). Products include:
Inapsine Injection 462

Enflurane (Possible additive effects which may include hypotension).
No products indexed under this heading.

Estazolam (Possible additive effects which may include hypotension). Products include:
ProSom Tablets 457

Ethchlorvynol (Possible additive effects which may include hypotension). Products include:
Placidyl Capsules 456

Ethinamate (Possible additive effects which may include hypotension).
No products indexed under this heading.

Fentanyl (Possible additive effects which may include hypotension). Products include:
Duragesic Transdermal System 1336

Fentanyl Citrate (Possible additive effects which may include hypotension). Products include:
Sublimaze Injection 463

Fluphenazine Decanoate (Possible additive effects which may include hypotension). Products include:
Prolixin Decanoate 510

Fluphenazine Enanthate (Possible additive effects which may include hypotension). Products include:
Prolixin Enanthate 510

Fluphenazine Hydrochloride (Possible additive effects which may include hypotension). Products include:
Prolixin 510

Flurazepam Hydrochloride (Possible additive effects which may include hypotension). Products include:
Dalmane Capsules 2329

Glutethimide (Possible additive effects which may include hypotension).
No products indexed under this heading.

Glycopyrrolate (Thiothixene possesses weak anticholinergic properties; concurrent use requires caution because of increased atropine-like effect). Products include:
Robinul Forte Tablets 2247
Robinul Injectable 2247
Robinul Tablets 2247

IMPORTANT NOTE: Always consult each drug listing in the patient's regimen for possible interactions.

Navane Oral — Interactions Index — 720

Haloperidol (Possible additive effects which may include hypotension). Products include:
- Haldol Injection, Tablets and Concentrate ... 1585

Haloperidol Decanoate (Possible additive effects which may include hypotension). Products include:
- Haldol Decanoate ... 1587

Hydrocodone Bitartrate (Possible additive effects which may include hypotension). Products include:
- Codiclear DH Syrup ... 808
- Duratuss HD Elixir ... 2750
- Histussin D Liquid ... 670
- Hycodan Tablets and Syrup ... 946
- Hycomine Compound Tablets ... 948
- Hycomine ... 947
- Hycotuss Expectorant Syrup ... 950
- Hydrocet Capsules ... 787
- Lorcet 10/650 Tablets ... 1016
- Lortab ... 2751
- Tussend ... 1830
- Tussend Expectorant ... 1831
- Vicodin Tablets ... 1404
- Vicodin ES Tablets ... 1405
- Vicodin HP Tablets ... 1403
- Vicodin Tuss Expectorant ... 1406
- Zydone Capsules ... 967

Hydrocodone Polistirex (Possible additive effects which may include hypotension). Products include:
- Tussionex Pennkinetic Extended-Release Suspension ... 1624

Hydroxyzine Hydrochloride (Possible additive effects which may include hypotension). Products include:
- Atarax Tablets & Syrup ... 1992
- Marax Tablets & DF Syrup ... 2015
- Vistaril Intramuscular Solution ... 2042

Hyoscyamine (Thiothixene possesses weak anticholinergic properties; concurrent use requires caution because of increased atropine-like effect). Products include:
- Cystospaz Tablets ... 2123
- Urised Tablets ... 2123

Hyoscyamine Sulfate (Thiothixene possesses weak anticholinergic properties; concurrent use requires caution because of increased atropine-like effect). Products include:
- Arco-Lase Plus Tablets ... 513
- Atrohist Plus Tablets ... 1605
- Cystospaz-M Capsules ... 2123
- Donnatal ... 2234
- Donnatal Extentabs ... 2234
- Donnatal Tablets ... 2234
- Kutrase Capsules ... 2546
- Levsin/Levsinex/Levbid ... 2549

Ipratropium Bromide (Thiothixene possesses weak anticholinergic properties; concurrent use requires caution because of increased atropine-like effect). Products include:
- Atrovent Inhalation Aerosol ... 674
- Atrovent Inhalation Solution ... 675
- Atrovent Nasal Spray 0.03% ... 676
- Atrovent Nasal Spray 0.06% ... 678

Isoflurane (Possible additive effects which may include hypotension).
- No products indexed under this heading.

Ketamine Hydrochloride (Possible additive effects which may include hypotension).
- No products indexed under this heading.

Levomethadyl Acetate Hydrochloride (Possible additive effects which may include hypotension). Products include:
- Orlaam Oral Solution ... 2361

Levorphanol Tartrate (Possible additive effects which may include hypotension). Products include:
- Levo-Dromoran ... 2297

Lorazepam (Possible additive effects which may include hypotension). Products include:
- Ativan Injection ... 2805
- Ativan Tablets ... 2807

Loxapine Hydrochloride (Possible additive effects which may include hypotension). Products include:
- Loxitane ... 1426

Loxapine Succinate (Possible additive effects which may include hypotension). Products include:
- Loxitane Capsules ... 1426

Mepenzolate Bromide (Thiothixene possesses weak anticholinergic properties; concurrent use requires caution because of increased atropine-like effect).
- No products indexed under this heading.

Meperidine Hydrochloride (Possible additive effects which may include hypotension). Products include:
- Demerol ... 2438
- Mepergan Injection ... 2859

Mephobarbital (Thiothixene potentiates the action of barbiturates, however, the dosage of anticonvulsant barbiturates should not be reduced since thiothixene is capable of precipitating convulsion). Products include:
- Mebaral Tablets ... 2452

Meprobamate (Possible additive effects which may include hypotension). Products include:
- Miltown Tablets ... 2780
- PMB 200 and PMB 400 ... 2890

Mesoridazine Besylate (Possible additive effects which may include hypotension). Products include:
- Serentil ... 689

Methadone Hydrochloride (Possible additive effects which may include hypotension). Products include:
- Methadone Hydrochloride Oral Concentrate ... 2356
- Methadone Hydrochloride Oral Solution & Tablets ... 2357

Methohexital Sodium (Possible additive effects which may include hypotension).
- No products indexed under this heading.

Methotrimeprazine (Possible additive effects which may include hypotension). Products include:
- Levoprome ... 1321

Methoxyflurane (Possible additive effects which may include hypotension).
- No products indexed under this heading.

Midazolam Hydrochloride (Possible additive effects which may include hypotension). Products include:
- Versed Injection ... 2324

Molindone Hydrochloride (Possible additive effects which may include hypotension). Products include:
- Moban Tablets and Concentrate ... 1036

Morphine Sulfate (Possible additive effects which may include hypotension). Products include:
- Astramorph/PF Injection, USP (Preservative-Free) ... 526
- Duramorph Injection ... 983
- Infumorph 200 and Infumorph 500 Sterile Solutions ... 985
- Kadian Capsules ... 2948
- MS Contin Tablets ... 2149
- MSIR ... 2152
- Oramorph SR (Morphine Sulfate Sustained Release Tablets) ... 2359
- RMS Suppositories CII ... 2766
- Roxanol ... 2365

Opium Alkaloids (Possible additive effects which may include hypotension).
- No products indexed under this heading.

Oxazepam (Possible additive effects which may include hypotension). Products include:
- Serax Capsules ... 2916
- Serax Tablets ... 2916

Oxybutynin Chloride (Thiothixene possesses weak anticholinergic properties; concurrent use requires caution because of increased atropine-like effect). Products include:
- Ditropan ... 1267

Oxycodone Hydrochloride (Possible additive effects which may include hypotension). Products include:
- OxyContin Tablets ... 2163
- OxyIR Capsules ... 2167
- Percocet Tablets ... 955
- Percodan Tablets ... 955
- Percodan-Demi Tablets ... 956
- Roxicodone Tablets, Oral Solution & Intensol (Oxycodone) ... 2366
- Tylox Capsules ... 1593

Pentobarbital Sodium (Thiothixene potentiates the action of barbiturates). Products include:
- Nembutal Sodium Capsules ... 440
- Nembutal Sodium Solution ... 442
- Nembutal Sodium Suppositories ... 444

Perphenazine (Possible additive effects which may include hypotension). Products include:
- Etrafon ... 2495
- Triavil Tablets ... 1800
- Trilafon ... 2532

Phenobarbital (Thiothixene potentiates the action of barbiturates, however, the dosage of anticonvulsant barbiturates should not be reduced since thiothixene is capable of precipitating convulsion). Products include:
- Arco-Lase Plus Tablets ... 513
- Bellergal-S Tablets ... 2375
- Donnatal ... 2234
- Donnatal Extentabs ... 2234
- Donnatal Tablets ... 2234
- Phenobarbital Elixir and Tablets ... 1523
- Quadrinal Tablets ... 1398

Prazepam (Possible additive effects which may include hypotension).
- No products indexed under this heading.

Prochlorperazine (Possible additive effects which may include hypotension). Products include:
- Compazine ... 2644

Procyclidine Hydrochloride (Thiothixene possesses weak anticholinergic properties; concurrent use requires caution because of increased atropine-like effect). Products include:
- Kemadrin Tablets ... 1105

Promethazine Hydrochloride (Possible additive effects which may include hypotension). Products include:
- Mepergan Injection ... 2859
- Phenergan with Codeine ... 2883
- Phenergan with Dextromethorphan ... 2885
- Phenergan Injection ... 2880
- Phenergan Suppositories ... 2882
- Phenergan Syrup ... 2881
- Phenergan Tablets ... 2882
- Phenergan VC ... 2886
- Phenergan VC with Codeine ... 2888

Propantheline Bromide (Thiothixene possesses weak anticholinergic properties; concurrent use requires caution because of increased atropine-like effect). Products include:
- Pro-Banthine Tablets ... 2226

Propofol (Possible additive effects which may include hypotension). Products include:
- Diprivan Injectable Emulsion ... 2939

Propoxyphene Hydrochloride (Possible additive effects which may include hypotension). Products include:
- Darvon ... 1475
- Wygesic Tablets ... 2930

Propoxyphene Napsylate (Possible additive effects which may include hypotension). Products include:
- Darvon-N/Darvocet-N ... 1473

Quazepam (Possible additive effects which may include hypotension). Products include:
- Doral Tablets ... 2773

Risperidone (Possible additive effects which may include hypotension). Products include:
- Risperdal Tablets ... 1348

Scopolamine (Thiothixene possesses weak anticholinergic properties; concurrent use requires caution because of increased atropine-like effect). Products include:
- Transderm Scōp Transdermal Therapeutic System ... 890

Scopolamine Hydrobromide (Thiothixene possesses weak anticholinergic properties; concurrent use requires caution because of increased atropine-like effect). Products include:
- Atrohist Plus Tablets ... 1605
- Donnatal ... 2234
- Donnatal Extentabs ... 2234
- Donnatal Tablets ... 2234

Secobarbital Sodium (Thiothixene potentiates the action of barbiturates). Products include:
- Seconal Sodium Pulvules ... 1529

Sevoflurane (Possible additive effects which may include hypotension).
- No products indexed under this heading.

Sufentanil Citrate (Possible additive effects which may include hypotension). Products include:
- Sufenta Injection ... 1355

Temazepam (Possible additive effects which may include hypotension). Products include:
- Restoril Capsules ... 2413

Thiamylal Sodium (Thiothixene potentiates the action of barbiturates).
- No products indexed under this heading.

Thioridazine Hydrochloride (Possible additive effects which may include hypotension). Products include:
- Mellaril ... 2398

Triazolam (Possible additive effects which may include hypotension). Products include:
- Halcion Tablets ... 2093

Tridihexethyl Chloride (Thiothixene possesses weak anticholinergic properties; concurrent use requires caution because of increased atropine-like effect).
- No products indexed under this heading.

721 **Interactions Index** **Navane Intramuscular**

Trifluoperazine Hydrochloride (Possible additive effects which may include hypotension). Products include:
- Stelazine ... 2692

Trihexyphenidyl Hydrochloride (Thiothixene possesses weak anticholinergic properties; concurrent use requires caution because of increased atropine-like effect). Products include:
- Artane ... 1418

Zolpidem Tartrate (Possible additive effects which may include hypotension). Products include:
- Ambien Tablets ... 2559

Food Interactions

Alcohol (Possible additive effects which may include hypotension).

NAVANE INTRAMUSCULAR

(Thiothixene) ... 2019

May interact with barbiturates, central nervous system depressants, anticholinergics, and certain other agents. Compounds in these categories include:

Alfentanil Hydrochloride (Possible additive effects which may include hypotension). Products include:
- Alfenta Injection ... 1334

Alprazolam (Possible additive effects which may include hypotension). Products include:
- Xanax Tablets ... 2115

Aprobarbital (Thiothixene potentiates the action of barbiturates).
- No products indexed under this heading.

Atropine Sulfate (Thiothixene possesses weak anticholinergic properties; concurrent use requires caution because of increased atropine-like effect). Products include:
- Arco-Lase Plus Tablets ... 513
- Atrohist Plus Tablets ... 1605
- Donnatal ... 2234
- Donnatal Extentabs ... 2234
- Donnatal Tablets ... 2234
- Lomotil ... 2591
- Motofen Tablets ... 789
- Urised Tablets ... 2123

Belladonna Alkaloids (Thiothixene possesses weak anticholinergic properties; concurrent use requires caution because of increased atropine-like effect). Products include:
- Bellergal-S Tablets ... 2375
- Hyland's Bedwetting Tablets ... 788
- Hyland's EnurAid Tablets ... 789
- Hyland's Headache Tablets ... 790
- Hyland's Teething Tablets ... 790
- Similasan Eye Drops #1 ... 769

Benztropine Mesylate (Thiothixene possesses weak anticholinergic properties; concurrent use requires caution because of increased atropine-like effect). Products include:
- Cogentin ... 1661

Biperiden Hydrochloride (Thiothixene possesses weak anticholinergic properties; concurrent use requires caution because of increased atropine-like effect). Products include:
- Akineton ... 1380

Buprenorphine (Possible additive effects which may include hypotension). Products include:
- Buprenex Injectable ... 2170

Buspirone Hydrochloride (Possible additive effects which may include hypotension). Products include:
- BuSpar Tablets ... 738

Butabarbital (Thiothixene potentiates the action of barbiturates).
- No products indexed under this heading.

Butalbital (Thiothixene potentiates the action of barbiturates). Products include:
- Axocet Capsules ... 2469
- Esgic-plus Capsules ... 1012
- Esgic-plus Tablets ... 1012
- Fioricet Tablets ... 2386
- Fioricet with Codeine Capsules ... 2387
- Fiorinal Capsules ... 2388
- Fiorinal with Codeine Capsules ... 2390
- Fiorinal Tablets ... 2388
- Phrenilin ... 790
- Sedapap Tablets 50 mg/650 mg .. 1826

Chlordiazepoxide (Possible additive effects which may include hypotension). Products include:
- Limbitrol ... 2333

Chlordiazepoxide Hydrochloride (Possible additive effects which may include hypotension). Products include:
- Librax Capsules ... 2330
- Librium Capsules ... 2331
- Librium Injectable ... 2332

Chlorpromazine (Possible additive effects which may include hypotension). Products include:
- Thorazine Suppositories ... 2701

Chlorpromazine Hydrochloride (Possible additive effects which may include hypotension). Products include:
- Thorazine ... 2701

Chlorprothixene (Possible additive effects which may include hypotension).
- No products indexed under this heading.

Chlorprothixene Hydrochloride (Possible additive effects which may include hypotension).
- No products indexed under this heading.

Chlorprothixene Lactate (Possible additive effects which may include hypotension).
- No products indexed under this heading.

Clidinium Bromide (Thiothixene possesses weak anticholinergic properties; concurrent use requires caution because of increased atropine-like effect). Products include:
- Librax Capsules ... 2330

Clorazepate Dipotassium (Possible additive effects which may include hypotension). Products include:
- Tranxene ... 459

Clozapine (Possible additive effects which may include hypotension). Products include:
- Clozaril Tablets ... 2377

Codeine Phosphate (Possible additive effects which may include hypotension). Products include:
- Brontex ... 2130
- Dimetane-DC Cough Syrup ... 2232
- Fioricet with Codeine Capsules ... 2387
- Fiorinal with Codeine Capsules ... 2390
- Nucofed ... 2225
- Phenergan with Codeine ... 2883
- Phenergan VC with Codeine ... 2888
- Robitussin A-C Syrup ... 2248
- Robitussin-DAC Syrup ... 2249
- Ryna ... 804
- Soma Compound w/Codeine Tablets ... 2784
- Tylenol with Codeine ... 1592

Desflurane (Possible additive effects which may include hypotension). Products include:
- Suprane (desflurane, USP) ... 1865

Dezocine (Possible additive effects which may include hypotension). Products include:
- Dalgan Injection ... 529

Diazepam (Possible additive effects which may include hypotension). Products include:
- Dizac (diazepam injectable emulsion) CIV ... 1862
- Valium Injectable ... 2336
- Valium Tablets ... 2335

Dicyclomine Hydrochloride (Thiothixene possesses weak anticholinergic properties; concurrent use requires caution because of increased atropine-like effect). Products include:
- Bentyl ... 1246

Droperidol (Possible additive effects which may include hypotension). Products include:
- Inapsine Injection ... 462

Enflurane (Possible additive effects which may include hypotension).
- No products indexed under this heading.

Estazolam (Possible additive effects which may include hypotension). Products include:
- ProSom Tablets ... 457

Ethchlorvynol (Possible additive effects which may include hypotension). Products include:
- Placidyl Capsules ... 456

Ethinamate (Possible additive effects which may include hypotension).
- No products indexed under this heading.

Fentanyl (Possible additive effects which may include hypotension). Products include:
- Duragesic Transdermal System ... 1336

Fentanyl Citrate (Possible additive effects which may include hypotension). Products include:
- Sublimaze Injection ... 463

Fluphenazine Decanoate (Possible additive effects which may include hypotension). Products include:
- Prolixin Decanoate ... 510

Fluphenazine Enanthate (Possible additive effects which may include hypotension). Products include:
- Prolixin Enanthate ... 510

Fluphenazine Hydrochloride (Possible additive effects which may include hypotension). Products include:
- Prolixin ... 510

Flurazepam Hydrochloride (Possible additive effects which may include hypotension). Products include:
- Dalmane Capsules ... 2329

Glutethimide (Possible additive effects which may include hypotension).
- No products indexed under this heading.

Glycopyrrolate (Thiothixene possesses weak anticholinergic properties; concurrent use requires caution because of increased atropine-like effect). Products include:
- Robinul Forte Tablets ... 2247
- Robinul Injectable ... 2247
- Robinul Tablets ... 2247

Haloperidol (Possible additive effects which may include hypotension). Products include:
- Haldol Injection, Tablets and Concentrate ... 1585

Haloperidol Decanoate (Possible additive effects which may include hypotension). Products include:
- Haldol Decanoate ... 1587

Hydrocodone Bitartrate (Possible additive effects which may include hypotension). Products include:
- Codiclear DH Syrup ... 808
- Duratuss HD Elixir ... 2750
- Histussin D Liquid ... 670
- Hycodan Tablets and Syrup ... 946
- Hycomine Compound Tablets ... 948
- Hycomine ... 947
- Hycotuss Expectorant Syrup ... 950
- Hydrocet Capsules ... 787
- Lorcet 10/650 Tablets ... 1016
- Lortab ... 2751
- Tussend ... 1830
- Tussend Expectorant ... 1831
- Vicodin Tablets ... 1404
- Vicodin ES Tablets ... 1405
- Vicodin HP Tablets ... 1403
- Vicodin Tuss Expectorant ... 1406
- Zydone Capsules ... 967

Hydrocodone Polistirex (Possible additive effects which may include hypotension). Products include:
- Tussionex Pennkinetic Extended-Release Suspension ... 1624

Hydroxyzine Hydrochloride (Possible additive effects which may include hypotension). Products include:
- Atarax Tablets & Syrup ... 1992
- Marax Tablets & DF Syrup ... 2015
- Vistaril Intramuscular Solution ... 2042

Hyoscyamine (Thiothixene possesses weak anticholinergic properties; concurrent use requires caution because of increased atropine-like effect). Products include:
- Cystospaz Tablets ... 2123
- Urised Tablets ... 2123

Hyoscyamine Sulfate (Thiothixene possesses weak anticholinergic properties; concurrent use requires caution because of increased atropine-like effect). Products include:
- Arco-Lase Plus Tablets ... 513
- Atrohist Plus Tablets ... 1605
- Cystospaz-M Capsules ... 2123
- Donnatal ... 2234
- Donnatal Extentabs ... 2234
- Donnatal Tablets ... 2234
- Kutrase Capsules ... 2546
- Levsin/Levsinex/Levbid ... 2549

Ipratropium Bromide (Thiothixene possesses weak anticholinergic properties; concurrent use requires caution because of increased atropine-like effect). Products include:
- Atrovent Inhalation Aerosol ... 674
- Atrovent Inhalation Solution ... 675
- Atrovent Nasal Spray 0.03% ... 676
- Atrovent Nasal Spray 0.06% ... 678

Isoflurane (Possible additive effects which may include hypotension).
- No products indexed under this heading.

Ketamine Hydrochloride (Possible additive effects which may include hypotension).
- No products indexed under this heading.

Levomethadyl Acetate Hydrochloride (Possible additive effects which may include hypotension). Products include:
- Orlaam Oral Solution ... 2361

Levorphanol Tartrate (Possible additive effects which may include hypotension). Products include:
- Levo-Dromoran ... 2297

Lorazepam (Possible additive effects which may include hypotension). Products include:
- Ativan Injection ... 2805

IMPORTANT NOTE: Always consult each drug listing in the patient's regimen for possible interactions.

Navane Intramuscular / Interactions Index — 722

Ativan Tablets 2807

Loxapine Hydrochloride (Possible additive effects which may include hypotension). Products include:
Loxitane 1426

Loxapine Succinate (Possible additive effects which may include hypotension). Products include:
Loxitane Capsules 1426

Mepenzolate Bromide (Thiothixene possesses weak anticholinergic properties; concurrent use requires caution because of increased atropine-like effect).
No products indexed under this heading.

Meperidine Hydrochloride (Possible additive effects which may include hypotension). Products include:
Demerol 2438
Mepergan Injection 2859

Mephobarbital (Thiothixene potentiates the action of barbiturates, however, the dosage of anticonvulsant barbiturates should not be reduced since thiothixene is capable of precipitating convulsion). Products include:
Mebaral Tablets 2452

Meprobamate (Possible additive effects which may include hypotension). Products include:
Miltown Tablets 2780
PMB 200 and PMB 400 2890

Mesoridazine Besylate (Possible additive effects which may include hypotension). Products include:
Serentil 689

Methadone Hydrochloride (Possible additive effects which may include hypotension). Products include:
Methadone Hydrochloride Oral Concentrate 2356
Methadone Hydrochloride Oral Solution & Tablets 2357

Methohexital Sodium (Possible additive effects which may include hypotension).
No products indexed under this heading.

Methotrimeprazine (Possible additive effects which may include hypotension). Products include:
Levoprome 1321

Methoxyflurane (Possible additive effects which may include hypotension).
No products indexed under this heading.

Midazolam Hydrochloride (Possible additive effects which may include hypotension). Products include:
Versed Injection 2324

Molindone Hydrochloride (Possible additive effects which may include hypotension). Products include:
Moban Tablets and Concentrate 1036

Morphine Sulfate (Possible additive effects which may include hypotension). Products include:
Astramorph/PF Injection, USP (Preservative-Free) 526
Duramorph Injection 983
Infumorph 200 and Infumorph 500 Sterile Solutions 985
Kadian Capsules 2948
MS Contin Tablets 2149
MSIR 2152
Oramorph SR (Morphine Sulfate Sustained Release Tablets) 2359
RMS Suppositories CII 2766
Roxanol 2365

Opium Alkaloids (Possible additive effects which may include hypotension).
No products indexed under this heading.

Oxazepam (Possible additive effects which may include hypotension). Products include:
Serax Capsules 2916
Serax Tablets 2916

Oxybutynin Chloride (Thiothixene possesses weak anticholinergic properties; concurrent use requires caution because of increased atropine-like effect). Products include:
Ditropan 1267

Oxycodone Hydrochloride (Possible additive effects which may include hypotension). Products include:
OxyContin Tablets 2163
OxyIR Capsules 2167
Percocet Tablets 955
Percodan Tablets 955
Percodan-Demi Tablets 956
Roxicodone Tablets, Oral Solution & Intensol (Oxycodone) 2366
Tylox Capsules 1593

Pentobarbital Sodium (Thiothixene potentiates the action of barbiturates). Products include:
Nembutal Sodium Capsules 440
Nembutal Sodium Solution 442
Nembutal Sodium Suppositories 444

Perphenazine (Possible additive effects which may include hypotension). Products include:
Etrafon 2495
Triavil Tablets 1800
Trilafon 2532

Phenobarbital (Thiothixene potentiates the action of barbiturates, however, the dosage of anticonvulsant barbiturates should not be reduced since thiothixene is capable of precipitating convulsion). Products include:
Arco-Lase Plus Tablets 513
Bellergal-S Tablets 2375
Donnatal 2234
Donnatal Extentabs 2234
Donnatal Tablets 2234
Phenobarbital Elixir and Tablets 1523
Quadrinal Tablets 1398

Prazepam (Possible additive effects which may include hypotension).
No products indexed under this heading.

Prochlorperazine (Possible additive effects which may include hypotension). Products include:
Compazine 2644

Procyclidine Hydrochloride (Thiothixene possesses weak anticholinergic properties; concurrent use requires caution because of increased atropine-like effect). Products include:
Kemadrin Tablets 1105

Promethazine Hydrochloride (Possible additive effects which may include hypotension). Products include:
Mepergan Injection 2859
Phenergan with Codeine 2883
Phenergan with Dextromethorphan .. 2885
Phenergan Injection 2880
Phenergan Suppositories 2882
Phenergan Syrup 2881
Phenergan Tablets 2882
Phenergan VC 2886
Phenergan VC with Codeine 2888

Propantheline Bromide (Thiothixene possesses weak anticholinergic properties; concurrent use requires caution because of increased atropine-like effect). Products include:
Pro-Banthine Tablets 2226

Propofol (Possible additive effects which may include hypotension). Products include:
Diprivan Injectable Emulsion 2939

Propoxyphene Hydrochloride (Possible additive effects which may include hypotension). Products include:
Darvon 1475
Wygesic Tablets 2930

Propoxyphene Napsylate (Possible additive effects which may include hypotension). Products include:
Darvon-N/Darvocet-N 1473

Quazepam (Possible additive effects which may include hypotension). Products include:
Doral Tablets 2773

Risperidone (Possible additive effects which may include hypotension). Products include:
Risperdal Tablets 1348

Scopolamine (Thiothixene possesses weak anticholinergic properties; concurrent use requires caution because of increased atropine-like effect). Products include:
Transderm Scōp Transdermal Therapeutic System 890

Scopolamine Hydrobromide (Thiothixene possesses weak anticholinergic properties; concurrent use requires caution because of increased atropine-like effect). Products include:
Atrohist Plus Tablets 1605
Donnatal 2234
Donnatal Extentabs 2234
Donnatal Tablets 2234

Secobarbital Sodium (Thiothixene potentiates the action of barbiturates). Products include:
Seconal Sodium Pulvules 1529

Sevoflurane (Possible additive effects which may include hypotension).
No products indexed under this heading.

Sufentanil Citrate (Possible additive effects which may include hypotension). Products include:
Sufenta Injection 1355

Temazepam (Possible additive effects which may include hypotension). Products include:
Restoril Capsules 2413

Thiamylal Sodium (Thiothixene potentiates the action of barbiturates).
No products indexed under this heading.

Thioridazine Hydrochloride (Possible additive effects which may include hypotension). Products include:
Mellaril 2398

Triazolam (Possible additive effects which may include hypotension). Products include:
Halcion Tablets 2093

Tridihexethyl Chloride (Thiothixene possesses weak anticholinergic properties; concurrent use requires caution because of increased atropine-like effect).
No products indexed under this heading.

Trifluoperazine Hydrochloride (Possible additive effects which may include hypotension). Products include:
Stelazine 2692

Trihexyphenidyl Hydrochloride (Thiothixene possesses weak anticholinergic properties; concurrent use requires caution because of increased atropine-like effect). Products include:
Artane 1418

Zolpidem Tartrate (Possible additive effects which may include hypotension). Products include:
Ambien Tablets 2559

Food Interactions

Alcohol (Possible additive effects which may include hypotension).

NAVELBINE INJECTION
(Vinorelbine Tartrate) 1212
May interact with:

Cisplatin (Potential for higher incidence of granulocytopenia with vinorelbine used in combination with cisplatin). Products include:
Platinol for Injection 717
Platinol-AQ Injection 719

Mitomycin (Mitomycin-C) (Acute pulmonary reactions have been reported with vinorelbine and other vinca alkaloids used in conjunction with mitomycin). Products include:
Mutamycin for Injection 712

NEBCIN VIALS, HYPORETS & ADD-VANTAGE
(Tobramycin Sulfate) 1518
May interact with aminoglycosides, cephalosporins, and certain other agents. Compounds in these categories include:

Amikacin Sulfate (Tobramycin has an inherent potential for causing nephrotoxicity and ototoxicity; concurrent and sequential use should be avoided). Products include:
Amikacin Sulfate Injection, USP 523
Amikacin Sulfate Injection, USP 981
Amikin Injectable 502

Cefaclor (Co-administration has resulted in an increased incidence of nephrotoxicity). Products include:
Ceclor Pulvules & Suspension ... 1470

Cefadroxil (Co-administration has resulted in an increased incidence of nephrotoxicity). Products include:
Duricef Capsules, Tablets, and Oral Suspension 750

Cefamandole Nafate (Co-administration has resulted in an increased incidence of nephrotoxicity). Products include:
Mandol Vials, Faspak & ADD-Vantage 1516

Cefazolin Sodium (Co-administration has resulted in an increased incidence of nephrotoxicity). Products include:
Ancef Injection 2632
Kefzol Vials, Faspak & ADD-Vantage 1511

Cefixime (Co-administration has resulted in an increased incidence of nephrotoxicity). Products include:
Suprax 1443

Cefmetazole Sodium (Co-administration has resulted in an increased incidence of nephrotoxicity).
No products indexed under this heading.

Cefonicid Sodium (Co-administration has resulted in an increased incidence of nephrotoxicity). Products include:
Monocid Injection 2674

(▣ Described in PDR For Nonprescription Drugs)   (◉ Described in PDR For Ophthalmology)

723 Interactions Index NegGram

Cefoperazone Sodium (Co-administration has resulted in an increased incidence of nephrotoxicity). Products include:

Cefobid Intravenous/Intramuscular 1996
Cefobid Pharmacy Bulk Package - Not for Direct Infusion 1999

Ceforanide (Co-administration has resulted in an increased incidence of nephrotoxicity).

No products indexed under this heading.

Cefotaxime Sodium (Co-administration has resulted in an increased incidence of nephrotoxicity). Products include:

Claforan Sterile and Injection 1259

Cefotetan (Co-administration has resulted in an increased incidence of nephrotoxicity). Products include:

Cefotan 2936

Cefoxitin Sodium (Co-administration has resulted in an increased incidence of nephrotoxicity). Products include:

Mefoxin 1734
Mefoxin Premixed Intravenous Solution 1737

Cefpodoxime Proxetil (Co-administration has resulted in an increased incidence of nephrotoxicity). Products include:

Vantin for Oral Suspension and Vantin Tablets 2112

Cefprozil (Co-administration has resulted in an increased incidence of nephrotoxicity). Products include:

Cefzil Tablets and Oral Suspension 747

Ceftazidime (Co-administration has resulted in an increased incidence of nephrotoxicity). Products include:

Ceptaz 1070
Fortaz 1092
Tazicef for Injection 2697
Tazidime Vials, Faspak & ADD-Vantage 1531

Ceftizoxime Sodium (Co-administration has resulted in an increased incidence of nephrotoxicity). Products include:

Cefizox for Intramuscular or Intravenous Use 1025

Ceftriaxone Sodium (Co-administration has resulted in an increased incidence of nephrotoxicity). Products include:

Rocephin Injectable Vials, ADD-Vantage, Galaxy Container 2305

Cefuroxime Axetil (Co-administration has resulted in an increased incidence of nephrotoxicity). Products include:

Ceftin 1067

Cefuroxime Sodium (Co-administration has resulted in an increased incidence of nephrotoxicity). Products include:

Kefurox Vials, Faspak & ADD-Vantage 1509
Zinacef 1184

Cephalexin (Co-administration has resulted in an increased incidence of nephrotoxicity). Products include:

Keflex Pulvules & Oral Suspension 930

Cephaloridine (Tobramycin has an inherent potential for causing nephrotoxicity and ototoxicity; concurrent and sequential use should be avoided).

Cephalothin Sodium (Co-administration has resulted in an increased incidence of nephrotoxicity).

Cephapirin Sodium (Co-administration has resulted in an increased incidence of nephrotoxicity).

No products indexed under this heading.

Cephradine (Co-administration has resulted in an increased incidence of nephrotoxicity).

No products indexed under this heading.

Cisplatin (Tobramycin has an inherent potential for causing nephrotoxicity and ototoxicity; concurrent and sequential use should be avoided). Products include:

Platinol for Injection 717
Platinol-AQ Injection 719

Colistin Sulfate (Tobramycin has an inherent potential for causing nephrotoxicity and ototoxicity; concurrent and sequential use should be avoided). Products include:

Coly-Mycin S Otic w/Neomycin & Hydrocortisone 1965

Ethacrynic Acid (Co-administration should be avoided; ethacrynic acid enhances aminoglycoside toxicity by altering antibiotic concentrations in serum and tissue; increased potential for ototoxicity). Products include:

Edecrin Tablets 1698

Furosemide (Co-administration should be avoided; furosemide enhances aminoglycoside toxicity by altering antibiotic concentrations in serum and tissue; increased potential for ototoxicity). Products include:

Lasix Injection, Oral Solution and Tablets 1267

Gentamicin Sulfate (Tobramycin has an inherent potential for causing nephrotoxicity and ototoxicity; concurrent and sequential use should be avoided). Products include:

Garamycin Cream 0.1% 2501
Garamycin Injectable 2502
Garamycin Ointment 0.1% 2501
Garamycin Ophthalmic 2501
Genoptic Sterile Ophthalmic Solution ◉ 241
Genoptic Sterile Ophthalmic Ointment ◉ 241
Gentak ◉ 209
Pred-G Liquifilm Sterile Ophthalmic Suspension ◉ 248
Pred-G S.O.P. Sterile Ophthalmic Ointment ◉ 249

Kanamycin Sulfate (Tobramycin has an inherent potential for causing nephrotoxicity and ototoxicity; concurrent and sequential use should be avoided).

No products indexed under this heading.

Loracarbef (Co-administration has resulted in an increased incidence of nephrotoxicity). Products include:

Lorabid Suspension and Pulvules 1513

Neomycin Sulfate (Tobramycin has an inherent potential for causing nephrotoxicity and ototoxicity; concurrent and sequential use should be avoided). Products include:

AK-Spore ◉ 205
AK-Trol Ointment & Suspension ◉ 205
Coly-Mycin S Otic w/Neomycin & Hydrocortisone 1965
Cortisporin Cream 1073
Cortisporin Ointment 1074
Cortisporin Ophthalmic Ointment Sterile 1074
Cortisporin Ophthalmic Suspension Sterile 1075
Cortisporin Otic Solution Sterile 1076
Cortisporin Otic Suspension Sterile 1077
Maxitrol Ophthalmic Ointment and Suspension ◉ 222
Mycitracin ▣ 803
NeoDecadron Sterile Ophthalmic Ointment 1755
NeoDecadron Sterile Ophthalmic Solution 1756
NeoDecadron Topical Cream 1757
Neosporin G.U. Irrigant Sterile 1130
Neosporin Ointment ▣ 821
Neosporin Plus Maximum Strength Cream ▣ 821
Neosporin Plus Maximum Strength Ointment ▣ 822
Neosporin Ophthalmic Ointment Sterile 1130
Neosporin Ophthalmic Solution Sterile 1131
Pediotic Suspension Sterile 1140
Poly-Pred Liquifilm ◉ 246

Paromomycin Sulfate (Tobramycin has an inherent potential for causing nephrotoxicity and ototoxicity; concurrent and sequential use should be avoided).

No products indexed under this heading.

Polymyxin B Sulfate (Tobramycin has an inherent potential for causing nephrotoxicity and ototoxicity; concurrent and sequential use should be avoided). Products include:

AK-Spore ◉ 205
AK-Trol Ointment & Suspension ◉ 205
Betadine Brand First Aid Antibiotics & Moisturizer Ointment 2144
Cortisporin Cream 1073
Cortisporin Ointment 1074
Cortisporin Ophthalmic Ointment Sterile 1074
Cortisporin Ophthalmic Suspension Sterile 1075
Cortisporin Otic Solution Sterile 1076
Cortisporin Otic Suspension Sterile 1077
Maxitrol Ophthalmic Ointment and Suspension ◉ 222
Mycitracin ▣ 803
Neosporin G.U. Irrigant Sterile 1130
Neosporin Ointment ▣ 821
Neosporin Plus Maximum Strength Cream ▣ 821
Neosporin Plus Maximum Strength Ointment ▣ 822
Neosporin Ophthalmic Ointment Sterile 1130
Neosporin Ophthalmic Solution Sterile 1131
Pediotic Suspension Sterile 1140
Poly-Pred Liquifilm ◉ 246
Polysporin Ointment ▣ 822
Polysporin Ophthalmic Ointment Sterile 1140
Polysporin Powder ▣ 823
Polytrim Ophthalmic Solution Sterile 479
TERAK Ointment ◉ 210
Terramycin with Polymyxin B Sulfate Ophthalmic Ointment 2035

Streptomycin Sulfate (Tobramycin has an inherent potential for causing nephrotoxicity and ototoxicity; concurrent and sequential use should be avoided). Products include:

Streptomycin Sulfate Injection 2031

Tobramycin (Tobramycin has an inherent potential for causing nephrotoxicity and ototoxicity; concurrent and sequential use should be avoided). Products include:

AKTOB ◉ 207
TobraDex Ophthalmic Suspension and Ointment 469
Tobrex Ophthalmic Ointment and Solution ◉ 226

Vancomycin Hydrochloride (Tobramycin has an inherent potential for causing nephrotoxicity and ototoxicity; concurrent and sequential use should be avoided). Products include:

Vancocin HCl, Oral Solution & Pulvules 1536
Vancocin HCl, Vials & ADD-Vantage 1534

Viomycin (Tobramycin has an inherent potential for causing nephrotoxicity and ototoxicity; concurrent and sequential use should be avoided).

NEGGRAM CAPLETS

(Nalidixic Acid) 2453

May interact with oral anticoagulants, xanthine bronchodilators, antacids containing aluminium, calcium and magnesium, iron containing oral preparations, and certain other agents. Compounds in these categories include:

Aluminum Carbonate (Co-administration with antacids may substantially interfere with the absorption of quinolones; these agents should not be given simultaneously or within two hours of the administration of quinolones). Products include:

Basaljel Capsules 2810
Basaljel Suspension 2810
Basaljel Tablets 2810

Aluminum Hydroxide (Co-administration with antacids may substantially interfere with the absorption of quinolones; these agents should not be given simultaneously or within two hours of the administration of quinolones). Products include:

ALternaGEL Liquid 1358
Maximum Strength Ascriptin ▣ 650
Cama Arthritis Pain Reliever ▣ 748
Gaviscon Extra Strength Relief Formula Antacid Tablets ▣ 778
Gaviscon Extra Strength Relief Formula Liquid Antacid ▣ 779
Gaviscon Liquid Antacid ▣ 779
Gelusil Antacid-Anti-gas Liquid ▣ 819
Gelusil Antacid-Anti-gas Tablets ▣ 819
Maalox Antacid/Anti-Gas Tablets 889
Maalox Heartburn Relief Suspension ▣ 658
Maalox Antacid Liquid 888
Extra Strength Maalox Antacid/Anti-Gas Liquid and Tablets 888
Mylanta 1359
Tempo Soft Antacid ▣ 799

Aluminum Hydroxide Gel (Co-administration with antacids may substantially interfere with the absorption of quinolones; these agents should not be given simultaneously or within two hours of the administration of quinolones). Products include:

ALternaGEL Liquid ▣ 675
Aludrox Oral Suspension ▣ 850
Amphojel Suspension 2802
Amphojel Suspension without Flavor 2802
Amphojel Tablets 2802
Ascriptin ▣ 650
Gaviscon Antacid Tablets ▣ 778
Gaviscon-2 Antacid Tablets ▣ 779
Mylanta Liquid ▣ 676
Mylanta Double Strength Liquid ▣ 676
Nephrox Suspension ▣ 671

Aminophylline (Co-administration with quinolones has shown to increase plasma theophylline levels; potential for theophylline-related side effects).

No products indexed under this heading.

Caffeine (Quinolones have shown to interfere with the metabolism of caffeine, this may lead to reduced clearance of caffeine and the prolongation of its half-life). Products include:

Arthritis Strength BC Powder ▣ 631
BC Powder ▣ 631
Cafergot 2376
DHCplus Capsules 2148
Darvon Compound-65 Pulvules 1475
Esgic-plus Capsules 1012
Esgic-plus Tablets 1012
Aspirin Free Excedrin Analgesic Caplets and Geltabs 734
Excedrin Extra-Strength Analgesic Tablets, Caplets, and Geltabs 734
Fioricet Tablets 2386
Fioricet with Codeine Capsules 2387
Fiorinal Capsules 2388
Fiorinal with Codeine Capsules 2390
Fiorinal Tablets 2388
Goody's Extra Strength Headache Powders ▣ 632
Goody's Extra Strength Pain Relief Tablets ▣ 632
Maximum Strength Multi-Symptom Formula Midol ▣ 621

IMPORTANT NOTE: Always consult each drug listing in the patient's regimen for possible interactions.

NegGram — **Interactions Index** — **724**

No Doz Maximum Strength Caplets ▣ 644
Norgesic 1554
Vanquish Analgesic Caplets ▣ 627
Wigraine Tablets 1884

Cyclosporine (Co-administration with other members of quinolone class has resulted in elevated cyclosporine serum levels). Products include:
Neoral 2405
Sandimmune 2416

Dicumarol (Quinolones, including nalidixic acid, may enhance the effects of oral anticoagulants).
No products indexed under this heading.

Digoxin (Enoxacin may raise serum digoxin levels in some patients). Products include:
Lanoxicaps 1110
Lanoxin Elixir Pediatric 1113
Lanoxin Injection 1116
Lanoxin Injection Pediatric 1119
Lanoxin Tablets 1121

Dyphylline (Co-administration with quinolones has shown to increase plasma theophylline levels; potential for theophylline-related side effects). Products include:
Lufyllin & Lufyllin-400 Tablets 2778
Lufyllin-GG Elixir & Tablets 2779

Ferrous Fumarate (Co-administration with oral iron-containing products may substantially interfere with the absorption of quinolones; these agents should not be given simultaneously or within two hours of the administration of quinolones). Products include:
Chromagen Capsules 2470
Chromagen FA 2471
Chromagen Forte 2471
Ferro-Sequels ▣ 684
Nephro-Fer Tablets 2168
Nephro-Fer Rx Tablets 2168
Nephro-Vite + Fe Tablets 2170
Stresstabs + Iron ▣ 685
Trinsicon Capsules 2759
Vitron-C Tablets ▣ 667

Ferrous Gluconate (Co-administration with oral iron-containing products may substantially interfere with the absorption of quinolones; these agents should not be given simultaneously or within two hours of the administration of quinolones). Products include:
Megadose 513

Ferrous Sulfate (Co-administration with oral iron-containing products may substantially interfere with the absorption of quinolones; these agents should not be given simultaneously or within two hours of the administration of quinolones). Products include:
Feosol Capsules ▣ 777
Feosol Elixir 2627
Feosol Tablets 2627
Fero-Folic-500 Filmtab 433
Fero-Grad-500 Filmtab 434
Fero-Gradumet Filmtab 434
Iberet Tablets 437
Iberet-500 Liquid 438
Iberet-Folic-500 Filmtab 433
Iberet-Liquid 438
Irospan 1000
Slow Fe Tablets 889
Slow Fe with Folic Acid 890

Iron (Co-administration with oral iron-containing products may substantially interfere with the absorption of quinolones; these agents should not be given simultaneously or within two hours of the administration of quinolones). Products include:
Feosol Caplets 2626

Magaldrate (Co-administration with antacids may substantially interfere with the absorption of quinolones; these agents should not be given simultaneously or within two hours of the administration of quinolones).
No products indexed under this heading.

Magnesium Hydroxide (Co-administration with antacids may substantially interfere with the absorption of quinolones; these agents should not be given simultaneously or within two hours of the administration of quinolones). Products include:
Aludrox Oral Suspension ▣ 850
Ascriptin ▣ 650
Di-Gel Antacid/Anti-Gas ▣ 762
Gelusil Antacid-Anti-gas Liquid ▣ 819
Gelusil Antacid-Anti-gas Tablets ▣ 819
Maalox Antacid/Anti-Gas Tablets 889
Maalox Antacid Liquid 888
Extra Strength Maalox Antacid/Anti-Gas Liquid and Tablets 888
Mylanta Fast-Acting 1359
Mylanta Gelcaps Antacid ▣ 678
Fast-Acting Mylanta Liquid Antacid 1359
Mylanta Tablets ▣ 677
Maximum-Strength Fast-Acting Mylanta Liquid Antacid 1359
Mylanta Double Strength Tablets ▣ 677
Phillips' Milk of Magnesia Liquid ▣ 627
Rolaids Antacid Tablets ▣ 807
Tempo Soft Antacid ▣ 799

Magnesium Oxide (Co-administration with antacids may substantially interfere with the absorption of quinolones; these agents should not be given simultaneously or within two hours of the administration of quinolones). Products include:
Beelith Tablets 632
Bufferin Analgesic Tablets ▣ 636
Arthritis Strength Bufferin Analgesic Caplets ▣ 637
Extra Strength Bufferin Analgesic Tablets ▣ 637
Caltrate PLUS ▣ 681
Cama Arthritis Pain Reliever ▣ 748
Mag-Ox 400 666
Uro-Mag 666

Nitrofurantoin (Interferes with the therapeutic action of nalidixic acid). Products include:
Macrodantin Capsules 2140

Nitrofurantoin Macrocrystals (Interferes with the therapeutic action of nalidixic acid).

Polysaccharide-Iron Complex (Co-administration with oral iron-containing products may substantially interfere with the absorption of quinolones; these agents should not be given simultaneously or within two hours of the administration of quinolones). Products include:
Niferex-150 Capsules 811
Niferex Elixir 811
Niferex-150 Forte Capsules 811
Niferex 811
Niferex-PN Tablets 811
Nu-Iron 150 Capsules 1826
Nu-Iron Elixir 1826

Sucralfate (Co-administration with sucralfate may substantially interfere with the absorption of quinolones; sucralfate should not be given simultaneously or within two hours of the administration of quinolones). Products include:
Carafate Suspension 1250
Carafate Tablets 1249

Theophylline (Co-administration with quinolones has shown to increase plasma theophylline levels; potential for theophylline-related side effects). Products include:
Marax Tablets & DF Syrup 2015
Quibron 2227

Theophylline Anhydrous (Co-administration with quinolones has shown to increase plasma theophylline levels; potential for theophylline-related side effects). Products include:
Aerolate 1003
Primatene Tablets ▣ 844
Respbid Tablets 687
Slo-bid Gyrocaps 2201
Theo-24 Extended Release Capsules 2753
Theo-Dur Extended-Release Tablets 1367
Theo-X Extended-Release Tablets 793
Uni-Dur Extended-Release Tablets 1374
Uniphyl 400 mg and 600 mg Tablets 2157

Theophylline Calcium Salicylate (Co-administration with quinolones has shown to increase plasma theophylline levels; potential for theophylline-related side effects). Products include:
Quadrinal Tablets 1398

Theophylline Sodium Glycinate (Co-administration with quinolones has shown to increase plasma theophylline levels; potential for theophylline-related side effects).
No products indexed under this heading.

Warfarin Sodium (Quinolones, including nalidixic acid, may enhance the effects of oral anticoagulants). Products include:
Coumadin 941

Zinc Sulfate (Co-administration with oral zinc-containing products may substantially interfere with the absorption of quinolones; these agents should not be given simultaneously or within two hours of the administration of quinolones). Products include:
Clear Eyes ACR Astringent/Lubricant Eye Redness Reliever Eye Drops ◉ 314
Visine A.C. Seasonal Relief From Pollen and Dust ◉ 301

NEGGRAM SUSPENSION
(Nalidixic Acid) 2453
See **NegGram Caplets**

NEMBUTAL SODIUM CAPSULES
(Pentobarbital Sodium) 440
May interact with central nervous system depressants, oral anticoagulants, corticosteroids, monoamine oxidase inhibitors, estrogens, and certain other agents. Compounds in these categories include:

Alfentanil Hydrochloride (Additive CNS depressant effects). Products include:
Alfenta Injection 1334

Alprazolam (Additive CNS depressant effects). Products include:
Xanax Tablets 2115

Aprobarbital (Additive CNS depressant effects).
No products indexed under this heading.

Betamethasone Acetate (Barbiturates enhance metabolism). Products include:
Celestone Soluspan Suspension 2484

Betamethasone Sodium Phosphate (Barbiturates enhance metabolism). Products include:
Celestone Soluspan Suspension 2484

Buprenorphine (Additive CNS depressant effects). Products include:
Buprenex Injectable 2170

Buspirone Hydrochloride (Additive CNS depressant effects). Products include:
BuSpar Tablets 738

Butabarbital (Additive CNS depressant effects).
No products indexed under this heading.

Butalbital (Additive CNS depressant effects). Products include:
Axocet Capsules 2469
Esgic-plus Capsules 1012
Esgic-plus Tablets 1012
Fioricet Tablets 2386
Fioricet with Codeine Capsules 2387
Fiorinal Capsules 2388
Fiorinal with Codeine Capsules 2390
Fiorinal Tablets 2388
Phrenilin 790
Sedapap Tablets 50 mg/650 mg 1826

Chlordiazepoxide (Additive CNS depressant effects). Products include:
Limbitrol 2333

Chlordiazepoxide Hydrochloride (Additive CNS depressant effects). Products include:
Librax Capsules 2330
Librium Capsules 2331
Librium Injectable 2332

Chlorotrianisene (Decreased effects of estrogens).
No products indexed under this heading.

Chlorpromazine (Additive CNS depressant effects). Products include:
Thorazine Suppositories 2701

Chlorprothixene (Additive CNS depressant effects).
No products indexed under this heading.

Chlorprothixene Hydrochloride (Additive CNS depressant effects).
No products indexed under this heading.

Chlorprothixene Lactate (Additive CNS depressant effects).
No products indexed under this heading.

Clorazepate Dipotassium (Additive CNS depressant effects). Products include:
Tranxene 459

Clozapine (Additive CNS depressant effects). Products include:
Clozaril Tablets 2377

Codeine Phosphate (Additive CNS depressant effects). Products include:
Brontex 2130
Dimetane-DC Cough Syrup 2232
Fioricet with Codeine Capsules 2387
Fiorinal with Codeine Capsules 2390
Nucofed 2225
Phenergan with Codeine 2883
Phenergan VC with Codeine 2888
Robitussin A-C Syrup 2248
Robitussin-DAC Syrup 2249
Ryna ▣ 804
Soma Compound w/Codeine Tablets 2784
Tylenol with Codeine 1592

Cortisone Acetate (Barbiturates enhance metabolism). Products include:
Cortone Acetate Sterile Suspension 1663
Cortone Acetate Tablets 1664

Desflurane (Additive CNS depressant effects). Products include:
Suprane (desflurane, USP) 1865

Dexamethasone (Barbiturates enchance metabolism). Products include:
AK-Trol Ointment & Suspension ◉ 205
Decadron Elixir 1676
Decadron Tablets 1678
Decaspray Topical Aerosol 1689
Maxitrol Ophthalmic Ointment and Suspension ◉ 222

(▣ Described in PDR For Nonprescription Drugs) (◉ Described in PDR For Ophthalmology)

Interactions Index

TobraDex Ophthalmic Suspension and Ointment................ 469

Dexamethasone Acetate (Barbiturates enhance metabolism). Products include:
Dalalone D.P. Injectable 1009
Decadron-LA Sterile Suspension...... 1687

Dexamethasone Sodium Phosphate (Barbiturates enhance metabolism). Products include:
Decadron Phosphate Injection 1680
Decadron Phosphate Sterile Ophthalmic Ointment 1684
Decadron Phosphate Sterile Ophthalmic Solution 1685
Decadron Phosphate Topical Cream 1686
Decadron Phosphate with Xylocaine Injection, Sterile 1683
Dexacort Phosphate in Respihaler .. 1606
Dexacort Phosphate in Turbinaire .. 1607
NeoDecadron Sterile Ophthalmic Ointment 1755
NeoDecadron Sterile Ophthalmic Solution 1756
NeoDecadron Topical Cream 1757

Dezocine (Additive CNS depressant effects). Products include:
Dalgan Injection............... 529

Diazepam (Additive CNS depressant effects). Products include:
Dizac (diazepam injectable emulsion) CIV 1862
Valium Injectable 2336
Valium Tablets 2335

Dicumarol (Increased metabolism, decreased anticoagulant response).
No products indexed under this heading.

Dienestrol (Decreased effects of estrogens). Products include:
Ortho Dienestrol Cream 1922

Diethylstilbestrol (Decreased effects of estrogens). Products include:
Diethylstilbestrol Tablets 1477

Doxycycline Calcium (Barbiturates shorten half-life of doxycycline). Products include:
Vibramycin Calcium Oral Suspension Syrup 2038

Doxycycline Hyclate (Barbiturates shorten half-life of doxycycline). Products include:
Doryx Capsules 1970
Vibramycin Hyclate Capsules 2038
Vibramycin Hyclate Intravenous 2040
Vibra-Tabs Film Coated Tablets 2038

Doxycycline Monohydrate (Barbiturates shorten half-life of doxycycline). Products include:
Monodox Capsules 1858
Vibramycin Monohydrate for Oral Suspension 2038

Droperidol (Additive CNS depressant effects). Products include:
Inapsine Injection............... 462

Enflurane (Additive CNS depressant effects).
No products indexed under this heading.

Estazolam (Additive CNS depressant effects). Products include:
ProSom Tablets 457

Estradiol (Decreased effects of estrogens). Products include:
Climara Transdermal System 640
Estrace Cream and Tablets 751
Estraderm Transdermal System 842
Estring Vaginal Ring 2086
Vivelle Transdermal System 880

Estrogens, Conjugated (Decreased effects of estrogens). Products include:
PMB 200 and PMB 400 2890
Premarin Intravenous 2893
Premarin Tablets 2896
Premarin Vaginal Cream 2898
Premphase 2900
Prempro 2905

Estrogens, Esterified (Decreased effects of estrogens). Products include:
ESTRATAB Tablets (0.3, 0.625, 1.25, 2.5 mg) 2715
Estratest 2718
Menest Tablets 2671

Estropipate (Decreased effects of estrogens). Products include:
Ogen Tablets 2103
Ogen Vaginal Cream 2106
Ortho-Est 1925

Ethchlorvynol (Additive CNS depressant effects). Products include:
Placidyl Capsules 456

Ethinamate (Additive CNS depressant effects).
No products indexed under this heading.

Ethinyl Estradiol (Decreased effects on estrogens). Products include:
Brevicon............... 2563
Demulen 2580
Desogen Tablets 1867
Levlen/Tri-Levlen 646
Lo/Ovral Tablets 2852
Lo/Ovral-28 Tablets 2857
Modicon 1928
Nordette-21 Tablets 2863
Nordette-28 Tablets 2866
Norinyl 2563
Ortho-Cept 1907
Ortho-Cyclen/Ortho-Tri-Cyclen 1914
Ortho-Novum 1928
Ortho-Cyclen/Ortho Tri-Cyclen 1914
Ovcon 765
Ovral Tablets 2877
Ovral-28 Tablets 2878
Levlen/Tri-Levlen 646
Tri-Norinyl 2607
Triphasil-21 Tablets 2919
Triphasil-28 Tablets 2924

Fentanyl (Additive CNS depressant effects). Products include:
Duragesic Transdermal System 1336

Fentanyl Citrate (Additive CNS depressant effects). Products include:
Sublimaze Injection............... 463

Fludrocortisone Acetate (Barbiturates enhance metabolism). Products include:
Florinef Acetate Tablets 506

Fluphenazine Decanoate (Additive CNS depressant effects). Products include:
Prolixin Decanoate 510

Fluphenazine Enanthate (Additive CNS depressant effects). Products include:
Prolixin Enanthate 510

Fluphenazine Hydrochloride (Additive CNS depressant effects). Products include:
Prolixin 510

Flurazepam Hydrochloride (Additive CNS depressant effects). Products include:
Dalmane Capsules 2329

Furazolidone (Prolongs effects of barbiturates). Products include:
Furoxone 2221

Glutethimide (Additive CNS depressant effects).
No products indexed under this heading.

Griseofulvin (Phenobarbital interferes with absorption). Products include:
Fulvicin P/G Tablets 2499
Fulvicin P/G 165 & 330 Tablets 2500
Grifulvin V (griseofulvin tablets) Microsize (griseofulvin oral suspension) Microsize 1944
Gris-PEG Tablets, 125 mg & 250 mg 476

Haloperidol (Additive CNS depressant effects). Products include:
Haldol Injection, Tablets and Concentrate 1585

Haloperidol Decanoate (Additive CNS depressant effects). Products include:
Haldol Decanoate............... 1587

Hydrocodone Bitartrate (Additive CNS depressant effects). Products include:
Codiclear DH Syrup 808
Duratuss HD Elixir 2750
Histussin D Liquid 670
Hycodan Tablets and Syrup 946
Hycomine Compound Tablets 948
Hycomine 947
Hycotuss Expectorant Syrup 950
Hydrocet Capsules 787
Lorcet 10/650 Tablets 1016
Lortab 2751
Tussend 1830
Tussend Expectorant 1831
Vicodin Tablets 1404
Vicodin ES Tablets 1405
Vicodin HP Tablets 1403
Vicodin Tuss Expectorant 1406
Zydone Capsules 967

Hydrocodone Polistirex (Additive CNS depressant effects). Products include:
Tussionex Pennkinetic Extended-Release Suspension 1624

Hydrocortisone (Barbiturates enhance metabolism). Products include:
Anusol-HC Cream 2.5 % 1953
Aquanil HC Lotion 1989
Maximum Strength Cortaid Spray ... 800
CORTENEMA 2713
Cortisporin Ointment 1074
Cortisporin Ophthalmic Ointment Sterile 1074
Cortisporin Ophthalmic Suspension Sterile 1075
Cortisporin Otic Solution Sterile 1076
Cortisporin Otic Suspension Sterile 1077
Cortizone-5 795
Cortizone-10 795
Hydrocortone Tablets 1715
Hytone 922
Hytone Ointment 2 ½ % 923
Massengill Medicated Soft Cloth Towelettes 2628
Pediotic Suspension Sterile 1140
Preparation H Hydrocortisone 1% Cream 843
ProctoCream-HC 2.5 % 2552
VōSoL HC Otic Solution 2786

Hydrocortisone Acetate (Barbiturates enhance metabolism). Products include:
Analpram-HC Rectal Cream 1% and 2.5 % 993
Anusol HC-1 Hydrocortisone Anti-Itch Ointment 810
Anusol-HC Suppositories 1954
Caldecort Anti-Itch Hydrocortisone Cream 651
Coly-Mycin S Otic w/Neomycin & Hydrocortisone 1965
Cortaid 800
Cortifoam 2540
Cortisporin Cream 1073
Epifoam 2543
Hydrocortone Acetate Sterile Suspension............... 1712
Mantadil Cream 1124
Nupercainal Hydrocortisone 1% Cream 661
Pramosone Cream, Lotion & Ointment 995
ProctoFoam-HC 2552
Terra-Cortril Ophthalmic Suspension 2033

Hydrocortisone Sodium Phosphate (Barbiturates enhance metabolism). Products include:
Hydrocortone Phosphate Injection, Sterile 1713

Hydrocortisone Sodium Succinate (Barbiturates enhance metabolism).
No products indexed under this heading.

Hydroxyzine Hydrochloride (Additive CNS depressant effects). Products include:
Atarax Tablets & Syrup 1992

Marax Tablets & DF Syrup............... 2015
Vistaril Intramuscular Solution........... 2042

Isocarboxazid (Prolongs effects of barbiturates).
No products indexed under this heading.

Isoflurane (Additive CNS depressant effects).
No products indexed under this heading.

Ketamine Hydrochloride (Additive CNS depressant effects).
No products indexed under this heading.

Levomethadyl Acetate Hydrochloride (Additive CNS depressant effects). Products include:
Orlaam Oral Solution 2361

Levorphanol Tartrate (Additive CNS depressant effects). Products include:
Levo-Dromoran 2297

Lorazepam (Additive CNS depressant effects). Products include:
Ativan Injection............... 2805
Ativan Tablets............... 2807

Loxapine Hydrochloride (Additive CNS depressant effects). Products include:
Loxitane 1426

Loxapine Succinate (Additive CNS depressant effects). Products include:
Loxitane Capsules 1426

Meperidine Hydrochloride (Additive CNS depressant effects). Products include:
Demerol 2438
Mepergan Injection 2859

Mephobarbital (Additive CNS depressant effects). Products include:
Mebaral Tablets 2452

Meprobamate (Additive CNS depressant effects). Products include:
Miltown Tablets 2780
PMB 200 and PMB 400 2890

Mesoridazine Besylate (Additive CNS depressant effects). Products include:
Serentil 689

Methadone Hydrochloride (Additive CNS depressant effects). Products include:
Methadone Hydrochloride Oral Concentrate 2356
Methadone Hydrochloride Oral Solution & Tablets 2357

Methohexital Sodium (Additive CNS depressant effects).
No products indexed under this heading.

Methotrimeprazine (Additive CNS depressant effects). Products include:
Levoprome 1321

Methoxyflurane (Additive CNS depressant effects).
No products indexed under this heading.

Methylprednisolone Acetate (Barbiturates enhance metabolism).
No products indexed under this heading.

Methylprednisolone Sodium Succinate (Barbiturates enhance metabolism).
No products indexed under this heading.

Midazolam Hydrochloride (Additive CNS depressant effects). Products include:
Versed Injection 2324

Molindone Hydrochloride (Additive CNS depressant effects). Products include:
Moban Tablets and Concentrate...... 1036

IMPORTANT NOTE: Always consult each drug listing in the patient's regimen for possible interactions.

Nembutal Sodium Capsules / Interactions Index

Morphine Sulfate (Additive CNS depressant effects). Products include:
- Astramorph/PF Injection, USP (Preservative-Free) 526
- Duramorph Injection 983
- Infumorph 200 and Infumorph 500 Sterile Solutions 985
- Kadian Capsules 2948
- MS Contin Tablets 2149
- MSIR 2152
- Oramorph SR (Morphine Sulfate Sustained Release Tablets) 2359
- RMS Suppositories CII 2766
- Roxanol 2365

Opium Alkaloids (Additive CNS depressant effects).
No products indexed under this heading.

Oxazepam (Additive CNS depressant effects). Products include:
- Serax Capsules 2916
- Serax Tablets 2916

Oxycodone Hydrochloride (Additive CNS depressant effects). Products include:
- OxyContin Tablets 2163
- OxyIR Capsules 2167
- Percocet Tablets 955
- Percodan Tablets 955
- Percodan-Demi Tablets 956
- Roxicodone Tablets, Oral Solution & Intensol (Oxycodone) 2366
- Tylox Capsules 1593

Perphenazine (Additive CNS depressant effects). Products include:
- Etrafon 2495
- Triavil Tablets 1800
- Trilafon 2532

Phenelzine Sulfate (Prolongs effects of barbiturates). Products include:
- Nardil 1977

Phenobarbital (Additive CNS depressant effects). Products include:
- Arco-Lase Plus Tablets 513
- Bellergal-S Tablets 2375
- Donnatal 2234
- Donnatal Extentabs 2234
- Donnatal Tablets 2234
- Phenobarbital Elixir and Tablets 1523
- Quadrinal Tablets 1398

Phenytoin (Variable effect on metabolism of phenytoin). Products include:
- Dilantin Infatabs 1967
- Dilantin-125 Suspension 1969

Phenytoin Sodium (Variable effect on metabolism of phenytoin). Products include:
- Dilantin Kapseals 1965

Polyestradiol Phosphate (Decreased effects of estrogens).
No products indexed under this heading.

Prazepam (Additive CNS depressant effects).
No products indexed under this heading.

Prednisolone Acetate (Barbiturates enhance metabolism). Products include:
- AK-CIDE .... ◉ 203
- AK-CIDE Ointment .... ◉ 203
- Blephamide Liquifilm Sterile Ophthalmic Suspension 472
- Blephamide Ointment .... ◉ 234
- Econopred & Econopred Plus Ophthalmic Suspensions .... ◉ 216
- Poly-Pred Liquifilm .... ◉ 246
- Pred Forte .... ◉ 247
- Pred Mild .... ◉ 250
- Pred-G Liquifilm Sterile Ophthalmic Suspension .... ◉ 248
- Pred-G S.O.P. Sterile Ophthalmic Ointment .... ◉ 249

Prednisolone Sodium Phosphate (Barbiturates enhance metabolism). Products include:
- AK-PRED .... ◉ 204
- Hydeltrasol Injection, Sterile 1708
- Pediapred Oral Solution 1618

Prednisolone Tebutate (Barbiturates enhance metabolism). Products include:
- Hydeltra-T.B.A. Sterile Suspension 1710

Prednisone (Barbiturates enhance metabolism).
No products indexed under this heading.

Prochlorperazine (Additive CNS depressant effects). Products include:
- Compazine 2644

Promethazine Hydrochloride (Additive CNS depressant effects). Products include:
- Mepergan Injection 2859
- Phenergan with Codeine 2883
- Phenergan with Dextromethorphan 2885
- Phenergan Injection 2880
- Phenergan Suppositories 2882
- Phenergan Syrup 2881
- Phenergan Tablets 2882
- Phenergan VC 2886
- Phenergan VC with Codeine 2888

Propofol (Additive CNS depressant effects). Products include:
- Diprivan Injectable Emulsion 2939

Propoxyphene Hydrochloride (Additive CNS depressant effects). Products include:
- Darvon 1475
- Wygesic Tablets 2930

Propoxyphene Napsylate (Additive CNS depressant effects). Products include:
- Darvon-N/Darvocet-N 1473

Quazepam (Additive CNS depressant effects). Products include:
- Doral Tablets 2773

Quinestrol (Decreased effects of estrogens).
No products indexed under this heading.

Risperidone (Additive CNS depressant effects). Products include:
- Risperdal Tablets 1348

Secobarbital Sodium (Additive CNS depressant effects). Products include:
- Seconal Sodium Pulvules 1529

Selegiline Hydrochloride (Prolongs effects of barbiturates). Products include:
- Eldepryl Capsules 2729

Sevoflurane (Additive CNS depressant effects).
No products indexed under this heading.

Sufentanil Citrate (Additive CNS depressant effects). Products include:
- Sufenta Injection 1355

Temazepam (Additive CNS depressant effects). Products include:
- Restoril Capsules 2413

Thiamylal Sodium (Additive CNS depressant effects).
No products indexed under this heading.

Thioridazine Hydrochloride (Additive CNS depressant effects). Products include:
- Mellaril 2398

Thiothixene (Additive CNS depressant effects). Products include:
- Navane Capsules and Concentrate 2018
- Navane Intramuscular 2019

Tranylcypromine Sulfate (Prolongs effects of barbiturates). Products include:
- Parnate Tablets 2679

Triamcinolone (Barbiturates enhance metabolism).
No products indexed under this heading.

Triamcinolone Acetonide (Barbiturates enhance metabolism). Products include:
- Azmacort Oral Inhaler 2175
- Nasacort AQ Nasal Spray 2191
- Nasacort Nasal Inhaler 2189

Triamcinolone Diacetate (Barbiturates enhance metabolism).
No products indexed under this heading.

Triamcinolone Hexacetonide (Barbiturates enhance metabolism).
No products indexed under this heading.

Triazolam (Additive CNS depressant effects). Products include:
- Halcion Tablets 2093

Trifluoperazine Hydrochloride (Additive CNS depressant effects). Products include:
- Stelazine 2692

Valproic Acid (Decreases barbiturate metabolism). Products include:
- Depakene 416

Warfarin Sodium (Increased metabolism, decreased anticoagulant response). Products include:
- Coumadin 941

Zolpidem Tartrate (Additive CNS depressant effects). Products include:
- Ambien Tablets 2559

NEMBUTAL SODIUM SOLUTION
(Pentobarbital Sodium) 442
May interact with central nervous system depressants, oral anticoagulants, corticosteroids, monoamine oxidase inhibitors, estrogens, and certain other agents. Compounds in these categories include:

Alfentanil Hydrochloride (Additive CNS depressant effects). Products include:
- Alfenta Injection 1334

Alprazolam (Additive CNS depressant effects). Products include:
- Xanax Tablets 2115

Aprobarbital (Additive CNS depressant effects).
No products indexed under this heading.

Betamethasone Acetate (Barbiturates enhance metabolism). Products include:
- Celestone Soluspan Suspension 2484

Betamethasone Sodium Phosphate (Barbiturates enhance metabolism). Products include:
- Celestone Soluspan Suspension 2484

Buprenorphine (Additive CNS depressant effects). Products include:
- Buprenex Injectable 2170

Buspirone Hydrochloride (Additive CNS depressant effects). Products include:
- BuSpar Tablets 738

Butabarbital (Additive CNS depressant effects).
No products indexed under this heading.

Butalbital (Additive CNS depressant effects). Products include:
- Axocet Capsules 2469
- Esgic-plus Capsules 1012
- Esgic-plus Tablets 1012
- Fioricet Tablets 2386
- Fioricet with Codeine Capsules 2387
- Fiorinal Capsules 2388
- Fiorinal with Codeine Capsules 2390
- Fiorinal Tablets 2388
- Phrenilin 790
- Sedapap Tablets 50 mg/650 mg 1826

Chlordiazepoxide (Additive CNS depressant effects). Products include:
- Limbitrol 2333

Chlordiazepoxide Hydrochloride (Additive CNS depressant effects). Products include:
- Librax Capsules 2330
- Librium Capsules 2331
- Librium Injectable 2332

Chlorotrianisene (Decreased effects of estrogens).
No products indexed under this heading.

Chlorpromazine (Additive CNS depressant effects). Products include:
- Thorazine Suppositories 2701

Chlorprothixene (Additive CNS depressant effects).
No products indexed under this heading.

Chlorprothixene Hydrochloride (Additive CNS depressant effects).
No products indexed under this heading.

Chlorprothixene Lactate (Additive CNS depressant effects).
No products indexed under this heading.

Clorazepate Dipotassium (Additive CNS depressant effects). Products include:
- Tranxene 459

Clozapine (Additive CNS depressant effects). Products include:
- Clozaril Tablets 2377

Codeine Phosphate (Additive CNS depressant effects). Products include:
- Brontex 2130
- Dimetane-DC Cough Syrup 2232
- Fioricet with Codeine Capsules 2387
- Fiorinal with Codeine Capsules 2390
- Nucofed 2225
- Phenergan with Codeine 2883
- Phenergan VC with Codeine 2888
- Robitussin A-C Syrup 2248
- Robitussin-DAC Syrup 2249
- Ryna .... ▣ 804
- Soma Compound w/Codeine Tablets 2784
- Tylenol with Codeine 1592

Cortisone Acetate (Barbiturates enhance metabolism). Products include:
- Cortone Acetate Sterile Suspension 1663
- Cortone Acetate Tablets 1664

Desflurane (Additive CNS depressant effects). Products include:
- Suprane (desflurane, USP) 1865

Dexamethasone (Barbiturates enchance metabolism). Products include:
- AK-Trol Ointment & Suspension .... ◉ 205
- Decadron Elixir 1676
- Decadron Tablets 1678
- Decaspray Topical Aerosol 1689
- Maxitrol Ophthalmic Ointment and Suspension .... ◉ 222
- TobraDex Ophthalmic Suspension and Ointment 469

Dexamethasone Acetate (Barbiturates enhance metabolism). Products include:
- Dalalone D.P. Injectable 1009
- Decadron-LA Sterile Suspension 1687

Dexamethasone Sodium Phosphate (Barbiturates enhance metabolism). Products include:
- Decadron Phosphate Injection 1680
- Decadron Phosphate Sterile Ophthalmic Ointment 1684
- Decadron Phosphate Sterile Ophthalmic Solution 1685
- Decadron Phosphate Topical Cream 1686
- Decadron Phosphate with Xylocaine Injection, Sterile 1683
- Dexacort Phosphate in Respihaler 1606
- Dexacort Phosphate in Turbinaire 1607

(▣ Described in PDR For Nonprescription Drugs)   (◉ Described in PDR For Ophthalmology)

NeoDecadron Sterile Ophthalmic Ointment ... 1755
NeoDecadron Sterile Ophthalmic Solution ... 1756
NeoDecadron Topical Cream ... 1757

Dezocine (Additive CNS depressant effects). Products include:
Dalgan Injection ... 529

Diazepam (Additive CNS depressant effects). Products include:
Dizac (diazepam injectable emulsion) CIV ... 1862
Valium Injectable ... 2336
Valium Tablets ... 2335

Dicumarol (Increased metabolism, decreased anticoagulant response).
No products indexed under this heading.

Dienestrol (Decreased effects of estrogens). Products include:
Ortho Dienestrol Cream ... 1922

Diethylstilbestrol (Decreased effects of estrogens). Products include:
Diethylstilbestrol Tablets ... 1477

Doxepin Hydrochloride (Phenobarbital shortens half-life). Products include:
Adapin Capsules ... 1542
Sinequan ... 2028
Zonalon Cream ... 1042

Doxycycline Calcium (Barbiturates shorten half-life of doxycycline). Products include:
Vibramycin Calcium Oral Suspension ... 2038

Doxycycline Hyclate (Barbiturates shorten half-life of doxycycline). Products include:
Doryx Capsules ... 1970
Vibramycin Hyclate Capsules ... 2038
Vibramycin Hyclate Intravenous ... 2040
Vibra-Tabs Film Coated Tablets ... 2038

Doxycycline Monohydrate (Barbiturates shorten half-life of doxycycline). Products include:
Monodox Capsules ... 1858
Vibramycin Monohydrate for Oral Suspension ... 2038

Droperidol (Additive CNS depressant effects). Products include:
Inapsine Injection ... 462

Enflurane (Additive CNS depressant effects).
No products indexed under this heading.

Estazolam (Additive CNS depressant effects). Products include:
ProSom Tablets ... 457

Estradiol (Decreased effects of estrogens). Products include:
Climara Transdermal System ... 640
Estrace Cream and Tablets ... 751
Estraderm Transdermal System ... 842
Estring Vaginal Ring ... 2086
Vivelle Transdermal System ... 880

Estrogens, Conjugated (Decreased effects of estrogens). Products include:
PMB 200 and PMB 400 ... 2890
Premarin Intravenous ... 2893
Premarin Tablets ... 2896
Premarin Vaginal Cream ... 2898
Premphase ... 2900
Prempro ... 2905

Estrogens, Esterified (Decreased effects of estrogens). Products include:
ESTRATAB Tablets (0.3, 0.625, 1.25, 2.5 mg) ... 2715
Estratest ... 2718
Menest Tablets ... 2671

Estropipate (Decreased effects of estrogens). Products include:
Ogen Tablets ... 2103
Ogen Vaginal Cream ... 2106
Ortho-Est ... 1925

Ethchlorvynol (Additive CNS depressant effects). Products include:
Placidyl Capsules ... 456

Ethinamate (Additive CNS depressant effects).
No products indexed under this heading.

Ethinyl Estradiol (Decreased effects of estrogens). Products include:
Brevicon ... 2563
Demulen ... 2580
Desogen Tablets ... 1867
Levlen/Tri-Levlen ... 646
Lo/Ovral Tablets ... 2852
Lo/Ovral-28 Tablets ... 2857
Modicon ... 1928
Nordette-21 Tablets ... 2863
Nordette-28 Tablets ... 2866
Norinyl ... 2563
Ortho-Cept ... 1907
Ortho-Cyclen/Ortho-Tri-Cyclen ... 1914
Ortho-Novum ... 1928
Ortho-Cyclen/Ortho Tri-Cyclen ... 1914
Ovcon ... 765
Ovral Tablets ... 2877
Ovral-28 Tablets ... 2878
Levlen/Tri-Levlen ... 646
Tri-Norinyl ... 2607
Triphasil-21 Tablets ... 2919
Triphasil-28 Tablets ... 2924

Fentanyl (Additive CNS depressant effects). Products include:
Duragesic Transdermal System ... 1336

Fentanyl Citrate (Additive CNS depressant effects). Products include:
Sublimaze Injection ... 463

Fludrocortisone Acetate (Barbiturates enhance metabolism). Products include:
Florinef Acetate Tablets ... 506

Fluphenazine Decanoate (Additive CNS depressant effects). Products include:
Prolixin Decanoate ... 510

Fluphenazine Enanthate (Additive CNS depressant effects). Products include:
Prolixin Enanthate ... 510

Fluphenazine Hydrochloride (Additive CNS depressant effects). Products include:
Prolixin ... 510

Flurazepam Hydrochloride (Additive CNS depressant effects). Products include:
Dalmane Capsules ... 2329

Furazolidone (Prolongs effects of barbiturates). Products include:
Furoxone ... 2221

Glutethimide (Additive CNS depressant effects).
No products indexed under this heading.

Griseofulvin (Phenobarbital interferes with absorption). Products include:
Fulvicin P/G Tablets ... 2499
Fulvicin P/G 165 & 330 Tablets ... 2500
Grifulvin V (griseofulvin tablets) Microsize (griseofulvin oral suspension) Microsize ... 1944
Gris-PEG Tablets, 125 mg & 250 mg ... 476

Haloperidol (Additive CNS depressant effects). Products include:
Haldol Injection, Tablets and Concentrate ... 1585

Haloperidol Decanoate (Additive CNS depressant effects). Products include:
Haldol Decanoate ... 1587

Hydrocodone Bitartrate (Additive CNS depressant effects). Products include:
Codiclear DH Syrup ... 808
Duratuss HD Elixir ... 2750
Histussin D Liquid ... 670
Hycodan Tablets and Syrup ... 946
Hycomine Compound Tablets ... 948
Hycomine ... 947
Hycotuss Expectorant Syrup ... 950
Hydrocet Capsules ... 787
Lorcet 10/650 Tablets ... 1016
Lortab ... 2751
Tussend ... 1830
Tussend Expectorant ... 1831
Vicodin Tablets ... 1404
Vicodin ES Tablets ... 1405
Vicodin HP Tablets ... 1403
Vicodin Tuss Expectorant ... 1406
Zydone Capsules ... 967

Hydrocodone Polistirex (Additive CNS depressant effects). Products include:
Tussionex Pennkinetic Extended-Release Suspension ... 1624

Hydrocortisone (Barbiturates enhance metabolism). Products include:
Anusol-HC Cream 2.5% ... 1953
Aquanil HC Lotion ... 1989
Maximum Strength Cortaid Spray ... 800
CORTENEMA ... 2713
Cortisporin Ointment ... 1074
Cortisporin Ophthalmic Ointment Sterile ... 1074
Cortisporin Ophthalmic Suspension Sterile ... 1075
Cortisporin Otic Solution Sterile ... 1076
Cortisporin Otic Suspension Sterile ... 1077
Cortizone-5 ... 795
Cortizone-10 ... 795
Hydrocortone Tablets ... 1715
Hytone ... 922
Hytone Ointment 2 ½% ... 923
Massengill Medicated Soft Cloth Towelettes ... 2628
Pediotic Suspension Sterile ... 1140
Preparation H Hydrocortisone 1% Cream ... 843
ProctoCream-HC 2.5% ... 2552
VōSoL HC Otic Solution ... 2786

Hydrocortisone Acetate (Barbiturates enhance metabolism). Products include:
Analpram-HC Rectal Cream 1% and 2.5% ... 993
Anusol HC-1 Hydrocortisone Anti-Itch Ointment ... 810
Anusol-HC Suppositories ... 1954
Caldecort Anti-Itch Hydrocortisone Cream ... 651
Coly-Mycin S Otic w/Neomycin & Hydrocortisone ... 1965
Cortaid ... 800
Cortifoam ... 2540
Cortisporin Cream ... 1073
Epifoam ... 2543
Hydrocortone Acetate Sterile Suspension ... 1712
Mantadil Cream ... 1124
Nupercainal Hydrocortisone 1% Cream ... 661
Pramosone Cream, Lotion & Ointment ... 995
ProctoFoam-HC ... 2552
Terra-Cortril Ophthalmic Suspension ... 2033

Hydrocortisone Sodium Phosphate (Barbiturates enhance metabolism). Products include:
Hydrocortone Phosphate Injection, Sterile ... 1713

Hydrocortisone Sodium Succinate (Barbiturates enhance metabolism).
No products indexed under this heading.

Hydroxyzine Hydrochloride (Additive CNS depressant effects). Products include:
Atarax Tablets & Syrup ... 1992
Marax Tablets & DF Syrup ... 2015
Vistaril Intramuscular Solution ... 2042

Isocarboxazid (Prolongs effects of barbiturates).
No products indexed under this heading.

Isoflurane (Additive CNS depressant effects).
No products indexed under this heading.

Ketamine Hydrochloride (Additive CNS depressant effects).
No products indexed under this heading.

Levomethadyl Acetate Hydrochloride (Additive CNS depressant effects). Products include:
Orlaam Oral Solution ... 2361

Levorphanol Tartrate (Additive CNS depressant effects). Products include:
Levo-Dromoran ... 2297

Lorazepam (Additive CNS depressant effects). Products include:
Ativan Injection ... 2805
Ativan Tablets ... 2807

Loxapine Hydrochloride (Additive CNS depressant effects). Products include:
Loxitane ... 1426

Loxapine Succinate (Additive CNS depressant effects). Products include:
Loxitane Capsules ... 1426

Meperidine Hydrochloride (Additive CNS depressant effects). Products include:
Demerol ... 2438
Mepergan Injection ... 2859

Mephobarbital (Additive CNS depressant effects). Products include:
Mebaral Tablets ... 2452

Meprobamate (Additive CNS depressant effects). Products include:
Miltown Tablets ... 2780
PMB 200 and PMB 400 ... 2890

Mesoridazine Besylate (Additive CNS depressant effects). Products include:
Serentil ... 689

Methadone Hydrochloride (Additive CNS depressant effects). Products include:
Methadone Hydrochloride Oral Concentrate ... 2356
Methadone Hydrochloride Oral Solution & Tablets ... 2357

Methohexital Sodium (Additive CNS depressant effects).
No products indexed under this heading.

Methotrimeprazine (Additive CNS depressant effects). Products include:
Levoprome ... 1321

Methoxyflurane (Additive CNS depressant effects).
No products indexed under this heading.

Methylprednisolone Acetate (Barbiturates enhance metabolism).
No products indexed under this heading.

Methylprednisolone Sodium Succinate (Barbiturates enhance metabolism).
No products indexed under this heading.

Midazolam Hydrochloride (Additive CNS depressant effects). Products include:
Versed Injection ... 2324

Molindone Hydrochloride (Additive CNS depressant effects). Products include:
Moban Tablets and Concentrate ... 1036

Morphine Sulfate (Additive CNS depressant effects). Products include:
Astramorph/PF Injection, USP (Preservative-Free) ... 526
Duramorph Injection ... 983
Infumorph 200 and Infumorph 500 Sterile Solutions ... 985
Kadian Capsules ... 2948
MS Contin Tablets ... 2149
MSIR ... 2152
Oramorph SR (Morphine Sulfate Sustained Release Tablets) ... 2359
RMS Suppositories CII ... 2766
Roxanol ... 2365

IMPORTANT NOTE: Always consult each drug listing in the patient's regimen for possible interactions.

Nembutal Sodium Solution / Interactions Index 728

Opium Alkaloids (Additive CNS depressant effects).
   No products indexed under this heading.

Oxazepam (Additive CNS depressant effects). Products include:
   Serax Capsules 2916
   Serax Tablets 2916

Oxycodone Hydrochloride (Additive CNS depressant effects). Products include:
   OxyContin Tablets 2163
   OxyIR Capsules 2167
   Percocet Tablets 955
   Percodan Tablets 955
   Percodan-Demi Tablets 956
   Roxicodone Tablets, Oral Solution & Intensol (Oxycodone) ... 2366
   Tylox Capsules 1593

Perphenazine (Additive CNS depressant effects). Products include:
   Etrafon 2495
   Triavil Tablets 1800
   Trilafon 2532

Phenelzine Sulfate (Prolongs effects of barbiturates). Products include:
   Nardil 1977

Phenobarbital (Additive CNS depressant effects). Products include:
   Arco-Lase Plus Tablets 513
   Bellergal-S Tablets 2375
   Donnatal 2234
   Donnatal Extentabs 2234
   Donnatal Tablets 2234
   Phenobarbital Elixir and Tablets ... 1523
   Quadrinal Tablets 1398

Phenytoin (Variable effect on metabolism of phenytoin). Products include:
   Dilantin Infatabs 1967
   Dilantin-125 Suspension 1969

Phenytoin Sodium (Variable effect on metabolism of phenytoin). Products include:
   Dilantin Kapseals 1965

Polyestradiol Phosphate (Decreased effects of estrogens).
   No products indexed under this heading.

Prazepam (Additive CNS depressant effects).
   No products indexed under this heading.

Prednisolone Acetate (Barbiturates enhance metabolism). Products include:
   AK-CIDE .... ⊚ 203
   AK-CIDE Ointment .... ⊚ 203
   Blephamide Liquifilm Sterile Ophthalmic Suspension 472
   Blephamide Ointment .... ⊚ 234
   Econopred & Econopred Plus Ophthalmic Suspensions .... ⊚ 216
   Poly-Pred Liquifilm .... ⊚ 246
   Pred Forte .... ⊚ 247
   Pred Mild .... ⊚ 250
   Pred-G Liquifilm Sterile Ophthalmic Suspension .... ⊚ 248
   Pred-G S.O.P. Sterile Ophthalmic Ointment .... ⊚ 249

Prednisolone Sodium Phosphate (Barbiturates enhance metabolism). Products include:
   AK-PRED .... ⊚ 204
   Hydeltrasol Injection, Sterile ... 1708
   Pediapred Oral Solution 1618

Prednisolone Tebutate (Barbiturates enhance metabolism). Products include:
   Hydeltra-T.B.A. Sterile Suspension ... 1710

Prednisone (Barbiturates enhance metabolism).
   No products indexed under this heading.

Prochlorperazine (Additive CNS depressant effects). Products include:
   Compazine 2644

Promethazine Hydrochloride (Additive CNS depressant effects). Products include:
   Mepergan Injection 2859
   Phenergan with Codeine 2883
   Phenergan with Dextromethorphan ... 2885
   Phenergan Injection 2880
   Phenergan Suppositories 2882
   Phenergan Syrup 2881
   Phenergan Tablets 2882
   Phenergan VC 2886
   Phenergan VC with Codeine 2888

Propofol (Additive CNS depressant effects). Products include:
   Diprivan Injectable Emulsion 2939

Propoxyphene Hydrochloride (Additive CNS depressant effects). Products include:
   Darvon 1475
   Wygesic Tablets 2930

Propoxyphene Napsylate (Additive CNS depressant effects). Products include:
   Darvon-N/Darvocet-N 1473

Quazepam (Additive CNS depressant effects). Products include:
   Doral Tablets 2773

Quinestrol (Decreased effects of estrogens).
   No products indexed under this heading.

Risperidone (Additive CNS depressant effects). Products include:
   Risperdal Tablets 1348

Secobarbital Sodium (Additive CNS depressant effects). Products include:
   Seconal Sodium Pulvules 1529

Selegiline Hydrochloride (Prolongs effects of barbiturates). Products include:
   Eldepryl Capsules 2729

Sevoflurane (Additive CNS depressant effects).
   No products indexed under this heading.

Sufentanil Citrate (Additive CNS depressant effects). Products include:
   Sufenta Injection 1355

Temazepam (Additive CNS depressant effects). Products include:
   Restoril Capsules 2413

Thiamylal Sodium (Additive CNS depressant effects).
   No products indexed under this heading.

Thioridazine Hydrochloride (Additive CNS depressant effects). Products include:
   Mellaril 2398

Thiothixene (Additive CNS depressant effects). Products include:
   Navane Capsules and Concentrate ... 2018
   Navane Intramuscular 2019

Tranylcypromine Sulfate (Prolongs effects of barbiturates). Products include:
   Parnate Tablets 2679

Triamcinolone (Barbiturates enhance metabolism).
   No products indexed under this heading.

Triamcinolone Acetonide (Barbiturates enhance metabolism). Products include:
   Azmacort Oral Inhaler 2175
   Nasacort AQ Nasal Spray 2191
   Nasacort Nasal Inhaler 2189

Triamcinolone Diacetate (Barbiturates enhance metabolism).
   No products indexed under this heading.

Triamcinolone Hexacetonide (Barbiturates enhance metabolism).
   No products indexed under this heading.

Triazolam (Additive CNS depressant effects). Products include:
   Halcion Tablets 2093

Trifluoperazine Hydrochloride (Additive CNS depressant effects). Products include:
   Stelazine 2692

Valproic Acid (Decreases barbiturate metabolism). Products include:
   Depakene 416

Warfarin Sodium (Decreased anticoagulant response). Products include:
   Coumadin 941

Zolpidem Tartrate (Additive CNS depressant effects). Products include:
   Ambien Tablets 2559

NEMBUTAL SODIUM SUPPOSITORIES
(Pentobarbital Sodium) 444
May interact with central nervous system depressants, oral anticoagulants, corticosteroids, monoamine oxidase inhibitors, estrogens, and certain other agents. Compounds in these categories include:

Alfentanil Hydrochloride (Additive CNS depressant effects). Products include:
   Alfenta Injection 1334

Alprazolam (Additive CNS depressant effects). Products include:
   Xanax Tablets 2115

Aprobarbital (Additive CNS depressant effects).
   No products indexed under this heading.

Betamethasone Acetate (Barbiturates enhance metabolism). Products include:
   Celestone Soluspan Suspension ... 2484

Betamethasone Sodium Phosphate (Barbiturates enhance metabolism). Products include:
   Celestone Soluspan Suspension ... 2484

Buprenorphine (Additive CNS depressant effects). Products include:
   Buprenex Injectable 2170

Buspirone Hydrochloride (Additive CNS depressant effects). Products include:
   BuSpar Tablets 738

Butabarbital (Additive CNS depressant effects).
   No products indexed under this heading.

Butalbital (Additive CNS depressant effects). Products include:
   Axocet Capsules 2469
   Esgic-plus Capsules 1012
   Esgic-plus Tablets 1012
   Fioricet Tablets 2386
   Fioricet with Codeine Capsules ... 2387
   Fiorinal Capsules 2388
   Fiorinal with Codeine Capsules ... 2390
   Fiorinal Tablets 2388
   Phrenilin 790
   Sedapap Tablets 50 mg/650 mg .. 1826

Chlordiazepoxide (Additive CNS depressant effects). Products include:
   Limbitrol 2333

Chlordiazepoxide Hydrochloride (Additive CNS depressant effects). Products include:
   Librax Capsules 2330
   Librium Capsules 2331
   Librium Injectable 2332

Chlorotrianisene (Decreased effects of estrogens).
   No products indexed under this heading.

Chlorpromazine (Additive CNS depressant effects). Products include:
   Thorazine Suppositories 2701

Chlorprothixene (Additive CNS depressant effects).
   No products indexed under this heading.

Chlorprothixene Hydrochloride (Additive CNS depressant effects).
   No products indexed under this heading.

Chlorprothixene Lactate (Additive CNS depressant effects).
   No products indexed under this heading.

Clorazepate Dipotassium (Additive CNS depressant effects). Products include:
   Tranxene 459

Clozapine (Additive CNS depressant effects). Products include:
   Clozaril Tablets 2377

Codeine Phosphate (Additive CNS depressant effects). Products include:
   Brontex 2130
   Dimetane-DC Cough Syrup 2232
   Fioricet with Codeine Capsules ... 2387
   Fiorinal with Codeine Capsules ... 2390
   Nucofed 2225
   Phenergan with Codeine 2883
   Phenergan VC with Codeine 2888
   Robitussin A-C Syrup 2248
   Robitussin-DAC Syrup 2249
   Ryna .... ⊞ 804
   Soma Compound w/Codeine Tablets ... 2784
   Tylenol with Codeine 1592

Cortisone Acetate (Barbiturates enhance metabolism). Products include:
   Cortone Acetate Sterile Suspension ... 1663
   Cortone Acetate Tablets 1664

Desflurane (Additive CNS depressant effects). Products include:
   Suprane (desflurane, USP) 1865

Dexamethasone (Barbiturates enhance metabolism). Products include:
   AK-Trol Ointment & Suspension ... ⊚ 205
   Decadron Elixir 1676
   Decadron Tablets 1678
   Decaspray Topical Aerosol 1689
   Maxitrol Ophthalmic Ointment and Suspension .... ⊚ 222
   TobraDex Ophthalmic Suspension and Ointment 469

Dexamethasone Acetate (Barbiturates enhance metabolism). Products include:
   Dalalone D.P. Injectable 1009
   Decadron-LA Sterile Suspension ... 1687

Dexamethasone Sodium Phosphate (Barbiturates enhance metabolism). Products include:
   Decadron Phosphate Injection 1680
   Decadron Phosphate Sterile Ophthalmic Ointment 1684
   Decadron Phosphate Sterile Ophthalmic Solution 1685
   Decadron Phosphate Topical Cream 1686
   Decadron Phosphate with Xylocaine Injection, Sterile 1683
   Dexacort Phosphate in Respihaler ... 1606
   Dexacort Phosphate in Turbinaire ... 1607
   NeoDecadron Sterile Ophthalmic Ointment 1755
   NeoDecadron Sterile Ophthalmic Solution 1756
   NeoDecadron Topical Cream 1757

Dezocine (Additive CNS depressant effects). Products include:
   Dalgan Injection 529

Diazepam (Additive CNS depressant effects). Products include:
   Dizac (diazepam injectable emulsion) CIV 1862
   Valium Injectable 2336
   Valium Tablets 2335

(⊞ Described in PDR For Nonprescription Drugs)   (⊚ Described in PDR For Ophthalmology)

729 **Interactions Index** **Nembutal Sodium Suppositories**

Dicumarol (Decreased anticoagulant response).
No products indexed under this heading.

Dienestrol (Decreased effects of estrogens). Products include:
Ortho Dienestrol Cream ... 1922

Diethylstilbestrol (Decreased effects of estrogens). Products include:
Diethylstilbestrol Tablets ... 1477

Doxepin Hydrochloride (Phenobarbital shortens half-life). Products include:
Adapin Capsules ... 1542
Sinequan ... 2028
Zonalon Cream ... 1042

Doxycycline Hyclate (Barbiturates shorten half-life of doxycycline). Products include:
Doryx Capsules ... 1970
Vibramycin Hyclate Capsules ... 2038
Vibramycin Hyclate Intravenous ... 2040
Vibra-Tabs Film Coated Tablets ... 2038

Doxycycline Monohydrate (Barbiturates shorten half-life of doxycycline). Products include:
Monodox Capsules ... 1858
Vibramycin Monohydrate for Oral Suspension ... 2038

Droperidol (Additive CNS depressant effects). Products include:
Inapsine Injection ... 462

Enflurane (Additive CNS depressant effects).
No products indexed under this heading.

Estazolam (Additive CNS depressant effects). Products include:
ProSom Tablets ... 457

Estradiol (Decreased effects of estrogens). Products include:
Climara Transdermal System ... 640
Estrace Cream and Tablets ... 751
Estraderm Transdermal System ... 842
Estring Vaginal Ring ... 2086
Vivelle Transdermal System ... 880

Estrogens, Conjugated (Decreased effects of estrogens). Products include:
PMB 200 and PMB 400 ... 2890
Premarin Intravenous ... 2893
Premarin Tablets ... 2896
Premarin Vaginal Cream ... 2898
Premphase ... 2900
Prempro ... 2905

Estrogens, Esterified (Decreased effects of estrogens). Products include:
ESTRATAB Tablets (0.3, 0.625, 1.25, 2.5 mg) ... 2715
Estratest ... 2718
Menest Tablets ... 2671

Estropipate (Decreased effects of estrogens). Products include:
Ogen Tablets ... 2103
Ogen Vaginal Cream ... 2106
Ortho-Est ... 1925

Ethchlorvynol (Additive CNS depressant effects). Products include:
Placidyl Capsules ... 456

Ethinamate (Additive CNS depressant effects).
No products indexed under this heading.

Ethinyl Estradiol (Decreased effects of estrogens). Products include:
Brevicon ... 2563
Demulen ... 2580
Desogen Tablets ... 1867
Levlen/Tri-Levlen ... 646
Lo/Ovral Tablets ... 2852
Lo/Ovral-28 Tablets ... 2857
Modicon ... 1928
Nordette-21 Tablets ... 2863
Nordette-28 Tablets ... 2866
Norinyl ... 2563
Ortho-Cept ... 1907
Ortho-Cyclen/Ortho-Tri-Cyclen ... 1914
Ortho-Novum ... 1928
Ortho-Cyclen/Ortho Tri-Cyclen ... 1914
Ovcon ... 765
Ovral Tablets ... 2877
Ovral-28 Tablets ... 2878
Levlen/Tri-Levlen ... 646
Tri-Norinyl ... 2607
Triphasil-21 Tablets ... 2919
Triphasil-28 Tablets ... 2924

Fentanyl (Additive CNS depressant effects). Products include:
Duragesic Transdermal System ... 1336

Fentanyl Citrate (Additive CNS depressant effects). Products include:
Sublimaze Injection ... 463

Fludrocortisone Acetate (Barbiturates enhance metabolism). Products include:
Florinef Acetate Tablets ... 506

Fluphenazine Decanoate (Additive CNS depressant effects). Products include:
Prolixin Decanoate ... 510

Fluphenazine Enanthate (Additive CNS depressant effects). Products include:
Prolixin Enanthate ... 510

Fluphenazine Hydrochloride (Additive CNS depressant effects). Products include:
Prolixin ... 510

Flurazepam Hydrochloride (Additive CNS depressant effects). Products include:
Dalmane Capsules ... 2329

Furazolidone (Prolongs effects of barbiturates). Products include:
Furoxone ... 2221

Glutethimide (Additive CNS depressant effects).
No products indexed under this heading.

Haloperidol (Additive CNS depressant effects). Products include:
Haldol Injection, Tablets and Concentrate ... 1585

Haloperidol Decanoate (Additive CNS depressant effects). Products include:
Haldol Decanoate ... 1587

Hydrocodone Bitartrate (Additive CNS depressant effects). Products include:
Codiclear DH Syrup ... 808
Duratuss HD Elixir ... 2750
Histussin D Liquid ... 670
Hycodan Tablets and Syrup ... 946
Hycomine Compound Tablets ... 948
Hycomine ... 947
Hycotuss Expectorant Syrup ... 950
Hydrocet Capsules ... 787
Lorcet 10/650 Tablets ... 1016
Lortab ... 2751
Tussend ... 1830
Tussend Expectorant ... 1831
Vicodin Tablets ... 1404
Vicodin ES Tablets ... 1405
Vicodin HP Tablets ... 1403
Vicodin Tuss Expectorant ... 1406
Zydone Capsules ... 967

Hydrocodone Polistirex (Additive CNS depressant effects). Products include:
Tussionex Pennkinetic Extended-Release Suspension ... 1624

Hydrocortisone (Barbiturates enhance metabolism). Products include:
Anusol-HC Cream 2.5% ... 1953
Aquanil HC Lotion ... 1989
Maximum Strength Cortaid Spray ... 800
CORTENEMA ... 2713
Cortisporin Ointment ... 1074
Cortisporin Ophthalmic Ointment Sterile ... 1074
Cortisporin Ophthalmic Suspension Sterile ... 1075
Cortisporin Otic Solution Sterile ... 1076
Cortisporin Otic Suspension Sterile ... 1077
Cortizone-5 ... 795
Cortizone-10 ... 795
Hydrocortone Tablets ... 1715
Hytone ... 922
Hytone Ointment 2 ½% ... 923
Massengill Medicated Soft Cloth Towelettes ... 2628
Pediotic Suspension Sterile ... 1140
Preparation H Hydrocortisone 1% Cream ... 843
ProctoCream-HC 2.5% ... 2552
VōSoL HC Otic Solution ... 2786

Hydrocortisone Acetate (Barbiturates enhance metabolism). Products include:
Analpram-HC Rectal Cream 1% and 2.5% ... 993
Anusol HC-1 Hydrocortisone Anti-Itch Ointment ... 810
Anusol-HC Suppositories ... 1954
Caldecort Anti-Itch Hydrocortisone Cream ... 651
Coly-Mycin S Otic w/Neomycin & Hydrocortisone ... 1965
Cortaid ... 800
Cortifoam ... 2540
Cortisporin Cream ... 1073
Epifoam ... 2543
Hydrocortone Acetate Sterile Suspension ... 1712
Mantadil Cream ... 1124
Nupercainal Hydrocortisone 1% Cream ... 661
Pramosone Cream, Lotion & Ointment ... 995
ProctoFoam-HC ... 2552
Terra-Cortril Ophthalmic Suspension ... 2033

Hydrocortisone Sodium Phosphate (Barbiturates enhance metabolism). Products include:
Hydrocortone Phosphate Injection, Sterile ... 1713

Hydrocortisone Sodium Succinate (Barbiturates enhance metabolism).
No products indexed under this heading.

Hydroxyzine Hydrochloride (Additive CNS depressant effects). Products include:
Atarax Tablets & Syrup ... 1992
Marax Tablets & DF Syrup ... 2015
Vistaril Intramuscular Solution ... 2042

Isocarboxazid (Prolongs effects of barbiturates).
No products indexed under this heading.

Isoflurane (Additive CNS depressant effects).
No products indexed under this heading.

Ketamine Hydrochloride (Additive CNS depressant effects).
No products indexed under this heading.

Levomethadyl Acetate Hydrochloride (Additive CNS depressant effects). Products include:
Orlaam Oral Solution ... 2361

Levorphanol Tartrate (Additive CNS depressant effects). Products include:
Levo-Dromoran ... 2297

Lorazepam (Additive CNS depressant effects). Products include:
Ativan Injection ... 2805
Ativan Tablets ... 2807

Loxapine Hydrochloride (Additive CNS depressant effects). Products include:
Loxitane ... 1426

Loxapine Succinate (Additive CNS depressant effects). Products include:
Loxitane Capsules ... 1426

Meperidine Hydrochloride (Additive CNS depressant effects). Products include:
Demerol ... 2438
Mepergan Injection ... 2859

Mephobarbital (Additive CNS depressant effects). Products include:
Mebaral Tablets ... 2452

Meprobamate (Additive CNS depressant effects). Products include:
Miltown Tablets ... 2780
PMB 200 and PMB 400 ... 2890

Mesoridazine Besylate (Additive CNS depressant effects). Products include:
Serentil ... 689

Methadone Hydrochloride (Additive CNS depressant effects). Products include:
Methadone Hydrochloride Oral Concentrate ... 2356
Methadone Hydrochloride Oral Solution & Tablets ... 2357

Methohexital Sodium (Additive CNS depressant effects).
No products indexed under this heading.

Methotrimeprazine (Additive CNS depressant effects). Products include:
Levoprome ... 1321

Methoxyflurane (Additive CNS depressant effects).
No products indexed under this heading.

Methylprednisolone Acetate (Barbiturates enhance metabolism).
No products indexed under this heading.

Methylprednisolone Sodium Succinate (Barbiturates enhance metabolism).
No products indexed under this heading.

Midazolam Hydrochloride (Additive CNS depressant effects). Products include:
Versed Injection ... 2324

Molindone Hydrochloride (Additive CNS depressant effects). Products include:
Moban Tablets and Concentrate ... 1036

Morphine Sulfate (Additive CNS depressant effects). Products include:
Astramorph/PF Injection, USP (Preservative-Free) ... 526
Duramorph Injection ... 983
Infumorph 200 and Infumorph 500 Sterile Solutions ... 985
Kadian Capsules ... 2948
MS Contin Tablets ... 2149
MSIR ... 2152
Oramorph SR (Morphine Sulfate Sustained Release Tablets) ... 2359
RMS Suppositories CII ... 2766
Roxanol ... 2365

Opium Alkaloids (Additive CNS depressant effects).
No products indexed under this heading.

Oxazepam (Additive CNS depressant effects). Products include:
Serax Capsules ... 2916
Serax Tablets ... 2916

Oxycodone Hydrochloride (Additive CNS depressant effects). Products include:
OxyContin Tablets ... 2163
OxyIR Capsules ... 2167
Percocet Tablets ... 955
Percodan Tablets ... 955
Percodan-Demi Tablets ... 956
Roxicodone Tablets, Oral Solution & Intensol (Oxycodone) ... 2366
Tylox Capsules ... 1593

Perphenazine (Additive CNS depressant effects). Products include:
Etrafon ... 2495
Triavil Tablets ... 1800
Trilafon ... 2532

Phenelzine Sulfate (Prolongs effects of barbiturates). Products include:
Nardil ... 1977

Phenobarbital (Additive CNS depressant effects). Products include:
Arco-Lase Plus Tablets ... 513
Bellergal-S Tablets ... 2375

IMPORTANT NOTE: Always consult each drug listing in the patient's regimen for possible interactions.

Nembutal Sodium Suppositories | Interactions Index | 730

Donnatal 2234
Donnatal Extentabs 2234
Donnatal Tablets 2234
Phenobarbital Elixir and Tablets 1523
Quadrinal Tablets 1398

Phenytoin (Variable effect on metabolism of phenytoin). Products include:
Dilantin Infatabs 1967
Dilantin-125 Suspension 1969

Phenytoin Sodium (Variable effect on metabolism of phenytoin). Products include:
Dilantin Kapseals 1965

Polyestradiol Phosphate (Decreased effects of estrogens).
No products indexed under this heading.

Prazepam (Additive CNS depressant effects).
No products indexed under this heading.

Prednisolone Acetate (Barbiturates enhance metabolism). Products include:
AK-CIDE .... ⊙ 203
AK-CIDE Ointment .... ⊙ 203
Blephamide Liquifilm Sterile Ophthalmic Suspension 472
Blephamide Ointment .... ⊙ 234
Econopred & Econopred Plus Ophthalmic Suspensions .... ⊙ 216
Poly-Pred Liquifilm .... ⊙ 246
Pred Forte .... ⊙ 247
Pred Mild .... ⊙ 250
Pred-G Liquifilm Sterile Ophthalmic Suspension .... ⊙ 248
Pred-G S.O.P. Sterile Ophthalmic Ointment .... ⊙ 249

Prednisolone Sodium Phosphate (Barbiturates enhance metabolism). Products include:
AK-PRED .... ⊙ 204
Hydeltrasol Injection, Sterile 1708
Pediapred Oral Solution 1618

Prednisolone Tebutate (Barbiturates enhance metabolism). Products include:
Hydeltra-T.B.A. Sterile Suspension 1710

Prednisone (Barbiturates enhance metabolism).
No products indexed under this heading.

Prochlorperazine (Additive CNS depressant effects). Products include:
Compazine 2644

Promethazine Hydrochloride (Additive CNS depressant effects). Products include:
Mepergan Injection 2859
Phenergan with Codeine 2883
Phenergan with Dextromethorphan 2885
Phenergan Injection 2880
Phenergan Suppositories 2882
Phenergan Syrup 2881
Phenergan Tablets 2882
Phenergan VC 2886
Phenergan VC with Codeine 2888

Propofol (Additive CNS depressant effects). Products include:
Diprivan Injectable Emulsion 2939

Propoxyphene Hydrochloride (Additive CNS depressant effects). Products include:
Darvon 1475
Wygesic Tablets 2930

Propoxyphene Napsylate (Additive CNS depressant effects). Products include:
Darvon-N/Darvocet-N 1473

Quazepam (Additive CNS depressant effects). Products include:
Doral Tablets 2773

Quinestrol (Decreased effects of estrogens).
No products indexed under this heading.

Risperidone (Additive CNS depressant effects). Products include:
Risperdal Tablets 1348

Secobarbital Sodium (Additive CNS depressant effects). Products include:
Seconal Sodium Pulvules 1529

Selegiline Hydrochloride (Prolongs effects of barbiturates). Products include:
Eldepryl Capsules 2729

Sevoflurane (Additive CNS depressant effects).
No products indexed under this heading.

Sufentanil Citrate (Additive CNS depressant effects). Products include:
Sufenta Injection 1355

Temazepam (Additive CNS depressant effects). Products include:
Restoril Capsules 2413

Thiamylal Sodium (Additive CNS depressant effects).
No products indexed under this heading.

Thioridazine Hydrochloride (Additive CNS depressant effects). Products include:
Mellaril 2398

Thiothixene (Additive CNS depressant effects). Products include:
Navane Capsules and Concentrate 2018
Navane Intramuscular 2019

Tranylcypromine Sulfate (Prolongs effects of barbiturates). Products include:
Parnate Tablets 2679

Triamcinolone (Barbiturates enhance metabolism).
No products indexed under this heading.

Triamcinolone Acetonide (Barbiturates enhance metabolism). Products include:
Azmacort Oral Inhaler 2175
Nasacort AQ Nasal Spray 2191
Nasacort Nasal Inhaler 2189

Triamcinolone Diacetate (Barbiturates enhance metabolism).
No products indexed under this heading.

Triamcinolone Hexacetonide (Barbiturates enhance metabolism).
No products indexed under this heading.

Triazolam (Additive CNS depressant effects). Products include:
Halcion Tablets 2093

Trifluoperazine Hydrochloride (Additive CNS depressant effects). Products include:
Stelazine 2692

Valproic Acid (Decreases barbiturates metabolism). Products include:
Depakene 416

Warfarin Sodium (Increased metabolism, decreased anticoagulant response). Products include:
Coumadin 941

Zolpidem Tartrate (Additive CNS depressant effects). Products include:
Ambien Tablets 2559

NEODECADRON STERILE OPHTHALMIC OINTMENT
(Neomycin Sulfate, Dexamethasone Sodium Phosphate) 1755
None cited in PDR database.

NEODECADRON STERILE OPHTHALMIC SOLUTION
(Neomycin Sulfate, Dexamethasone Sodium Phosphate) 1756
None cited in PDR database.

NEODECADRON TOPICAL CREAM
(Neomycin Sulfate, Dexamethasone Sodium Phosphate) 1757
None cited in PDR database.

NEORAL SOFT GELATIN CAPSULES FOR MICROEMULSION
(Cyclosporine) 2405
May interact with potassium sparing diuretics and certain other agents. Compounds in these categories include:

Allopurinol (Increases cyclosporine concentrations). Products include:
Zyloprim Tablets 1194

Amiloride Hydrochloride (Cyclosporine may cause hyperkalemia; concurrent use should be avoided). Products include:
Midamor Tablets 1746
Moduretic Tablets 1748

Amphotericin B (May potentiate renal dysfunction). Products include:
Abelcet Injection 1540
Fungizone Intravenous 507
Fungizone Oral Suspension 704

Azathioprine (May potentiate renal dysfunction). Products include:
Azathioprine Tablets 2349
Imuran 1103

Bromocriptine Mesylate (Increases cyclosporine concentrations). Products include:
Parlodel 2411

Carbamazepine (Decreases cyclosporine concentrations). Products include:
Atretol Tablets 569
Tegretol/Tegretol-XR 870

Cimetidine (May potentiate renal dysfunction). Products include:
Tagamet HB Tablets .... ▣ 786
Tagamet Tablets 2694

Cimetidine Hydrochloride (May potentiate renal dysfunction). Products include:
Tagamet 2694

Clarithromycin (Increases cyclosporine concentrations). Products include:
Biaxin 406

Danazol (Increases cyclosporine concentrations). Products include:
Danocrine Capsules 2437

Diclofenac Potassium (May potentiate renal dysfunction). Products include:
Cataflam Tablets 833

Diclofenac Sodium (May potentiate renal dysfunction). Products include:
Voltaren Ophthalmic Sterile Ophthalmic Solution .... ⊙ 264
Cataflam/Voltaren/Voltaren-XR 833

Digoxin (Reduced clearance of digoxin; decrease in the apparent volume of distribution of digoxin; severe digoxin toxicity can occur). Products include:
Lanoxicaps 1110
Lanoxin Elixir Pediatric 1113
Lanoxin Injection 1116
Lanoxin Injection Pediatric 1119
Lanoxin Tablets 1121

Diltiazem Hydrochloride (Increases cyclosporine concentrations). Products include:
Cardizem CD Capsules 1251
Cardizem SR Capsules 1255
Cardizem Injectable 1253
Cardizem Tablets 1257
Dilacor XR Extended-release Capsules 2183
Tiazac Capsules 1019

Erythromycin (Increases cyclosporine concentrations). Products include:
A/T/S 2% Acne Topical Gel 1244
A/T/S 2% Acne Topical Solution 1244
Benzamycin Topical Gel 919
E-Mycin Tablets 1388
Emgel 2% Topical Gel 1081
ERYC 1972
Erycette (erythromycin 2%) Topical Solution 1943
Ery-Tab Tablets 426
Erythromycin Base Filmtab 430
Erythromycin Delayed-Release Capsules, USP 431
Ilotycin Ophthalmic Ointment 928
PCE Dispertab Tablets 453
T-Stat 2.0% Topical Solution and Pads 2797
THERAMYCIN Z 2% Solution 1629

Erythromycin Estolate (Increases cyclosporine concentrations). Products include:
Ilosone 927

Erythromycin Ethylsuccinate (Increases cyclosporine concentrations). Products include:
E.E.S. 427
EryPed 425
Pediazole Suspension 2340

Erythromycin Gluceptate (Increases cyclosporine concentrations). Products include:
Ilotycin Gluceptate, IV, Vials 929

Erythromycin Lactobionate (Increases cyclosporine concentrations).
No products indexed under this heading.

Erythromycin Stearate (Increases cyclosporine concentrations). Products include:
Erythrocin Stearate Filmtab 429

Fluconazole (Increases cyclosporine concentrations). Products include:
Diflucan Tablets, Injection, and Oral Suspension 2003

Gentamicin Sulfate (May potentiate renal dysfunction). Products include:
Garamycin Cream 0.1% 2501
Garamycin Injectable 2502
Garamycin Ointment 0.1% 2501
Garamycin Ophthalmic 2501
Genoptic Sterile Ophthalmic Solution .... ⊙ 241
Genoptic Sterile Ophthalmic Ointment .... ⊙ 241
Gentak .... ⊙ 209
Pred-G Liquifilm Sterile Ophthalmic Suspension .... ⊙ 248
Pred-G S.O.P. Sterile Ophthalmic Ointment .... ⊙ 249

Itraconazole (Increases cyclosporine concentrations). Products include:
Sporanox Capsules 1352

Ketoconazole (May potentiate renal dysfunction; increases cyclosporine concentrations). Products include:
Nizoral 2% Cream 1344
Nizoral 2% Shampoo 1344
Nizoral Tablets 1345

Lovastatin (Reduced clearance of lovastatin; potential for mycositis). Products include:
Mevacor Tablets 1742

Melphalan (May potentiate renal dysfunction). Products include:
Alkeran Tablets 1198

Methylprednisolone (Increases cyclosporine concentrations; potential for convulsion with high doses of methylprednisolone).
No products indexed under this heading.

Methylprednisolone Acetate (Increases cyclosporine concentrations; potential for convulsion with high doses of methylprednisolone).
No products indexed under this heading.

(▣ Described in PDR For Nonprescription Drugs) (⊙ Described in PDR For Ophthalmology)

Methylprednisolone Sodium Succinate (Increases cyclosporine concentrations; potential for convulsion with high doses of methylprednisolone).
   No products indexed under this heading.

Metoclopramide Hydrochloride (Increases cyclosporine concentrations). Products include:
   Reglan 2243

Nafcillin Sodium (Decreases cyclosporine concentrations).
   No products indexed under this heading.

Nephrotoxic Drugs (Potential for increased nephrotoxicity; careful monitoring of renal function is required).

Nicardipine Hydrochloride (Increases cyclosporine concentrations). Products include:
   Cardene Capsules 2261
   Cardene I.V. 2815
   Cardene SR Capsules 2264

Nifedipine (Potential for frequent gingival hyperplasia). Products include:
   Adalat Capsules (10 mg and 20 mg) 580
   Adalat CC 582
   Procardia Capsules 2024
   Procardia XL Extended Release Tablets 2026

Octreotide Acetate (Decreases cyclosporine concentrations). Products include:
   Sandostatin Injection 2421

Phenobarbital (Decreases cyclosporine concentrations). Products include:
   Arco-Lase Plus Tablets 513
   Bellergal-S Tablets 2375
   Donnatal 2234
   Donnatal Extentabs 2234
   Donnatal Tablets 2234
   Phenobarbital Elixir and Tablets ... 1523
   Quadrinal Tablets 1398

Phenytoin (Decreases cyclosporine concentrations). Products include:
   Dilantin Infatabs 1967
   Dilantin-125 Suspension 1969

Phenytoin Sodium (Decreases cyclosporine concentrations). Products include:
   Dilantin Kapseals 1965

Prednisolone (Reduced clearance of prednisolone). Products include:
   Prelone Syrup 1834

Prednisolone Acetate (Reduced clearance of prednisolone). Products include:
   AK-CIDE .... ⓘ 203
   AK-CIDE Ointment .... ⓘ 203
   Blephamide Liquifilm Sterile Ophthalmic Suspension 472
   Blephamide Ointment .... ⓘ 234
   Econopred & Econopred Plus Ophthalmic Suspensions .... ⓘ 216
   Poly-Pred Liquifilm .... ⓘ 246
   Pred Forte .... ⓘ 247
   Pred Mild .... ⓘ 250
   Pred-G Liquifilm Sterile Ophthalmic Suspension .... ⓘ 248
   Pred-G S.O.P. Sterile Ophthalmic Ointment .... ⓘ 249

Prednisolone Sodium Phosphate (Reduced clearance of prednisolone). Products include:
   AK-PRED .... ⓘ 204
   Hydeltrasol Injection, Sterile 1708
   Pediapred Oral Solution 1618

Ranitidine Hydrochloride (May potentiate renal dysfunction). Products include:
   Zantac 1182
   Zantac Injection 1180
   Zantac Syrup 1182

Rifabutin (Caution should be exercised if used concurrently). Products include:
   Mycobutin Capsules 2101

Rifampin (Decreases cyclosporine concentrations). Products include:
   Rifadin 1276
   Rifamate Capsules 1278
   Rifater 1280
   Rimactane Capsules 865

Spironolactone (Cyclosporine may cause hyperkalemia; concurrent use should be avoided). Products include:
   Aldactazide Tablets 2556
   Aldactone Tablets 2558

Sulfamethoxazole (May potentiate renal dysfunction). Products include:
   Bactrim DS Tablets 2257
   Bactrim I.V. Infusion 2255
   Bactrim 2257
   Gantanol Tablets 2285
   Septra 1146
   Septra I.V. Infusion 1142
   Septra I.V. Infusion ADD-Vantage Vials 1144
   Septra 1146

Tacrolimus (May potentiate renal dysfunction). Products include:
   Prograf 1028

Ticlopidine Hydrochloride (Decreases cyclosporine concentrations). Products include:
   Ticlid Tablets 2317

Tobramycin (May potentiate renal dysfunction). Products include:
   AKTOB .... ⓘ 207
   TobraDex Ophthalmic Suspension and Ointment 469
   Tobrex Ophthalmic Ointment and Solution .... ⓘ 226

Tobramycin Sulfate (May potentiate renal dysfunction). Products include:
   Nebcin Vials, Hyporets & ADD-Vantage 1518

Triamterene (Cyclosporine may cause hyperkalemia; concurrent use should be avoided). Products include:
   Dyazide Capsules 2653
   Dyrenium Capsules 2655

Trimethoprim (May potentiate renal dysfunction). Products include:
   Bactrim DS Tablets 2257
   Bactrim I.V. Infusion 2255
   Bactrim 2257
   Proloprim Tablets 1141
   Septra 1146
   Septra I.V. Infusion 1142
   Septra I.V. Infusion ADD-Vantage Vials 1144
   Septra 1146
   Trimpex Tablets 2323

Vaccines (Live) (Vaccination may be less effective).

Vancomycin Hydrochloride (May potentiate renal dysfunction). Products include:
   Vancocin HCl, Oral Solution & Pulvules 1536
   Vancocin HCl, Vials & ADD-Vantage 1534

Verapamil Hydrochloride (Increases cyclosporine concentrations). Products include:
   Calan SR Caplets 2571
   Calan Tablets 2568
   Covera-HS Tablets 2573
   Isoptin Injectable 1391
   Isoptin Oral Tablets 1393
   Isoptin SR Tablets 1395
   Verelan Capsules 1455

Food Interactions

Diet, high-lipid (A high fat meal consumed within one-half hour before Neoral administration decreased the AUC by 13% and C_{max} by 33%).

Food, unspecified (Administration of food with Neoral decreases the AUC and C_{max}).

Grapefruit (Affects the metabolism of cyclosporine and should be avoided).

Grapefruit Juice (Affects the metabolism of cyclosporine and should be avoided).

NEORAL ORAL SOLUTION FOR MICROEMULSION
(Cyclosporine) 2405
  See **Neoral Soft Gelatin Capsules for Microemulsion**

NEOSPORIN G.U. IRRIGANT STERILE
(Neomycin Sulfate, Polymyxin B Sulfate) 1130
None cited in PDR database.

NEOSPORIN OINTMENT
(Bacitracin Zinc, Neomycin Sulfate, Polymyxin B Sulfate) .... ⓘ 821
None cited in PDR database.

NEOSPORIN PLUS MAXIMUM STRENGTH CREAM
(Polymyxin B Sulfate, Neomycin Sulfate, Lidocaine) .... ⓘ 821
None cited in PDR database.

NEOSPORIN PLUS MAXIMUM STRENGTH OINTMENT
(Polymyxin B Sulfate, Bacitracin Zinc, Neomycin Sulfate, Lidocaine) ⓘ 822
None cited in PDR database.

NEOSPORIN OPHTHALMIC OINTMENT STERILE
(Polymyxin B Sulfate, Bacitracin Zinc, Neomycin Sulfate) 1130
None cited in PDR database.

NEOSPORIN OPHTHALMIC SOLUTION STERILE
(Polymyxin B Sulfate, Neomycin Sulfate, Gramicidin) 1131
None cited in PDR database.

NEO-SYNEPHRINE MAXIMUM STRENGTH 12 HOUR NASAL SPRAY
(Oxymetazoline Hydrochloride) ⓘ 624
None cited in PDR database.

NEO-SYNEPHRINE MAXIMUM STRENGTH 12 HOUR EXTRA MOISTURIZING NASAL SPRAY
(Oxymetazoline Hydrochloride) ⓘ 624
None cited in PDR database.

NEO-SYNEPHRINE MAXIMUM STRENGTH 12 HOUR NASAL SPRAY PUMP
(Oxymetazoline Hydrochloride) ⓘ 624
None cited in PDR database.

NEO-SYNEPHRINE HYDROCHLORIDE 1% CARPUJECT
(Phenylephrine Hydrochloride) 2455
May interact with monoamine oxidase inhibitors, tricyclic antidepressants, oxytocic drugs, and certain other agents. Compounds in these categories include:

Amitriptyline Hydrochloride (Pressor response potentiated). Products include:
   Elavil 2945
   Etrafon 2495
   Limbitrol 2333
   Triavil Tablets 1800

Amoxapine (Pressor response potentiated). Products include:
   Asendin Tablets 1419

Clomipramine Hydrochloride (Pressor response potentiated). Products include:
   Anafranil Capsules 819

Desipramine Hydrochloride (Pressor response potentiated). Products include:
   Norpramin Tablets 1273

Doxepin Hydrochloride (Pressor response potentiated). Products include:
   Adapin Capsules 1542
   Sinequan 2028
   Zonalon Cream 1042

Ergonovine Maleate (Potentiates pressor effect).
   No products indexed under this heading.

Furazolidone (Potentiates effect of sympathomimetic pressor amines). Products include:
   Furoxone 2221

Halothane (May cause serious cardiac arrhythmias). Products include:
   Fluothane 2830

Imipramine Hydrochloride (Pressor response potentiated). Products include:
   Tofranil Ampuls 873
   Tofranil Tablets 875

Imipramine Pamoate (Pressor response potentiated). Products include:
   Tofranil-PM Capsules 876

Isocarboxazid (Potentiates effect of sympathomimetic pressor amines).
   No products indexed under this heading.

Methylergonovine Maleate (Potentiates pressor effect). Products include:
   Methergine 2401

Nortriptyline Hydrochloride (Pressor response potentiated). Products include:
   Pamelor 2409

Oxytocin (Potentiates pressor effect). Products include:
   Syntocinon Injection 2425

Phenelzine Sulfate (Potentiates effect of sympathomimetic pressor amines). Products include:
   Nardil 1977

Protriptyline Hydrochloride (Pressor response potentiated). Products include:
   Vivactil Tablets 1820

Selegiline Hydrochloride (Potentiates effect of sympathomimetic pressor amines). Products include:
   Eldepryl Capsules 2729

Tranylcypromine Sulfate (Potentiates effect of sympathomimetic pressor amines). Products include:
   Parnate Tablets 2679

Trimipramine Maleate (Pressor response potentiated). Products include:
   Surmontil Capsules 2917

NEO-SYNEPHRINE HYDROCHLORIDE 1% INJECTION
(Phenylephrine Hydrochloride) 2455
See **Neo-Synephrine Hydrochloride 1% Carpuject**

IMPORTANT NOTE: Always consult each drug listing in the patient's regimen for possible interactions.

Neo-Synephrine — Interactions Index

NEO-SYNEPHRINE HYDROCHLORIDE (OPHTHALMIC)
(Phenylephrine Hydrochloride) 2456
May interact with beta blockers, monoamine oxidase inhibitors, tricyclic antidepressants, inhalant anesthetics, and certain other agents. Compounds in these categories include:

Acebutolol Hydrochloride (Acute hypertension; ruptured congenital cerebral aneurysm may occur). Products include:
- Sectral Capsules 2914

Amitriptyline Hydrochloride (Pressor response potentiated). Products include:
- Elavil 2945
- Etrafon 2495
- Limbitrol 2333
- Triavil Tablets 1800

Amoxapine (Pressor response potentiated). Products include:
- Asendin Tablets 1419

Atenolol (Acute hypertension; ruptured congenital cerebral aneurysm may occur). Products include:
- Tenoretic Tablets 2963
- Tenormin Tablets and I.V. Injection 2965

Betaxolol Hydrochloride (Acute hypertension; ruptured congenital cerebral aneurysm may occur). Products include:
- Betoptic Ophthalmic Solution........... 465
- Betoptic S Ophthalmic Suspension... 467
- Kerlone Tablets 2588

Bisoprolol Fumarate (Acute hypertension; ruptured congenital cerebral aneurysm may occur). Products include:
- Zebeta Tablets 1457
- Ziac 1459

Carteolol Hydrochloride (Acute hypertension; ruptured congenital cerebral aneurysm may occur). Products include:
- Cartrol Tablets 413
- Ocupress Ophthalmic Solution, 1% Sterile......................... ⊙ 297

Clomipramine Hydrochloride (Pressor response potentiated). Products include:
- Anafranil Capsules 819

Desflurane (Neo-Synephrine may potentiate the cardiovascular depressant effects of potent inhalation anesthetic agents). Products include:
- Suprane (desflurane, USP) 1865

Desipramine Hydrochloride (Pressor response potentiated). Products include:
- Norpramin Tablets 1273

Doxepin Hydrochloride (Pressor response potentiated). Products include:
- Adapin Capsules 1542
- Sinequan 2028
- Zonalon Cream 1042

Enflurane (Neo-Synephrine may potentiate the cardiovascular depressant effects of potent inhalation anesthetic agents).
- No products indexed under this heading.

Esmolol Hydrochloride (Acute hypertension; ruptured congenital cerebral aneurysm may occur). Products include:
- Brevibloc (esmolol HCl) Injection 1860

Furazolidone (Exaggerated adrenergic effects may occur). Products include:
- Furoxone 2221

Guanethidine Monosulfate (Pressor response potentiated). Products include:
- Esimil Tablets 840
- Ismelin Tablets 845

Halothane (Neo-Synephrine may potentiate the cardiovascular depressant effects of potent inhalation anesthetic agents). Products include:
- Fluothane 2830

Imipramine Hydrochloride (Pressor response potentiated). Products include:
- Tofranil Ampuls 873
- Tofranil Tablets 875

Imipramine Pamoate (Pressor response potentiated). Products include:
- Tofranil-PM Capsules 876

Isocarboxazid (Exaggerated adrenergic effects may occur).
- No products indexed under this heading.

Isoflurane (Neo-Synephrine may potentiate the cardiovascular depressant effects of potent inhalation anesthetic agents).
- No products indexed under this heading.

Labetalol Hydrochloride (Acute hypertension; ruptured congenital cerebral aneurysm may occur). Products include:
- Normodyne Injection 2519
- Normodyne Tablets 2522
- Trandate 1158

Levobunolol Hydrochloride (Acute hypertension; ruptured congenital cerebral aneurysm may occur). Products include:
- Betagan .... ⊙ 230

Maprotiline Hydrochloride (Pressor response potentiated). Products include:
- Ludiomil Tablets 861

Methoxyflurane (Neo-Synephrine may potentiate the cardiovascular depressant effects of potent inhalation anesthetic agents).
- No products indexed under this heading.

Methyldopa (Pressor response potentiated). Products include:
- Aldoclor Tablets 1638
- Aldomet Oral 1640
- Aldoril Tablets 1644

Methyldopate Hydrochloride (Pressor response potentiated). Products include:
- Aldomet Ester HCl Injection ... 1642

Metipranolol Hydrochloride (Acute hypertension; ruptured congenital cerebral aneurysm may occur). Products include:
- OptiPranolol (Metipranolol 0.3%) Sterile Ophthalmic Solution ..... ⊙ 256

Metoprolol Succinate (Acute hypertension; ruptured congenital cerebral aneurysm may occur). Products include:
- Toprol-XL Tablets 560

Metoprolol Tartrate (Acute hypertension; ruptured congenital cerebral aneurysm may occur). Products include:
- Lopressor 848
- Lopressor HCT Tablets 850

Nadolol (Acute hypertension; ruptured congenital cerebral aneurysm may occur).
- No products indexed under this heading.

Nortriptyline Hydrochloride (Pressor response potentiated). Products include:
- Pamelor 2409

Penbutolol Sulfate (Acute hypertension; ruptured congenital cerebral aneurysm may occur). Products include:
- Levatol Tablets 2547

Phenelzine Sulfate (Exaggerated adrenergic effects may occur). Products include:
- Nardil 1977

Pindolol (Acute hypertension; ruptured congenital cerebral aneurysm may occur). Products include:
- Visken Tablets 2428

Propranolol Hydrochloride (Acute hypertension; ruptured congenital cerebral aneurysm may occur). Products include:
- Inderal 2834
- Inderal LA Long Acting Capsules 2836
- Inderide Tablets 2838
- Inderide LA Long Acting Capsules .. 2840

Protriptyline Hydrochloride (Pressor response potentiated). Products include:
- Vivactil Tablets 1820

Selegiline Hydrochloride (Exaggerated adrenergic effects may occur). Products include:
- Eldepryl Capsules 2729

Sotalol Hydrochloride (Acute hypertension; ruptured congenital cerebral aneurysm may occur). Products include:
- Betapace Tablets 637

Timolol Hemihydrate (Acute hypertension; ruptured congenital cerebral aneurysm may occur). Products include:
- Betimol 0.25%, 0.5% .... ⊙ 259

Timolol Maleate (Acute hypertension; ruptured congenital cerebral aneurysm may occur). Products include:
- Blocadren Tablets 1654
- Timolide Tablets 1791
- Timoptic in Ocudose 1796
- Timoptic Sterile Ophthalmic Solution 1794
- Timoptic-XE 1798

Tranylcypromine Sulfate (Exaggerated adrenergic effects may occur). Products include:
- Parnate Tablets 2679

Trimipramine Maleate (Pressor response potentiated). Products include:
- Surmontil Capsules 2917

NEO-SYNEPHRINE NASAL DROPS, PEDIATRIC, MILD, REGULAR & EXTRA STRENGTH
(Phenylephrine Hydrochloride) .... ■ 624
None cited in PDR database.

NEO-SYNEPHRINE NASAL SPRAYS, PEDIATRIC, MILD, REGULAR & EXTRA STRENGTH
(Phenylephrine Hydrochloride) .... ■ 624
None cited in PDR database.

NEPHRAMINE INJECTION
(Amino Acid Preparations) 2169
None cited in PDR database.

NEPHRO-CALCI TABLETS
(Calcium Carbonate) 2168
None cited in PDR database.

NEPHROCAPS
(Vitamins, Multiple) 1004
None cited in PDR database.

NEPHRO-FER TABLETS
(Ferrous Fumarate) 2168
None cited in PDR database.

NEPHRO-FER RX TABLETS
(Ferrous Fumarate, Folic Acid) 2168
None cited in PDR database.

NEPHRO-VITE + FE TABLETS
(Vitamins, Multiple, Ferrous Fumarate) 2170
None cited in PDR database.

NEPHRO-VITE RX TABLETS
(Vitamins with Minerals) 2170
None cited in PDR database.

NEPHROX SUSPENSION
(Aluminum Hydroxide Gel, Mineral Oil) .... ■ 671
None cited in PDR database.

NEPRO SPECIALIZED LIQUID NUTRITION
(Nutritional Supplement) 2339
None cited in PDR database.

NEPTAZANE TABLETS
(Methazolamide) .... ⊙ 320
May interact with corticosteroids and certain other agents. Compounds in these categories include:

Aspirin (Concomitant use of high-dose aspirin and carbonic anhydrase inhibitors may produce anorexia, tachypnea, lethargy, coma, and death). Products include:
- Alka-Seltzer Cherry Effervescent Antacid and Pain Reliever .... ■ 609
- Alka-Seltzer Extra Strength Effervescent Antacid and Pain Reliever .... ■ 609
- Alka-Seltzer Lemon Lime Effervescent Antacid and Pain Reliever .... ■ 609
- Alka-Seltzer Original Effervescent Antacid and Pain Reliever .... ■ 609
- Alka-Seltzer Plus .... ■ 611
- Alka-Seltzer Plus Sinus Medicine .. ■ 611
- Ascriptin .... ■ 650
- Arthritis Strength BC Powder ■ 631
- BC Cold Powder Multi-Symptom Formula (Cold-Sinus-Allergy) ■ 631
- BC Cold Powder Non-Drowsy Formula (Cold-Sinus) .... ■ 631
- BC Powder .... ■ 631
- Genuine Bayer Aspirin Tablets & Caplets .... ■ 618
- Extra Strength Bayer Arthritis Pain Regimen Formula .... ■ 615
- Extra Strength Bayer Aspirin Caplets & Tablets .... ■ 617
- Extended-Release Bayer 8-Hour Aspirin .... ■ 616
- Extra Strength Bayer Plus Aspirin Caplets .... ■ 617
- Extra Strength Bayer PM Aspirin Plus Sleep Aid .... ■ 617
- Aspirin Regimen Bayer 81 mg Tablets with Calcium .... ■ 615
- Aspirin Regimen Bayer Adult Low Strength 81 mg Tablets ..... ■ 613
- Aspirin Regimen Bayer Children's Chewable Aspirin .... ■ 616
- Aspirin Regimen Bayer Regular Strength 325 mg Caplets ..... ■ 613
- Bufferin Analgesic Tablets ..... ■ 636
- Arthritis Strength Bufferin Analgesic Caplets .... ■ 637
- Extra Strength Bufferin Analgesic Tablets .... ■ 637
- Cama Arthritis Pain Reliever.... ■ 748
- Darvon Compound-65 Pulvules .. 1475
- Easprin 1971
- Ecotrin 2625
- Ecotrin Enteric Coated Aspirin Maximum Strength Tablets and Caplets .... ■ 775
- Ecotrin Enteric Coated Aspirin Regular Strength Tablets 2625
- Empirin Aspirin Tablets .... ■ 818
- Excedrin Extra-Strength Analgesic Tablets, Caplets, and Geltabs 734
- Fiorinal Capsules 2388
- Fiorinal with Codeine Capsules ... 2390
- Fiorinal Tablets 2388
- Goody's Extra Strength Headache Powders .... ■ 632
- Goody's Extra Strength Pain Relief Tablets .... ■ 632
- Halfprin Tablets 1413
- Norgesic................................. 1554
- Percodan Tablets 955

(■ Described in PDR For Nonprescription Drugs)   (⊙ Described in PDR For Ophthalmology)

Percodan-Demi Tablets 956
Robaxisal Tablets 2246
Soma Compound w/Codeine Tablets 2784
Soma Compound Tablets 2783
St. Joseph Adult Chewable Aspirin (81 mg.) .... ▣ 768
Talwin Compound 2466
Vanquish Analgesic Caplets .... ▣ 627

Betamethasone Acetate (Potential for developing hypokalemia). Products include:
Celestone Soluspan Suspension 2484

Betamethasone Sodium Phosphate (Potential for developing hypokalemia). Products include:
Celestone Soluspan Suspension 2484

Cortisone Acetate (Potential for developing hypokalemia). Products include:
Cortone Acetate Sterile Suspension 1663
Cortone Acetate Tablets 1664

Dexamethasone (Potential for developing hypokalemia). Products include:
AK-Trol Ointment & Suspension .... ◉ 205
Decadron Elixir 1676
Decadron Tablets 1678
Decaspray Topical Aerosol 1689
Maxitrol Ophthalmic Ointment and Suspension .... ◉ 222
TobraDex Ophthalmic Suspension and Ointment 469

Dexamethasone Acetate (Potential for developing hypokalemia). Products include:
Dalalone D.P. Injectable 1009
Decadron-LA Sterile Suspension 1687

Dexamethasone Sodium Phosphate (Potential for developing hypokalemia). Products include:
Decadron Phosphate Injection 1680
Decadron Phosphate Sterile Ophthalmic Ointment 1684
Decadron Phosphate Sterile Ophthalmic Solution 1685
Decadron Phosphate Topical Cream 1686
Decadron Phosphate with Xylocaine Injection, Sterile 1683
Dexacort Phosphate in Respihaler .. 1606
Dexacort Phosphate in Turbinaire .. 1607
NeoDecadron Sterile Ophthalmic Ointment 1755
NeoDecadron Sterile Ophthalmic Solution 1756
NeoDecadron Topical Cream 1757

Fludrocortisone Acetate (Potential for developing hypokalemia). Products include:
Florinef Acetate Tablets 506

Hydrocortisone (Potential for developing hypokalemia). Products include:
Anusol-HC Cream 2.5% 1953
Aquanil HC Lotion 1989
Maximum Strength Cortaid Spray ▣ 800
CORTENEMA 2713
Cortisporin Ointment 1074
Cortisporin Ophthalmic Ointment Sterile 1074
Cortisporin Ophthalmic Suspension Sterile 1075
Cortisporin Otic Solution Sterile 1076
Cortisporin Otic Suspension Sterile 1077
Cortizone-5 .... ▣ 795
Cortizone-10 .... ▣ 795
Hydrocortone Tablets 1715
Hytone 922
Hytone Ointment 2 ½% 923
Massengill Medicated Soft Cloth Towelettes 2628
Pediotic Suspension Sterile 1140
Preparation H Hydrocortisone 1% Cream .... ▣ 843
ProctoCream-HC 2.5% 2552
VōSoL HC Otic Solution 2786

Hydrocortisone Acetate (Potential for developing hypokalemia). Products include:
Analpram-HC Rectal Cream 1% and 2.5% 993
Anusol HC-1 Hydrocortisone Anti-Itch Ointment .... ▣ 810
Anusol-HC Suppositories 1954
Caldecort Anti-Itch Hydrocortisone Cream .... ▣ 651
Coly-Mycin S Otic w/Neomycin & Hydrocortisone 1965
Cortaid .... ▣ 800
Cortifoam 2540
Cortisporin Cream 1073
Epifoam 2543
Hydrocortone Acetate Sterile Suspension 1712
Mantadil Cream 1124
Nupercainal Hydrocortisone 1% Cream .... ▣ 661
Pramosone Cream, Lotion & Ointment 995
ProctoFoam-HC 2552
Terra-Cortril Ophthalmic Suspension 2033

Hydrocortisone Sodium Phosphate (Potential for developing hypokalemia). Products include:
Hydrocortone Phosphate Injection, Sterile 1713

Hydrocortisone Sodium Succinate (Potential for developing hypokalemia).
No products indexed under this heading.

Methylprednisolone Acetate (Potential for developing hypokalemia).
No products indexed under this heading.

Methylprednisolone Sodium Succinate (Potential for developing hypokalemia).
No products indexed under this heading.

Prednisolone Acetate (Potential for developing hypokalemia). Products include:
AK-CIDE .... ◉ 203
AK-CIDE Ointment .... ◉ 203
Blephamide Liquifilm Sterile Ophthalmic Suspension 472
Blephamide Ointment .... ◉ 234
Econopred & Econopred Plus Ophthalmic Suspensions .... ◉ 216
Poly-Pred Liquifilm .... ◉ 246
Pred Forte .... ◉ 247
Pred Mild .... ◉ 250
Pred-G Liquifilm Sterile Ophthalmic Suspension .... ◉ 248
Pred-G S.O.P. Sterile Ophthalmic Ointment .... ◉ 249

Prednisolone Sodium Phosphate (Potential for developing hypokalemia). Products include:
AK-PRED .... ◉ 204
Hydeltrasol Injection, Sterile 1708
Pediapred Oral Solution 1618

Prednisolone Tebutate (Potential for developing hypokalemia). Products include:
Hydeltra-T.B.A. Sterile Suspension 1710

Prednisone (Potential for developing hypokalemia).
No products indexed under this heading.

Triamcinolone (Potential for developing hypokalemia).
No products indexed under this heading.

Triamcinolone Acetonide (Potential for developing hypokalemia). Products include:
Azmacort Oral Inhaler 2175
Nasacort AQ Nasal Spray 2191
Nasacort Nasal Inhaler 2189

Triamcinolone Diacetate (Potential for developing hypokalemia).
No products indexed under this heading.

Triamcinolone Hexacetonide (Potential for developing hypokalemia).
No products indexed under this heading.

NESACAINE INJECTIONS
(Chloroprocaine Hydrochloride) 549
May interact with monoamine oxidase inhibitors, phenothiazines, tricyclic antidepressants, ergot-type oxytocic drugs, and certain other agents. Compounds in these categories include:

Amitriptyline Hydrochloride (Co-administration of local anesthetic solutions containing epinephrine may produce severe, prolonged hypotension or hypertension; concurrent use should be avoided). Products include:
Elavil 2945
Etrafon 2495
Limbitrol 2333
Triavil Tablets 1800

Amoxapine (Co-administration of local anesthetic solutions containing epinephrine may produce severe, prolonged hypotension or hypertension; concurrent use should be avoided). Products include:
Asendin Tablets 1419

Chlorpromazine (Co-administration of local anesthetic solutions containing epinephrine may produce severe, prolonged hypotension or hypertension; concurrent use should be avoided). Products include:
Thorazine Suppositories 2701

Chlorpromazine Hydrochloride (Co-administration of local anesthetic solutions containing epinephrine may produce severe, prolonged hypotension or hypertension; concurrent use should be avoided). Products include:
Thorazine 2701

Clomipramine Hydrochloride (Co-administration of local anesthetic solutions containing epinephrine may produce severe, prolonged hypotension or hypertension; concurrent use should be avoided). Products include:
Anafranil Capsules 819

Desipramine Hydrochloride (Co-administration of local anesthetic solutions containing epinephrine may produce severe, prolonged hypotension or hypertension; concurrent use should be avoided). Products include:
Norpramin Tablets 1273

Doxepin Hydrochloride (Co-administration of local anesthetic solutions containing epinephrine may produce severe, prolonged hypotension or hypertension; concurrent use should be avoided). Products include:
Adapin Capsules 1542
Sinequan 2028
Zonalon Cream 1042

Fluphenazine Decanoate (Co-administration of local anesthetic solutions containing epinephrine may produce severe, prolonged hypotension or hypertension; concurrent use should be avoided). Products include:
Prolixin Decanoate 510

Fluphenazine Enanthate (Co-administration of local anesthetic solutions containing epinephrine may produce severe, prolonged hypotension or hypertension; concurrent use should be avoided). Products include:
Prolixin Enanthate 510

Fluphenazine Hydrochloride (Co-administration of local anesthetic solutions containing epinephrine may produce severe, prolonged hypotension or hypertension; concurrent use should be avoided). Products include:
Prolixin 510

Furazolidone (Co-administration of local anesthetic solutions containing epinephrine may produce severe, prolonged hypotension or hypertension; concurrent use should be avoided). Products include:
Furoxone 2221

Imipramine Hydrochloride (Co-administration of local anesthetic solutions containing epinephrine may produce severe, prolonged hypotension or hypertension; concurrent use should be avoided). Products include:
Tofranil Ampuls 873
Tofranil Tablets 875

Imipramine Pamoate (Co-administration of local anesthetic solutions containing epinephrine may produce severe, prolonged hypotension or hypertension; concurrent use should be avoided). Products include:
Tofranil-PM Capsules 876

Isocarboxazid (Co-administration of local anesthetic solutions containing epinephrine may produce severe, prolonged hypotension or hypertension; concurrent use should be avoided).
No products indexed under this heading.

Maprotiline Hydrochloride (Co-administration of local anesthetic solutions containing epinephrine may produce severe, prolonged hypotension or hypertension; concurrent use should be avoided). Products include:
Ludiomil Tablets 861

Mesoridazine Besylate (Co-administration of local anesthetic solutions containing epinephrine may produce severe, prolonged hypotension or hypertension; concurrent use should be avoided). Products include:
Serentil 689

Methotrimeprazine (Co-administration of local anesthetic solutions containing epinephrine may produce severe, prolonged hypotension or hypertension; concurrent use should be avoided). Products include:
Levoprome 1321

Methylergonovine Maleate (Co-administration of vasopressors (for the treatment of hypotension related to obstetrical blocks) and ergot-type oxytocic drugs may cause severe, persistent hypertension or cerebrovascular accidents). Products include:
Methergine 2401

Nortriptyline Hydrochloride (Co-administration of local anesthetic solutions containing epinephrine may produce severe, prolonged hypotension or hypertension; concurrent use should be avoided). Products include:
Pamelor 2409

Perphenazine (Co-administration of local anesthetic solutions containing epinephrine may produce severe, prolonged hypotension or hypertension; concurrent use should be avoided). Products include:
Etrafon 2495
Triavil Tablets 1800
Trilafon 2532

Phenelzine Sulfate (Co-administration of local anesthetic solutions containing epinephrine may produce severe, prolonged hypotension or hypertension; concurrent use should be avoided). Products include:
Nardil 1977

IMPORTANT NOTE: Always consult each drug listing in the patient's regimen for possible interactions.

Nescaine/Nescaine MPF | Interactions Index | 734

Prochlorperazine (Co-administration of local anesthetic solutions containing epinephrine may produce severe, prolonged hypotension or hypertension; concurrent use should be avoided). Products include:
- Compazine ... 2644

Promethazine Hydrochloride (Co-administration of local anesthetic solutions containing epinephrine may produce severe, prolonged hypotension or hypertension; concurrent use should be avoided). Products include:
- Mepergan Injection ... 2859
- Phenergan with Codeine ... 2883
- Phenergan with Dextromethorphan 2885
- Phenergan Injection ... 2880
- Phenergan Suppositories ... 2882
- Phenergan Syrup ... 2881
- Phenergan Tablets ... 2882
- Phenergan VC ... 2886
- Phenergan VC with Codeine ... 2888

Protriptyline Hydrochloride (Co-administration of local anesthetic solutions containing epinephrine may produce severe, prolonged hypotension or hypertension; concurrent use should be avoided). Products include:
- Vivactil Tablets ... 1820

Selegiline Hydrochloride (Co-administration of local anesthetic solutions containing epinephrine may produce severe, prolonged hypotension or hypertension; concurrent use should be avoided). Products include:
- Eldepryl Capsules ... 2729

Sulfamethizole (The para-aminobenzoic acid metabolite of chloroprocaine inhibits the action of sulfonamides; concurrent use should be avoided). Products include:
- Urobiotic-250 Capsules ... 2038

Sulfamethoxazole (The para-aminobenzoic acid metabolite of chloroprocaine inhibits the action of sulfonamides; concurrent use should be avoided). Products include:
- Bactrim DS Tablets ... 2257
- Bactrim I.V. Infusion ... 2255
- Bactrim ... 2257
- Gantanol Tablets ... 2285
- Septra ... 1146
- Septra I.V. Infusion ... 1142
- Septra I.V. Infusion ADD-Vantage Vials ... 1144
- Septra ... 1146

Sulfisoxazole (The para-aminobenzoic acid metabolite of chloroprocaine inhibits the action of sulfonamides; concurrent use should be avoided). Products include:
- Gantrisin Tablets ... 2286

Thioridazine Hydrochloride (Co-administration of local anesthetic solutions containing epinephrine may produce severe, prolonged hypotension or hypertension; concurrent use should be avoided). Products include:
- Mellaril ... 2398

Tranylcypromine Sulfate (Co-administration of local anesthetic solutions containing epinephrine may produce severe, prolonged hypotension or hypertension; concurrent use should be avoided). Products include:
- Parnate Tablets ... 2679

Trifluoperazine Hydrochloride (Co-administration of local anesthetic solutions containing epinephrine may produce severe, prolonged hypotension or hypertension; concurrent use should be avoided). Products include:
- Stelazine ... 2692

Trimipramine Maleate (Co-administration of local anesthetic solutions containing epinephrine may produce severe, prolonged hypotension or hypertension; concurrent use should be avoided). Products include:
- Surmontil Capsules ... 2917

NESACAINE-MPF INJECTIONS
(Chloroprocaine Hydrochloride) ... 549
See **Nesacaine Injections**

NESTABS FA TABLETS
(Vitamins with Minerals) ... 1000
None cited in PDR database.

NETROMYCIN INJECTION 100 MG/ML
(Netilmicin Sulfate) ... 2516
May interact with nondepolarizing neuromuscular blocking agents, diuretics, cephalosporins, penicillins, and certain other agents. Compounds in these categories include:

Acyclovir (Neurotoxicity and/or nephrotoxicity). Products include:
- Zovirax Capsules ... 1187
- Zovirax Ointment 5% ... 1190
- Zovirax ... 1187

Acyclovir Sodium (Neurotoxicity and/or nephrotoxicity). Products include:
- Zovirax Sterile Powder ... 1191

Amikacin Sulfate (Neurotoxicity and/or nephrotoxicity). Products include:
- Amikacin Sulfate Injection, USP ... 523
- Amikacin Sulfate Injection, USP ... 981
- Amikin Injectable ... 502

Amiloride Hydrochloride (Ototoxicity). Products include:
- Midamor Tablets ... 1746
- Moduretic Tablets ... 1748

Amoxicillin Trihydrate (Mutual inactivation). Products include:
- Amoxil ... 2631
- Augmentin ... 2637
- Augmentin Tablets ... 2640

Amphotericin B (Neurotoxicity and/or nephrotoxicity). Products include:
- Abelcet Injection ... 1540
- Fungizone Intravenous ... 507
- Fungizone Oral Suspension ... 704

Ampicillin Sodium (Mutual inactivation). Products include:
- Unasyn ... 2035

Atracurium Besylate (Potential for increased neuromuscular blockade and respiratory paralysis). Products include:
- Tracrium Injection ... 1155

Azlocillin Sodium (Mutual inactivation).
No products indexed under this heading.

Bacampicillin Hydrochloride (Mutual inactivation). Products include:
- Spectrobid Tablets ... 2030

Bacitracin (Neurotoxicity and/or nephrotoxicity).
No products indexed under this heading.

Bacitracin Zinc (Neurotoxicity and/or nephrotoxicity). Products include:
- AK-Spore Ointment ... ⊙ 205
- Betadine Brand First Aid Antibiotics & Moisturizer Ointment ... 2144
- Cortisporin Ointment ... 1074
- Cortisporin Ophthalmic Ointment Sterile ... 1074
- Mycitracin ... ▣ 803
- Neosporin Ointment ... ▣ 821
- Neosporin Plus Maximum Strength Ointment ... ▣ 822
- Neosporin Ophthalmic Ointment Sterile ... 1130
- Polysporin Ointment ... ▣ 822
- Polysporin Ophthalmic Ointment Sterile ... 1140
- Polysporin Powder ... ▣ 823

Bendroflumethiazide (Ototoxicity).
No products indexed under this heading.

Bumetanide (Ototoxicity). Products include:
- Bumex ... 2260

Carbenicillin Disodium (Mutual inactivation).
No products indexed under this heading.

Carbenicillin Indanyl Sodium (Mutual inactivation). Products include:
- Geocillin Tablets ... 2009

Cefaclor (Nephrotoxicity). Products include:
- Ceclor Pulvules & Suspension ... 1470

Cefadroxil (Nephrotoxicity). Products include:
- Duricef Capsules, Tablets, and Oral Suspension ... 750

Cefamandole Nafate (Nephrotoxicity). Products include:
- Mandol Vials, Faspak & ADD-Vantage ... 1516

Cefazolin Sodium (Nephrotoxicity). Products include:
- Ancef Injection ... 2632
- Kefzol Vials, Faspak & ADD-Vantage ... 1511

Cefixime (Nephrotoxicity). Products include:
- Suprax ... 1443

Cefmetazole Sodium (Nephrotoxicity).
No products indexed under this heading.

Cefonicid Sodium (Nephrotoxicity). Products include:
- Monocid Injection ... 2674

Cefoperazone Sodium (Nephrotoxicity). Products include:
- Cefobid Intravenous/Intramuscular 1996
- Cefobid Pharmacy Bulk Package - Not for Direct Infusion ... 1999

Ceforanide (Nephrotoxicity).
No products indexed under this heading.

Cefotaxime Sodium (Nephrotoxicity). Products include:
- Claforan Sterile and Injection ... 1259

Cefotetan (Nephrotoxicity). Products include:
- Cefotan ... 2936

Cefoxitin Sodium (Nephrotoxicity). Products include:
- Mefoxin ... 1734
- Mefoxin Premixed Intravenous Solution ... 1737

Cefpodoxime Proxetil (Nephrotoxicity). Products include:
- Vantin for Oral Suspension and Vantin Tablets ... 2112

Cefprozil (Nephrotoxicity). Products include:
- Cefzil Tablets and Oral Suspension 747

Ceftazidime (Nephrotoxicity). Products include:
- Ceptaz ... 1070
- Fortaz ... 1092
- Tazicef for Injection ... 2697
- Tazidime Vials, Faspak & ADD-Vantage ... 1531

Ceftizoxime Sodium (Nephrotoxicity). Products include:
- Cefizox for Intramuscular or Intravenous Use ... 1025

Ceftriaxone Sodium (Nephrotoxicity). Products include:
- Rocephin Injectable Vials, ADD-Vantage, Galaxy Container ... 2305

Cefuroxime Axetil (Nephrotoxicity). Products include:
- Ceftin ... 1067

Cefuroxime Sodium (Nephrotoxicity). Products include:
- Kefurox Vials, Faspak & ADD-Vantage ... 1509
- Zinacef ... 1184

Cephalexin (Nephrotoxicity). Products include:
- Keflex Pulvules & Oral Suspension 930

Cephalothin Sodium (Nephrotoxicity).

Cephapirin Sodium (Nephrotoxicity).
No products indexed under this heading.

Cephradine (Nephrotoxicity).
No products indexed under this heading.

Chlorothiazide (Ototoxicity). Products include:
- Aldoclor Tablets ... 1638
- Diupres Tablets ... 1691
- Diuril Oral ... 1694

Chlorothiazide Sodium (Ototoxicity). Products include:
- Diuril Sodium Intravenous ... 1693

Chlorthalidone (Ototoxicity). Products include:
- Combipres Tablets ... 682
- Tenoretic Tablets ... 2963
- Thalitone ... 1293

Cisatracurium Besylate (Potential for increased neuromuscular blockade and respiratory paralysis). Products include:
- Nimbex Injection ... 1131

Cisplatin (Neurotoxicity and/or nephrotoxicity). Products include:
- Platinol for Injection ... 717
- Platinol-AQ Injection ... 719

Colistin Sulfate (Neurotoxicity and/or nephrotoxicity). Products include:
- Coly-Mycin S Otic w/Neomycin & Hydrocortisone ... 1965

Decamethonium (Potential for increased neuromuscular blockade and respiratory paralysis).

Dicloxacillin Sodium (Mutual inactivation).
No products indexed under this heading.

Ethacrynic Acid (Ototoxicity). Products include:
- Edecrin Tablets ... 1698

Furosemide (Ototoxicity). Products include:
- Lasix Injection, Oral Solution and Tablets ... 1267

Gentamicin (Neurotoxicity and/or nephrotoxicity).
No products indexed under this heading.

Gentamicin Sulfate (Neurotoxicity and/or nephrotoxicity). Products include:
- Garamycin Cream 0.1% ... 2501
- Garamycin Injectable ... 2502
- Garamycin Ointment 0.1% ... 2501
- Garamycin Ophthalmic ... 2501
- Genoptic Sterile Ophthalmic Solution ... ⊙ 241
- Genoptic Sterile Ophthalmic Ointment ... ⊙ 241
- Gentak ... ⊙ 209
- Pred-G Liquifilm Sterile Ophthalmic Suspension ... ⊙ 248
- Pred-G S.O.P. Sterile Ophthalmic Ointment ... ⊙ 249

Hydrochlorothiazide (Ototoxicity). Products include:
- Aldactazide Tablets ... 2556
- Aldoril Tablets ... 1644
- Apresazide Capsules ... 824
- Capozide Tablets ... 744
- Dyazide Capsules ... 2653
- Esidrix Tablets ... 839
- Esimil Tablets ... 840

(▣ Described in PDR For Nonprescription Drugs) (⊙ Described in PDR For Ophthalmology)

735 **Interactions Index** **Neutrexin**

HydroDIURIL Tablets ... 1716
Hydropres Tablets ... 1718
Hyzaar Tablets ... 1720
Inderide Tablets ... 2838
Inderide LA Long Acting Capsules .. 2840
Lopressor HCT Tablets ... 850
Lotensin HCT Tablets ... 855
Moduretic Tablets ... 1748
Oretic Tablets ... 450
Prinzide Tablets ... 1780
Ser-Ap-Es Tablets ... 867
Timolide Tablets ... 1791
Vaseretic Tablets ... 1810
Zestoretic Tablets ... 2968
Ziac ... 1459

Hydroflumethiazide (Ototoxicity). Products include:
Diucardin Tablets ... 2824

Indapamide (Ototoxicity).
No products indexed under this heading.

Kanamycin Sulfate (Neurotoxicity and/or nephrotoxicity).
No products indexed under this heading.

Loracarbef (Nephrotoxicity). Products include:
Lorabid Suspension and Pulvules 1513

Methyclothiazide (Ototoxicity). Products include:
Enduron Tablets ... 424

Metocurine Iodide (Potential for increased neuromuscular blockade and respiratory paralysis). Products include:
Metubine Iodide Vials ... 932

Metolazone (Ototoxicity). Products include:
Mykrox Tablets ... 1617
Zaroxolyn Tablets ... 1625

Mezlocillin Sodium (Mutual inactivation). Products include:
Mezlin ... 594
Mezlin Pharmacy Bulk Package ... 597

Mivacurium Chloride (Potential for increased neuromuscular blockade and respiratory paralysis). Products include:
Mivacron ... 1125

Nafcillin Sodium (Mutual inactivation).
No products indexed under this heading.

Neomycin Sulfate (Neurotoxicity and/or nephrotoxicity). Products include:
AK-Spore ... ◉ 205
AK-Trol Ointment & Suspension .... ◉ 205
Coly-Mycin S Otic w/Neomycin & Hydrocortisone ... 1965
Cortisporin Cream ... 1073
Cortisporin Ointment ... 1074
Cortisporin Ophthalmic Ointment Sterile ... 1074
Cortisporin Ophthalmic Suspension Sterile ... 1075
Cortisporin Otic Solution Sterile ... 1076
Cortisporin Otic Suspension Sterile 1077
Maxitrol Ophthalmic Ointment and Suspension ... ◉ 222
Mycitracin ... ▣ 803
NeoDecadron Sterile Ophthalmic Ointment ... 1755
NeoDecadron Sterile Ophthalmic Solution ... 1756
NeoDecadron Topical Cream ... 1757
Neosporin G.U. Irrigant Sterile ... 1130
Neosporin Ointment ... ▣ 821
Neosporin Plus Maximum Strength Cream ... ▣ 821
Neosporin Plus Maximum Strength Ointment ... ▣ 822
Neosporin Ophthalmic Ointment Sterile ... 1130
Neosporin Ophthalmic Solution Sterile ... 1131
Pediotic Suspension Sterile ... 1140
Poly-Pred Liquifilm ... ◉ 246

Pancuronium Bromide (Potential for increased neuromuscular blockade and respiratory paralysis).
No products indexed under this heading.

Paromomycin Sulfate (Neurotoxicity and/or nephrotoxicity).
No products indexed under this heading.

Penicillin G Benzathine (Mutual inactivation). Products include:
Bicillin C-R Injection ... 2810
Bicillin C-R 900/300 Injection ... 2812
Bicillin L-A Injection ... 2813

Penicillin G Potassium (Mutual inactivation). Products include:
Pfizerpen for Injection ... 2022

Penicillin G Procaine (Mutual inactivation). Products include:
Bicillin C-R Injection ... 2810
Bicillin C-R 900/300 Injection ... 2812

Penicillin G Sodium (Mutual inactivation).
No products indexed under this heading.

Penicillin V Potassium (Mutual inactivation). Products include:
Pen•Vee K ... 2879

Polymyxin B Sulfate (Neurotoxicity and/or nephrotoxicity). Products include:
AK-Spore ... ◉ 205
AK-Trol Ointment & Suspension .... ◉ 205
Betadine Brand First Aid Antibiotics & Moisturizer Ointment ... 2144
Cortisporin Cream ... 1073
Cortisporin Ointment ... 1074
Cortisporin Ophthalmic Ointment Sterile ... 1074
Cortisporin Ophthalmic Suspension Sterile ... 1075
Cortisporin Otic Solution Sterile ... 1076
Cortisporin Otic Suspension Sterile 1077
Maxitrol Ophthalmic Ointment and Suspension ... ◉ 222
Mycitracin ... ▣ 803
Neosporin G.U. Irrigant Sterile ... 1130
Neosporin Ointment ... ▣ 821
Neosporin Plus Maximum Strength Cream ... ▣ 821
Neosporin Plus Maximum Strength Ointment ... ▣ 822
Neosporin Ophthalmic Ointment Sterile ... 1130
Neosporin Ophthalmic Solution Sterile ... 1131
Pediotic Suspension Sterile ... 1140
Poly-Pred Liquifilm ... ◉ 246
Polysporin Ointment ... ▣ 822
Polysporin Ophthalmic Ointment Sterile ... 1140
Polysporin Powder ... ▣ 823
Polytrim Ophthalmic Solution Sterile ... 479
TERAK Ointment ... ◉ 210
Terramycin with Polymyxin B Sulfate Ophthalmic Ointment ... 2035

Polythiazide (Ototoxicity). Products include:
Minizide Capsules ... 2016

Rocuronium Bromide (Potential for increased neuromuscular blockade and respiratory paralysis). Products include:
Zemuron Injection ... 1885

Spironolactone (Ototoxicity). Products include:
Aldactazide Tablets ... 2556
Aldactone Tablets ... 2558

Streptomycin Sulfate (Neurotoxicity and/or nephrotoxicity). Products include:
Streptomycin Sulfate Injection ... 2031

Succinylcholine Chloride (Potential for increased neuromuscular blockade and respiratory paralysis). Products include:
Anectine ... 1062

Ticarcillin Disodium (Mutual inactivation). Products include:
Ticar for Injection ... 2704
Timentin for Injection ... 2706

Tobramycin (Toxicity). Products include:
AKTOB ... ◉ 207
TobraDex Ophthalmic Suspension and Ointment ... 469
Tobrex Ophthalmic Ointment and Solution ... ◉ 226

Tobramycin Sulfate (Toxicity). Products include:
Nebcin Vials, Hyporets & ADD-Vantage ... 1518

Torsemide (Ototoxicity). Products include:
Demadex Tablets and Injection ... 691

Triamterene (Ototoxicity). Products include:
Dyazide Capsules ... 2653
Dyrenium Capsules ... 2655

Vancomycin Hydrochloride (Toxicity). Products include:
Vancocin HCl, Oral Solution & Pulvules ... 1536
Vancocin HCl, Vials & ADD-Vantage ... 1534

Vecuronium Bromide (Potential for increased neuromuscular blockade and respiratory paralysis). Products include:
Norcuron for Injection ... 1875

NEUPOGEN FOR INJECTION
(Filgrastim) ... 495
May interact with drugs which potentiate the release of neutrophils. Compounds in this category include:

Lithium Carbonate (Concurrent use should be undertaken with caution since lithium potentiates the release of neutrophils). Products include:
Eskalith ... 2658
Lithium Carbonate Capsules & Tablets ... 2352
Lithonate/Lithotabs/Lithobid ... 2721

Lithium Citrate (Concurrent use should be undertaken with caution since lithium potentiates the release of neutrophils).
No products indexed under this heading.

NEURONTIN CAPSULES
(Gabapentin) ... 1978
May interact with:

Aluminum Hydroxide (Coadministration reduces bioavailability of gabapentin by 20%; gabapentin should be taken at least 2 hours following antacid containing aluminum hydroxide and magnesium hydroxide). Products include:
ALternaGEL Liquid ... 1358
Maximum Strength Ascriptin ... ▣ 650
Cama Arthritis Pain Reliever ... ▣ 748
Gaviscon Extra Strength Relief Formula Antacid Tablets ... ▣ 778
Gaviscon Extra Strength Relief Formula Liquid Antacid ... ▣ 779
Gaviscon Liquid Antacid ... ▣ 779
Gelusil Antacid-Anti-gas Liquid ... ▣ 819
Gelusil Antacid-Anti-gas Tablets ... ▣ 819
Maalox Antacid/Anti-Gas Tablets 889
Maalox Heartburn Relief Suspension ... ▣ 658
Maalox Antacid Liquid ... 888
Extra Strength Maalox Antacid/Anti-Gas Liquid and Tablets ... 888
Mylanta ... 1359
Tempo Soft Antacid ... ▣ 799

Cimetidine (Alters renal clearance of gabapentin and creatinine; this small decrease in excretion of gabapentin is not expected to be of clinical importance). Products include:
Tagamet HB Tablets ... ▣ 786
Tagamet Tablets ... 2694

Cimetidine Hydrochloride (Alters renal clearance of gabapentin and creatinine; this small decrease in excretion of gabapentin is not expected to be of clinical importance). Products include:
Tagamet ... 2694

Magnesium Hydroxide (Coadministration reduces bioavailability of gabapentin by 20%; gabapentin should be taken at least 2 hours following antacid containing aluminum hydroxide and magnesium hydroxide). Products include:
Aludrox Oral Suspension ... ▣ 850
Ascriptin ... ▣ 650
Di-Gel Antacid/Anti-Gas ... ▣ 762
Gelusil Antacid-Anti-gas Liquid ... ▣ 819
Gelusil Antacid-Anti-gas Tablets ... ▣ 819
Maalox Antacid/Anti-Gas Tablets 889
Maalox Antacid Liquid ... 888
Extra Strength Maalox Antacid/Anti-Gas Liquid and Tablets ... 888
Mylanta Fast-Acting ... 1359
Mylanta Gelcaps Antacid ... ▣ 678
Fast-Acting Mylanta Liquid Antacid 1359
Mylanta Tablets ... ▣ 677
Maximum-Strength Fast-Acting Mylanta Liquid Antacid ... 1359
Mylanta Double Strength Tablets .. ▣ 677
Phillips' Milk of Magnesia Liquid .... ▣ 627
Rolaids Antacid Tablets ... ▣ 807
Tempo Soft Antacid ... ▣ 799

Norethindrone (The Cmax of norethindrone was 13% higher when it was coadministered with gabapentin; this interaction is not expected to be of clinical importance). Products include:
Brevicon ... 2563
Micronor Tablets ... 1903
Modicon ... 1928
Norinyl ... 2563
Nor-Q D Tablets ... 2598
Ortho-Novum ... 1928
Ovcon ... 765
Tri-Norinyl ... 2607

Norethindrone Acetate (The Cmax of norethindrone was 13% higher when it was coadministered with gabapentin; this interaction is not expected to be of clinical importance). Products include:
Aygestin Tablets ... 990

NEUTREXIN FOR INJECTION
(Trimetrexate Glucuronate) ... 2761
May interact with:

Acetaminophen (*In vitro* animal study indicates that acetaminophen alters the relative concentration of trimetrexate metabolites). Products include:
Actifed Cold & Sinus Caplets and Tablets ... ▣ 808
Actifed Sinus Daytime/Nighttime Tablets and Caplets ... ▣ 809
Alka-Seltzer Fast Relief Caplets ... ▣ 610
Alka-Seltzer Plus Liqui-Gels ... ▣ 612
Alka-Seltzer Plus Flu & Body Aches Effervescent Tablets ... ▣ 612
Alka-Seltzer Plus Flu & Body Aches Liqui-Gels Non-Drowsy Formula ... ▣ 613
Alka-Seltzer Plus Night-Time Cold Medicine Liqui-Gels ... ▣ 612
Allerest No Drowsiness ... ▣ 649
Allerest Sinus Pain Formula ... ▣ 649
Axocet Capsules ... 2469
Benadryl Allergy/Cold Tablets ... ▣ 811
Benadryl Allergy Sinus Headache Caplets ... ▣ 813
Children's TYLENOL acetaminophen Chewable Tablets, Elixir, Suspension Liquid, and Suspension Drops ... 1559
Children's TYLENOL Cold Multi-Symptom Chewable Tablets and Liquid ... 1559
Children's TYLENOL Cold Plus Cough Multi Symptom Chewable Tablets and Liquid ... 1560
Children's TYLENOL Flu Suspension Liquid ... 1560
Allergy-Sinus Comtrex Multi-Symptom Allergy-Sinus Formula Tablets and Caplets ... ▣ 639
Comtrex Multi-Symptom ... ▣ 638
Comtrex Non-Drowsy ... ▣ 640
Contac Day Allergy/Sinus Caplets ▣ 771
Contac Day & Night ... ▣ 772

IMPORTANT NOTE: Always consult each drug listing in the patient's regimen for possible interactions.

Neutrexin **Interactions Index** **736**

Contac Night Allergy/Sinus Caplets ■ 771
Contac Severe Cold and Flu Formula Caplets ■ 773
Contac Severe Cold & Flu Non-Drowsy ■ 774
Coricidin Cold + Flu Tablets ■ 760
Coricidin 'D' Decongestant Tablets ■ 760
DHCplus Capsules 2148
Darvon-N/Darvocet-N 1473
Dimetapp Allergy Sinus Caplets ■ 838
Dimetapp Cold & Fever Suspension ■ 839
Drixoral Cold and Flu Extended-Release Tablets ■ 764
Drixoral Cough + Sore Throat Liquid Caps ■ 763
Drixoral Allergy/Sinus Extended Release Tablets ■ 765
Esgic-plus Capsules 1012
Esgic-plus Tablets 1012
Aspirin Free Excedrin Analgesic Caplets and Geltabs 734
Excedrin Extra-Strength Analgesic Tablets, Caplets, and Geltabs 734
Excedrin P.M. Analgesic/Sleeping Aid Tablets, Caplets, Liquigels 735
Fioricet Tablets 2386
Fioricet with Codeine Capsules 2387
Goody's Extra Strength Headache Powders ■ 632
Goody's Extra Strength Pain Relief Tablets ■ 632
Hycomine Compound Tablets 948
Hydrocet Capsules 787
Infants' TYLENOL acetaminophen Suspension Drops 1559
Infants' TYLENOL Cold Decongestant & Fever-Reducer Drops 1561
Junior Strength TYLENOL acetaminophen Coated Caplets and Chewable Tablets 1562
Lorcet 10/650 Tablets 1016
Lortab 2751
Lurline PMS Tablets 1000
Maximum Strength Multi-Symptom Formula Midol ■ 621
PMS Multi-Symptom Formula Midol ■ 622
Maximum Strength Midol Teen Multi-Symptom Formula ■ 621
Midrin Capsules 788
Panodol Tablets and Caplets ■ 783
Children's Panadol Chewable Tablets, Liquid, Infant's Drops ■ 783
Percocet Tablets 955
Percogesic Analgesic Tablets ■ 727
Phrenilin 790
Pyrroxate Caplets ■ 742
Robitussin Cold, Cough & Flu Liqui-Gels ■ 844
Robitussin Night-Time Cold Formula ■ 847
Sedapap Tablets 50 mg/650 mg 1826
Sinarest ■ 663
Sine-Aid Maximum Strength Sinus Headache Gelcaps, Caplets and Tablets 1570
Sine-Off No Drowsiness Formula Caplets ■ 784
Sine-Off Sinus Medicine ■ 784
Singlet Tablets ■ 785
Sinulin Tablets 792
Sinutab Sinus Allergy Medication, Maximum Strength Tablets and Caplets ■ 823
Sinutab Sinus Medication, Maximum Strength Without Drowsiness Formula, Tablets & Caplets ■ 824
Sudafed Cold and Cough Liquid Caps ■ 826
Sudafed Severe Cold Formula Caplets ■ 828
Sudafed Severe Cold Formula Tablets ■ 828
Sudafed Sinus Caplets ■ 829
Sudafed Sinus Tablets ■ 829
Talacen Caplets 2464
TheraFlu Flu and Cold Medicine ■ 750
Theraflu Maximum Strength Flu and Cold Medicine For Sore Throat ■ 751
TheraFlu Flu, Cold and Cough Medicine ■ 750
TheraFlu Maximum Strength Nighttime Flu, Cold & Cough Medicine ■ 751
TheraFlu Maximum Strength Non-Drowsy Formula Flu, Cold & Cough Medicine ■ 751
TheraFlu Maximum Strength, Non-Drowsy Formula Flu, Cold and Cough Caplets ■ 752
Theraflu Maximum Strength Sinus Non-Drowsy Formula Caplets ■ 752
Triaminic Sore Throat Formula ■ 755
Triaminicin Tablets ■ 756
TYLENOL acetaminophen Extended Relief Caplets 1570
TYLENOL acetaminophen, Extra Strength Adult Liquid Pain Reliever 1570
TYLENOL acetaminophen, Extra Strength Gelcaps, Geltabs, Caplets, Tablets 1570
TYLENOL acetaminophen, Regular Strength Caplets and Tablets 1570
TYLENOL Allergy Sinus, Maximum Strength Caplets and Gelcaps 1571
TYLENOL Allergy Sinus NightTime, Maximum Strength Caplets 1571
TYLENOL Cold Medication, Multi-Symptom Formula Tablets and Caplets 1572
TYLENOL Cold Medication, Multi-Symptom Hot Liquid Packets 1572
TYLENOL Cold Medication, No Drowsiness Formula Caplets and Gelcaps 1572
TYLENOL Cold Severe Congestion Caplets 1573
TYLENOL Cough Medication, Multi Symptom 1574
TYLENOL Cough Medication with Decongestant, Multi Symptom 1574
TYLENOL Flu No Drowsiness Formula, Maximum Strength Gelcaps 1575
TYLENOL Flu NightTime, Maximum Strength Gelcaps 1575
TYLENOL Flu NightTime, Maximum Strength Hot Medication Packets 1575
TYLENOL Headache Plus Pain Reliever with Antacid, Extra Strength Caplets ■ 705
TYLENOL PM Pain Reliever/Sleep Aid, Extra Strength Gelcaps, Caplets, Geltabs 1576
TYLENOL Severe Allergy Medication Caplets 1571
TYLENOL Sinus, Maximum Strength Geltabs, Gelcaps, Caplets and Tablets 1576
Tylenol with Codeine 1592
Tylox Capsules 1593
Unisom With Pain Relief-Nighttime Sleep Aid and Pain Reliever 1991
Vanquish Analgesic Caplets ■ 627
Vicks 44 LiquiCaps Cough, Cold & Flu Relief ■ 728
Vicks 44M Cough, Cold & Flu Relief ■ 729
Vicks DayQuil LiquiCaps/Liquid Multi-Symptom Cold/Flu Relief ■ 734
Vicks Nyquil Hot Therapy ■ 735
Vicks NyQuil LiquiCaps/Liquid Multi-Symptom Cold/Flu Relief, Original and Cherry Flavors ■ 736
Vicodin Tablets 1404
Vicodin ES Tablets 1405
Vicodin HP Tablets 1403
Wygesic Tablets 2930
Zydone Capsules 967

Cimetidine (*In vitro* animal study indicates significant reduction in trimetrexate metabolism). Products include:
Tagamet HB Tablets ■ 786
Tagamet Tablets 2694

Cimetidine Hydrochloride (*In vitro* animal study indicates significant reduction in trimetrexate metabolism). Products include:
Tagamet 2694

Clotrimazole (Based on *in vitro* animal model, nitrogen substituted imidazole drugs were potent, non-competitive inhibitors of trimetrexate metabolism). Products include:
Prescription Strength Desenex AF Cream ■ 653
Lotrimin 2514
Lotrimin AF Antifungal Cream, Lotion and Solution ■ 766
Lotrisone Cream 2515
Mycelex OTC Cream Antifungal ■ 622
Mycelex Troches 601
Mycelex-7 Vaginal Cream Antifungal ■ 622
Mycelex-7 Vaginal Antifungal Cream with 7 Disposable Applicators ■ 623
Mycelex-7 Vaginal Inserts Antifungal ■ 623
Mycelex-7 Combination-Pack Vaginal Inserts & External Vulvar Cream ■ 623
Mycelex-G 500 mg Vaginal Tablets 602

Erythromycin (May alter trimetrexate plasma concentrations). Products include:
A/T/S 2% Acne Topical Gel 1244
A/T/S 2% Acne Topical Solution 1244
Benzamycin Topical Gel 919
E-Mycin Tablets 1388
Emgel 2% Topical Gel 1081
ERYC 1972
Erycette (erythromycin 2%) Topical Solution 1943
Ery-Tab Tablets 426
Erythromycin Base Filmtab 430
Erythromycin Delayed-Release Capsules, USP 431
Ilotycin Ophthalmic Ointment 928
PCE Dispertab Tablets 453
T-Stat 2.0% Topical Solution and Pads 2797
THERAMYCIN Z 2% Solution 1629

Erythromycin Estolate (May alter trimetrexate plasma concentrations). Products include:
Ilosone 927

Erythromycin Ethylsuccinate (May alter trimetrexate plasma concentrations). Products include:
E.E.S. 427
EryPed 425
Pediazole Suspension 2340

Erythromycin Gluceptate (May alter trimetrexate plasma concentrations). Products include:
Ilotycin Gluceptate, IV, Vials 929

Erythromycin Stearate (May alter trimetrexate plasma concentrations). Products include:
Erythrocin Stearate Filmtab 429

Fluconazole (May alter trimetrexate plasma concentrations). Products include:
Diflucan Tablets, Injection, and Oral Suspension 2003

Ketoconazole (May alter trimetrexate plasma concentrations; based on *in vitro* animal model, nitrogen substituted imidazole drugs were potent, non-competitive inhibitors of trimetrexate metabolism). Products include:
Nizoral 2% Cream 1344
Nizoral 2% Shampoo 1344
Nizoral Tablets 1345

Miconazole (Based on *in vitro* animal model, nitrogen substituted imidazole drugs were potent, non-competitive inhibitors of trimetrexate metabolism).
No products indexed under this heading.

Rifabutin (May alter trimetrexate plasma concentrations). Products include:
Mycobutin Capsules 2101

Rifampin (May alter trimetrexate plasma concentrations). Products include:
Rifadin 1276
Rifamate Capsules 1278
Rifater 1280
Rimactane Capsules 865

N'ICE MEDICATED SUGARLESS SORE THROAT AND COUGH LOZENGES
(Menthol) ■ 781
None cited in PDR database.

NICOTINEX ELIXIR
(Niacin) ■ 671
None cited in PDR database.

NICOTROL NS NICOTINE NASAL SPRAY
(Nicotine) 1565
May interact with insulin, beta blockers, xanthine bronchodilators, sympathomimetics, and certain other agents. Compounds in these categories include:

Acebutolol Hydrochloride (Deinduction of hepatic enzyme on smoking cessation; may require a decrease in dose at cessation of smoking). Products include:
Sectral Capsules 2914

Acetaminophen (Deinduction of hepatic enzyme on smoking cessation; may require a decrease in dose at cessation of smoking). Products include:
Actifed Cold & Sinus Caplets and Tablets ■ 808
Actifed Sinus Daytime/Nighttime Tablets and Caplets ■ 809
Alka-Seltzer Fast Relief Caplets ■ 610
Alka-Seltzer Plus Liqui-Gels ■ 612
Alka-Seltzer Plus Flu & Body Aches Effervescent Tablets ■ 612
Alka-Seltzer Plus Flu & Body Aches Liqui-Gels Non-Drowsy Formula ■ 613
Alka-Seltzer Plus Night-Time Cold Medicine Liqui-Gels ■ 612
Allerest No Drowsiness ■ 649
Allerest Sinus Pain Formula ■ 649
Axocet Capsules 2469
Benadryl Allergy/Cold Tablets ■ 811
Benadryl Allergy Sinus Headache Caplets ■ 813
Children's TYLENOL acetaminophen Chewable Tablets, Elixir, Suspension Liquid, and Suspension Drops 1559
Children's TYLENOL Cold Multi-Symptom Chewable Tablets and Liquid 1559
Children's TYLENOL Cold Plus Cough Multi Symptom Chewable Tablets and Liquid 1560
Children's TYLENOL Flu Suspension Liquid 1560
Allergy-Sinus Comtrex Multi-Symptom Allergy-Sinus Formula Tablets and Caplets ■ 639
Comtrex Multi-Symptom ■ 638
Comtrex Non-Drowsy ■ 640
Contac Day Allergy/Sinus Caplets ■ 771
Contac Day & Night ■ 772
Contac Night Allergy/Sinus Caplets ■ 771
Contac Severe Cold and Flu Formula Caplets ■ 773
Contac Severe Cold & Flu Non-Drowsy ■ 774
Coricidin Cold + Flu Tablets ■ 760
Coricidin 'D' Decongestant Tablets ■ 760
DHCplus Capsules 2148
Darvon-N/Darvocet-N 1473
Dimetapp Allergy Sinus Caplets ■ 838
Dimetapp Cold & Fever Suspension ■ 839
Drixoral Cold and Flu Extended-Release Tablets ■ 764
Drixoral Cough + Sore Throat Liquid Caps ■ 763
Drixoral Allergy/Sinus Extended Release Tablets ■ 765
Esgic-plus Capsules 1012
Esgic-plus Tablets 1012
Aspirin Free Excedrin Analgesic Caplets and Geltabs 734
Excedrin Extra-Strength Analgesic Tablets, Caplets, and Geltabs 734
Excedrin P.M. Analgesic/Sleeping Aid Tablets, Caplets, Liquigels 735
Fioricet Tablets 2386
Fioricet with Codeine Capsules 2387
Goody's Extra Strength Headache Powders ■ 632
Goody's Extra Strength Pain Relief Tablets ■ 632
Hycomine Compound Tablets 948
Hydrocet Capsules 787

(■ Described in PDR For Nonprescription Drugs) (◉ Described in PDR For Ophthalmology)

737 **Interactions Index** **Nicotrol NS**

Infants' TYLENOL acetaminophen Suspension Drops ... 1559
Infants' TYLENOL Cold Decongestant & Fever-Reducer Drops ... 1561
Junior Strength TYLENOL acetaminophen Coated Caplets and Chewable Tablets ... 1562
Lorcet 10/650 Tablets ... 1016
Lortab ... 2751
Lurline PMS Tablets ... 1000
Maximum Strength Multi-Symptom Formula Midol ... ▣ 621
PMS Multi-Symptom Formula Midol ... ▣ 622
Maximum Strength Midol Teen Multi-Symptom Formula ... ▣ 621
Midrin Capsules ... 788
Panodol Tablets and Caplets ... ▣ 783
Children's Panadol Chewable Tablets, Liquid, Infant's Drops ... ▣ 783
Percocet Tablets ... 955
Percogesic Analgesic Tablets ... ▣ 727
Phrenilin ... 790
Pyrroxate Caplets ... ▣ 742
Robitussin Cold, Cough & Flu Liqui-Gels ... ▣ 844
Robitussin Night-Time Cold Formula ... ▣ 847
Sedapap Tablets 50 mg/650 mg ... 1826
Sinarest ... ▣ 663
Sine-Aid Maximum Strength Sinus Headache Gelcaps, Caplets and Tablets ... 1570
Sine-Off No Drowsiness Formula Caplets ... ▣ 784
Sine-Off Sinus Medicine ... ▣ 784
Singlet Tablets ... ▣ 785
Sinulin Tablets ... 792
Sinutab Sinus Allergy Medication, Maximum Strength Tablets and Caplets ... ▣ 823
Sinutab Sinus Medication, Maximum Strength Without Drowsiness Formula, Tablets & Caplets ... ▣ 824
Sudafed Cold and Cough Liquid Caps ... ▣ 826
Sudafed Severe Cold Formula Caplets ... ▣ 828
Sudafed Severe Cold Formula Tablets ... ▣ 828
Sudafed Sinus Caplets ... ▣ 829
Sudafed Sinus Tablets ... ▣ 829
Talacen Caplets ... 2464
TheraFlu Flu and Cold Medicine ... ▣ 750
Theraflu Maximum Strength Flu and Cold Medicine For Sore Throat ... ▣ 751
TheraFlu Flu, Cold and Cough Medicine ... ▣ 750
TheraFlu Maximum Strength Nighttime Flu, Cold & Cough Medicine ... ▣ 751
TheraFlu Maximum Strength Non-Drowsy Formula Flu, Cold & Cough Medicine ... ▣ 751
TheraFlu Maximum Strength, Non-Drowsy Formula Flu, Cold and Cough Caplets ... ▣ 752
Theraflu Maximum Strength Sinus Non-Drowsy Formula Caplets ... ▣ 752
Triaminic Sore Throat Formula ... ▣ 755
Triaminicin Tablets ... ▣ 756
TYLENOL acetaminophen Extended Relief Caplets ... 1570
TYLENOL acetaminophen, Extra Strength Adult Liquid Pain Reliever ... 1570
TYLENOL acetaminophen, Extra Strength Gelcaps, Geltabs, Caplets, Tablets ... 1570
TYLENOL acetaminophen, Regular Strength Caplets and Tablets ... 1570
TYLENOL Allergy Sinus, Maximum Strength Caplets and Gelcaps ... 1571
TYLENOL Allergy Sinus NightTime, Maximum Strength Caplets ... 1571
TYLENOL Cold Medication, Multi-Symptom Formula Tablets and Caplets ... 1572
TYLENOL Cold Medication, Multi-Symptom Hot Liquid Packets ... 1572
TYLENOL Cold Medication, No Drowsiness Formula Caplets and Gelcaps ... 1572
TYLENOL Cold Severe Congestion Caplets ... 1573
TYLENOL Cough Medication, Multi Symptom ... 1574
TYLENOL Cough Medication with Decongestant, Multi Symptom ... 1574
TYLENOL Flu No Drowsiness Formula, Maximum Strength Gelcaps ... 1575
TYLENOL Flu NightTime, Maximum Strength Gelcaps ... 1575
TYLENOL Flu NightTime, Maximum Strength Hot Medication Packets ... 1575
TYLENOL Headache Plus Pain Reliever with Antacid, Extra Strength Caplets ... ▣ 705
TYLENOL PM Pain Reliever/Sleep Aid, Extra Strength Gelcaps, Caplets, Geltabs ... 1576
TYLENOL Severe Allergy Medication Caplets ... 1571
TYLENOL Sinus, Maximum Strength Geltabs, Gelcaps, Caplets and Tablets ... 1576
Tylenol with Codeine ... 1592
Tylox Capsules ... 1593
Unisom With Pain Relief-Nighttime Sleep Aid and Pain Reliever ... 1991
Vanquish Analgesic Caplets ... ▣ 627
Vicks 44 LiquiCaps Cough, Cold & Flu Relief ... ▣ 728
Vicks 44M Cough, Cold & Flu Relief ... ▣ 729
Vicks DayQuil LiquiCaps/Liquid Multi-Symptom Cold/Flu Relief ... ▣ 734
Vicks Nyquil Hot Therapy ... ▣ 735
Vicks NyQuil LiquiCaps/Liquid Multi-Symptom Cold/Flu Relief, Original and Cherry Flavors ... ▣ 736
Vicodin Tablets ... 1404
Vicodin ES Tablets ... 1405
Vicodin HP Tablets ... 1403
Wygesic Tablets ... 2930
Zydone Capsules ... 967

Albuterol (Decrease in circulating catecholamines with smoking cessation; may require an increase in dose at cessation of smoking). Products include:
Proventil Inhalation Aerosol ... 2524
Ventolin Inhalation Aerosol and Refill ... 1170

Albuterol Sulfate (Decrease in circulating catecholamines with smoking cessation; may require an increase in dose at cessation of smoking). Products include:
Airet Albuterol Sulfate Inhalation Solution ... 1602
Albuterol Sulfate, USP Solution for Inhalation, Arm-a-Med ... 522
Proventil Inhalation Solution 0.083% ... 2527
Proventil Repetabs Tablets ... 2529
Proventil Solution for Inhalation 0.5% ... 2525
Proventil Syrup ... 2528
Proventil Tablets ... 2529
Ventolin Inhalation Solution ... 1171
Ventolin Nebules Inhalation Solution ... 1172
Ventolin Rotacaps for Inhalation ... 1173
Ventolin Syrup ... 1175
Ventolin Tablets ... 1176
Volmax Extended-Release Tablets ... 1835

Aminophylline (Deinduction of hepatic enzyme on smoking cessation; may require a decrease in dose at cessation of smoking).
No products indexed under this heading.

Atenolol (Deinduction of hepatic enzyme on smoking cessation; may require a decrease in dose at cessation of smoking). Products include:
Tenoretic Tablets ... 2963
Tenormin Tablets and I.V. Injection ... 2965

Betaxolol Hydrochloride (Deinduction of hepatic enzyme on smoking cessation; may require a decrease in dose at cessation of smoking). Products include:
Betoptic Ophthalmic Solution ... 465
Betoptic S Ophthalmic Suspension ... 467
Kerlone Tablets ... 2588

Bisoprolol Fumarate (Deinduction of hepatic enzyme on smoking cessation; may require a decrease in dose at cessation of smoking). Products include:
Zebeta Tablets ... 1457
Ziac ... 1459

Caffeine (Deinduction of hepatic enzyme on smoking cessation; may require a decrease in dose at cessation of smoking). Products include:
Arthritis Strength BC Powder ... ▣ 631
BC Powder ... ▣ 631
Cafergot ... 2376
DHCplus Capsules ... 2148
Darvon Compound-65 Pulvules ... 1475
Esgic-plus Capsules ... 1012
Esgic-plus Tablets ... 1012
Aspirin Free Excedrin Analgesic Caplets and Geltabs ... 734
Excedrin Extra-Strength Analgesic Tablets, Caplets, and Geltabs ... 734
Fioricet Tablets ... 2386
Fioricet with Codeine Capsules ... 2387
Fiorinal Capsules ... 2388
Fiorinal with Codeine Capsules ... 2390
Fiorinal Tablets ... 2388
Goody's Extra Strength Headache Powders ... ▣ 632
Goody's Extra Strength Pain Relief Tablets ... ▣ 632
Maximum Strength Multi-Symptom Formula Midol ... ▣ 621
No Doz Maximum Strength Caplets ... ▣ 644
Norgesic ... 1554
Vanquish Analgesic Caplets ... ▣ 627
Wigraine Tablets ... 1884

Carteolol Hydrochloride (Deinduction of hepatic enzyme on smoking cessation; may require a decrease in dose at cessation of smoking). Products include:
Cartrol Tablets ... 413
Ocupress Ophthalmic Solution, 1% Sterile ... ◉ 297

Dobutamine Hydrochloride (Decrease in circulating catecholamines with smoking cessation; may require an increase in dose at cessation of smoking). Products include:
Dobutrex Solution Vials ... 1480

Dopamine Hydrochloride (Decrease in circulating catecholamines with smoking cessation; may require an increase in dose at cessation of smoking).
No products indexed under this heading.

Dyphylline (Deinduction of hepatic enzyme on smoking cessation; may require a decrease in dose at cessation of smoking). Products include:
Lufyllin & Lufyllin-400 Tablets ... 2778
Lufyllin-GG Elixir & Tablets ... 2779

Ephedrine Hydrochloride (Decrease in circulating catecholamines with smoking cessation; may require an increase in dose at cessation of smoking). Products include:
Primatene Tablets ... ▣ 844
Quadrinal Tablets ... 1398

Ephedrine Sulfate (Decrease in circulating catecholamines with smoking cessation; may require an increase in dose at cessation of smoking). Products include:
Marax Tablets & DF Syrup ... 2015

Ephedrine Tannate (Decrease in circulating catecholamines with smoking cessation; may require an increase in dose at cessation of smoking). Products include:
Rynatuss ... 2782

Epinephrine (Decrease in circulating catecholamines with smoking cessation; may require an increase in dose at cessation of smoking). Products include:
EPIFRIN ... ◉ 237
EpiPen ... 808
Marcaine with Epinephrine ... 2446
Primatene Mist ... ▣ 843
Sensorcaine with Epinephrine Injection ... 554
Sus-Phrine Injection ... 1017
Xylocaine with Epinephrine Injections ... 562

Epinephrine Bitartrate (Decrease in circulating catecholamines with smoking cessation; may require an increase in dose at cessation of smoking). Products include:
Sensorcaine-MPF with Epinephrine Injection ... 554

Epinephrine Hydrochloride (Decrease in circulating catecholamines with smoking cessation; may require an increase in dose at cessation of smoking). Products include:
Ana-Kit Anaphylaxis Emergency Treatment Kit ... 611

Esmolol Hydrochloride (Deinduction of hepatic enzyme on smoking cessation; may require a decrease in dose at cessation of smoking). Products include:
Brevibloc (esmolol HCl) Injection ... 1860

Imipramine Hydrochloride (Deinduction of hepatic enzyme on smoking cessation; may require a decrease in dose at cessation of smoking). Products include:
Tofranil Ampuls ... 873
Tofranil Tablets ... 875

Imipramine Pamoate (Deinduction of hepatic enzyme on smoking cessation; may require a decrease in dose at cessation of smoking). Products include:
Tofranil-PM Capsules ... 876

Insulin, Human (Increase of subcutaneous insulin absorption with smoking cessation; may require a decrease in dose at cessation of smoking).
No products indexed under this heading.

Insulin, Human Isophane Suspension (Increase of subcutaneous insulin absorption with smoking cessation; may require a decrease in dose at cessation of smoking). Products include:
Novolin N Human Insulin 10 ml Vials ... 1846

Insulin, Human NPH (Increase of subcutaneous insulin absorption with smoking cessation; may require a decrease in dose at cessation of smoking). Products include:
Humulin N, 100 Units ... 1495
Novolin N PenFill 1.5 ml Cartridges Durable Insulin Delivery System ... 1849
Novolin N Prefilled Syringe Disposable Insulin Delivery System ... 1850

Insulin, Human Regular (Increase of subcutaneous insulin absorption with smoking cessation; may require a decrease in dose at cessation of smoking). Products include:
Humulin R, 100 Units ... 1497
Novolin R Human Insulin 10 ml Vials ... 1846
Novolin R PenFill 1.5 ml Cartridges Durable Insulin Delivery System ... 1849
Novolin R Prefilled Syringe Disposable Insulin Delivery System ... 1850
Velosulin BR Human Insulin 10 ml Vials ... 1847

Insulin, Human, Zinc Suspension (Increase of subcutaneous insulin absorption with smoking cessation; may require a decrease in dose at cessation of smoking). Products include:
Humulin L, 100 Units ... 1494
Humulin U, 100 Units ... 1498
Novolin L Human Insulin 10 ml Vials ... 1846

IMPORTANT NOTE: Always consult each drug listing in the patient's regimen for possible interactions.

Nicotrol NS | Interactions Index | 738

Insulin Lispro, Human (Increase of subcutaneous insulin absorption with smoking cessation; may require a decrease in dose at cessation of smoking). Products include:
- Humalog Injection 1488

Insulin, NPH (Increase of subcutaneous insulin absorption with smoking cessation; may require a decrease in dose at cessation of smoking). Products include:
- NPH, 100 Units 1502
- Pork NPH, 100 Units 1506
- Purified Pork NPH Isophane Insulin 1852

Insulin, Regular (Increase of subcutaneous insulin absorption with smoking cessation; may require a decrease in dose at cessation of smoking). Products include:
- Regular, 100 Units 1503
- Pork Regular, 100 Units 1507
- Pork Regular (Concentrated), 500 Units 1508
- Purified Pork Regular Insulin 1852

Insulin, Zinc Crystals (Increase of subcutaneous insulin absorption with smoking cessation; may require a decrease in dose at cessation of smoking). Products include:
- NPH, 100 Units 1502

Insulin, Zinc Suspension (Increase of subcutaneous insulin absorption with smoking cessation; may require a decrease in dose at cessation of smoking). Products include:
- Iletin I 1501
- Lente, 100 Units 1501
- Iletin II 1504
- Pork Lente, 100 Units 1504
- Purified Pork Lente Insulin 1852

Isoproterenol Hydrochloride (Decrease in circulating catecholamines with smoking cessation; may require an increase in dose at cessation of smoking). Products include:
- Isuprel Hydrochloride Solution 2443
- Isuprel Injection 2441
- Isuprel Mistometer 2442

Isoproterenol Sulfate (Decrease in circulating catecholamines with smoking cessation; may require an increase in dose at cessation of smoking). Products include:
- Norisodrine with Calcium Iodide Syrup 446

Labetalol Hydrochloride (Decrease in circulating catecholamines with smoking cessation; may require a decrease in dose at cessation of smoking). Products include:
- Normodyne Injection 2519
- Normodyne Tablets 2522
- Trandate 1158

Levobunolol Hydrochloride (Deinduction of hepatic enzyme on smoking cessation; may require a decrease in dose at cessation of smoking). Products include:
- Betagan .... ⊙ 230

Metaproterenol Sulfate (Decrease in circulating catecholamines with smoking cessation; may require an increase in dose at cessation of smoking). Products include:
- Alupent 672
- Metaproterenol Sulfate Inhalation Solution, USP, Arm-a-Med 547

Metaraminol Bitartrate (Decrease in circulating catecholamines with smoking cessation; may require an increase in dose at cessation of smoking). Products include:
- Aramine Injection 1649

Methoxamine Hydrochloride (Decrease in circulating catecholamines with smoking cessation; may require an increase in dose at cessation of smoking). Products include:
- Vasoxyl Injection 1169

Metipranolol Hydrochloride (Deinduction of hepatic enzyme on smoking cessation; may require a decrease in dose at cessation of smoking). Products include:
- OptiPranolol (Metipranolol 0.3%) Sterile Ophthalmic Solution .... ⊙ 256

Metoprolol Succinate (Deinduction of hepatic enzyme on smoking cessation; may require a decrease in dose at cessation of smoking). Products include:
- Toprol-XL Tablets 560

Metoprolol Tartrate (Deinduction of hepatic enzyme on smoking cessation; may require a decrease in dose at cessation of smoking). Products include:
- Lopressor 848
- Lopressor HCT Tablets 850

Nadolol (Deinduction of hepatic enzyme on smoking cessation; may require a decrease in dose at cessation of smoking).
- No products indexed under this heading.

Norepinephrine Bitartrate (Decrease in circulating catecholamines with smoking cessation; may require an increase in dose at cessation of smoking). Products include:
- Levophed Bitartrate Injection 2445

Oxazepam (Deinduction of hepatic enzyme on smoking cessation; may require a decrease in dose at cessation of smoking). Products include:
- Serax Capsules 2916
- Serax Tablets 2916

Penbutolol Sulfate (Deinduction of hepatic enzyme on smoking cessation; may require a decrease in dose at cessation of smoking). Products include:
- Levatol Tablets 2547

Pentazocine Hydrochloride (Deinduction of hepatic enzyme on smoking cessation; may require a decrease in dose at cessation of smoking). Products include:
- Talacen Caplets 2464
- Talwin Compound 2466
- Talwin Nx Tablets 2467

Pentazocine Lactate (Deinduction of hepatic enzyme on smoking cessation; may require a decrease in dose at cessation of smoking). Products include:
- Talwin Injection 2465

Phenylephrine Bitartrate (Decrease in circulating catecholamines with smoking cessation; may require an increase in dose at cessation of smoking).
- No products indexed under this heading.

Phenylephrine Hydrochloride (Decrease in circulating catecholamines with smoking cessation; may require an increase in dose at cessation of smoking). Products include:
- Atrohist Plus Tablets 1605
- Cerose DM .... ▣ 853
- D.A. II Tablets 972
- D.A. Chewable Tablets 970
- Dura-Vent/DA Tablets 972
- Extendryl 1003
- 4-Way Fast Acting Nasal Spray (regular & mentholated) .... ▣ 644
- Hemorid .... ▣ 797
- Hycomine Compound Tablets 948
- Neo-Synephrine Hydrochloride 1% Carpuject 2455
- Neo-Synephrine Hydrochloride 1% Injection 2455
- Neo-Synephrine Hydrochloride (Ophthalmic) 2456
- Neo-Synephrine .... ▣ 624
- Novahistine Elixir .... ▣ 782
- Phenergan VC 2886
- Phenergan VC with Codeine 2888
- Preparation H .... ▣ 842
- Tympagesic Ear Drops 2476
- Vicks Sinex Nasal Spray and Ultra Fine Mist .... ▣ 738

Phenylephrine Tannate (Decrease in circulating catecholamines with smoking cessation; may require an increase in dose at cessation of smoking). Products include:
- Atrohist Pediatric Suspension 1604
- Atrohist Pediatric Suspension Dye-Free 1604
- Rynatan 2781
- Rynatuss 2782

Phenylpropanolamine Hydrochloride (Decrease in circulating catecholamines with smoking cessation; may require an increase in dose at cessation of smoking). Products include:
- Acutrim .... ▣ 648
- Atrohist Plus Tablets 1605
- BC Cold Powder Multi-Symptom Formula (Cold-Sinus-Allergy) .... ▣ 631
- BC Cold Powder Non-Drowsy Formula (Cold-Sinus) .... ▣ 631
- Cheracol Plus Head Cold/Cough Formula .... ▣ 741
- Comtrex Multi-Symptom Cold Reliever Liqui-Gels .... ▣ 638
- Comtrex Multi-Symptom Non-Drowsy Liqui-gels .... ▣ 640
- Contac Continuous Action Nasal Decongestant/Antihistamine 12 Hour Capsules .... ▣ 773
- Contac Maximum Strength Continuous Action Decongestant/Antihistamine 12 Hour Caplets .... ▣ 772
- Contac Severe Cold and Flu Formula Caplets .... ▣ 773
- Coricidin 'D' Decongestant Tablets .... ▣ 760
- Dexatrim .... ▣ 795
- Dexatrim Plus Vitamins Caplets .... ▣ 796
- Dimetane-DC Cough Syrup 2232
- Dimetapp Allergy Sinus Caplets .... ▣ 838
- Dimetapp Cold & Allergy Chewable Tablets .... ▣ 838
- Dimetapp Cold & Cough Liqui-Gels .... ▣ 839
- Dimetapp DM Elixir .... ▣ 840
- Dimetapp Elixir .... ▣ 840
- Dimetapp Extentabs .... ▣ 841
- Dimetapp Tablets/Liqui-Gels .... ▣ 841
- Dura-Vent Tablets 971
- Entex LA Tablets 972
- Exgest LA Tablets 787
- Hycomine 947
- Nolamine Timed-Release Tablets 790
- Ornade Spansule Capsules 2678
- Propagest Tablets 791
- Pyrroxate Caplets .... ▣ 742
- Robitussin-CF .... ▣ 846
- Sinulin Tablets 792
- Tavist-D 12 Hour Relief Tablets .... ▣ 750
- Teldrin 12 Hour Antihistamine/Nasal Decongestant Allergy Relief Capsules .... ▣ 786
- Triaminic Expectorant .... ▣ 753
- Triaminic Syrup .... ▣ 755
- Triaminic Triaminicol Cold & Cough .... ▣ 756
- Triaminic DM Syrup .... ▣ 756
- Triaminicin Tablets .... ▣ 756
- Vicks DayQuil Allergy Relief 12-Hour Extended Release Tablets .... ▣ 733
- Vicks DayQuil Allergy Relief 4-Hour Tablets .... ▣ 733
- Vicks DayQuil SINUS Pressure & CONGESTION Relief .... ▣ 734

Pindolol (Deinduction of hepatic enzyme on smoking cessation; may require a decrease in dose at cessation of smoking). Products include:
- Visken Tablets 2428

Pirbuterol Acetate (Decrease in circulating catecholamines with smoking cessation; may require an increase in dose at cessation of smoking). Products include:
- Maxair Autohaler 1550
- Maxair Inhaler 1552

Prazosin Hydrochloride (Decrease in circulating catecholamines with smoking cessation; may require a decrease in dose at cessation of smoking). Products include:
- Minipress Capsules 2015
- Minizide Capsules 2016

Propranolol Hydrochloride (Deinduction of hepatic enzyme on smoking cessation; may require a decrease in dose at cessation of smoking). Products include:
- Inderal 2834
- Inderal LA Long Acting Capsules 2836
- Inderide Tablets 2838
- Inderide LA Long Acting Capsules 2840

Pseudoephedrine Hydrochloride (Decrease in circulating catecholamines with smoking cessation; may require an increase in dose at cessation of smoking). Products include:
- Actifed Allergy Daytime/Nighttime Caplets .... ▣ 808
- Actifed Cold & Allergy Tablets .... ▣ 807
- Actifed Cold & Sinus Caplets and Tablets .... ▣ 808
- Actifed Sinus Daytime/Nighttime Tablets and Caplets .... ▣ 809
- Advil Cold and Sinus Caplets and Tablets .... ▣ 837
- Alka-Seltzer Plus Liqui-Gels .... ▣ 612
- Alka-Seltzer Plus Flu & Body Aches Liqui-Gels Non-Drowsy Formula .... ▣ 613
- Alka-Seltzer Plus Night-Time Cold Medicine Liqui-Gels .... ▣ 612
- Allerest Maximum Strength .... ▣ 649
- Allerest No Drowsiness .... ▣ 649
- Allerest Sinus Pain Formula .... ▣ 649
- Atrohist Pediatric Capsules 1603
- Benadryl Allergy/Cold Tablets .... ▣ 811
- Benadryl Allergy Decongestant Liquid Medication .... ▣ 812
- Benadryl Allergy Decongestant Tablets .... ▣ 812
- Benadryl Allergy Sinus Headache Caplets .... ▣ 813
- Benylin Multisymptom .... ▣ 816
- Bromfed Capsules (Extended-Release) 1832
- Bromfed Syrup .... ▣ 712
- Bromfed Tablets 1832
- Bromfed-DM Cough Syrup 1832
- Bromfed-PD Capsules (Extended-Release) 1832
- Children's TYLENOL Cold Multi-Symptom Chewable Tablets and Liquid 1559
- Children's TYLENOL Cold Plus Cough Multi Symptom Chewable Tablets and Liquid 1560
- Children's TYLENOL Flu Suspension Liquid 1560
- Children's Vicks DayQuil Allergy Relief .... ▣ 730
- Children's Vicks NyQuil Cold/Cough Relief .... ▣ 731
- Allergy-Sinus Comtrex Multi-Symptom Allergy-Sinus Formula Tablets and Caplets .... ▣ 639
- Comtrex Multi-Symptom .... ▣ 638
- Comtrex Multi-Symptom Non-Drowsy Caplets .... ▣ 640
- Congess 1003
- Contac Day Allergy/Sinus Caplets ▣ 771
- Contac Day & Night .... ▣ 772
- Contac Night Allergy/Sinus Caplets .... ▣ 771
- Contac Severe Cold & Flu Non-Drowsy .... ▣ 774
- Deconsal II Tablets 1605
- Dimetane-DX Cough Syrup 2233
- Dimetapp Cold & Fever Suspension .... ▣ 839
- Dimetapp Decongestant Pediatric Drops .... ▣ 840
- Dorcol Children's Cough Syrup .... ▣ 748
- Drixoral Cough + Congestion Liquid Caps .... ▣ 763
- Dura-Tap/PD Capsules 970
- Duratuss Tablets 2750
- Duratuss HD Elixir 2750
- Efidac/24 .... ▣ 655
- Entex PSE Tablets 973
- Fedahist Gyrocaps 2545
- Guaifed 1833

(▣ Described in PDR For Nonprescription Drugs) (⊙ Described in PDR For Ophthalmology)

739 **Interactions Index** **Nimbex**

Guaifed Syrup ... 712
Guaimax-D Tablets ... 809
Histussin D Liquid ... 670
Infants' TYLENOL Cold Decongestant & Fever-Reducer Drops ... 1561
Kronofed-A ... 994
Novahistine DMX ... 782
Nucofed ... 2225
PediaCare Cough-Cold Chewable Tablets and Liquid ... 1569
PediaCare Infants' Decongestant Drops ... 1569
PediaCare Infants' Drops Decongestant Plus Cough ... 1569
PediaCare NightRest Cough-Cold Liquid ... 1569
Pediatric Vicks 44d Cough & Head Congestion Relief ... 736
Pediatric Vicks 44m Cough & Cold Relief ... 737
Robitussin Cold & Cough Liqui-Gels ... 844
Robitussin Cold, Cough & Flu Liqui-Gels ... 844
Robitussin Maximum Strength Cough & Cold ... 847
Robitussin Night-Time Cold Formula ... 847
Robitussin Pediatric Cough & Cold Formula ... 848
Robitussin Pediatric Drops ... 849
Robitussin Severe Congestion Liqui-Gels ... 845
Robitussin-DAC Syrup ... 2249
Robitussin-PE ... 846
Rondec Oral Drops ... 974
Rondec Syrup ... 974
Rondec Tablet ... 974
Rondec Chewable Tablets ... 974
Rondec-TR Tablet ... 974
Ryna ... 804
Seldane-D Extended-Release Tablets ... 1286
Semprex-D Capsules ... 1620
Sinarest ... 663
Sine-Aid Maximum Strength Sinus Headache Gelcaps, Caplets and Tablets ... 1570
Sine-Off No Drowsiness Formula Caplets ... 784
Sine-Off Sinus Medicine ... 784
Singlet Tablets ... 785
Sinutab Non-Drying Liquid Caps ... 823
Sinutab Sinus Allergy Medication, Maximum Strength Tablets and Caplets ... 823
Sinutab Sinus Medication, Maximum Strength Without Drowsiness Formula, Tablets & Caplets ... 824
Sudafed Children's Cold & Cough Liquid Medication ... 825
Sudafed Children's Nasal Decongestant Liquid Medication ... 826
Sudafed Cold & Allergy Tablets ... 826
Sudafed Cold and Cough Liquid Caps ... 826
Sudafed Nasal Decongestant Tablets, 30 mg ... 825
Sudafed Nasal Decongestant Tablets, 60 mg ... 825
Sudafed Non-Drying Sinus Liquid Caps ... 827
Sudafed Pediatric Nasal Decongestant Liquid Oral Drops ... 827
Sudafed Severe Cold Formula Caplets ... 828
Sudafed Severe Cold Formula Tablets ... 828
Sudafed Sinus Caplets ... 829
Sudafed Sinus Tablets ... 829
Sudafed 12 Hour Caplets ... 824
Syn-Rx Tablets ... 1622
Syn-Rx DM Tablets ... 1623
TheraFlu Flu and Cold Medicine ... 750
Theraflu Maximum Strength Flu and Cold Medicine For Sore Throat ... 751
TheraFlu Flu, Cold and Cough Medicine ... 750
TheraFlu Maximum Strength Nighttime Flu, Cold & Cough Medicine ... 751
TheraFlu Maximum Strength Non-Drowsy Formula Flu, Cold & Cough Medicine ... 751
TheraFlu Maximum Strength, Non-Drowsy Formula Flu, Cold and Cough Caplets ... 752
Theraflu Maximum Strength Sinus Non-Drowsy Formula Caplets ... 752
Triaminic AM Cough and Decongestant Formula ... 753
Triaminic AM Decongestant Formula ... 753
Triaminic Infant Oral Decongestant Drops ... 754
Triaminic Night Time ... 754
Triaminic Sore Throat Formula ... 755
Tussend ... 1830
Tussend Expectorant ... 1831
TYLENOL Allergy Sinus, Maximum Strength Caplets and Gelcaps ... 1571
TYLENOL Allergy Sinus NightTime, Maximum Strength Caplets ... 1571
TYLENOL Cold Medication, Multi-Symptom Formula Tablets and Caplets ... 1572
TYLENOL Cold Medication, Multi-Symptom Hot Liquid Packets ... 1572
TYLENOL Cold Medication, No Drowsiness Formula Caplets and Gelcaps ... 1572
TYLENOL Cold Severe Congestion Caplets ... 1573
TYLENOL Cough Medication with Decongestant, Multi Symptom ... 1574
TYLENOL Flu No Drowsiness Formula, Maximum Strength Gelcaps ... 1575
TYLENOL Flu NightTime, Maximum Strength Gelcaps ... 1575
TYLENOL Flu NightTime, Maximum Strength Hot Medication Packets ... 1575
TYLENOL Sinus, Maximum Strength Geltabs, Gelcaps, Caplets and Tablets ... 1576
Vicks 44 LiquiCaps Cough, Cold & Flu Relief ... 728
Vicks 44 LiquiCaps Non-Drowsy Cough & Cold Relief ... 729
Vicks 44D Cough & Head Congestion Relief ... 728
Vicks 44M Cough, Cold & Flu Relief ... 729
Vicks DayQuil LiquiCaps/Liquid Multi-Symptom Cold/Flu Relief ... 734
Vicks DayQuil SINUS Pressure & PAIN Relief with IBUPROFEN ... 735
Vicks Nyquil Hot Therapy ... 735
Vicks NyQuil LiquiCaps/Liquid Multi-Symptom Cold/Flu Relief, Original and Cherry Flavors ... 736

Pseudoephedrine Sulfate (Decrease in circulating catecholamines with smoking cessation; may require an increase in dose at cessation of smoking). Products include:
Chlor-Trimeton Allergy Decongestant Tablets ... 759
Claritin-D Tablets ... 2487
Drixoral Cold and Allergy Sustained-Action Tablets ... 763
Drixoral Cold and Flu Extended-Release Tablets ... 764
Drixoral Non-Drowsy Formula Extended-Release Tablets ... 764
Drixoral Allergy/Sinus Extended Release Tablets ... 765
Trinalin Repetabs Tablets ... 1373

Salmeterol Xinafoate (Decrease in circulating catecholamines with smoking cessation; may require an increase in dose at cessation of smoking). Products include:
Serevent Inhalation Aerosol ... 1149

Sotalol Hydrochloride (Deinduction of hepatic enzyme on smoking cessation; may require a decrease in dose at cessation of smoking). Products include:
Betapace Tablets ... 637

Terbutaline Sulfate (Decrease in circulating catecholamines with smoking cessation; may require an increase in dose at cessation of smoking). Products include:
Brethaire Inhaler ... 830
Brethine Ampuls ... 832
Brethine Tablets ... 831
Bricanyl Subcutaneous Injection ... 1247
Bricanyl Tablets ... 1248

Theophylline (Deinduction of hepatic enzyme on smoking cessation; may require a decrease in dose at cessation of smoking). Products include:
Marax Tablets & DF Syrup ... 2015
Quibron ... 2227

Theophylline Anhydrous (Deinduction of hepatic enzyme on smoking cessation; may require a decrease in dose at cessation of smoking). Products include:
Aerolate ... 1003
Primatene Tablets ... 844
Respbid Tablets ... 687
Slo-bid Gyrocaps ... 2201
Theo-24 Extended Release Capsules ... 2753
Theo-Dur Extended-Release Tablets ... 1367
Theo-X Extended-Release Tablets ... 793
Uni-Dur Extended-Release Tablets ... 1374
Uniphyl 400 mg and 600 mg Tablets ... 2157

Theophylline Calcium Salicylate (Deinduction of hepatic enzyme on smoking cessation; may require a decrease in dose at cessation of smoking). Products include:
Quadrinal Tablets ... 1398

Theophylline Sodium Glycinate (Deinduction of hepatic enzyme on smoking cessation; may require a decrease in dose at cessation of smoking).
No products indexed under this heading.

Timolol Hemihydrate (Deinduction of hepatic enzyme on smoking cessation; may require a decrease in dose at cessation of smoking). Products include:
Betimol 0.25%, 0.5% ... ⊙ 259

Timolol Maleate (Deinduction of hepatic enzyme on smoking cessation; may require a decrease in dose at cessation of smoking). Products include:
Blocadren Tablets ... 1654
Timolide Tablets ... 1791
Timoptic in Ocudose ... 1796
Timoptic Sterile Ophthalmic Solution ... 1794
Timoptic-XE ... 1798

Xylometazoline Hydrochloride (The extent of absorption and peak plasma concentration is slightly reduced in patients with common cold/rhinitis; time to peak concentration is prolonged with the use of xylometazoline). Products include:
Otrivin ... 662

NICOTROL NICOTINE TRANSDERMAL SYSTEM
(Nicotine) ... 1568
None cited in PDR database.

NIFEREX-150 CAPSULES
(Polysaccharide-Iron Complex) ... 811
None cited in PDR database.

NIFEREX ELIXIR
(Polysaccharide-Iron Complex) ... 811
None cited in PDR database.

NIFEREX-150 FORTE CAPSULES
(Polysaccharide-Iron Complex, Folic Acid, Cyanocobalamin) ... 811
None cited in PDR database.

NIFEREX TABLETS
(Polysaccharide-Iron Complex) ... 811
None cited in PDR database.

NIFEREX W/VITAMIN C TABLETS
(Polysaccharide-Iron Complex, Vitamin C) ... 811
None cited in PDR database.

NIFEREX-PN TABLETS
(Vitamins with Iron) ... 811
None cited in PDR database.

NIMBEX INJECTION
(Cisatracurium Besylate) ... 1131
May interact with aminoglycosides, tetracyclines, lithium preparations, local anesthetics, and certain other agents. Compounds in these categories include:

Amikacin Sulfate (Enhances neuromuscular blocking action). Products include:
Amikacin Sulfate Injection, USP ... 523
Amikacin Sulfate Injection, USP ... 981
Amikin Injectable ... 502

Bacitracin (Enhances neuromuscular blocking action).
No products indexed under this heading.

Bupivacaine Hydrochloride (Enhances neuromuscular blocking action). Products include:
Marcaine ... 2446
Marcaine Spinal ... 2449
Sensorcaine ... 554

Carbamazepine (Chronic administration of carbamazepine may produce resistance to the neuromuscular blocking action; slightly shorter durations of neuromuscular block may be anticipated). Products include:
Atretol Tablets ... 569
Tegretol/Tegretol-XR ... 870

Chloroprocaine Hydrochloride (Enhances neuromuscular blocking action). Products include:
Nescaine/Nescaine MPF ... 549

Clindamycin Hydrochloride (Enhances neuromuscular blocking action).
No products indexed under this heading.

Clindamycin Palmitate Hydrochloride (Enhances neuromuscular blocking action).
No products indexed under this heading.

Clindamycin Phosphate (Enhances neuromuscular blocking action). Products include:
Cleocin Phosphate Injection ... 2068
Cleocin T Topical ... 2072
Cleocin Vaginal Cream ... 2070

Colistimethate Sodium (Enhances neuromuscular blocking action).
No products indexed under this heading.

Colistin Sulfate (Enhances neuromuscular blocking action). Products include:
Coly-Mycin S Otic w/Neomycin & Hydrocortisone ... 1965

Demeclocycline Hydrochloride (Enhances neuromuscular blocking action). Products include:
Declomycin Tablets ... 1421

Doxycycline Calcium (Enhances neuromuscular blocking action). Products include:
Vibramycin Calcium Oral Suspension Syrup ... 2038

Doxycycline Hyclate (Enhances neuromuscular blocking action). Products include:
Doryx Capsules ... 1970
Vibramycin Hyclate Capsules ... 2038
Vibramycin Hyclate Intravenous ... 2040
Vibra-Tabs Film Coated Tablets ... 2038

Doxycycline Monohydrate (Enhances neuromuscular blocking action). Products include:
Monodox Capsules ... 1858
Vibramycin Monohydrate for Oral Suspension ... 2038

IMPORTANT NOTE: Always consult each drug listing in the patient's regimen for possible interactions.

Nimbex | Interactions Index | 740

Enflurane (Enflurane administered with nitrous oxide/oxygen may prolong the clinically effective duration of action of initial and maintenance doses of cisatracurium and decrease the required infusion rate of cisatracurium).
- No products indexed under this heading.

Etidocaine Hydrochloride (Enhances neuromuscular blocking action). Products include:
- Duranest Injections 533

Gentamicin Sulfate (Enhances neuromuscular blocking action). Products include:
- Garamycin Cream 0.1% 2501
- Garamycin Injectable 2502
- Garamycin Ointment 0.1% 2501
- Garamycin Ophthalmic 2501
- Genoptic Sterile Ophthalmic Solution .... ⊙ 241
- Genoptic Sterile Ophthalmic Ointment .... ⊙ 241
- Gentak .... ⊙ 209
- Pred-G Liquifilm Sterile Ophthalmic Suspension .... ⊙ 248
- Pred-G S.O.P. Sterile Ophthalmic Ointment .... ⊙ 249

Isoflurane (Isoflurane administered with nitrous oxide/oxygen may prolong the clinically effective duration of action of initial and maintenance doses of cisatracurium and decrease the required infusion rate of cisatracurium).
- No products indexed under this heading.

Kanamycin Sulfate (Enhances neuromuscular blocking action).
- No products indexed under this heading.

Lidocaine Hydrochloride (Enhances neuromuscular blocking action). Products include:
- Decadron Phosphate with Xylocaine Injection, Sterile 1683
- Unguentine Plus .... ▣ 712
- Xylocaine Injections 562

Lincomycin Hydrochloride (Enhances neuromuscular blocking action).
- No products indexed under this heading.

Lithium Carbonate (Enhances neuromuscular blocking action). Products include:
- Eskalith 2658
- Lithium Carbonate Capsules & Tablets 2352
- Lithonate/Lithotabs/Lithobid 2721

Lithium Citrate (Enhances neuromuscular blocking action).
- No products indexed under this heading.

Magnesium Salts (Enhances neuromuscular blocking action).

Mepivacaine Hydrochloride Injection (Enhances neuromuscular blocking action). Products include:
- Carbocaine Injection 2432

Methacycline Hydrochloride (Enhances neuromuscular blocking action).
- No products indexed under this heading.

Minocycline Hydrochloride (Enhances neuromuscular blocking action). Products include:
- DYNACIN Capsules 1627
- Minocin Intravenous 1428
- Minocin Oral Suspension 1431
- Minocin Pellet-Filled Capsules 1429

Oxytetracycline Hydrochloride (Enhances neuromuscular blocking action). Products include:
- TERAK Ointment .... ⊙ 210
- Terra-Cortril Ophthalmic Suspension 2033
- Terramycin with Polymyxin B Sulfate Ophthalmic Ointment 2035
- Urobiotic-250 Capsules 2038

Phenytoin (Chronic administration of phenytoin may produce resistance to the neuromuscular blocking action; slightly shorter durations of neuromuscular block may be anticipated). Products include:
- Dilantin Infatabs 1967
- Dilantin-125 Suspension 1969

Phenytoin Sodium (Chronic administration of phenytoin may produce resistance to the neuromuscular blocking action; slightly shorter durations of neuromuscular block may be anticipated). Products include:
- Dilantin Kapseals 1965

Polymyxin Preparations (Enhances neuromuscular blocking action).

Procainamide Hydrochloride (Enhances neuromuscular blocking action). Products include:
- Procanbid Extended-Release Tablets 1983

Procaine Hydrochloride (Enhances neuromuscular blocking action). Products include:
- Novocain Hydrochloride for Spinal Anesthesia 2457

Quinidine Gluconate (Enhances neuromuscular blocking action). Products include:
- Quinaglute Dura-Tabs Tablets 644

Quinidine Polygalacturonate (Enhances neuromuscular blocking action). Products include:
- Cardioquin Tablets 2146

Quinidine Sulfate (Enhances neuromuscular blocking action). Products include:
- Quinidex Extentabs 2240

Streptomycin Sulfate (Enhances neuromuscular blocking action). Products include:
- Streptomycin Sulfate Injection 2031

Tetracaine Hydrochloride (Enhances neuromuscular blocking action). Products include:
- Cetacaine Topical Anesthetic 812
- Pontocaine Hydrochloride for Spinal Anesthesia 2460

Tetracycline Hydrochloride (Enhances neuromuscular blocking action). Products include:
- Achromycin V Capsules 1417
- Helidac Therapy 2135

Tobramycin (Enhances neuromuscular blocking action). Products include:
- AKTOB .... ⊙ 207
- TobraDex Ophthalmic Suspension and Ointment 469
- Tobrex Ophthalmic Ointment and Solution .... ⊙ 226

Tobramycin Sulfate (Enhances neuromuscular blocking action). Products include:
- Nebcin Vials, Hyporets & ADD-Vantage 1518

NIMOTOP CAPSULES
(Nimodipine) 603
May interact with antihypertensives, calcium channel blockers, and certain other agents. Compounds in these categories include:

Acebutolol Hydrochloride (Concomitant administration results in intensified effect). Products include:
- Sectral Capsules 2914

Amlodipine Besylate (Possibility of enhanced cardiovascular action). Products include:
- Lotrel Capsules 858
- Norvasc Tablets 2020

Atenolol (Concomitant administration results in intensified effect). Products include:
- Tenoretic Tablets 2963
- Tenormin Tablets and I.V. Injection 2965

Benazepril Hydrochloride (Concomitant administration results in intensified effect). Products include:
- Lotensin Tablets 852
- Lotensin HCT Tablets 855
- Lotrel Capsules 858

Bendroflumethiazide (Concomitant administration results in intensified effect).
- No products indexed under this heading.

Bepridil Hydrochloride (Possibility of enhanced cardiovascular action). Products include:
- Vascor Tablets (200 and 300 mg) 1597

Betaxolol Hydrochloride (Concomitant administration results in intensified effect). Products include:
- Betoptic Ophthalmic Solution 465
- Betoptic S Ophthalmic Suspension 467
- Kerlone Tablets 2588

Bisoprolol Fumarate (Concomitant administration results in intensified effect). Products include:
- Zebeta Tablets 1457
- Ziac 1459

Captopril (Concomitant administration results in intensified effect). Products include:
- Capoten Tablets 740
- Capozide Tablets 744

Carteolol Hydrochloride (Concomitant administration results in intensified effect). Products include:
- Cartrol Tablets 413
- Ocupress Ophthalmic Solution, 1% Sterile .... ⊙ 297

Chlorothiazide (Concomitant administration results in intensified effect). Products include:
- Aldoclor Tablets 1638
- Diupres Tablets 1691
- Diuril Oral 1694

Chlorothiazide Sodium (Concomitant administration results in intensified effect). Products include:
- Diuril Sodium Intravenous 1693

Chlorthalidone (Concomitant administration results in intensified effect). Products include:
- Combipres Tablets 682
- Tenoretic Tablets 2963
- Thalitone 1293

Cimetidine (May increase peak nimodipine plasma concentrations and AUC). Products include:
- Tagamet HB Tablets .... ▣ 786
- Tagamet Tablets 2694

Cimetidine Hydrochloride (May increase peak nimodipine plasma concentrations and AUC). Products include:
- Tagamet 2694

Clonidine (Concomitant administration results in intensified effect). Products include:
- Catapres-TTS 680

Clonidine Hydrochloride (Concomitant administration results in intensified effect). Products include:
- Catapres Tablets 679
- Combipres Tablets 682

Deserpidine (Concomitant administration results in intensified effect).
- No products indexed under this heading.

Diazoxide (Concomitant administration results in intensified effect). Products include:
- Hyperstat I.V. Injection 2504
- Proglycem 575

Diltiazem Hydrochloride (Possibility of enhanced cardiovascular action). Products include:
- Cardizem CD Capsules 1251
- Cardizem SR Capsules 1255
- Cardizem Injectable 1253
- Cardizem Tablets 1257
- Dilacor XR Extended-release Capsules 2183
- Tiazac Capsules 1019

Doxazosin Mesylate (Concomitant administration results in intensified effect). Products include:
- Cardura Tablets 1993

Enalapril Maleate (Concomitant administration results in intensified effect). Products include:
- Vaseretic Tablets 1810
- Vasotec Tablets 1816

Enalaprilat (Concomitant administration results in intensified effect). Products include:
- Vasotec I.V. 1814

Esmolol Hydrochloride (Concomitant administration results in intensified effect). Products include:
- Brevibloc (esmolol HCl) Injection 1860

Felodipine (Possibility of enhanced cardiovascular action). Products include:
- Plendil Extended-Release Tablets 514

Fosinopril Sodium (Concomitant administration results in intensified effect). Products include:
- Monopril Tablets 762

Furosemide (Concomitant administration results in intensified effect). Products include:
- Lasix Injection, Oral Solution and Tablets 1267

Guanabenz Acetate (Concomitant administration results in intensified effect).
- No products indexed under this heading.

Guanethidine Monosulfate (Concomitant administration results in intensified effect). Products include:
- Esimil Tablets 840
- Ismelin Tablets 845

Hydralazine Hydrochloride (Concomitant administration results in intensified effect). Products include:
- Apresazide Capsules 824
- Apresoline Hydrochloride Tablets 826
- Hydralazine Hydrochloride Injection USP 2712
- Ser-Ap-Es Tablets 867

Hydrochlorothiazide (Concomitant administration results in intensified effect). Products include:
- Aldactazide Tablets 2556
- Aldoril Tablets 1644
- Apresazide Capsules 824
- Capozide Tablets 744
- Dyazide Capsules 2653
- Esidrix Tablets 839
- Esimil Tablets 840
- HydroDIURIL Tablets 1716
- Hydropres Tablets 1718
- Hyzaar Tablets 1720
- Inderide Tablets 2838
- Inderide LA Long Acting Capsules 2840
- Lopressor HCT Tablets 850
- Lotensin HCT Tablets 855
- Moduretic Tablets 1748
- Oretic Tablets 450
- Prinzide Tablets 1780
- Ser-Ap-Es Tablets 867
- Timolide Tablets 1791
- Vaseretic Tablets 1810
- Zestoretic Tablets 2968
- Ziac 1459

Hydroflumethiazide (Concomitant administration results in intensified effect). Products include:
- Diucardin Tablets 2824

(▣ Described in PDR For Nonprescription Drugs) (⊙ Described in PDR For Ophthalmology)

Indapamide (Concomitant administration results in intensified effect).
No products indexed under this heading.

Isradipine (Possibility of enhanced cardiovascular action). Products include:
DynaCirc Capsules 2381
DynaCirc CR Tablets 2383

Labetalol Hydrochloride (Concomitant administration results in intensified effect). Products include:
Normodyne Injection 2519
Normodyne Tablets 2522
Trandate 1158

Lisinopril (Concomitant administration results in intensified effect). Products include:
Prinivil Tablets 1776
Prinzide Tablets 1780
Zestoretic Tablets 2968
Zestril Tablets 2972

Losartan Potassium (Possibility of enhanced cardiovascular action). Products include:
Cozaar Tablets 1668
Hyzaar Tablets 1720

Mecamylamine Hydrochloride (Concomitant administration results in intensified effect). Products include:
Inversine Tablets 1729

Methyclothiazide (Concomitant administration results in intensified effect). Products include:
Enduron Tablets 424

Methyldopa (Concomitant administration results in intensified effect). Products include:
Aldoclor Tablets 1638
Aldomet Oral 1640
Aldoril Tablets 1644

Methyldopate Hydrochloride (Concomitant administration results in intensified effect). Products include:
Aldomet Ester HCl Injection 1642

Metolazone (Concomitant administration results in intensified effect). Products include:
Mykrox Tablets 1617
Zaroxolyn Tablets 1625

Metoprolol Succinate (Concomitant administration results in intensified effect). Products include:
Toprol-XL Tablets 560

Metoprolol Tartrate (Concomitant administration results in intensified effect). Products include:
Lopressor 848
Lopressor HCT Tablets 850

Metyrosine (Concomitant administration results in intensified effect). Products include:
Demser Capsules 1690

Minoxidil (Concomitant administration results in intensified effect).
No products indexed under this heading.

Moexipril Hydrochloride (Possibility of enhanced cardiovascular action). Products include:
Univasc Tablets 2553

Nadolol (Concomitant administration results in intensified effect).
No products indexed under this heading.

Nicardipine Hydrochloride (Possibility of enhanced cardiovascular action). Products include:
Cardene Capsules 2261
Cardene I.V. 2815
Cardene SR Capsules 2264

Nifedipine (Possibility of enhanced cardiovascular action). Products include:
Adalat Capsules (10 mg and 20 mg) 580
Adalat CC 582
Procardia Capsules 2024
Procardia XL Extended Release Tablets 2026

Nisoldipine (Possibility of enhanced cardiovascular action). Products include:
Sular Tablets 2961

Nitroglycerin (Concomitant administration results in intensified effect). Products include:
Deponit NTG Transdermal Delivery System 2541
Nitro-Bid IV 1270
Nitro-Bid Ointment 1272
Nitro-Dur (nitroglycerin) Transdermal Infusion System 1365
Nitrolingual Spray 2193
Nitrostat Tablets 1981
Transderm-Nitro Transdermal Therapeutic System 878

Penbutolol Sulfate (Concomitant administration results in intensified effect). Products include:
Levatol Tablets 2547

Phenoxybenzamine Hydrochloride (Concomitant administration results in intensified effect). Products include:
Dibenzyline Capsules 2650

Phentolamine Mesylate (Concomitant administration results in intensified effect). Products include:
Regitine Vials 864

Phenytoin (Potential for phenytoin toxicity). Products include:
Dilantin Infatabs 1967
Dilantin-125 Suspension 1969

Phenytoin Sodium (Potential for phenytoin toxicity). Products include:
Dilantin Kapseals 1965

Pindolol (Concomitant administration results in intensified effect). Products include:
Visken Tablets 2428

Polythiazide (Concomitant administration results in intensified effect). Products include:
Minizide Capsules 2016

Prazosin Hydrochloride (Concomitant administration results in intensified effect). Products include:
Minipress Capsules 2015
Minizide Capsules 2016

Propranolol Hydrochloride (Concomitant administration results in intensified effect). Products include:
Inderal 2834
Inderal LA Long Acting Capsules 2836
Inderide Tablets 2838
Inderide LA Long Acting Capsules .. 2840

Quinapril Hydrochloride (Concomitant administration results in intensified effect). Products include:
Accupril Tablets 1950

Ramipril (Concomitant administration results in intensified effect). Products include:
Altace Capsules 1238

Rauwolfia Serpentina (Concomitant administration results in intensified effect).
No products indexed under this heading.

Rescinnamine (Concomitant administration results in intensified effect).
No products indexed under this heading.

Reserpine (Concomitant administration results in intensified effect). Products include:
Diupres Tablets 1691
Hydropres Tablets 1718
Ser-Ap-Es Tablets 867

Sodium Nitroprusside (Concomitant administration results in intensified effect).
No products indexed under this heading.

Sotalol Hydrochloride (Concomitant administration results in intensified effect). Products include:
Betapace Tablets 637

Spirapril Hydrochloride (Concomitant administration results in intensified effect).
No products indexed under this heading.

Terazosin Hydrochloride (Concomitant administration results in intensified effect). Products include:
Hytrin Capsules 434

Timolol Maleate (Concomitant administration results in intensified effect). Products include:
Blocadren Tablets 1654
Timolide Tablets 1791
Timoptic in Ocudose 1796
Timoptic Sterile Ophthalmic Solution 1794
Timoptic-XE 1798

Torsemide (Concomitant administration results in intensified effect). Products include:
Demadex Tablets and Injection 691

Trimethaphan Camsylate (Concomitant administration results in intensified effect).
No products indexed under this heading.

Verapamil Hydrochloride (Possibility of enhanced cardiovascular action). Products include:
Calan SR Caplets 2571
Calan Tablets 2568
Covera-HS Tablets 2573
Isoptin Injectable 1391
Isoptin Oral Tablets 1393
Isoptin SR Tablets 1395
Verelan Capsules 1455

Food Interactions

Meal, unspecified (Administration of nimodipine capsules following a standard breakfast resulted in 68% lower peak plasma concentration and 38% lower bioavailability).

NIPENT FOR INJECTION
(Pentostatin) 2733
May interact with:

Allopurinol (Both drugs are associated with skin rashes; concomitant therapy in one patient has resulted in a fatal hypersensitivity vasculitis). Products include:
Zyloprim Tablets 1194

Carmustine (BCNU) (Co-administration with high dose cyclophosphamide, carmustine, and etoposide has resulted in a report of acute pulmonary edema, hypotension, and death). Products include:
BiCNU 696

Cyclophosphamide (Co-administration with high dose cyclophosphamide, carmustine, and etoposide has resulted in a report of acute pulmonary edema, hypotension, and death). Products include:
Cytoxan 700

Etoposide (Co-administration with high dose cyclophosphamide, carmustine, and etoposide has resulted in a report of acute pulmonary edema, hypotension, and death). Products include:
Etoposide Injection 539
VePesid Capsules and Injection ... 727

Fludarabine Phosphate (Increased risk of fatal pulmonary toxicity; combined use is not recommended). Products include:
Fludara for Injection 658

Vidarabine (Enhanced effects of vidarabine and may result in increased adverse reactions associated with each drug). Products include:
Vira-A Ophthalmic Ointment, 3%.. © 299

NITRO-BID IV
(Nitroglycerin) 1270
May interact with vasodilators and certain other agents. Compounds in these categories include:

Diazoxide (Additive vasodilating effects). Products include:
Hyperstat I.V. Injection 2504
Proglycem 575

Epoprostenol Sodium (Additive vasodilating effects). Products include:
Flolan for Injection 1085

Heparin Calcium (Intravenous nitroglycerin may interfere with the anticoagulant effect of heparin).
No products indexed under this heading.

Heparin Sodium (Intravenous nitroglycerin may interfere with the anticoagulant effect of heparin). Products include:
Heparin Lock Flush Solution 2831
Heparin Sodium Injection 2832
Heparin Sodium Vials 1486

Hydralazine Hydrochloride (Additive vasodilating effects). Products include:
Apresazide Capsules 824
Apresoline Hydrochloride Tablets .. 826
Hydralazine Hydrochloride Injection USP 2712
Ser-Ap-Es Tablets 867

Minoxidil (Additive vasodilating effects).
No products indexed under this heading.

NITRO-BID OINTMENT
(Nitroglycerin) 1272
May interact with calcium channel blockers, vasodilators, and certain other agents. Compounds in these categories include:

Amlodipine Besylate (May produce marked symptomatic orthostatic hypotension). Products include:
Lotrel Capsules 858
Norvasc Tablets 2020

Bepridil Hydrochloride (May produce marked symptomatic orthostatic hypotension). Products include:
Vascor Tablets (200 and 300 mg) 1597

Diazoxide (Additive vasodilating effects). Products include:
Hyperstat I.V. Injection 2504
Proglycem 575

Diltiazem Hydrochloride (May produce marked symptomatic orthostatic hypotension). Products include:
Cardizem CD Capsules 1251
Cardizem SR Capsules 1255
Cardizem Injectable 1253
Cardizem Tablets 1257
Dilacor XR Extended-release Capsules 2183
Tiazac Capsules 1019

Epoprostenol Sodium (Additive vasodilating effects). Products include:
Flolan for Injection 1085

IMPORTANT NOTE: Always consult each drug listing in the patient's regimen for possible interactions.

Felodipine (May produce marked symptomatic orthostatic hypotension). Products include:
- Plendil Extended-Release Tablets.... 514

Hydralazine Hydrochloride (Additive vasodilating effects). Products include:
- Apresazide Capsules 824
- Apresoline Hydrochloride Tablets .. 826
- Hydralazine Hydrochloride Injection USP.......... 2712
- Ser-Ap-Es Tablets 867

Isradipine (May produce marked symptomatic orthostatic hypotension). Products include:
- DynaCirc Capsules 2381
- DynaCirc CR Tablets 2383

Minoxidil (Additive vasodilating effects).
- No products indexed under this heading.

Nicardipine Hydrochloride (May produce marked symptomatic orthostatic hypotension). Products include:
- Cardene Capsules 2261
- Cardene I.V. 2815
- Cardene SR Capsules.......... 2264

Nifedipine (May produce marked symptomatic orthostatic hypotension). Products include:
- Adalat Capsules (10 mg and 20 mg) 580
- Adalat CC 582
- Procardia Capsules.......... 2024
- Procardia XL Extended Release Tablets 2026

Nimodipine (May produce marked symptomatic orthostatic hypotension). Products include:
- Nimotop Capsules 603

Nisoldipine (May produce marked symptomatic orthostatic hypotension). Products include:
- Sular Tablets 2961

Verapamil Hydrochloride (May produce marked symptomatic orthostatic hypotension). Products include:
- Calan SR Caplets 2571
- Calan Tablets.......... 2568
- Covera-HS Tablets 2573
- Isoptin Injectable 1391
- Isoptin Oral Tablets 1393
- Isoptin SR Tablets 1395
- Verelan Capsules 1455

Food Interactions

Alcohol (Exhibits additive vasodilating effects).

NITRO-DUR (NITROGLYCERIN) TRANSDERMAL INFUSION SYSTEM

(Nitroglycerin) 1365

May interact with vasodilators. Compounds in this category include:

Diazoxide (Vasodilating effects of nitroglycerin may be additive with those of other vasodilators). Products include:
- Hyperstat I.V. Injection 2504
- Proglycem.......... 575

Epoprostenol Sodium (Vasodilating effects of nitroglycerin may be additive with those of other vasodilators). Products include:
- Flolan for Injection.......... 1085

Hydralazine Hydrochloride (Vasodilating effects of nitroglycerin may be additive with those of other vasodilators). Products include:
- Apresazide Capsules 824
- Apresoline Hydrochloride Tablets .. 826
- Hydralazine Hydrochloride Injection USP.......... 2712
- Ser-Ap-Es Tablets 867

Minoxidil (Vasodilating effects of nitroglycerin may be additive with those of other vasodilators).
- No products indexed under this heading.

Food Interactions

Alcohol (Enhances sensitivity to the hypotensive effects).

NITROLINGUAL SPRAY

(Nitroglycerin) 2193

May interact with calcium channel blockers and certain other agents. Compounds in these categories include:

Amlodipine Besylate (Marked symptomatic orthostatic hypotension). Products include:
- Lotrel Capsules.......... 858
- Norvasc Tablets 2020

Bepridil Hydrochloride (Marked symptomatic orthostatic hypotension). Products include:
- Vascor Tablets (200 and 300 mg) 1597

Diltiazem Hydrochloride (Marked symptomatic orthostatic hypotension). Products include:
- Cardizem CD Capsules 1251
- Cardizem SR Capsules 1255
- Cardizem Injectable 1253
- Cardizem Tablets.......... 1257
- Dilacor XR Extended-release Capsules 2183
- Tiazac Capsules 1019

Drugs Depending On Vascular Smooth Muscle (Decreased or increased effect).

Felodipine (Marked symptomatic orthostatic hypotension). Products include:
- Plendil Extended-Release Tablets.... 514

Isradipine (Marked symptomatic orthostatic hypotension). Products include:
- DynaCirc Capsules 2381
- DynaCirc CR Tablets 2383

Nicardipine Hydrochloride (Marked symptomatic orthostatic hypotension). Products include:
- Cardene Capsules 2261
- Cardene I.V. 2815
- Cardene SR Capsules.......... 2264

Nifedipine (Marked symptomatic orthostatic hypotension). Products include:
- Adalat Capsules (10 mg and 20 mg) 580
- Adalat CC 582
- Procardia Capsules.......... 2024
- Procardia XL Extended Release Tablets 2026

Nimodipine (Marked symptomatic orthostatic hypotension). Products include:
- Nimotop Capsules 603

Nisoldipine (Marked symptomatic orthostatic hypotension). Products include:
- Sular Tablets 2961

Verapamil Hydrochloride (Marked symptomatic orthostatic hypotension). Products include:
- Calan SR Caplets 2571
- Calan Tablets.......... 2568
- Covera-HS Tablets 2573
- Isoptin Injectable 1391
- Isoptin Oral Tablets 1393
- Isoptin SR Tablets 1395
- Verelan Capsules 1455

Food Interactions

Alcohol (Enhanced sensitivity to hypotensive effects).

NITROSTAT TABLETS

(Nitroglycerin) 1981

May interact with antihypertensives, phenothiazines, beta blockers, calcium channel blockers, and certain other agents. Compounds in these categories include:

Acebutolol Hydrochloride (Possible additive hypotensive effects). Products include:
- Sectral Capsules 2914

Amlodipine Besylate (Concomitant use has resulted in marked hypotension). Products include:
- Lotrel Capsules.......... 858
- Norvasc Tablets 2020

Aspirin (Decreases the clearance and enhances the hemodynamic effects of sublingual nitroglycerin). Products include:
- Alka-Seltzer Cherry Effervescent Antacid and Pain Reliever .... ▣ 609
- Alka-Seltzer Extra Strength Effervescent Antacid and Pain Reliever .... ▣ 609
- Alka-Seltzer Lemon Lime Effervescent Antacid and Pain Reliever .... ▣ 609
- Alka-Seltzer Original Effervescent Antacid and Pain Reliever .... ▣ 609
- Alka-Seltzer Plus .... ▣ 611
- Alka-Seltzer Plus Sinus Medicine .. ▣ 611
- Ascriptin .... ▣ 650
- Arthritis Strength BC Powder.......... ▣ 631
- BC Cold Powder Multi-Symptom Formula (Cold-Sinus-Allergy) ...... ▣ 631
- BC Cold Powder Non-Drowsy Formula (Cold-Sinus) .... ▣ 631
- BC Powder .... ▣ 631
- Genuine Bayer Aspirin Tablets & Caplets .... ▣ 618
- Extra Strength Bayer Arthritis Pain Regimen Formula .... ▣ 615
- Extra Strength Bayer Aspirin Caplets & Tablets .... ▣ 617
- Extended-Release Bayer 8-Hour Aspirin .... ▣ 616
- Extra Strength Bayer Plus Aspirin Caplets .... ▣ 617
- Extra Strength Bayer PM Aspirin Plus Sleep Aid .... ▣ 617
- Aspirin Regimen Bayer 81 mg Tablets with Calcium .... ▣ 615
- Aspirin Regimen Bayer Adult Low Strength 81 mg Tablets .... ▣ 613
- Aspirin Regimen Bayer Children's Chewable Aspirin .... ▣ 616
- Aspirin Regimen Bayer Regular Strength 325 mg Caplets .... ▣ 613
- Bufferin Analgesic Tablets.......... ▣ 636
- Arthritis Strength Bufferin Analgesic Caplets .... ▣ 637
- Extra Strength Bufferin Analgesic Tablets .... ▣ 637
- Cama Arthritis Pain Reliever.......... ▣ 748
- Darvon Compound-65 Pulvules 1475
- Easprin.......... 1971
- Ecotrin 2625
- Ecotrin Enteric Coated Aspirin Maximum Strength Tablets and Caplets .... ▣ 775
- Ecotrin Enteric Coated Aspirin Regular Strength Tablets 2625
- Empirin Aspirin Tablets .... ▣ 818
- Excedrin Extra-Strength Analgesic Tablets, Caplets, and Geltabs.......... 734
- Fiorinal Capsules 2388
- Fiorinal with Codeine Capsules 2390
- Fiorinal Tablets.......... 2388
- Goody's Extra Strength Headache Powders.......... ▣ 632
- Goody's Extra Strength Pain Relief Tablets .... ▣ 632
- Halfprin Tablets 1413
- Norgesic.......... 1554
- Percodan Tablets.......... 955
- Percodan-Demi Tablets.......... 956
- Robaxisal Tablets.......... 2246
- Soma Compound w/Codeine Tablets 2784
- Soma Compound Tablets.......... 2783
- St. Joseph Adult Chewable Aspirin (81 mg.) .... ▣ 768
- Talwin Compound 2466
- Vanquish Analgesic Caplets .... ▣ 627

Atenolol (Possible additive hypotensive effects). Products include:
- Tenoretic Tablets.......... 2963
- Tenormin Tablets and I.V. Injection 2965

Benazepril Hydrochloride (Possible additive hypotensive effects). Products include:
- Lotensin Tablets.......... 852
- Lotensin HCT Tablets 855
- Lotrel Capsules.......... 858

Bendroflumethiazide (Possible additive hypotensive effects).
- No products indexed under this heading.

Bepridil Hydrochloride (Concomitant use has resulted in marked hypotension). Products include:
- Vascor Tablets (200 and 300 mg) 1597

Betaxolol Hydrochloride (Possible additive hypotensive effects). Products include:
- Betoptic Ophthalmic Solution.......... 465
- Betoptic S Ophthalmic Suspension 467
- Kerlone Tablets.......... 2588

Bisoprolol Fumarate (Possible additive hypotensive effects). Products include:
- Zebeta Tablets 1457
- Ziac 1459

Captopril (Possible additive hypotensive effects). Products include:
- Capoten Tablets.......... 740
- Capozide Tablets.......... 744

Carteolol Hydrochloride (Possible additive hypotensive effects). Products include:
- Cartrol Tablets 413
- Ocupress Ophthalmic Solution, 1% Sterile.......... ⊙ 297

Chlorothiazide (Possible additive hypotensive effects). Products include:
- Aldoclor Tablets.......... 1638
- Diupres Tablets 1691
- Diuril Oral 1694

Chlorothiazide Sodium (Possible additive hypotensive effects). Products include:
- Diuril Sodium Intravenous 1693

Chlorpromazine (Possible additive hypotensive effects). Products include:
- Thorazine Suppositories.......... 2701

Chlorpromazine Hydrochloride (Possible additive hypotensive effects). Products include:
- Thorazine 2701

Chlorthalidone (Possible additive hypotensive effects). Products include:
- Combipres Tablets 682
- Tenoretic Tablets.......... 2963
- Thalitone 1293

Clonidine (Possible additive hypotensive effects). Products include:
- Catapres-TTS.......... 680

Clonidine Hydrochloride (Possible additive hypotensive effects). Products include:
- Catapres Tablets 679
- Combipres Tablets 682

Deserpidine (Possible additive hypotensive effects).
- No products indexed under this heading.

Diazoxide (Possible additive hypotensive effects). Products include:
- Hyperstat I.V. Injection 2504
- Proglycem.......... 575

Diltiazem Hydrochloride (Concomitant use has resulted in marked hypotension). Products include:
- Cardizem CD Capsules 1251
- Cardizem SR Capsules 1255
- Cardizem Injectable 1253
- Cardizem Tablets.......... 1257
- Dilacor XR Extended-release Capsules 2183
- Tiazac Capsules 1019

Doxazosin Mesylate (Possible additive hypotensive effects). Products include:
- Cardura Tablets 1993

(▣ Described in PDR For Nonprescription Drugs) (⊙ Described in PDR For Ophthalmology)

743 **Interactions Index** **Nitrostat Tablets**

Enalapril Maleate (Possible additive hypotensive effects). Products include:
- Vaseretic Tablets ... 1810
- Vasotec Tablets ... 1816

Enalaprilat (Possible additive hypotensive effects). Products include:
- Vasotec I.V. ... 1814

Esmolol Hydrochloride (Possible additive hypotensive effects). Products include:
- Brevibloc (esmolol HCl) Injection ... 1860

Felodipine (Concomitant use has resulted in marked hypotension). Products include:
- Plendil Extended-Release Tablets ... 514

Fluphenazine Decanoate (Possible additive hypotensive effects). Products include:
- Prolixin Decanoate ... 510

Fluphenazine Enanthate (Possible additive hypotensive effects). Products include:
- Prolixin Enanthate ... 510

Fluphenazine Hydrochloride (Possible additive hypotensive effects). Products include:
- Prolixin ... 510

Fosinopril Sodium (Possible additive hypotensive effects). Products include:
- Monopril Tablets ... 762

Furosemide (Possible additive hypotensive effects). Products include:
- Lasix Injection, Oral Solution and Tablets ... 1267

Guanabenz Acetate (Possible additive hypotensive effects).
- No products indexed under this heading.

Guanethidine Monosulfate (Possible additive hypotensive effects). Products include:
- Esimil Tablets ... 840
- Ismelin Tablets ... 845

Hydralazine Hydrochloride (Possible additive hypotensive effects). Products include:
- Apresazide Capsules ... 824
- Apresoline Hydrochloride Tablets ... 826
- Hydralazine Hydrochloride Injection USP ... 2712
- Ser-Ap-Es Tablets ... 867

Hydrochlorothiazide (Possible additive hypotensive effects). Products include:
- Aldactazide Tablets ... 2556
- Aldoril Tablets ... 1644
- Apresazide Capsules ... 824
- Capozide Tablets ... 744
- Dyazide Capsules ... 2653
- Esidrix Tablets ... 839
- Esimil Tablets ... 840
- HydroDIURIL Tablets ... 1716
- Hydropres Tablets ... 1718
- Hyzaar Tablets ... 1720
- Inderide Tablets ... 2838
- Inderide LA Long Acting Capsules ... 2840
- Lopressor HCT Tablets ... 850
- Lotensin HCT Tablets ... 855
- Moduretic Tablets ... 1748
- Oretic Tablets ... 450
- Prinzide Tablets ... 1780
- Ser-Ap-Es Tablets ... 867
- Timolide Tablets ... 1791
- Vaseretic Tablets ... 1810
- Zestoretic Tablets ... 2968
- Ziac ... 1459

Hydroflumethiazide (Possible additive hypotensive effects). Products include:
- Diucardin Tablets ... 2824

Indapamide (Possible additive hypotensive effects).
- No products indexed under this heading.

Isosorbide Dinitrate (A decrease in the therapeutic effects of sublingual nitroglycerin may result from use of long-acting nitrates). Products include:
- Dilatrate-SR Capsules ... 2542
- Isordil Sublingual Tablets ... 2845
- Isordil Tembids ... 2847
- Isordil Titradose Tablets ... 2848
- Sorbitrate ... 2959

Isosorbide Mononitrate (A decrease in the therapeutic effects of sublingual nitroglycerin may result from use of long-acting nitrates). Products include:
- Imdur ... 1362
- Ismo Tablets ... 2844
- Monoket Tablets ... 2550

Isradipine (Concomitant use has resulted in marked hypotension). Products include:
- DynaCirc Capsules ... 2381
- DynaCirc CR Tablets ... 2383

Labetalol Hydrochloride (Possible additive hypotensive effects). Products include:
- Normodyne Injection ... 2519
- Normodyne Tablets ... 2522
- Trandate ... 1158

Levobunolol Hydrochloride (Possible additive hypotensive effects). Products include:
- Betagan ... ◉ 230

Lisinopril (Possible additive hypotensive effects). Products include:
- Prinivil Tablets ... 1776
- Prinzide Tablets ... 1780
- Zestoretic Tablets ... 2968
- Zestril Tablets ... 2972

Losartan Potassium (Possible additive hypotensive effects). Products include:
- Cozaar Tablets ... 1668
- Hyzaar Tablets ... 1720

Mecamylamine Hydrochloride (Possible additive hypotensive effects). Products include:
- Inversine Tablets ... 1729

Mesoridazine Besylate (Possible additive hypotensive effects). Products include:
- Serentil ... 689

Methotrimeprazine (Possible additive hypotensive effects). Products include:
- Levoprome ... 1321

Methyclothiazide (Possible additive hypotensive effects). Products include:
- Enduron Tablets ... 424

Methyldopa (Possible additive hypotensive effects). Products include:
- Aldoclor Tablets ... 1638
- Aldomet Oral ... 1640
- Aldoril Tablets ... 1644

Methyldopate Hydrochloride (Possible additive hypotensive effects). Products include:
- Aldomet Ester HCl Injection ... 1642

Metipranolol Hydrochloride (Possible additive hypotensive effects). Products include:
- OptiPranolol (Metipranolol 0.3%) Sterile Ophthalmic Solution ... ◉ 256

Metolazone (Possible additive hypotensive effects). Products include:
- Mykrox Tablets ... 1617
- Zaroxolyn Tablets ... 1625

Metoprolol Succinate (Possible additive hypotensive effects). Products include:
- Toprol-XL Tablets ... 560

Metoprolol Tartrate (Possible additive hypotensive effects). Products include:
- Lopressor ... 848
- Lopressor HCT Tablets ... 850

Metyrosine (Possible additive hypotensive effects). Products include:
- Demser Capsules ... 1690

Minoxidil (Possible additive hypotensive effects).
- No products indexed under this heading.

Moexipril Hydrochloride (Possible additive hypotensive effects). Products include:
- Univasc Tablets ... 2553

Nadolol (Possible additive hypotensive effects).
- No products indexed under this heading.

Nicardipine Hydrochloride (Concomitant use has resulted in marked hypotension). Products include:
- Cardene Capsules ... 2261
- Cardene I.V. ... 2815
- Cardene SR Capsules ... 2264

Nifedipine (Concomitant use has resulted in marked hypotension). Products include:
- Adalat Capsules (10 mg and 20 mg) ... 580
- Adalat CC ... 582
- Procardia Capsules ... 2024
- Procardia XL Extended Release Tablets ... 2026

Nimodipine (Concomitant use has resulted in marked hypotension). Products include:
- Nimotop Capsules ... 603

Nisoldipine (Concomitant use has resulted in marked hypotension). Products include:
- Sular Tablets ... 2961

Nitroglycerin, long acting formulations (A decrease in the therapeutic effects of sublingual nitroglycerin may result from use of long-acting nitrates).

Penbutolol Sulfate (Possible additive hypotensive effects). Products include:
- Levatol Tablets ... 2547

Perphenazine (Possible additive hypotensive effects). Products include:
- Etrafon ... 2495
- Triavil Tablets ... 1800
- Trilafon ... 2532

Phenoxybenzamine Hydrochloride (Possible additive hypotensive effects). Products include:
- Dibenzyline Capsules ... 2650

Phentolamine Mesylate (Possible additive hypotensive effects). Products include:
- Regitine Vials ... 864

Pindolol (Possible additive hypotensive effects). Products include:
- Visken Tablets ... 2428

Polythiazide (Possible additive hypotensive effects). Products include:
- Minizide Capsules ... 2016

Prazosin Hydrochloride (Possible additive hypotensive effects). Products include:
- Minipress Capsules ... 2015
- Minizide Capsules ... 2016

Prochlorperazine (Possible additive hypotensive effects). Products include:
- Compazine ... 2644

Promethazine Hydrochloride (Possible additive hypotensive effects). Products include:
- Mepergan Injection ... 2859
- Phenergan with Codeine ... 2883
- Phenergan with Dextromethorphan ... 2885
- Phenergan Injection ... 2880
- Phenergan Suppositories ... 2882
- Phenergan Syrup ... 2881
- Phenergan Tablets ... 2882
- Phenergan VC ... 2886
- Phenergan VC with Codeine ... 2888

Propranolol Hydrochloride (Possible additive hypotensive effects). Products include:
- Inderal ... 2834
- Inderal LA Long Acting Capsules ... 2836
- Inderide Tablets ... 2838
- Inderide LA Long Acting Capsules ... 2840

Quinapril Hydrochloride (Possible additive hypotensive effects). Products include:
- Accupril Tablets ... 1950

Ramipril (Possible additive hypotensive effects). Products include:
- Altace Capsules ... 1238

Rauwolfia Serpentina (Possible additive hypotensive effects).
- No products indexed under this heading.

Rescinnamine (Possible additive hypotensive effects).
- No products indexed under this heading.

Reserpine (Possible additive hypotensive effects). Products include:
- Diupres Tablets ... 1691
- Hydropres Tablets ... 1718
- Ser-Ap-Es Tablets ... 867

Sodium Nitroprusside (Possible additive hypotensive effects).
- No products indexed under this heading.

Sotalol Hydrochloride (Possible additive hypotensive effects). Products include:
- Betapace Tablets ... 637

Spirapril Hydrochloride (Possible additive hypotensive effects).
- No products indexed under this heading.

Terazosin Hydrochloride (Possible additive hypotensive effects). Products include:
- Hytrin Capsules ... 434

Thioridazine Hydrochloride (Possible additive hypotensive effects). Products include:
- Mellaril ... 2398

Timolol Hemihydrate (Possible additive hypotensive effects). Products include:
- Betimol 0.25%, 0.5% ... ◉ 259

Timolol Maleate (Possible additive hypotensive effects). Products include:
- Blocadren Tablets ... 1654
- Timolide Tablets ... 1791
- Timoptic in Ocudose ... 1796
- Timoptic Sterile Ophthalmic Solution ... 1794
- Timoptic-XE ... 1798

Torsemide (Possible additive hypotensive effects). Products include:
- Demadex Tablets and Injection ... 691

Trifluoperazine Hydrochloride (Possible additive hypotensive effects). Products include:
- Stelazine ... 2692

Trimethaphan Camsylate (Possible additive hypotensive effects).
- No products indexed under this heading.

Verapamil Hydrochloride (Concomitant use has resulted in marked hypotension). Products include:
- Calan SR Caplets ... 2571
- Calan Tablets ... 2568
- Covera-HS Tablets ... 2573
- Isoptin Injectable ... 1391
- Isoptin Oral Tablets ... 1393
- Isoptin SR Tablets ... 1395
- Verelan Capsules ... 1455

Food Interactions

Alcohol (Concomitant use may cause hypotension).

IMPORTANT NOTE: Always consult each drug listing in the patient's regimen for possible interactions.

NIX CREME RINSE
(Permethrin) ▣ 822
None cited in PDR database.

NIZORAL 2% CREAM
(Ketoconazole) 1344
None cited in PDR database.

NIZORAL 2% SHAMPOO
(Ketoconazole) 1344
None cited in PDR database.

NIZORAL TABLETS
(Ketoconazole) 1345
May interact with oral anticoagulants, oral hypoglycemic agents, anticholinergics, histamine h2-receptor antagonists, antacids, and certain other agents. Compounds in these categories include:

Acarbose (Possibility of severe hypoglycemia cannot be ruled out). Products include:
- Precose 604

Aluminum Carbonate (Nizoral requires acidity for dissolution, antacids should be given at least two hours after Nizoral administration). Products include:
- Basaljel Capsules 2810
- Basaljel Suspension 2810
- Basaljel Tablets 2810

Aluminum Hydroxide (Nizoral requires acidity for dissolution, antacids should be given at least two hours after Nizoral administration). Products include:
- ALternaGEL Liquid 1358
- Maximum Strength Ascriptin ▣ 650
- Cama Arthritis Pain Reliever ▣ 748
- Gaviscon Extra Strength Relief Formula Antacid Tablets ▣ 778
- Gaviscon Extra Strength Relief Formula Liquid Antacid ▣ 779
- Gaviscon Liquid Antacid ▣ 779
- Gelusil Antacid-Anti-gas Liquid ▣ 819
- Gelusil Antacid-Anti-gas Tablets ▣ 819
- Maalox Antacid/Anti-Gas Tablets 889
- Maalox Heartburn Relief Suspension ▣ 658
- Maalox Antacid Liquid 888
- Extra Strength Maalox Antacid/Anti-Gas Liquid and Tablets 888
- Mylanta 1359
- Tempo Soft Antacid ▣ 799

Aluminum Hydroxide Gel (Nizoral requires acidity for dissolution, antacids should be given at least two hours after Nizoral administration). Products include:
- ALternaGEL Liquid ▣ 675
- Aludrox Oral Suspension ▣ 850
- Amphojel Suspension 2802
- Amphojel Suspension without Flavor 2802
- Amphojel Tablets 2802
- Ascriptin ▣ 650
- Gaviscon Antacid Tablets ▣ 778
- Gaviscon-2 Antacid Tablets ▣ 779
- Mylanta Liquid ▣ 676
- Mylanta Double Strength Liquid ▣ 676
- Nephrox Suspension ▣ 671

Astemizole (Coadministration is contraindicated; elevated plasma levels of astemizole resulting in prolonged QT intervals). Products include:
- Hismanal Tablets 1341

Atropine Sulfate (Nizoral requires acidity for dissolution, these drugs should be given at least two hours after Nizoral administration). Products include:
- Arco-Lase Plus Tablets 513
- Atrohist Plus Tablets 1605
- Donnatal 2234
- Donnatal Extentabs 2234
- Donnatal Tablets 2234
- Lomotil 2591
- Motofen Tablets 789
- Urised Tablets 2123

Belladonna Alkaloids (Nizoral requires acidity for dissolution, these drugs should be given at least two hours after Nizoral administration). Products include:
- Bellergal-S Tablets 2375
- Hyland's Bedwetting Tablets ▣ 788
- Hyland's EnurAid Tablets ▣ 789
- Hyland's Headache Tablets ▣ 790
- Hyland's Teething Tablets ▣ 790
- Similasan Eye Drops #1 ▣ 769

Benztropine Mesylate (Nizoral requires acidity for dissolution, these drugs should be given at least two hours after Nizoral administration). Products include:
- Cogentin 1661

Biperiden Hydrochloride (Nizoral requires acidity for dissolution, these drugs should be given at least two hours after Nizoral administration). Products include:
- Akineton 1380

Chlorpropamide (Possibility of severe hypoglycemia cannot be ruled out). Products include:
- Diabinese Tablets 2002

Cimetidine (Nizoral requires acidity for dissolution, these drugs should be given at least two hours after Nizoral administration). Products include:
- Tagamet HB Tablets ▣ 786
- Tagamet Tablets 2694

Cimetidine Hydrochloride (Nizoral requires acidity for dissolution, these drugs should be given at least two hours after Nizoral administration). Products include:
- Tagamet 2694

Cisapride (Co-administration has resulted in serious cardiovascular adverse events including ventricular tachycardia, ventricular fibrillation and torsade de pointes; concurrent use is contraindicated). Products include:
- Propulsid 1346

Clidinium Bromide (Nizoral requires acidity for dissolution, these drugs should be given at least two hours after Nizoral administration). Products include:
- Librax Capsules 2330

Cyclosporine (Co-administration may alter the metabolism of cyclosporine resulting in increased plasma concentration of cyclosporine). Products include:
- Neoral 2405
- Sandimmune 2416

Dicumarol (Anticoagulant effect enhanced).
No products indexed under this heading.

Dicyclomine Hydrochloride (Nizoral requires acidity for dissolution, these drugs should be given at least two hours after Nizoral administration). Products include:
- Bentyl 1246

Digoxin (Rare cases of elevated plasma concentrations of digoxin; monitor digoxin concentration). Products include:
- Lanoxicaps 1110
- Lanoxin Elixir Pediatric 1113
- Lanoxin Injection 1116
- Lanoxin Injection Pediatric 1119
- Lanoxin Tablets 1121

Famotidine (Nizoral requires acidity for dissolution, these drugs should be given at least two hours after Nizoral administration). Products include:
- Pepcid AC Acid Controller 1360
- Pepcid Injection 1765
- Pepcid 1763

Fosphenytoin Sodium (Co-administration may alter metabolism of one or both of the drugs). Products include:
- Cerebyx Injection 1956

Glimepiride (Possibility of severe hypoglycemia cannot be ruled out). Products include:
- Amaryl Tablets 1241

Glipizide (Possibility of severe hypoglycemia cannot be ruled out). Products include:
- Glucotrol Tablets 2011
- Glucotrol XL Extended Release Tablets 2012

Glyburide (Possibility of severe hypoglycemia cannot be ruled out). Products include:
- DiaBeta Tablets 1265
- Glynase PresTab Tablets 2091
- Micronase Tablets 2099

Glycopyrrolate (Nizoral requires acidity for dissolution, these drugs should be given at least two hours after Nizoral administration). Products include:
- Robinul Forte Tablets 2247
- Robinul Injectable 2247
- Robinul Tablets 2247

Hyoscyamine (Nizoral requires acidity for dissolution, these drugs should be given at least two hours after Nizoral administration). Products include:
- Cystospaz Tablets 2123
- Urised Tablets 2123

Hyoscyamine Sulfate (Nizoral requires acidity for dissolution, these drugs should be given at least two hours after Nizoral administration). Products include:
- Arco-Lase Plus Tablets 513
- Atrohist Plus Tablets 1605
- Cystospaz-M Capsules 2123
- Donnatal 2234
- Donnatal Extentabs 2234
- Donnatal Tablets 2234
- Kutrase Capsules 2546
- Levsin/Levsinex/Levbid 2549

Ipratropium Bromide (Nizoral requires acidity for dissolution, these drugs should be given at least two hours after Nizoral administration). Products include:
- Atrovent Inhalation Aerosol 674
- Atrovent Inhalation Solution 675
- Atrovent Nasal Spray 0.03% 676
- Atrovent Nasal Spray 0.06% 678

Isoniazid (Affects ketoconazole concentrations adversely). Products include:
- Nydrazid Injection 509
- Rifamate Capsules 1278
- Rifater 1280

Loratadine (AUC and C_{max} of loratadine averaged 302% and 251% respectively following coadministration; no cardiac changes were noted). Products include:
- Claritin Tablets 2485
- Claritin-D Tablets 2487

Magaldrate (Nizoral requires acidity for dissolution, antacids should be given at least two hours after Nizoral administration).
No products indexed under this heading.

Magnesium Hydroxide (Nizoral requires acidity for dissolution, antacids should be given at least two hours after Nizoral administration). Products include:
- Aludrox Oral Suspension ▣ 850
- Ascriptin ▣ 650
- Di-Gel Antacid/Anti-Gas ▣ 762
- Gelusil Antacid-Anti-gas Liquid ▣ 819
- Gelusil Antacid-Anti-gas Tablets ▣ 819
- Maalox Antacid/Anti-Gas Tablets 889
- Maalox Antacid Liquid 888
- Extra Strength Maalox Antacid/Anti-Gas Liquid and Tablets 888
- Mylanta Fast-Acting 1359
- Mylanta Gelcaps Antacid ▣ 678
- Fast-Acting Mylanta Liquid Antacid 1359
- Mylanta Tablets ▣ 677
- Maximum-Strength Fast-Acting Mylanta Liquid Antacid 1359
- Mylanta Double Strength Tablets ▣ 677
- Phillips' Milk of Magnesia Liquid ▣ 627
- Rolaids Antacid Tablets ▣ 807
- Tempo Soft Antacid ▣ 799

Magnesium Oxide (Nizoral requires acidity for dissolution, antacids should be given at least two hours after Nizoral administration). Products include:
- Beelith Tablets 632
- Bufferin Analgesic Tablets ▣ 636
- Arthritis Strength Bufferin Analgesic Caplets ▣ 637
- Extra Strength Bufferin Analgesic Tablets ▣ 637
- Caltrate PLUS ▣ 681
- Cama Arthritis Pain Reliever ▣ 748
- Mag-Ox 400 666
- Uro-Mag 666

Mepenzolate Bromide (Nizoral requires acidity for dissolution, these drugs should be given at least two hours after Nizoral administration).
No products indexed under this heading.

Metformin Hydrochloride (Possibility of severe hypoglycemia cannot be ruled out). Products include:
- Glucophage Tablets 754

Methylprednisolone (Co-administration may alter the metabolism of methylprednisolone resulting in increased plasma concentration; dosage of methylprednisolone may have to be adjusted).
No products indexed under this heading.

Methylprednisolone Acetate (Co-administration may alter the metabolism of methylprednisolone resulting in increased plasma concentration; dosage of methylprednisolone may have to be adjusted).
No products indexed under this heading.

Methylprednisolone Sodium Succinate (Co-administration may alter the metabolism of methylprednisolone resulting in increased plasma concentration; dosage of methylprednisolone may have to be adjusted).
No products indexed under this heading.

Midazolam Hydrochloride (Co-administration with oral midazolam has resulted in elevated plasma concentration of midazolam resulting in prolonged hypnotic and sedative effects; concurrent oral use should be avoided). Products include:
- Versed Injection 2324

Nizatidine (Nizoral requires acidity for dissolution, these drugs should be given at least two hours after Nizoral administration). Products include:
- Axid Pulvules 1468

Oxybutynin Chloride (Nizoral requires acidity for dissolution, these drugs should be given at least two hours after Nizoral administration). Products include:
- Ditropan 1267

Phenytoin (Co-administration may alter metabolism of one or both of the drugs). Products include:
- Dilantin Infatabs 1967
- Dilantin-125 Suspension 1969

Phenytoin Sodium (Co-administration may alter metabolism of one or both of the drugs). Products include:
- Dilantin Kapseals 1965

(▣ Described in PDR For Nonprescription Drugs) (◉ Described in PDR For Ophthalmology)

Procyclidine Hydrochloride (Nizoral requires acidity for dissolution, these drugs should be given at least two hours after Nizoral administration). Products include:
　Kemadrin Tablets 1105

Propantheline Bromide (Nizoral requires acidity for dissolution, these drugs should be given at least two hours after Nizoral administration). Products include:
　Pro-Banthine Tablets 2226

Ranitidine Hydrochloride (Nizoral requires acidity for dissolution, these drugs should be given at least two hours after Nizoral administration). Products include:
　Zantac 1182
　Zantac Injection 1180
　Zantac Syrup 1182

Rifampin (Reduces blood levels of ketoconazole). Products include:
　Rifadin 1276
　Rifamate Capsules 1278
　Rifater 1280
　Rimactane Capsules 865

Scopolamine (Nizoral requires acidity for dissolution, these drugs should be given at least two hours after Nizoral administration). Products include:
　Transderm Scōp Transdermal Therapeutic System 890

Scopolamine Hydrobromide (Nizoral requires acidity for dissolution, these drugs should be given at least two hours after Nizoral administration). Products include:
　Atrohist Plus Tablets 1605
　Donnatal 2234
　Donnatal Extentabs 2234
　Donnatal Tablets 2234

Sodium Bicarbonate (Nizoral requires acidity for dissolution, antacids should be given at least two hours after Nizoral administration). Products include:
　Alka-Seltzer Cherry Effervescent Antacid and Pain Reliever 609
　Alka-Seltzer Extra Strength Effervescent Antacid and Pain Reliever 609
　Alka-Seltzer Gold Effervescent Antacid 611
　Alka-Seltzer Lemon Lime Effervescent Antacid and Pain Reliever 609
　Alka-Seltzer Original Effervescent Antacid and Pain Reliever 609
　Arm & Hammer Pure Baking Soda 648
　Colyte and Colyte-flavored 2540
　GoLYTELY 694
　Massengill Disposable Douches ... 780
　Massengill Liquid Concentrate 780
　NuLYTELY 694
　Cherry Flavor NuLYTELY 694

Tacrolimus (Co-administration may alter the metabolism of tacrolimus resulting in increased plasma concentration; dosage of tacrolimus may have to be adjusted). Products include:
　Prograf 1028

Terfenadine (Co-administration has resulted in rare cases of serious cardiovascular adverse events including death, ventricular tachycardia, and torsade de pointes due to increased terfenadine concentrations caused by ketoconazole tablets; concurrent use is contraindicated). Products include:
　Seldane Tablets 1284
　Seldane-D Extended-Release Tablets 1286

Tolazamide (Possibility of severe hypoglycemia cannot be ruled out).
　No products indexed under this heading.

Tolbutamide (Possibility of severe hypoglycemia cannot be ruled out).
　No products indexed under this heading.

Triazolam (Co-administration has resulted in elevated plasma concentration of triazolam resulting in prolonged hypnotic and sedative effects; concurrent use with oral triazolam is contraindicated). Products include:
　Halcion Tablets 2093

Tridihexethyl Chloride (Nizoral requires acidity for dissolution, these drugs should be given at least two hours after Nizoral administration).
　No products indexed under this heading.

Trihexyphenidyl Hydrochloride (Nizoral requires acidity for dissolution, these drugs should be given at least two hours after Nizoral administration). Products include:
　Artane 1418

Warfarin Sodium (Anticoagulant effect enhanced). Products include:
　Coumadin 941

Food Interactions

Alcohol (Potential for disulfiram-like reaction to alcohol resulting in flushing, rash, peripheral edema, nausea and headache).

NO DOZ MAXIMUM STRENGTH CAPLETS
(Caffeine) 644
May interact with:

Caffeine-containing medications (May cause sleeplessness, irritability, nervousness and rapid heart beat).

Food Interactions
Beverages, caffeine-containing (May cause sleeplessness, irritability, nervousness and rapid heart beat).

Food, caffeine containing (May cause sleeplessness, irritability, nervousness and rapid heart beat).

NOLAHIST TABLETS
(Phenindamine Tartrate) 790
May interact with tranquilizers, hypnotics and sedatives, and certain other agents. Compounds in these categories include:

Alprazolam (May increase drowsiness effect). Products include:
　Xanax Tablets 2115

Buspirone Hydrochloride (May increase drowsiness effect). Products include:
　BuSpar Tablets 738

Chlordiazepoxide (May increase drowsiness effect). Products include:
　Limbitrol 2333

Chlordiazepoxide Hydrochloride (May increase drowsiness effect). Products include:
　Librax Capsules 2330
　Librium Capsules 2331
　Librium Injectable 2332

Chlorpromazine (May increase drowsiness effect). Products include:
　Thorazine Suppositories 2701

Chlorpromazine Hydrochloride (May increase drowsiness effect). Products include:
　Thorazine 2701

Chlorprothixene (May increase drowsiness effect).
　No products indexed under this heading.

Chlorprothixene Hydrochloride (May increase drowsiness effect).
　No products indexed under this heading.

Clorazepate Dipotassium (May increase drowsiness effect). Products include:
　Tranxene 459

Diazepam (May increase drowsiness effect). Products include:
　Dizac (diazepam injectable emulsion) CIV 1862
　Valium Injectable 2336
　Valium Tablets 2335

Droperidol (May increase drowsiness effect). Products include:
　Inapsine Injection 462

Estazolam (May increase drowsiness effect). Products include:
　ProSom Tablets 457

Ethchlorvynol (May increase drowsiness effect). Products include:
　Placidyl Capsules 456

Ethinamate (May increase drowsiness effect).
　No products indexed under this heading.

Fluphenazine Decanoate (May increase drowsiness effect). Products include:
　Prolixin Decanoate 510

Fluphenazine Enanthate (May increase drowsiness effect). Products include:
　Prolixin Enanthate 510

Fluphenazine Hydrochloride (May increase drowsiness effect). Products include:
　Prolixin 510

Flurazepam Hydrochloride (May increase drowsiness effect). Products include:
　Dalmane Capsules 2329

Glutethimide (May increase drowsiness effect).
　No products indexed under this heading.

Haloperidol (May increase drowsiness effect). Products include:
　Haldol Injection, Tablets and Concentrate 1585

Haloperidol Decanoate (May increase drowsiness effect). Products include:
　Haldol Decanoate 1587

Hydroxyzine Hydrochloride (May increase drowsiness effect). Products include:
　Atarax Tablets & Syrup 1992
　Marax Tablets & DF Syrup 2015
　Vistaril Intramuscular Solution 2042

Lorazepam (May increase drowsiness effect). Products include:
　Ativan Injection 2805
　Ativan Tablets 2807

Loxapine Hydrochloride (May increase drowsiness effect). Products include:
　Loxitane 1426

Loxapine Succinate (May increase drowsiness effect). Products include:
　Loxitane Capsules 1426

Meprobamate (May increase drowsiness effect). Products include:
　Miltown Tablets 2780
　PMB 200 and PMB 400 2890

Mesoridazine Besylate (May increase drowsiness effect). Products include:
　Serentil 689

Midazolam Hydrochloride (May increase drowsiness effect). Products include:
　Versed Injection 2324

Molindone Hydrochloride (May increase drowsiness effect). Products include:
　Moban Tablets and Concentrate ... 1036

Oxazepam (May increase drowsiness effect). Products include:
　Serax Capsules 2916
　Serax Tablets 2916

Perphenazine (May increase drowsiness effect). Products include:
　Etrafon 2495
　Triavil Tablets 1800
　Trilafon 2532

Prazepam (May increase drowsiness effect).
　No products indexed under this heading.

Prochlorperazine (May increase drowsiness effect). Products include:
　Compazine 2644

Promethazine Hydrochloride (May increase drowsiness effect). Products include:
　Mepergan Injection 2859
　Phenergan with Codeine 2883
　Phenergan with Dextromethorphan 2885
　Phenergan Injection 2880
　Phenergan Suppositories 2882
　Phenergan Syrup 2881
　Phenergan Tablets 2882
　Phenergan VC 2886
　Phenergan VC with Codeine 2888

Propofol (May increase drowsiness effect). Products include:
　Diprivan Injectable Emulsion 2939

Quazepam (May increase drowsiness effect). Products include:
　Doral Tablets 2773

Secobarbital Sodium (May increase drowsiness effect). Products include:
　Seconal Sodium Pulvules 1529

Temazepam (May increase drowsiness effect). Products include:
　Restoril Capsules 2413

Thioridazine Hydrochloride (May increase drowsiness effect). Products include:
　Mellaril 2398

Thiothixene (May increase drowsiness effect). Products include:
　Navane Capsules and Concentrate 2018
　Navane Intramuscular 2019

Triazolam (May increase drowsiness effect). Products include:
　Halcion Tablets 2093

Trifluoperazine Hydrochloride (May increase drowsiness effect). Products include:
　Stelazine 2692

Zolpidem Tartrate (May increase drowsiness effect). Products include:
　Ambien Tablets 2559

Food Interactions
Alcohol (Increased drowsiness).

NOLAMINE TIMED-RELEASE TABLETS
(Phenindamine Tartrate, Phenylpropanolamine Hydrochloride, Chlorpheniramine Maleate) 790
May interact with monoamine oxidase inhibitors. Compounds in this category include:

Furazolidone (Concurrent therapy contraindicated). Products include:
　Furoxone 2221

Isocarboxazid (Concurrent therapy contraindicated).
　No products indexed under this heading.

Phenelzine Sulfate (Concurrent therapy contraindicated). Products include:
　Nardil 1977

Selegiline Hydrochloride (Concurrent therapy contraindicated). Products include:
　Eldepryl Capsules 2729

IMPORTANT NOTE: Always consult each drug listing in the patient's regimen for possible interactions.

Interactions Index

Tranylcypromine Sulfate (Concurrent therapy contraindicated). Products include:
- Parnate Tablets 2679

NOLVADEX TABLETS
(Tamoxifen Citrate) 2957
May interact with oral anticoagulants, cytotoxic drugs, and certain other agents. Compounds in these categories include:

Bleomycin Sulfate (Increased incidence of thromboembolic events when cytotoxic agents are combined with Nolvadex). Products include:
- Blenoxane 697

Bromocriptine Mesylate (Concomitant therapy has been shown to elevate serum tamoxifen and N-desmethyl-tamoxifen). Products include:
- Parlodel 2411

Daunorubicin Hydrochloride (Increased incidence of thromboembolic events when cytotoxic agents are combined with Nolvadex). Products include:
- Cerubidine for Injection 634

Dicumarol (Increased anticoagulant effect; monitor patient's prothrombin time).
- No products indexed under this heading.

Doxorubicin Hydrochloride (Increased incidence of thromboembolic events when cytotoxic agents are combined with Nolvadex). Products include:
- Adriamycin PFS 2056
- Adriamycin RDF 2056
- Doxil 2613
- Doxorubicin Astra 531
- Rubex for Injection 721

Fluorouracil (Increased incidence of thromboembolic events when cytotoxic agents are combined with Nolvadex). Products include:
- Efudex 2280
- Fluoroplex Topical Solution & Cream 1% 475
- Fluorouracil Injection 2282

Hydroxyurea (Increased incidence of thromboembolic events when cytotoxic agents are combined with Nolvadex). Products include:
- Hydrea Capsules 705

Methotrexate Sodium (Increased incidence of thromboembolic events when cytotoxic agents are combined with Nolvadex). Products include:
- Methotrexate Sodium Tablets, Injection, for Injection and LPF Injection 1322

Mitotane (Increased incidence of thromboembolic events when cytotoxic agents are combined with Nolvadex). Products include:
- Lysodren Tablets 707

Mitoxantrone Hydrochloride (Increased incidence of thromboembolic events when cytotoxic agents are combined with Nolvadex). Products include:
- Novantrone for Injection 1327

Phenobarbital (Concomitant therapy in one patient resulted in lower steady state serum level of tamoxifen). Products include:
- Arco-Lase Plus Tablets 513
- Bellergal-S Tablets 2375
- Donnatal 2234
- Donnatal Extentabs 2234
- Donnatal Tablets 2234
- Phenobarbital Elixir and Tablets ..1523
- Quadrinal Tablets 1398

Procarbazine Hydrochloride (Increased incidence of thromboembolic events when cytotoxic agents are combined with Nolvadex). Products include:
- Matulane Capsules 2300

Vincristine Sulfate (Increased incidence of thromboembolic events when cytotoxic agents are combined with Nolvadex). Products include:
- Oncovin Solution Vials & Hyporets 1521

Warfarin Sodium (Increased anticoagulant effect; monitor patient's prothrombin time). Products include:
- Coumadin 941

NORCURON FOR INJECTION
(Vecuronium Bromide) 1875
May interact with nondepolarizing neuromuscular blocking agents, inhalant anesthetics, aminoglycosides, tetracyclines, and certain other agents. Compounds in these categories include:

Amikacin Sulfate (Possible prolongation of neuromuscular blockade). Products include:
- Amikacin Sulfate Injection, USP 523
- Amikacin Sulfate Injection, USP 981
- Amikin Injectable 502

Atracurium Besylate (Additive effect). Products include:
- Tracrium Injection 1155

Bacitracin (Possible prolongation of neuromuscular blockade).
- No products indexed under this heading.

Cisatracurium Besylate (Additive effect). Products include:
- Nimbex Injection 1131

Colistimethate Sodium (Possible prolongation of neuromuscular blockade).
- No products indexed under this heading.

Colistin Sulfate (Possible prolongation of neuromuscular blockade). Products include:
- Coly-Mycin S Otic w/Neomycin & Hydrocortisone 1965

Demeclocycline Hydrochloride (Possible prolongation of neuromuscular blockade). Products include:
- Declomycin Tablets 1421

Desflurane (Pronounced enhancement of neuromuscular blockade). Products include:
- Suprane (desflurane, USP) ... 1865

Doxycycline Calcium (Possible prolongation of neuromuscular blockade). Products include:
- Vibramycin Calcium Oral Suspension Syrup 2038

Doxycycline Hyclate (Possible prolongation of neuromuscular blockade). Products include:
- Doryx Capsules 1970
- Vibramycin Hyclate Capsules 2038
- Vibramycin Hyclate Intravenous ... 2040
- Vibra-Tabs Film Coated Tablets .. 2038

Doxycycline Monohydrate (Possible prolongation of neuromuscular blockade). Products include:
- Monodox Capsules 1858
- Vibramycin Monohydrate for Oral Suspension 2038

Enflurane (Pronounced enhancement of neuromuscular blockade).
- No products indexed under this heading.

Gentamicin Sulfate (Possible prolongation of neuromuscular blockade). Products include:
- Garamycin Cream 0.1% 2501
- Garamycin Injectable 2502
- Garamycin Ointment 0.1% ... 2501
- Garamycin Ophthalmic 2501

- Genoptic Sterile Ophthalmic Solution .... ◎ 241
- Genoptic Sterile Ophthalmic Ointment .... ◎ 241
- Gentak .... ◎ 209
- Pred-G Liquifilm Sterile Ophthalmic Suspension .... ◎ 248
- Pred-G S.O.P. Sterile Ophthalmic Ointment .... ◎ 249

Halothane (Pronounced enhancement of neuromuscular blockade). Products include:
- Fluothane 2830

Isoflurane (Pronounced enhancement of neuromuscular blockade).
- No products indexed under this heading.

Kanamycin Sulfate (Possible prolongation of neuromuscular blockade).
- No products indexed under this heading.

Magnesium Sulfate Injection (May enhance the neuromuscular blockade).

Methacycline Hydrochloride (Possible prolongation of neuromuscular blockade).
- No products indexed under this heading.

Methoxyflurane (Pronounced enhancement of neuromuscular blockade).
- No products indexed under this heading.

Metocurine Iodide (Additive effect). Products include:
- Metubine Iodide Vials 932

Minocycline Hydrochloride (Possible prolongation of neuromuscular blockade). Products include:
- DYNACIN Capsules 1627
- Minocin Intravenous 1428
- Minocin Oral Suspension 1431
- Minocin Pellet-Filled Capsules ... 1429

Mivacurium Chloride (Additive effect). Products include:
- Mivacron 1125

Neomycin, oral (Possible prolongation of neuromuscular blockade).

Oxytetracycline (Possible prolongation of neuromuscular blockade). Products include:
- Terramycin Intramuscular Solution 2034

Oxytetracycline Hydrochloride (Possible prolongation of neuromuscular blockade). Products include:
- TERAK Ointment .... ◎ 210
- Terra-Cortril Ophthalmic Suspension 2033
- Terramycin with Polymyxin B Sulfate Ophthalmic Ointment ... 2035
- Urobiotic-250 Capsules 2038

Pancuronium Bromide (Additive effect).
- No products indexed under this heading.

Polymyxin B Sulfate (Possible prolongation of neuromuscular blockade). Products include:
- AK-Spore .... ◎ 205
- AK-Trol Ointment & Suspension ... ◎ 205
- Betadine Brand First Aid Antibiotics & Moisturizer Ointment 2144
- Cortisporin Cream 1073
- Cortisporin Ointment 1074
- Cortisporin Ophthalmic Ointment Sterile 1074
- Cortisporin Ophthalmic Suspension Sterile 1075
- Cortisporin Otic Solution Sterile ... 1076
- Cortisporin Otic Suspension Sterile 1077
- Maxitrol Ophthalmic Ointment and Suspension .... ◎ 222
- Mycitracin .... ⊞ 803
- Neosporin G.U. Irrigant Sterile ... 1130
- Neosporin Ointment .... ⊞ 821
- Neosporin Plus Maximum Strength Cream .... ⊞ 821
- Neosporin Plus Maximum Strength Ointment .... ⊞ 822

- Neosporin Ophthalmic Ointment Sterile 1130
- Neosporin Ophthalmic Solution Sterile 1131
- Pediotic Suspension Sterile ..1140
- Poly-Pred Liquifilm .... ◎ 246
- Polysporin Ointment .... ⊞ 822
- Polysporin Ophthalmic Ointment Sterile 1140
- Polysporin Powder .... ⊞ 823
- Polytrim Ophthalmic Solution Sterile 479
- TERAK Ointment .... ◎ 210
- Terramycin with Polymyxin B Sulfate Ophthalmic Ointment ... 2035

Quinidine Gluconate (Possible recurrent paralysis). Products include:
- Quinaglute Dura-Tabs Tablets .. 644

Quinidine Polygalacturonate (Possible recurrent paralysis). Products include:
- Cardioquin Tablets 2146

Quinidine Sulfate (Possible recurrent paralysis). Products include:
- Quinidex Extentabs 2240

Rocuronium Bromide (Additive effect). Products include:
- Zemuron Injection 1885

Streptomycin Sulfate (Possible prolongation of neuromuscular blockade). Products include:
- Streptomycin Sulfate Injection ... 2031

Succinylcholine Chloride (Prior administration may enhance neuromuscular blocking effect and duration of action of Norcuron). Products include:
- Anectine 1062

Tetracycline Hydrochloride (Possible prolongation of neuromuscular blockade). Products include:
- Achromycin V Capsules 1417
- Helidac Therapy 2135

Tobramycin (Possible prolongation of neuromuscular blockade). Products include:
- AKTOB .... ◎ 207
- TobraDex Ophthalmic Suspension and Ointment 469
- Tobrex Ophthalmic Ointment and Solution .... ◎ 226

Tobramycin Sulfate (Possible prolongation of neuromuscular blockade). Products include:
- Nebcin Vials, Hyporets & ADD-Vantage 1518

NORDETTE-21 TABLETS
(Levonorgestrel, Ethinyl Estradiol) .. 2863
May interact with barbiturates and certain other agents. Compounds in these categories include:

Ampicillin Sodium (Reduced efficacy; increased incidence of breakthrough bleeding). Products include:
- Unasyn 2035

Aprobarbital (Reduced efficacy; increased incidence of breakthrough bleeding).
- No products indexed under this heading.

Butabarbital (Reduced efficacy; increased incidence of breakthrough bleeding).
- No products indexed under this heading.

Butalbital (Reduced efficacy; increased incidence of breakthrough bleeding). Products include:
- Axocet Capsules 2469
- Esgic-plus Capsules 1012
- Esgic-plus Tablets 1012
- Fioricet Tablets 2386
- Fioricet with Codeine Capsules .. 2387
- Fiorinal Capsules 2388
- Fiorinal with Codeine Capsules .. 2390
- Fiorinal Tablets 2388
- Phrenilin 790
- Sedapap Tablets 50 mg/650 mg .. 1826

(⊞ Described in PDR For Nonprescription Drugs)   (◎ Described in PDR For Ophthalmology)

Mephobarbital (Reduced efficacy; increased incidence of breakthrough bleeding). Products include:
- Mebaral Tablets ... 2452

Oxytetracycline (Reduced efficacy; increased incidence of breakthrough bleeding). Products include:
- Terramycin Intramuscular Solution 2034

Oxytetracycline Hydrochloride (Reduced efficacy; increased incidence of breakthrough bleeding). Products include:
- TERAK Ointment ... ◉ 210
- Terra-Cortril Ophthalmic Suspension ... 2033
- Terramycin with Polymyxin B Sulfate Ophthalmic Ointment ... 2035
- Urobiotic-250 Capsules ... 2038

Pentobarbital Sodium (Reduced efficacy; increased incidence of breakthrough bleeding). Products include:
- Nembutal Sodium Capsules ... 440
- Nembutal Sodium Solution ... 442
- Nembutal Sodium Suppositories ... 444

Phenobarbital (Reduced efficacy; increased incidence of breakthrough bleeding). Products include:
- Arco-Lase Plus Tablets ... 513
- Bellergal-S Tablets ... 2375
- Donnatal ... 2234
- Donnatal Extentabs ... 2234
- Donnatal Tablets ... 2234
- Phenobarbital Elixir and Tablets ... 1523
- Quadrinal Tablets ... 1398

Phenylbutazone (Reduced efficacy; increased incidence of breakthrough bleeding).
- No products indexed under this heading.

Phenytoin Sodium (Reduced efficacy; increased incidence of breakthrough bleeding). Products include:
- Dilantin Kapseals ... 1965

Rifampin (Reduced efficacy; increased incidence of breakthrough bleeding). Products include:
- Rifadin ... 1276
- Rifamate Capsules ... 1278
- Rifater ... 1280
- Rimactane Capsules ... 865

Secobarbital Sodium (Reduced efficacy; increased incidence of breakthrough bleeding). Products include:
- Seconal Sodium Pulvules ... 1529

Tetracycline Hydrochloride (Reduced efficacy; increased incidence of breakthrough bleeding). Products include:
- Achromycin V Capsules ... 1417
- Helidac Therapy ... 2135

Thiamylal Sodium (Reduced efficacy; increased incidence of breakthrough bleeding).
- No products indexed under this heading.

NORDETTE-28 TABLETS
(Levonorgestrel, Ethinyl Estradiol) ... 2866
See **Nordette-21 Tablets**

NORFLEX INJECTION
(Orphenadrine Citrate) ... 1554
See **Norflex Extended-Release Tablets**

NORFLEX EXTENDED-RELEASE TABLETS
(Orphenadrine Citrate) ... 1554
May interact with:

Propoxyphene Hydrochloride (Concomitant use results in confusion, anxiety and tremors). Products include:
- Darvon ... 1475
- Wygesic Tablets ... 2930

Propoxyphene Napsylate (Concomitant use results in confusion, anxiety and tremors). Products include:
- Darvon-N/Darvocet-N ... 1473

NORGESIC FORTE TABLETS
(Orphenadrine Citrate, Aspirin) ... 1554
See **Norgesic Tablets**

NORGESIC TABLETS
(Orphenadrine Citrate, Aspirin) ... 1554
May interact with:

Propoxyphene Hydrochloride (Potential for confusion, anxiety and tremors). Products include:
- Darvon ... 1475
- Wygesic Tablets ... 2930

Propoxyphene Napsylate (Potential for confusion, anxiety and tremors). Products include:
- Darvon-N/Darvocet-N ... 1473

NORINYL 1+35 21-DAY TABLETS
(Ethinyl Estradiol, Norethindrone) ... 2563
See **Brevicon 21-Day Tablets**

NORINYL 1+35 28-DAY TABLETS
(Norethindrone, Ethinyl Estradiol) ... 2563
See **Brevicon 21-Day Tablets**

NORINYL 1+50 21-DAY TABLETS
(Norethindrone, Mestranol) ... 2563
See **Brevicon 21-Day Tablets**

NORINYL 1+50 28-DAY TABLETS
(Norethindrone, Mestranol) ... 2563
See **Brevicon 21-Day Tablets**

NORISODRINE WITH CALCIUM IODIDE SYRUP
(Calcium Iodide, Isoproterenol Sulfate) ... 446
May interact with monoamine oxidase inhibitors, sympathomimetics, and certain other agents. Compounds in these categories include:

Albuterol (Co-administration with other adrenergic agent produces additive effects). Products include:
- Proventil Inhalation Aerosol ... 2524
- Ventolin Inhalation Aerosol and Refill ... 1170

Albuterol Sulfate (Co-administration with other adrenergic agent produces additive effects). Products include:
- Airet Albuterol Sulfate Inhalation Solution ... 1602
- Albuterol Sulfate, USP Solution for Inhalation, Arm-a-Med ... 522
- Proventil Inhalation Solution 0.083% ... 2527
- Proventil Repetabs Tablets ... 2529
- Proventil Solution for Inhalation 0.5% ... 2525
- Proventil Syrup ... 2528
- Proventil Tablets ... 2529
- Ventolin Inhalation Solution ... 1171
- Ventolin Nebules Inhalation Solution ... 1172
- Ventolin Rotacaps for Inhalation ... 1173
- Ventolin Syrup ... 1175
- Ventolin Tablets ... 1176
- Volmax Extended-Release Tablets ... 1835

Dobutamine Hydrochloride (Co-administration with other adrenergic agent produces additive effects). Products include:
- Dobutrex Solution Vials ... 1480

Dopamine Hydrochloride (Co-administration with other adrenergic agent produces additive effects).
- No products indexed under this heading.

Ephedrine Hydrochloride (Co-administration with other adrenergic agent produces additive effects). Products include:
- Primatene Tablets ... ▣ 844
- Quadrinal Tablets ... 1398

Ephedrine Sulfate (Co-administration with other adrenergic agent produces additive effects). Products include:
- Marax Tablets & DF Syrup ... 2015

Ephedrine Tannate (Co-administration with other adrenergic agent produces additive effects). Products include:
- Rynatuss ... 2782

Epinephrine (Co-administration with other adrenergic agent produces additive effects). Products include:
- EPIFRIN ... ◉ 237
- EpiPen ... 808
- Marcaine with Epinephrine ... 2446
- Primatene Mist ... ▣ 843
- Sensorcaine with Epinephrine Injection ... 554
- Sus-Phrine Injection ... 1017
- Xylocaine with Epinephrine Injections ... 562

Epinephrine Bitartrate (Co-administration with other adrenergic agent produces additive effects). Products include:
- Sensorcaine-MPF with Epinephrine Injection ... 554

Epinephrine Hydrochloride (Co-administration with other adrenergic agent produces additive effects). Products include:
- Ana-Kit Anaphylaxis Emergency Treatment Kit ... 611

Furazolidone (Co-administration may induce hypertensive crisis). Products include:
- Furoxone ... 2221

Isocarboxazid (Co-administration may induce hypertensive crisis).
- No products indexed under this heading.

Isoproterenol Hydrochloride (Co-administration with other adrenergic agent produces additive effects). Products include:
- Isuprel Hydrochloride Solution ... 2443
- Isuprel Injection ... 2441
- Isuprel Mistometer ... 2442

Lithium Carbonate (Concurrant use may enhance the hypothyroid and goitrogenic effects of either drug). Products include:
- Eskalith ... 2658
- Lithium Carbonate Capsules & Tablets ... 2352
- Lithonate/Lithotabs/Lithobid ... 2721

Metaproterenol Sulfate (Co-administration with other adrenergic agent produces additive effects). Products include:
- Alupent ... 672
- Metaproterenol Sulfate Inhalation Solution, USP, Arm-a-Med ... 547

Metaraminol Bitartrate (Co-administration with other adrenergic agent produces additive effects). Products include:
- Aramine Injection ... 1649

Methoxamine Hydrochloride (Co-administration with other adrenergic agent produces additive effects). Products include:
- Vasoxyl Injection ... 1169

Norepinephrine Bitartrate (Co-administration with other adrenergic agent produces additive effects). Products include:
- Levophed Bitartrate Injection ... 2445

Phenelzine Sulfate (Co-administration may induce hypertensive crisis). Products include:
- Nardil ... 1977

Phenylephrine Bitartrate (Co-administration with other adrenergic agent produces additive effects).
- No products indexed under this heading.

Phenylephrine Hydrochloride (Co-administration with other adrenergic agent produces additive effects). Products include:
- Atrohist Plus Tablets ... 1605
- Cerose DM ... ▣ 853
- D.A. II Tablets ... 972
- D.A. Chewable Tablets ... 970
- Dura-Vent/DA Tablets ... 972
- Extendryl ... 1003
- 4-Way Fast Acting Nasal Spray (regular & mentholated) ... ▣ 644
- Hemorid ... ▣ 797
- Hycomine Compound Tablets ... 948
- Neo-Synephrine Hydrochloride 1% Carpuject ... 2455
- Neo-Synephrine Hydrochloride 1% Injection ... 2455
- Neo-Synephrine Hydrochloride (Ophthalmic) ... 2456
- Neo-Synephrine ... ▣ 624
- Novahistine Elixir ... ▣ 782
- Phenergan VC ... 2886
- Phenergan VC with Codeine ... 2888
- Preparation H ... ▣ 842
- Tympagesic Ear Drops ... 2476
- Vicks Sinex Nasal Spray and Ultra Fine Mist ... ▣ 738

Phenylephrine Tannate (Co-administration with other adrenergic agent produces additive effects). Products include:
- Atrohist Pediatric Suspension ... 1604
- Atrohist Pediatric Suspension Dye-Free ... 1604
- Rynatan ... 2781
- Rynatuss ... 2782

Phenylpropanolamine Hydrochloride (Co-administration with other adrenergic agent produces additive effects). Products include:
- Acutrim ... ▣ 648
- Atrohist Plus Tablets ... 1605
- BC Cold Powder Multi-Symptom Formula (Cold-Sinus-Allergy) ... ▣ 631
- BC Cold Powder Non-Drowsy Formula (Cold-Sinus) ... ▣ 631
- Cheracol Plus Head Cold/Cough Formula ... ▣ 741
- Comtrex Multi-Symptom Cold Reliever Liqui-Gels ... ▣ 638
- Comtrex Multi-Symptom Non-Drowsy Liqui-gels ... ▣ 640
- Contac Continuous Action Nasal Decongestant/Antihistamine 12 Hour Capsules ... ▣ 773
- Contac Maximum Strength Continuous Action Decongestant/Antihistamine 12 Hour Caplets ... ▣ 772
- Contac Severe Cold and Flu Formula Caplets ... ▣ 773
- Coricidin 'D' Decongestant Tablets ... ▣ 760
- Dexatrim ... ▣ 795
- Dexatrim Plus Vitamins Caplets ... ▣ 796
- Dimetane-DC Cough Syrup ... 2232
- Dimetapp Allergy Sinus Caplets ... ▣ 838
- Dimetapp Cold & Allergy Chewable Tablets ... ▣ 838
- Dimetapp Cold & Cough Liqui-Gels ... ▣ 839
- Dimetapp DM Elixir ... ▣ 840
- Dimetapp Elixir ... ▣ 840
- Dimetapp Extentabs ... ▣ 841
- Dimetapp Tablets/Liqui-Gels ... ▣ 841
- Dura-Vent Tablets ... 971
- Entex LA Tablets ... 972
- Exgest LA Tablets ... 787
- Hycomine ... 947
- Nolamine Timed-Release Tablets ... 790
- Ornade Spansule Capsules ... 2678
- Propagest Tablets ... 791
- Pyrroxate Caplets ... ▣ 742
- Robitussin-CF ... ▣ 846
- Sinulin Tablets ... 792
- Tavist-D 12 Hour Relief Tablets ... ▣ 750
- Teldrin 12 Hour Antihistamine/Nasal Decongestant Allergy Relief Capsules ... ▣ 786
- Triaminic Expectorant ... ▣ 753
- Triaminic Syrup ... ▣ 755
- Triaminic Triaminicol Cold & Cough ... ▣ 756

IMPORTANT NOTE: Always consult each drug listing in the patient's regimen for possible interactions.

Norisodrine with Calcium Iodide — Interactions Index — 748

Triaminic DM Syrup ... 756
Triaminicin Tablets ... 756
Vicks DayQuil Allergy Relief 12-Hour Extended Release Tablets ... 733
Vicks DayQuil Allergy Relief 4-Hour Tablets ... 733
Vicks DayQuil SINUS Pressure & CONGESTION Relief ... 734

Pirbuterol Acetate (Co-administration with other adrenergic agent produces additive effects). Products include:
Maxair Autohaler ... 1550
Maxair Inhaler ... 1552

Propranolol Hydrochloride (Antagonizes isoproterenol). Products include:
Inderal ... 2834
Inderal LA Long Acting Capsules ... 2836
Inderide Tablets ... 2838
Inderide LA Long Acting Capsules ... 2840

Pseudoephedrine Hydrochloride (Co-administration with other adrenergic agent produces additive effects). Products include:
Actifed Allergy Daytime/Nighttime Caplets ... 808
Actifed Cold & Allergy Tablets ... 807
Actifed Cold & Sinus Caplets and Tablets ... 808
Actifed Sinus Daytime/Nighttime Tablets and Caplets ... 809
Advil Cold and Sinus Caplets and Tablets ... 837
Alka-Seltzer Plus Liqui-Gels ... 612
Alka-Seltzer Plus Flu & Body Aches Liqui-Gels Non-Drowsy Formula ... 613
Alka-Seltzer Plus Night-Time Cold Medicine Liqui-Gels ... 612
Allerest Maximum Strength ... 649
Allerest No Drowsiness ... 649
Allerest Sinus Pain Formula ... 649
Atrohist Pediatric Capsules ... 1603
Benadryl Allergy/Cold Tablets ... 811
Benadryl Allergy Decongestant Liquid Medication ... 812
Benadryl Allergy Decongestant Tablets ... 812
Benadryl Allergy Sinus Headache Caplets ... 813
Benylin Multisymptom ... 816
Bromfed Capsules (Extended-Release) ... 1832
Bromfed Syrup ... 712
Bromfed Tablets ... 1832
Bromfed-DM Cough Syrup ... 1832
Bromfed-PD Capsules (Extended-Release) ... 1832
Children's TYLENOL Cold Multi-Symptom Chewable Tablets and Liquid ... 1559
Children's TYLENOL Cold Plus Cough Multi Symptom Chewable Tablets and Liquid ... 1560
Children's TYLENOL Flu Suspension Liquid ... 1560
Children's Vicks DayQuil Allergy Relief ... 730
Children's Vicks NyQuil Cold/Cough Relief ... 731
Allergy-Sinus Comtrex Multi-Symptom Allergy-Sinus Formula Tablets and Caplets ... 639
Comtrex Multi-Symptom ... 638
Comtrex Multi-Symptom Non-Drowsy Caplets ... 640
Congess ... 1003
Contac Day Allergy/Sinus Caplets ... 771
Contac Day & Night ... 772
Contac Night Allergy/Sinus Caplets ... 771
Contac Severe Cold & Flu Non-Drowsy ... 774
Deconsal II Tablets ... 1605
Dimetane-DX Cough Syrup ... 2233
Dimetapp Cold & Fever Suspension ... 839
Dimetapp Decongestant Pediatric Drops ... 840
Dorcol Children's Cough Syrup ... 748
Drixoral Cough + Congestion Liquid Caps ... 763
Dura-Tap/PD Capsules ... 970
Duratuss Tablets ... 2750
Duratuss HD Elixir ... 2750
Efidac/24 ... 655
Entex PSE Tablets ... 973
Fedahist Gyrocaps ... 2545
Guaifed ... 1833
Guaifed Syrup ... 712
Guaimax-D Tablets ... 809
Histussin D Liquid ... 670
Infants' TYLENOL Cold Decongestant & Fever-Reducer Drops ... 1561
Kronofed-A ... 994
Novahistine DMX ... 782
Nucofed ... 2225
PediaCare Cough-Cold Chewable Tablets and Liquid ... 1569
PediaCare Infants' Decongestant Drops ... 1569
PediaCare Infants' Drops Decongestant Plus Cough ... 1569
PediaCare NightRest Cough-Cold Liquid ... 1569
Pediatric Vicks 44d Cough & Head Congestion Relief ... 736
Pediatric Vicks 44m Cough & Cold Relief ... 737
Robitussin Cold & Cough Liqui-Gels ... 844
Robitussin Cold, Cough & Flu Liqui-Gels ... 844
Robitussin Maximum Strength Cough & Cold ... 847
Robitussin Night-Time Cold Formula ... 847
Robitussin Pediatric Cough & Cold Formula ... 848
Robitussin Pediatric Drops ... 849
Robitussin Severe Congestion Liqui-Gels ... 845
Robitussin-DAC Syrup ... 2249
Robitussin-PE ... 846
Rondec Oral Drops ... 974
Rondec Syrup ... 974
Rondec Tablet ... 974
Rondec Chewable Tablets ... 974
Rondec-TR Tablet ... 974
Ryna ... 804
Seldane-D Extended-Release Tablets ... 1286
Semprex-D Capsules ... 1620
Sinarest ... 663
Sine-Aid Maximum Strength Sinus Headache Gelcaps, Caplets and Tablets ... 1570
Sine-Off No Drowsiness Formula Caplets ... 784
Sine-Off Sinus Medicine ... 784
Singlet Tablets ... 785
Sinutab Non-Drying Liquid Caps ... 823
Sinutab Sinus Allergy Medication, Maximum Strength Tablets and Caplets ... 823
Sinutab Sinus Medication, Maximum Strength Without Drowsiness Formula, Tablets & Caplets ... 824
Sudafed Children's Cold & Cough Liquid Medication ... 825
Sudafed Children's Nasal Decongestant Liquid Medication ... 826
Sudafed Cold & Allergy Tablets ... 826
Sudafed Cold and Cough Liquid Caps ... 826
Sudafed Nasal Decongestant Tablets, 30 mg ... 825
Sudafed Nasal Decongestant Tablets, 60 mg ... 825
Sudafed Non-Drying Sinus Liquid Caps ... 827
Sudafed Pediatric Nasal Decongestant Liquid Oral Drops ... 827
Sudafed Severe Cold Formula Caplets ... 828
Sudafed Severe Cold Formula Tablets ... 828
Sudafed Sinus Caplets ... 829
Sudafed Sinus Tablets ... 829
Sudafed 12 Hour Caplets ... 824
Syn-Rx Tablets ... 1622
Syn-Rx DM Tablets ... 1623
TheraFlu Flu and Cold Medicine ... 750
Theraflu Maximum Strength Flu and Cold Medicine For Sore Throat ... 751
TheraFlu Flu, Cold and Cough Medicine ... 750
TheraFlu Maximum Strength Nighttime Flu, Cold & Cough Medicine ... 751
TheraFlu Maximum Strength Non-Drowsy Formula Flu, Cold & Cough Medicine ... 751
TheraFlu Maximum Strength, Non-Drowsy Formula Flu, Cold and Cough Caplets ... 752
Theraflu Maximum Strength Sinus Non-Drowsy Formula Caplets ... 752
Triaminic AM Cough and Decongestant Formula ... 753
Triaminic AM Decongestant Formula ... 753
Triaminic Infant Oral Decongestant Drops ... 754
Triaminic Night Time ... 754
Triaminic Sore Throat Formula ... 755
Tussend ... 1830
Tussend Expectorant ... 1831
TYLENOL Allergy Sinus, Maximum Strength Caplets and Gelcaps ... 1571
TYLENOL Allergy Sinus NightTime, Maximum Strength Caplets ... 1571
TYLENOL Cold Medication, Multi-Symptom Formula Tablets and Caplets ... 1572
TYLENOL Cold Medication, Multi-Symptom Hot Liquid Packets ... 1572
TYLENOL Cold Medication, No Drowsiness Formula Caplets and Gelcaps ... 1572
TYLENOL Cold Severe Congestion Caplets ... 1573
TYLENOL Cough Medication with Decongestant, Multi Symptom ... 1574
TYLENOL Flu No Drowsiness Formula, Maximum Strength Gelcaps ... 1575
TYLENOL Flu NightTime, Maximum Strength Gelcaps ... 1575
TYLENOL Flu NightTime, Maximum Strength Hot Medication Packets ... 1575
TYLENOL Sinus, Maximum Strength Geltabs, Gelcaps, Caplets and Tablets ... 1576
Vicks 44 LiquiCaps Cough, Cold & Flu Relief ... 728
Vicks 44 LiquiCaps Non-Drowsy Cough & Cold Relief ... 729
Vicks 44D Cough & Head Congestion Relief ... 728
Vicks 44M Cough, Cold & Flu Relief ... 729
Vicks DayQuil LiquiCaps/Liquid Multi-Symptom Cold/Flu Relief ... 734
Vicks DayQuil SINUS Pressure & PAIN Relief with IBUPROFEN ... 735
Vicks Nyquil Hot Therapy ... 735
Vicks NyQuil LiquiCaps/Liquid Multi-Symptom Cold/Flu Relief, Original and Cherry Flavors ... 736

Pseudoephedrine Sulfate (Co-administration with other adrenergic agent produces additive effects). Products include:
Chlor-Trimeton Allergy Decongestant Tablets ... 759
Claritin-D Tablets ... 2487
Drixoral Cold and Allergy Sustained-Action Tablets ... 763
Drixoral Cold and Flu Extended-Release Tablets ... 764
Drixoral Non-Drowsy Formula Extended-Release Tablets ... 764
Drixoral Allergy/Sinus Extended Release Tablets ... 765
Trinalin Repetabs Tablets ... 1373

Salmeterol Xinafoate (Co-administration with other adrenergic agent produces additive effects). Products include:
Serevent Inhalation Aerosol ... 1149

Selegiline Hydrochloride (Co-administration may induce hypertensive crisis). Products include:
Eldepryl Capsules ... 2729

Terbutaline Sulfate (Co-administration with other adrenergic agent produces additive effects). Products include:
Brethaire Inhaler ... 830
Brethine Ampuls ... 832
Brethine Tablets ... 831
Bricanyl Subcutaneous Injection ... 1247
Bricanyl Tablets ... 1248

Tranylcypromine Sulfate (Co-administration may induce hypertensive crisis). Products include:
Parnate Tablets ... 2679

NORMODYNE INJECTION
(Labetalol Hydrochloride) ... 2519
May interact with oral hypoglycemic agents, insulin, tricyclic antidepressants, sympathomimetic bronchodilators, diphenylalkylamine-type calcium antagonists, and certain other agents. Compounds in these categories include:

Acarbose (Beta blockade may prevent the appearance of premonitory signs and symptoms of acute hypoglycemia; additionally, beta blockade reduces the release of insulin in response to hyperglycemia; it may be necessary to adjust the dosage of antidiabetic drugs). Products include:
Precose ... 604

Albuterol (Beta-blocker can blunt the bronchodilator effect of beta-receptor agonists in patients with bronchospasm; greater than normal anti-asthmatic dose of beta-agonist may be required). Products include:
Proventil Inhalation Aerosol ... 2524
Ventolin Inhalation Aerosol and Refill ... 1170

Albuterol Sulfate (Beta-blocker can blunt the bronchodilator effect of beta-receptor agonists in patients with bronchospasm; greater than normal anti-asthmatic dose of beta-agonist may be required). Products include:
Airet Albuterol Sulfate Inhalation Solution ... 1602
Albuterol Sulfate, USP Solution for Inhalation, Arm-a-Med ... 522
Proventil Inhalation Solution 0.083% ... 2527
Proventil Repetabs Tablets ... 2529
Proventil Solution for Inhalation 0.5% ... 2525
Proventil Syrup ... 2528
Proventil Tablets ... 2529
Ventolin Inhalation Solution ... 1171
Ventolin Nebules Inhalation Solution ... 1172
Ventolin Rotacaps for Inhalation ... 1173
Ventolin Syrup ... 1175
Ventolin Tablets ... 1176
Volmax Extended-Release Tablets ... 1835

Amitriptyline Hydrochloride (Potential for tremor). Products include:
Elavil ... 2945
Etrafon ... 2495
Limbitrol ... 2333
Triavil Tablets ... 1800

Amoxapine (Potential for tremor). Products include:
Asendin Tablets ... 1419

Bitolterol Mesylate (Beta-blocker can blunt the bronchodilator effect of beta-receptor agonists in patients with bronchospasm; greater than normal anti-asthmatic dose of beta-agonist may be required). Products include:
Tornalate Solution for Inhalation, 0.2% ... 976
Tornalate Metered Dose Inhaler ... 978

Chlorpropamide (Beta blockade may prevent the appearance of premonitory signs and symptoms of acute hypoglycemia; additionally, beta blockade reduces the release of insulin in response to hyperglycemia; it may be necessary to adjust the dosage of antidiabetic drugs). Products include:
Diabinese Tablets ... 2002

Cimetidine (Increases bioavailability of labetalol). Products include:
Tagamet HB Tablets ... 786
Tagamet Tablets ... 2694

Cimetidine Hydrochloride (Increases bioavailability of labetalol). Products include:
Tagamet ... 2694

(Described in PDR For Nonprescription Drugs) (⊚ Described in PDR For Ophthalmology)

749 **Interactions Index** **Normodyne Injection**

Clomipramine Hydrochloride (Potential for tremor). Products include:

Anafranil Capsules ... 819

Desipramine Hydrochloride (Potential for tremor). Products include:

Norpramin Tablets ... 1273

Doxepin Hydrochloride (Potential for tremor). Products include:

Adapin Capsules ... 1542
Sinequan ... 2028
Zonalon Cream ... 1042

Ephedrine Hydrochloride (Beta-blocker can blunt the bronchodilator effect of beta-receptor agonists in patients with bronchospasm; greater than normal anti-asthmatic dose of beta-agonist may be required). Products include:

Primatene Tablets ... 844
Quadrinal Tablets ... 1398

Ephedrine Sulfate (Beta-blocker can blunt the bronchodilator effect of beta-receptor agonists in patients with bronchospasm; greater than normal anti-asthmatic dose of beta-agonist may be required). Products include:

Marax Tablets & DF Syrup ... 2015

Ephedrine Tannate (Beta-blocker can blunt the bronchodilator effect of beta-receptor agonists in patients with bronchospasm; greater than normal anti-asthmatic dose of beta-agonist may be required). Products include:

Rynatuss ... 2782

Epinephrine (Beta-blocker can blunt the bronchodilator effect of beta-receptor agonists in patients with bronchospasm; greater than normal anti-asthmatic dose of beta-agonist may be required). Products include:

EPIFRIN ... 237
EpiPen ... 808
Marcaine with Epinephrine ... 2446
Primatene Mist ... 843
Sensorcaine with Epinephrine Injection ... 554
Sus-Phrine Injection ... 1017
Xylocaine with Epinephrine Injections ... 562

Epinephrine Hydrochloride (Beta-blocker can blunt the bronchodilator effect of beta-receptor agonists in patients with bronchospasm; greater than normal anti-asthmatic dose of beta-agonist may be required). Products include:

Ana-Kit Anaphylaxis Emergency Treatment Kit ... 611

Ethylnorepinephrine Hydrochloride (Beta-blocker can blunt the bronchodilator effect of beta-receptor agonists in patients with bronchospasm; greater than normal anti-asthmatic dose of beta-agonist may be required).

No products indexed under this heading.

Glimepiride (Beta blockade may prevent the appearance of premonitory signs and symptoms of acute hypoglycemia; additionally, beta blockade reduces the release of insulin in response to hyperglycemia; it may be necessary to adjust the dosage of antidiabetic drugs). Products include:

Amaryl Tablets ... 1241

Glipizide (Beta blockade may prevent the appearance of premonitory signs and symptoms of acute hypoglycemia; additionally, beta blockade reduces the release of insulin in response to hyperglycemia; it may be necessary to adjust the dosage of antidiabetic drugs). Products include:

Glucotrol Tablets ... 2011
Glucotrol XL Extended Release Tablets ... 2012

Glyburide (Beta blockade may prevent the appearance of premonitory signs and symptoms of acute hypoglycemia; additionally, beta blockade reduces the release of insulin in response to hyperglycemia; it may be necessary to adjust the dosage of antidiabetic drugs). Products include:

DiaBeta Tablets ... 1265
Glynase PresTab Tablets ... 2091
Micronase Tablets ... 2099

Halothane (Synergism has been reported between labetalol I.V. and halothane anesthesia; potential increased hypotensive effect, reduction in cardiac output and increase in central venous pressure). Products include:

Fluothane ... 2830

Imipramine Hydrochloride (Potential for tremor). Products include:

Tofranil Ampuls ... 873
Tofranil Tablets ... 875

Imipramine Pamoate (Potential for tremor). Products include:

Tofranil-PM Capsules ... 876

Insulin, Human (Beta blockade may prevent the appearance of premonitory signs and symptoms of acute hypoglycemia; additionally, beta blockade reduces the release of insulin in response to hyperglycemia; it may be necessary to adjust the dosage of insulin).

No products indexed under this heading.

Insulin, Human Isophane Suspension (Beta blockade may prevent the appearance of premonitory signs and symptoms of acute hypoglycemia; additionally, beta blockade reduces the release of insulin in response to hyperglycemia; it may be necessary to adjust the dosage of insulin). Products include:

Novolin N Human Insulin 10 ml Vials ... 1846

Insulin, Human NPH (Beta blockade may prevent the appearance of premonitory signs and symptoms of acute hypoglycemia; additionally, beta blockade reduces the release of insulin in response to hyperglycemia; it may be necessary to adjust the dosage of insulin). Products include:

Humulin N, 100 Units ... 1495
Novolin N PenFill 1.5 ml Cartridges Durable Insulin Delivery System ... 1849
Novolin N Prefilled Syringe Disposable Insulin Delivery System ... 1850

Insulin, Human Regular (Beta blockade may prevent the appearance of premonitory signs and symptoms of acute hypoglycemia; additionally, beta blockade reduces the release of insulin in response to hyperglycemia; it may be necessary to adjust the dosage of insulin). Products include:

Humulin R, 100 Units ... 1497
Novolin R Human Insulin 10 ml Vials ... 1846
Novolin R PenFill 1.5 ml Cartridges Durable Insulin Delivery System ... 1849
Novolin R Prefilled Syringe Disposable Insulin Delivery System ... 1850
Velosulin BR Human Insulin 10 ml Vials ... 1847

Insulin, Human, Zinc Suspension (Beta blockade may prevent the appearance of premonitory signs and symptoms of acute hypoglycemia; additionally, beta blockade reduces the release of insulin in response to hyperglycemia; it may be necessary to adjust the dosage of insulin). Products include:

Humulin L, 100 Units ... 1494
Humulin U, 100 Units ... 1498
Novolin L Human Insulin 10 ml Vials ... 1846

Insulin Lispro, Human (Beta blockade may prevent the appearance of premonitory signs and symptoms of acute hypoglycemia; additionally, beta blockade reduces the release of insulin in response to hyperglycemia; it may be necessary to adjust the dosage of insulin). Products include:

Humalog Injection ... 1488

Insulin, NPH (Beta blockade may prevent the appearance of premonitory signs and symptoms of acute hypoglycemia; additionally, beta blockade reduces the release of insulin in response to hyperglycemia; it may be necessary to adjust the dosage of insulin). Products include:

NPH, 100 Units ... 1502
Pork NPH, 100 Units ... 1506
Purified Pork NPH Isophane Insulin ... 1852

Insulin, Regular (Beta blockade may prevent the appearance of premonitory signs and symptoms of acute hypoglycemia; additionally, beta blockade reduces the release of insulin in response to hyperglycemia; it may be necessary to adjust the dosage of insulin). Products include:

Regular, 100 Units ... 1503
Pork Regular, 100 Units ... 1507
Pork Regular (Concentrated), 500 Units ... 1508
Purified Pork Regular Insulin ... 1852

Insulin, Zinc Crystals (Beta blockade may prevent the appearance of premonitory signs and symptoms of acute hypoglycemia; additionally, beta blockade reduces the release of insulin in response to hyperglycemia; it may be necessary to adjust the dosage of insulin). Products include:

NPH, 100 Units ... 1502

Insulin, Zinc Suspension (Beta blockade may prevent the appearance of premonitory signs and symptoms of acute hypoglycemia; additionally, beta blockade reduces the release of insulin in response to hyperglycemia; it may be necessary to adjust the dosage of insulin). Products include:

Iletin I ... 1501
Lente, 100 Units ... 1501
Iletin II ... 1504
Pork Lente, 100 Units ... 1504
Purified Pork Lente Insulin ... 1852

Isoetharine (Beta-blocker can blunt the bronchodilator effect of beta-receptor agonists in patients with bronchospasm; greater than normal anti-asthmatic dose of beta-agonist may be required). Products include:

Bronkometer Aerosol ... 2432
Bronkosol Solution ... 2432
Isoetharine Inhalation Solution, USP, Arm-a-Med ... 545

Isoproterenol Hydrochloride (Beta-blocker can blunt the bronchodilator effect of beta-receptor agonists in patients with bronchospasm; greater than normal anti-asthmatic dose of beta-agonist may be required). Products include:

Isuprel Hydrochloride Solution ... 2443
Isuprel Injection ... 2441
Isuprel Mistometer ... 2442

Isoproterenol Sulfate (Beta-blocker can blunt the bronchodilator effect of beta-receptor agonists in patients with bronchospasm; greater than normal anti-asthmatic dose of beta-agonist may be required). Products include:

Norisodrine with Calcium Iodide Syrup ... 446

Maprotiline Hydrochloride (Potential for tremor). Products include:

Ludiomil Tablets ... 861

Metaproterenol Sulfate (Beta-blocker can blunt the bronchodilator effect of beta-receptor agonists in patients with bronchospasm; greater than normal anti-asthmatic dose of beta-agonist may be required). Products include:

Alupent ... 672
Metaproterenol Sulfate Inhalation Solution, USP, Arm-a-Med ... 547

Metformin Hydrochloride (Beta blockade may prevent the appearance of premonitory signs and symptoms of acute hypoglycemia; additionally, beta blockade reduces the release of insulin in response to hyperglycemia; it may be necessary to adjust the dosage of antidiabetic drugs). Products include:

Glucophage Tablets ... 754

Nitroglycerin (Reflex tachycardia produced by nitroglycerin blunted). Products include:

Deponit NTG Transdermal Delivery System ... 2541
Nitro-Bid IV ... 1270
Nitro-Bid Ointment ... 1272
Nitro-Dur (nitroglycerin) Transdermal Infusion System ... 1365
Nitrolingual Spray ... 2193
Nitrostat Tablets ... 1981
Transderm-Nitro Transdermal Therapeutic System ... 878

Nortriptyline Hydrochloride (Potential for tremor). Products include:

Pamelor ... 2409

Pirbuterol Acetate (Beta-blocker can blunt the bronchodilator effect of beta-receptor agonists in patients with bronchospasm; greater than normal anti-asthmatic dose of beta-agonist may be required). Products include:

Maxair Autohaler ... 1550
Maxair Inhaler ... 1552

Protriptyline Hydrochloride (Potential for tremor). Products include:

Vivactil Tablets ... 1820

Salmeterol Xinafoate (Beta-blocker can blunt the bronchodilator effect of beta-receptor agonists in patients with bronchospasm; greater than normal anti-asthmatic dose of beta-agonist may be required). Products include:

Serevent Inhalation Aerosol ... 1149

Terbutaline Sulfate (Beta-blocker can blunt the bronchodilator effect of beta-receptor agonists in patients with bronchospasm; greater than normal anti-asthmatic dose of beta-agonist may be required). Products include:

Brethaire Inhaler ... 830
Brethine Ampuls ... 832
Brethine Tablets ... 831

IMPORTANT NOTE: Always consult each drug listing in the patient's regimen for possible interactions.

Normodyne Injection

Bricanyl Subcutaneous Injection 1247
Bricanyl Tablets 1248

Tolazamide (Beta blockade may prevent the appearance of premonitory signs and symptoms of acute hypoglycemia; additionally, beta blockade reduces the release of insulin in response to hyperglycemia; it may be necessary to adjust the dosage of antidiabetic drugs).
No products indexed under this heading.

Tolbutamide (Beta blockade may prevent the appearance of premonitory signs and symptoms of acute hypoglycemia; additionally, beta blockade reduces the release of insulin in response to hyperglycemia; it may be necessary to adjust the dosage of antidiabetic drugs).
No products indexed under this heading.

Trimipramine Maleate (Potential for tremor). Products include:
Surmontil Capsules 2917

Verapamil Hydrochloride (Care should be taken if coadministered; effects of concomitant use not specified). Products include:
Calan SR Caplets 2571
Calan Tablets 2568
Covera-HS Tablets 2573
Isoptin Injectable 1391
Isoptin Oral Tablets 1393
Isoptin SR Tablets 1395
Verelan Capsules 1455

NORMODYNE TABLETS
(Labetalol Hydrochloride) 2522
May interact with oral hypoglycemic agents, tricyclic antidepressants, sympathomimetic bronchodilators, diphenylalkylamine-type calcium antagonists, insulin, and certain other agents. Compounds in these categories include:

Acarbose (Beta blockade may prevent the appearance of premonitory signs and symptoms of acute hypoglycemia; additionally, beta blockade reduces the release of insulin in response to hyperglycemia; it may be necessary to adjust the dosage of antidiabetic drugs). Products include:
Precose 604

Albuterol (Beta-blocker can blunt the bronchodilator effect of beta-receptor agonists in patients with bronchospasm; greater than normal anti-asthmatic dose of beta-agonist may be required). Products include:
Proventil Inhalation Aerosol 2524
Ventolin Inhalation Aerosol and Refill 1170

Albuterol Sulfate (Beta-blocker can blunt the bronchodilator effect of beta-receptor agonists in patients with bronchospasm; greater than normal anti-asthmatic dose of beta-agonist may be required). Products include:
Airet Albuterol Sulfate Inhalation Solution 1602
Albuterol Sulfate, USP Solution for Inhalation, Arm-a-Med 522
Proventil Inhalation Solution 0.083% 2527
Proventil Repetabs Tablets 2529
Proventil Solution for Inhalation 0.5% 2525
Proventil Syrup 2528
Proventil Tablets 2529
Ventolin Inhalation Solution 1171
Ventolin Nebules Inhalation Solution 1172
Ventolin Rotacaps for Inhalation 1173
Ventolin Syrup 1175
Ventolin Tablets 1176
Volmax Extended-Release Tablets .. 1835

Amitriptyline Hydrochloride (Potential for tremor). Products include:
Elavil 2945
Etrafon 2495
Limbitrol 2333
Triavil Tablets 1800

Amoxapine (Potential for tremor). Products include:
Asendin Tablets 1419

Bitolterol Mesylate (Beta-blocker can blunt the bronchodilator effect of beta-receptor agonists in patients with bronchospasm; greater than normal anti-asthmatic dose of beta-agonist may be required). Products include:
Tornalate Solution for Inhalation, 0.2% 976
Tornalate Metered Dose Inhaler 978

Chlorpropamide (Beta blockade may prevent the appearance of premonitory signs and symptoms of acute hypoglycemia; additionally, beta blockade reduces the release of insulin in response to hyperglycemia; it may be necessary to adjust the dosage of antidiabetic drugs). Products include:
Diabinese Tablets 2002

Cimetidine (Increases bioavailability of labetalol). Products include:
Tagamet HB Tablets 786
Tagamet Tablets 2694

Cimetidine Hydrochloride (Increases bioavailability of labetalol). Products include:
Tagamet 2694

Clomipramine Hydrochloride (Potential for tremor). Products include:
Anafranil Capsules 819

Desipramine Hydrochloride (Potential for tremor). Products include:
Norpramin Tablets 1273

Doxepin Hydrochloride (Potential for tremor). Products include:
Adapin Capsules 1542
Sinequan 2028
Zonalon Cream 1042

Ephedrine Hydrochloride (Beta-blocker can blunt the bronchodilator effect of beta-receptor agonists in patients with bronchospasm; greater than normal anti-asthmatic dose of beta-agonist may be required). Products include:
Primatene Tablets 844
Quadrinal Tablets 1398

Ephedrine Sulfate (Beta-blocker can blunt the bronchodilator effect of beta-receptor agonists in patients with bronchospasm; greater than normal anti-asthmatic dose of beta-agonist may be required). Products include:
Marax Tablets & DF Syrup 2015

Ephedrine Tannate (Beta-blocker can blunt the bronchodilator effect of beta-receptor agonists in patients with bronchospasm; greater than normal anti-asthmatic dose of beta-agonist may be required). Products include:
Rynatuss 2782

Epinephrine (Potential for unresponsiveness to the usual dose of epinephrine to treat allergic reaction). Products include:
EPIFRIN 237
EpiPen 808
Marcaine with Epinephrine 2446
Primatene Mist 843
Sensorcaine with Epinephrine Injection 554
Sus-Phrine Injection 1017
Xylocaine with Epinephrine Injections 562

Interactions Index

Epinephrine Hydrochloride (Potential for unresponsiveness to the usual dose of epinephrine to treat allergic reaction). Products include:
Ana-Kit Anaphylaxis Emergency Treatment Kit 611

Ethylnorepinephrine Hydrochloride (Beta-blocker can blunt the bronchodilator effect of beta-receptor agonists in patients with bronchospasm; greater than normal anti-asthmatic dose of beta-agonist may be required).
No products indexed under this heading.

Glimepiride (Beta blockade may prevent the appearance of premonitory signs and symptoms of acute hypoglycemia; additionally, beta blockade reduces the release of insulin in response to hyperglycemia; it may be necessary to adjust the dosage of antidiabetic drugs). Products include:
Amaryl Tablets 1241

Glipizide (Beta blockade may prevent the appearance of premonitory signs and symptoms of acute hypoglycemia; additionally, beta blockade reduces the release of insulin in response to hyperglycemia; it may be necessary to adjust the dosage of antidiabetic drugs). Products include:
Glucotrol Tablets 2011
Glucotrol XL Extended Release Tablets 2012

Glyburide (Beta blockade may prevent the appearance of premonitory signs and symptoms of acute hypoglycemia; additionally, beta blockade reduces the release of insulin in response to hyperglycemia; it may be necessary to adjust the dosage of antidiabetic drugs). Products include:
DiaBeta Tablets 1265
Glynase PresTab Tablets 2091
Micronase Tablets 2099

Halothane (Synergism has been reported between labetalol I.V. and halothane anesthesia; potential increased hypotensive effect, reduction in cardiac output and increased in central venous pressure). Products include:
Fluothane 2830

Imipramine Hydrochloride (Potential for tremor). Products include:
Tofranil Ampuls 873
Tofranil Tablets 875

Imipramine Pamoate (Potential for tremor). Products include:
Tofranil-PM Capsules 876

Insulin, Human (Beta blockade may prevent the appearance of premonitory signs and symptoms of acute hypoglycemia; additionally, beta blockade reduces the release of insulin in response to hyperglycemia; it may be necessary to adjust the dosage of insulin).
No products indexed under this heading.

Insulin, Human Isophane Suspension (Beta blockade may prevent the appearance of premonitory signs and symptoms of acute hypoglycemia; additionally, beta blockade reduces the release of insulin in response to hyperglycemia; it may be necessary to adjust the dosage of insulin). Products include:
Novolin N Human Insulin 10 ml Vials 1846

Insulin, Human NPH (Beta blockade may prevent the appearance of premonitory signs and symptoms of acute hypoglycemia; additionally, beta blockade reduces the release of insulin in response to hyperglycemia; it may be necessary to adjust the dosage of insulin). Products include:
Humulin N, 100 Units 1495
Novolin N PenFill 1.5 ml Cartridges Durable Insulin Delivery System 1849
Novolin N Prefilled Syringe Disposable Insulin Delivery System 1850

Insulin, Human Regular (Beta blockade may prevent the appearance of premonitory signs and symptoms of acute hypoglycemia; additionally, beta blockade reduces the release of insulin in response to hyperglycemia; it may be necessary to adjust the dosage of insulin). Products include:
Humulin R, 100 Units 1497
Novolin R Human Insulin 10 ml Vials 1846
Novolin R PenFill 1.5 ml Cartridges Durable Insulin Delivery System 1849
Novolin R Prefilled Syringe Disposable Insulin Delivery System 1850
Velosulin BR Human Insulin 10 ml Vials 1847

Insulin, Human, Zinc Suspension (Beta blockade may prevent the appearance of premonitory signs and symptoms of acute hypoglycemia; additionally, beta blockade reduces the release of insulin in response to hyperglycemia; it may be necessary to adjust the dosage of insulin). Products include:
Humulin L, 100 Units 1494
Humulin U, 100 Units 1498
Novolin L Human Insulin 10 ml Vials 1846

Insulin Lispro, Human (Beta blockade may prevent the appearance of premonitory signs and symptoms of acute hypoglycemia; additionally, beta blockade reduces the release of insulin in response to hyperglycemia; it may be necessary to adjust the dosage of insulin). Products include:
Humalog Injection 1488

Insulin, NPH (Beta blockade may prevent the appearance of premonitory signs and symptoms of acute hypoglycemia; additionally, beta blockade reduces the release of insulin in response to hyperglycemia; it may be necessary to adjust the dosage of insulin). Products include:
NPH, 100 Units 1502
Pork NPH, 100 Units 1506
Purified Pork NPH Isophane Insulin 1852

Insulin, Regular (Beta blockade may prevent the appearance of premonitory signs and symptoms of acute hypoglycemia; additionally, beta blockade reduces the release of insulin in response to hyperglycemia; it may be necessary to adjust the dosage of insulin). Products include:
Regular, 100 Units 1503
Pork Regular, 100 Units 1507
Pork Regular (Concentrated), 500 Units 1508
Purified Pork Regular Insulin 1852

Insulin, Zinc Crystals (Beta blockade may prevent the appearance of premonitory signs and symptoms of acute hypoglycemia; additionally, beta blockade reduces the release of insulin in response to hyperglycemia; it may be necessary to adjust the dosage of insulin). Products include:
NPH, 100 Units 1502

(■ Described in PDR For Nonprescription Drugs) (◎ Described in PDR For Ophthalmology)

Interactions Index — Noroxin

Insulin, Zinc Suspension (Beta blockade may prevent the appearance of premonitory signs and symptoms of acute hypoglycemia; additionally, beta blockade reduces the release of insulin in response to hyperglycemia; it may be necessary to adjust the dosage of insulin). Products include:

Iletin I	1501
Lente, 100 Units	1501
Iletin II	1504
Pork Lente, 100 Units	1504
Purified Pork Lente Insulin	1852

Isoetharine (Beta-blocker can blunt the bronchodilator effect of beta-receptor agonists in patients with bronchospasm; greater than normal anti-asthmatic dose of beta-agonist may be required). Products include:

Bronkometer Aerosol	2432
Bronkosol Solution	2432
Isoetharine Inhalation Solution, USP, Arm-a-Med	545

Isoproterenol Hydrochloride (Beta-blocker can blunt the bronchodilator effect of beta-receptor agonists in patients with bronchospasm; greater than normal anti-asthmatic dose of beta-agonist may be required). Products include:

Isuprel Hydrochloride Solution	2443
Isuprel Injection	2441
Isuprel Mistometer	2442

Isoproterenol Sulfate (Beta-blocker can blunt the bronchodilator effect of beta-receptor agonists in patients with bronchospasm; greater than normal anti-asthmatic dose of beta-agonist may be required). Products include:

Norisodrine with Calcium Iodide Syrup	446

Maprotiline Hydrochloride (Potential for tremor). Products include:

Ludiomil Tablets	861

Metaproterenol Sulfate (Beta-blocker can blunt the bronchodilator effect of beta-receptor agonists in patients with bronchospasm; greater than normal anti-asthmatic dose of beta-agonist may be required). Products include:

Alupent	672
Metaproterenol Sulfate Inhalation Solution, USP, Arm-a-Med	547

Metformin Hydrochloride (Beta blockade may prevent the appearance of premonitory signs and symptoms of acute hypoglycemia; additionally, beta blockade reduces the release of insulin in response to hyperglycemia; it may be necessary to adjust the dosage of antidiabetic drugs). Products include:

Glucophage Tablets	754

Nitroglycerin (Reflex tachycardia produced by nitroglycerin blunted). Products include:

Deponit NTG Transdermal Delivery System	2541
Nitro-Bid IV	1270
Nitro-Bid Ointment	1272
Nitro-Dur (nitroglycerin) Transdermal Infusion System	1365
Nitrolingual Spray	2193
Nitrostat Tablets	1981
Transderm-Nitro Transdermal Therapeutic System	878

Nortriptyline Hydrochloride (Potential for tremor). Products include:

Pamelor	2409

Pirbuterol Acetate (Beta-blocker can blunt the bronchodilator effect of beta-receptor agonists in patients with bronchospasm; greater than normal anti-asthmatic dose of beta-agonist may be required). Products include:

Maxair Autohaler	1550
Maxair Inhaler	1552

Protriptyline Hydrochloride (Potential for tremor). Products include:

Vivactil Tablets	1820

Salmeterol Xinafoate (Beta-blocker can blunt the bronchodilator effect of beta-receptor agonists in patients with bronchospasm; greater than normal anti-asthmatic dose of beta-agonist may be required). Products include:

Serevent Inhalation Aerosol	1149

Terbutaline Sulfate (Beta-blocker can blunt the bronchodilator effect of beta-receptor agonists in patients with bronchospasm; greater than normal anti-asthmatic dose of beta-agonist may be required). Products include:

Brethaire Inhaler	830
Brethine Ampuls	832
Brethine Tablets	831
Bricanyl Subcutaneous Injection	1247
Bricanyl Tablets	1248

Tolazamide (Beta blockade may prevent the appearance of premonitory signs and symptoms of acute hypoglycemia; additionally, beta blockade reduces the release of insulin in response to hyperglycemia; it may be necessary to adjust the dosage of antidiabetic drugs).

No products indexed under this heading.

Tolbutamide (Beta blockade may prevent the appearance of premonitory signs and symptoms of acute hypoglycemia; additionally, beta blockade reduces the release of insulin in response to hyperglycemia; it may be necessary to adjust the dosage of antidiabetic drugs).

No products indexed under this heading.

Trimipramine Maleate (Potential for tremor). Products include:

Surmontil Capsules	2917

Verapamil Hydrochloride (Care should be taken if coadministered; effects of concomitant use not specified). Products include:

Calan SR Caplets	2571
Calan Tablets	2568
Covera-HS Tablets	2573
Isoptin Injectable	1391
Isoptin Oral Tablets	1393
Isoptin SR Tablets	1395
Verelan Capsules	1455

NOROXIN TABLETS
(Norfloxacin) 1758

May interact with xanthine bronchodilators, oral anticoagulants, iron containing oral preparations, antacids containing aluminium, calcium and magnesium, and certain other agents. Compounds in these categories include:

Aluminum Carbonate (May interfere with absorption resulting in lower serum and urine levels of norfloxacin; antacids should not be administered concomitantly with, or within two hours of, the administration of norfloxacin). Products include:

Basaljel Capsules	2810
Basaljel Suspension	2810
Basaljel Tablets	2810

Aluminum Hydroxide (May interfere with absorption resulting in lower serum and urine levels of norfloxacin; antacids should not be administered concomitantly with, or within two hours of, the administration of norfloxacin). Products include:

ALternaGEL Liquid	1358
Maximum Strength Ascriptin	650
Cama Arthritis Pain Reliever	748
Gaviscon Extra Strength Relief Formula Antacid Tablets	778
Gaviscon Extra Strength Relief Formula Liquid Antacid	779
Gaviscon Liquid Antacid	779
Gelusil Antacid-Anti-gas Liquid	819
Gelusil Antacid-Anti-gas Tablets	819
Maalox Antacid/Anti-Gas Tablets	889
Maalox Heartburn Relief Suspension	658
Maalox Antacid Liquid	888
Extra Strength Maalox Antacid/Anti-Gas Liquid and Tablets	888
Mylanta	1359
Tempo Soft Antacid	799

Aluminum Hydroxide Gel (May interfere with absorption resulting in lower serum and urine levels of norfloxacin; antacids should not be administered concomitantly with, or within two hours of, the administration of norfloxacin). Products include:

ALternaGEL Liquid	675
Aludrox Oral Suspension	850
Amphojel Suspension	2802
Amphojel Suspension without Flavor	2802
Amphojel Tablets	2802
Ascriptin	650
Gaviscon Antacid Tablets	778
Gaviscon-2 Antacid Tablets	779
Mylanta Liquid	676
Mylanta Double Strength Liquid	676
Nephrox Suspension	671

Aminophylline (Co-administration of quinolone with theophylline has resulted in elevated plasma levels of theophylline resulting in theophylline-related side effects).

No products indexed under this heading.

Caffeine (Some quinolones have been shown to interfere with the metabolism of caffeine leading to reduced clearance of caffeine and a prolongation of its plasma half-life). Products include:

Arthritis Strength BC Powder	631
BC Powder	631
Cafergot	2376
DHCplus Capsules	2148
Darvon Compound-65 Pulvules	1475
Esgic-plus Capsules	1012
Esgic-plus Tablets	1012
Aspirin Free Excedrin Analgesic Caplets and Geltabs	734
Excedrin Extra-Strength Analgesic Tablets, Caplets, and Geltabs	734
Fioricet Tablets	2386
Fioricet with Codeine Capsules	2387
Fiorinal Capsules	2388
Fiorinal with Codeine Capsules	2390
Fiorinal Tablets	2388
Goody's Extra Strength Headache Powders	632
Goody's Extra Strength Pain Relief Tablets	632
Maximum Strength Multi-Symptom Formula Midol	621
No Doz Maximum Strength Caplets	644
Norgesic	1554
Vanquish Analgesic Caplets	627
Wigraine Tablets	1884

Cyclosporine (Co-administration has resulted in elevated serum levels of cyclosporine). Products include:

Neoral	2405
Sandimmune	2416

Dicumarol (Co-administration may enhance the effects of oral anticoagulants).

No products indexed under this heading.

Dyphylline (Co-administration of quinolone with theophylline has resulted in elevated plasma levels of theophylline resulting in theophylline-related side effects). Products include:

Lufyllin & Lufyllin-400 Tablets	2778
Lufyllin-GG Elixir & Tablets	2779

Ferrous Fumarate (May interfere with absorption resulting in lower serum and urine levels of norfloxacin; iron containing products should not be administered concomitantly with, or within 2 hours of, the administration of norfloxacin). Products include:

Chromagen Capsules	2470
Chromagen FA	2471
Chromagen Forte	2471
Ferro-Sequels	684
Nephro-Fer Tablets	2168
Nephro-Fer Rx Tablets	2168
Nephro-Vite + Fe Tablets	2170
Stresstabs + Iron	685
Trinsicon Capsules	2759
Vitron-C Tablets	667

Ferrous Gluconate (May interfere with absorption resulting in lower serum and urine levels of norfloxacin; iron containing products should not be administered concomitantly with, or within 2 hours of, the administration of norfloxacin). Products include:

Megadose	513

Ferrous Sulfate (May interfere with absorption resulting in lower serum and urine levels of norfloxacin; iron containing products should not be administered concomitantly with, or within 2 hours of, the administration of norfloxacin). Products include:

Feosol Capsules	777
Feosol Elixir	2627
Feosol Tablets	2627
Fero-Folic-500 Filmtab	433
Fero-Grad-500 Filmtab	434
Fero-Gradumet Filmtab	434
Iberet Tablets	437
Iberet-500 Liquid	438
Iberet-Folic-500 Filmtab	433
Iberet-Liquid	438
Irospan	1000
Slow Fe Tablets	889
Slow Fe with Folic Acid	890

Magaldrate (May interfere with absorption resulting in lower serum and urine levels of norfloxacin; antacids should not be administered concomitantly with, or within two hours of, the administration of norfloxacin).

No products indexed under this heading.

Magnesium Hydroxide (May interfere with absorption resulting in lower serum and urine levels of norfloxacin; antacids should not be administered concomitantly with, or within two hours of, the administration of norfloxacin). Products include:

Aludrox Oral Suspension	850
Ascriptin	650
Di-Gel Antacid/Anti-Gas	762
Gelusil Antacid-Anti-gas Liquid	819
Gelusil Antacid-Anti-gas Tablets	819
Maalox Antacid/Anti-Gas Tablets	889
Maalox Antacid Liquid	888
Extra Strength Maalox Antacid/Anti-Gas Liquid and Tablets	888
Mylanta Fast-Acting	1359
Mylanta Gelcaps Antacid	678
Fast-Acting Mylanta Liquid Antacid	1359
Mylanta Tablets	677
Maximum-Strength Fast-Acting Mylanta Liquid Antacid	1359

IMPORTANT NOTE: Always consult each drug listing in the patient's regimen for possible interactions.

Noroxin **Interactions Index** 752

Mylanta Double Strength Tablets .. ■ 677
Phillips' Milk of Magnesia Liquid .... ■ 627
Rolaids Antacid Tablets ■ 807
Tempo Soft Antacid ■ 799

Magnesium Oxide (May interfere with absorption resulting in lower serum and urine levels of norfloxacin; antacids should not be administered concomitantly with, or within two hours of, the administration of norfloxacin). Products include:
Beelith Tablets 632
Bufferin Analgesic Tablets ■ 636
Arthritis Strength Bufferin Analgesic Caplets ■ 637
Extra Strength Bufferin Analgesic Tablets ■ 637
Caltrate PLUS ■ 681
Cama Arthritis Pain Reliever ■ 748
Mag-Ox 400 666
Uro-Mag 666

Nitrofurantoin (Nitrofurantoin may antagonize the antibacterial effect of norfloxacin in the urinary tract; concurrent use is not recommended). Products include:
Macrodantin Capsules 2140

Polysaccharide-Iron Complex (May interfere with absorption resulting in lower serum and urine levels of norfloxacin; iron containing products should not be administered concomitantly with, or within 2 hours of, the administration of norfloxacin). Products include:
Niferex-150 Capsules 811
Niferex Elixir 811
Niferex-150 Forte Capsules 811
Niferex 811
Niferex-PN Tablets 811
Nu-Iron 150 Capsules 1826
Nu-Iron Elixir 1826

Probenecid (Co-administration with probenecid has resulted in diminished urinary excretion). Products include:
Benemid Tablets 1651
ColBENEMID Tablets 1662

Sucralfate (May interfere with absorption resulting in lower serum and urine levels of norfloxacin; sucralfate should not be administered concomitantly with, or within 2 hours of, administration of norfloxacin). Products include:
Carafate Suspension 1250
Carafate Tablets 1249

Theophylline (Co-administration of quinolone with theophylline has resulted in elevated plasma levels of theophylline resulting in theophylline-related side effects). Products include:
Marax Tablets & DF Syrup 2015
Quibron 2227

Theophylline Anhydrous (Co-administration of quinolone with theophylline has resulted in elevated plasma levels of theophylline resulting in theophylline-related side effects). Products include:
Aerolate 1003
Primatene Tablets ■ 844
Respbid Tablets 687
Slo-bid Gyrocaps 2201
Theo-24 Extended Release Capsules 2753
Theo-Dur Extended-Release Tablets 1367
Theo-X Extended-Release Tablets .. 793
Uni-Dur Extended-Release Tablets .. 1374
Uniphyl 400 mg and 600 mg Tablets 2157

Theophylline Calcium Salicylate (Co-administration of quinolone with theophylline has resulted in elevated plasma levels of theophylline resulting in theophylline-related side effects). Products include:
Quadrinal Tablets 1398

Theophylline Sodium Glycinate (Co-administration of quinolone with theophylline has resulted in elevated plasma levels of theophylline resulting in theophylline-related side effects).
No products indexed under this heading.

Warfarin Sodium (Co-administration may enhance the effects of oral anticoagulants). Products include:
Coumadin 941

Zinc Sulfate (May interfere with absorption resulting in lower serum and urine levels of norfloxacin; zinc containing oral products should not be administered concomitantly with, or within 2 hours of, the administration of norfloxacin). Products include:
Clear Eyes ACR Astringent/Lubricant Eye Redness Reliever Eye Drops ◉ 314
Visine A.C. Seasonal Relief From Pollen and Dust ◉ 301

Food Interactions

Dairy products (Avoid simultaneous ingestion; administer norfloxacin at least one hour before or two hours after milk ingestion).

Food, unspecified (Co-administration may decrease the absorption of norfloxacin; administer at least one hour before or two hours after a meal).

NOROXIN TABLETS
(Norfloxacin) 2222
May interact with xanthine bronchodilators, oral anticoagulants, antacids containing aluminium, calcium and magnesium, iron containing oral preparations, and certain other agents. Compounds in these categories include:

Aluminum Carbonate (May interfere with absorption resulting in lower serum and urine levels of norfloxacin; antacids should not be administered concomitantly with, or within two hours of, the administration of norfloxacin). Products include:
Basaljel Capsules 2810
Basaljel Suspension 2810
Basaljel Tablets 2810

Aluminum Hydroxide (May interfere with absorption resulting in lower serum and urine levels of norfloxacin; antacids should not be administered concomitantly with, or within two hours of, the administration of norfloxacin). Products include:
ALternaGEL Liquid 1358
Maximum Strength Ascriptin ■ 650
Cama Arthritis Pain Reliever ■ 748
Gaviscon Extra Strength Relief Formula Antacid Tablets ■ 778
Gaviscon Extra Strength Relief Formula Liquid Antacid ■ 779
Gaviscon Liquid Antacid ■ 779
Gelusil Antacid-Anti-gas Liquid ■ 819
Gelusil Antacid-Anti-gas Tablets ■ 819
Maalox Antacid/Anti-Gas Tablets 889
Maalox Heartburn Relief Suspension ■ 658
Maalox Antacid Liquid 888
Extra Strength Maalox Antacid/Anti-Gas Liquid and Tablets 888
Mylanta 1359
Tempo Soft Antacid ■ 799

Aluminum Hydroxide Gel (May interfere with absorption resulting in lower serum and urine levels of norfloxacin; antacids should not be administered concomitantly with, or within two hours of, the administration of norfloxacin). Products include:
ALternaGEL Liquid ■ 675
Aludrox Oral Suspension ■ 850
Amphojel Suspension 2802
Amphojel Suspension without Flavor 2802
Amphojel Tablets 2802
Ascriptin ■ 650
Gaviscon Antacid Tablets ■ 778
Gaviscon-2 Antacid Tablets ■ 779
Mylanta Liquid ■ 676
Mylanta Double Strength Liquid .... ■ 676
Nephrox Suspension ■ 671

Aminophylline (Co-administration of quinolone with theophylline has resulted in elevated plasma levels of theophylline resulting in theophylline-related side effects).
No products indexed under this heading.

Caffeine (Some quinolones have been shown to interfere with the metabolism of caffeine leading to reduced clearance of caffeine and a prolongation of its plasma half-life). Products include:
Arthritis Strength BC Powder ■ 631
BC Powder ■ 631
Cafergot 2376
DHCplus Capsules 2148
Darvon Compound-65 Pulvules 1475
Esgic-plus Capsules 1012
Esgic-plus Tablets 1012
Aspirin Free Excedrin Analgesic Caplets and Geltabs 734
Excedrin Extra-Strength Analgesic Tablets, Caplets, and Geltabs 734
Fioricet Tablets 2386
Fioricet with Codeine Capsules 2387
Fiorinal Capsules 2388
Fiorinal with Codeine Capsules 2390
Fiorinal Tablets 2388
Goody's Extra Strength Headache Powders ■ 632
Goody's Extra Strength Pain Relief Tablets ■ 632
Maximum Strength Multi-Symptom Formula Midol ■ 621
No Doz Maximum Strength Caplets ■ 644
Norgesic 1554
Vanquish Analgesic Caplets ■ 627
Wigraine Tablets 1884

Cyclosporine (Co-administration has resulted in elevated serum levels of cyclosporine). Products include:
Neoral 2405
Sandimmune 2416

Dicumarol (Co-administration may enhance the effects of oral anticoagulants).
No products indexed under this heading.

Dyphylline (Co-administration of quinolone with theophylline has resulted in elevated plasma levels of theophylline resulting in theophylline-related side effects). Products include:
Lufyllin & Lufyllin-400 Tablets 2778
Lufyllin-GG Elixir & Tablets 2779

Ferrous Fumarate (May interfere with absorption resulting in lower serum and urine levels of norfloxacin; iron-containing products should not be administered concomitantly with, or within two hours of, the administration of norfloxacin). Products include:
Chromagen Capsules 2470
Chromagen FA 2471
Chromagen Forte 2471
Ferro-Sequels ■ 684
Nephro-Fer Tablets 2168
Nephro-Fer Rx Tablets 2168
Nephro-Vite + Fe Tablets 2170
Stresstabs + Iron ■ 685
Trinsicon Capsules 2759
Vitron-C Tablets ■ 667

Ferrous Gluconate (May interfere with absorption resulting in lower serum and urine levels of norfloxacin; iron-containing products should not be administered concomitantly with, or within two hours of, the administration of norfloxacin). Products include:
Megadose 513

Ferrous Sulfate (May interfere with absorption resulting in lower serum and urine levels of norfloxacin; iron-containing products should not be administered concomitantly with, or within two hours of, the administration of norfloxacin). Products include:
Feosol Capsules ■ 777
Feosol Elixir 2627
Feosol Tablets 2627
Fero-Folic-500 Filmtab 433
Fero-Grad-500 Filmtab 434
Fero-Gradumet Filmtab 434
Iberet Tablets 437
Iberet-500 Liquid 438
Iberet-Folic-500 Filmtab 433
Iberet-Liquid 438
Irospan 1000
Slow Fe Tablets 889
Slow Fe with Folic Acid 890

Magaldrate (May interfere with absorption resulting in lower serum and urine levels of norfloxacin; antacids should not be administered concomitantly with, or within two hours of, the administration of norfloxacin).
No products indexed under this heading.

Magnesium Hydroxide (May interfere with absorption resulting in lower serum and urine levels of norfloxacin; antacids should not be administered concomitantly with, or within two hours of, the administration of norfloxacin). Products include:
Aludrox Oral Suspension ■ 850
Ascriptin ■ 650
Di-Gel Antacid/Anti-Gas ■ 762
Gelusil Antacid-Anti-gas Liquid ■ 819
Gelusil Antacid-Anti-gas Tablets ■ 819
Maalox Antacid/Anti-Gas Tablets 889
Maalox Antacid Liquid 888
Extra Strength Maalox Antacid/Anti-Gas Liquid and Tablets 888
Mylanta Fast-Acting 1359
Mylanta Gelcaps Antacid ■ 678
Fast-Acting Mylanta Liquid Antacid 1359
Mylanta Tablets ■ 677
Maximum-Strength Fast-Acting Mylanta Liquid Antacid 1359
Mylanta Double Strength Tablets .. ■ 677
Phillips' Milk of Magnesia Liquid .... ■ 627
Rolaids Antacid Tablets ■ 807
Tempo Soft Antacid ■ 799

Magnesium Oxide (May interfere with absorption resulting in lower serum and urine levels of norfloxacin; antacids should not be administered concomitantly with, or within two hours of, the administration of norfloxacin). Products include:
Beelith Tablets 632
Bufferin Analgesic Tablets ■ 636
Arthritis Strength Bufferin Analgesic Caplets ■ 637
Extra Strength Bufferin Analgesic Tablets ■ 637
Caltrate PLUS ■ 681
Cama Arthritis Pain Reliever ■ 748
Mag-Ox 400 666
Uro-Mag 666

Nitrofurantoin (Nitrofurantoin may antagonize the antibacterial effect of norfloxacin in the urinary tract; concurrent use is not recommended). Products include:
Macrodantin Capsules 2140

(■ Described in PDR For Nonprescription Drugs) (◉ Described In PDR For Ophthalmology)

Polysaccharide-Iron Complex (May interfere with absorption resulting in lower serum and urine levels of norfloxacin; iron-containing products should not be administered concomitantly with, or within two hours of, the administration of norfloxacin). Products include:

Niferex-150 Capsules	811
Niferex Elixir	811
Niferex-150 Forte Capsules	811
Niferex	811
Niferex-PN Tablets	811
Nu-Iron 150 Capsules	1826
Nu-Iron Elixir	1826

Probenecid (Co-administration with probenecid has resulted in diminished urinary excretion). Products include:

Benemid Tablets	1651
ColBENEMID Tablets	1662

Sucralfate (May interfere with absorption resulting in lower serum and urine levels of norfloxacin; sucralfate should not be administered concomitantly with, or within two hours of, the administration of norfloxacin). Products include:

Carafate Suspension	1250
Carafate Tablets	1249

Theophylline (Co-administration of quinolone with theophylline has resulted in elevated plasma levels of theophylline resulting in theophylline-related side effects). Products include:

Marax Tablets & DF Syrup	2015
Quibron	2227

Theophylline Anhydrous (Co-administration of quinolone with theophylline has resulted in elevated plasma levels of theophylline resulting in theophylline-related side effects). Products include:

Aerolate	1003
Primatene Tablets	844
Respbid Tablets	687
Slo-bid Gyrocaps	2201
Theo-24 Extended Release Capsules	2753
Theo-Dur Extended-Release Tablets	1367
Theo-X Extended-Release Tablets	793
Uni-Dur Extended-Release Tablets	1374
Uniphyl 400 mg and 600 mg Tablets	2157

Theophylline Calcium Salicylate (Co-administration of quinolone with theophylline has resulted in elevated plasma levels of theophylline resulting in theophylline-related side effects). Products include:

Quadrinal Tablets	1398

Theophylline Sodium Glycinate (Co-administration of quinolone with theophylline has resulted in elevated plasma levels of theophylline resulting in theophylline-related side effects).

No products indexed under this heading.

Warfarin Sodium (Co-administration may enhance the effects of oral anticoagulants). Products include:

Coumadin	941

Zinc Sulfate (May interfere with absorption resulting in lower serum and urine levels of norfloxacin; zinc-containing oral products should not be administered concomitantly with, or within two hours of, the administration of norfloxacin). Products include:

Clear Eyes ACR Astringent/Lubricant Eye Redness Reliever Eye Drops	314
Visine A.C. Seasonal Relief From Pollen and Dust	301

Food Interactions

Dairy products (Avoid simultaneous ingestion; administer norfloxacin at least one hour before or two hours after milk ingestion).

Food, unspecified (Co-administration may decrease the absorption of norfloxacin; administer at least one hour before or two hours after a meal).

NORPACE CAPSULES

(Disopyramide Phosphate) 2596
May interact with antiarrhythmics, hepatic microsomal emzyme inducers, and certain other agents. Compounds in these categories include:

Acebutolol Hydrochloride (Excessive widening of QRS complex and prolongation of Q-T interval). Products include:

Sectral Capsules	2914

Adenosine (Excessive widening of QRS complex and prolongation of Q-T interval). Products include:

Adenocard Injection	1021
Adenoscan	1022

Amiodarone Hydrochloride (Excessive widening of QRS complex and prolongation of Q-T interval). Products include:

Cordarone Intravenous	2821
Cordarone Tablets	2818

Bretylium Tosylate (Excessive widening of QRS complex and prolongation of Q-T interval).

No products indexed under this heading.

Carbamazepine (Concurrent administration with hepatic enzyme inducers may lower plasma levels of disopyramide). Products include:

Atretol Tablets	569
Tegretol/Tegretol-XR	870

Chlorpropamide (Concurrent administration with hepatic enzyme inducers may lower plasma levels of disopyramide). Products include:

Diabinese Tablets	2002

Glipizide (Concurrent administration with hepatic enzyme inducers may lower plasma levels of disopyramide). Products include:

Glucotrol Tablets	2011
Glucotrol XL Extended Release Tablets	2012

Glyburide (Concurrent administration with hepatic enzyme inducers may lower plasma levels of disopyramide). Products include:

DiaBeta Tablets	1265
Glynase PresTab Tablets	2091
Micronase Tablets	2099

Lidocaine Hydrochloride (Excessive widening of QRS complex and prolongation of Q-T interval). Products include:

Decadron Phosphate with Xylocaine Injection, Sterile	1683
Unguentine Plus	712
Xylocaine Injections	562

Mexiletine Hydrochloride (Excessive widening of QRS complex and prolongation of Q-T interval). Products include:

Mexitil Capsules	684

Moricizine Hydrochloride (Excessive widening of QRS complex and prolongation of Q-T interval). Products include:

Ethmozine Tablets	2217

Phenobarbital (Concurrent administration with hepatic enzyme inducers may lower plasma levels of disopyramide). Products include:

Arco-Lase Plus Tablets	513
Bellergal-S Tablets	2375
Donnatal	2234
Donnatal Extentabs	2234
Donnatal Tablets	2234
Phenobarbital Elixir and Tablets	1523
Quadrinal Tablets	1398

Phenylbutazone (Concurrent administration with hepatic enzyme inducers may lower plasma levels of disopyramide).

No products indexed under this heading.

Phenytoin (Concurrent administration with hepatic enzyme inducers may lower plasma levels of disopyramide). Products include:

Dilantin Infatabs	1967
Dilantin-125 Suspension	1969

Phenytoin Sodium (Concurrent administration with hepatic enzyme inducers may lower plasma levels of disopyramide). Products include:

Dilantin Kapseals	1965

Procainamide Hydrochloride (Excessive widening of QRS complex and prolongation of Q-T interval). Products include:

Procanbid Extended-Release Tablets	1983

Propafenone Hydrochloride (Excessive widening of QRS complex and prolongation of Q-T interval). Products include:

Rythmol Tablets–150mg, 225mg, 300mg	1399

Propranolol Hydrochloride (Excessive widening of QRS complex and prolongation of Q-T interval). Products include:

Inderal	2834
Inderal LA Long Acting Capsules	2836
Inderide Tablets	2838
Inderide LA Long Acting Capsules	2840

Quinidine Gluconate (Excessive widening of QRS complex and prolongation of Q-T interval). Products include:

Quinaglute Dura-Tabs Tablets	644

Quinidine Polygalacturonate (Excessive widening of QRS complex and prolongation of Q-T interval). Products include:

Cardioquin Tablets	2146

Quinidine Sulfate (Excessive widening of QRS complex and prolongation of Q-T interval). Products include:

Quinidex Extentabs	2240

Rifampin (Concurrent administration with hepatic enzyme inducers may lower plasma levels of disopyramide). Products include:

Rifadin	1276
Rifamate Capsules	1278
Rifater	1280
Rimactane Capsules	865

Sotalol Hydrochloride (Excessive widening of QRS complex and prolongation of Q-T interval). Products include:

Betapace Tablets	637

Tocainide Hydrochloride (Excessive widening of QRS complex and prolongation of Q-T interval). Products include:

Tonocard Tablets	519

Tolazamide (Concurrent administration with hepatic enzyme inducers may lower plasma levels of disopyramide).

No products indexed under this heading.

Tolbutamide (Concurrent administration with hepatic enzyme inducers may lower plasma levels of disopyramide).

No products indexed under this heading.

Verapamil Hydrochloride (Excessive widening of QRS complex and prolongation of Q-T interval; disopyramide should not be administered within 48 hours before or 24 hours after verapamil administration). Products include:

Calan SR Caplets	2571
Calan Tablets	2568
Covera-HS Tablets	2573
Isoptin Injectable	1391
Isoptin Oral Tablets	1393
Isoptin SR Tablets	1395
Verelan Capsules	1455

NORPACE CR CAPSULES

(Disopyramide Phosphate) 2596
See **Norpace Capsules**

NORPLANT SYSTEM

(Levonorgestrel) 2868
May interact with:

Carbamazepine (Reduces efficacy (pregnancy)). Products include:

Atretol Tablets	569
Tegretol/Tegretol-XR	870

Phenytoin (Reduces efficacy (pregnancy)). Products include:

Dilantin Infatabs	1967
Dilantin-125 Suspension	1969

Phenytoin Sodium (Reduces efficacy (pregnancy)). Products include:

Dilantin Kapseals	1965

NORPRAMIN TABLETS

(Desipramine Hydrochloride) 1273
May interact with thyroid preparations, anticholinergics, sympathomimetics, phenothiazines, tranquilizers, hypnotics and sedatives, monoamine oxidase inhibitors, quinidine, antidepressant drugs, barbiturates, and certain other agents. Compounds in these categories include:

Albuterol (Tricyclic antidepressants may potentiate the effects of sympathomimetics; close supervision and careful adjustment of dosage are required). Products include:

Proventil Inhalation Aerosol	2524
Ventolin Inhalation Aerosol and Refill	1170

Albuterol Sulfate (Tricyclic antidepressants may potentiate the effects of sympathomimetics; close supervision and careful adjustment of dosage are required). Products include:

Airet Albuterol Sulfate Inhalation Solution	1602
Albuterol Sulfate, USP Solution for Inhalation, Arm-a-Med	522
Proventil Inhalation Solution 0.083%	2527
Proventil Repetabs Tablets	2529
Proventil Solution for Inhalation 0.5%	2525
Proventil Syrup	2528
Proventil Tablets	2529
Ventolin Inhalation Solution	1171
Ventolin Nebules Inhalation Solution	1172
Ventolin Rotacaps for Inhalation	1173
Ventolin Syrup	1175
Ventolin Tablets	1176
Volmax Extended-Release Tablets	1835

Alprazolam (Co-administration with tranquilizers may produce additive sedative and anticholinergic effects). Products include:

Xanax Tablets	2115

Amitriptyline Hydrochloride (Co-administration with substrates for P450 2D6, such as many other antidepressants, may make normal metabolizers resemble poor metabolizers resulting in higher than expected plasma levels of tricyclic antidepressants). Products include:

Elavil	2945
Etrafon	2495

IMPORTANT NOTE: Always consult each drug listing in the patient's regimen for possible interactions.

Norpramin **Interactions Index** **754**

Limbitrol 2333
Triavil Tablets 1800

Amoxapine (Co-administration with substrates for P450 2D6, such as many other antidepressants, may make normal metabolizers resemble poor metabolizers resulting in higher than expected plasma levels of tricyclic antidepressants). Products include:
Asendin Tablets 1419

Aprobarbital (Barbiturates induce liver enzyme activity and thereby reduce tricyclic antidepressant plasma levels; co-administration may produce additive sedative effects).
No products indexed under this heading.

Atropine Sulfate (Co-administration results in additive anticholinergic effects; close supervision and careful adjustment of dosage are required). Products include:
Arco-Lase Plus Tablets 513
Atrohist Plus Tablets 1605
Donnatal 2234
Donnatal Extentabs 2234
Donnatal Tablets 2234
Lomotil 2591
Motofen Tablets 789
Urised Tablets 2123

Belladonna Alkaloids (Co-administration results in additive anticholinergic effects; close supervision and careful adjustment of dosage are required). Products include:
Bellergal-S Tablets 2375
Hyland's Bedwetting Tablets .... ■ 788
Hyland's EnurAid Tablets .... ■ 789
Hyland's Headache Tablets .... ■ 790
Hyland's Teething Tablets .... ■ 790
Similasan Eye Drops # 1 .... ■ 769

Benztropine Mesylate (Co-administration results in additive anticholinergic effects; close supervision and careful adjustment of dosage are required). Products include:
Cogentin 1661

Biperiden Hydrochloride (Co-administration results in additive anticholinergic effects; close supervision and careful adjustment of dosage are required). Products include:
Akineton 1380

Bupropion Hydrochloride (Co-administration with substrates for P450 2D6, such as many other antidepressants, may make normal metabolizers resemble poor metabolizers resulting in higher than expected plasma levels of tricyclic antidepressants). Products include:
Wellbutrin Tablets 1177

Buspirone Hydrochloride (Co-administration with tranquilizers may produce additive sedative and anticholinergic effects). Products include:
BuSpar Tablets 738

Butabarbital (Barbiturates induce liver enzyme activity and thereby reduce tricyclic antidepressant plasma levels; co-administration may produce additive sedative effects).
No products indexed under this heading.

Butalbital (Barbiturates induce liver enzyme activity and thereby reduce tricyclic antidepressant plasma levels; co-administration may produce additive sedative effects). Products include:
Axocet Capsules 2469
Esgic-plus Capsules 1012
Esgic-plus Tablets 1012
Fioricet Tablets 2386
Fioricet with Codeine Capsules 2387
Fiorinal Capsules 2388
Fiorinal with Codeine Capsules 2390
Fiorinal Tablets 2388
Phrenilin 790
Sedapap Tablets 50 mg/650 mg .. 1826

Chlordiazepoxide (Co-administration with tranquilizers may produce additive sedative and anticholinergic effects). Products include:
Limbitrol 2333

Chlordiazepoxide Hydrochloride (Co-administration with tranquilizers may produce additive sedative and anticholinergic effects). Products include:
Librax Capsules 2330
Librium Capsules 2331
Librium Injectable 2332

Chlorpromazine (Phenothiazines are substrates for P450 2D6 and co-administration may make normal metabolizers resemble poor metabolizers resulting in higher than expected plasma levels of tricyclic antidepressants; co-administration with major tranquilizers may produce additive sedative and anticholinergic effects). Products include:
Thorazine Suppositories 2701

Chlorpromazine Hydrochloride (Phenothiazines are substrates for P450 2D6 and co-administration may make normal metabolizers resemble poor metabolizers resulting in higher than expected plasma levels of tricyclic antidepressants; co-administration with major tranquilizers may produce additive sedative and anticholinergic effects). Products include:
Thorazine 2701

Chlorprothixene (Co-administration with major tranquilizers may produce additive sedative and anticholinergic effects).
No products indexed under this heading.

Chlorprothixene Hydrochloride (Co-administration with major tranquilizers may produce additive sedative and anticholinergic effects).
No products indexed under this heading.

Cimetidine (Concurrent administration can produce clinically significant increase in the plasma concentrations of the tricyclic antidepressants through competition for the same metabolic enzyme systems; decreases in plasma levels of the TCA have been reported upon discontinuation of cimetidine, which may result in the loss of the therapeutic efficacy of TCA). Products include:
Tagamet HB Tablets .... ■ 786
Tagamet Tablets 2694

Cimetidine Hydrochloride (Concurrent administration can produce clinically significant increase in the plasma concentrations of the tricyclic antidepressants through competition for the same metabolic enzyme systems; decreases in plasma levels of the TCA have been reported upon discontinuation of cimetidine, which may result in the loss of the therapeutic efficacy of TCA). Products include:
Tagamet 2694

Clidinium Bromide (Co-administration results in additive anticholinergic effects; close supervision and careful adjustment of dosage are required). Products include:
Librax Capsules 2330

Clonidine (Desipramine may block the antihypertensive effects). Products include:
Catapres-TTS 680

Clonidine Hydrochloride (Desipramine may block the antihypertensive effects). Products include:
Catapres Tablets 679
Combipres Tablets 682

Clorazepate Dipotassium (Co-administration with tranquilizers may produce additive sedative and anticholinergic effects). Products include:
Tranxene 459

Diazepam (Co-administration with tranquilizers may produce additive sedative and anticholinergic effects). Products include:
Dizac (diazepam injectable emulsion) CIV 1862
Valium Injectable 2336
Valium Tablets 2335

Dicyclomine Hydrochloride (Co-administration results in additive anticholinergic effects; close supervision and careful adjustment of dosage are required). Products include:
Bentyl 1246

Dobutamine Hydrochloride (Tricyclic antidepressants may potentiate the effects of sympathomimetics; close supervision and careful adjustment of dosage are required). Products include:
Dobutrex Solution Vials 1480

Dopamine Hydrochloride (Tricyclic antidepressants may potentiate the effects of sympathomimetics; close supervision and careful adjustment of dosage are required).
No products indexed under this heading.

Doxepin Hydrochloride (Co-administration with substrates for P450 2D6, such as many other antidepressants, may make normal metabolizers resemble poor metabolizers resulting in higher than expected plasma levels of tricyclic antidepressants). Products include:
Adapin Capsules 1542
Sinequan 2028
Zonalon Cream 1042

Droperidol (Co-administration with tranquilizers may produce additive sedative and anticholinergic effects). Products include:
Inapsine Injection 462

Ephedrine Hydrochloride (Tricyclic antidepressants may potentiate the effects of sympathomimetics; close supervision and careful adjustment of dosage are required). Products include:
Primatene Tablets .... ■ 844
Quadrinal Tablets 1398

Ephedrine Sulfate (Tricyclic antidepressants may potentiate the effects of sympathomimetics; close supervision and careful adjustment of dosage are required). Products include:
Marax Tablets & DF Syrup 2015

Ephedrine Tannate (Tricyclic antidepressants may potentiate the effects of sympathomimetics; close supervision and careful adjustment of dosage are required). Products include:
Rynatuss 2782

Epinephrine (Tricyclic antidepressants may potentiate the effects of sympathomimetics; close supervision and careful adjustment of dosage are required). Products include:
EPIFRIN .... ◉ 237
EpiPen 808
Marcaine with Epinephrine 2446
Primatene Mist .... ■ 843
Sensorcaine with Epinephrine Injection 554
Sus-Phrine Injection 1017
Xylocaine with Epinephrine Injections 562

Epinephrine Bitartrate (Tricyclic antidepressants may potentiate the effects of sympathomimetics; close supervision and careful adjustment of dosage are required). Products include:
Sensorcaine-MPF with Epinephrine Injection 554

Epinephrine Hydrochloride (Tricyclic antidepressants may potentiate the effects of sympathomimetics; close supervision and careful adjustment of dosage are required). Products include:
Ana-Kit Anaphylaxis Emergency Treatment Kit 611

Estazolam (Co-administration may produce additive sedative effects). Products include:
ProSom Tablets 457

Ethchlorvynol (Co-administration may produce additive sedative effects). Products include:
Placidyl Capsules 456

Ethinamate (Co-administration may produce additive sedative effects).
No products indexed under this heading.

Flecainide Acetate (Co-administration with substrates for P450 2D6, such as flecainide, may make normal metabolizers resemble poor metabolizers resulting in higher than expected plasma levels of tricyclic antidepressants). Products include:
Tambocor Tablets 1555

Fluoxetine Hydrochloride (Selective serotonin reuptake inhibitors, such as fluoxetine, may have variable extent of inhibition of P450 2D6; potential for higher than expected plasma levels of tricyclic antidepressants; due to long half-life of fluoxetine, at least 5 weeks should elapse before initiating TCA treatment in a patient being withdrawn from fluoxetine). Products include:
Prozac Pulvules & Liquid, Oral Solution 935

Fluphenazine Decanoate (Phenothiazines are substrates for P450 2D6 and co-administration may make normal metabolizers resemble poor metabolizers resulting in higher than expected plasma levels of tricyclic antidepressants; co-administration with major tranquilizers may produce additive sedative and anticholinergic effects). Products include:
Prolixin Decanoate 510

Fluphenazine Enanthate (Phenothiazines are substrates for P450 2D6 and co-administration may make normal metabolizers resemble poor metabolizers resulting in higher than expected plasma levels of tricyclic antidepressants; co-administration with major tranquilizers may produce additive sedative and anticholinergic effects). Products include:
Prolixin Enanthate 510

Fluphenazine Hydrochloride (Phenothiazines are substrates for P450 2D6 and co-administration may make normal metabolizers resemble poor metabolizers resulting in higher than expected plasma levels of tricyclic antidepressants; co-administration with major tranquilizers may produce additive sedative and anticholinergic effects). Products include:
Prolixin 510

(■ Described in PDR For Nonprescription Drugs) (◉ Described in PDR For Ophthalmology)

Flurazepam Hydrochloride (Co-administration may produce additive sedative effects). Products include:
 Dalmane Capsules 2329
Furazolidone (Co-administration of tricyclic antidepressants and MAO inhibitor has produced hyperpyretic crises, severe convulsions, and deaths; concurrent and/or sequential use is contraindicated). Products include:
 Furoxone 2221
Glutethimide (Co-administration may produce additive sedative effects).
 No products indexed under this heading.
Glycopyrrolate (Co-administration results in additive anticholinergic effects; close supervision and careful adjustment of dosage are required). Products include:
 Robinul Forte Tablets 2247
 Robinul Injectable 2247
 Robinul Tablets 2247
Guanadrel Sulfate (Desipramine may block the antihypertensive effects). Products include:
 Hylorel Tablets 1613
Guanethidine Monosulfate (Desipramine may block the antihypertensive effects). Products include:
 Esimil Tablets 840
 Ismelin Tablets 845
Haloperidol (Co-administration with major tranquilizers may produce additive sedative and anticholinergic effects). Products include:
 Haldol Injection, Tablets and Concentrate 1585
Haloperidol Decanoate (Co-administration with major tranquilizers may produce additive sedative and anticholinergic effects). Products include:
 Haldol Decanoate 1587
Hydroxyzine Hydrochloride (Co-administration with tranquilizers may produce additive sedative and anticholinergic effects). Products include:
 Atarax Tablets & Syrup 1992
 Marax Tablets & DF Syrup 2015
 Vistaril Intramuscular Solution 2042
Hyoscyamine (Co-administration results in additive anticholinergic effects; close supervision and careful adjustment of dosage are required). Products include:
 Cystospaz Tablets 2123
 Urised Tablets 2123
Hyoscyamine Sulfate (Co-administration results in additive anticholinergic effects; close supervision and careful adjustment of dosage are required). Products include:
 Arco-Lase Plus Tablets 513
 Atrohist Plus Tablets 1605
 Cystospaz-M Capsules 2123
 Donnatal 2234
 Donnatal Extentabs 2234
 Donnatal Tablets 2234
 Kutrase Capsules 2546
 Levsin/Levsinex/Levbid 2549
Imipramine Hydrochloride (Co-administration with substrates for P450 2D6, such as many other antidepressants, may make normal metabolizers resemble poor metabolizers resulting in higher than expected plasma levels of tricyclic antidepressants). Products include:
 Tofranil Ampuls 873
 Tofranil Tablets 875

Imipramine Pamoate (Co-administration with substrates for P450 2D6, such as many other antidepressants, may make normal metabolizers resemble poor metabolizers resulting in higher than expected plasma levels of tricyclic antidepressants). Products include:
 Tofranil-PM Capsules 876
Ipratropium Bromide (Co-administration results in additive anticholinergic effects; close supervision and careful adjustment of dosage are required). Products include:
 Atrovent Inhalation Aerosol 674
 Atrovent Inhalation Solution 675
 Atrovent Nasal Spray 0.03% 676
 Atrovent Nasal Spray 0.06% 678
Isocarboxazid (Co-administration of tricyclic antidepressants and MAO inhibitor has produced hyperpyretic crises, severe convulsions, and deaths; concurrent and/or sequential use is contraindicated).
 No products indexed under this heading.
Isoproterenol Hydrochloride (Tricyclic antidepressants may potentiate the effects of sympathomimetics; close supervision and careful adjustment of dosage are required). Products include:
 Isuprel Hydrochloride Solution ... 2443
 Isuprel Injection 2441
 Isuprel Mistometer 2442
Isoproterenol Sulfate (Tricyclic antidepressants may potentiate the effects of sympathomimetics; close supervision and careful adjustment of dosage are required). Products include:
 Norisodrine with Calcium Iodide Syrup 446
Levothyroxine Sodium (Co-administration with thyroid medications may increase the possibility of cardiovascular toxicity, including arrhythmias). Products include:
 Eltroxin Tablets 2214
 Levothroid Tablets 1015
 Levothyroxine Sodium, USP for Injection 546
 Levoxyl Tablets 918
 Synthroid 1410
Liothyronine Sodium (Co-administration with thyroid medications may increase the possibility of cardiovascular toxicity, including arrhythmias). Products include:
 Cytomel Tablets 2647
 Triostat Injection 2708
Liotrix (Co-administration with thyroid medications may increase the possibility of cardiovascular toxicity, including arrhythmias).
 No products indexed under this heading.
Lorazepam (Co-administration with tranquilizers may produce additive sedative and anticholinergic effects). Products include:
 Ativan Injection 2805
 Ativan Tablets 2807
Loxapine Hydrochloride (Co-administration with major tranquilizers may produce additive sedative and anticholinergic effects). Products include:
 Loxitane 1426
Loxapine Succinate (Co-administration with major tranquilizers may produce additive sedative and anticholinergic effects). Products include:
 Loxitane Capsules 1426

Maprotiline Hydrochloride (Co-administration with substrates for P450 2D6, such as many other antidepressants, may make normal metabolizers resemble poor metabolizers resulting in higher than expected plasma levels of tricyclic antidepressants). Products include:
 Ludiomil Tablets 861
Mepenzolate Bromide (Co-administration results in additive anticholinergic effects; close supervision and careful adjustment of dosage are required).
 No products indexed under this heading.
Mephobarbital (Barbiturates induce liver enzyme activity and thereby reduce tricyclic antidepressant plasma levels; co-administration may produce additive sedative effects). Products include:
 Mebaral Tablets 2452
Meprobamate (Co-administration with tranquilizers may produce additive sedative and anticholinergic effects). Products include:
 Miltown Tablets 2780
 PMB 200 and PMB 400 2890
Mesoridazine Besylate (Phenothiazines are substrates for P450 2D6 and co-administration may make normal metabolizers resemble poor metabolizers resulting in higher than expected plasma levels of tricyclic antidepressants; co-administration with major tranquilizers may produce additive sedative and anticholinergic effects). Products include:
 Serentil 689
Metaproterenol Sulfate (Tricyclic antidepressants may potentiate the effects of sympathomimetics; close supervision and careful adjustment of dosage are required). Products include:
 Alupent 672
 Metaproterenol Sulfate Inhalation Solution, USP, Arm-a-Med 547
Metaraminol Bitartrate (Tricyclic antidepressants may potentiate the effects of sympathomimetics; close supervision and careful adjustment of dosage are required). Products include:
 Aramine Injection 1649
Methotrimeprazine (Phenothiazines are substrates for P450 2D6 and co-administration may make normal metabolizers resemble poor metabolizers resulting in higher than expected plasma levels of tricyclic antidepressants; co-administration with major tranquilizers may produce additive sedative and anticholinergic effects). Products include:
 Levoprome 1321
Methoxamine Hydrochloride (Tricyclic antidepressants may potentiate the effects of sympathomimetics; close supervision and careful adjustment of dosage are required). Products include:
 Vasoxyl Injection 1169
Midazolam Hydrochloride (Co-administration may produce additive sedative effects). Products include:
 Versed Injection 2324
Mirtazapine (Co-administration with substrates for P450 2D6, such as many other antidepressants, may make normal metabolizers resemble poor metabolizers resulting in higher than expected plasma levels of tricyclic antidepressants). Products include:
 Remeron Tablets 1878

Molindone Hydrochloride (Co-administration with major tranquilizers may produce additive sedative and anticholinergic effects). Products include:
 Moban Tablets and Concentrate 1036
Nefazodone Hydrochloride (Co-administration with substrates for P450 2D6, such as many other antidepressants, may make normal metabolizers resemble poor metabolizers resulting in higher than expected plasma levels of tricyclic antidepressants). Products include:
 Serzone Tablets 776
Norepinephrine Bitartrate (Tricyclic antidepressants may potentiate the effects of sympathomimetics; close supervision and careful adjustment of dosage are required). Products include:
 Levophed Bitartrate Injection 2445
Nortriptyline Hydrochloride (Co-administration with substrates for P450 2D6, such as many other antidepressants, may make normal metabolizers resemble poor metabolizers resulting in higher than expected plasma levels of tricyclic antidepressants). Products include:
 Pamelor 2409
Oxazepam (Co-administration with tranquilizers may produce additive sedative and anticholinergic effects). Products include:
 Serax Capsules 2916
 Serax Tablets 2916
Oxybutynin Chloride (Co-administration results in additive anticholinergic effects; close supervision and careful adjustment of dosage are required). Products include:
 Ditropan 1267
Paroxetine Hydrochloride (Selective serotonin reuptake inhibitors, such as paroxetine, may have variable extent of inhibition of P450 2D6; potential for higher than expected plasma levels of tricyclic antidepressants). Products include:
 Paxil Tablets 2681
Pentobarbital Sodium (Barbiturates induce liver enzyme activity and thereby reduce tricyclic antidepressant plasma levels; co-administration may produce additive sedative effects). Products include:
 Nembutal Sodium Capsules 440
 Nembutal Sodium Solution 442
 Nembutal Sodium Suppositories 444
Perphenazine (Phenothiazines are substrates for P450 2D6 and co-administration may make normal metabolizers resemble poor metabolizers resulting in higher than expected plasma levels of tricyclic antidepressants; co-administration with major tranquilizers may produce additive sedative and anticholinergic effects). Products include:
 Etrafon 2495
 Triavil Tablets 1800
 Trilafon 2532
Phenelzine Sulfate (Co-administration of tricyclic antidepressants and MAO inhibitor has produced hyperpyretic crises, severe convulsions, and deaths; concurrent and/or sequential use is contraindicated). Products include:
 Nardil 1977
Phenobarbital (Barbiturates induce liver enzyme activity and thereby reduce tricyclic antidepressant plasma levels; co-administration may produce additive sedative effects). Products include:
 Arco-Lase Plus Tablets 513

IMPORTANT NOTE: Always consult each drug listing in the patient's regimen for possible interactions.

Norpramin Interactions Index 756

Bellergal-S Tablets ... 2375
Donnatal ... 2234
Donnatal Extentabs ... 2234
Donnatal Tablets ... 2234
Phenobarbital Elixir and Tablets ... 1523
Quadrinal Tablets ... 1398

Phenylephrine Bitartrate (Tricyclic antidepressants may potentiate the effects of sympathomimetics; close supervision and careful adjustment of dosage are required).
No products indexed under this heading.

Phenylephrine Hydrochloride (Tricyclic antidepressants may potentiate the effects of sympathomimetics; close supervision and careful adjustment of dosage are required). Products include:
Atrohist Plus Tablets ... 1605
Cerose DM ... ▣ 853
D.A. II Tablets ... 972
D.A. Chewable Tablets ... 970
Dura-Vent/DA Tablets ... 972
Extendryl ... 1003
4-Way Fast Acting Nasal Spray (regular & mentholated) ... ▣ 644
Hemorid ... ▣ 797
Hycomine Compound Tablets ... 948
Neo-Synephrine Hydrochloride 1% Carpuject ... 2455
Neo-Synephrine Hydrochloride 1% Injection ... 2455
Neo-Synephrine Hydrochloride (Ophthalmic) ... 2456
Neo-Synephrine ... ▣ 624
Novahistine Elixir ... ▣ 782
Phenergan VC ... 2886
Phenergan VC with Codeine ... 2888
Preparation H ... ▣ 842
Tympagesic Ear Drops ... 2476
Vicks Sinex Nasal Spray and Ultra Fine Mist ... ▣ 738

Phenylephrine Tannate (Tricyclic antidepressants may potentiate the effects of sympathomimetics; close supervision and careful adjustment of dosage are required). Products include:
Atrohist Pediatric Suspension ... 1604
Atrohist Pediatric Suspension Dye-Free ... 1604
Rynatan ... 2781
Rynatuss ... 2782

Phenylpropanolamine Hydrochloride (Tricyclic antidepressants may potentiate the effects of sympathomimetics; close supervision and careful adjustment of dosage are required). Products include:
Acutrim ... ▣ 648
Atrohist Plus Tablets ... 1605
BC Cold Powder Multi-Symptom Formula (Cold-Sinus-Allergy) ... ▣ 631
BC Cold Powder Non-Drowsy Formula (Cold-Sinus) ... ▣ 631
Cheracol Plus Head Cold/Cough Formula ... ▣ 741
Comtrex Multi-Symptom Cold Reliever Liqui-Gels ... ▣ 638
Comtrex Multi-Symptom Non-Drowsy Liqui-gels ... ▣ 640
Contac Continuous Action Nasal Decongestant/Antihistamine 12 Hour Capsules ... ▣ 773
Contac Maximum Strength Continuous Action Decongestant/Antihistamine 12 Hour Caplets ... ▣ 772
Contac Severe Cold and Flu Formula Caplets ... ▣ 773
Coricidin 'D' Decongestant Tablets ... ▣ 760
Dexatrim ... ▣ 795
Dexatrim Plus Vitamins Caplets ... ▣ 796
Dimetane-DC Cough Syrup ... 2232
Dimetapp Allergy Sinus Caplets ... ▣ 838
Dimetapp Cold & Allergy Chewable Tablets ... ▣ 838
Dimetapp Cold & Cough Liqui-Gels ... ▣ 839
Dimetapp DM Elixir ... ▣ 840
Dimetapp Elixir ... ▣ 840
Dimetapp Extentabs ... ▣ 841
Dimetapp Tablets/Liqui-Gels ... ▣ 841
Dura-Vent Tablets ... 971
Entex LA Tablets ... 972
Exgest LA Tablets ... 787
Hycomine ... 947
Nolamine Timed-Release Tablets ... 790
Ornade Spansule Capsules ... 2678
Propagest Tablets ... 791
Pyrroxate Caplets ... ▣ 742
Robitussin-CF ... ▣ 846
Sinulin Tablets ... 792
Tavist-D 12 Hour Relief Tablets ... ▣ 750
Teldrin 12 Hour Antihistamine/Nasal Decongestant Allergy Relief Capsules ... ▣ 786
Triaminic Expectorant ... ▣ 753
Triaminic Syrup ... ▣ 755
Triaminic Triaminicol Cold & Cough ... ▣ 756
Triaminic DM Syrup ... ▣ 756
Triaminicin Tablets ... ▣ 756
Vicks DayQuil Allergy Relief 12-Hour Extended Release Tablets ... ▣ 733
Vicks DayQuil Allergy Relief 4-Hour Tablets ... ▣ 733
Vicks DayQuil SINUS Pressure & CONGESTION Relief ... ▣ 734

Pirbuterol Acetate (Tricyclic antidepressants may potentiate the effects of sympathomimetics; close supervision and careful adjustment of dosage are required). Products include:
Maxair Autohaler ... 1550
Maxair Inhaler ... 1552

Prazepam (Co-administration with tranquilizers may produce additive sedative and anticholinergic effects).
No products indexed under this heading.

Prochlorperazine (Phenothiazines are substrates for P450 2D6 and co-administration may make normal metabolizers resemble poor metabolizers resulting in higher than expected plasma levels of tricyclic antidepressants; co-administration with major tranquilizers may produce additive sedative and anticholinergic effects). Products include:
Compazine ... 2644

Procyclidine Hydrochloride (Co-administration results in additive anticholinergic effects; close supervision and careful adjustment of dosage are required). Products include:
Kemadrin Tablets ... 1105

Promethazine Hydrochloride (Phenothiazines are substrates for P450 2D6 and co-administration may make normal metabolizers resemble poor metabolizers resulting in higher than expected plasma levels of tricyclic antidepressants; co-administration with major tranquilizers may produce additive sedative and anticholinergic effects). Products include:
Mepergan Injection ... 2859
Phenergan with Codeine ... 2883
Phenergan with Dextromethorphan ... 2885
Phenergan Injection ... 2880
Phenergan Suppositories ... 2882
Phenergan Syrup ... 2881
Phenergan Tablets ... 2882
Phenergan VC ... 2886
Phenergan VC with Codeine ... 2888

Propafenone Hydrochloride (Co-administration with substrates for P450 2D6, such as propafenone, may make normal metabolizers resemble poor metabolizers resulting in higher than expected plasma levels of tricyclic antidepressants). Products include:
Rythmol Tablets–150mg, 225mg, 300mg ... 1399

Propantheline Bromide (Co-administration results in additive anticholinergic effects; close supervision and careful adjustment of dosage are required). Products include:
Pro-Banthine Tablets ... 2226

Propofol (Co-administration may produce additive sedative effects). Products include:
Diprivan Injectable Emulsion ... 2939

Protriptyline Hydrochloride (Co-administration with substrates for P450 2D6, such as many other antidepressants, may make normal metabolizers resemble poor metabolizers resulting in higher than expected plasma levels of tricyclic antidepressants). Products include:
Vivactil Tablets ... 1820

Pseudoephedrine Hydrochloride (Tricyclic antidepressants may potentiate the effects of sympathomimetics; close supervision and careful adjustment of dosage are required). Products include:
Actifed Allergy Daytime/Nighttime Caplets ... ▣ 808
Actifed Cold & Allergy Tablets ... ▣ 807
Actifed Cold & Sinus Caplets and Tablets ... ▣ 808
Actifed Sinus Daytime/Nighttime Tablets and Caplets ... ▣ 809
Advil Cold and Sinus Caplets and Tablets ... ▣ 837
Alka-Seltzer Plus Liqui-Gels ... ▣ 612
Alka-Seltzer Plus Flu & Body Aches Liqui-Gels Non-Drowsy Formula ... ▣ 613
Alka-Seltzer Plus Night-Time Cold Medicine Liqui-Gels ... ▣ 612
Allerest Maximum Strength ... ▣ 649
Allerest No Drowsiness ... ▣ 649
Allerest Sinus Pain Formula ... ▣ 649
Atrohist Pediatric Capsules ... 1603
Benadryl Allergy/Cold Tablets ... ▣ 811
Benadryl Allergy Decongestant Liquid Medication ... ▣ 812
Benadryl Allergy Decongestant Tablets ... ▣ 812
Benadryl Allergy Sinus Headache Caplets ... ▣ 813
Benylin Multisymptom ... ▣ 816
Bromfed Capsules (Extended-Release) ... 1832
Bromfed Syrup ... ▣ 712
Bromfed Tablets ... 1832
Bromfed-DM Cough Syrup ... 1832
Bromfed-PD Capsules (Extended-Release) ... 1832
Children's TYLENOL Cold Multi-Symptom Chewable Tablets and Liquid ... 1559
Children's TYLENOL Cold Plus Cough Multi Symptom Chewable Tablets and Liquid ... 1560
Children's TYLENOL Flu Suspension Liquid ... 1560
Children's Vicks DayQuil Allergy Relief ... ▣ 730
Children's Vicks NyQuil Cold/Cough Relief ... ▣ 731
Allergy-Sinus Comtrex Multi-Symptom Allergy-Sinus Formula Tablets and Caplets ... ▣ 639
Comtrex Multi-Symptom ... ▣ 638
Comtrex Multi-Symptom Non-Drowsy Caplets ... ▣ 640
Congess ... 1003
Contac Day Allergy/Sinus Caplets ▣ 771
Contac Day & Night ... ▣ 772
Contac Night Allergy/Sinus Caplets ... ▣ 771
Contac Severe Cold & Flu Non-Drowsy ... ▣ 774
Deconsal II Tablets ... 1605
Dimetane-DX Cough Syrup ... 2233
Dimetapp Cold & Fever Suspension ... ▣ 839
Dimetapp Decongestant Pediatric Drops ... ▣ 840
Dorcol Children's Cough Syrup ... ▣ 748
Drixoral Cough + Congestion Liquid Caps ... ▣ 763
Dura-Tap/PD Capsules ... 970
Duratuss Tablets ... 2750
Duratuss HD Elixir ... 2750
Efidac/24 ... ▣ 655
Entex PSE Tablets ... 973
Fedahist Gyrocaps ... 2545
Guaifed ... 1833
Guaifed Syrup ... ▣ 712
Guaimax-D Tablets ... 809
Histussin D Liquid ... 670
Infants' TYLENOL Cold Decongestant & Fever-Reducer Drops ... 1561
Kronofed-A ... 994
Novahistine DMX ... ▣ 782
Nucofed ... 2225
PediaCare Cough-Cold Chewable Tablets and Liquid ... 1569
PediaCare Infants' Decongestant Drops ... 1569
PediaCare Infants' Drops Decongestant Plus Cough ... 1569
PediaCare NightRest Cough-Cold Liquid ... 1569
Pediatric Vicks 44d Cough & Head Congestion Relief ... ▣ 736
Pediatric Vicks 44m Cough & Cold Relief ... ▣ 737
Robitussin Cold & Cough Liqui-Gels ... ▣ 844
Robitussin Cold, Cough & Flu Liqui-Gels ... ▣ 844
Robitussin Maximum Strength Cough & Cold ... ▣ 847
Robitussin Night-Time Cold Formula ... ▣ 847
Robitussin Pediatric Cough & Cold Formula ... ▣ 848
Robitussin Pediatric Drops ... ▣ 849
Robitussin Severe Congestion Liqui-Gels ... ▣ 845
Robitussin-DAC Syrup ... 2249
Robitussin-PE ... ▣ 846
Rondec Oral Drops ... 974
Rondec Syrup ... 974
Rondec Tablet ... 974
Rondec Chewable Tablets ... 974
Rondec-TR Tablet ... 974
Ryna ... ▣ 804
Seldane-D Extended-Release Tablets ... 1286
Semprex-D Capsules ... 1620
Sinarest ... ▣ 663
Sine-Aid Maximum Strength Sinus Headache Gelcaps, Caplets and Tablets ... 1570
Sine-Off No Drowsiness Formula Caplets ... ▣ 784
Sine-Off Sinus Medicine ... ▣ 784
Singlet Tablets ... ▣ 785
Sinutab Non-Drying Liquid Caps ... ▣ 823
Sinutab Sinus Allergy Medication, Maximum Strength Tablets and Caplets ... ▣ 823
Sinutab Sinus Medication, Maximum Strength Without Drowsiness Formula, Tablets & Caplets ... ▣ 824
Sudafed Children's Cold & Cough Liquid Medication ... ▣ 825
Sudafed Children's Nasal Decongestant Liquid Medication ... ▣ 826
Sudafed Cold & Allergy Tablets ... ▣ 826
Sudafed Cold and Cough Liquid Caps ... ▣ 826
Sudafed Nasal Decongestant Tablets, 30 mg ... ▣ 825
Sudafed Nasal Decongestant Tablets, 60 mg ... ▣ 825
Sudafed Non-Drying Sinus Liquid Caps ... ▣ 827
Sudafed Pediatric Nasal Decongestant Liquid Oral Drops ... ▣ 827
Sudafed Severe Cold Formula Caplets ... ▣ 828
Sudafed Severe Cold Formula Tablets ... ▣ 828
Sudafed Sinus Caplets ... ▣ 829
Sudafed Sinus Tablets ... ▣ 829
Sudafed 12 Hour Caplets ... ▣ 824
Syn-Rx Tablets ... 1622
Syn-Rx DM Tablets ... 1623
TheraFlu Flu and Cold Medicine ... ▣ 750
Theraflu Maximum Strength Flu and Cold Medicine For Sore Throat ... ▣ 751
TheraFlu Flu, Cold and Cough Medicine ... ▣ 750
TheraFlu Maximum Strength Nighttime Flu, Cold & Cough Medicine ... ▣ 751
TheraFlu Maximum Strength Non-Drowsy Formula Flu, Cold & Cough Medicine ... ▣ 751
TheraFlu Maximum Strength, Non-Drowsy Formula Flu, Cold and Cough Caplets ... ▣ 752
Theraflu Maximum Strength Sinus Non-Drowsy Formula Caplets ... ▣ 752
Triaminic AM Cough and Decongestant Formula ... ▣ 753

(▣ Described in PDR For Nonprescription Drugs) (◉ Described in PDR For Ophthalmology)

757 Interactions Index Nor-Q D

- Triaminic AM Decongestant Formula ... 753
- Triaminic Infant Oral Decongestant Drops ... 754
- Triaminic Night Time ... 754
- Triaminic Sore Throat Formula ... 755
- Tussend ... 1830
- Tussend Expectorant ... 1831
- TYLENOL Allergy Sinus, Maximum Strength Caplets and Gelcaps ... 1571
- TYLENOL Allergy Sinus NightTime, Maximum Strength Caplets ... 1571
- TYLENOL Cold Medication, Multi-Symptom Formula Tablets and Caplets ... 1572
- TYLENOL Cold Medication, Multi-Symptom Hot Liquid Packets ... 1572
- TYLENOL Cold Medication, No Drowsiness Formula Caplets and Gelcaps ... 1572
- TYLENOL Cold Severe Congestion Caplets ... 1573
- TYLENOL Cough Medication with Decongestant, Multi Symptom ... 1574
- TYLENOL Flu No Drowsiness Formula, Maximum Strength Gelcaps ... 1575
- TYLENOL Flu NightTime, Maximum Strength Gelcaps ... 1575
- TYLENOL Flu NightTime, Maximum Strength Hot Medication Packets ... 1575
- TYLENOL Sinus, Maximum Strength Geltabs, Gelcaps, Caplets and Tablets ... 1576
- Vicks 44 LiquiCaps Cough, Cold & Flu Relief ... 728
- Vicks 44 LiquiCaps Non-Drowsy Cough & Cold Relief ... 729
- Vicks 44D Cough & Head Congestion Relief ... 728
- Vicks 44M Cough, Cold & Flu Relief ... 729
- Vicks DayQuil LiquiCaps/Liquid Multi-Symptom Cold/Flu Relief ... 734
- Vicks DayQuil SINUS Pressure & PAIN Relief with IBUPROFEN ... 735
- Vicks Nyquil Hot Therapy ... 735
- Vicks NyQuil LiquiCaps/Liquid Multi-Symptom Cold/Flu Relief, Original and Cherry Flavors ... 736

Pseudoephedrine Sulfate (Tricyclic antidepressants may potentiate the effects of sympathomimetics; close supervision and careful adjustment of dosage are required). Products include:
- Chlor-Trimeton Allergy Decongestant Tablets ... 759
- Claritin-D Tablets ... 2487
- Drixoral Cold and Allergy Sustained-Action Tablets ... 763
- Drixoral Cold and Flu Extended-Release Tablets ... 764
- Drixoral Non-Drowsy Formula Extended-Release Tablets ... 764
- Drixoral Allergy/Sinus Extended Release Tablets ... 765
- Trinalin Repetabs Tablets ... 1373

Quazepam (Co-administration may produce additive sedative effects). Products include:
- Doral Tablets ... 2773

Quinidine Gluconate (May inhibit the activity of cytochrome P450 2D6 isoenzyme and may make normal metabolizers resemble poor metabolizers resulting in higher than expected plasma levels of tricyclic antidepressants). Products include:
- Quinaglute Dura-Tabs Tablets ... 644

Quinidine Polygalacturonate (May inhibit the activity of cytochrome P450 2D6 isoenzyme and may make normal metabolizers resemble poor metabolizers resulting in higher than expected plasma levels of tricyclic antidepressants). Products include:
- Cardioquin Tablets ... 2146

Quinidine Sulfate (May inhibit the activity of cytochrome P450 2D6 isoenzyme and may make normal metabolizers resemble poor metabolizers resulting in higher than expected plasma levels of tricyclic antidepressants). Products include:
- Quinidex Extentabs ... 2240

Salmeterol Xinafoate (Tricyclic antidepressants may potentiate the effects of sympathomimetics; close supervision and careful adjustment of dosage are required). Products include:
- Serevent Inhalation Aerosol ... 1149

Scopolamine (Co-administration results in additive anticholinergic effects; close supervision and careful adjustment of dosage are required). Products include:
- Transderm Scōp Transdermal Therapeutic System ... 890

Scopolamine Hydrobromide (Co-administration results in additive anticholinergic effects; close supervision and careful adjustment of dosage are required). Products include:
- Atrohist Plus Tablets ... 1605
- Donnatal ... 2234
- Donnatal Extentabs ... 2234
- Donnatal Tablets ... 2234

Secobarbital Sodium (Barbiturates induce liver enzyme activity and thereby reduce tricyclic antidepressant plasma levels; co-administration may produce additive sedative effects). Products include:
- Seconal Sodium Pulvules ... 1529

Selegiline Hydrochloride (Co-administration of tricyclic antidepressants and MAO inhibitor has produced hyperpyretic crises, severe convulsions, and deaths; concurrent and/or sequential use is contraindicated). Products include:
- Eldepryl Capsules ... 2729

Sertraline Hydrochloride (Selective serotonin reuptake inhibitors, such as sertraline, may have variable extent of inhibition of P450 2D6; potential for higher than expected plasma levels of tricyclic antidepressants). Products include:
- Zoloft Tablets ... 2051

Temazepam (Co-administration may produce additive sedative effects). Products include:
- Restoril Capsules ... 2413

Terbutaline Sulfate (Tricyclic antidepressants may potentiate the effects of sympathomimetics; close supervision and careful adjustment of dosage are required). Products include:
- Brethaire Inhaler ... 830
- Brethine Ampuls ... 832
- Brethine Tablets ... 831
- Bricanyl Subcutaneous Injection ... 1247
- Bricanyl Tablets ... 1248

Thiamylal Sodium (Barbiturates induce liver enzyme activity and thereby reduce tricyclic antidepressant plasma levels; co-administration may produce additive sedative effects).
- No products indexed under this heading.

Thioridazine Hydrochloride (Phenothiazines are substrates for P450 2D6 and co-administration may make normal metabolizers resemble poor metabolizers resulting in higher than expected plasma levels of tricyclic antidepressants; co-administration with major tranquilizers may produce additive sedative and anticholinergic effects). Products include:
- Mellaril ... 2398

Thiothixene (Co-administration with major tranquilizers may produce additive sedative and anticholinergic effects). Products include:
- Navane Capsules and Concentrate 2018
- Navane Intramuscular ... 2019

Thyroglobulin (Co-administration with thyroid medications may increase the possibility of cardiovascular toxicity, including arrhythmias).
- No products indexed under this heading.

Thyroid (Co-administration with thyroid medications may increase the possibility of cardiovascular toxicity, including arrhythmias).
- No products indexed under this heading.

Thyroxine (Co-administration with thyroid medications may increase the possibility of cardiovascular toxicity, including arrhythmias).
- No products indexed under this heading.

Thyroxine Sodium (Co-administration with thyroid medications may increase the possibility of cardiovascular toxicity, including arrhythmias).
- No products indexed under this heading.

Tranylcypromine Sulfate (Co-administration of tricyclic antidepressants and MAO inhibitor has produced hyperpyretic crises, severe convulsions, and deaths; concurrent and/or sequential use is contraindicated). Products include:
- Parnate Tablets ... 2679

Trazodone Hydrochloride (Co-administration with substrates for P450 2D6, such as many other antidepressants, may make normal metabolizers resemble poor metabolizers resulting in higher than expected plasma levels of tricyclic antidepressants). Products include:
- Desyrel and Desyrel Dividose ... 504

Triazolam (Co-administration may produce additive sedative effects). Products include:
- Halcion Tablets ... 2093

Tridihexethyl Chloride (Co-administration results in additive anticholinergic effects; close supervision and careful adjustment of dosage are required).
- No products indexed under this heading.

Trifluoperazine Hydrochloride (Phenothiazines are substrates for P450 2D6 and co-administration may make normal metabolizers resemble poor metabolizers resulting in higher than expected plasma levels of tricyclic antidepressants; co-administration with major tranquilizers may produce additive sedative and anticholinergic effects). Products include:
- Stelazine ... 2692

Trihexyphenidyl Hydrochloride (Co-administration results in additive anticholinergic effects; close supervision and careful adjustment of dosage are required). Products include:
- Artane ... 1418

Trimipramine Maleate (Co-administration with substrates for P450 2D6, such as many other antidepressants, may make normal metabolizers resemble poor metabolizers resulting in higher than expected plasma levels of tricyclic antidepressants). Products include:
- Surmontil Capsules ... 2917

Venlafaxine Hydrochloride (Co-administration with substrates for P450 2D6, such as many other antidepressants, may make normal metabolizers resemble poor metabolizers resulting in higher than expected plasma levels of tricyclic antidepressants). Products include:
- Effexor ... 2825

Zolpidem Tartrate (Co-administration may produce additive sedative effects). Products include:
- Ambien Tablets ... 2559

Food Interactions

Alcohol (Concurrent use results in exaggerated response to alcohol; alcohol induces liver enzyme activity and thereby reduces tricyclic antidepressant plasma levels).

NOR-Q D TABLETS
(Norethindrone) ... 2598

May interact with barbiturates, tetracyclines, and certain other agents. Compounds in these categories include:

Ampicillin (Potential for reduced efficacy and increased incidence of breakthrough bleeding and menstrual irregularities with concomitant use). Products include:
- Omnipen Capsules ... 2872
- Omnipen for Oral Suspension ... 2873

Ampicillin Sodium (Potential for reduced efficacy and increased incidence of breakthrough bleeding and menstrual irregularities with concomitant use). Products include:
- Unasyn ... 2035

Aprobarbital (Potential for reduced efficacy and increased incidence of breakthrough bleeding and menstrual irregularities with concomitant use).
- No products indexed under this heading.

Butabarbital (Potential for reduced efficacy and increased incidence of breakthrough bleeding and menstrual irregularities with concomitant use).
- No products indexed under this heading.

Butalbital (Potential for reduced efficacy and increased incidence of breakthrough bleeding and menstrual irregularities with concomitant use). Products include:
- Axocet Capsules ... 2469
- Esgic-plus Capsules ... 1012
- Esgic-plus Tablets ... 1012
- Fioricet Tablets ... 2386
- Fioricet with Codeine Capsules ... 2387
- Fiorinal Capsules ... 2388
- Fiorinal with Codeine Capsules ... 2390
- Fiorinal Tablets ... 2388
- Phrenilin ... 790
- Sedapap Tablets 50 mg/650 mg .. 1826

Demeclocycline Hydrochloride (Potential for reduced efficacy and increased incidence of breakthrough bleeding and menstrual irregularities with concomitant use). Products include:
- Declomycin Tablets ... 1421

Doxycycline Calcium (Potential for reduced efficacy and increased incidence of breakthrough bleeding and menstrual irregularities with concomitant use). Products include:
- Vibramycin Calcium Oral Suspension Syrup ... 2038

Doxycycline Hyclate (Potential for reduced efficacy and increased incidence of breakthrough bleeding and menstrual irregularities with concomitant use). Products include:
- Doryx Capsules ... 1970

IMPORTANT NOTE: Always consult each drug listing in the patient's regimen for possible interactions.

Vibramycin Hyclate Capsules 2038
Vibramycin Hyclate Intravenous 2040
Vibra-Tabs Film Coated Tablets 2038

Doxycycline Monohydrate (Potential for reduced efficacy and increased incidence of breakthrough bleeding and menstrual irregularities with concomitant use). Products include:

Monodox Capsules 1858
Vibramycin Monohydrate for Oral Suspension 2038

Fosphenytoin Sodium (Potential for reduced efficacy and increased incidence of breakthrough bleeding and menstrual irregularities with concomitant use). Products include:

Cerebyx Injection 1956

Griseofulvin (Potential for reduced efficacy and increased incidence of breakthrough bleeding and menstrual irregularities with concomitant use). Products include:

Fulvicin P/G Tablets 2499
Fulvicin P/G 165 & 330 Tablets 2500
Grifulvin V (griseofulvin tablets) Microsize (griseofulvin oral suspension) Microsize 1944
Gris-PEG Tablets, 125 mg & 250 mg 476

Mephobarbital (Potential for reduced efficacy and increased incidence of breakthrough bleeding and menstrual irregularities with concomitant use). Products include:

Mebaral Tablets 2452

Methacycline Hydrochloride (Potential for reduced efficacy and increased incidence of breakthrough bleeding and menstrual irregularities with concomitant use).

No products indexed under this heading.

Minocycline Hydrochloride (Potential for reduced efficacy and increased incidence of breakthrough bleeding and menstrual irregularities with concomitant use). Products include:

DYNACIN Capsules 1627
Minocin Intravenous 1428
Minocin Oral Suspension 1431
Minocin Pellet-Filled Capsules 1429

Oxytetracycline Hydrochloride (Potential for reduced efficacy and increased incidence of breakthrough bleeding and menstrual irregularities with concomitant use). Products include:

TERAK Ointment .... ◉ 210
Terra-Cortril Ophthalmic Suspension 2033
Terramycin with Polymyxin B Sulfate Ophthalmic Ointment 2035
Urobiotic-250 Capsules 2038

Pentobarbital Sodium (Potential for reduced efficacy and increased incidence of breakthrough bleeding and menstrual irregularities with concomitant use). Products include:

Nembutal Sodium Capsules 440
Nembutal Sodium Solution 442
Nembutal Sodium Suppositories...... 444

Phenobarbital (Potential for reduced efficacy and increased incidence of breakthrough bleeding and menstrual irregularities with concomitant use). Products include:

Arco-Lase Plus Tablets 513
Bellergal-S Tablets 2375
Donnatal 2234
Donnatal Extentabs........................ 2234
Donnatal Tablets 2234
Phenobarbital Elixir and Tablets...... 1523
Quadrinal Tablets 1398

Phenylbutazone (Potential for reduced efficacy and increased incidence of breakthrough bleeding and menstrual irregularities with concomitant use).

No products indexed under this heading.

Phenytoin (Potential for reduced efficacy and increased incidence of breakthrough bleeding and menstrual irregularities with concomitant use). Products include:

Dilantin Infatabs 1967
Dilantin-125 Suspension 1969

Phenytoin Sodium (Potential for reduced efficacy and increased incidence of breakthrough bleeding and menstrual irregularities with concomitant use). Products include:

Dilantin Kapseals 1965

Rifampin (Co-administration has been associated with reduced efficacy and increased incidence of breakthrough bleeding and menstrual irregularities). Products include:

Rifadin 1276
Rifamate Capsules 1278
Rifater........................ 1280
Rimactane Capsules 865

Secobarbital Sodium (Potential for reduced efficacy and increased incidence of breakthrough bleeding and menstrual irregularities with concomitant use). Products include:

Seconal Sodium Pulvules 1529

Tetracycline Hydrochloride (Potential for reduced efficacy and increased incidence of breakthrough bleeding and menstrual irregularities with concomitant use). Products include:

Achromycin V Capsules 1417
Helidac Therapy 2135

Thiamylal Sodium (Potential for reduced efficacy and increased incidence of breakthrough bleeding and menstrual irregularities with concomitant use).

No products indexed under this heading.

NORVASC TABLETS

(Amlodipine Besylate)........................2020
None cited in PDR database.

NORVIR CAPSULES

(Ritonavir)........................ 447

May interact with agents which increase cytochrome p4503a activity, tricyclic antidepressants, xanthine bronchodilators, highly metabolized sedatives and hypnotics, erythromycin, calcium channel blockers, and certain other agents. Compounds in these categories include:

Acebutolol Hydrochloride (Co-administration results in a possible increase in AUC of acebutolol; dosage adjustments may be required). Products include:

Sectral Capsules 2914

Albendazole (Co-administration results in a possible increase in AUC of albendazole; dosage adjustments may be required). Products include:

Albenza Tablets 2629

Alfentanil Hydrochloride (Co-administration results in a large increase (greater than 3x) in AUC of alfentanil; dosage adjustments may be required). Products include:

Alfenta Injection 1334

Alprazolam (Co-administration is likely to produce large increases in highly metabolized sedatives and hypnotics resulting in extreme sedation and respiratory depression; concurrent use is contraindicated). Products include:

Xanax Tablets 2115

Aminophylline (Co-administration results in the reduction of the average AUC of theophylline; increased dosage of theophylline may be required).

No products indexed under this heading.

Amiodarone Hydrochloride (Ritonavir is expected to produce a large increase in the plasma concentrations of amiodarone; concurrent use is contraindicated). Products include:

Cordarone Intravenous 2821
Cordarone Tablets........................ 2818

Amitriptyline Hydrochloride (Potential for moderate (1.5 to 3x) increase in the AUC; dosage adjustment of antidepressant may be required). Products include:

Elavil 2945
Etrafon 2495
Limbitrol 2333
Triavil Tablets 1800

Amlodipine Besylate (Co-administration results in a large increase (greater than 3x) in AUC of calcium channel blocker; dosage adjustments may be required). Products include:

Lotrel Capsules........................ 858
Norvasc Tablets 2020

Amoxapine (Potential for moderate (1.5 to 3x) increase in the AUC; dosage adjustment of antidepressant may be required). Products include:

Asendin Tablets 1419

Astemizole (Ritonavir is expected to produce a large increase in the plasma concentrations of astemizole; concurrent use is contraindicated). Products include:

Hismanal Tablets........................ 1341

Atovaquone (Ritonavir may increase the activity of glucuronosyl transferases; co-administration results in a decrease in AUC of atovaquone; dosage adjustments may be required). Products include:

Mepron Suspension 1206

Bepridil Hydrochloride (Ritonavir is expected to produce a large increase in the plasma concentrations of bepridil; concurrent use is contraindicated). Products include:

Vascor Tablets (200 and 300 mg) 1597

Betaxolol Hydrochloride (Co-administration results in a possible increase in AUC of betaxolol; dosage adjustments may be required). Products include:

Betoptic Ophthalmic Solution........... 465
Betoptic S Ophthalmic Suspension 467
Kerlone Tablets........................ 2588

Bupropion Hydrochloride (Ritonavir is expected to produce a large increase in the plasma concentrations of bupropion; concurrent use is contraindicated). Products include:

Wellbutrin Tablets 1177

Carbamazepine (Co-administration results in a large increase (greater than 3x) in AUC of carbamazepine; dosage adjustments may be required; potential for increase in the clearance of ritonavir resulting in decreased ritonavir plasma concentrations). Products include:

Atretol Tablets 569
Tegretol/Tegretol-XR 870

Chloroquine Hydrochloride (Co-administration results in a possible increase in AUC of chloroquine; dosage adjustments may be required). Products include:

Aralen Hydrochloride Injection 2430

Chloroquine Phosphate (Co-administration results in a possible increase in AUC of chloroquine; dosage adjustments may be required). Products include:

Aralen Phosphate Tablets 2431

Chlorpromazine (Co-administration results in a moderate increase (1.5 to 3x) in AUC of chlorpromazine; dosage adjustments may be required). Products include:

Thorazine Suppositories.................... 2701

Chlorpromazine Hydrochloride (Co-administration results in a moderate increase (1.5 to 3x) in AUC of chlorpromazine; dosage adjustments may be required). Products include:

Thorazine 2701

Cimetidine (Co-administration results in a possible increase in AUC of cimetidine; dosage adjustments may be required). Products include:

Tagamet HB Tablets........................ ▣ 786
Tagamet Tablets 2694

Cimetidine Hydrochloride (Co-administration results in a possible increase in AUC of cimetidine; dosage adjustments may be required). Products include:

Tagamet........................ 2694

Cisapride (Ritonavir is expected to produce a large increase in the plasma concentrations of cisapride; concurrent use is contraindicated). Products include:

Propulsid........................ 1346

Clarithromycin (Increased AUC of clarithromycin in the presence of ritonavir; dosage reduction may be required, especially in patients with renal impairment). Products include:

Biaxin 406

Clofibrate (Ritonavir may increase the activity of glucuronosyl transferases; co-administration results in a decrease in AUC of clofibrate; dosage adjustments may be required). Products include:

Atromid-S Capsules 2808

Clomipramine Hydrochloride (Potential for moderate (1.5 to 3x) increase in the AUC; dosage adjustment of antidepressant may be required). Products include:

Anafranil Capsules 819

Clonazepam (Co-administration results in a large increase (greater than 3x) in AUC of clonazepam; dosage adjustments may be required). Products include:

Klonopin Tablets 2294

Clorazepate Dipotassium (Co-administration is likely to produce large increases in highly metabolized sedatives and hypnotics resulting in extreme sedation and respiratory depression; concurrent use is contraindicated). Products include:

Tranxene 459

Clozapine (Ritonavir is expected to produce a large increase in the plasma concentrations of clozapine; concurrent use is contraindicated). Products include:

Clozaril Tablets........................ 2377

(▣ Described in PDR For Nonprescription Drugs) (◉ Described in PDR For Ophthalmology)

Codeine Phosphate (Ritonavir may increase the activity of glucuronosyl transferases; co-administration results in possible decrease in AUC of codeine; possible need for dosage alterations of codeine). Products include:

Brontex	2130
Dimetane-DC Cough Syrup	2232
Fioricet with Codeine Capsules	2387
Fiorinal with Codeine Capsules	2390
Nucofed	2225
Phenergan with Codeine	2883
Phenergan VC with Codeine	2888
Robitussin A-C Syrup	2248
Robitussin-DAC Syrup	2249
Ryna	804
Soma Compound w/Codeine Tablets	2784
Tylenol with Codeine	1592

Cyclophosphamide (Co-administration results in a possible increase in AUC of cyclophosphamide; dosage adjustments may be required). Products include:

Cytoxan	700

Cyclosporine (Co-administration results in a large increase (greater than 3x) in AUC of cyclosporine; dosage adjustments may be required). Products include:

Neoral	2405
Sandimmune	2416

Daunorubicin Hydrochloride (Co-administration results in a possible increase in AUC of daunorubicin; dosage adjustments may be required). Products include:

Cerubidine for Injection	634

Desipramine Hydrochloride (Co-administration results in a 145% mean increase in the AUC of desipramine; dosage reduction of desipramine should be considered). Products include:

Norpramin Tablets	1273

Dexamethasone (Co-administration results in a large increase (greater than 3x) in AUC of dexamethasone; dosage adjustments may be required; potential for increase in the clearance of ritonavir resulting in decreased ritonavir plasma concentrations). Products include:

AK-Trol Ointment & Suspension	205
Decadron Elixir	1676
Decadron Tablets	1678
Decaspray Topical Aerosol	1689
Maxitrol Ophthalmic Ointment and Suspension	222
TobraDex Ophthalmic Suspension and Ointment	469

Dexamethasone Acetate (Co-administration results in a large increase (greater than 3x) in AUC of dexamethasone; dosage adjustments may be required; potential for increase in the clearance of ritonavir resulting in decreased ritonavir plasma concentrations). Products include:

Dalalone D.P. Injectable	1009
Decadron-LA Sterile Suspension	1687

Dexamethasone Sodium Phosphate (Co-administration results in a large increase (greater than 3x) in AUC of dexamethasone; dosage adjustments may be required; potential for increase in the clearance of ritonavir resulting in decreased ritonavir plasma concentrations). Products include:

Decadron Phosphate Injection	1680
Decadron Phosphate Sterile Ophthalmic Ointment	1684
Decadron Phosphate Sterile Ophthalmic Solution	1685
Decadron Phosphate Topical Cream	1686
Decadron Phosphate with Xylocaine Injection, Sterile	1683
Dexacort Phosphate in Respihaler	1606
Dexacort Phosphate in Turbinaire	1607
NeoDecadron Sterile Ophthalmic Ointment	1755
NeoDecadron Sterile Ophthalmic Solution	1756
NeoDecadron Topical Cream	1757

Diazepam (Co-administration is likely to produce large increases in highly metabolized sedatives and hypnotics resulting in extreme sedation and respiratory depression; concurrent use is contraindicated). Products include:

Dizac (diazepam injectable emulsion) CIV	1862
Valium Injectable	2336
Valium Tablets	2335

Diclofenac Potassium (Co-administration results in a moderate (1.5 to 3x) increase or decrease in AUC of diclofenac). Products include:

Cataflam Tablets	833

Diclofenac Sodium (Co-administration results in a moderate (1.5 to 3x) increase or decrease in AUC of diclofenac). Products include:

Voltaren Ophthalmic Sterile Ophthalmic Solution	264
Cataflam/Voltaren/Voltaren-XR	833

Digoxin (Co-administration results in a possible increase in AUC of digoxin; dosage adjustments may be required). Products include:

Lanoxicaps	1110
Lanoxin Elixir Pediatric	1113
Lanoxin Injection	1116
Lanoxin Injection Pediatric	1119
Lanoxin Tablets	1121

Diltiazem Hydrochloride (Co-administration results in a large increase (greater than 3x) in AUC of calcium channel blocker; dosage adjustments may be required). Products include:

Cardizem CD Capsules	1251
Cardizem SR Capsules	1255
Cardizem Injectable	1253
Cardizem Tablets	1257
Dilacor XR Extended-release Capsules	2183
Tiazac Capsules	1019

Diphenoxylate Hydrochloride (Ritonavir may increase the activity of glucuronosyl transferases; co-administration results in a decrease in AUC of diphenoxylate; dosage adjustments may be required). Products include:

Lomotil	2591

Disopyramide Phosphate (Co-administration results in a large increase (greater than 3x) in AUC of disopyramide; dosage adjustments may be required). Products include:

Norpace	2596

Disulfiram (Potential for disulfiram-like reactions due to the presence of ethanol in the ritonavir formulations). Products include:

Antabuse Tablets	2802

Divalproex Sodium (Ritonavir may increase the activity of glucuronosyl transferases; co-administration results in a decrease in AUC of divalproex; dosage adjustments may be required). Products include:

Depakote Tablets	418

Doxazosin Mesylate (Co-administration results in a possible increase in AUC of doxazosin; dosage adjustments may be required). Products include:

Cardura Tablets	1993

Doxepin Hydrochloride (Co-administration results in a possible increase in the AUC of doxepine; dosage adjustment of doxepine may be required). Products include:

Adapin Capsules	1542
Sinequan	2028
Zonalon Cream	1042

Doxorubicin Hydrochloride (Co-administration results in a possible increase in AUC of doxorubicin; dosage adjustments may be required). Products include:

Adriamycin PFS	2056
Adriamycin RDF	2056
Doxil	2613
Doxorubicin Astra	531
Rubex for Injection	721

Dronabinol (Co-administration results in a large increase (greater than 3x) in AUC of dronabinol; dosage adjustments may be required). Products include:

Marinol (Dronabinol) Capsules	2353

Dyphylline (Co-administration results in the reduction of the average AUC of theophylline; increased dosage of theophylline may be required). Products include:

Lufyllin & Lufyllin-400 Tablets	2778
Lufyllin-GG Elixir & Tablets	2779

Encainide Hydrochloride (Ritonavir is expected to produce a large increase in the plasma concentrations of encainide; concurrent use is contraindicated).

No products indexed under this heading.

Erythromycin (Co-administration results in a large increase (greater than 3x) in AUC of erythromycin; dosage adjustments may be required). Products include:

A/T/S 2% Acne Topical Gel	1244
A/T/S 2% Acne Topical Solution	1244
Benzamycin Topical Gel	919
E-Mycin Tablets	1388
Emgel 2% Topical Gel	1081
ERYC	1972
Erycette (erythromycin 2%) Topical Solution	1943
Ery-Tab Tablets	426
Erythromycin Base Filmtab	430
Erythromycin Delayed-Release Capsules, USP	431
Ilotycin Ophthalmic Ointment	928
PCE Dispertab Tablets	453
T-Stat 2.0% Topical Solution and Pads	2797
THERAMYCIN Z 2% Solution	1629

Erythromycin Estolate (Co-administration results in a large increase (greater than 3x) in AUC of erythromycin; dosage adjustments may be required). Products include:

Ilosone	927

Erythromycin Ethylsuccinate (Co-administration results in a large increase (greater than 3x) in AUC of erythromycin; dosage adjustments may be required). Products include:

E.E.S.	427
EryPed	425
Pediazole Suspension	2340

Erythromycin Glucepate (Co-administration results in a large increase (greater than 3x) in AUC of erythromycin; dosage adjustments may be required). Products include:

Ilotycin Gluceptate, IV, Vials	929

Erythromycin Stearate (Co-administration results in a large increase (greater than 3x) in AUC of erythromycin; dosage adjustments may be required). Products include:

Erythrocin Stearate Filmtab	429

Estazolam (Co-administration is likely to produce large increases in highly metabolized sedatives and hypnotics resulting in extreme sedation and respiratory depression; concurrent use is contraindicated). Products include:

ProSom Tablets	457

Ethinyl Estradiol (Co-administration results in the reduction in the mean AUC of ethinyl estradiol, a component of oral contraceptives; dosage increase or alternate contraceptive measures should be considered). Products include:

Brevicon	2563
Demulen	2580
Desogen Tablets	1867
Levlen/Tri-Levlen	646
Lo/Ovral Tablets	2852
Lo/Ovral-28 Tablets	2857
Modicon	1928
Nordette-21 Tablets	2863
Nordette-28 Tablets	2866
Norinyl	2563
Ortho-Cept	1907
Ortho-Cyclen/Ortho Tri-Cyclen	1914
Ortho-Novum	1928
Ortho-Cyclen/Ortho Tri-Cyclen	1914
Ovcon	765
Ovral Tablets	2877
Ovral-28 Tablets	2878
Levlen/Tri-Levlen	646
Tri-Norinyl	2607
Triphasil-21 Tablets	2919
Triphasil-28 Tablets	2924

Ethosuximide (Co-administration results in a large increase (greater than 3x) in AUC of ethosuximide; dosage adjustments may be required). Products include:

Zarontin Capsules	1986
Zarontin Syrup	1986

Etoposide (Co-administration results in a large increase (greater than 3x) in AUC of etoposide; dosage adjustments may be required). Products include:

Etoposide Injection	539
VePesid Capsules and Injection	727

Felodipine (Co-administration results in a large increase (greater than 3x) in AUC of calcium channel blocker; dosage adjustments may be required). Products include:

Plendil Extended-Release Tablets	514

Fentanyl (Co-administration results in a large increase (greater than 3x) in AUC of fentanyl; dosage adjustments may be required). Products include:

Duragesic Transdermal System	1336

Fentanyl Citrate (Co-administration results in a large increase (greater than 3x) in AUC of fentanyl; dosage adjustments may be required). Products include:

Sublimaze Injection	463

Flecainide Acetate (Ritonavir is expected to produce a large increase in the plasma concentrations of flecainide; concurrent use is contraindicated). Products include:

Tambocor Tablets	1555

Fluoxetine Hydrochloride (Co-administration results in a moderate increase (1.5 to 3x) in AUC of fluoxetine; dosage adjustments may be required). Products include:

Prozac Pulvules & Liquid, Oral Solution	935

Flurazepam Hydrochloride (Co-administration is likely to produce large increases in highly metabolized sedatives and hypnotics resulting in extreme sedation and respiratory depression; concurrent use is contraindicated). Products include:

Dalmane Capsules	2329

Fluvastatin Sodium (Co-administration results in a possible increase in AUC of fluvastatin; dosage adjustments may be required). Products include:

Lescol Capsules	2395

IMPORTANT NOTE: Always consult each drug listing in the patient's regimen for possible interactions.

Norvir **Interactions Index** **760**

Fluvoxamine Maleate (Co-administration results in a possible increase in AUC of fluvoxamine; dosage adjustments may be required). Products include:
- LUVOX Tablets 2723

Fosphenytoin Sodium (Co-administration results in a moderate increase or decrease in AUC of phenytoin; dosage adjustments may be required; potential for increase in the clearance of ritonavir resulting in decrease ritonavir plasma concentrations). Products include:
- Cerebyx Injection 1956

Gemfibrozil (Co-administration results in a possible increase in AUC of gemfibrozil; dosage adjustments may be required). Products include:
- Lopid Tablets 1974

Glipizide (Co-administration results in a moderate increase or decrease in AUC of glipizide; dosage adjustments may be required). Products include:
- Glucotrol Tablets 2011
- Glucotrol XL Extended Release Tablets 2012

Glyburide (Co-administration results in a moderate increase or decrease in AUC of glyburide; dosage adjustments may be required). Products include:
- DiaBeta Tablets 1265
- Glynase PresTab Tablets 2091
- Micronase Tablets 2099

Haloperidol (Co-administration results in a moderate increase (1.5 to 3x) in AUC of haloperidol; dosage adjustments may be required). Products include:
- Haldol Injection, Tablets and Concentrate 1585

Haloperidol Decanoate (Co-administration results in a moderate increase (1.5 to 3x) in AUC of haloperidol; dosage adjustments may be required). Products include:
- Haldol Decanoate 1587

Hydrocodone Bitartrate (Co-administration results in a moderate increase (1.5 to 3x) in AUC of hydrocodone; dosage adjustments may be required). Products include:
- Codiclear DH Syrup 808
- Duratuss HD Elixir 2750
- Histussin D Liquid 670
- Hycodan Tablets and Syrup 946
- Hycomine Compound Tablets 948
- Hycomine 947
- Hycotuss Expectorant Syrup 950
- Hydrocet Capsules 787
- Lorcet 10/650 Tablets 1016
- Lortab 2751
- Tussend 1830
- Tussend Expectorant 1831
- Vicodin Tablets 1404
- Vicodin ES Tablets 1405
- Vicodin HP Tablets 1403
- Vicodin Tuss Expectorant 1406
- Zydone Capsules 967

Hydromorphone Hydrochloride (Ritonavir may increase the activity of glucuronosyl transferases; co-administration results in possible decrease in AUC of hydromorphone; possible need for dosage alterations of hydromorphone). Products include:
- Dilaudid Ampules 1382
- Dilaudid Cough Syrup 1383
- Dilaudid-HP Injection 1384
- Dilaudid-HP Lyophilized Powder 250 mg 1384
- Dilaudid 1382
- Dilaudid Oral Liquid 1386
- Dilaudid 1382
- Dilaudid Tablets - 8 mg 1386

Ibuprofen (Co-administration results in a moderate (1.5 to 3x) increase or decrease in AUC of ibuprofen). Products include:
- Advil Cold and Sinus Caplets and Tablets .... ▣ 837
- Advil Ibuprofen Tablets, Caplets and Gel Caplets .... ▣ 836
- Children's Motrin Ibuprofen Oral Suspension 1558
- IBU Tablets 1389
- Ibuprohm .... ▣ 713
- Motrin IB Caplets, Tablets, and Gelcaps .... ▣ 802
- Motrin Ibuprofen Suspension, Oral Drops, Chewable Tablets, Caplets 1563
- Nuprin Ibuprofen/Analgesic Tablets & Caplets .... ▣ 645
- Vicks DayQuil SINUS Pressure & PAIN Relief with IBUPROFEN .... ▣ 735

Imipramine Hydrochloride (Potential for moderate (1.5 to 3x) increase in the AUC; dosage adjustment of antidepressant may be required). Products include:
- Tofranil Ampuls 873
- Tofranil Tablets 875

Imipramine Pamoate (Potential for moderate (1.5 to 3x) increase in the AUC; dosage adjustment of antidepressant may be required). Products include:
- Tofranil-PM Capsules 876

Indomethacin (Co-administration results in a moderate (1.5 to 3x) increase or decrease in AUC of indomethacin). Products include:
- Indocin 1723

Isradipine (Co-administration results in a large increase (greater than 3x) in AUC of calcium channel blocker; dosage adjustments may be required). Products include:
- DynaCirc Capsules 2381
- DynaCirc CR Tablets 2383

Itraconazole (Co-administration results in a possible increase in AUC of itraconazole; dosage adjustments may be required). Products include:
- Sporanox Capsules 1352

Ketoconazole (Co-administration results in a possible increase in AUC of ketoconazole; dosage adjustments may be required). Products include:
- Nizoral 2% Cream 1344
- Nizoral 2% Shampoo 1344
- Nizoral Tablets 1345

Ketoprofen (Ritonavir may increase the activity of glucuronosyl transferases; co-administration results in possible decrease in AUC of ketoprofen; possible need for dosage alterations of ketoprofen). Products include:
- Actron Caplets and Tablets .... ▣ 608
- Orudis Capsules 2874
- Orudis KT .... ▣ 842
- Oruvail Capsules 2874

Ketorolac Tromethamine (Ritonavir may increase the activity of glucuronosyl transferases; co-administration results in possible decrease in AUC of ketorolac; possible need for dosage alterations of ketorolac). Products include:
- Acular Sterile Ophthalmic Solution 470
- Toradol 2319

Lamotrigine (Ritonavir may increase the activity of glucuronosyl transferases; co-administration results in a decrease in AUC of lamotrigine; dosage adjustments may be required). Products include:
- Lamictal Tablets 1105

Lansoprazole (Co-administration results in a moderate increase or decrease in AUC of lansoprazole; dosage adjustments may be required). Products include:
- Prevacid Delayed-Release Capsules 2746

Lidocaine Hydrochloride (Co-administration results in a large increase (greater than 3x) in AUC of lidocaine; dosage adjustments may be required). Products include:
- Decadron Phosphate with Xylocaine Injection, Sterile 1683
- Unguentine Plus .... ▣ 712
- Xylocaine Injections 562

Loratadine (Ritonavir is expected to produce a large increase (greater than 3x) in the plasma concentrations of loratadine; dosage adjustments may be required). Products include:
- Claritin Tablets 2485
- Claritin-D Tablets 2487

Lorazepam (Ritonavir may increase the activity of glucuronosyl transferases; co-administration results in a decrease in AUC of lorazepam; dosage adjustments may be required). Products include:
- Ativan Injection 2805
- Ativan Tablets 2807

Losartan Potassium (Co-administration results in a moderate increase or decrease in AUC of losartan; dosage adjustments may be required). Products include:
- Cozaar Tablets 1668
- Hyzaar Tablets 1720

Lovastatin (Co-administration results in a large increase (greater than 3x) in AUC of lovastatin; dosage adjustments may be required). Products include:
- Mevacor Tablets 1742

Maprotiline Hydrochloride (Potential for moderate (1.5 to 3x) increase in the AUC; dosage adjustment of antidepressant may be required). Products include:
- Ludiomil Tablets 861

Meperidine Hydrochloride (Ritonavir is expected to produce a large increase in the plasma concentrations of meperidine; concurrent use is contraindicated). Products include:
- Demerol 2438
- Mepergan Injection 2859

Methadone Hydrochloride (Co-administration results in possible increase in AUC of methadone). Products include:
- Methadone Hydrochloride Oral Concentrate 2356
- Methadone Hydrochloride Oral Solution & Tablets 2357

Methamphetamine Hydrochloride (Co-administration results in a moderate increase (1.5 to 3x) in AUC of methamphetamine; dosage adjustments may be required). Products include:
- Desoxyn Gradumet Tablets 422

Methylphenidate Hydrochloride (Co-administration results in a possible increase in AUC of methylphenidate; dosage adjustments may be required). Products include:
- Ritalin 866

Metoclopramide Hydrochloride (Ritonavir may increase the activity of glucuronosyl transferases; co-administration results in a decrease in AUC of metoclopramide; dosage adjustments may be required). Products include:
- Reglan 2243

Metoprolol Succinate (Co-administration results in a moderate increase (1.5 to 3x) in AUC of metoprolol; dosage adjustments may be required). Products include:
- Toprol-XL Tablets 560

Metoprolol Tartrate (Co-administration results in a moderate increase (1.5 to 3x) in AUC of metoprolol; dosage adjustments may be required). Products include:
- Lopressor 848
- Lopressor HCT Tablets 850

Metronidazole (Potential for disulfiram-like reactions due to the presence of ethanol in the ritonavir formulations; co-administration results in possible increase in metronidazole AUC). Products include:
- Flagyl 375 Capsules 2587
- Flagyl I.V. RTU 2373
- Helidac Therapy 2135
- MetroCream 1034
- MetroGel 1034
- MetroGel-Vaginal 917
- Protostat Tablets 1939

Metronidazole Hydrochloride (Potential for disulfiram-like reactions due to the presence of ethanol in the ritonavir formulations; co-administration results in possible increase in metronidazole AUC). Products include:
- Flagyl I.V. 2373

Mexiletine Hydrochloride (Co-administration results in a moderate increase (1.5 to 3x) in AUC of mexiletine; dosage adjustments may be required). Products include:
- Mexitil Capsules 684

Miconazole (Co-administration results in a possible increase in AUC of miconazole; dosage adjustments may be required).
- No products indexed under this heading.

Miconazole Nitrate (Co-administration results in a possible increase in AUC of miconazole; dosage adjustments may be required). Products include:
- Prescription Strength Desenex Spray Powder and Spray Liquid ▣ 653
- Lotrimin AF Antifungal Spray Liquid, Spray Powder, Spray Deodorant Powder, Powder and Jock Itch Spray Powder .... ▣ 766
- Monistat Dual-Pak 1906
- Monistat 3 Vaginal Suppositories 1905
- Monistat-Derm (miconazole nitrate 2%) Cream 1944
- Ting Antifungal Spray Powder .... ▣ 666

Midazolam Hydrochloride (Co-administration is likely to produce large increases in highly metabolized sedatives and hypnotics resulting in extreme sedation and respiratory depression; concurrent use is contraindicated). Products include:
- Versed Injection 2324

Morphine Sulfate (Ritonavir may increase the activity of glucuronosyl transferases; co-administration results in possible decrease in AUC of morphine; possible need for dosage alterations of morphine). Products include:
- Astramorph/PF Injection, USP (Preservative-Free) 526
- Duramorph Injection 983
- Infumorph 200 and Infumorph 500 Sterile Solutions 985
- Kadian Capsules 2948
- MS Contin Tablets 2149
- MSIR 2152
- Oramorph SR (Morphine Sulfate Sustained Release Tablets) 2359
- RMS Suppositories CII 2766
- Roxanol 2365

(▣ Described in PDR For Nonprescription Drugs) (◉ Described in PDR For Ophthalmology)

Nabumetone (Co-administration results in a possible increase in AUC of nabumetone). Products include:
Relafen Tablets 2688

Naproxen (Ritonavir may increase the activity of glucuronosyl transferases; co-administration results in possible decrease in AUC of naproxen; possible need for dosage alterations of naproxen). Products include:
Anaprox/Naprosyn 2277

Naproxen Sodium (Ritonavir may increase the activity of glucuronosyl transferases; co-administration results in possible decrease in AUC of naproxen; possible need for dosage alterations of naproxen). Products include:
Aleve 2124
Anaprox/Naprosyn 2277
Naprelan Tablets 2861

Nefazodone Hydrochloride (Co-administration results in a large increase (greater than 3x) in AUC of nefazodone; dosage adjustments may be required). Products include:
Serzone Tablets 776

Nicardipine Hydrochloride (Co-administration results in a large increase (greater than 3x) in AUC of calcium channel blocker; dosage adjustments may be required). Products include:
Cardene Capsules 2261
Cardene I.V. 2815
Cardene SR Capsules 2264

Nifedipine (Co-administration results in a large increase (greater than 3x) in AUC of calcium channel blocker; dosage adjustments may be required). Products include:
Adalat Capsules (10 mg and 20 mg) 580
Adalat CC 582
Procardia Capsules 2024
Procardia XL Extended Release Tablets 2026

Nimodipine (Co-administration results in a large increase (greater than 3x) in AUC of calcium channel blocker; dosage adjustments may be required). Products include:
Nimotop Capsules 603

Nisoldipine (Co-administration results in a large increase (greater than 3x) in AUC of calcium channel blocker; dosage adjustments may be required). Products include:
Sular Tablets 2961

Nortriptyline Hydrochloride (Potential for moderate (1.5 to 3x) increase in the AUC; dosage adjustment of antidepressant may be required). Products include:
Pamelor 2409

Omeprazole (Co-administration results in a moderate increase or decrease in AUC of omeprazole; dosage adjustments may be required). Products include:
Prilosec Delayed-Release Capsules 516

Ondansetron Hydrochloride (Co-administration results in a large increase (greater than 3x) in AUC of ondansetrone; dosage adjustments may be required). Products include:
Zofran Injection 1227
Zofran Tablets 1231

Oxazepam (Ritonavir may increase the activity of glucuronosyl transferases; co-administration results in a decrease in AUC of oxazepam; dosage adjustments may be required). Products include:
Serax Capsules 2916
Serax Tablets 2916

Oxycodone Hydrochloride (Co-administration results in a moderate increase (1.5 to 3x) in AUC of oxycodone; dosage adjustments may be required). Products include:
OxyContin Tablets 2163
OxyIR Capsules 2167
Percocet Tablets 955
Percodan Tablets 955
Percodan-Demi Tablets 956
Roxicodone Tablets, Oral Solution & Intensol (Oxycodone) 2366
Tylox Capsules 1593

Paclitaxel (Co-administration results in a large increase (greater than 3x) in AUC of paclitaxel; dosage adjustments may be required). Products include:
Taxol Injection 723

Paroxetine Hydrochloride (Co-administration results in a moderate increase (1.5 to 3x) in AUC of paroxetine; dosage adjustments may be required). Products include:
Paxil Tablets 2681

Penbutolol Sulfate (Co-administration results in a possible increase in AUC of penbutolol; dosage adjustments may be required). Products include:
Levatol Tablets 2547

Pentoxifylline (Co-administration results in a possible increase in AUC of pentoxifylline; dosage adjustments may be required). Products include:
Trental Tablets 1291

Perphenazine (Co-administration results in a moderate increase (1.5 to 3x) in AUC of perphenazine; dosage adjustments may be required). Products include:
Etrafon 2495
Triavil Tablets 1800
Trilafon 2532

Phenobarbital (Co-administration results in a possible increase in AUC of phenobarbital; dosage adjustments may be required; potential for increase in the clearance of ritonavir resulting in decreased ritonavir plasma concentrations). Products include:
Arco-Lase Plus Tablets 513
Bellergal-S Tablets 2375
Donnatal 2234
Donnatal Extentabs 2234
Donnatal Tablets 2234
Phenobarbital Elixir and Tablets 1523
Quadrinal Tablets 1398

Phenytoin (Co-administration results in a moderate increase or decrease in AUC of phenytoin; dosage adjustments may be required; potential for increase in the clearance of ritonavir resulting in decreased ritonavir plasma concentrations). Products include:
Dilantin Infatabs 1967
Dilantin-125 Suspension 1969

Phenytoin Sodium (Co-administration results in a moderate increase or decrease in AUC of phenytoin; dosage adjustments may be required; potential for increase in the clearance of ritonavir resulting in decreased ritonavir plasma concentrations). Products include:
Dilantin Kapseals 1965

Piroxicam (Ritonavir is expected to produce a large increase in the plasma concentrations of piroxicam; concurrent use is contraindicated). Products include:
Feldene Capsules 2008

Pravastatin Sodium (Co-administration results in a large increase (greater than 3x) in AUC of pravastatin; dosage adjustments may be required). Products include:
Pravachol Tablets 770

Prazosin Hydrochloride (Co-administration results in a possible increase in AUC of prazosin; dosage adjustments may be required). Products include:
Minipress Capsules 2015
Minizide Capsules 2016

Prednisone (Co-administration results in a large increase (greater than 3x) in AUC of prednisone; dosage adjustments may be required).
No products indexed under this heading.

Primaquine Phosphate (Co-administration results in a possible increase in AUC of primaquine; dosage adjustments may be required).
No products indexed under this heading.

Prochlorperazine (Co-administration results in a possible increase in AUC of prochlorperazine; dosage adjustments may be required). Products include:
Compazine 2644

Proguanil (Co-administration results in a moderate increase or decrease in AUC of proguanil; dosage adjustments may be required).
No products indexed under this heading.

Promethazine Hydrochloride (Co-administration results in a possible increase in AUC of promethazine; dosage adjustments may be required). Products include:
Mepergan Injection 2859
Phenergan with Codeine 2883
Phenergan with Dextromethorphan 2885
Phenergan Injection 2880
Phenergan Suppositories 2882
Phenergan Syrup 2881
Phenergan Tablets 2882
Phenergan VC 2886
Phenergan VC with Codeine 2888

Propafenone Hydrochloride (Ritonavir is expected to produce a large increase in the plasma concentrations of propafenone; concurrent use is contraindicated). Products include:
Rythmol Tablets-150mg, 225mg, 300mg 1399

Propofol (Ritonavir may increase the activity of glucuronosyl transferases; co-administration results in a decrease in AUC of propofol; dosage adjustments may be required). Products include:
Diprivan Injectable Emulsion 2939

Propoxyphene Hydrochloride (Ritonavir is expected to produce a large increase in the plasma concentrations of propoxyphene; concurrent use is contraindicated). Products include:
Darvon 1475
Wygesic Tablets 2930

Propoxyphene Napsylate (Ritonavir is expected to produce a large increase in the plasma concentrations of propoxyphene; concurrent use is contraindicated). Products include:
Darvon-N/Darvocet-N 1473

Propranolol Hydrochloride (Co-administration results in a moderate increase (1.5 to 3x) in AUC of propranolol; dosage adjustments may be required). Products include:
Inderal 2834
Inderal LA Long Acting Capsules 2836
Inderide Tablets 2838
Inderide LA Long Acting Capsules .. 2840

Protriptyline Hydrochloride (Potential for moderate (1.5 to 3x) increase in the AUC; dosage adjustment of antidepressant may be required). Products include:
Vivactil Tablets 1820

Pyrimethamine (Co-administration results in a possible increase in AUC of pyrimethamine; dosage adjustments may be required). Products include:
Daraprim Tablets 1199
Fansidar Tablets 2281

Quinidine Gluconate (Ritonavir is expected to produce a large increase in the plasma concentrations of quinidine; concurrent use is contraindicated). Products include:
Quinaglute Dura-Tabs Tablets 644

Quinidine Polygalacturonate (Ritonavir is expected to produce a large increase in the plasma concentrations of quinidine; concurrent use is contraindicated). Products include:
Cardioquin Tablets 2146

Quinidine Sulfate (Ritonavir is expected to produce a large increase in the plasma concentrations of quinidine; concurrent use is contraindicated). Products include:
Quinidex Extentabs 2240

Quinine Sulfate (Co-administration results in a large increase (greater than 3x) in AUC of quinine; dosage adjustments may be required).
No products indexed under this heading.

Rifabutin (Ritonavir is expected to produce a large increase in the plasma concentrations of rifabutin; potential for increase in the clearance of ritonavir resulting in decreased ritonavir plasma concentrations; concurrent use in contraindicated). Products include:
Mycobutin Capsules 2101

Rifampin (Co-administration results in a large increase (greater than 3x) in AUC of rifampin; dosage adjustments may be required; potential for increase in the clearance of ritonavir resulting in decreased ritonavir plasma concentrations). Products include:
Rifadin 1276
Rifamate Capsules 1278
Rifater 1280
Rimactane Capsules 865

Risperidone (Co-administration results in a moderate increase (1.5 to 3x) in AUC of risperidone; dosage adjustments may be required). Products include:
Risperdal Tablets 1348

Saquinavir Mesylate (Ritonavir extensively inhibits the metabolism of saquinavir resulting in a large (greater than 3x) increase in the AUC of saquinavir). Products include:
Invirase Capsules 2291

Sertraline Hydrochloride (Co-administration results in a large increase (greater than 3x) in AUC of sertraline; dosage adjustments may be required). Products include:
Zoloft Tablets 2051

Simvastatin (Co-administration results in a possible increase in AUC of simvastatin; dosage adjustments may be required). Products include:
Zocor Tablets 1821

Sulindac (Co-administration results in a possible increase in AUC of sulindac). Products include:
Clinoril Tablets 1658

IMPORTANT NOTE: Always consult each drug listing in the patient's regimen for possible interactions.

Tacrolimus (Co-administration results in a large increase (greater than 3x) in AUC of tacrolimus; dosage adjustments may be required). Products include:
- Prograf 1028

Tamoxifen Citrate (Co-administration results in a large increase (greater than 3x) in AUC of tamoxifen; dosage adjustments may be required). Products include:
- Nolvadex Tablets 2957

Temazepam (Ritonavir may increase the activity of glucuronosyl transferases; co-administration results in a decrease in AUC of temazepam; dosage adjustments may be required). Products include:
- Restoril Capsules 2413

Terazosin Hydrochloride (Co-administration results in a possible increase in AUC of terazosin; dosage adjustments may be required). Products include:
- Hytrin Capsules 434

Terfenadine (Ritonavir is expected to produce a large increase in the plasma concentrations of terfenadine; concurrent use is contraindicated). Products include:
- Seldane Tablets 1284
- Seldane-D Extended-Release Tablets 1286

Theophylline (Co-administration results in the reduction of the average AUC of theophylline; increased dosage of theophylline may be required). Products include:
- Marax Tablets & DF Syrup 2015
- Quibron 2227

Theophylline Anhydrous (Co-administration results in the reduction of the average AUC of theophylline; increased dosage of theophylline may be required). Products include:
- Aerolate 1003
- Primatene Tablets .... ▣ 844
- Respbid Tablets 687
- Slo-bid Gyrocaps 2201
- Theo-24 Extended Release Capsules 2753
- Theo-Dur Extended-Release Tablets 1367
- Theo-X Extended-Release Tablets .. 793
- Uni-Dur Extended-Release Tablets .. 1374
- Uniphyl 400 mg and 600 mg Tablets 2157

Theophylline Calcium Salicylate (Co-administration results in the reduction of the average AUC of theophylline; increased dosage of theophylline may be required). Products include:
- Quadrinal Tablets 1398

Theophylline Sodium Glycinate (Co-administration results in the reduction of the average AUC of theophylline; increased dosage of theophylline may be required).
- No products indexed under this heading.

Thioridazine Hydrochloride (Co-administration results in a moderate increase (1.5 to 3x) in AUC of thioridazine; dosage adjustments may be required). Products include:
- Mellaril 2398

Timolol Hemihydrate (Co-administration results in a moderate increase (1.5 to 3x) in AUC of timolol; dosage adjustments may be required). Products include:
- Betimol 0.25%, 0.5% .... ◉ 259

Timolol Maleate (Co-administration results in a moderate increase (1.5 to 3x) in AUC of timolol; dosage adjustments may be required). Products include:
- Blocadren Tablets 1654
- Timolide Tablets 1791
- Timoptic in Ocudose 1796
- Timoptic Sterile Ophthalmic Solution 1794
- Timoptic-XE 1798

Tocainide Hydrochloride (Co-administration results in a possible increase in AUC of tocainide; dosage adjustments may be required). Products include:
- Tonocard Tablets 519

Tolbutamide (Co-administration results in a moderate increase or decrease in AUC of tolbutamide; dosage adjustments may be required).
- No products indexed under this heading.

Tramadol Hydrochloride (Co-administration results in a moderate increase (1.5 to 3x) in AUC of tramadol; dosage adjustments may be required). Products include:
- Ultram Tablets (50 mg) 1594

Trazodone Hydrochloride (Co-administration results in a large increase (greater than 3x) in AUC of trazodone; dosage adjustments may be required). Products include:
- Desyrel and Desyrel Dividose 504

Triazolam (Co-administration is likely to produce large increases in highly metabolized sedatives and hypnotics resulting in extreme sedation and respiratory depression; concurrent use is contraindicated). Products include:
- Halcion Tablets 2093

Trimipramine Maleate (Potential for moderate (1.5 to 3x) increase in the AUC; dosage adjustment of antidepressant may be required). Products include:
- Surmontil Capsules 2917

Valproic Acid (Ritonavir may increase the activity of glucuronosyl transferases; co-administration results in a decrease in AUC of divalproex; dosage adjustments may be required). Products include:
- Depakene 416

Venlafaxine Hydrochloride (Co-administration results in a moderate increase (1.5 to 3x) in AUC of venlafaxine; dosage adjustments may be required). Products include:
- Effexor 2825

Verapamil Hydrochloride (Co-administration results in a large increase (greater than 3x) in AUC of calcium channel blocker; dosage adjustments may be required). Products include:
- Calan SR Caplets 2571
- Calan Tablets 2568
- Covera-HS Tablets 2573
- Isoptin Injectable 1391
- Isoptin Oral Tablets 1393
- Isoptin SR Tablets 1395
- Verelan Capsules 1455

Vinblastine Sulfate (Co-administration results in a large increase (greater than 3x) in AUC of vinblastine; dosage adjustments may be required). Products include:
- Velban Vials 1537

Vincristine Sulfate (Co-administration results in a large increase (greater than 3x) in AUC of vincristine; dosage adjustments may be required). Products include:
- Oncovin Solution Vials & Hyporets 1521

Warfarin Sodium (Co-administration results in a large increase (greater than 3x) in AUC of warfarin; therapeutic drug concentration monitoring is advised). Products include:
- Coumadin 941

Zolpidem Tartrate (Co-administration is likely to produce large increases in highly metabolized sedatives and hypnotics resulting in extreme sedation and respiratory depression; concurrent use is contraindicated). Products include:
- Ambien Tablets 2559

Food Interactions

Meal, unspecified (Relative to fasting conditions, the extent of absorption of ritonavir from capsule formulation was 15% higher when administered with a meal; decreased peak ritonavir concentrations when oral solution was given under non-fasting condition).

NORVIR ORAL SOLUTION
(Ritonavir) 447
See **Norvir Capsules**

12 HOUR NōSTRILLA
(Oxymetazoline Hydrochloride) ...... ▣ 660
None cited in PDR database.

NOVACET LOTION
(Sulfur, Sulfacetamide Sodium) 1041
None cited in PDR database.

NOVAHISTINE DMX
(Dextromethorphan Hydrobromide, Guaifenesin, Pseudoephedrine Hydrochloride) .... ▣ 782
May interact with monoamine oxidase inhibitors. Compounds in this category include:

Furazolidone (Concurrent and/or sequential use is contraindicated). Products include:
- Furoxone 2221

Isocarboxazid (Concurrent and/or sequential use is contraindicated).
- No products indexed under this heading.

Phenelzine Sulfate (Concurrent and/or sequential use is contraindicated). Products include:
- Nardil 1977

Selegiline Hydrochloride (Concurrent and/or sequential use is contraindicated). Products include:
- Eldepryl Capsules 2729

Tranylcypromine Sulfate (Concurrent and/or sequential use is contraindicated). Products include:
- Parnate Tablets 2679

NOVAHISTINE ELIXIR
(Chlorpheniramine Maleate, Phenylephrine Hydrochloride) .... ▣ 782
May interact with monoamine oxidase inhibitors, hypnotics and sedatives, tranquilizers, and certain other agents. Compounds in these categories include:

Alprazolam (May increase the drowsiness effect; avoid concurrent use). Products include:
- Xanax Tablets 2115

Buspirone Hydrochloride (May increase the drowsiness effect; avoid concurrent use). Products include:
- BuSpar Tablets 738

Chlordiazepoxide (May increase the drowsiness effect; avoid concurrent use). Products include:
- Limbitrol 2333

Chlordiazepoxide Hydrochloride (May increase the drowsiness effect; avoid concurrent use). Products include:
- Librax Capsules 2330
- Librium Capsules 2331
- Librium Injectable 2332

Chlorpromazine (May increase the drowsiness effect; avoid concurrent use). Products include:
- Thorazine Suppositories 2701

Chlorpromazine Hydrochloride (May increase the drowsiness effect; avoid concurrent use). Products include:
- Thorazine 2701

Chlorprothixene (May increase the drowsiness effect; avoid concurrent use).
- No products indexed under this heading.

Chlorprothixene Hydrochloride (May increase the drowsiness effect; avoid concurrent use).
- No products indexed under this heading.

Clorazepate Dipotassium (May increase the drowsiness effect; avoid concurrent use). Products include:
- Tranxene 459

Diazepam (May increase the drowsiness effect; avoid concurrent use). Products include:
- Dizac (diazepam injectable emulsion) CIV 1862
- Valium Injectable 2336
- Valium Tablets 2335

Droperidol (May increase the drowsiness effect; avoid concurrent use). Products include:
- Inapsine Injection 462

Estazolam (May increase the drowsiness effect; avoid concurrent use). Products include:
- ProSom Tablets 457

Ethchlorvynol (May increase the drowsiness effect; avoid concurrent use). Products include:
- Placidyl Capsules 456

Ethinamate (May increase the drowsiness effect; avoid concurrent use).
- No products indexed under this heading.

Fluphenazine Decanoate (May increase the drowsiness effect; avoid concurrent use). Products include:
- Prolixin Decanoate 510

Fluphenazine Enanthate (May increase the drowsiness effect; avoid concurrent use). Products include:
- Prolixin Enanthate 510

Fluphenazine Hydrochloride (May increase the drowsiness effect; avoid concurrent use). Products include:
- Prolixin 510

Flurazepam Hydrochloride (May increase the drowsiness effect; avoid concurrent use). Products include:
- Dalmane Capsules 2329

Furazolidone (Concurrent and/or sequential use is contraindicated). Products include:
- Furoxone 2221

Glutethimide (May increase the drowsiness effect; avoid concurrent use).
- No products indexed under this heading.

Haloperidol (May increase the drowsiness effect; avoid concurrent use). Products include:
- Haldol Injection, Tablets and Concentrate 1585

Haloperidol Decanoate (May increase the drowsiness effect; avoid concurrent use). Products include:
- Haldol Decanoate 1587

Hydroxyzine Hydrochloride (May increase the drowsiness effect; avoid concurrent use). Products include:
- Atarax Tablets & Syrup 1992
- Marax Tablets & DF Syrup 2015

(▣ Described in PDR For Nonprescription Drugs) (◉ Described in PDR For Ophthalmology)

Vistaril Intramuscular Solution.......... 2042

Isocarboxazid (Concurrent and/or sequential use is contraindicated).
No products indexed under this heading.

Lorazepam (May increase the drowsiness effect; avoid concurrent use). Products include:
Ativan Injection.......................... 2805
Ativan Tablets............................ 2807

Loxapine Hydrochloride (May increase the drowsiness effect; avoid concurrent use). Products include:
Loxitane..................................... 1426

Loxapine Succinate (May increase the drowsiness effect; avoid concurrent use). Products include:
Loxitane Capsules...................... 1426

Meprobamate (May increase the drowsiness effect; avoid concurrent use). Products include:
Miltown Tablets......................... 2780
PMB 200 and PMB 400............... 2890

Mesoridazine Besylate (May increase the drowsiness effect; avoid concurrent use). Products include:
Serentil....................................... 689

Midazolam Hydrochloride (May increase the drowsiness effect; avoid concurrent use). Products include:
Versed Injection......................... 2324

Molindone Hydrochloride (May increase the drowsiness effect; avoid concurrent use). Products include:
Moban Tablets and Concentrate.... 1036

Oxazepam (May increase the drowsiness effect; avoid concurrent use). Products include:
Serax Capsules.......................... 2916
Serax Tablets............................ 2916

Perphenazine (May increase the drowsiness effect; avoid concurrent use). Products include:
Etrafon...................................... 2495
Triavil Tablets........................... 1800
Trilafon..................................... 2532

Phenelzine Sulfate (Concurrent and/or sequential use is contraindicated). Products include:
Nardil....................................... 1977

Prazepam (May increase the drowsiness effect; avoid concurrent use).
No products indexed under this heading.

Prochlorperazine (May increase the drowsiness effect; avoid concurrent use). Products include:
Compazine................................ 2644

Promethazine Hydrochloride (May increase the drowsiness effect; avoid concurrent use). Products include:
Mepergan Injection................... 2859
Phenergan with Codeine............ 2883
Phenergan with Dextromethorphan 2885
Phenergan Injection................... 2880
Phenergan Suppositories........... 2882
Phenergan Syrup....................... 2881
Phenergan Tablets..................... 2882
Phenergan VC........................... 2886
Phenergan VC with Codeine....... 2888

Propofol (May increase the drowsiness effect; avoid concurrent use). Products include:
Diprivan Injectable Emulsion...... 2939

Quazepam (May increase the drowsiness effect; avoid concurrent use). Products include:
Doral Tablets............................ 2773

Secobarbital Sodium (May increase the drowsiness effect; avoid concurrent use). Products include:
Seconal Sodium Pulvules........... 1529

Selegiline Hydrochloride (Concurrent and/or sequential use is contraindicated). Products include:
Eldepryl Capsules..................... 2729

Temazepam (May increase the drowsiness effect; avoid concurrent use). Products include:
Restoril Capsules...................... 2413

Thioridazine Hydrochloride (May increase the drowsiness effect; avoid concurrent use). Products include:
Mellaril..................................... 2398

Thiothixene (May increase the drowsiness effect; avoid concurrent use). Products include:
Navane Capsules and Concentrate 2018
Navane Intramuscular................ 2019

Tranylcypromine Sulfate (Concurrent and/or sequential use is contraindicated). Products include:
Parnate Tablets......................... 2679

Triazolam (May increase the drowsiness effect; avoid concurrent use). Products include:
Halcion Tablets......................... 2093

Trifluoperazine Hydrochloride (May increase the drowsiness effect; avoid concurrent use). Products include:
Stelazine................................... 2692

Zolpidem Tartrate (May increase the drowsiness effect; avoid concurrent use). Products include:
Ambien Tablets......................... 2559

Food Interactions
Alcohol (May increase the drowsiness effect; avoid concurrent use).

NOVANTRONE FOR INJECTION
(Mitoxantrone Hydrochloride)...........1327
May interact with:

Daunorubicin Citrate (Increased risk of cardiac effects in patients previously treated with daunorubicin). Products include:
DaunoXome............................... 1842

Daunorubicin Hydrochloride (Increased risk of cardiac effects in patients previously treated with daunorubicin). Products include:
Cerubidine for Injection............ 634

Doxorubicin Hydrochloride (Increased risk of cardiac effects in patients previously treated with doxorubicin). Products include:
Adriamycin PFS......................... 2056
Adriamycin RDF........................ 2056
Doxil... 2613
Doxorubicin Astra..................... 531
Rubex for Injection................... 721

NOVOCAIN HYDROCHLORIDE FOR SPINAL ANESTHESIA
(Procaine Hydrochloride)................2457
May interact with sulfonamides. Compounds in this category include:

Sulfamethizole (Action of sulfonamides inhibited). Products include:
Urobiotic-250 Capsules............. 2038

Sulfamethoxazole (Action of sulfonamides inhibited). Products include:
Bactrim DS Tablets.................... 2257
Bactrim I.V. Infusion................. 2255
Bactrim..................................... 2257
Gantanol Tablets....................... 2285
Septra....................................... 1146
Septra I.V. Infusion................... 1142
Septra I.V. Infusion ADD-Vantage Vials.. 1144
Septra....................................... 1146

Sulfasalazine (Action of sulfonamides inhibited). Products include:
Azulfidine................................. 2059

Sulfinpyrazone (Action of sulfonamides inhibited). Products include:
Anturane................................... 823

Sulfisoxazole (Action of sulfonamides inhibited). Products include:
Gantrisin Tablets....................... 2286

Sulfisoxazole Diolamine (Action of sulfonamides inhibited).
No products indexed under this heading.

NOVOLIN L HUMAN INSULIN 10 ML VIALS
(Insulin, Human, Zinc Suspension) 1846
None cited in PDR database.

NOVOLIN N HUMAN INSULIN 10 ML VIALS
(Insulin, Human Isophane Suspension)...............................1846
None cited in PDR database.

NOVOLIN N PENFILL 1.5 ML CARTRIDGES DURABLE INSULIN DELIVERY SYSTEM
(Insulin, Human NPH)...............1849
None cited in PDR database.

NOVOLIN N PREFILLED SYRINGE DISPOSABLE INSULIN DELIVERY SYSTEM
(Insulin, Human NPH)...............1850
None cited in PDR database.

NOVOLIN 70/30 HUMAN INSULIN 10 ML VIALS
(Insulin, Human Regular and Human NPH Mixture)...........................1845
None cited in PDR database.

NOVOLIN 70/30 PENFILL 1.5 ML CARTRIDGES DURABLE INSULIN DELIVERY SYSTEM
(Insulin, Human Regular and Human NPH Mixture)...........................1848
None cited in PDR database.

NOVOLIN 70/30 PREFILLED DISPOSABLE INSULIN DELIVERY SYSTEM
(Insulin, Human Regular and Human NPH Mixture)...........................1850
None cited in PDR database.

NOVOLIN R HUMAN INSULIN 10 ML VIALS
(Insulin, Human Regular)...............1846
None cited in PDR database.

NOVOLIN R PENFILL 1.5 ML CARTRIDGES DURABLE INSULIN DELIVERY SYSTEM
(Insulin, Human Regular)...............1849
None cited in PDR database.

NOVOLIN R PREFILLED SYRINGE DISPOSABLE INSULIN DELIVERY SYSTEM
(Insulin, Human Regular)...............1850
None cited in PDR database.

NUBAIN INJECTION
(Nalbuphine Hydrochloride)............... 952
May interact with narcotic analgesics, anesthetics, phenothiazines, tranquilizers, hypnotics and sedatives, central nervous system depressants, general anesthetics, and certain other agents. Compounds in these categories include:

Alfentanil Hydrochloride (Additive CNS depression). Products include:
Alfenta Injection....................... 1334

Alprazolam (Additive CNS depression). Products include:
Xanax Tablets............................ 2115

Aprobarbital (Additive CNS depression).
No products indexed under this heading.

Buprenorphine (Additive CNS depression). Products include:
Buprenex Injectable.................. 2170

Buspirone Hydrochloride (Additive CNS depression). Products include:
BuSpar Tablets.......................... 738

Butabarbital (Additive CNS depression).
No products indexed under this heading.

Butalbital (Additive CNS depression). Products include:
Axocet Capsules........................ 2469
Esgic-plus Capsules................... 1012
Esgic-plus Tablets..................... 1012
Fioricet Tablets......................... 2386
Fioricet with Codeine Capsules... 2387
Fiorinal Capsules...................... 2388
Fiorinal with Codeine Capsules.. 2390
Fiorinal Tablets........................ 2388
Phrenilin................................... 790
Sedapap Tablets 50 mg/650 mg .. 1826

Chlordiazepoxide (Additive CNS depression). Products include:
Limbitrol.................................. 2333

Chlordiazepoxide Hydrochloride (Additive CNS depression). Products include:
Librax Capsules........................ 2330
Librium Capsules...................... 2331
Librium Injectable..................... 2332

Chlorpromazine (Additive CNS depression). Products include:
Thorazine Suppositories............ 2701

Chlorpromazine Hydrochloride (Additive CNS depression). Products include:
Thorazine.................................. 2701

Chlorprothixene (Additive CNS depression).
No products indexed under this heading.

Chlorprothixene Hydrochloride (Additive CNS depression).
No products indexed under this heading.

Chlorprothixene Lactate (Additive CNS depression).
No products indexed under this heading.

Clorazepate Dipotassium (Additive CNS depression). Products include:
Tranxene................................... 459

Clozapine (Additive CNS depression). Products include:
Clozaril Tablets......................... 2377

Codeine Phosphate (Additive CNS depression). Products include:
Brontex..................................... 2130
Dimetane-DC Cough Syrup........ 2232
Fioricet with Codeine Capsules... 2387
Fiorinal with Codeine Capsules.. 2390
Nucofed.................................... 2225
Phenergan with Codeine............ 2883
Phenergan VC with Codeine....... 2888
Robitussin A-C Syrup................ 2248
Robitussin-DAC Syrup............... 2249
Ryna... 804
Soma Compound w/Codeine Tablets.. 2784
Tylenol with Codeine................ 1592

Desflurane (Additive CNS depression). Products include:
Suprane (desflurane, USP)......... 1865

Dezocine (Additive CNS depression). Products include:
Dalgan Injection....................... 529

IMPORTANT NOTE: Always consult each drug listing in the patient's regimen for possible interactions.

Nubain Injection

Diazepam (Additive CNS depression). Products include:
- Dizac (diazepam injectable emulsion) CIV ... 1862
- Valium Injectable ... 2336
- Valium Tablets ... 2335

Droperidol (Additive CNS depression). Products include:
- Inapsine Injection ... 462

Enflurane (Additive CNS depression).
No products indexed under this heading.

Estazolam (Additive CNS depression). Products include:
- ProSom Tablets ... 457

Ethchlorvynol (Additive CNS depression). Products include:
- Placidyl Capsules ... 456

Ethinamate (Additive CNS depression).
No products indexed under this heading.

Fentanyl (Additive CNS depression). Products include:
- Duragesic Transdermal System ... 1336

Fentanyl Citrate (Additive CNS depression). Products include:
- Sublimaze Injection ... 463

Fluphenazine Decanoate (Additive CNS depression). Products include:
- Prolixin Decanoate ... 510

Fluphenazine Enanthate (Additive CNS depression). Products include:
- Prolixin Enanthate ... 510

Fluphenazine Hydrochloride (Additive CNS depression). Products include:
- Prolixin ... 510

Flurazepam Hydrochloride (Additive CNS depression). Products include:
- Dalmane Capsules ... 2329

Glutethimide (Additive CNS depression).
No products indexed under this heading.

Haloperidol (Additive CNS depression). Products include:
- Haldol Injection, Tablets and Concentrate ... 1585

Haloperidol Decanoate (Additive CNS depression). Products include:
- Haldol Decanoate ... 1587

Halothane (Additive CNS depression). Products include:
- Fluothane ... 2830

Hydrocodone Bitartrate (Additive CNS depression). Products include:
- Codiclear DH Syrup ... 808
- Duratuss HD Elixir ... 2750
- Histussin D Liquid ... 670
- Hycodan Tablets and Syrup ... 946
- Hycomine Compound Tablets ... 948
- Hycomine ... 947
- Hycotuss Expectorant Syrup ... 950
- Hydrocet Capsules ... 787
- Lorcet 10/650 Tablets ... 1016
- Lortab ... 2751
- Tussend ... 1830
- Tussend Expectorant ... 1831
- Vicodin Tablets ... 1404
- Vicodin ES Tablets ... 1405
- Vicodin HP Tablets ... 1403
- Vicodin Tuss Expectorant ... 1406
- Zydone Capsules ... 967

Hydrocodone Polistirex (Additive CNS depression). Products include:
- Tussionex Pennkinetic Extended-Release Suspension ... 1624

Hydromorphone Hydrochloride (Additive CNS depression). Products include:
- Dilaudid Ampules ... 1382
- Dilaudid Cough Syrup ... 1383
- Dilaudid-HP Injection ... 1384
- Dilaudid-HP Lyophilized Powder 250 mg ... 1384
- Dilaudid ... 1382
- Dilaudid Oral Liquid ... 1386
- Dilaudid ... 1382
- Dilaudid Tablets - 8 mg ... 1386

Hydroxyzine Hydrochloride (Additive CNS depression). Products include:
- Atarax Tablets & Syrup ... 1992
- Marax Tablets & DF Syrup ... 2015
- Vistaril Intramuscular Solution ... 2042

Isoflurane (Additive CNS depression).
No products indexed under this heading.

Ketamine Hydrochloride (Additive CNS depression).
No products indexed under this heading.

Levomethadyl Acetate Hydrochloride (Additive CNS depression). Products include:
- Orlaam Oral Solution ... 2361

Levorphanol Tartrate (Additive CNS depression). Products include:
- Levo-Dromoran ... 2297

Lorazepam (Additive CNS depression). Products include:
- Ativan Injection ... 2805
- Ativan Tablets ... 2807

Loxapine Hydrochloride (Additive CNS depression). Products include:
- Loxitane ... 1426

Loxapine Succinate (Additive CNS depression). Products include:
- Loxitane Capsules ... 1426

Meperidine Hydrochloride (Additive CNS depression). Products include:
- Demerol ... 2438
- Mepergan Injection ... 2859

Mephobarbital (Additive CNS depression). Products include:
- Mebaral Tablets ... 2452

Meprobamate (Additive CNS depression). Products include:
- Miltown Tablets ... 2780
- PMB 200 and PMB 400 ... 2890

Mesoridazine Besylate (Additive CNS depression). Products include:
- Serentil ... 689

Methadone Hydrochloride (Additive CNS depression). Products include:
- Methadone Hydrochloride Oral Concentrate ... 2356
- Methadone Hydrochloride Oral Solution & Tablets ... 2357

Methohexital Sodium (Additive CNS depression).
No products indexed under this heading.

Methotrimeprazine (Additive CNS depression). Products include:
- Levoprome ... 1321

Methoxyflurane (Additive CNS depression).
No products indexed under this heading.

Midazolam Hydrochloride (Additive CNS depression). Products include:
- Versed Injection ... 2324

Molindone Hydrochloride (Additive CNS depression). Products include:
- Moban Tablets and Concentrate ... 1036

Morphine Sulfate (Additive CNS depression). Products include:
- Astramorph/PF Injection, USP (Preservative-Free) ... 526
- Duramorph Injection ... 983
- Infumorph 200 and Infumorph 500 Sterile Solutions ... 985
- Kadian Capsules ... 2948
- MS Contin Tablets ... 2149
- MSIR ... 2152
- Oramorph SR (Morphine Sulfate Sustained Release Tablets) ... 2359
- RMS Suppositories CII ... 2766
- Roxanol ... 2365

Opium Alkaloids (Additive CNS depression).
No products indexed under this heading.

Oxazepam (Additive CNS depression). Products include:
- Serax Capsules ... 2916
- Serax Tablets ... 2916

Oxycodone Hydrochloride (Additive CNS depression). Products include:
- OxyContin Tablets ... 2163
- OxyIR Capsules ... 2167
- Percocet Tablets ... 955
- Percodan Tablets ... 955
- Percodan-Demi Tablets ... 956
- Roxicodone Tablets, Oral Solution & Intensol (Oxycodone) ... 2366
- Tylox Capsules ... 1593

Pentobarbital Sodium (Additive CNS depression). Products include:
- Nembutal Sodium Capsules ... 440
- Nembutal Sodium Solution ... 442
- Nembutal Sodium Suppositories ... 444

Perphenazine (Additive CNS depression). Products include:
- Etrafon ... 2495
- Triavil Tablets ... 1800
- Trilafon ... 2532

Phenobarbital (Additive CNS depression). Products include:
- Arco-Lase Plus Tablets ... 513
- Bellergal-S Tablets ... 2375
- Donnatal ... 2234
- Donnatal Extentabs ... 2234
- Donnatal Tablets ... 2234
- Phenobarbital Elixir and Tablets ... 1523
- Quadrinal Tablets ... 1398

Prazepam (Additive CNS depression).
No products indexed under this heading.

Prochlorperazine (Additive CNS depression). Products include:
- Compazine ... 2644

Promethazine Hydrochloride (Additive CNS depression). Products include:
- Mepergan Injection ... 2859
- Phenergan with Codeine ... 2883
- Phenergan with Dextromethorphan ... 2885
- Phenergan Injection ... 2880
- Phenergan Suppositories ... 2882
- Phenergan Syrup ... 2881
- Phenergan Tablets ... 2882
- Phenergan VC ... 2886
- Phenergan VC with Codeine ... 2888

Propofol (Additive CNS depression). Products include:
- Diprivan Injectable Emulsion ... 2939

Propoxyphene Hydrochloride (Additive CNS depression). Products include:
- Darvon ... 1475
- Wygesic Tablets ... 2930

Propoxyphene Napsylate (Additive CNS depression). Products include:
- Darvon-N/Darvocet-N ... 1473

Quazepam (Additive CNS depression). Products include:
- Doral Tablets ... 2773

Risperidone (Additive CNS depression). Products include:
- Risperdal Tablets ... 1348

Secobarbital Sodium (Additive CNS depression). Products include:
- Seconal Sodium Pulvules ... 1529

Sevoflurane (Additive CNS depression).
No products indexed under this heading.

Sufentanil Citrate (Additive CNS depression). Products include:
- Sufenta Injection ... 1355

Temazepam (Additive CNS depression). Products include:
- Restoril Capsules ... 2413

Thiamylal Sodium (Additive CNS depression).
No products indexed under this heading.

Thioridazine Hydrochloride (Additive CNS depression). Products include:
- Mellaril ... 2398

Thiothixene (Additive CNS depression). Products include:
- Navane Capsules and Concentrate ... 2018
- Navane Intramuscular ... 2019

Triazolam (Additive CNS depression). Products include:
- Halcion Tablets ... 2093

Trifluoperazine Hydrochloride (Additive CNS depression). Products include:
- Stelazine ... 2692

Zolpidem Tartrate (Additive CNS depression). Products include:
- Ambien Tablets ... 2559

Food Interactions

Alcohol (Additive CNS depression).

NUCOFED EXPECTORANT
(Codeine Phosphate, Pseudoephedrine Hydrochloride, Guaifenesin) ... 2225
See Nucofed Syrup and Capsules

NUCOFED PEDIATRIC EXPECTORANT
(Codeine Phosphate, Pseudoephedrine Hydrochloride, Guaifenesin) ... 2225
See Nucofed Syrup and Capsules

NUCOFED SYRUP AND CAPSULES
(Codeine Phosphate, Pseudoephedrine Hydrochloride) ... 2225
May interact with beta blockers, veratrum alkaloids, sympathomimetics, tricyclic antidepressants, central nervous system depressants, general anesthetics, anticholinergics, monoamine oxidase inhibitors, cardiac glycosides, and certain other agents. Compounds in these categories include:

Acebutolol Hydrochloride (Increased pressor effect of pseudoephedrine). Products include:
- Sectral Capsules ... 2914

Albuterol (Increased effect of either agent; increased potential for side effects). Products include:
- Proventil Inhalation Aerosol ... 2524
- Ventolin Inhalation Aerosol and Refill ... 1170

Albuterol Sulfate (Increased effect of either agent; increased potential for side effects). Products include:
- Airet Albuterol Sulfate Inhalation Solution ... 1602
- Albuterol Sulfate, USP Solution for Inhalation, Arm-a-Med ... 522
- Proventil Inhalation Solution 0.083% ... 2527
- Proventil Repetabs Tablets ... 2529
- Proventil Solution for Inhalation 0.5% ... 2525
- Proventil Syrup ... 2528
- Proventil Tablets ... 2529
- Ventolin Inhalation Solution ... 1171
- Ventolin Nebules Inhalation Solution ... 1172
- Ventolin Rotacaps for Inhalation ... 1173
- Ventolin Syrup ... 1175
- Ventolin Tablets ... 1176
- Volmax Extended-Release Tablets ... 1835

Alfentanil Hydrochloride (May increase the depressant effects of codeine). Products include:
- Alfenta Injection ... 1334

(⬛ Described in PDR For Nonprescription Drugs)   (⊙ Described in PDR For Ophthalmology)

Alprazolam (May increase the depressant effects of codeine). Products include:
- Xanax Tablets 2115

Amitriptyline Hydrochloride (May antagonize effects of pseudoephedrine; increased effects of antidepressants or the codeine). Products include:
- Elavil 2945
- Etrafon 2495
- Limbitrol 2333
- Triavil Tablets 1800

Amoxapine (May antagonize effects of pseudoephedrine; increased effects of antidepressants or the codeine). Products include:
- Asendin Tablets 1419

Aprobarbital (May increase the depressant effects of codeine).
- No products indexed under this heading.

Atenolol (Increased pressor effect of pseudoephedrine). Products include:
- Tenoretic Tablets 2963
- Tenormin Tablets and I.V. Injection 2965

Atropine Sulfate (Concurrent use may result in paralytic ileus). Products include:
- Arco-Lase Plus Tablets 513
- Atrohist Plus Tablets 1605
- Donnatal 2234
- Donnatal Extentabs 2234
- Donnatal Tablets 2234
- Lomotil 2591
- Motofen Tablets 789
- Urised Tablets 2123

Belladonna Alkaloids (Concurrent use may result in paralytic ileus). Products include:
- Bellergal-S Tablets 2375
- Hyland's Bedwetting Tablets 788
- Hyland's EnurAid Tablets 789
- Hyland's Headache Tablets 790
- Hyland's Teething Tablets 790
- Similasan Eye Drops #1 769

Benztropine Mesylate (Concurrent use may result in paralytic ileus). Products include:
- Cogentin 1661

Betaxolol Hydrochloride (Increased pressor effect of pseudoephedrine). Products include:
- Betoptic Ophthalmic Solution 465
- Betoptic S Ophthalmic Suspension 467
- Kerlone Tablets 2588

Biperiden Hydrochloride (Concurrent use may result in paralytic ileus). Products include:
- Akineton 1380

Bisoprolol Fumarate (Increased pressor effect of pseudoephedrine). Products include:
- Zebeta Tablets 1457
- Ziac 1459

Buprenorphine (May increase the depressant effects of codeine). Products include:
- Buprenex Injectable 2170

Buspirone Hydrochloride (May increase the depressant effects of codeine). Products include:
- BuSpar Tablets 738

Butabarbital (May increase the depressant effects of codeine).
- No products indexed under this heading.

Butalbital (May increase the depressant effects of codeine). Products include:
- Axocet Capsules 2469
- Esgic-plus Capsules 1012
- Esgic-plus Tablets 1012
- Fioricet Tablets 2386
- Fioricet with Codeine Capsules 2387
- Fiorinal Capsules 2388
- Fiorinal with Codeine Capsules 2390
- Fiorinal Tablets 2388
- Phrenilin 790
- Sedapap Tablets 50 mg/650 mg 1826

Carteolol Hydrochloride (Increased pressor effect of pseudoephedrine). Products include:
- Cartrol Tablets 413
- Ocupress Ophthalmic Solution, 1% Sterile 297

Chlordiazepoxide (May increase the depressant effects of codeine). Products include:
- Limbitrol 2333

Chlordiazepoxide Hydrochloride (May increase the depressant effects of codeine). Products include:
- Librax Capsules 2330
- Librium Capsules 2331
- Librium Injectable 2332

Chlorpromazine (May increase the depressant effects of codeine). Products include:
- Thorazine Suppositories 2701

Chlorpromazine Hydrochloride (May increase the depressant effects of codeine). Products include:
- Thorazine 2701

Chlorprothixene (May increase the depressant effects of codeine).
- No products indexed under this heading.

Chlorprothixene Hydrochloride (May increase the depressant effects of codeine).
- No products indexed under this heading.

Chlorprothixene Lactate (May increase the depressant effects of codeine).
- No products indexed under this heading.

Clidinium Bromide (Concurrent use may result in paralytic ileus). Products include:
- Librax Capsules 2330

Clomipramine Hydrochloride (May antagonize effects of pseudoephedrine; increased effects of antidepressants or the codeine). Products include:
- Anafranil Capsules 819

Clorazepate Dipotassium (May increase the depressant effects of codeine). Products include:
- Tranxene 459

Clozapine (May increase the depressant effects of codeine). Products include:
- Clozaril Tablets 2377

Cryptenamine Preparations (Decreased hypotensive effects).

Desflurane (May increase the depressant effects of codeine). Products include:
- Suprane (desflurane, USP) 1865

Desipramine Hydrochloride (May antagonize effects of pseudoephedrine; increased effects of antidepressants or the codeine). Products include:
- Norpramin Tablets 1273

Deslanoside (Possibility of cardiac arrhythmias).
- No products indexed under this heading.

Dezocine (May increase the depressant effects of codeine). Products include:
- Dalgan Injection 529

Diazepam (May increase the depressant effects of codeine). Products include:
- Dizac (diazepam injectable emulsion) CIV 1862
- Valium Injectable 2336
- Valium Tablets 2335

Dicyclomine Hydrochloride (Concurrent use may result in paralytic ileus). Products include:
- Bentyl 1246

Digitoxin (Possibility of cardiac arrhythmias). Products include:
- Crystodigin Tablets 1472

Digoxin (Possibility of cardiac arrhythmias). Products include:
- Lanoxicaps 1110
- Lanoxin Elixir Pediatric 1113
- Lanoxin Injection 1116
- Lanoxin Injection Pediatric 1119
- Lanoxin Tablets 1121

Dobutamine Hydrochloride (Increased effect of either agent; increased potential for side effects). Products include:
- Dobutrex Solution Vials 1480

Dopamine Hydrochloride (Increased effect of either agent; increased potential for side effects).
- No products indexed under this heading.

Doxepin Hydrochloride (May antagonize effects of pseudoephedrine; increased effects of antidepressants or the codeine). Products include:
- Adapin Capsules 1542
- Sinequan 2028
- Zonalon Cream 1042

Droperidol (May increase the depressant effects of codeine). Products include:
- Inapsine Injection 462

Enflurane (May increase the depressant effects of codeine).
- No products indexed under this heading.

Ephedrine Hydrochloride (Increased effect of either agent; increased potential for side effects). Products include:
- Primatene Tablets 844
- Quadrinal Tablets 1398

Ephedrine Sulfate (Increased effect of either agent; increased potential for side effects). Products include:
- Marax Tablets & DF Syrup 2015

Ephedrine Tannate (Increased effect of either agent; increased potential for side effects). Products include:
- Rynatuss 2782

Epinephrine (Increased effect of either agent; increased potential for side effects). Products include:
- EPIFRIN 237
- EpiPen 808
- Marcaine with Epinephrine 2446
- Primatene Mist 843
- Sensorcaine with Epinephrine Injection 554
- Sus-Phrine Injection 1017
- Xylocaine with Epinephrine Injections 562

Epinephrine Bitartrate (Increased effect of either agent; increased potential for side effects). Products include:
- Sensorcaine-MPF with Epinephrine Injection 554

Epinephrine Hydrochloride (Increased effect of either agent; increased potential for side effects). Products include:
- Ana-Kit Anaphylaxis Emergency Treatment Kit 611

Esmolol Hydrochloride (Increased pressor effect of pseudoephedrine). Products include:
- Brevibloc (esmolol HCl) Injection 1860

Estazolam (May increase the depressant effects of codeine). Products include:
- ProSom Tablets 457

Ethchlorvynol (May increase the depressant effects of codeine). Products include:
- Placidyl Capsules 456

Ethinamate (May increase the depressant effects of codeine).
- No products indexed under this heading.

Fentanyl (May increase the depressant effects of codeine). Products include:
- Duragesic Transdermal System 1336

Fentanyl Citrate (May increase the depressant effects of codeine). Products include:
- Sublimaze Injection 463

Fluphenazine Decanoate (May increase the depressant effects of codeine). Products include:
- Prolixin Decanoate 510

Fluphenazine Enanthate (May increase the depressant effects of codeine). Products include:
- Prolixin Enanthate 510

Fluphenazine Hydrochloride (May increase the depressant effects of codeine). Products include:
- Prolixin 510

Flurazepam Hydrochloride (May increase the depressant effects of codeine). Products include:
- Dalmane Capsules 2329

Furazolidone (Concurrent and/or sequential use is contraindicated; potential for hypertensive crisis). Products include:
- Furoxone 2221

Glutethimide (May increase the depressant effects of codeine).
- No products indexed under this heading.

Glycopyrrolate (Concurrent use may result in paralytic ileus). Products include:
- Robinul Forte Tablets 2247
- Robinul Injectable 2247
- Robinul Tablets 2247

Haloperidol (May increase the depressant effects of codeine). Products include:
- Haldol Injection, Tablets and Concentrate 1585

Haloperidol Decanoate (May increase the depressant effects of codeine). Products include:
- Haldol Decanoate 1587

Hydrocodone Bitartrate (May increase the depressant effects of codeine). Products include:
- Codiclear DH Syrup 808
- Duratuss HD Elixir 2750
- Histussin D Liquid 670
- Hycodan Tablets and Syrup 946
- Hycomine Compound Tablets 948
- Hycomine 947
- Hycotuss Expectorant Syrup 950
- Hydrocet Capsules 787
- Lorcet 10/650 Tablets 1016
- Lortab 2751
- Tussend 1830
- Tussend Expectorant 1831
- Vicodin Tablets 1404
- Vicodin ES Tablets 1405
- Vicodin HP Tablets 1403
- Vicodin Tuss Expectorant 1406
- Zydone Capsules 967

Hydrocodone Polistirex (May increase the depressant effects of codeine). Products include:
- Tussionex Pennkinetic Extended-Release Suspension 1624

Hydroxyzine Hydrochloride (May increase the depressant effects of codeine). Products include:
- Atarax Tablets & Syrup 1992
- Marax Tablets & DF Syrup 2015
- Vistaril Intramuscular Solution 2042

Hyoscyamine (Concurrent use may result in paralytic ileus). Products include:
- Cystospaz Tablets 2123
- Urised Tablets 2123

IMPORTANT NOTE: Always consult each drug listing in the patient's regimen for possible interactions.

Nucofed / Interactions Index   766

Hyoscyamine Sulfate (Concurrent use may result in paralytic ileus). Products include:
- Arco-Lase Plus Tablets 513
- Atrohist Plus Tablets 1605
- Cystospaz-M Capsules 2123
- Donnatal 2234
- Donnatal Extentabs 2234
- Donnatal Tablets 2234
- Kutrase Capsules 2546
- Levsin/Levsinex/Levbid 2549

Imipramine Hydrochloride (May antagonize effects of pseudoephedrine; increased effects of antidepressants or the codeine). Products include:
- Tofranil Ampuls 873
- Tofranil Tablets 875

Imipramine Pamoate (May antagonize effects of pseudoephedrine; increased effects of antidepressants or the codeine). Products include:
- Tofranil-PM Capsules 876

Ipratropium Bromide (Concurrent use may result in paralytic ileus). Products include:
- Atrovent Inhalation Aerosol 674
- Atrovent Inhalation Solution 675
- Atrovent Nasal Spray 0.03% 676
- Atrovent Nasal Spray 0.06% 678

Isocarboxazid (Concurrent and/or sequential use is contraindicated; potential for hypertensive crisis).
No products indexed under this heading.

Isoflurane (May increase the depressant effects of codeine).
No products indexed under this heading.

Isoproterenol Hydrochloride (Increased effect of either agent; increased potential for side effects). Products include:
- Isuprel Hydrochloride Solution 2443
- Isuprel Injection 2441
- Isuprel Mistometer 2442

Isoproterenol Sulfate (Increased effect of either agent; increased potential for side effects). Products include:
- Norisodrine with Calcium Iodide Syrup 446

Ketamine Hydrochloride (May increase the depressant effects of codeine).
No products indexed under this heading.

Labetalol Hydrochloride (Increased pressor effect of pseudoephedrine). Products include:
- Normodyne Injection 2519
- Normodyne Tablets 2522
- Trandate 1158

Levobunolol Hydrochloride (Increased pressor effect of pseudoephedrine). Products include:
- Betagan .... ⓞ 230

Levomethadyl Acetate Hydrochloride (May increase the depressant effects of codeine). Products include:
- Orlaam Oral Solution 2361

Levorphanol Tartrate (May increase the depressant effects of codeine). Products include:
- Levo-Dromoran 2297

Lorazepam (May increase the depressant effects of codeine). Products include:
- Ativan Injection 2805
- Ativan Tablets 2807

Loxapine Hydrochloride (May increase the depressant effects of codeine). Products include:
- Loxitane 1426

Loxapine Succinate (May increase the depressant effects of codeine). Products include:
- Loxitane Capsules 1426

Maprotiline Hydrochloride (May antagonize effects of pseudoephedrine; increased effects of antidepressants or the codeine). Products include:
- Ludiomil Tablets 861

Mepenzolate Bromide (Concurrent use may result in paralytic ileus).
No products indexed under this heading.

Meperidine Hydrochloride (May increase the depressant effects of codeine). Products include:
- Demerol 2438
- Mepergan Injection 2859

Mephobarbital (May increase the depressant effects of codeine). Products include:
- Mebaral Tablets 2452

Meprobamate (May increase the depressant effects of codeine). Products include:
- Miltown Tablets 2780
- PMB 200 and PMB 400 2890

Mesoridazine Besylate (May increase the depressant effects of codeine). Products include:
- Serentil 689

Metaproterenol Sulfate (Increased effect of either agent; increased potential for side effects). Products include:
- Alupent 672
- Metaproterenol Sulfate Inhalation Solution, USP, Arm-a-Med 547

Metaraminol Bitartrate (Increased effect of either agent; increased potential for side effects). Products include:
- Aramine Injection 1649

Methadone Hydrochloride (May increase the depressant effects of codeine). Products include:
- Methadone Hydrochloride Oral Concentrate 2356
- Methadone Hydrochloride Oral Solution & Tablets 2357

Methohexital Sodium (May increase the depressant effects of codeine).
No products indexed under this heading.

Methotrimeprazine (May increase the depressant effects of codeine). Products include:
- Levoprome 1321

Methoxamine Hydrochloride (Increased effect of either agent; increased potential for side effects). Products include:
- Vasoxyl Injection 1169

Methoxyflurane (May increase the depressant effects of codeine).
No products indexed under this heading.

Metipranolol Hydrochloride (Increased pressor effect of pseudoephedrine). Products include:
- OptiPranolol (Metipranolol 0.3%) Sterile Ophthalmic Solution .... ⓞ 256

Metoprolol Succinate (Increased pressor effect of pseudoephedrine). Products include:
- Toprol-XL Tablets 560

Metoprolol Tartrate (Increased pressor effect of pseudoephedrine). Products include:
- Lopressor 848
- Lopressor HCT Tablets 850

Midazolam Hydrochloride (May increase the depressant effects of codeine). Products include:
- Versed Injection 2324

Molindone Hydrochloride (May increase the depressant effects of codeine). Products include:
- Moban Tablets and Concentrate 1036

Morphine Sulfate (May increase the depressant effects of codeine). Products include:
- Astramorph/PF Injection, USP (Preservative-Free) 526
- Duramorph Injection 983
- Infumorph 200 and Infumorph 500 Sterile Solutions 985
- Kadian Capsules 2948
- MS Contin Tablets 2149
- MSIR 2152
- Oramorph SR (Morphine Sulfate Sustained Release Tablets) 2359
- RMS Suppositories CII 2766
- Roxanol 2365

Nadolol (Increased pressor effect of pseudoephedrine).
No products indexed under this heading.

Norepinephrine Bitartrate (Increased effect of either agent; increased potential for side effects). Products include:
- Levophed Bitartrate Injection 2445

Nortriptyline Hydrochloride (May antagonize effects of pseudoephedrine; increased effects of antidepressants or the codeine). Products include:
- Pamelor 2409

Opium Alkaloids (May increase the depressant effects of codeine).
No products indexed under this heading.

Oxazepam (May increase the depressant effects of codeine). Products include:
- Serax Capsules 2916
- Serax Capsules 2916

Oxybutynin Chloride (Concurrent use may result in paralytic ileus). Products include:
- Ditropan 1267

Oxycodone Hydrochloride (May increase the depressant effects of codeine). Products include:
- OxyContin Tablets 2163
- OxyIR Capsules 2167
- Percocet Tablets 955
- Percodan Tablets 955
- Percodan-Demi Tablets 956
- Roxicodone Tablets, Oral Solution & Intensol (Oxycodone) 2366
- Tylox Capsules 1593

Penbutolol Sulfate (Increased pressor effect of pseudoephedrine). Products include:
- Levatol Tablets 2547

Pentobarbital Sodium (May increase the depressant effects of codeine). Products include:
- Nembutal Sodium Capsules 440
- Nembutal Sodium Solution 442
- Nembutal Sodium Suppositories 444

Perphenazine (May increase the depressant effects of codeine). Products include:
- Etrafon 2495
- Triavil Tablets 1800
- Trilafon 2532

Phenelzine Sulfate (Concurrent and/or sequential use is contraindicated; potential for hypertensive crisis). Products include:
- Nardil 1977

Phenobarbital (May increase the depressant effects of codeine). Products include:
- Arco-Lase Plus Tablets 513
- Bellergal-S Tablets 2375
- Donnatal 2234
- Donnatal Extentabs 2234
- Donnatal Tablets 2234
- Phenobarbital Elixir and Tablets 1523
- Quadrinal Tablets 1398

Phenylephrine Bitartrate (Increased effect of either agent; increased potential for side effects).
No products indexed under this heading.

Phenylephrine Hydrochloride (Increased effect of either agent; increased potential for side effects). Products include:
- Atrohist Plus Tablets 1605
- Cerose DM .... ▣ 853
- D.A. II Tablets 972
- D.A. Chewable Tablets 970
- Dura-Vent/DA Tablets 972
- Extendryl 1003
- 4-Way Fast Acting Nasal Spray (regular & mentholated) .... ▣ 644
- Hemoril .... ▣ 797
- Hycomine Compound Tablets 948
- Neo-Synephrine Hydrochloride 1% Carpuject 2455
- Neo-Synephrine Hydrochloride 1% Injection 2455
- Neo-Synephrine Hydrochloride (Ophthalmic) 2456
- Neo-Synephrine .... ▣ 624
- Novahistine Elixir .... ▣ 782
- Phenergan VC 2886
- Phenergan VC with Codeine 2888
- Preparation H .... ▣ 842
- Tympagesic Ear Drops 2476
- Vicks Sinex Nasal Spray and Ultra Fine Mist .... ▣ 738

Phenylephrine Tannate (Increased effect of either agent; increased potential for side effects). Products include:
- Atrohist Pediatric Suspension 1604
- Atrohist Pediatric Suspension Dye-Free 1604
- Rynatan 2781
- Rynatuss 2782

Phenylpropanolamine Hydrochloride (Increased effect of either agent; increased potential for side effects). Products include:
- Acutrim .... ▣ 648
- Atrohist Plus Tablets 1605
- BC Cold Powder Multi-Symptom Formula (Cold-Sinus-Allergy) .... ▣ 631
- BC Cold Powder Non-Drowsy Formula (Cold-Sinus) .... ▣ 631
- Cheracol Plus Head Cold/Cough Formula .... ▣ 741
- Comtrex Multi-Symptom Cold Reliever Liqui-Gels .... ▣ 638
- Comtrex Multi-Symptom Non-Drowsy Liqui-gels .... ▣ 640
- Contac Continuous Action Nasal Decongestant/Antihistamine 12 Hour Capsules .... ▣ 773
- Contac Maximum Strength Continuous Action Decongestant/Antihistamine 12 Hour Caplets 772
- Contac Severe Cold and Flu Formula Caplets .... ▣ 773
- Coricidin 'D' Decongestant Tablets .... ▣ 760
- Dexatrim .... ▣ 795
- Dexatrim Plus Vitamins Caplets .... ▣ 796
- Dimetane-DC Cough Syrup 2232
- Dimetapp Allergy Sinus Caplets .... ▣ 838
- Dimetapp Cold & Allergy Chewable Tablets .... ▣ 838
- Dimetapp Cold & Cough Liqui-Gels .... ▣ 839
- Dimetapp DM Elixir .... ▣ 840
- Dimetapp Elixir .... ▣ 840
- Dimetapp Extentabs .... ▣ 841
- Dimetapp Tablets/Liqui-Gels .... ▣ 841
- Dura-Vent Tablets 971
- Entex LA Tablets 972
- Exgest LA Tablets 787
- Hycomine 947
- Nolamine Timed-Release Tablets 790
- Ornade Spansule Capsules 2678
- Propagest Tablets 791
- Pyrroxate Caplets .... ▣ 742
- Robitussin-CF .... ▣ 846
- Sinulin Tablets 792
- Tavist-D 12 Hour Relief Tablets .... ▣ 750
- Teldrin 12 Hour Antihistamine/Nasal Decongestant Allergy Relief Capsules .... ▣ 786
- Triaminic Expectorant .... ▣ 753
- Triaminic Syrup .... ▣ 755
- Triaminic Triaminicol Cold & Cough .... ▣ 756
- Triaminic DM Syrup .... ▣ 756
- Triaminicin Tablets .... ▣ 756
- Vicks DayQuil Allergy Relief 12-Hour Extended Release Tablets .... ▣ 733
- Vicks DayQuil Allergy Relief 4-Hour Tablets .... ▣ 733

(▣ Described in PDR For Nonprescription Drugs)   (ⓞ Described in PDR For Ophthalmology)

767 Interactions Index Numorphan Injection

Vicks DayQuil SINUS Pressure & CONGESTION Relief 734

Pindolol (Increased pressor effect of pseudoephedrine). Products include:

Visken Tablets 2428

Pirbuterol Acetate (Increased effect of either agent; increased potential for side effects). Products include:

Maxair Autohaler 1550
Maxair Inhaler 1552

Prazepam (May increase the depressant effects of codeine).

No products indexed under this heading.

Prochlorperazine (May increase the depressant effects of codeine). Products include:

Compazine 2644

Procyclidine Hydrochloride (Concurrent use may result in paralytic ileus). Products include:

Kemadrin Tablets 1105

Promethazine Hydrochloride (May increase the depressant effects of codeine). Products include:

Mepergan Injection 2859
Phenergan with Codeine 2883
Phenergan with Dextromethorphan 2885
Phenergan Injection 2880
Phenergan Suppositories 2882
Phenergan Syrup 2881
Phenergan Tablets 2882
Phenergan VC 2886
Phenergan VC with Codeine 2888

Propantheline Bromide (Concurrent use may result in paralytic ileus). Products include:

Pro-Banthine Tablets 2226

Propofol (May increase the depressant effects of codeine). Products include:

Diprivan Injectable Emulsion 2939

Propoxyphene Hydrochloride (May increase the depressant effects of codeine). Products include:

Darvon 1475
Wygesic Tablets 2930

Propoxyphene Napsylate (May increase the depressant effects of codeine). Products include:

Darvon-N/Darvocet-N 1473

Propranolol Hydrochloride (Increased pressor effect of pseudoephedrine). Products include:

Inderal 2834
Inderal LA Long Acting Capsules ... 2836
Inderide Tablets 2838
Inderide LA Long Acting Capsules .. 2840

Protriptyline Hydrochloride (May antagonize effects of pseudoephedrine; increased effects of antidepressants or the codeine). Products include:

Vivactil Tablets 1820

Pseudoephedrine Sulfate (Increased effect of either agent; increased potential for side effects). Products include:

Chlor-Trimeton Allergy Decongestant Tablets 759
Claritin-D Tablets 2487
Drixoral Cold and Allergy Sustained-Action Tablets 763
Drixoral Cold and Flu Extended-Release Tablets 764
Drixoral Non-Drowsy Formula Extended-Release Tablets 764
Drixoral Allergy/Sinus Extended Release Tablets 765
Trinalin Repetabs Tablets 1373

Quazepam (May increase the depressant effects of codeine). Products include:

Doral Tablets 2773

Risperidone (May increase the depressant effects of codeine). Products include:

Risperdal Tablets 1348

Salmeterol Xinafoate (Increased effect of either agent; increased potential for side effects). Products include:

Serevent Inhalation Aerosol 1149

Scopolamine (Concurrent use may result in paralytic ileus). Products include:

Transderm Scōp Transdermal Therapeutic System 890

Scopolamine Hydrobromide (Concurrent use may result in paralytic ileus). Products include:

Atrohist Plus Tablets 1605
Donnatal 2234
Donnatal Extentabs 2234
Donnatal Tablets 2234

Secobarbital Sodium (May increase the depressant effects of codeine). Products include:

Seconal Sodium Pulvules 1529

Selegiline Hydrochloride (Concurrent and/or sequential use is contraindicated; potential for hypertensive crisis). Products include:

Eldepryl Capsules 2729

Sevoflurane (May increase the depressant effects of codeine).

No products indexed under this heading.

Sotalol Hydrochloride (Increased pressor effect of pseudoephedrine). Products include:

Betapace Tablets 637

Sufentanil Citrate (May increase the depressant effects of codeine). Products include:

Sufenta Injection 1355

Temazepam (May increase the depressant effects of codeine). Products include:

Restoril Capsules 2413

Terbutaline Sulfate (Increased effect of either agent; increased potential for side effects). Products include:

Brethaire Inhaler 830
Brethine Ampuls 832
Brethine Tablets 831
Bricanyl Subcutaneous Injection 1247
Bricanyl Tablets 1248

Thiamylal Sodium (May increase the depressant effects of codeine).

No products indexed under this heading.

Thioridazine Hydrochloride (May increase the depressant effects of codeine). Products include:

Mellaril 2398

Thiothixene (May increase the depressant effects of codeine). Products include:

Navane Capsules and Concentrate 2018
Navane Intramuscular 2019

Timolol Maleate (Increased pressor effect of pseudoephedrine). Products include:

Blocadren Tablets 1654
Timolide Tablets 1791
Timoptic in Ocudose 1796
Timoptic Sterile Ophthalmic Solution 1794
Timoptic-XE 1798

Tranylcypromine Sulfate (Concurrent and/or sequential use is contraindicated; potential for hypertensive crisis). Products include:

Parnate Tablets 2679

Triazolam (May increase the depressant effects of codeine). Products include:

Halcion Tablets 2093

Tridihexethyl Chloride (Concurrent use may result in paralytic ileus).

No products indexed under this heading.

Trifluoperazine Hydrochloride (May increase the depressant effects of codeine). Products include:

Stelazine 2692

Trihexyphenidyl Hydrochloride (Concurrent use may result in paralytic ileus). Products include:

Artane 1418

Trimipramine Maleate (May antagonize effects of pseudoephedrine; increased effects of antidepressants or the codeine). Products include:

Surmontil Capsules 2917

Zolpidem Tartrate (May increase the depressant effects of codeine). Products include:

Ambien Tablets 2559

Food Interactions

Alcohol (May increase the depressant effects of codeine).

NU-IRON 150 CAPSULES

(Polysaccharide-Iron Complex) 1826
None cited in PDR database.

NU-IRON ELIXIR

(Polysaccharide-Iron Complex) 1826
None cited in PDR database.

NULYTELY

(Polyethylene Glycol, Sodium Bicarbonate, Sodium Chloride, Potassium Chloride) 694
May interact with:

Oral Medications, unspecified (Oral medications may not be absorbed if given within one hour).

Food Interactions

Food, unspecified (Solid food should not be given for at least two hours before the solution is given).

CHERRY FLAVOR NULYTELY

(Polyethylene Glycol, Sodium Bicarbonate, Sodium Chloride, Potassium Chloride) 694
See **NuLYTELY**

NUMORPHAN INJECTION

(Oxymorphone Hydrochloride) 953
May interact with narcotic analgesics, anesthetics, phenothiazines, tranquilizers, hypnotics and sedatives, central nervous system depressants, and certain other agents. Compounds in these categories include:

Alfentanil Hydrochloride (Additive CNS depression). Products include:

Alfenta Injection 1334

Alprazolam (Additive CNS depression). Products include:

Xanax Tablets 2115

Aprobarbital (Additive CNS depression).

No products indexed under this heading.

Buprenorphine (Additive CNS depression). Products include:

Buprenex Injectable 2170

Buspirone Hydrochloride (Additive CNS depression). Products include:

BuSpar Tablets 738

Butabarbital (Additive CNS depression).

No products indexed under this heading.

Butalbital (Additive CNS depression). Products include:

Axocet Capsules 2469
Esgic-plus Capsules 1012
Esgic-plus Tablets 1012
Fioricet Tablets 2386
Fioricet with Codeine Capsules 2387
Fiorinal Capsules 2388
Fiorinal with Codeine Capsules 2390
Fiorinal Tablets 2388
Phrenilin 790
Sedapap Tablets 50 mg/650 mg .. 1826

Chlordiazepoxide (Additive CNS depression). Products include:

Limbitrol 2333

Chlordiazepoxide Hydrochloride (Additive CNS depression). Products include:

Librax Capsules 2330
Librium Capsules 2331
Librium Injectable 2332

Chlorpromazine (Additive CNS depression). Products include:

Thorazine Suppositories 2701

Chlorprothixene (Additive CNS depression).

No products indexed under this heading.

Chlorprothixene Hydrochloride (Additive CNS depression).

No products indexed under this heading.

Chlorprothixene Lactate (Additive CNS depression).

No products indexed under this heading.

Clorazepate Dipotassium (Additive CNS depression). Products include:

Tranxene 459

Clozapine (Additive CNS depression). Products include:

Clozaril Tablets 2377

Codeine Phosphate (Additive CNS depression). Products include:

Brontex 2130
Dimetane-DC Cough Syrup 2232
Fioricet with Codeine Capsules 2387
Fiorinal with Codeine Capsules 2390
Nucofed 2225
Phenergan with Codeine 2883
Phenergan VC with Codeine 2888
Robitussin A-C Syrup 2248
Robitussin-DAC Syrup 2249
Ryna 804
Soma Compound w/Codeine Tablets 2784
Tylenol with Codeine 1592

Desflurane (Additive CNS depression). Products include:

Suprane (desflurane, USP) 1865

Dezocine (Additive CNS depression). Products include:

Dalgan Injection 529

Diazepam (Additive CNS depression). Products include:

Dizac (diazepam injectable emulsion) CIV 1862
Valium Injectable 2336
Valium Tablets 2335

Droperidol (Additive CNS depression). Products include:

Inapsine Injection 462

Enflurane (Additive CNS depression).

No products indexed under this heading.

Estazolam (Additive CNS depression). Products include:

ProSom Tablets 457

Ethchlorvynol (Additive CNS depression). Products include:

Placidyl Capsules 456

Ethinamate (Additive CNS depression).

No products indexed under this heading.

Fentanyl (Additive CNS depression). Products include:

Duragesic Transdermal System 1336

Fentanyl Citrate (Additive CNS depression). Products include:

Sublimaze Injection 463

IMPORTANT NOTE: Always consult each drug listing in the patient's regimen for possible interactions.

Numorphan Injection — Interactions Index

Fluphenazine Decanoate (Additive CNS depression). Products include:
- Prolixin Decanoate 510

Fluphenazine Enanthate (Additive CNS depression). Products include:
- Prolixin Enanthate 510

Fluphenazine Hydrochloride (Additive CNS depression). Products include:
- Prolixin 510

Flurazepam Hydrochloride (Additive CNS depression). Products include:
- Dalmane Capsules 2329

Glutethimide (Additive CNS depression).
- No products indexed under this heading.

Haloperidol (Additive CNS depression). Products include:
- Haldol Injection, Tablets and Concentrate 1585

Haloperidol Decanoate (Additive CNS depression). Products include:
- Haldol Decanoate 1587

Halothane (Additive CNS depression). Products include:
- Fluothane 2830

Hydrocodone Bitartrate (Additive CNS depression). Products include:
- Codiclear DH Syrup 808
- Duratuss HD Elixir 2750
- Histussin D Liquid 670
- Hycodan Tablets and Syrup 946
- Hycomine Compound Tablets 948
- Hycomine 947
- Hycotuss Expectorant Syrup 950
- Hydrocet Capsules 787
- Lorcet 10/650 Tablets 1016
- Lortab 2751
- Tussend 1830
- Tussend Expectorant 1831
- Vicodin Tablets 1404
- Vicodin ES Tablets 1405
- Vicodin HP Tablets 1403
- Vicodin Tuss Expectorant 1406
- Zydone Capsules 967

Hydrocodone Polistirex (Additive CNS depression). Products include:
- Tussionex Pennkinetic Extended-Release Suspension 1624

Hydromorphone Hydrochloride (Additive CNS depression). Products include:
- Dilaudid Ampules 1382
- Dilaudid Cough Syrup 1383
- Dilaudid-HP Injection 1384
- Dilaudid-HP Lyophilized Powder 250 mg 1384
- Dilaudid 1382
- Dilaudid Oral Liquid 1386
- Dilaudid 1382
- Dilaudid Tablets - 8 mg 1386

Hydroxyzine Hydrochloride (Additive CNS depression). Products include:
- Atarax Tablets & Syrup 1992
- Marax Tablets & DF Syrup 2015
- Vistaril Intramuscular Solution 2042

Isoflurane (Additive CNS depression).
- No products indexed under this heading.

Ketamine Hydrochloride (Additive CNS depression).
- No products indexed under this heading.

Levomethadyl Acetate Hydrochloride (Additive CNS depression). Products include:
- Orlaam Oral Solution 2361

Levorphanol Tartrate (Additive CNS depression). Products include:
- Levo-Dromoran 2297

Lorazepam (Additive CNS depression). Products include:
- Ativan Injection 2805
- Ativan Tablets 2807

Loxapine Hydrochloride (Additive CNS depression). Products include:
- Loxitane 1426

Loxapine Succinate (Additive CNS depression). Products include:
- Loxitane Capsules 1426

Meperidine Hydrochloride (Additive CNS depression). Products include:
- Demerol 2438
- Mepergan Injection 2859

Mephobarbital (Additive CNS depression). Products include:
- Mebaral Tablets 2452

Meprobamate (Additive CNS depression). Products include:
- Miltown Tablets 2780
- PMB 200 and PMB 400 2890

Mesoridazine Besylate (Additive CNS depression). Products include:
- Serentil 689

Methadone Hydrochloride (Additive CNS depression). Products include:
- Methadone Hydrochloride Oral Concentrate 2356
- Methadone Hydrochloride Oral Solution & Tablets 2357

Methohexital Sodium (Additive CNS depression).
- No products indexed under this heading.

Methotrimeprazine (Additive CNS depression). Products include:
- Levoprome 1321

Methoxyflurane (Additive CNS depression).
- No products indexed under this heading.

Midazolam Hydrochloride (Additive CNS depression). Products include:
- Versed Injection 2324

Molindone Hydrochloride (Additive CNS depression). Products include:
- Moban Tablets and Concentrate 1036

Morphine Sulfate (Additive CNS depression). Products include:
- Astramorph/PF Injection, USP (Preservative-Free) 526
- Duramorph Injection 983
- Infumorph 200 and Infumorph 500 Sterile Solutions 985
- Kadian Capsules 2948
- MS Contin Tablets 2149
- MSIR 2152
- Oramorph SR (Morphine Sulfate Sustained Release Tablets) 2359
- RMS Suppositories CII 2766
- Roxanol 2365

Opium Alkaloids (Additive CNS depression).
- No products indexed under this heading.

Oxazepam (Additive CNS depression). Products include:
- Serax Capsules 2916
- Serax Tablets 2916

Oxycodone Hydrochloride (Additive CNS depression). Products include:
- OxyContin Tablets 2163
- OxyIR Capsules 2167
- Percocet Tablets 955
- Percodan Tablets 955
- Percodan-Demi Tablets 956
- Roxicodone Tablets, Oral Solution & Intensol (Oxycodone) 2366
- Tylox Capsules 1593

Pentobarbital Sodium (Additive CNS depression). Products include:
- Nembutal Sodium Capsules 440
- Nembutal Sodium Solution 442
- Nembutal Sodium Suppositories 444

Perphenazine (Additive CNS depression). Products include:
- Etrafon 2495
- Triavil Tablets 1800
- Trilafon 2532

Phenobarbital (Additive CNS depression). Products include:
- Arco-Lase Plus Tablets 513
- Bellergal-S Tablets 2375
- Donnatal 2234
- Donnatal Extentabs 2234
- Donnatal Tablets 2234
- Phenobarbital Elixir and Tablets 1523
- Quadrinal Tablets 1398

Prazepam (Additive CNS depression).
- No products indexed under this heading.

Prochlorperazine (Additive CNS depression). Products include:
- Compazine 2644

Promethazine Hydrochloride (Additive CNS depression). Products include:
- Mepergan Injection 2859
- Phenergan with Codeine 2883
- Phenergan with Dextromethorphan 2885
- Phenergan Injection 2880
- Phenergan Suppositories 2882
- Phenergan Syrup 2881
- Phenergan Tablets 2882
- Phenergan VC 2886
- Phenergan VC with Codeine 2888

Propofol (Additive CNS depression). Products include:
- Diprivan Injectable Emulsion 2939

Propoxyphene Hydrochloride (Additive CNS depression). Products include:
- Darvon 1475
- Wygesic Tablets 2930

Propoxyphene Napsylate (Additive CNS depression). Products include:
- Darvon-N/Darvocet-N 1473

Quazepam (Additive CNS depression). Products include:
- Doral Tablets 2773

Risperidone (Additive CNS depression). Products include:
- Risperdal Tablets 1348

Secobarbital Sodium (Additive CNS depression). Products include:
- Seconal Sodium Pulvules 1529

Sevoflurane (Additive CNS depression).
- No products indexed under this heading.

Sufentanil Citrate (Additive CNS depression). Products include:
- Sufenta Injection 1355

Temazepam (Additive CNS depression). Products include:
- Restoril Capsules 2413

Thiamylal Sodium (Additive CNS depression).
- No products indexed under this heading.

Thioridazine Hydrochloride (Additive CNS depression). Products include:
- Mellaril 2398

Thiothixene (Additive CNS depression). Products include:
- Navane Capsules and Concentrate 2018
- Navane Intramuscular 2019

Triazolam (Additive CNS depression). Products include:
- Halcion Tablets 2093

Trifluoperazine Hydrochloride (Additive CNS depression). Products include:
- Stelazine 2692

Zolpidem Tartrate (Additive CNS depression). Products include:
- Ambien Tablets 2559

Food Interactions
Alcohol (Additive CNS depression).

NUMORPHAN SUPPOSITORIES
(Oxymorphone Hydrochloride) 953

May interact with narcotic analgesics, tranquilizers, hypnotics and sedatives, general anesthetics, phenothiazines, central nervous system depressants, and certain other agents. Compounds in these categories include:

Alfentanil Hydrochloride (Additive CNS depression). Products include:
- Alfenta Injection 1334

Alprazolam (Additive CNS depression). Products include:
- Xanax Tablets 2115

Aprobarbital (Additive CNS depression).
- No products indexed under this heading.

Buprenorphine (Additive CNS depression). Products include:
- Buprenex Injectable 2170

Buspirone Hydrochloride (Additive CNS depression). Products include:
- BuSpar Tablets 738

Butabarbital (Additive CNS depression).
- No products indexed under this heading.

Butalbital (Additive CNS depression). Products include:
- Axocet Capsules 2469
- Esgic-plus Capsules 1012
- Esgic-plus Tablets 1012
- Fioricet Tablets 2386
- Fioricet with Codeine Capsules 2387
- Fiorinal Capsules 2388
- Fiorinal with Codeine Capsules 2390
- Fiorinal Tablets 2388
- Phrenilin 790
- Sedapap Tablets 50 mg/650 mg 1826

Chlordiazepoxide (Additive CNS depression). Products include:
- Limbitrol 2333

Chlordiazepoxide Hydrochloride (Additive CNS depression). Products include:
- Librax Capsules 2330
- Librium Capsules 2331
- Librium Injectable 2332

Chlorpromazine (Additive CNS depression). Products include:
- Thorazine Suppositories 2701

Chlorprothixene (Additive CNS depression).
- No products indexed under this heading.

Chlorprothixene Hydrochloride (Additive CNS depression).
- No products indexed under this heading.

Chlorprothixene Lactate (Additive CNS depression).
- No products indexed under this heading.

Clorazepate Dipotassium (Additive CNS depression). Products include:
- Tranxene 459

Clozapine (Additive CNS depression). Products include:
- Clozaril Tablets 2377

Codeine Phosphate (Additive CNS depression). Products include:
- Brontex 2130
- Dimetane-DC Cough Syrup 2232
- Fioricet with Codeine Capsules 2387
- Fiorinal with Codeine Capsules 2390
- Nucofed 2225
- Phenergan with Codeine 2883
- Phenergan VC with Codeine 2888
- Robitussin A-C Syrup 2248
- Robitussin-DAC Syrup 2249
- Ryna 804
- Soma Compound w/Codeine Tablets 2784
- Tylenol with Codeine 1592

(◨ Described in PDR For Nonprescription Drugs)   (◉ Described in PDR For Ophthalmology)

Interactions Index

Desflurane (Additive CNS depression). Products include:
- Suprane (desflurane, USP) 1865

Dezocine (Additive CNS depression). Products include:
- Dalgan Injection 529

Diazepam (Additive CNS depression). Products include:
- Dizac (diazepam injectable emulsion) CIV 1862
- Valium Injectable 2336
- Valium Tablets 2335

Droperidol (Additive CNS depression). Products include:
- Inapsine Injection 462

Enflurane (Additive CNS depression).
- No products indexed under this heading.

Estazolam (Additive CNS depression). Products include:
- ProSom Tablets 457

Ethchlorvynol (Additive CNS depression). Products include:
- Placidyl Capsules 456

Ethinamate (Additive CNS depression).
- No products indexed under this heading.

Fentanyl (Additive CNS depression). Products include:
- Duragesic Transdermal System 1336

Fentanyl Citrate (Additive CNS depression). Products include:
- Sublimaze Injection 463

Fluphenazine Decanoate (Additive CNS depression). Products include:
- Prolixin Decanoate 510

Fluphenazine Enanthate (Additive CNS depression). Products include:
- Prolixin Enanthate 510

Fluphenazine Hydrochloride (Additive CNS depression). Products include:
- Prolixin 510

Flurazepam Hydrochloride (Additive CNS depression). Products include:
- Dalmane Capsules 2329

Glutethimide (Additive CNS depression).
- No products indexed under this heading.

Haloperidol (Additive CNS depression). Products include:
- Haldol Injection, Tablets and Concentrate 1585

Haloperidol Decanoate (Additive CNS depression). Products include:
- Haldol Decanoate 1587

Hydrocodone Bitartrate (Additive CNS depression). Products include:
- Codiclear DH Syrup 808
- Duratuss HD Elixir 2750
- Histussin D Liquid 670
- Hycodan Tablets and Syrup 946
- Hycomine Compound Tablets 948
- Hycomine 947
- Hycotuss Expectorant Syrup 950
- Hydrocet Capsules 787
- Lorcet 10/650 Tablets 1016
- Lortab 2751
- Tussend 1830
- Tussend Expectorant 1831
- Vicodin Tablets 1404
- Vicodin ES Tablets 1405
- Vicodin HP Tablets 1403
- Vicodin Tuss Expectorant 1406
- Zydone Capsules 967

Hydrocodone Polistirex (Additive CNS depression). Products include:
- Tussionex Pennkinetic Extended-Release Suspension 1624

Hydromorphone Hydrochloride (Additive CNS depression). Products include:
- Dilaudid Ampules 1382
- Dilaudid Cough Syrup 1383
- Dilaudid-HP Injection 1384
- Dilaudid-HP Lyophilized Powder 250 mg 1384
- Dilaudid 1382
- Dilaudid Oral Liquid 1386
- Dilaudid 1382
- Dilaudid Tablets - 8 mg 1386

Hydroxyzine Hydrochloride (Additive CNS depression). Products include:
- Atarax Tablets & Syrup 1992
- Marax Tablets & DF Syrup 2015
- Vistaril Intramuscular Solution 2042

Isoflurane (Additive CNS depression).
- No products indexed under this heading.

Ketamine Hydrochloride (Additive CNS depression).
- No products indexed under this heading.

Levomethadyl Acetate Hydrochloride (Additive CNS depression). Products include:
- Orlaam Oral Solution 2361

Levorphanol Tartrate (Additive CNS depression). Products include:
- Levo-Dromoran 2297

Lorazepam (Additive CNS depression). Products include:
- Ativan Injection 2805
- Ativan Tablets 2807

Loxapine Hydrochloride (Additive CNS depression). Products include:
- Loxitane 1426

Loxapine Succinate (Additive CNS depression). Products include:
- Loxitane Capsules 1426

Meperidine Hydrochloride (Additive CNS depression). Products include:
- Demerol 2438
- Mepergan Injection 2859

Mephobarbital (Additive CNS depression). Products include:
- Mebaral Tablets 2452

Meprobamate (Additive CNS depression). Products include:
- Miltown Tablets 2780
- PMB 200 and PMB 400 2890

Mesoridazine Besylate (Additive CNS depression). Products include:
- Serentil 689

Methadone Hydrochloride (Additive CNS depression). Products include:
- Methadone Hydrochloride Oral Concentrate 2356
- Methadone Hydrochloride Oral Solution & Tablets 2357

Methohexital Sodium (Additive CNS depression).
- No products indexed under this heading.

Methotrimeprazine (Additive CNS depression). Products include:
- Levoprome 1321

Methoxyflurane (Additive CNS depression).
- No products indexed under this heading.

Midazolam Hydrochloride (Additive CNS depression). Products include:
- Versed Injection 2324

Molindone Hydrochloride (Additive CNS depression). Products include:
- Moban Tablets and Concentrate ... 1036

Morphine Sulfate (Additive CNS depression). Products include:
- Astramorph/PF Injection, USP (Preservative-Free) 526

- Duramorph Injection 983
- Infumorph 200 and Infumorph 500 Sterile Solutions 985
- Kadian Capsules 2948
- MS Contin Tablets 2149
- MSIR 2152
- Oramorph SR (Morphine Sulfate Sustained Release Tablets) 2359
- RMS Suppositories CII 2766
- Roxanol 2365

Opium Alkaloids (Additive CNS depression).
- No products indexed under this heading.

Oxazepam (Additive CNS depression). Products include:
- Serax Capsules 2916
- Serax Tablets 2916

Oxycodone Hydrochloride (Additive CNS depression). Products include:
- OxyContin Tablets 2163
- OxyIR Capsules 2167
- Percocet Tablets 955
- Percodan Tablets 955
- Percodan-Demi Tablets 956
- Roxicodone Tablets, Oral Solution & Intensol (Oxycodone) 2366
- Tylox Capsules 1593

Pentobarbital Sodium (Additive CNS depression). Products include:
- Nembutal Sodium Capsules 440
- Nembutal Sodium Solution 442
- Nembutal Sodium Suppositories 444

Perphenazine (Additive CNS depression). Products include:
- Etrafon 2495
- Triavil Tablets 1800
- Trilafon 2532

Phenobarbital (Additive CNS depression). Products include:
- Arco-Lase Plus Tablets 513
- Bellergal-S Tablets 2375
- Donnatal 2234
- Donnatal Extentabs 2234
- Donnatal Tablets 2234
- Phenobarbital Elixir and Tablets ... 1523
- Quadrinal Tablets 1398

Prazepam (Additive CNS depression).
- No products indexed under this heading.

Prochlorperazine (Additive CNS depression). Products include:
- Compazine 2644

Promethazine Hydrochloride (Additive CNS depression). Products include:
- Mepergan Injection 2859
- Phenergan with Codeine 2883
- Phenergan with Dextromethorphan 2885
- Phenergan Injection 2880
- Phenergan Suppositories 2882
- Phenergan Syrup 2881
- Phenergan Tablets 2882
- Phenergan VC 2886
- Phenergan VC with Codeine 2888

Propofol (Additive CNS depression). Products include:
- Diprivan Injectable Emulsion 2939

Propoxyphene Hydrochloride (Additive CNS depression). Products include:
- Darvon 1475
- Wygesic Tablets 2930

Propoxyphene Napsylate (Additive CNS depression). Products include:
- Darvon-N/Darvocet-N 1473

Quazepam (Additive CNS depression). Products include:
- Doral Tablets 2773

Risperidone (Additive CNS depression). Products include:
- Risperdal Tablets 1348

Secobarbital Sodium (Additive CNS depression). Products include:
- Seconal Sodium Pulvules 1529

Sevoflurane (Additive CNS depression).
- No products indexed under this heading.

Sufentanil Citrate (Additive CNS depression). Products include:
- Sufenta Injection 1355

Temazepam (Additive CNS depression). Products include:
- Restoril Capsules 2413

Thiamylal Sodium (Additive CNS depression).
- No products indexed under this heading.

Thioridazine Hydrochloride (Additive CNS depression). Products include:
- Mellaril 2398

Thiothixene (Additive CNS depression). Products include:
- Navane Capsules and Concentrate 2018
- Navane Intramuscular 2019

Triazolam (Additive CNS depression). Products include:
- Halcion Tablets 2093

Trifluoperazine Hydrochloride (Additive CNS depression). Products include:
- Stelazine 2692

Zolpidem Tartrate (Additive CNS depression). Products include:
- Ambien Tablets 2559

Food Interactions

Alcohol (Additive CNS depression).

NUPERCAINAL HEMORRHOIDAL AND ANESTHETIC OINTMENT
(Dibucaine) 661
None cited in PDR database.

NUPERCAINAL HYDROCORTISONE 1% CREAM
(Hydrocortisone Acetate) 661
None cited in PDR database.

NUPERCAINAL PAIN RELIEF CREAM
(Dibucaine) 661
None cited in PDR database.

NUPERCAINAL SUPPOSITORIES
(Cocoa Butter, Zinc Oxide) 661
None cited in PDR database.

NUPRIN IBUPROFEN/ANALGESIC TABLETS & CAPLETS
(Ibuprofen) 645
May interact with aspirin and acetaminophen containing products. Compounds in this category include:

Acetaminophen (Concomitant administration recommended only under a doctor's direction). Products include:
- Actifed Cold & Sinus Caplets and Tablets 808
- Actifed Sinus Daytime/Nighttime Tablets and Caplets 809
- Alka-Seltzer Fast Relief Caplets ... 610
- Alka-Seltzer Plus Liqui-Gels 612
- Alka-Seltzer Plus Flu & Body Aches Effervescent Tablets 612
- Alka-Seltzer Plus Flu & Body Aches Liqui-Gels Non-Drowsy Formula 613
- Alka-Seltzer Plus Night-Time Cold Medicine Liqui-Gels 612
- Allerest No Drowsiness 649
- Allerest Sinus Pain Formula 649
- Axocet Capsules 2469
- Benadryl Allergy/Cold Tablets 811
- Benadryl Allergy Sinus Headache Caplets 813
- Children's TYLENOL acetaminophen Chewable Tablets, Elixir, Suspension Liquid, and Suspension Drops 1559

IMPORTANT NOTE: Always consult each drug listing in the patient's regimen for possible interactions.

Nuprin | Interactions Index | 770

Children's TYLENOL Cold Multi-Symptom Chewable Tablets and Liquid ... 1559
Children's TYLENOL Cold Plus Cough Multi Symptom Chewable Tablets and Liquid ... 1560
Children's TYLENOL Flu Suspension Liquid ... 1560
Allergy-Sinus Comtrex Multi-Symptom Allergy-Sinus Formula Tablets and Caplets ... ▣ 639
Comtrex Multi-Symptom ... ▣ 638
Comtrex Non-Drowsy ... ▣ 640
Contac Day Allergy/Sinus Caplets ▣ 771
Contac Day & Night ... ▣ 772
Contac Night Allergy/Sinus Caplets ... ▣ 771
Contac Severe Cold and Flu Formula Caplets ... ▣ 773
Contac Severe Cold & Flu Non-Drowsy ... ▣ 774
Coricidin Cold + Flu Tablets ... ▣ 760
Coricidin 'D' Decongestant Tablets ... ▣ 760
DHCplus Capsules ... 2148
Darvon-N/Darvocet-N ... 1473
Dimetapp Allergy Sinus Caplets ... ▣ 838
Dimetapp Cold & Fever Suspension ... ▣ 839
Drixoral Cold and Flu Extended-Release Tablets ... ▣ 764
Drixoral Cough + Sore Throat Liquid Caps ... ▣ 763
Drixoral Allergy/Sinus Extended Release Tablets ... ▣ 765
Esgic-plus Capsules ... 1012
Esgic-plus Tablets ... 1012
Aspirin Free Excedrin Analgesic Caplets and Geltabs ... 734
Excedrin Extra-Strength Analgesic Tablets, Caplets, and Geltabs ... 734
Excedrin P.M. Analgesic/Sleeping Aid Tablets, Caplets, Liquigels ... 735
Fioricet Tablets ... 2386
Fioricet with Codeine Capsules ... 2387
Goody's Extra Strength Headache Powders ... ▣ 632
Goody's Extra Strength Pain Relief Tablets ... ▣ 632
Hycomine Compound Tablets ... 948
Hydrocet Capsules ... 787
Infants' TYLENOL acetaminophen Suspension Drops ... 1559
Infants' TYLENOL Cold Decongestant & Fever-Reducer Drops ... 1561
Junior Strength TYLENOL acetaminophen Coated Caplets and Chewable Tablets ... 1562
Lorcet 10/650 Tablets ... 1016
Lortab ... 2751
Lurline PMS Tablets ... 1000
Maximum Strength Multi-Symptom Formula Midol ... ▣ 621
PMS Multi-Symptom Formula Midol ... ▣ 622
Maximum Strength Midol Teen Multi-Symptom Formula ... ▣ 621
Midrin Capsules ... 788
Panodol Tablets and Caplets ... ▣ 783
Children's Panadol Chewable Tablets, Liquid, Infant's Drops ... ▣ 783
Percocet Tablets ... 955
Percogesic Analgesic Tablets ... ▣ 727
Phrenilin ... 790
Pyrroxate Caplets ... ▣ 742
Robitussin Cold, Cough & Flu Liqui-Gels ... ▣ 844
Robitussin Night-Time Cold Formula ... ▣ 847
Sedapap Tablets 50 mg/650 mg ... 1826
Sinarest ... ▣ 663
Sine-Aid Maximum Strength Sinus Headache Gelcaps, Caplets and Tablets ... 1570
Sine-Off No Drowsiness Formula Caplets ... ▣ 784
Sine-Off Sinus Medicine ... ▣ 784
Singlet Tablets ... ▣ 785
Sinulin Tablets ... 792
Sinutab Sinus Allergy Medication, Maximum Strength Tablets and Caplets ... ▣ 823
Sinutab Sinus Medication, Maximum Strength Without Drowsiness Formula, Tablets & Caplets ... ▣ 824
Sudafed Cold and Cough Liquid Caps ... ▣ 826
Sudafed Severe Cold Formula Caplets ... ▣ 828
Sudafed Severe Cold Formula Tablets ... ▣ 828
Sudafed Sinus Caplets ... ▣ 829
Sudafed Sinus Tablets ... ▣ 829
Talacen Caplets ... 2464
TheraFlu Flu and Cold Medicine ... ▣ 750
Theraflu Maximum Strength Flu and Cold Medicine For Sore Throat ... ▣ 751
TheraFlu Flu, Cold and Cough Medicine ... ▣ 750
TheraFlu Maximum Strength Nighttime Flu, Cold & Cough Medicine ... ▣ 751
TheraFlu Maximum Strength Non-Drowsy Formula Flu, Cold & Cough Medicine ... ▣ 751
TheraFlu Maximum Strength, Non-Drowsy Formula Flu, Cold and Cough Caplets ... ▣ 752
Theraflu Maximum Strength Sinus Non-Drowsy Formula Caplets ... ▣ 752
Triaminic Sore Throat Formula ... ▣ 755
Triaminicin Tablets ... ▣ 756
TYLENOL acetaminophen Extended Relief Caplets ... 1570
TYLENOL acetaminophen, Extra Strength Adult Liquid Pain Reliever ... 1570
TYLENOL acetaminophen, Extra Strength Gelcaps, Geltabs, Caplets, Tablets ... 1570
TYLENOL acetaminophen, Regular Strength Caplets and Tablets ... 1570
TYLENOL Allergy Sinus, Maximum Strength Caplets and Gelcaps ... 1571
TYLENOL Allergy Sinus NightTime, Maximum Strength Caplets ... 1571
TYLENOL Cold Medication, Multi-Symptom Formula Tablets and Caplets ... 1572
TYLENOL Cold Medication, Multi-Symptom Hot Liquid Packets ... 1572
TYLENOL Cold Medication, No Drowsiness Formula Caplets and Gelcaps ... 1572
TYLENOL Cold Severe Congestion Caplets ... 1573
TYLENOL Cough Medication, Multi Symptom ... 1574
TYLENOL Cough Medication with Decongestant, Multi Symptom ... 1574
TYLENOL Flu No Drowsiness Formula, Maximum Strength Gelcaps ... 1575
TYLENOL Flu NightTime, Maximum Strength Gelcaps ... 1575
TYLENOL Flu NightTime, Maximum Strength Hot Medication Packets ... 1575
TYLENOL Headache Plus Pain Reliever with Antacid, Extra Strength Caplets ... ▣ 705
TYLENOL PM Pain Reliever/Sleep Aid, Extra Strength Gelcaps, Caplets, Geltabs ... 1576
TYLENOL Severe Allergy Medication Caplets ... 1571
TYLENOL Sinus, Maximum Strength Geltabs, Gelcaps, Caplets and Tablets ... 1576
Tylenol with Codeine ... 1592
Tylox Capsules ... 1593
Unisom With Pain Relief-Nighttime Sleep Aid and Pain Reliever ... 1991
Vanquish Analgesic Caplets ... ▣ 627
Vicks 44 LiquiCaps Cough, Cold & Flu Relief ... ▣ 728
Vicks 44M Cough, Cold & Flu Relief ... ▣ 729
Vicks DayQuil LiquiCaps/Liquid Multi-Symptom Cold/Flu Relief ... ▣ 734
Vicks Nyquil Hot Therapy ... ▣ 735
Vicks NyQuil LiquiCaps/Liquid Multi-Symptom Cold/Flu Relief, Original and Cherry Flavors ... ▣ 736
Vicodin Tablets ... 1404
Vicodin ES Tablets ... 1405
Vicodin HP Tablets ... 1403
Wygesic Tablets ... 2930
Zydone Capsules ... 967

Aspirin (Concomitant administration recommended only under a doctor's direction). Products include:

Alka-Seltzer Cherry Effervescent Antacid and Pain Reliever ... ▣ 609
Alka-Seltzer Extra Strength Effervescent Antacid and Pain Reliever ... ▣ 609
Alka-Seltzer Lemon Lime Effervescent Antacid and Pain Reliever ... ▣ 609
Alka-Seltzer Original Effervescent Antacid and Pain Reliever ... ▣ 609
Alka-Seltzer Plus ... ▣ 611
Alka-Seltzer Plus Sinus Medicine ... ▣ 611
Ascriptin ... ▣ 650
Arthritis Strength BC Powder ... ▣ 631
BC Cold Powder Multi-Symptom Formula (Cold-Sinus-Allergy) ... ▣ 631
BC Cold Powder Non-Drowsy Formula (Cold-Sinus) ... ▣ 631
BC Powder ... ▣ 631
Genuine Bayer Aspirin Tablets & Caplets ... ▣ 618
Extra Strength Bayer Arthritis Pain Regimen Formula ... ▣ 615
Extra Strength Bayer Aspirin Caplets & Tablets ... ▣ 617
Extended-Release Bayer 8-Hour Aspirin ... ▣ 616
Extra Strength Bayer Plus Aspirin Caplets ... ▣ 617
Extra Strength Bayer PM Aspirin Plus Sleep Aid ... ▣ 617
Aspirin Regimen Bayer 81 mg Tablets with Calcium ... ▣ 615
Aspirin Regimen Bayer Adult Low Strength 81 mg Tablets ... ▣ 613
Aspirin Regimen Bayer Children's Chewable Aspirin ... ▣ 616
Aspirin Regimen Bayer Regular Strength 325 mg Caplets ... ▣ 613
Bufferin Analgesic Tablets ... ▣ 636
Arthritis Strength Bufferin Analgesic Caplets ... ▣ 637
Extra Strength Bufferin Analgesic Tablets ... ▣ 637
Cama Arthritis Pain Reliever ... ▣ 748
Darvon Compound-65 Pulvules ... 1475
Easprin ... 1971
Ecotrin ... 2625
Ecotrin Enteric Coated Aspirin Maximum Strength Tablets and Caplets ... ▣ 775
Ecotrin Enteric Coated Aspirin Regular Strength Tablets ... 2625
Empirin Aspirin Tablets ... ▣ 818
Excedrin Extra-Strength Analgesic Tablets, Caplets, and Geltabs ... 734
Fiorinal Capsules ... 2388
Fiorinal with Codeine Capsules ... 2390
Fiorinal Tablets ... 2388
Goody's Extra Strength Headache Powders ... ▣ 632
Goody's Extra Strength Pain Relief Tablets ... ▣ 632
Halfprin Tablets ... 1413
Norgesic ... 1554
Percodan Tablets ... 955
Percodan-Demi Tablets ... 956
Robaxisal Tablets ... 2246
Soma Compound w/Codeine Tablets ... 2784
Soma Compound Tablets ... 2783
St. Joseph Adult Chewable Aspirin (81 mg.) ... ▣ 768
Talwin Compound ... 2466
Vanquish Analgesic Caplets ... ▣ 627

NUROMAX INJECTION

(Doxacurium Chloride) ... 1136

May interact with inhalant anesthetics, aminoglycosides, tetracyclines, lithium preparations, local anesthetics, and certain other agents. Compounds in these categories include:

Amikacin Sulfate (Enhances the neuromuscular blocking action). Products include:

Amikacin Sulfate Injection, USP ... 523
Amikacin Sulfate Injection, USP ... 981
Amikin Injectable ... 502

Bacitracin (Enhances the neuromuscular blocking action).

No products indexed under this heading.

Bupivacaine Hydrochloride (Enhances the neuromuscular blocking action). Products include:

Marcaine ... 2446
Marcaine Spinal ... 2449
Sensorcaine ... 554

Carbamazepine (The time of onset of neuromuscular block is lengthened and the duration of block is shortened). Products include:

Atretol Tablets ... 569
Tegretol/Tegretol-XR ... 870

Chloroprocaine Hydrochloride (Enhances the neuromuscular blocking action). Products include:

Nescaine/Nescaine MPF ... 549

Clindamycin Hydrochloride (Enhances the neuromuscular blocking action).

No products indexed under this heading.

Clindamycin Palmitate Hydrochloride (Enhances the neuromuscular blocking action).

No products indexed under this heading.

Clindamycin Phosphate (Enhances the neuromuscular blocking action). Products include:

Cleocin Phosphate Injection ... 2068
Cleocin T Topical ... 2072
Cleocin Vaginal Cream ... 2070

Colistimethate Sodium (Enhances the neuromuscular blocking action).

No products indexed under this heading.

Colistin Sulfate (Enhances the neuromuscular blocking action). Products include:

Coly-Mycin S Otic w/Neomycin & Hydrocortisone ... 1965

Demeclocycline Hydrochloride (Enhances the neuromuscular blocking action). Products include:

Declomycin Tablets ... 1421

Desflurane (Decreases the ED_{50} by 30% to 45%; prolongs the clinically effective duration of action by up to 25%). Products include:

Suprane (desflurane, USP) ... 1865

Doxycycline Calcium (Enhances the neuromuscular blocking action). Products include:

Vibramycin Calcium Oral Suspension Syrup ... 2038

Doxycycline Hyclate (Enhances the neuromuscular blocking action). Products include:

Doryx Capsules ... 1970
Vibramycin Hyclate Capsules ... 2038
Vibramycin Hyclate Intravenous ... 2040
Vibra-Tabs Film Coated Tablets ... 2038

Doxycycline Monohydrate (Enhances the neuromuscular blocking action). Products include:

Monodox Capsules ... 1858
Vibramycin Monohydrate for Oral Suspension ... 2038

Enflurane (Decreases the ED_{50} by 30% to 45%; prolongs the clinically effective duration of action by up to 25%).

No products indexed under this heading.

Etidocaine Hydrochloride (Enhances the neuromuscular blocking action). Products include:

Duranest Injections ... 533

Gentamicin Sulfate (Enhances the neuromuscular blocking action). Products include:

Garamycin Cream 0.1% ... 2501
Garamycin Injectable ... 2502
Garamycin Ointment 0.1% ... 2501
Garamycin Ophthalmic ... 2501
Genoptic Sterile Ophthalmic Solution ... ◉ 241
Genoptic Sterile Ophthalmic Ointment ... ◉ 241
Gentak ... ◉ 209
Pred-G Liquifilm Sterile Ophthalmic Suspension ... ◉ 248
Pred-G S.O.P. Sterile Ophthalmic Ointment ... ◉ 249

(▣ Described in PDR For Nonprescription Drugs) (◉ Described in PDR For Ophthalmology)

771 **Interactions Index** **Nutropin**

Halothane (Decreases the ED_{50} by 30% to 45%; prolongs the clinically effective duration of action by up to 25%). Products include:

Fluothane 2830

Isoflurane (Decreases the ED_{50} by 30% to 45%; prolongs the clinically effective duration of action by up to 25%).

No products indexed under this heading.

Kanamycin Sulfate (Enhances the neuromuscular blocking action).

No products indexed under this heading.

Lidocaine Hydrochloride (Enhances the neuromuscular blocking action). Products include:

Decadron Phosphate with Xylocaine Injection, Sterile 1683
Unguentine Plus ..... ▣ 712
Xylocaine Injections 562

Lincomycin Hydrochloride Monohydrate (Enhances the neuromuscular blocking action).

No products indexed under this heading.

Lithium Carbonate (Enhances the neuromuscular blocking action). Products include:

Eskalith 2658
Lithium Carbonate Capsules & Tablets 2352
Lithonate/Lithotabs/Lithobid 2721

Lithium Citrate (Enhances the neuromuscular blocking action).

No products indexed under this heading.

Magnesium Salts (Enhances the neuromuscular blocking action).

Mepivacaine Hydrochloride Injection (Enhances the neuromuscular blocking action). Products include:

Carbocaine Injection 2432

Methacycline Hydrochloride (Enhances the neuromuscular blocking action).

No products indexed under this heading.

Methoxyflurane (Decreases the ED_{50} by 30% to 45%; prolongs the clinically effective duration of action by up to 25%).

No products indexed under this heading.

Minocycline Hydrochloride (Enhances the neuromuscular blocking action). Products include:

DYNACIN Capsules 1627
Minocin Intravenous 1428
Minocin Oral Suspension 1431
Minocin Pellet-Filled Capsules 1429

Oxytetracycline Hydrochloride (Enhances the neuromuscular blocking action). Products include:

TERAK Ointment ..... ◉ 210
Terra-Cortril Ophthalmic Suspension 2033
Terramycin with Polymyxin B Sulfate Ophthalmic Ointment 2035
Urobiotic-250 Capsules 2038

Phenytoin (The time of onset of neuromuscular block is lengthened and the duration of block is shortened). Products include:

Dilantin Infatabs 1967
Dilantin-125 Suspension 1969

Phenytoin Sodium (The time of onset of neuromuscular block is lengthened and the duration of block is shortened). Products include:

Dilantin Kapseals 1965

Polymyxin Preparations (Enhances the neuromuscular blocking action).

Procainamide Hydrochloride (Enhances the neuromuscular blocking action). Products include:

Procanbid Extended-Release Tablets 1983

Procaine Hydrochloride (Enhances the neuromuscular blocking action). Products include:

Novocain Hydrochloride for Spinal Anesthesia 2457

Quinidine Gluconate (Enhances the neuromuscular blocking action). Products include:

Quinaglute Dura-Tabs Tablets 644

Quinidine Polygalacturonate (Enhances the neuromuscular blocking action). Products include:

Cardioquin Tablets 2146

Quinidine Sulfate (Enhances the neuromuscular blocking action). Products include:

Quinidex Extentabs 2240

Streptomycin Sulfate (Enhances the neuromuscular blocking action). Products include:

Streptomycin Sulfate Injection 2031

Tetracaine Hydrochloride (Enhances the neuromuscular blocking action). Products include:

Cetacaine Topical Anesthetic 812
Pontocaine Hydrochloride for Spinal Anesthesia 2460

Tetracycline Hydrochloride (Enhances the neuromuscular blocking action). Products include:

Achromycin V Capsules 1417
Helidac Therapy 2135

Tobramycin (Enhances the neuromuscular blocking action). Products include:

AKTOB ..... ◉ 207
TobraDex Ophthalmic Suspension and Ointment 469
Tobrex Ophthalmic Ointment and Solution ..... ◉ 226

Tobramycin Sulfate (Enhances the neuromuscular blocking action). Products include:

Nebcin Vials, Hyporets & ADD-Vantage 1518

NUTR-E-SOL

(Vitamin E) 461
None cited in PDR database.

NUTROPIN

(Somatropin) 1049
May interact with glucocorticoids. Compounds in this category include:

Betamethasone Acetate (Concomitant glucocorticoid therapy may inhibit the growth promoting effect, especially in patients with chronic renal failure). Products include:

Celestone Soluspan Suspension 2484

Betamethasone Sodium Phosphate (Concomitant glucocorticoid therapy may inhibit the growth promoting effect, especially in patients with chronic renal failure). Products include:

Celestone Soluspan Suspension 2484

Cortisone Acetate (Concomitant glucocorticoid therapy may inhibit the growth promoting effect, especially in patients with chronic renal failure). Products include:

Cortone Acetate Sterile Suspension 1663
Cortone Acetate Tablets 1664

Dexamethasone (Concomitant glucocorticoid therapy may inhibit the growth promoting effect, especially in patients with chronic renal failure). Products include:

AK-Trol Ointment & Suspension ..... ◉ 205
Decadron Elixir 1676
Decadron Tablets 1678
Decaspray Topical Aerosol 1689
Maxitrol Ophthalmic Ointment and Suspension ..... ◉ 222
TobraDex Ophthalmic Suspension and Ointment 469

Dexamethasone Acetate (Concomitant glucocorticoid therapy may inhibit the growth promoting effect, especially in patients with chronic renal failure). Products include:

Dalalone D.P. Injectable 1009
Decadron-LA Sterile Suspension 1687

Dexamethasone Sodium Phosphate (Concomitant glucocorticoid therapy may inhibit the growth promoting effect, especially in patients with chronic renal failure). Products include:

Decadron Phosphate Injection 1680
Decadron Phosphate Sterile Ophthalmic Ointment 1684
Decadron Phosphate Sterile Ophthalmic Solution 1685
Decadron Phosphate Topical Cream 1686
Decadron Phosphate with Xylocaine Injection, Sterile 1683
Dexacort Phosphate in Respihaler .. 1606
Dexacort Phosphate in Turbinaire .. 1607
NeoDecadron Sterile Ophthalmic Ointment 1755
NeoDecadron Sterile Ophthalmic Solution 1756
NeoDecadron Topical Cream 1757

Fludrocortisone Acetate (Concomitant glucocorticoid therapy may inhibit the growth promoting effect, especially in patients with chronic renal failure). Products include:

Florinef Acetate Tablets 506

Hydrocortisone (Concomitant glucocorticoid therapy may inhibit the growth promoting effect, especially in patients with chronic renal failure). Products include:

Anusol-HC Cream 2.5% 1953
Aquanil HC Lotion 1989
Maximum Strength Cortaid Spray ▣ 800
CORTENEMA 2713
Cortisporin Ointment 1074
Cortisporin Ophthalmic Ointment Sterile 1074
Cortisporin Ophthalmic Suspension Sterile 1075
Cortisporin Otic Solution Sterile 1076
Cortisporin Otic Suspension Sterile 1077
Cortizone-5 ..... ▣ 795
Cortizone-10 ..... ▣ 795
Hydrocortone Tablets 1715
Hytone 922
Hytone Ointment 2 ½% 923
Massengill Medicated Soft Cloth Towelettes 2628
Pediotic Suspension Sterile 1140
Preparation H Hydrocortisone 1% Cream ..... ▣ 843
ProctoCream-HC 2.5% 2552
VōSoL HC Otic Solution 2786

Hydrocortisone Acetate (Concomitant glucocorticoid therapy may inhibit the growth promoting effect, especially in patients with chronic renal failure). Products include:

Analpram-HC Rectal Cream 1% and 2.5% 993
Anusol HC-1 Hydrocortisone Anti-Itch Ointment ..... ▣ 810
Anusol-HC Suppositories 1954
Caldecort Anti-Itch Hydrocortisone Cream ..... ▣ 651
Coly-Mycin S Otic w/Neomycin & Hydrocortisone 1965
Cortaid ..... ▣ 800
Cortifoam 2540
Cortisporin Cream 1073
Epifoam 2543
Hydrocortone Acetate Sterile Suspension 1712
Mantadil Cream 1124
Nupercainal Hydrocortisone 1% Cream ..... ▣ 661
Pramosone Cream, Lotion & Ointment 995
ProctoFoam-HC 2552
Terra-Cortril Ophthalmic Suspension 2033

Hydrocortisone Sodium Phosphate (Concomitant glucocorticoid therapy may inhibit the growth promoting effect, especially in patients with chronic renal failure). Products include:

Hydrocortone Phosphate Injection, Sterile 1713

Hydrocortisone Sodium Succinate (Concomitant glucocorticoid therapy may inhibit the growth promoting effect, especially in patients with chronic renal failure).

No products indexed under this heading.

Methylprednisolone Acetate (Concomitant glucocorticoid therapy may inhibit the growth promoting effect, especially in patients with chronic renal failure).

No products indexed under this heading.

Methylprednisolone Sodium Succinate (Concomitant glucocorticoid therapy may inhibit the growth promoting effect, especially in patients with chronic renal failure).

No products indexed under this heading.

Prednisolone Acetate (Concomitant glucocorticoid therapy may inhibit the growth promoting effect, especially in patients with chronic renal failure). Products include:

AK-CIDE ..... ◉ 203
AK-CIDE Ointment ..... ◉ 203
Blephamide Liquifilm Sterile Ophthalmic Suspension 472
Blephamide Ointment ..... ◉ 234
Econopred & Econopred Plus Ophthalmic Suspensions ..... ◉ 216
Poly-Pred Liquifilm ..... ◉ 246
Pred Forte ..... ◉ 247
Pred Mild ..... ◉ 250
Pred-G Liquifilm Sterile Ophthalmic Suspension ..... ◉ 248
Pred-G S.O.P. Sterile Ophthalmic Ointment ..... ◉ 249

Prednisolone Sodium Phosphate (Concomitant glucocorticoid therapy may inhibit the growth promoting effect, especially in patients with chronic renal failure). Products include:

AK-PRED ..... ◉ 204
Hydeltrasol Injection, Sterile 1708
Pediapred Oral Solution 1618

Prednisolone Tebutate (Concomitant glucocorticoid therapy may inhibit the growth promoting effect, especially in patients with chronic renal failure). Products include:

Hydeltra-T.B.A. Sterile Suspension 1710

Prednisone (Concomitant glucocorticoid therapy may inhibit the growth promoting effect, especially in patients with chronic renal failure).

No products indexed under this heading.

Triamcinolone (Concomitant glucocorticoid therapy may inhibit the growth promoting effect, especially in patients with chronic renal failure).

No products indexed under this heading.

Triamcinolone Acetonide (Concomitant glucocorticoid therapy may inhibit the growth promoting effect, especially in patients with chronic renal failure). Products include:

Azmacort Oral Inhaler 2175
Nasacort AQ Nasal Spray 2191
Nasacort Nasal Inhaler 2189

IMPORTANT NOTE: Always consult each drug listing in the patient's regimen for possible interactions.

Nutropin | Interactions Index | 772

Triamcinolone Diacetate (Concomitant glucocorticoid therapy may inhibit the growth promoting effect, especially in patients with chronic renal failure).
No products indexed under this heading.

Triamcinolone Hexacetonide (Concomitant glucocorticoid therapy may inhibit the growth promoting effect, especially in patients with chronic renal failure).
No products indexed under this heading.

NUTROPIN AQ INJECTION
(Somatropin) 1051
May interact with glucocorticoids. Compounds in this category include:

Betamethasone Acetate (Concomitant glucocorticoid therapy may inhibit the growth promoting effect, especially in patients with chronic renal failure). Products include:
Celestone Soluspan Suspension 2484

Betamethasone Sodium Phosphate (Concomitant glucocorticoid therapy may inhibit the growth promoting effect, especially in patients with chronic renal failure). Products include:
Celestone Soluspan Suspension 2484

Cortisone Acetate (Concomitant glucocorticoid therapy may inhibit the growth promoting effect, especially in patients with chronic renal failure). Products include:
Cortone Acetate Sterile Suspension 1663
Cortone Acetate Tablets 1664

Dexamethasone (Concomitant glucocorticoid therapy may inhibit the growth promoting effect, especially in patients with chronic renal failure). Products include:
AK-Trol Ointment & Suspension .... ◉ 205
Decadron Elixir 1676
Decadron Tablets 1678
Decaspray Topical Aerosol 1689
Maxitrol Ophthalmic Ointment and Suspension .... ◉ 222
TobraDex Ophthalmic Suspension and Ointment 469

Dexamethasone Acetate (Concomitant glucocorticoid therapy may inhibit the growth promoting effect, especially in patients with chronic renal failure). Products include:
Dalalone D.P. Injectable 1009
Decadron-LA Sterile Suspension 1687

Dexamethasone Sodium Phosphate (Concomitant glucocorticoid therapy may inhibit the growth promoting effect, especially in patients with chronic renal failure). Products include:
Decadron Phosphate Injection 1680
Decadron Phosphate Sterile Ophthalmic Ointment 1684
Decadron Phosphate Sterile Ophthalmic Solution 1685
Decadron Phosphate Topical Cream 1686
Decadron Phosphate with Xylocaine Injection, Sterile 1683
Dexacort Phosphate in Respihaler ..1606
Dexacort Phosphate in Turbinaire ..1607
NeoDecadron Sterile Ophthalmic Ointment 1755
NeoDecadron Sterile Ophthalmic Solution 1756
NeoDecadron Topical Cream 1757

Fludrocortisone Acetate (Concomitant glucocorticoid therapy may inhibit the growth promoting effect, especially in patients with chronic renal failure). Products include:
Florinef Acetate Tablets 506

Hydrocortisone (Concomitant glucocorticoid therapy may inhibit the growth promoting effect, especially in patients with chronic renal failure). Products include:
Anusol-HC Cream 2.5% 1953
Aquanil HC Lotion 1989
Maximum Strength Cortaid Spray ▣ 800
CORTENEMA 2713
Cortisporin Ointment 1074
Cortisporin Ophthalmic Ointment Sterile 1074
Cortisporin Ophthalmic Suspension Sterile 1075
Cortisporin Otic Solution Sterile 1076
Cortisporin Otic Suspension Sterile 1077
Cortizone-5 .... ▣ 795
Cortizone-10 .... ▣ 795
Hydrocortone Tablets 1715
Hytone 922
Hytone Ointment 2 ½% 923
Massengill Medicated Soft Cloth Towelettes 2628
Pediotic Suspension Sterile 1140
Preparation H Hydrocortisone 1% Cream .... ▣ 843
ProctoCream-HC 2.5% 2552
VōSoL HC Otic Solution 2786

Hydrocortisone Acetate (Concomitant glucocorticoid therapy may inhibit the growth promoting effect, especially in patients with chronic renal failure). Products include:
Analpram-HC Rectal Cream 1% and 2.5% 993
Anusol HC-1 Hydrocortisone Anti-Itch Ointment .... ▣ 810
Anusol-HC Suppositories 1954
Caldecort Anti-Itch Hydrocortisone Cream .... ▣ 651
Coly-Mycin S Otic w/Neomycin & Hydrocortisone 1965
Cortaid .... ▣ 800
Cortifoam 2540
Cortisporin Cream 1073
Epifoam 2543
Hydrocortone Acetate Sterile Suspension 1712
Mantadil Cream 1124
Nupercainal Hydrocortisone 1% Cream .... ▣ 661
Pramosone Cream, Lotion & Ointment 995
ProctoFoam-HC 2552
Terra-Cortril Ophthalmic Suspension 2033

Hydrocortisone Sodium Phosphate (Concomitant glucocorticoid therapy may inhibit the growth promoting effect, especially in patients with chronic renal failure). Products include:
Hydrocortone Phosphate Injection, Sterile 1713

Hydrocortisone Sodium Succinate (Concomitant glucocorticoid therapy may inhibit the growth promoting effect, especially in patients with chronic renal failure).
No products indexed under this heading.

Methylprednisolone Acetate (Concomitant glucocorticoid therapy may inhibit the growth promoting effect, especially in patients with chronic renal failure).
No products indexed under this heading.

Methylprednisolone Sodium Succinate (Concomitant glucocorticoid therapy may inhibit the growth promoting effect, especially in patients with chronic renal failure).
No products indexed under this heading.

Prednisolone Acetate (Concomitant glucocorticoid therapy may inhibit the growth promoting effect, especially in patients with chronic renal failure). Products include:
AK-CIDE .... ◉ 203
AK-CIDE Ointment .... ◉ 203
Blephamide Liquifilm Sterile Ophthalmic Suspension 472
Blephamide Ointment .... ◉ 234
Econopred & Econopred Plus Ophthalmic Suspensions .... ◉ 216
Poly-Pred Liquifilm .... ◉ 246
Pred Forte .... ◉ 247
Pred Mild .... ◉ 250
Pred-G Liquifilm Sterile Ophthalmic Suspension .... ◉ 248
Pred-G S.O.P. Sterile Ophthalmic Ointment .... ◉ 249

Prednisolone Sodium Phosphate (Concomitant glucocorticoid therapy may inhibit the growth promoting effect, especially in patients with chronic renal failure). Products include:
AK-PRED .... ◉ 204
Hydeltrasol Injection, Sterile 1708
Pediapred Oral Solution 1618

Prednisolone Tebutate (Concomitant glucocorticoid therapy may inhibit the growth promoting effect, especially in patients with chronic renal failure). Products include:
Hydeltra-T.B.A. Sterile Suspension 1710

Prednisone (Concomitant glucocorticoid therapy may inhibit the growth promoting effect, especially in patients with chronic renal failure).
No products indexed under this heading.

Triamcinolone (Concomitant glucocorticoid therapy may inhibit the growth promoting effect, especially in patients with chronic renal failure).
No products indexed under this heading.

Triamcinolone Acetonide (Concomitant glucocorticoid therapy may inhibit the growth promoting effect, especially in patients with chronic renal failure). Products include:
Azmacort Oral Inhaler 2175
Nasacort AQ Nasal Spray 2191
Nasacort Nasal Inhaler 2189

Triamcinolone Diacetate (Concomitant glucocorticoid therapy may inhibit the growth promoting effect, especially in patients with chronic renal failure).
No products indexed under this heading.

Triamcinolone Hexacetonide (Concomitant glucocorticoid therapy may inhibit the growth promoting effect, especially in patients with chronic renal failure).
No products indexed under this heading.

NYDRAZID INJECTION
(Isoniazid) 509
May interact with:

Phenytoin (Co-administration may decrease the excretion of phenytoin resulting in enhanced effects and phenytoin intoxication; appropriate dosage adjustment of the anticonvulsant should be made). Products include:
Dilantin Infatabs 1967
Dilantin-125 Suspension 1969

Phenytoin Sodium (Co-administration may decrease the excretion of phenytoin resulting in enhanced effects and phenytoin intoxication; appropriate dosage adjustment of the anticonvulsant should be made). Products include:
Dilantin Kapseals 1965

Food Interactions

Alcohol (Daily ingestion of alcohol may be associated with a higher incidence of isoniazid hepatitis).

NYSTOP (NYSTATIN TOPICAL POWDER, USP)
(Nystatin) 1948
None cited in PDR database.

MAXIMUM STRENGTH NYTOL CAPLETS
(Doxylamine Succinate) .... ▣ 632

Food Interactions

Alcohol (When consuming alcohol, use Nytol with caution).

NYTOL QUICKCAPS CAPLETS
(Diphenhydramine Hydrochloride) .. ▣ 632
May interact with central nervous system depressants, monoamine oxidase inhibitors, and certain other agents. Compounds in these categories include:

Alfentanil Hydrochloride (Heightens depressant effect). Products include:
Alfenta Injection 1334

Alprazolam (Heightens depressant effect). Products include:
Xanax Tablets 2115

Aprobarbital (Heightens depressant effect).
No products indexed under this heading.

Buprenorphine (Heightens depressant effect). Products include:
Buprenex Injectable 2170

Buspirone Hydrochloride (Heightens depressant effect). Products include:
BuSpar Tablets 738

Butabarbital (Heightens depressant effect).
No products indexed under this heading.

Butalbital (Heightens depressant effect). Products include:
Axocet Capsules 2469
Esgic-plus Capsules 1012
Esgic-plus Tablets 1012
Fioricet Tablets 2386
Fioricet with Codeine Capsules 2387
Fiorinal Capsules 2388
Fiorinal with Codeine Capsules 2390
Fiorinal Tablets 2388
Phrenilin 790
Sedapap Tablets 50 mg/650 mg ..1826

Chlordiazepoxide (Heightens depressant effect). Products include:
Limbitrol 2333

Chlordiazepoxide Hydrochloride (Heightens depressant effect). Products include:
Librax Capsules 2330
Librium Capsules 2331
Librium Injectable 2332

Chlorpromazine (Heightens depressant effect). Products include:
Thorazine Suppositories 2701

Chlorpromazine Hydrochloride (Heightens depressant effect). Products include:
Thorazine 2701

Chlorprothixene (Heightens depressant effect).
No products indexed under this heading.

Chlorprothixene Hydrochloride (Heightens depressant effect).
No products indexed under this heading.

Chlorprothixene Lactate (Heightens depressant effect).
No products indexed under this heading.

Clorazepate Dipotassium (Heightens depressant effect). Products include:
Tranxene 459

(▣ Described in PDR For Nonprescription Drugs) (◉ Described in PDR For Ophthalmology)

Interactions Index

Clozapine (Heightens depressant effect). Products include:
- Clozaril Tablets ... 2377

Codeine Phosphate (Heightens depressant effect). Products include:
- Brontex ... 2130
- Dimetane-DC Cough Syrup ... 2232
- Fioricet with Codeine Capsules ... 2387
- Fiorinal with Codeine Capsules ... 2390
- Nucofed ... 2225
- Phenergan with Codeine ... 2883
- Phenergan VC with Codeine ... 2888
- Robitussin A-C Syrup ... 2248
- Robitussin-DAC Syrup ... 2249
- Ryna ... 804
- Soma Compound w/Codeine Tablets ... 2784
- Tylenol with Codeine ... 1592

Desflurane (Heightens depressant effect). Products include:
- Suprane (desflurane, USP) ... 1865

Dezocine (Heightens depressant effect). Products include:
- Dalgan Injection ... 529

Diazepam (Heightens depressant effect). Products include:
- Dizac (diazepam injectable emulsion) CIV ... 1862
- Valium Injectable ... 2336
- Valium Tablets ... 2335

Droperidol (Heightens depressant effect). Products include:
- Inapsine Injection ... 462

Enflurane (Heightens depressant effect).
- No products indexed under this heading.

Estazolam (Heightens depressant effect). Products include:
- ProSom Tablets ... 457

Ethchlorvynol (Heightens depressant effect). Products include:
- Placidyl Capsules ... 456

Ethinamate (Heightens depressant effect).
- No products indexed under this heading.

Fentanyl (Heightens depressant effect). Products include:
- Duragesic Transdermal System ... 1336

Fentanyl Citrate (Heightens depressant effect). Products include:
- Sublimaze Injection ... 463

Fluphenazine Decanoate (Heightens depressant effect). Products include:
- Prolixin Decanoate ... 510

Fluphenazine Enanthate (Heightens depressant effect). Products include:
- Prolixin Enanthate ... 510

Fluphenazine Hydrochloride (Heightens depressant effect). Products include:
- Prolixin ... 510

Flurazepam Hydrochloride (Heightens depressant effect). Products include:
- Dalmane Capsules ... 2329

Furazolidone (Prolongs and intensifies anticholinergic effects). Products include:
- Furoxone ... 2221

Glutethimide (Heightens depressant effect).
- No products indexed under this heading.

Haloperidol (Heightens depressant effect). Products include:
- Haldol Injection, Tablets and Concentrate ... 1585

Haloperidol Decanoate (Heightens depressant effect). Products include:
- Haldol Decanoate ... 1587

Hydrocodone Bitartrate (Heightens depressant effect). Products include:
- Codiclear DH Syrup ... 808
- Duratuss HD Elixir ... 2750
- Histussin D Liquid ... 670
- Hycodan Tablets and Syrup ... 946
- Hycomine Compound Tablets ... 948
- Hycomine ... 947
- Hycotuss Expectorant Syrup ... 950
- Hydrocet Capsules ... 787
- Lorcet 10/650 Tablets ... 1016
- Lortab ... 2751
- Tussend ... 1830
- Tussend Expectorant ... 1831
- Vicodin Tablets ... 1404
- Vicodin ES Tablets ... 1405
- Vicodin HP Tablets ... 1403
- Vicodin Tuss Expectorant ... 1406
- Zydone Tablets ... 967

Hydrocodone Polistirex (Heightens depressant effect). Products include:
- Tussionex Pennkinetic Extended-Release Suspension ... 1624

Hydroxyzine Hydrochloride (Heightens depressant effect). Products include:
- Atarax Tablets & Syrup ... 1992
- Marax Tablets & DF Syrup ... 2015
- Vistaril Intramuscular Solution ... 2042

Isocarboxazid (Prolongs and intensifies anticholinergic effects).
- No products indexed under this heading.

Isoflurane (Heightens depressant effect).
- No products indexed under this heading.

Ketamine Hydrochloride (Heightens depressant effect).
- No products indexed under this heading.

Levomethadyl Acetate Hydrochloride (Heightens depressant effect). Products include:
- Orlaam Oral Solution ... 2361

Levorphanol Tartrate (Heightens depressant effect). Products include:
- Levo-Dromoran ... 2297

Lorazepam (Heightens depressant effect). Products include:
- Ativan Injection ... 2805
- Ativan Tablets ... 2807

Loxapine Hydrochloride (Heightens depressant effect). Products include:
- Loxitane ... 1426

Loxapine Succinate (Heightens depressant effect). Products include:
- Loxitane Capsules ... 1426

Meperidine Hydrochloride (Heightens depressant effect). Products include:
- Demerol ... 2438
- Mepergan Injection ... 2859

Mephobarbital (Heightens depressant effect). Products include:
- Mebaral Tablets ... 2452

Meprobamate (Heightens depressant effect). Products include:
- Miltown Tablets ... 2780
- PMB 200 and PMB 400 ... 2890

Mesoridazine Besylate (Heightens depressant effect). Products include:
- Serentil ... 689

Methadone Hydrochloride (Heightens depressant effect). Products include:
- Methadone Hydrochloride Oral Concentrate ... 2356
- Methadone Hydrochloride Oral Solution & Tablets ... 2357

Methohexital Sodium (Heightens depressant effect).
- No products indexed under this heading.

Methotrimeprazine (Heightens depressant effect). Products include:
- Levoprome ... 1321

Methoxyflurane (Heightens depressant effect).
- No products indexed under this heading.

Midazolam Hydrochloride (Heightens depressant effect). Products include:
- Versed Injection ... 2324

Molindone Hydrochloride (Heightens depressant effect). Products include:
- Moban Tablets and Concentrate ... 1036

Morphine Sulfate (Heightens depressant effect). Products include:
- Astramorph/PF Injection, USP (Preservative-Free) ... 526
- Duramorph Injection ... 983
- Infumorph 200 and Infumorph 500 Sterile Solutions ... 985
- Kadian Capsules ... 2948
- MS Contin Tablets ... 2149
- MSIR ... 2152
- Oramorph SR (Morphine Sulfate Sustained Release Tablets) ... 2359
- RMS Suppositories CII ... 2766
- Roxanol ... 2365

Opium Alkaloids (Heightens depressant effect).
- No products indexed under this heading.

Oxazepam (Heightens depressant effect). Products include:
- Serax Capsules ... 2916
- Serax Tablets ... 2916

Oxycodone Hydrochloride (Heightens depressant effect). Products include:
- OxyContin Tablets ... 2163
- OxyIR Capsules ... 2167
- Percocet Tablets ... 955
- Percodan Tablets ... 955
- Percodan-Demi Tablets ... 956
- Roxicodone Tablets, Oral Solution & Intensol (Oxycodone) ... 2366
- Tylox Capsules ... 1593

Pentobarbital Sodium (Heightens depressant effect). Products include:
- Nembutal Sodium Capsules ... 440
- Nembutal Sodium Solution ... 442
- Nembutal Sodium Suppositories ... 444

Perphenazine (Heightens depressant effect). Products include:
- Etrafon ... 2495
- Triavil Tablets ... 1800
- Trilafon ... 2532

Phenelzine Sulfate (Prolongs and intensifies anticholinergic effects). Products include:
- Nardil ... 1977

Phenobarbital (Heightens depressant effect). Products include:
- Arco-Lase Plus Tablets ... 513
- Bellergal-S Tablets ... 2375
- Donnatal ... 2234
- Donnatal Extentabs ... 2234
- Donnatal Tablets ... 2234
- Phenobarbital Elixir and Tablets ... 1523
- Quadrinal Tablets ... 1398

Prazepam (Heightens depressant effect).
- No products indexed under this heading.

Prochlorperazine (Heightens depressant effect). Products include:
- Compazine ... 2644

Promethazine Hydrochloride (Heightens depressant effect). Products include:
- Mepergan Injection ... 2859
- Phenergan with Codeine ... 2883
- Phenergan with Dextromethorphan ... 2885
- Phenergan Injection ... 2880
- Phenergan Suppositories ... 2882
- Phenergan Syrup ... 2881
- Phenergan Tablets ... 2882
- Phenergan VC ... 2886
- Phenergan VC with Codeine ... 2888

Propofol (Heightens depressant effect). Products include:
- Diprivan Injectable Emulsion ... 2939

Propoxyphene Hydrochloride (Heightens depressant effect). Products include:
- Darvon ... 1475
- Wygesic Tablets ... 2930

Propoxyphene Napsylate (Heightens depressant effect). Products include:
- Darvon-N/Darvocet-N ... 1473

Quazepam (Heightens depressant effect). Products include:
- Doral Tablets ... 2773

Risperidone (Heightens depressant effect). Products include:
- Risperdal Tablets ... 1348

Secobarbital Sodium (Heightens depressant effect). Products include:
- Seconal Sodium Pulvules ... 1529

Selegiline Hydrochloride (Prolongs and intensifies anticholinergic effects). Products include:
- Eldepryl Capsules ... 2729

Sevoflurane (Heightens depressant effect).
- No products indexed under this heading.

Sufentanil Citrate (Heightens depressant effect). Products include:
- Sufenta Injection ... 1355

Temazepam (Heightens depressant effect). Products include:
- Restoril Capsules ... 2413

Thiamylal Sodium (Heightens depressant effect).
- No products indexed under this heading.

Thioridazine Hydrochloride (Heightens depressant effect). Products include:
- Mellaril ... 2398

Thiothixene (Heightens depressant effect). Products include:
- Navane Capsules and Concentrate ... 2018
- Navane Intramuscular ... 2019

Tranylcypromine Sulfate (Prolongs and intensifies anticholinergic effects). Products include:
- Parnate Tablets ... 2679

Triazolam (Heightens depressant effect). Products include:
- Halcion Tablets ... 2093

Trifluoperazine Hydrochloride (Heightens depressant effect). Products include:
- Stelazine ... 2692

Zolpidem Tartrate (Heightens depressant effect). Products include:
- Ambien Tablets ... 2559

Food Interactions

Alcohol (Heightens depressant effect).

OCCLUSAL-HP
(Salicylic Acid) ... 1041
None cited in PDR database.

OCUCOAT
(Hydroxypropyl Methylcellulose) ... 321
None cited in PDR database.

OCUCOAT AND OCUCOAT PF EYE DROPS
(Dextran 70, Hydroxypropyl Methylcellulose) ... 322
None cited in PDR database.

OCEAN NASAL MIST
(Sodium Chloride) ... 671
None cited in PDR database.

OCUFEN
(Flurbiprofen Sodium) ... 242
May interact with:

Acetylcholine Chloride (There have been reports that acetylcholine chloride is ineffective when used in patients treated with ophthalmic flurbiprofen). Products include:
- Miochol-E with Iocare Steri-Tags and Miochol-E System Pak ... 263

IMPORTANT NOTE: Always consult each drug listing in the patient's regimen for possible interactions.

Carbachol (There have been reports that carbachol is ineffective when used in patients treated with ophthalmic flurbiprofen). Products include:

- Carbastat Intraocular Solution .... ◉ 260
- Isopto Carbachol Ophthalmic Solution .... ◉ 221
- MIOSTAT Intraocular Solution .... ◉ 222

OCUFLOX OPHTHALMIC SOLUTION

(Ofloxacin) 478

May interact with oral anticoagulants, xanthine bronchodilators, and certain other agents. Compounds in these categories include:

Aminophylline (Systemic administration of quinolone has shown to elevate plasma theophylline levels; specific drug interactions studies have not been conducted with the ofloxacin ophthalmic solution).

No products indexed under this heading.

Caffeine-containing medications (Systemic administration of quinolone has shown to interfere with the metabolism of caffeine; specific drug interactions studies have not been conducted with the ofloxacin ophthalmic solution).

Cyclosporine (Systemic administration of quinolone has been associated with transient elevations in serum creatinine; specific drug interactions studies have not been conducted with the ofloxacin ophthalmic solution). Products include:

- Neoral 2405
- Sandimmune 2416

Dicumarol (Systemic administration of quinolone has shown to enhance the effects of oral anticoagulants; specific drug interactions studies have not been conducted with the ofloxacin ophthalmic solution).

No products indexed under this heading.

Dyphylline (Systemic administration of quinolone has shown to elevate plasma theophylline levels; specific drug interactions studies have not been conducted with the ofloxacin ophthalmic solution). Products include:

- Lufyllin & Lufyllin-400 Tablets 2778
- Lufyllin-GG Elixir & Tablets 2779

Theophylline (Systemic administration of quinolone has shown to elevate plasma theophylline levels; specific drug interactions studies have not been conducted with the ofloxacin ophthalmic solution). Products include:

- Marax Tablets & DF Syrup 2015
- Quibron 2227

Theophylline Anhydrous (Systemic administration of quinolone has shown to elevate plasma theophylline levels; specific drug interactions studies have not been conducted with the ofloxacin ophthalmic solution). Products include:

- Aerolate 1003
- Primatene Tablets .... ▣ 844
- Respbid Tablets 687
- Slo-bid Gyrocaps 2201
- Theo-24 Extended Release Capsules 2753
- Theo-Dur Extended-Release Tablets 1367
- Theo-X Extended-Release Tablets .. 793
- Uni-Dur Extended-Release Tablets .. 1374
- Uniphyl 400 mg and 600 mg Tablets 2157

Theophylline Calcium Salicylate (Systemic administration of quinolone has shown to elevate plasma theophylline levels; specific drug interactions studies have not been conducted with the ofloxacin ophthalmic solution). Products include:

- Quadrinal Tablets 1398

Theophylline Sodium Glycinate (Systemic administration of quinolone has shown to elevate plasma theophylline levels; specific drug interactions studies have not been conducted with the ofloxacin ophthalmic solution).

No products indexed under this heading.

Warfarin Sodium (Systemic administration of quinolone has shown to enhance the effects of oral anticoagulants; specific drug interactions studies have not been conducted with the ofloxacin ophthalmic solution). Products include:

- Coumadin 941

OCUHIST

(Naphazoline Hydrochloride, Pheniramine Maleate) .... ◉ 300

None cited in PDR database.

OCUPRESS OPHTHALMIC SOLUTION, 1% STERILE

(Carteolol Hydrochloride) .... ◉ 297

May interact with beta blockers and catecholamine depleting drugs. Compounds in these categories include:

Acebutolol Hydrochloride (Potential for additive effects). Products include:

- Sectral Capsules 2914

Atenolol (Potential for additive effects). Products include:

- Tenoretic Tablets 2963
- Tenormin Tablets and I.V. Injection 2965

Betaxolol Hydrochloride (Potential for additive effects). Products include:

- Betoptic Ophthalmic Solution 465
- Betoptic S Ophthalmic Suspension 467
- Kerlone Tablets 2588

Bisoprolol Fumarate (Potential for additive effects). Products include:

- Zebeta Tablets 1457
- Ziac 1459

Deserpidine (Possible additive effects and the production of hypotension and/or marked bradycardia).

No products indexed under this heading.

Esmolol Hydrochloride (Potential for additive effects). Products include:

- Brevibloc (esmolol HCl) Injection 1860

Guanethidine Monosulfate (Possible additive effects and the production of hypotension and/or marked bradycardia). Products include:

- Esimil Tablets 840
- Ismelin Tablets 845

Labetalol Hydrochloride (Potential for additive effects). Products include:

- Normodyne Injection 2519
- Normodyne Tablets 2522
- Trandate 1158

Levobunolol Hydrochloride (Potential for additive effects). Products include:

- Betagan .... ◉ 230

Metipranolol Hydrochloride (Potential for additive effects). Products include:

- OptiPranolol (Metipranolol 0.3%) Sterile Ophthalmic Solution .... ◉ 256

Metoprolol Succinate (Potential for additive effects). Products include:

- Toprol-XL Tablets 560

Metoprolol Tartrate (Potential for additive effects). Products include:

- Lopressor 848
- Lopressor HCT Tablets 850

Nadolol (Potential for additive effects).

No products indexed under this heading.

Penbutolol Sulfate (Potential for additive effects). Products include:

- Levatol Tablets 2547

Pindolol (Potential for additive effects). Products include:

- Visken Tablets 2428

Propranolol Hydrochloride (Potential for additive effects). Products include:

- Inderal 2834
- Inderal LA Long Acting Capsules 2836
- Inderide Tablets 2838
- Inderide LA Long Acting Capsules .. 2840

Rauwolfia Serpentina (Possible additive effects and the production of hypotension and/or marked bradycardia).

No products indexed under this heading.

Rescinnamine (Possible additive effects and the production of hypotension and/or marked bradycardia).

No products indexed under this heading.

Reserpine (Possible additive effects and the production of hypotension and/or marked bradycardia). Products include:

- Diupres Tablets 1691
- Hydropres Tablets 1718
- Ser-Ap-Es Tablets 867

Sotalol Hydrochloride (Potential for additive effects). Products include:

- Betapace Tablets 637

Timolol Hemihydrate (Potential for additive effects). Products include:

- Betimol 0.25%, 0.5% .... ◉ 259

Timolol Maleate (Potential for additive effects). Products include:

- Blocadren Tablets 1654
- Timolide Tablets 1791
- Timoptic in Ocudose 1796
- Timoptic Sterile Ophthalmic Solution 1794
- Timoptic-XE 1798

OCUSERT PILO-20 AND PILO-40 OCULAR THERAPEUTIC SYSTEMS

(Pilocarpine) .... ◉ 252

May interact with:

Epinephrine (Increased rate of absorption from the eye). Products include:

- EPIFRIN .... ◉ 237
- EpiPen 808
- Marcaine with Epinephrine 2446
- Primatene Mist .... ▣ 843
- Sensorcaine with Epinephrine Injection 554
- Sus-Phrine Injection 1017
- Xylocaine with Epinephrine Injections 562

Epinephrine Bitartrate (Increased rate of absorption from the eye). Products include:

- Sensorcaine-MPF with Epinephrine Injection 554

OCUVITE VITAMIN AND MINERAL SUPPLEMENT

(Vitamins with Minerals) .... ◉ 322

None cited in PDR database.

OCUVITE EXTRA VITAMIN AND MINERAL SUPPLEMENT

(Vitamins with Minerals) .... ◉ 322

None cited in PDR database.

OGEN TABLETS

(Estropipate) 2103

May interact with progestins. Compounds in this category include:

Desogestrel (Possible adverse effects on lipoprotein metabolism; impairment of glucose tolerance and possible enhancement of mitotic activity in breast epithelial tissues). Products include:

- Desogen Tablets 1867
- Ortho-Cept 1907

Medroxyprogesterone Acetate (Possible adverse effects on lipoprotein metabolism; impairment of glucose tolerance and possible enhancement of mitotic activity in breast epithelial tissues). Products include:

- Amen Tablets 785
- Cycrin Tablets 991
- Depo-Provera Contraceptive Injection 2079
- Depo-Provera Sterile Aqueous Suspension 2083
- Premphase 2900
- Prempro 2905
- Provera Tablets 2110

Megestrol Acetate (Possible adverse effects on lipoprotein metabolism; impairment of glucose tolerance and possible enhancement of mitotic activity in breast epithelial tissues). Products include:

- Megace Oral Suspension 708
- Megace Tablets 710

Norgestimate (Possible adverse effects on lipoprotein metabolism; impairment of glucose tolerance and possible enhancement of mitotic activity in breast epithelial tissues). Products include:

- Ortho-Cyclen/Ortho-Tri-Cyclen 1914
- Ortho-Cyclen/Ortho Tri-Cyclen 1914

OGEN VAGINAL CREAM

(Estropipate) 2106

May interact with progestins. Compounds in this category include:

Desogestrel (Potential for adverse effects on carbohydrate and lipid metabolism). Products include:

- Desogen Tablets 1867
- Ortho-Cept 1907

Medroxyprogesterone Acetate (Potential for adverse effects on carbohydrate and lipid metabolism). Products include:

- Amen Tablets 785
- Cycrin Tablets 991
- Depo-Provera Contraceptive Injection 2079
- Depo-Provera Sterile Aqueous Suspension 2083
- Premphase 2900
- Prempro 2905
- Provera Tablets 2110

Megestrol Acetate (Potential for adverse effects on carbohydrate and lipid metabolism). Products include:

- Megace Oral Suspension 708
- Megace Tablets 710

Norgestimate (Potential for adverse effects on carbohydrate and lipid metabolism). Products include:

- Ortho-Cyclen/Ortho-Tri-Cyclen 1914
- Ortho-Cyclen/Ortho Tri-Cyclen 1914

(▣ Described in PDR For Nonprescription Drugs) (◉ Described in PDR For Ophthalmology)

OIL OF OLAY DAILY UV PROTECTANT SPF 15 BEAUTY FLUID-ORIGINAL AND FRAGRANCE FREE (OLAY CO. INC.)
(Octyl Methoxycinnamate, Phenylbenzimidazole-5-Sulfonic Acid) ⊞ 725
None cited in PDR database.

OMNIHIB
(Haemophilus B Conjugate Vaccine) 2676
None cited in PDR database.

OMNIPEN CAPSULES
(Ampicillin) 2872
None cited in PDR database.

OMNIPEN FOR ORAL SUSPENSION
(Ampicillin) 2873
May interact with bacteriostatic antibiotics and oral contraceptives. Compounds in these categories include:

Allopurinol (Increased possibility of skin rash, particularly in hyperuricemic patients, may occur). Products include:
- Zyloprim Tablets 1194

Chloramphenicol (Bacteriostatic antibiotics may interfere with the bactericidal effect of penicillin; clinical significance of this interaction is not well-documented). Products include:
- Chloromycetin Ophthalmic Ointment, 1% ⊙ 298
- Chloromycetin Ophthalmic Solution ⊙ 299
- Chloroptic S.O.P. ⊙ 236
- Chloroptic Sterile Ophthalmic Solution ⊙ 236

Chloramphenicol Palmitate (Bacteriostatic antibiotics may interfere with the bactericidal effect of penicillin; clinical significance of this interaction is not well-documented).
- No products indexed under this heading.

Chloramphenicol Sodium Succinate (Bacteriostatic antibiotics may interfere with the bactericidal effect of penicillin; clinical significance of this interaction is not well-documented). Products include:
- Chloromycetin Sodium Succinate 1960

Demeclocycline Hydrochloride (Bacteriostatic antibiotics may interfere with the bactericidal effect of penicillin; clinical significance of this interaction is not well-documented). Products include:
- Declomycin Tablets 1421

Desogestrel (Oral contraceptives may be less effective and potential for increased breakthrough bleeding). Products include:
- Desogen Tablets 1867
- Ortho-Cept 1907

Doxycycline Calcium (Bacteriostatic antibiotics may interfere with the bactericidal effect of penicillin; clinical significance of this interaction is not well-documented). Products include:
- Vibramycin Calcium Oral Suspension Syrup 2038

Doxycycline Hyclate (Bacteriostatic antibiotics may interfere with the bactericidal effect of penicillin; clinical significance of this interaction is not well-documented). Products include:
- Doryx Capsules 1970
- Vibramycin Hyclate Capsules 2038
- Vibramycin Hyclate Intravenous 2040
- Vibra-Tabs Film Coated Tablets 2038

Doxycycline Monohydrate (Bacteriostatic antibiotics may interfere with the bactericidal effect of penicillin; clinical significance of this interaction is not well-documented). Products include:
- Monodox Capsules 1858
- Vibramycin Monohydrate for Oral Suspension 2038

Erythromycin (Bacteriostatic antibiotics may interfere with the bactericidal effect of penicillin; clinical significance of this interaction is not well-documented). Products include:
- A/T/S 2% Acne Topical Gel 1244
- A/T/S 2% Acne Topical Solution 1244
- Benzamycin Topical Gel 919
- E-Mycin Tablets 1388
- Emgel 2% Topical Gel 1081
- ERYC 1972
- Erycette (erythromycin 2%) Topical Solution 1943
- Ery-Tab Tablets 426
- Erythromycin Base Filmtab 430
- Erythromycin Delayed-Release Capsules, USP 431
- Ilotycin Ophthalmic Ointment 928
- PCE Dispertab Tablets 453
- T-Stat 2.0% Topical Solution and Pads 2797
- THERAMYCIN Z 2% Solution 1629

Erythromycin Estolate (Bacteriostatic antibiotics may interfere with the bactericidal effect of penicillin; clinical significance of this interaction is not well-documented). Products include:
- Ilosone 927

Erythromycin Ethylsuccinate (Bacteriostatic antibiotics may interfere with the bactericidal effect of penicillin; clinical significance of this interaction is not well-documented). Products include:
- E.E.S. 427
- EryPed 425
- Pediazole Suspension 2340

Erythromycin Gluceptate (Bacteriostatic antibiotics may interfere with the bactericidal effect of penicillin; clinical significance of this interaction is not well-documented). Products include:
- Ilotycin Gluceptate, IV, Vials 929

Erythromycin Stearate (Bacteriostatic antibiotics may interfere with the bactericidal effect of penicillin; clinical significance of this interaction is not well-documented). Products include:
- Erythrocin Stearate Filmtab 429

Ethinyl Estradiol (Oral contraceptives may be less effective and potential for increased breakthrough bleeding). Products include:
- Brevicon 2563
- Demulen 2580
- Desogen Tablets 1867
- Levlen/Tri-Levlen 646
- Lo/Ovral Tablets 2852
- Lo/Ovral-28 Tablets 2857
- Modicon 1928
- Nordette-21 Tablets 2863
- Nordette-28 Tablets 2866
- Norinyl 2563
- Ortho-Cept 1907
- Ortho-Cyclen/Ortho-Tri-Cyclen 1914
- Ortho-Novum 1928
- Ortho-Cyclen/Ortho Tri-Cyclen 1914
- Ovcon 765
- Ovral Tablets 2877
- Ovral-28 Tablets 2878
- Levlen/Tri-Levlen 646
- Tri-Norinyl 2607
- Triphasil-21 Tablets 2919
- Triphasil-28 Tablets 2924

Ethynodiol Diacetate (Oral contraceptives may be less effective and potential for increased breakthrough bleeding). Products include:
- Demulen 2580

Levonorgestrel (Oral contraceptives may be less effective and potential for increased breakthrough bleeding). Products include:
- Levlen/Tri-Levlen 646
- Nordette-21 Tablets 2863
- Nordette-28 Tablets 2866
- Norplant System 2868
- Levlen/Tri-Levlen 646
- Triphasil-21 Tablets 2919
- Triphasil-28 Tablets 2924

Mestranol (Oral contraceptives may be less effective and potential for increased breakthrough bleeding). Products include:
- Norinyl 2563
- Ortho-Novum 1928

Methacycline Hydrochloride (Bacteriostatic antibiotics may interfere with the bactericidal effect of penicillin; clinical significance of this interaction is not well-documented).
- No products indexed under this heading.

Minocycline Hydrochloride (Bacteriostatic antibiotics may interfere with the bactericidal effect of penicillin; clinical significance of this interaction is not well-documented). Products include:
- DYNACIN Capsules 1627
- Minocin Intravenous 1428
- Minocin Oral Suspension 1431
- Minocin Pellet-Filled Capsules 1429

Norethindrone (Oral contraceptives may be less effective and potential for increased breakthrough bleeding). Products include:
- Brevicon 2563
- Micronor Tablets 1903
- Modicon 1928
- Norinyl 2563
- Nor-Q D Tablets 2598
- Ortho-Novum 1928
- Ovcon 765
- Tri-Norinyl 2607

Norethynodrel (Oral contraceptives may be less effective and potential for increased breakthrough bleeding).
- No products indexed under this heading.

Norgestimate (Oral contraceptives may be less effective and potential for increased breakthrough bleeding). Products include:
- Ortho-Cyclen/Ortho-Tri-Cyclen 1914
- Ortho-Cyclen/Ortho Tri-Cyclen 1914

Norgestrel (Oral contraceptives may be less effective and potential for increased breakthrough bleeding). Products include:
- Lo/Ovral Tablets 2852
- Lo/Ovral-28 Tablets 2857
- Ovral Tablets 2877
- Ovral-28 Tablets 2878
- Ovrette Tablets 2878

Oxytetracycline Hydrochloride (Bacteriostatic antibiotics may interfere with the bactericidal effect of penicillin; clinical significance of this interaction is not well-documented). Products include:
- TERAK Ointment ⊙ 210
- Terra-Cortril Ophthalmic Suspension 2033
- Terramycin with Polymyxin B Sulfate Ophthalmic Ointment 2035
- Urobiotic-250 Capsules 2038

Probenecid (Decreases renal tubular secretion of ampicillin resulting in increased blood levels and/or ampicillin toxicity). Products include:
- Benemid Tablets 1651
- ColBENEMID Tablets 1662

Sulfamethizole (Bacteriostatic antibiotics may interfere with the bactericidal effect of penicillin; clinical significance of this interaction is not well-documented). Products include:
- Urobiotic-250 Capsules 2038

Sulfamethoxazole (Bacteriostatic antibiotics may interfere with the bactericidal effect of penicillin; clinical significance of this interaction is not well-documented). Products include:
- Bactrim DS Tablets 2257
- Bactrim I.V. Infusion 2255
- Bactrim 2257
- Gantanol Tablets 2285
- Septra 1146
- Septra I.V. Infusion 1142
- Septra I.V. Infusion ADD-Vantage Vials 1144
- Septra 1146

Sulfinpyrazone (Bacteriostatic antibiotics may interfere with the bactericidal effect of penicillin; clinical significance of this interaction is not well-documented). Products include:
- Anturane 823

Sulfisoxazole (Bacteriostatic antibiotics may interfere with the bactericidal effect of penicillin; clinical significance of this interaction is not well-documented). Products include:
- Gantrisin Tablets 2286

Tetracycline Hydrochloride (Bacteriostatic antibiotics may interfere with the bactericidal effect of penicillin; clinical significance of this interaction is not well-documented). Products include:
- Achromycin V Capsules 1417
- Helidac Therapy 2135

ONCASPAR
(Pegaspargase) 2194
May interact with anticoagulants, non-steroidal anti-inflammatory agents, antineoplastics, highly protein bound drugs (selected), and certain other agents. Compounds in these categories include:

Altretamine (Potential for unspecified unfavorable interactions). Products include:
- Hexalen Capsules 2760

Amiodarone Hydrochloride (Depletion of serum proteins by pegaspargase may increase the toxicity of other drugs which are protein bound). Products include:
- Cordarone Intravenous 2821
- Cordarone Tablets 2818

Amitriptyline Hydrochloride (Depletion of serum proteins by pegaspargase may increase the toxicity of other drugs which are protein bound). Products include:
- Elavil 2945
- Etrafon 2495
- Limbitrol 2333
- Triavil Tablets 1800

Anastrozole (Potential for unspecified unfavorable interactions). Products include:
- Arimidex Tablets 2932

Asparaginase (Potential for unspecified unfavorable interactions). Products include:
- Elspar 1700

Aspirin (Increased risk of bleeding and/or thrombosis). Products include:
- Alka-Seltzer Cherry Effervescent Antacid and Pain Reliever ⊞ 609
- Alka-Seltzer Extra Strength Effervescent Antacid and Pain Reliever ⊞ 609

IMPORTANT NOTE: Always consult each drug listing in the patient's regimen for possible interactions.

Oncaspar / Interactions Index

Alka-Seltzer Lemon Lime Effervescent Antacid and Pain Reliever ... ⃞ 609
Alka-Seltzer Original Effervescent Antacid and Pain Reliever ... ⃞ 609
Alka-Seltzer Plus ... ⃞ 611
Alka-Seltzer Plus Sinus Medicine ... ⃞ 611
Ascriptin ... ⃞ 650
Arthritis Strength BC Powder ... ⃞ 631
BC Cold Powder Multi-Symptom Formula (Cold-Sinus-Allergy) ... ⃞ 631
BC Cold Powder Non-Drowsy Formula (Cold-Sinus) ... ⃞ 631
BC Powder ... ⃞ 631
Genuine Bayer Aspirin Tablets & Caplets ... ⃞ 618
Extra Strength Bayer Arthritis Pain Regimen Formula ... ⃞ 615
Extra Strength Bayer Aspirin Caplets & Tablets ... ⃞ 617
Extended-Release Bayer 8-Hour Aspirin ... ⃞ 616
Extra Strength Bayer Plus Aspirin Caplets ... ⃞ 617
Extra Strength Bayer PM Aspirin Plus Sleep Aid ... ⃞ 617
Aspirin Regimen Bayer 81 mg Tablets with Calcium ... ⃞ 615
Aspirin Regimen Bayer Adult Low Strength 81 mg Tablets ... ⃞ 613
Aspirin Regimen Bayer Children's Chewable Aspirin ... ⃞ 616
Aspirin Regimen Bayer Regular Strength 325 mg Caplets ... ⃞ 613
Bufferin Analgesic Tablets ... ⃞ 636
Arthritis Strength Bufferin Analgesic Caplets ... ⃞ 637
Extra Strength Bufferin Analgesic Tablets ... ⃞ 637
Cama Arthritis Pain Reliever ... ⃞ 748
Darvon Compound-65 Pulvules ... 1475
Easprin ... 1971
Ecotrin ... 2625
Ecotrin Enteric Coated Aspirin Maximum Strength Tablets and Caplets ... ⃞ 775
Ecotrin Enteric Coated Aspirin Regular Strength Tablets ... 2625
Empirin Aspirin Tablets ... ⃞ 818
Excedrin Extra-Strength Analgesic Tablets, Caplets, and Geltabs ... 734
Fiorinal Capsules ... 2388
Fiorinal with Codeine Capsules ... 2390
Fiorinal Tablets ... 2388
Goody's Extra Strength Headache Powders ... ⃞ 632
Goody's Extra Strength Pain Relief Tablets ... ⃞ 632
Halfprin Tablets ... 1413
Norgesic ... 1554
Percodan Tablets ... 955
Percodan-Demi Tablets ... 956
Robaxisal Tablets ... 2246
Soma Compound w/Codeine Tablets ... 2784
Soma Compound Tablets ... 2783
St. Joseph Adult Chewable Aspirin (81 mg.) ... ⃞ 768
Talwin Compound ... 2466
Vanquish Analgesic Caplets ... ⃞ 627

Atovaquone (Depletion of serum proteins by pegaspargase may increase the toxicity of other drugs which are protein bound). Products include:
Mepron Suspension ... 1206

Bicalutamide (Potential for unspecified unfavorable interactions). Products include:
Casodex Tablets ... 2934

Bleomycin Sulfate (Potential for unspecified unfavorable interactions). Products include:
Blenoxane ... 697

Busulfan (Potential for unspecified unfavorable interactions). Products include:
Myleran Tablets ... 1209

Carboplatin (Potential for unspecified unfavorable interactions). Products include:
Paraplatin for Injection ... 713

Carmustine (BCNU) (Potential for unspecified unfavorable interactions). Products include:
BiCNU ... 696

Cefonicid Sodium (Depletion of serum proteins by pegaspargase may increase the toxicity of other drugs which are protein bound). Products include:
Monocid Injection ... 2674

Chlorambucil (Potential for unspecified unfavorable interactions). Products include:
Leukeran Tablets ... 1205

Chlordiazepoxide (Depletion of serum proteins by pegaspargase may increase the toxicity of other drugs which are protein bound). Products include:
Limbitrol ... 2333

Chlordiazepoxide Hydrochloride (Depletion of serum proteins by pegaspargase may increase the toxicity of other drugs which are protein bound). Products include:
Librax Capsules ... 2330
Librium Capsules ... 2331
Librium Injectable ... 2332

Chlorpromazine (Depletion of serum proteins by pegaspargase may increase the toxicity of other drugs which are protein bound). Products include:
Thorazine Suppositories ... 2701

Chlorpromazine Hydrochloride (Depletion of serum proteins by pegaspargase may increase the toxicity of other drugs which are protein bound). Products include:
Thorazine ... 2701

Cisplatin (Potential for unspecified unfavorable interactions). Products include:
Platinol for Injection ... 717
Platinol-AQ Injection ... 719

Clomipramine Hydrochloride (Depletion of serum proteins by pegaspargase may increase the toxicity of other drugs which are protein bound). Products include:
Anafranil Capsules ... 819

Clozapine (Depletion of serum proteins by pegaspargase may increase the toxicity of other drugs which are protein bound). Products include:
Clozaril Tablets ... 2377

Cyclophosphamide (Potential for unspecified unfavorable interactions). Products include:
Cytoxan ... 700

Cyclosporine (Depletion of serum proteins by pegaspargase may increase the toxicity of other drugs which are protein bound). Products include:
Neoral ... 2405
Sandimmune ... 2416

Dacarbazine (Potential for unspecified unfavorable interactions). Products include:
DTIC-Dome ... 593

Dalteparin Sodium (Increased risk of bleeding and/or thrombosis). Products include:
Fragmin Injection ... 2088

Daunorubicin Citrate (Potential for unspecified unfavorable interactions). Products include:
DaunoXome ... 1842

Daunorubicin Hydrochloride (Potential for unspecified unfavorable interactions). Products include:
Cerubidine for Injection ... 634

Diazepam (Depletion of serum proteins by pegaspargase may increase the toxicity of other drugs which are protein bound). Products include:
Dizac (diazepam injectable emulsion) CIV ... 1862

Valium Injectable ... 2336
Valium Tablets ... 2335

Diclofenac Potassium (Depletion of serum proteins by pegaspargase may increase the toxicity of other drugs which are protein bound; increased risk of bleeding and/or thrombosis). Products include:
Cataflam Tablets ... 833

Diclofenac Sodium (Depletion of serum proteins by pegaspargase may increase the toxicity of other drugs which are protein bound; increased risk of bleeding and/or thrombosis). Products include:
Voltaren Ophthalmic Sterile Ophthalmic Solution ... ⊚ 264
Cataflam/Voltaren/Voltaren-XR ... 833

Dicumarol (Increased risk of bleeding and/or thrombosis).
No products indexed under this heading.

Dipyridamole (Increased risk of bleeding and/or thrombosis). Products include:
Persantine Tablets ... 686

Docetaxel (Potential for unspecified unfavorable interactions). Products include:
Taxotere for Injection Concentrate ... 2204

Doxorubicin Hydrochloride (Potential for unspecified unfavorable interactions). Products include:
Adriamycin PFS ... 2056
Adriamycin RDF ... 2056
Doxil ... 2613
Doxorubicin Astra ... 531
Rubex for Injection ... 721

Enoxaparin (Increased risk of bleeding and/or thrombosis). Products include:
Lovenox Injection ... 2187

Estramustine Phosphate Sodium (Potential for unspecified unfavorable interactions). Products include:
Emcyt Capsules ... 2085

Etodolac (Increased risk of bleeding and/or thrombosis). Products include:
Lodine Capsules and Tablets ... 2849

Etoposide (Potential for unspecified unfavorable interactions). Products include:
Etoposide Injection ... 539
VePesid Capsules and Injection ... 727

Fenoprofen Calcium (Depletion of serum proteins by pegaspargase may increase the toxicity of other drugs which are protein bound; increased risk of bleeding and/or thrombosis). Products include:
Nalfon 200 Pulvules & Nalfon Tablets ... 933

Floxuridine (Potential for unspecified unfavorable interactions). Products include:
Sterile FUDR ... 2284

Fluorouracil (Potential for unspecified unfavorable interactions). Products include:
Efudex ... 2280
Fluoroplex Topical Solution & Cream 1% ... 475
Fluorouracil Injection ... 2282

Flurazepam Hydrochloride (Depletion of serum proteins by pegaspargase may increase the toxicity of other drugs which are protein bound). Products include:
Dalmane Capsules ... 2329

Flurbiprofen (Depletion of serum proteins by pegaspargase may increase the toxicity of other drugs which are protein bound; increased risk of bleeding and/or thrombosis).
No products indexed under this heading.

Flutamide (Potential for unspecified unfavorable interactions). Products include:
Eulexin Capsules ... 2498

Gemcitabine Hydrochloride (Potential for unspecified unfavorable interactions). Products include:
Gemzar for Injection ... 1482

Glipizide (Depletion of serum proteins by pegaspargase may increase the toxicity of other drugs which are protein bound). Products include:
Glucotrol Tablets ... 2011
Glucotrol XL Extended Release Tablets ... 2012

Heparin Calcium (Increased risk of bleeding and/or thrombosis).
No products indexed under this heading.

Heparin Sodium (Increased risk of bleeding and/or thrombosis). Products include:
Heparin Lock Flush Solution ... 2831
Heparin Sodium Injection ... 2832
Heparin Sodium Vials ... 1486

Hydroxyurea (Potential for unspecified unfavorable interactions). Products include:
Hydrea Capsules ... 705

Ibuprofen (Depletion of serum proteins by pegaspargase may increase the toxicity of other drugs which are protein bound; increased risk of bleeding and/or thrombosis). Products include:
Advil Cold and Sinus Caplets and Tablets ... ⃞ 837
Advil Ibuprofen Tablets, Caplets and Gel Caplets ... ⃞ 836
Children's Motrin Ibuprofen Oral Suspension ... 1558
IBU Tablets ... 1389
Ibuprohm ... 713
Motrin IB Caplets, Tablets, and Gelcaps ... ⃞ 802
Motrin Ibuprofen Suspension, Oral Drops, Chewable Tablets, Caplets ... 1563
Nuprin Ibuprofen/Analgesic Tablets & Caplets ... ⃞ 645
Vicks DayQuil SINUS Pressure & PAIN Relief with IBUPROFEN ... ⃞ 735

Idarubicin Hydrochloride (Potential for unspecified unfavorable interactions). Products include:
Idamycin Injection ... 2096

Ifosfamide (Potential for unspecified unfavorable interactions). Products include:
IFEX ... 706

Imipramine Hydrochloride (Depletion of serum proteins by pegaspargase may increase the toxicity of other drugs which are protein bound). Products include:
Tofranil Ampuls ... 873
Tofranil Tablets ... 875

Imipramine Pamoate (Depletion of serum proteins by pegaspargase may increase the toxicity of other drugs which are protein bound). Products include:
Tofranil-PM Capsules ... 876

Indomethacin (Depletion of serum proteins by pegaspargase may increase the toxicity of other drugs which are protein bound; increased risk of bleeding and/or thrombosis). Products include:
Indocin ... 1723

Indomethacin Sodium Trihydrate (Depletion of serum proteins by pegaspargase may increase the toxicity of other drugs which are protein bound; increased risk of bleeding and/or thrombosis). Products include:
Indocin I.V. ... 1727

(⃞ Described in PDR For Nonprescription Drugs) (⊚ Described in PDR For Ophthalmology)

Interferon alfa-2A, Recombinant (Potential for unspecified unfavorable interactions). Products include:
Roferon-A Injection 2308
Interferon alfa-2B, Recombinant (Potential for unspecified unfavorable interactions). Products include:
Intron A for Injection 2506
Irinotecan Hydrochloride (Potential for unspecified unfavorable interactions).
No products indexed under this heading.
Ketoprofen (Depletion of serum proteins by pegaspargase may increase the toxicity of other drugs which are protein bound; increased risk of bleeding and/or thrombosis). Products include:
Actron Caplets and Tablets........... 608
Orudis Capsules 2874
Orudis KT 842
Oruvail Capsules 2874
Ketorolac Tromethamine (Depletion of serum proteins by pegaspargase may increase the toxicity of other drugs which are protein bound; increased risk of bleeding and/or thrombosis). Products include:
Acular Sterile Ophthalmic Solution ... 470
Toradol 2319
Levamisole Hydrochloride (Potential for unspecified unfavorable interactions). Products include:
Ergamisol Tablets 1340
Lomustine (CCNU) (Potential for unspecified unfavorable interactions). Products include:
CeeNU Capsules 699
Mechlorethamine Hydrochloride (Potential for unspecified unfavorable interactions). Products include:
Mustargen 1752
Meclofenamate Sodium (Depletion of serum proteins by pegaspargase may increase the toxicity of other drugs which are protein bound; increased risk of bleeding and/or thrombosis).
No products indexed under this heading.
Mefenamic Acid (Depletion of serum proteins by pegaspargase may increase the toxicity of other drugs which are protein bound; increased risk of bleeding and/or thrombosis). Products include:
Ponstel 1982
Megestrol Acetate (Potential for unspecified unfavorable interactions). Products include:
Megace Oral Suspension 708
Megace Tablets 710
Melphalan (Potential for unspecified unfavorable interactions). Products include:
Alkeran Tablets 1198
Mercaptopurine (Potential for unspecified unfavorable interactions). Products include:
Purinethol Tablets 1214
Methotrexate Sodium (Pegaspargase inhibits protein synthesis and cell replication and thus interferes with the action of methotrexate which requires cell replication for its lethal effect; potential for unspecified unfavorable interactions). Products include:
Methotrexate Sodium Tablets, Injection, for Injection and LPF Injection 1322

Midazolam Hydrochloride (Depletion of serum proteins by pegaspargase may increase the toxicity of other drugs which are protein bound). Products include:
Versed Injection 2324
Mitomycin (Mitomycin-C) (Potential for unspecified unfavorable interactions). Products include:
Mutamycin for Injection 712
Mitotane (Potential for unspecified unfavorable interactions). Products include:
Lysodren Tablets 707
Mitoxantrone Hydrochloride (Potential for unspecified unfavorable interactions). Products include:
Novantrone for Injection 1327
Nabumetone (Increased risk of bleeding and/or thrombosis). Products include:
Relafen Tablets 2688
Naproxen (Depletion of serum proteins by pegaspargase may increase the toxicity of other drugs which are protein bound; increased risk of bleeding and/or thrombosis). Products include:
Anaprox/Naprosyn 2277
Naproxen Sodium (Depletion of serum proteins by pegaspargase may increase the toxicity of other drugs which are protein bound; increased risk of bleeding and/or thrombosis). Products include:
Aleve 2124
Anaprox/Naprosyn 2277
Naprelan Tablets 2861
Nortriptyline Hydrochloride (Depletion of serum proteins by pegaspargase may increase the toxicity of other drugs which are protein bound). Products include:
Pamelor 2409
Oxaprozin (Depletion of serum proteins by pegaspargase may increase the toxicity of other drugs which are protein bound; increased risk of bleeding and/or thrombosis). Products include:
Daypro Caplets 2578
Oxazepam (Depletion of serum proteins by pegaspargase may increase the toxicity of other drugs which are protein bound). Products include:
Serax Capsules 2916
Serax Tablets 2916
Paclitaxel (Potential for unspecified unfavorable interactions). Products include:
Taxol Injection 723
Phenylbutazone (Depletion of serum proteins by pegaspargase may increase the toxicity of other drugs which are protein bound; increased risk of bleeding and/or thrombosis).
No products indexed under this heading.
Piroxicam (Depletion of serum proteins by pegaspargase may increase the toxicity of other drugs which are protein bound; increased risk of bleeding and/or thrombosis). Products include:
Feldene Capsules 2008
Procarbazine Hydrochloride (Potential for unspecified unfavorable interactions). Products include:
Matulane Capsules 2300
Propranolol Hydrochloride (Depletion of serum proteins by pegaspargase may increase the toxicity of other drugs which are protein bound). Products include:
Inderal 2834
Inderal LA Long Acting Capsules 2836

Inderide Tablets 2838
Inderide LA Long Acting Capsules .. 2840
Streptozocin (Potential for unspecified unfavorable interactions). Products include:
Zanosar Sterile Powder 2119
Sulindac (Depletion of serum proteins by pegaspargase may increase the toxicity of other drugs which are protein bound; increased risk of bleeding and/or thrombosis). Products include:
Clinoril Tablets 1658
Tamoxifen Citrate (Potential for unspecified unfavorable interactions). Products include:
Nolvadex Tablets 2957
Temazepam (Depletion of serum proteins by pegaspargase may increase the toxicity of other drugs which are protein bound). Products include:
Restoril Capsules 2413
Teniposide (Potential for unspecified unfavorable interactions). Products include:
Vumon for Injection 729
Thioguanine (Potential for unspecified unfavorable interactions). Products include:
Thioguanine Tablets, Tabloid Brand 1225
Thiotepa (Potential for unspecified unfavorable interactions). Products include:
Thioplex (Thiotepa For Injection) 1329
Tolbutamide (Depletion of serum proteins by pegaspargase may increase the toxicity of other drugs which are protein bound).
No products indexed under this heading.
Tolmetin Sodium (Depletion of serum proteins by pegaspargase may increase the toxicity of other drugs which are protein bound; increased risk of bleeding and/or thrombosis). Products include:
Tolectin (200, 400 and 600 mg) .. 1591
Topotecan Hydrochloride (Potential for unspecified unfavorable interactions). Products include:
Hycamtin for Injection 2665
Trimipramine Maleate (Depletion of serum proteins by pegaspargase may increase the toxicity of other drugs which are protein bound). Products include:
Surmontil Capsules 2917
Vincristine Sulfate (Potential for unspecified unfavorable interactions). Products include:
Oncovin Solution Vials & Hyporets 1521
Vinorelbine Tartrate (Potential for unspecified unfavorable interactions). Products include:
Navelbine Injection 1212
Warfarin Sodium (Depletion of serum proteins by pegaspargase may increase the toxicity of other drugs which are protein bound; increased risk of bleeding and/or thrombosis). Products include:
Coumadin 941

ONCOVIN SOLUTION VIALS & HYPORETS
(Vincristine Sulfate) 1521
May interact with:

Fosphenytoin Sodium (Increased seizure activity due to reduced phenytoin blood levels). Products include:
Cerebyx Injection 1956

Ketoconazole (Co-administration with a known inhibitor of the metabolic pathway, ketoconazole, has been reported to cause an earlier onset and/or an increased severity of neuromuscular side effects). Products include:
Nizoral 2% Cream 1344
Nizoral 2% Shampoo 1344
Nizoral Tablets 1345
Mitomycin (Mitomycin-C) (Acute shortness of breath; severe bronchospasm). Products include:
Mutamycin for Injection 712
Neurotoxic Drugs (Potential for increased neurotoxicity).
Phenytoin (Increased seizure activity due to reduced phenytoin blood levels). Products include:
Dilantin Infatabs 1967
Dilantin-125 Suspension 1969
Phenytoin Sodium (Increased seizure activity due to reduced phenytoin blood levels). Products include:
Dilantin Kapseals 1965

ONE-A-DAY ANTIOXIDANT PLUS
(Vitamin A, Vitamin C, Vitamin E, Zinc Oxide) 625
None cited in PDR database.

ONE-A-DAY CALCIUM PLUS
(Calcium Carbonate, Magnesium Carbonate, Vitamin D) 625
None cited in PDR database.

ONE-A-DAY ESSENTIAL VITAMINS WITH BETA CAROTENE
(Vitamins with Minerals) 625
None cited in PDR database.

ONE-A-DAY GARLIC SOFTGELS
(Garlic Extract) 626
None cited in PDR database.

ONE-A-DAY MAXIMUM
(Vitamins with Minerals) 626
None cited in PDR database.

ONE-A-DAY MEN'S
(Vitamins, Multiple) 626
None cited in PDR database.

ONE-A-DAY WOMEN'S
(Vitamins with Minerals) 626
None cited in PDR database.

ONE-A-DAY 55 PLUS
(Vitamins with Minerals) 624
None cited in PDR database.

OPHTHALGAN
(Glycerin) 323
None cited in PDR database.

OPHTHETIC
(Proparacaine Hydrochloride) 244
None cited in PDR database.

OPTIPRANOLOL (METIPRANOLOL 0.3%) STERILE OPHTHALMIC SOLUTION
(Metipranolol Hydrochloride) 256
May interact with beta blockers, adrenergic augmenting psychotropics, calcium channel blockers, cardiac glycosides, and certain other agents. Compounds in these categories include:

Acebutolol Hydrochloride (Co-administration with oral beta blockers may result in additive effects on

IMPORTANT NOTE: Always consult each drug listing in the patient's regimen for possible interactions.

systemic beta blockade). Products include:
- Sectral Capsules ... 2914

Amlodipine Besylate (Co-administration with oral or intravenous calcium channel antagonists may result in possible precipitation of left ventricular failure, and hypotension). Products include:
- Lotrel Capsules ... 858
- Norvasc Tablets ... 2020

Atenolol (Co-administration with oral beta blockers may result in additive effects on systemic beta blockade). Products include:
- Tenoretic Tablets ... 2963
- Tenormin Tablets and I.V. Injection 2965

Bepridil Hydrochloride (Co-administration with oral or intravenous calcium channel antagonists may result in possible precipitation of left ventricular failure, and hypotension). Products include:
- Vascor Tablets (200 and 300 mg) 1597

Betaxolol Hydrochloride (Co-administration with oral beta blockers may result in additive effects on systemic beta blockade). Products include:
- Betoptic Ophthalmic Solution ... 465
- Betoptic S Ophthalmic Suspension 467
- Kerlone Tablets ... 2588

Bisoprolol Fumarate (Co-administration with oral beta blockers may result in additive effects on systemic beta blockade). Products include:
- Zebeta Tablets ... 1457
- Ziac ... 1459

Carteolol Hydrochloride (Co-administration with oral beta blockers may result in additive effects on systemic beta blockade). Products include:
- Cartrol Tablets ... 413
- Ocupress Ophthalmic Solution, 1% Sterile ... ◉ 297

Deserpidine (Possible additive effects and production of hypotension and/or bradycardia when beta blocker is used concurrently with catecholamine depleting drugs).
- No products indexed under this heading.

Deslanoside (Concomitant use of beta blockers with digitalis and calcium channel blockers may result in additive effects in prolonging atrioventricular conduction time).
- No products indexed under this heading.

Digitoxin (Concomitant use of beta blockers with digitalis and calcium channel blockers may result in additive effects in prolonging atrioventricular conduction time). Products include:
- Crystodigin Tablets ... 1472

Digoxin (Concomitant use of beta blockers with digitalis and calcium channel blockers may result in additive effects in prolonging atrioventricular conduction time). Products include:
- Lanoxicaps ... 1110
- Lanoxin Elixir Pediatric ... 1113
- Lanoxin Injection ... 1116
- Lanoxin Injection Pediatric ... 1119
- Lanoxin Tablets ... 1121

Diltiazem Hydrochloride (Co-administration with oral or intravenous calcium channel antagonists may result in possible precipitation of left ventricular failure, and hypotension). Products include:
- Cardizem CD Capsules ... 1251
- Cardizem SR Capsules ... 1255
- Cardizem Injectable ... 1253
- Cardizem Tablets ... 1257
- Dilacor XR Extended-release Capsules ... 2183
- Tiazac Capsules ... 1019

Epinephrine (Concurrent use in patients with history of atopy or severe anaphylactic reaction to allergens may be unresponsive to the usual doses of epinephrine used to treat anaphylactic reaction). Products include:
- EPIFRIN ... ◉ 237
- EpiPen ... 808
- Marcaine with Epinephrine ... 2446
- Primatene Mist ... ▣ 843
- Sensorcaine with Epinephrine Injection ... 554
- Sus-Phrine Injection ... 1017
- Xylocaine with Epinephrine Injections ... 562

Epinephrine Hydrochloride (Concurrent use in patients with history of atopy or severe anaphylactic reaction to allergens may be unresponsive to the usual doses of epinephrine used to treat anaphylactic reaction). Products include:
- Ana-Kit Anaphylaxis Emergency Treatment Kit ... 611

Esmolol Hydrochloride (Co-administration with oral beta blockers may result in additive effects on systemic beta blockade). Products include:
- Brevibloc (esmolol HCl) Injection ... 1860

Felodipine (Co-administration with oral or intravenous calcium channel antagonists may result in possible precipitation of left ventricular failure, and hypotension). Products include:
- Plendil Extended-Release Tablets ... 514

Isocarboxazid (Exercise caution when using concurrently with adrenergic psychotropic drugs).
- No products indexed under this heading.

Isradipine (Co-administration with oral or intravenous calcium channel antagonists may result in possible precipitation of left ventricular failure, and hypotension). Products include:
- DynaCirc Capsules ... 2381
- DynaCirc CR Tablets ... 2383

Labetalol Hydrochloride (Co-administration with oral beta blockers may result in additive effects on systemic beta blockade). Products include:
- Normodyne Injection ... 2519
- Normodyne Tablets ... 2522
- Trandate ... 1158

Levobunolol Hydrochloride (Co-administration with oral beta blockers may result in additive effects on systemic beta blockade). Products include:
- Betagan ... ◉ 230

Metoprolol Succinate (Co-administration with oral beta blockers may result in additive effects on systemic beta blockade). Products include:
- Toprol-XL Tablets ... 560

Metoprolol Tartrate (Co-administration with oral beta blockers may result in additive effects on systemic beta blockade). Products include:
- Lopressor ... 848
- Lopressor HCT Tablets ... 850

Nadolol (Co-administration with oral beta blockers may result in additive effects on systemic beta blockade).
- No products indexed under this heading.

Nicardipine Hydrochloride (Co-administration with oral or intravenous calcium channel antagonists may result in possible precipitation of left ventricular failure, and hypotension). Products include:
- Cardene Capsules ... 2261
- Cardene I.V. ... 2815
- Cardene SR Capsules ... 2264

Nifedipine (Co-administration with oral or intravenous calcium channel antagonists may result in possible precipitation of left ventricular failure, and hypotension). Products include:
- Adalat Capsules (10 mg and 20 mg) ... 580
- Adalat CC ... 582
- Procardia Capsules ... 2024
- Procardia XL Extended Release Tablets ... 2026

Nimodipine (Co-administration with oral or intravenous calcium channel antagonists may result in possible precipitation of left ventricular failure, and hypotension). Products include:
- Nimotop Capsules ... 603

Nisoldipine (Co-administration with oral or intravenous calcium channel antagonists may result in possible precipitation of left ventricular failure, and hypotension). Products include:
- Sular Tablets ... 2961

Pargyline Hydrochloride (Exercise caution when using concurrently with adrenergic psychotropic drugs).
- No products indexed under this heading.

Penbutolol Sulfate (Co-administration with oral beta blockers may result in additive effects on systemic beta blockade). Products include:
- Levatol Tablets ... 2547

Phenelzine Sulfate (Exercise caution when using concurrently with adrenergic psychotropic drugs). Products include:
- Nardil ... 1977

Pindolol (Co-administration with oral beta blockers may result in additive effects on systemic beta blockade). Products include:
- Visken Tablets ... 2428

Propranolol Hydrochloride (Co-administration with oral beta blockers may result in additive effects on systemic beta blockade). Products include:
- Inderal ... 2834
- Inderal LA Long Acting Capsules ... 2836
- Inderide Tablets ... 2838
- Inderide LA Long Acting Capsules .. 2840

Rauwolfia Serpentina (Possible additive effects and production of hypotension and/or bradycardia when beta blocker is used concurrently with catecholamine depleting drugs).
- No products indexed under this heading.

Rescinnamine (Possible additive effects and production of hypotension and/or bradycardia when beta blocker is used concurrently with catecholamine depleting drugs).
- No products indexed under this heading.

Reserpine (Possible additive effects and production of hypotension and/or bradycardia when beta blocker is used concurrently with catecholamine depleting drugs). Products include:
- Diupres Tablets ... 1691
- Hydropres Tablets ... 1718
- Ser-Ap-Es Tablets ... 867

Sotalol Hydrochloride (Co-administration with oral beta blockers may result in additive effects on systemic beta blockade). Products include:
- Betapace Tablets ... 637

Timolol Hemihydrate (Co-administration with oral beta blockers may result in additive effects on systemic beta blockade). Products include:
- Betimol 0.25%, 0.5% ... ◉ 259

Timolol Maleate (Co-administration with oral beta blockers may result in additive effects on systemic beta blockade). Products include:
- Blocadren Tablets ... 1654
- Timolide Tablets ... 1791
- Timoptic in Ocudose ... 1796
- Timoptic Sterile Ophthalmic Solution ... 1794
- Timoptic-XE ... 1798

Tranylcypromine Sulfate (Exercise caution when using concurrently with adrenergic psychotropic drugs). Products include:
- Parnate Tablets ... 2679

Verapamil Hydrochloride (Co-administration with oral or intravenous calcium channel antagonists may result in possible precipitation of left ventricular failure, and hypotension). Products include:
- Calan SR Caplets ... 2571
- Calan Tablets ... 2568
- Covera-HS Tablets ... 2573
- Isoptin Injectable ... 1391
- Isoptin Oral Tablets ... 1393
- Isoptin SR Tablets ... 1395
- Verelan Capsules ... 1455

BABY ORAJEL TEETHING PAIN MEDICINE
(Benzocaine) ... ▣ 667
None cited in PDR database.

BABY ORAJEL TOOTH & GUM CLEANSER
(Simethicone) ... ▣ 668
None cited in PDR database.

ORAJEL COVERMED TINTED COLD SORE MEDICINE
(Allantoin, Dyclonine Hydrochloride) ... ▣ 668
None cited in PDR database.

ORAJEL MAXIMUM STRENGTH TOOTHACHE MEDICATION
(Benzocaine) ... ▣ 668
None cited in PDR database.

ORAJEL MOUTH-AID FOR CANKER AND COLD SORES
(Benzocaine, Benzalkonium Chloride, Zinc Chloride) ... ▣ 668
None cited in PDR database.

ORAJEL PERIOSEPTIC OXYGENATING LIQUID
(Carbamide Peroxide) ... ▣ 669
None cited in PDR database.

ORAMORPH SR (MORPHINE SULFATE SUSTAINED RELEASE TABLETS)
(Morphine Sulfate) ... 2359
May interact with central nervous system depressants, hypnotics and sedatives, antihistamines, psychotropics, and certain other agents. Compounds in these categories include:

Acrivastine (CNS depressant ef-

(▣ Described in PDR For Nonprescription Drugs) (◉ Described in PDR For Ophthalmology)

779 Interactions Index Oramorph SR

fects are potentiated). Products include:

Semprex-D Capsules ... 1620

Alfentanil Hydrochloride (CNS depressant effects are potentiated). Products include:

Alfenta Injection ... 1334

Alprazolam (CNS depressant effects are potentiated). Products include:

Xanax Tablets ... 2115

Amitriptyline Hydrochloride (CNS depressant effects are potentiated). Products include:

Elavil ... 2945
Etrafon ... 2495
Limbitrol ... 2333
Triavil Tablets ... 1800

Amoxapine (CNS depressant effects are potentiated). Products include:

Asendin Tablets ... 1419

Aprobarbital (CNS depressant effects are potentiated).

No products indexed under this heading.

Astemizole (CNS depressant effects are potentiated). Products include:

Hismanal Tablets ... 1341

Azatadine Maleate (CNS depressant effects are potentiated). Products include:

Trinalin Repetabs Tablets ... 1373

Bromodiphenhydramine Hydrochloride (CNS depressant effects are potentiated).

No products indexed under this heading.

Brompheniramine Maleate (CNS depressant effects are potentiated). Products include:

Alka-Seltzer Plus Sinus Medicine ... 611
Bromfed Capsules (Extended-Release) ... 1832
Bromfed Syrup ... 712
Bromfed Tablets ... 1832
Bromfed-DM Cough Syrup ... 1832
Bromfed-PD Capsules (Extended-Release) ... 1832
Dimetane-DC Cough Syrup ... 2232
Dimetane-DX Cough Syrup ... 2233
Dimetapp Allergy Dye-Free Elixir ... 838
Dimetapp Allergy Sinus Caplets ... 838
Dimetapp Cold & Allergy Chewable Tablets ... 838
Dimetapp Cold & Cough Liqui-Gels ... 839
Dimetapp Cold & Fever Suspension ... 839
Dimetapp DM Elixir ... 840
Dimetapp Elixir ... 840
Dimetapp Extentabs ... 841
Dimetapp Tablets/Liqui-Gels ... 841
Rondec Chewable Tablets ... 974
Vicks DayQuil Allergy Relief 12-Hour Extended Release Tablets ... 733
Vicks DayQuil Allergy Relief 4-Hour Tablets ... 733

Buprenorphine (CNS depressant effects are potentiated; may alter analgesic effect or may precipitate withdrawal symptoms). Products include:

Buprenex Injectable ... 2170

Buspirone Hydrochloride (CNS depressant effects are potentiated). Products include:

BuSpar Tablets ... 738

Butabarbital (CNS depressant effects are potentiated).

No products indexed under this heading.

Butalbital (CNS depressant effects are potentiated). Products include:

Axocet Capsules ... 2469
Esgic-plus Capsules ... 1012
Esgic-plus Tablets ... 1012
Fioricet Tablets ... 2386
Fioricet with Codeine Capsules ... 2387
Fiorinal Capsules ... 2388
Fiorinal with Codeine Capsules ... 2390
Fiorinal Tablets ... 2388
Phrenilin ... 790
Sedapap Tablets 50 mg/650 mg ... 1826

Butorphanol Tartrate (May alter analgesic effect or may precipitate withdrawal symptoms). Products include:

Stadol ... 779

Cetirizine Hydrochloride (CNS depressant effects are potentiated). Products include:

Zyrtec Tablets ... 2053

Chlordiazepoxide (CNS depressant effects are potentiated). Products include:

Limbitrol ... 2333

Chlordiazepoxide Hydrochloride (CNS depressant effects are potentiated). Products include:

Librax Capsules ... 2330
Librium Capsules ... 2331
Librium Injectable ... 2332

Chlorpheniramine Maleate (CNS depressant effects are potentiated). Products include:

Alka-Seltzer Plus Cold Medicine ... 611
Alka-Seltzer Plus Cold Medicine Liqui-Gels ... 612
Alka-Seltzer Plus Cold & Cough Medicine ... 611
Alka-Seltzer Plus Cold & Cough Medicine Liqui-Gels ... 612
Alka-Seltzer Plus Flu & Body Aches Effervescent Tablets ... 612
Allerest Maximum Strength ... 649
Allerest Sinus Pain Formula ... 649
Ana-Kit Anaphylaxis Emergency Treatment Kit ... 611
Atrohist Pediatric Capsules ... 1603
Atrohist Plus Tablets ... 1605
BC Cold Powder Multi-Symptom Formula (Cold-Sinus-Allergy) ... 631
Cerose DM ... 853
Cheracol Plus Head Cold/Cough Formula ... 741
Children's TYLENOL Cold Multi-Symptom Chewable Tablets and Liquid ... 1559
Children's TYLENOL Cold Plus Cough Multi Symptom Chewable Tablets and Liquid ... 1560
Children's TYLENOL Flu Suspension Liquid ... 1560
Children's Vicks DayQuil Allergy Relief ... 730
Children's Vicks NyQuil Cold/Cough Relief ... 731
Chlor-Trimeton Allergy Decongestant Tablets ... 759
Chlor-Trimeton Allergy Tablets ... 758
Allergy-Sinus Comtrex Multi-Symptom Allergy-Sinus Formula Tablets and Caplets ... 639
Comtrex Multi-Symptom ... 638
Contac Continuous Action Nasal Decongestant/Antihistamine 12 Hour Capsules ... 773
Contac Maximum Strength Continuous Action Decongestant/Antihistamine 12 Hour Caplets ... 772
Contac Severe Cold and Flu Formula Caplets ... 773
Coricidin Cold + Flu Tablets ... 760
Coricidin Cough + Cold Tablets ... 760
Coricidin 'D' Decongestant Tablets ... 760
D.A. II Tablets ... 972
D.A. Chewable Tablets ... 970
Dura-Tap/PD Capsules ... 970
Dura-Vent/DA Tablets ... 972
Efidac 24 Chlorpheniramine ... 655
Extendryl ... 1003
Fedahist Gyrocaps ... 2545
Hycomine Compound Tablets ... 948
Kronofed-A ... 994
Nolamine Timed-Release Tablets ... 790
Novahistine Elixir ... 782
Ornade Spansule Capsules ... 2678
PediaCare Cough-Cold Chewable Tablets and Liquid ... 1569
PediaCare NightRest Cough-Cold Liquid ... 1569
Pediatric Vicks 44m Cough & Cold Relief ... 737
Pyrroxate Caplets ... 742
Ryna ... 804
Sinarest ... 663
Sine-Off Sinus Medicine ... 784
Singlet Tablets ... 785
Sinulin Tablets ... 792
Sinutab Sinus Allergy Medication, Maximum Strength Tablets and Caplets ... 823
Sudafed Cold & Allergy Tablets ... 826
Teldrin 12 Hour Antihistamine/Nasal Decongestant Allergy Relief Capsules ... 786
TheraFlu Flu and Cold Medicine ... 750
Theraflu Maximum Strength Flu and Cold Medicine For Sore Throat ... 751
TheraFlu Flu, Cold and Cough Medicine ... 750
TheraFlu Maximum Strength Nighttime Flu, Cold & Cough Medicine ... 751
Triaminic Night Time ... 754
Triaminic Syrup ... 755
Triaminic Triaminicol Cold & Cough ... 756
Triaminicin Tablets ... 756
Tussend ... 1830
TYLENOL Allergy Sinus, Maximum Strength Caplets and Gelcaps ... 1571
TYLENOL Cold Medication, Multi-Symptom Formula Tablets and Caplets ... 1572
TYLENOL Cold Medication, Multi-Symptom Hot Liquid Packets ... 1572
Vicks 44 LiquiCaps Cough, Cold & Flu Relief ... 728
Vicks 44M Cough, Cold & Flu Relief ... 729

Chlorpheniramine Polistirex (CNS depressant effects are potentiated). Products include:

Tussionex Pennkinetic Extended-Release Suspension ... 1624

Chlorpheniramine Tannate (CNS depressant effects are potentiated). Products include:

Atrohist Pediatric Suspension ... 1604
Atrohist Pediatric Suspension Dye-Free ... 1604
Rynatan ... 2781
Rynatuss ... 2782

Chlorpromazine (CNS depressant effects are potentiated). Products include:

Thorazine Suppositories ... 2701

Chlorprothixene (CNS depressant effects are potentiated).

No products indexed under this heading.

Chlorprothixene Hydrochloride (CNS depressant effects are potentiated).

No products indexed under this heading.

Chlorprothixene Lactate (CNS depressant effects are potentiated).

No products indexed under this heading.

Clemastine Fumarate (CNS depressant effects are potentiated). Products include:

Tavist Syrup ... 2426
Tavist Tablets ... 2427
Tavist-1 12 Hour Relief Tablets ... 749
Tavist-D 12 Hour Relief Tablets ... 750

Clorazepate Dipotassium (CNS depressant effects are potentiated). Products include:

Tranxene ... 459

Clozapine (CNS depressant effects are potentiated). Products include:

Clozaril Tablets ... 2377

Codeine Phosphate (CNS depressant effects are potentiated). Products include:

Brontex ... 2130
Dimetane-DC Cough Syrup ... 2232
Fioricet with Codeine Capsules ... 2387
Fiorinal with Codeine Capsules ... 2390
Nucofed ... 2225
Phenergan with Codeine ... 2883
Phenergan VC with Codeine ... 2888
Robitussin A-C Syrup ... 2248
Robitussin-DAC Syrup ... 2249
Ryna ... 804
Soma Compound w/Codeine Tablets ... 2784
Tylenol with Codeine ... 1592

Cyproheptadine Hydrochloride (CNS depressant effects are potentiated). Products include:

Periactin ... 1767

Desflurane (CNS depressant effects are potentiated). Products include:

Suprane (desflurane, USP) ... 1865

Desipramine Hydrochloride (CNS depressant effects are potentiated). Products include:

Norpramin Tablets ... 1273

Dexchlorpheniramine Maleate (CNS depressant effects are potentiated).

No products indexed under this heading.

Dezocine (CNS depressant effects are potentiated). Products include:

Dalgan Injection ... 529

Diazepam (CNS depressant effects are potentiated). Products include:

Dizac (diazepam injectable emulsion) CIV ... 1862
Valium Injectable ... 2336
Valium Tablets ... 2335

Diphenhydramine Citrate (CNS depressant effects are potentiated). Products include:

Excedrin P.M. Analgesic/Sleeping Aid Tablets, Caplets, Liquigels ... 735

Diphenhydramine Hydrochloride (CNS depressant effects are potentiated). Products include:

Actifed Allergy Daytime/Nighttime Caplets ... 808
Actifed Sinus Daytime/Nighttime Tablets and Caplets ... 809
Extra Strength Bayer PM Aspirin Plus Sleep Aid ... 617
Benadryl Allergy Chewables ... 811
Benadryl Allergy/Cold Tablets ... 811
Benadryl Allergy Decongestant Liquid Medication ... 812
Benadryl Allergy Decongestant Tablets ... 812
Benadryl Allergy Liquid Medication ... 813
Benadryl Allergy ... 811
Benadryl Allergy Sinus Headache Caplets ... 813
Benadryl Dye-Free Allergy Liquigel Softgels ... 813
Benadryl Dye-Free Allergy Liquid Medication ... 814
Benadryl Itch Relief Stick Extra Strength ... 814
Benadryl Cream ... 814
Benadryl Gel ... 815
Benadryl Spray ... 815
Benadryl Injection ... 1955
Contac Day & Night Cold/Flu Night Caplets ... 772
Contac Night Allergy/Sinus Caplets ... 771
Extra Strength Doan's P.M. ... 653
Excedrin P.M. Analgesic/Sleeping Aid Tablets, Caplets, Liquigels ... 643
Nytol QuickCaps Caplets ... 632
Sleepinal Night-time Sleep Aid Capsules and Softgels ... 798
TYLENOL Allergy Sinus NightTime, Maximum Strength Caplets ... 1571
TYLENOL Flu NightTime, Maximum Strength Gelcaps ... 1575
TYLENOL Flu NightTime, Maximum Strength Hot Medication Packets ... 1575
TYLENOL PM Pain Reliever/Sleep Aid, Extra Strength Gelcaps, Caplets, Geltabs ... 1576
TYLENOL Severe Allergy Medication Caplets ... 1571
Maximum Strength Unisom Sleepgels ... 1990
Unisom With Pain Relief-Nighttime Sleep Aid and Pain Reliever ... 1991

Doxepin Hydrochloride (CNS depressant effects are potentiated). Products include:

Adapin Capsules ... 1542
Sinequan ... 2028
Zonalon Cream ... 1042

IMPORTANT NOTE: Always consult each drug listing in the patient's regimen for possible interactions.

Droperidol (CNS depressant effects are potentiated). Products include:
   Inapsine Injection 462

Enflurane (CNS depressant effects are potentiated).
   No products indexed under this heading.

Estazolam (CNS depressant effects are potentiated). Products include:
   ProSom Tablets 457

Ethchlorvynol (CNS depressant effects are potentiated). Products include:
   Placidyl Capsules 456

Ethinamate (CNS depressant effects are potentiated).
   No products indexed under this heading.

Fentanyl (CNS depressant effects are potentiated). Products include:
   Duragesic Transdermal System 1336

Fentanyl Citrate (CNS depressant effects are potentiated). Products include:
   Sublimaze Injection 463

Fluphenazine Decanoate (CNS depressant effects are potentiated). Products include:
   Prolixin Decanoate 510

Fluphenazine Enanthate (CNS depressant effects are potentiated). Products include:
   Prolixin Enanthate 510

Fluphenazine Hydrochloride (CNS depressant effects are potentiated). Products include:
   Prolixin 510

Flurazepam Hydrochloride (CNS depressant effects are potentiated). Products include:
   Dalmane Capsules 2329

Glutethimide (CNS depressant effects are potentiated).
   No products indexed under this heading.

Haloperidol (CNS depressant effects are potentiated). Products include:
   Haldol Injection, Tablets and Concentrate 1585

Haloperidol Decanoate (CNS depressant effects are potentiated). Products include:
   Haldol Decanoate 1587

Hydrocodone Bitartrate (CNS depressant effects are potentiated). Products include:
   Codiclear DH Syrup 808
   Duratuss HD Elixir 2750
   Histussin D Liquid 670
   Hycodan Tablets and Syrup 946
   Hycomine Compound Tablets 948
   Hycomine 947
   Hycotuss Expectorant Syrup 950
   Hydrocet Capsules 787
   Lorcet 10/650 Tablets 1016
   Lortab 2751
   Tussend 1830
   Tussend Expectorant 1831
   Vicodin Tablets 1404
   Vicodin ES Tablets 1405
   Vicodin HP Tablets 1403
   Vicodin Tuss Expectorant 1406
   Zydone Capsules 967

Hydrocodone Polistirex (CNS depressant effects are potentiated). Products include:
   Tussionex Pennkinetic Extended-Release Suspension 1624

Hydroxyzine Hydrochloride (CNS depressant effects are potentiated). Products include:
   Atarax Tablets & Syrup 1992
   Marax Tablets & DF Syrup 2015
   Vistaril Intramuscular Solution 2042

Imipramine Hydrochloride (CNS depressant effects are potentiated). Products include:
   Tofranil Ampuls 873
   Tofranil Tablets 875

Imipramine Pamoate (CNS depressant effects are potentiated). Products include:
   Tofranil-PM Capsules 876

Isocarboxazid (CNS depressant effects are potentiated).
   No products indexed under this heading.

Isoflurane (CNS depressant effects are potentiated).
   No products indexed under this heading.

Ketamine Hydrochloride (CNS depressant effects are potentiated).
   No products indexed under this heading.

Levomethadyl Acetate Hydrochloride (CNS depressant effects are potentiated). Products include:
   Orlaam Oral Solution 2361

Levorphanol Tartrate (CNS depressant effects are potentiated). Products include:
   Levo-Dromoran 2297

Lithium Carbonate (CNS depressant effects are potentiated). Products include:
   Eskalith 2658
   Lithium Carbonate Capsules & Tablets 2352
   Lithonate/Lithotabs/Lithobid 2721

Lithium Citrate (CNS depressant effects are potentiated).
   No products indexed under this heading.

Loratadine (CNS depressant effects are potentiated). Products include:
   Claritin Tablets 2485
   Claritin-D Tablets 2487

Lorazepam (CNS depressant effects are potentiated). Products include:
   Ativan Injection 2805
   Ativan Tablets 2807

Loxapine Hydrochloride (CNS depressant effects are potentiated). Products include:
   Loxitane 1426

Loxapine Succinate (CNS depressant effects are potentiated). Products include:
   Loxitane Capsules 1426

Maprotiline Hydrochloride (CNS depressant effects are potentiated). Products include:
   Ludiomil Tablets 861

Meperidine Hydrochloride (CNS depressant effects are potentiated). Products include:
   Demerol 2438
   Mepergan Injection 2859

Mephobarbital (CNS depressant effects are potentiated). Products include:
   Mebaral Tablets 2452

Meprobamate (CNS depressant effects are potentiated). Products include:
   Miltown Tablets 2780
   PMB 200 and PMB 400 2890

Mesoridazine Besylate (CNS depressant effects are potentiated). Products include:
   Serentil 689

Methadone Hydrochloride (CNS depressant effects are potentiated). Products include:
   Methadone Hydrochloride Oral Concentrate 2356
   Methadone Hydrochloride Oral Solution & Tablets 2357

Methdilazine Hydrochloride (CNS depressant effects are potentiated).
   No products indexed under this heading.

Methohexital Sodium (CNS depressant effects are potentiated).
   No products indexed under this heading.

Methotrimeprazine (CNS depressant effects are potentiated). Products include:
   Levoprome 1321

Methoxyflurane (CNS depressant effects are potentiated).
   No products indexed under this heading.

Midazolam Hydrochloride (CNS depressant effects are potentiated). Products include:
   Versed Injection 2324

Molindone Hydrochloride (CNS depressant effects are potentiated). Products include:
   Moban Tablets and Concentrate 1036

Nalbuphine Hydrochloride (May alter analgesic effect or may precipitate withdrawal symptoms). Products include:
   Nubain Injection 952

Nortriptyline Hydrochloride (CNS depressant effects are potentiated). Products include:
   Pamelor 2409

Opium Alkaloids (CNS depressant effects are potentiated).
   No products indexed under this heading.

Oxazepam (CNS depressant effects are potentiated). Products include:
   Serax Capsules 2916
   Serax Tablets 2916

Oxycodone Hydrochloride (CNS depressant effects are potentiated). Products include:
   OxyContin Tablets 2163
   OxyIR Capsules 2167
   Percocet Tablets 955
   Percodan Tablets 955
   Percodan-Demi Tablets 956
   Roxicodone Tablets, Oral Solution & Intensol (Oxycodone) 2366
   Tylox Capsules 1593

Pentazocine Hydrochloride (May alter analgesic effect or may precipitate withdrawal symptoms). Products include:
   Talacen Caplets 2464
   Talwin Compound 2466
   Talwin Nx Tablets 2467

Pentazocine Lactate (May alter analgesic effect or may precipitate withdrawal symptoms). Products include:
   Talwin Injection 2465

Pentobarbital Sodium (CNS depressant effects are potentiated). Products include:
   Nembutal Sodium Capsules 440
   Nembutal Sodium Solution 442
   Nembutal Sodium Suppositories 444

Perphenazine (CNS depressant effects are potentiated). Products include:
   Etrafon 2495
   Triavil Tablets 1800
   Trilafon 2532

Phenelzine Sulfate (CNS depressant effects are potentiated). Products include:
   Nardil 1977

Phenobarbital (CNS depressant effects are potentiated). Products include:
   Arco-Lase Plus Tablets 513
   Bellergal-S Tablets 2375
   Donnatal 2234
   Donnatal Extentabs 2234
   Donnatal Tablets 2234
   Phenobarbital Elixir and Tablets 1523
   Quadrinal Tablets 1398

Prazepam (CNS depressant effects are potentiated).
   No products indexed under this heading.

Prochlorperazine (CNS depressant effects are potentiated). Products include:
   Compazine 2644

Promethazine Hydrochloride (CNS depressant effects are potentiated). Products include:
   Mepergan Injection 2859
   Phenergan with Codeine 2883
   Phenergan with Dextromethorphan ... 2885
   Phenergan Injection 2880
   Phenergan Suppositories 2882
   Phenergan Syrup 2881
   Phenergan Tablets 2882
   Phenergan VC 2886
   Phenergan VC with Codeine 2888

Propofol (CNS depressant effects are potentiated). Products include:
   Diprivan Injectable Emulsion 2939

Propoxyphene Hydrochloride (CNS depressant effects are potentiated). Products include:
   Darvon 1475
   Wygesic Tablets 2930

Propoxyphene Napsylate (CNS depressant effects are potentiated). Products include:
   Darvon-N/Darvocet-N 1473

Protriptyline Hydrochloride (CNS depressant effects are potentiated). Products include:
   Vivactil Tablets 1820

Pyrilamine Maleate (CNS depressant effects are potentiated). Products include:
   4-Way Fast Acting Nasal Spray (regular & mentholated) .... ■ 644
   Maximum Strength Multi-Symptom Formula Midol .... ■ 621
   PMS Multi-Symptom Formula Midol .... ■ 622

Pyrilamine Tannate (CNS depressant effects are potentiated). Products include:
   Atrohist Pediatric Suspension 1604
   Atrohist Pediatric Suspension Dye-Free 1604
   Rynatan 2781

Quazepam (CNS depressant effects are potentiated). Products include:
   Doral Tablets 2773

Risperidone (CNS depressant effects are potentiated). Products include:
   Risperdal Tablets 1348

Secobarbital Sodium (CNS depressant effects are potentiated). Products include:
   Seconal Sodium Pulvules 1529

Sevoflurane (CNS depressant effects are potentiated).
   No products indexed under this heading.

Sufentanil Citrate (CNS depressant effects are potentiated). Products include:
   Sufenta Injection 1355

Temazepam (CNS depressant effects are potentiated). Products include:
   Restoril Capsules 2413

Terfenadine (CNS depressant effects are potentiated). Products include:
   Seldane Tablets 1284
   Seldane-D Extended-Release Tablets 1286

Thiamylal Sodium (CNS depressant effects are potentiated).
   No products indexed under this heading.

(■ Described in PDR For Nonprescription Drugs)   (⊙ Described in PDR For Ophthalmology)

Interactions Index — Orap Tablets

Thioridazine Hydrochloride (CNS depressant effects are potentiated). Products include:
- Mellaril 2398

Thiothixene (CNS depressant effects are potentiated). Products include:
- Navane Capsules and Concentrate ... 2018
- Navane Intramuscular 2019

Tranylcypromine Sulfate (CNS depressant effects are potentiated). Products include:
- Parnate Tablets 2679

Triazolam (CNS depressant effects are potentiated). Products include:
- Halcion Tablets 2093

Trifluoperazine Hydrochloride (CNS depressant effects are potentiated). Products include:
- Stelazine 2692

Trimeprazine Tartrate (CNS depressant effects are potentiated).
No products indexed under this heading.

Trimipramine Maleate (CNS depressant effects are potentiated). Products include:
- Surmontil Capsules 2917

Tripelennamine Hydrochloride (CNS depressant effects are potentiated). Products include:
- PBZ Tablets 863
- PBZ-SR Tablets 862

Triprolidine Hydrochloride (CNS depressant effects are potentiated). Products include:
- Actifed Cold & Allergy Tablets 807
- Actifed Cold & Sinus Caplets and Tablets 808

Zolpidem Tartrate (CNS depressant effects are potentiated). Products include:
- Ambien Tablets 2559

Food Interactions
Alcohol (CNS depressant effects are potentiated).

ORAP TABLETS
(Pimozide) 1037
May interact with phenothiazines, tricyclic antidepressants, antiarrhythmics, hypnotics and sedatives, narcotic analgesics, tranquilizers, central nervous system depressants, macrolide antibiotics, and certain other agents. Compounds in these categories include:

Acebutolol Hydrochloride (Additive effect on QT prolongation). Products include:
- Sectral Capsules 2914

Adenosine (Additive effect on QT prolongation). Products include:
- Adenocard Injection 1021
- Adenoscan 1022

Alfentanil Hydrochloride (CNS depression potentiated). Products include:
- Alfenta Injection 1334

Alprazolam (CNS depression potentiated). Products include:
- Xanax Tablets 2115

Amiodarone Hydrochloride (Additive effect on QT prolongation). Products include:
- Cordarone Intravenous 2821
- Cordarone Tablets 2818

Amitriptyline Hydrochloride (Additive effect on QT prolongation; CNS depression potentiated). Products include:
- Elavil 2945
- Etrafon 2495
- Limbitrol 2333
- Triavil Tablets 1800

Amoxapine (Additive effect on QT prolongation; CNS depression potentiated). Products include:
- Asendin Tablets 1419

Aprobarbital (CNS depression potentiated).
No products indexed under this heading.

Azithromycin (Ventricular arrhythmias have been rarely associated with the use of macrolide antibiotics in patients with prolonged QT intervals; two sudden deaths have been reported with clarithromycin co-administration; combined therapy with macrolide antibiotics is contraindicated). Products include:
- Zithromax 2043
- Zithromax Tablets 2046

Bretylium Tosylate (Additive effect on QT prolongation).
No products indexed under this heading.

Buprenorphine (CNS depression potentiated). Products include:
- Buprenex Injectable 2170

Buspirone Hydrochloride (CNS depression potentiated). Products include:
- BuSpar Tablets 738

Butabarbital (CNS depression potentiated).
No products indexed under this heading.

Butalbital (CNS depression potentiated). Products include:
- Axocet Capsules 2469
- Esgic-plus Capsules 1012
- Esgic-plus Tablets 1012
- Fioricet Tablets 2386
- Fioricet with Codeine Capsules 2387
- Fiorinal Capsules 2388
- Fiorinal with Codeine Capsules 2390
- Fiorinal Tablets 2388
- Phrenilin 790
- Sedapap Tablets 50 mg/650 mg .. 1826

Chlordiazepoxide (CNS depression potentiated). Products include:
- Limbitrol 2333

Chlordiazepoxide Hydrochloride (CNS depression potentiated). Products include:
- Librax Capsules 2330
- Librium Capsules 2331
- Librium Injectable 2332

Chlorpromazine (Additive effect on QT prolongation; CNS depression potentiated). Products include:
- Thorazine Suppositories 2701

Chlorpromazine Hydrochloride (Additive effect on QT prolongation; CNS depression potentiated). Products include:
- Thorazine 2701

Chlorprothixene (CNS depression potentiated).
No products indexed under this heading.

Chlorprothixene Hydrochloride (CNS depression potentiated).
No products indexed under this heading.

Chlorprothixene Lactate (CNS depression potentiated).
No products indexed under this heading.

Clarithromycin (Ventricular arrhythmias have been rarely associated with the use of macrolide antibiotics in patients with prolonged QT intervals; two sudden deaths have been reported with clarithromycin co-administration; combined therapy with macrolide antibiotics is contraindicated). Products include:
- Biaxin 406

Clomipramine Hydrochloride (Additive effect on QT prolongation; CNS depression potentiated). Products include:
- Anafranil Capsules 819

Clorazepate Dipotassium (CNS depression potentiated). Products include:
- Tranxene 459

Clozapine (CNS depression potentiated). Products include:
- Clozaril Tablets 2377

Codeine Phosphate (CNS depression potentiated). Products include:
- Brontex 2130
- Dimetane-DC Cough Syrup 2232
- Fioricet with Codeine Capsules 2387
- Fiorinal with Codeine Capsules 2390
- Nucofed 2225
- Phenergan with Codeine 2883
- Phenergan VC with Codeine 2888
- Robitussin A-C Syrup 2248
- Robitussin-DAC Syrup 2249
- Ryna 804
- Soma Compound w/Codeine Tablets 2784
- Tylenol with Codeine 1592

Desflurane (CNS depression potentiated). Products include:
- Suprane (desflurane, USP) 1865

Desipramine Hydrochloride (Additive effect on QT prolongation; CNS depression potentiated). Products include:
- Norpramin Tablets 1273

Dezocine (CNS depression potentiated). Products include:
- Dalgan Injection 529

Diazepam (CNS depression potentiated). Products include:
- Dizac (diazepam injectable emulsion) CIV 1862
- Valium Injectable 2336
- Valium Tablets 2335

Dirithromycin (Ventricular arrhythmias have been rarely associated with the use of macrolide antibiotics in patients with prolonged QT intervals; two sudden deaths have been reported with clarithromycin co-administration; combined therapy with macrolide antibiotics is contraindicated). Products include:
- Dynabac 668

Disopyramide Phosphate (Additive effect on QT prolongation). Products include:
- Norpace 2596

Doxepin Hydrochloride (Additive effect on QT prolongation; CNS depression potentiated). Products include:
- Adapin Capsules 1542
- Sinequan 2028
- Zonalon Cream 1042

Droperidol (CNS depression potentiated). Products include:
- Inapsine Injection 462

Enflurane (CNS depression potentiated).
No products indexed under this heading.

Erythromycin (Ventricular arrhythmias have been rarely associated with the use of macrolide antibiotics in patients with prolonged QT intervals; two sudden deaths have been reported with clarithromycin co-administration; combined therapy with macrolide antibiotics is contraindicated). Products include:
- A/T/S 2% Acne Topical Gel 1244
- A/T/S 2% Acne Topical Solution ... 1244
- Benzamycin Topical Gel 919
- E-Mycin Tablets 1388
- Emgel 2% Topical Gel 1081
- ERYC 1972
- Erycette (erythromycin 2%) Topical Solution 1943
- Ery-Tab Tablets 426
- Erythromycin Base Filmtab 430
- Erythromycin Delayed-Release Capsules, USP 431
- Ilotycin Ophthalmic Ointment 928
- PCE Dispertab Tablets 453
- T-Stat 2.0% Topical Solution and Pads 2797
- THERAMYCIN Z 2% Solution 1629

Erythromycin Estolate (Ventricular arrhythmias have been rarely associated with the use of macrolide antibiotics in patients with prolonged QT intervals; two sudden deaths have been reported with clarithromycin co-administration; combined therapy with macrolide antibiotics is contraindicated). Products include:
- Ilosone 927

Erythromycin Ethylsuccinate (Ventricular arrhythmias have been rarely associated with the use of macrolide antibiotics in patients with prolonged QT intervals; two sudden deaths have been reported with clarithromycin co-administration; combined therapy with macrolide antibiotics is contraindicated). Products include:
- E.E.S. 427
- EryPed 425
- Pediazole Suspension 2340

Erythromycin Gluceptate (Ventricular arrhythmias have been rarely associated with the use of macrolide antibiotics in patients with prolonged QT intervals; two sudden deaths have been reported with clarithromycin co-administration; combined therapy with macrolide antibiotics is contraindicated). Products include:
- Ilotycin Gluceptate, IV, Vials 929

Erythromycin Stearate (Ventricular arrhythmias have been rarely associated with the use of macrolide antibiotics in patients with prolonged QT intervals; two sudden deaths have been reported with clarithromycin co-administration; combined therapy with macrolide antibiotics is contraindicated). Products include:
- Erythrocin Stearate Filmtab 429

Estazolam (CNS depression potentiated). Products include:
- ProSom Tablets 457

Ethchlorvynol (CNS depression potentiated). Products include:
- Placidyl Capsules 456

Ethinamate (CNS depression potentiated).
No products indexed under this heading.

Fentanyl (CNS depression potentiated). Products include:
- Duragesic Transdermal System 1336

Fentanyl Citrate (CNS depression potentiated). Products include:
- Sublimaze Injection 463

Flecainide Acetate (Additive effect on QT prolongation). Products include:
- Tambocor Tablets 1555

Fluphenazine Decanoate (Additive effect on QT prolongation; CNS depression potentiated). Products include:
- Prolixin Decanoate 510

Fluphenazine Enanthate (Additive effect on QT prolongation; CNS depression potentiated). Products include:
- Prolixin Enanthate 510

Fluphenazine Hydrochloride (Additive effect on QT prolongation; CNS depression potentiated). Products include:
- Prolixin 510

IMPORTANT NOTE: Always consult each drug listing in the patient's regimen for possible interactions.

Orap Tablets — Interactions Index

Flurazepam Hydrochloride (CNS depression potentiated). Products include:
- Dalmane Capsules 2329

Glutethimide (CNS depression potentiated).
No products indexed under this heading.

Haloperidol (CNS depression potentiated). Products include:
- Haldol Injection, Tablets and Concentrate 1585

Haloperidol Decanoate (CNS depression potentiated). Products include:
- Haldol Decanoate 1587

Hydrocodone Bitartrate (CNS depression potentiated). Products include:
- Codiclear DH Syrup 808
- Duratuss HD Elixir 2750
- Histussin D Liquid 670
- Hycodan Tablets and Syrup 946
- Hycomine Compound Tablets 948
- Hycomine 947
- Hycotuss Expectorant Syrup 950
- Hydrocet Capsules 787
- Lorcet 10/650 Tablets 1016
- Lortab 2751
- Tussend 1830
- Tussend Expectorant 1831
- Vicodin Tablets 1404
- Vicodin ES Tablets 1405
- Vicodin HP Tablets 1403
- Vicodin Tuss Expectorant 1406
- Zydone Capsules 967

Hydrocodone Polistirex (CNS depression potentiated). Products include:
- Tussionex Pennkinetic Extended-Release Suspension 1624

Hydromorphone Hydrochloride (CNS depression potentiated). Products include:
- Dilaudid Ampules 1382
- Dilaudid Cough Syrup 1383
- Dilaudid-HP Injection 1384
- Dilaudid-HP Lyophilized Powder 250 mg 1384
- Dilaudid 1382
- Dilaudid Oral Liquid 1386
- Dilaudid 1382
- Dilaudid Tablets - 8 mg 1386

Hydroxyzine Hydrochloride (CNS depression potentiated). Products include:
- Atarax Tablets & Syrup 1992
- Marax Tablets & DF Syrup 2015
- Vistaril Intramuscular Solution 2042

Imipramine Hydrochloride (Additive effect on QT prolongation; CNS depression potentiated). Products include:
- Tofranil Ampuls 873
- Tofranil Tablets 875

Imipramine Pamoate (Additive effect on QT prolongation; CNS depression potentiated). Products include:
- Tofranil-PM Capsules 876

Isoflurane (CNS depression potentiated).
No products indexed under this heading.

Ketamine Hydrochloride (CNS depression potentiated).
No products indexed under this heading.

Levomethadyl Acetate Hydrochloride (CNS depression potentiated). Products include:
- Orlaam Oral Solution 2361

Levorphanol Tartrate (CNS depression potentiated). Products include:
- Levo-Dromoran 2297

Lidocaine Hydrochloride (Additive effect on QT prolongation). Products include:
- Decadron Phosphate with Xylocaine Injection, Sterile 1683
- Unguentine Plus .... ⊞ 712
- Xylocaine Injections 562

Lorazepam (CNS depression potentiated). Products include:
- Ativan Injection 2805
- Ativan Tablets 2807

Loxapine Hydrochloride (CNS depression potentiated). Products include:
- Loxitane 1426

Loxapine Succinate (CNS depression potentiated). Products include:
- Loxitane Capsules 1426

Maprotiline Hydrochloride (Additive effect on QT prolongation; CNS depression potentiated). Products include:
- Ludiomil Tablets 861

Meperidine Hydrochloride (CNS depression potentiated). Products include:
- Demerol 2438
- Mepergan Injection 2859

Mephobarbital (CNS depression potentiated). Products include:
- Mebaral Tablets 2452

Meprobamate (CNS depression potentiated). Products include:
- Miltown Tablets 2780
- PMB 200 and PMB 400 2890

Mesoridazine Besylate (Additive effect on QT prolongation; CNS depression potentiated). Products include:
- Serentil 689

Methadone Hydrochloride (CNS depression potentiated). Products include:
- Methadone Hydrochloride Oral Concentrate 2356
- Methadone Hydrochloride Oral Solution & Tablets 2357

Methohexital Sodium (CNS depression potentiated).
No products indexed under this heading.

Methotrimeprazine (Additive effect on QT prolongation; CNS depression potentiated). Products include:
- Levoprome 1321

Methoxyflurane (CNS depression potentiated).
No products indexed under this heading.

Mexiletine Hydrochloride (Additive effect on QT prolongation). Products include:
- Mexitil Capsules 684

Midazolam Hydrochloride (CNS depression potentiated). Products include:
- Versed Injection 2324

Molindone Hydrochloride (CNS depression potentiated). Products include:
- Moban Tablets and Concentrate 1036

Moricizine Hydrochloride (Additive effect on QT prolongation). Products include:
- Ethmozine Tablets 2217

Morphine Sulfate (CNS depression potentiated). Products include:
- Astramorph/PF Injection, USP (Preservative-Free) 526
- Duramorph Injection 983
- Infumorph 200 and Infumorph 500 Sterile Solutions 985
- Kadian Capsules 2948
- MS Contin Tablets 2149
- MSIR 2152
- Oramorph SR (Morphine Sulfate Sustained Release Tablets) 2359
- RMS Suppositories CII 2766
- Roxanol 2365

Nortriptyline Hydrochloride (Additive effect on QT prolongation; CNS depression potentiated). Products include:
- Pamelor 2409

Opium Alkaloids (CNS depression potentiated).
No products indexed under this heading.

Oxazepam (CNS depression potentiated). Products include:
- Serax Capsules 2916
- Serax Tablets 2916

Oxycodone Hydrochloride (CNS depression potentiated). Products include:
- OxyContin Tablets 2163
- OxyIR Capsules 2167
- Percocet Tablets 955
- Percodan Tablets 955
- Percodan-Demi Tablets 956
- Roxicodone Tablets, Oral Solution & Intensol (Oxycodone) 2366
- Tylox Capsules 1593

Pentobarbital Sodium (CNS depression potentiated). Products include:
- Nembutal Sodium Capsules 440
- Nembutal Sodium Solution 442
- Nembutal Sodium Suppositories 444

Perphenazine (Additive effect on QT prolongation; CNS depression potentiated). Products include:
- Etrafon 2495
- Triavil Tablets 1800
- Trilafon 2532

Phenobarbital (CNS depression potentiated). Products include:
- Arco-Lase Plus Tablets 513
- Bellergal-S Tablets 2375
- Donnatal 2234
- Donnatal Extentabs 2234
- Donnatal Tablets 2234
- Phenobarbital Elixir and Tablets 1523
- Quadrinal Tablets 1398

Prazepam (CNS depression potentiated).
No products indexed under this heading.

Procainamide Hydrochloride (Additive effect on QT prolongation). Products include:
- Procanbid Extended-Release Tablets 1983

Prochlorperazine (Additive effect on QT prolongation; CNS depression potentiated). Products include:
- Compazine 2644

Promethazine Hydrochloride (Additive effect on QT prolongation; CNS depression potentiated). Products include:
- Mepergan Injection 2859
- Phenergan with Codeine 2883
- Phenergan with Dextromethorphan 2885
- Phenergan Injection 2880
- Phenergan Suppositories 2882
- Phenergan Syrup 2881
- Phenergan Tablets 2882
- Phenergan VC 2886
- Phenergan VC with Codeine 2888

Propafenone Hydrochloride (Additive effect on QT prolongation). Products include:
- Rythmol Tablets—150mg, 225mg, 300mg 1399

Propofol (CNS depression potentiated). Products include:
- Diprivan Injectable Emulsion 2939

Propoxyphene Hydrochloride (CNS depression potentiated). Products include:
- Darvon 1475
- Wygesic Tablets 2930

Propoxyphene Napsylate (CNS depression potentiated). Products include:
- Darvon-N/Darvocet-N 1473

Propranolol Hydrochloride (Additive effect on QT prolongation). Products include:
- Inderal 2834
- Inderal LA Long Acting Capsules 2836
- Inderide Tablets 2838
- Inderide LA Long Acting Capsules 2840

Protriptyline Hydrochloride (Additive effect on QT prolongation; CNS depression potentiated). Products include:
- Vivactil Tablets 1820

Quazepam (CNS depression potentiated). Products include:
- Doral Tablets 2773

Quinidine Gluconate (Additive effect on QT prolongation). Products include:
- Quinaglute Dura-Tabs Tablets 644

Quinidine Polygalacturonate (Additive effect on QT prolongation). Products include:
- Cardioquin Tablets 2146

Quinidine Sulfate (Additive effect on QT prolongation). Products include:
- Quinidex Extentabs 2240

Risperidone (CNS depression potentiated). Products include:
- Risperdal Tablets 1348

Secobarbital Sodium (CNS depression potentiated). Products include:
- Seconal Sodium Pulvules 1529

Sevoflurane (CNS depression potentiated).
No products indexed under this heading.

Sotalol Hydrochloride (Additive effect on QT prolongation). Products include:
- Betapace Tablets 637

Sufentanil Citrate (CNS depression potentiated). Products include:
- Sufenta Injection 1355

Temazepam (CNS depression potentiated). Products include:
- Restoril Capsules 2413

Thiamylal Sodium (CNS depression potentiated).
No products indexed under this heading.

Thioridazine Hydrochloride (Additive effect on QT prolongation; CNS depression potentiated). Products include:
- Mellaril 2398

Thiothixene (CNS depression potentiated). Products include:
- Navane Capsules and Concentrate 2018
- Navane Intramuscular 2019

Tocainide Hydrochloride (Additive effect on QT prolongation). Products include:
- Tonocard Tablets 519

Triazolam (CNS depression potentiated). Products include:
- Halcion Tablets 2093

Trifluoperazine Hydrochloride (Additive effect on QT prolongation; CNS depression potentiated). Products include:
- Stelazine 2692

Trimipramine Maleate (Additive effect on QT prolongation; CNS depression potentiated). Products include:
- Surmontil Capsules 2917

Troleandomycin (Ventricular arrhythmias have been rarely associated with the use of macrolide antibiotics in patients with prolonged QT intervals; two sudden deaths have been reported with clarithromycin co-administration; combined therapy with macrolide antibiotics is contraindicated). Products include:
- Tao Capsules 2033

(⊞ Described in PDR For Nonprescription Drugs)   (◉ Described in PDR For Ophthalmology)

Verapamil Hydrochloride (Additive effect on QT prolongation). Products include:
- Calan SR Caplets ... 2571
- Calan Tablets ... 2568
- Covera-HS Tablets ... 2573
- Isoptin Injectable ... 1391
- Isoptin Oral Tablets ... 1393
- Isoptin SR Tablets ... 1395
- Verelan Capsules ... 1455

Zolpidem Tartrate (CNS depression potentiated). Products include:
- Ambien Tablets ... 2559

Food Interactions

Alcohol (CNS depression potentiated).

ORCHID FRESH II PERINEAL/OSTOMY CLEANSER
(Benzethonium Chloride) ... ▣ 647
None cited in PDR database.

ORETIC TABLETS
(Hydrochlorothiazide) ... 450
May interact with antihypertensives, ganglionic blocking agents, peripheral adrenergic blockers, corticosteroids, cardiac glycosides, insulin, barbiturates, narcotic analgesics, and certain other agents. Compounds in these categories include:

Acebutolol Hydrochloride (Additive or potentiative effects). Products include:
- Sectral Capsules ... 2914

ACTH (Potential for intensified electrolyte depletion, particularly hypokalemia).
No products indexed under this heading.

Alfentanil Hydrochloride (May aggravate orthostatic hypotension). Products include:
- Alfenta Injection ... 1334

Amlodipine Besylate (Additive or potentiative effects). Products include:
- Lotrel Capsules ... 858
- Norvasc Tablets ... 2020

Aprobarbital (May aggravate orthostatic hypotension).
No products indexed under this heading.

Atenolol (Additive or potentiative effects). Products include:
- Tenoretic Tablets ... 2963
- Tenormin Tablets and I.V. Injection ... 2965

Benazepril Hydrochloride (Additive or potentiative effects). Products include:
- Lotensin Tablets ... 852
- Lotensin HCT Tablets ... 855
- Lotrel Capsules ... 858

Bendroflumethiazide (Additive or potentiative effects).
No products indexed under this heading.

Betamethasone Acetate (Potential for intensified electrolyte depletion, particularly hypokalemia). Products include:
- Celestone Soluspan Suspension ... 2484

Betamethasone Sodium Phosphate (Potential for intensified electrolyte depletion, particularly hypokalemia). Products include:
- Celestone Soluspan Suspension ... 2484

Betaxolol Hydrochloride (Additive or potentiative effects). Products include:
- Betoptic Ophthalmic Solution ... 465
- Betoptic S Ophthalmic Suspension ... 467
- Kerlone Tablets ... 2588

Bisoprolol Fumarate (Additive or potentiative effects). Products include:
- Zebeta Tablets ... 1457
- Ziac ... 1459

Buprenorphine (May aggravate orthostatic hypotension). Products include:
- Buprenex Injectable ... 2170

Butabarbital (May aggravate orthostatic hypotension).
No products indexed under this heading.

Butalbital (May aggravate orthostatic hypotension). Products include:
- Axocet Capsules ... 2469
- Esgic-plus Capsules ... 1012
- Esgic-plus Capsules ... 1012
- Fioricet Tablets ... 2386
- Fioricet with Codeine Capsules ... 2387
- Fiorinal Capsules ... 2388
- Fiorinal with Codeine Capsules ... 2390
- Fiorinal Tablets ... 2388
- Phrenilin ... 790
- Sedapap Tablets 50 mg/650 mg ... 1826

Captopril (Additive or potentiative effects). Products include:
- Capoten Tablets ... 740
- Capozide Tablets ... 744

Carteolol Hydrochloride (Additive or potentiative effects). Products include:
- Cartrol Tablets ... 413
- Ocupress Ophthalmic Solution, 1% Sterile ... ▣ 297

Chlorothiazide (Additive or potentiative effects). Products include:
- Aldoclor Tablets ... 1638
- Diupres Tablets ... 1691
- Diuril Oral ... 1694

Chlorothiazide Sodium (Additive or potentiative effects). Products include:
- Diuril Sodium Intravenous ... 1693

Chlorthalidone (Additive or potentiative effects). Products include:
- Combipres Tablets ... 682
- Tenoretic Tablets ... 2963
- Thalitone ... 1293

Clonidine (Additive or potentiative effects). Products include:
- Catapres-TTS ... 680

Clonidine Hydrochloride (Additive or potentiative effects). Products include:
- Catapres Tablets ... 679
- Combipres Tablets ... 682

Codeine Phosphate (May aggravate orthostatic hypotension). Products include:
- Brontex ... 2130
- Dimetane-DC Cough Syrup ... 2232
- Fioricet with Codeine Capsules ... 2387
- Fiorinal with Codeine Capsules ... 2390
- Nucofed ... 2225
- Phenergan with Codeine ... 2883
- Phenergan VC with Codeine ... 2888
- Robitussin A-C Syrup ... 2248
- Robitussin-DAC Syrup ... 2249
- Ryna ... ▣ 804
- Soma Compound w/Codeine Tablets ... 2784
- Tylenol with Codeine ... 1592

Cortisone Acetate (Potential for intensified electrolyte depletion, particularly hypokalemia). Products include:
- Cortone Acetate Sterile Suspension ... 1663
- Cortone Acetate Tablets ... 1664

Deserpidine (Potentiation occurs).
No products indexed under this heading.

Deslanoside (Thiazide-induced hypokalemia may exaggerate or sensitize the response of the heart to toxic effects of digitalis).
No products indexed under this heading.

Dexamethasone (Potential for intensified electrolyte depletion, particularly hypokalemia). Products include:
- AK-Trol Ointment & Suspension ... ▣ 205
- Decadron Elixir ... 1676
- Decadron Tablets ... 1678
- Decaspray Topical Aerosol ... 1689
- Maxitrol Ophthalmic Ointment and Suspension ... ▣ 222
- TobraDex Ophthalmic Suspension and Ointment ... 469

Dexamethasone Acetate (Potential for intensified electrolyte depletion, particularly hypokalemia). Products include:
- Dalalone D.P. Injectable ... 1009
- Decadron-LA Sterile Suspension ... 1687

Dexamethasone Sodium Phosphate (Potential for intensified electrolyte depletion, particularly hypokalemia). Products include:
- Decadron Phosphate Injection ... 1680
- Decadron Phosphate Sterile Ophthalmic Ointment ... 1684
- Decadron Phosphate Sterile Ophthalmic Solution ... 1685
- Decadron Phosphate Topical Cream ... 1686
- Decadron Phosphate with Xylocaine Injection, Sterile ... 1683
- Dexacort Phosphate in Respihaler ... 1606
- Dexacort Phosphate in Turbinaire ... 1607
- NeoDecadron Sterile Ophthalmic Ointment ... 1755
- NeoDecadron Sterile Ophthalmic Solution ... 1756
- NeoDecadron Topical Cream ... 1757

Dezocine (May aggravate orthostatic hypotension). Products include:
- Dalgan Injection ... 529

Diazoxide (Additive or potentiative effects). Products include:
- Hyperstat I.V. Injection ... 2504
- Proglycem ... 575

Digitoxin (Thiazide-induced hypokalemia may exaggerate or sensitize the response of the heart to toxic effects of digitalis). Products include:
- Crystodigin Tablets ... 1472

Digoxin (Thiazide-induced hypokalemia may exaggerate or sensitize the response of the heart to toxic effects of digitalis). Products include:
- Lanoxicaps ... 1110
- Lanoxin Elixir Pediatric ... 1113
- Lanoxin Injection ... 1116
- Lanoxin Injection Pediatric ... 1119
- Lanoxin Tablets ... 1121

Diltiazem Hydrochloride (Additive or potentiative effects). Products include:
- Cardizem CD Capsules ... 1251
- Cardizem SR Capsules ... 1255
- Cardizem Injectable ... 1253
- Cardizem Tablets ... 1257
- Dilacor XR Extended-release Capsules ... 2183
- Tiazac Capsules ... 1019

Doxazosin Mesylate (Additive or potentiative effects). Products include:
- Cardura Tablets ... 1993

Enalapril Maleate (Additive or potentiative effects). Products include:
- Vaseretic Tablets ... 1810
- Vasotec Tablets ... 1816

Enalaprilat (Additive or potentiative effects). Products include:
- Vasotec I.V. ... 1814

Esmolol Hydrochloride (Additive or potentiative effects). Products include:
- Brevibloc (esmolol HCl) Injection ... 1860

Felodipine (Additive or potentiative effects). Products include:
- Plendil Extended-Release Tablets ... 514

Fentanyl (May aggravate orthostatic hypotension). Products include:
- Duragesic Transdermal System ... 1336

Fentanyl Citrate (May aggravate orthostatic hypotension). Products include:
- Sublimaze Injection ... 463

Fludrocortisone Acetate (Potential for intensified electrolyte depletion, particularly hypokalemia). Products include:
- Florinef Acetate Tablets ... 506

Fosinopril Sodium (Additive or potentiative effects). Products include:
- Monopril Tablets ... 762

Furosemide (Additive or potentiative effects). Products include:
- Lasix Injection, Oral Solution and Tablets ... 1267

Guanabenz Acetate (Additive or potentiative effects).
No products indexed under this heading.

Guanethidine Monosulfate (Potentiation occurs). Products include:
- Esimil Tablets ... 840
- Ismelin Tablets ... 845

Hydralazine Hydrochloride (Additive or potentiative effects). Products include:
- Apresazide Capsules ... 824
- Apresoline Hydrochloride Tablets ... 826
- Hydralazine Hydrochloride Injection USP ... 2712
- Ser-Ap-Es Tablets ... 867

Hydrocodone Bitartrate (May aggravate orthostatic hypotension). Products include:
- Codiclear DH Syrup ... 808
- Duratuss HD Elixir ... 2750
- Histussin D Liquid ... 670
- Hycodan Tablets and Syrup ... 946
- Hycomine Compound Tablets ... 948
- Hycomine ... 947
- Hycotuss Expectorant Syrup ... 950
- Hydrocet Capsules ... 787
- Lorcet 10/650 Tablets ... 1016
- Lortab ... 2751
- Tussend ... 1830
- Tussend Expectorant ... 1831
- Vicodin Tablets ... 1404
- Vicodin ES Tablets ... 1405
- Vicodin HP Tablets ... 1403
- Vicodin Tuss Expectorant ... 1406
- Zydone Capsules ... 967

Hydrocodone Polistirex (May aggravate orthostatic hypotension). Products include:
- Tussionex Pennkinetic Extended-Release Suspension ... 1624

Hydrocortisone (Potential for intensified electrolyte depletion, particularly hypokalemia). Products include:
- Anusol-HC Cream 2.5% ... 1953
- Aquanil HC Lotion ... 1989
- Maximum Strength Cortaid Spray ▣ 800
- CORTENEMA ... 2713
- Cortisporin Ointment ... 1074
- Cortisporin Ophthalmic Ointment Sterile ... 1074
- Cortisporin Ophthalmic Suspension Sterile ... 1075
- Cortisporin Otic Solution Sterile ... 1076
- Cortisporin Otic Suspension Sterile ... 1077
- Cortizone-5 ... ▣ 795
- Cortizone-10 ... ▣ 795
- Hydrocortone Tablets ... 1715
- Hytone ... 922
- Hytone Ointment 2½% ... 923
- Massengill Medicated Soft Cloth Towelettes ... 2628
- Pediotic Suspension Sterile ... 1140
- Preparation H Hydrocortisone 1% Cream ... ▣ 843
- ProctoCream-HC 2.5% ... 2552
- VōSoL HC Otic Solution ... 2786

Hydrocortisone Acetate (Potential for intensified electrolyte depletion, particularly hypokalemia). Products include:
- Analpram-HC Rectal Cream 1% and 2.5% ... 993
- Anusol HC-1 Hydrocortisone Anti-Itch Ointment ... ▣ 810
- Anusol-HC Suppositories ... 1954

IMPORTANT NOTE: Always consult each drug listing in the patient's regimen for possible interactions.

Oretic · Interactions Index · 784

Caldecort Anti-Itch Hydrocortisone Cream ■■ 651
Coly-Mycin S Otic w/Neomycin & Hydrocortisone 1965
Cortaid ■■ 800
Cortifoam 2540
Cortisporin Cream 1073
Epifoam 2543
Hydrocortone Acetate Sterile Suspension 1712
Mantadil Cream 1124
Nupercainal Hydrocortisone 1% Cream ■■ 661
Pramosone Cream, Lotion & Ointment 995
ProctoFoam-HC 2552
Terra-Cortril Ophthalmic Suspension 2033

Hydrocortisone Sodium Phosphate (Potential for intensified electrolyte depletion, particularly hypokalemia). Products include:
Hydrocortone Phosphate Injection, Sterile 1713

Hydrocortisone Sodium Succinate (Potential for intensified electrolyte depletion, particularly hypokalemia).
No products indexed under this heading.

Hydroflumethiazide (Additive or potentiative effects). Products include:
Diucardin Tablets 2824

Hydromorphone Hydrochloride (May aggravate orthostatic hypotension). Products include:
Dilaudid Ampules 1382
Dilaudid Cough Syrup 1383
Dilaudid-HP Injection 1384
Dilaudid-HP Lyophilized Powder 250 mg 1384
Dilaudid 1382
Dilaudid Oral Liquid 1386
Dilaudid 1382
Dilaudid Tablets - 8 mg 1386

Indapamide (Additive or potentiative effects).
No products indexed under this heading.

Insulin, Human (Increased or decreased insulin requirements).
No products indexed under this heading.

Insulin, Human Isophane Suspension (Increased or decreased insulin requirements). Products include:
Novolin N Human Insulin 10 ml Vials 1846

Insulin, Human NPH (Increased or decreased insulin requirements). Products include:
Humulin N, 100 Units 1495
Novolin N PenFill 1.5 ml Cartridges Durable Insulin Delivery System 1849
Novolin N Prefilled Syringe Disposable Insulin Delivery System 1850

Insulin, Human Regular (Increased or decreased insulin requirements). Products include:
Humulin R, 100 Units 1497
Novolin R Human Insulin 10 ml Vials 1846
Novolin R PenFill 1.5 ml Cartridges Durable Insulin Delivery System 1849
Novolin R Prefilled Syringe Disposable Insulin Delivery System 1850
Velosulin BR Human Insulin 10 ml Vials 1847

Insulin, Human, Zinc Suspension (Increased or decreased insulin requirements). Products include:
Humulin L, 100 Units 1494
Humulin U, 100 Units 1498
Novolin L Human Insulin 10 ml Vials 1846

Insulin Lispro, Human (Increased or decreased insulin requirements). Products include:
Humalog Injection 1488

Insulin, NPH (Increased or decreased insulin requirements). Products include:
NPH, 100 Units 1502
Pork NPH, 100 Units 1506
Purified Pork NPH Isophane Insulin 1852

Insulin, Regular (Increased or decreased insulin requirements). Products include:
Regular, 100 Units 1503
Pork Regular, 100 Units 1507
Pork Regular (Concentrated), 500 Units 1508
Purified Pork Regular Insulin 1852

Insulin, Zinc Crystals (Increased or decreased insulin requirements). Products include:
NPH, 100 Units 1502

Insulin, Zinc Suspension (Increased or decreased insulin requirements). Products include:
Iletin I 1501
Lente, 100 Units 1501
Iletin II 1504
Pork Lente, 100 Units 1504
Purified Pork Lente Insulin 1852

Isradipine (Additive or potentiative effects). Products include:
DynaCirc Capsules 2381
DynaCirc CR Tablets 2383

Labetalol Hydrochloride (Additive or potentiative effects). Products include:
Normodyne Injection 2519
Normodyne Tablets 2522
Trandate 1158

Levorphanol Tartrate (May aggravate orthostatic hypotension). Products include:
Levo-Dromoran 2297

Lisinopril (Additive or potentiative effects). Products include:
Prinivil Tablets 1776
Prinzide Tablets 1780
Zestoretic Tablets 2968
Zestril Tablets 2972

Losartan Potassium (Additive or potentiative effects). Products include:
Cozaar Tablets 1668
Hyzaar Tablets 1720

Mecamylamine Hydrochloride (Potentiation occurs). Products include:
Inversine Tablets 1729

Meperidine Hydrochloride (May aggravate orthostatic hypotension). Products include:
Demerol 2438
Mepergan Injection 2859

Mephobarbital (May aggravate orthostatic hypotension). Products include:
Mebaral Tablets 2452

Methadone Hydrochloride (May aggravate orthostatic hypotension). Products include:
Methadone Hydrochloride Oral Concentrate 2356
Methadone Hydrochloride Oral Solution & Tablets 2357

Methyclothiazide (Additive or potentiative effects). Products include:
Enduron Tablets 424

Methyldopa (Additive or potentiative effects). Products include:
Aldoclor Tablets 1638
Aldomet Oral 1640
Aldoril Tablets 1644

Methyldopate Hydrochloride (Additive or potentiated effects). Products include:
Aldomet Ester HCl Injection 1642

Methylprednisolone Acetate (Potential for intensified electrolyte depletion, particularly hypokalemia).
No products indexed under this heading.

Methylprednisolone Sodium Succinate (Potential for intensified electrolyte depletion, particularly hypokalemia).
No products indexed under this heading.

Metolazone (Additive or potentiative effects). Products include:
Mykrox Tablets 1617
Zaroxolyn Tablets 1625

Metoprolol Succinate (Additive or potentiative effects). Products include:
Toprol-XL Tablets 560

Metoprolol Tartrate (Additive or potentiative effects). Products include:
Lopressor 848
Lopressor HCT Tablets 850

Metyrosine (Additive or potentiative effects). Products include:
Demser Capsules 1690

Minoxidil (Additive or potentiative effects).
No products indexed under this heading.

Moexipril Hydrochloride (Additive or potentiative effects). Products include:
Univasc Tablets 2553

Morphine Sulfate (May aggravate orthostatic hypotension). Products include:
Astramorph/PF Injection, USP (Preservative-Free) 526
Duramorph Injection 983
Infumorph 200 and Infumorph 500 Sterile Solutions 985
Kadian Capsules 2948
MS Contin Tablets 2149
MSIR 2152
Oramorph SR (Morphine Sulfate Sustained Release Tablets) 2359
RMS Suppositories CII 2766
Roxanol 2365

Nadolol (Additive or potentiative effects).
No products indexed under this heading.

Nicardipine Hydrochloride (Additive or potentiative effects). Products include:
Cardene Capsules 2261
Cardene I.V. 2815
Cardene SR Capsules 2264

Nifedipine (Additive or potentiative effects). Products include:
Adalat Capsules (10 mg and 20 mg) 580
Adalat CC 582
Procardia Capsules 2024
Procardia XL Extended Release Tablets 2026

Nisoldipine (Additive or potentiative effects). Products include:
Sular Tablets 2961

Nitroglycerin (Additive or potentiative effects). Products include:
Deponit NTG Transdermal Delivery System 2541
Nitro-Bid IV 1270
Nitro-Bid Ointment 1272
Nitro-Dur (nitroglycerin) Transdermal Infusion System 1365
Nitrolingual Spray 2193
Nitrostat Tablets 1981
Transderm-Nitro Transdermal Therapeutic System 878

Norepinephrine Bitartrate (Decreased arterial responsiveness). Products include:
Levophed Bitartrate Injection 2445

Opium Alkaloids (May aggravate orthostatic hypotension).
No products indexed under this heading.

Oxycodone Hydrochloride (May aggravate orthostatic hypotension). Products include:
OxyContin Tablets 2163
OxyIR Capsules 2167
Percocet Tablets 955
Percodan Tablets 955
Percodan-Demi Tablets 956
Roxicodone Tablets, Oral Solution & Intensol (Oxycodone) 2366
Tylox Capsules 1593

Penbutolol Sulfate (Additive or potentiative effects). Products include:
Levatol Tablets 2547

Pentobarbital Sodium (May aggravate orthostatic hypotension). Products include:
Nembutal Sodium Capsules 440
Nembutal Sodium Solution 442
Nembutal Sodium Suppositories 444

Phenobarbital (May aggravate orthostatic hypotension). Products include:
Arco-Lase Plus Tablets 513
Bellergal-S Tablets 2375
Donnatal 2234
Donnatal Extentabs 2234
Donnatal Tablets 2234
Phenobarbital Elixir and Tablets 1523
Quadrinal Tablets 1398

Phenoxybenzamine Hydrochloride (Additive or potentiative effects). Products include:
Dibenzyline Capsules 2650

Phentolamine Mesylate (Additive or potentiative effects). Products include:
Regitine Vials 864

Pindolol (Additive or potentiative effects). Products include:
Visken Tablets 2428

Polythiazide (Additive or potentiative effects). Products include:
Minizide Capsules 2016

Prazosin Hydrochloride (Potentiation occurs). Products include:
Minipress Capsules 2015
Minizide Capsules 2016

Prednisolone Acetate (Potential for intensified electrolyte depletion, particularly hypokalemia). Products include:
AK-CIDE ◉ 203
AK-CIDE Ointment ◉ 203
Blephamide Liquifilm Sterile Ophthalmic Suspension 472
Blephamide Ointment ◉ 234
Econopred & Econopred Plus Ophthalmic Suspensions ◉ 216
Poly-Pred Liquifilm ◉ 246
Pred Forte ◉ 247
Pred Mild ◉ 250
Pred-G Liquifilm Sterile Ophthalmic Suspension ◉ 248
Pred-G S.O.P. Sterile Ophthalmic Ointment ◉ 249

Prednisolone Sodium Phosphate (Potential for intensified electrolyte depletion, particularly hypokalemia). Products include:
AK-PRED ◉ 204
Hydeltrasol Injection, Sterile 1708
Pediapred Oral Solution 1618

Prednisolone Tebutate (Potential for intensified electrolyte depletion, particularly hypokalemia). Products include:
Hydeltra-T.B.A. Sterile Suspension 1710

Prednisone (Potential for intensified electrolyte depletion, particularly hypokalemia).
No products indexed under this heading.

Propoxyphene Hydrochloride (May aggravate orthostatic hypotension). Products include:
Darvon 1475
Wygesic Tablets 2930

Propoxyphene Napsylate (May aggravate orthostatic hypotension). Products include:
Darvon-N/Darvocet-N 1473

(■■ Described in PDR For Nonprescription Drugs) (◉ Described in PDR For Ophthalmology)

Propranolol Hydrochloride (Additive or potentiative effects). Products include:
- Inderal ... 2834
- Inderal LA Long Acting Capsules ... 2836
- Inderide Tablets ... 2838
- Inderide LA Long Acting Capsules ... 2840

Quinapril Hydrochloride (Additive or potentiative effects). Products include:
- Accupril Tablets ... 1950

Ramipril (Additive or potentiative effects). Products include:
- Altace Capsules ... 1238

Rauwolfia Serpentina (Potentiation occurs).
- No products indexed under this heading.

Rescinnamine (Potentiation occurs).
- No products indexed under this heading.

Reserpine (Potentiation occurs). Products include:
- Diupres Tablets ... 1691
- Hydropres Tablets ... 1718
- Ser-Ap-Es Tablets ... 867

Secobarbital Sodium (May aggravate orthostatic hypotension). Products include:
- Seconal Sodium Pulvules ... 1529

Sodium Nitroprusside (Additive or potentiative effects).
- No products indexed under this heading.

Sotalol Hydrochloride (Additive or potentiative effects). Products include:
- Betapace Tablets ... 637

Spirapril Hydrochloride (Additive or potentiative effects).
- No products indexed under this heading.

Sufentanil Citrate (May aggravate orthostatic hypotension). Products include:
- Sufenta Injection ... 1355

Terazosin Hydrochloride (Additive or potentiative effects). Products include:
- Hytrin Capsules ... 434

Thiamylal Sodium (May aggravate orthostatic hypotension).
- No products indexed under this heading.

Timolol Maleate (Additive or potentiative effects). Products include:
- Blocadren Tablets ... 1654
- Timolide Tablets ... 1791
- Timoptic in Ocudose ... 1796
- Timoptic Sterile Ophthalmic Solution ... 1794
- Timoptic-XE ... 1798

Torsemide (Additive or potentiative effects). Products include:
- Demadex Tablets and Injection ... 691

Triamcinolone (Potential for intensified electrolyte depletion, particularly hypokalemia).
- No products indexed under this heading.

Triamcinolone Acetonide (Potential for intensified electrolyte depletion, particularly hypokalemia). Products include:
- Azmacort Oral Inhaler ... 2175
- Nasacort AQ Nasal Spray ... 2191
- Nasacort Nasal Inhaler ... 2189

Triamcinolone Diacetate (Potential for intensified electrolyte depletion, particularly hypokalemia).
- No products indexed under this heading.

Triamcinolone Hexacetonide (Potential for intensified electrolyte depletion, particularly hypokalemia).
- No products indexed under this heading.

Trimethaphan Camsylate (Potentiation occurs).
- No products indexed under this heading.

Tubocurarine Chloride (Increased responsiveness).
- No products indexed under this heading.

Verapamil Hydrochloride (Additive or potentiative effects). Products include:
- Calan SR Caplets ... 2571
- Calan Tablets ... 2568
- Covera-HS Tablets ... 2573
- Isoptin Injectable ... 1391
- Isoptin Oral Tablets ... 1393
- Isoptin SR Tablets ... 1395
- Verelan Capsules ... 1455

Food Interactions

Alcohol (May aggravate orthostatic hypotension).

ORGANIDIN NR TABLETS AND LIQUID

(Guaifenesin) ... 2781
None cited in PDR database.

ORIGINAL VICKS COUGH DROPS, MENTHOL AND CHERRY FLAVORS

(Menthol) ... ⊡ 733
None cited in PDR database.

ORIMUNE

(Poliovirus Vaccine, Live, Oral, Trivalent, Types 1,2,3 (Sabin)) ... 1433
May interact with antineoplastics and corticosteroids. Compounds in these categories include:

Altretamine (Contraindicated). Products include:
- Hexalen Capsules ... 2760

Anastrozole (Contraindicated). Products include:
- Arimidex Tablets ... 2932

Asparaginase (Contraindicated). Products include:
- Elspar ... 1700

Betamethasone Acetate (Contraindicated). Products include:
- Celestone Soluspan Suspension ... 2484

Betamethasone Sodium Phosphate (Contraindicated). Products include:
- Celestone Soluspan Suspension ... 2484

Bicalutamide (Contraindicated). Products include:
- Casodex Tablets ... 2934

Bleomycin Sulfate (Contraindicated). Products include:
- Blenoxane ... 697

Busulfan (Contraindicated). Products include:
- Myleran Tablets ... 1209

Carboplatin (Contraindicated). Products include:
- Paraplatin for Injection ... 713

Carmustine (BCNU) (Contraindicated). Products include:
- BiCNU ... 696

Chlorambucil (Contraindicated). Products include:
- Leukeran Tablets ... 1205

Cisplatin (Contraindicated). Products include:
- Platinol for Injection ... 717
- Platinol-AQ Injection ... 719

Cortisone Acetate (Contraindicated). Products include:
- Cortone Acetate Sterile Suspension ... 1663
- Cortone Acetate Tablets ... 1664

Cyclophosphamide (Contraindicated). Products include:
- Cytoxan ... 700

Dacarbazine (Contraindicated). Products include:
- DTIC-Dome ... 593

Daunorubicin Citrate (Contraindicated). Products include:
- DaunoXome ... 1842

Daunorubicin Hydrochloride (Contraindicated). Products include:
- Cerubidine for Injection ... 634

Dexamethasone (Contraindicated). Products include:
- AK-Trol Ointment & Suspension ... ◎ 205
- Decadron Elixir ... 1676
- Decadron Tablets ... 1678
- Decaspray Topical Aerosol ... 1689
- Maxitrol Ophthalmic Ointment and Suspension ... ◎ 222
- TobraDex Ophthalmic Suspension and Ointment ... 469

Dexamethasone Acetate (Contraindicated). Products include:
- Dalalone D.P. Injectable ... 1009
- Decadron-LA Sterile Suspension ... 1687

Dexamethasone Sodium Phosphate (Contraindicated). Products include:
- Decadron Phosphate Injection ... 1680
- Decadron Phosphate Sterile Ophthalmic Ointment ... 1684
- Decadron Phosphate Sterile Ophthalmic Solution ... 1685
- Decadron Phosphate Topical Cream ... 1686
- Decadron Phosphate with Xylocaine Injection, Sterile ... 1683
- Dexacort Phosphate in Respihaler ... 1606
- Dexacort Phosphate in Turbinaire ... 1607
- NeoDecadron Sterile Ophthalmic Ointment ... 1755
- NeoDecadron Sterile Ophthalmic Solution ... 1756
- NeoDecadron Topical Cream ... 1757

Docetaxel (Contraindicated). Products include:
- Taxotere for Injection Concentrate 2204

Doxorubicin Hydrochloride (Contraindicated). Products include:
- Adriamycin PFS ... 2056
- Adriamycin RDF ... 2056
- Doxil ... 2613
- Doxorubicin Astra ... 531
- Rubex for Injection ... 721

Estramustine Phosphate Sodium (Contraindicated). Products include:
- Emcyt Capsules ... 2085

Etoposide (Contraindicated). Products include:
- Etoposide Injection ... 539
- VePesid Capsules and Injection ... 727

Floxuridine (Contraindicated). Products include:
- Sterile FUDR ... 2284

Fludrocortisone Acetate (Contraindicated). Products include:
- Florinef Acetate Tablets ... 506

Fluorouracil (Contraindicated). Products include:
- Efudex ... 2280
- Fluoroplex Topical Solution & Cream 1% ... 475
- Fluorouracil Injection ... 2282

Flutamide (Contraindicated). Products include:
- Eulexin Capsules ... 2498

Gemcitabine Hydrochloride (Contraindicated). Products include:
- Gemzar for Injection ... 1482

Hydrocortisone (Contraindicated). Products include:
- Anusol-HC Cream 2.5% ... 1953
- Aquanil HC Lotion ... 1989
- Maximum Strength Cortaid Spray ⊡ 800
- CORTENEMA ... 2713
- Cortisporin Ointment ... 1074
- Cortisporin Ophthalmic Ointment Sterile ... 1074
- Cortisporin Ophthalmic Suspension Sterile ... 1075
- Cortisporin Otic Solution Sterile ... 1076
- Cortisporin Otic Suspension Sterile 1077
- Cortizone-5 ... ⊡ 795
- Cortizone-10 ... ⊡ 795
- Hydrocortone Tablets ... 1715
- Hytone ... 922
- Hytone Ointment 2 ½% ... 923
- Massengill Medicated Soft Cloth Towelettes ... 2628
- Pediotic Suspension Sterile ... 1140
- Preparation H Hydrocortisone 1% Cream ... ⊡ 843
- ProctoCream-HC 2.5% ... 2552
- VōSoL HC Otic Solution ... 2786

Hydrocortisone Acetate (Contraindicated). Products include:
- Analpram-HC Rectal Cream 1% and 2.5% ... 993
- Anusol HC-1 Hydrocortisone Anti-Itch Ointment ... ⊡ 810
- Anusol-HC Suppositories ... 1954
- Caldecort Anti-Itch Hydrocortisone Cream ... ⊡ 651
- Coly-Mycin S Otic w/Neomycin & Hydrocortisone ... 1965
- Cortaid ... ⊡ 800
- Cortifoam ... 2540
- Cortisporin Cream ... 1073
- Epifoam ... 2543
- Hydrocortone Acetate Sterile Suspension ... 1712
- Mantadil Cream ... 1124
- Nupercainal Hydrocortisone 1% Cream ... ⊡ 661
- Pramosone Cream, Lotion & Ointment ... 995
- ProctoFoam-HC ... 2552
- Terra-Cortril Ophthalmic Suspension ... 2033

Hydrocortisone Sodium Phosphate (Contraindicated). Products include:
- Hydrocortone Phosphate Injection, Sterile ... 1713

Hydrocortisone Sodium Succinate (Contraindicated).
- No products indexed under this heading.

Hydroxyurea (Contraindicated). Products include:
- Hydrea Capsules ... 705

Idarubicin Hydrochloride (Contraindicated). Products include:
- Idamycin Injection ... 2096

Ifosfamide (Contraindicated). Products include:
- IFEX ... 706

Interferon alfa-2A, Recombinant (Contraindicated). Products include:
- Roferon-A Injection ... 2308

Interferon alfa-2B, Recombinant (Contraindicated). Products include:
- Intron A for Injection ... 2506

Irinotecan Hydrochloride (Contraindicated).
- No products indexed under this heading.

Levamisole Hydrochloride (Contraindicated). Products include:
- Ergamisol Tablets ... 1340

Lomustine (CCNU) (Contraindicated). Products include:
- CeeNU Capsules ... 699

Mechlorethamine Hydrochloride (Contraindicated). Products include:
- Mustargen ... 1752

Megestrol Acetate (Contraindicated). Products include:
- Megace Oral Suspension ... 708
- Megace Tablets ... 710

Melphalan (Contraindicated). Products include:
- Alkeran Tablets ... 1198

Mercaptopurine (Contraindicated). Products include:
- Purinethol Tablets ... 1214

Methotrexate Sodium (Contraindicated). Products include:
- Methotrexate Sodium Tablets, Injection, for Injection and LPF Injection ... 1322

IMPORTANT NOTE: Always consult each drug listing in the patient's regimen for possible interactions.

Orimune Interactions Index 786

Methylprednisolone Acetate (Contraindicated).
No products indexed under this heading.

Methylprednisolone Sodium Succinate (Contraindicated).
No products indexed under this heading.

Mitomycin (Mitomycin-C) (Contraindicated). Products include:
Mutamycin for Injection 712

Mitotane (Contraindicated). Products include:
Lysodren Tablets 707

Mitoxantrone Hydrochloride (Contraindicated). Products include:
Novantrone for Injection 1327

Paclitaxel (Contraindicated). Products include:
Taxol Injection 723

Prednisolone Acetate (Contraindicated). Products include:
AK-CIDE .... ◉ 203
AK-CIDE Ointment .... ◉ 203
Blephamide Liquifilm Sterile Ophthalmic Suspension 472
Blephamide Ointment .... ◉ 234
Econopred & Econopred Plus Ophthalmic Suspensions .... ◉ 216
Poly-Pred Liquifilm .... ◉ 246
Pred Forte .... ◉ 247
Pred Mild .... ◉ 250
Pred-G Liquifilm Sterile Ophthalmic Suspension .... ◉ 248
Pred-G S.O.P. Sterile Ophthalmic Ointment .... ◉ 249

Prednisolone Sodium Phosphate (Contraindicated). Products include:
AK-PRED .... ◉ 204
Hydeltrasol Injection, Sterile 1708
Pediapred Oral Solution 1618

Prednisolone Tebutate (Contraindicated). Products include:
Hydeltra-T.B.A. Sterile Suspension 1710

Prednisone (Contraindicated).
No products indexed under this heading.

Procarbazine Hydrochloride (Contraindicated). Products include:
Matulane Capsules 2300

Streptozocin (Contraindicated). Products include:
Zanosar Sterile Powder 2119

Tamoxifen Citrate (Contraindicated). Products include:
Nolvadex Tablets 2957

Teniposide (Contraindicated). Products include:
Vumon for Injection 729

Thioguanine (Contraindicated). Products include:
Thioguanine Tablets, Tabloid Brand 1225

Thiotepa (Contraindicated). Products include:
Thioplex (Thiotepa For Injection) 1329

Topotecan Hydrochloride (Contraindicated). Products include:
Hycamtin for Injection 2665

Triamcinolone (Contraindicated).
No products indexed under this heading.

Triamcinolone Acetonide (Contraindicated). Products include:
Azmacort Oral Inhaler 2175
Nasacort AQ Nasal Spray 2191
Nasacort Nasal Inhaler 2189

Triamcinolone Diacetate (Contraindicated).
No products indexed under this heading.

Triamcinolone Hexacetonide (Contraindicated).
No products indexed under this heading.

Vincristine Sulfate (Contraindicated). Products include:
Oncovin Solution Vials & Hyporets 1521

Vinorelbine Tartrate (Contraindicated). Products include:
Navelbine Injection 1212

ORLAAM ORAL SOLUTION
(Levomethadyl Acetate Hydrochloride) 2361
May interact with mixed agonist/antagonist opioid analgesics, hypnotics and sedatives, narcotic analgesics, antihistamines, benzodiazepines, tranquilizers, phenothiazines, antidepressant drugs, central nervous system depressants, and certain other agents. Compounds in these categories include:

Acrivastine (Potential for serious side effects, including respiratory depression, hypotension, profound sedation and coma, if used concurrently). Products include:
Semprex-D Capsules 1620

Alfentanil Hydrochloride (Potential for serious side effects, including respiratory depression, hypotension, profound sedation and coma, if used concurrently). Products include:
Alfenta Injection 1334

Alprazolam (Potential for serious side effects, including respiratory depression, hypotension, profound sedation and coma, if used concurrently). Products include:
Xanax Tablets 2115

Amitriptyline Hydrochloride (Potential for serious side effects, including respiratory depression, hypotension, profound sedation and coma, if used concurrently). Products include:
Elavil 2945
Etrafon 2495
Limbitrol 2333
Triavil Tablets 1800

Amoxapine (Potential for serious side effects, including respiratory depression, hypotension, profound sedation and coma, if used concurrently). Products include:
Asendin Tablets 1419

Aprobarbital (Potential for serious side effects, including respiratory depression, hypotension, profound sedation and coma, if used concurrently).
No products indexed under this heading.

Astemizole (Potential for serious side effects, including respiratory depression, hypotension, profound sedation and coma, if used concurrently). Products include:
Hismanal Tablets 1341

Azatadine Maleate (Potential for serious side effects, including respiratory depression, hypotension, profound sedation and coma, if used concurrently). Products include:
Trinalin Repetabs Tablets 1373

Bromodiphenhydramine Hydrochloride (Potential for serious side effects, including respiratory depression, hypotension, profound sedation and coma, if used concurrently).
No products indexed under this heading.

Brompheniramine Maleate (Potential for serious side effects, including respiratory depression, hypotension, profound sedation and coma, if used concurrently). Products include:
Alka-Seltzer Plus Sinus Medicine .. ▣ 611
Bromfed Capsules (Extended-Release) 1832
Bromfed Syrup .... ▣ 712
Bromfed Tablets 1832
Bromfed-DM Cough Syrup 1832
Bromfed-PD Capsules (Extended-Release) 1832
Dimetane-DC Cough Syrup 2232
Dimetane-DX Cough Syrup 2233
Dimetapp Allergy Dye-Free Elixir.... ▣ 838
Dimetapp Allergy Sinus Caplets .... ▣ 838
Dimetapp Cold & Allergy Chewable Tablets .... ▣ 838
Dimetapp Cold & Cough Liqui-Gels .... ▣ 839
Dimetapp Cold & Fever Suspension .... ▣ 839
Dimetapp DM Elixir .... ▣ 840
Dimetapp Elixir .... ▣ 840
Dimetapp Extentabs .... ▣ 841
Dimetapp Tablets/Liqui-Gels .... ▣ 841
Rondec Chewable Tablets 974
Vicks DayQuil Allergy Relief 12-Hour Extended Release Tablets.. ▣ 733
Vicks DayQuil Allergy Relief 4-Hour Tablets .... ▣ 733

Buprenorphine (Potential for serious side effects, including respiratory depression, hypotension, profound sedation and coma, if used concurrently; patients maintained on levomethadyl acetate hydrochloride may experience withdrawal symptoms when administered mixed agonists/antagonists). Products include:
Buprenex Injectable 2170

Bupropion Hydrochloride (Potential for serious side effects, including respiratory depression, hypotension, profound sedation and coma, if used concurrently). Products include:
Wellbutrin Tablets 1177

Buspirone Hydrochloride (Potential for serious side effects, including respiratory depression, hypotension, profound sedation and coma, if used concurrently). Products include:
BuSpar Tablets 738

Butabarbital (Potential for serious side effects, including respiratory depression, hypotension, profound sedation and coma, if used concurrently).
No products indexed under this heading.

Butalbital (Potential for serious side effects, including respiratory depression, hypotension, profound sedation and coma, if used concurrently). Products include:
Axocet Capsules 2469
Esgic-plus Capsules 1012
Esgic-plus Tablets 1012
Fioricet Tablets 2386
Fioricet with Codeine Capsules 2387
Fiorinal Capsules 2388
Fiorinal with Codeine Capsules 2390
Fiorinal Tablets 2388
Phrenilin 790
Sedapap Tablets 50 mg/650 mg .. 1826

Butorphanol Tartrate (Patients maintained on levomethadyl acetate hydrochloride may experience withdrawal symptoms when administered mixed agonists/antagonists). Products include:
Stadol 779

Carbamazepine (May increase levomethadyl acetate hydrochloride's peak activity and/or shorten its duration of action). Products include:
Atretol Tablets 569
Tegretol/Tegretol-XR 870

Cetirizine Hydrochloride (Potential for serious side effects, including respiratory depression, hypotension, profound sedation and coma, if used concurrently). Products include:
Zyrtec Tablets 2053

Chlordiazepoxide (Potential for serious side effects, including respiratory depression, hypotension, profound sedation and coma, if used concurrently). Products include:
Limbitrol 2333

Chlordiazepoxide Hydrochloride (Potential for serious side effects, including respiratory depression, hypotension, profound sedation and coma, if used concurrently). Products include:
Librax Capsules 2330
Librium Capsules 2331
Librium Injectable 2332

Chlorpheniramine Maleate (Potential for serious side effects, including respiratory depression, hypotension, profound sedation and coma, if used concurrently). Products include:
Alka-Seltzer Plus Cold Medicine .... ▣ 611
Alka-Seltzer Plus Cold Medicine Liqui-Gels .... ▣ 612
Alka-Seltzer Plus Cold & Cough Medicine .... ▣ 611
Alka-Seltzer Plus Cold & Cough Medicine Liqui-Gels .... ▣ 612
Alka-Seltzer Plus Flu & Body Aches Effervescent Tablets .... ▣ 612
Allerest Maximum Strength .... ▣ 649
Allerest Sinus Pain Formula .... ▣ 649
Ana-Kit Anaphylaxis Emergency Treatment Kit 611
Atrohist Pediatric Capsules 1603
Atrohist Plus Tablets 1605
BC Cold Powder Multi-Symptom Formula (Cold-Sinus-Allergy) .... ▣ 631
Cerose DM .... ▣ 853
Cheracol Plus Head Cold/Cough Formula .... ▣ 741
Children's TYLENOL Cold Multi-Symptom Chewable Tablets and Liquid 1559
Children's TYLENOL Cold Plus Cough Multi Symptom Chewable Tablets and Liquid 1560
Children's TYLENOL Flu Suspension Liquid 1560
Children's Vicks DayQuil Allergy Relief .... ▣ 730
Children's Vicks NyQuil Cold/Cough Relief .... ▣ 731
Chlor-Trimeton Allergy Decongestant Tablets .... ▣ 759
Chlor-Trimeton Allergy Tablets .... ▣ 758
Allergy-Sinus Comtrex Multi-Symptom Allergy-Sinus Formula Tablets and Caplets .... ▣ 639
Comtrex Multi-Symptom .... ▣ 638
Contac Continuous Action Nasal Decongestant/Antihistamine 12 Hour Capsules .... ▣ 773
Contac Maximum Strength Continuous Action Decongestant/Antihistamine 12 Hour Caplets.. ▣ 772
Contac Severe Cold and Flu Formula Caplets .... ▣ 773
Coricidin Cold + Flu Tablets .... ▣ 760
Coricidin Cough + Cold Tablets .... ▣ 760
Coricidin 'D' Decongestant Tablets .... ▣ 760
D.A. II Tablets 972
D.A. Chewable Tablets 970
Dura-Tap/PD Capsules 970
Dura-Vent/DA Tablets 972
Efidac 24 Chlorpheniramine .... ▣ 655
Extendryl 1003
Fedahist Gyrocaps 2545
Hycomine Compound Tablets 948
Kronofed-A 994
Nolamine Timed-Release Tablets 790
Novahistine Elixir .... ▣ 782
Ornade Spansule Capsules 2678
PediaCare Cough-Cold Chewable Tablets and Liquid 1569
PediaCare NightRest Cough-Cold Liquid 1569
Pediatric Vicks 44m Cough & Cold Relief .... ▣ 737
Pyrroxate Caplets .... ▣ 742
Ryna .... ▣ 804
Sinarest .... ▣ 663
Sine-Off Sinus Medicine .... ▣ 784
Singlet Tablets .... ▣ 785
Sinulin Tablets 792

(▣ Described in PDR For Nonprescription Drugs) (◉ Described in PDR For Ophthalmology)

Sinutab Sinus Allergy Medication, Maximum Strength Tablets and Caplets ... 823
Sudafed Cold & Allergy Tablets ... 826
Teldrin 12 Hour Antihistamine/Nasal Decongestant Allergy Relief Capsules ... 786
TheraFlu Flu and Cold Medicine ... 750
Theraflu Maximum Strength Flu and Cold Medicine For Sore Throat ... 751
TheraFlu Flu, Cold and Cough Medicine ... 750
TheraFlu Maximum Strength Nighttime Flu, Cold & Cough Medicine ... 751
Triaminic Night Time ... 754
Triaminic Syrup ... 755
Triaminic Triaminicol Cold & Cough ... 756
Triaminicin Tablets ... 756
Tussend ... 1830
TYLENOL Allergy Sinus, Maximum Strength Caplets and Gelcaps ... 1571
TYLENOL Cold Medication, Multi-Symptom Formula Tablets and Caplets ... 1572
TYLENOL Cold Medication, Multi-Symptom Hot Liquid Packets ... 1572
Vicks 44 LiquiCaps Cough, Cold & Flu Relief ... 728
Vicks 44M Cough, Cold & Flu Relief ... 729

Chlorpheniramine Polistirex (Potential for serious side effects, including respiratory depression, hypotension, profound sedation and coma, if used concurrently). Products include:
Tussionex Pennkinetic Extended-Release Suspension ... 1624

Chlorpheniramine Tannate (Potential for serious side effects, including respiratory depression, hypotension, profound sedation and coma, if used concurrently). Products include:
Atrohist Pediatric Suspension ... 1604
Atrohist Pediatric Suspension Dye-Free ... 1604
Rynatan ... 2781
Rynatuss ... 2782

Chlorpromazine (Potential for serious side effects, including respiratory depression, hypotension, profound sedation and coma, if used concurrently). Products include:
Thorazine Suppositories ... 2701

Chlorpromazine Hydrochloride (Potential for serious side effects, including respiratory depression, hypotension, profound sedation and coma, if used concurrently). Products include:
Thorazine ... 2701

Chlorprothixene (Potential for serious side effects, including respiratory depression, hypotension, profound sedation and coma, if used concurrently).
No products indexed under this heading.

Chlorprothixene Hydrochloride (Potential for serious side effects, including respiratory depression, hypotension, profound sedation and coma, if used concurrently).
No products indexed under this heading.

Chlorprothixene Lactate (Potential for serious side effects, including respiratory depression, hypotension, profound sedation and coma, if used concurrently).
No products indexed under this heading.

Cimetidine (May slow the onset, lower the activity and/or increase the duration of action of levomethadyl acetate hydrochloride). Products include:
Tagamet HB Tablets ... 786
Tagamet Tablets ... 2694

Cimetidine Hydrochloride (May slow the onset, lower the activity and/or increase the duration of action of levomethadyl acetate hydrochloride). Products include:
Tagamet ... 2694

Clemastine Fumarate (Potential for serious side effects, including respiratory depression, hypotension, profound sedation and coma, if used concurrently). Products include:
Tavist Syrup ... 2426
Tavist Tablets ... 2427
Tavist-1 12 Hour Relief Tablets ... 749
Tavist-D 12 Hour Relief Tablets ... 750

Clorazepate Dipotassium (Potential for serious side effects, including respiratory depression, hypotension, profound sedation and coma, if used concurrently). Products include:
Tranxene ... 459

Clozapine (Potential for serious side effects, including respiratory depression, hypotension, profound sedation and coma, if used concurrently). Products include:
Clozaril Tablets ... 2377

Codeine Phosphate (Potential for serious side effects, including respiratory depression, hypotension, profound sedation and coma, if used concurrently). Products include:
Brontex ... 2130
Dimetane-DC Cough Syrup ... 2232
Fioricet with Codeine Capsules ... 2387
Fiorinal with Codeine Capsules ... 2390
Nucofed ... 2225
Phenergan with Codeine ... 2883
Phenergan VC with Codeine ... 2888
Robitussin A-C Syrup ... 2248
Robitussin-DAC Syrup ... 2249
Ryna ... 804
Soma Compound w/Codeine Tablets ... 2784
Tylenol with Codeine ... 1592

Cyproheptadine Hydrochloride (Potential for serious side effects, including respiratory depression, hypotension, profound sedation and coma, if used concurrently). Products include:
Periactin ... 1767

Desflurane (Potential for serious side effects, including respiratory depression, hypotension, profound sedation and coma, if used concurrently). Products include:
Suprane (desflurane, USP) ... 1865

Desipramine Hydrochloride (Potential for serious side effects, including respiratory depression, hypotension, profound sedation and coma, if used concurrently). Products include:
Norpramin Tablets ... 1273

Dexchlorpheniramine Maleate (Potential for serious side effects, including respiratory depression, hypotension, profound sedation and coma, if used concurrently).
No products indexed under this heading.

Dezocine (Potential for serious side effects, including respiratory depression, hypotension, profound sedation and coma, if used concurrently). Products include:
Dalgan Injection ... 529

Diazepam (Potential for serious side effects, including respiratory depression, hypotension, profound sedation and coma, if used concurrently). Products include:
Dizac (diazepam injectable emulsion) CIV ... 1862
Valium Injectable ... 2336
Valium Tablets ... 2335

Diphenhydramine Citrate (Potential for serious side effects, including respiratory depression, hypotension, profound sedation and coma, if used concurrently). Products include:
Excedrin P.M. Analgesic/Sleeping Aid Tablets, Caplets, Liquigels ... 735

Diphenhydramine Hydrochloride (Potential for serious side effects, including respiratory depression, hypotension, profound sedation and coma, if used concurrently). Products include:
Actifed Allergy Daytime/Nighttime Caplets ... 808
Actifed Sinus Daytime/Nighttime Tablets and Caplets ... 809
Extra Strength Bayer PM Aspirin Plus Sleep Aid ... 617
Benadryl Allergy Chewables ... 811
Benadryl Allergy/Cold Tablets ... 811
Benadryl Allergy Decongestant Liquid Medication ... 812
Benadryl Allergy Decongestant Tablets ... 812
Benadryl Allergy Liquid Medication ... 813
Benadryl Allergy Tablets ... 811
Benadryl Allergy Sinus Headache Caplets ... 813
Benadryl Dye-Free Allergy Liquigel Softgels ... 813
Benadryl Dye-Free Allergy Liquid Medication ... 814
Benadryl Itch Relief Stick Extra Strength ... 814
Benadryl Cream ... 814
Benadryl Gel ... 815
Benadryl Spray ... 815
Benadryl Injection ... 1955
Contac Day & Night Cold/Flu Night Caplets ... 772
Contac Night Allergy/Sinus Caplets ... 771
Extra Strength Doan's P.M. ... 653
Excedrin P.M. Analgesic/Sleeping Aid Tablets, Caplets, Liquigels ... 643
Nytol QuickCaps Caplets ... 632
Sleepinal Night-time Sleep Aid Capsules and Softgels ... 798
TYLENOL Allergy Sinus NightTime, Maximum Strength Caplets ... 1571
TYLENOL Flu NightTime, Maximum Strength Gelcaps ... 1575
TYLENOL Flu NightTime, Maximum Strength Hot Medication Packets ... 1575
TYLENOL PM Pain Reliever/Sleep Aid, Extra Strength Gelcaps, Caplets, Geltabs ... 1576
TYLENOL Severe Allergy Medication Caplets ... 1571
Maximum Strength Unisom Sleepgels ... 1990
Unisom With Pain Relief-Nighttime Sleep Aid and Pain Reliever ... 1991

Diphenylpyraline Hydrochloride (Potential for serious side effects, including respiratory depression, hypotension, profound sedation and coma, if used concurrently).
No products indexed under this heading.

Doxepin Hydrochloride (Potential for serious side effects, including respiratory depression, hypotension, profound sedation and coma, if used concurrently). Products include:
Adapin Capsules ... 1542
Sinequan ... 2028
Zonalon Cream ... 1042

Droperidol (Potential for serious side effects, including respiratory depression, hypotension, profound sedation and coma, if used concurrently). Products include:
Inapsine Injection ... 462

Enflurane (Potential for serious side effects, including respiratory depression, hypotension, profound sedation and coma, if used concurrently).
No products indexed under this heading.

Erythromycin (May slow the onset, lower the activity and/or increase the duration of action of levomethadyl acetate hydrochloride). Products include:
A/T/S 2% Acne Topical Gel ... 1244
A/T/S 2% Acne Topical Solution ... 1244
Benzamycin Topical Gel ... 919
E-Mycin Tablets ... 1388
Emgel 2% Topical Gel ... 1081
ERYC ... 1972
Erycette (erythromycin 2%) Topical Solution ... 1943
Ery-Tab Tablets ... 426
Erythromycin Base Filmtab ... 430
Erythromycin Delayed-Release Capsules, USP ... 431
Ilotycin Ophthalmic Ointment ... 928
PCE Dispertab Tablets ... 453
T-Stat 2.0% Topical Solution and Pads ... 2797
THERAMYCIN Z 2% Solution ... 1629

Erythromycin Estolate (May slow the onset, lower the activity and/or increase the duration of action of levomethadyl acetate hydrochloride). Products include:
Ilosone ... 927

Erythromycin Ethylsuccinate (May slow the onset, lower the activity and/or increase the duration of action of levomethadyl acetate hydrochloride). Products include:
E.E.S. ... 427
EryPed ... 425
Pediazole Suspension ... 2340

Erythromycin Glucaptate (May slow the onset, lower the activity and/or increase the duration of action of levomethadyl acetate hydrochloride). Products include:
Ilotycin Gluceptate, IV, Vials ... 929

Erythromycin Lactobionate (May slow the onset, lower the activity and/or increase the duration of action of levomethadyl acetate hydrochloride).
No products indexed under this heading.

Erythromycin Stearate (May slow the onset, lower the activity and/or increase the duration of action of levomethadyl acetate hydrochloride). Products include:
Erythrocin Stearate Filmtab ... 429

Estazolam (Potential for serious side effects, including respiratory depression, hypotension, profound sedation and coma, if used concurrently). Products include:
ProSom Tablets ... 457

Ethchlorvynol (Potential for serious side effects, including respiratory depression, hypotension, profound sedation and coma, if used concurrently). Products include:
Placidyl Capsules ... 456

Ethinamate (Potential for serious side effects, including respiratory depression, hypotension, profound sedation and coma, if used concurrently).
No products indexed under this heading.

Fentanyl (Potential for serious side effects, including respiratory depression, hypotension, profound sedation and coma, if used concurrently). Products include:
Duragesic Transdermal System ... 1336

Fentanyl Citrate (Potential for serious side effects, including respiratory depression, hypotension, profound sedation and coma, if used concurrently). Products include:
Sublimaze Injection ... 463

IMPORTANT NOTE: Always consult each drug listing in the patient's regimen for possible interactions.

Orlaam — Interactions Index

Fluoxetine Hydrochloride (Potential for serious side effects, including respiratory depression, hypotension, profound sedation and coma, if used concurrently). Products include:
- Prozac Pulvules & Liquid, Oral Solution 935

Fluphenazine Decanoate (Potential for serious side effects, including respiratory depression, hypotension, profound sedation and coma, if used concurrently). Products include:
- Prolixin Decanoate 510

Fluphenazine Enanthate (Potential for serious side effects, including respiratory depression, hypotension, profound sedation and coma, if used concurrently). Products include:
- Prolixin Enanthate 510

Fluphenazine Hydrochloride (Potential for serious side effects, including respiratory depression, hypotension, profound sedation and coma, if used concurrently). Products include:
- Prolixin 510

Flurazepam Hydrochloride (Potential for serious side effects, including respiratory depression, hypotension, profound sedation and coma, if used concurrently). Products include:
- Dalmane Capsules 2329

Glutethimide (Potential for serious side effects, including respiratory depression, hypotension, profound sedation and coma, if used concurrently).
- No products indexed under this heading.

Halazepam (Potential for serious side effects, including respiratory depression, hypotension, profound sedation and coma, if used concurrently).
- No products indexed under this heading.

Haloperidol (Potential for serious side effects, including respiratory depression, hypotension, profound sedation and coma, if used concurrently). Products include:
- Haldol Injection, Tablets and Concentrate 1585

Haloperidol Decanoate (Potential for serious side effects, including respiratory depression, hypotension, profound sedation and coma, if used concurrently). Products include:
- Haldol Decanoate 1587

Hydrocodone Bitartrate (Potential for serious side effects, including respiratory depression, hypotension, profound sedation and coma, if used concurrently). Products include:
- Codiclear DH Syrup 808
- Duratuss HD Elixir 2750
- Histussin D Liquid 670
- Hycodan Tablets and Syrup 946
- Hycomine Compound Tablets 948
- Hycomine 947
- Hycotuss Expectorant Syrup 950
- Hydrocet Capsules 787
- Lorcet 10/650 Tablets 1016
- Lortab 2751
- Tussend 1830
- Tussend Expectorant 1831
- Vicodin Tablets 1404
- Vicodin ES Tablets 1405
- Vicodin HP Tablets 1403
- Vicodin Tuss Expectorant 1406
- Zydone Capsules 967

Hydrocodone Polistirex (Potential for serious side effects, including respiratory depression, hypotension, profound sedation and coma, if used concurrently). Products include:
- Tussionex Pennkinetic Extended-Release Suspension 1624

Hydromorphone Hydrochloride (Potential for serious side effects, including respiratory depression, hypotension, profound sedation and coma, if used concurrently). Products include:
- Dilaudid Ampules 1382
- Dilaudid Cough Syrup 1383
- Dilaudid-HP Injection 1384
- Dilaudid-HP Lyophilized Powder 250 mg 1384
- Dilaudid 1382
- Dilaudid Oral Liquid 1386
- Dilaudid 1382
- Dilaudid Tablets - 8 mg 1386

Hydroxyzine Hydrochloride (Potential for serious side effects, including respiratory depression, hypotension, profound sedation and coma, if used concurrently). Products include:
- Atarax Tablets & Syrup 1992
- Marax Tablets & DF Syrup 2015
- Vistaril Intramuscular Solution 2042

Imipramine Hydrochloride (Potential for serious side effects, including respiratory depression, hypotension, profound sedation and coma, if used concurrently). Products include:
- Tofranil Ampuls 873
- Tofranil Tablets 875

Imipramine Pamoate (Potential for serious side effects, including respiratory depression, hypotension, profound sedation and coma, if used concurrently). Products include:
- Tofranil-PM Capsules 876

Isocarboxazid (Potential for serious side effects, including respiratory depression, hypotension, profound sedation and coma, if used concurrently).
- No products indexed under this heading.

Isoflurane (Potential for serious side effects, including respiratory depression, hypotension, profound sedation and coma, if used concurrently).
- No products indexed under this heading.

Ketamine Hydrochloride (Potential for serious side effects, including respiratory depression, hypotension, profound sedation and coma, if used concurrently).
- No products indexed under this heading.

Ketoconazole (May slow the onset, lower the activity and/or increase the duration of action of levomethadyl acetate hydrochloride). Products include:
- Nizoral 2% Cream 1344
- Nizoral 2% Shampoo 1344
- Nizoral Tablets 1345

Levorphanol Tartrate (Potential for serious side effects, including respiratory depression, hypotension, profound sedation and coma, if used concurrently). Products include:
- Levo-Dromoran 2297

Loratadine (Potential for serious side effects, including respiratory depression, hypotension, profound sedation and coma, if used concurrently). Products include:
- Claritin Tablets 2485
- Claritin-D Tablets 2487

Lorazepam (Potential for serious side effects, including respiratory depression, hypotension, profound sedation and coma, if used concurrently). Products include:
- Ativan Injection 2805
- Ativan Tablets 2807

Loxapine Hydrochloride (Potential for serious side effects, including respiratory depression, hypotension, profound sedation and coma, if used concurrently). Products include:
- Loxitane 1426

Loxapine Succinate (Potential for serious side effects, including respiratory depression, hypotension, profound sedation and coma, if used concurrently). Products include:
- Loxitane Capsules 1426

Maprotiline Hydrochloride (Potential for serious side effects, including respiratory depression, hypotension, profound sedation and coma, if used concurrently). Products include:
- Ludiomil Tablets 861

Meperidine Hydrochloride (Agonists, such as meperidine, should not be used concurrently because they would be ineffective unless given at high doses; potential for serious side effects, including respiratory depression, hypotension, profound sedation and coma, if used concurrently). Products include:
- Demerol 2438
- Mepergan Injection 2859

Mephobarbital (Potential for serious side effects, including respiratory depression, hypotension, profound sedation and coma, if used concurrently). Products include:
- Mebaral Tablets 2452

Meprobamate (Potential for serious side effects, including respiratory depression, hypotension, profound sedation and coma, if used concurrently). Products include:
- Miltown Tablets 2780
- PMB 200 and PMB 400 2890

Mesoridazine Besylate (Potential for serious side effects, including respiratory depression, hypotension, profound sedation and coma, if used concurrently). Products include:
- Serentil 689

Methadone Hydrochloride (Potential for serious side effects, including respiratory depression, hypotension, profound sedation and coma, if used concurrently). Products include:
- Methadone Hydrochloride Oral Concentrate 2356
- Methadone Hydrochloride Oral Solution & Tablets 2357

Methdilazine Hydrochloride (Potential for serious side effects, including respiratory depression, hypotension, profound sedation and coma, if used concurrently).
- No products indexed under this heading.

Methohexital Sodium (Potential for serious side effects, including respiratory depression, hypotension, profound sedation and coma, if used concurrently).
- No products indexed under this heading.

Methotrimeprazine (Potential for serious side effects, including respiratory depression, hypotension, profound sedation and coma, if used concurrently). Products include:
- Levoprome 1321

Methoxyflurane (Potential for serious side effects, including respiratory depression, hypotension, profound sedation and coma, if used concurrently).
- No products indexed under this heading.

Midazolam Hydrochloride (Potential for serious side effects, including respiratory depression, hypotension, profound sedation and coma, if used concurrently). Products include:
- Versed Injection 2324

Molindone Hydrochloride (Potential for serious side effects, including respiratory depression, hypotension, profound sedation and coma, if used concurrently). Products include:
- Moban Tablets and Concentrate 1036

Morphine Sulfate (Potential for serious side effects, including respiratory depression, hypotension, profound sedation and coma, if used concurrently). Products include:
- Astramorph/PF Injection, USP (Preservative-Free) 526
- Duramorph Injection 983
- Infumorph 200 and Infumorph 500 Sterile Solutions 985
- Kadian Capsules 2948
- MS Contin Tablets 2149
- MSIR 2152
- Oramorph SR (Morphine Sulfate Sustained Release Tablets) 2359
- RMS Suppositories CII 2766
- Roxanol 2365

Nalbuphine Hydrochloride (Patients maintained on levomethadyl acetate hydrochloride may experience withdrawal symptoms when administered mixed agonists/antagonists). Products include:
- Nubain Injection 952

Naloxone Hydrochloride (Patients maintained on levomethadyl acetate hydrochloride may experience withdrawal symptoms when administered naloxone). Products include:
- Narcan Injection 950
- Talwin Nx Tablets 2467

Naltrexone Hydrochloride (Patients maintained on levomethadyl acetate hydrochloride may experience withdrawal symptoms when administered naltrexone). Products include:
- ReVia Tablets 957

Nefazodone Hydrochloride (Potential for serious side effects, including respiratory depression, hypotension, profound sedation and coma, if used concurrently). Products include:
- Serzone Tablets 776

Nortriptyline Hydrochloride (Potential for serious side effects, including respiratory depression, hypotension, profound sedation and coma, if used concurrently). Products include:
- Pamelor 2409

Opium Alkaloids (Potential for serious side effects, including respiratory depression, hypotension, profound sedation and coma, if used concurrently).
- No products indexed under this heading.

Oxazepam (Potential for serious side effects, including respiratory depression, hypotension, profound sedation and coma, if used concurrently). Products include:
- Serax Capsules 2916
- Serax Tablets 2916

Oxycodone Hydrochloride (Potential for serious side effects, including respiratory depression, hypotension, profound sedation and coma, if used concurrently). Products include:

- OxyContin Tablets ... 2163
- OxyIR Capsules ... 2167
- Percocet Tablets ... 955
- Percodan Tablets ... 955
- Percodan-Demi Tablets ... 956
- Roxicodone Tablets, Oral Solution & Intensol (Oxycodone) ... 2366
- Tylox Capsules ... 1593

Paroxetine Hydrochloride (Potential for serious side effects, including respiratory depression, hypotension, profound sedation and coma, if used concurrently). Products include:

- Paxil Tablets ... 2681

Pentazocine Hydrochloride (Patients maintained on levomethadyl acetate hydrochloride may experience withdrawal symptoms when administered mixed agonists/antagonists). Products include:

- Talacen Caplets ... 2464
- Talwin Compound ... 2466
- Talwin Nx Tablets ... 2467

Pentazocine Lactate (Patients maintained on levomethadyl acetate hydrochloride may experience withdrawal symptoms when administered mixed agonists/antagonists). Products include:

- Talwin Injection ... 2465

Pentobarbital Sodium (Potential for serious side effects, including respiratory depression, hypotension, profound sedation and coma, if used concurrently). Products include:

- Nembutal Sodium Capsules ... 440
- Nembutal Sodium Solution ... 442
- Nembutal Sodium Suppositories ... 444

Perphenazine (Potential for serious side effects, including respiratory depression, hypotension, profound sedation and coma, if used concurrently). Products include:

- Etrafon ... 2495
- Triavil Tablets ... 1800
- Trilafon ... 2532

Phenelzine Sulfate (Potential for serious side effects, including respiratory depression, hypotension, profound sedation and coma, if used concurrently). Products include:

- Nardil ... 1977

Phenobarbital (May increase levomethadyl acetate hydrochloride's peak activity and/or shorten its duration of action). Products include:

- Arco-Lase Plus Tablets ... 513
- Bellergal-S Tablets ... 2375
- Donnatal ... 2234
- Donnatal Extentabs ... 2234
- Donnatal Tablets ... 2234
- Phenobarbital Elixir and Tablets ... 1523
- Quadrinal Tablets ... 1398

Phenytoin (May increase levomethadyl acetate hydrochloride's peak activity and/or shorten its duration of action). Products include:

- Dilantin Infatabs ... 1967
- Dilantin-125 Suspension ... 1969

Phenytoin Sodium (May increase levomethadyl acetate hydrochloride's peak activity and/or shorten its duration of action). Products include:

- Dilantin Kapseals ... 1965

Prazepam (Potential for serious side effects, including respiratory depression, hypotension, profound sedation and coma, if used concurrently).

No products indexed under this heading.

Prochlorperazine (Potential for serious side effects, including respiratory depression, hypotension, profound sedation and coma, if used concurrently). Products include:

- Compazine ... 2644

Promethazine Hydrochloride (Potential for serious side effects, including respiratory depression, hypotension, profound sedation and coma, if used concurrently). Products include:

- Mepergan Injection ... 2859
- Phenergan with Codeine ... 2883
- Phenergan with Dextromethorphan 2885
- Phenergan Injection ... 2880
- Phenergan Suppositories ... 2882
- Phenergan Syrup ... 2881
- Phenergan Tablets ... 2882
- Phenergan VC ... 2886
- Phenergan VC with Codeine ... 2888

Propofol (Potential for serious side effects, including respiratory depression, hypotension, profound sedation and coma, if used concurrently). Products include:

- Diprivan Injectable Emulsion ... 2939

Propoxyphene Hydrochloride (Agonists, such as propoxyphene, should not be used concurrently because they would be ineffective unless given at high doses; potential for serious side effects, including respiratory depression, hypotension, profound sedation and coma, if used concurrently). Products include:

- Darvon ... 1475
- Wygesic Tablets ... 2930

Propoxyphene Napsylate (Agonists, such as propoxyphene, should not be used concurrently because they would be ineffective unless given at high doses; potential for serious side effects, including respiratory depression, hypotension, profound sedation and coma, if used concurrently). Products include:

- Darvon-N/Darvocet-N ... 1473

Protriptyline Hydrochloride (Potential for serious side effects, including respiratory depression, hypotension, profound sedation and coma, if used concurrently). Products include:

- Vivactil Tablets ... 1820

Pyrilamine Maleate (Potential for serious side effects, including respiratory depression, hypotension, profound sedation and coma, if used concurrently). Products include:

- 4-Way Fast Acting Nasal Spray (regular & mentholated) ... 644
- Maximum Strength Multi-Symptom Formula Midol ... 621
- PMS Multi-Symptom Formula Midol ... 622

Pyrilamine Tannate (Potential for serious side effects, including respiratory depression, hypotension, profound sedation and coma, if used concurrently). Products include:

- Atrohist Pediatric Suspension ... 1604
- Atrohist Pediatric Suspension Dye-Free ... 1604
- Rynatan ... 2781

Quazepam (Potential for serious side effects, including respiratory depression, hypotension, profound sedation and coma, if used concurrently). Products include:

- Doral Tablets ... 2773

Rifampin (May increase levomethadyl acetate hydrochloride's peak activity and/or shorten its duration of action). Products include:

- Rifadin ... 1276
- Rifamate Capsules ... 1278
- Rifater ... 1280
- Rimactane Capsules ... 865

Risperidone (Potential for serious side effects, including respiratory depression, hypotension, profound sedation and coma, if used concurrently). Products include:

- Risperdal Tablets ... 1348

Secobarbital Sodium (Potential for serious side effects, including respiratory depression, hypotension, profound sedation and coma, if used concurrently). Products include:

- Seconal Sodium Pulvules ... 1529

Sertraline Hydrochloride (Potential for serious side effects, including respiratory depression, hypotension, profound sedation and coma, if used concurrently). Products include:

- Zoloft Tablets ... 2051

Sevoflurane (Potential for serious side effects, including respiratory depression, hypotension, profound sedation and coma, if used concurrently).

No products indexed under this heading.

Sufentanil Citrate (Potential for serious side effects, including respiratory depression, hypotension, profound sedation and coma, if used concurrently). Products include:

- Sufenta Injection ... 1355

Temazepam (Potential for serious side effects, including respiratory depression, hypotension, profound sedation and coma, if used concurrently). Products include:

- Restoril Capsules ... 2413

Terfenadine (Potential for serious side effects, including respiratory depression, hypotension, profound sedation and coma, if used concurrently). Products include:

- Seldane Tablets ... 1284
- Seldane-D Extended-Release Tablets ... 1286

Thiamylal Sodium (Potential for serious side effects, including respiratory depression, hypotension, profound sedation and coma, if used concurrently).

No products indexed under this heading.

Thioridazine Hydrochloride (Potential for serious side effects, including respiratory depression, hypotension, profound sedation and coma, if used concurrently). Products include:

- Mellaril ... 2398

Thiothixene (Potential for serious side effects, including respiratory depression, hypotension, profound sedation and coma, if used concurrently). Products include:

- Navane Capsules and Concentrate 2018
- Navane Intramuscular ... 2019

Tranylcypromine Sulfate (Potential for serious side effects, including respiratory depression, hypotension, profound sedation and coma, if used concurrently). Products include:

- Parnate Tablets ... 2679

Trazodone Hydrochloride (Potential for serious side effects, including respiratory depression, hypotension, profound sedation and coma, if used concurrently). Products include:

- Desyrel and Desyrel Dividose ... 504

Triazolam (Potential for serious side effects, including respiratory depression, hypotension, profound sedation and coma, if used concurrently). Products include:

- Halcion Tablets ... 2093

Trifluoperazine Hydrochloride (Potential for serious side effects, including respiratory depression, hypotension, profound sedation and coma, if used concurrently). Products include:

- Stelazine ... 2692

Trimeprazine Tartrate (Potential for serious side effects, including respiratory depression, hypotension, profound sedation and coma, if used concurrently).

No products indexed under this heading.

Trimipramine Maleate (Potential for serious side effects, including respiratory depression, hypotension, profound sedation and coma, if used concurrently). Products include:

- Surmontil Capsules ... 2917

Tripelennamine Hydrochloride (Potential for serious side effects, including respiratory depression, hypotension, profound sedation and coma, if used concurrently). Products include:

- PBZ Tablets ... 863
- PBZ-SR Tablets ... 862

Triprolidine Hydrochloride (Potential for serious side effects, including respiratory depression, hypotension, profound sedation and coma, if used concurrently). Products include:

- Actifed Cold & Allergy Tablets ... 807
- Actifed Cold & Sinus Caplets and Tablets ... 808

Venlafaxine Hydrochloride (Potential for serious side effects, including respiratory depression, hypotension, profound sedation and coma, if used concurrently). Products include:

- Effexor ... 2825

Zolpidem Tartrate (Potential for serious side effects, including respiratory depression, hypotension, profound sedation and coma, if used concurrently). Products include:

- Ambien Tablets ... 2559

Food Interactions

Alcohol (Potential for serious side effects, including respiratory depression, hypotension, profound sedation and coma, if used concurrently).

ORNADE SPANSULE CAPSULES

(Phenylpropanolamine Hydrochloride, Chlorpheniramine Maleate) ... 2678

May interact with monoamine oxidase inhibitors, central nervous system depressants, hypnotics and sedatives, tranquilizers, oral anticoagulants, anticholinergics, tricyclic antidepressants, beta blockers, corticosteroids, phenothiazines, and certain other agents. Compounds in these categories include:

Acebutolol Hydrochloride (Beta adrenergic blockers may be antagonized by antihistamines). Products include:

- Sectral Capsules ... 2914

Alfentanil Hydrochloride (Concurrent use results in potentiation of CNS depressant effects). Products include:

- Alfenta Injection ... 1334

Alprazolam (Concurrent use results in potentiation of CNS depressant effects). Products include:

- Xanax Tablets ... 2115

IMPORTANT NOTE: Always consult each drug listing in the patient's regimen for possible interactions.

Ornade Spansule — Interactions Index

Amitriptyline Hydrochloride (Co-administration of antihistamines with other drugs possessing anticholinergic action, such as tricyclic antidepressants, may result in xerostomia). Products include:
- Elavil 2945
- Etrafon 2495
- Limbitrol 2333
- Triavil Tablets 1800

Amoxapine (Co-administration of antihistamines with other drugs possessing anticholinergic action, such as tricyclic antidepressants, may result in xerostomia). Products include:
- Asendin Tablets 1419

Amphetamine Resins (Ornade may have additive effects when taken simultaneously with amphetamines).
- No products indexed under this heading.

Aprobarbital (Concurrent use results in potentiation of CNS depressant effects).
- No products indexed under this heading.

Atenolol (Beta adrenergic blockers may be antagonized by antihistamines). Products include:
- Tenoretic Tablets 2963
- Tenormin Tablets and I.V. Injection ... 2965

Atropine Sulfate (The CNS depressant and atropine-like effects (e.g., xerostomia) of anticholinergics may be potentiated by concomitant use of antihistamines). Products include:
- Arco-Lase Plus Tablets 513
- Atrohist Plus Tablets 1605
- Donnatal 2234
- Donnatal Extentabs 2234
- Donnatal 2234
- Lomotil 2591
- Motofen Tablets 789
- Urised Tablets 2123

Belladonna Alkaloids (The CNS depressant and atropine-like effects (e.g., xerostomia) of anticholinergics may be potentiated by concomitant use of antihistamines). Products include:
- Bellergal-S Tablets 2375
- Hyland's Bedwetting Tablets ... ⊞ 788
- Hyland's EnurAid Tablets ..... ⊞ 789
- Hyland's Headache Tablets .... ⊞ 790
- Hyland's Teething Tablets .... ⊞ 790
- Similasan Eye Drops #1 .... ⊞ 769

Benztropine Mesylate (The CNS depressant and atropine-like effects (e.g., xerostomia) of anticholinergics may be potentiated by concomitant use of antihistamines). Products include:
- Cogentin 1661

Betamethasone Acetate (Co-administration of corticosteroids with antihistamines may decrease the effects of corticosteroids by enzyme induction). Products include:
- Celestone Soluspan Suspension ... 2484

Betamethasone Sodium Phosphate (Co-administration of corticosteroids with antihistamines may decrease the effects of corticosteroids by enzyme induction). Products include:
- Celestone Soluspan Suspension ... 2484

Betaxolol Hydrochloride (Beta adrenergic blockers may be antagonized by antihistamines). Products include:
- Betoptic Ophthalmic Solution ... 465
- Betoptic S Ophthalmic Suspension ... 467
- Kerlone Tablets 2588

Biperiden Hydrochloride (The CNS depressant and atropine-like effects (e.g., xerostomia) of anticholinergics may be potentiated by concomitant use of antihistamines). Products include:
- Akineton 1380

Bisoprolol Fumarate (Beta adrenergic blockers may be antagonized by antihistamines). Products include:
- Zebeta Tablets 1457
- Ziac 1459

Buprenorphine (Concurrent use results in potentiation of CNS depressant effects). Products include:
- Buprenex Injectable 2170

Buspirone Hydrochloride (Concurrent use results in potentiation of CNS depressant effects). Products include:
- BuSpar Tablets 738

Butabarbital (Concurrent use results in potentiation of CNS depressant effects). Products include:
- No products indexed under this heading.

Butalbital (Concurrent use results in potentiation of CNS depressant effects). Products include:
- Axocet Capsules 2469
- Esgic-plus Capsules 1012
- Esgic-plus Tablets 1012
- Fioricet Tablets 2386
- Fioricet with Codeine Capsules ... 2387
- Fiorinal Capsules 2388
- Fiorinal with Codeine Capsules ... 2390
- Fiorinal Tablets 2388
- Phrenilin 790
- Sedapap Tablets 50 mg/650 mg ... 1826

Carteolol Hydrochloride (Beta adrenergic blockers may be antagonized by antihistamines). Products include:
- Cartrol Tablets 413
- Ocupress Ophthalmic Solution, 1% Sterile ... ⊙ 297

Chlordiazepoxide (Concurrent use results in potentiation of CNS depressant effects). Products include:
- Limbitrol 2333

Chlordiazepoxide Hydrochloride (Concurrent use results in potentiation of CNS depressant effects). Products include:
- Librax Capsules 2330
- Librium Capsules 2331
- Librium Injectable 2332

Chlorpromazine (Concomitant use of antihistamines and phenothiazines may produce an additive CNS depressant effect and may cause urinary retention or glaucoma). Products include:
- Thorazine Suppositories 2701

Chlorpromazine Hydrochloride (Concomitant use of antihistamines and phenothiazines may produce an additive CNS depressant effect and may cause urinary retention or glaucoma). Products include:
- Thorazine 2701

Chlorprothixene (Concurrent use results in potentiation of CNS depressant effects).
- No products indexed under this heading.

Chlorprothixene Hydrochloride (Concurrent use results in potentiation of CNS depressant effects).
- No products indexed under this heading.

Chlorprothixene Lactate (Concurrent use results in potentiation of CNS depressant effects).
- No products indexed under this heading.

Clidinium Bromide (The CNS depressant and atropine-like effects (e.g., xerostomia) of anticholinergics may be potentiated by concomitant use of antihistamines). Products include:
- Librax Capsules 2330

Clomipramine Hydrochloride (Co-administration of antihistamines with other drugs possessing anticholinergic action, such as tricyclic antidepressants, may result in xerostomia). Products include:
- Anafranil Capsules 819

Clorazepate Dipotassium (Concurrent use results in potentiation of CNS depressant effects). Products include:
- Tranxene 459

Clozapine (Concurrent use results in potentiation of CNS depressant effects). Products include:
- Clozaril Tablets 2377

Codeine Phosphate (Concurrent use results in potentiation of CNS depressant effects). Products include:
- Brontex 2130
- Dimetane-DC Cough Syrup ... 2232
- Fioricet with Codeine Capsules ... 2387
- Fiorinal with Codeine Capsules ... 2390
- Nucofed 2225
- Phenergan with Codeine 2883
- Phenergan VC with Codeine ... 2888
- Robitussin A-C Syrup 2248
- Robitussin-DAC Syrup 2249
- Ryna .... ⊞ 804
- Soma Compound w/Codeine Tablets ... 2784
- Tylenol with Codeine 1592

Cortisone Acetate (Co-administration of corticosteroids with antihistamines may decrease the effects of corticosteroids by enzyme induction). Products include:
- Cortone Acetate Sterile Suspension ... 1663
- Cortone Acetate Tablets 1664

Desflurane (Concurrent use results in potentiation of CNS depressant effects). Products include:
- Suprane (desflurane, USP) ... 1865

Desipramine Hydrochloride (Co-administration of antihistamines with other drugs possessing anticholinergic action, such as tricyclic antidepressants, may result in xerostomia). Products include:
- Norpramin Tablets 1273

Dexamethasone (Co-administration of corticosteroids with antihistamines may decrease the effects of corticosteroids by enzyme induction). Products include:
- AK-Trol Ointment & Suspension ... ⊙ 205
- Decadron Elixir 1676
- Decadron Tablets 1678
- Decaspray Topical Aerosol ... 1689
- Maxitrol Ophthalmic Ointment and Suspension ... ⊙ 222
- TobraDex Ophthalmic Suspension and Ointment ... 469

Dexamethasone Acetate (Co-administration of corticosteroids with antihistamines may decrease the effects of corticosteroids by enzyme induction). Products include:
- Dalalone D.P. Injectable 1009
- Decadron-LA Sterile Suspension ... 1687

Dexamethasone Sodium Phosphate (Co-administration of corticosteroids with antihistamines may decrease the effects of corticosteroids by enzyme induction). Products include:
- Decadron Phosphate Injection ... 1680
- Decadron Phosphate Sterile Ophthalmic Ointment ... 1684
- Decadron Phosphate Sterile Ophthalmic Solution ... 1685
- Decadron Phosphate Topical Cream ... 1686
- Decadron Phosphate with Xylocaine Injection, Sterile ... 1683
- Dexacort Phosphate in Respihaler ... 1606
- Dexacort Phosphate in Turbinaire ... 1607
- NeoDecadron Sterile Ophthalmic Ointment ... 1755
- NeoDecadron Sterile Ophthalmic Solution ... 1756
- NeoDecadron Topical Cream ... 1757

Dextroamphetamine Sulfate (Ornade may have additive effects when taken simultaneously with amphetamines). Products include:
- Adderall Tablets 2209
- Dexedrine 2648
- DextroStat-Dextroamphetamine Sulfate Tablets ... 2211

Dezocine (Concurrent use results in potentiation of CNS depressant effects). Products include:
- Dalgan Injection 529

Diazepam (Concurrent use results in potentiation of CNS depressant effects). Products include:
- Dizac (diazepam injectable emulsion) CIV ... 1862
- Valium Injectable 2336
- Valium Tablets 2335

Dicumarol (The action of oral anticoagulants may be inhibited by antihistamines).
- No products indexed under this heading.

Dicyclomine Hydrochloride (The CNS depressant and atropine-like effects (e.g., xerostomia) of anticholinergics may be potentiated by concomitant use of antihistamines). Products include:
- Bentyl 1246

Doxepin Hydrochloride (Co-administration of antihistamines with other drugs possessing anticholinergic action, such as tricyclic antidepressants, may result in xerostomia). Products include:
- Adapin Capsules 1542
- Sinequan 2028
- Zonalon Cream 1042

Droperidol (Concurrent use results in potentiation of CNS depressant effects). Products include:
- Inapsine Injection 462

Enflurane (Concurrent use results in potentiation of CNS depressant effects).
- No products indexed under this heading.

Esmolol Hydrochloride (Beta adrenergic blockers may be antagonized by antihistamines). Products include:
- Brevibloc (esmolol HCl) Injection ... 1860

Estazolam (Concurrent use results in potentiation of CNS depressant effects). Products include:
- ProSom Tablets 457

Ethchlorvynol (Concurrent use results in potentiation of CNS depressant effects). Products include:
- Placidyl Capsules 456

Ethinamate (Concurrent use results in potentiation of CNS depressant effects).
- No products indexed under this heading.

Fentanyl (Concurrent use results in potentiation of CNS depressant effects). Products include:
- Duragesic Transdermal System ... 1336

Fentanyl Citrate (Concurrent use results in potentiation of CNS depressant effects). Products include:
- Sublimaze Injection 463

(⊞ Described in PDR For Nonprescription Drugs)   (⊙ Described in PDR For Ophthalmology)

791 **Interactions Index** **Ornade Spansule**

Fludrocortisone Acetate (Co-administration of corticosteroids with antihistamines may decrease the effects of corticosteroids by enzyme induction). Products include:
- Florinef Acetate Tablets ... 506

Fluphenazine Decanoate (Concomitant use of antihistamines and phenothiazines may produce an additive CNS depressant effect and may cause urinary retention or glaucoma). Products include:
- Prolixin Decanoate ... 510

Fluphenazine Enanthate (Concomitant use of antihistamines and phenothiazines may produce an additive CNS depressant effect and may cause urinary retention or glaucoma). Products include:
- Prolixin Enanthate ... 510

Fluphenazine Hydrochloride (Concomitant use of antihistamines and phenothiazines may produce an additive CNS depressant effect and may cause urinary retention or glaucoma). Products include:
- Prolixin ... 510

Flurazepam Hydrochloride (Concurrent use results in potentiation of CNS depressant effects). Products include:
- Dalmane Capsules ... 2329

Furazolidone (MAO inhibitors prolong and intensify the anticholinergic effects of antihistamines and potentiate the pressor effects of sympathomimetics; concurrent use is contraindicated). Products include:
- Furoxone ... 2221

Glutethimide (Concurrent use results in potentiation of CNS depressant effects).
- No products indexed under this heading.

Glycopyrrolate (The CNS depressant and atropine-like effects (e.g., xerostomia) of anticholinergics may be potentiated by concomitant use of antihistamines). Products include:
- Robinul Forte Tablets ... 2247
- Robinul Injectable ... 2247
- Robinul Tablets ... 2247

Guanethidine Monosulfate (Phenylpropanolamine antagonizes the hypotensive action). Products include:
- Esimil Tablets ... 840
- Ismelin Tablets ... 845

Haloperidol (Concurrent use results in potentiation of CNS depressant effects). Products include:
- Haldol Injection, Tablets and Concentrate ... 1585

Haloperidol Decanoate (Concurrent use results in potentiation of CNS depressant effects). Products include:
- Haldol Decanoate ... 1587

Hydrocodone Bitartrate (Concurrent use results in potentiation of CNS depressant effects). Products include:
- Codiclear DH Syrup ... 808
- Duratuss HD Elixir ... 2750
- Histussin D Liquid ... 670
- Hycodan Tablets and Syrup ... 946
- Hycomine Compound Tablets ... 948
- Hycomine ... 947
- Hycotuss Expectorant Syrup ... 950
- Hydrocet Capsules ... 787
- Lorcet 10/650 Tablets ... 1016
- Lortab ... 2751
- Tussend ... 1830
- Tussend Expectorant ... 1831
- Vicodin Tablets ... 1404
- Vicodin ES Tablets ... 1405
- Vicodin HP Tablets ... 1403
- Vicodin Tuss Expectorant ... 1406
- Zydone Capsules ... 967

Hydrocodone Polistirex (Concurrent use results in potentiation of CNS depressant effects). Products include:
- Tussionex Pennkinetic Extended-Release Suspension ... 1624

Hydrocortisone (Co-administration of corticosteroids with antihistamines may decrease the effects of corticosteroids by enzyme induction). Products include:
- Anusol-HC Cream 2.5% ... 1953
- Aquanil HC Lotion ... 1989
- Maximum Strength Cortaid Spray ... 800
- CORTENEMA ... 2713
- Cortisporin Ointment ... 1074
- Cortisporin Ophthalmic Ointment Sterile ... 1074
- Cortisporin Ophthalmic Suspension Sterile ... 1075
- Cortisporin Otic Solution Sterile ... 1076
- Cortisporin Otic Suspension Sterile ... 1077
- Cortizone-5 ... 795
- Cortizone-10 ... 795
- Hydrocortone Tablets ... 1715
- Hytone ... 922
- Hytone Ointment 2 ½% ... 923
- Massengill Medicated Soft Cloth Towelettes ... 2628
- Pediotic Suspension Sterile ... 1140
- Preparation H Hydrocortisone 1% Cream ... 843
- ProctoCream-HC 2.5% ... 2552
- VōSoL HC Otic Solution ... 2786

Hydrocortisone Acetate (Co-administration of corticosteroids with antihistamines may decrease the effects of corticosteroids by enzyme induction). Products include:
- Analpram-HC Rectal Cream 1% and 2.5% ... 993
- Anusol HC-1 Hydrocortisone Anti-Itch Ointment ... 810
- Anusol-HC Suppositories ... 1954
- Caldecort Anti-Itch Hydrocortisone Cream ... 651
- Coly-Mycin S Otic w/Neomycin & Hydrocortisone ... 1965
- Cortaid ... 800
- Cortifoam ... 2540
- Cortisporin Cream ... 1073
- Epifoam ... 2543
- Hydrocortone Acetate Sterile Suspension ... 1712
- Mantadil Cream ... 1124
- Nupercainal Hydrocortisone 1% Cream ... 661
- Pramosone Cream, Lotion & Ointment ... 995
- ProctoFoam-HC ... 2552
- Terra-Cortril Ophthalmic Suspension ... 2033

Hydrocortisone Sodium Phosphate (Co-administration of corticosteroids with antihistamines may decrease the effects of corticosteroids by enzyme induction). Products include:
- Hydrocortone Phosphate Injection, Sterile ... 1713

Hydrocortisone Sodium Succinate (Co-administration of corticosteroids with antihistamines may decrease the effects of corticosteroids by enzyme induction).
- No products indexed under this heading.

Hydroxyzine Hydrochloride (Concurrent use results in potentiation of CNS depressant effects). Products include:
- Atarax Tablets & Syrup ... 1992
- Marax Tablets & DF Syrup ... 2015
- Vistaril Intramuscular Solution ... 2042

Hyoscyamine (The CNS depressant and atropine-like effects (e.g., xerostomia) of anticholinergics may be potentiated by concomitant use of antihistamines). Products include:
- Cystospaz Tablets ... 2123
- Urised Tablets ... 2123

Hyoscyamine Sulfate (The CNS depressant and atropine-like effects (e.g., xerostomia) of anticholinergics may be potentiated by concomitant use of antihistamines). Products include:
- Arco-Lase Plus Tablets ... 513
- Atrohist Plus Tablets ... 1605
- Cystospaz-M Capsules ... 2123
- Donnatal ... 2234
- Donnatal Extentabs ... 2234
- Donnatal Tablets ... 2234
- Kutrase Capsules ... 2546
- Levsin/Levsinex/Levbid ... 2549

Imipramine Hydrochloride (Co-administration of antihistamines with other drugs possessing anticholinergic action, such as tricyclic antidepressants, may result in xerostomia). Products include:
- Tofranil Ampuls ... 873
- Tofranil Tablets ... 875

Imipramine Pamoate (Co-administration of antihistamines with other drugs possessing anticholinergic action, such as tricyclic antidepressants, may result in xerostomia). Products include:
- Tofranil-PM Capsules ... 876

Ipratropium Bromide (The CNS depressant and atropine-like effects (e.g., xerostomia) of anticholinergics may be potentiated by concomitant use of antihistamines). Products include:
- Atrovent Inhalation Aerosol ... 674
- Atrovent Inhalation Solution ... 675
- Atrovent Nasal Spray 0.03% ... 676
- Atrovent Nasal Spray 0.06% ... 678

Isocarboxazid (MAO inhibitors prolong and intensify the anticholinergic effects of antihistamines and potentiate the pressor effects of sympathomimetics; concurrent use is contraindicated).
- No products indexed under this heading.

Isoflurane (Concurrent use results in potentiation of CNS depressant effects).
- No products indexed under this heading.

Ketamine Hydrochloride (Concurrent use results in potentiation of CNS depressant effects).
- No products indexed under this heading.

Labetalol Hydrochloride (Beta adrenergic blockers may be antagonized by antihistamines). Products include:
- Normodyne Injection ... 2519
- Normodyne Tablets ... 2522
- Trandate ... 1158

Levobunolol Hydrochloride (Beta adrenergic blockers may be antagonized by antihistamines). Products include:
- Betagan ... ◎ 230

Levomethadyl Acetate Hydrochloride (Concurrent use results in potentiation of CNS depressant effects). Products include:
- Orlaam Oral Solution ... 2361

Levorphanol Tartrate (Concurrent use results in potentiation of CNS depressant effects). Products include:
- Levo-Dromoran ... 2297

Lorazepam (Concurrent use results in potentiation of CNS depressant effects). Products include:
- Ativan Injection ... 2805
- Ativan Tablets ... 2807

Loxapine Hydrochloride (Concurrent use results in potentiation of CNS depressant effects). Products include:
- Loxitane ... 1426

Loxapine Succinate (Concurrent use results in potentiation of CNS depressant effects). Products include:
- Loxitane Capsules ... 1426

Maprotiline Hydrochloride (Co-administration of antihistamines with other drugs possessing anticholinergic action, such as tricyclic antidepressants, may result in xerostomia). Products include:
- Ludiomil Tablets ... 861

Mecamylamine Hydrochloride (Mecamylamine, a ganglionic blocking drug, potentiates reactions of sympathomimetics). Products include:
- Inversine Tablets ... 1729

Mepenzolate Bromide (The CNS depressant and atropine-like effects (e.g., xerostomia) of anticholinergics may be potentiated by concomitant use of antihistamines).
- No products indexed under this heading.

Meperidine Hydrochloride (Concurrent use results in potentiation of CNS depressant effects). Products include:
- Demerol ... 2438
- Mepergan Injection ... 2859

Mephobarbital (Concurrent use results in potentiation of CNS depressant effects). Products include:
- Mebaral Tablets ... 2452

Meprobamate (Concurrent use results in potentiation of CNS depressant effects). Products include:
- Miltown Tablets ... 2780
- PMB 200 and PMB 400 ... 2890

Mesoridazine Besylate (Concomitant use of antihistamines and phenothiazines may produce an additive CNS depressant effect and may cause urinary retention or glaucoma). Products include:
- Serentil ... 689

Methadone Hydrochloride (Concurrent use results in potentiation of CNS depressant effects). Products include:
- Methadone Hydrochloride Oral Concentrate ... 2356
- Methadone Hydrochloride Oral Solution & Tablets ... 2357

Methamphetamine Hydrochloride (Ornade may have additive effects when taken simultaneously with amphetamines). Products include:
- Desoxyn Gradumet Tablets ... 422

Methohexital Sodium (Concurrent use results in potentiation of CNS depressant effects).
- No products indexed under this heading.

Methotrimeprazine (Concomitant use of antihistamines and phenothiazines may produce an additive CNS depressant effect and may cause urinary retention or glaucoma). Products include:
- Levoprome ... 1321

Methoxyflurane (Concurrent use results in potentiation of CNS depressant effects).
- No products indexed under this heading.

Methylprednisolone Acetate (Co-administration of corticosteroids with antihistamines may decrease the effects of corticosteroids by enzyme induction).
- No products indexed under this heading.

IMPORTANT NOTE: Always consult each drug listing in the patient's regimen for possible interactions.

Ornade Spansule
Interactions Index
792

Methylprednisolone Sodium Succinate (Co-administration of corticosteroids with antihistamines may decrease the effects of corticosteroids by enzyme induction).
No products indexed under this heading.

Metipranolol Hydrochloride (Beta adrenergic blockers may be antagonized by antihistamines). Products include:
OptiPranolol (Metipranolol 0.3%) Sterile Ophthalmic Solution ⊙ 256

Metoprolol Succinate (Beta adrenergic blockers may be antagonized by antihistamines). Products include:
Toprol-XL Tablets 560

Metoprolol Tartrate (Beta adrenergic blockers may be antagonized by antihistamines). Products include:
Lopressor 848
Lopressor HCT Tablets 850

Midazolam Hydrochloride (Concurrent use results in potentiation of CNS depressant effects). Products include:
Versed Injection 2324

Molindone Hydrochloride (Concurrent use results in potentiation of CNS depressant effects). Products include:
Moban Tablets and Concentrate 1036

Morphine Sulfate (Concurrent use results in potentiation of CNS depressant effects). Products include:
Astramorph/PF Injection, USP (Preservative-Free) 526
Duramorph Injection 983
Infumorph 200 and Infumorph 500 Sterile Solutions 985
Kadian Capsules 2948
MS Contin Tablets 2149
MSIR 2152
Oramorph SR (Morphine Sulfate Sustained Release Tablets) 2359
RMS Suppositories CII 2766
Roxanol 2365

Nadolol (Beta adrenergic blockers may be antagonized by antihistamines).
No products indexed under this heading.

Norepinephrine Bitartrate (Antihistamines inhibit norepinephrine reuptake by tissues and therefore potentiate the cardiovascular effects of norepinephrine). Products include:
Levophed Bitartrate Injection 2445

Nortriptyline Hydrochloride (Co-administration of antihistamines with other drugs possessing anticholinergic action, such as tricyclic antidepressants, may result in xerostomia). Products include:
Pamelor 2409

Opium Alkaloids (Concurrent use results in potentiation of CNS depressant effects).
No products indexed under this heading.

Oxazepam (Concurrent use results in potentiation of CNS depressant effects). Products include:
Serax Capsules 2916
Serax Tablets 2916

Oxybutynin Chloride (The CNS depressant and atropine-like effects (e.g., xerostomia) of anticholinergics may be potentiated by concomitant use of antihistamines). Products include:
Ditropan 1267

Oxycodone Hydrochloride (Concurrent use results in potentiation of CNS depressant effects). Products include:
OxyContin Tablets 2163
OxyIR Capsules 2167
Percocet Tablets 955
Percodan Tablets 955
Percodan-Demi Tablets 956
Roxicodone Tablets, Oral Solution & Intensol (Oxycodone) 2366
Tylox Capsules 1593

Penbutolol Sulfate (Beta adrenergic blockers may be antagonized by antihistamines). Products include:
Levatol Tablets 2547

Pentobarbital Sodium (Concurrent use results in potentiation of CNS depressant effects). Products include:
Nembutal Sodium Capsules 440
Nembutal Sodium Solution 442
Nembutal Sodium Suppositories 444

Perphenazine (Concomitant use of antihistamines and phenothiazines may produce an additive CNS depressant effect and may cause urinary retention or glaucoma). Products include:
Etrafon 2495
Triavil Tablets 1800
Trilafon 2532

Phenelzine Sulfate (MAO inhibitors prolong and intensify the anticholinergic effects of antihistamines and potentiate the pressor effects of sympathomimetics; concurrent use is contraindicated). Products include:
Nardil 1977

Phenobarbital (Concurrent use results in potentiation of CNS depressant effects). Products include:
Arco-Lase Plus Tablets 513
Bellergal-S Tablets 2375
Donnatal 2234
Donnatal Extentabs 2234
Donnatal Tablets 2234
Phenobarbital Elixir and Tablets 1523
Quadrinal Tablets 1398

Phenylpropanolamine Containing Anorectics (Ornade may have additive effects when taken simultaneously with other phenylpropanolamine-containing products).

Pindolol (Beta adrenergic blockers may be antagonized by antihistamines). Products include:
Visken Tablets 2428

Prazepam (Concurrent use results in potentiation of CNS depressant effects).
No products indexed under this heading.

Prednisolone Acetate (Co-administration of corticosteroids with antihistamines may decrease the effects of corticosteroids by enzyme induction). Products include:
AK-CIDE ⊙ 203
AK-CIDE Ointment ⊙ 203
Blephamide Liquifilm Sterile Ophthalmic Suspension 472
Blephamide Ointment ⊙ 234
Econopred & Econopred Plus Ophthalmic Suspensions ⊙ 216
Poly-Pred Liquifilm ⊙ 246
Pred Forte ⊙ 247
Pred Mild ⊙ 250
Pred-G Liquifilm Sterile Ophthalmic Suspension ⊙ 248
Pred-G S.O.P. Sterile Ophthalmic Ointment ⊙ 249

Prednisolone Sodium Phosphate (Co-administration of corticosteroids with antihistamines may decrease the effects of corticosteroids by enzyme induction). Products include:
AK-PRED ⊙ 204
Hydeltrasol Injection, Sterile 1708
Pediapred Oral Solution 1618

Prednisolone Tebutate (Co-administration of corticosteroids with antihistamines may decrease the effects of corticosteroids by enzyme induction). Products include:
Hydeltra-T.B.A. Sterile Suspension 1710

Prednisone (Co-administration of corticosteroids with antihistamines may decrease the effects of corticosteroids by enzyme induction).
No products indexed under this heading.

Prochlorperazine (Concomitant use of antihistamines and phenothiazines may produce an additive CNS depressant effect and may cause urinary retention or glaucoma). Products include:
Compazine 2644

Procyclidine Hydrochloride (The CNS depressant and atropine-like effects (e.g., xerostomia) of anticholinergics may be potentiated by concomitant use of antihistamines). Products include:
Kemadrin Tablets 1105

Promethazine Hydrochloride (Concomitant use of antihistamines and phenothiazines may produce an additive CNS depressant effect and may cause urinary retention or glaucoma). Products include:
Mepergan Injection 2859
Phenergan with Codeine 2883
Phenergan with Dextromethorphan 2885
Phenergan Injection 2880
Phenergan Suppositories 2882
Phenergan Syrup 2881
Phenergan Tablets 2882
Phenergan VC 2886
Phenergan VC with Codeine 2888

Propantheline Bromide (The CNS depressant and atropine-like effects (e.g., xerostomia) of anticholinergics may be potentiated by concomitant use of antihistamines). Products include:
Pro-Banthine Tablets 2226

Propofol (Concurrent use results in potentiation of CNS depressant effects). Products include:
Diprivan Injectable Emulsion 2939

Propoxyphene Hydrochloride (Concurrent use results in potentiation of CNS depressant effects). Products include:
Darvon 1475
Wygesic Tablets 2930

Propoxyphene Napsylate (Concurrent use results in potentiation of CNS depressant effects). Products include:
Darvon-N/Darvocet-N 1473

Propranolol Hydrochloride (Beta adrenergic blockers may be antagonized by antihistamines). Products include:
Inderal 2834
Inderal LA Long Acting Capsules 2836
Inderide Tablets 2838
Inderide LA Long Acting Capsules 2840

Protriptyline Hydrochloride (Co-administration of antihistamines with other drugs possessing anticholinergic action, such as tricyclic antidepressants, may result in xerostomia). Products include:
Vivactil Tablets 1820

Quazepam (Concurrent use results in potentiation of CNS depressant effects). Products include:
Doral Tablets 2773

Risperidone (Concurrent use results in potentiation of CNS depressant effects). Products include:
Risperdal Tablets 1348

Scopolamine (The CNS depressant and atropine-like effects (e.g., xerostomia) of anticholinergics may be potentiated by concomitant use of antihistamines). Products include:
Transderm Scōp Transdermal Therapeutic System 890

Scopolamine Hydrobromide (The CNS depressant and atropine-like effects (e.g., xerostomia) of anticholinergics may be potentiated by concomitant use of antihistamines). Products include:
Atrohist Plus Tablets 1605
Donnatal 2234
Donnatal Extentabs 2234
Donnatal Tablets 2234

Secobarbital Sodium (Concurrent use results in potentiation of CNS depressant effects). Products include:
Seconal Sodium Pulvules 1529

Selegiline Hydrochloride (MAO inhibitors prolong and intensify the anticholinergic effects of antihistamines and potentiate the pressor effects of sympathomimetics; concurrent use is contraindicated). Products include:
Eldepryl Capsules 2729

Sevoflurane (Concurrent use results in potentiation of CNS depressant effects).
No products indexed under this heading.

Sotalol Hydrochloride (Beta adrenergic blockers may be antagonized by antihistamines). Products include:
Betapace Tablets 637

Sufentanil Citrate (Concurrent use results in potentiation of CNS depressant effects). Products include:
Sufenta Injection 1355

Temazepam (Concurrent use results in potentiation of CNS depressant effects). Products include:
Restoril Capsules 2413

Thiamylal Sodium (Concurrent use results in potentiation of CNS depressant effects).
No products indexed under this heading.

Thioridazine Hydrochloride (Concomitant use of antihistamines and phenothiazines may produce an additive CNS depressant effect and may cause urinary retention or glaucoma). Products include:
Mellaril 2398

Thiothixene (Concurrent use results in potentiation of CNS depressant effects). Products include:
Navane Capsules and Concentrate 2018
Navane Intramuscular 2019

Timolol Hemihydrate (Beta adrenergic blockers may be antagonized by antihistamines). Products include:
Betimol 0.25%, 0.5% ⊙ 259

Timolol Maleate (Beta adrenergic blockers may be antagonized by antihistamines). Products include:
Blocadren Tablets 1654
Timolide Tablets 1791
Timoptic in Ocudose 1796
Timoptic Sterile Ophthalmic Solution 1794
Timoptic-XE 1798

Tranylcypromine Sulfate (MAO inhibitors prolong and intensify the anticholinergic effects of antihistamines and potentiate the pressor effects of sympathomimetics; concurrent use is contraindicated). Products include:
Parnate Tablets 2679

Triamcinolone (Co-administration of corticosteroids with antihistamines may decrease the effects of corticosteroids by enzyme induction).
  No products indexed under this heading.

Triamcinolone Acetonide (Co-administration of corticosteroids with antihistamines may decrease the effects of corticosteroids by enzyme induction). Products include:
  Azmacort Oral Inhaler 2175
  Nasacort AQ Nasal Spray 2191
  Nasacort Nasal Inhaler 2189

Triamcinolone Diacetate (Co-administration of corticosteroids with antihistamines may decrease the effects of corticosteroids by enzyme induction).
  No products indexed under this heading.

Triamcinolone Hexacetonide (Co-administration of corticosteroids with antihistamines may decrease the effects of corticosteroids by enzyme induction).
  No products indexed under this heading.

Triazolam (Concurrent use results in potentiation of CNS depressant effects). Products include:
  Halcion Tablets 2093

Tridihexethyl Chloride (The CNS depressant and atropine-like effects (e.g., xerostomia) of anticholinergics may be potentiated by concomitant use of antihistamines).
  No products indexed under this heading.

Trifluoperazine Hydrochloride (Concomitant use of antihistamines and phenothiazines may produce an additive CNS depressant effect and may cause urinary retention or glaucoma). Products include:
  Stelazine 2692

Trihexyphenidyl Hydrochloride (The CNS depressant and atropine-like effects (e.g., xerostomia) of anticholinergics may be potentiated by concomitant use of antihistamines). Products include:
  Artane 1418

Trimipramine Maleate (Co-administration of antihistamines with other drugs possessing anticholinergic action, such as tricyclic antidepressants, may result in xerostomia). Products include:
  Surmontil Capsules 2917

Warfarin Sodium (The action of oral anticoagulants may be inhibited by antihistamines). Products include:
  Coumadin 941

Zolpidem Tartrate (Concurrent use results in potentiation of CNS depressant effects). Products include:
  Ambien Tablets 2559

Food Interactions
Alcohol (Concurrent use results in potentiation of CNS depressant effects).

ORTHO-CEPT 21 TABLETS
(Desogestrel, Ethinyl Estradiol) 1907
May interact with barbiturates, tetracyclines, and certain other agents. Compounds in these categories include:

Ampicillin (Potential for reduced efficacy and increased incidence of breakthrough bleeding and menstrual irregularities with concomitant use). Products include:
  Omnipen Capsules 2872
  Omnipen for Oral Suspension 2873

Ampicillin Sodium (Potential for reduced efficacy and increased incidence of breakthrough bleeding and menstrual irregularities with concomitant use). Products include:
  Unasyn 2035

Aprobarbital (Potential for reduced efficacy and increased incidence of breakthrough bleeding and menstrual irregularities with concomitant use).
  No products indexed under this heading.

Butabarbital (Potential for reduced efficacy and increased incidence of breakthrough bleeding and menstrual irregularities with concomitant use).
  No products indexed under this heading.

Butalbital (Potential for reduced efficacy and increased incidence of breakthrough bleeding and menstrual irregularities with concomitant use). Products include:
  Axocet Capsules 2469
  Esgic-plus Capsules 1012
  Esgic-plus Tablets 1012
  Fioricet Tablets 2386
  Fioricet with Codeine Capsules 2387
  Fiorinal Capsules 2388
  Fiorinal with Codeine Capsules ... 2390
  Fiorinal Tablets 2388
  Phrenilin 790
  Sedapap Tablets 50 mg/650 mg .. 1826

Carbamazepine (Potential for reduced efficacy and increased incidence of breakthrough bleeding and menstrual irregularities with concomitant use). Products include:
  Atretol Tablets 569
  Tegretol/Tegretol-XR 870

Demeclocycline Hydrochloride (Potential for reduced efficacy and increased incidence of breakthrough bleeding and menstrual irregularities with concomitant use). Products include:
  Declomycin Tablets 1421

Doxycycline Calcium (Potential for reduced efficacy and increased incidence of breakthrough bleeding and menstrual irregularities with concomitant use). Products include:
  Vibramycin Calcium Oral Suspension Syrup 2038

Doxycycline Hyclate (Potential for reduced efficacy and increased incidence of breakthrough bleeding and menstrual irregularities with concomitant use). Products include:
  Doryx Capsules 1970
  Vibramycin Hyclate Capsules 2038
  Vibramycin Hyclate Intravenous .. 2040
  Vibra-Tabs Film Coated Tablets ... 2038

Doxycycline Monohydrate (Potential for reduced efficacy and increased incidence of breakthrough bleeding and menstrual irregularities with concomitant use). Products include:
  Monodox Capsules 1858
  Vibramycin Monohydrate for Oral Suspension 2038

Fosphenytoin Sodium (Potential for reduced efficacy and increased incidence of breakthrough bleeding and menstrual irregularities with concomitant use). Products include:
  Cerebyx Injection 1956

Griseofulvin (Potential for reduced efficacy and increased incidence of breakthrough bleeding and menstrual irregularities with concomitant use). Products include:
  Fulvicin P/G Tablets 2499
  Fulvicin P/G 165 & 330 Tablets ... 2500
  Grifulvin V (griseofulvin tablets) Microsize (griseofulvin oral suspension) Microsize 1944
  Gris-PEG Tablets, 125 mg & 250 mg 476

Mephobarbital (Potential for reduced efficacy and increased incidence of breakthrough bleeding and menstrual irregularities with concomitant use). Products include:
  Mebaral Tablets 2452

Methacycline Hydrochloride (Potential for reduced efficacy and increased incidence of breakthrough bleeding and menstrual irregularities with concomitant use).
  No products indexed under this heading.

Minocycline Hydrochloride (Potential for reduced efficacy and increased incidence of breakthrough bleeding and menstrual irregularities with concomitant use). Products include:
  DYNACIN Capsules 1627
  Minocin Intravenous 1428
  Minocin Oral Suspension 1431
  Minocin Pellet-Filled Capsules ... 1429

Oxytetracycline Hydrochloride (Potential for reduced efficacy and increased incidence of breakthrough bleeding and menstrual irregularities with concomitant use). Products include:
  TERAK Ointment 210
  Terra-Cortril Ophthalmic Suspension 2033
  Terramycin with Polymyxin B Sulfate Ophthalmic Ointment 2035
  Urobiotic-250 Capsules 2038

Pentobarbital Sodium (Potential for reduced efficacy and increased incidence of breakthrough bleeding and menstrual irregularities with concomitant use). Products include:
  Nembutal Sodium Capsules 440
  Nembutal Sodium Solution 442
  Nembutal Sodium Suppositories .. 444

Phenobarbital (Potential for reduced efficacy and increased incidence of breakthrough bleeding and menstrual irregularities with concomitant use). Products include:
  Arco-Lase Plus Tablets 513
  Bellergal-S Tablets 2375
  Donnatal 2234
  Donnatal Extentabs 2234
  Donnatal Tablets 2234
  Phenobarbital Elixir and Tablets .. 1523
  Quadrinal Tablets 1398

Phenylbutazone (Potential for reduced efficacy and increased incidence of breakthrough bleeding and menstrual irregularities with concomitant use).
  No products indexed under this heading.

Phenytoin (Potential for reduced efficacy and increased incidence of breakthrough bleeding and menstrual irregularities with concomitant use). Products include:
  Dilantin Infatabs 1967
  Dilantin-125 Suspension 1969

Phenytoin Sodium (Potential for reduced efficacy and increased incidence of breakthrough bleeding and menstrual irregularities with concomitant use). Products include:
  Dilantin Kapseals 1965

Rifampin (Co-administration has been associated with reduced efficacy and increased incidence of breakthrough bleeding and menstrual irregularities). Products include:
  Rifadin 1276
  Rifamate Capsules 1278
  Rifater 1280
  Rimactane Capsules 865

Secobarbital Sodium (Potential for reduced efficacy and increased incidence of breakthrough bleeding and menstrual irregularities with concomitant use). Products include:
  Seconal Sodium Pulvules 1529

Tetracycline Hydrochloride (Potential for reduced efficacy and increased incidence of breakthrough bleeding and menstrual irregularities with concomitant use). Products include:
  Achromycin V Capsules 1417
  Helidac Therapy 2135

Thiamylal Sodium (Potential for reduced efficacy and increased incidence of breakthrough bleeding and menstrual irregularities with concomitant use).
  No products indexed under this heading.

ORTHO-CEPT 28 TABLETS
(Desogestrel, Ethinyl Estradiol) 1907
See **Ortho-Cept 21 Tablets**

ORTHO-CYCLEN 21 TABLETS
(Norgestimate, Ethinyl Estradiol) 1914
May interact with barbiturates, tetracyclines, and certain other agents. Compounds in these categories include:

Ampicillin (Potential for reduced efficacy and increased incidence of breakthrough bleeding and menstrual irregularities with concomitant use). Products include:
  Omnipen Capsules 2872
  Omnipen for Oral Suspension 2873

Ampicillin Sodium (Potential for reduced efficacy and increased incidence of breakthrough bleeding and menstrual irregularities with concomitant use). Products include:
  Unasyn 2035

Aprobarbital (Potential for reduced efficacy and increased incidence of breakthrough bleeding and menstrual irregularities with concomitant use).
  No products indexed under this heading.

Butabarbital (Potential for reduced efficacy and increased incidence of breakthrough bleeding and menstrual irregularities with concomitant use).
  No products indexed under this heading.

Butalbital (Potential for reduced efficacy and increased incidence of breakthrough bleeding and menstrual irregularities with concomitant use). Products include:
  Axocet Capsules 2469
  Esgic-plus Capsules 1012
  Esgic-plus Tablets 1012
  Fioricet Tablets 2386
  Fioricet with Codeine Capsules 2387
  Fiorinal Capsules 2388
  Fiorinal with Codeine Capsules ... 2390
  Fiorinal Tablets 2388
  Phrenilin 790
  Sedapap Tablets 50 mg/650 mg .. 1826

Carbamazepine (Potential for reduced efficacy and increased incidence of breakthrough bleeding and menstrual irregularities with concomitant use). Products include:
  Atretol Tablets 569
  Tegretol/Tegretol-XR 870

Demeclocycline Hydrochloride (Potential for reduced efficacy and increased incidence of breakthrough bleeding and menstrual irregularities with concomitant use). Products include:
  Declomycin Tablets 1421

IMPORTANT NOTE: Always consult each drug listing in the patient's regimen for possible interactions.

Ortho-Cyclen/Ortho-Tri-Cyclen — Interactions Index

Doxycycline Calcium (Potential for reduced efficacy and increased incidence of breakthrough bleeding and menstrual irregularities with concomitant use). Products include:
- Vibramycin Calcium Oral Suspension Syrup 2038

Doxycycline Hyclate (Potential for reduced efficacy and increased incidence of breakthrough bleeding and menstrual irregularities with concomitant use). Products include:
- Doryx Capsules 1970
- Vibramycin Hyclate Capsules 2038
- Vibramycin Hyclate Intravenous 2040
- Vibra-Tabs Film Coated Tablets 2038

Doxycycline Monohydrate (Potential for reduced efficacy and increased incidence of breakthrough bleeding and menstrual irregularities with concomitant use). Products include:
- Monodox Capsules 1858
- Vibramycin Monohydrate for Oral Suspension 2038

Fosphenytoin Sodium (Potential for reduced efficacy and increased incidence of breakthrough bleeding and menstrual irregularities with concomitant use). Products include:
- Cerebyx Injection 1956

Griseofulvin (Potential for reduced efficacy and increased incidence of breakthrough bleeding and menstrual irregularities with concomitant use). Products include:
- Fulvicin P/G Tablets 2499
- Fulvicin P/G 165 & 330 Tablets 2500
- Grifulvin V (griseofulvin tablets) Microsize (griseofulvin oral suspension) Microsize 1944
- Gris-PEG Tablets, 125 mg & 250 mg 476

Mephobarbital (Potential for reduced efficacy and increased incidence of breakthrough bleeding and menstrual irregularities with concomitant use). Products include:
- Mebaral Tablets 2452

Methacycline Hydrochloride (Potential for reduced efficacy and increased incidence of breakthrough bleeding and menstrual irregularities with concomitant use).
No products indexed under this heading.

Minocycline Hydrochloride (Potential for reduced efficacy and increased incidence of breakthrough bleeding and menstrual irregularities with concomitant use). Products include:
- DYNACIN Capsules 1627
- Minocin Intravenous 1428
- Minocin Oral Suspension 1431
- Minocin Pellet-Filled Capsules 1429

Oxytetracycline Hydrochloride (Potential for reduced efficacy and increased incidence of breakthrough bleeding and menstrual irregularities with concomitant use). Products include:
- TERAK Ointment .... ⊚ 210
- Terra-Cortril Ophthalmic Suspension 2033
- Terramycin with Polymyxin B Sulfate Ophthalmic Ointment 2035
- Urobiotic-250 Capsules 2038

Pentobarbital Sodium (Potential for reduced efficacy and increased incidence of breakthrough bleeding and menstrual irregularities with concomitant use). Products include:
- Nembutal Sodium Capsules 440
- Nembutal Sodium Solution 442
- Nembutal Sodium Suppositories...... 444

Phenobarbital (Potential for reduced efficacy and increased incidence of breakthrough bleeding and menstrual irregularities with concomitant use). Products include:
- Arco-Lase Plus Tablets 513
- Bellergal-S Tablets 2375
- Donnatal 2234
- Donnatal Extentabs 2234
- Donnatal Tablets 2234
- Phenobarbital Elixir and Tablets 1523
- Quadrinal Tablets 1398

Phenylbutazone (Potential for reduced efficacy and increased incidence of breakthrough bleeding and menstrual irregularities with concomitant use).
No products indexed under this heading.

Phenytoin (Potential for reduced efficacy and increased incidence of breakthrough bleeding and menstrual irregularities with concomitant use). Products include:
- Dilantin Infatabs 1967
- Dilantin-125 Suspension 1969

Phenytoin Sodium (Potential for reduced efficacy and increased incidence of breakthrough bleeding and menstrual irregularities with concomitant use). Products include:
- Dilantin Kapseals 1965

Rifampin (Co-administration has been associated with reduced efficacy and increased incidence of breakthrough bleeding and menstrual irregularities). Products include:
- Rifadin 1276
- Rifamate Capsules 1278
- Rifater 1280
- Rimactane Capsules 865

Secobarbital Sodium (Potential for reduced efficacy and increased incidence of breakthrough bleeding and menstrual irregularities with concomitant use). Products include:
- Seconal Sodium Pulvules 1529

Tetracycline Hydrochloride (Potential for reduced efficacy and increased incidence of breakthrough bleeding and menstrual irregularities with concomitant use). Products include:
- Achromycin V Capsules 1417
- Helidac Therapy 2135

Thiamylal Sodium (Potential for reduced efficacy and increased incidence of breakthrough bleeding and menstrual irregularities with concomitant use).
No products indexed under this heading.

ORTHO-CYCLEN 28 TABLETS
(Norgestimate, Ethinyl Estradiol)........1914
See Ortho-Cyclen 21 Tablets

ORTHO DIAPHRAGM KITS—ALL-FLEX ARCING SPRING; ORTHO COIL SPRING; ORTHO-WHITE FLAT SPRING
(Diaphragm)............1921
None cited in PDR database.

ORTHO DIAPHRAGM KIT-COIL SPRING
(Diaphragm)............1921
None cited in PDR database.

ORTHO DIENESTROL CREAM
(Dienestrol)............1922
None cited in PDR database.

ORTHO-EST .625 TABLETS
(Estropipate)............1925
May interact with progestins. Compounds in this category include:

Desogestrel (Potential risk of adverse effects on carbohydrate and lipid metabolism; the choice of progestin and dosage may be important in minimizing these adverse effects). Products include:
- Desogen Tablets 1867
- Ortho-Cept 1907

Medroxyprogesterone Acetate (Potential risk of adverse effects on carbohydrate and lipid metabolism; the choice of progestin and dosage may be important in minimizing these adverse effects). Products include:
- Amen Tablets 785
- Cycrin Tablets 991
- Depo-Provera Contraceptive Injection 2079
- Depo-Provera Sterile Aqueous Suspension 2083
- Premphase 2900
- Prempro 2905
- Provera Tablets 2110

Megestrol Acetate (Potential risk of adverse effects on carbohydrate and lipid metabolism; the choice of progestin and dosage may be important in minimizing these adverse effects). Products include:
- Megace Oral Suspension 708
- Megace Tablets 710

Norgestimate (Potential risk of adverse effects on carbohydrate and lipid metabolism; the choice of progestin and dosage may be important in minimizing these adverse effects). Products include:
- Ortho-Cyclen/Ortho-Tri-Cyclen 1914
- Ortho-Cyclen/Ortho-Tri-Cyclen 1914

ORTHO-EST 1.25 TABLETS
(Estropipate)............1925
See Ortho-Est .625 Tablets

ORTHO-NOVUM 1/35□21 TABLETS
(Norethindrone, Ethinyl Estradiol)......1928
See Ortho-Novum 7/7/7 □21 Tablets

ORTHO-NOVUM 1/35□28 TABLETS
(Norethindrone, Ethinyl Estradiol)......1928
See Ortho-Novum 7/7/7 □21 Tablets

ORTHO-NOVUM 1/50□21 TABLETS
(Norethindrone, Mestranol)............1928
See Ortho-Novum 7/7/7 □21 Tablets

ORTHO-NOVUM 1/50□28 TABLETS
(Norethindrone, Mestranol)............1928
See Ortho-Novum 7/7/7 □21 Tablets

ORTHO-NOVUM 7/7/7 □21 TABLETS
(Norethindrone, Ethinyl Estradiol)......1928
May interact with tetracyclines, barbiturates, and certain other agents. Compounds in these categories include:

Ampicillin (Potential for reduced efficacy and increased incidence of breakthrough bleeding and menstrual irregularities with concomitant use). Products include:
- Omnipen Capsules 2872
- Omnipen for Oral Suspension 2873

Ampicillin Sodium (Potential for reduced efficacy and increased incidence of breakthrough bleeding and menstrual rregularities with concomitent use1). Products include:
- Unasyn 2035

Aprobarbital (Potential for reduced efficacy and increased incidence of breakthrough bleeding and menstrual irregularities with concomitant use).
No products indexed under this heading.

Butabarbital (Potential for reduced efficacy and increased incidence of breakthrough bleeding and menstrual irregularities with concomitant use).
No products indexed under this heading.

Butalbital (Potential for reduced efficacy and increased incidence of breakthrough bleeding and menstrual irregularities with concomitant use). Products include:
- Axocet Capsules 2469
- Esgic-plus Capsules 1012
- Esgic-plus Tablets 1012
- Fioricet Tablets 2386
- Fioricet with Codeine Capsules 2387
- Fiorinal Capsules 2388
- Fiorinal with Codeine Capsules 2390
- Fiorinal Tablets 2388
- Phrenilin 790
- Sedapap Tablets 50 mg/650 mg .. 1826

Carbamazepine (Potential for reduced efficacy and increased incidence of breakthrough bleeding and menstrual irregularities with concomitant use). Products include:
- Atretol Tablets 569
- Tegretol/Tegretol-XR 870

Demeclocycline Hydrochloride (Potential for reduced efficacy and increased incidence of breakthrough bleeding and menstrual irregularities with concomitant use). Products include:
- Declomycin Tablets............ 1421

Doxycycline Calcium (Potential for reduced efficacy and increased incidence of breakthrough bleeding and menstrual irregularities with concomitant use). Products include:
- Vibramycin Calcium Oral Suspension Syrup 2038

Doxycycline Hyclate (Potential for reduced efficacy and increased incidence of breakthrough bleeding and menstrual irregularities with concomitant use). Products include:
- Doryx Capsules 1970
- Vibramycin Hyclate Capsules 2038
- Vibramycin Hyclate Intravenous 2040
- Vibra-Tabs Film Coated Tablets 2038

Doxycycline Monohydrate (Potential for reduced efficacy and increased incidence of breakthrough bleeding and menstrual irregularities with concomitant use). Products include:
- Monodox Capsules 1858
- Vibramycin Monohydrate for Oral Suspension 2038

Fosphenytoin Sodium (Potential for reduced efficacy and increased incidence of breakthrough bleeding and menstrual irregularities with concomitant use). Products include:
- Cerebyx Injection 1956

Griseofulvin (Potential for reduced efficacy and increased incidence of breakthrough bleeding and menstrual irregularities with concomitant use). Products include:
- Fulvicin P/G Tablets 2499
- Fulvicin P/G 165 & 330 Tablets 2500
- Grifulvin V (griseofulvin tablets) Microsize (griseofulvin oral suspension) Microsize 1944

(▣ Described in PDR For Nonprescription Drugs)   (⊚ Described in PDR For Ophthalmology)

Gris-PEG Tablets, 125 mg & 250 mg 476

Mephobarbital (Potential for reduced efficacy and increased incidence of breakthrough bleeding and menstrual irregularities with concomitant use). Products include:
Mebaral Tablets 2452

Methacycline Hydrochloride (Potential for reduced efficacy and increased incidence of breakthrough bleeding and menstrual irregularities with concomitant use).
No products indexed under this heading.

Minocycline Hydrochloride (Potential for reduced efficacy and increased incidence of breakthrough bleeding and menstrual irregularities with concomitant use). Products include:
DYNACIN Capsules 1627
Minocin Intravenous 1428
Minocin Oral Suspension 1431
Minocin Pellet-Filled Capsules 1429

Oxytetracycline Hydrochloride (Potential for reduced efficacy and increased incidence of breakthrough bleeding and menstrual irregularities with concomitant use). Products include:
TERAK Ointment .... ⓧ 210
Terra-Cortril Ophthalmic Suspension 2033
Terramycin with Polymyxin B Sulfate Ophthalmic Ointment 2035
Urobiotic-250 Capsules 2038

Pentobarbital Sodium (Potential for reduced efficacy and increased incidence of breakthrough bleeding and menstrual irregularities with concomitant use). Products include:
Nembutal Sodium Capsules 440
Nembutal Sodium Solution 442
Nembutal Sodium Suppositories..... 444

Phenobarbital (Potential for reduced efficacy and increased incidence of breakthrough bleeding and menstrual irregularities with concomitant use). Products include:
Arco-Lase Plus Tablets 513
Bellergal-S Tablets 2375
Donnatal 2234
Donnatal Extentabs 2234
Donnatal Tablets 2234
Phenobarbital Elixir and Tablets 1523
Quadrinal Tablets 1398

Phenylbutazone (Potential for reduced efficacy and increased incidence of breakthrough bleeding and menstrual irregularities with concomitant use).
No products indexed under this heading.

Phenytoin (Potential for reduced efficacy and increased incidence of breakthrough bleeding and menstrual irregularities with concomitant use). Products include:
Dilantin Infatabs 1967
Dilantin-125 Suspension 1969

Phenytoin Sodium (Potential for reduced efficacy and increased incidence of breakthrough bleeding and menstrual irregularities with concomitant use). Products include:
Dilantin Kapseals 1965

Rifampin (Co-administration has been associated with reduced efficacy and increased incidence of breakthrough bleeding and menstrual irregularities with concomitant use). Products include:
Rifadin 1276
Rifamate Capsules 1278
Rifater 1280
Rimactane Capsules 865

Secobarbital Sodium (Potential for reduced efficacy and increased incidence of breakthrough bleeding and menstrual irregularities with concomitant use). Products include:
Seconal Sodium Pulvules 1529

Tetracycline Hydrochloride (Potential for reduced efficacy and increased incidence of breakthrough bleeding and menstrual irregularities with concomitant use). Products include:
Achromycin V Capsules 1417
Helidac Therapy 2135

Thiamylal Sodium (Potential for reduced efficacy and increased incidence of breakthrough bleeding and menstrual irregularities with concomitant use).
No products indexed under this heading.

ORTHO-NOVUM 7/7/7 ☐28 TABLETS
(Norethindrone, Ethinyl Estradiol)......1928
See **Ortho-Novum 7/7/7 ☐21 Tablets**

ORTHO-NOVUM 10/11☐21 TABLETS
(Norethindrone, Ethinyl Estradiol)......1928
See **Ortho-Novum 7/7/7 ☐21 Tablets**

ORTHO-NOVUM 10/11☐28 TABLETS
(Norethindrone, Ethinyl Estradiol)......1928
See **Ortho-Novum 7/7/7 ☐21 Tablets**

ORTHO TRI-CYCLEN 21 TABLETS
(Norgestimate, Ethinyl Estradiol)........1914
See **Ortho-Cyclen 21 Tablets**

ORTHO TRI-CYCLEN 28 TABLETS
(Norgestimate, Ethinyl Estradiol)........1914
See **Ortho-Cyclen 21 Tablets**

ORTHO-WHITE DIAPHRAGM KIT-FLAT SPRING (SEE ALSO ORTHO DIAPHRAGM KITS)
(Diaphragm)............................1921
None cited in PDR database.

ORTHOCLONE OKT3 STERILE SOLUTION
(Muromonab-CD3) 1892
May interact with corticosteroids and certain other agents. Compounds in these categories include:

Azathioprine (Infection or malignancies have been reported with azathioprine alone and in conjunction with muromonab-CD3). Products include:
Azathioprine Tablets 2349
Imuran 1103

Betamethasone Acetate (Psychosis and infection have been reported in patients treated with corticosteroids alone and in conjunction with muromonab-CD3). Products include:
Celestone Soluspan Suspension 2484

Betamethasone Sodium Phosphate (Psychosis and infection have been reported in patients treated with corticosteroids alone and in conjunction with muromonab-CD3). Products include:
Celestone Soluspan Suspension 2484

Cortisone Acetate (Psychosis and infection have been reported in patients treated with corticosteroids alone and in conjunction with muromonab-CD3). Products include:
Cortone Acetate Sterile Suspension 1663
Cortone Acetate Tablets 1664

Cyclosporine (Seizures, encephalopathy, infections, malignancies, and thrombotic events have been reported in patients receiving cyclosporine alone and in conjunction with muromonab-CD3). Products include:
Neoral 2405
Sandimmune 2416

Dexamethasone (Psychosis and infection have been reported in patients treated with corticosteroids alone and in conjunction with muromonab-CD3). Products include:
AK-Trol Ointment & Suspension .... ⓧ 205
Decadron Elixir 1676
Decadron Tablets 1678
Decaspray Topical Aerosol 1689
Maxitrol Ophthalmic Ointment and Suspension .... ⓧ 222
TobraDex Ophthalmic Suspension and Ointment.......... 469

Dexamethasone Acetate (Psychosis and infection have been reported in patients treated with corticosteroids alone and in conjunction with muromonab-CD3). Products include:
Dalalone D.P. Injectable 1009
Decadron-LA Sterile Suspension 1687

Dexamethasone Sodium Phosphate (Psychosis and infection have been reported in patients treated with corticosteroids alone and in conjunction with muromonab-CD3). Products include:
Decadron Phosphate Injection 1680
Decadron Phosphate Sterile Ophthalmic Ointment 1684
Decadron Phosphate Sterile Ophthalmic Solution 1685
Decadron Phosphate Topical Cream 1686
Decadron Phosphate with Xylocaine Injection, Sterile 1683
Dexacort Phosphate in Respihaler .. 1606
Dexacort Phosphate in Turbinaire .. 1607
NeoDecadron Sterile Ophthalmic Ointment 1755
NeoDecadron Sterile Ophthalmic Solution 1756
NeoDecadron Topical Cream ... 1757

Fludrocortisone Acetate (Psychosis and infection have been reported in patients treated with corticosteroids alone and in conjunction with muromonab-CD-3). Products include:
Florinef Acetate Tablets 506

Hydrocortisone (Psychosis and infection have been reported in patients treated with corticosteroids alone and in conjunction with muromonab-CD3). Products include:
Anusol-HC Cream 2.5% 1953
Aquanil HC Lotion 1989
Maximum Strength Cortaid Spray ⓧ 800
CORTENEMA 2713
Cortisporin Ointment 1074
Cortisporin Ophthalmic Ointment Sterile 1074
Cortisporin Ophthalmic Suspension Sterile 1075
Cortisporin Otic Solution Sterile 1076
Cortisporin Otic Suspension Sterile ... 1077
Cortizone-5 .... ⓧ 795
Cortizone-10 .... ⓧ 795
Hydrocortone Tablets 1715
Hytone 922
Hytone Ointment 2 ½% 923
Massengill Medicated Soft Cloth Towelettes 2628
Pediotic Suspension Sterile ... 1140
Preparation H Hydrocortisone 1% Cream .... ⓧ 843
ProctoCream-HC 2.5% 2552
VōSoL HC Otic Solution 2786

Hydrocortisone Acetate (Psychosis and infection have been reported in patients treated with corticosteroids alone and in conjunction with muromonab-CD3). Products include:
Analpram-HC Rectal Cream 1% and 2.5% 993
Anusol HC-1 Hydrocortisone Anti-Itch Ointment .... ⓧ 810
Anusol-HC Suppositories 1954
Caldecort Anti-Itch Hydrocortisone Cream .... ⓧ 651
Coly-Mycin S Otic w/Neomycin & Hydrocortisone 1965
Cortaid .... ⓧ 800
Cortifoam 2540
Cortisporin Cream 1073
Epifoam 2543
Hydrocortone Acetate Sterile Suspension 1712
Mantadil Cream 1124
Nupercainal Hydrocortisone 1% Cream .... ⓧ 661
Pramosone Cream, Lotion & Ointment 995
ProctoFoam-HC 2552
Terra-Cortril Ophthalmic Suspension 2033

Hydrocortisone Sodium Phosphate (Psychosis and infection have been reported in patients treated with corticosteroids alone and in conjunction with muromonab-CD3). Products include:
Hydrocortone Phosphate Injection, Sterile 1713

Hydrocortisone Sodium Succinate (Psychosis and infection have been reported in patients treated with corticosteroids alone and in conjunction with muromonab-CD3).
No products indexed under this heading.

Indomethacin (Encephalopathy and other CNS effects have been reported in patients treated with indomethacin alone and in conjunction with muromonab-CD3). Products include:
Indocin 1723

Indomethacin Sodium Trihydrate (Encephalopathy and other CNS effects have been reported in patients treated with indomethacin alone and in conjunction with muromonab-CD3). Products include:
Indocin I.V. 1727

Methylprednisolone Acetate (Psychosis and infection have been reported in patients treated with corticosteroids alone and in conjunction with muromonab-CD3).
No products indexed under this heading.

Methylprednisolone Sodium Succinate (Psychosis and infection have been reported in patients treated with corticosteroids alone and in conjunction with muromonab-CD3).
No products indexed under this heading.

Prednisolone Acetate (Psychosis and infection have been reported in patients treated with corticosteroids alone and in conjunction with muromonab-CD3). Products include:
AK-CIDE .... ⓧ 203
AK-CIDE Ointment .... ⓧ 203
Blephamide Liquifilm Sterile Ophthalmic Suspension 472
Blephamide Ointment .... ⓧ 234
Econopred & Econopred Plus Ophthalmic Suspensions .. ⓧ 216
Poly-Pred Liquifilm .... ⓧ 246
Pred Forte .... ⓧ 247
Pred Mild .... ⓧ 250
Pred-G Liquifilm Sterile Ophthalmic Suspension .... ⓧ 248
Pred-G S.O.P. Sterile Ophthalmic Ointment .... ⓧ 249

IMPORTANT NOTE: Always consult each drug listing in the patient's regimen for possible interactions.

Prednisolone Sodium Phosphate (Psychosis and infection have been reported in patients treated with corticosteroids alone and in conjunction with muromonab-CD3). Products include:

- AK-PRED ⊙ 204
- Hydeltrasol Injection, Sterile 1708
- Pediapred Oral Solution 1618

Prednisolone Tebutate (Psychosis and infection have been reported in patients treated with corticosteroids alone and in conjunction with muromonab-CD3). Products include:

- Hydeltra-T.B.A. Sterile Suspension 1710

Prednisone (Psychosis and infection have been reported in patients treated with corticosteroids alone and in conjunction with muromonab-CD3).

No products indexed under this heading.

Triamcinolone (Psychosis and infection have been reported in patients treated with corticosteroids alone and in conjunction with muromonab-CD3).

No products indexed under this heading.

Triamcinolone Acetonide (Psychosis and infection have been reported in patients treated with corticosteroids alone and in conjunction with muromonab-CD3). Products include:

- Azmacort Oral Inhaler 2175
- Nasacort AQ Nasal Spray 2191
- Nasacort Nasal Inhaler 2189

Triamcinolone Diacetate (Psychosis and infection have been reported in patients treated with corticosteroids alone and in conjunction with muromonab-CD3).

No products indexed under this heading.

Triamcinolone Hexacetonide (Psychosis and infection have been reported in patients treated with corticosteroids alone and in conjunction with muromonab-CD3).

No products indexed under this heading.

ORUDIS CAPSULES

(Ketoprofen) 2874

May interact with lithium preparations, diuretics, and certain other agents. Compounds in these categories include:

Amiloride Hydrochloride (Reduced urinary potassium and chloride excretion). Products include:

- Midamor Tablets 1746
- Moduretic Tablets 1748

Aspirin (Decreased protein-binding and increased plasma clearance of ketoprofen). Products include:

- Alka-Seltzer Cherry Effervescent Antacid and Pain Reliever ▣ 609
- Alka-Seltzer Extra Strength Effervescent Antacid and Pain Reliever ▣ 609
- Alka-Seltzer Lemon Lime Effervescent Antacid and Pain Reliever ▣ 609
- Alka-Seltzer Original Effervescent Antacid and Pain Reliever ▣ 609
- Alka-Seltzer Plus ▣ 611
- Alka-Seltzer Plus Sinus Medicine ▣ 611
- Ascriptin ▣ 650
- Arthritis Strength BC Powder ▣ 631
- BC Cold Powder Multi-Symptom Formula (Cold-Sinus-Allergy) ▣ 631
- BC Cold Powder Non-Drowsy Formula (Cold-Sinus) ▣ 631
- BC Powder ▣ 631
- Genuine Bayer Aspirin Tablets & Caplets ▣ 618
- Extra Strength Bayer Arthritis Pain Regimen Formula ▣ 615
- Extra Strength Bayer Aspirin Caplets & Tablets ▣ 617
- Extended-Release Bayer 8-Hour Aspirin ▣ 616
- Extra Strength Bayer Plus Aspirin Caplets ▣ 617
- Extra Strength Bayer PM Aspirin Plus Sleep Aid ▣ 617
- Aspirin Regimen Bayer 81 mg Tablets with Calcium ▣ 615
- Aspirin Regimen Bayer Adult Low Strength 81 mg Tablets ▣ 613
- Aspirin Regimen Bayer Children's Chewable Aspirin ▣ 616
- Aspirin Regimen Bayer Regular Strength 325 mg Caplets ▣ 613
- Bufferin Analgesic Tablets ▣ 636
- Arthritis Strength Bufferin Analgesic Caplets ▣ 637
- Extra Strength Bufferin Analgesic Tablets ▣ 637
- Cama Arthritis Pain Reliever ▣ 748
- Darvon Compound-65 Pulvules 1475
- Easprin 1971
- Ecotrin 2625
- Ecotrin Enteric Coated Aspirin Maximum Strength Tablets and Caplets ▣ 775
- Ecotrin Enteric Coated Aspirin Regular Strength Tablets 2625
- Empirin Aspirin Tablets ▣ 818
- Excedrin Extra-Strength Analgesic Tablets, Caplets, and Geltabs 734
- Fiorinal Capsules 2388
- Fiorinal with Codeine Capsules 2390
- Fiorinal Tablets 2388
- Goody's Extra Strength Headache Powders ▣ 632
- Goody's Extra Strength Pain Relief Tablets ▣ 632
- Halfprin Tablets 1413
- Norgesic 1554
- Percodan Tablets 955
- Percodan-Demi Tablets 956
- Robaxisal Tablets 2246
- Soma Compound w/Codeine Tablets 2784
- Soma Compound Tablets 2783
- St. Joseph Adult Chewable Aspirin (81 mg.) ▣ 768
- Talwin Compound 2466
- Vanquish Analgesic Caplets ▣ 627

Bendroflumethiazide (Reduced urinary potassium and chloride excretion).

No products indexed under this heading.

Bumetanide (Reduced urinary potassium and chloride excretion). Products include:

- Bumex 2260

Chlorothiazide (Reduced urinary potassium and chloride excretion). Products include:

- Aldoclor Tablets 1638
- Diupres Tablets 1691
- Diuril Oral 1694

Chlorothiazide Sodium (Reduced urinary potassium and chloride excretion). Products include:

- Diuril Sodium Intravenous 1693

Chlorthalidone (Reduced urinary potassium and chloride excretion). Products include:

- Combipres Tablets 682
- Tenoretic Tablets 2963
- Thalitone 1293

Ethacrynic Acid (Reduced urinary potassium and chloride excretion). Products include:

- Edecrin Tablets 1698

Furosemide (Reduced urinary potassium and chloride excretion). Products include:

- Lasix Injection, Oral Solution and Tablets 1267

Hydrochlorothiazide (Reduced urinary potassium and chloride excretion). Products include:

- Aldactazide Tablets 2556
- Aldoril Tablets 1644
- Apresazide Capsules 824
- Capozide Tablets 744
- Dyazide Capsules 2653
- Esidrix Tablets 839
- Esimil Tablets 840
- HydroDIURIL Tablets 1716
- Hydropres Tablets 1718
- Hyzaar Tablets 1720
- Inderide Tablets 2838
- Inderide LA Long Acting Capsules 2840
- Lopressor HCT Tablets 850
- Lotensin HCT Tablets 855
- Moduretic Tablets 1748
- Oretic Tablets 450
- Prinzide Tablets 1780
- Ser-Ap-Es Tablets 867
- Timolide Tablets 1791
- Vaseretic Tablets 1810
- Zestoretic Tablets 2968
- Ziac 1459

Hydroflumethiazide (Reduced urinary potassium and chloride excretion). Products include:

- Diucardin Tablets 2824

Indapamide (Reduced urinary potassium and chloride excretion).

No products indexed under this heading.

Lithium Carbonate (Increased steady-state plasma lithium levels). Products include:

- Eskalith 2658
- Lithium Carbonate Capsules & Tablets 2352
- Lithonate/Lithotabs/Lithobid 2721

Lithium Citrate (Increased steady-state plasma lithium levels).

No products indexed under this heading.

Methotrexate Sodium (Increased toxicity; avoid coadministration). Products include:

- Methotrexate Sodium Tablets, Injection, for Injection and LPF Injection 1322

Methyclothiazide (Reduced urinary potassium and chloride excretion). Products include:

- Enduron Tablets 424

Metolazone (Reduced urinary potassium and chloride excretion). Products include:

- Mykrox Tablets 1617
- Zaroxolyn Tablets 1625

Polythiazide (Reduced urinary potassium and chloride excretion). Products include:

- Minizide Capsules 2016

Probenecid (Decreased protein-binding and increased plasma clearance of ketoprofen). Products include:

- Benemid Tablets 1651
- ColBENEMID Tablets 1662

Spironolactone (Reduced urinary potassium and chloride excretion). Products include:

- Aldactazide Tablets 2556
- Aldactone Tablets 2558

Torsemide (Reduced urinary potassium and chloride excretion). Products include:

- Demadex Tablets and Injection 691

Triamterene (Reduced urinary potassium and chloride excretion). Products include:

- Dyazide Capsules 2653
- Dyrenium Capsules 2655

Warfarin Sodium (Concurrent therapy requires close monitoring of patients on both drugs). Products include:

- Coumadin 941

Food Interactions

Food, unspecified (Slows rate of absorption resulting in delayed and reduced peak concentrations).

ORUDIS KT

(Ketoprofen) ▣ 842

Food Interactions

Alcohol (Patients consuming three or more alcohol-containing drinks should consult doctor for advice on when and how they should take Orudis KT).

ORUVAIL CAPSULES

(Ketoprofen) 2874

See **Orudis Capsules**

OSCILLOCOCCINUM

(Homeopathic Medications) ▣ 635

None cited in PDR database.

OSMOGLYN ORAL OSMOTIC AGENT

(Glycerin) ⊙ 225

None cited in PDR database.

OSMOLITE ISOTONIC LIQUID NUTRITION

(Nutritional Supplement) 2339

None cited in PDR database.

OSMOLITE HN HIGH NITROGEN ISOTONIC LIQUID NUTRITION

(Nutritional Supplement) 2339

None cited in PDR database.

OSMOLITE HN PLUS 1.2 CAL/ML, HIGH-NITROGEN LIQUID NUTRITION

(Nutritional Supplement) 2340

None cited in PDR database.

OTIC DOMEBORO SOLUTION

(Acetic Acid) 604

None cited in PDR database.

OTRIVIN NASAL DROPS

(Xylometazoline Hydrochloride) ▣ 662

None cited in PDR database.

OTRIVIN PEDIATRIC NASAL DROPS

(Xylometazoline Hydrochloride) ▣ 662

None cited in PDR database.

OTRIVIN NASAL SPRAY

(Xylometazoline Hydrochloride) ▣ 662

None cited in PDR database.

OVCON 35 TABLETS

(Norethindrone, Ethinyl Estradiol) 765

May interact with barbiturates, tetracyclines, and certain other agents. Compounds in these categories include:

Ampicillin (Potential for reduced efficacy and increased incidence of breakthrough bleeding and menstrual irregularities with concomitant use). Products include:

- Omnipen Capsules 2872
- Omnipen for Oral Suspension 2873

Ampicillin Sodium (Potential for reduced efficacy and increased incidence of breakthrough bleeding and menstrual irregularities with concomitant use). Products include:

- Unasyn 2035

Aprobarbital (Potential for reduced efficacy and increased incidence of breakthrough bleeding and menstrual irregularities with concomitant use).

No products indexed under this heading.

Butabarbital (Potential for reduced efficacy and increased incidence of breakthrough bleeding and menstrual irregularities with concomitant use).

No products indexed under this heading.

Butalbital (Potential for reduced efficacy and increased incidence of breakthrough bleeding and menstrual irregularities with concomitant use). Products include:

- Axocet Capsules 2469

(▣ Described in PDR For Nonprescription Drugs) (⊙ Described in PDR For Ophthalmology)

Esgic-plus Capsules 1012
Esgic-plus Tablets 1012
Fioricet Tablets 2386
Fioricet with Codeine Capsules 2387
Fiorinal Capsules 2388
Fiorinal with Codeine Capsules 2390
Fiorinal Tablets 2388
Phrenilin 790
Sedapap Tablets 50 mg/650 mg .. 1826

Demeclocycline Hydrochloride (Potential for reduced efficacy and increased incidence of breakthrough bleeding and menstrual irregularities with concomitant use). Products include:
Declomycin Tablets 1421

Doxycycline Calcium (Potential for reduced efficacy and increased incidence of breakthrough bleeding and menstrual irregularities with concomitant use). Products include:
Vibramycin Calcium Oral Suspension Syrup 2038

Doxycycline Hyclate (Potential for reduced efficacy and increased incidence of breakthrough bleeding and menstrual irregularities with concomitant use). Products include:
Doryx Capsules 1970
Vibramycin Hyclate Capsules 2038
Vibramycin Hyclate Intravenous 2040
Vibra-Tabs Film Coated Tablets 2038

Doxycycline Monohydrate (Potential for reduced efficacy and increased incidence of breakthrough bleeding and menstrual irregularities with concomitant use). Products include:
Monodox Capsules 1858
Vibramycin Monohydrate for Oral Suspension 2038

Fosphenytoin Sodium (Potential for reduced efficacy and increased incidence of breakthrough bleeding and menstrual irregularities with concomitant use). Products include:
Cerebyx Injection 1956

Griseofulvin (Potential for reduced efficacy and increased incidence of breakthrough bleeding and menstrual irregularities with concomitant use). Products include:
Fulvicin P/G Tablets 2499
Fulvicin P/G 165 & 330 Tablets 2500
Grifulvin V (griseofulvin tablets) Microsize (griseofulvin oral suspension) Microsize 1944
Gris-PEG Tablets, 125 mg & 250 mg 476

Mephobarbital (Potential for reduced efficacy and increased incidence of breakthrough bleeding and menstrual irregularities with concomitant use). Products include:
Mebaral Tablets 2452

Methacycline Hydrochloride (Potential for reduced efficacy and increased incidence of breakthrough bleeding and menstrual irregularities with concomitant use).
No products indexed under this heading.

Minocycline Hydrochloride (Potential for reduced efficacy and increased incidence of breakthrough bleeding and menstrual irregularities with concomitant use). Products include:
DYNACIN Capsules 1627
Minocin Intravenous 1428
Minocin Oral Suspension 1431
Minocin Pellet-Filled Capsules 1429

Oxytetracycline Hydrochloride (Potential for reduced efficacy and increased incidence of breakthrough bleeding and menstrual irregularities with concomitant use). Products include:
TERAK Ointment .... ◉ 210
Terra-Cortril Ophthalmic Suspension 2033
Terramycin with Polymyxin B Sulfate Ophthalmic Ointment 2035
Urobiotic-250 Capsules 2038

Pentobarbital Sodium (Potential for reduced efficacy and increased incidence of breakthrough bleeding and menstrual irregularities with concomitant use). Products include:
Nembutal Sodium Capsules 440
Nembutal Sodium Solution 442
Nembutal Sodium Suppositories 444

Phenobarbital (Potential for reduced efficacy and increased incidence of breakthrough bleeding and menstrual irregularities with concomitant use). Products include:
Arco-Lase Plus Tablets 513
Bellergal-S Tablets 2375
Donnatal 2234
Donnatal Extentabs 2234
Donnatal Tablets 2234
Phenobarbital Elixir and Tablets 1523
Quadrinal Tablets 1398

Phenylbutazone (Potential for reduced efficacy and increased incidence of breakthrough bleeding and menstrual irregularities with concomitant use).
No products indexed under this heading.

Phenytoin (Potential for reduced efficacy and increased incidence of breakthrough bleeding and menstrual irregularities with concomitant use). Products include:
Dilantin Infatabs 1967
Dilantin-125 Suspension 1969

Phenytoin Sodium (Potential for reduced efficacy and increased incidence of breakthrough bleeding and menstrual irregularities with concomitant use). Products include:
Dilantin Kapseals 1965

Rifampin (Co-administration has been associated with reduced efficacy and increased incidence of breakthrough bleeding and menstrual irregularities). Products include:
Rifadin 1276
Rifamate Capsules 1278
Rifater 1280
Rimactane Capsules 865

Secobarbital Sodium (Potential for reduced efficacy and increased incidence of breakthrough bleeding and menstrual irregularities with concomitant use). Products include:
Seconal Sodium Pulvules 1529

Tetracycline Hydrochloride (Possibility for reduced efficacy and increased incidence of breakthrough bleeding and menstrual irregularities with concomitant use). Products include:
Achromycin V Capsules 1417
Helidac Therapy 2135

Thiamylal Sodium (Potential for reduced efficacy and increased incidence of breakthrough bleeding and menstrual irregularities with concomitant use).
No products indexed under this heading.

OVCON 50 TABLETS
(Norethindrone, Ethinyl Estradiol) 765
See **Ovcon 35 Tablets**

OVRAL TABLETS
(Norgestrel, Ethinyl Estradiol) 2877
See **Lo/Ovral Tablets**

OVRAL-28 TABLETS
(Norgestrel, Ethinyl Estradiol) 2878
See **Lo/Ovral Tablets**

OVRETTE TABLETS
(Norgestrel) 2878
See **Lo/Ovral Tablets**

OXANDRIN
(Oxandrolone) 783
May interact with oral anticoagulants, oral hypoglycemic agents, corticosteroids, and certain other agents. Compounds in these categories include:

Acarbose (Oxandrolone may inhibit the metabolism of oral hypoglycemic agents). Products include:
Precose 604

ACTH (Increased risk of edema).
No products indexed under this heading.

Betamethasone Acetate (Increased risk of edema). Products include:
Celestone Soluspan Suspension 2484

Betamethasone Sodium Phosphate (Increased risk of edema). Products include:
Celestone Soluspan Suspension 2484

Chlorpropamide (Oxandrolone may inhibit the metabolism of oral hypoglycemic agents). Products include:
Diabinese Tablets 2002

Cortisone Acetate (Increased risk of edema). Products include:
Cortone Acetate Sterile Suspension 1663
Cortone Acetate Tablets 1664

Dexamethasone (Increased risk of edema). Products include:
AK-Trol Ointment & Suspension .... ◉ 205
Decadron Elixir 1676
Decadron Tablets 1678
Decaspray Topical Aerosol 1689
Maxitrol Ophthalmic Ointment and Suspension .... ◉ 222
TobraDex Ophthalmic Suspension and Ointment 469

Dexamethasone Acetate (Increased risk of edema). Products include:
Dalalone D.P. Injectable 1009
Decadron-LA Sterile Suspension 1687

Dexamethasone Sodium Phosphate (Increased risk of edema). Products include:
Decadron Phosphate Injection 1680
Decadron Phosphate Sterile Ophthalmic Ointment 1684
Decadron Phosphate Sterile Ophthalmic Solution 1685
Decadron Phosphate Topical Cream 1686
Decadron Phosphate with Xylocaine Injection, Sterile 1683
Dexacort Phosphate in Respihaler .. 1606
Dexacort Phosphate in Turbinaire .. 1607
NeoDecadron Sterile Ophthalmic Ointment 1755
NeoDecadron Sterile Ophthalmic Solution 1756
NeoDecadron Topical Cream 1757

Dicumarol (Anabolic steroids may increase the sensitivity to oral anticoagulants; dosage of the anticoagulants may have to be decreased in order to maintain desired prothrombin time).
No products indexed under this heading.

Fludrocortisone Acetate (Increased risk of edema). Products include:
Florinef Acetate Tablets 506

Glimepiride (Oxandrolone may inhibit the metabolism of oral hypoglycemic agents). Products include:
Amaryl Tablets 1241

Glipizide (Oxandrolone may inhibit the metabolism of oral hypoglycemic agents). Products include:
Glucotrol Tablets 2011
Glucotrol XL Extended Release Tablets 2012

Glyburide (Oxandrolone may inhibit the metabolism of oral hypoglycemic agents). Products include:
DiaBeta Tablets 1265
Glynase PresTab Tablets 2091
Micronase Tablets 2099

Hydrocortisone (Increased risk of edema). Products include:
Anusol-HC Cream 2.5% 1953
Aquanil HC Lotion 1989
Maximum Strength Cortaid Spray ▣ 800
CORTENEMA 2713
Cortisporin Ointment 1074
Cortisporin Ophthalmic Ointment Sterile 1074
Cortisporin Ophthalmic Suspension Sterile 1075
Cortisporin Otic Solution Sterile 1076
Cortisporin Otic Suspension Sterile 1077
Cortizone-5 .... ▣ 795
Cortizone-10 .... ▣ 795
Hydrocortone Tablets 1715
Hytone 922
Hytone Ointment 2 ½% 923
Massengill Medicated Soft Cloth Towelettes 2628
Pediotic Suspension Sterile 1140
Preparation H Hydrocortisone 1% Cream .... ▣ 843
ProctoCream-HC 2.5% 2552
VōSoL HC Otic Solution 2786

Hydrocortisone Acetate (Increased risk of edema). Products include:
Analpram-HC Rectal Cream 1% and 2.5% 993
Anusol HC-1 Hydrocortisone Anti-Itch Ointment .... ▣ 810
Anusol-HC Suppositories 1954
Caldecort Anti-Itch Hydrocortisone Cream .... ▣ 651
Coly-Mycin S Otic w/Neomycin & Hydrocortisone 1965
Cortaid .... ▣ 800
Cortifoam 2540
Cortisporin Cream 1073
Epifoam 2543
Hydrocortone Acetate Sterile Suspension 1712
Mantadil Cream 1124
Nupercainal Hydrocortisone 1% Cream .... ▣ 661
Pramosone Cream, Lotion & Ointment 995
ProctoFoam-HC 2552
Terra-Cortril Ophthalmic Suspension 2033

Hydrocortisone Sodium Phosphate (Increased risk of edema). Products include:
Hydrocortone Phosphate Injection, Sterile 1713

Hydrocortisone Sodium Succinate (Increased risk of edema).
No products indexed under this heading.

Metformin Hydrochloride (Oxandrolone may inhibit the metabolism of oral hypoglycemic agents). Products include:
Glucophage Tablets 754

Methylprednisolone Acetate (Increased risk of edema).
No products indexed under this heading.

Methylprednisolone Sodium Succinate (Increased risk of edema).
No products indexed under this heading.

Prednisolone Acetate (Increased risk of edema). Products include:
AK-CIDE .... ◉ 203
AK-CIDE Ointment .... ◉ 203
Blephamide Liquifilm Sterile Ophthalmic Suspension 472
Blephamide Ointment .... ◉ 234
Econopred & Econopred Plus Ophthalmic Suspensions .... ◉ 216
Poly-Pred Liquifilm .... ◉ 246
Pred Forte .... ◉ 247
Pred Mild .... ◉ 250
Pred-G Liquifilm Sterile Ophthalmic Suspension .... ◉ 248
Pred-G S.O.P. Sterile Ophthalmic Ointment .... ◉ 249

IMPORTANT NOTE: Always consult each drug listing in the patient's regimen for possible interactions.

Oxandrin / Interactions Index

Prednisolone Sodium Phosphate (Increased risk of edema). Products include:
- AK-PRED ... ⓞ 204
- Hydeltrasol Injection, Sterile ... 1708
- Pediapred Oral Solution ... 1618

Prednisolone Tebutate (Increased risk of edema). Products include:
- Hydeltra-T.B.A. Sterile Suspension ... 1710

Prednisone (Increased risk of edema).
- No products indexed under this heading.

Tolazamide (Oxandrolone may inhibit the metabolism of oral hypoglycemic agents).
- No products indexed under this heading.

Tolbutamide (Oxandrolone may inhibit the metabolism of oral hypoglycemic agents).
- No products indexed under this heading.

Triamcinolone (Increased risk of edema).
- No products indexed under this heading.

Triamcinolone Acetonide (Increased risk of edema). Products include:
- Azmacort Oral Inhaler ... 2175
- Nasacort AQ Nasal Spray ... 2191
- Nasacort Nasal Inhaler ... 2189

Triamcinolone Diacetate (Increased risk of edema).
- No products indexed under this heading.

Triamcinolone Hexacetonide (Increased risk of edema).
- No products indexed under this heading.

Warfarin Sodium (Anabolic steroids may increase the sensitivity to oral anticoagulants; dosage of the anticoagulants may have to be decreased in order to maintain desired prothrombin time). Products include:
- Coumadin ... 941

OXISTAT CREAM
(Oxiconazole Nitrate) ... 1139
None cited in PDR database.

OXISTAT LOTION
(Oxiconazole Nitrate) ... 1139
None cited in PDR database.

OXSORALEN LOTION 1%
(Methoxsalen) ... 1301
May interact with phenothiazines, sulfonamides, tetracyclines, thiazides, and certain other agents. Compounds in these categories include:

Anthralin (Possible photosensitivity effects). Products include:
- Drithocreme 0.1%, 0.25%, 0.5%, 1.0% (HP) ... 920
- Dritho-Scalp 0.25%, 0.5% ... 921

Bendroflumethiazide (Possible photosensitivity effects).
- No products indexed under this heading.

Chlorothiazide (Possible photosensitivity effects). Products include:
- Aldoclor Tablets ... 1638
- Diupres Tablets ... 1691
- Diuril Oral ... 1694

Chlorothiazide Sodium (Possible photosensitivity effects). Products include:
- Diuril Sodium Intravenous ... 1693

Chlorpromazine (Possible photosensitivity effects). Products include:
- Thorazine Suppositories ... 2701

Coal Tar (Possible photosensitivity effects). Products include:
- DHS ... 1989
- Fototar Cream ... 1300
- MG 217 ... ⓝ 800
- Pentrax Shampoo ... 1042
- Tegrin Dandruff Shampoo ... ⓝ 634
- Tegrin Skin Cream & Tegrin Medicated Soap ... ⓝ 634

Demeclocycline Hydrochloride (Possible photosensitivity effects). Products include:
- Declomycin Tablets ... 1421

Doxycycline Calcium (Possible photosensitivity effects). Products include:
- Vibramycin Calcium Oral Suspension Syrup ... 2038

Doxycycline Hyclate (Possible photosensitivity effects). Products include:
- Doryx Capsules ... 1970
- Vibramycin Hyclate Capsules ... 2038
- Vibramycin Hyclate Intravenous ... 2040
- Vibra-Tabs Film Coated Tablets ... 2038

Doxycycline Monohydrate (Possible photosensitivity effects). Products include:
- Monodox Capsules ... 1858
- Vibramycin Monohydrate for Oral Suspension ... 2038

Fluphenazine Decanoate (Possible photosensitivity effects). Products include:
- Prolixin Decanoate ... 510

Fluphenazine Enanthate (Possible photosensitivity effects). Products include:
- Prolixin Enanthate ... 510

Fluphenazine Hydrochloride (Possible photosensitivity effects). Products include:
- Prolixin ... 510

Griseofulvin (Possible photosensitivity effects). Products include:
- Fulvicin P/G Tablets ... 2499
- Fulvicin P/G 165 & 330 Tablets ... 2500
- Grifulvin V (griseofulvin tablets) Microsize (griseofulvin oral suspension) Microsize ... 1944
- Gris-PEG Tablets, 125 mg & 250 mg ... 476

Hydrochlorothiazide (Possible photosensitivity effects). Products include:
- Aldactazide Tablets ... 2556
- Aldoril Tablets ... 1644
- Apresazide Capsules ... 824
- Capozide Tablets ... 744
- Dyazide Capsules ... 2653
- Esidrix Tablets ... 839
- Esimil Tablets ... 840
- HydroDIURIL Tablets ... 1716
- Hydropres Tablets ... 1718
- Hyzaar Tablets ... 1720
- Inderide Tablets ... 2838
- Inderide LA Long Acting Capsules ... 2840
- Lopressor HCT Tablets ... 850
- Lotensin HCT Tablets ... 855
- Moduretic Tablets ... 1748
- Oretic Tablets ... 450
- Prinzide Tablets ... 1780
- Ser-Ap-Es Tablets ... 867
- Timolide Tablets ... 1791
- Vaseretic Tablets ... 1810
- Zestoretic Tablets ... 2968
- Ziac ... 1459

Hydroflumethiazide (Possible photosensitivity effects). Products include:
- Diucardin Tablets ... 2824

Mesoridazine Besylate (Possible photosensitivity effects). Products include:
- Serentil ... 689

Methacycline Hydrochloride (Possible photosensitivity effects).
- No products indexed under this heading.

Methotrimeprazine (Possible photosensitivity effects). Products include:
- Levoprome ... 1321

Methyclothiazide (Possible photosensitivity effects). Products include:
- Enduron Tablets ... 424

Methylene Blue (Possible photosensitivity effects). Products include:
- Urised Tablets ... 2123

Minocycline Hydrochloride (Possible photosensitivity effects). Products include:
- DYNACIN Capsules ... 1627
- Minocin Intravenous ... 1428
- Minocin Oral Suspension ... 1431
- Minocin Pellet-Filled Capsules ... 1429

Nalidixic Acid (Possible photosensitivity effects). Products include:
- NegGram ... 2453

Oxytetracycline (Possible photosensitivity effects). Products include:
- Terramycin Intramuscular Solution ... 2034

Oxytetracycline Hydrochloride (Possible photosensitivity effects). Products include:
- TERAK Ointment ... ⓞ 210
- Terra-Cortril Ophthalmic Suspension ... 2033
- Terramycin with Polymyxin B Sulfate Ophthalmic Ointment ... 2035
- Urobiotic-250 Capsules ... 2038

Perphenazine (Possible photosensitivity effects). Products include:
- Etrafon ... 2495
- Triavil Tablets ... 1800
- Trilafon ... 2532

Polythiazide (Possible photosensitivity effects). Products include:
- Minizide Capsules ... 2016

Prochlorperazine (Possible photosensitivity effects). Products include:
- Compazine ... 2644

Promethazine Hydrochloride (Possible photosensitivity effects). Products include:
- Mepergan Injection ... 2859
- Phenergan with Codeine ... 2883
- Phenergan with Dextromethorphan ... 2885
- Phenergan Injection ... 2880
- Phenergan Suppositories ... 2882
- Phenergan Syrup ... 2881
- Phenergan Tablets ... 2882
- Phenergan VC ... 2886
- Phenergan VC with Codeine ... 2888

Sulfamethizole (Possible photosensitivity effects). Products include:
- Urobiotic-250 Capsules ... 2038

Sulfamethoxazole (Possible photosensitivity effects). Products include:
- Bactrim DS Tablets ... 2257
- Bactrim I.V. Infusion ... 2255
- Bactrim ... 2257
- Gantanol Tablets ... 2285
- Septra ... 1146
- Septra I.V. Infusion ... 1142
- Septra I.V. Infusion ADD-Vantage Vials ... 1144
- Septra ... 1146

Sulfasalazine (Possible photosensitivity effects). Products include:
- Azulfidine ... 2059

Sulfinpyrazone (Possible photosensitivity effects). Products include:
- Anturane ... 823

Sulfisoxazole (Possible photosensitivity effects). Products include:
- Gantrisin Tablets ... 2286

Sulfisoxazole Diolamine (Possible photosensitivity effects).
- No products indexed under this heading.

Tetracycline Hydrochloride (Possible photosensitivity effects). Products include:
- Achromycin V Capsules ... 1417
- Helidac Therapy ... 2135

Thioridazine Hydrochloride (Possible photosensitivity effects). Products include:
- Mellaril ... 2398

Trifluoperazine Hydrochloride (Possible photosensitivity effects). Products include:
- Stelazine ... 2692

OXSORALEN-ULTRA CAPSULES
(Methoxsalen) ... 1302
May interact with phenothiazines, sulfonamides, tetracyclines, thiazides, and certain other agents. Compounds in these categories include:

Anthralin (Possible photosensitivity effects). Products include:
- Drithocreme 0.1%, 0.25%, 0.5%, 1.0% (HP) ... 920
- Dritho-Scalp 0.25%, 0.5% ... 921

Bendroflumethiazide (Possible photosensitivity effects).
- No products indexed under this heading.

Chlorothiazide (Possible photosensitivity effects). Products include:
- Aldoclor Tablets ... 1638
- Diupres Tablets ... 1691
- Diuril Oral ... 1694

Chlorothiazide Sodium (Possible photosensitivity effects). Products include:
- Diuril Sodium Intravenous ... 1693

Chlorpromazine (Possible photosensitivity effects). Products include:
- Thorazine Suppositories ... 2701

Coal Tar (Possible photosensitivity effects). Products include:
- DHS ... 1989
- Fototar Cream ... 1300
- MG 217 ... ⓝ 800
- Pentrax Shampoo ... 1042
- Tegrin Dandruff Shampoo ... ⓝ 634
- Tegrin Skin Cream & Tegrin Medicated Soap ... ⓝ 634

Demeclocycline Hydrochloride (Possible photosensitivity effects). Products include:
- Declomycin Tablets ... 1421

Doxycycline Calcium (Possible photosensitivity effects). Products include:
- Vibramycin Calcium Oral Suspension Syrup ... 2038

Doxycycline Hyclate (Possible photosensitivity effects). Products include:
- Doryx Capsules ... 1970
- Vibramycin Hyclate Capsules ... 2038
- Vibramycin Hyclate Intravenous ... 2040
- Vibra-Tabs Film Coated Tablets ... 2038

Doxycycline Monohydrate (Possible photosensitivity effects). Products include:
- Monodox Capsules ... 1858
- Vibramycin Monohydrate for Oral Suspension ... 2038

Fluphenazine Decanoate (Possible photosensitivity effects). Products include:
- Prolixin Decanoate ... 510

Fluphenazine Enanthate (Possible photosensitivity effects). Products include:
- Prolixin Enanthate ... 510

Fluphenazine Hydrochloride (Possible photosensitivity effects). Products include:
- Prolixin ... 510

Griseofulvin (Possible photosensitivity effects). Products include:
- Fulvicin P/G Tablets ... 2499
- Fulvicin P/G 165 & 330 Tablets ... 2500
- Grifulvin V (griseofulvin tablets) Microsize (griseofulvin oral suspension) Microsize ... 1944
- Gris-PEG Tablets, 125 mg & 250 mg ... 476

Hydrochlorothiazide (Possible photosensitivity effects). Products include:
- Aldactazide Tablets ... 2556

(ⓝ Described in PDR For Nonprescription Drugs) (ⓞ Described in PDR For Ophthalmology)

799 **Interactions Index** **OxyContin**

Aldoril Tablets 1644
Apresazide Capsules 824
Capozide Tablets 744
Dyazide Capsules 2653
Esidrix Tablets 839
Esimil Tablets 840
HydroDIURIL Tablets 1716
Hydropres Tablets 1718
Hyzaar Tablets 1720
Inderide Tablets 2838
Inderide LA Long Acting Capsules 2840
Lopressor HCT Tablets 850
Lotensin HCT Tablets 855
Moduretic Tablets 1748
Oretic Tablets 450
Prinzide Tablets 1780
Ser-Ap-Es Tablets 867
Timolide Tablets 1791
Vaseretic Tablets 1810
Zestoretic Tablets 2968
Ziac 1459

Hydroflumethiazide (Possible photosensitivity effects). Products include:
Diucardin Tablets 2824

Mesoridazine Besylate (Possible photosensitivity effects). Products include:
Serentil 689

Methacycline Hydrochloride (Possible photosensitivity effects).
No products indexed under this heading.

Methotrimeprazine (Possible photosensitivity effects). Products include:
Levoprome 1321

Methyclothiazide (Possible photosensitivity effects). Products include:
Enduron Tablets 424

Methylene Blue (Possible photosensitivity effects). Products include:
Urised Tablets 2123

Minocycline Hydrochloride (Possible photosensitivity effects). Products include:
DYNACIN Capsules 1627
Minocin Intravenous 1428
Minocin Oral Suspension 1431
Minocin Pellet-Filled Capsules 1429

Nalidixic Acid (Possible photosensitivity effects). Products include:
NegGram 2453

Oxytetracycline (Possible photosensitivity effects). Products include:
Terramycin Intramuscular Solution 2034

Oxytetracycline Hydrochloride (Possible photosensitivity effects). Products include:
TERAK Ointment ⊙ 210
Terra-Cortril Ophthalmic Suspension 2033
Terramycin with Polymyxin B Sulfate Ophthalmic Ointment 2035
Urobiotic-250 Capsules 2038

Perphenazine (Possible photosensitivity effects). Products include:
Etrafon 2495
Triavil Tablets 1800
Trilafon 2532

Polythiazide (Possible photosensitivity effects). Products include:
Minizide Capsules 2016

Prochlorperazine (Possible photosensitivity effects). Products include:
Compazine 2644

Promethazine Hydrochloride (Possible photosensitivity effects). Products include:
Mepergan Injection 2859
Phenergan with Codeine 2883
Phenergan with Dextromethorphan 2885
Phenergan Injection 2880
Phenergan Suppositories 2882
Phenergan Syrup 2881
Phenergan Tablets 2882
Phenergan VC 2886
Phenergan VC with Codeine 2888

Sulfamethizole (Possible photosensitivity effects). Products include:
Urobiotic-250 Capsules 2038

Sulfamethoxazole (Possible photosensitivity effects). Products include:
Bactrim DS Tablets 2257
Bactrim I.V. Infusion 2255
Bactrim 2257
Gantanol Tablets 2285
Septra 1146
Septra I.V. Infusion 1142
Septra I.V. Infusion ADD-Vantage Vials 1144
Septra 1146

Sulfasalazine (Possible photosensitivity effects). Products include:
Azulfidine 2059

Sulfinpyrazone (Possible photosensitivity effects). Products include:
Anturane 823

Sulfisoxazole (Possible photosensitivity effects). Products include:
Gantrisin Tablets 2286

Sulfisoxazole Diolamine (Possible photosensitivity effects).
No products indexed under this heading.

Tetracycline Hydrochloride (Possible photosensitivity effects). Products include:
Achromycin V Capsules 1417
Helidac Therapy 2135

Thioridazine Hydrochloride (Possible photosensitivity effects). Products include:
Mellaril 2398

Trifluoperazine Hydrochloride (Possible photosensitivity effects). Products include:
Stelazine 2692

OXYCONTIN TABLETS
(Oxycodone Hydrochloride) 2163
May interact with central nervous system depressants, hypnotics and sedatives, general anesthetics, phenothiazines, tranquilizers, mixed agonist/antagonist opioid analgesics, and certain other agents. Compounds in these categories include:

Alfentanil Hydrochloride (Concurrent use with the usual dose of OxyContin may result in respiratory depression, profound sedation or coma; reduced dosage (1/3 to ½ of the usual dosage) may be necessary). Products include:
Alfenta Injection 1334

Alprazolam (Concurrent use with the usual dose of OxyContin may result in respiratory depression, profound sedation or coma; reduced dosage (1/3 to ½ of the usual dosage) may be necessary). Products include:
Xanax Tablets 2115

Aprobarbital (Concurrent use with the usual dose of OxyContin may result in respiratory depression, profound sedation or coma; reduced dosage (1/3 to ½ of the usual dosage) may be necessary).
No products indexed under this heading.

Buprenorphine (Mixed agonist/antagonist analgesics may reduce the analgesic effect of oxycodone and/or may precipitate withdrawal symptoms). Products include:
Buprenex Injectable 2170

Buspirone Hydrochloride (Concurrent use with the usual dose of OxyContin may result in respiratory depression, profound sedation or coma; reduced dosage (1/3 to ½ of the usual dosage) may be necessary). Products include:
BuSpar Tablets 738

Butabarbital (Concurrent use with the usual dose of OxyContin may result in respiratory depression, profound sedation or coma; reduced dosage (1/3 to ½ of the usual dosage) may be necessary).
No products indexed under this heading.

Butalbital (Concurrent use with the usual dose of OxyContin may result in respiratory depression, profound sedation or coma; reduced dosage (1/3 to ½ of the usual dosage) may be necessary). Products include:
Axocet Capsules 2469
Esgic-plus Capsules 1012
Esgic-plus Tablets 1012
Fioricet Tablets 2386
Fioricet with Codeine Capsules 2387
Fiorinal Capsules 2388
Fiorinal with Codeine Capsules 2390
Fiorinal Tablets 2388
Phrenilin 790
Sedapap Tablets 50 mg/650 mg 1826

Butorphanol Tartrate (Mixed agonist/antagonist analgesics may reduce the analgesic effect of oxycodone and/or may precipitate withdrawal symptoms). Products include:
Stadol 779

Chlordiazepoxide (Concurrent use with the usual dose of OxyContin may result in respiratory depression, profound sedation or coma; reduced dosage (1/3 to ½ of the usual dosage) may be necessary). Products include:
Limbitrol 2333

Chlordiazepoxide Hydrochloride (Concurrent use with the usual dose of OxyContin may result in respiratory depression, profound sedation or coma; reduced dosage (1/3 to ½ of the usual dosage) may be necessary). Products include:
Librax Capsules 2330
Librium Capsules 2331
Librium Injectable 2332

Chlorpromazine (Concurrent use with the usual dose of OxyContin may result in respiratory depression, profound sedation or coma; reduced dosage (1/3 to ½ of the usual dosage) may be necessary). Products include:
Thorazine Suppositories 2701

Chlorpromazine Hydrochloride (Concurrent use with the usual dose of OxyContin may result in respiratory depression, profound sedation or coma; reduced dosage (1/3 to ½ of the usual dosage) may be necessary). Products include:
Thorazine 2701

Chlorprothixene (Concurrent use with the usual dose of OxyContin may result in respiratory depression, profound sedation or coma; reduced dosage (1/3 to ½ of the usual dosage) may be necessary).
No products indexed under this heading.

Chlorprothixene Hydrochloride (Concurrent use with the usual dose of OxyContin may result in respiratory depression, profound sedation or coma; reduced dosage (1/3 to ½ of the usual dosage) may be necessary).
No products indexed under this heading.

Chlorprothixene Lactate (Concurrent use with the usual dose of OxyContin may result in respiratory depression, profound sedation or coma; reduced dosage (1/3 to ½ of the usual dosage) may be necessary).
No products indexed under this heading.

Clorazepate Dipotassium (Concurrent use with the usual dose of OxyContin may result in respiratory depression, profound sedation or coma; reduced dosage (1/3 to ½ of the usual dosage) may be necessary). Products include:
Tranxene 459

Clozapine (Concurrent use with the usual dose of OxyContin may result in respiratory depression, profound sedation or coma; reduced dosage (1/3 to ½ of the usual dosage) may be necessary). Products include:
Clozaril Tablets 2377

Codeine Phosphate (Concurrent use with the usual dose of OxyContin may result in respiratory depression, profound sedation or coma; reduced dosage (1/3 to ½ of the usual dosage) may be necessary). Products include:
Brontex 2130
Dimetane-DC Cough Syrup 2232
Fioricet with Codeine Capsules 2387
Fiorinal with Codeine Capsules 2390
Nucofed 2225
Phenergan with Codeine 2883
Phenergan VC with Codeine 2888
Robitussin A-C Syrup 2248
Robitussin-DAC Syrup 2249
Ryna 804
Soma Compound w/Codeine Tablets 2784
Tylenol with Codeine 1592

Desflurane (Concurrent use with the usual dose of OxyContin may result in respiratory depression, profound sedation or coma; reduced dosage (1/3 to ½ of the usual dosage) may be necessary). Products include:
Suprane (desflurane, USP) 1865

Dezocine (Concurrent use with the usual dose of OxyContin may result in respiratory depression, profound sedation or coma; reduced dosage (1/3 to ½ of the usual dosage) may be necessary). Products include:
Dalgan Injection 529

Diazepam (Concurrent use with the usual dose of OxyContin may result in respiratory depression, profound sedation or coma; reduced dosage (1/3 to ½ of the usual dosage) may be necessary). Products include:
Dizac (diazepam injectable emulsion) CIV 1862
Valium Injectable 2336
Valium Tablets 2335

Droperidol (Concurrent use with the usual dose of OxyContin may result in respiratory depression, profound sedation or coma; reduced dosage (1/3 to ½ of the usual dosage) may be necessary). Products include:
Inapsine Injection 462

Enflurane (Concurrent use with the usual dose of OxyContin may result in respiratory depression, profound sedation or coma; reduced dosage (1/3 to ½ of the usual dosage) may be necessary).
No products indexed under this heading.

Estazolam (Concurrent use with the usual dose of OxyContin may result in respiratory depression, profound sedation or coma; reduced dosage (1/3 to ½ of the usual dosage) may be necessary). Products include:
ProSom Tablets 457

IMPORTANT NOTE: Always consult each drug listing in the patient's regimen for possible interactions.

OxyContin — Interactions Index

Ethchlorvynol (Concurrent use with the usual dose of OxyContin may result in respiratory depression, profound sedation or coma; reduced dosage (1/3 to 1/2 of the usual dosage) may be necessary). Products include:
- Placidyl Capsules 456

Ethinamate (Concurrent use with the usual dose of OxyContin may result in respiratory depression, profound sedation or coma; reduced dosage (1/3 to 1/2 of the usual dosage) may be necessary).
- No products indexed under this heading.

Fentanyl (Concurrent use with the usual dose of OxyContin may result in respiratory depression, profound sedation or coma; reduced dosage (1/3 to 1/2 of the usual dosage) may be necessary). Products include:
- Duragesic Transdermal System 1336

Fentanyl Citrate (Concurrent use with the usual dose of OxyContin may result in respiratory depression, profound sedation or coma; reduced dosage (1/3 to 1/2 of the usual dosage) may be necessary). Products include:
- Sublimaze Injection 463

Fluphenazine Decanoate (Concurrent use with the usual dose of OxyContin may result in respiratory depression, profound sedation or coma; reduced dosage (1/3 to 1/2 of the usual dosage) may be necessary). Products include:
- Prolixin Decanoate 510

Fluphenazine Enanthate (Concurrent use with the usual dose of OxyContin may result in respiratory depression, profound sedation or coma; reduced dosage (1/3 to 1/2 of the usual dosage) may be necessary). Products include:
- Prolixin Enanthate 510

Fluphenazine Hydrochloride (Concurrent use with the usual dose of OxyContin may result in respiratory depression, profound sedation or coma; reduced dosage (1/3 to 1/2 of the usual dosage) may be necessary). Products include:
- Prolixin 510

Flurazepam Hydrochloride (Concurrent use with the usual dose of OxyContin may result in respiratory depression, profound sedation or coma; reduced dosage (1/3 to 1/2 of the usual dosage) may be necessary). Products include:
- Dalmane Capsules 2329

Glutethimide (Concurrent use with the usual dose of OxyContin may result in respiratory depression, profound sedation or coma; reduced dosage (1/3 to 1/2 of the usual dosage) may be necessary).
- No products indexed under this heading.

Haloperidol (Concurrent use with the usual dose of OxyContin may result in respiratory depression, profound sedation or coma; reduced dosage (1/3 to 1/2 of the usual dosage) may be necessary). Products include:
- Haldol Injection, Tablets and Concentrate 1585

Haloperidol Decanoate (Concurrent use with the usual dose of OxyContin may result in respiratory depression, profound sedation or coma; reduced dosage (1/3 to 1/2 of the usual dosage) may be necessary). Products include:
- Haldol Decanoate 1587

Hydrocodone Bitartrate (Concurrent use with the usual dose of OxyContin may result in respiratory depression, profound sedation or coma; reduced dosage (1/3 to 1/2 of the usual dosage) may be necessary). Products include:
- Codiclear DH Syrup 808
- Duratuss HD Elixir 2750
- Histussin D Liquid 670
- Hycodan Tablets and Syrup 946
- Hycomine Compound Tablets 948
- Hycomine 947
- Hycotuss Expectorant Syrup 950
- Hydrocet Capsules 787
- Lorcet 10/650 Tablets 1016
- Lortab 2751
- Tussend 1830
- Tussend Expectorant 1831
- Vicodin Tablets 1404
- Vicodin ES Tablets 1405
- Vicodin HP Tablets 1403
- Vicodin Tuss Expectorant 1406
- Zydone Capsules 967

Hydrocodone Polistirex (Concurrent use with the usual dose of OxyContin may result in respiratory depression, profound sedation or coma; reduced dosage (1/3 to 1/2 of the usual dosage) may be necessary). Products include:
- Tussionex Pennkinetic Extended-Release Suspension 1624

Hydromorphone Hydrochloride (Concurrent use with the usual dose of OxyContin may result in respiratory depression, profound sedation or coma; reduced dosage (1/3 to 1/2 of the usual dosage) may be necessary). Products include:
- Dilaudid Ampules 1382
- Dilaudid Cough Syrup 1383
- Dilaudid-HP Injection 1384
- Dilaudid-HP Lyophilized Powder 250 mg 1384
- Dilaudid 1382
- Dilaudid Oral Liquid 1386
- Dilaudid 1382
- Dilaudid Tablets - 8 mg 1386

Hydroxyzine Hydrochloride (Concurrent use with the usual dose of OxyContin may result in respiratory depression, profound sedation or coma; reduced dosage (1/3 to 1/2 of the usual dosage) may be necessary). Products include:
- Atarax Tablets & Syrup 1992
- Marax Tablets & DF Syrup 2015
- Vistaril Intramuscular Solution 2042

Isoflurane (Concurrent use with the usual dose of OxyContin may result in respiratory depression, profound sedation or coma; reduced dosage (1/3 to 1/2 of the usual dosage) may be necessary).
- No products indexed under this heading.

Ketamine Hydrochloride (Concurrent use with the usual dose of OxyContin may result in respiratory depression, profound sedation or coma; reduced dosage (1/3 to 1/2 of the usual dosage) may be necessary).
- No products indexed under this heading.

Levomethadyl Acetate Hydrochloride (Concurrent use with the usual dose of OxyContin may result in respiratory depression, profound sedation or coma; reduced dosage (1/3 to 1/2 of the usual dosage) may be necessary). Products include:
- Orlaam Oral Solution 2361

Levorphanol Tartrate (Concurrent use with the usual dose of OxyContin may result in respiratory depression, profound sedation or coma; reduced dosage (1/3 to 1/2 of the usual dosage) may be necessary). Products include:
- Levo-Dromoran 2297

Lorazepam (Concurrent use with the usual dose of OxyContin may result in respiratory depression, profound sedation or coma; reduced dosage (1/3 to 1/2 of the usual dosage) may be necessary). Products include:
- Ativan Injection 2805
- Ativan Tablets 2807

Loxapine Hydrochloride (Concurrent use with the usual dose of OxyContin may result in respiratory depression, profound sedation or coma; reduced dosage (1/3 to 1/2 of the usual dosage) may be necessary). Products include:
- Loxitane 1426

Loxapine Succinate (Concurrent use with the usual dose of OxyContin may result in respiratory depression, profound sedation or coma; reduced dosage (1/3 to 1/2 of the usual dosage) may be necessary). Products include:
- Loxitane Capsules 1426

Meperidine Hydrochloride (Concurrent use with the usual dose of OxyContin may result in respiratory depression, profound sedation or coma; reduced dosage (1/3 to 1/2 of the usual dosage) may be necessary). Products include:
- Demerol 2438
- Mepergan Injection 2859

Mephobarbital (Concurrent use with the usual dose of OxyContin may result in respiratory depression, profound sedation or coma; reduced dosage (1/3 to 1/2 of the usual dosage) may be necessary). Products include:
- Mebaral Tablets 2452

Meprobamate (Concurrent use with the usual dose of OxyContin may result in respiratory depression, profound sedation or coma; reduced dosage (1/3 to 1/2 of the usual dosage) may be necessary). Products include:
- Miltown Tablets 2780
- PMB 200 and PMB 400 2890

Mesoridazine Besylate (Concurrent use with the usual dose of OxyContin may result in respiratory depression, profound sedation or coma; reduced dosage (1/3 to 1/2 of the usual dosage) may be necessary). Products include:
- Serentil 689

Methadone Hydrochloride (Concurrent use with the usual dose of OxyContin may result in respiratory depression, profound sedation or coma; reduced dosage (1/3 to 1/2 of the usual dosage) may be necessary). Products include:
- Methadone Hydrochloride Oral Concentrate 2356
- Methadone Hydrochloride Oral Solution & Tablets 2357

Methohexital Sodium (Concurrent use with the usual dose of OxyContin may result in respiratory depression, profound sedation or coma; reduced dosage (1/3 to 1/2 of the usual dosage) may be necessary).
- No products indexed under this heading.

Methotrimeprazine (Concurrent use with the usual dose of OxyContin may result in respiratory depression, profound sedation or coma; reduced dosage (1/3 to 1/2 of the usual dosage) may be necessary). Products include:
- Levoprome 1321

Methoxyflurane (Concurrent use with the usual dose of OxyContin may result in respiratory depression, profound sedation or coma; reduced dosage (1/3 to 1/2 of the usual dosage) may be necessary).
- No products indexed under this heading.

Midazolam Hydrochloride (Concurrent use with the usual dose of OxyContin may result in respiratory depression, profound sedation or coma; reduced dosage (1/3 to 1/2 of the usual dosage) may be necessary). Products include:
- Versed Injection 2324

Molindone Hydrochloride (Concurrent use with the usual dose of OxyContin may result in respiratory depression, profound sedation or coma; reduced dosage (1/3 to 1/2 of the usual dosage) may be necessary). Products include:
- Moban Tablets and Concentrate 1036

Morphine Sulfate (Concurrent use with the usual dose of OxyContin may result in respiratory depression, profound sedation or coma; reduced dosage (1/3 to 1/2 of the usual dosage) may be necessary). Products include:
- Astramorph/PF Injection, USP (Preservative-Free) 526
- Duramorph Injection 983
- Infumorph 200 and Infumorph 500 Sterile Solutions 985
- Kadian Capsules 2948
- MS Contin Tablets 2149
- MSIR 2152
- Oramorph SR (Morphine Sulfate Sustained Release Tablets) 2359
- RMS Suppositories CII 2766
- Roxanol 2365

Nalbuphine Hydrochloride (Mixed agonist/antagonist analgesics may reduce the analgesic effect of oxycodone and/or may precipitate withdrawal symptoms). Products include:
- Nubain Injection 952

Opium Alkaloids (Concurrent use with the usual dose of OxyContin may result in respiratory depression, profound sedation or coma; reduced dosage (1/3 to 1/2 of the usual dosage) may be necessary).
- No products indexed under this heading.

Oxazepam (Concurrent use with the usual dose of OxyContin may result in respiratory depression, profound sedation or coma; reduced dosage (1/3 to 1/2 of the usual dosage) may be necessary). Products include:
- Serax Capsules 2916
- Serax Tablets 2916

Pentazocine Hydrochloride (Mixed agonist/antagonist analgesics may reduce the analgesic effect of oxycodone and/or may precipitate withdrawal symptoms). Products include:
- Talacen Caplets 2464
- Talwin Compound 2466
- Talwin Nx Tablets 2467

Pentazocine Lactate (Mixed agonist/antagonist analgesics may reduce the analgesic effect of oxycodone and/or may precipitate withdrawal symptoms). Products include:
- Talwin Injection 2465

Pentobarbital Sodium (Concurrent use with the usual dose of OxyContin may result in respiratory depression, profound sedation or coma; reduced dosage (1/3 to 1/2 of the usual dosage) may be necessary). Products include:
- Nembutal Sodium Capsules 440

(◫ Described in PDR For Nonprescription Drugs) (⊙ Described in PDR For Ophthalmology)

Nembutal Sodium Solution 442
Nembutal Sodium Suppositories...... 444

Perphenazine (Concurrent use with the usual dose of OxyContin may result in respiratory depression, profound sedation or coma; reduced dosage (1/3 to ½ of the usual dosage) may be necessary). Products include:
Etrafon 2495
Triavil Tablets 1800
Trilafon... 2532

Phenobarbital (Concurrent use with the usual dose of OxyContin may result in respiratory depression, profound sedation or coma; reduced dosage (1/3 to ½ of the usual dosage) may be necessary). Products include:
Arco-Lase Plus Tablets 513
Bellergal-S Tablets 2375
Donnatal 2234
Donnatal Extentabs......................... 2234
Donnatal Tablets 2234
Phenobarbital Elixir and Tablets...... 1523
Quadrinal Tablets 1398

Prazepam (Concurrent use with the usual dose of OxyContin may result in respiratory depression, profound sedation or coma; reduced dosage (1/3 to ½ of the usual dosage) may be necessary).
No products indexed under this heading.

Prochlorperazine (Concurrent use with the usual dose of OxyContin may result in respiratory depression, profound sedation or coma; reduced dosage (1/3 to ½ of the usual dosage) may be necessary). Products include:
Compazine 2644

Promethazine Hydrochloride (Concurrent use with the usual dose of OxyContin may result in respiratory depression, profound sedation or coma; reduced dosage (1/3 to ½ of the usual dosage) may be necessary). Products include:
Mepergan Injection 2859
Phenergan with Codeine 2883
Phenergan with Dextromethorphan 2885
Phenergan Injection 2880
Phenergan Suppositories 2882
Phenergan Syrup 2881
Phenergan Tablets 2882
Phenergan VC 2886
Phenergan VC with Codeine 2888

Propofol (Concurrent use with the usual dose of OxyContin may result in respiratory depression, profound sedation or coma; reduced dosage (1/3 to ½ of the usual dosage) may be necessary). Products include:
Diprivan Injectable Emulsion 2939

Propoxyphene Hydrochloride (Concurrent use with the usual dose of OxyContin may result in respiratory depression, profound sedation or coma; reduced dosage (1/3 to ½ of the usual dosage) may be necessary). Products include:
Darvon 1475
Wygesic Tablets 2930

Propoxyphene Napsylate (Concurrent use with the usual dose of OxyContin may result in respiratory depression, profound sedation or coma; reduced dosage (1/3 to ½ of the usual dosage) may be necessary). Products include:
Darvon-N/Darvocet-N 1473

Quazepam (Concurrent use with the usual dose of OxyContin may result in respiratory depression, profound sedation or coma; reduced dosage (1/3 to ½ of the usual dosage) may be necessary). Products include:
Doral Tablets 2773

Risperidone (Concurrent use with the usual dose of OxyContin may result in respiratory depression, profound sedation or coma; reduced dosage (1/3 to ½ of the usual dosage) may be necessary). Products include:
Risperdal Tablets 1348

Secobarbital Sodium (Concurrent use with the usual dose of OxyContin may result in respiratory depression, profound sedation or coma; reduced dosage (1/3 to ½ of the usual dosage) may be necessary). Products include:
Seconal Sodium Pulvules 1529

Sevoflurane (Concurrent use with the usual dose of OxyContin may result in respiratory depression, profound sedation or coma; reduced dosage (1/3 to ½ of the usual dosage) may be necessary).
No products indexed under this heading.

Sufentanil Citrate (Concurrent use with the usual dose of OxyContin may result in respiratory depression, profound sedation or coma; reduced dosage (1/3 to ½ of the usual dosage) may be necessary). Products include:
Sufenta Injection 1355

Temazepam (Concurrent use with the usual dose of OxyContin may result in respiratory depression, profound sedation or coma; reduced dosage (1/3 to ½ of the usual dosage) may be necessary). Products include:
Restoril Capsules 2413

Thiamylal Sodium (Concurrent use with the usual dose of OxyContin may result in respiratory depression, profound sedation or coma; reduced dosage (1/3 to ½ of the usual dosage) may be necessary).
No products indexed under this heading.

Thioridazine Hydrochloride (Concurrent use with the usual dose of OxyContin may result in respiratory depression, profound sedation or coma; reduced dosage (1/3 to ½ of the usual dosage) may be necessary). Products include:
Mellaril 2398

Thiothixene (Concurrent use with the usual dose of OxyContin may result in respiratory depression, profound sedation or coma; reduced dosage (1/3 to ½ of the usual dosage) may be necessary). Products include:
Navane Capsules and Concentrate 2018
Navane Intramuscular 2019

Triazolam (Concurrent use with the usual dose of OxyContin may result in respiratory depression, profound sedation or coma; reduced dosage (1/3 to ½ of the usual dosage) may be necessary). Products include:
Halcion Tablets 2093

Trifluoperazine Hydrochloride (Concurrent use with the usual dose of OxyContin may result in respiratory depression, profound sedation or coma; reduced dosage (1/3 to ½ of the usual dosage) may be necessary). Products include:
Stelazine 2692

Zolpidem Tartrate (Concurrent use with the usual dose of OxyContin may result in respiratory depression, profound sedation or coma; reduced dosage (1/3 to ½ of the usual dosage) may be necessary). Products include:
Ambien Tablets 2559

Food Interactions

Alcohol (Concurrent use with the usual dose of OxyContin may result in respiratory depression, profound sedation or coma).

OXYIR CAPSULES

(Oxycodone Hydrochloride) 2167
May interact with central nervous system depressants, narcotic analgesics, general anesthetics, phenothiazines, tranquilizers, hypnotics and sedatives, and certain other agents. Compounds in these categories include:

Alfentanil Hydrochloride (Concomitant use may exhibit an additive CNS depression). Products include:
Alfenta Injection 1334

Alprazolam (Concomitant use may exhibit an additive CNS depression). Products include:
Xanax Tablets 2115

Aprobarbital (Concomitant use may exhibit an additive CNS depression).
No products indexed under this heading.

Buprenorphine (Concomitant use may exhibit an additive CNS depression). Products include:
Buprenex Injectable 2170

Buspirone Hydrochloride (Concomitant use may exhibit an additive CNS depression). Products include:
BuSpar Tablets 738

Butabarbital (Concomitant use may exhibit an additive CNS depression).
No products indexed under this heading.

Butalbital (Concomitant use may exhibit an additive CNS depression). Products include:
Axocet Capsules 2469
Esgic-plus Capsules 1012
Esgic-plus Tablets 1012
Fioricet Tablets 2386
Fioricet with Codeine Capsules 2387
Fiorinal Capsules 2388
Fiorinal with Codeine Capsules 2390
Fiorinal Tablets 2388
Phrenilin 790
Sedapap Tablets 50 mg/650 mg .. 1826

Chlordiazepoxide (Concomitant use may exhibit an additive CNS depression). Products include:
Limbitrol 2333

Chlordiazepoxide Hydrochloride (Concomitant use may exhibit an additive CNS depression). Products include:
Librax Capsules 2330
Librium Capsules 2331
Librium Injectable 2332

Chlorpromazine (Concomitant use may exhibit an additive CNS depression). Products include:
Thorazine Suppositories 2701

Chlorpromazine Hydrochloride (Concomitant use may exhibit an additive CNS depression). Products include:
Thorazine 2701

Chlorprothixene (Concomitant use may exhibit an additive CNS depression).
No products indexed under this heading.

Chlorprothixene Hydrochloride (Concomitant use may exhibit an additive CNS depression).
No products indexed under this heading.

Chlorprothixene Lactate (Concomitant use may exhibit an additive CNS depression).
No products indexed under this heading.

Clorazepate Dipotassium (Concomitant use may exhibit an additive CNS depression). Products include:
Tranxene 459

Clozapine (Concomitant use may exhibit an additive CNS depression). Products include:
Clozaril Tablets 2377

Codeine Phosphate (Concomitant use may exhibit an additive CNS depression). Products include:
Brontex 2130
Dimetane-DC Cough Syrup 2232
Fioricet with Codeine Capsules 2387
Fiorinal with Codeine Capsules 2390
Nucofed 2225
Phenergan with Codeine 2883
Phenergan VC with Codeine 2888
Robitussin A-C Syrup 2248
Robitussin-DAC Syrup 2249
Ryna 804
Soma Compound w/Codeine Tablets 2784
Tylenol with Codeine 1592

Desflurane (Concomitant use may exhibit an additive CNS depression). Products include:
Suprane (desflurane, USP) 1865

Dezocine (Concomitant use may exhibit an additive CNS depression). Products include:
Dalgan Injection 529

Diazepam (Concomitant use may exhibit an additive CNS depression). Products include:
Dizac (diazepam injectable emulsion) CIV 1862
Valium Injectable 2336
Valium Tablets 2335

Droperidol (Concomitant use may exhibit an additive CNS depression). Products include:
Inapsine Injection 462

Enflurane (Concomitant use may exhibit an additive CNS depression).
No products indexed under this heading.

Estazolam (Concomitant use may exhibit an additive CNS depression). Products include:
ProSom Tablets 457

Ethchlorvynol (Concomitant use may exhibit an additive CNS depression). Products include:
Placidyl Capsules 456

Ethinamate (Concomitant use may exhibit an additive CNS depression).
No products indexed under this heading.

Fentanyl (Concomitant use may exhibit an additive CNS depression). Products include:
Duragesic Transdermal System........ 1336

Fentanyl Citrate (Concomitant use may exhibit an additive CNS depression). Products include:
Sublimaze Injection 463

Fluphenazine Decanoate (Concomitant use may exhibit an additive CNS depression). Products include:
Prolixin Decanoate 510

Fluphenazine Enanthate (Concomitant use may exhibit an additive CNS depression). Products include:
Prolixin Enanthate 510

IMPORTANT NOTE: Always consult each drug listing in the patient's regimen for possible interactions.

Fluphenazine Hydrochloride (Concomitant use may exhibit an additive CNS depression). Products include:
   Prolixin 510

Flurazepam Hydrochloride (Concomitant use may exhibit an additive CNS depression). Products include:
   Dalmane Capsules 2329

Glutethimide (Concomitant use may exhibit an additive CNS depression).
   No products indexed under this heading.

Haloperidol (Concomitant use may exhibit an additive CNS depression). Products include:
   Haldol Injection, Tablets and Concentrate 1585

Haloperidol Decanoate (Concomitant use may exhibit an additive CNS depression). Products include:
   Haldol Decanoate 1587

Hydrocodone Bitartrate (Concomitant use may exhibit an additive CNS depression). Products include:
   Codiclear DH Syrup 808
   Duratuss HD Elixir 2750
   Histussin D Liquid 670
   Hycodan Tablets and Syrup ... 946
   Hycomine Compound Tablets .. 948
   Hycomine 947
   Hycotuss Expectorant Syrup .. 950
   Hydrocet Capsules 787
   Lorcet 10/650 Tablets 1016
   Lortab 2751
   Tussend 1830
   Tussend Expectorant 1831
   Vicodin Tablets 1404
   Vicodin ES Tablets 1405
   Vicodin HP Tablets 1403
   Vicodin Tuss Expectorant 1406
   Zydone Capsules 967

Hydrocodone Polistirex (Concomitant use may exhibit an additive CNS depression). Products include:
   Tussionex Pennkinetic Extended-Release Suspension 1624

Hydromorphone Hydrochloride (Concomitant use may exhibit an additive CNS depression). Products include:
   Dilaudid Ampules 1382
   Dilaudid Cough Syrup 1383
   Dilaudid-HP Injection 1384
   Dilaudid-HP Lyophilized Powder 250 mg 1384
   Dilaudid 1382
   Dilaudid Oral Liquid 1386
   Dilaudid 1382
   Dilaudid Tablets - 8 mg. 1386

Hydroxyzine Hydrochloride (Concomitant use may exhibit an additive CNS depression). Products include:
   Atarax Tablets & Syrup 1992
   Marax Tablets & DF Syrup 2015
   Vistaril Intramuscular Solution .. 2042

Isoflurane (Concomitant use may exhibit an additive CNS depression).
   No products indexed under this heading.

Ketamine Hydrochloride (Concomitant use may exhibit an additive CNS depression).
   No products indexed under this heading.

Levomethadyl Acetate Hydrochloride (Concomitant use may exhibit an additive CNS depression). Products include:
   Orlaam Oral Solution 2361

Levorphanol Tartrate (Concomitant use may exhibit an additive CNS depression). Products include:
   Levo-Dromoran 2297

Lorazepam (Concomitant use may exhibit an additive CNS depression). Products include:
   Ativan Injection 2805
   Ativan Tablets 2807

Loxapine Hydrochloride (Concomitant use may exhibit an additive CNS depression). Products include:
   Loxitane 1426

Loxapine Succinate (Concomitant use may exhibit an additive CNS depression). Products include:
   Loxitane Capsules 1426

Meperidine Hydrochloride (Concomitant use may exhibit an additive CNS depression). Products include:
   Demerol 2438
   Mepergan Injection 2859

Mephobarbital (Concomitant use may exhibit an additive CNS depression). Products include:
   Mebaral Tablets 2452

Meprobamate (Concomitant use may exhibit an additive CNS depression). Products include:
   Miltown Tablets 2780
   PMB 200 and PMB 400 2890

Mesoridazine Besylate (Concomitant use may exhibit an additive CNS depression). Products include:
   Serentil 689

Methadone Hydrochloride (Concomitant use may exhibit an additive CNS depression). Products include:
   Methadone Hydrochloride Oral Concentrate 2356
   Methadone Hydrochloride Oral Solution & Tablets............. 2357

Methohexital Sodium (Concomitant use may exhibit an additive CNS depression).
   No products indexed under this heading.

Methotrimeprazine (Concomitant use may exhibit an additive CNS depression). Products include:
   Levoprome 1321

Methoxyflurane (Concomitant use may exhibit an additive CNS depression).
   No products indexed under this heading.

Midazolam Hydrochloride (Concomitant use may exhibit an additive CNS depression). Products include:
   Versed Injection 2324

Molindone Hydrochloride (Concomitant use may exhibit an additive CNS depression). Products include:
   Moban Tablets and Concentrate ... 1036

Morphine Sulfate (Concomitant use may exhibit an additive CNS depression). Products include:
   Astramorph/PF Injection, USP (Preservative-Free) 526
   Duramorph Injection 983
   Infumorph 200 and Infumorph 500 Sterile Solutions 985
   Kadian Capsules 2948
   MS Contin Tablets 2149
   MSIR 2152
   Oramorph SR (Morphine Sulfate Sustained Release Tablets) ... 2359
   RMS Suppositories CII 2766
   Roxanol 2365

Opium Alkaloids (Concomitant use may exhibit an additive CNS depression).
   No products indexed under this heading.

Oxazepam (Concomitant use may exhibit an additive CNS depression). Products include:
   Serax Capsules 2916
   Serax Tablets 2916

Pentobarbital Sodium (Concomitant use may exhibit an additive CNS depression). Products include:
   Nembutal Sodium Capsules ... 440
   Nembutal Sodium Solution 442
   Nembutal Sodium Suppositories .. 444

Perphenazine (Concomitant use may exhibit an additive CNS depression). Products include:
   Etrafon 2495
   Triavil Tablets 1800
   Trilafon 2532

Phenobarbital (Concomitant use may exhibit an additive CNS depression). Products include:
   Arco-Lase Plus Tablets 513
   Bellergal-S Tablets 2375
   Donnatal 2234
   Donnatal Extentabs 2234
   Donnatal Tablets 2234
   Phenobarbital Elixir and Tablets .. 1523
   Quadrinal Tablets 1398

Prazepam (Concomitant use may exhibit an additive CNS depression).
   No products indexed under this heading.

Prochlorperazine (Concomitant use may exhibit an additive CNS depression). Products include:
   Compazine 2644

Promethazine Hydrochloride (Concomitant use may exhibit an additive CNS depression). Products include:
   Mepergan Injection 2859
   Phenergan with Codeine 2883
   Phenergan with Dextromethorphan .. 2885
   Phenergan Injection 2880
   Phenergan Suppositories 2882
   Phenergan Syrup 2881
   Phenergan Tablets 2882
   Phenergan VC 2886
   Phenergan VC with Codeine . 2888

Propofol (Concomitant use may exhibit an additive CNS depression). Products include:
   Diprivan Injectable Emulsion .. 2939

Propoxyphene Hydrochloride (Concomitant use may exhibit an additive CNS depression). Products include:
   Darvon 1475
   Wygesic Tablets 2930

Propoxyphene Napsylate (Concomitant use may exhibit an additive CNS depression). Products include:
   Darvon-N/Darvocet-N 1473

Quazepam (Concomitant use may exhibit an additive CNS depression). Products include:
   Doral Tablets 2773

Risperidone (Concomitant use may exhibit an additive CNS depression). Products include:
   Risperdal Tablets 1348

Secobarbital Sodium (Concomitant use may exhibit an additive CNS depression). Products include:
   Seconal Sodium Pulvules 1529

Sevoflurane (Concomitant use may exhibit an additive CNS depression).
   No products indexed under this heading.

Sufentanil Citrate (Concomitant use may exhibit an additive CNS depression). Products include:
   Sufenta Injection 1355

Temazepam (Concomitant use may exhibit an additive CNS depression). Products include:
   Restoril Capsules 2413

Thiamylal Sodium (Concomitant use may exhibit an additive CNS depression).
   No products indexed under this heading.

Thioridazine Hydrochloride (Concomitant use may exhibit an additive CNS depression). Products include:
   Mellaril 2398

Thiothixene (Concomitant use may exhibit an additive CNS depression). Products include:
   Navane Capsules and Concentrate 2018
   Navane Intramuscular 2019

Triazolam (Concomitant use may exhibit an additive CNS depression). Products include:
   Halcion Tablets 2093

Trifluoperazine Hydrochloride (Concomitant use may exhibit an additive CNS depression). Products include:
   Stelazine 2692

Zolpidem Tartrate (Concomitant use may exhibit an additive CNS depression). Products include:
   Ambien Tablets 2559

Food Interactions

Alcohol (Concomitant use may exhibit an additive CNS depression).

PBZ TABLETS

(Tripelennamine Hydrochloride) 863
May interact with central nervous system depressants and certain other agents. Compounds in these categories include:

Alfentanil Hydrochloride (CNS effects may be additive). Products include:
   Alfenta Injection 1334

Alprazolam (CNS effects may be additive). Products include:
   Xanax Tablets 2115

Aprobarbital (CNS effects may be additive).
   No products indexed under this heading.

Buprenorphine (CNS effects may be additive). Products include:
   Buprenex Injectable 2170

Buspirone Hydrochloride (CNS effects may be additive). Products include:
   BuSpar Tablets 738

Butabarbital (CNS effects may be additive).
   No products indexed under this heading.

Butalbital (CNS effects may be additive). Products include:
   Axocet Capsules 2469
   Esgic-plus Capsules 1012
   Esgic-plus Tablets 1012
   Fioricet Tablets 2386
   Fioricet with Codeine Capsules .. 2387
   Fiorinal Capsules 2388
   Fiorinal with Codeine Capsules .. 2390
   Fiorinal Tablets 2388
   Phrenilin 790
   Sedapap Tablets 50 mg/650 mg .. 1826

Chlordiazepoxide (CNS effects may be additive). Products include:
   Limbitrol 2333

Chlordiazepoxide Hydrochloride (CNS effects may be additive). Products include:
   Librax Capsules 2330
   Librium Capsules 2331
   Librium Injectable 2332

Chlorpromazine (CNS effects may be additive). Products include:
   Thorazine Suppositories 2701

Chlorprothixene (CNS effects may be additive).
   No products indexed under this heading.

Chlorprothixene Hydrochloride (CNS effects may be additive).
   No products indexed under this heading.

Chlorprothixene Lactate (CNS effects may be additive).
   No products indexed under this heading.

Clorazepate Dipotassium (CNS effects may be additive). Products include:
Tranxene ... 459

Clozapine (CNS effects may be additive). Products include:
Clozaril Tablets ... 2377

Codeine Phosphate (CNS effects may be additive). Products include:
Brontex ... 2130
Dimetane-DC Cough Syrup ... 2232
Fioricet with Codeine Capsules ... 2387
Fiorinal with Codeine Capsules ... 2390
Nucofed ... 2225
Phenergan with Codeine ... 2883
Phenergan VC with Codeine ... 2888
Robitussin A-C Syrup ... 2248
Robitussin-DAC Syrup ... 2249
Ryna ... 804
Soma Compound w/Codeine Tablets ... 2784
Tylenol with Codeine ... 1592

Desflurane (CNS effects may be additive). Products include:
Suprane (desflurane, USP) ... 1865

Dezocine (CNS effects may be additive). Products include:
Dalgan Injection ... 529

Diazepam (CNS effects may be additive). Products include:
Dizac (diazepam injectable emulsion) CIV ... 1862
Valium Injectable ... 2336
Valium Tablets ... 2335

Droperidol (CNS effects may be additive). Products include:
Inapsine Injection ... 462

Enflurane (CNS effects may be additive).
No products indexed under this heading.

Estazolam (CNS effects may be additive). Products include:
ProSom Tablets ... 457

Ethchlorvynol (CNS effects may be additive). Products include:
Placidyl Capsules ... 456

Ethinamate (CNS effects may be additive).
No products indexed under this heading.

Fentanyl (CNS effects may be additive). Products include:
Duragesic Transdermal System ... 1336

Fentanyl Citrate (CNS effects may be additive). Products include:
Sublimaze Injection ... 463

Fluphenazine Decanoate (CNS effects may be additive). Products include:
Prolixin Decanoate ... 510

Fluphenazine Enanthate (CNS effects may be additive). Products include:
Prolixin Enanthate ... 510

Fluphenazine Hydrochloride (CNS effects may be additive). Products include:
Prolixin ... 510

Flurazepam Hydrochloride (CNS effects may be additive). Products include:
Dalmane Capsules ... 2329

Glutethimide (CNS effects may be additive).
No products indexed under this heading.

Haloperidol (CNS effects may be additive). Products include:
Haldol Injection, Tablets and Concentrate ... 1585

Haloperidol Decanoate (CNS effects may be additive). Products include:
Haldol Decanoate ... 1587

Hydrocodone Bitartrate (CNS effects may be additive). Products include:
Codiclear DH Syrup ... 808
Duratuss HD Elixir ... 2750
Histussin D Liquid ... 670
Hycodan Tablets and Syrup ... 946
Hycomine Compound Tablets ... 948
Hycomine ... 947
Hycotuss Expectorant Syrup ... 950
Hydrocet Capsules ... 787
Lorcet 10/650 Tablets ... 1016
Lortab ... 2751
Tussend ... 1830
Tussend Expectorant ... 1831
Vicodin Tablets ... 1404
Vicodin ES Tablets ... 1405
Vicodin HP Tablets ... 1403
Vicodin Tuss Expectorant ... 1406
Zydone Capsules ... 967

Hydrocodone Polistirex (CNS effects may be additive). Products include:
Tussionex Pennkinetic Extended-Release Suspension ... 1624

Hydroxyzine Hydrochloride (CNS effects may be additive). Products include:
Atarax Tablets & Syrup ... 1992
Marax Tablets & DF Syrup ... 2015
Vistaril Intramuscular Solution ... 2042

Isoflurane (CNS effects may be additive).
No products indexed under this heading.

Ketamine Hydrochloride (CNS effects may be additive).
No products indexed under this heading.

Levomethadyl Acetate Hydrochloride (CNS effects may be additive). Products include:
Orlaam Oral Solution ... 2361

Levorphanol Tartrate (CNS effects may be additive). Products include:
Levo-Dromoran ... 2297

Lorazepam (CNS effects may be additive). Products include:
Ativan Injection ... 2805
Ativan Tablets ... 2807

Loxapine Hydrochloride (CNS effects may be additive). Products include:
Loxitane ... 1426

Loxapine Succinate (CNS effects may be additive). Products include:
Loxitane Capsules ... 1426

Meperidine Hydrochloride (CNS effects may be additive). Products include:
Demerol ... 2438
Mepergan Injection ... 2859

Mephobarbital (CNS effects may be additive). Products include:
Mebaral Tablets ... 2452

Meprobamate (CNS effects may be additive). Products include:
Miltown Tablets ... 2780
PMB 200 and PMB 400 ... 2890

Mesoridazine Besylate (CNS effects may be additive). Products include:
Serentil ... 689

Methadone Hydrochloride (CNS effects may be additive). Products include:
Methadone Hydrochloride Oral Concentrate ... 2356
Methadone Hydrochloride Oral Solution & Tablets ... 2357

Methohexital Sodium (CNS effects may be additive).
No products indexed under this heading.

Methotrimeprazine (CNS effects may be additive). Products include:
Levoprome ... 1321

Methoxyflurane (CNS effects may be additive).
No products indexed under this heading.

Midazolam Hydrochloride (CNS effects may be additive). Products include:
Versed Injection ... 2324

Molindone Hydrochloride (CNS effects may be additive). Products include:
Moban Tablets and Concentrate ... 1036

Morphine Sulfate (CNS effects may be additive). Products include:
Astramorph/PF Injection, USP (Preservative-Free) ... 526
Duramorph Injection ... 983
Infumorph 200 and Infumorph 500 Sterile Solutions ... 985
Kadian Capsules ... 2948
MS Contin Tablets ... 2149
MSIR ... 2152
Oramorph SR (Morphine Sulfate Sustained Release Tablets) ... 2359
RMS Suppositories CII ... 2766
Roxanol ... 2365

Opium Alkaloids (CNS effects may be additive).
No products indexed under this heading.

Oxazepam (CNS effects may be additive). Products include:
Serax Capsules ... 2916
Serax Tablets ... 2916

Oxycodone Hydrochloride (CNS effects may be additive). Products include:
OxyContin Tablets ... 2163
OxyIR Capsules ... 2167
Percocet Tablets ... 955
Percodan Tablets ... 955
Percodan-Demi Tablets ... 956
Roxicodone Tablets, Oral Solution & Intensol (Oxycodone) ... 2366
Tylox Capsules ... 1593

Pentobarbital Sodium (CNS effects may be additive). Products include:
Nembutal Sodium Capsules ... 440
Nembutal Sodium Solution ... 442
Nembutal Sodium Suppositories ... 444

Perphenazine (CNS effects may be additive). Products include:
Etrafon ... 2495
Triavil Tablets ... 1800
Trilafon ... 2532

Phenobarbital (CNS effects may be additive). Products include:
Arco-Lase Plus Tablets ... 513
Bellergal-S Tablets ... 2375
Donnatal ... 2234
Donnatal Extentabs ... 2234
Donnatal Tablets ... 2234
Phenobarbital Elixir and Tablets ... 1523
Quadrinal Tablets ... 1398

Prazepam (CNS effects may be additive).
No products indexed under this heading.

Prochlorperazine (CNS effects may be additive). Products include:
Compazine ... 2644

Promethazine Hydrochloride (CNS effects may be additive). Products include:
Mepergan Injection ... 2859
Phenergan with Codeine ... 2883
Phenergan with Dextromethorphan ... 2885
Phenergan Injection ... 2880
Phenergan Suppositories ... 2882
Phenergan Syrup ... 2881
Phenergan Tablets ... 2882
Phenergan VC ... 2886
Phenergan VC with Codeine ... 2888

Propofol (CNS effects may be additive). Products include:
Diprivan Injectable Emulsion ... 2939

Propoxyphene Hydrochloride (CNS effects may be additive). Products include:
Darvon ... 1475
Wygesic Tablets ... 2930

Propoxyphene Napsylate (CNS effects may be additive). Products include:
Darvon-N/Darvocet-N ... 1473

Quazepam (CNS effects may be additive). Products include:
Doral Tablets ... 2773

Risperidone (CNS effects may be additive). Products include:
Risperdal Tablets ... 1348

Secobarbital Sodium (CNS effects may be additive). Products include:
Seconal Sodium Pulvules ... 1529

Sevoflurane (CNS effects may be additive).
No products indexed under this heading.

Sufentanil Citrate (CNS effects may be additive). Products include:
Sufenta Injection ... 1355

Temazepam (CNS effects may be additive). Products include:
Restoril Capsules ... 2413

Thiamylal Sodium (CNS effects may be additive).
No products indexed under this heading.

Thioridazine Hydrochloride (CNS effects may be additive). Products include:
Mellaril ... 2398

Thiothixene (CNS effects may be additive). Products include:
Navane Capsules and Concentrate ... 2018
Navane Intramuscular ... 2019

Triazolam (CNS effects may be additive). Products include:
Halcion Tablets ... 2093

Trifluoperazine Hydrochloride (CNS effects may be additive). Products include:
Stelazine ... 2692

Zolpidem Tartrate (CNS effects may be additive). Products include:
Ambien Tablets ... 2559

Food Interactions

Alcohol (CNS effects may be additive).

PBZ-SR TABLETS
(Tripelennamine Hydrochloride) ... 862
May interact with central nervous system depressants, monoamine oxidase inhibitors, and certain other agents. Compounds in these categories include:

Alfentanil Hydrochloride (CNS effects may be additive). Products include:
Alfenta Injection ... 1334

Alprazolam (CNS effects may be additive). Products include:
Xanax Tablets ... 2115

Aprobarbital (CNS effects may be additive).
No products indexed under this heading.

Buprenorphine (CNS effects may be additive). Products include:
Buprenex Injectable ... 2170

Buspirone Hydrochloride (CNS effects may be additive). Products include:
BuSpar Tablets ... 738

Butabarbital (CNS effects may be additive).
No products indexed under this heading.

Butalbital (CNS effects may be additive). Products include:
Axocet Capsules ... 2469
Esgic-plus Capsules ... 1012
Esgic-plus Tablets ... 1012
Fioricet Tablets ... 2386
Fioricet with Codeine Capsules ... 2387
Fiorinal Capsules ... 2388
Fiorinal with Codeine Capsules ... 2390
Fiorinal Tablets ... 2388
Phrenilin ... 790
Sedapap Tablets 50 mg/650 mg ... 1826

IMPORTANT NOTE: Always consult each drug listing in the patient's regimen for possible interactions.

PBZ-SR **Interactions Index** 804

Chlordiazepoxide (CNS effects may be additive). Products include:
- Limbitrol 2333

Chlordiazepoxide Hydrochloride (CNS effects may be additive). Products include:
- Librax Capsules 2330
- Librium Capsules 2331
- Librium Injectable 2332

Chlorpromazine (CNS effects may be additive). Products include:
- Thorazine Suppositories 2701

Chlorprothixene (CNS effects may be additive).
- No products indexed under this heading.

Chlorprothixene Hydrochloride (CNS effects may be additive).
- No products indexed under this heading.

Chlorprothixene Lactate (CNS effects may be additive).
- No products indexed under this heading.

Clorazepate Dipotassium (CNS effects may be additive). Products include:
- Tranxene 459

Clozapine (CNS effects may be additive). Products include:
- Clozaril Tablets 2377

Codeine Phosphate (CNS effects may be additive). Products include:
- Brontex 2130
- Dimetane-DC Cough Syrup 2232
- Fioricet with Codeine Capsules 2387
- Fiorinal with Codeine Capsules 2390
- Nucofed 2225
- Phenergan with Codeine 2883
- Phenergan VC with Codeine 2888
- Robitussin A-C Syrup 2248
- Robitussin-DAC Syrup 2249
- Ryna .... ▣ 804
- Soma Compound w/Codeine Tablets 2784
- Tylenol with Codeine 1592

Desflurane (CNS effects may be additive). Products include:
- Suprane (desflurane, USP) 1865

Dezocine (CNS effects may be additive). Products include:
- Dalgan Injection 529

Diazepam (CNS effects may be additive). Products include:
- Dizac (diazepam injectable emulsion) CIV 1862
- Valium Injectable 2336
- Valium Tablets 2335

Droperidol (CNS effects may be additive). Products include:
- Inapsine Injection 462

Enflurane (CNS effects may be additive).
- No products indexed under this heading.

Estazolam (CNS effects may be additive). Products include:
- ProSom Tablets 457

Ethchlorvynol (CNS effects may be additive). Products include:
- Placidyl Capsules 456

Ethinamate (CNS effects may be additive).
- No products indexed under this heading.

Fentanyl (CNS effects may be additive). Products include:
- Duragesic Transdermal System 1336

Fentanyl Citrate (CNS effects may be additive). Products include:
- Sublimaze Injection 463

Fluphenazine Decanoate (CNS effects may be additive). Products include:
- Prolixin Decanoate 510

Fluphenazine Enanthate (CNS effects may be additive). Products include:
- Prolixin Enanthate 510

Fluphenazine Hydrochloride (CNS effects may be additive). Products include:
- Prolixin 510

Flurazepam Hydrochloride (CNS effects may be additive). Products include:
- Dalmane Capsules 2329

Furazolidone (Concurrent use contraindicated). Products include:
- Furoxone 2221

Glutethimide (CNS effects may be additive).
- No products indexed under this heading.

Haloperidol (CNS effects may be additive). Products include:
- Haldol Injection, Tablets and Concentrate 1585

Haloperidol Decanoate (CNS effects may be additive). Products include:
- Haldol Decanoate 1587

Hydrocodone Bitartrate (CNS effects may be additive). Products include:
- Codiclear DH Syrup 808
- Duratuss HD Elixir 2750
- Histussin D Liquid 670
- Hycodan Tablets and Syrup 946
- Hycomine Compound Tablets 948
- Hycomine 947
- Hycotuss Expectorant Syrup 950
- Hydrocet Capsules 787
- Lorcet 10/650 Tablets 1016
- Lortab 2751
- Tussend 1830
- Tussend Expectorant 1831
- Vicodin Tablets 1404
- Vicodin ES Tablets 1405
- Vicodin HP Tablets 1403
- Vicodin Tuss Expectorant 1406
- Zydone Capsules 967

Hydrocodone Polistirex (CNS effects may be additive). Products include:
- Tussionex Pennkinetic Extended-Release Suspension 1624

Hydroxyzine Hydrochloride (CNS effects may be additive). Products include:
- Atarax Tablets & Syrup 1992
- Marax Tablets & DF Syrup 2015
- Vistaril Intramuscular Solution 2042

Isocarboxazid (Concurrent use contraindicated).
- No products indexed under this heading.

Isoflurane (CNS effects may be additive).
- No products indexed under this heading.

Ketamine Hydrochloride (CNS effects may be additive).
- No products indexed under this heading.

Levomethadyl Acetate Hydrochloride (CNS effects may be additive). Products include:
- Orlaam Oral Solution 2361

Levorphanol Tartrate (CNS effects may be additive). Products include:
- Levo-Dromoran 2297

Lorazepam (CNS effects may be additive). Products include:
- Ativan Injection 2805
- Ativan Tablets 2807

Loxapine Hydrochloride (CNS effects may be additive). Products include:
- Loxitane 1426

Loxapine Succinate (CNS effects may be additive). Products include:
- Loxitane Capsules 1426

Meperidine Hydrochloride (CNS effects may be additive). Products include:
- Demerol 2438
- Mepergan Injection 2859

Mephobarbital (CNS effects may be additive). Products include:
- Mebaral Tablets 2452

Meprobamate (CNS effects may be additive). Products include:
- Miltown Tablets 2780
- PMB 200 and PMB 400 2890

Mesoridazine Besylate (CNS effects may be additive). Products include:
- Serentil 689

Methadone Hydrochloride (CNS effects may be additive). Products include:
- Methadone Hydrochloride Oral Concentrate 2356
- Methadone Hydrochloride Oral Solution & Tablets 2357

Methohexital Sodium (CNS effects may be additive).
- No products indexed under this heading.

Methotrimeprazine (CNS effects may be additive). Products include:
- Levoprome 1321

Methoxyflurane (CNS effects may be additive).
- No products indexed under this heading.

Midazolam Hydrochloride (CNS effects may be additive). Products include:
- Versed Injection 2324

Molindone Hydrochloride (CNS effects may be additive). Products include:
- Moban Tablets and Concentrate 1036

Morphine Sulfate (CNS effects may be additive). Products include:
- Astramorph/PF Injection, USP (Preservative-Free) 526
- Duramorph Injection 983
- Infumorph 200 and Infumorph 500 Sterile Solutions 985
- Kadian Capsules 2948
- MS Contin Tablets 2149
- MSIR 2152
- Oramorph SR (Morphine Sulfate Sustained Release Tablets) 2359
- RMS Suppositories CII 2766
- Roxanol 2365

Opium Alkaloids (CNS effects may be additive).
- No products indexed under this heading.

Oxazepam (CNS effects may be additive). Products include:
- Serax Capsules 2916
- Serax Tablets 2916

Oxycodone Hydrochloride (CNS effects may be additive). Products include:
- OxyContin Tablets 2163
- OxyIR Capsules 2167
- Percocet Tablets 955
- Percodan Tablets 955
- Percodan-Demi Tablets 956
- Roxicodone Tablets, Oral Solution & Intensol (Oxycodone) 2366
- Tylox Capsules 1593

Pentobarbital Sodium (CNS effects may be additive). Products include:
- Nembutal Sodium Capsules 440
- Nembutal Sodium Solution 442
- Nembutal Sodium Suppositories 444

Perphenazine (CNS effects may be additive). Products include:
- Etrafon 2495
- Triavil Tablets 1800
- Trilafon 2532

Phenelzine Sulfate (Concurrent use contraindicated). Products include:
- Nardil 1977

Phenobarbital (CNS effects may be additive). Products include:
- Arco-Lase Plus Tablets 513
- Bellergal-S Tablets 2375
- Donnatal 2234
- Donnatal Extentabs 2234
- Donnatal Tablets 2234
- Phenobarbital Elixir and Tablets 1523
- Quadrinal Tablets 1398

Prazepam (CNS effects may be additive).
- No products indexed under this heading.

Prochlorperazine (CNS effects may be additive). Products include:
- Compazine 2644

Promethazine Hydrochloride (CNS effects may be additive). Products include:
- Mepergan Injection 2859
- Phenergan with Codeine 2883
- Phenergan with Dextromethorphan 2885
- Phenergan Injection 2880
- Phenergan Suppositories 2882
- Phenergan Syrup 2881
- Phenergan Tablets 2882
- Phenergan VC 2886
- Phenergan VC with Codeine 2888

Propofol (CNS effects may be additive). Products include:
- Diprivan Injectable Emulsion 2939

Propoxyphene Hydrochloride (CNS effects may be additive). Products include:
- Darvon 1475
- Wygesic Tablets 2930

Propoxyphene Napsylate (CNS effects may be additive). Products include:
- Darvon-N/Darvocet-N 1473

Quazepam (CNS effects may be additive). Products include:
- Doral Tablets 2773

Risperidone (CNS effects may be additive). Products include:
- Risperdal Tablets 1348

Secobarbital Sodium (CNS effects may be additive). Products include:
- Seconal Sodium Pulvules 1529

Selegiline Hydrochloride (Concurrent use contraindicated). Products include:
- Eldepryl Capsules 2729

Sevoflurane (CNS effects may be additive).
- No products indexed under this heading.

Sufentanil Citrate (CNS effects may be additive). Products include:
- Sufenta Injection 1355

Temazepam (CNS effects may be additive). Products include:
- Restoril Capsules 2413

Thiamylal Sodium (CNS effects may be additive).
- No products indexed under this heading.

Thioridazine Hydrochloride (CNS effects may be additive). Products include:
- Mellaril 2398

Thiothixene (CNS effects may be additive). Products include:
- Navane Capsules and Concentrate 2018
- Navane Intramuscular 2019

Tranylcypromine Sulfate (Concurrent use contraindicated). Products include:
- Parnate Tablets 2679

Triazolam (CNS effects may be additive). Products include:
- Halcion Tablets 2093

Trifluoperazine Hydrochloride (CNS effects may be additive). Products include:
- Stelazine 2692

Zolpidem Tartrate (CNS effects may be additive). Products include:
- Ambien Tablets 2559

Food Interactions

Alcohol (CNS effects may be additive).

PCE DISPERTAB TABLETS
(Erythromycin) 453
May interact with oral anticoagulants, xanthine bronchodilators, and certain other agents. Compounds in these categories include:

Alfentanil Hydrochloride (Co-administration is associated with elevation in alfentanil serum levels). Products include:
Alfenta Injection 1334

Aminophylline (Concomitant administration with high doses of theophylline may be associated with increased theophylline levels and potential toxicity).
No products indexed under this heading.

Bromocriptine Mesylate (Co-administration is associated with elevation in bromocriptine serum levels). Products include:
Parlodel 2411

Carbamazepine (Co-administration is associated with elevation in carbamazepine serum levels). Products include:
Atretol Tablets 569
Tegretol/Tegretol-XR 870

Cyclosporine (Co-administration is associated with elevation in cyclosporine serum levels). Products include:
Neoral 2405
Sandimmune 2416

Dicumarol (Increased anticoagulant effects).
No products indexed under this heading.

Digoxin (Elevated digoxin serum levels). Products include:
Lanoxicaps 1110
Lanoxin Elixir Pediatric 1113
Lanoxin Injection 1116
Lanoxin Injection Pediatric 1119
Lanoxin Tablets 1121

Dihydroergotamine Mesylate (Potential for acute ergot toxicity characterized by severe peripheral vasospasm and dysesthesia). Products include:
D.H.E. 45 Injection 2381

Disopyramide Phosphate (Co-administration is associated with elevation in disopyramide serum levels). Products include:
Norpace 2596

Dyphylline (Concomitant administration with high doses of theophylline may be associated with increased theophylline levels and potential toxicity). Products include:
Lufyllin & Lufyllin-400 Tablets 2778
Lufyllin-GG Elixir & Tablets 2779

Ergotamine Tartrate (Potential for acute ergot toxicity characterized by severe peripheral vasospasm and dysesthesia). Products include:
Bellergal-S Tablets 2375
Cafergot 2376
Ergomar Tablets 1543
Wigraine Tablets 1884

Hexobarbital (Co-administration is associated with elevation in hexobarbital serum levels).

Lovastatin (Co-administration is associated with elevation in lovastatin serum levels; combined therapy has resulted in rhabdomyolysis with or without renal impairment). Products include:
Mevacor Tablets 1742

Midazolam Hydrochloride (Decreased clearance of midazolam and increase in the pharmacologic effect of midazolam). Products include:
Versed Injection 2324

Phenytoin (Co-administration is associated with elevation in phenytoin serum levels). Products include:
Dilantin Infatabs 1967
Dilantin-125 Suspension 1969

Phenytoin Sodium (Co-administration is associated with elevation in phenytoin serum levels). Products include:
Dilantin Kapseals 1965

Terfenadine (Concomitant use alters the metabolism of terfenadine; rare cases of serious cardiovascular adverse events, including deaths, cardiac arrest, torsades de pointes, and other ventricular arrhythmias; concurrent use is contraindicated). Products include:
Seldane Tablets 1284
Seldane-D Extended-Release Tablets 1286

Theophylline (Concomitant administration with high doses of theophylline may be associated with increased theophylline levels and potential toxicity). Products include:
Marax Tablets & DF Syrup 2015
Quibron 2227

Theophylline Anhydrous (Concomitant administration with high doses of theophylline may be associated with increased theophylline levels and potential toxicity). Products include:
Aerolate 1003
Primatene Tablets 844
Respbid Tablets 687
Slo-bid Gyrocaps 2201
Theo-24 Extended Release Capsules 2753
Theo-Dur Extended-Release Tablets 1367
Theo-X Extended-Release Tablets ... 793
Uni-Dur Extended-Release Tablets .. 1374
Uniphyl 400 mg and 600 mg Tablets 2157

Theophylline Calcium Salicylate (Concomitant administration with high doses of theophylline may be associated with increased theophylline levels and potential toxicity). Products include:
Quadrinal Tablets 1398

Theophylline Sodium Glycinate (Concomitant administration with high doses of theophylline may be associated with increased theophylline levels and potential toxicity).
No products indexed under this heading.

Triazolam (Decreased clearance of triazolam and increase in the pharmacologic effect of triazolam). Products include:
Halcion Tablets 2093

Warfarin Sodium (Increased anticoagulant effects; effect more pronounced in elderly). Products include:
Coumadin 941

Food Interactions
Meal, unspecified (Optimal blood levels are obtained when PCE is given in the fasting state).

PHISOHEX
(Hexachlorophene) 2458
None cited in PDR database.

PAMELOR CAPSULES
(Nortriptyline Hydrochloride) 2409
May interact with anticholinergics, sympathomimetics, monoamine oxidase inhibitors, thyroid preparations, drugs that inhibit cytochrome p450iid6, antidepressant drugs, phenothiazines, selective serotonin reuptake inhibitors, and certain other agents. Compounds in these categories include:

Albuterol (Effects of concurrent use not specified; careful adjustment of dosage and close supervision are required). Products include:
Proventil Inhalation Aerosol 2524
Ventolin Inhalation Aerosol and Refill 1170

Albuterol Sulfate (Effects of concurrent use not specified; careful adjustment of dosage and close supervision are required). Products include:
Airet Albuterol Sulfate Inhalation Solution 1602
Albuterol Sulfate, USP Solution for Inhalation, Arm-a-Med 522
Proventil Inhalation Solution 0.083% 2527
Proventil Repetabs Tablets 2529
Proventil Solution for Inhalation 0.5% 2525
Proventil Syrup 2528
Proventil Tablets 2529
Ventolin Inhalation Solution 1171
Ventolin Nebules Inhalation Solution 1172
Ventolin Rotacaps for Inhalation ... 1173
Ventolin Syrup 1175
Ventolin Tablets 1176
Volmax Extended-Release Tablets .. 1835

Amitriptyline Hydrochloride (Concurrent use with drugs that are substrate for cytochrome $P_{450}IID_6$ may make normal metabolizer resemble poor metabolizer leading to higher than expectd plasma concentrations of TCA with resultant toxicity). Products include:
Elavil 2945
Etrafon 2495
Limbitrol 2333
Triavil Tablets 1800

Amoxapine (Concurrent use with drugs that are substrate for cytochrome $P_{450}IID_6$ may make normal metabolizer resemble poor metabolizer leading to higher than expectd plasma concentrations of TCA with resultant toxicity). Products include:
Asendin Tablets 1419

Atropine Sulfate (Effects of concurrent use not specified; careful adjustment of dosage and close supervision are required). Products include:
Arco-Lase Plus Tablets 513
Atrohist Plus Tablets 1605
Donnatal 2234
Donnatal Extentabs 2234
Donnatal Tablets 2234
Lomotil 2591
Motofen Tablets 789
Urised Tablets 2123

Belladonna Alkaloids (Effects of concurrent use not specified; careful adjustment of dosage and close supervision are required). Products include:
Bellergal-S Tablets 2375
Hyland's Bedwetting Tablets 788
Hyland's EnurAid Tablets 789
Hyland's Headache Tablets 790
Hyland's Teething Tablets 790
Similasan Eye Drops #1 769

Benztropine Mesylate (Effects of concurrent use not specified; careful adjustment of dosage and close supervision are required). Products include:
Cogentin 1661

Biperiden Hydrochloride (Effects of concurrent use not specified; careful adjustment of dosage and close supervision are required). Products include:
Akineton 1380

Bupropion Hydrochloride (Concurrent use with drugs that are substrate for cytochrome $P_{450}IID_6$ may make normal metabolizer resemble poor metabolizer leading to higher than expected plasma concentrations of TCA with resultant toxicity). Products include:
Wellbutrin Tablets 1177

Chlorpromazine (Concurrent use with drugs that are substrate for cytochrome $P_{450}IID_6$ may make normal metabolizer resemble poor metabolizer leading to higher than expected plasma concentrations of TCA with resultant toxicity). Products include:
Thorazine Suppositories 2701

Chlorpromazine Hydrochloride (Concurrent use with drugs that are substrate for cytochrome $P_{450}IID_6$ may make normal metabolizer resemble poor metabolizer leading to higher than expected plasma concentrations of TCA with resultant toxicity). Products include:
Thorazine 2701

Chlorpropamide (Potential for significant hypoglycemia in type II diabetics). Products include:
Diabinese Tablets 2002

Cimetidine (Concurrent administration can produce clinically significant increases in the plasma concentrations of the tricyclic antidepressant). Products include:
Tagamet HB Tablets 786
Tagamet Tablets 2694

Cimetidine Hydrochloride (Concurrent administration can produce clinically significant increases in the plasma concentrations of the tricyclic antidepressant). Products include:
Tagamet 2694

Clidinium Bromide (Effects of concurrent use not specified; careful adjustment of dosage and close supervision are required). Products include:
Librax Capsules 2330

Clonidine (Protryptyline may block the antihypertensive effect). Products include:
Catapres-TTS 680

Clonidine Hydrochloride (Protryptyline may block the antihypertensive effect). Products include:
Catapres Tablets 679
Combipres Tablets 682

Desipramine Hydrochloride (Concurrent use with drugs that are substrate for cytochrome $P_{450}IID_6$ may make normal metabolizer resemble poor metabolizer leading to higher than expected plasma concentrations of TCA with resultant toxicity). Products include:
Norpramin Tablets 1273

Dicyclomine Hydrochloride (Effects of concurrent use not specified; careful adjustment of dosage and close supervision are required). Products include:
Bentyl 1246

Dobutamine Hydrochloride (Effects of concurrent use not specified; careful adjustment of dosage and close supervision are required). Products include:
Dobutrex Solution Vials 1480

Dopamine Hydrochloride (Effects of concurrent use not specified; careful adjustment of dosage and close supervision are required).
No products indexed under this heading.

IMPORTANT NOTE: Always consult each drug listing in the patient's regimen for possible interactions.

Pamelor | Interactions Index | 806

Doxepin Hydrochloride (Concurrent use with drugs that are substrate for cytochrome $P_{450}IID_6$ may make normal metabolizer resemble poor metabolizer leading to higher than expected plasma concentrations of TCA with resultant toxicity). Products include:

Adapin Capsules 1542
Sinequan 2028
Zonalon Cream 1042

Ephedrine Hydrochloride (Effects of concurrent use not specified; careful adjustment of dosage and close supervision are required). Products include:

Primatene Tablets .... ⊡ 844
Quadrinal Tablets 1398

Ephedrine Sulfate (Effects of concurrent use not specified; careful adjustment of dosage and close supervision are required). Products include:

Marax Tablets & DF Syrup 2015

Ephedrine Tannate (Effects of concurrent use not specified; careful adjustment of dosage and close supervision are required). Products include:

Rynatuss 2782

Epinephrine (Effects of concurrent use not specified; careful adjustment of dosage and close supervision are required). Products include:

EPIFRIN .... ⊙ 237
EpiPen 808
Marcaine with Epinephrine 2446
Primatene Mist .... ⊡ 843
Sensorcaine with Epinephrine Injection 554
Sus-Phrine Injection 1017
Xylocaine with Epinephrine Injections 562

Epinephrine Bitartrate (Effects of concurrent use not specified; careful adjustment of dosage and close supervision are required). Products include:

Sensorcaine-MPF with Epinephrine Injection 554

Epinephrine Hydrochloride (Effects of concurrent use not specified; careful adjustment of dosage and close supervision are required). Products include:

Ana-Kit Anaphylaxis Emergency Treatment Kit 611

Flecainide Acetate (Concurrent use with drugs that are substrate for cytochrome $P_{450}IID_6$ may make normal metabolizer resemble poor metabolizer leading to higher than expected plasma concentrations of TCA with resultant toxicity). Products include:

Tambocor Tablets 1555

Fluoxetine Hydrochloride (Concurrent use with drugs that are substrate for cytochrome $P_{450}IID_6$ may make normal matabolizer resemble poor metabolizer leading to higher than expected plasma concentrations of TCA with resultant toxicity; due to variation in the extent of inhibition of $P_{450}IID_6$ and long half-life of fluoxetine and active metabolite sufficient time must elapse, at least 5 weeks, before switching to TCA). Products include:

Prozac Pulvules & Liquid, Oral Solution 935

Fluphenazine Decanoate (Concurrent use with drugs that are substrate for cytochrome $P_{450}IID_6$ may make normal metabolizer resemble poor metabolizer leading to higher than expected plasma concentrations of TCA with resultant toxicity). Products include:

Prolixin Decanoate 510

Fluphenazine Enanthate (Concurrent use with drugs that are substrate for cytochrome $P_{450}IID_6$ may make normal metabolizer resemble poor metabolizer leading to higher than expected plasma concentrations of TCA with resultant toxicity). Products include:

Prolixin Enanthate 510

Fluphenazine Hydrochloride (Concurrent use with drugs that are substrate for cytochrome $P_{450}IID_6$ may make normal metabolizer resemble poor metabolizer leading to higher than expected plasma concentrations of TCA with resultant toxicity). Products include:

Prolixin 510

Fluvoxamine Maleate (Concurrent use with drugs that are substrate for cytochrome $P_{450}IID_6$ may make normal metabolizer resemble poor metabolizer leading to higher than expected plasma concentrations of TCA with resultant toxicity). Products include:

LUVOX Tablets 2723

Furazolidone (Potential for hyperpyretic crises, severe convulsions, and fatalities; concurrent and/or sequential use is contraindicated). Products include:

Furoxone 2221

Glycopyrrolate (Effects of concurrent use not specified; careful adjustment of dosage and close supervision are required). Products include:

Robinul Forte Tablets 2247
Robinul Injectable 2247
Robinul Tablets 2247

Guanadrel Sulfate (Protryptyline may block the antihypertensive effect). Products include:

Hylorel Tablets 1613

Guanethidine Monosulfate (Protryptyline may block the antihypertensive effect of guanethidine or similarly acting compounds). Products include:

Esimil Tablets 840
Ismelin Tablets 845

Hyoscyamine (Effects of concurrent use not specified; careful adjustment of dosage and close supervision are required). Products include:

Cystospaz Tablets 2123
Urised Tablets 2123

Hyoscyamine Sulfate (Effects of concurrent use not specified; careful adjustment of dosage and close supervision are required). Products include:

Arco-Lase Plus Tablets 513
Atrohist Plus Tablets 1605
Cystospaz-M Capsules 2123
Donnatal 2234
Donnatal Extentabs 2234
Donnatal Tablets 2234
Kutrase Capsules 2546
Levsin/Levsinex/Levbid 2549

Imipramine Hydrochloride (Concurrent use with drugs that are substrate for cytochrome $P_{450}IID_6$ may make normal metabolizer resemble poor metabolizer leading to higher than expected plasma concentrations of TCA with resultant toxicity). Products include:

Tofranil Ampuls 873
Tofranil Tablets 875

Imipramine Pamoate (Concurrent use with drugs that are substrate for cytochrome $P_{450}IID_6$ may make normal metabolizer resemble poor metabolizer leading to higher than expected plasma concentrations of TCA with resultant toxicity). Products include:

Tofranil-PM Capsules 876

Ipratropium Bromide (Effects of concurrent use not specified; careful adjustment of dosage and close supervision are required). Products include:

Atrovent Inhalation Aerosol 674
Atrovent Inhalation Solution 675
Atrovent Nasal Spray 0.03% 676
Atrovent Nasal Spray 0.06% 678

Isocarboxazid (Potential for hyperpyretic crises, severe convulsions, and fatalities; concurrent and/or sequential use is contraindicated).

No products indexed under this heading.

Isoproterenol Hydrochloride (Effects of concurrent use not specified; careful adjustment of dosage and close supervision are required). Products include:

Isuprel Hydrochloride Solution 2443
Isuprel Injection 2441
Isuprel Mistometer 2442

Isoproterenol Sulfate (Effects of concurrent use not specified; careful adjustment of dosage and close supervision are required). Products include:

Norisodrine with Calcium Iodide Syrup 446

Levothyroxine Sodium (Co-administration may produce cardiac arrhythmias). Products include:

Eltroxin Tablets 2214
Levothroid Tablets 1015
Levothyroxine Sodium, USP for Injection 546
Levoxyl Tablets 918
Synthroid 1410

Liothyronine Sodium (Co-administration may produce cardiac arrhythmias). Products include:

Cytomel Tablets 2647
Triostat Injection 2708

Liotrix (Co-administration may produce cardiac arrhythmias).

No products indexed under this heading.

Maprotiline Hydrochloride (Concurrent use with drugs that are substrate for cytochrome $P_{450}IID_6$ may make normal metabolizer resemble poor metabolizer leading to higher than expected plasma concentrations of TCA with resultant toxicity). Products include:

Ludiomil Tablets 861

Mepenzolate Bromide (Effects of concurrent use not specified; careful adjustment of dosage and close supervision are required).

No products indexed under this heading.

Mesoridazine Besylate (Concurrent use with drugs that are substrate for cytochrome $P_{450}IID_6$ may make normal metabolizer resemble poor metabolizer leading to higher than expected plasma concentrations of TCA with resultant toxicity). Products include:

Serentil 689

Metaproterenol Sulfate (Effects of concurrent use not specified; careful adjustment of dosage and close supervision are required). Products include:

Alupent 672
Metaproterenol Sulfate Inhalation Solution, USP, Arm-a-Med 547

Metaraminol Bitartrate (Effects of concurrent use not specified; careful adjustment of dosage and close supervision are required). Products include:

Aramine Injection 1649

Methotrimeprazine (Concurrent use with drugs that are substrate for cytochrome $P_{450}IID_6$ may make normal metabolizer resemble poor metabolizer leading to higher than expected plasma concentrations of TCA with resultant toxicity). Products include:

Levoprome 1321

Methoxamine Hydrochloride (Effects of concurrent use not specified; careful adjustment of dosage and close supervision are required). Products include:

Vasoxyl Injection 1169

Nefazodone Hydrochloride (Concurrent use with drugs that are substrate for cytochrome $P_{450}IID_6$ may make normal metabolizer resemble poor metabolizer leading to higher than expected plasma concentrations of TCA with resultant toxicity). Products include:

Serzone Tablets 776

Norepinephrine Bitartrate (Effects of concurrent use not specified; careful adjustment of dosage and close supervision are required). Products include:

Levophed Bitartrate Injection 2445

Oxybutynin Chloride (Effects of concurrent use not specified; careful adjustment of dosage and close supervision are required). Products include:

Ditropan 1267

Paroxetine Hydrochloride (Concurrent use with drugs that are substrate for cytochrome $P_{450}IID_6$ may make normal metabolizer resemble poor metabolizer leading to higher than expected plasma concentrations of TCA with resultant toxicity; due to variation in the extent of inhibition of $P_{450}IID_6$ caution is indicated; if co-administered sufficient time should elapse before switching to TCA). Products include:

Paxil Tablets 2681

Perphenazine (Concurrent use with drugs that are substrate for cytochrome $P_{450}IID_6$ may make normal metabolizer resemble poor metabolizer leading to higher than expected plasma concentrations of TCA with resultant toxicity). Products include:

Etrafon 2495
Triavil Tablets 1800
Trilafon 2532

(⊡ Described in PDR For Nonprescription Drugs) (⊙ Described in PDR For Ophthalmology)

807 **Interactions Index** **Pamelor**

Phenelzine Sulfate (Potential for hyperpyretic crises, severe convulsions, and fatalities; concurrent and/or sequential use is contraindicated). Products include:

Nardil 1977

Phenylephrine Bitartrate (Effects of concurrent use not specified; careful adjustment of dosage and close supervision are required).

No products indexed under this heading.

Phenylephrine Hydrochloride (Effects of concurrent use not specified; careful adjustment of dosage and close supervision are required). Products include:

Atrohist Plus Tablets 1605
Cerose DM 853
D.A. II Tablets 972
D.A. Chewable Tablets 970
Dura-Vent/DA Tablets 972
Extendryl 1003
4-Way Fast Acting Nasal Spray (regular & mentholated) 644
Hemorid 797
Hycomine Compound Tablets 948
Neo-Synephrine Hydrochloride 1% Carpuject 2455
Neo-Synephrine Hydrochloride 1% Injection 2455
Neo-Synephrine Hydrochloride (Ophthalmic) 2456
Neo-Synephrine 624
Novahistine Elixir 782
Phenergan VC 2886
Phenergan VC with Codeine 2888
Preparation H 842
Tympagesic Ear Drops 2476
Vicks Sinex Nasal Spray and Ultra Fine Mist 738

Phenylephrine Tannate (Effects of concurrent use not specified; careful adjustment of dosage and close supervision are required). Products include:

Atrohist Pediatric Suspension 1604
Atrohist Pediatric Suspension Dye-Free 1604
Rynatan 2781
Rynatuss 2782

Phenylpropanolamine Hydrochloride (Effects of concurrent use not specified; careful adjustment of dosage and close supervision are required). Products include:

Acutrim 648
Atrohist Plus Tablets 1605
BC Cold Powder Multi-Symptom Formula (Cold-Sinus-Allergy) 631
BC Cold Powder Non-Drowsy Formula (Cold-Sinus) 631
Cheracol Plus Head Cold/Cough Formula 741
Comtrex Multi-Symptom Cold Reliever Liqui-Gels 638
Comtrex Multi-Symptom Non-Drowsy Liqui-gels 640
Contac Continuous Action Nasal Decongestant/Antihistamine 12 Hour Capsules 773
Contac Maximum Strength Continuous Action Decongestant/Antihistamine 12 Hour Caplets 772
Contac Severe Cold and Flu Formula Caplets 773
Coricidin 'D' Decongestant Tablets 760
Dexatrim 795
Dexatrim Plus Vitamins Caplets 796
Dimetane-DC Cough Syrup 2232
Dimetapp Allergy Sinus Caplets 838
Dimetapp Cold & Allergy Chewable Tablets 838
Dimetapp Cold & Cough Liqui-Gels 839
Dimetapp DM Elixir 840
Dimetapp Elixir 840
Dimetapp Extentabs 841
Dimetapp Tablets/Liqui-Gels 841
Dura-Vent Tablets 971
Entex LA Tablets 972
Exgest LA Tablets 787
Hycomine 947
Nolamine Timed-Release Tablets 790
Ornade Spansule Capsules 2678
Propagest Tablets 791
Pyrroxate Caplets 742
Robitussin-CF 846
Sinulin Tablets 792
Tavist-D 12 Hour Relief Tablets 750
Teldrin 12 Hour Antihistamine/Nasal Decongestant Allergy Relief Capsules 786
Triaminic Expectorant 753
Triaminic Syrup 755
Triaminic Triaminicol Cold & Cough 756
Triaminic DM Syrup 756
Triaminicin Tablets 756
Vicks DayQuil Allergy Relief 12-Hour Extended Release Tablets 733
Vicks DayQuil Allergy Relief 4-Hour Tablets 733
Vicks DayQuil SINUS Pressure & CONGESTION Relief 734

Pirbuterol Acetate (Effects of concurrent use not specified; careful adjustment of dosage and close supervision are required). Products include:

Maxair Autohaler 1550
Maxair Inhaler 1552

Prochlorperazine (Concurrent use with drugs that are substrate for cytochrome $P_{450}IID_6$ may make normal metabolizer resemble poor metabolizer leading to higher than expected plasma concentrations of TCA with resultant toxicity). Products include:

Compazine 2644

Procyclidine Hydrochloride (Effects of concurrent use not specified; careful adjustment of dosage and close supervision are required). Products include:

Kemadrin Tablets 1105

Promethazine Hydrochloride (Concurrent use with drugs that are substrate for cytochrome $P_{450}IID_6$ may make normal metabolizer resemble poor metabolizer leading to higher than expected plasma concentrations of TCA with resultant toxicity). Products include:

Mepergan Injection 2859
Phenergan with Codeine 2883
Phenergan with Dextromethorphan 2885
Phenergan Injection 2880
Phenergan Suppositories 2882
Phenergan Syrup 2881
Phenergan Tablets 2882
Phenergan VC 2886
Phenergan VC with Codeine 2888

Propafenone Hydrochloride (Concurrent use with drugs that are substrate for cytochrome $P_{450}IID_6$ may make normal metabolizer resemble poor metabolizer leading to higher than expected plasma concentrations of TCA with resultant toxicity). Products include:

Rythmol Tablets–150mg, 225mg, 300mg 1399

Propantheline Bromide (Effects of concurrent use not specified; careful adjustment of dosage and close supervision are required). Products include:

Pro-Banthine Tablets 2226

Protriptyline Hydrochloride (Concurrent use with drugs that are substrate for cytochrome $P_{450}IID_6$ may make normal metabolizer resemble poor metabolizer leading to higher than expected plasma concentrations of TCA with resultant toxicity). Products include:

Vivactil Tablets 1820

Pseudoephedrine Hydrochloride (Effects of concurrent use not specified; careful adjustment of dosage and close supervision are required). Products include:

Actifed Allergy Daytime/Nighttime Caplets 808
Actifed Cold & Allergy Tablets 807
Actifed Cold & Sinus Caplets and Tablets 808
Actifed Sinus Daytime/Nighttime Tablets and Caplets 809
Advil Cold and Sinus Caplets and Tablets 837
Alka-Seltzer Plus Liqui-Gels 612
Alka-Seltzer Plus Flu & Body Aches Liqui-Gels Non-Drowsy Formula 613
Alka-Seltzer Plus Night-Time Cold Medicine Liqui-Gels 612
Allerest Maximum Strength 649
Allerest No Drowsiness 649
Allerest Sinus Pain Formula 649
Atrohist Pediatric Capsules 1603
Benadryl Allergy/Cold Tablets 811
Benadryl Allergy Decongestant Liquid Medication 812
Benadryl Allergy Decongestant Tablets 812
Benadryl Allergy Sinus Headache Caplets 813
Benylin Multisymptom 816
Bromfed Capsules (Extended-Release) 1832
Bromfed Syrup 712
Bromfed Tablets 1832
Bromfed-DM Cough Syrup 1832
Bromfed-PD Capsules (Extended-Release) 1832
Children's TYLENOL Cold Multi-Symptom Chewable Tablets and Liquid 1559
Children's TYLENOL Cold Plus Cough Multi Symptom Chewable Tablets and Liquid 1560
Children's TYLENOL Flu Suspension Liquid 1560
Children's Vicks DayQuil Allergy Relief 730
Children's Vicks NyQuil Cold/Cough Relief 731
Allergy-Sinus Comtrex Multi-Symptom Allergy-Sinus Formula Tablets and Caplets 639
Comtrex Multi-Symptom 638
Comtrex Multi-Symptom Non-Drowsy Caplets 640
Congess 1003
Contac Day Allergy/Sinus Caplets 771
Contac Day & Night 772
Contac Night Allergy/Sinus Caplets 771
Contac Severe Cold & Flu Non-Drowsy 774
Deconsal II Tablets 1605
Dimetane-DX Cough Syrup 2233
Dimetapp Cold & Fever Suspension 839
Dimetapp Decongestant Pediatric Drops 840
Dorcol Children's Cough Syrup 748
Drixoral Cough + Congestion Liquid Caps 763
Dura-Tap/PD Capsules 970
Duratuss Tablets 2750
Duratuss HD Elixir 2750
Efidac/24 655
Entex PSE Tablets 973
Fedahist Gyrocaps 2545
Guaifed 1833
Guaifed Syrup 712
Guaimax-D Tablets 809
Histussin D Liquid 670
Infants' TYLENOL Cold Decongestant & Fever-Reducer Drops 1561
Kronofed-A 994
Novahistine DMX 782
Nucofed 2225
PediaCare Cough-Cold Chewable Tablets and Liquid 1569
PediaCare Infants' Decongestant Drops 1569
PediaCare Infants' Drops Decongestant Plus Cough 1569
PediaCare NightRest Cough-Cold Liquid 1569
Pediatric Vicks 44d Cough & Head Congestion Relief 736
Pediatric Vicks 44m Cough & Cold Relief 737
Robitussin Cold & Cough Liqui-Gels 844
Robitussin Cold, Cough & Flu Liqui-Gels 844
Robitussin Maximum Strength Cough & Cold 847
Robitussin Night-Time Cold Formula 847
Robitussin Pediatric Cough & Cold Formula 848
Robitussin Pediatric Drops 849
Robitussin Severe Congestion Liqui-Gels 845
Robitussin-DAC Syrup 2249
Robitussin-PE 846
Rondec Oral Drops 974
Rondec Syrup 974
Rondec Tablet 974
Rondec Chewable Tablets 974
Rondec-TR Tablet 974
Ryna 804
Seldane-D Extended-Release Tablets 1286
Semprex-D Capsules 1620
Sinarest 663
Sine-Aid Maximum Strength Sinus Headache Gelcaps, Caplets and Tablets 1570
Sine-Off No Drowsiness Formula Caplets 784
Sine-Off Sinus Medicine 784
Singlet Tablets 785
Sinutab Non-Drying Liquid Caps 823
Sinutab Sinus Allergy Medication, Maximum Strength Tablets and Caplets 823
Sinutab Sinus Medication, Maximum Strength Without Drowsiness Formula, Tablets & Caplets 824
Sudafed Children's Cold & Cough Liquid Medication 825
Sudafed Children's Nasal Decongestant Liquid Medication 826
Sudafed Cold & Allergy Tablets 826
Sudafed Cold and Cough Liquid Caps 826
Sudafed Nasal Decongestant Tablets, 30 mg 825
Sudafed Nasal Decongestant Tablets, 60 mg 825
Sudafed Non-Drying Sinus Liquid Caps 827
Sudafed Pediatric Nasal Decongestant Liquid Oral Drops 827
Sudafed Severe Cold Formula Caplets 828
Sudafed Severe Cold Formula Tablets 828
Sudafed Sinus Caplets 829
Sudafed Sinus Tablets 829
Sudafed 12 Hour Caplets 824
Syn-Rx Tablets 1622
Syn-Rx DM Tablets 1623
TheraFlu Flu and Cold Medicine 750
Theraflu Maximum Strength Flu and Cold Medicine For Sore Throat 751
TheraFlu Flu, Cold and Cough Medicine 750
TheraFlu Maximum Strength Nighttime Flu, Cold & Cough Medicine 751
TheraFlu Maximum Strength Non-Drowsy Formula Flu, Cold & Cough Medicine 751
TheraFlu Maximum Strength, Non-Drowsy Formula Flu, Cold and Cough Caplets 752
Theraflu Maximum Strength Sinus Non-Drowsy Formula Caplets 752
Triaminic AM Cough and Decongestant Formula 753
Triaminic AM Decongestant Formula 753
Triaminic Infant Oral Decongestant Drops 754
Triaminic Night Time 754
Triaminic Sore Throat Formula 755
Tussend 1830
Tussend Expectorant 1831
TYLENOL Allergy Sinus, Maximum Strength Caplets and Gelcaps 1571
TYLENOL Allergy Sinus NightTime, Maximum Strength Caplets 1571
TYLENOL Cold Medication, Multi-Symptom Formula Tablets and Caplets 1572
TYLENOL Cold Medication, Multi-Symptom Hot Liquid Packets 1572
TYLENOL Cold Medication, No Drowsiness Formula Caplets and Gelcaps 1572
TYLENOL Cold Severe Congestion Caplets 1573
TYLENOL Cough Medication with Decongestant, Multi Symptom 1574

IMPORTANT NOTE: Always consult each drug listing in the patient's regimen for possible interactions.

Pamelor Interactions Index 808

TYLENOL Flu No Drowsiness Formula, Maximum Strength Gelcaps 1575
TYLENOL Flu NightTime, Maximum Strength Gelcaps 1575
TYLENOL Flu NightTime, Maximum Strength Hot Medication Packets 1575
TYLENOL Sinus, Maximum Strength Geltabs, Gelcaps, Caplets and Tablets 1576
Vicks 44 LiquiCaps Cough, Cold & Flu Relief ..... ▣ 728
Vicks 44 LiquiCaps Non-Drowsy Cough & Cold Relief ..... ▣ 729
Vicks 44D Cough & Head Congestion Relief ..... ▣ 728
Vicks 44M Cough, Cold & Flu Relief ..... ▣ 729
Vicks DayQuil LiquiCaps/Liquid Multi-Symptom Cold/Flu Relief .. ▣ 734
Vicks DayQuil SINUS Pressure & PAIN Relief with IBUPROFEN ..... ▣ 735
Vicks Nyquil Hot Therapy ..... ▣ 735
Vicks NyQuil LiquiCaps/Liquid Multi-Symptom Cold/Flu Relief, Original and Cherry Flavors ..... ▣ 736

Pseudoephedrine Sulfate (Effects of concurrent use not specified; careful adjustment of dosage and close supervision are required). Products include:

Chlor-Trimeton Allergy Decongestant Tablets ..... ▣ 759
Claritin-D Tablets 2487
Drixoral Cold and Allergy Sustained-Action Tablets ..... ▣ 763
Drixoral Cold and Flu Extended-Release Tablets ..... ▣ 764
Drixoral Non-Drowsy Formula Extended-Release Tablets ..... ▣ 764
Drixoral Allergy/Sinus Extended Release Tablets ..... ▣ 765
Trinalin Repetabs Tablets 1373

Quinidine Gluconate (Co-administration may result in longer plasma half-life, higher AUC and lower clearance of nortriptyline). Products include:

Quinaglute Dura-Tabs Tablets 644

Quinidine Polygalacturonate (Co-administration may result in longer plasma half-life, higher AUC and lower clearance of nortriptyline). Products include:

Cardioquin Tablets 2146

Quinidine Sulfate (Co-administration may result in longer plasma half-life, higher AUC and lower clearance of nortriptyline). Products include:

Quinidex Extentabs 2240

Reserpine (Co-administration may produce a "stimulating" effect in some depressed patients). Products include:

Diupres Tablets 1691
Hydropres Tablets 1718
Ser-Ap-Es Tablets 867

Salmeterol Xinafoate (Effects of concurrent use not specified; careful adjustment of dosage and close supervision are required). Products include:

Serevent Inhalation Aerosol 1149

Scopolamine (Effects of concurrent use not specified; careful adjustment of dosage and close supervision are required). Products include:

Transderm Scōp Transdermal Therapeutic System 890

Scopolamine Hydrobromide (Effects of concurrent use not specified; careful adjustment of dosage and close supervision are required). Products include:

Atrohist Plus Tablets 1605
Donnatal 2234
Donnatal Extentabs 2234
Donnatal Tablets 2234

Selegiline Hydrochloride (Potential for hyperpyretic crises, severe convulsions, and fatalities; concurrent and/or sequential use is contraindicated). Products include:

Eldepryl Capsules 2729

Sertraline Hydrochloride (Concurrent use with drugs that are substrate for cytochrome $P_{450}IID_6$ may make normal metabolizer resemble poor metabolizer leading to higher than expected plasma concentrations of TCA with resultant toxicity; due to variation in the extent of inhibition of $P_{450}IID_6$ caution is indicated; if co-administered sufficient time should elapse before switching to TCA). Products include:

Zoloft Tablets 2051

Terbutaline Sulfate (Effects of concurrent use not specified; careful adjustment of dosage and close supervision are required). Products include:

Brethaire Inhaler 830
Brethine Ampuls 832
Brethine Tablets 831
Bricanyl Subcutaneous Injection 1247
Bricanyl Tablets 1248

Thioridazine Hydrochloride (Concurrent use with drugs that are substrate for cytochrome $P_{450}IID_6$ may make normal metabolizer resemble poor metabolizer leading to higher than expected plasma concentrations of TCA with resultant toxicity). Products include:

Mellaril 2398

Thyroglobulin (Co-administration may produce cardiac arrhythmias).

No products indexed under this heading.

Thyroid (Co-administration may produce cardiac arrhythmias).

No products indexed under this heading.

Thyroxine (Co-administration may produce cardiac arrhythmias).

No products indexed under this heading.

Thyroxine Sodium (Co-administration may produce cardiac arrhythmias).

No products indexed under this heading.

Tranylcypromine Sulfate (Potential for hyperpyretic crises, severe convulsions, and fatalities; concurrent and/or sequential use is contraindicated). Products include:

Parnate Tablets 2679

Trazodone Hydrochloride (Concurrent use with drugs that are substrate for cytochrome $P_{450}IID_6$ may make normal metabolizer resemble poor metabolizer leading to higher than expected plasma concentrations of TCA with resultant toxicity). Products include:

Desyrel and Desyrel Dividose 504

Tridihexethyl Chloride (Effects of concurrent use not specified; careful adjustment of dosage and close supervision are required).

No products indexed under this heading.

Trifluoperazine Hydrochloride (Concurrent use with drugs that are substrate for cytochrome $P_{450}IID_6$ may make normal metabolizer resemble poor metabolizer leading to higher than expected plasma concentrations of TCA with resultant toxicity). Products include:

Stelazine 2692

Trihexyphenidyl Hydrochloride (Effects of concurrent use not specified; careful adjustment of dosage and close supervision are required). Products include:

Artane 1418

Trimipramine Maleate (Concurrent use with drugs that are substrate for cytochrome $P_{450}IID_6$ may make normal metabolizer resemble poor metabolizer leading to higher than expected plasma concentrations of TCA with resultant toxicity). Products include:

Surmontil Capsules 2917

Venlafaxine Hydrochloride (Concurrent use with drugs that are substrate for cytochrome $P_{450}IID_6$ may make normal metabolizer resemble poor metabolizer leading to higher than expected plasma concentrations of TCA with resultant toxicity; due to variation in the extent of inhibition of $P_{450}IID_6$ caution is indicated; if co-administered sufficient time should elapse before switching to TCA). Products include:

Effexor 2825

Food Interactions

Alcohol (Excessive consumption of alcohol with nortriptyline may have a potentiating effect and exaggerated response to alcohol).

PAMELOR SOLUTION
(Nortriptyline Hydrochloride) 2409
See **Pamelor Capsules**

PANODOL TABLETS AND CAPLETS
(Acetaminophen) ..... ▣ 783
None cited in PDR database.

CHILDREN'S PANADOL CHEWABLE TABLETS, LIQUID, INFANT'S DROPS
(Acetaminophen) ..... ▣ 783
None cited in PDR database.

PANAFIL OINTMENT
(Papain, Chlorophyllin Copper Complex, Urea) 2372
May interact with:

Heavy metal salts, unspecified (Papain may be inactivated by the salts of heavy metals).

Hydrogen Peroxide (May inactivate papain).

No products indexed under this heading.

PANAFIL-WHITE OINTMENT
(Papain, Urea) 2372
May interact with:

Heavy metal salts, unspecified (Papain may be inactivated by the salts of heavy metals).

Hydrogen Peroxide (May inactivate papain).

No products indexed under this heading.

PANCREASE CAPSULES
(Pancrelipase) 1589
None cited in PDR database.

PANCREASE MT CAPSULES
(Pancrelipase) 1589
None cited in PDR database.

PANDEL CREAM, 0.1%
(Hydrocortisone Buteprate) 2475
None cited in PDR database.

PANHEMATIN
(Hemin For Injection) 452
May interact with oral anticoagulants, estrogens, and barbiturates. Compounds in these categories include:

Aprobarbital (Increases delta-aminolevalinic acid synthetase).

No products indexed under this heading.

Butabarbital (Increases delta-aminolevalinic acid synthetase).

No products indexed under this heading.

Butalbital (Increases delta-aminolevalinic acid synthetase). Products include:

Axocet Capsules 2469
Esgic-plus Capsules 1012
Esgic-plus Tablets 1012
Fioricet Tablets 2386
Fioricet with Codeine Capsules 2387
Fiorinal Capsules 2388
Fiorinal with Codeine Capsules 2390
Fiorinal Tablets 2388
Phrenilin 790
Sedapap Tablets 50 mg/650 mg .. 1826

Chlorotrianisene (Increases delta-aminolevalinic acid synthetase).

No products indexed under this heading.

Dicumarol (Hypocoagulable state).

No products indexed under this heading.

Dienestrol (Increases delta-aminolevalinic acid synthetase). Products include:

Ortho Dienestrol Cream 1922

Diethylstilbestrol (Increases delta-aminolevalinic acid synthetase). Products include:

Diethylstilbestrol Tablets 1477

Estradiol (Increases delta-aminolevalinic acid synthetase). Products include:

Climara Transdermal System 640
Estrace Cream and Tablets 751
Estraderm Transdermal System 842
Estring Vaginal Ring 2086
Vivelle Transdermal System 880

Estrogens, Conjugated (Increases delta-aminolevalinic acid synthetase). Products include:

PMB 200 and PMB 400 2890
Premarin Intravenous 2893
Premarin Tablets 2896
Premarin Vaginal Cream 2898
Premphase 2900
Prempro 2905

Estrogens, Esterified (Increases delta-aminolevalinic acid synthetase). Products include:

ESTRATAB Tablets (0.3, 0.625, 1.25, 2.5 mg) 2715
Estratest 2718
Menest Tablets 2671

Estropipate (Increases delta-aminolevalinic acid synthetase). Products include:

Ogen Tablets 2103
Ogen Vaginal Cream 2106
Ortho-Est 1925

Ethinyl Estradiol (Increases delta-aminolevalinic acid synthetase). Products include:

Brevicon 2563
Demulen 2580
Desogen Tablets 1867
Levlen/Tri-Levlen 646
Lo/Ovral Tablets 2852
Lo/Ovral-28 Tablets 2857
Modicon 1928
Nordette-21 Tablets 2863
Nordette-28 Tablets 2866
Norinyl 2563
Ortho-Cept 1907
Ortho-Cyclen/Ortho-Tri-Cyclen 1914
Ortho-Novum 1928
Ortho-Cyclen/Ortho Tri-Cyclen 1914
Ovcon 765
Ovral Tablets 2877
Ovral-28 Tablets 2878

(▣ Described in PDR For Nonprescription Drugs) (◉ Described in PDR For Ophthalmology)

Levlen/Tri-Levlen	646
Tri-Norinyl	2607
Triphasil-21 Tablets	2919
Triphasil-28 Tablets	2924

Mephobarbital (Increases delta-aminolevalinic acid synthetase). Products include:

Mebaral Tablets	2452

Pentobarbital Sodium (Increases delta-aminolevalinic acid synthetase). Products include:

Nembutal Sodium Capsules	440
Nembutal Sodium Solution	442
Nembutal Sodium Suppositories	444

Phenobarbital (Increases delta-aminolevalinic acid synthetase). Products include:

Arco-Lase Plus Tablets	513
Bellergal-S Tablets	2375
Donnatal	2234
Donnatal Extentabs	2234
Donnatal Tablets	2234
Phenobarbital Elixir and Tablets	1523
Quadrinal Tablets	1398

Polyestradiol Phosphate (Increases delta-aminolevalinic acid synthetase).
No products indexed under this heading.

Quinestrol (Increases delta-aminolevalinic acid synthetase).
No products indexed under this heading.

Secobarbital Sodium (Increases delta-aminolevalinic acid synthetase). Products include:

Seconal Sodium Pulvules	1529

Thiamylal Sodium (Increases delta-aminolevalinic acid synthetase).
No products indexed under this heading.

Warfarin Sodium (Hypocoagulable state). Products include:

Coumadin	941

PAPAVERINE HYDROCHLORIDE VIALS AND AMPOULES
(Papaverine Hydrochloride) 1523
None cited in PDR database.

PARAFON FORTE DSC CAPLETS
(Chlorzoxazone) 1590
May interact with central nervous system depressants and certain other agents. Compounds in these categories include:

Alfentanil Hydrochloride (May produce additive effect). Products include:

Alfenta Injection	1334

Alprazolam (May produce additive effect). Products include:

Xanax Tablets	2115

Aprobarbital (May produce additive effect).
No products indexed under this heading.

Buprenorphine (May produce additive effect). Products include:

Buprenex Injectable	2170

Buspirone Hydrochloride (May produce additive effect). Products include:

BuSpar Tablets	738

Butabarbital (May produce additive effect).
No products indexed under this heading.

Butalbital (May produce additive effect). Products include:

Axocet Capsules	2469
Esgic-plus Capsules	1012
Esgic-plus Tablets	1012
Fioricet Tablets	2386
Fioricet with Codeine Capsules	2387
Fiorinal Capsules	2388
Fiorinal with Codeine Capsules	2390
Fiorinal Tablets	2388
Phrenilin	790
Sedapap Tablets 50 mg / 650 mg	1826

Chlordiazepoxide (May produce additive effect). Products include:

Limbitrol	2333

Chlordiazepoxide Hydrochloride (May produce additive effect). Products include:

Librax Capsules	2330
Librium Capsules	2331
Librium Injectable	2332

Chlorpromazine (May produce additive effect). Products include:

Thorazine Suppositories	2701

Chlorpromazine Hydrochloride (May produce additive effect). Products include:

Thorazine	2701

Chlorprothixene (May produce additive effect).
No products indexed under this heading.

Chlorprothixene Hydrochloride (May produce additive effect).
No products indexed under this heading.

Chlorprothixene Lactate (May produce additive effect).
No products indexed under this heading.

Clorazepate Dipotassium (May produce additive effect). Products include:

Tranxene	459

Clozapine (May produce additive effect). Products include:

Clozaril Tablets	2377

Codeine Phosphate (May produce additive effect). Products include:

Brontex	2130
Dimetane-DC Cough Syrup	2232
Fioricet with Codeine Capsules	2387
Fiorinal with Codeine Capsules	2390
Nucofed	2225
Phenergan with Codeine	2883
Phenergan VC with Codeine	2888
Robitussin A-C Syrup	2248
Robitussin-DAC Syrup	2249
Ryna	804
Soma Compound w/Codeine Tablets	2784
Tylenol with Codeine	1592

Desflurane (May produce additive effect). Products include:

Suprane (desflurane, USP)	1865

Dezocine (May produce additive effect). Products include:

Dalgan Injection	529

Diazepam (May produce additive effect). Products include:

Dizac (diazepam injectable emulsion) CIV	1862
Valium Injectable	2336
Valium Tablets	2335

Droperidol (May produce additive effect). Products include:

Inapsine Injection	462

Enflurane (May produce additive effect).
No products indexed under this heading.

Estazolam (May produce additive effect). Products include:

ProSom Tablets	457

Ethchlorvynol (May produce additive effect). Products include:

Placidyl Capsules	456

Ethinamate (May produce additive effect).
No products indexed under this heading.

Fentanyl (May produce additive effect). Products include:

Duragesic Transdermal System	1336

Fentanyl Citrate (May produce additive effect). Products include:

Sublimaze Injection	463

Fluphenazine Decanoate (May produce additive effect). Products include:

Prolixin Decanoate	510

Fluphenazine Enanthate (May produce additive effect). Products include:

Prolixin Enanthate	510

Fluphenazine Hydrochloride (May produce additive effect). Products include:

Prolixin	510

Flurazepam Hydrochloride (May produce additive effect). Products include:

Dalmane Capsules	2329

Glutethimide (May produce additive effect).
No products indexed under this heading.

Haloperidol (May produce additive effect). Products include:

Haldol Injection, Tablets and Concentrate	1585

Haloperidol Decanoate (May produce additive effect). Products include:

Haldol Decanoate	1587

Hydrocodone Bitartrate (May produce additive effect). Products include:

Codiclear DH Syrup	808
Duratuss HD Elixir	2750
Histussin D Liquid	670
Hycodan Tablets and Syrup	946
Hycomine Compound Tablets	948
Hycomine	947
Hycotuss Expectorant Syrup	950
Hydrocet Capsules	787
Lorcet 10/650 Tablets	1016
Lortab	2751
Tussend	1830
Tussend Expectorant	1831
Vicodin Tablets	1404
Vicodin ES Tablets	1405
Vicodin HP Tablets	1403
Vicodin Tuss Expectorant	1406
Zydone Capsules	967

Hydrocodone Polistirex (May produce additive effect). Products include:

Tussionex Pennkinetic Extended-Release Suspension	1624

Hydromorphone Hydrochloride (May produce additive effect). Products include:

Dilaudid Ampules	1382
Dilaudid Cough Syrup	1383
Dilaudid-HP Injection	1384
Dilaudid-HP Lyophilized Powder 250 mg	1384
Dilaudid	1382
Dilaudid Oral Liquid	1386
Dilaudid	1382
Dilaudid Tablets - 8 mg	1386

Hydroxyzine Hydrochloride (May produce additive effect). Products include:

Atarax Tablets & Syrup	1992
Marax Tablets & DF Syrup	2015
Vistaril Intramuscular Solution	2042

Isoflurane (May produce additive effect).
No products indexed under this heading.

Ketamine Hydrochloride (May produce additive effect).
No products indexed under this heading.

Levomethadyl Acetate Hydrochloride (May produce additive effect). Products include:

Orlaam Oral Solution	2361

Levorphanol Tartrate (May produce additive effect). Products include:

Levo-Dromoran	2297

Lorazepam (May produce additive effect). Products include:

Ativan Injection	2805
Ativan Tablets	2807

Loxapine Hydrochloride (May produce additive effect). Products include:

Loxitane	1426

Loxapine Succinate (May produce additive effect). Products include:

Loxitane Capsules	1426

Meperidine Hydrochloride (May produce additive effect). Products include:

Demerol	2438
Mepergan Injection	2859

Mephobarbital (May produce additive effect). Products include:

Mebaral Tablets	2452

Meprobamate (May produce additive effect). Products include:

Miltown Tablets	2780
PMB 200 and PMB 400	2890

Mesoridazine Besylate (May produce additive effect). Products include:

Serentil	689

Methadone Hydrochloride (May produce additive effect). Products include:

Methadone Hydrochloride Oral Concentrate	2356
Methadone Hydrochloride Oral Solution & Tablets	2357

Methohexital Sodium (May produce additive effect).
No products indexed under this heading.

Methotrimeprazine (May produce additive effect). Products include:

Levoprome	1321

Methoxyflurane (May produce additive effect).
No products indexed under this heading.

Midazolam Hydrochloride (May produce additive effect). Products include:

Versed Injection	2324

Molindone Hydrochloride (May produce additive effect). Products include:

Moban Tablets and Concentrate	1036

Morphine Sulfate (May produce additive effect). Products include:

Astramorph/PF Injection, USP (Preservative-Free)	526
Duramorph Injection	983
Infumorph 200 and Infumorph 500 Sterile Solutions	985
Kadian Capsules	2948
MS Contin Tablets	2149
MSIR	2152
Oramorph SR (Morphine Sulfate Sustained Release Tablets)	2359
RMS Suppositories CII	2766
Roxanol	2365

Opium Alkaloids (May produce additive effect).
No products indexed under this heading.

Oxazepam (May produce additive effect). Products include:

Serax Capsules	2916
Serax Tablets	2916

Oxycodone Hydrochloride (May produce additive effect). Products include:

OxyContin Tablets	2163
OxyIR Capsules	2167
Percocet Tablets	955
Percodan Tablets	955
Percodan-Demi Tablets	956
Roxicodone Tablets, Oral Solution & Intensol (Oxycodone)	2366
Tylox Capsules	1593

Pentobarbital Sodium (May produce additive effect). Products include:

Nembutal Sodium Capsules	440
Nembutal Sodium Solution	442
Nembutal Sodium Suppositories	444

IMPORTANT NOTE: Always consult each drug listing in the patient's regimen for possible interactions.

Parafon Forte DSC — Interactions Index

Perphenazine (May produce additive effect). Products include:
- Etrafon 2495
- Triavil Tablets 1800
- Trilafon 2532

Phenobarbital (May produce additive effect). Products include:
- Arco-Lase Plus Tablets 513
- Bellergal-S Tablets 2375
- Donnatal 2234
- Donnatal Extentabs 2234
- Donnatal Tablets 2234
- Phenobarbital Elixir and Tablets 1523
- Quadrinal Tablets 1398

Prazepam (May produce additive effect).
- No products indexed under this heading.

Prochlorperazine (May produce additive effect). Products include:
- Compazine 2644

Promethazine Hydrochloride (May produce additive effect). Products include:
- Meperidine Injection 2859
- Phenergan with Codeine 2883
- Phenergan with Dextromethorphan ... 2885
- Phenergan Injection 2880
- Phenergan Suppositories 2882
- Phenergan Syrup 2881
- Phenergan Tablets 2882
- Phenergan VC 2886
- Phenergan VC with Codeine 2888

Propofol (May produce additive effect). Products include:
- Diprivan Injectable Emulsion 2939

Propoxyphene Hydrochloride (May produce additive effect). Products include:
- Darvon 1475
- Wygesic Tablets 2930

Propoxyphene Napsylate (May produce additive effect). Products include:
- Darvon-N/Darvocet-N 1473

Quazepam (May produce additive effect). Products include:
- Doral Tablets 2773

Risperidone (May produce additive effect). Products include:
- Risperdal Tablets 1348

Secobarbital Sodium (May produce additive effect). Products include:
- Seconal Sodium Pulvules 1529

Sevoflurane (May produce additive effect).
- No products indexed under this heading.

Sufentanil Citrate (May produce additive effect). Products include:
- Sufenta Injection 1355

Temazepam (May produce additive effect). Products include:
- Restoril Capsules 2413

Thiamylal Sodium (May produce additive effect).
- No products indexed under this heading.

Thioridazine Hydrochloride (May produce additive effect). Products include:
- Mellaril 2398

Thiothixene (May produce additive effect). Products include:
- Navane Capsules and Concentrate ... 2018
- Navane Intramuscular 2019

Triazolam (May produce additive effect). Products include:
- Halcion Tablets 2093

Trifluoperazine Hydrochloride (May produce additive effect). Products include:
- Stelazine 2692

Zolpidem Tartrate (May produce additive effect). Products include:
- Ambien Tablets 2559

Food Interactions
Alcohol (May produce additive effect).

PARAGARD T 380A INTRAUTERINE COPPER CONTRACEPTIVE
(Intrauterine device) 1936
None cited in PDR database.

PARAPLATIN FOR INJECTION
(Carboplatin) 713
May interact with aminoglycosides and certain other agents. Compounds in these categories include:

Amikacin Sulfate (Concomitant treatment has resulted in increased renal and/or audiologic toxicity). Products include:
- Amikacin Sulfate Injection, USP 523
- Amikacin Sulfate Injection, USP 981
- Amikin Injectable 502

Gentamicin Sulfate (Concomitant treatment has resulted in increased renal and/or audiologic toxicity). Products include:
- Garamycin Cream 0.1% 2501
- Garamycin Injectable 2502
- Garamycin Ointment 0.1% 2501
- Garamycin Ophthalmic 2501
- Genoptic Sterile Ophthalmic Solution .... ⊙ 241
- Genoptic Sterile Ophthalmic Ointment .... ⊙ 241
- Gentak .... ⊙ 209
- Pred-G Liquifilm Sterile Ophthalmic Suspension .... ⊙ 248
- Pred-G S.O.P. Sterile Ophthalmic Ointment .... ⊙ 249

Kanamycin Sulfate (Concomitant treatment has resulted in increased renal and/or audiologic toxicity).
- No products indexed under this heading.

Nephrotoxic Drugs (Renal effects may be potentiated).

Streptomycin Sulfate (Concomitant treatment has resulted in increased renal and/or audiologic toxicity). Products include:
- Streptomycin Sulfate Injection 2031

Tobramycin (Concomitant treatment has resulted in increased renal and/or audiologic toxicity). Products include:
- AKTOB .... ⊙ 207
- TobraDex Ophthalmic Suspension and Ointment 469
- Tobrex Ophthalmic Ointment and Solution .... ⊙ 226

Tobramycin Sulfate (Concomitant treatment has resulted in increased renal and/or audiologic toxicity). Products include:
- Nebcin Vials, Hyporets & ADD-Vantage 1518

PAREMYD
(Hydroxyamphetamine Hydrobromide, Tropicamide) .... ⊙ 244
None cited in PDR database.

PARLODEL CAPSULES
(Bromocriptine Mesylate) 2411
May interact with dopamine antagonists, butyrophenones, ergot-containing drugs, and certain other agents. Compounds in these categories include:

Chlorpromazine (Potential for decreased efficacy of bromocriptine). Products include:
- Thorazine Suppositories 2701

Chlorpromazine Hydrochloride (Potential for decreased efficacy of bromocriptine). Products include:
- Thorazine 2701

Clozapine (Potential for decreased efficacy of bromocriptine). Products include:
- Clozaril Tablets 2377

Dihydroergotamine Mesylate (Co-administration with ergot alkaloids is not recommended). Products include:
- D.H.E. 45 Injection 2381

Ergotamine Tartrate (Co-administration with ergot alkaloids is not recommended). Products include:
- Bellergal-S Tablets 2375
- Cafergot 2376
- Ergomar Tablets 1543
- Wigraine Tablets 1884

Fluphenazine Decanoate (Potential for decreased efficacy of bromocriptine). Products include:
- Prolixin Decanoate 510

Fluphenazine Enanthate (Potential for decreased efficacy of bromocriptine). Products include:
- Prolixin Enanthate 510

Fluphenazine Hydrochloride (Potential for decreased efficacy of bromocriptine). Products include:
- Prolixin 510

Haloperidol (Potential for decreased efficacy of bromocriptine). Products include:
- Haldol Injection, Tablets and Concentrate 1585

Haloperidol Decanoate (Potential for decreased efficacy of bromocriptine). Products include:
- Haldol Decanoate 1587

Mesoridazine Besylate (Potential for decreased efficacy of bromocriptine). Products include:
- Serentil 689

Methotrimeprazine (Potential for decreased efficacy of bromocriptine). Products include:
- Levoprome 1321

Methylergonovine Maleate (Co-administration with ergot alkaloids is not recommended). Products include:
- Methergine 2401

Methysergide Maleate (Co-administration with ergot alkaloids is not recommended). Products include:
- Sansert Tablets 2424

Metoclopramide Hydrochloride (Potential for decreased efficacy of bromocriptine). Products include:
- Reglan 2243

Perphenazine (Potential for decreased efficacy of bromocriptine). Products include:
- Etrafon 2495
- Triavil Tablets 1800
- Trilafon 2532

Pimozide (Potential for decreased efficacy of bromocriptine). Products include:
- Orap Tablets 1037

Prochlorperazine (Potential for decreased efficacy of bromocriptine). Products include:
- Compazine 2644

Promethazine Hydrochloride (Potential for decreased efficacy of bromocriptine). Products include:
- Meperidine Injection 2859
- Phenergan with Codeine 2883
- Phenergan with Dextromethorphan ... 2885
- Phenergan Injection 2880
- Phenergan Suppositories 2882
- Phenergan Syrup 2881
- Phenergan Tablets 2882
- Phenergan VC 2886
- Phenergan VC with Codeine 2888

Thioridazine Hydrochloride (Potential for decreased efficacy of bromocriptine). Products include:
- Mellaril 2398

Trifluoperazine Hydrochloride (Potential for decreased efficacy of bromocriptine). Products include:
- Stelazine 2692

Food Interactions
Alcohol (Alcohol may potentiate the side effects of bromocriptine).

PARLODEL SNAPTABS
(Bromocriptine Mesylate) 2411
See **Parlodel Capsules**

PARNATE TABLETS
(Tranylcypromine Sulfate) 2679
May interact with dibenzazepines, tricyclic antidepressants, monoamine oxidase inhibitors, selective serotonin reuptake inhibitors, sympathomimetics, amphetamines, anorexiants, antihypertensives, narcotic analgesics, anticholinergic-type antiparkinsonism drugs, phenothiazines, oral hypoglycemic agents, insulin, hypnotics and sedatives, alpha adrenergic stimulants, antihistamines, anesthetics, diuretics, and certain other agents. Compounds in these categories include:

Acarbose (Some MAO inhibitors have contributed to hypoglycemic episodes in diabetic patients receiving oral hypoglycemic agents). Products include:
- Precose 604

Acebutolol Hydrochloride (Concurrent use with hypotensive agents is contraindicated; a marked potentiating effect on these classes of drugs has been reported). Products include:
- Sectral Capsules 2914

Acrivastine (Concurrent use is contraindicated). Products include:
- Semprex-D Capsules 1620

Albuterol (Concurrent and/or sequential use is contraindicated; combination therapy may precipitate hypertension, headache and related symptoms). Products include:
- Proventil Inhalation Aerosol 2524
- Ventolin Inhalation Aerosol and Refill 1170

Albuterol Sulfate (Concurrent and/or sequential use is contraindicated; combination therapy may precipitate hypertension, headache and related symptoms). Products include:
- Airet Albuterol Sulfate Inhalation Solution 1602
- Albuterol Sulfate, USP Solution for Inhalation, Arm-a-Med 522
- Proventil Inhalation Solution 0.083% 2527
- Proventil Repetabs Tablets 2529
- Proventil Solution for Inhalation 0.5% 2525
- Proventil Syrup 2528
- Proventil Tablets 2529
- Ventolin Inhalation Solution 1171
- Ventolin Nebules Inhalation Solution 1172
- Ventolin Rotacaps for Inhalation ... 1173
- Ventolin Syrup 1175
- Ventolin Tablets 1176
- Volmax Extended-Release Tablets .. 1835

Alfentanil Hydrochloride (Concurrent use is contraindicated; a marked potentiating effect on these classes of drugs has been reported). Products include:
- Alfenta Injection 1334

Amiloride Hydrochloride (Concurrent use with hypotensive agents is contraindicated; a marked potentiating effect on these classes of drugs has been reported). Products include:
- Midamor Tablets 1746
- Moduretic Tablets 1748

(▣ Described in PDR For Nonprescription Drugs)   (⊙ Described in PDR For Ophthalmology)

Interactions Index — Parnate

Amitriptyline Hydrochloride (Concurrent use with tricyclic antidepressants may result in hypertensive crises or severe convulsive seizures; concurrent and/or sequential use is contraindicated). Products include:
- Elavil ... 2945
- Etrafon ... 2495
- Limbitrol ... 2333
- Triavil Tablets ... 1800

Amlodipine Besylate (Concurrent use with hypotensive agents is contraindicated; a marked potentiating effect on these classes of drugs has been reported). Products include:
- Lotrel Capsules ... 858
- Norvasc Tablets ... 2020

Amoxapine (Concurrent use with tricyclic antidepressants may result in hypertensive crises or severe convulsive seizures; concurrent and/or sequential use is contraindicated). Products include:
- Asendin Tablets ... 1419

Amphetamine Resins (Concurrent and/or sequential use is contraindicated).
- No products indexed under this heading.

Amphetamine Sulfate (Concurrent and/or sequential use is contraindicated). Products include:
- Adderall Tablets ... 2209

Astemizole (Concurrent use is contraindicated). Products include:
- Hismanal Tablets ... 1341

Atenolol (Concurrent use with hypotensive agents is contraindicated; a marked potentiating effect on these classes of drugs has been reported). Products include:
- Tenoretic Tablets ... 2963
- Tenormin Tablets and I.V. Injection ... 2965

Azatadine Maleate (Concurrent use is contraindicated). Products include:
- Trinalin Repetabs Tablets ... 1373

Benazepril Hydrochloride (Concurrent use is contraindicated; a marked potentiating effect on these classes of drugs has been reported). Products include:
- Lotensin Tablets ... 852
- Lotensin HCT Tablets ... 855
- Lotrel Capsules ... 858

Bendroflumethiazide (Concurrent use with hypotensive agents is contraindicated; a marked potentiating effect on these classes of drugs has been reported).
- No products indexed under this heading.

Benzphetamine Hydrochloride (Concurrent and/or sequential use is contraindicated).
- No products indexed under this heading.

Benztropine Mesylate (Anti-Parkinsonism drugs should be used with caution in patients receiving Parnate since severe reactions have been reported). Products include:
- Cogentin ... 1661

Betaxolol Hydrochloride (Concurrent use with hypotensive agents is contraindicated; a marked potentiating effect on these classes of drugs has been reported). Products include:
- Betoptic Ophthalmic Solution ... 465
- Betoptic S Ophthalmic Suspension ... 467
- Kerlone Tablets ... 2588

Biperiden Hydrochloride (Anti-Parkinsonism drugs should be used with caution in patients receiving Parnate since severe reactions have been reported). Products include:
- Akineton ... 1380

Bisoprolol Fumarate (Concurrent use with hypotensive agents is contraindicated; a marked potentiating effect on these classes of drugs has been reported). Products include:
- Zebeta Tablets ... 1457
- Ziac ... 1459

Bromodiphenhydramine Hydrochloride (Concurrent use is contraindicated).
- No products indexed under this heading.

Brompheniramine Maleate (Concurrent use is contraindicated). Products include:
- Alka-Seltzer Plus Sinus Medicine ... 611
- Bromfed Capsules (Extended-Release) ... 1832
- Bromfed Syrup ... 712
- Bromfed Tablets ... 1832
- Bromfed-DM Cough Syrup ... 1832
- Bromfed-PD Capsules (Extended-Release) ... 1832
- Dimetane-DC Cough Syrup ... 2232
- Dimetane-DX Cough Syrup ... 2233
- Dimetapp Allergy Dye-Free Elixir ... 838
- Dimetapp Allergy Sinus Caplets ... 838
- Dimetapp Cold & Allergy Chewable Tablets ... 838
- Dimetapp Cold & Cough Liqui-Gels ... 839
- Dimetapp Cold & Fever Suspension ... 839
- Dimetapp DM Elixir ... 840
- Dimetapp Elixir ... 840
- Dimetapp Extentabs ... 841
- Dimetapp Tablets/Liqui-Gels ... 841
- Rondec Chewable Tablets ... 974
- Vicks DayQuil Allergy Relief 12-Hour Extended Release Tablets ... 733
- Vicks DayQuil Allergy Relief 4-Hour Tablets ... 733

Bumetanide (Concurrent use with hypotensive agents is contraindicated; a marked potentiating effect on these classes of drugs has been reported). Products include:
- Bumex ... 2260

Buprenorphine (Concurrent use is contraindicated; a marked potentiating effect on these classes of drugs has been reported). Products include:
- Buprenex Injectable ... 2170

Bupropion Hydrochloride (Concurrent use is contraindicated; at least 14 days should elapse between discontinuation of an MAO inhibitor and initiation of treatment with bupropion). Products include:
- Wellbutrin Tablets ... 1177

Buspirone Hydrochloride (Concurrent use of buspirone and MAO inhibitor has resulted in several cases of hypertension; concurrent use is contraindicated; at least 10 days should elapse between the discontinuation of Parnate and the institution of buspirone). Products include:
- BuSpar Tablets ... 738

Caffeine (Excessive use of caffeine in any form is contraindicated). Products include:
- Arthritis Strength BC Powder ... 631
- BC Powder ... 631
- Cafergot ... 2376
- DHCplus Capsules ... 2148
- Darvon Compound-65 Pulvules ... 1475
- Esgic-plus Capsules ... 1012
- Esgic-plus Tablets ... 1012
- Aspirin Free Excedrin Analgesic Caplets and Geltabs ... 734
- Excedrin Extra-Strength Analgesic Tablets, Caplets, and Geltabs ... 734
- Fioricet Tablets ... 2386
- Fioricet with Codeine Capsules ... 2387
- Fiorinal Capsules ... 2388
- Fiorinal with Codeine Capsules ... 2390
- Fiorinal Tablets ... 2388
- Goody's Extra Strength Headache Powders ... 632
- Goody's Extra Strength Pain Relief Tablets ... 632
- Maximum Strength Multi-Symptom Formula Midol ... 621
- No Doz Maximum Strength Caplets ... 644
- Norgesic ... 1554
- Vanquish Analgesic Caplets ... 627
- Wigraine Tablets ... 1884

Captopril (Concurrent use with hypotensive agents is contraindicated; a marked potentiating effect on these classes of drugs has been reported). Products include:
- Capoten Tablets ... 740
- Capozide Tablets ... 744

Carbamazepine (Concurrent use with dibenzazeprine-related entities may result in hypertensive crises or severe convulsive seizures; concurrent and/or sequential use is contraindicated). Products include:
- Atretol Tablets ... 569
- Tegretol/Tegretol-XR ... 870

Carteolol Hydrochloride (Concurrent use with hypotensive agents is contraindicated; a marked potentiating effect on these classes of drugs has been reported). Products include:
- Cartrol Tablets ... 413
- Ocupress Ophthalmic Solution, 1% Sterile ... 297

Cetirizine Hydrochloride (Concurrent use is contraindicated). Products include:
- Zyrtec Tablets ... 2053

Chlorothiazide (Concurrent use with hypotensive agents is contraindicated; a marked potentiating effect on these classes of drugs has been reported). Products include:
- Aldoclor Tablets ... 1638
- Diupres Tablets ... 1691
- Diuril Oral ... 1694

Chlorothiazide Sodium (Concurrent use with hypotensive agents is contraindicated; a marked potentiating effect on these classes of drugs has been reported). Products include:
- Diuril Sodium Intravenous ... 1693

Chlorpheniramine Maleate (Concurrent use is contraindicated). Products include:
- Alka-Seltzer Plus Cold Medicine ... 611
- Alka-Seltzer Plus Cold Medicine Liqui-Gels ... 612
- Alka-Seltzer Plus Cold & Cough Medicine ... 611
- Alka-Seltzer Plus Cold & Cough Medicine Liqui-Gels ... 612
- Alka-Seltzer Plus Flu & Body Aches Effervescent Tablets ... 612
- Allerest Maximum Strength ... 649
- Allerest Sinus Pain Formula ... 649
- Ana-Kit Anaphylaxis Emergency Treatment Kit ... 611
- Atrohist Pediatric Capsules ... 1603
- Atrohist Plus Tablets ... 1605
- BC Cold Powder Multi-Symptom Formula (Cold-Sinus-Allergy) ... 631
- Cerose DM ... 853
- Cheracol Plus Head Cold/Cough Formula ... 741
- Children's TYLENOL Cold Multi-Symptom Chewable Tablets and Liquid ... 1559
- Children's TYLENOL Cold Plus Cough Multi Symptom Chewable Tablets and Liquid ... 1560
- Children's TYLENOL Flu Suspension Liquid ... 1560
- Children's Vicks DayQuil Allergy Relief ... 730
- Children's Vicks NyQuil Cold/Cough Relief ... 731
- Chlor-Trimeton Allergy Decongestant Tablets ... 759
- Chlor-Trimeton Allergy Tablets ... 758
- Allergy-Sinus Comtrex Multi-Symptom Allergy-Sinus Formula Tablets and Caplets ... 639
- Comtrex Multi-Symptom ... 638
- Contac Continuous Action Nasal Decongestant/Antihistamine 12 Hour Capsules ... 773
- Contac Maximum Strength Continuous Action Decongestant/Antihistamine 12 Hour Caplets ... 772
- Contac Severe Cold and Flu Formula Caplets ... 773
- Coricidin Cold + Flu Tablets ... 760
- Coricidin Cough + Cold Tablets ... 760
- Coricidin 'D' Decongestant Tablets ... 760
- D.A. II Tablets ... 972
- D.A. Chewable Tablets ... 970
- Dura-Tap/PD Capsules ... 970
- Dura-Vent/DA Tablets ... 972
- Efidac 24 Chlorpheniramine ... 655
- Extendryl ... 1003
- Fedahist Gyrocaps ... 2545
- Hycomine Compound Tablets ... 948
- Kronofed-A ... 994
- Nolamine Timed-Release Tablets ... 790
- Novahistine Elixir ... 782
- Ornade Spansule Capsules ... 2678
- PediaCare Cough-Cold Chewable Tablets and Liquid ... 1569
- PediaCare NightRest Cough-Cold Liquid ... 1569
- Pediatric Vicks 44m Cough & Cold Relief ... 737
- Pyrroxate Caplets ... 742
- Ryna ... 804
- Sinarest ... 663
- Sine-Off Sinus Medicine ... 784
- Singlet Tablets ... 785
- Sinulin Tablets ... 792
- Sinutab Sinus Allergy Medication, Maximum Strength Tablets and Caplets ... 823
- Sudafed Cold & Allergy Tablets ... 826
- Teldrin 12 Hour Antihistamine/Nasal Decongestant Allergy Relief Capsules ... 786
- TheraFlu Flu and Cold Medicine ... 750
- Theraflu Maximum Strength Flu and Cold Medicine For Sore Throat ... 751
- TheraFlu Flu, Cold and Cough Medicine ... 750
- TheraFlu Maximum Strength Nighttime Flu, Cold & Cough Medicine ... 751
- Triaminic Night Time ... 754
- Triaminic Syrup ... 755
- Triaminic Triaminicol Cold & Cough ... 756
- Triaminicin Tablets ... 756
- Tussend ... 1830
- TYLENOL Allergy Sinus, Maximum Strength Caplets and Gelcaps ... 1571
- TYLENOL Cold Medication, Multi-Symptom Formula Tablets and Caplets ... 1572
- TYLENOL Cold Medication, Multi-Symptom Hot Liquid Packets ... 1572
- Vicks 44 LiquiCaps Cough, Cold & Flu Relief ... 728
- Vicks 44M Cough, Cold & Flu Relief ... 729

Chlorpheniramine Polistirex (Concurrent use is contraindicated). Products include:
- Tussionex Pennkinetic Extended-Release Suspension ... 1624

Chlorpheniramine Tannate (Concurrent use is contraindicated). Products include:
- Atrohist Pediatric Suspension ... 1604
- Atrohist Pediatric Suspension Dye-Free ... 1604
- Rynatan ... 2781
- Rynatuss ... 2782

Chlorpromazine (Possibility of additive hypotensive effects). Products include:
- Thorazine Suppositories ... 2701

Chlorpromazine Hydrochloride (Possibility of additive hypotensive effects). Products include:
- Thorazine ... 2701

IMPORTANT NOTE: Always consult each drug listing in the patient's regimen for possible interactions.

Parnate **Interactions Index** **812**

Chlorpropamide (Some MAO inhibitors have contributed to hypoglycemic episodes in diabetic patients receiving oral hypoglycemic agents). Products include:
- Diabinese Tablets ... 2002

Chlorthalidone (Concurrent use with hypotensive agents is contraindicated; a marked potentiating effect on these classes of drugs has been reported). Products include:
- Combipres Tablets ... 682
- Tenoretic Tablets ... 2963
- Thalitone ... 1293

Clemastine Fumarate (Concurrent use is contraindicated). Products include:
- Tavist Syrup ... 2426
- Tavist Tablets ... 2427
- Tavist-1 12 Hour Relief Tablets ... ▣ 749
- Tavist-D 12 Hour Relief Tablets ... ▣ 750

Clomipramine Hydrochloride (Concurrent use with tricyclic antidepressants may result in hypertensive crises or severe convulsive seizures; concurrent and/or sequential use is contraindicated). Products include:
- Anafranil Capsules ... 819

Clonidine (Concurrent use with hypotensive agents is contraindicated; a marked potentiating effect on these classes of drugs has been reported). Products include:
- Catapres-TTS ... 680

Clonidine Hydrochloride (Concurrent use with hypotensive agents is contraindicated; a marked potentiating effect on these classes of drugs has been reported). Products include:
- Catapres Tablets ... 679
- Combipres Tablets ... 682

Clozapine (Concurrent use with dibenzazepine-related entities may result in hypertensive crises or severe convulsive seizures; concurrent and/or sequential use is contraindicated). Products include:
- Clozaril Tablets ... 2377

Cocaine Hydrochloride (Concurrent use is contraindicated). Products include:
- Cocaine Hydrochloride Topical Solutions ... 529

Codeine Phosphate (Concurrent use is contraindicated; a marked potentiating effect on these classes of drugs has been reported). Products include:
- Brontex ... 2130
- Dimetane-DC Cough Syrup ... 2232
- Fioricet with Codeine Capsules ... 2387
- Fiorinal with Codeine Capsules ... 2390
- Nucofed ... 2225
- Phenergan with Codeine ... 2883
- Phenergan VC with Codeine ... 2888
- Robitussin A-C Syrup ... 2248
- Robitussin-DAC Syrup ... 2249
- Ryna ... ▣ 804
- Soma Compound w/Codeine Tablets ... 2784
- Tylenol with Codeine ... 1592

Cyclobenzaprine Hydrochloride (Concurrent use with dibenzazepine-related entities may result in hypertensive crises or severe convulsive seizures; concurrent and/or sequential use is contraindicated). Products include:
- Flexeril Tablets ... 1701

Cyproheptadine Hydrochloride (Concurrent use is contraindicated). Products include:
- Periactin ... 1767

Deserpidine (Concurrent use with hypotensive agents is contraindicated; a marked potentiating effect on these classes of drugs has been reported).
- No products indexed under this heading.

Desipramine Hydrochloride (Concurrent use with tricyclic antidepressants may result in hypertensive crises or severe convulsive seizures; concurrent and/or sequential use is contraindicated). Products include:
- Norpramin Tablets ... 1273

Dextroamphetamine Sulfate (Concurrent and/or sequential use is contraindicated).

Dexchlorpheniramine Maleate (Concurrent use is contraindicated).
- No products indexed under this heading.

Dextroamphetamine Sulfate (Concurrent and/or sequential use is contraindicated). Products include:
- Adderall Tablets ... 2209
- Dexedrine ... 2648
- DextroStat-Dextroamphetamine Sulfate Tablets ... 2211

Dextromethorphan Hydrobromide (The combination of dextromethorphan and MAO inhibitors have been reported to cause brief episodes of psychosis or bizzare behavior; concurrent use is contraindicated). Products include:
- Alka-Seltzer Plus Cold & Cough Medicine ... ▣ 611
- Alka-Seltzer Plus Cold & Cough Medicine Liqui-Gels ... ▣ 612
- Alka-Seltzer Plus Flu & Body Aches Effervescent Tablets ... ▣ 612
- Alka-Seltzer Plus Flu & Body Aches Liqui-Gels Non-Drowsy Formula ... ▣ 613
- Alka-Seltzer Plus Night-Time Cold Medicine ... ▣ 611
- Alka-Seltzer Plus Night-Time Cold Medicine Liqui-Gels ... ▣ 612
- Benylin Adult Formula Cough Suppressant ... ▣ 817
- Benylin Expectorant ... ▣ 816
- Benylin Multisymptom ... ▣ 816
- Benylin Pediatric Cough Suppressant ... ▣ 817
- Bromfed-DM Cough Syrup ... 1832
- Cerose DM ... ▣ 853
- Cheracol D Cough Formula ... ▣ 740
- Cheracol Plus Head Cold/Cough Formula ... ▣ 741
- Children's TYLENOL Cold Plus Cough Multi Symptom Chewable Tablets and Liquid ... 1560
- Children's TYLENOL Flu Suspension Liquid ... 1560
- Children's Vicks NyQuil Cold/Cough Relief ... ▣ 731
- Comtrex Multi-Symptom ... ▣ 638
- Comtrex Non-Drowsy ... ▣ 640
- Contac Day & Night Cold/Flu Caplets ... ▣ 772
- Contac Severe Cold and Flu Formula Caplets ... ▣ 773
- Contac Severe Cold & Flu Non-Drowsy ... ▣ 774
- Coricidin Cough + Cold Tablets ... ▣ 760
- Cough-X Lozenges ... ▣ 606
- Diabe-Tuss DM Syrup ... 1948
- Dimetane-DX Cough Syrup ... 2233
- Dimetapp Cold & Cough Liqui-Gels ... ▣ 839
- Dimetapp DM Elixir ... ▣ 840
- Dorcol Children's Cough Syrup ... ▣ 748
- Drixoral Cough Liquid Caps ... ▣ 762
- Drixoral Cough + Congestion Liquid Caps ... ▣ 763
- Drixoral Cough + Sore Throat Liquid Caps ... ▣ 763
- Humibid DM Tablets ... 1612
- Novahistine DMX ... ▣ 782
- PediaCare Cough-Cold Chewable Tablets and Liquid ... 1569
- PediaCare Infants' Drops Decongestant Plus Cough ... 1569
- PediaCare NightRest Cough-Cold Liquid ... 1569
- Pediatric Vicks 44d Cough & Head Congestion Relief ... ▣ 736
- Pediatric Vicks 44e Cough & Chest Congestion Relief ... ▣ 737
- Pediatric Vicks 44m Cough & Cold Relief ... ▣ 737
- Pertussin Adult Extra Strength ... ▣ 630
- Pertussin Children's Strength ... ▣ 630
- Phenergan with Dextromethorphan 2885
- Robitussin Cold & Cough Liqui-Gels ... ▣ 844
- Robitussin Cold, Cough & Flu Liqui-Gels ... ▣ 844
- Robitussin Maximum Strength Cough Suppressant ... ▣ 847
- Robitussin Maximum Strength Cough & Cold ... ▣ 847
- Robitussin Night-Time Cold Formula ... ▣ 847
- Robitussin Pediatric Cough & Cold Formula ... ▣ 848
- Robitussin Pediatric Cough Suppressant ... ▣ 848
- Robitussin Pediatric Drops ... ▣ 849
- Robitussin-CF ... ▣ 846
- Robitussin-DM ... ▣ 846
- Safe Tussin 30 Liquid ... 1413
- Sucrets 4-Hour Cough Suppressant ... ▣ 785
- Sudafed Children's Cold & Cough Liquid Medication ... ▣ 825
- Sudafed Cold and Cough Liquid Caps ... ▣ 826
- Sudafed Severe Cold Formula Caplets ... ▣ 828
- Sudafed Severe Cold Formula Tablets ... ▣ 828
- Syn-Rx DM Tablets ... 1623
- TheraFlu Flu, Cold and Cough Medicine ... ▣ 750
- TheraFlu Maximum Strength Nighttime Flu, Cold & Cough Medicine ... ▣ 751
- TheraFlu Maximum Strength Non-Drowsy Formula Flu, Cold & Cough Medicine ... ▣ 751
- TheraFlu Maximum Strength, Non-Drowsy Formula Flu, Cold and Cough Caplets ... ▣ 752
- Triaminic AM Cough and Decongestant Formula ... ▣ 753
- Triaminic Night Time ... ▣ 754
- Triaminic Sore Throat Formula ... ▣ 755
- Triaminic Triaminicol Cold & Cough ... ▣ 756
- Triaminic DM Syrup ... ▣ 756
- Tussi-Organidin DM NR Liquid and DM-S NR Liquid ... 2786
- TYLENOL Cold Medication, Multi-Symptom Formula Tablets and Caplets ... 1572
- TYLENOL Cold Medication, Multi-Symptom Hot Liquid Packets ... 1572
- TYLENOL Cold Medication, No Drowsiness Formula Caplets and Gelcaps ... 1572
- TYLENOL Cold Severe Congestion Caplets ... 1573
- TYLENOL Cough Medication, Multi Symptom ... 1574
- TYLENOL Cough Medication with Decongestant, Multi Symptom ... 1574
- TYLENOL Flu No Drowsiness Formula, Maximum Strength Gelcaps ... 1575
- Vicks 44 Cough Relief ... ▣ 728
- Vicks 44 LiquiCaps Cough, Cold & Flu Relief ... ▣ 728
- Vicks 44 LiquiCaps Non-Drowsy Cough & Cold Relief ... ▣ 729
- Vicks 44D Cough & Head Congestion Relief ... ▣ 728
- Vicks 44E Cough & Chest Congestion Relief ... ▣ 729
- Vicks 44M Cough, Cold & Flu Relief ... ▣ 729
- Vicks DayQuil LiquiCaps/Liquid Multi-Symptom Cold/Flu Relief ... ▣ 734
- Vicks Nyquil Hot Therapy ... ▣ 735
- Vicks NyQuil LiquiCaps/Liquid Multi-Symptom Cold/Flu Relief, Original and Cherry Flavors ... ▣ 736

Dextromethorphan Polistirex (The combination of dextromethorphan and MAO inhibitors have been reported to cause brief episodes of psychosis or bizarre behavior; concurrent use is contraindicated). Products include:
- Delsym Extended-Release Suspension ... ▣ 670

Dezocine (Concurrent use is contraindicated; a marked potentiating effect on these classes of drugs has been reported). Products include:
- Dalgan Injection ... 529

Diazoxide (Concurrent use with hypotensive agents is contraindicated; a marked potentiating effect on these classes of drugs has been reported). Products include:
- Hyperstat I.V. Injection ... 2504
- Proglycem ... 575

Diethylpropion Hydrochloride (Concurrent and/or sequential use is contraindicated).
- No products indexed under this heading.

Diltiazem Hydrochloride (Concurrent use with hypotensive agents is contraindicated; a marked potentiating effect on these classes of drugs has been reported). Products include:
- Cardizem CD Capsules ... 1251
- Cardizem SR Capsules ... 1255
- Cardizem Injectable ... 1253
- Cardizem Tablets ... 1257
- Dilacor XR Extended-release Capsules ... 2183
- Tiazac Capsules ... 1019

Diphenhydramine Citrate (Concurrent use is contraindicated). Products include:
- Excedrin P.M. Analgesic/Sleeping Aid Tablets, Caplets, Liquigels ... 735

Diphenhydramine Hydrochloride (Concurrent use is contraindicated). Products include:
- Actifed Allergy Daytime/Nighttime Caplets ... ▣ 808
- Actifed Sinus Daytime/Nighttime Tablets and Caplets ... ▣ 809
- Extra Strength Bayer PM Aspirin Plus Sleep Aid ... ▣ 617
- Benadryl Allergy Chewables ... ▣ 811
- Benadryl Allergy/Cold Tablets ... ▣ 811
- Benadryl Allergy Decongestant Liquid Medication ... ▣ 812
- Benadryl Allergy Decongestant Tablets ... ▣ 812
- Benadryl Allergy Liquid Medication ... ▣ 813
- Benadryl Allergy ... ▣ 811
- Benadryl Allergy Sinus Headache Caplets ... ▣ 813
- Benadryl Dye-Free Allergy Liquigel Softgels ... ▣ 813
- Benadryl Dye-Free Allergy Liquid Medication ... ▣ 814
- Benadryl Itch Relief Stick Extra Strength ... ▣ 814
- Benadryl Cream ... ▣ 814
- Benadryl Gel ... ▣ 815
- Benadryl Spray ... ▣ 815
- Benadryl Injection ... 1955
- Contac Day & Night Cold/Flu Night Caplets ... ▣ 772
- Contac Night Allergy/Sinus Caplets ... ▣ 771
- Extra Strength Doan's P.M. ... ▣ 653
- Excedrin P.M. Analgesic/Sleeping Aid Tablets, Caplets, Liquigels ... ▣ 643
- Nytol QuickCaps Caplets ... ▣ 632
- Sleepinal Night-time Sleep Aid Capsules and Softgels ... ▣ 798
- TYLENOL Allergy Sinus NightTime, Maximum Strength Caplets ... 1571
- TYLENOL Flu NightTime, Maximum Strength Gelcaps ... 1575
- TYLENOL Flu NightTime, Maximum Strength Hot Medication Packets ... 1575
- TYLENOL PM Pain Reliever/Sleep Aid, Extra Strength Gelcaps, Caplets, Geltabs ... 1576
- TYLENOL Severe Allergy Medication Caplets ... 1571
- Maximum Strength Unisom Sleepgels ... 1990
- Unisom With Pain Relief-Nighttime Sleep Aid and Pain Reliever ... 1991

Diphenylpyraline Hydrochloride (Concurrent use is contraindicated).
- No products indexed under this heading.

(▣ Described in PDR For Nonprescription Drugs) (◉ Described in PDR For Ophthalmology)

813 **Interactions Index** **Parnate**

Disulfiram (Concurrent use requires caution; co-administration in animal models has resulted in severe toxicity including convulsions and death). Products include:

Antabuse Tablets ... 2802

Dobutamine Hydrochloride (Concurrent and/or sequential use is contraindicated; combination therapy may precipitate hypertension, headache and related symptoms). Products include:

Dobutrex Solution Vials ... 1480

Dopamine Hydrochloride (Concurrent and/or sequential use is contraindicated; combination therapy may precipitate hypertension, headache and related symptoms).

No products indexed under this heading.

Doxazosin Mesylate (Concurrent use with hypotensive agents is contraindicated; a marked potentiating effect on these classes of drugs has been reported). Products include:

Cardura Tablets ... 1993

Doxepin Hydrochloride (Concurrent use with tricyclic antidepressants may result in hypertensive crises or severe convulsive seizures; concurrent and/or sequential use is contraindicated). Products include:

Adapin Capsules ... 1542
Sinequan ... 2028
Zonalon Cream ... 1042

Enalapril Maleate (Concurrent use with hypotensive agents is contraindicated; a marked potentiating effect on these classes of drugs has been reported). Products include:

Vaseretic Tablets ... 1810
Vasotec Tablets ... 1816

Enalaprilat (Concurrent use with hypotensive agents is contraindicated; a marked potentiating effect on these classes of drugs has been reported). Products include:

Vasotec I.V. ... 1814

Enflurane (Concurrent use is contraindicated).

No products indexed under this heading.

Ephedrine Hydrochloride (Concurrent and/or sequential use is contraindicated; combination therapy may precipitate hypertension, headache and related symptoms). Products include:

Primatene Tablets ... 844
Quadrinal Tablets ... 1398

Ephedrine Sulfate (Concurrent and/or sequential use is contraindicated; combination therapy may precipitate hypertension, headache and related symptoms). Products include:

Marax Tablets & DF Syrup ... 2015

Ephedrine Tannate (Concurrent and/or sequential use is contraindicated; combination therapy may precipitate hypertension, headache and related symptoms). Products include:

Rynatuss ... 2782

Epinephrine (Concurrent and/or sequential use is contraindicated; combination therapy may precipitate hypertension, headache and related symptoms). Products include:

EPIFRIN ... 237
EpiPen ... 808
Marcaine with Epinephrine ... 2446
Primatene Mist ... 843
Sensorcaine with Epinephrine Injection ... 554
Sus-Phrine Injection ... 1017
Xylocaine with Epinephrine Injections ... 562

Epinephrine Bitartrate (Concurrent and/or sequential use is contraindicated; combination therapy may precipitate hypertension, headache and related symptoms). Products include:

Sensorcaine-MPF with Epinephrine Injection ... 554

Epinephrine Hydrochloride (Concurrent and/or sequential use is contraindicated; combination therapy may precipitate hypertension, headache and related symptoms). Products include:

Ana-Kit Anaphylaxis Emergency Treatment Kit ... 611

Esmolol Hydrochloride (Concurrent use with hypotensive agents is contraindicated; a marked potentiating effect on these classes of drugs has been reported). Products include:

Brevibloc (esmolol HCl) Injection ... 1860

Estazolam (Concurrent use is contraindicated). Products include:

ProSom Tablets ... 457

Ethacrynic Acid (Concurrent use with hypotensive agents is contraindicated; a marked potentiating effect on these classes of drugs has been reported). Products include:

Edecrin Tablets ... 1698

Ethchlorvynol (Concurrent use is contraindicated). Products include:

Placidyl Capsules ... 456

Ethinamate (Concurrent use is contraindicated).

No products indexed under this heading.

Felodipine (Concurrent use with hypotensive agents is contraindicated; a marked potentiating effect on these classes of drugs has been reported). Products include:

Plendil Extended-Release Tablets ... 514

Fenfluramine Hydrochloride (Concurrent and/or sequential use is contraindicated). Products include:

Pondimin Tablets ... 2239

Fentanyl (Concurrent use is contraindicated; a marked potentiating effect on these classes of drugs has been reported). Products include:

Duragesic Transdermal System ... 1336

Fentanyl Citrate (Concurrent use is contraindicated; a marked potentiating effect on these classes of drugs has been reported). Products include:

Sublimaze Injection ... 463

Fluoxetine Hydrochloride (Concurrent use has resulted in serious, sometimes fatal, reactions including hyperthermia, rigidity, myoclonus, autonomic instability with possible rapid fluctuations of vital signs and mental status; concurrent use is contraindicated; at least 5 weeks should be allowed after stopping fluoxetine before starting an MAO inhibitor). Products include:

Prozac Pulvules & Liquid, Oral Solution ... 935

Fluphenazine Decanoate (Possibility of additive hypotensive effects). Products include:

Prolixin Decanoate ... 510

Fluphenazine Enanthate (Possibility of additive hypotensive effects). Products include:

Prolixin Enanthate ... 510

Fluphenazine Hydrochloride (Possibility of additive hypotensive effects). Products include:

Prolixin ... 510

Flurazepam Hydrochloride (Concurrent use is contraindicated). Products include:

Dalmane Capsules ... 2329

Fluvoxamine Maleate (Concurrent and/or sequential use is contraindicated; potential for serious, sometimes fatal, reactions including hyperthermia, rigidity, myoclonus, and other toxicities). Products include:

LUVOX Tablets ... 2723

Fosinopril Sodium (Concurrent use with hypotensive agents is contraindicated; a marked potentiating effect on these classes of drugs has been reported). Products include:

Monopril Tablets ... 762

Furazolidone (Concurrent use with another MAO inhibitor may result in hypertensive crises or severe convulsive seizures; concurrent and/or sequential use is contraindicated). Products include:

Furoxone ... 2221

Furosemide (Concurrent use with hypotensive agents is contraindicated; a marked potentiating effect on these classes of drugs has been reported). Products include:

Lasix Injection, Oral Solution and Tablets ... 1267

Glimepiride (Some MAO inhibitors have contributed to hypoglycemic episodes in diabetic patients receiving oral hypoglycemic agents). Products include:

Amaryl Tablets ... 1241

Glipizide (Some MAO inhibitors have contributed to hypoglycemic episodes in diabetic patients receiving oral hypoglycemic agents). Products include:

Glucotrol Tablets ... 2011
Glucotrol XL Extended Release Tablets ... 2012

Glutethimide (Concurrent use is contraindicated).

No products indexed under this heading.

Glyburide (Some MAO inhibitors have contributed to hypoglycemic episodes in diabetic patients receiving oral hypoglycemic agents). Products include:

DiaBeta Tablets ... 1265
Glynase PresTab Tablets ... 2091
Micronase Tablets ... 2099

Guanabenz Acetate (Concurrent use with hypotensive agents is contraindicated; a marked potentiating effect on these classes of drugs has been reported).

No products indexed under this heading.

Guanethidine Monosulfate (Concurrent and/or sequential use is contraindicated; combination therapy may precipitate hypertension, headache and related symptoms). Products include:

Esimil Tablets ... 840
Ismelin Tablets ... 845

Halothane (Concurrent use is contraindicated). Products include:

Fluothane ... 2830

Hydralazine Hydrochloride (Concurrent use with hypotensive agents is contraindicated; a marked potentiating effect on these classes of drugs has been reported). Products include:

Apresazide Capsules ... 824
Apresoline Hydrochloride Tablets .. 826
Hydralazine Hydrochloride Injection USP ... 2712
Ser-Ap-Es Tablets ... 867

Hydrochlorothiazide (Concurrent use with hypotensive agents is contraindicated; a marked potentiating effect on these classes of drugs has been reported). Products include:

Aldactazide Tablets ... 2556
Aldoril Tablets ... 1644
Apresazide Capsules ... 824
Capozide Tablets ... 744
Dyazide Capsules ... 2653
Esidrix Tablets ... 839
Esimil Tablets ... 840
HydroDIURIL Tablets ... 1716
Hydropres Tablets ... 1718
Hyzaar Tablets ... 1720
Inderide Tablets ... 2838
Inderide LA Long Acting Capsules .. 2840
Lopressor HCT Tablets ... 850
Lotensin HCT Tablets ... 855
Moduretic Tablets ... 1748
Oretic Tablets ... 450
Prinzide Tablets ... 1780
Ser-Ap-Es Tablets ... 867
Timolide Tablets ... 1791
Vaseretic Tablets ... 1810
Zestoretic Tablets ... 2968
Ziac ... 1459

Hydrocodone Bitartrate (Concurrent use is contraindicated; a marked potentiating effect on these classes of drugs has been reported). Products include:

Codiclear DH Syrup ... 808
Duratuss HD Elixir ... 2750
Histussin D Liquid ... 670
Hycodan Tablets and Syrup ... 946
Hycomine Compound Tablets ... 948
Hycomine ... 947
Hycotuss Expectorant Syrup ... 950
Hydrocet Capsules ... 787
Lorcet 10/650 Tablets ... 1016
Lortab ... 2751
Tussend ... 1830
Tussend Expectorant ... 1831
Vicodin Tablets ... 1404
Vicodin ES Tablets ... 1405
Vicodin HP Tablets ... 1403
Vicodin Tuss Expectorant ... 1406
Zydone Capsules ... 967

Hydrocodone Polistirex (Concurrent use is contraindicated; a marked potentiating effect on these classes of drugs has been reported). Products include:

Tussionex Pennkinetic Extended-Release Suspension ... 1624

Hydroflumethiazide (Concurrent use with hypotensive agents is contraindicated; a marked potentiating effect on these classes of drugs has been reported). Products include:

Diucardin Tablets ... 2824

Hydromorphone Hydrochloride (Concurrent use is contraindicated; a marked potentiating effect on these classes of drugs has been reported). Products include:

Dilaudid Ampules ... 1382
Dilaudid Cough Syrup ... 1383
Dilaudid-HP Injection ... 1384
Dilaudid-HP Lyophilized Powder 250 mg ... 1384
Dilaudid ... 1382
Dilaudid Oral Liquid ... 1386
Dilaudid ... 1382
Dilaudid Tablets - 8 mg ... 1386

Imipramine Hydrochloride (Concurrent use with tricyclic antidepressants may result in hypertensive crises or severe convulsive seizures; concurrent and/or sequential use is contraindicated). Products include:

Tofranil Ampuls ... 873
Tofranil Tablets ... 875

Imipramine Pamoate (Concurrent use with tricyclic antidepressants may result in hypertensive crises or severe convulsive seizures; concurrent and/or sequential use is contraindicated). Products include:

Tofranil-PM Capsules ... 876

IMPORTANT NOTE: Always consult each drug listing in the patient's regimen for possible interactions.

Parnate
Interactions Index
814

Indapamide (Concurrent use with hypotensive agents is contraindicated; a marked potentiating effect on these classes of drugs has been reported).
No products indexed under this heading.

Insulin, Human (Some MAO inhibitors have contributed to hypoglycemic episodes in diabetic patients receiving insulin).
No products indexed under this heading.

Insulin, Human Isophane Suspension (Some MAO inhibitors have contributed to hypoglycemic episodes in diabetic patients receiving insulin). Products include:
Novolin N Human Insulin 10 ml Vials 1846

Insulin, Human NPH (Some MAO inhibitors have contributed to hypoglycemic episodes in diabetic patients receiving insulin). Products include:
Humulin N, 100 Units 1495
Novolin N PenFill 1.5 ml Cartridges Durable Insulin Delivery System 1849
Novolin N Prefilled Syringe Disposable Insulin Delivery System 1850

Insulin, Human Regular (Some MAO inhibitors have contributed to hypoglycemic episodes in diabetic patients receiving insulin). Products include:
Humulin R, 100 Units 1497
Novolin R Human Insulin 10 ml Vials 1846
Novolin R PenFill 1.5 ml Cartridges Durable Insulin Delivery System 1849
Novolin R Prefilled Syringe Disposable Insulin Delivery System 1850
Velosulin BR Human Insulin 10 ml Vials 1847

Insulin, Human, Zinc Suspension (Some MAO inhibitors have contributed to hypoglycemic episodes in diabetic patients receiving insulin). Products include:
Humulin L, 100 Units 1494
Humulin U, 100 Units 1498
Novolin L Human Insulin 10 ml Vials 1846

Insulin Lispro, Human (Some MAO inhibitors have contributed to hypoglycemic episodes in diabetic patients receiving insulin). Products include:
Humalog Injection 1488

Insulin, NPH (Some MAO inhibitors have contributed to hypoglycemic episodes in diabetic patients receiving insulin). Products include:
NPH, 100 Units 1502
Pork NPH, 100 Units 1506
Purified Pork NPH Isophane Insulin 1852

Insulin, Regular (Some MAO inhibitors have contributed to hypoglycemic episodes in diabetic patients receiving insulin). Products include:
Regular, 100 Units 1503
Pork Regular, 100 Units 1507
Pork Regular (Concentrated), 500 Units 1508
Purified Pork Regular Insulin 1852

Insulin, Zinc Crystals (Some MAO inhibitors have contributed to hypoglycemic episodes in diabetic patients receiving insulin). Products include:
NPH, 100 Units 1502

Insulin, Zinc Suspension (Some MAO inhibitors have contributed to hypoglycemic episodes in diabetic patients receiving insulin). Products include:
Iletin I 1501
Lente, 100 Units 1501
Iletin II 1504
Pork Lente, 100 Units 1504
Purified Pork Lente Insulin 1852

Isocarboxazid (Concurrent use with another MAO inhibitor may result in hypertensive crises or severe convulsive seizures; concurrent and/or sequential use is contraindicated).
No products indexed under this heading.

Isoflurane (Concurrent use is contraindicated).
No products indexed under this heading.

Isoproterenol Hydrochloride (Concurrent and/or sequential use is contraindicated; combination therapy may precipitate hypertension, headache and related symptoms). Products include:
Isuprel Hydrochloride Solution 2443
Isuprel Injection 2441
Isuprel Mistometer 2442

Isoproterenol Sulfate (Concurrent and/or sequential use is contraindicated; combination therapy may precipitate hypertension, headache and related symptoms). Products include:
Norisodrine with Calcium Iodide Syrup 446

Isradipine (Concurrent use with hypotensive agents is contraindicated; a marked potentiating effect on these classes of drugs has been reported). Products include:
DynaCirc Capsules 2381
DynaCirc CR Tablets 2383

Ketamine Hydrochloride (Concurrent use is contraindicated).
No products indexed under this heading.

Labetalol Hydrochloride (Concurrent use with hypotensive agents is contraindicated; a marked potentiating effect on these classes of drugs has been reported). Products include:
Normodyne Injection 2519
Normodyne Tablets 2522
Trandate 1158

Levodopa (Concurrent and/or sequential use is contraindicated; combination therapy may precipitate hypertension, headache and related symptoms). Products include:
Atamet Tablets 567
Larodopa Tablets 2296
Sinemet Tablets 959
Sinemet CR Tablets 961

Levorphanol Tartrate (Concurrent use is contraindicated; a marked potentiating effect on these classes of drugs has been reported). Products include:
Levo-Dromoran 2297

Lisinopril (Concurrent use with hypotensive agents is contraindicated; a marked potentiating effect on these classes of drugs has been reported). Products include:
Prinivil Tablets 1776
Prinzide Tablets 1780
Zestoretic Tablets 2968
Zestril Tablets 2972

Loratadine (Concurrent use is contraindicated). Products include:
Claritin Tablets 2485
Claritin-D Tablets 2487

Lorazepam (Concurrent use is contraindicated). Products include:
Ativan Injection 2805
Ativan Tablets 2807

Losartan Potassium (Concurrent use with hypotensive agents is contraindicated; a marked potentiating effect on these classes of drugs has been reported). Products include:
Cozaar Tablets 1668
Hyzaar Tablets 1720

Maprotiline Hydrochloride (Concurrent use with tricyclic antidepressants may result in hypertensive crises or severe convulsive seizures; concurrent and/or sequential use is contraindicated). Products include:
Ludiomil Tablets 861

Mazindol (Concurrent and/or sequential use is contraindicated). Products include:
Sanorex Tablets 2423

Mecamylamine Hydrochloride (Concurrent use with hypotensive agents is contraindicated; a marked potentiating effect on these classes of drugs has been reported). Products include:
Inversine Tablets 1729

Meperidine Hydrochloride (Concomitant use or within 2 or 3 weeks following MAOI therapy is contraindicated; serious reactions including coma, severe hypertension or hypotension, convulsion, severe respiratory depression, malignant hyperpyrexia, excitation, peripheral vascular collapse, and death have been reported with combined use). Products include:
Demerol 2438
Mepergan Injection 2859

Mesoridazine Besylate (Possibility of additive hypotensive effects). Products include:
Serentil 689

Metaproterenol Sulfate (Concurrent and/or sequential use is contraindicated; combination therapy may precipitate hypertension, headache and related symptoms). Products include:
Alupent 672
Metaproterenol Sulfate Inhalation Solution, USP, Arm-a-Med 547

Metaraminol Bitartrate (Concurrent and/or sequential use is contraindicated; combination therapy may precipitate hypertension, headache and related symptoms). Products include:
Aramine Injection 1649

Metformin Hydrochloride (Some MAO inhibitors have contributed to hypoglycemic episodes in diabetic patients receiving oral hypoglycemic agents). Products include:
Glucophage Tablets 754

Methadone Hydrochloride (Concurrent use is contraindicated; a marked potentiating effect on these classes of drugs has been reported). Products include:
Methadone Hydrochloride Oral Concentrate 2356
Methadone Hydrochloride Oral Solution & Tablets 2357

Methamphetamine Hydrochloride (Concurrent and/or sequential use is contraindicated). Products include:
Desoxyn Gradumet Tablets 422

Methdilazine Hydrochloride (Concurrent use is contraindicated).
No products indexed under this heading.

Methohexital Sodium (Concurrent use is contraindicated).
No products indexed under this heading.

Methotrimeprazine (Possibility of additive hypotensive effects). Products include:
Levoprome 1321

Methoxamine Hydrochloride (Concurrent and/or sequential use is contraindicated; combination therapy may precipitate hypertension, headache and related symptoms). Products include:
Vasoxyl Injection 1169

Methyclothiazide (Concurrent use with hypotensive agents is contraindicated; a marked potentiating effect on these classes of drugs has been reported). Products include:
Enduron Tablets 424

Methyldopa (Concurrent and/or sequential use is contraindicated; combination therapy may precipitate hypertension, headache and related symptoms). Products include:
Aldoclor Tablets 1638
Aldomet Oral 1640
Aldoril Tablets 1644

Methyldopate Hydrochloride (Concurrent and/or sequential use is contraindicated; combination therapy may precipitate hypertension, headache and related symptoms). Products include:
Aldomet Ester HCl Injection 1642

Metolazone (Concurrent use with hypotensive agents is contraindicated; a marked potentiating effect on these classes of drugs has been reported). Products include:
Mykrox Tablets 1617
Zaroxolyn Tablets 1625

Metoprolol Succinate (Concurrent use with hypotensive agents is contraindicated; a marked potentiating effect on these classes of drugs has been reported). Products include:
Toprol-XL Tablets 560

Metoprolol Tartrate (Concurrent use with hypotensive agents is contraindicated; a marked potentiating effect on these classes of drugs has been reported). Products include:
Lopressor 848
Lopressor HCT Tablets 850

Metrizamide (Concurrent use with drugs which lower seizure threshold, including MAO inhibitors, should not be used with metrizamide).

Metyrosine (Concurrent use with hypotensive agents is contraindicated; a marked potentiating effect on these classes of drugs has been reported). Products include:
Demser Capsules 1690

Midazolam Hydrochloride (Concurrent use is contraindicated). Products include:
Versed Injection 2324

Minoxidil (Concurrent use with hypotensive agents is contraindicated; a marked potentiating effect on these classes of drugs has been reported).
No products indexed under this heading.

Moexipril Hydrochloride (Concurrent use with hypotensive agents is contraindicated; a marked potentiating effect on these classes of drugs has been reported). Products include:
Univasc Tablets 2553

Morphine Sulfate (Concurrent use is contraindicated; a marked potentiating effect on these classes of drugs has been reported). Products include:
Astramorph/PF Injection, USP (Preservative-Free) 526
Duramorph Injection 983
Infumorph 200 and Infumorph 500 Sterile Solutions 985
Kadian Capsules 2948
MS Contin Tablets 2149

(Described in PDR For Nonprescription Drugs)
(Described in PDR For Ophthalmology)

MSIR 2152
Oramorph SR (Morphine Sulfate Sustained Release Tablets) 2359
RMS Suppositories CII 2766
Roxanol 2365

Nadolol (Concurrent use with hypotensive agents is contraindicated; a marked potentiating effect on these classes of drugs has been reported).
No products indexed under this heading.

Naphazoline Hydrochloride (Concurrent and/or sequential use is contraindicated; combination therapy may precipitate hypertension, headache and related symptoms). Products include:
Albalon Solution with Liquifilm .... ◉ 229
Clear Eyes ACR Astringent/Lubricant Eye Redness Reliever Eye Drops .... ◉ 314
Clear Eyes Lubricant Eye Redness Reliever .... ◉ 314
4-Way Fast Acting Nasal Spray (regular & mentholated) .... [MD] 644
Naphcon-A Ophthalmic Solution 469
OcuHist .... ◉ 300
Privine .... [MD] 663
Vasocon-A .... ◉ 263

Nicardipine Hydrochloride (Concurrent use with hypotensive agents is contraindicated; a marked potentiating effect on these classes of drugs has been reported). Products include:
Cardene Capsules 2261
Cardene I.V. 2815
Cardene SR Capsules 2264

Nifedipine (Concurrent use with hypotensive agents is contraindicated; a marked potentiating effect on these classes of drugs has been reported). Products include:
Adalat Capsules (10 mg and 20 mg) 580
Adalat CC 582
Procardia Capsules 2024
Procardia XL Extended Release Tablets 2026

Nisoldipine (Concurrent use with hypotensive agents is contraindicated; a marked potentiating effect on these classes of drugs has been reported). Products include:
Sular Tablets 2961

Nitroglycerin (Concurrent use with hypotensive agents is contraindicated; a marked potentiating effect on these classes of drugs has been reported). Products include:
Deponit NTG Transdermal Delivery System 2541
Nitro-Bid IV 1270
Nitro-Bid Ointment 1272
Nitro-Dur (nitroglycerin) Transdermal Infusion System 1365
Nitrolingual Spray 2193
Nitrostat Tablets 1981
Transderm-Nitro Transdermal Therapeutic System 878

Norepinephrine Bitartrate (Concurrent and/or sequential use is contraindicated; combination therapy may precipitate hypertension, headache and related symptoms). Products include:
Levophed Bitartrate Injection 2445

Nortriptyline Hydrochloride (Concurrent use with tricyclic antidepressants may result in hypertensive crises or severe convulsive seizures; concurrent and/or sequential use is contraindicated). Products include:
Pamelor 2409

Opium Alkaloids (Concurrent use is contraindicated; a marked potentiating effect on these classes of drugs has been reported).
No products indexed under this heading.

Oxycodone Hydrochloride (Concurrent use is contraindicated; a marked potentiating effect on these classes of drugs has been reported). Products include:
OxyContin Tablets 2163
OxyIR Capsules 2167
Percocet Tablets 955
Percodan Tablets 955
Percodan-Demi Tablets 956
Roxicodone Tablets, Oral Solution & Intensol (Oxycodone) 2366
Tylox Capsules 1593

Oxymetazoline Hydrochloride (Concurrent and/or sequential use is contraindicated; combination therapy may precipitate hypertension, headache and related symptoms). Products include:
Afrin .... [MD] 757
Duration 12 Hour Nasal Spray .... [MD] 766
4-Way 12 Hour Nasal Spray .... [MD] 644
Neo-Synephrine Maximum Strength 12 Hour Nasal Spray .... [MD] 624
Neo-Synephrine 12 Hour .... [MD] 624
12 Hour Nōstrilla .... [MD] 660
Vicks Sinex 12-Hour Nasal Decongestant Spray and Ultra Fine Mist .... [MD] 738
Visine L.R. Eye Drops .... [MD] 719
Visine L.R. Eye Drops .... ◉ 301

Paroxetine Hydrochloride (Concurrent and/or sequential use is contraindicated; potential for serious, sometimes fatal, reactions including hyperthermia, rigidity, myoclonus, and other toxicities; at least 2 weeks should be allowed after stopping paroxetine before starting an MAO inhibitor). Products include:
Paxil Tablets 2681

Penbutolol Sulfate (Concurrent use with hypotensive agents is contraindicated; a marked potentiating effect on these classes of drugs has been reported). Products include:
Levatol Tablets 2547

Perphenazine (Possibility of additive hypotensive effects). Products include:
Etrafon 2495
Triavil Tablets 1800
Trilafon 2532

Phendimetrazine Tartrate (Concurrent and/or sequential use is contraindicated). Products include:
Bontril Slow-Release Capsules 786
Prelu-2 Timed Release Capsules 687

Phenelzine Sulfate (Concurrent use with another MAO inhibitor may result in hypertensive crises or severe convulsive seizures; concurrent and/or sequential use is contraindicated). Products include:
Nardil 1977

Phenmetrazine Hydrochloride (Concurrent and/or sequential use is contraindicated).
No products indexed under this heading.

Phenoxybenzamine Hydrochloride (Concurrent use with hypotensive agents is contraindicated; a marked potentiating effect on these classes of drugs has been reported). Products include:
Dibenzyline Capsules 2650

Phentolamine Mesylate (Concurrent use with hypotensive agents is contraindicated; a marked potentiating effect on these classes of drugs has been reported). Products include:
Regitine Vials 864

Phenylephrine Bitartrate (Concurrent and/or sequential use is contraindicated; combination therapy may precipitate hypertension, headache and related symptoms).
No products indexed under this heading.

Phenylephrine Hydrochloride (Concurrent and/or sequential use is contraindicated; combination therapy may precipitate hypertension, headache and related symptoms). Products include:
Atrohist Plus Tablets 1605
Cerose DM .... [MD] 853
D.A. II Tablets 972
D.A. Chewable Tablets 970
Dura-Vent/DA Tablets 972
Extendryl 1003
4-Way Fast Acting Nasal Spray (regular & mentholated) .... [MD] 644
Hemorid .... [MD] 797
Hycomine Compound Tablets 948
Neo-Synephrine Hydrochloride 1% Carpuject 2455
Neo-Synephrine Hydrochloride 1% Injection 2455
Neo-Synephrine Hydrochloride (Ophthalmic) 2456
Neo-Synephrine .... [MD] 624
Novahistine Elixir .... [MD] 782
Phenergan VC 2886
Phenergan VC with Codeine 2888
Preparation H .... [MD] 842
Tympagesic Ear Drops 2476
Vicks Sinex Nasal Spray and Ultra Fine Mist .... [MD] 738

Phenylephrine Tannate (Concurrent and/or sequential use is contraindicated; combination therapy may precipitate hypertension, headache and related symptoms). Products include:
Atrohist Pediatric Suspension 1604
Atrohist Pediatric Suspension Dye-Free 1604
Rynatan 2781
Rynatuss 2782

Phenylpropanolamine Hydrochloride (Concurrent and/or sequential use is contraindicated; combination therapy may precipitate hypertension, headache and related symptoms). Products include:
Acutrim .... [MD] 648
Atrohist Plus Tablets 1605
BC Cold Powder Multi-Symptom Formula (Cold-Sinus-Allergy) .... [MD] 631
BC Cold Powder Non-Drowsy Formula (Cold-Sinus) .... [MD] 631
Cheracol Plus Head Cold/Cough Formula .... [MD] 741
Comtrex Multi-Symptom Cold Reliever Liqui-Gels .... [MD] 638
Comtrex Multi-Symptom Non-Drowsy Liqui-gels .... [MD] 640
Contac Continuous Action Nasal Decongestant/Antihistamine 12 Hour Capsules .... [MD] 773
Contac Maximum Strength Continuous Action Decongestant/Antihistamine 12 Hour Caplets .... [MD] 772
Contac Severe Cold and Flu Formula Caplets .... [MD] 773
Coricidin 'D' Decongestant Tablets .... [MD] 760
Dexatrim .... [MD] 795
Dexatrim Plus Vitamins Caplets .... [MD] 796
Dimetane-DC Cough Syrup 2232
Dimetapp Allergy Sinus Caplets .... [MD] 838
Dimetapp Cold & Allergy Chewable Tablets .... [MD] 838
Dimetapp Cold & Cough Liqui-Gels .... [MD] 839
Dimetapp DM Elixir .... [MD] 840
Dimetapp Elixir .... [MD] 840
Dimetapp Extentabs .... [MD] 841
Dimetapp Tablets/Liqui-Gels .... [MD] 841
Dura-Vent Tablets 971
Entex LA Tablets 972
Exgest LA Tablets 787
Hycomine 947
Nolamine Timed-Release Tablets 790
Ornade Spansule Capsules 2678
Propagest Tablets 791
Pyrroxate Caplets .... [MD] 742
Robitussin-CF .... [MD] 846
Sinulin Tablets 792
Tavist-D 12 Hour Relief Tablets .... [MD] 750
Teldrin 12 Hour Antihistamine/Nasal Decongestant Allergy Relief Capsules .... [MD] 786
Triaminic Expectorant .... [MD] 753
Triaminic Syrup .... [MD] 755
Triaminic Triaminicol Cold & Cough .... [MD] 756
Triaminic DM Syrup .... [MD] 756
Triaminicin Tablets .... [MD] 756
Vicks DayQuil Allergy Relief 12-Hour Extended Release Tablets .... [MD] 733
Vicks DayQuil Allergy Relief 4-Hour Tablets .... [MD] 733
Vicks DayQuil SINUS Pressure & CONGESTION Relief .... [MD] 734

Pindolol (Concurrent use with hypotensive agents is contraindicated; a marked potentiating effect on these classes of drugs has been reported). Products include:
Visken Tablets 2428

Pirbuterol Acetate (Concurrent and/or sequential use is contraindicated; combination therapy may precipitate hypertension, headache and related symptoms). Products include:
Maxair Autohaler 1550
Maxair Inhaler 1552

Polythiazide (Concurrent use with hypotensive agents is contraindicated; a marked potentiating effect on these classes of drugs has been reported). Products include:
Minizide Capsules 2016

Prazosin Hydrochloride (Concurrent use with hypotensive agents is contraindicated; a marked potentiating effect on these classes of drugs has been reported). Products include:
Minipress Capsules 2015
Minizide Capsules 2016

Prochlorperazine (Possibility of additive hypotensive effects). Products include:
Compazine 2644

Procyclidine Hydrochloride (Anti-Parkinsonism drugs should be used with caution in patients receiving Parnate since severe reactions have been reported). Products include:
Kemadrin Tablets 1105

Promethazine Hydrochloride (Possibility of additive hypotensive effects). Products include:
Mepergan Injection 2859
Phenergan with Codeine 2883
Phenergan with Dextromethorphan 2885
Phenergan Injection 2880
Phenergan Suppositories 2882
Phenergan Syrup 2881
Phenergan Tablets 2882
Phenergan VC 2886
Phenergan VC with Codeine 2888

Propofol (Concurrent use is contraindicated). Products include:
Diprivan Injectable Emulsion 2939

Propoxyphene Hydrochloride (Concurrent use is contraindicated; a marked potentiating effect on these classes of drugs has been reported). Products include:
Darvon 1475
Wygesic Tablets 2930

Propoxyphene Napsylate (Concurrent use is contraindicated; a marked potentiating effect on these classes of drugs has been reported). Products include:
Darvon-N/Darvocet-N 1473

Propranolol Hydrochloride (Concurrent use with hypotensive agents is contraindicated; a marked potentiating effect on these classes of drugs has been reported). Products include:
Inderal 2834

IMPORTANT NOTE: Always consult each drug listing in the patient's regimen for possible interactions.

Parnate | **Interactions Index** | **816**

Inderal LA Long Acting Capsules 2836
Inderide Tablets 2838
Inderide LA Long Acting Capsules .. 2840

Protriptyline Hydrochloride (Concurrent use with tricyclic antidepressants may result in hypertensive crises or severe convulsive seizures; concurrent and/or sequential use is contraindicated). Products include:
Vivactil Tablets 1820

Pseudoephedrine Hydrochloride (Concurrent and/or sequential use is contraindicated; combination therapy may precipitate hypertension, headache and related symptoms). Products include:
Actifed Allergy Daytime/Nighttime Caplets .... ▣ 808
Actifed Cold & Allergy Tablets .... ▣ 807
Actifed Cold & Sinus Caplets and Tablets .... ▣ 808
Actifed Sinus Daytime/Nighttime Tablets and Caplets .... ▣ 809
Advil Cold and Sinus Caplets and Tablets .... ▣ 837
Alka-Seltzer Plus Liqui-Gels .... ▣ 612
Alka-Seltzer Plus Flu & Body Aches Liqui-Gels Non-Drowsy Formula .... ▣ 613
Alka-Seltzer Plus Night-Time Cold Medicine Liqui-Gels .... ▣ 612
Allerest Maximum Strength .... ▣ 649
Allerest No Drowsiness .... ▣ 649
Allerest Sinus Pain Formula .... ▣ 649
Atrohist Pediatric Capsules 1603
Benadryl Allergy/Cold Tablets .... ▣ 811
Benadryl Allergy Decongestant Liquid Medication .... ▣ 812
Benadryl Allergy Decongestant Tablets .... ▣ 812
Benadryl Allergy Sinus Headache Caplets .... ▣ 813
Benylin Multisymptom .... ▣ 816
Bromfed Capsules (Extended-Release) 1832
Bromfed Syrup .... ▣ 712
Bromfed Tablets 1832
Bromfed-DM Cough Syrup 1832
Bromfed-PD Capsules (Extended-Release) 1832
Children's TYLENOL Cold Multi-Symptom Chewable Tablets and Liquid 1559
Children's TYLENOL Cold Plus Cough Multi Symptom Chewable Tablets and Liquid 1560
Children's TYLENOL Flu Suspension Liquid 1560
Children's Vicks DayQuil Allergy Relief .... ▣ 730
Children's Vicks NyQuil Cold/Cough Relief .... ▣ 731
Allergy-Sinus Comtrex Multi-Symptom Allergy-Sinus Formula Tablets and Caplets .... ▣ 639
Comtrex Multi-Symptom .... ▣ 638
Comtrex Multi-Symptom Non-Drowsy Caplets .... ▣ 640
Congess 1003
Contac Day Allergy/Sinus Caplets ▣ 771
Contac Day & Night .... ▣ 772
Contac Night Allergy/Sinus Caplets .... ▣ 771
Contac Severe Cold & Flu Non-Drowsy .... ▣ 774
Deconsal II Tablets 1605
Dimetane-DX Cough Syrup 2233
Dimetapp Cold & Fever Suspension .... ▣ 839
Dimetapp Decongestant Pediatric Drops .... ▣ 840
Dorcol Children's Cough Syrup .... ▣ 748
Drixoral Cough + Congestion Liquid Caps .... ▣ 763
Dura-Tap/PD Capsules 970
Duratuss Tablets 2750
Duratuss HD Elixir 2750
Efidac/24 .... ▣ 655
Entex PSE Tablets 973
Fedahist Gyrocaps 2545
Guaifed 1833
Guaifed Syrup .... ▣ 712
Guaimax-D Tablets 809
Histussin D Liquid 670
Infants' TYLENOL Cold Decongestant & Fever-Reducer Drops 1561
Kronofed-A 994
Novahistine DMX .... ▣ 782
Nucofed 2225
PediaCare Cough-Cold Chewable Tablets and Liquid 1569
PediaCare Infants' Decongestant Drops 1569
PediaCare Infants' Drops Decongestant Plus Cough 1569
PediaCare NightRest Cough-Cold Liquid 1569
Pediatric Vicks 44d Cough & Head Congestion Relief .... ▣ 736
Pediatric Vicks 44m Cough & Cold Relief .... ▣ 737
Robitussin Cold & Cough Liqui-Gels .... ▣ 844
Robitussin Cold, Cough & Flu Liqui-Gels .... ▣ 844
Robitussin Maximum Strength Cough & Cold .... ▣ 847
Robitussin Night-Time Cold Formula .... ▣ 847
Robitussin Pediatric Cough & Cold Formula .... ▣ 848
Robitussin Pediatric Drops .... ▣ 849
Robitussin Severe Congestion Liqui-Gels .... ▣ 845
Robitussin-DAC Syrup 2249
Robitussin-PE .... ▣ 846
Rondec Oral Drops 974
Rondec Syrup 974
Rondec Tablet 974
Rondec Chewable Tablets 974
Rondec-TR Tablet 974
Ryna .... ▣ 804
Seldane-D Extended-Release Tablets 1286
Semprex-D Capsules 1620
Sinarest .... ▣ 663
Sine-Aid Maximum Strength Sinus Headache Gelcaps, Caplets and Tablets 1570
Sine-Off No Drowsiness Formula Caplets .... ▣ 784
Sine-Off Sinus Medicine .... ▣ 784
Singlet Tablets .... ▣ 785
Sinutab Non-Drying Liquid Caps .... ▣ 823
Sinutab Sinus Allergy Medication, Maximum Strength Tablets and Caplets .... ▣ 823
Sinutab Sinus Medication, Maximum Strength Without Drowsiness Formula, Tablets & Caplets .... ▣ 824
Sudafed Children's Cold & Cough Liquid Medication .... ▣ 825
Sudafed Children's Nasal Decongestant Liquid Medication .... ▣ 826
Sudafed Cold & Allergy Tablets .... ▣ 826
Sudafed Cold and Cough Liquid Caps .... ▣ 826
Sudafed Nasal Decongestant Tablets, 30 mg .... ▣ 825
Sudafed Nasal Decongestant Tablets, 60 mg .... ▣ 825
Sudafed Non-Drying Sinus Liquid Caps .... ▣ 827
Sudafed Pediatric Nasal Decongestant Liquid Oral Drops .... ▣ 827
Sudafed Severe Cold Formula Caplets .... ▣ 828
Sudafed Severe Cold Formula Tablets .... ▣ 828
Sudafed Sinus Caplets .... ▣ 829
Sudafed Sinus Tablets .... ▣ 829
Sudafed 12 Hour Caplets .... ▣ 824
Syn-Rx Tablets 1622
Syn-Rx DM Tablets 1623
TheraFlu Flu and Cold Medicine .... ▣ 750
Theraflu Maximum Strength Flu and Cold Medicine For Sore Throat .... ▣ 751
TheraFlu Flu, Cold and Cough Medicine .... ▣ 750
TheraFlu Maximum Strength Nighttime Flu, Cold & Cough Medicine .... ▣ 751
TheraFlu Maximum Strength Non-Drowsy Formula Flu, Cold & Cough Medicine .... ▣ 751
TheraFlu Maximum Strength, Non-Drowsy Formula Flu, Cold and Cough Caplets .... ▣ 752
Theraflu Maximum Strength Sinus Non-Drowsy Formula Caplets .... ▣ 752
Triaminic AM Cough and Decongestant Formula .... ▣ 753
Triaminic AM Decongestant Formula .... ▣ 753
Triaminic Infant Oral Decongestant Drops .... ▣ 754
Triaminic Night Time .... ▣ 754
Triaminic Sore Throat Formula .... ▣ 755
Tussend 1830
Tussend Expectorant 1831
TYLENOL Allergy Sinus, Maximum Strength Caplets and Gelcaps 1571
TYLENOL Allergy Sinus NightTime, Maximum Strength Caplets 1571
TYLENOL Cold Medication, Multi-Symptom Formula Tablets and Caplets 1572
TYLENOL Cold Medication, Multi-Symptom Hot Liquid Packets 1572
TYLENOL Cold Medication, No Drowsiness Formula Caplets and Gelcaps 1572
TYLENOL Cold Severe Congestion Caplets 1573
TYLENOL Cough Medication with Decongestant, Multi Symptom 1574
TYLENOL Flu No Drowsiness Formula, Maximum Strength Gelcaps 1575
TYLENOL Flu NightTime, Maximum Strength Gelcaps 1575
TYLENOL Flu NightTime, Maximum Strength Hot Medication Packets 1575
TYLENOL Sinus, Maximum Strength Geltabs, Gelcaps, Caplets and Tablets 1576
Vicks 44 LiquiCaps Cough, Cold & Flu Relief .... ▣ 728
Vicks 44 LiquiCaps Non-Drowsy Cough & Cold Relief .... ▣ 729
Vicks 44D Cough & Head Congestion Relief .... ▣ 728
Vicks 44M Cough, Cold & Flu Relief .... ▣ 729
Vicks DayQuil LiquiCaps/Liquid Multi-Symptom Cold/Flu Relief .. ▣ 734
Vicks DayQuil SINUS Pressure & PAIN Relief with IBUPROFEN .... ▣ 735
Vicks Nyquil Hot Therapy .... ▣ 735
Vicks NyQuil LiquiCaps/Liquid Multi-Symptom Cold/Flu Relief, Original and Cherry Flavors .... ▣ 736

Pseudoephedrine Sulfate (Concurrent and/or sequential use is contraindicated; combination therapy may precipitate hypertension, headache and related symptoms). Products include:
Chlor-Trimeton Allergy Decongestant Tablets .... ▣ 759
Claritin-D Tablets 2487
Drixoral Cold and Allergy Sustained-Action Tablets .... ▣ 763
Drixoral Cold and Flu Extended-Release Tablets .... ▣ 764
Drixoral Non-Drowsy Formula Extended-Release Tablets .... ▣ 764
Drixoral Allergy/Sinus Extended Release Tablets .... ▣ 765
Trinalin Repetabs Tablets 1373

Pyrilamine Maleate (Concurrent use is contraindicated). Products include:
4-Way Fast Acting Nasal Spray (regular & mentholated) .... ▣ 644
Maximum Strength Multi-Symptom Formula Midol .... ▣ 621
PMS Multi-Symptom Formula Midol .... ▣ 622

Pyrilamine Tannate (Concurrent use is contraindicated). Products include:
Atrohist Pediatric Suspension 1604
Atrohist Pediatric Suspension Dye-Free 1604
Rynatan 2781

Quazepam (Concurrent use is contraindicated). Products include:
Doral Tablets 2773

Quinapril Hydrochloride (Concurrent use with hypotensive agents is contraindicated; a marked potentiating effect on these classes of drugs has been reported). Products include:
Accupril Tablets 1950

Ramipril (Concurrent use with hypotensive agents is contraindicated; a marked potentiating effect on these classes of drugs has been reported). Products include:
Altace Capsules 1238

Rauwolfia Serpentina (Concurrent use with hypotensive agents is contraindicated; a marked potentiating effect on these classes of drugs has been reported).
No products indexed under this heading.

Rescinnamine (Concurrent use with hypotensive agents is contraindicated; a marked potentiating effect on these classes of drugs has been reported).
No products indexed under this heading.

Reserpine (Concurrent and/or sequential use is contraindicated; combination therapy may precipitate hypertension, headache and related symptoms). Products include:
Diupres Tablets 1691
Hydropres Tablets 1718
Ser-Ap-Es Tablets 867

Salmeterol Xinafoate (Concurrent and/or sequential use is contraindicated; combination therapy may precipitate hypertension, headache and related symptoms). Products include:
Serevent Inhalation Aerosol 1149

Secobarbital Sodium (Concurrent use is contraindicated). Products include:
Seconal Sodium Pulvules 1529

Selegiline Hydrochloride (Concurrent use with another MAO inhibitor may result in hypertensive crises or severe convulsive seizures; concurrent and/or sequential use is contraindicated). Products include:
Eldepryl Capsules 2729

Sertraline Hydrochloride (Concurrent and/or sequential use is contraindicated; potential for serious, sometimes fatal, reactions including hyperthermia, rigidity, myoclonus, and other toxicities; at least 2 weeks should be allowed after stopping sertraline before starting an MAO inhibitor). Products include:
Zoloft Tablets 2051

Sodium Nitroprusside (Concurrent use with hypotensive agents is contraindicated; a marked potentiating effect on these classes of drugs has been reported).
No products indexed under this heading.

Sotalol Hydrochloride (Concurrent use with hypotensive agents is contraindicated; a marked potentiating effect on these classes of drugs has been reported). Products include:
Betapace Tablets 637

Spirapril Hydrochloride (Concurrent use with hypotensive agents is contraindicated; a marked potentiating effect on these classes of drugs has been reported).
No products indexed under this heading.

Spironolactone (Concurrent use with hypotensive agents is contraindicated; a marked potentiating effect on these classes of drugs has been reported). Products include:
Aldactazide Tablets 2556
Aldactone Tablets 2558

Sufentanil Citrate (Concurrent use is contraindicated; a marked potentiating effect on these classes of drugs has been reported). Products include:
Sufenta Injection 1355

Temazepam (Concurrent use is contraindicated). Products include:
Restoril Capsules 2413

(▣ Described in PDR For Nonprescription Drugs) (⊚ Described in PDR For Ophthalmology)

Terazosin Hydrochloride (Concurrent use with hypotensive agents is contraindicated; a marked potentiating effect on these classes of drugs has been reported). Products include:
- Hytrin Capsules 434

Terbutaline Sulfate (Concurrent and/or sequential use is contraindicated; combination therapy may precipitate hypertension, headache and related symptoms). Products include:
- Brethaire Inhaler 830
- Brethine Ampuls 832
- Brethine Tablets 831
- Bricanyl Subcutaneous Injection 1247
- Bricanyl Tablets 1248

Terfenadine (Concurrent use is contraindicated). Products include:
- Seldane Tablets 1284
- Seldane-D Extended-Release Tablets 1286

Tetrahydrozoline Hydrochloride (Concurrent and/or sequential use is contraindicated; combination therapy may precipitate hypertension, headache and related symptoms). Products include:
- Collyrium Fresh .... ◉ 316
- Murine Tears Plus Lubricant Redness Reliever Eye Drops .... ▣ 744
- Murine Tears Plus Lubricant Redness Reliever Eye Drops .... ◉ 315
- Visine A.C. Seasonal Relief From Pollen and Dust .... ◉ 301
- Visine Moisturizing Eye Drops .... ◉ 301
- Visine Original Eye Drops .... ◉ 301

Thiamylal Sodium (Concurrent use is contraindicated).
- No products indexed under this heading.

Thioridazine Hydrochloride (Possibility of additive hypotensive effects). Products include:
- Mellaril 2398

Timolol Maleate (Concurrent use with hypotensive agents is contraindicated; a marked potentiating effect on these classes of drugs has been reported). Products include:
- Blocadren Tablets 1654
- Timolide Tablets 1791
- Timoptic in Ocudose 1796
- Timoptic Sterile Ophthalmic Solution 1794
- Timoptic-XE 1798

Tolazamide (Some MAO inhibitors have contributed to hypoglycemic episodes in diabetic patients receiving oral hypoglycemic agents).
- No products indexed under this heading.

Tolbutamide (Some MAO inhibitors have contributed to hypoglycemic episodes in diabetic patients receiving oral hypoglycemic agents).
- No products indexed under this heading.

Torsemide (Concurrent use with hypotensive agents is contraindicated; a marked potentiating effect on these classes of drugs has been reported). Products include:
- Demadex Tablets and Injection 691

Triamterene (Concurrent use with hypotensive agents is contraindicated; a marked potentiating effect on these classes of drugs has been reported). Products include:
- Dyazide Capsules 2653
- Dyrenium Capsules 2655

Triazolam (Concurrent use is contraindicated). Products include:
- Halcion Tablets 2093

Tridihexethyl Chloride (Anti-Parkinsonism drugs should be used with caution in patients receiving Parnate since severe reactions have been reported).
- No products indexed under this heading.

Trifluoperazine Hydrochloride (Possibility of additive hypotensive effects). Products include:
- Stelazine 2692

Trihexyphenidyl Hydrochloride (Anti-Parkinsonism drugs should be used with caution in patients receiving Parnate since severe reactions have been reported). Products include:
- Artane 1418

Trimeprazine Tartrate (Concurrent use is contraindicated).
- No products indexed under this heading.

Trimethaphan Camsylate (Concurrent use with hypotensive agents is contraindicated; a marked potentiating effect on these classes of drugs has been reported).
- No products indexed under this heading.

Trimipramine Maleate (Concurrent use with tricyclic antidepressants may result in hypertensive crises or severe convulsive seizures; concurrent and/or sequential use is contraindicated). Products include:
- Surmontil Capsules 2917

Tripelennamine Hydrochloride (Concurrent use is contraindicated). Products include:
- PBZ Tablets 863
- PBZ-SR Tablets 862

Triprolidine Hydrochloride (Concurrent use is contraindicated). Products include:
- Actifed Cold & Allergy Tablets .... ▣ 807
- Actifed Cold & Sinus Caplets and Tablets .... ▣ 808

L-Tryptophan (Concurrent and/or sequential use is contraindicated; combination therapy may precipitate hypertension, disorientation, memory impairment, other neurologic and behavioral changes, headache and related symptoms).
- No products indexed under this heading.

Tyramine (Concurrent use is contraindicated).

Venlafaxine Hydrochloride (Concurrent and/or sequential use is contraindicated; potential for serious, sometimes fatal, reactions including hyperthermia, rigidity, myoclonus, and other toxicities). Products include:
- Effexor 2825

Verapamil Hydrochloride (Concurrent use with hypotensive agents is contraindicated; a marked potentiating effect on these classes of drugs has been reported). Products include:
- Calan SR Caplets 2571
- Calan Tablets 2568
- Covera-HS Tablets 2573
- Isoptin Injectable 1391
- Isoptin Oral Tablets 1393
- Isoptin SR Tablets 1395
- Verelan Capsules 1455

Zolpidem Tartrate (Concurrent use is contraindicated). Products include:
- Ambien Tablets 2559

Food Interactions

Alcohol (Concurrent use is contraindicated; a marked potentiating effect on alcohol has been reported).

Anchovies (Potential for hypertensive crisis; concurrent use is contraindicated).

Avocados (Potential for hypertensive crisis; concurrent use is contraindicated).

Bananas (Potential for hypertensive crisis; concurrent use is contraindicated).

Beans, broad (Potential for hypertensive crisis; concurrent use is contraindicated).

Beans, Fava (Potential for hypertensive crisis; concurrent use is contraindicated).

Beer, alcohol-free (Potential for hypertensive crisis; concurrent use is contraindicated).

Beer, unspecified (Potential for hypertensive crisis; concurrent use is contraindicated).

Beverages, caffeine-containing (Potential for hypertensive crisis; concurrent use is contraindicated).

Caviar (Potential for hypertensive crisis; concurrent use is contraindicated).

Cheese, aged (Potential for hypertensive crisis; concurrent use is contraindicated).

Cheese, strong, unpasteurized (Potential for hypertensive crisis; concurrent use is contraindicated).

Cheese, unspecified (Potential for hypertensive crisis; concurrent use is contraindicated).

Chocolate (Potential for hypertensive crisis; concurrent use is contraindicated).

Cream, sour (Potential for hypertensive crisis; concurrent use is contraindicated).

Figs, canned (Potential for hypertensive crisis; concurrent use is contraindicated).

Food with high concentration of tyramine (Potential for hypertensive crisis; concurrent use is contraindicated).

Herring, pickled (Potential for hypertensive crisis; concurrent use is contraindicated).

Liqueurs (Potential for hypertensive crisis; concurrent use is contraindicated).

Liver (Potential for hypertensive crisis; concurrent use is contraindicated).

Meat extracts (Potential for hypertensive crisis; concurrent use is contraindicated).

Meat prepared with tenderizers (Potential for hypertensive crisis; concurrent use is contraindicated).

Raisins (Potential for hypertensive crisis; concurrent use is contraindicated).

Sauerkraut (Potential for hypertensive crisis; concurrent use is contraindicated).

Sherry (Potential for hypertensive crisis; concurrent use is contraindicated).

Soy sauce (Potential for hypertensive crisis; concurrent use is contraindicated).

Wine, Chianti (Potential for hypertensive crisis; concurrent use is contraindicated).

Yeast extract (Potential for hypertensive crisis; concurrent use is contraindicated).

Yogurt (Potential for hypertensive crisis; concurrent use is contraindicated).

PASER GRANULES

(Aminosalicylic Acid) 1333
May interact with:

Digoxin (Potential for reduced digoxin levels). Products include:
- Lanoxicaps 1110
- Lanoxin Elixir Pediatric 1113
- Lanoxin Injection 1116
- Lanoxin Injection Pediatric 1119
- Lanoxin Tablets 1121

Isoniazid (Concurrent use with a rapidly available form of aminosalicylic acid has been reported to produce a 20% reduction in the acetylation of INH; the lower serum levels produced by delayed release preparation will result in a reduced effect on the acetylation of INH). Products include:
- Nydrazid Injection 509
- Rifamate Capsules 1278
- Rifater 1280

Rifampin (May block the absorption of rifampin; PASER granules do not contain excipient that blocks the absorption). Products include:
- Rifadin 1276
- Rifamate Capsules 1278
- Rifater 1280
- Rimactane Capsules 865

Vitamin B_{12} (Reduced absorption of vitamin B_{12} with clinically significant erythrocyte abnormalities developing after depletion). Products include:
- Chromagen Capsules 2470
- Chromagen FA 2471
- Chromagen Forte 2471
- Mega-B 513
- Niferex-150 Forte Capsules 811
- Trinsicon Capsules 2759

PAXIL TABLETS

(Paroxetine Hydrochloride) 2681
May interact with:

Aminophylline (There have been reports of elevated theophylline levels associated with co-administration).
- No products indexed under this heading.

Amiodarone Hydrochloride (Paroxetine is highly protein bound to plasma protein, co-administration may result in displacement from binding sites of either drug resulting in increased adverse effects). Products include:
- Cordarone Intravenous 2821
- Cordarone Tablets 2818

Amitriptyline Hydrochloride (Co-administration may result in inhibition of tricyclic antidepressants by paroxetine; monitor plasma concentration of tricyclic antidepressant). Products include:
- Elavil 2945
- Etrafon 2495
- Limbitrol 2333
- Triavil Tablets 1800

Amoxapine (Co-administration may result in inhibition of tricyclic antidepressants by paroxetine; monitor plasma concentration of tricyclic antidepressant). Products include:
- Asendin Tablets 1419

Atovaquone (Paroxetine is highly protein bound to plasma protein, co-administration may result in displacement from binding sites of either drug resulting in increased adverse effects). Products include:
- Mepron Suspension 1206

Bupropion Hydrochloride (Paroxetine may significantly inhibit the activity of cytochrome isoenzyme $P_{450}IID_6$; co-administration should be approached with caution). Products include:
- Wellbutrin Tablets 1177

Cefonicid Sodium (Paroxetine is highly protein bound to plasma protein, co-administration may result in displacement from binding sites of either drug resulting in increased adverse effects). Products include:
- Monocid Injection 2674

IMPORTANT NOTE: Always consult each drug listing in the patient's regimen for possible interactions.

Paxil Interactions Index 818

Chlordiazepoxide (Paroxetine is highly protein bound to plasma protein, co-administration may result in displacement from binding sites of either drug resulting in increased adverse effects). Products include:

Limbitrol 2330

Chlordiazepoxide Hydrochloride (Paroxetine is highly protein bound to plasma protein, co-administration may result in displacement from binding sites of either drug resulting in increased adverse effects). Products include:

Librax Capsules 2330
Librium Capsules 2331
Librium Injectable 2332

Chlorpromazine (Paroxetine may significantly inhibit the activity of cytochrome isoenzyme $P_{450}IID_6$; co-administration should be approached with caution). Products include:

Thorazine Suppositories 2701

Chlorpromazine Hydrochloride (Paroxetine may significantly inhibit the activity of cytochrome isoenzyme $P_{450}IID_6$; co-administration should be approached with caution). Products include:

Thorazine 2701

Cimetidine (Co-administration with oral cimetidine has resulted in an increase in steady-state plasma concentrations of paroxetine). Products include:

Tagamet HB Tablets .... ▣ 786
Tagamet Tablets 2694

Cimetidine Hydrochloride (Co-administration with oral cimetidine has resulted in an increase in steady-state plasma concentrations of paroxetine). Products include:

Tagamet 2694

Clomipramine Hydrochloride (Co-administration may result in inhibition of tricyclic antidepressants by paroxetine; monitor plasma concentration of tricyclic antidepressant). Products include:

Anafranil Capsules 819

Clozapine (Paroxetine is highly protein bound to plasma protein, co-administration may result in displacement from binding sites of either drug resulting in increased adverse effects). Products include:

Clozaril Tablets 2377

Cyclosporine (Paroxetine is highly protein bound to plasma protein, co-administration may result in displacement from binding sites of either drug resulting in increased adverse effects). Products include:

Neoral 2405
Sandimmune 2416

Desipramine Hydrochloride (Co-administration with desipramine has resulted in an increase in C_{max}, AUC and $T^1/_2$ by an average of approximately two-, five- and three-fold respectively). Products include:

Norpramin Tablets 1273

Diazepam (Under steady-state conditions, diazepam does not appear to affect paroxetine kinetics, however, paroxetine is highly protein bound to plasma protein; co-administration may result in displacement from binding sites of either drug resulting in increased adverse effects). Products include:

Dizac (diazepam injectable emulsion) CIV 1862
Valium Injectable 2336
Valium Tablets 2335

Diclofenac Potassium (Paroxetine is highly protein bound to plasma protein, co-administration may result in displacement from binding sites of either drug resulting in increased adverse effects). Products include:

Cataflam Tablets 833

Diclofenac Sodium (Paroxetine is highly protein bound to plasma protein, co-administration may result in displacement from binding sites of either drug resulting in increased adverse effects). Products include:

Voltaren Ophthalmic Sterile Ophthalmic Solution .... ⊙ 264
Cataflam/Voltaren/Voltaren-XR 833

Digoxin (Potential for decrease in mean digoxin AUC). Products include:

Lanoxicaps 1110
Lanoxin Elixir Pediatric 1113
Lanoxin Injection 1116
Lanoxin Injection Pediatric 1119
Lanoxin Tablets 1121

Dipyridamole (Paroxetine is highly protein bound to plasma protein, co-administration may result in displacement from binding sites of either drug resulting in increased adverse effects). Products include:

Persantine Tablets 686

Disopyramide Phosphate (Paroxetine may significantly inhibit the activity of cytochrome isoenzyme $P_{450}IID_6$; co-administration should be approached with caution). Products include:

Norpace 2596

Doxepin Hydrochloride (Co-administration may result in inhibition of tricyclic antidepressants by paroxetine; monitor plasma concentration of tricyclic antidepressant). Products include:

Adapin Capsules 1542
Sinequan 2028
Zonalon Cream 1042

Dyphylline (There have been reports of elevated theophylline levels associated with co-administration). Products include:

Lufyllin & Lufyllin-400 Tablets 2778
Lufyllin-GG Elixir & Tablets 2779

Fenoprofen Calcium (Paroxetine is highly protein bound to plasma protein, co-administration may result in displacement from binding sites of either drug resulting in increased adverse effects). Products include:

Nalfon 200 Pulvules & Nalfon Tablets 933

Fluoxetine Hydrochloride (Paroxetine may significantly inhibit the activity of cytochrome isoenzyme P_{450} IID_6; co-administration should be approached with caution). Products include:

Prozac Pulvules & Liquid, Oral Solution 935

Fluphenazine Decanoate (Paroxetine may significantly inhibit the activity of cytochrome isoenzyme $P_{450}IID_6$; co-administration should be approached with caution). Products include:

Prolixin Decanoate 510

Fluphenazine Enanthate (Paroxetine may significantly inhibit the activity of cytochrome isoenzyme $P_{450}IID_6$; co-administration should be approached with caution). Products include:

Prolixin Enanthate 510

Fluphenazine Hydrochloride (Paroxetine may significantly inhibit the activity of cytochrome isoenzyme $P_{450}IID_6$; co-administration should be approached with caution). Products include:

Prolixin 510

Flurazepam Hydrochloride (Paroxetine is highly protein bound to plasma protein, co-administration may result in displacement from binding sites of either drug resulting in increased adverse effects). Products include:

Dalmane Capsules 2329

Flurbiprofen (Paroxetine is highly protein bound to plasma protein, co-administration may result in displacement from binding sites of either drug resulting in increased adverse effects).

No products indexed under this heading.

Furazolidone (Potential for serious and fatal reactions including hyperthermia, rigidity, myoclonus and other serious reactions; concurrent and/or sequential use is contraindicated). Products include:

Furoxone 2221

Glipizide (Paroxetine is highly protein bound to plasma protein, co-administration may result in displacement from binding sites of either drug resulting in increased adverse effects). Products include:

Glucotrol Tablets 2011
Glucotrol XL Extended Release Tablets 2012

Ibuprofen (Paroxetine is highly protein bound to plasma protein, co-administration may result in displacement from binding sites of either drug resulting in increased adverse effects). Products include:

Advil Cold and Sinus Caplets and Tablets .... ▣ 837
Advil Ibuprofen Tablets, Caplets and Gel Caplets .... ▣ 836
Children's Motrin Ibuprofen Oral Suspension 1558
IBU Tablets 1389
Ibuprohm .... ▣ 713
Motrin IB Caplets, Tablets, and Gelcaps .... ▣ 802
Motrin Ibuprofen Suspension, Oral Drops, Chewable Tablets, Caplets 1563
Nuprin Ibuprofen/Analgesic Tablets & Caplets .... ▣ 645
Vicks DayQuil SINUS Pressure & PAIN Relief with IBUPROFEN .... ▣ 735

Imipramine Hydrochloride (Co-administration may result in inhibition of tricyclic antidepressants by paroxetine; monitor plasma concentration of tricyclic antidepressant). Products include:

Tofranil Ampuls 873
Tofranil Tablets 875

Imipramine Pamoate (Co-administration may result in inhibition of tricyclic antidepressants by paroxetine; monitor plasma concentration of tricyclic antidepressant). Products include:

Tofranil-PM Capsules 876

Indomethacin (Paroxetine is highly protein bound to plasma protein, co-administration may result in displacement from binding sites of either drug resulting in increased adverse effects). Products include:

Indocin 1723

Indomethacin Sodium Trihydrate (Paroxetine is highly protein bound to plasma protein, co-administration may result in displacement from binding sites of either drug resulting in increased adverse effects). Products include:

Indocin I.V. 1727

Isocarboxazid (Potential for serious and fatal reactions including hyperthermia, rigidity, myoclonus and other serious reactions; concurrent and/or sequential use is contraindicated).

No products indexed under this heading.

Ketoprofen (Paroxetine is highly protein bound to plasma protein, co-administration may result in displacement from binding sites of either drug resulting in increased adverse effects). Products include:

Actron Caplets and Tablets .... ▣ 608
Orudis Capsules 2874
Orudis KT .... ▣ 842
Oruvail Capsules 2874

Ketorolac Tromethamine (Paroxetine is highly protein bound to plasma protein, co-administration may result in displacement from binding sites of either drug resulting in increased adverse effects). Products include:

Acular Sterile Ophthalmic Solution 470
Toradol 2319

Lithium Carbonate (Concurrent administration should be undertaken with caution). Products include:

Eskalith 2658
Lithium Carbonate Capsules & Tablets 2352
Lithonate/Lithotabs/Lithobid 2721

Lithium Citrate (Concurrent administration should be undertaken with caution).

No products indexed under this heading.

Maprotiline Hydrochloride (Co-administration may result in inhibition of tricyclic antidepressants by paroxetine; monitor plasma concentration of tricyclic antidepressant). Products include:

Ludiomil Tablets 861

Meclofenamate Sodium (Paroxetine is highly protein bound to plasma protein, co-administration may result in displacement from binding sites of either drug resulting in increased adverse effects).

No products indexed under this heading.

Mefenamic Acid (Paroxetine is highly protein bound to plasma protein, co-administration may result in displacement from binding sites of either drug resulting in increased adverse effects). Products include:

Ponstel 1982

Mesoridazine Besylate (Paroxetine may significantly inhibit the activity of cytochrome isoenzyme $P_{450}IID_6$; co-administration should be approached with caution). Products include:

Serentil 689

Methotrimeprazine (Paroxetine may significantly inhibit the activity of cytochrome isoenzyme $P_{450}IID_6$; co-administration should be approached with caution). Products include:

Levoprome 1321

Metoprolol Succinate (There has been a case report of severe hypotension when paroxetine was added to chronic metoprolol treatment). Products include:

Toprol-XL Tablets 560

(▣ Described in PDR For Nonprescription Drugs) (⊙ Described in PDR For Ophthalmology)

Metoprolol Tartrate (There has been a case report of severe hypotension when paroxetine was added to chronic metoprolol treatment). Products include:

Lopressor ... 848
Lopressor HCT Tablets ... 850

Midazolam Hydrochloride (Paroxetine is highly protein bound to plasma protein, co-administration may result in displacement from binding sites of either drug resulting in increased adverse effects). Products include:

Versed Injection ... 2324

Moricizine Hydrochloride (Paroxetine may significantly inhibit the activity of cytochrome isoenzyme $P_{450}IID_6$; co-administration should be approached with caution). Products include:

Ethmozine Tablets ... 2217

Naproxen (Paroxetine is highly protein bound to plasma protein, co-administration may result in displacement from binding sites of either drug resulting in increased adverse effects). Products include:

Anaprox/Naprosyn ... 2277

Naproxen Sodium (Paroxetine is highly protein bound to plasma protein, co-administration may result in displacement from binding sites of either drug resulting in increased adverse effects). Products include:

Aleve ... 2124
Anaprox/Naprosyn ... 2277
Naprelan Tablets ... 2861

Nortriptyline Hydrochloride (Co-administration may result in inhibition of tricyclic antidepressants by paroxetine; monitor plasma concentration of tricyclic antidepressant). Products include:

Pamelor ... 2409

Oxaprozin (Paroxetine is highly protein bound to plasma protein, co-administration may result in displacement from binding sites of either drug resulting in increased adverse effects). Products include:

Daypro Caplets ... 2578

Oxazepam (Paroxetine is highly protein bound to plasma protein, co-administration may result in displacement from binding sites of either drug resulting in increased adverse effects). Products include:

Serax Capsules ... 2916
Serax Tablets ... 2916

Perphenazine (Paroxetine may significantly inhibit the activity of cytochrome isoenzyme $P_{450}IID_6$; co-administration should be approached with caution). Products include:

Etrafon ... 2495
Triavil Tablets ... 1800
Trilafon ... 2532

Phenelzine Sulfate (Potential for serious and fatal reactions including hyperthermia, rigidity, myoclonus and other serious reactions; concurrent and/or sequential use is contraindicated). Products include:

Nardil ... 1977

Phenobarbital (Co-administration has resulted in reduction of paroxetine AUC and T½). Products include:

Arco-Lase Plus Tablets ... 513
Bellergal-S Tablets ... 2375
Donnatal ... 2234
Donnatal Extentabs ... 2234
Donnatal Tablets ... 2234
Phenobarbital Elixir and Tablets ... 1523
Quadrinal Tablets ... 1398

Phenylbutazone (Paroxetine is highly protein bound to plasma protein, co-administration may result in displacement from binding sites of either drug resulting in increased adverse effects).

No products indexed under this heading.

Phenytoin (Co-administration has resulted in reduction of paroxetine AUC and T½; potential for elevated phenytoin levels or slight reduction in phenytoin AUC). Products include:

Dilantin Infatabs ... 1967
Dilantin-125 Suspension ... 1969

Phenytoin Sodium (Co-administration has resulted in reduction of paroxetine AUC and T½; potential for elevated phenytoin levels or slight reduction in phenytoin AUC). Products include:

Dilantin Kapseals ... 1965

Pimozide (Concomitant use has been associated with extrapyramidal symptoms including dystonia, akathesia, bradykinesia, cogwheel rigidity, hypertonia, and oculogyric crisis). Products include:

Orap Tablets ... 1037

Piroxicam (Paroxetine is highly protein bound to plasma protein, co-administration may result in displacement from binding sites of either drug resulting in increased adverse effects). Products include:

Feldene Capsules ... 2008

Procainamide Hydrochloride (Paroxetine may significantly inhibit the activity of cytochrome isoenzyme $P_{450}IID_6$; co-administration should be approached with caution). Products include:

Procanbid Extended-Release Tablets ... 1983

Prochlorperazine (Paroxetine may significantly inhibit the activity of cytochrome isoenzyme $P_{450}IID_6$; co-administration should be approached with caution). Products include:

Compazine ... 2644

Procyclidine Hydrochloride (Increased steady-state AUC, C_{max} and C_{min} values of procyclidine with concurrent use). Products include:

Kemadrin Tablets ... 1105

Promethazine Hydrochloride (Paroxetine may significantly inhibit the activity of cytochrome isoenzyme $P_{450}IID_6$; co-administration should be approached with caution). Products include:

Mepergan Injection ... 2859
Phenergan with Codeine ... 2883
Phenergan with Dextromethorphan ... 2885
Phenergan Injection ... 2880
Phenergan Suppositories ... 2882
Phenergan Syrup ... 2881
Phenergan Tablets ... 2882
Phenergan VC ... 2886
Phenergan VC with Codeine ... 2888

Propafenone Hydrochloride (Paroxetine may significantly inhibit the activity of cytochrome isoenzyme $P_{450}IID_6$; co-administration should be approached with caution). Products include:

Rythmol Tablets–150mg, 225mg, 300mg ... 1399

Propranolol Hydrochloride (Paroxetine is highly protein bound to plasma protein, co-administration may result in displacement from binding sites of either drug resulting in increased adverse effects). Products include:

Inderal ... 2834
Inderal LA Long Acting Capsules ... 2836
Inderide Tablets ... 2838
Inderide LA Long Acting Capsules ... 2840

Protriptyline Hydrochloride (Co-administration may result in inhibition of tricyclic antidepressants by paroxetine; monitor plasma concentration of tricyclic antidepressant). Products include:

Vivactil Tablets ... 1820

Quinidine Gluconate (Paroxetine may significantly inhibit the activity of cytochrome isoenzyme $P_{450}IID_6$; co-administration should be approached with caution). Products include:

Quinaglute Dura-Tabs Tablets ... 644

Quinidine Polygalacturonate (Paroxetine may significantly inhibit the activity of cytochrome isoenzyme $P_{450}IID_6$; co-administration should be approached with caution). Products include:

Cardioquin Tablets ... 2146

Quinidine Sulfate (Paroxetine may significantly inhibit the activity of cytochrome isoenzyme $P_{450}IID_6$; co-administration should be approached with caution). Products include:

Quinidex Extentabs ... 2240

Selegiline Hydrochloride (Potential for serious and fatal reactions including hyperthermia, rigidity, myoclonus and other serious reactions; concurrent and/or sequential use is contraindicated). Products include:

Eldepryl Capsules ... 2729

Sertraline Hydrochloride (Paroxetine may significantly inhibit the activity of cytochrome isoenzyme $P_{450}IID_6$; co-administration should be approached with caution). Products include:

Zoloft Tablets ... 2051

Sulindac (Paroxetine is highly protein bound to plasma protein, co-administration may result in displacement from binding sites of either drug resulting in increased adverse effects). Products include:

Clinoril Tablets ... 1658

Temazepam (Paroxetine is highly protein bound to plasma protein, co-administration may result in displacement from binding sites of either drug resulting in increased adverse effects). Products include:

Restoril Capsules ... 2413

Theophylline (There have been reports of elevated theophylline levels associated with co-administration). Products include:

Marax Tablets & DF Syrup ... 2015
Quibron ... 2227

Theophylline Anhydrous (There have been reports of elevated theophylline levels associated with co-administration). Products include:

Aerolate ... 1003
Primatene Tablets ... 844
Respbid Tablets ... 687
Slo-bid Gyrocaps ... 2201
Theo-24 Extended Release Capsules ... 2753
Theo-Dur Extended-Release Tablets ... 1367
Theo-X Extended-Release Tablets ... 793
Uni-Dur Extended-Release Tablets ... 1374
Uniphyl 400 mg and 600 mg Tablets ... 2157

Theophylline Calcium Salicylate (There have been reports of elevated theophylline levels associated with co-administration). Products include:

Quadrinal Tablets ... 1398

Theophylline Sodium Glycinate (There have been reports of elevated theophylline levels associated with co-administration).

No products indexed under this heading.

Thioridazine Hydrochloride (Paroxetine may significantly inhibit the activity of cytochrome isoenzyme $P_{450}IID_6$; co-administration should be approached with caution). Products include:

Mellaril ... 2398

Tolbutamide (Paroxetine is highly protein bound to plasma protein, co-administration may result in displacement from binding sites of either drug resulting in increased adverse effects).

No products indexed under this heading.

Tolmetin Sodium (Paroxetine is highly protein bound to plasma protein, co-administration may result in displacement from binding sites of either drug resulting in increased adverse effects). Products include:

Tolectin (200, 400 and 600 mg) ... 1591

Tranylcypromine Sulfate (Potential for serious and fatal reactions including hyperthermia, rigidity, myoclonus and other serious reactions; concurrent and/or sequential use is contraindicated). Products include:

Parnate Tablets ... 2679

Trazodone Hydrochloride (Paroxetine may significantly inhibit the activity of cytochrome isoenzyme $P_{450}IID_6$; co-administration should be approached with caution). Products include:

Desyrel and Desyrel Dividose ... 504

Trifluoperazine Hydrochloride (Paroxetine may significantly inhibit the activity of cytochrome isoenzyme $P_{450}IID_6$; co-administration should be approached with caution). Products include:

Stelazine ... 2692

Trimipramine Maleate (Co-administration may result in inhibition of tricyclic antidepressants by paroxetine; monitor plasma concentration of tricyclic antidepressant). Products include:

Surmontil Capsules ... 2917

L-Tryptophan (Potential for headache, nausea, sweating and dizziness; concomitant use is not recommended).

No products indexed under this heading.

Venlafaxine Hydrochloride (Potential for increase in adverse effects of either drug; Paroxetine may significantly inhibit the activity of cytochrome isoenzyme $P_{450}IID_6$; co-administration should be approached with caution). Products include:

Effexor ... 2825

Warfarin Sodium (Potential for pharmacodynamic interaction that causes an increased bleeding diathesis in the face of unaltered prothrombin time). Products include:

Coumadin ... 941

Food Interactions

Alcohol (Concurrent use should be avoided).

IMPORTANT NOTE: Always consult each drug listing in the patient's regimen for possible interactions.

Pediacare | Interactions Index

PEDIACARE COUGH-COLD CHEWABLE TABLETS AND LIQUID
(Pseudoephedrine Hydrochloride, Chlorpheniramine Maleate, Dextromethorphan Hydrobromide) 1569
   See **PediaCare NightRest Cough-Cold Liquid**

PEDIACARE INFANTS' DECONGESTANT DROPS
(Pseudoephedrine Hydrochloride) 1569
   See **PediaCare NightRest Cough-Cold Liquid**

PEDIACARE INFANTS' DROPS DECONGESTANT PLUS COUGH
(Dextromethorphan Hydrobromide, Pseudoephedrine Hydrochloride) 1569
   See **PediaCare NightRest Cough-Cold Liquid**

PEDIACARE NIGHTREST COUGH-COLD LIQUID
(Chlorpheniramine Maleate, Dextromethorphan Hydrobromide, Pseudoephedrine Hydrochloride) 1569
May interact with monoamine oxidase inhibitors, hypnotics and sedatives, and tranquilizers. Compounds in these categories include:

Alprazolam (Increases the drowsiness effect). Products include:
   Xanax Tablets 2115

Buspirone Hydrochloride (Increases the drowsiness effect). Products include:
   BuSpar Tablets 738

Chlordiazepoxide (Increases the drowsiness effect). Products include:
   Limbitrol 2333

Chlordiazepoxide Hydrochloride (Increases the drowsiness effect). Products include:
   Librax Capsules 2330
   Librium Capsules 2331
   Librium Injectable 2332

Chlorpromazine (Increases the drowsiness effect). Products include:
   Thorazine Suppositories 2701

Chlorpromazine Hydrochloride (Increases the drowsiness effect). Products include:
   Thorazine 2701

Chlorprothixene (Increases the drowsiness effect).
   No products indexed under this heading.

Chlorprothixene Hydrochloride (Increases the drowsiness effect).
   No products indexed under this heading.

Clorazepate Dipotassium (Increases the drowsiness effect). Products include:
   Tranxene 459

Diazepam (Increases the drowsiness effect). Products include:
   Dizac (diazepam injectable emulsion) CIV 1862
   Valium Injectable 2336
   Valium Tablets 2335

Droperidol (Increases the drowsiness effect). Products include:
   Inapsine Injection 462

Estazolam (Increases the drowsiness effect). Products include:
   ProSom Tablets 457

Ethchlorvynol (Increases the drowsiness effect). Products include:
   Placidyl Capsules 456

Ethinamate (Increases the drowsiness effect).
   No products indexed under this heading.

Fluphenazine Decanoate (Increases the drowsiness effect). Products include:
   Prolixin Decanoate 510

Fluphenazine Enanthate (Increases the drowsiness effect). Products include:
   Prolixin Enanthate 510

Fluphenazine Hydrochloride (Increases the drowsiness effect). Products include:
   Prolixin 510

Flurazepam Hydrochloride (Increases the drowsiness effect). Products include:
   Dalmane Capsules 2329

Furazolidone (Concurrent and/or sequential use is not recommended). Products include:
   Furoxone 2221

Glutethimide (Increases the drowsiness effect).
   No products indexed under this heading.

Haloperidol (Increases the drowsiness effect). Products include:
   Haldol Injection, Tablets and Concentrate 1585

Haloperidol Decanoate (Increases the drowsiness effect). Products include:
   Haldol Decanoate 1587

Hydroxyzine Hydrochloride (Increases the drowsiness effect). Products include:
   Atarax Tablets & Syrup 1992
   Marax Tablets & DF Syrup 2015
   Vistaril Intramuscular Solution 2042

Isocarboxazid (Concurrent and/or sequential use is not recommended).
   No products indexed under this heading.

Lorazepam (Increases the drowsiness effect). Products include:
   Ativan Injection 2805
   Ativan Tablets 2807

Loxapine Hydrochloride (Increases the drowsiness effect). Products include:
   Loxitane 1426

Loxapine Succinate (Increases the drowsiness effect). Products include:
   Loxitane Capsules 1426

Meprobamate (Increases the drowsiness effect). Products include:
   Miltown Tablets 2780
   PMB 200 and PMB 400 2890

Mesoridazine Besylate (Increases the drowsiness effect). Products include:
   Serentil 689

Midazolam Hydrochloride (Increases the drowsiness effect). Products include:
   Versed Injection 2324

Molindone Hydrochloride (Increases the drowsiness effect). Products include:
   Moban Tablets and Concentrate 1036

Oxazepam (Increases the drowsiness effect). Products include:
   Serax Capsules 2916
   Serax Tablets 2916

Perphenazine (Increases the drowsiness effect). Products include:
   Etrafon 2495
   Triavil Tablets 1800
   Trilafon 2532

Phenelzine Sulfate (Concurrent and/or sequential use is not recommended). Products include:
   Nardil 1977

Prazepam (Increases the drowsiness effect).
   No products indexed under this heading.

Prochlorperazine (Increases the drowsiness effect). Products include:
   Compazine 2644

Promethazine Hydrochloride (Increases the drowsiness effect). Products include:
   Mepergan Injection 2859
   Phenergan with Codeine 2883
   Phenergan with Dextromethorphan 2885
   Phenergan Injection 2880
   Phenergan Suppositories 2882
   Phenergan Syrup 2881
   Phenergan Tablets 2882
   Phenergan VC 2886
   Phenergan VC with Codeine 2888

Propofol (Increases the drowsiness effect). Products include:
   Diprivan Injectable Emulsion 2939

Quazepam (Increases the drowsiness effect). Products include:
   Doral Tablets 2773

Secobarbital Sodium (Increases the drowsiness effect). Products include:
   Seconal Sodium Pulvules 1529

Selegiline Hydrochloride (Concurrent and/or sequential use is not recommended). Products include:
   Eldepryl Capsules 2729

Temazepam (Increases the drowsiness effect). Products include:
   Restoril Capsules 2413

Thioridazine Hydrochloride (Increases the drowsiness effect). Products include:
   Mellaril 2398

Thiothixene (Increases the drowsiness effect). Products include:
   Navane Capsules and Concentrate 2018
   Navane Intramuscular 2019

Tranylcypromine Sulfate (Concurrent and/or sequential use is not recommended). Products include:
   Parnate Tablets 2679

Triazolam (Increases the drowsiness effect). Products include:
   Halcion Tablets 2093

Trifluoperazine Hydrochloride (Increases the drowsiness effect). Products include:
   Stelazine 2692

Zolpidem Tartrate (Increases the drowsiness effect). Products include:
   Ambien Tablets 2559

PEDIALYTE ORAL ELECTROLYTE MAINTENANCE SOLUTION
(Electrolyte Supplement) 2340
None cited in PDR database.

PEDIAPRED ORAL SOLUTION
(Prednisolone Sodium Phosphate) 1618
May interact with barbiturates, oral hypoglycemic agents, insulin, and certain other agents. Compounds in these categories include:

Acarbose (Increased requirement of hypoglycemic agents in diabetes). Products include:
   Precose 604

Aprobarbital (Induces hepatic microsomal drug metabolizing enzyme activity which may result in enhanced metabolism of prednisolone; dosage of prednisolone may need to be increased).
   No products indexed under this heading.

Aspirin (Aspirin should be used cautiously in conjunction with corticosteroids in hypoprothrombinemia). Products include:
   Alka-Seltzer Cherry Effervescent Antacid and Pain Reliever ..... ◫ 609
   Alka-Seltzer Extra Strength Effervescent Antacid and Pain Reliever ..... ◫ 609
   Alka-Seltzer Lemon Lime Effervescent Antacid and Pain Reliever ..... ◫ 609
   Alka-Seltzer Original Effervescent Antacid and Pain Reliever ..... ◫ 609
   Alka-Seltzer Plus ..... ◫ 611
   Alka-Seltzer Plus Sinus Medicine ..... ◫ 611
   Ascriptin 650
   Arthritis Strength BC Powder ..... ◫ 631
   BC Cold Powder Multi-Symptom Formula (Cold-Sinus-Allergy) ..... ◫ 631
   BC Cold Powder Non-Drowsy Formula (Cold-Sinus) ..... ◫ 631
   BC Powder ..... ◫ 631
   Genuine Bayer Aspirin Tablets & Caplets ..... ◫ 618
   Extra Strength Bayer Arthritis Pain Regimen Formula ..... ◫ 615
   Extra Strength Bayer Aspirin Caplets & Tablets ..... ◫ 617
   Extended-Release Bayer 8-Hour Aspirin ..... ◫ 616
   Extra Strength Bayer Plus Aspirin Caplets ..... ◫ 617
   Extra Strength Bayer PM Aspirin Plus Sleep Aid ..... ◫ 617
   Aspirin Regimen Bayer 81 mg Tablets with Calcium ..... ◫ 615
   Aspirin Regimen Bayer Adult Low Strength 81 mg Tablets ..... ◫ 613
   Aspirin Regimen Bayer Children's Chewable Aspirin ..... ◫ 616
   Aspirin Regimen Bayer Regular Strength 325 mg Caplets ..... ◫ 613
   Bufferin Analgesic Tablets ..... ◫ 636
   Arthritis Strength Bufferin Analgesic Caplets ..... ◫ 637
   Extra Strength Bufferin Analgesic Tablets ..... ◫ 637
   Cama Arthritis Pain Reliever ..... ◫ 748
   Darvon Compound-65 Pulvules 1475
   Easprin 1971
   Ecotrin 2625
   Ecotrin Enteric Coated Aspirin Maximum Strength Tablets and Caplets ..... ◫ 775
   Ecotrin Enteric Coated Aspirin Regular Strength Tablets 2625
   Empirin Aspirin Tablets ..... ◫ 818
   Excedrin Extra-Strength Analgesic Tablets, Caplets, and Geltabs 734
   Fiorinal Capsules 2388
   Fiorinal with Codeine Capsules 2390
   Fiorinal Tablets 2388
   Goody's Extra Strength Headache Powders ..... ◫ 632
   Goody's Extra Strength Pain Relief Tablets ..... ◫ 632
   Halfprin Tablets 1413
   Norgesic 1554
   Percodan Tablets 955
   Percodan-Demi Tablets 956
   Robaxisal Tablets 2246
   Soma Compound w/Codeine Tablets 2784
   Soma Compound Tablets 2783
   St. Joseph Adult Chewable Aspirin (81 mg.) ..... ◫ 768
   Talwin Compound 2466
   Vanquish Analgesic Caplets ..... ◫ 627

Butabarbital (Induces hepatic microsomal drug metabolizing enzyme activity which may result in enhanced metabolism of prednisolone; dosage of prednisolone may need to be increased).
   No products indexed under this heading.

Butalbital (Induces hepatic microsomal drug metabolizing enzyme activity which may result in enhanced metabolism of prednisolone; dosage of prednisolone may need to be increased). Products include:
   Axocet Capsules 2469
   Esgic-plus Capsules 1012
   Esgic-plus Tablets 1012
   Fioricet Tablets 2386
   Fioricet with Codeine Capsules 2387
   Fiorinal Capsules 2388
   Fiorinal with Codeine Capsules 2390
   Fiorinal Tablets 2388
   Phrenilin 790
   Sedapap Tablets 50 mg/650 mg 1826

(◫ Described in PDR For Nonprescription Drugs)   (⊚ Described in PDR For Ophthalmology)

Chlorpropamide (Increased requirement of hypoglycemic agents in diabetes). Products include:
Diabinese Tablets 2002
Glimepiride (Increased requirement of hypoglycemic agents in diabetes). Products include:
Amaryl Tablets 1241
Glipizide (Increased requirement of hypoglycemic agents in diabetes). Products include:
Glucotrol Tablets 2011
Glucotrol XL Extended Release Tablets 2012
Glyburide (Increased requirement of hypoglycemic agents in diabetes). Products include:
DiaBeta Tablets 1265
Glynase PresTab Tablets 2091
Micronase Tablets 2099
Insulin, Human (Increased requirement of insulin in diabetes).
No products indexed under this heading.
Insulin, Human Isophane Suspension (Increased requirement of insulin in diabetes). Products include:
Novolin N Human Insulin 10 ml Vials 1846
Insulin, Human NPH (Increased requirement of insulin in diabetes). Products include:
Humulin N, 100 Units 1495
Novolin N PenFill 1.5 ml Cartridges Durable Insulin Delivery System 1849
Novolin N Prefilled Syringe Disposable Insulin Delivery System ... 1850
Insulin, Human Regular (Increased requirement of insulin in diabetes). Products include:
Humulin R, 100 Units 1497
Novolin R Human Insulin 10 ml Vials 1846
Novolin R PenFill 1.5 ml Cartridges Durable Insulin Delivery System 1849
Novolin R Prefilled Syringe Disposable Insulin Delivery System ... 1850
Velosulin BR Human Insulin 10 ml Vials 1847
Insulin, Human, Zinc Suspension (Increased requirement of insulin in diabetes). Products include:
Humulin L, 100 Units 1494
Humulin U, 100 Units 1498
Novolin L Human Insulin 10 ml Vials 1846
Insulin Lispro, Human (Increased requirement of insulin in diabetes). Products include:
Humalog Injection 1488
Insulin, NPH (Increased requirement of insulin in diabetes). Products include:
NPH, 100 Units 1502
Pork NPH, 100 Units 1506
Purified Pork NPH Isophane Insulin 1852
Insulin, Regular (Increased requirement of insulin in diabetes). Products include:
Regular, 100 Units 1503
Pork Regular, 100 Units 1507
Pork Regular (Concentrated), 500 Units 1508
Purified Pork Regular Insulin 1852
Insulin, Zinc Crystals (Increased requirement of insulin in diabetes). Products include:
NPH, 100 Units 1502
Insulin, Zinc Suspension (Increased requirement of insulin in diabetes). Products include:
Iletin I 1501
Lente, 100 Units 1501
Iletin II 1504
Pork Lente, 100 Units 1504
Purified Pork Lente Insulin 1852

Mephobarbital (Induces hepatic microsomal drug metabolizing enzyme activity which may result in enhanced metabolism of prednisolone; dosage of prednisolone may need to be increased). Products include:
Mebaral Tablets 2452
Metformin Hydrochloride (Increased requirement of hypoglycemic agents in diabetes). Products include:
Glucophage Tablets 754
Pentobarbital Sodium (Induces hepatic microsomal drug metabolizing enzyme activity which may result in enhanced metabolism of prednisolone; dosage of prednisolone may need to be increased). Products include:
Nembutal Sodium Capsules 440
Nembutal Sodium Solution 442
Nembutal Sodium Suppositories.. 444
Phenobarbital (Induces hepatic microsomal drug metabolizing enzyme activity which may result in enhanced metabolism of prednisolone; dosage of prednisolone may need to be increased). Products include:
Arco-Lase Plus Tablets 513
Bellergal-S Tablets 2375
Donnatal 2234
Donnatal Extentabs 2234
Donnatal Tablets 2234
Phenobarbital Elixir and Tablets 1523
Quadrinal Tablets 1398
Secobarbital Sodium (Induces hepatic microsomal drug metabolizing enzyme activity which may result in enhanced metabolism of prednisolone; dosage of prednisolone may need to be increased). Products include:
Seconal Sodium Pulvules 1529
Thiamylal Sodium (Induces hepatic microsomal drug metabolizing enzyme activity which may result in enhanced metabolism of prednisolone; dosage of prednisolone may need to be increased).
No products indexed under this heading.
Tolazamide (Increased requirement of hypoglycemic agents in diabetes).
No products indexed under this heading.
Tolbutamide (Increased requirement of hypoglycemic agents in diabetes).
No products indexed under this heading.

PEDIASURE COMPLETE LIQUID NUTRITION
(Nutritional Supplement) 2342
None cited in PDR database.

PEDIASURE WITH FIBER COMPLETE LIQUID NUTRITION
(Nutritional Supplement) 2343
None cited in PDR database.

PEDIATRIC VICKS 44D COUGH & HEAD CONGESTION RELIEF
(Dextromethorphan Hydrobromide, Pseudoephedrine Hydrochloride) 736
May interact with monoamine oxidase inhibitors. Compounds in this category include:
Furazolidone (Concurrent and/or sequential use is not recommended). Products include:
Furoxone 2221

Isocarboxazid (Concurrent and/or sequential use is not recommended).
No products indexed under this heading.
Phenelzine Sulfate (Concurrent and/or sequential use is not recommended). Products include:
Nardil 1977
Selegiline Hydrochloride (Concurrent and/or sequential use is not recommended). Products include:
Eldepryl Capsules 2729
Tranylcypromine Sulfate (Concurrent and/or sequential use is not recommended). Products include:
Parnate Tablets 2679

PEDIATRIC VICKS 44E COUGH & CHEST CONGESTION RELIEF
(Dextromethorphan Hydrobromide, Guaifenesin) 737
May interact with monoamine oxidase inhibitors. Compounds in this category include:
Furazolidone (Concurrent and/or sequential use is not recommended). Products include:
Furoxone 2221
Isocarboxazid (Concurrent and/or sequential use is not recommended).
No products indexed under this heading.
Phenelzine Sulfate (Concurrent and/or sequential use is not recommended). Products include:
Nardil 1977
Selegiline Hydrochloride (Concurrent and/or sequential use is not recommended). Products include:
Eldepryl Capsules 2729
Tranylcypromine Sulfate (Concurrent and/or sequential use is not recommended). Products include:
Parnate Tablets 2679

PEDIATRIC VICKS 44M COUGH & COLD RELIEF
(Chlorpheniramine Maleate, Dextromethorphan Hydrobromide, Pseudoephedrine Hydrochloride) 737
May interact with hypnotics and sedatives, tranquilizers, monoamine oxidase inhibitors, and certain other agents. Compounds in these categories include:
Alprazolam (May increase drowsiness effect). Products include:
Xanax Tablets 2115
Buspirone Hydrochloride (May increase drowsiness effect). Products include:
BuSpar Tablets 738
Chlordiazepoxide (May increase drowsiness effect). Products include:
Limbitrol 2333
Chlordiazepoxide Hydrochloride (May increase drowsiness effect). Products include:
Librax Capsules 2330
Librium Capsules 2331
Librium Injectable 2332
Chlorpromazine (May increase drowsiness effect). Products include:
Thorazine Suppositories 2701
Chlorpromazine Hydrochloride (May increase drowsiness effect). Products include:
Thorazine 2701
Chlorprothixene (May increase drowsiness effect).
No products indexed under this heading.
Chlorprothixene Hydrochloride (May increase drowsiness effect).
No products indexed under this heading.

Clorazepate Dipotassium (May increase drowsiness effect). Products include:
Tranxene 459
Diazepam (May increase drowsiness effect). Products include:
Dizac (diazepam injectable emulsion) CIV 1862
Valium Injectable 2336
Valium Tablets 2335
Droperidol (May increase drowsiness effect). Products include:
Inapsine Injection 462
Estazolam (May increase drowsiness effect). Products include:
ProSom Tablets 457
Ethchlorvynol (May increase drowsiness effect). Products include:
Placidyl Capsules 456
Ethinamate (May increase drowsiness effect).
No products indexed under this heading.
Fluphenazine Decanoate (May increase drowsiness effect). Products include:
Prolixin Decanoate 510
Fluphenazine Enanthate (May increase drowsiness effect). Products include:
Prolixin Enanthate 510
Fluphenazine Hydrochloride (May increase drowsiness effect). Products include:
Prolixin 510
Flurazepam Hydrochloride (May increase drowsiness effect). Products include:
Dalmane Capsules 2329
Furazolidone (Concurrent and/or sequential use is not recommended). Products include:
Furoxone 2221
Glutethimide (May increase drowsiness effect).
No products indexed under this heading.
Haloperidol (May increase drowsiness effect). Products include:
Haldol Injection, Tablets and Concentrate 1585
Haloperidol Decanoate (May increase drowsiness effect). Products include:
Haldol Decanoate 1587
Hydroxyzine Hydrochloride (May increase drowsiness effect). Products include:
Atarax Tablets & Syrup 1992
Marax Tablets & DF Syrup 2015
Vistaril Intramuscular Solution 2042
Isocarboxazid (Concurrent and/or sequential use is not recommended).
No products indexed under this heading.
Lorazepam (May increase drowsiness effect). Products include:
Ativan Injection 2805
Ativan Tablets 2807
Loxapine Hydrochloride (May increase drowsiness effect). Products include:
Loxitane 1426
Loxapine Succinate (May increase drowsiness effect). Products include:
Loxitane Capsules 1426
Meprobamate (May increase drowsiness effect). Products include:
Miltown Tablets 2780
PMB 200 and PMB 400 2890
Mesoridazine Besylate (May increase drowsiness effect). Products include:
Serentil 689

IMPORTANT NOTE: Always consult each drug listing in the patient's regimen for possible interactions.

Vicks Pediatric 44m C & C

Midazolam Hydrochloride (May increase drowsiness effect). Products include:
  Versed Injection 2324
Molindone Hydrochloride (May increase drowsiness effect). Products include:
  Moban Tablets and Concentrate...... 1036
Oxazepam (May increase drowsiness effect). Products include:
  Serax Capsules 2916
  Serax Tablets 2916
Perphenazine (May increase drowsiness effect). Products include:
  Etrafon 2495
  Triavil Tablets 1800
  Trilafon 2532
Phenelzine Sulfate (Concurrent and/or sequential use is not recommended). Products include:
  Nardil 1977
Prazepam (May increase drowsiness effect).
  No products indexed under this heading.
Prochlorperazine (May increase drowsiness effect). Products include:
  Compazine 2644
Promethazine Hydrochloride (May increase drowsiness effect). Products include:
  Mepergan Injection 2859
  Phenergan with Codeine 2883
  Phenergan with Dextromethorphan 2885
  Phenergan Injection 2880
  Phenergan Suppositories 2882
  Phenergan Syrup 2881
  Phenergan Tablets 2882
  Phenergan VC 2886
  Phenergan VC with Codeine 2888
Propofol (May increase drowsiness effect). Products include:
  Diprivan Injectable Emulsion 2939
Quazepam (May increase drowsiness effect). Products include:
  Doral Tablets 2773
Secobarbital Sodium (May increase drowsiness effect). Products include:
  Seconal Sodium Pulvules 1529
Selegiline Hydrochloride (Concurrent and/or sequential use is not recommended). Products include:
  Eldepryl Capsules 2729
Temazepam (May increase drowsiness effect). Products include:
  Restoril Capsules 2413
Thioridazine Hydrochloride (May increase drowsiness effect). Products include:
  Mellaril 2398
Thiothixene (May increase drowsiness effect). Products include:
  Navane Capsules and Concentrate   2018
  Navane Intramuscular 2019
Tranylcypromine Sulfate (Concurrent and/or sequential use is not recommended). Products include:
  Parnate Tablets 2679
Triazolam (May increase drowsiness effect). Products include:
  Halcion Tablets 2093
Trifluoperazine Hydrochloride (May increase drowsiness effect). Products include:
  Stelazine 2692
Zolpidem Tartrate (May increase drowsiness effect). Products include:
  Ambien Tablets 2559

Food Interactions
Alcohol (May increase drowsiness effect).

PEDIAZOLE SUSPENSION
(Erythromycin Ethylsuccinate, Sulfisoxazole Acetyl) 2340
May interact with xanthine bronchodilators and certain other agents. Compounds in these categories include:

Alfentanil Hydrochloride (Co-administration is associated with elevation in alfentanil serum levels). Products include:
  Alfenta Injection 1334
Aminophylline (Erythromycin use in patients who are receiving high doses of theophylline may be associated with an increase in serum theophylline levels and potential theophylline toxicity).
  No products indexed under this heading.
Bromocriptine Mesylate (Co-administration is associated with elevation in bromocriptine serum levels). Products include:
  Parlodel 2411
Carbamazepine (Co-administration is associated with elevation in carbamazepine serum levels). Products include:
  Atretol Tablets 569
  Tegretol/Tegretol-XR 870
Chlorpropamide (Sulfisoxazole can potentiate the blood-sugar-lowering activity of sulfonylureas). Products include:
  Diabinese Tablets 2002
Cyclosporine (Co-administration is associated with elevation in cyclosporine serum levels). Products include:
  Neoral 2405
  Sandimmune 2416
Dicumarol (Co-administration of erythromycin and oral anticoagulants has resulted in increased anticoagulant effects; sulfisoxazole may prolong the prothrombin time with concurrent use).
  No products indexed under this heading.
Digoxin (Co-administration has been reported to result in elevated digoxin serum levels). Products include:
  Lanoxicaps 1110
  Lanoxin Elixir Pediatric 1113
  Lanoxin Injection 1116
  Lanoxin Injection Pediatric....... 1119
  Lanoxin Tablets 1121
Dihydroergotamine Mesylate (Co-administration has been associated with acute ergot toxicity characterized by severe peripheral vasospasm and dysesthesia). Products include:
  D.H.E. 45 Injection 2381
Disopyramide Phosphate (Co-administration is associated with elevation in disopyramide serum levels). Products include:
  Norpace 2596
Dyphylline (Erythromycin use in patients who are receiving high doses of theophylline may be associated with an increase in serum theophylline levels and potential theophylline toxicity). Products include:
  Lufyllin & Lufyllin-400 Tablets .. 2778
  Lufyllin-GG Elixir & Tablets 2779
Ergotamine Tartrate (Co-administration has been associated with acute ergot toxicity characterized by severe peripheral vasospasm and dysesthesia). Products include:
  Bellergal-S Tablets 2375
  Cafergot 2376
  Ergomar Tablets 1543
  Wigraine Tablets 1884

Fosphenytoin Sodium (Co-administration is associated with elevation in phenytoin serum levels). Products include:
  Cerebyx Injection 1956
Glimepiride (Sulfisoxazole can potentiate the blood-sugar-lowering activity of sulfonylureas). Products include:
  Amaryl Tablets 1241
Glipizide (Sulfisoxazole can potentiate the blood-sugar-lowering activity of sulfonylureas). Products include:
  Glucotrol Tablets 2011
  Glucotrol XL Extended Release Tablets 2012
Glyburide (Sulfisoxazole can potentiate the blood-sugar-lowering activity of sulfonylureas). Products include:
  DiaBeta Tablets 1265
  Glynase PresTab Tablets 2091
  Micronase Tablets 2099
Hexobarbital (Co-administration is associated with elevation in hexobarbital serum levels).
Lovastatin (Co-administration is associated with elevation in lovastatin serum levels; combined therapy has resulted in rhabdomyolysis with or without renal impairment in seriously ill patients; carefully monitor creatine kinase and serum transaminase levels). Products include:
  Mevacor Tablets 1742
Methotrexate Sodium (Sulfonamides can displace methotrexate from plasma binding sites, thus increasing free methotrexate concentrations). Products include:
  Methotrexate Sodium Tablets, Injection, for Injection and LPF Injection 1322
Midazolam Hydrochloride (Erythromycin has been reported to decrease the clearance of midazolam and thus may increase the pharmacological effect of midazolam). Products include:
  Versed Injection 2324
Phenytoin (Co-administration is associated with elevation in phenytoin serum levels). Products include:
  Dilantin Infatabs 1967
  Dilantin-125 Suspension 1969
Phenytoin Sodium (Co-administration is associated with elevation in phenytoin serum levels). Products include:
  Dilantin Kapseals 1965
Sodium Thiopental (Sulfisoxazole competes with thiopental for plasma protein binding resulting in a decrease in the amount of thiopental required for anesthesia).
  No products indexed under this heading.
Terfenadine (Concomitant use significantly alters the metabolism of terfenadine metabolism; rare cases of serious cardiovascular adverse events, including cardiac arrest, torsade de pointes, other ventricular arrhythmias, and death have been observed; concurrent use is contraindicated). Products include:
  Seldane Tablets 1284
  Seldane-D Extended-Release Tablets 1286
Theophylline (Erythromycin use in patients who are receiving high doses of theophylline may be associated with an increase in serum theophylline levels and potential theophylline toxicity). Products include:
  Marax Tablets & DF Syrup......... 2015
  Quibron 2227

Theophylline Anhydrous (Erythromycin use in patients who are receiving high doses of theophylline may be associated with an increase in serum theophylline levels and potential theophylline toxicity). Products include:
  Aerolate 1003
  Primatene Tablets 844
  Respbid Tablets 687
  Slo-bid Gyrocaps 2201
  Theo-24 Extended Release Capsules 2753
  Theo-Dur Extended-Release Tablets 1367
  Theo-X Extended-Release Tablets .. 793
  Uni-Dur Extended-Release Tablets. 1374
  Uniphyl 400 mg and 600 mg Tablets 2157
Theophylline Calcium Salicylate (Erythromycin use in patients who are receiving high doses of theophylline may be associated with an increase in serum theophylline levels and potential theophylline toxicity). Products include:
  Quadrinal Tablets 1398
Theophylline Sodium Glycinate (Erythromycin use in patients who are receiving high doses of theophylline may be associated with an increase in serum theophylline levels and potential theophylline toxicity).
  No products indexed under this heading.
Tolazamide (Sulfisoxazole can potentiate the blood-sugar-lowering activity of sulfonylureas).
  No products indexed under this heading.
Tolbutamide (Sulfisoxazole can potentiate the blood-sugar-lowering activity of sulfonylureas).
  No products indexed under this heading.
Triazolam (Erythromycin has been reported to decrease the clearance of triazolam and thus may increase the pharmacological effect of triazolam). Products include:
  Halcion Tablets 2093
Warfarin Sodium (Co-administration of erythromycin and oral anticoagulants has resulted in increased anticoagulant effects; sulfisoxazole may prolong the prothrombin time with concurrent use). Products include:
  Coumadin 941

PEDIOTIC SUSPENSION STERILE
(Polymyxin B Sulfate, Neomycin Sulfate, Hydrocortisone).................1140
None cited in PDR database.

PEDVAXHIB
(Haemophilus B Conjugate Vaccine)..1761
May interact with immunosuppressive agents. Compounds in this category include:

Azathioprine (Expected immune response may not be observed). Products include:
  Azathioprine Tablets 2349
  Imuran 1103
Cyclosporine (Expected immune response may not be observed). Products include:
  Neoral 2405
  Sandimmune 2416
Immune Globulin (Human) (Expected immune response may not be observed).
  No products indexed under this heading.
Immune Globulin Intravenous (Human) (Expected immune response may not be observed).

(▣ Described in PDR For Nonprescription Drugs)   (◎ Described in PDR For Ophthalmology)

Muromonab-CD3 (Expected immune response may not be observed). Products include:

Orthoclone OKT3 Sterile Solution ... 1892

Mycophenolate Mofetil (Expected immune response may not be observed). Products include:

CellCept Capsules ... 2265

Tacrolimus (Expected immune response may not be observed). Products include:

Prograf ... 1028

PEGANONE TABLETS

(Ethotoin) ... 455

May interact with oral anticoagulants and certain other agents. Compounds in these categories include:

Dicumarol (Possible interactions, not yet documented).

No products indexed under this heading.

Folic Acid (Interferes with folic acid metabolism). Products include:

Cefol Filmtab ... 415
Chromagen FA ... 2471
Chromagen Forte ... 2471
Fero-Folic-500 Filmtab ... 433
Iberet-Folic-500 Filmtab ... 433
Materna Tablets ... 1427
Mega-B ... 513
Megadose ... 513
Nephro-Fer Rx Tablets ... 2168
Nephro-Vite + Fe Tablets ... 2170
Nephro-Vite Rx Tablets ... 2170
Niferex-150 Forte Capsules ... 811
Slow Fe with Folic Acid ... 890
Trinsicon Capsules ... 2759

Phenacemide (Paranoid symptoms). Products include:

Phenurone Tablets ... 455

Warfarin Sodium (Possible interactions, not yet documented). Products include:

Coumadin ... 941

PEN•VEE K FOR ORAL SOLUTION

(Penicillin V Potassium) ... 2879

None cited in PDR database.

PEN•VEE K TABLETS

(Penicillin V Potassium) ... 2879

None cited in PDR database.

PENETREX TABLETS

(Enoxacin) ... 2196

May interact with xanthine bronchodilators, antacids containing aluminium, calcium and magnesium, iron containing oral preparations, and certain other agents. Compounds in these categories include:

Aluminum Carbonate (Co-administration with antacids reduces the oral absorption of enoxacin by 75%; these agents should not be taken for 8 hours before or for 2 hours after enoxacin administration). Products include:

Basaljel Capsules ... 2810
Basaljel Suspension ... 2810
Basaljel Tablets ... 2810

Aluminum Hydroxide (Co-administration with antacids reduces the oral absorption of enoxacin by 75%; these agents should not be taken for 8 hours before or for 2 hours after enoxacin administration). Products include:

ALternaGEL Liquid ... 1358
Maximum Strength Ascriptin ... 650
Cama Arthritis Pain Reliever ... 748
Gaviscon Extra Strength Relief Formula Antacid Tablets ... 778
Gaviscon Extra Strength Relief Formula Liquid Antacid ... 779
Gaviscon Liquid Antacid ... 779
Gelusil Antacid-Anti-gas Liquid ... 819
Gelusil Antacid-Anti-gas Tablets ... 819
Maalox Antacid/Anti-Gas Tablets ... 889
Maalox Heartburn Relief Suspension ... 658
Maalox Antacid Liquid ... 888
Extra Strength Maalox Antacid/Anti-Gas Liquid and Tablets ... 888
Mylanta ... 1359
Tempo Soft Antacid ... 799

Aluminum Hydroxide Gel (Co-administration with antacids reduces the oral absorption of enoxacin by 75%; these agents should not be taken for 8 hours before or for 2 hours after enoxacin administration). Products include:

ALternaGEL Liquid ... 675
Aludrox Oral Suspension ... 850
Amphojel Suspension ... 2802
Amphojel Suspension without Flavor ... 2802
Amphojel Tablets ... 2802
Ascriptin ... 650
Gaviscon Antacid Tablets ... 778
Gaviscon-2 Antacid Tablets ... 779
Mylanta Liquid ... 676
Mylanta Double Strength Liquid ... 676
Nephrox Suspension ... 671

Aminophylline (Enoxacin, a potent inhibitor of the cytochrome P450 isoenzyme, interferes with the metabolism of methylxanthines resulting in 42% to 74% dose-related decrease in theophylline clearance and a subsequent 260% to 350% increase in serum theophylline levels).

No products indexed under this heading.

Bismuth Subsalicylate (Bismuth subsalicylate given concomitantly with enoxacin or 60 minutes following enoxacin administration, decreased enoxacin bioavailability by approximately 25%; co-administration should be avoided). Products include:

Helidac Therapy ... 2135
Pepto-Bismol Original Liquid, Original and Cherry Tablets and Easy-To-Swallow Caplets ... 2126
Pepto-Bismol Maximum Strength Liquid ... 2126

Caffeine (Enoxacin, a potent inhibitor of the cytochrome P450 isoenzyme, causes a dose-related increase in the mean elimination half-life of caffeine by up to 80% leading to a five-fold increase in the AUC and the half-life of caffeine; caffeine-related adverse effects have occurred). Products include:

Arthritis Strength BC Powder ... 631
BC Powder ... 631
Cafergot ... 2376
DHCplus Capsules ... 2148
Darvon Compound-65 Pulvules ... 1475
Esgic-plus Capsules ... 1012
Esgic-plus Tablets ... 1012
Aspirin Free Excedrin Analgesic Caplets and Geltabs ... 734
Excedrin Extra-Strength Analgesic Tablets, Caplets, and Geltabs ... 734
Fioricet Tablets ... 2386
Fioricet with Codeine Capsules ... 2387
Fiorinal Capsules ... 2388
Fiorinal with Codeine Capsules ... 2390
Fiorinal Tablets ... 2388
Goody's Extra Strength Headache Powders ... 632
Goody's Extra Strength Pain Relief Tablets ... 632
Maximum Strength Multi-Symptom Formula Midol ... 621
No Doz Maximum Strength Caplets ... 644
Norgesic ... 1554
Vanquish Analgesic Caplets ... 627
Wigraine Tablets ... 1884

Cyclosporine (Co-administration with other members of quinolone class has resulted in elevated cyclosporine serum levels). Products include:

Neoral ... 2405
Sandimmune ... 2416

Digoxin (Enoxacin may raise serum digoxin levels in some patients). Products include:

Lanoxicaps ... 1110
Lanoxin Elixir Pediatric ... 1113
Lanoxin Injection ... 1116
Lanoxin Injection Pediatric ... 1119
Lanoxin Tablets ... 1121

Dyphylline (Enoxacin, a potent inhibitor of the cytochrome P450 isoenzyme, interferes with the metabolism of methylxanthines resulting in 42% to 74% dose-related decrease in theophylline clearance and a subsequent 260% to 350% increase in serum theophylline levels). Products include:

Lufyllin & Lufyllin-400 Tablets ... 2778
Lufyllin-GG Elixir & Tablets ... 2779

Fenbufen (Co-administration has resulted in seizures).

Ferrous Fumarate (Oral iron preparations may substantially interfere with enoxacin absorption, resulting in insufficient plasma and tissue quinolone concentration; these agents should not be taken for 8 hours before or for 2 hours after enoxacin administration). Products include:

Chromagen Capsules ... 2470
Chromagen FA ... 2471
Chromagen Forte ... 2471
Ferro-Sequels ... 684
Nephro-Fer Tablets ... 2168
Nephro-Fer Rx Tablets ... 2168
Nephro-Vite + Fe Tablets ... 2170
Stresstabs + Iron ... 685
Trinsicon Capsules ... 2759
Vitron-C Tablets ... 667

Ferrous Gluconate (Oral iron preparations may substantially interfere with enoxacin absorption, resulting in insufficient plasma and tissue quinolone concentration; these agents should not be taken for 8 hours before or for 2 hours after enoxacin administration). Products include:

Megadose ... 513

Ferrous Sulfate (Oral iron preparations may substantially interfere with enoxacin absorption, resulting in insufficient plasma and tissue quinolone concentration; these agents should not be taken for 8 hours before or for 2 hours after enoxacin administration). Products include:

Feosol Capsules ... 777
Feosol Elixir ... 2627
Feosol Tablets ... 2627
Fero-Folic-500 Filmtab ... 433
Fero-Grad-500 Filmtab ... 434
Fero-Gradumet Filmtab ... 434
Iberet Tablets ... 437
Iberet-500 Liquid ... 438
Iberet-Folic-500 Filmtab ... 433
Iberet-Liquid ... 438
Irospan ... 1000
Slow Fe Tablets ... 889
Slow Fe with Folic Acid ... 890

Iron (Oral iron preparations may substantially interfere with enoxacin absorption, resulting in insufficient plasma and tissue quinolone concentration; these agents should not be taken for 8 hours before or for 2 hours after enoxacin administration). Products include:

Feosol Caplets ... 2626

Magaldrate (Co-administration with antacids reduces the oral absorption of enoxacin by 75%; these agents should not be taken for 8 hours before or for 2 hours after enoxacin administration).

No products indexed under this heading.

Magnesium Hydroxide (Co-administration with antacids reduces the oral absorption of enoxacin by 75%; these agents should not be taken for 8 hours before or for 2 hours after enoxacin administration). Products include:

Aludrox Oral Suspension ... 850
Ascriptin ... 650
Di-Gel Antacid/Anti-Gas ... 762
Gelusil Antacid-Anti-gas Liquid ... 819
Gelusil Antacid-Anti-gas Tablets ... 819
Maalox Antacid/Anti-Gas Tablets ... 889
Maalox Antacid Liquid ... 888
Extra Strength Maalox Antacid/Anti-Gas Liquid and Tablets ... 888
Mylanta Fast-Acting ... 1359
Mylanta Gelcaps Antacid ... 678
Fast-Acting Mylanta Liquid Antacid 1359
Mylanta Tablets ... 677
Maximum-Strength Fast-Acting Mylanta Liquid Antacid ... 1359
Mylanta Double Strength Tablets ... 677
Phillips' Milk of Magnesia Liquid ... 627
Rolaids Antacid Tablets ... 807
Tempo Soft Antacid ... 799

Magnesium Oxide (Co-administration with antacids reduces the oral absorption of enoxacin by 75%; these agents should not be taken for 8 hours before or for 2 hours after enoxacin administration). Products include:

Beelith Tablets ... 632
Bufferin Analgesic Tablets ... 636
Arthritis Strength Bufferin Analgesic Caplets ... 637
Extra Strength Bufferin Analgesic Tablets ... 637
Caltrate PLUS ... 681
Cama Arthritis Pain Reliever ... 748
Mag-Ox 400 ... 666
Uro-Mag ... 666

Polysaccharide-Iron Complex (Oral iron preparations may substantially interfere with enoxacin absorption, resulting in insufficient plasma and tissue quinolone concentration; these agents should not be taken for 8 hours before or for 2 hours after enoxacin administration). Products include:

Niferex-150 Capsules ... 811
Niferex Elixir ... 811
Niferex-150 Forte Capsules ... 811
Niferex ... 811
Niferex-PN Tablets ... 811
Nu-Iron 150 Capsules ... 1826
Nu-Iron Elixir ... 1826

Ranitidine Hydrochloride (Co-administration reduces oral bioavailability of enoxacin by 60%; ranitidine should not be taken for 8 hours before or for 2 hours after enoxacin administration). Products include:

Zantac ... 1182
Zantac Injection ... 1180
Zantac Syrup ... 1182

Sucralfate (May substantially interfere with enoxacin absorption, resulting in insufficient plasma and tissue quinolone concentration; these agents should not be taken for 8 hours before or for 2 hours after enoxacin administration). Products include:

Carafate Suspension ... 1250
Carafate Tablets ... 1249

Theophylline (Enoxacin, a potent inhibitor of the cytochrome P450 isoenzyme, interferes with the metabolism of methylxanthines resulting in 42% to 74% dose-related decrease in theophylline clearance and a subsequent 260% to 350% increase in serum theophylline levels). Products include:

Marax Tablets & DF Syrup ... 2015
Quibron ... 2227

IMPORTANT NOTE: Always consult each drug listing in the patient's regimen for possible interactions.

Penetrex

Theophylline Anhydrous (Enoxacin, a potent inhibitor of the cytochrome P450 isoenzyme, interferes with the metabolism of methylxanthines resulting in 42% to 74% dose-related decrease in theophylline clearance and a subsequent 260% to 350% increase in serum theophylline levels). Products include:
- Aerolate 1003
- Primatene Tablets 844
- Respbid Tablets 687
- Slo-bid Gyrocaps 2201
- Theo-24 Extended Release Capsules 2753
- Theo-Dur Extended-Release Tablets 1367
- Theo-X Extended-Release Tablets .. 793
- Uni-Dur Extended-Release Tablets . 1374
- Uniphyl 400 mg and 600 mg Tablets 2157

Theophylline Calcium Salicylate (Enoxacin, a potent inhibitor of the cytochrome P450 isoenzyme, interferes with the metabolism of methylxanthines resulting in 42% to 74% dose-related decrease in theophylline clearance and a subsequent 260% to 350% increase in serum theophylline levels). Products include:
- Quadrinal Tablets 1398

Theophylline Sodium Glycinate (Enoxacin, a potent inhibitor of the cytochrome P450 isoenzyme, interferes with the metabolism of methylxanthines resulting in 42% to 74% dose-related decrease in theophylline clearance and a subsequent 260% to 350% increase in serum theophylline levels).
No products indexed under this heading.

Warfarin Sodium (Decreased clearance of R-warfarin, the less active isomer of warfarin; change in clotting time has not been observed). Products include:
- Coumadin 941

Zinc Sulfate (Oral zinc preparations may substantially interfere with enoxacin absorption, resulting in insufficient plasma and tissue quinolone concentration; these agents should not be taken for 8 hours before or for 2 hours after enoxacin administration). Products include:
- Clear Eyes ACR Astringent/Lubricant Eye Redness Reliever Eye Drops 314
- Visine A.C. Seasonal Relief From Pollen and Dust 301

Food Interactions
Beverages, caffeine-containing (Enoxacin causes a dose-related increase in the mean elimination half-life of caffeine leading to caffeine-related adverse effects; consumption of caffeine-containing products should be avoided).

Chocolate (Enoxacin causes a dose-related increase in the mean elimination half-life of caffeine leading to caffeine-related adverse effects; consumption of caffeine-containing products should be avoided).

Cola (Enoxacin causes a dose-related increase in the mean elimination half-life of caffeine leading to caffeine-related adverse effects; consumption of caffeine-containing products should be avoided).

PENTASA
(Mesalamine) 1275
None cited in PDR database.

PENTASPAN INJECTION
(Pentastarch) 954
None cited in PDR database.

PENTRAX SHAMPOO
(Coal Tar) 1042
None cited in PDR database.

PEPCID AC ACID CONTROLLER
(Famotidine) 1360
None cited in PDR database.

PEPCID INJECTION
(Famotidine) 1765
None cited in PDR database.

PEPCID INJECTION PREMIXED
(Famotidine) 1765
None cited in PDR database.

PEPCID ORAL SUSPENSION
(Famotidine) 1763
May interact with antacids and certain other agents. Compounds in these categories include:

Aluminum Carbonate (Bioavailability may be slightly decreased by antacids). Products include:
- Basaljel Capsules 2810
- Basaljel Suspension 2810
- Basaljel Tablets 2810

Aluminum Hydroxide (Bioavailability may be slightly decreased by antacids). Products include:
- ALternaGEL Liquid 1358
- Maximum Strength Ascriptin ... 650
- Cama Arthritis Pain Reliever ... 748
- Gaviscon Extra Strength Relief Formula Antacid Tablets ... 778
- Gaviscon Extra Strength Relief Formula Liquid Antacid ... 779
- Gaviscon Liquid Antacid ... 779
- Gelusil Antacid-Anti-gas Liquid ... 819
- Gelusil Antacid-Anti-gas Tablets ... 819
- Maalox Antacid/Anti-Gas Tablets ... 889
- Maalox Heartburn Relief Suspension ... 658
- Maalox Suspension 888
- Extra Strength Maalox Antacid/Anti-Gas Liquid and Tablets ... 888
- Mylanta 1359
- Tempo Soft Antacid 799

Aluminum Hydroxide Gel (Bioavailability may be slightly decreased by antacids). Products include:
- ALternaGEL Liquid 675
- Aludrox Oral Suspension ... 850
- Amphojel Suspension ... 2802
- Amphojel Suspension without Flavor ... 2802
- Amphojel Tablets 2802
- Ascriptin 650
- Gaviscon Antacid Tablets ... 778
- Gaviscon-2 Antacid Tablets ... 779
- Mylanta Liquid 676
- Mylanta Double Strength Liquid ... 676
- Nephrox Suspension 671

Magaldrate (Bioavailability may be slightly decreased by antacids).
No products indexed under this heading.

Magnesium Hydroxide (Bioavailability may be slightly decreased by antacids). Products include:
- Aludrox Oral Suspension ... 850
- Ascriptin 650
- Di-Gel Antacid/Anti-Gas ... 762
- Gelusil Antacid-Anti-gas Liquid ... 819
- Gelusil Antacid-Anti-gas Tablets ... 819
- Maalox Antacid/Anti-Gas Tablets ... 889
- Maalox Antacid Liquid ... 888
- Extra Strength Maalox Antacid/Anti-Gas Liquid and Tablets ... 888
- Mylanta Fast-Acting 1359
- Mylanta Gelcaps Antacid ... 678
- Fast-Acting Mylanta Liquid Antacid ... 1359
- Mylanta Tablets 677
- Maximum-Strength Fast-Acting Mylanta Liquid Antacid ... 1359
- Mylanta Double Strength Tablets ... 677
- Phillips' Milk of Magnesia Liquid ... 627
- Rolaids Antacid Tablets ... 807
- Tempo Soft Antacid 799

Interactions Index

Magnesium Oxide (Bioavailability may be slightly decreased by antacids). Products include:
- Beelith Tablets 632
- Bufferin Analgesic Tablets ... 636
- Arthritis Strength Bufferin Analgesic Caplets 637
- Extra Strength Bufferin Analgesic Tablets 637
- Caltrate PLUS 681
- Cama Arthritis Pain Reliever ... 748
- Mag-Ox 400 666
- Uro-Mag 666

Sodium Bicarbonate (Bioavailability may be slightly decreased by antacids). Products include:
- Alka-Seltzer Cherry Effervescent Antacid and Pain Reliever ... 609
- Alka-Seltzer Extra Strength Effervescent Antacid and Pain Reliever ... 609
- Alka-Seltzer Gold Effervescent Antacid 611
- Alka-Seltzer Lemon Lime Effervescent Antacid and Pain Reliever ... 609
- Alka-Seltzer Original Effervescent Antacid and Pain Reliever ... 609
- Arm & Hammer Pure Baking Soda 609
- Colyte and Colyte-flavored ... 2540
- GoLYTELY 694
- Massengill Disposable Douches ... 780
- Massengill Liquid Concentrate ... 780
- NuLYTELY 694
- Cherry Flavor NuLYTELY ... 694

Food Interactions
Food, unspecified (Bioavailability may be slightly increased by antacids).

PEPCID TABLETS
(Famotidine) 1763
See **Pepcid Oral Suspension**

PEPTAVLON
(Pentagastrin) 2997
None cited in PDR database.

PEPTO-BISMOL ORIGINAL LIQUID, ORIGINAL AND CHERRY TABLETS AND EASY-TO-SWALLOW CAPLETS
(Bismuth Subsalicylate) ... 2126
May interact with oral anticoagulants, oral hypoglycemic agents, and antigout agents. Compounds in these categories include:

Acarbose (Use cautiously). Products include:
- Precose 604

Allopurinol (Use cautiously). Products include:
- Zyloprim Tablets 1194

Chlorpropamide (Use cautiously). Products include:
- Diabinese Tablets 2002

Dicumarol (Use cautiously).
No products indexed under this heading.

Glimepiride (Use cautiously). Products include:
- Amaryl Tablets 1241

Glipizide (Use cautiously). Products include:
- Glucotrol Tablets 2011
- Glucotrol XL Extended Release Tablets 2012

Glyburide (Use cautiously). Products include:
- DiaBeta Tablets 1265
- Glynase PresTab Tablets ... 2091
- Micronase Tablets 2099

Metformin Hydrochloride (Use cautiously). Products include:
- Glucophage Tablets 754

Probenecid (Use cautiously). Products include:
- Benemid Tablets 1651
- ColBENEMID Tablets 1662

Sulfinpyrazone (Use cautiously). Products include:
- Anturane 823

Tolazamide (Use cautiously).
No products indexed under this heading.

Tolbutamide (Use cautiously).
No products indexed under this heading.

Warfarin Sodium (Use cautiously). Products include:
- Coumadin 941

PEPTO-BISMOL MAXIMUM STRENGTH LIQUID
(Bismuth Subsalicylate) ... 2126
May interact with oral anticoagulants, antigout agents, and oral hypoglycemic agents. Compounds in these categories include:

Acarbose (Use cautiously). Products include:
- Precose 604

Allopurinol (Use cautiously). Products include:
- Zyloprim Tablets 1194

Chlorpropamide (Use cautiously). Products include:
- Diabinese Tablets 2002

Dicumarol (Use cautiously).
No products indexed under this heading.

Glimepiride (Use cautiously). Products include:
- Amaryl Tablets 1241

Glipizide (Use cautiously). Products include:
- Glucotrol Tablets 2011
- Glucotrol XL Extended Release Tablets 2012

Glyburide (Use cautiously). Products include:
- DiaBeta Tablets 1265
- Glynase PresTab Tablets ... 2091
- Micronase Tablets 2099

Metformin Hydrochloride (Use cautiously). Products include:
- Glucophage Tablets 754

Probenecid (Use cautiously). Products include:
- Benemid Tablets 1651
- ColBENEMID Tablets 1662

Sulfinpyrazone (Use cautiously). Products include:
- Anturane 823

Tolazamide (Use cautiously).
No products indexed under this heading.

Tolbutamide (Use cautiously).
No products indexed under this heading.

Warfarin Sodium (Use cautiously). Products include:
- Coumadin 941

PEPTO DIARRHEA CONTROL
(Loperamide Hydrochloride) ... 2127
May interact with:

Antibiotics, unspecified (Effect not specified).

PERATIVE SPECIALIZED LIQUID NUTRITION
(Nutritional Beverage) 2343
None cited in PDR database.

PERCOCET TABLETS
(Oxycodone Hydrochloride, Acetaminophen) 955
May interact with narcotic analgesics, general anesthetics, phenothiazines, tranquilizers, hypnotics and sedatives, central nervous system depressants, monoamine oxidase inhibitors, tricyclic antidepressants, anticholinergics, and certain other

---

Described in PDR For Nonprescription Drugs | Described in PDR For Ophthalmology

825 **Interactions Index** **Percocet**

agents. Compounds in these categories include:

Alfentanil Hydrochloride (Additive CNS depression; dose of one or both agents should be reduced). Products include:
Alfenta Injection ... 1334

Alprazolam (Additive CNS depression; dose of one or both agents should be reduced). Products include:
Xanax Tablets ... 2115

Amitriptyline Hydrochloride (Increased effect of antidepressant or oxycodone). Products include:
Elavil ... 2945
Etrafon ... 2495
Limbitrol ... 2333
Triavil Tablets ... 1800

Amoxapine (Increased effect of antidepressant or oxycodone). Products include:
Asendin Tablets ... 1419

Aprobarbital (Additive CNS depression; dose of one or both agents should be reduced).
No products indexed under this heading.

Atropine Sulfate (May produce paralytic ileus). Products include:
Arco-Lase Plus Tablets ... 513
Atrohist Plus Tablets ... 1605
Donnatal ... 2234
Donnatal Extentabs ... 2234
Donnatal Tablets ... 2234
Lomotil ... 2591
Motofen Tablets ... 789
Urised Tablets ... 2123

Belladonna Alkaloids (May produce paralytic ileus). Products include:
Bellergal-S Tablets ... 2375
Hyland's Bedwetting Tablets ... 788
Hyland's EnurAid Tablets ... 789
Hyland's Headache Tablets ... 790
Hyland's Teething Tablets ... 790
Similasan Eye Drops #1 ... 769

Benztropine Mesylate (May produce paralytic ileus). Products include:
Cogentin ... 1661

Biperiden Hydrochloride (May produce paralytic ileus). Products include:
Akineton ... 1380

Buprenorphine (Additive CNS depression; dose of one or both agents should be reduced). Products include:
Buprenex Injectable ... 2170

Buspirone Hydrochloride (Additive CNS depression; dose of one or both agents should be reduced). Products include:
BuSpar Tablets ... 738

Butabarbital (Additive CNS depression; dose of one or both agents should be reduced).
No products indexed under this heading.

Butalbital (Additive CNS depression; dose of one or both agents should be reduced). Products include:
Axocet Capsules ... 2469
Esgic-plus Capsules ... 1012
Esgic-plus Tablets ... 1012
Fioricet Tablets ... 2386
Fioricet with Codeine Capsules ... 2387
Fiorinal Capsules ... 2388
Fiorinal with Codeine Capsules ... 2390
Fiorinal Tablets ... 2388
Phrenilin ... 790
Sedapap Tablets 50 mg/650 mg ... 1826

Chlordiazepoxide (Additive CNS depression; dose of one or both agents should be reduced). Products include:
Limbitrol ... 2333

Chlordiazepoxide Hydrochloride (Additive CNS depression; dose of one or both agents should be reduced). Products include:
Librax Capsules ... 2330
Librium Capsules ... 2331
Librium Injectable ... 2332

Chlorpromazine (Additive CNS depression; dose of one or both agents should be reduced). Products include:
Thorazine Suppositories ... 2701

Chlorpromazine Hydrochloride (Additive CNS depression; dose of one or both agents should be reduced). Products include:
Thorazine ... 2701

Chlorprothixene (Additive CNS depression; dose of one or both agents should be reduced).
No products indexed under this heading.

Chlorprothixene Hydrochloride (Additive CNS depression; dose of one or both agents should be reduced).
No products indexed under this heading.

Chlorprothixene Lactate (Additive CNS depression; dose of one or both agents should be reduced).
No products indexed under this heading.

Clidinium Bromide (May produce paralytic ileus). Products include:
Librax Capsules ... 2330

Clomipramine Hydrochloride (Increased effect of antidepressant or oxycodone). Products include:
Anafranil Capsules ... 819

Clorazepate Dipotassium (Additive CNS depression; dose of one or both agents should be reduced). Products include:
Tranxene ... 459

Clozapine (Additive CNS depression; dose of one or both agents should be reduced). Products include:
Clozaril Tablets ... 2377

Codeine Phosphate (Additive CNS depression; dose of one or both agents should be reduced). Products include:
Brontex ... 2130
Dimetane-DC Cough Syrup ... 2232
Fioricet with Codeine Capsules ... 2387
Fiorinal with Codeine Capsules ... 2390
Nucofed ... 2225
Phenergan with Codeine ... 2883
Phenergan VC with Codeine ... 2888
Robitussin A-C Syrup ... 2248
Robitussin-DAC Syrup ... 2249
Ryna ... 804
Soma Compound w/Codeine Tablets ... 2784
Tylenol with Codeine ... 1592

Desflurane (Additive CNS depression; dose of one or both agents should be reduced). Products include:
Suprane (desflurane, USP) ... 1865

Desipramine Hydrochloride (Increased effect of antidepressant or oxycodone). Products include:
Norpramin Tablets ... 1273

Dezocine (Additive CNS depression; dose of one or both agents should be reduced). Products include:
Dalgan Injection ... 529

Diazepam (Additive CNS depression; dose of one or both agents should be reduced). Products include:
Dizac (diazepam injectable emulsion) CIV ... 1862
Valium Injectable ... 2336
Valium Tablets ... 2335

Dicyclomine Hydrochloride (May produce paralytic ileus). Products include:
Bentyl ... 1246

Doxepin Hydrochloride (Increased effect of antidepressant or oxycodone). Products include:
Adapin Capsules ... 1542
Sinequan ... 2028
Zonalon Cream ... 1042

Droperidol (Additive CNS depression; dose of one or both agents should be reduced). Products include:
Inapsine Injection ... 462

Enflurane (Additive CNS depression; dose of one or both agents should be reduced).
No products indexed under this heading.

Estazolam (Additive CNS depression; dose of one or both agents should be reduced). Products include:
ProSom Tablets ... 457

Ethchlorvynol (Additive CNS depression; dose of one or both agents should be reduced). Products include:
Placidyl Capsules ... 456

Ethinamate (Additive CNS depression; dose of one or both agents should be reduced).
No products indexed under this heading.

Ethopropazine Hydrochloride (May produce paralytic ileus).

Fentanyl (Additive CNS depression; dose of one or both agents should be reduced). Products include:
Duragesic Transdermal System ... 1336

Fentanyl Citrate (Additive CNS depression; dose of one or both agents should be reduced). Products include:
Sublimaze Injection ... 463

Fluphenazine Decanoate (Additive CNS depression; dose of one or both agents should be reduced). Products include:
Prolixin Decanoate ... 510

Fluphenazine Enanthate (Additive CNS depression; dose of one or both agents should be reduced). Products include:
Prolixin Enanthate ... 510

Fluphenazine Hydrochloride (Additive CNS depression; dose of one or both agents should be reduced). Products include:
Prolixin ... 510

Flurazepam Hydrochloride (Additive CNS depression; dose of one or both agents should be reduced). Products include:
Dalmane Capsules ... 2329

Furazolidone (Increased effect of either oxycodone or MAO inhibitor). Products include:
Furoxone ... 2221

Glutethimide (Additive CNS depression; dose of one or both agents should be reduced).
No products indexed under this heading.

Glycopyrrolate (May produce paralytic ileus). Products include:
Robinul Forte Tablets ... 2247
Robinul Injectable ... 2247
Robinul Tablets ... 2247

Haloperidol (Additive CNS depression; dose of one or both agents should be reduced). Products include:
Haldol Injection, Tablets and Concentrate ... 1585

Haloperidol Decanoate (Additive CNS depression; dose of one or both agents should be reduced). Products include:
Haldol Decanoate ... 1587

Hydrocodone Bitartrate (Additive CNS depression; dose of one or both agents should be reduced). Products include:
Codiclear DH Syrup ... 808
Duratuss HD Elixir ... 2750
Histussin D Liquid ... 670
Hycodan Tablets and Syrup ... 946
Hycomine Compound Tablets ... 948
Hycomine ... 947
Hycotuss Expectorant Syrup ... 950
Hydrocet Capsules ... 787
Lorcet 10/650 Tablets ... 1016
Lortab ... 2751
Tussend ... 1830
Tussend Expectorant ... 1831
Vicodin Tablets ... 1404
Vicodin ES Tablets ... 1405
Vicodin HP Tablets ... 1403
Vicodin Tuss Expectorant ... 1406
Zydone Capsules ... 967

Hydrocodone Polistirex (Additive CNS depression; dose of one or both agents should be reduced). Products include:
Tussionex Pennkinetic Extended-Release Suspension ... 1624

Hydromorphone Hydrochloride (Additive CNS depression; dose of one or both agents should be reduced). Products include:
Dilaudid Ampules ... 1382
Dilaudid Cough Syrup ... 1383
Dilaudid-HP Injection ... 1384
Dilaudid-HP Lyophilized Powder 250 mg ... 1384
Dilaudid ... 1382
Dilaudid Oral Liquid ... 1386
Dilaudid ... 1382
Dilaudid Tablets - 8 mg ... 1386

Hydroxyzine Hydrochloride (Additive CNS depression; dose of one or both agents should be reduced). Products include:
Atarax Tablets & Syrup ... 1992
Marax Tablets & DF Syrup ... 2015
Vistaril Intramuscular Solution ... 2042

Hyoscyamine (May produce paralytic ileus). Products include:
Cystospaz Tablets ... 2123
Urised Tablets ... 2123

Hyoscyamine Sulfate (May produce paralytic ileus). Products include:
Arco-Lase Plus Tablets ... 513
Atrohist Plus Tablets ... 1605
Cystospaz-M Capsules ... 2123
Donnatal ... 2234
Donnatal Extentabs ... 2234
Donnatal Tablets ... 2234
Kutrase Capsules ... 2546
Levsin/Levsinex/Levbid ... 2549

Imipramine Hydrochloride (Increased effect of antidepressant or oxycodone). Products include:
Tofranil Ampuls ... 873
Tofranil Tablets ... 875

Imipramine Pamoate (Increased effect of antidepressant or oxycodone). Products include:
Tofranil-PM Capsules ... 876

Ipratropium Bromide (May produce paralytic ileus). Products include:
Atrovent Inhalation Aerosol ... 674
Atrovent Inhalation Solution ... 675
Atrovent Nasal Spray 0.03% ... 676
Atrovent Nasal Spray 0.06% ... 678

Isocarboxazid (Increased effect of either oxycodone or MAO inhibitor).
No products indexed under this heading.

Isoflurane (Additive CNS depression; dose of one or both agents should be reduced).
No products indexed under this heading.

IMPORTANT NOTE: Always consult each drug listing in the patient's regimen for possible interactions.

Percocet — Interactions Index

Ketamine Hydrochloride (Additive CNS depression; dose of one or both agents should be reduced.)
    No products indexed under this heading.

Levomethadyl Acetate Hydrochloride (Additive CNS depression; dose of one or both agents should be reduced). Products include:
    Orlaam Oral Solution 2361

Levorphanol Tartrate (Additive CNS depression; dose of one or both agents should be reduced). Products include:
    Levo-Dromoran 2297

Lorazepam (Additive CNS depression; dose of one or both agents should be reduced). Products include:
    Ativan Injection 2805
    Ativan Tablets 2807

Loxapine Hydrochloride (Additive CNS depression; dose of one or both agents should be reduced). Products include:
    Loxitane 1426

Loxapine Succinate (Additive CNS depression; dose of one or both agents should be reduced). Products include:
    Loxitane Capsules 1426

Maprotiline Hydrochloride (Increased effect of antidepressant or oxycodone). Products include:
    Ludiomil Tablets 861

Mepenzolate Bromide (May produce paralytic ileus).
    No products indexed under this heading.

Meperidine Hydrochloride (Additive CNS depression; dose of one or both agents should be reduced). Products include:
    Demerol 2438
    Mepergan Injection 2859

Mephobarbital (Additive CNS depression; dose of one or both agents should be reduced). Products include:
    Mebaral Tablets 2452

Meprobamate (Additive CNS depression; dose of one or both agents should be reduced). Products include:
    Miltown Tablets 2780
    PMB 200 and PMB 400 2890

Mesoridazine Besylate (Additive CNS depression; dose of one or both agents should be reduced). Products include:
    Serentil 689

Methadone Hydrochloride (Additive CNS depression; dose of one or both agents should be reduced). Products include:
    Methadone Hydrochloride Oral Concentrate 2356
    Methadone Hydrochloride Oral Solution & Tablets 2357

Methohexital Sodium (Additive CNS depression; dose of one or both agents should be reduced).
    No products indexed under this heading.

Methotrimeprazine (Additive CNS depression; dose of one or both agents should be reduced). Products include:
    Levoprome 1321

Methoxyflurane (Additive CNS depression; dose of one or both agents should be reduced).
    No products indexed under this heading.

Midazolam Hydrochloride (Additive CNS depression; dose of one or both agents should be reduced). Products include:
    Versed Injection 2324

Molindone Hydrochloride (Additive CNS depression; dose of one or both agents should be reduced). Products include:
    Moban Tablets and Concentrate 1036

Morphine Sulfate (Additive CNS depression; dose of one or both agents should be reduced). Products include:
    Astramorph/PF Injection, USP (Preservative-Free) 526
    Duramorph Injection 983
    Infumorph 200 and Infumorph 500 Sterile Solutions 985
    Kadian Capsules 2948
    MS Contin Tablets 2149
    MSIR 2152
    Oramorph SR (Morphine Sulfate Sustained Release Tablets) 2359
    RMS Suppositories CII 2766
    Roxanol 2365

Nortriptyline Hydrochloride (Increased effect of antidepressant or oxycodone). Products include:
    Pamelor 2409

Opium Alkaloids (Additive CNS depression; dose of one or both agents should be reduced).
    No products indexed under this heading.

Oxazepam (Additive CNS depression; dose of one or both agents should be reduced; increased effect of antidepressant). Products include:
    Serax Capsules 2916
    Serax Tablets 2916

Oxybutynin Chloride (May produce paralytic ileus). Products include:
    Ditropan 1267

Oxyphenonium Bromide (May produce paralytic ileus).

Pentobarbital Sodium (Additive CNS depression; dose of one or both agents should be reduced). Products include:
    Nembutal Sodium Capsules 440
    Nembutal Sodium Solution 442
    Nembutal Sodium Suppositories ... 444

Perphenazine (Additive CNS depression; dose of one or both agents should be reduced). Products include:
    Etrafon 2495
    Triavil Tablets 1800
    Trilafon 2532

Phenelzine Sulfate (Increased effect of either oxycodone or MAO inhibitor). Products include:
    Nardil 1977

Phenobarbital (Additive CNS depression; dose of one or both agents should be reduced). Products include:
    Arco-Lase Plus Tablets 513
    Bellergal-S Tablets 2375
    Donnatal 2234
    Donnatal Extentabs 2234
    Donnatal Tablets 2234
    Phenobarbital Elixir and Tablets 1523
    Quadrinal Tablets 1398

Prazepam (Additive CNS depression; dose of one or both agents should be reduced).
    No products indexed under this heading.

Prochlorperazine (Additive CNS depression; dose of one or both agents should be reduced). Products include:
    Compazine 2644

Procyclidine Hydrochloride (May produce paralytic ileus). Products include:
    Kemadrin Tablets 1105

Promethazine Hydrochloride (Additive CNS depression; dose of one or both agents should be reduced). Products include:
    Mepergan Injection 2859
    Phenergan with Codeine 2883
    Phenergan with Dextromethorphan 2885
    Phenergan Injection 2880
    Phenergan Suppositories 2882
    Phenergan Syrup 2881
    Phenergan Tablets 2882
    Phenergan VC 2886
    Phenergan VC with Codeine 2888

Propantheline Bromide (May produce paralytic ileus). Products include:
    Pro-Banthine Tablets 2226

Propofol (Additive CNS depression; dose of one or both agents should be reduced). Products include:
    Diprivan Injectable Emulsion 2939

Propoxyphene Hydrochloride (Additive CNS depression; dose of one or both agents should be reduced). Products include:
    Darvon 1475
    Wygesic Tablets 2930

Propoxyphene Napsylate (Additive CNS depression; dose of one or both agents should be reduced). Products include:
    Darvon-N/Darvocet-N 1473

Protriptyline Hydrochloride (Increased effect of antidepressant or oxycodone). Products include:
    Vivactil Tablets 1820

Quazepam (Additive CNS depression; dose of one or both agents should be reduced). Products include:
    Doral Tablets 2773

Risperidone (Additive CNS depression; dose of one or both agents should be reduced). Products include:
    Risperdal Tablets 1348

Scopolamine (May produce paralytic ileus). Products include:
    Transderm Scōp Transdermal Therapeutic System 890

Scopolamine Hydrobromide (May produce paralytic ileus). Products include:
    Atrohist Plus Tablets 1605
    Donnatal 2234
    Donnatal Extentabs 2234
    Donnatal Tablets 2234

Secobarbital Sodium (Additive CNS depression; dose of one or both agents should be reduced). Products include:
    Seconal Sodium Pulvules 1529

Selegiline Hydrochloride (Increased effect of either oxycodone or MAO inhibitor). Products include:
    Eldepryl Capsules 2729

Sevoflurane (Additive CNS depression; dose of one or both agents should be reduced).
    No products indexed under this heading.

Sufentanil Citrate (Additive CNS depression; dose of one or both agents should be reduced). Products include:
    Sufenta Injection 1355

Temazepam (Additive CNS depression; dose of one or both agents should be reduced). Products include:
    Restoril Capsules 2413

Thiamylal Sodium (Additive CNS depression; dose of one or both agents should be reduced).
    No products indexed under this heading.

Thioridazine Hydrochloride (Additive CNS depression; dose of one or both agents should be reduced). Products include:
    Mellaril 2398

Thiothixene (Additive CNS depression; dose of one or both agents should be reduced). Products include:
    Navane Capsules and Concentrate 2018
    Navane Intramuscular 2019

Tranylcypromine Sulfate (Increased effect of either oxycodone or MAO inhibitor). Products include:
    Parnate Tablets 2679

Triazolam (Additive CNS depression; dose of one or both agents should be reduced). Products include:
    Halcion Tablets 2093

Tridihexethyl Chloride (May produce paralytic ileus).
    No products indexed under this heading.

Trifluoperazine Hydrochloride (Additive CNS depression; dose of one or both agents should be reduced). Products include:
    Stelazine 2692

Trihexyphenidyl Hydrochloride (May produce paralytic ileus). Products include:
    Artane 1418

Trimipramine Maleate (Increased effect of antidepressant or oxycodone). Products include:
    Surmontil Capsules 2917

Zolpidem Tartrate (Additive CNS depression; dose of one or both agents should be reduced). Products include:
    Ambien Tablets 2559

Food Interactions
Alcohol (Additive CNS depression).

PERCODAN TABLETS
(Oxycodone Hydrochloride, Oxycodone Terephthalate, Aspirin) 955
May interact with narcotic analgesics, general anesthetics, phenothiazines, tranquilizers, hypnotics and sedatives, anticoagulants, central nervous system depressants, and certain other agents. Compounds in these categories include:

Alfentanil Hydrochloride (Additive CNS depression). Products include:
    Alfenta Injection 1334

Alprazolam (Additive CNS depression). Products include:
    Xanax Tablets 2115

Aprobarbital (Additive CNS depression).
    No products indexed under this heading.

Buprenorphine (Additive CNS depression). Products include:
    Buprenex Injectable 2170

Buspirone Hydrochloride (Additive CNS depression). Products include:
    BuSpar Tablets 738

Butabarbital (Additive CNS depression).
    No products indexed under this heading.

Butalbital (Additive CNS depression). Products include:
    Axocet Capsules 2469
    Esgic-plus Capsules 1012
    Esgic-plus Tablets 1012
    Fioricet Tablets 2386
    Fioricet with Codeine Capsules 2387
    Fiorinal Capsules 2388
    Fiorinal with Codeine Capsules 2390
    Fiorinal Tablets 2388
    Phrenilin 790

(◼ Described in PDR For Nonprescription Drugs)   (⊚ Described in PDR For Ophthalmology)

827 **Interactions Index** **Percodan**

Sedapap Tablets 50 mg/650 mg .. 1826

Chlordiazepoxide (Additive CNS depression). Products include:
Limbitrol ... 2333

Chlordiazepoxide Hydrochloride (Additive CNS depression). Products include:
Librax Capsules ... 2330
Librium Capsules ... 2331
Librium Injectable ... 2332

Chlorpromazine (Additive CNS depression). Products include:
Thorazine Suppositories ... 2701

Chlorpromazine Hydrochloride (Additive CNS depression). Products include:
Thorazine ... 2701

Chlorprothixene (Additive CNS depression).
No products indexed under this heading.

Chlorprothixene Hydrochloride (Additive CNS depression).
No products indexed under this heading.

Chlorprothixene Lactate (Additive CNS depression).
No products indexed under this heading.

Clorazepate Dipotassium (Additive CNS depression). Products include:
Tranxene ... 459

Clozapine (Additive CNS depression). Products include:
Clozaril Tablets ... 2377

Codeine Phosphate (Additive CNS depression). Products include:
Brontex ... 2130
Dimetane-DC Cough Syrup ... 2232
Fioricet with Codeine Capsules ... 2387
Fiorinal with Codeine Capsules ... 2390
Nucofed ... 2225
Phenergan with Codeine ... 2883
Phenergan VC with Codeine ... 2888
Robitussin A-C Syrup ... 2248
Robitussin-DAC Syrup ... 2249
Ryna ... 804
Soma Compound w/Codeine Tablets ... 2784
Tylenol with Codeine ... 1592

Dalteparin Sodium (Enhanced effect of anticoagulant). Products include:
Fragmin Injection ... 2088

Desflurane (Additive CNS depression). Products include:
Suprane (desflurane, USP) ... 1865

Dezocine (Additive CNS depression). Products include:
Dalgan Injection ... 529

Diazepam (Additive CNS depression). Products include:
Dizac (diazepam injectable emulsion) CIV ... 1862
Valium Injectable ... 2336
Valium Tablets ... 2335

Dicumarol (Enhanced effect of anticoagulant).
No products indexed under this heading.

Droperidol (Additive CNS depression). Products include:
Inapsine Injection ... 462

Enflurane (Additive CNS depression).
No products indexed under this heading.

Enoxaparin (Enhanced effect of anticoagulant). Products include:
Lovenox Injection ... 2187

Estazolam (Additive CNS depression). Products include:
ProSom Tablets ... 457

Ethchlorvynol (Additive CNS depression). Products include:
Placidyl Capsules ... 456

Ethinamate (Additive CNS depression).
No products indexed under this heading.

Fentanyl (Additive CNS depression). Products include:
Duragesic Transdermal System ... 1336

Fentanyl Citrate (Additive CNS depression). Products include:
Sublimaze Injection ... 463

Fluphenazine Decanoate (Additive CNS depression). Products include:
Prolixin Decanoate ... 510

Fluphenazine Enanthate (Additive CNS depression). Products include:
Prolixin Enanthate ... 510

Fluphenazine Hydrochloride (Additive CNS depression). Products include:
Prolixin ... 510

Flurazepam Hydrochloride (Additive CNS depression). Products include:
Dalmane Capsules ... 2329

Glutethimide (Additive CNS depression).
No products indexed under this heading.

Haloperidol (Additive CNS depression). Products include:
Haldol Injection, Tablets and Concentrate ... 1585

Haloperidol Decanoate (Additive CNS depression). Products include:
Haldol Decanoate ... 1587

Heparin Calcium (Enhanced effect of anticoagulant).
No products indexed under this heading.

Heparin Sodium (Enhanced effect of anticoagulant). Products include:
Heparin Lock Flush Solution ... 2831
Heparin Sodium Injection ... 2832
Heparin Sodium Vials ... 1486

Hydrocodone Bitartrate (Additive CNS depression). Products include:
Codiclear DH Syrup ... 808
Duratuss HD Elixir ... 2750
Histussin D Liquid ... 670
Hycodan Tablets and Syrup ... 946
Hycomine Compound Tablets ... 948
Hycomine ... 947
Hycotuss Expectorant Syrup ... 950
Hydrocet Capsules ... 787
Lorcet 10/650 Tablets ... 1016
Lortab ... 2751
Tussend ... 1830
Tussend Expectorant ... 1831
Vicodin Tablets ... 1404
Vicodin ES Tablets ... 1405
Vicodin HP Tablets ... 1403
Vicodin Tuss Expectorant ... 1406
Zydone Capsules ... 967

Hydrocodone Polistirex (Additive CNS depression). Products include:
Tussionex Pennkinetic Extended-Release Suspension ... 1624

Hydromorphone Hydrochloride (Additive CNS depression). Products include:
Dilaudid Ampules ... 1382
Dilaudid Cough Syrup ... 1383
Dilaudid-HP Injection ... 1384
Dilaudid-HP Lyophilized Powder 250 mg ... 1384
Dilaudid ... 1382
Dilaudid Oral Liquid ... 1386
Dilaudid ... 1382
Dilaudid Tablets - 8 mg ... 1386

Hydroxyzine Hydrochloride (Additive CNS depression). Products include:
Atarax Tablets & Syrup ... 1992
Marax Tablets & DF Syrup ... 2015
Vistaril Intramuscular Solution ... 2042

Isoflurane (Additive CNS depression).
No products indexed under this heading.

Ketamine Hydrochloride (Additive CNS depression).
No products indexed under this heading.

Levomethadyl Acetate Hydrochloride (Additive CNS depression). Products include:
Orlaam Oral Solution ... 2361

Levorphanol Tartrate (Additive CNS depression). Products include:
Levo-Dromoran ... 2297

Lorazepam (Additive CNS depression). Products include:
Ativan Injection ... 2805
Ativan Tablets ... 2807

Loxapine Hydrochloride (Additive CNS depression). Products include:
Loxitane ... 1426

Loxapine Succinate (Additive CNS depression). Products include:
Loxitane Capsules ... 1426

Meperidine Hydrochloride (Additive CNS depression). Products include:
Demerol ... 2438
Mepergan Injection ... 2859

Mephobarbital (Additive CNS depression). Products include:
Mebaral Tablets ... 2452

Meprobamate (Additive CNS depression). Products include:
Miltown Tablets ... 2780
PMB 200 and PMB 400 ... 2890

Mesoridazine Besylate (Additive CNS depression). Products include:
Serentil ... 689

Methadone Hydrochloride (Additive CNS depression). Products include:
Methadone Hydrochloride Oral Concentrate ... 2356
Methadone Hydrochloride Oral Solution & Tablets ... 2357

Methohexital Sodium (Additive CNS depression).
No products indexed under this heading.

Methotrimeprazine (Additive CNS depression). Products include:
Levoprome ... 1321

Methoxyflurane (Additive CNS depression).
No products indexed under this heading.

Midazolam Hydrochloride (Additive CNS depression). Products include:
Versed Injection ... 2324

Molindone Hydrochloride (Additive CNS depression). Products include:
Moban Tablets and Concentrate ... 1036

Morphine Sulfate (Additive CNS depression). Products include:
Astramorph/PF Injection, USP (Preservative-Free) ... 526
Duramorph Injection ... 983
Infumorph 200 and Infumorph 500 Sterile Solutions ... 985
Kadian Capsules ... 2948
MS Contin Tablets ... 2149
MSIR ... 2152
Oramorph SR (Morphine Sulfate Sustained Release Tablets) ... 2359
RMS Suppositories CII ... 2766
Roxanol ... 2365

Opium Alkaloids (Additive CNS depression).
No products indexed under this heading.

Oxazepam (Additive CNS depression). Products include:
Serax Capsules ... 2916
Serax Tablets ... 2916

Pentobarbital Sodium (Additive CNS depression). Products include:
Nembutal Sodium Capsules ... 440
Nembutal Sodium Solution ... 442
Nembutal Sodium Suppositories ... 444

Perphenazine (Additive CNS depression). Products include:
Etrafon ... 2495
Triavil Tablets ... 1800
Trilafon ... 2532

Phenobarbital (Additive CNS depression). Products include:
Arco-Lase Plus Tablets ... 513
Bellergal-S Tablets ... 2375
Donnatal ... 2234
Donnatal Extentabs ... 2234
Donnatal Tablets ... 2234
Phenobarbital Elixir and Tablets ... 1523
Quadrinal Tablets ... 1398

Prazepam (Additive CNS depression).
No products indexed under this heading.

Probenecid (Aspirin may inhibit the uricosuric effects). Products include:
Benemid Tablets ... 1651
ColBENEMID Tablets ... 1662

Prochlorperazine (Additive CNS depression). Products include:
Compazine ... 2644

Promethazine Hydrochloride (Additive CNS depression). Products include:
Mepergan Injection ... 2859
Phenergan with Codeine ... 2883
Phenergan with Dextromethorphan 2885
Phenergan Injection ... 2880
Phenergan Suppositories ... 2882
Phenergan Syrup ... 2881
Phenergan Tablets ... 2882
Phenergan VC ... 2886
Phenergan VC with Codeine ... 2888

Propofol (Additive CNS depression). Products include:
Diprivan Injectable Emulsion ... 2939

Propoxyphene Hydrochloride (Additive CNS depression). Products include:
Darvon ... 1475
Wygesic Tablets ... 2930

Propoxyphene Napsylate (Additive CNS depression). Products include:
Darvon-N/Darvocet-N ... 1473

Quazepam (Additive CNS depression). Products include:
Doral Tablets ... 2773

Risperidone (Additive CNS depression). Products include:
Risperdal Tablets ... 1348

Secobarbital Sodium (Additive CNS depression). Products include:
Seconal Sodium Pulvules ... 1529

Sevoflurane (Additive CNS depression).
No products indexed under this heading.

Sufentanil Citrate (Additive CNS depression). Products include:
Sufenta Injection ... 1355

Sulfinpyrazone (Aspirin may inhibit the uricosuric effects). Products include:
Anturane ... 823

Temazepam (Additive CNS depression). Products include:
Restoril Capsules ... 2413

Thiamylal Sodium (Additive CNS depression).
No products indexed under this heading.

Thioridazine Hydrochloride (Additive CNS depression). Products include:
Mellaril ... 2398

Thiothixene (Additive CNS depression). Products include:
Navane Capsules and Concentrate 2018
Navane Intramuscular ... 2019

IMPORTANT NOTE: Always consult each drug listing in the patient's regimen for possible interactions.

Percodan / Interactions Index

Triazolam (Additive CNS depression). Products include:
- Halcion Tablets 2093

Trifluoperazine Hydrochloride (Additive CNS depression). Products include:
- Stelazine 2692

Warfarin Sodium (Enhanced effect of anticoagulant). Products include:
- Coumadin 941

Zolpidem Tartrate (Additive CNS depression). Products include:
- Ambien Tablets 2559

Food Interactions
Alcohol (Additive CNS depression).

PERCODAN-DEMI TABLETS
(Oxycodone Hydrochloride, Oxycodone Terephthalate, Aspirin) 956
May interact with central nervous system depressants, anticoagulants, antigout agents, general anesthetics, hypnotics and sedatives, tranquilizers, phenothiazines, and certain other agents. Compounds in these categories include:

Alfentanil Hydrochloride (CNS depressant effects of Percodan-Demi may be additive). Products include:
- Alfenta Injection 1334

Allopurinol (Aspirin inhibits the uricosuric effect of uricosuric agents). Products include:
- Zyloprim Tablets 1194

Alprazolam (CNS depressant effects of Percodan-Demi may be additive). Products include:
- Xanax Tablets 2115

Aprobarbital (CNS depressant effects of Percodan-Demi may be additive).
- No products indexed under this heading.

Buprenorphine (CNS depressant effects of Percodan-Demi may be additive). Products include:
- Buprenex Injectable 2170

Buspirone Hydrochloride (CNS depressant effects of Percodan-Demi may be additive). Products include:
- BuSpar Tablets 738

Butabarbital (CNS depressant effects of Percodan-Demi may be additive).
- No products indexed under this heading.

Butalbital (CNS depressant effects of Percodan-Demi may be additive). Products include:
- Axocet Capsules 2469
- Esgic-plus Capsules 1012
- Esgic-plus Tablets 1012
- Fioricet Tablets 2386
- Fioricet with Codeine Capsules 2387
- Fiorinal Capsules 2388
- Fiorinal with Codeine Capsules 2390
- Fiorinal Tablets 2388
- Phrenilin 790
- Sedapap Tablets 50 mg/650 mg .. 1826

Chlordiazepoxide (CNS depressant effects of Percodan-Demi may be additive). Products include:
- Limbitrol 2333

Chlordiazepoxide Hydrochloride (CNS depressant effects of Percodan-Demi may be additive). Products include:
- Librax Capsules 2330
- Librium Capsules 2331
- Librium Injectable 2332

Chlorpromazine (CNS depressant effects of Percodan-Demi may be additive). Products include:
- Thorazine Suppositories 2701

Chlorpromazine Hydrochloride (CNS depressant effects of Percodan-Demi may be additive). Products include:
- Thorazine 2701

Chlorprothixene (CNS depressant effects of Percodan-Demi may be additive).
- No products indexed under this heading.

Chlorprothixene Hydrochloride (CNS depressant effects of Percodan-Demi may be additive).
- No products indexed under this heading.

Chlorprothixene Lactate (CNS depressant effects of Percodan-Demi may be additive).
- No products indexed under this heading.

Clorazepate Dipotassium (CNS depressant effects of Percodan-Demi may be additive). Products include:
- Tranxene 459

Clozapine (CNS depressant effects of Percodan-Demi may be additive). Products include:
- Clozaril Tablets 2377

Codeine Phosphate (CNS depressant effects of Percodan-Demi may be additive). Products include:
- Brontex 2130
- Dimetane-DC Cough Syrup 2232
- Fioricet with Codeine Capsules 2387
- Fiorinal with Codeine Capsules 2390
- Nucofed 2225
- Phenergan with Codeine 2883
- Phenergan VC with Codeine 2888
- Robitussin A-C Syrup 2248
- Robitussin-DAC Syrup 2249
- Ryna .... ⊠ 804
- Soma Compound w/Codeine Tablets 2784
- Tylenol with Codeine 1592

Dalteparin Sodium (Enhanced effect of anticoagulants). Products include:
- Fragmin Injection 2088

Desflurane (CNS depressant effects of Percodan-Demi may be additive). Products include:
- Suprane (desflurane, USP) .. 1865

Dezocine (CNS depressant effects of Percodan-Demi may be additive). Products include:
- Dalgan Injection 529

Diazepam (CNS depressant effects of Percodan-Demi may be additive). Products include:
- Dizac (diazepam injectable emulsion) CIV 1862
- Valium Injectable 2336
- Valium Tablets 2335

Dicumarol (Enhanced effect of anticoagulants).
- No products indexed under this heading.

Droperidol (CNS depressant effects of Percodan-Demi may be additive). Products include:
- Inapsine Injection 462

Enflurane (CNS depressant effects of Percodan-Demi may be additive).
- No products indexed under this heading.

Enoxaparin (Enhanced effect of anticoagulants). Products include:
- Lovenox Injection 2187

Estazolam (CNS depressant effects of Percodan-Demi may be additive). Products include:
- ProSom Tablets 457

Ethchlorvynol (CNS depressant effects of Percodan-Demi may be additive). Products include:
- Placidyl Capsules 456

Ethinamate (CNS depressant effects of Percodan-Demi may be additive).
- No products indexed under this heading.

Fentanyl (CNS depressant effects of Percodan-Demi may be additive). Products include:
- Duragesic Transdermal System 1336

Fentanyl Citrate (CNS depressant effects of Percodan-Demi may be additive). Products include:
- Sublimaze Injection 463

Fluphenazine Decanoate (CNS depressant effects of Percodan-Demi may be additive). Products include:
- Prolixin Decanoate 510

Fluphenazine Enanthate (CNS depressant effects of Percodan-Demi may be additive). Products include:
- Prolixin Enanthate 510

Fluphenazine Hydrochloride (CNS depressant effects of Percodan-Demi may be additive). Products include:
- Prolixin 510

Flurazepam Hydrochloride (CNS depressant effects of Percodan-Demi may be additive). Products include:
- Dalmane Capsules 2329

Glutethimide (CNS depressant effects of Percodan-Demi may be additive).
- No products indexed under this heading.

Haloperidol (CNS depressant effects of Percodan-Demi may be additive). Products include:
- Haldol Injection, Tablets and Concentrate 1585

Haloperidol Decanoate (CNS depressant effects of Percodan-Demi may be additive). Products include:
- Haldol Decanoate 1587

Heparin Calcium (Enhanced effect of anticoagulants).
- No products indexed under this heading.

Heparin Sodium (Enhanced effect of anticoagulants). Products include:
- Heparin Lock Flush Solution 2831
- Heparin Sodium Injection 2832
- Heparin Sodium Vials 1486

Hydrocodone Bitartrate (CNS depressant effects of Percodan-Demi may be additive). Products include:
- Codiclear DH Syrup 808
- Duratuss HD Elixir 2750
- Histussin D Liquid 670
- Hycodan Tablets and Syrup 946
- Hycomine Compound Tablets 948
- Hycomine 947
- Hycotuss Expectorant Syrup 950
- Hydrocet Capsules 787
- Lorcet 10/650 Tablets 1016
- Lortab 2751
- Tussend 1830
- Tussend Expectorant 1831
- Vicodin Tablets 1404
- Vicodin ES Tablets 1405
- Vicodin HP Tablets 1403
- Vicodin Tuss Expectorant .. 1406
- Zydone Capsules 967

Hydrocodone Polistirex (CNS depressant effects of Percodan-Demi may be additive). Products include:
- Tussionex Pennkinetic Extended-Release Suspension 1624

Hydroxyzine Hydrochloride (CNS depressant effects of Percodan-Demi may be additive). Products include:
- Atarax Tablets & Syrup 1992
- Marax Tablets & DF Syrup 2015
- Vistaril Intramuscular Solution 2042

Isoflurane (CNS depressant effects of Percodan-Demi may be additive).
- No products indexed under this heading.

Ketamine Hydrochloride (CNS depressant effects of Percodan-Demi may be additive).
- No products indexed under this heading.

Levomethadyl Acetate Hydrochloride (CNS depressant effects of Percodan-Demi may be additive). Products include:
- Orlaam Oral Solution 2361

Levorphanol Tartrate (CNS depressant effects of Percodan-Demi may be additive). Products include:
- Levo-Dromoran 2297

Lorazepam (CNS depressant effects of Percodan-Demi may be additive). Products include:
- Ativan Injection 2805
- Ativan Tablets 2807

Loxapine Hydrochloride (CNS depressant effects of Percodan-Demi may be additive). Products include:
- Loxitane 1426

Loxapine Succinate (CNS depressant effects of Percodan-Demi may be additive). Products include:
- Loxitane Capsules 1426

Meperidine Hydrochloride (CNS depressant effects of Percodan-Demi may be additive). Products include:
- Demerol 2438
- Mepergan Injection 2859

Mephobarbital (CNS depressant effects of Percodan-Demi may be additive). Products include:
- Mebaral Tablets 2452

Meprobamate (CNS depressant effects of Percodan-Demi may be additive). Products include:
- Miltown Tablets 2780
- PMB 200 and PMB 400 2890

Mesoridazine Besylate (CNS depressant effects of Percodan-Demi may be additive). Products include:
- Serentil 689

Methadone Hydrochloride (CNS depressant effects of Percodan-Demi may be additive). Products include:
- Methadone Hydrochloride Oral Concentrate 2356
- Methadone Hydrochloride Oral Solution & Tablets 2357

Methohexital Sodium (CNS depressant effects of Percodan-Demi may be additive).
- No products indexed under this heading.

Methotrimeprazine (CNS depressant effects of Percodan-Demi may be additive). Products include:
- Levoprome 1321

Methoxyflurane (CNS depressant effects of Percodan-Demi may be additive).
- No products indexed under this heading.

Midazolam Hydrochloride (CNS depressant effects of Percodan-Demi may be additive). Products include:
- Versed Injection 2324

Molindone Hydrochloride (CNS depressant effects of Percodan-Demi may be additive). Products include:
- Moban Tablets and Concentrate 1036

Morphine Sulfate (CNS depressant effects of Percodan-Demi may be additive). Products include:
- Astramorph/PF Injection, USP (Preservative-Free) 526
- Duramorph Injection 983
- Infumorph 200 and Infumorph 500 Sterile Solutions 985
- Kadian Capsules 2948
- MS Contin Tablets 2149
- MSIR 2152
- Oramorph SR (Morphine Sulfate Sustained Release Tablets) ... 2359
- RMS Suppositories CII 2766
- Roxanol 2365

(⊠ Described in PDR For Nonprescription Drugs)   (⊙ Described in PDR For Ophthalmology)

Opium Alkaloids (CNS depressant effects of Percodan-Demi may be additive).
No products indexed under this heading.

Oxazepam (CNS depressant effects of Percodan-Demi may be additive). Products include:
Serax Capsules ... 2916
Serax Tablets ... 2916

Pentobarbital Sodium (CNS depressant effects of Percodan-Demi may be additive). Products include:
Nembutal Sodium Capsules ... 440
Nembutal Sodium Solution ... 442
Nembutal Sodium Suppositories ... 444

Perphenazine (CNS depressant effects of Percodan-Demi may be additive). Products include:
Etrafon ... 2495
Triavil Tablets ... 1800
Trilafon ... 2532

Phenobarbital (CNS depressant effects of Percodan-Demi may be additive). Products include:
Arco-Lase Plus Tablets ... 513
Bellergal-S Tablets ... 2375
Donnatal ... 2234
Donnatal Extentabs ... 2234
Donnatal Tablets ... 2234
Phenobarbital Elixir and Tablets ... 1523
Quadrinal Tablets ... 1398

Prazepam (CNS depressant effects of Percodan-Demi may be additive).
No products indexed under this heading.

Probenecid (Aspirin inhibits the uricosuric effect of uricosuric agents). Products include:
Benemid Tablets ... 1651
ColBENEMID Tablets ... 1662

Prochlorperazine (CNS depressant effects of Percodan-Demi may be additive). Products include:
Compazine ... 2644

Promethazine Hydrochloride (CNS depressant effects of Percodan-Demi may be additive). Products include:
Mepergan Injection ... 2859
Phenergan with Codeine ... 2883
Phenergan with Dextromethorphan 2885
Phenergan Injection ... 2880
Phenergan Suppositories ... 2882
Phenergan Syrup ... 2881
Phenergan Tablets ... 2882
Phenergan VC ... 2886
Phenergan VC with Codeine ... 2888

Propofol (CNS depressant effects of Percodan-Demi may be additive). Products include:
Diprivan Injectable Emulsion ... 2939

Propoxyphene Hydrochloride (CNS depressant effects of Percodan-Demi may be additive). Products include:
Darvon ... 1475
Wygesic Tablets ... 2930

Propoxyphene Napsylate (CNS depressant effects of Percodan-Demi may be additive). Products include:
Darvon-N/Darvocet-N ... 1473

Quazepam (CNS depressant effects of Percodan-Demi may be additive). Products include:
Doral Tablets ... 2773

Risperidone (CNS depressant effects of Percodan-Demi may be additive). Products include:
Risperdal Tablets ... 1348

Secobarbital Sodium (CNS depressant effects of Percodan-Demi may be additive). Products include:
Seconal Sodium Pulvules ... 1529

Sevoflurane (CNS depressant effects of Percodan-Demi may be additive).
No products indexed under this heading.

Sufentanil Citrate (CNS depressant effects of Percodan-Demi may be additive). Products include:
Sufenta Injection ... 1355

Sulfinpyrazone (Aspirin inhibits the uricosuric effect of uricosuric agents). Products include:
Anturane ... 823

Temazepam (CNS depressant effects of Percodan-Demi may be additive). Products include:
Restoril Capsules ... 2413

Thiamylal Sodium (CNS depressant effects of Percodan-Demi may be additive).
No products indexed under this heading.

Thioridazine Hydrochloride (CNS depressant effects of Percodan-Demi may be additive). Products include:
Mellaril ... 2398

Thiothixene (CNS depressant effects of Percodan-Demi may be additive). Products include:
Navane Capsules and Concentrate 2018
Navane Intramuscular ... 2019

Triazolam (CNS depressant effects of Percodan-Demi may be additive). Products include:
Halcion Tablets ... 2093

Trifluoperazine Hydrochloride (CNS depressant effects of Percodan-Demi may be additive). Products include:
Stelazine ... 2692

Warfarin Sodium (Enhanced effect of anticoagulants). Products include:
Coumadin ... 941

Zolpidem Tartrate (CNS depressant effects of Percodan-Demi may be additive). Products include:
Ambien Tablets ... 2559

Food Interactions

Alcohol (CNS depressant effects of Percodan-Demi may be additive).

PERCOGESIC ANALGESIC TABLETS

(Acetaminophen, Phenyltoloxamine Citrate) ... 727
May interact with tranquilizers, hypnotics and sedatives, and certain other agents. Compounds in these categories include:

Alprazolam (May increase the drowsiness effect). Products include:
Xanax Tablets ... 2115

Buspirone Hydrochloride (May increase the drowsiness effect). Products include:
BuSpar Tablets ... 738

Chlordiazepoxide (May increase the drowsiness effect). Products include:
Limbitrol ... 2333

Chlordiazepoxide Hydrochloride (May increase the drowsiness effect). Products include:
Librax Capsules ... 2330
Librium Capsules ... 2331
Librium Injectable ... 2332

Chlorpromazine (May increase the drowsiness effect). Products include:
Thorazine Suppositories ... 2701

Chlorprothixene (May increase the drowsiness effect).
No products indexed under this heading.

Chlorprothixene Hydrochloride (May increase the drowsiness effect).
No products indexed under this heading.

Clorazepate Dipotassium (May increase the drowsiness effect). Products include:
Tranxene ... 459

Diazepam (May increase the drowsiness effect). Products include:
Dizac (diazepam injectable emulsion) CIV ... 1862
Valium Injectable ... 2336
Valium Tablets ... 2335

Droperidol (May increase the drowsiness effect). Products include:
Inapsine Injection ... 462

Estazolam (May increase the drowsiness effect). Products include:
ProSom Tablets ... 457

Ethchlorvynol (May increase the drowsiness effect). Products include:
Placidyl Capsules ... 456

Ethinamate (May increase the drowsiness effect).
No products indexed under this heading.

Fluphenazine Decanoate (May increase the drowsiness effect). Products include:
Prolixin Decanoate ... 510

Fluphenazine Enanthate (May increase the drowsiness effect). Products include:
Prolixin Enanthate ... 510

Fluphenazine Hydrochloride (May increase the drowsiness effect). Products include:
Prolixin ... 510

Flurazepam Hydrochloride (May increase the drowsiness effect). Products include:
Dalmane Capsules ... 2329

Glutethimide (May increase the drowsiness effect).
No products indexed under this heading.

Haloperidol (May increase the drowsiness effect). Products include:
Haldol Injection, Tablets and Concentrate ... 1585

Haloperidol Decanoate (May increase the drowsiness effect). Products include:
Haldol Decanoate ... 1587

Hydroxyzine Hydrochloride (May increase the drowsiness effect). Products include:
Atarax Tablets & Syrup ... 1992
Marax Tablets & DF Syrup ... 2015
Vistaril Intramuscular Solution ... 2042

Lorazepam (May increase the drowsiness effect). Products include:
Ativan Injection ... 2805
Ativan Tablets ... 2807

Loxapine Hydrochloride (May increase the drowsiness effect). Products include:
Loxitane ... 1426

Loxapine Succinate (May increase the drowsiness effect). Products include:
Loxitane Capsules ... 1426

Meprobamate (May increase the drowsiness effect). Products include:
Miltown Tablets ... 2780
PMB 200 and PMB 400 ... 2890

Mesoridazine Besylate (May increase the drowsiness effect). Products include:
Serentil ... 689

Midazolam Hydrochloride (May increase the drowsiness effect). Products include:
Versed Injection ... 2324

Molindone Hydrochloride (May increase the drowsiness effect). Products include:
Moban Tablets and Concentrate ... 1036

Oxazepam (May increase the drowsiness effect). Products include:
Serax Capsules ... 2916
Serax Tablets ... 2916

Perphenazine (May increase the drowsiness effect). Products include:
Etrafon ... 2495
Triavil Tablets ... 1800
Trilafon ... 2532

Prazepam (May increase the drowsiness effect).
No products indexed under this heading.

Prochlorperazine (May increase the drowsiness effect). Products include:
Compazine ... 2644

Promethazine Hydrochloride (May increase the drowsiness effect). Products include:
Mepergan Injection ... 2859
Phenergan with Codeine ... 2883
Phenergan with Dextromethorphan 2885
Phenergan Injection ... 2880
Phenergan Suppositories ... 2882
Phenergan Syrup ... 2881
Phenergan Tablets ... 2882
Phenergan VC ... 2886
Phenergan VC with Codeine ... 2888

Propofol (May increase the drowsiness effect). Products include:
Diprivan Injectable Emulsion ... 2939

Quazepam (May increase the drowsiness effect). Products include:
Doral Tablets ... 2773

Secobarbital Sodium (May increase the drowsiness effect). Products include:
Seconal Sodium Pulvules ... 1529

Temazepam (May increase the drowsiness effect). Products include:
Restoril Capsules ... 2413

Thioridazine Hydrochloride (May increase the drowsiness effect). Products include:
Mellaril ... 2398

Thiothixene (May increase the drowsiness effect). Products include:
Navane Capsules and Concentrate 2018
Navane Intramuscular ... 2019

Triazolam (May increase the drowsiness effect). Products include:
Halcion Tablets ... 2093

Trifluoperazine Hydrochloride (May increase the drowsiness effect). Products include:
Stelazine ... 2692

Zolpidem Tartrate (May increase the drowsiness effect). Products include:
Ambien Tablets ... 2559

Food Interactions

Alcohol (May increase the drowsiness effect).

PERDIEM

(Psyllium Preparations, Senna Concentrates) ... 889
None cited in PDR database.

PERDIEM FIBER

(Psyllium Preparations) ... 889
None cited in PDR database.

PERGONAL (MENOTROPINS FOR INJECTION, USP)

(Menotropins) ... 2618
None cited in PDR database.

PERIACTIN SYRUP

(Cyproheptadine Hydrochloride) ... 1767
May interact with central nervous system depressants and monoamine oxidase inhibitors. Compounds in these categories include:

Alfentanil Hydrochloride (Additive effects). Products include:

IMPORTANT NOTE: Always consult each drug listing in the patient's regimen for possible interactions.

Periactin — Interactions Index

Alfenta Injection 1334
Alprazolam (Additive effects). Products include:
  Xanax Tablets 2115
Aprobarbital (Additive effects). No products indexed under this heading.
Buprenorphine (Additive effects). Products include:
  Buprenex Injectable 2170
Buspirone Hydrochloride (Additive effects). Products include:
  BuSpar Tablets 738
Butabarbital (Additive effects). No products indexed under this heading.
Butalbital (Additive effects). Products include:
  Axocet Capsules 2469
  Esgic-plus Capsules 1012
  Esgic-plus Tablets 1012
  Fioricet Tablets 2386
  Fioricet with Codeine Capsules 2387
  Fiorinal Capsules 2388
  Fiorinal with Codeine Capsules 2390
  Fiorinal Tablets 2388
  Phrenilin 790
  Sedapap Tablets 50 mg/650 mg .. 1826
Chlordiazepoxide (Additive effects). Products include:
  Limbitrol 2333
Chlordiazepoxide Hydrochloride (Additive effects). Products include:
  Librax Capsules 2330
  Librium Capsules 2331
  Librium Injectable 2332
Chlorpromazine (Additive effects). Products include:
  Thorazine Suppositories 2701
Chlorprothixene (Additive effects). No products indexed under this heading.
Chlorprothixene Hydrochloride (Additive effects). No products indexed under this heading.
Chlorprothixene Lactate (Additive effects). No products indexed under this heading.
Clorazepate Dipotassium (Additive effects). Products include:
  Tranxene 459
Clozapine (Additive effects). Products include:
  Clozaril Tablets 2377
Codeine Phosphate (Additive effects). Products include:
  Brontex 2130
  Dimetane-DC Cough Syrup 2232
  Fioricet with Codeine Capsules 2387
  Fiorinal with Codeine Capsules 2390
  Nucofed 2225
  Phenergan with Codeine 2883
  Phenergan VC with Codeine 2888
  Robitussin A-C Syrup 2248
  Robitussin-DAC Syrup 2249
  Ryna .... ▣ 804
  Soma Compound w/Codeine Tablets 2784
  Tylenol with Codeine 1592
Desflurane (Additive effects). Products include:
  Suprane (desflurane, USP) 1865
Dezocine (Additive effects). Products include:
  Dalgan Injection 529
Diazepam (Additive effects). Products include:
  Dizac (diazepam injectable emulsion) CIV 1862
  Valium Injectable 2336
  Valium Tablets 2335
Droperidol (Additive effects). Products include:
  Inapsine Injection 462

Enflurane (Additive effects). No products indexed under this heading.
Estazolam (Additive effects). Products include:
  ProSom Tablets 457
Ethchlorvynol (Additive effects). Products include:
  Placidyl Capsules 456
Ethinamate (Additive effects). No products indexed under this heading.
Fentanyl (Additive effects). Products include:
  Duragesic Transdermal System 1336
Fentanyl Citrate (Additive effects). Products include:
  Sublimaze Injection 463
Fluphenazine Decanoate (Additive effects). Products include:
  Prolixin Decanoate 510
Fluphenazine Enanthate (Additive effects). Products include:
  Prolixin Enanthate 510
Fluphenazine Hydrochloride (Additive effects). Products include:
  Prolixin 510
Flurazepam Hydrochloride (Additive effects). Products include:
  Dalmane Capsules 2329
Furazolidone (Contraindication; anticholinergic effects of antihistamines prolonged and intensified). Products include:
  Furoxone 2221
Glutethimide (Additive effects). No products indexed under this heading.
Haloperidol (Additive effects). Products include:
  Haldol Injection, Tablets and Concentrate 1585
Haloperidol Decanoate (Additive effects). Products include:
  Haldol Decanoate 1587
Hydrocodone Bitartrate (Additive effects). Products include:
  Codiclear DH Syrup 808
  Duratuss HD Elixir 2750
  Histussin D Liquid 670
  Hycodan Tablets and Syrup 946
  Hycomine Compound Tablets 948
  Hycomine 947
  Hycotuss Expectorant Syrup 950
  Hydrocet Capsules 787
  Lorcet 10/650 Tablets 1016
  Lortab 2751
  Tussend 1830
  Tussend Expectorant 1831
  Vicodin Tablets 1404
  Vicodin ES Tablets 1405
  Vicodin HP Tablets 1403
  Vicodin Tuss Expectorant 1406
  Zydone Capsules 967
Hydrocodone Polistirex (Additive effects). Products include:
  Tussionex Pennkinetic Extended-Release Suspension 1624
Hydroxyzine Hydrochloride (Additive effects). Products include:
  Atarax Tablets & Syrup 1992
  Marax Tablets & DF Syrup 2015
  Vistaril Intramuscular Solution 2042
Isocarboxazid (Contraindication; anticholinergic effects of antihistamines prolonged and intensified). No products indexed under this heading.
Isoflurane (Additive effects). No products indexed under this heading.
Ketamine Hydrochloride (Additive effects). No products indexed under this heading.
Levomethadyl Acetate Hydrochloride (Additive effects). Products include:
  Orlaam Oral Solution 2361

Levorphanol Tartrate (Additive effects). Products include:
  Levo-Dromoran 2297
Lorazepam (Additive effects). Products include:
  Ativan Injection 2805
  Ativan Tablets 2807
Loxapine Hydrochloride (Additive effects). Products include:
  Loxitane 1426
Loxapine Succinate (Additive effects). Products include:
  Loxitane Capsules 1426
Meperidine Hydrochloride (Additive effects). Products include:
  Demerol 2438
  Mepergan Injection 2859
Mephobarbital (Additive effects). Products include:
  Mebaral Tablets 2452
Meprobamate (Additive effects). Products include:
  Miltown Tablets 2780
  PMB 200 and PMB 400 2890
Mesoridazine Besylate (Additive effects). Products include:
  Serentil 689
Methadone Hydrochloride (Additive effects). Products include:
  Methadone Hydrochloride Oral Concentrate 2356
  Methadone Hydrochloride Oral Solution & Tablets 2357
Methohexital Sodium (Additive effects). No products indexed under this heading.
Methotrimeprazine (Additive effects). Products include:
  Levoprome 1321
Methoxyflurane (Additive effects). No products indexed under this heading.
Midazolam Hydrochloride (Additive effects). Products include:
  Versed Injection 2324
Molindone Hydrochloride (Additive effects). Products include:
  Moban Tablets and Concentrate 1036
Morphine Sulfate (Additive effects). Products include:
  Astramorph/PF Injection, USP (Preservative-Free) 526
  Duramorph Injection 983
  Infumorph 200 and Infumorph 500 Sterile Solutions 985
  Kadian Capsules 2948
  MS Contin Tablets 2149
  MSIR 2152
  Oramorph SR (Morphine Sulfate Sustained Release Tablets) 2359
  RMS Suppositories CII 2766
  Roxanol 2365
Opium Alkaloids (Additive effects). No products indexed under this heading.
Oxazepam (Additive effects). Products include:
  Serax Capsules 2916
  Serax Tablets 2916
Oxycodone Hydrochloride (Additive effects). Products include:
  OxyContin Tablets 2163
  OxyIR Capsules 2167
  Percocet Tablets 955
  Percodan Tablets 955
  Percodan-Demi Tablets 956
  Roxicodone Tablets, Oral Solution & Intensol (Oxycodone) 2366
  Tylox Capsules 1593
Pentobarbital Sodium (Additive effects). Products include:
  Nembutal Sodium Capsules 440
  Nembutal Sodium Solution 442
  Nembutal Sodium Suppositories 444
Perphenazine (Additive effects). Products include:
  Etrafon 2495

  Triavil Tablets 1800
  Trilafon 2532
Phenelzine Sulfate (Contraindication; anticholinergic effects of antihistamines prolonged and intensified). Products include:
  Nardil 1977
Phenobarbital (Additive effects). Products include:
  Arco-Lase Plus Tablets 513
  Bellergal-S Tablets 2375
  Donnatal 2234
  Donnatal Extentabs 2234
  Donnatal Tablets 2234
  Phenobarbital Elixir and Tablets 1523
  Quadrinal Tablets 1398
Prazepam (Additive effects). No products indexed under this heading.
Prochlorperazine (Additive effects). Products include:
  Compazine 2644
Promethazine Hydrochloride (Additive effects). Products include:
  Mepergan Injection 2859
  Phenergan with Codeine 2883
  Phenergan with Dextromethorphan 2885
  Phenergan Injection 2882
  Phenergan Suppositories 2882
  Phenergan Syrup 2881
  Phenergan Tablets 2882
  Phenergan VC 2886
  Phenergan VC with Codeine 2888
Propofol (Additive effects). Products include:
  Diprivan Injectable Emulsion 2939
Propoxyphene Hydrochloride (Additive effects). Products include:
  Darvon 1475
  Wygesic Tablets 2930
Propoxyphene Napsylate (Additive effects). Products include:
  Darvon-N/Darvocet-N 1473
Quazepam (Additive effects). Products include:
  Doral Tablets 2773
Risperidone (Additive effects). Products include:
  Risperdal Tablets 1348
Secobarbital Sodium (Additive effects). Products include:
  Seconal Sodium Pulvules 1529
Selegiline Hydrochloride (Contraindication; anticholinergic effects of antihistamines prolonged and intensified). Products include:
  Eldepryl Capsules 2729
Sevoflurane (Additive effects). No products indexed under this heading.
Sufentanil Citrate (Additive effects). Products include:
  Sufenta Injection 1355
Temazepam (Additive effects). Products include:
  Restoril Capsules 2413
Thiamylal Sodium (Additive effects). No products indexed under this heading.
Thioridazine Hydrochloride (Additive effects). Products include:
  Mellaril 2398
Thiothixene (Additive effects). Products include:
  Navane Capsules and Concentrate 2018
  Navane Intramuscular 2019
Tranylcypromine Sulfate (Contraindication; anticholinergic effects of antihistamines prolonged and intensified). Products include:
  Parnate Tablets 2679
Triazolam (Additive effects). Products include:
  Halcion Tablets 2093
Trifluoperazine Hydrochloride (Additive effects). Products include:
  Stelazine 2692

(▣ Described in PDR For Nonprescription Drugs)   (◎ Described in PDR For Ophthalmology)

Zolpidem Tartrate (Additive effects). Products include:
  Ambien Tablets............................. 2559

Food Interactions
Alcohol (Additive effects).

PERIACTIN TABLETS
(Cyproheptadine Hydrochloride) 1767
See **Periactin Syrup**

PERI-COLACE CAPSULES AND SYRUP
(Casanthranol, Docusate Sodium).....2226
None cited in PDR database.

PERIDEX
(Chlorhexidine Gluconate) 2127
None cited in PDR database.

PERIOGARD ORAL RINSE
(Chlorhexidine Gluconate) 892
None cited in PDR database.

PERMAX TABLETS
(Pergolide Mesylate) 571
May interact with dopamine antagonists, highly protein bound drugs (selected), and certain other agents. Compounds in these categories include:

Amiodarone Hydrochloride (Caution should be exercised if coadministered). Products include:
  Cordarone Intravenous 2821
  Cordarone Tablets........................... 2818

Amitriptyline Hydrochloride (Caution should be exercised if coadministered). Products include:
  Elavil 2945
  Etrafon 2495
  Limbitrol 2333
  Triavil Tablets 1800

Atovaquone (Caution should be exercised if coadministered). Products include:
  Mepron Suspension 1206

Cefonicid Sodium (Caution should be exercised if coadministered). Products include:
  Monocid Injection 2674

Chlordiazepoxide (Caution should be exercised if coadministered). Products include:
  Limbitrol 2333

Chlordiazepoxide Hydrochloride (Caution should be exercised if coadministered). Products include:
  Librax Capsules 2330
  Librium Capsules 2331
  Librium Injectable 2332

Chlorpromazine (May diminish the effectiveness of Permax; caution should be exercised if coadministered). Products include:
  Thorazine Suppositories 2701

Clomipramine Hydrochloride (Caution should be exercised if coadministered). Products include:
  Anafranil Capsules 819

Clozapine (May diminish the effectiveness of Permax). Products include:
  Clozaril Tablets 2377

Cyclosporine (Caution should be exercised if coadministered). Products include:
  Neoral 2405
  Sandimmune 2416

Diazepam (Caution should be exercised if coadministered). Products include:
  Dizac (diazepam injectable emulsion) CIV 1862
  Valium Injectable 2336
  Valium Tablets 2335

Diclofenac Potassium (Caution should be exercised if coadministered). Products include:
  Cataflam Tablets 833

Diclofenac Sodium (Caution should be exercised if coadministered). Products include:
  Voltaren Ophthalmic Sterile Ophthalmic Solution .... ⊚ 264
  Cataflam/Voltaren/Voltaren-XR 833

Dipyridamole (Caution should be exercised if coadministered). Products include:
  Persantine Tablets 686

Fenoprofen Calcium (Caution should be exercised if coadministered). Products include:
  Nalfon 200 Pulvules & Nalfon Tablets 933

Fluphenazine Decanoate (May diminish the effectiveness of Permax). Products include:
  Prolixin Decanoate 510

Fluphenazine Enanthate (May diminish the effectiveness of Permax). Products include:
  Prolixin Enanthate 510

Fluphenazine Hydrochloride (May diminish the effectiveness of Permax). Products include:
  Prolixin 510

Flurazepam Hydrochloride (Caution should be exercised if coadministered). Products include:
  Dalmane Capsules 2329

Flurbiprofen (Caution should be exercised if coadministered).
  No products indexed under this heading.

Glipizide (Caution should be exercised if coadministered). Products include:
  Glucotrol Tablets 2011
  Glucotrol XL Extended Release Tablets 2012

Haloperidol (May diminish the effectiveness of Permax). Products include:
  Haldol Injection, Tablets and Concentrate 1585

Haloperidol Decanoate (May diminish the effectiveness of Permax). Products include:
  Haldol Decanoate 1587

Ibuprofen (Caution should be exercised if coadministered). Products include:
  Advil Cold and Sinus Caplets and Tablets .... ⊞ 837
  Advil Ibuprofen Tablets, Caplets and Gel Caplets .... ⊞ 836
  Children's Motrin Ibuprofen Oral Suspension 1558
  IBU Tablets 1389
  Ibuprohm .... ⊞ 713
  Motrin IB Caplets, Tablets, and Gelcaps 802
  Motrin Ibuprofen Suspension, Oral Drops, Chewable Tablets, Caplets 1563
  Nuprin Ibuprofen/Analgesic Tablets & Caplets 645
  Vicks DayQuil SINUS Pressure & PAIN Relief with IBUPROFEN ..... ⊞ 735

Imipramine Hydrochloride (Caution should be exercised if coadministered). Products include:
  Tofranil Ampuls 873
  Tofranil Tablets 875

Imipramine Pamoate (Caution should be exercised if coadministered). Products include:
  Tofranil-PM Capsules 876

Indomethacin (Caution should be exercised if coadministered). Products include:
  Indocin 1723

Indomethacin Sodium Trihydrate (Caution should be exercised if coadministered). Products include:
  Indocin I.V. 1727

Ketoprofen (Caution should be exercised if coadministered). Products include:
  Actron Caplets and Tablets........ ⊞ 608
  Orudis Capsules 2874
  Orudis KT .... ⊞ 842
  Oruvail Capsules 2874

Ketorolac Tromethamine (Caution should be exercised if coadministered). Products include:
  Acular Sterile Ophthalmic Solution . 470
  Toradol 2319

Levodopa (Concomitant use may cause and/or exacerbate preexisting states of confusion and hallucination). Products include:
  Atamet Tablets 567
  Larodopa Tablets 2296
  Sinemet Tablets 959
  Sinemet CR Tablets 961

Meclofenamate Sodium (Caution should be exercised if coadministered).
  No products indexed under this heading.

Mefenamic Acid (Caution should be exercised if coadministered). Products include:
  Ponstel 1982

Mesoridazine Besylate (May diminish the effectiveness of Permax). Products include:
  Serentil 689

Metoclopramide Hydrochloride (May diminish the effectiveness of Permax). Products include:
  Reglan 2243

Midazolam Hydrochloride (Caution should be exercised if coadministered). Products include:
  Versed Injection 2324

Naproxen (Caution should be exercised if coadministered). Products include:
  Anaprox/Naprosyn 2277

Naproxen Sodium (Caution should be exercised if coadministered). Products include:
  Aleve 2124
  Anaprox/Naprosyn 2277
  Naprelan Tablets 2861

Nortriptyline Hydrochloride (Caution should be exercised if coadministered). Products include:
  Pamelor 2409

Oxaprozin (Caution should be exercised if coadministered). Products include:
  Daypro Caplets 2578

Oxazepam (Caution should be exercised if coadministered). Products include:
  Serax Capsules 2916
  Serax Tablets 2916

Perphenazine (May diminish the effectiveness of Permax). Products include:
  Etrafon 2495
  Triavil Tablets 1800
  Trilafon 2532

Phenylbutazone (Caution should be exercised if coadministered).
  No products indexed under this heading.

Pimozide (May diminish the effectiveness of Permax). Products include:
  Orap Tablets 1037

Piroxicam (Caution should be exercised if coadministered). Products include:
  Feldene Capsules 2008

Prochlorperazine (May diminish the effectiveness of Permax). Products include:
  Compazine 2644

Promethazine Hydrochloride (May diminish the effectiveness of Permax). Products include:
  Mepergan Injection 2859
  Phenergan with Codeine 2883
  Phenergan with Dextromethorphan 2885
  Phenergan Injection 2880
  Phenergan Suppositories 2882
  Phenergan Syrup 2881
  Phenergan Tablets 2882
  Phenergan VC 2886
  Phenergan VC with Codeine 2888

Propranolol Hydrochloride (Caution should be exercised if coadministered). Products include:
  Inderal 2834
  Inderal LA Long Acting Capsules 2836
  Inderide Tablets 2838
  Inderide LA Long Acting Capsules .. 2840

Sulindac (Caution should be exercised if coadministered). Products include:
  Clinoril Tablets 1658

Temazepam (Caution should be exercised if coadministered). Products include:
  Restoril Capsules 2413

Thioridazine Hydrochloride (May diminish the effectiveness of Permax). Products include:
  Mellaril 2398

Thiothixene (May diminish the effectiveness of Permax). Products include:
  Navane Capsules and Concentrate 2018
  Navane Intramuscular 2019

Tolbutamide (Caution should be exercised if coadministered).
  No products indexed under this heading.

Tolmetin Sodium (Caution should be exercised if coadministered). Products include:
  Tolectin (200, 400 and 600 mg) .. 1591

Trifluoperazine Hydrochloride (May diminish the effectiveness of Permax). Products include:
  Stelazine 2692

Trimipramine Maleate (Caution should be exercised if coadministered). Products include:
  Surmontil Capsules 2917

Warfarin Sodium (Caution should be exercised if coadministered). Products include:
  Coumadin 941

PERSANTINE TABLETS
(Dipyridamole) 686
None cited in PDR database.

PERTUSSIN ADULT EXTRA STRENGTH
(Dextromethorphan Hydrobromide) .... ⊞ 630
May interact with monoamine oxidase inhibitors. Compounds in this category include:

Furazolidone (Concurrent and/or sequential use is not recommended). Products include:
  Furoxone 2221

Isocarboxazid (Concurrent and/or sequential use is not recommended).
  No products indexed under this heading.

Phenelzine Sulfate (Concurrent and/or sequential use is not recommended). Products include:
  Nardil 1977

Selegiline Hydrochloride (Concurrent and/or sequential use is not recommended). Products include:
  Eldepryl Capsules 2729

IMPORTANT NOTE: Always consult each drug listing in the patient's regimen for possible interactions.

Interactions Index

Tranylcypromine Sulfate (Concurrent and/or sequential use is not recommended). Products include:
Parnate Tablets 2679

PERTUSSIN CHILDREN'S STRENGTH
(Dextromethorphan Hydrobromide) 630
May interact with monoamine oxidase inhibitors. Compounds in this category include:

Furazolidone (Concurrent and/or sequential use is not recommended). Products include:
Furoxone 2221

Isocarboxazid (Concurrent and/or sequential use is not recommended).
No products indexed under this heading.

Phenelzine Sulfate (Concurrent and/or sequential use is not recommended). Products include:
Nardil 1977

Selegiline Hydrochloride (Concurrent and/or sequential use is not recommended). Products include:
Eldepryl Capsules 2729

Tranylcypromine Sulfate (Concurrent and/or sequential use is not recommended). Products include:
Parnate Tablets 2679

PFIZERPEN FOR INJECTION
(Penicillin G Potassium) 2022
May interact with tetracyclines and certain other agents. Compounds in these categories include:

Demeclocycline Hydrochloride (May diminish bactericidal effects of penicillins). Products include:
Declomycin Tablets 1421

Doxycycline Calcium (May diminish bactericidal effects of penicillins). Products include:
Vibramycin Calcium Oral Suspension Syrup 2038

Doxycycline Hyclate (May diminish bactericidal effects of penicillins). Products include:
Doryx Capsules 1970
Vibramycin Hyclate Capsules 2038
Vibramycin Hyclate Intravenous 2040
Vibra-Tabs Film Coated Tablets 2038

Doxycycline Monohydrate (May diminish bactericidal effects of penicillins). Products include:
Monodox Capsules 1858
Vibramycin Monohydrate for Oral Suspension 2038

Erythromycin (May diminish bactericidal effects of penicillin). Products include:
A/T/S 2% Acne Topical Gel 1244
A/T/S 2% Acne Topical Solution 1244
Benzamycin Topical Gel 919
E-Mycin Tablets 1388
Emgel 2% Topical Gel 1081
ERYC 1972
Erycette (erythromycin 2%) Topical Solution 1943
Ery-Tab Tablets 426
Erythromycin Base Filmtab 430
Erythromycin Delayed-Release Capsules, USP 431
Ilotycin Ophthalmic Ointment 928
PCE Dispertab Tablets 453
T-Stat 2.0% Topical Solution and Pads 2797
THERAMYCIN Z 2% Solution 1629

Erythromycin Estolate (May diminish bactericidal effects of penicillin). Products include:
Ilosone 927

Erythromycin Ethylsuccinate (May diminish bactericidal effects of penicillin). Products include:
E.E.S. 427

EryPed 425
Pediazole Suspension 2340

Erythromycin Gluceptate (May diminish bactericidal effects of penicillin). Products include:
Ilotycin Gluceptate, IV, Vials 929

Erythromycin Stearate (May diminish bactericidal effects of penicillin). Products include:
Erythrocin Stearate Filmtab 429

Methacycline Hydrochloride (May diminish bactericidal effects of penicillins).
No products indexed under this heading.

Minocycline Hydrochloride (May diminish bactericidal effects of penicillins). Products include:
DYNACIN Capsules 1627
Minocin Intravenous 1428
Minocin Oral Suspension 1431
Minocin Pellet-Filled Capsules 1429

Oxytetracycline Hydrochloride (May diminish bactericidal effects of penicillins). Products include:
TERAK Ointment 210
Terra-Cortril Ophthalmic Suspension 2033
Terramycin with Polymyxin B Sulfate Ophthalmic Ointment 2035
Urobiotic-250 Capsules 2038

Probenecid (Penicillin blood levels may be prolonged). Products include:
Benemid Tablets 1651
ColBENEMID Tablets 1662

Tetracycline Hydrochloride (May diminish bactericidal effects of penicillins). Products include:
Achromycin V Capsules 1417
Helidac Therapy 2135

PHAZYME DROPS
(Simethicone) 633
None cited in PDR database.

PHAZYME-95 TABLETS
(Simethicone) 633
None cited in PDR database.

PHAZYME-125 CHEWABLE TABLETS
(Simethicone) 633
None cited in PDR database.

PHAZYME-125 SOFTGELS MAXIMUM STRENGTH
(Simethicone) 633
None cited in PDR database.

PHENERGAN WITH CODEINE
(Codeine Phosphate, Promethazine Hydrochloride) 2883
May interact with narcotic analgesics, hypnotics and sedatives, tricyclic antidepressants, tranquilizers, monoamine oxidase inhibitors, and certain other agents. Compounds in these categories include:

Alfentanil Hydrochloride (Additive sedative effects). Products include:
Alfenta Injection 1334

Alprazolam (Additive sedative effects). Products include:
Xanax Tablets 2115

Amitriptyline Hydrochloride (Additive sedative effects). Products include:
Elavil 2945
Etrafon 2495
Limbitrol 2333
Triavil Tablets 1800

Amoxapine (Additive sedative effects). Products include:
Asendin Tablets 1419

Buprenorphine (Additive sedative effects). Products include:
Buprenex Injectable 2170

Buspirone Hydrochloride (Additive sedative effects). Products include:
BuSpar Tablets 738

Chlordiazepoxide (Additive sedative effects). Products include:
Limbitrol 2333

Chlordiazepoxide Hydrochloride (Additive sedative effects). Products include:
Librax Capsules 2330
Librium Capsules 2331
Librium Injectable 2332

Chlorpromazine (Additive sedative effects). Products include:
Thorazine Suppositories 2701

Chlorprothixene (Additive sedative effects).
No products indexed under this heading.

Chlorprothixene Hydrochloride (Additive sedative effects).
No products indexed under this heading.

Clomipramine Hydrochloride (Additive sedative effects). Products include:
Anafranil Capsules 819

Clorazepate Dipotassium (Additive sedative effects). Products include:
Tranxene 459

Desipramine Hydrochloride (Additive sedative effects). Products include:
Norpramin Tablets 1273

Dezocine (Additive sedative effects). Products include:
Dalgan Injection 529

Diazepam (Additive sedative effects). Products include:
Dizac (diazepam injectable emulsion) CIV 1862
Valium Injection 2336
Valium Tablets 2335

Doxepin Hydrochloride (Additive sedative effects). Products include:
Adapin Capsules 1542
Sinequan 2028
Zonalon Cream 1042

Droperidol (Additive sedative effects). Products include:
Inapsine Injection 462

Estazolam (Additive sedative effects). Products include:
ProSom Tablets 457

Ethchlorvynol (Additive sedative effects). Products include:
Placidyl Capsules 456

Ethinamate (Additive sedative effects).
No products indexed under this heading.

Fentanyl (Additive sedative effects). Products include:
Duragesic Transdermal System 1336

Fentanyl Citrate (Additive sedative effects). Products include:
Sublimaze Injection 463

Fluphenazine Decanoate (Additive sedative effects). Products include:
Prolixin Decanoate 510

Fluphenazine Enanthate (Additive sedative effects). Products include:
Prolixin Enanthate 510

Fluphenazine Hydrochloride (Additive sedative effects). Products include:
Prolixin 510

Flurazepam Hydrochloride (Additive sedative effects). Products include:
Dalmane Capsules 2329

Furazolidone (Excessive narcotic effects). Products include:
Furoxone 2221

Glutethimide (Additive sedative effects).
No products indexed under this heading.

Haloperidol (Additive sedative effects). Products include:
Haldol Injection, Tablets and Concentrate 1585

Haloperidol Decanoate (Additive sedative effects). Products include:
Haldol Decanoate 1587

Hydrocodone Bitartrate (Additive sedative effects). Products include:
Codiclear DH Syrup 808
Duratuss HD Elixir 2750
Histussin D Liquid 670
Hycodan Tablets and Syrup 946
Hycomine Compound Tablets 948
Hycomine 947
Hycotuss Expectorant Syrup 950
Hydrocet Capsules 787
Lorcet 10/650 Tablets 1016
Lortab 2751
Tussend 1830
Tussend Expectorant 1831
Vicodin Tablets 1404
Vicodin ES Tablets 1405
Vicodin HP Tablets 1403
Vicodin Tuss Expectorant 1406
Zydone Capsules 967

Hydrocodone Polistirex (Additive sedative effects). Products include:
Tussionex Pennkinetic Extended-Release Suspension 1624

Hydromorphone Hydrochloride (Additive sedative effects). Products include:
Dilaudid Ampules 1382
Dilaudid Cough Syrup 1383
Dilaudid-HP Injection 1384
Dilaudid-HP Lyophilized Powder 250 mg 1384
Dilaudid 1382
Dilaudid Oral Liquid 1386
Dilaudid 1382
Dilaudid Tablets - 8 mg 1386

Hydroxyzine Hydrochloride (Additive sedative effects). Products include:
Atarax Tablets & Syrup 1992
Marax Tablets & DF Syrup 2015
Vistaril Intramuscular Solution 2042

Imipramine Hydrochloride (Additive sedative effects). Products include:
Tofranil Ampuls 873
Tofranil Tablets 875

Imipramine Pamoate (Additive sedative effects). Products include:
Tofranil-PM Capsules 876

Isocarboxazid (Excessive narcotic effects).
No products indexed under this heading.

Levorphanol Tartrate (Additive sedative effects). Products include:
Levo-Dromoran 2297

Lorazepam (Additive sedative effects). Products include:
Ativan Injection 2805
Ativan Tablets 2807

Loxapine Hydrochloride (Additive sedative effects). Products include:
Loxitane 1426

Maprotiline Hydrochloride (Additive sedative effects). Products include:
Ludiomil Tablets 861

Meperidine Hydrochloride (Additive sedative effects). Products include:
Demerol 2438
Mepergan Injection 2859

Meprobamate (Additive sedative effects). Products include:
Miltown Tablets 2780
PMB 200 and PMB 400 2890

Mesoridazine Besylate (Additive sedative effects). Products include:
Serentil ... 689

Methadone Hydrochloride (Additive sedative effects). Products include:
Methadone Hydrochloride Oral Concentrate ... 2356
Methadone Hydrochloride Oral Solution & Tablets ... 2357

Midazolam Hydrochloride (Additive sedative effects). Products include:
Versed Injection ... 2324

Molindone Hydrochloride (Additive sedative effects). Products include:
Moban Tablets and Concentrate ... 1036

Morphine Sulfate (Additive sedative effects). Products include:
Astramorph/PF Injection, USP (Preservative-Free) ... 526
Duramorph Injection ... 983
Infumorph 200 and Infumorph 500 Sterile Solutions ... 985
Kadian Capsules ... 2948
MS Contin Tablets ... 2149
MSIR ... 2152
Oramorph SR (Morphine Sulfate Sustained Release Tablets) ... 2359
RMS Suppositories CII ... 2766
Roxanol ... 2365

Nortriptyline Hydrochloride (Additive sedative effects). Products include:
Pamelor ... 2409

Opium Alkaloids (Additive sedative effects).
No products indexed under this heading.

Oxazepam (Additive sedative effects). Products include:
Serax Capsules ... 2916
Serax Tablets ... 2916

Oxycodone Hydrochloride (Additive sedative effects). Products include:
OxyContin Tablets ... 2163
OxyIR Capsules ... 2167
Percocet Tablets ... 955
Percodan Tablets ... 955
Percodan-Demi Tablets ... 956
Roxicodone Tablets, Oral Solution & Intensol (Oxycodone) ... 2366
Tylox Capsules ... 1593

Perphenazine (Additive sedative effects). Products include:
Etrafon ... 2495
Triavil Tablets ... 1800
Trilafon ... 2532

Phenelzine Sulfate (Excessive narcotic effects). Products include:
Nardil ... 1977

Prazepam (Additive sedative effects).
No products indexed under this heading.

Prochlorperazine (Additive sedative effects). Products include:
Compazine ... 2644

Propofol (Additive sedative effects). Products include:
Diprivan Injectable Emulsion ... 2939

Propoxyphene Hydrochloride (Additive sedative effects). Products include:
Darvon ... 1475
Wygesic Tablets ... 2930

Propoxyphene Napsylate (Additive sedative effects). Products include:
Darvon-N/Darvocet-N ... 1473

Protriptyline Hydrochloride (Additive sedative effects). Products include:
Vivactil Tablets ... 1820

Quazepam (Additive sedative effects). Products include:
Doral Tablets ... 2773

Secobarbital Sodium (Additive sedative effects). Products include:
Seconal Sodium Pulvules ... 1529

Selegiline Hydrochloride (Excessive narcotic effects). Products include:
Eldepryl Capsules ... 2729

Sufentanil Citrate (Additive sedative effects). Products include:
Sufenta Injection ... 1355

Temazepam (Additive sedative effects). Products include:
Restoril Capsules ... 2413

Thioridazine Hydrochloride (Additive sedative effects). Products include:
Mellaril ... 2398

Thiothixene (Additive sedative effects). Products include:
Navane Capsules and Concentrate ... 2018
Navane Intramuscular ... 2019

Tranylcypromine Sulfate (Excessive narcotic effects). Products include:
Parnate Tablets ... 2679

Triazolam (Additive sedative effects). Products include:
Halcion Tablets ... 2093

Trifluoperazine Hydrochloride (Additive sedative effects). Products include:
Stelazine ... 2692

Trimipramine Maleate (Additive sedative effects). Products include:
Surmontil Capsules ... 2917

Zolpidem Tartrate (Additive sedative effects). Products include:
Ambien Tablets ... 2559

Food Interactions
Alcohol (Additive sedative effects).

PHENERGAN WITH DEXTROMETHORPHAN
(Promethazine Hydrochloride, Dextromethorphan Hydrobromide) ... 2885
May interact with narcotic analgesics, hypnotics and sedatives, tricyclic antidepressants, tranquilizers, and certain other agents. Compounds in these categories include:

Alfentanil Hydrochloride (Additive sedative effects). Products include:
Alfenta Injection ... 1334

Alprazolam (Additive sedative effects). Products include:
Xanax Tablets ... 2115

Amitriptyline Hydrochloride (Additive sedative effects). Products include:
Elavil ... 2945
Etrafon ... 2495
Limbitrol ... 2333
Triavil Tablets ... 1800

Amoxapine (Additive sedative effects). Products include:
Asendin Tablets ... 1419

Buprenorphine (Additive sedative effects). Products include:
Buprenex Injectable ... 2170

Buspirone Hydrochloride (Additive sedative effects). Products include:
BuSpar Tablets ... 738

Chlordiazepoxide (Additive sedative effects). Products include:
Limbitrol ... 2333

Chlordiazepoxide Hydrochloride (Additive sedative effects). Products include:
Librax Capsules ... 2330
Librium Capsules ... 2331
Librium Injectable ... 2332

Chlorpromazine (Additive sedative effects). Products include:
Thorazine Suppositories ... 2701

Clomipramine Hydrochloride (Additive sedative effects). Products include:
Anafranil Capsules ... 819

Clorazepate Dipotassium (Additive sedative effects). Products include:
Tranxene ... 459

Codeine Phosphate (Additive sedative effects). Products include:
Brontex ... 2130
Dimetane-DC Cough Syrup ... 2232
Fioricet with Codeine Capsules ... 2387
Fiorinal with Codeine Capsules ... 2390
Nucofed ... 2225
Phenergan with Codeine ... 2883
Phenergan VC with Codeine ... 2888
Robitussin A-C Syrup ... 2248
Robitussin-DAC Syrup ... 2249
Ryna ... 804
Soma Compound w/Codeine Tablets ... 2784
Tylenol with Codeine ... 1592

Desipramine Hydrochloride (Additive sedative effects). Products include:
Norpramin Tablets ... 1273

Dezocine (Additive sedative effects). Products include:
Dalgan Injection ... 529

Diazepam (Additive sedative effects). Products include:
Dizac (diazepam injectable emulsion) CIV ... 1862
Valium Injectable ... 2336
Valium Tablets ... 2335

Doxepin Hydrochloride (Additive sedative effects). Products include:
Adapin Capsules ... 1542
Sinequan ... 2028
Zonalon Cream ... 1042

Droperidol (Additive sedative effects). Products include:
Inapsine Injection ... 462

Estazolam (Additive sedative effects). Products include:
ProSom Tablets ... 457

Ethchlorvynol (Additive sedative effects). Products include:
Placidyl Capsules ... 456

Ethinamate (Additive sedative effects).
No products indexed under this heading.

Fentanyl (Additive sedative effects). Products include:
Duragesic Transdermal System ... 1336

Fentanyl Citrate (Additive sedative effects). Products include:
Sublimaze Injection ... 463

Fluphenazine Decanoate (Additive sedative effects). Products include:
Prolixin Decanoate ... 510

Fluphenazine Enanthate (Additive sedative effects). Products include:
Prolixin Enanthate ... 510

Fluphenazine Hydrochloride (Additive sedative effects). Products include:
Prolixin ... 510

Flurazepam Hydrochloride (Additive sedative effects). Products include:
Dalmane Capsules ... 2329

Glutethimide (Additive sedative effects).
No products indexed under this heading.

Haloperidol (Additive sedative effects). Products include:
Haldol Injection, Tablets and Concentrate ... 1585

Haloperidol Decanoate (Additive sedative effects). Products include:
Haldol Decanoate ... 1587

Hydrocodone Bitartrate (Additive sedative effects). Products include:
Codiclear DH Syrup ... 808
Duratuss HD Elixir ... 2750
Histussin D Liquid ... 670
Hycodan Tablets and Syrup ... 946
Hycomine Compound Tablets ... 948
Hycomine ... 947
Hycotuss Expectorant Syrup ... 950
Hydrocet Capsules ... 787
Lorcet 10/650 Tablets ... 1016
Lortab ... 2751
Tussend ... 1830
Tussend Expectorant ... 1831
Vicodin Tablets ... 1404
Vicodin ES Tablets ... 1405
Vicodin HP Tablets ... 1403
Vicodin Tuss Expectorant ... 1406
Zydone Capsules ... 967

Hydrocodone Polistirex (Additive sedative effects). Products include:
Tussionex Pennkinetic Extended-Release Suspension ... 1624

Hydromorphone Hydrochloride (Additive sedative effects). Products include:
Dilaudid Ampules ... 1382
Dilaudid Cough Syrup ... 1383
Dilaudid-HP Injection ... 1384
Dilaudid-HP Lyophilized Powder 250 mg ... 1384
Dilaudid ... 1382
Dilaudid Oral Liquid ... 1386
Dilaudid ... 1382
Dilaudid Tablets - 8 mg ... 1386

Hydroxyzine Hydrochloride (Additive sedative effects). Products include:
Atarax Tablets & Syrup ... 1992
Marax Tablets & DF Syrup ... 2015
Vistaril Intramuscular Solution ... 2042

Imipramine Hydrochloride (Additive sedative effects). Products include:
Tofranil Ampuls ... 873
Tofranil Tablets ... 875

Imipramine Pamoate (Additive sedative effects). Products include:
Tofranil-PM Capsules ... 876

Levorphanol Tartrate (Additive sedative effects). Products include:
Levo-Dromoran ... 2297

Lorazepam (Additive sedative effects). Products include:
Ativan Injection ... 2805
Ativan Tablets ... 2807

Loxapine Hydrochloride (Additive sedative effects). Products include:
Loxitane ... 1426

Maprotiline Hydrochloride (Additive sedative effects). Products include:
Ludiomil Tablets ... 861

Meperidine Hydrochloride (Additive sedative effects). Products include:
Demerol ... 2438
Mepergan Injection ... 2859

Meprobamate (Additive sedative effects). Products include:
Miltown Tablets ... 2780
PMB 200 and PMB 400 ... 2890

Mesoridazine Besylate (Additive sedative effects). Products include:
Serentil ... 689

Methadone Hydrochloride (Additive sedative effects). Products include:
Methadone Hydrochloride Oral Concentrate ... 2356
Methadone Hydrochloride Oral Solution & Tablets ... 2357

Midazolam Hydrochloride (Additive sedative effects). Products include:
Versed Injection ... 2324

IMPORTANT NOTE: Always consult each drug listing in the patient's regimen for possible interactions.

Molindone Hydrochloride (Additive sedative effects). Products include:
  Moban Tablets and Concentrate 1036

Morphine Sulfate (Additive sedative effects). Products include:
  Astramorph/PF Injection, USP (Preservative-Free) 526
  Duramorph Injection 983
  Infumorph 200 and Infumorph 500 Sterile Solutions 985
  Kadian Capsules 2948
  MS Contin Tablets 2149
  MSIR 2152
  Oramorph SR (Morphine Sulfate Sustained Release Tablets) 2359
  RMS Suppositories CII 2766
  Roxanol 2365

Nortriptyline Hydrochloride (Additive sedative effects). Products include:
  Pamelor 2409

Opium Alkaloids (Additive sedative effects).
  No products indexed under this heading.

Oxazepam (Additive sedative effects). Products include:
  Serax Capsules 2916
  Serax Tablets 2916

Oxycodone Hydrochloride (Additive sedative effects). Products include:
  OxyContin Tablets 2163
  OxyIR Capsules 2167
  Percocet Tablets 955
  Percodan Tablets 955
  Percodan-Demi Tablets 956
  Roxicodone Tablets, Oral Solution & Intensol (Oxycodone) 2366
  Tylox Capsules 1593

Perphenazine (Additive sedative effects). Products include:
  Etrafon 2495
  Triavil Tablets 1800
  Trilafon 2532

Prazepam (Additive sedative effects).
  No products indexed under this heading.

Prochlorperazine (Additive sedative effects). Products include:
  Compazine 2644

Propofol (Additive sedative effects). Products include:
  Diprivan Injectable Emulsion 2939

Propoxyphene Hydrochloride (Additive sedative effects). Products include:
  Darvon 1475
  Wygesic Tablets 2930

Propoxyphene Napsylate (Additive sedative effects). Products include:
  Darvon-N/Darvocet-N 1473

Protriptyline Hydrochloride (Additive sedative effects). Products include:
  Vivactil Tablets 1820

Quazepam (Additive sedative effects). Products include:
  Doral Tablets 2773

Secobarbital Sodium (Additive sedative effects). Products include:
  Seconal Sodium Pulvules 1529

Sufentanil Citrate (Additive sedative effects). Products include:
  Sufenta Injection 1355

Temazepam (Additive sedative effects). Products include:
  Restoril Capsules 2413

Thioridazine Hydrochloride (Additive sedative effects). Products include:
  Mellaril 2398

Thiothixene (Additive sedative effects). Products include:
  Navane Capsules and Concentrate 2018
  Navane Intramuscular 2019

Triazolam (Additive sedative effects). Products include:
  Halcion Tablets 2093

Trifluoperazine Hydrochloride (Additive sedative effects). Products include:
  Stelazine 2692

Trimipramine Maleate (Additive sedative effects). Products include:
  Surmontil Capsules 2917

Zolpidem Tartrate (Additive sedative effects). Products include:
  Ambien Tablets 2559

Food Interactions

Alcohol (Additive sedative effects).

PHENERGAN INJECTION
(Promethazine Hydrochloride) 2880
May interact with narcotic analgesics, barbiturates, hypnotics and sedatives, general anesthetics, tranquilizers, central nervous system depressants, monoamine oxidase inhibitors, and certain other agents. Compounds in these categories include:

Alfentanil Hydrochloride (Additive sedative effects). Products include:
  Alfenta Injection 1334

Alprazolam (Additive sedative effects). Products include:
  Xanax Tablets 2115

Aprobarbital (Additive sedative effects).
  No products indexed under this heading.

Buprenorphine (Additive sedative effects). Products include:
  Buprenex Injectable 2170

Buspirone Hydrochloride (Additive sedative effects). Products include:
  BuSpar Tablets 738

Butabarbital (Additive sedative effects).
  No products indexed under this heading.

Butalbital (Additive sedative effects). Products include:
  Axocet Capsules 2469
  Esgic-plus Capsules 1012
  Esgic-plus Tablets 1012
  Fioricet Tablets 2386
  Fioricet with Codeine Capsules 2387
  Fiorinal Capsules 2388
  Fiorinal with Codeine Capsules 2390
  Fiorinal Tablets 2388
  Phrenilin 790
  Sedapap Tablets 50 mg/650 mg 1826

Chlordiazepoxide (Additive sedative effects). Products include:
  Limbitrol 2333

Chlordiazepoxide Hydrochloride (Additive sedative effects). Products include:
  Librax Capsules 2330
  Librium Capsules 2331
  Librium Injectable 2332

Chlorpromazine (Additive sedative effects). Products include:
  Thorazine Suppositories 2701

Chlorprothixene (Additive sedative effects).
  No products indexed under this heading.

Chlorprothixene Hydrochloride (Additive sedative effects).
  No products indexed under this heading.

Chlorprothixene Lactate (Additive sedative effects).
  No products indexed under this heading.

Clorazepate Dipotassium (Additive sedative effects). Products include:
  Tranxene 459

Clozapine (Additive sedative effects). Products include:
  Clozaril Tablets 2377

Codeine Phosphate (Additive sedative effects). Products include:
  Brontex 2130
  Dimetane-DC Cough Syrup 2232
  Fioricet with Codeine Capsules 2387
  Fiorinal with Codeine Capsules 2390
  Nucofed 2225
  Phenergan with Codeine 2883
  Phenergan VC with Codeine 2888
  Robitussin A-C Syrup 2248
  Robitussin-DAC Syrup 2249
  Ryna ...... ▣ 804
  Soma Compound w/Codeine Tablets 2784
  Tylenol with Codeine 1592

Desflurane (Additive sedative effects). Products include:
  Suprane (desflurane, USP) 1865

Dezocine (Additive sedative effects). Products include:
  Dalgan Injection 529

Diazepam (Additive sedative effects). Products include:
  Dizac (diazepam injectable emulsion) CIV 1862
  Valium Injectable 2336
  Valium Tablets 2335

Droperidol (Additive sedative effects). Products include:
  Inapsine Injection 462

Enflurane (Additive sedative effects).
  No products indexed under this heading.

Epinephrine Hydrochloride (Potential for reversal of the vasopressor effect). Products include:
  Ana-Kit Anaphylaxis Emergency Treatment Kit 611

Estazolam (Additive sedative effects). Products include:
  ProSom Tablets 457

Ethchlorvynol (Additive sedative effects). Products include:
  Placidyl Capsules 456

Ethinamate (Additive sedative effects).
  No products indexed under this heading.

Fentanyl (Additive sedative effects). Products include:
  Duragesic Transdermal System 1336

Fentanyl Citrate (Additive sedative effects). Products include:
  Sublimaze Injection 463

Fluphenazine Decanoate (Additive sedative effects). Products include:
  Prolixin Decanoate 510

Fluphenazine Enanthate (Additive sedative effects). Products include:
  Prolixin Enanthate 510

Fluphenazine Hydrochloride (Additive sedative effects). Products include:
  Prolixin 510

Flurazepam Hydrochloride (Additive sedative effects). Products include:
  Dalmane Capsules 2329

Furazolidone (Possibility of increased incidence of extrapyramidal effects). Products include:
  Furoxone 2221

Glutethimide (Additive sedative effects).
  No products indexed under this heading.

Haloperidol (Additive sedative effects). Products include:
  Haldol Injection, Tablets and Concentrate 1585

Haloperidol Decanoate (Additive sedative effects). Products include:
  Haldol Decanoate 1587

Hydrocodone Bitartrate (Additive sedative effects). Products include:
  Codiclear DH Syrup 808
  Duratuss HD Elixir 2750
  Histussin D Liquid 670
  Hycodan Tablets and Syrup 946
  Hycomine Compound Tablets 948
  Hycomine 947
  Hycotuss Expectorant Syrup 950
  Hydrocet Capsules 787
  Lorcet 10/650 Tablets 1016
  Lortab 2751
  Tussend 1830
  Tussend Expectorant 1831
  Vicodin Tablets 1404
  Vicodin ES Tablets 1405
  Vicodin HP Tablets 1403
  Vicodin Tuss Expectorant 1406
  Zydone Capsules 967

Hydrocodone Polistirex (Additive sedative effects). Products include:
  Tussionex Pennkinetic Extended-Release Suspension 1624

Hydromorphone Hydrochloride (Additive sedative effects). Products include:
  Dilaudid Ampules 1382
  Dilaudid Cough Syrup 1383
  Dilaudid-HP Injection 1384
  Dilaudid-HP Lyophilized Powder 250 mg 1384
  Dilaudid 1382
  Dilaudid Oral Liquid 1386
  Dilaudid 1382
  Dilaudid Tablets - 8 mg 1386

Hydroxyzine Hydrochloride (Additive sedative effects). Products include:
  Atarax Tablets & Syrup 1992
  Marax Tablets & DF Syrup 2015
  Vistaril Intramuscular Solution 2042

Isocarboxazid (Possibility of increased incidence of extrapyramidal effects).
  No products indexed under this heading.

Isoflurane (Additive sedative effects).
  No products indexed under this heading.

Ketamine Hydrochloride (Additive sedative effects).
  No products indexed under this heading.

Levomethadyl Acetate Hydrochloride (Additive sedative effects). Products include:
  Orlaam Oral Solution 2361

Levorphanol Tartrate (Additive sedative effects). Products include:
  Levo-Dromoran 2297

Lorazepam (Additive sedative effects). Products include:
  Ativan Injection 2805
  Ativan Tablets 2807

Loxapine Hydrochloride (Additive sedative effects). Products include:
  Loxitane 1426

Loxapine Succinate (Additive sedative effects). Products include:
  Loxitane Capsules 1426

Meperidine Hydrochloride (Additive sedative effects). Products include:
  Demerol 2438
  Mepergan Injection 2859

Mephobarbital (Additive sedative effects). Products include:
  Mebaral Tablets 2452

Meprobamate (Additive sedative effects). Products include:
  Miltown Tablets 2780
  PMB 200 and PMB 400 2890

(▣ Described in PDR For Nonprescription Drugs)   (⊙ Described in PDR For Ophthalmology)

Mesoridazine Besylate (Additive sedative effects). Products include:
Serentil 689

Methadone Hydrochloride (Additive sedative effects). Products include:
Methadone Hydrochloride Oral Concentrate 2356
Methadone Hydrochloride Oral Solution & Tablets 2357

Methohexital Sodium (Additive sedative effects).
No products indexed under this heading.

Methotrimeprazine (Additive sedative effects). Products include:
Levoprome 1321

Methoxyflurane (Additive sedative effects).
No products indexed under this heading.

Midazolam Hydrochloride (Additive sedative effects). Products include:
Versed Injection 2324

Molindone Hydrochloride (Additive sedative effects). Products include:
Moban Tablets and Concentrate 1036

Morphine Sulfate (Additive sedative effects). Products include:
Astramorph/PF Injection, USP (Preservative-Free) 526
Duramorph Injection 983
Infumorph 200 and Infumorph 500 Sterile Solutions 985
Kadian Capsules 2948
MS Contin Tablets 2149
MSIR 2152
Oramorph SR (Morphine Sulfate Sustained Release Tablets) 2359
RMS Suppositories CII 2766
Roxanol 2365

Opium Alkaloids (Additive sedative effects).
No products indexed under this heading.

Oxazepam (Additive sedative effects). Products include:
Serax Capsules 2916
Serax Tablets 2916

Oxycodone Hydrochloride (Additive sedative effects). Products include:
OxyContin Tablets 2163
OxyIR Capsules 2167
Percocet Tablets 955
Percodan Tablets 955
Percodan-Demi Tablets 956
Roxicodone Tablets, Oral Solution & Intensol (Oxycodone) 2366
Tylox Capsules 1593

Pentobarbital Sodium (Additive sedative effects). Products include:
Nembutal Sodium Capsules 440
Nembutal Sodium Solution 442
Nembutal Sodium Suppositories 444

Perphenazine (Additive sedative effects). Products include:
Etrafon 2495
Triavil Tablets 1800
Trilafon 2532

Phenelzine Sulfate (Possibility of increased incidence of extrapyramidal effects). Products include:
Nardil 1977

Phenobarbital (Additive sedative effects). Products include:
Arco-Lase Plus Tablets 513
Bellergal-S Tablets 2375
Donnatal 2234
Donnatal Extentabs 2234
Donnatal Tablets 2234
Phenobarbital Elixir and Tablets 1523
Quadrinal Tablets 1398

Prazepam (Additive sedative effects).
No products indexed under this heading.

Prochlorperazine (Additive sedative effects). Products include:
Compazine 2644

Propofol (Additive sedative effects). Products include:
Diprivan Injectable Emulsion 2939

Propoxyphene Hydrochloride (Additive sedative effects). Products include:
Darvon 1475
Wygesic Tablets 2930

Propoxyphene Napsylate (Additive sedative effects). Products include:
Darvon-N/Darvocet-N 1473

Quazepam (Additive sedative effects). Products include:
Doral Tablets 2773

Risperidone (Additive sedative effects). Products include:
Risperdal Tablets 1348

Secobarbital Sodium (Additive sedative effects). Products include:
Seconal Sodium Pulvules 1529

Selegiline Hydrochloride (Possibility of increased incidence of extrapyramidal effects). Products include:
Eldepryl Capsules 2729

Sevoflurane (Additive sedative effects).
No products indexed under this heading.

Sufentanil Citrate (Additive sedative effects). Products include:
Sufenta Injection 1355

Temazepam (Additive sedative effects). Products include:
Restoril Capsules 2413

Thiamylal Sodium (Additive sedative effects).
No products indexed under this heading.

Thioridazine Hydrochloride (Additive sedative effects). Products include:
Mellaril 2398

Thiothixene (Additive sedative effects). Products include:
Navane Capsules and Concentrate 2018
Navane Intramuscular 2019

Tranylcypromine Sulfate (Possibility of increased incidence of extrapyramidal effects). Products include:
Parnate Tablets 2679

Triazolam (Additive sedative effects). Products include:
Halcion Tablets 2093

Trifluoperazine Hydrochloride (Additive sedative effects). Products include:
Stelazine 2692

Zolpidem Tartrate (Additive sedative effects). Products include:
Ambien Tablets 2559

Food Interactions

Alcohol (Additive sedative effects).

PHENERGAN SUPPOSITORIES

(Promethazine Hydrochloride) 2882
May interact with narcotic analgesics, hypnotics and sedatives, tricyclic antidepressants, tranquilizers, central nervous system depressants, barbiturates, and certain other agents. Compounds in these categories include:

Alfentanil Hydrochloride (Additive sedative effects). Products include:
Alfenta Injection 1334

Alprazolam (Additive sedative effects). Products include:
Xanax Tablets 2115

Amitriptyline Hydrochloride (Additive sedative effects). Products include:
Elavil 2945
Etrafon 2495
Limbitrol 2333
Triavil Tablets 1800

Amoxapine (Additive sedative effects). Products include:
Asendin Tablets 1419

Aprobarbital (Additive sedative effects; reduce the dose of barbiturate by one-half).
No products indexed under this heading.

Buprenorphine (Additive sedative effects). Products include:
Buprenex Injectable 2170

Buspirone Hydrochloride (Additive sedative effects). Products include:
BuSpar Tablets 738

Butabarbital (Additive sedative effects; reduce the dose of barbiturate by one-half).
No products indexed under this heading.

Butalbital (Additive sedative effects; reduce the dose of barbiturate by one-half). Products include:
Axocet Capsules 2469
Esgic-plus Capsules 1012
Esgic-plus Tablets 1012
Fioricet Tablets 2386
Fioricet with Codeine Capsules 2387
Fiorinal Capsules 2388
Fiorinal with Codeine Capsules 2390
Fiorinal Tablets 2388
Phrenilin 790
Sedapap Tablets 50 mg/650 mg .. 1826

Chlordiazepoxide (Additive sedative effects). Products include:
Limbitrol 2333

Chlordiazepoxide Hydrochloride (Additive sedative effects). Products include:
Librax Capsules 2330
Librium Capsules 2331
Librium Injectable 2332

Chlorpromazine (Additive sedative effects). Products include:
Thorazine Suppositories 2701

Chlorprothixene (Additive sedative effects).
No products indexed under this heading.

Chlorprothixene Hydrochloride (Additive sedative effects).
No products indexed under this heading.

Chlorprothixene Lactate (Additive sedative effects).
No products indexed under this heading.

Clomipramine Hydrochloride (Additive sedative effects). Products include:
Anafranil Capsules 819

Clorazepate Dipotassium (Additive sedative effects). Products include:
Tranxene 459

Clozapine (Additive sedative effects). Products include:
Clozaril Tablets 2377

Codeine Phosphate (Additive sedative effects). Products include:
Brontex 2130
Dimetane-DC Cough Syrup 2232
Fioricet with Codeine Capsules 2387
Fiorinal with Codeine Capsules 2390
Nucofed 2225
Phenergan with Codeine 2883
Phenergan VC with Codeine 2888
Robitussin A-C Syrup 2248
Robitussin-DAC Syrup 2249
Ryna 804
Soma Compound w/Codeine Tablets 2784
Tylenol with Codeine 1592

Desflurane (Additive sedative effects). Products include:
Suprane (desflurane, USP) 1865

Desipramine Hydrochloride (Additive sedative effects). Products include:
Norpramin Tablets 1273

Dezocine (Additive sedative effects). Products include:
Dalgan Injection 529

Diazepam (Additive sedative effects). Products include:
Dizac (diazepam injectable emulsion) CIV 1862
Valium Injectable 2336
Valium Tablets 2335

Doxepin Hydrochloride (Additive sedative effects). Products include:
Adapin Capsules 1542
Sinequan 2028
Zonalon Cream 1042

Droperidol (Additive sedative effects). Products include:
Inapsine Injection 462

Enflurane (Additive sedative effects).
No products indexed under this heading.

Epinephrine (Potential for reversal of the vasopressor effect). Products include:
EPIFRIN .... ◉ 237
EpiPen 808
Marcaine with Epinephrine 2446
Primatene Mist 843
Sensorcaine with Epinephrine Injection 554
Sus-Phrine Injection 1017
Xylocaine with Epinephrine Injections 562

Estazolam (Additive sedative effects). Products include:
ProSom Tablets 457

Ethchlorvynol (Additive sedative effects). Products include:
Placidyl Capsules 456

Ethinamate (Additive sedative effects).
No products indexed under this heading.

Fentanyl (Additive sedative effects). Products include:
Duragesic Transdermal System 1336

Fentanyl Citrate (Additive sedative effects). Products include:
Sublimaze Injection 463

Fluphenazine Decanoate (Additive sedative effects). Products include:
Prolixin Decanoate 510

Fluphenazine Enanthate (Additive sedative effects). Products include:
Prolixin Enanthate 510

Fluphenazine Hydrochloride (Additive sedative effects). Products include:
Prolixin 510

Flurazepam Hydrochloride (Additive sedative effects). Products include:
Dalmane Capsules 2329

Glutethimide (Additive sedative effects).
No products indexed under this heading.

Haloperidol (Additive sedative effects). Products include:
Haldol Injection, Tablets and Concentrate 1585

Haloperidol Decanoate (Additive sedative effects). Products include:
Haldol Decanoate 1587

Hydrocodone Bitartrate (Additive sedative effects). Products include:
Codiclear DH Syrup 808
Duratuss HD Elixir 2750
Histussin D Liquid 670

IMPORTANT NOTE: Always consult each drug listing in the patient's regimen for possible interactions.

Phenergan — Interactions Index

Hycodan Tablets and Syrup 946
Hycomine Compound Tablets 948
Hycomine 947
Hycotuss Expectorant Syrup 950
Hydrocet Capsules 787
Lorcet 10/650 Tablets 1016
Lortab 2751
Tussend 1830
Tussend Expectorant 1831
Vicodin Tablets 1404
Vicodin ES Tablets 1405
Vicodin HP Tablets 1403
Vicodin Tuss Expectorant 1406
Zydone Capsules 967

Hydrocodone Polistirex (Additive sedative effects). Products include:
Tussionex Pennkinetic Extended-Release Suspension 1624

Hydromorphone Hydrochloride (Additive sedative effects). Products include:
Dilaudid Ampules 1382
Dilaudid Cough Syrup 1383
Dilaudid-HP Injection 1384
Dilaudid-HP Lyophilized Powder 250 mg 1384
Dilaudid 1382
Dilaudid Oral Liquid 1386
Dilaudid 1382
Dilaudid Tablets - 8 mg. 1386

Hydroxyzine Hydrochloride (Additive sedative effects). Products include:
Atarax Tablets & Syrup 1992
Marax Tablets & DF Syrup 2015
Vistaril Intramuscular Solution 2042

Imipramine Hydrochloride (Additive sedative effects). Products include:
Tofranil Ampuls 873
Tofranil Tablets 875

Imipramine Pamoate (Additive sedative effects). Products include:
Tofranil-PM Capsules 876

Isoflurane (Additive sedative effects).
No products indexed under this heading.

Ketamine Hydrochloride (Additive sedative effects).
No products indexed under this heading.

Levomethadyl Acetate Hydrochloride (Additive sedative effects). Products include:
Orlaam Oral Solution 2361

Levorphanol Tartrate (Additive sedative effects). Products include:
Levo-Dromoran 2297

Lorazepam (Additive sedative effects). Products include:
Ativan Injection 2805
Ativan Tablets 2807

Loxapine Hydrochloride (Additive sedative effects). Products include:
Loxitane 1426

Loxapine Succinate (Additive sedative effects). Products include:
Loxitane Capsules 1426

Maprotiline Hydrochloride (Additive sedative effects). Products include:
Ludiomil Tablets 861

Meperidine Hydrochloride (Additive sedative effects; reduce meperidine dose by one-fourth to one-half). Products include:
Demerol 2438
Mepergan Injection 2859

Mephobarbital (Additive sedative effects; reduce the dose of barbiturate by one-half). Products include:
Mebaral Tablets 2452

Meprobamate (Additive sedative effects). Products include:
Miltown Tablets 2780
PMB 200 and PMB 400 2890

Mesoridazine Besylate (Additive sedative effects). Products include:
Serentil 689

Methadone Hydrochloride (Additive sedative effects). Products include:
Methadone Hydrochloride Oral Concentrate 2356
Methadone Hydrochloride Oral Solution & Tablets 2357

Methohexital Sodium (Additive sedative effects).
No products indexed under this heading.

Methotrimeprazine (Additive sedative effects). Products include:
Levoprome 1321

Methoxyflurane (Additive sedative effects).
No products indexed under this heading.

Midazolam Hydrochloride (Additive sedative effects). Products include:
Versed Injection 2324

Molindone Hydrochloride (Additive sedative effects). Products include:
Moban Tablets and Concentrate 1036

Morphine Sulfate (Additive sedative effects; reduce the dose of morphine by one-fourth to one-half). Products include:
Astramorph/PF Injection, USP (Preservative-Free) 526
Duramorph Injection 983
Infumorph 200 and Infumorph 500 Sterile Solutions 985
Kadian Capsules 2948
MS Contin Tablets 2149
MSIR 2152
Oramorph SR (Morphine Sulfate Sustained Release Tablets) 2359
RMS Suppositories CII 2766
Roxanol 2365

Nortriptyline Hydrochloride (Additive sedative effects). Products include:
Pamelor 2409

Opium Alkaloids (Additive sedative effects).
No products indexed under this heading.

Oxazepam (Additive sedative effects). Products include:
Serax Capsules 2916
Serax Tablets 2916

Oxycodone Hydrochloride (Additive sedative effects). Products include:
OxyContin Tablets 2163
OxyIR Capsules 2167
Percocet Tablets 955
Percodan Tablets 955
Percodan-Demi Tablets 956
Roxicodone Tablets, Oral Solution & Intensol (Oxycodone) 2366
Tylox Capsules 1593

Pentobarbital Sodium (Additive sedative effects; reduce the dose of barbiturate by one-half). Products include:
Nembutal Sodium Capsules 440
Nembutal Sodium Solution 442
Nembutal Sodium Suppositories 444

Perphenazine (Additive sedative effects). Products include:
Etrafon 2495
Triavil Tablets 1800
Trilafon 2532

Phenobarbital (Additive sedative effects; reduce the dose of barbiturate by one-half). Products include:
Arco-Lase Plus Tablets 513
Bellergal-S Tablets 2375
Donnatal 2234
Donnatal Extentabs 2234
Donnatal Tablets 2234
Phenobarbital Elixir and Tablets 1523
Quadrinal Tablets 1398

Prazepam (Additive sedative effects).
No products indexed under this heading.

Prochlorperazine (Additive sedative effects). Products include:
Compazine 2644

Propofol (Additive sedative effects). Products include:
Diprivan Injectable Emulsion 2939

Propoxyphene Hydrochloride (Additive sedative effects). Products include:
Darvon 1475
Wygesic Tablets 2930

Propoxyphene Napsylate (Additive sedative effects). Products include:
Darvon-N/Darvocet-N 1473

Protriptyline Hydrochloride (Additive sedative effects). Products include:
Vivactil Tablets 1820

Quazepam (Additive sedative effects). Products include:
Doral Tablets 2773

Risperidone (Additive sedative effects). Products include:
Risperdal Tablets 1348

Secobarbital Sodium (Additive sedative effects; reduce the dose of barbiturate by one-half). Products include:
Seconal Sodium Pulvules 1529

Sevoflurane (Additive sedative effects).
No products indexed under this heading.

Sufentanil Citrate (Additive sedative effects). Products include:
Sufenta Injection 1355

Temazepam (Additive sedative effects). Products include:
Restoril Capsules 2413

Thiamylal Sodium (Additive sedative effects; reduce the dose of barbiturate by one-half).
No products indexed under this heading.

Thioridazine Hydrochloride (Additive sedative effects). Products include:
Mellaril 2398

Thiothixene (Additive sedative effects). Products include:
Navane Capsules and Concentrate 2018
Navane Intramuscular 2019

Triazolam (Additive sedative effects). Products include:
Halcion Tablets 2093

Trifluoperazine Hydrochloride (Additive sedative effects). Products include:
Stelazine 2692

Trimipramine Maleate (Additive sedative effects). Products include:
Surmontil Capsules 2917

Zolpidem Tartrate (Additive sedative effects). Products include:
Ambien Tablets 2559

Food Interactions

Alcohol (Additive sedative effects).

PHENERGAN SYRUP FORTIS

(Promethazine Hydrochloride) 2881
May interact with narcotic analgesics, hypnotics and sedatives, tricyclic antidepressants, tranquilizers, and certain other agents. Compounds in these categories include:

Alfentanil Hydrochloride (Additive sedative effects). Products include:
Alfenta Injection 1334

Alprazolam (Additive sedative effects). Products include:
Xanax Tablets 2115

Amitriptyline Hydrochloride (Additive sedative effects). Products include:
Elavil 2945
Etrafon 2495
Limbitrol 2333
Triavil Tablets 1800

Amoxapine (Additive sedative effects). Products include:
Asendin Tablets 1419

Buprenorphine (Additive sedative effects). Products include:
Buprenex Injectable 2170

Buspirone Hydrochloride (Additive sedative effects). Products include:
BuSpar Tablets 738

Chlordiazepoxide (Additive sedative effects). Products include:
Limbitrol 2333

Chlordiazepoxide Hydrochloride (Additive sedative effects). Products include:
Librax Capsules 2330
Librium Capsules 2331
Librium Injectable 2332

Chlorpromazine (Additive sedative effects). Products include:
Thorazine Suppositories 2701

Chlorprothixene (Additive sedative effects).
No products indexed under this heading.

Chlorprothixene Hydrochloride (Additive sedative effects).
No products indexed under this heading.

Clomipramine Hydrochloride (Additive sedative effects). Products include:
Anafranil Capsules 819

Clorazepate Dipotassium (Additive sedative effects). Products include:
Tranxene 459

Codeine Phosphate (Additive sedative effects). Products include:
Brontex 2130
Dimetane-DC Cough Syrup 2232
Fioricet with Codeine Capsules 2387
Fiorinal with Codeine Capsules 2390
Nucofed 2225
Phenergan with Codeine 2883
Phenergan VC with Codeine 2888
Robitussin A-C Syrup 2248
Robitussin-DAC Syrup 2249
Ryna .... ▣ 804
Soma Compound w/Codeine Tablets 2784
Tylenol with Codeine 1592

Desipramine Hydrochloride (Additive sedative effects). Products include:
Norpramin Tablets 1273

Dezocine (Additive sedative effects). Products include:
Dalgan Injection 529

Diazepam (Additive sedative effects). Products include:
Dizac (diazepam injectable emulsion) CIV 1862
Valium Injectable 2336
Valium Tablets 2335

Doxepin Hydrochloride (Additive sedative effects). Products include:
Adapin Capsules 1542
Sinequan 2028
Zonalon Cream 1042

Droperidol (Additive sedative effects). Products include:
Inapsine Injection 462

Estazolam (Additive sedative effects). Products include:
ProSom Tablets 457

Ethchlorvynol (Additive sedative effects). Products include:
Placidyl Capsules 456

(▣ Described in PDR For Nonprescription Drugs) (⊙ Described in PDR For Ophthalmology)

Ethinamate (Additive sedative effects).
No products indexed under this heading.

Fentanyl (Additive sedative effects). Products include:
Duragesic Transdermal System 1336

Fentanyl Citrate (Additive sedative effects). Products include:
Sublimaze Injection 463

Fluphenazine Decanoate (Additive sedative effects). Products include:
Prolixin Decanoate 510

Fluphenazine Enanthate (Additive sedative effects). Products include:
Prolixin Enanthate 510

Fluphenazine Hydrochloride (Additive sedative effects). Products include:
Prolixin 510

Flurazepam Hydrochloride (Additive sedative effects). Products include:
Dalmane Capsules 2329

Glutethimide (Additive sedative effects).
No products indexed under this heading.

Haloperidol (Additive sedative effects). Products include:
Haldol Injection, Tablets and Concentrate 1585

Haloperidol Decanoate (Additive sedative effects). Products include:
Haldol Decanoate 1587

Hydrocodone Bitartrate (Additive sedative effects). Products include:
Codiclear DH Syrup 808
Duratuss HD Elixir 2750
Histussin D Liquid 670
Hycodan Tablets and Syrup 946
Hycomine Compound Tablets 948
Hycomine 947
Hycotuss Expectorant Syrup 950
Hydrocet Capsules 787
Lorcet 10/650 Tablets 1016
Lortab 2751
Tussend 1830
Tussend Expectorant 1831
Vicodin Tablets 1404
Vicodin ES Tablets 1405
Vicodin HP Tablets 1403
Vicodin Tuss Expectorant 1406
Zydone Capsules 967

Hydrocodone Polistirex (Additive sedative effects). Products include:
Tussionex Pennkinetic Extended-Release Suspension 1624

Hydromorphone Hydrochloride (Additive sedative effects). Products include:
Dilaudid Ampules 1382
Dilaudid Cough Syrup 1383
Dilaudid-HP Injection 1384
Dilaudid-HP Lyophilized Powder 250 mg 1384
Dilaudid 1382
Dilaudid Oral Liquid 1386
Dilaudid 1382
Dilaudid Tablets - 8 mg 1386

Hydroxyzine Hydrochloride (Additive sedative effects). Products include:
Atarax Tablets & Syrup 1992
Marax Tablets & DF Syrup 2015
Vistaril Intramuscular Solution 2042

Imipramine Hydrochloride (Additive sedative effects). Products include:
Tofranil Ampuls 873
Tofranil Tablets 875

Imipramine Pamoate (Additive sedative effects). Products include:
Tofranil-PM Capsules 876

Levorphanol Tartrate (Additive sedative effects). Products include:
Levo-Dromoran 2297

Lorazepam (Additive sedative effects). Products include:
Ativan Injection 2805
Ativan Tablets 2807

Loxapine Hydrochloride (Additive sedative effects). Products include:
Loxitane 1426

Loxapine Succinate (Additive sedative effects). Products include:
Loxitane Capsules 1426

Maprotiline Hydrochloride (Additive sedative effects). Products include:
Ludiomil Tablets 861

Meperidine Hydrochloride (Additive sedative effects). Products include:
Demerol 2438
Mepergan Injection 2859

Meprobamate (Additive sedative effects). Products include:
Miltown Tablets 2780
PMB 200 and PMB 400 2890

Mesoridazine Besylate (Additive sedative effects). Products include:
Serentil 689

Methadone Hydrochloride (Additive sedative effects). Products include:
Methadone Hydrochloride Oral Concentrate 2356
Methadone Hydrochloride Oral Solution & Tablets 2357

Midazolam Hydrochloride (Additive sedative effects). Products include:
Versed Injection 2324

Molindone Hydrochloride (Additive sedative effects). Products include:
Moban Tablets and Concentrate 1036

Morphine Sulfate (Additive sedative effects). Products include:
Astramorph/PF Injection, USP (Preservative-Free) 526
Duramorph Injection 983
Infumorph 200 and Infumorph 500 Sterile Solutions 985
Kadian Capsules 2948
MS Contin Tablets 2149
MSIR 2152
Oramorph SR (Morphine Sulfate Sustained Release Tablets) 2359
RMS Suppositories CII 2766
Roxanol 2365

Nortriptyline Hydrochloride (Additive sedative effects). Products include:
Pamelor 2409

Opium Alkaloids (Additive sedative effects).
No products indexed under this heading.

Oxazepam (Additive sedative effects). Products include:
Serax Capsules 2916
Serax Tablets 2916

Oxycodone Hydrochloride (Additive sedative effects). Products include:
OxyContin Tablets 2163
OxyIR Capsules 2167
Percocet Tablets 955
Percodan Tablets 955
Percodan-Demi Tablets 956
Roxicodone Tablets, Oral Solution & Intensol (Oxycodone) 2366
Tylox Capsules 1593

Perphenazine (Additive sedative effects). Products include:
Etrafon 2495
Triavil Tablets 1800
Trilafon 2532

Prazepam (Additive sedative effects).
No products indexed under this heading.

Prochlorperazine (Additive sedative effects). Products include:
Compazine 2644

Propofol (Additive sedative effects). Products include:
Diprivan Injectable Emulsion 2939

Propoxyphene Hydrochloride (Additive sedative effects). Products include:
Darvon 1475
Wygesic Tablets 2930

Propoxyphene Napsylate (Additive sedative effects). Products include:
Darvon-N/Darvocet-N 1473

Protriptyline Hydrochloride (Additive sedative effects). Products include:
Vivactil Tablets 1820

Quazepam (Additive sedative effects). Products include:
Doral Tablets 2773

Secobarbital Sodium (Additive sedative effects). Products include:
Seconal Sodium Pulvules 1529

Sufentanil Citrate (Additive sedative effects). Products include:
Sufenta Injection 1355

Temazepam (Additive sedative effects). Products include:
Restoril Capsules 2413

Thioridazine Hydrochloride (Additive sedative effects). Products include:
Mellaril 2398

Thiothixene (Additive sedative effects). Products include:
Navane Capsules and Concentrate 2018
Navane Intramuscular 2019

Triazolam (Additive sedative effects). Products include:
Halcion Tablets 2093

Trifluoperazine Hydrochloride (Additive sedative effects). Products include:
Stelazine 2692

Trimipramine Maleate (Additive sedative effects). Products include:
Surmontil Capsules 2917

Zolpidem Tartrate (Additive sedative effects). Products include:
Ambien Tablets 2559

Food Interactions

Alcohol (Additive sedative effects).

PHENERGAN SYRUP PLAIN
(Promethazine Hydrochloride) 2881
See **Phenergan Syrup Fortis**

PHENERGAN TABLETS
(Promethazine Hydrochloride) 2882
See **Phenergan Suppositories**

PHENERGAN VC
(Promethazine Hydrochloride, Phenylephrine Hydrochloride) 2886

May interact with narcotic analgesics, hypnotics and sedatives, tricyclic antidepressants, tranquilizers, monoamine oxidase inhibitors, sympathomimetics, sympathomimetic bronchodilators, beta blockers, alpha adrenergic blockers, and certain other agents. Compounds in these categories include:

Acebutolol Hydrochloride (Cardiostimulating effects blocked). Products include:
Sectral Capsules 2914

Albuterol (Tachycardia or arrhythmias may occur). Products include:
Proventil Inhalation Aerosol 2524
Ventolin Inhalation Aerosol and Refill 1170

Albuterol Sulfate (Tachycardia or arrhythmias may occur). Products include:
Airet Albuterol Sulfate Inhalation Solution 1602
Albuterol Sulfate, USP Solution for Inhalation, Arm-a-Med 522
Proventil Inhalation Solution 0.083% 2527
Proventil Repetabs Tablets 2529
Proventil Solution for Inhalation 0.5% 2525
Proventil Syrup 2528
Proventil Tablets 2529
Ventolin Inhalation Solution 1171
Ventolin Nebules Inhalation Solution 1172
Ventolin Rotacaps for Inhalation 1173
Ventolin Syrup 1175
Ventolin Tablets 1176
Volmax Extended-Release Tablets .. 1835

Alfentanil Hydrochloride (Additive sedative effects). Products include:
Alfenta Injection 1334

Alprazolam (Additive sedative effects). Products include:
Xanax Tablets 2115

Amitriptyline Hydrochloride (Additive sedative effects; increased pressor response). Products include:
Elavil 2945
Etrafon 2495
Limbitrol 2333
Triavil Tablets 1800

Amoxapine (Additive sedative effects; increased pressor response). Products include:
Asendin Tablets 1419

Amphetamine Aspartate (Synergistic adrenergic response). Products include:
Adderall Tablets 2209

Amphetamine Resins (Synergistic adrenergic response).
No products indexed under this heading.

Amphetamine Sulfate (Synergistic adrenergic response). Products include:
Adderall Tablets 2209

Atenolol (Cardiostimulating effects blocked). Products include:
Tenoretic Tablets 2963
Tenormin Tablets and I.V. Injection 2965

Atropine Sulfate (Enhanced pressor response; reflex bradycardia blocked). Products include:
Arco-Lase Plus Tablets 513
Atrohist Plus Tablets 1605
Donnatal 2234
Donnatal Extentabs 2234
Donnatal Tablets 2234
Lomotil 2591
Motofen Tablets 789
Urised Tablets 2123

Betaxolol Hydrochloride (Cardiostimulating effects blocked). Products include:
Betoptic Ophthalmic Solution 465
Betoptic S Ophthalmic Suspension 467
Kerlone Tablets 2588

Bisoprolol Fumarate (Cardiostimulating effects blocked). Products include:
Zebeta Tablets 1457
Ziac 1459

Bitolterol Mesylate (Tachycardia or arrhythmias may occur). Products include:
Tornalate Solution for Inhalation, 0.2% 976
Tornalate Metered Dose Inhaler 978

Buprenorphine (Additive sedative effects). Products include:
Buprenex Injectable 2170

Buspirone Hydrochloride (Additive sedative effects). Products include:
BuSpar Tablets 738

IMPORTANT NOTE: Always consult each drug listing in the patient's regimen for possible interactions.

Phenergan VC — Interactions Index — 838

Carteolol Hydrochloride (Cardiostimulating effects blocked). Products include:
- Cartrol Tablets ... 413
- Ocupress Ophthalmic Solution, 1% Sterile ... ◉ 297

Chlordiazepoxide (Additive sedative effects). Products include:
- Limbitrol ... 2333

Chlordiazepoxide Hydrochloride (Additive sedative effects). Products include:
- Librax Capsules ... 2330
- Librium Capsules ... 2331
- Librium Injectable ... 2332

Chlorpromazine (Additive sedative effects). Products include:
- Thorazine Suppositories ... 2701

Chlorprothixene (Additive sedative effects).
- No products indexed under this heading.

Chlorprothixene Hydrochloride (Additive sedative effects).
- No products indexed under this heading.

Clomipramine Hydrochloride (Additive sedative effects; increased pressor response). Products include:
- Anafranil Capsules ... 819

Clorazepate Dipotassium (Additive sedative effects). Products include:
- Tranxene ... 459

Codeine Phosphate (Additive sedative effects). Products include:
- Brontex ... 2130
- Dimetane-DC Cough Syrup ... 2232
- Fioricet with Codeine Capsules ... 2387
- Fiorinal with Codeine Capsules ... 2390
- Nucofed ... 2225
- Phenergan with Codeine ... 2883
- Phenergan VC with Codeine ... 2888
- Robitussin A-C Syrup ... 2248
- Robitussin-DAC Syrup ... 2249
- Ryna ... ▣ 804
- Soma Compound w/Codeine Tablets ... 2784
- Tylenol with Codeine ... 1592

Desipramine Hydrochloride (Additive sedative effects; increased pressor response). Products include:
- Norpramin Tablets ... 1273

Dezocine (Additive sedative effects). Products include:
- Dalgan Injection ... 529

Diazepam (Additive sedative effects). Products include:
- Dizac (diazepam injectable emulsion) CIV ... 1862
- Valium Injectable ... 2336
- Valium Tablets ... 2335

Dobutamine Hydrochloride (Tachycardia or arrhythmias may occur). Products include:
- Dobutrex Solution Vials ... 1480

Dopamine Hydrochloride (Tachycardia or arrhythmias may occur).
- No products indexed under this heading.

Doxazosin Mesylate (Decreased pressor response). Products include:
- Cardura Tablets ... 1993

Doxepin Hydrochloride (Additive sedative effects; increased pressor response). Products include:
- Adapin Capsules ... 1542
- Sinequan ... 2028
- Zonalon Cream ... 1042

Droperidol (Additive sedative effects). Products include:
- Inapsine Injection ... 462

Ephedrine Hydrochloride (Tachycardia or arrhythmias may occur). Products include:
- Primatene Tablets ... ▣ 844
- Quadrinal Tablets ... 1398

Ephedrine Sulfate (Tachycardia or arrhythmias may occur). Products include:
- Marax Tablets & DF Syrup ... 2015

Ephedrine Tannate (Tachycardia or arrhythmias may occur). Products include:
- Rynatuss ... 2782

Epinephrine (Tachycardia or arrhythmias may occur). Products include:
- EPIFRIN ... ◉ 237
- EpiPen ... 808
- Marcaine with Epinephrine ... 2446
- Primatene Mist ... ▣ 843
- Sensorcaine with Epinephrine Injection ... 554
- Sus-Phrine Injection ... 1017
- Xylocaine with Epinephrine Injections ... 562

Epinephrine Bitartrate (Tachycardia or arrhythmias may occur). Products include:
- Sensorcaine-MPF with Epinephrine Injection ... 554

Epinephrine Hydrochloride (Tachycardia or arrhythmias may occur). Products include:
- Ana-Kit Anaphylaxis Emergency Treatment Kit ... 611

Ergotamine Tartrate (Excessive rise in blood pressure). Products include:
- Bellergal-S Tablets ... 2375
- Cafergot ... 2376
- Ergomar Tablets ... 1543
- Wigraine Tablets ... 1884

Esmolol Hydrochloride (Cardiostimulating effects blocked). Products include:
- Brevibloc (esmolol HCl) Injection ... 1860

Estazolam (Additive sedative effects). Products include:
- ProSom Tablets ... 457

Ethchlorvynol (Additive sedative effects). Products include:
- Placidyl Capsules ... 456

Ethinamate (Additive sedative effects).
- No products indexed under this heading.

Ethylnorepinephrine Hydrochloride (Tachycardia or arrhythmias may occur).
- No products indexed under this heading.

Fentanyl (Additive sedative effects). Products include:
- Duragesic Transdermal System ... 1336

Fentanyl Citrate (Additive sedative effects). Products include:
- Sublimaze Injection ... 463

Fluphenazine Decanoate (Additive sedative effects). Products include:
- Prolixin Decanoate ... 510

Fluphenazine Enanthate (Additive sedative effects). Products include:
- Prolixin Enanthate ... 510

Fluphenazine Hydrochloride (Additive sedative effects). Products include:
- Prolixin ... 510

Flurazepam Hydrochloride (Additive sedative effects). Products include:
- Dalmane Capsules ... 2329

Furazolidone (Acute hypertensive crisis; concurrent use is contraindicated). Products include:
- Furoxone ... 2221

Glutethimide (Additive sedative effects).
- No products indexed under this heading.

Haloperidol (Additive sedative effects). Products include:
- Haldol Injection, Tablets and Concentrate ... 1585

Haloperidol Decanoate (Additive sedative effects). Products include:
- Haldol Decanoate ... 1587

Hydrocodone Bitartrate (Additive sedative effects). Products include:
- Codiclear DH Syrup ... 808
- Duratuss HD Elixir ... 2750
- Histussin D Liquid ... 670
- Hycodan Tablets and Syrup ... 946
- Hycomine Compound Tablets ... 948
- Hycomine ... 947
- Hycotuss Expectorant Syrup ... 950
- Hydrocet Capsules ... 787
- Lorcet 10/650 Tablets ... 1016
- Lortab ... 2751
- Tussend ... 1830
- Tussend Expectorant ... 1831
- Vicodin Tablets ... 1404
- Vicodin ES Tablets ... 1405
- Vicodin HP Tablets ... 1403
- Vicodin Tuss Expectorant ... 1406
- Zydone Capsules ... 967

Hydrocodone Polistirex (Additive sedative effects). Products include:
- Tussionex Pennkinetic Extended-Release Suspension ... 1624

Hydromorphone Hydrochloride (Additive sedative effects). Products include:
- Dilaudid Ampules ... 1382
- Dilaudid Cough Syrup ... 1383
- Dilaudid-HP Injection ... 1384
- Dilaudid-HP Lyophilized Powder 250 mg ... 1384
- Dilaudid ... 1382
- Dilaudid Oral Liquid ... 1386
- Dilaudid ... 1382
- Dilaudid Tablets - 8 mg ... 1386

Hydroxyzine Hydrochloride (Additive sedative effects). Products include:
- Atarax Tablets & Syrup ... 1992
- Marax Tablets & DF Syrup ... 2015
- Vistaril Intramuscular Solution ... 2042

Imipramine Hydrochloride (Additive sedative effects; increased pressor response). Products include:
- Tofranil Ampuls ... 873
- Tofranil Tablets ... 875

Imipramine Pamoate (Additive sedative effects; increased pressor response). Products include:
- Tofranil-PM Capsules ... 876

Isocarboxazid (Acute hypertensive crisis; concurrent use is contraindicated).
- No products indexed under this heading.

Isoetharine (Tachycardia or arrhythmias may occur). Products include:
- Bronkometer Aerosol ... 2432
- Bronkosol Solution ... 2432
- Isoetharine Inhalation Solution, USP, Arm-a-Med ... 545

Isoproterenol Hydrochloride (Tachycardia or arrhythmias may occur). Products include:
- Isuprel Hydrochloride Solution ... 2443
- Isuprel Injection ... 2441
- Isuprel Mistometer ... 2442

Isoproterenol Sulfate (Tachycardia or arrhythmias may occur). Products include:
- Norisodrine with Calcium Iodide Syrup ... 446

Labetalol Hydrochloride (Cardiostimulating effects blocked). Products include:
- Normodyne Injection ... 2519
- Normodyne Tablets ... 2522
- Trandate ... 1158

Levobunolol Hydrochloride (Cardiostimulating effects blocked). Products include:
- Betagan ... ◉ 230

Levorphanol Tartrate (Additive sedative effects). Products include:
- Levo-Dromoran ... 2297

Lorazepam (Additive sedative effects). Products include:
- Ativan Injection ... 2805
- Ativan Tablets ... 2807

Loxapine Hydrochloride (Additive sedative effects). Products include:
- Loxitane ... 1426

Maprotiline Hydrochloride (Additive sedative effects; increased pressor response). Products include:
- Ludiomil Tablets ... 861

Meperidine Hydrochloride (Additive sedative effects). Products include:
- Demerol ... 2438
- Mepergan Injection ... 2859

Meprobamate (Additive sedative effects). Products include:
- Miltown Tablets ... 2780
- PMB 200 and PMB 400 ... 2890

Mesoridazine Besylate (Additive sedative effects). Products include:
- Serentil ... 689

Metaproterenol Sulfate (Tachycardia or arrhythmias may occur). Products include:
- Alupent ... 672
- Metaproterenol Sulfate Inhalation Solution, USP, Arm-a-Med ... 547

Metaraminol Bitartrate (Tachycardia or arrhythmias may occur). Products include:
- Aramine Injection ... 1649

Methadone Hydrochloride (Additive sedative effects). Products include:
- Methadone Hydrochloride Oral Concentrate ... 2356
- Methadone Hydrochloride Oral Solution & Tablets ... 2357

Methoxamine Hydrochloride (Tachycardia or arrhythmias may occur). Products include:
- Vasoxyl Injection ... 1169

Metipranolol Hydrochloride (Cardiostimulating effects blocked). Products include:
- OptiPranolol (Metipranolol 0.3%) Sterile Ophthalmic Solution ... ◉ 256

Metoprolol Succinate (Cardiostimulating effects blocked). Products include:
- Toprol-XL Tablets ... 560

Metoprolol Tartrate (Cardiostimulating effects blocked). Products include:
- Lopressor ... 848
- Lopressor HCT Tablets ... 850

Midazolam Hydrochloride (Additive sedative effects). Products include:
- Versed Injection ... 2324

Molindone Hydrochloride (Additive sedative effects). Products include:
- Moban Tablets and Concentrate ... 1036

Morphine Sulfate (Additive sedative effects). Products include:
- Astramorph/PF Injection, USP (Preservative-Free) ... 526
- Duramorph Injection ... 983
- Infumorph 200 and Infumorph 500 Sterile Solutions ... 985
- Kadian Capsules ... 2948
- MS Contin Tablets ... 2149
- MSIR ... 2152
- Oramorph SR (Morphine Sulfate Sustained Release Tablets) ... 2359
- RMS Suppositories CII ... 2766
- Roxanol ... 2365

Nadolol (Cardiostimulating effects blocked).
- No products indexed under this heading.

(▣ Described in PDR For Nonprescription Drugs) (◉ Described in PDR For Ophthalmology)

839 **Interactions Index** **Phenergan VC**

Norepinephrine Bitartrate (Tachycardia or arrhythmias may occur). Products include:
- Levophed Bitartrate Injection 2445

Nortriptyline Hydrochloride (Additive sedative effects; increased pressor response). Products include:
- Pamelor 2409

Opium Alkaloids (Additive sedative effects).
- No products indexed under this heading.

Oxazepam (Additive sedative effects). Products include:
- Serax Capsules 2916
- Serax Tablets 2916

Oxycodone Hydrochloride (Additive sedative effects). Products include:
- OxyContin Tablets 2163
- OxyIR Capsules 2167
- Percocet Tablets 955
- Percodan Tablets 955
- Percodan-Demi Tablets 956
- Roxicodone Tablets, Oral Solution & Intensol (Oxycodone) 2366
- Tylox Capsules 1593

Penbutolol Sulfate (Cardiostimulating effects blocked). Products include:
- Levatol Tablets 2547

Perphenazine (Additive sedative effects). Products include:
- Etrafon 2495
- Triavil Tablets 1800
- Trilafon 2532

Phenelzine Sulfate (Acute hypertensive crisis; concurrent use is contraindicated). Products include:
- Nardil 1977

Phentolamine Mesylate (Decreased pressor response). Products include:
- Regitine Vials 864

Phenylephrine Bitartrate (Tachycardia or arrhythmias may occur).
- No products indexed under this heading.

Phenylephrine Tannate (Tachycardia or arrhythmias may occur). Products include:
- Atrohist Pediatric Suspension 1604
- Atrohist Pediatric Suspension Dye-Free 1604
- Rynatan 2781
- Rynatuss 2782

Phenylpropanolamine Hydrochloride (Tachycardia or arrhythmias may occur). Products include:
- Acutrim 648
- Atrohist Plus Tablets 1605
- BC Cold Powder Multi-Symptom Formula (Cold-Sinus-Allergy) 631
- BC Cold Powder Non-Drowsy Formula (Cold-Sinus) 631
- Cheracol Plus Head Cold/Cough Formula 741
- Comtrex Multi-Symptom Cold Reliever Liqui-Gels 638
- Comtrex Multi-Symptom Non-Drowsy Liqui-gels 640
- Contac Continuous Action Nasal Decongestant/Antihistamine 12 Hour Capsules 773
- Contac Maximum Strength Continuous Action Decongestant/Antihistamine 12 Hour Caplets 772
- Contac Severe Cold and Flu Formula Caplets 773
- Coricidin 'D' Decongestant Tablets 760
- Dexatrim 795
- Dexatrim Plus Vitamins Caplets 796
- Dimetane-DC Cough Syrup 2232
- Dimetapp Allergy Sinus Caplets 838
- Dimetapp Cold & Allergy Chewable Tablets 838
- Dimetapp Cold & Cough Liqui-Gels 839
- Dimetapp DM Elixir 840
- Dimetapp Elixir 840
- Dimetapp Extentabs 841
- Dimetapp Tablets/Liqui-Gels 841
- Dura-Vent Tablets 971
- Entex LA Tablets 972
- Exgest LA Tablets 787
- Hycomine 947
- Nolamine Timed-Release Tablets 790
- Ornade Spansule Capsules 2678
- Propagest Tablets 791
- Pyrroxate Caplets 742
- Robitussin-CF 846
- Sinulin Tablets 792
- Tavist-D 12 Hour Relief Tablets 750
- Teldrin 12 Hour Antihistamine/Nasal Decongestant Allergy Relief Capsules 786
- Triaminic Expectorant 753
- Triaminic Syrup 755
- Triaminic Triaminicol Cold & Cough 756
- Triaminic DM Syrup 756
- Triaminicin Tablets 756
- Vicks DayQuil Allergy Relief 12-Hour Extended Release Tablets 733
- Vicks DayQuil Allergy Relief 4-Hour Tablets 733
- Vicks DayQuil SINUS Pressure & CONGESTION Relief 734

Pindolol (Cardiostimulating effects blocked). Products include:
- Visken Tablets 2428

Pirbuterol Acetate (Tachycardia or arrhythmias may occur). Products include:
- Maxair Autohaler 1550
- Maxair Inhaler 1552

Prazepam (Additive sedative effects).
- No products indexed under this heading.

Prazosin Hydrochloride (Decreased pressor response). Products include:
- Minipress Capsules 2015
- Minizide Capsules 2016

Prochlorperazine (Additive sedative effects). Products include:
- Compazine 2644

Propofol (Additive sedative effects). Products include:
- Diprivan Injectable Emulsion 2939

Propoxyphene Hydrochloride (Additive sedative effects). Products include:
- Darvon 1475
- Wygesic Tablets 2930

Propoxyphene Napsylate (Additive sedative effects). Products include:
- Darvon-N/Darvocet-N 1473

Propranolol Hydrochloride (Cardiostimulating effects blocked). Products include:
- Inderal 2834
- Inderal LA Long Acting Capsules 2836
- Inderide Tablets 2838
- Inderide LA Long Acting Capsules 2840

Protriptyline Hydrochloride (Additive sedative effects; increased pressor response). Products include:
- Vivactil Tablets 1820

Pseudoephedrine Hydrochloride (Tachycardia or arrhythmias may occur). Products include:
- Actifed Allergy Daytime/Nighttime Caplets 808
- Actifed Cold & Allergy Tablets 807
- Actifed Cold & Sinus Caplets and Tablets 808
- Actifed Sinus Daytime/Nighttime Tablets and Caplets 809
- Advil Cold and Sinus Caplets and Tablets 837
- Alka-Seltzer Plus Liqui-Gels 612
- Alka-Seltzer Plus Flu & Body Aches Liqui-Gels Non-Drowsy Formula 613
- Alka-Seltzer Plus Night-Time Cold Medicine Liqui-Gels 612
- Allerest Maximum Strength 649
- Allerest No Drowsiness 649
- Allerest Sinus Pain Formula 649
- Atrohist Pediatric Capsules 1603
- Benadryl Allergy/Cold Tablets 811
- Benadryl Allergy Decongestant Liquid Medication 812
- Benadryl Allergy Decongestant Tablets 812
- Benadryl Allergy Sinus Headache Caplets 813
- Benylin Multisymptom 816
- Bromfed Capsules (Extended-Release) 1832
- Bromfed Syrup 712
- Bromfed Tablets 1832
- Bromfed-DM Cough Syrup 1832
- Bromfed-PD Capsules (Extended-Release) 1832
- Children's TYLENOL Cold Multi-Symptom Chewable Tablets and Liquid 1559
- Children's TYLENOL Cold Plus Cough Multi Symptom Chewable Tablets and Liquid 1560
- Children's TYLENOL Flu Suspension Liquid 1560
- Children's Vicks DayQuil Allergy Relief 730
- Children's Vicks NyQuil Cold/Cough Relief 731
- Allergy-Sinus Comtrex Multi-Symptom Allergy-Sinus Formula Tablets and Caplets 639
- Comtrex Multi-Symptom 638
- Comtrex Multi-Symptom Non-Drowsy Caplets 640
- Congess 1003
- Contac Day Allergy/Sinus Caplets 771
- Contac Day & Night 772
- Contac Night Allergy/Sinus Caplets 771
- Contac Severe Cold & Flu Non-Drowsy 774
- Deconsal II Tablets 1605
- Dimetane-DX Cough Syrup 2233
- Dimetapp Cold & Fever Suspension 839
- Dimetapp Decongestant Pediatric Drops 840
- Dorcol Children's Cough Syrup 748
- Drixoral Cough + Congestion Liquid Caps 763
- Dura-Tap/PD Capsules 970
- Duratuss Tablets 2750
- Duratuss HD Elixir 2750
- Efidac/24 655
- Entex PSE Tablets 973
- Fedahist Gyrocaps 2545
- Guaifed 1833
- Guaifed Syrup 712
- Guaimax-D Tablets 809
- Histussin D Liquid 670
- Infants' TYLENOL Cold Decongestant & Fever-Reducer Drops 1561
- Kronofed-A 994
- Novahistine DMX 782
- Nucofed 2225
- PediaCare Cough-Cold Chewable Tablets and Liquid 1569
- PediaCare Infants' Decongestant Drops 1569
- PediaCare Infants' Drops Decongestant Plus Cough 1569
- PediaCare NightRest Cough-Cold Liquid 1569
- Pediatric Vicks 44d Cough & Head Congestion Relief 736
- Pediatric Vicks 44m Cough & Cold Relief 737
- Robitussin Cold & Cough Liqui-Gels 844
- Robitussin Cold, Cough & Flu Liqui-Gels 844
- Robitussin Maximum Strength Cough & Cold 847
- Robitussin Night-Time Cold Formula 847
- Robitussin Pediatric Cough & Cold Formula 848
- Robitussin Pediatric Drops 849
- Robitussin Severe Congestion Liqui-Gels 845
- Robitussin-DAC Syrup 2249
- Robitussin-PE 846
- Rondec Oral Drops 974
- Rondec Syrup 974
- Rondec Tablet 974
- Rondec Chewable Tablets 974
- Rondec-TR Tablet 974
- Ryna 804
- Seldane-D Extended-Release Tablets 1286
- Semprex-D Capsules 1620
- Sinarest 663
- Sine-Aid Maximum Strength Sinus Headache Gelcaps, Caplets and Tablets 1570
- Sine-Off No Drowsiness Formula Caplets 784
- Sine-Off Sinus Medicine 784
- Singlet Tablets 785
- Sinutab Non-Drying Liquid Caps 823
- Sinutab Sinus Allergy Medication, Maximum Strength Tablets and Caplets 823
- Sinutab Sinus Medication, Maximum Strength Without Drowsiness Formula, Tablets & Caplets 824
- Sudafed Children's Cold & Cough Liquid Medication 825
- Sudafed Children's Nasal Decongestant Liquid Medication 826
- Sudafed Cold & Allergy Tablets 826
- Sudafed Cold and Cough Liquid Caps 826
- Sudafed Nasal Decongestant Tablets, 30 mg 825
- Sudafed Nasal Decongestant Tablets, 60 mg 825
- Sudafed Non-Drying Sinus Liquid Caps 827
- Sudafed Pediatric Nasal Decongestant Liquid Oral Drops 827
- Sudafed Severe Cold Formula Caplets 828
- Sudafed Severe Cold Formula Tablets 828
- Sudafed Sinus Caplets 829
- Sudafed Sinus Tablets 829
- Sudafed 12 Hour Caplets 824
- Syn-Rx Tablets 1622
- Syn-Rx DM Tablets 1623
- TheraFlu Flu and Cold Medicine 750
- Theraflu Maximum Strength Flu and Cold Medicine For Sore Throat 751
- TheraFlu Flu, Cold and Cough Medicine 750
- TheraFlu Maximum Strength Nighttime Flu, Cold & Cough Medicine 751
- TheraFlu Maximum Strength Non-Drowsy Formula Flu, Cold & Cough Medicine 751
- TheraFlu Maximum Strength, Non-Drowsy Formula Flu, Cold and Cough Caplets 752
- Theraflu Maximum Strength Sinus Non-Drowsy Formula Caplets 752
- Triaminic AM Cough and Decongestant Formula 753
- Triaminic AM Decongestant Formula 753
- Triaminic Infant Oral Decongestant Drops 754
- Triaminic Night Time 754
- Triaminic Sore Throat Formula 755
- Tussend 1830
- Tussend Expectorant 1831
- TYLENOL Allergy Sinus, Maximum Strength Caplets and Gelcaps 1571
- TYLENOL Allergy Sinus NightTime, Maximum Strength Caplets 1571
- TYLENOL Cold Medication, Multi-Symptom Formula Tablets and Caplets 1572
- TYLENOL Cold Medication, Multi-Symptom Hot Liquid Packets 1572
- TYLENOL Cold Medication, No Drowsiness Formula Caplets and Gelcaps 1572
- TYLENOL Cold Severe Congestion Caplets 1573
- TYLENOL Cough Medication with Decongestant, Multi Symptom 1574
- TYLENOL Flu No Drowsiness Formula, Maximum Strength Gelcaps 1575
- TYLENOL Flu NightTime, Maximum Strength Gelcaps 1575
- TYLENOL Flu NightTime, Maximum Strength Hot Medication Packets 1575
- TYLENOL Sinus, Maximum Strength Geltabs, Gelcaps, Caplets and Tablets 1576
- Vicks 44 LiquiCaps Cough, Cold & Flu Relief 728
- Vicks 44 LiquiCaps Non-Drowsy Cough & Cold Relief 729
- Vicks 44D Cough & Head Congestion Relief 728
- Vicks 44M Cough, Cold & Flu Relief 729
- Vicks DayQuil LiquiCaps/Liquid Multi-Symptom Cold/Flu Relief 734
- Vicks DayQuil SINUS Pressure & PAIN Relief with IBUPROFEN 735
- Vicks Nyquil Hot Therapy 735

IMPORTANT NOTE: Always consult each drug listing in the patient's regimen for possible interactions.

Phenergan VC Interactions Index 840

Vicks NyQuil LiquiCaps/Liquid Multi-Symptom Cold/Flu Relief, Original and Cherry Flavors ▣ 736

Pseudoephedrine Sulfate (Tachycardia or arrhythmias may occur). Products include:
- Chlor-Trimeton Allergy Decongestant Tablets ▣ 759
- Claritin-D Tablets 2487
- Drixoral Cold and Allergy Sustained-Action Tablets ▣ 763
- Drixoral Cold and Flu Extended-Release Tablets ▣ 764
- Drixoral Non-Drowsy Formula Extended-Release Tablets ▣ 764
- Drixoral Allergy/Sinus Extended Release Tablets ▣ 765
- Trinalin Repetabs Tablets 1373

Quazepam (Additive sedative effects). Products include:
- Doral Tablets 2773

Salmeterol Xinafoate (Tachycardia or arrhythmias may occur). Products include:
- Serevent Inhalation Aerosol 1149

Secobarbital Sodium (Additive sedative effects). Products include:
- Seconal Sodium Pulvules 1529

Selegiline Hydrochloride (Acute hypertensive crisis; concurrent use is contraindicated). Products include:
- Eldepryl Capsules 2729

Sotalol Hydrochloride (Cardiostimulating effects blocked). Products include:
- Betapace Tablets 637

Sufentanil Citrate (Additive sedative effects). Products include:
- Sufenta Injection 1355

Temazepam (Additive sedative effects). Products include:
- Restoril Capsules 2413

Terazosin Hydrochloride (Decreased pressor response). Products include:
- Hytrin Capsules 434

Terbutaline Sulfate (Tachycardia or arrhythmias may occur). Products include:
- Brethaire Inhaler 830
- Brethine Ampuls 832
- Brethine Tablets 831
- Bricanyl Subcutaneous Injection 1247
- Bricanyl Tablets 1248

Thioridazine Hydrochloride (Additive sedative effects). Products include:
- Mellaril 2398

Thiothixene (Additive sedative effects). Products include:
- Navane Capsules and Concentrate 2018
- Navane Intramuscular 2019

Timolol Hemihydrate (Cardiostimulating effects blocked). Products include:
- Betimol 0.25%, 0.5% ◉ 259

Timolol Maleate (Cardiostimulating effects blocked). Products include:
- Blocadren Tablets 1654
- Timolide Tablets 1791
- Timoptic in Ocudose 1796
- Timoptic Sterile Ophthalmic Solution 1794
- Timoptic-XE 1798

Tranylcypromine Sulfate (Acute hypertensive crisis; concurrent use is contraindicated). Products include:
- Parnate Tablets 2679

Triazolam (Additive sedative effects). Products include:
- Halcion Tablets 2093

Trifluoperazine Hydrochloride (Additive sedative effects). Products include:
- Stelazine 2692

Trimipramine Maleate (Additive sedative effects; increased pressor response). Products include:
- Surmontil Capsules 2917

Zolpidem Tartrate (Additive sedative effects). Products include:
- Ambien Tablets 2559

Food Interactions

Alcohol (Additive sedative effects).

PHENERGAN VC WITH CODEINE

(Codeine Phosphate, Promethazine Hydrochloride, Phenylephrine Hydrochloride) 2888

May interact with narcotic analgesics, hypnotics and sedatives, tricyclic antidepressants, tranquilizers, monoamine oxidase inhibitors, sympathomimetics, sympathomimetic bronchodilators, beta blockers, alpha adrenergic blockers, and certain other agents. Compounds in these categories include:

Acebutolol Hydrochloride (Cardiostimulating effects blocked). Products include:
- Sectral Capsules 2914

Albuterol (Tachycardia or arrhythmias may occur). Products include:
- Proventil Inhalation Aerosol 2524
- Ventolin Inhalation Aerosol and Refill 1170

Albuterol Sulfate (Tachycardia or arrhythmias may occur). Products include:
- Airet Albuterol Sulfate Inhalation Solution 1602
- Albuterol Sulfate, USP Solution for Inhalation, Arm-a-Med 522
- Proventil Inhalation Solution 0.083% 2527
- Proventil Repetabs Tablets 2529
- Proventil Solution for Inhalation 0.5% 2525
- Proventil Syrup 2528
- Proventil Tablets 2529
- Ventolin Inhalation Solution 1171
- Ventolin Nebules Inhalation Solution 1172
- Ventolin Rotacaps for Inhalation 1173
- Ventolin Syrup 1175
- Ventolin Tablets 1176
- Volmax Extended-Release Tablets 1835

Alfentanil Hydrochloride (Additive sedative effects). Products include:
- Alfenta Injection 1334

Alprazolam (Additive sedative effects). Products include:
- Xanax Tablets 2115

Amitriptyline Hydrochloride (Additive sedative effects; increased pressor response). Products include:
- Elavil 2945
- Etrafon 2495
- Limbitrol 2333
- Triavil Tablets 1800

Amoxapine (Additive sedative effects; increased pressor response). Products include:
- Asendin Tablets 1419

Atenolol (Cardiostimulating effects blocked). Products include:
- Tenoretic Tablets 2963
- Tenormin Tablets and I.V. Injection 2965

Atropine Sulfate (Enhanced pressor response; reflex bradycardia blocked). Products include:
- Arco-Lase Plus Tablets 513
- Atrohist Plus Tablets 1605
- Donnatal 2234
- Donnatal Extentabs 2234
- Donnatal Tablets 2234
- Lomotil 2591
- Motofen Tablets 789
- Urised Tablets 2123

Betaxolol Hydrochloride (Cardiostimulating effects blocked). Products include:
- Betoptic Ophthalmic Solution 465
- Betoptic S Ophthalmic Suspension 467
- Kerlone Tablets 2588

Bisoprolol Fumarate (Cardiostimulating effects blocked). Products include:
- Zebeta Tablets 1457
- Ziac 1459

Bitolterol Mesylate (Tachycardia or arrhythmias may occur). Products include:
- Tornalate Solution for Inhalation, 0.2% 976
- Tornalate Metered Dose Inhaler 978

Buprenorphine (Additive sedative effects). Products include:
- Buprenex Injectable 2170

Buspirone Hydrochloride (Additive sedative effects). Products include:
- BuSpar Tablets 738

Carteolol Hydrochloride (Cardiostimulating effects blocked). Products include:
- Cartrol Tablets 413
- Ocupress Ophthalmic Solution, 1% Sterile ◉ 297

Chlordiazepoxide (Additive sedative effects). Products include:
- Limbitrol 2333

Chlordiazepoxide Hydrochloride (Additive sedative effects). Products include:
- Librax Capsules 2330
- Librium Capsules 2331
- Librium Injectable 2332

Chlorpromazine (Additive sedative effects). Products include:
- Thorazine Suppositories 2701

Chlorprothixene (Additive sedative effects).
- No products indexed under this heading.

Chlorprothixene Hydrochloride (Additive sedative effects).
- No products indexed under this heading.

Clomipramine Hydrochloride (Additive sedative effects; increased pressor response). Products include:
- Anafranil Capsules 819

Clorazepate Dipotassium (Additive sedative effects). Products include:
- Tranxene 459

Desipramine Hydrochloride (Additive sedative effects; increased pressor response). Products include:
- Norpramin Tablets 1273

Dezocine (Additive sedative effects). Products include:
- Dalgan Injection 529

Diazepam (Additive sedative effects). Products include:
- Dizac (diazepam injectable emulsion) CIV 1862
- Valium Injectable 2336
- Valium Tablets 2335

Dobutamine Hydrochloride (Tachycardia or arrhythmias may occur). Products include:
- Dobutrex Solution Vials 1480

Dopamine Hydrochloride (Tachycardia or arrhythmias may occur).
- No products indexed under this heading.

Doxazosin Mesylate (Pressor response decreased). Products include:
- Cardura Tablets 1993

Doxepin Hydrochloride (Additive sedative effects; increased pressor response). Products include:
- Adapin Capsules 1542
- Sinequan 2028
- Zonalon Cream 1042

Droperidol (Additive sedative effects). Products include:
- Inapsine Injection 462

Ephedrine Hydrochloride (Tachycardia or arrhythmias may occur). Products include:
- Primatene Tablets ▣ 844
- Quadrinal Tablets 1398

Ephedrine Sulfate (Tachycardia or arrhythmias may occur). Products include:
- Marax Tablets & DF Syrup 2015

Ephedrine Tannate (Tachycardia or arrhythmias may occur). Products include:
- Rynatuss 2782

Epinephrine (Tachycardia or arrhythmias may occur). Products include:
- EPIFRIN ◉ 237
- EpiPen 808
- Marcaine with Epinephrine 2446
- Primatene Mist ▣ 843
- Sensorcaine with Epinephrine Injection 554
- Sus-Phrine Injection 1017
- Xylocaine with Epinephrine Injections 562

Epinephrine Bitartrate (Tachycardia or arrhythmias may occur). Products include:
- Sensorcaine-MPF with Epinephrine Injection 554

Epinephrine Hydrochloride (Tachycardia or arrhythmias may occur). Products include:
- Ana-Kit Anaphylaxis Emergency Treatment Kit 611

Ergotamine Tartrate (Excessive rise in blood pressure). Products include:
- Bellergal-S Tablets 2375
- Cafergot 2376
- Ergomar Tablets 1543
- Wigraine Tablets 1884

Esmolol Hydrochloride (Cardiostimulating effects blocked). Products include:
- Brevibloc (esmolol HCl) Injection 1860

Estazolam (Additive sedative effects). Products include:
- ProSom Tablets 457

Ethchlorvynol (Additive sedative effects). Products include:
- Placidyl Capsules 456

Ethinamate (Additive sedative effects).
- No products indexed under this heading.

Ethylnorepinephrine Hydrochloride (Tachycardia or arrhythmias may occur).
- No products indexed under this heading.

Fentanyl (Additive sedative effects). Products include:
- Duragesic Transdermal System 1336

Fentanyl Citrate (Additive sedative effects). Products include:
- Sublimaze Injection 463

Fluphenazine Decanoate (Additive sedative effects). Products include:
- Prolixin Decanoate 510

Fluphenazine Enanthate (Additive sedative effects). Products include:
- Prolixin Enanthate 510

Fluphenazine Hydrochloride (Additive sedative effects). Products include:
- Prolixin 510

Flurazepam Hydrochloride (Additive sedative effects). Products include:
- Dalmane Capsules 2329

Furazolidone (Acute hypertensive crisis; concurrent use is contraindicated). Products include:
- Furoxone 2221

(▣ Described in PDR For Nonprescription Drugs) (◉ Described in PDR For Ophthalmology)

841 **Interactions Index** **Phenergan VC with Codeine**

Glutethimide (Additive sedative effects).
No products indexed under this heading.

Haloperidol (Additive sedative effects). Products include:
Haldol Injection, Tablets and Concentrate 1585

Haloperidol Decanoate (Additive sedative effects). Products include:
Haldol Decanoate 1587

Hydrocodone Bitartrate (Additive sedative effects). Products include:
Codiclear DH Syrup 808
Duratuss HD Elixir 2750
Histussin D Liquid 670
Hycodan Tablets and Syrup 946
Hycomine Compound Tablets 948
Hycomine 947
Hycotuss Expectorant Syrup 950
Hydrocet Capsules 787
Lorcet 10/650 Tablets 1016
Lortab 2751
Tussend 1830
Tussend Expectorant 1831
Vicodin Tablets 1404
Vicodin ES Tablets 1405
Vicodin HP Tablets 1403
Vicodin Tuss Expectorant 1406
Zydone Capsules 967

Hydrocodone Polistirex (Additive sedative effects). Products include:
Tussionex Pennkinetic Extended-Release Suspension 1624

Hydromorphone Hydrochloride (Additive sedative effects). Products include:
Dilaudid Ampules 1382
Dilaudid Cough Syrup 1383
Dilaudid-HP Injection 1384
Dilaudid-HP Lyophilized Powder 250 mg 1384
Dilaudid 1382
Dilaudid Oral Liquid 1386
Dilaudid 1382
Dilaudid Tablets - 8 mg 1386

Hydroxyzine Hydrochloride (Additive sedative effects). Products include:
Atarax Tablets & Syrup 1992
Marax Tablets & DF Syrup 2015
Vistaril Intramuscular Solution 2042

Imipramine Hydrochloride (Additive sedative effects; increased pressor response). Products include:
Tofranil Ampuls 873
Tofranil Tablets 875

Imipramine Pamoate (Additive sedative effects; increased pressor response). Products include:
Tofranil-PM Capsules 876

Isocarboxazid (Acute hypertensive crisis; concurrent use is contraindicated).
No products indexed under this heading.

Isoetharine (Tachycardia or arrhythmias may occur). Products include:
Bronkometer Aerosol 2432
Bronkosol Solution 2432
Isoetharine Inhalation Solution, USP, Arm-a-Med 545

Isoproterenol Hydrochloride (Tachycardia or arrhythmias may occur). Products include:
Isuprel Hydrochloride Solution 2443
Isuprel Injection 2441
Isuprel Mistometer 2442

Isoproterenol Sulfate (Tachycardia or arrhythmias may occur). Products include:
Norisodrine with Calcium Iodide Syrup 446

Labetalol Hydrochloride (Cardiostimulating effects blocked). Products include:
Normodyne Injection 2519
Normodyne Tablets 2522
Trandate 1158

Levobunolol Hydrochloride (Cardiostimulating effects blocked). Products include:
Betagan .... ◉ 230

Levorphanol Tartrate (Additive sedative effects). Products include:
Levo-Dromoran 2297

Lorazepam (Additive sedative effects). Products include:
Ativan Injection 2805
Ativan Tablets 2807

Loxapine Hydrochloride (Additive sedative effects). Products include:
Loxitane 1426

Maprotiline Hydrochloride (Additive sedative effects; increased pressor response). Products include:
Ludiomil Tablets 861

Meperidine Hydrochloride (Additive sedative effects). Products include:
Demerol 2438
Mepergan Injection 2859

Meprobamate (Additive sedative effects). Products include:
Miltown Tablets 2780
PMB 200 and PMB 400 2890

Mesoridazine Besylate (Additive sedative effects). Products include:
Serentil 689

Metaproterenol Sulfate (Tachycardia or arrhythmias may occur). Products include:
Alupent 672
Metaproterenol Sulfate Inhalation Solution, USP, Arm-a-Med 547

Metaraminol Bitartrate (Tachycardia or arrhythmias may occur). Products include:
Aramine Injection 1649

Methadone Hydrochloride (Additive sedative effects). Products include:
Methadone Hydrochloride Oral Concentrate 2356
Methadone Hydrochloride Oral Solution & Tablets 2357

Methoxamine Hydrochloride (Tachycardia or arrhythmias may occur). Products include:
Vasoxyl Injection 1169

Metipranolol Hydrochloride (Cardiostimulating effects blocked). Products include:
OptiPranolol (Metipranolol 0.3%) Sterile Ophthalmic Solution .... ◉ 256

Metoprolol Succinate (Cardiostimulating effects blocked). Products include:
Toprol-XL Tablets 560

Metoprolol Tartrate (Cardiostimulating effects blocked). Products include:
Lopressor 848
Lopressor HCT Tablets 850

Midazolam Hydrochloride (Additive sedative effects). Products include:
Versed Injection 2324

Molindone Hydrochloride (Additive sedative effects). Products include:
Moban Tablets and Concentrate 1036

Morphine Sulfate (Additive sedative effects). Products include:
Astramorph/PF Injection, USP (Preservative-Free) 526
Duramorph Injection 983
Infumorph 200 and Infumorph 500 Sterile Solutions 985
Kadian Capsules 2948
MS Contin Tablets 2149
MSIR 2152
Oramorph SR (Morphine Sulfate Sustained Release Tablets) 2359
RMS Suppositories CII 2766
Roxanol 2365

Nadolol (Cardiostimulating effects blocked).
No products indexed under this heading.

Norepinephrine Bitartrate (Tachycardia or arrhythmias may occur). Products include:
Levophed Bitartrate Injection 2445

Nortriptyline Hydrochloride (Additive sedative effects; increased pressor response). Products include:
Pamelor 2409

Opium Alkaloids (Additive sedative effects).
No products indexed under this heading.

Oxazepam (Additive sedative effects). Products include:
Serax Capsules 2916
Serax Tablets 2916

Oxycodone Hydrochloride (Additive sedative effects). Products include:
OxyContin Tablets 2163
OxyIR Capsules 2167
Percocet Tablets 955
Percodan Tablets 955
Percodan-Demi Tablets 956
Roxicodone Tablets, Oral Solution & Intensol (Oxycodone) 2366
Tylox Capsules 1593

Penbutolol Sulfate (Cardiostimulating effects blocked). Products include:
Levatol Tablets 2547

Perphenazine (Additive sedative effects). Products include:
Etrafon 2495
Triavil Tablets 1800
Trilafon 2532

Phenelzine Sulfate (Acute hypertensive crisis; concurrent use is contraindicated). Products include:
Nardil 1977

Phentolamine Mesylate (Decreased pressor response). Products include:
Regitine Vials 864

Phenylephrine Bitartrate (Tachycardia or arrhythmias may occur).
No products indexed under this heading.

Phenylephrine Tannate (Tachycardia or arrhythmias may occur). Products include:
Atrohist Pediatric Suspension 1604
Atrohist Pediatric Suspension Dye-Free 1604
Rynatan 2781
Rynatuss 2782

Phenylpropanolamine Hydrochloride (Tachycardia or arrhythmias may occur). Products include:
Acutrim .... ⊡ 648
Atrohist Plus Tablets 1605
BC Cold Powder Multi-Symptom Formula (Cold-Sinus-Allergy) .... ⊡ 631
BC Cold Powder Non-Drowsy Formula (Cold-Sinus) .... ⊡ 631
Cheracol Plus Head Cold/Cough Formula .... ⊡ 741
Comtrex Multi-Symptom Cold Reliever Liqui-Gels .... ⊡ 638
Comtrex Multi-Symptom Non-Drowsy Liqui-gels .... ⊡ 640
Contac Continuous Action Nasal Decongestant/Antihistamine 12 Hour Capsules .... ⊡ 773
Contac Maximum Strength Continuous Action Decongestant/Antihistamine 12 Hour Caplets .... ⊡ 772
Contac Severe Cold and Flu Formula Caplets .... ⊡ 773
Coricidin 'D' Decongestant Tablets .... ⊡ 760
Dexatrim .... ⊡ 795
Dexatrim Plus Vitamins Caplets .... ⊡ 796
Dimetane-DC Cough Syrup 2232
Dimetapp Allergy Sinus Caplets .... ⊡ 838
Dimetapp Cold & Allergy Chewable Tablets .... ⊡ 838
Dimetapp Cold & Cough Liqui-Gels .... ⊡ 839
Dimetapp DM Elixir .... ⊡ 840
Dimetapp Elixir .... ⊡ 840
Dimetapp Extentabs .... ⊡ 841
Dimetapp Tablets/Liqui-Gels .... ⊡ 841
Dura-Vent Tablets 971
Entex LA Tablets 972
Exgest LA Tablets 787
Hycomine 947
Nolamine Timed-Release Tablets 790
Ornade Spansule Capsules 2678
Propagest Tablets 791
Pyrroxate Caplets .... ⊡ 742
Robitussin-CF .... ⊡ 846
Sinulin Tablets 792
Tavist-D 12 Hour Relief Tablets .... ⊡ 750
Teldrin 12 Hour Antihistamine/Nasal Decongestant Allergy Relief Capsules .... ⊡ 786
Triaminic Expectorant .... ⊡ 753
Triaminic Syrup .... ⊡ 755
Triaminic Triaminicol Cold & Cough .... ⊡ 756
Triaminic DM Syrup .... ⊡ 756
Triaminicin Tablets .... ⊡ 756
Vicks DayQuil Allergy Relief 12-Hour Extended Release Tablets .... ⊡ 733
Vicks DayQuil Allergy Relief 4-Hour Tablets .... ⊡ 733
Vicks DayQuil SINUS Pressure & CONGESTION Relief .... ⊡ 734

Pindolol (Cardiostimulating effects blocked). Products include:
Visken Tablets 2428

Pirbuterol Acetate (Tachycardia or arrhythmias may occur). Products include:
Maxair Autohaler 1550
Maxair Inhaler 1552

Prazepam (Additive sedative effects).
No products indexed under this heading.

Prazosin Hydrochloride (Pressor response decreased). Products include:
Minipress Capsules 2015
Minizide Capsules 2016

Prochlorperazine (Additive sedative effects). Products include:
Compazine 2644

Propofol (Additive sedative effects). Products include:
Diprivan Injectable Emulsion 2939

Propoxyphene Hydrochloride (Additive sedative effects). Products include:
Darvon 1475
Wygesic Tablets 2930

Propoxyphene Napsylate (Additive sedative effects). Products include:
Darvon-N/Darvocet-N 1473

Propranolol Hydrochloride (Cardiostimulating effects blocked). Products include:
Inderal 2834
Inderal LA Long Acting Capsules 2836
Inderide Tablets 2838
Inderide LA Long Acting Capsules 2840

Protriptyline Hydrochloride (Additive sedative effects; increased pressor response). Products include:
Vivactil Tablets 1820

Pseudoephedrine Hydrochloride (Tachycardia or arrhythmias may occur). Products include:
Actifed Allergy Daytime/Nighttime Caplets .... ⊡ 808
Actifed Cold & Allergy Tablets .... ⊡ 807
Actifed Cold & Sinus Caplets and Tablets .... ⊡ 808
Actifed Sinus Daytime/Nighttime Tablets and Caplets .... ⊡ 809
Advil Cold and Sinus Caplets and Tablets .... ⊡ 837
Alka-Seltzer Plus Liqui-Gels .... ⊡ 612
Alka-Seltzer Plus Flu & Body Aches Liqui-Gels Non-Drowsy Formula .... ⊡ 613
Alka-Seltzer Plus Night-Time Cold Medicine Liqui-Gels .... ⊡ 612
Allerest Maximum Strength .... ⊡ 649
Allerest No Drowsiness .... ⊡ 649
Allerest Sinus Pain Formula .... ⊡ 649
Atrohist Pediatric Capsules 1603

IMPORTANT NOTE: Always consult each drug listing in the patient's regimen for possible interactions.

Benadryl Allergy/Cold Tablets 811	Sine-Aid Maximum Strength Sinus Headache Gelcaps, Caplets and Tablets 1570	Vicks DayQuil LiquiCaps/Liquid Multi-Symptom Cold/Flu Relief ... 734	Trifluoperazine Hydrochloride (Additive sedative effects). Products include:
Benadryl Allergy Decongestant Liquid Medication 812	Sine-Off No Drowsiness Formula Caplets 784	Vicks DayQuil SINUS Pressure & PAIN Relief with IBUPROFEN 735	Stelazine 2692
Benadryl Allergy Decongestant Tablets 812	Sine-Off Sinus Medicine 784	Vicks Nyquil Hot Therapy 735	Trimipramine Maleate (Additive sedative effects; increased pressor response). Products include:
Benadryl Allergy Sinus Headache Caplets 813	Singlet Tablets 785	Vicks NyQuil LiquiCaps/Liquid Multi-Symptom Cold/Flu Relief, Original and Cherry Flavors 736	Surmontil Capsules 2917
Benylin Multisymptom 816	Sinutab Non-Drying Liquid Caps 823		Zolpidem Tartrate (Additive sedative effects). Products include:
Bromfed Capsules (Extended-Release) 1832	Sinutab Sinus Allergy Medication, Maximum Strength Tablets and Caplets 823	**Pseudoephedrine Sulfate** (Tachycardia or arrhythmias may occur). Products include:	Ambien Tablets 2559
Bromfed Syrup 712	Sinutab Sinus Medication, Maximum Strength Without Drowsiness Formula, Tablets & Caplets 824	Chlor-Trimeton Allergy Decongestant Tablets 759	**Food Interactions**
Bromfed Tablets 1832		Claritin-D Tablets 2487	**Alcohol** (Additive sedative effects).
Bromfed-DM Cough Syrup 1832	Sudafed Children's Cold & Cough Liquid Medication 825	Drixoral Cold and Allergy Sustained-Action Tablets 763	
Bromfed-PD Capsules (Extended-Release) 1832	Sudafed Children's Nasal Decongestant Liquid Medication 826	Drixoral Cold and Flu Extended-Release Tablets 764	**PHENOBARBITAL ELIXIR AND TABLETS**
Children's TYLENOL Cold Multi-Symptom Chewable Tablets and Liquid 1559	Sudafed Cold & Allergy Tablets 826	Drixoral Non-Drowsy Formula Extended-Release Tablets 764	(Phenobarbital) .... 1523 May interact with oral anticoagulants, corticosteroids, central nervous system depressants, antihistamines, tranquilizers, monoamine oxidase inhibitors, oral contraceptives, hypnotics and sedatives, and certain other agents. Compounds in these categories include:
Children's TYLENOL Cold Plus Cough Multi Symptom Chewable Tablets and Liquid 1560	Sudafed Cold and Cough Liquid Caps 826	Drixoral Allergy/Sinus Extended Release Tablets 765	
Children's TYLENOL Flu Suspension Liquid 1560	Sudafed Nasal Decongestant Tablets, 30 mg 825	Trinalin Repetabs Tablets 1373	
Children's Vicks DayQuil Allergy Relief 730	Sudafed Nasal Decongestant Tablets, 60 mg 825	**Quazepam** (Additive sedative effects). Products include:	
Children's Vicks NyQuil Cold/Cough Relief 731	Sudafed Non-Drying Sinus Liquid Caps 827	Doral Tablets 2773	**Acrivastine** (Additive depressant effects). Products include:
Allergy-Sinus Comtrex Multi-Symptom Allergy-Sinus Formula Tablets and Caplets 639	Sudafed Pediatric Nasal Decongestant Liquid Oral Drops 827	**Salmeterol Xinafoate** (Tachycardia or arrhythmias may occur). Products include:	Semprex-D Capsules 1620
Comtrex Multi-Symptom 638	Sudafed Severe Cold Formula Caplets 828	Serevent Inhalation Aerosol 1149	**Alfentanil Hydrochloride** (Additive depressant effects). Products include:
Comtrex Multi-Symptom Non-Drowsy Caplets 640	Sudafed Severe Cold Formula Tablets 828	**Secobarbital Sodium** (Additive sedative effects). Products include:	Alfenta Injection 1334
Congess 1003	Sudafed Sinus Caplets 829	Seconal Sodium Pulvules 1529	**Alprazolam** (Additive depressant effects). Products include:
Contac Day Allergy/Sinus Caplets ... 771	Sudafed Sinus Tablets 829	**Selegiline Hydrochloride** (Acute hypertensive crisis; concurrent use is contraindicated). Products include:	Xanax Tablets 2115
Contac Day & Night 772	Sudafed 12 Hour Caplets 824		**Aprobarbital** (Additive depressant effects).
Contac Night Allergy/Sinus Caplets 771	Syn-Rx Tablets 1622	Eldepryl Capsules 2729	No products indexed under this heading.
Contac Severe Cold & Flu Non-Drowsy 774	Syn-Rx DM Tablets 1623	**Sotalol Hydrochloride** (Cardiostimulating effects blocked). Products include:	**Astemizole** (Additive depressant effects). Products include:
Deconsal II Tablets 1605	TheraFlu Flu and Cold Medicine 750	Betapace Tablets 637	Hismanal Tablets 1341
Dimetane-DX Cough Syrup 2233	Theraflu Maximum Strength Flu and Cold Medicine For Sore Throat 751	**Sufentanil Citrate** (Additive sedative effects). Products include:	**Azatadine Maleate** (Additive depressant effects). Products include:
Dimetapp Cold & Fever Suspension 839		Sufenta Injection 1355	Trinalin Repetabs Tablets 1373
Dimetapp Decongestant Pediatric Drops 840	TheraFlu Flu, Cold and Cough Medicine 750	**Temazepam** (Additive sedative effects). Products include:	**Betamethasone Acetate** (Enhanced metabolism of exogenous corticosteroids). Products include:
Dorcol Children's Cough Syrup 748	TheraFlu Maximum Strength Nighttime Flu, Cold & Cough Medicine 751	Restoril Capsules 2413	Celestone Soluspan Suspension 2484
Drixoral Cough + Congestion Liquid Caps 763		**Terazosin Hydrochloride** (Pressor response decreased). Products include:	**Betamethasone Sodium Phosphate** (Enhanced metabolism of exogenous corticosteroids). Products include:
Dura-Tap/PD Capsules 970	TheraFlu Maximum Strength Non-Drowsy Formula Flu, Cold & Cough Medicine 751	Hytrin Capsules 434	
Duratuss Tablets 2750		**Terbutaline Sulfate** (Tachycardia or arrhythmias may occur). Products include:	Celestone Soluspan Suspension 2484
Duratuss HD Elixir 2750	TheraFlu Maximum Strength, Non-Drowsy Formula Flu, Cold and Cough Caplets 752		**Bromodiphenhydramine Hydrochloride** (Additive depressant effects).
Efidac/24 655		Brethaire Inhaler 830	No products indexed under this heading.
Entex PSE Tablets 973	Theraflu Maximum Strength Sinus Non-Drowsy Formula Caplets 752	Brethine Ampuls 832	
Fedahist Gyrocaps 2545	Triaminic AM Cough and Decongestant Formula 753	Brethine Tablets 831	**Brompheniramine Maleate** (Additive depressant effects). Products include:
Guaifed 1833		Bricanyl Subcutaneous Injection 1247	
Guaifed Syrup 712	Triaminic AM Decongestant Formula 753	Bricanyl Tablets 1248	Alka-Seltzer Plus Sinus Medicine 611
Guaimax-D Tablets 809		**Thioridazine Hydrochloride** (Additive sedative effects). Products include:	Bromfed Capsules (Extended-Release) 1832
Histussin D Liquid 670	Triaminic Infant Oral Decongestant Drops 754		
Infants' TYLENOL Cold Decongestant & Fever-Reducer Drops 1561	Triaminic Night Time 754	Mellaril 2398	Bromfed Syrup 712
Kronofed-A 994	Triaminic Sore Throat Formula 755	**Thiothixene** (Additive sedative effects). Products include:	Bromfed Tablets 1832
Novahistine DMX 782	Tussend 1830		Bromfed-DM Cough Syrup 1832
Nucofed 2225	Tussend Expectorant 1831	Navane Capsules and Concentrate 2018	Bromfed-PD Capsules (Extended-Release) 1832
PediaCare Cough-Cold Chewable Tablets and Liquid 1569	TYLENOL Allergy Sinus, Maximum Strength Caplets and Gelcaps 1571	Navane Intramuscular 2019	Dimetane-DC Cough Syrup 2232
PediaCare Infants' Decongestant Drops 1569	TYLENOL Allergy Sinus NightTime, Maximum Strength Caplets 1571	**Timolol Hemihydrate** (Cardiostimulating effects blocked). Products include:	Dimetane-DX Cough Syrup 2233
PediaCare Infants' Drops Decongestant Plus Cough 1569	TYLENOL Cold Medication, Multi-Symptom Formula Tablets and Caplets 1572		Dimetapp Allergy Dye-Free Elixir ... 838
PediaCare NightRest Cough-Cold Liquid 1569		Betimol 0.25%, 0.5% 259	Dimetapp Allergy Sinus Caplets 838
Pediatric Vicks 44d Cough & Head Congestion Relief 736	TYLENOL Cold Medication, Multi-Symptom Hot Liquid Packets 1572	**Timolol Maleate** (Cardiostimulating effects blocked). Products include:	Dimetapp Cold & Allergy Chewable Tablets 838
Pediatric Vicks 44m Cough & Cold Relief 737	TYLENOL Cold Medication, No Drowsiness Formula Caplets and Gelcaps 1572	Blocadren Tablets 1654	Dimetapp Cold & Cough Liqui-Gels 839
Robitussin Cold & Cough Liqui-Gels 844		Timolide Tablets 1791	
Robitussin Cold, Cough & Flu Liqui-Gels 844	TYLENOL Cold Severe Congestion Caplets 1573	Timoptic in Ocudose 1796	Dimetapp Cold & Fever Suspension 839
Robitussin Maximum Strength Cough & Cold 847	TYLENOL Cough Medication with Decongestant, Multi Symptom 1574	Timoptic Sterile Ophthalmic Solution 1794	Dimetapp DM Elixir 840
Robitussin Night-Time Cold Formula 847	TYLENOL Flu No Drowsiness Formula, Maximum Strength Gelcaps 1575	Timoptic-XE 1798	Dimetapp Elixir 840
Robitussin Pediatric Cough & Cold Formula 848		**Tranylcypromine Sulfate** (Acute hypertensive crisis; concurrent use is contraindicated). Products include:	Dimetapp Extentabs 841
Robitussin Pediatric Drops 849	TYLENOL Flu NightTime, Maximum Strength Gelcaps 1575		Dimetapp Tablets/Liqui-Gels 841
Robitussin Severe Congestion Liqui-Gels 845	TYLENOL Flu NightTime, Maximum Strength Hot Medication Packets 1575	Parnate Tablets 2679	Rondec Chewable Tablets 974
Robitussin-DAC Syrup 2249		**Triazolam** (Additive sedative effects). Products include:	Vicks DayQuil Allergy Relief 12-Hour Extended Release Tablets ... 733
Robitussin-PE 846	TYLENOL Sinus, Maximum Strength Geltabs, Gelcaps, Caplets and Tablets 1576		
Rondec Oral Drops 974		Halcion Tablets 2093	Vicks DayQuil Allergy Relief 4-Hour Tablets 733
Rondec Syrup 974	Vicks 44 LiquiCaps Cough, Cold & Flu Relief 728		
Rondec Tablet 974	Vicks 44 LiquiCaps Non-Drowsy Cough & Cold Relief 729		
Rondec Chewable Tablets 974	Vicks 44D Cough & Head Congestion Relief 728		
Rondec-TR Tablet 974	Vicks 44M Cough, Cold & Flu Relief 729		
Ryna 804			
Seldane-D Extended-Release Tablets 1286			
Semprex-D Capsules 1620			
Sinarest 663			

(▣ Described in PDR For Nonprescription Drugs) (◎ Described in PDR For Ophthalmology)

843 **Interactions Index** Phenobarbital

Buprenorphine (Additive depressant effects). Products include:
Buprenex Injectable 2170
Buspirone Hydrochloride (Additive depressant effects). Products include:
BuSpar Tablets 738
Butabarbital (Additive depressant effects).
No products indexed under this heading.
Butalbital (Additive depressant effects). Products include:
Axocet Capsules 2469
Esgic-plus Capsules 1012
Esgic-plus Tablets 1012
Fioricet Tablets 2386
Fioricet with Codeine Capsules 2387
Fiorinal Capsules 2388
Fiorinal with Codeine Capsules 2390
Fiorinal Tablets 2388
Phrenilin 790
Sedapap Tablets 50 mg/650 mg 1826
Cetirizine Hydrochloride (Additive depressant effects). Products include:
Zyrtec Tablets 2053
Chlordiazepoxide (Additive depressant effects). Products include:
Limbitrol 2333
Chlordiazepoxide Hydrochloride (Additive depressant effects). Products include:
Librax Capsules 2330
Librium Capsules 2331
Librium Injectable 2332
Chlorpheniramine Maleate (Additive depressant effects). Products include:
Alka-Seltzer Plus Cold Medicine 611
Alka-Seltzer Plus Cold Medicine Liqui-Gels 612
Alka-Seltzer Plus Cold & Cough Medicine 611
Alka-Seltzer Plus Cold & Cough Medicine Liqui-Gels 612
Alka-Seltzer Plus Flu & Body Aches Effervescent Tablets 612
Allerest Maximum Strength 649
Allerest Sinus Pain Formula 649
Ana-Kit Anaphylaxis Emergency Treatment Kit 611
Atrohist Pediatric Capsules 1603
Atrohist Plus Tablets 1605
BC Cold Powder Multi-Symptom Formula (Cold-Sinus-Allergy) 631
Cerose DM 853
Cheracol Plus Head Cold/Cough Formula 741
Children's TYLENOL Cold Multi-Symptom Chewable Tablets and Liquid 1559
Children's TYLENOL Cold Plus Cough Multi Symptom Chewable Tablets and Liquid 1560
Children's TYLENOL Flu Suspension Liquid 1560
Children's Vicks DayQuil Allergy Relief 730
Children's Vicks NyQuil Cold/Cough Relief 731
Chlor-Trimeton Allergy Decongestant Tablets 759
Chlor-Trimeton Allergy Tablets 758
Allergy-Sinus Comtrex Multi-Symptom Allergy-Sinus Formula Tablets and Caplets 639
Comtrex Multi-Symptom 638
Contac Continuous Action Nasal Decongestant/Antihistamine 12 Hour Capsules 773
Contac Maximum Strength Continuous Action Decongestant/Antihistamine 12 Hour Caplets 772
Contac Severe Cold and Flu Formula Caplets 773
Coricidin Cold + Flu Tablets 760
Coricidin Cough + Cold Tablets 760
Coricidin 'D' Decongestant Tablets 760
D.A. II Tablets 972
D.A. Chewable Tablets 970
Dura-Tap/PD Capsules 970
Dura-Vent/DA Tablets 972
Efidac 24 Chlorpheniramine 655
Extendryl 1003
Fedahist Gyrocaps 2545
Hycomine Compound Tablets 948
Kronofed-A 994
Nolamine Timed-Release Tablets 790
Novahistine Elixir 782
Ornade Spansule Capsules 2678
PediaCare Cough-Cold Chewable Tablets and Liquid 1569
PediaCare NightRest Cough-Cold Liquid 1569
Pediatric Vicks 44m Cough & Cold Relief 737
Pyrroxate Caplets 742
Ryna 804
Sinarest 663
Sine-Off Sinus Medicine 784
Singlet Tablets 785
Sinulin Tablets 792
Sinutab Sinus Allergy Medication, Maximum Strength Tablets and Caplets 823
Sudafed Cold & Allergy Tablets 826
Teldrin 12 Hour Antihistamine/Nasal Decongestant Allergy Relief Capsules 786
TheraFlu Flu and Cold Medicine 750
Theraflu Maximum Strength Flu and Cold Medicine For Sore Throat 751
TheraFlu Flu, Cold and Cough Medicine 750
TheraFlu Maximum Strength Nighttime Flu, Cold & Cough Medicine 751
Triaminic Night Time 754
Triaminic Syrup 755
Triaminic Triaminicol Cold & Cough 756
Triaminicin Tablets 756
Tussend 1830
TYLENOL Allergy Sinus, Maximum Strength Caplets and Gelcaps 1571
TYLENOL Cold Medication, Multi-Symptom Formula Tablets and Caplets 1572
TYLENOL Cold Medication, Multi-Symptom Hot Liquid Packets 1572
Vicks 44 LiquiCaps Cough, Cold & Flu Relief 728
Vicks 44M Cough, Cold & Flu Relief 729
Chlorpheniramine Polistirex (Additive depressant effects). Products include:
Tussionex Pennkinetic Extended-Release Suspension 1624
Chlorpheniramine Tannate (Additive depressant effects). Products include:
Atrohist Pediatric Suspension 1604
Atrohist Pediatric Suspension Dye-Free 1604
Rynatan 2781
Rynatuss 2782
Chlorpromazine (Additive depressant effects). Products include:
Thorazine Suppositories 2701
Chlorprothixene (Additive depressant effects).
No products indexed under this heading.
Chlorprothixene Hydrochloride (Additive depressant effects).
No products indexed under this heading.
Chlorprothixene Lactate (Additive depressant effects).
No products indexed under this heading.
Clemastine Fumarate (Additive depressant effects). Products include:
Tavist Syrup 2426
Tavist Tablets 2427
Tavist-1 12 Hour Relief Tablets 749
Tavist-D 12 Hour Relief Tablets 750
Clorazepate Dipotassium (Additive depressant effects). Products include:
Tranxene 459
Clozapine (Additive depressant effects). Products include:
Clozaril Tablets 2377
Codeine Phosphate (Additive depressant effects). Products include:
Brontex 2130
Dimetane-DC Cough Syrup 2232
Fioricet with Codeine Capsules 2387
Fiorinal with Codeine Capsules 2390
Nucofed 2225
Phenergan with Codeine 2883
Phenergan VC with Codeine 2888
Robitussin A-C Syrup 2248
Robitussin-DAC Syrup 2249
Ryna 804
Soma Compound w/Codeine Tablets 2784
Tylenol with Codeine 1592
Cortisone Acetate (Enhanced metabolism of exogenous corticosteroids). Products include:
Cortone Acetate Sterile Suspension 1663
Cortone Acetate Tablets 1664
Cyproheptadine Hydrochloride (Additive depressant effects). Products include:
Periactin 1767
Desflurane (Additive depressant effects). Products include:
Suprane (desflurane, USP) 1865
Desogestrel (Decreased estrogen effect). Products include:
Desogen Tablets 1867
Ortho-Cept 1907
Dexamethasone (Enhanced metabolism of exogenous corticosteroids). Products include:
AK-Trol Ointment & Suspension ◉ 205
Decadron Elixir 1676
Decadron Tablets 1678
Decaspray Topical Aerosol 1689
Maxitrol Ophthalmic Ointment and Suspension ◉ 222
TobraDex Ophthalmic Suspension and Ointment 469
Dexamethasone Acetate (Enhanced metabolism of exogenous corticosteroids). Products include:
Dalalone D.P. Injectable 1009
Decadron-LA Sterile Suspension 1687
Dexamethasone Sodium Phosphate (Enhanced metabolism of exogenous corticosteroids). Products include:
Decadron Phosphate Injection 1680
Decadron Phosphate Sterile Ophthalmic Ointment 1684
Decadron Phosphate Sterile Ophthalmic Solution 1685
Decadron Phosphate Topical Cream 1686
Decadron Phosphate with Xylocaine Injection, Sterile 1683
Dexacort Phosphate in Respihaler 1606
Dexacort Phosphate in Turbinaire 1607
NeoDecadron Sterile Ophthalmic Ointment 1755
NeoDecadron Sterile Ophthalmic Solution 1756
NeoDecadron Topical Cream 1757
Dexchlorpheniramine Maleate (Additive depressant effects).
No products indexed under this heading.
Dezocine (Additive depressant effects). Products include:
Dalgan Injection 529
Diazepam (Additive depressant effects). Products include:
Dizac (diazepam injectable emulsion) CIV 1862
Valium Injectable 2336
Valium Tablets 2335
Dicumarol (Lowered plasma levels and decreased anticoagulant activity).
No products indexed under this heading.
Diphenhydramine Citrate (Additive depressant effects). Products include:
Excedrin P.M. Analgesic/Sleeping Aid Tablets, Caplets, Liquigels 735
Diphenhydramine Hydrochloride (Additive depressant effects). Products include:
Actifed Allergy Daytime/Nighttime Caplets 808
Actifed Sinus Daytime/Nighttime Tablets and Caplets 809
Extra Strength Bayer PM Aspirin Plus Sleep Aid 617
Benadryl Allergy Chewables 811
Benadryl Allergy/Cold Tablets 811
Benadryl Allergy Decongestant Liquid Medication 812
Benadryl Allergy Decongestant Tablets 812
Benadryl Allergy Liquid Medication 813
Benadryl Allergy 811
Benadryl Allergy Sinus Headache Caplets 813
Benadryl Dye-Free Allergy Liqui-gel Softgels 813
Benadryl Dye-Free Allergy Liquid Medication 814
Benadryl Itch Relief Stick Extra Strength 814
Benadryl Cream 814
Benadryl Gel 815
Benadryl Spray 815
Benadryl Injection 1955
Contac Day & Night Cold/Flu Night Caplets 772
Contac Night Allergy/Sinus Caplets 771
Extra Strength Doan's P.M. 653
Excedrin P.M. Analgesic/Sleeping Aid Tablets, Caplets, Liquigels 643
Nytol QuickCaps Caplets 632
Sleepinal Night-time Sleep Aid Capsules and Softgels 798
TYLENOL Allergy Sinus NightTime, Maximum Strength Caplets 1571
TYLENOL Flu NightTime, Maximum Strength Gelcaps 1575
TYLENOL Flu NightTime, Maximum Strength Hot Medication Packets 1575
TYLENOL PM Pain Reliever/Sleep Aid, Extra Strength Gelcaps, Caplets, Geltabs 1576
TYLENOL Severe Allergy Medication Caplets 1571
Maximum Strength Unisom Sleepgels 1990
Unisom With Pain Relief-Nighttime Sleep Aid and Pain Reliever 1991
Divalproex Sodium (Increases the phenobarbital serum levels). Products include:
Depakote Tablets 418
Doxycycline Calcium (Shortened half-life of doxycycline). Products include:
Vibramycin Calcium Oral Suspension Syrup 2038
Doxycycline Hyclate (Shortened half-life of doxycycline). Products include:
Doryx Capsules 1970
Vibramycin Hyclate Capsules 2038
Vibramycin Hyclate Intravenous 2040
Vibra-Tabs Film Coated Tablets 2038
Doxycycline Monohydrate (Shortened half-life of doxycycline). Products include:
Monodox Capsules 1858
Vibramycin Monohydrate for Oral Suspension 2038
Droperidol (Additive depressant effects). Products include:
Inapsine Injection 462
Enflurane (Additive depressant effects).
No products indexed under this heading.
Estazolam (Additive depressant effects). Products include:
ProSom Tablets 457
Ethchlorvynol (Additive depressant effects). Products include:
Placidyl Capsules 456
Ethinamate (Additive depressant effects).
No products indexed under this heading.

IMPORTANT NOTE: Always consult each drug listing in the patient's regimen for possible interactions.

Phenobarbital / Interactions Index

Ethinyl Estradiol (Decreased estrogen effect). Products include:
- Brevicon ... 2563
- Demulen ... 2580
- Desogen Tablets ... 1867
- Levlen/Tri-Levlen ... 646
- Lo/Ovral Tablets ... 2852
- Lo/Ovral-28 Tablets ... 2857
- Modicon ... 1928
- Nordette-21 Tablets ... 2863
- Nordette-28 Tablets ... 2866
- Norinyl ... 2563
- Ortho-Cept ... 1907
- Ortho-Cyclen/Ortho-Tri-Cyclen ... 1914
- Ortho-Novum ... 1928
- Ortho-Cyclen/Ortho Tri-Cyclen ... 1914
- Ovcon ... 765
- Ovral Tablets ... 2877
- Ovral-28 Tablets ... 2878
- Levlen/Tri-Levlen ... 646
- Tri-Norinyl ... 2607
- Triphasil-21 Tablets ... 2919
- Triphasil-28 Tablets ... 2924

Ethynodiol Diacetate (Decreased estrogen effect). Products include:
- Demulen ... 2580

Fentanyl (Additive depressant effects). Products include:
- Duragesic Transdermal System ... 1336

Fentanyl Citrate (Additive depressant effects). Products include:
- Sublimaze Injection ... 463

Fludrocortisone Acetate (Enhanced metabolism of exogenous corticosteroids). Products include:
- Florinef Acetate Tablets ... 506

Fluphenazine Decanoate (Additive depressant effects). Products include:
- Prolixin Decanoate ... 510

Fluphenazine Enanthate (Additive depressant effects). Products include:
- Prolixin Enanthate ... 510

Fluphenazine Hydrochloride (Additive depressant effects). Products include:
- Prolixin ... 510

Flurazepam Hydrochloride (Additive depressant effects). Products include:
- Dalmane Capsules ... 2329

Furazolidone (Prolongs the effects of barbiturates). Products include:
- Furoxone ... 2221

Glutethimide (Additive depressant effects).
- No products indexed under this heading.

Griseofulvin (Interference with griseofulvin absorption; decreased blood levels). Products include:
- Fulvicin P/G Tablets ... 2499
- Fulvicin P/G 165 & 330 Tablets ... 2500
- Grifulvin V (griseofulvin tablets) Microsize (griseofulvin oral suspension) Microsize ... 1944
- Gris-PEG Tablets, 125 mg & 250 mg ... 476

Haloperidol (Additive depressant effects). Products include:
- Haldol Injection, Tablets and Concentrate ... 1585

Haloperidol Decanoate (Additive depressant effects). Products include:
- Haldol Decanoate ... 1587

Hydrocodone Bitartrate (Additive depressant effects). Products include:
- Codiclear DH Syrup ... 808
- Duratuss HD Elixir ... 2750
- Histussin D Liquid ... 670
- Hycodan Tablets and Syrup ... 946
- Hycomine Compound Tablets ... 948
- Hycomine ... 947
- Hycotuss Expectorant Syrup ... 950
- Hydrocet Capsules ... 787
- Lorcet 10/650 Tablets ... 1016
- Lortab ... 2751
- Tussend ... 1830
- Tussend Expectorant ... 1831

- Vicodin Tablets ... 1404
- Vicodin ES Tablets ... 1405
- Vicodin HP Tablets ... 1403
- Vicodin Tuss Expectorant ... 1406
- Zydone Capsules ... 967

Hydrocodone Polistirex (Additive depressant effects). Products include:
- Tussionex Pennkinetic Extended-Release Suspension ... 1624

Hydrocortisone (Enhanced metabolism of exogenous corticosteroids). Products include:
- Anusol-HC Cream 2.5% ... 1953
- Aquanil HC Lotion ... 1989
- Maximum Strength Cortaid Spray ... 800
- CORTENEMA ... 2713
- Cortisporin Ointment ... 1074
- Cortisporin Ophthalmic Ointment Sterile ... 1074
- Cortisporin Ophthalmic Suspension Sterile ... 1075
- Cortisporin Otic Solution Sterile ... 1076
- Cortisporin Otic Suspension Sterile ... 1077
- Cortizone-5 ... 795
- Cortizone-10 ... 795
- Hydrocortone Tablets ... 1715
- Hytone ... 922
- Hytone Ointment 2 ½ % ... 923
- Massengill Medicated Soft Cloth Towelettes ... 2628
- Pediotic Suspension Sterile ... 1140
- Preparation H Hydrocortisone 1% Cream ... 843
- ProctoCream-HC 2.5% ... 2552
- VōSoL HC Otic Solution ... 2786

Hydrocortisone Acetate (Enhanced metabolism of exogenous corticosteroids). Products include:
- Analpram-HC Rectal Cream 1% and 2.5% ... 993
- Anusol HC-1 Hydrocortisone Anti-Itch Ointment ... 810
- Anusol-HC Suppositories ... 1954
- Caldecort Anti-Itch Hydrocortisone Cream ... 651
- Coly-Mycin S Otic w/Neomycin & Hydrocortisone ... 1965
- Cortaid ... 800
- Cortifoam ... 2540
- Cortisporin Cream ... 1073
- Epifoam ... 2543
- Hydrocortone Acetate Sterile Suspension ... 1712
- Mantadil Cream ... 1124
- Nupercainal Hydrocortisone 1% Cream ... 661
- Pramosone Cream, Lotion & Ointment ... 995
- ProctoFoam-HC ... 2552
- Terra-Cortril Ophthalmic Suspension ... 2033

Hydrocortisone Sodium Phosphate (Enhanced metabolism of exogenous corticosteroids). Products include:
- Hydrocortone Phosphate Injection, Sterile ... 1713

Hydrocortisone Sodium Succinate (Enhanced metabolism of exogenous corticosteroids).
- No products indexed under this heading.

Hydroxyzine Hydrochloride (Additive depressant effects). Products include:
- Atarax Tablets & Syrup ... 1992
- Marax Tablets & DF Syrup ... 2015
- Vistaril Intramuscular Solution ... 2042

Isocarboxazid (Prolongs the effects of barbiturates).
- No products indexed under this heading.

Isoflurane (Additive depressant effects).
- No products indexed under this heading.

Ketamine Hydrochloride (Additive depressant effects).
- No products indexed under this heading.

Levomethadyl Acetate Hydrochloride (Additive depressant effects). Products include:
- Orlaam Oral Solution ... 2361

Levonorgestrel (Decreased estrogen effect). Products include:
- Levlen/Tri-Levlen ... 646
- Nordette-21 Tablets ... 2863
- Nordette-28 Tablets ... 2866
- Norplant System ... 2868
- Levlen/Tri-Levlen ... 646
- Triphasil-21 Tablets ... 2919
- Triphasil-28 Tablets ... 2924

Levorphanol Tartrate (Additive depressant effects). Products include:
- Levo-Dromoran ... 2297

Loratadine (Additive depressant effects). Products include:
- Claritin ... 2485
- Claritin-D Tablets ... 2487

Lorazepam (Additive depressant effects). Products include:
- Ativan Injection ... 2805
- Ativan Tablets ... 2807

Loxapine Hydrochloride (Additive depressant effects). Products include:
- Loxitane ... 1426

Loxapine Succinate (Additive depressant effects). Products include:
- Loxitane Capsules ... 1426

Meperidine Hydrochloride (Additive depressant effects). Products include:
- Demerol ... 2438
- Mepergan Injection ... 2859

Mephobarbital (Additive depressant effects). Products include:
- Mebaral Tablets ... 2452

Meprobamate (Additive depressant effects). Products include:
- Miltown Tablets ... 2780
- PMB 200 and PMB 400 ... 2890

Mesoridazine Besylate (Additive depressant effects). Products include:
- Serentil ... 689

Mestranol (Decreased estrogen effect). Products include:
- Norinyl ... 2563
- Ortho-Novum ... 1928

Methadone Hydrochloride (Additive depressant effects). Products include:
- Methadone Hydrochloride Oral Concentrate ... 2356
- Methadone Hydrochloride Oral Solution & Tablets ... 2357

Methdilazine Hydrochloride (Additive depressant effects).
- No products indexed under this heading.

Methohexital Sodium (Additive depressant effects).
- No products indexed under this heading.

Methotrimeprazine (Additive depressant effects). Products include:
- Levoprome ... 1321

Methoxyflurane (Additive depressant effects).
- No products indexed under this heading.

Methylprednisolone Acetate (Enhanced metabolism of exogenous corticosteroids).
- No products indexed under this heading.

Methylprednisolone Sodium Succinate (Enhanced metabolism of exogenous corticosteroids).
- No products indexed under this heading.

Midazolam Hydrochloride (Additive depressant effects). Products include:
- Versed Injection ... 2324

Molindone Hydrochloride (Additive depressant effects). Products include:
- Moban Tablets and Concentrate ... 1036

Morphine Sulfate (Additive depressant effects). Products include:
- Astramorph/PF Injection, USP (Preservative-Free) ... 526
- Duramorph Injection ... 983
- Infumorph 200 and Infumorph 500 Sterile Solutions ... 985
- Kadian Capsules ... 2948
- MS Contin Tablets ... 2149
- MSIR ... 2152
- Oramorph SR (Morphine Sulfate Sustained Release Tablets) ... 2359
- RMS Suppositories CII ... 2766
- Roxanol ... 2365

Norethindrone (Decreased estrogen effect). Products include:
- Brevicon ... 2563
- Micronor Tablets ... 1903
- Modicon ... 1928
- Norinyl ... 2563
- Nor-Q D Tablets ... 2598
- Ortho-Novum ... 1928
- Ovcon ... 765
- Tri-Norinyl ... 2607

Norethynodrel (Decreased estrogen effect).
- No products indexed under this heading.

Norgestimate (Decreased estrogen effect). Products include:
- Ortho-Cyclen/Ortho-Tri-Cyclen ... 1914
- Ortho-Cyclen/Ortho Tri-Cyclen ... 1914

Norgestrel (Decreased estrogen effect). Products include:
- Lo/Ovral Tablets ... 2852
- Lo/Ovral-28 Tablets ... 2857
- Ovral Tablets ... 2877
- Ovral-28 Tablets ... 2878
- Ovrette Tablets ... 2878

Opium Alkaloids (Additive depressant effects).
- No products indexed under this heading.

Oxazepam (Additive depressant effects). Products include:
- Serax Capsules ... 2916
- Serax Tablets ... 2916

Oxycodone Hydrochloride (Additive depressant effects). Products include:
- OxyContin Tablets ... 2163
- OxyIR Capsules ... 2167
- Percocet Tablets ... 955
- Percodan Tablets ... 955
- Percodan-Demi Tablets ... 956
- Roxicodone Tablets, Oral Solution & Intensol (Oxycodone) ... 2366
- Tylox Capsules ... 1593

Pentobarbital Sodium (Additive depressant effects). Products include:
- Nembutal Sodium Capsules ... 440
- Nembutal Sodium Solution ... 442
- Nembutal Sodium Suppositories ... 444

Perphenazine (Additive depressant effects). Products include:
- Etrafon ... 2495
- Triavil Tablets ... 1800
- Trilafon ... 2532

Phenelzine Sulfate (Prolongs the effects of barbiturates). Products include:
- Nardil ... 1977

Phenytoin (Variable effect on the metabolism of phenytoin). Products include:
- Dilantin Infatabs ... 1967
- Dilantin-125 Suspension ... 1969

Phenytoin Sodium (Variable effect on the metabolism of phenytoin). Products include:
- Dilantin Kapseals ... 1965

Prazepam (Additive depressant effects).
- No products indexed under this heading.

(▣ Described in PDR For Nonprescription Drugs)   (ⓞ Described in PDR For Ophthalmology)

845 **Interactions Index** **PhosLo**

Prednisolone Acetate (Enhanced metabolism of exogenous corticosteroids). Products include:
- AK-CIDE ⊙ 203
- AK-CIDE Ointment ⊙ 203
- Blephamide Liquifilm Sterile Ophthalmic Suspension 472
- Blephamide Ointment ⊙ 234
- Econopred & Econopred Plus Ophthalmic Suspensions ⊙ 216
- Poly-Pred Liquifilm ⊙ 246
- Pred Forte ⊙ 247
- Pred Mild ⊙ 250
- Pred-G Liquifilm Sterile Ophthalmic Suspension ⊙ 248
- Pred-G S.O.P. Sterile Ophthalmic Ointment ⊙ 249

Prednisolone Sodium Phosphate (Enhanced metabolism of exogenous corticosteroids). Products include:
- AK-PRED ⊙ 204
- Hydeltrasol Injection, Sterile 1708
- Pediapred Oral Solution 1618

Prednisolone Tebutate (Enhanced metabolism of exogenous corticosteroids). Products include:
- Hydeltra-T.B.A. Sterile Suspension 1710

Prednisone (Enhanced metabolism of exogenous corticosteroids).
- No products indexed under this heading.

Prochlorperazine (Additive depressant effects). Products include:
- Compazine 2644

Promethazine Hydrochloride (Additive depressant effects). Products include:
- Mepergan Injection 2859
- Phenergan with Codeine 2883
- Phenergan with Dextromethorphan 2885
- Phenergan Injection 2880
- Phenergan Suppositories 2882
- Phenergan Syrup 2881
- Phenergan Tablets 2882
- Phenergan VC 2886
- Phenergan VC with Codeine 2888

Propofol (Additive depressant effects). Products include:
- Diprivan Injectable Emulsion 2939

Propoxyphene Hydrochloride (Additive depressant effects). Products include:
- Darvon 1475
- Wygesic Tablets 2930

Propoxyphene Napsylate (Additive depressant effects). Products include:
- Darvon-N/Darvocet-N 1473

Pyrilamine Maleate (Additive depressant effects). Products include:
- 4-Way Fast Acting Nasal Spray (regular & mentholated) ▣ 644
- Maximum Strength Multi-Symptom Formula Midol ▣ 621
- PMS Multi-Symptom Formula Midol ▣ 622

Pyrilamine Tannate (Additive depressant effects). Products include:
- Atrohist Pediatric Suspension 1604
- Atrohist Pediatric Suspension Dye-Free 1604
- Rynatan 2781

Quazepam (Additive depressant effects). Products include:
- Doral Tablets 2773

Risperidone (Additive depressant effects). Products include:
- Risperdal Tablets 1348

Secobarbital Sodium (Additive depressant effects). Products include:
- Seconal Sodium Pulvules 1529

Selegiline Hydrochloride (Prolongs the effects of barbiturates). Products include:
- Eldepryl Capsules 2729

Sevoflurane (Additive depressant effects).
- No products indexed under this heading.

Sodium Valproate (Increases the phenobarbital serum levels).

Sufentanil Citrate (Additive depressant effects). Products include:
- Sufenta Injection 1355

Temazepam (Additive depressant effects). Products include:
- Restoril Capsules 2413

Terfenadine (Additive depressant effects). Products include:
- Seldane Tablets 1284
- Seldane-D Extended-Release Tablets 1286

Thiamylal Sodium (Additive depressant effects).
- No products indexed under this heading.

Thioridazine Hydrochloride (Additive depressant effects). Products include:
- Mellaril 2398

Thiothixene (Additive depressant effects). Products include:
- Navane Capsules and Concentrate 2018
- Navane Intramuscular 2019

Tranylcypromine Sulfate (Prolongs the effects of barbiturates). Products include:
- Parnate Tablets 2679

Triamcinolone (Enhanced metabolism of exogenous corticosteroids).
- No products indexed under this heading.

Triamcinolone Acetonide (Enhanced metabolism of exogenous corticosteroids). Products include:
- Azmacort Oral Inhaler 2175
- Nasacort AQ Nasal Spray 2191
- Nasacort Nasal Inhaler 2189

Triamcinolone Diacetate (Enhanced metabolism of exogenous corticosteroids).
- No products indexed under this heading.

Triamcinolone Hexacetonide (Enhanced metabolism of exogenous corticosteroids).
- No products indexed under this heading.

Triazolam (Additive depressant effects). Products include:
- Halcion Tablets 2093

Trifluoperazine Hydrochloride (Additive depressant effects). Products include:
- Stelazine 2692

Trimeprazine Tartrate (Additive depressant effects).
- No products indexed under this heading.

Tripelennamine Hydrochloride (Additive depressant effects). Products include:
- PBZ Tablets 863
- PBZ-SR Tablets 862

Triprolidine Hydrochloride (Additive depressant effects). Products include:
- Actifed Cold & Allergy Tablets ▣ 807
- Actifed Cold & Sinus Caplets and Tablets ▣ 808

Valproic Acid (Increases the phenobarbital serum levels). Products include:
- Depakene 416

Warfarin Sodium (Lowered plasma levels and decreased anticoagulant activity). Products include:
- Coumadin 941

Zolpidem Tartrate (Additive depressant effects). Products include:
- Ambien Tablets 2559

Food Interactions

Alcohol (Additive depressant effects).

PHENURONE TABLETS
(Phenacemide) 455
May interact with anticonvulsants and certain other agents. Compounds in these categories include:

Carbamazepine (Concurrent use requires extreme caution). Products include:
- Atretol Tablets 569
- Tegretol/Tegretol-XR 870

Divalproex Sodium (Concurrent use requires extreme caution). Products include:
- Depakote Tablets 418

Ethosuximide (Concurrent use requires extreme caution). Products include:
- Zarontin Capsules 1986
- Zarontin Syrup 1986

Ethotoin (May result in paranoid symptoms). Products include:
- Peganone Tablets 455

Felbamate (Concurrent use requires extreme caution). Products include:
- Felbatol 2774

Lamotrigine (Concurrent use requires extreme caution). Products include:
- Lamictal Tablets 1105

Mephenytoin (Concurrent use requires extreme caution). Products include:
- Mesantoin Tablets 2400

Methsuximide (Concurrent use requires extreme caution). Products include:
- Celontin Kapseals 1955

Paramethadione (Concurrent use requires extreme caution).
- No products indexed under this heading.

Phenobarbital (Concurrent use requires extreme caution). Products include:
- Arco-Lase Plus Tablets 513
- Bellergal-S Tablets 2375
- Donnatal 2234
- Donnatal Extentabs 2234
- Donnatal Tablets 2234
- Phenobarbital Elixir and Tablets 1523
- Quadrinal Tablets 1398

Phensuximide (Concurrent use requires extreme caution).
- No products indexed under this heading.

Phenytoin (Concurrent use requires extreme caution). Products include:
- Dilantin Infatabs 1967
- Dilantin-125 Suspension 1969

Phenytoin Sodium (Concurrent use requires extreme caution). Products include:
- Dilantin Kapseals 1965

Primidone (Concurrent use requires extreme caution). Products include:
- Mysoline 2860

Trimethadione (Concurrent use requires extreme caution).
- No products indexed under this heading.

Valproic Acid (Concurrent use requires extreme caution). Products include:
- Depakene 416

PHILLIPS' GELCAPS
(Docusate Sodium, Phenolphthalein) ▣ 627
May interact with:

Mineral Oil (Concurrent oral use is not recommended). Products include:
- Alpha Keri Moisture Rich Body Oil ▣ 635
- Anusol Hemorrhoidal Ointment ▣ 810
- Aquaphor Healing Ointment 636
- Aquaphor Healing Ointment, Original Formula 636
- Eucerin Original Moisturizing Creme (Unscented) 636
- Eucerin Original Moisturizing Lotion 636
- Eucerin Plus Dry Skin Care Moisturizing Lotion 636
- Eucerin Plus Moisturizing Creme 636
- Fleet Mineral Oil Enema 1001
- Hemorid ▣ 797
- HypoTears Ointment ⊙ 262
- Keri Lotion - Original Formula ▣ 644
- Kondremul ▣ 656
- Lubriderm Bath and Shower Oil ▣ 821
- Nephrox Suspension ▣ 671
- Preparation H Hemorrhoidal Ointment ▣ 842
- Refresh PM Lubricant Eye Ointment ⊙ 252
- Replens Vaginal Moisturizer ▣ 823
- Tears Renewed Ointment ⊙ 210

PHILLIPS' MILK OF MAGNESIA LIQUID
(Magnesium Hydroxide) ▣ 627
May interact with:

Prescription Drugs, unspecified (Effect not specified).

PHOSCHOL CONCENTRATE
(Phosphatidylcholine) 488
None cited in PDR database.

PHOSCHOL 900 SOFTGELS
(Phosphatidylcholine) 488
None cited in PDR database.

PHOSLO TABLETS
(Calcium Acetate) 695
May interact with cardiac glycosides, tetracyclines, and certain other agents. Compounds in these categories include:

Antacids, unspecified (Concurrent use should be avoided).

Demeclocycline Hydrochloride (Bioavailability of oral tetracyclines may be decreased). Products include:
- Declomycin Tablets 1421

Deslanoside (Hypercalcemia may precipitate cardiac arrhythmia).
- No products indexed under this heading.

Digitoxin (Hypercalcemia may precipitate cardiac arrhythmia). Products include:
- Crystodigin Tablets 1472

Digoxin (Hypercalcemia may precipitate cardiac arrhythmia). Products include:
- Lanoxicaps 1110
- Lanoxin Elixir Pediatric 1113
- Lanoxin Injection 1116
- Lanoxin Injection Pediatric 1119
- Lanoxin Tablets 1121

Doxycycline Calcium (Bioavailability of oral tetracyclines may be decreased). Products include:
- Vibramycin Calcium Oral Suspension Syrup 2038

Doxycycline Hyclate (Bioavailability of oral tetracyclines may be decreased). Products include:
- Doryx Capsules 1970
- Vibramycin Hyclate Capsules 2038
- Vibramycin Hyclate Intravenous 2040

IMPORTANT NOTE: Always consult each drug listing in the patient's regimen for possible interactions.

PhosLo | Interactions Index | 846

Vibra-Tabs Film Coated Tablets ... 2038

Doxycycline Monohydrate (Bioavailability of oral tetracyclines may be decreased). Products include:
- Monodox Capsules ... 1858
- Vibramycin Monohydrate for Oral Suspension ... 2038

Methacycline Hydrochloride (Bioavailability of oral tetracyclines may be decreased).
- No products indexed under this heading.

Minocycline Hydrochloride (Bioavailability of oral tetracyclines may be decreased). Products include:
- DYNACIN Capsules ... 1627
- Minocin Intravenous ... 1428
- Minocin Oral Suspension ... 1431
- Minocin Pellet-Filled Capsules ... 1429

Oxytetracycline Hydrochloride (Bioavailability of oral tetracyclines may be decreased). Products include:
- TERAK Ointment ... ◉ 210
- Terra-Cortril Ophthalmic Suspension ... 2033
- Terramycin with Polymyxin B Sulfate Ophthalmic Ointment ... 2035
- Urobiotic-250 Capsules ... 2038

Tetracycline Hydrochloride (Bioavailability of oral tetracyclines may be decreased). Products include:
- Achromycin V Capsules ... 1417
- Helidac Therapy ... 2135

PHOSPHOLINE IODIDE

(Echothiophate Iodide) ... ◉ 323

May interact with:

Succinylcholine Chloride (Possible additive effects). Products include:
- Anectine ... 1062

PHRENILIN FORTE CAPSULES

(Butalbital, Acetaminophen) ... 790

May interact with monoamine oxidase inhibitors, central nervous system depressants, narcotic analgesics, general anesthetics, tranquilizers, hypnotics and sedatives, and certain other agents. Compounds in these categories include:

Alfentanil Hydrochloride (Potential for increased CNS depression). Products include:
- Alfenta Injection ... 1334

Alprazolam (Potential for increased CNS depression). Products include:
- Xanax Tablets ... 2115

Aprobarbital (Potential for increased CNS depression).
- No products indexed under this heading.

Buprenorphine (Potential for increased CNS depression). Products include:
- Buprenex Injectable ... 2170

Buspirone Hydrochloride (Potential for increased CNS depression). Products include:
- BuSpar Tablets ... 738

Butabarbital (Potential for increased CNS depression).
- No products indexed under this heading.

Chlordiazepoxide (Potential for increased CNS depression). Products include:
- Limbitrol ... 2333

Chlordiazepoxide Hydrochloride (Potential for increased CNS depression). Products include:
- Librax Capsules ... 2330
- Librium Capsules ... 2331
- Librium Injectable ... 2332

Chlorpromazine (Potential for increased CNS depression). Products include:
- Thorazine Suppositories ... 2701

Chlorpromazine Hydrochloride (Potential for levels of both drugs). Products include:
- Thorazine ... 2701

Chlorprothixene (Potential for increased CNS depression).
- No products indexed under this heading.

Chlorprothixene Hydrochloride (Potential for increased CNS depression).
- No products indexed under this heading.

Chlorprothixene Lactate (Potential for increased CNS depression).
- No products indexed under this heading.

Clorazepate Dipotassium (Potential for increased CNS depression). Products include:
- Tranxene ... 459

Clozapine (Potential for increased CNS depression). Products include:
- Clozaril Tablets ... 2377

Codeine Phosphate (Potential for increased CNS depression). Products include:
- Brontex ... 2130
- Dimetane-DC Cough Syrup ... 2232
- Fioricet with Codeine Capsules ... 2387
- Fiorinal with Codeine Capsules ... 2390
- Nucofed ... 2225
- Phenergan with Codeine ... 2883
- Phenergan VC with Codeine ... 2888
- Robitussin A-C Syrup ... 2248
- Robitussin-DAC Syrup ... 2249
- Ryna ... ▣ 804
- Soma Compound w/Codeine Tablets ... 2784
- Tylenol with Codeine ... 1592

Desflurane (Potential for increased CNS depression). Products include:
- Suprane (desflurane, USP) ... 1865

Dezocine (Potential for increased CNS depression). Products include:
- Dalgan Injection ... 529

Diazepam (Potential for increased CNS depression). Products include:
- Dizac (diazepam injectable emulsion) CIV ... 1862
- Valium Injectable ... 2336
- Valium Tablets ... 2335

Droperidol (Potential for increased CNS depression). Products include:
- Inapsine Injection ... 462

Enflurane (Potential for increased CNS depression).
- No products indexed under this heading.

Estazolam (Potential for increased CNS depression). Products include:
- ProSom Tablets ... 457

Ethchlorvynol (Potential for increased CNS depression). Products include:
- Placidyl Capsules ... 456

Ethinamate (Potential for increased CNS depression).
- No products indexed under this heading.

Fentanyl (Potential for increased CNS depression). Products include:
- Duragesic Transdermal System ... 1336

Fentanyl Citrate (Potential for increased CNS depression). Products include:
- Sublimaze Injection ... 463

Fluphenazine Decanoate (Potential for increased CNS depression). Products include:
- Prolixin Decanoate ... 510

Fluphenazine Enanthate (Potential for increased CNS depression). Products include:
- Prolixin Enanthate ... 510

Fluphenazine Hydrochloride (Potential for increased CNS depression). Products include:
- Prolixin ... 510

Flurazepam Hydrochloride (Potential for increased CNS depression). Products include:
- Dalmane Capsules ... 2329

Furazolidone (Enhances the CNS effects of butalbital). Products include:
- Furoxone ... 2221

Glutethimide (Potential for increased CNS depression).
- No products indexed under this heading.

Haloperidol (Potential for increased CNS depression). Products include:
- Haldol Injection, Tablets and Concentrate ... 1585

Haloperidol Decanoate (Potential for increased CNS depression). Products include:
- Haldol Decanoate ... 1587

Hydrocodone Bitartrate (Potential for increased CNS depression). Products include:
- Codiclear DH Syrup ... 808
- Duratuss HD Elixir ... 2750
- Histussin D Liquid ... 670
- Hycodan Tablets and Syrup ... 946
- Hycomine Compound Tablets ... 948
- Hycomine ... 947
- Hycotuss Expectorant Syrup ... 950
- Hydrocet Capsules ... 787
- Lorcet 10/650 Tablets ... 1016
- Lortab ... 2751
- Tussend ... 1830
- Tussend Expectorant ... 1831
- Vicodin Tablets ... 1404
- Vicodin ES Tablets ... 1405
- Vicodin HP Tablets ... 1403
- Vicodin Tuss Expectorant ... 1406
- Zydone Capsules ... 967

Hydrocodone Polistirex (Potential for increased CNS depression). Products include:
- Tussionex Pennkinetic Extended-Release Suspension ... 1624

Hydromorphone Hydrochloride (Potential for increased CNS depression). Products include:
- Dilaudid Ampules ... 1382
- Dilaudid Cough Syrup ... 1383
- Dilaudid-HP Injection ... 1384
- Dilaudid-HP Lyophilized Powder 250 mg ... 1384
- Dilaudid ... 1382
- Dilaudid Oral Liquid ... 1386
- Dilaudid ... 1382
- Dilaudid Tablets - 8 mg ... 1386

Hydroxyzine Hydrochloride (Potential for increased CNS depression). Products include:
- Atarax Tablets & Syrup ... 1992
- Marax Tablets & DF Syrup ... 2015
- Vistaril Intramuscular Solution ... 2042

Isocarboxazid (Enhances the CNS effects of butalbital).
- No products indexed under this heading.

Isoflurane (Potential for increased CNS depression).
- No products indexed under this heading.

Ketamine Hydrochloride (Potential for increased CNS depression).
- No products indexed under this heading.

Levomethadyl Acetate Hydrochloride (Potential for increased CNS depression). Products include:
- Orlaam Oral Solution ... 2361

Levorphanol Tartrate (Potential for increased CNS depression). Products include:
- Levo-Dromoran ... 2297

Lorazepam (Potential for increased CNS depression). Products include:
- Ativan Injection ... 2805
- Ativan Tablets ... 2807

Loxapine Hydrochloride (Potential for increased CNS depression). Products include:
- Loxitane ... 1426

Loxapine Succinate (Potential for increased CNS depression). Products include:
- Loxitane Capsules ... 1426

Meperidine Hydrochloride (Potential for increased CNS depression). Products include:
- Demerol ... 2438
- Mepergan Injection ... 2859

Mephobarbital (Potential for increased CNS depression). Products include:
- Mebaral Tablets ... 2452

Meprobamate (Potential for increased CNS depression). Products include:
- Miltown Tablets ... 2780
- PMB 200 and PMB 400 ... 2890

Mesoridazine Besylate (Potential for increased CNS depression). Products include:
- Serentil ... 689

Methadone Hydrochloride (Potential for increased CNS depression). Products include:
- Methadone Hydrochloride Oral Concentrate ... 2356
- Methadone Hydrochloride Oral Solution & Tablets ... 2357

Methohexital Sodium (Potential for increased CNS depression).
- No products indexed under this heading.

Methotrimeprazine (Potential for increased CNS depression). Products include:
- Levoprome ... 1321

Methoxyflurane (Potential for increased CNS depression).
- No products indexed under this heading.

Midazolam Hydrochloride (Potential for increased CNS depression). Products include:
- Versed Injection ... 2324

Molindone Hydrochloride (Potential for increased CNS depression). Products include:
- Moban Tablets and Concentrate ... 1036

Morphine Sulfate (Potential for increased CNS depression). Products include:
- Astramorph/PF Injection, USP (Preservative-Free) ... 526
- Duramorph Injection ... 983
- Infumorph 200 and Infumorph 500 Sterile Solutions ... 985
- Kadian Capsules ... 2948
- MS Contin Tablets ... 2149
- MSIR ... 2152
- Oramorph SR (Morphine Sulfate Sustained Release Tablets) ... 2359
- RMS Suppositories CII ... 2766
- Roxanol ... 2365

Opium Alkaloids (Potential for increased CNS depression).
- No products indexed under this heading.

Oxazepam (Potential for increased CNS depression). Products include:
- Serax Capsules ... 2916
- Serax Tablets ... 2916

Oxycodone Hydrochloride (Potential for increased CNS depression). Products include:
- OxyContin Tablets ... 2163
- OxyIR Capsules ... 2167
- Percocet Tablets ... 955
- Percodan Tablets ... 955
- Percodan-Demi Tablets ... 956

(▣ Described in PDR For Nonprescription Drugs) (◉ Described in PDR For Ophthalmology)

Roxicodone Tablets, Oral Solution
  & Intensol (Oxycodone) 2366
Tylox Capsules 1593

Pentobarbital Sodium (Potential for increased CNS depression). Products include:
Nembutal Sodium Capsules 440
Nembutal Sodium Solution 442
Nembutal Sodium Suppositories 444

Perphenazine (Potential for increased CNS depression). Products include:
Etrafon 2495
Triavil Tablets 1800
Trilafon 2532

Phenelzine Sulfate (Enhances the CNS effects of butalbital). Products include:
Nardil 1977

Phenobarbital (Potential for increased CNS depression). Products include:
Arco-Lase Plus Tablets 513
Bellergal-S Tablets 2375
Donnatal 2234
Donnatal Extentabs 2234
Donnatal Tablets 2234
Phenobarbital Elixir and Tablets 1523
Quadrinal Tablets 1398

Prazepam (Potential for increased CNS depression).
No products indexed under this heading.

Prochlorperazine (Potential for increased CNS depression). Products include:
Compazine 2644

Promethazine Hydrochloride (Potential for increased CNS depression). Products include:
Mepergan Injection 2859
Phenergan with Codeine 2883
Phenergan with Dextromethorphan 2885
Phenergan Injection 2880
Phenergan Suppositories 2882
Phenergan Syrup 2881
Phenergan Tablets 2882
Phenergan VC 2886
Phenergan VC with Codeine 2888

Propofol (Potential for increased CNS depression). Products include:
Diprivan Injectable Emulsion 2939

Propoxyphene Hydrochloride (Potential for increased CNS depression). Products include:
Darvon 1475
Wygesic Tablets 2930

Propoxyphene Napsylate (Potential for increased CNS depression). Products include:
Darvon-N/Darvocet-N 1473

Quazepam (Potential for increased CNS depression). Products include:
Doral Tablets 2773

Risperidone (Potential for increased CNS depression). Products include:
Risperdal Tablets 1348

Secobarbital Sodium (Potential for increased CNS depression). Products include:
Seconal Sodium Pulvules 1529

Selegiline Hydrochloride (Enhances the CNS effects of butalbital). Products include:
Eldepryl Capsules 2729

Sevoflurane (Potential for increased CNS depression).
No products indexed under this heading.

Sufentanil Citrate (Potential for increased CNS depression). Products include:
Sufenta Injection 1355

Temazepam (Potential for increased CNS depression). Products include:
Restoril Capsules 2413

Thiamylal Sodium (Potential for increased CNS depression).
No products indexed under this heading.

Thioridazine Hydrochloride (Potential for increased CNS depression). Products include:
Mellaril 2398

Thiothixene (Potential for increased CNS depression). Products include:
Navane Capsules and Concentrate 2018
Navane Intramuscular 2019

Tranylcypromine Sulfate (Enhances the CNS effects of butalbital). Products include:
Parnate Tablets 2679

Triazolam (Potential for increased CNS depression). Products include:
Halcion Tablets 2093

Trifluoperazine Hydrochloride (Potential for increased CNS depression). Products include:
Stelazine 2692

Zolpidem Tartrate (Potential for increased CNS depression). Products include:
Ambien Tablets 2559

Food Interactions

Alcohol (Potential for increased CNS depression).

PHRENILIN TABLETS
(Butalbital, Acetaminophen) 790
See **Phrenilin Forte Capsules**

PHYTO-VITE
(Vitamins with Minerals) 835
None cited in PDR database.

PILAGAN LIQUIFILM STERILE OPHTHALMIC SOLUTION
(Pilocarpine Nitrate) 245
None cited in PDR database.

PILAGAN LIQUIFILM STERILE OPHTHALMIC SOLUTION WITH C CAP COMPLIANCE CAP
(Pilocarpine Nitrate) 245
None cited in PDR database.

PILOPINE HS OPHTHALMIC GEL
(Pilocarpine Hydrochloride) 224
None cited in PDR database.

PIMA SYRUP
(Potassium Iodide) 1004
None cited in PDR database.

PIN-X PINWORM TREATMENT
(Pyrantel Pamoate) 670
None cited in PDR database.

PIPRACIL
(Piperacillin Sodium) 1435
May interact with aminoglycosides, nondepolarizing neuromuscular blocking agents, and certain other agents. Compounds in these categories include:

Amikacin Sulfate (Substantial inactivation of aminoglycosides in vitro). Products include:
Amikacin Sulfate Injection, USP 523
Amikacin Sulfate Injection, USP 981
Amikin Injectable 502

Atracurium Besylate (Co-administration with vecuronium has been implicated in the prolongation of the neuromuscular blockage; due to similar mechanism of action, same interaction can be expected with other non-depolarizing muscle relaxants). Products include:
Tracrium Injection 1155

Cisatracurium Besylate (Co-administration with vecuronium has been implicated in the prolongation of the neuromuscular blockage; due to similar mechanism of action, same interaction can be expected with other non-depolarizing muscle relaxants). Products include:
Nimbex Injection 1131

Gentamicin Sulfate (Substantial inactivation of aminoglycosides in vitro). Products include:
Garamycin Cream 0.1% 2501
Garamycin Injectable 2502
Garamycin Ointment 0.1% 2501
Garamycin Ophthalmic 2501
Genoptic Sterile Ophthalmic Solution 241
Genoptic Sterile Ophthalmic Ointment 241
Gentak 209
Pred-G Liquifilm Sterile Ophthalmic Suspension 248
Pred-G S.O.P. Sterile Ophthalmic Ointment 249

Kanamycin Sulfate (Substantial inactivation of aminoglycosides in vitro).
No products indexed under this heading.

Metocurine Iodide (Co-administration with vecuronium has been implicated in the prolongation of the neuromuscular blockage; due to similar mechanism of action, same interaction can be expected with other non-depolarizing muscle relaxants). Products include:
Metubine Iodide Vials 932

Mivacurium Chloride (Co-administration with vecuronium has been implicated in the prolongation of the neuromuscular blockage; due to similar mechanism of action, same interaction can be expected with other non-depolarizing muscle relaxants). Products include:
Mivacron 1125

Pancuronium Bromide (Co-administration with vecuronium has been implicated in the prolongation of the neuromuscular blockage; due to similar mechanism of action, same interaction can be expected with other non-depolarizing muscle relaxants).
No products indexed under this heading.

Probenecid (Increases peak serum level and area under the curve). Products include:
Benemid Tablets 1651
ColBENEMID Tablets 1662

Rocuronium Bromide (Co-administration with vecuronium has been implicated in the prolongation of the neuromuscular blockage; due to similar mechanism of action, same interaction can be expected with other non-depolarizing muscle relaxants). Products include:
Zemuron Injection 1885

Streptomycin Sulfate (Substantial inactivation of aminoglycosides in vitro). Products include:
Streptomycin Sulfate Injection 2031

Tobramycin Sulfate (Substantial inactivation of aminoglycosides in vitro). Products include:
Nebcin Vials, Hyporets & ADD-Vantage 1518

Vecuronium Bromide (Co-administration with vecuronium has been implicated in the prolongation of the neuromuscular blockage; due to similar mechanism of action, same interaction can be expected with other non-depolarizing muscle relaxants). Products include:
Norcuron for Injection 1875

PLACIDYL CAPSULES
(Ethchlorvynol) 456
May interact with central nervous system depressants, monoamine oxidase inhibitors, oral anticoagulants, and tricyclic antidepressants. Compounds in these categories include:

Alfentanil Hydrochloride (Exaggerated depressant effects). Products include:
Alfenta Injection 1334

Alprazolam (Exaggerated depressant effects). Products include:
Xanax Tablets 2115

Amitriptyline Hydrochloride (Transient delirium). Products include:
Elavil 2945
Etrafon 2495
Limbitrol 2333
Triavil Tablets 1800

Amoxapine (Transient delirium). Products include:
Asendin Tablets 1419

Aprobarbital (Exaggerated depressant effects).
No products indexed under this heading.

Buprenorphine (Exaggerated depressant effects). Products include:
Buprenex Injectable 2170

Buspirone Hydrochloride (Exaggerated depressant effects). Products include:
BuSpar Tablets 738

Butabarbital (Exaggerated depressant effects).
No products indexed under this heading.

Butalbital (Exaggerated depressant effects). Products include:
Axocet Capsules 2469
Esgic-plus Capsules 1012
Esgic-plus Tablets 1012
Fioricet Tablets 2386
Fioricet with Codeine Capsules 2387
Fiorinal Capsules 2388
Fiorinal with Codeine Capsules ... 2390
Fiorinal Tablets 2388
Phrenilin 790
Sedapap Tablets 50 mg/650 mg .. 1826

Chlordiazepoxide (Exaggerated depressant effects). Products include:
Limbitrol 2333

Chlordiazepoxide Hydrochloride (Exaggerated depressant effects). Products include:
Librax Capsules 2330
Librium Capsules 2331
Librium Injectable 2332

Chlorpromazine (Exaggerated depressant effects). Products include:
Thorazine Suppositories 2701

Chlorpromazine Hydrochloride (Exaggerated depressant effects). Products include:
Thorazine 2701

IMPORTANT NOTE: Always consult each drug listing in the patient's regimen for possible interactions.

Placidyl — Interactions Index — 848

Chlorprothixene (Exaggerated depressant effects).
No products indexed under this heading.

Chlorprothixene Hydrochloride (Exaggerated depressant effects).
No products indexed under this heading.

Chlorprothixene Lactate (Exaggerated depressant effects).
No products indexed under this heading.

Clomipramine Hydrochloride (Transient delirium). Products include:
- Anafranil Capsules ... 819

Clorazepate Dipotassium (Exaggerated depressant effects). Products include:
- Tranxene ... 459

Clozapine (Exaggerated depressant effects). Products include:
- Clozaril Tablets ... 2377

Codeine Phosphate (Exaggerated depressant effects). Products include:
- Brontex ... 2130
- Dimetane-DC Cough Syrup ... 2232
- Fioricet with Codeine Capsules ... 2387
- Fiorinal with Codeine Capsules ... 2390
- Nucofed ... 2225
- Phenergan with Codeine ... 2883
- Phenergan VC with Codeine ... 2888
- Robitussin A-C Syrup ... 2248
- Robitussin-DAC Syrup ... 2249
- Ryna ... ⊡ 804
- Soma Compound w/Codeine Tablets ... 2784
- Tylenol with Codeine ... 1592

Desflurane (Exaggerated depressant effects). Products include:
- Suprane (desflurane, USP) ... 1865

Desipramine Hydrochloride (Transient delirium). Products include:
- Norpramin Tablets ... 1273

Dezocine (Exaggerated depressant effects). Products include:
- Dalgan Injection ... 529

Diazepam (Exaggerated depressant effects). Products include:
- Dizac (diazepam injectable emulsion) CIV ... 1862
- Valium Injectable ... 2336
- Valium Tablets ... 2335

Dicumarol (Decreased prothrombin time response).
No products indexed under this heading.

Doxepin Hydrochloride (Transient delirium). Products include:
- Adapin Capsules ... 1542
- Sinequan ... 2028
- Zonalon Cream ... 1042

Droperidol (Exaggerated depressant effects). Products include:
- Inapsine Injection ... 462

Enflurane (Exaggerated depressant effects).
No products indexed under this heading.

Estazolam (Exaggerated depressant effects). Products include:
- ProSom Tablets ... 457

Ethinamate (Exaggerated depressant effects).
No products indexed under this heading.

Fentanyl (Exaggerated depressant effects). Products include:
- Duragesic Transdermal System ... 1336

Fentanyl Citrate (Exaggerated depressant effects). Products include:
- Sublimaze Injection ... 463

Fluphenazine Decanoate (Exaggerated depressant effects). Products include:
- Prolixin Decanoate ... 510

Fluphenazine Enanthate (Exaggerated depressant effects). Products include:
- Prolixin Enanthate ... 510

Fluphenazine Hydrochloride (Exaggerated depressant effects). Products include:
- Prolixin ... 510

Flurazepam Hydrochloride (Exaggerated depressant effects). Products include:
- Dalmane Capsules ... 2329

Furazolidone (Exaggerated depressant effects). Products include:
- Furoxone ... 2221

Glutethimide (Exaggerated depressant effects).
No products indexed under this heading.

Haloperidol (Exaggerated depressant effects). Products include:
- Haldol Injection, Tablets and Concentrate ... 1585

Haloperidol Decanoate (Exaggerated depressant effects). Products include:
- Haldol Decanoate ... 1587

Hydrocodone Bitartrate (Exaggerated depressant effects). Products include:
- Codiclear DH Syrup ... 808
- Duratuss HD Elixir ... 2750
- Histussin D Liquid ... 670
- Hycodan Tablets and Syrup ... 946
- Hycomine Compound Tablets ... 948
- Hycomine ... 947
- Hycotuss Expectorant Syrup ... 950
- Hydrocet Capsules ... 787
- Lorcet 10/650 Tablets ... 1016
- Lortab ... 2751
- Tussend ... 1830
- Tussend Expectorant ... 1831
- Vicodin Tablets ... 1404
- Vicodin ES Tablets ... 1405
- Vicodin HP Tablets ... 1403
- Vicodin Tuss Expectorant ... 1406
- Zydone Capsules ... 967

Hydrocodone Polistirex (Exaggerated depressant effects). Products include:
- Tussionex Pennkinetic Extended-Release Suspension ... 1624

Hydroxyzine Hydrochloride (Exaggerated depressant effects). Products include:
- Atarax Tablets & Syrup ... 1992
- Marax Tablets & DF Syrup ... 2015
- Vistaril Intramuscular Solution ... 2042

Imipramine Hydrochloride (Transient delirium). Products include:
- Tofranil Ampuls ... 873
- Tofranil Tablets ... 875

Imipramine Pamoate (Transient delirium). Products include:
- Tofranil-PM Capsules ... 876

Isocarboxazid (Exaggerated depressant effects).
No products indexed under this heading.

Isoflurane (Exaggerated depressant effects).
No products indexed under this heading.

Ketamine Hydrochloride (Exaggerated depressant effects).
No products indexed under this heading.

Levomethadyl Acetate Hydrochloride (Exaggerated depressant effects). Products include:
- Orlaam Oral Solution ... 2361

Levorphanol Tartrate (Exaggerated depressant effects). Products include:
- Levo-Dromoran ... 2297

Lorazepam (Exaggerated depressant effects). Products include:
- Ativan Injection ... 2805
- Ativan Tablets ... 2807

Loxapine Hydrochloride (Exaggerated depressant effects). Products include:
- Loxitane ... 1426

Loxapine Succinate (Exaggerated depressant effects). Products include:
- Loxitane Capsules ... 1426

Maprotiline Hydrochloride (Transient delirium). Products include:
- Ludiomil Tablets ... 861

Meperidine Hydrochloride (Exaggerated depressant effects). Products include:
- Demerol ... 2438
- Mepergan Injection ... 2859

Mephobarbital (Exaggerated depressant effects). Products include:
- Mebaral Tablets ... 2452

Meprobamate (Exaggerated depressant effects). Products include:
- Miltown Tablets ... 2780
- PMB 200 and PMB 400 ... 2890

Mesoridazine Besylate (Exaggerated depressant effects). Products include:
- Serentil ... 689

Methadone Hydrochloride (Exaggerated depressant effects). Products include:
- Methadone Hydrochloride Oral Concentrate ... 2356
- Methadone Hydrochloride Oral Solution & Tablets ... 2357

Methohexital Sodium (Exaggerated depressant effects).
No products indexed under this heading.

Methotrimeprazine (Exaggerated depressant effects). Products include:
- Levoprome ... 1321

Methoxyflurane (Exaggerated depressant effects).
No products indexed under this heading.

Midazolam Hydrochloride (Exaggerated depressant effects). Products include:
- Versed Injection ... 2324

Molindone Hydrochloride (Exaggerated depressant effects). Products include:
- Moban Tablets and Concentrate ... 1036

Morphine Sulfate (Exaggerated depressant effects). Products include:
- Astramorph/PF Injection, USP (Preservative-Free) ... 526
- Duramorph Injection ... 983
- Infumorph 200 and Infumorph 500 Sterile Solutions ... 985
- Kadian Capsules ... 2948
- MS Contin Tablets ... 2149
- MSIR ... 2152
- Oramorph SR (Morphine Sulfate Sustained Release Tablets) ... 2359
- RMS Suppositories CII ... 2766
- Roxanol ... 2365

Nortriptyline Hydrochloride (Transient delirium). Products include:
- Pamelor ... 2409

Opium Alkaloids (Exaggerated depressant effects).
No products indexed under this heading.

Oxazepam (Exaggerated depressant effects). Products include:
- Serax Capsules ... 2916
- Serax Tablets ... 2916

Oxycodone Hydrochloride (Exaggerated depressant effects). Products include:
- OxyContin Tablets ... 2163
- OxyIR Capsules ... 2167
- Percocet Tablets ... 955
- Percodan Tablets ... 955
- Percodan-Demi Tablets ... 956
- Roxicodone Tablets, Oral Solution & Intensol (Oxycodone) ... 2366
- Tylox Capsules ... 1593

Pentobarbital Sodium (Exaggerated depressant effects). Products include:
- Nembutal Sodium Capsules ... 440
- Nembutal Sodium Solution ... 442
- Nembutal Sodium Suppositories ... 444

Perphenazine (Exaggerated depressant effects). Products include:
- Etrafon ... 2495
- Triavil Tablets ... 1800
- Trilafon ... 2532

Phenelzine Sulfate (Exaggerated depressant effects). Products include:
- Nardil ... 1977

Phenobarbital (Exaggerated depressant effects). Products include:
- Arco-Lase Plus Tablets ... 513
- Bellergal-S Tablets ... 2375
- Donnatal ... 2234
- Donnatal Extentabs ... 2234
- Donnatal Tablets ... 2234
- Phenobarbital Elixir and Tablets ... 1523
- Quadrinal Tablets ... 1398

Prazepam (Exaggerated depressant effects).
No products indexed under this heading.

Prochlorperazine (Exaggerated depressant effects). Products include:
- Compazine ... 2644

Promethazine Hydrochloride (Exaggerated depressant effects). Products include:
- Mepergan Injection ... 2859
- Phenergan with Codeine ... 2883
- Phenergan with Dextromethorphan ... 2885
- Phenergan Injection ... 2880
- Phenergan Suppositories ... 2882
- Phenergan Syrup ... 2881
- Phenergan Tablets ... 2882
- Phenergan VC ... 2886
- Phenergan VC with Codeine ... 2888

Propofol (Exaggerated depressant effects). Products include:
- Diprivan Injectable Emulsion ... 2939

Propoxyphene Hydrochloride (Exaggerated depressant effects). Products include:
- Darvon ... 1475
- Wygesic Tablets ... 2930

Propoxyphene Napsylate (Exaggerated depressant effects). Products include:
- Darvon-N/Darvocet-N ... 1473

Protriptyline Hydrochloride (Transient delirium). Products include:
- Vivactil Tablets ... 1820

Quazepam (Exaggerated depressant effects). Products include:
- Doral Tablets ... 2773

Risperidone (Exaggerated depressant effects). Products include:
- Risperdal Tablets ... 1348

Secobarbital Sodium (Exaggerated depressant effects). Products include:
- Seconal Sodium Pulvules ... 1529

Selegiline Hydrochloride (Exaggerated depressant effects). Products include:
- Eldepryl Capsules ... 2729

Sevoflurane (Exaggerated depressant effects).
No products indexed under this heading.

Sufentanil Citrate (Exaggerated depressant effects). Products include:
- Sufenta Injection ... 1355

Temazepam (Exaggerated depressant effects). Products include:
- Restoril Capsules ... 2413

(⊡ Described in PDR For Nonprescription Drugs)   (⊙ Described in PDR For Ophthalmology)

849 **Interactions Index** **Plendil**

Thiamylal Sodium (Exaggerated depressant effects).
No products indexed under this heading.
Thioridazine Hydrochloride (Exaggerated depressant effects). Products include:
Mellaril 2398
Thiothixene (Exaggerated depressant effects). Products include:
Navane Capsules and Concentrate 2018
Navane Intramuscular 2019
Tranylcypromine Sulfate (Exaggerated depressant effects). Products include:
Parnate Tablets 2679
Triazolam (Exaggerated depressant effects). Products include:
Halcion Tablets 2093
Trifluoperazine Hydrochloride (Exaggerated depressant effects). Products include:
Stelazine 2692
Trimipramine Maleate (Transient delirium). Products include:
Surmontil Capsules 2917
Warfarin Sodium (Decreased prothrombin time response). Products include:
Coumadin 941
Zolpidem Tartrate (Exaggerated depressant effects). Products include:
Ambien Tablets 2559

PLAQUENIL SULFATE TABLETS
(Hydroxychloroquine Sulfate) 2459
May interact with:

Hepatotoxic Drugs, unspecified (Use with caution).

PLASMA-PLEX, PLASMA PROTEIN FRACTION (HUMAN) U.S.P. 5% SOLUTION HEAT-TREATED
(Plasma Protein Fraction (Human)) .. 806
None cited in PDR database.

PLATINOL FOR INJECTION
(Cisplatin) 717
May interact with aminoglycosides, anticonvulsants, and certain other agents. Compounds in these categories include:

Amikacin Sulfate (Potentiation of cumulative nephrotoxicity). Products include:
Amikacin Sulfate Injection, USP 523
Amikacin Sulfate Injection, USP 981
Amikin Injectable 502
Carbamazepine (Plasma levels of anticonvulsant agents may become subtherapeutic). Products include:
Atretol Tablets 569
Tegretol/Tegretol-XR 870
Divalproex Sodium (Plasma levels of anticonvulsant agents may become subtherapeutic). Products include:
Depakote Tablets 418
Ethosuximide (Plasma levels of anticonvulsant agents may become subtherapeutic). Products include:
Zarontin Capsules 1986
Zarontin Syrup 1986
Ethotoin (Plasma levels of anticonvulsant agents may become subtherapeutic). Products include:
Peganone Tablets 455
Felbamate (Plasma levels of anticonvulsant agents may become subtherapeutic). Products include:
Felbatol 2774
Gentamicin Sulfate (Potentiation of cumulative nephrotoxicity). Products include:
Garamycin Cream 0.1% 2501
Garamycin Injectable 2502
Garamycin Ointment 0.1% 2501
Garamycin Ophthalmic 2501
Genoptic Sterile Ophthalmic Solution .... ◉ 241
Genoptic Sterile Ophthalmic Ointment .... ◉ 241
Gentak .... ◉ 209
Pred-G Liquifilm Sterile Ophthalmic Suspension .... ◉ 248
Pred-G S.O.P. Sterile Ophthalmic Ointment .... ◉ 249
Kanamycin Sulfate (Potentiation of cumulative nephrotoxicity).
No products indexed under this heading.
Lamotrigine (Plasma levels of anticonvulsant agents may become subtherapeutic). Products include:
Lamictal Tablets 1105
Mephenytoin (Plasma levels of anticonvulsant agents may become subtherapeutic). Products include:
Mesantoin Tablets 2400
Methsuximide (Plasma levels of anticonvulsant agents may become subtherapeutic). Products include:
Celontin Kapseals 1955
Paramethadione (Plasma levels of anticonvulsant agents may become subtherapeutic).
No products indexed under this heading.
Phenacemide (Plasma levels of anticonvulsant agents may become subtherapeutic). Products include:
Phenurone Tablets 455
Phenobarbital (Plasma levels of anticonvulsant agents may become subtherapeutic). Products include:
Arco-Lase Plus Tablets 513
Bellergal-S Tablets 2375
Donnatal 2234
Donnatal Extentabs 2234
Donnatal Tablets 2234
Phenobarbital Elixir and Tablets 1523
Quadrinal Tablets 1398
Phensuximide (Plasma levels of anticonvulsant agents may become subtherapeutic).
No products indexed under this heading.
Phenytoin (Plasma levels of anticonvulsant agents may become subtherapeutic). Products include:
Dilantin Infatabs 1967
Dilantin-125 Suspension 1969
Phenytoin Sodium (Plasma levels of anticonvulsant agents may become subtherapeutic). Products include:
Dilantin Kapseals 1965
Primidone (Plasma levels of anticonvulsant agents may become subtherapeutic). Products include:
Mysoline 2860
Pyridoxine Hydrochloride (Response duration may be adversely affected when pyridoxine is used in combination with altretamine and Platinol).
No products indexed under this heading.
Streptomycin Sulfate (Potentiation of cumulative nephrotoxicity). Products include:
Streptomycin Sulfate Injection 2031
Tobramycin (Potentiation of cumulative nephrotoxicity). Products include:
AKTOB .... ◉ 207
TobraDex Ophthalmic Suspension and Ointment 469
Tobrex Ophthalmic Ointment and Solution .... ◉ 226
Tobramycin Sulfate (Potentiation of cumulative nephrotoxicity). Products include:
Nebcin Vials, Hyporets & ADD-Vantage 1518
Trimethadione (Plasma levels of anticonvulsant agents may become subtherapeutic).
No products indexed under this heading.
Valproic Acid (Plasma levels of anticonvulsant agents may become subtherapeutic). Products include:
Depakene 416

PLATINOL-AQ INJECTION
(Cisplatin) 719
May interact with aminoglycosides, anticonvulsants, and certain other agents. Compounds in these categories include:

Amikacin Sulfate (Concomitant administration potentiates nephrotoxicity). Products include:
Amikacin Sulfate Injection, USP 523
Amikacin Sulfate Injection, USP 981
Amikin Injectable 502
Carbamazepine (Plasma levels of anticonvulsant agents may become subtherapeutic). Products include:
Atretol Tablets 569
Tegretol/Tegretol-XR 870
Divalproex Sodium (Plasma levels of anticonvulsant agents may become subtherapeutic). Products include:
Depakote Tablets 418
Ethosuximide (Plasma levels of anticonvulsant agents may become subtherapeutic). Products include:
Zarontin Capsules 1986
Zarontin Syrup 1986
Ethotoin (Plasma levels of anticonvulsant agents may become subtherapeutic). Products include:
Peganone Tablets 455
Felbamate (Plasma levels of anticonvulsant agents may become subtherapeutic). Products include:
Felbatol 2774
Gentamicin Sulfate (Concomitant administration potentiates nephrotoxicity). Products include:
Garamycin Cream 0.1% 2501
Garamycin Injectable 2502
Garamycin Ointment 0.1% 2501
Garamycin Ophthalmic 2501
Genoptic Sterile Ophthalmic Solution .... ◉ 241
Genoptic Sterile Ophthalmic Ointment .... ◉ 241
Gentak .... ◉ 209
Pred-G Liquifilm Sterile Ophthalmic Suspension .... ◉ 248
Pred-G S.O.P. Sterile Ophthalmic Ointment .... ◉ 249
Kanamycin Sulfate (Concomitant administration potentiates nephrotoxicity).
No products indexed under this heading.
Lamotrigine (Plasma levels of anticonvulsant agents may become subtherapeutic). Products include:
Lamictal Tablets 1105
Mephenytoin (Plasma levels of anticonvulsant agents may become subtherapeutic). Products include:
Mesantoin Tablets 2400
Methsuximide (Plasma levels of anticonvulsant agents may become subtherapeutic). Products include:
Celontin Kapseals 1955
Paramethadione (Plasma levels of anticonvulsant agents may become subtherapeutic).
No products indexed under this heading.
Phenacemide (Plasma levels of anticonvulsant agents may become subtherapeutic). Products include:
Phenurone Tablets 455
Phenobarbital (Plasma levels of anticonvulsant agents may become subtherapeutic). Products include:
Arco-Lase Plus Tablets 513
Bellergal-S Tablets 2375
Donnatal 2234
Donnatal Extentabs 2234
Donnatal Tablets 2234
Phenobarbital Elixir and Tablets 1523
Quadrinal Tablets 1398
Phensuximide (Plasma levels of anticonvulsant agents may become subtherapeutic).
No products indexed under this heading.
Phenytoin (Plasma levels of anticonvulsant agents may become subtherapeutic). Products include:
Dilantin Infatabs 1967
Dilantin-125 Suspension 1969
Phenytoin Sodium (Plasma levels of anticonvulsant agents may become subtherapeutic). Products include:
Dilantin Kapseals 1965
Primidone (Plasma levels of anticonvulsant agents may become subtherapeutic). Products include:
Mysoline 2860
Pyridoxine Hydrochloride (Response duration may be adversely affected when pyridoxine is used in combination with altretamine and Platinol).
No products indexed under this heading.
Streptomycin Sulfate (Concomitant administration potentiates nephrotoxicity). Products include:
Streptomycin Sulfate Injection 2031
Tobramycin (Concomitant administration potentiates nephrotoxicity). Products include:
AKTOB .... ◉ 207
TobraDex Ophthalmic Suspension and Ointment 469
Tobrex Ophthalmic Ointment and Solution .... ◉ 226
Tobramycin Sulfate (Concomitant administration potentiates nephrotoxicity). Products include:
Nebcin Vials, Hyporets & ADD-Vantage 1518
Trimethadione (Plasma levels of anticonvulsant agents may become subtherapeutic).
No products indexed under this heading.
Valproic Acid (Plasma levels of anticonvulsant agents may become subtherapeutic). Products include:
Depakene 416

PLENDIL EXTENDED-RELEASE TABLETS
(Felodipine) 514
May interact with anticonvulsants, beta blockers, and certain other agents. Compounds in these categories include:

Acebutolol Hydrochloride (Caution should be exercised when using Plendil in patients with heart failure or compromised ventricular function, particularly in combination with beta blocker). Products include:
Sectral Capsules 2914

IMPORTANT NOTE: Always consult each drug listing in the patient's regimen for possible interactions.

Plendil | Interactions Index | 850

Atenolol (Caution should be exercised when using Plendil in patients with heart failure or compromised ventricular function, particularly in combination with beta blocker). Products include:
- Tenoretic Tablets ... 2963
- Tenormin Tablets and I.V. Injection 2965

Betaxolol Hydrochloride (Caution should be exercised when using Plendil in patients with heart failure or compromised ventricular function, particularly in combination with beta blocker). Products include:
- Betoptic Ophthalmic Solution ... 465
- Betoptic S Ophthalmic Suspension 467
- Kerlone Tablets ... 2588

Bisoprolol Fumarate (Caution should be exercised when using Plendil in patients with heart failure or compromised ventricular function, particularly in combination with beta blocker). Products include:
- Zebeta Tablets ... 1457
- Ziac ... 1459

Carbamazepine (Potential for low maximum plasma concentrations of felodipine in epileptic patients on long-term anticonvulsant therapy). Products include:
- Atretol Tablets ... 569
- Tegretol/Tegretol-XR ... 870

Carteolol Hydrochloride (Caution should be exercised when using Plendil in patients with heart failure or compromised ventricular function, particularly in combination with beta blocker). Products include:
- Cartrol Tablets ... 413
- Ocupress Ophthalmic Solution, 1% Sterile ... ⊙ 297

Cimetidine (Increases AUC and C_{max} by approximately 50%; low doses of Plendil should be used). Products include:
- Tagamet HB Tablets ... ▣ 786
- Tagamet Tablets ... 2694

Cimetidine Hydrochloride (Increases AUC and C_{max} by approximately 50%; low doses of Plendil should be used). Products include:
- Tagamet ... 2694

Digoxin (Co-administration does not significantly alter the pharmacokinetics of digoxin in patients with heart failure). Products include:
- Lanoxicaps ... 1110
- Lanoxin Elixir Pediatric ... 1113
- Lanoxin Injection ... 1116
- Lanoxin Injection Pediatric ... 1119
- Lanoxin Tablets ... 1121

Divalproex Sodium (Potential for low maximum plasma concentrations of felodipine in epileptic patients on long-term anticonvulsant therapy). Products include:
- Depakote Tablets ... 418

Esmolol Hydrochloride (Caution should be exercised when using Plendil in 31% with 38% respectively compromised ventricular function, particularly in combination with beta blocker). Products include:
- Brevibloc (esmolol HCl) Injection ... 1860

Ethosuximide (Potential for low maximum plasma concentrations of felodipine in epileptic patients on long-term anticonvulsant therapy). Products include:
- Zarontin Capsules ... 1986
- Zarontin Syrup ... 1986

Ethotoin (Potential for low maximum plasma concentrations of felodipine in epileptic patients on long-term anticonvulsant therapy). Products include:
- Peganone Tablets ... 455

Felbamate (Potential for low maximum plasma concentrations of felodipine in epileptic patients on long-term anticonvulsant therapy). Products include:
- Felbatol ... 2774

Fosphenytoin Sodium (Potential for low maximum plasma concentrations of felodipine in epileptic patients on long-term anticonvulsant therapy). Products include:
- Cerebyx Injection ... 1956

Labetalol Hydrochloride (Caution should be exercised when using Plendil in patients with heart failure or compromised ventricular function, particularly in combination with beta blocker). Products include:
- Normodyne Injection ... 2519
- Normodyne Tablets ... 2522
- Trandate ... 1158

Lamotrigine (Potential for low maximum plasma concentrations of felodipine in epileptic patients on long-term anticonvulsant therapy). Products include:
- Lamictal Tablets ... 1105

Levobunolol Hydrochloride (Caution should be exercised when using Plendil in patients with heart failure or compromised ventricular function, particularly in combination with beta blocker). Products include:
- Betagan ... ⊙ 230

Mephenytoin (Potential for low maximum plasma concentrations of felodipine in epileptic patients on long-term anticonvulsant therapy). Products include:
- Mesantoin Tablets ... 2400

Methsuximide (Potential for low maximum plasma concentrations of felodipine in epileptic patients on long-term anticonvulsant therapy). Products include:
- Celontin Kapseals ... 1955

Metipranolol Hydrochloride (Caution should be exercised when using Plendil in patients with heart failure or compromised ventricular function, particularly in combination with beta blocker). Products include:
- OptiPranolol (Metipranolol 0.3%) Sterile Ophthalmic Solution ... ⊙ 256

Metoprolol Succinate (Increased AUC and C_{max} of metoprolol approximately 31% and 38% respectively). Products include:
- Toprol-XL Tablets ... 560

Metoprolol Tartrate (Increased AUC and C_{max} of metoprolol approximately 31% and 38% respectively). Products include:
- Lopressor ... 848
- Lopressor HCT Tablets ... 850

Nadolol (Caution should be exercised when using Plendil in patients with heart failure or compromised ventricular function, particularly in combination with beta blocker).
- No products indexed under this heading.

Paramethadione (Potential for low maximum plasma concentrations of felodipine in epileptic patients on long-term anticonvulsant therapy).
- No products indexed under this heading.

Penbutolol Sulfate (Caution should be exercised when using Plendil in patients with heart failure or compromised ventricular function, particularly in combination with beta blocker). Products include:
- Levatol Tablets ... 2547

Phenacemide (Potential for low maximum plasma concentrations of felodipine in epileptic patients on long-term anticonvulsant therapy). Products include:
- Phenurone Tablets ... 455

Phenobarbital (Potential for low maximum plasma concentrations of felodipine in epileptic patients on long-term anticonvulsant therapy). Products include:
- Arco-Lase Plus Tablets ... 513
- Bellergal-S Tablets ... 2375
- Donnatal ... 2234
- Donnatal Extentabs ... 2234
- Donnatal Tablets ... 2234
- Phenobarbital Elixir and Tablets ... 1523
- Quadrinal Tablets ... 1398

Phensuximide (Potential for low maximum plasma concentrations of felodipine in epileptic patients on long-term anticonvulsant therapy).
- No products indexed under this heading.

Phenytoin (Potential for low maximum plasma concentrations of felodipine in epileptic patients on long-term anticonvulsant therapy). Products include:
- Dilantin Infatabs ... 1967
- Dilantin-125 Suspension ... 1969

Phenytoin Sodium (Potential for low maximum plasma concentrations of felodipine in epileptic patients on long-term anticonvulsant therapy). Products include:
- Dilantin Kapseals ... 1965

Pindolol (Caution should be exercised when using Plendil in patients with heart failure or compromised ventricular function, particularly in combination with beta blocker). Products include:
- Visken Tablets ... 2428

Primidone (Potential for low maximum plasma concentrations of felodipine in epileptic patients on long-term anticonvulsant therapy). Products include:
- Mysoline ... 2860

Propranolol Hydrochloride (Caution should be exercised when using Plendil in patients with heart failure or compromised ventricular function, particularly in combination with beta blocker). Products include:
- Inderal ... 2834
- Inderal LA Long Acting Capsules ... 2836
- Inderide Tablets ... 2838
- Inderide LA Long Acting Capsules .. 2840

Sotalol Hydrochloride (Caution should be exercised when using Plendil in patients with heart failure or compromised ventricular function, particularly in combination with beta blocker). Products include:
- Betapace Tablets ... 637

Timolol Hemihydrate (Caution should be exercised when using Plendil in patients with heart failure or compromised ventricular function, particularly in combination with beta blocker). Products include:
- Betimol 0.25%, 0.5% ... ⊙ 259

Timolol Maleate (Caution should be exercised when using Plendil in patients with heart failure or compromised ventricular function, particularly in combination with beta blocker). Products include:
- Blocadren Tablets ... 1654
- Timolide Tablets ... 1791
- Timoptic in Ocudose ... 1796
- Timoptic Sterile Ophthalmic Solution ... 1794
- Timoptic-XE ... 1798

Trimethadione (Potential for low maximum plasma concentrations of felodipine in epileptic patients on long-term anticonvulsant therapy).
- No products indexed under this heading.

Valproic Acid (Potential for low maximum plasma concentrations of felodipine in epileptic patients on long-term anticonvulsant therapy). Products include:
- Depakene ... 416

Food Interactions

Grapefruit juice, doubly concentrated (Increases bioavailability more than two-fold).

PMB 200 AND PMB 400 (Estrogens, Conjugated, Meprobamate) ... 2890

May interact with central nervous system depressants, psychotropics, narcotic analgesics, progestins, and certain other agents. Compounds in these categories include:

Alfentanil Hydrochloride (Additive effects). Products include:
- Alfenta Injection ... 1334

Alprazolam (Additive effects). Products include:
- Xanax Tablets ... 2115

Amitriptyline Hydrochloride (Additive effects). Products include:
- Elavil ... 2945
- Etrafon ... 2495
- Limbitrol ... 2333
- Triavil Tablets ... 1800

Amoxapine (Additive effects). Products include:
- Asendin Tablets ... 1419

Aprobarbital (Additive effects).
- No products indexed under this heading.

Buprenorphine (Additive effects). Products include:
- Buprenex Injectable ... 2170

Buspirone Hydrochloride (Additive effects). Products include:
- BuSpar Tablets ... 738

Butabarbital (Additive effects).
- No products indexed under this heading.

Butalbital (Additive effects). Products include:
- Axocet Capsules ... 2469
- Esgic-plus Capsules ... 1012
- Esgic-plus Tablets ... 1012
- Fioricet Tablets ... 2386
- Fioricet with Codeine Capsules ... 2387
- Fiorinal Capsules ... 2388
- Fiorinal with Codeine Capsules ... 2390
- Fiorinal Tablets ... 2388
- Phrenilin ... 790
- Sedapap Tablets 50 mg/650 mg .. 1826

Chlordiazepoxide (Additive effects). Products include:
- Limbitrol ... 2333

Chlordiazepoxide Hydrochloride (Additive effects). Products include:
- Librax Capsules ... 2330
- Librium Capsules ... 2331
- Librium Injectable ... 2332

Chlorpromazine (Additive effects). Products include:
- Thorazine Suppositories ... 2701

Chlorprothixene (Additive effects).
- No products indexed under this heading.

Chlorprothixene Hydrochloride (Additive effects).
- No products indexed under this heading.

Chlorprothixene Lactate (Additive effects).
- No products indexed under this heading.

(▣ Described in PDR For Nonprescription Drugs) (⊙ Described in PDR For Ophthalmology)

Interactions Index

Clonidine (Additive effects). Products include:
- Catapres-TTS ... 680

Clonidine Hydrochloride (Additive effects). Products include:
- Catapres Tablets ... 679
- Combipres Tablets ... 682

Clorazepate Dipotassium (Additive effects). Products include:
- Tranxene ... 459

Clozapine (Additive effects). Products include:
- Clozaril Tablets ... 2377

Codeine Phosphate (Additive effects). Products include:
- Brontex ... 2130
- Dimetane-DC Cough Syrup ... 2232
- Fioricet with Codeine Capsules ... 2387
- Fiorinal with Codeine Capsules ... 2390
- Nucofed ... 2225
- Phenergan with Codeine ... 2883
- Phenergan VC with Codeine ... 2888
- Robitussin A-C Syrup ... 2248
- Robitussin-DAC Syrup ... 2249
- Ryna ... 804
- Soma Compound w/Codeine Tablets ... 2784
- Tylenol with Codeine ... 1592

Desflurane (Additive effects). Products include:
- Suprane (desflurane, USP) ... 1865

Desipramine Hydrochloride (Additive effects). Products include:
- Norpramin Tablets ... 1273

Desogestrel (Adverse effects on carbohydrate and lipid metabolism). Products include:
- Desogen Tablets ... 1867
- Ortho-Cept ... 1907

Dezocine (Additive effects). Products include:
- Dalgan Injection ... 529

Diazepam (Additive effects). Products include:
- Dizac (diazepam injectable emulsion) CIV ... 1862
- Valium Injectable ... 2336
- Valium Tablets ... 2335

Doxepin Hydrochloride (Additive effects). Products include:
- Adapin Capsules ... 1542
- Sinequan ... 2028
- Zonalon Cream ... 1042

Droperidol (Additive effects). Products include:
- Inapsine Injection ... 462

Enflurane (Additive effects).
No products indexed under this heading.

Estazolam (Additive effects). Products include:
- ProSom Tablets ... 457

Ethchlorvynol (Additive effects). Products include:
- Placidyl Capsules ... 456

Ethinamate (Additive effects).
No products indexed under this heading.

Fentanyl (Additive effects). Products include:
- Duragesic Transdermal System ... 1336

Fentanyl Citrate (Additive effects). Products include:
- Sublimaze Injection ... 463

Fluphenazine Decanoate (Additive effects). Products include:
- Prolixin Decanoate ... 510

Fluphenazine Enanthate (Additive effects). Products include:
- Prolixin Enanthate ... 510

Fluphenazine Hydrochloride (Additive effects). Products include:
- Prolixin ... 510

Flurazepam Hydrochloride (Additive effects). Products include:
- Dalmane Capsules ... 2329

Glutethimide (Additive effects).
No products indexed under this heading.

Haloperidol (Additive effects). Products include:
- Haldol Injection, Tablets and Concentrate ... 1585

Haloperidol Decanoate (Additive effects). Products include:
- Haldol Decanoate ... 1587

Hydrocodone Bitartrate (Additive effects). Products include:
- Codiclear DH Syrup ... 808
- Duratuss HD Elixir ... 2750
- Histussin D Liquid ... 670
- Hycodan Tablets and Syrup ... 946
- Hycomine Compound Tablets ... 948
- Hycomine ... 947
- Hycotuss Expectorant Syrup ... 950
- Hydrocet Capsules ... 787
- Lorcet 10/650 Tablets ... 1016
- Lortab ... 2751
- Tussend ... 1830
- Tussend Expectorant ... 1831
- Vicodin Tablets ... 1404
- Vicodin ES Tablets ... 1405
- Vicodin HP Tablets ... 1403
- Vicodin Tuss Expectorant ... 1406
- Zydone Capsules ... 967

Hydrocodone Polistirex (Additive effects). Products include:
- Tussionex Pennkinetic Extended-Release Suspension ... 1624

Hydromorphone Hydrochloride (Additive effects). Products include:
- Dilaudid Ampules ... 1382
- Dilaudid Cough Syrup ... 1383
- Dilaudid-HP Injection ... 1384
- Dilaudid-HP Lyophilized Powder 250 mg ... 1384
- Dilaudid ... 1382
- Dilaudid Oral Liquid ... 1386
- Dilaudid ... 1382
- Dilaudid Tablets - 8 mg. ... 1386

Hydroxyzine Hydrochloride (Additive effects). Products include:
- Atarax Tablets & Syrup ... 1992
- Marax Tablets & DF Syrup ... 2015
- Vistaril Intramuscular Solution ... 2042

Imipramine Hydrochloride (Additive effects). Products include:
- Tofranil Ampuls ... 873
- Tofranil Tablets ... 875

Imipramine Pamoate (Additive effects). Products include:
- Tofranil-PM Capsules ... 876

Isocarboxazid (Additive effects).
No products indexed under this heading.

Isoflurane (Additive effects).
No products indexed under this heading.

Ketamine Hydrochloride (Additive effects).
No products indexed under this heading.

Levomethadyl Acetate Hydrochloride (Additive effects). Products include:
- Orlaam Oral Solution ... 2361

Levorphanol Tartrate (Additive effects). Products include:
- Levo-Dromoran ... 2297

Lithium Carbonate (Additive effects). Products include:
- Eskalith ... 2658
- Lithium Carbonate Capsules & Tablets ... 2352
- Lithonate/Lithotabs/Lithobid ... 2721

Lithium Citrate (Additive effects).
No products indexed under this heading.

Lorazepam (Additive effects). Products include:
- Ativan Injection ... 2805
- Ativan Tablets ... 2807

Loxapine Hydrochloride (Additive effects). Products include:
- Loxitane ... 1426

Loxapine Succinate (Additive effects). Products include:
- Loxitane Capsules ... 1426

Maprotiline Hydrochloride (Additive effects). Products include:
- Ludiomil Tablets ... 861

Medroxyprogesterone Acetate (Adverse effects on carbohydrate and lipid metabolism). Products include:
- Amen Tablets ... 785
- Cycrin Tablets ... 991
- Depo-Provera Contraceptive Injection ... 2079
- Depo-Provera Sterile Aqueous Suspension ... 2083
- Premphase ... 2900
- Prempro ... 2905
- Provera Tablets ... 2110

Megestrol Acetate (Adverse effects on carbohydrate and lipid metabolism). Products include:
- Megace Oral Suspension ... 708
- Megace Tablets ... 710

Meperidine Hydrochloride (Additive effects). Products include:
- Demerol ... 2438
- Mepergan Injection ... 2859

Mephobarbital (Additive effects). Products include:
- Mebaral Tablets ... 2452

Mesoridazine Besylate (Additive effects). Products include:
- Serentil ... 689

Methadone Hydrochloride (Additive effects). Products include:
- Methadone Hydrochloride Oral Concentrate ... 2356
- Methadone Hydrochloride Oral Solution & Tablets ... 2357

Methohexital Sodium (Additive effects).
No products indexed under this heading.

Methotrimeprazine (Additive effects). Products include:
- Levoprome ... 1321

Methoxyflurane (Additive effects).
No products indexed under this heading.

Midazolam Hydrochloride (Additive effects). Products include:
- Versed Injection ... 2324

Molindone Hydrochloride (Additive effects). Products include:
- Moban Tablets and Concentrate ... 1036

Morphine Sulfate (Additive effects). Products include:
- Astramorph/PF Injection, USP (Preservative-Free) ... 526
- Duramorph Injection ... 983
- Infumorph 200 and Infumorph 500 Sterile Solutions ... 985
- Kadian Capsules ... 2948
- MS Contin Tablets ... 2149
- MSIR ... 2152
- Oramorph SR (Morphine Sulfate Sustained Release Tablets) ... 2359
- RMS Suppositories CII ... 2766
- Roxanol ... 2365

Norgestimate (Adverse effects on carbohydrate and lipid metabolism). Products include:
- Ortho-Cyclen/Ortho-Tri-Cyclen ... 1914
- Ortho-Cyclen/Ortho Tri-Cyclen ... 1914

Nortriptyline Hydrochloride (Additive effects). Products include:
- Pamelor ... 2409

Opium Alkaloids (Additive effects).
No products indexed under this heading.

Oxazepam (Additive effects). Products include:
- Serax Capsules ... 2916
- Serax Tablets ... 2916

Oxycodone Hydrochloride (Additive effects). Products include:
- OxyContin Tablets ... 2163
- OxyIR Capsules ... 2167
- Percocet Tablets ... 955
- Percodan Tablets ... 955
- Percodan-Demi Tablets ... 956
- Roxicodone Tablets, Oral Solution & Intensol (Oxycodone) ... 2366
- Tylox Capsules ... 1593

Pentobarbital Sodium (Additive effects). Products include:
- Nembutal Sodium Capsules ... 440
- Nembutal Sodium Solution ... 442
- Nembutal Sodium Suppositories ... 444

Perphenazine (Additive effects). Products include:
- Etrafon ... 2495
- Triavil Tablets ... 1800
- Trilafon ... 2532

Phenelzine Sulfate (Additive effects). Products include:
- Nardil ... 1977

Phenobarbital (Additive effects). Products include:
- Arco-Lase Plus Tablets ... 513
- Bellergal-S Tablets ... 2375
- Donnatal ... 2234
- Donnatal Extentabs ... 2234
- Donnatal ... 2234
- Phenobarbital Elixir and Tablets ... 1523
- Quadrinal Tablets ... 1398

Prazepam (Additive effects).
No products indexed under this heading.

Prochlorperazine (Additive effects). Products include:
- Compazine ... 2644

Promethazine Hydrochloride (Additive effects). Products include:
- Mepergan Injection ... 2859
- Phenergan with Codeine ... 2883
- Phenergan with Dextromethorphan ... 2885
- Phenergan Injection ... 2880
- Phenergan Suppositories ... 2882
- Phenergan Syrup ... 2881
- Phenergan Tablets ... 2882
- Phenergan VC ... 2886
- Phenergan VC with Codeine ... 2888

Propofol (Additive effects). Products include:
- Diprivan Injectable Emulsion ... 2939

Propoxyphene Hydrochloride (Additive effects). Products include:
- Darvon ... 1475
- Wygesic Tablets ... 2930

Propoxyphene Napsylate (Additive effects). Products include:
- Darvon-N/Darvocet-N ... 1473

Protriptyline Hydrochloride (Additive effects). Products include:
- Vivactil Tablets ... 1820

Quazepam (Additive effects). Products include:
- Doral Tablets ... 2773

Risperidone (Additive effects). Products include:
- Risperdal Tablets ... 1348

Secobarbital Sodium (Additive effects). Products include:
- Seconal Sodium Pulvules ... 1529

Sevoflurane (Additive effects).
No products indexed under this heading.

Sufentanil Citrate (Additive effects). Products include:
- Sufenta Injection ... 1355

Temazepam (Additive effects). Products include:
- Restoril Capsules ... 2413

Thiamylal Sodium (Additive effects).
No products indexed under this heading.

Thioridazine Hydrochloride (Additive effects). Products include:
- Mellaril ... 2398

Thiothixene (Additive effects). Products include:
- Navane Capsules and Concentrate ... 2018
- Navane Intramuscular ... 2019

Tranylcypromine Sulfate (Additive effects). Products include:
- Parnate Tablets ... 2679

Triazolam (Additive effects). Products include:
- Halcion Tablets ... 2093

IMPORTANT NOTE: Always consult each drug listing in the patient's regimen for possible interactions.

PMB **Interactions Index** 852

Trifluoperazine Hydrochloride (Additive effects). Products include:
- Stelazine 2692

Trimipramine Maleate (Additive effects). Products include:
- Surmontil Capsules 2917

Zolpidem Tartrate (Additive effects). Products include:
- Ambien Tablets 2559

Food Interactions

Alcohol (Additive effects).

PNEUMOVAX 23
(Pneumococcal Vaccine, Polyvalent)..1768
May interact with immunosuppressive agents. Compounds in this category include:

Azathioprine (Expected serum antibody response may not be obtained). Products include:
- Azathioprine Tablets 2349
- Imuran 1103

Cyclosporine (Expected serum antibody response may not be obtained). Products include:
- Neoral 2405
- Sandimmune 2416

Immune Globulin (Human) (Expected serum antibody response may not be obtained).
- No products indexed under this heading.

Immune Globulin Intravenous (Human) (Expected serum antibody response may not be obtained).

Muromonab-CD3 (Expected serum antibody response may not be obtained). Products include:
- Orthoclone OKT3 Sterile Solution .. 1892

Mycophenolate Mofetil (Expected serum antibody response may not be obtained). Products include:
- CellCept Capsules 2265

Tacrolimus (Expected serum antibody response may not be obtained). Products include:
- Prograf 1028

PNU-IMUNE 23
(Pneumococcal Vaccine, Polyvalent)..1437
May interact with immunosuppressive agents and antineoplastics. Compounds in these categories include:

Altretamine (Possible impaired serum antibody response to vaccine). Products include:
- Hexalen Capsules 2760

Anastrozole (Possible impaired serum antibody response to vaccine). Products include:
- Arimidex Tablets 2932

Asparaginase (Possible impaired serum antibody response to vaccine). Products include:
- Elspar 1700

Azathioprine (Reduction of antibody levels). Products include:
- Azathioprine Tablets 2349
- Imuran 1103

Bicalutamide (Possible impaired serum antibody response to vaccine). Products include:
- Casodex Tablets 2934

Bleomycin Sulfate (Possible impaired serum antibody response to vaccine). Products include:
- Blenoxane 697

Busulfan (Possible impaired serum antibody response to vaccine). Products include:
- Myleran Tablets 1209

Carboplatin (Possible impaired serum antibody response to vaccine). Products include:
- Paraplatin for Injection 713

Carmustine (BCNU) (Possible impaired serum antibody response to vaccine). Products include:
- BiCNU 696

Chlorambucil (Possible impaired serum antibody response to vaccine). Products include:
- Leukeran Tablets 1205

Cisplatin (Possible impaired serum antibody response to vaccine). Products include:
- Platinol for Injection 717
- Platinol-AQ Injection 719

Cyclophosphamide (Possible impaired serum antibody response to vaccine). Products include:
- Cytoxan 700

Cyclosporine (Reduction of antibody levels). Products include:
- Neoral 2405
- Sandimmune 2416

Dacarbazine (Possible impaired serum antibody response to vaccine). Products include:
- DTIC-Dome 593

Daunorubicin Citrate (Possible impaired serum antibody response to vaccine). Products include:
- DaunoXome 1842

Daunorubicin Hydrochloride (Possible impaired serum antibody response to vaccine). Products include:
- Cerubidine for Injection 634

Docetaxel (Possible impaired serum antibody response to vaccine). Products include:
- Taxotere for Injection Concentrate 2204

Doxorubicin Hydrochloride (Possible impaired serum antibody response to vaccine). Products include:
- Adriamycin PFS 2056
- Adriamycin RDF 2056
- Doxil 2613
- Doxorubicin Astra 531
- Rubex for Injection 721

Estramustine Phosphate Sodium (Possible impaired serum antibody response to vaccine). Products include:
- Emcyt Capsules 2085

Etoposide (Possible impaired serum antibody response to vaccine). Products include:
- Etoposide Injection 539
- VePesid Capsules and Injection 727

Floxuridine (Possible impaired serum antibody response to vaccine). Products include:
- Sterile FUDR 2284

Fluorouracil (Possible impaired serum antibody response to vaccine). Products include:
- Efudex 2280
- Fluoroplex Topical Solution & Cream 1% 475
- Fluorouracil Injection 2282

Flutamide (Possible impaired serum antibody response to vaccine). Products include:
- Eulexin Capsules 2498

Gemcitabine Hydrochloride (Possible impaired serum antibody response to vaccine). Products include:
- Gemzar for Injection 1482

Hydroxyurea (Possible impaired serum antibody response to vaccine). Products include:
- Hydrea Capsules 705

Idarubicin Hydrochloride (Possible impaired serum antibody response to vaccine). Products include:
- Idamycin Injection 2096

Ifosfamide (Possible impaired serum antibody response to vaccine). Products include:
- IFEX 706

Immune Globulin (Human) (Reduction of antibody levels).
- No products indexed under this heading.

Immune Globulin Intravenous (Human) (Reduction of antibody levels).

Interferon alfa-2A, Recombinant (Possible impaired serum antibody response to vaccine). Products include:
- Roferon-A Injection 2308

Interferon alfa-2B, Recombinant (Possible impaired serum antibody response to vaccine). Products include:
- Intron A for Injection 2506

Irinotecan Hydrochloride (Possible impaired serum antibody response to vaccine).
- No products indexed under this heading.

Levamisole Hydrochloride (Possible impaired serum antibody response to vaccine). Products include:
- Ergamisol Tablets 1340

Lomustine (CCNU) (Possible impaired serum antibody response to vaccine). Products include:
- CeeNU Capsules 699

Mechlorethamine Hydrochloride (Possible impaired serum antibody response to vaccine). Products include:
- Mustargen 1752

Megestrol Acetate (Possible impaired serum antibody response to vaccine). Products include:
- Megace Oral Suspension 708
- Megace Tablets 710

Melphalan (Possible impaired serum antibody response to vaccine). Products include:
- Alkeran Tablets 1198

Mercaptopurine (Possible impaired serum antibody response to vaccine). Products include:
- Purinethol Tablets 1214

Methotrexate Sodium (Possible impaired serum antibody response to vaccine). Products include:
- Methotrexate Sodium Tablets, Injection, for Injection and LPF Injection 1322

Mitomycin (Mitomycin-C) (Possible impaired serum antibody response to vaccine). Products include:
- Mutamycin for Injection 712

Mitotane (Possible impaired serum antibody response to vaccine). Products include:
- Lysodren Tablets 707

Mitoxantrone Hydrochloride (Possible impaired serum antibody response to vaccine). Products include:
- Novantrone for Injection 1327

Muromonab-CD3 (Reduction of antibody levels). Products include:
- Orthoclone OKT3 Sterile Solution .. 1892

Mycophenolate Mofetil (Reduction of antibody levels). Products include:
- CellCept Capsules 2265

Paclitaxel (Possible impaired serum antibody response to vaccine). Products include:
- Taxol Injection 723

Procarbazine Hydrochloride (Possible impaired serum antibody response to vaccine). Products include:
- Matulane Capsules 2300

Streptozocin (Possible impaired serum antibody response to vaccine). Products include:
- Zanosar Sterile Powder 2119

Tacrolimus (Reduction of antibody levels). Products include:
- Prograf 1028

Tamoxifen Citrate (Possible impaired serum antibody response to vaccine). Products include:
- Nolvadex Tablets 2957

Teniposide (Possible impaired serum antibody response to vaccine). Products include:
- Vumon for Injection 729

Thioguanine (Possible impaired serum antibody response to vaccine). Products include:
- Thioguanine Tablets, Tabloid Brand 1225

Thiotepa (Possible impaired serum antibody response to vaccine). Products include:
- Thioplex (Thiotepa For Injection) 1329

Topotecan Hydrochloride (Possible impaired serum antibody response to vaccine). Products include:
- Hycamtin for Injection 2665

Vincristine Sulfate (Possible impaired serum antibody response to vaccine). Products include:
- Oncovin Solution Vials & Hyporets 1521

Vinorelbine Tartrate (Possible impaired serum antibody response to vaccine). Products include:
- Navelbine Injection 1212

PODOCON-25
(Podophyllin) 1949
None cited in PDR database.

POLYCITRA SYRUP
(Potassium Citrate, Sodium Citrate, Citric Acid) 574
May interact with potassium preparations, potassium sparing diuretics, cardiac glycosides, ACE inhibitors, and certain other agents. Compounds in these categories include:

Aluminum Carbonate (Patients with low urinary output or reduced glomerular filtration rates should avoid concomitant use of aluminum-based antacids). Products include:
- Basaljel Capsules 2810
- Basaljel Suspension 2810
- Basaljel Tablets 2810

Aluminum Hydroxide (Patients with low urinary output or reduced glomerular filtration rates should avoid concomitant use of aluminum-based antacids). Products include:
- ALternaGEL Liquid 1358
- Maximum Strength Ascriptin .... ▣ 650
- Cama Arthritis Pain Reliever .... ▣ 748
- Gaviscon Extra Strength Relief Formula Antacid Tablets .... ▣ 778
- Gaviscon Extra Strength Relief Formula Liquid Antacid .... ▣ 779
- Gaviscon Liquid Antacid .... ▣ 779
- Gelusil Antacid-Anti-gas Liquid .... ▣ 819
- Gelusil Antacid-Anti-gas Tablets .... ▣ 819
- Maalox Antacid/Anti-Gas Tablets 889
- Maalox Heartburn Relief Suspension .... ▣ 658
- Maalox Antacid Liquid 888
- Extra Strength Maalox Antacid/Anti-Gas Liquid and Tablets 888
- Mylanta 1359
- Tempo Soft Antacid .... ▣ 799

Aluminum Hydroxide Gel (Patients with low urinary output or reduced glomerular filtration rates should avoid concomitant use of aluminum-based antacids). Products include:
ALternaGEL Liquid	675
Aludrox Oral Suspension	850
Amphojel Suspension	2802
Amphojel Suspension without Flavor	2802
Amphojel Tablets	2802
Ascriptin	650
Gaviscon Antacid Tablets	778
Gaviscon-2 Antacid Tablets	779
Mylanta Liquid	676
Mylanta Double Strength Liquid	676
Nephrox Suspension	671

Amiloride Hydrochloride (Potential toxicity). Products include:
Midamor Tablets	1746
Moduretic Tablets	1748

Benazepril Hydrochloride (Potential toxicity). Products include:
Lotensin Tablets	852
Lotensin HCT Tablets	855
Lotrel Capsules	858

Captopril (Potential toxicity). Products include:
Capoten Tablets	740
Capozide Tablets	744

Deslanoside (Potential toxicity).
No products indexed under this heading.

Digitoxin (Potential toxicity). Products include:
Crystodigin Tablets	1472

Digoxin (Potential toxicity). Products include:
Lanoxicaps	1110
Lanoxin Elixir Pediatric	1113
Lanoxin Injection	1116
Lanoxin Injection Pediatric	1119
Lanoxin Tablets	1121

Enalapril Maleate (Potential toxicity). Products include:
Vaseretic Tablets	1810
Vasotec Tablets	1816

Enalaprilat (Potential toxicity). Products include:
Vasotec I.V.	1814

Fosinopril Sodium (Potential toxicity). Products include:
Monopril Tablets	762

Lisinopril (Potential toxicity). Products include:
Prinivil Tablets	1776
Prinzide Tablets	1780
Zestoretic Tablets	2968
Zestril Tablets	2972

Moexipril Hydrochloride (Potential toxicity). Products include:
Univasc Tablets	2553

Potassium Acid Phosphate (Potential toxicity). Products include:
K-Phos Original Formula 'Sodium Free' Tablets	633

Potassium Bicarbonate (Potential toxicity). Products include:
Alka-Seltzer Gold Effervescent Antacid	611

Potassium Chloride (Potential toxicity). Products include:
Chlor-3 Condiment	1003
Colyte and Colyte-flavored	2540
GoLYTELY	694
K-Dur Microburst Release System (potassium chloride, USP) E.R. Tablets	1364
K-Lor Powder Packets	438
K-Norm Capsules	1615
K-Tab Filmtab	439
Micro-K	2237
Micro-K LS Packets	2238
NuLYTELY	694
Cherry Flavor NuLYTELY	694
Rum-K Syrup	1004
Slow-K Extended-Release Tablets	869

Potassium Gluconate (Potential toxicity).
No products indexed under this heading.

Potassium Phosphate, Dibasic (Potential toxicity).
No products indexed under this heading.

Potassium Phosphate, Monobasic (Potential toxicity). Products include:
K-Phos Neutral Tablets	633
K-Phos Original Formula 'Sodium Free' Tablets	633

Quinapril Hydrochloride (Potential toxicity). Products include:
Accupril Tablets	1950

Ramipril (Potential toxicity). Products include:
Altace Capsules	1238

Spirapril Hydrochloride (Potential toxicity).
No products indexed under this heading.

Spironolactone (Potential toxicity). Products include:
Aldactazide Tablets	2556
Aldactone Tablets	2558

Trandolapril (Potential toxicity). Products include:
Mavik Tablets	1407

Triamterene (Potential toxicity). Products include:
Dyazide Capsules	2653
Dyrenium Capsules	2655

POLYCITRA-K CRYSTALS
(Potassium Citrate, Citric Acid) 574
May interact with potassium preparations, potassium sparing diuretics, ACE inhibitors, and cardiac glycosides. Compounds in these categories include:

Amiloride Hydrochloride (Potential toxicity). Products include:
Midamor Tablets	1746
Moduretic Tablets	1748

Benazepril Hydrochloride (Potential toxicity). Products include:
Lotensin Tablets	852
Lotensin HCT Tablets	855
Lotrel Capsules	858

Captopril (Potential toxicity). Products include:
Capoten Tablets	740
Capozide Tablets	744

Deslanoside (Potential toxicity).
No products indexed under this heading.

Digitoxin (Potential toxicity). Products include:
Crystodigin Tablets	1472

Digoxin (Potential toxicity). Products include:
Lanoxicaps	1110
Lanoxin Elixir Pediatric	1113
Lanoxin Injection	1116
Lanoxin Injection Pediatric	1119
Lanoxin Tablets	1121

Enalapril Maleate (Potential toxicity). Products include:
Vaseretic Tablets	1810
Vasotec Tablets	1816

Enalaprilat (Potential toxicity). Products include:
Vasotec I.V.	1814

Fosinopril Sodium (Potential toxicity). Products include:
Monopril Tablets	762

Lisinopril (Potential toxicity). Products include:
Prinivil Tablets	1776
Prinzide Tablets	1780
Zestoretic Tablets	2968
Zestril Tablets	2972

Moexipril Hydrochloride (Potential toxicity). Products include:
Univasc Tablets	2553

Potassium Acid Phosphate (Potential toxicity). Products include:
K-Phos Original Formula 'Sodium Free' Tablets	633

Potassium Bicarbonate (Potential toxicity). Products include:
Alka-Seltzer Gold Effervescent Antacid	611

Potassium Chloride (Potential toxicity). Products include:
Chlor-3 Condiment	1003
Colyte and Colyte-flavored	2540
GoLYTELY	694
K-Dur Microburst Release System (potassium chloride, USP) E.R. Tablets	1364
K-Lor Powder Packets	438
K-Norm Capsules	1615
K-Tab Filmtab	439
Micro-K	2237
Micro-K LS Packets	2238
NuLYTELY	694
Cherry Flavor NuLYTELY	694
Rum-K Syrup	1004
Slow-K Extended-Release Tablets	869

Potassium Gluconate (Potential toxicity).
No products indexed under this heading.

Potassium Phosphate, Dibasic (Potential toxicity).
No products indexed under this heading.

Potassium Phosphate, Monobasic (Potential toxicity). Products include:
K-Phos Neutral Tablets	633
K-Phos Original Formula 'Sodium Free' Tablets	633

Quinapril Hydrochloride (Potential toxicity). Products include:
Accupril Tablets	1950

Ramipril (Potential toxicity). Products include:
Altace Capsules	1238

Spirapril Hydrochloride (Potential toxicity).
No products indexed under this heading.

Spironolactone (Potential toxicity). Products include:
Aldactazide Tablets	2556
Aldactone Tablets	2558

Trandolapril (Potential toxicity). Products include:
Mavik Tablets	1407

Triamterene (Potential toxicity). Products include:
Dyazide Capsules	2653
Dyrenium Capsules	2655

POLYCITRA-K ORAL SOLUTION
(Potassium Citrate, Citric Acid) 575
May interact with ACE inhibitors, potassium sparing diuretics, potassium preparations, and cardiac glycosides. Compounds in these categories include:

Amiloride Hydrochloride (Increased risk of hyperkalemia). Products include:
Midamor Tablets	1746
Moduretic Tablets	1748

Benazepril Hydrochloride (Increased risk of hyperkalemia). Products include:
Lotensin Tablets	852
Lotensin HCT Tablets	855
Lotrel Capsules	858

Captopril (Increased risk of hyperkalemia). Products include:
Capoten Tablets	740
Capozide Tablets	744

Deslanoside (Increased risk of hyperkalemia).
No products indexed under this heading.

Digitoxin (Increased risk of hyperkalemia). Products include:
Crystodigin Tablets	1472

Digoxin (Increased risk of hyperkalemia). Products include:
Lanoxicaps	1110
Lanoxin Elixir Pediatric	1113
Lanoxin Injection	1116
Lanoxin Injection Pediatric	1119
Lanoxin Tablets	1121

Enalapril Maleate (Increased risk of hyperkalemia). Products include:
Vaseretic Tablets	1810
Vasotec Tablets	1816

Enalaprilat (Increased risk of hyperkalemia). Products include:
Vasotec I.V.	1814

Fosinopril Sodium (Increased risk of hyperkalemia). Products include:
Monopril Tablets	762

Lisinopril (Increased risk of hyperkalemia). Products include:
Prinivil Tablets	1776
Prinzide Tablets	1780
Zestoretic Tablets	2968
Zestril Tablets	2972

Moexipril Hydrochloride (Increased risk of hyperkalemia). Products include:
Univasc Tablets	2553

Potassium Acid Phosphate (Increased risk of hyperkalemia). Products include:
K-Phos Original Formula 'Sodium Free' Tablets	633

Potassium Bicarbonate (Increased risk of hyperkalemia). Products include:
Alka-Seltzer Gold Effervescent Antacid	611

Potassium Chloride (Increased risk of hyperkalemia). Products include:
Chlor-3 Condiment	1003
Colyte and Colyte-flavored	2540
GoLYTELY	694
K-Dur Microburst Release System (potassium chloride, USP) E.R. Tablets	1364
K-Lor Powder Packets	438
K-Norm Capsules	1615
K-Tab Filmtab	439
Micro-K	2237
Micro-K LS Packets	2238
NuLYTELY	694
Cherry Flavor NuLYTELY	694
Rum-K Syrup	1004
Slow-K Extended-Release Tablets	869

Potassium Gluconate (Increased risk of hyperkalemia).
No products indexed under this heading.

Potassium Phosphate, Dibasic (Increased risk of hyperkalemia).
No products indexed under this heading.

Potassium Phosphate, Monobasic (Increased risk of hyperkalemia). Products include:
K-Phos Neutral Tablets	633
K-Phos Original Formula 'Sodium Free' Tablets	633

Quinapril Hydrochloride (Increased risk of hyperkalemia). Products include:
Accupril Tablets	1950

Ramipril (Increased risk of hyperkalemia). Products include:
Altace Capsules	1238

Spirapril Hydrochloride (Increased risk of hyperkalemia).
No products indexed under this heading.

Spironolactone (Increased risk of hyperkalemia). Products include:
Aldactazide Tablets	2556
Aldactone Tablets	2558

Trandolapril (Increased risk of hyperkalemia). Products include:
Mavik Tablets	1407

Triamterene (Increased risk of hyperkalemia). Products include:
Dyazide Capsules	2653
Dyrenium Capsules	2655

IMPORTANT NOTE: Always consult each drug listing in the patient's regimen for possible interactions.

Interactions Index

POLYCITRA-LC
(Potassium Citrate, Citric Acid, Sodium Citrate) 574
See Polycitra Syrup

POLYCOSE GLUCOSE POLYMERS
(Glucose Polymers) 2343
None cited in PDR database.

POLY-PRED LIQUIFILM
(Neomycin Sulfate, Polymyxin B Sulfate, Prednisolone Acetate) .... ⊚ 246
None cited in PDR database.

POLYSPORIN OINTMENT
(Bacitracin Zinc, Polymyxin B Sulfate) .... ▣ 822
None cited in PDR database.

POLYSPORIN OPHTHALMIC OINTMENT STERILE
(Polymyxin B Sulfate, Bacitracin Zinc) 1140
None cited in PDR database.

POLYSPORIN POWDER
(Bacitracin Zinc, Polymyxin B Sulfate) .... ▣ 823
None cited in PDR database.

POLYTRIM OPHTHALMIC SOLUTION STERILE
(Polymyxin B Sulfate, Trimethoprim Sulfate) 479
None cited in PDR database.

POLY-VI-FLOR DROPS
(Vitamins with Fluoride) 1600
None cited in PDR database.

POLY-VI-FLOR TABLETS
(Vitamins with Fluoride) 1600
None cited in PDR database.

PONDIMIN TABLETS
(Fenfluramine Hydrochloride) 2239
May interact with central nervous system depressants, monoamine oxidase inhibitors, and certain other agents. Compounds in these categories include:

Alfentanil Hydrochloride (Possible additive effects of CNS depressants). Products include:
  Alfenta Injection 1334

Alprazolam (Possible additive effects of CNS depressants). Products include:
  Xanax Tablets 2115

Aprobarbital (Possible additive effects of CNS depressants).
  No products indexed under this heading.

Buprenorphine (Possible additive effects of CNS depressants). Products include:
  Buprenex Injectable 2170

Buspirone Hydrochloride (Possible additive effects of CNS depressants). Products include:
  BuSpar Tablets 738

Butabarbital (Possible additive effects of CNS depressants).
  No products indexed under this heading.

Butalbital (Possible additive effects of CNS depressants). Products include:
  Axocet Capsules 2469
  Esgic-plus Capsules 1012
  Esgic-plus Tablets 1012
  Fioricet Tablets 2386
  Fioricet with Codeine Capsules 2387
  Fiorinal Capsules 2388
  Fiorinal with Codeine Capsules 2390
  Fiorinal Tablets 2388

Phrenilin 790
Sedapap Tablets 50 mg/650 mg .. 1826

Chlordiazepoxide (Possible additive effects of CNS depressants). Products include:
  Limbitrol 2333

Chlordiazepoxide Hydrochloride (Possible additive effects of CNS depressants). Products include:
  Librax Capsules 2330
  Librium Capsules 2331
  Librium Injectable 2332

Chlorpromazine (Possible additive effects of CNS depressants). Products include:
  Thorazine Suppositories 2701

Chlorprothixene (Possible additive effects of CNS depressants).
  No products indexed under this heading.

Chlorprothixene Hydrochloride (Possible additive effects of CNS depressants).
  No products indexed under this heading.

Chlorprothixene Lactate (Possible additive effects of CNS depressants).
  No products indexed under this heading.

Clorazepate Dipotassium (Possible additive effects of CNS depressants). Products include:
  Tranxene 459

Clozapine (Possible additive effects of CNS depressants). Products include:
  Clozaril Tablets 2377

Codeine Phosphate (Possible additive effects of CNS depressants). Products include:
  Brontex 2130
  Dimetane-DC Cough Syrup 2232
  Fioricet with Codeine Capsules 2387
  Fiorinal with Codeine Capsules 2390
  Nucofed 2225
  Phenergan with Codeine 2883
  Phenergan VC with Codeine 2888
  Robitussin A-C Syrup 2248
  Robitussin-DAC Syrup 2249
  Ryna .... ▣ 804
  Soma Compound w/Codeine Tablets 2784
  Tylenol with Codeine 1592

Deserpidine (Increased effect of hypertensives).
  No products indexed under this heading.

Desflurane (Possible additive effects of CNS depressants). Products include:
  Suprane (desflurane, USP) 1865

Dezocine (Possible additive effects of CNS depressants). Products include:
  Dalgan Injection 529

Diazepam (Possible additive effects of CNS depressants). Products include:
  Dizac (diazepam injectable emulsion) CIV 1862
  Valium Injectable 2336
  Valium Tablets 2335

Droperidol (Possible additive effects of CNS depressants). Products include:
  Inapsine Injection 462

Enflurane (Possible additive effects of CNS depressants).
  No products indexed under this heading.

Estazolam (Possible additive effects of CNS depressants). Products include:
  ProSom Tablets 457

Ethchlorvynol (Possible additive effects of CNS depressants). Products include:
  Placidyl Capsules 456

Ethinamate (Possible additive effects of CNS depressants).
  No products indexed under this heading.

Fentanyl (Possible additive effects of CNS depressants). Products include:
  Duragesic Transdermal System 1336

Fentanyl Citrate (Possible additive effects of CNS depressants). Products include:
  Sublimaze Injection 463

Fluphenazine Decanoate (Possible additive effects of CNS depressants). Products include:
  Prolixin Decanoate 510

Fluphenazine Enanthate (Possible additive effects of CNS depressants). Products include:
  Prolixin Enanthate 510

Fluphenazine Hydrochloride (Possible additive effects of CNS depressants). Products include:
  Prolixin 510

Flurazepam Hydrochloride (Possible additive effects of CNS depressants). Products include:
  Dalmane Capsules 2329

Furazolidone (Hypertensive crisis may result). Products include:
  Furoxone 2221

Glutethimide (Possible additive effects of CNS depressants).
  No products indexed under this heading.

Guanadrel Sulfate (Increased effect of hypertensives). Products include:
  Hylorel Tablets 1613

Guanethidine Monosulfate (Potential for slight increase in antihypertensive effect). Products include:
  Esimil Tablets 840
  Ismelin Tablets 845

Haloperidol (Possible additive effects of CNS depressants). Products include:
  Haldol Injection, Tablets and Concentrate 1585

Haloperidol Decanoate (Possible additive effects of CNS depressants). Products include:
  Haldol Decanoate 1587

Hydrocodone Bitartrate (Possible additive effects of CNS depressants). Products include:
  Codiclear DH Syrup 808
  Duratuss HD Elixir 2750
  Histussin D Liquid 670
  Hycodan Tablets and Syrup 946
  Hycomine Compound Tablets 948
  Hycomine 947
  Hycotuss Expectorant Syrup 950
  Hydrocet Capsules 787
  Lorcet 10/650 Tablets 1016
  Lortab 2751
  Tussend 1830
  Tussend Expectorant 1831
  Vicodin Tablets 1404
  Vicodin ES Tablets 1405
  Vicodin HP Tablets 1403
  Vicodin Tuss Expectorant 1406
  Zydone Capsules 967

Hydrocodone Polistirex (Possible additive effects of CNS depressants). Products include:
  Tussionex Pennkinetic Extended-Release Suspension 1624

Hydromorphone Hydrochloride (Possible additive effects of CNS depressants). Products include:
  Dilaudid Ampules 1382
  Dilaudid Cough Syrup 1383
  Dilaudid-HP Injection 1384
  Dilaudid-HP Lyophilized Powder 250 mg 1384
  Dilaudid 1382
  Dilaudid Oral Liquid 1386
  Dilaudid 1382
  Dilaudid Tablets - 8 mg. 1386

Hydroxyzine Hydrochloride (Possible additive effects of CNS depressants). Products include:
  Atarax Tablets & Syrup 1992
  Marax Tablets & DF Syrup 2015
  Vistaril Intramuscular Solution 2042

Isocarboxazid (Hypertensive crisis may result; concurrent or sequential use within 14 days is contraindicated).
  No products indexed under this heading.

Isoflurane (Possible additive effects of CNS depressants).
  No products indexed under this heading.

Ketamine Hydrochloride (Possible additive effects of CNS depressants).
  No products indexed under this heading.

Levomethadyl Acetate Hydrochloride (Possible additive effects of CNS depressants). Products include:
  Orlaam Oral Solution 2361

Levorphanol Tartrate (Possible additive effects of CNS depressants). Products include:
  Levo-Dromoran 2297

Lorazepam (Possible additive effects of CNS depressants). Products include:
  Ativan Injection 2805
  Ativan Tablets 2807

Loxapine Hydrochloride (Possible additive effects of CNS depressants). Products include:
  Loxitane 1426

Loxapine Succinate (Possible additive effects of CNS depressants). Products include:
  Loxitane Capsules 1426

Meperidine Hydrochloride (Possible additive effects of CNS depressants). Products include:
  Demerol 2438
  Mepergan Injection 2859

Mephobarbital (Possible additive effects of CNS depressants). Products include:
  Mebaral Tablets 2452

Meprobamate (Possible additive effects of CNS depressants). Products include:
  Miltown Tablets 2780
  PMB 200 and PMB 400 2890

Mesoridazine Besylate (Possible additive effects of CNS depressants). Products include:
  Serentil 689

Methadone Hydrochloride (Possible additive effects of CNS depressants). Products include:
  Methadone Hydrochloride Oral Concentrate 2356
  Methadone Hydrochloride Oral Solution & Tablets 2357

Methohexital Sodium (Possible additive effects of CNS depressants).
  No products indexed under this heading.

Methotrimeprazine (Possible additive effects of CNS depressants). Products include:
  Levoprome 1321

Methoxyflurane (Possible additive effects of CNS depressants).
  No products indexed under this heading.

Methyldopa (Potential for slight increase in antihypertensive effect). Products include:
  Aldoclor Tablets 1638
  Aldomet Oral 1640
  Aldoril Tablets 1644

(▣ Described in PDR For Nonprescription Drugs)   (⊚ Described in PDR For Ophthalmology)

Interactions Index

Methyldopate Hydrochloride (Potential for slight increase in antihypertensive effect). Products include:
- Aldomet Ester HCl Injection ... 1642

Midazolam Hydrochloride (Possible additive effects of CNS depressants). Products include:
- Versed Injection ... 2324

Molindone Hydrochloride (Possible additive effects of CNS depressants). Products include:
- Moban Tablets and Concentrate ... 1036

Morphine Sulfate (Possible additive effects of CNS depressants). Products include:
- Astramorph/PF Injection, USP (Preservative-Free) ... 526
- Duramorph Injection ... 983
- Infumorph 200 and Infumorph 500 Sterile Solutions ... 985
- Kadian Capsules ... 2948
- MS Contin Tablets ... 2149
- MSIR ... 2152
- Oramorph SR (Morphine Sulfate Sustained Release Tablets) ... 2359
- RMS Suppositories CII ... 2766
- Roxanol ... 2365

Opium Alkaloids (Possible additive effects of CNS depressants).
- No products indexed under this heading.

Oxazepam (Possible additive effects of CNS depressants). Products include:
- Serax Capsules ... 2916
- Serax Tablets ... 2916

Oxycodone Hydrochloride (Possible additive effects of CNS depressants). Products include:
- OxyContin Tablets ... 2163
- OxyIR Capsules ... 2167
- Percocet Tablets ... 955
- Percodan Tablets ... 955
- Percodan-Demi Tablets ... 956
- Roxicodone Tablets, Oral Solution & Intensol (Oxycodone) ... 2366
- Tylox Capsules ... 1593

Pentobarbital Sodium (Possible additive effects of CNS depressants). Products include:
- Nembutal Sodium Capsules ... 440
- Nembutal Sodium Solution ... 442
- Nembutal Sodium Suppositories ... 444

Perphenazine (Possible additive effects of CNS depressants). Products include:
- Etrafon ... 2495
- Triavil Tablets ... 1800
- Trilafon ... 2532

Phenelzine Sulfate (Hypertensive crisis may result; concurrent or sequential use within 14 days is contraindicated). Products include:
- Nardil ... 1977

Phenobarbital (Possible additive effects of CNS depressants). Products include:
- Arco-Lase Plus Tablets ... 513
- Bellergal-S Tablets ... 2375
- Donnatal ... 2234
- Donnatal Extentabs ... 2234
- Donnatal Tablets ... 2234
- Phenobarbital Elixir and Tablets ... 1523
- Quadrinal Tablets ... 1398

Prazepam (Possible additive effects of CNS depressants).
- No products indexed under this heading.

Prochlorperazine (Possible additive effects of CNS depressants). Products include:
- Compazine ... 2644

Promethazine Hydrochloride (Possible additive effects of CNS depressants). Products include:
- Mepergan Injection ... 2859
- Phenergan with Codeine ... 2883
- Phenergan with Dextromethorphan ... 2885
- Phenergan Injection ... 2880
- Phenergan Suppositories ... 2882
- Phenergan Syrup ... 2881
- Phenergan Tablets ... 2882
- Phenergan VC ... 2886
- Phenergan VC with Codeine ... 2888

Propofol (Possible additive effects of CNS depressants). Products include:
- Diprivan Injectable Emulsion ... 2939

Propoxyphene Hydrochloride (Possible additive effects of CNS depressants). Products include:
- Darvon ... 1475
- Wygesic Tablets ... 2930

Propoxyphene Napsylate (Possible additive effects of CNS depressants). Products include:
- Darvon-N/Darvocet-N ... 1473

Quazepam (Possible additive effects of CNS depressants). Products include:
- Doral Tablets ... 2773

Rauwolfia Serpentina (Potential for slight increase in antihypertensive effect).
- No products indexed under this heading.

Rescinnamine (Potential for slight increase in antihypertensive effect).
- No products indexed under this heading.

Reserpine (Potential for slight increase in antihypertensive effect). Products include:
- Diupres Tablets ... 1691
- Hydropres Tablets ... 1718
- Ser-Ap-Es Tablets ... 867

Risperidone (Possible additive effects of CNS depressants). Products include:
- Risperdal Tablets ... 1348

Secobarbital Sodium (Possible additive effects of CNS depressants). Products include:
- Seconal Sodium Pulvules ... 1529

Selegiline Hydrochloride (Hypertensive crisis may result; concurrent or sequential use within 14 days is contraindicated). Products include:
- Eldepryl Capsules ... 2729

Sevoflurane (Possible additive effects of CNS depressants).
- No products indexed under this heading.

Sufentanil Citrate (Possible additive effects of CNS depressants). Products include:
- Sufenta Injection ... 1355

Temazepam (Possible additive effects of CNS depressants). Products include:
- Restoril Capsules ... 2413

Thiamylal Sodium (Possible additive effects of CNS depressants).
- No products indexed under this heading.

Thioridazine Hydrochloride (Possible additive effects of CNS depressants). Products include:
- Mellaril ... 2398

Thiothixene (Possible additive effects of CNS depressants). Products include:
- Navane Capsules and Concentrate ... 2018
- Navane Intramuscular ... 2019

Tranylcypromine Sulfate (Hypertensive crisis may result; concurrent or sequential use within 14 days is contraindicated). Products include:
- Parnate Tablets ... 2679

Triazolam (Possible additive effects of CNS depressants). Products include:
- Halcion Tablets ... 2093

Trifluoperazine Hydrochloride (Possible additive effects of CNS depressants). Products include:
- Stelazine ... 2692

Zolpidem Tartrate (Possible additive effects of CNS depressants). Products include:
- Ambien Tablets ... 2559

Food Interactions

Alcohol (Possible additive effects of CNS depressants; avoid alcoholic beverages).

PONSTEL
(Mefenamic Acid) ... 1982
May interact with oral anticoagulants. Compounds in this category include:

Dicumarol (Prolonged prothrombin time).
- No products indexed under this heading.

Warfarin Sodium (Prolonged prothrombin time). Products include:
- Coumadin ... 941

PONTOCAINE HYDROCHLORIDE FOR SPINAL ANESTHESIA
(Tetracaine Hydrochloride) ... 2460
May interact with sulfonamides. Compounds in this category include:

Sulfamethizole (Inhibited sulfonamide action). Products include:
- Urobiotic-250 Capsules ... 2038

Sulfamethoxazole (Inhibited sulfonamide action). Products include:
- Bactrim DS Tablets ... 2257
- Bactrim I.V. Infusion ... 2255
- Bactrim ... 2257
- Gantanol Tablets ... 2285
- Septra ... 1146
- Septra I.V. Infusion ... 1142
- Septra I.V. Infusion ADD-Vantage Vials ... 1144
- Septra ... 1146

Sulfasalazine (Inhibited sulfonamide action). Products include:
- Azulfidine ... 2059

Sulfinpyrazone (Inhibited sulfonamide action). Products include:
- Anturane ... 823

Sulfisoxazole (Inhibited sulfonamide action). Products include:
- Gantrisin Tablets ... 2286

Sulfisoxazole Diolamine (Inhibited sulfonamide action).
- No products indexed under this heading.

POTABA CAPSULES, ENVULES, POWDER, AND TABLETS
(Aminobenzoate Potassium) ... 1234
May interact with sulfonamides. Compounds in this category include:

Bendroflumethiazide (Concurrent administration contraindicated).
- No products indexed under this heading.

Chlorothiazide (Concurrent administration contraindicated). Products include:
- Aldoclor Tablets ... 1638
- Diupres Tablets ... 1691
- Diuril Oral ... 1694

Chlorothiazide Sodium (Concurrent administration contraindicated). Products include:
- Diuril Sodium Intravenous ... 1693

Chlorpropamide (Concurrent administration contraindicated). Products include:
- Diabinese Tablets ... 2002

Glipizide (Concurrent administration contraindicated). Products include:
- Glucotrol Tablets ... 2011
- Glucotrol XL Extended Release Tablets ... 2012

Glyburide (Concurrent administration contraindicated). Products include:
- DiaBeta Tablets ... 1265
- Glynase PresTab Tablets ... 2091
- Micronase Tablets ... 2099

Hydrochlorothiazide (Concurrent administration contraindicated). Products include:
- Aldactazide Tablets ... 2556
- Aldoril Tablets ... 1644
- Apresazide Capsules ... 824
- Capozide Tablets ... 744
- Dyazide Capsules ... 2653
- Esidrix Tablets ... 839
- Esimil Tablets ... 840
- HydroDIURIL Tablets ... 1716
- Hydropres Tablets ... 1718
- Hyzaar Tablets ... 1720
- Inderide Tablets ... 2838
- Inderide LA Long Acting Capsules ... 2840
- Lopressor HCT Tablets ... 850
- Lotensin HCT Tablets ... 855
- Moduretic Tablets ... 1748
- Oretic Tablets ... 450
- Prinzide Tablets ... 1780
- Ser-Ap-Es Tablets ... 867
- Timolide Tablets ... 1791
- Vaseretic Tablets ... 1810
- Zestoretic Tablets ... 2968
- Ziac ... 1459

Hydroflumethiazide (Concurrent administration contraindicated). Products include:
- Diucardin Tablets ... 2824

Methyclothiazide (Concurrent administration contraindicated). Products include:
- Enduron Tablets ... 424

Polythiazide (Concurrent administration contraindicated). Products include:
- Minizide Capsules ... 2016

Sulfamethizole (Concurrent administration contraindicated). Products include:
- Urobiotic-250 Capsules ... 2038

Sulfamethoxazole (Concurrent administration contraindicated). Products include:
- Bactrim DS Tablets ... 2257
- Bactrim I.V. Infusion ... 2255
- Bactrim ... 2257
- Gantanol Tablets ... 2285
- Septra ... 1146
- Septra I.V. Infusion ... 1142
- Septra I.V. Infusion ADD-Vantage Vials ... 1144
- Septra ... 1146

Sulfasalazine (Concurrent administration contraindicated). Products include:
- Azulfidine ... 2059

Sulfinpyrazone (Concurrent administration contraindicated). Products include:
- Anturane ... 823

Sulfisoxazole (Concurrent administration contraindicated). Products include:
- Gantrisin Tablets ... 2286

Sulfisoxazole Diolamine (Concurrent administration contraindicated).
- No products indexed under this heading.

Tolazamide (Concurrent administration contraindicated).
- No products indexed under this heading.

Tolbutamide (Concurrent administration contraindicated).
- No products indexed under this heading.

PPD TINE TEST
(Tuberculin, Purified Protein Derivative, Multiple Puncture Device) ... 2993
May interact with corticosteroids and

IMPORTANT NOTE: Always consult each drug listing in the patient's regimen for possible interactions.

immunosuppressive agents. Compounds in these categories include:

Azathioprine (Reactivity to the test may be suppressed). Products include:
- Azathioprine Tablets ... 2349
- Imuran ... 1103

Betamethasone Acetate (Reactivity to the test may be suppressed). Products include:
- Celestone Soluspan Suspension ... 2484

Betamethasone Sodium Phosphate (Reactivity to the test may be suppressed). Products include:
- Celestone Soluspan Suspension ... 2484

Cortisone Acetate (Reactivity to the test may be suppressed). Products include:
- Cortone Acetate Sterile Suspension ... 1663
- Cortone Acetate Tablets ... 1664

Cyclosporine (Reactivity to the test may be suppressed). Products include:
- Neoral ... 2405
- Sandimmune ... 2416

Desoximetasone (Reactivity to the test may be suppressed). Products include:
- Topicort Emollient Cream 0.25% .. 1289
- Topicort Gel 0.05% ... 1290
- Topicort LP Emollient Cream 0.05% ... 1289
- Topicort Ointment 0.25% ... 1291

Dexamethasone Acetate (Reactivity to the test may be suppressed). Products include:
- Dalalone D.P. Injectable ... 1009
- Decadron-LA Sterile Suspension ... 1687

Dexamethasone Sodium Phosphate (Reactivity to the test may be suppressed). Products include:
- Decadron Phosphate Injection ... 1680
- Decadron Phosphate Sterile Ophthalmic Ointment ... 1684
- Decadron Phosphate Sterile Ophthalmic Solution ... 1685
- Decadron Phosphate Topical Cream ... 1686
- Decadron Phosphate with Xylocaine Injection, Sterile ... 1683
- Dexacort Phosphate in Respihaler .. 1606
- Dexacort Phosphate in Turbinaire .. 1607
- NeoDecadron Sterile Ophthalmic Ointment ... 1755
- NeoDecadron Sterile Ophthalmic Solution ... 1756
- NeoDecadron Topical Cream ... 1757

Fludrocortisone Acetate (Reactivity to the test may be suppressed). Products include:
- Florinef Acetate Tablets ... 506

Hydrocortisone (Reactivity to the test may be suppressed). Products include:
- Anusol-HC Cream 2.5% ... 1953
- Aquanil HC Lotion ... 1989
- Maximum Strength Cortaid Spray ▣ 800
- CORTENEMA ... 2713
- Cortisporin Ointment ... 1074
- Cortisporin Ophthalmic Ointment Sterile ... 1074
- Cortisporin Ophthalmic Suspension Sterile ... 1075
- Cortisporin Otic Solution Sterile ... 1076
- Cortisporin Otic Suspension Sterile 1077
- Cortizone-5 ... ▣ 795
- Cortizone-10 ... ▣ 795
- Hydrocortone Tablets ... 1715
- Hytone ... 922
- Hytone Ointment 2 ½% ... 923
- Massengill Medicated Soft Cloth Towelettes ... 2628
- Pediotic Suspension Sterile ... 1140
- Preparation H Hydrocortisone 1% Cream ... ▣ 843
- ProctoCream-HC 2.5% ... 2552
- VōSoL HC Otic Solution ... 2786

Hydrocortisone Acetate (Reactivity to the test may be suppressed). Products include:
- Analpram-HC Rectal Cream 1% and 2.5% ... 993
- Anusol HC-1 Hydrocortisone Anti-Itch Ointment ... ▣ 810
- Anusol-HC Suppositories ... 1954
- Caldecort Anti-Itch Hydrocortisone Cream ... ▣ 651
- Coly-Mycin S Otic w/Neomycin & Hydrocortisone ... 1965
- Cortaid ... ▣ 800
- Cortifoam ... 2540
- Cortisporin Cream ... 1073
- Epifoam ... 2543
- Hydrocortone Acetate Sterile Suspension ... 1712
- Mantadil Cream ... 1124
- Nupercainal Hydrocortisone 1% Cream ... ▣ 661
- Pramosone Cream, Lotion & Ointment ... 995
- ProctoFoam-HC ... 2552
- Terra-Cortril Ophthalmic Suspension ... 2033

Hydrocortisone Sodium Phosphate (Reactivity to the test may be suppressed). Products include:
- Hydrocortone Phosphate Injection, Sterile ... 1713

Hydrocortisone Sodium Succinate (Reactivity to the test may be suppressed).
- No products indexed under this heading.

Immune Globulin (Human) (Reactivity to the test may be suppressed).
- No products indexed under this heading.

Immune Globulin Intravenous (Human) (Reactivity to the test may be suppressed).

Methylprednisolone Acetate (Reactivity to the test may be suppressed).
- No products indexed under this heading.

Methylprednisolone Sodium Succinate (Reactivity to the test may be suppressed).
- No products indexed under this heading.

Muromonab-CD3 (Reactivity to the test may be suppressed). Products include:
- Orthoclone OKT3 Sterile Solution .. 1892

Mycophenolate Mofetil (Reactivity to the test may be suppressed). Products include:
- CellCept Capsules ... 2265

Prednisolone Acetate (Reactivity to the test may be suppressed). Products include:
- AK-CIDE ... ⊙ 203
- AK-CIDE Ointment ... ⊙ 203
- Blephamide Liquifilm Sterile Ophthalmic Suspension ... 472
- Blephamide Ointment ... ⊙ 234
- Econopred & Econopred Plus Ophthalmic Suspensions ... ⊙ 216
- Poly-Pred Liquifilm ... ⊙ 246
- Pred Forte ... ⊙ 247
- Pred Mild ... ⊙ 250
- Pred-G Liquifilm Sterile Ophthalmic Suspension ... ⊙ 248
- Pred-G S.O.P. Sterile Ophthalmic Ointment ... ⊙ 249

Prednisolone Sodium Phosphate (Reactivity to the test may be suppressed). Products include:
- AK-PRED ... ⊙ 204
- Hydeltrasol Injection, Sterile ... 1708
- Pediapred Oral Solution ... 1618

Prednisolone Tebutate (Reactivity to the test may be suppressed). Products include:
- Hydeltra-T.B.A. Sterile Suspension 1710

Prednisone (Reactivity to the test may be suppressed).
- No products indexed under this heading.

Tacrolimus (Reactivity to the test may be suppressed). Products include:
- Prograf ... 1028

Triamcinolone (Reactivity to the test may be suppressed).
- No products indexed under this heading.

Triamcinolone Acetonide (Reactivity to the test may be suppressed). Products include:
- Azmacort Oral Inhaler ... 2175
- Nasacort AQ Nasal Spray ... 2191
- Nasacort Nasal Inhaler ... 2189

Triamcinolone Diacetate (Reactivity to the test may be suppressed).
- No products indexed under this heading.

Triamcinolone Hexacetonide (Reactivity to the test may be suppressed).
- No products indexed under this heading.

PRAMEGEL
(Pramoxine Hydrochloride) ... 1042
None cited in PDR database.

PRAMOSONE CREAM, LOTION & OINTMENT
(Hydrocortisone Acetate, Pramoxine Hydrochloride) ... 995
None cited in PDR database.

PRAVACHOL TABLETS
(Pravastatin Sodium) ... 770
May interact with fibrates, erythromycin, and certain other agents. Compounds in these categories include:

Cholestyramine (Co-administration has resulted in an approximately 40% to 50% decrease in the mean AUC of pravastatin; Pravachol should be given either 1 hour or more before or at least 4 hours following the resin). Products include:
- Questran ... 774

Clofibrate (The risk of myopathy during treatment with another HMG-CoA reductase inhibitor has increased with concurrent therapy; combined therapy should be avoided). Products include:
- Atromid-S Capsules ... 2808

Colestipol Hydrochloride (Co-administration has resulted in an approximately 40% to 50% decrease in the mean AUC of pravastatin; Pravachol should be given either 1 hour or more before or at least 4 hours following the resin). Products include:
- Colestid ... 2073

Cyclosporine (The risk of myopathy during treatment with another HMG-CoA reductase inhibitor has increased with concurrent therapy; in one single-dose study, pravastatin levels were found to be increased with concurrent therapy in cardiac transplant patients). Products include:
- Neoral ... 2405
- Sandimmune ... 2416

Digoxin (Co-administration indicates that the bioavailability parameters of digoxin are not affected, however, the AUC of pravastatin tends to increase, but the overall bioavailability of pravastatin plus its metabolites are not affected). Products include:
- Lanoxicaps ... 1110
- Lanoxin Elixir Pediatric ... 1113
- Lanoxin Injection ... 1116
- Lanoxin Injection Pediatric ... 1119
- Lanoxin Tablets ... 1121

Erythromycin (The risk of myopathy during treatment with another HMG-CoA reductase inhibitor has increased with concurrent therapy). Products include:
- A/T/S 2% Acne Topical Gel ... 1244
- A/T/S 2% Acne Topical Solution ... 1244
- Benzamycin Topical Gel ... 919
- E-Mycin Tablets ... 1388
- Emgel 2% Topical Gel ... 1081
- ERYC ... 1972
- Erycette (erythromycin 2%) Topical Solution ... 1943
- Ery-Tab Tablets ... 426
- Erythromycin Base Filmtab ... 430
- Erythromycin Delayed-Release Capsules, USP ... 431
- Ilotycin Ophthalmic Ointment ... 928
- PCE Dispertab Tablets ... 453
- T-Stat 2.0% Topical Solution and Pads ... 2797
- THERAMYCIN Z 2% Solution ... 1629

Erythromycin Estolate (The risk of myopathy during treatment with another HMG-CoA reductase inhibitor has increased with concurrent therapy). Products include:
- Ilosone ... 927

Erythromycin Ethylsuccinate (The risk of myopathy during treatment with another HMG-CoA reductase inhibitor has increased with concurrent therapy). Products include:
- E.E.S. ... 427
- EryPed ... 425
- Pediazole Suspension ... 2340

Erythromycin Gluceptate (The risk of myopathy during treatment with another HMG-CoA reductase inhibitor has increased with concurrent therapy). Products include:
- Ilotycin Gluceptate, IV, Vials ... 929

Erythromycin Stearate (The risk of myopathy during treatment with another HMG-CoA reductase inhibitor has increased with concurrent therapy). Products include:
- Erythrocin Stearate Filmtab ... 429

Gemfibrozil (Co-administration has resulted in a significant decrease in urinary excretion and protein binding; significant increase in AUC, C_{max}, and T_{max} for pravastatin metabolite; combined therapy is generally not recommended due to potential for increased risk of myopathy). Products include:
- Lopid Tablets ... 1974

Niacin (The risk of myopathy during treatment with another HMG-CoA reductase inhibitor has increased with concurrent therapy). Products include:
- Kyo-Chrome ... ▣ 680
- Nicotinex Elixir ... ▣ 671
- Slo-Niacin Tablets ... 2767

Warfarin Sodium (The risk of bleeding and extreme prolongation of prothrombin time has been reported with another HMG-CoA reductase inhibitor; monitor prothrombin times closely if used concurrently). Products include:
- Coumadin ... 941

PRECOSE
(Acarbose) ... 604
May interact with thiazides, corticosteroids, phenothiazines, thyroid preparations, oral contraceptives, estrogens, sympathomimetics, calcium channel blockers, and certain

(▣ Described in PDR For Nonprescription Drugs) (⊙ Described in PDR For Ophthalmology)

Interactions Index

other agents. Compounds in these categories include:

Albuterol (Sympathomimetics tend to produce hyperglycemia leading to loss of control; patients on concurrent therapy should be closely observed for loss of control). Products include:

Proventil Inhalation Aerosol	2524
Ventolin Inhalation Aerosol and Refill	1170

Albuterol Sulfate (Sympathomimetics tend to produce hyperglycemia leading to loss of control; patients on concurrent therapy should be closely observed for loss of control). Products include:

Airet Albuterol Sulfate Inhalation Solution	1602
Albuterol Sulfate, USP Solution for Inhalation, Arm-a-Med	522
Proventil Inhalation Solution 0.083%	2527
Proventil Repetabs Tablets	2529
Proventil Solution for Inhalation 0.5%	2525
Proventil Syrup	2528
Proventil Tablets	2529
Ventolin Inhalation Solution	1171
Ventolin Nebules Inhalation Solution	1172
Ventolin Rotacaps for Inhalation	1173
Ventolin Syrup	1175
Ventolin Tablets	1176
Volmax Extended-Release Tablets	1835

Amlodipine Besylate (Calcium channel blockers tend to produce hyperglycemia leading to loss of control; patients on concurrent therapy should be closely observed for loss of control). Products include:

Lotrel Capsules	858
Norvasc Tablets	2020

Amylase (Amylase, a carbohydrate splitting enzyme, may reduce the effect of acarbose and should not be taken concurrently). Products include:

Arco-Lase Plus Tablets	513
Arco-Lase Tablets	513
Cotazym Capsules	1866
Donnazyme Tablets	2235
Kutrase Capsules	2546
Ku-Zyme Capsules	2546
Ku-Zyme HP Capsules	2547

Bendroflumethiazide (Thiazide diuretics tend to produce hyperglycemia leading to loss of control; patients on concurrent therapy should be closely observed for loss of control).
No products indexed under this heading.

Bepridil Hydrochloride (Calcium channel blockers tend to produce hyperglycemia leading to loss of control; patients on concurrent therapy should be closely observed for loss of control). Products include:

Vascor Tablets (200 and 300 mg)	1597

Betamethasone Acetate (Corticosteroids tend to produce hyperglycemia leading to loss of control; patients on concurrent therapy should be closely observed for loss of control). Products include:

Celestone Soluspan Suspension	2484

Betamethasone Sodium Phosphate (Corticosteroids tend to produce hyperglycemia leading to loss of control; patients on concurrent therapy should be closely observed for loss of control). Products include:

Celestone Soluspan Suspension	2484

Charcoal, Activated (Charcoal, an intestinal adsorbent, may reduce the effect of acarbose and should not be taken concurrently). Products include:

CharcoAid 2000	740

CharcoCaps	740

Chlorothiazide (Thiazide diuretics tend to produce hyperglycemia leading to loss of control; patients on concurrent therapy should be closely observed for loss of control). Products include:

Aldoclor Tablets	1638
Diupres Tablets	1691
Diuril Oral	1694

Chlorothiazide Sodium (Thiazide diuretics tend to produce hyperglycemia leading to loss of control; patients on concurrent therapy should be closely observed for loss of control). Products include:

Diuril Sodium Intravenous	1693

Chlorotrianisene (Estrogens tend to produce hyperglycemia leading to loss of control; patients on concurrent therapy should be closely observed for loss of control).
No products indexed under this heading.

Chlorpromazine (Phenothiazines tend to produce hyperglycemia leading to loss of control; patients on concurrent therapy should be closely observed for loss of control). Products include:

Thorazine Suppositories	2701

Chlorpromazine Hydrochloride (Phenothiazines tend to produce hyperglycemia leading to loss of control; patients on concurrent therapy should be closely observed for loss of control). Products include:

Thorazine	2701

Cortisone Acetate (Corticosteroids tend to produce hyperglycemia leading to loss of control; patients on concurrent therapy should be closely observed for loss of control). Products include:

Cortone Acetate Sterile Suspension	1663
Cortone Acetate Tablets	1664

Desogestrel (Oral contraceptives tend to produce hyperglycemia leading to loss of control; patients on concurrent therapy should be closely observed for loss of control). Products include:

Desogen Tablets	1867
Ortho-Cept	1907

Dexamethasone (Corticosteroids tend to produce hyperglycemia leading to loss of control; patients on concurrent therapy should be closely observed for loss of control). Products include:

AK-Trol Ointment & Suspension	205
Decadron Elixir	1676
Decadron Tablets	1678
Decaspray Topical Aerosol	1689
Maxitrol Ophthalmic Ointment and Suspension	222
TobraDex Ophthalmic Suspension and Ointment	469

Dexamethasone Acetate (Corticosteroids tend to produce hyperglycemia leading to loss of control; patients on concurrent therapy should be closely observed for loss of control). Products include:

Dalalone D.P. Injectable	1009
Decadron-LA Sterile Suspension	1687

Dexamethasone Sodium Phosphate (Corticosteroids tend to produce hyperglycemia leading to loss of control; patients on concurrent therapy should be closely observed for loss of control). Products include:

Decadron Phosphate Injection	1680
Decadron Phosphate Sterile Ophthalmic Ointment	1684
Decadron Phosphate Sterile Ophthalmic Solution	1685
Decadron Phosphate Topical Cream	1686
Decadron Phosphate with Xylocaine Injection, Sterile	1683
Dexacort Phosphate in Respihaler	1606
Dexacort Phosphate in Turbinaire	1607
NeoDecadron Sterile Ophthalmic Ointment	1755
NeoDecadron Sterile Ophthalmic Solution	1756
NeoDecadron Topical Cream	1757

Dienestrol (Estrogens tend to produce hyperglycemia leading to loss of control; patients on concurrent therapy should be closely observed for loss of control). Products include:

Ortho Dienestrol Cream	1922

Diethylstilbestrol (Estrogens tend to produce hyperglycemia leading to loss of control; patients on concurrent therapy should be closely observed for loss of control). Products include:

Diethylstilbestrol Tablets	1477

Diltiazem Hydrochloride (Calcium channel blockers tend to produce hyperglycemia leading to loss of control; patients on concurrent therapy should be closely observed for loss of control). Products include:

Cardizem CD Capsules	1251
Cardizem SR Capsules	1255
Cardizem Injectable	1253
Cardizem Tablets	1257
Dilacor XR Extended-release Capsules	2183
Tiazac Capsules	1019

Dobutamine Hydrochloride (Sympathomimetics tend to produce hyperglycemia leading to loss of control; patients on concurrent therapy should be closely observed for loss of control). Products include:

Dobutrex Solution Vials	1480

Dopamine Hydrochloride (Sympathomimetics tend to produce hyperglycemia leading to loss of control; patients on concurrent therapy should be closely observed for loss of control).
No products indexed under this heading.

Ephedrine Hydrochloride (Sympathomimetics tend to produce hyperglycemia leading to loss of control; patients on concurrent therapy should be closely observed for loss of control). Products include:

Primatene Tablets	844
Quadrinal Tablets	1398

Ephedrine Sulfate (Sympathomimetics tend to produce hyperglycemia leading to loss of control; patients on concurrent therapy should be closely observed for loss of control). Products include:

Marax Tablets & DF Syrup	2015

Ephedrine Tannate (Sympathomimetics tend to produce hyperglycemia leading to loss of control; patients on concurrent therapy should be closely observed for loss of control). Products include:

Rynatuss	2782

Epinephrine (Sympathomimetics tend to produce hyperglycemia leading to loss of control; patients on concurrent therapy should be closely observed for loss of control). Products include:

EPIFRIN	237
EpiPen	808
Marcaine with Epinephrine	2446
Primatene Mist	843
Sensorcaine with Epinephrine Injection	554
Sus-Phrine Injection	1017
Xylocaine with Epinephrine Injections	562

Epinephrine Bitartrate (Sympathomimetics tend to produce hyperglycemia leading to loss of control; patients on concurrent therapy should be closely observed for loss of control). Products include:

Sensorcaine-MPF with Epinephrine Injection	554

Epinephrine Hydrochloride (Sympathomimetics tend to produce hyperglycemia leading to loss of control; patients on concurrent therapy should be closely observed for loss of control). Products include:

Ana-Kit Anaphylaxis Emergency Treatment Kit	611

Estradiol (Estrogens tend to produce hyperglycemia leading to loss of control; patients on concurrent therapy should be closely observed for loss of control). Products include:

Climara Transdermal System	640
Estrace Cream and Tablets	751
Estraderm Transdermal System	842
Estring Vaginal Ring	2086
Vivelle Transdermal System	880

Estrogens, Conjugated (Estrogens tend to produce hyperglycemia leading to loss of control; patients on concurrent therapy should be closely observed for loss of control). Products include:

PMB 200 and PMB 400	2890
Premarin Intravenous	2893
Premarin Tablets	2896
Premarin Vaginal Cream	2898
Premphase	2900
Prempro	2905

Estrogens, Esterified (Estrogens tend to produce hyperglycemia leading to loss of control; patients on concurrent therapy should be closely observed for loss of control). Products include:

ESTRATAB Tablets (0.3, 0.625, 1.25, 2.5 mg)	2715
Estratest	2718
Menest Tablets	2671

Estropipate (Estrogens tend to produce hyperglycemia leading to loss of control; patients on concurrent therapy should be closely observed for loss of control). Products include:

Ogen Tablets	2103
Ogen Vaginal Cream	2106
Ortho-Est	1925

Ethinyl Estradiol (Estrogens tend to produce hyperglycemia leading to loss of control; patients on concurrent therapy should be closely observed for loss of control). Products include:

Brevicon	2563
Demulen	2580
Desogen Tablets	1867
Levlen/Tri-Levlen	646
Lo/Ovral Tablets	2852
Lo/Ovral-28 Tablets	2857
Modicon	1928
Nordette-21 Tablets	2863
Nordette-28 Tablets	2866
Norinyl	2563
Ortho-Cept	1907
Ortho-Cyclen/Ortho-Tri-Cyclen	1914
Ortho-Novum	1928
Ortho-Cyclen/Ortho Tri-Cyclen	1914
Ovcon	765
Ovral Tablets	2877
Ovral-28 Tablets	2878
Levlen/Tri-Levlen	646
Tri-Norinyl	2607
Triphasil-21 Tablets	2919
Triphasil-28 Tablets	2924

Ethynodiol Diacetate (Oral contraceptives tend to produce hyperglycemia leading to loss of control; patients on concurrent therapy should be closely observed for loss of control). Products include:

Demulen	2580

IMPORTANT NOTE: Always consult each drug listing in the patient's regimen for possible interactions.

Felodipine (Calcium channel blockers tend to produce hyperglycemia leading to loss of control; patients on concurrent therapy should be closely observed for loss of control). Products include:

Plendil Extended-Release Tablets 514

Fludrocortisone Acetate (Corticosteroids tend to produce hyperglycemia leading to loss of control; patients on concurrent therapy should be closely observed for loss of control). Products include:

Florinef Acetate Tablets 506

Fluphenazine Decanoate (Phenothiazines tend to produce hyperglycemia leading to loss of control; patients on concurrent therapy should be closely observed for loss of control). Products include:

Prolixin Decanoate 510

Fluphenazine Enanthate (Phenothiazines tend to produce hyperglycemia leading to loss of control; patients on concurrent therapy should be closely observed for loss of control). Products include:

Prolixin Enanthate 510

Fluphenazine Hydrochloride (Phenothiazines tend to produce hyperglycemia leading to loss of control; patients on concurrent therapy should be closely observed for loss of control). Products include:

Prolixin 510

Hydrochlorothiazide (Thiazide diuretics tend to produce hyperglycemia leading to loss of control; patients on concurrent therapy should be closely observed for loss of control). Products include:

Aldactazide Tablets 2556
Aldoril Tablets 1644
Apresazide Capsules 824
Capozide Tablets 744
Dyazide Capsules 2653
Esidrix Tablets 839
Esimil Tablets 840
HydroDIURIL Tablets 1716
Hydropres Tablets 1718
Hyzaar Tablets 1720
Inderide Tablets 2838
Inderide LA Long Acting Capsules .. 2840
Lopressor HCT Tablets 850
Lotensin HCT Tablets 855
Moduretic Tablets 1748
Oretic Tablets 450
Prinzide Tablets 1780
Ser-Ap-Es Tablets 867
Timolide Tablets 1791
Vaseretic Tablets 1810
Zestoretic Tablets 2968
Ziac 1459

Hydrocortisone (Corticosteroids tend to produce hyperglycemia leading to loss of control; patients on concurrent therapy should be closely observed for loss of control). Products include:

Anusol-HC Cream 2.5% 1953
Aquanil HC Lotion 1989
Maximum Strength Cortaid Spray ▣ 800
CORTENEMA 2713
Cortisporin Ointment 1074
Cortisporin Ophthalmic Ointment Sterile 1074
Cortisporin Ophthalmic Suspension Sterile 1075
Cortisporin Otic Solution Sterile 1076
Cortisporin Otic Suspension Sterile 1077
Cortizone-5 .... ▣ 795
Cortizone-10 .... ▣ 795
Hydrocortone Tablets 1715
Hytone 922
Hytone Ointment 2 ½% 923
Massengill Medicated Soft Cloth Towelettes 2628
Pediotic Suspension Sterile 1140
Preparation H Hydrocortisone 1% Cream .... ▣ 843
ProctoCream-HC 2.5% 2552
VōSoL HC Otic Solution 2786

Hydrocortisone Acetate (Corticosteroids tend to produce hyperglycemia leading to loss of control; patients on concurrent therapy should be closely observed for loss of control). Products include:

Analpram-HC Rectal Cream 1% and 2.5% 993
Anusol HC-1 Hydrocortisone Anti-Itch Ointment .... ▣ 810
Anusol-HC Suppositories 1954
Caldecort Anti-Itch Hydrocortisone Cream .... ▣ 651
Coly-Mycin S Otic w/Neomycin & Hydrocortisone 1965
Cortaid .... ▣ 800
Cortifoam 2540
Cortisporin Cream 1073
Epifoam 2543
Hydrocortone Acetate Sterile Suspension 1712
Mantadil Cream 1124
Nupercainal Hydrocortisone 1% Cream .... ▣ 661
Pramosone Cream, Lotion & Ointment 995
ProctoFoam-HC 2552
Terra-Cortril Ophthalmic Suspension 2033

Hydrocortisone Sodium Phosphate (Corticosteroids tend to produce hyperglycemia leading to loss of control; patients on concurrent therapy should be closely observed for loss of control). Products include:

Hydrocortone Phosphate Injection, Sterile 1713

Hydrocortisone Sodium Succinate (Corticosteroids tend to produce hyperglycemia leading to loss of control; patients on concurrent therapy should be closely observed for loss of control).

No products indexed under this heading.

Hydroflumethiazide (Thiazide diuretics tend to produce hyperglycemia leading to loss of control; patients on concurrent therapy should be closely observed for loss of control). Products include:

Diucardin Tablets 2824

Isoniazid (Isoniazid tends to produce hyperglycemia leading to loss of control; patients on concurrent therapy should be closely observed for loss of control). Products include:

Nydrazid Injection 509
Rifamate Capsules 1278
Rifater 1280

Isoproterenol Hydrochloride (Sympathomimetics tend to produce hyperglycemia leading to loss of control; patients on concurrent therapy should be closely observed for loss of control). Products include:

Isuprel Hydrochloride Solution 2443
Isuprel Injection 2441
Isuprel Mistometer 2442

Isoproterenol Sulfate (Sympathomimetics tend to produce hyperglycemia leading to loss of control; patients on concurrent therapy should be closely observed for loss of control). Products include:

Norisodrine with Calcium Iodide Syrup 446

Isradipine (Calcium channel blockers tend to produce hyperglycemia leading to loss of control; patients on concurrent therapy should be closely observed for loss of control). Products include:

DynaCirc Capsules 2381
DynaCirc CR Tablets 2383

Levonorgestrel (Oral contraceptives tend to produce hyperglycemia leading to loss of control; patients on concurrent therapy should be closely observed for loss of control). Products include:

Levlen/Tri-Levlen 646
Nordette-21 Tablets 2863
Nordette-28 Tablets 2866
Norplant System 2868
Levlen/Tri-Levlen 646
Triphasil-21 Tablets 2919
Triphasil-28 Tablets 2924

Levothyroxine Sodium (Thyroid products tend to produce hyperglycemia leading to loss of control; patients on concurrent therapy should be closely observed for loss of control). Products include:

Eltroxin Tablets 2214
Levothroid Tablets 1015
Levothyroxine Sodium, USP for Injection 546
Levoxyl Tablets 918
Synthroid 1410

Liothyronine Sodium (Thyroid products tend to produce hyperglycemia leading to loss of control; patients on concurrent therapy should be closely observed for loss of control). Products include:

Cytomel Tablets 2647
Triostat Injection 2708

Liotrix (Thyroid products tend to produce hyperglycemia leading to loss of control; patients on concurrent therapy should be closely observed for loss of control).

No products indexed under this heading.

Mesoridazine Besylate (Phenothiazines tend to produce hyperglycemia leading to loss of control; patients on concurrent therapy should be closely observed for loss of control). Products include:

Serentil 689

Mestranol (Oral contraceptives tend to produce hyperglycemia leading to loss of control; patients on concurrent therapy should be closely observed for loss of control). Products include:

Norinyl 2563
Ortho-Novum 1928

Metaproterenol Sulfate (Sympathomimetics tend to produce hyperglycemia leading to loss of control; patients on concurrent therapy should be closely observed for loss of control). Products include:

Alupent 672
Metaproterenol Sulfate Inhalation Solution, USP, Arm-a-Med 547

Metaraminol Bitartrate (Sympathomimetics tend to produce hyperglycemia leading to loss of control; patients on concurrent therapy should be closely observed for loss of control). Products include:

Aramine Injection 1649

Methotrimeprazine (Phenothiazines tend to produce hyperglycemia leading to loss of control; patients on concurrent therapy should be closely observed for loss of control). Products include:

Levoprome 1321

Methoxamine Hydrochloride (Sympathomimetics tend to produce hyperglycemia leading to loss of control; patients on concurrent therapy should be closely observed for loss of control). Products include:

Vasoxyl Injection 1169

Methyclothiazide (Thiazide diuretics tend to produce hyperglycemia leading to loss of control; patients on concurrent therapy should be closely observed for loss of control). Products include:

Enduron Tablets 424

Methylprednisolone Acetate (Corticosteroids tend to produce hyperglycemia leading to loss of control; patients on concurrent therapy should be closely observed for loss of control).

No products indexed under this heading.

Methylprednisolone Sodium Succinate (Corticosteroids tend to produce hyperglycemia leading to loss of control; patients on concurrent therapy should be closely observed for loss of control).

No products indexed under this heading.

Nicardipine Hydrochloride (Calcium channel blockers tend to produce hyperglycemia leading to loss of control; patients on concurrent therapy should be closely observed for loss of control). Products include:

Cardene Capsules 2261
Cardene I.V. 2815
Cardene SR Capsules 2264

Nicotinic Acid (Nicotinic acid tends to produce hyperglycemia leading to loss of control; patients on concurrent therapy should be closely observed for loss of control).

No products indexed under this heading.

Nifedipine (Calcium channel blockers tend to produce hyperglycemia leading to loss of control; patients on concurrent therapy should be closely observed for loss of control). Products include:

Adalat Capsules (10 mg and 20 mg) 580
Adalat CC 582
Procardia Capsules 2024
Procardia XL Extended Release Tablets 2026

Nimodipine (Calcium channel blockers tend to produce hyperglycemia leading to loss of control; patients on concurrent therapy should be closely observed for loss of control). Products include:

Nimotop Capsules 603

Nisoldipine (Calcium channel blockers tend to produce hyperglycemia leading to loss of control; patients on concurrent therapy should be closely observed for loss of control). Products include:

Sular Tablets 2961

Norepinephrine Bitartrate (Sympathomimetics tend to produce hyperglycemia leading to loss of control; patients on concurrent therapy should be closely observed for loss of control). Products include:

Levophed Bitartrate Injection 2445

Norethindrone (Oral contraceptives tend to produce hyperglycemia leading to loss of control; patients on concurrent therapy should be closely observed for loss of control). Products include:

Brevicon 2563
Micronor Tablets 1903
Modicon 1928
Norinyl 2563
Nor-Q D Tablets 2598
Ortho-Novum 1928
Ovcon 765
Tri-Norinyl 2607

(▣ Described in PDR For Nonprescription Drugs) (◉ Described in PDR For Ophthalmology)

859 Interactions Index Precose

Norethynodrel (Oral contraceptives tend to produce hyperglycemia leading to loss of control; patients on concurrent therapy should be closely observed for loss of control).
No products indexed under this heading.

Norgestimate (Oral contraceptives tend to produce hyperglycemia leading to loss of control; patients on concurrent therapy should be closely observed for loss of control). Products include:
Ortho-Cyclen/Ortho-Tri-Cyclen 1914
Ortho-Cyclen/Ortho Tri-Cyclen 1914

Norgestrel (Oral contraceptives tend to produce hyperglycemia leading to loss of control; patients on concurrent therapy should be closely observed for loss of control). Products include:
Lo/Ovral Tablets 2852
Lo/Ovral-28 Tablets 2857
Ovral Tablets 2877
Ovral-28 Tablets 2878
Ovrette Tablets 2878

Pancreatin (Pancreatin, a carbohydrate splitting enzyme, may reduce the effect of acarbose and should not be taken concurrently). Products include:
Donnazyme Tablets 2235

Perphenazine (Phenothiazines tend to produce hyperglycemia leading to loss of control; patients on concurrent therapy should be closely observed for loss of control). Products include:
Etrafon 2495
Triavil Tablets 1800
Trilafon 2532

Phenylephrine Bitartrate (Sympathomimetics tend to produce hyperglycemia leading to loss of control; patients on concurrent therapy should be closely observed for loss of control).
No products indexed under this heading.

Phenylephrine Hydrochloride (Sympathomimetics tend to produce hyperglycemia leading to loss of control; patients on concurrent therapy should be closely observed for loss of control). Products include:
Atrohist Plus Tablets 1605
Cerose DM 853
D.A. II Tablets 972
D.A. Chewable Tablets 970
Dura-Vent/DA Tablets 972
Extendryl 1003
4-Way Fast Acting Nasal Spray (regular & mentholated) 644
Hemorid 797
Hycomine Compound Tablets 948
Neo-Synephrine Hydrochloride 1% Carpuject 2455
Neo-Synephrine Hydrochloride 1% Injection 2455
Neo-Synephrine Hydrochloride (Ophthalmic) 2456
Neo-Synephrine 624
Novahistine Elixir 782
Phenergan VC 2886
Phenergan VC with Codeine 2888
Preparation H 842
Tympagesic Ear Drops 2476
Vicks Sinex Nasal Spray and Ultra Fine Mist 738

Phenylephrine Tannate (Sympathomimetics tend to produce hyperglycemia leading to loss of control; patients on concurrent therapy should be closely observed for loss of control). Products include:
Atrohist Pediatric Suspension 1604
Atrohist Pediatric Suspension Dye-Free 1604
Rynatan 2781
Rynatuss 2782

Phenylpropanolamine Hydrochloride (Sympathomimetics tend to produce hyperglycemia leading to loss of control; patients on concurrent therapy should be closely observed for loss of control). Products include:
Acutrim 648
Atrohist Plus Tablets 1605
BC Cold Powder Multi-Symptom Formula (Cold-Sinus-Allergy) 631
BC Cold Powder Non-Drowsy Formula (Cold-Sinus) 631
Cheracol Plus Head Cold/Cough Formula 741
Comtrex Multi-Symptom Cold Reliever Liqui-Gels 638
Comtrex Multi-Symptom Non-Drowsy Liqui-gels 640
Contac Continuous Action Nasal Decongestant/Antihistamine 12 Hour Capsules 773
Contac Maximum Strength Continuous Action Decongestant/Antihistamine 12 Hour Caplets 772
Contac Severe Cold and Flu Formula Caplets 773
Coricidin 'D' Decongestant Tablets 760
Dexatrim 795
Dexatrim Plus Vitamins Caplets 796
Dimetane-DC Cough Syrup 2232
Dimetapp Allergy Sinus Caplets 838
Dimetapp Cold & Allergy Chewable Tablets 838
Dimetapp Cold & Cough Liqui-Gels 839
Dimetapp DM Elixir 840
Dimetapp Elixir 840
Dimetapp Extentabs 841
Dimetapp Tablets/Liqui-Gels 841
Dura-Vent Tablets 971
Entex LA Tablets 972
Exgest LA Tablets 787
Hycomine 947
Nolamine Timed-Release Tablets 790
Ornade Spansule Capsules 2678
Propagest Tablets 791
Pyrroxate Caplets 742
Robitussin-CF 846
Sinulin Tablets 792
Tavist-D 12 Hour Relief Tablets 750
Teldrin 12 Hour Antihistamine/Nasal Decongestant Allergy Relief Capsules 786
Triaminic Expectorant 753
Triaminic Syrup 755
Triaminic Triaminicol Cold & Cough 756
Triaminic DM Syrup 756
Triaminicin Tablets 756
Vicks DayQuil Allergy Relief 12-Hour Extended Release Tablets 733
Vicks DayQuil Allergy Relief 4-Hour Tablets 733
Vicks DayQuil SINUS Pressure & CONGESTION Relief 734

Phenytoin (Phenytoin tends to produce hyperglycemia leading to loss of control; patients on concurrent therapy should be closely observed for loss of control). Products include:
Dilantin Infatabs 1967
Dilantin-125 Suspension 1969

Phenytoin Sodium (Phenytoin tends to produce hyperglycemia leading to loss of control; patients on concurrent therapy should be closely observed for loss of control). Products include:
Dilantin Kapseals 1965

Pirbuterol Acetate (Sympathomimetics tend to produce hyperglycemia leading to loss of control; patients on concurrent therapy should be closely observed for loss of control). Products include:
Maxair Autohaler 1550
Maxair Inhaler 1552

Polyestradiol Phosphate (Estrogens tend to produce hyperglycemia leading to loss of control; patients on concurrent therapy should be closely observed for loss of control).
No products indexed under this heading.

Polythiazide (Thiazide diuretics tend to produce hyperglycemia leading to loss of control; patients on concurrent therapy should be closely observed for loss of control). Products include:
Minizide Capsules 2016

Prednisolone Acetate (Corticosteroids tend to produce hyperglycemia leading to loss of control; patients on concurrent therapy should be closely observed for loss of control). Products include:
AK-CIDE .... ⊙ 203
AK-CIDE Ointment .... ⊙ 203
Blephamide Liquifilm Sterile Ophthalmic Suspension 472
Blephamide Ointment .... ⊙ 234
Econopred & Econopred Plus Ophthalmic Suspensions .... ⊙ 216
Poly-Pred Liquifilm .... ⊙ 246
Pred Forte .... ⊙ 247
Pred Mild .... ⊙ 250
Pred-G Liquifilm Sterile Ophthalmic Suspension .... ⊙ 248
Pred-G S.O.P. Sterile Ophthalmic Ointment .... ⊙ 249

Prednisolone Sodium Phosphate (Corticosteroids tend to produce hyperglycemia leading to loss of control; patients on concurrent therapy should be closely observed for loss of control). Products include:
AK-PRED .... ⊙ 204
Hydeltrasol Injection, Sterile 1708
Pediapred Oral Solution 1618

Prednisolone Tebutate (Corticosteroids tend to produce hyperglycemia leading to loss of control; patients on concurrent therapy should be closely observed for loss of control). Products include:
Hydeltra-T.B.A. Sterile Suspension 1710

Prednisone (Corticosteroids tend to produce hyperglycemia leading to loss of control; patients on concurrent therapy should be closely observed for loss of control).
No products indexed under this heading.

Prochlorperazine (Phenothiazines tend to produce hyperglycemia leading to loss of control; patients on concurrent therapy should be closely observed for loss of control). Products include:
Compazine 2644

Promethazine Hydrochloride (Phenothiazines tend to produce hyperglycemia leading to loss of control; patients on concurrent therapy should be closely observed for loss of control). Products include:
Mepergan Injection 2859
Phenergan with Codeine 2883
Phenergan with Dextromethorphan 2885
Phenergan Injection 2880
Phenergan Suppositories 2882
Phenergan Syrup 2881
Phenergan Tablets 2882
Phenergan VC 2886
Phenergan VC with Codeine 2888

Pseudoephedrine Hydrochloride (Sympathomimetics tend to produce hyperglycemia leading to loss of control; patients on concurrent therapy should be closely observed for loss of control). Products include:
Actifed Allergy Daytime/Nighttime Caplets 808
Actifed Cold & Allergy Tablets 807
Actifed Cold & Sinus Caplets and Tablets 808
Actifed Sinus Daytime/Nighttime Tablets and Caplets 809
Advil Cold and Sinus Caplets and Tablets 837
Alka-Seltzer Plus Liqui-Gels 612
Alka-Seltzer Plus Flu & Body Aches Liqui-Gels Non-Drowsy Formula 613
Alka-Seltzer Plus Night-Time Cold Medicine Liqui-Gels 612
Allerest Maximum Strength 649
Allerest No Drowsiness 649
Allerest Sinus Pain Formula 649
Atrohist Pediatric Capsules 1603
Benadryl Allergy/Cold Tablets 811
Benadryl Allergy Decongestant Liquid Medication 812
Benadryl Allergy Decongestant Tablets 812
Benadryl Allergy Sinus Headache Caplets 813
Benylin Multisymptom 816
Bromfed Capsules (Extended-Release) 1832
Bromfed Syrup 712
Bromfed Tablets 1832
Bromfed-DM Cough Syrup 1832
Bromfed-PD Capsules (Extended-Release) 1832
Children's TYLENOL Cold Multi-Symptom Chewable Tablets and Liquid 1559
Children's TYLENOL Cold Plus Cough Multi Symptom Chewable Tablets and Liquid 1560
Children's TYLENOL Flu Suspension Liquid 1560
Children's Vicks DayQuil Allergy Relief 730
Children's Vicks NyQuil Cold/Cough Relief 731
Allergy-Sinus Comtrex Multi-Symptom Allergy-Sinus Formula Tablets and Caplets 639
Comtrex Multi-Symptom 638
Comtrex Multi-Symptom Non-Drowsy Caplets 640
Congess 1003
Contac Day Allergy/Sinus Caplets 771
Contac Day & Night 772
Contac Night Allergy/Sinus Caplets 771
Contac Severe Cold & Flu Non-Drowsy 774
Deconsal II Tablets 1605
Dimetane-DX Cough Syrup 2233
Dimetapp Cold & Fever Suspension 839
Dimetapp Decongestant Pediatric Drops 840
Dorcol Children's Cough Syrup 748
Drixoral Cough + Congestion Liquid Caps 763
Dura-Tap/PD Capsules 970
Duratuss Tablets 2750
Duratuss HD Elixir 2750
Efidac/24 655
Entex PSE Tablets 973
Fedahist Gyrocaps 2545
Guaifed 1833
Guaifed Syrup 712
Guaimax-D Tablets 809
Histussin D Liquid 670
Infants' TYLENOL Cold Decongestant & Fever-Reducer Drops 1561
Kronofed-A 994
Novahistine DMX 782
Nucofed 2225
PediaCare Cough-Cold Chewable Tablets and Liquid 1569
PediaCare Infants' Decongestant Drops 1569
PediaCare Infants' Drops Decongestant Plus Cough 1569
PediaCare NightRest Cough-Cold Liquid 1569
Pediatric Vicks 44d Cough & Head Congestion Relief 736
Pediatric Vicks 44m Cough & Cold Relief 737
Robitussin Cold & Cough Liqui-Gels 844
Robitussin Cold, Cough & Flu Liqui-Gels 844
Robitussin Maximum Strength Cough & Cold 847
Robitussin Night-Time Cold Formula 847
Robitussin Pediatric Cough & Cold Formula 848
Robitussin Pediatric Drops 849

IMPORTANT NOTE: Always consult each drug listing in the patient's regimen for possible interactions.

Precose | Interactions Index | 860

Robitussin Severe Congestion Liqui-Gels ▣ 845
Robitussin-DAC Syrup 2249
Robitussin-PE ▣ 846
Rondec Oral Drops 974
Rondec Syrup 974
Rondec Tablet 974
Rondec Chewable Tablets 974
Rondec-TR Tablet 974
Ryna ▣ 804
Seldane-D Extended-Release Tablets 1286
Semprex-D Capsules 1620
Sinarest ▣ 663
Sine-Aid Maximum Strength Sinus Headache Gelcaps, Caplets and Tablets 1570
Sine-Off No Drowsiness Formula Caplets ▣ 784
Sine-Off Sinus Medicine ▣ 784
Singlet Tablets ▣ 785
Sinutab Non-Drying Liquid Caps ▣ 823
Sinutab Sinus Allergy Medication, Maximum Strength Tablets and Caplets ▣ 823
Sinutab Sinus Medication, Maximum Strength Without Drowsiness Formula, Tablets & Caplets ▣ 824
Sudafed Children's Cold & Cough Liquid Medication ▣ 825
Sudafed Children's Nasal Decongestant Liquid Medication ▣ 826
Sudafed Cold & Allergy Tablets ▣ 826
Sudafed Cold and Cough Liquid Caps ▣ 826
Sudafed Nasal Decongestant Tablets, 30 mg ▣ 825
Sudafed Nasal Decongestant Tablets, 60 mg ▣ 825
Sudafed Non-Drying Sinus Liquid Caps ▣ 827
Sudafed Pediatric Nasal Decongestant Liquid Oral Drops ▣ 827
Sudafed Severe Cold Formula Caplets ▣ 828
Sudafed Severe Cold Formula Tablets ▣ 828
Sudafed Sinus Caplets ▣ 829
Sudafed Sinus Tablets ▣ 829
Sudafed 12 Hour Caplets ▣ 824
Syn-Rx Tablets 1622
Syn-Rx DM Tablets 1623
TheraFlu Flu and Cold Medicine ▣ 750
Theraflu Maximum Strength Flu and Cold Medicine For Sore Throat ▣ 751
TheraFlu Flu, Cold and Cough Medicine ▣ 750
TheraFlu Maximum Strength Nighttime Flu, Cold & Cough Medicine ▣ 751
TheraFlu Maximum Strength Non-Drowsy Formula Flu, Cold & Cough Medicine ▣ 751
TheraFlu Maximum Strength, Non-Drowsy Formula Flu, Cold and Cough Caplets ▣ 752
Theraflu Maximum Strength Sinus Non-Drowsy Formula Caplets ▣ 752
Triaminic AM Cough and Decongestant Formula ▣ 753
Triaminic AM Decongestant Formula ▣ 753
Triaminic Infant Oral Decongestant Drops ▣ 754
Triaminic Night Time ▣ 754
Triaminic Sore Throat Formula ▣ 755
Tussend 1830
Tussend Expectorant 1831
TYLENOL Allergy Sinus, Maximum Strength Caplets and Gelcaps 1571
TYLENOL Allergy Sinus NightTime, Maximum Strength Caplets 1571
TYLENOL Cold Medication, Multi-Symptom Formula Tablets and Caplets 1572
TYLENOL Cold Medication, Multi-Symptom Hot Liquid Packets 1572
TYLENOL Cold Medication, No Drowsiness Formula Caplets and Gelcaps 1572
TYLENOL Cold Severe Congestion Caplets 1573
TYLENOL Cough Medication with Decongestant, Multi Symptom 1574
TYLENOL Flu No Drowsiness Formula, Maximum Strength Gelcaps 1575
TYLENOL Flu NightTime, Maximum Strength Gelcaps 1575
TYLENOL Flu NightTime, Maximum Strength Hot Medication Packets 1575
TYLENOL Sinus, Maximum Strength Geltabs, Gelcaps, Caplets and Tablets 1576
Vicks 44 LiquiCaps Cough, Cold & Flu Relief ▣ 728
Vicks 44 LiquiCaps Non-Drowsy Cough & Cold Relief ▣ 729
Vicks 44D Cough & Head Congestion Relief ▣ 728
Vicks 44M Cough, Cold & Flu Relief ▣ 729
Vicks DayQuil LiquiCaps/Liquid Multi-Symptom Cold/Flu Relief ▣ 734
Vicks DayQuil SINUS Pressure & PAIN Relief with IBUPROFEN ▣ 735
Vicks Nyquil Hot Therapy ▣ 735
Vicks NyQuil LiquiCaps/Liquid Multi-Symptom Cold/Flu Relief, Original and Cherry Flavors ▣ 736

Pseudoephedrine Sulfate (Sympathomimetics tend to produce hyperglycemia leading to loss of control; patients on concurrent therapy should be closely observed for loss of control). Products include:
Chlor-Trimeton Allergy Decongestant Tablets ▣ 759
Claritin-D Tablets 2487
Drixoral Cold and Allergy Sustained-Action Tablets ▣ 763
Drixoral Cold and Flu Extended-Release Tablets ▣ 764
Drixoral Non-Drowsy Formula Extended-Release Tablets ▣ 764
Drixoral Allergy/Sinus Extended Release Tablets ▣ 765
Trinalin Repetabs Tablets 1373

Quinestrol (Estrogens tend to produce hyperglycemia leading to loss of control; patients on concurrent therapy should be closely observed for loss of control).
No products indexed under this heading.

Salmeterol Xinafoate (Sympathomimetics tend to produce hyperglycemia leading to loss of control; patients on concurrent therapy should be closely observed for loss of control). Products include:
Serevent Inhalation Aerosol 1149

Terbutaline Sulfate (Sympathomimetics tend to produce hyperglycemia leading to loss of control; patients on concurrent therapy should be closely observed for loss of control). Products include:
Brethaire Inhaler 830
Brethine Ampuls 832
Brethine Tablets 831
Bricanyl Subcutaneous Injection 1247
Bricanyl Tablets 1248

Thioridazine Hydrochloride (Phenothiazines tend to produce hyperglycemia leading to loss of control; patients on concurrent therapy should be closely observed for loss of control). Products include:
Mellaril 2398

Thyroglobulin (Thyroid products tend to produce hyperglycemia leading to loss of control; patients on concurrent therapy should be closely observed for loss of control).
No products indexed under this heading.

Thyroid (Thyroid products tend to produce hyperglycemia leading to loss of control; patients on concurrent therapy should be closely observed for loss of control).
No products indexed under this heading.

Thyroxine (Thyroid products tend to produce hyperglycemia leading to loss of control; patients on concurrent therapy should be closely observed for loss of control).
No products indexed under this heading.

Thyroxine Sodium (Thyroid products tend to produce hyperglycemia leading to loss of control; patients on concurrent therapy should be closely observed for loss of control).
No products indexed under this heading.

Triamcinolone (Corticosteroids tend to produce hyperglycemia leading to loss of control; patients on concurrent therapy should be closely observed for loss of control).
No products indexed under this heading.

Triamcinolone Acetonide (Corticosteroids tend to produce hyperglycemia leading to loss of control; patients on concurrent therapy should be closely observed for loss of control). Products include:
Azmacort Oral Inhaler 2175
Nasacort AQ Nasal Spray 2191
Nasacort Nasal Inhaler 2189

Triamcinolone Diacetate (Corticosteroids tend to produce hyperglycemia leading to loss of control; patients on concurrent therapy should be closely observed for loss of control).
No products indexed under this heading.

Triamcinolone Hexacetonide (Corticosteroids tend to produce hyperglycemia leading to loss of control; patients on concurrent therapy should be closely observed for loss of control).
No products indexed under this heading.

Trifluoperazine Hydrochloride (Phenothiazines tend to produce hyperglycemia leading to loss of control; patients on concurrent therapy should be closely observed for loss of control). Products include:
Stelazine 2692

Verapamil Hydrochloride (Calcium channel blockers tend to produce hyperglycemia leading to loss of control; patients on concurrent therapy should be closely observed for loss of control). Products include:
Calan SR Caplets 2571
Calan Tablets 2568
Covera-HS Tablets 2573
Isoptin Injectable 1391
Isoptin Oral Tablets 1393
Isoptin SR Tablets 1395
Verelan Capsules 1455

PRECARE PRENATAL MULTI-VITAMIN/MINERAL
(Vitamins with Minerals) 2753
None cited in PDR database.

PRED FORTE
(Prednisolone Acetate) ◉ 247
None cited in PDR database.

PRED MILD
(Prednisolone Acetate) ◉ 250
None cited in PDR database.

PRED-G LIQUIFILM STERILE OPHTHALMIC SUSPENSION
(Gentamicin Sulfate, Prednisolone Acetate) ◉ 248
None cited in PDR database.

PRED-G S.O.P. STERILE OPHTHALMIC OINTMENT
(Gentamicin Sulfate, Prednisolone Acetate) ◉ 249
None cited in PDR database.

PREGNYL FOR INJECTION
(Chorionic Gonadotropin) 1878
None cited in PDR database.

PRELONE SYRUP
(Prednisolone) 1834
May interact with oral hypoglycemic agents, insulin, and certain other agents. Compounds in these categories include:

Acarbose (Potential for increased requirements of oral hypoglycemic agents). Products include:
Precose 604

Aspirin (Aspirin should be used cautiously in conjunction with corticosteroids in hypoprothrombinemia). Products include:
Alka-Seltzer Cherry Effervescent Antacid and Pain Reliever ▣ 609
Alka-Seltzer Extra Strength Effervescent Antacid and Pain Reliever ▣ 609
Alka-Seltzer Lemon Lime Effervescent Antacid and Pain Reliever ▣ 609
Alka-Seltzer Original Effervescent Antacid and Pain Reliever ▣ 609
Alka-Seltzer Plus ▣ 611
Alka-Seltzer Plus Sinus Medicine ▣ 611
Ascriptin ▣ 650
Arthritis Strength BC Powder ▣ 631
BC Cold Powder Multi-Symptom Formula (Cold-Sinus-Allergy) ▣ 631
BC Cold Powder Non-Drowsy Formula (Cold-Sinus) ▣ 631
BC Powder ▣ 631
Genuine Bayer Aspirin Tablets & Caplets ▣ 618
Extra Strength Bayer Arthritis Pain Regimen Formula ▣ 615
Extra Strength Bayer Aspirin Caplets & Tablets ▣ 617
Extended-Release Bayer 8-Hour Aspirin ▣ 616
Extra Strength Bayer Plus Aspirin Caplets ▣ 617
Extra Strength Bayer PM Aspirin Plus Sleep Aid ▣ 617
Aspirin Regimen Bayer 81 mg Tablets with Calcium ▣ 615
Aspirin Regimen Bayer Adult Low Strength 81 mg Tablets ▣ 613
Aspirin Regimen Bayer Children's Chewable Aspirin ▣ 616
Aspirin Regimen Bayer Regular Strength 325 mg Caplets ▣ 613
Bufferin Analgesic Tablets ▣ 636
Arthritis Strength Bufferin Analgesic Caplets ▣ 637
Extra Strength Bufferin Analgesic Tablets ▣ 637
Cama Arthritis Pain Reliever ▣ 748
Darvon Compound-65 Pulvules 1475
Easprin 1971
Ecotrin 2625
Ecotrin Enteric Coated Aspirin Maximum Strength Tablets and Caplets ▣ 775
Ecotrin Enteric Coated Aspirin Regular Strength Tablets 2625
Empirin Aspirin Tablets ▣ 818
Excedrin Extra-Strength Analgesic Tablets, Caplets, and Geltabs 734
Fiorinal Capsules 2388
Fiorinal with Codeine Capsules 2390
Fiorinal Tablets 2388
Goody's Extra Strength Headache Powders ▣ 632
Goody's Extra Strength Pain Relief Tablets ▣ 632
Halfprin Tablets 1413
Norgesic 1554
Percodan Tablets 955
Percodan-Demi Tablets 956
Robaxisal Tablets 2246
Soma Compound w/Codeine Tablets 2784
Soma Compound Tablets 2783
St. Joseph Adult Chewable Aspirin (81 mg.) ▣ 768
Talwin Compound 2466
Vanquish Analgesic Caplets ▣ 627

Chlorpropamide (Potential for increased requirements of oral hypoglycemic agents). Products include:
Diabinese Tablets 2002

Glimepiride (Potential for increased requirements of oral hypoglycemic agents). Products include:
Amaryl Tablets 1241

(▣ Described in PDR For Nonprescription Drugs) (◉ Described in PDR For Ophthalmology)

861 **Interactions Index** **Prepidil**

Glipizide (Potential for increased requirements of oral hypoglycemic agents). Products include:
- Glucotrol Tablets 2011
- Glucotrol XL Extended Release Tablets 2012

Glyburide (Potential for increased requirements of oral hypoglycemic agents). Products include:
- DiaBeta Tablets 1265
- Glynase PresTab Tablets 2091
- Micronase Tablets 2099

Insulin, Human (Potential for increased requirements of insulin).
- No products indexed under this heading.

Insulin, Human Isophane Suspension (Potential for increased requirements of insulin). Products include:
- Novolin N Human Insulin 10 ml Vials 1846

Insulin, Human NPH (Potential for increased requirements of insulin). Products include:
- Humulin N, 100 Units 1495
- Novolin N PenFill 1.5 ml Cartridges Durable Insulin Delivery System 1849
- Novolin N Prefilled Syringe Disposable Insulin Delivery System 1850

Insulin, Human Regular (Potential for increased requirements of insulin). Products include:
- Humulin R, 100 Units 1497
- Novolin R Human Insulin 10 ml Vials 1846
- Novolin R PenFill 1.5 ml Cartridges Durable Insulin Delivery System 1849
- Novolin R Prefilled Syringe Disposable Insulin Delivery System 1850
- Velosulin BR Human Insulin 10 ml Vials 1847

Insulin, Human, Zinc Suspension (Potential for increased requirements of insulin). Products include:
- Humulin L, 100 Units 1494
- Humulin U, 100 Units 1498
- Novolin L Human Insulin 10 ml Vials 1846

Insulin Lispro, Human (Potential for increased requirements of insulin). Products include:
- Humalog Injection 1488

Insulin, NPH (Potential for increased requirements of insulin). Products include:
- NPH, 100 Units 1502
- Pork NPH, 100 Units 1506
- Purified Pork NPH Isophane Insulin 1852

Insulin, Regular (Potential for increased requirements of insulin). Products include:
- Regular, 100 Units 1503
- Pork Regular, 100 Units 1507
- Pork Regular (Concentrated), 500 Units 1508
- Purified Pork Regular Insulin 1852

Insulin, Zinc Crystals (Potential for increased requirements of insulin). Products include:
- NPH, 100 Units 1502

Insulin, Zinc Suspension (Potential for increased requirements of insulin). Products include:
- Iletin I 1501
- Lente, 100 Units 1501
- Iletin II 1504
- Pork Lente, 100 Units 1504
- Purified Pork Lente Insulin 1852

Metformin Hydrochloride (Potential for increased requirements of oral hypoglycemic agents). Products include:
- Glucophage Tablets 754

Tolazamide (Potential for increased requirements of oral hypoglycemic agents).
- No products indexed under this heading.

Tolbutamide (Potential for increased requirements of oral hypoglycemic agents).
- No products indexed under this heading.

PRELU-2 TIMED RELEASE CAPSULES
(Phendimetrazine Tartrate) 687
May interact with monoamine oxidase inhibitors, insulin, and certain other agents. Compounds in these categories include:

Furazolidone (Contraindicated; hypertensive crises may result). Products include:
- Furoxone 2221

Guanethidine Monosulfate (Decreased hypotensive effect). Products include:
- Esimil Tablets 840
- Ismelin Tablets 845

Insulin, Human (Altered insulin requirements).
- No products indexed under this heading.

Insulin, Human Isophane Suspension (Altered insulin requirements). Products include:
- Novolin N Human Insulin 10 ml Vials 1846

Insulin, Human NPH (Altered insulin requirements). Products include:
- Humulin N, 100 Units 1495
- Novolin N PenFill 1.5 ml Cartridges Durable Insulin Delivery System 1849
- Novolin N Prefilled Syringe Disposable Insulin Delivery System 1850

Insulin, Human Regular (Altered insulin requirements). Products include:
- Humulin R, 100 Units 1497
- Novolin R Human Insulin 10 ml Vials 1846
- Novolin R PenFill 1.5 ml Cartridges Durable Insulin Delivery System 1849
- Novolin R Prefilled Syringe Disposable Insulin Delivery System 1850
- Velosulin BR Human Insulin 10 ml Vials 1847

Insulin, Human, Zinc Suspension (Altered insulin requirements). Products include:
- Humulin L, 100 Units 1494
- Humulin U, 100 Units 1498
- Novolin L Human Insulin 10 ml Vials 1846

Insulin Lispro, Human (Altered insulin requirements). Products include:
- Humalog Injection 1488

Insulin, NPH (Altered insulin requirements). Products include:
- NPH, 100 Units 1502
- Pork NPH, 100 Units 1506
- Purified Pork NPH Isophane Insulin 1852

Insulin, Regular (Altered insulin requirements). Products include:
- Regular, 100 Units 1503
- Pork Regular, 100 Units 1507
- Pork Regular (Concentrated), 500 Units 1508
- Purified Pork Regular Insulin 1852

Insulin, Zinc Crystals (Altered insulin requirements). Products include:
- NPH, 100 Units 1502

Insulin, Zinc Suspension (Altered insulin requirements). Products include:
- Iletin I 1501
- Lente, 100 Units 1501
- Iletin II 1504
- Pork Lente, 100 Units 1504
- Purified Pork Lente Insulin 1852

Isocarboxazid (Contraindicated; hypertensive crises may result).
- No products indexed under this heading.

Phenelzine Sulfate (Contraindicated; hypertensive crises may result). Products include:
- Nardil 1977

Selegiline Hydrochloride (Contraindicated; hypertensive crises may result). Products include:
- Eldepryl Capsules 2729

Tranylcypromine Sulfate (Contraindicated; hypertensive crises may result). Products include:
- Parnate Tablets 2679

PREMARIN INTRAVENOUS
(Estrogens, Conjugated) 2893
None cited in PDR database.

PREMARIN TABLETS
(Estrogens, Conjugated) 2896
May interact with progestins. Compounds in this category include:

Desogestrel (Potential adverse effects on carbohydrate and lipid metabolism). Products include:
- Desogen Tablets 1867
- Ortho-Cept 1907

Medroxyprogesterone Acetate (Potential adverse effects on carbohydrate and lipid metabolism). Products include:
- Amen Tablets 785
- Cycrin Tablets 991
- Depo-Provera Contraceptive Injection 2079
- Depo-Provera Sterile Aqueous Suspension 2083
- Premphase 2900
- Prempro 2905
- Provera Tablets 2110

Megestrol Acetate (Potential adverse effects on carbohydrate and lipid metabolism). Products include:
- Megace Oral Suspension 708
- Megace Tablets 710

Norgestimate (Potential adverse effects on carbohydrate and lipid metabolism). Products include:
- Ortho-Cyclen/Ortho-Tri-Cyclen 1914
- Ortho-Cyclen/Ortho Tri-Cyclen 1914

PREMARIN VAGINAL CREAM
(Estrogens, Conjugated) 2898
May interact with progestins. Compounds in this category include:

Desogestrel (Potential adverse effects on carbohydrate and lipid metabolism). Products include:
- Desogen Tablets 1867
- Ortho-Cept 1907

Medroxyprogesterone Acetate (Potential adverse effects on carbohydrate and lipid metabolism). Products include:
- Amen Tablets 785
- Cycrin Tablets 991
- Depo-Provera Contraceptive Injection 2079
- Depo-Provera Sterile Aqueous Suspension 2083
- Premphase 2900
- Prempro 2905
- Provera Tablets 2110

Megestrol Acetate (Potential adverse effects on carbohydrate and lipid metabolism). Products include:
- Megace Oral Suspension 708
- Megace Tablets 710

Norgestimate (Potential adverse effects on carbohydrate and lipid metabolism). Products include:
- Ortho-Cyclen/Ortho-Tri-Cyclen 1914
- Ortho-Cyclen/Ortho Tri-Cyclen 1914

PREMPHASE
(Estrogens, Conjugated, Medroxyprogesterone Acetate) 2900
May interact with:

Aminoglutethimide (Aminoglutethimide administered concomitantly with medroxyprogesterone acetate (MPA) may significantly depress the bioavailability of MPA). Products include:
- Cytadren Tablets 837

Food Interactions

Food, unspecified (Administration with a high-fat breakfast decreased total estrone C_{max} and increased total equilin C_{max} compared to fasting state, no other effect on rate or extent of absorption; administration with food doubles MPA C_{max} and increases MPA AUC).

PREMPRO
(Estrogens, Conjugated, Medroxyprogesterone Acetate) 2905
May interact with:

Aminoglutethimide (Aminoglutethimide administered concomitantly with medroxyprogesterone acetate (MPA) may significantly depress the bioavailability of MPA). Products include:
- Cytadren Tablets 837

Food Interactions

Food, unspecified (Administration with food decreased C_{max} of total estrone compared to fasting state, no other effect on rate or extent of absorption; administration with food doubles MPA C_{max} and increases MPA AUC).

PREPARATION H HEMORRHOIDAL CREAM
(Glycerin, Petrolatum, Phenylephrine Hydrochloride, Shark Liver Oil) 842
None cited in PDR database.

PREPARATION H HEMORRHOIDAL OINTMENT
(Mineral Oil, Petrolatum, Phenylephrine Hydrochloride, Shark Liver Oil) 842
None cited in PDR database.

PREPARATION H HEMORRHOIDAL SUPPOSITORIES
(Yeast Cell Derivative, Live) 842
None cited in PDR database.

PREPARATION H HYDROCORTISONE 1% CREAM
(Hydrocortisone) 843
None cited in PDR database.

PREPIDIL GEL
(Dinoprostone) 2108
May interact with oxytocic drugs. Compounds in this category include:

Ergonovine Maleate (Prepidil may augment the activity of other oxytocic drugs; co-administration is not recommended).
- No products indexed under this heading.

Methylergonovine Maleate (Prepidil may augment the activity of other oxytocic drugs; co-administration is not recommended). Products include:
- Methergine 2401

IMPORTANT NOTE: Always consult each drug listing in the patient's regimen for possible interactions.

Prepidil **Interactions Index** **862**

Oxytocin (Prepidil may augment the activity of other oxytocic drugs; co-administration is not recommended; allow a 6–12 hour dosing interval for sequential use of oxytocin). Products include:
Syntocinon Injection 2425

PREVACID DELAYED-RELEASE CAPSULES
(Lansoprazole) 2746
May interact with absorption of drugs where gastric ph is an important determinant in their bioavailability, xanthine bronchodilators, and certain other agents. Compounds in these categories include:

Aminophylline (Co-administration has resulted in a minor increase (10%) in the clearance of theophylline; this interaction is unlikely to be of clinical concern, nonetheless monitor blood levels).
No products indexed under this heading.

Bacampicillin Hydrochloride (Lansoprazole causes a profound and long lasting inhibition of gastric acid secretion; therefore, it is theoretically possible that it may interfere with the oral absorption of drugs where gastric pH is an important determinant of bioavailability). Products include:
Spectrobid Tablets 2030

Digoxin (Lansoprazole causes a profound and long lasting inhibition of gastric acid secretion; therefore, it is theoretically possible that it may interfere with the oral absorption of drugs where gastric pH is an important determinant of bioavailability, such as digoxin). Products include:
Lanoxicaps 1110
Lanoxin Elixir Pediatric 1113
Lanoxin Injection 1116
Lanoxin Injection Pediatric 1119
Lanoxin Tablets 1121

Dyphylline (Co-administration has resulted in a minor increase (10%) in the clearance of theophylline; this interaction is unlikely to be of clinical concern, nonetheless monitor blood levels). Products include:
Lufyllin & Lufyllin-400 Tablets 2778
Lufyllin-GG Elixir & Tablets 2779

Ferrous Fumarate (Lansoprazole causes a profound and long lasting inhibition of gastric acid secretion; therefore, it is theoretically possible that it may interfere with the oral absorption of drugs where gastric pH is an important determinant of bioavailability). Products include:
Chromagen Capsules 2470
Chromagen FA 2471
Chromagen Forte 2471
Ferro-Sequels .... ■ 684
Nephro-Fer Tablets 2168
Nephro-Fer Rx Tablets 2168
Nephro-Vite + Fe Tablets 2170
Stresstabs + Iron .... ■ 685
Trinsicon Capsules 2759
Vitron-C Tablets .... ■ 667

Ferrous Gluconate (Lansoprazole causes a profound and long lasting inhibition of gastric acid secretion; therefore, it is theoretically possible that it may interfere with the oral absorption of drugs where gastric pH is an important determinant of bioavailability). Products include:
Megadose 513

Ferrous Sulfate (Lansoprazole causes a profound and long lasting inhibition of gastric acid secretion; therefore, it is theoretically possible that it may interfere with the oral absorption of drugs where gastric pH is an important determinant of bioavailability). Products include:
Feosol Capsules .... ■ 777
Feosol Elixir 2627
Feosol Tablets 2627
Fero-Folic-500 Filmtab 433
Fero-Grad-500 Filmtab 434
Fero-Gradumet Filmtab 434
Iberet Tablets 437
Iberet-500 Liquid 438
Iberet-Folic-500 Filmtab 433
Iberet-Liquid 438
Irospan 1000
Slow Fe Tablets 889
Slow Fe with Folic Acid 890

Ketoconazole (Lansoprazole causes a profound and long lasting inhibition of gastric acid secretion; therefore, it is theoretically possible that it may interfere with the oral absorption of drugs where gastric pH is an important determinant of bioavailability). Products include:
Nizoral 2% Cream 1344
Nizoral 2% Shampoo 1344
Nizoral Tablets 1345

Sucralfate (Co-administration delays absorption and reduces bioavailability of lansoprazole by about 30%, therefore lansoprazole should be taken at least 30 minutes prior to sucralfate). Products include:
Carafate Suspension 1250
Carafate Tablets 1249

Theophylline (Co-administration has resulted in a minor increase (10%) in the clearance of theophylline; this interaction is unlikely to be of clinical concern, nonetheless monitor blood levels). Products include:
Marax Tablets & DF Syrup 2015
Quibron 2227

Theophylline Anhydrous (Co-administration has resulted in a minor increase (10%) in the clearance of theophylline; this interaction is unlikely to be of clinical concern, nonetheless monitor blood levels). Products include:
Aerolate 1003
Primatene Tablets .... ■ 844
Respbid Tablets 687
Slo-bid Gyrocaps 2201
Theo-24 Extended Release Capsules 2753
Theo-Dur Extended-Release Tablets 1367
Theo-X Extended-Release Tablets .. 793
Uni-Dur Extended-Release Tablets .. 1374
Uniphyl 400 mg and 600 mg Tablets 2157

Theophylline Calcium Salicylate (Co-administration has resulted in a minor increase (10%) in the clearance of theophylline; this interaction is unlikely to be of clinical concern, nonetheless monitor blood levels). Products include:
Quadrinal Tablets 1398

Theophylline Sodium Glycinate (Co-administration has resulted in a minor increase (10%) in the clearance of theophylline; this interaction is unlikely to be of clinical concern, nonetheless monitor blood levels).
No products indexed under this heading.

Food Interactions

Food, unspecified (Cmax and AUC are diminished by about 50% if the drug is given 30 minutes after food as opposed to the fasting condition; Prevacid should be taken before eating).

PREVIDENT 5000 PLUS CREAM
(Sodium Fluoride) 893
None cited in PDR database.

PRILOSEC DELAYED-RELEASE CAPSULES
(Omeprazole) 516
May interact with absorption of drugs where gastric ph is an important determinant in their bioavailability, benzodiazepines, and certain other agents. Compounds in these categories include:

Alprazolam (Potential for metabolism interaction via cytochrome P-450 system). Products include:
Xanax Tablets 2115

Bacampicillin Hydrochloride (Omeprazole may interfere with the gastric absorption). Products include:
Spectrobid Tablets 2030

Chlordiazepoxide (Potential for metabolism interaction via cytochrome P-450 system). Products include:
Limbitrol 2333

Chlordiazepoxide Hydrochloride (Potential for metabolism interaction via cytochrome P-450 system). Products include:
Librax Capsules 2330
Librium Capsules 2331
Librium Injectable 2332

Clarithromycin (Co-administration may result in increases in plasma levels of omeprazole, clarithromycin, and 14-hydroxy-clarithromycin; co-administration also results in increased clarithromycin concentrations in gastric tissue and mucus). Products include:
Biaxin 406

Clonazepam (Potential for metabolism interaction via cytochrome P-450 system). Products include:
Klonopin Tablets 2294

Clorazepate Dipotassium (Potential for metabolism interaction via cytochrome P-450 system). Products include:
Tranxene 459

Cyclosporine (Potential of metabolism interaction via the cytochrome P-450 system). Products include:
Neoral 2405
Sandimmune 2416

Diazepam (Potential for metabolism interaction via cytochrome P-450 system; prolonged elimination of diazepam). Products include:
Dizac (diazepam injectable emulsion) CIV 1862
Valium Injectable 2336
Valium Tablets 2335

Disulfiram (Potential of metabolism interaction via the cytochrome P-450 system). Products include:
Antabuse Tablets 2802

Drugs which undergo biotransformation by cytochrome P-450 mixed function oxidase (Potential of metabolism interaction via the cytochrome P-450 system).

Estazolam (Potential for metabolism interaction via cytochrome P-450 system). Products include:
ProSom Tablets 457

Ferrous Fumarate (Omeprazole may interfere with the gastric absorption). Products include:
Chromagen Capsules 2470
Chromagen FA 2471
Chromagen Forte 2471
Ferro-Sequels .... ■ 684
Nephro-Fer Tablets 2168
Nephro-Fer Rx Tablets 2168
Nephro-Vite + Fe Tablets 2170
Stresstabs + Iron .... ■ 685
Trinsicon Capsules 2759
Vitron-C Tablets .... ■ 667

Ferrous Gluconate (Omeprazole may interfere with the gastric absorption). Products include:
Megadose 513

Ferrous Sulfate (Omeprazole may interfere with the gastric absorption). Products include:
Feosol Capsules .... ■ 777
Feosol Elixir 2627
Feosol Tablets 2627
Fero-Folic-500 Filmtab 433
Fero-Grad-500 Filmtab 434
Fero-Gradumet Filmtab 434
Iberet Tablets 437
Iberet-500 Liquid 438
Iberet-Folic-500 Filmtab 433
Iberet-Liquid 438
Irospan 1000
Slow Fe Tablets 889
Slow Fe with Folic Acid 890

Flurazepam Hydrochloride (Potential for metabolism interaction via cytochrome P-450 system). Products include:
Dalmane Capsules 2329

Fosphenytoin Sodium (Prolonged elimination of phenytoin). Products include:
Cerebyx Injection 1956

Halazepam (Potential for metabolism interaction via cytochrome P-450 system).
No products indexed under this heading.

Ketoconazole (Omeprazole may interfere with the gastric absorption). Products include:
Nizoral 2% Cream 1344
Nizoral 2% Shampoo 1344
Nizoral Tablets 1345

Lorazepam (Potential for metabolism interaction via cytochrome P-450 system). Products include:
Ativan Injection 2805
Ativan Tablets 2807

Midazolam Hydrochloride (Potential for metabolism interaction via cytochrome P-450 system). Products include:
Versed Injection 2324

Oxazepam (Potential for metabolism interaction via cytochrome P-450 system). Products include:
Serax Capsules 2916
Serax Tablets 2916

Phenytoin (Prolonged elimination of phenytoin). Products include:
Dilantin Infatabs 1967
Dilantin-125 Suspension 1969

Phenytoin Sodium (Prolonged elimination of phenytoin). Products include:
Dilantin Kapseals 1965

Prazepam (Potential for metabolism interaction via cytochrome P-450 system).
No products indexed under this heading.

Quazepam (Potential for metabolism interaction via cytochrome P-450 system). Products include:
Doral Tablets 2773

Temazepam (Potential for metabolism interaction via cytochrome P-450 system). Products include:
Restoril Capsules 2413

Triazolam (Potential for metabolism interaction via cytochrome P-450 system). Products include:
Halcion Tablets 2093

Warfarin Sodium (Prolonged elimination of warfarin). Products include:
Coumadin 941

(■ Described in PDR For Nonprescription Drugs) (◉ Described in PDR For Ophthalmology)

863 **Interactions Index** **Prinzide**

PRIMACOR INJECTION
(Milrinone Lactate) 2461
May interact with:

Furosemide (Immediate chemical interaction which is evidenced by the formation of a precipitate when furosemide is injected into IV line of an infusion of Primacor). Products include:
- Lasix Injection, Oral Solution and Tablets 1267

PRIMATENE MIST
(Epinephrine) 843
May interact with monoamine oxidase inhibitors. Compounds in this category include:

Furazolidone (Concurrent and/or sequential use is not recommended). Products include:
- Furoxone 2221

Isocarboxazid (Concurrent and/or sequential use is not recommended).
- No products indexed under this heading.

Phenelzine Sulfate (Concurrent and/or sequential use is not recommended). Products include:
- Nardil 1977

Selegiline Hydrochloride (Concurrent and/or sequential use is not recommended). Products include:
- Eldepryl Capsules 2729

Tranylcypromine Sulfate (Concurrent and/or sequential use is not recommended). Products include:
- Parnate Tablets 2679

PRIMATENE TABLETS
(Theophylline Anhydrous, Ephedrine Hydrochloride) 844
May interact with monoamine oxidase inhibitors. Compounds in this category include:

Furazolidone (Concurrent and/or sequential use is not recommended). Products include:
- Furoxone 2221

Isocarboxazid (Concurrent and/or sequential use is not recommended).
- No products indexed under this heading.

Phenelzine Sulfate (Concurrent and/or sequential use is not recommended). Products include:
- Nardil 1977

Selegiline Hydrochloride (Concurrent and/or sequential use is not recommended). Products include:
- Eldepryl Capsules 2729

Tranylcypromine Sulfate (Concurrent and/or sequential use is not recommended). Products include:
- Parnate Tablets 2679

PRIMAXIN I.M.
(Cilastatin Sodium, Imipenem) 1770
May interact with:

Probenecid (Concomitant administration results in only minimal increase in plasma levels of imipenem). Products include:
- Benemid Tablets 1651
- ColBENEMID Tablets 1662

PRIMAXIN I.V.
(Cilastatin Sodium, Imipenem) 1772
May interact with:

Ganciclovir Sodium (Concomitant administration may result in generalized seizures). Products include:
- Cytovene-IV 2270

Probenecid (Concomitant administration results in only minimal increase in plasma levels of imipenem; concomitant administration not recommended). Products include:
- Benemid Tablets 1651
- ColBENEMID Tablets 1662

PRINIVIL TABLETS
(Lisinopril) 1776
May interact with diuretics, potassium sparing diuretics, potassium preparations, thiazides, lithium preparations, and certain other agents. Compounds in these categories include:

Amiloride Hydrochloride (Potential for significant hyperkalemia; possibility of excessive reduction in blood pressure). Products include:
- Midamor Tablets 1746
- Moduretic Tablets 1748

Bendroflumethiazide (Thiazide-induced potassium loss attenuated; possibility of excessive reduction in blood pressure).
- No products indexed under this heading.

Bumetanide (Possibility of excessive reduction in blood pressure). Products include:
- Bumex 2260

Chlorothiazide (Thiazide-induced potassium loss attenuated; possibility of excessive reduction in blood pressure). Products include:
- Aldoclor Tablets 1638
- Diupres Tablets 1691
- Diuril Oral 1694

Chlorothiazide Sodium (Thiazide-induced potassium loss attenuated; possibility of excessive reduction in blood pressure). Products include:
- Diuril Sodium Intravenous 1693

Chlorthalidone (Possibility of excessive reduction in blood pressure). Products include:
- Combipres Tablets 682
- Tenoretic Tablets 2963
- Thalitone 1293

Ethacrynic Acid (Possibility of excessive reduction in blood pressure). Products include:
- Edecrin Tablets 1698

Furosemide (Possibility of excessive reduction in blood pressure). Products include:
- Lasix Injection, Oral Solution and Tablets 1267

Hydrochlorothiazide (Thiazide-induced potassium loss attenuated; possibility of excessive reduction in blood pressure). Products include:
- Aldactazide Tablets 2556
- Aldoril Tablets 1644
- Apresazide Capsules 824
- Capozide Tablets 744
- Dyazide Capsules 2653
- Esidrix Tablets 839
- Esimil Tablets 840
- HydroDIURIL Tablets 1716
- Hydropres Tablets 1718
- Hyzaar Tablets 1720
- Inderide Tablets 2838
- Inderide LA Long Acting Capsules .. 2840
- Lopressor HCT Tablets 850
- Lotensin HCT Tablets 855
- Moduretic Tablets 1748
- Oretic Tablets 450
- Prinzide Tablets 1780
- Ser-Ap-Es Tablets 867
- Timolide Tablets 1791
- Vaseretic Tablets 1810
- Zestoretic Tablets 2968
- Ziac 1459

Hydroflumethiazide (Thiazide-induced potassium loss attenuated; possibility of excessive reduction in blood pressure). Products include:
- Diucardin Tablets 2824

Indapamide (Possibility of excessive reduction in blood pressure).
- No products indexed under this heading.

Indomethacin (Reduces antihypertensive effect). Products include:
- Indocin 1723

Indomethacin Sodium Trihydrate (Reduces antihypertensive effect). Products include:
- Indocin I.V. 1727

Lithium Carbonate (Potential for reversible lithium toxicity; frequent monitoring of lithium levels is recommended). Products include:
- Eskalith 2658
- Lithium Carbonate Capsules & Tablets 2352
- Lithonate/Lithotabs/Lithobid 2721

Lithium Citrate (Potential for reversible lithium toxicity; frequent monitoring of lithium levels is recommended).
- No products indexed under this heading.

Methyclothiazide (Thiazide-induced potassium loss attenuated; possibility of excessive reduction in blood pressure). Products include:
- Enduron Tablets 424

Metolazone (Possibility of excessive reduction in blood pressure). Products include:
- Mykrox Tablets 1617
- Zaroxolyn Tablets 1625

Polythiazide (Thiazide-induced potassium loss attenuated; possibility of excessive reduction in blood pressure). Products include:
- Minizide Capsules 2016

Potassium Acid Phosphate (Potential for significant hyperkalemia). Products include:
- K-Phos Original Formula 'Sodium Free' Tablets 633

Potassium Bicarbonate (Potential for significant hyperkalemia). Products include:
- Alka-Seltzer Gold Effervescent Antacid 611

Potassium Chloride (Potential for significant hyperkalemia). Products include:
- Chlor-3 Condiment 1003
- Colyte and Colyte-flavored 2540
- GoLYTELY 694
- K-Dur Microburst Release System (potassium chloride, USP) E.R. Tablets 1364
- K-Lor Powder Packets 438
- K-Norm Capsules 1615
- K-Tab Filmtab 439
- Micro-K 2237
- Micro-K LS Packets 2238
- NuLYTELY 694
- Cherry Flavor NuLYTELY 694
- Rum-K Syrup 1004
- Slow-K Extended-Release Tablets 869

Potassium Citrate (Potential for significant hyperkalemia). Products include:
- Polycitra Syrup 574
- Polycitra-K Crystals 574
- Polycitra-K Oral Solution 575
- Polycitra-LC 574
- Urocit-K Tablets 1828

Potassium Gluconate (Potential for significant hyperkalemia).
- No products indexed under this heading.

Potassium Phosphate, Dibasic (Potential for significant hyperkalemia).
- No products indexed under this heading.

Potassium Phosphate, Monobasic (Potential for significant hyperkalemia). Products include:
- K-Phos Neutral Tablets 633
- K-Phos Original Formula 'Sodium Free' Tablets 633

Spironolactone (Potential for significant hyperkalemia; possibility of excessive reduction in blood pressure). Products include:
- Aldactazide Tablets 2556
- Aldactone Tablets 2558

Torsemide (Possibility of excessive reduction in blood pressure). Products include:
- Demadex Tablets and Injection 691

Triamterene (Potential for significant hyperkalemia; possibility of excessive reduction in blood pressure). Products include:
- Dyazide Capsules 2653
- Dyrenium Capsules 2655

PRINZIDE TABLETS
(Lisinopril, Hydrochlorothiazide) 1780
May interact with barbiturates, narcotic analgesics, potassium sparing diuretics, potassium preparations, antihypertensives, corticosteroids, lithium preparations, non-steroidal anti-inflammatory agents, diuretics, insulin, oral hypoglycemic agents, nondepolarizing neuromuscular blocking agents, bile acid sequestering agents, and certain other agents. Compounds in these categories include:

Acarbose (Dosage adjustment of the antidiabetic drug may be required). Products include:
- Precose 604

Acebutolol Hydrochloride (Additive effect or potentiation). Products include:
- Sectral Capsules 2914

ACTH (Intensified electrolyte depletion, particularly hypokalemia).
- No products indexed under this heading.

Alfentanil Hydrochloride (Potentiates orthostatic hypotension). Products include:
- Alfenta Injection 1334

Amiloride Hydrochloride (Concomitant therapy may lead to hyperkalemia). Products include:
- Midamor Tablets 1746
- Moduretic Tablets 1748

Amlodipine Besylate (Additive effect or potentiation). Products include:
- Lotrel Capsules 858
- Norvasc Tablets 2020

Aprobarbital (Potentiates orthostatic hypotension).
- No products indexed under this heading.

Atenolol (Additive effect or potentiation). Products include:
- Tenoretic Tablets 2963
- Tenormin Tablets and I.V. Injection 2965

Atracurium Besylate (Possible increased responsiveness to the muscle relaxant). Products include:
- Tracrium Injection 1155

Benazepril Hydrochloride (Additive effect or potentiation). Products include:
- Lotensin Tablets 852
- Lotensin HCT Tablets 855
- Lotrel Capsules 858

Bendroflumethiazide (Additive effect or potentiation).
- No products indexed under this heading.

Betamethasone Acetate (Intensified electrolyte depletion, particularly hypokalemia). Products include:
- Celestone Soluspan Suspension 2484

Betamethasone Sodium Phosphate (Intensified electrolyte depletion, particularly hypokalemia). Products include:
- Celestone Soluspan Suspension 2484

IMPORTANT NOTE: Always consult each drug listing in the patient's regimen for possible interactions.

Prinzide **Interactions Index** **864**

Betaxolol Hydrochloride (Additive effect or potentiation). Products include:
- Betoptic Ophthalmic Solution ... 465
- Betoptic S Ophthalmic Suspension ... 467
- Kerlone Tablets ... 2588

Bisoprolol Fumarate (Additive effect or potentiation). Products include:
- Zebeta Tablets ... 1457
- Ziac ... 1459

Buprenorphine (Potentiates orthostatic hypotension). Products include:
- Buprenex Injectable ... 2170

Butabarbital (Potentiates orthostatic hypotension).
- No products indexed under this heading.

Butalbital (Potentiates orthostatic hypotension). Products include:
- Axocet Capsules ... 2469
- Esgic-plus Capsules ... 1012
- Esgic-plus Tablets ... 1012
- Fioricet Tablets ... 2386
- Fioricet with Codeine Capsules ... 2387
- Fiorinal Capsules ... 2388
- Fiorinal with Codeine Capsules ... 2390
- Fiorinal Tablets ... 2388
- Phrenilin ... 790
- Sedapap Tablets 50 mg/650 mg ... 1826

Captopril (Additive effect or potentiation). Products include:
- Capoten Tablets ... 740
- Capozide Tablets ... 744

Carteolol Hydrochloride (Additive effect or potentiation). Products include:
- Cartrol Tablets ... 413
- Ocupress Ophthalmic Solution, 1% Sterile ... ⊙ 297

Chlorothiazide (Additive effect or potentiation). Products include:
- Aldoclor Tablets ... 1638
- Diupres Tablets ... 1691
- Diuril Oral ... 1694

Chlorothiazide Sodium (Additive effect or potentiation). Products include:
- Diuril Sodium Intravenous ... 1693

Chlorpropamide (Dosage adjustment of the antidiabetic drug may be required). Products include:
- Diabinese Tablets ... 2002

Chlorthalidone (Additive effect or potentiation). Products include:
- Combipres Tablets ... 682
- Tenoretic Tablets ... 2963
- Thalitone ... 1293

Cholestyramine (Binds the hydrochlorothiazide and reduces its absorption by 85% from the gastrointestinal tract). Products include:
- Questran ... 774

Cisatracurium Besylate (Possible increased responsiveness to the muscle relaxant). Products include:
- Nimbex Injection ... 1131

Clonidine (Additive effect or potentiation). Products include:
- Catapres-TTS ... 680

Clonidine Hydrochloride (Additive effect or potentiation). Products include:
- Catapres Tablets ... 679
- Combipres Tablets ... 682

Codeine Phosphate (Potentiates orthostatic hypotension). Products include:
- Brontex ... 2130
- Dimetane-DC Cough Syrup ... 2232
- Fioricet with Codeine Capsules ... 2387
- Fiorinal with Codeine Capsules ... 2390
- Nucofed ... 2225
- Phenergan with Codeine ... 2883
- Phenergan VC with Codeine ... 2888
- Robitussin A-C Syrup ... 2248
- Robitussin-DAC Syrup ... 2249
- Ryna ... ▣ 804
- Soma Compound w/Codeine Tablets ... 2784
- Tylenol with Codeine ... 1592

Colestipol Hydrochloride (Binds the hydrochlorothiazide and reduces its absorption by 43% from the gastrointestinal tract). Products include:
- Colestid ... 2073

Cortisone Acetate (Intensified electrolyte depletion, particularly hypokalemia). Products include:
- Cortone Acetate Sterile Suspension ... 1663
- Cortone Acetate Tablets ... 1664

Deserpidine (Additive effect or potentiation).
- No products indexed under this heading.

Dexamethasone (Intensified electrolyte depletion, particularly hypokalemia). Products include:
- AK-Trol Ointment & Suspension ... ⊙ 205
- Decadron Elixir ... 1676
- Decadron Tablets ... 1678
- Decaspray Topical Aerosol ... 1689
- Maxitrol Ophthalmic Ointment and Suspension ... ⊙ 222
- TobraDex Ophthalmic Suspension and Ointment ... 469

Dexamethasone Acetate (Intensified electrolyte depletion, particularly hypokalemia). Products include:
- Dalalone D.P. Injectable ... 1009
- Decadron-LA Sterile Suspension ... 1687

Dexamethasone Sodium Phosphate (Intensified electrolyte depletion, particularly hypokalemia). Products include:
- Decadron Phosphate Injection ... 1680
- Decadron Phosphate Sterile Ophthalmic Ointment ... 1684
- Decadron Phosphate Sterile Ophthalmic Solution ... 1685
- Decadron Phosphate Topical Cream ... 1686
- Decadron Phosphate with Xylocaine Injection, Sterile ... 1683
- Dexacort Phosphate in Respihaler ... 1606
- Dexacort Phosphate in Turbinaire ... 1607
- NeoDecadron Sterile Ophthalmic Ointment ... 1755
- NeoDecadron Sterile Ophthalmic Solution ... 1756
- NeoDecadron Topical Cream ... 1757

Dezocine (Potentiates orthostatic hypotension). Products include:
- Dalgan Injection ... 529

Diazoxide (Additive effect or potentiation). Products include:
- Hyperstat I.V. Injection ... 2504
- Proglycem ... 575

Diclofenac Potassium (Reduces the diuretic, naturetic, and antihypertensive effects of thiazides). Products include:
- Cataflam Tablets ... 833

Diclofenac Sodium (Reduces the diuretic, naturetic, and antihypertensive effects of thiazides). Products include:
- Voltaren Ophthalmic Sterile Ophthalmic Solution ... ⊙ 264
- Cataflam/Voltaren/Voltaren-XR ... 833

Diltiazem Hydrochloride (Additive effect or potentiation). Products include:
- Cardizem CD Capsules ... 1251
- Cardizem SR Capsules ... 1255
- Cardizem Injectable ... 1253
- Cardizem Tablets ... 1257
- Dilacor XR Extended-release Capsules ... 2183
- Tiazac Capsules ... 1019

Doxazosin Mesylate (Additive effect or potentiation). Products include:
- Cardura Tablets ... 1993

Enalapril Maleate (Additive effect or potentiation). Products include:
- Vaseretic Tablets ... 1810
- Vasotec Tablets ... 1816

Enalaprilat (Additive effect or potentiation). Products include:
- Vasotec I.V. ... 1814

Esmolol Hydrochloride (Additive effect or potentiation). Products include:
- Brevibloc (esmolol HCl) Injection ... 1860

Etodolac (Reduces the diuretic, naturetic, and antihypertensive effects of thiazides). Products include:
- Lodine Capsules and Tablets ... 2849

Felodipine (Additive effect or potentiation). Products include:
- Plendil Extended-Release Tablets ... 514

Fenoprofen Calcium (Reduces the diuretic, naturetic, and antihypertensive effects of thiazides). Products include:
- Nalfon 200 Pulvules & Nalfon Tablets ... 933

Fentanyl (Potentiates orthostatic hypotension). Products include:
- Duragesic Transdermal System ... 1336

Fentanyl Citrate (Potentiates orthostatic hypotension). Products include:
- Sublimaze Injection ... 463

Fludrocortisone Acetate (Intensified electrolyte depletion, particularly hypokalemia). Products include:
- Florinef Acetate Tablets ... 506

Flurbiprofen (Reduces the diuretic, naturetic, and antihypertensive effects of thiazides).
- No products indexed under this heading.

Fosinopril Sodium (Additive effect or potentiation). Products include:
- Monopril Tablets ... 762

Furosemide (Additive effect or potentiation). Products include:
- Lasix Injection, Oral Solution and Tablets ... 1267

Glimepiride (Dosage adjustment of the antidiabetic drug may be required). Products include:
- Amaryl Tablets ... 1241

Glipizide (Dosage adjustment of the antidiabetic drug may be required). Products include:
- Glucotrol Tablets ... 2011
- Glucotrol XL Extended Release Tablets ... 2012

Glyburide (Dosage adjustment of the antidiabetic drug may be required). Products include:
- DiaBeta Tablets ... 1265
- Glynase PresTab Tablets ... 2091
- Micronase Tablets ... 2099

Guanabenz Acetate (Additive effect or potentiation).
- No products indexed under this heading.

Guanethidine Monosulfate (Additive effect or potentiation). Products include:
- Esimil Tablets ... 840
- Ismelin Tablets ... 845

Hydralazine Hydrochloride (Additive effect or potentiation). Products include:
- Apresazide Capsules ... 824
- Apresoline Hydrochloride Tablets ... 826
- Hydralazine Hydrochloride Injection USP ... 2712
- Ser-Ap-Es Tablets ... 867

Hydrocodone Bitartrate (Potentiates orthostatic hypotension). Products include:
- Codiclear DH Syrup ... 808
- Duratuss HD Elixir ... 2750
- Histussin D Liquid ... 670
- Hycodan Tablets and Syrup ... 946
- Hycomine Compound Tablets ... 948
- Hycomine ... 947
- Hycotuss Expectorant Syrup ... 950
- Hydrocet Capsules ... 787
- Lorcet 10/650 Tablets ... 1016
- Lortab ... 2751
- Tussend ... 1830
- Tussend Expectorant ... 1831
- Vicodin Tablets ... 1404
- Vicodin ES Tablets ... 1405
- Vicodin HP Tablets ... 1403
- Vicodin Tuss Expectorant ... 1406
- Zydone Capsules ... 967

Hydrocodone Polistirex (Potentiates orthostatic hypotension). Products include:
- Tussionex Pennkinetic Extended-Release Suspension ... 1624

Hydrocortisone (Intensified electrolyte depletion, particularly hypokalemia). Products include:
- Anusol-HC Cream 2.5% ... 1953
- Aquanil HC Lotion ... 1989
- Maximum Strength Cortaid Spray ... ▣ 800
- CORTENEMA ... 2713
- Cortisporin Ointment ... 1074
- Cortisporin Ophthalmic Ointment Sterile ... 1074
- Cortisporin Ophthalmic Suspension Sterile ... 1075
- Cortisporin Otic Solution Sterile ... 1076
- Cortisporin Otic Suspension Sterile ... 1077
- Cortizone-5 ... ▣ 795
- Cortizone-10 ... ▣ 795
- Hydrocortone Tablets ... 1715
- Hytone ... 922
- Hytone Ointment 2 ½% ... 923
- Massengill Medicated Soft Cloth Towelettes ... 2628
- Pediotic Suspension Sterile ... 1140
- Preparation H Hydrocortisone 1% Cream ... ▣ 843
- ProctoCream-HC 2.5% ... 2552
- VōSoL HC Otic Solution ... 2786

Hydrocortisone Acetate (Intensified electrolyte depletion, particularly hypokalemia). Products include:
- Analpram-HC Rectal Cream 1% and 2.5% ... 993
- Anusol HC-1 Hydrocortisone Anti-Itch Ointment ... ▣ 810
- Anusol-HC Suppositories ... 1954
- Caldecort Anti-Itch Hydrocortisone Cream ... ▣ 651
- Coly-Mycin S Otic w/Neomycin & Hydrocortisone ... 1965
- Cortaid ... ▣ 800
- Cortifoam ... 2540
- Cortisporin Cream ... 1073
- Epifoam ... 2543
- Hydrocortone Acetate Sterile Suspension ... 1712
- Mantadil Cream ... 1124
- Nupercainal Hydrocortisone 1% Cream ... ▣ 661
- Pramosone Cream, Lotion & Ointment ... 995
- ProctoFoam-HC ... 2552
- Terra-Cortril Ophthalmic Suspension ... 2033

Hydrocortisone Sodium Phosphate (Intensified electrolyte depletion, particularly hypokalemia). Products include:
- Hydrocortone Phosphate Injection, Sterile ... 1713

Hydrocortisone Sodium Succinate (Intensified electrolyte depletion, particularly hypokalemia).
- No products indexed under this heading.

Hydroflumethiazide (Additive effect or potentiation). Products include:
- Diucardin Tablets ... 2824

Hydromorphone Hydrochloride (Potentiates orthostatic hypotension). Products include:
- Dilaudid Ampules ... 1382
- Dilaudid Cough Syrup ... 1383
- Dilaudid-HP Injection ... 1384
- Dilaudid-HP Lyophilized Powder 250 mg ... 1384
- Dilaudid ... 1382
- Dilaudid Oral Liquid ... 1386
- Dilaudid ... 1382
- Dilaudid Tablets - 8 mg ... 1386

(▣ Described in PDR For Nonprescription Drugs) (⊙ Described in PDR For Ophthalmology)

865 **Interactions Index** **Prinzide**

Ibuprofen (Reduces the diuretic, naturetic, and antihypertensive effects of thiazides). Products include:
- Advil Cold and Sinus Caplets and Tablets ... 837
- Advil Ibuprofen Tablets, Caplets and Gel Caplets ... 836
- Children's Motrin Ibuprofen Oral Suspension ... 1558
- IBU Tablets ... 1389
- Ibuprohm ... 713
- Motrin IB Caplets, Tablets, and Gelcaps ... 802
- Motrin Ibuprofen Suspension, Oral Drops, Chewable Tablets, Caplets ... 1563
- Nuprin Ibuprofen/Analgesic Tablets & Caplets ... 645
- Vicks DayQuil SINUS Pressure & PAIN Relief with IBUPROFEN ... 735

Indapamide (Additive effect or potentiation).
- No products indexed under this heading.

Indomethacin (Reduces lisinopril effects; reduces the diuretic, naturetic and antihypertensive effects of thiazides). Products include:
- Indocin ... 1723

Indomethacin Sodium Trihydrate (Reduces the diuretic, naturetic, and antihypertensive effects of thiazides; reduces lisinopril effects). Products include:
- Indocin I.V. ... 1727

Insulin, Human (Dosage adjustment of the antidiabetic drug may be required).
- No products indexed under this heading.

Insulin, Human Isophane Suspension (Dosage adjustment of the antidiabetic drug may be required). Products include:
- Novolin N Human Insulin 10 ml Vials ... 1846

Insulin, Human NPH (Dosage adjustment of the antidiabetic drug may be required). Products include:
- Humulin N, 100 Units ... 1495
- Novolin N PenFill 1.5 ml Cartridges Durable Insulin Delivery System ... 1849
- Novolin N Prefilled Syringe Disposable Insulin Delivery System ... 1850

Insulin, Human Regular (Dosage adjustment of the antidiabetic drug may be required). Products include:
- Humulin R, 100 Units ... 1497
- Novolin R Human Insulin 10 ml Vials ... 1846
- Novolin R PenFill 1.5 ml Cartridges Durable Insulin Delivery System ... 1849
- Novolin R Prefilled Syringe Disposable Insulin Delivery System ... 1850
- Velosulin BR Human Insulin 10 ml Vials ... 1847

Insulin, Human, Zinc Suspension (Dosage adjustment of the antidiabetic drug may be required). Products include:
- Humulin L, 100 Units ... 1494
- Humulin U, 100 Units ... 1498
- Novolin L Human Insulin 10 ml Vials ... 1846

Insulin Lispro, Human (Dosage adjustment of the antidiabetic drug may be required). Products include:
- Humalog Injection ... 1488

Insulin, NPH (Dosage adjustment of the antidiabetic drug may be required). Products include:
- NPH, 100 Units ... 1502
- Pork NPH, 100 Units ... 1506
- Purified Pork NPH Isophane Insulin ... 1852

Insulin, Regular (Dosage adjustment of the antidiabetic drug may be required). Products include:
- Regular, 100 Units ... 1503
- Pork Regular, 100 Units ... 1507
- Pork Regular (Concentrated), 500 Units ... 1508
- Purified Pork Regular Insulin ... 1852

Insulin, Zinc Crystals (Dosage adjustment of the antidiabetic drug may be required). Products include:
- NPH, 100 Units ... 1502

Insulin, Zinc Suspension (Dosage adjustment of the antidiabetic drug may be required). Products include:
- Iletin I ... 1501
- Lente, 100 Units ... 1501
- Iletin II ... 1504
- Pork Lente, 100 Units ... 1504
- Purified Pork Lente Insulin ... 1852

Isradipine (Additive effect or potentiation). Products include:
- DynaCirc Capsules ... 2381
- DynaCirc CR Tablets ... 2383

Ketoprofen (Reduces the diuretic, naturetic, and antihypertensive effects of thiazides). Products include:
- Actron Caplets and Tablets ... 608
- Orudis Capsules ... 2874
- Orudis KT ... 842
- Oruvail Capsules ... 2874

Ketorolac Tromethamine (Reduces the diuretic, naturetic, and antihypertensive effects of thiazides). Products include:
- Acular Sterile Ophthalmic Solution ... 470
- Toradol ... 2319

Labetalol Hydrochloride (Additive effect or potentiation). Products include:
- Normodyne Injection ... 2519
- Normodyne Tablets ... 2522
- Trandate ... 1158

Levorphanol Tartrate (Potentiates orthostatic hypotension). Products include:
- Levo-Dromoran ... 2297

Lithium Carbonate (Potential for lithium toxicity; monitor lithium levels frequently). Products include:
- Eskalith ... 2658
- Lithium Carbonate Capsules & Tablets ... 2352
- Lithonate/Lithotabs/Lithobid ... 2721

Lithium Citrate (Potential for lithium toxicity; monitor lithium levels frequently).
- No products indexed under this heading.

Losartan Potassium (Additive effect or potentiation). Products include:
- Cozaar Tablets ... 1668
- Hyzaar Tablets ... 1720

Mecamylamine Hydrochloride (Additive effect or potentiation). Products include:
- Inversine Tablets ... 1729

Meclofenamate Sodium (Reduces the diuretic, naturetic, and antihypertensive effects of thiazides).
- No products indexed under this heading.

Mefenamic Acid (Reduces the diuretic, naturetic, and antihypertensive effects of thiazides). Products include:
- Ponstel ... 1982

Meperidine Hydrochloride (Potentiates orthostatic hypotension). Products include:
- Demerol ... 2438
- Mepergan Injection ... 2859

Mephobarbital (Potentiates orthostatic hypotension). Products include:
- Mebaral Tablets ... 2452

Metformin Hydrochloride (Dosage adjustment of the antidiabetic drug may be required). Products include:
- Glucophage Tablets ... 754

Methadone Hydrochloride (Potentiates orthostatic hypotension). Products include:
- Methadone Hydrochloride Oral Concentrate ... 2356
- Methadone Hydrochloride Oral Solution & Tablets ... 2357

Methyclothiazide (Additive effect or potentiation). Products include:
- Enduron Tablets ... 424

Methyldopa (Additive effect or potentiation). Products include:
- Aldoclor Tablets ... 1638
- Aldomet Oral ... 1640
- Aldoril Tablets ... 1644

Methyldopate Hydrochloride (Additive effect or potentiation). Products include:
- Aldomet Ester HCl Injection ... 1642

Methylprednisolone Acetate (Intensified electrolyte depletion, particularly hypokalemia).
- No products indexed under this heading.

Methylprednisolone Sodium Succinate (Intensified electrolyte depletion, particularly hypokalemia).
- No products indexed under this heading.

Metocurine Iodide (Possible increased responsiveness to the muscle relaxant). Products include:
- Metubine Iodide Vials ... 932

Metolazone (Additive effect or potentiation). Products include:
- Mykrox Tablets ... 1617
- Zaroxolyn Tablets ... 1625

Metoprolol Succinate (Additive effect or potentiation). Products include:
- Toprol-XL Tablets ... 560

Metoprolol Tartrate (Additive effect or potentiation). Products include:
- Lopressor ... 848
- Lopressor HCT Tablets ... 850

Metyrosine (Additive effect or potentiation). Products include:
- Demser Capsules ... 1690

Minoxidil (Additive effect or potentiation).
- No products indexed under this heading.

Mivacurium Chloride (Possible increased responsiveness to the muscle relaxant). Products include:
- Mivacron ... 1125

Moexipril Hydrochloride (Additive effect or potentiation). Products include:
- Univasc Tablets ... 2553

Morphine Sulfate (Potentiates orthostatic hypotension). Products include:
- Astramorph/PF Injection, USP (Preservative-Free) ... 526
- Duramorph Injection ... 983
- Infumorph 200 and Infumorph 500 Sterile Solutions ... 985
- Kadian Capsules ... 2948
- MS Contin Tablets ... 2149
- MSIR ... 2152
- Oramorph SR (Morphine Sulfate Sustained Release Tablets) ... 2359
- RMS Suppositories CII ... 2766
- Roxanol ... 2365

Nabumetone (Reduces the diuretic, naturetic, and antihypertensive effects of thiazides). Products include:
- Relafen Tablets ... 2688

Nadolol (Additive effect or potentiation).
- No products indexed under this heading.

Naproxen (Reduces the diuretic, naturetic, and antihypertensive effects of thiazides). Products include:
- Anaprox/Naprosyn ... 2277

Naproxen Sodium (Reduces the diuretic, naturetic, and antihypertensive effects of thiazides). Products include:
- Aleve ... 2124
- Anaprox/Naprosyn ... 2277
- Naprelan Tablets ... 2861

Nicardipine Hydrochloride (Additive effect or potentiation). Products include:
- Cardene Capsules ... 2261
- Cardene I.V. ... 2815
- Cardene SR Capsules ... 2264

Nifedipine (Additive effect or potentiation). Products include:
- Adalat Capsules (10 mg and 20 mg) ... 580
- Adalat CC ... 582
- Procardia Capsules ... 2024
- Procardia XL Extended Release Tablets ... 2026

Nisoldipine (Additive effect or potentiation). Products include:
- Sular Tablets ... 2961

Nitroglycerin (Additive effect or potentiation). Products include:
- Deponit NTG Transdermal Delivery System ... 2541
- Nitro-Bid IV ... 1270
- Nitro-Bid Ointment ... 1272
- Nitro-Dur (nitroglycerin) Transdermal Infusion System ... 1365
- Nitrolingual Spray ... 2193
- Nitrostat Tablets ... 1981
- Transderm-Nitro Transdermal Therapeutic System ... 878

Norepinephrine Bitartrate (Possible decreased response to pressor amines). Products include:
- Levophed Bitartrate Injection ... 2445

Opium Alkaloids (Potentiates orthostatic hypotension).
- No products indexed under this heading.

Oxaprozin (Reduces the diuretic, naturetic, and antihypertensive effects of thiazides). Products include:
- Daypro Caplets ... 2578

Oxycodone Hydrochloride (Potentiates orthostatic hypotension). Products include:
- OxyContin Tablets ... 2163
- OxyIR Capsules ... 2167
- Percocet Tablets ... 955
- Percodan Tablets ... 955
- Percodan-Demi Tablets ... 956
- Roxicodone Tablets, Oral Solution & Intensol (Oxycodone) ... 2366
- Tylox Capsules ... 1593

Pancuronium Bromide (Possible increased responsiveness to the muscle relaxant).
- No products indexed under this heading.

Penbutolol Sulfate (Additive effect or potentiation). Products include:
- Levatol Tablets ... 2547

Pentobarbital Sodium (Potentiates orthostatic hypotension). Products include:
- Nembutal Sodium Capsules ... 440
- Nembutal Sodium Solution ... 442
- Nembutal Sodium Suppositories ... 444

Phenobarbital (Potentiates orthostatic hypotension). Products include:
- Arco-Lase Plus Tablets ... 513
- Bellergal-S Tablets ... 2375
- Donnatal ... 2234
- Donnatal Extentabs ... 2234
- Donnatal Tablets ... 2234
- Phenobarbital Elixir and Tablets ... 1523
- Quadrinal Tablets ... 1398

Phenoxybenzamine Hydrochloride (Additive effect or potentiation). Products include:
- Dibenzyline Capsules ... 2650

IMPORTANT NOTE: Always consult each drug listing in the patient's regimen for possible interactions.

Prinzide | Interactions Index | 866

Phentolamine Mesylate (Additive effect or potentiation). Products include:
- Regitine Vials 864

Phenylbutazone (Reduces the diuretic, naturetic, and antihypertensive effects of thiazides).
- No products indexed under this heading.

Pindolol (Additive effect or potentiation). Products include:
- Visken Tablets 2428

Piroxicam (Reduces the diuretic, naturetic, and antihypertensive effects of thiazides). Products include:
- Feldene Capsules 2008

Polythiazide (Additive effect or potentiation). Products include:
- Minizide Capsules 2016

Potassium Acid Phosphate (Concomitant therapy may lead to hyperkalemia). Products include:
- K-Phos Original Formula 'Sodium Free' Tablets 633

Potassium Bicarbonate (Concomitant therapy may lead to hyperkalemia). Products include:
- Alka-Seltzer Gold Effervescent Antacid .... ▣ 611

Potassium Chloride (Concomitant therapy may lead to hyperkalemia). Products include:
- Chlor-3 Condiment 1003
- Colyte and Colyte-flavored 2540
- GoLYTELY 694
- K-Dur Microburst Release System (potassium chloride, USP) E.R. Tablets 1364
- K-Lor Powder Packets 438
- K-Norm Capsules 1615
- K-Tab Filmtab 439
- Micro-K 2237
- Micro-K LS Packets 2238
- NuLYTELY 694
- Cherry Flavor NuLYTELY 694
- Rum-K Syrup 1004
- Slow-K Extended-Release Tablets 869

Potassium Citrate (Concomitant therapy may lead to hyperkalemia). Products include:
- Polycitra Syrup 574
- Polycitra-K Crystals 574
- Polycitra-K Oral Solution 575
- Polycitra-LC 574
- Urocit-K Tablets 1828

Potassium Gluconate (Concomitant therapy may lead to hyperkalemia).
- No products indexed under this heading.

Potassium Phosphate, Dibasic (Concomitant therapy may lead to hyperkalemia).
- No products indexed under this heading.

Potassium Phosphate, Monobasic (Concomitant therapy may lead to hyperkalemia). Products include:
- K-Phos Neutral Tablets 633
- K-Phos Original Formula 'Sodium Free' Tablets 633

Prazosin Hydrochloride (Additive effect or potentiation). Products include:
- Minipress Capsules 2015
- Minizide Capsules 2016

Prednisolone Acetate (Intensified electrolyte depletion, particularly hypokalemia). Products include:
- AK-CIDE .... ◉ 203
- AK-CIDE Ointment .... ◉ 203
- Blephamide Liquifilm Sterile Ophthalmic Suspension 472
- Blephamide Ointment .... ◉ 234
- Econopred & Econopred Plus Ophthalmic Suspensions .... ◉ 216
- Poly-Pred Liquifilm .... ◉ 246
- Pred Forte .... ◉ 247
- Pred Mild .... ◉ 250
- Pred-G Liquifilm Sterile Ophthalmic Suspension .... ◉ 248
- Pred-G S.O.P. Sterile Ophthalmic Ointment .... ◉ 249

Prednisolone Sodium Phosphate (Intensified electrolyte depletion, particularly hypokalemia). Products include:
- AK-PRED .... ◉ 204
- Hydeltrasol Injection, Sterile 1708
- Pediapred Oral Solution 1618

Prednisolone Tebutate (Intensified electrolyte depletion, particularly hypokalemia). Products include:
- Hydeltra-T.B.A. Sterile Suspension 1710

Prednisone (Intensified electrolyte depletion, particularly hypokalemia).
- No products indexed under this heading.

Propoxyphene Hydrochloride (Potentiates orthostatic hypotension). Products include:
- Darvon 1475
- Wygesic Tablets 2930

Propoxyphene Napsylate (Potentiates orthostatic hypotension). Products include:
- Darvon-N/Darvocet-N 1473

Propranolol Hydrochloride (Additive effect or potentiation). Products include:
- Inderal 2834
- Inderal LA Long Acting Capsules 2836
- Inderide Tablets 2838
- Inderide LA Long Acting Capsules .. 2840

Quinapril Hydrochloride (Additive effect or potentiation). Products include:
- Accupril Tablets 1950

Ramipril (Additive effect or potentiation). Products include:
- Altace Capsules 1238

Rauwolfia Serpentina (Additive effect or potentiation).
- No products indexed under this heading.

Rescinnamine (Additive effect or potentiation).
- No products indexed under this heading.

Reserpine (Additive effect or potentiation). Products include:
- Diupres Tablets 1691
- Hydropres Tablets 1718
- Ser-Ap-Es Tablets 867

Rocuronium Bromide (Possible increased responsiveness to the muscle relaxant). Products include:
- Zemuron Injection 1885

Secobarbital Sodium (Potentiates orthostatic hypotension). Products include:
- Seconal Sodium Pulvules 1529

Sodium Nitroprusside (Additive effect or potentiation).
- No products indexed under this heading.

Sotalol Hydrochloride (Additive effect or potentiation). Products include:
- Betapace Tablets 637

Spirapril Hydrochloride (Additive effect or potentiation).
- No products indexed under this heading.

Spironolactone (Concomitant therapy may lead to hyperkalemia). Products include:
- Aldactazide Tablets 2556
- Aldactone Tablets 2558

Sufentanil Citrate (Potentiates orthostatic hypotension). Products include:
- Sufenta Injection 1355

Sulindac (Reduces the diuretic, naturetic, and antihypertensive effects of thiazides). Products include:
- Clinoril Tablets 1658

Terazosin Hydrochloride (Additive effect or potentiation). Products include:
- Hytrin Capsules 434

Thiamylal Sodium (Potentiates orthostatic hypotension).
- No products indexed under this heading.

Timolol Maleate (Additive effect or potentiation). Products include:
- Blocadren Tablets 1654
- Timolide Tablets 1791
- Timoptic in Ocudose 1796
- Timoptic Sterile Ophthalmic Solution 1794
- Timoptic-XE 1798

Tolazamide (Dosage adjustment of the antidiabetic drug may be required).
- No products indexed under this heading.

Tolbutamide (Dosage adjustment of the antidiabetic drug may be required).
- No products indexed under this heading.

Tolmetin Sodium (Reduces the diuretic, naturetic, and antihypertensive effects of thiazides). Products include:
- Tolectin (200, 400 and 600 mg) .. 1591

Torsemide (Additive effect or potentiation). Products include:
- Demadex Tablets and Injection 691

Trandolapril (Additive effect or potentiation). Products include:
- Mavik Tablets 1407

Triamcinolone (Intensified electrolyte depletion, particularly hypokalemia).
- No products indexed under this heading.

Triamcinolone Acetonide (Intensified electrolyte depletion, particularly hypokalemia). Products include:
- Azmacort Oral Inhaler 2175
- Nasacort AQ Nasal Spray 2191
- Nasacort Nasal Inhaler 2189

Triamcinolone Diacetate (Intensified electrolyte depletion, particularly hypokalemia).
- No products indexed under this heading.

Triamcinolone Hexacetonide (Intensified electrolyte depletion, particularly hypokalemia).
- No products indexed under this heading.

Triamterene (Concomitant therapy may lead to hyperkalemia). Products include:
- Dyazide Capsules 2653
- Dyrenium Capsules 2655

Trimethaphan Camsylate (Additive effect or potentiation).
- No products indexed under this heading.

Vecuronium Bromide (Possible increased responsiveness to the muscle relaxant). Products include:
- Norcuron for Injection 1875

Verapamil Hydrochloride (Additive effect or potentiation). Products include:
- Calan SR Caplets 2571
- Calan Tablets 2568
- Covera-HS Tablets 2573
- Isoptin Injectable 1391
- Isoptin Oral Tablets 1393
- Isoptin SR Tablets 1395
- Verelan Capsules 1455

Food Interactions

Alcohol (Potentiates orthostatic hypotension).

PRISCOLINE HYDROCHLORIDE AMPULS
(Tolazoline Hydrochloride) 864
None cited in PDR database.

PRIVINE NASAL DROPS
(Naphazoline Hydrochloride) .... ▣ 663
None cited in PDR database.

PRIVINE NASAL SPRAY
(Naphazoline Hydrochloride) .... ▣ 663
None cited in PDR database.

PRO-BANTHINE TABLETS
(Propantheline Bromide) 2226
May interact with antiarrhythmics, antihistamines, phenothiazines, tricyclic antidepressants, corticosteroids, anticholinergics, belladonna products, narcotic analgesics, and certain other agents. Compounds in these categories include:

Acebutolol Hydrochloride (Excessive cholinergic blockade). Products include:
- Sectral Capsules 2914

Acrivastine (Excessive cholinergic blockade). Products include:
- Semprex-D Capsules 1620

Adenosine (Excessive cholinergic blockade). Products include:
- Adenocard Injection 1021
- Adenoscan 1022

Alfentanil Hydrochloride (Excessive cholinergic blockade). Products include:
- Alfenta Injection 1334

Amiodarone Hydrochloride (Excessive cholinergic blockade). Products include:
- Cordarone Intravenous 2821
- Cordarone Tablets 2818

Amitriptyline Hydrochloride (Excessive cholinergic blockade). Products include:
- Elavil 2945
- Etrafon 2495
- Limbitrol 2333
- Triavil Tablets 1800

Amoxapine (Excessive cholinergic blockade). Products include:
- Asendin Tablets 1419

Astemizole (Excessive cholinergic blockade). Products include:
- Hismanal Tablets 1341

Atropine Sulfate (Excessive cholinergic blockade; increased intraocular pressure). Products include:
- Arco-Lase Plus Tablets 513
- Atrohist Plus Tablets 1605
- Donnatal 2234
- Donnatal Extentabs 2234
- Donnatal Tablets 2234
- Lomotil 2591
- Motofen Tablets 789
- Urised Tablets 2123

Azatadine Maleate (Excessive cholinergic blockade). Products include:
- Trinalin Repetabs Tablets 1373

Belladonna Alkaloids (Excessive cholinergic blockade; increased intraocular pressure). Products include:
- Bellergal-S Tablets 2375
- Hyland's Bedwetting Tablets .... ▣ 788
- Hyland's EnurAid Tablets .... ▣ 789
- Hyland's Headache Tablets .... ▣ 790
- Hyland's Teething Tablets .... ▣ 790
- Similasan Eye Drops #1 .... ▣ 769

Benztropine Mesylate (Excessive cholinergic blockade; increased intraocular pressure). Products include:
- Cogentin 1661

(▣ Described in PDR For Nonprescription Drugs) (◉ Described in PDR For Ophthalmology)

Betamethasone Acetate (Increased intraocular pressure). Products include:
- Celestone Soluspan Suspension 2484

Betamethasone Sodium Phosphate (Increased intraocular pressure). Products include:
- Celestone Soluspan Suspension 2484

Biperiden Hydrochloride (Excessive cholinergic blockade; increased intraocular pressure). Products include:
- Akineton 1380

Bretylium Tosylate (Excessive cholinergic blockade).
- No products indexed under this heading.

Bromodiphenhydramine Hydrochloride (Excessive cholinergic blockade).
- No products indexed under this heading.

Brompheniramine Maleate (Excessive cholinergic blockade). Products include:
- Alka-Seltzer Plus Sinus Medicine .. 611
- Bromfed Capsules (Extended-Release) 1832
- Bromfed Syrup 712
- Bromfed Tablets 1832
- Bromfed-DM Cough Syrup 1832
- Bromfed-PD Capsules (Extended-Release) 1832
- Dimetane-DC Cough Syrup 2232
- Dimetane-DX Cough Syrup 2233
- Dimetapp Allergy Dye-Free Elixir .. 838
- Dimetapp Allergy Sinus Caplets 838
- Dimetapp Cold & Allergy Chewable Tablets 838
- Dimetapp Cold & Cough Liqui-Gels 839
- Dimetapp Cold & Fever Suspension 839
- Dimetapp DM Elixir 840
- Dimetapp Elixir 840
- Dimetapp Extentabs 841
- Dimetapp Tablets/Liqui-Gels 841
- Rondec Chewable Tablets 974
- Vicks DayQuil Allergy Relief 12-Hour Extended Release Tablets.. 733
- Vicks DayQuil Allergy Relief 4-Hour Tablets 733

Buprenorphine (Excessive cholinergic blockade). Products include:
- Buprenex Injectable 2170

Cetirizine Hydrochloride (Excessive cholinergic blockade). Products include:
- Zyrtec Tablets 2053

Chlorpheniramine Maleate (Excessive cholinergic blockade). Products include:
- Alka-Seltzer Plus Cold Medicine 611
- Alka-Seltzer Plus Cold Medicine Liqui-Gels 612
- Alka-Seltzer Plus Cold & Cough Medicine 611
- Alka-Seltzer Plus Cold & Cough Medicine Liqui-Gels 612
- Alka-Seltzer Plus Flu & Body Aches Effervescent Tablets......... 612
- Allerest Maximum Strength 649
- Allerest Sinus Pain Formula 649
- Ana-Kit Anaphylaxis Emergency Treatment Kit 611
- Atrohist Pediatric Capsules....... 1603
- Atrohist Plus Tablets 1605
- BC Cold Powder Multi-Symptom Formula (Cold-Sinus-Allergy) 631
- Cerose DM 853
- Cheracol Plus Head Cold/Cough Formula 741
- Children's TYLENOL Cold Multi-Symptom Chewable Tablets and Liquid 1559
- Children's TYLENOL Cold Plus Cough Multi Symptom Chewable Tablets and Liquid 1560
- Children's TYLENOL Flu Suspension Liquid 1560
- Children's Vicks DayQuil Allergy Relief 730
- Children's Vicks NyQuil Cold/Cough Relief 731

- Chlor-Trimeton Allergy Decongestant Tablets 759
- Chlor-Trimeton Allergy Tablets 758
- Allergy-Sinus Comtrex Multi-Symptom Allergy-Sinus Formula Tablets and Caplets 639
- Comtrex Multi-Symptom 638
- Contac Continuous Action Nasal Decongestant/Antihistamine 12 Hour Capsules 773
- Contac Maximum Strength Continuous Action Decongestant/Antihistamine 12 Hour Caplets.. 772
- Contac Severe Cold and Flu Formula Caplets 773
- Coricidin Cold + Flu Tablets........... 760
- Coricidin Cough + Cold Tablets 760
- Coricidin 'D' Decongestant Tablets 760
- D.A. II Tablets 972
- D.A. Chewable Tablets 970
- Dura-Tap/PD Capsules 970
- Dura-Vent/DA Tablets 972
- Efidac 24 Chlorpheniramine....... 655
- Extendryl 1003
- Fedahist Gyrocaps.................. 2545
- Hycomine Compound Tablets 948
- Kronofed-A 994
- Nolamine Timed-Release Tablets 790
- Novahistine Elixir 782
- Ornade Spansule Capsules 2678
- PediaCare Cough-Cold Chewable Tablets and Liquid............... 1569
- PediaCare NightRest Cough-Cold Liquid 1569
- Pediatric Vicks 44m Cough & Cold Relief 737
- Pyrroxate Caplets 742
- Ryna 804
- Sinarest 663
- Sine-Off Sinus Medicine 784
- Singlet Tablets 785
- Sinulin Tablets 792
- Sinutab Sinus Allergy Medication, Maximum Strength Tablets and Caplets 823
- Sudafed Cold & Allergy Tablets...... 826
- Teldrin 12 Hour Antihistamine/ Nasal Decongestant Allergy Relief Capsules 786
- TheraFlu Flu and Cold Medicine 750
- Theraflu Maximum Strength Flu and Cold Medicine For Sore Throat 751
- TheraFlu Flu, Cold and Cough Medicine 750
- TheraFlu Maximum Strength Nighttime Flu, Cold & Cough Medicine 751
- Triaminic Night Time 754
- Triaminic Syrup 755
- Triaminic Triaminicol Cold & Cough 756
- Triaminicin Tablets 756
- Tussend 1830
- TYLENOL Allergy Sinus, Maximum Strength Caplets and Gelcaps ... 1571
- TYLENOL Cold Medication, Multi-Symptom Formula Tablets and Caplets 1572
- TYLENOL Cold Medication, Multi-Symptom Hot Liquid Packets 1572
- Vicks 44 LiquiCaps Cough, Cold & Flu Relief 728
- Vicks 44M Cough, Cold & Flu Relief 729

Chlorpheniramine Polistirex (Excessive cholinergic blockade). Products include:
- Tussionex Pennkinetic Extended-Release Suspension 1624

Chlorpheniramine Tannate (Excessive cholinergic blockade). Products include:
- Atrohist Pediatric Suspension 1604
- Atrohist Pediatric Suspension Dye-Free 1604
- Rynatan 2781
- Rynatuss 2782

Chlorpromazine (Excessive cholinergic blockade; potentiated sedative effect). Products include:
- Thorazine Suppositories........... 2701

Chlorpromazine Hydrochloride (Excessive cholinergic blockade; potentiated sedative effect). Products include:
- Thorazine 2701

Clemastine Fumarate (Excessive cholinergic blockade). Products include:
- Tavist Syrup 2426
- Tavist Tablets 2427
- Tavist-1 12 Hour Relief Tablets 749
- Tavist-D 12 Hour Relief Tablets 750

Clidinium Bromide (Excessive cholinergic blockade; increased intraocular pressure). Products include:
- Librax Capsules 2330

Clomipramine Hydrochloride (Excessive cholinergic blockade). Products include:
- Anafranil Capsules 819

Codeine Phosphate (Excessive cholinergic blockade). Products include:
- Brontex 2130
- Dimetane-DC Cough Syrup 2232
- Fioricet with Codeine Capsules 2387
- Fiorinal with Codeine Capsules 2390
- Nucofed 2225
- Phenergan with Codeine 2883
- Phenergan VC with Codeine 2888
- Robitussin A-C Syrup 2248
- Robitussin-DAC Syrup 2249
- Ryna 804
- Soma Compound w/Codeine Tablets 2784
- Tylenol with Codeine 1592

Cortisone Acetate (Increased intraocular pressure). Products include:
- Cortone Acetate Sterile Suspension 1663
- Cortone Acetate Tablets 1664

Cyproheptadine Hydrochloride (Excessive cholinergic blockade). Products include:
- Periactin 1767

Desipramine Hydrochloride (Excessive cholinergic blockade). Products include:
- Norpramin Tablets 1273

Dexamethasone (Increased intraocular pressure). Products include:
- AK-Trol Ointment & Suspension 205
- Decadron Elixir 1676
- Decadron Tablets 1678
- Decaspray Topical Aerosol 1689
- Maxitrol Ophthalmic Ointment and Suspension 222
- TobraDex Ophthalmic Suspension and Ointment 469

Dexamethasone Acetate (Increased intraocular pressure). Products include:
- Dalalone D.P. Injectable 1009
- Decadron-LA Sterile Suspension 1687

Dexamethasone Sodium Phosphate (Increased intraocular pressure). Products include:
- Decadron Phosphate Injection 1680
- Decadron Phosphate Sterile Ophthalmic Ointment 1684
- Decadron Phosphate Sterile Ophthalmic Solution 1685
- Decadron Phosphate Topical Cream 1686
- Decadron Phosphate with Xylocaine Injection, Sterile 1683
- Dexacort Phosphate in Respihaler .. 1606
- Dexacort Phosphate in Turbinaire ... 1607
- NeoDecadron Sterile Ophthalmic Ointment 1755
- NeoDecadron Sterile Ophthalmic Solution 1756
- NeoDecadron Topical Cream 1757

Dexchlorpheniramine Maleate (Excessive cholinergic blockade).
- No products indexed under this heading.

Dezocine (Excessive cholinergic blockade). Products include:
- Dalgan Injection 529

Dicyclomine Hydrochloride (Excessive cholinergic blockade; increased intraocular pressure). Products include:
- Bentyl 1246

Digoxin (Increased serum digoxin levels in patients who are taking slow-dissolving tablets of digoxin). Products include:
- Lanoxicaps 1110
- Lanoxin Elixir Pediatric 1113
- Lanoxin Injection 1116
- Lanoxin Injection Pediatric 1119
- Lanoxin Tablets 1121

Diphenhydramine Citrate (Excessive cholinergic blockade). Products include:
- Excedrin P.M. Analgesic/Sleeping Aid Tablets, Caplets, Liquigels 735

Diphenhydramine Hydrochloride (Excessive cholinergic blockade). Products include:
- Actifed Allergy Daytime/Nighttime Caplets............................ 808
- Actifed Sinus Daytime/Nighttime Tablets and Caplets 809
- Extra Strength Bayer PM Aspirin Plus Sleep Aid 617
- Benadryl Allergy Chewables 811
- Benadryl Allergy/Cold Tablets 811
- Benadryl Allergy Decongestant Liquid Medication 812
- Benadryl Allergy Decongestant Tablets 812
- Benadryl Allergy Liquid Medication 813
- Benadryl Allergy 811
- Benadryl Allergy Sinus Headache Caplets 813
- Benadryl Dye-Free Allergy Liquigel Softgels 813
- Benadryl Dye-Free Allergy Liquid Medication 814
- Benadryl Itch Relief Stick Extra Strength 814
- Benadryl Cream 814
- Benadryl Gel 815
- Benadryl Spray 815
- Benadryl Injection 1955
- Contac Day & Night Cold/Flu Night Caplets 772
- Contac Night Allergy/Sinus Caplets 771
- Extra Strength Doan's P.M. 653
- Excedrin P.M. Analgesic/Sleeping Aid Tablets, Caplets, Liquigels 643
- Nytol QuickCaps Caplets 632
- Sleepinal Night-time Sleep Aid Capsules and Softgels 798
- TYLENOL Allergy Sinus NightTime, Maximum Strength Caplets........... 1571
- TYLENOL Flu NightTime, Maximum Strength Gelcaps 1575
- TYLENOL Flu NightTime, Maximum Strength Hot Medication Packets 1575
- TYLENOL PM Pain Reliever/Sleep Aid, Extra Strength Gelcaps, Caplets, Geltabs 1576
- TYLENOL Severe Allergy Medication Caplets 1571
- Maximum Strength Unisom Sleepgels 1990
- Unisom With Pain Relief-Nighttime Sleep Aid and Pain Reliever......... 1991

Diphenylpyraline Hydrochloride (Excessive cholinergic blockade).
- No products indexed under this heading.

Disopyramide Phosphate (Excessive cholinergic blockade). Products include:
- Norpace 2596

Doxepin Hydrochloride (Excessive cholinergic blockade). Products include:
- Adapin Capsules 1542
- Sinequan 2028
- Zonalon Cream 1042

Drugs, Oral, unspecified (Delayed absorption of other medications given concomitantly).

Fentanyl (Excessive cholinergic blockade). Products include:
- Duragesic Transdermal System ... 1336

Fentanyl Citrate (Excessive cholinergic blockade). Products include:
- Sublimaze Injection 463

IMPORTANT NOTE: Always consult each drug listing in the patient's regimen for possible interactions.

Pro-Banthine **Interactions Index** **868**

Flecainide Acetate (Excessive cholinergic blockade). Products include:
- Tambocor Tablets ... 1555

Fludrocortisone Acetate (Increased intraocular pressure). Products include:
- Florinef Acetate Tablets ... 506

Fluphenazine Decanoate (Excessive cholinergic blockade; potentiated sedative effect). Products include:
- Prolixin Decanoate ... 510

Fluphenazine Enanthate (Excessive cholinergic blockade; potentiated sedative effect). Products include:
- Prolixin Enanthate ... 510

Fluphenazine Hydrochloride (Excessive cholinergic blockade; potentiated sedative effect). Products include:
- Prolixin ... 510

Glycopyrrolate (Excessive cholinergic blockade; increased intraocular pressure). Products include:
- Robinul Forte Tablets ... 2247
- Robinul Injectable ... 2247
- Robinul Tablets ... 2247

Hydrocodone Bitartrate (Excessive cholinergic blockade). Products include:
- Codiclear DH Syrup ... 808
- Duratuss HD Elixir ... 2750
- Histussin D Liquid ... 670
- Hycodan Tablets and Syrup ... 946
- Hycomine Compound Tablets ... 948
- Hycomine ... 947
- Hycotuss Expectorant Syrup ... 950
- Hydrocet Capsules ... 787
- Lorcet 10/650 Tablets ... 1016
- Lortab ... 2751
- Tussend ... 1830
- Tussend Expectorant ... 1831
- Vicodin Tablets ... 1404
- Vicodin ES Tablets ... 1405
- Vicodin HP Tablets ... 1403
- Vicodin Tuss Expectorant ... 1406
- Zydone Capsules ... 967

Hydrocodone Polistirex (Excessive cholinergic blockade). Products include:
- Tussionex Pennkinetic Extended-Release Suspension ... 1624

Hydrocortisone (Increased intraocular pressure). Products include:
- Anusol-HC Cream 2.5% ... 1953
- Aquanil HC Lotion ... 1989
- Maximum Strength Cortaid Spray ▣ 800
- CORTENEMA ... 2713
- Cortisporin Ointment ... 1074
- Cortisporin Ophthalmic Ointment Sterile ... 1074
- Cortisporin Ophthalmic Suspension Sterile ... 1075
- Cortisporin Otic Solution Sterile ... 1076
- Cortisporin Otic Suspension Sterile 1077
- Cortizone-5 ... ▣ 795
- Cortizone-10 ... ▣ 795
- Hydrocortone Tablets ... 1715
- Hytone ... 922
- Hytone Ointment 2 ½% ... 923
- Massengill Medicated Soft Cloth Towelettes ... 2628
- Pediotic Suspension Sterile ... 1140
- Preparation H Hydrocortisone 1% Cream ... ▣ 843
- ProctoCream-HC 2.5% ... 2552
- VōSoL HC Otic Solution ... 2786

Hydrocortisone Acetate (Increased intraocular pressure). Products include:
- Analpram-HC Rectal Cream 1% and 2.5% ... 993
- Anusol HC-1 Hydrocortisone Anti-Itch Ointment ... ▣ 810
- Anusol-HC Suppositories ... 1954
- Caldecort Anti-Itch Hydrocortisone Cream ... ▣ 651
- Coly-Mycin S Otic w/Neomycin & Hydrocortisone ... 1965
- Cortaid ... ▣ 800
- Cortifoam ... 2540
- Cortisporin Cream ... 1073
- Epifoam ... 2543
- Hydrocortone Acetate Sterile Suspension ... 1712
- Mantadil Cream ... 1124
- Nupercainal Hydrocortisone 1% Cream ... ▣ 661
- Pramosone Cream, Lotion & Ointment ... 995
- ProctoFoam-HC ... 2552
- Terra-Cortril Ophthalmic Suspension ... 2033

Hydrocortisone Sodium Phosphate (Increased intraocular pressure). Products include:
- Hydrocortone Phosphate Injection, Sterile ... 1713

Hydrocortisone Sodium Succinate (Increased intraocular pressure).
- No products indexed under this heading.

Hydromorphone Hydrochloride (Excessive cholinergic blockade). Products include:
- Dilaudid Ampules ... 1382
- Dilaudid Cough Syrup ... 1383
- Dilaudid-HP Injection ... 1384
- Dilaudid-HP Lyophilized Powder 250 mg ... 1384
- Dilaudid ... 1382
- Dilaudid Oral Liquid ... 1386
- Dilaudid ... 1382
- Dilaudid Tablets - 8 mg ... 1386

Hyoscyamine (Excessive cholinergic blockade; increased intraocular pressure). Products include:
- Cystospaz Tablets ... 2123
- Urised Tablets ... 2123

Hyoscyamine Sulfate (Excessive cholinergic blockade; increased intraocular pressure). Products include:
- Arco-Lase Plus Tablets ... 513
- Atrohist Plus Tablets ... 1605
- Cystospaz-M Capsules ... 2123
- Donnatal ... 2234
- Donnatal Extentabs ... 2234
- Donnatal Tablets ... 2234
- Kutrase Capsules ... 2546
- Levsin/Levsinex/Levbid ... 2549

Imipramine Hydrochloride (Excessive cholinergic blockade). Products include:
- Tofranil Ampuls ... 873
- Tofranil Tablets ... 875

Imipramine Pamoate (Excessive cholinergic blockade). Products include:
- Tofranil-PM Capsules ... 876

Ipratropium Bromide (Excessive cholinergic blockade; increased intraocular pressure). Products include:
- Atrovent Inhalation Aerosol ... 674
- Atrovent Inhalation Solution ... 675
- Atrovent Nasal Spray 0.03% ... 676
- Atrovent Nasal Spray 0.06% ... 678

Levorphanol Tartrate (Excessive cholinergic blockade). Products include:
- Levo-Dromoran ... 2297

Lidocaine Hydrochloride (Excessive cholinergic blockade). Products include:
- Decadron Phosphate with Xylocaine Injection, Sterile ... 1683
- Unguentine Plus ... ▣ 712
- Xylocaine Injections ... 562

Loratadine (Excessive cholinergic blockade). Products include:
- Claritin Tablets ... 2485
- Claritin-D Tablets ... 2487

Maprotiline Hydrochloride (Excessive cholinergic blockade). Products include:
- Ludiomil Tablets ... 861

Mepenzolate Bromide (Excessive cholinergic blockade; increased intraocular pressure).
- No products indexed under this heading.

Meperidine Hydrochloride (Excessive cholinergic blockade). Products include:
- Demerol ... 2438
- Mepergan Injection ... 2859

Mesoridazine Besylate (Excessive cholinergic blockade; potentiated sedative effect). Products include:
- Serentil ... 689

Methadone Hydrochloride (Excessive cholinergic blockade). Products include:
- Methadone Hydrochloride Oral Concentrate ... 2356
- Methadone Hydrochloride Oral Solution & Tablets ... 2357

Methdilazine Hydrochloride (Excessive cholinergic blockade).
- No products indexed under this heading.

Methotrimeprazine (Excessive cholinergic blockade; potentiated sedative effect). Products include:
- Levoprome ... 1321

Methylprednisolone Acetate (Increased intraocular pressure).
- No products indexed under this heading.

Methylprednisolone Sodium Succinate (Increased intraocular pressure).
- No products indexed under this heading.

Mexiletine Hydrochloride (Excessive cholinergic blockade). Products include:
- Mexitil Capsules ... 684

Moricizine Hydrochloride (Excessive cholinergic blockade). Products include:
- Ethmozine Tablets ... 2217

Morphine Sulfate (Excessive cholinergic blockade). Products include:
- Astramorph/PF Injection, USP (Preservative-Free) ... 526
- Duramorph Injection ... 983
- Infumorph 200 and Infumorph 500 Sterile Solutions ... 985
- Kadian Capsules ... 2948
- MS Contin Tablets ... 2149
- MSIR ... 2152
- Oramorph SR (Morphine Sulfate Sustained Release Tablets) ... 2359
- RMS Suppositories CII ... 2766
- Roxanol ... 2365

Nortriptyline Hydrochloride (Excessive cholinergic blockade). Products include:
- Pamelor ... 2409

Opium Alkaloids (Excessive cholinergic blockade).
- No products indexed under this heading.

Oxybutynin Chloride (Excessive cholinergic blockade; increased intraocular pressure). Products include:
- Ditropan ... 1267

Oxycodone Hydrochloride (Excessive cholinergic blockade). Products include:
- OxyContin Tablets ... 2163
- OxyIR Capsules ... 2167
- Percocet Tablets ... 955
- Percodan Tablets ... 955
- Percodan-Demi Tablets ... 956
- Roxicodone Tablets, Oral Solution & Intensol (Oxycodone) ... 2366
- Tylox Capsules ... 1593

Perphenazine (Excessive cholinergic blockade; potentiated sedative effect). Products include:
- Etrafon ... 2495
- Triavil Tablets ... 1800
- Trilafon ... 2532

Prednisolone Acetate (Increased intraocular pressure). Products include:
- AK-CIDE ... ⊙ 203
- AK-CIDE Ointment ... ⊙ 203
- Blephamide Liquifilm Sterile Ophthalmic Suspension ... 472
- Blephamide Ointment ... ⊙ 234
- Econopred & Econopred Plus Ophthalmic Suspensions ... ⊙ 216
- Poly-Pred Liquifilm ... ⊙ 246
- Pred Forte ... ⊙ 247
- Pred Mild ... ⊙ 250
- Pred-G Liquifilm Sterile Ophthalmic Suspension ... ⊙ 248
- Pred-G S.O.P. Sterile Ophthalmic Ointment ... ⊙ 249

Prednisolone Sodium Phosphate (Increased intraocular pressure). Products include:
- AK-PRED ... ⊙ 204
- Hydeltrasol Injection, Sterile ... 1708
- Pediapred Oral Solution ... 1618

Prednisolone Tebutate (Increased intraocular pressure). Products include:
- Hydeltra-T.B.A. Sterile Suspension 1710

Prednisone (Increased intraocular pressure).
- No products indexed under this heading.

Procainamide Hydrochloride (Excessive cholinergic blockade). Products include:
- Procanbid Extended-Release Tablets ... 1983

Prochlorperazine (Excessive cholinergic blockade; potentiated sedative effect). Products include:
- Compazine ... 2644

Procyclidine Hydrochloride (Excessive cholinergic blockade; increased intraocular pressure). Products include:
- Kemadrin Tablets ... 1105

Promethazine Hydrochloride (Excessive cholinergic blockade; potentiated sedative effect). Products include:
- Mepergan Injection ... 2859
- Phenergan with Codeine ... 2883
- Phenergan with Dextromethorphan 2885
- Phenergan Injection ... 2880
- Phenergan Suppositories ... 2882
- Phenergan Syrup ... 2881
- Phenergan Tablets ... 2882
- Phenergan VC ... 2886
- Phenergan VC with Codeine ... 2888

Propafenone Hydrochloride (Excessive cholinergic blockade). Products include:
- Rythmol Tablets–150mg, 225mg, 300mg ... 1399

Propoxyphene Hydrochloride (Excessive cholinergic blockade). Products include:
- Darvon ... 1475
- Wygesic Tablets ... 2930

Propoxyphene Napsylate (Excessive cholinergic blockade). Products include:
- Darvon-N/Darvocet-N ... 1473

Propranolol Hydrochloride (Excessive cholinergic blockade). Products include:
- Inderal ... 2834
- Inderal LA Long Acting Capsules ... 2836
- Inderide Tablets ... 2838
- Inderide LA Long Acting Capsules .. 2840

Protriptyline Hydrochloride (Excessive cholinergic blockade). Products include:
- Vivactil Tablets ... 1820

Pyrilamine Maleate (Excessive cholinergic blockade). Products include:
- 4-Way Fast Acting Nasal Spray (regular & mentholated) ... ▣ 644
- Maximum Strength Multi-Symptom Formula Midol ... ▣ 621
- PMS Multi-Symptom Formula Midol ... ▣ 622

Pyrilamine Tannate (Excessive cholinergic blockade). Products include:
- Atrohist Pediatric Suspension ... 1604

(▣ Described in PDR For Nonprescription Drugs) (⊙ Described in PDR For Ophthalmology)

Interactions Index — Procanbid

Atrohist Pediatric Suspension Dye-Free 1604
Rynatan 2781

Quinidine Gluconate (Excessive cholinergic blockade). Products include:
Quinaglute Dura-Tabs Tablets 644

Quinidine Polygalacturonate (Excessive cholinergic blockade). Products include:
Cardioquin Tablets 2146

Quinidine Sulfate (Excessive cholinergic blockade). Products include:
Quinidex Extentabs 2240

Scopolamine (Excessive cholinergic blockade; increased intraocular pressure). Products include:
Transderm Scōp Transdermal Therapeutic System 890

Scopolamine Hydrobromide (Excessive cholinergic blockade; increased intraocular pressure). Products include:
Atrohist Plus Tablets 1605
Donnatal 2234
Donnatal Extentabs 2234
Donnatal Tablets 2234

Sotalol Hydrochloride (Excessive cholinergic blockade). Products include:
Betapace Tablets 637

Sufentanil Citrate (Excessive cholinergic blockade). Products include:
Sufenta Injection 1355

Terfenadine (Excessive cholinergic blockade). Products include:
Seldane Tablets 1284
Seldane-D Extended-Release Tablets 1286

Thioridazine Hydrochloride (Excessive cholinergic blockade; potentiated sedative effect). Products include:
Mellaril 2398

Tocainide Hydrochloride (Excessive cholinergic blockade). Products include:
Tonocard Tablets 519

Triamcinolone (Increased intraocular pressure).
No products indexed under this heading.

Triamcinolone Acetonide (Increased intraocular pressure). Products include:
Azmacort Oral Inhaler 2175
Nasacort AQ Nasal Spray 2191
Nasacort Nasal Inhaler 2189

Triamcinolone Diacetate (Increased intraocular pressure).
No products indexed under this heading.

Triamcinolone Hexacetonide (Increased intraocular pressure).
No products indexed under this heading.

Tridihexethyl Chloride (Excessive cholinergic blockade; increased intraocular pressure).
No products indexed under this heading.

Trifluoperazine Hydrochloride (Excessive cholinergic blockade; potentiated sedative effect). Products include:
Stelazine 2692

Trihexyphenidyl Hydrochloride (Excessive cholinergic blockade; increased intraocular pressure). Products include:
Artane 1418

Trimeprazine Tartrate (Excessive cholinergic blockade).
No products indexed under this heading.

Trimipramine Maleate (Excessive cholinergic blockade). Products include:
Surmontil Capsules 2917

Tripelennamine Hydrochloride (Excessive cholinergic blockade). Products include:
PBZ Tablets 863
PBZ-SR Tablets 862

Triprolidine Hydrochloride (Excessive cholinergic blockade). Products include:
Actifed Cold & Allergy Tablets 807
Actifed Cold & Sinus Caplets and Tablets 808

Verapamil Hydrochloride (Excessive cholinergic blockade). Products include:
Calan SR Caplets 2571
Calan Tablets 2568
Covera-HS Tablets 2573
Isoptin Injectable 1391
Isoptin Oral Tablets 1393
Isoptin SR Tablets 1395
Verelan Capsules 1455

PROCANBID EXTENDED-RELEASE TABLETS

(Procainamide Hydrochloride) 1983
May interact with antiarrhythmics, type 1 antiarrhythmic drugs, anticholinergics, cardiac glycosides, neuromuscular blocking agents, and certain other agents. Compounds in these categories include:

Acebutolol Hydrochloride (Additive cardiac effects). Products include:
Sectral Capsules 2914

Adenosine (Additive cardiac effects). Products include:
Adenocard Injection 1021
Adenoscan 1022

Amiodarone Hydrochloride (Co-administration may result in higher plasma PA concentration). Products include:
Cordarone Intravenous 2821
Cordarone Tablets 2818

Atracurium Besylate (Co-administration may require less than usual doses of the neuromuscular blocking agent due to PA effects of reducing acetylcholine release). Products include:
Tracrium Injection 1155

Atropine Sulfate (May produce additive antivagal effects on A-V nodal conduction). Products include:
Arco-Lase Plus Tablets 513
Atrohist Plus Tablets 1605
Donnatal 2234
Donnatal Extentabs 2234
Donnatal Tablets 2234
Lomotil 2591
Motofen Tablets 789
Urised Tablets 2123

Belladonna Alkaloids (May produce additive antivagal effects on A-V nodal conduction). Products include:
Bellergal-S Tablets 2375
Hyland's Bedwetting Tablets 788
Hyland's EnurAid Tablets 789
Hyland's Headache Tablets 790
Hyland's Teething Tablets 790
Similasan Eye Drops #1 769

Benztropine Mesylate (May produce additive antivagal effects on A-V nodal conduction). Products include:
Cogentin 1661

Biperiden Hydrochloride (May produce additive antivagal effects on A-V nodal conduction). Products include:
Akineton 1380

Bretylium Tosylate (Additive cardiac effects).
No products indexed under this heading.

Cimetidine (Co-administration decreases renal clearance of procainamide, potentially leading to clinically significant increases in plasma concentrations). Products include:
Tagamet HB Tablets 786
Tagamet Tablets 2694

Cimetidine Hydrochloride (Co-administration decreases renal clearance of procainamide, potentially leading to clinically significant increases in plasma concentrations). Products include:
Tagamet 2694

Cisatracurium Besylate (Co-administration may require less than usual doses of the neuromuscular blocking agent due to PA effects of reducing acetylcholine release). Products include:
Nimbex Injection 1131

Clidinium Bromide (May produce additive antivagal effects on A-V nodal conduction). Products include:
Librax Capsules 2330

Deslanoside (Potential for additional disturbance of conduction, ventricular asystole or fibrillation in patients with concomitant marked disturbance of A-V conduction).
No products indexed under this heading.

Dicyclomine Hydrochloride (May produce additive antivagal effects on A-V nodal conduction). Products include:
Bentyl 1246

Digitoxin (Potential for additional disturbance of conduction, ventricular asystole or fibrillation in patients with concomitant marked disturbance of A-V conduction). Products include:
Crystodigin Tablets 1472

Digoxin (Potential for additional disturbance of conduction, ventricular asystole or fibrillation in patients with concomitant marked disturbance of A-V conduction). Products include:
Lanoxicaps 1110
Lanoxin Elixir Pediatric 1113
Lanoxin Injection 1116
Lanoxin Injection Pediatric 1119
Lanoxin Tablets 1121

Disopyramide Phosphate (Concurrent use with other Group 1A antiarrhythmic agents may produce enhanced prolongation of conduction or depression of contractility and hypotension, especially in patients with cardiac decompensation). Products include:
Norpace 2596

Doxacurium Chloride (Co-administration may require less than usual doses of the neuromuscular blocking agent due to PA effects of reducing acetylcholine release). Products include:
Nuromax Injection 1136

Flecainide Acetate (Additive cardiac effects). Products include:
Tambocor Tablets 1555

Glycopyrrolate (May produce additive antivagal effects on A-V nodal conduction). Products include:
Robinul Forte Tablets 2247
Robinul Injectable 2247
Robinul Tablets 2247

Hyoscyamine (May produce additive antivagal effects on A-V nodal conduction). Products include:
Cystospaz Tablets 2123
Urised Tablets 2123

Hyoscyamine Sulfate (May produce additive antivagal effects on A-V nodal conduction). Products include:
Arco-Lase Plus Tablets 513
Atrohist Plus Tablets 1605
Cystospaz-M Capsules 2123
Donnatal 2234
Donnatal Extentabs 2234
Donnatal Tablets 2234
Kutrase Capsules 2546
Levsin/Levsinex/Levbid 2549

Ipratropium Bromide (May produce additive antivagal effects on A-V nodal conduction). Products include:
Atrovent Inhalation Aerosol 674
Atrovent Inhalation Solution 675
Atrovent Nasal Spray 0.03% 676
Atrovent Nasal Spray 0.06% 678

Lidocaine Hydrochloride (Additive cardiac effects). Products include:
Decadron Phosphate with Xylocaine Injection, Sterile 1683
Unguentine Plus 712
Xylocaine Injections 562

Mepenzolate Bromide (May produce additive antivagal effects on A-V nodal conduction).
No products indexed under this heading.

Metocurine Iodide (Co-administration may require less than usual doses of the neuromuscular blocking agent due to PA effects of reducing acetylcholine release). Products include:
Metubine Iodide Vials 932

Mexiletine Hydrochloride (Additive cardiac effects). Products include:
Mexitil Capsules 684

Mivacurium Chloride (Co-administration may require less than usual doses of the neuromuscular blocking agent due to PA effects of reducing acetylcholine release). Products include:
Mivacron 1125

Moricizine Hydrochloride (Concurrent use with other Group 1A antiarrhythmic agents may produce enhanced prolongation of conduction or depression of contractility and hypotension, especially in patients with cardiac decompensation). Products include:
Ethmozine Tablets 2217

Oxybutynin Chloride (May produce additive antivagal effects on A-V nodal conduction). Products include:
Ditropan 1267

Pancuronium Bromide (Co-administration may require less than usual doses of the neuromuscular blocking agent due to PA effects of reducing acetylcholine release).
No products indexed under this heading.

Procyclidine Hydrochloride (May produce additive antivagal effects on A-V nodal conduction). Products include:
Kemadrin Tablets 1105

IMPORTANT NOTE: Always consult each drug listing in the patient's regimen for possible interactions.

Procanbid | Interactions Index | 870

Propafenone Hydrochloride (Concurrent use with other Group 1A antiarrhythmic agents may produce enhanced prolongation of conduction or depression of contractility and hypotension, especially in patients with cardiac decompensation). Products include:
- Rythmol Tablets–150mg, 225mg, 300mg ... 1399

Propantheline Bromide (May produce additive antivagal effects on A-V nodal conduction). Products include:
- Pro-Banthine Tablets ... 2226

Propranolol Hydrochloride (Additive cardiac effects). Products include:
- Inderal ... 2834
- Inderal LA Long Acting Capsules ... 2836
- Inderide Tablets ... 2838
- Inderide LA Long Acting Capsules ... 2840

Quinidine Gluconate (Concurrent use with other Group 1A antiarrhythmic agents may produce enhanced prolongation of conduction or depression of contractility and hypotension, especially in patients with cardiac decompensation). Products include:
- Quinaglute Dura-Tabs Tablets ... 644

Quinidine Polygalacturonate (Concurrent use with other Group 1A antiarrhythmic agents may produce enhanced prolongation of conduction or depression of contractility and hypotension, especially in patients with cardiac decompensation). Products include:
- Cardioquin Tablets ... 2146

Quinidine Sulfate (Concurrent use with other Group 1A antiarrhythmic agents may produce enhanced prolongation of conduction or depression of contractility and hypotension, especially in patients with cardiac decompensation). Products include:
- Quinidex Extentabs ... 2240

Ranitidine Hydrochloride (Co-administration at large (greater than 300 mg/day) doses of ranitidine may decrease renal clearance of procainamide). Products include:
- Zantac ... 1182
- Zantac Injection ... 1180
- Zantac Syrup ... 1182

Rocuronium Bromide (Co-administration may require less than usual doses of the neuromuscular blocking agent due to PA effects of reducing acetylcholine release). Products include:
- Zemuron Injection ... 1885

Scopolamine (May produce additive antivagal effects on A-V nodal conduction). Products include:
- Transderm Scōp Transdermal Therapeutic System ... 890

Scopolamine Hydrobromide (May produce additive antivagal effects on A-V nodal conduction). Products include:
- Atrohist Plus Tablets ... 1605
- Donnatal ... 2234
- Donnatal Extentabs ... 2234
- Donnatal Tablets ... 2234

Sotalol Hydrochloride (Additive cardiac effects). Products include:
- Betapace Tablets ... 637

Succinylcholine Chloride (Co-administration may require less than usual doses of the neuromuscular blocking agent due to PA effects of reducing acetylcholine release). Products include:
- Anectine ... 1062

Tocainide Hydrochloride (Additive cardiac effects). Products include:
- Tonocard Tablets ... 519

Tridihexethyl Chloride (May produce additive antivagal effects on A-V nodal conduction).
- No products indexed under this heading.

Trihexyphenidyl Hydrochloride (May produce additive antivagal effects on A-V nodal conduction). Products include:
- Artane ... 1418

Trimethoprim (Co-administration may result in higher plasma PA concentration). Products include:
- Bactrim DS Tablets ... 2257
- Bactrim I.V. Infusion ... 2255
- Bactrim ... 2257
- Proloprim Tablets ... 1141
- Septra ... 1146
- Septra I.V. Infusion ... 1142
- Septra I.V. Infusion ADD-Vantage Vials ... 1144
- Septra ... 1146
- Trimpex Tablets ... 2323

Vecuronium Bromide (Co-administration may require less than usual doses of the neuromuscular blocking agent due to PA effects of reducing acetylcholine release). Products include:
- Norcuron for Injection ... 1875

Verapamil Hydrochloride (Additive cardiac effects). Products include:
- Calan SR Caplets ... 2571
- Calan Tablets ... 2568
- Covera-HS Tablets ... 2573
- Isoptin Injectable ... 1391
- Isoptin Oral Tablets ... 1393
- Isoptin SR Tablets ... 1395
- Verelan Capsules ... 1455

Food Interactions

Alcohol (Alcohol consumption tends to decrease the half-life of procainamide in the blood through induction of its acetylation to NAPA).

PROCARDIA CAPSULES
(Nifedipine) ... 2024

May interact with beta blockers, oral anticoagulants, cardiac glycosides, narcotic analgesics, and certain other agents. Compounds in these categories include:

Acebutolol Hydrochloride (Increased likelihood of congestive heart failure, severe hypotension or exacerbation of angina). Products include:
- Sectral Capsules ... 2914

Alfentanil Hydrochloride (Co-administration may result in the possibility of severe hypotension and/or increased fluid volume requirements in surgical procedures). Products include:
- Alfenta Injection ... 1334

Atenolol (Increased likelihood of congestive heart failure, severe hypotension or exacerbation of angina). Products include:
- Tenoretic Tablets ... 2963
- Tenormin Tablets and I.V. Injection 2965

Betaxolol Hydrochloride (Increased likelihood of congestive heart failure, severe hypotension or exacerbation of angina). Products include:
- Betoptic Ophthalmic Solution ... 465
- Betoptic S Ophthalmic Suspension 467
- Kerlone Tablets ... 2588

Bisoprolol Fumarate (Increased likelihood of congestive heart failure, severe hypotension or exacerbation of angina). Products include:
- Zebeta Tablets ... 1457
- Ziac ... 1459

Buprenorphine (Co-administration may result in the possibility of severe hypotension and/or increased fluid volume requirements in surgical procedures). Products include:
- Buprenex Injectable ... 2170

Carteolol Hydrochloride (Increased likelihood of congestive heart failure, severe hypotension or exacerbation of angina). Products include:
- Cartrol Tablets ... 413
- Ocupress Ophthalmic Solution, 1% Sterile ... ◉ 297

Cimetidine (A significant increase in peak nifedipine plasma levels (80%) and AUC (74%) after a one week course of cimetidine at 1000 mg per day and 40 mg nifedipine has been reported). Products include:
- Tagamet HB Tablets ... ■ 786
- Tagamet Tablets ... 2694

Cimetidine Hydrochloride (A significant increase in peak nifedipine plasma levels (80%) and AUC (74%) after a one week course of cimetidine at 1000 mg per day and 40 mg nifedipine has been reported). Products include:
- Tagamet ... 2694

Codeine Phosphate (Co-administration may result in the possibility of severe hypotension and/or increased fluid volume requirements in surgical procedures). Products include:
- Brontex ... 2130
- Dimetane-DC Cough Syrup ... 2232
- Fioricet with Codeine Capsules ... 2387
- Fiorinal with Codeine Capsules ... 2390
- Nucofed ... 2225
- Phenergan with Codeine ... 2883
- Phenergan VC with Codeine ... 2888
- Robitussin A-C Syrup ... 2248
- Robitussin-DAC Syrup ... 2249
- Ryna ... ■ 804
- Soma Compound w/Codeine Tablets ... 2784
- Tylenol with Codeine ... 1592

Deslanoside (Potential for increased digoxin levels).
- No products indexed under this heading.

Dezocine (Co-administration may result in the possibility of severe hypotension and/or increased fluid volume requirements in surgical procedures). Products include:
- Dalgan Injection ... 529

Dicumarol (Increased prothrombin time).
- No products indexed under this heading.

Digitoxin (Potential for increased digoxin levels). Products include:
- Crystodigin Tablets ... 1472

Digoxin (Potential for increased digoxin levels). Products include:
- Lanoxicaps ... 1110
- Lanoxin Elixir Pediatric ... 1113
- Lanoxin Injection ... 1116
- Lanoxin Injection Pediatric ... 1119
- Lanoxin Tablets ... 1121

Esmolol Hydrochloride (Increased likelihood of congestive heart failure, severe hypotension or exacerbation of angina). Products include:
- Brevibloc (esmolol HCl) Injection ... 1860

Fentanyl (Co-administration may result in the possibility of severe hypotension and/or increased fluid volume requirements in surgical procedures). Products include:
- Duragesic Transdermal System ... 1336

Fentanyl Citrate (Co-administration may result in the possibility of severe hypotension and/or increased fluid volume requirements in surgical procedures). Products include:
- Sublimaze Injection ... 463

Hydrocodone Bitartrate (Co-administration may result in the possibility of severe hypotension and/or increased fluid volume requirements in surgical procedures). Products include:
- Codiclear DH Syrup ... 808
- Duratuss HD Elixir ... 2750
- Histussin D Liquid ... 670
- Hycodan Tablets and Syrup ... 946
- Hycomine Compound Tablets ... 948
- Hycomine ... 947
- Hycotuss Expectorant Syrup ... 950
- Hydrocet Capsules ... 787
- Lorcet 10/650 Tablets ... 1016
- Lortab ... 2751
- Tussend ... 1830
- Tussend Expectorant ... 1831
- Vicodin Tablets ... 1404
- Vicodin ES Tablets ... 1405
- Vicodin HP Tablets ... 1403
- Vicodin Tuss Expectorant ... 1406
- Zydone Capsules ... 967

Hydrocodone Polistirex (Co-administration may result in the possibility of severe hypotension and/or increased fluid volume requirements in surgical procedures). Products include:
- Tussionex Pennkinetic Extended-Release Suspension ... 1624

Hydromorphone Hydrochloride (Co-administration may result in the possibility of severe hypotension and/or increased fluid volume requirements in surgical procedures). Products include:
- Dilaudid Ampules ... 1382
- Dilaudid Cough Syrup ... 1383
- Dilaudid-HP Injection ... 1384
- Dilaudid-HP Lyophilized Powder 250 mg ... 1384
- Dilaudid ... 1382
- Dilaudid Oral Liquid ... 1386
- Dilaudid ... 1382
- Dilaudid Tablets - 8 mg ... 1386

Labetalol Hydrochloride (Increased likelihood of congestive heart failure, severe hypotension or exacerbation of angina). Products include:
- Normodyne Injection ... 2519
- Normodyne Tablets ... 2522
- Trandate ... 1158

Levobunolol Hydrochloride (Increased likelihood of congestive heart failure, severe hypotension or exacerbation of angina). Products include:
- Betagan ... ◉ 230

Levorphanol Tartrate (Co-administration may result in the possibility of severe hypotension and/or increased fluid volume requirements in surgical procedures). Products include:
- Levo-Dromoran ... 2297

Meperidine Hydrochloride (Co-administration may result in the possibility of severe hypotension and/or increased fluid volume requirements in surgical procedures). Products include:
- Demerol ... 2438
- Mepergan Injection ... 2859

Methadone Hydrochloride (Co-administration may result in the possibility of severe hypotension and/or increased fluid volume requirements in surgical procedures). Products include:
- Methadone Hydrochloride Oral Concentrate ... 2356
- Methadone Hydrochloride Oral Solution & Tablets ... 2357

(■ Described in PDR For Nonprescription Drugs) (◉ Described in PDR For Ophthalmology)

Procardia XL

Metipranolol Hydrochloride (Increased likelihood of congestive heart failure, severe hypotension or exacerbation of angina). Products include:
OptiPranolol (Metipranolol 0.3%) Sterile Ophthalmic Solution........... ⊚ 256

Metoprolol Succinate (Increased likelihood of congestive heart failure, severe hypotension or exacerbation of angina). Products include:
Toprol-XL Tablets 560

Metoprolol Tartrate (Increased likelihood of congestive heart failure, severe hypotension or exacerbation of angina). Products include:
Lopressor 848
Lopressor HCT Tablets 850

Morphine Sulfate (Co-administration may result in the possibility of severe hypotension and/or increased fluid volume requirements in surgical procedures). Products include:
Astramorph/PF Injection, USP (Preservative-Free) 526
Duramorph Injection 983
Infumorph 200 and Infumorph 500 Sterile Solutions 985
Kadian Capsules...................... 2948
MS Contin Tablets 2149
MSIR 2152
Oramorph SR (Morphine Sulfate Sustained Release Tablets) .. 2359
RMS Suppositories CII 2766
Roxanol 2365

Nadolol (Increased likelihood of congestive heart failure, severe hypotension or exacerbation of angina).
No products indexed under this heading.

Opium Alkaloids (Co-administration may result in the possibility of severe hypotension and/or increased fluid volume requirements in surgical procedures).
No products indexed under this heading.

Oxycodone Hydrochloride (Co-administration may result in the possibility of severe hypotension and/or increased fluid volume requirements in surgical procedures). Products include:
OxyContin Tablets 2163
OxyIR Capsules 2167
Percocet Tablets 955
Percodan Tablets 955
Percodan-Demi Tablets........... 956
Roxicodone Tablets, Oral Solution & Intensol (Oxycodone) 2366
Tylox Capsules 1593

Penbutolol Sulfate (Increased likelihood of congestive heart failure, severe hypotension or exacerbation of angina). Products include:
Levatol Tablets 2547

Pindolol (Increased likelihood of congestive heart failure, severe hypotension or exacerbation of angina). Products include:
Visken Tablets.......................... 2428

Propoxyphene Hydrochloride (Co-administration may result in the possibility of severe hypotension and/or increased fluid volume requirements in surgical procedures). Products include:
Darvon 1475
Wygesic Tablets 2930

Propoxyphene Napsylate (Co-administration may result in the possibility of severe hypotension and/or increased fluid volume requirements in surgical procedures). Products include:
Darvon-N/Darvocet-N 1473

Propranolol Hydrochloride (Increased likelihood of congestive heart failure, severe hypotension or exacerbation of angina). Products include:
Inderal 2834
Inderal LA Long Acting Capsules 2836
Inderide Tablets 2838
Inderide LA Long Acting Capsules .. 2840

Quinidine Gluconate (Co-administration has resulted in decreased plasma level of quinidine in rare cases). Products include:
Quinaglute Dura-Tabs Tablets 644

Quinidine Polygalacturonate (Co-administration has resulted in decreased plasma level of quinidine in rare cases). Products include:
Cardioquin Tablets 2146

Quinidine Sulfate (Co-administration has resulted in decreased plasma level of quinidine in rare cases). Products include:
Quinidex Extentabs 2240

Ranitidine Hydrochloride (Co-administration produces smaller non-significant increases in nifedipine level). Products include:
Zantac 1182
Zantac Injection 1180
Zantac Syrup 1182

Sotalol Hydrochloride (Increased likelihood of congestive heart failure, severe hypotension or exacerbation of angina). Products include:
Betapace Tablets 637

Sufentanil Citrate (Co-administration may result in the possibility of severe hypotension and/or increased fluid volume requirements in surgical procedures). Products include:
Sufenta Injection 1355

Timolol Hemihydrate (Increased likelihood of congestive heart failure, severe hypotension or exacerbation of angina). Products include:
Betimol 0.25%, 0.5% .... ⊚ 259

Timolol Maleate (Increased likelihood of congestive heart failure, severe hypotension or exacerbation of angina). Products include:
Blocadren Tablets 1654
Timolide Tablets....................... 1791
Timoptic in Ocudose 1796
Timoptic Sterile Ophthalmic Solution 1794
Timoptic-XE 1798

Warfarin Sodium (Increased prothrombin time). Products include:
Coumadin 941

PROCARDIA XL EXTENDED RELEASE TABLETS
(Nifedipine) 2026
May interact with beta blockers, oral anticoagulants, diuretics, cardiac glycosides, narcotic analgesics, and certain other agents. Compounds in these categories include:

Acebutolol Hydrochloride (Combination therapy may increase the likelihood of congestive heart failure, severe hypotension, or exacerbation of angina). Products include:
Sectral Capsules 2914

Alfentanil Hydrochloride (Severe hypotension and/or increased fluid volume requirements have been reported in patients receiving nifedipine with beta blocker who underwent coronary artery bypass surgery using high-dose fentanyl anesthesia; possibility of this interaction cannot be ruled out with other narcotic analgesics or in other surgical procedures). Products include:
Alfenta Injection 1334

Amiloride Hydrochloride (Concomitant diuretic therapy has resulted in slight decrease in serum potassium; serum potassium was unchanged in the absence of diuretic). Products include:
Midamor Tablets 1746
Moduretic Tablets 1748

Atenolol (Combination therapy may increase the likelihood of congestive heart failure, severe hypotension, or exacerbation of angina). Products include:
Tenoretic Tablets..................... 2963
Tenormin Tablets and I.V. Injection 2965

Bendroflumethiazide (Concomitant diuretic therapy has resulted in slight decrease in serum potassium; serum potassium was unchanged in the absence of diuretic).
No products indexed under this heading.

Betaxolol Hydrochloride (Combination therapy may increase the likelihood of congestive heart failure, severe hypotension, or exacerbation of angina). Products include:
Betoptic Ophthalmic Solution........... 465
Betoptic S Ophthalmic Suspension .. 467
Kerlone Tablets 2588

Bisoprolol Fumarate (Combination therapy may increase the likelihood of congestive heart failure, severe hypotension, or exacerbation of angina). Products include:
Zebeta Tablets 1457
Ziac 1459

Bumetanide (Concomitant diuretic therapy has resulted in slight decrease in serum potassium; serum potassium was unchanged in the absence of diuretic). Products include:
Bumex 2260

Buprenorphine (Severe hypotension and/or increased fluid volume requirements have been reported in patients receiving nifedipine with beta blocker who underwent coronary artery bypass surgery using high-dose fentanyl anesthesia; possibility of this interaction cannot be ruled out with other narcotic analgesics or in other surgical procedures). Products include:
Buprenex Injectable 2170

Carteolol Hydrochloride (Combination therapy may increase the likelihood of congestive heart failure, severe hypotension, or exacerbation of angina). Products include:
Cartrol Tablets 413
Ocupress Ophthalmic Solution, 1% Sterile............................. ⊚ 297

Chlorothiazide (Concomitant diuretic therapy has resulted in slight decrease in serum potassium; serum potassium was unchanged in the absence of diuretic). Products include:
Aldoclor Tablets 1638
Diupres Tablets 1691
Diuril Oral 1694

Chlorothiazide Sodium (Concomitant diuretic therapy has resulted in slight decrease in serum potassium; serum potassium was unchanged in the absence of diuretic). Products include:
Diuril Sodium Intravenous 1693

Chlorthalidone (Concomitant diuretic therapy has resulted in slight decrease in serum potassium; serum potassium was unchanged in the absence of diuretic). Products include:
Combipres Tablets 682
Tenoretic Tablets..................... 2963
Thalitone 1293

Cimetidine (Significant increase in peak nifedipine plasma levels and AUC). Products include:
Tagamet HB Tablets............... ⊚ 786
Tagamet Tablets 2694

Cimetidine Hydrochloride (Significant increase in peak nifedipine plasma levels and AUC). Products include:
Tagamet.................................... 2694

Codeine Phosphate (Severe hypotension and/or increased fluid volume requirements have been reported in patients receiving nifedipine with beta blocker who underwent coronary artery bypass surgery using high-dose fentanyl anesthesia; possibility of this interaction cannot be ruled out with other narcotic analgesics or in other surgical procedures). Products include:
Brontex 2130
Dimetane-DC Cough Syrup 2232
Fioricet with Codeine Capsules 2387
Fiorinal with Codeine Capsules 2390
Nucofed 2225
Phenergan with Codeine 2883
Phenergan VC with Codeine .. 2888
Robitussin A-C Syrup 2248
Robitussin-DAC Syrup 2249
Ryna .... ⊚ 804
Soma Compound w/Codeine Tablets 2784
Tylenol with Codeine 1592

Deslanoside (Co-administration has resulted in isolated reports of increased digoxin blood levels).
No products indexed under this heading.

Dezocine (Severe hypotension and/or increased fluid volume requirements have been reported in patients receiving nifedipine with beta blocker who underwent coronary artery bypass surgery using high-dose fentanyl anesthesia; possibility of this interaction cannot be ruled out with other narcotic analgesics or in other surgical procedures). Products include:
Dalgan Injection 529

Dicumarol (Co-administration has resulted in rare reports of increased prothrombin time; relationship to nifedipine therapy is uncertain).
No products indexed under this heading.

Digitoxin (Co-administration has resulted in isolated reports of increased digoxin blood levels). Products include:
Crystodigin Tablets 1472

Digoxin (Co-administration has resulted in isolated reports of increased digoxin blood levels). Products include:
Lanoxicaps 1110
Lanoxin Elixir Pediatric 1113
Lanoxin Injection 1116
Lanoxin Injection Pediatric 1119
Lanoxin Tablets 1121

IMPORTANT NOTE: Always consult each drug listing in the patient's regimen for possible interactions.

Procardia XL Interactions Index 872

Esmolol Hydrochloride (Combination therapy may increase the likelihood of congestive heart failure, severe hypotension, or exacerbation of angina). Products include:
Brevibloc (esmolol HCl) Injection 1860

Ethacrynic Acid (Concomitant diuretic therapy has resulted in slight decrease in serum potassium; serum potassium was unchanged in the absence of diuretic). Products include:
Edecrin Tablets ... 1698

Fentanyl (Severe hypotension and/or increased fluid volume requirements have been reported in patients receiving nifedipine with beta blocker who underwent coronary artery bypass surgery using high-dose fentanyl anesthesia; possibility of this interaction cannot be ruled out with low dose fentanyl or in other surgical procedures). Products include:
Duragesic Transdermal System ... 1336

Fentanyl Citrate (Severe hypotension and/or increased fluid volume requirements have been reported in patients receiving nifedipine with beta blocker who underwent coronary artery bypass surgery using high-dose fentanyl anesthesia; possibility of this interaction cannot be ruled out with low dose fentanyl or in other surgical procedures). Products include:
Sublimaze Injection ... 463

Furosemide (Concomitant diuretic therapy has resulted in slight decrease in serum potassium; serum potassium was unchanged in the absence of diuretic). Products include:
Lasix Injection, Oral Solution and Tablets ... 1267

Hydrochlorothiazide (Concomitant diuretic therapy has resulted in slight decrease in serum potassium; serum potassium was unchanged in the absence of diuretic). Products include:
Aldactazide Tablets ... 2556
Aldoril Tablets ... 1644
Apresazide Capsules ... 824
Capozide Tablets ... 744
Dyazide Capsules ... 2653
Esidrix Tablets ... 839
Esimil Tablets ... 840
HydroDIURIL Tablets ... 1716
Hydropres Tablets ... 1718
Hyzaar Tablets ... 1720
Inderide Tablets ... 2838
Inderide LA Long Acting Capsules .. 2840
Lopressor HCT Tablets ... 850
Lotensin HCT Tablets ... 855
Moduretic Tablets ... 1748
Oretic Tablets ... 450
Prinzide Tablets ... 1780
Ser-Ap-Es Tablets ... 867
Timolide Tablets ... 1791
Vaseretic Tablets ... 1810
Zestoretic Tablets ... 2968
Ziac ... 1459

Hydrocodone Bitartrate (Severe hypotension and/or increased fluid volume requirements have been reported in patients receiving nifedipine with beta blocker who underwent coronary artery bypass surgery using high-dose fentanyl anesthesia; possibility of this interaction cannot be ruled out with other narcotic analgesics or in other surgical procedures). Products include:
Codiclear DH Syrup ... 808
Duratuss HD Elixir ... 2750
Histussin D Liquid ... 670
Hycodan Tablets and Syrup ... 946
Hycomine Compound Tablets ... 948
Hycomine ... 947
Hycotuss Expectorant Syrup ... 950
Hydrocet Capsules ... 787
Lorcet 10/650 Tablets ... 1016
Lortab ... 2751
Tussend ... 1830
Tussend Expectorant ... 1831
Vicodin Tablets ... 1404
Vicodin ES Tablets ... 1405
Vicodin HP Tablets ... 1403
Vicodin Tuss Expectorant ... 1406
Zydone Capsules ... 967

Hydrocodone Polistirex (Severe hypotension and/or increased fluid volume requirements have been reported in patients receiving nifedipine with beta blocker who underwent coronary artery bypass surgery using high-dose fentanyl anesthesia; possibility of this interaction cannot be ruled out with other narcotic analgesics or in other surgical procedures). Products include:
Tussionex Pennkinetic Extended-Release Suspension ... 1624

Hydroflumethiazide (Concomitant diuretic therapy has resulted in slight decrease in serum potassium; serum potassium was unchanged in the absence of diuretic). Products include:
Diucardin Tablets ... 2824

Hydromorphone Hydrochloride (Severe hypotension and/or increased fluid volume requirements have been reported in patients receiving nifedipine with beta blocker who underwent coronary artery bypass surgery using high-dose fentanyl anesthesia; possibility of this interaction cannot be ruled out with other narcotic analgesics or in other surgical procedures). Products include:
Dilaudid Ampules ... 1382
Dilaudid Cough Syrup ... 1383
Dilaudid-HP Injection ... 1384
Dilaudid-HP Lyophilized Powder 250 mg ... 1384
Dilaudid ... 1382
Dilaudid Oral Liquid ... 1386
Dilaudid ... 1382
Dilaudid Tablets - 8 mg ... 1386

Indapamide (Concomitant diuretic therapy has resulted in slight decrease in serum potassium; serum potassium was unchanged in the absence of diuretic).
No products indexed under this heading.

Labetalol Hydrochloride (Combination therapy may increase the likelihood of congestive heart failure, severe hypotension, or exacerbation of angina). Products include:
Normodyne Injection ... 2519
Normodyne Tablets ... 2522
Trandate ... 1158

Levobunolol Hydrochloride (Combination therapy may increase the likelihood of congestive heart failure, severe hypotension, or exacerbation of angina). Products include:
Betagan ... ◉ 230

Levorphanol Tartrate (Severe hypotension and/or increased fluid volume requirements have been reported in patients receiving nifedipine with beta blocker who underwent coronary artery bypass surgery using high-dose fentanyl anesthesia; possibility of this interaction cannot be ruled out with other narcotic analgesics or in other surgical procedures). Products include:
Levo-Dromoran ... 2297

Meperidine Hydrochloride (Severe hypotension and/or increased fluid volume requirements have been reported in patients receiving nifedipine with beta blocker who underwent coronary artery bypass surgery using high-dose fentanyl anesthesia; possibility of this interaction cannot be ruled out with other narcotic analgesics or in other surgical procedures). Products include:
Demerol ... 2438
Mepergan Injection ... 2859

Methadone Hydrochloride (Severe hypotension and/or increased fluid volume requirements have been reported in patients receiving nifedipine with beta blocker who underwent coronary artery bypass surgery using high-dose fentanyl anesthesia; possibility of this interaction cannot be ruled out with other narcotic analgesics or in other surgical procedures). Products include:
Methadone Hydrochloride Oral Concentrate ... 2356
Methadone Hydrochloride Oral Solution & Tablets ... 2357

Methyclothiazide (Concomitant diuretic therapy has resulted in slight decrease in serum potassium; serum potassium was unchanged in the absence of diuretic). Products include:
Enduron Tablets ... 424

Metipranolol Hydrochloride (Combination therapy may increase the likelihood of congestive heart failure, severe hypotension, or exacerbation of angina). Products include:
OptiPranolol (Metipranolol 0.3%) Sterile Ophthalmic Solution ... ◉ 256

Metolazone (Concomitant diuretic therapy has resulted in slight decrease in serum potassium; serum potassium was unchanged in the absence of diuretic). Products include:
Mykrox Tablets ... 1617
Zaroxolyn Tablets ... 1625

Metoprolol Succinate (Combination therapy may increase the likelihood of congestive heart failure, severe hypotension, or exacerbation of angina). Products include:
Toprol-XL Tablets ... 560

Metoprolol Tartrate (Combination therapy may increase the likelihood of congestive heart failure, severe hypotension, or exacerbation of angina). Products include:
Lopressor ... 848
Lopressor HCT Tablets ... 850

Morphine Sulfate (Severe hypotension and/or increased fluid volume requirements have been reported in patients receiving nifedipine with beta blocker who underwent coronary artery bypass surgery using high-dose fentanyl anesthesia; possibility of this interaction cannot be ruled out with other narcotic analgesics or in other surgical procedures). Products include:
Astramorph/PF Injection, USP (Preservative-Free) ... 526
Duramorph Injection ... 983
Infumorph 200 and Infumorph 500 Sterile Solutions ... 985
Kadian Capsules ... 2948
MS Contin Tablets ... 2149
MSIR ... 2152
Oramorph SR (Morphine Sulfate Sustained Release Tablets) ... 2359
RMS Suppositories CII ... 2766
Roxanol ... 2365

Nadolol (Combination therapy may increase the likelihood of congestive heart failure, severe hypotension, or exacerbation of angina).
No products indexed under this heading.

Opium Alkaloids (Severe hypotension and/or increased fluid volume requirements have been reported in patients receiving nifedipine with beta blocker who underwent coronary artery bypass surgery using high-dose fentanyl anesthesia; possibility of this interaction cannot be ruled out with other narcotic analgesics or in other surgical procedures).
No products indexed under this heading.

Oxycodone Hydrochloride (Severe hypotension and/or increased fluid volume requirements have been reported in patients receiving nifedipine with beta blocker who underwent coronary artery bypass surgery using high-dose fentanyl anesthesia; possibility of this interaction cannot be ruled out with other narcotic analgesics or in other surgical procedures). Products include:
OxyContin Tablets ... 2163
OxyIR Capsules ... 2167
Percocet Tablets ... 955
Percodan Tablets ... 955
Percodan-Demi Tablets ... 956
Roxicodone Tablets, Oral Solution & Intensol (Oxycodone) ... 2366
Tylox Capsules ... 1593

Penbutolol Sulfate (Combination therapy may increase the likelihood of congestive heart failure, severe hypotension, or exacerbation of angina). Products include:
Levatol Tablets ... 2547

Pindolol (Combination therapy may increase the likelihood of congestive heart failure, severe hypotension, or exacerbation of angina). Products include:
Visken Tablets ... 2428

Polythiazide (Concomitant diuretic therapy has resulted in slight decrease in serum potassium; serum potassium was unchanged in the absence of diuretic). Products include:
Minizide Capsules ... 2016

Propoxyphene Hydrochloride (Severe hypotension and/or increased fluid volume requirements have been reported in patients receiving nifedipine with beta blocker who underwent coronary artery bypass surgery using high-dose fentanyl anesthesia; possibility of this interaction cannot be ruled out with other narcotic analgesics or in other surgical procedures). Products include:
Darvon ... 1475
Wygesic Tablets ... 2930

Propoxyphene Napsylate (Severe hypotension and/or increased fluid volume requirements have been reported in patients receiving nifedipine with beta blocker who underwent coronary artery bypass surgery using high-dose fentanyl anesthesia; possibility of this interaction cannot be ruled out with other narcotic analgesics or in other surgical procedures). Products include:
Darvon-N/Darvocet-N ... 1473

Propranolol Hydrochloride (Combination therapy may increase the likelihood of congestive heart failure, severe hypotension, or exacerbation of angina). Products include:
Inderal ... 2834

(▣ Described in PDR For Nonprescription Drugs) (◉ Described in PDR For Ophthalmology)

Inderal LA Long Acting Capsules 2836
Inderide Tablets 2838
Inderide LA Long Acting Capsules .. 2840

Ranitidine Hydrochloride (Co-administration produces smaller non-significant increases in nifedipine level). Products include:
Zantac 1182
Zantac Injection 1180
Zantac Syrup 1182

Sotalol Hydrochloride (Combination therapy may increase the likelihood of congestive heart failure, severe hypotension, or exacerbation of angina). Products include:
Betapace Tablets 637

Spironolactone (Concomitant diuretic therapy has resulted in slight decrease in serum potassium; serum potassium was unchanged in the absence of diuretic). Products include:
Aldactazide Tablets 2556
Aldactone Tablets 2558

Sufentanil Citrate (Severe hypotension and/or increased fluid volume requirements have been reported in patients receiving nifedipine with beta blocker who underwent coronary artery bypass surgery using high-dose fentanyl anesthesia; possibility of this interaction cannot be ruled out with other narcotic analgesics or in other surgical procedures). Products include:
Sufenta Injection 1355

Timolol Hemihydrate (Combination therapy may increase the likelihood of congestive heart failure, severe hypotension, or exacerbation of angina). Products include:
Betimol 0.25%, 0.5% .... ◉ 259

Timolol Maleate (Combination therapy may increase the likelihood of congestive heart failure, severe hypotension, or exacerbation of angina). Products include:
Blocadren Tablets 1654
Timolide Tablets 1791
Timoptic in Ocudose 1796
Timoptic Sterile Ophthalmic Solution 1794
Timoptic-XE 1798

Torsemide (Concomitant diuretic therapy has resulted in slight decrease in serum potassium; serum potassium was unchanged in the absence of diuretic). Products include:
Demadex Tablets and Injection 691

Triamterene (Concomitant diuretic therapy has resulted in slight decrease in serum potassium; serum potassium was unchanged in the absence of diuretic). Products include:
Dyazide Capsules 2653
Dyrenium Capsules 2655

Warfarin Sodium (Co-administration has resulted in rare reports of increased prothrombin time; relationship to nifedipine therapy is uncertain). Products include:
Coumadin 941

Food Interactions

Food, unspecified (Presence of food slightly alters the early rate of drug absorption).

PROCRIT FOR INJECTION
(Epoetin Alfa) 1896
None cited in PDR database.

PROCTOCREAM-HC 2.5%
(Hydrocortisone) 2552
None cited in PDR database.

PROCTOFOAM-HC
(Hydrocortisone Acetate, Pramoxine Hydrochloride) 2552
None cited in PDR database.

PRODIUM
(Phenazopyridine Hydrochloride) 695
None cited in PDR database.

PROFASI (CHORIONIC GONADOTROPIN FOR INJECTION, USP)
(Chorionic Gonadotropin) 2620
None cited in PDR database.

PROGLYCEM CAPSULES
(Diazoxide) 575
May interact with oral anticoagulants, thiazides, diuretics, and certain other agents. Compounds in these categories include:

Amiloride Hydrochloride (Concomitant administration may potentiate the hyperglycemic and hyperuricemic effects of diazoxide). Products include:
Midamor Tablets 1746
Moduretic Tablets 1748

Bendroflumethiazide (Concomitant administration may potentiate the hyperglycemic and hyperuricemic effects of diazoxide).
No products indexed under this heading.

Bumetanide (Concomitant administration may potentiate the hyperglycemic and hyperuricemic effects of diazoxide). Products include:
Bumex 2260

Chlorothiazide (Concomitant administration may potentiate the hyperglycemic and hyperuricemic effects of diazoxide). Products include:
Aldoclor Tablets 1638
Diupres Tablets 1691
Diuril Oral 1694

Chlorothiazide Sodium (Concomitant administration may potentiate the hyperglycemic and hyperuricemic effects of diazoxide). Products include:
Diuril Sodium Intravenous 1693

Chlorthalidone (Concomitant administration may potentiate the hyperglycemic and hyperuricemic effects of diazoxide). Products include:
Combipres Tablets 682
Tenoretic Tablets 2963
Thalitone 1293

Dicumarol (Increased blood levels of coumarin derivatives).
No products indexed under this heading.

Ethacrynic Acid (Concomitant administration may potentiate the hyperglycemic and hyperuricemic effects of diazoxide). Products include:
Edecrin Tablets 1698

Furosemide (Concomitant administration may potentiate the hyperglycemic and hyperuricemic effects of diazoxide). Products include:
Lasix Injection, Oral Solution and Tablets 1267

Hydrochlorothiazide (Concomitant administration may potentiate the hyperglycemic and hyperuricemic effects of diazoxide). Products include:
Aldactazide Tablets 2556
Aldoril Tablets 1644
Apresazide Capsules 824
Capozide Tablets 744
Dyazide Capsules 2653
Esidrix Tablets 839
Esimil Tablets 840
HydroDIURIL Tablets 1716
Hydropres Tablets 1718
Hyzaar Tablets 1720
Inderide Tablets 2838
Inderide LA Long Acting Capsules .. 2840
Lopressor HCT Tablets 850
Lotensin HCT Tablets 855
Moduretic Tablets 1748
Oretic Tablets 450
Prinzide Tablets 1780
Ser-Ap-Es Tablets 867
Timolide Tablets 1791
Vaseretic Tablets 1810
Zestoretic Tablets 2968
Ziac 1459

Hydroflumethiazide (Concomitant administration may potentiate the hyperglycemic and hyperuricemic effects of diazoxide). Products include:
Diucardin Tablets 2824

Indapamide (Concomitant administration may potentiate the hyperglycemic and hyperuricemic effects of diazoxide).
No products indexed under this heading.

Methyclothiazide (Concomitant administration may potentiate the hyperglycemic and hyperuricemic effects of diazoxide). Products include:
Enduron Tablets 424

Metolazone (Concomitant administration may potentiate the hyperglycemic and hyperuricemic effects of diazoxide). Products include:
Mykrox Tablets 1617
Zaroxolyn Tablets 1625

Phenytoin (Concomitant administration with oral diazoxide may result in a loss of seizure control). Products include:
Dilantin Infatabs 1967
Dilantin-125 Suspension 1969

Phenytoin Sodium (Concomitant administration with oral diazoxide may result in a loss of seizure control). Products include:
Dilantin Kapseals 1965

Polythiazide (Concomitant administration may potentiate the hyperglycemic and hyperuricemic effects of diazoxide). Products include:
Minizide Capsules 2016

Spironolactone (Concomitant administration may potentiate the hyperglycemic and hyperuricemic effects of diazoxide). Products include:
Aldactazide Tablets 2556
Aldactone Tablets 2558

Torsemide (Concomitant administration may potentiate the hyperglycemic and hyperuricemic effects of diazoxide). Products include:
Demadex Tablets and Injection 691

Triamterene (Concomitant administration may potentiate the hyperglycemic and hyperuricemic effects of diazoxide). Products include:
Dyazide Capsules 2653
Dyrenium Capsules 2655

Warfarin Sodium (Increased blood levels of coumarin derivatives). Products include:
Coumadin 941

PROGLYCEM SUSPENSION
(Diazoxide) 575
May interact with oral anticoagulants and diuretics. Compounds in these categories include:

Amiloride Hydrochloride (Co-administration of thiazides or other commonly used diuretics may potentiate the hyperglycemic and hyperuricemic effects of diazoxide). Products include:
Midamor Tablets 1746
Moduretic Tablets 1748

Bendroflumethiazide (Co-administration of thiazides or other commonly used diuretics may potentiate the hyperglycemic and hyperuricemic effects of diazoxide).
No products indexed under this heading.

Bumetanide (Co-administration of thiazides or other commonly used diuretics may potentiate the hyperglycemic and hyperuricemic effects of diazoxide). Products include:
Bumex 2260

Chlorothiazide (Co-administration of thiazides or other commonly used diuretics may potentiate the hyperglycemic and hyperuricemic effects of diazoxide). Products include:
Aldoclor Tablets 1638
Diupres Tablets 1691
Diuril Oral 1694

Chlorothiazide Sodium (Co-administration of thiazides or other commonly used diuretics may potentiate the hyperglycemic and hyperuricemic effects of diazoxide). Products include:
Diuril Sodium Intravenous 1693

Chlorthalidone (Co-administration of thiazides or other commonly used diuretics may potentiate the hyperglycemic and hyperuricemic effects of diazoxide). Products include:
Combipres Tablets 682
Tenoretic Tablets 2963
Thalitone 1293

Dicumarol (Diazoxide is highly protein bound and co-administration may result in higher blood levels of coumarin derivatives).
No products indexed under this heading.

Ethacrynic Acid (Co-administration of thiazides or other commonly used diuretics may potentiate the hyperglycemic and hyperuricemic effects of diazoxide). Products include:
Edecrin Tablets 1698

Fosphenytoin Sodium (Co-administration of oral diazoxide and diphenylhydantoin may result in a loss of seizure control). Products include:
Cerebyx Injection 1956

Furosemide (Co-administration of thiazides or other commonly used diuretics may potentiate the hyperglycemic and hyperuricemic effects of diazoxide). Products include:
Lasix Injection, Oral Solution and Tablets 1267

Hydrochlorothiazide (Co-administration of thiazides or other commonly used diuretics may potentiate the hyperglycemic and hyperuricemic effects of diazoxide). Products include:
Aldactazide Tablets 2556
Aldoril Tablets 1644
Apresazide Capsules 824
Capozide Tablets 744
Dyazide Capsules 2653
Esidrix Tablets 839
Esimil Tablets 840
HydroDIURIL Tablets 1716
Hydropres Tablets 1718
Hyzaar Tablets 1720
Inderide Tablets 2838
Inderide LA Long Acting Capsules .. 2840
Lopressor HCT Tablets 850
Lotensin HCT Tablets 855
Moduretic Tablets 1748
Oretic Tablets 450
Prinzide Tablets 1780
Ser-Ap-Es Tablets 867
Timolide Tablets 1791
Vaseretic Tablets 1810
Zestoretic Tablets 2968
Ziac 1459

IMPORTANT NOTE: Always consult each drug listing in the patient's regimen for possible interactions.

Hydroflumethiazide (Co-administration of thiazides or other commonly used diuretics may potentiate the hyperglycemic and hyperuricemic effects of diazoxide). Products include:

Diucardin Tablets 2824

Indapamide (Co-administration of thiazides or other commonly used diuretics may potentiate the hyperglycemic and hyperuricemic effects of diazoxide).

No products indexed under this heading.

Methyclothiazide (Co-administration of thiazides or other commonly used diuretics may potentiate the hyperglycemic and hyperuricemic effects of diazoxide). Products include:

Enduron Tablets 424

Metolazone (Co-administration of thiazides or other commonly used diuretics may potentiate the hyperglycemic and hyperuricemic effects of diazoxide). Products include:

Mykrox Tablets 1617
Zaroxolyn Tablets 1625

Phenytoin (Co-administration of oral diazoxide and diphenylhydantoin may result in a loss of seizure control). Products include:

Dilantin Infatabs 1967
Dilantin-125 Suspension 1969

Phenytoin Sodium (Co-administration of oral diazoxide and diphenylhydantoin may result in a loss of seizure control). Products include:

Dilantin Kapseals 1965

Polythiazide (Co-administration of thiazides or other commonly used diuretics may potentiate the hyperglycemic and hyperuricemic effects of diazoxide). Products include:

Minizide Capsules 2016

Spironolactone (Co-administration of thiazides or other commonly used diuretics may potentiate the hyperglycemic and hyperuricemic effects of diazoxide). Products include:

Aldactazide Tablets 2556
Aldactone Tablets 2558

Torsemide (Co-administration of thiazides or other commonly used diuretics may potentiate the hyperglycemic and hyperuricemic effects of diazoxide). Products include:

Demadex Tablets and Injection 691

Triamterene (Co-administration of thiazides or other commonly used diuretics may potentiate the hyperglycemic and hyperuricemic effects of diazoxide). Products include:

Dyazide Capsules 2653
Dyrenium Capsules 2655

Warfarin Sodium (Diazoxide is highly protein bound and co-administration may result in higher blood levels of coumarin derivatives). Products include:

Coumadin 941

PROGRAF

(Tacrolimus) 1028

May interact with potassium sparing diuretics, aminoglycosides, and certain other agents. Compounds in these categories include:

Amikacin Sulfate (Potential for additive or synergistic impairment of renal function). Products include:

Amikacin Sulfate Injection, USP 523
Amikacin Sulfate Injection, USP 981
Amikin Injectable 502

Amiloride Hydrochloride (Mild to severe hyperkalemia has been reported with tacrolimus; concurrent use with potassium sparing diuretics should be avoided). Products include:

Midamor Tablets 1746
Moduretic Tablets 1748

Amphotericin B (Potential for additive or synergistic impairment of renal function). Products include:

Abelcet Injection 1540
Fungizone Intravenous 507
Fungizone Oral Suspension 704

Bromocriptine Mesylate (May increase tacrolimus blood levels). Products include:

Parlodel 2411

Carbamazepine (May decrease tacrolimus blood levels). Products include:

Atretol Tablets 569
Tegretol/Tegretol-XR 870

Cimetidine (May increase tacrolimus blood levels). Products include:

Tagamet HB Tablets .... ⊞ 786
Tagamet Tablets 2694

Cimetidine Hydrochloride (May increase tacrolimus blood levels). Products include:

Tagamet 2694

Cisplatin (Potential for additive or synergistic impairment of renal function). Products include:

Platinol for Injection 717
Platinol-AQ Injection 719

Clarithromycin (May increase tacrolimus blood levels). Products include:

Biaxin 406

Clotrimazole (May increase tacrolimus blood levels). Products include:

Prescription Strength Desenex AF Cream .... ⊞ 653
Lotrimin 2514
Lotrimin AF Antifungal Cream, Lotion and Solution .... ⊞ 766
Lotrisone Cream 2515
Mycelex OTC Cream Antifungal .... ⊞ 622
Mycelex Troches 601
Mycelex-7 Vaginal Cream Antifungal .... ⊞ 622
Mycelex-7 Vaginal Antifungal Cream with 7 Disposable Applicators .... ⊞ 623
Mycelex-7 Vaginal Inserts Antifungal .... ⊞ 623
Mycelex-7 Combination-Pack Vaginal Inserts & External Vulvar Cream .... ⊞ 623
Mycelex-G 500 mg Vaginal Tablets 602

Cyclosporine (Increases tacrolimus blood levels resulting in additive/synergistic nephrotoxicity; Prograf should not be used simultaneously with cyclosporine; Prograf or cyclosporine should be discontinued at least 24 hours or more prior to initiating the other). Products include:

Neoral 2405
Sandimmune 2416

Danazol (May increase tacrolimus blood levels). Products include:

Danocrine Capsules 2437

Diltiazem Hydrochloride (May increase tacrolimus blood levels). Products include:

Cardizem CD Capsules 1251
Cardizem SR Capsules 1255
Cardizem Injectable 1253
Cardizem Tablets 1257
Dilacor XR Extended-release Capsules 2183
Tiazac Capsules 1019

Erythromycin (May increase tacrolimus blood levels). Products include:

A/T/S 2% Acne Topical Gel 1244
A/T/S 2% Acne Topical Solution 1244
Benzamycin Topical Gel 919
E-Mycin Tablets 1388
Emgel 2% Topical Gel 1081
ERYC 1972
Erycette (erythromycin 2%) Topical Solution 1943
Ery-Tab Tablets 426
Erythromycin Base Filmtab 430
Erythromycin Delayed-Release Capsules, USP 431
Ilotycin Ophthalmic Ointment 928
PCE Dispertab Tablets 453
T-Stat 2.0% Topical Solution and Pads 2797
THERAMYCIN Z 2% Solution 1629

Erythromycin Estolate (May increase tacrolimus blood levels). Products include:

Ilosone 927

Erythromycin Ethylsuccinate (May increase tacrolimus blood levels). Products include:

E.E.S. 427
EryPed 425
Pediazole Suspension 2340

Erythromycin Gluceptate (May increase tacrolimus blood levels). Products include:

Ilotycin Gluceptate, IV, Vials 929

Erythromycin Stearate (May increase tacrolimus blood levels). Products include:

Erythrocin Stearate Filmtab 429

Fluconazole (May increase tacrolimus blood levels). Products include:

Diflucan Tablets, Injection, and Oral Suspension 2003

Gentamicin Sulfate (Potential for additive or synergistic impairment of renal function). Products include:

Garamycin Cream 0.1% 2501
Garamycin Injectable 2502
Garamycin Ointment 0.1% 2501
Garamycin Ophthalmic 2501
Genoptic Sterile Ophthalmic Solution .... ⊙ 241
Genoptic Sterile Ophthalmic Ointment .... ⊙ 241
Gentak .... ⊙ 209
Pred-G Liquifilm Sterile Ophthalmic Suspension .... ⊙ 248
Pred-G S.O.P. Sterile Ophthalmic Ointment .... ⊙ 249

Itraconazole (May increase tacrolimus blood levels). Products include:

Sporanox Capsules 1352

Kanamycin Sulfate (Potential for additive or synergistic impairment of renal function).

No products indexed under this heading.

Ketoconazole (May increase tacrolimus blood levels). Products include:

Nizoral 2% Cream 1344
Nizoral 2% Shampoo 1344
Nizoral Tablets 1345

Measles Virus Vaccine Live (During treatment with tacrolimus, vaccination may be less effective). Products include:

Attenuvax 1650

Measles & Rubella Virus Vaccine Live (During treatment with tacrolimus, vaccination may be less effective). Products include:

M-R-VAX II 1732

Measles, Mumps & Rubella Virus Vaccine Live (During treatment with tacrolimus, vaccination may be less effective). Products include:

M-M-R II 1730

Methylprednisolone (May increase tacrolimus blood levels).

No products indexed under this heading.

Methylprednisolone Acetate (May increase tacrolimus blood levels).

No products indexed under this heading.

Methylprednisolone Sodium Succinate (May increase tacrolimus blood levels).

No products indexed under this heading.

Metoclopramide Hydrochloride (May increase tacrolimus blood levels). Products include:

Reglan 2243

Nicardipine Hydrochloride (May increase tacrolimus blood levels). Products include:

Cardene Capsules 2261
Cardene I.V. 2815
Cardene SR Capsules 2264

Phenobarbital (May decrease tacrolimus blood levels). Products include:

Arco-Lase Plus Tablets 513
Bellergal-S Tablets 2375
Donnatal 2234
Donnatal Extentabs 2234
Donnatal Tablets 2234
Phenobarbital Elixir and Tablets 1523
Quadrinal Tablets 1398

Phenytoin (May decrease tacrolimus blood levels). Products include:

Dilantin Infatabs 1967
Dilantin-125 Suspension 1969

Phenytoin Sodium (May decrease tacrolimus blood levels). Products include:

Dilantin Kapseals 1965

Poliovirus Vaccine Inactivated, Trivalent Types 1,2,3 (During treatment with tacrolimus, vaccination may be less effective). Products include:

IPOL Poliovirus Vaccine Inactivated 903

Poliovirus Vaccine, Live, Oral, Trivalent, Types 1,2,3 (Sabin) (During treatment with tacrolimus, vaccination may be less effective). Products include:

Orimune 1433

Rifabutin (May decrease tacrolimus blood levels). Products include:

Mycobutin Capsules 2101

Rifampin (May decrease tacrolimus blood levels). Products include:

Rifadin 1276
Rifamate Capsules 1278
Rifater 1280
Rimactane Capsules 865

Spironolactone (Mild to severe hyperkalemia has been reported with tacrolimus; concurrent use with potassium sparing diuretics should be avoided). Products include:

Aldactazide Tablets 2556
Aldactone Tablets 2558

Streptomycin Sulfate (Potential for additive or synergistic impairment of renal function). Products include:

Streptomycin Sulfate Injection 2031

Tobramycin (Potential for additive or synergistic impairment of renal function). Products include:

AKTOB .... ⊙ 207
TobraDex Ophthalmic Suspension and Ointment 469
Tobrex Ophthalmic Ointment and Solution .... ⊙ 226

Tobramycin Sulfate (Potential for additive or synergistic impairment of renal function). Products include:

Nebcin Vials, Hyporets & ADD-Vantage 1518

(⊞ Described in PDR For Nonprescription Drugs) (⊙ Described in PDR For Ophthalmology)

875 **Interactions Index** **Proleukin**

Triamterene (Mild to severe hyperkalemia has been reported with tacrolimus; concurrent use with potassium sparing diuretics should be avoided). Products include:
- Dyazide Capsules ... 2653
- Dyrenium Capsules ... 2655

Troleandomycin (Increases tacrolimus blood levels). Products include:
- Tao Capsules ... 2033

Typhoid Vaccine Live Oral TY21a (During treatment with tacrolimus, vaccination may be less effective). Products include:
- Vivotif Berna ... 660

Vaccines (Live) (During treatment with tacrolimus, vaccination may be less effective).

Verapamil Hydrochloride (May increase tacrolimus blood levels). Products include:
- Calan SR Caplets ... 2571
- Calan Tablets ... 2568
- Covera-HS Tablets ... 2573
- Isoptin Injectable ... 1391
- Isoptin Oral Tablets ... 1393
- Isoptin SR Tablets ... 1395
- Verelan Capsules ... 1455

Yellow Fever Vaccine (During treatment with tacrolimus, vaccination may be less effective).
- No products indexed under this heading.

Food Interactions

Meal, unspecified (The presence of food reduces the absorption of tacrolimus (decrease in AUC and C_{max}, and increase in T_{max}).

PRO-HEPATONE CAPSULES
(Vitamins with Minerals, Amino Acid Preparations) ... 1558
None cited in PDR database.

PROLASTIN ALPHA$_1$-PROTEINASE INHIBITOR (HUMAN)
(Alpha$_1$-Proteinase Inhibitor (Human)) ... 629
None cited in PDR database.

PROLEUKIN FOR INJECTION
(Aldesleukin) ... 812
May interact with beta blockers, antihypertensives, narcotic analgesics, hypnotics and sedatives, tranquilizers, aminoglycosides, radiographic iodinated contrast media, cytotoxic drugs, glucocorticoids, and certain other agents. Compounds in these categories include:

Acebutolol Hydrochloride (May potentiate the hypotension seen with aldesleukin). Products include:
- Sectral Capsules ... 2914

Alfentanil Hydrochloride (Potential for unspecified effect on central nervous function). Products include:
- Alfenta Injection ... 1334

Alprazolam (Potential for unspecified effect on central nervous function). Products include:
- Xanax Tablets ... 2115

Amikacin Sulfate (Potential for increased nephrotoxicity). Products include:
- Amikacin Sulfate Injection, USP ... 523
- Amikacin Sulfate Injection, USP ... 981
- Amikin Injectable ... 502

Amlodipine Besylate (May potentiate the hypotension seen with aldesleukin). Products include:
- Lotrel Capsules ... 858
- Norvasc Tablets ... 2020

Asparaginase (Potential for increased hepatic toxicity). Products include:
- Elspar ... 1700

Atenolol (May potentiate the hypotension seen with aldesleukin). Products include:
- Tenoretic Tablets ... 2963
- Tenormin Tablets and I.V. Injection 2965

Benazepril Hydrochloride (May potentiate the hypotension seen with aldesleukin). Products include:
- Lotensin Tablets ... 852
- Lotensin HCT Tablets ... 855
- Lotrel Capsules ... 858

Bendroflumethiazide (May potentiate the hypotension seen with aldesleukin).
- No products indexed under this heading.

Betamethasone Acetate (May reduce the antitumor effectiveness of aldesleukin). Products include:
- Celestone Soluspan Suspension ... 2484

Betamethasone Sodium Phosphate (May reduce the antitumor effectiveness of aldesleukin). Products include:
- Celestone Soluspan Suspension ... 2484

Betaxolol Hydrochloride (May potentiate the hypotension seen with aldesleukin). Products include:
- Betoptic Ophthalmic Solution ... 465
- Betoptic S Ophthalmic Suspension 467
- Kerlone Tablets ... 2588

Bisoprolol Fumarate (May potentiate the hypotension seen with aldesleukin). Products include:
- Zebeta Tablets ... 1457
- Ziac ... 1459

Bleomycin Sulfate (Potential for increased myelotoxicity). Products include:
- Blenoxane ... 697

Buprenorphine (Potential for unspecified effect on central nervous function). Products include:
- Buprenex Injectable ... 2170

Buspirone Hydrochloride (Potential for unspecified effect on central nervous function). Products include:
- BuSpar Tablets ... 738

Captopril (May potentiate the hypotension seen with aldesleukin). Products include:
- Capoten Tablets ... 740
- Capozide Tablets ... 744

Carteolol Hydrochloride (May potentiate the hypotension seen with aldesleukin). Products include:
- Cartrol Tablets ... 413
- Ocupress Ophthalmic Solution, 1% Sterile ... ◉ 297

Chlordiazepoxide (Potential for unspecified effect on central nervous function). Products include:
- Limbitrol ... 2333

Chlordiazepoxide Hydrochloride (Potential for unspecified effect on central nervous function). Products include:
- Librax Capsules ... 2330
- Librium Capsules ... 2331
- Librium Injectable ... 2332

Chlorothiazide (May potentiate the hypotension seen with aldesleukin). Products include:
- Aldoclor Tablets ... 1638
- Diupres Tablets ... 1691
- Diuril Oral ... 1694

Chlorothiazide Sodium (May potentiate the hypotension seen with aldesleukin). Products include:
- Diuril Sodium Intravenous ... 1693

Chlorpromazine (Potential for unspecified effect on central nervous function). Products include:
- Thorazine Suppositories ... 2701

Chlorprothixene (Potential for unspecified effect on central nervous function).
- No products indexed under this heading.

Chlorprothixene Hydrochloride (Potential for unspecified effect on central nervous function).
- No products indexed under this heading.

Chlorthalidone (May potentiate the hypotension seen with aldesleukin). Products include:
- Combipres Tablets ... 682
- Tenoretic Tablets ... 2963
- Thalitone ... 1293

Clonidine (May potentiate the hypotension seen with aldesleukin). Products include:
- Catapres-TTS ... 680

Clonidine Hydrochloride (May potentiate the hypotension seen with aldesleukin). Products include:
- Catapres Tablets ... 679
- Combipres Tablets ... 682

Clorazepate Dipotassium (Potential for unspecified effect on central nervous function). Products include:
- Tranxene ... 459

Codeine Phosphate (Potential for unspecified effect on central nervous function). Products include:
- Brontex ... 2130
- Dimetane-DC Cough Syrup ... 2232
- Fioricet with Codeine Capsules ... 2387
- Fiorinal with Codeine Capsules ... 2390
- Nucofed ... 2225
- Phenergan with Codeine ... 2883
- Phenergan VC with Codeine ... 2888
- Robitussin A-C Syrup ... 2248
- Robitussin-DAC Syrup ... 2249
- Ryna ... 804
- Soma Compound w/Codeine Tablets ... 2784
- Tylenol with Codeine ... 1592

Cortisone Acetate (May reduce the antitumor effectiveness of aldesleukin). Products include:
- Cortone Acetate Sterile Suspension ... 1663
- Cortone Acetate Tablets ... 1664

Daunorubicin Hydrochloride (Potential for increased myelotoxicity). Products include:
- Cerubidine for Injection ... 634

Deserpidine (May potentiate the hypotension seen with aldesleukin).
- No products indexed under this heading.

Dexamethasone (May reduce the antitumor effectiveness of aldesleukin). Products include:
- AK-Trol Ointment & Suspension ... ◉ 205
- Decadron Elixir ... 1676
- Decadron Tablets ... 1678
- Decaspray Topical Aerosol ... 1689
- Maxitrol Ophthalmic Ointment and Suspension ... ◉ 222
- TobraDex Ophthalmic Suspension and Ointment ... 469

Dexamethasone Acetate (May reduce the antitumor effectiveness of aldesleukin). Products include:
- Dalalone D.P. Injectable ... 1009
- Decadron-LA Sterile Suspension ... 1687

Dexamethasone Sodium Phosphate (May reduce the antitumor effectiveness of aldesleukin). Products include:
- Decadron Phosphate Injection ... 1680
- Decadron Phosphate Sterile Ophthalmic Ointment ... 1684
- Decadron Phosphate Sterile Ophthalmic Solution ... 1685
- Decadron Phosphate Topical Cream ... 1686
- Decadron Phosphate with Xylocaine Injection, Sterile ... 1683
- Dexacort Phosphate in Respihaler .. 1606
- Dexacort Phosphate in Turbinaire .. 1607
- NeoDecadron Sterile Ophthalmic Ointment ... 1755
- NeoDecadron Sterile Ophthalmic Solution ... 1756
- NeoDecadron Topical Cream ... 1757

Dezocine (Potential for unspecified effect on central nervous function). Products include:
- Dalgan Injection ... 529

Diatrizoate Meglumine (Potential for delayed adverse reactions to iodinated contrast media including fever, chills, nausea, vomiting, pruritus, rash, diarrhea, hypotension, edema, and oliguria).

Diatrizoate Sodium (Potential for delayed adverse reactions to iodinated contrast media including fever, chills, nausea, vomiting, pruritus, rash, diarrhea, hypotension, edema, and oliguria).

Diazepam (Potential for unspecified effect on central nervous function). Products include:
- Dizac (diazepam injectable emulsion) CIV ... 1862
- Valium Injectable ... 2336
- Valium Tablets ... 2335

Diazoxide (May potentiate the hypotension seen with aldesleukin). Products include:
- Hyperstat I.V. Injection ... 2504
- Proglycem ... 575

Diltiazem Hydrochloride (May potentiate the hypotension seen with aldesleukin). Products include:
- Cardizem CD Capsules ... 1251
- Cardizem SR Capsules ... 1255
- Cardizem Injectable ... 1253
- Cardizem Tablets ... 1257
- Dilacor XR Extended-release Capsules ... 2183
- Tiazac Capsules ... 1019

Doxazosin Mesylate (May potentiate the hypotension seen with aldesleukin). Products include:
- Cardura Tablets ... 1993

Doxorubicin Hydrochloride (Potential for increased cardiotoxicity and myelotoxicity). Products include:
- Adriamycin PFS ... 2056
- Adriamycin RDF ... 2056
- Doxil ... 2613
- Doxorubicin Astra ... 531
- Rubex for Injection ... 721

Droperidol (Potential for unspecified effect on central nervous function). Products include:
- Inapsine Injection ... 462

Enalapril Maleate (May potentiate the hypotension seen with aldesleukin). Products include:
- Vaseretic Tablets ... 1810
- Vasotec Tablets ... 1816

Enalaprilat (May potentiate the hypotension seen with aldesleukin). Products include:
- Vasotec I.V. ... 1814

Esmolol Hydrochloride (May potentiate the hypotension seen with aldesleukin). Products include:
- Brevibloc (esmolol HCl) Injection ... 1860

Estazolam (Potential for unspecified effect on central nervous function). Products include:
- ProSom Tablets ... 457

Ethchlorvynol (Potential for unspecified effect on central nervous function). Products include:
- Placidyl Capsules ... 456

Ethinamate (Potential for unspecified effect on central nervous function).
- No products indexed under this heading.

IMPORTANT NOTE: Always consult each drug listing in the patient's regimen for possible interactions.

Proleukin **Interactions Index** **876**

Ethiodized Oil (Potential for delayed adverse reactions to iodinated contrast media including fever, chills, nausea, vomiting, pruritus, rash, diarrhea, hypotension, edema, and oliguria).
No products indexed under this heading.

Felodipine (May potentiate the hypotension seen with aldesleukin). Products include:
Plendil Extended-Release Tablets.... 514

Fentanyl (Potential for unspecified effect on central nervous function). Products include:
Duragesic Transdermal System........ 1336

Fentanyl Citrate (Potential for unspecified effect on central nervous function). Products include:
Sublimaze Injection.... 463

Fludrocortisone Acetate (May reduce the antitumor effectiveness of aldesleukin). Products include:
Florinef Acetate Tablets 506

Fluorouracil (Potential for increased myelotoxicity). Products include:
Efudex 2280
Fluoroplex Topical Solution & Cream 1% 475
Fluorouracil Injection 2282

Fluphenazine Decanoate (Potential for unspecified effect on central nervous function). Products include:
Prolixin Decanoate 510

Fluphenazine Enanthate (Potential for unspecified effect on central nervous function). Products include:
Prolixin Enanthate.... 510

Fluphenazine Hydrochloride (Potential for unspecified effect on central nervous function). Products include:
Prolixin.... 510

Flurazepam Hydrochloride (Potential for unspecified effect on central nervous function). Products include:
Dalmane Capsules.... 2329

Fosinopril Sodium (May potentiate the hypotension seen with aldesleukin). Products include:
Monopril Tablets 762

Furosemide (May potentiate the hypotension seen with aldesleukin). Products include:
Lasix Injection, Oral Solution and Tablets 1267

Gadopentetate Dimeglumine (Potential for delayed adverse reactions to iodinated contrast media including fever, chills, nausea, vomiting, pruritus, rash, diarrhea, hypotension, edema, and oliguria).
No products indexed under this heading.

Gentamicin Sulfate (Potential for increased nephrotoxicity). Products include:
Garamycin Cream 0.1% 2501
Garamycin Injectable 2502
Garamycin Ointment 0.1%.... 2501
Garamycin Ophthalmic 2501
Genoptic Sterile Ophthalmic Solution.... ⊙ 241
Genoptic Sterile Ophthalmic Ointment .... ⊙ 241
Gentak .... ⊙ 209
Pred-G Liquifilm Sterile Ophthalmic Suspension .... ⊙ 248
Pred-G S.O.P. Sterile Ophthalmic Ointment .... ⊙ 249

Glutethimide (Potential for unspecified effect on central nervous function).
No products indexed under this heading.

Guanabenz Acetate (May potentiate the hypotension seen with aldesleukin).
No products indexed under this heading.

Guanethidine Monosulfate (May potentiate the hypotension seen with aldesleukin). Products include:
Esimil Tablets 840
Ismelin Tablets 845

Haloperidol (Potential for unspecified effect on central nervous function). Products include:
Haldol Injection, Tablets and Concentrate 1585

Haloperidol Decanoate (Potential for unspecified effect on central nervous function). Products include:
Haldol Decanoate.... 1587

Hepatotoxic Drugs, unspecified (Potential for increased hepatic toxicity).

Hydralazine Hydrochloride (May potentiate the hypotension seen with aldesleukin). Products include:
Apresazide Capsules 824
Apresoline Hydrochloride Tablets .. 826
Hydralazine Hydrochloride Injection USP.... 2712
Ser-Ap-Es Tablets 867

Hydrochlorothiazide (May potentiate the hypotension seen with aldesleukin). Products include:
Aldactazide Tablets 2556
Aldoril Tablets.... 1644
Apresazide Capsules 824
Capozide Tablets 744
Dyazide Capsules.... 2653
Esidrix Tablets 839
Esimil Tablets 840
HydroDIURIL Tablets 1716
Hydropres Tablets.... 1718
Hyzaar Tablets 1720
Inderide Tablets 2838
Inderide LA Long Acting Capsules .. 2840
Lopressor HCT Tablets 850
Lotensin HCT Tablets 855
Moduretic Tablets 1748
Oretic Tablets 450
Prinzide Tablets 1780
Ser-Ap-Es Tablets 867
Timolide Tablets.... 1791
Vaseretic Tablets.... 1810
Zestoretic Tablets 2968
Ziac 1459

Hydrocodone Bitartrate (Potential for unspecified effect on central nervous function). Products include:
Codiclear DH Syrup 808
Duratuss HD Elixir.... 2750
Histussin D Liquid 670
Hycodan Tablets and Syrup 946
Hycomine Compound Tablets 948
Hycomine 947
Hycotuss Expectorant Syrup 950
Hydrocet Capsules 787
Lorcet 10/650 Tablets 1016
Lortab.... 2751
Tussend.... 1830
Tussend Expectorant.... 1831
Vicodin Tablets.... 1404
Vicodin ES Tablets 1405
Vicodin HP Tablets 1403
Vicodin Tuss Expectorant 1406
Zydone Capsules 967

Hydrocodone Polistirex (Potential for unspecified effect on central nervous function). Products include:
Tussionex Pennkinetic Extended-Release Suspension 1624

Hydrocortisone (May reduce the antitumor effectiveness of aldesleukin). Products include:
Anusol-HC Cream 2.5%.... 1953
Aquanil HC Lotion 1989
Maximum Strength Cortaid Spray ▣ 800
CORTENEMA.... 2713
Cortisporin Ointment.... 1074
Cortisporin Ophthalmic Ointment Sterile 1074
Cortisporin Ophthalmic Suspension Sterile 1075
Cortisporin Otic Solution Sterile 1076
Cortisporin Otic Suspension Sterile 1077
Cortizone-5 .... ▣ 795
Cortizone-10 .... ▣ 795
Hydrocortone Tablets 1715
Hytone 922
Hytone Ointment 2 ½%.... 923
Massengill Medicated Soft Cloth Towelettes.... 2628
Pediotic Suspension Sterile.... 1140
Preparation H Hydrocortisone 1% Cream .... ▣ 843
ProctoCream-HC 2.5%.... 2552
VōSoL HC Otic Solution.... 2786

Hydrocortisone Acetate (May reduce the antitumor effectiveness of aldesleukin). Products include:
Analpram-HC Rectal Cream 1% and 2.5% 993
Anusol HC-1 Hydrocortisone Anti-Itch Ointment .... ▣ 810
Anusol-HC Suppositories 1954
Caldecort Anti-Itch Hydrocortisone Cream .... ▣ 651
Coly-Mycin S Otic w/Neomycin & Hydrocortisone.... 1965
Cortaid .... ▣ 800
Cortifoam 2540
Cortisporin Cream.... 1073
Epifoam 2543
Hydrocortone Acetate Sterile Suspension.... 1712
Mantadil Cream 1124
Nupercainal Hydrocortisone 1% Cream.... ▣ 661
Pramosone Cream, Lotion & Ointment 995
ProctoFoam-HC 2552
Terra-Cortril Ophthalmic Suspension 2033

Hydrocortisone Sodium Phosphate (May reduce the antitumor effectiveness of aldesleukin). Products include:
Hydrocortone Phosphate Injection, Sterile 1713

Hydrocortisone Sodium Succinate (May reduce the antitumor effectiveness of aldesleukin).
No products indexed under this heading.

Hydroflumethiazide (May potentiate the hypotension seen with aldesleukin). Products include:
Diucardin Tablets.... 2824

Hydromorphone Hydrochloride (Potential for unspecified effect on central nervous function). Products include:
Dilaudid Ampules.... 1382
Dilaudid Cough Syrup 1383
Dilaudid-HP Injection 1384
Dilaudid-HP Lyophilized Powder 250 mg 1384
Dilaudid 1382
Dilaudid Oral Liquid 1386
Dilaudid 1382
Dilaudid Tablets - 8 mg.... 1386

Hydroxyurea (Potential for increased myelotoxicity). Products include:
Hydrea Capsules 705

Hydroxyzine Hydrochloride (Potential for unspecified effect on central nervous function). Products include:
Atarax Tablets & Syrup.... 1992
Marax Tablets & DF Syrup.... 2015
Vistaril Intramuscular Solution.... 2042

Indapamide (May potentiate the hypotension seen with aldesleukin).
No products indexed under this heading.

Indomethacin (Potential for increased nephrotoxicity). Products include:
Indocin 1723

Iodamide Meglumine (Potential for delayed adverse reactions to iodinated contrast media including fever, chills, nausea, vomiting, pruritus, rash, diarrhea, hypotension, edema, and oliguria).
No products indexed under this heading.

Iohexol (Potential for delayed adverse reactions to iodinated contrast media including fever, chills, nausea, vomiting, pruritus, rash, diarrhea, hypotension, edema, and oliguria).
No products indexed under this heading.

Iopamidol (Potential for delayed adverse reactions to iodinated contrast media including fever, chills, nausea, vomiting, pruritus, rash, diarrhea, hypotension, edema, and oliguria).
No products indexed under this heading.

Iothalamate Meglumine (Potential for delayed adverse reactions to iodinated contrast media including fever, chills, nausea, vomiting, pruritus, rash, diarrhea, hypotension, edema, and oliguria).
No products indexed under this heading.

Iopanoic Acid (Potential for delayed adverse reactions to iodinated contrast media including fever, chills, nausea, vomiting, pruritus, rash, diarrhea, hypotension, edema, and oliguria).

Ioxaglate Meglumine (Potential for delayed adverse reactions to iodinated contrast media including fever, chills, nausea, vomiting, pruritus, rash, diarrhea, hypotension, edema, and oliguria).
No products indexed under this heading.

Ioxaglate Sodium (Potential for delayed adverse reactions to iodinated contrast media including fever, chills, nausea, vomiting, pruritus, rash, diarrhea, hypotension, edema, and oliguria).
No products indexed under this heading.

Isradipine (May potentiate the hypotension seen with aldesleukin). Products include:
DynaCirc Capsules 2381
DynaCirc CR Tablets 2383

Kanamycin Sulfate (Potential for increased nephrotoxicity).
No products indexed under this heading.

Labetalol Hydrochloride (May potentiate the hypotension seen with aldesleukin). Products include:
Normodyne Injection 2519
Normodyne Tablets 2522
Trandate 1158

Levobunolol Hydrochloride (May potentiate the hypotension seen with aldesleukin). Products include:
Betagan .... ⊙ 230

Levorphanol Tartrate (Potential for unspecified effect on central nervous function). Products include:
Levo-Dromoran.... 2297

Lisinopril (May potentiate the hypotension seen with aldesleukin). Products include:
Prinivil Tablets 1776
Prinzide Tablets 1780
Zestoretic Tablets 2968
Zestril Tablets 2972

Lorazepam (Potential for unspecified effect on central nervous function). Products include:
Ativan Injection.... 2805
Ativan Tablets.... 2807

Losartan Potassium (May potentiate the hypotension seen with aldesleukin). Products include:
Cozaar Tablets 1668
Hyzaar Tablets 1720

(▣ Described in PDR For Nonprescription Drugs) (⊙ Described in PDR For Ophthalmology)

877 **Interactions Index** **Proleukin**

Loxapine Hydrochloride (Potential for unspecified effect on central nervous function). Products include:
- Loxitane 1426

Loxapine Succinate (Potential for unspecified effect on central nervous function). Products include:
- Loxitane Capsules 1426

Mecamylamine Hydrochloride (May potentiate the hypotension seen with aldesleukin). Products include:
- Inversine Tablets 1729

Meperidine Hydrochloride (Potential for unspecified effect on central nervous function). Products include:
- Demerol 2438
- Mepergan Injection 2859

Meprobamate (Potential for unspecified effect on central nervous function). Products include:
- Miltown Tablets 2780
- PMB 200 and PMB 400 2890

Mesoridazine Besylate (Potential for unspecified effect on central nervous function). Products include:
- Serentil 689

Methadone Hydrochloride (Potential for unspecified effect on central nervous function). Products include:
- Methadone Hydrochloride Oral Concentrate 2356
- Methadone Hydrochloride Oral Solution & Tablets 2357

Methotrexate Sodium (Potential for increased hepatic toxicity and myelotoxicity). Products include:
- Methotrexate Sodium Tablets, Injection, for Injection and LPF Injection 1322

Methyclothiazide (May potentiate the hypotension seen with aldesleukin). Products include:
- Enduron Tablets 424

Methyldopa (May potentiate the hypotension seen with aldesleukin). Products include:
- Aldoclor Tablets 1638
- Aldomet Oral 1640
- Aldoril Tablets 1644

Methyldopate Hydrochloride (May potentiate the hypotension seen with aldesleukin). Products include:
- Aldomet Ester HCl Injection 1642

Methylprednisolone Acetate (May reduce the antitumor effectiveness of aldesleukin).
- No products indexed under this heading.

Methylprednisolone Sodium Succinate (May reduce the antitumor effectiveness of aldesleukin).
- No products indexed under this heading.

Metipranolol Hydrochloride (May potentiate the hypotension seen with aldesleukin). Products include:
- OptiPranolol (Metipranolol 0.3%) Sterile Ophthalmic Solution........ ◉ 256

Metolazone (May potentiate the hypotension seen with aldesleukin). Products include:
- Mykrox Tablets 1617
- Zaroxolyn Tablets 1625

Metoprolol Succinate (May potentiate the hypotension seen with aldesleukin). Products include:
- Toprol-XL Tablets 560

Metoprolol Tartrate (May potentiate the hypotension seen with aldesleukin). Products include:
- Lopressor 848
- Lopressor HCT Tablets 850

Metyrosine (May potentiate the hypotension seen with aldesleukin). Products include:
- Demser Capsules 1690

Midazolam Hydrochloride (Potential for unspecified effect on central nervous function). Products include:
- Versed Injection 2324

Minoxidil (May potentiate the hypotension seen with aldesleukin).
- No products indexed under this heading.

Mitotane (Potential for increased myelotoxicity). Products include:
- Lysodren Tablets 707

Mitoxantrone Hydrochloride (Potential for increased myelotoxicity). Products include:
- Novantrone for Injection 1327

Moexipril Hydrochloride (May potentiate the hypotension seen with aldesleukin). Products include:
- Univasc Tablets 2553

Molindone Hydrochloride (Potential for unspecified effect on central nervous function). Products include:
- Moban Tablets and Concentrate 1036

Morphine Sulfate (Potential for unspecified effect on central nervous function). Products include:
- Astramorph/PF Injection, USP (Preservative-Free) 526
- Duramorph Injection 983
- Infumorph 200 and Infumorph 500 Sterile Solutions 985
- Kadian Capsules 2948
- MS Contin Tablets 2149
- MSIR 2152
- Oramorph SR (Morphine Sulfate Sustained Release Tablets) 2359
- RMS Suppositories CII 2766
- Roxanol 2365

Nadolol (May potentiate the hypotension seen with aldesleukin).
- No products indexed under this heading.

Nephrotoxic Drugs (Potential for increased nephrotoxicity).

Nicardipine Hydrochloride (May potentiate the hypotension seen with aldesleukin). Products include:
- Cardene Capsules 2261
- Cardene I.V. 2815
- Cardene SR Capsules 2264

Nifedipine (May potentiate the hypotension seen with aldesleukin). Products include:
- Adalat Capsules (10 mg and 20 mg) 580
- Adalat CC 582
- Procardia Capsules 2024
- Procardia XL Extended Release Tablets 2026

Nisoldipine (May potentiate the hypotension seen with aldesleukin). Products include:
- Sular Tablets 2961

Nitroglycerin (May potentiate the hypotension seen with aldesleukin). Products include:
- Deponit NTG Transdermal Delivery System 2541
- Nitro-Bid IV 1270
- Nitro-Bid Ointment 1272
- Nitro-Dur (nitroglycerin) Transdermal Infusion System 1365
- Nitrolingual Spray 2193
- Nitrostat Tablets 1981
- Transderm-Nitro Transdermal Therapeutic System 878

Opium Alkaloids (Potential for unspecified effect on central nervous function).
- No products indexed under this heading.

Oxazepam (Potential for unspecified effect on central nervous function). Products include:
- Serax Capsules 2916
- Serax Tablets 2916

Oxycodone Hydrochloride (Potential for unspecified effect on central nervous function). Products include:
- OxyContin Tablets 2163
- OxyIR Capsules 2167
- Percocet Tablets 955
- Percodan Tablets 955
- Percodan-Demi Tablets 956
- Roxicodone Tablets, Oral Solution & Intensol (Oxycodone) 2366
- Tylox Capsules 1593

Penbutolol Sulfate (May potentiate the hypotension seen with aldesleukin). Products include:
- Levatol Tablets 2547

Perphenazine (Potential for unspecified effect on central nervous function). Products include:
- Etrafon 2495
- Triavil Tablets 1800
- Trilafon 2532

Phenoxybenzamine Hydrochloride (May potentiate the hypotension seen with aldesleukin). Products include:
- Dibenzyline Capsules 2650

Phentolamine Mesylate (May potentiate the hypotension seen with aldesleukin). Products include:
- Regitine Vials 864

Pindolol (May potentiate the hypotension seen with aldesleukin). Products include:
- Visken Tablets 2428

Polythiazide (May potentiate the hypotension seen with aldesleukin). Products include:
- Minizide Capsules 2016

Prazepam (Potential for unspecified effect on central nervous function).
- No products indexed under this heading.

Prazosin Hydrochloride (May potentiate the hypotension seen with aldesleukin). Products include:
- Minipress Capsules 2015
- Minizide Capsules 2016

Prednisolone Acetate (May reduce the antitumor effectiveness of aldesleukin). Products include:
- AK-CIDE .... ◉ 203
- AK-CIDE Ointment .... ◉ 203
- Blephamide Liquifilm Sterile Ophthalmic Suspension 472
- Blephamide Ointment .... ◉ 234
- Econopred & Econopred Plus Ophthalmic Suspensions .... ◉ 216
- Poly-Pred Liquifilm .... ◉ 246
- Pred Forte .... ◉ 247
- Pred Mild .... ◉ 250
- Pred-G Liquifilm Sterile Ophthalmic Suspension .... ◉ 248
- Pred-G S.O.P. Sterile Ophthalmic Ointment .... ◉ 249

Prednisolone Sodium Phosphate (May reduce the antitumor effectiveness of aldesleukin). Products include:
- AK-PRED .... ◉ 204
- Hydeltrasol Injection, Sterile 1708
- Pediapred Oral Solution 1618

Prednisolone Tebutate (May reduce the antitumor effectiveness of aldesleukin). Products include:
- Hydeltra-T.B.A. Sterile Suspension 1710

Prednisone (May reduce the antitumor effectiveness of aldesleukin).
- No products indexed under this heading.

Procarbazine Hydrochloride (Potential for increased myelotoxicity). Products include:
- Matulane Capsules 2300

Prochlorperazine (Potential for unspecified effect on central nervous function). Products include:
- Compazine 2644

Promethazine Hydrochloride (Potential for unspecified effect on central nervous function). Products include:
- Mepergan Injection 2859
- Phenergan with Codeine 2883
- Phenergan with Dextromethorphan 2885
- Phenergan Injection 2880
- Phenergan Suppositories 2882
- Phenergan Syrup 2881
- Phenergan Tablets 2882
- Phenergan VC 2886
- Phenergan VC with Codeine 2888

Propofol (Potential for unspecified effect on central nervous function). Products include:
- Diprivan Injectable Emulsion 2939

Propoxyphene Hydrochloride (Potential for unspecified effect on central nervous function). Products include:
- Darvon 1475
- Wygesic Tablets 2930

Propoxyphene Napsylate (Potential for unspecified effect on central nervous function). Products include:
- Darvon-N/Darvocet-N 1473

Propranolol Hydrochloride (May potentiate the hypotension seen with aldesleukin). Products include:
- Inderal 2834
- Inderal LA Long Acting Capsules 2836
- Inderide Tablets 2838
- Inderide LA Long Acting Capsules .. 2840

Quazepam (Potential for unspecified effect on central nervous function). Products include:
- Doral Tablets 2773

Quinapril Hydrochloride (May potentiate the hypotension seen with aldesleukin). Products include:
- Accupril Tablets 1950

Ramipril (May potentiate the hypotension seen with aldesleukin). Products include:
- Altace Capsules 1238

Rauwolfia Serpentina (May potentiate the hypotension seen with aldesleukin).
- No products indexed under this heading.

Rescinnamine (May potentiate the hypotension seen with aldesleukin).
- No products indexed under this heading.

Reserpine (May potentiate the hypotension seen with aldesleukin). Products include:
- Diupres Tablets 1691
- Hydropres Tablets 1718
- Ser-Ap-Es Tablets 867

Secobarbital Sodium (Potential for unspecified effect on central nervous function). Products include:
- Seconal Sodium Pulvules 1529

Sodium Nitroprusside (May potentiate the hypotension seen with aldesleukin).
- No products indexed under this heading.

Sotalol Hydrochloride (May potentiate the hypotension seen with aldesleukin). Products include:
- Betapace Tablets 637

Spirapril Hydrochloride (May potentiate the hypotension seen with aldesleukin).
- No products indexed under this heading.

Streptomycin Sulfate (Potential for increased nephrotoxicity). Products include:
- Streptomycin Sulfate Injection 2031

IMPORTANT NOTE: Always consult each drug listing in the patient's regimen for possible interactions.

Proleukin **Interactions Index** 878

Sufentanil Citrate (Potential for unspecified effect on central nervous function). Products include:
Sufenta Injection ... 1355

Tamoxifen Citrate (Potential for increased myelotoxicity). Products include:
Nolvadex Tablets ... 2957

Temazepam (Potential for unspecified effect on central nervous function). Products include:
Restoril Capsules ... 2413

Terazosin Hydrochloride (May potentiate the hypotension seen with aldesleukin). Products include:
Hytrin Capsules ... 434

Thioridazine Hydrochloride (Potential for unspecified effect on central nervous function). Products include:
Mellaril ... 2398

Thiothixene (Potential for unspecified effect on central nervous function). Products include:
Navane Capsules and Concentrate 2018
Navane Intramuscular ... 2019

Timolol Hemihydrate (May potentiate the hypotension seen with aldesleukin). Products include:
Betimol 0.25%, 0.5% ... ⊚ 259

Timolol Maleate (May potentiate the hypotension seen with aldesleukin). Products include:
Blocadren Tablets ... 1654
Timolide Tablets ... 1791
Timoptic in Ocudose ... 1796
Timoptic Sterile Ophthalmic Solution ... 1794
Timoptic-XE ... 1798

Tobramycin (Potential for increased nephrotoxicity). Products include:
AKTOB ... ⊚ 207
TobraDex Ophthalmic Suspension and Ointment ... 469
Tobrex Ophthalmic Ointment and Solution ... ⊚ 226

Tobramycin Sulfate (Potential for increased nephrotoxicity). Products include:
Nebcin Vials, Hyporets & ADD-Vantage ... 1518

Torsemide (May potentiate the hypotension seen with aldesleukin). Products include:
Demadex Tablets and Injection ... 691

Triamcinolone (May reduce the antitumor effectiveness of aldesleukin).
No products indexed under this heading.

Triamcinolone Acetonide (May reduce the antitumor effectiveness of aldesleukin). Products include:
Azmacort Oral Inhaler ... 2175
Nasacort AQ Nasal Spray ... 2191
Nasacort Nasal Inhaler ... 2189

Triamcinolone Diacetate (May reduce the antitumor effectiveness of aldesleukin).
No products indexed under this heading.

Triamcinolone Hexacetonide (May reduce the antitumor effectiveness of aldesleukin).
No products indexed under this heading.

Triazolam (Potential for unspecified effect on central nervous function). Products include:
Halcion Tablets ... 2093

Trifluoperazine Hydrochloride (Potential for unspecified effect on central nervous function). Products include:
Stelazine ... 2692

Trimethaphan Camsylate (May potentiate the hypotension seen with aldesleukin).
No products indexed under this heading.

Tyropanoate Sodium (Potential for delayed adverse reactions to iodinated contrast media including fever, chills, nausea, vomiting, pruritus, rash, diarrhea, hypotension, edema, and oliguria).
No products indexed under this heading.

Verapamil Hydrochloride (May potentiate the hypotension seen with aldesleukin). Products include:
Calan SR Caplets ... 2571
Calan Tablets ... 2568
Covera-HS Tablets ... 2573
Isoptin Injectable ... 1391
Isoptin Oral Tablets ... 1393
Isoptin SR Tablets ... 1395
Verelan Capsules ... 1455

Vincristine Sulfate (Potential for increased myelotoxicity). Products include:
Oncovin Solution Vials & Hyporets 1521

Zolpidem Tartrate (Potential for unspecified effect on central nervous function). Products include:
Ambien Tablets ... 2559

PROLIXIN DECANOATE
(Fluphenazine Decanoate) ... 510
May interact with central nervous system depressants, narcotic analgesics, antihistamines, barbiturates, and certain other agents. Compounds in these categories include:

Acrivastine (Potentiation of CNS depressant effect may occur). Products include:
Semprex-D Capsules ... 1620

Alfentanil Hydrochloride (Potentiation of CNS depressant effect may occur). Products include:
Alfenta Injection ... 1334

Alprazolam (Potentiation of CNS depressant effect may occur). Products include:
Xanax Tablets ... 2115

Aprobarbital (Potentiation of CNS depressant effect may occur).
No products indexed under this heading.

Astemizole (Potentiation of CNS depressant effect may occur). Products include:
Hismanal Tablets ... 1341

Atropine Sulfate (Additive anticholinergic effects). Products include:
Arco-Lase Plus Tablets ... 513
Atrohist Plus Tablets ... 1605
Donnatal ... 2234
Donnatal Extentabs ... 2234
Donnatal Tablets ... 2234
Lomotil ... 2591
Motofen Tablets ... 789
Urised Tablets ... 2123

Azatadine Maleate (Potentiation of CNS depressant effect may occur). Products include:
Trinalin Repetabs Tablets ... 1373

Bromodiphenhydramine Hydrochloride (Potentiation of CNS depressant effect may occur).
No products indexed under this heading.

Brompheniramine Maleate (Potentiation of CNS depressant effect may occur). Products include:
Alka-Seltzer Plus Sinus Medicine .. ▣ 611
Bromfed Capsules (Extended-Release) ... 1832
Bromfed Syrup ... ▣ 712
Bromfed Tablets ... 1832
Bromfed-DM Cough Syrup ... 1832
Bromfed-PD Capsules (Extended-Release) ... 1832
Dimetane-DC Cough Syrup ... 2232
Dimetane-DX Cough Syrup ... 2233
Dimetapp Allergy Dye-Free Elixir ... ▣ 838
Dimetapp Allergy Sinus Caplets ... ▣ 838
Dimetapp Cold & Allergy Chewable Tablets ... ▣ 838
Dimetapp Cold & Cough Liqui-Gels ... ▣ 839
Dimetapp Cold & Fever Suspension ... ▣ 839
Dimetapp DM Elixir ... ▣ 840
Dimetapp Elixir ... ▣ 840
Dimetapp Extentabs ... ▣ 841
Dimetapp Tablets/Liqui-Gels ... ▣ 841
Rondec Chewable Tablets ... 974
Vicks DayQuil Allergy Relief 12-Hour Extended Release Tablets .. ▣ 733
Vicks DayQuil Allergy Relief 4-Hour Tablets ... ▣ 733

Buprenorphine (Potentiation of CNS depressant effect may occur). Products include:
Buprenex Injectable ... 2170

Buspirone Hydrochloride (Potentiation of CNS depressant effect may occur). Products include:
BuSpar Tablets ... 738

Butabarbital (Potentiation of CNS depressant effect may occur).
No products indexed under this heading.

Butalbital (Potentiation of CNS depressant effect may occur). Products include:
Axocet Capsules ... 2469
Esgic-plus Capsules ... 1012
Esgic-plus Tablets ... 1012
Fioricet Tablets ... 2386
Fioricet with Codeine Capsules ... 2387
Fiorinal Capsules ... 2388
Fiorinal with Codeine Capsules ... 2390
Fiorinal Tablets ... 2388
Phrenilin ... 790
Sedapap Tablets 50 mg/650 mg .. 1826

Cetirizine Hydrochloride (Potentiation of CNS depressant effect may occur). Products include:
Zyrtec Tablets ... 2053

Chlordiazepoxide (Potentiation of CNS depressant effect may occur). Products include:
Limbitrol ... 2333

Chlordiazepoxide Hydrochloride (Potentiation of CNS depressant effect may occur). Products include:
Librax Capsules ... 2330
Librium Capsules ... 2331
Librium Injectable ... 2332

Chlorpheniramine Maleate (Potentiation of CNS depressant effect may occur). Products include:
Alka-Seltzer Plus Cold Medicine ... ▣ 611
Alka-Seltzer Plus Cold Medicine Liqui-Gels ... ▣ 612
Alka-Seltzer Plus Cold & Cough Medicine ... ▣ 611
Alka-Seltzer Plus Cold & Cough Medicine Liqui-Gels ... ▣ 612
Alka-Seltzer Plus Flu & Body Aches Effervescent Tablets ... ▣ 612
Allerest Maximum Strength ... ▣ 649
Allerest Sinus Pain Formula ... ▣ 649
Ana-Kit Anaphylaxis Emergency Treatment Kit ... 611
Atrohist Pediatric Capsules ... 1603
Atrohist Plus Tablets ... 1605
BC Cold Powder Multi-Symptom Formula (Cold-Sinus-Allergy) ... ▣ 631
Cerose DM ... ▣ 853
Cheracol Plus Head Cold/Cough Formula ... ▣ 741
Children's TYLENOL Cold Multi-Symptom Chewable Tablets and Liquid ... 1559
Children's TYLENOL Cold Plus Cough Multi Symptom Chewable Tablets and Liquid ... 1560
Children's TYLENOL Flu Suspension Liquid ... 1560
Children's Vicks DayQuil Allergy Relief ... ▣ 730
Children's Vicks NyQuil Cold/Cough Relief ... ▣ 731
Chlor-Trimeton Allergy Decongestant Tablets ... ▣ 759
Chlor-Trimeton Allergy Tablets ... ▣ 758
Allergy-Sinus Comtrex Multi-Symptom Allergy-Sinus Formula Tablets and Caplets ... ▣ 639
Comtrex Multi-Symptom ... ▣ 638
Contac Continuous Action Nasal Decongestant/Antihistamine 12 Hour Capsules ... ▣ 773
Contac Maximum Strength Continuous Action Decongestant/Antihistamine 12 Hour Caplets .. ▣ 772
Contac Severe Cold and Flu Formula Caplets ... ▣ 773
Coricidin Cold + Flu Tablets ... ▣ 760
Coricidin Cough + Cold Tablets ... ▣ 760
Coricidin 'D' Decongestant Tablets ... ▣ 760
D.A. II Tablets ... 972
D.A. Chewable Tablets ... 970
Dura-Tap/PD Capsules ... 970
Dura-Vent/DA Tablets ... 972
Efidac 24 Chlorpheniramine ... ▣ 655
Extendryl ... 1003
Fedahist Gyrocaps ... 2545
Hycomine Compound Tablets ... 948
Kronofed-A ... 994
Nolamine Timed-Release Tablets ... 790
Novahistine Elixir ... ▣ 782
Ornade Spansule Capsules ... 2678
PediaCare Cough-Cold Chewable Tablets and Liquid ... 1569
PediaCare NightRest Cough-Cold Liquid ... 1569
Pediatric Vicks 44m Cough & Cold Relief ... ▣ 737
Pyrroxate Caplets ... ▣ 742
Ryna ... ▣ 804
Sinarest ... ▣ 663
Sine-Off Sinus Medicine ... ▣ 784
Singlet Tablets ... ▣ 785
Sinulin Tablets ... 792
Sinutab Sinus Allergy Medication, Maximum Strength Tablets and Caplets ... ▣ 823
Sudafed Cold & Allergy Tablets ... ▣ 826
Teldrin 12 Hour Antihistamine/Nasal Decongestant Allergy Relief Capsules ... ▣ 786
TheraFlu Flu and Cold Medicine ... ▣ 750
Theraflu Maximum Strength Flu and Cold Medicine For Sore Throat ... ▣ 751
TheraFlu Flu, Cold and Cough Medicine ... ▣ 750
TheraFlu Maximum Strength Nighttime Flu, Cold & Cough Medicine ... ▣ 751
Triaminic Night Time ... ▣ 754
Triaminic Syrup ... ▣ 755
Triaminic Triaminicol Cold & Cough ... ▣ 756
Triaminicin Tablets ... ▣ 756
Tussend ... 1830
TYLENOL Allergy Sinus, Maximum Strength Caplets and Gelcaps ... 1571
TYLENOL Cold Medication, Multi-Symptom Formula Tablets and Caplets ... 1572
TYLENOL Cold Medication, Multi-Symptom Hot Liquid Packets ... 1572
Vicks 44 LiquiCaps Cough, Cold & Flu Relief ... ▣ 728
Vicks 44M Cough, Cold & Flu Relief ... ▣ 729

Chlorpheniramine Polistirex (Potentiation of CNS depressant effect may occur). Products include:
Tussionex Pennkinetic Extended-Release Suspension ... 1624

Chlorpheniramine Tannate (Potentiation of CNS depressant effect may occur). Products include:
Atrohist Pediatric Suspension ... 1604
Atrohist Pediatric Suspension Dye-Free ... 1604
Rynatan ... 2781
Rynatuss ... 2782

Chlorpromazine (Potentiation of CNS depressant effect may occur). Products include:
Thorazine Suppositories ... 2701

Chlorprothixene (Potentiation of CNS depressant effect may occur).
No products indexed under this heading.

(▣ Described in PDR For Nonprescription Drugs) (⊚ Described in PDR For Ophthalmology)

879 Interactions Index Prolixin

Chlorprothixene Hydrochloride (Potentiation of CNS depressant effect may occur).
No products indexed under this heading.

Chlorprothixene Lactate (Potentiation of CNS depressant effect may occur).
No products indexed under this heading.

Clemastine Fumarate (Potentiation of CNS depressant effect may occur). Products include:
- Tavist Syrup 2426
- Tavist Tablets 2427
- Tavist-1 12 Hour Relief Tablets 749
- Tavist-D 12 Hour Relief Tablets 750

Clorazepate Dipotassium (Potentiation of CNS depressant effect may occur). Products include:
- Tranxene 459

Clozapine (Potentiation of CNS depressant effect may occur). Products include:
- Clozaril Tablets 2377

Codeine Phosphate (Potentiation of CNS depressant effect may occur). Products include:
- Brontex 2130
- Dimetane-DC Cough Syrup 2232
- Fioricet with Codeine Capsules 2387
- Fiorinal with Codeine Capsules 2390
- Nucofed 2225
- Phenergan with Codeine 2883
- Phenergan VC with Codeine 2888
- Robitussin A-C Syrup 2248
- Robitussin-DAC Syrup 2249
- Ryna 804
- Soma Compound w/Codeine Tablets 2784
- Tylenol with Codeine 1592

Cyproheptadine Hydrochloride (Potentiation of CNS depressant effect may occur). Products include:
- Periactin 1767

Desflurane (Potentiation of CNS depressant effect may occur). Products include:
- Suprane (desflurane, USP) 1865

Dexchlorpheniramine Maleate (Potentiation of CNS depressant effect may occur).
No products indexed under this heading.

Dezocine (Potentiation of CNS depressant effect may occur). Products include:
- Dalgan Injection 529

Diazepam (Potentiation of CNS depressant effect may occur). Products include:
- Dizac (diazepam injectable emulsion) CIV 1862
- Valium Injectable 2336
- Valium Tablets 2335

Diphenhydramine Citrate (Potentiation of CNS depressant effect may occur). Products include:
- Excedrin P.M. Analgesic/Sleeping Aid Tablets, Caplets, Liquigels 735

Diphenhydramine Hydrochloride (Potentiation of CNS depressant effect may occur). Products include:
- Actifed Allergy Daytime/Nighttime Caplets 808
- Actifed Sinus Daytime/Nighttime Tablets and Caplets 809
- Extra Strength Bayer PM Aspirin Plus Sleep Aid 617
- Benadryl Allergy Chewables 811
- Benadryl Allergy/Cold Tablets 811
- Benadryl Allergy Decongestant Liquid Medication 812
- Benadryl Allergy Decongestant Tablets 812
- Benadryl Allergy Liquid Medication 813
- Benadryl Allergy 811
- Benadryl Allergy Sinus Headache Caplets 813
- Benadryl Dye-Free Allergy Liquigel Softgels 813
- Benadryl Dye-Free Allergy Liquid Medication 814
- Benadryl Itch Relief Stick Extra Strength 814
- Benadryl Cream 814
- Benadryl Gel 815
- Benadryl Spray 815
- Benadryl Injection 1955
- Contac Day & Night Cold/Flu Night Caplets 772
- Contac Night Allergy/Sinus Caplets 771
- Extra Strength Doan's P.M. 653
- Excedrin P.M. Analgesic/Sleeping Aid Tablets, Caplets, Liquigels 643
- Nytol QuickCaps Caplets 632
- Sleepinal Night-time Sleep Aid Capsules and Softgels 798
- TYLENOL Allergy Sinus NightTime, Maximum Strength Caplets 1571
- TYLENOL Flu NightTime, Maximum Strength Gelcaps 1575
- TYLENOL Flu NightTime, Maximum Strength Hot Medication Packets 1575
- TYLENOL PM Pain Reliever/Sleep Aid, Extra Strength Gelcaps, Caplets, Geltabs 1576
- TYLENOL Severe Allergy Medication Caplets 1571
- Maximum Strength Unisom Sleepgels 1990
- Unisom With Pain Relief-Nighttime Sleep Aid and Pain Reliever 1991

Diphenylpyraline Hydrochloride (Potentiation of CNS depressant effect may occur).
No products indexed under this heading.

Droperidol (Potentiation of CNS depressant effect may occur). Products include:
- Inapsine Injection 462

Enflurane (Potentiation of CNS depressant effect may occur).
No products indexed under this heading.

Estazolam (Potentiation of CNS depressant effect may occur). Products include:
- ProSom Tablets 457

Ethchlorvynol (Potentiation of CNS depressant effect may occur). Products include:
- Placidyl Capsules 456

Ethinamate (Potentiation of CNS depressant effect may occur).
No products indexed under this heading.

Fentanyl (Potentiation of CNS depressant effect may occur). Products include:
- Duragesic Transdermal System 1336

Fentanyl Citrate (Potentiation of CNS depressant effect may occur). Products include:
- Sublimaze Injection 463

Fluphenazine Enanthate (Potentiation of CNS depressant effect may occur). Products include:
- Prolixin Enanthate 510

Fluphenazine Hydrochloride (Potentiation of CNS depressant effect may occur). Products include:
- Prolixin 510

Flurazepam Hydrochloride (Potentiation of CNS depressant effect may occur). Products include:
- Dalmane Capsules 2329

Glutethimide (Potentiation of CNS depressant effect may occur).
No products indexed under this heading.

Haloperidol (Potentiation of CNS depressant effect may occur). Products include:
- Haldol Injection, Tablets and Concentrate 1585

Haloperidol Decanoate (Potentiation of CNS depressant effect may occur). Products include:
- Haldol Decanoate 1587

Hydrocodone Bitartrate (Potentiation of CNS depressant effect may occur). Products include:
- Codiclear DH Syrup 808
- Duratuss HD Elixir 2750
- Histussin D Liquid 670
- Hycodan Tablets and Syrup 946
- Hycomine Compound Tablets 948
- Hycomine 947
- Hycotuss Expectorant Syrup 950
- Hydrocet Capsules 787
- Lorcet 10/650 Tablets 1016
- Lortab 2751
- Tussend 1830
- Tussend Expectorant 1831
- Vicodin Tablets 1404
- Vicodin ES Tablets 1405
- Vicodin HP Tablets 1403
- Vicodin Tuss Expectorant 1406
- Zydone Capsules 967

Hydrocodone Polistirex (Potentiation of CNS depressant effect may occur). Products include:
- Tussionex Pennkinetic Extended-Release Suspension 1624

Hydromorphone Hydrochloride (Potentiation of CNS depressant effect may occur). Products include:
- Dilaudid Ampules 1382
- Dilaudid Cough Syrup 1383
- Dilaudid-HP Injection 1384
- Dilaudid-HP Lyophilized Powder 250 mg 1384
- Dilaudid 1382
- Dilaudid Oral Liquid 1386
- Dilaudid 1382
- Dilaudid Tablets - 8 mg 1386

Hydroxyzine Hydrochloride (Potentiation of CNS depressant effect may occur). Products include:
- Atarax Tablets & Syrup 1992
- Marax Tablets & DF Syrup 2015
- Vistaril Intramuscular Solution 2042

Isoflurane (Potentiation of CNS depressant effect may occur).
No products indexed under this heading.

Ketamine Hydrochloride (Potentiation of CNS depressant effect may occur).
No products indexed under this heading.

Levomethadyl Acetate Hydrochloride (Potentiation of CNS depressant effect may occur). Products include:
- Orlaam Oral Solution 2361

Levorphanol Tartrate (Potentiation of CNS depressant effect may occur). Products include:
- Levo-Dromoran 2297

Loratadine (Potentiation of CNS depressant effect may occur). Products include:
- Claritin Tablets 2485
- Claritin-D Tablets 2487

Lorazepam (Potentiation of CNS depressant effect may occur). Products include:
- Ativan Injection 2805
- Ativan Tablets 2807

Loxapine Hydrochloride (Potentiation of CNS depressant effect may occur). Products include:
- Loxitane 1426

Loxapine Succinate (Potentiation of CNS depressant effect may occur). Products include:
- Loxitane Capsules 1426

Meperidine Hydrochloride (Potentiation of CNS depressant effect may occur). Products include:
- Demerol 2438
- Mepergan Injection 2859

Mephobarbital (Potentiation of CNS depressant effect may occur). Products include:
- Mebaral Tablets 2452

Meprobamate (Potentiation of CNS depressant effect may occur). Products include:
- Miltown Tablets 2780
- PMB 200 and PMB 400 2890

Mesoridazine Besylate (Potentiation of CNS depressant effect may occur). Products include:
- Serentil 689

Methadone Hydrochloride (Potentiation of CNS depressant effect may occur). Products include:
- Methadone Hydrochloride Oral Concentrate 2356
- Methadone Hydrochloride Oral Solution & Tablets 2357

Methdilazine Hydrochloride (Potentiation of CNS depressant effect may occur).
No products indexed under this heading.

Methohexital Sodium (Potentiation of CNS depressant effect may occur).
No products indexed under this heading.

Methotrimeprazine (Potentiation of CNS depressant effect may occur). Products include:
- Levoprome 1321

Methoxyflurane (Potentiation of CNS depressant effect may occur).
No products indexed under this heading.

Midazolam Hydrochloride (Potentiation of CNS depressant effect may occur). Products include:
- Versed Injection 2324

Molindone Hydrochloride (Potentiation of CNS depressant effect may occur). Products include:
- Moban Tablets and Concentrate 1036

Morphine Sulfate (Potentiation of CNS depressant effect may occur). Products include:
- Astramorph/PF Injection, USP (Preservative-Free) 526
- Duramorph Injection 983
- Infumorph 200 and Infumorph 500 Sterile Solutions 985
- Kadian Capsules 2948
- MS Contin Tablets 2149
- MSIR 2152
- Oramorph SR (Morphine Sulfate Sustained Release Tablets) 2359
- RMS Suppositories CII 2766
- Roxanol 2365

Opium Alkaloids (Potentiation of CNS depressant effect may occur).
No products indexed under this heading.

Oxazepam (Potentiation of CNS depressant effect may occur). Products include:
- Serax Capsules 2916
- Serax Tablets 2916

Oxycodone Hydrochloride (Potentiation of CNS depressant effect may occur). Products include:
- OxyContin Tablets 2163
- OxyIR Capsules 2167
- Percocet Tablets 955
- Percodan Tablets 955
- Percodan-Demi Tablets 956
- Roxicodone Tablets, Oral Solution & Intensol (Oxycodone) 2366
- Tylox Capsules 1593

Pentobarbital Sodium (Potentiation of CNS depressant effect may occur). Products include:
- Nembutal Sodium Capsules 440
- Nembutal Sodium Solution 442
- Nembutal Sodium Suppositories 444

IMPORTANT NOTE: Always consult each drug listing in the patient's regimen for possible interactions.

Prolixin / Interactions Index

Perphenazine (Potentiation of CNS depressant effect may occur). Products include:
- Etrafon 2495
- Triavil Tablets 1800
- Trilafon 2532

Phenobarbital (Potentiation of CNS depressant effect may occur). Products include:
- Arco-Lase Plus Tablets 513
- Bellergal-S Tablets 2375
- Donnatal 2234
- Donnatal Extentabs 2234
- Donnatal Tablets 2234
- Phenobarbital Elixir and Tablets 1523
- Quadrinal Tablets 1398

Prazepam (Potentiation of CNS depressant effect may occur).
- No products indexed under this heading.

Prochlorperazine (Potentiation of CNS depressant effect may occur). Products include:
- Compazine 2644

Promethazine Hydrochloride (Potentiation of CNS depressant effect may occur). Products include:
- Mepergan Injection 2859
- Phenergan with Codeine 2883
- Phenergan with Dextromethorphan 2885
- Phenergan Injection 2880
- Phenergan Suppositories 2882
- Phenergan Syrup 2881
- Phenergan Tablets 2882
- Phenergan VC 2886
- Phenergan VC with Codeine 2888

Propofol (Potentiation of CNS depressant effect may occur). Products include:
- Diprivan Injectable Emulsion 2939

Propoxyphene Hydrochloride (Potentiation of CNS depressant effect may occur). Products include:
- Darvon 1475
- Wygesic Tablets 2930

Propoxyphene Napsylate (Potentiation of CNS depressant effect may occur). Products include:
- Darvon-N/Darvocet-N 1473

Pyrilamine Maleate (Potentiation of CNS depressant effect may occur). Products include:
- 4-Way Fast Acting Nasal Spray (regular & mentholated) 644
- Maximum Strength Multi-Symptom Formula Midol 621
- PMS Multi-Symptom Formula Midol 622

Pyrilamine Tannate (Potentiation of CNS depressant effect may occur). Products include:
- Atrohist Pediatric Suspension 1604
- Atrohist Pediatric Suspension Dye-Free 1604
- Rynatan 2781

Quazepam (Potentiation of CNS depressant effect may occur). Products include:
- Doral Tablets 2773

Risperidone (Potentiation of CNS depressant effect may occur). Products include:
- Risperdal Tablets 1348

Secobarbital Sodium (Potentiation of CNS depressant effect may occur). Products include:
- Seconal Sodium Pulvules 1529

Sevoflurane (Potentiation of CNS depressant effect may occur).
- No products indexed under this heading.

Sufentanil Citrate (Potentiation of CNS depressant effect may occur). Products include:
- Sufenta Injection 1355

Temazepam (Potentiation of CNS depressant effect may occur). Products include:
- Restoril Capsules 2413

Terfenadine (Potentiation of CNS depressant effect may occur). Products include:
- Seldane Tablets 1284
- Seldane-D Extended-Release Tablets 1286

Thiamylal Sodium (Potentiation of CNS depressant effect may occur).
- No products indexed under this heading.

Thioridazine Hydrochloride (Potentiation of CNS depressant effect may occur). Products include:
- Mellaril 2398

Thiothixene (Potentiation of CNS depressant effect may occur). Products include:
- Navane Capsules and Concentrate 2018
- Navane Intramuscular 2019

Triazolam (Potentiation of CNS depressant effect may occur). Products include:
- Halcion Tablets 2093

Trifluoperazine Hydrochloride (Potentiation of CNS depressant effect may occur). Products include:
- Stelazine 2692

Trimeprazine Tartrate (Potentiation of CNS depressant effect may occur).
- No products indexed under this heading.

Tripelennamine Hydrochloride (Potentiation of CNS depressant effect may occur). Products include:
- PBZ Tablets 863
- PBZ-SR Tablets 862

Triprolidine Hydrochloride (Potentiation of CNS depressant effect may occur). Products include:
- Actifed Cold & Allergy Tablets 807
- Actifed Cold & Sinus Caplets and Tablets 808

Zolpidem Tartrate (Potentiation of CNS depressant effect may occur). Products include:
- Ambien Tablets 2559

Food Interactions

Alcohol (Potentiation of the effect of alcohol may occur).

PROLIXIN ELIXIR
(Fluphenazine Hydrochloride) 510
See **Prolixin Decanoate**

PROLIXIN ENANTHATE
(Fluphenazine Enanthate) 510
See **Prolixin Decanoate**

PROLIXIN INJECTION
(Fluphenazine Hydrochloride) 510
See **Prolixin Decanoate**

PROLIXIN ORAL CONCENTRATE
(Fluphenazine Hydrochloride) 510
See **Prolixin Decanoate**

PROLOPRIM TABLETS
(Trimethoprim) 1141
May interact with:

Phenytoin (Increased phenytoin half-life and decreased phenytoin metabolic clearance rate; possible excessive phenytoin effect). Products include:
- Dilantin Infatabs 1967
- Dilantin-125 Suspension 1969

Phenytoin Sodium (Increased phenytoin half-life and decreased phenytoin metabolic clearance rate; possible excessive phenytoin effect). Products include:
- Dilantin Kapseals 1965

PROMISE SENSITIVE TOOTHPASTE
(Potassium Nitrate, Sodium Monofluorophosphate) 633
None cited in PDR database.

PROMOTE HIGH PROTEIN LIQUID NUTRITION
(Nutritional Supplement) 2343
None cited in PDR database.

PROMOTE WITH FIBER, HIGH-PROTEIN LIQUID NUTRITION
(Nutritional Beverage) 2343
None cited in PDR database.

PRONTO LICE KILLING SHAMPOO & CONDITIONER IN ONE KIT
(Pyrethrins, Piperonyl Butoxide) 669
None cited in PDR database.

PROPAGEST TABLETS
(Phenylpropanolamine Hydrochloride) 791
May interact with antihypertensives and antidepressant drugs. Compounds in these categories include:

Acebutolol Hydrochloride (Concurrent administration is not recommended). Products include:
- Sectral Capsules 2914

Amitriptyline Hydrochloride (Concurrent administration is not recommended). Products include:
- Elavil 2945
- Etrafon 2495
- Limbitrol 2333
- Triavil Tablets 1800

Amlodipine Besylate (Concurrent administration is not recommended). Products include:
- Lotrel Capsules 858
- Norvasc Tablets 2020

Amoxapine (Concurrent administration is not recommended). Products include:
- Asendin Tablets 1419

Atenolol (Concurrent administration is not recommended). Products include:
- Tenoretic Tablets 2963
- Tenormin Tablets and I.V. Injection 2965

Benazepril Hydrochloride (Concurrent administration is not recommended). Products include:
- Lotensin Tablets 852
- Lotensin HCT Tablets 855
- Lotrel Capsules 858

Bendroflumethiazide (Concurrent administration is not recommended).
- No products indexed under this heading.

Betaxolol Hydrochloride (Concurrent administration is not recommended). Products include:
- Betoptic Ophthalmic Solution 465
- Betoptic S Ophthalmic Suspension 467
- Kerlone Tablets 2588

Bisoprolol Fumarate (Concurrent administration is not recommended). Products include:
- Zebeta Tablets 1457
- Ziac 1459

Bupropion Hydrochloride (Concurrent administration is not recommended). Products include:
- Wellbutrin Tablets 1177

Captopril (Concurrent administration is not recommended). Products include:
- Capoten Tablets 740
- Capozide Tablets 744

Carteolol Hydrochloride (Concurrent administration is not recommended). Products include:
- Cartrol Tablets 413
- Ocupress Ophthalmic Solution, 1% Sterile 297

Chlorothiazide (Concurrent administration is not recommended). Products include:
- Aldoclor Tablets 1638
- Diupres Tablets 1691
- Diuril Oral 1694

Chlorothiazide Sodium (Concurrent administration is not recommended). Products include:
- Diuril Sodium Intravenous 1693

Chlorthalidone (Concurrent administration is not recommended). Products include:
- Combipres Tablets 682
- Tenoretic Tablets 2963
- Thalitone 1293

Clonidine (Concurrent administration is not recommended). Products include:
- Catapres-TTS 680

Clonidine Hydrochloride (Concurrent administration is not recommended). Products include:
- Catapres Tablets 679
- Combipres Tablets 682

Deserpidine (Concurrent administration is not recommended).
- No products indexed under this heading.

Desipramine Hydrochloride (Concurrent administration is not recommended). Products include:
- Norpramin Tablets 1273

Diazoxide (Concurrent administration is not recommended). Products include:
- Hyperstat I.V. Injection 2504
- Proglycem 575

Diltiazem Hydrochloride (Concurrent administration is not recommended). Products include:
- Cardizem CD Capsules 1251
- Cardizem SR Capsules 1255
- Cardizem Injectable 1253
- Cardizem Tablets 1257
- Dilacor XR Extended-release Capsules 2183
- Tiazac Capsules 1019

Doxazosin Mesylate (Concurrent administration is not recommended). Products include:
- Cardura Tablets 1993

Doxepin Hydrochloride (Concurrent administration is not recommended). Products include:
- Adapin Capsules 1542
- Sinequan 2028
- Zonalon Cream 1042

Enalapril Maleate (Concurrent administration is not recommended). Products include:
- Vaseretic Tablets 1810
- Vasotec Tablets 1816

Enalaprilat (Concurrent administration is not recommended). Products include:
- Vasotec I.V. 1814

Esmolol Hydrochloride (Concurrent administration is not recommended). Products include:
- Brevibloc (esmolol HCl) Injection 1860

Felodipine (Concurrent administration is not recommended). Products include:
- Plendil Extended-Release Tablets 514

Fluoxetine Hydrochloride (Concurrent administration is not recommended). Products include:
- Prozac Pulvules & Liquid, Oral Solution 935

(Described in PDR For Nonprescription Drugs)   (Described in PDR For Ophthalmology)

Interactions Index — Propulsid

Fosinopril Sodium (Concurrent administration is not recommended). Products include:
- Monopril Tablets 762

Furosemide (Concurrent administration is not recommended). Products include:
- Lasix Injection, Oral Solution and Tablets 1267

Guanabenz Acetate (Concurrent administration is not recommended).
- No products indexed under this heading.

Guanethidine Monosulfate (Concurrent administration is not recommended). Products include:
- Esimil Tablets 840
- Ismelin Tablets 845

Hydralazine Hydrochloride (Concurrent administration is not recommended). Products include:
- Apresazide Capsules 824
- Apresoline Hydrochloride Tablets .. 826
- Hydralazine Hydrochloride Injection USP 2712
- Ser-Ap-Es Tablets 867

Hydrochlorothiazide (Concurrent administration is not recommended). Products include:
- Aldactazide Tablets 2556
- Aldoril Tablets 1644
- Apresazide Capsules 824
- Capozide Tablets 744
- Dyazide Capsules 2653
- Esidrix Tablets 839
- Esimil Tablets 840
- HydroDIURIL Tablets 1716
- Hydropres Tablets 1718
- Hyzaar Tablets 1720
- Inderide Tablets 2838
- Inderide LA Long Acting Capsules .. 2840
- Lopressor HCT Tablets 850
- Lotensin HCT Tablets 855
- Moduretic Tablets 1748
- Oretic Tablets 450
- Prinzide Tablets 1780
- Ser-Ap-Es Tablets 867
- Timolide Tablets 1791
- Vaseretic Tablets 1810
- Zestoretic Tablets 2968
- Ziac 1459

Hydroflumethiazide (Concurrent administration is not recommended). Products include:
- Diucardin Tablets 2824

Imipramine Hydrochloride (Concurrent administration is not recommended). Products include:
- Tofranil Ampuls 873
- Tofranil Tablets 875

Imipramine Pamoate (Concurrent administration is not recommended). Products include:
- Tofranil-PM Capsules 876

Indapamide (Concurrent administration is not recommended).
- No products indexed under this heading.

Isocarboxazid (Concurrent administration is not recommended).
- No products indexed under this heading.

Isradipine (Concurrent administration is not recommended). Products include:
- DynaCirc Capsules 2381
- DynaCirc CR Tablets 2383

Labetalol Hydrochloride (Concurrent administration is not recommended). Products include:
- Normodyne Injection 2519
- Normodyne Tablets 2522
- Trandate 1158

Lisinopril (Concurrent administration is not recommended). Products include:
- Prinivil Tablets 1776
- Prinzide Tablets 1780
- Zestoretic Tablets 2968
- Zestril Tablets 2972

Losartan Potassium (Concurrent administration is not recommended). Products include:
- Cozaar Tablets 1668
- Hyzaar Tablets 1720

Maprotiline Hydrochloride (Concurrent administration is not recommended). Products include:
- Ludiomil Tablets 861

Mecamylamine Hydrochloride (Concurrent administration is not recommended). Products include:
- Inversine Tablets 1729

Methyclothiazide (Concurrent administration is not recommended). Products include:
- Enduron Tablets 424

Methyldopa (Concurrent administration is not recommended). Products include:
- Aldoclor Tablets 1638
- Aldomet Oral 1640
- Aldoril Tablets 1644

Methyldopate Hydrochloride (Concurrent administration is not recommended). Products include:
- Aldomet Ester HCl Injection 1642

Metolazone (Concurrent administration is not recommended). Products include:
- Mykrox Tablets 1617
- Zaroxolyn Tablets 1625

Metoprolol Succinate (Concurrent administration is not recommended). Products include:
- Toprol-XL Tablets 560

Metoprolol Tartrate (Concurrent administration is not recommended). Products include:
- Lopressor 848
- Lopressor HCT Tablets 850

Metyrosine (Concurrent administration is not recommended). Products include:
- Demser Capsules 1690

Minoxidil (Concurrent administration is not recommended).
- No products indexed under this heading.

Moexipril Hydrochloride (Concurrent administration is not recommended). Products include:
- Univasc Tablets 2553

Nadolol (Concurrent administration is not recommended).
- No products indexed under this heading.

Nefazodone Hydrochloride (Concurrent administration is not recommended). Products include:
- Serzone Tablets 776

Nicardipine Hydrochloride (Concurrent administration is not recommended). Products include:
- Cardene Capsules 2261
- Cardene I.V. 2815
- Cardene SR Capsules 2264

Nifedipine (Concurrent administration is not recommended). Products include:
- Adalat Capsules (10 mg and 20 mg) 580
- Adalat CC 582
- Procardia Capsules 2024
- Procardia XL Extended Release Tablets 2026

Nisoldipine (Concurrent administration is not recommended). Products include:
- Sular Tablets 2961

Nitroglycerin (Concurrent administration is not recommended). Products include:
- Deponit NTG Transdermal Delivery System 2541
- Nitro-Bid IV 1270
- Nitro-Bid Ointment 1272
- Nitro-Dur (nitroglycerin) Transdermal Infusion System 1365
- Nitrolingual Spray 2193
- Nitrostat Tablets 1981
- Transderm-Nitro Transdermal Therapeutic System 878

Nortriptyline Hydrochloride (Concurrent administration is not recommended). Products include:
- Pamelor 2409

Paroxetine Hydrochloride (Concurrent administration is not recommended). Products include:
- Paxil Tablets 2681

Penbutolol Sulfate (Concurrent administration is not recommended). Products include:
- Levatol Tablets 2547

Phenelzine Sulfate (Concurrent administration is not recommended). Products include:
- Nardil 1977

Phenoxybenzamine Hydrochloride (Concurrent administration is not recommended). Products include:
- Dibenzyline Capsules 2650

Phentolamine Mesylate (Concurrent administration is not recommended). Products include:
- Regitine Vials 864

Pindolol (Concurrent administration is not recommended). Products include:
- Visken Tablets 2428

Polythiazide (Concurrent administration is not recommended). Products include:
- Minizide Capsules 2016

Prazosin Hydrochloride (Concurrent administration is not recommended). Products include:
- Minipress Capsules 2015
- Minizide Capsules 2016

Propranolol Hydrochloride (Concurrent administration is not recommended). Products include:
- Inderal 2834
- Inderal LA Long Acting Capsules 2836
- Inderide Tablets 2838
- Inderide LA Long Acting Capsules .. 2840

Protriptyline Hydrochloride (Concurrent administration is not recommended). Products include:
- Vivactil Tablets 1820

Quinapril Hydrochloride (Concurrent administration is not recommended). Products include:
- Accupril Tablets 1950

Ramipril (Concurrent administration is not recommended). Products include:
- Altace Capsules 1238

Rauwolfia Serpentina (Concurrent administration is not recommended).
- No products indexed under this heading.

Rescinnamine (Concurrent administration is not recommended).
- No products indexed under this heading.

Reserpine (Concurrent administration is not recommended). Products include:
- Diupres Tablets 1691
- Hydropres Tablets 1718
- Ser-Ap-Es Tablets 867

Sertraline Hydrochloride (Concurrent administration is not recommended). Products include:
- Zoloft Tablets 2051

Sodium Nitroprusside (Concurrent administration is not recommended).
- No products indexed under this heading.

Sotalol Hydrochloride (Concurrent administration is not recommended). Products include:
- Betapace Tablets 637

Spirapril Hydrochloride (Concurrent administration is not recommended).
- No products indexed under this heading.

Terazosin Hydrochloride (Concurrent administration is not recommended). Products include:
- Hytrin Capsules 434

Timolol Maleate (Concurrent administration is not recommended). Products include:
- Blocadren Tablets 1654
- Timolide Tablets 1791
- Timoptic in Ocudose 1796
- Timoptic Sterile Ophthalmic Solution 1794
- Timoptic-XE 1798

Torsemide (Concurrent administration is not recommended). Products include:
- Demadex Tablets and Injection 691

Tranylcypromine Sulfate (Concurrent administration is not recommended). Products include:
- Parnate Tablets 2679

Trazodone Hydrochloride (Concurrent administration is not recommended). Products include:
- Desyrel and Desyrel Dividose 504

Trimethaphan Camsylate (Concurrent administration is not recommended).
- No products indexed under this heading.

Trimipramine Maleate (Concurrent administration is not recommended). Products include:
- Surmontil Capsules 2917

Venlafaxine Hydrochloride (Concurrent administration is not recommended). Products include:
- Effexor 2825

Verapamil Hydrochloride (Concurrent administration is not recommended). Products include:
- Calan SR Caplets 2571
- Calan Tablets 2568
- Covera-HS Tablets 2573
- Isoptin Injectable 1391
- Isoptin Oral Tablets 1393
- Isoptin SR Tablets 1395
- Verelan Capsules 1455

PROPHYLLIN CCC TOPICAL EMOLLIENT OINTMENT
(Petrolatum, White) 2372
None cited in PDR database.

PROPINE WITH C CAP COMPLIANCE CAP
(Dipivefrin Hydrochloride) .... ⊙ 251
None cited in PDR database.

PROPULSID TABLETS
(Cisapride) 1346

May interact with benzodiazepines, erythromycin, anticholinergics, oral anticoagulants, and certain other agents. Compounds in these categories include:

Alprazolam (Sedative effects of benzodiazepines may be accelerated). Products include:
- Xanax Tablets 2115

Atropine Sulfate (Concurrent use of anticholinergic compounds would be expected to compromise the beneficial effects of cisapride). Products include:
- Arco-Lase Plus Tablets 513
- Atrohist Plus Tablets 1605
- Donnatal 2234
- Donnatal Extentabs 2234
- Donnatal Tablets 2234
- Lomotil 2591
- Motofen Tablets 789
- Urised Tablets 2123

IMPORTANT NOTE: Always consult each drug listing in the patient's regimen for possible interactions.

Propulsid — Interactions Index

Belladonna Alkaloids (Concurrent use of anticholinergic compounds would be expected to compromise the beneficial effects of cisapride). Products include:
- Bellergal-S Tablets 2375
- Hyland's Bedwetting Tablets 788
- Hyland's EnurAid Tablets 789
- Hyland's Headache Tablets 790
- Hyland's Teething Tablets 790
- Similasan Eye Drops #1 769

Benztropine Mesylate (Concurrent use of anticholinergic compounds would be expected to compromise the beneficial effects of cisapride). Products include:
- Cogentin 1661

Biperiden Hydrochloride (Concurrent use of anticholinergic compounds would be expected to compromise the beneficial effects of cisapride). Products include:
- Akineton 1380

Chlordiazepoxide (Sedative effects of benzodiazepines may be accelerated). Products include:
- Limbitrol 2333

Chlordiazepoxide Hydrochloride (Sedative effects of benzodiazepines may be accelerated). Products include:
- Librax Capsules 2330
- Librium Capsules 2331
- Librium Injectable 2332

Cimetidine (Co-administration leads to an increased peak plasma concentration and AUC of cisapride; GI absorption of cimetidine is accelerated when co-administered). Products include:
- Tagamet HB Tablets 786
- Tagamet Tablets 2694

Cimetidine Hydrochloride (Co-administration leads to an increased peak plasma concentration and AUC of cisapride; GI absorption of cimetidine is accelerated when co-administered). Products include:
- Tagamet 2694

Clarithromycin (Rare cases of serious cardiac arrhythmias, including ventricular arrhythmias and torsade de pointes associated with QT prolongation have been reported during concomitant therapy due to inhibition of hepatic cytochrome P4503A4 isoenzyme by clarithromycin; concurrent use is contraindicated). Products include:
- Biaxin 406

Clidinium Bromide (Concurrent use of anticholinergic compounds would be expected to compromise the beneficial effects of cisapride). Products include:
- Librax Capsules 2330

Clonazepam (Sedative effects of benzodiazepines may be accelerated). Products include:
- Klonopin Tablets 2294

Clorazepate Dipotassium (Sedative effects of benzodiazepines may be accelerated). Products include:
- Tranxene 459

Diazepam (Sedative effects of benzodiazepines may be accelerated). Products include:
- Dizac (diazepam injectable emulsion) CIV 1862
- Valium Injectable 2336
- Valium Tablets 2335

Dicumarol (Concurrent use results in increased coagulation times in some cases).
No products indexed under this heading.

Dicyclomine Hydrochloride (Concurrent use of anticholinergic compounds would be expected to compromise the beneficial effects of cisapride). Products include:
- Bentyl 1246

Erythromycin (Rare cases of serious cardiac arrhythmias, including ventricular arrhythmias and torsade de pointes associated with QT prolongation have been reported during concomitant therapy due to inhibition of hepatic cytochrome P4503A4 isoenzyme by erythromycin; concurrent use is contraindicated). Products include:
- A/T/S 2% Acne Topical Gel 1244
- A/T/S 2% Acne Topical Solution 1244
- Benzamycin Topical Gel 919
- E-Mycin Tablets 1388
- Emgel 2% Topical Gel 1081
- ERYC 1972
- Erycette (erythromycin 2%) Topical Solution 1943
- Ery-Tab Tablets 426
- Erythromycin Base Filmtab 430
- Erythromycin Delayed-Release Capsules, USP 431
- Ilotycin Ophthalmic Ointment ... 928
- PCE Dispertab Tablets 453
- T-Stat 2.0% Topical Solution and Pads 2797
- THERAMYCIN Z 2% Solution 1629

Erythromycin Estolate (Rare cases of serious cardiac arrhythmias, including ventricular arrhythmias and torsade de pointes associated with QT prolongation have been reported during concomitant therapy due to inhibition of hepatic cytochrome P4503A4 isoenzyme by erythromycin; concurrent use is contraindicated). Products include:
- Ilosone 927

Erythromycin Ethylsuccinate (Rare cases of serious cardiac arrhythmias, including ventricular arrhythmias and torsade de pointes associated with QT prolongation have been reported during concomitant therapy due to inhibition of hepatic cytochrome P4503A4 isoenzyme by erythromycin; concurrent use is contraindicated). Products include:
- E.E.S. 427
- EryPed 425
- Pediazole Suspension 2340

Erythromycin Gluceptate (Rare cases of serious cardiac arrhythmias, including ventricular arrhythmias and torsade de pointes associated with QT prolongation have been reported during concomitant therapy due to inhibition of hepatic cytochrome P4503A4 isoenzyme by erythromycin; concurrent use is contraindicated). Products include:
- Ilotycin Gluceptate, IV, Vials ... 929

Erythromycin Stearate (Rare cases of serious cardiac arrhythmias, including ventricular arrhythmias and torsade de pointes associated with QT prolongation have been reported during concomitant therapy due to inhibition of hepatic cytochrome P4503A4 isoenzyme by erythromycin; concurrent use is contraindicated). Products include:
- Erythrocin Stearate Filmtab 429

Estazolam (Sedative effects of benzodiazepines may be accelerated). Products include:
- ProSom Tablets 457

Fluconazole (Rare cases of serious cardiac arrhythmias, including ventricular arrhythmias and torsade de pointes associated with QT prolongation have been reported during concomitant therapy due to inhibition of hepatic cytochrome P4503A4 isoenzyme by fluconazole; concurrent use is contraindicated). Products include:
- Diflucan Tablets, Injection, and Oral Suspension 2003

Flurazepam Hydrochloride (Sedative effects of benzodiazepines may be accelerated). Products include:
- Dalmane Capsules 2329

Glycopyrrolate (Concurrent use of anticholinergic compounds would be expected to compromise the beneficial effects of cisapride). Products include:
- Robinul Forte Tablets 2247
- Robinul Injectable 2247
- Robinul Tablets 2247

Halazepam (Sedative effects of benzodiazepines may be accelerated).
No products indexed under this heading.

Hyoscyamine (Concurrent use of anticholinergic compounds would be expected to compromise the beneficial effects of cisapride). Products include:
- Cystospaz Tablets 2123
- Urised Tablets 2123

Hyoscyamine Sulfate (Concurrent use of anticholinergic compounds would be expected to compromise the beneficial effects of cisapride). Products include:
- Arco-Lase Plus Tablets 513
- Atrohist Plus Tablets 1605
- Cystospaz-M Capsules 2123
- Donnatal 2234
- Donnatal Extentabs 2234
- Donnatal Tablets 2234
- Kutrase Capsules 2546
- Levsin/Levsinex/Levbid 2549

Ipratropium Bromide (Concurrent use of anticholinergic compounds would be expected to compromise the beneficial effects of cisapride). Products include:
- Atrovent Inhalation Aerosol 674
- Atrovent Inhalation Solution 675
- Atrovent Nasal Spray 0.03% 676
- Atrovent Nasal Spray 0.06% 678

Itraconazole (Rare cases of serious cardiac arrhythmias, including ventricular arrhythmias and torsade de pointes associated with QT prolongation have been reported during concomitant therapy due to inhibition of hepatic cytochrome P4503A4 isoenzyme by itraconazole; concurrent use is contraindicated). Products include:
- Sporanox Capsules 1352

Ketoconazole (Rare cases of serious cardiac arrhythmias, including ventricular arrhythmias and torsade de pointes associated with QT prolongation have been reported during concomitant therapy due to inhibition of hepatic cytochrome P4503A4 isoenzyme by ketoconazole; concurrent use with oral ketoconazole is contraindicated). Products include:
- Nizoral 2% Cream 1344
- Nizoral 2% Shampoo 1344
- Nizoral Tablets 1345

Lorazepam (Sedative effects of benzodiazepines may be accelerated). Products include:
- Ativan Injection 2805
- Ativan Tablets 2807

Mepenzolate Bromide (Concurrent use of anticholinergic compounds would be expected to compromise the beneficial effects of cisapride).
No products indexed under this heading.

Miconazole (Rare cases of serious cardiac arrhythmias, including ventricular arrhythmias and torsade de pointes associated with QT prolongation have been reported during concomitant therapy due to inhibition of hepatic cytochrome P4503A4 isoenzyme by miconazole; concurrent use is contraindicated).
No products indexed under this heading.

Midazolam Hydrochloride (Sedative effects of benzodiazepines may be accelerated). Products include:
- Versed Injection 2324

Oxazepam (Sedative effects of benzodiazepines may be accelerated). Products include:
- Serax Capsules 2916
- Serax Tablets 2916

Oxybutynin Chloride (Concurrent use of anticholinergic compounds would be expected to compromise the beneficial effects of cisapride). Products include:
- Ditropan 1267

Prazepam (Sedative effects of benzodiazepines may be accelerated).
No products indexed under this heading.

Procyclidine Hydrochloride (Concurrent use of anticholinergic compounds would be expected to compromise the beneficial effects of cisapride). Products include:
- Kemadrin Tablets 1105

Propantheline Bromide (Concurrent use of anticholinergic compounds would be expected to compromise the beneficial effects of cisapride). Products include:
- Pro-Banthine Tablets 2226

Quazepam (Sedative effects of benzodiazepines may be accelerated). Products include:
- Doral Tablets 2773

Ranitidine Hydrochloride (GI absorption of ranitidine is accelerated when co-administered). Products include:
- Zantac 1182
- Zantac Injection 1180
- Zantac Syrup 1182

Scopolamine (Concurrent use of anticholinergic compounds would be expected to compromise the beneficial effects of cisapride). Products include:
- Transderm Scōp Transdermal Therapeutic System 890

Scopolamine Hydrobromide (Concurrent use of anticholinergic compounds would be expected to compromise the beneficial effects of cisapride). Products include:
- Atrohist Plus Tablets 1605
- Donnatal 2234
- Donnatal Extentabs 2234
- Donnatal Tablets 2234

Temazepam (Sedative effects of benzodiazepines may be accelerated). Products include:
- Restoril Capsules 2413

Triazolam (Sedative effects of benzodiazepines may be accelerated). Products include:
- Halcion Tablets 2093

(▣ Described in PDR For Nonprescription Drugs)   (⊚ Described in PDR For Ophthalmology)

883 **Interactions Index** **ProSom**

Tridihexethyl Chloride (Concurrent use of anticholinergic compounds would be expected to compromise the beneficial effects of cisapride).
No products indexed under this heading.

Trihexyphenidyl Hydrochloride (Concurrent use of anticholinergic compounds would be expected to compromise the beneficial effects of cisapride). Products include:
Artane 1418

Troleandomycin (Rare cases of serious cardiac arrhythmias, including ventricular arrhythmias and torsade de pointes associated with QT prolongation have been reported during concomitant therapy due to inhibition of hepatic cytochrome P4503A4 isoenzyme by troleandomycin; concurrent use is contraindicated). Products include:
Tao Capsules 2033

Warfarin Sodium (Concurrent use results in increased coagulation times in some cases). Products include:
Coumadin 941

Food Interactions

Alcohol (Sedative effects of alcohol may be accelerated).

PROPULSID SUSPENSION
(Cisapride) 1346
See **Propulsid Tablets**

PROSCAR TABLETS
(Finasteride) 1784
May interact with xanthine bronchodilators. Compounds in this category include:

Aminophylline (Increased theophylline clearance by 7% and decreased its half-life by 10%).
No products indexed under this heading.

Dyphylline (Increased theophylline clearance by 7% and decreased its half-life by 10%). Products include:
Lufyllin & Lufyllin-400 Tablets 2778
Lufyllin-GG Elixir & Tablets 2779

Theophylline (Increased theophylline clearance by 7% and decreased its half-life by 10%). Products include:
Marax Tablets & DF Syrup 2015
Quibron 2227

Theophylline Anhydrous (Increased theophylline clearance by 7% and decreased its half-life by 10%). Products include:
Aerolate 1003
Primatene Tablets 844
Respbid Tablets 687
Slo-bid Gyrocaps 2201
Theo-24 Extended Release Capsules 2753
Theo-Dur Extended-Release Tablets 1367
Theo-X Extended-Release Tablets .. 793
Uni-Dur Extended-Release Tablets .. 1374
Uniphyl 400 mg and 600 mg Tablets 2157

Theophylline Calcium Salicylate (Increased theophylline clearance by 7% and decreased its half-life by 10%). Products include:
Quadrinal Tablets 1398

Theophylline Sodium Glycinate (Increased theophylline clearance by 7% and decreased its half-life by 10%).
No products indexed under this heading.

PROSOM TABLETS
(Estazolam) 457
May interact with central nervous system depressants, anticonvulsants, antihistamines, barbiturates, monoamine oxidase inhibitors, narcotic analgesics, phenothiazines, and certain other agents. Compounds in these categories include:

Acrivastine (Co-administration results in increased CNS depression). Products include:
Semprex-D Capsules 1620

Alfentanil Hydrochloride (Co-administration results in increased CNS depression). Products include:
Alfenta Injection 1334

Alprazolam (Co-administration results in increased CNS depression). Products include:
Xanax Tablets 2115

Aprobarbital (Co-administration results in increased CNS depression).
No products indexed under this heading.

Astemizole (Co-administration results in increased CNS depression). Products include:
Hismanal Tablets 1341

Azatadine Maleate (Co-administration results in increased CNS depression). Products include:
Trinalin Repetabs Tablets 1373

Bromodiphenhydramine Hydrochloride (Co-administration results in increased CNS depression).
No products indexed under this heading.

Brompheniramine Maleate (Co-administration results in increased CNS depression). Products include:
Alka-Seltzer Plus Sinus Medicine .. 611
Bromfed Capsules (Extended-Release) 1832
Bromfed Syrup 712
Bromfed Tablets 1832
Bromfed-DM Cough Syrup 1832
Bromfed-PD Capsules (Extended-Release) 1832
Dimetane-DC Cough Syrup 2232
Dimetane-DX Cough Syrup 2233
Dimetapp Allergy Dye-Free Elixir.... 838
Dimetapp Allergy Sinus Caplets 838
Dimetapp Cold & Allergy Chewable Tablets 838
Dimetapp Cold & Cough Liqui-Gels 839
Dimetapp Cold & Fever Suspension 839
Dimetapp DM Elixir 840
Dimetapp Elixir 840
Dimetapp Extentabs 841
Dimetapp Tablets/Liqui-Gels 841
Rondec Chewable Tablets 974
Vicks DayQuil Allergy Relief 12-Hour Extended Release Tablets.. 733
Vicks DayQuil Allergy Relief 4-Hour Tablets 733

Buprenorphine (Co-administration results in increased CNS depression). Products include:
Buprenex Injectable 2170

Buspirone Hydrochloride (Co-administration results in increased CNS depression). Products include:
BuSpar Tablets 738

Butabarbital (Co-administration results in increased CNS depression).
No products indexed under this heading.

Butalbital (Co-administration results in increased CNS depression). Products include:
Axocet Capsules 2469
Esgic-plus Capsules 1012
Esgic-plus Tablets 1012
Fioricet Tablets 2386
Fioricet with Codeine Capsules 2387
Fiorinal Capsules 2388
Fiorinal with Codeine Capsules 2390
Fiorinal Tablets 2388
Phrenilin 790
Sedapap Tablets 50 mg/650 mg .. 1826

Carbamazepine (Co-administration results in increased CNS depression). Products include:
Atretol Tablets 569
Tegretol/Tegretol-XR 870

Cetirizine Hydrochloride (Co-administration results in increased CNS depression). Products include:
Zyrtec Tablets 2053

Chlordiazepoxide (Co-administration results in increased CNS depression). Products include:
Limbitrol 2333

Chlordiazepoxide Hydrochloride (Co-administration results in increased CNS depression). Products include:
Librax Capsules 2330
Librium Capsules 2331
Librium Injectable 2332

Chlorpheniramine Maleate (Co-administration results in increased CNS depression). Products include:
Alka-Seltzer Plus Cold Medicine 611
Alka-Seltzer Plus Cold Medicine Liqui-Gels 612
Alka-Seltzer Plus Cold & Cough Medicine 611
Alka-Seltzer Plus Cold & Cough Medicine Liqui-Gels 612
Alka-Seltzer Plus Flu & Body Aches Effervescent Tablets 612
Allerest Maximum Strength 649
Allerest Sinus Pain Formula 649
Ana-Kit Anaphylaxis Emergency Treatment Kit 611
Atrohist Pediatric Capsules 1603
Atrohist Plus Tablets 1605
BC Cold Powder Multi-Symptom Formula (Cold-Sinus-Allergy) 631
Cerose DM 853
Cheracol Plus Head Cold/Cough Formula 741
Children's TYLENOL Cold Multi-Symptom Chewable Tablets and Liquid 1559
Children's TYLENOL Cold Plus Cough Multi Symptom Chewable Tablets and Liquid 1560
Children's TYLENOL Flu Suspension Liquid 1560
Children's Vicks DayQuil Allergy Relief 730
Children's Vicks NyQuil Cold/Cough Relief 731
Chlor-Trimeton Allergy Decongestant Tablets 759
Chlor-Trimeton Allergy Tablets 758
Allergy-Sinus Comtrex Multi-Symptom Allergy-Sinus Formula Tablets and Caplets 639
Comtrex Multi-Symptom 638
Contac Continuous Action Nasal Decongestant/Antihistamine 12 Hour Capsules 773
Contac Maximum Strength Continuous Action Decongestant/Antihistamine 12 Hour Caplets.. 772
Contac Severe Cold and Flu Formula Caplets 773
Coricidin Cold + Flu Tablets 760
Coricidin Cough + Cold Tablets 760
Coricidin 'D' Decongestant Tablets 760
D.A. II Tablets 972
D.A. Chewable Tablets 970
Dura-Tap/PD Capsules 970
Dura-Vent/DA Tablets 972
Efidac 24 Chlorpheniramine 655
Extendryl 1003
Fedahist Gyrocaps 2545
Hycomine Compound Tablets 948
Kronofed-A 994
Nolamine Timed-Release Tablets 790
Novahistine Elixir 782
Ornade Spansule Capsules 2678
PediaCare Cough-Cold Chewable Tablets and Liquid 1569
PediaCare NightRest Cough-Cold Liquid 1569
Pediatric Vicks 44m Cough & Cold Relief 737
Pyrroxate Caplets 742
Ryna 804
Sinarest 663
Sine-Off Sinus Medicine 784
Singlet Tablets 785
Sinulin Tablets 792
Sinutab Sinus Allergy Medication, Maximum Strength Tablets and Caplets 823
Sudafed Cold & Allergy Tablets 826
Teldrin 12 Hour Antihistamine/Nasal Decongestant Allergy Relief Capsules 786
TheraFlu Flu and Cold Medicine 750
Theraflu Maximum Strength Flu and Cold Medicine For Sore Throat 751
TheraFlu Flu, Cold and Cough Medicine 750
TheraFlu Maximum Strength Nighttime Flu, Cold & Cough Medicine 751
Triaminic Night Time 754
Triaminic Syrup 755
Triaminic Triaminicol Cold & Cough 756
Triaminicin Tablets 756
Tussend 1830
TYLENOL Allergy Sinus, Maximum Strength Caplets and Gelcaps 1571
TYLENOL Cold Medication, Multi-Symptom Formula Tablets and Caplets 1572
TYLENOL Cold Medication, Multi-Symptom Hot Liquid Packets 1572
Vicks 44 LiquiCaps Cough, Cold & Flu Relief 728
Vicks 44M Cough, Cold & Flu Relief 729

Chlorpheniramine Polistirex (Co-administration results in increased CNS depression). Products include:
Tussionex Pennkinetic Extended-Release Suspension 1624

Chlorpheniramine Tannate (Co-administration results in increased CNS depression). Products include:
Atrohist Pediatric Suspension 1604
Atrohist Pediatric Suspension Dye-Free 1604
Rynatan 2781
Rynatuss 2782

Chlorpromazine (Co-administration results in increased CNS depression). Products include:
Thorazine Suppositories 2701

Chlorpromazine Hydrochloride (Co-administration results in increased CNS depression). Products include:
Thorazine 2701

Chlorprothixene (Co-administration results in increased CNS depression).
No products indexed under this heading.

Chlorprothixene Hydrochloride (Co-administration results in increased CNS depression).
No products indexed under this heading.

Chlorprothixene Lactate (Co-administration results in increased CNS depression).
No products indexed under this heading.

Clemastine Fumarate (Co-administration results in increased CNS depression). Products include:
Tavist Syrup 2426
Tavist Tablets 2427
Tavist-1 12 Hour Relief Tablets 749
Tavist-D 12 Hour Relief Tablets 750

Clonazepam (Co-administration results in increased CNS depression). Products include:
Klonopin Tablets 2294

Clorazepate Dipotassium (Co-administration results in increased CNS depression). Products include:
Tranxene 459

Clozapine (Co-administration results in increased CNS depression). Products include:
Clozaril Tablets 2377

IMPORTANT NOTE: Always consult each drug listing in the patient's regimen for possible interactions.

Codeine Phosphate (Co-administration results in increased CNS depression). Products include:
- Brontex ... 2130
- Dimetane-DC Cough Syrup ... 2232
- Fioricet with Codeine Capsules ... 2387
- Fiorinal with Codeine Capsules ... 2390
- Nucofed ... 2225
- Phenergan with Codeine ... 2883
- Phenergan VC with Codeine ... 2888
- Robitussin A-C Syrup ... 2248
- Robitussin-DAC Syrup ... 2249
- Ryna ... 804
- Soma Compound w/Codeine Tablets ... 2784
- Tylenol with Codeine ... 1592

Cyproheptadine Hydrochloride (Co-administration results in increased CNS depression). Products include:
- Periactin ... 1767

Desflurane (Co-administration results in increased CNS depression). Products include:
- Suprane (desflurane, USP) ... 1865

Dexchlorpheniramine Maleate (Co-administration results in increased CNS depression).
- No products indexed under this heading.

Dezocine (Co-administration results in increased CNS depression). Products include:
- Dalgan Injection ... 529

Diazepam (Co-administration results in increased CNS depression). Products include:
- Dizac (diazepam injectable emulsion) CIV ... 1862
- Valium Injectable ... 2336
- Valium Tablets ... 2335

Diphenhydramine Citrate (Co-administration results in increased CNS depression). Products include:
- Excedrin P.M. Analgesic/Sleeping Aid Tablets, Caplets, Liquigels ... 735

Diphenhydramine Hydrochloride (Co-administration results in increased CNS depression). Products include:
- Actifed Allergy Daytime/Nighttime Caplets ... 808
- Actifed Sinus Daytime/Nighttime Tablets and Caplets ... 809
- Extra Strength Bayer PM Aspirin Plus Sleep Aid ... 617
- Benadryl Allergy Chewables ... 811
- Benadryl Allergy/Cold Caplets ... 811
- Benadryl Allergy Decongestant Liquid Medication ... 812
- Benadryl Allergy Decongestant Tablets ... 812
- Benadryl Allergy Liquid Medication ... 813
- Benadryl Allergy ... 811
- Benadryl Allergy Sinus Headache Caplets ... 813
- Benadryl Dye-Free Allergy Liquigel Softgels ... 813
- Benadryl Dye-Free Allergy Liquid Medication ... 814
- Benadryl Itch Relief Stick Extra Strength ... 814
- Benadryl Cream ... 814
- Benadryl Gel ... 815
- Benadryl Spray ... 815
- Benadryl Injection ... 1955
- Contac Day & Night Cold/Flu Night Caplets ... 772
- Contac Night Allergy/Sinus Caplets ... 771
- Extra Strength Doan's P.M. ... 653
- Excedrin P.M. Analgesic/Sleeping Aid Tablets, Caplets, Liquigels ... 643
- Nytol QuickCaps Caplets ... 632
- Sleepinal Night-time Sleep Aid Capsules and Softgels ... 798
- TYLENOL Allergy Sinus NightTime, Maximum Strength Caplets ... 1571
- TYLENOL Flu NightTime, Maximum Strength Gelcaps ... 1575
- TYLENOL Flu NightTime, Maximum Strength Hot Medication Packets ... 1575
- TYLENOL PM Pain Reliever/Sleep Aid, Extra Strength Gelcaps, Caplets, Geltabs ... 1576
- TYLENOL Severe Allergy Medication Caplets ... 1571
- Maximum Strength Unisom Sleepgels ... 1990
- Unisom With Pain Relief-Nighttime Sleep Aid and Pain Reliever ... 1991

Diphenylpyraline Hydrochloride (Co-administration results in increased CNS depression).
- No products indexed under this heading.

Divalproex Sodium (Co-administration results in increased CNS depression). Products include:
- Depakote Tablets ... 418

Droperidol (Co-administration results in increased CNS depression). Products include:
- Inapsine Injection ... 462

Enflurane (Co-administration results in increased CNS depression).
- No products indexed under this heading.

Ethchlorvynol (Co-administration results in increased CNS depression). Products include:
- Placidyl Capsules ... 456

Ethinamate (Co-administration results in increased CNS depression).
- No products indexed under this heading.

Ethosuximide (Co-administration results in increased CNS depression). Products include:
- Zarontin Capsules ... 1986
- Zarontin Syrup ... 1986

Ethotoin (Co-administration results in increased CNS depression). Products include:
- Peganone Tablets ... 455

Felbamate (Co-administration results in increased CNS depression). Products include:
- Felbatol ... 2774

Fentanyl (Co-administration results in increased CNS depression). Products include:
- Duragesic Transdermal System ... 1336

Fentanyl Citrate (Co-administration results in increased CNS depression). Products include:
- Sublimaze Injection ... 463

Fluphenazine Decanoate (Co-administration results in increased CNS depression). Products include:
- Prolixin Decanoate ... 510

Fluphenazine Enanthate (Co-administration results in increased CNS depression). Products include:
- Prolixin Enanthate ... 510

Fluphenazine Hydrochloride (Co-administration results in increased CNS depression). Products include:
- Prolixin ... 510

Flurazepam Hydrochloride (Co-administration results in increased CNS depression). Products include:
- Dalmane Capsules ... 2329

Furazolidone (Co-administration results in increased CNS depression). Products include:
- Furoxone ... 2221

Glutethimide (Co-administration results in increased CNS depression).
- No products indexed under this heading.

Haloperidol (Co-administration results in increased CNS depression). Products include:
- Haldol Injection, Tablets and Concentrate ... 1585

Haloperidol Decanoate (Co-administration results in increased CNS depression). Products include:
- Haldol Decanoate ... 1587

Hydrocodone Bitartrate (Co-administration results in increased CNS depression). Products include:
- Codiclear DH Syrup ... 808
- Duratuss HD Elixir ... 2750
- Histussin D Liquid ... 670
- Hycodan Tablets and Syrup ... 946
- Hycomine Compound Tablets ... 948
- Hycomine ... 947
- Hycotuss Expectorant Syrup ... 950
- Hydrocet Capsules ... 787
- Lorcet 10/650 Tablets ... 1016
- Lortab ... 2751
- Tussend ... 1830
- Tussend Expectorant ... 1831
- Vicodin Tablets ... 1404
- Vicodin ES Tablets ... 1405
- Vicodin HP Tablets ... 1403
- Vicodin Tuss Expectorant ... 1406
- Zydone Capsules ... 967

Hydrocodone Polistirex (Co-administration results in increased CNS depression). Products include:
- Tussionex Pennkinetic Extended-Release Suspension ... 1624

Hydromorphone Hydrochloride (Co-administration results in increased CNS depression). Products include:
- Dilaudid Ampules ... 1382
- Dilaudid Cough Syrup ... 1383
- Dilaudid-HP Injection ... 1384
- Dilaudid-HP Lyophilized Powder 250 mg ... 1384
- Dilaudid ... 1382
- Dilaudid Oral Liquid ... 1386
- Dilaudid ... 1382
- Dilaudid Tablets - 8 mg. ... 1386

Hydroxyzine Hydrochloride (Co-administration results in increased CNS depression). Products include:
- Atarax Tablets & Syrup ... 1992
- Marax Tablets & DF Syrup ... 2015
- Vistaril Intramuscular Solution ... 2042

Isocarboxazid (Co-administration results in increased CNS depression).
- No products indexed under this heading.

Isoflurane (Co-administration results in increased CNS depression).
- No products indexed under this heading.

Ketamine Hydrochloride (Co-administration results in increased CNS depression).
- No products indexed under this heading.

Lamotrigine (Co-administration results in increased CNS depression). Products include:
- Lamictal Tablets ... 1105

Levomethadyl Acetate Hydrochloride (Co-administration results in increased CNS depression). Products include:
- Orlaam Oral Solution ... 2361

Levorphanol Tartrate (Co-administration results in increased CNS depression). Products include:
- Levo-Dromoran ... 2297

Loratadine (Co-administration results in increased CNS depression). Products include:
- Claritin Tablets ... 2485
- Claritin-D Tablets ... 2487

Lorazepam (Co-administration results in increased CNS depression). Products include:
- Ativan Injection ... 2805
- Ativan Tablets ... 2807

Loxapine Hydrochloride (Co-administration results in increased CNS depression). Products include:
- Loxitane ... 1426

Loxapine Succinate (Co-administration results in increased CNS depression). Products include:
- Loxitane Capsules ... 1426

Meperidine Hydrochloride (Co-administration results in increased CNS depression). Products include:
- Demerol ... 2438
- Mepergan Injection ... 2859

Mephenytoin (Co-administration results in increased CNS depression). Products include:
- Mesantoin Tablets ... 2400

Mephobarbital (Co-administration results in increased CNS depression). Products include:
- Mebaral Tablets ... 2452

Meprobamate (Co-administration results in increased CNS depression). Products include:
- Miltown Tablets ... 2780
- PMB 200 and PMB 400 ... 2890

Mesoridazine Besylate (Co-administration results in increased CNS depression). Products include:
- Serentil ... 689

Methadone Hydrochloride (Co-administration results in increased CNS depression). Products include:
- Methadone Hydrochloride Oral Concentrate ... 2356
- Methadone Hydrochloride Oral Solution & Tablets ... 2357

Methdilazine Hydrochloride (Co-administration results in increased CNS depression).
- No products indexed under this heading.

Methohexital Sodium (Co-administration results in increased CNS depression).
- No products indexed under this heading.

Methotrimeprazine (Co-administration results in increased CNS depression). Products include:
- Levoprome ... 1321

Methoxyflurane (Co-administration results in increased CNS depression).
- No products indexed under this heading.

Methsuximide (Co-administration results in increased CNS depression). Products include:
- Celontin Kapseals ... 1955

Midazolam Hydrochloride (Co-administration results in increased CNS depression). Products include:
- Versed Injection ... 2324

Molindone Hydrochloride (Co-administration results in increased CNS depression). Products include:
- Moban Tablets and Concentrate ... 1036

Morphine Sulfate (Co-administration results in increased CNS depression). Products include:
- Astramorph/PF Injection, USP (Preservative-Free) ... 526
- Duramorph Injection ... 983
- Infumorph 200 and Infumorph 500 Sterile Solutions ... 985
- Kadian Capsules ... 2948
- MS Contin Tablets ... 2149
- MSIR ... 2152
- Oramorph SR (Morphine Sulfate Sustained Release Tablets) ... 2359
- RMS Suppositories CII ... 2766
- Roxanol ... 2365

Opium Alkaloids (Co-administration results in increased CNS depression).
- No products indexed under this heading.

Oxazepam (Co-administration results in increased CNS depression). Products include:
- Serax Capsules ... 2916
- Serax Tablets ... 2916

885 **Interactions Index** **Prostep**

Oxycodone Hydrochloride (Co-administration results in increased CNS depression). Products include:
- OxyContin Tablets ... 2163
- OxyIR Capsules ... 2167
- Percocet Tablets ... 955
- Percodan Tablets ... 955
- Percodan-Demi Tablets ... 956
- Roxicodone Tablets, Oral Solution & Intensol (Oxycodone) ... 2366
- Tylox Capsules ... 1593

Paramethadione (Co-administration results in increased CNS depression).
- No products indexed under this heading.

Pentobarbital Sodium (Co-administration results in increased CNS depression). Products include:
- Nembutal Sodium Capsules ... 440
- Nembutal Sodium Solution ... 442
- Nembutal Sodium Suppositories ... 444

Perphenazine (Co-administration results in increased CNS depression). Products include:
- Etrafon ... 2495
- Triavil Tablets ... 1800
- Trilafon ... 2532

Phenacemide (Co-administration results in increased CNS depression). Products include:
- Phenurone Tablets ... 455

Phenelzine Sulfate (Co-administration results in increased CNS depression). Products include:
- Nardil ... 1977

Phenobarbital (Co-administration results in increased CNS depression). Products include:
- Arco-Lase Plus Tablets ... 513
- Bellergal-S Tablets ... 2375
- Donnatal ... 2234
- Donnatal Extentabs ... 2234
- Donnatal Tablets ... 2234
- Phenobarbital Elixir and Tablets ... 1523
- Quadrinal Tablets ... 1398

Phensuximide (Co-administration results in increased CNS depression).
- No products indexed under this heading.

Phenytoin (Co-administration results in increased CNS depression). Products include:
- Dilantin Infatabs ... 1967
- Dilantin-125 Suspension ... 1969

Phenytoin Sodium (Co-administration results in increased CNS depression). Products include:
- Dilantin Kapseals ... 1965

Prazepam (Co-administration results in increased CNS depression).
- No products indexed under this heading.

Primidone (Co-administration results in increased CNS depression). Products include:
- Mysoline ... 2860

Prochlorperazine (Co-administration results in increased CNS depression). Products include:
- Compazine ... 2644

Promethazine Hydrochloride (Co-administration results in increased CNS depression). Products include:
- Mepergan Injection ... 2859
- Phenergan with Codeine ... 2883
- Phenergan with Dextromethorphan ... 2885
- Phenergan Injection ... 2880
- Phenergan Suppositories ... 2882
- Phenergan Syrup ... 2881
- Phenergan Tablets ... 2882
- Phenergan VC ... 2886
- Phenergan VC with Codeine ... 2888

Propofol (Co-administration results in increased CNS depression). Products include:
- Diprivan Injectable Emulsion ... 2939

Propoxyphene Hydrochloride (Co-administration results in increased CNS depression). Products include:
- Darvon ... 1475
- Wygesic Tablets ... 2930

Propoxyphene Napsylate (Co-administration results in increased CNS depression). Products include:
- Darvon-N/Darvocet-N ... 1473

Pyrilamine Maleate (Co-administration results in increased CNS depression). Products include:
- 4-Way Fast Acting Nasal Spray (regular & mentholated) ... 644
- Maximum Strength Multi-Symptom Formula Midol ... 621
- PMS Multi-Symptom Formula Midol ... 622

Pyrilamine Tannate (Co-administration results in increased CNS depression). Products include:
- Atrohist Pediatric Suspension ... 1604
- Atrohist Pediatric Suspension Dye-Free ... 1604
- Rynatan ... 2781

Quazepam (Co-administration results in increased CNS depression). Products include:
- Doral Tablets ... 2773

Risperidone (Co-administration results in increased CNS depression). Products include:
- Risperdal Tablets ... 1348

Secobarbital Sodium (Co-administration results in increased CNS depression). Products include:
- Seconal Sodium Pulvules ... 1529

Selegiline Hydrochloride (Co-administration results in increased CNS depression). Products include:
- Eldepryl Capsules ... 2729

Sevoflurane (Co-administration results in increased CNS depression).
- No products indexed under this heading.

Sufentanil Citrate (Co-administration results in increased CNS depression). Products include:
- Sufenta Injection ... 1355

Temazepam (Co-administration results in increased CNS depression). Products include:
- Restoril Capsules ... 2413

Terfenadine (Co-administration results in increased CNS depression). Products include:
- Seldane Tablets ... 1284
- Seldane-D Extended-Release Tablets ... 1286

Thiamylal Sodium (Co-administration results in increased CNS depression).
- No products indexed under this heading.

Thioridazine Hydrochloride (Co-administration results in increased CNS depression). Products include:
- Mellaril ... 2398

Thiothixene (Co-administration results in increased CNS depression). Products include:
- Navane Capsules and Concentrate ... 2018
- Navane Intramuscular ... 2019

Tranylcypromine Sulfate (Co-administration results in increased CNS depression). Products include:
- Parnate Tablets ... 2679

Triazolam (Co-administration results in increased CNS depression). Products include:
- Halcion Tablets ... 2093

Trifluoperazine Hydrochloride (Co-administration results in increased CNS depression). Products include:
- Stelazine ... 2692

Trimeprazine Tartrate (Co-administration results in increased CNS depression).
- No products indexed under this heading.

Trimethadione (Co-administration results in increased CNS depression).
- No products indexed under this heading.

Tripelennamine Hydrochloride (Co-administration results in increased CNS depression). Products include:
- PBZ Tablets ... 863
- PBZ-SR Tablets ... 862

Triprolidine Hydrochloride (Co-administration results in increased CNS depression). Products include:
- Actifed Cold & Allergy Tablets ... 807
- Actifed Cold & Sinus Caplets and Tablets ... 808

Valproic Acid (Co-administration results in increased CNS depression). Products include:
- Depakene ... 416

Zolpidem Tartrate (Co-administration results in increased CNS depression). Products include:
- Ambien Tablets ... 2559

Food Interactions

Alcohol (Co-administration results in increased CNS depression).

PROSTEP (NICOTINE TRANSDERMAL SYSTEM)
(Nicotine) ... 1439
May interact with xanthine bronchodilators, insulin, and certain other agents. Compounds in these categories include:

Acetaminophen (Deinduction of hepatic enzymes on smoking cessation; may require a decrease in dose at cessation of smoking). Products include:
- Actifed Cold & Sinus Caplets and Tablets ... 808
- Actifed Sinus Daytime/Nighttime Tablets and Caplets ... 809
- Alka-Seltzer Fast Relief Caplets ... 610
- Alka-Seltzer Plus Liqui-Gels ... 612
- Alka-Seltzer Plus Flu & Body Aches Effervescent Tablets ... 612
- Alka-Seltzer Plus Flu & Body Aches Liqui-Gels Non-Drowsy Formula ... 613
- Alka-Seltzer Plus Night-Time Cold Medicine Liqui-Gels ... 612
- Allerest No Drowsiness ... 649
- Allerest Sinus Pain Formula ... 649
- Axocet Capsules ... 2469
- Benadryl Allergy/Cold Tablets ... 811
- Benadryl Allergy Sinus Headache Caplets ... 813
- Children's TYLENOL acetaminophen Chewable Tablets, Elixir, Suspension Liquid, and Suspension Drops ... 1559
- Children's TYLENOL Cold Multi-Symptom Chewable Tablets and Liquid ... 1559
- Children's TYLENOL Cold Plus Cough Multi Symptom Chewable Tablets and Liquid ... 1560
- Children's TYLENOL Flu Suspension Liquid ... 1560
- Allergy-Sinus Comtrex Multi-Symptom Allergy-Sinus Formula Tablets and Caplets ... 639
- Comtrex Multi-Symptom ... 638
- Comtrex Non-Drowsy ... 640
- Contac Day Allergy/Sinus Caplets ... 771
- Contac Day & Night ... 772
- Contac Night Allergy/Sinus Caplets ... 771
- Contac Severe Cold and Flu Formula Caplets ... 773
- Contac Severe Cold & Flu Non-Drowsy ... 774
- Coricidin Cold + Flu Tablets ... 760
- Coricidin 'D' Decongestant Tablets ... 760
- DHCplus Capsules ... 2148
- Darvon-N/Darvocet-N ... 1473
- Dimetapp Allergy Sinus Caplets ... 838
- Dimetapp Cold & Fever Suspension ... 839
- Drixoral Cold and Flu Extended-Release Tablets ... 764
- Drixoral Cough + Sore Throat Liquid Caps ... 763
- Drixoral Allergy/Sinus Extended Release Tablets ... 765
- Esgic-plus Capsules ... 1012
- Esgic-plus Tablets ... 1012
- Aspirin Free Excedrin Analgesic Caplets and Geltabs ... 734
- Excedrin Extra-Strength Analgesic Tablets, Caplets, and Geltabs ... 734
- Excedrin P.M. Analgesic/Sleeping Aid Tablets, Caplets, Liquigels ... 735
- Fioricet Tablets ... 2386
- Fioricet with Codeine Capsules ... 2387
- Goody's Extra Strength Headache Powders ... 632
- Goody's Extra Strength Pain Relief Tablets ... 632
- Hycomine Compound Tablets ... 948
- Hydrocet Capsules ... 787
- Infants' TYLENOL acetaminophen Suspension Drops ... 1559
- Infants' TYLENOL Cold Decongestant & Fever-Reducer Drops ... 1561
- Junior Strength TYLENOL acetaminophen Coated Caplets and Chewable Tablets ... 1562
- Lorcet 10/650 Tablets ... 1016
- Lortab ... 2751
- Lurline PMS Tablets ... 1000
- Maximum Strength Multi-Symptom Formula Midol ... 621
- PMS Multi-Symptom Formula Midol ... 622
- Maximum Strength Midol Teen Multi-Symptom Formula ... 621
- Midrin Capsules ... 788
- Panadol Tablets and Caplets ... 783
- Children's Panadol Chewable Tablets, Liquid, Infant's Drops ... 783
- Percocet Tablets ... 955
- Percogesic Analgesic Tablets ... 727
- Phrenilin ... 790
- Pyrroxate Caplets ... 742
- Robitussin Cold, Cough & Flu Liqui-Gels ... 844
- Robitussin Night-Time Cold Formula ... 847
- Sedapap Tablets 50 mg/650 mg ... 1826
- Sinarest ... 663
- Sine-Aid Maximum Strength Sinus Headache Gelcaps, Caplets and Tablets ... 1570
- Sine-Off No Drowsiness Formula Caplets ... 784
- Sine-Off Sinus Medicine ... 784
- Singlet Tablets ... 785
- Sinulin Tablets ... 792
- Sinutab Sinus Allergy Medication, Maximum Strength Tablets and Caplets ... 823
- Sinutab Sinus Medication, Maximum Strength Without Drowsiness Formula, Tablets & Caplets ... 824
- Sudafed Cold and Cough Liquid Caps ... 826
- Sudafed Severe Cold Formula Caplets ... 828
- Sudafed Severe Cold Formula Tablets ... 828
- Sudafed Sinus Caplets ... 829
- Sudafed Sinus Tablets ... 829
- Talacen Caplets ... 2464
- TheraFlu Flu and Cold Medicine ... 750
- Theraflu Maximum Strength Flu and Cold Medicine For Sore Throat ... 751
- TheraFlu Flu, Cold and Cough Medicine ... 750
- TheraFlu Maximum Strength Nighttime Flu, Cold & Cough Medicine ... 751
- TheraFlu Maximum Strength Non-Drowsy Formula Flu, Cold & Cough Medicine ... 751
- TheraFlu Maximum Strength, Non-Drowsy Formula Flu, Cold and Cough Caplets ... 752
- Theraflu Maximum Strength Sinus Non-Drowsy Formula Caplets ... 752
- Triaminic Sore Throat Formula ... 755
- Triaminicin Tablets ... 756

IMPORTANT NOTE: Always consult each drug listing in the patient's regimen for possible interactions.

TYLENOL acetaminophen Extended Relief Caplets 1570
TYLENOL acetaminophen, Extra Strength Adult Liquid Pain Reliever 1570
TYLENOL acetaminophen, Extra Strength Gelcaps, Geltabs, Caplets, Tablets 1570
TYLENOL acetaminophen, Regular Strength Caplets and Tablets 1570
TYLENOL Allergy Sinus, Maximum Strength Caplets and Gelcaps 1571
TYLENOL Allergy Sinus NightTime, Maximum Strength Caplets 1571
TYLENOL Cold Medication, Multi-Symptom Formula Tablets and Caplets 1572
TYLENOL Cold Medication, Multi-Symptom Hot Liquid Packets 1572
TYLENOL Cold Medication, No Drowsiness Formula Caplets and Gelcaps 1572
TYLENOL Cold Severe Congestion Caplets 1573
TYLENOL Cough Medication, Multi Symptom 1574
TYLENOL Cough Medication with Decongestant, Multi Symptom 1574
TYLENOL Flu No Drowsiness Formula, Maximum Strength Gelcaps 1575
TYLENOL Flu NightTime, Maximum Strength Gelcaps 1575
TYLENOL Flu NightTime, Maximum Strength Hot Medication Packets 1575
TYLENOL Headache Plus Pain Reliever with Antacid, Extra Strength Caplets ...... 🆎 705
TYLENOL PM Pain Reliever/Sleep Aid, Extra Strength Gelcaps, Caplets, Geltabs 1576
TYLENOL Severe Allergy Medication Caplets 1571
TYLENOL Sinus, Maximum Strength Geltabs, Gelcaps, Caplets and Tablets 1576
Tylenol with Codeine 1592
Tylox Capsules 1593
Unisom With Pain Relief-Nighttime Sleep Aid and Pain Reliever 1991
Vanquish Analgesic Caplets ...... 🆎 627
Vicks 44 LiquiCaps Cough, Cold & Flu Relief ...... 🆎 728
Vicks 44M Cough, Cold & Flu Relief ...... 🆎 729
Vicks DayQuil LiquiCaps/Liquid Multi-Symptom Cold/Flu Relief .. 🆎 734
Vicks Nyquil Hot Therapy ...... 🆎 735
Vicks NyQuil LiquiCaps/Liquid Multi-Symptom Cold/Flu Relief, Original and Cherry Flavors ...... 🆎 736
Vicodin Tablets 1404
Vicodin ES Tablets 1405
Vicodin HP Tablets 1403
Wygesic Tablets 2930
Zydone Capsules 967

Aminophylline (Deinduction of hepatic enzymes on smoking cessation; may require a decrease in dose at cessation of smoking).
No products indexed under this heading.

Caffeine (Deinduction of hepatic enzymes on smoking cessation; may require a decrease in dose at cessation of smoking). Products include:
Arthritis Strength BC Powder ...... 🆎 631
BC Powder ...... 🆎 631
Cafergot 2376
DHCplus Capsules 2148
Darvon Compound-65 Pulvules 1475
Esgic-plus Capsules 1012
Esgic-plus Tablets 1012
Aspirin Free Excedrin Analgesic Caplets and Geltabs 734
Excedrin Extra-Strength Analgesic Tablets, Caplets, and Geltabs 734
Fioricet 2386
Fioricet with Codeine Capsules 2387
Fiorinal Capsules 2388
Fiorinal with Codeine Capsules 2390
Fiorinal Tablets 2388
Goody's Extra Strength Headache Powders ...... 🆎 632
Goody's Extra Strength Pain Relief Tablets ...... 🆎 632
Maximum Strength Multi-Symptom Formula Midol ...... 🆎 621
No Doz Maximum Strength Caplets ...... 🆎 644
Norgesic 1554
Vanquish Analgesic Caplets ...... 🆎 627
Wigraine Tablets 1884

Caffeine Anhydrous (Deinduction of hepatic enzymes on smoking cessation; may require a decrease in dose at cessation of smoking).
No products indexed under this heading.

Caffeine Citrate (Deinduction of hepatic enzymes on smoking cessation; may require a decrease in dose at cessation of smoking).
No products indexed under this heading.

Caffeine Sodium Benzoate (Deinduction of hepatic enzymes on smoking cessation; may require a decrease in dose at cessation of smoking).
No products indexed under this heading.

Dyphylline (Deinduction of hepatic enzymes on smoking cessation; may require a decrease in dose at cessation of smoking). Products include:
Lufyllin & Lufyllin-400 Tablets 2778
Lufyllin-GG Elixir & Tablets 2779

Imipramine Hydrochloride (Deinduction of hepatic enzymes on smoking cessation; may require a decrease in dose at cessation of smoking). Products include:
Tofranil Ampuls 873
Tofranil Tablets 875

Imipramine Pamoate (Deinduction of hepatic enzymes on smoking cessation; may require a decrease in dose at cessation of smoking). Products include:
Tofranil-PM Capsules 876

Insulin, Human (Increased subcutaneous insulin absorption with smoking cessation).
No products indexed under this heading.

Insulin, Human Isophane Suspension (Increased subcutaneous insulin absorption with smoking cessation). Products include:
Novolin N Human Insulin 10 ml Vials 1846

Insulin, Human NPH (Increased subcutaneous insulin absorption with smoking cessation). Products include:
Humulin N, 100 Units 1495
Novolin N PenFill 1.5 ml Cartridges Durable Insulin Delivery System 1849
Novolin N Prefilled Syringe Disposable Insulin Delivery System 1850

Insulin, Human Regular (Increased subcutaneous insulin absorption with smoking cessation). Products include:
Humulin R, 100 Units 1497
Novolin R Human Insulin 10 ml Vials 1846
Novolin R PenFill 1.5 ml Cartridges Durable Insulin Delivery System 1849
Novolin R Prefilled Syringe Disposable Insulin Delivery System 1850
Velosulin BR Human Insulin 10 ml Vials 1847

Insulin, Human, Zinc Suspension (Increased subcutaneous insulin absorption with smoking cessation). Products include:
Humulin L, 100 Units 1494
Humulin U, 100 Units 1498
Novolin L Human Insulin 10 ml Vials 1846

Insulin Lispro, Human (Increased subcutaneous insulin absorption with smoking cessation). Products include:
Humalog Injection 1488

Insulin, NPH (Increased subcutaneous insulin absorption with smoking cessation). Products include:
NPH, 100 Units 1502
Pork NPH, 100 Units 1506
Purified Pork NPH Isophane Insulin 1852

Insulin, Regular (Increased subcutaneous insulin absorption with smoking cessation). Products include:
Regular, 100 Units 1503
Pork Regular, 100 Units 1507
Pork Regular (Concentrated), 500 Units 1508
Purified Pork Regular Insulin 1852

Insulin, Zinc Crystals (Increased subcutaneous insulin absorption with smoking cessation). Products include:
NPH, 100 Units 1502

Insulin, Zinc Suspension (Increased subcutaneous insulin absorption with smoking cessation). Products include:
Iletin I 1501
Lente, 100 Units 1501
Iletin II 1504
Pork Lente, 100 Units 1504
Purified Pork Lente Insulin 1852

Isoproterenol Hydrochloride (Decrease in circulating catecholamines with smoking cessation). Products include:
Isuprel Hydrochloride Solution 2443
Isuprel Injection 2441
Isuprel Mistometer 2442

Labetalol Hydrochloride (Decrease in circulating catecholamines with smoking cessation). Products include:
Normodyne Injection 2519
Normodyne Tablets 2522
Trandate 1158

Oxazepam (Deinduction of hepatic enzymes on smoking cessation; may require a decrease in dose at cessation of smoking). Products include:
Serax Capsules 2916
Serax Tablets 2916

Pentazocine Hydrochloride (Deinduction of hepatic enzymes on smoking cessation; may require a decrease in dose at cessation of smoking). Products include:
Talacen Caplets 2464
Talwin Compound 2466
Talwin Nx Tablets 2467

Pentazocine Lactate (Deinduction of hepatic enzymes on smoking cessation; may require a decrease in dose at cessation of smoking). Products include:
Talwin Injection 2465

Phenylephrine Hydrochloride (Decrease in circulating catecholamines with smoking cessation). Products include:
Atrohist Plus Tablets 1605
Cerose DM ...... 🆎 853
D.A. II Tablets 972
D.A. Chewable Tablets 970
Dura-Vent/DA Tablets 972
Extendryl 1003
4-Way Fast Acting Nasal Spray (regular & mentholated) ...... 🆎 644
Hemorid ...... 🆎 797
Hycomine Compound Tablets 948
Neo-Synephrine Hydrochloride 1% Carpuject 2455
Neo-Synephrine Hydrochloride 1% Injection 2455
Neo-Synephrine Hydrochloride (Ophthalmic) 2456
Neo-Synephrine ...... 🆎 624
Novahistine Elixir ...... 🆎 782
Phenergan VC 2886
Phenergan VC with Codeine 2888
Preparation H ...... 🆎 842
Tympagesic Ear Drops 2476
Vicks Sinex Nasal Spray and Ultra Fine Mist ...... 🆎 738

Prazosin Hydrochloride (Decrease in circulating catecholamines with smoking cessation). Products include:
Minipress Capsules 2015
Minizide Capsules 2016

Propranolol Hydrochloride (Deinduction of hepatic enzymes on smoking cessation; may require a decrease in dose at cessation of smoking). Products include:
Inderal 2834
Inderal LA Long Acting Capsules 2836
Inderide Tablets 2838
Inderide LA Long Acting Capsules .. 2840

Theophylline (Deinduction of hepatic enzymes on smoking cessation; may require a decrease in dose at cessation of smoking). Products include:
Marax Tablets & DF Syrup 2015
Quibron 2227

Theophylline Anhydrous (Deinduction of hepatic enzymes on smoking cessation; may require a decrease in dose at cessation of smoking). Products include:
Aerolate 1003
Primatene Tablets ...... 🆎 844
Respbid Tablets 687
Slo-bid Gyrocaps 2201
Theo-24 Extended Release Capsules 2753
Theo-Dur Extended-Release Tablets 1367
Theo-X Extended-Release Tablets .. 793
Uni-Dur Extended-Release Tablets .. 1374
Uniphyl 400 mg and 600 mg Tablets 2157

Theophylline Calcium Salicylate (Deinduction of hepatic enzymes on smoking cessation; may require a decrease in dose at cessation of smoking). Products include:
Quadrinal Tablets 1398

Theophylline Sodium Glycinate (Deinduction of hepatic enzymes on smoking cessation; may require a decrease in dose at cessation of smoking).
No products indexed under this heading.

PROSTIGMIN INJECTABLE
(Neostigmine Methylsulfate) 1305
May interact with antiarrhythmics, general anesthetics, and certain other agents. Compounds in these categories include:

Acebutolol Hydrochloride (Interferes with neuromuscular transmission). Products include:
Sectral Capsules 2914

Adenosine (Interferes with neuromuscular transmission). Products include:
Adenocard Injection 1021
Adenoscan 1022

Amiodarone Hydrochloride (Interferes with neuromuscular transmission). Products include:
Cordarone Intravenous 2821
Cordarone Tablets 2818

Bretylium Tosylate (Interferes with neuromuscular transmission).
No products indexed under this heading.

Decamethonium (Phase I block of depolarizing muscle relaxants may be prolonged).

Disopyramide Phosphate (Interferes with neuromuscular transmission). Products include:
Norpace 2596

Enflurane (Caution should be exercised if used concurrently in myasthenia gravis).
No products indexed under this heading.

(🆎 Described in PDR For Nonprescription Drugs)   (ⓞ Described in PDR For Ophthalmology)

887 **Interactions Index** **Prostin E2**

Isoflurane (Caution should be exercised if used concurrently in myasthenia gravis).
No products indexed under this heading.
Kanamycin Sulfate (May accentuate neuromuscular block).
No products indexed under this heading.
Ketamine Hydrochloride (Caution should be exercised if used concurrently in myasthenia gravis).
No products indexed under this heading.
Lidocaine Hydrochloride (Interferes with neuromuscular transmission). Products include:
Decadron Phosphate with Xylocaine Injection, Sterile ... 1683
Unguentine Plus ... ⊞ 712
Xylocaine Injections ... 562
Local Anesthetics (Prostigmin dosage increase may be required).
Methohexital Sodium (Caution should be exercised if used concurrently in myasthenia gravis).
No products indexed under this heading.
Methoxyflurane (Caution should be exercised if used concurrently in myasthenia gravis).
No products indexed under this heading.
Mexiletine Hydrochloride (Interferes with neuromuscular transmission). Products include:
Mexitil Capsules ... 684
Moricizine Hydrochloride (Interferes with neuromuscular transmission). Products include:
Ethmozine Tablets ... 2217
Neomycin Sulfate (May accentuate neuromuscular block). Products include:
AK-Spore ... ◉ 205
AK-Trol Ointment & Suspension ... ◉ 205
Coly-Mycin S Otic w/Neomycin & Hydrocortisone ... 1965
Cortisporin Cream ... 1073
Cortisporin Ointment ... 1074
Cortisporin Ophthalmic Ointment Sterile ... 1074
Cortisporin Ophthalmic Suspension Sterile ... 1075
Cortisporin Otic Solution Sterile ... 1076
Cortisporin Otic Suspension Sterile 1077
Maxitrol Ophthalmic Ointment and Suspension ... ◉ 222
Mycitracin ... ⊞ 803
NeoDecadron Sterile Ophthalmic Ointment ... 1755
NeoDecadron Sterile Ophthalmic Solution ... 1756
NeoDecadron Topical Cream ... 1757
Neosporin G.U. Irrigant Sterile ... 1130
Neosporin Ointment ... ⊞ 821
Neosporin Plus Maximum Strength Cream ... ⊞ 821
Neosporin Plus Maximum Strength Ointment ... ⊞ 822
Neosporin Ophthalmic Ointment Sterile ... 1130
Neosporin Ophthalmic Solution Sterile ... 1131
Pediotic Suspension Sterile ... 1140
Poly-Pred Liquifilm ... ◉ 246
Procainamide Hydrochloride (Interferes with neuromuscular transmission). Products include:
Procanbid Extended-Release Tablets ... 1983
Propafenone Hydrochloride (Interferes with neuromuscular transmission). Products include:
Rythmol Tablets–150mg, 225mg, 300mg ... 1399
Propofol (Caution should be exercised if used concurrently in myasthenia gravis). Products include:
Diprivan Injectable Emulsion ... 2939
Propranolol Hydrochloride (Interferes with neuromuscular transmission). Products include:
Inderal ... 2834
Inderal LA Long Acting Capsules ... 2836
Inderide Tablets ... 2838
Inderide LA Long Acting Capsules ... 2840
Quinidine Gluconate (Interferes with neuromuscular transmission). Products include:
Quinaglute Dura-Tabs Tablets ... 644
Quinidine Polygalacturonate (Interferes with neuromuscular transmission). Products include:
Cardioquin Tablets ... 2146
Quinidine Sulfate (Interferes with neuromuscular transmission). Products include:
Quinidex Extentabs ... 2240
Sevoflurane (Caution should be exercised if used concurrently in myasthenia gravis).
No products indexed under this heading.
Sotalol Hydrochloride (Interferes with neuromuscular transmission). Products include:
Betapace Tablets ... 637
Streptomycin Sulfate (May accentuate neuromuscular block). Products include:
Streptomycin Sulfate Injection ... 2031
Succinylcholine Chloride (Phase I block of depolarizing muscle relaxants may be prolonged). Products include:
Anectine ... 1062
Tocainide Hydrochloride (Interferes with neuromuscular transmission). Products include:
Tonocard Tablets ... 519
Verapamil Hydrochloride (Interferes with neuromuscular transmission). Products include:
Calan SR Caplets ... 2571
Calan Tablets ... 2568
Covera-HS Tablets ... 2573
Isoptin Injectable ... 1391
Isoptin Oral Tablets ... 1393
Isoptin SR Tablets ... 1395
Verelan Capsules ... 1455

PROSTIGMIN TABLETS
(Neostigmine Bromide) ... 1306
May interact with anticholinergics, antiarrhythmics, and certain other agents. Compounds in these categories include:

Acebutolol Hydrochloride (Interferes with neuromuscular transmission). Products include:
Sectral Capsules ... 2914
Adenosine (Interferes with neuromuscular transmission). Products include:
Adenocard Injection ... 1021
Adenoscan ... 1022
Amiodarone Hydrochloride (Interferes with neuromuscular transmission). Products include:
Cordarone Intravenous ... 2821
Cordarone Tablets ... 2818
Atropine Sulfate (Decreased intestinal motility). Products include:
Arco-Lase Plus Tablets ... 513
Atrohist Plus Tablets ... 1605
Donnatal ... 2234
Donnatal Extentabs ... 2234
Donnatal Tablets ... 2234
Lomotil ... 2591
Motofen Tablets ... 789
Urised Tablets ... 2123
Belladonna Alkaloids (Decreased intestinal motility). Products include:
Bellergal-S Tablets ... 2375
Hyland's Bedwetting Tablets ... ⊞ 788
Hyland's EnurAid Tablets ... ⊞ 789
Hyland's Headache Tablets ... ⊞ 790
Hyland's Teething Tablets ... ⊞ 790
Similasan Eye Drops #1 ... ⊞ 769
Benztropine Mesylate (Decreased intestinal motility). Products include:
Cogentin ... 1661
Biperiden Hydrochloride (Decreased intestinal motility). Products include:
Akineton ... 1380
Bretylium Tosylate (Interferes with neuromuscular transmission).
No products indexed under this heading.
Clidinium Bromide (Decreased intestinal motility). Products include:
Librax Capsules ... 2330
Dicyclomine Hydrochloride (Decreased intestinal motility). Products include:
Bentyl ... 1246
Disopyramide Phosphate (Interferes with neuromuscular transmission). Products include:
Norpace ... 2596
Ethopropazine Hydrochloride (Decreased intestinal motility).
Glycopyrrolate (Decreased intestinal motility). Products include:
Robinul Forte Tablets ... 2247
Robinul Injectable ... 2247
Robinul Tablets ... 2247
Hyoscyamine (Decreased intestinal motility). Products include:
Cystospaz Tablets ... 2123
Urised Tablets ... 2123
Hyoscyamine Sulfate (Decreased intestinal motility). Products include:
Arco-Lase Plus Tablets ... 513
Atrohist Plus Tablets ... 1605
Cystospaz-M Capsules ... 2123
Donnatal ... 2234
Donnatal Extentabs ... 2234
Donnatal Tablets ... 2234
Kutrase Capsules ... 2546
Levsin/Levsinex/Levbid ... 2549
Ipratropium Bromide (Decreased intestinal motility). Products include:
Atrovent Inhalation Aerosol ... 674
Atrovent Inhalation Solution ... 675
Atrovent Nasal Spray 0.03% ... 676
Atrovent Nasal Spray 0.06% ... 678
Kanamycin Sulfate (May accentuate neuromuscular block).
No products indexed under this heading.
Lidocaine Hydrochloride (Interferes with neuromuscular transmission). Products include:
Decadron Phosphate with Xylocaine Injection, Sterile ... 1683
Unguentine Plus ... ⊞ 712
Xylocaine Injections ... 562
Local Anesthetics (Prostigmin dosage increase may be required).
Mepenzolate Bromide (Decreased intestinal motility).
No products indexed under this heading.
Mexiletine Hydrochloride (Interferes with neuromuscular transmission). Products include:
Mexitil Capsules ... 684
Moricizine Hydrochloride (Interferes with neuromuscular transmission). Products include:
Ethmozine Tablets ... 2217
Oxybutynin Chloride (Decreased intestinal motility). Products include:
Ditropan ... 1267
Oxyphenonium Bromide (Decreased intestinal motility).
Procainamide Hydrochloride (Interferes with neuromuscular transmission). Products include:
Procanbid Extended-Release Tablets ... 1983
Procyclidine Hydrochloride (Decreased intestinal motility). Products include:
Kemadrin Tablets ... 1105
Propafenone Hydrochloride (Interferes with neuromuscular transmission). Products include:
Rythmol Tablets–150mg, 225mg, 300mg ... 1399
Propantheline Bromide (Decreased intestinal motility). Products include:
Pro-Banthine Tablets ... 2226
Propranolol Hydrochloride (Interferes with neuromuscular transmission). Products include:
Inderal ... 2834
Inderal LA Long Acting Capsules ... 2836
Inderide Tablets ... 2838
Inderide LA Long Acting Capsules ... 2840
Quinidine Gluconate (Interferes with neuromuscular transmission). Products include:
Quinaglute Dura-Tabs Tablets ... 644
Quinidine Polygalacturonate (Interferes with neuromuscular transmission). Products include:
Cardioquin Tablets ... 2146
Quinidine Sulfate (Interferes with neuromuscular transmission). Products include:
Quinidex Extentabs ... 2240
Scopolamine (Decreased intestinal motility). Products include:
Transderm Scōp Transdermal Therapeutic System ... 890
Scopolamine Hydrobromide (Decreased intestinal motility). Products include:
Atrohist Plus Tablets ... 1605
Donnatal ... 2234
Donnatal Extentabs ... 2234
Donnatal Tablets ... 2234
Sotalol Hydrochloride (Interferes with neuromuscular transmission). Products include:
Betapace Tablets ... 637
Streptomycin Sulfate (May accentuate neuromuscular block). Products include:
Streptomycin Sulfate Injection ... 2031
Tocainide Hydrochloride (Interferes with neuromuscular transmission). Products include:
Tonocard Tablets ... 519
Tridihexethyl Chloride (Decreased intestinal motility).
No products indexed under this heading.
Trihexyphenidyl Hydrochloride (Decreased intestinal motility). Products include:
Artane ... 1418
Verapamil Hydrochloride (Interferes with neuromuscular transmission). Products include:
Calan SR Caplets ... 2571
Calan Tablets ... 2568
Covera-HS Tablets ... 2573
Isoptin Injectable ... 1391
Isoptin Oral Tablets ... 1393
Isoptin SR Tablets ... 1395
Verelan Capsules ... 1455

PROSTIN E2 SUPPOSITORY
(Dinoprostone) ... 2109
May interact with oxytocic drugs. Compounds in this category include:

Ergonovine Maleate (Prostin E2 may augment the activity of other oxytocic drugs; coadministration is not recommended).
No products indexed under this heading.
Methylergonovine Maleate (Prostin E2 may augment the activity of other oxytocic drugs; coadministration is not recommended). Products include:
Methergine ... 2401

IMPORTANT NOTE: Always consult each drug listing in the patient's regimen for possible interactions.

Prostin E2 — Interactions Index — 888

Oxytocin (Prostin E2 may augment the activity of other oxytocic drugs; coadministration is not recommended). Products include:
- Syntocinon Injection 2425

PROTAMINE SULFATE VIALS
(Protamine Sulfate) 1526
May interact with:

Antibiotics, unspecified (Incompatible with unspecified cephalosporins and penicillins in vitro).

PROTEGRA ANTIOXIDANT VITAMIN & MINERAL SUPPLEMENT
(Vitamin C, Vitamin E, Beta Carotene) .... ⊠ 685
None cited in PDR database.

PROTOPAM CHLORIDE FOR INJECTION
(Pralidoxime Chloride) 2909
May interact with barbiturates, xanthine bronchodilators, phenothiazines, and certain other agents. Compounds in these categories include:

Aminophylline (Concurrent use should be avoided in patients with organophosphate poisoning).
No products indexed under this heading.

Aprobarbital (Barbiturates are potentiated by the anticholinesterases, they should be used cautiously in the treatment of convulsions).
No products indexed under this heading.

Atropine Nitrate, Methyl (Signs of atropinization may occur earlier than expected).
No products indexed under this heading.

Atropine Sulfate (Signs of atropinization may occur earlier than expected). Products include:
- Arco-Lase Plus Tablets 513
- Atrohist Plus Tablets 1605
- Donnatal 2234
- Donnatal Extentabs 2234
- Donnatal Tablets 2234
- Lomotil 2591
- Motofen Tablets 789
- Urised Tablets 2123

Butabarbital (Barbiturates are potentiated by the anticholinesterases, they should be used cautiously in the treatment of convulsions).
No products indexed under this heading.

Butalbital (Barbiturates are potentiated by the anticholinesterases, they should be used cautiously in the treatment of convulsions). Products include:
- Axocet Capsules 2469
- Esgic-plus Capsules 1012
- Esgic-plus Tablets 1012
- Fioricet Tablets 2386
- Fioricet with Codeine Capsules 2387
- Fiorinal Capsules 2388
- Fiorinal with Codeine Capsules 2390
- Fiorinal Tablets 2388
- Phrenilin 790
- Sedapap Tablets 50 mg/650 mg .. 1826

Chlorpromazine (Concurrent use should be avoided in patients with organophosphate poisoning). Products include:
- Thorazine Suppositories 2701

Dyphylline (Concurrent use should be avoided in patients with organophosphate poisoning). Products include:
- Lufyllin & Lufyllin-400 Tablets 2778
- Lufyllin-GG Elixir & Tablets 2779

Fluphenazine Decanoate (Concurrent use should be avoided in patients with organophosphate poisoning). Products include:
- Prolixin Decanoate 510

Fluphenazine Enanthate (Concurrent use should be avoided in patients with organophosphate poisoning). Products include:
- Prolixin Enanthate 510

Fluphenazine Hydrochloride (Concurrent use should be avoided in patients with organophosphate poisoning). Products include:
- Prolixin 510

Mephobarbital (Barbiturates are potentiated by the anticholinesterases, they should be used cautiously in the treatment of convulsions). Products include:
- Mebaral Tablets 2452

Mesoridazine Besylate (Concurrent use should be avoided in patients with organophosphate poisoning). Products include:
- Serentil 689

Methotrimeprazine (Concurrent use should be avoided in patients with organophosphate poisoning). Products include:
- Levoprome 1321

Morphine Sulfate (Concurrent use should be avoided in patients with organophosphate poisoning). Products include:
- Astramorph/PF Injection, USP (Preservative-Free) 526
- Duramorph Injection 983
- Infumorph 200 and Infumorph 500 Sterile Solutions 985
- Kadian Capsules 2948
- MS Contin Tablets 2149
- MSIR 2152
- Oramorph SR (Morphine Sulfate Sustained Release Tablets) 2359
- RMS Suppositories CII 2766
- Roxanol 2365

Pentobarbital Sodium (Barbiturates are potentiated by the anticholinesterases, they should be used cautiously in the treatment of convulsions). Products include:
- Nembutal Sodium Capsules 440
- Nembutal Sodium Solution 442
- Nembutal Sodium Suppositories 444

Perphenazine (Concurrent use should be avoided in patients with organophosphate poisoning). Products include:
- Etrafon 2495
- Triavil Tablets 1800
- Trilafon 2532

Phenobarbital (Barbiturates are potentiated by the anticholinesterases, they should be used cautiously in the treatment of convulsions). Products include:
- Arco-Lase Plus Tablets 513
- Bellergal-S Tablets 2375
- Donnatal 2234
- Donnatal Extentabs 2234
- Donnatal Tablets 2234
- Phenobarbital Elixir and Tablets 1523
- Quadrinal Tablets 1398

Prochlorperazine (Concurrent use should be avoided in patients with organophosphate poisoning). Products include:
- Compazine 2644

Promethazine Hydrochloride (Concurrent use should be avoided in patients with organophosphate poisoning). Products include:
- Mepergan Injection 2859
- Phenergan with Codeine 2883
- Phenergan with Dextromethorphan 2885
- Phenergan Injection 2880
- Phenergan Suppositories 2882
- Phenergan Syrup 2881
- Phenergan Tablets 2882
- Phenergan VC 2886

Phenergan VC with Codeine 2888

Reserpine (Concurrent use should be avoided in patients with organophosphate poisoning). Products include:
- Diupres Tablets 1691
- Hydropres Tablets 1718
- Ser-Ap-Es Tablets 867

Secobarbital Sodium (Barbiturates are potentiated by the anticholinesterases, they should be used cautiously in the treatment of convulsions). Products include:
- Seconal Sodium Pulvules 1529

Succinylcholine Chloride (Concurrent use should be avoided in patients with organophosphate poisoning). Products include:
- Anectine 1062

Theophylline (Concurrent use should be avoided in patients with organophosphate poisoning). Products include:
- Marax Tablets & DF Syrup 2015
- Quibron 2227

Theophylline Anhydrous (Concurrent use should be avoided in patients with organophosphate poisoning). Products include:
- Aerolate 1003
- Primatene Tablets .... ⊠ 844
- Respbid Tablets 687
- Slo-bid Gyrocaps 2201
- Theo-24 Extended Release Capsules 2753
- Theo-Dur Extended-Release Tablets 1367
- Theo-X Extended-Release Tablets 793
- Uni-Dur Extended-Release Tablets 1374
- Uniphyl 400 mg and 600 mg Tablets 2157

Theophylline Calcium Salicylate (Concurrent use should be avoided in patients with organophosphate poisoning). Products include:
- Quadrinal Tablets 1398

Theophylline Sodium Glycinate (Concurrent use should be avoided in patients with organophosphate poisoning).
No products indexed under this heading.

Thiamylal Sodium (Barbiturates are potentiated by the anticholinesterases, they should be used cautiously in the treatment of convulsions).
No products indexed under this heading.

Thioridazine Hydrochloride (Concurrent use should be avoided in patients with organophosphate poisoning). Products include:
- Mellaril 2398

Trifluoperazine Hydrochloride (Concurrent use should be avoided in patients with organophosphate poisoning). Products include:
- Stelazine 2692

PROTOSTAT TABLETS
(Metronidazole) 1939
May interact with oral anticoagulants, lithium preparations, and certain other agents. Compounds in these categories include:

Cimetidine (Prolongs the half-life and decreases plasma clearance of metronidazole). Products include:
- Tagamet HB Tablets .... ⊠ 786
- Tagamet Tablets 2694

Cimetidine Hydrochloride (Prolongs the half-life and decreases plasma clearance of metronidazole). Products include:
- Tagamet 2694

Dicumarol (Potentiation of anticoagulant effect).
No products indexed under this heading.

Disulfiram (Potential for psychotic reactions in alcoholic patients who are using metronidazole and disulfiram concurrently). Products include:
- Antabuse Tablets 2802

Lithium Carbonate (Elevated serum lithium levels and potential for Lithium toxicity). Products include:
- Eskalith 2658
- Lithium Carbonate Capsules & Tablets 2352
- Lithonate/Lithotabs/Lithobid 2721

Lithium Citrate (Elevated serum lithium levels and potential for Lithium toxicity).
No products indexed under this heading.

Phenobarbital (May accelerate the elimination of metronidazole reduced plasma levels). Products include:
- Arco-Lase Plus Tablets 513
- Bellergal-S Tablets 2375
- Donnatal 2234
- Donnatal Extentabs 2234
- Donnatal Tablets 2234
- Phenobarbital Elixir and Tablets 1523
- Quadrinal Tablets 1398

Phenytoin (May accelerate the elimination of metronidazole reduced plasma levels). Products include:
- Dilantin Infatabs 1967
- Dilantin-125 Suspension 1969

Phenytoin Sodium (May accelerate the elimination of metronidazole reduced plasma levels). Products include:
- Dilantin Kapseals 1965

Warfarin Sodium (Potentiation of anticoagulant effect). Products include:
- Coumadin 941

Food Interactions

Alcohol (Abdominal cramps, nausea, vomiting, headache, and flushing may occur; alcohol should not be consumed during and for at least one day after therapy).

PROTROPIN
(Somatrem) 1053
May interact with glucocorticoids. Compounds in this category include:

Betamethasone Acetate (May inhibit growth-promoting effect of Protropin growth hormone). Products include:
- Celestone Soluspan Suspension 2484

Betamethasone Sodium Phosphate (May inhibit growth-promoting effect of Protropin growth hormone). Products include:
- Celestone Soluspan Suspension 2484

Cortisone Acetate (May inhibit growth-promoting effect of Protropin growth hormone). Products include:
- Cortone Acetate Sterile Suspension 1663
- Cortone Acetate Tablets 1664

Dexamethasone (May inhibit growth-promoting effect of Protropin growth hormone). Products include:
- AK-Trol Ointment & Suspension .... ⊙ 205
- Decadron Elixir 1676
- Decadron Tablets 1678
- Decaspray Topical Aerosol 1689
- Maxitrol Ophthalmic Ointment and Suspension .... ⊙ 222
- TobraDex Ophthalmic Suspension and Ointment 469

Dexamethasone Acetate (May inhibit growth-promoting effect of Protropin growth hormone). Products include:
- Dalalone D.P. Injectable 1009
- Decadron-LA Sterile Suspension 1687

(⊠ Described in PDR For Nonprescription Drugs)   (⊙ Described in PDR For Ophthalmology)

Dexamethasone Sodium Phosphate (May inhibit growth-promoting effect of Protropin growth hormone). Products include:

Decadron Phosphate Injection	1680
Decadron Phosphate Sterile Ophthalmic Ointment	1684
Decadron Phosphate Sterile Ophthalmic Solution	1685
Decadron Phosphate Topical Cream	1686
Decadron Phosphate with Xylocaine Injection, Sterile	1683
Dexacort Phosphate in Respihaler	1606
Dexacort Phosphate in Turbinaire	1607
NeoDecadron Sterile Ophthalmic Ointment	1755
NeoDecadron Sterile Ophthalmic Solution	1756
NeoDecadron Topical Cream	1757

Fludrocortisone Acetate (May inhibit growth-promoting effect of Protropin growth hormone). Products include:

Florinef Acetate Tablets	506

Hydrocortisone (May inhibit growth-promoting effect of Protropin growth hormone). Products include:

Anusol-HC Cream 2.5%	1953
Aquanil HC Lotion	1989
Maximum Strength Cortaid Spray	800
CORTENEMA	2713
Cortisporin Ointment	1074
Cortisporin Ophthalmic Ointment Sterile	1074
Cortisporin Ophthalmic Suspension Sterile	1075
Cortisporin Otic Solution Sterile	1076
Cortisporin Otic Suspension Sterile	1077
Cortizone-5	795
Cortizone-10	795
Hydrocortone Tablets	1715
Hytone	922
Hytone Ointment 2 ½%	923
Massengill Medicated Soft Cloth Towelettes	2628
Pediotic Suspension Sterile	1140
Preparation H Hydrocortisone 1% Cream	843
ProctoCream-HC 2.5%	2552
VōSoL HC Otic Solution	2786

Hydrocortisone Acetate (May inhibit growth-promoting effect of Protropin growth hormone). Products include:

Analpram-HC Rectal Cream 1% and 2.5%	993
Anusol HC-1 Hydrocortisone Anti-Itch Ointment	810
Anusol-HC Suppositories	1954
Caldecort Anti-Itch Hydrocortisone Cream	651
Coly-Mycin S Otic w/Neomycin & Hydrocortisone	1965
Cortaid	800
Cortifoam	2540
Cortisporin Cream	1073
Epifoam	2543
Hydrocortone Acetate Sterile Suspension	1712
Mantadil Cream	1124
Nupercainal Hydrocortisone 1% Cream	661
Pramosone Cream, Lotion & Ointment	995
ProctoFoam-HC	2552
Terra-Cortril Ophthalmic Suspension	2033

Hydrocortisone Sodium Phosphate (May inhibit growth-promoting effect of Protropin growth hormone). Products include:

Hydrocortone Phosphate Injection, Sterile	1713

Hydrocortisone Sodium Succinate (May inhibit growth-promoting effect of Protropin growth hormone). Products include:

No products indexed under this heading.

Methylprednisolone Acetate (May inhibit growth-promoting effect of Protropin growth hormone). Products include:

No products indexed under this heading.

Methylprednisolone Sodium Succinate (May inhibit growth-promoting effect of Protropin growth hormone).

No products indexed under this heading.

Prednisolone Acetate (May inhibit growth-promoting effect of Protropin growth hormone). Products include:

AK-CIDE	203
AK-CIDE Ointment	203
Blephamide Liquifilm Sterile Ophthalmic Suspension	472
Blephamide Ointment	234
Econopred & Econopred Plus Ophthalmic Suspensions	216
Poly-Pred Liquifilm	246
Pred Forte	247
Pred Mild	250
Pred-G Liquifilm Sterile Ophthalmic Suspension	248
Pred-G S.O.P. Sterile Ophthalmic Ointment	249

Prednisolone Sodium Phosphate (May inhibit growth-promoting effect of Protropin growth hormone). Products include:

AK-PRED	204
Hydeltrasol Injection, Sterile	1708
Pediapred Oral Solution	1618

Prednisolone Tebutate (May inhibit growth-promoting effect of Protropin growth hormone). Products include:

Hydeltra-T.B.A. Sterile Suspension	1710

Prednisone (May inhibit growth-promoting effect of Protropin growth hormone).

No products indexed under this heading.

Triamcinolone (May inhibit growth-promoting effect of Protropin growth hormone).

No products indexed under this heading.

Triamcinolone Acetonide (May inhibit growth-promoting effect of Protropin growth hormone). Products include:

Azmacort Oral Inhaler	2175
Nasacort AQ Nasal Spray	2191
Nasacort Nasal Inhaler	2189

Triamcinolone Diacetate (May inhibit growth-promoting effect of Protropin growth hormone).

No products indexed under this heading.

Triamcinolone Hexacetonide (May inhibit growth-promoting effect of Protropin growth hormone).

No products indexed under this heading.

PROVENTIL INHALATION AEROSOL

(Albuterol) 2524

May interact with sympathomimetic aerosol bronchodilators, monoamine oxidase inhibitors, tricyclic antidepressants, drugs which lower serum potassium (selected), and beta blockers. Compounds in these categories include:

Acebutolol Hydrochloride (Inhibited effects of both drugs). Products include:

Sectral Capsules	2914

Amitriptyline Hydrochloride (Potentiates albuterol's effects on the vascular system). Products include:

Elavil	2945
Etrafon	2495
Limbitrol	2333
Triavil Tablets	1800

Amoxapine (Potentiates albuterol's effects on the vascular system). Products include:

Asendin Tablets	1419

Atenolol (Inhibited effects of both drugs). Products include:

Tenoretic Tablets	2963
Tenormin Tablets and I.V. Injection	2965

Bendroflumethiazide (Potential for additive hypokalemic effect with concurrent use).

No products indexed under this heading.

Betamethasone Acetate (Potential for additive hypokalemic effect with concurrent use). Products include:

Celestone Soluspan Suspension	2484

Betamethasone Sodium Phosphate (Potential for additive hypokalemic effect with concurrent use). Products include:

Celestone Soluspan Suspension	2484

Betaxolol Hydrochloride (Inhibited effects of both drugs). Products include:

Betoptic Ophthalmic Solution	465
Betoptic S Ophthalmic Suspension	467
Kerlone Tablets	2588

Bisoprolol Fumarate (Inhibited effects of both drugs). Products include:

Zebeta Tablets	1457
Ziac	1459

Bitolterol Mesylate (Potentiates cardiovascular effects). Products include:

Tornalate Solution for Inhalation, 0.2%	976
Tornalate Metered Dose Inhaler	978

Carteolol Hydrochloride (Inhibited effects of both drugs). Products include:

Cartrol Tablets	413
Ocupress Ophthalmic Solution, 1% Sterile	297

Chlorothiazide (Potential for additive hypokalemic effect with concurrent use). Products include:

Aldoclor Tablets	1638
Diupres Tablets	1691
Diuril Oral	1694

Chlorothiazide Sodium (Potential for additive hypokalemic effect with concurrent use). Products include:

Diuril Sodium Intravenous	1693

Clomipramine Hydrochloride (Potentiates albuterol's effects on the vascular system). Products include:

Anafranil Capsules	819

Cortisone Acetate (Potential for additive hypokalemic effect with concurrent use). Products include:

Cortone Acetate Sterile Suspension	1663
Cortone Acetate Tablets	1664

Desipramine Hydrochloride (Potentiates albuterol's effects on the vascular system). Products include:

Norpramin Tablets	1273

Dexamethasone (Potential for additive hypokalemic effect with concurrent use). Products include:

AK-Trol Ointment & Suspension	205
Decadron Elixir	1676
Decadron Tablets	1678
Decaspray Topical Aerosol	1689
Maxitrol Ophthalmic Ointment and Suspension	222
TobraDex Ophthalmic Suspension and Ointment	469

Dexamethasone Acetate (Potential for additive hypokalemic effect with concurrent use). Products include:

Dalalone D.P. Injectable	1009
Decadron-LA Sterile Suspension	1687

Dexamethasone Sodium Phosphate (Potential for additive hypokalemic effect with concurrent use). Products include:

Decadron Phosphate Injection	1680
Decadron Phosphate Sterile Ophthalmic Ointment	1684
Decadron Phosphate Sterile Ophthalmic Solution	1685
Decadron Phosphate Topical Cream	1686
Decadron Phosphate with Xylocaine Injection, Sterile	1683
Dexacort Phosphate in Respihaler	1606
Dexacort Phosphate in Turbinaire	1607
NeoDecadron Sterile Ophthalmic Ointment	1755
NeoDecadron Sterile Ophthalmic Solution	1756
NeoDecadron Topical Cream	1757

Doxepin Hydrochloride (Potentiates albuterol's effects on the vascular system). Products include:

Adapin Capsules	1542
Sinequan	2028
Zonalon Cream	1042

Furazolidone (Potentiates albuterol's effects on the vascular system). Products include:

Furoxone	2221

Hydrochlorothiazide (Potential for additive hypokalemic effect with concurrent use). Products include:

Aldactazide Tablets	2556
Aldoril Tablets	1644
Apresazide Capsules	824
Capozide Tablets	744
Dyazide Capsules	2653
Esidrix Tablets	839
Esimil Tablets	840
HydroDIURIL Tablets	1716
Hydropres Tablets	1718
Hyzaar Tablets	1720
Inderide Tablets	2838
Inderide LA Long Acting Capsules	2840
Lopressor HCT Tablets	850
Lotensin HCT Tablets	855
Moduretic Tablets	1748
Oretic Tablets	450
Prinzide Tablets	1780
Ser-Ap-Es Tablets	867
Timolide Tablets	1791
Vaseretic Tablets	1810
Zestoretic Tablets	2968
Ziac	1459

Hydrocortisone (Potential for additive hypokalemic effect with concurrent use). Products include:

Anusol-HC Cream 2.5%	1953
Aquanil HC Lotion	1989
Maximum Strength Cortaid Spray	800
CORTENEMA	2713
Cortisporin Ointment	1074
Cortisporin Ophthalmic Ointment Sterile	1074
Cortisporin Ophthalmic Suspension Sterile	1075
Cortisporin Otic Solution Sterile	1076
Cortisporin Otic Suspension Sterile	1077
Cortizone-5	795
Cortizone-10	795
Hydrocortone Tablets	1715
Hytone	922
Hytone Ointment 2 ½%	923
Massengill Medicated Soft Cloth Towelettes	2628
Pediotic Suspension Sterile	1140
Preparation H Hydrocortisone 1% Cream	843
ProctoCream-HC 2.5%	2552
VōSoL HC Otic Solution	2786

Hydrocortisone Acetate (Potential for additive hypokalemic effect with concurrent use). Products include:

Analpram-HC Rectal Cream 1% and 2.5%	993
Anusol HC-1 Hydrocortisone Anti-Itch Ointment	810
Anusol-HC Suppositories	1954
Caldecort Anti-Itch Hydrocortisone Cream	651
Coly-Mycin S Otic w/Neomycin & Hydrocortisone	1965
Cortaid	800
Cortifoam	2540
Cortisporin Cream	1073

IMPORTANT NOTE: Always consult each drug listing in the patient's regimen for possible interactions.

Proventil Inhaler   **Interactions Index**   890

Epifoam 2543
Hydrocortone Acetate Sterile Suspension................................. 1712
Mantadil Cream 1124
Nupercainal Hydrocortisone 1% Cream .... ▣ 661
Pramosone Cream, Lotion & Ointment 995
ProctoFoam-HC 2552
Terra-Cortril Ophthalmic Suspension 2033

Hydrocortisone Sodium Phosphate (Potential for additive hypokalemic effect with concurrent use). Products include:
Hydrocortone Phosphate Injection, Sterile 1713

Hydrocortisone Sodium Succinate (Potential for additive hypokalemic effect with concurrent use).
No products indexed under this heading.

Hydroflumethiazide (Potential for additive hypokalemic effect with concurrent use). Products include:
Diucardin Tablets..................... 2824

Imipramine Hydrochloride (Potentiates albuterol's effects on the vascular system). Products include:
Tofranil Ampuls 873
Tofranil Tablets 875

Imipramine Pamoate (Potentiates albuterol's effects on the vascular system). Products include:
Tofranil-PM Capsules 876

Isocarboxazid (Potentiates albuterol's effects on the vascular system).
No products indexed under this heading.

Isoetharine (Potentiates cardiovascular effects). Products include:
Bronkometer Aerosol 2432
Bronkosol Solution 2432
Isoetharine Inhalation Solution, USP, Arm-a-Med 545

Isoproterenol Hydrochloride (Potentiates cardiovascular effects). Products include:
Isuprel Hydrochloride Solution ... 2443
Isuprel Injection 2441
Isuprel Mistometer 2442

Labetalol Hydrochloride (Inhibited effects of both drugs). Products include:
Normodyne Injection 2519
Normodyne Tablets 2522
Trandate 1158

Levobunolol Hydrochloride (Inhibited effects of both drugs). Products include:
Betagan .... ⊙ 230

Maprotiline Hydrochloride (Potentiates albuterol's effects on the vascular system). Products include:
Ludiomil Tablets...................... 861

Metaproterenol Sulfate (Potentiates cardiovascular effects). Products include:
Alupent 672
Metaproterenol Sulfate Inhalation Solution, USP, Arm-a-Med 547

Methyclothiazide (Potential for additive hypokalemic effect with concurrent use). Products include:
Enduron Tablets 424

Methylprednisolone Acetate (Potential for additive hypokalemic effect with concurrent use).
No products indexed under this heading.

Methylprednisolone Sodium Succinate (Potential for additive hypokalemic effect with concurrent use).
No products indexed under this heading.

Metipranolol Hydrochloride (Inhibited effects of both drugs). Products include:
OptiPranolol (Metipranolol 0.3%) Sterile Ophthalmic Solution........ ⊙ 256

Metoprolol Succinate (Inhibited effects of both drugs). Products include:
Toprol-XL Tablets 560

Metoprolol Tartrate (Inhibited effects of both drugs). Products include:
Lopressor 848
Lopressor HCT Tablets 850

Nadolol (Inhibited effects of both drugs).
No products indexed under this heading.

Nortriptyline Hydrochloride (Potentiates albuterol's effects on the vascular system). Products include:
Pamelor 2409

Penbutolol Sulfate (Inhibited effects of both drugs). Products include:
Levatol Tablets 2547

Phenelzine Sulfate (Potentiates albuterol's effects on the vascular system). Products include:
Nardil 1977

Pindolol (Inhibited effects of both drugs). Products include:
Visken Tablets 2428

Pirbuterol Acetate (Potentiates cardiovascular effects). Products include:
Maxair Autohaler 1550
Maxair Inhaler 1552

Polythiazide (Potential for additive hypokalemic effect with concurrent use). Products include:
Minizide Capsules 2016

Prednisolone Acetate (Potential for additive hypokalemic effect with concurrent use). Products include:
AK-CIDE .... ⊙ 203
AK-CIDE Ointment................. ⊙ 203
Blephamide Liquifilm Sterile Ophthalmic Suspension................ 472
Blephamide Ointment .... ⊙ 234
Econopred & Econopred Plus Ophthalmic Suspensions ...... ⊙ 216
Poly-Pred Liquifilm .... ⊙ 246
Pred Forte .... ⊙ 247
Pred Mild .... ⊙ 250
Pred-G Liquifilm Sterile Ophthalmic Suspension .... ⊙ 248
Pred-G S.O.P. Sterile Ophthalmic Ointment .... ⊙ 249

Prednisolone Sodium Phosphate (Potential for additive hypokalemic effect with concurrent use). Products include:
AK-PRED .... ⊙ 204
Hydeltrasol Injection, Sterile...... 1708
Pediapred Oral Solution 1618

Prednisolone Tebutate (Potential for additive hypokalemic effect with concurrent use). Products include:
Hydeltra-T.B.A. Sterile Suspension ... 1710

Prednisone (Potential for additive hypokalemic effect with concurrent use).
No products indexed under this heading.

Propranolol Hydrochloride (Inhibited effects of both drugs). Products include:
Inderal 2834
Inderal LA Long Acting Capsules 2836
Inderide Tablets 2838
Inderide LA Long Acting Capsules .. 2840

Protriptyline Hydrochloride (Potentiates albuterol's effects on the vascular system). Products include:
Vivactil Tablets 1820

Salmeterol Xinafoate (Potentiates cardiovascular effects). Products include:
Serevent Inhalation Aerosol........ 1149

Selegiline Hydrochloride (Potentiates albuterol's effects on the vascular system). Products include:
Eldepryl Capsules 2729

Sotalol Hydrochloride (Inhibited effects of both drugs). Products include:
Betapace Tablets 637

Terbutaline Sulfate (Potentiates cardiovascular effects). Products include:
Brethaire Inhaler 830
Brethine Ampuls 832
Brethine Tablets 831
Bricanyl Subcutaneous Injection ... 1247
Bricanyl Tablets 1248

Timolol Hemihydrate (Inhibited effects of both drugs). Products include:
Betimol 0.25%, 0.5% .... ⊙ 259

Timolol Maleate (Inhibited effects of both drugs). Products include:
Blocadren Tablets 1654
Timolide Tablets..................... 1791
Timoptic in Ocudose 1796
Timoptic Sterile Ophthalmic Solution 1794
Timoptic-XE 1798

Tranylcypromine Sulfate (Potentiates albuterol's effects on the vascular system). Products include:
Parnate Tablets 2679

Triamcinolone (Potential for additive hypokalemic effect with concurrent use).
No products indexed under this heading.

Triamcinolone Acetonide (Potential for additive hypokalemic effect with concurrent use). Products include:
Azmacort Oral Inhaler 2175
Nasacort AQ Nasal Spray 2191
Nasacort Nasal Inhaler 2189

Triamcinolone Diacetate (Potential for additive hypokalemic effect with concurrent use).
No products indexed under this heading.

Triamcinolone Hexacetonide (Potential for additive hypokalemic effect with concurrent use).
No products indexed under this heading.

Trimipramine Maleate (Potentiates albuterol's effects on the vascular system). Products include:
Surmontil Capsules................ 2917

PROVENTIL INHALATION SOLUTION 0.083%
(Albuterol Sulfate)..................2527
May interact with sympathomimetic aerosol bronchodilators, monoamine oxidase inhibitors, tricyclic antidepressants, drugs which lower serum potassium (selected), and beta blockers. Compounds in these categories include:

Acebutolol Hydrochloride (Effects of both drugs inhibited). Products include:
Sectral Capsules 2914

Albuterol (Effect not specified; concurrent use should be avoided). Products include:
Proventil Inhalation Aerosol 2524
Ventolin Inhalation Aerosol and Refill 1170

Amitriptyline Hydrochloride (Action of albuterol on the vascular system may be potentiated). Products include:
Elavil 2945

Etrafon 2495
Limbitrol 2333
Triavil Tablets 1800

Amoxapine (Action of albuterol on the vascular system may be potentiated). Products include:
Asendin Tablets 1419

Atenolol (Effects of both drugs inhibited). Products include:
Tenoretic Tablets 2963
Tenormin Tablets and I.V. Injection 2965

Bendroflumethiazide (Potential for additive hypokalemic effect with concurrent use).
No products indexed under this heading.

Betamethasone Acetate (Potential for additive hypokalemic effect with concurrent use). Products include:
Celestone Soluspan Suspension 2484

Betamethasone Sodium Phosphate (Potential for additive hypokalemic effect with concurrent use). Products include:
Celestone Soluspan Suspension 2484

Betaxolol Hydrochloride (Effects of both drugs inhibited). Products include:
Betoptic Ophthalmic Solution........... 465
Betoptic S Ophthalmic Suspension ... 467
Kerlone Tablets 2588

Bisoprolol Fumarate (Effects of both drugs inhibited). Products include:
Zebeta Tablets 1457
Ziac 1459

Bitolterol Mesylate (Effect not specified; concurrent use should be avoided). Products include:
Tornalate Solution for Inhalation, 0.2% 976
Tornalate Metered Dose Inhaler 978

Carteolol Hydrochloride (Effects of both drugs inhibited). Products include:
Cartrol Tablets 413
Ocupress Ophthalmic Solution, 1% Sterile......................... ⊙ 297

Chlorothiazide (Potential for additive hypokalemic effect with concurrent use). Products include:
Aldoclor Tablets 1638
Diupres Tablets 1691
Diuril Oral 1694

Chlorothiazide Sodium (Potential for additive hypokalemic effect with concurrent use). Products include:
Diuril Sodium Intravenous 1693

Clomipramine Hydrochloride (Action of albuterol on the vascular system may be potentiated). Products include:
Anafranil Capsules 819

Cortisone Acetate (Potential for additive hypokalemic effect with concurrent use). Products include:
Cortone Acetate Sterile Suspension 1663
Cortone Acetate Tablets........ 1664

Desipramine Hydrochloride (Action of albuterol on the vascular system may be potentiated). Products include:
Norpramin Tablets 1273

Dexamethasone (Potential for additive hypokalemic effect with concurrent use). Products include:
AK-Trol Ointment & Suspension .... ⊙ 205
Decadron Elixir 1676
Decadron Tablets 1678
Decaspray Topical Aerosol ... 1689
Maxitrol Ophthalmic Ointment and Suspension .... ⊙ 222
TobraDex Ophthalmic Suspension and Ointment......................... 469

(▣ Described in PDR For Nonprescription Drugs)   (⊙ Described in PDR For Ophthalmology)

Dexamethasone Acetate (Potential for additive hypokalemic effect with concurrent use). Products include:
- Dalalone D.P. Injectable 1009
- Decadron-LA Sterile Suspension 1687

Dexamethasone Sodium Phosphate (Potential for additive hypokalemic effect with concurrent use). Products include:
- Decadron Phosphate Injection 1680
- Decadron Phosphate Sterile Ophthalmic Ointment 1684
- Decadron Phosphate Sterile Ophthalmic Solution 1685
- Decadron Phosphate Topical Cream 1686
- Decadron Phosphate with Xylocaine Injection, Sterile 1683
- Dexacort Phosphate in Respihaler .. 1606
- Dexacort Phosphate in Turbinaire .. 1607
- NeoDecadron Sterile Ophthalmic Ointment 1755
- NeoDecadron Sterile Ophthalmic Solution 1756
- NeoDecadron Topical Cream 1757

Doxepin Hydrochloride (Action of albuterol on the vascular system may be potentiated). Products include:
- Adapin Capsules 1542
- Sinequan 2028
- Zonalon Cream 1042

Esmolol Hydrochloride (Effects of both drugs inhibited). Products include:
- Brevibloc (esmolol HCl) Injection 1860

Furazolidone (Action of albuterol on the vascular system may be potentiated). Products include:
- Furoxone 2221

Hydrochlorothiazide (Potential for additive hypokalemic effect with concurrent use). Products include:
- Aldactazide Tablets 2556
- Aldoril Tablets 1644
- Apresazide Capsules 824
- Capozide Tablets 744
- Dyazide Capsules 2653
- Esidrix Tablets 839
- Esimil Tablets 840
- HydroDIURIL Tablets 1716
- Hydropres Tablets 1718
- Hyzaar Tablets 1720
- Inderide Tablets 2838
- Inderide LA Long Acting Capsules .. 2840
- Lopressor HCT Tablets 850
- Lotensin HCT Tablets 855
- Moduretic Tablets 1748
- Oretic Tablets 450
- Prinzide Tablets 1780
- Ser-Ap-Es Tablets 867
- Timolide Tablets 1791
- Vaseretic Tablets 1810
- Zestoretic Tablets 2968
- Ziac 1459

Hydrocortisone (Potential for additive hypokalemic effect with concurrent use). Products include:
- Anusol-HC Cream 2.5% 1953
- Aquanil HC Lotion 1989
- Maximum Strength Cortaid Spray 800
- CORTENEMA 2713
- Cortisporin Ointment 1074
- Cortisporin Ophthalmic Ointment Sterile 1074
- Cortisporin Ophthalmic Suspension Sterile 1075
- Cortisporin Otic Solution Sterile 1076
- Cortisporin Otic Suspension Sterile 1077
- Cortizone-5 795
- Cortizone-10 795
- Hydrocortone Tablets 1715
- Hytone 922
- Hytone Ointment 2 ½% 923
- Massengill Medicated Soft Cloth Towelettes 2628
- Pediotic Suspension Sterile 1140
- Preparation H Hydrocortisone 1% Cream 843
- ProctoCream-HC 2.5% 2552
- VōSoL HC Otic Solution 2786

Hydrocortisone Acetate (Potential for additive hypokalemic effect with concurrent use). Products include:
- Analpram-HC Rectal Cream 1% and 2.5% 993
- Anusol HC-1 Hydrocortisone Anti-Itch Ointment 810
- Anusol-HC Suppositories 1954
- Caldecort Anti-Itch Hydrocortisone Cream 651
- Coly-Mycin S Otic w/Neomycin & Hydrocortisone 1965
- Cortaid 800
- Cortifoam 2540
- Cortisporin Cream 1073
- Epifoam 2543
- Hydrocortone Acetate Sterile Suspension 1712
- Mantadil Cream 1124
- Nupercainal Hydrocortisone 1% Cream 661
- Pramosone Cream, Lotion & Ointment 995
- ProctoFoam-HC 2552
- Terra-Cortril Ophthalmic Suspension 2033

Hydrocortisone Sodium Phosphate (Potential for additive hypokalemic effect with concurrent use). Products include:
- Hydrocortone Phosphate Injection, Sterile 1713

Hydrocortisone Sodium Succinate (Potential for additive hypokalemic effect with concurrent use).
No products indexed under this heading.

Hydroflumethiazide (Potential for additive hypokalemic effect with concurrent use). Products include:
- Diucardin Tablets 2824

Imipramine Hydrochloride (Action of albuterol on the vascular system may be potentiated). Products include:
- Tofranil Ampuls 873
- Tofranil Tablets 875

Imipramine Pamoate (Action of albuterol on the vascular system may be potentiated). Products include:
- Tofranil-PM Capsules 876

Isocarboxazid (Action of albuterol on the vascular system may be potentiated).
No products indexed under this heading.

Isoetharine (Effect not specified; concurrent use should be avoided). Products include:
- Bronkometer Aerosol 2432
- Bronkosol Solution 2432
- Isoetharine Inhalation Solution, USP, Arm-a-Med 545

Isoproterenol Hydrochloride (Effect not specified; concurrent use should be avoided). Products include:
- Isuprel Hydrochloride Solution 2443
- Isuprel Injection 2441
- Isuprel Mistometer 2442

Labetalol Hydrochloride (Effects of both drugs inhibited). Products include:
- Normodyne Injection 2519
- Normodyne Tablets 2522
- Trandate 1158

Levobunolol Hydrochloride (Effects of both drugs inhibited). Products include:
- Betagan 230

Maprotiline Hydrochloride (Action of albuterol on the vascular system may be potentiated). Products include:
- Ludiomil Tablets 861

Metaproterenol Sulfate (Effect not specified; concurrent use should be avoided). Products include:
- Alupent 672
- Metaproterenol Sulfate Inhalation Solution, USP, Arm-a-Med 547

Methyclothiazide (Potential for additive hypokalemic effect with concurrent use). Products include:
- Enduron Tablets 424

Methylprednisolone Acetate (Potential for additive hypokalemic effect with concurrent use).
No products indexed under this heading.

Methylprednisolone Sodium Succinate (Potential for additive hypokalemic effect with concurrent use).
No products indexed under this heading.

Metipranolol Hydrochloride (Effects of both drugs inhibited). Products include:
- OptiPranolol (Metipranolol 0.3%) Sterile Ophthalmic Solution 256

Metoprolol Succinate (Effects of both drugs inhibited). Products include:
- Toprol-XL Tablets 560

Metoprolol Tartrate (Effects of both drugs inhibited). Products include:
- Lopressor 848
- Lopressor HCT Tablets 850

Nadolol (Effects of both drugs inhibited).
No products indexed under this heading.

Nortriptyline Hydrochloride (Action of albuterol on the vascular system may be potentiated). Products include:
- Pamelor 2409

Penbutolol Sulfate (Effects of both drugs inhibited). Products include:
- Levatol Tablets 2547

Phenelzine Sulfate (Action of albuterol on the vascular system may be potentiated). Products include:
- Nardil 1977

Pindolol (Effects of both drugs inhibited). Products include:
- Visken Tablets 2428

Pirbuterol Acetate (Effect not specified; concurrent use should be avoided). Products include:
- Maxair Autohaler 1550
- Maxair Inhaler 1552

Polythiazide (Potential for additive hypokalemic effect with concurrent use). Products include:
- Minizide Capsules 2016

Prednisolone Acetate (Potential for additive hypokalemic effect with concurrent use). Products include:
- AK-CIDE 203
- AK-CIDE Ointment 203
- Blephamide Liquifilm Sterile Ophthalmic Suspension 472
- Blephamide Ointment 234
- Econopred & Econopred Plus Ophthalmic Suspensions 216
- Poly-Pred Liquifilm 246
- Pred Forte 247
- Pred Mild 250
- Pred-G Liquifilm Sterile Ophthalmic Suspension 248
- Pred-G S.O.P. Sterile Ophthalmic Ointment 249

Prednisolone Sodium Phosphate (Potential for additive hypokalemic effect with concurrent use). Products include:
- AK-PRED 204
- Hydeltrasol Injection, Sterile 1708
- Pediapred Oral Solution 1618

Prednisolone Tebutate (Potential for additive hypokalemic effect with concurrent use). Products include:
- Hydeltra-T.B.A. Sterile Suspension 1710

Prednisone (Potential for additive hypokalemic effect with concurrent use).
No products indexed under this heading.

Propranolol Hydrochloride (Effects of both drugs inhibited). Products include:
- Inderal 2834
- Inderal LA Long Acting Capsules 2836
- Inderide Tablets 2838
- Inderide LA Long Acting Capsules .. 2840

Protriptyline Hydrochloride (Action of albuterol on the vascular system may be potentiated). Products include:
- Vivactil Tablets 1820

Salmeterol Xinafoate (Effect not specified; concurrent use should be avoided). Products include:
- Serevent Inhalation Aerosol 1149

Selegiline Hydrochloride (Action of albuterol on the vascular system may be potentiated). Products include:
- Eldepryl Capsules 2729

Sotalol Hydrochloride (Effects of both drugs inhibited). Products include:
- Betapace Tablets 637

Terbutaline Sulfate (Effect not specified; concurrent use should be avoided). Products include:
- Brethaire Inhaler 830
- Brethine Ampuls 832
- Brethine Tablets 831
- Bricanyl Subcutaneous Injection 1247
- Bricanyl Tablets 1248

Timolol Hemihydrate (Effects of both drugs inhibited). Products include:
- Betimol 0.25%, 0.5% 259

Timolol Maleate (Effects of both drugs inhibited). Products include:
- Blocadren Tablets 1654
- Timolide Tablets 1791
- Timoptic in Ocudose 1796
- Timoptic Sterile Ophthalmic Solution 1794
- Timoptic-XE 1798

Tranylcypromine Sulfate (Action of albuterol on the vascular system may be potentiated). Products include:
- Parnate Tablets 2679

Triamcinolone (Potential for additive hypokalemic effect with concurrent use).
No products indexed under this heading.

Triamcinolone Acetonide (Potential for additive hypokalemic effect with concurrent use). Products include:
- Azmacort Oral Inhaler 2175
- Nasacort AQ Nasal Spray 2191
- Nasacort Nasal Inhaler 2189

Triamcinolone Diacetate (Potential for additive hypokalemic effect with concurrent use).
No products indexed under this heading.

Triamcinolone Hexacetonide (Potential for additive hypokalemic effect with concurrent use).
No products indexed under this heading.

Trimipramine Maleate (Action of albuterol on the vascular system may be potentiated). Products include:
- Surmontil Capsules 2917

PROVENTIL REPETABS TABLETS
(Albuterol Sulfate) 2529
May interact with sympathomimetic bronchodilators, monoamine oxidase inhibitors, tricyclic antidepressants, beta blockers, drugs which lower

---

IMPORTANT NOTE: Always consult each drug listing in the patient's regimen for possible interactions.

Proventil | Interactions Index | 892

serum potassium (selected), and certain other agents. Compounds in these categories include:

Acebutolol Hydrochloride (Effect of both drugs inhibited). Products include:
- Sectral Capsules 2914

Amitriptyline Hydrochloride (Potentiation of albuterol's action on vascular system). Products include:
- Elavil 2945
- Etrafon 2495
- Limbitrol 2333
- Triavil Tablets 1800

Amoxapine (Potentiation of albuterol's action on vascular system). Products include:
- Asendin Tablets 1419

Atenolol (Effect of both drugs inhibited). Products include:
- Tenoretic Tablets 2963
- Tenormin Tablets and I.V. Injection 2965

Bendroflumethiazide (Potential for additive hypokalemic effect with concurrent use).
- No products indexed under this heading.

Betamethasone Acetate (Potential for additive hypokalemic effect with concurrent use). Products include:
- Celestone Soluspan Suspension 2484

Betamethasone Sodium Phosphate (Potential for additive hypokalemic effect with concurrent use). Products include:
- Celestone Soluspan Suspension 2484

Betaxolol Hydrochloride (Effect of both drugs inhibited). Products include:
- Betoptic Ophthalmic Solution.......... 465
- Betoptic S Ophthalmic Suspension 467
- Kerlone Tablets.......... 2588

Bisoprolol Fumarate (Effect of both drugs inhibited). Products include:
- Zebeta Tablets 1457
- Ziac 1459

Bitolterol Mesylate (Deleterious cardiovascular effects). Products include:
- Tornalate Solution for Inhalation, 0.2% 976
- Tornalate Metered Dose Inhaler 978

Carteolol Hydrochloride (Effect of both drugs inhibited). Products include:
- Cartrol Tablets 413
- Ocupress Ophthalmic Solution, 1% Sterile.......... ◉ 297

Chlorothiazide (Potential for additive hypokalemic effect with concurrent use). Products include:
- Aldoclor Tablets 1638
- Diupres Tablets 1691
- Diuril Oral 1694

Chlorothiazide Sodium (Potential for additive hypokalemic effect with concurrent use). Products include:
- Diuril Sodium Intravenous 1693

Clomipramine Hydrochloride (Potentiation of albuterol's action on vascular system). Products include:
- Anafranil Capsules 819

Cortisone Acetate (Potential for additive hypokalemic effect with concurrent use). Products include:
- Cortone Acetate Sterile Suspension 1663
- Cortone Acetate Tablets.......... 1664

Desipramine Hydrochloride (Potentiation of albuterol's action on vascular system). Products include:
- Norpramin Tablets 1273

Dexamethasone (Potential for additive hypokalemic effect with concurrent use). Products include:
- AK-Trol Ointment & Suspension .... ◉ 205
- Decadron Elixir 1676
- Decadron Tablets.......... 1678
- Decaspray Topical Aerosol 1689
- Maxitrol Ophthalmic Ointment and Suspension .... ◉ 222
- TobraDex Ophthalmic Suspension and Ointment.......... 469

Dexamethasone Acetate (Potential for additive hypokalemic effect with concurrent use). Products include:
- Dalalone D.P. Injectable 1009
- Decadron-LA Sterile Suspension.......... 1687

Dexamethasone Sodium Phosphate (Potential for additive hypokalemic effect with concurrent use). Products include:
- Decadron Phosphate Injection 1680
- Decadron Phosphate Sterile Ophthalmic Ointment.......... 1684
- Decadron Phosphate Sterile Ophthalmic Solution 1685
- Decadron Phosphate Topical Cream 1686
- Decadron Phosphate with Xylocaine Injection, Sterile 1683
- Dexacort Phosphate in Respihaler .. 1606
- Dexacort Phosphate in Turbinaire .. 1607
- NeoDecadron Sterile Ophthalmic Ointment 1755
- NeoDecadron Sterile Ophthalmic Solution 1756
- NeoDecadron Topical Cream 1757

Digoxin (Decreased serum digoxin levels (16%-22%); the clinical significance of these findings for patients with COPD who are concurrently taking these drugs on a chronic basis is unclear). Products include:
- Lanoxicaps 1110
- Lanoxin Elixir Pediatric 1113
- Lanoxin Injection 1116
- Lanoxin Injection Pediatric.......... 1119
- Lanoxin Tablets 1121

Doxepin Hydrochloride (Potentiation of albuterol's action on vascular system). Products include:
- Adapin Capsules 1542
- Sinequan 2028
- Zonalon Cream 1042

Ephedrine Hydrochloride (Deleterious cardiovascular effects). Products include:
- Primatene Tablets .... ▣ 844
- Quadrinal Tablets 1398

Ephedrine Sulfate (Deleterious cardiovascular effects). Products include:
- Marax Tablets & DF Syrup.......... 2015

Ephedrine Tannate (Deleterious cardiovascular effects). Products include:
- Rynatuss 2782

Epinephrine (Deleterious cardiovascular effects). Products include:
- EPIFRIN .... ◉ 237
- EpiPen 808
- Marcaine with Epinephrine 2446
- Primatene Mist.......... ▣ 843
- Sensorcaine with Epinephrine Injection.......... 554
- Sus-Phrine Injection 1017
- Xylocaine with Epinephrine Injections.......... 562

Epinephrine Bitartrate (Deleterious cardiovascular effects). Products include:
- Sensorcaine-MPF with Epinephrine Injection.......... 554

Epinephrine Hydrochloride (Deleterious cardiovascular effects). Products include:
- Ana-Kit Anaphylaxis Emergency Treatment Kit 611

Esmolol Hydrochloride (Effect of both drugs inhibited). Products include:
- Brevibloc (esmolol HCl) Injection 1860

Ethylnorepinephrine Hydrochloride (Deleterious cardiovascular effects).
- No products indexed under this heading.

Furazolidone (Potentiation of albuterol's action on vascular system). Products include:
- Furoxone 2221

Hydrochlorothiazide (Potential for additive hypokalemic effect with concurrent use). Products include:
- Aldactazide Tablets 2556
- Aldoril Tablets.......... 1644
- Apresazide Capsules 824
- Capozide Tablets 744
- Dyazide Capsules.......... 2653
- Esidrix Tablets 839
- Esimil Tablets 840
- HydroDIURIL Tablets 1716
- Hydropres Tablets.......... 1718
- Hyzaar Tablets 1720
- Inderide Tablets 2838
- Inderide LA Long Acting Capsules .. 2840
- Lopressor HCT Tablets 850
- Lotensin HCT Tablets 855
- Moduretic Tablets 1748
- Oretic Tablets 450
- Prinzide Tablets 1780
- Ser-Ap-Es Tablets 867
- Timolide Tablets.......... 1791
- Vaseretic Tablets.......... 1810
- Zestoretic Tablets 2968
- Ziac 1459

Hydrocortisone (Potential for additive hypokalemic effect with concurrent use). Products include:
- Anusol-HC Cream 2.5% 1953
- Aquanil HC Lotion 1989
- Maximum Strength Cortaid Spray ▣ 800
- CORTENEMA.......... 2713
- Cortisporin Ointment.......... 1074
- Cortisporin Ophthalmic Ointment Sterile 1074
- Cortisporin Ophthalmic Suspension Sterile 1075
- Cortisporin Otic Solution Sterile 1076
- Cortisporin Otic Suspension Sterile 1077
- Cortizone-5 .... ▣ 795
- Cortizone-10 .... ▣ 795
- Hydrocortone Tablets 1715
- Hytone 922
- Hytone Ointment 2 ½% 923
- Massengill Medicated Soft Cloth Towelettes.......... 2628
- Pediotic Suspension Sterile.......... 1140
- Preparation H Hydrocortisone 1% Cream .... ▣ 843
- ProctoCream-HC 2.5%.......... 2552
- VōSoL HC Otic Solution.......... 2786

Hydrocortisone Acetate (Potential for additive hypokalemic effect with concurrent use). Products include:
- Analpram-HC Rectal Cream 1% and 2.5% 993
- Anusol HC-1 Hydrocortisone Anti-Itch Ointment .... ▣ 810
- Anusol-HC Suppositories 1954
- Caldecort Anti-Itch Hydrocortisone Cream .... ▣ 651
- Coly-Mycin S Otic w/Neomycin & Hydrocortisone.......... 1965
- Cortaid .... ▣ 800
- Cortifoam 2540
- Cortisporin Cream.......... 1073
- Epifoam 2543
- Hydrocortone Acetate Sterile Suspension.......... 1712
- Mantadil Cream 1124
- Nupercainal Hydrocortisone 1% Cream.......... ▣ 661
- Pramosone Cream, Lotion & Ointment 995
- ProctoFoam-HC 2552
- Terra-Cortril Ophthalmic Suspension 2033

Hydrocortisone Sodium Phosphate (Potential for additive hypokalemic effect with concurrent use). Products include:
- Hydrocortone Phosphate Injection, Sterile 1713

Hydrocortisone Sodium Succinate (Potential for additive hypokalemic effect with concurrent use).
- No products indexed under this heading.

Hydroflumethiazide (Potential for additive hypokalemic effect with concurrent use). Products include:
- Diucardin Tablets.......... 2824

Imipramine Hydrochloride (Potentiation of albuterol's action on vascular system). Products include:
- Tofranil Ampuls 873
- Tofranil Tablets 875

Imipramine Pamoate (Potentiation of albuterol's action on vascular system). Products include:
- Tofranil-PM Capsules.......... 876

Isocarboxazid (Potentiation of albuterol's action on vascular system).
- No products indexed under this heading.

Isoetharine (Deleterious cardiovascular effects). Products include:
- Bronkometer Aerosol.......... 2432
- Bronkosol Solution 2432
- Isoetharine Inhalation Solution, USP, Arm-a-Med.......... 545

Isoproterenol Hydrochloride (Deleterious cardiovascular effects). Products include:
- Isuprel Hydrochloride Solution 2443
- Isuprel Injection 2441
- Isuprel Mistometer 2442

Isoproterenol Sulfate (Deleterious cardiovascular effects). Products include:
- Norisodrine with Calcium Iodide Syrup.......... 446

Labetalol Hydrochloride (Effect of both drugs inhibited). Products include:
- Normodyne Injection 2519
- Normodyne Tablets 2522
- Trandate 1158

Levobunolol Hydrochloride (Effect of both drugs inhibited). Products include:
- Betagan .... ◉ 230

Maprotiline Hydrochloride (Potentiation of albuterol's action on vascular system). Products include:
- Ludiomil Tablets.......... 861

Metaproterenol Sulfate (Deleterious cardiovascular effects). Products include:
- Alupent.......... 672
- Metaproterenol Sulfate Inhalation Solution, USP, Arm-a-Med 547

Methyclothiazide (Potential for additive hypokalemic effect with concurrent use). Products include:
- Enduron Tablets.......... 424

Methylprednisolone Acetate (Potential for additive hypokalemic effect with concurrent use).
- No products indexed under this heading.

Methylprednisolone Sodium Succinate (Potential for additive hypokalemic effect with concurrent use).
- No products indexed under this heading.

Metipranolol Hydrochloride (Effect of both drugs inhibited). Products include:
- OptiPranolol (Metipranolol 0.3%) Sterile Ophthalmic Solution.......... ◉ 256

Metoprolol Succinate (Effect of both drugs inhibited). Products include:
- Toprol-XL Tablets 560

Metoprolol Tartrate (Effect of both drugs inhibited). Products include:
- Lopressor 848
- Lopressor HCT Tablets 850

(▣ Described in PDR For Nonprescription Drugs) (◉ Described in PDR For Ophthalmology)

893 **Interactions Index** **Proventil Solution 0.5%**

Nadolol (Effect of both drugs inhibited).
No products indexed under this heading.

Nortriptyline Hydrochloride (Potentiation of albuterol's action on vascular system). Products include:
Pamelor 2409

Penbutolol Sulfate (Effect of both drugs inhibited). Products include:
Levatol Tablets 2547

Phenelzine Sulfate (Potentiation of albuterol's action on vascular system). Products include:
Nardil 1977

Pindolol (Effect of both drugs inhibited). Products include:
Visken Tablets 2428

Pirbuterol Acetate (Deleterious cardiovascular effects). Products include:
Maxair Autohaler 1550
Maxair Inhaler 1552

Polythiazide (Potential for additive hypokalemic effect with concurrent use). Products include:
Minizide Capsules 2016

Prednisolone Acetate (Potential for additive hypokalemic effect with concurrent use). Products include:
AK-CIDE .... ◉ 203
AK-CIDE Ointment .... ◉ 203
Blephamide Liquifilm Sterile Ophthalmic Suspension 472
Blephamide Ointment .... ◉ 234
Econopred & Econopred Plus Ophthalmic Suspensions .... ◉ 216
Poly-Pred Liquifilm .... ◉ 246
Pred Forte .... ◉ 247
Pred Mild .... ◉ 250
Pred-G Liquifilm Sterile Ophthalmic Suspension .... ◉ 248
Pred-G S.O.P. Sterile Ophthalmic Ointment .... ◉ 249

Prednisolone Sodium Phosphate (Potential for additive hypokalemic effect with concurrent use). Products include:
AK-PRED .... ◉ 204
Hydeltrasol Injection, Sterile 1708
Pediapred Oral Solution 1618

Prednisolone Tebutate (Potential for additive hypokalemic effect with concurrent use). Products include:
Hydeltra-T.B.A. Sterile Suspension 1710

Prednisone (Potential for additive hypokalemic effect with concurrent use).
No products indexed under this heading.

Propranolol Hydrochloride (Effect of both drugs inhibited). Products include:
Inderal 2834
Inderal LA Long Acting Capsules 2836
Inderide Tablets 2838
Inderide LA Long Acting Capsules .. 2840

Protriptyline Hydrochloride (Potentiation of albuterol's action on vascular system). Products include:
Vivactil Tablets 1820

Salmeterol Xinafoate (Deleterious cardiovascular effects). Products include:
Serevent Inhalation Aerosol 1149

Selegiline Hydrochloride (Potentiation of albuterol's action on vascular system). Products include:
Eldepryl Capsules 2729

Sotalol Hydrochloride (Effect of both drugs inhibited). Products include:
Betapace Tablets 637

Terbutaline Sulfate (Deleterious cardiovascular effects). Products include:
Brethaire Inhaler 830
Brethine Ampuls 832
Brethine Tablets 831
Bricanyl Subcutaneous Injection 1247
Bricanyl Tablets 1248

Timolol Hemihydrate (Effect of both drugs inhibited). Products include:
Betimol 0.25%, 0.5% .... ◉ 259

Timolol Maleate (Effect of both drugs inhibited). Products include:
Blocadren Tablets 1654
Timolide Tablets 1791
Timoptic in Ocudose 1796
Timoptic Sterile Ophthalmic Solution 1794
Timoptic-XE 1798

Tranylcypromine Sulfate (Potentiation of albuterol's action on vascular system). Products include:
Parnate Tablets 2679

Triamcinolone (Potential for additive hypokalemic effect with concurrent use).
No products indexed under this heading.

Triamcinolone Acetonide (Potential for additive hypokalemic effect with concurrent use). Products include:
Azmacort Oral Inhaler 2175
Nasacort AQ Nasal Spray 2191
Nasacort Nasal Inhaler 2189

Triamcinolone Diacetate (Potential for additive hypokalemic effect with concurrent use).
No products indexed under this heading.

Triamcinolone Hexacetonide (Potential for additive hypokalemic effect with concurrent use).
No products indexed under this heading.

Trimipramine Maleate (Potentiation of albuterol's action on vascular system). Products include:
Surmontil Capsules 2917

PROVENTIL SOLUTION FOR INHALATION 0.5%
(Albuterol Sulfate) 2525
May interact with sympathomimetic aerosol bronchodilators, monoamine oxidase inhibitors, tricyclic antidepressants, beta blockers, and drugs which lower serum potassium (selected). Compounds in these categories include:

Acebutolol Hydrochloride (Effects of both drugs inhibited). Products include:
Sectral Capsules 2914

Albuterol (Effect not specified; concurrent use should be avoided). Products include:
Proventil Inhalation Aerosol 2524
Ventolin Inhalation Aerosol and Refill 1170

Amitriptyline Hydrochloride (Potentiation of albuterol's action on vascular system). Products include:
Elavil 2945
Etrafon 2495
Limbitrol 2333
Triavil Tablets 1800

Amoxapine (Potentiation of albuterol's action on vascular system). Products include:
Asendin Tablets 1419

Atenolol (Effects of both drugs inhibited). Products include:
Tenoretic Tablets 2963
Tenormin Tablets and I.V. Injection 2965

Bendroflumethiazide (Potential for additive hypokalemic effect with concurrent use).
No products indexed under this heading.

Betamethasone Acetate (Potential for additive hypokalemic effect with concurrent use). Products include:
Celestone Soluspan Suspension 2484

Betamethasone Sodium Phosphate (Potential for additive hypokalemic effect with concurrent use). Products include:
Celestone Soluspan Suspension 2484

Betaxolol Hydrochloride (Effects of both drugs inhibited). Products include:
Betoptic Ophthalmic Solution 465
Betoptic S Ophthalmic Suspension 467
Kerlone Tablets 2588

Bisoprolol Fumarate (Effects of both drugs inhibited). Products include:
Zebeta Tablets 1457
Ziac 1459

Bitolterol Mesylate (Effect not specified; concurrent use should be avoided). Products include:
Tornalate Solution for Inhalation, 0.2% 976
Tornalate Metered Dose Inhaler 978

Carteolol Hydrochloride (Effects of both drugs inhibited). Products include:
Cartrol Tablets 413
Ocupress Ophthalmic Solution, 1% Sterile .... ◉ 297

Chlorothiazide (Potential for additive hypokalemic effect with concurrent use). Products include:
Aldoclor Tablets 1638
Diupres Tablets 1691
Diuril Oral 1694

Chlorothiazide Sodium (Potential for additive hypokalemic effect with concurrent use). Products include:
Diuril Sodium Intravenous 1693

Clomipramine Hydrochloride (Potentiation of albuterol's action on vascular system). Products include:
Anafranil Capsules 819

Cortisone Acetate (Potential for additive hypokalemic effect with concurrent use). Products include:
Cortone Acetate Sterile Suspension 1663
Cortone Acetate Tablets 1664

Desipramine Hydrochloride (Potentiation of albuterol's action on vascular system). Products include:
Norpramin Tablets 1273

Dexamethasone (Potential for additive hypokalemic effect with concurrent use). Products include:
AK-Trol Ointment & Suspension .... ◉ 205
Decadron Elixir 1676
Decadron Tablets 1678
Decaspray Topical Aerosol 1689
Maxitrol Ophthalmic Ointment and Suspension .... ◉ 222
TobraDex Ophthalmic Suspension and Ointment 469

Dexamethasone Acetate (Potential for additive hypokalemic effect with concurrent use). Products include:
Dalalone D.P. Injectable 1009
Decadron-LA Sterile Suspension 1687

Dexamethasone Sodium Phosphate (Potential for additive hypokalemic effect with concurrent use). Products include:
Decadron Phosphate Injection 1680
Decadron Phosphate Sterile Ophthalmic Ointment 1684
Decadron Phosphate Sterile Ophthalmic Solution 1685
Decadron Phosphate Topical Cream 1686
Decadron Phosphate with Xylocaine Injection, Sterile 1683
Dexacort Phosphate in Respihaler .. 1606
Dexacort Phosphate in Turbinaire .. 1607
NeoDecadron Sterile Ophthalmic Ointment 1755
NeoDecadron Sterile Ophthalmic Solution 1756
NeoDecadron Topical Cream 1757

Doxepin Hydrochloride (Potentiation of albuterol's action on vascular system). Products include:
Adapin Capsules 1542
Sinequan 2028
Zonalon Cream 1042

Epinephrine (Should not be used concomitantly). Products include:
EPIFRIN .... ◉ 237
EpiPen 808
Marcaine with Epinephrine 2446
Primatene Mist .... ND 843
Sensorcaine with Epinephrine Injection 554
Sus-Phrine Injection 1017
Xylocaine with Epinephrine Injections 562

Epinephrine Hydrochloride (Should not be used concomitantly). Products include:
Ana-Kit Anaphylaxis Emergency Treatment Kit 611

Esmolol Hydrochloride (Effects of both drugs inhibited). Products include:
Brevibloc (esmolol HCl) Injection 1860

Ethylnorepinephrine Hydrochloride (Should not be used concomitantly).
No products indexed under this heading.

Furazolidone (Potentiation of albuterol's action on vascular system). Products include:
Furoxone 2221

Hydrochlorothiazide (Potential for additive hypokalemic effect with concurrent use). Products include:
Aldactazide Tablets 2556
Aldoril Tablets 1644
Apresazide Capsules 824
Capozide Tablets 744
Dyazide Capsules 2653
Esidrix Tablets 839
Esimil Tablets 840
HydroDIURIL Tablets 1716
Hydropres Tablets 1718
Hyzaar Tablets 1720
Inderide Tablets 2838
Inderide LA Long Acting Capsules .. 2840
Lopressor HCT Tablets 850
Lotensin HCT Tablets 855
Moduretic Tablets 1748
Oretic Tablets 450
Prinzide Tablets 1780
Ser-Ap-Es Tablets 867
Timolide Tablets 1791
Vaseretic Tablets 1810
Zestoretic Tablets 2968
Ziac 1459

Hydrocortisone (Potential for additive hypokalemic effect with concurrent use). Products include:
Anusol-HC Cream 2.5% 1953
Aquanil HC Lotion 1989
Maximum Strength Cortaid Spray ND 800
CORTENEMA 2713
Cortisporin Ointment 1074
Cortisporin Ophthalmic Ointment Sterile 1074
Cortisporin Ophthalmic Suspension Sterile 1075
Cortisporin Otic Solution Sterile 1076
Cortisporin Otic Suspension Sterile 1077
Cortizone-5 .... ND 795
Cortizone-10 .... ND 795
Hydrocortone Tablets 1715
Hytone 922
Hytone Ointment 2 ½% 923
Massengill Medicated Soft Cloth Towelettes 2628
Pediotic Suspension Sterile 1140
Preparation H Hydrocortisone 1% Cream .... ND 843
ProctoCream-HC 2.5% 2552
VōSoL HC Otic Solution 2786

IMPORTANT NOTE: Always consult each drug listing in the patient's regimen for possible interactions.

Proventil Solution 0.5%   **Interactions Index**

Hydrocortisone Acetate (Potential for additive hypokalemic effect with concurrent use). Products include:
- Analpram-HC Rectal Cream 1% and 2.5% ... 993
- Anusol HC-1 Hydrocortisone Anti-Itch Ointment ... 810
- Anusol-HC Suppositories ... 1954
- Caldecort Anti-Itch Hydrocortisone Cream ... 651
- Coly-Mycin S Otic w/Neomycin & Hydrocortisone ... 1965
- Cortaid ... 800
- Cortifoam ... 2540
- Cortisporin Cream ... 1073
- Epifoam ... 2543
- Hydrocortone Acetate Sterile Suspension ... 1712
- Mantadil Cream ... 1124
- Nupercainal Hydrocortisone 1% Cream ... 661
- Pramosone Cream, Lotion & Ointment ... 995
- ProctoFoam-HC ... 2552
- Terra-Cortril Ophthalmic Suspension ... 2033

Hydrocortisone Sodium Phosphate (Potential for additive hypokalemic effect with concurrent use). Products include:
- Hydrocortone Phosphate Injection, Sterile ... 1713

Hydrocortisone Sodium Succinate (Potential for additive hypokalemic effect with concurrent use).
- No products indexed under this heading.

Hydroflumethiazide (Potential for additive hypokalemic effect with concurrent use). Products include:
- Diucardin Tablets ... 2824

Imipramine Hydrochloride (Potentiation of albuterol's action on vascular system). Products include:
- Tofranil Ampuls ... 873
- Tofranil Tablets ... 875

Imipramine Pamoate (Potentiation of albuterol's action on vascular system). Products include:
- Tofranil-PM Capsules ... 876

Isocarboxazid (Potentiation of albuterol's action on vascular system).
- No products indexed under this heading.

Isoetharine (Effect not specified; concurrent use should be avoided). Products include:
- Bronkometer Aerosol ... 2432
- Bronkosol Solution ... 2432
- Isoetharine Inhalation Solution, USP, Arm-a-Med ... 545

Isoproterenol Hydrochloride (Effect not specified; concurrent use should be avoided). Products include:
- Isuprel Hydrochloride Solution ... 2443
- Isuprel Injection ... 2441
- Isuprel Mistometer ... 2442

Labetalol Hydrochloride (Effects of both drugs inhibited). Products include:
- Normodyne Injection ... 2519
- Normodyne Tablets ... 2522
- Trandate ... 1158

Levobunolol Hydrochloride (Effects of both drugs inhibited). Products include:
- Betagan ... 230

Maprotiline Hydrochloride (Potentiation of albuterol's action on vascular system). Products include:
- Ludiomil Tablets ... 861

Metaproterenol Sulfate (Effect not specified; concurrent use should be avoided). Products include:
- Alupent ... 672
- Metaproterenol Sulfate Inhalation Solution, USP, Arm-a-Med ... 547

Methyclothiazide (Potential for additive hypokalemic effect with concurrent use). Products include:
- Enduron Tablets ... 424

Methylprednisolone Acetate (Potential for additive hypokalemic effect with concurrent use).
- No products indexed under this heading.

Methylprednisolone Sodium Succinate (Potential for additive hypokalemic effect with concurrent use).
- No products indexed under this heading.

Metipranolol Hydrochloride (Effects of both drugs inhibited). Products include:
- OptiPranolol (Metipranolol 0.3%) Sterile Ophthalmic Solution ... 256

Metoprolol Succinate (Effects of both drugs inhibited). Products include:
- Toprol-XL Tablets ... 560

Metoprolol Tartrate (Effects of both drugs inhibited). Products include:
- Lopressor ... 848
- Lopressor HCT Tablets ... 850

Nadolol (Effects of both drugs inhibited).
- No products indexed under this heading.

Nortriptyline Hydrochloride (Potentiation of albuterol's action on vascular system). Products include:
- Pamelor ... 2409

Penbutolol Sulfate (Effects of both drugs inhibited). Products include:
- Levatol Tablets ... 2547

Phenelzine Sulfate (Potentiation of albuterol's action on vascular system). Products include:
- Nardil ... 1977

Pindolol (Effects of both drugs inhibited). Products include:
- Visken Tablets ... 2428

Pirbuterol Acetate (Effect not specified; concurrent use should be avoided). Products include:
- Maxair Autohaler ... 1550
- Maxair Inhaler ... 1552

Polythiazide (Potential for additive hypokalemic effect with concurrent use). Products include:
- Minizide Capsules ... 2016

Prednisolone Acetate (Potential for additive hypokalemic effect with concurrent use). Products include:
- AK-CIDE ... 203
- AK-CIDE Ointment ... 203
- Blephamide Liquifilm Sterile Ophthalmic Suspension ... 472
- Blephamide Ointment ... 234
- Econopred & Econopred Plus Ophthalmic Suspensions ... 216
- Poly-Pred Liquifilm ... 246
- Pred Forte ... 247
- Pred Mild ... 250
- Pred-G Liquifilm Sterile Ophthalmic Suspension ... 248
- Pred-G S.O.P. Sterile Ophthalmic Ointment ... 249

Prednisolone Sodium Phosphate (Potential for additive hypokalemic effect with concurrent use). Products include:
- AK-PRED ... 204
- Hydeltrasol Injection, Sterile ... 1708
- Pediapred Oral Solution ... 1618

Prednisolone Tebutate (Potential for additive hypokalemic effect with concurrent use). Products include:
- Hydeltra-T.B.A. Sterile Suspension ... 1710

Prednisone (Potential for additive hypokalemic effect with concurrent use).
- No products indexed under this heading.

Propranolol Hydrochloride (Effects of both drugs inhibited). Products include:
- Inderal ... 2834
- Inderal LA Long Acting Capsules ... 2836
- Inderide Tablets ... 2838
- Inderide LA Long Acting Capsules ... 2840

Protriptyline Hydrochloride (Potentiation of albuterol's action on vascular system). Products include:
- Vivactil Tablets ... 1820

Salmeterol Xinafoate (Effect not specified; concurrent use should be avoided). Products include:
- Serevent Inhalation Aerosol ... 1149

Selegiline Hydrochloride (Potentiation of albuterol's action on vascular system). Products include:
- Eldepryl Tablets ... 2729

Sotalol Hydrochloride (Effects of both drugs inhibited). Products include:
- Betapace Tablets ... 637

Terbutaline Sulfate (Effect not specified; concurrent use should be avoided). Products include:
- Brethaire Inhaler ... 830
- Brethine Ampuls ... 832
- Brethine Tablets ... 831
- Bricanyl Subcutaneous Injection ... 1247
- Bricanyl Tablets ... 1248

Timolol Hemihydrate (Effects of both drugs inhibited). Products include:
- Betimol 0.25%, 0.5% ... 259

Timolol Maleate (Effects of both drugs inhibited). Products include:
- Blocadren Tablets ... 1654
- Timolide Tablets ... 1791
- Timoptic in Ocudose ... 1796
- Timoptic Sterile Ophthalmic Solution ... 1794
- Timoptic-XE ... 1798

Tranylcypromine Sulfate (Potentiation of albuterol's action on vascular system). Products include:
- Parnate Tablets ... 2679

Triamcinolone (Potential for additive hypokalemic effect with concurrent use).
- No products indexed under this heading.

Triamcinolone Acetonide (Potential for additive hypokalemic effect with concurrent use). Products include:
- Azmacort Oral Inhaler ... 2175
- Nasacort AQ Nasal Spray ... 2191
- Nasacort Nasal Inhaler ... 2189

Triamcinolone Diacetate (Potential for additive hypokalemic effect with concurrent use).
- No products indexed under this heading.

Triamcinolone Hexacetonide (Potential for additive hypokalemic effect with concurrent use).
- No products indexed under this heading.

Trimipramine Maleate (Potentiation of albuterol's action on vascular system). Products include:
- Surmontil Capsules ... 2917

PROVENTIL SYRUP
(Albuterol Sulfate) ... 2528
May interact with monoamine oxidase inhibitors, tricyclic antidepressants, beta blockers, sympathomimetics, drugs which lower serum potassium (selected), and certain other agents. Compounds in these categories include:

Acebutolol Hydrochloride (Effects of both drugs inhibited). Products include:
- Sectral Capsules ... 2914

Albuterol (Concomitant use with other oral sympathomimetic agents is not recommended since such use may lead to deleterious cardiovascular effects). Products include:
- Proventil Inhalation Aerosol ... 2524
- Ventolin Inhalation Aerosol and Refill ... 1170

Amitriptyline Hydrochloride (Potentiation of albuterol's action on vascular system). Products include:
- Elavil ... 2945
- Etrafon ... 2495
- Limbitrol ... 2333
- Triavil Tablets ... 1800

Amoxapine (Potentiation of albuterol's action on vascular system). Products include:
- Asendin Tablets ... 1419

Atenolol (Effects of both drugs inhibited). Products include:
- Tenoretic Tablets ... 2963
- Tenormin Tablets and I.V. Injection ... 2965

Bendroflumethiazide (Potential for additive hypokalemic effect with concurrent use).
- No products indexed under this heading.

Betamethasone Acetate (Potential for additive hypokalemic effect with concurrent use). Products include:
- Celestone Soluspan Suspension ... 2484

Betamethasone Sodium Phosphate (Potential for additive hypokalemic effect with concurrent use). Products include:
- Celestone Soluspan Suspension ... 2484

Betaxolol Hydrochloride (Effects of both drugs inhibited). Products include:
- Betoptic Ophthalmic Solution ... 465
- Betoptic S Ophthalmic Suspension ... 467
- Kerlone Tablets ... 2588

Bisoprolol Fumarate (Effects of both drugs inhibited). Products include:
- Zebeta Tablets ... 1457
- Ziac ... 1459

Carteolol Hydrochloride (Effects of both drugs inhibited). Products include:
- Cartrol Tablets ... 413
- Ocupress Ophthalmic Solution, 1% Sterile ... 297

Chlorothiazide (Potential for additive hypokalemic effect with concurrent use). Products include:
- Aldoclor Tablets ... 1638
- Diupres Tablets ... 1691
- Diuril Oral ... 1694

Chlorothiazide Sodium (Potential for additive hypokalemic effect with concurrent use). Products include:
- Diuril Sodium Intravenous ... 1693

Clomipramine Hydrochloride (Potentiation of albuterol's action on vascular system). Products include:
- Anafranil Capsules ... 819

Cortisone Acetate (Potential for additive hypokalemic effect with concurrent use). Products include:
- Cortone Acetate Sterile Suspension ... 1663
- Cortone Acetate Tablets ... 1664

Desipramine Hydrochloride (Potentiation of albuterol's action on vascular system). Products include:
- Norpramin Tablets ... 1273

(▣ Described in PDR For Nonprescription Drugs)   (◉ Described in PDR For Ophthalmology)

895 Interactions Index Proventil Syrup

Dexamethasone (Potential for additive hypokalemic effect with concurrent use). Products include:
- AK-Trol Ointment & Suspension .... ◉ 205
- Decadron Elixir 1676
- Decadron Tablets 1678
- Decaspray Topical Aerosol 1689
- Maxitrol Ophthalmic Ointment and Suspension .... ◉ 222
- TobraDex Ophthalmic Suspension and Ointment 469

Dexamethasone Acetate (Potential for additive hypokalemic effect with concurrent use). Products include:
- Dalalone D.P. Injectable 1009
- Decadron-LA Sterile Suspension 1687

Dexamethasone Sodium Phosphate (Potential for additive hypokalemic effect with concurrent use). Products include:
- Decadron Phosphate Injection 1680
- Decadron Phosphate Sterile Ophthalmic Ointment 1684
- Decadron Phosphate Sterile Ophthalmic Solution 1685
- Decadron Phosphate Topical Cream 1686
- Decadron Phosphate with Xylocaine Injection, Sterile 1683
- Dexacort Phosphate in Respihaler .. 1606
- Dexacort Phosphate in Turbinaire .. 1607
- NeoDecadron Sterile Ophthalmic Ointment 1755
- NeoDecadron Sterile Ophthalmic Solution 1756
- NeoDecadron Topical Cream 1757

Digoxin (Decreased serum digoxin levels (16%-22%); the clinical significance of these findings for patients with COPD who are concurrently taking these drugs on a chronic basis is unclear). Products include:
- Lanoxicaps 1110
- Lanoxin Elixir Pediatric 1113
- Lanoxin Injection 1116
- Lanoxin Injection Pediatric 1119
- Lanoxin Tablets 1121

Dobutamine Hydrochloride (Concomitant use with other oral sympathomimetic agents is not recommended since such use may lead to deleterious cardiovascular effects). Products include:
- Dobutrex Solution Vials 1480

Dopamine Hydrochloride (Concomitant use with other oral sympathomimetic agents is not recommended since such use may lead to deleterious cardiovascular effects).
- No products indexed under this heading.

Doxepin Hydrochloride (Potentiation of albuterol's action on vascular system). Products include:
- Adapin Capsules 1542
- Sinequan 2028
- Zonalon Cream 1042

Ephedrine Hydrochloride (Concomitant use with other oral sympathomimetic agents is not recommended since such use may lead to deleterious cardiovascular effects). Products include:
- Primatene Tablets .... ▣ 844
- Quadrinal Tablets 1398

Ephedrine Sulfate (Concomitant use with other oral sympathomimetic agents is not recommended since such use may lead to deleterious cardiovascular effects). Products include:
- Marax Tablets & DF Syrup 2015

Ephedrine Tannate (Concomitant use with other oral sympathomimetic agents is not recommended since such use may lead to deleterious cardiovascular effects). Products include:
- Rynatuss 2782

Esmolol Hydrochloride (Effects of both drugs inhibited). Products include:
- Brevibloc (esmolol HCl) Injection 1860

Furazolidone (Potentiation of albuterol's action on vascular system). Products include:
- Furoxone 2221

Hydrochlorothiazide (Potential for additive hypokalemic effect with concurrent use). Products include:
- Aldactazide Tablets 2556
- Aldoril Tablets 1644
- Apresazide Capsules 824
- Capozide Tablets 744
- Dyazide Capsules 2653
- Esidrix Tablets 839
- Esimil Tablets 840
- HydroDIURIL Tablets 1716
- Hydropres Tablets 1718
- Hyzaar Tablets 1720
- Inderide Tablets 2838
- Inderide LA Long Acting Capsules .. 2840
- Lopressor HCT Tablets 850
- Lotensin HCT Tablets 855
- Moduretic Tablets 1748
- Oretic Tablets 450
- Prinzide Tablets 1780
- Ser-Ap-Es Tablets 867
- Timolide Tablets 1791
- Vaseretic Tablets 1810
- Zestoretic Tablets 2968
- Ziac 1459

Hydrocortisone (Potential for additive hypokalemic effect with concurrent use). Products include:
- Anusol-HC Cream 2.5% 1953
- Aquanil HC Lotion 1989
- Maximum Strength Cortaid Spray ▣ 800
- CORTENEMA 2713
- Cortisporin Ointment 1074
- Cortisporin Ophthalmic Ointment Sterile 1074
- Cortisporin Ophthalmic Suspension Sterile 1075
- Cortisporin Otic Solution Sterile 1076
- Cortisporin Otic Suspension Sterile 1077
- Cortizone-5 .... ▣ 795
- Cortizone-10 .... ▣ 795
- Hydrocortone Tablets 1715
- Hytone 922
- Hytone Ointment 2 ½% 923
- Massengill Medicated Soft Cloth Towelettes 2628
- Pediotic Suspension Sterile 1140
- Preparation H Hydrocortisone 1% Cream .... ▣ 843
- ProctoCream-HC 2.5% 2552
- VōSoL HC Otic Solution 2786

Hydrocortisone Acetate (Potential for additive hypokalemic effect with concurrent use). Products include:
- Analpram-HC Rectal Cream 1% and 2.5% 993
- Anusol HC-1 Hydrocortisone Anti-Itch Ointment .... ▣ 810
- Anusol-HC Suppositories 1954
- Caldecort Anti-Itch Hydrocortisone Cream .... ▣ 651
- Coly-Mycin S Otic w/Neomycin & Hydrocortisone 1965
- Cortaid .... ▣ 800
- Cortifoam 2540
- Cortisporin Cream 1073
- Epifoam 2543
- Hydrocortone Acetate Sterile Suspension 1712
- Mantadil Cream 1124
- Nupercainal Hydrocortisone 1% Cream .... ▣ 661
- Pramosone Cream, Lotion & Ointment 995
- ProctoFoam-HC 2552
- Terra-Cortril Ophthalmic Suspension 2033

Hydrocortisone Sodium Phosphate (Potential for additive hypokalemic effect with concurrent use). Products include:
- Hydrocortone Phosphate Injection, Sterile 1713

Hydrocortisone Sodium Succinate (Potential for additive hypokalemic effect with concurrent use).
- No products indexed under this heading.

Hydroflumethiazide (Potential for additive hypokalemic effect with concurrent use). Products include:
- Diucardin Tablets 2824

Imipramine Hydrochloride (Potentiation of albuterol's action on vascular system). Products include:
- Tofranil Ampuls 873
- Tofranil Tablets 875

Imipramine Pamoate (Potentiation of albuterol's action on vascular system). Products include:
- Tofranil-PM Capsules 876

Isocarboxazid (Potentiation of albuterol's action on vascular system).
- No products indexed under this heading.

Isoproterenol Sulfate (Concomitant use with other oral sympathomimetic agents is not recommended since such use may lead to deleterious cardiovascular effects). Products include:
- Norisodrine with Calcium Iodide Syrup 446

Labetalol Hydrochloride (Effects of both drugs inhibited). Products include:
- Normodyne Injection 2519
- Normodyne Tablets 2522
- Trandate 1158

Levobunolol Hydrochloride (Effects of both drugs inhibited). Products include:
- Betagan .... ◉ 230

Maprotiline Hydrochloride (Potentiation of albuterol's action on vascular system). Products include:
- Ludiomil Tablets 861

Metaproterenol Sulfate (Concomitant use with other oral sympathomimetic agents is not recommended since such use may lead to deleterious cardiovascular effects). Products include:
- Alupent 672
- Metaproterenol Sulfate Inhalation Solution, USP, Arm-a-Med 547

Methyclothiazide (Potential for additive hypokalemic effect with concurrent use). Products include:
- Enduron Tablets 424

Methylprednisolone Acetate (Potential for additive hypokalemic effect with concurrent use).
- No products indexed under this heading.

Methylprednisolone Sodium Succinate (Potential for additive hypokalemic effect with concurrent use).
- No products indexed under this heading.

Metipranolol Hydrochloride (Effects of both drugs inhibited). Products include:
- OptiPranolol (Metipranolol 0.3%) Sterile Ophthalmic Solution .... ◉ 256

Metoprolol Succinate (Effects of both drugs inhibited). Products include:
- Toprol-XL Tablets 560

Metoprolol Tartrate (Effects of both drugs inhibited). Products include:
- Lopressor 848
- Lopressor HCT Tablets 850

Nadolol (Effects of both drugs inhibited).
- No products indexed under this heading.

Nortriptyline Hydrochloride (Potentiation of albuterol's action on vascular system). Products include:
- Pamelor 2409

Penbutolol Sulfate (Effects of both drugs inhibited). Products include:
- Levatol Tablets 2547

Phenelzine Sulfate (Potentiation of albuterol's action on vascular system). Products include:
- Nardil 1977

Phenylephrine Bitartrate (Concomitant use with other oral sympathomimetic agents is not recommended since such use may lead to deleterious cardiovascular effects).
- No products indexed under this heading.

Phenylephrine Hydrochloride (Concomitant use with other oral sympathomimetic agents is not recommended since such use may lead to deleterious cardiovascular effects). Products include:
- Atrohist Plus Tablets 1605
- Cerose DM .... ▣ 853
- D.A. II Tablets 972
- D.A. Chewable Tablets 970
- Dura-Vent/DA Tablets 972
- Extendryl 1003
- 4-Way Fast Acting Nasal Spray (regular & mentholated) .... ▣ 644
- Hemorid .... ▣ 797
- Hycomine Compound Tablets 948
- Neo-Synephrine Hydrochloride 1% Carpuject 2455
- Neo-Synephrine Hydrochloride 1% Injection 2455
- Neo-Synephrine Hydrochloride (Ophthalmic) 2456
- Neo-Synephrine .... ▣ 624
- Novahistine Elixir .... ▣ 782
- Phenergan VC 2886
- Phenergan VC with Codeine 2888
- Preparation H .... ▣ 842
- Tympagesic Ear Drops 2476
- Vicks Sinex Nasal Spray and Ultra Fine Mist .... ▣ 738

Phenylephrine Tannate (Concomitant use with other oral sympathomimetic agents is not recommended since such use may lead to deleterious cardiovascular effects). Products include:
- Atrohist Pediatric Suspension 1604
- Atrohist Pediatric Suspension Dye-Free 1604
- Rynatan 2781
- Rynatuss 2782

Phenylpropanolamine Hydrochloride (Concomitant use with other oral sympathomimetic agents is not recommended since such use may lead to deleterious cardiovascular effects). Products include:
- Acutrim .... ▣ 648
- Atrohist Plus Tablets 1605
- BC Cold Powder Multi-Symptom Formula (Cold-Sinus-Allergy) .... ▣ 631
- BC Cold Powder Non-Drowsy Formula (Cold-Sinus) .... ▣ 631
- Cheracol Plus Head Cold/Cough Formula .... ▣ 741
- Comtrex Multi-Symptom Cold Reliever Liqui-Gels .... ▣ 638
- Comtrex Multi-Symptom Non-Drowsy Liqui-gels .... ▣ 640
- Contac Continuous Action Nasal Decongestant/Antihistamine 12 Hour Capsules .... ▣ 773
- Contac Maximum Strength Continuous Action Decongestant/Antihistamine 12 Hour Caplets .. ▣ 772
- Contac Severe Cold and Flu Formula Caplets .... ▣ 773
- Coricidin 'D' Decongestant Tablets .... ▣ 760
- Dexatrim .... ▣ 795
- Dexatrim Plus Vitamins Caplets .... ▣ 796
- Dimetane-DC Cough Syrup 2232
- Dimetapp Allergy Sinus Caplets .... ▣ 838
- Dimetapp Cold & Allergy Chewable Tablets .... ▣ 838

IMPORTANT NOTE: Always consult each drug listing in the patient's regimen for possible interactions.

Proventil Syrup / Interactions Index

Dimetapp Cold & Cough Liqui-Gels	⬛ 839	
Dimetapp DM Elixir	840	
Dimetapp Elixir	840	
Dimetapp Extentabs	841	
Dimetapp Tablets/Liqui-Gels	⬛ 841	
Dura-Vent Tablets	971	
Entex LA Tablets	972	
Exgest LA Tablets	787	
Hycomine	947	
Nolamine Timed-Release Tablets	790	
Ornade Spansule Capsules	2678	
Propagest Tablets	791	
Pyrroxate Caplets	742	
Robitussin-CF	846	
Sinulin Tablets	792	
Tavist-D 12 Hour Relief Tablets	⬛ 750	
Teldrin 12 Hour Antihistamine/Nasal Decongestant Allergy Relief Capsules	786	
Triaminic Expectorant	753	
Triaminic Syrup	755	
Triaminic Triaminicol Cold & Cough	756	
Triaminic DM Syrup	756	
Triaminicin Tablets	756	
Vicks DayQuil Allergy Relief 12-Hour Extended Release Tablets	⬛ 733	
Vicks DayQuil Allergy Relief 4-Hour Tablets	⬛ 733	
Vicks DayQuil SINUS Pressure & CONGESTION Relief	⬛ 734	

Pindolol (Effects of both drugs inhibited). Products include:
- Visken Tablets ... 2428

Polythiazide (Potential for additive hypokalemic effect with concurrent use). Products include:
- Minizide Capsules ... 2016

Prednisolone Acetate (Potential for additive hypokalemic effect with concurrent use). Products include:
- AK-CIDE ... ⓞ 203
- AK-CIDE Ointment ... ⓞ 203
- Blephamide Liquifilm Sterile Ophthalmic Suspension ... 472
- Blephamide Ointment ... ⓞ 234
- Econopred & Econopred Plus Ophthalmic Suspensions ... ⓞ 216
- Poly-Pred Liquifilm ... ⓞ 246
- Pred Forte ... ⓞ 247
- Pred Mild ... ⓞ 250
- Pred-G Liquifilm Sterile Ophthalmic Suspension ... ⓞ 248
- Pred-G S.O.P. Sterile Ophthalmic Ointment ... ⓞ 249

Prednisolone Sodium Phosphate (Potential for additive hypokalemic effect with concurrent use). Products include:
- AK-PRED ... ⓞ 204
- Hydeltrasol Injection, Sterile ... 1708
- Pediapred Oral Solution ... 1618

Prednisolone Tebutate (Potential for additive hypokalemic effect with concurrent use). Products include:
- Hydeltra-T.B.A. Sterile Suspension ... 1710

Prednisone (Potential for additive hypokalemic effect with concurrent use).
No products indexed under this heading.

Propranolol Hydrochloride (Effects of both drugs inhibited). Products include:
- Inderal ... 2834
- Inderal LA Long Acting Capsules ... 2836
- Inderide ... 2838
- Inderide LA Long Acting Capsules ... 2840

Protriptyline Hydrochloride (Potentiation of albuterol's action on vascular system). Products include:
- Vivactil Tablets ... 1820

Pseudoephedrine Hydrochloride (Concomitant use with other oral sympathomimetic agents is not recommended since such use may lead to deleterious cardiovascular effects). Products include:
- Actifed Allergy Daytime/Nighttime Caplets ... ⬛ 808
- Actifed Cold & Allergy Tablets ... ⬛ 807
- Actifed Cold & Sinus Caplets and Tablets ... ⬛ 808
- Actifed Sinus Daytime/Nighttime Tablets and Caplets ... ⬛ 809
- Advil Cold and Sinus Caplets and Tablets ... ⬛ 837
- Alka-Seltzer Plus Liqui-Gels ... ⬛ 612
- Alka-Seltzer Plus Flu & Body Aches Liqui-Gels Non-Drowsy Formula ... ⬛ 613
- Alka-Seltzer Plus Night-Time Cold Medicine Liqui-Gels ... ⬛ 612
- Allerest Maximum Strength ... ⬛ 649
- Allerest No Drowsiness ... ⬛ 649
- Allerest Sinus Pain Formula ... ⬛ 649
- Atrohist Pediatric Capsules ... 1603
- Benadryl Allergy/Cold Tablets ... ⬛ 811
- Benadryl Allergy Decongestant Liquid Medication ... ⬛ 812
- Benadryl Allergy Decongestant Tablets ... ⬛ 812
- Benadryl Allergy Sinus Headache Caplets ... ⬛ 813
- Benylin Multisymptom ... ⬛ 816
- Bromfed Capsules (Extended-Release) ... 1832
- Bromfed Syrup ... 712
- Bromfed Tablets ... 1832
- Bromfed-DM Cough Syrup ... 1832
- Bromfed-PD Capsules (Extended-Release) ... 1832
- Children's TYLENOL Cold Multi-Symptom Chewable Tablets and Liquid ... 1559
- Children's TYLENOL Cold Plus Cough Multi Symptom Chewable Tablets and Liquid ... 1560
- Children's TYLENOL Flu Suspension Liquid ... 1560
- Children's Vicks DayQuil Allergy Relief ... ⬛ 730
- Children's Vicks NyQuil Cold/Cough Relief ... ⬛ 731
- Allergy-Sinus Comtrex Multi-Symptom Allergy-Sinus Formula Tablets and Caplets ... ⬛ 639
- Comtrex Multi-Symptom ... ⬛ 638
- Comtrex Multi-Symptom Non-Drowsy Caplets ... ⬛ 640
- Congess ... 1003
- Contac Day Allergy/Sinus Caplets ... ⬛ 771
- Contac Day & Night ... ⬛ 772
- Contac Night Allergy/Sinus Caplets ... ⬛ 771
- Contac Severe Cold & Flu Non-Drowsy ... ⬛ 774
- Deconsal II Tablets ... 1605
- Dimetane-DX Cough Syrup ... 2233
- Dimetapp Cold & Fever Suspension ... ⬛ 839
- Dimetapp Decongestant Pediatric Drops ... ⬛ 840
- Dorcol Children's Cough Syrup ... ⬛ 748
- Drixoral Cough + Congestion Liquid Caps ... ⬛ 763
- Dura-Tap/PD Capsules ... 970
- Duratuss Tablets ... 2750
- Duratuss HD Elixir ... 2750
- Efidac/24 ... 655
- Entex PSE Tablets ... 973
- Fedahist Gyrocaps ... 2545
- Guaifed ... 1833
- Guaifed Syrup ... 712
- Guaimax-D Tablets ... 809
- Histussin D Liquid ... 670
- Infants' TYLENOL Cold Decongestant & Fever-Reducer Drops ... 1561
- Kronofed-A ... 994
- Novahistine DMX ... ⬛ 782
- Nucofed ... 2225
- PediaCare Cough-Cold Chewable Tablets and Liquid ... 1569
- PediaCare Infants' Decongestant Drops ... 1569
- PediaCare Infants' Drops Decongestant Plus Cough ... 1569
- PediaCare NightRest Cough-Cold Liquid ... 1569
- Pediatric Vicks 44d Cough & Head Congestion Relief ... ⬛ 736
- Pediatric Vicks 44m Cough & Cold Relief ... ⬛ 737
- Robitussin Cold & Cough Liqui-Gels ... ⬛ 844
- Robitussin Cold, Cough & Flu Liqui-Gels ... ⬛ 844
- Robitussin Maximum Strength Cough & Cold ... ⬛ 847
- Robitussin Night-Time Cold Formula ... ⬛ 847
- Robitussin Pediatric Cough & Cold Formula ... ⬛ 848
- Robitussin Pediatric Drops ... ⬛ 849
- Robitussin Severe Congestion Liqui-Gels ... ⬛ 845
- Robitussin-DAC Syrup ... 2249
- Robitussin-PE ... ⬛ 846
- Rondec Oral Drops ... 974
- Rondec Syrup ... 974
- Rondec Tablet ... 974
- Rondec Chewable Tablets ... 974
- Rondec-TR Tablet ... 974
- Ryna ... 804
- Seldane-D Extended-Release Tablets ... 1286
- Semprex-D Capsules ... 1620
- Sinarest ... 663
- Sine-Aid Maximum Strength Sinus Headache Gelcaps, Caplets and Tablets ... 1570
- Sine-Off No Drowsiness Formula Caplets ... 784
- Sine-Off Sinus Medicine ... 784
- Singlet Tablets ... ⬛ 785
- Sinutab Non-Drying Liquid Caps ... ⬛ 823
- Sinutab Sinus Allergy Medication, Maximum Strength Tablets and Caplets ... ⬛ 823
- Sinutab Sinus Medication, Maximum Strength Without Drowsiness Formula, Tablets & Caplets ... ⬛ 824
- Sudafed Children's Cold & Cough Liquid Medication ... ⬛ 825
- Sudafed Children's Nasal Decongestant Liquid Medication ... ⬛ 826
- Sudafed Cold & Allergy Tablets ... ⬛ 826
- Sudafed Cold and Cough Liquid Caps ... ⬛ 826
- Sudafed Nasal Decongestant Tablets, 30 mg ... ⬛ 825
- Sudafed Nasal Decongestant Tablets, 60 mg ... ⬛ 825
- Sudafed Non-Drying Sinus Liquid Caps ... ⬛ 827
- Sudafed Pediatric Nasal Decongestant Liquid Oral Drops ... ⬛ 827
- Sudafed Severe Cold Formula Caplets ... ⬛ 828
- Sudafed Severe Cold Formula Tablets ... ⬛ 828
- Sudafed Sinus Caplets ... ⬛ 829
- Sudafed Sinus Tablets ... ⬛ 829
- Sudafed 12 Hour Caplets ... ⬛ 824
- Syn-Rx Tablets ... 1622
- Syn-Rx DM Tablets ... 1623
- TheraFlu Flu and Cold Medicine ... ⬛ 750
- TheraFlu Maximum Strength Flu and Cold Medicine For Sore Throat ... ⬛ 751
- TheraFlu Flu, Cold and Cough Medicine ... ⬛ 750
- TheraFlu Maximum Strength Nighttime Flu, Cold & Cough Medicine ... ⬛ 751
- TheraFlu Maximum Strength Non-Drowsy Formula Flu, Cold & Cough Medicine ... ⬛ 751
- TheraFlu Maximum Strength, Non-Drowsy Formula Flu, Cold and Cough Caplets ... ⬛ 752
- Theraflu Maximum Strength Sinus Non-Drowsy Formula Caplets ... ⬛ 752
- Triaminic AM Cough and Decongestant Formula ... ⬛ 753
- Triaminic AM Decongestant Formula ... ⬛ 753
- Triaminic Infant Oral Decongestant Drops ... ⬛ 754
- Triaminic Night Time ... ⬛ 754
- Triaminic Sore Throat Formula ... ⬛ 755
- Tussend ... 1830
- Tussend Expectorant ... 1831
- TYLENOL Allergy Sinus, Maximum Strength Caplets and Gelcaps ... 1571
- TYLENOL Allergy Sinus NightTime, Maximum Strength Caplets ... 1571
- TYLENOL Cold Medication, Multi-Symptom Formula Tablets and Caplets ... 1572
- TYLENOL Cold Medication, Multi-Symptom Hot Liquid Packets ... 1572
- TYLENOL Cold Medication, No Drowsiness Formula Caplets and Gelcaps ... 1572
- TYLENOL Cold Severe Congestion Caplets ... 1573
- TYLENOL Cough Medication with Decongestant, Multi Symptom ... 1574
- TYLENOL Flu No Drowsiness Formula, Maximum Strength Gelcaps ... 1575
- TYLENOL Flu NightTime, Maximum Strength Gelcaps ... 1575
- TYLENOL Flu NightTime, Maximum Strength Hot Medication Packets ... 1575
- TYLENOL Sinus, Maximum Strength Geltabs, Gelcaps, Caplets and Tablets ... 1576
- Vicks 44 LiquiCaps Cough, Cold & Flu Relief ... ⬛ 728
- Vicks 44 LiquiCaps Non-Drowsy Cough & Cold Relief ... ⬛ 729
- Vicks 44D Cough & Head Congestion Relief ... ⬛ 728
- Vicks 44M Cough, Cold & Flu Relief ... ⬛ 729
- Vicks DayQuil LiquiCaps/Liquid Multi-Symptom Cold/Flu Relief ... ⬛ 734
- Vicks DayQuil SINUS Pressure & PAIN Relief with IBUPROFEN ... ⬛ 735
- Vicks Nyquil Hot Therapy ... ⬛ 735
- Vicks NyQuil LiquiCaps/Liquid Multi-Symptom Cold/Flu Relief, Original and Cherry Flavors ... ⬛ 736

Pseudoephedrine Sulfate (Concomitant use with other oral sympathomimetic agents is not recommended since such use may lead to deleterious cardiovascular effects). Products include:
- Chlor-Trimeton Allergy Decongestant Tablets ... ⬛ 759
- Claritin-D Tablets ... 2487
- Drixoral Cold and Allergy Sustained-Action Tablets ... ⬛ 763
- Drixoral Cold and Flu Extended-Release Tablets ... ⬛ 764
- Drixoral Non-Drowsy Formula Extended-Release Tablets ... ⬛ 764
- Drixoral Allergy/Sinus Extended Release Tablets ... ⬛ 765
- Trinalin Repetabs Tablets ... 1373

Salmeterol Xinafoate (Concomitant use with other oral sympathomimetic agents is not recommended since such use may lead to deleterious cardiovascular effects). Products include:
- Serevent Inhalation Aerosol ... 1149

Selegiline Hydrochloride (Potentiation of albuterol's action on vascular system). Products include:
- Eldepryl Capsules ... 2729

Sotalol Hydrochloride (Effects of both drugs inhibited). Products include:
- Betapace Tablets ... 637

Terbutaline Sulfate (Concomitant use with other oral sympathomimetic agents is not recommended since such use may lead to deleterious cardiovascular effects). Products include:
- Brethaire Inhaler ... 830
- Brethine Ampuls ... 832
- Brethine Tablets ... 831
- Bricanyl Subcutaneous Injection ... 1247
- Bricanyl Tablets ... 1248

Timolol Hemihydrate (Effects of both drugs inhibited). Products include:
- Betimol 0.25%, 0.5% ... ⓞ 259

Timolol Maleate (Effects of both drugs inhibited). Products include:
- Blocadren Tablets ... 1654
- Timolide Tablets ... 1791
- Timoptic in Ocudose ... 1796
- Timoptic Sterile Ophthalmic Solution ... 1794
- Timoptic-XE ... 1798

Tranylcypromine Sulfate (Potentiation of albuterol's action on vascular system). Products include:
- Parnate Tablets ... 2679

Triamcinolone (Potential for additive hypokalemic effect with concurrent use).
No products indexed under this heading.

Triamcinolone Acetonide (Potential for additive hypokalemic effect with concurrent use). Products include:
- Azmacort Oral Inhaler ... 2175
- Nasacort AQ Nasal Spray ... 2191

(⬛ Described in PDR For Nonprescription Drugs)   (ⓞ Described in PDR For Ophthalmology)

Nasacort Nasal Inhaler 2189

Triamcinolone Diacetate (Potential for additive hypokalemic effect with concurrent use).
No products indexed under this heading.

Triamcinolone Hexacetonide (Potential for additive hypokalemic effect with concurrent use).
No products indexed under this heading.

Trimipramine Maleate (Potentiation of albuterol's action on vascular system). Products include:
Surmontil Capsules 2917

PROVENTIL TABLETS
(Albuterol Sulfate) 2529
See Proventil Repetabs Tablets

PROVERA TABLETS
(Medroxyprogesterone Acetate) 2110
May interact with estrogens and certain other agents. Compounds in these categories include:

Aminoglutethimide (Significantly depresses the bioavailability of Provera). Products include:
Cytadren Tablets 837

Chlorotrianisene (Potential for adverse effects on carbohydrate and lipid metabolism).
No products indexed under this heading.

Dienestrol (Potential for adverse effects on carbohydrate and lipid metabolism). Products include:
Ortho Dienestrol Cream 1922

Diethylstilbestrol (Potential for adverse effects on carbohydrate and lipid metabolism). Products include:
Diethylstilbestrol Tablets 1477

Estradiol (Potential for adverse effects on carbohydrate and lipid metabolism). Products include:
Climara Transdermal System 640
Estrace Cream and Tablets 751
Estraderm Transdermal System 842
Estring Vaginal Ring 2086
Vivelle Transdermal System 880

Estrogens, Conjugated (Potential for adverse effects on carbohydrate and lipid metabolism). Products include:
PMB 200 and PMB 400 2890
Premarin Intravenous 2893
Premarin Tablets 2896
Premarin Vaginal Cream.......... 2898
Premphase 2900
Prempro 2905

Estrogens, Esterified (Potential for adverse effects on carbohydrate and lipid metabolism). Products include:
ESTRATAB Tablets (0.3, 0.625, 1.25, 2.5 mg) 2715
Estratest 2718
Menest Tablets 2671

Estropipate (Potential for adverse effects on carbohydrate and lipid metabolism). Products include:
Ogen Tablets 2103
Ogen Vaginal Cream 2106
Ortho-Est 1925

Ethinyl Estradiol (Potential for adverse effects on carbohydrate and lipid metabolism). Products include:
Brevicon 2563
Demulen 2580
Desogen Tablets 1867
Levlen/Tri-Levlen 646
Lo/Ovral Tablets 2852
Lo/Ovral-28 Tablets 2857
Modicon 1928
Nordette-21 Tablets 2863
Nordette-28 Tablets 2866
Norinyl 2563
Ortho-Cept 1907
Ortho-Cyclen/Ortho-Tri-Cyclen 1914
Ortho-Novum 1928
Ortho-Cyclen/Ortho Tri-Cyclen 1914
Ovcon 765
Ovral Tablets 2877
Ovral-28 Tablets 2878
Levlen/Tri-Levlen 646
Tri-Norinyl 2607
Triphasil-21 Tablets 2919
Triphasil-28 Tablets 2924

Polyestradiol Phosphate (Potential for adverse effects on carbohydrate and lipid metabolism).
No products indexed under this heading.

Quinestrol (Potential for adverse effects on carbohydrate and lipid metabolism).
No products indexed under this heading.

PROZAC PULVULES & LIQUID, ORAL SOLUTION
(Fluoxetine Hydrochloride) 935
May interact with monoamine oxidase inhibitors, insulin, oral hypoglycemic agents, tricyclic antidepressants, lithium preparations, and certain other agents. Compounds in these categories include:

Acarbose (Hyperglycemia has occurred during therapy with fluoxetine and glycemic control may be altered; dosage of hypoglycemic agents may need to be adjusted). Products include:
Precose 604

Amitriptyline Hydrochloride (Inhibition of the activity of isoenzyme p450iid6 making normal metabolizers resemble "poor metabolizers"; therapy with drugs that are predominantly metabolized by the p450iid6 and have relatively narrow therapeutic index should be initiated at low end of the dose range if a patient is receiving Prozac concurrently or has taken it in the previous 5 weeks). Products include:
Elavil 2945
Etrafon 2495
Limbitrol 2333
Triavil Tablets 1800

Amoxapine (Inhibition of the activity of isoenzyme p450iid6 making normal metabolizers resemble "poor metabolizers"; therapy with drugs that are predominantly metabolized by the p450iid6 and have relatively narrow therapeutic index should be initiated at low end of the dose range if a patient is receiving Prozac concurrently or has taken it in the previous 5 weeks). Products include:
Asendin Tablets 1419

Carbamazepine (Inhibition of the activity of isoenzyme p450iid6 making normal metabolizers resemble "poor metabolizers"; therapy with drugs that are predominantly metabolized by the p450iid6 and have relatively narrow therapeutic index should be initiated at low end of the dose range if a patient is receiving Prozac concurrently or has taken it in the previous 5 weeks). Products include:
Atretol Tablets 569
Tegretol/Tegretol-XR 870

Chlorpropamide (Hyperglycemia has occurred during therapy with fluoxetine and glycemic control may be altered; dosage of hypoglycemic agents may need to be adjusted). Products include:
Diabinese Tablets 2002

Clomipramine Hydrochloride (Inhibition of the activity of isoenzyme p450iid6 making normal metabolizers resemble "poor metabolizers"; therapy with drugs that are predominantly metabolized by the p450iid6 and have relatively narrow therapeutic index should be initiated at low end of the dose range if a patient is receiving Prozac concurrently or has taken it in the previous 5 weeks). Products include:
Anafranil Capsules 819

Desipramine Hydrochloride (Co-administration in patients with previously stable plasma levels of desipramine has resulted in 2 to 10-fold elevation in plasma levels when fluoxetine was added; this influence continues for three weeks or longer; desipramine dose may need to be reduced). Products include:
Norpramin Tablets 1273

Diazepam (Co-administration results in prolonged half-life of diazepam). Products include:
Dizac (diazepam injectable emulsion) CIV 1862
Valium Injectable 2336
Valium Tablets 2335

Digitoxin (Fluoxetine is tightly bound to protein, co-administration may cause shift in plasma concentrations resulting in potential adverse effects). Products include:
Crystodigin Tablets 1472

Doxepin Hydrochloride (Inhibition of the activity of isoenzyme p450iid6 making normal metabolizers resemble "poor metabolizers"; therapy with drugs that are predominantly metabolized by the p450iid6 and have relatively narrow therapeutic index should be initiated at low end of the dose range if a patient is receiving Prozac concurrently or has taken it in the previous 5 weeks). Products include:
Adapin Capsules 1542
Sinequan 2028
Zonalon Cream 1042

Flecainide Acetate (Inhibition of the activity of isoenzyme p450iid6 making normal metabolizers resemble "poor metabolizers"; therapy with drugs that are predominantly metabolized by the p450iid6 and have relatively narrow therapeutic index should be initiated at low end of the dose range if a patient is receiving Prozac concurrently or has taken it in the previous 5 weeks). Products include:
Tambocor Tablets 1555

Fosphenytoin Sodium (Patients on stable doses of phenytoin have developed elevated plasma phenytoin concentrations and clinical phenytoin toxicity following initiation of fluoxetine treatment). Products include:
Cerebyx Injection 1956

Furazolidone (Co-administration with MAO inhibitors has resulted in serious, sometimes fatal, reactions including hyperthermia, rigidity, extreme agitation, delirium, coma, and features resembling neuroleptic malignant syndrome; concurrent and/or sequential use is contraindicated). Products include:
Furoxone 2221

Glimepiride (Hyperglycemia has occurred during therapy with fluoxetine and glycemic control may be altered; dosage of hypoglycemic agents may need to be adjusted). Products include:
Amaryl Tablets 1241

Glipizide (Hyperglycemia has occurred during therapy with fluoxetine and glycemic control may be altered; dosage of hypoglycemic agents may need to be adjusted). Products include:
Glucotrol Tablets 2011
Glucotrol XL Extended Release Tablets 2012

Glyburide (Hyperglycemia has occurred during therapy with fluoxetine and glycemic control may be altered; dosage of hypoglycemic agents may need to be adjusted). Products include:
DiaBeta Tablets 1265
Glynase PresTab Tablets 2091
Micronase Tablets 2099

Imipramine Hydrochloride (Co-administration in patients with previously stable plasma levels of imipramine has resulted in 2 to 10-fold elevation in plasma levels when fluoxetine was added; this influence continues for three weeks or longer; imipramine dose may need to be reduced). Products include:
Tofranil Ampuls 873
Tofranil Tablets 875

Imipramine Pamoate (Inhibition of the activity of isoenzyme p450iid6 making normal metabolizers resemble "poor metabolizers"; therapy with drugs that are predominantly metabolized by the p450iid6 and have relatively narrow therapeutic index should be initiated at low end of the dose range if a patient is receiving Prozac concurrently or has taken it in the previous 5 weeks). Products include:
Tofranil-PM Capsules 876

Insulin, Human (Hyperglycemia has occurred during therapy with fluoxetine and glycemic control may be altered; dosage of insulin may need to be adjusted).
No products indexed under this heading.

Insulin, Human Isophane Suspension (Hyperglycemia has occurred during therapy with fluoxetine and glycemic control may be altered; dosage of insulin may need to be adjusted). Products include:
Novolin N Human Insulin 10 ml Vials 1846

Insulin, Human NPH (Hyperglycemia has occurred during therapy with fluoxetine and glycemic control may be altered; dosage of insulin may need to be adjusted). Products include:
Humulin N, 100 Units 1495
Novolin N PenFill 1.5 ml Cartridges Durable Insulin Delivery System 1849
Novolin N Prefilled Syringe Disposable Insulin Delivery System 1850

Insulin, Human Regular (Hyperglycemia has occurred during therapy with fluoxetine and glycemic control may be altered; dosage of insulin may need to be adjusted). Products include:
Humulin R, 100 Units 1497
Novolin R Human Insulin 10 ml Vials 1846
Novolin R PenFill 1.5 ml Cartridges Durable Insulin Delivery System 1849
Novolin R Prefilled Syringe Disposable Insulin Delivery System 1850

IMPORTANT NOTE: Always consult each drug listing in the patient's regimen for possible interactions.

Prozac — Interactions Index

Velosulin BR Human Insulin 10 ml Vials 1847

Insulin, Human, Zinc Suspension (Hyperglycemia has occurred during therapy with fluoxetine and glycemic control may be altered; dosage of insulin may need to be adjusted). Products include:
Humulin L, 100 Units 1494
Humulin U, 100 Units 1498
Novolin L Human Insulin 10 ml Vials 1846

Insulin Lispro, Human (Hyperglycemia has occurred during therapy with fluoxetine and glycemic control may be altered; dosage of insulin may need to be adjusted). Products include:
Humalog Injection 1488

Insulin, NPH (Hyperglycemia has occurred during therapy with fluoxetine and glycemic control may be altered; dosage of insulin may need to be adjusted). Products include:
NPH, 100 Units 1502
Pork NPH, 100 Units 1506
Purified Pork NPH Isophane Insulin 1852

Insulin, Regular (Hyperglycemia has occurred during therapy with fluoxetine and glycemic control may be altered; dosage of insulin may need to be adjusted). Products include:
Regular, 100 Units 1503
Pork Regular, 100 Units 1507
Pork Regular (Concentrated), 500 Units 1508
Purified Pork Regular Insulin 1852

Insulin, Zinc Crystals (Hyperglycemia has occurred during therapy with fluoxetine and glycemic control may be altered; dosage of insulin may need to be adjusted). Products include:
NPH, 100 Units 1502

Insulin, Zinc Suspension (Hyperglycemia has occurred during therapy with fluoxetine and glycemic control may be altered; dosage of insulin may need to be adjusted). Products include:
Iletin I 1501
Lente, 100 Units 1501
Iletin II 1504
Pork Lente, 100 Units 1504
Purified Pork Lente Insulin 1852

Isocarboxazid (Co-administration with MAO inhibitors has resulted in serious, sometimes fatal, reactions including hyperthermia, rigidity, extreme agitation, delirium, coma, and features resembling neuroleptic malignant syndrome; concurrent and/or sequential use is contraindicated).
No products indexed under this heading.

Lithium Carbonate (Co-administration has resulted in reports of both increased and decreased lithium levels; cases of lithium toxicity have been reported). Products include:
Eskalith 2658
Lithium Carbonate Capsules & Tablets 2352
Lithonate/Lithotabs/Lithobid 2721

Lithium Citrate (Co-administration has resulted in reports of both increased and decreased lithium levels; cases of lithium toxicity have been reported).
No products indexed under this heading.

Maprotiline Hydrochloride (Inhibition of the activity of isoenzyme p450iid6 making normal metabolizers resemble "poor metabolizers"; therapy with drugs that are predominantly metabolized by the p450iid6 and have relatively narrow therapeutic index should be initiated at low end of the dose range if a patient is receiving Prozac concurrently or has taken it in the previous 5 weeks). Products include:
Ludiomil Tablets 861

Metformin Hydrochloride (Hyperglycemia has occurred during therapy with fluoxetine and glycemic control may be altered; dosage of hypoglycemic agents may need to be adjusted). Products include:
Glucophage Tablets 754

Mirtazapine (Inhibition of the activity of isoenzyme p450iid6 making normal metabolizers resemble "poor metabolizers"; therapy with drugs that are predominantly metabolized by the p450iid6 and have relatively narrow therapeutic index should be initiated at low end of the dose range if a patient is receiving Prozac concurrently or has taken it in the previous 5 weeks). Products include:
Remeron Tablets 1878

Nortriptyline Hydrochloride (Inhibition of the activity of isoenzyme p450iid6 making normal metabolizers resemble "poor metabolizers"; therapy with drugs that are predominantly metabolized by the p450iid6 and have relatively narrow therapeutic index should be initiated at low end of the dose range if a patient is receiving Prozac concurrently or has taken it in the previous 5 weeks). Products include:
Pamelor 2409

Phenelzine Sulfate (Co-administration with MAO inhibitors has resulted in serious, sometimes fatal, reactions including hyperthermia, rigidity, extreme agitation, delirium, coma, and features resembling neuroleptic malignant syndrome; concurrent and/or sequential use is contraindicated). Products include:
Nardil 1977

Phenytoin (Patients on stable doses of phenytoin have developed elevated plasma phenytoin concentrations and clinical phenytoin toxicity following initiation of fluoxetine treatment). Products include:
Dilantin Infatabs 1967
Dilantin-125 Suspension 1969

Phenytoin Sodium (Patients on stable doses of phenytoin have developed elevated plasma phenytoin concentrations and clinical phenytoin toxicity following initiation of fluoxetine treatment). Products include:
Dilantin Kapseals 1965

Protriptyline Hydrochloride (Inhibition of the activity of isoenzyme p450iid6 making normal metabolizers resemble "poor metabolizers"; therapy with drugs that are predominantly metabolized by the p450iid6 and have relatively narrow therapeutic index should be initiated at low end of the dose range if a patient is receiving Prozac concurrently or has taken it in the previous 5 weeks). Products include:
Vivactil Tablets 1820

Selegiline Hydrochloride (Co-administration with MAO inhibitors has resulted in serious, sometimes fatal, reactions including hyperthermia, rigidity, extreme agitation, delirium, coma, and features resembling neuroleptic malignant syndrome; concurrent and/or sequential use is contraindicated). Products include:
Eldepryl Capsules 2729

Tolazamide (Hyperglycemia has occurred during therapy with fluoxetine and glycemic control may be altered; dosage of hypoglycemic agents may need to be adjusted).
No products indexed under this heading.

Tolbutamide (Hyperglycemia has occurred during therapy with fluoxetine and glycemic control may be altered; dosage of hypoglycemic agents may need to be adjusted).
No products indexed under this heading.

Tranylcypromine Sulfate (Co-administration with MAO inhibitors has resulted in serious, sometimes fatal, reactions including hyperthermia, rigidity, extreme agitation, delirium, coma, and features resembling neuroleptic malignant syndrome; concurrent and/or sequential use is contraindicated). Products include:
Parnate Tablets 2679

Trimipramine Maleate (Inhibition of the activity of isoenzyme p450iid6 making normal metabolizers resemble "poor metabolizers"; therapy with drugs that are predominantly metabolized by the p450iid6 and have relatively narrow therapeutic index should be initiated at low end of the dose range if a patient is receiving Prozac concurrently or has taken it in the previous 5 weeks). Products include:
Surmontil Capsules 2917

L-Tryptophan (Co-administration has resulted in adverse reactions, including agitation, restlessness, and gastrointestinal distress).
No products indexed under this heading.

Vinblastine Sulfate (Inhibition of the activity of isoenzyme p450iid6 making normal metabolizers resemble "poor metabolizers"; therapy with drugs that are predominantly metabolized by the p450iid6 and have relatively narrow therapeutic index should be initiated at low end of the dose range if a patient is receiving Prozac concurrently or has taken it in the previous 5 weeks). Products include:
Velban Vials 1537

Warfarin Sodium (Fluoxetine is tightly bound to protein, co-administration may cause shift in plasma concentrations resulting in potential adverse effects). Products include:
Coumadin 941

Food Interactions
Alcohol (Concurrent use with CNS active agents, such as alcohol, requires caution).
Food, unspecified (May delay absorption of fluoxetine inconsequentially).

PSORCON CREAM 0.05%
(Diflorasone Diacetate) 924
None cited in PDR database.

PSORCON OINTMENT 0.05%
(Diflorasone Diacetate) 923
None cited in PDR database.

PULMOCARE SPECIALIZED NUTRITION FOR PULMONARY PATIENTS
(Nutritional Supplement) 2344
None cited in PDR database.

PULMOZYME INHALATION
(Dornase Alfa) 1054
None cited in PDR database.

PURGE CONCENTRATE
(Castor Oil) 671
None cited in PDR database.

PURIFIED PORK LENTE INSULIN
(Insulin, Zinc Suspension) 1852
None cited in PDR database.

PURINETHOL TABLETS
(Mercaptopurine) 1214
May interact with:

Allopurinol (Concomitant use at the regular dose results in delayed catabolism of mercaptopurine; substantial dosage reductions may be required to avoid the development of life-threatening bone marrow depression). Products include:
Zyloprim Tablets 1194

Doxorubicin Hydrochloride (Potential for increased hepatotoxicity). Products include:
Adriamycin PFS 2056
Adriamycin RDF 2056
Doxil 2613
Doxorubicin Astra 531
Rubex for Injection 721

Hepatotoxic Drugs, unspecified (Hepatotoxicity).

Sulfamethoxazole (Enhanced bone marrow suppression has been noted in some of the patients also receiving trimethoprim-sulfamethoxazole). Products include:
Bactrim DS Tablets 2257
Bactrim I.V. Infusion 2255
Bactrim 2257
Gantanol Tablets 2285
Septra 1146
Septra I.V. Infusion 1142
Septra I.V. Infusion ADD-Vantage Vials 1144
Septra 1146

Thioguanine (Complete cross-resistance). Products include:
Thioguanine Tablets, Tabloid Brand 1225

Trimethoprim (Enhanced bone marrow suppression has been noted in some of the patients also receiving trimethoprim-sulfamethoxazole). Products include:
Bactrim DS Tablets 2257
Bactrim I.V. Infusion 2255
Bactrim 2257
Proloprim Tablets 1141
Septra 1146
Septra I.V. Infusion 1142
Septra I.V. Infusion ADD-Vantage Vials 1144
Septra 1146
Trimpex Tablets 2323

PYRAZINAMIDE TABLETS
(Pyrazinamide) 1442
None cited in PDR database.

PYRIDIUM
(Phenazopyridine Hydrochloride) 1985
None cited in PDR database.

PYRROXATE CAPLETS
(Acetaminophen, Chlorpheniramine Maleate, Phenylpropanolamine Hydrochloride) 742
May interact with monoamine oxidase inhibitors and certain other

agents. Compounds in these categories include:

Furazolidone (Product labeling recommends physician's supervision for concurrent administration of these drugs). Products include:
Furoxone 2221

Isocarboxazid (Product labeling recommends physician's supervision for concurrent administration of these drugs).
No products indexed under this heading.

Phenelzine Sulfate (Product labeling recommends physician's supervision for concurrent administration of these drugs). Products include:
Nardil 1977

Selegiline Hydrochloride (Product labeling recommends physician's supervision for concurrent administration of these drugs). Products include:
Eldepryl Capsules 2729

Tranylcypromine Sulfate (Product labeling recommends physician's supervision for concurrent administration of these drugs). Products include:
Parnate Tablets 2679

Food Interactions

Alcohol (Concurrent use not recommended).

QUADRINAL TABLETS
(Ephedrine Hydrochloride, Phenobarbital, Potassium Iodide, Theophylline Calcium Salicylate) 1398
May interact with central nervous system depressants, general anesthetics, monoamine oxidase inhibitors, sympathomimetics, tricyclic antidepressants, lithium preparations, oral anticoagulants, corticosteroids, cardiac glycosides, erythromycin, and certain other agents. Compounds in these categories include:

Albuterol (Co-administration of ephedrine with sympathomimetic agent results in increased effects of either medication). Products include:
Proventil Inhalation Aerosol 2524
Ventolin Inhalation Aerosol and Refill 1170

Albuterol Sulfate (Co-administration of ephedrine with sympathomimetic agent results in increased effects of either medication). Products include:
Airet Albuterol Sulfate Inhalation Solution 1602
Albuterol Sulfate, USP Solution for Inhalation, Arm-a-Med 522
Proventil Inhalation Solution 0.083% 2527
Proventil Repetabs Tablets 2529
Proventil Solution for Inhalation 0.5% 2525
Proventil Syrup 2528
Proventil Tablets 2529
Ventolin Inhalation Solution............. 1171
Ventolin Nebules Inhalation Solution 1172
Ventolin Rotacaps for Inhalation 1173
Ventolin Syrup 1175
Ventolin Tablets 1176
Volmax Extended-Release Tablets .. 1835

Alfentanil Hydrochloride (Co-administration of phenobarbital with CNS depressant results in increased effects of either medication). Products include:
Alfenta Injection 1334

Alprazolam (Co-administration of phenobarbital with CNS depressant results in increased effects of either medication). Products include:
Xanax Tablets 2115

Amitriptyline Hydrochloride (Co-administration of ephedrine with tricyclic antidepressant (TCA) may antagonize the pressor action of ephedrine; use of phenobarbital and TCA results in decreased effects of TCA). Products include:
Elavil 2945
Etrafon 2495
Limbitrol 2333
Triavil Tablets 1800

Amoxapine (Co-administration of ephedrine with tricyclic antidepressant (TCA) may antagonize the pressor action of ephedrine; use of phenobarbital and TCA results in decreased effects of TCA). Products include:
Asendin Tablets 1419

Aprobarbital (Co-administration of phenobarbital with CNS depressant results in increased effects of either medication).
No products indexed under this heading.

Betamethasone Acetate (Concurrent use of phenobarbital and corticosteroid results in decreased corticosteroid effects). Products include:
Celestone Soluspan Suspension 2484

Betamethasone Sodium Phosphate (Concurrent use of phenobarbital and corticosteroid results in decreased corticosteroid effects). Products include:
Celestone Soluspan Suspension 2484

Buprenorphine (Co-administration of phenobarbital with CNS depressant results in increased effects of either medication). Products include:
Buprenex Injectable 2170

Buspirone Hydrochloride (Co-administration of phenobarbital with CNS depressant results in increased effects of either medication). Products include:
BuSpar Tablets 738

Butabarbital (Co-administration of phenobarbital with CNS depressant results in increased effects of either medication).
No products indexed under this heading.

Butalbital (Co-administration of phenobarbital with CNS depressant results in increased effects of either medication). Products include:
Axocet Capsules................................ 2469
Esgic-plus Capsules 1012
Esgic-plus Tablets 1012
Fioricet Tablets 2386
Fioricet with Codeine Capsules 2387
Fiorinal Capsules 2388
Fiorinal with Codeine Capsules 2390
Fiorinal Tablets 2388
Phrenilin 790
Sedapap Tablets 50 mg/650 mg .. 1826

Chlordiazepoxide (Co-administration of theophylline and chlordiazepoxide results in chlordiazepoxide-induced fatty acid mobilization; concurrent use of phenobarbital with CNS depressant results in increased effects of either medication). Products include:
Limbitrol 2333

Chlordiazepoxide Hydrochloride (Co-administration of theophylline and chlordiazepoxide results in chlordiazepoxide-induced fatty acid mobilization; concurrent use of phenobarbital with CNS depressant results in increased effects of either medication). Products include:
Librax Capsules 2330
Librium Capsules 2331
Librium Injectable 2332

Chlorpromazine (Co-administration of phenobarbital with CNS depressant results in increased effects of either medication). Products include:
Thorazine Suppositories................... 2701

Chlorpromazine Hydrochloride (Co-administration of phenobarbital with CNS depressant results in increased effects of either medication). Products include:
Thorazine 2701

Chlorprothixene (Co-administration of phenobarbital with CNS depressant results in increased effects of either medication).
No products indexed under this heading.

Chlorprothixene Hydrochloride (Co-administration of phenobarbital with CNS depressant results in increased effects of either medication).
No products indexed under this heading.

Chlorprothixene Lactate (Co-administration of phenobarbital with CNS depressant results in increased effects of either medication).
No products indexed under this heading.

Cimetidine (Concurrent use with cimetidine results in increased theophylline blood levels). Products include:
Tagamet HB Tablets......................... 786
Tagamet Tablets 2694

Cimetidine Hydrochloride (Concurrent use with cimetidine results in increased theophylline blood levels). Products include:
Tagamet... 2694

Clindamycin Hydrochloride (Concurrent use of theophylline and clindamycin results in increased theophylline levels).
No products indexed under this heading.

Clindamycin Palmitate Hydrochloride (Concurrent use of theophylline and clindamycin results in increased theophylline levels).
No products indexed under this heading.

Clindamycin Phosphate (Concurrent use of theophylline and clindamycin results in increased theophylline levels). Products include:
Cleocin Phosphate Injection 2068
Cleocin T Topical 2072
Cleocin Vaginal Cream.................... 2070

Clomipramine Hydrochloride (Co-administration of ephedrine with tricyclic antidepressant (TCA) may antagonize the pressor action of ephedrine; use of phenobarbital and TCA results in decreased effects of TCA). Products include:
Anafranil Capsules 819

Clorazepate Dipotassium (Co-administration of phenobarbital with CNS depressant results in increased effects of either medication). Products include:
Tranxene 459

Clozapine (Co-administration of phenobarbital with CNS depressant results in increased effects of either medication). Products include:
Clozaril Tablets 2377

Codeine Phosphate (Co-administration of phenobarbital with CNS depressant results in increased effects of either medication). Products include:
Brontex 2130
Dimetane-DC Cough Syrup 2232
Fioricet with Codeine Capsules 2387
Fiorinal with Codeine Capsules 2390
Nucofed 2225
Phenergan with Codeine.................. 2883
Phenergan VC with Codeine 2888
Robitussin A-C Syrup 2248
Robitussin-DAC Syrup 2249
Ryna 804
Soma Compound w/Codeine Tablets 2784
Tylenol with Codeine 1592

Cortisone Acetate (Concurrent use of phenobarbital and corticosteroid results in decreased corticosteroid effects). Products include:
Cortone Acetate Sterile Suspension 1663
Cortone Acetate Tablets................... 1664

Desflurane (Co-administration of phenobarbital with CNS depressant results in increased effects of either medication). Products include:
Suprane (desflurane, USP) 1865

Desipramine Hydrochloride (Co-administration of ephedrine with tricyclic antidepressant (TCA) may antagonize the pressor action of ephedrine; use of phenobarbital and TCA results in decreased effects of TCA). Products include:
Norpramin Tablets 1273

Deslanoside (Concurrent use of ephedrine and digitalis may cause cardiac arrhythmias; phenobarbital decreases effects of digitalis).
No products indexed under this heading.

Dexamethasone (Concurrent use of phenobarbital and corticosteroid results in decreased corticosteroid effects). Products include:
AK-Trol Ointment & Suspension 205
Decadron Elixir 1676
Decadron Tablets.............................. 1678
Decaspray Topical Aerosol 1689
Maxitrol Ophthalmic Ointment and Suspension 222
TobraDex Ophthalmic Suspension and Ointment............................ 469

Dexamethasone Acetate (Concurrent use of phenobarbital and corticosteroid results in decreased corticosteroid effects). Products include:
Dalalone D.P. Injectable 1009
Decadron-LA Sterile Suspension...... 1687

Dexamethasone Sodium Phosphate (Concurrent use of phenobarbital and corticosteroid results in decreased corticosteroid effects). Products include:
Decadron Phosphate Injection 1680
Decadron Phosphate Sterile Ophthalmic Ointment 1684
Decadron Phosphate Sterile Ophthalmic Solution 1685
Decadron Phosphate Topical Cream... 1686
Decadron Phosphate with Xylocaine Injection, Sterile 1683
Dexacort Phosphate in Respihaler .. 1606
Dexacort Phosphate in Turbinaire .. 1607
NeoDecadron Sterile Ophthalmic Ointment....................................... 1755
NeoDecadron Sterile Ophthalmic Solution 1756
NeoDecadron Topical Cream 1757

IMPORTANT NOTE: Always consult each drug listing in the patient's regimen for possible interactions.

Quadrinal **Interactions Index** **900**

Dezocine (Co-administration of phenobarbital with CNS depressant results in increased effects of either medication). Products include:

Dalgan Injection 529

Diazepam (Co-administration of phenobarbital with CNS depressant results in increased effects of either medication). Products include:

Dizac (diazepam injectable emulsion) CIV 1862
Valium Injectable 2336
Valium Tablets 2335

Dicumarol (Concurrent use of phenobarbital and oral anticoagulant results in decreased anticoagulant effects).

No products indexed under this heading.

Digitoxin (Concurrent use of ephedrine and digitalis may cause cardiac arrhythmias; phenobarbital decreases effects of digitalis). Products include:

Crystodigin Tablets 1472

Digoxin (Concurrent use of ephedrine and digitalis may cause cardiac arrhythmias; phenobarbital decreases effects of digitalis). Products include:

Lanoxicaps 1110
Lanoxin Elixir Pediatric 1113
Lanoxin Injection 1116
Lanoxin Injection Pediatric 1119
Lanoxin Tablets 1121

Dobutamine Hydrochloride (Co-administration of ephedrine with sympathomimetic agent results in increased effects of either medication). Products include:

Dobutrex Solution Vials 1480

Dopamine Hydrochloride (Co-administration of ephedrine with sympathomimetic agent results in increased effects of either medication).

No products indexed under this heading.

Doxepin Hydrochloride (Co-administration of ephedrine with tricyclic antidepressant (TCA) may antagonize the pressor action of ephedrine; use of phenobarbital and TCA results in decreased effects of TCA). Products include:

Adapin Capsules 1542
Sinequan 2028
Zonalon Cream 1042

Doxycycline Calcium (Concurrent use of phenobarbital and doxycycline results in decreased doxycycline effects). Products include:

Vibramycin Calcium Oral Suspension Syrup 2038

Doxycycline Hyclate (Concurrent use of phenobarbital and doxycycline results in decreased doxycycline effects). Products include:

Doryx Capsules 1970
Vibramycin Hyclate Capsules 2038
Vibramycin Hyclate Intravenous 2040
Vibra-Tabs Film Coated Tablets 2038

Doxycycline Monohydrate (Concurrent use of phenobarbital and doxycycline results in decreased doxycycline effects). Products include:

Monodox Capsules 1858
Vibramycin Monohydrate for Oral Suspension 2038

Droperidol (Co-administration of phenobarbital with CNS depressant results in increased effects of either medication). Products include:

Inapsine Injection 462

Enflurane (Co-administration of phenobarbital with general anesthetic results in increased effects of either medication; concurrent use of ephedrine and anesthetics may cause cardiac arrhythmias).

No products indexed under this heading.

Ephedrine Sulfate (Co-administration of ephedrine with sympathomimetic agent results in increased effects of either medication). Products include:

Marax Tablets & DF Syrup 2015

Ephedrine Tannate (Co-administration of ephedrine with sympathomimetic agent results in increased effects of either medication). Products include:

Rynatuss 2782

Epinephrine (Co-administration of ephedrine with sympathomimetic agent results in increased effects of either medication). Products include:

EPIFRIN .... ◉ 237
EpiPen 808
Marcaine with Epinephrine 2446
Primatene Mist .... ▣ 843
Sensorcaine with Epinephrine Injection 554
Sus-Phrine Injection 1017
Xylocaine with Epinephrine Injections 562

Epinephrine Bitartrate (Co-administration of ephedrine with sympathomimetic agent results in increased effects of either medication). Products include:

Sensorcaine-MPF with Epinephrine Injection 554

Epinephrine Hydrochloride (Co-administration of ephedrine with sympathomimetic agent results in increased effects of either medication). Products include:

Ana-Kit Anaphylaxis Emergency Treatment Kit 611

Ergonovine Maleate (Use of ephedrine with ergonovine results in hypertension).

No products indexed under this heading.

Erythromycin (Concurrent use of theophylline and erythromycin results in increased theophylline levels). Products include:

A/T/S 2% Acne Topical Gel 1244
A/T/S 2% Acne Topical Solution 1244
Benzamycin Topical Gel 919
E-Mycin Tablets 1388
Emgel 2% Topical Gel 1081
ERYC 1972
Erycette (erythromycin 2%) Topical Solution 1943
Ery-Tab Tablets 426
Erythromycin Base Filmtab 430
Erythromycin Delayed-Release Capsules, USP 431
Ilotycin Ophthalmic Ointment 928
PCE Dispertab Tablets 453
T-Stat 2.0% Topical Solution and Pads 2797
THERAMYCIN Z 2% Solution 1629

Erythromycin Estolate (Concurrent use of theophylline and erythromycin results in increased theophylline levels). Products include:

Ilosone 927

Erythromycin Ethylsuccinate (Concurrent use of theophylline and erythromycin results in increased theophylline levels). Products include:

E.E.S. 427
EryPed 425
Pediazole Suspension 2340

Erythromycin Gluceptate (Concurrent use of theophylline and erythromycin results in increased theophylline levels). Products include:

Ilotycin Gluceptate, IV, Vials 929

Erythromycin Stearate (Concurrent use of theophylline and erythromycin results in increased theophylline levels). Products include:

Erythrocin Stearate Filmtab 429

Estazolam (Co-administration of phenobarbital with CNS depressant results in increased effects of either medication). Products include:

ProSom Tablets 457

Ethchlorvynol (Co-administration of phenobarbital with CNS depressant results in increased effects of either medication). Products include:

Placidyl Capsules 456

Ethinamate (Co-administration of phenobarbital with CNS depressant results in increased effects of either medication).

No products indexed under this heading.

Fentanyl (Co-administration of phenobarbital with CNS depressant results in increased effects of either medication). Products include:

Duragesic Transdermal System 1336

Fentanyl Citrate (Co-administration of phenobarbital with CNS depressant results in increased effects of either medication). Products include:

Sublimaze Injection 463

Fludrocortisone Acetate (Concurrent use of phenobarbital and corticosteroid results in decreased corticosteroid effects). Products include:

Florinef Acetate Tablets 506

Fluphenazine Decanoate (Co-administration of phenobarbital with CNS depressant results in increased effects of either medication). Products include:

Prolixin Decanoate 510

Fluphenazine Enanthate (Co-administration of phenobarbital with CNS depressant results in increased effects of either medication). Products include:

Prolixin Enanthate 510

Fluphenazine Hydrochloride (Co-administration of phenobarbital with CNS depressant results in increased effects of either medication). Products include:

Prolixin 510

Flurazepam Hydrochloride (Co-administration of phenobarbital with CNS depressant results in increased effects of either medication). Products include:

Dalmane Capsules 2329

Furazolidone (Co-administration of phenobarbital with MAO inhibitor results in increased effects of either medication; potentiation of pressor effect of ephedrine). Products include:

Furoxone 2221

Furosemide (Concurrent use of theophylline and furosemide results in increased diuresis). Products include:

Lasix Injection, Oral Solution and Tablets 1267

Glutethimide (Co-administration of phenobarbital with CNS depressant results in increased effects of either medication).

No products indexed under this heading.

Griseofulvin (Concurrent use of phenobarbital and doxycycline results in decreased griseofulvin effects). Products include:

Fulvicin P/G Tablets 2499
Fulvicin P/G 165 & 330 Tablets 2500
Grifulvin V (griseofulvin tablets) Microsize (griseofulvin oral suspension) Microsize 1944
Gris-PEG Tablets, 125 mg & 250 mg 476

Guanethidine Monosulfate (Co-administration of ephedrine with guanethidine results in decreased hypotensive effect). Products include:

Esimil Tablets 840
Ismelin Tablets 845

Haloperidol (Co-administration of phenobarbital with CNS depressant results in increased effects of either medication). Products include:

Haldol Injection, Tablets and Concentrate 1585

Haloperidol Decanoate (Co-administration of phenobarbital with CNS depressant results in increased effects of either medication). Products include:

Haldol Decanoate 1587

Hexamethonium (Concurrent use of theophylline and hexamethonium results in decreased hexamethonium-induced chronotropic effect).

Hydrocodone Bitartrate (Co-administration of phenobarbital with CNS depressant results in increased effects of either medication). Products include:

Codiclear DH Syrup 808
Duratuss HD Elixir 2750
Histussin D Liquid 670
Hycodan Tablets and Syrup 946
Hycomine Compound Tablets 948
Hycomine 947
Hycotuss Expectorant Syrup 950
Hydrocet Capsules 787
Lorcet 10/650 Tablets 1016
Lortab 2751
Tussend 1830
Tussend Expectorant 1831
Vicodin Tablets 1404
Vicodin ES Tablets 1405
Vicodin HP Tablets 1403
Vicodin Tuss Expectorant 1406
Zydone Capsules 967

Hydrocodone Polistirex (Co-administration of phenobarbital with CNS depressant results in increased effects of either medication). Products include:

Tussionex Pennkinetic Extended-Release Suspension 1624

Hydrocortisone (Concurrent use of phenobarbital and corticosteroid results in decreased corticosteroid effects). Products include:

Anusol-HC Cream 2.5% 1953
Aquanil HC Lotion 1989
Maximum Strength Cortaid Spray .... ▣ 800
CORTENEMA 2713
Cortisporin Ointment 1074
Cortisporin Ophthalmic Ointment Sterile 1074
Cortisporin Ophthalmic Suspension Sterile 1075
Cortisporin Otic Solution Sterile 1076
Cortisporin Otic Suspension Sterile 1077
Cortizone-5 .... ▣ 795
Cortizone-10 .... ▣ 795
Hydrocortone Tablets 1715
Hytone 922
Hytone Ointment 2 ½% 923
Massengill Medicated Soft Cloth Towelettes 2628
Pediotic Suspension Sterile 1140
Preparation H Hydrocortisone 1% Cream .... ▣ 843
ProctoCream-HC 2.5% 2552
VōSoL HC Otic Solution 2786

(▣ Described in PDR For Nonprescription Drugs) (◉ Described in PDR For Ophthalmology)

Hydrocortisone Acetate (Concurrent use of phenobarbital and corticosteroid results in decreased corticosteroid effects). Products include:
- Analpram-HC Rectal Cream 1% and 2.5% 993
- Anusol HC-1 Hydrocortisone Anti-Itch Ointment 810
- Anusol-HC Suppositories 1954
- Caldecort Anti-Itch Hydrocortisone Cream 651
- Coly-Mycin S Otic w/Neomycin & Hydrocortisone 1965
- Cortaid 800
- Cortifoam 2540
- Cortisporin Cream 1073
- Epifoam 2543
- Hydrocortone Acetate Sterile Suspension 1712
- Mantadil Cream 1124
- Nupercainal Hydrocortisone 1% Cream 661
- Pramosone Cream, Lotion & Ointment 995
- ProctoFoam-HC 2552
- Terra-Cortril Ophthalmic Suspension 2033

Hydrocortisone Sodium Phosphate (Concurrent use of phenobarbital and corticosteroid results in decreased corticosteroid effects). Products include:
- Hydrocortone Phosphate Injection, Sterile 1713

Hydrocortisone Sodium Succinate (Concurrent use of phenobarbital and corticosteroid results in decreased corticosteroid effects).
No products indexed under this heading.

Hydroxyzine Hydrochloride (Co-administration of phenobarbital with CNS depressant results in increased effects of either medication). Products include:
- Atarax Tablets & Syrup 1992
- Marax Tablets & DF Syrup 2015
- Vistaril Intramuscular Solution 2042

Imipramine Hydrochloride (Co-administration of ephedrine with tricyclic antidepressant (TCA) may antagonize the pressor action of ephedrine; use of phenobarbital and TCA results in decreased effects of TCA). Products include:
- Tofranil Ampuls 873
- Tofranil Tablets 875

Imipramine Pamoate (Co-administration of ephedrine with tricyclic antidepressant (TCA) may antagonize the pressor action of ephedrine; use of phenobarbital and TCA results in decreased effects of TCA). Products include:
- Tofranil-PM Capsules 876

Isocarboxazid (Co-administration of phenobarbital with MAO inhibitor results in increased effects of either medication; potentiation of pressor effect of ephedrine).
No products indexed under this heading.

Isoflurane (Co-administration of phenobarbital with general anesthetic results in increased effects of either medication; concurrent use of ephedrine and anesthetics may cause cardiac arrhythmias).
No products indexed under this heading.

Isoproterenol Hydrochloride (Co-administration of ephedrine with sympathomimetic agent results in increased effects of either medication). Products include:
- Isuprel Hydrochloride Solution 2443
- Isuprel Injection 2441
- Isuprel Mistometer 2442

Isoproterenol Sulfate (Co-administration of ephedrine with sympathomimetic agent results in increased effects of either medication). Products include:
- Norisodrine with Calcium Iodide Syrup 446

Ketamine Hydrochloride (Co-administration of phenobarbital with general anesthetic results in increased effects of either medication; concurrent use of ephedrine and anesthetics may cause cardiac arrhythmias).
No products indexed under this heading.

Levomethadyl Acetate Hydrochloride (Co-administration of phenobarbital with CNS depressant results in increased effects of either medication). Products include:
- Orlaam Oral Solution 2361

Levorphanol Tartrate (Co-administration of phenobarbital with CNS depressant results in increased effects of either medication). Products include:
- Levo-Dromoran 2297

Lincomycin Hydrochloride Monohydrate (Concurrent use of theophylline and lincomycin results in increased theophylline levels).
No products indexed under this heading.

Lithium Carbonate (Concurrent use of potassium iodide and lithium results in increased hypothyroid and goiterogenic effects; use of lithium carbonate and aminophylline has resulted in increased excretion of lithium carbonate). Products include:
- Eskalith 2658
- Lithium Carbonate Capsules & Tablets 2352
- Lithonate/Lithotabs/Lithobid 2721

Lithium Citrate (Concurrent use of potassium iodide and lithium results in increased hypothyroid and goiterogenic effects).
No products indexed under this heading.

Lorazepam (Co-administration of phenobarbital with CNS depressant results in increased effects of either medication). Products include:
- Ativan Injection 2805
- Ativan Tablets 2807

Loxapine Hydrochloride (Co-administration of phenobarbital with CNS depressant results in increased effects of either medication). Products include:
- Loxitane 1426

Loxapine Succinate (Co-administration of phenobarbital with CNS depressant results in increased effects of either medication). Products include:
- Loxitane Capsules 1426

Maprotiline Hydrochloride (Co-administration of ephedrine with tricyclic antidepressant (TCA) may antagonize the pressor action of ephedrine; use of phenobarbital and TCA results in decreased effects of TCA). Products include:
- Ludiomil Tablets 861

Meperidine Hydrochloride (Co-administration of phenobarbital with CNS depressant results in increased effects of either medication). Products include:
- Demerol 2438
- Mepergan Injection 2859

Mephobarbital (Co-administration of phenobarbital with CNS depressant results in increased effects of either medication). Products include:
- Mebaral Tablets 2452

Meprobamate (Co-administration of phenobarbital with CNS depressant results in increased effects of either medication). Products include:
- Miltown Tablets 2780
- PMB 200 and PMB 400 2890

Mesoridazine Besylate (Co-administration of phenobarbital with CNS depressant results in increased effects of either medication). Products include:
- Serentil 689

Metaproterenol Sulfate (Co-administration of ephedrine with sympathomimetic agent results in increased effects of either medication). Products include:
- Alupent 672
- Metaproterenol Sulfate Inhalation Solution, USP, Arm-a-Med 547

Metaraminol Bitartrate (Co-administration of ephedrine with sympathomimetic agent results in increased effects of either medication). Products include:
- Aramine Injection 1649

Methadone Hydrochloride (Co-administration of phenobarbital with CNS depressant results in increased effects of either medication). Products include:
- Methadone Hydrochloride Oral Concentrate 2356
- Methadone Hydrochloride Oral Solution & Tablets 2357

Methohexital Sodium (Co-administration of phenobarbital with general anesthetic results in increased effects of either medication; concurrent use of ephedrine and anesthetics may cause cardiac arrhythmias).
No products indexed under this heading.

Methotrimeprazine (Co-administration of phenobarbital with CNS depressant results in increased effects of either medication). Products include:
- Levoprome 1321

Methoxamine Hydrochloride (Co-administration of ephedrine with sympathomimetic agent results in increased effects of either medication). Products include:
- Vasoxyl Injection 1169

Methoxyflurane (Co-administration of phenobarbital with general anesthetic results in increased effects of either medication; concurrent use of ephedrine and anesthetics may cause cardiac arrhythmias).
No products indexed under this heading.

Methylergonovine Maleate (Use of ephedrine with methylergonovine results in hypertension). Products include:
- Methergine 2401

Methylprednisolone Acetate (Concurrent use of phenobarbital and corticosteroid results in decreased corticosteroid effects).
No products indexed under this heading.

Methylprednisolone Sodium Succinate (Concurrent use of phenobarbital and corticosteroid results in decreased corticosteroid effects).
No products indexed under this heading.

Midazolam Hydrochloride (Co-administration of phenobarbital with CNS depressant results in increased effects of either medication). Products include:
- Versed Injection 2324

Molindone Hydrochloride (Co-administration of phenobarbital with CNS depressant results in increased effects of either medication). Products include:
- Moban Tablets and Concentrate 1036

Morphine Sulfate (Co-administration of phenobarbital with CNS depressant results in increased effects of either medication). Products include:
- Astramorph/PF Injection, USP (Preservative-Free) 526
- Duramorph Injection 983
- Infumorph 200 and Infumorph 500 Sterile Solutions 985
- Kadian Capsules 2948
- MS Contin Tablets 2149
- MSIR 2152
- Oramorph SR (Morphine Sulfate Sustained Release Tablets) 2359
- RMS Suppositories CII 2766
- Roxanol 2365

Norepinephrine Bitartrate (Co-administration of ephedrine with sympathomimetic agent results in increased effects of either medication). Products include:
- Levophed Bitartrate Injection 2445

Nortriptyline Hydrochloride (Co-administration of ephedrine with tricyclic antidepressant (TCA) may antagonize the pressor action of ephedrine; use of phenobarbital and TCA results in decreased effects of TCA). Products include:
- Pamelor 2409

Opium Alkaloids (Co-administration of phenobarbital with CNS depressant results in increased effects of either medication).
No products indexed under this heading.

Oxazepam (Co-administration of phenobarbital with CNS depressant results in increased effects of either medication). Products include:
- Serax Capsules 2916
- Serax Tablets 2916

Oxycodone Hydrochloride (Co-administration of phenobarbital with CNS depressant results in increased effects of either medication). Products include:
- OxyContin Tablets 2163
- OxyIR Capsules 2167
- Percocet Tablets 955
- Percodan Tablets 955
- Percodan-Demi Tablets 956
- Roxicodone Tablets, Oral Solution & Intensol (Oxycodone) 2366
- Tylox Capsules 1593

Oxytocin (Use of ephedrine with oxytocin results in hypertension). Products include:
- Syntocinon Injection 2425

Pentobarbital Sodium (Co-administration of phenobarbital with CNS depressant results in increased effects of either medication). Products include:
- Nembutal Sodium Capsules 440
- Nembutal Sodium Solution 442
- Nembutal Sodium Suppositories 444

Perphenazine (Co-administration of phenobarbital with CNS depressant results in increased effects of either medication). Products include:
- Etrafon 2495
- Triavil Tablets 1800
- Trilafon 2532

IMPORTANT NOTE: Always consult each drug listing in the patient's regimen for possible interactions.

Quadrinal | Interactions Index | 902

Phenelzine Sulfate (Co-administration of phenobarbital with MAO inhibitor results in increased effects of either medication; potentiation of pressor effect of ephedrine). Products include:

Nardil 1977

Phenylephrine Bitartrate (Co-administration of ephedrine with sympathomimetic agent results in increased effects of either medication).

No products indexed under this heading.

Phenylephrine Hydrochloride (Co-administration of ephedrine with sympathomimetic agent results in increased effects of either medication). Products include:

Atrohist Plus Tablets 1605
Cerose DM .... ▣ 853
D.A. II Tablets 972
D.A. Chewable Tablets 970
Dura-Vent/DA Tablets 972
Extendryl 1003
4-Way Fast Acting Nasal Spray (regular & mentholated) .... ▣ 644
Hemorid .... ▣ 797
Hycomine Compound Tablets 948
Neo-Synephrine Hydrochloride 1% Carpuject 2455
Neo-Synephrine Hydrochloride 1% Injection 2455
Neo-Synephrine Hydrochloride (Ophthalmic) 2456
Neo-Synephrine .... ▣ 624
Novahistine Elixir .... ▣ 782
Phenergan VC 2886
Phenergan VC with Codeine 2888
Preparation H .... ▣ 842
Tympagesic Ear Drops 2476
Vicks Sinex Nasal Spray and Ultra Fine Mist .... ▣ 738

Phenylephrine Tannate (Co-administration of ephedrine with sympathomimetic agent results in increased effects of either medication). Products include:

Atrohist Pediatric Suspension 1604
Atrohist Pediatric Suspension Dye-Free 1604
Rynatan 2781
Rynatuss 2782

Phenylpropanolamine Hydrochloride (Co-administration of ephedrine with sympathomimetic agent results in increased effects of either medication). Products include:

Acutrim .... ▣ 648
Atrohist Plus Tablets 1605
BC Cold Powder Multi-Symptom Formula (Cold-Sinus-Allergy) .... ▣ 631
BC Cold Powder Non-Drowsy Formula (Cold-Sinus) .... ▣ 631
Cheracol Plus Head Cold/Cough Formula .... ▣ 741
Comtrex Multi-Symptom Cold Reliever Liqui-Gels .... ▣ 638
Comtrex Multi-Symptom Non-Drowsy Liqui-gels .... ▣ 640
Contac Continuous Action Nasal Decongestant/Antihistamine 12 Hour Capsules .... ▣ 773
Contac Maximum Strength Continuous Action Decongestant/Antihistamine 12 Hour Caplets .... ▣ 772
Contac Severe Cold and Flu Formula Caplets .... ▣ 773
Coricidin 'D' Decongestant Tablets .... ▣ 760
Dexatrim .... ▣ 795
Dexatrim Plus Vitamins Caplets .... ▣ 796
Dimetane-DC Cough Syrup 2232
Dimetapp Allergy Sinus Caplets .... ▣ 838
Dimetapp Cold & Allergy Chewable Tablets .... ▣ 838
Dimetapp Cold & Cough Liqui-Gels .... ▣ 839
Dimetapp DM Elixir .... ▣ 840
Dimetapp Elixir .... ▣ 840
Dimetapp Extentabs .... ▣ 841
Dimetapp Tablets/Liqui-Gels .... ▣ 841
Dura-Vent Tablets 971
Entex LA Tablets 972
Exgest LA Tablets 787
Hycomine 947
Nolamine Timed-Release Tablets 790
Ornade Spansule Capsules 2678
Propagest Tablets 791
Pyrroxate Caplets .... ▣ 742
Robitussin-CF .... ▣ 846
Sinulin Tablets 792
Tavist-D 12 Hour Relief Tablets .... ▣ 750
Teldrin 12 Hour Antihistamine/Nasal Decongestant Allergy Relief Capsules .... ▣ 786
Triaminic Expectorant .... ▣ 753
Triaminic Syrup .... ▣ 755
Triaminic Triaminicol Cold & Cough .... ▣ 756
Triaminic DM Syrup .... ▣ 756
Triaminicin Tablets .... ▣ 756
Vicks DayQuil Allergy Relief 12-Hour Extended Release Tablets .... ▣ 733
Vicks DayQuil Allergy Relief 4-Hour Tablets .... ▣ 733
Vicks DayQuil SINUS Pressure & CONGESTION Relief .... ▣ 734

Phenytoin (Phenobarbital decreases effects of phenytoin; theophylline decreases phenytoin levels). Products include:

Dilantin Infatabs 1967
Dilantin-125 Suspension 1969

Phenytoin Sodium (Phenobarbital decreases effects of phenytoin; theophylline decreases phenytoin levels). Products include:

Dilantin Kapseals 1965

Pirbuterol Acetate (Co-administration of ephedrine with sympathomimetic agent results in increased effects of either medication). Products include:

Maxair Autohaler 1550
Maxair Inhaler 1552

Prazepam (Co-administration of phenobarbital with CNS depressant results in increased effects of either medication).

No products indexed under this heading.

Prednisolone Acetate (Concurrent use of phenobarbital and corticosteroid results in decreased corticosteroid effects). Products include:

AK-CIDE .... ⊙ 203
AK-CIDE Ointment .... ⊙ 203
Blephamide Liquifilm Sterile Ophthalmic Suspension 472
Blephamide Ointment .... ⊙ 234
Econopred & Econopred Plus Ophthalmic Suspensions .... ⊙ 216
Poly-Pred Liquifilm .... ⊙ 246
Pred Forte .... ⊙ 247
Pred Mild .... ⊙ 250
Pred-G Liquifilm Sterile Ophthalmic Suspension .... ⊙ 248
Pred-G S.O.P. Sterile Ophthalmic Ointment .... ⊙ 249

Prednisolone Sodium Phosphate (Concurrent use of phenobarbital and corticosteroid results in decreased corticosteroid effects). Products include:

AK-PRED .... ⊙ 204
Hydeltrasol Injection, Sterile 1708
Pediapred Oral Solution 1618

Prednisolone Tebutate (Concurrent use of phenobarbital and corticosteroid results in decreased corticosteroid effects). Products include:

Hydeltra-T.B.A. Sterile Suspension 1710

Prednisone (Concurrent use of phenobarbital and corticosteroid results in decreased corticosteroid effects).

No products indexed under this heading.

Prochlorperazine (Co-administration of phenobarbital with CNS depressant results in increased effects of either medication). Products include:

Compazine 2644

Promethazine Hydrochloride (Co-administration of phenobarbital with CNS depressant results in increased effects of either medication). Products include:

Mepergan Injection 2859
Phenergan with Codeine 2883
Phenergan with Dextromethorphan 2885
Phenergan Injection 2880
Phenergan Suppositories 2882
Phenergan Syrup 2881
Phenergan Tablets 2882
Phenergan VC 2886
Phenergan VC with Codeine 2888

Propofol (Co-administration of phenobarbital with general anesthetic results in increased effects of either medication; concurrent use of ephedrine and anesthetics may cause cardiac arrhythmias). Products include:

Diprivan Injectable Emulsion 2939

Propoxyphene Hydrochloride (Co-administration of phenobarbital with CNS depressant results in increased effects of either medication). Products include:

Darvon 1475
Wygesic Tablets 2930

Propoxyphene Napsylate (Co-administration of phenobarbital with CNS depressant results in increased effects of either medication). Products include:

Darvon-N/Darvocet-N 1473

Propranolol Hydrochloride (Concurrent use of propranolol and aminophylline has resulted in antagonism of propranolol effect). Products include:

Inderal 2834
Inderal LA Long Acting Capsules 2836
Inderide Tablets 2838
Inderide LA Long Acting Capsules 2840

Protriptyline Hydrochloride (Co-administration of ephedrine with tricyclic antidepressant (TCA) may antagonize the pressor action of ephedrine; use of phenobarbital and TCA results in decreased effects of TCA). Products include:

Vivactil Tablets 1820

Pseudoephedrine Hydrochloride (Co-administration of ephedrine with sympathomimetic agent results in increased effects of either medication). Products include:

Actifed Allergy Daytime/Nighttime Caplets .... ▣ 808
Actifed Cold & Allergy Tablets .... ▣ 807
Actifed Cold & Sinus Caplets and Tablets .... ▣ 808
Actifed Sinus Daytime/Nighttime Tablets and Caplets .... ▣ 809
Advil Cold and Sinus Caplets and Tablets .... ▣ 837
Alka-Seltzer Plus Liqui-Gels .... ▣ 612
Alka-Seltzer Plus Flu & Body Aches Liqui-Gels Non-Drowsy Formula .... ▣ 613
Alka-Seltzer Plus Night-Time Cold Medicine Liqui-Gels .... ▣ 612
Allerest Maximum Strength .... ▣ 649
Allerest No Drowsiness .... ▣ 649
Allerest Sinus Pain Formula .... ▣ 649
Atrohist Pediatric Capsules 1603
Benadryl Allergy/Cold Tablets .... ▣ 811
Benadryl Allergy Decongestant Liquid Medication .... ▣ 812
Benadryl Allergy Decongestant Tablets .... ▣ 812
Benadryl Allergy Sinus Headache Caplets .... ▣ 813
Benylin Multisymptom .... ▣ 816
Bromfed Capsules (Extended-Release) 1832
Bromfed Syrup .... ▣ 712
Bromfed Tablets 1832
Bromfed-DM Cough Syrup 1832
Bromfed-PD Capsules (Extended-Release) 1832
Children's TYLENOL Cold Multi-Symptom Chewable Tablets and Liquid 1559
Children's TYLENOL Cold Plus Cough Multi Symptom Chewable Tablets and Liquid 1560
Children's TYLENOL Flu Suspension Liquid 1560
Children's Vicks DayQuil Allergy Relief .... ▣ 730
Children's Vicks NyQuil Cold/Cough Relief .... ▣ 731
Allergy-Sinus Comtrex Multi-Symptom Allergy-Sinus Formula Tablets and Caplets .... ▣ 639
Comtrex Multi-Symptom .... ▣ 638
Comtrex Multi-Symptom Non-Drowsy Caplets .... ▣ 640
Congess 1003
Contac Day Allergy/Sinus Caplets ▣ 771
Contac Day & Night .... ▣ 772
Contac Night Allergy/Sinus Caplets .... ▣ 771
Contac Severe Cold & Flu Non-Drowsy .... ▣ 774
Deconsal II Tablets 1605
Dimetane-DX Cough Syrup 2233
Dimetapp Cold & Fever Suspension .... ▣ 839
Dimetapp Decongestant Pediatric Drops .... ▣ 840
Dorcol Children's Cough Syrup .... ▣ 748
Drixoral Cough + Congestion Liquid Caps .... ▣ 763
Dura-Tap/PD Capsules 970
Duratuss Tablets 2750
Duratuss HD Elixir 2750
Efidac/24 .... ▣ 655
Entex PSE Tablets 973
Fedahist Gyrocaps 2545
Guaifed 1833
Guaifed Syrup .... ▣ 712
Guaimax-D Tablets 809
Histussin D Liquid 670
Infants' TYLENOL Cold Decongestant & Fever-Reducer Drops 1561
Kronofed-A 994
Novahistine DMX .... ▣ 782
Nucofed 2225
PediaCare Cough-Cold Chewable Tablets and Liquid 1569
PediaCare Infants' Decongestant Drops 1569
PediaCare Infants' Drops Decongestant Plus Cough 1569
PediaCare NightRest Cough-Cold Liquid 1569
Pediatric Vicks 44d Cough & Head Congestion Relief .... ▣ 736
Pediatric Vicks 44m Cough & Cold Relief .... ▣ 737
Robitussin Cold & Cough Liqui-Gels .... ▣ 844
Robitussin Cold, Cough & Flu Liqui-Gels .... ▣ 844
Robitussin Maximum Strength Cough & Cold .... ▣ 847
Robitussin Night-Time Cold Formula .... ▣ 847
Robitussin Pediatric Cough & Cold Formula .... ▣ 848
Robitussin Pediatric Drops .... ▣ 849
Robitussin Severe Congestion Liqui-Gels .... ▣ 845
Robitussin-DAC Syrup 2249
Robitussin-PE .... ▣ 846
Rondec Oral Drops 974
Rondec Syrup 974
Rondec Tablet 974
Rondec Chewable Tablets 974
Rondec-TR Tablet 974
Ryna .... ▣ 804
Seldane-D Extended-Release Tablets 1286
Semprex-D Capsules 1620
Sinarest .... ▣ 663
Sine-Aid Maximum Strength Sinus Headache Gelcaps, Caplets and Tablets 1570
Sine-Off No Drowsiness Formula Caplets .... ▣ 784
Sine-Off Sinus Medicine .... ▣ 784
Singlet Tablets .... ▣ 785
Sinutab Non-Drying Liquid Caps .... ▣ 823
Sinutab Sinus Allergy Medication, Maximum Strength Tablets and Caplets .... ▣ 823
Sinutab Sinus Medication, Maximum Strength Without Drowsiness Formula, Tablets & Caplets .... ▣ 824
Sudafed Children's Cold & Cough Liquid Medication .... ▣ 825

(▣ Described in PDR For Nonprescription Drugs) (⊙ Described in PDR For Ophthalmology)

Interactions Index

Sudafed Children's Nasal Decongestant Liquid Medication 826
Sudafed Cold & Allergy Tablets...... 826
Sudafed Cold and Cough Liquid Caps 826
Sudafed Nasal Decongestant Tablets, 30 mg 825
Sudafed Nasal Decongestant Tablets, 60 mg 825
Sudafed Non-Drying Sinus Liquid Caps 827
Sudafed Pediatric Nasal Decongestant Liquid Oral Drops 827
Sudafed Severe Cold Formula Caplets 828
Sudafed Severe Cold Formula Tablets 828
Sudafed Sinus Caplets 829
Sudafed Sinus Tablets 829
Sudafed 12 Hour Caplets 824
Syn-Rx Tablets 1622
Syn-Rx DM Tablets 1623
TheraFlu Flu and Cold Medicine 750
TheraFlu Maximum Strength Flu and Cold Medicine For Sore Throat 751
TheraFlu Flu, Cold and Cough Medicine 750
TheraFlu Maximum Strength Nighttime Flu, Cold & Cough Medicine 751
TheraFlu Maximum Strength Non-Drowsy Formula Flu, Cold & Cough Medicine 751
TheraFlu Maximum Strength, Non-Drowsy Formula Flu, Cold and Cough Caplets 752
Theraflu Maximum Strength Sinus Non-Drowsy Formula Caplets ... 752
Triaminic AM Cough and Decongestant Formula 753
Triaminic AM Decongestant Formula 753
Triaminic Infant Oral Decongestant Drops 754
Triaminic Night Time 754
Triaminic Sore Throat Formula 755
Tussend 1830
Tussend Expectorant 1831
TYLENOL Allergy Sinus, Maximum Strength Caplets and Gelcaps 1571
TYLENOL Allergy Sinus NightTime, Maximum Strength Caplets.......... 1571
TYLENOL Cold Medication, Multi-Symptom Formula Tablets and Caplets 1572
TYLENOL Cold Medication, Multi-Symptom Hot Liquid Packets 1572
TYLENOL Cold Medication, No Drowsiness Formula Caplets and Gelcaps 1572
TYLENOL Cold Severe Congestion Caplets 1573
TYLENOL Cough Medication with Decongestant, Multi Symptom..... 1574
TYLENOL Flu No Drowsiness Formula, Maximum Strength Gelcaps 1575
TYLENOL Flu NightTime, Maximum Strength Gelcaps 1575
TYLENOL Flu NightTime, Maximum Strength Hot Medication Packets 1575
TYLENOL Sinus, Maximum Strength Geltabs, Gelcaps, Caplets and Tablets 1576
Vicks 44 LiquiCaps Cough, Cold & Flu Relief 728
Vicks 44 LiquiCaps Non-Drowsy Cough & Cold Relief 729
Vicks 44D Cough & Head Congestion Relief 728
Vicks 44M Cough, Cold & Flu Relief 729
Vicks DayQuil LiquiCaps/Liquid Multi-Symptom Cold/Flu Relief .. 734
Vicks DayQuil SINUS Pressure & PAIN Relief with IBUPROFEN 735
Vicks Nyquil Hot Therapy 735
Vicks NyQuil LiquiCaps/Liquid Multi-Symptom Cold/Flu Relief, Original and Cherry Flavors......... 736

Pseudoephedrine Sulfate (Co-administration of ephedrine with sympathomimetic agent results in increased effects of either medication). Products include:
Chlor-Trimeton Allergy Decongestant Tablets 759
Claritin-D Tablets 2487

Drixoral Cold and Allergy Sustained-Action Tablets 763
Drixoral Cold and Flu Extended-Release Tablets 764
Drixoral Non-Drowsy Formula Extended-Release Tablets 764
Drixoral Allergy/Sinus Extended Release Tablets 765
Trinalin Repetabs Tablets 1373

Quazepam (Co-administration of phenobarbital with CNS depressant results in increased effects of either medication). Products include:
Doral Tablets 2773

Reserpine (Co-administration of theophylline and reserpine results in an increase in reserpine-induced tachycardia; use of ephedrine and reserpine results in decreased pressor effect of ephedrine). Products include:
Diupres Tablets 1691
Hydropres Tablets 1718
Ser-Ap-Es Tablets 867

Risperidone (Co-administration of phenobarbital with CNS depressant results in increased effects of either medication). Products include:
Risperdal Tablets 1348

Salmeterol Xinafoate (Co-administration of ephedrine with sympathomimetic agent results in increased effects of either medication). Products include:
Serevent Inhalation Aerosol............. 1149

Secobarbital Sodium (Co-administration of phenobarbital with CNS depressant results in increased effects of either medication). Products include:
Seconal Sodium Pulvules 1529

Selegiline Hydrochloride (Co-administration of phenobarbital with MAO inhibitor results in increased effects of either medication; potentiation of pressor effect of ephedrine). Products include:
Eldepryl Capsules 2729

Sevoflurane (Co-administration of phenobarbital with general anesthetic results in increased effects of either medication; concurrent use of ephedrine and anesthetics may cause cardiac arrhythmias).
No products indexed under this heading.

Sufentanil Citrate (Co-administration of phenobarbital with CNS depressant results in increased effects of either medication). Products include:
Sufenta Injection 1355

Temazepam (Co-administration of phenobarbital with CNS depressant results in increased effects of either medication). Products include:
Restoril Capsules 2413

Terbutaline Sulfate (Co-administration of ephedrine with sympathomimetic agent results in increased effects of either medication). Products include:
Brethaire Inhaler 830
Brethine Ampuls 832
Brethine Tablets 831
Bricanyl Subcutaneous Injection 1247
Bricanyl Tablets 1248

Thiamylal Sodium (Co-administration of phenobarbital with CNS depressant results in increased effects of either medication).
No products indexed under this heading.

Thioridazine Hydrochloride (Co-administration of phenobarbital with CNS depressant results in increased effects of either medication). Products include:
Mellaril Tablets 2398

Thiothixene (Co-administration of phenobarbital with CNS depressant results in increased effects of either medication). Products include:
Navane Capsules and Concentrate ... 2018
Navane Intramuscular 2019

Tranylcypromine Sulfate (Co-administration of phenobarbital with MAO inhibitor results in increased effects of either medication; potentiation of pressor effect of ephedrine). Products include:
Parnate Tablets 2679

Triamcinolone (Concurrent use of phenobarbital and corticosteroid results in decreased corticosteroid effects).
No products indexed under this heading.

Triamcinolone Acetonide (Concurrent use of phenobarbital and corticosteroid results in decreased corticosteroid effects). Products include:
Azmacort Oral Inhaler 2175
Nasacort AQ Nasal Spray 2191
Nasacort Nasal Inhaler 2189

Triamcinolone Diacetate (Concurrent use of phenobarbital and corticosteroid results in decreased corticosteroid effects).
No products indexed under this heading.

Triamcinolone Hexacetonide (Concurrent use of phenobarbital and corticosteroid results in decreased corticosteroid effects).
No products indexed under this heading.

Triazolam (Co-administration of phenobarbital with CNS depressant results in increased effects of either medication). Products include:
Halcion Tablets 2093

Trifluoperazine Hydrochloride (Co-administration of phenobarbital with CNS depressant results in increased effects of either medication). Products include:
Stelazine 2692

Trimipramine Maleate (Co-administration of ephedrine with tricyclic antidepressant (TCA) may antagonize the pressor action of ephedrine; use of phenobarbital and TCA results in decreased effects of TCA). Products include:
Surmontil Capsules 2917

Troleandomycin (Concurrent use of theophylline and troleandomycin results in increased theophylline levels). Products include:
Tao Capsules 2033

Warfarin Sodium (Concurrent use of phenobarbital and oral anticoagulant results in decreased anticoagulant effects). Products include:
Coumadin 941

Zolpidem Tartrate (Co-administration of phenobarbital with CNS depressant results in increased effects of either medication). Products include:
Ambien Tablets 2559

Food Interactions

Alcohol (Co-administration of phenobarbital with alcohol results in increased effects of either agent).

QUESTRAN LIGHT FOR ORAL SUSPENSION
(Cholestyramine) 774
See Questran Powder for Oral Suspension

QUESTRAN POWDER FOR ORAL SUSPENSION
(Cholestyramine) 774
May interact with cardiac glycosides, tetracyclines, hmg-coa reductase inhibitors, estrogens, progestins, thiazides, and certain other agents. Compounds in these categories include:

Bendroflumethiazide (Cholestyramine may delay or reduce absorption of concomitant oral thiazide diuretics (acidic); it is recommended that patients take these drugs at least one hour before or 4 to 6 hours after cholestyramine administration).
No products indexed under this heading.

Chlorothiazide (Cholestyramine may delay or reduce absorption of concomitant oral thiazide diuretics (acidic); it is recommended that patients take these drugs at least one hour before or 4 to 6 hours after cholestyramine administration). Products include:
Aldoclor Tablets 1638
Diupres Tablets 1691
Diuril Oral 1694

Chlorothiazide Sodium (Cholestyramine may delay or reduce absorption of concomitant oral thiazide diuretics (acidic); it is recommended that patients take these drugs at least one hour before or 4 to 6 hours after cholestyramine administration). Products include:
Diuril Sodium Intravenous 1693

Chlorotrianisene (Cholestyramine may delay or reduce absorption of concomitant oral estrogens; it is recommended that patients take estrogens at least one hour before or 4 to 6 hours after cholestyramine administration).
No products indexed under this heading.

Demeclocycline Hydrochloride (Cholestyramine may delay or reduce absorption of concomitant oral tetracycline; it is recommended that patients take tetracycline at least one hour before or 4 to 6 hours after cholestyramine administration). Products include:
Declomycin Tablets 1421

Deslanoside (Cholestyramine may delay or reduce absorption of concomitant oral digitalis; it is recommended that patients take digitalis at least one hour before or 4 to 6 hours after cholestyramine administration).
No products indexed under this heading.

Desogestrel (Cholestyramine may delay or reduce absorption of concomitant oral progestins; it is recommended that patients take progestin at least one hour before or 4 to 6 hours after cholestyramine administration). Products include:
Desogen Tablets 1867
Ortho-Cept 1907

Dienestrol (Cholestyramine may delay or reduce absorption of concomitant oral estrogens; it is recommended that patients take estrogens at least one hour before or 4 to 6 hours after cholestyramine administration). Products include:
Ortho Dienestrol Cream 1922

IMPORTANT NOTE: Always consult each drug listing in the patient's regimen for possible interactions.

Diethylstilbestrol (Cholestyramine may delay or reduce absorption of concomitant oral estrogens; it is recommended that patients take estrogens at least one hour before or 4 to 6 hours after cholestyramine administration). Products include:
Diethylstilbestrol Tablets 1477

Digitoxin (Cholestyramine may delay or reduce absorption of concomitant oral digitalis; it is recommended that patients take digitalis at least one hour before or 4 to 6 hours after cholestyramine administration). Products include:
Crystodigin Tablets 1472

Digoxin (Cholestyramine may delay or reduce absorption of concomitant oral digitalis; it is recommended that patients take digitalis at least one hour before or 4 to 6 hours after cholestyramine administration). Products include:
Lanoxicaps 1110
Lanoxin Elixir Pediatric 1113
Lanoxin Injection 1116
Lanoxin Injection Pediatric 1119
Lanoxin Tablets 1121

Doxycycline Calcium (Cholestyramine may delay or reduce absorption of concomitant oral tetracycline; it is recommended that patients take tetracycline at least one hour before or 4 to 6 hours after cholestyramine administration). Products include:
Vibramycin Calcium Oral Suspension Syrup 2038

Doxycycline Hyclate (Cholestyramine may delay or reduce absorption of concomitant oral tetracycline; it is recommended that patients take tetracycline at least one hour before or 4 to 6 hours after cholestyramine administration). Products include:
Doryx Capsules 1970
Vibramycin Hyclate Capsules 2038
Vibramycin Hyclate Intravenous 2040
Vibra-Tabs Film Coated Tablets 2038

Doxycycline Monohydrate (Cholestyramine may delay or reduce absorption of concomitant oral tetracycline; it is recommended that patients take tetracycline at least one hour before or 4 to 6 hours after cholestyramine administration). Products include:
Monodox Capsules 1858
Vibramycin Monohydrate for Oral Suspension 2038

Estradiol (Cholestyramine may delay or reduce absorption of concomitant oral estrogens; it is recommended that patients take estrogens at least one hour before or 4 to 6 hours after cholestyramine administration). Products include:
Climara Transdermal System 640
Estrace Cream and Tablets 751
Estraderm Transdermal System 842
Estring Vaginal Ring 2086
Vivelle Transdermal System 880

Estrogens, Conjugated (Cholestyramine may delay or reduce absorption of concomitant oral estrogens; it is recommended that patients take estrogens at least one hour before or 4 to 6 hours after cholestyramine administration). Products include:
PMB 200 and PMB 400 2890
Premarin Intravenous 2893
Premarin Tablets 2896
Premarin Vaginal Cream 2898
Premphase 2900
Prempro 2905

Estrogens, Esterified (Cholestyramine may delay or reduce absorption of concomitant oral estrogens; it is recommended that patients take estrogens at least one hour before or 4 to 6 hours after cholestyramine administration). Products include:
ESTRATAB Tablets (0.3, 0.625, 1.25, 2.5 mg) 2715
Estratest 2718
Menest Tablets 2671

Estropipate (Cholestyramine may delay or reduce absorption of concomitant oral estrogens; it is recommended that patients take estrogens at least one hour before or 4 to 6 hours after cholestyramine administration). Products include:
Ogen Tablets 2103
Ogen Vaginal Cream 2106
Ortho-Est 1925

Ethinyl Estradiol (Cholestyramine may delay or reduce absorption of concomitant oral estrogens; it is recommended that patients take estrogens at least one hour before or 4 to 6 hours after cholestyramine administration). Products include:
Brevicon 2563
Demulen 2580
Desogen Tablets 1867
Levlen/Tri-Levlen 646
Lo/Ovral Tablets 2852
Lo/Ovral-28 Tablets 2857
Modicon 1928
Nordette-21 Tablets 2863
Nordette-28 Tablets 2866
Norinyl 2563
Ortho-Cept 1907
Ortho-Cyclen/Ortho-Tri-Cyclen 1914
Ortho-Novum 1928
Ortho-Cyclen/Ortho Tri-Cyclen 1914
Ovcon 765
Ovral Tablets 2877
Ovral-28 Tablets 2878
Levlen/Tri-Levlen 646
Tri-Norinyl 2607
Triphasil-21 Tablets 2919
Triphasil-28 Tablets 2924

Fluvastatin Sodium (Lipid-lowering effects of cholestyramine are enhanced when combined with HMG-CoA reductase inhibitors; it is recommended that patients take HMG CoA reductase inhibitors at least one hour before or 4 to 6 hours after cholestyramine administration). Products include:
Lescol Capsules 2395

Hydrochlorothiazide (Cholestyramine may delay or reduce absorption of concomitant oral thiazide diuretics (acidic); it is recommended that patients take these drugs at least one hour before or 4 to 6 hours after cholestyramine administration). Products include:
Aldactazide Tablets 2556
Aldoril Tablets 1644
Apresazide Capsules 824
Capozide Tablets 744
Dyazide Capsules 2653
Esidrix Tablets 839
Esimil Tablets 840
HydroDIURIL Tablets 1716
Hydropres Tablets 1718
Hyzaar Tablets 1720
Inderide Tablets 2838
Inderide LA Long Acting Capsules .. 2840
Lopressor HCT Tablets 850
Lotensin HCT Tablets 855
Moduretic Tablets 1748
Oretic Tablets 450
Prinzide Tablets 1780
Ser-Ap-Es Tablets 867
Timolide Tablets 1791
Vaseretic Tablets 1810
Zestoretic Tablets 2968
Ziac 1459

Hydroflumethiazide (Cholestyramine may delay or reduce absorption of concomitant oral thiazide diuretics (acidic); it is recommended that patients take these drugs at least one hour before or 4 to 6 hours after cholestyramine administration). Products include:
Diucardin Tablets 2824

Levothyroxine Sodium (Cholestyramine may delay or reduce absorption of concomitant oral thyroid; it is recommended that patients take thyroid at least one hour before or 4 to 6 hours after cholestyramine administration). Products include:
Eltroxin Tablets 2214
Levothroid Tablets 1015
Levothyroxine Sodium, USP for Injection 546
Levoxyl Tablets 918
Synthroid 1410

Liothyronine Sodium (Cholestyramine may delay or reduce absorption of concomitant oral thyroid; it is recommended that patients take thyroid at least one hour before or 4 to 6 hours after cholestyramine administration). Products include:
Cytomel Tablets 2647
Triostat Injection 2708

Lovastatin (Lipid-lowering effects of cholestyramine are enhanced when combined with HMG-CoA reductase inhibitors; it is recommended that patients take HMG CoA reductase inhibitors at least one hour before or 4 to 6 hours after cholestyramine administration). Products include:
Mevacor Tablets 1742

Medroxyprogesterone Acetate (Cholestyramine may delay or reduce absorption of concomitant oral progestins; it is recommended that patients take progestin at least one hour before or 4 to 6 hours after cholestyramine administration). Products include:
Amen Tablets 785
Cycrin Tablets 991
Depo-Provera Contraceptive Injection 2079
Depo-Provera Sterile Aqueous Suspension 2083
Premphase 2900
Prempro 2905
Provera Tablets 2110

Megestrol Acetate (Cholestyramine may delay or reduce absorption of concomitant oral progestins; it is recommended that patients take progestin at least one hour before or 4 to 6 hours after cholestyramine administration). Products include:
Megace Oral Suspension 708
Megace Tablets 710

Methacycline Hydrochloride (Cholestyramine may delay or reduce absorption of concomitant oral tetracycline; it is recommended that patients take tetracycline at least one hour before or 4 to 6 hours after cholestyramine administration).
No products indexed under this heading.

Methyclothiazide (Cholestyramine may delay or reduce absorption of concomitant oral thiazide diuretics (acidic); it is recommended that patients take these drugs at least one hour before or 4 to 6 hours after cholestyramine administration). Products include:
Enduron Tablets 424

Minocycline Hydrochloride (Cholestyramine may delay or reduce absorption of concomitant oral tetracycline; it is recommended that patients take tetracycline at least one hour before or 4 to 6 hours after cholestyramine administration). Products include:
DYNACIN Capsules 1627
Minocin Intravenous 1428
Minocin Oral Suspension 1431
Minocin Pellet-Filled Capsules 1429

Nicotinic Acid (Lipid-lowering effects of cholestyramine are enhanced when combined with nicotinic acid; it is recommended that patients take nicotinic acid at least one hour before or 4 to 6 hours after cholestyramine administration).
No products indexed under this heading.

Norgestimate (Cholestyramine may delay or reduce absorption of concomitant oral progestins; it is recommended that patients take progestin at least one hour before or 4 to 6 hours after cholestyramine administration). Products include:
Ortho-Cyclen/Ortho-Tri-Cyclen 1914
Ortho-Cyclen/Ortho Tri-Cyclen 1914

Oxytetracycline Hydrochloride (Cholestyramine may delay or reduce absorption of concomitant oral tetracycline; it is recommended that patients take tetracycline at least one hour before or 4 to 6 hours after cholestyramine administration). Products include:
TERAK Ointment .... ⊙ 210
Terra-Cortril Ophthalmic Suspension 2033
Terramycin with Polymyxin B Sulfate Ophthalmic Ointment 2035
Urobiotic-250 Capsules 2038

Penicillin G Potassium (Cholestyramine may delay or reduce absorption of concomitant oral penicillin G; it is recommended that patients take penicillin G at least one hour before or 4 to 6 hours after cholestyramine administration). Products include:
Pfizerpen for Injection 2022

Phenobarbital (Cholestyramine may delay or reduce absorption of concomitant oral phenobarbital; it is recommended that patients take phenobarbital at least one hour before or 4 to 6 hours after cholestyramine administration). Products include:
Arco-Lase Plus Tablets 513
Bellergal-S Tablets 2375
Donnatal 2234
Donnatal Extentabs 2234
Donnatal Tablets 2234
Phenobarbital Elixir and Tablets 1523
Quadrinal Tablets 1398

Phenylbutazone (Cholestyramine may delay or reduce absorption of concomitant oral phenylbutazone; it is recommended that patients take phenylbutazone at least one hour before or 4 to 6 hours after cholestyramine administration).
No products indexed under this heading.

Polyestradiol Phosphate (Cholestyramine may delay or reduce absorption of concomitant oral estrogens; it is recommended that patients take estrogens at least one hour before or 4 to 6 hours after cholestyramine administration).
No products indexed under this heading.

(▣ Described in PDR For Nonprescription Drugs) (⊙ Described in PDR For Ophthalmology)

905 **Interactions Index** **Quibron**

Polythiazide (Cholestyramine may delay or reduce absorption of concomitant oral thiazide diuretics (acidic); it is recommended that patients take these drugs at least one hour before or 4 to 6 hours after cholestyramine administration). Products include:
- Minizide Capsules ... 2016

Potassium Phosphate, Monobasic (Possible interference with the absorption of oral phosphate supplements). Products include:
- K-Phos Neutral Tablets ... 633
- K-Phos Original Formula 'Sodium Free' Tablets ... 633

Pravastatin Sodium (Lipid-lowering effects of cholestyramine are enhanced when combined with HMG-CoA reductase inhibitors; it is recommended that patients take HMG CoA reductase inhibitors at least one hour before or 4 to 6 hours after cholestyramine administration). Products include:
- Pravachol Tablets ... 770

Propranolol Hydrochloride (Cholestyramine may delay or reduce absorption of concomitant oral propranolol (basic); it is recommended that patients take propranolol at least one hour before or 4 to 6 hours after cholestyramine administration). Products include:
- Inderal ... 2834
- Inderal LA Long Acting Capsules ... 2836
- Inderide Tablets ... 2838
- Inderide LA Long Acting Capsules .. 2840

Quinestrol (Cholestyramine may delay or reduce absorption of concomitant oral estrogens; it is recommended that patients take estrogens at least one hour before or 4 to 6 hours after cholestyramine administration).
- No products indexed under this heading.

Simvastatin (Lipid-lowering effects of cholestyramine are enhanced when combined with HMG-CoA reductase inhibitors; it is recommended that patients take HMG CoA reductase inhibitors at least one hour before or 4 to 6 hours after cholestyramine administration). Products include:
- Zocor Tablets ... 1821

Tetracycline Hydrochloride (Cholestyramine may delay or reduce absorption of concomitant oral tetracycline; it is recommended that patients take tetracycline at least one hour before or 4 to 6 hours after cholestyramine administration). Products include:
- Achromycin V Capsules ... 1417
- Helidac Therapy ... 2135

Vitamin A (Cholestyramine may interfere with normal fat digestion and absorption and this may prevent oral absorption of fat soluble vitamins). Products include:
- Aquasol A Vitamin A Capsules, USP ... 525
- Aquasol A Parenteral ... 526
- Breath + Plus ... 603
- Materna Tablets ... 1427
- Megadose ... 513
- One-A-Day Antioxidant Plus ... 625

Vitamin D (Cholestyramine may interfere with normal fat digestion and absorption and this may prevent oral absorption of fat soluble vitamins). Products include:
- Caltrate PLUS ... 681
- Caltrate 600 + D ... 681
- Dical-D Tablets & Wafers ... 424
- Materna Tablets ... 1427
- Megadose ... 513
- One-A-Day Calcium Plus ... 625

Vitamin E (Cholestyramine may interfere with normal fat digestion and absorption and this may prevent oral absorption of fat soluble vitamins). Products include:
- ACES Antioxidant Soft Gels ... 647
- Breath + Plus ... 603
- Cefol Filmtab ... 415
- Materna Tablets ... 1427
- Megadose ... 513
- Nutr-E-Sol ... 461
- One-A-Day Antioxidant Plus ... 625
- Protegra Antioxidant Vitamin & Mineral Supplement ... 685
- StePHan Essential ... 834
- StePHan Feminine ... 834
- Stresstabs ... 685
- Unique E Vitamin E Capsules ... 1236

Vitamin K_1 (Cholestyramine may interfere with normal fat digestion and absorption and this may prevent absorption of fat soluble vitamins). Products include:
- AquaMEPHYTON Injection ... 1648
- Mephyton Tablets ... 1739

Warfarin Sodium (Cholestyramine may delay or reduce absorption of concomitant oral warfarin; it is recommended that patients take warfarin at least one hour before or 4 to 6 hours after cholestyramine administration). Products include:
- Coumadin ... 941

QUIBRON CAPSULES
(Theophylline, Guaifenesin) ...2227
See **Quibron-T/SR Tablets**

QUIBRON-300 CAPSULES
(Theophylline, Guaifenesin) ...2227
See **Quibron-T/SR Tablets**

QUIBRON-T TABLETS
(Theophylline) ...2227
See **Quibron-T/SR Tablets**

QUIBRON-T/SR TABLETS
(Theophylline) ...2227
May interact with oral contraceptives, sympathomimetic bronchodilators, and certain other agents. Compounds in these categories include:

Albuterol (Toxic synergism may occur). Products include:
- Proventil Inhalation Aerosol ... 2524
- Ventolin Inhalation Aerosol and Refill ... 1170

Albuterol Sulfate (Toxic synergism may occur). Products include:
- Airet Albuterol Sulfate Inhalation Solution ... 1602
- Albuterol Sulfate, USP Solution for Inhalation, Arm-a-Med ... 522
- Proventil Inhalation Solution 0.083% ... 2527
- Proventil Repetabs Tablets ... 2529
- Proventil Solution for Inhalation 0.5% ... 2525
- Proventil Syrup ... 2528
- Proventil Tablets ... 2529
- Ventolin Inhalation Solution ... 1171
- Ventolin Nebules Inhalation Solution ... 1172
- Ventolin Rotacaps for Inhalation ... 1173
- Ventolin Syrup ... 1175
- Ventolin Tablets ... 1176
- Volmax Extended-Release Tablets .. 1835

Allopurinol (High doses of allopurinol increase serum theophylline levels). Products include:
- Zyloprim Tablets ... 1194

Bitolterol Mesylate (Toxic synergism may occur). Products include:
- Tornalate Solution for Inhalation, 0.2% ... 976
- Tornalate Metered Dose Inhaler ... 978

Cimetidine (Increases serum theophylline levels). Products include:
- Tagamet HB Tablets ... 786
- Tagamet Tablets ... 2694

Cimetidine Hydrochloride (Increases serum theophylline levels). Products include:
- Tagamet ... 2694

Ciprofloxacin (Increases serum theophylline levels). Products include:
- Cipro I.V. ... 587
- Cipro I.V. Pharmacy Bulk Package .. 590

Ciprofloxacin Hydrochloride (Increases serum theophylline levels). Products include:
- Ciloxan Ophthalmic Solution ... 468
- Cipro Tablets ... 584

Desogestrel (Increases serum theophylline levels). Products include:
- Desogen Tablets ... 1867
- Ortho-Cept ... 1907

Ephedrine Hydrochloride (Toxic synergism may occur). Products include:
- Primatene Tablets ... 844
- Quadrinal Tablets ... 1398

Ephedrine Sulfate (Toxic synergism may occur). Products include:
- Marax Tablets & DF Syrup ... 2015

Ephedrine Tannate (Toxic synergism may occur). Products include:
- Rynatuss ... 2782

Epinephrine (Toxic synergism may occur). Products include:
- EPIFRIN ... 237
- EpiPen ... 808
- Marcaine with Epinephrine ... 2446
- Primatene Mist ... 843
- Sensorcaine with Epinephrine Injection ... 554
- Sus-Phrine Injection ... 1017
- Xylocaine with Epinephrine Injections ... 562

Epinephrine Hydrochloride (Toxic synergism may occur). Products include:
- Ana-Kit Anaphylaxis Emergency Treatment Kit ... 611

Erythromycin (Increases serum theophylline levels). Products include:
- A/T/S 2% Acne Topical Gel ... 1244
- A/T/S 2% Acne Topical Solution ... 1244
- Benzamycin Topical Gel ... 919
- E-Mycin Tablets ... 1388
- Emgel 2% Topical Gel ... 1081
- ERYC ... 1972
- Erycette (erythromycin 2%) Topical Solution ... 1943
- Ery-Tab Tablets ... 426
- Erythromycin Base Filmtab ... 430
- Erythromycin Delayed-Release Capsules, USP ... 431
- Ilotycin Ophthalmic Ointment ... 928
- PCE Dispertab Tablets ... 453
- T-Stat 2.0% Topical Solution and Pads ... 2797
- THERAMYCIN Z 2% Solution ... 1629

Erythromycin Estolate (Increases serum theophylline levels). Products include:
- Ilosone ... 927

Erythromycin Ethylsuccinate (Increases serum theophylline levels). Products include:
- E.E.S. ... 427
- EryPed ... 425
- Pediazole Suspension ... 2340

Erythromycin Gluceptate (Increases serum theophylline levels). Products include:
- Ilotycin Gluceptate, IV, Vials ... 929

Erythromycin Stearate (Increases serum theophylline levels). Products include:
- Erythrocin Stearate Filmtab ... 429

Ethinyl Estradiol (Increases serum theophylline levels). Products include:
- Brevicon ... 2563
- Demulen ... 2580
- Desogen Tablets ... 1867
- Levlen/Tri-Levlen ... 646
- Lo/Ovral Tablets ... 2852
- Lo/Ovral-28 Tablets ... 2857
- Modicon ... 1928
- Nordette-21 Tablets ... 2863
- Nordette-28 Tablets ... 2866
- Norinyl ... 2563
- Ortho-Cept ... 1907
- Ortho-Cyclen/Ortho-Tri-Cyclen ... 1914
- Ortho-Novum ... 1928
- Ortho-Cyclen/Ortho Tri-Cyclen ... 1914
- Ovcon ... 765
- Ovral Tablets ... 2877
- Ovral-28 Tablets ... 2878
- Levlen/Tri-Levlen ... 646
- Tri-Norinyl ... 2607
- Triphasil-21 Tablets ... 2919
- Triphasil-28 Tablets ... 2924

Ethylnorepinephrine Hydrochloride (Toxic synergism may occur).
- No products indexed under this heading.

Ethynodiol Diacetate (Increases serum theophylline levels). Products include:
- Demulen ... 2580

Isoetharine (Toxic synergism may occur). Products include:
- Bronkometer Aerosol ... 2432
- Bronkosol Solution ... 2432
- Isoetharine Inhalation Solution, USP, Arm-a-Med ... 545

Isoproterenol Hydrochloride (Toxic synergism may occur). Products include:
- Isuprel Hydrochloride Solution ... 2443
- Isuprel Injection ... 2441
- Isuprel Mistometer ... 2442

Isoproterenol Sulfate (Toxic synergism may occur). Products include:
- Norisodrine with Calcium Iodide Syrup ... 446

Levonorgestrel (Increases serum theophylline levels). Products include:
- Levlen/Tri-Levlen ... 646
- Nordette-21 Tablets ... 2863
- Nordette-28 Tablets ... 2866
- Norplant System ... 2868
- Levlen/Tri-Levlen ... 646
- Triphasil-21 Tablets ... 2919
- Triphasil-28 Tablets ... 2924

Lithium Carbonate (Increased renal excretion of lithium). Products include:
- Eskalith ... 2658
- Lithium Carbonate Capsules & Tablets ... 2352
- Lithonate/Lithotabs/Lithobid ... 2721

Mestranol (Increases serum theophylline levels). Products include:
- Norinyl ... 2563
- Ortho-Novum ... 1928

Metaproterenol Sulfate (Toxic synergism may occur). Products include:
- Alupent ... 672
- Metaproterenol Sulfate Inhalation Solution, USP, Arm-a-Med ... 547

Norethindrone (Increases serum theophylline levels). Products include:
- Brevicon ... 2563
- Micronor Tablets ... 1903
- Modicon ... 1928
- Norinyl ... 2563
- Nor-Q D Tablets ... 2598
- Ortho-Novum ... 1928
- Ovcon ... 765
- Tri-Norinyl ... 2607

Norethynodrel (Increases serum theophylline levels).
- No products indexed under this heading.

Norgestimate (Increases serum theophylline levels). Products include:
- Ortho-Cyclen/Ortho-Tri-Cyclen ... 1914
- Ortho-Cyclen/Ortho Tri-Cyclen ... 1914

Norgestrel (Increases serum theophylline levels). Products include:
- Lo/Ovral Tablets ... 2852
- Lo/Ovral-28 Tablets ... 2857

IMPORTANT NOTE: Always consult each drug listing in the patient's regimen for possible interactions.

Quibron

Ovral Tablets	2877
Ovral-28 Tablets	2878
Ovrette Tablets	2878

Phenytoin (Decreased theophylline and phenytoin serum levels). Products include:

Dilantin Infatabs	1967
Dilantin-125 Suspension	1969

Phenytoin Sodium (Decreased theophylline and phenytoin serum levels). Products include:

Dilantin Kapseals	1965

Pirbuterol Acetate (Toxic synergism may occur). Products include:

Maxair Autohaler	1550
Maxair Inhaler	1552

Propranolol Hydrochloride (Increases serum theophylline levels). Products include:

Inderal	2834
Inderal LA Long Acting Capsules	2836
Inderide Tablets	2838
Inderide LA Long Acting Capsules	2840

Rifampin (Decreased serum theophylline levels). Products include:

Rifadin	1276
Rifamate Capsules	1278
Rifater	1280
Rimactane Capsules	865

Salmeterol Xinafoate (Toxic synergism may occur). Products include:

Serevent Inhalation Aerosol	1149

Terbutaline Sulfate (Toxic synergism may occur). Products include:

Brethaire Inhaler	830
Brethine Ampuls	832
Brethine Tablets	831
Bricanyl Subcutaneous Injection	1247
Bricanyl Tablets	1248

Troleandomycin (Increases serum theophylline levels). Products include:

Tao Capsules	2033

Food Interactions

Food, unspecified (Food ingestion may influence the absorption characteristics of some or all theophylline controlled-release products).

QUINAGLUTE DURA-TABS TABLETS

(Quinidine Gluconate) 644

May interact with carbonic anhydrase inhibitors, thiazides, phenothiazines, tricyclic antidepressants, neuromuscular blocking agents, anticholinergics, negative inotropic agents, vasodilators, cholinergic agents, vasopressors, and certain other agents. Compounds in these categories include:

Acebutolol Hydrochloride (Quinidine's negative inotropic actions may be additive to those of other similar agents). Products include:

Sectral Capsules	2914

Acetazolamide (Reduces renal elimination of quinidine by alkalinizing the urine). Products include:

Diamox Sequels (Sustained Release)	⊚ 318
Diamox Tablets	⊚ 317

Amiodarone Hydrochloride (Co-administration may increase quinidine levels). Products include:

Cordarone Intravenous	2821
Cordarone Tablets	2818

Amitriptyline Hydrochloride (Therapeutic serum levels of quinidine inhibit the action of cytochrome P45OIID6 and most polycyclic antidepressants are metabolized by this enzyme; caution should be exercised). Products include:

Elavil	2945
Etrafon	2495
Limbitrol	2333
Triavil Tablets	1800

Amoxapine (Therapeutic serum levels of quinidine inhibit the action of cytochrome P45OIID6 and most polycyclic antidepressants are metabolized by this enzyme; caution should be exercised). Products include:

Asendin Tablets	1419

Atenolol (Quinidine's negative inotropic actions may be additive to those of other similar agents). Products include:

Tenoretic Tablets	2963
Tenormin Tablets and I.V. Injection	2965

Atracurium Besylate (Quinidine potentiates the action of neuromuscular blocking agents). Products include:

Tracrium Injection	1155

Atropine Sulfate (Quinidine's anticholinergic actions may be additive to those of other anticholinergic drugs). Products include:

Arco-Lase Plus Tablets	513
Atrohist Plus Tablets	1605
Donnatal	2234
Donnatal Extentabs	2234
Donnatal Tablets	2234
Lomotil	2591
Motofen Tablets	789
Urised Tablets	2123

Belladonna Alkaloids (Quinidine's anticholinergic actions may be additive to those of other anticholinergic drugs). Products include:

Bellergal-S Tablets	2375
Hyland's Bedwetting Tablets	▣ 788
Hyland's EnurAid Tablets	▣ 789
Hyland's Headache Tablets	▣ 790
Hyland's Teething Tablets	▣ 790
Similasan Eye Drops #1	▣ 769

Bendroflumethiazide (Reduces renal elimination of quinidine by alkalinizing the urine).
No products indexed under this heading.

Benztropine Mesylate (Quinidine's anticholinergic actions may be additive to those of other anticholinergic drugs). Products include:

Cogentin	1661

Betaxolol Hydrochloride (Quinidine's negative inotropic actions may be additive to those of other similar agents). Products include:

Betoptic Ophthalmic Solution	465
Betoptic S Ophthalmic Suspension	467
Kerlone Tablets	2588

Biperiden Hydrochloride (Quinidine's anticholinergic actions may be additive to those of other anticholinergic drugs). Products include:

Akineton	1380

Carteolol Hydrochloride (Quinidine's negative inotropic actions may be additive to those of other similar agents). Products include:

Cartrol Tablets	413
Ocupress Ophthalmic Solution, 1% Sterile	⊚ 297

Chlorothiazide (Reduces renal elimination of quinidine by alkalinizing the urine). Products include:

Aldoclor Tablets	1638
Diupres Tablets	1691
Diuril Oral	1694

Chlorothiazide Sodium (Reduces renal elimination of quinidine by alkalinizing the urine). Products include:

Diuril Sodium Intravenous	1693

Chlorpromazine (Therapeutic serum levels of quinidine inhibit the action of cytochrome P45OIID6 and certain unspecified phenothiazines are metabolized by this enzyme; caution should be exercised). Products include:

Thorazine Suppositories	2701

Chlorpromazine Hydrochloride (Therapeutic serum levels of quinidine inhibit the action of cytochrome P45OIID6 and certain unspecified phenothiazines are metabolized by this enzyme; caution should be exercised). Products include:

Thorazine	2701

Cimetidine (Co-administration may increase quinidine levels). Products include:

Tagamet HB Tablets	▣ 786
Tagamet Tablets	2694

Cimetidine Hydrochloride (Co-administration may increase quinidine levels). Products include:

Tagamet	2694

Cisatracurium Besylate (Quinidine potentiates the action of neuromuscular blocking agents). Products include:

Nimbex Injection	1131

Clidinium Bromide (Quinidine's anticholinergic actions may be additive to those of other anticholinergic drugs). Products include:

Librax Capsules	2330

Clomipramine Hydrochloride (Therapeutic serum levels of quinidine inhibit the action of cytochrome P45OIID6 and most polycyclic antidepressants are metabolized by this enzyme; caution should be exercised). Products include:

Anafranil Capsules	819

Decamethonium (Quinidine potentiates the action of neuromuscular blocking agent).

Desipramine Hydrochloride (Therapeutic serum levels of quinidine inhibit the action of cytochrome P45OIID6 and most polycyclic antidepressants are metabolized by this enzyme; caution should be exercised). Products include:

Norpramin Tablets	1273

Diazoxide (Quinidine's vasodilating actions may be additive to those of other vasodilators). Products include:

Hyperstat I.V. Injection	2504
Proglycem	575

Dichlorphenamide (Reduces renal elimination of quinidine by alkalinizing the urine). Products include:

Daranide Tablets	1676

Dicyclomine Hydrochloride (Quinidine's anticholinergic actions may be additive to those of other anticholinergic drugs). Products include:

Bentyl	1246

Digitoxin (Quinidine slows the elimination of digitoxin resulting in the elevation of serum levels of digitoxin when co-administered, although the effect appears to be smaller). Products include:

Crystodigin Tablets	1472

Digoxin (Quinidine slows the elimination of digoxin and simultaneously reduces digoxin's apparent volume of distribution resulting in elevated serum digoxin levels). Products include:

Lanoxicaps	1110
Lanoxin Elixir Pediatric	1113
Lanoxin Injection	1116
Lanoxin Injection Pediatric	1119
Lanoxin Tablets	1121

Dopamine Hydrochloride (Quinidine's vasodilating actions may be antagonistic to those of vasopressors).
No products indexed under this heading.

Dorzolamide Hydrochloride (Reduces renal elimination of quinidine by alkalinizing the urine). Products include:

Trusopt Sterile Ophthalmic Solution	1803

Doxacurium Chloride (Quinidine potentiates the action of neuromuscular blocking agents). Products include:

Nuromax Injection	1136

Doxepin Hydrochloride (Therapeutic serum levels of quinidine inhibit the action of cytochrome P45OIID6 and most polycyclic antidepressants are metabolized by this enzyme; caution should be exercised). Products include:

Adapin Capsules	1542
Sinequan	2028
Zonalon Cream	1042

Edrophonium Chloride (Quinidine's anticholinergic actions may be antagonistic to those of cholinergic agents). Products include:

Tensilon Injectable	1307

Epinephrine Bitartrate (Quinidine's vasodilating actions may be antagonistic to those of vasopressors). Products include:

Sensorcaine-MPF with Epinephrine Injection	554

Epinephrine Hydrochloride (Quinidine's vasodilating actions may be antagonistic to those of vasopressors). Products include:

Ana-Kit Anaphylaxis Emergency Treatment Kit	611

Epoprostenol Sodium (Quinidine's vasodilating actions may be additive to those of other vasodilators). Products include:

Flolan for Injection	1085

Esmolol Hydrochloride (Quinidine's negative inotropic actions may be additive to those of other similar agents). Products include:

Brevibloc (esmolol HCl) Injection	1860

Felodipine (Potential for variable slowing of the metabolism of felodipine). Products include:

Plendil Extended-Release Tablets	514

Fluphenazine Decanoate (Therapeutic serum levels of quinidine inhibit the action of cytochrome P45OIID6 and certain unspecified phenothiazines are metabolized by this enzyme; caution should be exercised). Products include:

Prolixin Decanoate	510

Fluphenazine Enanthate (Therapeutic serum levels of quinidine inhibit the action of cytochrome P45OIID6 and certain unspecified phenothiazines are metabolized by this enzyme; caution should be exercised). Products include:

Prolixin Enanthate	510

Fluphenazine Hydrochloride (Therapeutic serum levels of quinidine inhibit the action of cytochrome P45OIID6 and certain unspecified phenothiazines are metabolized by this enzyme; caution should be exercised). Products include:

Prolixin	510

Fosphenytoin Sodium (Hepatic elimination of quinidine may be accelerated by co-administration). Products include:

Cerebyx Injection	1956

Glycopyrrolate (Quinidine's anticholinergic actions may be additive to those of other anticholinergic drugs). Products include:

Robinul Forte Tablets	2247
Robinul Injectable	2247
Robinul Tablets	2247

(▣ Described in PDR For Nonprescription Drugs) (⊚ Described in PDR For Ophthalmology)

Haloperidol (Serum levels of haloperidol are increased when quinidine is co-administered). Products include:
   Haldol Injection, Tablets and Concentrate 1585

Haloperidol Decanoate (Serum levels of haloperidol are increased when quinidine is co-administered). Products include:
   Haldol Decanoate 1587

Hydralazine Hydrochloride (Quinidine's vasodilating actions may be additive to those of other vasodilators). Products include:
   Apresazide Capsules 824
   Apresoline Hydrochloride Tablets .. 826
   Hydralazine Hydrochloride Injection USP 2712
   Ser-Ap-Es Tablets 867

Hydrochlorothiazide (Reduces renal elimination of quinidine by alkalinizing the urine). Products include:
   Aldactazide Tablets 2556
   Aldoril Tablets 1644
   Apresazide Capsules 824
   Capozide Tablets 744
   Dyazide Capsules 2653
   Esidrix Tablets 839
   Esimil Tablets 840
   HydroDIURIL Tablets 1716
   Hydropres Tablets 1718
   Hyzaar Tablets 1720
   Inderide Tablets 2838
   Inderide LA Long Acting Capsules .. 2840
   Lopressor HCT Tablets 850
   Lotensin HCT Tablets 855
   Moduretic Tablets 1748
   Oretic Tablets 450
   Prinzide Tablets 1780
   Ser-Ap-Es Tablets 867
   Timolide Tablets 1791
   Vaseretic Tablets 1810
   Zestoretic Tablets 2968
   Ziac 1459

Hydroflumethiazide (Reduces renal elimination of quinidine by alkalinizing the urine). Products include:
   Diucardin Tablets 2824

Hyoscyamine (Quinidine's anticholinergic actions may be additive to those of other anticholinergic drugs). Products include:
   Cystospaz Tablets 2123
   Urised Tablets 2123

Hyoscyamine Sulfate (Quinidine's anticholinergic actions may be additive to those of other anticholinergic drugs). Products include:
   Arco-Lase Plus Tablets 513
   Atrohist Plus Tablets 1605
   Cystospaz-M Capsules 2123
   Donnatal 2234
   Donnatal Extentabs 2234
   Donnatal Tablets 2234
   Kutrase Capsules 2546
   Levsin/Levsinex/Levbid 2549

Imipramine Hydrochloride (Therapeutic serum levels of quinidine inhibit the action of cytochrome P450IID6 and most polycyclic antidepressants are metabolized by this enzyme; caution should be exercised). Products include:
   Tofranil Ampuls 873
   Tofranil Tablets 875

Imipramine Pamoate (Therapeutic serum levels of quinidine inhibit the action of cytochrome P450IID6 and most polycyclic antidepressants are metabolized by this enzyme; caution should be exercised). Products include:
   Tofranil-PM Capsules 876

Ipratropium Bromide (Quinidine's anticholinergic actions may be additive to those of other anticholinergic drugs). Products include:
   Atrovent Inhalation Aerosol 674
   Atrovent Inhalation Solution 675
   Atrovent Nasal Spray 0.03% 676
   Atrovent Nasal Spray 0.06% 678

Ketoconazole (Co-administration may increase quinidine levels). Products include:
   Nizoral 2% Cream 1344
   Nizoral 2% Shampoo 1344
   Nizoral Tablets 1345

Labetalol Hydrochloride (Quinidine's negative inotropic actions may be additive to those of other similar agents). Products include:
   Normodyne Injection 2519
   Normodyne Tablets 2522
   Trandate 1158

Maprotiline Hydrochloride (Therapeutic serum levels of quinidine inhibit the action of cytochrome P450IID6 and most polycyclic antidepressants are metabolized by this enzyme; caution should be exercised). Products include:
   Ludiomil Tablets 861

Mepenzolate Bromide (Quinidine's anticholinergic actions may be additive to those of other anticholinergic drugs).
   No products indexed under this heading.

Mesoridazine Besylate (Therapeutic serum levels of quinidine inhibit the action of cytochrome P450IID6 and certain unspecified phenothiazines are metabolized by this enzyme; caution should be exercised). Products include:
   Serentil 689

Metaraminol Bitartrate (Quinidine's vasodilating actions may be antagonistic to those of vasopressors). Products include:
   Aramine Injection 1649

Methazolamide (Reduces renal elimination of quinidine by alkalinizing the urine). Products include:
   GlaucTabs .... ⓘ 209
   Neptazane Tablets .... ⓘ 320

Methotrimeprazine (Therapeutic serum levels of quinidine inhibit the action of cytochrome P450IID6 and certain unspecified phenothiazines are metabolized by this enzyme; caution should be exercised). Products include:
   Levoprome 1321

Methoxamine Hydrochloride (Quinidine's vasodilating actions may be antagonistic to those of vasopressors). Products include:
   Vasoxyl Injection 1169

Methyclothiazide (Reduces renal elimination of quinidine by alkalinizing the urine). Products include:
   Enduron Tablets 424

Metocurine Iodide (Quinidine potentiates the action of neuromuscular blocking agents). Products include:
   Metubine Iodide Vials 932

Metoprolol Tartrate (Quinidine's negative inotropic actions may be additive to those of other similar agents). Products include:
   Lopressor 848
   Lopressor HCT Tablets 850

Mexiletine Hydrochloride (Therapeutic serum levels of quinidine inhibit the action of cytochrome P450IID6 and mexiletine is metabolized by this enzyme; caution should be exercised). Products include:
   Mexitil Capsules 684

Minoxidil (Quinidine's vasodilating actions may be additive to those of other vasodilators).
   No products indexed under this heading.

Mivacurium Chloride (Quinidine potentiates the action of neuromuscular blocking agents). Products include:
   Mivacron 1125

Nadolol (Quinidine's negative inotropic actions may be additive to those of other similar agents).
   No products indexed under this heading.

Neostigmine Bromide (Quinidine's anticholinergic actions may be antagonistic to those of cholinergic agents). Products include:
   Prostigmin Tablets 1306

Neostigmine Methylsulfate (Quinidine's anticholinergic actions may be antagonistic to those of cholinergic agents). Products include:
   Prostigmin Injectable 1305

Nicardipine Hydrochloride (Potential for variable slowing of the metabolism of nicardipine). Products include:
   Cardene Capsules 2261
   Cardene I.V. 2815
   Cardene SR Capsules 2264

Nifedipine (Very rarely co-administration may decrease quinidine levels; quinidine causes variable slowing of the metabolism of nifedipine). Products include:
   Adalat Capsules (10 mg and 20 mg) 580
   Adalat CC 582
   Procardia Capsules 2024
   Procardia XL Extended Release Tablets 2026

Nimodipine (Potential for variable slowing of the metabolism of nimodipine). Products include:
   Nimotop Capsules 603

Norepinephrine Bitartrate (Quinidine's vasodilating actions may be antagonistic to those of vasopressors). Products include:
   Levophed Bitartrate Injection 2445

Nortriptyline Hydrochloride (Therapeutic serum levels of quinidine inhibit the action of cytochrome P450IID6 and most polycyclic antidepressants are metabolized by this enzyme; caution should be exercised). Products include:
   Pamelor 2409

Oxybutynin Chloride (Quinidine's anticholinergic actions may be additive to those of other anticholinergic drugs). Products include:
   Ditropan 1267

Pancuronium Bromide (Quinidine potentiates the action of neuromuscular blocking agents).
   No products indexed under this heading.

Penbutolol Sulfate (Quinidine's negative inotropic actions may be additive to those of other similar agents). Products include:
   Levatol Tablets 2547

Perphenazine (Therapeutic serum levels of quinidine inhibit the action of cytochrome P450IID6 and certain unspecified phenothiazines are metabolized by this enzyme; caution should be exercised). Products include:
   Etrafon 2495
   Triavil Tablets 1800
   Trilafon 2532

Phenobarbital (Hepatic elimination of quinidine may be accelerated by co-administration). Products include:
   Arco-Lase Plus Tablets 513
   Bellergal-S Tablets 2375
   Donnatal 2234
   Donnatal Extentabs 2234

   Donnatal Tablets 2234
   Phenobarbital Elixir and Tablets 1523
   Quadrinal Tablets 1398

Phenylephrine Hydrochloride (Quinidine's vasodilating actions may be antagonistic to those of vasopressors). Products include:
   Atrohist Plus Tablets 1605
   Cerose DM .... ⓘ 853
   D.A. II Tablets 972
   D.A. Chewable Tablets 970
   Dura-Vent/DA Tablets 972
   Extendryl 1003
   4-Way Fast Acting Nasal Spray (regular & mentholated) .... ⓘ 644
   Hemoril 797
   Hycomine Compound Tablets 948
   Neo-Synephrine Hydrochloride 1% Carpuject 2455
   Neo-Synephrine Hydrochloride 1% Injection 2455
   Neo-Synephrine Hydrochloride (Ophthalmic) 2456
   Neo-Synephrine .... ⓘ 624
   Novahistine Elixir .... ⓘ 782
   Phenergan VC 2886
   Phenergan VC with Codeine 2888
   Preparation H .... ⓘ 842
   Tympagesic Ear Drops 2476
   Vicks Sinex Nasal Spray and Ultra Fine Mist .... ⓘ 738

Phenytoin (Hepatic elimination of quinidine may be accelerated by co-administration). Products include:
   Dilantin Infatabs 1967
   Dilantin-125 Suspension 1969

Phenytoin Sodium (Hepatic elimination of quinidine may be accelerated by co-administration). Products include:
   Dilantin Kapseals 1965

Pindolol (Quinidine's negative inotropic actions may be additive to those of other similar agents). Products include:
   Visken Tablets 2428

Polythiazide (Reduces renal elimination of quinidine by alkalinizing the urine). Products include:
   Minizide Capsules 2016

Procainamide Hydrochloride (Co-administration causes an increase in serum levels of procainamide). Products include:
   Procanbid Extended-Release Tablets 1983

Prochlorperazine (Therapeutic serum levels of quinidine inhibit the action of cytochrome P450IID6 and certain unspecified phenothiazines are metabolized by this enzyme; caution should be exercised). Products include:
   Compazine 2644

Procyclidine Hydrochloride (Quinidine's anticholinergic actions may be additive to those of other anticholinergic drugs). Products include:
   Kemadrin Tablets 1105

Promethazine Hydrochloride (Therapeutic serum levels of quinidine inhibit the action of cytochrome P450IID6 and certain unspecified phenothiazines are metabolized by this enzyme; caution should be exercised). Products include:
   Mepergan Injection 2859
   Phenergan with Codeine 2883
   Phenergan with Dextromethorphan 2885
   Phenergan Injection 2880
   Phenergan Suppositories 2882
   Phenergan Syrup 2881
   Phenergan Tablets 2882
   Phenergan VC 2886
   Phenergan VC with Codeine 2888

Propantheline Bromide (Quinidine's anticholinergic actions may be additive to those of other anticholinergic drugs). Products include:
   Pro-Banthine Tablets 2226

IMPORTANT NOTE: Always consult each drug listing in the patient's regimen for possible interactions.

Quinaglute — Interactions Index

Propranolol Hydrochloride (Co-administration may cause increase in the peak serum levels of quinidine; decrease in quinidine's volume of distribution, and decrease in total quinidine clearance). Products include:
- Inderal ... 2834
- Inderal LA Long Acting Capsules ... 2836
- Inderide Tablets ... 2838
- Inderide LA Long Acting Capsules ... 2840

Protriptyline Hydrochloride (Therapeutic serum levels of quinidine inhibit the action of cytochrome P450IID6 and most polycyclic antidepressants are metabolized by this enzyme; caution should be exercised). Products include:
- Vivactil Tablets ... 1820

Pyridostigmine Bromide (Quinidine's anticholinergic actions may be antagonistic to those of cholinergic agents). Products include:
- Mestinon Injectable ... 1300
- Mestinon ... 1300

Rifampin (Hepatic elimination of quinidine may be accelerated by co-administration). Products include:
- Rifadin ... 1276
- Rifamate Capsules ... 1278
- Rifater ... 1280
- Rimactane Capsules ... 865

Rocuronium Bromide (Quinidine potentiates the action of neuromuscular blocking agents). Products include:
- Zemuron Injection ... 1885

Scopolamine (Quinidine's anticholinergic actions may be additive to those of other anticholinergic drugs). Products include:
- Transderm Scōp Transdermal Therapeutic System ... 890

Scopolamine Hydrobromide (Quinidine's anticholinergic actions may be additive to those of other anticholinergic drugs). Products include:
- Atrohist Plus Tablets ... 1605
- Donnatal ... 2234
- Donnatal Extentabs ... 2234
- Donnatal Tablets ... 2234

Sodium Bicarbonate (Systemic sodium bicarbonate reduces renal elimination of quinidine by alkalinizing the urine). Products include:
- Alka-Seltzer Cherry Effervescent Antacid and Pain Reliever ... 609
- Alka-Seltzer Extra Strength Effervescent Antacid and Pain Reliever ... 609
- Alka-Seltzer Gold Effervescent Antacid ... 611
- Alka-Seltzer Lemon Lime Effervescent Antacid and Pain Reliever ... 609
- Alka-Seltzer Original Effervescent Antacid and Pain Reliever ... 609
- Arm & Hammer Pure Baking Soda ... 648
- Colyte and Colyte-flavored ... 2540
- GoLYTELY ... 694
- Massengill Disposable Douches ... 780
- Massengill Liquid Concentrate ... 780
- NuLYTELY ... 694
- Cherry Flavor NuLYTELY ... 694

Succinylcholine Chloride (Quinidine potentiates the action of neuromuscular blocking agents). Products include:
- Anectine ... 1062

Thioridazine Hydrochloride (Therapeutic serum levels of quinidine inhibit the action of cytochrome P450IID6 and certain unspecified phenothiazines are metabolized by this enzyme; caution should be exercised). Products include:
- Mellaril ... 2398

Timolol Maleate (Quinidine's negative inotropic actions may be additive to those of other similar agents). Products include:
- Blocadren Tablets ... 1654
- Timolide Tablets ... 1791
- Timoptic in Ocudose ... 1796
- Timoptic Sterile Ophthalmic Solution ... 1794
- Timoptic-XE ... 1798

Trazodone Hydrochloride (Therapeutic serum levels of quinidine inhibit the action of cytochrome P450IID6 and most polycyclic antidepressants are metabolized by this enzyme; caution should be exercised). Products include:
- Desyrel and Desyrel Dividose ... 504

Tridihexethyl Chloride (Quinidine's anticholinergic actions may be additive to those of other anticholinergic drugs).
No products indexed under this heading.

Trifluoperazine Hydrochloride (Therapeutic serum levels of quinidine inhibit the action of cytochrome P450IID6 and certain unspecified phenothiazines are metabolized by this enzyme; caution should be exercised). Products include:
- Stelazine ... 2692

Trihexyphenidyl Hydrochloride (Quinidine's anticholinergic actions may be additive to those of other anticholinergic drugs). Products include:
- Artane ... 1418

Trimipramine Maleate (Therapeutic serum levels of quinidine inhibit the action of cytochrome P450IID6 and most polycyclic antidepressants are metabolized by this enzyme; caution should be exercised). Products include:
- Surmontil Capsules ... 2917

Tubocurarine Chloride (Potentiation of neuromuscular blockade).
No products indexed under this heading.

Vecuronium Bromide (Quinidine potentiates the action of neuromuscular blocking agents). Products include:
- Norcuron for Injection ... 1875

Verapamil Hydrochloride (Hepatic clearance of quinidine is significantly reduced with co-administration resulting in corresponding increase in serum levels and half-life). Products include:
- Calan SR Caplets ... 2571
- Calan Tablets ... 2568
- Covera-HS Tablets ... 2573
- Isoptin Injectable ... 1391
- Isoptin Oral Tablets ... 1393
- Isoptin SR Tablets ... 1395
- Verelan Capsules ... 1455

Warfarin Sodium (Quinidine may potentiate anticoagulant action of warfarin). Products include:
- Coumadin ... 941

Food Interactions

Food, unspecified (Increases absorption of quinidine in both rate (27%) and extent (17%)).

QUINIDEX EXTENTABS

(Quinidine Sulfate) ... 2240
May interact with carbonic anhydrase inhibitors, thiazides, oral anticoagulants, phenothiazines, and certain other agents. Compounds in these categories include:

Acetazolamide (Co-administration with drugs that alkalinize the urine, such as carbonic anhydrase inhibitors, may reduce renal elimination of quinidine). Products include:
- Diamox Sequels (Sustained Release) ... 318
- Diamox Tablets ... 317

Amiodarone Hydrochloride (Co-administration with amiodarone increases quinidine levels). Products include:
- Cordarone Intravenous ... 2821
- Cordarone Tablets ... 2818

Amitriptyline Hydrochloride (Therapeutic serum levels of quinidine inhibit the action of cytochrome P450IID6; for most polycyclic antidepressants, this enzyme is critical to the metabolic pathway; potential exists for alteration in serum levels). Products include:
- Elavil ... 2945
- Etrafon ... 2495
- Limbitrol ... 2333
- Triavil Tablets ... 1800

Amoxapine (Therapeutic serum levels of quinidine inhibit the action of cytochrome P450IID6; for most polycyclic antidepressants, this enzyme is critical to the metabolic pathway; potential exists for alteration in serum levels). Products include:
- Asendin Tablets ... 1419

Bendroflumethiazide (Co-administration with drugs that alkalinize the urine, such as thiazide diuretics, may reduce renal elimination of quinidine).
No products indexed under this heading.

Chlorothiazide (Co-administration with drugs that alkalinize the urine, such as thiazide diuretics, may reduce renal elimination of quinidine). Products include:
- Aldoclor Tablets ... 1638
- Diupres Tablets ... 1691
- Diuril Oral ... 1694

Chlorothiazide Sodium (Co-administration with drugs that alkalinize the urine, such as thiazide diuretics, may reduce renal elimination of quinidine). Products include:
- Diuril Sodium Intravenous ... 1693

Chlorpromazine (Therapeutic serum levels of quinidine inhibit the action of cytochrome P450IID6; for some phenothiazines, this enzyme is critical to the metabolic pathway; potential exists for alteration in serum levels). Products include:
- Thorazine Suppositories ... 2701

Chlorpromazine Hydrochloride (Therapeutic serum levels of quinidine inhibit the action of cytochrome P450IID6; for some phenothiazines, this enzyme is critical to the metabolic pathway; potential exists for alteration in serum levels). Products include:
- Thorazine ... 2701

Cimetidine (Co-administration with cimetidine increases quinidine levels). Products include:
- Tagamet HB Tablets ... 786
- Tagamet Tablets ... 2694

Cimetidine Hydrochloride (Co-administration with cimetidine increases quinidine levels). Products include:
- Tagamet ... 2694

Clomipramine Hydrochloride (Therapeutic serum levels of quinidine inhibit the action of cytochrome P450IID6; for most polycyclic antidepressants, this enzyme is critical to the metabolic pathway; potential exists for alteration in serum levels). Products include:
- Anafranil Capsules ... 819

Codeine Phosphate (Therapeutic serum levels of quinidine inhibit the action of cytochrome P450IID6; for codeine, the analgesic/antitussive action may be mediated by this enzyme; it may not be possible to achieve the desired clinical benefits with concurrent use). Products include:
- Brontex ... 2130
- Dimetane-DC Cough Syrup ... 2232
- Fioricet with Codeine Capsules ... 2387
- Fiorinal with Codeine Capsules ... 2390
- Nucofed ... 2225
- Phenergan with Codeine ... 2883
- Phenergan VC with Codeine ... 2888
- Robitussin A-C Syrup ... 2248
- Robitussin-DAC Syrup ... 2249
- Ryna ... 804
- Soma Compound w/Codeine Tablets ... 2784
- Tylenol with Codeine ... 1592

Desipramine Hydrochloride (Therapeutic serum levels of quinidine inhibit the action of cytochrome P450IID6; for most polycyclic antidepressants, this enzyme is critical to the metabolic pathway; potential exists for alteration in serum levels). Products include:
- Norpramin Tablets ... 1273

Dichlorphenamide (Co-administration with drugs that alkalinize the urine, such as carbonic anhydrase inhibitors, may reduce renal elimination of quinidine). Products include:
- Daranide Tablets ... 1676

Digitoxin (Co-administration lowers digitoxin serum levels). Products include:
- Crystodigin Tablets ... 1472

Digoxin (Quinidine slows the elimination of digoxin and simultaneously reduces digoxin's apparent volume of distribution resulting in doubling in digoxin serum levels; digoxin dose may need to be reduced). Products include:
- Lanoxicaps ... 1110
- Lanoxin Elixir Pediatric ... 1113
- Lanoxin Injection ... 1116
- Lanoxin Injection Pediatric ... 1119
- Lanoxin Tablets ... 1121

Dorzolamide Hydrochloride (Co-administration with drugs that alkalinize the urine, such as carbonic anhydrase inhibitors, may reduce renal elimination of quinidine). Products include:
- Trusopt Sterile Ophthalmic Solution ... 1803

Doxepin Hydrochloride (Therapeutic serum levels of quinidine inhibit the action of cytochrome P450IID6; for most polycyclic antidepressants, this enzyme is critical to the metabolic pathway; potential exists for alteration in serum levels). Products include:
- Adapin Capsules ... 1542
- Sinequan ... 2028
- Zonalon Cream ... 1042

Felodipine (Quinidine may cause slowing of the metabolism of felodipine). Products include:
- Plendil Extended-Release Tablets ... 514

(⊡ Described in PDR For Nonprescription Drugs)   (⊙ Described in PDR For Ophthalmology)

Fluphenazine Decanoate (Therapeutic serum levels of quinidine inhibit the action of cytochrome P450IID6; for some phenothiazines, this enzyme is critical to the metabolic pathway; potential exists for alteration in serum levels). Products include:
Prolixin Decanoate 510

Fluphenazine Enanthate (Therapeutic serum levels of quinidine inhibit the action of cytochrome P450IID6; for some phenothiazines, this enzyme is critical to the metabolic pathway; potential exists for alteration in serum levels). Products include:
Prolixin Enanthate 510

Fluphenazine Hydrochloride (Therapeutic serum levels of quinidine inhibit the action of cytochrome P450IID6; for some phenothiazines, this enzyme is critical to the metabolic pathway; potential exists for alteration in serum levels). Products include:
Prolixin 510

Fosphenytoin Sodium (Hepatic elimination of quinidine may be accelerated by co-administration of drugs that induce production of cytochrome P450IIIA4, such as phenytoin). Products include:
Cerebyx Injection 1956

Haloperidol (Serum levels of haloperidol are increased when co-administered). Products include:
Haldol Injection, Tablets and Concentrate 1585

Haloperidol Decanoate (Serum levels of haloperidol are increased when co-administered). Products include:
Haldol Decanoate 1587

Hydrochlorothiazide (Co-administration with drugs that alkalinize the urine, such as thiazide diuretics, may reduce renal elimination of quinidine). Products include:
Aldactazide Tablets 2556
Aldoril Tablets 1644
Apresazide Capsules 824
Capozide Tablets 744
Dyazide Capsules 2653
Esidrix Tablets 839
Esimil Tablets 840
HydroDIURIL Tablets 1716
Hydropres Tablets 1718
Hyzaar Tablets 1720
Inderide Tablets 2838
Inderide LA Long Acting Capsules .. 2840
Lopressor HCT Tablets 850
Lotensin HCT Tablets 855
Moduretic Tablets 1748
Oretic Tablets 450
Prinzide Tablets 1780
Ser-Ap-Es Tablets 867
Timolide Tablets 1791
Vaseretic Tablets 1810
Zestoretic Tablets 2968
Ziac 1459

Hydrocodone Bitartrate (Therapeutic serum levels of quinidine inhibit the action of cytochrome P450IID6; for hydrocodone, the analgesic/antitussive action is mediated by this enzyme; it may not be possible to achieve the desired clinical benefits with concurrent use). Products include:
Codiclear DH Syrup 808
Duratuss HD Elixir 2750
Histussin D Liquid 670
Hycodan Tablets and Syrup 946
Hycomine Compound Tablets 948
Hycomine 947
Hycotuss Expectorant Syrup 950
Hydrocet Capsules 787
Lorcet 10/650 Tablets 1016
Lortab 2751
Tussend 1830
Tussend Expectorant 1831
Vicodin Tablets 1404
Vicodin ES Tablets 1405
Vicodin HP Tablets 1403
Vicodin Tuss Expectorant 1406
Zydone Capsules 967

Hydrocodone Polistirex (Therapeutic serum levels of quinidine inhibit the action of cytochrome P450IID6; for hydrocodone, the analgesic/antitussive action is mediated by this enzyme; it may not be possible to achieve the desired clinical benefits with concurrent use). Products include:
Tussionex Pennkinetic Extended-Release Suspension 1624

Hydroflumethiazide (Co-administration with drugs that alkalinize the urine, such as thiazide diuretics, may reduce renal elimination of quinidine). Products include:
Diucardin Tablets 2824

Imipramine Hydrochloride (Therapeutic serum levels of quinidine inhibit the action of cytochrome P450IID6; for most polycyclic antidepressants, this enzyme is critical to the metabolic pathway; potential exists for alteration in serum levels). Products include:
Tofranil Ampuls 873
Tofranil Tablets 875

Imipramine Pamoate (Therapeutic serum levels of quinidine inhibit the action of cytochrome P450IID6; for most polycyclic antidepressants, this enzyme is critical to the metabolic pathway; potential exists for alteration in serum levels). Products include:
Tofranil-PM Capsules 876

Ketoconazole (Co-administration results in an increase in quinidine levels due to competition for the P450IIIA4 metabolic pathway). Products include:
Nizoral 2% Cream 1344
Nizoral 2% Shampoo 1344
Nizoral Tablets 1345

Maprotiline Hydrochloride (Therapeutic serum levels of quinidine inhibit the action of cytochrome P450IID6; for most polycyclic antidepressants, this enzyme is critical to the metabolic pathway; potential exists for alteration in serum levels). Products include:
Ludiomil Tablets 861

Mesoridazine Besylate (Therapeutic serum levels of quinidine inhibit the action of cytochrome P450IID6; for some phenothiazines, this enzyme is critical to the metabolic pathway; potential exists for alteration in serum levels). Products include:
Serentil 689

Methazolamide (Co-administration with drugs that alkalinize the urine, such as carbonic anhydrase inhibitors, may reduce renal elimination of quinidine). Products include:
GlaucTabs 209
Neptazane Tablets 320

Methotrimeprazine (Therapeutic serum levels of quinidine inhibit the action of cytochrome P450IID6; for some phenothiazines, this enzyme is critical to the metabolic pathway; potential exists for alteration in serum levels). Products include:
Levoprome 1321

Methyclothiazide (Co-administration with drugs that alkalinize the urine, such as thiazide diuretics, may reduce renal elimination of quinidine). Products include:
Enduron Tablets 424

Mexiletine Hydrochloride (Therapeutic serum levels of quinidine inhibit the action of cytochrome P450IID6; for mexiletine, this enzyme is critical to the metabolic pathway; potential exists for alteration in serum levels). Products include:
Mexitil Capsules 684

Nicardipine Hydrochloride (Quinidine may cause slowing of the metabolism of nicardipine). Products include:
Cardene Capsules 2261
Cardene I.V. 2815
Cardene SR Capsules 2264

Nifedipine (Co-administration with nifedipine decreases quinidine levels; variable slowing of the metabolism of nifedipine). Products include:
Adalat Capsules (10 mg and 20 mg) 580
Adalat CC 582
Procardia Capsules 2024
Procardia XL Extended Release Tablets 2026

Nimodipine (Quinidine may cause slowing of the metabolism of nimodipine). Products include:
Nimotop Capsules 603

Nortriptyline Hydrochloride (Therapeutic serum levels of quinidine inhibit the action of cytochrome P450IID6; for most polycyclic antidepressants, this enzyme is critical to the metabolic pathway; potential exists for alteration in serum levels). Products include:
Pamelor 2409

Pancuronium Bromide (Quinidine potentiates the actions of nondepolarizing neuromuscular blocking agents).
No products indexed under this heading.

Perphenazine (Therapeutic serum levels of quinidine inhibit the action of cytochrome P450IID6; for some phenothiazines, this enzyme is critical to the metabolic pathway; potential exists for alteration in serum levels). Products include:
Etrafon 2495
Triavil Tablets 1800
Trilafon 2532

Phenobarbital (Hepatic elimination of quinidine may be accelerated by co-administration of drugs that induce production of cytochrome P450IIIA4, such as phenobarbital). Products include:
Arco-Lase Plus Tablets 513
Bellergal-S Tablets 2375
Donnatal 2234
Donnatal Extentabs 2234
Donnatal Tablets 2234
Phenobarbital Elixir and Tablets ... 1523
Quadrinal Tablets 1398

Phenytoin (Hepatic elimination of quinidine may be accelerated by co-administration of drugs that induce production of cytochrome P450IIIA4, such as phenytoin). Products include:
Dilantin Infatabs 1967
Dilantin-125 Suspension 1969

Phenytoin Sodium (Hepatic elimination of quinidine may be accelerated by co-administration of drugs that induce production of cytochrome P450IIIA4, such as phenytoin). Products include:
Dilantin Kapseals 1965

Polythiazide (Co-administration with drugs that alkalinize the urine, such as thiazide diuretics, may reduce renal elimination of quinidine). Products include:
Minizide Capsules 2016

Procainamide Hydrochloride (Co-administration causes an increase in serum levels of procainamide due to competition for pathways of renal clearance). Products include:
Procanbid Extended-Release Tablets 1983

Prochlorperazine (Therapeutic serum levels of quinidine inhibit the action of cytochrome P450IID6; for some phenothiazines, this enzyme is critical to the metabolic pathway; potential exists for alteration in serum levels). Products include:
Compazine 2644

Promethazine Hydrochloride (Therapeutic serum levels of quinidine inhibit the action of cytochrome P450IID6; for some phenothiazines, this enzyme is critical to the metabolic pathway; potential exists for alteration in serum levels). Products include:
Mepergan Injection 2859
Phenergan with Codeine 2883
Phenergan with Dextromethorphan 2885
Phenergan Injection 2880
Phenergan Suppositories 2882
Phenergan Syrup 2881
Phenergan Tablets 2882
Phenergan VC 2886
Phenergan VC with Codeine 2888

Propranolol Hydrochloride (Co-administration may cause an increase in the peak serum levels of quinidine, decrease in quinidine's volume of distribution, and decrease in total quinidine clearance). Products include:
Inderal 2834
Inderal LA Long Acting Capsules 2836
Inderide Tablets 2838
Inderide LA Long Acting Capsules .. 2840

Protriptyline Hydrochloride (Therapeutic serum levels of quinidine inhibit the action of cytochrome P450IID6; for most polycyclic antidepressants, this enzyme is critical to the metabolic pathway; potential exists for alteration in serum levels). Products include:
Vivactil Tablets 1820

Rifampin (Hepatic elimination of quinidine may be accelerated by co-administration of drugs that induce production of cytochrome P450IIIA4, such as rifampin). Products include:
Rifadin 1276
Rifamate Capsules 1278
Rifater 1280
Rimactane Capsules 865

Sodium Bicarbonate (Co-administration with drugs that alkalinize the urine, such as systemic sodium bicarbonate, may reduce renal elimination of quinidine). Products include:
Alka-Seltzer Cherry Effervescent Antacid and Pain Reliever 609
Alka-Seltzer Extra Strength Effervescent Antacid and Pain Reliever 609
Alka-Seltzer Gold Effervescent Antacid 611
Alka-Seltzer Lemon Lime Effervescent Antacid and Pain Reliever 609
Alka-Seltzer Original Effervescent Antacid and Pain Reliever 609
Arm & Hammer Pure Baking Soda 648
Colyte and Colyte-flavored 2540
GoLYTELY 694
Massengill Disposable Douches ... 780
Massengill Liquid Concentrate 780
NuLYTELY 694
Cherry Flavor NuLYTELY 694

IMPORTANT NOTE: Always consult each drug listing in the patient's regimen for possible interactions.

Quinidex — Interactions Index

Succinylcholine Chloride (Quinidine potentiates the actions of depolarizing neuromuscular blocking agents). Products include:
- Anectine 1062

Thioridazine Hydrochloride (Therapeutic serum levels of quinidine inhibit the action of cytochrome P450IID6; for some phenothiazines, this enzyme is critical to the metabolic pathway; potential exists for alteration in serum levels). Products include:
- Mellaril 2398

Trifluoperazine Hydrochloride (Therapeutic serum levels of quinidine inhibit the action of cytochrome P450IID6; for some phenothiazines, this enzyme is critical to the metabolic pathway; potential exists for alteration in serum levels). Products include:
- Stelazine 2692

Trimipramine Maleate (Therapeutic serum levels of quinidine inhibit the action of cytochrome P450IID6; for most polycyclic antidepressants, this enzyme is critical to the metabolic pathway; potential exists for alteration in serum levels). Products include:
- Surmontil Capsules 2917

Tubocurarine Chloride (Quinidine potentiates the actions of non-depolarizing neuromuscular blocking agents).
- No products indexed under this heading.

Verapamil Hydrochloride (Hepatic clearance of quinidine is significantly reduced during co-administration of verapamil, with corresponding increases in serum levels and half-life; potential for hypotension due to additive peripheral alpha blockade). Products include:
- Calan SR Caplets 2571
- Calan Tablets 2568
- Covera-HS Tablets 2573
- Isoptin Injectable 1391
- Isoptin Oral Tablets 1393
- Isoptin SR Tablets 1395
- Verelan Capsules 1455

Warfarin Sodium (Quinidine potentiates the anticoagulatory action of warfarin, and the anticoagulant dosage may need to be reduced). Products include:
- Coumadin 941

Food Interactions

Food, unspecified (Peak serum quinidine levels obtained from immediate-release quinidine sulfate are known to be delayed by nearly an hour without change in total absorption when these products are taken with food).

PURIFIED PORK NPH ISOPHANE INSULIN
(Insulin, NPH) 1852
None cited in PDR database.

PURIFIED PORK REGULAR INSULIN
(Insulin, Regular) 1852
None cited in PDR database.

RMS SUPPOSITORIES CII
(Morphine Sulfate) 2766
May interact with narcotic analgesics, general anesthetics, antihistamines, phenothiazines, barbiturates, tranquilizers, hypnotics and sedatives, tricyclic antidepressants, central nervous system depressants, and certain other agents. Compounds in these categories include:

Acrivastine (Additive CNS depressant effect). Products include:
- Semprex-D Capsules 1620

Alfentanil Hydrochloride (Additive CNS depressant effect). Products include:
- Alfenta Injection 1334

Alprazolam (Additive CNS depressant effect). Products include:
- Xanax Tablets 2115

Amitriptyline Hydrochloride (Additive CNS depressant effect). Products include:
- Elavil 2945
- Etrafon 2495
- Limbitrol 2333
- Triavil Tablets 1800

Amoxapine (Additive CNS depressant effect). Products include:
- Asendin Tablets 1419

Aprobarbital (Additive CNS depressant effect).
- No products indexed under this heading.

Astemizole (Additive CNS depressant effect). Products include:
- Hismanal Tablets 1341

Azatadine Maleate (Additive CNS depressant effect). Products include:
- Trinalin Repetabs Tablets 1373

Bromodiphenhydramine Hydrochloride (Additive CNS depressant effect).
- No products indexed under this heading.

Brompheniramine Maleate (Additive CNS depressant effect). Products include:
- Alka-Seltzer Plus Sinus Medicine .. 611
- Bromfed Capsules (Extended-Release) 1832
- Bromfed Syrup 712
- Bromfed Tablets 1832
- Bromfed-DM Cough Syrup 1832
- Bromfed-PD Capsules (Extended-Release) 1832
- Dimetane-DC Cough Syrup 2232
- Dimetane-DX Cough Syrup 2233
- Dimetapp Allergy Dye-Free Elixir 838
- Dimetapp Allergy Sinus Caplets 838
- Dimetapp Cold & Allergy Chewable Tablets 838
- Dimetapp Cold & Cough Liqui-Gels 839
- Dimetapp Cold & Fever Suspension 839
- Dimetapp DM Elixir 840
- Dimetapp Elixir 840
- Dimetapp Extentabs 841
- Dimetapp Tablets/Liqui-Gels 841
- Rondec Chewable Tablets 974
- Vicks DayQuil Allergy Relief 12-Hour Extended Release Tablets.. 733
- Vicks DayQuil Allergy Relief 4-Hour Tablets 733

Buprenorphine (Additive CNS depressant effect). Products include:
- Buprenex Injectable 2170

Buspirone Hydrochloride (Additive CNS depressant effect). Products include:
- BuSpar Tablets 738

Butabarbital (Additive CNS depressant effect).
- No products indexed under this heading.

Butalbital (Additive CNS depressant effect). Products include:
- Axocet Capsules 2469
- Esgic-plus Capsules 1012
- Esgic-plus Tablets 1012
- Fioricet Tablets 2386
- Fioricet with Codeine Capsules 2387
- Fiorinal Capsules 2388
- Fiorinal with Codeine Capsules 2390
- Fiorinal Tablets 2388
- Phrenilin 790
- Sedapap Tablets 50 mg/650 mg .. 1826

Cetirizine Hydrochloride (Additive CNS depressant effect). Products include:
- Zyrtec Tablets 2053

Chlordiazepoxide (Additive CNS depressant effect). Products include:
- Limbitrol 2333

Chlordiazepoxide Hydrochloride (Additive CNS depressant effect). Products include:
- Librax Capsules 2330
- Librium Capsules 2331
- Librium Injectable 2332

Chlorpheniramine Maleate (Additive CNS depressant effect). Products include:
- Alka-Seltzer Plus Cold Medicine 611
- Alka-Seltzer Plus Cold Medicine Liqui-Gels 612
- Alka-Seltzer Plus Cold & Cough Medicine 611
- Alka-Seltzer Plus Cold & Cough Medicine Liqui-Gels 612
- Alka-Seltzer Plus Flu & Body Aches Effervescent Tablets 612
- Allerest Maximum Strength 649
- Allerest Sinus Pain Formula 649
- Ana-Kit Anaphylaxis Emergency Treatment Kit 611
- Atrohist Pediatric Capsules 1603
- Atrohist Plus Tablets 1605
- BC Cold Powder Multi-Symptom Formula (Cold-Sinus-Allergy) 631
- Cerose DM 853
- Cheracol Plus Head Cold/Cough Formula 741
- Children's TYLENOL Cold Multi-Symptom Chewable Tablets and Liquid 1559
- Children's TYLENOL Cold Plus Cough Multi Symptom Chewable Tablets and Liquid 1560
- Children's TYLENOL Flu Suspension Liquid 1560
- Children's Vicks DayQuil Allergy Relief 730
- Children's Vicks NyQuil Cold/Cough Relief 731
- Chlor-Trimeton Allergy Decongestant Tablets 759
- Chlor-Trimeton Allergy Tablets 758
- Allergy-Sinus Comtrex Multi-Symptom Allergy-Sinus Formula Tablets and Caplets 639
- Comtrex Multi-Symptom 638
- Contac Continuous Action Nasal Decongestant/Antihistamine 12 Hour Capsules 773
- Contac Maximum Strength Continuous Action Decongestant/Antihistamine 12 Hour Caplets.. 772
- Contac Severe Cold and Flu Formula Caplets 773
- Coricidin + Cold Tablets 760
- Coricidin Cough + Cold Tablets 760
- Coricidin 'D' Decongestant Tablets 760
- D.A. II Tablets 972
- D.A. Chewable Tablets 970
- Dura-Tap/PD Capsules 970
- Dura-Vent/DA Tablets 972
- Efidac 24 Chlorpheniramine 655
- Extendryl 1003
- Fedahist Gyrocaps 2545
- Hycomine Compound Tablets 948
- Kronofed-A 994
- Nolamine Timed-Release Tablets 790
- Novahistine Elixir 782
- Ornade Spansule Capsules 2678
- PediaCare Cough-Cold Chewable Tablets and Liquid 1569
- PediaCare NightRest Cough-Cold Liquid 1569
- Pediatric Vicks 44m Cough & Cold Relief 737
- Pyrroxate Caplets 742
- Ryna 804
- Sinarest 663
- Sine-Off Sinus Medicine 784
- Singlet Tablets 785
- Sinulin Tablets 792
- Sinutab Sinus Allergy Medication, Maximum Strength Tablets and Caplets 823
- Sudafed Cold & Allergy Tablets 826
- Teldrin 12 Hour Antihistamine/Nasal Decongestant Allergy Relief Capsules 786
- TheraFlu Flu and Cold Medicine 750
- Theraflu Maximum Strength Flu and Cold Medicine For Sore Throat 751
- TheraFlu Flu, Cold and Cough Medicine 750
- TheraFlu Maximum Strength Nighttime Flu, Cold & Cough Medicine 751
- Triaminic Night Time 754
- Triaminic Syrup 755
- Triaminic Triaminicol Cold & Cough 756
- Triaminicin Tablets 756
- Tussend 1830
- TYLENOL Allergy Sinus, Maximum Strength Caplets and Gelcaps 1571
- TYLENOL Cold Medication, Multi-Symptom Formula Tablets and Caplets 1572
- TYLENOL Cold Medication, Multi-Symptom Hot Liquid Packets 1572
- Vicks 44 LiquiCaps Cough, Cold & Flu Relief 728
- Vicks 44M Cough, Cold & Flu Relief 729

Chlorpheniramine Polistirex (Additive CNS depressant effect). Products include:
- Tussionex Pennkinetic Extended-Release Suspension 1624

Chlorpheniramine Tannate (Additive CNS depressant effect). Products include:
- Atrohist Pediatric Suspension 1604
- Atrohist Pediatric Suspension Dye-Free 1604
- Rynatan 2781
- Rynatuss 2782

Chlorpromazine (Additive CNS depressant effect). Products include:
- Thorazine Suppositories 2701

Chlorpromazine Hydrochloride (Additive CNS depressant effect). Products include:
- Thorazine 2701

Chlorprothixene (Additive CNS depressant effect).
- No products indexed under this heading.

Chlorprothixene Hydrochloride (Additive CNS depressant effect).
- No products indexed under this heading.

Chlorprothixene Lactate (Additive CNS depressant effect).
- No products indexed under this heading.

Clemastine Fumarate (Additive CNS depressant effect). Products include:
- Tavist Syrup 2426
- Tavist Tablets 2427
- Tavist-1 12 Hour Relief Tablets 749
- Tavist-D 12 Hour Relief Tablets 750

Clomipramine Hydrochloride (Additive CNS depressant effect). Products include:
- Anafranil Capsules 819

Clorazepate Dipotassium (Additive CNS depressant effect). Products include:
- Tranxene 459

Clozapine (Additive CNS depressant effect). Products include:
- Clozaril Tablets 2377

Codeine Phosphate (Additive CNS depressant effect). Products include:
- Brontex 2130
- Dimetane-DC Cough Syrup 2232
- Fioricet with Codeine Capsules 2387
- Fiorinal with Codeine Capsules 2390
- Nucofed 2225
- Phenergan with Codeine 2883
- Phenergan VC with Codeine 2888
- Robitussin A-C Syrup 2248
- Robitussin-DAC Syrup 2249
- Ryna 804
- Soma Compound w/Codeine Tablets 2784
- Tylenol with Codeine 1592

Interactions Index

Cyproheptadine Hydrochloride (Additive CNS depressant effect). Products include:
- Periactin 1767

Desflurane (Additive CNS depressant effect). Products include:
- Suprane (desflurane, USP) 1865

Desipramine Hydrochloride (Additive CNS depressant effect). Products include:
- Norpramin Tablets 1273

Dexchlorpheniramine Maleate (Additive CNS depressant effect).
- No products indexed under this heading.

Dezocine (Additive CNS depressant effect). Products include:
- Dalgan Injection 529

Diazepam (Additive CNS depressant effect). Products include:
- Dizac (diazepam injectable emulsion) CIV 1862
- Valium Injectable 2336
- Valium Tablets 2335

Diphenhydramine Citrate (Additive CNS depressant effect). Products include:
- Excedrin P.M. Analgesic/Sleeping Aid Tablets, Caplets, Liquigels 735

Diphenhydramine Hydrochloride (Additive CNS depressant effect). Products include:
- Actifed Allergy Daytime/Nighttime Caplets 808
- Actifed Allergy Daytime/Nighttime Tablets and Caplets 809
- Extra Strength Bayer PM Aspirin Plus Sleep Aid 617
- Benadryl Allergy Chewables 811
- Benadryl Allergy/Cold Tablets 811
- Benadryl Allergy Decongestant Liquid Medication 812
- Benadryl Allergy Decongestant Tablets 812
- Benadryl Allergy Liquid Medication 813
- Benadryl Allergy 811
- Benadryl Allergy Sinus Headache Caplets 813
- Benadryl Dye-Free Allergy Liquigel Softgels 813
- Benadryl Dye-Free Allergy Liquid Medication 814
- Benadryl Itch Relief Stick Extra Strength 814
- Benadryl Cream 814
- Benadryl Gel 815
- Benadryl Spray 815
- Benadryl Injection 1955
- Contac Day & Night Cold/Flu Night Caplets 772
- Contac Night Allergy/Sinus Caplets 771
- Extra Strength Doan's P.M. 653
- Excedrin P.M. Analgesic/Sleeping Aid Tablets, Caplets, Liquigels 643
- Nytol QuickCaps Caplets 632
- Sleepinal Night-time Sleep Aid Capsules and Softgels 798
- TYLENOL Allergy Sinus NightTime, Maximum Strength Caplets 1571
- TYLENOL Flu NightTime, Maximum Strength Gelcaps 1575
- TYLENOL Flu NightTime, Maximum Strength Hot Medication Packets 1575
- TYLENOL PM Pain Reliever/Sleep Aid, Extra Strength Gelcaps, Caplets, Geltabs 1576
- TYLENOL Severe Allergy Medication Caplets 1571
- Maximum Strength Unisom Sleepgels 1990
- Unisom With Pain Relief-Nighttime Sleep Aid and Pain Reliever 1991

Diphenylpyraline Hydrochloride (Additive CNS depressant effect).
- No products indexed under this heading.

Doxepin Hydrochloride (Additive CNS depressant effect). Products include:
- Adapin Capsules 1542
- Sinequan 2028
- Zonalon Cream 1042

Droperidol (Additive CNS depressant effect). Products include:
- Inapsine Injection 462

Enflurane (Additive CNS depressant effect).
- No products indexed under this heading.

Estazolam (Additive CNS depressant effect). Products include:
- ProSom Tablets 457

Ethchlorvynol (Additive CNS depressant effect). Products include:
- Placidyl Capsules 456

Ethinamate (Additive CNS depressant effect).
- No products indexed under this heading.

Fentanyl (Additive CNS depressant effect). Products include:
- Duragesic Transdermal System 1336

Fentanyl Citrate (Additive CNS depressant effect). Products include:
- Sublimaze Injection 463

Fluphenazine Decanoate (Additive CNS depressant effect). Products include:
- Prolixin Decanoate 510

Fluphenazine Enanthate (Additive CNS depressant effect). Products include:
- Prolixin Enanthate 510

Fluphenazine Hydrochloride (Additive CNS depressant effect). Products include:
- Prolixin 510

Flurazepam Hydrochloride (Additive CNS depressant effect). Products include:
- Dalmane Capsules 2329

Glutethimide (Additive CNS depressant effect).
- No products indexed under this heading.

Haloperidol (Additive CNS depressant effect). Products include:
- Haldol Injection, Tablets and Concentrate 1585

Haloperidol Decanoate (Additive CNS depressant effect). Products include:
- Haldol Decanoate 1587

Hydrocodone Bitartrate (Additive CNS depressant effect). Products include:
- Codiclear DH Syrup 808
- Duratuss HD Elixir 2750
- Histussin D Liquid 670
- Hycodan Tablets and Syrup 946
- Hycomine Compound Tablets 948
- Hycomine 947
- Hycotuss Expectorant Syrup 950
- Hydrocet Capsules 787
- Lorcet 10/650 Tablets 1016
- Lortab 2751
- Tussend 1830
- Tussend Expectorant 1831
- Vicodin Tablets 1404
- Vicodin ES Tablets 1405
- Vicodin HP Tablets 1403
- Vicodin Tuss Expectorant 1406
- Zydone Capsules 967

Hydrocodone Polistirex (Additive CNS depressant effect). Products include:
- Tussionex Pennkinetic Extended-Release Suspension 1624

Hydromorphone Hydrochloride (Additive CNS depressant effect). Products include:
- Dilaudid Ampules 1382
- Dilaudid Cough Syrup 1383
- Dilaudid-HP Injection 1384
- Dilaudid-HP Lyophilized Powder 250 mg 1384
- Dilaudid 1382
- Dilaudid Oral Liquid 1386
- Dilaudid 1382
- Dilaudid Tablets - 8 mg 1386

Hydroxyzine Hydrochloride (Additive CNS depressant effect). Products include:
- Atarax Tablets & Syrup 1992
- Marax Tablets & DF Syrup 2015
- Vistaril Intramuscular Solution 2042

Imipramine Hydrochloride (Additive CNS depressant effect). Products include:
- Tofranil Ampuls 873
- Tofranil Tablets 875

Imipramine Pamoate (Additive CNS depressant effect). Products include:
- Tofranil-PM Capsules 876

Isoflurane (Additive CNS depressant effect).
- No products indexed under this heading.

Ketamine Hydrochloride (Additive CNS depressant effect).
- No products indexed under this heading.

Levomethadyl Acetate Hydrochloride (Additive CNS depressant effect). Products include:
- Orlaam Oral Solution 2361

Levorphanol Tartrate (Additive CNS depressant effect). Products include:
- Levo-Dromoran 2297

Loratadine (Additive CNS depressant effect). Products include:
- Claritin Tablets 2485
- Claritin-D Tablets 2487

Lorazepam (Additive CNS depressant effect). Products include:
- Ativan Injection 2805
- Ativan Tablets 2807

Loxapine Hydrochloride (Additive CNS depressant effect). Products include:
- Loxitane 1426

Loxapine Succinate (Additive CNS depressant effect). Products include:
- Loxitane Capsules 1426

Maprotiline Hydrochloride (Additive CNS depressant effect). Products include:
- Ludiomil Tablets 861

Meperidine Hydrochloride (Additive CNS depressant effect). Products include:
- Demerol 2438
- Mepergan Injection 2859

Mephobarbital (Additive CNS depressant effect). Products include:
- Mebaral Tablets 2452

Meprobamate (Additive CNS depressant effect). Products include:
- Miltown Tablets 2780
- PMB 200 and PMB 400 2890

Mesoridazine Besylate (Additive CNS depressant effect). Products include:
- Serentil 689

Methadone Hydrochloride (Additive CNS depressant effect). Products include:
- Methadone Hydrochloride Oral Concentrate 2356
- Methadone Hydrochloride Oral Solution & Tablets 2357

Methdilazine Hydrochloride (Additive CNS depressant effect).
- No products indexed under this heading.

Methohexital Sodium (Additive CNS depressant effect).
- No products indexed under this heading.

Methotrimeprazine (Additive CNS depressant effect). Products include:
- Levoprome 1321

Methoxyflurane (Additive CNS depressant effect).
- No products indexed under this heading.

Midazolam Hydrochloride (Additive CNS depressant effect). Products include:
- Versed Injection 2324

Molindone Hydrochloride (Additive CNS depressant effect). Products include:
- Moban Tablets and Concentrate 1036

Nortriptyline Hydrochloride (Additive CNS depressant effect). Products include:
- Pamelor 2409

Opium Alkaloids (Additive CNS depressant effect).
- No products indexed under this heading.

Oxazepam (Additive CNS depressant effect). Products include:
- Serax Capsules 2916
- Serax Tablets 2916

Oxycodone Hydrochloride (Additive CNS depressant effect). Products include:
- OxyContin Tablets 2163
- OxyIR Capsules 2167
- Percocet Tablets 955
- Percodan Tablets 955
- Percodan-Demi Tablets 956
- Roxicodone Tablets, Oral Solution & Intensol (Oxycodone) 2366
- Tylox Capsules 1593

Pentobarbital Sodium (Additive CNS depressant effect). Products include:
- Nembutal Sodium Capsules 440
- Nembutal Sodium Solution 442
- Nembutal Sodium Suppositories 444

Perphenazine (Additive CNS depressant effect). Products include:
- Etrafon 2495
- Triavil Tablets 1800
- Trilafon 2532

Phenobarbital (Additive CNS depressant effect). Products include:
- Arco-Lase Plus Tablets 513
- Bellergal-S Tablets 2375
- Donnatal 2234
- Donnatal Extentabs 2234
- Donnatal Tablets 2234
- Phenobarbital Elixir and Tablets 1523
- Quadrinal Tablets 1398

Prazepam (Additive CNS depressant effect).
- No products indexed under this heading.

Prochlorperazine (Additive CNS depressant effect). Products include:
- Compazine 2644

Promethazine Hydrochloride (Additive CNS depressant effect). Products include:
- Mepergan Injection 2859
- Phenergan with Codeine 2883
- Phenergan with Dextromethorphan 2885
- Phenergan Injection 2880
- Phenergan Suppositories 2882
- Phenergan Syrup 2881
- Phenergan Tablets 2882
- Phenergan VC 2886
- Phenergan VC with Codeine 2888

Propofol (Additive CNS depressant effect). Products include:
- Diprivan Injectable Emulsion 2939

Propoxyphene Hydrochloride (Additive CNS depressant effect). Products include:
- Darvon 1475
- Wygesic Tablets 2930

Propoxyphene Napsylate (Additive CNS depressant effect). Products include:
- Darvon-N/Darvocet-N 1473

Protriptyline Hydrochloride (Additive CNS depressant effect). Products include:
- Vivactil Tablets 1820

IMPORTANT NOTE: Always consult each drug listing in the patient's regimen for possible interactions.

Pyrilamine Maleate (Additive CNS depressant effect). Products include:
   4-Way Fast Acting Nasal Spray (regular & mentholated) 644
   Maximum Strength Multi-Symptom Formula Midol 621
   PMS Multi-Symptom Formula Midol 622

Pyrilamine Tannate (Additive CNS depressant effect). Products include:
   Atrohist Pediatric Suspension 1604
   Atrohist Pediatric Suspension Dye-Free 1604
   Rynatan 2781

Quazepam (Additive CNS depressant effect). Products include:
   Doral Tablets 2773

Risperidone (Additive CNS depressant effect). Products include:
   Risperdal Tablets 1348

Secobarbital Sodium (Additive CNS depressant effect). Products include:
   Seconal Sodium Pulvules 1529

Sevoflurane (Additive CNS depressant effect).
   No products indexed under this heading.

Sufentanil Citrate (Additive CNS depressant effect). Products include:
   Sufenta Injection 1355

Temazepam (Additive CNS depressant effect). Products include:
   Restoril Capsules 2413

Terfenadine (Additive CNS depressant effect). Products include:
   Seldane Tablets 1284
   Seldane-D Extended-Release Tablets 1286

Thiamylal Sodium (Additive CNS depressant effect).
   No products indexed under this heading.

Thioridazine Hydrochloride (Additive CNS depressant effect). Products include:
   Mellaril 2398

Thiothixene (Additive CNS depressant effect). Products include:
   Navane Capsules and Concentrate ... 2018
   Navane Intramuscular 2019

Triazolam (Additive CNS depressant effect). Products include:
   Halcion Tablets 2093

Trifluoperazine Hydrochloride (Additive CNS depressant effect). Products include:
   Stelazine 2692

Trimeprazine Tartrate (Additive CNS depressant effect).
   No products indexed under this heading.

Trimipramine Maleate (Additive CNS depressant effect). Products include:
   Surmontil Capsules 2917

Tripelennamine Hydrochloride (Additive CNS depressant effect). Products include:
   PBZ Tablets 863
   PBZ-SR Tablets 862

Triprolidine Hydrochloride (Additive CNS depressant effect). Products include:
   Actifed Cold & Allergy Tablets 807
   Actifed Cold & Sinus Caplets and Tablets 808

Zolpidem Tartrate (Additive CNS depressant effect). Products include:
   Ambien Tablets 2559

Food Interactions

Alcohol (Additive CNS depressant effect).

RABIES VACCINE ADSORBED
(Rabies Vaccine) 2686
May interact with immunosuppressive agents. Compounds in this category include:

Azathioprine (Interferes with development of active immunity and may reduce the effectiveness of rabies vaccine). Products include:
   Azathioprine Tablets 2349
   Imuran 1103

Cyclosporine (Interferes with development of active immunity and may reduce the effectiveness of rabies vaccine). Products include:
   Neoral 2405
   Sandimmune 2416

Immune Globulin (Human) (Interferes with development of active immunity and may reduce the effectiveness of rabies vaccine).
   No products indexed under this heading.

Immune Globulin Intravenous (Human) (Interferes with development of active immunity and may reduce the effectiveness of rabies vaccine).
   No products indexed under this heading.

Muromonab-CD3 (Interferes with development of active immunity and may reduce the effectiveness of rabies vaccine). Products include:
   Orthoclone OKT3 Sterile Solution .. 1892

Mycophenolate Mofetil (Interferes with development of active immunity and may reduce the effectiveness of rabies vaccine). Products include:
   CellCept Capsules 2265

Tacrolimus (Interferes with development of active immunity and may reduce the effectiveness of rabies vaccine). Products include:
   Prograf 1028

RABIES VACCINE, IMOVAX RABIES I.D.
(Rabies Vaccine) 901
May interact with:

Chloroquine Hydrochloride (Reduced antibody response). Products include:
   Aralen Hydrochloride Injection 2430

Chloroquine Phosphate (Reduced antibody response). Products include:
   Aralen Phosphate Tablets 2431

RECOMBIVAX HB
(Hepatitis B Vaccine) 1787
None cited in PDR database.

RED CROSS TOOTHACHE MEDICATION
(Eugenol) 711
None cited in PDR database.

REDUX CAPSULES
(Dexfenfluramine Hydrochloride) 2911
May interact with monoamine oxidase inhibitors, serotoninergic agents, antimigraine drugs, anorexiants, and certain other agents. Compounds in these categories include:

Amphetamine Resins (Concomitant use with other weight-loss agents is not recommended).
   No products indexed under this heading.

Benzphetamine Hydrochloride (Concomitant use with other weight-loss agents is not recommended).
   No products indexed under this heading.

Dextroamphetamine Sulfate (Concomitant use with other weight-loss agents is not recommended). Products include:
   Adderall Tablets 2209
   Dexedrine 2648
   DextroStat-Dextroamphetamine Sulfate Tablets 2211

Diethylpropion Hydrochloride (Concomitant use with other weight-loss agents is not recommended).
   No products indexed under this heading.

Dihydroergotamine Mesylate ("Serotonin syndrome", a rare, but serious, constellation of symptoms has been reported with the concurrent use of SSRIs and agents for migraine; Redux is a serotonin releaser and reuptake inhibitor, the possibility for serotonin syndrome exists). Products include:
   D.H.E. 45 Injection 2381

Ergotamine Tartrate ("Serotonin syndrome", a rare, but serious, constellation of symptoms has been reported with the concurrent use of SSRIs and agents for migraine; Redux is a serotonin releaser and reuptake inhibitor, the possibility for serotonin syndrome exists). Products include:
   Bellergal-S Tablets 2375
   Cafergot 2376
   Ergomar Tablets 1543
   Wigraine Tablets 1884

Fenfluramine Hydrochloride (Concomitant use with other weight-loss agents is not recommended). Products include:
   Pondimin Tablets 2239

Fluoxetine Hydrochloride (Concurrent and/or sequential use is not recommended with other serotoninergic agents). Products include:
   Prozac Pulvules & Liquid, Oral Solution 935

Fluvoxamine Maleate (Concurrent and/or sequential use is not recommended with other serotoninergic agents). Products include:
   LUVOX Tablets 2723

Furazolidone (Concurrent and/or sequential use is contraindicated). Products include:
   Furoxone 2221

Isocarboxazid (Concurrent and/or sequential use is contraindicated).
   No products indexed under this heading.

Mazindol (Concomitant use with other weight-loss agents is not recommended). Products include:
   Sanorex Tablets 2423

Methamphetamine Hydrochloride (Concomitant use with other weight-loss agents is not recommended). Products include:
   Desoxyn Gradumet Tablets 422

Methysergide Maleate ("Serotonin syndrome", a rare, but serious, constellation of symptoms has been reported with the concurrent use of SSRIs and agents for migraine; Redux is a serotonin releaser and reuptake inhibitor, the possibility for serotonin syndrome exists). Products include:
   Sansert Tablets 2424

Paroxetine Hydrochloride (Concurrent and/or sequential use is not recommended with other serotoninergic agents). Products include:
   Paxil Tablets 2681

Phendimetrazine Tartrate (Concomitant use with other weight-loss agents is not recommended). Products include:
   Bontril Slow-Release Capsules 786
   Prelu-2 Timed Release Capsules 687

Phenelzine Sulfate (Concurrent and/or sequential use is contraindicated). Products include:
   Nardil 1977

Phenmetrazine Hydrochloride (Concomitant use with other weight-loss agents is not recommended).
   No products indexed under this heading.

Selegiline Hydrochloride (Concurrent and/or sequential use is contraindicated). Products include:
   Eldepryl Capsules 2729

Sertraline Hydrochloride (Concurrent and/or sequential use is not recommended with other serotoninergic agents). Products include:
   Zoloft Tablets 2051

Sumatriptan Succinate ("Serotonin syndrome", a rare, but serious, constellation of symptoms has been reported with the concurrent use of SSRIs and agents for migraine; Redux is a serotonin releaser and reuptake inhibitor, the possibility for "serotonin syndrome" exists). Products include:
   Imitrex Injection 1095
   Imitrex Tablets 1099

Tranylcypromine Sulfate (Concurrent and/or sequential use is contraindicated). Products include:
   Parnate Tablets 2679

Venlafaxine Hydrochloride (Concurrent and/or sequential use is not recommended with other serotoninergic agents). Products include:
   Effexor 2825

REFRESH PLUS LUBRICANT EYE DROPS
(Carboxymethylcellulose Sodium) .. 252
None cited in PDR database.

REFRESH PM LUBRICANT EYE OINTMENT
(Petrolatum, White, Mineral Oil) 252
None cited in PDR database.

REGITINE VIALS
(Phentolamine Mesylate) 864
May interact with:

Withhold all medications, except those deemed essential, for at least 24 hours prior to Regitine blocking test for pheochromocytoma.

REGLAN INJECTABLE
(Metoclopramide Hydrochloride) 2243
May interact with anticholinergics, narcotic analgesics, central nervous system depressants, hypnotics and sedatives, tranquilizers, cardiac glycosides, insulin, monoamine oxidase inhibitors, and certain other agents. Compounds in these categories include:

Acetaminophen (Increased rate and/or extent of absorption from the small bowel). Products include:
   Actifed Cold & Sinus Caplets and Tablets 808
   Actifed Sinus Daytime/Nighttime Tablets and Caplets 809
   Alka-Seltzer Fast Relief Caplets 610
   Alka-Seltzer Plus Liqui-Gels 612
   Alka-Seltzer Plus Flu & Body Aches Effervescent Tablets 612
   Alka-Seltzer Plus Flu & Body Aches Liqui-Gels Non-Drowsy Formula 613
   Alka-Seltzer Plus Night-Time Cold Medicine Liqui-Gels 612
   Allerest No Drowsiness 649
   Allerest Sinus Pain Formula 649
   Axocet Capsules 2469
   Benadryl Allergy/Cold Tablets 811

(Described in PDR For Nonprescription Drugs)   (Described in PDR For Ophthalmology)

Benadryl Allergy Sinus Headache Caplets ... 813
Children's TYLENOL acetaminophen Chewable Tablets, Elixir, Suspension Liquid, and Suspension Drops ... 1559
Children's TYLENOL Cold Multi-Symptom Chewable Tablets and Liquid ... 1559
Children's TYLENOL Cold Plus Cough Multi Symptom Chewable Tablets and Liquid ... 1560
Children's TYLENOL Flu Suspension Liquid ... 1560
Allergy-Sinus Comtrex Multi-Symptom Allergy-Sinus Formula Tablets and Caplets ... 639
Comtrex Multi-Symptom ... 638
Comtrex Non-Drowsy ... 640
Contac Day Allergy/Sinus Caplets ... 771
Contac Day & Night ... 772
Contac Night Allergy/Sinus Caplets ... 771
Contac Severe Cold and Flu Formula Caplets ... 773
Contac Severe Cold & Flu Non-Drowsy ... 774
Coricidin Cold + Flu Tablets ... 760
Coricidin 'D' Decongestant Tablets ... 760
DHCplus Capsules ... 2148
Darvon-N/Darvocet-N ... 1473
Dimetapp Allergy Sinus Caplets ... 838
Dimetapp Cold & Fever Suspension ... 839
Drixoral Cold and Flu Extended-Release Tablets ... 764
Drixoral Cough + Sore Throat Liquid Caps ... 763
Drixoral Allergy/Sinus Extended Release Tablets ... 765
Esgic-plus Capsules ... 1012
Esgic-plus Tablets ... 1012
Aspirin Free Excedrin Analgesic Caplets and Geltabs ... 734
Excedrin Extra-Strength Analgesic Tablets, Caplets, and Geltabs ... 734
Excedrin P.M. Analgesic/Sleeping Aid Tablets, Caplets, Liquigels ... 735
Fioricet Tablets ... 2386
Fioricet with Codeine Capsules ... 2387
Goody's Extra Strength Headache Powders ... 632
Goody's Extra Strength Pain Relief Tablets ... 632
Hycomine Compound Tablets ... 948
Hydrocet Capsules ... 787
Infants' TYLENOL acetaminophen Suspension Drops ... 1559
Infants' TYLENOL Cold Decongestant & Fever-Reducer Drops ... 1561
Junior Strength TYLENOL acetaminophen Coated Caplets and Chewable Tablets ... 1562
Lorcet 10/650 Tablets ... 1016
Lortab ... 2751
Lurline PMS Tablets ... 1000
Maximum Strength Multi-Symptom Formula Midol ... 621
PMS Multi-Symptom Formula Midol ... 622
Maximum Strength Midol Teen Multi-Symptom Formula ... 621
Midrin Capsules ... 788
Panodol Tablets and Caplets ... 783
Children's Panadol Chewable Tablets, Liquid, Infant's Drops ... 783
Percocet Tablets ... 955
Percogesic Analgesic Tablets ... 727
Phrenilin ... 790
Pyrroxate Caplets ... 742
Robitussin Cold, Cough & Flu Liqui-Gels ... 844
Robitussin Night-Time Cold Formula ... 847
Sedapap Tablets 50 mg/650 mg ... 1826
Sinarest ... 663
Sine-Aid Maximum Strength Sinus Headache Gelcaps, Caplets and Tablets ... 1570
Sine-Off No Drowsiness Formula Caplets ... 784
Sine-Off Sinus Medicine ... 784
Singlet Tablets ... 785
Sinulin Tablets ... 792
Sinutab Sinus Allergy Medication, Maximum Strength Tablets and Caplets ... 823
Sinutab Sinus Medication, Maximum Strength Without Drowsiness Formula, Tablets & Caplets ... 824
Sudafed Cold and Cough Liquid Caps ... 826
Sudafed Severe Cold Formula Caplets ... 828
Sudafed Severe Cold Formula Tablets ... 828
Sudafed Sinus Caplets ... 829
Sudafed Sinus Tablets ... 829
Talacen Caplets ... 2464
TheraFlu Flu and Cold Medicine ... 750
Theraflu Maximum Strength Flu and Cold Medicine For Sore Throat ... 751
TheraFlu Flu, Cold and Cough Medicine ... 750
TheraFlu Maximum Strength Nighttime Flu, Cold & Cough Medicine ... 751
TheraFlu Maximum Strength Non-Drowsy Formula Flu, Cold & Cough Medicine ... 751
TheraFlu Maximum Strength, Non-Drowsy Formula Flu, Cold and Cough Caplets ... 752
Theraflu Maximum Strength Sinus Non-Drowsy Formula Caplets ... 752
Triaminic Sore Throat Formula ... 755
Triaminicin Tablets ... 756
TYLENOL acetaminophen Extended Relief Caplets ... 1570
TYLENOL acetaminophen, Extra Strength Adult Liquid Pain Reliever ... 1570
TYLENOL acetaminophen, Extra Strength Gelcaps, Geltabs, Caplets, Tablets ... 1570
TYLENOL acetaminophen, Regular Strength Caplets and Tablets ... 1570
TYLENOL Allergy Sinus, Maximum Strength Caplets and Gelcaps ... 1571
TYLENOL Allergy Sinus NightTime, Maximum Strength Caplets ... 1571
TYLENOL Cold Medication, Multi-Symptom Formula Tablets and Caplets ... 1572
TYLENOL Cold Medication, Multi-Symptom Hot Liquid Packets ... 1572
TYLENOL Cold Medication, No Drowsiness Formula Caplets and Gelcaps ... 1572
TYLENOL Cold Severe Congestion Caplets ... 1573
TYLENOL Cough Medication, Multi Symptom ... 1574
TYLENOL Cough Medication with Decongestant, Multi Symptom ... 1574
TYLENOL Flu No Drowsiness Formula, Maximum Strength Gelcaps ... 1575
TYLENOL Flu NightTime, Maximum Strength Gelcaps ... 1575
TYLENOL Flu NightTime, Maximum Strength Hot Medication Packets ... 1575
TYLENOL Headache Plus Pain Reliever with Antacid, Extra Strength Caplets ... 705
TYLENOL PM Pain Reliever/Sleep Aid, Extra Strength Gelcaps, Caplets, Geltabs ... 1576
TYLENOL Severe Allergy Medication Caplets ... 1571
TYLENOL Sinus, Maximum Strength Geltabs, Gelcaps, Caplets and Tablets ... 1576
Tylenol with Codeine ... 1592
Tylox Capsules ... 1593
Unisom With Pain Relief-Nighttime Sleep Aid and Pain Reliever ... 1991
Vanquish Analgesic Caplets ... 627
Vicks 44 LiquiCaps Cough, Cold & Flu Relief ... 728
Vicks 44M Cough, Cold & Flu Relief ... 729
Vicks DayQuil LiquiCaps/Liquid Multi-Symptom Cold/Flu Relief ... 734
Vicks Nyquil Hot Therapy ... 735
Vicks NyQuil LiquiCaps/Liquid Multi-Symptom Cold/Flu Relief, Original and Cherry Flavors ... 736
Vicodin Tablets ... 1404
Vicodin ES Tablets ... 1405
Vicodin HP Tablets ... 1403
Wygesic Tablets ... 2930
Zydone Capsules ... 967

Alfentanil Hydrochloride (Additive sedative effects; antagonizes gastrointestinal motility effects). Products include:
Alfenta Injection ... 1334

Alprazolam (Additive sedative effects). Products include:
Xanax Tablets ... 2115

Aprobarbital (Additive sedative effects).
No products indexed under this heading.

Atropine Sulfate (Antagonizes gastrointestinal motility effects). Products include:
Arco-Lase Plus Tablets ... 513
Atrohist Plus Tablets ... 1605
Donnatal ... 2234
Donnatal Extentabs ... 2234
Donnatal Tablets ... 2234
Lomotil ... 2591
Motofen Tablets ... 789
Urised Tablets ... 2123

Belladonna Alkaloids (Antagonizes gastrointestinal motility effects). Products include:
Bellergal-S Tablets ... 2375
Hyland's Bedwetting Tablets ... 788
Hyland's EnurAid Tablets ... 789
Hyland's Headache Tablets ... 790
Hyland's Teething Tablets ... 790
Similasan Eye Drops #1 ... 769

Benztropine Mesylate (Antagonizes gastrointestinal motility effects). Products include:
Cogentin ... 1661

Biperiden Hydrochloride (Antagonizes gastrointestinal motility effects). Products include:
Akineton ... 1380

Buprenorphine (Additive sedative effects; antagonizes gastrointestinal motility effects). Products include:
Buprenex Injectable ... 2170

Buspirone Hydrochloride (Additive sedative effects). Products include:
BuSpar Tablets ... 738

Butabarbital (Additive sedative effects).
No products indexed under this heading.

Butalbital (Additive sedative effects). Products include:
Axocet Capsules ... 2469
Esgic-plus Capsules ... 1012
Esgic-plus Tablets ... 1012
Fioricet Tablets ... 2386
Fioricet with Codeine Capsules ... 2387
Fiorinal Capsules ... 2388
Fiorinal with Codeine Capsules ... 2390
Fiorinal Tablets ... 2388
Phrenilin ... 790
Sedapap Tablets 50 mg/650 mg ... 1826

Chlordiazepoxide (Additive sedative effects). Products include:
Limbitrol ... 2333

Chlordiazepoxide Hydrochloride (Additive sedative effects). Products include:
Librax Capsules ... 2330
Librium Capsules ... 2331
Librium Injectable ... 2332

Chlorpromazine (Additive sedative effects). Products include:
Thorazine Suppositories ... 2701

Chlorpromazine Hydrochloride (Additive sedative effects). Products include:
Thorazine ... 2701

Chlorprothixene (Additive sedative effects).
No products indexed under this heading.

Chlorprothixene Hydrochloride (Additive sedative effects).
No products indexed under this heading.

Chlorprothixene Lactate (Additive sedative effects; antagonizes gastrointestinal motility effects).
No products indexed under this heading.

Clidinium Bromide (Antagonizes gastrointestinal motility effects). Products include:
Librax Capsules ... 2330

Clorazepate Dipotassium (Additive sedative effects). Products include:
Tranxene ... 459

Clozapine (Additive sedative effects; antagonizes gastrointestinal motility effects). Products include:
Clozaril Tablets ... 2377

Codeine Phosphate (Additive sedative effects; antagonizes gastrointestinal motility effects). Products include:
Brontex ... 2130
Dimetane-DC Cough Syrup ... 2232
Fioricet with Codeine Capsules ... 2387
Fiorinal with Codeine Capsules ... 2390
Nucofed ... 2225
Phenergan with Codeine ... 2883
Phenergan VC with Codeine ... 2888
Robitussin A-C Syrup ... 2248
Robitussin-DAC Syrup ... 2249
Ryna ... 804
Soma Compound w/Codeine Tablets ... 2784
Tylenol with Codeine ... 1592

Cyclosporine (Increased rate and/or extent of absorption from the small bowel). Products include:
Neoral ... 2405
Sandimmune ... 2416

Desflurane (Additive sedative effects; antagonizes gastrointestinal motility effects). Products include:
Suprane (desflurane, USP) ... 1865

Deslanoside (Diminished absorption from the stomach).
No products indexed under this heading.

Dezocine (Additive sedative effects; antagonizes gastrointestinal motility effects). Products include:
Dalgan Injection ... 529

Diazepam (Additive sedative effects). Products include:
Dizac (diazepam injectable emulsion) CIV ... 1862
Valium Injectable ... 2336
Valium Tablets ... 2335

Dicyclomine Hydrochloride (Antagonizes gastrointestinal motility effects). Products include:
Bentyl ... 1246

Digitoxin (Diminished absorption from the stomach). Products include:
Crystodigin Tablets ... 1472

Digoxin (Diminished absorption from the stomach). Products include:
Lanoxicaps ... 1110
Lanoxin Elixir Pediatric ... 1113
Lanoxin Injection ... 1116
Lanoxin Injection Pediatric ... 1119
Lanoxin Tablets ... 1121

Droperidol (Additive sedative effects). Products include:
Inapsine Injection ... 462

Enflurane (Additive sedative effects).
No products indexed under this heading.

Estazolam (Additive sedative effects; antagonizes gastrointestinal motility effects). Products include:
ProSom Tablets ... 457

Ethchlorvynol (Additive sedative effects). Products include:
Placidyl Capsules ... 456

IMPORTANT NOTE: Always consult each drug listing in the patient's regimen for possible interactions.

Reglan Interactions Index 914

Ethinamate (Additive sedative effects).
No products indexed under this heading.
Fentanyl (Additive sedative effects; antagonizes gastrointestinal motility effects). Products include:
Duragesic Transdermal System........ 1336
Fentanyl Citrate (Additive sedative effects; antagonizes gastrointestinal motility effects). Products include:
Sublimaze Injection........ 463
Fluphenazine Decanoate (Additive sedative effects). Products include:
Prolixin Decanoate........ 510
Fluphenazine Enanthate (Additive sedative effects). Products include:
Prolixin Enanthate........ 510
Fluphenazine Hydrochloride (Additive sedative effects). Products include:
Prolixin........ 510
Flurazepam Hydrochloride (Additive sedative effects). Products include:
Dalmane Capsules........ 2329
Furazolidone (Metoclopramide releases catecholamines in patients with essential hypertension hence it should be used cautiously in patients receiving MAO inhibitors). Products include:
Furoxone........ 2221
Glutethimide (Additive sedative effects).
No products indexed under this heading.
Glycopyrrolate (Antagonizes gastrointestinal motility effects). Products include:
Robinul Forte Tablets........ 2247
Robinul Injectable........ 2247
Robinul Tablets........ 2247
Haloperidol (Additive sedative effects). Products include:
Haldol Injection, Tablets and Concentrate........ 1585
Haloperidol Decanoate (Additive sedative effects). Products include:
Haldol Decanoate........ 1587
Hydrocodone Bitartrate (Additive sedative effects; antagonizes gastrointestinal motility effects). Products include:
Codiclear DH Syrup........ 808
Duratuss HD Elixir........ 2750
Histussin D Liquid........ 670
Hycodan Tablets and Syrup........ 946
Hycomine Compound Tablets........ 948
Hycomine........ 947
Hycotuss Expectorant Syrup........ 950
Hydrocet Capsules........ 787
Lorcet 10/650 Tablets........ 1016
Lortab........ 2751
Tussend........ 1830
Tussend Expectorant........ 1831
Vicodin Tablets........ 1404
Vicodin ES Tablets........ 1405
Vicodin HP Tablets........ 1403
Vicodin Tuss Expectorant........ 1406
Zydone Capsules........ 967
Hydrocodone Polistirex (Additive sedative effects; antagonizes gastrointestinal motility effects). Products include:
Tussionex Pennkinetic Extended-Release Suspension........ 1624
Hydromorphone Hydrochloride (Additive sedative effects; antagonizes gastrointestinal motility effects). Products include:
Dilaudid Ampules........ 1382
Dilaudid Cough Syrup........ 1383
Dilaudid-HP Injection........ 1384
Dilaudid-HP Lyophilized Powder 250 mg........ 1384
Dilaudid........ 1382
Dilaudid Oral Liquid........ 1386
Dilaudid........ 1382
Dilaudid Tablets - 8 mg........ 1386
Hydroxyzine Hydrochloride (Additive sedative effects). Products include:
Atarax Tablets & Syrup........ 1992
Marax Tablets & DF Syrup........ 2015
Vistaril Intramuscular Solution........ 2042
Hyoscyamine (Antagonizes gastrointestinal motility effects). Products include:
Cystospaz Tablets........ 2123
Urised Tablets........ 2123
Hyoscyamine Sulfate (Antagonizes gastrointestinal motility effects). Products include:
Arco-Lase Plus Tablets........ 513
Atrohist Plus Tablets........ 1605
Cystospaz-M Capsules........ 2123
Donnatal........ 2234
Donnatal Extentabs........ 2234
Donnatal Tablets........ 2234
Kutrase Capsules........ 2546
Levsin/Levsinex/Levbid........ 2549
Insulin, Human (Exogenous insulin may begin to act before food has left the stomach and lead to hypoglycemia in diabetic patients with gastroparesis; insulin dosage or timing of dosage may require adjustment).
No products indexed under this heading.
Insulin, Human Isophane Suspension (Exogenous insulin may begin to act before food has left the stomach and lead to hypoglycemia in diabetic patients with gastroparesis; insulin dosage or timing of dosage may require adjustment). Products include:
Novolin N Human Insulin 10 ml Vials........ 1846
Insulin, Human NPH (Exogenous insulin may begin to act before food has left the stomach and lead to hypoglycemia in diabetic patients with gastroparesis; insulin dosage or timing of dosage may require adjustment). Products include:
Humulin N, 100 Units........ 1495
Novolin N PenFill 1.5 ml Cartridges Durable Insulin Delivery System........ 1849
Novolin N Prefilled Syringe Disposable Insulin Delivery System........ 1850
Insulin, Human Regular (Exogenous insulin may begin to act before food has left the stomach and lead to hypoglycemia in diabetic patients with gastroparesis; insulin dosage or timing of dosage may require adjustment). Products include:
Humulin R, 100 Units........ 1497
Novolin R Human Insulin 10 ml Vials........ 1846
Novolin R PenFill 1.5 ml Cartridges Durable Insulin Delivery System........ 1849
Novolin R Prefilled Syringe Disposable Insulin Delivery System........ 1850
Velosulin BR Human Insulin 10 ml Vials........ 1847
Insulin, Human, Zinc Suspension (Exogenous insulin may begin to act before food has left the stomach and lead to hypoglycemia in diabetic patients with gastroparesis; insulin dosage or timing of dosage may require adjustment). Products include:
Humulin L, 100 Units........ 1494
Humulin U, 100 Units........ 1498
Novolin L Human Insulin 10 ml Vials........ 1846
Insulin Lispro, Human (Exogenous insulin may begin to act before food has left the stomach and lead to hypoglycemia in diabetic patients with gastroparesis; insulin dosage or timing of dosage may require adjustment). Products include:
Humalog Injection........ 1488
Insulin, NPH (Exogenous insulin may begin to act before food has left the stomach and lead to hypoglycemia in diabetic patients with gastroparesis; insulin dosage or timing of dosage may require adjustment). Products include:
NPH, 100 Units........ 1502
Pork NPH, 100 Units........ 1506
Purified Pork NPH Isophane Insulin........ 1852
Insulin, Regular (Exogenous insulin may begin to act before food has left the stomach and lead to hypoglycemia in diabetic patients with gastroparesis; insulin dosage or timing of dosage may require adjustment). Products include:
Regular, 100 Units........ 1503
Pork Regular, 100 Units........ 1507
Pork Regular (Concentrated), 500 Units........ 1508
Purified Pork Regular Insulin........ 1852
Insulin, Zinc Crystals (Exogenous insulin may begin to act before food has left the stomach and lead to hypoglycemia in diabetic patients with gastroparesis; insulin dosage or timing of dosage may require adjustment). Products include:
NPH, 100 Units........ 1502
Insulin, Zinc Suspension (Exogenous insulin may begin to act before food has left the stomach and lead to hypoglycemia in diabetic patients with gastroparesis; insulin dosage or timing of dosage may require adjustment). Products include:
Iletin I........ 1501
Lente, 100 Units........ 1501
Iletin II........ 1504
Pork Lente, 100 Units........ 1504
Purified Pork Lente Insulin........ 1852
Ipratropium Bromide (Antagonizes gastrointestinal motility effects). Products include:
Atrovent Inhalation Aerosol........ 674
Atrovent Inhalation Solution........ 675
Atrovent Nasal Spray 0.03%........ 676
Atrovent Nasal Spray 0.06%........ 678
Isocarboxazid (Metoclopramide releases catecholamines in patients with essential hypertension hence it should be used cautiously in patients receiving MAO inhibitors).
No products indexed under this heading.
Ketamine Hydrochloride (Additive sedative effects; antagonizes gastrointestinal motility effects).
No products indexed under this heading.
Levodopa (Increased rate and/or extent of absorption from the small bowel). Products include:
Atamet Tablets........ 567
Larodopa Tablets........ 2296
Sinemet Tablets........ 959
Sinemet CR Tablets........ 961
Levomethadyl Acetate Hydrochloride (Additive sedative effects; antagonizes gastrointestinal motility effects). Products include:
Orlaam Oral Solution........ 2361
Levorphanol Tartrate (Additive sedative effects; antagonizes gastrointestinal motility effects). Products include:
Levo-Dromoran........ 2297
Lorazepam (Additive sedative effects). Products include:
Ativan Injection........ 2805
Ativan Tablets........ 2807
Loxapine Hydrochloride (Additive sedative effects). Products include:
Loxitane........ 1426
Loxapine Succinate (Additive sedative effects; antagonizes gastrointestinal motility effects). Products include:
Loxitane Capsules........ 1426
Mepenzolate Bromide (Antagonizes gastrointestinal motility effects).
No products indexed under this heading.
Meperidine Hydrochloride (Additive sedative effects; antagonizes gastrointestinal motility effects). Products include:
Demerol........ 2438
Mepergan Injection........ 2859
Mephobarbital (Additive sedative effects). Products include:
Mebaral Tablets........ 2452
Meprobamate (Additive sedative effects). Products include:
Miltown Tablets........ 2780
PMB 200 and PMB 400........ 2890
Mesoridazine Besylate (Additive sedative effects). Products include:
Serentil........ 689
Methadone Hydrochloride (Additive sedative effects; antagonizes gastrointestinal motility effects). Products include:
Methadone Hydrochloride Oral Concentrate........ 2356
Methadone Hydrochloride Oral Solution & Tablets........ 2357
Methohexital Sodium (Additive sedative effects).
No products indexed under this heading.
Methotrimeprazine (Additive sedative effects; antagonizes gastrointestinal motility effects). Products include:
Levoprome........ 1321
Methoxyflurane (Additive sedative effects).
No products indexed under this heading.
Midazolam Hydrochloride (Additive sedative effects). Products include:
Versed Injection........ 2324
Molindone Hydrochloride (Additive sedative effects). Products include:
Moban Tablets and Concentrate........ 1036
Morphine Sulfate (Additive sedative effects; antagonizes gastrointestinal motility effects). Products include:
Astramorph/PF Injection, USP (Preservative-Free)........ 526
Duramorph Injection........ 983
Infumorph 200 and Infumorph 500 Sterile Solutions........ 985
Kadian Capsules........ 2948
MS Contin Tablets........ 2149
MSIR........ 2152
Oramorph SR (Morphine Sulfate Sustained Release Tablets)........ 2359
RMS Suppositories CII........ 2766
Roxanol........ 2365
Opium Alkaloids (Additive sedative effects; antagonizes gastrointestinal motility effects).
No products indexed under this heading.
Oxazepam (Additive sedative effects). Products include:
Serax Capsules........ 2916
Serax Tablets........ 2916
Oxybutynin Chloride (Antagonizes gastrointestinal motility effects). Products include:
Ditropan........ 1267
Oxycodone Hydrochloride (Additive sedative effects; antagonizes gastrointestinal motility effects). Products include:
OxyContin Tablets........ 2163

OxyIR Capsules 2167
Percocet Tablets 955
Percodan Tablets 955
Percodan-Demi Tablets 956
Roxicodone Tablets, Oral Solution
 & Intensol (Oxycodone) 2366
Tylox Capsules 1593

Pentobarbital Sodium (Additive sedative effects). Products include:
Nembutal Sodium Capsules 440
Nembutal Sodium Solution 442
Nembutal Sodium Suppositories ... 444

Perphenazine (Additive sedative effects). Products include:
Etrafon 2495
Triavil Tablets 1800
Trilafon 2532

Phenelzine Sulfate (Metoclopramide releases catecholamines in patients with essential hypertension hence it should be used cautiously in patients receiving MAO inhibitors). Products include:
Nardil 1977

Phenobarbital (Additive sedative effects). Products include:
Arco-Lase Plus Tablets 513
Bellergal-S Tablets 2375
Donnatal 2234
Donnatal Extentabs 2234
Donnatal Tablets 2234
Phenobarbital Elixir and Tablets 1523
Quadrinal Tablets 1398

Prazepam (Additive sedative effects).
No products indexed under this heading.

Prochlorperazine (Additive sedative effects). Products include:
Compazine 2644

Procyclidine Hydrochloride (Antagonizes gastrointestinal motility effects). Products include:
Kemadrin Tablets 1105

Promethazine Hydrochloride (Additive sedative effects). Products include:
Mepergan Injection 2859
Phenergan with Codeine 2883
Phenergan with Dextromethorphan 2885
Phenergan Injection 2880
Phenergan Suppositories 2882
Phenergan Syrup 2881
Phenergan Tablets 2882
Phenergan VC 2886
Phenergan VC with Codeine 2888

Propantheline Bromide (Antagonizes gastrointestinal motility effects). Products include:
Pro-Banthine Tablets 2226

Propofol (Additive sedative effects; antagonizes gastrointestinal motility effects). Products include:
Diprivan Injectable Emulsion 2939

Propoxyphene Hydrochloride (Additive sedative effects; antagonizes gastrointestinal motility effects). Products include:
Darvon 1475
Wygesic Tablets 2930

Propoxyphene Napsylate (Additive sedative effects; antagonizes gastrointestinal motility effects). Products include:
Darvon-N/Darvocet-N 1473

Quazepam (Additive sedative effects; antagonizes gastrointestinal motility effects). Products include:
Doral Tablets 2773

Risperidone (Additive sedative effects; antagonizes gastrointestinal motility effects). Products include:
Risperdal Tablets 1348

Scopolamine (Antagonizes gastrointestinal motility effects). Products include:
Transderm Scōp Transdermal Therapeutic System 890

Scopolamine Hydrobromide (Antagonizes gastrointestinal motility effects). Products include:
Atrohist Plus Tablets 1605
Donnatal 2234
Donnatal Extentabs 2234
Donnatal Tablets 2234

Secobarbital Sodium (Additive sedative effects; antagonizes gastrointestinal motility effects). Products include:
Seconal Sodium Pulvules 1529

Selegiline Hydrochloride (Metoclopramide releases catecholamines in patients with essential hypertension hence it should be used cautiously in patients receiving MAO inhibitors). Products include:
Eldepryl Capsules 2729

Sevoflurane (Additive sedative effects; antagonizes gastrointestinal motility effects).
No products indexed under this heading.

Sufentanil Citrate (Additive sedative effects; antagonizes gastrointestinal motility effects). Products include:
Sufenta Injection 1355

Temazepam (Additive sedative effects). Products include:
Restoril Capsules 2413

Tetracycline Hydrochloride (Increased rate and/or extent of absorption from the small bowel). Products include:
Achromycin V Capsules 1417
Helidac Therapy 2135

Thiamylal Sodium (Additive sedative effects).
No products indexed under this heading.

Thioridazine Hydrochloride (Additive sedative effects). Products include:
Mellaril 2398

Thiothixene (Additive sedative effects). Products include:
Navane Capsules and Concentrate 2018
Navane Intramuscular 2019

Tranylcypromine Sulfate (Metoclopramide releases catecholamines in patients with essential hypertension hence it should be used cautiously in patients receiving MAO inhibitors). Products include:
Parnate Tablets 2679

Triazolam (Additive sedative effects). Products include:
Halcion Tablets 2093

Tridihexethyl Chloride (Antagonizes gastrointestinal motility effects).
No products indexed under this heading.

Trifluoperazine Hydrochloride (Additive sedative effects). Products include:
Stelazine 2692

Trihexyphenidyl Hydrochloride (Antagonizes gastrointestinal motility effects). Products include:
Artane 1418

Zolpidem Tartrate (Additive sedative effects; antagonizes gastrointestinal motility effects). Products include:
Ambien Tablets 2559

Food Interactions

Alcohol (Increased rate and/or extent of absorption from the small bowel; additive sedative effects).

REGLAN SYRUP
(Metoclopramide Hydrochloride) 2243
See Reglan Injectable

REGLAN TABLETS
(Metoclopramide Hydrochloride) 2243
See Reglan Injectable

REHYDRALYTE ORAL ELECTROLYTE REHYDRATION SOLUTION
(Electrolyte Supplement) 2344
None cited in PDR database.

REJUVEX
(Vitamins with Minerals) 791
None cited in PDR database.

RELAFEN TABLETS
(Nabumetone) 2688
May interact with highly protein bound drugs (selected). Compounds in this category include:

Amiodarone Hydrochloride (In vitro studies have shown that 6 MNA, an active metabolite of nabumetone, may displace other protein bound drugs from their binding site). Products include:
Cordarone Intravenous 2821
Cordarone Tablets 2818

Amitriptyline Hydrochloride (In vitro studies have shown that 6 MNA, an active metabolite of nabumetone, may displace other protein bound drugs from their binding site). Products include:
Elavil 2945
Etrafon 2495
Limbitrol 2333
Triavil Tablets 1800

Atovaquone (In vitro studies have shown that 6 MNA, an active metabolite of nabumetone, may displace other protein bound drugs from their binding site). Products include:
Mepron Suspension 1206

Cefonicid Sodium (In vitro studies have shown that 6 MNA, an active metabolite of nabumetone, may displace other protein bound drugs from their binding site). Products include:
Monocid Injection 2674

Chlordiazepoxide (In vitro studies have shown that 6 MNA, an active metabolite of nabumetone, may displace other protein bound drugs from their binding site). Products include:
Limbitrol 2333

Chlordiazepoxide Hydrochloride (In vitro studies have shown that 6 MNA, an active metabolite of nabumetone, may displace other protein bound drugs from their binding site). Products include:
Librax Capsules 2330
Librium Capsules 2331
Librium Injectable 2332

Chlorpromazine (In vitro studies have shown that 6 MNA, an active metabolite of nabumetone, may displace other protein bound drugs from their binding site). Products include:
Thorazine Suppositories 2701

Chlorpromazine Hydrochloride (In vitro studies have shown that 6 MNA, an active metabolite of nabumetone, may displace other protein bound drugs from their binding site). Products include:
Thorazine 2701

Clomipramine Hydrochloride (In vitro studies have shown that 6 MNA, an active metabolite of nabumetone, may displace other protein bound drugs from their binding site). Products include:
Anafranil Capsules 819

Clozapine (In vitro studies have shown that 6 MNA, an active metabolite of nabumetone, may displace other protein bound drugs from their binding site). Products include:
Clozaril Tablets 2377

Cyclosporine (In vitro studies have shown that 6 MNA, an active metabolite of nabumetone, may displace other protein bound drugs from their binding site). Products include:
Neoral 2405
Sandimmune 2416

Diazepam (In vitro studies have shown that 6 MNA, an active metabolite of nabumetone, may displace other protein bound drugs from their binding site). Products include:
Dizac (diazepam injectable emulsion) CIV 1862
Valium Injectable 2336
Valium Tablets 2335

Diclofenac Potassium (In vitro studies have shown that 6 MNA, an active metabolite of nabumetone, may displace other protein bound drugs from their binding site). Products include:
Cataflam Tablets 833

Diclofenac Sodium (In vitro studies have shown that 6 MNA, an active metabolite of nabumetone, may displace other protein bound drugs from their binding site). Products include:
Voltaren Ophthalmic Sterile Ophthalmic Solution 264
Cataflam/Voltaren/Voltaren-XR ... 833

Dipyridamole (In vitro studies have shown that 6 MNA, an active metabolite of nabumetone, may displace other protein bound drugs from their binding site). Products include:
Persantine Tablets 686

Fenoprofen Calcium (In vitro studies have shown that 6 MNA, an active metabolite of nabumetone, may displace other protein bound drugs from their binding site). Products include:
Nalfon 200 Pulvules & Nalfon Tablets 933

Flurazepam Hydrochloride (In vitro studies have shown that 6 MNA, an active metabolite of nabumetone, may displace other protein bound drugs from their binding site). Products include:
Dalmane Capsules 2329

Flurbiprofen (In vitro studies have shown that 6 MNA, an active metabolite of nabumetone, may displace other protein bound drugs from their binding site).
No products indexed under this heading.

Glipizide (In vitro studies have shown that 6 MNA, an active metabolite of nabumetone, may displace other protein bound drugs from their binding site). Products include:
Glucotrol Tablets 2011
Glucotrol XL Extended Release Tablets 2012

Ibuprofen (In vitro studies have shown that 6 MNA, an active metabolite of nabumetone, may displace other protein bound drugs from their binding site). Products include:
Advil Cold and Sinus Caplets and Tablets 837
Advil Ibuprofen Tablets, Caplets and Gel Caplets 836
Children's Motrin Ibuprofen Oral Suspension 1558
IBU Tablets 1389
Ibuprohm 713

IMPORTANT NOTE: Always consult each drug listing in the patient's regimen for possible interactions.

Motrin IB Caplets, Tablets, and Gelcaps ▣ 802
Motrin Ibuprofen Suspension, Oral Drops, Chewable Tablets, Caplets 1563
Nuprin Ibuprofen/Analgesic Tablets & Caplets ▣ 645
Vicks DayQuil SINUS Pressure & PAIN Relief with IBUPROFEN ▣ 735

Imipramine Hydrochloride (In vitro studies have shown that 6 MNA, an active metabolite of nabumetone, may displace other protein bound drugs from their binding site). Products include:
Tofranil Ampuls 873
Tofranil Tablets 875

Imipramine Pamoate (In vitro studies have shown that 6 MNA, an active metabolite of nabumetone, may displace other protein bound drugs from their binding site). Products include:
Tofranil-PM Capsules 876

Indomethacin (In vitro studies have shown that 6 MNA, an active metabolite of nabumetone, may displace other protein bound drugs from their binding site). Products include:
Indocin 1723

Indomethacin Sodium Trihydrate (In vitro studies have shown that 6 MNA, an active metabolite of nabumetone, may displace other protein bound drugs from their binding site). Products include:
Indocin I.V. 1727

Ketoprofen (In vitro studies have shown that 6 MNA, an active metabolite of nabumetone, may displace other protein bound drugs from their binding site). Products include:
Actron Caplets and Tablets ▣ 608
Orudis Capsules 2874
Orudis KT ▣ 842
Oruvail Capsules 2874

Ketorolac Tromethamine (In vitro studies have shown that 6 MNA, an active metabolite of nabumetone, may displace other protein bound drugs from their binding site). Products include:
Acular Sterile Ophthalmic Solution 470
Toradol 2319

Meclofenamate Sodium (In vitro studies have shown that 6 MNA, an active metabolite of nabumetone, may displace other protein bound drugs from their binding site).
No products indexed under this heading.

Mefenamic Acid (In vitro studies have shown that 6 MNA, an active metabolite of nabumetone, may displace other protein bound drugs from their binding site). Products include:
Ponstel 1982

Midazolam Hydrochloride (In vitro studies have shown that 6 MNA, an active metabolite of nabumetone, may displace other protein bound drugs from their binding site). Products include:
Versed Injection 2324

Naproxen (In vitro studies have shown that 6 MNA, an active metabolite of nabumetone, may displace other protein bound drugs from their binding site). Products include:
Anaprox/Naprosyn 2277

Naproxen Sodium (In vitro studies have shown that 6 MNA, an active metabolite of nabumetone, may displace other protein bound drugs from their binding site). Products include:
Aleve 2124
Anaprox/Naprosyn 2277
Naprelan Tablets 2861

Nortriptyline Hydrochloride (In vitro studies have shown that 6 MNA, an active metabolite of nabumetone, may displace other protein bound drugs from their binding site). Products include:
Pamelor 2409

Oxaprozin (In vitro studies have shown that 6 MNA, an active metabolite of nabumetone, may displace other protein bound drugs from their binding site). Products include:
Daypro Caplets 2578

Oxazepam (In vitro studies have shown that 6 MNA, an active metabolite of nabumetone, may displace other protein bound drugs from their binding site). Products include:
Serax Capsules 2916
Serax Tablets 2916

Phenylbutazone (In vitro studies have shown that 6 MNA, an active metabolite of nabumetone, may displace other protein bound drugs from their binding site).
No products indexed under this heading.

Piroxicam (In vitro studies have shown that 6 MNA, an active metabolite of nabumetone, may displace other protein bound drugs from their binding site). Products include:
Feldene Capsules 2008

Propranolol Hydrochloride (In vitro studies have shown that 6 MNA, an active metabolite of nabumetone, may displace other protein bound drugs from their binding site). Products include:
Inderal 2834
Inderal LA Long Acting Capsules 2836
Inderide Tablets 2838
Inderide LA Long Acting Capsules 2840

Sulindac (In vitro studies have shown that 6 MNA, an active metabolite of nabumetone, may displace other protein bound drugs from their binding site). Products include:
Clinoril Tablets 1658

Temazepam (In vitro studies have shown that 6 MNA, an active metabolite of nabumetone, may displace other protein bound drugs from their binding site). Products include:
Restoril Capsules 2413

Tolbutamide (In vitro studies have shown that 6 MNA, an active metabolite of nabumetone, may displace other protein bound drugs from their binding site).
No products indexed under this heading.

Tolmetin Sodium (In vitro studies have shown that 6 MNA, an active metabolite of nabumetone, may displace other protein bound drugs from their binding site). Products include:
Tolectin (200, 400 and 600 mg) 1591

Trimipramine Maleate (In vitro studies have shown that 6 MNA, an active metabolite of nabumetone, may displace other protein bound drugs from their binding site). Products include:
Surmontil Capsules 2917

Warfarin Sodium (Effects not specified; caution should be exercised; in vitro studies have shown that 6 MNA, an active metabolite of nabumetone, may displace other protein bound drugs from their binding site). Products include:
Coumadin 941

Food Interactions

Dairy products (Potential for more rapid absorption, however, the total amount of GMNA in the plasma is unchanged).

Food, unspecified (Potential for more rapid absorption, however, the total amount of GMNA in the plasma is unchanged).

REMERON TABLETS

(Mirtazapine) 1878
May interact with central nervous system depressants, monoamine oxidase inhibitors, and certain other agents. Compounds in these categories include:

Alfentanil Hydrochloride (Co-administration may result in an additive impairment of motor skills). Products include:
Alfenta Injection 1334

Alprazolam (Co-administration may result in an additive impairment of motor skills). Products include:
Xanax Tablets 2115

Aprobarbital (Co-administration may result in an additive impairment of motor skills).
No products indexed under this heading.

Buprenorphine (Co-administration may result in an additive impairment of motor skills). Products include:
Buprenex Injectable 2170

Buspirone Hydrochloride (Co-administration may result in an additive impairment of motor skills). Products include:
BuSpar Tablets 738

Butabarbital (Co-administration may result in an additive impairment of motor skills).
No products indexed under this heading.

Butalbital (Co-administration may result in an additive impairment of motor skills). Products include:
Axocet Capsules 2469
Esgic-plus Capsules 1012
Esgic-plus Tablets 1012
Fioricet Tablets 2386
Fioricet with Codeine Capsules 2387
Fiorinal Capsules 2388
Fiorinal with Codeine Capsules 2390
Fiorinal Tablets 2388
Phrenilin 790
Sedapap Tablets 50 mg/650 mg 1826

Chlordiazepoxide (Co-administration may result in an additive impairment of motor skills). Products include:
Limbitrol 2333

Chlordiazepoxide Hydrochloride (Co-administration may result in an additive impairment of motor skills). Products include:
Librax Capsules 2330
Librium Capsules 2331
Librium Injectable 2332

Chlorpromazine (Co-administration may result in an additive impairment of motor skills). Products include:
Thorazine Suppositories 2701

Chlorpromazine Hydrochloride (Co-administration may result in an additive impairment of motor skills). Products include:
Thorazine 2701

Chlorprothixene (Co-administration may result in an additive impairment of motor skills).
No products indexed under this heading.

Chlorprothixene Hydrochloride (Co-administration may result in an additive impairment of motor skills).
No products indexed under this heading.

Chlorprothixene Lactate (Co-administration may result in an additive impairment of motor skills).
No products indexed under this heading.

Clorazepate Dipotassium (Co-administration may result in an additive impairment of motor skills). Products include:
Tranxene 459

Clozapine (Co-administration may result in an additive impairment of motor skills). Products include:
Clozaril Tablets 2377

Codeine Phosphate (Co-administration may result in an additive impairment of motor skills). Products include:
Brontex 2130
Dimetane-DC Cough Syrup 2232
Fioricet with Codeine Capsules 2387
Fiorinal with Codeine Capsules 2390
Nucofed 2225
Phenergan with Codeine 2883
Phenergan VC with Codeine 2888
Robitussin A-C Syrup 2248
Robitussin-DAC Syrup 2249
Ryna ▣ 804
Soma Compound w/Codeine Tablets 2784
Tylenol with Codeine 1592

Desflurane (Co-administration may result in an additive impairment of motor skills). Products include:
Suprane (desflurane, USP) 1865

Dezocine (Co-administration may result in an additive impairment of motor skills). Products include:
Dalgan Injection 529

Diazepam (Co-administration has shown to result in an additive impairment of motor skills). Products include:
Dizac (diazepam injectable emulsion) CIV 1862
Valium Injectable 2336
Valium Tablets 2335

Droperidol (Co-administration may result in an additive impairment of motor skills). Products include:
Inapsine Injection 462

Enflurane (Co-administration may result in an additive impairment of motor skills).
No products indexed under this heading.

Estazolam (Co-administration may result in an additive impairment of motor skills). Products include:
ProSom Tablets 457

Ethchlorvynol (Co-administration may result in an additive impairment of motor skills). Products include:
Placidyl Capsules 456

Ethinamate (Co-administration may result in an additive impairment of motor skills).
No products indexed under this heading.

Fentanyl (Co-administration may result in an additive impairment of motor skills). Products include:
Duragesic Transdermal System 1336

Fentanyl Citrate (Co-administration may result in an additive impairment of motor skills). Products include:
Sublimaze Injection 463

Fluphenazine Decanoate (Co-administration may result in an additive impairment of motor skills). Products include:
Prolixin Decanoate 510

(▣ Described in PDR For Nonprescription Drugs) (◉ Described in PDR For Ophthalmology)

917 **Interactions Index** **Remeron**

Fluphenazine Enanthate (Co-administration may result in an additive impairment of motor skills). Products include:
Prolixin Enanthate 510

Fluphenazine Hydrochloride (Co-administration may result in an additive impairment of motor skills). Products include:
Prolixin 510

Flurazepam Hydrochloride (Co-administration may result in an additive impairment of motor skills). Products include:
Dalmane Capsules 2329

Furazolidone (Co-administration of antidepressants and MAO inhibitors has resulted in serious, and sometimes fatal, reactions including hyperthermia, autonomic instability, seizures, agitation, and coma; concurrent and/or sequential use is contraindicated). Products include:
Furoxone 2221

Glutethimide (Co-administration may result in an additive impairment of motor skills).
No products indexed under this heading.

Haloperidol (Co-administration may result in an additive impairment of motor skills). Products include:
Haldol Injection, Tablets and Concentrate 1585

Haloperidol Decanoate (Co-administration may result in an additive impairment of motor skills). Products include:
Haldol Decanoate 1587

Hydrocodone Bitartrate (Co-administration may result in an additive impairment of motor skills). Products include:
Codiclear DH Syrup 808
Duratuss HD Elixir 2750
Histussin D Liquid 670
Hycodan Tablets and Syrup 946
Hycomine Compound Tablets 948
Hycomine 947
Hycotuss Expectorant Syrup 950
Hydrocet Capsules 787
Lorcet 10/650 Tablets 1016
Lortab 2751
Tussend 1830
Tussend Expectorant 1831
Vicodin Tablets 1404
Vicodin ES Tablets 1405
Vicodin HP Tablets 1403
Vicodin Tuss Expectorant 1406
Zydone Capsules 967

Hydrocodone Polistirex (Co-administration may result in an additive impairment of motor skills). Products include:
Tussionex Pennkinetic Extended-Release Suspension 1624

Hydromorphone Hydrochloride (Co-administration may result in an additive impairment of motor skills). Products include:
Dilaudid Ampules 1382
Dilaudid Cough Syrup 1383
Dilaudid-HP Injection 1384
Dilaudid-HP Lyophilized Powder 250 mg 1384
Dilaudid 1382
Dilaudid Oral Liquid 1386
Dilaudid 1382
Dilaudid Tablets - 8 mg 1386

Hydroxyzine Hydrochloride (Co-administration may result in an additive impairment of motor skills). Products include:
Atarax Tablets & Syrup 1992
Marax Tablets & DF Syrup 2015
Vistaril Intramuscular Solution 2042

Isocarboxazid (Co-administration of antidepressants and MAO inhibitors has resulted in serious, and sometimes fatal, reactions including hyperthermia, autonomic instability, seizures, agitation, and coma; concurrent and/or sequential use is contraindicated).
No products indexed under this heading.

Isoflurane (Co-administration may result in an additive impairment of motor skills).
No products indexed under this heading.

Ketamine Hydrochloride (Co-administration may result in an additive impairment of motor skills).
No products indexed under this heading.

Levomethadyl Acetate Hydrochloride (Co-administration may result in an additive impairment of motor skills). Products include:
Orlaam Oral Solution 2361

Levorphanol Tartrate (Co-administration may result in an additive impairment of motor skills). Products include:
Levo-Dromoran 2297

Lorazepam (Co-administration may result in an additive impairment of motor skills). Products include:
Ativan Injection 2805
Ativan Tablets 2807

Loxapine Hydrochloride (Co-administration may result in an additive impairment of motor skills). Products include:
Loxitane 1426

Loxapine Succinate (Co-administration may result in an additive impairment of motor skills). Products include:
Loxitane Capsules 1426

Meperidine Hydrochloride (Co-administration may result in an additive impairment of motor skills). Products include:
Demerol 2438
Mepergan Injection 2859

Mephobarbital (Co-administration may result in an additive impairment of motor skills). Products include:
Mebaral Tablets 2452

Meprobamate (Co-administration may result in an additive impairment of motor skills). Products include:
Miltown Tablets 2780
PMB 200 and PMB 400 2890

Mesoridazine Besylate (Co-administration may result in an additive impairment of motor skills). Products include:
Serentil 689

Methadone Hydrochloride (Co-administration may result in an additive impairment of motor skills). Products include:
Methadone Hydrochloride Oral Concentrate 2356
Methadone Hydrochloride Oral Solution & Tablets 2357

Methohexital Sodium (Co-administration may result in an additive impairment of motor skills).
No products indexed under this heading.

Methotrimeprazine (Co-administration may result in an additive impairment of motor skills). Products include:
Levoprome 1321

Methoxyflurane (Co-administration may result in an additive impairment of motor skills).
No products indexed under this heading.

Midazolam Hydrochloride (Co-administration may result in an additive impairment of motor skills). Products include:
Versed Injection 2324

Molindone Hydrochloride (Co-administration may result in an additive impairment of motor skills). Products include:
Moban Tablets and Concentrate 1036

Morphine Sulfate (Co-administration may result in an additive impairment of motor skills). Products include:
Astramorph/PF Injection, USP (Preservative-Free) 526
Duramorph Injection 983
Infumorph 200 and Infumorph 500 Sterile Solutions 985
Kadian Capsules 2948
MS Contin Tablets 2149
MSIR 2152
Oramorph SR (Morphine Sulfate Sustained Release Tablets) 2359
RMS Suppositories CII 2766
Roxanol 2365

Opium Alkaloids (Co-administration may result in an additive impairment of motor skills).
No products indexed under this heading.

Oxazepam (Co-administration may result in an additive impairment of motor skills). Products include:
Serax Capsules 2916
Serax Tablets 2916

Oxycodone Hydrochloride (Co-administration may result in an additive impairment of motor skills). Products include:
OxyContin Tablets 2163
OxyIR Capsules 2167
Percocet Tablets 955
Percodan Tablets 955
Percodan-Demi Tablets 956
Roxicodone Tablets, Oral Solution & Intensol (Oxycodone) 2366
Tylox Capsules 1593

Pentobarbital Sodium (Co-administration may result in an additive impairment of motor skills). Products include:
Nembutal Sodium Capsules 440
Nembutal Sodium Solution 442
Nembutal Sodium Suppositories 444

Perphenazine (Co-administration may result in an additive impairment of motor skills). Products include:
Etrafon 2495
Triavil Tablets 1800
Trilafon 2532

Phenelzine Sulfate (Co-administration of antidepressants and MAO inhibitors has resulted in serious, and sometimes fatal, reactions including hyperthermia, autonomic instability, seizures, agitation, and coma; concurrent and/or sequential use is contraindicated). Products include:
Nardil 1977

Phenobarbital (Co-administration may result in an additive impairment of motor skills). Products include:
Arco-Lase Plus Tablets 513
Bellergal-S Tablets 2375
Donnatal 2234
Donnatal Extentabs 2234
Donnatal Tablets 2234
Phenobarbital Elixir and Tablets 1523
Quadrinal Tablets 1398

Prazepam (Co-administration may result in an additive impairment of motor skills).
No products indexed under this heading.

Prochlorperazine (Co-administration may result in an additive impairment of motor skills). Products include:
Compazine 2644

Promethazine Hydrochloride (Co-administration may result in an additive impairment of motor skills). Products include:
Mepergan Injection 2859
Phenergan with Codeine 2883
Phenergan with Dextromethorphan 2885
Phenergan Injection 2880
Phenergan Suppositories 2882
Phenergan Syrup 2881
Phenergan Tablets 2882
Phenergan VC 2886
Phenergan VC with Codeine 2888

Propofol (Co-administration may result in an additive impairment of motor skills). Products include:
Diprivan Injectable Emulsion 2939

Propoxyphene Hydrochloride (Co-administration may result in an additive impairment of motor skills). Products include:
Darvon 1475
Wygesic Tablets 2930

Propoxyphene Napsylate (Co-administration may result in an additive impairment of motor skills). Products include:
Darvon-N/Darvocet-N 1473

Quazepam (Co-administration may result in an additive impairment of motor skills). Products include:
Doral Tablets 2773

Risperidone (Co-administration may result in an additive impairment of motor skills). Products include:
Risperdal Tablets 1348

Secobarbital Sodium (Co-administration may result in an additive impairment of motor skills). Products include:
Seconal Sodium Pulvules 1529

Selegiline Hydrochloride (Co-administration of antidepressants and MAO inhibitors has resulted in serious, and sometimes fatal, reactions including hyperthermia, autonomic instability, seizures, agitation, and coma; concurrent and/or sequential use is contraindicated). Products include:
Eldepryl Capsules 2729

Sevoflurane (Co-administration may result in an additive impairment of motor skills).
No products indexed under this heading.

Sufentanil Citrate (Co-administration may result in an additive impairment of motor skills). Products include:
Sufenta Injection 1355

Temazepam (Co-administration may result in an additive impairment of motor skills). Products include:
Restoril Capsules 2413

Thiamylal Sodium (Co-administration may result in an additive impairment of motor skills).
No products indexed under this heading.

Thioridazine Hydrochloride (Co-administration may result in an additive impairment of motor skills). Products include:
Mellaril 2398

Thiothixene (Co-administration may result in an additive impairment of motor skills). Products include:
Navane Capsules and Concentrate 2018
Navane Intramuscular 2019

IMPORTANT NOTE: Always consult each drug listing in the patient's regimen for possible interactions.

Remeron / Interactions Index

Tranylcypromine Sulfate (Co-administration of antidepressants and MAO inhibitors has resulted in serious, and sometimes fatal, reactions including hyperthermia, autonomic instability, seizures, agitation, and coma; concurrent and/or sequential use is contraindicated). Products include:
- Parnate Tablets 2679

Triazolam (Co-administration may result in an additive impairment of motor skills). Products include:
- Halcion Tablets 2093

Trifluoperazine Hydrochloride (Co-administration may result in an additive impairment of motor skills). Products include:
- Stelazine 2692

Zolpidem Tartrate (Co-administration may result in an additive impairment of motor skills). Products include:
- Ambien Tablets 2559

Food Interactions

Alcohol (Co-administration has shown to result in an additive impairment of cognitive and motor skills).

Food, unspecified (The presence of food in the stomach has a minimal effect on both the rate and extent of absorption and does not require a dosage adjustment).

RENOVA (TRETINOIN EMOLLIENT CREAM) 0.05%
(Tretinoin) 1945
May interact with drugs known to be photosensitizers and certain other agents. Compounds in these categories include:

Bendroflumethiazide (Concurrent use should be avoided because of the possibility of augmented phototoxicity).
No products indexed under this heading.

Chlorothiazide (Concurrent use should be avoided because of the possibility of augmented phototoxicity). Products include:
- Aldoclor Tablets 1638
- Diupres Tablets 1691
- Diuril Oral 1694

Chlorothiazide Sodium (Concurrent use should be avoided because of the possibility of augmented phototoxicity). Products include:
- Diuril Sodium Intravenous 1693

Chlorpromazine (Concurrent use should be avoided because of the possibility of augmented phototoxicity). Products include:
- Thorazine Suppositories 2701

Chlorpromazine Hydrochloride (Concurrent use should be avoided because of the possibility of augmented phototoxicity). Products include:
- Thorazine 2701

Chlorpropamide (Concurrent use should be avoided because of the possibility of augmented phototoxicity). Products include:
- Diabinese Tablets 2002

Ciprofloxacin (Concurrent use should be avoided because of the possibility of augmented phototoxicity). Products include:
- Cipro I.V. 587
- Cipro I.V. Pharmacy Bulk Package .. 590

Ciprofloxacin Hydrochloride (Concurrent use should be avoided because of the possibility of augmented phototoxicity). Products include:
- Ciloxan Ophthalmic Solution 468
- Cipro Tablets 584

Demeclocycline Hydrochloride (Concurrent use should be avoided because of the possibility of augmented phototoxicity). Products include:
- Declomycin Tablets 1421

Doxycycline Calcium (Concurrent use should be avoided because of the possibility of augmented phototoxicity). Products include:
- Vibramycin Calcium Oral Suspension Syrup 2038

Doxycycline Hyclate (Concurrent use should be avoided because of the possibility of augmented phototoxicity). Products include:
- Doryx Capsules 1970
- Vibramycin Hyclate Capsules 2038
- Vibramycin Hyclate Intravenous 2040
- Vibra-Tabs Film Coated Tablets 2038

Doxycycline Monohydrate (Concurrent use should be avoided because of the possibility of augmented phototoxicity). Products include:
- Monodox Capsules 1858
- Vibramycin Monohydrate for Oral Suspension 2038

Enoxacin (Concurrent use should be avoided because of the possibility of augmented phototoxicity). Products include:
- Penetrex Tablets 2196

Fluphenazine Decanoate (Concurrent use should be avoided because of the possibility of augmented phototoxicity). Products include:
- Prolixin Decanoate 510

Fluphenazine Enanthate (Concurrent use should be avoided because of the possibility of augmented phototoxicity). Products include:
- Prolixin Enanthate 510

Fluphenazine Hydrochloride (Concurrent use should be avoided because of the possibility of augmented phototoxicity). Products include:
- Prolixin 510

Glipizide (Concurrent use should be avoided because of the possibility of augmented phototoxicity). Products include:
- Glucotrol Tablets 2011
- Glucotrol XL Extended Release Tablets 2012

Glyburide (Concurrent use should be avoided because of the possibility of augmented phototoxicity). Products include:
- DiaBeta Tablets 1265
- Glynase PresTab Tablets 2091
- Micronase Tablets 2099

Hydrochlorothiazide (Concurrent use should be avoided because of the possibility of augmented phototoxicity). Products include:
- Aldactazide Tablets 2556
- Aldoril Tablets 1644
- Apresazide Capsules 824
- Capozide Tablets 744
- Dyazide Capsules 2653
- Esidrix Tablets 839
- Esimil Tablets 840
- HydroDIURIL Tablets 1716
- Hydropres Tablets 1718
- Hyzaar Tablets 1720
- Inderide Tablets 2838
- Inderide LA Long Acting Capsules .. 2840
- Lopressor HCT Tablets 850
- Lotensin HCT Tablets 855
- Moduretic Tablets 1748
- Oretic Tablets 450
- Prinzide Tablets 1780
- Ser-Ap-Es Tablets 867
- Timolide Tablets 1791
- Vaseretic Tablets 1810
- Zestoretic Tablets 2968
- Ziac 1459

Hydroflumethiazide (Concurrent use should be avoided because of the possibility of augmented phototoxicity). Products include:
- Diucardin Tablets 2824

Lomefloxacin Hydrochloride (Concurrent use should be avoided because of the possibility of augmented phototoxicity). Products include:
- Maxaquin Tablets 2593

Mesoridazine Besylate (Concurrent use should be avoided because of the possibility of augmented phototoxicity). Products include:
- Serentil 689

Methacycline Hydrochloride (Concurrent use should be avoided because of the possibility of augmented phototoxicity).
No products indexed under this heading.

Methotrimeprazine (Concurrent use should be avoided because of the possibility of augmented phototoxicity). Products include:
- Levoprome 1321

Methyclothiazide (Concurrent use should be avoided because of the possibility of augmented phototoxicity). Products include:
- Enduron Tablets 424

Minocycline Hydrochloride (Concurrent use should be avoided because of the possibility of augmented phototoxicity). Products include:
- DYNACIN Capsules 1627
- Minocin Intravenous 1428
- Minocin Oral Suspension 1431
- Minocin Pellet-Filled Capsules 1429

Norfloxacin (Concurrent use should be avoided because of the possibility of augmented phototoxicity). Products include:
- Chibroxin Sterile Ophthalmic Solution 1657
- Noroxin Tablets 1758
- Noroxin Tablets 2222

Ofloxacin (Concurrent use should be avoided because of the possibility of augmented phototoxicity). Products include:
- Floxin I.V. 1580
- Floxin Tablets (200 mg, 300 mg, 400 mg) 1577
- Ocuflox Ophthalmic Solution 478
- Ocuflox .... ⓞ 242

Oxytetracycline Hydrochloride (Concurrent use should be avoided because of the possibility of augmented phototoxicity). Products include:
- TERAK Ointment .... ⓞ 210
- Terra-Cortril Ophthalmic Suspension 2033
- Terramycin with Polymyxin B Sulfate Ophthalmic Ointment 2035
- Urobiotic-250 Capsules 2038

Perphenazine (Concurrent use should be avoided because of the possibility of augmented phototoxicity). Products include:
- Etrafon 2495
- Triavil Tablets 1800
- Trilafon 2532

Polythiazide (Concurrent use should be avoided because of the possibility of augmented phototoxicity). Products include:
- Minizide Capsules 2016

Prochlorperazine (Concurrent use should be avoided because of the possibility of augmented phototoxicity). Products include:
- Compazine 2644

Promethazine Hydrochloride (Concurrent use should be avoided because of the possibility of augmented phototoxicity). Products include:
- Mepergan Injection 2859
- Phenergan with Codeine 2883
- Phenergan with Dextromethorphan 2885
- Phenergan Injection 2880
- Phenergan Suppositories 2882
- Phenergan Syrup 2881
- Phenergan Tablets 2882
- Phenergan VC 2886
- Phenergan VC with Codeine 2888

Sulfamethizole (Concurrent use should be avoided because of the possibility of augmented phototoxicity). Products include:
- Urobiotic-250 Capsules 2038

Sulfamethoxazole (Concurrent use should be avoided because of the possibility of augmented phototoxicity). Products include:
- Bactrim DS Tablets 2257
- Bactrim I.V. Infusion 2255
- Bactrim 2257
- Gantanol Tablets 2285
- Septra I.V. Infusion 1146
- Septra I.V. Infusion 1142
- Septra I.V. Infusion ADD-Vantage Vials 1144
- Septra 1146

Sulfasalazine (Concurrent use should be avoided because of the possibility of augmented phototoxicity). Products include:
- Azulfidine 2059

Sulfinpyrazone (Concurrent use should be avoided because of the possibility of augmented phototoxicity). Products include:
- Anturane 823

Sulfisoxazole (Concurrent use should be avoided because of the possibility of augmented phototoxicity). Products include:
- Gantrisin Tablets 2286

Sulfisoxazole Diolamine (Concurrent use should be avoided because of the possibility of augmented phototoxicity).
No products indexed under this heading.

Tetracycline Hydrochloride (Concurrent use should be avoided because of the possibility of augmented phototoxicity). Products include:
- Achromycin V Capsules 1417
- Helidac Therapy 2135

Thioridazine Hydrochloride (Concurrent use should be avoided because of the possibility of augmented phototoxicity). Products include:
- Mellaril 2398

Tolazamide (Concurrent use should be avoided because of the possibility of augmented phototoxicity).
No products indexed under this heading.

Tolbutamide (Concurrent use should be avoided because of the possibility of augmented phototoxicity).
No products indexed under this heading.

Trifluoperazine Hydrochloride (Concurrent use should be avoided because of the possibility of augmented phototoxicity). Products include:
- Stelazine 2692

(ⓝ Described in PDR For Nonprescription Drugs)   (ⓞ Described in PDR For Ophthalmology)

919 Interactions Index ReoPro

REOPRO VIALS
(Abciximab) 1526
May interact with non-steroidal anti-inflammatory agents, anticoagulants, thrombolytics, and platelet inhibitors. Compounds in these categories include:

Alteplase, Recombinant (Abciximab inhibits platelet aggregation; concurrent use may be associated with an increase in bleeding). Products include:
- Activase 1045

Anistreplase (Abciximab inhibits platelet aggregation; concurrent use may be associated with an increase in bleeding). Products include:
- Eminase 2215

Aspirin (Abciximab inhibits platelet aggregation; concurrent use may be associated with an increase in bleeding). Products include:
- Alka-Seltzer Cherry Effervescent Antacid and Pain Reliever .... ▣ 609
- Alka-Seltzer Extra Strength Effervescent Antacid and Pain Reliever .... ▣ 609
- Alka-Seltzer Lemon Lime Effervescent Antacid and Pain Reliever .... ▣ 609
- Alka-Seltzer Original Effervescent Antacid and Pain Reliever .... ▣ 609
- Alka-Seltzer Plus .... ▣ 611
- Alka-Seltzer Plus Sinus Medicine .. ▣ 611
- Ascriptin .... ▣ 650
- Arthritis Strength BC Powder .... ▣ 631
- BC Cold Powder Multi-Symptom Formula (Cold-Sinus-Allergy) .... ▣ 631
- BC Cold Powder Non-Drowsy Formula (Cold-Sinus) .... ▣ 631
- BC Powder .... ▣ 631
- Genuine Bayer Aspirin Tablets & Caplets .... ▣ 618
- Extra Strength Bayer Arthritis Pain Regimen Formula .... ▣ 615
- Extra Strength Bayer Aspirin Caplets & Tablets .... ▣ 617
- Extended-Release Bayer 8-Hour Aspirin .... ▣ 616
- Extra Strength Bayer Plus Aspirin Caplets .... ▣ 617
- Extra Strength Bayer PM Aspirin Plus Sleep Aid .... ▣ 617
- Aspirin Regimen Bayer 81 mg Tablets with Calcium .... ▣ 615
- Aspirin Regimen Bayer Adult Low Strength 81 mg Tablets .... ▣ 613
- Aspirin Regimen Bayer Children's Chewable Aspirin .... ▣ 616
- Aspirin Regimen Bayer Regular Strength 325 mg Caplets .... ▣ 613
- Bufferin Analgesic Tablets .... ▣ 636
- Arthritis Strength Bufferin Analgesic Caplets .... ▣ 637
- Extra Strength Bufferin Analgesic Tablets .... ▣ 637
- Cama Arthritis Pain Reliever .... ▣ 748
- Darvon Compound-65 Pulvules 1475
- Easprin 1971
- Ecotrin 2625
- Ecotrin Enteric Coated Aspirin Maximum Strength Tablets and Caplets .... ▣ 775
- Ecotrin Enteric Coated Aspirin Regular Strength Tablets 2625
- Empirin Aspirin Tablets .... ▣ 818
- Excedrin Extra-Strength Analgesic Tablets, Caplets, and Geltabs 734
- Fiorinal Capsules 2388
- Fiorinal with Codeine Capsules 2390
- Fiorinal Tablets 2388
- Goody's Extra Strength Headache Powders .... ▣ 632
- Goody's Extra Strength Pain Relief Tablets .... ▣ 632
- Halfprin Tablets 1413
- Norgesic 1554
- Percodan Tablets 955
- Percodan-Demi Tablets 956
- Robaxisal Tablets 2246
- Soma Compound w/Codeine Tablets 2784
- Soma Compound Tablets 2783
- St. Joseph Adult Chewable Aspirin (81 mg.) .... ▣ 768
- Talwin Compound 2466
- Vanquish Analgesic Caplets .... ▣ 627

Azlocillin Sodium (Abciximab inhibits platelet aggregation; concurrent use may be associated with an increase in bleeding).
No products indexed under this heading.

Carbenicillin Indanyl Sodium (Abciximab inhibits platelet aggregation; concurrent use may be associated with an increase in bleeding). Products include:
- Geocillin Tablets 2009

Choline Magnesium Trisalicylate (Abciximab inhibits platelet aggregation; concurrent use may be associated with an increase in bleeding). Products include:
- Trilisate 2155

Dalteparin Sodium (Abciximab inhibits platelet aggregation; concurrent use may be associated with an increase in bleeding). Products include:
- Fragmin Injection 2088

Diclofenac Potassium (Abciximab inhibits platelet aggregation; concurrent use may be associated with an increase in bleeding). Products include:
- Cataflam Tablets 833

Diclofenac Sodium (Abciximab inhibits platelet aggregation; concurrent use may be associated with an increase in bleeding). Products include:
- Voltaren Ophthalmic Sterile Ophthalmic Solution .... ⊙ 264
- Cataflam/Voltaren/Voltaren-XR 833

Dicumarol (Abciximab inhibits platelet aggregation; concurrent use may be associated with an increase in bleeding).
No products indexed under this heading.

Diflunisal (Abciximab inhibits platelet aggregation; concurrent use may be associated with an increase in bleeding). Products include:
- Dolobid Tablets 1695

Dipyridamole (Abciximab inhibits platelet aggregation; concurrent use may be associated with an increase in bleeding). Products include:
- Persantine Tablets 686

Enoxaparin (Abciximab inhibits platelet aggregation; concurrent use may be associated with an increase in bleeding). Products include:
- Lovenox Injection 2187

Etodolac (Abciximab inhibits platelet aggregation; concurrent use may be associated with an increase in bleeding). Products include:
- Lodine Capsules and Tablets 2849

Fenoprofen Calcium (Abciximab inhibits platelet aggregation; concurrent use may be associated with an increase in bleeding). Products include:
- Nalfon 200 Pulvules & Nalfon Tablets 933

Flurbiprofen (Abciximab inhibits platelet aggregation; concurrent use may be associated with an increase in bleeding).
No products indexed under this heading.

Heparin Calcium (Abciximab inhibits platelet aggregation; concurrent use may be associated with an increase in bleeding).
No products indexed under this heading.

Heparin Sodium (Abciximab inhibits platelet aggregation; concurrent use may be associated with an increase in bleeding). Products include:
- Heparin Lock Flush Solution 2831
- Heparin Sodium Injection 2832
- Heparin Sodium Vials 1486

Ibuprofen (Abciximab inhibits platelet aggregation; concurrent use may be associated with an increase in bleeding). Products include:
- Advil Cold and Sinus Caplets and Tablets .... ▣ 837
- Advil Ibuprofen Tablets, Caplets and Gel Caplets .... ▣ 836
- Children's Motrin Ibuprofen Oral Suspension 1558
- IBU Tablets 1389
- Ibuprohm .... ▣ 713
- Motrin IB Caplets, Tablets, and Gelcaps .... ▣ 802
- Motrin Ibuprofen Suspension, Oral Drops, Chewable Tablets, Caplets 1563
- Nuprin Ibuprofen/Analgesic Tablets & Caplets .... ▣ 645
- Vicks DayQuil SINUS Pressure & PAIN Relief with IBUPROFEN .... ▣ 735

Indomethacin (Abciximab inhibits platelet aggregation; concurrent use may be associated with an increase in bleeding). Products include:
- Indocin 1723

Indomethacin Sodium Trihydrate (Abciximab inhibits platelet aggregation; concurrent use may be associated with an increase in bleeding). Products include:
- Indocin I.V. 1727

Ketoprofen (Abciximab inhibits platelet aggregation; concurrent use may be associated with an increase in bleeding). Products include:
- Actron Caplets and Tablets .... ▣ 608
- Orudis Capsules 2874
- Orudis KT .... ▣ 842
- Oruvail Capsules 2874

Ketorolac Tromethamine (Abciximab inhibits platelet aggregation; concurrent use may be associated with an increase in bleeding). Products include:
- Acular Sterile Ophthalmic Solution 470
- Toradol 2319

Magnesium Salicylate (Abciximab inhibits platelet aggregation; concurrent use may be associated with an increase in bleeding). Products include:
- Backache Caplets .... ▣ 635
- Doan's Extra-Strength Analgesic .... ▣ 653
- Extra Strength Doan's P.M. .... ▣ 653
- Doan's Regular Strength Analgesic .... ▣ 654
- Mobigesic Tablets .... ▣ 607

Meclofenamate Sodium (Abciximab inhibits platelet aggregation; concurrent use may be associated with an increase in bleeding).
No products indexed under this heading.

Mefenamic Acid (Abciximab inhibits platelet aggregation; concurrent use may be associated with an increase in bleeding). Products include:
- Ponstel 1982

Mezlocillin Sodium (Abciximab inhibits platelet aggregation; concurrent use may be associated with an increase in bleeding). Products include:
- Mezlin 594
- Mezlin Pharmacy Bulk Package 597

Nabumetone (Abciximab inhibits platelet aggregation; concurrent use may be associated with an increase in bleeding). Products include:
- Relafen Tablets 2688

Nafcillin Sodium (Abciximab inhibits platelet aggregation; concurrent use may be associated with an increase in bleeding).
No products indexed under this heading.

Naproxen (Abciximab inhibits platelet aggregation; concurrent use may be associated with an increase in bleeding). Products include:
- Anaprox/Naprosyn 2277

Naproxen Sodium (Abciximab inhibits platelet aggregation; concurrent use may be associated with an increase in bleeding). Products include:
- Aleve 2124
- Anaprox/Naprosyn 2277
- Naprelan Tablets 2861

Oxaprozin (Abciximab inhibits platelet aggregation; concurrent use may be associated with an increase in bleeding). Products include:
- Daypro Caplets 2578

Penicillin G Benzathine (Abciximab inhibits platelet aggregation; concurrent use may be associated with an increase in bleeding). Products include:
- Bicillin C-R Injection 2810
- Bicillin C-R 900/300 Injection 2812
- Bicillin L-A Injection 2813

Penicillin G Procaine (Abciximab inhibits platelet aggregation; concurrent use may be associated with an increase in bleeding). Products include:
- Bicillin C-R Injection 2810
- Bicillin C-R 900/300 Injection 2812

Phenylbutazone (Abciximab inhibits platelet aggregation; concurrent use may be associated with an increase in bleeding).
No products indexed under this heading.

Piroxicam (Abciximab inhibits platelet aggregation; concurrent use may be associated with an increase in bleeding). Products include:
- Feldene Capsules 2008

Salsalate (Abciximab inhibits platelet aggregation; concurrent use may be associated with an increase in bleeding). Products include:
- Disalcid 1549
- Mono-Gesic Tablets 810
- Salflex Tablets 791

Streptokinase (Abciximab inhibits platelet aggregation; concurrent use may be associated with an increase in bleeding). Products include:
- Streptase for Infusion 557

Sulindac (Abciximab inhibits platelet aggregation; concurrent use may be associated with an increase in bleeding). Products include:
- Clinoril Tablets 1658

Ticarcillin Disodium (Abciximab inhibits platelet aggregation; concurrent use may be associated with an increase in bleeding). Products include:
- Ticar for Injection 2704
- Timentin for Injection 2706

Ticlopidine Hydrochloride (Abciximab inhibits platelet aggregation; concurrent use may be associated with an increase in bleeding). Products include:
- Ticlid Tablets 2317

Tolmetin Sodium (Abciximab inhibits platelet aggregation; concurrent use may be associated with an increase in bleeding). Products include:
- Tolectin (200, 400 and 600 mg) .. 1591

IMPORTANT NOTE: Always consult each drug listing in the patient's regimen for possible interactions.

ReoPro — Interactions Index

Urokinase (Abciximab inhibits platelet aggregation; concurrent use may be associated with an increase in bleeding). Products include:
Abbokinase ... 403
Abbokinase Open-Cath ... 405

Warfarin Sodium (Abciximab inhibits platelet aggregation; concurrent use may be associated with an increase in bleeding). Products include:
Coumadin ... 941

REPLENS VAGINAL MOISTURIZER
(Glycerin, Lubricant) ... 823
None cited in PDR database.

RESPBID TABLETS
(Theophylline Anhydrous) ... 687
May interact with sympathomimetic bronchodilators, oral contraceptives, macrolide antibiotics, and certain other agents. Compounds in these categories include:

Albuterol (Toxic synergism). Products include:
Proventil Inhalation Aerosol ... 2524
Ventolin Inhalation Aerosol and Refill ... 1170

Albuterol Sulfate (Toxic synergism). Products include:
Airet Albuterol Sulfate Inhalation Solution ... 1602
Albuterol Sulfate, USP Solution for Inhalation, Arm-a-Med ... 522
Proventil Inhalation Solution 0.083% ... 2527
Proventil Repetabs Tablets ... 2529
Proventil Solution for Inhalation 0.5% ... 2525
Proventil Syrup ... 2528
Proventil Tablets ... 2529
Ventolin Inhalation Solution ... 1171
Ventolin Nebules Inhalation Solution ... 1172
Ventolin Rotacaps for Inhalation ... 1173
Ventolin Syrup ... 1175
Ventolin Tablets ... 1176
Volmax Extended-Release Tablets ... 1835

Allopurinol (Increased serum theophylline levels with high-dose allopurinol). Products include:
Zyloprim Tablets ... 1194

Azithromycin (Increases theophylline blood levels). Products include:
Zithromax ... 2043
Zithromax Tablets ... 2046

Bitolterol Mesylate (Toxic synergism). Products include:
Tornalate Solution for Inhalation, 0.2% ... 976
Tornalate Metered Dose Inhaler ... 978

Cimetidine (Increased theophylline blood levels). Products include:
Tagamet HB Tablets ... 786
Tagamet Tablets ... 2694

Ciprofloxacin (Increased serum theophylline levels). Products include:
Cipro I.V. ... 587
Cipro I.V. Pharmacy Bulk Package ... 590

Ciprofloxacin Hydrochloride (Increased serum theophylline levels). Products include:
Ciloxan Ophthalmic Solution ... 468
Cipro Tablets ... 584

Clarithromycin (Increases theophylline blood levels). Products include:
Biaxin ... 406

Desogestrel (Increased serum theophylline levels). Products include:
Desogen Tablets ... 1867
Ortho-Cept ... 1907

Dirithromycin (Increases theophylline blood levels). Products include:
Dynabac ... 668

Ephedrine Hydrochloride (Toxic synergism). Products include:
Primatene Tablets ... 844
Quadrinal Tablets ... 1398

Ephedrine Sulfate (Toxic synergism). Products include:
Marax Tablets & DF Syrup ... 2015

Ephedrine Tannate (Toxic synergism). Products include:
Rynatuss ... 2782

Epinephrine (Toxic synergism). Products include:
EPIFRIN ... 237
EpiPen ... 808
Marcaine with Epinephrine ... 2446
Primatene Mist ... 843
Sensorcaine with Epinephrine Injection ... 554
Sus-Phrine Injection ... 1017
Xylocaine with Epinephrine Injections ... 562

Epinephrine Bitartrate (Toxic synergism). Products include:
Sensorcaine-MPF with Epinephrine Injection ... 554

Epinephrine Hydrochloride (Toxic synergism). Products include:
Ana-Kit Anaphylaxis Emergency Treatment Kit ... 611

Erythromycin (Increases theophylline blood levels). Products include:
A/T/S 2% Acne Topical Gel ... 1244
A/T/S 2% Acne Topical Solution ... 1244
Benzamycin Topical Gel ... 919
E-Mycin Tablets ... 1388
Emgel 2% Topical Gel ... 1081
ERYC ... 1972
Erycette (erythromycin 2%) Topical Solution ... 1943
Ery-Tab Tablets ... 426
Erythromycin Base Filmtab ... 430
Erythromycin Delayed-Release Capsules, USP ... 431
Ilotycin Ophthalmic Ointment ... 928
PCE Dispertab Tablets ... 453
T-Stat 2.0% Topical Solution and Pads ... 2797
THERAMYCIN Z 2% Solution ... 1629

Erythromycin Estolate (Increases theophylline blood levels). Products include:
Ilosone ... 927

Erythromycin Ethylsuccinate (Increases theophylline blood levels). Products include:
E.E.S. ... 427
EryPed ... 425
Pediazole Suspension ... 2340

Erythromycin Gluceptate (Increases theophylline blood levels). Products include:
Ilotycin Gluceptate, IV, Vials ... 929

Erythromycin Stearate (Increases theophylline blood levels). Products include:
Erythrocin Stearate Filmtab ... 429

Ethinyl Estradiol (Increased serum theophylline levels). Products include:
Brevicon ... 2563
Demulen ... 2580
Desogen Tablets ... 1867
Levlen/Tri-Levlen ... 646
Lo/Ovral Tablets ... 2852
Lo/Ovral-28 Tablets ... 2857
Modicon ... 1928
Nordette-21 Tablets ... 2863
Nordette-28 Tablets ... 2866
Norinyl ... 2563
Ortho-Cept ... 1907
Ortho-Cyclen/Ortho-Tri-Cyclen ... 1914
Ortho-Novum ... 1928
Ortho-Cyclen/Ortho Tri-Cyclen ... 1914
Ovcon ... 765
Ovral Tablets ... 2877
Ovral-28 Tablets ... 2878
Levlen/Tri-Levlen ... 646
Tri-Norinyl ... 2607
Triphasil-21 Tablets ... 2919
Triphasil-28 Tablets ... 2924

Ethylnorepinephrine Hydrochloride (Toxic synergism).
No products indexed under this heading.

Ethynodiol Diacetate (Increased serum theophylline levels). Products include:
Demulen ... 2580

Isoetharine (Toxic synergism). Products include:
Bronkometer Aerosol ... 2432
Bronkosol Solution ... 2432
Isoetharine Inhalation Solution, USP, Arm-a-Med ... 545

Isoproterenol Hydrochloride (Toxic synergism). Products include:
Isuprel Hydrochloride Solution ... 2443
Isuprel Injection ... 2441
Isuprel Mistometer ... 2442

Isoproterenol Sulfate (Toxic synergism). Products include:
Norisodrine with Calcium Iodide Syrup ... 446

Levonorgestrel (Increased serum theophylline levels). Products include:
Levlen/Tri-Levlen ... 646
Nordette-21 Tablets ... 2863
Nordette-28 Tablets ... 2866
Norplant System ... 2868
Levlen/Tri-Levlen ... 646
Triphasil-21 Tablets ... 2919
Triphasil-28 Tablets ... 2924

Lithium Carbonate (Increased excretion of lithium carbonate). Products include:
Eskalith ... 2658
Lithium Carbonate Capsules & Tablets ... 2352
Lithonate/Lithotabs/Lithobid ... 2721

Mestranol (Increased serum theophylline levels). Products include:
Norinyl ... 2563
Ortho-Novum ... 1928

Metaproterenol Sulfate (Toxic synergism). Products include:
Alupent ... 672
Metaproterenol Sulfate Inhalation Solution, USP, Arm-a-Med ... 547

Norethindrone (Increased serum theophylline levels). Products include:
Brevicon ... 2563
Micronor Tablets ... 1903
Modicon ... 1928
Norinyl ... 2563
Nor-Q D Tablets ... 2598
Ortho-Novum ... 1928
Ovcon ... 765
Tri-Norinyl ... 2607

Norethynodrel (Increased serum theophylline levels).
No products indexed under this heading.

Norgestimate (Increased serum theophylline levels). Products include:
Ortho-Cyclen/Ortho-Tri-Cyclen ... 1914
Ortho-Cyclen/Ortho Tri-Cyclen ... 1914

Norgestrel (Increased serum theophylline levels). Products include:
Lo/Ovral Tablets ... 2852
Lo/Ovral-28 Tablets ... 2857
Ovral Tablets ... 2877
Ovral-28 Tablets ... 2878
Ovrette Tablets ... 2878

Phenytoin (Decreased theophylline and phenytoin serum levels). Products include:
Dilantin Infatabs ... 1967
Dilantin-125 Suspension ... 1969

Phenytoin Sodium (Decreased theophylline and phenytoin serum levels). Products include:
Dilantin Kapseals ... 1965

Pirbuterol Acetate (Toxic synergism). Products include:
Maxair Autohaler ... 1550
Maxair Inhaler ... 1552

Propranolol Hydrochloride (Increases serum theophylline levels). Products include:
Inderal ... 2834
Inderal LA Long Acting Capsules ... 2836
Inderide Tablets ... 2838

Inderide LA Long Acting Capsules ... 2840

Rifampin (Decreases serum theophylline levels). Products include:
Rifadin ... 1276
Rifamate Capsules ... 1278
Rifater ... 1280
Rimactane Capsules ... 865

Salmeterol Xinafoate (Toxic synergism). Products include:
Serevent Inhalation Aerosol ... 1149

Terbutaline Sulfate (Toxic synergism). Products include:
Brethaire Inhaler ... 830
Brethine Ampuls ... 832
Brethine Tablets ... 831
Bricanyl Subcutaneous Injection ... 1247
Bricanyl Tablets ... 1248

Troleandomycin (Increases theophylline blood levels). Products include:
Tao Capsules ... 2033

Food Interactions

Beverages, caffeine-containing (Avoid large quantities; increased side effects).

Chocolate (Eating large quantity of chocolate increases theophylline side effects).

Cola (Drinking large quantity of cola increases theophylline side effects).

Diet, high-lipid (Reduced plasma concentration levels; delay in time of peak plasma levels).

RESPIGAM
(Immune Globulin Intravenous (Human)) ... 1631
May interact with:

Mumps Virus Vaccine, Live (Antibodies present in immune globulin may interfere with the immune response to vaccine). Products include:
Mumpsvax ... 1751

Rubella & Mumps Virus Vaccine Live (Antibodies present in immune globulin may interfere with the immune response to vaccine). Products include:
Biavax II ... 1653

RESTORIL CAPSULES
(Temazepam) ... 2413
May interact with central nervous system depressants, hypnotics and sedatives, and certain other agents. Compounds in these categories include:

Alfentanil Hydrochloride (Additive effects). Products include:
Alfenta Injection ... 1334

Alprazolam (Additive effects). Products include:
Xanax Tablets ... 2115

Aprobarbital (Additive effects).
No products indexed under this heading.

Buprenorphine (Additive effects). Products include:
Buprenex Injectable ... 2170

Buspirone Hydrochloride (Additive effects). Products include:
BuSpar Tablets ... 738

Butabarbital (Additive effects).
No products indexed under this heading.

Butalbital (Additive effects). Products include:
Axocet Capsules ... 2469
Esgic-plus Capsules ... 1012
Esgic-plus Tablets ... 1012
Fioricet Tablets ... 2386
Fioricet with Codeine Capsules ... 2387
Fiorinal Capsules ... 2388
Fiorinal with Codeine Capsules ... 2390
Fiorinal Tablets ... 2388
Phrenilin ... 790
Sedapap Tablets 50 mg/650 mg ... 1826

(▣ Described in PDR For Nonprescription Drugs)   (◉ Described in PDR For Ophthalmology)

Interactions Index

Chlordiazepoxide (Additive effects). Products include:
- Limbitrol ... 2333

Chlordiazepoxide Hydrochloride (Additive effects). Products include:
- Librax Capsules ... 2330
- Librium Capsules ... 2331
- Librium Injectable ... 2332

Chlorpromazine (Additive effects). Products include:
- Thorazine Suppositories ... 2701

Chlorprothixene (Additive effects).
No products indexed under this heading.

Chlorprothixene Hydrochloride (Additive effects).
No products indexed under this heading.

Chlorprothixene Lactate (Additive effects).
No products indexed under this heading.

Clorazepate Dipotassium (Additive effects). Products include:
- Tranxene ... 459

Clozapine (Additive effects). Products include:
- Clozaril Tablets ... 2377

Codeine Phosphate (Additive effects). Products include:
- Brontex ... 2130
- Dimetane-DC Cough Syrup ... 2232
- Fioricet with Codeine Capsules ... 2387
- Fiorinal with Codeine Capsules ... 2390
- Nucofed ... 2225
- Phenergan with Codeine ... 2883
- Phenergan VC with Codeine ... 2888
- Robitussin A-C Syrup ... 2248
- Robitussin-DAC Syrup ... 2249
- Ryna ... 804
- Soma Compound w/Codeine Tablets ... 2784
- Tylenol with Codeine ... 1592

Desflurane (Additive effects). Products include:
- Suprane (desflurane, USP) ... 1865

Dezocine (Additive effects). Products include:
- Dalgan Injection ... 529

Diazepam (Additive effects). Products include:
- Dizac (diazepam injectable emulsion) CIV ... 1862
- Valium Injectable ... 2336
- Valium Tablets ... 2335

Diphenhydramine Hydrochloride (Synergistic effect is possible). Products include:
- Actifed Allergy Daytime/Nighttime Caplets ... 808
- Actifed Sinus Daytime/Nighttime Tablets and Caplets ... 809
- Extra Strength Bayer PM Aspirin Plus Sleep Aid ... 617
- Benadryl Allergy Chewables ... 811
- Benadryl Allergy/Cold Tablets ... 811
- Benadryl Allergy Decongestant Liquid Medication ... 812
- Benadryl Allergy Decongestant Tablets ... 812
- Benadryl Allergy Liquid Medication ... 813
- Benadryl Allergy ... 811
- Benadryl Allergy Sinus Headache Caplets ... 813
- Benadryl Dye-Free Allergy Liquigel Softgels ... 813
- Benadryl Dye-Free Allergy Liquid Medication ... 814
- Benadryl Itch Relief Stick Extra Strength ... 814
- Benadryl Cream ... 814
- Benadryl Gel ... 815
- Benadryl Spray ... 815
- Benadryl Injection ... 1955
- Contac Day & Night Cold/Flu Night Caplets ... 772
- Contac Night Allergy/Sinus Caplets ... 771
- Extra Strength Doan's P.M. ... 653
- Excedrin P.M. Analgesic/Sleeping Aid Tablets, Caplets, Liquigels ... 643
- Nytol QuickCaps Caplets ... 632
- Sleepinal Night-time Sleep Aid Capsules and Softgels ... 798
- TYLENOL Allergy Sinus NightTime, Maximum Strength Caplets ... 1571
- TYLENOL Flu NightTime, Maximum Strength Gelcaps ... 1575
- TYLENOL Flu NightTime, Maximum Strength Hot Medication Packets ... 1575
- TYLENOL PM Pain Reliever/Sleep Aid, Extra Strength Gelcaps, Caplets, Geltabs ... 1576
- TYLENOL Severe Allergy Medication Caplets ... 1571
- Maximum Strength Unisom Sleepgels ... 1990
- Unisom With Pain Relief-Nighttime Sleep Aid and Pain Reliever ... 1991

Droperidol (Additive effects). Products include:
- Inapsine Injection ... 462

Enflurane (Additive effects).
No products indexed under this heading.

Estazolam (Additive effects). Products include:
- ProSom Tablets ... 457

Ethchlorvynol (Additive effects). Products include:
- Placidyl Capsules ... 456

Ethinamate (Additive effects).
No products indexed under this heading.

Fentanyl (Additive effects). Products include:
- Duragesic Transdermal System ... 1336

Fentanyl Citrate (Additive effects). Products include:
- Sublimaze Injection ... 463

Fluphenazine Decanoate (Additive effects). Products include:
- Prolixin Decanoate ... 510

Fluphenazine Enanthate (Additive effects). Products include:
- Prolixin Enanthate ... 510

Fluphenazine Hydrochloride (Additive effects). Products include:
- Prolixin ... 510

Flurazepam Hydrochloride (Additive effects). Products include:
- Dalmane Capsules ... 2329

Glutethimide (Additive effects).
No products indexed under this heading.

Haloperidol (Additive effects). Products include:
- Haldol Injection, Tablets and Concentrate ... 1585

Haloperidol Decanoate (Additive effects). Products include:
- Haldol Decanoate ... 1587

Hydrocodone Bitartrate (Additive effects). Products include:
- Codiclear DH Syrup ... 808
- Duratuss HD Elixir ... 2750
- Histussin D Liquid ... 670
- Hycodan Tablets and Syrup ... 946
- Hycomine Compound Tablets ... 948
- Hycomine ... 947
- Hycotuss Expectorant Syrup ... 950
- Hydrocet Capsules ... 787
- Lorcet 10/650 Tablets ... 1016
- Lortab ... 2751
- Tussend ... 1830
- Tussend Expectorant ... 1831
- Vicodin Tablets ... 1404
- Vicodin ES Tablets ... 1405
- Vicodin HP Tablets ... 1403
- Vicodin Tuss Expectorant ... 1406
- Zydone Capsules ... 967

Hydrocodone Polistirex (Additive effects). Products include:
- Tussionex Pennkinetic Extended-Release Suspension ... 1624

Hydroxyzine Hydrochloride (Additive effects). Products include:
- Atarax Tablets & Syrup ... 1992
- Marax Tablets & DF Syrup ... 2015
- Vistaril Intramuscular Solution ... 2042

Isoflurane (Additive effects).
No products indexed under this heading.

Ketamine Hydrochloride (Additive effects).
No products indexed under this heading.

Levomethadyl Acetate Hydrochloride (Additive effects). Products include:
- Orlaam Oral Solution ... 2361

Levorphanol Tartrate (Additive effects). Products include:
- Levo-Dromoran ... 2297

Lorazepam (Additive effects). Products include:
- Ativan Injection ... 2805
- Ativan Tablets ... 2807

Loxapine Hydrochloride (Additive effects). Products include:
- Loxitane ... 1426

Loxapine Succinate (Additive effects). Products include:
- Loxitane Capsules ... 1426

Meperidine Hydrochloride (Additive effects). Products include:
- Demerol ... 2438
- Mepergan Injection ... 2859

Mephobarbital (Additive effects). Products include:
- Mebaral Tablets ... 2452

Meprobamate (Additive effects). Products include:
- Miltown Tablets ... 2780
- PMB 200 and PMB 400 ... 2890

Mesoridazine Besylate (Additive effects). Products include:
- Serentil ... 689

Methadone Hydrochloride (Additive effects). Products include:
- Methadone Hydrochloride Oral Concentrate ... 2356
- Methadone Hydrochloride Oral Solution & Tablets ... 2357

Methohexital Sodium (Additive effects).
No products indexed under this heading.

Methotrimeprazine (Additive effects). Products include:
- Levoprome ... 1321

Methoxyflurane (Additive effects).
No products indexed under this heading.

Midazolam Hydrochloride (Additive effects). Products include:
- Versed Injection ... 2324

Molindone Hydrochloride (Additive effects). Products include:
- Moban Tablets and Concentrate ... 1036

Morphine Sulfate (Additive effects). Products include:
- Astramorph/PF Injection, USP (Preservative-Free) ... 526
- Duramorph Injection ... 983
- Infumorph 200 and Infumorph 500 Sterile Solutions ... 985
- Kadian Capsules ... 2948
- MS Contin Tablets ... 2149
- MSIR ... 2152
- Oramorph SR (Morphine Sulfate Sustained Release Tablets) ... 2359
- RMS Suppositories CII ... 2766
- Roxanol ... 2365

Opium Alkaloids (Additive effects).
No products indexed under this heading.

Oxazepam (Additive effects). Products include:
- Serax Capsules ... 2916
- Serax Capsules ... 2916

Oxycodone Hydrochloride (Additive effects). Products include:
- OxyContin Tablets ... 2163
- OxyIR Capsules ... 2167
- Percocet Tablets ... 955
- Percodan Tablets ... 955
- Percodan-Demi Tablets ... 956
- Roxicodone Tablets, Oral Solution & Intensol (Oxycodone) ... 2366
- Tylox Capsules ... 1593

Pentobarbital Sodium (Additive effects). Products include:
- Nembutal Sodium Capsules ... 440
- Nembutal Sodium Solution ... 442
- Nembutal Sodium Suppositories ... 444

Perphenazine (Additive effects). Products include:
- Etrafon ... 2495
- Triavil Tablets ... 1800
- Trilafon ... 2532

Phenobarbital (Additive effects). Products include:
- Arco-Lase Plus Tablets ... 513
- Bellergal-S Tablets ... 2375
- Donnatal ... 2234
- Donnatal Extentabs ... 2234
- Donnatal Tablets ... 2234
- Phenobarbital Elixir and Tablets ... 1523
- Quadrinal Tablets ... 1398

Prazepam (Additive effects).
No products indexed under this heading.

Prochlorperazine (Additive effects). Products include:
- Compazine ... 2644

Promethazine Hydrochloride (Additive effects). Products include:
- Mepergan Injection ... 2859
- Phenergan with Codeine ... 2883
- Phenergan with Dextromethorphan ... 2885
- Phenergan Injection ... 2880
- Phenergan Suppositories ... 2882
- Phenergan Syrup ... 2881
- Phenergan Tablets ... 2882
- Phenergan VC ... 2886
- Phenergan VC with Codeine ... 2888

Propofol (Additive effects). Products include:
- Diprivan Injectable Emulsion ... 2939

Propoxyphene Hydrochloride (Additive effects). Products include:
- Darvon ... 1475
- Wygesic Tablets ... 2930

Propoxyphene Napsylate (Additive effects). Products include:
- Darvon-N/Darvocet-N ... 1473

Quazepam (Additive effects). Products include:
- Doral Tablets ... 2773

Risperidone (Additive effects). Products include:
- Risperdal Tablets ... 1348

Secobarbital Sodium (Additive effects). Products include:
- Seconal Sodium Pulvules ... 1529

Sevoflurane (Additive effects).
No products indexed under this heading.

Sufentanil Citrate (Additive effects). Products include:
- Sufenta Injection ... 1355

Thiamylal Sodium (Additive effects).
No products indexed under this heading.

Thioridazine Hydrochloride (Additive effects). Products include:
- Mellaril ... 2398

Thiothixene (Additive effects). Products include:
- Navane Capsules and Concentrate ... 2018
- Navane Intramuscular ... 2019

Triazolam (Additive effects). Products include:
- Halcion Tablets ... 2093

Trifluoperazine Hydrochloride (Additive effects). Products include:
- Stelazine ... 2692

Zolpidem Tartrate (Additive effects). Products include:
- Ambien Tablets ... 2559

Food Interactions

Alcohol (Additive effects).

IMPORTANT NOTE: Always consult each drug listing in the patient's regimen for possible interactions.

RETIN-A (TRETINOIN) CREAM/GEL/LIQUID

(Tretinoin) 1947

May interact with:

Concomitant Topical Acne Therapy (Effect not specified).

Resorcinol (Caution should be exercised). Products include:

- BiCozene Creme .... ■ 747

Salicylic Acid (Caution should be exercised). Products include:

- DHS Sal Shampoo 1989
- DuoFilm Liquid Wart Remover .... ■ 765
- DuoFilm Patch Wart Remover .... ■ 765
- DuoPlant Gel Plantar Wart Remover .... ■ 765
- Exact Pore Treatment Gel .... ■ 722
- MG 217 .... ■ 800
- Occlusal-HP 1041
- SalAc 1042
- Wart-Off Wart Remover .... ■ 720

Sulfur (Caution should be exercised). Products include:

- CharcoCaps .... ■ 740
- MG 217 Medicated Tar-Free Shampoo .... ■ 800
- Novacet Lotion 1041
- Sulfacet-R Lotion 925
- Sulfacet-R Tint Free Lotion 925

Topical Medications (Effect not specified).

RETROVIR CAPSULES

(Zidovudine) 1216

May interact with aspirin and acetaminophen containing products, cytotoxic drugs, experimental nucleoside analogues (selected) for aids and arc, and certain other agents. Compounds in these categories include:

Acetaminophen (May competitively inhibit glucuronidation; possible increased incidence of granulocytopenia). Products include:

- Actifed Cold & Sinus Caplets and Tablets .... ■ 808
- Actifed Sinus Daytime/Nighttime Tablets and Caplets .... ■ 809
- Alka-Seltzer Fast Relief Caplets .... ■ 610
- Alka-Seltzer Plus Liqui-Gels .... ■ 612
- Alka-Seltzer Plus Flu & Body Aches Effervescent Tablets .... ■ 612
- Alka-Seltzer Plus Flu & Body Aches Liqui-Gels Non-Drowsy Formula .... ■ 613
- Alka-Seltzer Plus Night-Time Cold Medicine Liqui-Gels .... ■ 612
- Allerest No Drowsiness .... ■ 649
- Allerest Sinus Pain Formula .... ■ 649
- Axocet Capsules 2469
- Benadryl Allergy/Cold Tablets .... ■ 811
- Benadryl Allergy Sinus Headache Caplets .... ■ 813
- Children's TYLENOL acetaminophen Chewable Tablets, Elixir, Suspension Liquid, and Suspension Drops 1559
- Children's TYLENOL Cold Multi-Symptom Chewable Tablets and Liquid 1559
- Children's TYLENOL Cold Plus Cough Multi Symptom Chewable Tablets and Liquid 1560
- Children's TYLENOL Flu Suspension Liquid 1560
- Allergy-Sinus Comtrex Multi-Symptom Allergy-Sinus Formula Tablets and Caplets .... ■ 639
- Comtrex Multi-Symptom .... ■ 638
- Comtrex Non-Drowsy .... ■ 640
- Contac Day Allergy/Sinus Caplets .... ■ 771
- Contac Day & Night .... ■ 772
- Contac Night Allergy/Sinus Caplets .... ■ 771
- Contac Severe Cold and Flu Formula Caplets .... ■ 773
- Contac Severe Cold & Flu Non-Drowsy .... ■ 774
- Coricidin Cold + Flu Tablets .... ■ 760
- Coricidin 'D' Decongestant Tablets .... ■ 760
- DHCplus Capsules 2148
- Darvon-N/Darvocet-N 1473
- Dimetapp Allergy Sinus Caplets .... ■ 838
- Dimetapp Cold & Fever Suspension .... ■ 839
- Drixoral Cold and Flu Extended-Release Tablets .... ■ 764
- Drixoral Cough + Sore Throat Liquid Caps .... ■ 763
- Drixoral Allergy/Sinus Extended Release Tablets .... ■ 765
- Esgic-plus Capsules 1012
- Esgic-plus Tablets 1012
- Aspirin Free Excedrin Analgesic Caplets and Geltabs 734
- Excedrin Extra-Strength Analgesic Tablets, Caplets, and Geltabs 734
- Excedrin P.M. Analgesic/Sleeping Aid Tablets, Caplets, Liquigels 735
- Fioricet Tablets 2386
- Fioricet with Codeine Capsules 2387
- Goody's Extra Strength Headache Powders .... ■ 632
- Goody's Extra Strength Pain Relief Tablets .... ■ 632
- Hycomine Compound Tablets 948
- Hydrocet Capsules 787
- Infants' TYLENOL acetaminophen Suspension Drops 1559
- Infants' TYLENOL Cold Decongestant & Fever-Reducer Drops 1561
- Junior Strength TYLENOL acetaminophen Coated Caplets and Chewable Tablets 1562
- Lorcet 10/650 Tablets 1016
- Lortab 2751
- Lurline PMS Tablets 1000
- Maximum Strength Multi-Symptom Formula Midol .... ■ 621
- PMS Multi-Symptom Formula Midol .... ■ 622
- Maximum Strength Midol Teen Multi-Symptom Formula .... ■ 621
- Midrin Capsules 788
- Panodol Tablets and Caplets .... ■ 783
- Children's Panadol Chewable Tablets, Liquid, Infant's Drops .... ■ 783
- Percocet Tablets 955
- Percogesic Analgesic Tablets .... ■ 727
- Phrenilin 790
- Pyrroxate Caplets .... ■ 742
- Robitussin Cold, Cough & Flu Liqui-Gels .... ■ 844
- Robitussin Night-Time Cold Formula .... ■ 847
- Sedapap Tablets 50 mg/650 mg 1826
- Sinarest .... ■ 663
- Sine-Aid Maximum Strength Sinus Headache Gelcaps, Caplets and Tablets 1570
- Sine-Off No Drowsiness Formula Caplets .... ■ 784
- Sine-Off Sinus Medicine .... ■ 784
- Singlet Tablets .... ■ 785
- Sinulin Tablets 792
- Sinutab Sinus Allergy Medication, Maximum Strength Tablets and Caplets .... ■ 823
- Sinutab Sinus Medication, Maximum Strength Without Drowsiness Formula, Tablets & Caplets .... ■ 824
- Sudafed Cold and Cough Liquid Caps .... ■ 826
- Sudafed Severe Cold Formula Caplets .... ■ 828
- Sudafed Severe Cold Formula Tablets .... ■ 828
- Sudafed Sinus Caplets .... ■ 829
- Sudafed Sinus Tablets .... ■ 829
- Talacen Caplets 2464
- TheraFlu Flu and Cold Medicine .... ■ 750
- Theraflu Maximum Strength Flu and Cold Medicine For Sore Throat .... ■ 751
- TheraFlu Flu, Cold and Cough Medicine .... ■ 750
- TheraFlu Maximum Strength Nighttime Flu, Cold & Cough Medicine .... ■ 751
- TheraFlu Maximum Strength Non-Drowsy Formula Flu, Cold & Cough Medicine .... ■ 751
- TheraFlu Maximum Strength, Non-Drowsy Formula Flu, Cold and Cough Caplets .... ■ 752
- Theraflu Maximum Strength Sinus Non-Drowsy Formula Caplets .... ■ 752
- Triaminic Sore Throat Formula .... ■ 755
- Triaminicin Tablets .... ■ 756
- TYLENOL acetaminophen Extended Relief Caplets 1570
- TYLENOL acetaminophen, Extra Strength Adult Liquid Pain Reliever 1570
- TYLENOL acetaminophen, Extra Strength Gelcaps, Geltabs, Caplets, Tablets 1570
- TYLENOL acetaminophen, Regular Strength Caplets and Tablets 1570
- TYLENOL Allergy Sinus, Maximum Strength Caplets and Gelcaps 1571
- TYLENOL Allergy Sinus NightTime, Maximum Strength Caplets 1571
- TYLENOL Cold Medication, Multi-Symptom Formula Tablets and Caplets 1572
- TYLENOL Cold Medication, Multi-Symptom Hot Liquid Packets 1572
- TYLENOL Cold Medication, No Drowsiness Formula Caplets and Gelcaps 1572
- TYLENOL Cold Severe Congestion Caplets 1573
- TYLENOL Cough Medication, Multi Symptom 1574
- TYLENOL Cough Medication with Decongestant, Multi Symptom 1574
- TYLENOL Flu No Drowsiness Formula, Maximum Strength Gelcaps 1575
- TYLENOL Flu NightTime, Maximum Strength Gelcaps 1575
- TYLENOL Flu NightTime, Maximum Strength Hot Medication Packets 1575
- TYLENOL Headache Plus Pain Reliever with Antacid, Extra Strength Caplets .... ■ 705
- TYLENOL PM Pain Reliever/Sleep Aid, Extra Strength Gelcaps, Caplets, Geltabs 1576
- TYLENOL Severe Allergy Medication Caplets 1571
- TYLENOL Sinus, Maximum Strength Geltabs, Gelcaps, Caplets and Tablets 1576
- Tylenol with Codeine 1592
- Tylox Capsules 1593
- Unisom With Pain Relief-Nighttime Sleep Aid and Pain Reliever 1991
- Vanquish Analgesic Caplets .... ■ 627
- Vicks 44 LiquiCaps Cough, Cold & Flu Relief .... ■ 728
- Vicks 44M Cough, Cold & Flu Relief .... ■ 729
- Vicks DayQuil LiquiCaps/Liquid Multi-Symptom Cold/Flu Relief .... ■ 734
- Vicks Nyquil Hot Therapy .... ■ 735
- Vicks NyQuil LiquiCaps/Liquid Multi-Symptom Cold/Flu Relief, Original and Cherry Flavors .... ■ 736
- Vicodin Tablets 1404
- Vicodin ES Tablets 1405
- Vicodin HP Tablets 1403
- Wygesic Tablets 2930
- Zydone Capsules 967

Acyclovir (Concomitant use may result in neurotoxicity (profound lethargy)). Products include:

- Zovirax Capsules 1187
- Zovirax Ointment 5% 1190
- Zovirax 1187

Acyclovir Sodium (Concomitant use may result in neurotoxicity (profound lethargy)). Products include:

- Zovirax Sterile Powder 1191

Amphotericin B (Increased risk of nephrotoxicity). Products include:

- Abelcet Injection 1540
- Fungizone Intravenous 507
- Fungizone Oral Suspension 704

Aspirin (May competitively inhibit glucuronidation; possible increased incidence of granulocytopenia). Products include:

- Alka-Seltzer Cherry Effervescent Antacid and Pain Reliever .... ■ 609
- Alka-Seltzer Extra Strength Effervescent Antacid and Pain Reliever .... ■ 609
- Alka-Seltzer Lemon Lime Effervescent Antacid and Pain Reliever .... ■ 609
- Alka-Seltzer Original Effervescent Antacid and Pain Reliever .... ■ 609
- Alka-Seltzer Plus .... ■ 611
- Alka-Seltzer Plus Sinus Medicine .... ■ 611
- Ascriptin .... ■ 650
- Arthritis Strength BC Powder .... ■ 631
- BC Cold Powder Multi-Symptom Formula (Cold-Sinus-Allergy) .... ■ 631
- BC Cold Powder Non-Drowsy Formula (Cold-Sinus) .... ■ 631
- BC Powder .... ■ 631
- Genuine Bayer Aspirin Tablets & Caplets .... ■ 618
- Extra Strength Bayer Arthritis Pain Regimen Formula .... ■ 615
- Extra Strength Bayer Aspirin Caplets & Tablets .... ■ 617
- Extended-Release Bayer 8-Hour Aspirin .... ■ 616
- Extra Strength Bayer Plus Aspirin Caplets .... ■ 617
- Extra Strength Bayer PM Aspirin Plus Sleep Aid .... ■ 617
- Aspirin Regimen Bayer 81 mg Tablets with Calcium .... ■ 615
- Aspirin Regimen Bayer Adult Low Strength 81 mg Tablets .... ■ 613
- Aspirin Regimen Bayer Children's Chewable Aspirin .... ■ 616
- Aspirin Regimen Bayer Regular Strength 325 mg Caplets .... ■ 613
- Bufferin Analgesic Tablets .... ■ 636
- Arthritis Strength Bufferin Analgesic Caplets .... ■ 637
- Extra Strength Bufferin Analgesic Tablets .... ■ 637
- Cama Arthritis Pain Reliever .... ■ 748
- Darvon Compound-65 Pulvules 1475
- Easprin 1971
- Ecotrin 2625
- Ecotrin Enteric Coated Aspirin Maximum Strength Tablets and Caplets .... ■ 775
- Ecotrin Enteric Coated Aspirin Regular Strength Tablets 2625
- Empirin Aspirin Tablets .... ■ 818
- Excedrin Extra-Strength Analgesic Tablets, Caplets, and Geltabs 734
- Fiorinal Capsules 2388
- Fiorinal with Codeine Capsules 2390
- Fiorinal Tablets 2388
- Goody's Extra Strength Headache Powders .... ■ 632
- Goody's Extra Strength Pain Relief Tablets .... ■ 632
- Halfprin Tablets 1413
- Norgesic 1554
- Percodan Tablets 955
- Percodan-Demi Tablets 956
- Robaxisal Tablets 2246
- Soma Compound w/Codeine Tablets 2784
- Soma Compound Tablets 2783
- St. Joseph Adult Chewable Aspirin (81 mg.) .... ■ 768
- Talwin Compound 2466
- Vanquish Analgesic Caplets .... ■ 627

Atovaquone (Co-administration shows a 24% +/- 12% decrease in zidovudine oral clearance, leading to a 35% +/- 23% increase in plasma zidovudine AUC; this effect is minor and would not expect to produce clinically significant events). Products include:

- Mepron Suspension 1206

Bleomycin Sulfate (Increased risk of hematological toxicity). Products include:

- Blenoxane 697

Dapsone (Increased risk of hematological toxicity). Products include:

- Dapsone Tablets USP 1331

Daunorubicin Hydrochloride (Increased risk of hematological toxicity). Products include:

- Cerubidine for Injection 634

Divalproex Sodium (Increases the oral bioavailability of zidovudine through the inhibition of first-pass hepatic metabolism; patients should be monitored more closely for a possible increase in zidovudine-related adverse effects). Products include:

- Depakote Tablets 418

Doxorubicin Hydrochloride (Increased risk of hematological toxicity). Products include:

- Adriamycin PFS 2056
- Adriamycin RDF 2056
- Doxil 2613

(■ Described in PDR For Nonprescription Drugs) (◉ Described in PDR For Ophthalmology)

Doxorubicin Astra 531
Rubex for Injection 721

Fluconazole (Co-administration may interfere with the oral clearance and metabolism of zidovudine). Products include:
Diflucan Tablets, Injection, and Oral Suspension 2003

Flucytosine (Increased risk of hematological toxicity). Products include:
Ancobon Capsules 2254

Fluorouracil (Increased risk of hematological toxicity). Products include:
Efudex 2280
Fluoroplex Topical Solution & Cream 1% 475
Fluorouracil Injection 2282

Ganciclovir Sodium (May increase the potential for hematological toxicity). Products include:
Cytovene-IV 2270

Hydroxyurea (Increased risk of hematological toxicity). Products include:
Hydrea Capsules 705

Indomethacin (Inhibits glucuronidation of Retrovir). Products include:
Indocin 1723

Indomethacin Sodium Trihydrate (Inhibits glucuronidation of Retrovir). Products include:
Indocin I.V. 1727

Interferon alfa-2A, Recombinant (Increased risk of hematological toxicity). Products include:
Roferon-A Injection 2308

Interferon alfa-2B, Recombinant (Increased risk of hematological toxicity). Products include:
Intron A for Injection 2506

Methadone Hydrochloride (Elevates plasma levels in some patients while remaining unchanged in others). Products include:
Methadone Hydrochloride Oral Concentrate 2356
Methadone Hydrochloride Oral Solution & Tablets 2357

Methotrexate Sodium (Increased risk of hematological toxicity). Products include:
Methotrexate Sodium Tablets, Injection, for Injection and LPF Injection 1322

Mitotane (Increased risk of toxicity). Products include:
Lysodren Tablets 707

Mitoxantrone Hydrochloride (Increased risk of hematological toxicity). Products include:
Novantrone for Injection 1327

Nephrotoxic Drugs (Increased risk of toxicity).

Pentamidine Isethionate (Increased risk of toxicity).
No products indexed under this heading.

Phenytoin (Possible alteration in the phenytoin plasma levels; low levels in some patients; high level documented in one case). Products include:
Dilantin Infatabs 1967
Dilantin-125 Suspension 1969

Phenytoin Sodium (Possible alteration in the phenytoin plasma levels; low levels in some patients; high level documented in one case). Products include:
Dilantin Kapseals 1965

Probenecid (Inhibits glucuronidation of Retrovir; may reduce renal excretion of Retrovir; concomitant use may result in flu-like symptoms consisting of myalgia, malaise and/or fever and maculopapular rash). Products include:
Benemid Tablets 1651
ColBENEMID Tablets 1662

Procarbazine Hydrochloride (Increased risk of hematological toxicity). Products include:
Matulane Capsules 2300

Ribavirin (Some experimental nucleoside analogues affecting DNA replication, such as ribavirin, antagonizes the *in vitro* antiviral activity of Retrovir against HIV and thus concomitant use of such drugs should be avoided). Products include:
Virazole 1310

Rifampin (Co-administration decreases the area under the plasma concentration curve by an average of 48% +/- 34%). Products include:
Rifadin 1276
Rifamate Capsules 1278
Rifater 1280
Rimactane Capsules 865

Tamoxifen Citrate (Increased risk of hematological toxicity). Products include:
Nolvadex Tablets 2957

Valproic Acid (Increases the oral bioavailability of zidovudine through the inhibition of first-pass hepatic metabolism; patients should be monitored closely for zidovudine-related adverse effects). Products include:
Depakene 416

Vinblastine Sulfate (Increased risk of hematological toxicity). Products include:
Velban Vials 1537

Vincristine Sulfate (Increased risk of hematological toxicity). Products include:
Oncovin Solution Vials & Hyporets 1521

Food Interactions

Food, unspecified (Administration of Retrovir Capsules with food decreased peak plasma concentrations by greater than 50%, however, bioavailability as determined by AUC may not be affected).

RETROVIR I.V. INFUSION

(Zidovudine) 1221
May interact with cytotoxic drugs, aspirin and acetaminophen containing products, experimental nucleoside analogues (selected) for aids and arc, and certain other agents. Compounds in these categories include:

Acetaminophen (May competitively inhibit glucuronidation; possible increased incidence of granulocytopenia). Products include:
Actifed Cold & Sinus Caplets and Tablets 808
Actifed Sinus Daytime/Nighttime Tablets and Caplets 809
Alka-Seltzer Fast Relief Caplets 610
Alka-Seltzer Plus Liqui-Gels 612
Alka-Seltzer Plus Flu & Body Aches Effervescent Tablets 612
Alka-Seltzer Plus Flu & Body Aches Liqui-Gels Non-Drowsy Formula 613
Alka-Seltzer Plus Night-Time Cold Medicine Liqui-Gels 612
Allerest No Drowsiness 649
Allerest Sinus Pain Formula 649
Axocet Capsules 2469
Benadryl Allergy/Cold Tablets 811
Benadryl Allergy Sinus Headache Caplets 813
Children's TYLENOL acetaminophen Chewable Tablets, Elixir, Suspension Liquid, and Suspension Drops 1559
Children's TYLENOL Cold Multi-Symptom Chewable Tablets and Liquid 1559
Children's TYLENOL Cold Plus Cough Multi Symptom Chewable Tablets and Liquid 1560
Children's TYLENOL Flu Suspension Liquid 1560
Allergy-Sinus Comtrex Multi-Symptom Allergy-Sinus Formula Tablets and Caplets 639
Comtrex Multi-Symptom 638
Comtrex Non-Drowsy 640
Contac Day Allergy/Sinus Caplets 771
Contac Day & Night 772
Contac Night Allergy/Sinus Caplets 771
Contac Severe Cold and Flu Formula Caplets 773
Contac Severe Cold & Flu Non-Drowsy 774
Coricidin Cold + Flu Tablets 760
Coricidin 'D' Decongestant Tablets 760
DHCplus Capsules 2148
Darvon-N/Darvocet-N 1473
Dimetapp Allergy Sinus Caplets 838
Dimetapp Cold & Fever Suspension 839
Drixoral Cold and Flu Extended-Release Tablets 764
Drixoral Cough + Sore Throat Liquid Caps 763
Drixoral Allergy/Sinus Extended Release Tablets 765
Esgic-plus Capsules 1012
Esgic-plus Tablets 1012
Aspirin Free Excedrin Analgesic Caplets and Geltabs 734
Excedrin Extra-Strength Analgesic Tablets, Caplets, and Geltabs 734
Excedrin P.M. Analgesic/Sleeping Aid Tablets, Caplets, Liquigels 735
Fioricet Tablets 2386
Fioricet with Codeine Capsules 2387
Goody's Extra Strength Headache Powders 632
Goody's Extra Strength Pain Relief Tablets 632
Hycomine Compound Tablets 948
Hydrocet Capsules 787
Infants' TYLENOL acetaminophen Suspension Drops 1559
Infants' TYLENOL Cold Decongestant & Fever-Reducer Drops 1561
Junior Strength TYLENOL acetaminophen Coated Caplets and Chewable Tablets 1562
Lorcet 10/650 Tablets 1016
Lortab 2751
Lurline PMS Tablets 1000
Maximum Strength Multi-Symptom Formula Midol 621
PMS Multi-Symptom Formula Midol 622
Maximum Strength Midol Teen Multi-Symptom Formula 621
Midrin Capsules 788
Panodol Tablets and Caplets 783
Children's Panadol Chewable Tablets, Liquid, Infant's Drops 783
Percocet Tablets 955
Percogesic Analgesic Tablets 727
Phrenilin 790
Pyrroxate Caplets 742
Robitussin Cold, Cough & Flu Liqui-Gels 844
Robitussin Night-Time Cold Formula 847
Sedapap Tablets 50 mg/650 mg .. 1826
Sinarest 663
Sine-Aid Maximum Strength Sinus Headache Gelcaps, Caplets and Tablets 1570
Sine-Off No Drowsiness Formula Caplets 784
Sine-Off Sinus Medicine 784
Singlet Tablets 785
Sinulin Tablets 792
Sinutab Sinus Allergy Medication, Maximum Strength Tablets and Caplets 823
Sinutab Sinus Medication, Maximum Strength Without Drowsiness Formula, Tablets & Caplets 824
Sudafed Cold and Cough Liquid Caps 826
Sudafed Severe Cold Formula Caplets 828
Sudafed Severe Cold Formula Tablets 828
Sudafed Sinus Caplets 829
Sudafed Sinus Tablets 829
Talacen Caplets 2464
TheraFlu Flu and Cold Medicine 750
Theraflu Maximum Strength Flu and Cold Medicine For Sore Throat 751
TheraFlu Flu, Cold and Cough Medicine 750
TheraFlu Maximum Strength Nighttime Flu, Cold & Cough Medicine 751
TheraFlu Maximum Strength Non-Drowsy Formula Flu, Cold & Cough Medicine 751
TheraFlu Maximum Strength, Non-Drowsy Formula Flu, Cold and Cough Caplets 752
Theraflu Maximum Strength Sinus Non-Drowsy Formula Caplets 752
Triaminic Sore Throat Formula 755
Triaminicin Tablets 756
TYLENOL acetaminophen Extended Relief Caplets 1570
TYLENOL acetaminophen, Extra Strength Adult Liquid Pain Reliever 1570
TYLENOL acetaminophen, Extra Strength Gelcaps, Geltabs, Caplets, Tablets 1570
TYLENOL acetaminophen, Regular Strength Caplets and Tablets 1570
TYLENOL Allergy Sinus, Maximum Strength Caplets and Gelcaps 1571
TYLENOL Allergy Sinus NightTime, Maximum Strength Caplets 1571
TYLENOL Cold Medication, Multi-Symptom Formula Tablets and Caplets 1572
TYLENOL Cold Medication, Multi-Symptom Hot Liquid Packets 1572
TYLENOL Cold Medication, No Drowsiness Formula Caplets and Gelcaps 1572
TYLENOL Cold Severe Congestion Caplets 1573
TYLENOL Cough Medication, Multi Symptom 1574
TYLENOL Cough Medication with Decongestant, Multi Symptom 1574
TYLENOL Flu No Drowsiness Formula, Maximum Strength Gelcaps 1575
TYLENOL Flu NightTime, Maximum Strength Gelcaps 1575
TYLENOL Flu NightTime, Maximum Strength Hot Medication Packets 1575
TYLENOL Headache Plus Pain Reliever with Antacid, Extra Strength Caplets 705
TYLENOL PM Pain Reliever/Sleep Aid, Extra Strength Gelcaps, Caplets, Geltabs 1576
TYLENOL Severe Allergy Medication Caplets 1571
TYLENOL Sinus, Maximum Strength Geltabs, Gelcaps, Caplets and Tablets 1576
Tylenol with Codeine 1592
Tylox Capsules 1593
Unisom With Pain Relief-Nighttime Sleep Aid and Pain Reliever 1991
Vanquish Analgesic Caplets 627
Vicks 44 LiquiCaps Cough, Cold & Flu Relief 728
Vicks 44M Cough, Cold & Flu Relief 729
Vicks DayQuil LiquiCaps/Liquid Multi-Symptom Cold/Flu Relief .. 734
Vicks Nyquil Hot Therapy 735
Vicks NyQuil LiquiCaps/Liquid Multi-Symptom Cold/Flu Relief, Original and Cherry Flavors 736
Vicodin Tablets 1404
Vicodin ES Tablets 1405
Vicodin HP Tablets 1403
Wygesic Tablets 2930
Zydone Capsules 967

Acyclovir (Concomitant use has resulted in neurotoxicity, profound lethargy). Products include:
Zovirax Capsules 1187
Zovirax Ointment 5% 1190
Zovirax 1187

IMPORTANT NOTE: Always consult each drug listing in the patient's regimen for possible interactions.

Retrovir I.V. — Interactions Index

Amphotericin B (Increased risk of nephrotoxicity). Products include:
- Abelcet Injection 1540
- Fungizone Intravenous 507
- Fungizone Oral Suspension 704

Aspirin (May competitively inhibit glucuronidation; possible increased incidence of granulocytopenia). Products include:
- Alka-Seltzer Cherry Effervescent Antacid and Pain Reliever 609
- Alka-Seltzer Extra Strength Effervescent Antacid and Pain Reliever 609
- Alka-Seltzer Lemon Lime Effervescent Antacid and Pain Reliever 609
- Alka-Seltzer Original Effervescent Antacid and Pain Reliever 609
- Alka-Seltzer Plus 611
- Alka-Seltzer Plus Sinus Medicine 611
- Ascriptin 650
- Arthritis Strength BC Powder 631
- BC Cold Powder Multi-Symptom Formula (Cold-Sinus-Allergy) 631
- BC Cold Powder Non-Drowsy Formula (Cold-Sinus) 631
- BC Powder 631
- Genuine Bayer Aspirin Tablets & Caplets 618
- Extra Strength Bayer Arthritis Pain Regimen Formula 615
- Extra Strength Bayer Aspirin Caplets & Tablets 617
- Extended-Release Bayer 8-Hour Aspirin 616
- Extra Strength Bayer Plus Aspirin Caplets 617
- Extra Strength Bayer PM Aspirin Plus Sleep Aid 617
- Aspirin Regimen Bayer 81 mg Tablets with Calcium 615
- Aspirin Regimen Bayer Adult Low Strength 81 mg Tablets 613
- Aspirin Regimen Bayer Children's Chewable Aspirin 616
- Aspirin Regimen Bayer Regular Strength 325 mg Caplets 613
- Bufferin Analgesic Tablets 636
- Arthritis Strength Bufferin Analgesic Caplets 637
- Extra Strength Bufferin Analgesic Tablets 637
- Cama Arthritis Pain Reliever 748
- Darvon Compound-65 Pulvules 1475
- Easprin 1971
- Ecotrin 2625
- Ecotrin Enteric Coated Aspirin Maximum Strength Tablets and Caplets 775
- Ecotrin Enteric Coated Aspirin Regular Strength Tablets 2625
- Empirin Aspirin Tablets 818
- Excedrin Extra-Strength Analgesic Tablets, Caplets, and Geltabs 734
- Fiorinal Capsules 2388
- Fiorinal with Codeine Capsules 2390
- Fiorinal Tablets 2388
- Goody's Extra Strength Headache Powders 632
- Goody's Extra Strength Pain Relief Tablets 632
- Halfprin Tablets 1413
- Norgesic 1554
- Percodan Tablets 955
- Percodan-Demi Tablets 956
- Robaxisal Tablets 2246
- Soma Compound w/Codeine Tablets 2784
- Soma Compound Tablets 2783
- St. Joseph Adult Chewable Aspirin (81 mg.) 768
- Talwin Compound 2466
- Vanquish Analgesic Caplets 627

Atovaquone (Co-administration shows a 24% +/- 12% decrease in zidovudine oral clearance, leading to a 35% +/- 23% increase in plasma zidovudine AUC; this effect is minor and would not expect to produce clinically significant events). Products include:
- Mepron Suspension 1206

Bleomycin Sulfate (Increased risk of hematological toxicity). Products include:
- Blenoxane 697

Dapsone (Increased risk of hematological toxicity). Products include:
- Dapsone Tablets USP 1331

Daunorubicin Hydrochloride (Increased risk of hematological toxicity). Products include:
- Cerubidine for Injection 634

Divalproex Sodium (Increases the oral bioavailability of zidovudine through the inhibition of first-pass hepatic metabolism; patients should be monitored more closely for a possible increase in zidovudine-related adverse effects). Products include:
- Depakote Tablets 418

Doxorubicin Hydrochloride (Increased risk of hematological toxicity). Products include:
- Adriamycin PFS 2056
- Adriamycin RDF 2056
- Doxil 2613
- Doxorubicin Astra 531
- Rubex for Injection 721

Fluconazole (Co-administration may interfere with the oral clearance and metabolism of zidovudine). Products include:
- Diflucan Tablets, Injection, and Oral Suspension 2003

Flucytosine (Increased risk of hematological toxicity). Products include:
- Ancobon Capsules 2254

Fluorouracil (Increased risk of hematological toxicity). Products include:
- Efudex 2280
- Fluoroplex Topical Solution & Cream 1% 475
- Fluorouracil Injection 2282

Ganciclovir Sodium (May increase the potential for hematological toxicity). Products include:
- Cytovene-IV 2270

Hydroxyurea (Increased risk of hematological toxicity). Products include:
- Hydrea Capsules 705

Indomethacin (May competitively inhibit glucuronidation). Products include:
- Indocin 1723

Indomethacin Sodium Trihydrate (May competitively inhibit glucuronidation). Products include:
- Indocin I.V. 1727

Interferon alfa-2A, Recombinant (Increased risk of hematological toxicity). Products include:
- Roferon-A Injection 2308

Interferon alfa-2B, Recombinant (Increased risk of hematological toxicity). Products include:
- Intron A Injection 2506

Methadone Hydrochloride (Mean zidovudine AUC may be elevated in some patients; no change in the pharmacokinetics of methadone). Products include:
- Methadone Hydrochloride Oral Concentrate 2356
- Methadone Hydrochloride Oral Solution & Tablets 2357

Methotrexate Sodium (Increased risk of hematological toxicity). Products include:
- Methotrexate Sodium Tablets, Injection, for Injection and LPF 1322

Mitotane (Increased risk of hematological toxicity). Products include:
- Lysodren Tablets 707

Mitoxantrone Hydrochloride (Increased risk of hematological toxicity). Products include:
- Novantrone for Injection 1327

Nephrotoxic Drugs (Increased risk of toxicity).

Pentamidine Isethionate (Increased risk of toxicity).
No products indexed under this heading.

Phenytoin (Low phenytoin levels reported in some patients; high level documented in one case). Products include:
- Dilantin Infatabs 1967
- Dilantin-125 Suspension 1969

Phenytoin Sodium (Low phenytoin levels reported in some patients; high level documented in one case). Products include:
- Dilantin Kapseals 1965

Probenecid (May increase zidovudine levels by inhibiting glucuronidation and/or reducing renal excretion of zidovudine; some patients have developed flu-like symptoms consisting of fever, myalgia, malaise, and rash). Products include:
- Benemid Tablets 1651
- ColBENEMID Tablets 1662

Procarbazine Hydrochloride (Increased risk of hematological toxicity). Products include:
- Matulane Capsules 2300

Rifampin (Co-administration may decrease the area under the plasma concentration curve of zidovudine). Products include:
- Rifadin 1276
- Rifamate Capsules 1278
- Rifater 1280
- Rimactane Capsules 865

Tamoxifen Citrate (Increased risk of hematological toxicity). Products include:
- Nolvadex Tablets 2957

Valproic Acid (Increases the oral bioavailability of zidovudine through the inhibition of first-pass hepatic metabolism; patients should be monitored more closely for a possible increase in zidovudine-related adverse effects). Products include:
- Depakene 416

Vinblastine Sulfate (Increased risk of hematological toxicity). Products include:
- Velban Vials 1537

Vincristine Sulfate (Increased risk of hematological toxicity). Products include:
- Oncovin Solution Vials & Hyporets 1521

RETROVIR SYRUP
(Zidovudine) 1216
See **Retrovir Capsules**

REV-EYES OPHTHALMIC EYEDROPS 0.5%
(Dapiprazole Hydrochloride) 324
None cited in PDR database.

REVEX (NALMEFENE HYDROCHLORIDE INJECTION)
(Nalmefene Hydrochloride) 1863
May interact with:

Flumazenil (Physicians should remain aware of the potential risk, based on animal studies, of seizures from agents in these classes). Products include:
- Romazicon 2311

REVIA TABLETS
(Naltrexone Hydrochloride) 957
May interact with narcotic analgesics and certain other agents. Compounds in these categories include:

Alfentanil Hydrochloride (Concurrent use is contraindicated; if an opioid analgesic is co-administered, the amount required may be greater than usual, and the resulting respiratory depression may be deeper and more prolonged). Products include:
- Alfenta Injection 1334

Buprenorphine (Concurrent use is contraindicated; if an opioid analgesic is co-administered, the amount required may be greater than usual, and the resulting respiratory depression may be deeper and more prolonged). Products include:
- Buprenex Injectable 2170

Codeine Phosphate (Concurrent use is contraindicated; if an opioid analgesic is co-administered, the amount required may be greater than usual, and the resulting respiratory depression may be deeper and more prolonged). Products include:
- Brontex 2130
- Dimetane-DC Cough Syrup 2232
- Fioricet with Codeine Capsules 2387
- Fiorinal with Codeine Capsules 2390
- Nucofed 2225
- Phenergan with Codeine 2883
- Phenergan VC with Codeine 2888
- Robitussin A-C Syrup 2248
- Robitussin-DAC Syrup 2249
- Ryna 804
- Soma Compound w/Codeine Tablets 2784
- Tylenol with Codeine 1592

Dezocine (Concurrent use is contraindicated; if an opioid analgesic is co-administered, the amount required may be greater than usual, and the resulting respiratory depression may be deeper and more prolonged). Products include:
- Dalgan Injection 529

Difenoxin Hydrochloride (Patients may not benefit from opioid-containing antidiarrheal preparations). Products include:
- Motofen Tablets 789

Diphenoxylate Hydrochloride (Patients may not benefit from opioid-containing antidiarrheal preparations). Products include:
- Lomotil 2591

Disulfiram (Co-administration of two potentially hepatotoxic agents is not recommended unless the probable benefits outweigh the known risks). Products include:
- Antabuse Tablets 2802

Fentanyl (Concurrent use is contraindicated; if an opioid analgesic is co-administered, the amount required may be greater than usual, and the resulting respiratory depression may be deeper and more prolonged). Products include:
- Duragesic Transdermal System 1336

Fentanyl Citrate (Concurrent use is contraindicated; if an opioid analgesic is co-administered, the amount required may be greater than usual, and the resulting respiratory depression may be deeper and more prolonged). Products include:
- Sublimaze Injection 463

Hydrocodone Bitartrate (Concurrent use is contraindicated; if an opioid analgesic is co-administered, the amount required may be greater than usual, and the resulting respiratory depression may be deeper and more prolonged). Products include:
- Codiclear DH Syrup 808
- Duratuss HD Elixir 2750
- Histussin D Liquid 670

(▣ Described in PDR For Nonprescription Drugs)   (◉ Described in PDR For Ophthalmology)

Interactions Index — Rifadin

Hycodan Tablets and Syrup 946
Hycomine Compound Tablets 948
Hycomine 947
Hycotuss Expectorant Syrup 950
Hydrocet Capsules 787
Lorcet 10/650 Tablets 1016
Lortab 2751
Tussend 1830
Tussend Expectorant 1831
Vicodin Tablets 1404
Vicodin ES Tablets 1405
Vicodin HP Tablets 1403
Vicodin Tuss Expectorant 1406
Zydone Capsules 967

Hydrocodone Polistirex (Concurrent use is contraindicated; if an opioid analgesic is co-administered, the amount required may be greater than usual, and the resulting respiratory depression may be deeper and more prolonged). Products include:

Tussionex Pennkinetic Extended-Release Suspension 1624

Hydromorphone Hydrochloride (Concurrent use is contraindicated; if an opioid analgesic is co-administered, the amount required may be greater than usual, and the resulting respiratory depression may be deeper and more prolonged). Products include:

Dilaudid Ampules 1382
Dilaudid Cough Syrup 1383
Dilaudid-HP Injection 1384
Dilaudid-HP Lyophilized Powder 250 mg 1384
Dilaudid 1382
Dilaudid Oral Liquid 1386
Dilaudid 1382
Dilaudid Tablets - 8 mg 1386

Levorphanol Tartrate (Concurrent use is contraindicated; if an opioid analgesic is co-administered, the amount required may be greater than usual, and the resulting respiratory depression may be deeper and more prolonged). Products include:

Levo-Dromoran 2297

Meperidine Hydrochloride (Concurrent use is contraindicated; if an opioid analgesic is co-administered, the amount required may be greater than usual, and the resulting respiratory depression may be deeper and more prolonged). Products include:

Demerol 2438
Mepergan Injection 2859

Methadone Hydrochloride (Concurrent use is contraindicated; if an opioid analgesic is co-administered, the amount required may be greater than usual, and the resulting respiratory depression may be deeper and more prolonged). Products include:

Methadone Hydrochloride Oral Concentrate 2356
Methadone Hydrochloride Oral Solution & Tablets 2357

Morphine Sulfate (Concurrent use is contraindicated; if an opioid analgesic is co-administered, the amount required may be greater than usual, and the resulting respiratory depression may be deeper and more prolonged). Products include:

Astramorph/PF Injection, USP (Preservative-Free) 526
Duramorph Injection 983
Infumorph 200 and Infumorph 500 Sterile Solutions 985
Kadian Capsules 2948
MS Contin Tablets 2149
MSIR 2152

Oramorph SR (Morphine Sulfate Sustained Release Tablets) 2359
RMS Suppositories CII 2766
Roxanol 2365

Opium Alkaloids (Concurrent use is contraindicated; if an opioid analgesic is co-administered, the amount required may be greater than usual, and the resulting respiratory depression may be deeper and more prolonged).

No products indexed under this heading.

Oxycodone Hydrochloride (Concurrent use is contraindicated; if an opioid analgesic is co-administered, the amount required may be greater than usual, and the resulting respiratory depression may be deeper and more prolonged). Products include:

OxyContin Tablets 2163
OxyIR Capsules 2167
Percocet Tablets 955
Percodan Tablets 955
Percodan-Demi Tablets 956
Roxicodone Tablets, Oral Solution & Intensol (Oxycodone) 2366
Tylox Capsules 1593

Propoxyphene Hydrochloride (Concurrent use is contraindicated; if an opioid analgesic is co-administered, the amount required may be greater than usual, and the resulting respiratory depression may be deeper and more prolonged). Products include:

Darvon 1475
Wygesic Tablets 2930

Propoxyphene Napsylate (Concurrent use is contraindicated; if an opioid analgesic is co-administered, the amount required may be greater than usual, and the resulting respiratory depression may be deeper and more prolonged). Products include:

Darvon-N/Darvocet-N 1473

Sufentanil Citrate (Concurrent use is contraindicated; if an opioid analgesic is co-administered, the amount required may be greater than usual, and the resulting respiratory depression may be deeper and more prolonged). Products include:

Sufenta Injection 1355

Thioridazine Hydrochloride (Lethargy and somnolence have been reported following doses of ReVia and thioridazine). Products include:

Mellaril 2398

RHEABAN MAXIMUM STRENGTH FAST ACTING CAPLETS
(Attapulgite, Activated) 716
None cited in PDR database.

RHINOCORT NASAL INHALER
(Budesonide) 552
None cited in PDR database.

RHOGAM RH₀(D) IMMUNE GLOBULIN (HUMAN)
(Immune Globulin (Human)) 1902
None cited in PDR database.

RID LICE CONTROL SPRAY
(Permethrin) 716
None cited in PDR database.

RID LICE KILLING SHAMPOO
(Pyrethrum Extract, Piperonyl Butoxide) 717
None cited in PDR database.

RIDAURA CAPSULES
(Auranofin) 2691
May interact with:

Phenytoin (Increased phenytoin blood levels). Products include:
Dilantin Infatabs 1967
Dilantin-125 Suspension 1969

Phenytoin Sodium (Increased phenytoin blood levels). Products include:
Dilantin Kapseals 1965

RIFADIN CAPSULES
(Rifampin) 1276
May interact with corticosteroids, cardiac glycosides, oral contraceptives, narcotic analgesics, barbiturates, beta blockers, anticonvulsants, xanthine bronchodilators, progestins, quinidine, sulfonylureas, and certain other agents. Compounds in these categories include:

Acebutolol Hydrochloride (Rifampin has been reported to diminish the effects of concurrently administered beta blockers). Products include:
Sectral Capsules 2914

Alfentanil Hydrochloride (Rifampin has liver enzyme-inducing properties and may reduce the activity of narcotics). Products include:
Alfenta Injection 1334

Aminophylline (Rifampin has been reported to diminish the effects of concurrently administered theophylline).
No products indexed under this heading.

Aprobarbital (Rifampin has been reported to diminish the effects of concurrently administered barbiturates).
No products indexed under this heading.

Atenolol (Rifampin has been reported to diminish the effects of concurrently administered beta blockers). Products include:
Tenoretic Tablets 2963
Tenormin Tablets and I.V. Injection 2965

Betamethasone Acetate (Rifampin has liver enzyme-inducing properties and may reduce the activity of corticosteroids). Products include:
Celestone Soluspan Suspension 2484

Betamethasone Sodium Phosphate (Rifampin has liver enzyme-inducing properties and may reduce the activity of corticosteroids). Products include:
Celestone Soluspan Suspension 2484

Betaxolol Hydrochloride (Rifampin has been reported to diminish the effects of concurrently administered beta blockers). Products include:
Betoptic Ophthalmic Solution 465
Betoptic S Ophthalmic Suspension 467
Kerlone Tablets 2588

Bisoprolol Fumarate (Rifampin has been reported to diminish the effects of concurrently administered beta blockers). Products include:
Zebeta Tablets 1457
Ziac 1459

Buprenorphine (Rifampin has liver enzyme-inducing properties and may reduce the activity of narcotics). Products include:
Buprenex Injectable 2170

Butabarbital (Rifampin has been reported to diminish the effects of concurrently administered barbiturates).
No products indexed under this heading.

Butalbital (Rifampin has been reported to diminish the effects of concurrently administered barbiturates). Products include:
Axocet Capsules 2469
Esgic-plus Capsules 1012
Esgic-plus Tablets 1012
Fioricet Tablets 2386
Fioricet with Codeine Capsules 2387
Fiorinal Capsules 2388
Fiorinal with Codeine Capsules 2390
Fiorinal Tablets 2388
Phrenilin 790
Sedapap Tablets 50 mg/650 mg 1826

Carbamazepine (Rifampin has liver enzyme-inducing properties and may reduce the activity of anticonvulsants). Products include:
Atretol Tablets 569
Tegretol/Tegretol-XR 870

Carteolol Hydrochloride (Rifampin has been reported to diminish the effects of concurrently administered beta blockers). Products include:
Cartrol Tablets 413
Ocupress Ophthalmic Solution, 1% Sterile 297

Chloramphenicol (Rifampin has been reported to diminish the effects of concurrently administered chloramphenicol). Products include:
Chloromycetin Ophthalmic Ointment, 1% 298
Chloromycetin Ophthalmic Solution 299
Chloroptic S.O.P. 236
Chloroptic Sterile Ophthalmic Solution 236

Chloramphenicol Palmitate (Rifampin has been reported to diminish the effects of concurrently administered chloramphenicol).
No products indexed under this heading.

Chloramphenicol Sodium Succinate (Rifampin has been reported to diminish the effects of concurrently administered chloramphenicol). Products include:
Chloromycetin Sodium Succinate 1960

Chlorpropamide (Rifampin has liver enzyme-inducing properties and may reduce the activity of sulfonylureas). Products include:
Diabinese Tablets 2002

Clofibrate (Rifampin has been reported to diminish the effects of concurrently administered clofibrate). Products include:
Atromid-S Capsules 2808

Codeine Phosphate (Rifampin has liver enzyme-inducing properties and may reduce the activity of narcotics). Products include:
Brontex 2130
Dimetane-DC Cough Syrup 2232
Fioricet with Codeine Capsules 2387
Fiorinal with Codeine Capsules 2390
Nucofed 2225
Phenergan with Codeine 2883
Phenergan VC with Codeine 2888
Robitussin A-C Syrup 2248
Robitussin-DAC Syrup 2249
Ryna 804
Soma Compound w/Codeine Tablets 2784
Tylenol with Codeine 1592

Cortisone Acetate (Rifampin has liver enzyme-inducing properties and may reduce the activity of corticosteroids). Products include:
Cortone Acetate Sterile Suspension 1663
Cortone Acetate Tablets 1664

Cyclosporine (Rifampin has liver enzyme-inducing properties and may reduce the activity of cyclosporine). Products include:
Neoral 2405
Sandimmune 2416

IMPORTANT NOTE: Always consult each drug listing in the patient's regimen for possible interactions.

Rifadin — Interactions Index

Dapsone (Rifampin has liver enzyme-inducing properties and may reduce the activity of dapsone). Products include:
- Dapsone Tablets USP ... 1331

Deslanoside (Rifampin has liver enzyme-inducing properties and may reduce the activity of cardiac glycosides).
- No products indexed under this heading.

Desogestrel (Rifampin has liver enzyme-inducing properties and may reduce the activity of oral contraceptives; nonhormonal methods of contraception during therapy with rifampin is recommended). Products include:
- Desogen Tablets ... 1867
- Ortho-Cept ... 1907

Dexamethasone (Rifampin has liver enzyme-inducing properties and may reduce the activity of corticosteroids). Products include:
- AK-Trol Ointment & Suspension ... ⊙ 205
- Decadron Elixir ... 1676
- Decadron Tablets ... 1678
- Decaspray Topical Aerosol ... 1689
- Maxitrol Ophthalmic Ointment and Suspension ... ⊙ 222
- TobraDex Ophthalmic Suspension and Ointment ... 469

Dexamethasone Acetate (Rifampin has liver enzyme-inducing properties and may reduce the activity of corticosteroids). Products include:
- Dalalone D.P. Injectable ... 1009
- Decadron-LA Sterile Suspension ... 1687

Dexamethasone Sodium Phosphate (Rifampin has liver enzyme-inducing properties and may reduce the activity of corticosteroids). Products include:
- Decadron Phosphate Injection ... 1680
- Decadron Phosphate Sterile Ophthalmic Ointment ... 1684
- Decadron Phosphate Sterile Ophthalmic Solution ... 1685
- Decadron Phosphate Topical Cream ... 1686
- Decadron Phosphate with Xylocaine Injection, Sterile ... 1683
- Dexacort Phosphate in Respihaler ... 1606
- Dexacort Phosphate in Turbinaire ... 1607
- NeoDecadron Sterile Ophthalmic Ointment ... 1755
- NeoDecadron Sterile Ophthalmic Solution ... 1756
- NeoDecadron Topical Cream ... 1757

Dezocine (Rifampin has liver enzyme-inducing properties and may reduce the activity of narcotics). Products include:
- Dalgan Injection ... 529

Diazepam (Rifampin has been reported to diminish the effects of concurrently administered diazepam). Products include:
- Dizac (diazepam injectable emulsion) CIV ... 1862
- Valium Injectable ... 2336
- Valium Tablets ... 2335

Digitoxin (Rifampin has liver enzyme-inducing properties and may reduce the activity of cardiac glycosides). Products include:
- Crystodigin Tablets ... 1472

Digoxin (Rifampin has liver enzyme-inducing properties and may reduce the activity of cardiac glycosides). Products include:
- Lanoxicaps ... 1110
- Lanoxin Elixir Pediatric ... 1113
- Lanoxin Injection ... 1116
- Lanoxin Injection Pediatric ... 1119
- Lanoxin Tablets ... 1121

Disopyramide Phosphate (Rifampin has been reported to diminish the effects of concurrently administered disopyramide). Products include:
- Norpace ... 2596

Divalproex Sodium (Rifampin has liver enzyme-inducing properties and may reduce the activity of anticonvulsants). Products include:
- Depakote Tablets ... 418

Dyphylline (Rifampin has been reported to diminish the effects of concurrently administered theophylline). Products include:
- Lufyllin & Lufyllin-400 Tablets ... 2778
- Lufyllin-GG Elixir & Tablets ... 2779

Esmolol Hydrochloride (Rifampin has been reported to diminish the effects of concurrently administered beta blockers). Products include:
- Brevibloc (esmolol HCl) Injection ... 1860

Ethinyl Estradiol (Rifampin has liver enzyme-inducing properties and may reduce the activity of oral contraceptives; nonhormonal methods of contraception during therapy with rifampin is recommended). Products include:
- Brevicon ... 2563
- Demulen ... 2580
- Desogen Tablets ... 1867
- Levlen/Tri-Levlen ... 646
- Lo/Ovral Tablets ... 2852
- Lo/Ovral-28 Tablets ... 2857
- Modicon ... 1928
- Nordette-21 Tablets ... 2863
- Nordette-28 Tablets ... 2866
- Norinyl ... 2563
- Ortho-Cept ... 1907
- Ortho-Cyclen/Ortho-Tri-Cyclen ... 1914
- Ortho-Novum ... 1928
- Ortho-Cyclen/Ortho Tri-Cyclen ... 1914
- Ovcon ... 765
- Ovral Tablets ... 2877
- Ovral-28 Tablets ... 2878
- Levlen/Tri-Levlen ... 646
- Tri-Norinyl ... 2607
- Triphasil-21 Tablets ... 2919
- Triphasil-28 Tablets ... 2924

Ethosuximide (Rifampin has liver enzyme-inducing properties and may reduce the activity of anticonvulsants). Products include:
- Zarontin Capsules ... 1986
- Zarontin Syrup ... 1986

Ethotoin (Rifampin has liver enzyme-inducing properties and may reduce the activity of anticonvulsants). Products include:
- Peganone Tablets ... 455

Ethynodiol Diacetate (Rifampin has liver enzyme-inducing properties and may reduce the activity of oral contraceptives; nonhormonal methods of contraception during therapy with rifampin is recommended). Products include:
- Demulen ... 2580

Felbamate (Rifampin has liver enzyme-inducing properties and may reduce the activity of anticonvulsants). Products include:
- Felbatol ... 2774

Fentanyl (Rifampin has liver enzyme-inducing properties and may reduce the activity of narcotics). Products include:
- Duragesic Transdermal System ... 1336

Fentanyl Citrate (Rifampin has liver enzyme-inducing properties and may reduce the activity of narcotics). Products include:
- Sublimaze Injection ... 463

Fludrocortisone Acetate (Rifampin has liver enzyme-inducing properties and may reduce the activity of corticosteroids). Products include:
- Florinef Acetate Tablets ... 506

Fosphenytoin Sodium (Rifampin has liver enzyme-inducing properties and may reduce the activity of anticonvulsants). Products include:
- Cerebyx Injection ... 1956

Glimepiride (Rifampin has liver enzyme-inducing properties and may reduce the activity of sulfonylureas). Products include:
- Amaryl Tablets ... 1241

Glipizide (Rifampin has liver enzyme-inducing properties and may reduce the activity of sulfonylureas). Products include:
- Glucotrol Tablets ... 2011
- Glucotrol XL Extended Release Tablets ... 2012

Glyburide (Rifampin has liver enzyme-inducing properties and may reduce the activity of sulfonylureas). Products include:
- DiaBeta Tablets ... 1265
- Glynase PresTab Tablets ... 2091
- Micronase Tablets ... 2099

Halothane (Co-administration has been reported to increase the hepatic toxicity of both drugs). Products include:
- Fluothane ... 2830

Hydrocodone Bitartrate (Rifampin has liver enzyme-inducing properties and may reduce the activity of narcotics). Products include:
- Codiclear DH Syrup ... 808
- Duratuss HD Elixir ... 2750
- Histussin D Liquid ... 670
- Hycodan Tablets and Syrup ... 946
- Hycomine Compound Tablets ... 948
- Hycomine ... 947
- Hycotuss Expectorant Syrup ... 950
- Hydrocet Capsules ... 787
- Lorcet 10/650 Tablets ... 1016
- Lortab ... 2751
- Tussend ... 1830
- Tussend Expectorant ... 1831
- Vicodin Tablets ... 1404
- Vicodin ES Tablets ... 1405
- Vicodin HP Tablets ... 1403
- Vicodin Tuss Expectorant ... 1406
- Zydone Capsules ... 967

Hydrocodone Polistirex (Rifampin has liver enzyme-inducing properties and may reduce the activity of narcotics). Products include:
- Tussionex Pennkinetic Extended-Release Suspension ... 1624

Hydrocortisone (Rifampin has liver enzyme-inducing properties and may reduce the activity of corticosteroids). Products include:
- Anusol-HC Cream 2.5% ... 1953
- Aquanil HC Lotion ... 1989
- Maximum Strength Cortaid Spray ... ▣ 800
- CORTENEMA ... 2713
- Cortisporin Ointment ... 1074
- Cortisporin Ophthalmic Ointment Sterile ... 1074
- Cortisporin Ophthalmic Suspension Sterile ... 1075
- Cortisporin Otic Solution Sterile ... 1076
- Cortisporin Otic Suspension Sterile ... 1077
- Cortizone-5 ... ▣ 795
- Cortizone-10 ... ▣ 795
- Hydrocortone Tablets ... 1715
- Hytone ... 922
- Hytone Ointment 2 ½ % ... 923
- Massengill Medicated Soft Cloth Towelettes ... 2628
- Pediotic Suspension Sterile ... 1140
- Preparation H Hydrocortisone 1% Cream ... ▣ 843
- ProctoCream-HC 2.5% ... 2552
- VōSoL HC Otic Solution ... 2786

Hydrocortisone Acetate (Rifampin has liver enzyme-inducing properties and may reduce the activity of corticosteroids). Products include:
- Analpram-HC Rectal Cream 1% and 2.5% ... 993
- Anusol HC-1 Hydrocortisone Anti-Itch Ointment ... ▣ 810
- Anusol-HC Suppositories ... 1954
- Caldecort Anti-Itch Hydrocortisone Cream ... ▣ 651
- Coly-Mycin S Otic w/Neomycin & Hydrocortisone ... 1965
- Cortaid ... ▣ 800
- Cortifoam ... 2540
- Cortisporin Cream ... 1073
- Epifoam ... 2543
- Hydrocortone Acetate Sterile Suspension ... 1712
- Mantadil Cream ... 1124
- Nupercainal Hydrocortisone 1% Cream ... ▣ 661
- Pramosone Cream, Lotion & Ointment ... 995
- ProctoFoam-HC ... 2552
- Terra-Cortril Ophthalmic Suspension ... 2033

Hydrocortisone Sodium Phosphate (Rifampin has liver enzyme-inducing properties and may reduce the activity of corticosteroids). Products include:
- Hydrocortone Phosphate Injection, Sterile ... 1713

Hydrocortisone Sodium Succinate (Rifampin has liver enzyme-inducing properties and may reduce the activity of corticosteroids).
- No products indexed under this heading.

Hydromorphone Hydrochloride (Rifampin has liver enzyme-inducing properties and may reduce the activity of narcotics). Products include:
- Dilaudid Ampules ... 1382
- Dilaudid Cough Syrup ... 1383
- Dilaudid-HP Injection ... 1384
- Dilaudid-HP Lyophilized Powder 250 mg ... 1384
- Dilaudid ... 1382
- Dilaudid Oral Liquid ... 1386
- Dilaudid ... 1382
- Dilaudid Tablets - 8 mg. ... 1386

Ketoconazole (Co-administration has been reported to diminish the serum concentration of both drugs). Products include:
- Nizoral 2% Cream ... 1344
- Nizoral 2% Shampoo ... 1344
- Nizoral Tablets ... 1345

Labetalol Hydrochloride (Rifampin has been reported to diminish the effects of concurrently administered beta blockers). Products include:
- Normodyne Injection ... 2519
- Normodyne Tablets ... 2522
- Trandate ... 1158

Lamotrigine (Rifampin has liver enzyme-inducing properties and may reduce the activity of anticonvulsants). Products include:
- Lamictal Tablets ... 1105

Levobunolol Hydrochloride (Rifampin has been reported to diminish the effects of concurrently administered beta blockers). Products include:
- Betagan ... ⊙ 230

Levonorgestrel (Rifampin has liver enzyme-inducing properties and may reduce the activity of oral contraceptives; nonhormonal methods of contraception during therapy with rifampin is recommended). Products include:
- Levlen/Tri-Levlen ... 646
- Nordette-21 Tablets ... 2863
- Nordette-28 Tablets ... 2866
- Norplant System ... 2868
- Levlen/Tri-Levlen ... 646
- Triphasil-21 Tablets ... 2919
- Triphasil-28 Tablets ... 2924

Levorphanol Tartrate (Rifampin has liver enzyme-inducing properties and may reduce the activity of narcotics). Products include:
- Levo-Dromoran ... 2297

(▣ Described in PDR For Nonprescription Drugs) (⊙ Described in PDR For Ophthalmology)

Medroxyprogesterone Acetate (Rifampin has been reported to diminish the effects of concurrently administered progestins). Products include:
- Amen Tablets 785
- Cycrin Tablets 991
- Depo-Provera Contraceptive Injection 2079
- Depo-Provera Sterile Aqueous Suspension 2083
- Premphase 2900
- Prempro 2905
- Provera Tablets 2110

Megestrol Acetate (Rifampin has been reported to diminish the effects of concurrently administered progestins). Products include:
- Megace Oral Suspension 708
- Megace Tablets 710

Meperidine Hydrochloride (Rifampin has liver enzyme-inducing properties and may reduce the activity of narcotics). Products include:
- Demerol 2438
- Mepergan Injection 2859

Mephenytoin (Rifampin has liver enzyme-inducing properties and may reduce the activity of anticonvulsants). Products include:
- Mesantoin Tablets 2400

Mephobarbital (Rifampin has been reported to diminish the effects of concurrently administered barbiturates). Products include:
- Mebaral Tablets 2452

Mestranol (Rifampin has liver enzyme-inducing properties and may reduce the activity of oral contraceptives; nonhormonal methods of contraception during therapy with rifampin is recommended). Products include:
- Norinyl 2563
- Ortho-Novum 1928

Methadone Hydrochloride (Rifampin has been reported to diminish the effects of concurrently administered methadone). Products include:
- Methadone Hydrochloride Oral Concentrate 2356
- Methadone Hydrochloride Oral Solution & Tablets 2357

Methsuximide (Rifampin has liver enzyme-inducing properties and may reduce the activity of anticonvulsants). Products include:
- Celontin Kapseals 1955

Methylprednisolone Acetate (Rifampin has liver enzyme-inducing properties and may reduce the activity of corticosteroids).
- No products indexed under this heading.

Methylprednisolone Sodium Succinate (Rifampin has liver enzyme-inducing properties and may reduce the activity of corticosteroids).
- No products indexed under this heading.

Metipranolol Hydrochloride (Rifampin has been reported to diminish the effects of concurrently administered beta blockers). Products include:
- OptiPranolol (Metipranolol 0.3%) Sterile Ophthalmic Solution .... ⊛ 256

Metoprolol Succinate (Rifampin has been reported to diminish the effects of concurrently administered beta blockers). Products include:
- Toprol-XL Tablets 560

Metoprolol Tartrate (Rifampin has been reported to diminish the effects of concurrently administered beta blockers). Products include:
- Lopressor 848
- Lopressor HCT Tablets 850

Mexiletine Hydrochloride (Rifampin has been reported to diminish the effects of concurrently administered mexiletine). Products include:
- Mexitil Capsules 684

Morphine Sulfate (Rifampin has liver enzyme-inducing properties and may reduce the activity of narcotics). Products include:
- Astramorph/PF Injection, USP (Preservative-Free) 526
- Duramorph Injection 983
- Infumorph 200 and Infumorph 500 Sterile Solutions 985
- Kadian Capsules 2948
- MS Contin Tablets 2149
- MSIR 2152
- Oramorph SR (Morphine Sulfate Sustained Release Tablets) 2359
- RMS Suppositories CII 2766
- Roxanol 2365

Nadolol (Rifampin has been reported to diminish the effects of concurrently administered beta blockers).
- No products indexed under this heading.

Norethindrone (Rifampin has liver enzyme-inducing properties and may reduce the activity of oral contraceptives; nonhormonal methods of contraception during therapy with rifampin is recommended). Products include:
- Brevicon 2563
- Micronor Tablets 1903
- Modicon 1928
- Norinyl 2563
- Nor-Q D Tablets 2598
- Ortho-Novum 1928
- Ovcon 765
- Tri-Norinyl 2607

Norethynodrel (Rifampin has liver enzyme-inducing properties and may reduce the activity of oral contraceptives; nonhormonal methods of contraception during therapy with rifampin is recommended).
- No products indexed under this heading.

Norgestimate (Rifampin has liver enzyme-inducing properties and may reduce the activity of oral contraceptives; nonhormonal methods of contraception during therapy with rifampin is recommended). Products include:
- Ortho-Cyclen/Ortho-Tri-Cyclen 1914
- Ortho-Cyclen/Ortho Tri-Cyclen 1914

Norgestrel (Rifampin has liver enzyme-inducing properties and may reduce the activity of oral contraceptives; nonhormonal methods of contraception during therapy with rifampin is recommended). Products include:
- Lo/Ovral Tablets 2852
- Lo/Ovral-28 Tablets 2857
- Ovral Tablets 2877
- Ovral-28 Tablets 2878
- Ovrette Tablets 2878

Opium Alkaloids (Rifampin has liver enzyme-inducing properties and may reduce the activity of narcotics).
- No products indexed under this heading.

Oxycodone Hydrochloride (Rifampin has liver enzyme-inducing properties and may reduce the activity of narcotics). Products include:
- OxyContin Tablets 2163
- OxyIR Capsules 2167
- Percocet Tablets 955
- Percodan Tablets 955
- Percodan-Demi Tablets 956
- Roxicodone Tablets, Oral Solution & Intensol (Oxycodone) 2366
- Tylox Capsules 1593

Para-Aminosalicylic Acid (Coadministration may decrease rifampin serum levels; these drugs should be taken at least 8 hours apart).

Paramethadione (Rifampin has liver enzyme-inducing properties and may reduce the activity of anticonvulsants).
- No products indexed under this heading.

Penbutolol Sulfate (Rifampin has been reported to diminish the effects of concurrently administered beta blockers). Products include:
- Levatol Tablets 2547

Pentobarbital Sodium (Rifampin has been reported to diminish the effects of concurrently administered barbiturates). Products include:
- Nembutal Sodium Capsules 440
- Nembutal Sodium Solution 442
- Nembutal Sodium Suppositories 444

Phenacemide (Rifampin has liver enzyme-inducing properties and may reduce the activity of anticonvulsants). Products include:
- Phenurone Tablets 455

Phenobarbital (Rifampin has liver enzyme-inducing properties and may reduce the activity of anticonvulsants). Products include:
- Arco-Lase Plus Tablets 513
- Bellergal-S Tablets 2375
- Donnatal 2234
- Donnatal Extentabs 2234
- Donnatal Tablets 2234
- Phenobarbital Elixir and Tablets 1523
- Quadrinal Tablets 1398

Phensuximide (Rifampin has liver enzyme-inducing properties and may reduce the activity of anticonvulsants).
- No products indexed under this heading.

Phenytoin (Rifampin has liver enzyme-inducing properties and may reduce the activity of anticonvulsants). Products include:
- Dilantin Infatabs 1967
- Dilantin-125 Suspension 1969

Phenytoin Sodium (Rifampin has liver enzyme-inducing properties and may reduce the activity of anticonvulsants). Products include:
- Dilantin Kapseals 1965

Pindolol (Rifampin has been reported to diminish the effects of concurrently administered beta blockers). Products include:
- Visken Tablets 2428

Prednisolone Acetate (Rifampin has liver enzyme-inducing properties and may reduce the activity of corticosteroids). Products include:
- AK-CIDE .... ⊛ 203
- AK-CIDE Ointment .... ⊛ 203
- Blephamide Liquifilm Sterile Ophthalmic Suspension 472
- Blephamide Ointment .... ⊛ 234
- Econopred & Econopred Plus Ophthalmic Suspensions .... ⊛ 216
- Poly-Pred Liquifilm .... ⊛ 246
- Pred Forte .... ⊛ 247
- Pred Mild .... ⊛ 250
- Pred-G Liquifilm Sterile Ophthalmic Suspension .... ⊛ 248
- Pred-G S.O.P. Sterile Ophthalmic Ointment .... ⊛ 249

Prednisolone Sodium Phosphate (Rifampin has liver enzyme-inducing properties and may reduce the activity of corticosteroids). Products include:
- AK-PRED .... ⊛ 204
- Hydeltrasol Injection, Sterile 1708
- Pediapred Oral Solution 1618

Prednisolone Tebutate (Rifampin has liver enzyme-inducing properties and may reduce the activity of corticosteroids). Products include:
- Hydeltra-T.B.A. Sterile Suspension 1710

Prednisone (Rifampin has liver enzyme-inducing properties and may reduce the activity of corticosteroids).
- No products indexed under this heading.

Primidone (Rifampin has liver enzyme-inducing properties and may reduce the activity of anticonvulsants). Products include:
- Mysoline 2860

Probenecid (Increases rifampin blood levels). Products include:
- Benemid Tablets 1651
- ColBENEMID Tablets 1662

Propoxyphene Hydrochloride (Rifampin has liver enzyme-inducing properties and may reduce the activity of narcotics). Products include:
- Darvon 1475
- Wygesic Tablets 2930

Propoxyphene Napsylate (Rifampin has liver enzyme-inducing properties and may reduce the activity of narcotics). Products include:
- Darvon-N/Darvocet-N 1473

Propranolol Hydrochloride (Rifampin has been reported to diminish the effects of concurrently administered beta blockers). Products include:
- Inderal 2834
- Inderal LA Long Acting Capsules 2836
- Inderide Tablets 2838
- Inderide LA Long Acting Capsules 2840

Quinidine Gluconate (Rifampin has liver enzyme-inducing properties and may reduce the activity of quinidine). Products include:
- Quinaglute Dura-Tabs Tablets 644

Quinidine Polygalacturonate (Rifampin has liver enzyme-inducing properties and may reduce the activity of quinidine). Products include:
- Cardioquin Tablets 2146

Quinidine Sulfate (Rifampin has liver enzyme-inducing properties and may reduce the activity of quinidine). Products include:
- Quinidex Extentabs 2240

Secobarbital Sodium (Rifampin has been reported to diminish the effects of concurrently administered barbiturates). Products include:
- Seconal Sodium Pulvules 1529

Sotalol Hydrochloride (Rifampin has been reported to diminish the effects of concurrently administered beta blockers). Products include:
- Betapace Tablets 637

Sufentanil Citrate (Rifampin has liver enzyme-inducing properties and may reduce the activity of narcotics). Products include:
- Sufenta Injection 1355

Theophylline (Rifampin has been reported to diminish the effects of concurrently administered theophylline). Products include:
- Marax Tablets & DF Syrup 2015
- Quibron 2227

Theophylline Anhydrous (Rifampin has been reported to diminish the effects of concurrently administered theophylline). Products include:
- Aerolate 1003
- Primatene Tablets 844
- Respbid Tablets 687
- Slo-bid Gyrocaps 2201
- Theo-24 Extended Release Capsules 2753
- Theo-Dur Extended-Release Tablets 1367
- Theo-X Extended-Release Tablets 793
- Uni-Dur Extended-Release Tablets 1374
- Uniphyl 400 mg and 600 mg Tablets 2157

IMPORTANT NOTE: Always consult each drug listing in the patient's regimen for possible interactions.

Rifadin Interactions Index 928

Theophylline Calcium Salicylate (Rifampin has been reported to diminish the effects of concurrently administered theophylline). Products include:
Quadrinal Tablets ... 1398
Theophylline Sodium Glycinate (Rifampin has been reported to diminish the effects of concurrently administered theophylline).
No products indexed under this heading.
Thiamylal Sodium (Rifampin has been reported to diminish the effects of concurrently administered barbiturates).
No products indexed under this heading.
Timolol Hemihydrate (Rifampin has been reported to diminish the effects of concurrently administered beta blockers). Products include:
Betimol 0.25%, 0.5% ... ◉ 259
Timolol Maleate (Rifampin has been reported to diminish the effects of concurrently administered beta blockers). Products include:
Blocadren Tablets ... 1654
Timolide Tablets ... 1791
Timoptic in Ocudose ... 1796
Timoptic Sterile Ophthalmic Solution ... 1794
Timoptic-XE ... 1798
Tolazamide (Rifampin has liver enzyme-inducing properties and may reduce the activity of sulfonylureas).
No products indexed under this heading.
Tolbutamide (Rifampin has liver enzyme-inducing properties and may reduce the activity of sulfonylureas).
No products indexed under this heading.
Triamcinolone (Rifampin has liver enzyme-inducing properties and may reduce the activity of corticosteroids).
No products indexed under this heading.
Triamcinolone Acetonide (Rifampin has liver enzyme-inducing properties and may reduce the activity of corticosteroids). Products include:
Azmacort Oral Inhaler ... 2175
Nasacort AQ Nasal Spray ... 2191
Nasacort Nasal Inhaler ... 2189
Triamcinolone Diacetate (Rifampin has liver enzyme-inducing properties and may reduce the activity of corticosteroids).
No products indexed under this heading.
Triamcinolone Hexacetonide (Rifampin has liver enzyme-inducing properties and may reduce the activity of corticosteroids).
No products indexed under this heading.
Trimethadione (Rifampin has liver enzyme-inducing properties and may reduce the activity of anticonvulsants).
No products indexed under this heading.
Valproic Acid (Rifampin has liver enzyme-inducing properties and may reduce the activity of anticonvulsants). Products include:
Depakene ... 416
Verapamil Hydrochloride (Rifampin has been reported to diminish the effects of concurrently administered verapamil). Products include:
Calan SR Caplets ... 2571
Calan Tablets ... 2568
Covera-HS Tablets ... 2573
Isoptin Injectable ... 1391
Isoptin Oral Tablets ... 1393
Isoptin SR Tablets ... 1395
Verelan Capsules ... 1455
Vitamin D (An interaction has been reported with rifampin-isoniazid and vitamin D). Products include:
Caltrate PLUS ... ▣ 681
Caltrate 600 + D ... ▣ 681
Dical-D Tablets & Wafers ... 424
Materna Tablets ... 1427
Megadose ... 513
One-A-Day Calcium Plus ... ▣ 625

RIFADIN I.V.
(Rifampin) ... 1276
See **Rifadin Capsules**

RIFAMATE CAPSULES
(Rifampin, Isoniazid) ... 1278
May interact with oral anticoagulants, oral contraceptives, oral hypoglycemic agents, corticosteroids, and certain other agents. Compounds in these categories include:
Acarbose (Rifampin given in combination with other antituberculosis drugs may decrease the pharmacologic activity of oral hypoglycemic agents; dosage adjustment may be required). Products include:
Precose ... 604
Betamethasone Acetate (Rifampin given in combination with other antituberculosis drugs may decrease the pharmacologic activity of corticosteroids; dosage adjustment may be required). Products include:
Celestone Soluspan Suspension ... 2484
Betamethasone Sodium Phosphate (Rifampin given in combination with other antituberculosis drugs may decrease the pharmacologic activity of corticosteroids; dosage adjustment may be required). Products include:
Celestone Soluspan Suspension ... 2484
Chlorpropamide (Rifampin given in combination with other antituberculosis drugs may decrease the pharmacologic activity of oral hypoglycemic agents; dosage adjustment may be required). Products include:
Diabinese Tablets ... 2002
Cortisone Acetate (Rifampin given in combination with other antituberculosis drugs may decrease the pharmacologic activity of corticosteroids; dosage adjustment may be required). Products include:
Cortone Acetate Sterile Suspension ... 1663
Cortone Acetate Tablets ... 1664
Dapsone (Rifampin given in combination with other antituberculosis drugs may decrease the pharmacologic activity of dapsone; dosage adjustment may be required). Products include:
Dapsone Tablets USP ... 1331
Desogestrel (Rifampin given in combination with other antituberculosis drugs may affect the reliability of oral contraceptives; alternative contraceptive measures may need to be considered). Products include:
Desogen Tablets ... 1867
Ortho-Cept ... 1907
Dexamethasone (Rifampin given in combination with other antituberculosis drugs may decrease the pharmacologic activity of corticosteroids; dosage adjustment may be required). Products include:
AK-Trol Ointment & Suspension ... ◉ 205
Decadron Elixir ... 1676
Decadron Tablets ... 1678
Decaspray Topical Aerosol ... 1689
Maxitrol Ophthalmic Ointment and Suspension ... ◉ 222
TobraDex Ophthalmic Suspension and Ointment ... 469
Dexamethasone Acetate (Rifampin given in combination with other antituberculosis drugs may decrease the pharmacologic activity of corticosteroids; dosage adjustment may be required). Products include:
Dalalone D.P. Injectable ... 1009
Decadron-LA Sterile Suspension ... 1687
Dexamethasone Sodium Phosphate (Rifampin given in combination with other antituberculosis drugs may decrease the pharmacologic activity of corticosteroids; dosage adjustment may be required). Products include:
Decadron Phosphate Injection ... 1680
Decadron Phosphate Sterile Ophthalmic Ointment ... 1684
Decadron Phosphate Sterile Ophthalmic Solution ... 1685
Decadron Phosphate Topical Cream ... 1686
Decadron Phosphate with Xylocaine Injection, Sterile ... 1683
Dexacort Phosphate in Respihaler ... 1606
Dexacort Phosphate in Turbinaire ... 1607
NeoDecadron Sterile Ophthalmic Ointment ... 1755
NeoDecadron Sterile Ophthalmic Solution ... 1756
NeoDecadron Topical Cream ... 1757
Dicumarol (Rifampin has been observed to increase the requirements of coumarin-type anticoagulant; it is recommended that prothrombin time be performed frequently and dosage adjustment may be required).
No products indexed under this heading.
Digitoxin (Rifampin given in combination with other antituberculosis drugs may decrease the pharmacologic activity of digitoxin; dosage adjustment may be required). Products include:
Crystodigin Tablets ... 1472
Disopyramide Phosphate (Rifampin given in combination with other antituberculosis drugs may decrease the pharmacologic activity of disopyramide; dosage adjustment may be required). Products include:
Norpace ... 2596
Ethinyl Estradiol (Rifampin given in combination with other antituberculosis drugs may affect the reliability of oral contraceptives; alternative contraceptive measures may need to be considered). Products include:
Brevicon ... 2563
Demulen ... 2580
Desogen Tablets ... 1867
Levlen/Tri-Levlen ... 646
Lo/Ovral Tablets ... 2852
Lo/Ovral-28 Tablets ... 2857
Modicon ... 1928
Nordette-21 Tablets ... 2863
Nordette-28 Tablets ... 2866
Norinyl ... 2563
Ortho-Cept ... 1907
Ortho-Cyclen/Ortho-Tri-Cyclen ... 1914
Ortho-Novum ... 1928
Ortho-Cyclen/Ortho Tri-Cyclen ... 1914
Ovcon ... 765
Ovral Tablets ... 2877
Ovral-28 Tablets ... 2878
Levlen/Tri-Levlen ... 646
Tri-Norinyl ... 2607
Triphasil-21 Tablets ... 2919
Triphasil-28 Tablets ... 2924
Ethynodiol Diacetate (Rifampin given in combination with other antituberculosis drugs may affect the reliability of oral contraceptives; alternative contraceptive measures may need to be considered). Products include:
Demulen ... 2580
Fludrocortisone Acetate (Rifampin given in combination with other antituberculosis drugs may decrease the pharmacologic activity of corticosteroids; dosage adjustment may be required). Products include:
Florinef Acetate Tablets ... 506
Glimepiride (Rifampin given in combination with other antituberculosis drugs may decrease the pharmacologic activity of oral hypoglycemic agents; dosage adjustment may be required). Products include:
Amaryl Tablets ... 1241
Glipizide (Rifampin given in combination with other antituberculosis drugs may decrease the pharmacologic activity of oral hypoglycemic agents; dosage adjustment may be required). Products include:
Glucotrol Tablets ... 2011
Glucotrol XL Extended Release Tablets ... 2012
Glyburide (Rifampin given in combination with other antituberculosis drugs may decrease the pharmacologic activity of oral hypoglycemic agents; dosage adjustment may be required). Products include:
DiaBeta Tablets ... 1265
Glynase PresTab Tablets ... 2091
Micronase Tablets ... 2099
Hydrocortisone (Rifampin given in combination with other antituberculosis drugs may decrease the pharmacologic activity of corticosteroids; dosage adjustment may be required). Products include:
Anusol-HC Cream 2.5% ... 1953
Aquanil HC Lotion ... 1989
Maximum Strength Cortaid Spray ▣ 800
CORTENEMA ... 2713
Cortisporin Ointment ... 1074
Cortisporin Ophthalmic Ointment Sterile ... 1074
Cortisporin Ophthalmic Suspension Sterile ... 1075
Cortisporin Otic Solution Sterile ... 1076
Cortisporin Otic Suspension Sterile 1077
Cortizone-5 ... ▣ 795
Cortizone-10 ... ▣ 795
Hydrocortone Tablets ... 1715
Hytone ... 922
Hytone Ointment 2 ½% ... 923
Massengill Medicated Soft Cloth Towelettes ... 2628
Pediotic Suspension Sterile ... 1140
Preparation H Hydrocortisone 1% Cream ... ▣ 843
ProctoCream-HC 2.5% ... 2552
VōSoL HC Otic Solution ... 2786
Hydrocortisone Acetate (Rifampin given in combination with other antituberculosis drugs may decrease the pharmacologic activity of corticosteroids; dosage adjustment may be required). Products include:
Analpram-HC Rectal Cream 1% and 2.5% ... 993
Anusol HC-1 Hydrocortisone Anti-Itch Ointment ... ▣ 810
Anusol-HC Suppositories ... 1954
Caldecort Anti-Itch Hydrocortisone Cream ... ▣ 651
Coly-Mycin S Otic w/Neomycin & Hydrocortisone ... 1965
Cortaid ... ▣ 800
Cortifoam ... 2540
Cortisporin Cream ... 1073
Epifoam ... 2543
Hydrocortone Acetate Sterile Suspension ... 1712
Mantadil Cream ... 1124
Nupercainal Hydrocortisone 1% Cream ... ▣ 661
Pramosone Cream, Lotion & Ointment ... 995
ProctoFoam-HC ... 2552
Terra-Cortril Ophthalmic Suspension ... 2033

(▣ Described in PDR For Nonprescription Drugs) (◉ Described in PDR For Ophthalmology)

Hydrocortisone Sodium Phosphate (Rifampin given in combination with other antituberculosis drugs may decrease the pharmacologic activity of corticosteroids; dosage adjustment may be required). Products include:

Hydrocortone Phosphate Injection, Sterile 1713

Hydrocortisone Sodium Succinate (Rifampin given in combination with other antituberculosis drugs may decrease the pharmacologic activity of corticosteroids; dosage adjustment may be required).

No products indexed under this heading.

Levonorgestrel (Rifampin given in combination with other antituberculosis drugs may affect the reliability of oral contraceptives; alternative contraceptive measures may need to be considered). Products include:

Levlen/Tri-Levlen 646
Nordette-21 Tablets 2863
Nordette-28 Tablets 2866
Norplant System 2868
Levlen/Tri-Levlen 646
Triphasil-21 Tablets 2919
Triphasil-28 Tablets 2924

Mestranol (Rifampin given in combination with other antituberculosis drugs may affect the reliability of oral contraceptives; alternative contraceptive measures may need to be considered). Products include:

Norinyl 2563
Ortho-Novum 1928

Metformin Hydrochloride (Rifampin given in combination with other antituberculosis drugs may decrease the pharmacologic activity of oral hypoglycemic agents; dosage adjustment may be required). Products include:

Glucophage Tablets 754

Methadone Hydrochloride (Rifampin given in combination with other antituberculosis drugs may decrease the pharmacologic activity of methadone; dosage adjustment may be required). Products include:

Methadone Hydrochloride Oral Concentrate 2356
Methadone Hydrochloride Oral Solution & Tablets 2357

Methylprednisolone Acetate (Rifampin given in combination with other antituberculosis drugs may decrease the pharmacologic activity of corticosteroids; dosage adjustment may be required).

No products indexed under this heading.

Methylprednisolone Sodium Succinate (Rifampin given in combination with other antituberculosis drugs may decrease the pharmacologic activity of corticosteroids; dosage adjustment may be required).

No products indexed under this heading.

Norethindrone (Rifampin given in combination with other antituberculosis drugs may affect the reliability of oral contraceptives; alternative contraceptive measures may need to be considered). Products include:

Brevicon 2563
Micronor Tablets 1903
Modicon 1928
Norinyl 2563
Nor-Q D Tablets 2598
Ortho-Novum 1928
Ovcon 765
Tri-Norinyl 2607

Norethynodrel (Rifampin given in combination with other antituberculosis drugs may affect the reliability of oral contraceptives; alternative contraceptive measures may need to be considered).

No products indexed under this heading.

Norgestimate (Rifampin given in combination with other antituberculosis drugs may affect the reliability of oral contraceptives; alternative contraceptive measures may need to be considered). Products include:

Ortho-Cyclen/Ortho-Tri-Cyclen 1914
Ortho-Cyclen/Ortho Tri-Cyclen 1914

Norgestrel (Rifampin given in combination with other antituberculosis drugs may affect the reliability of oral contraceptives; alternative contraceptive measures may need to be considered). Products include:

Lo/Ovral Tablets 2852
Lo/Ovral-28 Tablets 2857
Ovral Tablets 2877
Ovral-28 Tablets 2878
Ovrette Tablets 2878

Phenytoin (Isoniazid may decrease the excretion of phenytoin or may enhance its effects; dosage adjustment may be required). Products include:

Dilantin Infatabs 1967
Dilantin-125 Suspension 1969

Phenytoin Sodium (Isoniazid may decrease the excretion of phenytoin or may enhance its effects; dosage adjustment may be required). Products include:

Dilantin Kapseals 1965

Prednisolone Acetate (Rifampin given in combination with other antituberculosis drugs may decrease the pharmacologic activity of corticosteroids; dosage adjustment may be required). Products include:

AK-CIDE .... ⊚ 203
AK-CIDE Ointment .... ⊚ 203
Blephamide Liquifilm Sterile Ophthalmic Suspension 472
Blephamide Ointment .... ⊚ 234
Econopred & Econopred Plus Ophthalmic Suspensions .... ⊚ 216
Poly-Pred Liquifilm .... ⊚ 246
Pred Forte .... ⊚ 247
Pred Mild .... ⊚ 250
Pred-G Liquifilm Sterile Ophthalmic Suspension .... ⊚ 248
Pred-G S.O.P. Sterile Ophthalmic Ointment .... ⊚ 249

Prednisolone Sodium Phosphate (Rifampin given in combination with other antituberculosis drugs may decrease the pharmacologic activity of corticosteroids; dosage adjustment may be required). Products include:

AK-PRED .... ⊚ 204
Hydeltrasol Injection, Sterile 1708
Pediapred Oral Solution 1618

Prednisolone Tebutate (Rifampin given in combination with other antituberculosis drugs may decrease the pharmacologic activity of corticosteroids; dosage adjustment may be required). Products include:

Hydeltra-T.B.A. Sterile Suspension 1710

Prednisone (Rifampin given in combination with other antituberculosis drugs may decrease the pharmacologic activity of corticosteroids; dosage adjustment may be required).

No products indexed under this heading.

Quinidine Gluconate (Rifampin given in combination with other antituberculosis drugs may decrease the pharmacologic activity of quinidine; dosage adjustment may be required). Products include:

Quinaglute Dura-Tabs Tablets 644

Quinidine Polygalacturonate (Rifampin given in combination with other antituberculosis drugs may decrease the pharmacologic activity of quinidine; dosage adjustment may be required). Products include:

Cardioquin Tablets 2146

Quinidine Sulfate (Rifampin given in combination with other antituberculosis drugs may decrease the pharmacologic activity of quinidine; dosage adjustment may be required). Products include:

Quinidex Extentabs 2240

Tolazamide (Rifampin given in combination with other antituberculosis drugs may decrease the pharmacologic activity of oral hypoglycemic agents; dosage adjustment may be required).

No products indexed under this heading.

Tolbutamide (Rifampin given in combination with other antituberculosis drugs may decrease the pharmacologic activity of oral hypoglycemic agents; dosage adjustment may be required).

No products indexed under this heading.

Triamcinolone (Rifampin given in combination with other antituberculosis drugs may decrease the pharmacologic activity of corticosteroids; dosage adjustment may be required).

No products indexed under this heading.

Triamcinolone Acetonide (Rifampin given in combination with other antituberculosis drugs may decrease the pharmacologic activity of corticosteroids; dosage adjustment may be required). Products include:

Azmacort Oral Inhaler 2175
Nasacort AQ Nasal Spray 2191
Nasacort Nasal Inhaler 2189

Triamcinolone Diacetate (Rifampin given in combination with other antituberculosis drugs may decrease the pharmacologic activity of corticosteroids; dosage adjustment may be required).

No products indexed under this heading.

Triamcinolone Hexacetonide (Rifampin given in combination with other antituberculosis drugs may decrease the pharmacologic activity of corticosteroids; dosage adjustment may be required).

No products indexed under this heading.

Warfarin Sodium (Rifampin has been observed to increase the requirements of coumarin-type anticoagulant; it is recommended that prothrombin time be performed frequently and dosage adjustment may be required). Products include:

Coumadin 941

Food Interactions

Alcohol (Daily ingestion of alcohol may be associated with a higher incidence of isoniazid hepatitis).

RIFATER

(Rifampin, Isoniazid, Pyrazinamide) ..1280
May interact with barbiturates, oral anticoagulants, beta blockers, narcotic analgesics, xanthine bronchodilators, oral hypoglycemic agents, oral contraceptives, cardiac glycosides, corticosteroids, progestins, antacids, and certain other agents. Compounds in these categories include:

Acarbose (Rifampin accelerates the metabolism of oral hypoglycemic agent; isoniazid may produce hyperglycemia and lead to loss of glucose control; dosage adjustment may be required when starting or stopping concomitantly administered rifampin). Products include:

Precose 604

Acebutolol Hydrochloride (Rifampin accelerates the metabolism of beta blocker; dosage adjustment may be required when starting or stopping concomitantly administered rifampin). Products include:

Sectral Capsules 2914

Alfentanil Hydrochloride (Rifampin accelerates the metabolism of narcotic; dosage adjustment may be required when starting or stopping concomitantly administered rifampin). Products include:

Alfenta Injection 1334

Aluminum Carbonate (Reduces absorption of rifampin and isoniazid). Products include:

Basaljel Capsules 2810
Basaljel Suspension 2810
Basaljel Tablets 2810

Aluminum Hydroxide (Reduces absorption of rifampin and isoniazid). Products include:

ALternaGEL Liquid 1358
Maximum Strength Ascriptin .... ▣ 650
Cama Arthritis Pain Reliever .... ▣ 748
Gaviscon Extra Strength Relief Formula Antacid Tablets .... ▣ 778
Gaviscon Extra Strength Relief Formula Liquid Antacid .... ▣ 779
Gaviscon Liquid Antacid .... ▣ 779
Gelusil Antacid-Anti-gas Liquid .... ▣ 819
Gelusil Antacid-Anti-gas Tablets .... ▣ 819
Maalox Antacid/Anti-Gas Tablets 889
Maalox Heartburn Relief Suspension .... ▣ 658
Maalox Antacid Liquid 888
Extra Strength Maalox Antacid/Anti-Gas Liquid and Tablets 888
Mylanta 1359
Tempo Soft Antacid .... ▣ 799

Aluminum Hydroxide Gel (Reduces absorption of rifampin and isoniazid). Products include:

ALternaGEL Liquid .... ▣ 675
Aludrox Oral Suspension .... ▣ 850
Amphojel Suspension 2802
Amphojel Suspension without Flavor 2802
Amphojel Tablets 2802
Ascriptin .... ▣ 650
Gaviscon Antacid Tablets .... ▣ 778
Gaviscon-2 Antacid Tablets .... ▣ 779
Mylanta Liquid .... ▣ 676
Mylanta Double Strength Liquid .... ▣ 676
Nephrox Suspension .... ▣ 671

Aminosalicylic Acid (Increases the plasma concentration and elimination half-life of isoniazid). Products include:

PASER Granules 1333

Aminophylline (Rifampin accelerates the metabolism of theophylline and isoniazid inhibits the metabolism; dosage adjustment may be required when starting stopping concomitantly administered rifampin).

No products indexed under this heading.

IMPORTANT NOTE: Always consult each drug listing in the patient's regimen for possible interactions.

Aprobarbital (Rifampin accelerates the metabolism of barbiturates; dosage adjustment may be required when starting or stopping concomitantly administered rifampin).
No products indexed under this heading.

Atenolol (Rifampin accelerates the metabolism of beta blocker; dosage adjustment may be required when starting or stopping concomitantly administered rifampin). Products include:
Tenoretic Tablets 2963
Tenormin Tablets and I.V. Injection 2965

Betamethasone Acetate (Rifampin accelerates the metabolism of corticosteroid; dosage adjustment may be required when starting or stopping concomitantly administered rifampin). Products include:
Celestone Soluspan Suspension 2484

Betamethasone Sodium Phosphate (Rifampin accelerates the metabolism of corticosteroid; dosage adjustment may be required when starting or stopping concomitantly administered rifampin). Products include:
Celestone Soluspan Suspension 2484

Betaxolol Hydrochloride (Rifampin accelerates the metabolism of beta blocker; dosage adjustment may be required when starting or stopping concomitantly administered rifampin). Products include:
Betoptic Ophthalmic Solution 465
Betoptic S Ophthalmic Suspension 467
Kerlone Tablets 2588

Bisoprolol Fumarate (Rifampin accelerates the metabolism of beta blocker; dosage adjustment may be required when starting or stopping concomitantly administered rifampin). Products include:
Zebeta Tablets 1457
Ziac 1459

Buprenorphine (Rifampin accelerates the metabolism of narcotic; dosage adjustment may be required when starting or stopping concomitantly administered rifampin). Products include:
Buprenex Injectable 2170

Butabarbital (Rifampin accelerates the metabolism of barbiturates; dosage adjustment may be required when starting or stopping concomitantly administered rifampin).
No products indexed under this heading.

Butalbital (Rifampin accelerates the metabolism of barbiturates; dosage adjustment may be required when starting or stopping concomitantly administered rifampin). Products include:
Axocet Capsules 2469
Esgic-plus Capsules 1012
Esgic-plus Tablets 1012
Fioricet Tablets 2386
Fioricet with Codeine Capsules 2387
Fiorinal Capsules 2388
Fiorinal with Codeine Capsules 2390
Fiorinal Tablets 2388
Phrenilin 790
Sedapap Tablets 50 mg/650 mg .. 1826

Carbamazepine (Isoniazid inhibits the metabolism of carbamazepine). Products include:
Atretol Tablets 569
Tegretol/Tegretol-XR 870

Carteolol Hydrochloride (Rifampin accelerates the metabolism of beta blocker; dosage adjustment may be required when starting or stopping concomitantly administered rifampin). Products include:
Cartrol Tablets 413
Ocupress Ophthalmic Solution, 1% Sterile .... ◉ 297

Chloramphenicol (Rifampin accelerates the metabolism of chloramphenicol; dosage adjustment may be required when starting or stopping concomitantly administered rifampin). Products include:
Chloromycetin Ophthalmic Ointment, 1% .... ◉ 298
Chloromycetin Ophthalmic Solution .... ◉ 299
Chloroptic S.O.P. .... ◉ 236
Chloroptic Sterile Ophthalmic Solution .... ◉ 236

Chloramphenicol Palmitate (Rifampin accelerates the metabolism of chloramphenicol; dosage adjustment may be required when starting or stopping concomitantly administered rifampin).
No products indexed under this heading.

Chloramphenicol Sodium Succinate (Rifampin accelerates the metabolism of chloramphenicol; dosage adjustment may be required when starting or stopping concomitantly administered rifampin). Products include:
Chloromycetin Sodium Succinate.... 1960

Chlorpropamide (Rifampin accelerates the metabolism of oral hypoglycemic agent; isoniazid may produce hyperglycemia and lead to loss of glucose control; dosage adjustment may be required when starting or stopping concomitantly administered rifampin). Products include:
Diabinese Tablets 2002

Ciprofloxacin (Rifampin accelerates the metabolism of ciprofloxacin; dosage adjustment may be required when starting or stopping concomitantly administered rifampin). Products include:
Cipro I.V. 587
Cipro I.V. Pharmacy Bulk Package.. 590

Ciprofloxacin Hydrochloride (Rifampin accelerates the metabolism of ciprofloxacin; dosage adjustment may be required when starting or stopping concomitantly administered rifampin). Products include:
Ciloxan Ophthalmic Solution 468
Cipro Tablets 584

Clofibrate (Rifampin accelerates the metabolism of clofibrate; dosage adjustment may be required when starting or stopping concomitantly administered rifampin). Products include:
Atromid-S Capsules 2808

Codeine Phosphate (Rifampin accelerates the metabolism of narcotic; dosage adjustment may be required when starting or stopping concomitantly administered rifampin). Products include:
Brontex 2130
Dimetane-DC Cough Syrup 2232
Fioricet with Codeine Capsules 2387
Fiorinal with Codeine Capsules 2390
Nucofed 2225
Phenergan with Codeine 2883
Phenergan VC with Codeine 2888
Robitussin A-C Syrup 2248
Robitussin-DAC Syrup 2249
Ryna .... ▣ 804
Soma Compound w/Codeine Tablets 2784
Tylenol with Codeine 1592

Cortisone Acetate (Rifampin accelerates the metabolism of corticosteroid; dosage adjustment may be required when starting or stopping concomitantly administered rifampin). Products include:
Cortone Acetate Sterile Suspension 1663
Cortone Acetate Tablets 1664

Cycloserine (Rifater exaggerates drowsiness and dizziness). Products include:
Seromycin Capsules 975

Cyclosporine (Rifampin accelerates the metabolism of cyclosporine; dosage adjustment may be required when starting or stopping concomitantly administered rifampin). Products include:
Neoral 2405
Sandimmune 2416

Deslanoside (Rifampin accelerates the metabolism of cardiac glycosides; dosage adjustment may be required when starting or stopping concomitantly administered rifampin).
No products indexed under this heading.

Desogestrel (Rifampin accelerates the metabolism of oral contraceptive or progestin; dosage adjustment may be required when starting or stopping concomitantly administered rifampin). Products include:
Desogen Tablets 1867
Ortho-Cept 1907

Dexamethasone (Rifampin accelerates the metabolism of corticosteroid; dosage adjustment may be required when starting or stopping concomitantly administered rifampin). Products include:
AK-Trol Ointment & Suspension .... ◉ 205
Decadron Elixir 1676
Decadron Tablets 1678
Decaspray Topical Aerosol 1689
Maxitrol Ophthalmic Ointment and Suspension .... ◉ 222
TobraDex Ophthalmic Suspension and Ointment 469

Dexamethasone Acetate (Rifampin accelerates the metabolism of corticosteroid; dosage adjustment may be required when starting or stopping concomitantly administered rifampin). Products include:
Dalalone D.P. Injectable 1009
Decadron-LA Sterile Suspension 1687

Dexamethasone Sodium Phosphate (Rifampin accelerates the metabolism of corticosteroid; dosage adjustment may be required when starting or stopping concomitantly administered rifampin). Products include:
Decadron Phosphate Injection 1680
Decadron Phosphate Sterile Ophthalmic Ointment 1684
Decadron Phosphate Sterile Ophthalmic Solution 1685
Decadron Phosphate Topical Cream 1686
Decadron Phosphate with Xylocaine Injection, Sterile 1683
Dexacort Phosphate in Respihaler .. 1606
Dexacort Phosphate in Turbinaire .. 1607
NeoDecadron Sterile Ophthalmic Ointment 1755
NeoDecadron Sterile Ophthalmic Solution 1756
NeoDecadron Topical Cream 1757

Dezocine (Rifampin accelerates the metabolism of narcotic; dosage adjustment may be required when starting or stopping concomitantly administered rifampin). Products include:
Dalgan Injection 529

Diazepam (Rifampin accelerates the metabolism of diazepam and isoniazid inhibits the metabolism of diazepam; dosage adjustment may be required when starting or stopping concomitantly administered rifampin). Products include:
Dizac (diazepam injectable emulsion) CIV 1862
Valium Injectable 2336
Valium Tablets 2335

Dicumarol (Rifampin accelerates the metabolism of anticoagulants and isoniazid inhibits the metabolism; increased requirements of coumarin type anticoagulant; dosage adjustment may be required when starting or stopping concomitantly administered rifampin).
No products indexed under this heading.

Digitoxin (Rifampin accelerates the metabolism of cardiac glycosides; dosage adjustment may be required when starting or stopping concomitantly administered rifampin). Products include:
Crystodigin Tablets 1472

Digoxin (Rifampin accelerates the metabolism of cardiac glycosides; dosage adjustment may be required when starting or stopping concomitantly administered rifampin). Products include:
Lanoxicaps 1110
Lanoxin Elixir Pediatric 1113
Lanoxin Injection 1116
Lanoxin Injection Pediatric 1119
Lanoxin Tablets 1121

Diltiazem Hydrochloride (Rifampin accelerates the metabolism of diltiazem; dosage adjustment may be required when starting or stopping concomitantly administered rifampin). Products include:
Cardizem CD Capsules 1251
Cardizem SR Capsules 1255
Cardizem Injectable 1253
Cardizem Tablets 1257
Dilacor XR Extended-release Capsules 2183
Tiazac Capsules 1019

Disopyramide Phosphate (Rifampin accelerates the metabolism of disopyramide; dosage adjustment may be required when starting or stopping concomitantly administered rifampin). Products include:
Norpace 2596

Disulfiram (Rifater exaggerates acute behavioral and coordination changes). Products include:
Antabuse Tablets 2802

Divalproex Sodium (Isoniazid inhibits the metabolism of valproic acid). Products include:
Depakote Tablets 418

Dyphylline (Rifampin accelerates the metabolism of theophylline and isoniazid inhibits the metabolism; dosage adjustment may be required when starting or stopping concomitantly administered rifampin). Products include:
Lufyllin & Lufyllin-400 Tablets 2778
Lufyllin-GG Elixir & Tablets 2779

Enalapril Maleate (Concurrent use results in decreased concentrations of enalaprilat, the active metabolite). Products include:
Vaseretic Tablets 1810
Vasotec Tablets 1816

Enflurane (Fast acetylation of isoniazid may produce high concentrations of hydrazine which facilitate defloration).
No products indexed under this heading.

Esmolol Hydrochloride (Rifampin accelerates the metabolism of beta blocker; dosage adjustment may be required when starting or stopping concomitantly administered rifampin). Products include:
Brevibloc (esmolol HCl) Injection 1860

(▣ Described in PDR For Nonprescription Drugs) (◉ Described in PDR For Ophthalmology)

Ethinyl Estradiol (Rifampin accelerates the metabolism of oral contraceptive; dosage adjustment may be required when starting or stopping concomitantly administered rifampin). Products include:

Brevicon ... 2563
Demulen ... 2580
Desogen Tablets ... 1867
Levlen/Tri-Levlen ... 646
Lo/Ovral Tablets ... 2852
Lo/Ovral-28 Tablets ... 2857
Modicon ... 1928
Nordette-21 Tablets ... 2863
Nordette-28 Tablets ... 2866
Norinyl ... 2563
Ortho-Cept ... 1907
Ortho-Cyclen/Ortho-Tri-Cyclen ... 1914
Ortho-Novum ... 1928
Ortho-Cyclen/Ortho Tri-Cyclen ... 1914
Ovcon ... 765
Ovral Tablets ... 2877
Ovral-28 Tablets ... 2878
Levlen/Tri-Levlen ... 646
Tri-Norinyl ... 2607
Triphasil-21 Tablets ... 2919
Triphasil-28 Tablets ... 2924

Ethynodiol Diacetate (Rifampin accelerates the metabolism of oral contraceptive; dosage adjustment may be required when starting or stopping concomitantly administered rifampin). Products include:

Demulen ... 2580

Fentanyl (Rifampin accelerates the metabolism of narcotic; dosage adjustment may be required when starting or stopping concomitantly administered rifampin). Products include:

Duragesic Transdermal System ... 1336

Fentanyl Citrate (Rifampin accelerates the metabolism of narcotic; dosage adjustment may be required when starting or stopping concomitantly administered rifampin). Products include:

Sublimaze Injection ... 463

Fluconazole (Rifampin accelerates the metabolism of fluconazole; dosage adjustment may be required when starting or stopping concomitantly administered rifampin). Products include:

Diflucan Tablets, Injection, and Oral Suspension ... 2003

Fludrocortisone Acetate (Rifampin accelerates the metabolism of corticosteroid; dosage adjustment may be required when starting or stopping concomitantly administered rifampin). Products include:

Florinef Acetate Tablets ... 506

Glimepiride (Rifampin accelerates the metabolism of oral hypoglycemic agent; isoniazid may produce hyperglycemia and lead to loss of glucose control; dosage adjustment may be required when starting or stopping concomitantly administered rifampin). Products include:

Amaryl Tablets ... 1241

Glipizide (Rifampin accelerates the metabolism of oral hypoglycemic agent; isoniazid may produce hyperglycemia and lead to loss of glucose control; dosage adjustment may be required when starting or stopping concomitantly administered rifampin). Products include:

Glucotrol Tablets ... 2011
Glucotrol XL Extended Release Tablets ... 2012

Glyburide (Rifampin accelerates the metabolism of oral hypoglycemic agent; isoniazid may produce hyperglycemia and lead to loss of glucose control; dosage adjustment may be required when starting or stopping concomitantly administered rifampin). Products include:

DiaBeta Tablets ... 1265
Glynase PresTab Tablets ... 2091
Micronase Tablets ... 2099

Haloperidol (Rifampin accelerates the metabolism of haloperidol and isoniazid inhibits the metabolism of haloperidol; dosage adjustment may be required when starting or stopping concomitantly administered rifampin). Products include:

Haldol Injection, Tablets and Concentrate ... 1585

Haloperidol Decanoate (Rifampin accelerates the metabolism of haloperidol and isoniazid inhibits the metabolism of haloperidol; dosage adjustment may be required when starting or stopping concomitantly administered rifampin). Products include:

Haldol Decanoate ... 1587

Halothane (Incresed potential for hepatotoxicity). Products include:

Fluothane ... 2830

Hydrocodone Bitartrate (Rifampin accelerates the metabolism of narcotic; dosage adjustment may be required when starting or stopping concomitantly administered rifampin). Products include:

Codiclear DH Syrup ... 808
Duratuss HD Elixir ... 2750
Histussin D Liquid ... 670
Hycodan Tablets and Syrup ... 946
Hycomine Compound Tablets ... 948
Hycomine ... 947
Hycotuss Expectorant Syrup ... 950
Hydrocet Capsules ... 787
Lorcet 10/650 Tablets ... 1016
Lortab ... 2751
Tussend ... 1830
Tussend Expectorant ... 1831
Vicodin Tablets ... 1404
Vicodin ES Tablets ... 1405
Vicodin HP Tablets ... 1403
Vicodin Tuss Expectorant ... 1406
Zydone Capsules ... 967

Hydrocodone Polistirex (Rifampin accelerates the metabolism of narcotic; dosage adjustment may be required when starting or stopping concomitantly administered rifampin). Products include:

Tussionex Pennkinetic Extended-Release Suspension ... 1624

Hydrocortisone (Rifampin accelerates the metabolism of corticosteroid; dosage adjustment may be required when starting or stopping concomitantly administered rifampin). Products include:

Anusol-HC Cream 2.5% ... 1953
Aquanil HC Lotion ... 1989
Maximum Strength Cortaid Spray ◙ 800
CORTENEMA ... 2713
Cortisporin Ointment ... 1074
Cortisporin Ophthalmic Ointment Sterile ... 1074
Cortisporin Ophthalmic Suspension Sterile ... 1075
Cortisporin Otic Solution Sterile ... 1076
Cortisporin Otic Suspension Sterile 1077
Cortizone-5 ... ◙ 795
Cortizone-10 ... ◙ 795
Hydrocortone Tablets ... 1715
Hytone ... 922
Hytone Ointment 2 ½% ... 923
Massengill Medicated Soft Cloth Towelettes ... 2628
Pediotic Suspension Sterile ... 1140
Preparation H Hydrocortisone 1% Cream ... ◙ 843
ProctoCream-HC 2.5% ... 2552
VōSoL HC Otic Solution ... 2786

Hydrocortisone Acetate (Rifampin accelerates the metabolism of corticosteroid; dosage adjustment may be required when starting or stopping concomitantly administered rifampin). Products include:

Analpram-HC Rectal Cream 1% and 2.5% ... 993
Anusol HC-1 Hydrocortisone Anti-Itch Ointment ... ◙ 810
Anusol-HC Suppositories ... 1954
Caldecort Anti-Itch Hydrocortisone Cream ... ◙ 651
Coly-Mycin S Otic w/Neomycin & Hydrocortisone ... 1965
Cortaid ... ◙ 800
Cortifoam ... 2540
Cortisporin Cream ... 1073
Epifoam ... 2543
Hydrocortone Acetate Sterile Suspension ... 1712
Mantadil Cream ... 1124
Nupercainal Hydrocortisone 1% Cream ... ◙ 661
Pramosone Cream, Lotion & Ointment ... 995
ProctoFoam-HC ... 2552
Terra-Cortril Ophthalmic Suspension ... 2033

Hydrocortisone Sodium Phosphate (Rifampin accelerates the metabolism of corticosteroid; dosage adjustment may be required when starting or stopping concomitantly administered rifampin). Products include:

Hydrocortone Phosphate Injection, Sterile ... 1713

Hydrocortisone Sodium Succinate (Rifampin accelerates the metabolism of corticosteroid; dosage adjustment may be required when starting or stopping concomitantly administered rifampin).

No products indexed under this heading.

Hydromorphone Hydrochloride (Rifampin accelerates the metabolism of narcotic; dosage adjustment may be required when starting or stopping concomitantly administered rifampin). Products include:

Dilaudid Ampules ... 1382
Dilaudid Cough Syrup ... 1383
Dilaudid-HP Injection ... 1384
Dilaudid-HP Lyophilized Powder 250 mg ... 1384
Dilaudid ... 1382
Dilaudid Oral Liquid ... 1386
Dilaudid ... 1382
Dilaudid Tablets - 8 mg ... 1386

Itraconazole (Rifampin accelerates the metabolism of itraconazole; dosage adjustment may be required when starting or stopping concomitantly administered rifampin). Products include:

Sporanox Capsules ... 1352

Ketoconazole (Rifampin accelerates the metabolism of ketoconazole; dosage adjustment may be required when starting or stopping concomitantly administered rifampin). Products include:

Nizoral 2% Cream ... 1344
Nizoral 2% Shampoo ... 1344
Nizoral Tablets ... 1345

Labetalol Hydrochloride (Rifampin accelerates the metabolism of beta blocker; dosage adjustment may be required when starting or stopping concomitantly administered rifampin). Products include:

Normodyne Injection ... 2519
Normodyne Tablets ... 2522
Trandate ... 1158

Levobunolol Hydrochloride (Rifampin accelerates the metabolism of beta blocker; dosage adjustment may be required when starting or stopping concomitantly administered rifampin). Products include:

Betagan ... ⊙ 230

Levodopa (Concurrent use may produce symptoms of excess catecholamine stimulation (agitation, flushing, palpitations) or lack of levodopa effect). Products include:

Atamet Tablets ... 567
Larodopa Tablets ... 2296
Sinemet Tablets ... 959
Sinemet CR Tablets ... 961

Levonorgestrel (Rifampin accelerates the metabolism of oral contraceptive; dosage adjustment may be required when starting or stopping concomitantly administered rifampin). Products include:

Levlen/Tri-Levlen ... 646
Nordette-21 Tablets ... 2863
Nordette-28 Tablets ... 2866
Norplant System ... 2868
Levlen/Tri-Levlen ... 646
Triphasil-21 Tablets ... 2919
Triphasil-28 Tablets ... 2924

Levorphanol Tartrate (Rifampin accelerates the metabolism of narcotic; dosage adjustment may be required when starting or stopping concomitantly administered rifampin). Products include:

Levo-Dromoran ... 2297

Magaldrate (Reduces absorption of rifampin and isoniazid).

No products indexed under this heading.

Magnesium Hydroxide (Reduces absorption of rifampin and isoniazid). Products include:

Aludrox Oral Suspension ... ◙ 850
Ascriptin ... ◙ 650
Di-Gel Antacid/Anti-Gas ... ◙ 762
Gelusil Antacid-Anti-gas Liquid ... ◙ 819
Gelusil Antacid-Anti-gas Tablets ... ◙ 819
Maalox Antacid/Anti-Gas Tablets ... 889
Maalox Antacid Liquid ... 888
Extra Strength Maalox Antacid/Anti-Gas Liquid and Tablets ... 888
Mylanta Fast-Acting ... 1359
Mylanta Gelcaps Antacid ... ◙ 678
Fast-Acting Mylanta Liquid Antacid 1359
Mylanta Tablets ... ◙ 677
Maximum-Strength Fast-Acting Mylanta Liquid Antacid ... 1359
Mylanta Double Strength Tablets .. ◙ 677
Phillips' Milk of Magnesia Liquid ... ◙ 627
Rolaids Antacid Tablets ... ◙ 807
Tempo Soft Antacid ... ◙ 799

Magnesium Oxide (Reduces absorption of rifampin and isoniazid). Products include:

Beelith Tablets ... 632
Bufferin Analgesic Tablets ... ◙ 636
Arthritis Strength Bufferin Analgesic Caplets ... ◙ 637
Extra Strength Bufferin Analgesic Tablets ... ◙ 637
Caltrate PLUS ... ◙ 681
Cama Arthritis Pain Reliever ... ◙ 748
Mag-Ox 400 ... 666
Uro-Mag ... 666

Medroxyprogesterone Acetate (Rifampin accelerates the metabolism of progestin; dosage adjustment may be required when starting or stopping concomitantly administered rifampin). Products include:

Amen Tablets ... 785
Cycrin Tablets ... 991
Depo-Provera Contraceptive Injection ... 2079
Depo-Provera Sterile Aqueous Suspension ... 2083
Premphase ... 2900
Prempro ... 2905
Provera Tablets ... 2110

IMPORTANT NOTE: Always consult each drug listing in the patient's regimen for possible interactions.

Rifater — Interactions Index

Megestrol Acetate (Rifampin accelerates the metabolism of progestin; dosage adjustment may be required when starting or stopping concomitantly administered rifampin). Products include:
- Megace Oral Suspension ... 708
- Megace Tablets ... 710

Meperidine Hydrochloride (Rifampin accelerates the metabolism of narcotic; dosage adjustment may be required when starting or stopping concomitantly administered rifampin; Rifater exaggerates drowsiness). Products include:
- Demerol ... 2438
- Mepergan Injection ... 2859

Mephobarbital (Rifampin accelerates the metabolism of barbiturates; dosage adjustment may be required when starting or stopping concomitantly administered rifampin). Products include:
- Mebaral Tablets ... 2452

Mestranol (Rifampin accelerates the metabolism of oral contraceptive; dosage adjustment may be required when starting or stopping concomitantly administered rifampin). Products include:
- Norinyl ... 2563
- Ortho-Novum ... 1928

Metformin Hydrochloride (Rifampin accelerates the metabolism of oral hypoglycemic agent; isoniazid may produce hyperglycemia and lead to loss of glucose control; dosage adjustment may be required when starting or stopping concomitantly administered rifampin). Products include:
- Glucophage Tablets ... 754

Methadone Hydrochloride (Rifampin accelerates the metabolism of narcotic; dosage adjustment may be required when starting or stopping concomitantly administered rifampin). Products include:
- Methadone Hydrochloride Oral Concentrate ... 2356
- Methadone Hydrochloride Oral Solution & Tablets ... 2357

Methylprednisolone Acetate (Rifampin accelerates the metabolism of corticosteroid; dosage adjustment may be required when starting or stopping concomitantly administered rifampin).
No products indexed under this heading.

Methylprednisolone Sodium Succinate (Rifampin accelerates the metabolism of corticosteroid; dosage adjustment may be required when starting or stopping concomitantly administered rifampin).
No products indexed under this heading.

Metipranolol Hydrochloride (Rifampin accelerates the metabolism of beta blocker; dosage adjustment may be required when starting or stopping concomitantly administered rifampin). Products include:
- OptiPranolol (Metipranolol 0.3%) Sterile Ophthalmic Solution ... ⊚ 256

Metoprolol Succinate (Rifampin accelerates the metabolism of beta blocker; dosage adjustment may be required when starting or stopping concomitantly administered rifampin). Products include:
- Toprol-XL Tablets ... 560

Metoprolol Tartrate (Rifampin accelerates the metabolism of beta blocker; dosage adjustment may be required when starting or stopping concomitantly administered rifampin). Products include:
- Lopressor ... 848
- Lopressor HCT Tablets ... 850

Mexiletine Hydrochloride (Rifampin accelerates the metabolism of mexiletine; dosage adjustment may be required when starting or stopping concomitantly administered rifampin). Products include:
- Mexitil Capsules ... 684

Morphine Sulfate (Rifampin accelerates the metabolism of narcotic; dosage adjustment may be required when starting or stopping concomitantly administered rifampin). Products include:
- Astramorph/PF Injection, USP (Preservative-Free) ... 526
- Duramorph Injection ... 983
- Infumorph 200 and Infumorph 500 Sterile Solutions ... 985
- Kadian Capsules ... 2948
- MS Contin Tablets ... 2149
- MSIR ... 2152
- Oramorph SR (Morphine Sulfate Sustained Release Tablets) ... 2359
- RMS Suppositories CII ... 2766
- Roxanol ... 2365

Nadolol (Rifampin accelerates the metabolism of beta blocker; dosage adjustment may be required when starting or stopping concomitantly administered rifampin).
No products indexed under this heading.

Nifedipine (Rifampin accelerates the metabolism of nifedipine; dosage adjustment may be required when starting or stopping concomitantly administered rifampin). Products include:
- Adalat Capsules (10 mg and 20 mg) ... 580
- Adalat CC ... 582
- Procardia Capsules ... 2024
- Procardia XL Extended Release Tablets ... 2026

Norethindrone (Rifampin accelerates the metabolism of oral contraceptive; dosage adjustment may be required when starting or stopping concomitantly administered rifampin). Products include:
- Brevicon ... 2563
- Micronor Tablets ... 1903
- Modicon ... 1928
- Norinyl ... 2563
- Nor-Q D Tablets ... 2598
- Ortho-Novum ... 1928
- Ovcon ... 765
- Tri-Norinyl ... 2607

Norethynodrel (Rifampin accelerates the metabolism of oral contraceptive; dosage adjustment may be required when starting or stopping concomitantly administered rifampin).
No products indexed under this heading.

Norgestimate (Rifampin accelerates the metabolism of oral contraceptive or progestin; dosage adjustment may be required when starting or stopping concomitantly administered rifampin). Products include:
- Ortho-Cyclen/Ortho-Tri-Cyclen ... 1914
- Ortho-Cyclen/Ortho Tri-Cyclen ... 1914

Norgestrel (Rifampin accelerates the metabolism of oral contraceptive; dosage adjustment may be required when starting or stopping concomitantly administered rifampin). Products include:
- Lo/Ovral Tablets ... 2852
- Lo/Ovral-28 Tablets ... 2857
- Ovral Tablets ... 2877
- Ovral-28 Tablets ... 2878
- Ovrette Tablets ... 2878

Nortriptyline Hydrochloride (Rifampin accelerates the metabolism of nortriptyline; dosage adjustment may be required when starting or stopping concomitantly administered rifampin). Products include:
- Pamelor ... 2409

Opium Alkaloids (Rifampin accelerates the metabolism of narcotic; dosage adjustment may be required when starting or stopping concomitantly administered rifampin).
No products indexed under this heading.

Oxycodone Hydrochloride (Rifampin accelerates the metabolism of narcotic; dosage adjustment may be required when starting or stopping concomitantly administered rifampin). Products include:
- OxyContin Tablets ... 2163
- OxyIR Capsules ... 2167
- Percocet Tablets ... 955
- Percodan Tablets ... 955
- Percodan-Demi Tablets ... 956
- Roxicodone Tablets, Oral Solution & Intensol (Oxycodone) ... 2366
- Tylox Capsules ... 1593

Para-Aminosalicylic Acid (Increases the plasma concentration and elimination half-life of isoniazid).

Penbutolol Sulfate (Rifampin accelerates the metabolism of beta blocker; dosage adjustment may be required when starting or stopping concomitantly administered rifampin). Products include:
- Levatol Tablets ... 2547

Pentobarbital Sodium (Rifampin accelerates the metabolism of barbiturates; dosage adjustment may be required when starting or stopping concomitantly administered rifampin). Products include:
- Nembutal Sodium Capsules ... 440
- Nembutal Sodium Solution ... 442
- Nembutal Sodium Suppositories ... 444

Phenobarbital (Rifampin accelerates the metabolism of barbiturates; dosage adjustment may be required when starting or stopping concomitantly administered rifampin). Products include:
- Arco-Lase Plus Tablets ... 513
- Bellergal-S Tablets ... 2375
- Donnatal ... 2234
- Donnatal Extentabs ... 2234
- Donnatal Tablets ... 2234
- Phenobarbital Elixir and Tablets ... 1523
- Quadrinal Tablets ... 1398

Phenytoin (Rifampin accelerates the metabolism and isoniazid inhibits the metabolism of phenytoin; dosage adjustment may be required when starting or stopping concomitantly administered rifampin). Products include:
- Dilantin Infatabs ... 1967
- Dilantin-125 Suspension ... 1969

Phenytoin Sodium (Rifampin accelerates the metabolism and isoniazid inhibits the metabolism of phenytoin; dosage adjustment may be required when starting or stopping concomitantly administered rifampin). Products include:
- Dilantin Kapseals ... 1965

Pindolol (Rifampin accelerates the metabolism of beta blocker; dosage adjustment may be required when starting or stopping concomitantly administered rifampin). Products include:
- Visken Tablets ... 2428

Prednisolone Acetate (Rifampin accelerates the metabolism of corticosteroid; dosage adjustment may be required when starting or stopping concomitantly administered rifampin; may increase the serum concentration of isoniazid by increasing acetylation rate and/or renal clearance). Products include:
- AK-CIDE ... ⊚ 203
- AK-CIDE Ointment ... ⊚ 203
- Blephamide Liquifilm Sterile Ophthalmic Suspension ... 472
- Blephamide Ointment ... ⊚ 234
- Econopred & Econopred Plus Ophthalmic Suspensions ... ⊚ 216
- Poly-Pred Liquifilm ... ⊚ 246
- Pred Forte ... ⊚ 247
- Pred Mild ... ⊚ 250
- Pred-G Liquifilm Sterile Ophthalmic Suspension ... ⊚ 248
- Pred-G S.O.P. Sterile Ophthalmic Ointment ... ⊚ 249

Prednisolone Sodium Phosphate (Rifampin accelerates the metabolism of corticosteroid; dosage adjustment may be required when starting or stopping concomitantly administered rifampin; may increase the serum concentration of isoniazid by increasing acetylation rate and/or renal clearance). Products include:
- AK-PRED ... ⊚ 204
- Hydeltrasol Injection, Sterile ... 1708
- Pediapred Oral Solution ... 1618

Prednisolone Tebutate (Rifampin accelerates the metabolism of corticosteroid; dosage adjustment may be required when starting or stopping concomitantly administered rifampin; may increase the serum concentration of isoniazid by increasing acetylation rate and/or renal clearance). Products include:
- Hydeltra-T.B.A. Sterile Suspension ... 1710

Prednisone (Rifampin accelerates the metabolism of corticosteroid; dosage adjustment may be required when starting or stopping concomitantly administered rifampin).
No products indexed under this heading.

Primidone (Isoniazid inhibits the metabolism of primidone). Products include:
- Mysoline ... 2860

Probenecid (Increases blood levels of rifampin). Products include:
- Benemid Tablets ... 1651
- ColBENEMID Tablets ... 1662

Propoxyphene Hydrochloride (Rifampin accelerates the metabolism of narcotic; dosage adjustment may be required when starting or stopping concomitantly administered rifampin). Products include:
- Darvon ... 1475
- Wygesic Tablets ... 2930

Propoxyphene Napsylate (Rifampin accelerates the metabolism of narcotic; dosage adjustment may be required when starting or stopping concomitantly administered rifampin). Products include:
- Darvon-N/Darvocet-N ... 1473

Propranolol Hydrochloride (Rifampin accelerates the metabolism of beta blocker; dosage adjustment may be required when starting or stopping concomitantly administered rifampin). Products include:
- Inderal ... 2834
- Inderal LA Long Acting Capsules ... 2836
- Inderide Tablets ... 2838
- Inderide LA Long Acting Capsules ... 2840

(▣ Described in PDR For Nonprescription Drugs) (⊚ Described in PDR For Ophthalmology)

Quinidine Gluconate (Rifampin accelerates the metabolism of quinidine; dosage adjustment may be required when starting or stopping concomitantly administered rifampin). Products include:
Quinaglute Dura-Tabs Tablets 644

Quinidine Polygalacturonate (Rifampin accelerates the metabolism of quinidine; dosage adjustment may be required when starting or stopping concomitantly administered rifampin). Products include:
Cardioquin Tablets 2146

Quinidine Sulfate (Rifampin accelerates the metabolism of tocainide; dosage adjustment may be required when starting or stopping concomitantly administered rifampin). Products include:
Quinidex Extentabs 2240

Secobarbital Sodium (Rifampin accelerates the metabolism of barbiturates; dosage adjustment may be required when starting or stopping concomitantly administered rifampin). Products include:
Seconal Sodium Pulvules 1529

Sodium Bicarbonate (Reduces absorption of rifampin and isoniazid). Products include:
Alka-Seltzer Cherry Effervescent Antacid and Pain Reliever 609
Alka-Seltzer Extra Strength Effervescent Antacid and Pain Reliever 609
Alka-Seltzer Gold Effervescent Antacid 611
Alka-Seltzer Lemon Lime Effervescent Antacid and Pain Reliever 609
Alka-Seltzer Original Effervescent Antacid and Pain Reliever 609
Arm & Hammer Pure Baking Soda 648
Colyte and Colyte-flavored 2540
GoLYTELY 694
Massengill Disposable Douches 780
Massengill Liquid Concentrate 780
NuLYTELY 694
Cherry Flavor NuLYTELY 694

Sotalol Hydrochloride (Rifampin accelerates the metabolism of beta blocker; dosage adjustment may be required when starting or stopping concomitantly administered rifampin). Products include:
Betapace Tablets 637

Sufentanil Citrate (Rifampin accelerates the metabolism of narcotic; dosage adjustment may be required when starting or stopping concomitantly administered rifampin). Products include:
Sufenta Injection 1355

Sulfamethoxazole (Increases blood levels of rifampin). Products include:
Bactrim DS Tablets 2257
Bactrim I.V. Infusion 2255
Bactrim 2257
Gantanol Tablets 2285
Septra 1146
Septra I.V. Infusion 1142
Septra I.V. Infusion ADD-Vantage Vials 1144
Septra 1146

Sulfasalazine (Reduced plasma concentration of sulfapyridine by rifampin due to alteration in colonic bacteria responsible for reduction of sulfasalazine to sulfapyridine). Products include:
Azulfidine 2059

Theophylline (Rifampin accelerates the metabolism of theophylline and isoniazid inhibits the metabolism; dosage adjustment may be required when starting or stopping concomitantly administered rifampin). Products include:
Marax Tablets & DF Syrup 2015
Quibron 2227

Theophylline Anhydrous (Rifampin accelerates the metabolism of theophylline and isoniazid inhibits the metabolism; dosage adjustment may be required when starting or stopping concomitantly administered rifampin). Products include:
Aerolate 1003
Primatene Tablets 844
Respbid Tablets 687
Slo-bid Gyrocaps 2201
Theo-24 Extended Release Capsules 2753
Theo-Dur Extended-Release Tablets 1367
Theo-X Extended-Release Tablets 793
Uni-Dur Extended-Release Tablets 1374
Uniphyl 400 mg and 600 mg Tablets 2157

Theophylline Calcium Salicylate (Rifampin accelerates the metabolism of theophylline and isoniazid inhibits the metabolism; dosage adjustment may be required when starting or stopping concomitantly administered rifampin). Products include:
Quadrinal Tablets 1398

Theophylline Sodium Glycinate (Rifampin accelerates the metabolism of theophylline and isoniazid inhibits the metabolism; dosage adjustment may be required when starting or stopping concomitantly administered rifampin).
No products indexed under this heading.

Thiamylal Sodium (Rifampin accelerates the metabolism of barbiturates; dosage adjustment may be required when starting or stopping concomitantly administered rifampin).
No products indexed under this heading.

Timolol Hemihydrate (Rifampin accelerates the metabolism of beta blocker; dosage adjustment may be required when starting or stopping concomitantly administered rifampin). Products include:
Betimol 0.25%, 0.5% 259

Timolol Maleate (Rifampin accelerates the metabolism of beta blocker; dosage adjustment may be required when starting or stopping concomitantly administered rifampin). Products include:
Blocadren Tablets 1654
Timolide Tablets 1791
Timoptic in Ocudose 1796
Timoptic Sterile Ophthalmic Solution 1794
Timoptic-XE 1798

Tocainide Hydrochloride (Rifampin accelerates the metabolism of tocainide; dosage adjustment may be required when starting or stopping concomitantly administered rifampin). Products include:
Tonocard Tablets 519

Tolazamide (Rifampin accelerates the metabolism of oral hypoglycemic agent; isoniazid may produce hyperglycemia and lead to loss of glucose control; dosage adjustment may be required when starting or stopping concomitantly administered rifampin).
No products indexed under this heading.

Tolbutamide (Rifampin accelerates the metabolism of oral hypoglycemic agent; isoniazid may produce hyperglycemia and lead to loss of glucose control; dosage adjustment may be required when starting or stopping concomitantly administered rifampin).
No products indexed under this heading.

Triamcinolone (Rifampin accelerates the metabolism of corticosteroid; dosage adjustment may be required when starting or stopping concomitantly administered rifampin).
No products indexed under this heading.

Triamcinolone Acetonide (Rifampin accelerates the metabolism of corticosteroid; dosage adjustment may be required when starting or stopping concomitantly administered rifampin). Products include:
Azmacort Oral Inhaler 2175
Nasacort AQ Nasal Spray 2191
Nasacort Nasal Inhaler 2189

Triamcinolone Diacetate (Rifampin accelerates the metabolism of corticosteroid; dosage adjustment may be required when starting or stopping concomitantly administered rifampin).
No products indexed under this heading.

Triamcinolone Hexacetonide (Rifampin accelerates the metabolism of corticosteroid; dosage adjustment may be required when starting or stopping concomitantly administered rifampin).
No products indexed under this heading.

Trimethoprim (Increases blood levels of rifampin). Products include:
Bactrim DS Tablets 2257
Bactrim I.V. Infusion 2255
Bactrim 2257
Proloprim Tablets 1141
Septra 1146
Septra I.V. Infusion 1142
Septra I.V. Infusion ADD-Vantage Vials 1144
Septra 1146
Trimpex Tablets 2323

Valproic Acid (Isoniazid inhibits the metabolism of valproic acid). Products include:
Depakene 416

Verapamil Hydrochloride (Rifampin accelerates the metabolism of verapamil; dosage adjustment may be required when starting or stopping concomitantly administered rifampin). Products include:
Calan SR Caplets 2571
Calan Tablets 2568
Covera-HS Tablets 2573
Isoptin Injectable 1391
Isoptin Oral Tablets 1393
Isoptin SR Tablets 1395
Verelan Capsules 1455

Warfarin Sodium (Rifampin accelerates the metabolism of anticoagulants and isoniazid inhibits the metabolism; increased requirements of coumarin type anticoagulant; dosage adjustment may be required when starting or stopping concomitantly administered rifampin). Products include:
Coumadin 941

Food Interactions

Alcohol (Daily ingestion of alcohol may be associated with higher incidence of isoniazid hepatitis).

Cheese, unspecified (Isoniazid has some MAO inhibiting activity, an interaction with tyramine-containing food may occur).

Fish, tropical (Isoniazid may inhibit diamine oxidase, causing exaggerated response (headache, sweating, palpitations, flushing, hypotension) to food containing histamine).

Food with high concentration of tyramine (Isoniazid has some MAO inhibiting activity, an interaction with tyramine-containing food may occur).

Skipjack fish (Isoniazid may inhibit diamine oxidase, causing exaggerated response (headache, sweating, palpitations, flushing, hypotension) to food containing histamine).

Tuna fish (Isoniazid may inhibit diamine oxidase, causing exaggerated response (headache, sweating, palpitations, flushing, hypotension) to food containing histamine).

Wine, red (Isoniazid has some MAO inhibiting activity, an interaction with tyramine-containing food may occur).

RILUTEK TABLETS
(Riluzole) 2198
May interact with xanthine bronchodilators, quinolones, and certain other agents. Compounds in these categories include:

Allopurinol (Riluzole induces hepatic injury; ALS patients on concomitant hepatotoxic drugs, such as allopurinol, were excluded in the clinical trials; if such combination is used, practitioner should exercise caution). Products include:
Zyloprim Tablets 1194

Aminophylline (Potential inhibitors of CYP1A2, such as theophylline, could decrease the rate of riluzole elimination).
No products indexed under this heading.

Amitriptyline Hydrochloride (Potential inhibitors of CYP1A2, such as amitriptyline, could decrease the rate of riluzole elimination). Products include:
Elavil 2945
Etrafon 2495
Limbitrol 2333
Triavil Tablets 1800

Caffeine (Potential inhibitors of CYP1A2, such as caffeine, could decrease the rate of riluzole elimination). Products include:
Arthritis Strength BC Powder 631
BC Powder 631
Cafergot 2376
DHCplus Capsules 2148
Darvon Compound-65 Pulvules 1475
Esgic-plus Capsules 1012
Esgic-plus Tablets 1012
Aspirin Free Excedrin Analgesic Caplets and Geltabs 734
Excedrin Extra-Strength Analgesic Tablets, Caplets, and Geltabs 734
Fioricet Tablets 2386
Fioricet with Codeine Capsules 2387
Fiorinal Capsules 2388
Fiorinal with Codeine Capsules 2390
Fiorinal Tablets 2388
Goody's Extra Strength Headache Powders 632
Goody's Extra Strength Pain Relief Tablets 632
Maximum Strength Multi-Symptom Formula Midol 621
No Doz Maximum Strength Caplets 644
Norgesic 1554
Vanquish Analgesic Caplets 627
Wigraine Tablets 1884

Ciprofloxacin (Potential inhibitors of CYP1A2, such as quinolones, could decrease the rate of riluzole elimination). Products include:
Cipro I.V. 587
Cipro I.V. Pharmacy Bulk Package 590

IMPORTANT NOTE: Always consult each drug listing in the patient's regimen for possible interactions.

Ciprofloxacin Hydrochloride (Potential inhibitors of CYP1A2, such as quinolones, could decrease the rate of riluzole elimination). Products include:
- Ciloxan Ophthalmic Solution 468
- Cipro Tablets 584

Dyphylline (Potential inhibitors of CYP1A2, such as theophylline, could decrease the rate of riluzole elimination). Products include:
- Lufyllin & Lufyllin-400 Tablets 2778
- Lufyllin-GG Elixir & Tablets 2779

Enoxacin (Potential inhibitors of CYP1A2, such as quinolones, could decrease the rate of riluzole elimination). Products include:
- Penetrex Tablets 2196

Lomefloxacin Hydrochloride (Potential inhibitors of CYP1A2, such as quinolones, could decrease the rate of riluzole elimination). Products include:
- Maxaquin Tablets 2593

Methyldopa (Riluzole induces hepatic injury; ALS patients on concomitant hepatotoxic drugs, such as methyldopa, were excluded in the clinical trials; if such combination is used, practitioner should exercise caution). Products include:
- Aldoclor Tablets 1638
- Aldomet Oral 1640
- Aldoril Tablets 1644

Norfloxacin (Potential inhibitors of CYP1A2, such as quinolones, could decrease the rate of riluzole elimination). Products include:
- Chibroxin Sterile Ophthalmic Solution 1657
- Noroxin Tablets 1758
- Noroxin Tablets 2222

Ofloxacin (Potential inhibitors of CYP1A2, such as quinolones, could decrease the rate of riluzole elimination). Products include:
- Floxin I.V. 1580
- Floxin Tablets (200 mg, 300 mg, 400 mg) 1577
- Ocuflox Ophthalmic Solution 478
- Ocuflox ..... ⊚ 242

Omeprazole (Potential inducers of CYP1A2, such as theophylline, could increase the rate of riluzole elimination). Products include:
- Prilosec Delayed-Release Capsules 516

Phenacetin (Potential inhibitors of CYP1A2, such as phenacetin, could decrease the rate of riluzole elimination).

Rifampin (Potential inducers of CYP1A2, such as theophylline, could increase the rate of riluzole elimination). Products include:
- Rifadin 1276
- Rifamate Capsules 1278
- Rifater 1280
- Rimactane Capsules 865

Sulfasalazine (Riluzole induces hepatic injury; ALS patients on concomitant hepatotoxic drugs, such as sulfasalazine, were excluded in the clinical trials; if such combination is used, practitioner should exercise caution). Products include:
- Azulfidine 2059

Tacrine Hydrochloride (CYP1A2 is the principal isoenzyme involved in the initial oxidative metabolism of riluzole; potential interaction may occur when co-administered with other agents, such as tacrine, which are also metabolized primarily by CYP1A2). Products include:
- Cognex Capsules 1961

Theophylline (Potential inhibitors of CYP1A2, such as theophylline, could decrease the rate of riluzole elimination). Products include:
- Marax Tablets & DF Syrup 2015
- Quibron 2227

Theophylline Anhydrous (Potential inhibitors of CYP1A2, such as theophylline, could decrease the rate of riluzole elimination). Products include:
- Aerolate 1003
- Primatene Tablets ..... ▣ 844
- Respbid Tablets 687
- Slo-bid Gyrocaps 2201
- Theo-24 Extended Release Capsules 2753
- Theo-Dur Extended-Release Tablets 1367
- Theo-X Extended-Release Tablets .. 793
- Uni-Dur Extended-Release Tablets .. 1374
- Uniphyl 400 mg and 600 mg Tablets 2157

Theophylline Calcium Salicylate (Potential inhibitors of CYP1A2, such as theophylline, could decrease the rate of riluzole elimination). Products include:
- Quadrinal Tablets 1398

Theophylline Sodium Glycinate (Potential inhibitors of CYP1A2, such as theophylline, could decrease the rate of riluzole elimination).
- No products indexed under this heading.

Food Interactions

Alcohol (Alcohol may increase the risk of hepatotoxicity; patients on riluzole should be discouraged from drinking excessive amounts of alcohol).

Diet, high-lipid (Co-administration with high-fat meal decreases absorption, reduces AUC by about 20% and peak blood levels by about 45%).

Food, charcoal-broiled (Potential inducers of CYP1A2, such as charcoal-broiled food, could increase the rate of riluzole elimination).

RIMACTANE CAPSULES

(Rifampin) 865

May interact with oral anticoagulants, oral contraceptives, oral hypoglycemic agents, corticosteroids, and cardiac glycosides. Compounds in these categories include:

Acarbose (Diminished effects). Products include:
- Precose 604

Betamethasone Acetate (Diminished effects). Products include:
- Celestone Soluspan Suspension 2484

Betamethasone Sodium Phosphate (Diminished effects). Products include:
- Celestone Soluspan Suspension 2484

Chlorpropamide (Diminished effects). Products include:
- Diabinese Tablets 2002

Cortisone Acetate (Diminished effects). Products include:
- Cortone Acetate Sterile Suspension 1663
- Cortone Acetate Tablets 1664

Dapsone (Diminished effects). Products include:
- Dapsone Tablets USP 1331

Deslanoside (Diminished effects).
- No products indexed under this heading.

Desogestrel (Reliability of oral contraceptive affected). Products include:
- Desogen Tablets 1867
- Ortho-Cept 1907

Dexamethasone (Diminished effects). Products include:
- AK-Trol Ointment & Suspension ..... ⊚ 205
- Decadron Elixir 1676
- Decadron Tablets 1678
- Decaspray Topical Aerosol 1689
- Maxitrol Ophthalmic Ointment and Suspension ..... ⊚ 222
- TobraDex Ophthalmic Suspension and Ointment 469

Dexamethasone Acetate (Diminished effects). Products include:
- Dalalone D.P. Injectable 1009
- Decadron-LA Sterile Suspension 1687

Dexamethasone Sodium Phosphate (Diminished effects). Products include:
- Decadron Phosphate Injection 1680
- Decadron Phosphate Sterile Ophthalmic Ointment 1684
- Decadron Phosphate Sterile Ophthalmic Solution 1685
- Decadron Phosphate Topical Cream 1686
- Decadron Phosphate with Xylocaine Injection, Sterile 1683
- Dexacort Phosphate in Respihaler .. 1606
- Dexacort Phosphate in Turbinaire .. 1607
- NeoDecadron Sterile Ophthalmic Ointment 1755
- NeoDecadron Sterile Ophthalmic Solution 1756
- NeoDecadron Topical Cream 1757

Dicumarol (Increased requirements).
- No products indexed under this heading.

Digitoxin (Diminished effects). Products include:
- Crystodigin Tablets 1472

Digoxin (Diminished effects). Products include:
- Lanoxicaps 1110
- Lanoxin Elixir Pediatric 1113
- Lanoxin Injection 1116
- Lanoxin Injection Pediatric 1119
- Lanoxin Tablets 1121

Ethambutol Hydrochloride (Potential for thrombocytopenia). Products include:
- Myambutol Tablets 1432

Ethinyl Estradiol (Reliability of oral contraceptive affected). Products include:
- Brevicon 2563
- Demulen 2580
- Desogen Tablets 1867
- Levlen/Tri-Levlen 646
- Lo/Ovral Tablets 2852
- Lo/Ovral-28 Tablets 2857
- Modicon 1928
- Nordette-21 Tablets 2863
- Nordette-28 Tablets 2866
- Norinyl 2563
- Ortho-Cept 1907
- Ortho-Cyclen/Ortho-Tri-Cyclen 1914
- Ortho-Novum 1928
- Ortho-Cyclen/Ortho Tri-Cyclen 1914
- Ovcon 765
- Ovral Tablets 2877
- Ovral-28 Tablets 2878
- Levlen/Tri-Levlen 646
- Tri-Norinyl 2607
- Triphasil-21 Tablets 2919
- Triphasil-28 Tablets 2924

Ethynodiol Diacetate (Reliability of oral contraceptive affected). Products include:
- Demulen 2580

Fludrocortisone Acetate (Diminished effects). Products include:
- Florinef Acetate Tablets 506

Glimepiride (Diminished effects). Products include:
- Amaryl Tablets 1241

Glipizide (Diminished effects). Products include:
- Glucotrol Tablets 2011
- Glucotrol XL Extended Release Tablets 2012

Glyburide (Diminished effects). Products include:
- DiaBeta Tablets 1265
- Glynase PresTab Tablets 2091
- Micronase Tablets 2099

Hepatotoxic Drugs, unspecified (Increased risk of liver toxicity).

Hydrocortisone (Diminished effects). Products include:
- Anusol-HC Cream 2.5% 1953
- Aquanil HC Lotion 1989
- Maximum Strength Cortaid Spray ▣ 800
- CORTENEMA 2713
- Cortisporin Ointment 1074
- Cortisporin Ophthalmic Ointment Sterile 1074
- Cortisporin Ophthalmic Suspension Sterile 1075
- Cortisporin Otic Solution Sterile 1076
- Cortisporin Otic Suspension Sterile 1077
- Cortizone-5 ..... ▣ 795
- Cortizone-10 ..... ▣ 795
- Hydrocortone Tablets 1715
- Hytone 922
- Hytone Ointment 2 ½% 923
- Massengill Medicated Soft Cloth Towelettes 2628
- Pediotic Suspension Sterile 1140
- Preparation H Hydrocortisone 1% Cream ..... ▣ 843
- ProctoCream-HC 2.5% 2552
- VōSoL HC Otic Solution 2786

Hydrocortisone Acetate (Diminished effects). Products include:
- Analpram-HC Rectal Cream 1% and 2.5% 993
- Anusol HC-1 Hydrocortisone Anti-Itch Ointment ..... ▣ 810
- Anusol-HC Suppositories 1954
- Caldecort Anti-Itch Hydrocortisone Cream ..... ▣ 651
- Coly-Mycin S Otic w/Neomycin & Hydrocortisone 1965
- Cortaid ..... ▣ 800
- Cortifoam 2540
- Cortisporin Cream 1073
- Epifoam 2543
- Hydrocortone Acetate Sterile Suspension 1712
- Mantadil Cream 1124
- Nupercainal Hydrocortisone 1% Cream ..... ▣ 661
- Pramosone Cream, Lotion & Ointment 995
- ProctoFoam-HC 2552
- Terra-Cortril Ophthalmic Suspension 2033

Hydrocortisone Sodium Phosphate (Diminished effects). Products include:
- Hydrocortone Phosphate Injection, Sterile 1713

Hydrocortisone Sodium Succinate (Diminished effects).
- No products indexed under this heading.

Levonorgestrel (Reliability of oral contraceptive affected). Products include:
- Levlen/Tri-Levlen 646
- Nordette-21 Tablets 2863
- Nordette-28 Tablets 2866
- Norplant System 2868
- Levlen/Tri-Levlen 646
- Triphasil-21 Tablets 2919
- Triphasil-28 Tablets 2924

Mestranol (Reliability of oral contraceptive affected). Products include:
- Norinyl 2563
- Ortho-Novum 1928

Metformin Hydrochloride (Diminished effects). Products include:
- Glucophage Tablets 754

Methadone Hydrochloride (Diminished effects). Products include:
- Methadone Hydrochloride Oral Concentrate 2356
- Methadone Hydrochloride Oral Solution & Tablets 2357

Methylprednisolone Acetate (Diminished effects).
- No products indexed under this heading.

Methylprednisolone Sodium Succinate (Diminished effects).
- No products indexed under this heading.

Norethindrone (Reliability of oral contraceptive affected). Products include:
- Brevicon 2563

(▣ Described in PDR For Nonprescription Drugs) (⊚ Described in PDR For Ophthalmology)

935 **Interactions Index** **Risperdal**

Micronor Tablets 1903
Modicon 1928
Norinyl 2563
Nor-Q D Tablets 2598
Ortho-Novum 1928
Ovcon 765
Tri-Norinyl 2607

Norethynodrel (Reliability of oral contraceptive affected).
No products indexed under this heading.

Norgestimate (Reliability of oral contraceptive affected). Products include:
Ortho-Cyclen/Ortho-Tri-Cyclen 1914
Ortho-Cyclen/Ortho Tri-Cyclen 1914

Norgestrel (Reliability of oral contraceptive affected). Products include:
Lo/Ovral Tablets 2852
Lo/Ovral-28 Tablets 2857
Ovral Tablets 2877
Ovral-28 Tablets 2878
Ovrette Tablets 2878

Prednisolone Acetate (Diminished effects). Products include:
AK-CIDE .... ⊛ 203
AK-CIDE Ointment .... ⊛ 203
Blephamide Liquifilm Sterile Ophthalmic Suspension 472
Blephamide Ointment .... ⊛ 234
Econopred & Econopred Plus Ophthalmic Suspensions .... ⊛ 216
Poly-Pred Liquifilm .... ⊛ 246
Pred Forte .... ⊛ 247
Pred Mild .... ⊛ 250
Pred-G Liquifilm Sterile Ophthalmic Suspension .... ⊛ 248
Pred-G S.O.P. Sterile Ophthalmic Ointment .... ⊛ 249

Prednisolone Sodium Phosphate (Diminished effects). Products include:
AK-PRED .... ⊛ 204
Hydeltrasol Injection, Sterile 1708
Pediapred Oral Solution 1618

Prednisolone Tebutate (Diminished effects). Products include:
Hydeltra-T.B.A. Sterile Suspension 1710

Prednisone (Diminished effects).
No products indexed under this heading.

Tolazamide (Diminished effects).
No products indexed under this heading.

Tolbutamide (Diminished effects).
No products indexed under this heading.

Triamcinolone (Diminished effects).
No products indexed under this heading.

Triamcinolone Acetonide (Diminished effects). Products include:
Azmacort Oral Inhaler 2175
Nasacort AQ Nasal Spray 2191
Nasacort Nasal Inhaler 2189

Triamcinolone Diacetate (Diminished effects).
No products indexed under this heading.

Triamcinolone Hexacetonide (Diminished effects).
No products indexed under this heading.

Verapamil Hydrochloride (Reduced bioavailability and efficacy). Products include:
Calan SR Caplets 2571
Calan Tablets 2568
Covera-HS Tablets 2573
Isoptin Injectable 1391
Isoptin Oral Tablets 1393
Isoptin SR Tablets 1395
Verelan Capsules 1455

Warfarin Sodium (Increased requirements). Products include:
Coumadin 941

RISPERDAL TABLETS
(Risperidone) 1348
May interact with antihypertensives, dopamine agonists, central nervous system depressants, drugs that inhibit cytochrome p450iid6 and other p450 isoenzymes, and certain other agents. Compounds in these categories include:

Acebutolol Hydrochloride (Co-administration with antihypertensive agents has resulted in clinically significant hypotension). Products include:
Sectral Capsules 2914

Alfentanil Hydrochloride (Effects not specified; caution should be used when used concurrently). Products include:
Alfenta Injection 1334

Alprazolam (Effects not specified; caution should be used when used concurrently). Products include:
Xanax Tablets 2115

Amitriptyline Hydrochloride (Inhibitors of cytochrome P450IID6 could interfere with the conversion of risperidone to 9-hydroxyrisperidone). Products include:
Elavil 2945
Etrafon 2495
Limbitrol 2333
Triavil Tablets 1800

Amlodipine Besylate (Co-administration with antihypertensive agents has resulted in clinically significant hypotension). Products include:
Lotrel Capsules 858
Norvasc Tablets 2020

Aprobarbital (Effects not specified; caution should be used when used concurrently).
No products indexed under this heading.

Atenolol (Co-administration with antihypertensive agents has resulted in clinically significant hypotension). Products include:
Tenoretic Tablets 2963
Tenormin Tablets and I.V. Injection 2965

Benazepril Hydrochloride (Co-administration with antihypertensive agents has resulted in clinically significant hypotension). Products include:
Lotensin Tablets 852
Lotensin HCT Tablets 855
Lotrel Capsules 858

Bendroflumethiazide (Co-administration with antihypertensive agents has resulted in clinically significant hypotension).
No products indexed under this heading.

Betaxolol Hydrochloride (Co-administration with antihypertensive agents has resulted in clinically significant hypotension). Products include:
Betoptic Ophthalmic Solution 465
Betoptic S Ophthalmic Suspension 467
Kerlone Tablets 2588

Bisoprolol Fumarate (Co-administration with antihypertensive agents has resulted in clinically significant hypotension). Products include:
Zebeta Tablets 1457
Ziac 1459

Bromocriptine Mesylate (Risperidone may antagonize the effect of dopamine agonists). Products include:
Parlodel 2411

Buprenorphine (Effects not specified; caution should be used when used concurrently). Products include:
Buprenex Injectable 2170

Buspirone Hydrochloride (Effects not specified; caution should be used when used concurrently). Products include:
BuSpar Tablets 738

Butabarbital (Effects not specified; caution should be used when used concurrently).
No products indexed under this heading.

Butalbital (Effects not specified; caution should be used when used concurrently). Products include:
Axocet Capsules 2469
Esgic-plus Capsules 1012
Esgic-plus Tablets 1012
Fioricet Tablets 2386
Fioricet with Codeine Capsules 2387
Fiorinal Capsules 2388
Fiorinal with Codeine Capsules 2390
Fiorinal Tablets 2388
Phrenilin 790
Sedapap Tablets 50 mg/650 mg .. 1826

Captopril (Co-administration with antihypertensive agents has resulted in clinically significant hypotension). Products include:
Capoten Tablets 740
Capozide Tablets 744

Carbamazepine (Chronic administration of carbamazepine may increase the clearance of risperidone). Products include:
Atretol Tablets 569
Tegretol/Tegretol-XR 870

Carteolol Hydrochloride (Co-administration with antihypertensive agents has resulted in clinically significant hypotension). Products include:
Cartrol Tablets 413
Ocupress Ophthalmic Solution, 1% Sterile .... ⊛ 297

Chlordiazepoxide (Effects not specified; caution should be used when used concurrently). Products include:
Limbitrol 2333

Chlordiazepoxide Hydrochloride (Effects not specified; caution should be used when used concurrently). Products include:
Librax Capsules 2330
Librium Capsules 2331
Librium Injectable 2332

Chlorothiazide (Co-administration with antihypertensive agents has resulted in clinically significant hypotension). Products include:
Aldoclor Tablets 1638
Diupres Tablets 1691
Diuril Oral 1694

Chlorothiazide Sodium (Co-administration with antihypertensive agents has resulted in clinically significant hypotension). Products include:
Diuril Sodium Intravenous 1693

Chlorpromazine (Inhibitors of cytochrome P450IID6 could interfere with the conversion of risperidone to 9-hydroxyrisperidone; caution should be used when used concurrently). Products include:
Thorazine Suppositories 2701

Chlorpromazine Hydrochloride (Inhibitors of cytochrome P450IID6 could interfere with the conversion of risperidone to 9-hydroxyrisperidone; caution should be used when used concurrently). Products include:
Thorazine 2701

Chlorprothixene (Effects not specified; caution should be used when used concurrently).
No products indexed under this heading.

Chlorprothixene Hydrochloride (Effects not specified; caution should be used when used concurrently).
No products indexed under this heading.

Chlorprothixene Lactate (Effects not specified; caution should be used when used concurrently).
No products indexed under this heading.

Chlorthalidone (Co-administration with antihypertensive agents has resulted in clinically significant hypotension). Products include:
Combipres Tablets 682
Tenoretic Tablets 2963
Thalitone 1293

Clonidine (Co-administration with antihypertensive agents has resulted in clinically significant hypotension). Products include:
Catapres-TTS 680

Clonidine Hydrochloride (Co-administration with antihypertensive agents has resulted in clinically significant hypotension). Products include:
Catapres Tablets 679
Combipres Tablets 682

Clorazepate Dipotassium (Effects not specified; caution should be used when used concurrently). Products include:
Tranxene 459

Clozapine (Chronic administration of clozapine with risperidone may decrease the clearance of risperidone; caution should be used when used concurrently). Products include:
Clozaril Tablets 2377

CNS-Active Drugs, unspecified (Effects not specified; caution should be used when used concurrently).

Codeine Phosphate (Effects not specified; caution should be used when used concurrently). Products include:
Brontex 2130
Dimetane-DC Cough Syrup 2232
Fioricet with Codeine Capsules 2387
Fiorinal with Codeine Capsules 2390
Nucofed 2225
Phenergan with Codeine 2883
Phenergan VC with Codeine 2888
Robitussin A-C Syrup 2248
Robitussin-DAC Syrup 2249
Ryna 804
Soma Compound w/Codeine Tablets 2784
Tylenol with Codeine 1592

Deserpidine (Co-administration with antihypertensive agents has resulted in clinically significant hypotension).
No products indexed under this heading.

Dezocine (Effects not specified; caution should be used when used concurrently). Products include:
Dalgan Injection 529

Diazepam (Effects not specified; caution should be used when used concurrently). Products include:
Dizac (diazepam injectable emulsion) CIV 1862
Valium Injectable 2336
Valium Tablets 2335

Diazoxide (Co-administration with antihypertensive agents has resulted in clinically significant hypotension). Products include:
Hyperstat I.V. Injection 2504
Proglycem 575

Diltiazem Hydrochloride (Co-administration with antihypertensive agents has resulted in clinically significant hypotension). Products include:
Cardizem CD Capsules 1251

IMPORTANT NOTE: Always consult each drug listing in the patient's regimen for possible interactions.

Risperdal | Interactions Index | 936

Cardizem SR Capsules 1255
Cardizem Injectable 1253
Cardizem Tablets 1257
Dilacor XR Extended-release Capsules 2183
Tiazac Capsules 1019

Dopamine Hydrochloride (Risperidone may antagonize the effect of dopamine agonists).
No products indexed under this heading.

Doxazosin Mesylate (Co-administration with antihypertensive agents has resulted in clinically significant hypotension). Products include:
Cardura Tablets 1993

Droperidol (Effects not specified; caution should be used when used concurrently). Products include:
Inapsine Injection 462

Enalapril Maleate (Co-administration with antihypertensive agents has resulted in clinically significant hypotension). Products include:
Vaseretic Tablets 1810
Vasotec Tablets 1816

Enalaprilat (Co-administration with antihypertensive agents has resulted in clinically significant hypotension). Products include:
Vasotec I.V. 1814

Enflurane (Effects not specified; caution should be used when used concurrently).
No products indexed under this heading.

Esmolol Hydrochloride (Co-administration with antihypertensive agents has resulted in clinically significant hypotension). Products include:
Brevibloc (esmolol HCl) Injection 1860

Estazolam (Effects not specified; caution should be used when used concurrently). Products include:
ProSom Tablets 457

Ethchlorvynol (Effects not specified; caution should be used when used concurrently). Products include:
Placidyl Capsules 456

Ethinamate (Effects not specified; caution should be used when used concurrently).
No products indexed under this heading.

Felodipine (Co-administration with antihypertensive agents has resulted in clinically significant hypotension). Products include:
Plendil Extended-Release Tablets 514

Fentanyl (Effects not specified; caution should be used when used concurrently). Products include:
Duragesic Transdermal System 1336

Fentanyl Citrate (Effects not specified; caution should be used when used concurrently). Products include:
Sublimaze Injection 463

Fluoxetine Hydrochloride (Inhibitors of cytochrome P450IID6 could interfere with the conversion of risperidone to 9-hydroxyrisperidone). Products include:
Prozac Pulvules & Liquid, Oral Solution 935

Fluphenazine Decanoate (Effects not specified; caution should be used when used concurrently). Products include:
Prolixin Decanoate 510

Fluphenazine Enanthate (Effects not specified; caution should be used when used concurrently). Products include:
Prolixin Enanthate 510

Fluphenazine Hydrochloride (Effects not specified; caution should be used when used concurrently). Products include:
Prolixin 510

Flurazepam Hydrochloride (Effects not specified; caution should be used when used concurrently). Products include:
Dalmane Capsules 2329

Fosinopril Sodium (Co-administration with antihypertensive agents has resulted in clinically significant hypotension). Products include:
Monopril Tablets 762

Furosemide (Co-administration with antihypertensive agents has resulted in clinically significant hypotension). Products include:
Lasix Injection, Oral Solution and Tablets 1267

Glutethimide (Effects not specified; caution should be used when used concurrently).
No products indexed under this heading.

Guanabenz Acetate (Co-administration with antihypertensive agents has resulted in clinically significant hypotension).
No products indexed under this heading.

Guanethidine Monosulfate (Co-administration with antihypertensive agents has resulted in clinically significant hypotension). Products include:
Esimil Tablets 840
Ismelin Tablets 845

Haloperidol (Inhibitors of cytochrome P450IID6 could interfere with the conversion of risperidone to 9-hydroxyrisperidone; caution should be used when used concurrently). Products include:
Haldol Injection, Tablets and Concentrate 1585

Haloperidol Decanoate (Inhibitors of cytochrome P450IID6 could interfere with the conversion of risperidone to 9-hydroxyrisperidone; caution should be used when used concurrently). Products include:
Haldol Decanoate 1587

Hydralazine Hydrochloride (Co-administration with antihypertensive agents has resulted in clinically significant hypotension). Products include:
Apresazide Capsules 824
Apresoline Hydrochloride Tablets 826
Hydralazine Hydrochloride Injection USP 2712
Ser-Ap-Es Tablets 867

Hydrochlorothiazide (Co-administration with antihypertensive agents has resulted in clinically significant hypotension). Products include:
Aldactazide Tablets 2556
Aldoril Tablets 1644
Apresazide Capsules 824
Capozide Tablets 744
Dyazide Capsules 2653
Esidrix Tablets 839
Esimil Tablets 840
HydroDIURIL Tablets 1716
Hydropres Tablets 1718
Hyzaar Tablets 1720
Inderide Tablets 2838
Inderide LA Long Acting Capsules 2840
Lopressor HCT Tablets 850
Lotensin HCT Tablets 855
Moduretic Tablets 1748
Oretic Tablets 450
Prinzide Tablets 1780
Ser-Ap-Es Tablets 867
Timolide Tablets 1791
Vaseretic Tablets 1810
Zestoretic Tablets 2968
Ziac 1459

Hydrocodone Bitartrate (Effects not specified; caution should be used when used concurrently). Products include:
Codiclear DH Syrup 808
Duratuss HD Elixir 2750
Histussin D Liquid 670
Hycodan Tablets and Syrup 946
Hycomine Compound Tablets 948
Hycomine 947
Hycotuss Expectorant Syrup 950
Hydrocet Capsules 787
Lorcet 10/650 Tablets 1016
Lortab 2751
Tussend 1830
Tussend Expectorant 1831
Vicodin Tablets 1404
Vicodin ES Tablets 1405
Vicodin HP Tablets 1403
Vicodin Tuss Expectorant 1406
Zydone Capsules 967

Hydrocodone Polistirex (Effects not specified; caution should be used when used concurrently). Products include:
Tussionex Pennkinetic Extended-Release Suspension 1624

Hydroflumethiazide (Co-administration with antihypertensive agents has resulted in clinically significant hypotension). Products include:
Diucardin Tablets 2824

Hydroxyzine Hydrochloride (Effects not specified; caution should be used when used concurrently). Products include:
Atarax Tablets & Syrup 1992
Marax Tablets & DF Syrup 2015
Vistaril Intramuscular Solution 2042

Imipramine Hydrochloride (Inhibitors of cytochrome P450IID6 could interfere with the conversion of risperidone to 9-hydroxyrisperidone). Products include:
Tofranil Ampuls 873
Tofranil Tablets 875

Indapamide (Co-administration with antihypertensive agents has resulted in clinically significant hypotension).
No products indexed under this heading.

Isoflurane (Effects not specified; caution should be used when used concurrently).
No products indexed under this heading.

Isradipine (Co-administration with antihypertensive agents has resulted in clinically significant hypotension). Products include:
DynaCirc Capsules 2381
DynaCirc CR Tablets 2383

Ketamine Hydrochloride (Effects not specified; caution should be used when used concurrently).
No products indexed under this heading.

Labetalol Hydrochloride (Co-administration with antihypertensive agents has resulted in clinically significant hypotension). Products include:
Normodyne Injection 2519
Normodyne Tablets 2522
Trandate 1158

Levodopa (Risperidone may antagonize the effect of levodopa). Products include:
Atamet Tablets 567
Larodopa Tablets 2296
Sinemet Tablets 959
Sinemet CR Tablets 961

Levorphanol Tartrate (Effects not specified; caution should be used when used concurrently). Products include:
Levo-Dromoran 2297

Lisinopril (Co-administration with antihypertensive agents has resulted in clinically significant hypotension). Products include:
Prinivil Tablets 1776
Prinzide Tablets 1780
Zestoretic Tablets 2968
Zestril Tablets 2972

Lorazepam (Effects not specified; caution should be used when used concurrently). Products include:
Ativan Injection 2805
Ativan Tablets 2807

Losartan Potassium (Co-administration with antihypertensive agents has resulted in clinically significant hypotension). Products include:
Cozaar Tablets 1668
Hyzaar Tablets 1720

Loxapine Hydrochloride (Effects not specified; caution should be used when used concurrently). Products include:
Loxitane 1426

Loxapine Succinate (Effects not specified; caution should be used when used concurrently). Products include:
Loxitane Capsules 1426

Mecamylamine Hydrochloride (Co-administration with antihypertensive agents has resulted in clinically significant hypotension). Products include:
Inversine Tablets 1729

Meperidine Hydrochloride (Effects not specified; caution should be used when used concurrently). Products include:
Demerol 2438
Mepergan Injection 2859

Mephobarbital (Effects not specified; caution should be used when used concurrently). Products include:
Mebaral Tablets 2452

Meprobamate (Effects not specified; caution should be used when used concurrently). Products include:
Miltown Tablets 2780
PMB 200 and PMB 400 2890

Mesoridazine Besylate (Effects not specified; caution should be used when used concurrently). Products include:
Serentil 689

Methadone Hydrochloride (Effects not specified; caution should be used when used concurrently). Products include:
Methadone Hydrochloride Oral Concentrate 2356
Methadone Hydrochloride Oral Solution & Tablets 2357

Methohexital Sodium (Effects not specified; caution should be used when used concurrently).
No products indexed under this heading.

Methotrimeprazine (Effects not specified; caution should be used when used concurrently). Products include:
Levoprome 1321

Methoxyflurane (Effects not specified; caution should be used when used concurrently).
No products indexed under this heading.

Methyclothiazide (Co-administration with antihypertensive agents has resulted in clinically significant hypotension). Products include:
Enduron Tablets 424

(▣ Described in PDR For Nonprescription Drugs) (◉ Described in PDR For Ophthalmology)

Methyldopa (Co-administration with antihypertensive agents has resulted in clinically significant hypotension). Products include:
Aldoclor Tablets 1638
Aldomet Oral 1640
Aldoril Tablets 1644

Methyldopate Hydrochloride (Co-administration with antihypertensive agents has resulted in clinically significant hypotension). Products include:
Aldomet Ester HCl Injection 1642

Metolazone (Co-administration with antihypertensive agents has resulted in clinically significant hypotension). Products include:
Mykrox Tablets 1617
Zaroxolyn Tablets 1625

Metoprolol Succinate (Co-administration with antihypertensive agents has resulted in clinically significant hypotension). Products include:
Toprol-XL Tablets 560

Metoprolol Tartrate (Co-administration with antihypertensive agents has resulted in clinically significant hypotension). Products include:
Lopressor 848
Lopressor HCT Tablets 850

Metyrosine (Co-administration with antihypertensive agents has resulted in clinically significant hypotension). Products include:
Demser Capsules 1690

Midazolam Hydrochloride (Effects not specified; caution should be used when used concurrently). Products include:
Versed Injection 2324

Minoxidil (Co-administration with antihypertensive agents has resulted in clinically significant hypotension).
No products indexed under this heading.

Moexipril Hydrochloride (Co-administration with antihypertensive agents has resulted in clinically significant hypotension). Products include:
Univasc Tablets 2553

Molindone Hydrochloride (Effects not specified; caution should be used when used concurrently). Products include:
Moban Tablets and Concentrate 1036

Morphine Sulfate (Effects not specified; caution should be used when used concurrently). Products include:
Astramorph/PF Injection, USP (Preservative-Free) 526
Duramorph Injection 983
Infumorph 200 and Infumorph 500 Sterile Solutions 985
Kadian Capsules 2948
MS Contin Tablets 2149
MSIR 2152
Oramorph SR (Morphine Sulfate Sustained Release Tablets) 2359
RMS Suppositories CII 2766
Roxanol 2365

Nadolol (Co-administration with antihypertensive agents has resulted in clinically significant hypotension).
No products indexed under this heading.

Nicardipine Hydrochloride (Co-administration with antihypertensive agents has resulted in clinically significant hypotension). Products include:
Cardene Capsules 2261
Cardene I.V. 2815
Cardene SR Capsules 2264

Nifedipine (Co-administration with antihypertensive agents has resulted in clinically significant hypotension). Products include:
Adalat Capsules (10 mg and 20 mg) 580
Adalat CC 582
Procardia Capsules 2024
Procardia XL Extended Release Tablets 2026

Nisoldipine (Co-administration with antihypertensive agents has resulted in clinically significant hypotension). Products include:
Sular Tablets 2961

Nitroglycerin (Co-administration with antihypertensive agents has resulted in clinically significant hypotension). Products include:
Deponit NTG Transdermal Delivery System 2541
Nitro-Bid IV 1270
Nitro-Bid Ointment 1272
Nitro-Dur (nitroglycerin) Transdermal Infusion System 1365
Nitrolingual Spray 2193
Nitrostat Tablets 1981
Transderm-Nitro Transdermal Therapeutic System 878

Opium Alkaloids (Effects not specified; caution should be used when used concurrently).
No products indexed under this heading.

Oxazepam (Effects not specified; caution should be used when used concurrently). Products include:
Serax Capsules 2916
Serax Tablets 2916

Oxycodone Hydrochloride (Effects not specified; caution should be used when used concurrently). Products include:
OxyContin Tablets 2163
OxyIR Capsules 2167
Percocet Tablets 955
Percodan Tablets 955
Percodan-Demi Tablets 956
Roxicodone Tablets, Oral Solution & Intensol (Oxycodone) 2366
Tylox Capsules 1593

Penbutolol Sulfate (Co-administration with antihypertensive agents has resulted in clinically significant hypotension). Products include:
Levatol Tablets 2547

Pentobarbital Sodium (Effects not specified; caution should be used when used concurrently). Products include:
Nembutal Sodium Capsules 440
Nembutal Sodium Solution 442
Nembutal Sodium Suppositories 444

Pergolide Mesylate (Risperidone may antagonize the effect of dopamine agonists). Products include:
Permax Tablets 571

Perphenazine (Effects not specified; caution should be used when used concurrently). Products include:
Etrafon 2495
Triavil Tablets 1800
Trilafon 2532

Phenobarbital (Effects not specified; caution should be used when used concurrently). Products include:
Arco-Lase Plus Tablets 513
Bellergal-S Tablets 2375
Donnatal 2234
Donnatal Extentabs 2234
Donnatal Tablets 2234
Phenobarbital Elixir and Tablets 1523
Quadrinal Tablets 1398

Phenoxybenzamine Hydrochloride (Co-administration with antihypertensive agents has resulted in clinically significant hypotension). Products include:
Dibenzyline Capsules 2650

Phentolamine Mesylate (Co-administration with antihypertensive agents has resulted in clinically significant hypotension). Products include:
Regitine Vials 864

Pindolol (Co-administration with antihypertensive agents has resulted in clinically significant hypotension). Products include:
Visken Tablets 2428

Polythiazide (Co-administration with antihypertensive agents has resulted in clinically significant hypotension). Products include:
Minizide Capsules 2016

Prazepam (Effects not specified; caution should be used when used concurrently).
No products indexed under this heading.

Prazosin Hydrochloride (Co-administration with antihypertensive agents has resulted in clinically significant hypotension). Products include:
Minipress Capsules 2015
Minizide Capsules 2016

Prochlorperazine (Effects not specified; caution should be used when used concurrently). Products include:
Compazine 2644

Promethazine Hydrochloride (Effects not specified; caution should be used when used concurrently). Products include:
Mepergan Injection 2859
Phenergan with Codeine 2883
Phenergan with Dextromethorphan 2885
Phenergan Injection 2880
Phenergan Suppositories 2882
Phenergan Syrup 2881
Phenergan Tablets 2882
Phenergan VC 2886
Phenergan VC with Codeine 2888

Propofol (Effects not specified; caution should be used when used concurrently). Products include:
Diprivan Injectable Emulsion 2939

Propoxyphene Hydrochloride (Effects not specified; caution should be used when used concurrently). Products include:
Darvon 1475
Wygesic Tablets 2930

Propoxyphene Napsylate (Effects not specified; caution should be used when used concurrently). Products include:
Darvon-N/Darvocet-N 1473

Propranolol Hydrochloride (Co-administration with antihypertensive agents has resulted in clinically significant hypotension). Products include:
Inderal 2834
Inderal LA Long Acting Capsules 2836
Inderide Tablets 2838
Inderide LA Long Acting Capsules .. 2840

Quazepam (Effects not specified; caution should be used when used concurrently). Products include:
Doral Tablets 2773

Quinapril Hydrochloride (Co-administration with antihypertensive agents has resulted in clinically significant hypotension). Products include:
Accupril Tablets 1950

Quinidine Gluconate (Inhibitors of cytochrome P450IID6 could interfere with the conversion of risperidone to 9-hydroxyrisperidone). Products include:
Quinaglute Dura-Tabs Tablets 644

Quinidine Polygalacturonate (Inhibitors of cytochrome P450IID6 could interfere with the conversion of risperidone to 9-hydroxyrisperidone). Products include:
Cardioquin Tablets 2146

Quinidine Sulfate (Inhibitors of cytochrome P450IID6 could interfere with the conversion of risperidone to 9-hydroxyrisperidone). Products include:
Quinidex Extentabs 2240

Ramipril (Co-administration with antihypertensive agents has resulted in clinically significant hypotension). Products include:
Altace Capsules 1238

Rauwolfia Serpentina (Co-administration with antihypertensive agents has resulted in clinically significant hypotension).
No products indexed under this heading.

Rescinnamine (Co-administration with antihypertensive agents has resulted in clinically significant hypotension).
No products indexed under this heading.

Reserpine (Co-administration with antihypertensive agents has resulted in clinically significant hypotension). Products include:
Diupres Tablets 1691
Hydropres Tablets 1718
Ser-Ap-Es Tablets 867

Secobarbital Sodium (Effects not specified; caution should be used when used concurrently). Products include:
Seconal Sodium Pulvules 1529

Sevoflurane (Effects not specified; caution should be used when used concurrently).
No products indexed under this heading.

Sodium Nitroprusside (Co-administration with antihypertensive agents has resulted in clinically significant hypotension).
No products indexed under this heading.

Sotalol Hydrochloride (Co-administration with antihypertensive agents has resulted in clinically significant hypotension). Products include:
Betapace Tablets 637

Spirapril Hydrochloride (Co-administration with antihypertensive agents has resulted in clinically significant hypotension).
No products indexed under this heading.

Sufentanil Citrate (Effects not specified; caution should be used when used concurrently). Products include:
Sufenta Injection 1355

Temazepam (Effects not specified; caution should be used when used concurrently). Products include:
Restoril Capsules 2413

Terazosin Hydrochloride (Co-administration with antihypertensive agents has resulted in clinically significant hypotension). Products include:
Hytrin Capsules 434

Thiamylal Sodium (Effects not specified; caution should be used when used concurrently).
No products indexed under this heading.

IMPORTANT NOTE: Always consult each drug listing in the patient's regimen for possible interactions.

Thioridazine Hydrochloride (Effects not specified; caution should be used when used concurrently). Products include:
Mellaril 2398

Thiothixene (Effects not specified; caution should be used when used concurrently). Products include:
Navane Capsules and Concentrate 2018
Navane Intramuscular 2019

Timolol Maleate (Co-administration with antihypertensive agents has resulted in clinically significant hypotension). Products include:
Blocadren Tablets 1654
Timolide Tablets 1791
Timoptic in Ocudose 1796
Timoptic Sterile Ophthalmic Solution 1794
Timoptic-XE 1798

Torsemide (Co-administration with antihypertensive agents has resulted in clinically significant hypotension). Products include:
Demadex Tablets and Injection 691

Trandolapril (Co-administration with antihypertensive agents has resulted in clinically significant hypotension). Products include:
Mavik Tablets 1407

Triazolam (Effects not specified; caution should be used when used concurrently). Products include:
Halcion Tablets 2093

Trifluoperazine Hydrochloride (Effects not specified; caution should be used when used concurrently). Products include:
Stelazine 2692

Trimethaphan Camsylate (Co-administration with antihypertensive agents has resulted in clinically significant hypotension).
No products indexed under this heading.

Verapamil Hydrochloride (Co-administration with antihypertensive agents has resulted in clinically significant hypotension). Products include:
Calan SR Caplets 2571
Calan Tablets 2568
Covera-HS Tablets 2573
Isoptin Injectable 1391
Isoptin Oral Tablets 1393
Isoptin SR Tablets 1395
Verelan Capsules 1455

Zolpidem Tartrate (Effects not specified; caution should be used when used concurrently). Products include:
Ambien Tablets 2559

Food Interactions
Alcohol (Effects not specified; concurrent use should be avoided).

RITALIN HYDROCHLORIDE TABLETS
(Methylphenidate Hydrochloride) 866
May interact with oral anticoagulants, vasopressors, monoamine oxidase inhibitors, tricyclic antidepressants, and certain other agents. Compounds in these categories include:

Amitriptyline Hydrochloride (Methylphenidate may inhibit the metabolism of tricyclic antidepressants; downward dosage adjustments may be required if used concomitantly). Products include:
Elavil 2945
Etrafon 2495
Limbitrol 2333
Triavil Tablets 1800

Amoxapine (Methylphenidate may inhibit the metabolism of tricyclic antidepressants; downward dosage adjustments may be required if used concomitantly). Products include:
Asendin Tablets 1419

Clomipramine Hydrochloride (Methylphenidate may inhibit the metabolism of tricyclic antidepressants; downward dosage adjustments may be required if used concomitantly). Products include:
Anafranil Capsules 819

Desipramine Hydrochloride (Methylphenidate may inhibit the metabolism of tricyclic antidepressants; downward dosage adjustments may be required if used concomitantly). Products include:
Norpramin Tablets 1273

Dicumarol (Methylphenidate may inhibit the metabolism of coumarin anticoagulants; downward dosage adjustments may be required if used concomitantly).
No products indexed under this heading.

Dopamine Hydrochloride (Resultant effect of concurrent use with pressor agent is not specified; caution is advised if used concomitantly).
No products indexed under this heading.

Doxepin Hydrochloride (Methylphenidate may inhibit the metabolism of tricyclic antidepressants; downward dosage adjustments may be required if used concomitantly). Products include:
Adapin Capsules 1542
Sinequan 2028
Zonalon Cream 1042

Epinephrine Bitartrate (Resultant effect of concurrent use with pressor agent is not specified; caution is advised if used concomitantly). Products include:
Sensorcaine-MPF with Epinephrine Injection 554

Epinephrine Hydrochloride (Resultant effect of concurrent use with pressor agent is not specified; caution is advised if used concomitantly). Products include:
Ana-Kit Anaphylaxis Emergency Treatment Kit 611

Furazolidone (Resultant effects of concurrent use not specified; caution is advised if used concomitantly). Products include:
Furoxone 2221

Guanethidine Monosulfate (Methylphenidate may decrease the hypotensive effect of guanethidine). Products include:
Esimil Tablets 840
Ismelin Tablets 845

Imipramine Hydrochloride (Methylphenidate may inhibit the metabolism of tricyclic antidepressants; downward dosage adjustments may be required if used concomitantly). Products include:
Tofranil Ampuls 873
Tofranil Tablets 875

Imipramine Pamoate (Methylphenidate may inhibit the metabolism of tricyclic antidepressants; downward dosage adjustments may be required if used concomitantly). Products include:
Tofranil-PM Capsules 876

Isocarboxazid (Resultant effects of concurrent use not specified; caution is advised if used concomitantly).
No products indexed under this heading.

Maprotiline Hydrochloride (Methylphenidate may inhibit the metabolism of tricyclic antidepressants; downward dosage adjustments may be required if used concomitantly). Products include:
Ludiomil Tablets 861

Metaraminol Bitartrate (Resultant effect of concurrent use with pressor agent is not specified; caution is advised if used concomitantly). Products include:
Aramine Injection 1649

Methoxamine Hydrochloride (Resultant effect of concurrent use with pressor agent is not specified; caution is advised if used concomitantly). Products include:
Vasoxyl Injection 1169

Norepinephrine Bitartrate (Resultant effect of concurrent use with pressor agent is not specified; caution is advised if used concomitantly). Products include:
Levophed Bitartrate Injection 2445

Nortriptyline Hydrochloride (Methylphenidate may inhibit the metabolism of tricyclic antidepressants; downward dosage adjustments may be required if used concomitantly). Products include:
Pamelor 2409

Phenelzine Sulfate (Resultant effects of concurrent use not specified; caution is advised if used concomitantly). Products include:
Nardil 1977

Phenobarbital (Methylphenidate may inhibit the metabolism of phenobarbital; downward dosage adjustments may be required if used concomitantly). Products include:
Arco-Lase Plus Tablets 513
Bellergal-S Tablets 2375
Donnatal 2234
Donnatal Extentabs 2234
Donnatal Tablets 2234
Phenobarbital Elixir and Tablets ... 1523
Quadrinal Tablets 1398

Phenylbutazone (Methylphenidate may inhibit the metabolism of phenylbutazone; downward dosage adjustments may be required if used concomitantly).
No products indexed under this heading.

Phenylephrine Hydrochloride (Resultant effect of concurrent use with pressor agent is not specified; caution is advised if used concomitantly). Products include:
Atrohist Plus Tablets 1605
Cerose DM 853
D.A. II Tablets 972
D.A. Chewable Tablets 970
Dura-Vent/DA Tablets 972
Extendryl 1003
4-Way Fast Acting Nasal Spray (regular & mentholated) 644
Hemoril 797
Hycomine Compound Tablets .. 948
Neo-Synephrine Hydrochloride 1% Carpuject 2455
Neo-Synephrine Hydrochloride 1% Injection 2455
Neo-Synephrine Hydrochloride (Ophthalmic) 2456
Neo-Synephrine 624
Novahistine Elixir 782
Phenergan VC 2886
Phenergan VC with Codeine .. 2888
Preparation H 842
Tympagesic Ear Drops 2476
Vicks Sinex Nasal Spray and Ultra Fine Mist 738

Phenytoin (Methylphenidate may inhibit the metabolism of diphenhydantoin; downward dosage adjustments may be required if used concomitantly). Products include:
Dilantin Infatabs 1967
Dilantin-125 Suspension 1969

Phenytoin Sodium (Methylphenidate may inhibit the metabolism of diphenhydantoin; downward dosage adjustments may be required if used concomitantly). Products include:
Dilantin Kapseals 1965

Primidone (Methylphenidate may inhibit the metabolism of primidone; downward dosage adjustments may be required if used concomitantly). Products include:
Mysoline 2860

Protriptyline Hydrochloride (Methylphenidate may inhibit the metabolism of tricyclic antidepressants; downward dosage adjustments may be required if used concomitantly). Products include:
Vivactil Tablets 1820

Selegiline Hydrochloride (Resultant effects of concurrent use not specified; caution is advised if used concomitantly). Products include:
Eldepryl Capsules 2729

Tranylcypromine Sulfate (Resultant effects of concurrent use not specified; caution is advised if used concomitantly). Products include:
Parnate Tablets 2679

Trimipramine Maleate (Methylphenidate may inhibit the metabolism of tricyclic antidepressants; downward dosage adjustments may be required if used concomitantly). Products include:
Surmontil Capsules 2917

Warfarin Sodium (Methylphenidate may inhibit the metabolism of coumarin anticoagulants; downward dosage adjustments may be required if used concomitantly). Products include:
Coumadin 941

RITALIN-SR TABLETS
(Methylphenidate Hydrochloride) 866
See **Ritalin Hydrochloride Tablets**

ROBAXIN INJECTABLE
(Methocarbamol) 2245
May interact with central nervous system depressants and certain other agents. Compounds in these categories include:

Alfentanil Hydrochloride (Increased CNS depressant effect). Products include:
Alfenta Injection 1334

Alprazolam (Increased CNS depressant effect). Products include:
Xanax Tablets 2115

Aprobarbital (Increased CNS depressant effect).
No products indexed under this heading.

Buprenorphine (Increased CNS depressant effect). Products include:
Buprenex Injectable 2170

Buspirone Hydrochloride (Increased CNS depressant effect). Products include:
BuSpar Tablets 738

Butabarbital (Increased CNS depressant effect).
No products indexed under this heading.

Butalbital (Increased CNS depressant effect). Products include:
Axocet Capsules 2469
Esgic-plus Capsules 1012
Esgic-plus Tablets 1012
Fioricet Tablets 2386
Fioricet with Codeine Capsules 2387
Fiorinal Capsules 2388
Fiorinal with Codeine Capsules 2390
Fiorinal Tablets 2388
Phrenilin 790
Sedapap Tablets 50 mg/650 mg .. 1826

Interactions Index — Robaxin Tablets

Chlordiazepoxide (Increased CNS depressant effect). Products include:
Limbitrol ... 2333

Chlordiazepoxide Hydrochloride (Increased CNS depressant effect). Products include:
Librax Capsules ... 2330
Librium Capsules ... 2331
Librium Injectable ... 2332

Chlorpromazine (Increased CNS depressant effect). Products include:
Thorazine Suppositories ... 2701

Chlorprothixene (Increased CNS depressant effect).
No products indexed under this heading.

Chlorprothixene Hydrochloride (Increased CNS depressant effect).
No products indexed under this heading.

Chlorprothixene Lactate (Increased CNS depressant effect).
No products indexed under this heading.

Clorazepate Dipotassium (Increased CNS depressant effect). Products include:
Tranxene ... 459

Clozapine (Increased CNS depressant effect). Products include:
Clozaril Tablets ... 2377

Codeine Phosphate (Increased CNS depressant effect). Products include:
Brontex ... 2130
Dimetane-DC Cough Syrup ... 2232
Fioricet with Codeine Capsules ... 2387
Fiorinal with Codeine Capsules ... 2390
Nucofed ... 2225
Phenergan with Codeine ... 2883
Phenergan VC with Codeine ... 2888
Robitussin A-C Syrup ... 2248
Robitussin-DAC Syrup ... 2249
Ryna ... 804
Soma Compound w/Codeine Tablets ... 2784
Tylenol with Codeine ... 1592

Desflurane (Increased CNS depressant effect). Products include:
Suprane (desflurane, USP) ... 1865

Dezocine (Increased CNS depressant effect). Products include:
Dalgan Injection ... 529

Diazepam (Increased CNS depressant effect). Products include:
Dizac (diazepam injectable emulsion) CIV ... 1862
Valium Injectable ... 2336
Valium Tablets ... 2335

Droperidol (Increased CNS depressant effect). Products include:
Inapsine Injection ... 462

Enflurane (Increased CNS depressant effect).
No products indexed under this heading.

Estazolam (Increased CNS depressant effect). Products include:
ProSom Tablets ... 457

Ethchlorvynol (Increased CNS depressant effect). Products include:
Placidyl Capsules ... 456

Ethinamate (Increased CNS depressant effect).
No products indexed under this heading.

Fentanyl (Increased CNS depressant effect). Products include:
Duragesic Transdermal System ... 1336

Fentanyl Citrate (Increased CNS depressant effect). Products include:
Sublimaze Injection ... 463

Fluphenazine Decanoate (Increased CNS depressant effect). Products include:
Prolixin Decanoate ... 510

Fluphenazine Enanthate (Increased CNS depressant effect). Products include:
Prolixin Enanthate ... 510

Fluphenazine Hydrochloride (Increased CNS depressant effect). Products include:
Prolixin ... 510

Flurazepam Hydrochloride (Increased CNS depressant effect). Products include:
Dalmane Capsules ... 2329

Glutethimide (Increased CNS depressant effect).
No products indexed under this heading.

Haloperidol (Increased CNS depressant effect). Products include:
Haldol Injection, Tablets and Concentrate ... 1585

Haloperidol Decanoate (Increased CNS depressant effect). Products include:
Haldol Decanoate ... 1587

Hydrocodone Bitartrate (Increased CNS depressant effect). Products include:
Codiclear DH Syrup ... 808
Duratuss HD Elixir ... 2750
Histussin D Liquid ... 670
Hycodan Tablets and Syrup ... 946
Hycomine Compound Tablets ... 948
Hycomine ... 947
Hycotuss Expectorant Syrup ... 950
Hydrocet Capsules ... 787
Lorcet 10/650 Tablets ... 1016
Lortab ... 2751
Tussend ... 1830
Tussend Expectorant ... 1831
Vicodin Tablets ... 1404
Vicodin ES Tablets ... 1405
Vicodin HP Tablets ... 1403
Vicodin Tuss Expectorant ... 1406
Zydone Capsules ... 967

Hydrocodone Polistirex (Increased CNS depressant effect). Products include:
Tussionex Pennkinetic Extended-Release Suspension ... 1624

Hydroxyzine Hydrochloride (Increased CNS depressant effect). Products include:
Atarax Tablets & Syrup ... 1992
Marax Tablets & DF Syrup ... 2015
Vistaril Intramuscular Solution ... 2042

Isoflurane (Increased CNS depressant effect).
No products indexed under this heading.

Ketamine Hydrochloride (Increased CNS depressant effect).
No products indexed under this heading.

Levomethadyl Acetate Hydrochloride (Increased CNS depressant effect). Products include:
Orlaam Oral Solution ... 2361

Levorphanol Tartrate (Increased CNS depressant effect). Products include:
Levo-Dromoran ... 2297

Lorazepam (Increased CNS depressant effect). Products include:
Ativan Injection ... 2805
Ativan Tablets ... 2807

Loxapine Hydrochloride (Increased CNS depressant effect). Products include:
Loxitane ... 1426

Loxapine Succinate (Increased CNS depressant effect). Products include:
Loxitane Capsules ... 1426

Meperidine Hydrochloride (Increased CNS depressant effect). Products include:
Demerol ... 2438
Mepergan Injection ... 2859

Mephobarbital (Increased CNS depressant effect). Products include:
Mebaral Tablets ... 2452

Meprobamate (Increased CNS depressant effect). Products include:
Miltown Tablets ... 2780
PMB 200 and PMB 400 ... 2890

Mesoridazine Besylate (Increased CNS depressant effect). Products include:
Serentil ... 689

Methadone Hydrochloride (Increased CNS depressant effect). Products include:
Methadone Hydrochloride Oral Concentrate ... 2356
Methadone Hydrochloride Oral Solution & Tablets ... 2357

Methohexital Sodium (Increased CNS depressant effect).
No products indexed under this heading.

Methotrimeprazine (Increased CNS depressant effect). Products include:
Levoprome ... 1321

Methoxyflurane (Increased CNS depressant effect).
No products indexed under this heading.

Midazolam Hydrochloride (Increased CNS depressant effect). Products include:
Versed Injection ... 2324

Molindone Hydrochloride (Increased CNS depressant effect). Products include:
Moban Tablets and Concentrate ... 1036

Morphine Sulfate (Increased CNS depressant effect). Products include:
Astramorph/PF Injection, USP (Preservative-Free) ... 526
Duramorph Injection ... 983
Infumorph 200 and Infumorph 500 Sterile Solutions ... 985
Kadian Capsules ... 2948
MS Contin Tablets ... 2149
MSIR ... 2152
Oramorph SR (Morphine Sulfate Sustained Release Tablets) ... 2359
RMS Suppositories CII ... 2766
Roxanol ... 2365

Opium Alkaloids (Increased CNS depressant effect).
No products indexed under this heading.

Oxazepam (Increased CNS depressant effect). Products include:
Serax Capsules ... 2916
Serax Tablets ... 2916

Oxycodone Hydrochloride (Increased CNS depressant effect). Products include:
OxyContin Tablets ... 2163
OxyIR Capsules ... 2167
Percocet Tablets ... 955
Percodan Tablets ... 955
Percodan-Demi Tablets ... 956
Roxicodone Tablets, Oral Solution & Intensol (Oxycodone) ... 2366
Tylox Capsules ... 1593

Pentobarbital Sodium (Increased additive effect). Products include:
Nembutal Sodium Capsules ... 440
Nembutal Sodium Solution ... 442
Nembutal Sodium Suppositories ... 444

Perphenazine (Increased CNS depressant effect). Products include:
Etrafon ... 2495
Triavil Tablets ... 1800
Trilafon ... 2532

Phenobarbital (Increased CNS depressant effect). Products include:
Arco-Lase Plus Tablets ... 513
Bellergal-S Tablets ... 2375
Donnatal ... 2234
Donnatal Extentabs ... 2234
Donnatal Tablets ... 2234
Phenobarbital Elixir and Tablets ... 1523
Quadrinal Tablets ... 1398

Prazepam (Increased CNS depressant effect).
No products indexed under this heading.

Prochlorperazine (Increased CNS depressant effect). Products include:
Compazine ... 2644

Promethazine Hydrochloride (Increased CNS depressant effect). Products include:
Mepergan Injection ... 2859
Phenergan with Codeine ... 2883
Phenergan with Dextromethorphan ... 2885
Phenergan Injection ... 2880
Phenergan Suppositories ... 2882
Phenergan Syrup ... 2881
Phenergan Tablets ... 2882
Phenergan VC ... 2886
Phenergan VC with Codeine ... 2888

Propofol (Increased CNS depressant effect). Products include:
Diprivan Injectable Emulsion ... 2939

Propoxyphene Hydrochloride (Increased CNS depressant effect). Products include:
Darvon ... 1475
Wygesic Tablets ... 2930

Propoxyphene Napsylate (Increased CNS depressant effect). Products include:
Darvon-N/Darvocet-N ... 1473

Quazepam (Increased CNS depressant effect). Products include:
Doral Tablets ... 2773

Risperidone (Increased CNS depressant effect). Products include:
Risperdal Tablets ... 1348

Secobarbital Sodium (Increased CNS depressant effect). Products include:
Seconal Sodium Pulvules ... 1529

Sevoflurane (Increased CNS depressant effect).
No products indexed under this heading.

Sufentanil Citrate (Increased CNS depressant effect). Products include:
Sufenta Injection ... 1355

Temazepam (Increased CNS depressant effect). Products include:
Restoril Capsules ... 2413

Thiamylal Sodium (Increased CNS depressant effect).
No products indexed under this heading.

Thioridazine Hydrochloride (Increased CNS depressant effect). Products include:
Mellaril ... 2398

Thiothixene (Increased CNS depressant effect). Products include:
Navane Capsules and Concentrate ... 2018
Navane Intramuscular ... 2019

Triazolam (Increased CNS depressant effect). Products include:
Halcion Tablets ... 2093

Trifluoperazine Hydrochloride (Increased CNS depressant effect). Products include:
Stelazine ... 2692

Zolpidem Tartrate (Increased CNS depressant effect). Products include:
Ambien Tablets ... 2559

Food Interactions
Alcohol (Increased depressant effect).

ROBAXIN TABLETS
(Methocarbamol) ... 2246
May interact with central nervous system depressants and certain other agents. Compounds in these categories include:

Alfentanil Hydrochloride (Increased CNS depressant effect). Products include:
Alfenta Injection ... 1334

IMPORTANT NOTE: Always consult each drug listing in the patient's regimen for possible interactions.

Robaxin Tablets
Interactions Index
940

Alprazolam (Increased CNS depressant effect). Products include:
Xanax Tablets ... 2115

Aprobarbital (Increased CNS depressant effect).
No products indexed under this heading.

Buprenorphine (Increased CNS depressant effect). Products include:
Buprenex Injectable ... 2170

Buspirone Hydrochloride (Increased CNS depressant effect). Products include:
BuSpar Tablets ... 738

Butabarbital (Increased CNS depressant effect).
No products indexed under this heading.

Butalbital (Increased CNS depressant effect). Products include:
Axocet Capsules ... 2469
Esgic-plus Capsules ... 1012
Esgic-plus Tablets ... 1012
Fioricet Tablets ... 2386
Fioricet with Codeine Capsules ... 2387
Fiorinal Capsules ... 2388
Fiorinal with Codeine Capsules ... 2390
Fiorinal Tablets ... 2388
Phrenilin ... 790
Sedapap Tablets 50 mg/650 mg .. 1826

Chlordiazepoxide (Increased CNS depressant effect). Products include:
Limbitrol ... 2333

Chlordiazepoxide Hydrochloride (Increased CNS depressant effect). Products include:
Librax Capsules ... 2330
Librium Capsules ... 2331
Librium Injectable ... 2332

Chlorpromazine (Increased CNS depressant effect). Products include:
Thorazine Suppositories ... 2701

Chlorprothixene (Increased CNS depressant effect).
No products indexed under this heading.

Chlorprothixene Hydrochloride (Increased CNS depressant effect).
No products indexed under this heading.

Chlorprothixene Lactate (Increased CNS depressant effect).
No products indexed under this heading.

Clorazepate Dipotassium (Increased CNS depressant effect). Products include:
Tranxene ... 459

Clozapine (Increased CNS depressant effect). Products include:
Clozaril Tablets ... 2377

Codeine Phosphate (Increased CNS depressant effect). Products include:
Brontex ... 2130
Dimetane-DC Cough Syrup ... 2232
Fioricet with Codeine Capsules ... 2387
Fiorinal with Codeine Capsules ... 2390
Nucofed ... 2225
Phenergan with Codeine ... 2883
Phenergan VC with Codeine ... 2888
Robitussin A-C Syrup ... 2248
Robitussin-DAC Syrup ... 2249
Ryna ... ⊞ 804
Soma Compound w/Codeine Tablets ... 2784
Tylenol with Codeine ... 1592

Desflurane (Increased CNS depressant effect). Products include:
Suprane (desflurane, USP) ... 1865

Dezocine (Increased CNS depressant effect). Products include:
Dalgan Injection ... 529

Diazepam (Increased CNS depressant effect). Products include:
Dizac (diazepam injectable emulsion) CIV ... 1862
Valium Injectable ... 2336
Valium Tablets ... 2335

Droperidol (Increased CNS depressant effect). Products include:
Inapsine Injection ... 462

Enflurane (Increased CNS depressant effect).
No products indexed under this heading.

Estazolam (Increased CNS depressant effect). Products include:
ProSom Tablets ... 457

Ethchlorvynol (Increased CNS depressant effect). Products include:
Placidyl Capsules ... 456

Ethinamate (Increased CNS depressant effect).
No products indexed under this heading.

Fentanyl (Increased CNS depressant effect). Products include:
Duragesic Transdermal System ... 1336

Fentanyl Citrate (Increased CNS depressant effect). Products include:
Sublimaze Injection ... 463

Fluphenazine Decanoate (Increased CNS depressant effect). Products include:
Prolixin Decanoate ... 510

Fluphenazine Enanthate (Increased CNS depressant effect). Products include:
Prolixin Enanthate ... 510

Fluphenazine Hydrochloride (Increased CNS depressant effect). Products include:
Prolixin ... 510

Flurazepam Hydrochloride (Increased CNS depressant effect). Products include:
Dalmane Capsules ... 2329

Glutethimide (Increased CNS depressant effect).
No products indexed under this heading.

Haloperidol (Increased CNS depressant effect). Products include:
Haldol Injection, Tablets and Concentrate ... 1585

Haloperidol Decanoate (Increased CNS depressant effect). Products include:
Haldol Decanoate ... 1587

Hydrocodone Bitartrate (Increased CNS depressant effect). Products include:
Codiclear DH Syrup ... 808
Duratuss HD Elixir ... 2750
Histussin D Liquid ... 670
Hycodan Tablets and Syrup ... 946
Hycomine Compound Tablets ... 948
Hycomine ... 947
Hycotuss Expectorant Syrup ... 950
Hydrocet Capsules ... 787
Lorcet 10/650 Tablets ... 1016
Lortab ... 2751
Tussend ... 1830
Tussend Expectorant ... 1831
Vicodin Tablets ... 1404
Vicodin ES Tablets ... 1405
Vicodin HP Tablets ... 1403
Vicodin Tuss Expectorant ... 1406
Zydone Capsules ... 967

Hydrocodone Polistirex (Increased CNS depressant effect). Products include:
Tussionex Pennkinetic Extended-Release Suspension ... 1624

Hydroxyzine Hydrochloride (Increased CNS depressant effect). Products include:
Atarax Tablets & Syrup ... 1992
Marax Tablets & DF Syrup ... 2015
Vistaril Intramuscular Solution ... 2042

Isoflurane (Increased CNS depressant effect).
No products indexed under this heading.

Ketamine Hydrochloride (Increased CNS depressant effect).
No products indexed under this heading.

Levomethadyl Acetate Hydrochloride (Increased CNS depressant effect). Products include:
Orlaam Oral Solution ... 2361

Levorphanol Tartrate (Increased CNS depressant effect). Products include:
Levo-Dromoran ... 2297

Lorazepam (Increased CNS depressant effect). Products include:
Ativan Injection ... 2805
Ativan Tablets ... 2807

Loxapine Hydrochloride (Increased CNS depressant effect). Products include:
Loxitane ... 1426

Loxapine Succinate (Increased CNS depressant effect). Products include:
Loxitane Capsules ... 1426

Meperidine Hydrochloride (Increased CNS depressant effect). Products include:
Demerol ... 2438
Mepergan Injection ... 2859

Mephobarbital (Increased CNS depressant effect). Products include:
Mebaral Tablets ... 2452

Meprobamate (Increased CNS depressant effect). Products include:
Miltown Tablets ... 2780
PMB 200 and PMB 400 ... 2890

Mesoridazine Besylate (Increased CNS depressant effect). Products include:
Serentil ... 689

Methadone Hydrochloride (Increased CNS depressant effect). Products include:
Methadone Hydrochloride Oral Concentrate ... 2356
Methadone Hydrochloride Oral Solution & Tablets ... 2357

Methohexital Sodium (Increased CNS depressant effect).
No products indexed under this heading.

Methotrimeprazine (Increased CNS depressant effect). Products include:
Levoprome ... 1321

Methoxyflurane (Increased CNS depressant effect).
No products indexed under this heading.

Midazolam Hydrochloride (Increased CNS depressant effect). Products include:
Versed Injection ... 2324

Molindone Hydrochloride (Increased CNS depressant effect). Products include:
Moban Tablets and Concentrate ... 1036

Morphine Sulfate (Increased CNS depressant effect). Products include:
Astramorph/PF Injection, USP (Preservative-Free) ... 526
Duramorph Injection ... 983
Infumorph 200 and Infumorph 500 Sterile Solutions ... 985
Kadian Capsules ... 2948
MS Contin Tablets ... 2149
MSIR ... 2152
Oramorph SR (Morphine Sulfate Sustained Release Tablets) ... 2359
RMS Suppositories CII ... 2766
Roxanol ... 2365

Opium Alkaloids (Increased CNS depressant effect).
No products indexed under this heading.

Oxazepam (Increased CNS depressant effect). Products include:
Serax Capsules ... 2916
Serax Tablets ... 2916

Oxycodone Hydrochloride (Increased CNS depressant effect). Products include:
OxyContin Tablets ... 2163
OxyIR Capsules ... 2167
Percocet Tablets ... 955
Percodan Tablets ... 955
Percodan-Demi Tablets ... 956
Roxicodone Tablets, Oral Solution & Intensol (Oxycodone) ... 2366
Tylox Capsules ... 1593

Pentobarbital Sodium (Increased CNS depressant effect). Products include:
Nembutal Sodium Capsules ... 440
Nembutal Sodium Solution ... 442
Nembutal Sodium Suppositories ... 444

Perphenazine (Increased CNS depressant effect). Products include:
Etrafon ... 2495
Triavil Tablets ... 1800
Trilafon ... 2532

Phenobarbital (Increased CNS depressant effect). Products include:
Arco-Lase Plus Tablets ... 513
Bellergal-S Tablets ... 2375
Donnatal ... 2234
Donnatal Extentabs ... 2234
Donnatal Tablets ... 2234
Phenobarbital Elixir and Tablets ... 1523
Quadrinal Tablets ... 1398

Prazepam (Increased CNS depressant effect).
No products indexed under this heading.

Prochlorperazine (Increased CNS depressant effect). Products include:
Compazine ... 2644

Promethazine Hydrochloride (Increased CNS depressant effect). Products include:
Mepergan Injection ... 2859
Phenergan with Codeine ... 2883
Phenergan with Dextromethorphan 2885
Phenergan Injection ... 2880
Phenergan Suppositories ... 2882
Phenergan Syrup ... 2881
Phenergan Tablets ... 2882
Phenergan VC ... 2886
Phenergan VC with Codeine ... 2888

Propofol (Increased CNS depressant effect). Products include:
Diprivan Injectable Emulsion ... 2939

Propoxyphene Hydrochloride (Increased CNS depressant effect). Products include:
Darvon ... 1475
Wygesic Tablets ... 2930

Propoxyphene Napsylate (Increased CNS depressant effect). Products include:
Darvon-N/Darvocet-N ... 1473

Quazepam (Increased CNS depressant effect). Products include:
Doral Tablets ... 2773

Risperidone (Increased CNS depressant effect). Products include:
Risperdal Tablets ... 1348

Secobarbital Sodium (Increased CNS depressant effect). Products include:
Seconal Sodium Pulvules ... 1529

Sevoflurane (Increased CNS depressant effect).
No products indexed under this heading.

Sufentanil Citrate (Increased CNS depressant effect). Products include:
Sufenta Injection ... 1355

Temazepam (Increased CNS depressant effect). Products include:
Restoril Capsules ... 2413

Thiamylal Sodium (Increased CNS depressant effect).
No products indexed under this heading.

Thioridazine Hydrochloride (Increased CNS depressant effect). Products include:
Mellaril ... 2398

Thiothixene (Increased CNS depressant effect). Products include:
Navane Capsules and Concentrate 2018
Navane Intramuscular ... 2019

(⊞ Described in PDR For Nonprescription Drugs)
(◉ Described in PDR For Ophthalmology)

Triazolam (Increased CNS depressant effect). Products include:
Halcion Tablets 2093
Trifluoperazine Hydrochloride (Increased CNS depressant effect). Products include:
Stelazine 2692
Zolpidem Tartrate (Increased CNS depressant effect). Products include:
Ambien Tablets 2559

Food Interactions

Alcohol (Increased CNS depressant effect).

ROBAXIN-750 TABLETS
(Methocarbamol) 2246
See Robaxin Tablets

ROBAXISAL TABLETS
(Methocarbamol, Aspirin) 2246
May interact with central nervous system depressants, anticoagulants, and certain other agents. Compounds in these categories include:

Alfentanil Hydrochloride (Increased depressant effect). Products include:
Alfenta Injection 1334
Alprazolam (Increased depressant effect). Products include:
Xanax Tablets 2115
Aprobarbital (Increased depressant effect). Products include:
No products indexed under this heading.
Buprenorphine (Increased depressant effect). Products include:
Buprenex Injectable 2170
Buspirone Hydrochloride (Increased depressant effect). Products include:
BuSpar Tablets 738
Butabarbital (Increased depressant effect). Products include:
No products indexed under this heading.
Butalbital (Increased depressant effect). Products include:
Axocet Capsules 2469
Esgic-plus Capsules 1012
Esgic-plus Tablets 1012
Fioricet Tablets 2386
Fioricet with Codeine Capsules ... 2387
Fiorinal Capsules 2388
Fiorinal with Codeine Capsules .. 2390
Fiorinal Tablets 2388
Phrenilin 790
Sedapap Tablets 50 mg/650 mg .. 1826
Chlordiazepoxide (Increased depressant effect). Products include:
Limbitrol 2333
Chlordiazepoxide Hydrochloride (Increased depressant effect). Products include:
Librax Capsules 2330
Librium Capsules 2331
Librium Injectable 2332
Chlorpromazine (Increased depressant effect). Products include:
Thorazine Suppositories 2701
Chlorprothixene (Increased depressant effect). Products include:
No products indexed under this heading.
Chlorprothixene Hydrochloride (Increased depressant effect). Products include:
No products indexed under this heading.
Chlorprothixene Lactate (Increased depressant effect). Products include:
No products indexed under this heading.
Clorazepate Dipotassium (Increased depressant effect). Products include:
Tranxene 459

Clozapine (Increased depressant effect). Products include:
Clozaril Tablets 2377
Codeine Phosphate (Increased depressant effect). Products include:
Brontex 2130
Dimetane-DC Cough Syrup 2232
Fioricet with Codeine Capsules ... 2387
Fiorinal with Codeine Capsules ... 2390
Nucofed 2225
Phenergan with Codeine 2883
Phenergan VC with Codeine 2888
Robitussin A-C Syrup 2248
Robitussin-DAC Syrup 2248
Ryna 804
Soma Compound w/Codeine Tablets 2784
Tylenol with Codeine 1592
Dalteparin Sodium (Increased anticoagulant effect). Products include:
Fragmin Injection 2088
Desflurane (Increased depressant effect). Products include:
Suprane (desflurane, USP) 1865
Dezocine (Increased depressant effect). Products include:
Dalgan Injection 529
Diazepam (Increased depressant effect). Products include:
Dizac (diazepam injectable emulsion) CIV 1862
Valium Injectable 2336
Valium Tablets 2335
Dicumarol (Increased anticoagulant effect). Products include:
No products indexed under this heading.
Droperidol (Increased depressant effect). Products include:
Inapsine Injection 462
Enflurane (Increased depressant effect). Products include:
No products indexed under this heading.
Enoxaparin (Increased anticoagulant effect). Products include:
Lovenox Injection 2187
Estazolam (Increased depressant effect). Products include:
ProSom Tablets 457
Ethchlorvynol (Increased depressant effect). Products include:
Placidyl Capsules 456
Ethinamate (Increased depressant effect). Products include:
No products indexed under this heading.
Fentanyl (Increased depressant effect). Products include:
Duragesic Transdermal System ... 1336
Fentanyl Citrate (Increased depressant effect). Products include:
Sublimaze Injection 463
Fluphenazine Decanoate (Increased depressant effect). Products include:
Prolixin Decanoate 510
Fluphenazine Enanthate (Increased depressant effect). Products include:
Prolixin Enanthate 510
Fluphenazine Hydrochloride (Increased depressant effect). Products include:
Prolixin 510
Flurazepam Hydrochloride (Increased depressant effect). Products include:
Dalmane Capsules 2329
Glutethimide (Increased depressant effect). Products include:
No products indexed under this heading.
Haloperidol (Increased depressant effect). Products include:
Haldol Injection, Tablets and Concentrate 1585

Haloperidol Decanoate (Increased depressant effect). Products include:
Haldol Decanoate 1587
Heparin Calcium (Increased anticoagulant effect).
No products indexed under this heading.
Heparin Sodium (Increased anticoagulant effect). Products include:
Heparin Lock Flush Solution ... 2831
Heparin Sodium Injection 2832
Heparin Sodium Vials 1486
Hydrocodone Bitartrate (Increased depressant effect). Products include:
Codiclear DH Syrup 808
Duratuss HD Elixir 2750
Histussin D Liquid 670
Hycodan Tablets and Syrup 946
Hycomine Compound Tablets .. 948
Hycomine 947
Hycotuss Expectorant Syrup 950
Hydrocet Capsules 787
Lorcet 10/650 Tablets 1016
Lortab 2751
Tussend 1830
Tussend Expectorant 1831
Vicodin Tablets 1404
Vicodin ES Tablets 1405
Vicodin HP Tablets 1403
Vicodin Tuss Expectorant 1406
Zydone Capsules 967
Hydrocodone Polistirex (Increased depressant effect). Products include:
Tussionex Pennkinetic Extended-Release Suspension 1624
Hydroxyzine Hydrochloride (Increased depressant effect). Products include:
Atarax Tablets & Syrup 1992
Marax Tablets & DF Syrup 2015
Vistaril Intramuscular Solution .. 2042
Isoflurane (Increased depressant effect).
No products indexed under this heading.
Ketamine Hydrochloride (Increased depressant effect).
No products indexed under this heading.
Levomethadyl Acetate Hydrochloride (Increased depressant effect). Products include:
Orlaam Oral Solution 2361
Levorphanol Tartrate (Increased depressant effect). Products include:
Levo-Dromoran 2297
Lorazepam (Increased depressant effect). Products include:
Ativan Injection 2805
Ativan Tablets 2807
Loxapine Hydrochloride (Increased depressant effect). Products include:
Loxitane 1426
Loxapine Succinate (Increased depressant effect). Products include:
Loxitane Capsules 1426
Meperidine Hydrochloride (Increased depressant effect). Products include:
Demerol 2438
Mepergan Injection 2859
Mephobarbital (Increased depressant effect). Products include:
Mebaral Tablets 2452
Meprobamate (Increased depressant effect). Products include:
Miltown Tablets 2780
PMB 200 and PMB 400 2890
Mesoridazine Besylate (Increased depressant effect). Products include:
Serentil 689

Methadone Hydrochloride (Increased depressant effect). Products include:
Methadone Hydrochloride Oral Concentrate 2356
Methadone Hydrochloride Oral Solution & Tablets 2357
Methohexital Sodium (Increased depressant effect). Products include:
No products indexed under this heading.
Methotrimeprazine (Increased depressant effect). Products include:
Levoprome 1321
Methoxyflurane (Increased depressant effect). Products include:
No products indexed under this heading.
Midazolam Hydrochloride (Increased depressant effect). Products include:
Versed Injection 2324
Molindone Hydrochloride (Increased depressant effect). Products include:
Moban Tablets and Concentrate .. 1036
Morphine Sulfate (Increased depressant effect). Products include:
Astramorph/PF Injection, USP (Preservative-Free) 526
Duramorph Injection 983
Infumorph 200 and Infumorph 500 Sterile Solutions 985
Kadian Capsules 2948
MS Contin Tablets 2149
MSIR 2152
Oramorph SR (Morphine Sulfate Sustained Release Tablets) ... 2359
RMS Suppositories CII 2766
Roxanol 2365
Opium Alkaloids (Increased depressant effect).
No products indexed under this heading.
Oxazepam (Increased depressant effect). Products include:
Serax Capsules 2916
Serax Tablets 2916
Oxycodone Hydrochloride (Increased depressant effect). Products include:
OxyContin Tablets 2163
OxyIR Capsules 2167
Percocet Tablets 955
Percodan Tablets 955
Percodan-Demi Tablets 956
Roxicodone Tablets, Oral Solution & Intensol (Oxycodone) .. 2366
Tylox Capsules 1593
Pentobarbital Sodium (Increased depressant effect). Products include:
Nembutal Sodium Capsules 440
Nembutal Sodium Solution 442
Nembutal Sodium Suppositories ... 444
Perphenazine (Increased depressant effect). Products include:
Etrafon 2495
Triavil Tablets 1800
Trilafon 2532
Phenobarbital (Increased depressant effect). Products include:
Arco-Lase Plus Tablets 513
Bellergal-S Tablets 2375
Donnatal 2234
Donnatal Extentabs 2234
Donnatal Tablets 2234
Phenobarbital Elixir and Tablets .. 1523
Quadrinal Tablets 1398
Prazepam (Increased depressant effect).
No products indexed under this heading.
Prochlorperazine (Increased depressant effect). Products include:
Compazine 2644
Promethazine Hydrochloride (Increased depressant effect). Products include:
Mepergan Injection 2859
Phenergan with Codeine 2883
Phenergan with Dextromethorphan .. 2885
Phenergan Injection 2880

IMPORTANT NOTE: Always consult each drug listing in the patient's regimen for possible interactions.

Robaxisal

Phenergan Suppositories 2882
Phenergan Syrup 2881
Phenergan Tablets 2882
Phenergan VC 2886
Phenergan VC with Codeine ... 2888

Propofol (Increased depressant effect). Products include:
Diprivan Injectable Emulsion ... 2939

Propoxyphene Hydrochloride (Increased depressant effect). Products include:
Darvon 1475
Wygesic Tablets 2930

Propoxyphene Napsylate (Increased depressant effect). Products include:
Darvon-N/Darvocet-N 1473

Quazepam (Increased depressant effect). Products include:
Doral Tablets 2773

Risperidone (Increased depressant effect). Products include:
Risperdal Tablets 1348

Secobarbital Sodium (Increased depressant effect). Products include:
Seconal Sodium Pulvules 1529

Sevoflurane (Increased depressant effect).
No products indexed under this heading.

Sufentanil Citrate (Increased depressant effect). Products include:
Sufenta Injection 1355

Temazepam (Increased depressant effect). Products include:
Restoril Capsules 2413

Thiamylal Sodium (Increased depressant effect).
No products indexed under this heading.

Thioridazine Hydrochloride (Increased depressant effect). Products include:
Mellaril 2398

Thiothixene (Increased depressant effect). Products include:
Navane Capsules and Concentrate 2018
Navane Intramuscular 2019

Triazolam (Increased depressant effect). Products include:
Halcion Tablets 2093

Trifluoperazine Hydrochloride (Increased depressant effect). Products include:
Stelazine 2692

Warfarin Sodium (Increased anticoagulant effect). Products include:
Coumadin 941

Zolpidem Tartrate (Increased depressant effect). Products include:
Ambien Tablets 2559

Food Interactions
Alcohol (Increased depressant effect).

ROBINUL FORTE TABLETS
(Glycopyrrolate) 2247
None cited in PDR database.

ROBINUL INJECTABLE
(Glycopyrrolate) 2247
May interact with:

Cyclopropane (Potential ventricular arrhythmias).

ROBINUL TABLETS
(Glycopyrrolate) 2247
None cited in PDR database.

ROBITUSSIN
(Guaifenesin) .... ▣ 845
None cited in PDR database.

ROBITUSSIN A-C SYRUP
(Codeine Phosphate, Guaifenesin) 2248
May interact with hypnotics and sedatives, tranquilizers, and monoamine oxidase inhibitors. Compounds in these categories include:

Alprazolam (Concurrent therapy may cause greater sedation). Products include:
Xanax Tablets 2115

Buspirone Hydrochloride (Concurrent therapy may cause greater sedation). Products include:
BuSpar Tablets 738

Chlordiazepoxide (Concurrent therapy may cause greater sedation). Products include:
Limbitrol 2333

Chlordiazepoxide Hydrochloride (Concurrent therapy may cause greater sedation). Products include:
Librax Capsules 2330
Librium Capsules 2331
Librium Injectable 2332

Chlorpromazine (Concurrent therapy may cause greater sedation). Products include:
Thorazine Suppositories 2701

Chlorprothixene (Concurrent therapy may cause greater sedation).
No products indexed under this heading.

Chlorprothixene Hydrochloride (Concurrent therapy may cause greater sedation).
No products indexed under this heading.

Clorazepate Dipotassium (Concurrent therapy may cause greater sedation). Products include:
Tranxene 459

Diazepam (Concurrent therapy may cause greater sedation). Products include:
Dizac (diazepam injectable emulsion) CIV 1862
Valium Injectable 2336
Valium Tablets 2335

Droperidol (Concurrent therapy may cause greater sedation). Products include:
Inapsine Injection 462

Estazolam (Concurrent therapy may cause greater sedation). Products include:
ProSom Tablets 457

Ethchlorvynol (Concurrent therapy may cause greater sedation). Products include:
Placidyl Capsules 456

Ethinamate (Concurrent therapy may cause greater sedation).
No products indexed under this heading.

Fluphenazine Decanoate (Concurrent therapy may cause greater sedation). Products include:
Prolixin Decanoate 510

Fluphenazine Enanthate (Concurrent therapy may cause greater sedation). Products include:
Prolixin Enanthate 510

Fluphenazine Hydrochloride (Concurrent therapy may cause greater sedation). Products include:
Prolixin 510

Flurazepam Hydrochloride (Concurrent therapy may cause greater sedation). Products include:
Dalmane Capsules 2329

Furazolidone (Concurrent therapy may cause greater sedation). Products include:
Furoxone 2221

Glutethimide (Concurrent therapy may cause greater sedation).
No products indexed under this heading.

Interactions Index

Haloperidol (Concurrent therapy may cause greater sedation). Products include:
Haldol Injection, Tablets and Concentrate 1585

Haloperidol Decanoate (Concurrent therapy may cause greater sedation). Products include:
Haldol Decanoate 1587

Hydroxyzine Hydrochloride (Concurrent therapy may cause greater sedation). Products include:
Atarax Tablets & Syrup 1992
Marax Tablets & DF Syrup ... 2015
Vistaril Intramuscular Solution 2042

Isocarboxazid (Concurrent therapy may cause greater sedation).
No products indexed under this heading.

Lorazepam (Concurrent therapy may cause greater sedation). Products include:
Ativan Injection 2805
Ativan Tablets 2807

Loxapine Hydrochloride (Concurrent therapy may cause greater sedation). Products include:
Loxitane 1426

Loxapine Succinate (Concurrent therapy may cause greater sedation). Products include:
Loxitane Capsules 1426

Meprobamate (Concurrent therapy may cause greater sedation). Products include:
Miltown Tablets 2780
PMB 200 and PMB 400 2890

Mesoridazine Besylate (Concurrent therapy may cause greater sedation). Products include:
Serentil 689

Midazolam Hydrochloride (Concurrent therapy may cause greater sedation). Products include:
Versed Injection 2324

Molindone Hydrochloride (Concurrent therapy may cause greater sedation). Products include:
Moban Tablets and Concentrate 1036

Oxazepam (Concurrent therapy may cause greater sedation). Products include:
Serax Capsules 2916
Serax Tablets 2916

Perphenazine (Concurrent therapy may cause greater sedation). Products include:
Etrafon 2495
Triavil Tablets 1800
Trilafon 2532

Phenelzine Sulfate (Concurrent therapy may cause greater sedation). Products include:
Nardil 1977

Prazepam (Concurrent therapy may cause greater sedation).
No products indexed under this heading.

Prochlorperazine (Concurrent therapy may cause greater sedation). Products include:
Compazine 2644

Promethazine Hydrochloride (Concurrent therapy may cause greater sedation). Products include:
Mepergan Injection 2859
Phenergan with Codeine 2883
Phenergan with Dextromethorphan 2885
Phenergan Injection 2880
Phenergan Suppositories 2882
Phenergan Syrup 2881
Phenergan Tablets 2882
Phenergan VC 2886
Phenergan VC with Codeine .. 2888

Propofol (Concurrent therapy may cause greater sedation). Products include:
Diprivan Injectable Emulsion ... 2939

Quazepam (Concurrent therapy may cause greater sedation). Products include:
Doral Tablets 2773

Secobarbital Sodium (Concurrent therapy may cause greater sedation). Products include:
Seconal Sodium Pulvules 1529

Selegiline Hydrochloride (Concurrent therapy may cause greater sedation). Products include:
Eldepryl Capsules 2729

Temazepam (Concurrent therapy may cause greater sedation). Products include:
Restoril Capsules 2413

Thioridazine Hydrochloride (Concurrent therapy may cause greater sedation). Products include:
Mellaril 2398

Thiothixene (Concurrent therapy may cause greater sedation). Products include:
Navane Capsules and Concentrate 2018
Navane Intramuscular 2019

Tranylcypromine Sulfate (Concurrent therapy may cause greater sedation). Products include:
Parnate Tablets 2679

Triazolam (Concurrent therapy may cause greater sedation). Products include:
Halcion Tablets 2093

Trifluoperazine Hydrochloride (Concurrent therapy may cause greater sedation). Products include:
Stelazine 2692

Zolpidem Tartrate (Concurrent therapy may cause greater sedation). Products include:
Ambien Tablets 2559

ROBITUSSIN COLD & COUGH LIQUI-GELS
(Guaifenesin, Dextromethorphan Hydrobromide, Pseudoephedrine Hydrochloride) .... ▣ 844
May interact with monoamine oxidase inhibitors. Compounds in this category include:

Furazolidone (Concurrent and/or sequential use is not recommended). Products include:
Furoxone 2221

Isocarboxazid (Concurrent and/or sequential use is not recommended).
No products indexed under this heading.

Phenelzine Sulfate (Concurrent and/or sequential use is not recommended). Products include:
Nardil 1977

Selegiline Hydrochloride (Concurrent and/or sequential use is not recommended). Products include:
Eldepryl Capsules 2729

Tranylcypromine Sulfate (Concurrent and/or sequential use is not recommended). Products include:
Parnate Tablets 2679

ROBITUSSIN COLD, COUGH & FLU LIQUI-GELS
(Acetaminophen, Dextromethorphan Hydrobromide, Guaifenesin, Pseudoephedrine Hydrochloride) .... ▣ 844
May interact with monoamine oxidase inhibitors. Compounds in this category include:

Furazolidone (Concurrent and/or sequential use is not recommended). Products include:
Furoxone 2221

(▣ Described in PDR For Nonprescription Drugs)   (⊙ Described in PDR For Ophthalmology)

943 Interactions Index Robitussin Pediatric Cough

Isocarboxazid (Concurrent and/or sequential use is not recommended).
No products indexed under this heading.
Phenelzine Sulfate (Concurrent and/or sequential use is not recommended). Products include:
Nardil 1977
Selegiline Hydrochloride (Concurrent and/or sequential use is not recommended). Products include:
Eldepryl Capsules 2729
Tranylcypromine Sulfate (Concurrent and/or sequential use is not recommended). Products include:
Parnate Tablets 2679

ROBITUSSIN MAXIMUM STRENGTH COUGH & COLD
(Dextromethorphan Hydrobromide, Pseudoephedrine Hydrochloride) .... ⊞ 847
May interact with monoamine oxidase inhibitors. Compounds in this category include:

Furazolidone (Concurrent and/or sequential use is not recommended). Products include:
Furoxone 2221
Isocarboxazid (Concurrent and/or sequential use is not recommended).
No products indexed under this heading.
Phenelzine Sulfate (Concurrent and/or sequential use is not recommended). Products include:
Nardil 1977
Selegiline Hydrochloride (Concurrent and/or sequential use is not recommended). Products include:
Eldepryl Capsules 2729
Tranylcypromine Sulfate (Concurrent and/or sequential use is not recommended). Products include:
Parnate Tablets 2679

ROBITUSSIN MAXIMUM STRENGTH COUGH SUPPRESSANT
(Dextromethorphan Hydrobromide) .... ⊞ 847
May interact with monoamine oxidase inhibitors. Compounds in this category include:

Furazolidone (Concurrent and/or sequential use is not recommended). Products include:
Furoxone 2221
Isocarboxazid (Concurrent and/or sequential use is not recommended).
No products indexed under this heading.
Phenelzine Sulfate (Concurrent and/or sequential use is not recommended). Products include:
Nardil 1977
Selegiline Hydrochloride (Concurrent and/or sequential use is not recommended). Products include:
Eldepryl Capsules 2729
Tranylcypromine Sulfate (Concurrent and/or sequential use is not recommended). Products include:
Parnate Tablets 2679

ROBITUSSIN NIGHT-TIME COLD FORMULA
(Acetaminophen, Dextromethorphan Hydrobromide, Doxylamine Succinate, Phenylpropanolamine Hydrochloride) .... ⊞ 847
May interact with monoamine oxidase inhibitors, tranquilizers, hypnotics and sedatives, and certain other agents. Compounds in these categories include:

Alprazolam (May increase drowsiness effect). Products include:
Xanax Tablets 2115
Buspirone Hydrochloride (May increase drowsiness effect). Products include:
BuSpar Tablets 738
Chlordiazepoxide (May increase drowsiness effect). Products include:
Limbitrol 2333
Chlordiazepoxide Hydrochloride (May increase drowsiness effect). Products include:
Librax Capsules 2330
Librium Capsules 2331
Librium Injectable 2332
Chlorpromazine (May increase drowsiness effect). Products include:
Thorazine Suppositories 2701
Chlorpromazine Hydrochloride (May increase drowsiness effect). Products include:
Thorazine 2701
Chlorprothixene (May increase drowsiness effect).
No products indexed under this heading.
Chlorprothixene Hydrochloride (May increase drowsiness effect).
No products indexed under this heading.
Clorazepate Dipotassium (May increase drowsiness effect). Products include:
Tranxene 459
Diazepam (May increase drowsiness effect). Products include:
Dizac (diazepam injectable emulsion) CIV 1862
Valium Injectable 2336
Valium Tablets 2335
Droperidol (May increase drowsiness effect). Products include:
Inapsine Injection 462
Estazolam (May increase drowsiness effect). Products include:
ProSom Tablets 457
Ethchlorvynol (May increase drowsiness effect). Products include:
Placidyl Capsules 456
Ethinamate (May increase drowsiness effect).
No products indexed under this heading.
Fluphenazine Decanoate (May increase drowsiness effect). Products include:
Prolixin Decanoate 510
Fluphenazine Enanthate (May increase drowsiness effect). Products include:
Prolixin Enanthate 510
Fluphenazine Hydrochloride (May increase drowsiness effect). Products include:
Prolixin 510
Flurazepam Hydrochloride (May increase drowsiness effect). Products include:
Dalmane Capsules 2329
Furazolidone (Concurrent and/or sequential use is not recommended). Products include:
Furoxone 2221
Glutethimide (May increase drowsiness effect).
No products indexed under this heading.
Haloperidol (May increase drowsiness effect). Products include:
Haldol Injection, Tablets and Concentrate 1585
Haloperidol Decanoate (May increase drowsiness effect). Products include:
Haldol Decanoate 1587
Hydroxyzine Hydrochloride (May increase drowsiness effect). Products include:
Atarax Tablets & Syrup 1992
Marax Tablets & DF Syrup 2015
Vistaril Intramuscular Solution 2042
Isocarboxazid (Concurrent and/or sequential use is not recommended).
No products indexed under this heading.
Lorazepam (May increase drowsiness effect). Products include:
Ativan Injection 2805
Ativan Tablets 2807
Loxapine Hydrochloride (May increase drowsiness effect). Products include:
Loxitane 1426
Loxapine Succinate (May increase drowsiness effect). Products include:
Loxitane Capsules 1426
Meprobamate (May increase drowsiness effect). Products include:
Miltown Tablets 2780
PMB 200 and PMB 400 2890
Mesoridazine Besylate (May increase drowsiness effect). Products include:
Serentil 689
Midazolam Hydrochloride (May increase drowsiness effect). Products include:
Versed Injection 2324
Molindone Hydrochloride (May increase drowsiness effect). Products include:
Moban Tablets and Concentrate 1036
Oxazepam (May increase drowsiness effect). Products include:
Serax Capsules 2916
Serax Tablets 2916
Perphenazine (May increase drowsiness effect). Products include:
Etrafon 2495
Triavil Tablets 1800
Trilafon 2532
Phenelzine Sulfate (Concurrent and/or sequential use is not recommended). Products include:
Nardil 1977
Prazepam (May increase drowsiness effect).
No products indexed under this heading.
Prochlorperazine (May increase drowsiness effect). Products include:
Compazine 2644
Promethazine Hydrochloride (May increase drowsiness effect). Products include:
Mepergan Injection 2859
Phenergan with Codeine 2883
Phenergan with Dextromethorphan 2885
Phenergan Injection 2880
Phenergan Suppositories 2882
Phenergan Syrup 2881
Phenergan Tablets 2882
Phenergan VC 2886
Phenergan VC with Codeine 2888
Propofol (May increase drowsiness effect). Products include:
Diprivan Injectable Emulsion 2939
Quazepam (May increase drowsiness effect). Products include:
Doral Tablets 2773
Secobarbital Sodium (May increase drowsiness effect). Products include:
Seconal Sodium Pulvules 1529
Selegiline Hydrochloride (Concurrent and/or sequential use is not recommended). Products include:
Eldepryl Capsules 2729
Temazepam (May increase drowsiness effect). Products include:
Restoril Capsules 2413
Thioridazine Hydrochloride (May increase drowsiness effect). Products include:
Mellaril 2398
Thiothixene (May increase drowsiness effect). Products include:
Navane Capsules and Concentrate 2018
Navane Intramuscular 2019
Tranylcypromine Sulfate (Concurrent and/or sequential use is not recommended). Products include:
Parnate Tablets 2679
Triazolam (May increase drowsiness effect). Products include:
Halcion Tablets 2093
Trifluoperazine Hydrochloride (May increase drowsiness effect). Products include:
Stelazine 2692
Zolpidem Tartrate (May increase drowsiness effect). Products include:
Ambien Tablets 2559

Food Interactions
Alcohol (May increase drowsiness effect).

ROBITUSSIN PEDIATRIC COUGH & COLD FORMULA
(Dextromethorphan Hydrobromide, Pseudoephedrine Hydrochloride) .... ⊞ 848
May interact with monoamine oxidase inhibitors. Compounds in this category include:

Furazolidone (Concurrent and/or sequential use should be avoided). Products include:
Furoxone 2221
Isocarboxazid (Concurrent and/or sequential use should be avoided).
No products indexed under this heading.
Phenelzine Sulfate (Concurrent and/or sequential use should be avoided). Products include:
Nardil 1977
Selegiline Hydrochloride (Concurrent and/or sequential use should be avoided). Products include:
Eldepryl Capsules 2729
Tranylcypromine Sulfate (Concurrent and/or sequential use should be avoided). Products include:
Parnate Tablets 2679

ROBITUSSIN PEDIATRIC COUGH SUPPRESSANT
(Dextromethorphan Hydrobromide) .... ⊞ 848
May interact with monoamine oxidase inhibitors. Compounds in this category include:

Furazolidone (Concurrent and/or sequential use should be avoided). Products include:
Furoxone 2221
Isocarboxazid (Concurrent and/or sequential use should be avoided).
No products indexed under this heading.
Phenelzine Sulfate (Concurrent and/or sequential use should be avoided). Products include:
Nardil 1977
Selegiline Hydrochloride (Concurrent and/or sequential use should be avoided). Products include:
Eldepryl Capsules 2729
Tranylcypromine Sulfate (Concurrent and/or sequential use should be avoided). Products include:
Parnate Tablets 2679

IMPORTANT NOTE: Always consult each drug listing in the patient's regimen for possible interactions.

ROBITUSSIN PEDIATRIC DROPS
(Dextromethorphan Hydrobromide, Guaifenesin, Pseudoephedrine Hydrochloride) .... ▣ 849
May interact with monoamine oxidase inhibitors. Compounds in this category include:

Furazolidone (Concurrent and/or sequential use is not recommended). Products include:
Furoxone 2221

Isocarboxazid (Concurrent and/or sequential use is not recommended).
No products indexed under this heading.

Phenelzine Sulfate (Concurrent and/or sequential use is not recommended). Products include:
Nardil 1977

Selegiline Hydrochloride (Concurrent and/or sequential use is not recommended). Products include:
Eldepryl Capsules 2729

Tranylcypromine Sulfate (Concurrent and/or sequential use is not recommended). Products include:
Parnate Tablets 2679

ROBITUSSIN SEVERE CONGESTION LIQUI-GELS
(Guaifenesin, Pseudoephedrine Hydrochloride) .... ▣ 845
May interact with monoamine oxidase inhibitors. Compounds in this category include:

Furazolidone (Concurrent and/or sequential use is not recommended). Products include:
Furoxone 2221

Isocarboxazid (Concurrent and/or sequential use is not recommended).
No products indexed under this heading.

Phenelzine Sulfate (Concurrent and/or sequential use is not recommended). Products include:
Nardil 1977

Selegiline Hydrochloride (Concurrent and/or sequential use is not recommended). Products include:
Eldepryl Capsules 2729

Tranylcypromine Sulfate (Concurrent and/or sequential use is not recommended). Products include:
Parnate Tablets 2679

ROBITUSSIN-CF
(Dextromethorphan Hydrobromide, Guaifenesin, Phenylpropanolamine Hydrochloride) .... ▣ 846
May interact with monoamine oxidase inhibitors. Compounds in this category include:

Furazolidone (Concurrent and/or sequential use is not recommended). Products include:
Furoxone 2221

Isocarboxazid (Concurrent and/or sequential use is not recommended).
No products indexed under this heading.

Phenelzine Sulfate (Concurrent and/or sequential use is not recommended). Products include:
Nardil 1977

Selegiline Hydrochloride (Concurrent and/or sequential use is not recommended). Products include:
Eldepryl Capsules 2729

Tranylcypromine Sulfate (Concurrent and/or sequential use is not recommended). Products include:
Parnate Tablets 2679

ROBITUSSIN-DAC SYRUP
(Codeine Phosphate, Guaifenesin, Pseudoephedrine Hydrochloride) 2249
May interact with monoamine oxidase inhibitors. Compounds in this category include:

Furazolidone (Concurrent use is not recommended). Products include:
Furoxone 2221

Isocarboxazid (Concurrent use is not recommended).
No products indexed under this heading.

Phenelzine Sulfate (Concurrent use is not recommended). Products include:
Nardil 1977

Selegiline Hydrochloride (Concurrent use is not recommended). Products include:
Eldepryl Capsules 2729

Tranylcypromine Sulfate (Concurrent use is not recommended). Products include:
Parnate Tablets 2679

ROBITUSSIN-DM
(Dextromethorphan Hydrobromide, Guaifenesin) .... ▣ 846
May interact with monoamine oxidase inhibitors. Compounds in this category include:

Furazolidone (Concurrent and/or sequential use is not recommended). Products include:
Furoxone 2221

Isocarboxazid (Concurrent and/or sequential use is not recommended).
No products indexed under this heading.

Phenelzine Sulfate (Concurrent and/or sequential use is not recommended). Products include:
Nardil 1977

Selegiline Hydrochloride (Concurrent and/or sequential use is not recommended). Products include:
Eldepryl Capsules 2729

Tranylcypromine Sulfate (Concurrent and/or sequential use is not recommended). Products include:
Parnate Tablets 2679

ROBITUSSIN-PE
(Guaifenesin, Pseudoephedrine Hydrochloride) .... ▣ 846
May interact with monoamine oxidase inhibitors. Compounds in this category include:

Furazolidone (Concurrent and/or sequential use is not recommended). Products include:
Furoxone 2221

Isocarboxazid (Concurrent and/or sequential use is not recommended).
No products indexed under this heading.

Phenelzine Sulfate (Concurrent and/or sequential use is not recommended). Products include:
Nardil 1977

Selegiline Hydrochloride (Concurrent and/or sequential use is not recommended). Products include:
Eldepryl Capsules 2729

Tranylcypromine Sulfate (Concurrent and/or sequential use is not recommended). Products include:
Parnate Tablets 2679

ROCALTROL CAPSULES
(Calcitriol) 2303
May interact with cardiac glycosides, magnesium-containing antacids, and certain other agents. Compounds in these categories include:

Cholestyramine (Reduced intestinal absorption of Rocaltrol). Products include:
Questran 774

Deslanoside (Increased risk of cardiac arrhythmias).
No products indexed under this heading.

Digitoxin (Increased risk of cardiac arrhythmias). Products include:
Crystodigin Tablets 1472

Digoxin (Increased risk of cardiac arrhythmias). Products include:
Lanoxicaps 1110
Lanoxin Elixir Pediatric 1113
Lanoxin Injection 1116
Lanoxin Injection Pediatric 1119
Lanoxin Tablets 1121

Magaldrate (Potential for hypermagnesemia in patients on chronic renal dialysis).
No products indexed under this heading.

Magnesium Carbonate (Potential for hypermagnesemia in patients on chronic renal dialysis). Products include:
Bufferin Analgesic Tablets .... ▣ 636
Arthritis Strength Bufferin Analgesic Caplets .... ▣ 637
Extra Strength Bufferin Analgesic Tablets .... ▣ 637
Gaviscon Extra Strength Relief Formula Antacid Tablets .... ▣ 778
Gaviscon Extra Strength Relief Formula Liquid Antacid .... ▣ 779
Gaviscon Liquid Antacid .... ▣ 779
Maalox Antacid Caplets .... ▣ 657
Maalox Heartburn Relief Suspension .... ▣ 658
Mag-Carb Capsules 2168
Marblen .... ▣ 671
One-A-Day Calcium Plus .... ▣ 625

Magnesium Hydroxide (Potential for hypermagnesemia in patients on chronic renal dialysis). Products include:
Aludrox Oral Suspension .... ▣ 850
Ascriptin .... ▣ 650
Di-Gel Antacid/Anti-Gas .... ▣ 762
Gelusil Antacid-Anti-gas Liquid .... ▣ 819
Gelusil Antacid-Anti-gas Tablets .... ▣ 819
Maalox Antacid/Anti-Gas Tablets 889
Maalox Antacid Liquid 888
Extra Strength Maalox Antacid/Anti-Gas Liquid and Tablets 888
Mylanta Fast-Acting 1359
Mylanta Gelcaps Antacid .... ▣ 678
Fast-Acting Mylanta Liquid Antacid 1359
Mylanta Tablets .... ▣ 677
Maximum-Strength Fast-Acting Mylanta Liquid Antacid 1359
Mylanta Double Strength Tablets .... ▣ 677
Phillips' Milk of Magnesia Liquid .... ▣ 627
Rolaids Antacid Tablets .... ▣ 807
Tempo Soft Antacid .... ▣ 799

Magnesium Trisilicate (Potential for hypermagnesemia in patients on chronic renal dialysis). Products include:
Gaviscon Antacid Tablets .... ▣ 778
Gaviscon-2 Antacid Tablets .... ▣ 779

Vitamin D (Possible additive effect and hypercalcemia). Products include:
Caltrate PLUS .... ▣ 681
Caltrate 600 + D .... ▣ 681
Dical-D Tablets & Wafers 424
Materna Tablets 1427
Megadose 513
One-A-Day Calcium Plus .... ▣ 625

ROCEPHIN INJECTABLE VIALS, ADD-VANTAGE, GALAXY CONTAINER
(Ceftriaxone Sodium) 2305
None cited in PDR database.

ROFERON-A INJECTION
(Interferon alfa-2A, Recombinant) 2308
May interact with:

Aldesleukin (Co-administration with interleukin-2 may potentiate risks of renal failure). Products include:
Proleukin for Injection 812

Aminophylline (Reduced clearance of theophylline).
No products indexed under this heading.

Bone Marrow Depressants, unspecified (Caution should be exercised when administered concomitantly with myelosuppressive agents).

Dyphylline (Reduced clearance of theophylline). Products include:
Lufyllin & Lufyllin-400 Tablets 2778
Lufyllin-GG Elixir & Tablets 2779

Theophylline (Reduced clearance of theophylline). Products include:
Marax Tablets & DF Syrup 2015
Quibron 2227

Theophylline Anhydrous (Reduced clearance of theophylline). Products include:
Aerolate 1003
Primatene Tablets .... ▣ 844
Respbid Tablets 687
Slo-bid Gyrocaps 2201
Theo-24 Extended Release Capsules 2753
Theo-Dur Extended-Release Tablets 1367
Theo-X Extended-Release Tablets 793
Uni-Dur Extended-Release Tablets 1374
Uniphyl 400 mg and 600 mg Tablets 2157

Theophylline Calcium Salicylate (Reduced clearance of theophylline). Products include:
Quadrinal Tablets 1398

Theophylline Sodium Glycinate (Reduced clearance of theophylline).
No products indexed under this heading.

Zidovudine (Concomitant therapy may result in synergistic toxicity). Products include:
Retrovir Capsules 1216
Retrovir I.V. Infusion 1221
Retrovir Syrup 1216

ROLAIDS ANTACID TABLETS
(Calcium Carbonate, Magnesium Hydroxide) .... ▣ 807
May interact with:

Drugs, Oral, unspecified (Antacids may interact with certain unspecified prescription drugs).

ROLAIDS ANTACID CALCIUM RICH/SODIUM FREE TABLETS
(Calcium Carbonate) .... ▣ 807
May interact with:

Drugs, Oral, unspecified (Antacids may interact with certain unspecified prescription drugs).

ROMAZICON
(Flumazenil) 2311
May interact with antidepressant drugs, neuromuscular blocking agents, and certain other agents. Compounds in these categories include:

Amitriptyline Hydrochloride (Toxic effects of cyclic antidepressant may emerge with the reversal of the benzodiazepine effect). Products include:
Elavil 2945
Etrafon 2495
Limbitrol 2333
Triavil Tablets 1800

(▣ Described in PDR For Nonprescription Drugs)   (◉ Described in PDR For Ophthalmology)

Interactions Index

Amoxapine (Toxic effects of cyclic antidepressant may emerge with the reversal of the benzodiazepine effect). Products include:
Asendin Tablets 1419

Atracurium Besylate (Romazicon should not be used until the effects of neuromuscular blockade have been fully reversed). Products include:
Tracrium Injection 1155

Cisatracurium Besylate (Romazicon should not be used until the effects of neuromuscular blockade have been fully reversed). Products include:
Nimbex Injection 1131

Desipramine Hydrochloride (Toxic effects of cyclic antidepressant may emerge with the reversal of the benzodiazepine effect). Products include:
Norpramin Tablets 1273

Doxacurium Chloride (Romazicon should not be used until the effects of neuromuscular blockade have been fully reversed). Products include:
Nuromax Injection 1136

Doxepin Hydrochloride (Toxic effects of cyclic antidepressant may emerge with the reversal of the benzodiazepine effect). Products include:
Adapin Capsules 1542
Sinequan 2028
Zonalon Cream 1042

Imipramine Hydrochloride (Toxic effects of cyclic antidepressant may emerge with the reversal of the benzodiazepine effect). Products include:
Tofranil Ampuls 873
Tofranil Tablets 875

Imipramine Pamoate (Toxic effects of cyclic antidepressant may emerge with the reversal of the benzodiazepine effect). Products include:
Tofranil-PM Capsules 876

Maprotiline Hydrochloride (Toxic effects of cyclic antidepressant may emerge with the reversal of the benzodiazepine effect). Products include:
Ludiomil Tablets 861

Metocurine Iodide (Romazicon should not be used until the effects of neuromuscular blockade have been fully reversed). Products include:
Metubine Iodide Vials 932

Mivacurium Chloride (Romazicon should not be used until the effects of neuromuscular blockade have been fully reversed). Products include:
Mivacron 1125

Nefazodone Hydrochloride (Toxic effects of cyclic antidepressant may emerge with the reversal of the benzodiazepine effect). Products include:
Serzone Tablets 776

Nortriptyline Hydrochloride (Toxic effects of cyclic antidepressant may emerge with the reversal of the benzodiazepine effect). Products include:
Pamelor 2409

Pancuronium Bromide (Romazicon should not be used until the effects of neuromuscular blockade have been fully reversed).
No products indexed under this heading.

Paroxetine Hydrochloride (Toxic effects of cyclic antidepressant may emerge with the reversal of the benzodiazepine effect). Products include:
Paxil Tablets 2681

Protriptyline Hydrochloride (Toxic effects of cyclic antidepressant may emerge with the reversal of the benzodiazepine effect). Products include:
Vivactil Tablets 1820

Rocuronium Bromide (Romazicon should not be used until the effects of neuromuscular blockade have been fully reversed). Products include:
Zemuron Injection 1885

Sertraline Hydrochloride (Toxic effects of cyclic antidepressant may emerge with the reversal of the benzodiazepine effect). Products include:
Zoloft Tablets 2051

Succinylcholine Chloride (Romazicon should not be used until the effects of neuromuscular blockade have been fully reversed). Products include:
Anectine 1062

Trazodone Hydrochloride (Toxic effects of cyclic antidepressant may emerge with the reversal of the benzodiazepine effect). Products include:
Desyrel and Desyrel Dividose 504

Trimipramine Maleate (Toxic effects of cyclic antidepressant may emerge with the reversal of the benzodiazepine effect). Products include:
Surmontil Capsules 2917

Vecuronium Bromide (Romazicon should not be used until the effects of neuromuscular blockade have been fully reversed). Products include:
Norcuron for Injection 1875

Venlafaxine Hydrochloride (Toxic effects of cyclic antidepressant may emerge with the reversal of the benzodiazepine effect). Products include:
Effexor 2825

Food Interactions

Alcohol (Concurrent use should be avoided).

RONDEC ORAL DROPS
(Carbinoxamine Maleate, Pseudoephedrine Hydrochloride) 974
May interact with tricyclic antidepressants, central nervous system depressants, monoamine oxidase inhibitors, veratrum alkaloids, beta blockers, and certain other agents. Compounds in these categories include:

Acebutolol Hydrochloride (Effects of sympathomimetics increased). Products include:
Sectral Capsules 2914

Alfentanil Hydrochloride (Enhanced effects of CNS depressants). Products include:
Alfenta Injection 1334

Alprazolam (Enhanced effects of CNS depressants). Products include:
Xanax Tablets 2115

Amitriptyline Hydrochloride (Enhanced effects of tricyclic antidepressants). Products include:
Elavil 2945
Etrafon 2495
Limbitrol 2333
Triavil Tablets 1800

Amoxapine (Enhanced effects of tricyclic antidepressants). Products include:
Asendin Tablets 1419

Aprobarbital (Enhanced effects of CNS depressants).
No products indexed under this heading.

Atenolol (Effects of sympathomimetics increased). Products include:
Tenoretic Tablets 2963
Tenormin Tablets and I.V. Injection 2965

Betaxolol Hydrochloride (Effects of sympathomimetics increased). Products include:
Betoptic Ophthalmic Solution 465
Betoptic S Ophthalmic Suspension 467
Kerlone Tablets 2588

Bisoprolol Fumarate (Effects of sympathomimetics increased). Products include:
Zebeta Tablets 1457
Ziac 1459

Buprenorphine (Enhanced effects of CNS depressants). Products include:
Buprenex Injectable 2170

Buspirone Hydrochloride (Enhanced effects of CNS depressants). Products include:
BuSpar Tablets 738

Butabarbital (Enhanced effects of CNS depressants).
No products indexed under this heading.

Butalbital (Enhanced effects of CNS depressants). Products include:
Axocet Capsules 2469
Esgic-plus Capsules 1012
Esgic-plus Tablets 1012
Fioricet Tablets 2386
Fioricet with Codeine Capsules 2387
Fiorinal Capsules 2388
Fiorinal with Codeine Capsules 2390
Fiorinal Tablets 2388
Phrenilin 790
Sedapap Tablets 50 mg/650 mg 1826

Carteolol Hydrochloride (Effects of sympathomimetics increased). Products include:
Cartrol Tablets 413
Ocupress Ophthalmic Solution, 1% Sterile 297

Chlordiazepoxide (Enhanced effects of CNS depressants). Products include:
Limbitrol 2333

Chlordiazepoxide Hydrochloride (Enhanced effects of CNS depressants). Products include:
Librax Capsules 2330
Librium Capsules 2331
Librium Injectable 2332

Chlorpromazine (Enhanced effects of CNS depressants). Products include:
Thorazine Suppositories 2701

Chlorprothixene (Enhanced effects of CNS depressants).
No products indexed under this heading.

Chlorprothixene Hydrochloride (Enhanced effects of CNS depressants).
No products indexed under this heading.

Chlorprothixene Lactate (Enhanced effects of CNS depressants).
No products indexed under this heading.

Clomipramine Hydrochloride (Enhanced effects of tricyclic antidepressants). Products include:
Anafranil Capsules 819

Clorazepate Dipotassium (Enhanced effects of CNS depressants). Products include:
Tranxene 459

Clozapine (Enhanced effects of CNS depressants). Products include:
Clozaril Tablets 2377

Codeine Phosphate (Enhanced effects of CNS depressants). Products include:
Brontex 2130
Dimetane-DC Cough Syrup 2232
Fioricet with Codeine Capsules 2387
Fiorinal with Codeine Capsules 2390
Nucofed 2225
Phenergan with Codeine 2883
Phenergan VC with Codeine 2888
Robitussin A-C Syrup 2248
Robitussin-DAC Syrup 2249
Ryna 804
Soma Compound w/Codeine Tablets 2784
Tylenol with Codeine 1592

Cryptenamine Preparations (Reduced antihypertensive effects).

Desflurane (Enhanced effects of CNS depressants). Products include:
Suprane (desflurane, USP) 1865

Desipramine Hydrochloride (Enhanced effects of tricyclic antidepressants). Products include:
Norpramin Tablets 1273

Dezocine (Enhanced effects of CNS depressants). Products include:
Dalgan Injection 529

Diazepam (Enhanced effects of CNS depressants). Products include:
Dizac (diazepam injectable emulsion) CIV 1862
Valium Injectable 2336
Valium Tablets 2335

Doxepin Hydrochloride (Enhanced effects of tricyclic antidepressants). Products include:
Adapin Capsules 1542
Sinequan 2028
Zonalon Cream 1042

Droperidol (Enhanced effects of CNS depressants). Products include:
Inapsine Injection 462

Enflurane (Enhanced effects of CNS depressants).
No products indexed under this heading.

Esmolol Hydrochloride (Effects of sympathomimetics increased). Products include:
Brevibloc (esmolol HCl) Injection 1860

Estazolam (Enhanced effects of CNS depressants). Products include:
ProSom Tablets 457

Ethchlorvynol (Enhanced effects of CNS depressants). Products include:
Placidyl Capsules 456

Ethinamate (Enhanced effects of CNS depressants).
No products indexed under this heading.

Fentanyl (Enhanced effects of CNS depressants). Products include:
Duragesic Transdermal System 1336

Fentanyl Citrate (Enhanced effects of CNS depressants). Products include:
Sublimaze Injection 463

Fluphenazine Decanoate (Enhanced effects of CNS depressants). Products include:
Prolixin Decanoate 510

Fluphenazine Enanthate (Enhanced effects of CNS depressants). Products include:
Prolixin Enanthate 510

Fluphenazine Hydrochloride (Enhanced effects of CNS depressants). Products include:
Prolixin 510

Flurazepam Hydrochloride (Enhanced effects of CNS depressants). Products include:
Dalmane Capsules 2329

IMPORTANT NOTE: Always consult each drug listing in the patient's regimen for possible interactions.

Rondec **Interactions Index** 946

Furazolidone (Effects of sympathomimetics increased; anticholinergic effects of antihistamines prolonged and intensified; concurrent use is contraindicated). Products include:

Furoxone ... 2221

Glutethimide (Enhanced effects of CNS depressants).

No products indexed under this heading.

Haloperidol (Enhanced effects of CNS depressants). Products include:

Haldol Injection, Tablets and Concentrate ... 1585

Haloperidol Decanoate (Enhanced effects of CNS depressants). Products include:

Haldol Decanoate ... 1587

Hydrocodone Bitartrate (Enhanced effects of CNS depressants). Products include:

Codiclear DH Syrup ... 808
Duratuss HD Elixir ... 2750
Histussin D Liquid ... 670
Hycodan Tablets and Syrup ... 946
Hycomine Compound Tablets ... 948
Hycomine ... 947
Hycotuss Expectorant Syrup ... 950
Hydrocet Capsules ... 787
Lorcet 10/650 Tablets ... 1016
Lortab ... 2751
Tussend ... 1830
Tussend Expectorant ... 1831
Vicodin Tablets ... 1404
Vicodin ES Tablets ... 1405
Vicodin HP Tablets ... 1403
Vicodin Tuss Expectorant ... 1406
Zydone Capsules ... 967

Hydrocodone Polistirex (Enhanced effects of CNS depressants). Products include:

Tussionex Pennkinetic Extended-Release Suspension ... 1624

Hydroxyzine Hydrochloride (Enhanced effects of CNS depressants). Products include:

Atarax Tablets & Syrup ... 1992
Marax Tablets & DF Syrup ... 2015
Vistaril Intramuscular Solution ... 2042

Imipramine Hydrochloride (Enhanced effects of tricyclic antidepressants). Products include:

Tofranil Ampuls ... 873
Tofranil Tablets ... 875

Imipramine Pamoate (Enhanced effects of tricyclic antidepressants). Products include:

Tofranil-PM Capsules ... 876

Isocarboxazid (Effects of sympathomimetics increased; anticholinergic effects of antihistamines prolonged and intensified; concurrent use is contraindicated).

No products indexed under this heading.

Isoflurane (Enhanced effects of CNS depressants).

No products indexed under this heading.

Ketamine Hydrochloride (Enhanced effects of CNS depressants).

No products indexed under this heading.

Labetalol Hydrochloride (Effects of sympathomimetics increased). Products include:

Normodyne Injection ... 2519
Normodyne Tablets ... 2522
Trandate ... 1158

Levobunolol Hydrochloride (Effects of sympathomimetics increased). Products include:

Betagan ... ⊙ 230

Levorphanol Tartrate (Enhanced effects of CNS depressants). Products include:

Levo-Dromoran ... 2297

Lorazepam (Enhanced effects of CNS depressants). Products include:

Ativan Injection ... 2805
Ativan Tablets ... 2807

Loxapine Hydrochloride (Enhanced effects of CNS depressants). Products include:

Loxitane ... 1426

Loxapine Succinate (Enhanced effects of CNS depressants). Products include:

Loxitane Capsules ... 1426

Maprotiline Hydrochloride (Enhanced effects of tricyclic antidepressants). Products include:

Ludiomil Tablets ... 861

Mecamylamine Hydrochloride (Reduced antihypertensive effects). Products include:

Inversine Tablets ... 1729

Meperidine Hydrochloride (Enhanced effects of CNS depressants). Products include:

Demerol ... 2438
Mepergan Injection ... 2859

Mephobarbital (Enhanced effects of CNS depressants). Products include:

Mebaral Tablets ... 2452

Meprobamate (Enhanced effects of CNS depressants). Products include:

Miltown Tablets ... 2780
PMB 200 and PMB 400 ... 2890

Mesoridazine Besylate (Enhanced effects of CNS depressants). Products include:

Serentil ... 689

Methadone Hydrochloride (Enhanced effects of CNS depressants). Products include:

Methadone Hydrochloride Oral Concentrate ... 2356
Methadone Hydrochloride Oral Solution & Tablets ... 2357

Methohexital Sodium (Enhanced effects of CNS depressants).

No products indexed under this heading.

Methotrimeprazine (Enhanced effects of CNS depressants). Products include:

Levoprome ... 1321

Methoxyflurane (Enhanced effects of CNS depressants).

No products indexed under this heading.

Methyldopa (Reduced antihypertensive effects). Products include:

Aldoclor Tablets ... 1638
Aldomet Oral ... 1640
Aldoril Tablets ... 1644

Metipranolol Hydrochloride (Effects of sympathomimetics increased). Products include:

OptiPranolol (Metipranolol 0.3%) Sterile Ophthalmic Solution ... ⊙ 256

Metoprolol Succinate (Effects of sympathomimetics increased). Products include:

Toprol-XL Tablets ... 560

Metoprolol Tartrate (Effects of sympathomimetics increased). Products include:

Lopressor ... 848
Lopressor HCT Tablets ... 850

Midazolam Hydrochloride (Enhanced effects of CNS depressants). Products include:

Versed Injection ... 2324

Molindone Hydrochloride (Enhanced effects of CNS depressants). Products include:

Moban Tablets and Concentrate ... 1036

Morphine Sulfate (Enhanced effects of CNS depressants). Products include:

Astramorph/PF Injection, USP (Preservative-Free) ... 526
Duramorph Injection ... 983
Infumorph 200 and Infumorph 500 Sterile Solutions ... 985
Kadian Capsules ... 2948
MS Contin Tablets ... 2149
MSIR ... 2152
Oramorph SR (Morphine Sulfate Sustained Release Tablets) ... 2359
RMS Suppositories CII ... 2766
Roxanol ... 2365

Nadolol (Effects of sympathomimetics increased).

No products indexed under this heading.

Nortriptyline Hydrochloride (Enhanced effects of tricyclic antidepressants). Products include:

Pamelor ... 2409

Opium Alkaloids (Enhanced effects of CNS depressants).

No products indexed under this heading.

Oxazepam (Enhanced effects of CNS depressants). Products include:

Serax Capsules ... 2916
Serax Tablets ... 2916

Oxycodone Hydrochloride (Enhanced effects of CNS depressants). Products include:

OxyContin Tablets ... 2163
OxyIR Capsules ... 2167
Percocet Tablets ... 955
Percodan Tablets ... 955
Percodan-Demi Tablets ... 956
Roxicodone Tablets, Oral Solution & Intensol (Oxycodone) ... 2366
Tylox Capsules ... 1593

Penbutolol Sulfate (Effects of sympathomimetics increased). Products include:

Levatol Tablets ... 2547

Pentobarbital Sodium (Enhanced effects of CNS depressants). Products include:

Nembutal Sodium Capsules ... 440
Nembutal Sodium Solution ... 442
Nembutal Sodium Suppositories ... 444

Perphenazine (Enhanced effects of CNS depressants). Products include:

Etrafon ... 2495
Triavil Tablets ... 1800
Trilafon ... 2532

Phenelzine Sulfate (Effects of sympathomimetics increased; anticholinergic effects of antihistamines prolonged and intensified; concurrent use is contraindicated). Products include:

Nardil ... 1977

Phenobarbital (Enhanced effects of CNS depressants). Products include:

Arco-Lase Plus Tablets ... 513
Bellergal-S Tablets ... 2375
Donnatal ... 2234
Donnatal Extentabs ... 2234
Donnatal Tablets ... 2234
Phenobarbital Elixir and Tablets ... 1523
Quadrinal Tablets ... 1398

Pindolol (Effects of sympathomimetics increased). Products include:

Visken Tablets ... 2428

Prazepam (Enhanced effects of CNS depressants).

No products indexed under this heading.

Prochlorperazine (Enhanced effects of CNS depressants). Products include:

Compazine ... 2644

Promethazine Hydrochloride (Enhanced effects of CNS depressants). Products include:

Mepergan Injection ... 2859
Phenergan with Codeine ... 2883
Phenergan with Dextromethorphan ... 2885
Phenergan Injection ... 2880
Phenergan Suppositories ... 2882
Phenergan Syrup ... 2881
Phenergan Tablets ... 2882
Phenergan VC ... 2886
Phenergan VC with Codeine ... 2888

Propofol (Enhanced effects of CNS depressants). Products include:

Diprivan Injectable Emulsion ... 2939

Propoxyphene Hydrochloride (Enhanced effects of CNS depressants). Products include:

Darvon ... 1475
Wygesic Tablets ... 2930

Propoxyphene Napsylate (Enhanced effects of CNS depressants). Products include:

Darvon-N/Darvocet-N ... 1473

Propranolol Hydrochloride (Effects of sympathomimetics increased). Products include:

Inderal ... 2834
Inderal LA Long Acting Capsules ... 2836
Inderide Tablets ... 2838
Inderide LA Long Acting Capsules ... 2840

Protriptyline Hydrochloride (Enhanced effects of tricyclic antidepressants). Products include:

Vivactil Tablets ... 1820

Quazepam (Enhanced effects of CNS depressants). Products include:

Doral Tablets ... 2773

Reserpine (Reduced antihypertensive effects). Products include:

Diupres Tablets ... 1691
Hydropres Tablets ... 1718
Ser-Ap-Es Tablets ... 867

Risperidone (Enhanced effects of CNS depressants). Products include:

Risperdal Tablets ... 1348

Secobarbital Sodium (Enhanced effects of CNS depressants). Products include:

Seconal Sodium Pulvules ... 1529

Selegiline Hydrochloride (Effects of sympathomimetics increased; anticholinergic effects of antihistamines prolonged and intensified; concurrent use is contraindicated). Products include:

Eldepryl Capsules ... 2729

Sevoflurane (Enhanced effects of CNS depressants).

No products indexed under this heading.

Sotalol Hydrochloride (Effects of sympathomimetics increased). Products include:

Betapace Tablets ... 637

Sufentanil Citrate (Enhanced effects of CNS depressants). Products include:

Sufenta Injection ... 1355

Temazepam (Enhanced effects of CNS depressants). Products include:

Restoril Capsules ... 2413

Thiamylal Sodium (Enhanced effects of CNS depressants).

No products indexed under this heading.

Thioridazine Hydrochloride (Enhanced effects of CNS depressants). Products include:

Mellaril ... 2398

Thiothixene (Enhanced effects of CNS depressants). Products include:

Navane Capsules and Concentrate ... 2018
Navane Intramuscular ... 2019

Timolol Maleate (Effects of sympathomimetics increased). Products include:

Blocadren Tablets ... 1654
Timolide Tablets ... 1791
Timoptic in Ocudose ... 1796
Timoptic Sterile Ophthalmic Solution ... 1794
Timoptic-XE ... 1798

(Described in PDR For Nonprescription Drugs) (⊙ Described in PDR For Ophthalmology)

Tranylcypromine Sulfate (Effects of sympathomimetics increased; anticholinergic effects of antihistamines prolonged and intensified; concurrent use is contraindicated). Products include:
Parnate Tablets 2679
Triazolam (Enhanced effects of CNS depressants). Products include:
Halcion Tablets 2093
Trifluoperazine Hydrochloride (Enhanced effects of CNS depressants). Products include:
Stelazine 2692
Trimipramine Maleate (Enhanced effects of tricyclic antidepressants). Products include:
Surmontil Capsules 2917
Zolpidem Tartrate (Enhanced effects of CNS depressants). Products include:
Ambien Tablets 2559

Food Interactions
Alcohol (Enhanced effects of alcohol).

RONDEC SYRUP
(Carbinoxamine Maleate, Pseudoephedrine Hydrochloride) 974
See **Rondec Oral Drops**

RONDEC TABLET
(Carbinoxamine Maleate, Pseudoephedrine Hydrochloride) 974
See **Rondec Oral Drops**

RONDEC CHEWABLE TABLETS
(Brompheniramine Maleate, Pseudoephedrine Hydrochloride) 974
May interact with central nervous system depressants, beta blockers, monoamine oxidase inhibitors, and certain other agents. Compounds in these categories include:

Acebutolol Hydrochloride (Increases the effects of sympathomimetics). Products include:
Sectral Capsules 2914
Alfentanil Hydrochloride (Concomitant use of antihistamines with CNS depressants may have an additive effect). Products include:
Alfenta Injection 1334
Alprazolam (Concomitant use of antihistamines with CNS depressants may have an additive effect). Products include:
Xanax Tablets 2115
Aprobarbital (Concomitant use of antihistamines with CNS depressants may have an additive effect).
No products indexed under this heading.
Atenolol (Increases the effects of sympathomimetics). Products include:
Tenoretic Tablets 2963
Tenormin Tablets and I.V. Injection 2965
Betaxolol Hydrochloride (Increases the effects of sympathomimetics). Products include:
Betoptic Ophthalmic Solution........... 465
Betoptic S Ophthalmic Suspension 467
Kerlone Tablets 2588
Bisoprolol Fumarate (Increases the effects of sympathomimetics). Products include:
Zebeta Tablets 1457
Ziac 1459
Buprenorphine (Concomitant use of antihistamines with CNS depressants may have an additive effect). Products include:
Buprenex Injectable 2170

Buspirone Hydrochloride (Concomitant use of antihistamines with CNS depressants may have an additive effect). Products include:
BuSpar Tablets 738
Butabarbital (Concomitant use of antihistamines with CNS depressants may have an additive effect).
No products indexed under this heading.
Butalbital (Concomitant use of antihistamines with CNS depressants may have an additive effect). Products include:
Axocet Capsules 2469
Esgic-plus Capsules 1012
Esgic-plus Tablets 1012
Fioricet Tablets 2386
Fioricet with Codeine Capsules 2387
Fiorinal Capsules 2388
Fiorinal with Codeine Capsules 2390
Fiorinal Tablets 2388
Phrenilin 790
Sedapap Tablets 50 mg/650 mg .. 1826
Carteolol Hydrochloride (Increases the effects of sympathomimetics). Products include:
Cartrol Tablets 413
Ocupress Ophthalmic Solution, 1 % Sterile 297
Chlordiazepoxide (Concomitant use of antihistamines with CNS depressants may have an additive effect). Products include:
Limbitrol 2333
Chlordiazepoxide Hydrochloride (Concomitant use of antihistamines with CNS depressants may have an additive effect). Products include:
Librax Capsules 2330
Librium Capsules 2331
Librium Injectable 2332
Chlorpromazine (Concomitant use of antihistamines with CNS depressants may have an additive effect). Products include:
Thorazine Suppositories 2701
Chlorpromazine Hydrochloride (Concomitant use of antihistamines with CNS depressants may have an additive effect). Products include:
Thorazine 2701
Chlorprothixene (Concomitant use of antihistamines with CNS depressants may have an additive effect).
No products indexed under this heading.
Chlorprothixene Hydrochloride (Concomitant use of antihistamines with CNS depressants may have an additive effect).
No products indexed under this heading.
Chlorprothixene Lactate (Concomitant use of antihistamines with CNS depressants may have an additive effect).
No products indexed under this heading.
Clorazepate Dipotassium (Concomitant use of antihistamines with CNS depressants may have an additive effect). Products include:
Tranxene 459
Clozapine (Concomitant use of antihistamines with CNS depressants may have an additive effect). Products include:
Clozaril Tablets 2377
Codeine Phosphate (Concomitant use of antihistamines with CNS depressants may have an additive effect). Products include:
Brontex 2130
Dimetane-DC Cough Syrup 2232
Fioricet with Codeine Capsules 2387

Fiorinal with Codeine Capsules 2390
Nucofed 2225
Phenergan with Codeine 2883
Phenergan VC with Codeine 2888
Robitussin A-C Syrup 2248
Robitussin-DAC Syrup 2249
Ryna 804
Soma Compound w/Codeine Tablets 2784
Tylenol with Codeine 1592
Desflurane (Concomitant use of antihistamines with CNS depressants may have an additive effect). Products include:
Suprane (desflurane, USP) 1865
Dezocine (Concomitant use of antihistamines with CNS depressants may have an additive effect). Products include:
Dalgan Injection 529
Diazepam (Concomitant use of antihistamines with CNS depressants may have an additive effect). Products include:
Dizac (diazepam injectable emulsion) CIV 1862
Valium Injectable 2336
Valium Tablets 2335
Droperidol (Concomitant use of antihistamines with CNS depressants may have an additive effect). Products include:
Inapsine Injection 462
Enflurane (Concomitant use of antihistamines with CNS depressants may have an additive effect).
No products indexed under this heading.
Esmolol Hydrochloride (Increases the effects of sympathomimetics). Products include:
Brevibloc (esmolol HCl) Injection 1860
Estazolam (Concomitant use of antihistamines with CNS depressants may have an additive effect). Products include:
ProSom Tablets 457
Ethchlorvynol (Concomitant use of antihistamines with CNS depressants may have an additive effect). Products include:
Placidyl Capsules 456
Ethinamate (Concomitant use of antihistamines with CNS depressants may have an additive effect).
No products indexed under this heading.
Fentanyl (Concomitant use of antihistamines with CNS depressants may have an additive effect). Products include:
Duragesic Transdermal System........ 1336
Fentanyl Citrate (Concomitant use of antihistamines with CNS depressants may have an additive effect). Products include:
Sublimaze Injection 463
Fluphenazine Decanoate (Concomitant use of antihistamines with CNS depressants may have an additive effect). Products include:
Prolixin Decanoate 510
Fluphenazine Enanthate (Concomitant use of antihistamines with CNS depressants may have an additive effect). Products include:
Prolixin Enanthate 510
Fluphenazine Hydrochloride (Concomitant use of antihistamines with CNS depressants may have an additive effect). Products include:
Prolixin 510
Flurazepam Hydrochloride (Concomitant use of antihistamines with CNS depressants may have an additive effect). Products include:
Dalmane Capsules 2329

Furazolidone (Increases the effects of sympathomimetics; concurrent and/or sequential use is contraindicated). Products include:
Furoxone 2221
Glutethimide (Concomitant use of antihistamines with CNS depressants may have an additive effect).
No products indexed under this heading.
Haloperidol (Concomitant use of antihistamines with CNS depressants may have an additive effect). Products include:
Haldol Injection, Tablets and Concentrate 1585
Haloperidol Decanoate (Concomitant use of antihistamines with CNS depressants may have an additive effect). Products include:
Haldol Decanoate..................... 1587
Hydrocodone Bitartrate (Concomitant use of antihistamines with CNS depressants may have an additive effect). Products include:
Codiclear DH Syrup 808
Duratuss HD Elixir 2750
Histussin D Liquid 670
Hycodan Tablets and Syrup 946
Hycomine Compound Tablets 948
Hycomine 947
Hycotuss Expectorant Syrup 950
Hydrocet Capsules 787
Lorcet 10/650 Tablets 1016
Lortab 2751
Tussend 1830
Tussend Expectorant 1831
Vicodin Tablets 1404
Vicodin ES Tablets 1405
Vicodin HP Tablets 1403
Vicodin Tuss Expectorant 1406
Zydone Capsules 967
Hydrocodone Polistirex (Concomitant use of antihistamines with CNS depressants may have an additive effect). Products include:
Tussionex Pennkinetic Extended-Release Suspension 1624
Hydroxyzine Hydrochloride (Concomitant use of antihistamines with CNS depressants may have an additive effect). Products include:
Atarax Tablets & Syrup 1992
Marax Tablets & DF Syrup 2015
Vistaril Intramuscular Solution........ 2042
Isocarboxazid (Increases the effects of sympathomimetics; concurrent and/or sequential use is contraindicated).
No products indexed under this heading.
Isoflurane (Concomitant use of antihistamines with CNS depressants may have an additive effect).
No products indexed under this heading.
Ketamine Hydrochloride (Concomitant use of antihistamines with CNS depressants may have an additive effect).
No products indexed under this heading.
Labetalol Hydrochloride (Increases the effects of sympathomimetics). Products include:
Normodyne Injection 2519
Normodyne Tablets 2522
Trandate 1158
Levobunolol Hydrochloride (Increases the effects of sympathomimetics). Products include:
Betagan 230
Levomethadyl Acetate Hydrochloride (Concomitant use of antihistamines with CNS depressants may have an additive effect). Products include:
Orlaam Oral Solution 2361

IMPORTANT NOTE: Always consult each drug listing in the patient's regimen for possible interactions.

Interactions Index

Levorphanol Tartrate (Concomitant use of antihistamines with CNS depressants may have an additive effect). Products include:
- Levo-Dromoran 2297

Lorazepam (Concomitant use of antihistamines with CNS depressants may have an additive effect). Products include:
- Ativan Injection 2805
- Ativan Tablets 2807

Loxapine Hydrochloride (Concomitant use of antihistamines with CNS depressants may have an additive effect). Products include:
- Loxitane 1426

Loxapine Succinate (Concomitant use of antihistamines with CNS depressants may have an additive effect). Products include:
- Loxitane Capsules 1426

Mecamylamine Hydrochloride (Sympathomimetics may reduce the antihypertensive effects). Products include:
- Inversine Tablets 1729

Meperidine Hydrochloride (Concomitant use of antihistamines with CNS depressants may have an additive effect). Products include:
- Demerol 2438
- Mepergan Injection 2859

Mephobarbital (Concomitant use of antihistamines with CNS depressants may have an additive effect). Products include:
- Mebaral Tablets 2452

Meprobamate (Concomitant use of antihistamines with CNS depressants may have an additive effect). Products include:
- Miltown Tablets 2780
- PMB 200 and PMB 400 2890

Mesoridazine Besylate (Concomitant use of antihistamines with CNS depressants may have an additive effect). Products include:
- Serentil 689

Methadone Hydrochloride (Concomitant use of antihistamines with CNS depressants may have an additive effect). Products include:
- Methadone Hydrochloride Oral Concentrate 2356
- Methadone Hydrochloride Oral Solution & Tablets 2357

Methohexital Sodium (Concomitant use of antihistamines with CNS depressants may have an additive effect).
- No products indexed under this heading.

Methotrimeprazine (Concomitant use of antihistamines with CNS depressants may have an additive effect). Products include:
- Levoprome 1321

Methoxyflurane (Concomitant use of antihistamines with CNS depressants may have an additive effect).
- No products indexed under this heading.

Methyldopa (Sympathomimetics may reduce the antihypertensive effects). Products include:
- Aldoclor Tablets 1638
- Aldomet Oral 1640
- Aldoril Tablets 1644

Methyldopate Hydrochloride (Sympathomimetics may reduce the antihypertensive effects). Products include:
- Aldomet Ester HCl Injection 1642

Metipranolol Hydrochloride (Increases the effects of sympathomimetics). Products include:
- OptiPranolol (Metipranolol 0.3%) Sterile Ophthalmic Solution ...... ⊚ 256

Metoprolol Succinate (Increases the effects of sympathomimetics). Products include:
- Toprol-XL Tablets 560

Metoprolol Tartrate (Increases the effects of sympathomimetics). Products include:
- Lopressor 848
- Lopressor HCT Tablets 850

Midazolam Hydrochloride (Concomitant use of antihistamines with CNS depressants may have an additive effect). Products include:
- Versed Injection 2324

Molindone Hydrochloride (Concomitant use of antihistamines with CNS depressants may have an additive effect). Products include:
- Moban Tablets and Concentrate 1036

Morphine Sulfate (Concomitant use of antihistamines with CNS depressants may have an additive effect). Products include:
- Astramorph/PF Injection, USP (Preservative-Free) 526
- Duramorph Injection 983
- Infumorph 200 and Infumorph 500 Sterile Solutions 985
- Kadian Capsules 2948
- MS Contin Tablets 2149
- MSIR 2152
- Oramorph SR (Morphine Sulfate Sustained Release Tablets) 2359
- RMS Suppositories CII 2766
- Roxanol 2365

Nadolol (Increases the effects of sympathomimetics).
- No products indexed under this heading.

Opium Alkaloids (Concomitant use of antihistamines with CNS depressants may have an additive effect).
- No products indexed under this heading.

Oxazepam (Concomitant use of antihistamines with CNS depressants may have an additive effect). Products include:
- Serax Capsules 2916
- Serax Tablets 2916

Oxycodone Hydrochloride (Concomitant use of antihistamines with CNS depressants may have an additive effect). Products include:
- OxyContin Tablets 2163
- OxyIR Capsules 2167
- Percocet Tablets 955
- Percodan Tablets 955
- Percodan-Demi Tablets 956
- Roxicodone Tablets, Oral Solution & Intensol (Oxycodone) 2366
- Tylox Capsules 1593

Penbutolol Sulfate (Increases the effects of sympathomimetics). Products include:
- Levatol Tablets 2547

Pentobarbital Sodium (Concomitant use of antihistamines with CNS depressants may have an additive effect). Products include:
- Nembutal Sodium Capsules 440
- Nembutal Sodium Solution 442
- Nembutal Sodium Suppositories 444

Perphenazine (Concomitant use of antihistamines with CNS depressants may have an additive effect). Products include:
- Etrafon 2495
- Triavil Tablets 1800
- Trilafon 2532

Phenelzine Sulfate (Increases the effects of sympathomimetics; concurrent and/or sequential use is contraindicated). Products include:
- Nardil 1977

Phenobarbital (Concomitant use of antihistamines with CNS depressants may have an additive effect). Products include:
- Arco-Lase Plus Tablets 513
- Bellergal-S Tablets 2375
- Donnatal 2234
- Donnatal Extentabs 2234
- Donnatal Tablets 2234
- Phenobarbital Elixir and Tablets 1523
- Quadrinal Tablets 1398

Pindolol (Increases the effects of sympathomimetics). Products include:
- Visken Tablets 2428

Prazepam (Concomitant use of antihistamines with CNS depressants may have an additive effect).
- No products indexed under this heading.

Prochlorperazine (Concomitant use of antihistamines with CNS depressants may have an additive effect). Products include:
- Compazine 2644

Promethazine Hydrochloride (Concomitant use of antihistamines with CNS depressants may have an additive effect). Products include:
- Meperigan Injection 2859
- Phenergan with Codeine 2883
- Phenergan with Dextromethorphan 2885
- Phenergan Injection 2880
- Phenergan Suppositories 2882
- Phenergan Syrup 2881
- Phenergan Tablets 2882
- Phenergan VC 2886
- Phenergan VC with Codeine 2888

Propofol (Concomitant use of antihistamines with CNS depressants may have an additive effect). Products include:
- Diprivan Injectable Emulsion 2939

Propoxyphene Hydrochloride (Concomitant use of antihistamines with CNS depressants may have an additive effect). Products include:
- Darvon 1475
- Wygesic Tablets 2930

Propoxyphene Napsylate (Concomitant use of antihistamines with CNS depressants may have an additive effect). Products include:
- Darvon-N/Darvocet-N 1473

Propranolol Hydrochloride (Increases the effects of sympathomimetics). Products include:
- Inderal 2834
- Inderal LA Long Acting Capsules 2836
- Inderide Tablets 2838
- Inderide LA Long Acting Capsules 2840

Quazepam (Concomitant use of antihistamines with CNS depressants may have an additive effect). Products include:
- Doral Tablets 2773

Reserpine (Sympathomimetics may reduce the antihypertensive effects). Products include:
- Diupres Tablets 1691
- Hydropres Tablets 1718
- Ser-Ap-Es Tablets 867

Risperidone (Concomitant use of antihistamines with CNS depressants may have an additive effect). Products include:
- Risperdal Tablets 1348

Secobarbital Sodium (Concomitant use of antihistamines with CNS depressants may have an additive effect). Products include:
- Seconal Sodium Pulvules 1529

Selegiline Hydrochloride (Increases the effects of sympathomimetics; concurrent and/or sequential use is contraindicated). Products include:
- Eldepryl Capsules 2729

Sevoflurane (Concomitant use of antihistamines with CNS depressants may have an additive effect).
- No products indexed under this heading.

Sotalol Hydrochloride (Increases the effects of sympathomimetics). Products include:
- Betapace Tablets 637

Sufentanil Citrate (Concomitant use of antihistamines with CNS depressants may have an additive effect). Products include:
- Sufenta Injection 1355

Temazepam (Concomitant use of antihistamines with CNS depressants may have an additive effect). Products include:
- Restoril Capsules 2413

Thiamylal Sodium (Concomitant use of antihistamines with CNS depressants may have an additive effect).
- No products indexed under this heading.

Thioridazine Hydrochloride (Concomitant use of antihistamines with CNS depressants may have an additive effect). Products include:
- Mellaril 2398

Thiothixene (Concomitant use of antihistamines with CNS depressants may have an additive effect). Products include:
- Navane Capsules and Concentrate 2018
- Navane Intramuscular 2019

Timolol Hemihydrate (Increases the effects of sympathomimetics). Products include:
- Betimol 0.25%, 0.5% .... ⊚ 259

Timolol Maleate (Increases the effects of sympathomimetics). Products include:
- Blocadren Tablets 1654
- Timolide Tablets 1791
- Timoptic in Ocudose 1796
- Timoptic Sterile Ophthalmic Solution 1794
- Timoptic-XE 1798

Tranylcypromine Sulfate (Increases the effects of sympathomimetics; concurrent and/or sequential use is contraindicated). Products include:
- Parnate Tablets 2679

Triazolam (Concomitant use of antihistamines with CNS depressants may have an additive effect). Products include:
- Halcion Tablets 2093

Trifluoperazine Hydrochloride (Concomitant use of antihistamines with CNS depressants may have an additive effect). Products include:
- Stelazine 2692

Zolpidem Tartrate (Concomitant use of antihistamines with CNS depressants may have an additive effect). Products include:
- Ambien Tablets 2559

Food Interactions

Alcohol (Concomitant use of antihistamines with alcohol may have an additive effect).

RONDEC-TR TABLET
(Carbinoxamine Maleate, Pseudoephedrine Hydrochloride) 974
See Rondec Oral Drops

ROWASA RECTAL SUPPOSITORIES, 500 MG
(Mesalamine) 2727
See ROWASA Rectal Suspension Enema 4.0 grams/unit (60 mL)

(⊡ Described in PDR For Nonprescription Drugs)   (⊚ Described in PDR For Ophthalmology)

949 Interactions Index Roxanol

ROWASA RECTAL SUSPENSION ENEMA 4.0 GRAMS/UNIT (60 ML)
(Mesalamine) 2727
May interact with:

Sulfasalazine (Patients on concurrent oral products which liberate mesalamine should be carefully monitored with urinalysis). Products include:
Azulfidine 2059

ROXANOL (MORPHINE SULFATE CONCENTRATED ORAL SOLUTION)
(Morphine Sulfate) 2365
May interact with tricyclic antidepressants, central nervous system depressants, urinary alkalizing agents, monoamine oxidase inhibitors, antihistamines, beta blockers, anticoagulants, and certain other agents. Compounds in these categories include:

Acebutolol Hydrochloride (Depressant effects of morphine may be enhanced). Products include:
Sectral Capsules 2914

Acrivastine (Depressant effects of morphine may be enhanced). Products include:
Semprex-D Capsules 1620

Alfentanil Hydrochloride (Respiratory depression, hypotension, and profound sedation or coma may result; depressant effects of morphine may be enhanced). Products include:
Alfenta Injection 1334

Alprazolam (Respiratory depression, hypotension, and profound sedation or coma may result; depressant effects of morphine may be enhanced). Products include:
Xanax Tablets 2115

Amitriptyline Hydrochloride (Respiratory depression, hypotension, and profound sedation or coma may result). Products include:
Elavil 2945
Etrafon 2495
Limbitrol 2333
Triavil Tablets 1800

Amoxapine (Respiratory depression, hypotension, and profound sedation or coma may result). Products include:
Asendin Tablets 1419

Aprobarbital (Respiratory depression, hypotension, and profound sedation or coma may result; depressant effects of morphine may be enhanced).
No products indexed under this heading.

Astemizole (Depressant effects of morphine may be enhanced). Products include:
Hismanal Tablets 1341

Atenolol (Depressant effects of morphine may be enhanced). Products include:
Tenoretic Tablets 2963
Tenormin Tablets and I.V. Injection 2965

Azatadine Maleate (Depressant effects of morphine may be enhanced). Products include:
Trinalin Repetabs Tablets 1373

Betaxolol Hydrochloride (Depressant effects of morphine may be enhanced). Products include:
Betoptic Ophthalmic Solution....... 465
Betoptic S Ophthalmic Suspension 467
Kerlone Tablets....... 2588

Bisoprolol Fumarate (Depressant effects of morphine may be enhanced). Products include:
Zebeta Tablets 1457
Ziac 1459

Bromodiphenhydramine Hydrochloride (Depressant effects of morphine may be enhanced).
No products indexed under this heading.

Brompheniramine Maleate (Depressant effects of morphine may be enhanced). Products include:
Alka-Seltzer Plus Sinus Medicine 611
Bromfed Capsules (Extended-Release) 1832
Bromfed Syrup 712
Bromfed Tablets 1832
Bromfed-DM Cough Syrup....... 1832
Bromfed-PD Capsules (Extended-Release) 1832
Dimetane-DC Cough Syrup 2232
Dimetane-DX Cough Syrup 2233
Dimetapp Allergy Dye-Free Elixir....... 838
Dimetapp Allergy Sinus Caplets 838
Dimetapp Cold & Allergy Chewable Tablets 838
Dimetapp Cold & Cough Liqui-Gels 839
Dimetapp Cold & Fever Suspension 839
Dimetapp DM Elixir....... 840
Dimetapp Elixir....... 840
Dimetapp Extentabs....... 841
Dimetapp Tablets/Liqui-Gels 841
Rondec Chewable Tablets 974
Vicks DayQuil Allergy Relief 12-Hour Extended Release Tablets....... 733
Vicks DayQuil Allergy Relief 4-Hour Tablets 733

Buprenorphine (Respiratory depression, hypotension, and profound sedation or coma may result; depressant effects of morphine may be enhanced). Products include:
Buprenex Injectable 2170

Buspirone Hydrochloride (Respiratory depression, hypotension, and profound sedation or coma may result; depressant effects of morphine may be enhanced). Products include:
BuSpar Tablets 738

Butabarbital (Respiratory depression, hypotension, and profound sedation or coma may result; depressant effects of morphine may be enhanced).
No products indexed under this heading.

Butalbital (Respiratory depression, hypotension, and profound sedation or coma may result; depressant effects of morphine may be enhanced). Products include:
Axocet Capsules....... 2469
Esgic-plus Capsules 1012
Esgic-plus Tablets 1012
Fioricet Tablets 2386
Fioricet with Codeine Capsules 2387
Fiorinal Capsules 2388
Fiorinal with Codeine Capsules 2390
Fiorinal Tablets 2388
Phrenilin 790
Sedapap Tablets 50 mg/650 mg .. 1826

Carteolol Hydrochloride (Depressant effects of morphine may be enhanced). Products include:
Cartrol Tablets 413
Ocupress Ophthalmic Solution, 1% Sterile....... ◉ 297

Cetirizine Hydrochloride (Depressant effects of morphine may be enhanced). Products include:
Zyrtec Tablets 2053

Chloral Hydrate (Depressant effects of morphine may be enhanced).
No products indexed under this heading.

Chlordiazepoxide (Respiratory depression, hypotension, and profound sedation or coma may result; depressant effects of morphine may be enhanced). Products include:
Limbitrol 2333

Chlordiazepoxide Hydrochloride (Respiratory depression, hypotension, and profound sedation or coma may result; depressant effects of morphine may be enhanced). Products include:
Librax Capsules 2330
Librium Capsules....... 2331
Librium Injectable 2332

Chlorpheniramine Maleate (Depressant effects of morphine may be enhanced). Products include:
Alka-Seltzer Plus Cold Medicine 611
Alka-Seltzer Plus Cold Medicine Liqui-Gels 612
Alka-Seltzer Plus Cold & Cough Medicine 611
Alka-Seltzer Plus Cold & Cough Medicine Liqui-Gels....... 612
Alka-Seltzer Plus Flu & Body Aches Effervescent Tablets....... 612
Allerest Maximum Strength....... 649
Allerest Sinus Pain Formula 649
Ana-Kit Anaphylaxis Emergency Treatment Kit 611
Atrohist Pediatric Capsules....... 1603
Atrohist Plus Tablets 1605
BC Cold Powder Multi-Symptom Formula (Cold-Sinus-Allergy) 631
Cerose DM 853
Cheracol Plus Head Cold/Cough Formula 741
Children's TYLENOL Cold Multi-Symptom Chewable Tablets and Liquid 1559
Children's TYLENOL Cold Plus Cough Multi Symptom Chewable Tablets and Liquid....... 1560
Children's TYLENOL Flu Suspension Liquid 1560
Children's Vicks DayQuil Allergy Relief....... 730
Children's Vicks NyQuil Cold/Cough Relief....... 731
Chlor-Trimeton Allergy Decongestant Tablets 759
Chlor-Trimeton Allergy Tablets 758
Allergy-Sinus Comtrex Multi-Symptom Allergy-Sinus Formula Tablets and Caplets 639
Comtrex Multi-Symptom....... 638
Contac Continuous Action Nasal Decongestant/Antihistamine 12 Hour Capsules....... 773
Contac Maximum Strength Continuous Action Decongestant/Antihistamine 12 Hour Caplets....... 772
Contac Severe Cold and Flu Formula Caplets 773
Coricidin Cold + Flu Tablets....... 760
Coricidin Cough + Cold Tablets 760
Coricidin 'D' Decongestant Tablets 760
D.A. II Tablets 972
D.A. Chewable Tablets....... 970
Dura-Tap/PD Capsules 970
Dura-Vent/DA Tablets 972
Efidac 24 Chlorpheniramine....... 655
Extendryl 1003
Fedahist Gyrocaps....... 2545
Hycomine Compound Tablets 948
Kronofed-A 994
Nolamine Timed-Release Tablets 790
Novahistine Elixir 782
Ornade Spansule Capsules 2678
PediaCare Cough-Cold Chewable Tablets and Liquid....... 1569
PediaCare NightRest Cough-Cold Liquid 1569
Pediatric Vicks 44m Cough & Cold Relief 737
Pyrroxate Caplets 742
Ryna 804
Sinarest 663
Sine-Off Sinus Medicine 784
Singlet Tablets 785
Sinulin Tablets 792
Sinutab Sinus Allergy Medication, Maximum Strength Tablets and Caplets 823
Sudafed Cold & Allergy Tablets....... 826
Teldrin 12 Hour Antihistamine/Nasal Decongestant Allergy Relief Capsules 786
TheraFlu Flu and Cold Medicine 750
Theraflu Maximum Strength Flu and Cold Medicine For Sore Throat....... 751
TheraFlu Flu, Cold and Cough Medicine 750
TheraFlu Maximum Strength Nighttime Flu, Cold & Cough Medicine 751
Triaminic Night Time 754
Triaminic Syrup 755
Triaminic Triaminicol Cold & Cough 756
Triaminicin Tablets 756
Tussend 1830
TYLENOL Allergy Sinus, Maximum Strength Caplets and Gelcaps 1571
TYLENOL Cold Medication, Multi-Symptom Formula Tablets and Caplets 1572
TYLENOL Cold Medication, Multi-Symptom Hot Liquid Packets....... 1572
Vicks 44 LiquiCaps Cough, Cold & Flu Relief....... 728
Vicks 44M Cough, Cold & Flu Relief....... 729

Chlorpheniramine Polistirex (Depressant effects of morphine may be enhanced). Products include:
Tussionex Pennkinetic Extended-Release Suspension 1624

Chlorpheniramine Tannate (Depressant effects of morphine may be enhanced). Products include:
Atrohist Pediatric Suspension 1604
Atrohist Pediatric Suspension Dye-Free 1604
Rynatan 2781
Rynatuss 2782

Chlorpromazine (Respiratory depression, hypotension, and profound sedation or coma may result; depressant effects of morphine may be enhanced; analgesic effect of morphine potentiated). Products include:
Thorazine Suppositories....... 2701

Chlorprothixene (Respiratory depression, hypotension, and profound sedation or coma may result; depressant effects of morphine may be enhanced).
No products indexed under this heading.

Chlorprothixene Hydrochloride (Respiratory depression, hypotension, and profound sedation or coma may result; depressant effects of morphine may be enhanced).
No products indexed under this heading.

Chlorprothixene Lactate (Respiratory depression, hypotension, and profound sedation or coma may result; depressant effects of morphine may be enhanced).
No products indexed under this heading.

Clemastine Fumarate (Depressant effects of morphine may be enhanced). Products include:
Tavist Syrup....... 2426
Tavist Tablets 2427
Tavist-1 12 Hour Relief Tablets 749
Tavist-D 12 Hour Relief Tablets 750

Clomipramine Hydrochloride (Respiratory depression, hypotension, and profound sedation or coma may result). Products include:
Anafranil Capsules 819

Clorazepate Dipotassium (Respiratory depression, hypotension, and profound sedation or coma may result; depressant effects of morphine may be enhanced). Products include:
Tranxene 459

IMPORTANT NOTE: Always consult each drug listing in the patient's regimen for possible interactions.

Roxanol / Interactions Index 950

Clozapine (Respiratory depression, hypotension, and profound sedation or coma may result; depressant effects of morphine may be enhanced). Products include:
- Clozaril Tablets 2377

Codeine Phosphate (Respiratory depression, hypotension, and profound sedation or coma may result; depressant effects of morphine may be enhanced). Products include:
- Brontex 2130
- Dimetane-DC Cough Syrup 2232
- Fioricet with Codeine Capsules 2387
- Fiorinal with Codeine Capsules 2390
- Nucofed 2225
- Phenergan with Codeine 2883
- Phenergan VC with Codeine 2888
- Robitussin A-C Syrup 2248
- Robitussin-DAC Syrup 2249
- Ryna 804
- Soma Compound w/Codeine Tablets 2784
- Tylenol with Codeine 1592

Cyproheptadine Hydrochloride (Depressant effects of morphine may be enhanced). Products include:
- Periactin 1767

Dalteparin Sodium (Anticoagulant activity may be increased). Products include:
- Fragmin Injection 2088

Desflurane (Respiratory depression, hypotension, and profound sedation or coma may result; depressant effects of morphine may be enhanced). Products include:
- Suprane (desflurane, USP) 1865

Desipramine Hydrochloride (Respiratory depression, hypotension, and profound sedation or coma may result). Products include:
- Norpramin Tablets 1273

Dexchlorpheniramine Maleate (Depressant effects of morphine may be enhanced).
- No products indexed under this heading.

Dezocine (Respiratory depression, hypotension, and profound sedation or coma may result; depressant effects of morphine may be enhanced). Products include:
- Dalgan Injection 529

Diazepam (Respiratory depression, hypotension, and profound sedation or coma may result; depressant effects of morphine may be enhanced). Products include:
- Dizac (diazepam injectable emulsion) CIV 1862
- Valium Injectable 2336
- Valium Tablets 2335

Dicumarol (Anticoagulant activity may be increased).
- No products indexed under this heading.

Diphenhydramine Citrate (Depressant effects of morphine may be enhanced). Products include:
- Excedrin P.M. Analgesic/Sleeping Aid Tablets, Caplets, Liquigels 735

Diphenhydramine Hydrochloride (Depressant effects of morphine may be enhanced). Products include:
- Actifed Allergy Daytime/Nighttime Caplets 808
- Actifed Sinus Daytime/Nighttime Tablets and Caplets 809
- Extra Strength Bayer PM Aspirin Plus Sleep Aid 617
- Benadryl Allergy Chewables 811
- Benadryl Allergy/Cold Tablets 811
- Benadryl Allergy Decongestant Liquid Medication 812
- Benadryl Allergy Decongestant Tablets 812
- Benadryl Allergy Liquid Medication 813
- Benadryl Allergy 811
- Benadryl Allergy Sinus Headache Caplets 813
- Benadryl Dye-Free Allergy Liquigel Softgels 813
- Benadryl Dye-Free Allergy Liquid Medication 814
- Benadryl Itch Relief Stick Extra Strength 814
- Benadryl Cream 814
- Benadryl Gel 815
- Benadryl Spray 815
- Benadryl Injection 1955
- Contac Day & Night Cold/Flu Night Caplets 772
- Contac Night Allergy/Sinus Caplets 771
- Extra Strength Doan's P.M. 653
- Excedrin P.M. Analgesic/Sleeping Aid Tablets, Caplets, Liquigels 643
- Nytol QuickCaps Caplets 632
- Sleepinal Night-time Sleep Aid Capsules and Softgels 798
- TYLENOL Allergy Sinus NightTime, Maximum Strength Caplets 1571
- TYLENOL Flu NightTime, Maximum Strength Gelcaps 1575
- TYLENOL Flu NightTime, Maximum Strength Hot Medication Packets 1575
- TYLENOL PM Pain Reliever/Sleep Aid, Extra Strength Gelcaps, Caplets, Geltabs 1576
- TYLENOL Severe Allergy Medication Caplets 1571
- Maximum Strength Unisom Sleepgels 1990
- Unisom With Pain Relief-Nighttime Sleep Aid and Pain Reliever 1991

Diphenylpyraline Hydrochloride (Depressant effects of morphine may be enhanced).
- No products indexed under this heading.

Doxepin Hydrochloride (Respiratory depression, hypotension, and profound sedation or coma may result). Products include:
- Adapin Capsules 1542
- Sinequan 2028
- Zonalon Cream 1042

Droperidol (Respiratory depression, hypotension, and profound sedation or coma may result; depressant effects of morphine may be enhanced). Products include:
- Inapsine Injection 462

Enflurane (Respiratory depression, hypotension, and profound sedation or coma may result; depressant effects of morphine may be enhanced).
- No products indexed under this heading.

Enoxaparin (Anticoagulant activity may be increased). Products include:
- Lovenox Injection 2187

Esmolol Hydrochloride (Depressant effects of morphine may be enhanced). Products include:
- Brevibloc (esmolol HCl) Injection 1860

Estazolam (Respiratory depression, hypotension, and profound sedation or coma may result; depressant effects of morphine may be enhanced). Products include:
- ProSom Tablets 457

Ethchlorvynol (Respiratory depression, hypotension, and profound sedation or coma may result; depressant effects of morphine may be enhanced). Products include:
- Placidyl Capsules 456

Ethinamate (Respiratory depression, hypotension, and profound sedation or coma may result; depressant effects of morphine may be enhanced).
- No products indexed under this heading.

Fentanyl (Respiratory depression, hypotension, and profound sedation or coma may result; depressant effects of morphine may be enhanced). Products include:
- Duragesic Transdermal System 1336

Fentanyl Citrate (Respiratory depression, hypotension, and profound sedation or coma may result; depressant effects of morphine may be enhanced). Products include:
- Sublimaze Injection 463

Fluphenazine Decanoate (Respiratory depression, hypotension, and profound sedation or coma may result; depressant effects of morphine may be enhanced). Products include:
- Prolixin Decanoate 510

Fluphenazine Enanthate (Respiratory depression, hypotension, and profound sedation or coma may result; depressant effects of morphine may be enhanced). Products include:
- Prolixin Enanthate 510

Fluphenazine Hydrochloride (Respiratory depression, hypotension, and profound sedation or coma may result; depressant effects of morphine may be enhanced). Products include:
- Prolixin 510

Flurazepam Hydrochloride (Respiratory depression, hypotension, and profound sedation or coma may result; depressant effects of morphine may be enhanced). Products include:
- Dalmane Capsules 2329

Furazolidone (Depressant effects of morphine may be enhanced). Products include:
- Furoxone 2221

Glutethimide (Respiratory depression, hypotension, and profound sedation or coma may result; depressant effects of morphine may be enhanced).
- No products indexed under this heading.

Haloperidol (Respiratory depression, hypotension, and profound sedation or coma may result; depressant effects of morphine may be enhanced). Products include:
- Haldol Injection, Tablets and Concentrate 1585

Haloperidol Decanoate (Respiratory depression, hypotension, and profound sedation or coma may result; depressant effects of morphine may be enhanced). Products include:
- Haldol Decanoate 1587

Heparin Calcium (Anticoagulant activity may be increased).
- No products indexed under this heading.

Heparin Sodium (Anticoagulant activity may be increased). Products include:
- Heparin Lock Flush Solution 2831
- Heparin Sodium Injection 2832
- Heparin Sodium Vials 1486

Hydrocodone Bitartrate (Respiratory depression, hypotension, and profound sedation or coma may result; depressant effects of morphine may be enhanced). Products include:
- Codiclear DH Syrup 808
- Duratuss HD Elixir 2750
- Histussin D Liquid 670
- Hycodan Tablets and Syrup 946
- Hycomine Compound Tablets 948
- Hycomine 947
- Hycotuss Expectorant Syrup 950
- Hydrocet Capsules 787
- Lorcet 10/650 Tablets 1016
- Lortab 2751
- Tussend 1830
- Tussend Expectorant 1831
- Vicodin Tablets 1404
- Vicodin ES Tablets 1405
- Vicodin HP Tablets 1403
- Vicodin Tuss Expectorant 1406
- Zydone Capsules 967

Hydrocodone Polistirex (Respiratory depression, hypotension, and profound sedation or coma may result; depressant effects of morphine may be enhanced). Products include:
- Tussionex Pennkinetic Extended-Release Suspension 1624

Hydroxyzine Hydrochloride (Respiratory depression, hypotension, and profound sedation or coma may result; depressant effects of morphine may be enhanced). Products include:
- Atarax Tablets & Syrup 1992
- Marax Tablets & DF Syrup 2015
- Vistaril Intramuscular Solution 2042

Imipramine Hydrochloride (Respiratory depression, hypotension, and profound sedation or coma may result). Products include:
- Tofranil Ampuls 873
- Tofranil Tablets 875

Imipramine Pamoate (Respiratory depression, hypotension, and profound sedation or coma may result). Products include:
- Tofranil-PM Capsules 876

Isocarboxazid (Depressant effects of morphine may be enhanced).
- No products indexed under this heading.

Isoflurane (Respiratory depression, hypotension, and profound sedation or coma may result; depressant effects of morphine may be enhanced).
- No products indexed under this heading.

Ketamine Hydrochloride (Respiratory depression, hypotension, and profound sedation or coma may result; depressant effects of morphine may be enhanced).
- No products indexed under this heading.

Labetalol Hydrochloride (Depressant effects of morphine may be enhanced). Products include:
- Normodyne Injection 2519
- Normodyne Tablets 2522
- Trandate 1158

Levobunolol Hydrochloride (Depressant effects of morphine may be enhanced). Products include:
- Betagan 230

Levomethadyl Acetate Hydrochloride (Respiratory depression, hypotension, and profound sedation or coma may result; depressant effects of morphine may be enhanced). Products include:
- Orlaam Oral Solution 2361

Levorphanol Tartrate (Respiratory depression, hypotension, and profound sedation or coma may result; depressant effects of morphine may be enhanced). Products include:
- Levo-Dromoran 2297

Loratadine (Depressant effects of morphine may be enhanced). Products include:
- Claritin Tablets 2485
- Claritin-D Tablets 2487

Lorazepam (Respiratory depression, hypotension, and profound sedation or coma may result; depressant effects of morphine may be enhanced). Products include:
- Ativan Injection 2805

(▣ Described in PDR For Nonprescription Drugs) (⊙ Described in PDR For Ophthalmology)

Ativan Tablets 2807

Loxapine Hydrochloride (Respiratory depression, hypotension, and profound sedation or coma may result; depressant effects of morphine may be enhanced). Products include:
Loxitane 1426

Loxapine Succinate (Respiratory depression, hypotension, and profound sedation or coma may result; depressant effects of morphine may be enhanced). Products include:
Loxitane Capsules 1426

Maprotiline Hydrochloride (Respiratory depression, hypotension, and profound sedation or coma may result). Products include:
Ludiomil Tablets 861

Meperidine Hydrochloride (Respiratory depression, hypotension, and profound sedation or coma may result; depressant effects of morphine may be enhanced). Products include:
Demerol 2438
Mepergan Injection 2859

Mephobarbital (Respiratory depression, hypotension, and profound sedation or coma may result; depressant effects of morphine may be enhanced). Products include:
Mebaral Tablets 2452

Meprobamate (Respiratory depression, hypotension, and profound sedation or coma may result; depressant effects of morphine may be enhanced). Products include:
Miltown Tablets 2780
PMB 200 and PMB 400 2890

Mesoridazine Besylate (Respiratory depression, hypotension, and profound sedation or coma may result; depressant effects of morphine may be enhanced). Products include:
Serentil 689

Methadone Hydrochloride (Respiratory depression, hypotension, and profound sedation or coma may result; depressant effects of morphine may be enhanced). Products include:
Methadone Hydrochloride Oral Concentrate 2356
Methadone Hydrochloride Oral Solution & Tablets 2357

Methdilazine Hydrochloride (Depressant effects of morphine may be enhanced).
No products indexed under this heading.

Methocarbamol (Analgesic effect of morphine potentiated). Products include:
Robaxin Injectable 2245
Robaxin Tablets 2246
Robaxisal Tablets 2246

Methohexital Sodium (Respiratory depression, hypotension, and profound sedation or coma may result; depressant effects of morphine may be enhanced).
No products indexed under this heading.

Methotrimeprazine (Respiratory depression, hypotension, and profound sedation or coma may result; depressant effects of morphine may be enhanced). Products include:
Levoprome 1321

Methoxyflurane (Respiratory depression, hypotension, and profound sedation or coma may result; depressant effects of morphine may be enhanced).
No products indexed under this heading.

Metipranolol Hydrochloride (Depressant effects of morphine may be enhanced). Products include:
OptiPranolol (Metipranolol 0.3%) Sterile Ophthalmic Solution ...... © 256

Metoprolol Succinate (Depressant effects of morphine may be enhanced). Products include:
Toprol-XL Tablets 560

Metoprolol Tartrate (Depressant effects of morphine may be enhanced). Products include:
Lopressor 848
Lopressor HCT Tablets 850

Midazolam Hydrochloride (Respiratory depression, hypotension, and profound sedation or coma may result; depressant effects of morphine may be enhanced). Products include:
Versed Injection 2324

Molindone Hydrochloride (Respiratory depression, hypotension, and profound sedation or coma may result; depressant effects of morphine may be enhanced). Products include:
Moban Tablets and Concentrate 1036

Nadolol (Depressant effects of morphine may be enhanced).
No products indexed under this heading.

Nortriptyline Hydrochloride (Respiratory depression, hypotension, and profound sedation or coma may result). Products include:
Pamelor 2409

Opium Alkaloids (Respiratory depression hypotension, and profound sedation or coma may result; depressant effects of morphine may be enhanced).
No products indexed under this heading.

Oxazepam (Respiratory depression, hypotension, and profound sedation or coma may result; depressant effects of morphine may be enhanced). Products include:
Serax Capsules 2916
Serax Tablets 2916

Oxycodone Hydrochloride (Respiratory depression, hypotension, and profound sedation or coma may result; depressant effects of morphine may be enhanced). Products include:
OxyContin Tablets 2163
OxyIR Capsules 2167
Percocet Tablets 955
Percodan Tablets 955
Percodan-Demi Tablets 956
Roxicodone Tablets, Oral Solution & Intensol (Oxycodone) 2366
Tylox Capsules 1593

Penbutolol Sulfate (Depressant effects of morphine may be enhanced). Products include:
Levatol Tablets 2547

Pentobarbital Sodium (Respiratory depression, hypotension, and profound sedation or coma may result; depressant effects of morphine sulfate may be enhanced). Products include:
Nembutal Sodium Capsules 440
Nembutal Sodium Solution 442
Nembutal Sodium Suppositories ... 444

Perphenazine (Respiratory depression, hypotension, and profound sedation or coma may result; depressant effects of morphine may be enhanced). Products include:
Etrafon 2495
Triavil Tablets 1800
Trilafon 2532

Phenelzine Sulfate (Depressant effects of morphine may be enhanced). Products include:
Nardil 1977

Phenobarbital (Respiratory depression, hypotension, and profound sedation or coma may result; depressant effects of morphine may be enhanced). Products include:
Arco-Lase Plus Tablets 513
Bellergal-S Tablets 2375
Donnatal 2234
Donnatal Extentabs 2234
Donnatal Tablets 2234
Phenobarbital Elixir and Tablets 1523
Quadrinal Tablets 1398

Pindolol (Depressant effects of morphine may be enhanced). Products include:
Visken Tablets 2428

Potassium Acid Phosphate (Effects of morphine may be antagonized). Products include:
K-Phos Original Formula 'Sodium Free' Tablets 633

Potassium Citrate (Effects of morphine may be potentiated). Products include:
Polycitra Syrup 574
Polycitra-K Crystals 574
Polycitra-K Oral Solution 575
Polycitra-LC 574
Urocit-K Tablets 1828

Prazepam (Respiratory depression, hypotension, and profound sedation or coma may result; depressant effects of morphine may be enhanced).
No products indexed under this heading.

Procarbazine Hydrochloride (Depressant effects of morphine may be enhanced). Products include:
Matulane Capsules 2300

Prochlorperazine (Respiratory depression, hypotension, and profound sedation or coma may result; depressant effects of morphine may be enhanced; analgesic effect of morphine potentiated). Products include:
Compazine 2644

Promethazine Hydrochloride (Respiratory depression, hypotension, and profound sedation or coma may result; depressant effects of morphine may be enhanced). Products include:
Mepergan Injection 2859
Phenergan with Codeine 2883
Phenergan with Dextromethorphan 2885
Phenergan Injection 2880
Phenergan Suppositories 2882
Phenergan Syrup 2881
Phenergan Tablets 2882
Phenergan VC 2886
Phenergan VC with Codeine 2888

Propofol (Respiratory depression, hypotension, and profound sedation or coma may result; depressant effects of morphine may be enhanced). Products include:
Diprivan Injectable Emulsion 2939

Propoxyphene Hydrochloride (Respiratory depression, hypotension, and profound sedation or coma may result; depressant effects of morphine may be enhanced). Products include:
Darvon 1475
Wygesic Tablets 2930

Propoxyphene Napsylate (Respiratory depression, hypotension, and profound sedation or coma may result; depressant effects of morphine may be enhanced). Products include:
Darvon-N/Darvocet-N 1473

Propranolol Hydrochloride (Depressant effects of morphine may be enhanced). Products include:
Inderal 2834
Inderal LA Long Acting Capsules 2836
Inderide Tablets 2838
Inderide LA Long Acting Capsules .. 2840

Protriptyline Hydrochloride (Respiratory depression, hypotension, and profound sedation or coma may result). Products include:
Vivactil Tablets 1820

Pyrilamine Maleate (Depressant effects of morphine may be enhanced). Products include:
4-Way Fast Acting Nasal Spray (regular & mentholated) .... © 644
Maximum Strength Multi-Symptom Formula Midol .... © 621
PMS Multi-Symptom Formula Midol .... © 622

Pyrilamine Tannate (Depressant effects of morphine may be enhanced). Products include:
Atrohist Pediatric Suspension 1604
Atrohist Pediatric Suspension Dye-Free 1604
Rynatan 2781

Quazepam (Respiratory depression, hypotension, and profound sedation or coma may result; depressant effects of morphine may be enhanced). Products include:
Doral Tablets 2773

Risperidone (Respiratory depression, hypotension, and profound sedation or coma may result; depressant effects of morphine may be enhanced). Products include:
Risperdal Tablets 1348

Secobarbital Sodium (Respiratory depression, hypotension, and profound sedation or coma may result; depressant effects of morphine may be enhanced). Products include:
Seconal Sodium Pulvules 1529

Selegiline Hydrochloride (Depressant effects of morphine may be enhanced). Products include:
Eldepryl Capsules 2729

Sevoflurane (Respiratory depression, hypotension, and profound sedation or coma may result; depressant effects of morphine may be enhanced).
No products indexed under this heading.

Sodium Acid Phosphate (Effects of morphine may be antagonized). Products include:
Uroqid-Acid No. 2 Tablets 633

Sodium Citrate (Effects of morphine may be potentiated). Products include:
Bicitra 573
Polycitra 574
Salix SST Lozenges Saliva Stimulant .... © 757

Sotalol Hydrochloride (Depressant effects of morphine may be enhanced). Products include:
Betapace Tablets 637

Sufentanil Citrate (Respiratory depression, hypotension, and profound sedation or coma may result; depressant effects of morphine may be enhanced). Products include:
Sufenta Injection 1355

Temazepam (Respiratory depression, hypotension, and profound sedation or coma may result; depressant effects of morphine may be enhanced). Products include:
Restoril Capsules 2413

Terfenadine (Depressant effects of morphine may be enhanced). Products include:
Seldane Tablets 1284

IMPORTANT NOTE: Always consult each drug listing in the patient's regimen for possible interactions.

Roxanol — Interactions Index

Seldane-D Extended-Release Tablets 1286

Thiamylal Sodium (Respiratory depression, hypotension, and profound sedation or coma may result; depressant effects of morphine may be enhanced).
 No products indexed under this heading.

Thioridazine Hydrochloride (Respiratory depression, hypotension, and profound sedation or coma may result; depressant effects of morphine may be enhanced). Products include:
 Mellaril 2398

Thiothixene (Respiratory depression, hypotension, and profound sedation or coma may result; depressant effects of morphine may be enhanced). Products include:
 Navane Capsules and Concentrate .. 2018
 Navane Intramuscular 2019

Timolol Hemihydrate (Depressant effects of morphine may be enhanced). Products include:
 Betimol 0.25%, 0.5% .... ⊚ 259

Timolol Maleate (Depressant effects of morphine may be enhanced). Products include:
 Blocadren Tablets 1654
 Timolide Tablets 1791
 Timoptic in Ocudose 1796
 Timoptic Sterile Ophthalmic Solution 1794
 Timoptic-XE 1798

Tranylcypromine Sulfate (Depressant effects of morphine may be enhanced). Products include:
 Parnate Tablets 2679

Triazolam (Respiratory depression, hypotension, and profound sedation or coma may result; depressant effects of morphine may be enhanced). Products include:
 Halcion Tablets 2093

Trifluoperazine Hydrochloride (Respiratory depression, hypotension, and profound sedation or coma may result; depressant effects of morphine may be enhanced). Products include:
 Stelazine 2692

Trimeprazine Tartrate (Depressant effects of morphine may be enhanced).
 No products indexed under this heading.

Trimipramine Maleate (Respiratory depression, hypotension, and profound sedation or coma may result). Products include:
 Surmontil Capsules 2917

Tripelennamine Hydrochloride (Depressant effects of morphine may be enhanced). Products include:
 PBZ Tablets 863
 PBZ-SR Tablets 862

Triprolidine Hydrochloride (Depressant effects of morphine may be enhanced). Products include:
 Actifed Cold & Allergy Tablets ..... ▣ 807
 Actifed Cold & Sinus Caplets and Tablets .... ▣ 808

Warfarin Sodium (Anticoagulant activity may be increased). Products include:
 Coumadin 941

Zolpidem Tartrate (Respiratory depression, hypotension, and profound sedation or coma may result; depressant effects of morphine may be enhanced). Products include:
 Ambien Tablets 2559

Food Interactions

Alcohol (Respiratory depression, hypotension, and profound sedation or coma

may result; depressant effects of morphine may be enhanced).

ROXANOL 100 (MORPHINE SULFATE CONCENTRATED ORAL SOLUTION)
(Morphine Sulfate) 2365
 See **Roxanol (Morphine Sulfate Concentrated Oral Solution)**

ROXICODONE TABLETS, ORAL SOLUTION & INTENSOL (OXYCODONE)
(Oxycodone Hydrochloride) 2366
May interact with central nervous system depressants and certain other agents. Compounds in these categories include:

Alfentanil Hydrochloride (Possible additive CNS depression). Products include:
 Alfenta Injection 1334

Alprazolam (Possible additive CNS depression). Products include:
 Xanax Tablets 2115

Aprobarbital (Possible additive CNS depression).
 No products indexed under this heading.

Buprenorphine (Possible additive CNS depression). Products include:
 Buprenex Injectable 2170

Buspirone Hydrochloride (Possible additive CNS depression). Products include:
 BuSpar Tablets 738

Butabarbital (Possible additive CNS depression).
 No products indexed under this heading.

Butalbital (Possible additive CNS depression). Products include:
 Axocet Capsules 2469
 Esgic-plus Capsules 1012
 Esgic-plus Tablets 1012
 Fioricet Tablets 2386
 Fioricet with Codeine Capsules 2387
 Fiorinal Capsules 2388
 Fiorinal with Codeine Capsules 2390
 Fiorinal Tablets 2388
 Phrenilin 790
 Sedapap Tablets 50 mg/650 mg ... 1826

Chlordiazepoxide (Possible additive CNS depression). Products include:
 Limbitrol 2333

Chlordiazepoxide Hydrochloride (Possible additive CNS depression). Products include:
 Librax Capsules 2330
 Librium Capsules 2331
 Librium Injectable 2332

Chlorpromazine (Possible additive CNS depression). Products include:
 Thorazine Suppositories 2701

Chlorprothixene (Possible additive CNS depression).
 No products indexed under this heading.

Chlorprothixene Hydrochloride (Possible additive CNS depression).
 No products indexed under this heading.

Chlorprothixene Lactate (Possible additive CNS depression).
 No products indexed under this heading.

Clorazepate Dipotassium (Possible additive CNS depression). Products include:
 Tranxene 459

Clozapine (Possible additive CNS depression). Products include:
 Clozaril Tablets 2377

Codeine Phosphate (Possible additive CNS depression). Products include:
 Brontex 2130
 Dimetane-DC Cough Syrup 2232
 Fioricet with Codeine Capsules 2387
 Fiorinal with Codeine Capsules 2390
 Nucofed 2225
 Phenergan with Codeine 2883
 Phenergan VC with Codeine 2888
 Robitussin A-C Syrup 2248
 Robitussin-DAC Syrup 2249
 Ryna .... ▣ 804
 Soma Compound w/Codeine Tablets 2784
 Tylenol with Codeine 1592

Desflurane (Possible additive CNS depression). Products include:
 Suprane (desflurane, USP) 1865

Dezocine (Possible additive CNS depression). Products include:
 Dalgan Injection 529

Diazepam (Possible additive CNS depression). Products include:
 Dizac (diazepam injectable emulsion) CIV 1862
 Valium Injectable 2336
 Valium Tablets 2335

Droperidol (Possible additive CNS depression). Products include:
 Inapsine Injection 462

Enflurane (Possible additive CNS depression).
 No products indexed under this heading.

Estazolam (Possible additive CNS depression). Products include:
 ProSom Tablets 457

Ethchlorvynol (Possible additive CNS depression). Products include:
 Placidyl Capsules 456

Ethinamate (Possible additive CNS depression).
 No products indexed under this heading.

Fentanyl (Possible additive CNS depression). Products include:
 Duragesic Transdermal System 1336

Fentanyl Citrate (Possible additive CNS depression). Products include:
 Sublimaze Injection 463

Fluphenazine Decanoate (Possible additive CNS depression). Products include:
 Prolixin Decanoate 510

Fluphenazine Enanthate (Possible additive CNS depression). Products include:
 Prolixin Enanthate 510

Fluphenazine Hydrochloride (Possible additive CNS depression). Products include:
 Prolixin 510

Flurazepam Hydrochloride (Possible additive CNS depression). Products include:
 Dalmane Capsules 2329

Glutethimide (Possible additive CNS depression).
 No products indexed under this heading.

Haloperidol (Possible additive CNS depression). Products include:
 Haldol Injection, Tablets and Concentrate 1585

Haloperidol Decanoate (Possible additive CNS depression). Products include:
 Haldol Decanoate 1587

Hydrocodone Bitartrate (Possible additive CNS depression). Products include:
 Codiclear DH Syrup 808
 Duratuss HD Elixir 2750
 Histussin D Liquid 670
 Hycodan Tablets and Syrup 946
 Hycomine Compound Tablets 948
 Hycomine 947
 Hycotuss Expectorant Syrup 950
 Hydrocet Capsules 787
 Lorcet 10/650 Tablets 1016
 Lortab 2751
 Tussend 1830
 Tussend Expectorant 1831
 Vicodin Tablets 1404
 Vicodin ES Tablets 1405
 Vicodin HP Tablets 1403
 Vicodin Tuss Expectorant 1406
 Zydone Capsules 967

Hydrocodone Polistirex (Possible additive CNS depression). Products include:
 Tussionex Pennkinetic Extended-Release Suspension 1624

Hydroxyzine Hydrochloride (Possible additive CNS depression). Products include:
 Atarax Tablets & Syrup 1992
 Marax Tablets & DF Syrup 2015
 Vistaril Intramuscular Solution 2042

Isoflurane (Possible additive CNS depression).
 No products indexed under this heading.

Ketamine Hydrochloride (Possible additive CNS depression).
 No products indexed under this heading.

Levomethadyl Acetate Hydrochloride (Possible additive CNS depression). Products include:
 Orlaam Oral Solution 2361

Levorphanol Tartrate (Possible additive CNS depression). Products include:
 Levo-Dromoran 2297

Lorazepam (Possible additive CNS depression). Products include:
 Ativan Injection 2805
 Ativan Tablets 2807

Loxapine Hydrochloride (Possible additive CNS depression). Products include:
 Loxitane 1426

Loxapine Succinate (Possible additive CNS depression). Products include:
 Loxitane Capsules 1426

Meperidine Hydrochloride (Possible additive CNS depression). Products include:
 Demerol 2438
 Mepergan Injection 2859

Mephobarbital (Possible additive CNS depression). Products include:
 Mebaral Tablets 2452

Meprobamate (Possible additive CNS depression). Products include:
 Miltown Tablets 2780
 PMB 200 and PMB 400 2890

Mesoridazine Besylate (Possible additive CNS depression). Products include:
 Serentil 689

Methadone Hydrochloride (Possible additive CNS depression). Products include:
 Methadone Hydrochloride Oral Concentrate 2356
 Methadone Hydrochloride Oral Solution & Tablets 2357

Methohexital Sodium (Possible additive CNS depression).
 No products indexed under this heading.

Methotrimeprazine (Possible additive CNS depression). Products include:
 Levoprome 1321

Methoxyflurane (Possible additive CNS depression).
 No products indexed under this heading.

Midazolam Hydrochloride (Possible additive CNS depression). Products include:
 Versed Injection 2324

(▣ Described in PDR For Nonprescription Drugs) (⊚ Described in PDR For Ophthalmology)

Molindone Hydrochloride (Possible additive CNS depression). Products include:
  Moban Tablets and Concentrate 1036
Morphine Sulfate (Possible additive CNS depression). Products include:
  Astramorph/PF Injection, USP (Preservative-Free) 526
  Duramorph Injection 983
  Infumorph 200 and Infumorph 500 Sterile Solutions 985
  Kadian Capsules 2948
  MS Contin Tablets 2149
  MSIR 2152
  Oramorph SR (Morphine Sulfate Sustained Release Tablets) 2359
  RMS Suppositories CII 2766
  Roxanol 2365
Opium Alkaloids (Possible additive CNS depression).
  No products indexed under this heading.
Oxazepam (Possible additive CNS depression). Products include:
  Serax Capsules 2916
  Serax Tablets 2916
Pentobarbital Sodium (Possible additive CNS depression). Products include:
  Nembutal Sodium Capsules 440
  Nembutal Sodium Solution 442
  Nembutal Sodium Suppositories 444
Perphenazine (Possible additive CNS depression). Products include:
  Etrafon 2495
  Triavil Tablets 1800
  Trilafon 2532
Phenobarbital (Possible additive CNS depression). Products include:
  Arco-Lase Plus Tablets 513
  Bellergal-S Tablets 2375
  Donnatal 2234
  Donnatal Extentabs 2234
  Donnatal Tablets 2234
  Phenobarbital Elixir and Tablets 1523
  Quadrinal Tablets 1398
Prazepam (Possible additive CNS depression).
  No products indexed under this heading.
Prochlorperazine (Possible additive CNS depression). Products include:
  Compazine 2644
Promethazine Hydrochloride (Possible additive CNS depression). Products include:
  Mepergan Injection 2859
  Phenergan with Codeine 2883
  Phenergan with Dextromethorphan 2885
  Phenergan Injection 2880
  Phenergan Suppositories 2882
  Phenergan Syrup 2881
  Phenergan Tablets 2882
  Phenergan VC 2886
  Phenergan VC with Codeine 2888
Propofol (Possible additive CNS depression). Products include:
  Diprivan Injectable Emulsion 2939
Propoxyphene Hydrochloride (Possible additive CNS depression). Products include:
  Darvon 1475
  Wygesic Tablets 2930
Propoxyphene Napsylate (Possible additive CNS depression). Products include:
  Darvon-N/Darvocet-N 1473
Quazepam (Possible additive CNS depression). Products include:
  Doral Tablets 2773
Risperidone (Possible additive CNS depression). Products include:
  Risperdal Tablets 1348
Secobarbital Sodium (Possible additive CNS depression). Products include:
  Seconal Sodium Pulvules 1529

Sevoflurane (Possible additive CNS depression).
  No products indexed under this heading.
Sufentanil Citrate (Possible additive CNS depression). Products include:
  Sufenta Injection 1355
Temazepam (Possible additive CNS depression). Products include:
  Restoril Capsules 2413
Thiamylal Sodium (Possible additive CNS depression).
  No products indexed under this heading.
Thioridazine Hydrochloride (Possible additive CNS depression). Products include:
  Mellaril 2398
Thiothixene (Possible additive CNS depression). Products include:
  Navane Capsules and Concentrate 2018
  Navane Intramuscular 2019
Triazolam (Possible additive CNS depression). Products include:
  Halcion Tablets 2093
Trifluoperazine Hydrochloride (Possible additive CNS depression). Products include:
  Stelazine 2692
Zolpidem Tartrate (Possible additive CNS depression). Products include:
  Ambien Tablets 2559

Food Interactions
Alcohol (Possible additive CNS depression).

RUBEX FOR INJECTION
(Doxorubicin Hydrochloride) 721
May interact with antineoplastics, calcium channel blockers, and certain other agents. Compounds in these categories include:

Altretamine (Doxorubicin may potentiate the toxicity of other anticancer therapies). Products include:
  Hexalen Capsules 2760
Amlodipine Besylate (Co-administration with calcium channel entry blockers may increase the risk of doxorubicin-induced cardiotoxicity). Products include:
  Lotrel Capsules 858
  Norvasc Tablets 2020
Anastrozole (Doxorubicin may potentiate the toxicity of other anticancer therapies). Products include:
  Arimidex Tablets 2932
Asparaginase (Doxorubicin may potentiate the toxicity of other anticancer therapies). Products include:
  Elspar 1700
Bepridil Hydrochloride (Co-administration with calcium channel entry blockers may increase the risk of doxorubicin-induced cardiotoxicity). Products include:
  Vascor Tablets (200 and 300 mg) 1597
Bicalutamide (Doxorubicin may potentiate the toxicity of other anticancer therapies). Products include:
  Casodex Tablets 2934
Bleomycin Sulfate (Doxorubicin may potentiate the toxicity of other anticancer therapies). Products include:
  Blenoxane 697
Busulfan (Doxorubicin may potentiate the toxicity of other anticancer therapies). Products include:
  Myleran Tablets 1209
Carboplatin (Doxorubicin may potentiate the toxicity of other anticancer therapies). Products include:
  Paraplatin for Injection 713

Carmustine (BCNU) (Doxorubicin may potentiate the toxicity of other anticancer therapies). Products include:
  BiCNU 696
Chlorambucil (Doxorubicin may potentiate the toxicity of other anticancer therapies). Products include:
  Leukeran Tablets 1205
Cisplatin (Doxorubicin may potentiate the toxicity of other anticancer therapies). Products include:
  Platinol for Injection 717
  Platinol-AQ Injection 719
Cyclophosphamide (Doxorubicin may potentiate the toxicity of other anticancer therapies; serious irreversible myocardial toxicity; exacerbation of cyclopyhosphamide-induced hemorrhagic cystitis). Products include:
  Cytoxan 700
Cyclosporine (Co-administration may result in coma and/or seizures). Products include:
  Neoral 2405
  Sandimmune 2416
Cytarabine (Combination therapy results in necrotizing colitis, typhilitis, bloody stools and severe infections). Products include:
  Cytosar-U Sterile Powder 2077
Dacarbazine (Doxorubicin may potentiate the toxicity of other anticancer therapies). Products include:
  DTIC-Dome 593
Daunorubicin Citrate (Doxorubicin may potentiate the toxicity of other anticancer therapies; concurrent use is contraindicated in patients who have received previous treatment with complete cumulative doses of daunorubicin). Products include:
  DaunoXome 1842
Daunorubicin Hydrochloride (Doxorubicin may potentiate the toxicity of other anticancer therapies; concurrent use is contraindicated in patients who have received previous treatment with complete cumulative doses of daunorubicin). Products include:
  Cerubidine for Injection 634
Diltiazem Hydrochloride (Co-administration with calcium channel entry blockers may increase the risk of doxorubicin-induced cardiotoxicity). Products include:
  Cardizem CD Capsules 1251
  Cardizem SR Capsules 1255
  Cardizem Injectable 1253
  Cardizem Tablets 1257
  Dilacor XR Extended-release Capsules 2183
  Tiazac Capsules 1019
Docetaxel (Doxorubicin may potentiate the toxicity of other anticancer therapies). Products include:
  Taxotere for Injection Concentrate 2204
Estramustine Phosphate Sodium (Doxorubicin may potentiate the toxicity of other anticancer therapies). Products include:
  Emcyt Capsules 2085
Etoposide (Doxorubicin may potentiate the toxicity of other anticancer therapies). Products include:
  Etoposide Injection 539
  VePesid Capsules and Injection 727
Felodipine (Co-administration with calcium channel entry blockers may increase the risk of doxorubicin-induced cardiotoxicity). Products include:
  Plendil Extended-Release Tablets 514

Floxuridine (Doxorubicin may potentiate the toxicity of other anticancer therapies). Products include:
  Sterile FUDR 2284
Fluorouracil (Doxorubicin may potentiate the toxicity of other anticancer therapies). Products include:
  Efudex 2280
  Fluoroplex Topical Solution & Cream 1% 475
  Fluorouracil Injection 2282
Flutamide (Doxorubicin may potentiate the toxicity of other anticancer therapies). Products include:
  Eulexin Capsules 2498
Fosphenytoin Sodium (Co-administration may result in decreased phenytoin levels). Products include:
  Cerebyx Injection 1956
Gemcitabine Hydrochloride (Doxorubicin may potentiate the toxicity of other anticancer therapies). Products include:
  Gemzar for Injection 1482
Hydroxyurea (Doxorubicin may potentiate the toxicity of other anticancer therapies). Products include:
  Hydrea Capsules 705
Idarubicin Hydrochloride (Doxorubicin may potentiate the toxicity of other anticancer therapies; concurrent use is contraindicated in patients who have received previous treatment with complete cumulative doses of idarubicin). Products include:
  Idamycin Injection 2096
Ifosfamide (Doxorubicin may potentiate the toxicity of other anticancer therapies). Products include:
  IFEX 706
Interferon alfa-2A, Recombinant (Doxorubicin may potentiate the toxicity of other anticancer therapies). Products include:
  Roferon-A Injection 2308
Interferon alfa-2B, Recombinant (Doxorubicin may potentiate the toxicity of other anticancer therapies). Products include:
  Intron A for Injection 2506
Irinotecan Hydrochloride (Doxorubicin may potentiate the toxicity of other anticancer therapies).
  No products indexed under this heading.
Isradipine (Co-administration with calcium channel entry blockers may increase the risk of doxorubicin-induced cardiotoxicity). Products include:
  DynaCirc Capsules 2381
  DynaCirc CR Tablets 2383
Levamisole Hydrochloride (Doxorubicin may potentiate the toxicity of other anticancer therapies). Products include:
  Ergamisol Tablets 1340
Live Virus Vaccines (Administration of live vaccine to immunosuppressed patients may be hazardous).
Lomustine (CCNU) (Doxorubicin may potentiate the toxicity of other anticancer therapies). Products include:
  CeeNU Capsules 699
Mechlorethamine Hydrochloride (Doxorubicin may potentiate the toxicity of other anticancer therapies). Products include:
  Mustargen 1752
Megestrol Acetate (Doxorubicin may potentiate the toxicity of other anticancer therapies). Products include:
  Megace Oral Suspension 708
  Megace Tablets 710

IMPORTANT NOTE: Always consult each drug listing in the patient's regimen for possible interactions.

Melphalan (Doxorubicin may potentiate the toxicity of other anticancer therapies). Products include:
Alkeran Tablets ... 1198

Mercaptopurine (Doxorubicin may potentiate the toxicity of other anticancer therapies; enhanced hepatotoxicity of 6-mercaptopurine). Products include:
Purinethol Tablets ... 1214

Methotrexate Sodium (Doxorubicin may potentiate the toxicity of other anticancer therapies). Products include:
Methotrexate Sodium Tablets, Injection, for Injection and LPF Injection ... 1322

Mitomycin (Mitomycin-C) (Doxorubicin may potentiate the toxicity of other anticancer therapies). Products include:
Mutamycin for Injection ... 712

Mitotane (Doxorubicin may potentiate the toxicity of other anticancer therapies). Products include:
Lysodren Tablets ... 707

Mitoxantrone Hydrochloride (Doxorubicin may potentiate the toxicity of other anticancer therapies). Products include:
Novantrone for Injection ... 1327

Nicardipine Hydrochloride (Co-administration with calcium channel entry blockers may increase the risk of doxorubicin-induced cardiotoxicity). Products include:
Cardene Capsules ... 2261
Cardene I.V. ... 2815
Cardene SR Capsules ... 2264

Nifedipine (Co-administration with calcium channel entry blockers may increase the risk of doxorubicin-induced cardiotoxicity). Products include:
Adalat Capsules (10 mg and 20 mg) ... 580
Adalat CC ... 582
Procardia Capsules ... 2024
Procardia XL Extended Release Tablets ... 2026

Nimodipine (Co-administration with calcium channel entry blockers may increase the risk of doxorubicin-induced cardiotoxicity). Products include:
Nimotop Capsules ... 603

Nisoldipine (Co-administration with calcium channel entry blockers may increase the risk of doxorubicin-induced cardiotoxicity). Products include:
Sular Tablets ... 2961

Paclitaxel (Doxorubicin may potentiate the toxicity of other anticancer therapies). Products include:
Taxol Injection ... 723

Phenobarbital (Increases the elimination of doxorubicin). Products include:
Arco-Lase Plus Tablets ... 513
Bellergal-S Tablets ... 2375
Donnatal ... 2234
Donnatal Extentabs ... 2234
Donnatal Tablets ... 2234
Phenobarbital Elixir and Tablets ... 1523
Quadrinal Tablets ... 1398

Phenytoin (Co-administration may result in decreased phenytoin levels). Products include:
Dilantin Infatabs ... 1967
Dilantin-125 Suspension ... 1969

Phenytoin Sodium (Co-administration may result in decreased phenytoin levels). Products include:
Dilantin Kapseals ... 1965

Procarbazine Hydrochloride (Doxorubicin may potentiate the toxicity of other anticancer therapies). Products include:
Matulane Capsules ... 2300

Streptozocin (May inhibit hepatic metabolism; doxorubicin may potentiate the toxicity of other anticancer therapies). Products include:
Zanosar Sterile Powder ... 2119

Tamoxifen Citrate (Doxorubicin may potentiate the toxicity of other anticancer therapies). Products include:
Nolvadex Tablets ... 2957

Teniposide (Doxorubicin may potentiate the toxicity of other anticancer therapies). Products include:
Vumon for Injection ... 729

Thioguanine (Doxorubicin may potentiate the toxicity of other anticancer therapies). Products include:
Thioguanine Tablets, Tabloid Brand ... 1225

Thiotepa (Doxorubicin may potentiate the toxicity of other anticancer therapies). Products include:
Thioplex (Thiotepa For Injection) ... 1329

Topotecan Hydrochloride (Doxorubicin may potentiate the toxicity of other anticancer therapies). Products include:
Hycamtin for Injection ... 2665

Verapamil Hydrochloride (Co-administration with calcium channel entry blockers may increase the risk of doxorubicin-induced cardiotoxicity). Products include:
Calan SR Caplets ... 2571
Calan Tablets ... 2568
Covera-HS Tablets ... 2573
Isoptin Injectable ... 1391
Isoptin Oral Tablets ... 1393
Isoptin SR Tablets ... 1395
Verelan Capsules ... 1455

Vincristine Sulfate (Doxorubicin may potentiate the toxicity of other anticancer therapies). Products include:
Oncovin Solution Vials & Hyporets 1521

Vinorelbine Tartrate (Doxorubicin may potentiate the toxicity of other anticancer therapies). Products include:
Navelbine Injection ... 1212

RUM-K SYRUP
(Potassium Chloride) ... 1004
None cited in PDR database.

RYNA LIQUID
(Chlorpheniramine Maleate, Pseudoephedrine Hydrochloride) ... 804
May interact with:

Furazolidone (Concurrent and/or sequential use is not recommended). Products include:
Furoxone ... 2221

Isocarboxazid (Concurrent and/or sequential use is not recommended).
No products indexed under this heading.

Phenelzine Sulfate (Concurrent and/or sequential use is not recommended). Products include:
Nardil ... 1977

Selegiline Hydrochloride (Concurrent and/or sequential use is not recommended). Products include:
Eldepryl Capsules ... 2729

Tranylcypromine Sulfate (Concurrent and/or sequential use is not recommended). Products include:
Parnate Tablets ... 2679

RYNA-C LIQUID
(Chlorpheniramine Maleate, Codeine Phosphate, Pseudoephedrine Hydrochloride) ... 804
May interact with monoamine oxidase inhibitors and certain other agents. Compounds in these categories include:

Furazolidone (Concurrent and/or sequential use is not recommended). Products include:
Furoxone ... 2221

Isocarboxazid (Concurrent and/or sequential use is not recommended).
No products indexed under this heading.

Phenelzine Sulfate (Concurrent and/or sequential use is not recommended). Products include:
Nardil ... 1977

Selegiline Hydrochloride (Concurrent and/or sequential use is not recommended). Products include:
Eldepryl Capsules ... 2729

Tranylcypromine Sulfate (Concurrent and/or sequential use is not recommended). Products include:
Parnate Tablets ... 2679

Food Interactions

Alcohol (May increase drowsiness effect).

RYNA-CX LIQUID
(Codeine Phosphate, Guaifenesin, Pseudoephedrine Hydrochloride) ... 804
See **Ryna-C Liquid**

RYNATAN TABLETS
(Chlorpheniramine Tannate, Pyrilamine Tannate, Phenylephrine Tannate) ... 2781
See **Rynatan-S Pediatric Suspension**

RYNATAN-S PEDIATRIC SUSPENSION
(Phenylephrine Tannate, Chlorpheniramine Tannate, Pyrilamine Tannate) ... 2781
May interact with monoamine oxidase inhibitors, central nervous system depressants, hypnotics and sedatives, tranquilizers, and certain other agents. Compounds in these categories include:

Alfentanil Hydrochloride (Antihistamines cause drowsiness and co-administration may increase drowsiness effect). Products include:
Alfenta Injection ... 1334

Alprazolam (Antihistamines cause drowsiness and co-administration may increase drowsiness effect). Products include:
Xanax Tablets ... 2115

Aprobarbital (Antihistamines cause drowsiness and co-administration may increase drowsiness effect).
No products indexed under this heading.

Buprenorphine (Antihistamines cause drowsiness and co-administration may increase drowsiness effect). Products include:
Buprenex Injectable ... 2170

Buspirone Hydrochloride (Antihistamines cause drowsiness and co-administration may increase drowsiness effect). Products include:
BuSpar Tablets ... 738

Butabarbital (Antihistamines cause drowsiness and co-administration may increase drowsiness effect).
No products indexed under this heading.

Butalbital (Antihistamines cause drowsiness and co-administration may increase drowsiness effect). Products include:
Axocet Capsules ... 2469
Esgic-plus Capsules ... 1012
Esgic-plus Tablets ... 1012
Fioricet Tablets ... 2386
Fioricet with Codeine Capsules ... 2387
Fiorinal Capsules ... 2388
Fiorinal with Codeine Capsules ... 2390
Fiorinal Tablets ... 2388
Phrenilin ... 790
Sedapap Tablets 50 mg/650 mg .. 1826

Chlordiazepoxide (Antihistamines cause drowsiness and co-administration may increase drowsiness effect). Products include:
Limbitrol ... 2333

Chlordiazepoxide Hydrochloride (Antihistamines cause drowsiness and co-administration may increase drowsiness effect). Products include:
Librax Capsules ... 2330
Librium Capsules ... 2331
Librium Injectable ... 2332

Chlorpromazine (Antihistamines cause drowsiness and co-administration may increase drowsiness effect). Products include:
Thorazine Suppositories ... 2701

Chlorpromazine Hydrochloride (Antihistamines cause drowsiness and co-administration may increase drowsiness effect). Products include:
Thorazine ... 2701

Chlorprothixene (Antihistamines cause drowsiness and co-administration may increase drowsiness effect).
No products indexed under this heading.

Chlorprothixene Hydrochloride (Antihistamines cause drowsiness and co-administration may increase drowsiness effect).
No products indexed under this heading.

Chlorprothixene Lactate (Antihistamines cause drowsiness and co-administration may increase drowsiness effect).
No products indexed under this heading.

Clorazepate Dipotassium (Antihistamines cause drowsiness and co-administration may increase drowsiness effect). Products include:
Tranxene ... 459

Clozapine (Antihistamines cause drowsiness and co-administration may increase drowsiness effect). Products include:
Clozaril Tablets ... 2377

Codeine Phosphate (Antihistamines cause drowsiness and co-administration may increase drowsiness effect). Products include:
Brontex ... 2130
Dimetane-DC Cough Syrup ... 2232
Fioricet with Codeine Capsules ... 2387
Fiorinal with Codeine Capsules ... 2390
Nucofed ... 2225
Phenergan with Codeine ... 2883
Phenergan VC with Codeine ... 2888
Robitussin A-C Syrup ... 2248
Robitussin-DAC Syrup ... 2249
Ryna ... 804
Soma Compound w/Codeine Tablets ... 2784
Tylenol with Codeine ... 1592

Desflurane (Antihistamines cause drowsiness and co-administration may increase drowsiness effect). Products include:
Suprane (desflurane, USP) ... 1865

Dezocine (Antihistamines cause drowsiness and co-administration may increase drowsiness effect). Products include:
Dalgan Injection ... 529

(Described in PDR For Nonprescription Drugs) (⊚ Described in PDR For Ophthalmology)

955 **Interactions Index** **Rynatan-S**

Diazepam (Antihistamines cause drowsiness and co-administration may increase drowsiness effect). Products include:
- Dizac (diazepam injectable emulsion) CIV ... 1862
- Valium Injectable ... 2336
- Valium Tablets ... 2335

Droperidol (Antihistamines cause drowsiness and co-administration may increase drowsiness effect). Products include:
- Inapsine Injection ... 462

Enflurane (Antihistamines cause drowsiness and co-administration may increase drowsiness effect).
- No products indexed under this heading.

Estazolam (Antihistamines cause drowsiness and co-administration may increase drowsiness effect). Products include:
- ProSom Tablets ... 457

Ethchlorvynol (Antihistamines cause drowsiness and co-administration may increase drowsiness effect). Products include:
- Placidyl Capsules ... 456

Ethinamate (Antihistamines cause drowsiness and co-administration may increase drowsiness effect).
- No products indexed under this heading.

Fentanyl (Antihistamines cause drowsiness and co-administration may increase drowsiness effect). Products include:
- Duragesic Transdermal System ... 1336

Fentanyl Citrate (Antihistamines cause drowsiness and co-administration may increase drowsiness effect). Products include:
- Sublimaze Injection ... 463

Fluphenazine Decanoate (Antihistamines cause drowsiness and co-administration may increase drowsiness effect). Products include:
- Prolixin Decanoate ... 510

Fluphenazine Enanthate (Antihistamines cause drowsiness and co-administration may increase drowsiness effect). Products include:
- Prolixin Enanthate ... 510

Fluphenazine Hydrochloride (Antihistamines cause drowsiness and co-administration may increase drowsiness effect). Products include:
- Prolixin ... 510

Flurazepam Hydrochloride (Antihistamines cause drowsiness and co-administration may increase drowsiness effect). Products include:
- Dalmane Capsules ... 2329

Furazolidone (MAO inhibitors prolong and intensify the anticholinergic effects of antihistamines and the overall effects of sympathomimetics; concurrent and/or sequential use is not recommended). Products include:
- Furoxone ... 2221

Glutethimide (Antihistamines cause drowsiness and co-administration may increase drowsiness effect).
- No products indexed under this heading.

Haloperidol (Antihistamines cause drowsiness and co-administration may increase drowsiness effect). Products include:
- Haldol Injection, Tablets and Concentrate ... 1585

Haloperidol Decanoate (Antihistamines cause drowsiness and co-administration may increase drowsiness effect). Products include:
- Haldol Decanoate ... 1587

Hydrocodone Bitartrate (Antihistamines cause drowsiness and co-administration may increase drowsiness effect). Products include:
- Codiclear DH Syrup ... 808
- Duratuss HD Elixir ... 2750
- Histussin D Liquid ... 670
- Hycodan Tablets and Syrup ... 946
- Hycomine Compound Tablets ... 948
- Hycomine ... 947
- Hycotuss Expectorant Syrup ... 950
- Hydrocet Capsules ... 787
- Lorcet 10/650 Tablets ... 1016
- Lortab ... 2751
- Tussend ... 1830
- Tussend Expectorant ... 1831
- Vicodin Tablets ... 1404
- Vicodin ES Tablets ... 1405
- Vicodin HP Tablets ... 1403
- Vicodin Tuss Expectorant ... 1406
- Zydone Capsules ... 967

Hydrocodone Polistirex (Antihistamines cause drowsiness and co-administration may increase drowsiness effect). Products include:
- Tussionex Pennkinetic Extended-Release Suspension ... 1624

Hydromorphone Hydrochloride (Antihistamines cause drowsiness and co-administration may increase drowsiness effect). Products include:
- Dilaudid Ampules ... 1382
- Dilaudid Cough Syrup ... 1383
- Dilaudid-HP Injection ... 1384
- Dilaudid-HP Lyophilized Powder 250 mg ... 1384
- Dilaudid ... 1382
- Dilaudid Oral Liquid ... 1386
- Dilaudid ... 1382
- Dilaudid Tablets - 8 mg ... 1386

Hydroxyzine Hydrochloride (Antihistamines cause drowsiness and co-administration may increase drowsiness effect). Products include:
- Atarax Tablets & Syrup ... 1992
- Marax Tablets & DF Syrup ... 2015
- Vistaril Intramuscular Solution ... 2042

Isocarboxazid (MAO inhibitors prolong and intensify the anticholinergic effects of antihistamines and the overall effects of sympathomimetics; concurrent and/or sequential use is not recommended).
- No products indexed under this heading.

Isoflurane (Antihistamines cause drowsiness and co-administration may increase drowsiness effect).
- No products indexed under this heading.

Ketamine Hydrochloride (Antihistamines cause drowsiness and co-administration may increase drowsiness effect).
- No products indexed under this heading.

Levomethadyl Acetate Hydrochloride (Antihistamines cause drowsiness and co-administration may increase drowsiness effect). Products include:
- Orlaam Oral Solution ... 2361

Levorphanol Tartrate (Antihistamines cause drowsiness and co-administration may increase drowsiness effect). Products include:
- Levo-Dromoran ... 2297

Lorazepam (Antihistamines cause drowsiness and co-administration may increase drowsiness effect). Products include:
- Ativan Injection ... 2805
- Ativan Tablets ... 2807

Loxapine Hydrochloride (Antihistamines cause drowsiness and co-administration may increase drowsiness effect). Products include:
- Loxitane ... 1426

Loxapine Succinate (Antihistamines cause drowsiness and co-administration may increase drowsiness effect). Products include:
- Loxitane Capsules ... 1426

Meperidine Hydrochloride (Antihistamines cause drowsiness and co-administration may increase drowsiness effect). Products include:
- Demerol ... 2438
- Mepergan Injection ... 2859

Mephobarbital (Antihistamines cause drowsiness and co-administration may increase drowsiness effect). Products include:
- Mebaral Tablets ... 2452

Meprobamate (Antihistamines cause drowsiness and co-administration may increase drowsiness effect). Products include:
- Miltown Tablets ... 2780
- PMB 200 and PMB 400 ... 2890

Mesoridazine Besylate (Antihistamines cause drowsiness and co-administration may increase drowsiness effect). Products include:
- Serentil ... 689

Methadone Hydrochloride (Antihistamines cause drowsiness and co-administration may increase drowsiness effect). Products include:
- Methadone Hydrochloride Oral Concentrate ... 2356
- Methadone Hydrochloride Oral Solution & Tablets ... 2357

Methohexital Sodium (Antihistamines cause drowsiness and co-administration may increase drowsiness effect).
- No products indexed under this heading.

Methotrimeprazine (Antihistamines cause drowsiness and co-administration may increase drowsiness effect). Products include:
- Levoprome ... 1321

Methoxyflurane (Antihistamines cause drowsiness and co-administration may increase drowsiness effect).
- No products indexed under this heading.

Midazolam Hydrochloride (Antihistamines cause drowsiness and co-administration may increase drowsiness effect). Products include:
- Versed Injection ... 2324

Molindone Hydrochloride (Antihistamines cause drowsiness and co-administration may increase drowsiness effect). Products include:
- Moban Tablets and Concentrate ... 1036

Morphine Sulfate (Antihistamines cause drowsiness and co-administration may increase drowsiness effect). Products include:
- Astramorph/PF Injection, USP (Preservative-Free) ... 526
- Duramorph Injection ... 983
- Infumorph 200 and Infumorph 500 Sterile Solutions ... 985
- Kadian Capsules ... 2948
- MS Contin Tablets ... 2149
- MSIR ... 2152
- Oramorph SR (Morphine Sulfate Sustained Release Tablets) ... 2359
- RMS Suppositories CII ... 2766
- Roxanol ... 2365

Opium Alkaloids (Antihistamines cause drowsiness and co-administration may increase drowsiness effect).
- No products indexed under this heading.

Oxazepam (Antihistamines cause drowsiness and co-administration may increase drowsiness effect). Products include:
- Serax Capsules ... 2916
- Serax Tablets ... 2916

Oxycodone Hydrochloride (Antihistamines cause drowsiness and co-administration may increase drowsiness effect). Products include:
- OxyContin Tablets ... 2163
- OxyIR Capsules ... 2167
- Percocet Tablets ... 955
- Percodan Tablets ... 955
- Percodan-Demi Tablets ... 956
- Roxicodone Tablets, Oral Solution & Intensol (Oxycodone) ... 2366
- Tylox Capsules ... 1593

Pentobarbital Sodium (Antihistamines cause drowsiness and co-administration may increase drowsiness effect). Products include:
- Nembutal Sodium Capsules ... 440
- Nembutal Sodium Solution ... 442
- Nembutal Sodium Suppositories ... 444

Perphenazine (Antihistamines cause drowsiness and co-administration may increase drowsiness effect). Products include:
- Etrafon ... 2495
- Triavil Tablets ... 1800
- Trilafon ... 2532

Phenelzine Sulfate (MAO inhibitors prolong and intensify the anticholinergic effects of antihistamines and the overall effects of sympathomimetics; concurrent and/or sequential use is not recommended). Products include:
- Nardil ... 1977

Phenobarbital (Antihistamines cause drowsiness and co-administration may increase drowsiness effect). Products include:
- Arco-Lase Plus Tablets ... 513
- Bellergal-S Tablets ... 2375
- Donnatal ... 2234
- Donnatal Extentabs ... 2234
- Donnatal Tablets ... 2234
- Phenobarbital Elixir and Tablets ... 1523
- Quadrinal Tablets ... 1398

Prazepam (Antihistamines cause drowsiness and co-administration may increase drowsiness effect).
- No products indexed under this heading.

Prochlorperazine (Antihistamines cause drowsiness and co-administration may increase drowsiness effect). Products include:
- Compazine ... 2644

Promethazine Hydrochloride (Antihistamines cause drowsiness and co-administration may increase drowsiness effect). Products include:
- Mepergan Injection ... 2859
- Phenergan with Codeine ... 2883
- Phenergan with Dextromethorphan ... 2885
- Phenergan Injection ... 2880
- Phenergan Suppositories ... 2882
- Phenergan Syrup ... 2881
- Phenergan Tablets ... 2882
- Phenergan VC ... 2886
- Phenergan VC with Codeine ... 2888

Propofol (Antihistamines cause drowsiness and co-administration may increase drowsiness effect). Products include:
- Diprivan Injectable Emulsion ... 2939

Propoxyphene Hydrochloride (Antihistamines cause drowsiness and co-administration may increase drowsiness effect). Products include:
- Darvon ... 1475
- Wygesic Tablets ... 2930

Propoxyphene Napsylate (Antihistamines cause drowsiness and co-administration may increase drowsiness effect). Products include:
- Darvon-N/Darvocet-N ... 1473

Quazepam (Antihistamines cause drowsiness and co-administration may increase drowsiness effect). Products include:
- Doral Tablets ... 2773

IMPORTANT NOTE: Always consult each drug listing in the patient's regimen for possible interactions.

Risperidone (Antihistamines cause drowsiness and co-administration may increase drowsiness effect). Products include:
  Risperdal Tablets 1348
Secobarbital Sodium (Antihistamines cause drowsiness and co-administration may increase drowsiness effect). Products include:
  Seconal Sodium Pulvules 1529
Selegiline Hydrochloride (MAO inhibitors prolong and intensify the anticholinergic effects of antihistamines and the overall effects of sympathomimetics; concurrent and/or sequential use is not recommended). Products include:
  Eldepryl Capsules 2729
Sevoflurane (Antihistamines cause drowsiness and co-administration may increase drowsiness effect).
  No products indexed under this heading.
Sufentanil Citrate (Antihistamines cause drowsiness and co-administration may increase drowsiness effect). Products include:
  Sufenta Injection 1355
Temazepam (Antihistamines cause drowsiness and co-administration may increase drowsiness effect). Products include:
  Restoril Capsules 2413
Thiamylal Sodium (Antihistamines cause drowsiness and co-administration may increase drowsiness effect).
  No products indexed under this heading.
Thioridazine Hydrochloride (Antihistamines cause drowsiness and co-administration may increase drowsiness effect). Products include:
  Mellaril 2398
Thiothixene (Antihistamines cause drowsiness and co-administration may increase drowsiness effect). Products include:
  Navane Capsules and Concentrate 2018
  Navane Intramuscular 2019
Tranylcypromine Sulfate (MAO inhibitors prolong and intensify the anticholinergic effects of antihistamines and the overall effects of sympathomimetics; concurrent and/or sequential use is not recommended). Products include:
  Parnate Tablets 2679
Triazolam (Antihistamines cause drowsiness and co-administration may increase drowsiness effect). Products include:
  Halcion Tablets 2093
Trifluoperazine Hydrochloride (Antihistamines cause drowsiness and co-administration may increase drowsiness effect). Products include:
  Stelazine 2692
Zolpidem Tartrate (Antihistamines cause drowsiness and co-administration may increase drowsiness effect). Products include:
  Ambien Tablets 2559

Food Interactions
Alcohol (Antihistamines cause drowsiness and co-administration may increase drowsiness effect).

RYNATUSS PEDIATRIC SUSPENSION
(Carbetapentane Tannate, Chlorpheniramine Tannate, Ephedrine Tannate, Phenylephrine Tannate) 2782
May interact with monoamine oxidase inhibitors, hypnotics and sedatives, tranquilizers, central nervous system depressants, and certain other agents. Compounds in these categories include:

Alfentanil Hydrochloride (Antihistamines cause drowsiness and co-administration may increase drowsiness effect). Products include:
  Alfenta Injection 1334
Alprazolam (Antihistamines cause drowsiness and co-administration may increase drowsiness effect). Products include:
  Xanax Tablets 2115
Aprobarbital (Antihistamines cause drowsiness and co-administration may increase drowsiness effect).
  No products indexed under this heading.
Buprenorphine (Antihistamines cause drowsiness and co-administration may increase drowsiness effect). Products include:
  Buprenex Injectable 2170
Buspirone Hydrochloride (Antihistamines cause drowsiness and co-administration may increase drowsiness effect). Products include:
  BuSpar Tablets 738
Butabarbital (Antihistamines cause drowsiness and co-administration may increase drowsiness effect).
  No products indexed under this heading.
Butalbital (Antihistamines cause drowsiness and co-administration may increase drowsiness effect). Products include:
  Axocet Capsules 2469
  Esgic-plus Capsules 1012
  Esgic-plus Tablets 1012
  Fioricet Tablets 2386
  Fioricet with Codeine Capsules .. 2387
  Fiorinal Capsules 2388
  Fiorinal with Codeine Capsules .. 2390
  Fiorinal Tablets 2388
  Phrenilin 790
  Sedapap Tablets 50 mg/650 mg .. 1826
Chlordiazepoxide (Antihistamines cause drowsiness and co-administration may increase drowsiness effect). Products include:
  Limbitrol 2333
Chlordiazepoxide Hydrochloride (Antihistamines cause drowsiness and co-administration may increase drowsiness effect). Products include:
  Librax Capsules 2330
  Librium Capsules 2331
  Librium Injectable 2332
Chlorpromazine (Antihistamines cause drowsiness and co-administration may increase drowsiness effect). Products include:
  Thorazine Suppositories 2701
Chlorpromazine Hydrochloride (Antihistamines cause drowsiness and co-administration may increase drowsiness effect). Products include:
  Thorazine 2701
Chlorprothixene (Antihistamines cause drowsiness and co-administration may increase drowsiness effect).
  No products indexed under this heading.
Chlorprothixene Hydrochloride (Antihistamines cause drowsiness and co-administration may increase drowsiness effect).
  No products indexed under this heading.
Chlorprothixene Lactate (Antihistamines cause drowsiness and co-administration may increase drowsiness effect).
  No products indexed under this heading.

Clorazepate Dipotassium (Antihistamines cause drowsiness and co-administration may increase drowsiness effect). Products include:
  Tranxene 459
Clozapine (Antihistamines cause drowsiness and co-administration may increase drowsiness effect). Products include:
  Clozaril Tablets 2377
Codeine Phosphate (Antihistamines cause drowsiness and co-administration may increase drowsiness effect). Products include:
  Brontex 2130
  Dimetane-DC Cough Syrup 2232
  Fioricet with Codeine Capsules .. 2387
  Fiorinal with Codeine Capsules .. 2390
  Nucofed 2225
  Phenergan with Codeine 2883
  Phenergan VC with Codeine 2888
  Robitussin A-C Syrup 2248
  Robitussin-DAC Syrup 2249
  Ryna 804
  Soma Compound w/Codeine Tablets 2784
  Tylenol with Codeine 1592
Desflurane (Antihistamines cause drowsiness and co-administration may increase drowsiness effect). Products include:
  Suprane (desflurane, USP) 1865
Dezocine (Antihistamines cause drowsiness and co-administration may increase drowsiness effect). Products include:
  Dalgan Injection 529
Diazepam (Antihistamines cause drowsiness and co-administration may increase drowsiness effect). Products include:
  Dizac (diazepam injectable emulsion) CIV 1862
  Valium Injectable 2336
  Valium Tablets 2335
Droperidol (Antihistamines cause drowsiness and co-administration may increase drowsiness effect). Products include:
  Inapsine Injection 462
Enflurane (Antihistamines cause drowsiness and co-administration may increase drowsiness effect).
  No products indexed under this heading.
Estazolam (Antihistamines cause drowsiness and co-administration may increase drowsiness effect). Products include:
  ProSom Tablets 457
Ethchlorvynol (Antihistamines cause drowsiness and co-administration may increase drowsiness effect). Products include:
  Placidyl Capsules 456
Ethinamate (Antihistamines cause drowsiness and co-administration may increase drowsiness effect).
  No products indexed under this heading.
Fentanyl (Antihistamines cause drowsiness and co-administration may increase drowsiness effect). Products include:
  Duragesic Transdermal System ... 1336
Fentanyl Citrate (Antihistamines cause drowsiness and co-administration may increase drowsiness effect). Products include:
  Sublimaze Injection 463
Fluphenazine Decanoate (Antihistamines cause drowsiness and co-administration may increase drowsiness effect). Products include:
  Prolixin Decanoate 510

Fluphenazine Enanthate (Antihistamines cause drowsiness and co-administration may increase drowsiness effect). Products include:
  Prolixin Enanthate 510
Fluphenazine Hydrochloride (Antihistamines cause drowsiness and co-administration may increase drowsiness effect). Products include:
  Prolixin 510
Flurazepam Hydrochloride (Antihistamines cause drowsiness and co-administration may increase drowsiness effect). Products include:
  Dalmane Capsules 2329
Furazolidone (MAO inhibitors prolong and intensify the anticholinergic effects of antihistamines and the overall effects of sympathomimetics; concurrent and/or sequential use is not recommended). Products include:
  Furoxone 2221
Glutethimide (Antihistamines cause drowsiness and co-administration may increase drowsiness effect).
  No products indexed under this heading.
Haloperidol (Antihistamines cause drowsiness and co-administration may increase drowsiness effect). Products include:
  Haldol Injection, Tablets and Concentrate 1585
Haloperidol Decanoate (Antihistamines cause drowsiness and co-administration may increase drowsiness effect). Products include:
  Haldol Decanoate 1587
Hydrocodone Bitartrate (Antihistamines cause drowsiness and co-administration may increase drowsiness effect). Products include:
  Codiclear DH Syrup 808
  Duratuss HD Elixir 2750
  Histussin D Liquid 670
  Hycodan Tablets and Syrup 946
  Hycomine Compound Tablets ... 948
  Hycomine 947
  Hycotuss Expectorant Syrup 950
  Hydrocet Capsules 787
  Lorcet 10/650 Tablets 1016
  Lortab 2751
  Tussend 1830
  Tussend Expectorant 1831
  Vicodin Tablets 1404
  Vicodin ES Tablets 1405
  Vicodin HP Tablets 1403
  Vicodin Tuss Expectorant 1406
  Zydone Capsules 967
Hydrocodone Polistirex (Antihistamines cause drowsiness and co-administration may increase drowsiness effect). Products include:
  Tussionex Pennkinetic Extended-Release Suspension 1624
Hydromorphone Hydrochloride (Antihistamines cause drowsiness and co-administration may increase drowsiness effect). Products include:
  Dilaudid Ampules 1382
  Dilaudid Cough Syrup 1383
  Dilaudid-HP Injection 1384
  Dilaudid-HP Lyophilized Powder 250 mg 1384
  Dilaudid 1382
  Dilaudid Oral Liquid 1386
  Dilaudid 1382
  Dilaudid Tablets - 8 mg 1386
Hydroxyzine Hydrochloride (Antihistamines cause drowsiness and co-administration may increase drowsiness effect). Products include:
  Atarax Tablets & Syrup 1992
  Marax Tablets & DF Syrup 2015
  Vistaril Intramuscular Solution ... 2042

957 **Interactions Index** **Rythmol**

Isocarboxazid (MAO inhibitors prolong and intensify the anticholinergic effects of antihistamines and the overall effects of sympathomimetics; concurrent and/or sequential use is not recommended).
No products indexed under this heading.

Isoflurane (Antihistamines cause drowsiness and co-administration may increase drowsiness effect).
No products indexed under this heading.

Ketamine Hydrochloride (Antihistamines cause drowsiness and co-administration may increase drowsiness effect).
No products indexed under this heading.

Levomethadyl Acetate Hydrochloride (Antihistamines cause drowsiness and co-administration may increase drowsiness effect). Products include:
Orlaam Oral Solution 2361

Levorphanol Tartrate (Antihistamines cause drowsiness and co-administration may increase drowsiness effect). Products include:
Levo-Dromoran 2297

Lorazepam (Antihistamines cause drowsiness and co-administration may increase drowsiness effect). Products include:
Ativan Injection 2805
Ativan Tablets 2807

Loxapine Hydrochloride (Antihistamines cause drowsiness and co-administration may increase drowsiness effect). Products include:
Loxitane 1426

Loxapine Succinate (Antihistamines cause drowsiness and co-administration may increase drowsiness effect). Products include:
Loxitane Capsules 1426

Meperidine Hydrochloride (Antihistamines cause drowsiness and co-administration may increase drowsiness effect). Products include:
Demerol 2438
Mepergan Injection 2859

Mephobarbital (Antihistamines cause drowsiness and co-administration may increase drowsiness effect). Products include:
Mebaral Tablets 2452

Meprobamate (Antihistamines cause drowsiness and co-administration may increase drowsiness effect). Products include:
Miltown Tablets 2780
PMB 200 and PMB 400 2890

Mesoridazine Besylate (Antihistamines cause drowsiness and co-administration may increase drowsiness effect). Products include:
Serentil 689

Methadone Hydrochloride (Antihistamines cause drowsiness and co-administration may increase drowsiness effect). Products include:
Methadone Hydrochloride Oral Concentrate 2356
Methadone Hydrochloride Oral Solution & Tablets 2357

Methohexital Sodium (Antihistamines cause drowsiness and co-administration may increase drowsiness effect).
No products indexed under this heading.

Methotrimeprazine (Antihistamines cause drowsiness and co-administration may increase drowsiness effect). Products include:
Levoprome 1321

Methoxyflurane (Antihistamines cause drowsiness and co-administration may increase drowsiness effect).
No products indexed under this heading.

Midazolam Hydrochloride (Antihistamines cause drowsiness and co-administration may increase drowsiness effect). Products include:
Versed Injection 2324

Molindone Hydrochloride (Antihistamines cause drowsiness and co-administration may increase drowsiness effect). Products include:
Moban Tablets and Concentrate 1036

Morphine Sulfate (Antihistamines cause drowsiness and co-administration may increase drowsiness effect). Products include:
Astramorph/PF Injection, USP (Preservative-Free) 526
Duramorph Injection 983
Infumorph 200 and Infumorph 500 Sterile Solutions 985
Kadian Capsules 2948
MS Contin Tablets 2149
MSIR 2152
Oramorph SR (Morphine Sulfate Sustained Release Tablets) 2359
RMS Suppositories CII 2766
Roxanol 2365

Opium Alkaloids (Antihistamines cause drowsiness and co-administration may increase drowsiness effect).
No products indexed under this heading.

Oxazepam (Antihistamines cause drowsiness and co-administration may increase drowsiness effect). Products include:
Serax Capsules 2916
Serax Tablets 2916

Oxycodone Hydrochloride (Antihistamines cause drowsiness and co-administration may increase drowsiness effect). Products include:
OxyContin Tablets 2163
OxyIR Capsules 2167
Percocet Tablets 955
Percodan Tablets 955
Percodan-Demi Tablets 956
Roxicodone Tablets, Oral Solution & Intensol (Oxycodone) 2366
Tylox Capsules 1593

Pentobarbital Sodium (Antihistamines cause drowsiness and co-administration may increase drowsiness effect). Products include:
Nembutal Sodium Capsules 440
Nembutal Sodium Solution 442
Nembutal Sodium Suppositories 444

Perphenazine (Antihistamines cause drowsiness and co-administration may increase drowsiness effect). Products include:
Etrafon 2495
Triavil Tablets 1800
Trilafon 2532

Phenelzine Sulfate (MAO inhibitors prolong and intensify the anticholinergic effects of antihistamines and the overall effects of sympathomimetics; concurrent and/or sequential use is not recommended). Products include:
Nardil 1977

Phenobarbital (Antihistamines cause drowsiness and co-administration may increase drowsiness effect). Products include:
Arco-Lase Plus Tablets 513
Bellergal-S Tablets 2375
Donnatal 2234
Donnatal Extentabs 2234
Donnatal Tablets 2234
Phenobarbital Elixir and Tablets 1523
Quadrinal Tablets 1398

Prazepam (Antihistamines cause drowsiness and co-administration may increase drowsiness effect).
No products indexed under this heading.

Prochlorperazine (Antihistamines cause drowsiness and co-administration may increase drowsiness effect). Products include:
Compazine 2644

Promethazine Hydrochloride (Antihistamines cause drowsiness and co-administration may increase drowsiness effect). Products include:
Mepergan Injection 2859
Phenergan with Codeine 2883
Phenergan with Dextromethorphan 2885
Phenergan Injection 2880
Phenergan Suppositories 2882
Phenergan Syrup 2881
Phenergan Tablets 2882
Phenergan VC 2886
Phenergan VC with Codeine 2888

Propofol (Antihistamines cause drowsiness and co-administration may increase drowsiness effect). Products include:
Diprivan Injectable Emulsion 2939

Propoxyphene Hydrochloride (Antihistamines cause drowsiness and co-administration may increase drowsiness effect). Products include:
Darvon 1475
Wygesic Tablets 2930

Propoxyphene Napsylate (Antihistamines cause drowsiness and co-administration may increase drowsiness effect). Products include:
Darvon-N/Darvocet-N 1473

Quazepam (Antihistamines cause drowsiness and co-administration may increase drowsiness effect). Products include:
Doral Tablets 2773

Risperidone (Antihistamines cause drowsiness and co-administration may increase drowsiness effect). Products include:
Risperdal Tablets 1348

Secobarbital Sodium (Antihistamines cause drowsiness and co-administration may increase drowsiness effect). Products include:
Seconal Sodium Pulvules 1529

Selegiline Hydrochloride (MAO inhibitors prolong and intensify the anticholinergic effects of antihistamines and the overall effects of sympathomimetics; concurrent and/or sequential use is not recommended). Products include:
Eldepryl Capsules 2729

Sevoflurane (Antihistamines cause drowsiness and co-administration may increase drowsiness effect).
No products indexed under this heading.

Sufentanil Citrate (Antihistamines cause drowsiness and co-administration may increase drowsiness effect). Products include:
Sufenta Injection 1355

Temazepam (Antihistamines cause drowsiness and co-administration may increase drowsiness effect). Products include:
Restoril Capsules 2413

Thiamylal Sodium (Antihistamines cause drowsiness and co-administration may increase drowsiness effect).
No products indexed under this heading.

Thioridazine Hydrochloride (Antihistamines cause drowsiness and co-administration may increase drowsiness effect). Products include:
Mellaril 2398

Thiothixene (Antihistamines cause drowsiness and co-administration may increase drowsiness effect). Products include:
Navane Capsules and Concentrate 2018
Navane Intramuscular 2019

Tranylcypromine Sulfate (MAO inhibitors prolong and intensify the anticholinergic effects of antihistamines and the overall effects of sympathomimetics; concurrent and/or sequential use is not recommended). Products include:
Parnate Tablets 2679

Triazolam (Antihistamines cause drowsiness and co-administration may increase drowsiness effect). Products include:
Halcion Tablets 2093

Trifluoperazine Hydrochloride (Antihistamines cause drowsiness and co-administration may increase drowsiness effect). Products include:
Stelazine 2692

Zolpidem Tartrate (Antihistamines cause drowsiness and co-administration may increase drowsiness effect). Products include:
Ambien Tablets 2559

Food Interactions

Alcohol (Antihistamines cause drowsiness and co-administration may increase drowsiness effect).

RYNATUSS TABLETS

(Chlorpheniramine Tannate, Carbetapentane Tannate, Phenylephrine Tannate, Ephedrine Tannate) 2782
See **Rynatuss Pediatric Suspension**

RYTHMOL TABLETS–150MG, 225MG, 300MG

(Propafenone Hydrochloride) 1399
May interact with beta blockers, cardiac glycosides, local anesthetics, and certain other agents. Compounds in these categories include:

Acebutolol Hydrochloride (Potential for increased plasma concentration and elimination half-life of beta blockers; dosage reduction of beta-antagonist may be necessary). Products include:
Sectral Capsules 2914

Atenolol (Potential for increased plasma concentration and elimination half-life of beta blockers; dosage reduction of beta-antagonist may be necessary). Products include:
Tenoretic Tablets 2963
Tenormin Tablets and I.V. Injection 2965

Betaxolol Hydrochloride (Potential for increased plasma concentration and elimination half-life of beta blockers; dosage reduction of beta-antagonist may be necessary). Products include:
Betoptic Ophthalmic Solution 465
Betoptic S Ophthalmic Suspension 467
Kerlone Tablets 2588

Bisoprolol Fumarate (Potential for increased plasma concentration and elimination half-life of beta blockers; dosage reduction of beta-antagonist may be necessary). Products include:
Zebeta Tablets 1457
Ziac 1459

Bupivacaine Hydrochloride (Concomitant use of local anesthetics may increase the risk of CNS side effects). Products include:
Marcaine 2446
Marcaine Spinal 2449
Sensorcaine 554

IMPORTANT NOTE: Always consult each drug listing in the patient's regimen for possible interactions.

Carteolol Hydrochloride (Potential for increased plasma concentration and elimination half-life of beta blockers; dosage reduction of beta-antagonist may be necessary). Products include:
   Cartrol Tablets 413
   Ocupress Ophthalmic Solution, 1% Sterile............................... ⊙ 297

Chloroprocaine Hydrochloride (Concomitant use of local anesthetics may increase the risk of CNS side effects). Products include:
   Nescaine/Nescaine MPF.............. 549

Cimetidine (Increases steady-state plasma concentrations with no detectable changes in electrocardiographic parameters). Products include:
   Tagamet HB Tablets................ ▣ 786
   Tagamet Tablets 2694

Cimetidine Hydrochloride (Increases steady-state plasma concentrations with no detectable changes in electrocardiographic parameters). Products include:
   Tagamet.. 2694

Deslanoside (Potential for elevated digoxin levels; dosage reduction of digitalis may be necessary).
   No products indexed under this heading.

Digitoxin (Potential for elevated digoxin levels; dosage reduction of digitalis may be necessary). Products include:
   Crystodigin Tablets 1472

Digoxin (Potential for elevated digoxin levels; dosage reduction of digitalis may be necessary). Products include:
   Lanoxicaps 1110
   Lanoxin Elixir Pediatric 1113
   Lanoxin Injection 1116
   Lanoxin Injection Pediatric........ 1119
   Lanoxin Tablets 1121

Esmolol Hydrochloride (Potential for increased plasma concentration and elimination half-life of beta blockers; dosage reduction of beta-antagonist may be necessary). Products include:
   Brevibloc (esmolol HCl) Injection 1860

Etidocaine Hydrochloride (Concomitant use of local anesthetics may increase the risk of CNS side effects). Products include:
   Duranest Injections 533

Labetalol Hydrochloride (Potential for increased plasma concentration and elimination half-life of beta blockers; dosage reduction of beta-antagonist may be necessary). Products include:
   Normodyne Injection 2519
   Normodyne Tablets 2522
   Trandate 1158

Levobunolol Hydrochloride (Potential for increased plasma concentration and elimination half-life of beta blockers; dosage reduction of beta-antagonist may be necessary). Products include:
   Betagan .... ⊙ 230

Lidocaine Hydrochloride (Concomitant use of local anesthetics may increase the risk of CNS side effects). Products include:
   Decadron Phosphate with Xylocaine Injection, Sterile 1683
   Unguentine Plus .... ▣ 712
   Xylocaine Injections 562

Mepivacaine Hydrochloride Injection (Concomitant use of local anesthetics may increase the risk of CNS side effects). Products include:
   Carbocaine Injection 2432

Metipranolol Hydrochloride (Potential for increased plasma concentration and elimination half-life of beta blockers; dosage reduction of beta-antagonist may be necessary). Products include:
   OptiPranolol (Metipranolol 0.3%) Sterile Ophthalmic Solution......... ⊙ 256

Metoprolol Succinate (Potential for increased plasma concentration and elimination half-life of beta blockers; dosage reduction of beta-antagonist may be necessary). Products include:
   Toprol-XL Tablets 560

Metoprolol Tartrate (Potential for increased plasma concentration and elimination half-life of beta blockers; dosage reduction of beta-antagonist may be necessary). Products include:
   Lopressor 848
   Lopressor HCT Tablets 850

Nadolol (Potential for increased plasma concentration and elimination half-life of beta blockers; dosage reduction of beta-antagonist may be necessary).
   No products indexed under this heading.

Penbutolol Sulfate (Potential for increased plasma concentration and elimination half-life of beta blockers; dosage reduction of beta-antagonist may be necessary). Products include:
   Levatol Tablets 2547

Pindolol (Potential for increased plasma concentration and elimination half-life of beta blockers; dosage reduction of beta-antagonist may be necessary). Products include:
   Visken Tablets 2428

Procaine Hydrochloride (Concomitant use of local anesthetics may increase the risk of CNS side effects). Products include:
   Novocain Hydrochloride for Spinal Anesthesia 2457

Propranolol Hydrochloride (Potential for increased plasma concentration and elimination half-life of beta blockers; dosage reduction of beta-antagonist may be necessary). Products include:
   Inderal 2834
   Inderal LA Long Acting Capsules 2836
   Inderide Tablets 2838
   Inderide LA Long Acting Capsules .. 2840

Quinidine Gluconate (Small doses of quinidine completely inhibit the hydroxylation metabolic pathway). Products include:
   Quinaglute Dura-Tabs Tablets 644

Quinidine Polygalacturonate (Small doses of quinidine completely inhibit the hydroxylation metabolic pathway). Products include:
   Cardioquin Tablets 2146

Quinidine Sulfate (Small doses of quinidine completely inhibit the hydroxylation metabolic pathway). Products include:
   Quinidex Extentabs 2240

Sotalol Hydrochloride (Potential for increased plasma concentration and elimination half-life of beta blockers; dosage reduction of beta-antagonist may be necessary). Products include:
   Betapace Tablets 637

Tetracaine Hydrochloride (Concomitant use of local anesthetics may increase the risk of CNS side effects). Products include:
   Cetacaine Topical Anesthetic 812
   Pontocaine Hydrochloride for Spinal Anesthesia 2460

Timolol Hemihydrate (Potential for increased plasma concentration and elimination half-life of beta blockers; dosage reduction of beta-antagonist may be necessary). Products include:
   Betimol 0.25%, 0.5% .... ⊙ 259

Timolol Maleate (Potential for increased plasma concentration and elimination half-life of beta blockers; dosage reduction of beta-antagonist may be necessary). Products include:
   Blocadren Tablets 1654
   Timolide Tablets 1791
   Timoptic in Ocudose 1796
   Timoptic Sterile Ophthalmic Solution 1794
   Timoptic-XE 1798

Warfarin Sodium (Increase in mean steady-state plasma levels of warfarin resulting in increased prothrombin time). Products include:
   Coumadin 941

Food Interactions

Food, unspecified (Increased peak blood level and bioavailability in a single dose study).

SSD CREAM
(Silver Sulfadiazine).....................1402
May interact with:

Cimetidine (Higher incidence of leukopenia). Products include:
   Tagamet HB Tablets................ ▣ 786
   Tagamet Tablets 2694

Cimetidine Hydrochloride (Higher incidence of leukopenia). Products include:
   Tagamet.. 2694

SSD AF CREAM
(Silver Sulfadiazine).....................1402
See SSD Cream

SSKI SOLUTION
(Potassium Iodide).......................2767
May interact with lithium preparations, antithyroid agents, ACE inhibitors, potassium preparations, and potassium sparing diuretics. Compounds in these categories include:

Amiloride Hydrochloride (Potential for hyperkalemia, cardiac arrhythmias or cardiac arrest). Products include:
   Midamor Tablets 1746
   Moduretic Tablets 1748

Benazepril Hydrochloride (Potential for hyperkalemia, cardiac arrhythmias or cardiac arrest). Products include:
   Lotensin Tablets 852
   Lotensin HCT Tablets 855
   Lotrel Capsules 858

Captopril (Potential for hyperkalemia, cardiac arrhythmias or cardiac arrest). Products include:
   Capoten Tablets 740
   Capozide Tablets 744

Enalapril Maleate (Potential for hyperkalemia, cardiac arrhythmias or cardiac arrest). Products include:
   Vaseretic Tablets 1810
   Vasotec Tablets 1816

Enalaprilat (Potential for hyperkalemia, cardiac arrhythmias or cardiac arrest). Products include:
   Vasotec I.V. 1814

Fosinopril Sodium (Potential for hyperkalemia, cardiac arrhythmias or cardiac arrest). Products include:
   Monopril Tablets 762

Lisinopril (Potential for hyperkalemia, cardiac arrhythmias or cardiac arrest). Products include:
   Prinivil Tablets 1776

   Prinzide Tablets 1780
   Zestoretic Tablets 2968
   Zestril Tablets 2972

Lithium Carbonate (Concurrent use may potentiate the hypothyroid and goitrogenic effect). Products include:
   Eskalith 2658
   Lithium Carbonate Capsules & Tablets 2352
   Lithonate/Lithotabs/Lithobid 2721

Lithium Citrate (Concurrent use may potentiate the hypothyroid and goitrogenic effect).
   No products indexed under this heading.

Methimazole (Concurrent use may potentiate the hypothyroid and goitrogenic effect). Products include:
   Tapazole Tablets 1361

Moexipril Hydrochloride (Potential for hyperkalemia, cardiac arrhythmias or cardiac arrest). Products include:
   Univasc Tablets 2553

Potassium Acid Phosphate (Potential for hyperkalemia, cardiac arrhythmias or cardiac arrest). Products include:
   K-Phos Original Formula 'Sodium Free' Tablets 633

Potassium Bicarbonate (Potential for hyperkalemia, cardiac arrhythmias or cardiac arrest). Products include:
   Alka-Seltzer Gold Effervescent Antacid .... ▣ 611

Potassium Chloride (Potential for hyperkalemia, cardiac arrhythmias or cardiac arrest). Products include:
   Chlor-3 Condiment 1003
   Colyte and Colyte-flavored......... 2540
   GoLYTELY 694
   K-Dur Microburst Release System (potassium chloride, USP) E.R. Tablets 1364
   K-Lor Powder Packets 438
   K-Norm Capsules 1615
   K-Tab Filmtab 439
   Micro-K 2237
   Micro-K LS Packets 2238
   NuLYTELY 694
   Cherry Flavor NuLYTELY 694
   Rum-K Syrup 1004
   Slow-K Extended-Release Tablets 869

Potassium Citrate (Potential for hyperkalemia, cardiac arrhythmias or cardiac arrest). Products include:
   Polycitra Syrup 574
   Polycitra-K Crystals 574
   Polycitra-K Oral Solution 575
   Polycitra-LC 574
   Urocit-K Tablets 1828

Potassium Gluconate (Potential for hyperkalemia, cardiac arrhythmias or cardiac arrest).
   No products indexed under this heading.

Potassium Phosphate, Dibasic (Potential for hyperkalemia, cardiac arrhythmias or cardiac arrest).
   No products indexed under this heading.

Potassium Phosphate, Monobasic (Potential for hyperkalemia, cardiac arrhythmias or cardiac arrest). Products include:
   K-Phos Neutral Tablets 633
   K-Phos Original Formula 'Sodium Free' Tablets 633

Quinapril Hydrochloride (Potential for hyperkalemia, cardiac arrhythmias or cardiac arrest). Products include:
   Accupril Tablets 1950

Ramipril (Potential for hyperkalemia, cardiac arrhythmias or cardiac arrest). Products include:
   Altace Capsules 1238

(▣ Described in PDR For Nonprescription Drugs)   (⊙ Described in PDR For Ophthalmology)

Spirapril Hydrochloride (Potential for hyperkalemia, cardiac arrhythmias or cardiac arrest).
No products indexed under this heading.

Spironolactone (Potential for hyperkalemia, cardiac arrhythmias or cardiac arrest). Products include:
Aldactazide Tablets 2556
Aldactone Tablets 2558

Trandolapril (Potential for hyperkalemia, cardiac arrhythmias or cardiac arrest). Products include:
Mavik Tablets 1407

Triamterene (Potential for hyperkalemia, cardiac arrhythmias or cardiac arrest). Products include:
Dyazide Capsules 2653
Dyrenium Capsules 2655

SAFE TUSSIN 30 LIQUID
(Dextromethorphan Hydrobromide, Guaifenesin) 1413
None cited in PDR database.

SALAC
(Salicylic Acid) 1042
None cited in PDR database.

SALAGEN TABLETS
(Pilocarpine Hydrochloride) 1546
May interact with beta blockers, parasympathomimetics, anticholinergics, and certain other agents. Compounds in these categories include:

Acebutolol Hydrochloride (Potential for conduction disturbances). Products include:
Sectral Capsules 2914

Atenolol (Potential for conduction disturbances). Products include:
Tenoretic Tablets 2963
Tenormin Tablets and I.V. Injection 2965

Atropine Sulfate (Pilocarpine might antagonize the anticholinergic effects of drugs used concomitantly). Products include:
Arco-Lase Plus Tablets 513
Atrohist Plus Tablets 1605
Donnatal 2234
Donnatal Extentabs 2234
Donnatal Tablets 2234
Lomotil 2591
Motofen Tablets 789
Urised Tablets 2123

Belladonna Alkaloids (Pilocarpine might antagonize the anticholinergic effects of drugs used concomitantly). Products include:
Bellergal-S Tablets 2375
Hyland's Bedwetting Tablets .... [PD] 788
Hyland's EnurAid Tablets .... [PD] 789
Hyland's Headache Tablets .... [PD] 790
Hyland's Teething Tablets .... [PD] 790
Similasan Eye Drops #1 .... [PD] 769

Benztropine Mesylate (Pilocarpine might antagonize the anticholinergic effects of drugs used concomitantly). Products include:
Cogentin 1661

Betaxolol Hydrochloride (Potential for conduction disturbances). Products include:
Betoptic Ophthalmic Solution 465
Betoptic S Ophthalmic Suspension 467
Kerlone Tablets 2588

Biperiden Hydrochloride (Pilocarpine might antagonize the anticholinergic effects of drugs used concomitantly). Products include:
Akineton 1380

Bisoprolol Fumarate (Potential for conduction disturbances). Products include:
Zebeta Tablets 1457
Ziac 1459

Carteolol Hydrochloride (Potential for conduction disturbances). Products include:
Cartrol Tablets 413
Ocupress Ophthalmic Solution, 1% Sterile .... ◉ 297

Clidinium Bromide (Pilocarpine might antagonize the anticholinergic effects of drugs used concomitantly). Products include:
Librax Capsules 2330

Dicyclomine Hydrochloride (Pilocarpine might antagonize the anticholinergic effects of drugs used concomitantly). Products include:
Bentyl 1246

Edrophonium Chloride (Additive pharmacologic effect). Products include:
Tensilon Injectable 1307

Esmolol Hydrochloride (Potential for conduction disturbances). Products include:
Brevibloc (esmolol HCl) Injection 1860

Glycopyrrolate (Pilocarpine might antagonize the anticholinergic effects of drugs used concomitantly). Products include:
Robinul Forte Tablets 2247
Robinul Injectable 2247
Robinul Tablets 2247

Hyoscyamine (Pilocarpine might antagonize the anticholinergic effects of drugs used concomitantly). Products include:
Cystospaz Tablets 2123
Urised Tablets 2123

Hyoscyamine Sulfate (Pilocarpine might antagonize the anticholinergic effects of drugs used concomitantly). Products include:
Arco-Lase Plus Tablets 513
Atrohist Plus Tablets 1605
Cystospaz-M Capsules 2123
Donnatal 2234
Donnatal Extentabs 2234
Donnatal Tablets 2234
Kutrase Capsules 2546
Levsin/Levsinex/Levbid 2549

Ipratropium Bromide (Pilocarpine might antagonize the anticholinergic effects of drugs used concomitantly). Products include:
Atrovent Inhalation Aerosol 674
Atrovent Inhalation Solution 675
Atrovent Nasal Spray 0.03% 676
Atrovent Nasal Spray 0.06% 678

Labetalol Hydrochloride (Potential for conduction disturbances). Products include:
Normodyne Injection 2519
Normodyne Tablets 2522
Trandate 1158

Levobunolol Hydrochloride (Potential for conduction disturbances). Products include:
Betagan .... ◉ 230

Mepenzolate Bromide (Pilocarpine might antagonize the anticholinergic effects of drugs used concomitantly).
No products indexed under this heading.

Metipranolol Hydrochloride (Potential for conduction disturbances). Products include:
OptiPranolol (Metipranolol 0.3%) Sterile Ophthalmic Solution .... ◉ 256

Metoprolol Succinate (Potential for conduction disturbances). Products include:
Toprol-XL Tablets 560

Metoprolol Tartrate (Potential for conduction disturbances). Products include:
Lopressor 848
Lopressor HCT Tablets 850

Nadolol (Potential for conduction disturbances).
No products indexed under this heading.

Neostigmine Bromide (Additive pharmacologic effect). Products include:
Prostigmin Tablets 1306

Neostigmine Methylsulfate (Additive pharmacologic effect). Products include:
Prostigmin Injectable 1305

Oxybutynin Chloride (Pilocarpine might antagonize the anticholinergic effects of drugs used concomitantly). Products include:
Ditropan 1267

Penbutolol Sulfate (Potential for conduction disturbances). Products include:
Levatol Tablets 2547

Pindolol (Potential for conduction disturbances). Products include:
Visken Tablets 2428

Procyclidine Hydrochloride (Pilocarpine might antagonize the anticholinergic effects of drugs used concomitantly). Products include:
Kemadrin Tablets 1105

Propantheline Bromide (Pilocarpine might antagonize the anticholinergic effects of drugs used concomitantly). Products include:
Pro-Banthine Tablets 2226

Propranolol Hydrochloride (Potential for conduction disturbances). Products include:
Inderal 2834
Inderal LA Long Acting Capsules 2836
Inderide Tablets 2838
Inderide LA Long Acting Capsules .. 2840

Pyridostigmine Bromide (Additive pharmacologic effect). Products include:
Mestinon Injectable 1300
Mestinon 1300

Scopolamine (Pilocarpine might antagonize the anticholinergic effects of drugs used concomitantly). Products include:
Transderm Scōp Transdermal Therapeutic System 890

Scopolamine Hydrobromide (Pilocarpine might antagonize the anticholinergic effects of drugs used concomitantly). Products include:
Atrohist Plus Tablets 1605
Donnatal 2234
Donnatal Extentabs 2234
Donnatal Tablets 2234

Sotalol Hydrochloride (Potential for conduction disturbances). Products include:
Betapace Tablets 637

Timolol Hemihydrate (Potential for conduction disturbances). Products include:
Betimol 0.25%, 0.5% .... ◉ 259

Timolol Maleate (Potential for conduction disturbances). Products include:
Blocadren Tablets 1654
Timolide Tablets 1791
Timoptic in Ocudose 1796
Timoptic Sterile Ophthalmic Solution 1794
Timoptic-XE 1798

Tridihexethyl Chloride (Pilocarpine might antagonize the anticholinergic effects of drugs used concomitantly).
No products indexed under this heading.

Trihexyphenidyl Hydrochloride (Pilocarpine might antagonize the anticholinergic effects of drugs used concomitantly). Products include:
Artane 1418

Food Interactions

Diet, high-lipid (Decrease in the rate of absorption of pilocarpine when taken with high fat meal).

SALFLEX TABLETS
(Salsalate) 791
May interact with antigout agents, salicylates, urinary alkalizing agents, oral anticoagulants, oral hypoglycemic agents, penicillins, corticosteroids, and certain other agents. Compounds in these categories include:

Acarbose (Hypoglycemic effect may be enhanced). Products include:
Precose 604

Allopurinol (Uricosuric action antagonized). Products include:
Zyloprim Tablets 1194

Amoxicillin Trihydrate (Competition for protein binding site). Products include:
Amoxil 2631
Augmentin 2637
Augmentin Tablets 2640

Ampicillin Sodium (Competition for protein binding site). Products include:
Unasyn 2035

Aspirin (Potential for additive effect and toxicity). Products include:
Alka-Seltzer Cherry Effervescent Antacid and Pain Reliever .... [PD] 609
Alka-Seltzer Extra Strength Effervescent Antacid and Pain Reliever .... [PD] 609
Alka-Seltzer Lemon Lime Effervescent Antacid and Pain Reliever .... [PD] 609
Alka-Seltzer Original Effervescent Antacid and Pain Reliever .... [PD] 609
Alka-Seltzer Plus .... [PD] 611
Alka-Seltzer Plus Sinus Medicine .. [PD] 611
Ascriptin .... [PD] 650
Arthritis Strength BC Powder .... [PD] 631
BC Cold Powder Multi-Symptom Formula (Cold-Sinus-Allergy) .... [PD] 631
BC Cold Powder Non-Drowsy Formula (Cold-Sinus) .... [PD] 631
BC Powder .... [PD] 631
Genuine Bayer Aspirin Tablets & Caplets .... [PD] 618
Extra Strength Bayer Arthritis Pain Regimen Formula .... [PD] 615
Extra Strength Bayer Aspirin Caplets & Tablets .... [PD] 617
Extended-Release Bayer 8-Hour Aspirin .... [PD] 616
Extra Strength Bayer Plus Aspirin Caplets .... [PD] 617
Extra Strength Bayer PM Aspirin Plus Sleep Aid .... [PD] 617
Aspirin Regimen Bayer 81 mg Tablets with Calcium .... [PD] 615
Aspirin Regimen Bayer Adult Low Strength 81 mg Tablets .... [PD] 613
Aspirin Regimen Bayer Children's Chewable Aspirin .... [PD] 616
Aspirin Regimen Bayer Regular Strength 325 mg Caplets .... [PD] 613
Bufferin Analgesic Tablets .... [PD] 636
Arthritis Strength Bufferin Analgesic Caplets .... [PD] 637
Extra Strength Bufferin Analgesic Tablets .... [PD] 637
Cama Arthritis Pain Reliever .... [PD] 748
Darvon Compound-65 Pulvules 1475
Easprin 1971
Ecotrin 2625
Ecotrin Enteric Coated Aspirin Maximum Strength Tablets and Caplets .... [PD] 775
Ecotrin Enteric Coated Aspirin Regular Strength Tablets 2625
Empirin Aspirin Tablets .... [PD] 818
Excedrin Extra-Strength Analgesic Tablets, Caplets, and Geltabs 734
Fiorinal Capsules 2388
Fiorinal with Codeine Capsules 2390
Fiorinal Tablets 2388
Goody's Extra Strength Headache Powders .... [PD] 632
Goody's Extra Strength Pain Relief Tablets .... [PD] 632
Halfprin Tablets 1413
Norgesic 1554

IMPORTANT NOTE: Always consult each drug listing in the patient's regimen for possible interactions.

Salflex — Interactions Index

Salflex
- Percodan Tablets 955
- Percodan-Demi Tablets 956
- Robaxisal Tablets 2246
- Soma Compound w/Codeine Tablets 2784
- Soma Compound Tablets 2783
- St. Joseph Adult Chewable Aspirin (81 mg.) 768
- Talwin Compound 2466
- Vanquish Analgesic Caplets 627

Azlocillin Sodium (Competition for protein binding site).
No products indexed under this heading.

Bacampicillin Hydrochloride (Competition for protein binding site). Products include:
- Spectrobid Tablets 2030

Betamethasone Acetate (Competition for protein binding sites). Products include:
- Celestone Soluspan Suspension 2484

Betamethasone Sodium Phosphate (Competition for protein binding sites). Products include:
- Celestone Soluspan Suspension 2484

Carbenicillin Disodium (Competition for protein binding site).
No products indexed under this heading.

Carbenicillin Indanyl Sodium (Competition for protein binding site). Products include:
- Geocillin Tablets 2009

Chlorpropamide (Hypoglycemic effect may be enhanced). Products include:
- Diabinese Tablets 2002

Choline Magnesium Trisalicylate (Potential for additive effect and toxicity). Products include:
- Trilisate 2155

Cortisone Acetate (Competition for protein binding sites). Products include:
- Cortone Acetate Sterile Suspension 1663
- Cortone Acetate Tablets 1664

Dexamethasone (Competition for protein binding sites). Products include:
- AK-Trol Ointment & Suspension 205
- Decadron Elixir 1676
- Decadron Tablets 1678
- Decaspray Topical Aerosol 1689
- Maxitrol Ophthalmic Ointment and Suspension 222
- TobraDex Ophthalmic Suspension and Ointment 469

Dexamethasone Acetate (Competition for protein binding sites). Products include:
- Dalalone D.P. Injectable 1009
- Decadron-LA Sterile Suspension 1687

Dexamethasone Sodium Phosphate (Competition for protein binding sites). Products include:
- Decadron Phosphate Injection 1680
- Decadron Phosphate Sterile Ophthalmic Ointment 1684
- Decadron Phosphate Sterile Ophthalmic Solution 1685
- Decadron Phosphate Topical Cream 1686
- Decadron Phosphate with Xylocaine Injection, Sterile 1683
- Dexacort Phosphate in Respihaler 1606
- Dexacort Phosphate in Turbinaire 1607
- NeoDecadron Sterile Ophthalmic Ointment 1755
- NeoDecadron Sterile Ophthalmic Solution 1756
- NeoDecadron Topical Cream 1757

Dicloxacillin Sodium (Competition for protein binding site).
No products indexed under this heading.

Dicumarol (Increased potential for systemic bleeding).
No products indexed under this heading.

Diflunisal (Potential for additive effect and toxicity). Products include:
- Dolobid Tablets 1695

Fludrocortisone Acetate (Competition for protein binding sites). Products include:
- Florinef Acetate Tablets 506

Glimepiride (Hypoglycemic effect may be enhanced). Products include:
- Amaryl Tablets 1241

Glipizide (Hypoglycemic effect may be enhanced). Products include:
- Glucotrol Tablets 2011
- Glucotrol XL Extended Release Tablets 2012

Glyburide (Hypoglycemic effect may be enhanced). Products include:
- DiaBeta Tablets 1265
- Glynase PresTab Tablets 2091
- Micronase Tablets 2099

Hydrocortisone (Competition for protein binding sites). Products include:
- Anusol-HC Cream 2.5% 1953
- Aquanil HC Lotion 1989
- Maximum Strength Cortaid Spray 800
- CORTENEMA 2713
- Cortisporin Ointment 1074
- Cortisporin Ophthalmic Ointment Sterile 1074
- Cortisporin Ophthalmic Suspension Sterile 1075
- Cortisporin Otic Solution Sterile 1076
- Cortisporin Otic Suspension Sterile 1077
- Cortizone-5 795
- Cortizone-10 795
- Hydrocortone Tablets 1715
- Hytone 922
- Hytone Ointment 2½% 923
- Massengill Medicated Soft Cloth Towelettes 2628
- Pediotic Suspension Sterile 1140
- Preparation H Hydrocortisone 1% Cream 843
- ProctoCream-HC 2.5% 2552
- VōSoL HC Otic Solution 2786

Hydrocortisone Acetate (Competition for protein binding sites). Products include:
- Analpram-HC Rectal Cream 1% and 2.5% 993
- Anusol-HC 1 Hydrocortisone Anti-Itch Ointment 810
- Anusol-HC Suppositories 1954
- Caldecort Anti-Itch Hydrocortisone Cream 651
- Coly-Mycin S Otic w/Neomycin & Hydrocortisone 1965
- Cortaid 800
- Cortifoam 2540
- Cortisporin Cream 1073
- Epifoam 2543
- Hydrocortone Acetate Sterile Suspension 1712
- Mantadil Cream 1124
- Nupercainal Hydrocortisone 1% Cream 661
- Pramosone Cream, Lotion & Ointment 995
- ProctoFoam-HC 2552
- Terra-Cortril Ophthalmic Suspension 2033

Hydrocortisone Sodium Phosphate (Competition for protein binding sites). Products include:
- Hydrocortone Phosphate Injection, Sterile 1713

Hydrocortisone Sodium Succinate (Competition for protein binding sites).
No products indexed under this heading.

Magnesium Salicylate (Potential for additive effect and toxicity). Products include:
- Backache Caplets 635
- Doan's Extra-Strength Analgesic 653
- Extra Strength Doan's P.M. 653
- Doan's Regular Strength Analgesic 654
- Mobigesic Tablets 607

Metformin Hydrochloride (Hypoglycemic effect may be enhanced). Products include:
- Glucophage Tablets 754

Methotrexate Sodium (Competition for protein binding sites). Products include:
- Methotrexate Sodium Tablets, Injection, for Injection and LPF Injection 1322

Methylprednisolone Acetate (Competition for protein binding sites).
No products indexed under this heading.

Methylprednisolone Sodium Succinate (Competition for protein binding sites).
No products indexed under this heading.

Mezlocillin Sodium (Competition for protein binding sites). Products include:
- Mezlin 594
- Mezlin Pharmacy Bulk Package 597

Nafcillin Sodium (Competition for protein binding site).
No products indexed under this heading.

Naproxen (Competition for protein binding sites). Products include:
- Anaprox/Naprosyn 2277

Naproxen Sodium (Competition for protein binding sites). Products include:
- Aleve 2124
- Anaprox/Naprosyn 2277
- Naprelan Tablets 2861

Penicillin G Benzathine (Competition for protein binding sites). Products include:
- Bicillin C-R Injection 2810
- Bicillin C-R 900/300 Injection 2812
- Bicillin L-A Injection 2813

Penicillin G Potassium (Competition for protein binding sites). Products include:
- Pfizerpen for Injection 2022

Penicillin G Procaine (Competition for protein binding sites). Products include:
- Bicillin C-R Injection 2810
- Bicillin C-R 900/300 Injection 2812

Penicillin G Sodium (Competition for protein binding site).
No products indexed under this heading.

Penicillin V Potassium (Competition for protein binding sites). Products include:
- Pen•Vee K 2879

Phenytoin (Competition for protein binding sites). Products include:
- Dilantin Infatabs 1967
- Dilantin-125 Suspension 1969

Phenytoin Sodium (Competition for protein binding sites). Products include:
- Dilantin Kapseals 1965

Potassium Citrate (Lowers plasma levels of salicylic acid). Products include:
- Polycitra Syrup 574
- Polycitra-K Crystals 574
- Polycitra-K Oral Solution 575
- Polycitra-LC 574
- Urocit-K Tablets 1828

Prednisolone Acetate (Competition for protein binding sites). Products include:
- AK-CIDE 203
- AK-CIDE Ointment 203
- Blephamide Liquifilm Sterile Ophthalmic Suspension 472
- Blephamide Ointment 234
- Econopred & Econopred Plus Ophthalmic Suspensions 216
- Poly-Pred Liquifilm 246
- Pred Forte 247
- Pred Mild 250
- Pred-G Liquifilm Sterile Ophthalmic Suspension 248
- Pred-G S.O.P. Sterile Ophthalmic Ointment 249

Prednisolone Sodium Phosphate (Competition for protein binding sites). Products include:
- AK-PRED 204
- Hydeltrasol Injection, Sterile 1708
- Pediapred Oral Solution 1618

Prednisolone Tebutate (Competition for protein binding sites). Products include:
- Hydeltra-T.B.A. Sterile Suspension 1710

Prednisone (Competition for protein binding sites).
No products indexed under this heading.

Probenecid (Uricosuric action antagonized). Products include:
- Benemid Tablets 1651
- ColBENEMID Tablets 1662

Sodium Citrate (Lowers plasma levels of salicylic acid). Products include:
- Bicitra 573
- Polycitra 574
- Salix SST Lozenges Saliva Stimulant 757

Sulfinpyrazone (Uricosuric action antagonized). Products include:
- Anturane 823

Thyroxine Sodium (Competition for protein binding sites).
No products indexed under this heading.

Ticarcillin Disodium (Competition for protein binding site). Products include:
- Ticar for Injection 2704
- Timentin for Injection 2706

Tolazamide (Hypoglycemic effect may be enhanced).
No products indexed under this heading.

Tolbutamide (Hypoglycemic effect may be enhanced).
No products indexed under this heading.

Triamcinolone (Competition for protein binding sites).
No products indexed under this heading.

Triamcinolone Acetonide (Competition for protein binding sites). Products include:
- Azmacort Oral Inhaler 2175
- Nasacort AQ Nasal Spray 2191
- Nasacort Nasal Inhaler 2189

Triamcinolone Diacetate (Competition for protein binding sites).
No products indexed under this heading.

Triamcinolone Hexacetonide (Competition for protein binding sites).
No products indexed under this heading.

l-Triiodothyronine (Competition for protein binding sites).

Warfarin Sodium (Increased potential for systemic bleeding; competition for protein binding site). Products include:
- Coumadin 941

Food Interactions

Food, unspecified (Slows the absorption).

SALINEX NASAL MIST AND DROPS
(Sodium Chloride) 713
None cited in PDR database.

SALIX SST LOZENGES SALIVA STIMULANT
(Sorbitol, Malic Acid, Sodium

(▩ Described in PDR For Nonprescription Drugs) (⊙ Described in PDR For Ophthalmology)

Citrate, Citric Acid, Dicalcium
Phosphate............................... ⊕ 757
None cited in PDR database.

SANDIMMUNE I.V. AMPULS FOR INFUSION
(Cyclosporine) 2416
May interact with immunosuppressive agents, potassium sparing diuretics, and certain other agents. Compounds in these categories include:

Amiloride Hydrochloride (Cyclosporine may cause hyperkalemia, concurrent use should be avoided). Products include:
- Midamor Tablets 1746
- Moduretic Tablets 1748

Amphotericin B (Potential synergies of nephrotoxicity may occur). Products include:
- Abelcet Injection 1540
- Fungizone Intravenous 507
- Fungizone Oral Suspension 704

Antibiotics, unspecified (Potential synergies of nephrotoxicity may occur).

Azapropazon (Potential nephrotoxic synergy).

Azathioprine (Increases susceptibility to infection). Products include:
- Azathioprine Tablets 2349
- Imuran 1103

Bromocriptine Mesylate (Increases cyclosporine levels; dosage adjustments are essential). Products include:
- Parlodel 2411

Carbamazepine (Decreases cyclosporine plasma concentrations; dosage adjustments are essential). Products include:
- Atretol Tablets 569
- Tegretol/Tegretol-XR 870

Cimetidine (Potential nephrotoxic synergy). Products include:
- Tagamet HB Tablets .... ⊕ 786
- Tagamet Tablets 2694

Cimetidine Hydrochloride (Potential nephrotoxic synergy). Products include:
- Tagamet 2694

Danazol (Increases cyclosporine plasma concentrations; dosage adjustments are essential). Products include:
- Danocrine Capsules 2437

Diclofenac Potassium (Potential nephrotoxic synergy). Products include:
- Cataflam Tablets 833

Diclofenac Sodium (Potential nephrotoxic synergy). Products include:
- Voltaren Ophthalmic Sterile Ophthalmic Solution .... ⊕ 264
- Cataflam/Voltaren/Voltaren-XR ... 833

Digoxin (Reduced clearance of digoxin and potential for severe digitalis toxicity). Products include:
- Lanoxicaps 1110
- Lanoxin Elixir Pediatric 1113
- Lanoxin Injection 1116
- Lanoxin Injection Pediatric 1119
- Lanoxin Tablets 1121

Diltiazem Hydrochloride (Increases cyclosporine plasma concentrations; dosage adjustments are essential). Products include:
- Cardizem CD Capsules 1251
- Cardizem SR Capsules 1255
- Cardizem Injectable 1253
- Cardizem Tablets 1257
- Dilacor XR Extended-release Capsules 2183
- Tiazac Capsules 1019

Erythromycin (Increases cyclosporine plasma concentrations; dosage adjustments are essential). Products include:
- A/T/S 2% Acne Topical Gel 1244
- A/T/S 2% Acne Topical Solution ... 1244
- Benzamycin Topical Gel 919
- E-Mycin Tablets 1388
- Emgel 2% Topical Gel 1081
- ERYC 1972
- Erycette (erythromycin 2%) Topical Solution 1943
- Ery-Tab Tablets 426
- Erythromycin Base Filmtab 430
- Erythromycin Delayed-Release Capsules, USP 431
- Ilotycin Ophthalmic Ointment ... 928
- PCE Dispertab Tablets 453
- T-Stat 2.0% Topical Solution and Pads 2797
- THERAMYCIN Z 2% Solution 1629

Erythromycin Estolate (Increases cyclosporine plasma concentrations; dosage adjustments are essential). Products include:
- Ilosone 927

Erythromycin Ethylsuccinate (Increases cyclosporine plasma concentrations; dosage adjustments are essential). Products include:
- E.E.S. 427
- EryPed 425
- Pediazole Suspension 2340

Erythromycin Gluceptate (Increases cyclosporine plasma concentrations; dosage adjustments are essential). Products include:
- Ilotycin Gluceptate, IV, Vials 929

Erythromycin Lactobionate (Increases cyclosporine plasma concentrations; dosage adjustments are essential).
- No products indexed under this heading.

Erythromycin Stearate (Increases cyclosporine plasma concentrations; dosage adjustments are essential). Products include:
- Erythrocin Stearate Filmtab 429

Fluconazole (Increases cyclosporine levels; dosage adjustments are essential). Products include:
- Diflucan Tablets, Injection, and Oral Suspension 2003

Gentamicin Sulfate (Potential synergies of nephrotoxicity may occur). Products include:
- Garamycin Cream 0.1% 2501
- Garamycin Injectable 2502
- Garamycin Ointment 0.1% 2501
- Garamycin Ophthalmic 2501
- Genoptic Sterile Ophthalmic Solution .... ⊕ 241
- Genoptic Sterile Ophthalmic Ointment .... ⊕ 241
- Gentak .... ⊕ 209
- Pred-G Liquifilm Sterile Ophthalmic Suspension .... ⊕ 248
- Pred-G S.O.P. Sterile Ophthalmic Ointment .... ⊕ 249

Immune Globulin (Human) (Increases susceptibility to infection).
- No products indexed under this heading.

Immune Globulin Intravenous (Human) (Increases susceptibility to infection).

Itraconazole (Increases cyclosporine levels; dosage adjustments are essential). Products include:
- Sporanox Capsules 1352

Ketoconazole (Potential nephrotoxic synergy; increases cyclosporine plasma concentrations; dosage adjustments are essential). Products include:
- Nizoral 2% Cream 1344
- Nizoral 2% Shampoo 1344
- Nizoral Tablets 1345

Lovastatin (Reduced clearance of lovastatin; concomitant administration associated with development of myositis). Products include:
- Mevacor Tablets 1742

Melphalan (Potential nephrotoxic synergy). Products include:
- Alkeran Tablets 1198

Methylprednisolone (Increases cyclosporine plasma concentrations; dosage adjustments are essential; convulsions have occurred with high dose methylprednisolone).
- No products indexed under this heading.

Methylprednisolone Acetate (Increases cyclosporine plasma concentrations; dosage adjustments are essential; convulsions have occurred with high dose methylprednisolone).
- No products indexed under this heading.

Methylprednisolone Sodium Succinate (Increases cyclosporine plasma concentrations; dosage adjustments are essential; convulsions have occurred with high dose methylprednisolone).
- No products indexed under this heading.

Metoclopramide Hydrochloride (Increases cyclosporine levels; dosage adjustments are essential). Products include:
- Reglan 2243

Muromonab-CD3 (Increased susceptibility to infection and increased risk for development of lymphomas and malignancies). Products include:
- Orthoclone OKT3 Sterile Solution .. 1892

Mycophenolate Mofetil (Increases susceptibility to infection). Products include:
- CellCept Capsules 2265

Nephrotoxic Drugs (Potential synergics of nephrotoxicity).

Nicardipine Hydrochloride (Increases cyclosporine plasma concentrations; dosage adjustments are essential). Products include:
- Cardene Capsules 2261
- Cardene I.V. 2815
- Cardene SR Capsules 2264

Nifedipine (Potential for frequent gingival hyperplasia). Products include:
- Adalat Capsules (10 mg and 20 mg) 580
- Adalat CC 582
- Procardia Capsules 2024
- Procardia XL Extended Release Tablets 2026

Phenobarbital (Decreases cyclosporine plasma levels; dosage adjustments are essential). Products include:
- Arco-Lase Plus Tablets 513
- Bellergal-S Tablets 2375
- Donnatal 2234
- Donnatal Extentabs 2234
- Donnatal Tablets 2234
- Phenobarbital Elixir and Tablets ... 1523
- Quadrinal Tablets 1398

Phenytoin (Decreases cyclosporine plasma levels; dosage adjustments are essential). Products include:
- Dilantin Infatabs 1967
- Dilantin-125 Suspension 1969

Phenytoin Sodium (Decreases cyclosporine plasma levels; dosage adjustments are essential). Products include:
- Dilantin Kapseals 1965

Prednisolone (Reduced clearance of prednisolone). Products include:
- Prelone Syrup 1834

Prednisolone Acetate (Reduced clearance of prednisolone). Products include:
- AK-CIDE .... ⊕ 203
- AK-CIDE Ointment .... ⊕ 203
- Blephamide Liquifilm Sterile Ophthalmic Suspension 472
- Blephamide Ointment .... ⊕ 234
- Econopred & Econopred Plus Ophthalmic Suspensions .... ⊕ 216
- Poly-Pred Liquifilm .... ⊕ 246
- Pred Forte .... ⊕ 247
- Pred Mild .... ⊕ 250
- Pred-G Liquifilm Sterile Ophthalmic Suspension .... ⊕ 248
- Pred-G S.O.P. Sterile Ophthalmic Ointment .... ⊕ 249

Prednisolone Sodium Phosphate (Reduced clearance of prednisolone). Products include:
- AK-PRED .... ⊕ 204
- Hydeltrasol Injection, Sterile 1708
- Pediapred Oral Solution 1618

Prednisolone Tebutate (Reduced clearance of prednisolone). Products include:
- Hydeltra-T.B.A. Sterile Suspension 1710

Ranitidine Hydrochloride (Potential nephrotoxic synergy). Products include:
- Zantac 1182
- Zantac Injection 1180
- Zantac Syrup 1182

Rifampin (Decreases cyclosporine plasma levels; dosage adjustments are essential). Products include:
- Rifadin 1276
- Rifamate Capsules 1278
- Rifater 1280
- Rimactane Capsules 865

Spironolactone (Cyclosporine may cause hyperkalemia, concurrent use should be avoided). Products include:
- Aldactazide Tablets 2556
- Aldactone Tablets 2558

Sulfamethoxazole (Potential nephrotoxic synergy; decreases cyclosporine plasma levels; dosage adjustments are essential). Products include:
- Bactrim DS Tablets 2257
- Bactrim I.V. Infusion 2255
- Bactrim 2257
- Gantanol Tablets 2285
- Septra 1146
- Septra I.V. Infusion 1142
- Septra I.V. Infusion ADD-Vantage Vials 1144
- Septra 1146

Tacrolimus (Increases susceptibility to infection). Products include:
- Prograf 1028

Tobramycin (Potential synergies of nephrotoxicity may occur). Products include:
- AKTOB .... ⊕ 207
- TobraDex Ophthalmic Suspension and Ointment 469
- Tobrex Ophthalmic Ointment and Solution .... ⊕ 226

Tobramycin Sulfate (Potential synergies of nephrotoxicity may occur). Products include:
- Nebcin Vials, Hyporets & ADD-Vantage 1518

Triamterene (Cyclosporine may cause hyperkalemia, concurrent use should be avoided). Products include:
- Dyazide Capsules 2653
- Dyrenium Capsules 2655

Trimethoprim (Potential nephrotoxic synergy; decreases cyclosporine plasma levels; dosage adjustments are essential). Products include:
- Bactrim DS Tablets 2257
- Bactrim I.V. Infusion 2255
- Bactrim 2257
- Proloprim Tablets 1141
- Septra 1146

IMPORTANT NOTE: Always consult each drug listing in the patient's regimen for possible interactions.

Sandimmune — Interactions Index

Septra I.V. Infusion 1142
Septra I.V. Infusion ADD-Vantage Vials 1144
Septra 1146
Trimpex Tablets 2323

Vancomycin Hydrochloride (Potential nephrotoxic synergy). Products include:
Vancocin HCl, Oral Solution & Pulvules 1536
Vancocin HCl, Vials & ADD-Vantage 1534

Verapamil Hydrochloride (Increases cyclosporine levels; dosage adjustments are essential). Products include:
Calan SR Caplets 2571
Calan Tablets 2568
Covera-HS Tablets 2573
Isoptin Injectable 1391
Isoptin Oral Tablets 1393
Isoptin SR Tablets 1395
Verelan Capsules 1455

SANDIMMUNE ORAL SOLUTION
(Cyclosporine) 2416
See Sandimmune I.V. Ampuls for Infusion

SANDIMMUNE SOFT GELATIN CAPSULES
(Cyclosporine) 2416
See Sandimmune I.V. Ampuls for Infusion

SANDOGLOBULIN I.V.
(Globulin, Immune (Human)) 2419
May interact with:

Measles, Mumps & Rubella Virus Vaccine Live (Antibodies in Immune Globulin may interfere with the response to live viral vaccines). Products include:
M-M-R II 1730

SANDOSTATIN INJECTION
(Octreotide Acetate) 2421
May interact with oral hypoglycemic agents, insulin, beta blockers, calcium channel blockers, and certain other agents. Compounds in these categories include:

Acarbose (Adjustment of the dosage of hypoglycemic agents may be required). Products include:
Precose 604

Acebutolol Hydrochloride (Adjustment of the dosage of beta blockers may be required). Products include:
Sectral Capsules 2914

Amlodipine Besylate (Adjustment of the dosage of calcium channel blocker may be required). Products include:
Lotrel Capsules 858
Norvasc Tablets 2020

Atenolol (Adjustment of the dosage of beta blockers may be required). Products include:
Tenoretic Tablets 2963
Tenormin Tablets and I.V. Injection .. 2965

Bepridil Hydrochloride (Adjustment of the dosage of calcium channel blocker may be required). Products include:
Vascor Tablets (200 and 300 mg) ... 1597

Betaxolol Hydrochloride (Adjustment of the dosage of beta blockers may be required). Products include:
Betoptic Ophthalmic Solution 465
Betoptic S Ophthalmic Suspension 467
Kerlone Tablets 2588

Bisoprolol Fumarate (Adjustment of the dosage of beta blockers may be required). Products include:
Zebeta Tablets 1457

Ziac 1459

Carteolol Hydrochloride (Adjustment of the dosage of beta blockers may be required). Products include:
Cartrol Tablets 413
Ocupress Ophthalmic Solution, 1% Sterile .... ⊚ 297

Chlorpropamide (Adjustment of the dosage of hypoglycemic agents may be required). Products include:
Diabinese Tablets 2002

Cyclosporine (Co-administration may decrease blood levels of cyclosporine and may result in transplant rejection). Products include:
Neoral 2405
Sandimmune 2416

Diazoxide (Adjustment of the dosage of diazoxide may be required). Products include:
Hyperstat I.V. Injection 2504
Proglycem 575

Diltiazem Hydrochloride (Adjustment of the dosage of calcium channel blocker may be required). Products include:
Cardizem CD Capsules 1251
Cardizem SR Capsules 1255
Cardizem Injectable 1253
Cardizem Tablets 1257
Dilacor XR Extended-release Capsules 2183
Tiazac Capsules 1019

Esmolol Hydrochloride (Adjustment of the dosage of beta blockers may be required). Products include:
Brevibloc (esmolol HCl) Injection 1860

Felodipine (Adjustment of the dosage of calcium channel blocker may be required). Products include:
Plendil Extended-Release Tablets 514

Glimepiride (Adjustment of the dosage of hypoglycemic agents may be required). Products include:
Amaryl Tablets 1241

Glipizide (Adjustment of the dosage of hypoglycemic agents may be required). Products include:
Glucotrol Tablets 2011
Glucotrol XL Extended Release Tablets 2012

Glyburide (Adjustment of the dosage of hypoglycemic agents may be required). Products include:
DiaBeta Tablets 1265
Glynase PresTab Tablets 2091
Micronase Tablets 2099

Insulin, Human (Adjustment of the dosage of insulin may be required).
No products indexed under this heading.

Insulin, Human Isophane Suspension (Adjustment of the dosage of insulin may be required). Products include:
Novolin N Human Insulin 10 ml Vials 1846

Insulin, Human NPH (Adjustment of the dosage of insulin may be required). Products include:
Humulin N, 100 Units 1495
Novolin N PenFill 1.5 ml Cartridges Durable Insulin Delivery System 1849
Novolin N Prefilled Syringe Disposable Insulin Delivery System 1850

Insulin, Human Regular (Adjustment of the dosage of insulin may be required). Products include:
Humulin R, 100 Units 1497
Novolin R Human Insulin 10 ml Vials 1846
Novolin R PenFill 1.5 ml Cartridges Durable Insulin Delivery System 1849
Novolin R Prefilled Syringe Disposable Insulin Delivery System 1850

Velosulin BR Human Insulin 10 ml Vials 1847

Insulin, Human, Zinc Suspension (Adjustment of the dosage of insulin may be required). Products include:
Humulin L, 100 Units 1494
Humulin U, 100 Units 1498
Novolin L Human Insulin 10 ml Vials 1846

Insulin Lispro, Human (Adjustment of the dosage of insulin may be required). Products include:
Humalog Injection 1488

Insulin, NPH (Adjustment of the dosage of insulin may be required). Products include:
NPH, 100 Units 1502
Pork NPH, 100 Units 1506
Purified Pork NPH Isophane Insulin 1852

Insulin, Regular (Adjustment of the dosage of insulin may be required). Products include:
Regular, 100 Units 1503
Pork Regular, 100 Units 1507
Pork Regular (Concentrated), 500 Units 1508
Purified Pork Regular Insulin 1852

Insulin, Zinc Crystals (Adjustment of the dosage of insulin may be required). Products include:
NPH, 100 Units 1502

Insulin, Zinc Suspension (Adjustment of the dosage of insulin may be required). Products include:
Iletin I 1501
Lente, 100 Units 1501
Iletin II 1504
Pork Lente, 100 Units 1504
Purified Pork Lente Insulin 1852

Isradipine (Adjustment of the dosage of calcium channel blocker may be required). Products include:
DynaCirc Capsules 2381
DynaCirc CR Tablets 2383

Labetalol Hydrochloride (Adjustment of the dosage of beta blockers may be required). Products include:
Normodyne Injection 2519
Normodyne Tablets 2522
Trandate 1158

Levobunolol Hydrochloride (Adjustment of the dosage of beta blockers may be required). Products include:
Betagan .... ⊚ 230

Metformin Hydrochloride (Adjustment of the dosage of hypoglycemic agents may be required). Products include:
Glucophage Tablets 754

Metipranolol Hydrochloride (Adjustment of the dosage of beta blockers may be required). Products include:
OptiPranolol (Metipranolol 0.3%) Sterile Ophthalmic Solution .... ⊚ 256

Metoprolol Succinate (Adjustment of the dosage of beta blockers may be required). Products include:
Toprol-XL Tablets 560

Metoprolol Tartrate (Adjustment of the dosage of beta blockers may be required). Products include:
Lopressor 848
Lopressor HCT Tablets 850

Nadolol (Adjustment of the dosage of beta blockers may be required).
No products indexed under this heading.

Nicardipine Hydrochloride (Adjustment of the dosage of calcium channel blocker may be required). Products include:
Cardene Capsules 2261

Cardene I.V. 2815
Cardene SR Capsules 2264

Nifedipine (Adjustment of the dosage of calcium channel blocker may be required). Products include:
Adalat Capsules (10 mg and 20 mg) 580
Adalat CC 582
Procardia Capsules 2024
Procardia XL Extended Release Tablets 2026

Nimodipine (Adjustment of the dosage of calcium channel blocker may be required). Products include:
Nimotop Capsules 603

Nisoldipine (Adjustment of the dosage of calcium channel blocker may be required). Products include:
Sular Tablets 2961

Penbutolol Sulfate (Adjustment of the dosage of beta blockers may be required). Products include:
Levatol Tablets 2547

Pindolol (Adjustment of the dosage of beta blockers may be required). Products include:
Visken Tablets 2428

Propranolol Hydrochloride (Adjustment of the dosage of beta blockers may be required). Products include:
Inderal 2834
Inderal LA Long Acting Capsules 2836
Inderide Tablets 2838
Inderide LA Long Acting Capsules .. 2840

Sotalol Hydrochloride (Adjustment of the dosage of beta blockers may be required). Products include:
Betapace Tablets 637

Timolol Hemihydrate (Adjustment of the dosage of beta blockers may be required). Products include:
Betimol 0.25%, 0.5% .... ⊚ 259

Timolol Maleate (Adjustment of the dosage of beta blockers may be required). Products include:
Blocadren Tablets 1654
Timolide Tablets 1791
Timoptic in Ocudose 1796
Timoptic Sterile Ophthalmic Solution 1794
Timoptic-XE 1798

Tolazamide (Adjustment of the dosage of hypoglycemic agents may be required).
No products indexed under this heading.

Tolbutamide (Adjustment of the dosage of hypoglycemic agents may be required).
No products indexed under this heading.

Verapamil Hydrochloride (Adjustment of the dosage of calcium channel blocker may be required). Products include:
Calan SR Caplets 2571
Calan Tablets 2568
Covera-HS Tablets 2573
Isoptin Injectable 1391
Isoptin Oral Tablets 1393
Isoptin SR Tablets 1395
Verelan Capsules 1455

SANOREX TABLETS
(Mazindol) 2423
May interact with monoamine oxidase inhibitors, insulin, vasopressors, sympathomimetics, and certain other agents. Compounds in these categories include:

Albuterol (Mazindol may potentiate blood pressure increases in those patients taking sympathomimetics). Products include:
Proventil Inhalation Aerosol 2524
Ventolin Inhalation Aerosol and Refill 1170

(⊞ Described in PDR For Nonprescription Drugs) (⊚ Described in PDR For Ophthalmology)

Albuterol Sulfate (Mazindol may potentiate blood pressure increases in those patients taking sympathomimetics). Products include:
- Airet Albuterol Sulfate Inhalation Solution ... 1602
- Albuterol Sulfate, USP Solution for Inhalation, Arm-a-Med ... 522
- Proventil Inhalation Solution 0.083% ... 2527
- Proventil Repetabs Tablets ... 2529
- Proventil Solution for Inhalation 0.5% ... 2525
- Proventil Syrup ... 2528
- Proventil Tablets ... 2529
- Ventolin Inhalation Solution ... 1171
- Ventolin Nebules Inhalation Solution ... 1172
- Ventolin Rotacaps for Inhalation ... 1173
- Ventolin Syrup ... 1175
- Ventolin Tablets ... 1176
- Volmax Extended-Release Tablets ... 1835

Dobutamine Hydrochloride (Mazindol may potentiate blood pressure increases in those patients taking sympathomimetics). Products include:
- Dobutrex Solution Vials ... 1480

Dopamine Hydrochloride (Potentiated pressor effects; Mazindol may potentiate blood pressure increases in those patients taking sympathomimetics).
No products indexed under this heading.

Ephedrine Hydrochloride (Mazindol may potentiate blood pressure increases in those patients taking sympathomimetics). Products include:
- Primatene Tablets ... 844
- Quadrinal Tablets ... 1398

Ephedrine Sulfate (Mazindol may potentiate blood pressure increases in those patients taking sympathomimetics). Products include:
- Marax Tablets & DF Syrup ... 2015

Ephedrine Tannate (Mazindol may potentiate blood pressure increases in those patients taking sympathomimetics). Products include:
- Rynatuss ... 2782

Epinephrine (Mazindol may potentiate blood pressure increases in those patients taking sympathomimetics). Products include:
- EPIFRIN ... 237
- EpiPen ... 808
- Marcaine with Epinephrine ... 2446
- Primatene Mist ... 843
- Sensorcaine with Epinephrine Injection ... 554
- Sus-Phrine Injection ... 1017
- Xylocaine with Epinephrine Injections ... 562

Epinephrine Bitartrate (Mazindol may potentiate blood pressure increases in those patients taking sympathomimetics). Products include:
- Sensorcaine-MPF with Epinephrine Injection ... 554

Epinephrine Hydrochloride (Potentiated pressor effects; Mazindol may potentiate blood pressure increases in those patients taking sympathomimetics). Products include:
- Ana-Kit Anaphylaxis Emergency Treatment Kit ... 611

Furazolidone (Concurrent use is contraindicated; potential for hypertensive crises). Products include:
- Furoxone ... 2221

Guanethidine Monosulfate (Decreased hypotensive effect). Products include:
- Esimil Tablets ... 840
- Ismelin Tablets ... 845

Insulin, Human (Altered insulin requirements).
No products indexed under this heading.

Insulin, Human Isophane Suspension (Altered insulin requirements). Products include:
- Novolin N Human Insulin 10 ml Vials ... 1846

Insulin, Human NPH (Altered insulin requirements). Products include:
- Humulin N, 100 Units ... 1495
- Novolin N PenFill 1.5 ml Cartridges Durable Insulin Delivery System ... 1849
- Novolin N Prefilled Syringe Disposable Insulin Delivery System ... 1850

Insulin, Human Regular (Altered insulin requirements). Products include:
- Humulin R, 100 Units ... 1497
- Novolin R Human Insulin 10 ml Vials ... 1846
- Novolin R PenFill 1.5 ml Cartridges Durable Insulin Delivery System ... 1849
- Novolin R Prefilled Syringe Disposable Insulin Delivery System ... 1850
- Velosulin BR Human Insulin 10 ml Vials ... 1847

Insulin, Human, Zinc Suspension (Altered insulin requirements). Products include:
- Humulin L, 100 Units ... 1494
- Humulin U, 100 Units ... 1498
- Novolin L Human Insulin 10 ml Vials ... 1846

Insulin Lispro, Human (Altered insulin requirements). Products include:
- Humalog Injection ... 1488

Insulin, NPH (Altered insulin requirements). Products include:
- NPH, 100 Units ... 1502
- Pork NPH, 100 Units ... 1506
- Purified Pork NPH Isophane Insulin ... 1852

Insulin, Regular (Altered insulin requirements). Products include:
- Regular, 100 Units ... 1503
- Pork Regular, 100 Units ... 1507
- Pork Regular (Concentrated), 500 Units ... 1508
- Purified Pork Regular Insulin ... 1852

Insulin, Zinc Crystals (Altered insulin requirements). Products include:
- NPH, 100 Units ... 1502

Insulin, Zinc Suspension (Altered insulin requirements). Products include:
- Iletin I ... 1501
- Lente, 100 Units ... 1501
- Iletin II ... 1504
- Pork Lente, 100 Units ... 1504
- Purified Pork Lente Insulin ... 1852

Isocarboxazid (Concurrent use is contraindicated; potential for hypertensive crises).
No products indexed under this heading.

Isoproterenol Hydrochloride (Mazindol may potentiate blood pressure increases in those patients taking sympathomimetics). Products include:
- Isuprel Hydrochloride Solution ... 2443
- Isuprel Injection ... 2441
- Isuprel Mistometer ... 2442

Isoproterenol Sulfate (Mazindol may potentiate blood pressure increases in those patients taking sympathomimetics). Products include:
- Norisodrine with Calcium Iodide Syrup ... 446

Metaproterenol Sulfate (Mazindol may potentiate blood pressure increases in those patients taking sympathomimetics). Products include:
- Alupent ... 672
- Metaproterenol Sulfate Inhalation Solution, USP, Arm-a-Med ... 547

Metaraminol Bitartrate (Potentiated pressor effects; Mazindol may potentiate blood pressure increases in those patients taking sympathomimetics). Products include:
- Aramine Injection ... 1649

Methoxamine Hydrochloride (Potentiated pressor effects; Mazindol may potentiate blood pressure increases in those patients taking sympathomimetics). Products include:
- Vasoxyl Injection ... 1169

Norepinephrine Bitartrate (Potentiated pressor effects; Mazindol may potentiate blood pressure increases in those patients taking sympathomimetics). Products include:
- Levophed Bitartrate Injection ... 2445

Phenelzine Sulfate (Concurrent use is contraindicated; potential for hypertensive crises). Products include:
- Nardil ... 1977

Phenylephrine Bitartrate (Mazindol may potentiate blood pressure increases in those patients taking sympathomimetics).
No products indexed under this heading.

Phenylephrine Hydrochloride (Potentiated pressor effects; Mazindol may potentiate blood pressure increases in those patients taking sympathomimetics). Products include:
- Atrohist Plus Tablets ... 1605
- Cerose DM ... 853
- D.A. II Tablets ... 972
- D.A. Chewable Tablets ... 970
- Dura-Vent/DA Tablets ... 972
- Extendryl ... 1003
- 4-Way Fast Acting Nasal Spray (regular & mentholated) ... 644
- Hemorid ... 797
- Hycomine Compound Tablets ... 948
- Neo-Synephrine Hydrochloride 1% Carpuject ... 2455
- Neo-Synephrine Hydrochloride 1% Injection ... 2455
- Neo-Synephrine Hydrochloride (Ophthalmic) ... 2456
- Neo-Synephrine ... 624
- Novahistine Elixir ... 782
- Phenergan VC ... 2886
- Phenergan VC with Codeine ... 2888
- Preparation H ... 842
- Tympagesic Ear Drops ... 2476
- Vicks Sinex Nasal Spray and Ultra Fine Mist ... 738

Phenylephrine Tannate (Mazindol may potentiate blood pressure increases in those patients taking sympathomimetics). Products include:
- Atrohist Pediatric Suspension ... 1604
- Atrohist Pediatric Suspension Dye-Free ... 1604
- Rynatan ... 2781
- Rynatuss ... 2782

Phenylpropanolamine Hydrochloride (Mazindol may potentiate blood pressure increases in those patients taking sympathomimetics). Products include:
- Acutrim ... 648
- Atrohist Plus Tablets ... 1605
- BC Cold Powder Multi-Symptom Formula (Cold-Sinus-Allergy) ... 631
- BC Cold Powder Non-Drowsy Formula (Cold-Sinus) ... 631
- Cheracol Plus Head Cold/Cough Formula ... 741
- Comtrex Multi-Symptom Cold Reliever Liqui-Gels ... 638
- Comtrex Multi-Symptom Non-Drowsy Liqui-gels ... 640
- Contac Continuous Action Nasal Decongestant/Antihistamine 12 Hour Capsules ... 773
- Contac Maximum Strength Continuous Action Decongestant/Antihistamine 12 Hour Caplets ... 772
- Contac Severe Cold and Flu Formula Caplets ... 773
- Coricidin 'D' Decongestant Tablets ... 760
- Dexatrim ... 795
- Dexatrim Plus Vitamins Caplets ... 796
- Dimetane-DC Cough Syrup ... 2232
- Dimetapp Allergy Sinus Caplets ... 838
- Dimetapp Cold & Allergy Chewable Tablets ... 838
- Dimetapp Cold & Cough Liqui-Gels ... 839
- Dimetapp DM Elixir ... 840
- Dimetapp Elixir ... 840
- Dimetapp Extentabs ... 841
- Dimetapp Tablets/Liqui-Gels ... 841
- Dura-Vent Tablets ... 971
- Entex LA Tablets ... 972
- Exgest LA Tablets ... 787
- Hycomine ... 947
- Nolamine Timed-Release Tablets ... 790
- Ornade Spansule Capsules ... 2678
- Propagest Tablets ... 791
- Pyrroxate Caplets ... 742
- Robitussin-CF ... 846
- Sinulin Tablets ... 792
- Tavist-D 12 Hour Relief Tablets ... 750
- Teldrin 12 Hour Antihistamine/Nasal Decongestant Allergy Relief Capsules ... 786
- Triaminic Expectorant ... 753
- Triaminic Syrup ... 755
- Triaminic Triaminicol Cold & Cough ... 756
- Triaminic DM Syrup ... 756
- Triaminicin Tablets ... 756
- Vicks DayQuil Allergy Relief 12-Hour Extended Release Tablets ... 733
- Vicks DayQuil Allergy Relief 4-Hour Tablets ... 733
- Vicks DayQuil SINUS Pressure & CONGESTION Relief ... 734

Pirbuterol Acetate (Mazindol may potentiate blood pressure increases in those patients taking sympathomimetics). Products include:
- Maxair Autohaler ... 1550
- Maxair Inhaler ... 1552

Pseudoephedrine Hydrochloride (Mazindol may potentiate blood pressure increases in those patients taking sympathomimetics). Products include:
- Actifed Allergy Daytime/Nighttime Caplets ... 808
- Actifed Cold & Allergy Tablets ... 807
- Actifed Cold & Sinus Caplets and Tablets ... 808
- Actifed Sinus Daytime/Nighttime Tablets and Caplets ... 809
- Advil Cold and Sinus Caplets and Tablets ... 837
- Alka-Seltzer Plus Liqui-Gels ... 612
- Alka-Seltzer Plus Flu & Body Aches Liqui-Gels Non-Drowsy Formula ... 613
- Alka-Seltzer Plus Night-Time Cold Medicine Liqui-Gels ... 612
- Allerest Maximum Strength ... 649
- Allerest No Drowsiness ... 649
- Allerest Sinus Pain Formula ... 649
- Atrohist Pediatric Capsules ... 1603
- Benadryl Allergy/Cold Tablets ... 811
- Benadryl Allergy Decongestant Liquid Medication ... 812
- Benadryl Allergy Decongestant Tablets ... 812
- Benadryl Allergy Sinus Headache Caplets ... 813
- Benylin Multisymptom ... 816
- Bromfed Capsules (Extended-Release) ... 1832
- Bromfed Syrup ... 712
- Bromfed Tablets ... 1832
- Bromfed-DM Cough Syrup ... 1832
- Bromfed-PD Capsules (Extended-Release) ... 1832
- Children's TYLENOL Cold Multi-Symptom Chewable Tablets and Liquid ... 1559

IMPORTANT NOTE: Always consult each drug listing in the patient's regimen for possible interactions.

Sanorex | Interactions Index | 964

Children's TYLENOL Cold Plus Cough Multi Symptom Chewable Tablets and Liquid 1560
Children's TYLENOL Flu Suspension Liquid 1560
Children's Vicks DayQuil Allergy Relief ..... ■ 730
Children's Vicks NyQuil Cold/Cough Relief ..... ■ 731
Allergy-Sinus Comtrex Multi-Symptom Allergy-Sinus Formula Tablets and Caplets ..... ■ 639
Comtrex Multi-Symptom ..... ■ 638
Comtrex Multi-Symptom Non-Drowsy Caplets ..... ■ 640
Congess 1003
Contac Day Allergy/Sinus Caplets ■ 771
Contac Day & Night ..... ■ 772
Contac Night Allergy/Sinus Caplets ..... ■ 771
Contac Severe Cold & Flu Non-Drowsy ..... ■ 774
Deconsal II Tablets 1605
Dimetane-DX Cough Syrup 2233
Dimetapp Cold & Fever Suspension ..... ■ 839
Dimetapp Decongestant Pediatric Drops ..... ■ 840
Dorcol Children's Cough Syrup ..... ■ 748
Drixoral Cough + Congestion Liquid Caps ..... ■ 763
Dura-Tap/PD Capsules 970
Duratuss Tablets 2750
Duratuss HD Elixir 2750
Efidac/24 ..... ■ 655
Entex PSE Tablets 973
Fedahist Gyrocaps 2545
Guaifed 1833
Guaifed Syrup ..... ■ 712
Guaimax-D Tablets 809
Histussin D Liquid 670
Infants' TYLENOL Cold Decongestant & Fever-Reducer Drops 1561
Kronofed-A 994
Novahistine DMX ..... ■ 782
Nucofed 2225
PediaCare Cough-Cold Chewable Tablets and Liquid 1569
PediaCare Infants' Decongestant Drops 1569
PediaCare Infants' Drops Decongestant Plus Cough 1569
PediaCare NightRest Cough-Cold Liquid 1569
Pediatric Vicks 44d Cough & Head Congestion Relief ..... ■ 736
Pediatric Vicks 44m Cough & Cold Relief ..... ■ 737
Robitussin Cold & Cough Liqui-Gels ..... ■ 844
Robitussin Cold, Cough & Flu Liqui-Gels ..... ■ 844
Robitussin Maximum Strength Cough & Cold ..... ■ 847
Robitussin Night-Time Cold Formula ..... ■ 847
Robitussin Pediatric Cough & Cold Formula ..... ■ 848
Robitussin Pediatric Drops ..... ■ 849
Robitussin Severe Congestion Liqui-Gels ..... ■ 845
Robitussin-DAC Syrup 2249
Robitussin-PE ..... ■ 846
Rondec Oral Drops 974
Rondec Syrup 974
Rondec Tablet 974
Rondec Chewable Tablets 974
Rondec-TR Tablet 974
Ryna ..... ■ 804
Seldane-D Extended-Release Tablets 1286
Semprex-D Capsules 1620
Sinarest ..... ■ 663
Sine-Aid Maximum Strength Sinus Headache Gelcaps, Caplets and Tablets 1570
Sine-Off No Drowsiness Formula Caplets ..... ■ 784
Sine-Off Sinus Medicine ..... ■ 784
Singlet Tablets ..... ■ 785
Sinutab Non-Drying Liquid Caps ..... ■ 823
Sinutab Sinus Allergy Medication, Maximum Strength Tablets and Caplets ..... ■ 823
Sinutab Sinus Medication, Maximum Strength Without Drowsiness Formula, Tablets & Caplets ..... ■ 824
Sudafed Children's Cold & Cough Liquid Medication ..... ■ 825
Sudafed Children's Nasal Decongestant Liquid Medication ..... ■ 826
Sudafed Cold & Allergy Tablets ..... ■ 826
Sudafed Cold and Cough Liquid Caps ..... ■ 826
Sudafed Nasal Decongestant Tablets, 30 mg ..... ■ 825
Sudafed Nasal Decongestant Tablets, 60 mg ..... ■ 825
Sudafed Non-Drying Sinus Liquid Caps ..... ■ 827
Sudafed Pediatric Nasal Decongestant Liquid Oral Drops ..... ■ 827
Sudafed Severe Cold Formula Caplets ..... ■ 828
Sudafed Severe Cold Formula Tablets ..... ■ 828
Sudafed Sinus Caplets ..... ■ 829
Sudafed Sinus Tablets ..... ■ 829
Sudafed 12 Hour Caplets ..... ■ 824
Syn-Rx Tablets 1622
Syn-Rx DM Tablets 1623
TheraFlu Flu and Cold Medicine ..... ■ 750
Theraflu Maximum Strength Flu and Cold Medicine For Sore Throat ..... ■ 751
TheraFlu Flu, Cold and Cough Medicine ..... ■ 750
TheraFlu Maximum Strength Nighttime Flu, Cold & Cough Medicine ..... ■ 751
TheraFlu Maximum Strength Non-Drowsy Formula Flu, Cold & Cough Medicine ..... ■ 751
TheraFlu Maximum Strength, Non-Drowsy Formula Flu, Cold and Cough Caplets ..... ■ 752
Theraflu Maximum Strength Sinus Non-Drowsy Formula Caplets ..... ■ 752
Triaminic AM Cough and Decongestant Formula ..... ■ 753
Triaminic AM Decongestant Formula ..... ■ 753
Triaminic Infant Oral Decongestant Drops ..... ■ 754
Triaminic Night Time ..... ■ 754
Triaminic Sore Throat Formula ..... ■ 755
Tussend 1830
Tussend Expectorant 1831
TYLENOL Allergy Sinus, Maximum Strength Caplets and Gelcaps 1571
TYLENOL Allergy Sinus NightTime, Maximum Strength Caplets 1571
TYLENOL Cold Medication, Multi-Symptom Formula Tablets and Caplets 1572
TYLENOL Cold Medication, Multi-Symptom Hot Liquid Packets 1572
TYLENOL Cold Medication, No Drowsiness Formula Caplets and Gelcaps 1572
TYLENOL Cold Severe Congestion Caplets 1573
TYLENOL Cough Medication with Decongestant, Multi Symptom 1574
TYLENOL Flu No Drowsiness Formula, Maximum Strength Gelcaps 1575
TYLENOL Flu NightTime, Maximum Strength Gelcaps 1575
TYLENOL Flu NightTime, Maximum Strength Hot Medication Packets 1575
TYLENOL Sinus, Maximum Strength Geltabs, Gelcaps, Caplets and Tablets 1576
Vicks 44 LiquiCaps Cough, Cold & Flu Relief ..... ■ 728
Vicks 44 LiquiCaps Non-Drowsy Cough & Cold Relief ..... ■ 729
Vicks 44D Cough & Head Congestion Relief ..... ■ 728
Vicks 44M Cough, Cold & Flu Relief ..... ■ 729
Vicks DayQuil LiquiCaps/Liquid Multi-Symptom Cold/Flu Relief ..... ■ 734
Vicks DayQuil SINUS Pressure & PAIN Relief with IBUPROFEN ..... ■ 735
Vicks Nyquil Hot Therapy ..... ■ 735
Vicks NyQuil LiquiCaps/Liquid Multi-Symptom Cold/Flu Relief, Original and Cherry Flavors ..... ■ 736

Pseudoephedrine Sulfate (Mazindol may potentiate blood pressure increases in those patients taking sympathomimetics). Products include:
Chlor-Trimeton Allergy Decongestant Tablets ..... ■ 759
Claritin-D Tablets 2487
Drixoral Cold and Allergy Sustained-Action Tablets ..... ■ 763
Drixoral Cold and Flu Extended-Release Tablets ..... ■ 764
Drixoral Non-Drowsy Formula Extended-Release Tablets ..... ■ 764
Drixoral Allergy/Sinus Extended Release Tablets ..... ■ 765
Trinalin Repetabs Tablets 1373

Salmeterol Xinafoate (Mazindol may potentiate blood pressure increases in those patients taking sympathomimetics). Products include:
Serevent Inhalation Aerosol 1149

Selegiline Hydrochloride (Concurrent use is contraindicated; potential for hypertensive crises). Products include:
Eldepryl Capsules 2729

Terbutaline Sulfate (Mazindol may potentiate blood pressure increases in those patients taking sympathomimetics). Products include:
Brethaire Inhaler 830
Brethine Ampuls 832
Brethine Tablets 831
Bricanyl Subcutaneous Injection 1247
Bricanyl Tablets 1248

Tranylcypromine Sulfate (Concurrent use is contraindicated; potential for hypertensive crises). Products include:
Parnate Tablets 2679

SANSERT TABLETS
(Methysergide Maleate) 2424
May interact with narcotic analgesics. Compounds in this category include:

Alfentanil Hydrochloride (Methysergide may reverse the analgesic activity of narcotic analgesics). Products include:
Alfenta Injection 1334

Buprenorphine (Methysergide may reverse the analgesic activity of narcotic analgesics). Products include:
Buprenex Injectable 2170

Codeine Phosphate (Methysergide may reverse the analgesic activity of narcotic analgesics). Products include:
Brontex 2130
Dimetane-DC Cough Syrup 2232
Fioricet with Codeine Capsules 2387
Fiorinal with Codeine Capsules 2390
Nucofed 2225
Phenergan with Codeine 2883
Phenergan VC with Codeine 2888
Robitussin A-C Syrup 2248
Robitussin-DAC Syrup 2249
Ryna ..... ■ 804
Soma Compound w/Codeine Tablets 2784
Tylenol with Codeine 1592

Dezocine (Methysergide may reverse the analgesic activity of narcotic analgesics). Products include:
Dalgan Injection 529

Fentanyl (Methysergide may reverse the analgesic activity of narcotic analgesics). Products include:
Duragesic Transdermal System 1336

Fentanyl Citrate (Methysergide may reverse the analgesic activity of narcotic analgesics). Products include:
Sublimaze Injection 463

Hydrocodone Bitartrate (Methysergide may reverse the analgesic activity of narcotic analgesics). Products include:
Codiclear DH Syrup 808
Duratuss HD Elixir 2750
Histussin D Liquid 670
Hycodan Tablets and Syrup 946
Hycomine Compound Tablets 948
Hycomine 947
Hycotuss Expectorant Syrup 950
Hydrocet Capsules 787
Lorcet 10/650 Tablets 1016
Lortab 2751
Tussend 1830
Tussend Expectorant 1831
Vicodin Tablets 1404
Vicodin ES Tablets 1405
Vicodin HP Tablets 1403
Vicodin Tuss Expectorant 1406
Zydone Capsules 967

Hydrocodone Polistirex (Methysergide may reverse the analgesic activity of narcotic analgesics). Products include:
Tussionex Pennkinetic Extended-Release Suspension 1624

Hydromorphone Hydrochloride (Methysergide may reverse the analgesic activity of narcotic analgesics). Products include:
Dilaudid Ampules 1382
Dilaudid Cough Syrup 1383
Dilaudid-HP Injection 1384
Dilaudid-HP Lyophilized Powder 250 mg 1384
Dilaudid 1382
Dilaudid Oral Liquid 1386
Dilaudid 1382
Dilaudid Tablets - 8 mg 1386

Levorphanol Tartrate (Methysergide may reverse the analgesic activity of narcotic analgesics). Products include:
Levo-Dromoran 2297

Meperidine Hydrochloride (Methysergide may reverse the analgesic activity of narcotic analgesics). Products include:
Demerol 2438
Mepergan Injection 2859

Methadone Hydrochloride (Methysergide may reverse the analgesic activity of narcotic analgesics). Products include:
Methadone Hydrochloride Oral Concentrate 2356
Methadone Hydrochloride Oral Solution & Tablets 2357

Morphine Sulfate (Methysergide may reverse the analgesic activity of narcotic analgesics). Products include:
Astramorph/PF Injection, USP (Preservative-Free) 526
Duramorph Injection 983
Infumorph 200 and Infumorph 500 Sterile Solutions 985
Kadian Capsules 2948
MS Contin Tablets 2149
MSIR 2152
Oramorph SR (Morphine Sulfate Sustained Release Tablets) 2359
RMS Suppositories CII 2766
Roxanol 2365

Opium Alkaloids (Methysergide may reverse the analgesic activity of narcotic analgesics).
No products indexed under this heading.

Oxycodone Hydrochloride (Methysergide may reverse the analgesic activity of narcotic analgesics). Products include:
OxyContin Tablets 2163
OxyIR Capsules 2167
Percocet Tablets 955
Percodan Tablets 955
Percodan-Demi Tablets 956
Roxicodone Tablets, Oral Solution & Intensol (Oxycodone) 2366
Tylox Capsules 1593

Propoxyphene Hydrochloride (Methysergide may reverse the analgesic activity of narcotic analgesics). Products include:
Darvon 1475
Wygesic Tablets 2930

Propoxyphene Napsylate (Methysergide may reverse the analgesic activity of narcotic analgesics). Products include:
Darvon-N/Darvocet-N 1473

(■ Described in PDR For Nonprescription Drugs) (⊙ Described in PDR For Ophthalmology)

Sufentanil Citrate (Methysergide may reverse the analgesic activity of narcotic analgesics). Products include:

Sufenta Injection 1355

SARAPIN
(Sarracenia purpurea, Pitcher Plant Distillate) 1237
None cited in PDR database.

SATIN ANTIMICROBIAL SKIN CLEANSER FOR DIABETIC/CANCER PATIENT CARE
(Chloroxylenol) 647
None cited in PDR database.

SCLEROMATE INJECTION
(Morrhuate Sodium) 1234
None cited in PDR database.

SECONAL SODIUM PULVULES
(Secobarbital Sodium) 1529
May interact with central nervous system depressants, narcotic analgesics, tranquilizers, antihistamines, oral anticoagulants, corticosteroids, monoamine oxidase inhibitors, oral contraceptives, and certain other agents. Compounds in these categories include:

Acrivastine (Concomitant use may produce additive CNS-depressant effects). Products include:
Semprex-D Capsules 1620

Alfentanil Hydrochloride (Concomitant use may produce additive CNS-depressant effects). Products include:
Alfenta Injection 1334

Alprazolam (Concomitant use may produce additive CNS-depressant effects). Products include:
Xanax Tablets 2115

Aprobarbital (Concomitant use may produce additive CNS-depressant effects).
No products indexed under this heading.

Astemizole (Concomitant use may produce additive CNS-depressant effects). Products include:
Hismanal Tablets 1341

Azatadine Maleate (Concomitant use may produce additive CNS-depressant effects). Products include:
Trinalin Repetabs Tablets 1373

Betamethasone Acetate (Enhanced metabolism of exogenous corticosteroids). Products include:
Celestone Soluspan Suspension 2484

Betamethasone Sodium Phosphate (Enhanced metabolism of exogenous corticosteroids). Products include:
Celestone Soluspan Suspension 2484

Bromodiphenhydramine Hydrochloride (Concomitant use may produce additive CNS-depressant effects).
No products indexed under this heading.

Brompheniramine Maleate (Concomitant use may produce additive CNS-depressant effects). Products include:
Alka-Seltzer Plus Sinus Medicine 611
Bromfed Capsules (Extended-Release) 1832
Bromfed Syrup 712
Bromfed Tablets 1832
Bromfed-DM Cough Syrup 1832
Bromfed-PD Capsules (Extended-Release) 1832
Dimetane-DC Cough Syrup 2232
Dimetane-DX Cough Syrup 2233
Dimetapp Allergy Dye-Free Elixir 838
Dimetapp Allergy Sinus Caplets 838
Dimetapp Cold & Allergy Chewable Tablets 838
Dimetapp Cold & Cough Liqui-Gels 839
Dimetapp Cold & Fever Suspension 839
Dimetapp DM Elixir 840
Dimetapp Elixir 840
Dimetapp Extentabs 841
Dimetapp Tablets/Liqui-Gels 841
Rondec Chewable Tablets 974
Vicks DayQuil Allergy Relief 12-Hour Extended Release Tablets 733
Vicks DayQuil Allergy Relief 4-Hour Tablets 733

Buprenorphine (Concomitant use may produce additive CNS-depressant effects). Products include:
Buprenex Injectable 2170

Buspirone Hydrochloride (Concomitant use may produce additive CNS-depressant effects). Products include:
BuSpar Tablets 738

Butabarbital (Concomitant use may produce additive CNS-depressant effects).
No products indexed under this heading.

Butalbital (Concomitant use may produce additive CNS-depressant effects). Products include:
Axocet Capsules 2469
Esgic-plus Capsules 1012
Esgic-plus Tablets 1012
Fioricet Tablets 2386
Fioricet with Codeine Capsules 2387
Fiorinal Capsules 2388
Fiorinal with Codeine Capsules 2390
Fiorinal Tablets 2388
Phrenilin 790
Sedapap Tablets 50 mg/650 mg 1826

Cetirizine Hydrochloride (Concomitant use may produce additive CNS-depressant effects). Products include:
Zyrtec Tablets 2053

Chlordiazepoxide (Concomitant use may produce additive CNS-depressant effects). Products include:
Limbitrol 2333

Chlordiazepoxide Hydrochloride (Concomitant use may produce additive CNS-depressant effects). Products include:
Librax Capsules 2330
Librium Capsules 2331
Librium Injectable 2332

Chlorpheniramine Maleate (Concomitant use may produce additive CNS-depressant effects). Products include:
Alka-Seltzer Plus Cold Medicine 611
Alka-Seltzer Plus Cold Medicine Liqui-Gels 612
Alka-Seltzer Plus Cold & Cough Medicine 611
Alka-Seltzer Plus Cold & Cough Medicine Liqui-Gels 612
Alka-Seltzer Plus Flu & Body Aches Effervescent Tablets 612
Allerest Maximum Strength 649
Allerest Sinus Pain Formula 649
Ana-Kit Anaphylaxis Emergency Treatment Kit 611
Atrohist Pediatric Capsules 1603
Atrohist Plus Tablets 1605
BC Cold Powder Multi-Symptom Formula (Cold-Sinus-Allergy) 631
Cerose DM 853
Cheracol Plus Head Cold/Cough Formula 741
Children's TYLENOL Cold Multi-Symptom Chewable Tablets and Liquid 1559
Children's TYLENOL Cold Plus Cough Multi Symptom Chewable Tablets and Liquid 1560
Children's TYLENOL Flu Suspension Liquid 1560
Children's Vicks DayQuil Allergy Relief 730
Children's Vicks NyQuil Cold/Cough Relief 731
Chlor-Trimeton Allergy Decongestant Tablets 759
Chlor-Trimeton Allergy Tablets 758
Allergy-Sinus Comtrex Multi-Symptom Allergy-Sinus Formula Tablets and Caplets 639
Comtrex Multi-Symptom 638
Contac Continuous Action Nasal Decongestant/Antihistamine 12 Hour Capsules 773
Contac Maximum Strength Continuous Action Decongestant/Antihistamine 12 Hour Caplets 772
Contac Severe Cold and Flu Formula Caplets 773
Coricidin Cold + Flu Tablets 760
Coricidin Cough + Cold Tablets 760
Coricidin 'D' Decongestant Tablets 760
D.A. II Tablets 972
D.A. Chewable Tablets 970
Dura-Tap/PD Capsules 970
Dura-Vent/DA Tablets 972
Efidac 24 Chlorpheniramine 655
Extendryl 1003
Fedahist Gyrocaps 2545
Hycomine Compound Tablets 948
Kronofed-A 994
Nolamine Timed-Release Tablets 790
Novahistine Elixir 782
Ornade Spansule Capsules 2678
PediaCare Cough-Cold Chewable Tablets and Liquid 1569
PediaCare NightRest Cough-Cold Liquid 1569
Pediatric Vicks 44m Cough & Cold Relief 737
Pyrroxate Caplets 742
Ryna 804
Sinarest 663
Sine-Off Sinus Medicine 784
Singlet Tablets 785
Sinulin Tablets 792
Sinutab Sinus Allergy Medication, Maximum Strength Tablets and Caplets 823
Sudafed Cold & Allergy Tablets 826
Teldrin 12 Hour Antihistamine/Nasal Decongestant Allergy Relief Capsules 786
TheraFlu Flu and Cold Medicine 750
Theraflu Maximum Strength Flu and Cold Medicine For Sore Throat 751
TheraFlu Flu, Cold and Cough Medicine 750
TheraFlu Maximum Strength Nighttime Flu, Cold & Cough Medicine 751
Triaminic Night Time 754
Triaminic Syrup 755
Triaminic Triaminicol Cold & Cough 756
Triaminicin Tablets 756
Tussend 1830
TYLENOL Allergy Sinus, Maximum Strength Caplets and Gelcaps 1571
TYLENOL Cold Medication, Multi-Symptom Formula Tablets and Caplets 1572
TYLENOL Cold Medication, Multi-Symptom Hot Liquid Packets 1572
Vicks 44 LiquiCaps Cough, Cold & Flu Relief 728
Vicks 44M Cough, Cold & Flu Relief 729

Chlorpheniramine Polistirex (Concomitant use may produce additive CNS-depressant effects). Products include:
Tussionex Pennkinetic Extended-Release Suspension 1624

Chlorpheniramine Tannate (Concomitant use may produce additive CNS-depressant effects). Products include:
Atrohist Pediatric Suspension 1604
Atrohist Pediatric Suspension Dye-Free 1604
Rynatan 2781
Rynatuss 2782

Chlorpromazine (Concomitant use may produce additive CNS-depressant effects). Products include:
Thorazine Suppositories 2701

Chlorprothixene (Concomitant use may produce additive CNS-depressant effects).
No products indexed under this heading.

Chlorprothixene Hydrochloride (Concomitant use may produce additive CNS-depressant effects).
No products indexed under this heading.

Chlorprothixene Lactate (Concomitant use may produce additive CNS-depressant effects).
No products indexed under this heading.

Clemastine Fumarate (Concomitant use may produce additive CNS-depressant effects). Products include:
Tavist Syrup 2426
Tavist Tablets 2427
Tavist-1 12 Hour Relief Tablets 749
Tavist-D 12 Hour Relief Tablets 750

Clorazepate Dipotassium (Concomitant use may produce additive CNS-depressant effects). Products include:
Tranxene 459

Clozapine (Concomitant use may produce additive CNS-depressant effects). Products include:
Clozaril Tablets 2377

Codeine Phosphate (Concomitant use may produce additive CNS-depressant effects). Products include:
Brontex 2130
Dimetane-DC Cough Syrup 2232
Fioricet with Codeine Capsules 2387
Fiorinal with Codeine Capsules 2390
Nucofed 2225
Phenergan with Codeine 2883
Phenergan VC with Codeine 2888
Robitussin A-C Syrup 2248
Robitussin-DAC Syrup 2249
Ryna 804
Soma Compound w/Codeine Tablets 2784
Tylenol with Codeine 1592

Cortisone Acetate (Enhanced metabolism of exogenous corticosteroids). Products include:
Cortone Acetate Sterile Suspension 1663
Cortone Acetate Tablets 1664

Cyproheptadine Hydrochloride (Concomitant use may produce additive CNS-depressant effects). Products include:
Periactin 1767

Desflurane (Concomitant use may produce additive CNS-depressant effects). Products include:
Suprane (desflurane, USP) 1865

Desogestrel (Decreased effect of estradiol by increasing its metabolism). Products include:
Desogen Tablets 1867
Ortho-Cept 1907

Dexamethasone (Enhanced metabolism of exogenous corticosteroids). Products include:
AK-Trol Ointment & Suspension ⊙ 205
Decadron Elixir 1676
Decadron Tablets 1678
Decaspray Topical Aerosol 1689
Maxitrol Ophthalmic Ointment and Suspension ⊙ 222
TobraDex Ophthalmic Suspension and Ointment 469

Dexamethasone Acetate (Enhanced metabolism of exogenous corticosteroids). Products include:
Dalalone D.P. Injectable 1009
Decadron-LA Sterile Suspension 1687

Dexamethasone Sodium Phosphate (Enhanced metabolism of exogenous corticosteroids). Products include:
Decadron Phosphate Injection 1680

IMPORTANT NOTE: Always consult each drug listing in the patient's regimen for possible interactions.

Seconal — **Interactions Index** — **966**

Decadron Phosphate Sterile Ophthalmic Ointment ... 1684
Decadron Phosphate Sterile Ophthalmic Solution ... 1685
Decadron Phosphate Topical Cream ... 1686
Decadron Phosphate with Xylocaine Injection, Sterile ... 1683
Dexacort Phosphate in Respihaler .. 1606
Dexacort Phosphate in Turbinaire .. 1607
NeoDecadron Sterile Ophthalmic Ointment ... 1755
NeoDecadron Sterile Ophthalmic Solution ... 1756
NeoDecadron Topical Cream ... 1757

Dexchlorpheniramine Maleate (Concomitant use may produce additive CNS-depressant effects).
No products indexed under this heading.

Dezocine (Concomitant use may produce additive CNS-depressant effects). Products include:
Dalgan Injection ... 529

Diazepam (Concomitant use may produce additive CNS-depressant effects). Products include:
Dizac (diazepam injectable emulsion) CIV ... 1862
Valium Injectable ... 2336
Valium Tablets ... 2335

Dicumarol (Barbiturates can induce hepatic microsomal enzymes, resulting in increased or decreased anticoagulant response).
No products indexed under this heading.

Diphenhydramine Citrate (Concomitant use may produce additive CNS-depressant effects). Products include:
Excedrin P.M. Analgesic/Sleeping Aid Tablets, Caplets, Liquigels ... 735

Diphenhydramine Hydrochloride (Concomitant use may produce additive CNS-depressant effects). Products include:
Actifed Allergy Daytime/Nighttime Caplets ... ▣ 808
Actifed Sinus Daytime/Nighttime Tablets and Caplets ... ▣ 809
Extra Strength Bayer PM Aspirin Plus Sleep Aid ... ▣ 617
Benadryl Allergy Chewables ... ▣ 811
Benadryl Allergy/Cold Tablets ... ▣ 811
Benadryl Allergy Decongestant Liquid Medication ... ▣ 812
Benadryl Allergy Decongestant Tablets ... ▣ 812
Benadryl Allergy Liquid Medication ... ▣ 813
Benadryl Allergy ... ▣ 811
Benadryl Allergy Sinus Headache Caplets ... ▣ 813
Benadryl Dye-Free Allergy Liquigel Softgels ... ▣ 813
Benadryl Dye-Free Allergy Liquid Medication ... ▣ 814
Benadryl Itch Relief Stick Extra Strength ... ▣ 814
Benadryl Cream ... ▣ 814
Benadryl Gel ... ▣ 815
Benadryl Spray ... ▣ 815
Benadryl Injection ... 1955
Contac Day & Night Cold/Flu Night Caplets ... ▣ 772
Contac Night Allergy/Sinus Caplets ... ▣ 771
Extra Strength Doan's P.M. ... ▣ 653
Excedrin P.M. Analgesic/Sleeping Aid Tablets, Caplets, Liquigels ... ▣ 643
Nytol QuickCaps Caplets ... ▣ 632
Sleepinal Night-time Sleep Aid Capsules and Softgels ... ▣ 798
TYLENOL Allergy Sinus NightTime, Maximum Strength Caplets ... 1571
TYLENOL Flu NightTime, Maximum Strength Gelcaps ... 1575
TYLENOL Flu NightTime, Maximum Strength Hot Medication Packets ... 1575
TYLENOL PM Pain Reliever/Sleep Aid, Extra Strength Gelcaps, Caplets, Geltabs ... 1576
TYLENOL Severe Allergy Medication Caplets ... 1571
Maximum Strength Unisom Sleepgels ... 1990
Unisom With Pain Relief-Nighttime Sleep Aid and Pain Reliever ... 1991

Divalproex Sodium (Increases blood levels of secobarbital sodium). Products include:
Depakote Tablets ... 418

Doxycycline Calcium (Half-life of doxycycline may be shortened). Products include:
Vibramycin Calcium Oral Suspension Syrup ... 2038

Doxycycline Hyclate (Half-life of doxycycline may be shortened). Products include:
Doryx Capsules ... 1970
Vibramycin Hyclate Capsules ... 2038
Vibramycin Hyclate Intravenous ... 2040
Vibra-Tabs Film Coated Tablets ... 2038

Doxycycline Monohydrate (Half-life of doxycycline may be shortened). Products include:
Monodox Capsules ... 1858
Vibramycin Monohydrate for Oral Suspension ... 2038

Droperidol (Concomitant use may produce additive CNS-depressant effects). Products include:
Inapsine Injection ... 462

Enflurane (Concomitant use may produce additive CNS-depressant effects).
No products indexed under this heading.

Estazolam (Concomitant use may produce additive CNS-depressant effects). Products include:
ProSom Tablets ... 457

Ethchlorvynol (Concomitant use may produce additive CNS-depressant effects). Products include:
Placidyl Capsules ... 456

Ethinamate (Concomitant use may produce additive CNS-depressant effects).
No products indexed under this heading.

Ethinyl Estradiol (Decreased effect of estradiol by increasing its metabolism). Products include:
Brevicon ... 2563
Demulen ... 2580
Desogen Tablets ... 1867
Levlen/Tri-Levlen ... 646
Lo/Ovral Tablets ... 2852
Lo/Ovral-28 Tablets ... 2857
Modicon ... 1928
Nordette-21 Tablets ... 2863
Nordette-28 Tablets ... 2866
Norinyl ... 2563
Ortho-Cept ... 1907
Ortho-Cyclen/Ortho-Tri-Cyclen ... 1914
Ortho-Novum ... 1928
Ortho-Cyclen/Ortho Tri-Cyclen ... 1914
Ovcon ... 765
Ovral Tablets ... 2877
Ovral-28 Tablets ... 2878
Levlen/Tri-Levlen ... 646
Tri-Norinyl ... 2607
Triphasil-21 Tablets ... 2919
Triphasil-28 Tablets ... 2924

Ethynodiol Diacetate (Decreased effect of estradiol by increasing its metabolism). Products include:
Demulen ... 2580

Fentanyl (Concomitant use may produce additive CNS-depressant effects). Products include:
Duragesic Transdermal System ... 1336

Fentanyl Citrate (Concomitant use may produce additive CNS-depressant effects). Products include:
Sublimaze Injection ... 463

Fludrocortisone Acetate (Enhanced metabolism of exogenous corticosteroids). Products include:
Florinef Acetate Tablets ... 506

Fluphenazine Decanoate (Concomitant use may produce additive CNS-depressant effects). Products include:
Prolixin Decanoate ... 510

Fluphenazine Enanthate (Concomitant use may produce additive CNS-depressant effects). Products include:
Prolixin Enanthate ... 510

Fluphenazine Hydrochloride (Concomitant use may produce additive CNS-depressant effects). Products include:
Prolixin ... 510

Flurazepam Hydrochloride (Concomitant use may produce additive CNS-depressant effects). Products include:
Dalmane Capsules ... 2329

Furazolidone (Prolongs the effects of barbiturates). Products include:
Furoxone ... 2221

Glutethimide (Concomitant use may produce additive CNS-depressant effects).
No products indexed under this heading.

Griseofulvin (Interference with absorption of orally administered griseofulvin, thus decreasing its blood level). Products include:
Fulvicin P/G Tablets ... 2499
Fulvicin P/G 165 & 330 Tablets ... 2500
Grifulvin V (griseofulvin tablets) Microsize (griseofulvin oral suspension) Microsize ... 1944
Gris-PEG Tablets, 125 mg & 250 mg ... 476

Haloperidol (Concomitant use may produce additive CNS-depressant effects). Products include:
Haldol Injection, Tablets and Concentrate ... 1585

Haloperidol Decanoate (Concomitant use may produce additive CNS-depressant effects). Products include:
Haldol Decanoate ... 1587

Hydrocodone Bitartrate (Concomitant use may produce additive CNS-depressant effects). Products include:
Codiclear DH Syrup ... 808
Duratuss HD Elixir ... 2750
Histussin D Liquid ... 670
Hycodan Tablets and Syrup ... 946
Hycomine Compound Tablets ... 948
Hycomine ... 947
Hycotuss Expectorant Syrup ... 950
Hydrocet Capsules ... 787
Lorcet 10/650 Tablets ... 1016
Lortab ... 2751
Tussend ... 1830
Tussend Expectorant ... 1831
Vicodin Tablets ... 1404
Vicodin ES Tablets ... 1405
Vicodin HP Tablets ... 1403
Vicodin Tuss Expectorant ... 1406
Zydone Capsules ... 967

Hydrocodone Polistirex (Concomitant use may produce additive CNS-depressant effects). Products include:
Tussionex Pennkinetic Extended-Release Suspension ... 1624

Hydrocortisone (Enhanced metabolism of exogenous corticosteroids). Products include:
Anusol-HC Cream 2.5% ... 1953
Aquanil HC Lotion ... 1989
Maximum Strength Cortaid Spray ▣ 800
CORTENEMA ... 2713
Cortisporin Ointment ... 1074
Cortisporin Ophthalmic Ointment Sterile ... 1074
Cortisporin Ophthalmic Suspension Sterile ... 1075
Cortisporin Otic Solution Sterile ... 1076
Cortisporin Otic Suspension Sterile 1077
Cortizone-5 ... ▣ 795
Cortizone-10 ... ▣ 795
Hydrocortone Tablets ... 1715
Hytone ... 922
Hytone Ointment 2 ½% ... 923
Massengill Medicated Soft Cloth Towelettes ... 2628
Pediotic Suspension Sterile ... 1140
Preparation H Hydrocortisone 1% Cream ... ▣ 843
ProctoCream-HC 2.5% ... 2552
VōSoL HC Otic Solution ... 2786

Hydrocortisone Acetate (Enhanced metabolism of exogenous corticosteroids). Products include:
Analpram-HC Rectal Cream 1% and 2.5% ... 993
Anusol HC-1 Hydrocortisone Anti-Itch Ointment ... ▣ 810
Anusol-HC Suppositories ... 1954
Caldecort Anti-Itch Hydrocortisone Cream ... ▣ 651
Coly-Mycin S Otic w/Neomycin & Hydrocortisone ... 1965
Cortaid ... ▣ 800
Cortifoam ... 2540
Cortisporin Cream ... 1073
Epifoam ... 2543
Hydrocortone Acetate Sterile Suspension ... 1712
Mantadil Cream ... 1124
Nupercainal Hydrocortisone 1% Cream ... ▣ 661
Pramosone Cream, Lotion & Ointment ... 995
ProctoFoam-HC ... 2552
Terra-Cortril Ophthalmic Suspension ... 2033

Hydrocortisone Sodium Phosphate (Enhanced metabolism of exogenous corticosteroids). Products include:
Hydrocortone Phosphate Injection, Sterile ... 1713

Hydrocortisone Sodium Succinate (Enhanced metabolism of exogenous corticosteroids).
No products indexed under this heading.

Hydromorphone Hydrochloride (Concomitant use may produce additive CNS-depressant effects). Products include:
Dilaudid Ampules ... 1382
Dilaudid Cough Syrup ... 1383
Dilaudid-HP Injection ... 1384
Dilaudid-HP Lyophilized Powder 250 mg ... 1384
Dilaudid ... 1382
Dilaudid Oral Liquid ... 1386
Dilaudid ... 1382
Dilaudid Tablets - 8 mg ... 1386

Hydroxyzine Hydrochloride (Concomitant use may produce additive CNS-depressant effects). Products include:
Atarax Tablets & Syrup ... 1992
Marax Tablets & DF Syrup ... 2015
Vistaril Intramuscular Solution ... 2042

Isocarboxazid (Prolongs the effects of barbiturates).
No products indexed under this heading.

Isoflurane (Concomitant use may produce additive CNS-depressant effects).
No products indexed under this heading.

Ketamine Hydrochloride (Concomitant use may produce additive CNS-depressant effects).
No products indexed under this heading.

Levomethadyl Acetate Hydrochloride (Concomitant use may produce additive CNS-depressant effects). Products include:
Orlaam Oral Solution ... 2361

Levonorgestrel (Decreased effect of estradiol by increasing its metabolism). Products include:
Levlen/Tri-Levlen ... 646
Nordette-21 Tablets ... 2863
Nordette-28 Tablets ... 2866
Norplant System ... 2868
Levlen/Tri-Levlen ... 646

(▣ Described in PDR For Nonprescription Drugs) (◉ Described in PDR For Ophthalmology)

Levorphanol Tartrate (Concomitant use may produce additive CNS-depressant effects). Products include:
Levo-Dromoran 2297

Loratadine (Concomitant use may produce additive CNS-depressant effects). Products include:
Claritin Tablets 2485
Claritin-D Tablets 2487

Lorazepam (Concomitant use may produce additive CNS-depressant effects). Products include:
Ativan Injection 2805
Ativan Tablets 2807

Loxapine Hydrochloride (Concomitant use may produce additive CNS-depressant effects). Products include:
Loxitane 1426

Loxapine Succinate (Concomitant use may produce additive CNS-depressant effects). Products include:
Loxitane Capsules 1426

Meperidine Hydrochloride (Concomitant use may produce additive CNS-depressant effects). Products include:
Demerol 2438
Mepergan Injection 2859

Mephobarbital (Concomitant use may produce additive CNS-depressant effects). Products include:
Mebaral Tablets 2452

Meprobamate (Concomitant use may produce additive CNS-depressant effects). Products include:
Miltown Tablets 2780
PMB 200 and PMB 400 2890

Mesoridazine Besylate (Concomitant use may produce additive CNS-depressant effects). Products include:
Serentil 689

Mestranol (Decreased effect of estradiol by increasing its metabolism). Products include:
Norinyl 2563
Ortho-Novum 1928

Methadone Hydrochloride (Concomitant use may produce additive CNS-depressant effects). Products include:
Methadone Hydrochloride Oral Concentrate 2356
Methadone Hydrochloride Oral Solution & Tablets ... 2357

Methdilazine Hydrochloride (Concomitant use may produce additive CNS-depressant effects).
No products indexed under this heading.

Methohexital Sodium (Concomitant use may produce additive CNS-depressant effects).
No products indexed under this heading.

Methotrimeprazine (Concomitant use may produce additive CNS-depressant effects). Products include:
Levoprome 1321

Methoxyflurane (Concomitant use may produce additive CNS-depressant effects).
No products indexed under this heading.

Methylprednisolone Acetate (Enhanced metabolism of exogenous corticosteroids).
No products indexed under this heading.

Methylprednisolone Sodium Succinate (Enhanced metabolism of exogenous corticosteroids).
No products indexed under this heading.

Triphasil-21 Tablets 2919
Triphasil-28 Tablets 2924

Midazolam Hydrochloride (Concomitant use may produce additive CNS-depressant effects). Products include:
Versed Injection 2324

Molindone Hydrochloride (Concomitant use may produce additive CNS-depressant effects). Products include:
Moban Tablets and Concentrate 1036

Morphine Sulfate (Concomitant use may produce additive CNS-depressant effects). Products include:
Astramorph/PF Injection, USP (Preservative-Free) 526
Duramorph Injection 983
Infumorph 200 and Infumorph 500 Sterile Solutions 985
Kadian Capsules 2948
MS Contin Tablets 2149
MSIR 2152
Oramorph SR (Morphine Sulfate Sustained Release Tablets) 2359
RMS Suppositories CII 2766
Roxanol 2365

Norethindrone (Decreased effect of estradiol by increasing its metabolism). Products include:
Brevicon 2563
Micronor Tablets 1903
Modicon 1928
Norinyl 2563
Nor-Q D Tablets 2598
Ortho-Novum 1928
Ovcon 765
Tri-Norinyl 2607

Norethynodrel (Decreased effect of estradiol by increasing its metabolism).
No products indexed under this heading.

Norgestimate (Decreased effect of estradiol by increasing its metabolism). Products include:
Ortho-Cyclen/Ortho Tri-Cyclen 1914
Ortho-Cyclen/Ortho Tri-Cyclen 1914

Norgestrel (Decreased effect of estradiol by increasing its metabolism). Products include:
Lo/Ovral Tablets 2852
Lo/Ovral-28 Tablets 2857
Ovral Tablets 2877
Ovral-28 Tablets 2878
Ovrette Tablets 2878

Opium Alkaloids (Concomitant use may produce additive CNS-depressant effects).
No products indexed under this heading.

Oxazepam (Concomitant use may produce additive CNS-depressant effects). Products include:
Serax Capsules 2916
Serax Tablets 2916

Oxycodone Hydrochloride (Concomitant use may produce additive CNS-depressant effects). Products include:
OxyContin Tablets 2163
OxyIR Capsules 2167
Percocet Tablets 955
Percodan Tablets 955
Percodan-Demi Tablets 956
Roxicodone Tablets, Oral Solution & Intensol (Oxycodone) ... 2366
Tylox Capsules 1593

Pentobarbital Sodium (Concomitant use may produce additive CNS-depressant effects). Products include:
Nembutal Sodium Capsules ... 440
Nembutal Sodium Solution 442
Nembutal Sodium Suppositories 444

Perphenazine (Concomitant use may produce additive CNS-depressant effects). Products include:
Etrafon 2495
Triavil Tablets 1800
Trilafon 2532

Phenelzine Sulfate (Prolongs the effects of barbiturates). Products include:
Nardil 1977

Phenobarbital (Concomitant use may produce additive CNS-depressant effects). Products include:
Arco-Lase Plus Tablets 513
Bellergal-S Tablets 2375
Donnatal 2234
Donnatal Extentabs 2234
Donnatal Tablets 2234
Phenobarbital Elixir and Tablets 1523
Quadrinal Tablets 1398

Phenytoin (Variable effect on the metabolism of phenytoin). Products include:
Dilantin Infatabs 1967
Dilantin-125 Suspension 1969

Phenytoin Sodium (Variable effect on the metabolism of phenytoin). Products include:
Dilantin Kapseals 1965

Prazepam (Concomitant use may produce additive CNS-depressant effects).
No products indexed under this heading.

Prednisolone Acetate (Enhanced metabolism of exogenous corticosteroids). Products include:
AK-CIDE .... ⊚ 203
AK-CIDE Ointment .... ⊚ 203
Blephamide Liquifilm Sterile Ophthalmic Suspension 472
Blephamide Ointment .... ⊚ 234
Econopred & Econopred Plus Ophthalmic Suspensions .. ⊚ 216
Poly-Pred Liquifilm .... ⊚ 246
Pred Forte .... ⊚ 247
Pred Mild .... ⊚ 250
Pred-G Liquifilm Sterile Ophthalmic Suspension .... ⊚ 248
Pred-G S.O.P. Sterile Ophthalmic Ointment .... ⊚ 249

Prednisolone Sodium Phosphate (Enhanced metabolism of exogenous corticosteroids). Products include:
AK-PRED .... ⊚ 204
Hydeltrasol Injection, Sterile .. 1708
Pediapred Oral Solution 1618

Prednisolone Tebutate (Enhanced metabolism of exogenous corticosteroids). Products include:
Hydeltra-T.B.A. Sterile Suspension 1710

Prednisone (Enhanced metabolism of exogenous corticosteroids).
No products indexed under this heading.

Prochlorperazine (Concomitant use may produce additive CNS-depressant effects). Products include:
Compazine 2644

Promethazine Hydrochloride (Concomitant use may produce additive CNS-depressant effects). Products include:
Mepergan Injection 2859
Phenergan with Codeine 2883
Phenergan with Dextromethorphan ... 2885
Phenergan Injection 2880
Phenergan Suppositories 2882
Phenergan Syrup 2881
Phenergan Tablets 2882
Phenergan VC 2886
Phenergan VC with Codeine .. 2888

Propofol (Concomitant use may produce additive CNS-depressant effects). Products include:
Diprivan Injectable Emulsion . 2939

Propoxyphene Hydrochloride (Concomitant use may produce additive CNS-depressant effects). Products include:
Darvon 1475
Wygesic Tablets 2930

Propoxyphene Napsylate (Concomitant use may produce additive CNS-depressant effects). Products include:
Darvon-N/Darvocet-N 1473

Pyrilamine Maleate (Concomitant use may produce additive CNS-depressant effects). Products include:
4-Way Fast Acting Nasal Spray (regular & mentholated) ... ⊚ 644
Maximum Strength Multi-Symptom Formula Midol .... ⊚ 621
PMS Multi-Symptom Formula Midol .... ⊚ 622

Pyrilamine Tannate (Concomitant use may produce additive CNS-depressant effects). Products include:
Atrohist Pediatric Suspension 1604
Atrohist Pediatric Suspension Dye-Free 1604
Rynatan 2781

Quazepam (Concomitant use may produce additive CNS-depressant effects). Products include:
Doral Tablets 2773

Risperidone (Concomitant use may produce additive CNS-depressant effects). Products include:
Risperdal Tablets 1348

Selegiline Hydrochloride (Prolongs the effects of barbiturates). Products include:
Eldepryl Capsules 2729

Sevoflurane (Concomitant use may produce additive CNS-depressant effects).
No products indexed under this heading.

Sufentanil Citrate (Concomitant use may produce additive CNS-depressant effects). Products include:
Sufenta Injection 1355

Temazepam (Concomitant use may produce additive CNS-depressant effects). Products include:
Restoril Capsules 2413

Terfenadine (Concomitant use may produce additive CNS-depressant effects). Products include:
Seldane Tablets 1284
Seldane-D Extended-Release Tablets 1286

Thiamylal Sodium (Concomitant use may produce additive CNS-depressant effects).
No products indexed under this heading.

Thioridazine Hydrochloride (Concomitant use may produce additive CNS-depressant effects). Products include:
Mellaril 2398

Thiothixene (Concomitant use may produce additive CNS-depressant effects). Products include:
Navane Capsules and Concentrate ... 2018
Navane Intramuscular 2019

Tranylcypromine Sulfate (Prolongs the effects of barbiturates). Products include:
Parnate Tablets 2679

Triamcinolone (Enhanced metabolism of exogenous corticosteroids).
No products indexed under this heading.

Triamcinolone Acetonide (Enhanced metabolism of exogenous corticosteroids). Products include:
Azmacort Oral Inhaler 2175
Nasacort AQ Nasal Spray 2191
Nasacort Nasal Inhaler 2189

Triamcinolone Diacetate (Enhanced metabolism of exogenous corticosteroids).
No products indexed under this heading.

IMPORTANT NOTE: Always consult each drug listing in the patient's regimen for possible interactions.

Seconal **Interactions Index** 968

Triamcinolone Hexacetonide (Enhanced metabolism of exogenous corticosteroids).
No products indexed under this heading.

Triazolam (Concomitant use may produce additive CNS-depressant effects). Products include:
Halcion Tablets ... 2093

Trifluoperazine Hydrochloride (Concomitant use may produce additive CNS-depressant effects). Products include:
Stelazine ... 2692

Trimeprazine Tartrate (Concomitant use may produce additive CNS-depressant effects).
No products indexed under this heading.

Tripelennamine Hydrochloride (Concomitant use may produce additive CNS-depressant effects). Products include:
PBZ Tablets ... 863
PBZ-SR Tablets ... 862

Triprolidine Hydrochloride (Concomitant use may produce additive CNS-depressant effects). Products include:
Actifed Cold & Allergy Tablets ... ⊡ 807
Actifed Cold & Sinus Caplets and Tablets ... ⊡ 808

Valproic Acid (Increases blood levels of secobarbital sodium). Products include:
Depakene ... 416

Warfarin Sodium (Barbiturates can induce hepatic microsomal enzymes, resulting in increased or decreased anticoagulant response). Products include:
Coumadin ... 941

Zolpidem Tartrate (Concomitant use may produce additive CNS-depressant effects). Products include:
Ambien Tablets ... 2559

Food Interactions

Alcohol (Concomitant use may produce additive CNS-depressant effects).

SECRETIN-FERRING
(Secretin) ... 2991
None cited in PDR database.

SECTRAL CAPSULES
(Acebutolol Hydrochloride) ... 2914
May interact with catecholamine depleting drugs, non-steroidal anti-inflammatory agents, alpha adrenergic stimulants, and insulin. Compounds in these categories include:

Deserpidine (Additive effect).
No products indexed under this heading.

Diclofenac Potassium (Blunting of the antihypertensive effect). Products include:
Cataflam Tablets ... 833

Diclofenac Sodium (Blunting of the antihypertensive effect). Products include:
Voltaren Ophthalmic Sterile Ophthalmic Solution ... ⊙ 264
Cataflam/Voltaren/Voltaren-XR ... 833

Etodolac (Blunting of the antihypertensive effect). Products include:
Lodine Capsules and Tablets ... 2849

Fenoprofen Calcium (Blunting of the antihypertensive effect). Products include:
Nalfon 200 Pulvules & Nalfon Tablets ... 933

Flurbiprofen (Blunting of the antihypertensive effect).
No products indexed under this heading.

Guanethidine Monosulfate (Additive effect). Products include:
Esimil Tablets ... 840
Ismelin Tablets ... 845

Ibuprofen (Blunting of the antihypertensive effect). Products include:
Advil Cold and Sinus Caplets and Tablets ... ⊡ 837
Advil Ibuprofen Tablets, Caplets and Gel Caplets ... ⊡ 836
Children's Motrin Ibuprofen Oral Suspension ... 1558
IBU Tablets ... 1389
Ibuprohm ... ⊡ 713
Motrin IB Caplets, Tablets, and Gelcaps ... ⊡ 802
Motrin Ibuprofen Suspension, Oral Drops, Chewable Tablets, Caplets ... 1563
Nuprin Ibuprofen/Analgesic Tablets & Caplets ... ⊡ 645
Vicks DayQuil SINUS Pressure & PAIN Relief with IBUPROFEN ... ⊡ 735

Indomethacin (Blunting of the antihypertensive effect). Products include:
Indocin ... 1723

Indomethacin Sodium Trihydrate (Blunting of the antihypertensive effect). Products include:
Indocin I.V. ... 1727

Insulin, Human (Beta-blockers may potentiate insulin-induced hypoglycemia).
No products indexed under this heading.

Insulin, Human Isophane Suspension (Beta-blockers may potentiate insulin-induced hypoglycemia). Products include:
Novolin N Human Insulin 10 ml Vials ... 1846

Insulin, Human NPH (Beta-blockers may potentiate insulin-induced hypoglycemia). Products include:
Humulin N, 100 Units ... 1495
Novolin N PenFill 1.5 ml Cartridges Durable Insulin Delivery System ... 1849
Novolin N Prefilled Syringe Disposable Insulin Delivery System ... 1850

Insulin, Human Regular (Beta-blockers may potentiate insulin-induced hypoglycemia). Products include:
Humulin R, 100 Units ... 1497
Novolin R Human Insulin 10 ml Vials ... 1846
Novolin R PenFill 1.5 ml Cartridges Durable Insulin Delivery System ... 1849
Novolin R Prefilled Syringe Disposable Insulin Delivery System ... 1850
Velosulin BR Human Insulin 10 ml Vials ... 1847

Insulin, Human, Zinc Suspension (Beta-blockers may potentiate insulin-induced hypoglycemia). Products include:
Humulin L, 100 Units ... 1494
Humulin U, 100 Units ... 1498
Novolin L Human Insulin 10 ml Vials ... 1846

Insulin Lispro, Human (Beta-blockers may potentiate insulin-induced hypoglycemia). Products include:
Humalog Injection ... 1488

Insulin, NPH (Beta-blockers may potentiate insulin-induced hypoglycemia). Products include:
NPH, 100 Units ... 1502
Pork NPH, 100 Units ... 1506
Purified Pork NPH Isophane Insulin ... 1852

Insulin, Regular (Beta-blockers may potentiate insulin-induced hypoglycemia). Products include:
Regular, 100 Units ... 1503
Pork Regular, 100 Units ... 1507
Pork Regular (Concentrated), 500 Units ... 1508
Purified Pork Regular Insulin ... 1852

Insulin, Zinc Crystals (Beta-blockers may potentiate insulin-induced hypoglycemia). Products include:
NPH, 100 Units ... 1502

Insulin, Zinc Suspension (Beta-blockers may potentiate insulin-induced hypoglycemia). Products include:
Iletin I ... 1501
Lente, 100 Units ... 1501
Iletin II ... 1504
Pork Lente, 100 Units ... 1504
Purified Pork Lente Insulin ... 1852

Ketoprofen (Blunting of the antihypertensive effect). Products include:
Actron Caplets and Tablets ... ⊡ 608
Orudis Capsules ... 2874
Orudis KT ... ⊡ 842
Oruvail Capsules ... 2874

Ketorolac Tromethamine (Blunting of the antihypertensive effect). Products include:
Acular Sterile Ophthalmic Solution 470
Toradol ... 2319

Meclofenamate Sodium (Blunting of the antihypertensive effect).
No products indexed under this heading.

Mefenamic Acid (Blunting of the antihypertensive effect). Products include:
Ponstel ... 1982

Nabumetone (Blunting of the antihypertensive effect). Products include:
Relafen Tablets ... 2688

Naphazoline Hydrochloride (Potential for exaggerated hypertensive response). Products include:
Albalon Solution with Liquifilm ... ⊙ 229
Clear Eyes ACR Astringent/Lubricant Eye Redness Reliever Eye Drops ... ⊙ 314
Clear Eyes Lubricant Eye Redness Reliever ... ⊙ 314
4-Way Fast Acting Nasal Spray (regular & mentholated) ... ⊡ 644
Naphcon-A Ophthalmic Solution ... 469
OcuHist ... ⊙ 300
Privine ... ⊡ 663
Vasocon-A ... ⊙ 263

Naproxen (Blunting of the antihypertensive effect). Products include:
Anaprox/Naprosyn ... 2277

Naproxen Sodium (Blunting of the antihypertensive effect). Products include:
Aleve ... 2124
Anaprox/Naprosyn ... 2277
Naprelan Tablets ... 2861

Oxaprozin (Blunting of the antihypertensive effect). Products include:
Daypro Caplets ... 2578

Oxymetazoline Hydrochloride (Potential for exaggerated hypertensive response). Products include:
Afrin ... ⊡ 757
Duration 12 Hour Nasal Spray ... ⊡ 766
4-Way 12 Hour Nasal Spray ... ⊡ 644
Neo-Synephrine Maximum Strength 12 Hour Nasal Spray ... ⊡ 624
Neo-Synephrine 12 Hour ... ⊡ 624
12 Hour Nōstrilla ... ⊡ 660
Vicks Sinex 12-Hour Nasal Decongestant Spray and Ultra Fine Mist ... ⊡ 738
Visine L.R. Eye Drops ... ⊡ 719
Visine L.R. Eye Drops ... ⊙ 301

Phenylbutazone (Blunting of the antihypertensive effect).
No products indexed under this heading.

Phenylephrine Hydrochloride (Potential for exaggerated hypertensive response). Products include:
Atrohist Plus Tablets ... 1605
Cerose DM ... ⊡ 853
D.A. II Tablets ... 972
D.A. Chewable Tablets ... 970
Dura-Vent/DA Tablets ... 972
Extendryl ... 1003
4-Way Fast Acting Nasal Spray (regular & mentholated) ... ⊡ 644
Hemorid ... ⊡ 797
Hycomine Compound Tablets ... 948
Neo-Synephrine Hydrochloride 1% Carpuject ... 2455
Neo-Synephrine Hydrochloride 1% Injection ... 2455
Neo-Synephrine Hydrochloride (Ophthalmic) ... 2456
Neo-Synephrine ... ⊡ 624
Novahistine Elixir ... ⊡ 782
Phenergan VC ... 2886
Phenergan VC with Codeine ... 2888
Preparation H ... ⊡ 842
Tympagesic Ear Drops ... 2476
Vicks Sinex Nasal Spray and Ultra Fine Mist ... ⊡ 738

Phenylpropanolamine Hydrochloride (Potential for exaggerated hypertensive response). Products include:
Acutrim ... ⊡ 648
Atrohist Plus Tablets ... 1605
BC Cold Powder Multi-Symptom Formula (Cold-Sinus-Allergy) ... ⊡ 631
BC Cold Powder Non-Drowsy Formula (Cold-Sinus) ... ⊡ 631
Cheracol Plus Head Cold/Cough Formula ... ⊡ 741
Comtrex Multi-Symptom Cold Reliever Liqui-Gels ... ⊡ 638
Comtrex Multi-Symptom Non-Drowsy Liqui-gels ... ⊡ 640
Contac Continuous Action Nasal Decongestant/Antihistamine 12 Hour Capsules ... ⊡ 773
Contac Maximum Strength Continuous Action Decongestant/Antihistamine 12 Hour Caplets ... ⊡ 772
Contac Severe Cold and Flu Formula Caplets ... ⊡ 773
Coricidin 'D' Decongestant Tablets ... ⊡ 760
Dexatrim ... ⊡ 795
Dexatrim Plus Vitamins Caplets ... ⊡ 796
Dimetane-DC Cough Syrup ... 2232
Dimetapp Allergy Sinus Caplets ... ⊡ 838
Dimetapp Cold & Allergy Chewable Tablets ... ⊡ 838
Dimetapp Cold & Cough Liqui-Gels ... ⊡ 839
Dimetapp DM Elixir ... ⊡ 840
Dimetapp Elixir ... ⊡ 840
Dimetapp Extentabs ... ⊡ 841
Dimetapp Tablets/Liqui-Gels ... ⊡ 841
Dura-Vent Tablets ... 971
Entex LA Tablets ... 972
Exgest LA Tablets ... 787
Hycomine ... 947
Nolamine Timed-Release Tablets ... 790
Ornade Spansule Capsules ... 2678
Propagest Tablets ... 791
Pyrroxate Caplets ... ⊡ 742
Robitussin-CF ... ⊡ 846
Sinulin Tablets ... 792
Tavist-D 12 Hour Relief Tablets ... ⊡ 750
Teldrin 12 Hour Antihistamine/Nasal Decongestant Allergy Relief Capsules ... ⊡ 786
Triaminic Expectorant ... ⊡ 753
Triaminic Syrup ... ⊡ 755
Triaminic Triaminicol Cold & Cough ... ⊡ 756
Triaminic DM Syrup ... ⊡ 756
Triaminicin Tablets ... ⊡ 756
Vicks DayQuil Allergy Relief 12-Hour Extended Release Tablets ... ⊡ 733
Vicks DayQuil Allergy Relief 4-Hour Tablets ... ⊡ 733
Vicks DayQuil SINUS Pressure & CONGESTION Relief ... ⊡ 734

Piroxicam (Blunting of the antihypertensive effect). Products include:
Feldene Capsules ... 2008

Pseudoephedrine Hydrochloride (Potential for exaggerated hypertensive response). Products include:
Actifed Allergy Daytime/Nighttime Caplets ... ⊡ 808
Actifed Cold & Allergy Tablets ... ⊡ 807
Actifed Cold & Sinus Caplets and Tablets ... ⊡ 808
Actifed Sinus Daytime/Nighttime Tablets and Caplets ... ⊡ 809
Advil Cold and Sinus Caplets and Tablets ... ⊡ 837
Alka-Seltzer Plus Liqui-Gels ... ⊡ 612

(⊡ Described in PDR For Nonprescription Drugs) (⊙ Described in PDR For Ophthalmology)

Alka-Seltzer Plus Flu & Body Aches Liqui-Gels Non-Drowsy Formula	▣ 613	Rondec Syrup	974
Alka-Seltzer Plus Night-Time Cold Medicine Liqui-Gels	▣ 612	Rondec Tablet	974
Allerest Maximum Strength	649	Rondec Chewable Tablets	974
Allerest No Drowsiness	649	Rondec-TR Tablet	974
Allerest Sinus Pain Formula	649	Ryna	▣ 804
Atrohist Pediatric Capsules	1603	Seldane-D Extended-Release Tablets	1286
Benadryl Allergy/Cold Tablets	▣ 811	Semprex-D Capsules	1620
Benadryl Allergy Decongestant Liquid Medication	▣ 812	Sinarest	▣ 663
Benadryl Allergy Decongestant Tablets	▣ 812	Sine-Aid Maximum Strength Sinus Headache Gelcaps, Caplets and Tablets	1570
Benadryl Allergy Sinus Headache Caplets	▣ 813	Sine-Off No Drowsiness Formula Caplets	▣ 784
Benylin Multisymptom	▣ 816	Sine-Off Sinus Medicine	▣ 784
Bromfed Capsules (Extended-Release)	1832	Singlet Tablets	▣ 785
Bromfed Syrup	▣ 712	Sinutab Non-Drying Liquid Caps	▣ 823
Bromfed Tablets	1832	Sinutab Sinus Allergy Medication, Maximum Strength Tablets and Caplets	▣ 823
Bromfed-DM Cough Syrup	1832	Sinutab Sinus Medication, Maximum Strength Without Drowsiness Formula, Tablets & Caplets	▣ 824
Bromfed-PD Capsules (Extended-Release)	1832	Sudafed Children's Cold & Cough Liquid Medication	▣ 825
Children's TYLENOL Cold Multi-Symptom Chewable Tablets and Liquid	1559	Sudafed Children's Nasal Decongestant Liquid Medication	▣ 826
Children's TYLENOL Cold Plus Cough Multi Symptom Chewable Tablets and Liquid	1560	Sudafed Cold & Allergy Tablets	▣ 825
Children's TYLENOL Flu Suspension Liquid	1560	Sudafed Cold and Cough Liquid Caps	▣ 826
Children's Vicks DayQuil Allergy Relief	▣ 730	Sudafed Nasal Decongestant Tablets, 30 mg	▣ 825
Children's Vicks NyQuil Cold/ Cough Relief	▣ 731	Sudafed Nasal Decongestant Tablets, 60 mg	▣ 825
Allergy-Sinus Comtrex Multi-Symptom Allergy-Sinus Formula Tablets and Caplets	▣ 639	Sudafed Non-Drying Sinus Liquid Caps	▣ 827
Comtrex Multi-Symptom	▣ 638	Sudafed Pediatric Nasal Decongestant Liquid Oral Drops	▣ 827
Comtrex Multi-Symptom Non-Drowsy Caplets	▣ 640	Sudafed Severe Cold Formula Caplets	▣ 828
Congess	1003	Sudafed Severe Cold Formula Tablets	▣ 828
Contac Day Allergy/Sinus Caplets	▣ 771	Sudafed Sinus Caplets	▣ 829
Contac Day & Night	▣ 772	Sudafed Sinus Tablets	▣ 829
Contac Night Allergy/Sinus Caplets	▣ 771	Sudafed 12 Hour Caplets	▣ 824
Contac Severe Cold & Flu Non-Drowsy	▣ 774	Syn-Rx Tablets	1622
Deconsal II Tablets	1605	Syn-Rx DM Tablets	1623
Dimetane-DX Cough Syrup	2233	TheraFlu and Cold Medicine	▣ 750
Dimetapp Cold & Fever Suspension	▣ 839	Theraflu Maximum Strength Flu and Cold Medicine For Sore Throat	▣ 751
Dimetapp Decongestant Pediatric Drops	▣ 840	TheraFlu Flu, Cold and Cough Medicine	▣ 750
Dorcol Children's Cough Syrup	▣ 748	TheraFlu Maximum Strength Nighttime Flu, Cold & Cough Medicine	▣ 751
Drixoral Cough + Congestion Liquid Caps	▣ 763	TheraFlu Maximum Strength Non-Drowsy Formula Flu, Cold & Cough Medicine	▣ 751
Dura-Tap/PD Capsules	970	TheraFlu Maximum Strength, Non-Drowsy Formula Flu, Cold and Cough Caplets	▣ 752
Duratuss Tablets	2750	Theraflu Maximum Strength Sinus Non-Drowsy Formula Caplets	▣ 752
Duratuss HD Elixir	2750	Triaminic AM Cough and Decongestant Formula	▣ 753
Efidac/24	▣ 655	Triaminic AM Decongestant Formula	▣ 753
Entex PSE Tablets	973	Triaminic Infant Oral Decongestant Drops	▣ 754
Fedahist Gyrocaps	2545	Triaminic Night Time	▣ 754
Guaifed	1833	Triaminic Sore Throat Formula	▣ 755
Guaifed Syrup	▣ 712	Tussend	1830
Guaimax-D Tablets	809	Tussend Expectorant	1831
Histussin D Liquid	670	TYLENOL Allergy Sinus, Maximum Strength Caplets and Gelcaps	1571
Infants' TYLENOL Cold Decongestant & Fever-Reducer Drops	1561	TYLENOL Allergy Sinus NightTime, Maximum Strength Caplets	1571
Kronofed-A	994	TYLENOL Cold Medication, Multi-Symptom Formula Tablets and Caplets	1572
Novahistine DMX	▣ 782	TYLENOL Cold Medication, Multi-Symptom Hot Liquid Packets	1572
Nucofed	2225	TYLENOL Cold Medication, No Drowsiness Formula Caplets and Gelcaps	1572
PediaCare Cough-Cold Chewable Tablets and Liquid	1569	TYLENOL Cold Severe Congestion Caplets	1573
PediaCare Infants' Decongestant Drops	1569	TYLENOL Cough Medication with Decongestant, Multi Symptom	1574
PediaCare Infants' Drops Decongestant Plus Cough	1569	TYLENOL Flu No Drowsiness Formula, Maximum Strength Gelcaps	1575
PediaCare NightRest Cough-Cold Liquid	1569	TYLENOL Flu NightTime, Maximum Strength Gelcaps	1575
Pediatric Vicks 44d Cough & Head Congestion Relief	▣ 736	TYLENOL Flu NightTime, Maximum Strength Hot Medication Packets	1575
Pediatric Vicks 44m Cough & Cold Relief	▣ 737	TYLENOL Sinus, Maximum Strength Geltabs, Gelcaps, Caplets and Tablets	1576
Robitussin Cold & Cough Liqui-Gels	▣ 844	Vicks 44 LiquiCaps Cough, Cold & Flu Relief	▣ 728
Robitussin Cold, Cough & Flu Liqui-Gels	▣ 844	Vicks 44 LiquiCaps Non-Drowsy Cough & Cold Relief	▣ 729
Robitussin Maximum Strength Cough & Cold	▣ 847	Vicks 44D Cough & Head Congestion Relief	▣ 728
Robitussin Night-Time Cold Formula	▣ 847	Vicks 44M Cough, Cold & Flu Relief	▣ 729
Robitussin Pediatric Cough & Cold Formula	▣ 848	Vicks DayQuil LiquiCaps/Liquid Multi-Symptom Cold/Flu Relief	▣ 734
Robitussin Pediatric Drops	▣ 849	Vicks DayQuil SINUS Pressure & PAIN Relief with IBUPROFEN	▣ 735
Robitussin Severe Congestion Liqui-Gels	▣ 845	Vicks Nyquil Hot Therapy	▣ 735
Robitussin-DAC Syrup	2249	Vicks NyQuil LiquiCaps/Liquid Multi-Symptom Cold/Flu Relief, Original and Cherry Flavors	▣ 736
Robitussin-PE	▣ 846		
Rondec Oral Drops	974		

Rauwolfia Serpentina (Additive effect).
No products indexed under this heading.

Rescinnamine (Additive effect).
No products indexed under this heading.

Reserpine (Additive effect). Products include:
Diupres Tablets 1691
Hydropres Tablets 1718
Ser-Ap-Es Tablets 867

Sulindac (Blunting of the antihypertensive effect). Products include:
Clinoril Tablets 1658

Tetrahydrozoline Hydrochloride (Potential for exaggerated hypertensive response). Products include:
Collyrium Fresh .... ⓞ 316
Murine Tears Plus Lubricant Redness Reliever Eye Drops ... ▣ 744
Murine Tears Plus Lubricant Redness Reliever Eye Drops ... ⓞ 315
Visine A.C. Seasonal Relief From Pollen and Dust .... ⓞ 301
Visine Moisturizing Eye Drops ... ⓞ 301
Visine Original Eye Drops .. ⓞ 301

Tolmetin Sodium (Blunting of the antihypertensive effect). Products include:
Tolectin (200, 400 and 600 mg) .. 1591

Food Interactions
Food, unspecified (Slightly decreases absorption and peak concentration).

SEDAPAP TABLETS 50 MG/650 MG
(Acetaminophen, Butalbital) 1826
May interact with central nervous system depressants, narcotic analgesics, tranquilizers, psychotropics, tricyclic antidepressants, monoamine oxidase inhibitors, general anesthetics, and certain other agents. Compounds in these categories include:

Alfentanil Hydrochloride (Additive CNS depression). Products include:
Alfenta Injection 1334

Alprazolam (Additive CNS depression). Products include:
Xanax Tablets 2115

Amitriptyline Hydrochloride (Additive CNS depression). Products include:
Elavil 2945
Etrafon 2495
Limbitrol 2333
Triavil Tablets 1800

Amoxapine (Additive CNS depression). Products include:
Asendin Tablets 1419

Aprobarbital (Additive CNS depression).
No products indexed under this heading.

Buprenorphine (Additive CNS depression). Products include:
Buprenex Injectable 2170

Buspirone Hydrochloride (Additive CNS depression). Products include:
BuSpar Tablets 738

Butabarbital (Additive CNS depression).
No products indexed under this heading.

Chlordiazepoxide (Additive CNS depression). Products include:
Limbitrol 2333

Chlordiazepoxide Hydrochloride (Additive CNS depression). Products include:
Librax Capsules 2330
Librium Capsules 2331
Librium Injectable 2332

Chlorpromazine (Additive CNS depression). Products include:
Thorazine Suppositories .. 2701

Chlorpromazine Hydrochloride (Additive CNS depression). Products include:
Thorazine 2701

Chlorprothixene (Additive CNS depression).
No products indexed under this heading.

Chlorprothixene Hydrochloride (Additive CNS depression).
No products indexed under this heading.

Chlorprothixene Lactate (Additive CNS depression).
No products indexed under this heading.

Clomipramine Hydrochloride (Additive CNS depression). Products include:
Anafranil Capsules 819

Clorazepate Dipotassium (Additive CNS depression). Products include:
Tranxene 459

Clozapine (Additive CNS depression). Products include:
Clozaril Tablets 2377

Codeine Phosphate (Additive CNS depression). Products include:
Brontex 2130
Dimetane-DC Cough Syrup ... 2232
Fioricet with Codeine Capsules ... 2387
Fiorinal with Codeine Capsules ... 2390
Nucofed 2225
Phenergan with Codeine ... 2883
Phenergan VC with Codeine ... 2888
Robitussin A-C Syrup 2248
Robitussin-DAC Syrup 2249
Ryna .... ▣ 804
Soma Compound w/Codeine Tablets 2784
Tylenol with Codeine 1592

Desflurane (Additive CNS depression). Products include:
Suprane (desflurane, USP) ... 1865

Desipramine Hydrochloride (Additive CNS depression). Products include:
Norpramin Tablets 1273

Dezocine (Additive CNS depression). Products include:
Dalgan Injection 529

Diazepam (Additive CNS depression). Products include:
Dizac (diazepam injectable emulsion) CIV 1862
Valium Injectable 2336
Valium Tablets 2335

Doxepin Hydrochloride (Additive CNS depression). Products include:
Adapin Capsules 1542
Sinequan 2028
Zonalon Cream 1042

Droperidol (Additive CNS depression). Products include:
Inapsine Injection 462

Enflurane (Additive CNS depression).
No products indexed under this heading.

IMPORTANT NOTE: Always consult each drug listing in the patient's regimen for possible interactions.

Sedapap / Interactions Index

Estazolam (Additive CNS depression). Products include:
- ProSom Tablets ... 457

Ethchlorvynol (Additive CNS depression). Products include:
- Placidyl Capsules ... 456

Ethinamate (Additive CNS depression).
- No products indexed under this heading.

Fentanyl (Additive CNS depression). Products include:
- Duragesic Transdermal System ... 1336

Fentanyl Citrate (Additive CNS depression). Products include:
- Sublimaze Injection ... 463

Fluphenazine Decanoate (Additive CNS depression). Products include:
- Prolixin Decanoate ... 510

Fluphenazine Enanthate (Additive CNS depression). Products include:
- Prolixin Enanthate ... 510

Fluphenazine Hydrochloride (Additive CNS depression). Products include:
- Prolixin ... 510

Flurazepam Hydrochloride (Additive CNS depression). Products include:
- Dalmane Capsules ... 2329

Furazolidone (Additive CNS depression). Products include:
- Furoxone ... 2221

Glutethimide (Additive CNS depression).
- No products indexed under this heading.

Haloperidol (Additive CNS depression). Products include:
- Haldol Injection, Tablets and Concentrate ... 1585

Haloperidol Decanoate (Additive CNS depression). Products include:
- Haldol Decanoate ... 1587

Hydrocodone Bitartrate (Additive CNS depression). Products include:
- Codiclear DH Syrup ... 808
- Duratuss HD Elixir ... 2750
- Histussin D Liquid ... 670
- Hycodan Tablets and Syrup ... 946
- Hycomine Compound Tablets ... 948
- Hycomine ... 947
- Hycotuss Expectorant Syrup ... 950
- Hydrocet Capsules ... 787
- Lorcet 10/650 Tablets ... 1016
- Lortab ... 2751
- Tussend ... 1830
- Tussend Expectorant ... 1831
- Vicodin Tablets ... 1404
- Vicodin ES Tablets ... 1405
- Vicodin HP Tablets ... 1403
- Vicodin Tuss Expectorant ... 1406
- Zydone Capsules ... 967

Hydrocodone Polistirex (Additive CNS depression). Products include:
- Tussionex Pennkinetic Extended-Release Suspension ... 1624

Hydromorphone Hydrochloride (Additive CNS depression). Products include:
- Dilaudid Ampules ... 1382
- Dilaudid Cough Syrup ... 1383
- Dilaudid-HP Injection ... 1384
- Dilaudid-HP Lyophilized Powder 250 mg ... 1384
- Dilaudid ... 1382
- Dilaudid Oral Liquid ... 1386
- Dilaudid ... 1382
- Dilaudid Tablets - 8 mg ... 1386

Hydroxyzine Hydrochloride (Additive CNS depression). Products include:
- Atarax Tablets & Syrup ... 1992
- Marax Tablets & DF Syrup ... 2015
- Vistaril Intramuscular Solution ... 2042

Imipramine Hydrochloride (Additive CNS depression). Products include:
- Tofranil Ampuls ... 873
- Tofranil Tablets ... 875

Imipramine Pamoate (Additive CNS depression). Products include:
- Tofranil-PM Capsules ... 876

Isocarboxazid (Additive CNS depression).
- No products indexed under this heading.

Isoflurane (Additive CNS depression).
- No products indexed under this heading.

Ketamine Hydrochloride (Additive CNS depression).
- No products indexed under this heading.

Levomethadyl Acetate Hydrochloride (Additive CNS depression). Products include:
- Orlaam Oral Solution ... 2361

Levorphanol Tartrate (Additive CNS depression). Products include:
- Levo-Dromoran ... 2297

Lithium Carbonate (Additive CNS depression). Products include:
- Eskalith ... 2658
- Lithium Carbonate Capsules & Tablets ... 2352
- Lithonate/Lithotabs/Lithobid ... 2721

Lithium Citrate (Additive CNS depression).
- No products indexed under this heading.

Lorazepam (Additive CNS depression). Products include:
- Ativan Injection ... 2805
- Ativan Tablets ... 2807

Loxapine Hydrochloride (Additive CNS depression). Products include:
- Loxitane ... 1426

Loxapine Succinate (Additive CNS depression). Products include:
- Loxitane Capsules ... 1426

Maprotiline Hydrochloride (Additive CNS depression). Products include:
- Ludiomil Tablets ... 861

Meperidine Hydrochloride (Additive CNS depression). Products include:
- Demerol ... 2438
- Mepergan Injection ... 2859

Mephobarbital (Additive CNS depression). Products include:
- Mebaral Tablets ... 2452

Meprobamate (Additive CNS depression). Products include:
- Miltown Tablets ... 2780
- PMB 200 and PMB 400 ... 2890

Mesoridazine Besylate (Additive CNS depression). Products include:
- Serentil ... 689

Methadone Hydrochloride (Additive CNS depression). Products include:
- Methadone Hydrochloride Oral Concentrate ... 2356
- Methadone Hydrochloride Oral Solution & Tablets ... 2357

Methohexital Sodium (Additive CNS depression).
- No products indexed under this heading.

Methotrimeprazine (Additive CNS depression). Products include:
- Levoprome ... 1321

Methoxyflurane (Additive CNS depression).
- No products indexed under this heading.

Midazolam Hydrochloride (Additive CNS depression). Products include:
- Versed Injection ... 2324

Molindone Hydrochloride (Additive CNS depression). Products include:
- Moban Tablets and Concentrate ... 1036

Morphine Sulfate (Additive CNS depression). Products include:
- Astramorph/PF Injection, USP (Preservative-Free) ... 526
- Duramorph Injection ... 983
- Infumorph 200 and Infumorph 500 Sterile Solutions ... 985
- Kadian Capsules ... 2948
- MS Contin Tablets ... 2149
- MSIR ... 2152
- Oramorph SR (Morphine Sulfate Sustained Release Tablets) ... 2359
- RMS Suppositories CII ... 2766
- Roxanol ... 2365

Nortriptyline Hydrochloride (Additive CNS depression). Products include:
- Pamelor ... 2409

Opium Alkaloids (Additive CNS depression).
- No products indexed under this heading.

Oxazepam (Additive CNS depression). Products include:
- Serax Capsules ... 2916
- Serax Tablets ... 2916

Oxycodone Hydrochloride (Additive CNS depression). Products include:
- OxyContin Tablets ... 2163
- OxyIR Capsules ... 2167
- Percocet Tablets ... 955
- Percodan Tablets ... 955
- Percodan-Demi Tablets ... 956
- Roxicodone Tablets, Oral Solution & Intensol (Oxycodone) ... 2366
- Tylox Capsules ... 1593

Pentobarbital Sodium (Additive CNS depression). Products include:
- Nembutal Sodium Capsules ... 440
- Nembutal Sodium Solution ... 442
- Nembutal Sodium Suppositories ... 444

Perphenazine (Additive CNS depression). Products include:
- Etrafon ... 2495
- Triavil Tablets ... 1800
- Trilafon ... 2532

Phenelzine Sulfate (Additive CNS depression). Products include:
- Nardil ... 1977

Phenobarbital (Additive CNS depression). Products include:
- Arco-Lase Plus Tablets ... 513
- Bellergal-S Tablets ... 2375
- Donnatal ... 2234
- Donnatal Extentabs ... 2234
- Donnatal Tablets ... 2234
- Phenobarbital Elixir and Tablets ... 1523
- Quadrinal Tablets ... 1398

Prazepam (Additive CNS depression).
- No products indexed under this heading.

Prochlorperazine (Additive CNS depression). Products include:
- Compazine ... 2644

Promethazine Hydrochloride (Additive CNS depression). Products include:
- Mepergan Injection ... 2859
- Phenergan with Codeine ... 2883
- Phenergan with Dextromethorphan ... 2885
- Phenergan Injection ... 2880
- Phenergan Suppositories ... 2882
- Phenergan Syrup ... 2881
- Phenergan Tablets ... 2882
- Phenergan VC ... 2886
- Phenergan VC with Codeine ... 2888

Propofol (Additive CNS depression). Products include:
- Diprivan Injectable Emulsion ... 2939

Propoxyphene Hydrochloride (Additive CNS depression). Products include:
- Darvon ... 1475
- Wygesic Tablets ... 2930

Propoxyphene Napsylate (Additive CNS depression). Products include:
- Darvon-N/Darvocet-N ... 1473

Protriptyline Hydrochloride (Additive CNS depression; decreased blood levels of the antidepressant). Products include:
- Vivactil Tablets ... 1820

Quazepam (Additive CNS depression). Products include:
- Doral Tablets ... 2773

Risperidone (Additive CNS depression). Products include:
- Risperdal Tablets ... 1348

Secobarbital Sodium (Additive CNS depression). Products include:
- Seconal Sodium Pulvules ... 1529

Selegiline Hydrochloride (Additive CNS depression). Products include:
- Eldepryl Capsules ... 2729

Sevoflurane (Additive CNS depression).
- No products indexed under this heading.

Sufentanil Citrate (Additive CNS depression). Products include:
- Sufenta Injection ... 1355

Temazepam (Additive CNS depression). Products include:
- Restoril Capsules ... 2413

Thiamylal Sodium (Additive CNS depression).
- No products indexed under this heading.

Thioridazine Hydrochloride (Additive CNS depression). Products include:
- Mellaril ... 2398

Thiothixene (Additive CNS depression). Products include:
- Navane Capsules and Concentrate ... 2018
- Navane Intramuscular ... 2019

Tranylcypromine Sulfate (Additive CNS depression). Products include:
- Parnate Tablets ... 2679

Triazolam (Additive CNS depression). Products include:
- Halcion Tablets ... 2093

Trifluoperazine Hydrochloride (Additive CNS depression). Products include:
- Stelazine ... 2692

Trimipramine Maleate (Additive CNS depression). Products include:
- Surmontil Capsules ... 2917

Zolpidem Tartrate (Additive CNS depression). Products include:
- Ambien Tablets ... 2559

Food Interactions

Alcohol (Additive CNS depression).

SELDANE TABLETS
(Terfenadine) ... 1284
May interact with macrolide antibiotics and certain other agents. Compounds in these categories include:

Azithromycin (Co-administration is contraindicated; potential for QT interval prolongation with ventricular arrhythmia including Torsades de pointes). Products include:
- Zithromax ... 2043
- Zithromax Tablets ... 2046

971 **Interactions Index** **Seldane-D**

Clarithromycin (Co-administration is contraindicated; potential for QT interval prolongation with ventricular arrhythmia including Torsades de pointes). Products include:

Biaxin ... 406

Dirithromycin (Co-administration is contraindicated; potential for QT interval prolongation with ventricular arrhythmia including Torsades de pointes). Products include:

Dynabac ... 668

Erythromycin (Co-administration is contraindicated; potential for QT interval prolongation with ventricular arrhythmia including Torsades de pointes). Products include:

A/T/S 2% Acne Topical Gel ... 1244
A/T/S 2% Acne Topical Solution ... 1244
Benzamycin Topical Gel ... 919
E-Mycin Tablets ... 1388
Emgel 2% Topical Gel ... 1081
ERYC ... 1972
Erycette (erythromycin 2%) Topical Solution ... 1943
Ery-Tab Tablets ... 426
Erythromycin Base Filmtab ... 430
Erythromycin Delayed-Release Capsules, USP ... 431
Ilotycin Ophthalmic Ointment ... 928
PCE Dispertab Tablets ... 453
T-Stat 2.0% Topical Solution and Pads ... 2797
THERAMYCIN Z 2% Solution ... 1629

Erythromycin Estolate (Co-administration is contraindicated; potential for QT interval prolongation with ventricular arrhythmia including Torsades de pointes). Products include:

Ilosone ... 927

Erythromycin Ethylsuccinate (Co-administration is contraindicated; potential for QT interval prolongation with ventricular arrhythmia including Torsades de pointes). Products include:

E.E.S. ... 427
EryPed ... 425
Pediazole Suspension ... 2340

Erythromycin Gluceptate (Co-administration is contraindicated; potential for QT interval prolongation with ventricular arrhythmia including Torsades de pointes). Products include:

Ilotycin Gluceptate, IV, Vials ... 929

Erythromycin Stearate (Co-administration is contraindicated; potential for QT interval prolongation with ventricular arrhythmia including Torsades de pointes). Products include:

Erythrocin Stearate Filmtab ... 429

Fluconazole (Co-administration is not recommended; due to chemical similarity of fluconazole to ketoconazole). Products include:

Diflucan Tablets, Injection, and Oral Suspension ... 2003

Itraconazole (Co-administration is contraindicated; potential for QT interval prolongation and rare serious cardiac events, e.g. death, cardiac arrest, and ventricular arrhythmia including Torsades de pointes). Products include:

Sporanox Capsules ... 1352

Ketoconazole (Co-administration is contraindicated; potential for QT interval prolongation and rare serious cardiac events, e.g. death, cardiac arrest, and ventricular arrhythmia including Torsade de pointes). Products include:

Nizoral 2% Cream ... 1344
Nizoral 2% Shampoo ... 1344
Nizoral Tablets ... 1345

Metronidazole (Co-administration is not recommended; due to chemical similarity of metronidazole to ketoconazole). Products include:

Flagyl 375 Capsules ... 2587
Flagyl I.V. RTU ... 2373
Helidac Therapy ... 2135
MetroCream ... 1034
MetroGel ... 1034
MetroGel-Vaginal ... 917
Protostat Tablets ... 1939

Metronidazole Hydrochloride (Co-administration is not recommended; due to chemical similarity of metronidazole to ketaconazole). Products include:

Flagyl I.V. ... 2373

Miconazole (Co-administration is not recommended; due to chemical similarity of miconazole to ketoconazole).

No products indexed under this heading.

Troleandomycin (Co-administration is contraindicated; potential for QT interval prolongation with ventricular arrhythmia including Torsades de pointes). Products include:

Tao Capsules ... 2033

SELDANE-D EXTENDED-RELEASE TABLETS

(Pseudoephedrine Hydrochloride, Terfenadine) ... 1286

May interact with monoamine oxidase inhibitors, beta blockers, sympathomimetics, and certain other agents. Compounds in these categories include:

Acebutolol Hydrochloride (Increases the effect of sympathomimetic amines). Products include:

Sectral Capsules ... 2914

Albuterol (Co-administration may produce combined harmful effects on cardiovascular system). Products include:

Proventil Inhalation Aerosol ... 2524
Ventolin Inhalation Aerosol and Refill ... 1170

Albuterol Sulfate (Co-administration may produce combined harmful effects on cardiovascular system). Products include:

Airet Albuterol Sulfate Inhalation Solution ... 1602
Albuterol Sulfate, USP Solution for Inhalation, Arm-a-Med ... 522
Proventil Inhalation Solution 0.083% ... 2527
Proventil Repetabs Tablets ... 2529
Proventil Solution for Inhalation 0.5% ... 2525
Proventil Syrup ... 2528
Proventil Tablets ... 2529
Ventolin Inhalation Solution ... 1171
Ventolin Nebules Inhalation Solution ... 1172
Ventolin Rotacaps for Inhalation ... 1173
Ventolin Syrup ... 1175
Ventolin Tablets ... 1176
Volmax Extended-Release Tablets .. 1835

Astemizole (Patients who may experience new or increased QT prolongation while receiving certain drugs, such as astemizole, may be at increased risk of ventricular tachyarrhythmias). Products include:

Hismanal Tablets ... 1341

Atenolol (Increases the effect of sympathomimetic amines). Products include:

Tenoretic Tablets ... 2963
Tenormin Tablets and I.V. Injection 2965

Azithromycin (Co-administration is contraindicated; potential for QT interval prolongation with ventricular arrhythmia including Torsades de pointes). Products include:

Zithromax ... 2043
Zithromax Tablets ... 2046

Bepridil Hydrochloride (Patients who may experience new or increased QT prolongation while receiving certain drugs, such as bepridil, may be at increased risk of ventricular tachyarrhythmias). Products include:

Vascor Tablets (200 and 300 mg) 1597

Betaxolol Hydrochloride (Increases the effect of sympathomimetic amines). Products include:

Betoptic Ophthalmic Solution ... 465
Betoptic S Ophthalmic Suspension 467
Kerlone Tablets ... 2588

Bisoprolol Fumarate (Increases the effect of sympathomimetic amines). Products include:

Zebeta Tablets ... 1457
Ziac ... 1459

Carteolol Hydrochloride (Increases the effect of sympathomimetic amines). Products include:

Cartrol Tablets ... 413
Ocupress Ophthalmic Solution, 1% Sterile ... ⊙ 297

Clarithromycin (Exerts an effect on terfenadine metabolism, probably by inhibiting isoenzyme, measurably decreases the clearance of terfenadine acid metabolite; co-administration has resulted in few spontaneous accounts of QT interval prolongation and with ventricular arrhythmias including torsade de pointes; concurrent use is contraindicated). Products include:

Biaxin ... 406

Deserpidine (Reduced antihypertensive effect).

No products indexed under this heading.

Dirithromycin (Co-administration is contraindicated; potential for QT interval prolongation with ventricular arrhythmia including Torsades de pointes). Products include:

Dynabac ... 668

Dobutamine Hydrochloride (Co-administration may produce combined harmful effects on cardiovascular system). Products include:

Dobutrex Solution Vials ... 1480

Dopamine Hydrochloride (Co-administration may produce combined harmful effects on cardiovascular system).

No products indexed under this heading.

Ephedrine Hydrochloride (Co-administration may produce combined harmful effects on cardiovascular system). Products include:

Primatene Tablets ... 844
Quadrinal Tablets ... 1398

Ephedrine Sulfate (Co-administration may produce combined harmful effects on cardiovascular system). Products include:

Marax Tablets & DF Syrup ... 2015

Ephedrine Tannate (Co-administration may produce combined harmful effects on cardiovascular system). Products include:

Rynatuss ... 2782

Epinephrine (Co-administration may produce combined harmful effects on cardiovascular system). Products include:

EPIFRIN ... ⊙ 237
EpiPen ... 808
Marcaine with Epinephrine ... 2446
Primatene Mist ... 843
Sensorcaine with Epinephrine Injection ... 554
Sus-Phrine Injection ... 1017
Xylocaine with Epinephrine Injections ... 562

Epinephrine Bitartrate (Co-administration may produce combined harmful effects on cardiovascular system). Products include:

Sensorcaine-MPF with Epinephrine Injection ... 554

Epinephrine Hydrochloride (Co-administration may produce combined harmful effects on cardiovascular system). Products include:

Ana-Kit Anaphylaxis Emergency Treatment Kit ... 611

Erythromycin (Exerts an effect on terfenadine metabolism, probably by inhibiting isoenzyme, measurably decreases the clearance of terfenadine acid metabolite; co-administration has resulted in few spontaneous accounts of QT interval prolongation and with ventricular arrhythmias including torsade de pointes; concurrent use is contraindicated). Products include:

A/T/S 2% Acne Topical Gel ... 1244
A/T/S 2% Acne Topical Solution ... 1244
Benzamycin Topical Gel ... 919
E-Mycin Tablets ... 1388
Emgel 2% Topical Gel ... 1081
ERYC ... 1972
Erycette (erythromycin 2%) Topical Solution ... 1943
Ery-Tab Tablets ... 426
Erythromycin Base Filmtab ... 430
Erythromycin Delayed-Release Capsules, USP ... 431
Ilotycin Ophthalmic Ointment ... 928
PCE Dispertab Tablets ... 453
T-Stat 2.0% Topical Solution and Pads ... 2797
THERAMYCIN Z 2% Solution ... 1629

Erythromycin Estolate (Exerts an effect on terfenadine metabolism, probably by inhibiting isoenzyme, measurably decreases the clearance of terfenadine acid metabolite; co-administration has resulted in few spontaneous accounts of QT interval prolongation and with ventricular arrhythmias including torsade de pointes; concurrent use is contraindicated). Products include:

Ilosone ... 927

Erythromycin Ethylsuccinate (Exerts an effect on terfenadine metabolism, probably by inhibiting isoenzyme, measurably decreases the clearance of terfenadine acid metabolite; co-administration has resulted in few spontaneous accounts of QT interval prolongation and with ventricular arrhythmias including torsade de pointes; concurrent use is contraindicated). Products include:

E.E.S. ... 427
EryPed ... 425
Pediazole Suspension ... 2340

Erythromycin Gluceptate (Exerts an effect on terfenadine metabolism, probably by inhibiting isoenzyme, measurably decreases the clearance of terfenadine acid metabolite; co-administration has resulted in few spontaneous accounts of QT interval prolongation and with ventricular arrhythmias including torsade de pointes; concurrent use is contraindicated). Products include:

Ilotycin Gluceptate, IV, Vials ... 929

Erythromycin Stearate (Exerts an effect on terfenadine metabolism, probably by inhibiting isoenzyme, measurably decreases the clearance of terfenadine acid metabolite; co-administration has resulted in few spontaneous accounts of QT interval prolongation and with ventricular arrhythmias including torsade de pointes; concurrent use is contraindicated). Products include:

Erythrocin Stearate Filmtab ... 429

IMPORTANT NOTE: Always consult each drug listing in the patient's regimen for possible interactions.

Seldane-D | Interactions Index | 972

Esmolol Hydrochloride (Increases the effect of sympathomimetic amines). Products include:

- Brevibloc (esmolol HCl) Injection 1860

Fluconazole (Co-administration is not recommended; due to chemical similarity of fluconazole to ketoconazole). Products include:

- Diflucan Tablets, Injection, and Oral Suspension 2003

Furazolidone (Concomitant therapy with MAO inhibitors increases the effect of sympathomimetic amines and prolongs and intensifies the effects of antihistamines; concurrent and/or sequential use is contraindicated). Products include:

- Furoxone 2221

Isocarboxazid (Concomitant therapy with MAO inhibitors increases the effect of sympathomimetic amines and prolongs and intensifies the effects of antihistamines; concurrent and/or sequential use is contraindicated).

No products indexed under this heading.

Isoproterenol Hydrochloride (Co-administration may produce combined harmful effects on cardiovascular system). Products include:

- Isuprel Hydrochloride Solution 2443
- Isuprel Injection 2441
- Isuprel Mistometer 2442

Isoproterenol Sulfate (Co-administration may produce combined harmful effects on cardiovascular system). Products include:

- Norisodrine with Calcium Iodide Syrup 446

Itraconazole (Inhibits the metabolism of terfenadine, resulting in elevated plasma terfenadine; co-administration has resulted in QT interval prolongation and rare serious cardiac events, e.g., cardiac arrest, and ventricular arrhythmias including torsade de pointes and death; concurrent use is contraindicated). Products include:

- Sporanox Capsules 1352

Ketoconazole (Markedly inhibits the metabolism of terfenadine, resulting in elevated plasma terfenadine; co-administration demonstrates QT interval prolongation and rare serious cardiac events, e.g., death, cardiac arrest, and ventricular arrhythmias including torsade de pointes; concurrent use is contraindicated). Products include:

- Nizoral 2% Cream 1344
- Nizoral 2% Shampoo 1344
- Nizoral Tablets 1345

Labetalol Hydrochloride (Increases the effect of sympathomimetic amines). Products include:

- Normodyne Injection 2519
- Normodyne Tablets 2522
- Trandate 1158

Levobunolol Hydrochloride (Increases the effect of sympathomimetic amines). Products include:

- Betagan .... ◉ 230

Mecamylamine Hydrochloride (Reduced antihypertensive effect). Products include:

- Inversine Tablets 1729

Metaproterenol Sulfate (Co-administration may produce combined harmful effects on cardiovascular system). Products include:

- Alupent 672
- Metaproterenol Sulfate Inhalation Solution, USP, Arm-a-Med 547

Metaraminol Bitartrate (Co-administration may produce combined harmful effects on cardiovascular system). Products include:

- Aramine Injection 1649

Methoxamine Hydrochloride (Co-administration may produce combined harmful effects on cardiovascular system). Products include:

- Vasoxyl Injection 1169

Methyldopa (Reduced antihypertensive effect). Products include:

- Aldoclor Tablets 1638
- Aldomet Oral 1640
- Aldoril Tablets 1644

Methyldopate Hydrochloride (Reduced antihypertensive effect). Products include:

- Aldomet Ester HCl Injection 1642

Metipranolol Hydrochloride (Increases the effect of sympathomimetic amines). Products include:

- OptiPranolol (Metipranolol 0.3%) Sterile Ophthalmic Solution .... ◉ 256

Metoprolol Succinate (Increases the effect of sympathomimetic amines). Products include:

- Toprol-XL Tablets 560

Metoprolol Tartrate (Increases the effect of sympathomimetic amines). Products include:

- Lopressor 848
- Lopressor HCT Tablets 850

Metronidazole (Co-administration is not recommended; due to chemical similarity of metronidazole to ketoconazole). Products include:

- Flagyl 375 Capsules 2587
- Flagyl I.V. RTU 2373
- Helidac Therapy 2135
- MetroCream 1034
- MetroGel 1034
- MetroGel-Vaginal 917
- Protostat Tablets 1939

Metronidazole Hydrochloride (Co-administration is not recommended; due to chemical similarity of metronidazole to ketaconazole). Products include:

- Flagyl I.V. 2373

Miconazole (Co-administration is not recommended; due to chemical similarity of miconazole to ketoconazole).

No products indexed under this heading.

Nadolol (Increases the effect of sympathomimetic amines).

No products indexed under this heading.

Norepinephrine Bitartrate (Co-administration may produce combined harmful effects on cardiovascular system). Products include:

- Levophed Bitartrate Injection 2445

Penbutolol Sulfate (Increases the effect of sympathomimetic amines). Products include:

- Levatol Tablets 2547

Phenelzine Sulfate (Concomitant therapy with MAO inhibitors increases the effect of sympathomimetic amines and prolongs and intensifies the effects of antihistamines; concurrent and/or sequential use is contraindicated). Products include:

- Nardil 1977

Phenylephrine Bitartrate (Co-administration may produce combined harmful effects on cardiovascular system).

No products indexed under this heading.

Phenylephrine Hydrochloride (Co-administration may produce combined harmful effects on cardiovascular system). Products include:

- Atrohist Plus Tablets 1605
- Cerose DM .... ▣ 853
- D.A. II Tablets 972
- D.A. Chewable Tablets 970
- Dura-Vent/DA Tablets 972
- Extendryl 1003
- 4-Way Fast Acting Nasal Spray (regular & mentholated) .... ▣ 644
- Hemorid .... ▣ 797
- Hycomine Compound Tablets 948
- Neo-Synephrine Hydrochloride 1% Carpuject 2455
- Neo-Synephrine Hydrochloride 1% Injection 2455
- Neo-Synephrine Hydrochloride (Ophthalmic) 2456
- Neo-Synephrine .... ▣ 624
- Novahistine Elixir .... ▣ 782
- Phenergan VC 2886
- Phenergan VC with Codeine 2888
- Preparation H .... ▣ 842
- Tympagesic Ear Drops 2476
- Vicks Sinex Nasal Spray and Ultra Fine Mist .... ▣ 738

Phenylephrine Tannate (Co-administration may produce combined harmful effects on cardiovascular system). Products include:

- Atrohist Pediatric Suspension 1604
- Atrohist Pediatric Suspension Dye-Free 1604
- Rynatan 2781
- Rynatuss 2782

Phenylpropanolamine Hydrochloride (Co-administration may produce combined harmful effects on cardiovascular system). Products include:

- Acutrim .... ▣ 648
- Atrohist Plus Tablets 1605
- BC Cold Powder Multi-Symptom Formula (Cold-Sinus-Allergy) .... ▣ 631
- BC Cold Powder Non-Drowsy Formula (Cold-Sinus) .... ▣ 631
- Cheracol Plus Head Cold/Cough Formula .... ▣ 741
- Comtrex Multi-Symptom Cold Reliever Liqui-Gels .... ▣ 638
- Comtrex Multi-Symptom Non-Drowsy Liqui-gels .... ▣ 640
- Contac Continuous Action Nasal Decongestant/Antihistamine 12 Hour Capsules .... ▣ 773
- Contac Maximum Strength Continuous Action Decongestant/Antihistamine 12 Hour Caplets .... ▣ 772
- Contac Severe Cold and Flu Formula Caplets .... ▣ 773
- Coricidin 'D' Decongestant Tablets .... ▣ 760
- Dexatrim .... ▣ 795
- Dexatrim Plus Vitamins Caplets .... ▣ 796
- Dimetane-DC Cough Syrup 2232
- Dimetapp Allergy Sinus Caplets .... ▣ 838
- Dimetapp Cold & Allergy Chewable Tablets .... ▣ 838
- Dimetapp Cold & Cough Liqui-Gels .... ▣ 839
- Dimetapp DM Elixir .... ▣ 840
- Dimetapp Elixir .... ▣ 840
- Dimetapp Extentabs .... ▣ 841
- Dimetapp Tablets/Liqui-Gels .... ▣ 841
- Dura-Vent Tablets 971
- Entex LA Tablets 972
- Exgest LA Tablets 787
- Hycomine 947
- Nolamine Timed-Release Tablets 790
- Ornade Spansule Capsules 2678
- Propagest Tablets 791
- Pyrroxate Caplets .... ▣ 742
- Robitussin-CF .... ▣ 846
- Sinulin Tablets 792
- Tavist-D 12 Hour Relief Tablets .... ▣ 750
- Teldrin 12 Hour Antihistamine/Nasal Decongestant Allergy Relief Capsules .... ▣ 786
- Triaminic Expectorant .... ▣ 753
- Triaminic Syrup .... ▣ 755
- Triaminic Triaminicol Cold & Cough .... ▣ 756
- Triaminic DM Syrup .... ▣ 756
- Triaminicin Tablets .... ▣ 756
- Vicks DayQuil Allergy Relief 12-Hour Extended Release Tablets .... ▣ 733
- Vicks DayQuil Allergy Relief 4-Hour Tablets .... ▣ 733
- Vicks DayQuil SINUS Pressure & CONGESTION Relief .... ▣ 734

Pindolol (Increases the effect of sympathomimetic amines). Products include:

- Visken Tablets 2428

Pirbuterol Acetate (Co-administration may produce combined harmful effects on cardiovascular system). Products include:

- Maxair Autohaler 1550
- Maxair Inhaler 1552

Probucol (Patients who may experience new or increased QT prolongation while receiving certain drugs, such as probucol, may be at increased risk of ventricular tachyarrhythmias).

No products indexed under this heading.

Propranolol Hydrochloride (Increases the effect of sympathomimetic amines). Products include:

- Inderal 2834
- Inderal LA Long Acting Capsules 2836
- Inderide Tablets 2838
- Inderide LA Long Acting Capsules 2840

Pseudoephedrine Sulfate (Co-administration may produce combined harmful effects on cardiovascular system). Products include:

- Chlor-Trimeton Allergy Decongestant Tablets .... ▣ 759
- Claritin-D Tablets 2487
- Drixoral Cold and Allergy Sustained-Action Tablets .... ▣ 763
- Drixoral Cold and Flu Extended-Release Tablets .... ▣ 764
- Drixoral Non-Drowsy Formula Extended-Release Tablets .... ▣ 764
- Drixoral Allergy/Sinus Extended Release Tablets .... ▣ 765
- Trinalin Repetabs Tablets 1373

Quinidine Gluconate (Patients who may experience new or increased QT prolongation while receiving certain drugs, such as quinidine, an antiarrhythmic, may be at increased risk of ventricular tachyarrhythmias). Products include:

- Quinaglute Dura-Tabs Tablets 644

Quinidine Polygalacturonate (Patients who may experience new or increased QT prolongation while receiving certain drugs, such as quinidine, an antiarrhythmic, may be at increased risk of ventricular tachyarrhythmias). Products include:

- Cardioquin Tablets 2146

Quinidine Sulfate (Patients who may experience new or increased QT prolongation while receiving certain drugs, such as quinidine, an antiarrhythmic, may be at increased risk of ventricular tachyarrhythmias). Products include:

- Quinidex Extentabs 2240

Rauwolfia Serpentina (Reduced antihypertensive effect).

No products indexed under this heading.

Rescinnamine (Reduced antihypertensive effect).

No products indexed under this heading.

Reserpine (Reduced antihypertensive effect). Products include:

- Diupres Tablets 1691
- Hydropres Tablets 1718
- Ser-Ap-Es Tablets 867

Salmeterol Xinafoate (Co-administration may produce combined harmful effects on cardiovascular system). Products include:

- Serevent Inhalation Aerosol 1149

(▣ Described in PDR For Nonprescription Drugs) (◉ Described in PDR For Ophthalmology)

Selegiline Hydrochloride (Concomitant therapy with MAO inhibitors increases the effect of sympathomimetic amines and prolongs and intensifies the effects of antihistamines; concurrent and/or sequential use is contraindicated). Products include:
Eldepryl Capsules 2729

Sotalol Hydrochloride (Increases the effect of sympathomimetic amines). Products include:
Betapace Tablets 637

Terbutaline Sulfate (Co-administration may produce combined harmful effects on cardiovascular system). Products include:
Brethaire Inhaler 830
Brethine Ampuls 832
Brethine Tablets 831
Bricanyl Subcutaneous Injection 1247
Bricanyl Tablets 1248

Timolol Hemihydrate (Increases the effect of sympathomimetic amines). Products include:
Betimol 0.25%, 0.5% .... ⊠ 259

Timolol Maleate (Increases the effect of sympathomimetic amines). Products include:
Blocadren Tablets 1654
Timolide Tablets 1791
Timoptic in Ocudose 1796
Timoptic Sterile Ophthalmic Solution ... 1794
Timoptic-XE 1798

Tocainide Hydrochloride (Patients who may experience new or increased QT prolongation while receiving certain drugs, such as tocainide an antiarrhythmic, may be at increased risk of ventricular tachyarrhythmias). Products include:
Tonocard Tablets 519

Tranylcypromine Sulfate (Concomitant therapy with MAO inhibitors increases the effect of sympathomimetic amines and prolongs and intensifies the effects of antihistamines; concurrent and/or sequential use is contraindicated). Products include:
Parnate Tablets 2679

Troleandomycin (Co-administration is contraindicated; potential for QT interval prolongation with ventricular arrhythmia including Torsades de pointes). Products include:
Tao Capsules 2033

SELSUN BLUE DANDRUFF SHAMPOO 2-IN-1 TREATMENT
(Selenium Sulfide) .... ⊠ 746
None cited in PDR database.

SELSUN BLUE DANDRUFF SHAMPOO BALANCED TREATMENT
(Selenium Sulfide) .... ⊠ 746
None cited in PDR database.

SELSUN BLUE DANDRUFF SHAMPOO MEDICATED TREATMENT
(Selenium Sulfide) .... ⊠ 746
None cited in PDR database.

SELSUN BLUE DANDRUFF SHAMPOO MOISTURIZING TREATMENT
(Selenium Sulfide) .... ⊠ 746
None cited in PDR database.

SELSUN RX 2.5% SELENIUM SULFIDE LOTION, USP
(Selenium Sulfide) 2345
None cited in PDR database.

SEMPREX-D CAPSULES
(Acrivastine, Pseudoephedrine Hydrochloride) 1620
May interact with monoamine oxidase inhibitors, sympathomimetics, central nervous system depressants, catecholamine depleting drugs, veratrum alkaloids, and certain other agents. Compounds in these categories include:

Albuterol (Beta-adrenergic agonists (other sympathomimetics) increase the effects of pseudoephedrine and combined effects on cardiovascular system may be harmful). Products include:
Proventil Inhalation Aerosol 2524
Ventolin Inhalation Aerosol and Refill 1170

Albuterol Sulfate (Beta-adrenergic agonists (other sympathomimetics) increase the effects of pseudoephedrine and combined effects on cardiovascular system may be harmful). Products include:
Airet Albuterol Sulfate Inhalation Solution 1602
Albuterol Sulfate, USP Solution for Inhalation, Arm-a-Med 522
Proventil Inhalation Solution 0.083% 2527
Proventil Repetabs Tablets 2529
Proventil Solution for Inhalation 0.5% 2525
Proventil Syrup 2528
Proventil Tablets 2529
Ventolin Inhalation Solution 1171
Ventolin Nebules Inhalation Solution 1172
Ventolin Rotacaps for Inhalation 1173
Ventolin Syrup 1175
Ventolin Tablets 1176
Volmax Extended-Release Tablets .. 1835

Alfentanil Hydrochloride (Co-administration may result in additional reduction in alertness and impairment of CNS performance and should be avoided). Products include:
Alfenta Injection 1334

Alprazolam (Co-administration may result in additional reduction in alertness and impairment of CNS performance and should be avoided). Products include:
Xanax Tablets 2115

Aprobarbital (Co-administration may result in additional reduction in alertness and impairment of CNS performance and should be avoided).
No products indexed under this heading.

Buprenorphine (Co-administration may result in additional reduction in alertness and impairment of CNS performance and should be avoided). Products include:
Buprenex Injectable 2170

Buspirone Hydrochloride (Co-administration may result in additional reduction in alertness and impairment of CNS performance and should be avoided). Products include:
BuSpar Tablets 738

Butabarbital (Co-administration may result in additional reduction in alertness and impairment of CNS performance and should be avoided).
No products indexed under this heading.

Butalbital (Co-administration may result in additional reduction in alertness and impairment of CNS performance and should be avoided). Products include:
Axocet Capsules 2469
Esgic-plus Capsules 1012
Esgic-plus Tablets 1012
Fioricet Tablets 2386
Fioricet with Codeine Capsules 2387
Fiorinal Capsules 2388
Fiorinal with Codeine Capsules 2390
Fiorinal Tablets 2388
Phrenilin 790
Sedapap Tablets 50 mg/650 mg .. 1826

Chlordiazepoxide (Co-administration may result in additional reduction in alertness and impairment of CNS performance and should be avoided). Products include:
Limbitrol 2333

Chlordiazepoxide Hydrochloride (Co-administration may result in additional reduction in alertness and impairment of CNS performance and should be avoided). Products include:
Librax Capsules 2330
Librium Capsules 2331
Librium Injectable 2332

Chlorpromazine (Co-administration may result in additional reduction in alertness and impairment of CNS performance and should be avoided). Products include:
Thorazine Suppositories 2701

Chlorpromazine Hydrochloride (Co-administration may result in additional reduction in alertness and impairment of CNS performance and should be avoided). Products include:
Thorazine 2701

Chlorprothixene (Co-administration may result in additional reduction in alertness and impairment of CNS performance and should be avoided).
No products indexed under this heading.

Chlorprothixene Hydrochloride (Co-administration may result in additional reduction in alertness and impairment of CNS performance and should be avoided).
No products indexed under this heading.

Chlorprothixene Lactate (Co-administration may result in additional reduction in alertness and impairment of CNS performance and should be avoided).
No products indexed under this heading.

Clorazepate Dipotassium (Co-administration may result in additional reduction in alertness and impairment of CNS performance and should be avoided). Products include:
Tranxene 459

Clozapine (Co-administration may result in additional reduction in alertness and impairment of CNS performance and should be avoided). Products include:
Clozaril Tablets 2377

Codeine Phosphate (Co-administration may result in additional reduction in alertness and impairment of CNS performance and should be avoided). Products include:
Brontex 2130
Dimetane-DC Cough Syrup 2232
Fioricet with Codeine Capsules 2387
Fiorinal with Codeine Capsules 2390
Nucofed 2225
Phenergan with Codeine 2883
Phenergan VC with Codeine 2888
Robitussin A-C Syrup 2248
Robitussin-DAC Syrup 2249
Ryna .... ⊠ 804
Soma Compound w/Codeine Tablets 2784
Tylenol with Codeine 1592

Cryptenamine Preparations (Reduced antihypertensive effects of drugs that interfere with sympathetic activity).

Deserpidine (Reduced antihypertensive effects of drugs that interfere with sympathetic activity).
No products indexed under this heading.

Desflurane (Co-administration may result in additional reduction in alertness and impairment of CNS performance and should be avoided). Products include:
Suprane (desflurane, USP) 1865

Dezocine (Co-administration may result in additional reduction in alertness and impairment of CNS performance and should be avoided). Products include:
Dalgan Injection 529

Diazepam (Co-administration may result in additional reduction in alertness and impairment of CNS performance and should be avoided). Products include:
Dizac (diazepam injectable emulsion) CIV 1862
Valium Injectable 2336
Valium Tablets 2335

Dobutamine Hydrochloride (Beta-adrenergic agonists (other sympathomimetics) increase the effects of pseudoephedrine and combined effects on cardiovascular system may be harmful). Products include:
Dobutrex Solution Vials 1480

Dopamine Hydrochloride (Beta-adrenergic agonists (other sympathomimetics) increase the effects of pseudoephedrine and combined effects on cardiovascular system may be harmful).
No products indexed under this heading.

Droperidol (Co-administration may result in additional reduction in alertness and impairment of CNS performance and should be avoided). Products include:
Inapsine Injection 462

Enflurane (Co-administration may result in additional reduction in alertness and impairment of CNS performance and should be avoided).
No products indexed under this heading.

Ephedrine Hydrochloride (Beta-adrenergic agonists (other sympathomimetics) increase the effects of pseudoephedrine and combined effects on cardiovascular system may be harmful). Products include:
Primatene Tablets .... ⊠ 844
Quadrinal Tablets 1398

Ephedrine Sulfate (Beta-adrenergic agonists (other sympathomimetics) increase the effects of pseudoephedrine and combined effects on cardiovascular system may be harmful). Products include:
Marax Tablets & DF Syrup 2015

Ephedrine Tannate (Beta-adrenergic agonists (other sympathomimetics) increase the effects of pseudoephedrine and combined effects on cardiovascular system may be harmful). Products include:
Rynatuss 2782

Epinephrine (Beta-adrenergic agonists (other sympathomimetics) increase the effects of pseudoephedrine and combined effects on cardiovascular system may be harmful). Products include:
EPIFRIN .... ⊠ 237
EpiPen 808
Marcaine with Epinephrine 2446
Primatene Mist .... ⊠ 843
Sensorcaine with Epinephrine Injection 554
Sus-Phrine Injection 1017

IMPORTANT NOTE: Always consult each drug listing in the patient's regimen for possible interactions.

Xylocaine with Epinephrine Injections... 562

Epinephrine Bitartrate (Beta-adrenergic agonists (other sympathomimetics) increase the effects of pseudoephedrine and combined effects on cardiovascular system may be harmful). Products include:
Sensorcaine-MPF with Epinephrine Injection 554

Epinephrine Hydrochloride (Beta-adrenergic agonists (other sympathomimetics) increase the effects of pseudoephedrine and combined effects on cardiovascular system may be harmful). Products include:
Ana-Kit Anaphylaxis Emergency Treatment Kit 611

Estazolam (Co-administration may result in additional reduction in alertness and impairment of CNS performance and should be avoided). Products include:
ProSom Tablets 457

Ethchlorvynol (Co-administration may result in additional reduction in alertness and impairment of CNS performance and should be avoided). Products include:
Placidyl Capsules 456

Ethinamate (Co-administration may result in additional reduction in alertness and impairment of CNS performance and should be avoided).
No products indexed under this heading.

Fentanyl (Co-administration may result in additional reduction in alertness and impairment of CNS performance and should be avoided). Products include:
Duragesic Transdermal System........ 1336

Fentanyl Citrate (Co-administration may result in additional reduction in alertness and impairment of CNS performance and should be avoided). Products include:
Sublimaze Injection 463

Fluphenazine Decanoate (Co-administration may result in additional reduction in alertness and impairment of CNS performance and should be avoided). Products include:
Prolixin Decanoate 510

Fluphenazine Enanthate (Co-administration may result in additional reduction in alertness and impairment of CNS performance and should be avoided). Products include:
Prolixin Enanthate 510

Fluphenazine Hydrochloride (Co-administration may result in additional reduction in alertness and impairment of CNS performance and should be avoided). Products include:
Prolixin 510

Flurazepam Hydrochloride (Co-administration may result in additional reduction in alertness and impairment of CNS performance and should be avoided). Products include:
Dalmane Capsules 2329

Furazolidone (Increases the effects of sympathomimetics; potential for hypertensive crisis; concurrent and/or sequential use is contraindicated for two weeks). Products include:
Furoxone 2221

Glutethimide (Co-administration may result in additional reduction in alertness and impairment of CNS performance and should be avoided).
No products indexed under this heading.

Guanethidine Monosulfate (Reduced antihypertensive effects of drugs that interfere with sympathetic activity). Products include:
Esimil Tablets 840
Ismelin Tablets 845

Haloperidol (Co-administration may result in additional reduction in alertness and impairment of CNS performance and should be avoided). Products include:
Haldol Injection, Tablets and Concentrate 1585

Haloperidol Decanoate (Co-administration may result in additional reduction in alertness and impairment of CNS performance and should be avoided). Products include:
Haldol Decanoate 1587

Hydrocodone Bitartrate (Co-administration may result in additional reduction in alertness and impairment of CNS performance and should be avoided). Products include:
Codiclear DH Syrup 808
Duratuss HD Elixir........................... 2750
Histussin D Liquid 670
Hycodan Tablets and Syrup 946
Hycomine Compound Tablets 948
Hycomine 947
Hycotuss Expectorant Syrup 950
Hydrocet Capsules 787
Lorcet 10/650 Tablets 1016
Lortab 2751
Tussend 1830
Tussend Expectorant 1831
Vicodin Tablets 1404
Vicodin ES Tablets 1405
Vicodin HP Tablets 1403
Vicodin Tuss Expectorant 1406
Zydone Capsules 967

Hydrocodone Polistirex (Co-administration may result in additional reduction in alertness and impairment of CNS performance and should be avoided). Products include:
Tussionex Pennkinetic Extended-Release Suspension 1624

Hydroxyzine Hydrochloride (Co-administration may result in additional reduction in alertness and impairment of CNS performance and should be avoided). Products include:
Atarax Tablets & Syrup..................... 1992
Marax Tablets & DF Syrup............... 2015
Vistaril Intramuscular Solution......... 2042

Isocarboxazid (Increases the effects of sympathomimetics; potential for hypertensive crisis; concurrent and/or sequential use is contraindicated for two weeks).
No products indexed under this heading.

Isoflurane (Co-administration may result in additional reduction in alertness and impairment of CNS performance and should be avoided).
No products indexed under this heading.

Isoproterenol Hydrochloride (Beta-adrenergic agonists (other sympathomimetics) increase the effects of pseudoephedrine and combined effects on cardiovascular system may be harmful). Products include:
Isuprel Hydrochloride Solution 2443
Isuprel Injection 2441

Isuprel Mistometer 2442

Ketamine Hydrochloride (Co-administration may result in additional reduction in alertness and impairment of CNS performance and should be avoided).
No products indexed under this heading.

Levomethadyl Acetate Hydrochloride (Co-administration may result in additional reduction in alertness and impairment of CNS performance and should be avoided). Products include:
Orlaam Oral Solution 2361

Levorphanol Tartrate (Co-administration may result in additional reduction in alertness and impairment of CNS performance and should be avoided). Products include:
Levo-Dromoran 2297

Lorazepam (Co-administration may result in additional reduction in alertness and impairment of CNS performance and should be avoided). Products include:
Ativan Injection 2805
Ativan Tablets 2807

Loxapine Hydrochloride (Co-administration may result in additional reduction in alertness and impairment of CNS performance and should be avoided). Products include:
Loxitane 1426

Loxapine Succinate (Co-administration may result in additional reduction in alertness and impairment of CNS performance and should be avoided). Products include:
Loxitane Capsules 1426

Mecamylamine Hydrochloride (Reduced antihypertensive effects of drugs that interfere with sympathetic activity). Products include:
Inversine Tablets 1729

Meperidine Hydrochloride (Co-administration may result in additional reduction in alertness and impairment of CNS performance and should be avoided). Products include:
Demerol 2438
Mepergan Injection 2859

Mephobarbital (Co-administration may result in additional reduction in alertness and impairment of CNS performance and should be avoided). Products include:
Mebaral Tablets 2452

Meprobamate (Co-administration may result in additional reduction in alertness and impairment of CNS performance and should be avoided). Products include:
Miltown Tablets 2780
PMB 200 and PMB 400 2890

Mesoridazine Besylate (Co-administration may result in additional reduction in alertness and impairment of CNS performance and should be avoided). Products include:
Serentil 689

Metaproterenol Sulfate (Beta-adrenergic agonists (other sympathomimetics) increase the effects of pseudoephedrine and combined effects on cardiovascular system may be harmful). Products include:
Alupent 672
Metaproterenol Sulfate Inhalation Solution, USP, Arm-a-Med 547

Metaraminol Bitartrate (Beta-adrenergic agohists (other sympathomimetics) increase the effects of pseudoephedrine and combined effects on cardiovascular system may be harmful). Products include:
Aramine Injection............................. 1649

Methadone Hydrochloride (Co-administration may result in additional reduction in alertness and impairment of CNS performance and should be avoided). Products include:
Methadone Hydrochloride Oral Concentrate 2356
Methadone Hydrochloride Oral Solution & Tablets....................... 2357

Methohexital Sodium (Co-administration may result in additional reduction in alertness and impairment of CNS performance and should be avoided).
No products indexed under this heading.

Methotrimeprazine (Co-administration may result in additional reduction in alertness and impairment of CNS performance and should be avoided). Products include:
Levoprome 1321

Methoxamine Hydrochloride (Beta-adrenergic agonists (other sympathomimetics) increase the effects of pseudoephedrine and combined effects on cardiovascular system may be harmful). Products include:
Vasoxyl Injection 1169

Methoxyflurane (Co-administration may result in additional reduction in alertness and impairment of CNS performance and should be avoided).
No products indexed under this heading.

Methyldopa (Reduced antihypertensive effects of drugs that interfere with sympathetic activity). Products include:
Aldoclor Tablets 1638
Aldomet Oral 1640
Aldoril Tablets 1644

Methyldopate Hydrochloride (Reduced antihypertensive effects of drugs that interfere with sympathetic activity). Products include:
Aldomet Ester HCl Injection 1642

Midazolam Hydrochloride (Co-administration may result in additional reduction in alertness and impairment of CNS performance and should be avoided). Products include:
Versed Injection 2324

Molindone Hydrochloride (Co-administration may result in additional reduction in alertness and impairment of CNS performance and should be avoided). Products include:
Moban Tablets and Concentrate...... 1036

Morphine Sulfate (Co-administration may result in additional reduction in alertness and impairment of CNS performance and should be avoided). Products include:
Astramorph/PF Injection, USP (Preservative-Free) 526
Duramorph Injection 983
Infumorph 200 and Infumorph 500 Sterile Solutions 985
Kadian Capsules.............................. 2948
MS Contin Tablets 2149
MSIR 2152
Oramorph SR (Morphine Sulfate Sustained Release Tablets) 2359
RMS Suppositories CII..................... 2766
Roxanol 2365

Norepinephrine Bitartrate (Beta-adrenergic agonists (other sympathomimetics) increase the effects of pseudoephedrine and combined effects on cardiovascular system may be harmful). Products include:
- Levophed Bitartrate Injection 2445

Opium Alkaloids (Co-administration may result in additional reduction in alertness and impairment of CNS performance and should be avoided).
- No products indexed under this heading.

Oxazepam (Co-administration may result in additional reduction in alertness and impairment of CNS performance and should be avoided). Products include:
- Serax Capsules 2916
- Serax Tablets 2916

Oxycodone Hydrochloride (Co-administration may result in additional reduction in alertness and impairment of CNS performance and should be avoided). Products include:
- OxyContin Tablets 2163
- OxyIR Capsules 2167
- Percocet Tablets 955
- Percodan Tablets 955
- Percodan-Demi Tablets 956
- Roxicodone Tablets, Oral Solution & Intensol (Oxycodone) 2366
- Tylox Capsules 1593

Pentobarbital Sodium (Co-administration may result in additional reduction in alertness and impairment of CNS performance and should be avoided). Products include:
- Nembutal Sodium Capsules 440
- Nembutal Sodium Solution 442
- Nembutal Sodium Suppositories 444

Perphenazine (Co-administration may result in additional reduction in alertness and impairment of CNS performance and should be avoided). Products include:
- Etrafon 2495
- Triavil Tablets 1800
- Trilafon 2532

Phenelzine Sulfate (Increases the effects of sympathomimetics; potential for hypertensive crisis; concurrent and/or sequential use is contraindicated for two weeks). Products include:
- Nardil 1977

Phenobarbital (Co-administration may result in additional reduction in alertness and impairment of CNS performance and should be avoided). Products include:
- Arco-Lase Plus Tablets 513
- Bellergal-S Tablets 2375
- Donnatal 2234
- Donnatal Extentabs 2234
- Donnatal Tablets 2234
- Phenobarbital Elixir and Tablets 1523
- Quadrinal Tablets 1398

Phenylephrine Bitartrate (Beta-adrenergic agonists (other sympathomimetics) increase the effects of pseudoephedrine and combined effects on cardiovascular system may be harmful).
- No products indexed under this heading.

Phenylephrine Hydrochloride (Beta-adrenergic agonists (other sympathomimetics) increase the effects of pseudoephedrine and combined effects on cardiovascular system may be harmful). Products include:
- Atrohist Plus Tablets 1605
- Cerose DM 853
- D.A. II Tablets 972
- D.A. Chewable Tablets 970
- Dura-Vent/DA Tablets 972
- Extendryl 1003
- 4-Way Fast Acting Nasal Spray (regular & mentholated) 644
- Hemorid 797
- Hycomine Compound Tablets 948
- Neo-Synephrine Hydrochloride 1% Carpuject 2455
- Neo-Synephrine Hydrochloride 1% Injection 2455
- Neo-Synephrine Hydrochloride (Ophthalmic) 2456
- Neo-Synephrine 624
- Novahistine Elixir 782
- Phenergan VC 2886
- Phenergan VC with Codeine 2888
- Preparation H 842
- Tympagesic Ear Drops 2476
- Vicks Sinex Nasal Spray and Ultra Fine Mist 738

Phenylephrine Tannate (Beta-adrenergic agonists (other sympathomimetics) increase the effects of pseudoephedrine and combined effects on cardiovascular system may be harmful). Products include:
- Atrohist Pediatric Suspension 1604
- Atrohist Pediatric Suspension Dye-Free 1604
- Rynatan 2781
- Rynatuss 2782

Phenylpropanolamine Hydrochloride (Beta-adrenergic agonists (other sympathomimetics) increase the effects of pseudoephedrine and combined effects on cardiovascular system may be harmful). Products include:
- Acutrim 648
- Atrohist Plus Tablets 1605
- BC Cold Powder Multi-Symptom Formula (Cold-Sinus-Allergy) 631
- BC Cold Powder Non-Drowsy Formula (Cold-Sinus) 631
- Cheracol Plus Head Cold/Cough Formula 741
- Comtrex Multi-Symptom Cold Reliever Liqui-Gels 638
- Comtrex Multi-Symptom Non-Drowsy Liqui-gels 640
- Contac Continuous Action Nasal Decongestant/Antihistamine 12 Hour Capsules 773
- Contac Maximum Strength Continuous Action Decongestant/Antihistamine 12 Hour Caplets 772
- Contac Severe Cold and Flu Formula Caplets 773
- Coricidin 'D' Decongestant Tablets 760
- Dexatrim 795
- Dexatrim Plus Vitamins Caplets 796
- Dimetane-DC Cough Syrup 2232
- Dimetapp Allergy Sinus Caplets 838
- Dimetapp Cold & Allergy Chewable Tablets 838
- Dimetapp Cold & Cough Liqui-Gels 839
- Dimetapp DM Elixir 840
- Dimetapp Elixir 840
- Dimetapp Extentabs 841
- Dimetapp Tablets/Liqui-Gels 841
- Dura-Vent Tablets 971
- Entex LA Tablets 972
- Exgest LA Tablets 787
- Hycomine 947
- Nolamine Timed-Release Tablets 790
- Ornade Spansule Capsules 2678
- Propagest Tablets 791
- Pyrroxate Caplets 742
- Robitussin-CF 846
- Sinulin Tablets 792
- Tavist-D 12 Hour Relief Tablets 750
- Teldrin 12 Hour Antihistamine/Nasal Decongestant Allergy Relief Capsules 786
- Triaminic Expectorant 753
- Triaminic Syrup 755
- Triaminic Triaminicol Cold & Cough 756
- Triaminic DM Syrup 756
- Triaminicin Tablets 756
- Vicks DayQuil Allergy Relief 12-Hour Extended Release Tablets 733
- Vicks DayQuil Allergy Relief 4-Hour Tablets 733
- Vicks DayQuil SINUS Pressure & CONGESTION Relief 734

Pirbuterol Acetate (Beta-adrenergic agonists (other sympathomimetics) increase the effects of pseudoephedrine and combined effects on cardiovascular system may be harmful). Products include:
- Maxair Autohaler 1550
- Maxair Inhaler 1552

Prazepam (Co-administration may result in additional reduction in alertness and impairment of CNS performance and should be avoided).
- No products indexed under this heading.

Prochlorperazine (Co-administration may result in additional reduction in alertness and impairment of CNS performance and should be avoided). Products include:
- Compazine 2644

Promethazine Hydrochloride (Co-administration may result in additional reduction in alertness and impairment of CNS performance and should be avoided). Products include:
- Mepergan Injection 2859
- Phenergan with Codeine 2883
- Phenergan with Dextromethorphan 2885
- Phenergan Injection 2880
- Phenergan Suppositories 2882
- Phenergan Syrup 2881
- Phenergan Tablets 2882
- Phenergan VC 2886
- Phenergan VC with Codeine 2888

Propofol (Co-administration may result in additional reduction in alertness and impairment of CNS performance and should be avoided). Products include:
- Diprivan Injectable Emulsion 2939

Propoxyphene Hydrochloride (Co-administration may result in additional reduction in alertness and impairment of CNS performance and should be avoided). Products include:
- Darvon 1475
- Wygesic Tablets 2930

Propoxyphene Napsylate (Co-administration may result in additional reduction in alertness and impairment of CNS performance and should be avoided). Products include:
- Darvon-N/Darvocet-N 1473

Pseudoephedrine Sulfate (Beta-adrenergic agonists (other sympathomimetics) increase the effects of pseudoephedrine and combined effects on cardiovascular system may be harmful). Products include:
- Chlor-Trimeton Allergy Decongestant Tablets 759
- Claritin-D Tablets 2487
- Drixoral Cold and Allergy Sustained-Action Tablets 763
- Drixoral Cold and Flu Extended-Release Tablets 764
- Drixoral Non-Drowsy Formula Extended-Release Tablets 764
- Drixoral Allergy/Sinus Extended Release Tablets 765
- Trinalin Repetabs Tablets 1373

Quazepam (Co-administration may result in additional reduction in alertness and impairment of CNS performance and should be avoided). Products include:
- Doral Tablets 2773

Rauwolfia Serpentina (Reduced antihypertensive effects of drugs that interfere with sympathetic activity).
- No products indexed under this heading.

Rescinnamine (Reduced antihypertensive effects of drugs that interfere with sympathetic activity).
- No products indexed under this heading.

Reserpine (Reduced antihypertensive effects of drugs that interfere with sympathetic activity). Products include:
- Diupres Tablets 1691
- Hydropres Tablets 1718
- Ser-Ap-Es Tablets 867

Risperidone (Co-administration may result in additional reduction in alertness and impairment of CNS performance and should be avoided). Products include:
- Risperdal Tablets 1348

Salmeterol Xinafoate (Beta-adrenergic agonists (other sympathomimetics) increase the effects of pseudoephedrine and combined effects on cardiovascular system may be harmful). Products include:
- Serevent Inhalation Aerosol 1149

Secobarbital Sodium (Co-administration may result in additional reduction in alertness and impairment of CNS performance and should be avoided). Products include:
- Seconal Sodium Pulvules 1529

Selegiline Hydrochloride (Increases the effects of sympathomimetics; potential for hypertensive crisis; concurrent and/or sequential use is contraindicated for two weeks). Products include:
- Eldepryl Capsules 2729

Sevoflurane (Co-administration may result in additional reduction in alertness and impairment of CNS performance and should be avoided).
- No products indexed under this heading.

Sufentanil Citrate (Co-administration may result in additional reduction in alertness and impairment of CNS performance and should be avoided). Products include:
- Sufenta Injection 1355

Temazepam (Co-administration may result in additional reduction in alertness and impairment of CNS performance and should be avoided). Products include:
- Restoril Capsules 2413

Terbutaline Sulfate (Beta-adrenergic agonists (other sympathomimetics) increase the effects of pseudoephedrine and combined effects on cardiovascular system may be harmful). Products include:
- Brethaire Inhaler 830
- Brethine Ampuls 832
- Brethine Tablets 831
- Bricanyl Subcutaneous Injection 1247
- Bricanyl Tablets 1248

Thiamylal Sodium (Co-administration may result in additional reduction in alertness and impairment of CNS performance and should be avoided).
- No products indexed under this heading.

Thioridazine Hydrochloride (Co-administration may result in additional reduction in alertness and impairment of CNS performance and should be avoided). Products include:
- Mellaril 2398

Thiothixene (Co-administration may result in additional reduction in alertness and impairment of CNS performance and should be avoided). Products include:
- Navane Capsules and Concentrate 2018
- Navane Intramuscular 2019

IMPORTANT NOTE: Always consult each drug listing in the patient's regimen for possible interactions.

Semprex-D | Interactions Index | 976

Tranylcypromine Sulfate (Increases the effects of sympathomimetics; potential for hypertensive crisis; concurrent and/or sequential use is contraindicated for two weeks). Products include:
   Parnate Tablets 2679

Triazolam (Co-administration may result in additional reduction in alertness and impairment of CNS performance and should be avoided). Products include:
   Halcion Tablets 2093

Trifluoperazine Hydrochloride (Co-administration may result in additional reduction in alertness and impairment of CNS performance and should be avoided). Products include:
   Stelazine 2692

Zolpidem Tartrate (Co-administration may result in additional reduction in alertness and impairment of CNS performance and should be avoided). Products include:
   Ambien Tablets 2559

Food Interactions

Alcohol (Co-administration may result in additional reduction in alertness and impairment of CNS performance and should be avoided).

SENNA X-PREP BOWEL EVACUANT LIQUID
(Senna Concentrates) 1236
None cited in PDR database.

SENOKOT CHILDREN'S SYRUP
(Senna) 2154
None cited in PDR database.

SENOKOT GRANULES
(Senna Concentrates) 2154
None cited in PDR database.

SENOKOT SYRUP
(Senna Concentrates) 2154
None cited in PDR database.

SENOKOT TABLETS
(Senna Concentrates) 2154
None cited in PDR database.

SENOKOTXTRA TABLETS
(Senna Concentrates) 2154
None cited in PDR database.

SENOKOT-S TABLETS
(Senna Concentrates, Docusate Sodium) 2154
None cited in PDR database.

COOL GEL SENSODYNE
(Potassium Nitrate, Sodium Fluoride) 634
None cited in PDR database.

FRESH MINT SENSODYNE TOOTHPASTE
(Potassium Nitrate, Sodium Monofluorophosphate) 634
None cited in PDR database.

ORIGINAL FORMULA SENSODYNE-SC TOOTHPASTE
(Strontium Chloride Hexahydrate) .. 634
None cited in PDR database.

SENSODYNE WITH BAKING SODA
(Potassium Nitrate, Sodium Fluoride) 634
None cited in PDR database.

SENSORCAINE WITH EPINEPHRINE INJECTION
(Bupivacaine Hydrochloride, Epinephrine Bitartrate) 554
May interact with phenothiazines, butyrophenones, inhalant anesthetics, monoamine oxidase inhibitors, tricyclic antidepressants, vasopressors, ergot-type oxytocic drugs, and certain other agents. Compounds in these categories include:

Amitriptyline Hydrochloride (May produce severe and prolonged hypertension). Products include:
   Elavil 2945
   Etrafon 2495
   Limbitrol 2333
   Triavil Tablets 1800

Amoxapine (May produce severe and prolonged hypertension). Products include:
   Asendin Tablets 1419

Chlorpromazine (Reduces or reverses the pressor effect of epinephrine). Products include:
   Thorazine Suppositories 2701

Clomipramine Hydrochloride (May produce severe and prolonged hypertension). Products include:
   Anafranil Capsules 819

Desflurane (Concurrent use may produce serious dose-related cardiac arrhythmias). Products include:
   Suprane (desflurane, USP) 1865

Desipramine Hydrochloride (May produce severe and prolonged hypertension). Products include:
   Norpramin Tablets 1273

Dopamine Hydrochloride (May produce severe and prolonged hypertension or cerebrovascular accidents).
   No products indexed under this heading.

Doxepin Hydrochloride (May produce severe and prolonged hypertension). Products include:
   Adapin Capsules 1542
   Sinequan 2028
   Zonalon Cream 1042

Enflurane (Concurrent use may produce serious dose-related cardiac arrhythmias).
   No products indexed under this heading.

Epinephrine Hydrochloride (May produce severe and prolonged hypertension or cerebrovascular accidents). Products include:
   Ana-Kit Anaphylaxis Emergency Treatment Kit 611

Fluphenazine Decanoate (Reduces or reverses the pressor effect of epinephrine). Products include:
   Prolixin Decanoate 510

Fluphenazine Enanthate (Reduces or reverses the pressor effect of epinephrine). Products include:
   Prolixin Enanthate 510

Fluphenazine Hydrochloride (Reduces or reverses the pressor effect of epinephrine). Products include:
   Prolixin 510

Furazolidone (May produce severe and prolonged hypertension). Products include:
   Furoxone 2221

Haloperidol (Reduces or reverses the pressor effect of epinephrine). Products include:
   Haldol Injection, Tablets and Concentrate 1585

Haloperidol Decanoate (Reduces or reverses the pressor effect of epinephrine). Products include:
   Haldol Decanoate 1587

Halothane (Concurrent use may produce serious dose-related cardiac arrhythmias). Products include:
   Fluothane 2830

Imipramine Hydrochloride (May produce severe and prolonged hypertension). Products include:
   Tofranil Ampuls 873
   Tofranil Tablets 875

Imipramine Pamoate (May produce severe and prolonged hypertension). Products include:
   Tofranil-PM Capsules 876

Isocarboxazid (May produce severe and prolonged hypertension).
   No products indexed under this heading.

Isoflurane (Concurrent use may produce serious dose-related cardiac arrhythmias).
   No products indexed under this heading.

Maprotiline Hydrochloride (May produce severe and prolonged hypertension). Products include:
   Ludiomil Tablets 861

Mesoridazine Besylate (Reduces or reverses the pressor effect of epinephrine). Products include:
   Serentil 689

Metaraminol Bitartrate (May produce severe and prolonged hypertension or cerebrovascular accidents). Products include:
   Aramine Injection 1649

Methotrimeprazine (Reduces or reverses the pressor effect of epinephrine). Products include:
   Levoprome 1321

Methoxamine Hydrochloride (May produce severe and prolonged hypertension or cerebrovascular accidents). Products include:
   Vasoxyl Injection 1169

Methoxyflurane (Concurrent use may produce serious dose-related cardiac arrhythmias).
   No products indexed under this heading.

Methylergonovine Maleate (May produce severe and prolonged hypertension or cerebrovascular accidents). Products include:
   Methergine 2401

Norepinephrine Bitartrate (May produce severe and prolonged hypertension or cerebrovascular accidents). Products include:
   Levophed Bitartrate Injection 2445

Nortriptyline Hydrochloride (May produce severe and prolonged hypertension). Products include:
   Pamelor 2409

Perphenazine (Reduces or reverses the pressor effect of epinephrine). Products include:
   Etrafon 2495
   Triavil Tablets 1800
   Trilafon 2532

Phenelzine Sulfate (May produce severe and prolonged hypertension). Products include:
   Nardil 1977

Phenylephrine Hydrochloride (May produce severe and prolonged hypertension or cerebrovascular accidents). Products include:
   Atrohist Plus Tablets 1605
   Cerose DM 853
   D.A. II Tablets 972
   D.A. Chewable Tablets 970
   Dura-Vent/DA Tablets 972
   Extendryl 1003
   4-Way Fast Acting Nasal Spray (regular & mentholated) 644
   Hemoril 797
   Hycomine Compound Tablets 948
   Neo-Synephrine Hydrochloride 1% Carpuject 2455
   Neo-Synephrine Hydrochloride 1% Injection 2455
   Neo-Synephrine Hydrochloride (Ophthalmic) 2456
   Neo-Synephrine 624
   Novahistine Elixir 782
   Phenergan VC 2886
   Phenergan VC with Codeine 2888
   Preparation H 842
   Tympagesic Ear Drops 2476
   Vicks Sinex Nasal Spray and Ultra Fine Mist 738

Prochlorperazine (Reduces or reverses the pressor effect of epinephrine). Products include:
   Compazine 2644

Promethazine Hydrochloride (Reduces or reverses the pressor effect of epinephrine). Products include:
   Mepergan Injection 2859
   Phenergan with Codeine 2883
   Phenergan with Dextromethorphan 2885
   Phenergan Injection 2880
   Phenergan Suppositories 2882
   Phenergan Syrup 2881
   Phenergan Tablets 2882
   Phenergan VC 2886
   Phenergan VC with Codeine 2888

Protriptyline Hydrochloride (May produce severe and prolonged hypertension). Products include:
   Vivactil Tablets 1820

Selegiline Hydrochloride (May produce severe and prolonged hypertension). Products include:
   Eldepryl Capsules 2729

Thioridazine Hydrochloride (Reduces or reverses the pressor effect of epinephrine). Products include:
   Mellaril 2398

Tranylcypromine Sulfate (May produce severe and prolonged hypertension). Products include:
   Parnate Tablets 2679

Trifluoperazine Hydrochloride (Reduces or reverses the pressor effect of epinephrine). Products include:
   Stelazine 2692

Trimipramine Maleate (May produce severe and prolonged hypertension). Products include:
   Surmontil Capsules 2917

SENSORCAINE INJECTION
(Bupivacaine Hydrochloride) 554
See **Sensorcaine with Epinephrine Injection**

SENSORCAINE-MPF WITH EPINEPHRINE INJECTION
(Bupivacaine Hydrochloride, Epinephrine Bitartrate) 554
See **Sensorcaine with Epinephrine Injection**

SENSORCAINE-MPF INJECTION
(Bupivacaine Hydrochloride) 554
See **Sensorcaine with Epinephrine Injection**

SEPTRA DS TABLETS
(Trimethoprim, Sulfamethoxazole) 1146
May interact with thiazides and certain other agents. Compounds in these categories include:

Bendroflumethiazide (Potential for thrombocytopenia with purpura in elderly).
   No products indexed under this heading.

Chlorothiazide (Potential for thrombocytopenia with purpura in elderly). Products include:
   Aldoclor Tablets 1638
   Diupres Tablets 1691
   Diuril Oral 1694

(▣ Described in PDR For Nonprescription Drugs)   (◉ Described in PDR For Ophthalmology)

Chlorothiazide Sodium (Potential for thrombocytopenia with purpura in elderly). Products include:
Diuril Sodium Intravenous 1693

Fosphenytoin Sodium (Hepatic metabolism of phenytoin may be inhibited resulting in increased phenytoin half-life and decreased metabolic clearance). Products include:
Cerebyx Injection 1956

Hydrochlorothiazide (Potential for thrombocytopenia with purpura in elderly). Products include:
Aldactazide Tablets 2556
Aldoril Tablets 1644
Apresazide Capsules 824
Capozide Tablets 744
Dyazide Capsules 2653
Esidrix Tablets 839
Esimil Tablets 840
HydroDIURIL Tablets 1716
Hydropres Tablets 1718
Hyzaar Tablets 1720
Inderide Tablets 2838
Inderide LA Long Acting Capsules .. 2840
Lopressor HCT Tablets 850
Lotensin HCT Tablets 855
Moduretic Tablets 1748
Oretic Tablets 450
Prinzide Tablets 1780
Ser-Ap-Es Tablets 867
Timolide Tablets 1791
Vaseretic Tablets 1810
Zestoretic Tablets 2968
Ziac 1459

Hydroflumethiazide (Potential for thrombocytopenia with purpura in elderly). Products include:
Diucardin Tablets 2824

Leucovorin Calcium (Co-administration for the acute treatment of *Pneumocystis carinii* pneumonia in patients with HIV infection is associated with increased rates of treatment failure and morbidity). Products include:
Leucovorin Calcium for Injection, Wellcovorin Brand 1203
Leucovorin Calcium for Injection 1313
Leucovorin Calcium Tablets, Wellcovorin Brand 1204
Leucovorin Calcium Tablets 1315

Methotrexate Sodium (Sulfonamides can displace methotrexate from plasma protein binding sites, thus increasing free methotrexate concentrations). Products include:
Methotrexate Sodium Tablets, Injection, for Injection and LPF Injection 1322

Methyclothiazide (Potential for thrombocytopenia with purpura in elderly). Products include:
Enduron Tablets 424

Phenytoin (Hepatic metabolism of phenytoin may be inhibited resulting in increased phenytoin half-life and decreased metabolic clearance). Products include:
Dilantin Infatabs 1967
Dilantin-125 Suspension 1969

Phenytoin Sodium (Hepatic metabolism of phenytoin may be inhibited resulting in increased phenytoin half-life and decreased metabolic clearance). Products include:
Dilantin Kapseals 1965

Polythiazide (Potential for thrombocytopenia with purpura in elderly). Products include:
Minizide Capsules 2016

Warfarin Sodium (Co-administration results in prolonged prothrombin time). Products include:
Coumadin 941

SEPTRA GRAPE SUSPENSION
(Trimethoprim, Sulfamethoxazole) 1146
See **Septra DS Tablets**

SEPTRA I.V. INFUSION
(Trimethoprim, Sulfamethoxazole) 1142
May interact with thiazides and certain other agents. Compounds in these categories include:

Bendroflumethiazide (Potential for thrombocytopenia with purpura in elderly).
No products indexed under this heading.

Chlorothiazide (Potential for thrombocytopenia with purpura in elderly patients). Products include:
Aldoclor Tablets 1638
Diupres Tablets 1691
Diuril Oral 1694

Chlorothiazide Sodium (Potential for thrombocytopenia with purpura in elderly). Products include:
Diuril Sodium Intravenous 1693

Fosphenytoin Sodium (Hepatic metabolism of phenytoin may be inhibited resulting in increased phenytoin half-life and decreased metabolic clearance). Products include:
Cerebyx Injection 1956

Hydrochlorothiazide (Potential for thrombocytopenia with purpura in elderly). Products include:
Aldactazide Tablets 2556
Aldoril Tablets 1644
Apresazide Capsules 824
Capozide Tablets 744
Dyazide Capsules 2653
Esidrix Tablets 839
Esimil Tablets 840
HydroDIURIL Tablets 1716
Hydropres Tablets 1718
Hyzaar Tablets 1720
Inderide Tablets 2838
Inderide LA Long Acting Capsules .. 2840
Lopressor HCT Tablets 850
Lotensin HCT Tablets 855
Moduretic Tablets 1748
Oretic Tablets 450
Prinzide Tablets 1780
Ser-Ap-Es Tablets 867
Timolide Tablets 1791
Vaseretic Tablets 1810
Zestoretic Tablets 2968
Ziac 1459

Hydroflumethiazide (Potential for thrombocytopenia with purpura in elderly). Products include:
Diucardin Tablets 2824

Leucovorin Calcium (Co-administration for the acute treatment of *Pneumocystis carinii* pneumonia in patients with HIV infection is associated with increased rates of treatment failure and morbidity). Products include:
Leucovorin Calcium for Injection, Wellcovorin Brand 1203
Leucovorin Calcium for Injection 1313
Leucovorin Calcium Tablets, Wellcovorin Brand 1204
Leucovorin Calcium Tablets 1315

Methotrexate Sodium (Sulfonamides can displace methotrexate from plasma protein binding sites, thus increasing free methotrexate concentrations). Products include:
Methotrexate Sodium Tablets, Injection, for Injection and LPF Injection 1322

Methyclothiazide (Potential for thrombocytopenia with purpura in elderly). Products include:
Enduron Tablets 424

Phenytoin (Hepatic metabolism of phenytoin may be inhibited resulting in increased phenytoin half-life and decreased metabolic clearance). Products include:
Dilantin Infatabs 1967
Dilantin-125 Suspension 1969

Phenytoin Sodium (Hepatic metabolism of phenytoin may be inhibited resulting in increased phenytoin half-life and decreased metabolic clearance). Products include:
Dilantin Kapseals 1965

Polythiazide (Potential for thrombocytopenia with purpura in elderly). Products include:
Minizide Capsules 2016

Warfarin Sodium (Co-administration results in prolonged prothrombin time). Products include:
Coumadin 941

SEPTRA I.V. INFUSION ADD-VANTAGE VIALS
(Trimethoprim, Sulfamethoxazole) 1144
May interact with thiazides and certain other agents. Compounds in these categories include:

Bendroflumethiazide (Potential for thrombocytopenia with purpura in elderly).
No products indexed under this heading.

Chlorothiazide (Potential for thrombocytopenia with purpura in elderly). Products include:
Aldoclor Tablets 1638
Diupres Tablets 1691
Diuril Oral 1694

Chlorothiazide Sodium (Potential for thrombocytopenia with purpura in elderly). Products include:
Diuril Sodium Intravenous 1693

Fosphenytoin Sodium (Decreased hepatic metabolism of phenytoin). Products include:
Cerebyx Injection 1956

Hydrochlorothiazide (Potential for thrombocytopenia with purpura in elderly). Products include:
Aldactazide Tablets 2556
Aldoril Tablets 1644
Apresazide Capsules 824
Capozide Tablets 744
Dyazide Capsules 2653
Esidrix Tablets 839
Esimil Tablets 840
HydroDIURIL Tablets 1716
Hydropres Tablets 1718
Hyzaar Tablets 1720
Inderide Tablets 2838
Inderide LA Long Acting Capsules .. 2840
Lopressor HCT Tablets 850
Lotensin HCT Tablets 855
Moduretic Tablets 1748
Oretic Tablets 450
Prinzide Tablets 1780
Ser-Ap-Es Tablets 867
Timolide Tablets 1791
Vaseretic Tablets 1810
Zestoretic Tablets 2968
Ziac 1459

Hydroflumethiazide (Potential for thrombocytopenia with purpura in elderly). Products include:
Diucardin Tablets 2824

Leucovorin Calcium (Co-administration for the acute treatment of *Pneumocystis carinii* pneumonia in patients with HIV infection is associated with increased rates of treatment failure and morbidity). Products include:
Leucovorin Calcium for Injection, Wellcovorin Brand 1203
Leucovorin Calcium for Injection 1313
Leucovorin Calcium Tablets, Wellcovorin Brand 1204
Leucovorin Calcium Tablets 1315

Methotrexate Sodium (Sulfonamides can displace methotrexate from plasma protein binding sites, thus increasing free methotrexate concentrations). Products include:
Methotrexate Sodium Tablets, Injection, for Injection and LPF Injection 1322

Phenytoin Sodium (Hepatic metabolism of phenytoin may be inhibited resulting in increased phenytoin half-life and decreased metabolic clearance). Products include:
Dilantin Kapseals 1965

Polythiazide (Potential for thrombocytopenia with purpura in elderly). Products include:
Minizide Capsules 2016

Warfarin Sodium (Co-administration results in prolonged prothrombin time). Products include:
Coumadin 941

SEPTRA SUSPENSION
(Trimethoprim, Sulfamethoxazole) 1146
See **Septra DS Tablets**

SEPTRA TABLETS
(Trimethoprim, Sulfamethoxazole) 1146
See **Septra DS Tablets**

SER-AP-ES TABLETS
(Hydralazine Hydrochloride, Hydrochlorothiazide, Reserpine) 867
May interact with oral hypoglycemic agents, insulin, corticosteroids, lithium preparations, direct-acting sympathomimetic amines, indirect-acting sympathomimetic amines, antihypertensives, barbiturates, narcotic analgesics, tricyclic antidepressants, cardiac glycosides, monoamine oxidase inhibitors, non-steroidal anti-inflammatory agents, quinidine, and certain other agents. Compounds in these categories include:

Acarbose (Hyperglycemia may occur with thiazide diuretics; dosage adjustment of the oral antidiabetic drug may be required). Products include:
Precose 604

Acebutolol Hydrochloride (Co-administration may result in additive or potentiating action). Products include:
Sectral Capsules 2914

ACTH (Intensified electrolyte depletion, particularly hypokalemia).
No products indexed under this heading.

Alfentanil Hydrochloride (Thiazide-induced orthostatic hypotension may be potentiated). Products include:
Alfenta Injection 1334

Amitriptyline Hydrochloride (Concurrent use may decrease the antihypertensive effect of reserpine). Products include:
Elavil 2945
Etrafon 2495
Limbitrol 2333
Triavil Tablets 1800

Amlodipine Besylate (Co-administration may result in additive or potentiating action). Products include:
Lotrel Capsules 858
Norvasc Tablets 2020

Amoxapine (Concurrent use may decrease the antihypertensive effect of reserpine). Products include:
Asendin Tablets 1419

Amphetamine Resins (The actions of indirect-acting sympathomimetic amines may be inhibited with concurrent use of reserpine).
No products indexed under this heading.

IMPORTANT NOTE: Always consult each drug listing in the patient's regimen for possible interactions.

Ser-Ap-Es | Interactions Index | 978

Aprobarbital (Thiazide-induced orthostatic hypotension may be potentiated).
No products indexed under this heading.

Atenolol (Co-administration may result in additive or potentiating action). Products include:
Tenoretic Tablets 2963
Tenormin Tablets and I.V. Injection 2965

Benazepril Hydrochloride (Co-administration may result in additive or potentiating action). Products include:
Lotensin Tablets 852
Lotensin HCT Tablets 855
Lotrel Capsules 858

Bendroflumethiazide (Co-administration may result in additive or potentiating action).
No products indexed under this heading.

Betamethasone Acetate (Intensified electrolyte depletion, particularly hypokalemia). Products include:
Celestone Soluspan Suspension 2484

Betamethasone Sodium Phosphate (Intensified electrolyte depletion, particularly hypokalemia). Products include:
Celestone Soluspan Suspension 2484

Betaxolol Hydrochloride (Co-administration may result in additive or potentiating action). Products include:
Betoptic Ophthalmic Solution 465
Betoptic S Ophthalmic Suspension 467
Kerlone Tablets 2588

Bisoprolol Fumarate (Co-administration may result in additive or potentiating action). Products include:
Zebeta Tablets 1457
Ziac 1459

Buprenorphine (Thiazide-induced orthostatic hypotension may be potentiated). Products include:
Buprenex Injectable 2170

Butabarbital (Thiazide-induced orthostatic hypotension may be potentiated).
No products indexed under this heading.

Butalbital (Thiazide-induced orthostatic hypotension may be potentiated). Products include:
Axocet Capsules 2469
Esgic-plus Capsules 1012
Esgic-plus Tablets 1012
Fioricet Tablets 2386
Fioricet with Codeine Capsules 2387
Fiorinal Capsules 2388
Fiorinal with Codeine Capsules 2390
Fiorinal Tablets 2388
Phrenilin 790
Sedapap Tablets 50 mg/650 mg 1826

Captopril (Co-administration may result in additive or potentiating action). Products include:
Capoten Tablets 740
Capozide Tablets 744

Carteolol Hydrochloride (Co-administration may result in additive or potentiating action). Products include:
Cartrol Tablets 413
Ocupress Ophthalmic Solution, 1% Sterile ⊚ 297

Chlorothiazide (Co-administration may result in additive or potentiating action). Products include:
Aldoclor Tablets 1638
Diupres Tablets 1691
Diuril Oral 1694

Chlorothiazide Sodium (Co-administration may result in additive or potentiating action). Products include:
Diuril Sodium Intravenous 1693

Chlorpropamide (Hyperglycemia may occur with thiazide diuretics; dosage adjustment of the oral antidiabetic drug may be required). Products include:
Diabinese Tablets 2002

Chlorthalidone (Co-administration may result in additive or potentiating action). Products include:
Combipres Tablets 682
Tenoretic Tablets 2963
Thalitone 1293

Cholestyramine (Anionic exchange resins impair the oral absorption of hydrochlorothiazide from gastrointestinal tract). Products include:
Questran 774

Clomipramine Hydrochloride (Concurrent use may decrease the antihypertensive effect of reserpine). Products include:
Anafranil Capsules 819

Clonidine (Co-administration may result in additive or potentiating action). Products include:
Catapres-TTS 680

Clonidine Hydrochloride (Co-administration may result in additive or potentiating action). Products include:
Catapres Tablets 679
Combipres Tablets 682

Codeine Phosphate (Thiazide-induced orthostatic hypotension may be potentiated). Products include:
Brontex 2130
Dimetane-DC Cough Syrup 2232
Fioricet with Codeine Capsules 2387
Fiorinal with Codeine Capsules 2390
Nucofed 2225
Phenergan with Codeine 2883
Phenergan VC with Codeine 2888
Robitussin A-C Syrup 2248
Robitussin-DAC Syrup 2249
Ryna ▣ 804
Soma Compound w/Codeine Tablets 2784
Tylenol with Codeine 1592

Colestipol Hydrochloride (Anionic exchange resins impair the oral absorption of hydrochlorothiazide from gastrointestinal tract). Products include:
Colestid 2073

Cortisone Acetate (Intensified electrolyte depletion, particularly hypokalemia). Products include:
Cortone Acetate Sterile Suspension 1663
Cortone Acetate Tablets 1664

Deserpidine (Co-administration may result in additive or potentiating action).
No products indexed under this heading.

Desipramine Hydrochloride (Concurrent use may decrease the antihypertensive effect of reserpine). Products include:
Norpramin Tablets 1273

Deslanoside (Thiazide-induced hypokalemia may exaggerate or sensitize the response of heart to the toxic effect of digitalis such as ventricular irritability; cardiac arrhythmias have occurred with rauwolfia; caution is required if co-administered).
No products indexed under this heading.

Dexamethasone (Intensified electrolyte depletion, particularly hypokalemia). Products include:
AK-Trol Ointment & Suspension ⊚ 205
Decadron Elixir 1676
Decadron Tablets 1678
Decaspray Topical Aerosol 1689
Maxitrol Ophthalmic Ointment and Suspension ⊚ 222
TobraDex Ophthalmic Suspension and Ointment 469

Dexamethasone Acetate (Intensified electrolyte depletion, particularly hypokalemia). Products include:
Dalalone D.P. Injectable 1009
Decadron-LA Sterile Suspension 1687

Dexamethasone Sodium Phosphate (Intensified electrolyte depletion, particularly hypokalemia). Products include:
Decadron Phosphate Injection 1680
Decadron Phosphate Sterile Ophthalmic Ointment 1684
Decadron Phosphate Sterile Ophthalmic Solution 1685
Decadron Phosphate Topical Cream 1686
Decadron Phosphate with Xylocaine Injection, Sterile 1683
Dexacort Phosphate in Respihaler 1606
Dexacort Phosphate in Turbinaire 1607
NeoDecadron Sterile Ophthalmic Ointment 1755
NeoDecadron Sterile Ophthalmic Solution 1756
NeoDecadron Topical Cream 1757

Dextroamphetamine Sulfate (The actions of indirect-acting sympathomimetic amines may be inhibited with concurrent use of reserpine). Products include:
Adderall Tablets 2209
Dexedrine 2648
DextroStat-Dextroamphetamine Sulfate Tablets 2211

Dezocine (Thiazide-induced orthostatic hypotension may be potentiated). Products include:
Dalgan Injection 529

Diazoxide (Co-administration of diazoxide and hydralazine has resulted in profound hypotensive episodes). Products include:
Hyperstat I.V. Injection 2504
Proglycem 575

Diclofenac Potassium (Concurrent use of some nonsteroidal anti-inflammatory agents may reduce the diuretic, natriuretic and antihypertensive effects of thiazide diuretics). Products include:
Cataflam Tablets 833

Diclofenac Sodium (Concurrent use of some nonsteroidal anti-inflammatory agents may reduce the diuretic, natriuretic and antihypertensive effects of thiazide diuretics). Products include:
Voltaren Ophthalmic Sterile Ophthalmic Solution ⊚ 264
Cataflam/Voltaren/Voltaren-XR 833

Digitoxin (Thiazide-induced hypokalemia may exaggerate or sensitize the response of heart to the toxic effect of digitalis such as ventricular irritability; cardiac arrhythmias have occurred with rauwolfia; caution is required if co-administered). Products include:
Crystodigin Tablets 1472

Digoxin (Thiazide-induced hypokalemia may exaggerate or sensitize the response of heart to the toxic effect of digitalis such as ventricular irritability; cardiac arrhythmias have occurred with rauwolfia; caution is required if co-administered). Products include:
Lanoxicaps 1110
Lanoxin Elixir Pediatric 1113
Lanoxin Injection 1116
Lanoxin Injection Pediatric 1119
Lanoxin Tablets 1121

Diltiazem Hydrochloride (Co-administration may result in additive or potentiating action). Products include:
Cardizem CD Capsules 1251
Cardizem SR Capsules 1255
Cardizem Injectable 1253
Cardizem Tablets 1257
Dilacor XR Extended-release Capsules 2183
Tiazac Capsules 1019

Doxazosin Mesylate (Co-administration may result in additive or potentiating action). Products include:
Cardura Tablets 1993

Doxepin Hydrochloride (Concurrent use may decrease the antihypertensive effect of reserpine). Products include:
Adapin Capsules 1542
Sinequan 2028
Zonalon Cream 1042

Enalapril Maleate (Co-administration may result in additive or potentiating action). Products include:
Vaseretic Tablets 1810
Vasotec Tablets 1816

Enalaprilat (Co-administration may result in additive or potentiating action). Products include:
Vasotec I.V. 1814

Ephedrine Hydrochloride (The actions of indirect-acting sympathomimetic amines may be inhibited with concurrent use of reserpine). Products include:
Primatene Tablets ▣ 844
Quadrinal Tablets 1398

Ephedrine Sulfate (The actions of indirect-acting sympathomimetic amines may be inhibited with concurrent use of reserpine). Products include:
Marax Tablets & DF Syrup 2015

Ephedrine Tannate (The actions of indirect-acting sympathomimetic amines may be inhibited with concurrent use of reserpine). Products include:
Rynatuss 2782

Epinephrine Hydrochloride (The actions of direct-acting sympathomimetic amines may be prolonged with concurrent use of reserpine). Products include:
Ana-Kit Anaphylaxis Emergency Treatment Kit 611

Esmolol Hydrochloride (Co-administration may result in additive or potentiating action). Products include:
Brevibloc (esmolol HCl) Injection 1860

Etodolac (Concurrent use of some nonsteroidal anti-inflammatory agents may reduce the diuretic, natriuretic and antihypertensive effects of thiazide diuretics). Products include:
Lodine Capsules and Tablets 2849

Felodipine (Co-administration may result in additive or potentiating action). Products include:
Plendil Extended-Release Tablets 514

Fenoprofen Calcium (Concurrent use of some nonsteroidal anti-inflammatory agents may reduce the diuretic, natriuretic and antihypertensive effects of thiazide diuretics). Products include:
Nalfon 200 Pulvules & Nalfon Tablets 933

Fentanyl (Thiazide-induced orthostatic hypotension may be potentiated). Products include:
Duragesic Transdermal System 1336

Fentanyl Citrate (Thiazide-induced orthostatic hypotension may be potentiated). Products include:
Sublimaze Injection 463

Fludrocortisone Acetate (Intensified electrolyte depletion, particularly hypokalemia). Products include:
Florinef Acetate Tablets 506

(▣ Described in PDR For Nonprescription Drugs) (⊚ Described in PDR For Ophthalmology)

Flurbiprofen (Concurrent use of some nonsteroidal anti-inflammatory agents may reduce the diuretic, natriuretic and antihypertensive effects of thiazide diuretics).
   No products indexed under this heading.

Fosinopril Sodium (Co-administration may result in additive or potentiating action). Products include:
   Monopril Tablets 762

Furazolidone (Concurrent use of an MAO inhibitor and reserpine or hydralazine should be avoided or used with extreme caution). Products include:
   Furoxone 2221

Furosemide (Co-administration may result in additive or potentiating action). Products include:
   Lasix Injection, Oral Solution and Tablets 1267

Glimepiride (Hyperglycemia may occur with thiazide diuretics; dosage adjustment of the oral antidiabetic drug may be required). Products include:
   Amaryl Tablets 1241

Glipizide (Hyperglycemia may occur with thiazide diuretics; dosage adjustment of the oral antidiabetic drug may be required). Products include:
   Glucotrol Tablets 2011
   Glucotrol XL Extended Release Tablets 2012

Glyburide (Hyperglycemia may occur with thiazide diuretics; dosage adjustment of the oral antidiabetic drug may be required). Products include:
   DiaBeta Tablets 1265
   Glynase PresTab Tablets 2091
   Micronase Tablets 2099

Guanabenz Acetate (Co-administration may result in additive or potentiating action).
   No products indexed under this heading.

Guanethidine Monosulfate (Co-administration may result in additive or potentiating action). Products include:
   Esimil Tablets 840
   Ismelin Tablets 845

Hydrocodone Bitartrate (Thiazide-induced orthostatic hypotension may be potentiated). Products include:
   Codiclear DH Syrup 808
   Duratuss HD Elixir 2750
   Histussin D Liquid 670
   Hycodan Tablets and Syrup .. 946
   Hycomine Compound Tablets .. 948
   Hycomine 947
   Hycotuss Expectorant Syrup .. 950
   Hydrocet Capsules 787
   Lorcet 10/650 Tablets 1016
   Lortab 2751
   Tussend 1830
   Tussend Expectorant 1831
   Vicodin Tablets 1404
   Vicodin ES Tablets 1405
   Vicodin HP Tablets 1403
   Vicodin Tuss Expectorant 1406
   Zydone Capsules 967

Hydrocodone Polistirex (Thiazide-induced orthostatic hypotension may be potentiated). Products include:
   Tussionex Pennkinetic Extended-Release Suspension 1624

Hydrocortisone (Intensified electrolyte depletion, particularly hypokalemia). Products include:
   Anusol-HC Cream 2.5% 1953
   Aquanil HC Lotion 1989
   Maximum Strength Cortaid Spray 800
   CORTENEMA 2713
   Cortisporin Ointment 1074
   Cortisporin Ophthalmic Ointment Sterile 1074
   Cortisporin Ophthalmic Suspension Sterile 1075
   Cortisporin Otic Solution Sterile .. 1076
   Cortisporin Otic Suspension Sterile .. 1077
   Cortizone-5 795
   Cortizone-10 795
   Hydrocortone Tablets 1715
   Hytone 922
   Hytone Ointment 2 ½ % 923
   Massengill Medicated Soft Cloth Towelettes 2628
   Pediotic Suspension Sterile .. 1140
   Preparation H Hydrocortisone 1% Cream 843
   ProctoCream-HC 2.5% 2552
   VōSoL HC Otic Solution 2786

Hydrocortisone Acetate (Intensified electrolyte depletion, particularly hypokalemia). Products include:
   Analpram-HC Rectal Cream 1% and 2.5% 993
   Anusol HC-1 Hydrocortisone Anti-Itch Ointment 810
   Anusol-HC Suppositories 1954
   Caldecort Anti-Itch Hydrocortisone Cream 651
   Coly-Mycin S Otic w/Neomycin & Hydrocortisone 1965
   Cortaid 800
   Cortifoam 2540
   Cortisporin Cream 1073
   Epifoam 2543
   Hydrocortone Acetate Sterile Suspension 1712
   Mantadil Cream 1124
   Nupercainal Hydrocortisone 1% Cream 661
   Pramosone Cream, Lotion & Ointment 995
   ProctoFoam-HC 2552
   Terra-Cortril Ophthalmic Suspension 2033

Hydrocortisone Sodium Phosphate (Intensified electrolyte depletion, particularly hypokalemia). Products include:
   Hydrocortone Phosphate Injection, Sterile 1713

Hydrocortisone Sodium Succinate (Intensified electrolyte depletion, particularly hypokalemia).
   No products indexed under this heading.

Hydroflumethiazide (Co-administration may result in additive or potentiating action). Products include:
   Diucardin Tablets 2824

Hydromorphone Hydrochloride (Thiazide-induced orthostatic hypotension may be potentiated). Products include:
   Dilaudid Ampules 1382
   Dilaudid Cough Syrup 1383
   Dilaudid-HP Injection 1384
   Dilaudid-HP Lyophilized Powder 250 mg 1384
   Dilaudid 1382
   Dilaudid Oral Liquid 1386
   Dilaudid 1382
   Dilaudid Tablets - 8 mg 1386

Ibuprofen (Concurrent use of some nonsteroidal anti-inflammatory agents may reduce the diuretic, natriuretic and antihypertensive effects of thiazide diuretics). Products include:
   Advil Cold and Sinus Caplets and Tablets 837
   Advil Ibuprofen Tablets, Caplets and Gel Caplets 836
   Children's Motrin Ibuprofen Oral Suspension 1558
   IBU Tablets 1389
   Ibuprohm 713
   Motrin IB Caplets, Tablets, and Gelcaps 802
   Motrin Ibuprofen Suspension, Oral Drops, Chewable Tablets, Caplets 1563
   Nuprin Ibuprofen/Analgesic Tablets & Caplets 645
   Vicks DayQuil SINUS Pressure & PAIN Relief with IBUPROFEN 735

Imipramine Hydrochloride (Concurrent use may decrease the antihypertensive effect of reserpine). Products include:
   Tofranil Ampuls 873
   Tofranil Tablets 875

Imipramine Pamoate (Concurrent use may decrease the antihypertensive effect of reserpine). Products include:
   Tofranil-PM Capsules 876

Indapamide (Co-administration may result in additive or potentiating action).
   No products indexed under this heading.

Indomethacin (Concurrent use of some nonsteroidal anti-inflammatory agents may reduce the diuretic, natriuretic and antihypertensive effects of thiazide diuretics). Products include:
   Indocin 1723

Indomethacin Sodium Trihydrate (Concurrent use of some nonsteroidal anti-inflammatory agents may reduce the diuretic, natriuretic and antihypertensive effects of thiazide diuretics). Products include:
   Indocin I.V. 1727

Insulin, Human (Hyperglycemia may occur with thiazide diuretics; dosage adjustment of insulin may be required).
   No products indexed under this heading.

Insulin, Human Isophane Suspension (Hyperglycemia may occur with thiazide diuretics; dosage adjustment of insulin may be required). Products include:
   Novolin N Human Insulin 10 ml Vials 1846

Insulin, Human NPH (Hyperglycemia may occur with thiazide diuretics; dosage adjustment of insulin may be required). Products include:
   Humulin N, 100 Units 1495
   Novolin N PenFill 1.5 ml Cartridges Durable Insulin Delivery System 1849
   Novolin N Prefilled Syringe Disposable Insulin Delivery System .. 1850

Insulin, Human Regular (Hyperglycemia may occur with thiazide diuretics; dosage adjustment of insulin may be required). Products include:
   Humulin R, 100 Units 1497
   Novolin R Human Insulin 10 ml Vials 1846
   Novolin R PenFill 1.5 ml Cartridges Durable Insulin Delivery System 1849
   Novolin R Prefilled Syringe Disposable Insulin Delivery System .. 1850
   Velosulin BR Human Insulin 10 ml Vials 1847

Insulin, Human, Zinc Suspension (Hyperglycemia may occur with thiazide diuretics; dosage adjustment of insulin may be required). Products include:
   Humulin L, 100 Units 1494
   Humulin U, 100 Units 1498
   Novolin L Human Insulin 10 ml Vials 1846

Insulin Lispro, Human (Hyperglycemia may occur with thiazide diuretics; dosage adjustment of insulin may be required). Products include:
   Humalog Injection 1488

Insulin, NPH (Hyperglycemia may occur with thiazide diuretics; dosage adjustment of insulin may be required). Products include:
   NPH, 100 Units 1502

   Pork NPH, 100 Units 1506
   Purified Pork NPH Isophane Insulin 1852

Insulin, Regular (Hyperglycemia may occur with thiazide diuretics; dosage adjustment of insulin may be required). Products include:
   Regular, 100 Units 1503
   Pork Regular, 100 Units 1507
   Pork Regular (Concentrated), 500 Units 1508
   Purified Pork Regular Insulin .. 1852

Insulin, Zinc Crystals (Hyperglycemia may occur with thiazide diuretics; dosage adjustment of insulin may be required). Products include:
   NPH, 100 Units 1502

Insulin, Zinc Suspension (Hyperglycemia may occur with thiazide diuretics; dosage adjustment of insulin may be required). Products include:
   Iletin I 1501
   Lente, 100 Units 1501
   Iletin II 1504
   Pork Lente, 100 Units 1504
   Purified Pork Lente Insulin .. 1852

Isocarboxazid (Concurrent use of an MAO inhibitor and reserpine or hydralazine should be avoided or used with extreme caution).
   No products indexed under this heading.

Isoproterenol Hydrochloride (The actions of direct-acting sympathomimetic amines may be prolonged with concurrent use of reserpine). Products include:
   Isuprel Hydrochloride Solution .. 2443
   Isuprel Injection 2441
   Isuprel Mistometer 2442

Isoproterenol Sulfate (The actions of direct-acting sympathomimetic amines may be prolonged with concurrent use of reserpine). Products include:
   Norisodrine with Calcium Iodide Syrup 446

Isradipine (Co-administration may result in additive or potentiating action). Products include:
   DynaCirc Capsules 2381
   DynaCirc CR Tablets 2383

Ketoprofen (Concurrent use of some nonsteroidal anti-inflammatory agents may reduce the diuretic, natriuretic and antihypertensive effects of thiazide diuretics). Products include:
   Actron Caplets and Tablets .. 608
   Orudis Capsules 2874
   Orudis KT 842
   Oruvail Capsules 2874

Ketorolac Tromethamine (Concurrent use of some nonsteroidal anti-inflammatory agents may reduce the diuretic, natriuretic and antihypertensive effects of thiazide diuretics). Products include:
   Acular Sterile Ophthalmic Solution 470
   Toradol 2319

Labetalol Hydrochloride (Co-administration may result in additive or potentiating action). Products include:
   Normodyne Injection 2519
   Normodyne Tablets 2522
   Trandate 1158

Levorphanol Tartrate (Thiazide-induced orthostatic hypotension may be potentiated). Products include:
   Levo-Dromoran 2297

Lisinopril (Co-administration may result in additive or potentiating action). Products include:
   Prinivil Tablets 1776
   Prinzide Tablets 1780
   Zestoretic Tablets 2968
   Zestril Tablets 2972

IMPORTANT NOTE: Always consult each drug listing in the patient's regimen for possible interactions.

Ser-Ap-Es **Interactions Index** 980

Lithium Carbonate (Diuretics reduce the renal clearance of lithium and add a high risk of lithium toxicity). Products include:
- Eskalith 2658
- Lithium Carbonate Capsules & Tablets 2352
- Lithonate/Lithotabs/Lithobid 2721

Lithium Citrate (Diuretics reduce the renal clearance of lithium and add a high risk of lithium toxicity).
- No products indexed under this heading.

Losartan Potassium (Co-administration may result in additive or potentiating action). Products include:
- Cozaar Tablets 1668
- Hyzaar Tablets 1720

Maprotiline Hydrochloride (Concurrent use may decrease the antihypertensive effect of reserpine). Products include:
- Ludiomil Tablets 861

Mecamylamine Hydrochloride (Co-administration may result in additive or potentiating action). Products include:
- Inversine Tablets 1729

Meclofenamate Sodium (Concurrent use of some nonsteroidal anti-inflammatory agents may reduce the diuretic, natriuretic and antihypertensive effects of thiazide diuretics).
- No products indexed under this heading.

Mefenamic Acid (Concurrent use of some nonsteroidal anti-inflammatory agents may reduce the diuretic, natriuretic and antihypertensive effects of thiazide diuretics). Products include:
- Ponstel 1982

Meperidine Hydrochloride (Thiazide-induced orthostatic hypotension may be potentiated). Products include:
- Demerol 2438
- Mepergan Injection 2859

Mephobarbital (Thiazide-induced orthostatic hypotension may be potentiated). Products include:
- Mebaral Tablets 2452

Metaraminol Bitartrate (The actions of direct-acting sympathomimetic amines may be prolonged with concurrent use of reserpine). Products include:
- Aramine Injection 1649

Metformin Hydrochloride (Hyperglycemia may occur with thiazide diuretics; dosage adjustment of the oral antidiabetic drug may be required). Products include:
- Glucophage Tablets 754

Methadone Hydrochloride (Thiazide-induced orthostatic hypotension may be potentiated). Products include:
- Methadone Hydrochloride Oral Concentrate 2356
- Methadone Hydrochloride Oral Solution & Tablets 2357

Methyclothiazide (Co-administration may result in additive or potentiating action). Products include:
- Enduron Tablets 424

Methyldopa (Co-administration of methyldopa and hydrochlorothiazide has resulted in rare reports of hemolytic anemia; concurrent use may result in additive or potentiating action). Products include:
- Aldoclor Tablets 1638
- Aldomet Oral 1640
- Aldoril Tablets 1644

Methyldopate Hydrochloride (Co-administration of methyldopa and hydrochlorothiazide has resulted in rare report of hemolytic anemia; concurrent use may result in additive or potentiating action). Products include:
- Aldomet Ester HCl Injection 1642

Methylprednisolone Acetate (Intensified electrolyte depletion, particularly hypokalemia).
- No products indexed under this heading.

Methylprednisolone Sodium Succinate (Intensified electrolyte depletion, particularly hypokalemia).
- No products indexed under this heading.

Metolazone (Co-administration may result in additive or potentiating action). Products include:
- Mykrox Tablets 1617
- Zaroxolyn Tablets 1625

Metoprolol Succinate (Co-administration may result in additive or potentiating action). Products include:
- Toprol-XL Tablets 560

Metoprolol Tartrate (Co-administration may result in additive or potentiating action). Products include:
- Lopressor 848
- Lopressor HCT Tablets 850

Metyrosine (Co-administration may result in additive or potentiating action). Products include:
- Demser Capsules 1690

Minoxidil (Co-administration may result in additive or potentiating action).
- No products indexed under this heading.

Moexipril Hydrochloride (Co-administration may result in additive or potentiating action). Products include:
- Univasc Tablets 2553

Morphine Sulfate (Thiazide-induced orthostatic hypotension may be potentiated). Products include:
- Astramorph/PF Injection, USP (Preservative-Free) 526
- Duramorph Injection 983
- Infumorph 200 and Infumorph 500 Sterile Solutions 985
- Kadian Capsules 2948
- MS Contin Tablets 2149
- MSIR 2152
- Oramorph SR (Morphine Sulfate Sustained Release Tablets) 2359
- RMS Suppositories CII 2766
- Roxanol 2365

Nabumetone (Concurrent use of some nonsteroidal anti-inflammatory agents may reduce the diuretic, natriuretic and antihypertensive effects of thiazide diuretics). Products include:
- Relafen Tablets 2688

Nadolol (Co-administration may result in additive or potentiating action).
- No products indexed under this heading.

Naproxen (Concurrent use of some nonsteroidal anti-inflammatory agents may reduce the diuretic, natriuretic and antihypertensive effects of thiazide diuretics). Products include:
- Anaprox/Naprosyn 2277

Naproxen Sodium (Concurrent use of some nonsteroidal anti-inflammatory agents may reduce the diuretic, natriuretic and antihypertensive effects of thiazide diuretics). Products include:
- Aleve 2124
- Anaprox/Naprosyn 2277
- Naprelan Tablets 2861

Nicardipine Hydrochloride (Co-administration may result in additive or potentiating action). Products include:
- Cardene Capsules 2261
- Cardene I.V. 2815
- Cardene SR Capsules 2264

Nifedipine (Co-administration may result in additive or potentiating action). Products include:
- Adalat Capsules (10 mg and 20 mg) 580
- Adalat CC 582
- Procardia Capsules 2024
- Procardia XL Extended Release Tablets 2026

Nisoldipine (Co-administration may result in additive or potentiating action). Products include:
- Sular Tablets 2961

Nitroglycerin (Co-administration may result in additive or potentiating action). Products include:
- Deponit NTG Transdermal Delivery System 2541
- Nitro-Bid IV 1270
- Nitro-Bid Ointment 1272
- Nitro-Dur (nitroglycerin) Transdermal Infusion System 1365
- Nitrolingual Spray 2193
- Nitrostat Tablets 1981
- Transderm-Nitro Transdermal Therapeutic System 878

Norepinephrine Bitartrate (Thiazides may decrease the arterial responsiveness to norepinephrine). Products include:
- Levophed Bitartrate Injection 2445

Norepinephrine Hydrochloride (The actions of direct-acting sympathomimetic amines may be prolonged with concurrent use of reserpine).
- No products indexed under this heading.

Nortriptyline Hydrochloride (Concurrent use may decrease the antihypertensive effect of reserpine). Products include:
- Pamelor 2409

Opium Alkaloids (Thiazide-induced orthostatic hypotension may be potentiated).
- No products indexed under this heading.

Oxaprozin (Concurrent use of some nonsteroidal anti-inflammatory agents may reduce the diuretic, natriuretic and antihypertensive effects of thiazide diuretics). Products include:
- Daypro Caplets 2578

Oxycodone Hydrochloride (Thiazide-induced orthostatic hypotension may be potentiated). Products include:
- OxyContin Tablets 2163
- OxyIR Capsules 2167
- Percocet Tablets 955
- Percodan Tablets 955
- Percodan-Demi Tablets 956
- Roxicodone Tablets, Oral Solution & Intensol (Oxycodone) 2366
- Tylox Capsules 1593

Penbutolol Sulfate (Co-administration may result in additive or potentiating action). Products include:
- Levatol Tablets 2547

Pentobarbital Sodium (Thiazide-induced orthostatic hypotension may be potentiated). Products include:
- Nembutal Sodium Capsules 440
- Nembutal Sodium Solution 442
- Nembutal Sodium Suppositories 444

Phenelzine Sulfate (Concurrent use of an MAO inhibitor and reserpine or hydralazine should be avoided or used with extreme caution). Products include:
- Nardil 1977

Phenobarbital (Thiazide-induced orthostatic hypotension may be potentiated). Products include:
- Arco-Lase Plus Tablets 513
- Bellergal-S Tablets 2375
- Donnatal 2234
- Donnatal Extentabs 2234
- Donnatal Tablets 2234
- Phenobarbital Elixir and Tablets 1523
- Quadrinal Tablets 1398

Phenoxybenzamine Hydrochloride (Co-administration may result in additive or potentiating action). Products include:
- Dibenzyline Capsules 2650

Phentolamine Mesylate (Co-administration may result in additive or potentiating action). Products include:
- Regitine Vials 864

Phenylbutazone (Concurrent use of some nonsteroidal anti-inflammatory agents may reduce the diuretic, natriuretic and antihypertensive effects of thiazide diuretics).
- No products indexed under this heading.

Phenylephrine Hydrochloride (The actions of direct-acting sympathomimetic amines may be prolonged with concurrent use of reserpine). Products include:
- Atrohist Plus Tablets 1605
- Cerose DM ..... ▣ 853
- D.A. II Tablets 972
- D.A. Chewable Tablets 970
- Dura-Vent/DA Tablets 972
- Extendryl 1003
- 4-Way Fast Acting Nasal Spray (regular & mentholated) ..... ▣ 644
- Hemorid ..... ▣ 797
- Hycomine Compound Tablets 948
- Neo-Synephrine Hydrochloride 1% Carpuject 2455
- Neo-Synephrine Hydrochloride 1% Injection 2455
- Neo-Synephrine Hydrochloride (Ophthalmic) 2456
- Neo-Synephrine ..... ▣ 624
- Novahistine Elixir ..... ▣ 782
- Phenergan VC 2886
- Phenergan VC with Codeine 2888
- Preparation H ..... ▣ 842
- Tympagesic Ear Drops 2476
- Vicks Sinex Nasal Spray and Ultra Fine Mist ..... ▣ 738

Phenylephrine Tannate (The actions of direct-acting sympathomimetic amines may be prolonged with concurrent use of reserpine). Products include:
- Atrohist Pediatric Suspension 1604
- Atrohist Pediatric Suspension Dye-Free 1604
- Rynatan 2781
- Rynatuss 2782

Pindolol (Co-administration may result in additive or potentiating action). Products include:
- Visken Tablets 2428

Piroxicam (Concurrent use of some nonsteroidal anti-inflammatory agents may reduce the diuretic, natriuretic and antihypertensive effects of thiazide diuretics). Products include:
- Feldene Capsules 2008

Polythiazide (Co-administration may result in additive or potentiating action). Products include:
- Minizide Capsules 2016

Prazosin Hydrochloride (Co-administration may result in additive or potentiating action). Products include:
- Minipress Capsules 2015
- Minizide Capsules 2016

Prednisolone Acetate (Intensified electrolyte depletion, particularly hypokalemia). Products include:
- AK-CIDE ..... ◉ 203
- AK-CIDE Ointment ..... ◉ 203

(▣ Described in PDR For Nonprescription Drugs) (◉ Described in PDR For Ophthalmology)

Blephamide Liquifilm Sterile Ophthalmic Suspension ... 472
Blephamide Ointment ... ⊚ 234
Econopred & Econopred Plus Ophthalmic Suspensions ... ⊚ 216
Poly-Pred Liquifilm ... ⊚ 246
Pred Forte ... ⊚ 247
Pred Mild ... ⊚ 250
Pred-G Liquifilm Sterile Ophthalmic Suspension ... ⊚ 248
Pred-G S.O.P. Sterile Ophthalmic Ointment ... ⊚ 249

Prednisolone Sodium Phosphate (Intensified electrolyte depletion, particularly hypokalemia). Products include:
AK-PRED ... ⊚ 204
Hydeltrasol Injection, Sterile ... 1708
Pediapred Oral Solution ... 1618

Prednisolone Tebutate (Intensified electrolyte depletion, particularly hypokalemia). Products include:
Hydeltra-T.B.A. Sterile Suspension ... 1710

Prednisone (Intensified electrolyte depletion, particularly hypokalemia).
No products indexed under this heading.

Propoxyphene Hydrochloride (Thiazide-induced orthostatic hypotension may be potentiated). Products include:
Darvon ... 1475
Wygesic Tablets ... 2930

Propoxyphene Napsylate (Thiazide-induced orthostatic hypotension may be potentiated). Products include:
Darvon-N/Darvocet-N ... 1473

Propranolol Hydrochloride (Co-administration may result in additive or potentiating action). Products include:
Inderal ... 2834
Inderal LA Long Acting Capsules ... 2836
Inderide Tablets ... 2838
Inderide LA Long Acting Capsules .. 2840

Protriptyline Hydrochloride (Concurrent use may decrease the antihypertensive effect of reserpine). Products include:
Vivactil Tablets ... 1820

Quinapril Hydrochloride (Co-administration may result in additive or potentiating action). Products include:
Accupril Tablets ... 1950

Quinidine Gluconate (Cardiac arrhythmias have occurred with rauwolfia; caution is required if co-administered). Products include:
Quinaglute Dura-Tabs Tablets ... 644

Quinidine Polygalacturonate (Cardiac arrhythmias have occurred with rauwolfia; caution is required if co-administered). Products include:
Cardioquin Tablets ... 2146

Quinidine Sulfate (Cardiac arrhythmias have occurred with rauwolfia; caution is required if co-administered). Products include:
Quinidex Extentabs ... 2240

Ramipril (Co-administration may result in additive or potentiating action). Products include:
Altace Capsules ... 1238

Rauwolfia Serpentina (Co-administration may result in additive or potentiating action).
No products indexed under this heading.

Rescinnamine (Co-administration may result in additive or potentiating action).
No products indexed under this heading.

Secobarbital Sodium (Thiazide-induced orthostatic hypotension may be potentiated). Products include:
Seconal Sodium Pulvules ... 1529

Selegiline Hydrochloride (Concurrent use of an MAO inhibitor and reserpine or hydralazine should be avoided or used with extreme caution). Products include:
Eldepryl Capsules ... 2729

Sodium Nitroprusside (Co-administration may result in additive or potentiating action).
No products indexed under this heading.

Sotalol Hydrochloride (Co-administration may result in additive or potentiating action). Products include:
Betapace Tablets ... 637

Spirapril Hydrochloride (Co-administration may result in additive or potentiating action).
No products indexed under this heading.

Sufentanil Citrate (Thiazide-induced orthostatic hypotension may be potentiated). Products include:
Sufenta Injection ... 1355

Sulindac (Concurrent use of some nonsteroidal anti-inflammatory agents may reduce the diuretic, natriuretic and antihypertensive effects of thiazide diuretics). Products include:
Clinoril Tablets ... 1658

Terazosin Hydrochloride (Co-administration may result in additive or potentiating action). Products include:
Hytrin Capsules ... 434

Thiamylal Sodium (Thiazide-induced orthostatic hypotension may be potentiated).
No products indexed under this heading.

Timolol Maleate (Co-administration may result in additive or potentiating action). Products include:
Blocadren Tablets ... 1654
Timolide Tablets ... 1791
Timoptic in Ocudose ... 1796
Timoptic Sterile Ophthalmic Solution ... 1794
Timoptic-XE ... 1798

Tolazamide (Hyperglycemia may occur with thiazide diuretics; dosage adjustment of the oral antidiabetic drug may be required).
No products indexed under this heading.

Tolbutamide (Hyperglycemia may occur with thiazide diuretics; dosage adjustment of the oral antidiabetic drug may be required).
No products indexed under this heading.

Tolmetin Sodium (Concurrent use of some nonsteroidal anti-inflammatory agents may reduce the diuretic, natriuretic and antihypertensive effects of thiazide diuretics). Products include:
Tolectin (200, 400 and 600 mg) .. 1591

Torsemide (Co-administration may result in additive or potentiating action). Products include:
Demadex Tablets and Injection ... 691

Tranylcypromine Sulfate (Concurrent use of an MAO inhibitor and reserpine or hydralazine should be avoided or used with extreme caution). Products include:
Parnate Tablets ... 2679

Triamcinolone (Intensified electrolyte depletion, particularly hypokalemia).
No products indexed under this heading.

Triamcinolone Acetonide (Intensified electrolyte depletion, particularly hypokalemia). Products include:
Azmacort Oral Inhaler ... 2175
Nasacort AQ Nasal Spray ... 2191
Nasacort Nasal Inhaler ... 2189

Triamcinolone Diacetate (Intensified electrolyte depletion, particularly hypokalemia).
No products indexed under this heading.

Triamcinolone Hexacetonide (Intensified electrolyte depletion, particularly hypokalemia).
No products indexed under this heading.

Trimethaphan Camsylate (Co-administration may result in additive or potentiating action).
No products indexed under this heading.

Trimipramine Maleate (Concurrent use may decrease the antihypertensive effect of reserpine). Products include:
Surmontil Capsules ... 2917

Tubocurarine Chloride (Thiazides may increase the responsiveness to tubocurarine).
No products indexed under this heading.

Verapamil Hydrochloride (Co-administration may result in additive or potentiating action). Products include:
Calan SR Caplets ... 2571
Calan Tablets ... 2568
Covera-HS Tablets ... 2573
Isoptin Injectable ... 1391
Isoptin Oral Tablets ... 1393
Isoptin SR Tablets ... 1395
Verelan Capsules ... 1455

Food Interactions

Alcohol (Thiazide-induced orthostatic hypotension may be potentiated).

Food, unspecified (Gastrointestinal absorption of hydrochlorothiazide is enhanced when administered with food).

SERAX CAPSULES
(Oxazepam) ... 2916
May interact with central nervous system depressants and certain other agents. Compounds in these categories include:

Alfentanil Hydrochloride (Effects may be additive). Products include:
Alfenta Injection ... 1334

Alprazolam (Effects may be additive). Products include:
Xanax Tablets ... 2115

Aprobarbital (Effects may be additive).
No products indexed under this heading.

Buprenorphine (Effects may be additive). Products include:
Buprenex Injectable ... 2170

Buspirone Hydrochloride (Effects may be additive). Products include:
BuSpar Tablets ... 738

Butabarbital (Effects may be additive).
No products indexed under this heading.

Butalbital (Effects may be additive). Products include:
Axocet Capsules ... 2469
Esgic-plus Capsules ... 1012
Esgic-plus Tablets ... 1012
Fioricet Tablets ... 2386
Fioricet with Codeine Capsules ... 2387
Fiorinal Capsules ... 2388
Fiorinal with Codeine Capsules ... 2390
Fiorinal Tablets ... 2388
Phrenilin ... 790
Sedapap Tablets 50 mg/650 mg .. 1826

Chlordiazepoxide (Effects may be additive). Products include:
Limbitrol ... 2333

Chlordiazepoxide Hydrochloride (Effects may be additive). Products include:
Librax Capsules ... 2330
Librium Capsules ... 2331
Librium Injectable ... 2332

Chlorpromazine (Effects may be additive). Products include:
Thorazine Suppositories ... 2701

Chlorprothixene (Effects may be additive).
No products indexed under this heading.

Chlorprothixene Hydrochloride (Effects may be additive).
No products indexed under this heading.

Chlorprothixene Lactate (Effects may be additive).
No products indexed under this heading.

Clorazepate Dipotassium (Effects may be additive). Products include:
Tranxene ... 459

Clozapine (Effects may be additive). Products include:
Clozaril Tablets ... 2377

Codeine Phosphate (Effects may be additive). Products include:
Brontex ... 2130
Dimetane-DC Cough Syrup ... 2232
Fioricet with Codeine Capsules ... 2387
Fiorinal with Codeine Capsules ... 2390
Nucofed ... 2225
Phenergan with Codeine ... 2883
Phenergan VC with Codeine ... 2888
Robitussin A-C Syrup ... 2248
Robitussin-DAC Syrup ... 2249
Ryna ... ⊡ 804
Soma Compound w/Codeine Tablets ... 2784
Tylenol with Codeine ... 1592

Desflurane (Effects may be additive). Products include:
Suprane (desflurane, USP) ... 1865

Dezocine (Effects may be additive). Products include:
Dalgan Injection ... 529

Diazepam (Effects may be additive). Products include:
Dizac (diazepam injectable emulsion) CIV ... 1862
Valium Injectable ... 2336
Valium Tablets ... 2335

Droperidol (Effects may be additive). Products include:
Inapsine Injection ... 462

Enflurane (Effects may be additive).
No products indexed under this heading.

Estazolam (Effects may be additive). Products include:
ProSom Tablets ... 457

Ethchlorvynol (Effects may be additive). Products include:
Placidyl Capsules ... 456

Ethinamate (Effects may be additive).
No products indexed under this heading.

Fentanyl (Effects may be additive). Products include:
Duragesic Transdermal System ... 1336

Fentanyl Citrate (Effects may be additive). Products include:
Sublimaze Injection ... 463

Fluphenazine Decanoate (Effects may be additive). Products include:
Prolixin Decanoate ... 510

IMPORTANT NOTE: Always consult each drug listing in the patient's regimen for possible interactions.

Serax Interactions Index 982

Fluphenazine Enanthate (Effects may be additive). Products include:
Prolixin Enanthate 510
Fluphenazine Hydrochloride (Effects may be additive). Products include:
Prolixin 510
Flurazepam Hydrochloride (Effects may be additive). Products include:
Dalmane Capsules 2329
Glutethimide (Effects may be additive).
No products indexed under this heading.
Haloperidol (Effects may be additive). Products include:
Haldol Injection, Tablets and Concentrate 1585
Haloperidol Decanoate (Effects may be additive). Products include:
Haldol Decanoate 1587
Hydrocodone Bitartrate (Effects may be additive). Products include:
Codiclear DH Syrup 808
Duratuss HD Elixir 2750
Histussin D Liquid 670
Hycodan Tablets and Syrup 946
Hycomine Compound Tablets 948
Hycomine 947
Hycotuss Expectorant Syrup 950
Hydrocet Capsules 787
Lorcet 10/650 Tablets 1016
Lortab 2751
Tussend 1830
Tussend Expectorant 1831
Vicodin Tablets 1404
Vicodin ES Tablets 1405
Vicodin HP Tablets 1403
Vicodin Tuss Expectorant 1406
Zydone Capsules 967
Hydrocodone Polistirex (Effects may be additive). Products include:
Tussionex Pennkinetic Extended-Release Suspension 1624
Hydroxyzine Hydrochloride (Effects may be additive). Products include:
Atarax Tablets & Syrup 1992
Marax Tablets & DF Syrup 2015
Vistaril Intramuscular Solution 2042
Isoflurane (Effects may be additive).
No products indexed under this heading.
Ketamine Hydrochloride (Effects may be additive).
No products indexed under this heading.
Levomethadyl Acetate Hydrochloride (Effects may be additive). Products include:
Orlaam Oral Solution 2361
Levorphanol Tartrate (Effects may be additive). Products include:
Levo-Dromoran 2297
Lorazepam (Effects may be additive). Products include:
Ativan Injection 2805
Ativan Tablets 2807
Loxapine Hydrochloride (Effects may be additive). Products include:
Loxitane 1426
Loxapine Succinate (Effects may be additive). Products include:
Loxitane Capsules 1426
Meperidine Hydrochloride (Effects may be additive). Products include:
Demerol 2438
Mepergan Injection 2859
Mephobarbital (Effects may be additive). Products include:
Mebaral Tablets 2452
Meprobamate (Effects may be additive). Products include:
Miltown Tablets 2780
PMB 200 and PMB 400 2890
Mesoridazine Besylate (Effects may be additive). Products include:
Serentil 689
Methadone Hydrochloride (Effects may be additive). Products include:
Methadone Hydrochloride Oral Concentrate 2356
Methadone Hydrochloride Oral Solution & Tablets 2357
Methohexital Sodium (Effects may be additive).
No products indexed under this heading.
Methotrimeprazine (Effects may be additive). Products include:
Levoprome 1321
Methoxyflurane (Effects may be additive).
No products indexed under this heading.
Midazolam Hydrochloride (Effects may be additive). Products include:
Versed Injection 2324
Molindone Hydrochloride (Effects may be additive). Products include:
Moban Tablets and Concentrate 1036
Morphine Sulfate (Effects may be additive). Products include:
Astramorph/PF Injection, USP (Preservative-Free) 526
Duramorph Injection 983
Infumorph 200 and Infumorph 500 Sterile Solutions 985
Kadian Capsules 2948
MS Contin Tablets 2149
MSIR 2152
Oramorph SR (Morphine Sulfate Sustained Release Tablets) 2359
RMS Suppositories CII 2766
Roxanol 2365
Opium Alkaloids (Effects may be additive).
No products indexed under this heading.
Oxycodone Hydrochloride (Effects may be additive). Products include:
OxyContin Tablets 2163
OxyIR Capsules 2167
Percocet Tablets 955
Percodan Tablets 955
Percodan-Demi Tablets 956
Roxicodone Tablets, Oral Solution & Intensol (Oxycodone) 2366
Tylox Capsules 1593
Pentobarbital Sodium (Effects may be additive). Products include:
Nembutal Sodium Capsules 440
Nembutal Sodium Solution 442
Nembutal Sodium Suppositories 444
Perphenazine (Effects may be additive). Products include:
Etrafon 2495
Triavil Tablets 1800
Trilafon 2532
Phenobarbital (Effects may be additive). Products include:
Arco-Lase Plus Tablets 513
Bellergal-S Tablets 2375
Donnatal 2234
Donnatal Extentabs 2234
Donnatal Tablets 2234
Phenobarbital Elixir and Tablets 1523
Quadrinal Tablets 1398
Prazepam (Effects may be additive).
No products indexed under this heading.
Prochlorperazine (Effects may be additive). Products include:
Compazine 2644
Promethazine Hydrochloride (Effects may be additive). Products include:
Mepergan Injection 2859
Phenergan with Codeine 2883
Phenergan with Dextromethorphan 2885
Phenergan Injection 2880
Phenergan Suppositories 2882
Phenergan Syrup 2881
Phenergan Tablets 2882
Phenergan VC 2886
Phenergan VC with Codeine 2888
Propofol (Effects may be additive). Products include:
Diprivan Injectable Emulsion 2939
Propoxyphene Hydrochloride (Effects may be additive). Products include:
Darvon 1475
Wygesic Tablets 2930
Propoxyphene Napsylate (Effects may be additive). Products include:
Darvon-N/Darvocet-N 1473
Quazepam (Effects may be additive). Products include:
Doral Tablets 2773
Risperidone (Effects may be additive). Products include:
Risperdal Tablets 1348
Secobarbital Sodium (Effects may be additive). Products include:
Seconal Sodium Pulvules 1529
Sevoflurane (Effects may be additive).
No products indexed under this heading.
Sufentanil Citrate (Effects may be additive). Products include:
Sufenta Injection 1355
Temazepam (Effects may be additive). Products include:
Restoril Capsules 2413
Thiamylal Sodium (Effects may be additive).
No products indexed under this heading.
Thioridazine Hydrochloride (Effects may be additive). Products include:
Mellaril 2398
Thiothixene (Effects may be additive). Products include:
Navane Capsules and Concentrate 2018
Navane Intramuscular 2019
Triazolam (Effects may be additive). Products include:
Halcion Tablets 2093
Trifluoperazine Hydrochloride (Effects may be additive). Products include:
Stelazine 2692
Zolpidem Tartrate (Effects may be additive). Products include:
Ambien Tablets 2559

Food Interactions
Alcohol (Effects may be additive).

SERAX TABLETS
(Oxazepam) 2916
See **Serax Capsules**

SERENTIL AMPULS
(Mesoridazine Besylate) 689
May interact with central nervous system depressants, barbiturates, general anesthetics, narcotic analgesics, and certain other agents. Compounds in these categories include:

Alfentanil Hydrochloride (Potentiation of central nervous system depressant). Products include:
Alfenta Injection 1334
Alprazolam (Potentiation of central nervous system depressant). Products include:
Xanax Tablets 2115
Aprobarbital (Potentiation of central nervous system depressant).
No products indexed under this heading.
Atropine Sulfate (Potentiation of central nervous system depressant). Products include:
Arco-Lase Plus Tablets 513
Atrohist Plus Tablets 1605
Donnatal 2234
Donnatal Extentabs 2234
Donnatal Tablets 2234
Lomotil 2591
Motofen Tablets 789
Urised Tablets 2123
Buprenorphine (Potentiation of central nervous system depressant). Products include:
Buprenex Injectable 2170
Buspirone Hydrochloride (Potentiation of central nervous system depressant). Products include:
BuSpar Tablets 738
Butabarbital (Potentiation of central nervous system depressant).
No products indexed under this heading.
Butalbital (Potentiation of central nervous system depressant). Products include:
Axocet Capsules 2469
Esgic-plus Capsules 1012
Esgic-plus Tablets 1012
Fioricet Tablets 2386
Fioricet with Codeine Capsules 2387
Fiorinal Capsules 2388
Fiorinal with Codeine Capsules 2390
Fiorinal Tablets 2388
Phrenilin 790
Sedapap Tablets 50 mg/650 mg 1826
Chlordiazepoxide (Potentiation of central nervous system depressant). Products include:
Limbitrol 2333
Chlordiazepoxide Hydrochloride (Potentiation of central nervous system depressant). Products include:
Librax Capsules 2330
Librium Capsules 2331
Librium Injectable 2332
Chlorpromazine (Potentiation of central nervous system depressant). Products include:
Thorazine Suppositories 2701
Chlorpromazine Hydrochloride (Potentiation of central nervous system depressant). Products include:
Thorazine 2701
Chlorprothixene (Potentiation of central nervous system depressant).
No products indexed under this heading.
Chlorprothixene Hydrochloride (Potentiation of central nervous system depressant).
No products indexed under this heading.
Chlorprothixene Lactate (Potentiation of central nervous system depressant).
No products indexed under this heading.
Clorazepate Dipotassium (Potentiation of central nervous system depressant). Products include:
Tranxene 459
Clozapine (Potentiation of central nervous system depressant). Products include:
Clozaril Tablets 2377
Codeine Phosphate (Potentiation of central nervous system depressant). Products include:
Brontex 2130
Dimetane-DC Cough Syrup 2232
Fioricet with Codeine Capsules 2387
Fiorinal with Codeine Capsules 2390
Nucofed 2225
Phenergan with Codeine 2883
Phenergan VC with Codeine 2888
Robitussin A-C Syrup 2248
Robitussin-DAC Syrup 2249
Ryna ▣ 804
Soma Compound w/Codeine Tablets 2784
Tylenol with Codeine 1592

(▣ Described in PDR For Nonprescription Drugs) (◉ Described in PDR For Ophthalmology)

983 **Interactions Index** **Serevent**

Desflurane (Potentiation of central nervous system depressant). Products include:
- Suprane (desflurane, USP) 1865

Dezocine (Potentiation of central nervous system depressant). Products include:
- Dalgan Injection 529

Diazepam (Potentiation of central nervous system depressant). Products include:
- Dizac (diazepam injectable emulsion) CIV 1862
- Valium Injectable 2336
- Valium Tablets 2335

Droperidol (Potentiation of central nervous system depressant). Products include:
- Inapsine Injection 462

Enflurane (Potentiation of central nervous system depressant).
- No products indexed under this heading.

Estazolam (Potentiation of central nervous system depressant). Products include:
- ProSom Tablets 457

Ethchlorvynol (Potentiation of central nervous system depressant). Products include:
- Placidyl Capsules 456

Ethinamate (Potentiation of central nervous system depressant).
- No products indexed under this heading.

Fentanyl (Potentiation of central nervous system depressant). Products include:
- Duragesic Transdermal System 1336

Fentanyl Citrate (Potentiation of central nervous system depressant). Products include:
- Sublimaze Injection 463

Fluphenazine Decanoate (Potentiation of central nervous system depressant). Products include:
- Prolixin Decanoate 510

Fluphenazine Enanthate (Potentiation of central nervous system depressant). Products include:
- Prolixin Enanthate 510

Fluphenazine Hydrochloride (Potentiation of central nervous system depressant). Products include:
- Prolixin 510

Flurazepam Hydrochloride (Potentiation of central nervous system depressant). Products include:
- Dalmane Capsules 2329

Glutethimide (Potentiation of central nervous system depressant).
- No products indexed under this heading.

Haloperidol (Potentiation of central nervous system depressant). Products include:
- Haldol Injection, Tablets and Concentrate 1585

Haloperidol Decanoate (Potentiation of central nervous system depressant). Products include:
- Haldol Decanoate 1587

Hydrocodone Bitartrate (Potentiation of central nervous system depressant). Products include:
- Codiclear DH Syrup 808
- Duratuss HD Elixir 2750
- Histussin D Liquid 670
- Hycodan Tablets and Syrup 946
- Hycomine Compound Tablets 948
- Hycomine 947
- Hycotuss Expectorant Syrup 950
- Hydrocet Capsules 787
- Lorcet 10/650 Tablets 1016
- Lortab 2751
- Tussend 1830
- Tussend Expectorant 1831
- Vicodin Tablets 1404
- Vicodin ES Tablets 1405
- Vicodin HP Tablets 1403
- Vicodin Tuss Expectorant 1406
- Zydone Capsules 967

Hydrocodone Polistirex (Potentiation of central nervous system depressant). Products include:
- Tussionex Pennkinetic Extended-Release Suspension 1624

Hydromorphone Hydrochloride (Potentiation of central nervous system depressant). Products include:
- Dilaudid Ampules 1382
- Dilaudid Cough Syrup 1383
- Dilaudid-HP Injection 1384
- Dilaudid-HP Lyophilized Powder 250 mg 1384
- Dilaudid 1382
- Dilaudid Oral Liquid 1386
- Dilaudid 1382
- Dilaudid Tablets - 8 mg 1386

Hydroxyzine Hydrochloride (Potentiation of central nervous system depressant). Products include:
- Atarax Tablets & Syrup 1992
- Marax Tablets & DF Syrup 2015
- Vistaril Intramuscular Solution 2042

Isoflurane (Potentiation of central nervous system depressant).
- No products indexed under this heading.

Ketamine Hydrochloride (Potentiation of central nervous system depressant).
- No products indexed under this heading.

Levomethadyl Acetate Hydrochloride (Potentiation of central nervous system depressant). Products include:
- Orlaam Oral Solution 2361

Levorphanol Tartrate (Potentiation of central nervous system depressant). Products include:
- Levo-Dromoran 2297

Lorazepam (Potentiation of central nervous system depressant). Products include:
- Ativan Injection 2805
- Ativan Tablets 2807

Loxapine Hydrochloride (Potentiation of central nervous system depressant). Products include:
- Loxitane 1426

Loxapine Succinate (Potentiation of central nervous system depressant). Products include:
- Loxitane Capsules 1426

Meperidine Hydrochloride (Potentiation of central nervous system depressant). Products include:
- Demerol 2438
- Mepergan Injection 2859

Mephobarbital (Potentiation of central nervous system depressant). Products include:
- Mebaral Tablets 2452

Meprobamate (Potentiation of central nervous system depressant). Products include:
- Miltown Tablets 2780
- PMB 200 and PMB 400 2890

Methadone Hydrochloride (Potentiation of central nervous system depressant). Products include:
- Methadone Hydrochloride Oral Concentrate 2356
- Methadone Hydrochloride Oral Solution & Tablets 2357

Methohexital Sodium (Potentiation of central nervous system depressant).
- No products indexed under this heading.

Methotrimeprazine (Potentiation of central nervous system depressant). Products include:
- Levoprome 1321

Methoxyflurane (Potentiation of central nervous system depressant).
- No products indexed under this heading.

Midazolam Hydrochloride (Potentiation of central nervous system depressant). Products include:
- Versed Injection 2324

Molindone Hydrochloride (Potentiation of central nervous system depressant). Products include:
- Moban Tablets and Concentrate 1036

Morphine Sulfate (Potentiation of central nervous system depressant). Products include:
- Astramorph/PF Injection, USP (Preservative-Free) 526
- Duramorph Injection 983
- Infumorph 200 and Infumorph 500 Sterile Solutions 985
- Kadian Capsules 2948
- MS Contin Tablets 2149
- MSIR 2152
- Oramorph SR (Morphine Sulfate Sustained Release Tablets) 2359
- RMS Suppositories CII 2766
- Roxanol 2365

Opium Alkaloids (Potentiation of central nervous system depressant).
- No products indexed under this heading.

Oxazepam (Potentiation of central nervous system depressant). Products include:
- Serax Capsules 2916
- Serax Tablets 2916

Oxycodone Hydrochloride (Potentiation of central nervous system depressant). Products include:
- OxyContin Tablets 2163
- OxyIR Capsules 2167
- Percocet Tablets 955
- Percodan Tablets 955
- Percodan-Demi Tablets 956
- Roxicodone Tablets, Oral Solution & Intensol (Oxycodone) 2366
- Tylox Capsules 1593

Pentobarbital Sodium (Potentiation of central nervous system depressant). Products include:
- Nembutal Sodium Capsules 440
- Nembutal Sodium Solution 442
- Nembutal Sodium Suppositories 444

Perphenazine (Potentiation of central nervous system depressant). Products include:
- Etrafon 2495
- Triavil Tablets 1800
- Trilafon 2532

Phenobarbital (Potentiation of central nervous system depressant). Products include:
- Arco-Lase Plus Tablets 513
- Bellergal-S Tablets 2375
- Donnatal 2234
- Donnatal Extentabs 2234
- Donnatal Tablets 2234
- Phenobarbital Elixir and Tablets 1523
- Quadrinal Tablets 1398

Prazepam (Potentiation of central nervous system depressant).
- No products indexed under this heading.

Prochlorperazine (Potentiation of central nervous system depressant). Products include:
- Compazine 2644

Promethazine Hydrochloride (Potentiation of central nervous system depressant). Products include:
- Mepergan Injection 2859
- Phenergan with Codeine 2883
- Phenergan with Dextromethorphan 2885
- Phenergan Injection 2880
- Phenergan Suppositories 2882
- Phenergan Syrup 2881
- Phenergan Tablets 2882
- Phenergan VC 2886
- Phenergan VC with Codeine 2888

Propofol (Potentiation of central nervous system depressant). Products include:
- Diprivan Injectable Emulsion 2939

Propoxyphene Hydrochloride (Potentiation of central nervous system depressant). Products include:
- Darvon 1475
- Wygesic Tablets 2930

Propoxyphene Napsylate (Potentiation of central nervous system depressant). Products include:
- Darvon-N/Darvocet-N 1473

Quazepam (Potentiation of central nervous system depressant). Products include:
- Doral Tablets 2773

Risperidone (Potentiation of central nervous system depressant). Products include:
- Risperdal Tablets 1348

Secobarbital Sodium (Potentiation of central nervous system depressant). Products include:
- Seconal Sodium Pulvules 1529

Sevoflurane (Potentiation of central nervous system depressant).
- No products indexed under this heading.

Sufentanil Citrate (Potentiation of central nervous system depressant). Products include:
- Sufenta Injection 1355

Temazepam (Potentiation of central nervous system depressant). Products include:
- Restoril Capsules 2413

Thiamylal Sodium (Potentiation of central nervous system depressant).
- No products indexed under this heading.

Thioridazine Hydrochloride (Potentiation of central nervous system depressant). Products include:
- Mellaril 2398

Thiothixene (Potentiation of central nervous system depressant). Products include:
- Navane Capsules and Concentrate 2018
- Navane Intramuscular 2019

Triazolam (Potentiation of central nervous system depressant). Products include:
- Halcion Tablets 2093

Trifluoperazine Hydrochloride (Potentiation of central nervous system depressant). Products include:
- Stelazine 2692

Zolpidem Tartrate (Potentiation of central nervous system depressant). Products include:
- Ambien Tablets 2559

Food Interactions

Alcohol (Potentiation of central nervous system depressant).

SERENTIL CONCENTRATE
(Mesoridazine Besylate) 689
See **Serentil Ampuls**

SERENTIL TABLETS
(Mesoridazine Besylate) 689
See **Serentil Ampuls**

SEREVENT INHALATION AEROSOL
(Salmeterol Xinafoate) 1149
May interact with monoamine oxidase inhibitors and tricyclic antide-

IMPORTANT NOTE: Always consult each drug listing in the patient's regimen for possible interactions.

Serevent / Interactions Index

pressants. Compounds in these categories include:

Amitriptyline Hydrochloride (The action of salmeterol on the vascular system may be potentiated by tricyclic antidepressant). Products include:
Elavil	2945
Etrafon	2495
Limbitrol	2333
Triavil Tablets	1800

Amoxapine (The action of salmeterol on the vascular system may be potentiated by tricyclic antidepressant). Products include:
Asendin Tablets	1419

Clomipramine Hydrochloride (The action of salmeterol on the vascular system may be potentiated by tricyclic antidepressant). Products include:
Anafranil Capsules	819

Desipramine Hydrochloride (The action of salmeterol on the vascular system may be potentiated by tricyclic antidepressant). Products include:
Norpramin Tablets	1273

Doxepin Hydrochloride (The action of salmeterol on the vascular system may be potentiated by tricyclic antidepressant). Products include:
Adapin Capsules	1542
Sinequan	2028
Zonalon Cream	1042

Furazolidone (The action of salmeterol on the vascular system may be potentiated by MAO inhibitor). Products include:
Furoxone	2221

Imipramine Hydrochloride (The action of salmeterol on the vascular system may be potentiated by tricyclic antidepressant). Products include:
Tofranil Ampuls	873
Tofranil Tablets	875

Imipramine Pamoate (The action of salmeterol on the vascular system may be potentiated by tricyclic antidepressant). Products include:
Tofranil-PM Capsules	876

Isocarboxazid (The action of salmeterol on the vascular system may be potentiated by MAO inhibitor).
No products indexed under this heading.

Maprotiline Hydrochloride (The action of salmeterol on the vascular system may be potentiated by tricyclic antidepressant). Products include:
Ludiomil Tablets	861

Nortriptyline Hydrochloride (The action of salmeterol on the vascular system may be potentiated by tricyclic antidepressant). Products include:
Pamelor	2409

Phenelzine Sulfate (The action of salmeterol on the vascular system may be potentiated by MAO inhibitor). Products include:
Nardil	1977

Protriptyline Hydrochloride (The action of salmeterol on the vascular system may be potentiated by tricyclic antidepressant). Products include:
Vivactil Tablets	1820

Selegiline Hydrochloride (The action of salmeterol on the vascular system may be potentiated by MAO inhibitor). Products include:
Eldepryl Capsules	2729

Tranylcypromine Sulfate (The action of salmeterol on the vascular system may be potentiated by MAO inhibitor). Products include:
Parnate Tablets	2679

Trimipramine Maleate (The action of salmeterol on the vascular system may be potentiated by tricyclic antidepressant). Products include:
Surmontil Capsules	2917

SEROMYCIN CAPSULES
(Cycloserine) 975
May interact with antituberculosis drugs and certain other agents. Compounds in these categories include:

Aminosalicylic Acid (Co-administration has been associated with a few instances of vitamin B_{12} and/or folic acid deficiency, megaloblastic anemia, and sideroblastic anemia). Products include:
PASER Granules	1333

p-Aminosalicylic Acid (Co-administration has been associated with a few instances of vitamin B_{12} and/or folic acid deficiency, megaloblastic anemia, and sideroblastic anemia).
No products indexed under this heading.

Ethambutol Hydrochloride (Co-administration has been associated with a few instances of vitamin B_{12} and/or folic acid deficiency, megaloblastic anemia, and sideroblastic anemia). Products include:
Myambutol Tablets	1432

Ethionamide (Co-administration has been reported to potentiate neurotoxic side effects). Products include:
Trecator-SC Tablets	2919

Isoniazid (Co-administration may result in increased incidence of CNS effects, such as dizziness or drowsiness). Products include:
Nydrazid Injection	509
Rifamate Capsules	1278
Rifater	1280

Pyrazinamide (Co-administration has been associated with a few instances of vitamin B_{12} and/or folic acid deficiency, megaloblastic anemia, and sideroblastic anemia). Products include:
Pyrazinamide Tablets	1442
Rifater	1280

Rifampin (Co-administration has been associated with a few instances of vitamin B_{12} and/or folic acid deficiency, megaloblastic anemia, and sideroblastic anemia). Products include:
Rifadin	1276
Rifamate Capsules	1278
Rifater	1280
Rimactane Capsules	865

Food Interactions
Alcohol (Concurrent use increases the possibility and risk of epileptic episodes).

SEROPHENE (CLOMIPHENE CITRATE TABLETS, USP)
(Clomiphene Citrate) 2621
None cited in PDR database.

SERZONE TABLETS
(Nefazodone Hydrochloride) 776
May interact with monoamine oxidase inhibitors, triazolobenzodiazepines, highly protein bound drugs (selected), and certain other agents. Compounds in these categories include:

Alprazolam (Co-administration may increase steady-state peak concentrations, AUC and half-life values; potentiated effects on psychomotor performance tests; reduction in initial dosage of triazolobenzodiazepines is required). Products include:
Xanax Tablets	2115

Amiodarone Hydrochloride (Nefazodone is highly bound to the plasma protein hence co-administration with another drug that is highly protein bound may cause increased free concentrations of other drug, potentially resulting in adverse events). Products include:
Cordarone Intravenous	2821
Cordarone Tablets	2818

Amitriptyline Hydrochloride (Nefazodone is highly bound to the plasma protein hence co-administration with another drug that is highly protein bound may cause increased free concentrations of other drug, potentially resulting in adverse events). Products include:
Elavil	2945
Etrafon	2495
Limbitrol	2333
Triavil Tablets	1800

Astemizole (Nefazodone has been shown in vitro to be inhibitor of cytochrome $P_{450}IIIA_4$ resulting in the potential for increased plasma concentration of astemizole leading to QT prolongation and rare cases of serious cardiovascular toxicity; concurrent use is contraindicated). Products include:
Hismanal Tablets	1341

Atovaquone (Nefazodone is highly bound to the plasma protein hence co-administration with another drug that is highly protein bound may cause increased free concentrations of other drug, potentially resulting in adverse events). Products include:
Mepron Suspension	1206

Cefonicid Sodium (Nefazodone is highly bound to the plasma protein hence co-administration with another drug that is highly protein bound may cause increased free concentrations of other drug, potentially resulting in adverse events). Products include:
Monocid Injection	2674

Chlordiazepoxide (Nefazodone is highly bound to the plasma protein hence co-administration with another drug that is highly protein bound may cause increased free concentrations of other drug, potentially resulting in adverse events). Products include:
Limbitrol	2333

Chlordiazepoxide Hydrochloride (Nefazodone is highly bound to the plasma protein hence co-administration with another drug that is highly protein bound may cause increased free concentrations of other drug, potentially resulting in adverse events). Products include:
Librax Capsules	2330
Librium Capsules	2331
Librium Injectable	2332

Chlorpromazine (Nefazodone is highly bound to the plasma protein hence co-administration with another drug that is highly protein bound may cause increased free concentrations of other drug, potentially resulting in adverse events). Products include:
Thorazine Suppositories	2701

Chlorpromazine Hydrochloride (Nefazodone is highly bound to the plasma protein hence co-administration with another drug that is highly protein bound may cause increased free concentrations of other drug, potentially resulting in adverse events). Products include:
Thorazine	2701

Cisapride (Nefazodone has been shown in vitro to be inhibitor of cytochrome $P_{450}IIIA_4$ resulting in the potential for increased plasma concentration of cisapride leading to QT prolongation and rare cases of serious cardiovascular toxicity; concurrent use is contraindicated). Products include:
Propulsid	1346

Clomipramine Hydrochloride (Nefazodone is highly bound to the plasma protein hence co-administration with another drug that is highly protein bound may cause increased free concentrations of other drug, potentially resulting in adverse events). Products include:
Anafranil Capsules	819

Clozapine (Nefazodone is highly bound to the plasma protein hence co-administration with another drug that is highly protein bound may cause increased free concentrations of other drug, potentially resulting in adverse events). Products include:
Clozaril Tablets	2377

Cyclosporine (Nefazodone is highly bound to the plasma protein hence co-administration with another drug that is highly protein bound may cause increased free concentrations of other drug, potentially resulting in adverse events). Products include:
Neoral	2405
Sandimmune	2416

Diazepam (Nefazodone is highly bound to the plasma protein hence co-administration with another drug that is highly protein bound may cause increased free concentrations of other drug, potentially resulting in adverse events). Products include:
Dizac (diazepam injectable emulsion) CIV	1862
Valium Injectable	2336
Valium Tablets	2335

Diclofenac Potassium (Nefazodone is highly bound to the plasma protein hence co-administration with another drug that is highly protein bound may cause increased free concentrations of other drug, potentially resulting in adverse events). Products include:
Cataflam Tablets	833

Diclofenac Sodium (Nefazodone is highly bound to the plasma protein hence co-administration with another drug that is highly protein bound may cause increased free concentrations of other drug, potentially resulting in adverse events). Products include:
Voltaren Ophthalmic Sterile Ophthalmic Solution	⊚ 264
Cataflam/Voltaren/Voltaren-XR	833

Digoxin (Potential for increased digoxin C_{max}, C_{min}, and AUC by 29%, 27%, and 15% respectively; caution should be exercised if used concurrently). Products include:
Lanoxicaps	1110
Lanoxin Elixir Pediatric	1113
Lanoxin Injection	1116
Lanoxin Injection Pediatric	1119
Lanoxin Tablets	1121

(■ Described in PDR For Nonprescription Drugs)   (⊚ Described in PDR For Ophthalmology)

Dipyridamole (Nefazodone is highly bound to the plasma protein hence co-administration with another drug that is highly protein bound may cause increased free concentrations of other drug, potentially resulting in adverse events). Products include:
   Persantine Tablets 686

Fenoprofen Calcium (Nefazodone is highly bound to the plasma protein hence co-administration with another drug that is highly protein bound may cause increased free concentrations of other drug, potentially resulting in adverse events). Products include:
   Nalfon 200 Pulvules & Nalfon Tablets 933

Flurazepam Hydrochloride (Nefazodone is highly bound to the plasma protein hence co-administration with another drug that is highly protein bound may cause increased free concentrations of other drug, potentially resulting in adverse events). Products include:
   Dalmane Capsules 2329

Flurbiprofen (Nefazodone is highly bound to the plasma protein hence co-administration with another drug that is highly protein bound may cause increased free concentrations of other drug, potentially resulting in adverse events).
   No products indexed under this heading.

Furazolidone (Potential for serious, sometimes fatal, reactions including hyperthermia, rigidity, myoclonus, extreme agitation progressing to delirium and coma; concurrent and/or sequential use is contraindicated). Products include:
   Furoxone 2221

Glipizide (Nefazodone is highly bound to the plasma protein hence co-administration with another drug that is highly protein bound may cause increased free concentrations of other drug, potentially resulting in adverse events). Products include:
   Glucotrol Tablets 2011
   Glucotrol XL Extended Release Tablets 2012

Haloperidol (Decreased haloperidol apparent clearance by 35% with no significant increase in peak plasma levels or time to peak; dosage adjustment may be required). Products include:
   Haldol Injection, Tablets and Concentrate 1585

Haloperidol Decanoate (Decreased haloperidol apparent clearance by 35% with no significant increase in peak plasma levels or time to peak; dosage adjustment may be required). Products include:
   Haldol Decanoate 1587

Ibuprofen (Nefazodone is highly bound to the plasma protein hence co-administration with another drug that is highly protein bound may cause increased free concentrations of other drug, potentially resulting in adverse events). Products include:
   Advil Cold and Sinus Caplets and Tablets 837
   Advil Ibuprofen Caplets, Caplets and Gel Caplets 836
   Children's Motrin Ibuprofen Oral Suspension 1558
   IBU Tablets 1389
   Ibuprohm 713
   Motrin IB Caplets, Tablets, and Gelcaps 802
   Motrin Ibuprofen Suspension, Oral Drops, Chewable Tablets, Caplets 1563
   Nuprin Ibuprofen/Analgesic Tablets & Caplets 645
   Vicks DayQuil SINUS Pressure & PAIN Relief with IBUPROFEN 735

Imipramine Hydrochloride (Nefazodone is highly bound to the plasma protein hence co-administration with another drug that is highly protein bound may cause increased free concentrations of other drug, potentially resulting in adverse events). Products include:
   Tofranil Ampuls 873
   Tofranil Tablets 875

Imipramine Pamoate (Nefazodone is highly bound to the plasma protein hence co-administration with another drug that is highly protein bound may cause increased free concentrations of other drug, potentially resulting in adverse events). Products include:
   Tofranil-PM Capsules 876

Indomethacin (Nefazodone is highly bound to the plasma protein hence co-administration with another drug that is highly protein bound may cause increased free concentrations of other drug, potentially resulting in adverse events). Products include:
   Indocin 1723

Indomethacin Sodium Trihydrate (Nefazodone is highly bound to the plasma protein hence co-administration with another drug that is highly protein bound may cause increased free concentrations of other drug, potentially resulting in adverse events). Products include:
   Indocin I.V. 1727

Isocarboxazid (Potential for serious, sometimes fatal, reactions including hyperthermia, rigidity, myoclonus, extreme agitation progressing to delirium and coma; concurrent and/or sequential use is contraindicated).
   No products indexed under this heading.

Ketoprofen (Nefazodone is highly bound to the plasma protein hence co-administration with another drug that is highly protein bound may cause increased free concentrations of other drug, potentially resulting in adverse events). Products include:
   Actron Caplets and Tablets 608
   Orudis Capsules 2874
   Orudis KT 842
   Oruvail Capsules 2874

Ketorolac Tromethamine (Nefazodone is highly bound to the plasma protein hence co-administration with another drug that is highly protein bound may cause increased free concentrations of other drug, potentially resulting in adverse events). Products include:
   Acular Sterile Ophthalmic Solution 470
   Toradol 2319

Meclofenamate Sodium (Nefazodone is highly bound to the plasma protein hence co-administration with another drug that is highly protein bound may cause increased free concentrations of other drug, potentially resulting in adverse events).
   No products indexed under this heading.

Mefenamic Acid (Nefazodone is highly bound to the plasma protein hence co-administration with another drug that is highly protein bound may cause increased free concentrations of other drug, potentially resulting in adverse events). Products include:
   Ponstel 1982

Midazolam Hydrochloride (Nefazodone is highly bound to the plasma protein hence co-administration with another drug that is highly protein bound may cause increased free concentrations of other drug, potentially resulting in adverse events). Products include:
   Versed Injection 2324

Naproxen (Nefazodone is highly bound to the plasma protein hence co-administration with another drug that is highly protein bound may cause increased free concentrations of other drug, potentially resulting in adverse events). Products include:
   Anaprox/Naprosyn 2277

Naproxen Sodium (Nefazodone is highly bound to the plasma protein hence co-administration with another drug that is highly protein bound may cause increased free concentrations of other drug, potentially resulting in adverse events). Products include:
   Aleve 2124
   Anaprox/Naprosyn 2277
   Naprelan Tablets 2861

Nortriptyline Hydrochloride (Nefazodone is highly bound to the plasma protein hence co-administration with another drug that is highly protein bound may cause increased free concentrations of other drug, potentially resulting in adverse events). Products include:
   Pamelor 2409

Oxaprozin (Nefazodone is highly bound to the plasma protein hence co-administration with another drug that is highly protein bound may cause increased free concentrations of other drug, potentially resulting in adverse events). Products include:
   Daypro Caplets 2578

Oxazepam (Nefazodone is highly bound to the plasma protein hence co-administration with another drug that is highly protein bound may cause increased free concentrations of other drug, potentially resulting in adverse events). Products include:
   Serax Capsules 2916
   Serax Tablets 2916

Phenelzine Sulfate (Potential for serious, sometimes fatal, reactions including hyperthermia, rigidity, myoclonus, extreme agitation progressing to delirium and coma; concurrent and/or sequential use is contraindicated). Products include:
   Nardil 1977

Phenylbutazone (Nefazodone is highly bound to the plasma protein hence co-administration with another drug that is highly protein bound may cause increased free concentrations of other drug, potentially resulting in adverse events).
   No products indexed under this heading.

Piroxicam (Nefazodone is highly bound to the plasma protein hence co-administration with another drug that is highly protein bound may cause increased free concentrations of other drug, potentially resulting in adverse events). Products include:
   Feldene Capsules 2008

Propranolol Hydrochloride (Potential for reduction in C_{max} and AUC of propranolol with no significant change in clinical outcome). Products include:
   Inderal 2834
   Inderal LA Long Acting Capsules 2836
   Inderide Tablets 2838
   Inderide LA Long Acting Capsules .. 2840

Selegiline Hydrochloride (Potential for serious, sometimes fatal, reactions including hyperthermia, rigidity, myoclonus, extreme agitation progressing to delirium and coma; concurrent and/or sequential use is contraindicated). Products include:
   Eldepryl Capsules 2729

Sulindac (Nefazodone is highly bound to the plasma protein hence co-administration with another drug that is highly protein bound may cause increased free concentrations of other drug, potentially resulting in adverse events). Products include:
   Clinoril Tablets 1658

Temazepam (Nefazodone is highly bound to the plasma protein hence co-administration with another drug that is highly protein bound may cause increased free concentrations of other drug, potentially resulting in adverse events). Products include:
   Restoril Capsules 2413

Terfenadine (Nefazodone has been shown *in vitro* to be inhibitor of cytochrome $P_{450}IIIA_4$ resulting in the potential for increased plasma concentration of terfenadine leading to QT prolongation and rare cases of serious cardiovascular toxicity; concurrent use is contraindicated). Products include:
   Seldane Tablets 1284
   Seldane-D Extended-Release Tablets 1286

Tolbutamide (Nefazodone is highly bound to the plasma protein hence co-administration with another drug that is highly protein bound may cause increased free concentrations of other drug, potentially resulting in adverse events).
   No products indexed under this heading.

Tolmetin Sodium (Nefazodone is highly bound to the plasma protein hence co-administration with another drug that is highly protein bound may cause increased free concentrations of other drug, potentially resulting in adverse events). Products include:
   Tolectin (200, 400 and 600 mg) .. 1591

Tranylcypromine Sulfate (Potential for serious, sometimes fatal, reactions including hyperthermia, rigidity, myoclonus, extreme agitation progressing to delirium and coma; concurrent and/or sequential use is contraindicated). Products include:
   Parnate Tablets 2679

Triazolam (Co-administration may increase steady-state peak concentrations, AUC and half-life values; potentiated effects on psychomotor performance tests; reduction in initial dosage of triazolobenzodiazepines is required). Products include:
   Halcion Tablets 2093

IMPORTANT NOTE: Always consult each drug listing in the patient's regimen for possible interactions.

Serzone

Trimipramine Maleate (Nefazodone is highly bound to the plasma protein hence co-administration with another drug that is highly protein bound may cause increased free concentrations of other drug, potentially resulting in adverse events). Products include:
Surmontil Capsules..................2917

Warfarin Sodium (Nefazodone is highly bound to the plasma protein hence co-administration with another drug that is highly protein bound may cause increased free concentrations of other drug, potentially resulting in adverse events). Products include:
Coumadin..................941

Food Interactions
Alcohol (Concomitant use should be avoided).
Food, unspecified (Food delays the absorption of nefazodone and decreases the bioavailability by approximately 20%).

SHADE GEL SPF 30 SUNBLOCK
(Ethylhexyl p-Methoxycinnamate, Oxybenzone, Homosalate)..................⊞ 767
None cited in PDR database.

SHADE LOTION SPF 45 SUNBLOCK
(Ethylhexyl p-Methoxycinnamate, Oxybenzone, 2-Ethylhexyl Salicylate, Homosalate)..................⊞ 767
None cited in PDR database.

SHADE UVAGUARD SPF 15 SUNCREEN LOTION
(Octyl Methoxycinnamate, Avobenzone, Oxybenzone)..................⊞ 768
None cited in PDR database.

SILVADENE CREAM 1%
(Silver Sulfadiazine)..................1288
May interact with:

Cimetidine (An increased incidence of leukopenia has been reported in patients treated concurrently with cimetidine). Products include:
Tagamet HB Tablets..................⊞ 786
Tagamet Tablets..................2694

Cimetidine Hydrochloride (An increased incidence of leukopenia has been reported in patients treated concurrently with cimetidine). Products include:
Tagamet..................2694

Protease (Concomitant use of topical proteolytic enzymes with silver sulfadiazine may result in inactivation of enzyme by silver). Products include:
Arco-Lase Plus Tablets..................513
Arco-Lase Tablets..................513
Cotazym Capsules..................1866
Donnazyme Tablets..................2235
Kutrase Capsules..................2546
Ku-Zyme Capsules..................2546
Ku-Zyme HP Capsules..................2547

SIMILAC TODDLER'S BEST NUTRITIONAL BEVERAGE WITH IRON
(Nutritional Beverage)..................⊞ 746
None cited in PDR database.

SIMILASAN EYE DROPS #1
(Belladonna Alkaloids, Homeopathic Medications)..................⊙ 316
None cited in PDR database.

SIMILASAN EYE DROPS #2
(Homeopathic Medications)..................⊙ 316
None cited in PDR database.

SINAREST TABLETS
(Acetaminophen, Chlorpheniramine Maleate, Pseudoephedrine Hydrochloride)..................⊞ 663
May interact with monoamine oxidase inhibitors, hypnotics and sedatives, tranquilizers, and certain other agents. Compounds in these categories include:

Alprazolam (May increase drowsiness effect). Products include:
Xanax Tablets..................2115

Buspirone Hydrochloride (May increase drowsiness effect). Products include:
BuSpar Tablets..................738

Chlordiazepoxide (May increase drowsiness effect). Products include:
Limbitrol..................2333

Chlordiazepoxide Hydrochloride (May increase drowsiness effect). Products include:
Librax Capsules..................2330
Librium Capsules..................2331
Librium Injectable..................2332

Chlorpromazine (May increase drowsiness effect). Products include:
Thorazine Suppositories..................2701

Chlorpromazine Hydrochloride (May increase drowsiness effect). Products include:
Thorazine..................2701

Chlorprothixene (May increase drowsiness effect).
No products indexed under this heading.

Chlorprothixene Hydrochloride (May increase drowsiness effect).
No products indexed under this heading.

Clorazepate Dipotassium (May increase drowsiness effect). Products include:
Tranxene..................459

Diazepam (May increase drowsiness effect). Products include:
Dizac (diazepam injectable emulsion) CIV..................1862
Valium Injectable..................2336
Valium Tablets..................2335

Droperidol (May increase drowsiness effect). Products include:
Inapsine Injection..................462

Estazolam (May increase drowsiness effect). Products include:
ProSom Tablets..................457

Ethchlorvynol (May increase drowsiness effect). Products include:
Placidyl Capsules..................456

Ethinamate (May increase drowsiness effect).
No products indexed under this heading.

Fluphenazine Decanoate (May increase drowsiness effect). Products include:
Prolixin Decanoate..................510

Fluphenazine Enanthate (May increase drowsiness effect). Products include:
Prolixin Enanthate..................510

Fluphenazine Hydrochloride (May increase drowsiness effect). Products include:
Prolixin..................510

Flurazepam Hydrochloride (May increase drowsiness effect). Products include:
Dalmane Capsules..................2329

Furazolidone (Concurrent and/or sequential use is not recommended). Products include:
Furoxone..................2221

Glutethimide (May increase drowsiness effect).
No products indexed under this heading.

Haloperidol (May increase drowsiness effect). Products include:
Haldol Injection, Tablets and Concentrate..................1585

Haloperidol Decanoate (May increase drowsiness effect). Products include:
Haldol Decanoate..................1587

Hydroxyzine Hydrochloride (May increase drowsiness effect). Products include:
Atarax Tablets & Syrup..................1992
Marax Tablets & DF Syrup..................2015
Vistaril Intramuscular Solution..................2042

Isocarboxazid (Concurrent and/or sequential use is not recommended).
No products indexed under this heading.

Lorazepam (May increase drowsiness effect). Products include:
Ativan Injection..................2805
Ativan Tablets..................2807

Loxapine Hydrochloride (May increase drowsiness effect). Products include:
Loxitane..................1426

Loxapine Succinate (May increase drowsiness effect). Products include:
Loxitane Capsules..................1426

Meprobamate (May increase drowsiness effect). Products include:
Miltown Tablets..................2780
PMB 200 and PMB 400..................2890

Mesoridazine Besylate (May increase drowsiness effect). Products include:
Serentil..................689

Midazolam Hydrochloride (May increase drowsiness effect). Products include:
Versed Injection..................2324

Molindone Hydrochloride (May increase drowsiness effect). Products include:
Moban Tablets and Concentrate..................1036

Oxazepam (May increase drowsiness effect). Products include:
Serax Capsules..................2916
Serax Tablets..................2916

Perphenazine (May increase drowsiness effect). Products include:
Etrafon..................2495
Triavil Tablets..................1800
Trilafon..................2532

Phenelzine Sulfate (Concurrent and/or sequential use is not recommended). Products include:
Nardil..................1977

Prazepam (May increase drowsiness effect).
No products indexed under this heading.

Prochlorperazine (May increase drowsiness effect). Products include:
Compazine..................2644

Promethazine Hydrochloride (May increase drowsiness effect). Products include:
Mepergan Injection..................2859
Phenergan with Codeine..................2883
Phenergan with Dextromethorphan..................2885
Phenergan Injection..................2880
Phenergan Suppositories..................2882
Phenergan Syrup..................2881
Phenergan Tablets..................2882
Phenergan VC..................2886
Phenergan VC with Codeine..................2888

Propofol (May increase drowsiness effect). Products include:
Diprivan Injectable Emulsion..................2939

Quazepam (May increase drowsiness effect). Products include:
Doral Tablets..................2773

Secobarbital Sodium (May increase drowsiness effect). Products include:
Seconal Sodium Pulvules..................1529

Selegiline Hydrochloride (Concurrent and/or sequential use is not recommended). Products include:
Eldepryl Capsules..................2729

Temazepam (May increase drowsiness effect). Products include:
Restoril Capsules..................2413

Thioridazine Hydrochloride (May increase drowsiness effect). Products include:
Mellaril..................2398

Thiothixene (May increase drowsiness effect). Products include:
Navane Capsules and Concentrate..................2018
Navane Intramuscular..................2019

Tranylcypromine Sulfate (Concurrent and/or sequential use is not recommended). Products include:
Parnate Tablets..................2679

Triazolam (May increase drowsiness effect). Products include:
Halcion Tablets..................2093

Trifluoperazine Hydrochloride (May increase drowsiness effect). Products include:
Stelazine..................2692

Zolpidem Tartrate (May increase drowsiness effect). Products include:
Ambien Tablets..................2559

Food Interactions
Alcohol (May increase drowsiness effect).

SINAREST EXTRA STRENGTH CAPLETS
(Acetaminophen, Chlorpheniramine Maleate, Pseudoephedrine Hydrochloride)..................⊞ 663
See Sinarest Tablets

SINAREST NO DROWSINESS CAPLETS
(Acetaminophen, Pseudoephedrine Hydrochloride)..................⊞ 663
See Sinarest Tablets

SINE-AID MAXIMUM STRENGTH SINUS HEADACHE GELCAPS, CAPLETS AND TABLETS
(Acetaminophen, Pseudoephedrine Hydrochloride)..................1570
May interact with monoamine oxidase inhibitors and certain other agents. Compounds in these categories include:

Furazolidone (Concurrent and/or sequential use is contraindicated). Products include:
Furoxone..................2221

Isocarboxazid (Concurrent and/or sequential use is contraindicated).
No products indexed under this heading.

Phenelzine Sulfate (Concurrent and/or sequential use is contraindicated). Products include:
Nardil..................1977

Selegiline Hydrochloride (Concurrent and/or sequential use is contraindicated). Products include:
Eldepryl Capsules..................2729

Tranylcypromine Sulfate (Concurrent and/or sequential use is contraindicated). Products include:
Parnate Tablets..................2679

Food Interactions
Alcohol (Chronic heavy alcohol abusers, 3 or more drinks per day, may be at increased risk of liver toxicity from acetaminophen use).

(⊞ Described in PDR For Nonprescription Drugs)   (⊙ Described in PDR For Ophthalmology)

SINE-OFF NO DROWSINESS FORMULA CAPLETS
(Acetaminophen, Pseudoephedrine Hydrochloride) ... 784
May interact with monoamine oxidase inhibitors. Compounds in this category include:

Furazolidone (Concurrent and/or sequential use is not recommended). Products include:
Furoxone ... 2221
Isocarboxazid (Concurrent and/or sequential use is not recommended).
No products indexed under this heading.
Phenelzine Sulfate (Concurrent and/or sequential use is not recommended). Products include:
Nardil ... 1977
Selegiline Hydrochloride (Concurrent and/or sequential use is not recommended). Products include:
Eldepryl Capsules ... 2729
Tranylcypromine Sulfate (Concurrent and/or sequential use is not recommended). Products include:
Parnate Tablets ... 2679

SINE-OFF SINUS MEDICINE
(Acetaminophen, Chlorpheniramine Maleate, Pseudoephedrine Hydrochloride) ... 784
May interact with monoamine oxidase inhibitors, hypnotics and sedatives, tranquilizers, and certain other agents. Compounds in these categories include:

Alprazolam (May increase drowsiness effect). Products include:
Xanax Tablets ... 2115
Buspirone Hydrochloride (May increase drowsiness effect). Products include:
BuSpar Tablets ... 738
Chlordiazepoxide (May increase drowsiness effect). Products include:
Limbitrol ... 2333
Chlordiazepoxide Hydrochloride (May increase drowsiness effect). Products include:
Librax Capsules ... 2330
Librium Capsules ... 2331
Librium Injectable ... 2332
Chlorpromazine (May increase drowsiness effect). Products include:
Thorazine Suppositories ... 2701
Chlorpromazine Hydrochloride (May increase drowsiness effect). Products include:
Thorazine ... 2701
Chlorprothixene (May increase drowsiness effect).
No products indexed under this heading.
Chlorprothixene Hydrochloride (May increase drowsiness effect).
No products indexed under this heading.
Clorazepate Dipotassium (May increase drowsiness effect). Products include:
Tranxene ... 459
Diazepam (May increase drowsiness effect). Products include:
Dizac (diazepam injectable emulsion) CIV ... 1862
Valium Injectable ... 2336
Valium Tablets ... 2335
Droperidol (May increase drowsiness effect). Products include:
Inapsine Injection ... 462
Estazolam (May increase drowsiness effect). Products include:
ProSom Tablets ... 457
Ethchlorvynol (May increase drowsiness effect). Products include:
Placidyl Capsules ... 456
Ethinamate (May increase drowsiness effect).
No products indexed under this heading.
Fluphenazine Decanoate (May increase drowsiness effect). Products include:
Prolixin Decanoate ... 510
Fluphenazine Enanthate (May increase drowsiness effect). Products include:
Prolixin Enanthate ... 510
Fluphenazine Hydrochloride (May increase drowsiness effect). Products include:
Prolixin ... 510
Flurazepam Hydrochloride (May increase drowsiness effect). Products include:
Dalmane Capsules ... 2329
Furazolidone (Concurrent and/or sequential use is not recommended). Products include:
Furoxone ... 2221
Glutethimide (May increase drowsiness effect).
No products indexed under this heading.
Haloperidol (May increase drowsiness effect). Products include:
Haldol Injection, Tablets and Concentrate ... 1585
Haloperidol Decanoate (May increase drowsiness effect). Products include:
Haldol Decanoate ... 1587
Hydroxyzine Hydrochloride (May increase drowsiness effect). Products include:
Atarax Tablets & Syrup ... 1992
Marax Tablets & DF Syrup ... 2015
Vistaril Intramuscular Solution ... 2042
Isocarboxazid (Concurrent and/or sequential use is not recommended).
No products indexed under this heading.
Lorazepam (May increase drowsiness effect). Products include:
Ativan Injection ... 2805
Ativan Tablets ... 2807
Loxapine Hydrochloride (May increase drowsiness effect). Products include:
Loxitane ... 1426
Loxapine Succinate (May increase drowsiness effect). Products include:
Loxitane Capsules ... 1426
Meprobamate (May increase drowsiness effect). Products include:
Miltown Tablets ... 2780
PMB 200 and PMB 400 ... 2890
Mesoridazine Besylate (May increase drowsiness effect). Products include:
Serentil ... 689
Midazolam Hydrochloride (May increase drowsiness effect). Products include:
Versed Injection ... 2324
Molindone Hydrochloride (May increase drowsiness effect). Products include:
Moban Tablets and Concentrate ... 1036
Oxazepam (May increase drowsiness effect). Products include:
Serax Capsules ... 2916
Serax Tablets ... 2916
Perphenazine (May increase drowsiness effect). Products include:
Etrafon ... 2495
Triavil Tablets ... 1800
Trilafon ... 2532
Phenelzine Sulfate (Concurrent and/or sequential use is not recommended). Products include:
Nardil ... 1977
Prazepam (May increase drowsiness effect).
No products indexed under this heading.
Prochlorperazine (May increase drowsiness effect). Products include:
Compazine ... 2644
Promethazine Hydrochloride (May increase drowsiness effect). Products include:
Mepergan Injection ... 2859
Phenergan with Codeine ... 2883
Phenergan with Dextromethorphan ... 2885
Phenergan Injection ... 2880
Phenergan Suppositories ... 2882
Phenergan Syrup ... 2881
Phenergan Tablets ... 2882
Phenergan VC ... 2886
Phenergan VC with Codeine ... 2888
Propofol (May increase drowsiness effect). Products include:
Diprivan Injectable Emulsion ... 2939
Quazepam (May increase drowsiness effect). Products include:
Doral Tablets ... 2773
Secobarbital Sodium (May increase drowsiness effect). Products include:
Seconal Sodium Pulvules ... 1529
Selegiline Hydrochloride (Concurrent and/or sequential use is not recommended). Products include:
Eldepryl Capsules ... 2729
Temazepam (May increase drowsiness effect). Products include:
Restoril Capsules ... 2413
Thioridazine Hydrochloride (May increase drowsiness effect). Products include:
Mellaril ... 2398
Thiothixene (May increase drowsiness effect). Products include:
Navane Capsules and Concentrate ... 2018
Navane Intramuscular ... 2019
Tranylcypromine Sulfate (Concurrent and/or sequential use is not recommended). Products include:
Parnate Tablets ... 2679
Triazolam (May increase drowsiness effect). Products include:
Halcion Tablets ... 2093
Trifluoperazine Hydrochloride (May increase drowsiness effect). Products include:
Stelazine ... 2692
Zolpidem Tartrate (May increase drowsiness effect). Products include:
Ambien Tablets ... 2559

Food Interactions

Alcohol (May increase drowsiness effect).

SINEMET TABLETS
(Carbidopa, Levodopa) ... 959
May interact with monoamine oxidase inhibitors, antihypertensives, tricyclic antidepressants, phenothiazines, butyrophenones, and certain other agents. Compounds in these categories include:

Acebutolol Hydrochloride (Symptomatic postural hypotension). Products include:
Sectral Capsules ... 2914
Amitriptyline Hydrochloride (Potential for rare adverse reactions, including hypertension and dyskinesia). Products include:
Elavil ... 2945
Etrafon ... 2495
Limbitrol ... 2333
Triavil Tablets ... 1800
Amlodipine Besylate (Symptomatic postural hypotension). Products include:
Lotrel Capsules ... 858
Norvasc Tablets ... 2020
Amoxapine (Potential for rare adverse reactions, including hypertension and dyskinesia). Products include:
Asendin Tablets ... 1419
Atenolol (Symptomatic postural hypotension). Products include:
Tenoretic Tablets ... 2963
Tenormin Tablets and I.V. Injection ... 2965
Benazepril Hydrochloride (Symptomatic postural hypotension). Products include:
Lotensin Tablets ... 852
Lotensin HCT Tablets ... 855
Lotrel Capsules ... 858
Bendroflumethiazide (Symptomatic postural hypotension).
No products indexed under this heading.
Betaxolol Hydrochloride (Symptomatic postural hypotension). Products include:
Betoptic Ophthalmic Solution ... 465
Betoptic S Ophthalmic Suspension ... 467
Kerlone Tablets ... 2588
Bisoprolol Fumarate (Symptomatic postural hypotension). Products include:
Zebeta Tablets ... 1457
Ziac ... 1459
Captopril (Symptomatic postural hypotension). Products include:
Capoten Tablets ... 740
Capozide Tablets ... 744
Carteolol Hydrochloride (Symptomatic postural hypotension). Products include:
Cartrol Tablets ... 413
Ocupress Ophthalmic Solution, 1% Sterile ... ⊙ 297
Chlorothiazide (Symptomatic postural hypotension). Products include:
Aldoclor Tablets ... 1638
Diupres Tablets ... 1691
Diuril Oral ... 1694
Chlorothiazide Sodium (Symptomatic postural hypotension). Products include:
Diuril Sodium Intravenous ... 1693
Chlorpromazine (Reduced therapeutic effects of levodopa). Products include:
Thorazine Suppositories ... 2701
Chlorthalidone (Symptomatic postural hypotension). Products include:
Combipres Tablets ... 682
Tenoretic Tablets ... 2963
Thalitone ... 1293
Clomipramine Hydrochloride (Potential for rare adverse reactions, including hypertension and dyskinesia). Products include:
Anafranil Capsules ... 819
Clonidine (Symptomatic postural hypotension). Products include:
Catapres-TTS ... 680
Clonidine Hydrochloride (Symptomatic postural hypotension). Products include:
Catapres Tablets ... 679
Combipres Tablets ... 682
Deserpidine (Symptomatic postural hypotension).
No products indexed under this heading.
Desipramine Hydrochloride (Potential for rare adverse reactions, including hypertension and dyskinesia). Products include:
Norpramin Tablets ... 1273

IMPORTANT NOTE: Always consult each drug listing in the patient's regimen for possible interactions.

Sinemet — Interactions Index

Diazoxide (Symptomatic postural hypotension). Products include:
- Hyperstat I.V. Injection 2504
- Proglycem 575

Diltiazem Hydrochloride (Symptomatic postural hypotension). Products include:
- Cardizem CD Capsules 1251
- Cardizem SR Capsules 1255
- Cardizem Injectable 1253
- Cardizem Tablets 1257
- Dilacor XR Extended-release Capsules 2183
- Tiazac Capsules 1019

Doxazosin Mesylate (Symptomatic postural hypotension). Products include:
- Cardura Tablets 1993

Doxepin Hydrochloride (Potential for rare adverse reactions, including hypertension and dyskinesia). Products include:
- Adapin Capsules 1542
- Sinequan 2028
- Zonalon Cream 1042

Enalapril Maleate (Symptomatic postural hypotension). Products include:
- Vaseretic Tablets 1810
- Vasotec Tablets 1816

Enalaprilat (Symptomatic postural hypotension). Products include:
- Vasotec I.V. 1814

Esmolol Hydrochloride (Symptomatic postural hypotension). Products include:
- Brevibloc (esmolol HCl) Injection 1860

Felodipine (Symptomatic postural hypotension). Products include:
- Plendil Extended-Release Tablets 514

Fluphenazine Decanoate (Reduced therapeutic effects of levodopa). Products include:
- Prolixin Decanoate 510

Fluphenazine Enanthate (Reduced therapeutic effects of levodopa). Products include:
- Prolixin Enanthate 510

Fluphenazine Hydrochloride (Reduced therapeutic effects of levodopa). Products include:
- Prolixin 510

Fosinopril Sodium (Symptomatic postural hypotension). Products include:
- Monopril Tablets 762

Furazolidone (Contraindication). Products include:
- Furoxone 2221

Furosemide (Symptomatic postural hypotension). Products include:
- Lasix Injection, Oral Solution and Tablets 1267

Guanabenz Acetate (Symptomatic postural hypotension).
No products indexed under this heading.

Guanethidine Monosulfate (Symptomatic postural hypotension). Products include:
- Esimil Tablets 840
- Ismelin Tablets 845

Haloperidol (Reduced therapeutic effects of levodopa). Products include:
- Haldol Injection, Tablets and Concentrate 1585

Haloperidol Decanoate (Reduced therapeutic effects of levodopa). Products include:
- Haldol Decanoate 1587

Hydralazine Hydrochloride (Symptomatic postural hypotension). Products include:
- Apresazide Capsules 824
- Apresoline Hydrochloride Tablets .. 826
- Hydralazine Hydrochloride Injection USP 2712
- Ser-Ap-Es Tablets 867

Hydrochlorothiazide (Symptomatic postural hypotension). Products include:
- Aldactazide Tablets 2556
- Aldoril Tablets 1644
- Apresazide Capsules 824
- Capozide Tablets 744
- Dyazide Capsules 2653
- Esidrix Tablets 839
- Esimil Tablets 840
- HydroDIURIL Tablets 1716
- Hydropres Tablets 1718
- Hyzaar Tablets 1720
- Inderide Tablets 2838
- Inderide LA Long Acting Capsules .. 2840
- Lopressor HCT Tablets 850
- Lotensin HCT Tablets 855
- Moduretic Tablets 1748
- Oretic Tablets 450
- Prinzide Tablets 1780
- Ser-Ap-Es Tablets 867
- Timolide Tablets 1791
- Vaseretic Tablets 1810
- Zestoretic Tablets 2968
- Ziac 1459

Hydroflumethiazide (Symptomatic postural hypotension). Products include:
- Diucardin Tablets 2824

Imipramine Hydrochloride (Potential for rare adverse reactions, including hypertension and dyskinesia). Products include:
- Tofranil Ampuls 873
- Tofranil Tablets 875

Imipramine Pamoate (Potential for rare adverse reactions, including hypertension and dyskinesia). Products include:
- Tofranil-PM Capsules 876

Indapamide (Symptomatic postural hypotension).
No products indexed under this heading.

Isocarboxazid (Contraindication).
No products indexed under this heading.

Isradipine (Symptomatic postural hypotension). Products include:
- DynaCirc Capsules 2381
- DynaCirc CR Tablets 2383

Labetalol Hydrochloride (Symptomatic postural hypotension). Products include:
- Normodyne Injection 2519
- Normodyne Tablets 2522
- Trandate 1158

Lisinopril (Symptomatic postural hypotension). Products include:
- Prinivil Tablets 1776
- Prinzide Tablets 1780
- Zestoretic Tablets 2968
- Zestril Tablets 2972

Losartan Potassium (Symptomatic postural hypotension). Products include:
- Cozaar Tablets 1668
- Hyzaar Tablets 1720

Maprotiline Hydrochloride (Potential for rare adverse reactions, including hypertension and dyskinesia). Products include:
- Ludiomil Tablets 861

Mecamylamine Hydrochloride (Symptomatic postural hypotension). Products include:
- Inversine Tablets 1729

Mesoridazine Besylate (Reduced therapeutic effects of levodopa). Products include:
- Serentil 689

Methotrimeprazine (Reduced therapeutic effects of levodopa). Products include:
- Levoprome 1321

Methyclothiazide (Symptomatic postural hypotension). Products include:
- Enduron Tablets 424

Methyldopa (Symptomatic postural hypotension). Products include:
- Aldoclor Tablets 1638
- Aldomet Oral 1640
- Aldoril Tablets 1644

Methyldopate Hydrochloride (Symptomatic postural hypotension). Products include:
- Aldomet Ester HCl Injection 1642

Metolazone (Symptomatic postural hypotension). Products include:
- Mykrox Tablets 1617
- Zaroxolyn Tablets 1625

Metoprolol Succinate (Symptomatic postural hypotension). Products include:
- Toprol-XL Tablets 560

Metoprolol Tartrate (Symptomatic postural hypotension). Products include:
- Lopressor 848
- Lopressor HCT Tablets 850

Metyrosine (Symptomatic postural hypotension). Products include:
- Demser Capsules 1690

Minoxidil (Symptomatic postural hypotension).
No products indexed under this heading.

Moexipril Hydrochloride (Symptomatic postural hypotension). Products include:
- Univasc Tablets 2553

Nadolol (Symptomatic postural hypotension).
No products indexed under this heading.

Nicardipine Hydrochloride (Symptomatic postural hypotension). Products include:
- Cardene Capsules 2261
- Cardene I.V. 2815
- Cardene SR Capsules 2264

Nifedipine (Symptomatic postural hypotension). Products include:
- Adalat Capsules (10 mg and 20 mg) 580
- Adalat CC 582
- Procardia Capsules 2024
- Procardia XL Extended Release Tablets 2026

Nisoldipine (Symptomatic postural hypotension). Products include:
- Sular Tablets 2961

Nitroglycerin (Symptomatic postural hypotension). Products include:
- Deponit NTG Transdermal Delivery System 2541
- Nitro-Bid IV 1270
- Nitro-Bid Ointment 1272
- Nitro-Dur (nitroglycerin) Transdermal Infusion System 1365
- Nitrolingual Spray 2193
- Nitrostat Tablets 1981
- Transderm-Nitro Transdermal Therapeutic System 878

Nortriptyline Hydrochloride (Potential for rare adverse reactions, including hypertension and dyskinesia). Products include:
- Pamelor 2409

Papaverine Hydrochloride (Beneficial effects of levodopa reversed in Parkinson's Disease). Products include:
- Papaverine Hydrochloride Vials and Ampoules 1523

Penbutolol Sulfate (Symptomatic postural hypotension). Products include:
- Levatol Tablets 2547

Perphenazine (Reduced therapeutic effects of levodopa). Products include:
- Etrafon 2495
- Triavil Tablets 1800
- Trilafon 2532

Phenelzine Sulfate (Contraindication). Products include:
- Nardil 1977

Phenoxybenzamine Hydrochloride (Symptomatic postural hypotension). Products include:
- Dibenzyline Capsules 2650

Phentolamine Mesylate (Symptomatic postural hypotension). Products include:
- Regitine Vials 864

Phenytoin (Beneficial effects of levodopa reversed in Parkinson's Disease). Products include:
- Dilantin Infatabs 1967
- Dilantin-125 Suspension 1969

Phenytoin Sodium (Beneficial effects of levodopa reversed in Parkinson's Disease). Products include:
- Dilantin Kapseals 1965

Pindolol (Symptomatic postural hypotension). Products include:
- Visken Tablets 2428

Polythiazide (Symptomatic postural hypotension). Products include:
- Minizide Capsules 2016

Prazosin Hydrochloride (Symptomatic postural hypotension). Products include:
- Minipress Capsules 2015
- Minizide Capsules 2016

Prochlorperazine (Reduced therapeutic effects of levodopa). Products include:
- Compazine 2644

Promethazine Hydrochloride (Reduced therapeutic effects of levodopa). Products include:
- Mepergan Injection 2859
- Phenergan with Codeine 2883
- Phenergan with Dextromethorphan .. 2885
- Phenergan Injection 2880
- Phenergan Suppositories 2882
- Phenergan Syrup 2881
- Phenergan Tablets 2882
- Phenergan VC 2886
- Phenergan VC with Codeine 2888

Propranolol Hydrochloride (Symptomatic postural hypotension). Products include:
- Inderal 2834
- Inderal LA Long Acting Capsules 2836
- Inderide Tablets 2838
- Inderide LA Long Acting Capsules .. 2840

Protriptyline Hydrochloride (Potential for rare adverse reactions, including hypertension and dyskinesia). Products include:
- Vivactil Tablets 1820

Quinapril Hydrochloride (Symptomatic postural hypotension). Products include:
- Accupril Tablets 1950

Ramipril (Symptomatic postural hypotension). Products include:
- Altace Capsules 1238

Rauwolfia Serpentina (Symptomatic postural hypotension).
No products indexed under this heading.

Rescinnamine (Symptomatic postural hypotension).
No products indexed under this heading.

Reserpine (Symptomatic postural hypotension). Products include:
- Diupres Tablets 1691
- Hydropres Tablets 1718
- Ser-Ap-Es Tablets 867

Sodium Nitroprusside (Symptomatic postural hypotension).
No products indexed under this heading.

Sotalol Hydrochloride (Symptomatic postural hypotension). Products include:
- Betapace Tablets 637

Spirapril Hydrochloride (Symptomatic postural hypotension).
No products indexed under this heading.

(◨ Described in PDR For Nonprescription Drugs) (◉ Described in PDR For Ophthalmology)

Terazosin Hydrochloride (Symptomatic postural hypotension). Products include:
- Hytrin Capsules 434

Thioridazine Hydrochloride (Reduced therapeutic effects of levodopa). Products include:
- Mellaril 2398

Timolol Maleate (Symptomatic postural hypotension). Products include:
- Blocadren Tablets 1654
- Timolide Tablets 1791
- Timoptic in Ocudose 1796
- Timoptic Sterile Ophthalmic Solution 1794
- Timoptic-XE 1798

Torsemide (Symptomatic postural hypotension). Products include:
- Demadex Tablets and Injection 691

Tranylcypromine Sulfate (Contraindication). Products include:
- Parnate Tablets 2679

Trifluoperazine Hydrochloride (Reduced therapeutic effects of levodopa). Products include:
- Stelazine 2692

Trimethaphan Camsylate (Symptomatic postural hypotension).
- No products indexed under this heading.

Trimipramine Maleate (Potential for rare adverse reactions, including hypertension and dyskinesia). Products include:
- Surmontil Capsules 2917

Verapamil Hydrochloride (Symptomatic postural hypotension). Products include:
- Calan SR Caplets 2571
- Calan Tablets 2568
- Covera-HS Tablets 2573
- Isoptin Injectable 1391
- Isoptin Oral Tablets 1393
- Isoptin SR Tablets 1395
- Verelan Capsules 1455

Food Interactions

Diet high in protein (Levodopa competes with certain amino acids, the absorption of levodopa may be impaired in some patients on a high protein diet).

SINEMET CR TABLETS

(Carbidopa, Levodopa) 961

May interact with antihypertensives, monoamine oxidase inhibitors, tricyclic antidepressants, phenothiazines, butyrophenones, and certain other agents. Compounds in these categories include:

Acebutolol Hydrochloride (Potential for postural hypertension). Products include:
- Sectral Capsules 2914

Amitriptyline Hydrochloride (Potential for hypertension and dyskinesia). Products include:
- Elavil 2945
- Etrafon 2495
- Limbitrol 2333
- Triavil Tablets 1800

Amlodipine Besylate (Potential for postural hypertension). Products include:
- Lotrel Capsules 858
- Norvasc Tablets 2020

Amoxapine (Potential for hypertension and dyskinesia). Products include:
- Asendin Tablets 1419

Atenolol (Potential for postural hypertension). Products include:
- Tenoretic Tablets 2963
- Tenormin Tablets and I.V. Injection 2965

Benazepril Hydrochloride (Potential for postural hypertension). Products include:
- Lotensin Tablets 852
- Lotensin HCT Tablets 855
- Lotrel Capsules 858

Bendroflumethiazide (Potential for postural hypertension).
- No products indexed under this heading.

Betaxolol Hydrochloride (Potential for postural hypertension). Products include:
- Betoptic Ophthalmic Solution 465
- Betoptic S Ophthalmic Suspension 467
- Kerlone Tablets 2588

Bisoprolol Fumarate (Potential for postural hypertension). Products include:
- Zebeta Tablets 1457
- Ziac 1459

Captopril (Potential for postural hypertension). Products include:
- Capoten Tablets 740
- Capozide Tablets 744

Carteolol Hydrochloride (Potential for postural hypertension). Products include:
- Cartrol Tablets 413
- Ocupress Ophthalmic Solution, 1% Sterile .... ◉ 297

Chlorothiazide (Potential for postural hypertension). Products include:
- Aldoclor Tablets 1638
- Diupres Tablets 1691
- Diuril Oral 1694

Chlorothiazide Sodium (Potential for postural hypertension). Products include:
- Diuril Sodium Intravenous 1693

Chlorpromazine (Reduces the therapeutic effects). Products include:
- Thorazine Suppositories 2701

Chlorthalidone (Potential for postural hypertension). Products include:
- Combipres Tablets 682
- Tenoretic Tablets 2963
- Thalitone 1293

Clomipramine Hydrochloride (Potential for hypertension and dyskinesia). Products include:
- Anafranil Capsules 819

Clonidine (Potential for postural hypertension). Products include:
- Catapres-TTS 680

Clonidine Hydrochloride (Potential for postural hypertension). Products include:
- Catapres Tablets 679
- Combipres Tablets 682

Deserpidine (Potential for postural hypertension).
- No products indexed under this heading.

Desipramine Hydrochloride (Potential for hypertension and dyskinesia). Products include:
- Norpramin Tablets 1273

Diazoxide (Potential for postural hypertension). Products include:
- Hyperstat I.V. Injection 2504
- Proglycem 575

Diltiazem Hydrochloride (Potential for postural hypertension). Products include:
- Cardizem CD Capsules 1251
- Cardizem SR Capsules 1255
- Cardizem Injectable 1253
- Cardizem Tablets 1257
- Dilacor XR Extended-release Capsules 2183
- Tiazac Capsules 1019

Doxazosin Mesylate (Potential for postural hypertension). Products include:
- Cardura Tablets 1993

Doxepin Hydrochloride (Potential for hypertension and dyskinesia). Products include:
- Adapin Capsules 1542
- Sinequan 2028
- Zonalon Cream 1042

Enalapril Maleate (Potential for postural hypertension). Products include:
- Vaseretic Tablets 1810
- Vasotec Tablets 1816

Enalaprilat (Potential for postural hypertension). Products include:
- Vasotec I.V. 1814

Esmolol Hydrochloride (Potential for postural hypertension). Products include:
- Brevibloc (esmolol HCl) Injection 1860

Felodipine (Potential for postural hypertension). Products include:
- Plendil Extended-Release Tablets 514

Fluphenazine Decanoate (Reduces the therapeutic effects). Products include:
- Prolixin Decanoate 510

Fluphenazine Enanthate (Reduces the therapeutic effects). Products include:
- Prolixin Enanthate 510

Fluphenazine Hydrochloride (Reduces the therapeutic effects). Products include:
- Prolixin 510

Fosinopril Sodium (Potential for postural hypertension). Products include:
- Monopril Tablets 762

Furazolidone (Concurrent administration is contraindicated). Products include:
- Furoxone 2221

Furosemide (Potential for postural hypertension). Products include:
- Lasix Injection, Oral Solution and Tablets 1267

Guanabenz Acetate (Potential for postural hypertension).
- No products indexed under this heading.

Guanethidine Monosulfate (Potential for postural hypertension). Products include:
- Esimil Tablets 840
- Ismelin Tablets 845

Haloperidol (Reduces the therapeutic effects). Products include:
- Haldol Injection, Tablets and Concentrate 1585

Haloperidol Decanoate (Reduces the therapeutic effects). Products include:
- Haldol Decanoate 1587

Hydralazine Hydrochloride (Potential for postural hypertension). Products include:
- Apresazide Capsules 824
- Apresoline Hydrochloride Tablets .. 826
- Hydralazine Hydrochloride Injection USP 2712
- Ser-Ap-Es Tablets 867

Hydrochlorothiazide (Potential for postural hypertension). Products include:
- Aldactazide Tablets 2556
- Aldoril Tablets 1644
- Apresazide Capsules 824
- Capozide Tablets 744
- Dyazide Capsules 2653
- Esidrix Tablets 839
- Esimil Tablets 840
- HydroDIURIL Tablets 1716
- Hydropres Tablets 1718
- Hyzaar Tablets 1720
- Inderide Tablets 2838
- Inderide LA Long Acting Capsules .. 2840
- Lopressor HCT Tablets 850
- Lotensin HCT Tablets 855
- Moduretic Tablets 1748
- Oretic Tablets 450
- Prinzide Tablets 1780
- Ser-Ap-Es Tablets 867
- Timolide Tablets 1791
- Vaseretic Tablets 1810
- Zestoretic Tablets 2968
- Ziac 1459

Hydroflumethiazide (Potential for postural hypertension). Products include:
- Diucardin Tablets 2824

Imipramine Hydrochloride (Potential for hypertension and dyskinesia). Products include:
- Tofranil Ampuls 873
- Tofranil Tablets 875

Imipramine Pamoate (Potential for hypertension and dyskinesia). Products include:
- Tofranil-PM Capsules 876

Indapamide (Potential for postural hypertension).
- No products indexed under this heading.

Isocarboxazid (Concurrent administration is contraindicated).
- No products indexed under this heading.

Isradipine (Potential for postural hypertension). Products include:
- DynaCirc Capsules 2381
- DynaCirc CR Tablets 2383

Labetalol Hydrochloride (Potential for postural hypertension). Products include:
- Normodyne Injection 2519
- Normodyne Tablets 2522
- Trandate 1158

Lisinopril (Potential for postural hypertension). Products include:
- Prinivil Tablets 1776
- Prinzide Tablets 1780
- Zestoretic Tablets 2968
- Zestril Tablets 2972

Losartan Potassium (Potential for postural hypertension). Products include:
- Cozaar Tablets 1668
- Hyzaar Tablets 1720

Maprotiline Hydrochloride (Potential for hypertension and dyskinesia). Products include:
- Ludiomil Tablets 861

Mecamylamine Hydrochloride (Potential for postural hypertension). Products include:
- Inversine Tablets 1729

Mesoridazine Besylate (Reduces the therapeutic effects). Products include:
- Serentil 689

Methotrimeprazine (Reduces the therapeutic effects). Products include:
- Levoprome 1321

Methyclothiazide (Potential for postural hypertension). Products include:
- Enduron Tablets 424

Methyldopa (Potential for postural hypertension). Products include:
- Aldoclor Tablets 1638
- Aldomet Oral 1640
- Aldoril Tablets 1644

Methyldopate Hydrochloride (Potential for postural hypertension). Products include:
- Aldomet Ester HCl Injection 1642

Metolazone (Potential for postural hypertension). Products include:
- Mykrox Tablets 1617
- Zaroxolyn Tablets 1625

Metoprolol Succinate (Potential for postural hypertension). Products include:
- Toprol-XL Tablets 560

Metoprolol Tartrate (Potential for postural hypertension). Products include:
- Lopressor 848
- Lopressor HCT Tablets 850

Metyrosine (Potential for postural hypertension). Products include:
- Demser Capsules 1690

IMPORTANT NOTE: Always consult each drug listing in the patient's regimen for possible interactions.

Sinemet CR / Interactions Index

Minoxidil (Potential for postural hypertension).
No products indexed under this heading.

Moexipril Hydrochloride (Potential for postural hypertension). Products include:
Univasc Tablets 2553

Nadolol (Potential for postural hypertension).
No products indexed under this heading.

Nicardipine Hydrochloride (Potential for postural hypertension). Products include:
Cardene Capsules 2261
Cardene I.V. 2815
Cardene SR Capsules 2264

Nifedipine (Potential for postural hypertension). Products include:
Adalat Capsules (10 mg and 20 mg) 580
Adalat CC 582
Procardia Capsules 2024
Procardia XL Extended Release Tablets 2026

Nisoldipine (Potential for postural hypertension). Products include:
Sular Tablets 2961

Nitroglycerin (Potential for postural hypertension). Products include:
Deponit NTG Transdermal Delivery System 2541
Nitro-Bid IV 1270
Nitro-Bid Ointment 1272
Nitro-Dur (nitroglycerin) Transdermal Infusion System 1365
Nitrolingual Spray 2193
Nitrostat Tablets 1981
Transderm-Nitro Transdermal Therapeutic System 878

Nortriptyline Hydrochloride (Potential for hypertension and dyskinesia). Products include:
Pamelor 2409

Papaverine Hydrochloride (Reverses beneficial effects of levodopa). Products include:
Papaverine Hydrochloride Vials and Ampoules 1523

Penbutolol Sulfate (Potential for postural hypertension). Products include:
Levatol Tablets 2547

Perphenazine (Reduces the therapeutic effects). Products include:
Etrafon 2495
Triavil Tablets 1800
Trilafon 2532

Phenelzine Sulfate (Concurrent administration is contraindicated). Products include:
Nardil 1977

Phenoxybenzamine Hydrochloride (Potential for postural hypertension). Products include:
Dibenzyline Capsules 2650

Phentolamine Mesylate (Potential for postural hypertension). Products include:
Regitine Vials 864

Phenytoin (Reverses beneficial effects of levodopa). Products include:
Dilantin Infatabs 1967
Dilantin-125 Suspension 1969

Phenytoin Sodium (Reverses beneficial effects of levodopa). Products include:
Dilantin Kapseals 1965

Pindolol (Potential for postural hypertension). Products include:
Visken Tablets 2428

Polythiazide (Potential for postural hypertension). Products include:
Minizide Capsules 2016

Prazosin Hydrochloride (Potential for postural hypertension). Products include:
Minipress Capsules 2015
Minizide Capsules 2016

Prochlorperazine (Reduces the therapeutic effects). Products include:
Compazine 2644

Promethazine Hydrochloride (Reduces the therapeutic effects). Products include:
Mepergan Injection 2859
Phenergan with Codeine 2883
Phenergan with Dextromethorphan 2885
Phenergan Injection 2880
Phenergan Suppositories 2882
Phenergan Syrup 2881
Phenergan Tablets 2882
Phenergan VC 2886
Phenergan VC with Codeine 2888

Propranolol Hydrochloride (Potential for postural hypertension). Products include:
Inderal 2834
Inderal LA Long Acting Capsules 2836
Inderide Tablets 2838
Inderide LA Long Acting Capsules 2840

Protriptyline Hydrochloride (Potential for hypertension and dyskinesia). Products include:
Vivactil Tablets 1820

Quinapril Hydrochloride (Potential for postural hypertension). Products include:
Accupril Tablets 1950

Ramipril (Potential for postural hypertension). Products include:
Altace Capsules 1238

Rauwolfia Serpentina (Potential for postural hypertension).
No products indexed under this heading.

Rescinnamine (Potential for postural hypertension).
No products indexed under this heading.

Reserpine (Potential for postural hypertension). Products include:
Diupres Tablets 1691
Hydropres Tablets 1718
Ser-Ap-Es Tablets 867

Sodium Nitroprusside (Potential for postural hypertension).
No products indexed under this heading.

Sotalol Hydrochloride (Potential for postural hypertension). Products include:
Betapace Tablets 637

Spirapril Hydrochloride (Potential for postural hypertension).
No products indexed under this heading.

Terazosin Hydrochloride (Potential for postural hypertension). Products include:
Hytrin Capsules 434

Thioridazine Hydrochloride (Reduces the therapeutic effects). Products include:
Mellaril 2398

Timolol Maleate (Potential for postural hypertension). Products include:
Blocadren Tablets 1654
Timolide Tablets 1791
Timoptic in Ocudose 1796
Timoptic Sterile Ophthalmic Solution 1794
Timoptic-XE 1798

Torsemide (Potential for postural hypertension). Products include:
Demadex Tablets and Injection 691

Tranylcypromine Sulfate (Concurrent administration is contraindicated). Products include:
Parnate Tablets 2679

Trifluoperazine Hydrochloride (Reduces the therapeutic effects). Products include:
Stelazine 2692

Trimethaphan Camsylate (Potential for postural hypertension).
No products indexed under this heading.

Trimipramine Maleate (Potential for hypertension and dyskinesia). Products include:
Surmontil Capsules 2917

Verapamil Hydrochloride (Potential for postural hypertension). Products include:
Calan SR Caplets 2571
Calan Tablets 2568
Covera-HS Tablets 2573
Isoptin Injectable 1391
Isoptin Oral Tablets 1393
Isoptin SR Tablets 1395
Verelan Capsules 1455

Food Interactions

Food, unspecified (Increases the extent of availability and peak concentrations of levodopa).

SINEQUAN CAPSULES

(Doxepin Hydrochloride) 2028
May interact with monoamine oxidase inhibitors, drugs that inhibit cytochrome p450iid6, antidepressant drugs, phenothiazines, selective serotonin reuptake inhibitors, anticholinergics, and certain other agents. Compounds in these categories include:

Amitriptyline Hydrochloride (Concurrent use with drugs that are substrate for cytochrome $P_{450}IID_6$ may make normal metabolizer resemble poor metabolizer leading to higher than expected plasma concentrations of TCA with resultant toxicity). Products include:
Elavil 2945
Etrafon 2495
Limbitrol 2333
Triavil Tablets 1800

Amoxapine (Concurrent use with drugs that are substrate for cytochrome $P_{450}IID_6$ may make normal metabolizer resemble poor metabolizer leading to higher than expected plasma concentrations of TCA with resultant toxicity). Products include:
Asendin Tablets 1419

Atropine Sulfate (Caution is advised when co-administered due to doxepine-induced anticholinergic effects). Products include:
Arco-Lase Plus Tablets 513
Atrohist Plus Tablets 1605
Donnatal 2234
Donnatal Extentabs 2234
Donnatal Tablets 2234
Lomotil 2591
Motofen Tablets 789
Urised Tablets 2123

Belladonna Alkaloids (Caution is advised when co-administered due to doxepine-induced anticholinergic effects). Products include:
Bellergal-S Tablets 2375
Hyland's Bedwetting Tablets .... ■□ 788
Hyland's EnurAid Tablets .... ■□ 789
Hyland's Headache Tablets .... ■□ 790
Hyland's Teething Tablets .... ■□ 790
Similasan Eye Drops # 1 .... ■□ 769

Benztropine Mesylate (Caution is advised when co-administered due to doxepine-induced anticholinergic effects). Products include:
Cogentin 1661

Biperiden Hydrochloride (Caution is advised when co-administered due to doxepine-induced anticholinergic effects). Products include:
Akineton 1380

Bupropion Hydrochloride (Concurrent use with drugs that are substrate for cytochrome $P_{450}IID_6$ may make normal metabolizer resemble poor metabolizer leading to higher than expected plasma concentrations of TCA with resultant toxicity). Products include:
Wellbutrin Tablets 1177

Chlorpromazine (Concurrent use with drugs that are substrate for cytochrome $P_{450}IID_6$ may make normal metabolizer resemble poor metabolizer leading to higher than expected plasma concentrations of TCA with resultant toxicity). Products include:
Thorazine Suppositories 2701

Chlorpromazine Hydrochloride (Concurrent use with drugs that are substrate for cytochrome $P_{450}IID_6$ may make normal metabolizer resemble poor metabolizer leading to higher than expected plasma concentrations of TCA with resultant toxicity). Products include:
Thorazine 2701

Cimetidine (Produces clinically significant fluctuations in steady-state serum concentrations of various tricyclic antidepressants resulting in frequency and severity of side effects, particularly anticholinergic). Products include:
Tagamet HB Tablets .... ■□ 786
Tagamet Tablets 2694

Cimetidine Hydrochloride (Produces clinically significant fluctuations in steady-state serum concentrations of various tricyclic antidepressants resulting in frequency and severity of side effects, particularly anticholinergic). Products include:
Tagamet 2694

Clidinium Bromide (Caution is advised when co-administered due to doxepine-induced anticholinergic effects). Products include:
Librax Capsules 2330

Desipramine Hydrochloride (Concurrent use with drugs that are substrate for cytochrome $P_{450}IID_6$ may make normal metabolizer resemble poor metabolizer leading to higher than expected plasma concentrations of TCA with resultant toxicity). Products include:
Norpramin Tablets 1273

Dicyclomine Hydrochloride (Caution is advised when co-administered due to doxepine-induced anticholinergic effects). Products include:
Bentyl 1246

Flecainide Acetate (Concurrent use with drugs that are substrate for cytochrome $P_{450}IID_6$ may make normal metabolizer resemble poor metabolizer leading to higher than expected plasma concentrations of TCA with resultant toxicity). Products include:
Tambocor Tablets 1555

(■□ Described in PDR For Nonprescription Drugs) (○ Described in PDR For Ophthalmology)

Interactions Index

Fluoxetine Hydrochloride (Concurrent use with drugs that are substrate for cytochrome $P_{450}IID_6$ may make normal metabolizer resemble poor metabolizer leading to higher than expected plasma concentrations of TCA with resultant toxicity; due to variation in the extent of inhibition of $P_{450}IID_6$ and long half-life of the parent (fluoxetine) and active metabolite sufficient time must elapse, at least 5 weeks before switching to TCA). Products include:
Prozac Pulvules & Liquid, Oral Solution 935

Fluphenazine Decanoate (Concurrent use with drugs that are substrate for cytochrome $P_{450}IID_6$ may make normal metabolizer resemble poor metabolizer leading to higher than expected plasma concentrations of TCA with resultant toxicity). Products include:
Prolixin Decanoate 510

Fluphenazine Enanthate (Concurrent use with drugs that are substrate for cytochrome $P_{450}IID_6$ may make normal metabolizer resemble poor metabolizer leading to higher than expected plasma concentrations of TCA with resultant toxicity). Products include:
Prolixin Enanthate 510

Fluphenazine Hydrochloride (Concurrent use with drugs that are substrate for cytochrome $P_{450}IID_6$ may make normal metabolizer resemble poor metabolizer leading to higher than expected plasma concentrations of TCA with resultant toxicity). Products include:
Prolixin 510

Fluvoxamine Maleate (Concurrent use with drugs that are substrate for cytochrome $P_{450}IID_6$ may make normal metabolizer resemble poor metabolizer leading to higher than expected plasma concentrations of TCA with resultant toxicity; due to variation in the extent of inhibition of $P_{450}IID_6$ caution is indicated if co-administered). Products include:
LUVOX Tablets 2723

Furazolidone (Concurrent use is not recommended; potential for serious adverse effects). Products include:
Furoxone 2221

Glycopyrrolate (Caution is advised when co-administered due to doxepine-induced anticholinergic effects). Products include:
Robinul Forte Tablets 2247
Robinul Injectable 2247
Robinul Tablets 2247

Hyoscyamine (Caution is advised when co-administered due to doxepine-induced anticholinergic effects). Products include:
Cystospaz Tablets 2123
Urised Tablets 2123

Hyoscyamine Sulfate (Caution is advised when co-administered due to doxepine-induced anticholinergic effects). Products include:
Arco-Lase Plus Tablets 513
Atrohist Plus Tablets 1605
Cystospaz-M Capsules 2123
Donnatal 2234
Donnatal Extentabs 2234
Donnatal Tablets 2234
Kutrase Capsules 2546
Levsin/Levsinex/Levbid 2549

Imipramine Hydrochloride (Concurrent use with drugs that are substrate for cytochrome $P_{450}IID_6$ may make normal metabolizer resemble poor metabolizer leading to higher than expected plasma concentrations of TCA with resultant toxicity). Products include:
Tofranil Ampuls 873
Tofranil Tablets 875

Imipramine Pamoate (Concurrent use with drugs that are substrate for cytochrome $P_{450}IID_6$ may make normal metabolizer resemble poor metabolizer leading to higher than expected plasma concentrations of TCA with resultant toxicity). Products include:
Tofranil-PM Capsules 876

Ipratropium Bromide (Caution is advised when co-administered due to doxepine-induced anticholinergic effects). Products include:
Atrovent Inhalation Aerosol 674
Atrovent Inhalation Solution 675
Atrovent Nasal Spray 0.03% 676
Atrovent Nasal Spray 0.06% 678

Isocarboxazid (Concurrent use is not recommended; potential for serious adverse effects).
No products indexed under this heading.

Maprotiline Hydrochloride (Concurrent use with drugs that are substrate for cytochrome $P_{450}IID_6$ may make normal metabolizer resemble poor metabolizer leading to higher than expected plasma concentrations of TCA with resultant toxicity). Products include:
Ludiomil Tablets 861

Mepenzolate Bromide (Caution is advised when co-administered due to doxepine-induced anticholinergic effects).
No products indexed under this heading.

Mesoridazine Besylate (Concurrent use with drugs that are substrate for cytochrome $P_{450}IID_6$ may make normal metabolizer resemble poor metabolizer leading to higher than expected plasma concentrations of TCA with resultant toxicity). Products include:
Serentil 689

Methotrimeprazine (Concurrent use with drugs that are substrate for cytochrome $P_{450}IID_6$ may make normal metabolizer resemble poor metabolizer leading to higher than expected plasma concentrations of TCA with resultant toxicity). Products include:
Levoprome 1321

Nefazodone Hydrochloride (Concurrent use with drugs that are substrate for cytochrome $P_{450}IID_6$ may make normal metabolizer resemble poor metabolizer leading to higher than expected plasma concentrations of TCA with resultant toxicity). Products include:
Serzone Tablets 776

Nortriptyline Hydrochloride (Concurrent use with drugs that are substrate for cytochrome $P_{450}IID_6$ may make normal metabolizer resemble poor metabolizer leading to higher than expected plasma concentrations of TCA with resultant toxicity). Products include:
Pamelor 2409

Oxybutynin Chloride (Caution is advised when co-administered due to doxepine-induced anticholinergic effects). Products include:
Ditropan 1267

Paroxetine Hydrochloride (Concurrent use with drugs that are substrate for cytochrome $P_{450}IID_6$ may make normal metabolizer resemble poor metabolizer leading to higher than expected plasma concentrations of TCA with resultant toxicity; due to variation in the extent of inhibition of $P_{450}IID_6$ caution is indicated if co-administered). Products include:
Paxil Tablets 2681

Perphenazine (Concurrent use with drugs that are substrate for cytochrome $P_{450}IID_6$ may make normal metabolizer resemble poor metabolizer leading to higher than expected plasma concentrations of TCA with resultant toxicity). Products include:
Etrafon 2495
Triavil Tablets 1800
Trilafon 2532

Phenelzine Sulfate (Concurrent use is not recommended; potential for serious adverse effects). Products include:
Nardil 1977

Prochlorperazine (Concurrent use with drugs that are substrate for cytochrome $P_{450}IID_6$ may make normal metabolizer resemble poor metabolizer leading to higher than expected plasma concentrations of TCA with resultant toxicity). Products include:
Compazine 2644

Procyclidine Hydrochloride (Caution is advised when co-administered due to doxepine-induced anticholinergic effects). Products include:
Kemadrin Tablets 1105

Promethazine Hydrochloride (Concurrent use with drugs that are substrate for cytochrome $P_{450}IID_6$ may make normal metabolizer resemble poor metabolizer leading to higher than expected plasma concentrations of TCA with resultant toxicity). Products include:
Mepergan Injection 2859
Phenergan with Codeine 2883
Phenergan with Dextromethorphan 2885
Phenergan Injection 2880
Phenergan Suppositories 2882
Phenergan Syrup 2881
Phenergan Tablets 2882
Phenergan VC 2886
Phenergan VC with Codeine 2888

Propafenone Hydrochloride (Concurrent use with drugs that are substrate for cytochrome $P_{450}IID_6$ may make normal metabolizer resemble poor metabolizer leading to higher than expected plasma concentrations of TCA with resultant toxicity). Products include:
Rythmol Tablets–150mg, 225mg, 300mg 1399

Propantheline Bromide (Caution is advised when co-administered due to doxepine-induced anticholinergic effects). Products include:
Pro-Banthine Tablets 2226

Protriptyline Hydrochloride (Concurrent use with drugs that are substrate for cytochrome $P_{450}IID_6$ may make normal metabolizer resemble poor metabolizer leading to higher than expected plasma concentrations of TCA with resultant toxicity). Products include:
Vivactil Tablets 1820

Quinidine Gluconate (Concurrent use with drugs that inhibit cytochrome $P_{450}IID_6$ may make normal metabolizer resemble poor metabolizer leading to higher than expected plasma concentrations of TCA with resultant toxicity). Products include:
Quinaglute Dura-Tabs Tablets 644

Quinidine Polygalacturonate (Concurrent use with drugs that inhibit cytochrome $P_{450}IID_6$ may make normal metabolizer resemble poor metabolizer leading to higher than expected plasma concentrations of TCA with resultant toxicity). Products include:
Cardioquin Tablets 2146

Quinidine Sulfate (Concurrent use with drugs that inhibit cytochrome $P_{450}IID_6$ may make normal metabolizer resemble poor metabolizer leading to higher than expected plasma concentrations of TCA with resultant toxicity). Products include:
Quinidex Extentabs 2240

Scopolamine (Caution is advised when co-administered due to doxepine-induced anticholinergic effects). Products include:
Transderm Scōp Transdermal Therapeutic System 890

Scopolamine Hydrobromide (Caution is advised when co-administered due to doxepine-induced anticholinergic effects). Products include:
Atrohist Plus Tablets 1605
Donnatal 2234
Donnatal Extentabs 2234
Donnatal Tablets 2234

Selegiline Hydrochloride (Concurrent use is not recommended; potential for serious adverse effects). Products include:
Eldepryl Capsules 2729

Sertraline Hydrochloride (Concurrent use with drugs that are substrate for cytochrome $P_{450}IID_6$ may make normal metabolizer resemble poor metabolizer leading to higher than expected plasma concentrations of TCA with resultant toxicity; due to variation in the extent of inhibition of $P_{450}IID_6$ caution is indicated if co-administered sufficient time must elapse). Products include:
Zoloft Tablets 2051

Thioridazine Hydrochloride (Concurrent use with drugs that are substrate for cytochrome $P_{450}IID_6$ may make normal metabolizer resemble poor metabolizer leading to higher than expected plasma concentrations of TCA with resultant toxicity). Products include:
Mellaril 2398

Tolazamide (A case of severe hypoglycemia has been reported in a type II diabetic patient maintained on tolazamide (1 gm/day) 11 days after the addition of doxepin (75 mg/day)).
No products indexed under this heading.

Tranylcypromine Sulfate (Concurrent use is not recommended; potential for serious adverse effects). Products include:
Parnate Tablets 2679

Trazodone Hydrochloride (Concurrent use with drugs that are substrate for cytochrome $P_{450}IID_6$ may make normal metabolizer resemble poor metabolizer leading to higher than expected plasma concentrations of TCA with resultant toxicity). Products include:
Desyrel and Desyrel Dividose 504

IMPORTANT NOTE: Always consult each drug listing in the patient's regimen for possible interactions.

Sinequan

Tridihexethyl Chloride (Caution is advised when co-administered due to doxepine-induced anticholinergic effects).
   No products indexed under this heading.

Trifluoperazine Hydrochloride (Concurrent use with drugs that are substrate for cytochrome $P_{450}IID_6$ may make normal metabolizer resemble poor metabolizer leading to higher than expected plasma concentrations of TCA with resultant toxicity). Products include:
   Stelazine 2692

Trihexyphenidyl Hydrochloride (Caution is advised when co-administered due to doxepine-induced anticholinergic effects). Products include:
   Artane 1418

Trimipramine Maleate (Concurrent use with drugs that are substrate for cytochrome $P_{450}IID_6$ may make normal metabolizer resemble poor metabolizer leading to higher than expected plasma concentrations of TCA with resultant toxicity). Products include:
   Surmontil Capsules 2917

Venlafaxine Hydrochloride (Concurrent use with drugs that are substrate for cytochrome $P_{450}IID_6$ may make normal metabolizer resemble poor metabolizer leading to higher than expected plasma concentrations of TCA with resultant toxicity; due to variation in the extent of inhibition of $P_{450}IID_6$ caution is indicated if co-administered). Products include:
   Effexor 2825

Food Interactions
Alcohol (Doxepin may enhance the response to alcohol).

SINEQUAN ORAL CONCENTRATE
(Doxepin Hydrochloride) 2028
   See **Sinequan Capsules**

SINGLET TABLETS
(Acetaminophen, Chlorpheniramine Maleate, Pseudoephedrine Hydrochloride) .... ⊞ 785
May interact with hypnotics and sedatives, tranquilizers, monoamine oxidase inhibitors, and certain other agents. Compounds in these categories include:

Alprazolam (May increase drowsiness effect). Products include:
   Xanax Tablets 2115

Buspirone Hydrochloride (May increase drowsiness effect). Products include:
   BuSpar Tablets 738

Chlordiazepoxide (May increase drowsiness effect). Products include:
   Limbitrol 2333

Chlordiazepoxide Hydrochloride (May increase drowsiness effect). Products include:
   Librax Capsules 2330
   Librium Capsules 2331
   Librium Injectable 2332

Chlorpromazine (May increase drowsiness effect). Products include:
   Thorazine Suppositories 2701

Chlorpromazine Hydrochloride (May increase drowsiness effect). Products include:
   Thorazine 2701

Chlorprothixene (May increase drowsiness effect).
   No products indexed under this heading.

Interactions Index

Chlorprothixene Hydrochloride (May increase drowsiness effect).
   No products indexed under this heading.

Clorazepate Dipotassium (May increase drowsiness effect). Products include:
   Tranxene 459

Diazepam (May increase drowsiness effect). Products include:
   Dizac (diazepam injectable emulsion) CIV 1862
   Valium Injectable 2336
   Valium Tablets 2335

Droperidol (May increase drowsiness effect). Products include:
   Inapsine Injection 462

Estazolam (May increase drowsiness effect). Products include:
   ProSom Tablets 457

Ethchlorvynol (May increase drowsiness effect). Products include:
   Placidyl Capsules 456

Ethinamate (May increase drowsiness effect).
   No products indexed under this heading.

Fluphenazine Decanoate (May increase drowsiness effect). Products include:
   Prolixin Decanoate 510

Fluphenazine Enanthate (May increase drowsiness effect). Products include:
   Prolixin Enanthate 510

Fluphenazine Hydrochloride (May increase drowsiness effect). Products include:
   Prolixin 510

Flurazepam Hydrochloride (May increase drowsiness effect). Products include:
   Dalmane Capsules 2329

Furazolidone (Concurrent and/or sequential use is not recommended). Products include:
   Furoxone 2221

Glutethimide (May increase drowsiness effect).
   No products indexed under this heading.

Haloperidol (May increase drowsiness effect). Products include:
   Haldol Injection, Tablets and Concentrate 1585

Haloperidol Decanoate (May increase drowsiness effect). Products include:
   Haldol Decanoate 1587

Hydroxyzine Hydrochloride (May increase drowsiness effect). Products include:
   Atarax Tablets & Syrup 1992
   Marax Tablets & DF Syrup 2015
   Vistaril Intramuscular Solution 2042

Isocarboxazid (Concurrent and/or sequential use is not recommended).
   No products indexed under this heading.

Lorazepam (May increase drowsiness effect). Products include:
   Ativan Injection 2805
   Ativan Tablets 2807

Loxapine Hydrochloride (May increase drowsiness effect). Products include:
   Loxitane 1426

Loxapine Succinate (May increase drowsiness effect). Products include:
   Loxitane Capsules 1426

Meprobamate (May increase drowsiness effect). Products include:
   Miltown Tablets 2780
   PMB 200 and PMB 400 2890

Mesoridazine Besylate (May increase drowsiness effect). Products include:
   Serentil 689

Midazolam Hydrochloride (May increase drowsiness effect). Products include:
   Versed Injection 2324

Molindone Hydrochloride (May increase drowsiness effect). Products include:
   Moban Tablets and Concentrate 1036

Nisoldipine (Effect not specified). Products include:
   Sular Tablets 2961

Nitroglycerin (Effect not specified). Products include:
   Deponit NTG Transdermal Delivery System 2541
   Nitro-Bid IV 1270
   Nitro-Bid Ointment 1272
   Nitro-Dur (nitroglycerin) Transdermal Infusion System 1365
   Nitrolingual Spray 2193
   Nitrostat Tablets 1981
   Transderm-Nitro Transdermal Therapeutic System 878

Nortriptyline Hydrochloride (Effect not specified). Products include:
   Pamelor 2409

Oxazepam (Increases drowsiness effect). Products include:
   Serax Capsules 2916
   Serax Tablets 2916

Paroxetine Hydrochloride (Effect not specified). Products include:
   Paxil Tablets 2681

Penbutolol Sulfate (Effect not specified). Products include:
   Levatol Tablets 2547

Perphenazine (Increases drowsiness effect). Products include:
   Etrafon 2495
   Triavil Tablets 1800
   Trilafon 2532

Phenelzine Sulfate (Concurrent and/or sequential use is not recommended). Products include:
   Nardil 1977

Prazepam (May increase drowsiness effect).
   No products indexed under this heading.

Prochlorperazine (May increase drowsiness effect). Products include:
   Compazine 2644

Promethazine Hydrochloride (May increase drowsiness effect). Products include:
   Mepergan Injection 2859
   Phenergan with Codeine 2883
   Phenergan with Dextromethorphan 2885
   Phenergan Injection 2880
   Phenergan Suppositories 2882
   Phenergan Syrup 2881
   Phenergan Tablets 2882
   Phenergan VC 2886
   Phenergan VC with Codeine .. 2888

Propofol (May increase drowsiness effect). Products include:
   Diprivan Injectable Emulsion 2939

Quazepam (May increase drowsiness effect). Products include:
   Doral Tablets 2773

Secobarbital Sodium (May increase drowsiness effect). Products include:
   Seconal Sodium Pulvules 1529

Selegiline Hydrochloride (Concurrent and/or sequential use is not recommended). Products include:
   Eldepryl Capsules 2729

Temazepam (May increase drowsiness effect). Products include:
   Restoril Capsules 2413

Thioridazine Hydrochloride (May increase drowsiness effect). Products include:
   Mellaril 2398

Thiothixene (May increase drowsiness effect). Products include:
   Navane Capsules and Concentrate 2018
   Navane Intramuscular 2019

Tranylcypromine Sulfate (Concurrent and/or sequential use is not recommended). Products include:
   Parnate Tablets 2679

Triazolam (May increase drowsiness effect). Products include:
   Halcion Tablets 2093

Trifluoperazine Hydrochloride (May increase drowsiness effect). Products include:
   Stelazine 2692

Zolpidem Tartrate (May increase drowsiness effect). Products include:
   Ambien Tablets 2559

Food Interactions
Alcohol (May increase drowsiness effect).

SINULIN TABLETS
(Acetaminophen, Phenylpropanolamine Hydrochloride, Chlorpheniramine Maleate) 792
May interact with antihypertensives, antidepressant drugs, tranquilizers, hypnotics and sedatives, and certain other agents. Compounds in these categories include:

Acebutolol Hydrochloride (Effects not specified). Products include:
   Sectral Capsules 2914

Alprazolam (May increase drowsiness effect). Products include:
   Xanax Tablets 2115

Amitriptyline Hydrochloride (Effects not specified). Products include:
   Elavil 2945
   Etrafon 2495
   Limbitrol 2333
   Triavil Tablets 1800

Amlodipine Besylate (Effects not specified). Products include:
   Lotrel Capsules 858
   Norvasc Tablets 2020

Amoxapine (Effects not specified). Products include:
   Asendin Tablets 1419

Atenolol (Effects not specified). Products include:
   Tenoretic Tablets 2963
   Tenormin Tablets and I.V. Injection 2965

Benazepril Hydrochloride (Effects not specified). Products include:
   Lotensin Tablets 852
   Lotensin HCT Tablets 855
   Lotrel Capsules 858

Betaxolol Hydrochloride (Effects not specified). Products include:
   Betoptic Ophthalmic Solution 465
   Betoptic S Ophthalmic Suspension 467
   Kerlone Tablets 2588

Bisoprolol Fumarate (Effects not specified). Products include:
   Zebeta Tablets 1457
   Ziac 1459

Bupropion Hydrochloride (Effects not specified). Products include:
   Wellbutrin Tablets 1177

Buspirone Hydrochloride (May increase drowsiness effect). Products include:
   BuSpar Tablets 738

Captopril (Effects not specified). Products include:
   Capoten Tablets 740
   Capozide Tablets 744

(⊞ Described in PDR For Nonprescription Drugs)   (⊚ Described in PDR For Ophthalmology)

993 Interactions Index Sinulin

Carteolol Hydrochloride (Effects not specified). Products include:
- Cartrol Tablets ... 413
- Ocupress Ophthalmic Solution, 1% Sterile ... ◉ 297

Chlordiazepoxide (May increase drowsiness effect). Products include:
- Limbitrol ... 2333

Chlordiazepoxide Hydrochloride (May increase drowsiness effect). Products include:
- Librax Capsules ... 2330
- Librium Capsules ... 2331
- Librium Injectable ... 2332

Chlorpromazine (May increase drowsiness effect). Products include:
- Thorazine Suppositories ... 2701

Chlorpromazine Hydrochloride (May increase drowsiness effect). Products include:
- Thorazine ... 2701

Chlorprothixene (May increase drowsiness effect).
- No products indexed under this heading.

Chlorprothixene Hydrochloride (May increase drowsiness effect).
- No products indexed under this heading.

Clonidine (Effects not specified). Products include:
- Catapres-TTS ... 680

Clonidine Hydrochloride (Effects not specified). Products include:
- Catapres Tablets ... 679
- Combipres Tablets ... 682

Clorazepate Dipotassium (May increase drowsiness effect). Products include:
- Tranxene ... 459

Deserpidine (Effects not specified).
- No products indexed under this heading.

Desipramine Hydrochloride (Effects not specified). Products include:
- Norpramin Tablets ... 1273

Diazepam (May increase drowsiness effect). Products include:
- Dizac (diazepam injectable emulsion) CIV ... 1862
- Valium Injectable ... 2336
- Valium Tablets ... 2335

Diazoxide (Effects not specified). Products include:
- Hyperstat I.V. Injection ... 2504
- Proglycem ... 575

Diltiazem Hydrochloride (Effects not specified). Products include:
- Cardizem CD Capsules ... 1251
- Cardizem SR Capsules ... 1255
- Cardizem Injectable ... 1253
- Cardizem Tablets ... 1257
- Dilacor XR Extended-release Capsules ... 2183
- Tiazac Capsules ... 1019

Doxazosin Mesylate (Effects not specified). Products include:
- Cardura Tablets ... 1993

Doxepin Hydrochloride (Effects not specified). Products include:
- Adapin Capsules ... 1542
- Sinequan ... 2028
- Zonalon Cream ... 1042

Droperidol (May increase drowsiness effect). Products include:
- Inapsine Injection ... 462

Enalapril Maleate (Effects not specified). Products include:
- Vaseretic Tablets ... 1810
- Vasotec Tablets ... 1816

Enalaprilat (Effects not specified). Products include:
- Vasotec I.V. ... 1814

Esmolol Hydrochloride (Effects not specified). Products include:
- Brevibloc (esmolol HCl) Injection ... 1860

Estazolam (May increase drowsiness effect). Products include:
- ProSom Tablets ... 457

Ethchlorvynol (May increase drowsiness effect). Products include:
- Placidyl Capsules ... 456

Ethinamate (May increase drowsiness effect).
- No products indexed under this heading.

Felodipine (Effects not specified). Products include:
- Plendil Extended-Release Tablets ... 514

Fluoxetine Hydrochloride (Effects not specified). Products include:
- Prozac Pulvules & Liquid, Oral Solution ... 935

Fluphenazine Decanoate (May increase drowsiness effect). Products include:
- Prolixin Decanoate ... 510

Fluphenazine Enanthate (May increase drowsiness effect). Products include:
- Prolixin Enanthate ... 510

Fluphenazine Hydrochloride (May increase drowsiness effect). Products include:
- Prolixin ... 510

Flurazepam Hydrochloride (May increase drowsiness effect). Products include:
- Dalmane Capsules ... 2329

Fosinopril Sodium (Effects not specified). Products include:
- Monopril Tablets ... 762

Glutethimide (May increase drowsiness effect).
- No products indexed under this heading.

Guanabenz Acetate (Effects not specified).
- No products indexed under this heading.

Guanethidine Monosulfate (Effects not specified). Products include:
- Esimil Tablets ... 840
- Ismelin Tablets ... 845

Haloperidol (May increase drowsiness effect). Products include:
- Haldol Injection, Tablets and Concentrate ... 1585

Haloperidol Decanoate (May increase drowsiness effect). Products include:
- Haldol Decanoate ... 1587

Hydralazine Hydrochloride (Effects not specified). Products include:
- Apresazide Capsules ... 824
- Apresoline Hydrochloride Tablets ... 826
- Hydralazine Hydrochloride Injection USP ... 2712
- Ser-Ap-Es Tablets ... 867

Hydroxyzine Hydrochloride (May increase drowsiness effect). Products include:
- Atarax Tablets & Syrup ... 1992
- Marax Tablets & DF Syrup ... 2015
- Vistaril Intramuscular Solution ... 2042

Imipramine Hydrochloride (Effects not specified). Products include:
- Tofranil Ampuls ... 873
- Tofranil Tablets ... 875

Imipramine Pamoate (Effects not specified). Products include:
- Tofranil-PM Capsules ... 876

Indapamide (Effects not specified).
- No products indexed under this heading.

Isocarboxazid (Effects not specified).
- No products indexed under this heading.

Isradipine (Effects not specified). Products include:
- DynaCirc Capsules ... 2381
- DynaCirc CR Tablets ... 2383

Labetalol Hydrochloride (Effects not specified). Products include:
- Normodyne Injection ... 2519
- Normodyne Tablets ... 2522
- Trandate ... 1158

Lisinopril (Effects not specified). Products include:
- Prinivil Tablets ... 1776
- Prinzide Tablets ... 1780
- Zestoretic Tablets ... 2968
- Zestril Tablets ... 2972

Lorazepam (May increase drowsiness effect). Products include:
- Ativan Injection ... 2805
- Ativan Tablets ... 2807

Losartan Potassium (Effects not specified). Products include:
- Cozaar Tablets ... 1668
- Hyzaar Tablets ... 1720

Loxapine Hydrochloride (May increase drowsiness effect). Products include:
- Loxitane ... 1426

Loxapine Succinate (May increase drowsiness effect). Products include:
- Loxitane Capsules ... 1426

Maprotiline Hydrochloride (Effects not specified). Products include:
- Ludiomil Tablets ... 861

Mecamylamine Hydrochloride (Effects not specified). Products include:
- Inversine Tablets ... 1729

Meprobamate (May increase drowsiness effect). Products include:
- Miltown Tablets ... 2780
- PMB 200 and PMB 400 ... 2890

Mesoridazine Besylate (May increase drowsiness effect). Products include:
- Serentil ... 689

Methyclothiazide (Effects not specified). Products include:
- Enduron Tablets ... 424

Methyldopa (Effects not specified). Products include:
- Aldoclor Tablets ... 1638
- Aldomet Oral ... 1640
- Aldoril Tablets ... 1644

Methyldopate Hydrochloride (Effects not specified). Products include:
- Aldomet Ester HCl Injection ... 1642

Metolazone (Effects not specified). Products include:
- Mykrox Tablets ... 1617
- Zaroxolyn Tablets ... 1625

Metoprolol Succinate (Effects not specified). Products include:
- Toprol-XL Tablets ... 560

Metoprolol Tartrate (Effects not specified). Products include:
- Lopressor ... 848
- Lopressor HCT Tablets ... 850

Metyrosine (Effects not specified). Products include:
- Demser Capsules ... 1690

Midazolam Hydrochloride (May increase drowsiness effect). Products include:
- Versed Injection ... 2324

Minoxidil (Effects not specified).
- No products indexed under this heading.

Moexipril Hydrochloride (Effects not specified). Products include:
- Univasc Tablets ... 2553

Molindone Hydrochloride (May increase drowsiness effect). Products include:
- Moban Tablets and Concentrate ... 1036

Nadolol (Effects not specified).
- No products indexed under this heading.

Nefazodone Hydrochloride (Effects not specified). Products include:
- Serzone Tablets ... 776

Nicardipine Hydrochloride (Effects not specified). Products include:
- Cardene Capsules ... 2261
- Cardene I.V. ... 2815
- Cardene SR Capsules ... 2264

Nifedipine (Effects not specified). Products include:
- Adalat Capsules (10 mg and 20 mg) ... 580
- Adalat CC ... 582
- Procardia Capsules ... 2024
- Procardia XL Extended Release Tablets ... 2026

Nisoldipine (Effects not specified). Products include:
- Sular Tablets ... 2961

Nitroglycerin (Effects not specified). Products include:
- Deponit NTG Transdermal Delivery System ... 2541
- Nitro-Bid IV ... 1270
- Nitro-Bid Ointment ... 1272
- Nitro-Dur (nitroglycerin) Transdermal Infusion System ... 1365
- Nitrolingual Spray ... 2193
- Nitrostat Tablets ... 1981
- Transderm-Nitro Transdermal Therapeutic System ... 878

Nortriptyline Hydrochloride (Effects not specified). Products include:
- Pamelor ... 2409

Oxazepam (May increase drowsiness effect). Products include:
- Serax Capsules ... 2916
- Serax Tablets ... 2916

Paroxetine Hydrochloride (Effects not specified). Products include:
- Paxil Tablets ... 2681

Penbutolol Sulfate (Effects not specified). Products include:
- Levatol Tablets ... 2547

Perphenazine (May increase drowsiness effect). Products include:
- Etrafon ... 2495
- Triavil Tablets ... 1800
- Trilafon ... 2532

Phenelzine Sulfate (Effects not specified). Products include:
- Nardil ... 1977

Phenoxybenzamine Hydrochloride (Effects not specified). Products include:
- Dibenzyline Capsules ... 2650

Phentolamine Mesylate (Effects not specified). Products include:
- Regitine Vials ... 864

Pindolol (Effects not specified). Products include:
- Visken Tablets ... 2428

Prazepam (May increase drowsiness effect).
- No products indexed under this heading.

Prazosin Hydrochloride (Effects not specified). Products include:
- Minipress Capsules ... 2015
- Minizide Capsules ... 2016

Prochlorperazine (May increase drowsiness effect). Products include:
- Compazine ... 2644

IMPORTANT NOTE: Always consult each drug listing in the patient's regimen for possible interactions.

Promethazine Hydrochloride
(May increase drowsiness effect).
Products include:
  Mepergan Injection 2859
  Phenergan with Codeine 2883
  Phenergan with Dextromethorphan 2885
  Phenergan Injection 2880
  Phenergan Suppositories 2882
  Phenergan Syrup 2881
  Phenergan Tablets 2882
  Phenergan VC 2886
  Phenergan VC with Codeine 2888

Propofol (May increase drowsiness effect). Products include:
  Diprivan Injectable Emulsion 2939

Propranolol Hydrochloride (Effects not specified). Products include:
  Inderal 2834
  Inderal LA Long Acting Capsules 2836
  Inderide Tablets 2838
  Inderide LA Long Acting Capsules .. 2840

Protriptyline Hydrochloride (Effects not specified). Products include:
  Vivactil Tablets 1820

Quazepam (May increase drowsiness effect). Products include:
  Doral Tablets 2773

Quinapril Hydrochloride (Effects not specified). Products include:
  Accupril Tablets 1950

Ramipril (Effects not specified). Products include:
  Altace Capsules 1238

Rauwolfia Serpentina (Effects not specified).
  No products indexed under this heading.

Rescinnamine (Effects not specified).
  No products indexed under this heading.

Reserpine (Effects not specified). Products include:
  Diupres Tablets 1691
  Hydropres Tablets 1718
  Ser-Ap-Es Tablets 867

Secobarbital Sodium (May increase drowsiness effect). Products include:
  Seconal Sodium Pulvules 1529

Sertraline Hydrochloride (Effects not specified). Products include:
  Zoloft Tablets 2051

Sodium Nitroprusside (Effects not specified).
  No products indexed under this heading.

Sotalol Hydrochloride (Effects not specified). Products include:
  Betapace Tablets 637

Spirapril Hydrochloride (Effects not specified).
  No products indexed under this heading.

Temazepam (May increase drowsiness effect). Products include:
  Restoril Capsules 2413

Terazosin Hydrochloride (Effects not specified). Products include:
  Hytrin Capsules 434

Thioridazine Hydrochloride (May increase drowsiness effect). Products include:
  Mellaril 2398

Thiothixene (May increase drowsiness effect). Products include:
  Navane Capsules and Concentrate 2018
  Navane Intramuscular 2019

Timolol Maleate (Effects not specified). Products include:
  Blocadren Tablets 1654
  Timolide Tablets 1791
  Timoptic in Ocudose 1796
  Timoptic Sterile Ophthalmic Solution .. 1794
  Timoptic-XE 1798

Torsemide (Effects not specified). Products include:
  Demadex Tablets and Injection ... 691

Tranylcypromine Sulfate (Effects not specified). Products include:
  Parnate Tablets 2679

Trazodone Hydrochloride (Effects not specified). Products include:
  Desyrel and Desyrel Dividose 504

Triazolam (May increase drowsiness effect). Products include:
  Halcion Tablets 2093

Trifluoperazine Hydrochloride (May increase drowsiness effect). Products include:
  Stelazine 2692

Trimethaphan Camsylate (Effects not specified).
  No products indexed under this heading.

Trimipramine Maleate (Effects not specified). Products include:
  Surmontil Capsules 2917

Venlafaxine Hydrochloride (Effects not specified). Products include:
  Effexor 2825

Verapamil Hydrochloride (Effects not specified). Products include:
  Calan SR Caplets 2571
  Calan Tablets 2568
  Covera-HS Tablets 2573
  Isoptin Injectable 1391
  Isoptin Oral Tablets 1393
  Isoptin SR Tablets 1395
  Verelan Capsules 1455

Zolpidem Tartrate (May increase drowsiness effect). Products include:
  Ambien Tablets 2559

Food Interactions

Alcohol (Increased drowsiness).

SINUTAB NON-DRYING LIQUID CAPS
(Pseudoephedrine Hydrochloride, Guaifenesin) .... ⊡ 823
May interact with monoamine oxidase inhibitors. Compounds in this category include:

Furazolidone (Concurrent and/or sequential use not recommended). Products include:
  Furoxone 2221

Isocarboxazid (Concurrent and/or sequential use not recommended).
  No products indexed under this heading.

Phenelzine Sulfate (Concurrent and/or sequential use not recommended). Products include:
  Nardil 1977

Selegiline Hydrochloride (Concurrent and/or sequential use not recommended). Products include:
  Eldepryl Capsules 2729

Tranylcypromine Sulfate (Concurrent and/or sequential use not recommended). Products include:
  Parnate Tablets 2679

SINUTAB SINUS ALLERGY MEDICATION, MAXIMUM STRENGTH TABLETS AND CAPLETS
(Acetaminophen, Chlorpheniramine Maleate, Pseudoephedrine Hydrochloride) .... ⊡ 823
May interact with monoamine oxidase inhibitors, hypnotics and sedatives, tranquilizers, and certain other agents. Compounds in these categories include:

Alprazolam (May increase drowsiness effect). Products include:
  Xanax Tablets 2115

Buspirone Hydrochloride (May increase drowsiness effect). Products include:
  BuSpar Tablets 738

Chlordiazepoxide (May increase drowsiness effect). Products include:
  Limbitrol 2333

Chlordiazepoxide Hydrochloride (May increase drowsiness effect). Products include:
  Librax Capsules 2330
  Librium Capsules 2331
  Librium Injectable 2332

Chlorpromazine (May increase drowsiness effect). Products include:
  Thorazine Suppositories 2701

Chlorpromazine Hydrochloride (May increase drowsiness effect). Products include:
  Thorazine 2701

Chlorprothixene (May increase drowsiness effect).
  No products indexed under this heading.

Chlorprothixene Hydrochloride (May increase drowsiness effect). Products include:
  No products indexed under this heading.

Clorazepate Dipotassium (May increase drowsiness effect). Products include:
  Tranxene 459

Diazepam (May increase drowsiness effect). Products include:
  Dizac (diazepam injectable emulsion) CIV 1862
  Valium Injectable 2336
  Valium Tablets 2335

Droperidol (May increase drowsiness effect). Products include:
  Inapsine Injection 462

Estazolam (May increase drowsiness effect). Products include:
  ProSom Tablets 457

Ethchlorvynol (May increase drowsiness effect). Products include:
  Placidyl Capsules 456

Ethinamate (May increase drowsiness effect).
  No products indexed under this heading.

Fluphenazine Decanoate (May increase drowsiness effect). Products include:
  Prolixin Decanoate 510

Fluphenazine Enanthate (May increase drowsiness effect). Products include:
  Prolixin Enanthate 510

Fluphenazine Hydrochloride (May increase drowsiness effect). Products include:
  Prolixin 510

Flurazepam Hydrochloride (May increase drowsiness effect). Products include:
  Dalmane Capsules 2329

Furazolidone (Concurrent and/or sequential use is not recommended). Products include:
  Furoxone 2221

Glutethimide (May increase drowsiness effect).
  No products indexed under this heading.

Haloperidol (May increase drowsiness effect). Products include:
  Haldol Injection, Tablets and Concentrate 1585

Haloperidol Decanoate (May increase drowsiness effect). Products include:
  Haldol Decanoate 1587

Hydroxyzine Hydrochloride (May increase drowsiness effect). Products include:
  Atarax Tablets & Syrup 1992
  Marax Tablets & DF Syrup 2015
  Vistaril Intramuscular Solution .. 2042

Isocarboxazid (Concurrent and/or sequential use is not recommended).
  No products indexed under this heading.

Lorazepam (May increase drowsiness effect). Products include:
  Ativan Injection 2805
  Ativan Tablets 2807

Loxapine Hydrochloride (May increase drowsiness effect). Products include:
  Loxitane 1426

Loxapine Succinate (May increase drowsiness effect). Products include:
  Loxitane Capsules 1426

Meprobamate (May increase drowsiness effect). Products include:
  Miltown Tablets 2780
  PMB 200 and PMB 400 2890

Mesoridazine Besylate (May increase drowsiness effect). Products include:
  Serentil 689

Midazolam Hydrochloride (May increase drowsiness effect). Products include:
  Versed Injection 2324

Molindone Hydrochloride (May increase drowsiness effect). Products include:
  Moban Tablets and Concentrate 1036

Oxazepam (May increase drowsiness effect). Products include:
  Serax Capsules 2916
  Serax Tablets 2916

Perphenazine (May increase drowsiness effect). Products include:
  Etrafon 2495
  Triavil Tablets 1800
  Trilafon 2532

Phenelzine Sulfate (Concurrent and/or sequential use is not recommended). Products include:
  Nardil 1977

Prazepam (May increase drowsiness effect).
  No products indexed under this heading.

Prochlorperazine (May increase drowsiness effect). Products include:
  Compazine 2644

Promethazine Hydrochloride (May increase drowsiness effect). Products include:
  Mepergan Injection 2859
  Phenergan with Codeine 2883
  Phenergan with Dextromethorphan 2885
  Phenergan Injection 2880
  Phenergan Suppositories 2882
  Phenergan Syrup 2881
  Phenergan Tablets 2882
  Phenergan VC 2886
  Phenergan VC with Codeine 2888

Propofol (May increase drowsiness effect). Products include:
  Diprivan Injectable Emulsion 2939

Quazepam (May increase drowsiness effect). Products include:
  Doral Tablets 2773

Secobarbital Sodium (May increase drowsiness effect). Products include:
  Seconal Sodium Pulvules 1529

Selegiline Hydrochloride (Concurrent and/or sequential use is not recommended). Products include:
  Eldepryl Capsules 2729

(⊡ Described in PDR For Nonprescription Drugs) (⊚ Described in PDR For Ophthalmology)

Temazepam (May increase drowsiness effect). Products include:
Restoril Capsules 2413
Thioridazine Hydrochloride (May increase drowsiness effect). Products include:
Mellaril 2398
Thiothixene (May increase drowsiness effect). Products include:
Navane Capsules and Concentrate 2018
Navane Intramuscular 2019
Tranylcypromine Sulfate (Concurrent and/or sequential use is not recommended). Products include:
Parnate Tablets 2679
Triazolam (May increase drowsiness effect). Products include:
Halcion Tablets 2093
Trifluoperazine Hydrochloride (May increase drowsiness effect). Products include:
Stelazine 2692
Zolpidem Tartrate (May increase drowsiness effect). Products include:
Ambien Tablets 2559

Food Interactions
Alcohol (May increase drowsiness effect).

SINUTAB SINUS MEDICATION, MAXIMUM STRENGTH WITHOUT DROWSINESS FORMULA, TABLETS & CAPLETS
(Acetaminophen, Pseudoephedrine Hydrochloride) 824
May interact with monoamine oxidase inhibitors. Compounds in this category include:

Furazolidone (Concurrent and/or sequential use is not recommended). Products include:
Furoxone 2221
Isocarboxazid (Concurrent and/or sequential use is not recommended).
No products indexed under this heading.
Phenelzine Sulfate (Concurrent and/or sequential use is not recommended). Products include:
Nardil 1977
Selegiline Hydrochloride (Concurrent and/or sequential use is not recommended). Products include:
Eldepryl Capsules 2729
Tranylcypromine Sulfate (Concurrent and/or sequential use is not recommended). Products include:
Parnate Tablets 2679

SKELAXIN TABLETS
(Metaxalone) 793
None cited in PDR database.

SLEEPINAL NIGHT-TIME SLEEP AID CAPSULES AND SOFTGELS
(Diphenhydramine Hydrochloride) .. 798
May interact with hypnotics and sedatives, tranquilizers, and certain other agents. Compounds in these categories include:

Alprazolam (Concomitant use is not recommended). Products include:
Xanax Tablets 2115
Buspirone Hydrochloride (Concomitant use is not recommended). Products include:
BuSpar Tablets 738
Chlordiazepoxide (Concomitant use is not recommended). Products include:
Limbitrol 2333

Chlordiazepoxide Hydrochloride (Concomitant use is not recommended). Products include:
Librax Capsules 2330
Librium Capsules 2331
Librium Injectable 2332
Chlorpromazine (Concomitant use is not recommended). Products include:
Thorazine Suppositories 2701
Chlorprothixene (Concomitant use is not recommended).
No products indexed under this heading.
Chlorprothixene Hydrochloride (Concomitant use is not recommended).
No products indexed under this heading.
Clorazepate Dipotassium (Concomitant use is not recommended). Products include:
Tranxene 459
Diazepam (Concomitant use is not recommended). Products include:
Dizac (diazepam injectable emulsion) CIV 1862
Valium Injectable 2336
Valium Tablets 2335
Droperidol (Concomitant use is not recommended). Products include:
Inapsine Injection 462
Estazolam (Concomitant use is not recommended). Products include:
ProSom Tablets 457
Ethchlorvynol (Concomitant use is not recommended). Products include:
Placidyl Capsules 456
Ethinamate (Concomitant use is not recommended).
No products indexed under this heading.
Fluphenazine Decanoate (Concomitant use is not recommended). Products include:
Prolixin Decanoate 510
Fluphenazine Enanthate (Concomitant use is not recommended). Products include:
Prolixin Enanthate 510
Fluphenazine Hydrochloride (Concomitant use is not recommended). Products include:
Prolixin 510
Flurazepam Hydrochloride (Concomitant use is not recommended). Products include:
Dalmane Capsules 2329
Glutethimide (Concomitant use is not recommended).
No products indexed under this heading.
Haloperidol (Concomitant use is not recommended). Products include:
Haldol Injection, Tablets and Concentrate 1585
Haloperidol Decanoate (Concomitant use is not recommended). Products include:
Haldol Decanoate 1587
Hydroxyzine Hydrochloride (Concomitant use is not recommended). Products include:
Atarax Tablets & Syrup 1992
Marax Tablets & DF Syrup 2015
Vistaril Intramuscular Solution 2042
Lorazepam (Concomitant use is not recommended). Products include:
Ativan Injection 2805
Ativan Tablets 2807
Loxapine Hydrochloride (Concomitant use is not recommended). Products include:
Loxitane 1426

Loxapine Succinate (Concomitant use is not recommended). Products include:
Loxitane Capsules 1426
Meprobamate (Concomitant use is not recommended). Products include:
Miltown Tablets 2780
PMB 200 and PMB 400 2890
Mesoridazine Besylate (Concomitant use is not recommended). Products include:
Serentil 689
Midazolam Hydrochloride (Concomitant use is not recommended). Products include:
Versed Injection 2324
Molindone Hydrochloride (Concomitant use is not recommended). Products include:
Moban Tablets and Concentrate 1036
Oxazepam (Concomitant use is not recommended). Products include:
Serax Capsules 2916
Serax Tablets 2916
Perphenazine (Concomitant use is not recommended). Products include:
Etrafon 2495
Triavil Tablets 1800
Trilafon 2532
Prazepam (Concomitant use is not recommended).
No products indexed under this heading.
Prochlorperazine (Concomitant use is not recommended). Products include:
Compazine 2644
Promethazine Hydrochloride (Concomitant use is not recommended). Products include:
Mepergan Injection 2859
Phenergan with Codeine 2883
Phenergan with Dextromethorphan 2885
Phenergan Injection 2880
Phenergan Suppositories 2882
Phenergan Syrup 2881
Phenergan Tablets 2882
Phenergan VC 2886
Phenergan VC with Codeine 2888
Propofol (Concomitant use is not recommended). Products include:
Diprivan Injectable Emulsion 2939
Quazepam (Concomitant use is not recommended). Products include:
Doral Tablets 2773
Secobarbital Sodium (Concomitant use is not recommended). Products include:
Seconal Sodium Pulvules 1529
Temazepam (Concomitant use is not recommended). Products include:
Restoril Capsules 2413
Thioridazine Hydrochloride (Concomitant use is not recommended). Products include:
Mellaril 2398
Thiothixene (Concomitant use is not recommended). Products include:
Navane Capsules and Concentrate 2018
Navane Intramuscular 2019
Triazolam (Concomitant use is not recommended). Products include:
Halcion Tablets 2093
Trifluoperazine Hydrochloride (Concomitant use is not recommended). Products include:
Stelazine 2692
Zolpidem Tartrate (Concomitant use is not recommended). Products include:
Ambien Tablets 2559

Food Interactions
Alcohol (Avoid alcoholic beverages).

SLO-BID GYROCAPS
(Theophylline Anhydrous) 2201
May interact with sympathomimetic bronchodilators, macrolide antibiotics, oral contraceptives, corticosteroids, thiazides, beta$_2$ agonists, and certain other agents. Compounds in these categories include:

Albuterol (Possible toxic synergism; xanthines can potentiate hypokalemia resulting from beta$_2$ agonist therapy). Products include:
Proventil Inhalation Aerosol 2524
Ventolin Inhalation Aerosol and Refill 1170
Albuterol Sulfate (Possible toxic synergism; xanthines can potentiate hypokalemia resulting from beta$_2$ agonist therapy). Products include:
Airet Albuterol Sulfate Inhalation Solution 1602
Albuterol Sulfate, USP Solution for Inhalation, Arm-a-Med 522
Proventil Inhalation Solution 0.083% 2527
Proventil Repetabs Tablets 2529
Proventil Solution for Inhalation 0.5% 2525
Proventil Syrup 2528
Proventil Tablets 2529
Ventolin Inhalation Solution 1171
Ventolin Nebules Inhalation Solution 1172
Ventolin Rotacaps for Inhalation 1173
Ventolin Syrup 1175
Ventolin Tablets 1176
Volmax Extended-Release Tablets 1835
Allopurinol (Allopurinol in high doses increases serum theophylline levels). Products include:
Zyloprim Tablets 1194
Azithromycin (Increased theophylline serum concentrations). Products include:
Zithromax 2043
Zithromax Tablets 2046
Bendroflumethiazide (Xanthines can potentiate hypokalemic effects).
No products indexed under this heading.
Betamethasone Acetate (Xanthines can potentiate hypokalemic effects). Products include:
Celestone Soluspan Suspension 2484
Betamethasone Sodium Phosphate (Xanthines can potentiate hypokalemic effects). Products include:
Celestone Soluspan Suspension 2484
Bitolterol Mesylate (Possible toxic synergism; xanthines can potentiate hypokalemia resulting from beta$_2$ agonist therapy). Products include:
Tornalate Solution for Inhalation, 0.2% 976
Tornalate Metered Dose Inhaler 978
Chlorothiazide (Xanthines can potentiate hypokalemic effects). Products include:
Aldoclor Tablets 1638
Diupres Tablets 1691
Diuril Oral 1694
Chlorothiazide Sodium (Xanthines can potentiate hypokalemic effects). Products include:
Diuril Sodium Intravenous 1693
Cimetidine (Increased theophylline serum concentrations). Products include:
Tagamet HB Tablets 786
Tagamet Tablets 2694
Cimetidine Hydrochloride (Increased theophylline serum concentrations). Products include:
Tagamet 2694
Ciprofloxacin (Increased serum theophylline levels). Products include:
Cipro I.V. 587

IMPORTANT NOTE: Always consult each drug listing in the patient's regimen for possible interactions.

Slo-bid **Interactions Index** 996

Cipro I.V. Pharmacy Bulk Package.. 590

Ciprofloxacin Hydrochloride (Increased serum theophylline levels). Products include:

Ciloxan Ophthalmic Solution 468
Cipro Tablets 584

Clarithromycin (Increased theophylline serum concentrations). Products include:

Biaxin 406

Cortisone Acetate (Xanthines can potentiate hypokalemic effects). Products include:

Cortone Acetate Sterile Suspension 1663
Cortone Acetate Tablets 1664

Desogestrel (Increased serum theophylline levels). Products include:

Desogen Tablets 1867
Ortho-Cept 1907

Dexamethasone (Xanthines can potentiate hypokalemic effects). Products include:

AK-Trol Ointment & Suspension .... ⊙ 205
Decadron Elixir 1676
Decadron Tablets 1678
Decaspray Topical Aerosol 1689
Maxitrol Ophthalmic Ointment and Suspension .... ⊙ 222
TobraDex Ophthalmic Suspension and Ointment 469

Dexamethasone Acetate (Xanthines can potentiate hypokalemic effects). Products include:

Dalalone D.P. Injectable 1009
Decadron-LA Sterile Suspension 1687

Dexamethasone Sodium Phosphate (Xanthines can potentiate hypokalemic effects). Products include:

Decadron Phosphate Injection 1680
Decadron Phosphate Sterile Ophthalmic Ointment 1684
Decadron Phosphate Sterile Ophthalmic Solution 1685
Decadron Phosphate Topical Cream 1686
Decadron Phosphate with Xylocaine Injection, Sterile 1683
Dexacort Phosphate in Respihaler .. 1606
Dexacort Phosphate in Turbinaire .. 1607
NeoDecadron Sterile Ophthalmic Ointment 1755
NeoDecadron Sterile Ophthalmic Solution 1756
NeoDecadron Topical Cream 1757

Dirithromycin (Increased theophylline serum concentrations). Products include:

Dynabac 668

Ephedrine Hydrochloride (Possible toxic synergism; xanthines can potentiate hypokalemia resulting from $beta_2$ agonist therapy). Products include:

Primatene Tablets .... ▣ 844
Quadrinal Tablets 1398

Ephedrine Sulfate (Possible toxic synergism; xanthines can potentiate hypokalemia resulting from $beta_2$ agonist therapy). Products include:

Marax Tablets & DF Syrup 2015

Ephedrine Tannate (Possible toxic synergism; xanthines can potentiate hypokalemia resulting from $beta_2$ agonist therapy). Products include:

Rynatuss 2782

Epinephrine (Possible toxic synergism; xanthines can potentiate hypokalemia resulting from $beta_2$ agonist therapy). Products include:

EPIFRIN .... ⊙ 237
EpiPen 808
Marcaine with Epinephrine 2446
Primatene Mist .... ▣ 843
Sensorcaine with Epinephrine Injection 554
Sus-Phrine Injection 1017
Xylocaine with Epinephrine Injections 562

Epinephrine Hydrochloride (Possible toxic synergism; xanthines can potentiate hypokalemia resulting from $beta_2$ agonist therapy). Products include:

Ana-Kit Anaphylaxis Emergency Treatment Kit 611

Erythromycin (Increased theophylline serum concentrations). Products include:

A/T/S 2% Acne Topical Gel 1244
A/T/S 2% Acne Topical Solution 1244
Benzamycin Topical Gel 919
E-Mycin Tablets 1388
Emgel 2% Topical Gel 1081
ERYC 1972
Erycette (erythromycin 2%) Topical Solution 1943
Ery-Tab Tablets 426
Erythromycin Base Filmtab 430
Erythromycin Delayed-Release Capsules, USP 431
Ilotycin Ophthalmic Ointment 928
PCE Dispertab Tablets 453
T-Stat 2.0% Topical Solution and Pads 2797
THERAMYCIN Z 2% Solution 1629

Erythromycin Estolate (Increased theophylline serum concentrations). Products include:

Ilosone 927

Erythromycin Ethylsuccinate (Increased theophylline serum concentrations). Products include:

E.E.S. 427
EryPed 425
Pediazole Suspension 2340

Erythromycin Gluceptate (Increased theophylline serum concentrations). Products include:

Ilotycin Gluceptate, IV, Vials 929

Erythromycin Stearate (Increased theophylline serum concentrations). Products include:

Erythrocin Stearate Filmtab 429

Ethinyl Estradiol (Increased serum theophylline levels). Products include:

Brevicon 2563
Demulen 2580
Desogen Tablets 1867
Levlen/Tri-Levlen 646
Lo/Ovral Tablets 2852
Lo/Ovral-28 Tablets 2857
Modicon 1928
Nordette-21 Tablets 2863
Nordette-28 Tablets 2866
Norinyl 2563
Ortho-Cept 1907
Ortho-Cyclen/Ortho-Tri-Cyclen 1914
Ortho-Novum 1928
Ortho-Cyclen/Ortho Tri-Cyclen 1914
Ovcon 765
Ovral Tablets 2877
Ovral-28 Tablets 2878
Levlen/Tri-Levlen 646
Tri-Norinyl 2607
Triphasil-21 Tablets 2919
Triphasil-28 Tablets 2924

Ethylnorepinephrine Hydrochloride (Possible toxic synergism; xanthines can potentiate hypokalemia resulting from $beta_2$ agonist therapy).

No products indexed under this heading.

Ethynodiol Diacetate (Increased serum theophylline levels). Products include:

Demulen 2580

Fludrocortisone Acetate (Xanthines can potentiate hypokalemic effects). Products include:

Florinef Acetate Tablets 506

Hydrochlorothiazide (Xanthines can potentiate hypokalemic effects). Products include:

Aldactazide Tablets 2556
Aldoril Tablets 1644
Apresazide Capsules 824
Capozide Tablets 744
Dyazide Capsules 2653
Esidrix Tablets 839
Esimil Tablets 840
HydroDIURIL Tablets 1716
Hydropres Tablets 1718
Hyzaar Tablets 1720
Inderide Tablets 2838
Inderide LA Long Acting Capsules .. 2840
Lopressor HCT Tablets 850
Lotensin HCT Tablets 855
Moduretic Tablets 1748
Oretic Tablets 450
Prinzide Tablets 1780
Ser-Ap-Es Tablets 867
Timolide Tablets 1791
Vaseretic Tablets 1810
Zestoretic Tablets 2968
Ziac 1459

Hydrocortisone (Xanthines can potentiate hypokalemic effects). Products include:

Anusol-HC Cream 2.5% 1953
Aquanil HC Lotion 1989
Maximum Strength Cortaid Spray ▣ 800
CORTENEMA 2713
Cortisporin Ointment 1074
Cortisporin Ophthalmic Ointment Sterile 1074
Cortisporin Ophthalmic Suspension Sterile 1075
Cortisporin Otic Solution Sterile 1076
Cortisporin Otic Suspension Sterile 1077
Cortizone-5 .... ▣ 795
Cortizone-10 .... ▣ 795
Hydrocortone Tablets 1715
Hytone 922
Hytone Ointment 2 ½% 923
Massengill Medicated Soft Cloth Towelettes 2628
Pediotic Suspension Sterile 1140
Preparation H Hydrocortisone 1% Cream .... ▣ 843
ProctoCream-HC 2.5% 2552
VōSoL HC Otic Solution 2786

Hydrocortisone Acetate (Xanthines can potentiate hypokalemic effects). Products include:

Analpram-HC Rectal Cream 1% and 2.5% 993
Anusol HC-1 Hydrocortisone Anti-Itch Ointment .... ▣ 810
Anusol-HC Suppositories 1954
Caldecort Anti-Itch Hydrocortisone Cream .... ▣ 651
Coly-Mycin S Otic w/Neomycin & Hydrocortisone 1965
Cortaid .... ▣ 800
Cortifoam 2540
Cortisporin Cream 1073
Epifoam 2543
Hydrocortone Acetate Sterile Suspension 1712
Mantadil Cream 1124
Nupercainal Hydrocortisone 1% Cream .... ▣ 661
Pramosone Cream, Lotion & Ointment 995
ProctoFoam-HC 2552
Terra-Cortril Ophthalmic Suspension 2033

Hydrocortisone Sodium Phosphate (Xanthines can potentiate hypokalemic effects). Products include:

Hydrocortone Phosphate Injection, Sterile 1713

Hydrocortisone Sodium Succinate (Xanthines can potentiate hypokalemic effects).

No products indexed under this heading.

Hydroflumethiazide (Xanthines can potentiate hypokalemic effects). Products include:

Diucardin Tablets 2824

Influenza Virus Vaccine (Decreases theophylline clearance). Products include:

Fluvirin (Influenza Virus Vaccine) 1608
Influenza Virus Vaccine, Trivalent, Types A and B (chromatograph- and filter-purified subviron antigen) FluShield, 1996-1997 Formula 2842

Isoetharine (Possible toxic synergism; xanthines can potentiate hypokalemia resulting from $beta_2$ agonist therapy). Products include:

Bronkometer Aerosol 2432
Bronkosol Solution 2432
Isoetharine Inhalation Solution, USP, Arm-a-Med 545

Isoproterenol Hydrochloride (Possible toxic synergism; xanthines can potentiate hypokalemia resulting from $beta_2$ agonist therapy). Products include:

Isuprel Hydrochloride Solution 2443
Isuprel Injection 2441
Isuprel Mistometer 2442

Isoproterenol Sulfate (Possible toxic synergism; xanthines can potentiate hypokalemia resulting from $beta_2$ agonist therapy). Products include:

Norisodrine with Calcium Iodide Syrup 446

Levonorgestrel (Increased serum theophylline levels). Products include:

Levlen/Tri-Levlen 646
Nordette-21 Tablets 2863
Nordette-28 Tablets 2866
Norplant System 2868
Levlen/Tri-Levlen 646
Triphasil-21 Tablets 2919
Triphasil-28 Tablets 2924

Lithium Carbonate (Increased excretion of lithium carbonate). Products include:

Eskalith 2658
Lithium Carbonate Capsules & Tablets 2352
Lithonate/Lithotabs/Lithobid 2721

Mestranol (Increased serum theophylline levels). Products include:

Norinyl 2563
Ortho-Novum 1928

Metaproterenol Sulfate (Possible toxic synergism; xanthines can potentiate hypokalemia resulting from $beta_2$ agonist therapy). Products include:

Alupent 672
Metaproterenol Sulfate Inhalation Solution, USP, Arm-a-Med 547

Methyclothiazide (Xanthines can potentiate hypokalemic effects). Products include:

Enduron Tablets 424

Methylprednisolone Acetate (Xanthines can potentiate hypokalemic effects).

No products indexed under this heading.

Methylprednisolone Sodium Succinate (Xanthines can potentiate hypokalemic effects).

No products indexed under this heading.

Norethindrone (Increased serum theophylline levels). Products include:

Brevicon 2563
Micronor Tablets 1903
Modicon 1928
Norinyl 2563
Nor-Q D Tablets 2598
Ortho-Novum 1928
Ovcon 765
Tri-Norinyl 2607

Norethynodrel (Increased serum theophylline levels).

No products indexed under this heading.

Norgestimate (Increased serum theophylline levels). Products include:

Ortho-Cyclen/Ortho-Tri-Cyclen 1914
Ortho-Cyclen/Ortho Tri-Cyclen 1914

Norgestrel (Increased serum theophylline levels). Products include:

Lo/Ovral Tablets 2852
Lo/Ovral-28 Tablets 2857
Ovral Tablets 2877

(▣ Described in PDR For Nonprescription Drugs) (⊙ Described in PDR For Ophthalmology)

997 Interactions Index Slo-Niacin

Ovral-28 Tablets 2878
Ovrette Tablets 2878

Phenytoin (Serum levels of both drugs decreased). Products include:
Dilantin Infatabs 1967
Dilantin-125 Suspension 1969

Phenytoin Sodium (Serum levels of both drugs decreased). Products include:
Dilantin Kapseals 1965

Pirbuterol Acetate (Possible toxic synergism; xanthines can potentiate hypokalemia resulting from $beta_2$ agonist therapy). Products include:
Maxair Autohaler 1550
Maxair Inhaler 1552

Polythiazide (Xanthines can potentiate hypokalemic effects). Products include:
Minizide Capsules 2016

Prednisolone Acetate (Xanthines can potentiate hypokalemic effects). Products include:
AK-CIDE .... ◉ 203
AK-CIDE Ointment .... ◉ 203
Blephamide Liquifilm Sterile Ophthalmic Suspension 472
Blephamide Ointment .... ◉ 234
Econopred & Econopred Plus Ophthalmic Suspensions .... ◉ 216
Poly-Pred Liquifilm .... ◉ 246
Pred Forte .... ◉ 247
Pred Mild .... ◉ 250
Pred-G Liquifilm Sterile Ophthalmic Suspension .... ◉ 248
Pred-G S.O.P. Sterile Ophthalmic Ointment .... ◉ 249

Prednisolone Sodium Phosphate (Xanthines can potentiate hypokalemic effects). Products include:
AK-PRED .... ◉ 204
Hydeltrasol Injection, Sterile 1708
Pediapred Oral Solution 1618

Prednisolone Tebutate (Xanthines can potentiate hypokalemic effects). Products include:
Hydeltra-T.B.A. Sterile Suspension 1710

Prednisone (Xanthines can potentiate hypokalemic effects).
No products indexed under this heading.

Propranolol Hydrochloride (Increased theophylline levels). Products include:
Inderal 2834
Inderal LA Long Acting Capsules 2836
Inderide Tablets 2838
Inderide LA Long Acting Capsules .. 2840

Rifampin (Decreased serum theophylline levels). Products include:
Rifadin 1276
Rifamate Capsules 1278
Rifater 1280
Rimactane Capsules 865

Salmeterol Xinafoate (Possible toxic synergism; xanthines can potentiate hypokalemia resulting from $beta_2$ agonist therapy). Products include:
Serevent Inhalation Aerosol 1149

Terbutaline Sulfate (Possible toxic synergism; xanthines can potentiate hypokalemia resulting from $beta_2$ agonist therapy). Products include:
Brethaire Inhaler 830
Brethine Ampuls 832
Brethine Tablets 831
Bricanyl Subcutaneous Injection 1247
Bricanyl Tablets 1248

Triamcinolone (Xanthines can potentiate hypokalemic effects).
No products indexed under this heading.

Triamcinolone Acetonide (Xanthines can potentiate hypokalemic effects). Products include:
Azmacort Oral Inhaler 2175
Nasacort AQ Nasal Spray 2191
Nasacort Nasal Inhaler 2189

Triamcinolone Diacetate (Xanthines can potentiate hypokalemic effects).
No products indexed under this heading.

Triamcinolone Hexacetonide (Xanthines can potentiate hypokalemic effects).
No products indexed under this heading.

Troleandomycin (Increased theophylline serum concentrations). Products include:
Tao Capsules 2033

Food Interactions

Diet, high-lipid (Decreases in the rate of absorption, but with no significant difference in the extent of absorption).

SLO-NIACIN TABLETS (Niacin) 2767
May interact with antihypertensives and lipid-lowering drugs. Compounds in these categories include:

Acebutolol Hydrochloride (Persons taking antihypertensives should contact their physicians before taking niacin because of unspecified interactions). Products include:
Sectral Capsules 2914

Amlodipine Besylate (Persons taking antihypertensives should contact their physicians before taking niacin because of unspecified interactions). Products include:
Lotrel Capsules 858
Norvasc Tablets 2020

Atenolol (Persons taking antihypertensives should contact their physicians before taking niacin because of unspecified interactions). Products include:
Tenoretic Tablets 2963
Tenormin Tablets and I.V. Injection 2965

Benazepril Hydrochloride (Persons taking antihypertensives should contact their physicians before taking niacin because of unspecified interactions). Products include:
Lotensin Tablets 852
Lotensin HCT Tablets 855
Lotrel Capsules 858

Bendroflumethiazide (Persons taking antihypertensives should contact their physicians before taking niacin because of unspecified interactions).
No products indexed under this heading.

Betaxolol Hydrochloride (Persons taking antihypertensives should contact their physicians before taking niacin because of unspecified interactions). Products include:
Betoptic Ophthalmic Solution 465
Betoptic S Ophthalmic Suspension 467
Kerlone Tablets 2588

Bisoprolol Fumarate (Persons taking antihypertensives should contact their physicians before taking niacin because of unspecified interactions). Products include:
Zebeta Tablets 1457
Ziac 1459

Captopril (Persons taking antihypertensives should contact their physicians before taking niacin because of unspecified interactions). Products include:
Capoten Tablets 740
Capozide Tablets 744

Carteolol Hydrochloride (Persons taking antihypertensives should contact their physicians before taking niacin because of unspecified interactions). Products include:
Cartrol Tablets 413
Ocupress Ophthalmic Solution, 1% Sterile .... ◉ 297

Chlorothiazide (Persons taking antihypertensives should contact their physicians before taking niacin because of unspecified interactions). Products include:
Aldoclor Tablets 1638
Diupres Tablets 1691
Diuril Oral 1694

Chlorothiazide Sodium (Persons taking antihypertensives should contact their physicians before taking niacin because of unspecified interactions). Products include:
Diuril Sodium Intravenous 1693

Chlorthalidone (Persons taking antihypertensives should contact their physicians before taking niacin because of unspecified interactions). Products include:
Combipres Tablets 682
Tenoretic Tablets 2963
Thalitone 1293

Cholestyramine (Persons taking cholesterol-lowering drugs should contact their physicians before taking niacin because of unspecified interactions). Products include:
Questran 774

Clofibrate (Persons taking cholesterol-lowering drugs should contact their physicians before taking niacin because of unspecified interactions). Products include:
Atromid-S Capsules 2808

Clonidine (Persons taking antihypertensives should contact their physicians before taking niacin because of unspecified interactions). Products include:
Catapres-TTS 680

Clonidine Hydrochloride (Persons taking antihypertensives should contact their physicians before taking niacin because of unspecified interactions). Products include:
Catapres Tablets 679
Combipres Tablets 682

Colestipol Hydrochloride (Persons taking cholesterol-lowering drugs should contact their physicians before taking niacin because of unspecified interactions). Products include:
Colestid 2073

Deserpidine (Persons taking antihypertensives should contact their physicians before taking niacin because of unspecified interactions).
No products indexed under this heading.

Diazoxide (Persons taking antihypertensives should contact their physicians before taking niacin because of unspecified interactions). Products include:
Hyperstat I.V. Injection 2504
Proglycem 575

Diltiazem Hydrochloride (Persons taking antihypertensives should contact their physicians before taking niacin because of unspecified interactions). Products include:
Cardizem CD Capsules 1251
Cardizem SR Capsules 1255
Cardizem Injectable 1253
Cardizem Tablets 1257
Dilacor XR Extended-release Capsules 2183
Tiazac Capsules 1019

Doxazosin Mesylate (Persons taking antihypertensives should contact their physicians before taking niacin because of unspecified interactions). Products include:
Cardura Tablets 1993

Enalapril Maleate (Persons taking antihypertensives should contact their physicians before taking niacin because of unspecified interactions). Products include:
Vaseretic Tablets 1810
Vasotec Tablets 1816

Enalaprilat (Persons taking antihypertensives should contact their physicians before taking niacin because of unspecified interactions). Products include:
Vasotec I.V. 1814

Esmolol Hydrochloride (Persons taking antihypertensives should contact their physicians before taking niacin because of unspecified interactions). Products include:
Brevibloc (esmolol HCl) Injection 1860

Felodipine (Persons taking antihypertensives should contact their physicians before taking niacin because of unspecified interactions). Products include:
Plendil Extended-Release Tablets 514

Fluvastatin Sodium (Persons taking cholesterol-lowering drugs should contact their physicians before taking niacin because of unspecified interactions). Products include:
Lescol Capsules 2395

Fosinopril Sodium (Persons taking antihypertensives should contact their physicians before taking niacin because of unspecified interactions). Products include:
Monopril Tablets 762

Furosemide (Persons taking antihypertensives should contact their physicians before taking niacin because of unspecified interactions). Products include:
Lasix Injection, Oral Solution and Tablets 1267

Gemfibrozil (Persons taking cholesterol-lowering drugs should contact their physicians before taking niacin because of unspecified interactions). Products include:
Lopid Tablets 1974

Guanabenz Acetate (Persons taking antihypertensives should contact their physicians before taking niacin because of unspecified interactions).
No products indexed under this heading.

Guanethidine Monosulfate (Persons taking antihypertensives should contact their physicians before taking niacin because of unspecified interactions). Products include:
Esimil Tablets 840
Ismelin Tablets 845

Hydralazine Hydrochloride (Persons taking antihypertensives should contact their physicians before taking niacin because of unspecified interactions). Products include:
Apresazide Capsules 824
Apresoline Hydrochloride Tablets .. 826
Hydralazine Hydrochloride Injection USP 2712
Ser-Ap-Es Tablets 867

Hydrochlorothiazide (Persons taking antihypertensives should contact their physicians before taking niacin because of unspecified interactions). Products include:
Aldactazide Tablets 2556
Aldoril Tablets 1644
Apresazide Capsules 824
Capozide Tablets 744
Dyazide Capsules 2653
Esidrix Tablets 839
Esimil Tablets 840
HydroDIURIL Tablets 1716

IMPORTANT NOTE: Always consult each drug listing in the patient's regimen for possible interactions.

Slo-Niacin — Interactions Index — 998

Hydropres Tablets ... 1718
Hyzaar Tablets ... 1720
Inderide Tablets ... 2838
Inderide LA Long Acting Capsules .. 2840
Lopressor HCT Tablets ... 850
Lotensin HCT Tablets ... 855
Moduretic Tablets ... 1748
Oretic Tablets ... 450
Prinzide Tablets ... 1780
Ser-Ap-Es Tablets ... 867
Timolide Tablets ... 1791
Vaseretic Tablets ... 1810
Zestoretic Tablets ... 2968
Ziac ... 1459

Hydroflumethiazide (Persons taking antihypertensives should contact their physicians before taking niacin because of unspecified interactions). Products include:
Diucardin Tablets ... 2824

Indapamide (Persons taking antihypertensives should contact their physicians before taking niacin because of unspecified interactions).
No products indexed under this heading.

Isradipine (Persons taking antihypertensives should contact their physicians before taking niacin because of unspecified interactions). Products include:
DynaCirc Capsules ... 2381
DynaCirc CR Tablets ... 2383

Labetalol Hydrochloride (Persons taking antihypertensives should contact their physicians before taking niacin because of unspecified interactions). Products include:
Normodyne Injection ... 2519
Normodyne Tablets ... 2522
Trandate ... 1158

Lisinopril (Persons taking antihypertensives should contact their physicians before taking niacin because of unspecified interactions). Products include:
Prinivil Tablets ... 1776
Prinzide Tablets ... 1780
Zestoretic Tablets ... 2968
Zestril Tablets ... 2972

Losartan Potassium (Persons taking antihypertensives should contact their physicians before taking niacin because of unspecified interactions). Products include:
Cozaar Tablets ... 1668
Hyzaar Tablets ... 1720

Lovastatin (Persons taking cholesterol-lowering drugs should contact their physicians before taking niacin because of unspecified interactions). Products include:
Mevacor Tablets ... 1742

Mecamylamine Hydrochloride (Persons taking antihypertensives should contact their physicians before taking niacin because of unspecified interactions). Products include:
Inversine Tablets ... 1729

Methyclothiazide (Persons taking antihypertensives should contact their physicians before taking niacin because of unspecified interactions). Products include:
Enduron Tablets ... 424

Methyldopa (Persons taking antihypertensives should contact their physicians before taking niacin because of unspecified interactions). Products include:
Aldoclor Tablets ... 1638
Aldomet Oral ... 1640
Aldoril Tablets ... 1644

Methyldopate Hydrochloride (Persons taking antihypertensives should contact their physicians before taking niacin because of unspecified interactions). Products include:
Aldomet Ester HCl Injection ... 1642

Metolazone (Persons taking antihypertensives should contact their physicians before taking niacin because of unspecified interactions). Products include:
Mykrox Tablets ... 1617
Zaroxolyn Tablets ... 1625

Metoprolol Succinate (Persons taking antihypertensives should contact their physicians before taking niacin because of unspecified interactions). Products include:
Toprol-XL Tablets ... 560

Metoprolol Tartrate (Persons taking antihypertensives should contact their physicians before taking niacin because of unspecified interactions). Products include:
Lopressor ... 848
Lopressor HCT Tablets ... 850

Metyrosine (Persons taking antihypertensives should contact their physicians before taking niacin because of unspecified interactions). Products include:
Demser Capsules ... 1690

Minoxidil (Persons taking antihypertensives should contact their physicians before taking niacin because of unspecified interactions).
No products indexed under this heading.

Moexipril Hydrochloride (Persons taking antihypertensives should contact their physicians before taking niacin because of unspecified interactions). Products include:
Univasc Tablets ... 2553

Nadolol (Persons taking antihypertensives should contact their physicians before taking niacin because of unspecified interactions).
No products indexed under this heading.

Nicardipine Hydrochloride (Persons taking antihypertensives should contact their physicians before taking niacin because of unspecified interactions). Products include:
Cardene Capsules ... 2261
Cardene I.V. ... 2815
Cardene SR Capsules ... 2264

Nifedipine (Persons taking antihypertensives should contact their physicians before taking niacin because of unspecified interactions). Products include:
Adalat Capsules (10 mg and 20 mg) ... 580
Adalat CC ... 582
Procardia Capsules ... 2024
Procardia XL Extended Release Tablets ... 2026

Nisoldipine (Persons taking antihypertensives should contact their physicians before taking niacin because of unspecified interactions). Products include:
Sular Tablets ... 2961

Nitroglycerin (Persons taking antihypertensives should contact their physicians before taking niacin because of unspecified interactions). Products include:
Deponit NTG Transdermal Delivery System ... 2541
Nitro-Bid IV ... 1270
Nitro-Bid Ointment ... 1272
Nitro-Dur (nitroglycerin) Transdermal Infusion System ... 1365
Nitrolingual Spray ... 2193
Nitrostat Tablets ... 1981
Transderm-Nitro Transdermal Therapeutic System ... 878

Penbutolol Sulfate (Persons taking antihypertensives should contact their physicians before taking niacin because of unspecified interactions). Products include:
Levatol Tablets ... 2547

Phenoxybenzamine Hydrochloride (Persons taking antihypertensives should contact their physicians before taking niacin because of unspecified interactions). Products include:
Dibenzyline Capsules ... 2650

Phentolamine Mesylate (Persons taking antihypertensives should contact their physicians before taking niacin because of unspecified interactions). Products include:
Regitine Vials ... 864

Pindolol (Persons taking antihypertensives should contact their physicians before taking niacin because of unspecified interactions). Products include:
Visken Tablets ... 2428

Polythiazide (Persons taking antihypertensives should contact their physicians before taking niacin because of unspecified interactions). Products include:
Minizide Capsules ... 2016

Pravastatin Sodium (Persons taking cholesterol-lowering drugs should contact their physicians before taking niacin because of unspecified interactions). Products include:
Pravachol Tablets ... 770

Prazosin Hydrochloride (Persons taking antihypertensives should contact their physicians before taking niacin because of unspecified interactions). Products include:
Minipress Capsules ... 2015
Minizide Capsules ... 2016

Probucol (Persons taking cholesterol-lowering drugs should contact their physicians before taking niacin because of unspecified interactions).
No products indexed under this heading.

Propranolol Hydrochloride (Persons taking antihypertensives should contact their physicians before taking niacin because of unspecified interactions). Products include:
Inderal ... 2834
Inderal LA Long Acting Capsules 2836
Inderide Tablets ... 2838
Inderide LA Long Acting Capsules .. 2840

Quinapril Hydrochloride (Persons taking antihypertensives should contact their physicians before taking niacin because of unspecified interactions). Products include:
Accupril Tablets ... 1950

Ramipril (Persons taking antihypertensives should contact their physicians before taking niacin because of unspecified interactions). Products include:
Altace Capsules ... 1238

Rauwolfia Serpentina (Persons taking antihypertensives should contact their physicians before taking niacin because of unspecified interactions).
No products indexed under this heading.

Rescinnamine (Persons taking antihypertensives should contact their physicians before taking niacin because of unspecified interactions).
No products indexed under this heading.

Reserpine (Persons taking antihypertensives should contact their physicians before taking niacin because of unspecified interactions). Products include:
Diupres Tablets ... 1691
Hydropres Tablets ... 1718
Ser-Ap-Es Tablets ... 867

Simvastatin (Persons taking cholesterol-lowering drugs should contact their physicians before taking niacin because of unspecified interactions). Products include:
Zocor Tablets ... 1821

Sodium Nitroprusside (Persons taking antihypertensives should contact their physicians before taking niacin because of unspecified interactions).
No products indexed under this heading.

Sotalol Hydrochloride (Persons taking antihypertensives should contact their physicians before taking niacin because of unspecified interactions). Products include:
Betapace Tablets ... 637

Spirapril Hydrochloride (Persons taking antihypertensives should contact their physicians before taking niacin because of unspecified interactions).
No products indexed under this heading.

Terazosin Hydrochloride (Persons taking antihypertensives should contact their physicians before taking niacin because of unspecified interactions). Products include:
Hytrin Capsules ... 434

Timolol Maleate (Persons taking antihypertensives should contact their physicians before taking niacin because of unspecified interactions). Products include:
Blocadren Tablets ... 1654
Timolide Tablets ... 1791
Timoptic in Ocudose ... 1796
Timoptic Sterile Ophthalmic Solution ... 1794
Timoptic-XE ... 1798

Torsemide (Persons taking antihypertensives should contact their physicians before taking niacin because of unspecified interactions). Products include:
Demadex Tablets and Injection ... 691

Trimethaphan Camsylate (Persons taking antihypertensives should contact their physicians before taking niacin because of unspecified interactions).
No products indexed under this heading.

Verapamil Hydrochloride (Persons taking antihypertensives should contact their physicians before taking niacin because of unspecified interactions). Products include:
Calan SR Caplets ... 2571
Calan Tablets ... 2568
Covera-HS Tablets ... 2573
Isoptin Injectable ... 1391
Isoptin Oral Tablets ... 1393
Isoptin SR Tablets ... 1395
Verelan Capsules ... 1455

SLOW FE TABLETS
(Ferrous Sulfate) ... 889
May interact with tetracyclines. Compounds in this category include:

Demeclocycline Hydrochloride (Absorption of oral tetracycline impaired). Products include:
Declomycin Tablets ... 1421

Doxycycline Calcium (Absorption of oral tetracycline impaired). Products include:
Vibramycin Calcium Oral Suspension Syrup ... 2038

Doxycycline Hyclate (Absorption of oral tetracycline impaired). Products include:
Doryx Capsules ... 1970
Vibramycin Hyclate Capsules ... 2038
Vibramycin Hyclate Intravenous ... 2040
Vibra-Tabs Film Coated Tablets ... 2038

(▣ Described in PDR For Nonprescription Drugs) (◉ Described in PDR For Ophthalmology)

Doxycycline Monohydrate (Absorption of oral tetracycline impaired). Products include:
- Monodox Capsules 1858
- Vibramycin Monohydrate for Oral Suspension 2038

Methacycline Hydrochloride (Absorption of oral tetracycline impaired).
- No products indexed under this heading.

Minocycline Hydrochloride (Absorption of oral tetracycline impaired). Products include:
- DYNACIN Capsules 1627
- Minocin Intravenous 1428
- Minocin Oral Suspension 1431
- Minocin Pellet-Filled Capsules 1429

Oxytetracycline (Absorption of oral tetracycline impaired). Products include:
- Terramycin Intramuscular Solution 2034

Oxytetracycline Hydrochloride (Absorption of oral tetracycline impaired). Products include:
- TERAK Ointment .... ⓟ 210
- Terra-Cortril Ophthalmic Suspension 2033
- Terramycin with Polymyxin B Sulfate Ophthalmic Ointment 2035
- Urobiotic-250 Capsules 2038

Tetracycline Hydrochloride (Absorption of oral tetracycline impaired). Products include:
- Achromycin V Capsules 1417
- Helidac Therapy 2135

SLOW FE WITH FOLIC ACID
(Ferrous Sulfate, Folic Acid) 890
May interact with tetracyclines. Compounds in this category include:

Demeclocycline Hydrochloride (Oral iron products interfere with oral absorption of tetracycline; do not take within two hours of each other). Products include:
- Declomycin Tablets 1421

Doxycycline Calcium (Oral iron products interfere with oral absorption of tetracycline; do not take within two hours of each other). Products include:
- Vibramycin Calcium Oral Suspension Syrup 2038

Doxycycline Hyclate (Oral iron products interfere with oral absorption of tetracycline; do not take within two hours of each other). Products include:
- Doryx Capsules 1970
- Vibramycin Hyclate Capsules 2038
- Vibramycin Hyclate Intravenous 2040
- Vibra-Tabs Film Coated Tablets 2038

Doxycycline Monohydrate (Oral iron products interfere with oral absorption of tetracycline; do not take within two hours of each other). Products include:
- Monodox Capsules 1858
- Vibramycin Monohydrate for Oral Suspension 2038

Methacycline Hydrochloride (Oral iron products interfere with oral absorption of tetracycline; do not take within two hours of each other).
- No products indexed under this heading.

Minocycline Hydrochloride (Oral iron products interfere with oral absorption of tetracycline; do not take within two hours of each other). Products include:
- DYNACIN Capsules 1627
- Minocin Intravenous 1428
- Minocin Oral Suspension 1431
- Minocin Pellet-Filled Capsules 1429

Oxytetracycline Hydrochloride (Oral iron products interfere with oral absorption of tetracycline; do not take within two hours of each other). Products include:
- TERAK Ointment .... ⓟ 210
- Terra-Cortril Ophthalmic Suspension 2033
- Terramycin with Polymyxin B Sulfate Ophthalmic Ointment 2035
- Urobiotic-250 Capsules 2038

Tetracycline Hydrochloride (Oral iron products interfere with oral absorption of tetracycline; do not take within two hours of each other). Products include:
- Achromycin V Capsules 1417
- Helidac Therapy 2135

SLOW-K EXTENDED-RELEASE TABLETS
(Potassium Chloride) 869
May interact with potassium sparing diuretics. Compounds in this category include:

Amiloride Hydrochloride (Co-administration of these agents can produce severe hyperkalemia; concurrent use is not recommended). Products include:
- Midamor Tablets 1746
- Moduretic Tablets 1748

Spironolactone (Co-administration of these agents can produce severe hyperkalemia; concurrent use is not recommended). Products include:
- Aldactazide Tablets 2556
- Aldactone Tablets 2558

Triamterene (Co-administration of these agents can produce severe hyperkalemia; concurrent use is not recommended). Products include:
- Dyazide Capsules 2653
- Dyrenium Capsules 2655

SODIUM CHLORIDE STERILE WATER FOR INHALATION, ARM-A-VIAL
(Sodium Chloride) 557
None cited in PDR database.

SODIUM POLYSTYRENE SULFONATE SUSPENSION
(Sodium Polystyrene Sulfonate) 2367
May interact with cardiac glycosides, antacids containing aluminium, calcium and magnesium, and certain other agents. Compounds in these categories include:

Aluminum Carbonate (Potential for systemic alkalosis). Products include:
- Basaljel Capsules 2810
- Basaljel Suspension 2810
- Basaljel Tablets 2810

Aluminum Hydroxide (Potential for systemic alkalosis). Products include:
- ALternaGEL Liquid 1358
- Maximum Strength Ascriptin .... ⓟ 650
- Cama Arthritis Pain Reliever .... ⓟ 748
- Gaviscon Extra Strength Relief Formula Antacid Tablets .... ⓟ 778
- Gaviscon Extra Strength Relief Formula Liquid Antacid .... ⓟ 779
- Gaviscon Liquid Antacid .... ⓟ 779
- Gelusil Antacid-Anti-gas Liquid .... ⓟ 819
- Gelusil Antacid-Anti-gas Tablets .... ⓟ 819
- Maalox Antacid/Anti-Gas Tablets 889
- Maalox Heartburn Relief Suspension .... ⓟ 658
- Maalox Antacid Liquid 888
- Extra Strength Maalox Antacid/Anti-Gas Liquid and Tablets 888
- Mylanta 1359
- Tempo Soft Antacid 799

Aluminum Hydroxide Gel (Potential for systemic alkalosis). Products include:
- ALternaGEL Liquid .... ⓟ 675
- Aludrox Oral Suspension .... ⓟ 850
- Amphojel Suspension 2802
- Amphojel Suspension without Flavor 2802
- Amphojel Tablets 2802
- Ascriptin .... ⓟ 650
- Gaviscon Antacid Tablets .... ⓟ 778
- Gaviscon-2 Antacid Tablets .... ⓟ 779
- Mylanta Liquid .... ⓟ 676
- Mylanta Double Strength Liquid .... ⓟ 676
- Nephrox Suspension .... ⓟ 671

Deslanoside (Potential for digitalis toxicity exaggerated by hypokalemia).
- No products indexed under this heading.

Digitoxin (Potential for digitalis toxicity exaggerated by hypokalemia). Products include:
- Crystodigin Tablets 1472

Digoxin (Potential for digitalis toxicity exaggerated by hypokalemia). Products include:
- Lanoxicaps 1110
- Lanoxin Elixir Pediatric 1113
- Lanoxin Injection 1116
- Lanoxin Injection Pediatric 1119
- Lanoxin Tablets 1121

Magaldrate (Potential for systemic alkalosis).
- No products indexed under this heading.

Magnesium Hydroxide (Should not be administered concomitantly; potential for systemic alkalosis; one case of grand mal seizure has been reported). Products include:
- Aludrox Oral Suspension .... ⓟ 850
- Ascriptin .... ⓟ 650
- Di-Gel Antacid/Anti-Gas .... ⓟ 762
- Gelusil Antacid-Anti-gas Liquid .... ⓟ 819
- Gelusil Antacid-Anti-gas Tablets .... ⓟ 819
- Maalox Antacid/Anti-Gas Tablets 889
- Maalox Antacid Liquid 888
- Extra Strength Maalox Antacid/Anti-Gas Liquid and Tablets 888
- Mylanta Fast-Acting 1359
- Mylanta Gelcaps Antacid .... ⓟ 678
- Fast-Acting Mylanta Liquid Antacid 1359
- Mylanta Tablets .... ⓟ 677
- Maximum-Strength Fast-Acting Mylanta Liquid Antacid 1359
- Mylanta Double Strength Tablets .... ⓟ 677
- Phillips' Milk of Magnesia Liquid .... ⓟ 627
- Rolaids Antacid Tablets .... ⓟ 807
- Tempo Soft Antacid .... ⓟ 799

Magnesium Oxide (Potential for systemic alkalosis). Products include:
- Beelith Tablets 632
- Bufferin Analgesic Tablets .... ⓟ 636
- Arthritis Strength Bufferin Analgesic Caplets .... ⓟ 637
- Extra Strength Bufferin Analgesic Tablets .... ⓟ 637
- Caltrate PLUS .... ⓟ 681
- Cama Arthritis Pain Reliever .... ⓟ 748
- Mag-Ox 400 666
- Uro-Mag 666

SOLAQUIN FORTE 4% CREAM
(Hydroquinone) 1299
None cited in PDR database.

SOLAQUIN FORTE 4% GEL
(Hydroquinone) 1299
None cited in PDR database.

SOLBAR PF ULTRA CREAM SPF 50 (PABA FREE)
(Oxybenzone) 1989
None cited in PDR database.

SOLBAR PF ULTRA LIQUID SPF 30
(Octyl Methoxycinnamate, Oxybenzone) 1989
None cited in PDR database.

SOLGANAL SUSPENSION
(Aurothioglucose) 2530
May interact with antimalarials, immunosuppressive agents, and certain other agents. Compounds in these categories include:

Azathioprine (Safety of coadministration has not been established). Products include:
- Azathioprine Tablets 2349
- Imuran 1103

Chloroquine Hydrochloride (Concurrent use is contraindicated). Products include:
- Aralen Hydrochloride Injection 2430

Chloroquine Phosphate (Concurrent use is contraindicated). Products include:
- Aralen Phosphate Tablets 2431

Cyclosporine (Safety of coadministration has not been established). Products include:
- Neoral 2405
- Sandimmune 2416

Immune Globulin (Human) (Safety of coadministration has not been established).
- No products indexed under this heading.

Immune Globulin Intravenous (Human) (Safety of coadministration has not been established).
- No products indexed under this heading.

Mefloquine Hydrochloride (Concurrent use is contraindicated). Products include:
- Lariam Tablets 2295

Muromonab-CD3 (Safety of coadministration has not been established). Products include:
- Orthoclone OKT3 Sterile Solution .. 1892

Mycophenolate Mofetil (Safety of coadministration has not been established). Products include:
- CellCept Capsules 2265

Penicillamine (Concurrent use is contraindicated). Products include:
- Cuprimine Capsules 1673
- Depen Titratable Tablets 2770

Pyrimethamine (Concurrent use is contraindicated). Products include:
- Daraprim Tablets 1199
- Fansidar Tablets 2281

Tacrolimus (Safety of coadministration has not been established). Products include:
- Prograf 1028

SOMA COMPOUND W/CODEINE TABLETS
(Carisoprodol, Aspirin, Codeine Phosphate) 2784
May interact with central nervous system depressants, psychotropics, oral anticoagulants, oral hypoglycemic agents, antacids, corticosteroids, and certain other agents. Compounds in these categories include:

Acarbose (Possible enhancement of hypoglycemia). Products include:
- Precose 604

Alfentanil Hydrochloride (Additive effects). Products include:
- Alfenta Injection 1334

Alprazolam (Additive effects). Products include:
- Xanax Tablets 2115

Aluminum Carbonate (May substantially decrease plasma salicylate concentration). Products include:
- Basaljel Capsules 2810
- Basaljel Suspension 2810
- Basaljel Tablets 2810

Aluminum Hydroxide (May substantially decrease plasma salicylate concentration). Products include:
- ALternaGEL Liquid 1358

IMPORTANT NOTE: Always consult each drug listing in the patient's regimen for possible interactions.

Soma Compound with Codeine — Interactions Index

Maximum Strength Ascriptin 650
Cama Arthritis Pain Reliever............ 748
Gaviscon Extra Strength Relief Formula Antacid Tablets............ 778
Gaviscon Extra Strength Relief Formula Liquid Antacid............ 779
Gaviscon Liquid Antacid 779
Gelusil Antacid-Anti-gas Liquid 819
Gelusil Antacid-Anti-gas Tablets 819
Maalox Antacid/Anti-Gas Tablets 889
Maalox Heartburn Relief Suspension 658
Maalox Antacid Liquid 888
Extra Strength Maalox Antacid/Anti-Gas Liquid and Tablets 888
Mylanta 1359
Tempo Soft Antacid 799

Aluminum Hydroxide Gel (May substantially decrease plasma salicylate concentration). Products include:
ALternaGEL Liquid 675
Aludrox Oral Suspension 850
Amphojel Suspension 2802
Amphojel Suspension without Flavor 2802
Amphojel Tablets 2802
Ascriptin 650
Gaviscon Antacid Tablets 778
Gaviscon-2 Antacid Tablets 779
Mylanta Liquid 676
Mylanta Double Strength Liquid 676
Nephrox Suspension 671

Amitriptyline Hydrochloride (Additive effects). Products include:
Elavil 2945
Etrafon 2495
Limbitrol 2333
Triavil Tablets 1800

Ammonium Chloride (Elevated plasma salicylate concentrations).
No products indexed under this heading.

Amoxapine (Additive effects). Products include:
Asendin Tablets 1419

Aprobarbital (Additive effects).
No products indexed under this heading.

Betamethasone Acetate (May decrease salicylate plasma levels). Products include:
Celestone Soluspan Suspension 2484

Betamethasone Sodium Phosphate (May decrease salicylate plasma levels). Products include:
Celestone Soluspan Suspension 2484

Buprenorphine (Additive effects). Products include:
Buprenex Injectable 2170

Buspirone Hydrochloride (Additive effects). Products include:
BuSpar Tablets 738

Butabarbital (Additive effects).
No products indexed under this heading.

Butalbital (Additive effects). Products include:
Axocet Capsules 2469
Esgic-plus Capsules 1012
Esgic-plus Tablets 1012
Fioricet Tablets 2386
Fioricet with Codeine Capsules 2387
Fiorinal Capsules 2388
Fiorinal with Codeine Capsules 2390
Fiorinal Tablets 2388
Phrenilin 790
Sedapap Tablets 50 mg/650 mg .. 1826

Chlordiazepoxide (Additive effects). Products include:
Limbitrol 2333

Chlordiazepoxide Hydrochloride (Additive effects). Products include:
Librax Capsules 2330
Librium Capsules 2331
Librium Injectable 2332

Chlorpromazine (Additive effects). Products include:
Thorazine Suppositories 2701

Chlorpropamide (Possible enhancement of hypoglycemia). Products include:
Diabinese Tablets 2002

Chlorprothixene (Additive effects).
No products indexed under this heading.

Chlorprothixene Hydrochloride (Additive effects).
No products indexed under this heading.

Chlorprothixene Lactate (Additive effects).
No products indexed under this heading.

Clorazepate Dipotassium (Additive effects). Products include:
Tranxene 459

Clozapine (Additive effects). Products include:
Clozaril Tablets 2377

Cortisone Acetate (May decrease salicylate plasma levels). Products include:
Cortone Acetate Sterile Suspension 1663
Cortone Acetate Tablets 1664

Desflurane (Additive effects). Products include:
Suprane (desflurane, USP) 1865

Desipramine Hydrochloride (Additive effects). Products include:
Norpramin Tablets 1273

Dexamethasone (May decrease salicylate plasma levels). Products include:
AK-Trol Ointment & Suspension 205
Decadron Elixir 1676
Decadron Tablets 1678
Decaspray Topical Aerosol 1689
Maxitrol Ophthalmic Ointment and Suspension 222
TobraDex Ophthalmic Suspension and Ointment 469

Dexamethasone Acetate (May decrease salicylate plasma levels). Products include:
Dalalone D.P. Injectable 1009
Decadron-LA Sterile Suspension 1687

Dexamethasone Sodium Phosphate (May decrease salicylate plasma levels). Products include:
Decadron Phosphate Injection 1680
Decadron Phosphate Sterile Ophthalmic Ointment 1684
Decadron Phosphate Sterile Ophthalmic Solution 1685
Decadron Phosphate Topical Cream 1686
Decadron Phosphate with Xylocaine Injection, Sterile 1683
Dexacort Phosphate in Respihaler .. 1606
Dexacort Phosphate in Turbinaire .. 1607
NeoDecadron Sterile Ophthalmic Ointment 1755
NeoDecadron Sterile Ophthalmic Solution 1756
NeoDecadron Topical Cream 1757

Dezocine (Additive effects). Products include:
Dalgan Injection 529

Diazepam (Additive effects). Products include:
Dizac (diazepam injectable emulsion) CIV 1862
Valium Injectable 2336
Valium Tablets 2335

Dicumarol (Enhanced potential for bleeding).
No products indexed under this heading.

Doxepin Hydrochloride (Additive effects). Products include:
Adapin Capsules 1542
Sinequan 2028
Zonalon Cream 1042

Droperidol (Additive effects). Products include:
Inapsine Injection 462

Enflurane (Additive effects).
No products indexed under this heading.

Estazolam (Additive effects). Products include:
ProSom Tablets 457

Ethchlorvynol (Additive effects). Products include:
Placidyl Capsules 456

Ethinamate (Additive effects).
No products indexed under this heading.

Fentanyl (Additive effects). Products include:
Duragesic Transdermal System 1336

Fentanyl Citrate (Additive effects). Products include:
Sublimaze Injection 463

Fludrocortisone Acetate (May decrease salicylate plasma levels). Products include:
Florinef Acetate Tablets 506

Fluphenazine Decanoate (Additive effects). Products include:
Prolixin Decanoate 510

Fluphenazine Enanthate (Additive effects). Products include:
Prolixin Enanthate 510

Fluphenazine Hydrochloride (Additive effects). Products include:
Prolixin 510

Flurazepam Hydrochloride (Additive effects). Products include:
Dalmane Capsules 2329

Glimepiride (Possible enhancement of hypoglycemia). Products include:
Amaryl Tablets 1241

Glipizide (Possible enhancement of hypoglycemia). Products include:
Glucotrol Tablets 2011
Glucotrol XL Extended Release Tablets 2012

Glutethimide (Additive effects).
No products indexed under this heading.

Glyburide (Possible enhancement of hypoglycemia). Products include:
DiaBeta Tablets 1265
Glynase PresTab Tablets 2091
Micronase Tablets 2099

Haloperidol (Additive effects). Products include:
Haldol Injection, Tablets and Concentrate 1585

Haloperidol Decanoate (Additive effects). Products include:
Haldol Decanoate 1587

Hydrocodone Bitartrate (Additive effects). Products include:
Codiclear DH Syrup 808
Duratuss HD Elixir 2750
Histussin D Liquid 670
Hycodan Tablets and Syrup 946
Hycomine Compound Tablets 948
Hycomine 947
Hycotuss Expectorant Syrup 950
Hydrocet Capsules 787
Lorcet 10/650 Tablets 1016
Lortab 2751
Tussend 1830
Tussend Expectorant 1831
Vicodin Tablets 1404
Vicodin ES Tablets 1405
Vicodin HP Tablets 1403
Vicodin Tuss Expectorant 1406
Zydone Capsules 967

Hydrocodone Polistirex (Additive effects). Products include:
Tussionex Pennkinetic Extended-Release Suspension 1624

Hydrocortisone (May decrease salicylate plasma levels). Products include:
Anusol-HC Cream 2.5% 1953
Aquanil HC Lotion 1989
Maximum Strength Cortaid Spray .. 800
CORTENEMA 2713
Cortisporin Ointment 1074

Cortisporin Ophthalmic Ointment Sterile 1074
Cortisporin Ophthalmic Suspension Sterile 1075
Cortisporin Otic Solution Sterile 1076
Cortisporin Otic Suspension Sterile 1077
Cortizone-5 795
Cortizone-10 795
Hydrocortone Tablets 1715
Hytone 922
Hytone Ointment 2 ½% 923
Massengill Medicated Soft Cloth Towelettes 2628
Pediotic Suspension Sterile 1140
Preparation H Hydrocortisone 1% Cream 843
ProctoCream-HC 2.5% 2552
VōSoL HC Otic Solution 2786

Hydrocortisone Acetate (May decrease salicylate plasma levels). Products include:
Analpram-HC Rectal Cream 1% and 2.5% 993
Anusol HC-1 Hydrocortisone Anti-Itch Ointment 810
Anusol-HC Suppositories 1954
Caldecort Anti-Itch Hydrocortisone Cream 651
Coly-Mycin S Otic w/Neomycin & Hydrocortisone 1965
Cortaid 800
Cortifoam 2540
Cortisporin Cream 1073
Epifoam 2543
Hydrocortone Acetate Sterile Suspension 1712
Mantadil Cream 1124
Nupercainal Hydrocortisone 1% Cream 661
Pramosone Cream, Lotion & Ointment 995
ProctoFoam-HC 2552
Terra-Cortril Ophthalmic Suspension 2033

Hydrocortisone Sodium Phosphate (May decrease salicylate plasma levels). Products include:
Hydrocortone Phosphate Injection, Sterile 1713

Hydrocortisone Sodium Succinate (May decrease salicylate plasma levels).
No products indexed under this heading.

Hydroxyzine Hydrochloride (Additive effects). Products include:
Atarax Tablets & Syrup 1992
Marax Tablets & DF Syrup 2015
Vistaril Intramuscular Solution 2042

Imipramine Hydrochloride (Additive effects). Products include:
Tofranil Ampuls 873
Tofranil Tablets 875

Imipramine Pamoate (Additive effects). Products include:
Tofranil-PM Capsules 876

Isocarboxazid (Additive effects).
No products indexed under this heading.

Isoflurane (Additive effects).
No products indexed under this heading.

Ketamine Hydrochloride (Additive effects).
No products indexed under this heading.

Levomethadyl Acetate Hydrochloride (Additive effects). Products include:
Orlaam Oral Solution 2361

Levorphanol Tartrate (Additive effects). Products include:
Levo-Dromoran 2297

Lithium Carbonate (Additive effects). Products include:
Eskalith 2658
Lithium Carbonate Capsules & Tablets 2352
Lithonate/Lithotabs/Lithobid 2721

Lithium Citrate (Additive effects).
No products indexed under this heading.

(▣ Described in PDR For Nonprescription Drugs) (⊙ Described in PDR For Ophthalmology)

Lorazepam (Additive effects). Products include:
- Ativan Injection 2805
- Ativan Tablets 2807

Loxapine Hydrochloride (Additive effects). Products include:
- Loxitane 1426

Loxapine Succinate (Additive effects). Products include:
- Loxitane Capsules 1426

Magaldrate (May substantially decrease plasma salicylate concentration).
- No products indexed under this heading.

Magnesium Hydroxide (May substantially decrease plasma salicylate concentration). Products include:
- Aludrox Oral Suspension 850
- Ascriptin 650
- Di-Gel Antacid/Anti-Gas 762
- Gelusil Antacid-Anti-gas Liquid .. 819
- Gelusil Antacid-Anti-gas Tablets .. 819
- Maalox Antacid/Anti-Gas Tablets .. 889
- Maalox Antacid Liquid 888
- Extra Strength Maalox Antacid/Anti-Gas Liquid and Tablets 888
- Mylanta Fast-Acting 1359
- Mylanta Gelcaps Antacid 678
- Fast-Acting Mylanta Liquid Antacid 1359
- Mylanta Tablets 677
- Maximum-Strength Fast-Acting Mylanta Liquid Antacid 1359
- Mylanta Double Strength Tablets .. 677
- Phillips' Milk of Magnesia Liquid .. 627
- Rolaids Antacid Tablets 807
- Tempo Soft Antacid 799

Magnesium Oxide (May substantially decrease plasma salicylate concentration). Products include:
- Beelith Tablets 632
- Bufferin Analgesic Tablets 636
- Arthritis Strength Bufferin Analgesic Caplets 637
- Extra Strength Bufferin Analgesic Tablets 637
- Caltrate PLUS 681
- Cama Arthritis Pain Reliever 748
- Mag-Ox 400 666
- Uro-Mag 666

Maprotiline Hydrochloride (Additive effects). Products include:
- Ludiomil Tablets 861

Meperidine Hydrochloride (Additive effects). Products include:
- Demerol 2438
- Mepergan Injection 2859

Mephobarbital (Additive effects). Products include:
- Mebaral Tablets 2452

Meprobamate (Additive effects). Products include:
- Miltown Tablets 2780
- PMB 200 and PMB 400 2890

Mesoridazine Besylate (Additive effects). Products include:
- Serentil 689

Metformin Hydrochloride (Possible enhancement of hypoglycemia). Products include:
- Glucophage Tablets 754

Methadone Hydrochloride (Additive effects). Products include:
- Methadone Hydrochloride Oral Concentrate 2356
- Methadone Hydrochloride Oral Solution & Tablets 2357

Methohexital Sodium (Additive effects).
- No products indexed under this heading.

Methotrexate Sodium (Toxic effects of methotrexate enhanced). Products include:
- Methotrexate Sodium Tablets, Injection, for Injection and LPF Injection 1322

Methotrimeprazine (Additive effects). Products include:
- Levoprome 1321

Methoxyflurane (Additive effects).
- No products indexed under this heading.

Methylprednisolone Acetate (May decrease salicylate plasma levels).
- No products indexed under this heading.

Methylprednisolone Sodium Succinate (May decrease salicylate plasma levels).
- No products indexed under this heading.

Midazolam Hydrochloride (Additive effects). Products include:
- Versed Injection 2324

Molindone Hydrochloride (Additive effects). Products include:
- Moban Tablets and Concentrate .. 1036

Morphine Sulfate (Additive effects). Products include:
- Astramorph/PF Injection, USP (Preservative-Free) 526
- Duramorph Injection 983
- Infumorph 200 and Infumorph 500 Sterile Solutions 985
- Kadian Capsules 2948
- MS Contin Tablets 2149
- MSIR 2152
- Oramorph SR (Morphine Sulfate Sustained Release Tablets) 2359
- RMS Suppositories CII 2766
- Roxanol 2365

Nortriptyline Hydrochloride (Additive effects). Products include:
- Pamelor 2409

Opium Alkaloids (Additive effects).
- No products indexed under this heading.

Oxazepam (Additive effects). Products include:
- Serax Capsules 2916
- Serax Tablets 2916

Oxycodone Hydrochloride (Additive effects). Products include:
- OxyContin Tablets 2163
- OxyIR Capsules 2167
- Percocet Tablets 955
- Percodan Tablets 955
- Percodan-Demi Tablets 956
- Roxicodone Tablets, Oral Solution & Intensol (Oxycodone) 2366
- Tylox Capsules 1593

Pentobarbital Sodium (Additive effects). Products include:
- Nembutal Sodium Capsules 440
- Nembutal Sodium Solution 442
- Nembutal Sodium Suppositories .. 444

Perphenazine (Additive effects). Products include:
- Etrafon 2495
- Triavil Tablets 1800
- Trilafon 2532

Phenelzine Sulfate (Additive effects). Products include:
- Nardil 1977

Phenobarbital (Additive effects). Products include:
- Arco-Lase Plus Tablets 513
- Bellergal-S Tablets 2375
- Donnatal 2234
- Donnatal Extentabs 2234
- Donnatal Tablets 2234
- Phenobarbital Elixir and Tablets .. 1523
- Quadrinal Tablets 1398

Potassium Acid Phosphate (Elevated plasma salicylate concentrations). Products include:
- K-Phos Original Formula 'Sodium Free' Tablets 633

Prazepam (Additive effects).
- No products indexed under this heading.

Prednisolone Acetate (May decrease salicylate plasma levels). Products include:
- AK-CIDE 203
- AK-CIDE Ointment 203
- Blephamide Liquifilm Sterile Ophthalmic Suspension 472

Blephamide Ointment 234
- Econopred & Econopred Plus Ophthalmic Suspensions 216
- Poly-Pred Liquifilm 246
- Pred Forte 247
- Pred Mild 250
- Pred-G Liquifilm Sterile Ophthalmic Suspension 248
- Pred-G S.O.P. Sterile Ophthalmic Ointment 249

Prednisolone Sodium Phosphate (May decrease salicylate plasma levels). Products include:
- AK-PRED 204
- Hydeltrasol Injection, Sterile ... 1708
- Pediapred Oral Solution 1618

Prednisolone Tebutate (May decrease salicylate plasma levels). Products include:
- Hydeltra-T.B.A. Sterile Suspension 1710

Prednisone (May decrease salicylate plasma levels).
- No products indexed under this heading.

Probenecid (Possible reduced renal excretion of salicylate). Products include:
- Benemid Tablets 1651
- ColBENEMID Tablets 1662

Prochlorperazine (Additive effects). Products include:
- Compazine 2644

Promethazine Hydrochloride (Additive effects). Products include:
- Mepergan Injection 2859
- Phenergan with Codeine 2883
- Phenergan with Dextromethorphan 2885
- Phenergan Injection 2880
- Phenergan Suppositories 2882
- Phenergan Syrup 2881
- Phenergan Tablets 2882
- Phenergan VC 2886
- Phenergan VC with Codeine 2888

Propofol (Additive effects). Products include:
- Diprivan Injectable Emulsion 2939

Propoxyphene Hydrochloride (Additive effects). Products include:
- Darvon 1475
- Wygesic Tablets 2930

Propoxyphene Napsylate (Additive effects). Products include:
- Darvon-N/Darvocet-N 1473

Protriptyline Hydrochloride (Additive effects). Products include:
- Vivactil Tablets 1820

Quazepam (Additive effects). Products include:
- Doral Tablets 2773

Risperidone (Additive effects). Products include:
- Risperdal Tablets 1348

Secobarbital Sodium (Additive effects). Products include:
- Seconal Sodium Pulvules 1529

Sevoflurane (Additive effects).
- No products indexed under this heading.

Sodium Acid Phosphate (Elevated plasma salicylate concentrations). Products include:
- Uroqid-Acid No. 2 Tablets 633

Sodium Bicarbonate (May substantially decrease plasma salicylate concentration). Products include:
- Alka-Seltzer Cherry Effervescent Antacid and Pain Reliever 609
- Alka-Seltzer Extra Strength Effervescent Antacid and Pain Reliever 609
- Alka-Seltzer Gold Effervescent Antacid 611
- Alka-Seltzer Lemon Lime Effervescent Antacid and Pain Reliever 609
- Alka-Seltzer Original Effervescent Antacid and Pain Reliever 609
- Arm & Hammer Pure Baking Soda 648
- Colyte and Colyte-flavored 2540
- GoLYTELY 694
- Massengill Disposable Douches .. 780

Massengill Liquid Concentrate 780
- NuLYTELY 694
- Cherry Flavor NuLYTELY 694

Sufentanil Citrate (Additive effects). Products include:
- Sufenta Injection 1355

Sulfinpyrazone (Reduced uricosuric effect of both drugs; possible reduced renal excretion of salicylate). Products include:
- Anturane 823

Temazepam (Additive effects). Products include:
- Restoril Capsules 2413

Thiamylal Sodium (Additive effects).
- No products indexed under this heading.

Thioridazine Hydrochloride (Additive effects). Products include:
- Mellaril 2398

Thiothixene (Additive effects). Products include:
- Navane Capsules and Concentrate 2018
- Navane Intramuscular 2019

Tolazamide (Possible enhancement of hypoglycemia).
- No products indexed under this heading.

Tolbutamide (Possible enhancement of hypoglycemia).
- No products indexed under this heading.

Tranylcypromine Sulfate (Additive effects). Products include:
- Parnate Tablets 2679

Triamcinolone (May decrease salicylate plasma levels).
- No products indexed under this heading.

Triamcinolone Acetonide (May decrease salicylate plasma levels). Products include:
- Azmacort Oral Inhaler 2175
- Nasacort AQ Nasal Spray 2191
- Nasacort Nasal Inhaler 2189

Triamcinolone Diacetate (May decrease salicylate plasma levels).
- No products indexed under this heading.

Triamcinolone Hexacetonide (May decrease salicylate plasma levels).
- No products indexed under this heading.

Triazolam (Additive effects). Products include:
- Halcion Tablets 2093

Trifluoperazine Hydrochloride (Additive effects). Products include:
- Stelazine 2692

Trimipramine Maleate (Additive effects). Products include:
- Surmontil Capsules 2917

Warfarin Sodium (Enhanced potential for bleeding). Products include:
- Coumadin 941

Zolpidem Tartrate (Additive effects). Products include:
- Ambien Tablets 2559

Food Interactions
Alcohol (Additive effects including gastrointestinal bleeding).

SOMA COMPOUND TABLETS
(Carisoprodol, Aspirin) 2783
May interact with central nervous system depressants, psychotropics, oral anticoagulants, oral hypoglycemic agents, antacids, corticosteroids, and certain other agents. Compounds in these categories include:

Acarbose (Possible enhancement of hypoglycemia). Products include:
- Precose 604

IMPORTANT NOTE: Always consult each drug listing in the patient's regimen for possible interactions.

Soma Compound **Interactions Index** **1002**

Alfentanil Hydrochloride (Additive effects). Products include:
- Alfenta Injection ... 1334

Alprazolam (Additive effects). Products include:
- Xanax Tablets ... 2115

Aluminum Carbonate (May substantially decrease plasma salicylate concentration). Products include:
- Basaljel Capsules ... 2810
- Basaljel Suspension ... 2810
- Basaljel Tablets ... 2810

Aluminum Hydroxide (May substantially decrease plasma salicylate concentration). Products include:
- ALternaGEL Liquid ... 1358
- Maximum Strength Ascriptin ... ▣ 650
- Cama Arthritis Pain Reliever ... ▣ 748
- Gaviscon Extra Strength Relief Formula Antacid Tablets ... ▣ 778
- Gaviscon Extra Strength Relief Formula Liquid Antacid ... ▣ 779
- Gaviscon Liquid Antacid ... ▣ 779
- Gelusil Antacid-Anti-gas Liquid ... ▣ 819
- Gelusil Antacid-Anti-gas Tablets ... ▣ 819
- Maalox Antacid/Anti-Gas Tablets ... 889
- Maalox Heartburn Relief Suspension ... ▣ 658
- Maalox Antacid Liquid ... 888
- Extra Strength Maalox Antacid/Anti-Gas Liquid and Tablets ... 888
- Mylanta ... 1359
- Tempo Soft Antacid ... ▣ 799

Aluminum Hydroxide Gel (May substantially decrease plasma salicylate concentration). Products include:
- ALternaGEL Liquid ... ▣ 675
- Aludrox Oral Suspension ... ▣ 850
- Amphojel Suspension ... 2802
- Amphojel Suspension without Flavor ... 2802
- Amphojel Tablets ... 2802
- Ascriptin ... ▣ 650
- Gaviscon Antacid Tablets ... ▣ 778
- Gaviscon-2 Antacid Tablets ... ▣ 779
- Mylanta Liquid ... ▣ 676
- Mylanta Double Strength Liquid ... ▣ 676
- Nephrox Suspension ... ▣ 671

Amitriptyline Hydrochloride (Additive effects). Products include:
- Elavil ... 2945
- Etrafon ... 2495
- Limbitrol ... 2333
- Triavil Tablets ... 1800

Ammonium Chloride (Elevated plasma salicylate concentrations).
- No products indexed under this heading.

Amoxapine (Additive effects). Products include:
- Asendin Tablets ... 1419

Aprobarbital (Additive effects).
- No products indexed under this heading.

Betamethasone Acetate (May decrease salicylate plasma levels). Products include:
- Celestone Soluspan Suspension ... 2484

Betamethasone Sodium Phosphate (May decrease salicylate plasma levels). Products include:
- Celestone Soluspan Suspension ... 2484

Buprenorphine (Additive effects). Products include:
- Buprenex Injectable ... 2170

Buspirone Hydrochloride (Additive effects). Products include:
- BuSpar Tablets ... 738

Butabarbital (Additive effects).
- No products indexed under this heading.

Butalbital (Additive effects). Products include:
- Axocet Capsules ... 2469
- Esgic-plus Capsules ... 1012
- Esgic-plus Tablets ... 1012
- Fioricet Tablets ... 2386
- Fioricet with Codeine Capsules ... 2387
- Fiorinal Capsules ... 2388
- Fiorinal with Codeine Capsules ... 2390
- Fiorinal Tablets ... 2388
- Phrenilin ... 790
- Sedapap Tablets 50 mg/650 mg ... 1826

Chlordiazepoxide (Additive effects). Products include:
- Limbitrol ... 2333

Chlordiazepoxide Hydrochloride (Additive effects). Products include:
- Librax Capsules ... 2330
- Librium Capsules ... 2331
- Librium Injectable ... 2332

Chlorpromazine (Additive effects). Products include:
- Thorazine Suppositories ... 2701

Chlorpromazine Hydrochloride (Additive effects). Products include:
- Thorazine ... 2701

Chlorpropamide (Possible enhancement of hypoglycemia). Products include:
- Diabinese Tablets ... 2002

Chlorprothixene (Additive effects).
- No products indexed under this heading.

Chlorprothixene Hydrochloride (Additive effects).
- No products indexed under this heading.

Chlorprothixene Lactate (Additive effects).
- No products indexed under this heading.

Clorazepate Dipotassium (Additive effects). Products include:
- Tranxene ... 459

Clozapine (Additive effects). Products include:
- Clozaril Tablets ... 2377

Codeine Phosphate (Additive effects). Products include:
- Brontex ... 2130
- Dimetane-DC Cough Syrup ... 2232
- Fioricet with Codeine Capsules ... 2387
- Fiorinal with Codeine Capsules ... 2390
- Nucofed ... 2225
- Phenergan with Codeine ... 2883
- Phenergan VC with Codeine ... 2888
- Robitussin A-C Syrup ... 2248
- Robitussin-DAC Syrup ... 2249
- Ryna ... ▣ 804
- Soma Compound w/Codeine Tablets ... 2784
- Tylenol with Codeine ... 1592

Cortisone Acetate (May decrease salicylate plasma levels). Products include:
- Cortone Acetate Sterile Suspension ... 1663
- Cortone Acetate Tablets ... 1664

Desflurane (Additive effects). Products include:
- Suprane (desflurane, USP) ... 1865

Desipramine Hydrochloride (Additive effects). Products include:
- Norpramin Tablets ... 1273

Dexamethasone (May decrease salicylate plasma levels). Products include:
- AK-Trol Ointment & Suspension ... ⊙ 205
- Decadron Elixir ... 1676
- Decadron Tablets ... 1678
- Decaspray Topical Aerosol ... 1689
- Maxitrol Ophthalmic Ointment and Suspension ... ⊙ 222
- TobraDex Ophthalmic Suspension and Ointment ... 469

Dexamethasone Acetate (May decrease salicylate plasma levels). Products include:
- Dalalone D.P. Injectable ... 1009
- Decadron-LA Sterile Suspension ... 1687

Dexamethasone Sodium Phosphate (May decrease salicylate plasma levels). Products include:
- Decadron Phosphate Injection ... 1680
- Decadron Phosphate Sterile Ophthalmic Ointment ... 1684
- Decadron Phosphate Sterile Ophthalmic Solution ... 1685
- Decadron Phosphate Topical Cream ... 1686
- Decadron Phosphate with Xylocaine Injection, Sterile ... 1683
- Dexacort Phosphate in Respihaler ... 1606
- Dexacort Phosphate in Turbinaire ... 1607
- NeoDecadron Sterile Ophthalmic Ointment ... 1755
- NeoDecadron Sterile Ophthalmic Solution ... 1756
- NeoDecadron Topical Cream ... 1757

Dezocine (Additive effects). Products include:
- Dalgan Injection ... 529

Diazepam (Additive effects). Products include:
- Dizac (diazepam injectable emulsion) CIV ... 1862
- Valium Injectable ... 2336
- Valium Tablets ... 2335

Dicumarol (Enhanced potential for bleeding).
- No products indexed under this heading.

Doxepin Hydrochloride (Additive effects). Products include:
- Adapin Capsules ... 1542
- Sinequan ... 2028
- Zonalon Cream ... 1042

Droperidol (Additive effects). Products include:
- Inapsine Injection ... 462

Enflurane (Additive effects).
- No products indexed under this heading.

Estazolam (Additive effects). Products include:
- ProSom Tablets ... 457

Ethchlorvynol (Additive effects). Products include:
- Placidyl Capsules ... 456

Ethinamate (Additive effects).
- No products indexed under this heading.

Fentanyl (Additive effects). Products include:
- Duragesic Transdermal System ... 1336

Fentanyl Citrate (Additive effects). Products include:
- Sublimaze Injection ... 463

Fludrocortisone Acetate (May decrease salicylate plasma levels). Products include:
- Florinef Acetate Tablets ... 506

Fluphenazine Decanoate (Additive effects). Products include:
- Prolixin Decanoate ... 510

Fluphenazine Enanthate (Additive effects). Products include:
- Prolixin Enanthate ... 510

Fluphenazine Hydrochloride (Additive effects). Products include:
- Prolixin ... 510

Flurazepam Hydrochloride (Additive effects). Products include:
- Dalmane Capsules ... 2329

Glimepiride (Possible enhancement of hypoglycemia). Products include:
- Amaryl Tablets ... 1241

Glipizide (Possible enhancement of hypoglycemia). Products include:
- Glucotrol Tablets ... 2011
- Glucotrol XL Extended Release Tablets ... 2012

Glutethimide (Additive effects).
- No products indexed under this heading.

Glyburide (Possible enhancement of hypoglycemia). Products include:
- DiaBeta Tablets ... 1265
- Glynase PresTab Tablets ... 2091
- Micronase Tablets ... 2099

Haloperidol (Additive effects). Products include:
- Haldol Injection, Tablets and Concentrate ... 1585

Haloperidol Decanoate (Additive effects). Products include:
- Haldol Decanoate ... 1587

Hydrocodone Bitartrate (Additive effects). Products include:
- Codiclear DH Syrup ... 808
- Duratuss HD Elixir ... 2750
- Histussin D Liquid ... 670
- Hycodan Tablets and Syrup ... 946
- Hycomine Compound Tablets ... 948
- Hycomine ... 947
- Hycotuss Expectorant Syrup ... 950
- Hydrocet Capsules ... 787
- Lorcet 10/650 Tablets ... 1016
- Lortab ... 2751
- Tussend ... 1830
- Tussend Expectorant ... 1831
- Vicodin Tablets ... 1404
- Vicodin ES Tablets ... 1405
- Vicodin HP Tablets ... 1403
- Vicodin Tuss Expectorant ... 1406
- Zydone Capsules ... 967

Hydrocodone Polistirex (Additive effects). Products include:
- Tussionex Pennkinetic Extended-Release Suspension ... 1624

Hydrocortisone (May decrease salicylate plasma levels). Products include:
- Anusol-HC Cream 2.5% ... 1953
- Aquanil HC Lotion ... 1989
- Maximum Strength Cortaid Spray ▣ 800
- CORTENEMA ... 2713
- Cortisporin Ointment ... 1074
- Cortisporin Ophthalmic Ointment Sterile ... 1074
- Cortisporin Ophthalmic Suspension Sterile ... 1075
- Cortisporin Otic Solution Sterile ... 1076
- Cortisporin Otic Suspension Sterile 1077
- Cortizone-5 ... ▣ 795
- Cortizone-10 ... ▣ 795
- Hydrocortone Tablets ... 1715
- Hytone ... 922
- Hytone Ointment 2 ½% ... 923
- Massengill Medicated Soft Cloth Towelettes ... 2628
- Pediotic Suspension Sterile ... 1140
- Preparation H Hydrocortisone 1% Cream ... ▣ 843
- ProctoCream-HC 2.5% ... 2552
- VōSoL HC Otic Solution ... 2786

Hydrocortisone Acetate (May decrease salicylate plasma levels). Products include:
- Analpram-HC Rectal Cream 1% and 2.5% ... 993
- Anusol HC-1 Hydrocortisone Anti-Itch Ointment ... ▣ 810
- Anusol-HC Suppositories ... 1954
- Caldecort Anti-Itch Hydrocortisone Cream ... ▣ 651
- Coly-Mycin S Otic w/Neomycin & Hydrocortisone ... 1965
- Cortaid ... ▣ 800
- Cortifoam ... 2540
- Cortisporin Cream ... 1073
- Epifoam ... 2543
- Hydrocortone Acetate Sterile Suspension ... 1712
- Mantadil Cream ... 1124
- Nupercainal Hydrocortisone 1% Cream ... ▣ 661
- Pramosone Cream, Lotion & Ointment ... 995
- ProctoFoam-HC ... 2552
- Terra-Cortril Ophthalmic Suspension ... 2033

Hydrocortisone Sodium Phosphate (May decrease salicylate plasma levels). Products include:
- Hydrocortone Phosphate Injection, Sterile ... 1713

Hydrocortisone Sodium Succinate (May decrease salicylate plasma levels).
- No products indexed under this heading.

Hydroxyzine Hydrochloride (Additive effects). Products include:
- Atarax Tablets & Syrup ... 1992
- Marax Tablets & DF Syrup ... 2015
- Vistaril Intramuscular Solution ... 2042

Imipramine Hydrochloride (Additive effects). Products include:
- Tofranil Ampuls ... 873

(▣ Described in PDR For Nonprescription Drugs) (⊙ Described in PDR For Ophthalmology)

1003 Interactions Index Soma Compound

Tofranil Tablets 875
Imipramine Pamoate (Additive effects). Products include:
Tofranil-PM Capsules 876
Isocarboxazid (Additive effects).
No products indexed under this heading.
Isoflurane (Additive effects).
No products indexed under this heading.
Ketamine Hydrochloride (Additive effects).
No products indexed under this heading.
Levomethadyl Acetate Hydrochloride (Additive effects). Products include:
Orlaam Oral Solution 2361
Levorphanol Tartrate (Additive effects). Products include:
Levo-Dromoran 2297
Lithium Carbonate (Additive effects). Products include:
Eskalith 2658
Lithium Carbonate Capsules & Tablets 2352
Lithonate/Lithotabs/Lithobid 2721
Lithium Citrate (Additive effects).
No products indexed under this heading.
Lorazepam (Additive effects). Products include:
Ativan Injection 2805
Ativan Tablets 2807
Loxapine Hydrochloride (Additive effects). Products include:
Loxitane 1426
Loxapine Succinate (Additive effects). Products include:
Loxitane Capsules 1426
Magaldrate (May substantially decrease plasma salicylate concentration).
No products indexed under this heading.
Magnesium Hydroxide (May substantially decrease plasma salicylate concentration). Products include:
Aludrox Oral Suspension .... ▣ 850
Ascriptin .... ▣ 650
Di-Gel Antacid/Anti-Gas .... ▣ 762
Gelusil Antacid-Anti-gas Liquid .... ▣ 819
Gelusil Antacid-Anti-gas Tablets .... ▣ 819
Maalox Antacid/Anti-Gas Tablets 889
Maalox Antacid Liquid 888
Extra Strength Maalox Antacid/Anti-Gas Liquid and Tablets 888
Mylanta Fast-Acting 1359
Mylanta Gelcaps Antacid .... ▣ 678
Fast-Acting Mylanta Liquid Antacid 1359
Mylanta Tablets .... ▣ 677
Maximum-Strength Fast-Acting Mylanta Liquid Antacid 1359
Mylanta Double Strength Tablets .... ▣ 677
Phillips' Milk of Magnesia Liquid .... ▣ 627
Rolaids Antacid Tablets .... ▣ 807
Tempo Soft Antacid .... ▣ 799
Magnesium Oxide (May substantially decrease plasma salicylate concentration). Products include:
Beelith Tablets 632
Bufferin Analgesic Tablets .... ▣ 636
Arthritis Strength Bufferin Analgesic Caplets .... ▣ 637
Extra Strength Bufferin Analgesic Tablets .... ▣ 637
Caltrate PLUS .... ▣ 681
Cama Arthritis Pain Reliever .... ▣ 748
Mag-Ox 400 666
Uro-Mag 666
Maprotiline Hydrochloride (Additive effects). Products include:
Ludiomil Tablets 861
Meperidine Hydrochloride (Additive effects). Products include:
Demerol 2438
Mepergan Injection 2859
Mephobarbital (Additive effects). Products include:
Mebaral Tablets 2452
Meprobamate (Additive effects). Products include:
Miltown Tablets 2780
PMB 200 and PMB 400 2890
Mesoridazine Besylate (Additive effects). Products include:
Serentil 689
Metformin Hydrochloride (Possible enhancement of hypoglycemia). Products include:
Glucophage Tablets 754
Methadone Hydrochloride (Additive effects). Products include:
Methadone Hydrochloride Oral Concentrate 2356
Methadone Hydrochloride Oral Solution & Tablets 2357
Methohexital Sodium (Additive effects).
No products indexed under this heading.
Methotrexate Sodium (Toxic effects of metotrexate enhanced). Products include:
Methotrexate Sodium Tablets, Injection, for Injection and LPF Injection 1322
Methotrimeprazine (Additive effects). Products include:
Levoprome 1321
Methoxyflurane (Additive effects).
No products indexed under this heading.
Methylprednisolone Acetate (May decrease salicylate plasma levels).
No products indexed under this heading.
Methylprednisolone Sodium Succinate (May decrease salicylate plasma levels).
No products indexed under this heading.
Midazolam Hydrochloride (Additive effects). Products include:
Versed Injection 2324
Molindone Hydrochloride (Additive effects). Products include:
Moban Tablets and Concentrate 1036
Morphine Sulfate (Additive effects). Products include:
Astramorph/PF Injection, USP (Preservative-Free) 526
Duramorph Injection 983
Infumorph 200 and Infumorph 500 Sterile Solutions 985
Kadian Capsules 2948
MS Contin Tablets 2149
MSIR 2152
Oramorph SR (Morphine Sulfate Sustained Release Tablets) 2359
RMS Suppositories CII 2766
Roxanol 2365
Nortriptyline Hydrochloride (Additive effects). Products include:
Pamelor 2409
Opium Alkaloids (Additive effects).
No products indexed under this heading.
Oxazepam (Additive effects). Products include:
Serax Capsules 2916
Serax Tablets 2916
Oxycodone Hydrochloride (Additive effects). Products include:
OxyContin Tablets 2163
OxyIR Capsules 2167
Percocet Tablets 955
Percodan Tablets 955
Percodan-Demi Tablets 956
Roxicodone Tablets, Oral Solution & Intensol (Oxycodone) 2366
Tylox Capsules 1593
Pentobarbital Sodium (Additive effects). Products include:
Nembutal Sodium Capsules 440
Nembutal Sodium Solution 442
Nembutal Sodium Suppositories 444
Perphenazine (Additive effects). Products include:
Etrafon 2495
Triavil Tablets 1800
Trilafon 2532
Phenelzine Sulfate (Additive effects). Products include:
Nardil 1977
Phenobarbital (Additive effects). Products include:
Arco-Lase Plus Tablets 513
Bellergal-S Tablets 2375
Donnatal 2234
Donnatal Extentabs 2234
Donnatal Tablets 2234
Phenobarbital Elixir and Tablets 1523
Quadrinal Tablets 1398
Potassium Acid Phosphate (Elevated plasma salicylate concentrations). Products include:
K-Phos Original Formula 'Sodium Free' Tablets 633
Prazepam (Additive effects).
No products indexed under this heading.
Prednisolone Acetate (May decrease salicylate plasma levels). Products include:
AK-CIDE .... ◉ 203
AK-CIDE Ointment .... ◉ 203
Blephamide Liquifilm Sterile Ophthalmic Suspension 472
Blephamide Ointment .... ◉ 234
Econopred & Econopred Plus Ophthalmic Suspensions .... ◉ 216
Poly-Pred Liquifilm .... ◉ 246
Pred Forte .... ◉ 247
Pred Mild .... ◉ 250
Pred-G Liquifilm Sterile Ophthalmic Suspension .... ◉ 248
Pred-G S.O.P. Sterile Ophthalmic Ointment .... ◉ 249
Prednisolone Sodium Phosphate (May decrease salicylate plasma levels). Products include:
AK-PRED .... ◉ 204
Hydeltrasol Injection, Sterile 1708
Pediapred Oral Solution 1618
Prednisolone Tebutate (May decrease salicylate plasma levels). Products include:
Hydeltra-T.B.A. Sterile Suspension 1710
Prednisone (May decrease salicylate plasma levels).
No products indexed under this heading.
Probenecid (Reduced uricosuric effect of both drugs; possible reduced renal excretion of salicylate). Products include:
Benemid Tablets 1651
ColBENEMID Tablets 1662
Prochlorperazine (Additive effects). Products include:
Compazine 2644
Promethazine Hydrochloride (Additive effects). Products include:
Mepergan Injection 2859
Phenergan with Codeine 2883
Phenergan with Dextromethorphan 2885
Phenergan Injection 2880
Phenergan Suppositories 2882
Phenergan Syrup 2881
Phenergan Tablets 2882
Phenergan VC 2886
Phenergan VC with Codeine 2888
Propofol (Additive effects). Products include:
Diprivan Injectable Emulsion 2939
Propoxyphene Hydrochloride (Additive effects). Products include:
Darvon 1475
Wygesic Tablets 2930
Propoxyphene Napsylate (Additive effects). Products include:
Darvon-N/Darvocet-N 1473
Protriptyline Hydrochloride (Additive effects). Products include:
Vivactil Tablets 1820
Quazepam (Additive effects). Products include:
Doral Tablets 2773
Risperidone (Additive effects). Products include:
Risperdal Tablets 1348
Secobarbital Sodium (Additive effects). Products include:
Seconal Sodium Pulvules 1529
Sevoflurane (Additive effects).
No products indexed under this heading.
Sodium Acid Phosphate (Elevated plasma salicylate concentrations). Products include:
Uroqid-Acid No. 2 Tablets 633
Sodium Bicarbonate (May substantially decrease plasma salicylate concentration). Products include:
Alka-Seltzer Cherry Effervescent Antacid and Pain Reliever .... ▣ 609
Alka-Seltzer Extra Strength Effervescent Antacid and Pain Reliever .... ▣ 609
Alka-Seltzer Gold Effervescent Antacid .... ▣ 611
Alka-Seltzer Lemon Lime Effervescent Antacid and Pain Reliever .... ▣ 609
Alka-Seltzer Original Effervescent Antacid and Pain Reliever .... ▣ 609
Arm & Hammer Pure Baking Soda .... ▣ 648
Colyte and Colyte-flavored 2540
GoLYTELY 694
Massengill Disposable Douches .... ▣ 780
Massengill Liquid Concentrate .... ▣ 780
NuLYTELY 694
Cherry Flavor NuLYTELY 694
Sufentanil Citrate (Additive effects). Products include:
Sufenta Injection 1355
Sulfinpyrazone (Reduced uricosuric effect of both drugs; possible reduced renal excretion of salicylate). Products include:
Anturane 823
Temazepam (Additive effects). Products include:
Restoril Capsules 2413
Thiamylal Sodium (Additive effects).
No products indexed under this heading.
Thioridazine Hydrochloride (Additive effects). Products include:
Mellaril 2398
Thiothixene (Additive effects). Products include:
Navane Capsules and Concentrate 2018
Navane Intramuscular 2019
Tolazamide (Possible enhancement of hypoglycemia).
No products indexed under this heading.
Tolbutamide (Possible enhancement of hypoglycemia).
No products indexed under this heading.
Tranylcypromine Sulfate (Additive effects). Products include:
Parnate Tablets 2679
Triamcinolone (May decrease salicylate plasma levels).
No products indexed under this heading.
Triamcinolone Acetonide (May decrease salicylate plasma levels). Products include:
Azmacort Oral Inhaler 2175
Nasacort AQ Nasal Spray 2191
Nasacort Nasal Inhaler 2189
Triamcinolone Diacetate (May decrease salicylate plasma levels).
No products indexed under this heading.
Triamcinolone Hexacetonide (May decrease salicylate plasma levels).
No products indexed under this heading.

IMPORTANT NOTE: Always consult each drug listing in the patient's regimen for possible interactions.

Soma Compound — Interactions Index — 1004

Triazolam (Additive effects). Products include:
Halcion Tablets ... 2093
Trifluoperazine Hydrochloride (Additive effects). Products include:
Stelazine ... 2692
Trimipramine Maleate (Additive effects). Products include:
Surmontil Capsules ... 2917
Warfarin Sodium (Enhanced potential for bleeding). Products include:
Coumadin ... 941
Zolpidem Tartrate (Additive effects). Products include:
Ambien Tablets ... 2559

Food Interactions

Alcohol (Additive effects including enhanced aspirin-induced fecal blood loss).

SOMA TABLETS
(Carisoprodol) ... 2782
May interact with central nervous system depressants and certain other agents. Compounds in these categories include:

Alfentanil Hydrochloride (Carisoprodol causes drowsiness and co-administration may increase drowsiness effect). Products include:
Alfenta Injection ... 1334
Alprazolam (Carisoprodol causes drowsiness and co-administration may increase drowsiness effect). Products include:
Xanax Tablets ... 2115
Aprobarbital (Carisoprodol causes drowsiness and co-administration may increase drowsiness effect).
No products indexed under this heading.
Buprenorphine (Carisoprodol causes drowsiness and co-administration may increase drowsiness effect). Products include:
Buprenex Injectable ... 2170
Buspirone Hydrochloride (Carisoprodol causes drowsiness and co-administration may increase drowsiness effect). Products include:
BuSpar Tablets ... 738
Butabarbital (Carisoprodol causes drowsiness and co-administration may increase drowsiness effect).
No products indexed under this heading.
Butalbital (Carisoprodol causes drowsiness and co-administration may increase drowsiness effect). Products include:
Axocet Capsules ... 2469
Esgic-plus Capsules ... 1012
Esgic-plus Tablets ... 1012
Fioricet Tablets ... 2386
Fioricet with Codeine Capsules ... 2387
Fiorinal Capsules ... 2388
Fiorinal with Codeine Capsules ... 2390
Fiorinal Tablets ... 2388
Phrenilin ... 790
Sedapap Tablets 50 mg/650 mg .. 1826
Chlordiazepoxide (Carisoprodol causes drowsiness and co-administration may increase drowsiness effect). Products include:
Limbitrol ... 2333
Chlordiazepoxide Hydrochloride (Carisoprodol causes drowsiness and co-administration may increase drowsiness effect). Products include:
Librax Capsules ... 2330
Librium Capsules ... 2331
Librium Injectable ... 2332
Chlorpromazine (Carisoprodol causes drowsiness and co-administration may increase drowsiness effect). Products include:
Thorazine Suppositories ... 2701
Chlorpromazine Hydrochloride (Carisoprodol causes drowsiness and co-administration may increase drowsiness effect). Products include:
Thorazine ... 2701
Chlorprothixene (Carisoprodol causes drowsiness and co-administration may increase drowsiness effect).
No products indexed under this heading.
Chlorprothixene Hydrochloride (Carisoprodol causes drowsiness and co-administration may increase drowsiness effect).
No products indexed under this heading.
Chlorprothixene Lactate (Carisoprodol causes drowsiness and co-administration may increase drowsiness effect).
No products indexed under this heading.
Clorazepate Dipotassium (Carisoprodol causes drowsiness and co-administration may increase drowsiness effect). Products include:
Tranxene ... 459
Clozapine (Carisoprodol causes drowsiness and co-administration may increase drowsiness effect). Products include:
Clozaril Tablets ... 2377
Codeine Phosphate (Carisoprodol causes drowsiness and co-administration may increase drowsiness effect). Products include:
Brontex ... 2130
Dimetane-DC Cough Syrup ... 2232
Fioricet with Codeine Capsules ... 2387
Fiorinal with Codeine Capsules ... 2390
Nucofed ... 2225
Phenergan with Codeine ... 2883
Phenergan VC with Codeine ... 2888
Robitussin A-C Syrup ... 2248
Robitussin-DAC Syrup ... 2249
Ryna ... ▣ 804
Soma Compound w/Codeine Tablets ... 2784
Tylenol with Codeine ... 1592
Desflurane (Carisoprodol causes drowsiness and co-administration may increase drowsiness effect). Products include:
Suprane (desflurane, USP) ... 1865
Dezocine (Carisoprodol causes drowsiness and co-administration may increase drowsiness effect). Products include:
Dalgan Injection ... 529
Diazepam (Carisoprodol causes drowsiness and co-administration may increase drowsiness effect). Products include:
Dizac (diazepam injectable emulsion) CIV ... 1862
Valium Injectable ... 2336
Valium Tablets ... 2335
Droperidol (Carisoprodol causes drowsiness and co-administration may increase drowsiness effect). Products include:
Inapsine Injection ... 462
Enflurane (Carisoprodol causes drowsiness and co-administration may increase drowsiness effect).
No products indexed under this heading.
Estazolam (Carisoprodol causes drowsiness and co-administration may increase drowsiness effect). Products include:
ProSom Tablets ... 457
Ethchlorvynol (Carisoprodol causes drowsiness and co-administration may increase drowsiness effect). Products include:
Placidyl Capsules ... 456
Ethinamate (Carisoprodol causes drowsiness and co-administration may increase drowsiness effect).
No products indexed under this heading.
Fentanyl (Carisoprodol causes drowsiness and co-administration may increase drowsiness effect). Products include:
Duragesic Transdermal System ... 1336
Fentanyl Citrate (Carisoprodol causes drowsiness and co-administration may increase drowsiness effect). Products include:
Sublimaze Injection ... 463
Fluphenazine Decanoate (Carisoprodol causes drowsiness and co-administration may increase drowsiness effect). Products include:
Prolixin Decanoate ... 510
Fluphenazine Enanthate (Carisoprodol causes drowsiness and co-administration may increase drowsiness effect). Products include:
Prolixin Enanthate ... 510
Fluphenazine Hydrochloride (Carisoprodol causes drowsiness and co-administration may increase drowsiness effect). Products include:
Prolixin ... 510
Flurazepam Hydrochloride (Carisoprodol causes drowsiness and co-administration may increase drowsiness effect). Products include:
Dalmane Capsules ... 2329
Glutethimide (Carisoprodol causes drowsiness and co-administration may increase drowsiness effect).
No products indexed under this heading.
Haloperidol (Carisoprodol causes drowsiness and co-administration may increase drowsiness effect). Products include:
Haldol Injection, Tablets and Concentrate ... 1585
Haloperidol Decanoate (Carisoprodol causes drowsiness and co-administration may increase drowsiness effect). Products include:
Haldol Decanoate ... 1587
Hydrocodone Bitartrate (Carisoprodol causes drowsiness and co-administration may increase drowsiness effect). Products include:
Codiclear DH Syrup ... 808
Duratuss HD Elixir ... 2750
Histussin D Liquid ... 670
Hycodan Tablets and Syrup ... 946
Hycomine Compound Tablets ... 948
Hycomine ... 947
Hycotuss Expectorant Syrup ... 950
Hydrocet Capsules ... 787
Lorcet 10/650 Tablets ... 1016
Lortab ... 2751
Tussend ... 1830
Tussend Expectorant ... 1831
Vicodin Tablets ... 1404
Vicodin ES Tablets ... 1405
Vicodin HP Tablets ... 1403
Vicodin Tuss Expectorant ... 1406
Zydone Capsules ... 967
Hydrocodone Polistirex (Carisoprodol causes drowsiness and co-administration may increase drowsiness effect). Products include:
Tussionex Pennkinetic Extended-Release Suspension ... 1624
Hydromorphone Hydrochloride (Carisoprodol causes drowsiness and co-administration may increase drowsiness effect). Products include:
Dilaudid Ampules ... 1382
Dilaudid Cough Syrup ... 1383
Dilaudid-HP Injection ... 1384
Dilaudid-HP Lyophilized Powder 250 mg ... 1384
Dilaudid ... 1382
Dilaudid Oral Liquid ... 1386
Dilaudid ... 1382
Dilaudid Tablets - 8 mg ... 1386
Hydroxyzine Hydrochloride (Carisoprodol causes drowsiness and co-administration may increase drowsiness effect). Products include:
Atarax Tablets & Syrup ... 1992
Marax Tablets & DF Syrup ... 2015
Vistaril Intramuscular Solution ... 2042
Isoflurane (Carisoprodol causes drowsiness and co-administration may increase drowsiness effect).
No products indexed under this heading.
Ketamine Hydrochloride (Carisoprodol causes drowsiness and co-administration may increase drowsiness effect).
No products indexed under this heading.
Levomethadyl Acetate Hydrochloride (Carisoprodol causes drowsiness and co-administration may increase drowsiness effect). Products include:
Orlaam Oral Solution ... 2361
Levorphanol Tartrate (Carisoprodol causes drowsiness and co-administration may increase drowsiness effect). Products include:
Levo-Dromoran ... 2297
Lorazepam (Carisoprodol causes drowsiness and co-administration may increase drowsiness effect). Products include:
Ativan Injection ... 2805
Ativan Tablets ... 2807
Loxapine Succinate (Carisoprodol causes drowsiness and co-administration may increase drowsiness effect). Products include:
Loxitane Capsules ... 1426
Meperidine Hydrochloride (Carisoprodol causes drowsiness and co-administration may increase drowsiness effect). Products include:
Demerol ... 2438
Mepergan Injection ... 2859
Mephobarbital (Carisoprodol causes drowsiness and co-administration may increase drowsiness effect). Products include:
Mebaral Tablets ... 2452
Meprobamate (Carisoprodol causes drowsiness and co-administration may increase drowsiness effect). Products include:
Miltown Tablets ... 2780
PMB 200 and PMB 400 ... 2890
Mesoridazine Besylate (Carisoprodol causes drowsiness and co-administration may increase drowsiness effect). Products include:
Serentil ... 689
Methadone Hydrochloride (Carisoprodol causes drowsiness and co-administration may increase drowsiness effect). Products include:
Methadone Hydrochloride Oral Concentrate ... 2356
Methadone Hydrochloride Oral Solution & Tablets ... 2357
Methohexital Sodium (Carisoprodol causes drowsiness and co-administration may increase drowsiness effect).
No products indexed under this heading.

(▣ Described in PDR For Nonprescription Drugs) (◉ Described in PDR For Ophthalmology)

Methotrimeprazine (Carisoprodol causes drowsiness and co-administration may increase drowsiness effect). Products include:

Levoprome 1321

Methoxyflurane (Carisoprodol causes drowsiness and co-administration may increase drowsiness effect).

No products indexed under this heading.

Midazolam Hydrochloride (Carisoprodol causes drowsiness and co-administration may increase drowsiness effect). Products include:

Versed Injection 2324

Molindone Hydrochloride (Carisoprodol causes drowsiness and co-administration may increase drowsiness effect). Products include:

Moban Tablets and Concentrate 1036

Morphine Sulfate (Carisoprodol causes drowsiness and co-administration may increase drowsiness effect). Products include:

Astramorph/PF Injection, USP (Preservative-Free) 526
Duramorph Injection 983
Infumorph 200 and Infumorph 500 Sterile Solutions 985
Kadian Capsules 2948
MS Contin Tablets 2149
MSIR 2152
Oramorph SR (Morphine Sulfate Sustained Release Tablets) 2359
RMS Suppositories CII 2766
Roxanol 2365

Opium Alkaloids (Carisoprodol causes drowsiness and co-administration may increase drowsiness effect).

No products indexed under this heading.

Oxazepam (Carisoprodol causes drowsiness and co-administration may increase drowsiness effect). Products include:

Serax Capsules 2916
Serax Tablets 2916

Oxycodone Hydrochloride (Carisoprodol causes drowsiness and co-administration may increase drowsiness effect). Products include:

OxyContin Tablets 2163
OxyIR Capsules 2167
Percocet Tablets 955
Percodan Tablets 955
Percodan-Demi Tablets 956
Roxicodone Tablets, Oral Solution & Intensol (Oxycodone) 2366
Tylox Capsules 1593

Pentobarbital Sodium (Carisoprodol causes drowsiness and co-administration may increase drowsiness effect). Products include:

Nembutal Sodium Capsules 440
Nembutal Sodium Solution 442
Nembutal Sodium Suppositories 444

Perphenazine (Carisoprodol causes drowsiness and co-administration may increase drowsiness effect). Products include:

Etrafon 2495
Triavil Tablets 1800
Trilafon 2532

Phenobarbital (Carisoprodol causes drowsiness and co-administration may increase drowsiness effect). Products include:

Arco-Lase Plus Tablets 513
Bellergal-S Tablets 2375
Donnatal 2234
Donnatal Extentabs 2234
Donnatal Tablets 2234
Phenobarbital Elixir and Tablets 1523
Quadrinal Tablets 1398

Prazepam (Carisoprodol causes drowsiness and co-administration may increase drowsiness effect).

No products indexed under this heading.

Prochlorperazine (Carisoprodol causes drowsiness and co-administration may increase drowsiness effect). Products include:

Compazine 2644

Promethazine Hydrochloride (Carisoprodol causes drowsiness and co-administration may increase drowsiness effect). Products include:

Mepergan Injection 2859
Phenergan with Codeine 2883
Phenergan with Dextromethorphan 2885
Phenergan Injection 2880
Phenergan Suppositories 2882
Phenergan Syrup 2881
Phenergan Tablets 2882
Phenergan VC 2886
Phenergan VC with Codeine 2888

Propofol (Carisoprodol causes drowsiness and co-administration may increase drowsiness effect). Products include:

Diprivan Injectable Emulsion 2939

Propoxyphene Hydrochloride (Carisoprodol causes drowsiness and co-administration may increase drowsiness effect). Products include:

Darvon 1475
Wygesic Tablets 2930

Propoxyphene Napsylate (Carisoprodol causes drowsiness and co-administration may increase drowsiness effect). Products include:

Darvon-N/Darvocet-N 1473

Quazepam (Carisoprodol causes drowsiness and co-administration may increase drowsiness effect). Products include:

Doral Tablets 2773

Risperidone (Carisoprodol causes drowsiness and co-administration may increase drowsiness effect). Products include:

Risperdal Tablets 1348

Secobarbital Sodium (Carisoprodol causes drowsiness and co-administration may increase drowsiness effect). Products include:

Seconal Sodium Pulvules 1529

Sevoflurane (Carisoprodol causes drowsiness and co-administration may increase drowsiness effect).

No products indexed under this heading.

Sufentanil Citrate (Carisoprodol causes drowsiness and co-administration may increase drowsiness effect). Products include:

Sufenta Injection 1355

Temazepam (Carisoprodol causes drowsiness and co-administration may increase drowsiness effect). Products include:

Restoril Capsules 2413

Thiamylal Sodium (Carisoprodol causes drowsiness and co-administration may increase drowsiness effect).

No products indexed under this heading.

Thioridazine Hydrochloride (Carisoprodol causes drowsiness and co-administration may increase drowsiness effect). Products include:

Mellaril 2398

Thiothixene (Carisoprodol causes drowsiness and co-administration may increase drowsiness effect). Products include:

Navane Capsules and Concentrate 2018
Navane Intramuscular 2019

Triazolam (Carisoprodol causes drowsiness and co-administration may increase drowsiness effect). Products include:

Halcion Tablets 2093

Trifluoperazine Hydrochloride (Carisoprodol causes drowsiness and co-administration may increase drowsiness effect). Products include:

Stelazine 2692

Zolpidem Tartrate (Carisoprodol causes drowsiness and co-administration may increase drowsiness effect). Products include:

Ambien Tablets 2559

Food Interactions

Alcohol (Carisoprodol causes drowsiness and co-administration may increase drowsiness effect).

SORBITRATE CHEWABLE TABLETS

(Isosorbide Dinitrate) 2959

May interact with calcium channel blockers and certain other agents. Compounds in these categories include:

Amlodipine Besylate (Combination therapy of calcium channel blockers and organic nitrates may result in marked symptomatic orthostatic hypotension; dose adjustment of either class of agent may be necessary). Products include:

Lotrel Capsules 858
Norvasc Tablets 2020

Bepridil Hydrochloride (Combination therapy of calcium channel blockers and organic nitrates may result in marked symptomatic orthostatic hypotension; dose adjustment of either class of agent may be necessary). Products include:

Vascor Tablets (200 and 300 mg) 1597

Diltiazem Hydrochloride (Combination therapy of calcium channel blockers and organic nitrates may result in marked symptomatic orthostatic hypotension; dose adjustment of either class of agent may be necessary). Products include:

Cardizem CD Capsules 1251
Cardizem SR Capsules 1255
Cardizem Injectable 1253
Cardizem Tablets 1257
Dilacor XR Extended-release Capsules 2183
Tiazac Capsules 1019

Drugs Depending On Vascular Smooth Muscle (Possible decreased or increased effect depending on the agent that depends on vascular smooth muscle as the final common path).

Felodipine (Combination therapy of calcium channel blockers and organic nitrates may result in marked symptomatic orthostatic hypotension; dose adjustment of either class of agent may be necessary). Products include:

Plendil Extended-Release Tablets 514

Isradipine (Combination therapy of calcium channel blockers and organic nitrates may result in marked symptomatic orthostatic hypotension; dose adjustment of either class of agent may be necessary). Products include:

DynaCirc Capsules 2381
DynaCirc CR Tablets 2383

Nicardipine Hydrochloride (Combination therapy of calcium channel blockers and organic nitrates may result in marked symptomatic orthostatic hypotension; dose adjustment of either class of agent may be necessary). Products include:

Cardene Capsules 2261
Cardene I.V. 2815
Cardene SR Capsules 2264

Nifedipine (Combination therapy of calcium channel blockers and organic nitrates may result in marked symptomatic orthostatic hypotension; dose adjustment of either class of agent may be necessary). Products include:

Adalat Capsules (10 mg and 20 mg) 580
Adalat CC 582
Procardia Capsules 2024
Procardia XL Extended Release Tablets 2026

Nimodipine (Combination therapy of calcium channel blockers and organic nitrates may result in marked symptomatic orthostatic hypotension; dose adjustment of either class of agent may be necessary). Products include:

Nimotop Capsules 603

Nisoldipine (Combination therapy of calcium channel blockers and organic nitrates may result in marked symptomatic orthostatic hypotension; dose adjustment of either class of agent may be necessary). Products include:

Sular Tablets 2961

Verapamil Hydrochloride (Combination therapy of calcium channel blockers and organic nitrates may result in marked symptomatic orthostatic hypotension; dose adjustment of either class of agent may be necessary). Products include:

Calan SR Caplets 2571
Calan Tablets 2568
Covera-HS Tablets 2573
Isoptin Injectable 1391
Isoptin Oral Tablets 1393
Isoptin SR Tablets 1395
Verelan Capsules 1455

Food Interactions

Alcohol (Enhances sensitivity to hypotensive activity of nitrates).

SORBITRATE ORAL TABLETS

(Isosorbide Dinitrate) 2959

See **Sorbitrate Chewable Tablets**

SORBITRATE SUBLINGUAL TABLETS

(Isosorbide Dinitrate) 2959

See **Sorbitrate Chewable Tablets**

SOTRADECOL (SODIUM TETRADECYL SULFATE INJECTION)

(Sodium Tetradecyl Sulfate) 987

May interact with oral contraceptives and certain other agents. Compounds in these categories include:

Desogestrel (Use caution prior to initiating treatment with Sotradecol). Products include:

Desogen Tablets 1867
Ortho-Cept 1907

Ethinyl Estradiol (Use caution prior to initiating treatment with Sotradecol). Products include:

Brevicon 2563
Demulen 2580
Desogen Tablets 1867
Levlen/Tri-Levlen 646
Lo/Ovral Tablets 2852
Lo/Ovral-28 Tablets 2857
Modicon 1928
Nordette-21 Tablets 2863
Nordette-28 Tablets 2866
Norinyl 2563
Ortho-Cept 1907
Ortho-Cyclen/Ortho-Tri-Cyclen 1914
Ortho-Novum 1928
Ortho-Cyclen/Ortho Tri-Cyclen 1914
Ovcon 765
Ovral Tablets 2877
Ovral-28 Tablets 2878
Levlen/Tri-Levlen 646

IMPORTANT NOTE: Always consult each drug listing in the patient's regimen for possible interactions.

Sotradecol **Interactions Index** 1006

Tri-Norinyl 2607
Triphasil-21 Tablets 2919
Triphasil-28 Tablets 2924

Ethynodiol Diacetate (Use caution prior to initiating treatment with Sotradecol). Products include:
Demulen 2580

Heparin Calcium (*In Vitro* incompatibilities).
No products indexed under this heading.

Heparin Sodium (*In Vitro* incompatibilities). Products include:
Heparin Lock Flush Solution 2831
Heparin Sodium Injection 2832
Heparin Sodium Vials 1486

Levonorgestrel (Use caution prior to initiating treatment with Sotradecol). Products include:
Levlen/Tri-Levlen 646
Nordette-21 Tablets 2863
Nordette-28 Tablets 2866
Norplant System 2868
Levlen/Tri-Levlen 646
Triphasil-21 Tablets 2919
Triphasil-28 Tablets 2924

Mestranol (Use caution prior to initiating treatment with Sotradecol). Products include:
Norinyl 2563
Ortho-Novum 1928

Norethindrone (Use caution prior to initiating treatment with Sotradecol). Products include:
Brevicon 2563
Micronor Tablets 1903
Modicon 1928
Norinyl 2563
Nor-Q D Tablets 2598
Ortho-Novum 1928
Ovcon 765
Tri-Norinyl 2607

Norethynodrel (Use caution prior to initiating treatment with Sotradecol).
No products indexed under this heading.

Norgestimate (Use caution prior to initiating treatment with Sotradecol). Products include:
Ortho-Cyclen/Ortho-Tri-Cyclen 1914
Ortho-Cyclen/Ortho Tri-Cyclen 1914

Norgestrel (Use caution prior to initiating treatment with Sotradecol). Products include:
Lo/Ovral Tablets 2852
Lo/Ovral-28 Tablets 2857
Ovral Tablets 2877
Ovral-28 Tablets 2878
Ovrette Tablets 2878

SPECTAZOLE (ECONAZOLE NITRATE 1%) CREAM
(Econazole Nitrate) 1947
None cited in PDR database.

SPECTROBID TABLETS
(Bacampicillin Hydrochloride) 2030
May interact with:

Allopurinol (Increased incidence of rashes). Products include:
Zyloprim Tablets 1194

Disulfiram (Spectrobid should not be co-administered). Products include:
Antabuse Tablets 2802

SPORANOX CAPSULES
(Itraconazole) 1352
May interact with oral anticoagulants, oral hypoglycemic agents, histamine h2-receptor antagonists, dihydropyridine calcium channel blockers, antacids, proton pump inhibitor, and certain other agents. Compounds in these categories include:

Acarbose (Potential for severe hypoglycemia). Products include:
Precose 604

Aluminum Carbonate (Absorption of itraconazole is impaired when gastric acidity is decreased; antacid should not be administered for at least two hours after itraconazole administration). Products include:
Basaljel Capsules 2810
Basaljel Suspension 2810
Basaljel Tablets 2810

Aluminum Hydroxide (Absorption of itraconazole is impaired when gastric acidity is decreased; antacid should not be administered for at least two hours after itraconazole administration). Products include:
ALternaGEL Liquid 1358
Maximum Strength Ascriptin .... ▣ 650
Cama Arthritis Pain Reliever .... ▣ 748
Gaviscon Extra Strength Relief Formula Antacid Tablets .... ▣ 778
Gaviscon Extra Strength Relief Formula Liquid Antacid .... ▣ 779
Gaviscon Liquid Antacid .... ▣ 779
Gelusil Antacid-Anti-gas Liquid .... ▣ 819
Gelusil Antacid-Anti-gas Tablets .... ▣ 819
Maalox Antacid/Anti-Gas Tablets 889
Maalox Heartburn Relief Suspension .... ▣ 658
Maalox Antacid Liquid 888
Extra Strength Maalox Antacid/Anti-Gas Liquid and Tablets 888
Mylanta 1359
Tempo Soft Antacid .... ▣ 799

Aluminum Hydroxide Gel (Absorption of itraconazole is impaired when gastric acidity is decreased; antacid should not be administered for at least two hours after itraconazole administration). Products include:
ALternaGEL Liquid .... ▣ 675
Aludrox Oral Suspension .... ▣ 850
Amphojel Suspension 2802
Amphojel Suspension without Flavor 2802
Amphojel Tablets 2802
Ascriptin .... ▣ 650
Gaviscon Antacid Tablets .... ▣ 778
Gaviscon-2 Antacid Tablets .... ▣ 779
Mylanta Liquid .... ▣ 676
Mylanta Double Strength Liquid .... ▣ 676
Nephrox Suspension .... ▣ 671

Amlodipine Besylate (Co-administration with dihydropyridine calcium channel blockers may result in edema). Products include:
Lotrel Capsules 858
Norvasc Tablets 2020

Amphotericin B (In vivo studies suggest that the activity of amphotericin B may be suppressed by azole antifungal therapy; clinical significance of this interaction is unknown). Products include:
Abelcet Injection 1540
Fungizone Intravenous 507
Fungizone Oral Suspension 704

Astemizole (Co-administration is contraindicated; potential for prolonged QT intervals). Products include:
Hismanal Tablets 1341

Chlorpropamide (Potential for severe hypoglycemia). Products include:
Diabinese Tablets 2002

Cimetidine (Potential for reduced plasma levels of itraconazole; absorption of oral itraconazole is enhanced when administered with a cola beverage in patients taking acid suppressors, e.g., H_2 inhibitors). Products include:
Tagamet HB Tablets .... ▣ 786
Tagamet Tablets 2694

Cimetidine Hydrochloride (Potential for reduced plasma levels of itraconazole; absorption of oral itraconazole is enhanced when administered with a cola beverage in patients taking acid suppressors, e.g., H_2 inhibitors). Products include:
Tagamet 2694

Cisapride (Itraconazole is expected to markedly raise cisapride plasma concentrations due to its chemical similarities to ketoconazole; potential for prolonged QT interval, ventricular arrhythmias and torsade de pointes; concurrent use is contraindicated). Products include:
Propulsid 1346

Cyclosporine (Co-administration results in increased plasma concentration of cyclosporine; dosage of cyclosporine may have to be reduced; rare reports of rhabdomyolysis involving renal transplant patients on concurrent therapy with HMG-CoA, cyclosporine and itraconazole). Products include:
Neoral 2405
Sandimmune 2416

Dicumarol (Enhanced anticoagulant effect).
No products indexed under this heading.

Digoxin (Elevated plasma concentrations of digoxin; monitor digoxin concentration and, if needed, reduce the dosage accordingly). Products include:
Lanoxicaps 1110
Lanoxin Elixir Pediatric 1113
Lanoxin Injection 1116
Lanoxin Injection Pediatric 1119
Lanoxin Tablets 1121

Famotidine (Potential for reduced plasma levels of itraconazole; absorption of oral itraconazole is enhanced when administered with a cola beverage in patients taking acid suppressors, e.g., H_2 inhibitors). Products include:
Pepcid AC Acid Controller 1360
Pepcid Injection 1765
Pepcid 1763

Felodipine (Co-administration with dihydropyridine calcium channel blockers may result in edema). Products include:
Plendil Extended-Release Tablets 514

Glimepiride (Potential for severe hypoglycemia). Products include:
Amaryl Tablets 1241

Glipizide (Potential for severe hypoglycemia). Products include:
Glucotrol Tablets 2011
Glucotrol XL Extended Release Tablets 2012

Glyburide (Potential for severe hypoglycemia). Products include:
DiaBeta Tablets 1265
Glynase PresTab Tablets 2091
Micronase Tablets 2099

Isoniazid (Co-administration may reduce plasma levels of azole antifungal agents). Products include:
Nydrazid Injection 509
Rifamate Capsules 1278
Rifater 1280

Isradipine (Co-administration with dihydropyridine calcium channel blockers may result in edema). Products include:
DynaCirc Capsules 2381
DynaCirc CR Tablets 2383

Lansoprazole (Absorption of oral itraconazole is enhanced when administered with a cola beverage in patients taking acid suppressors, e.g., proton pump inhibitors). Products include:
Prevacid Delayed-Release Capsules 2746

Lovastatin (Rare reports of rhabdomyolysis involving renal transplant patients on concurrent therapy with simvastatin, cyclosporine and itraconazole). Products include:
Mevacor Tablets 1742

Magaldrate (Absorption of itraconazole is impaired when gastric acidity is decreased; antacid should not be administered for at least two hours after itraconazole administration).
No products indexed under this heading.

Magnesium Hydroxide (Absorption of itraconazole is impaired when gastric acidity is decreased; antacid should not be administered for at least two hours after itraconazole administration). Products include:
Aludrox Oral Suspension .... ▣ 850
Ascriptin .... ▣ 650
Di-Gel Antacid/Anti-Gas .... ▣ 762
Gelusil Antacid-Anti-gas Liquid .... ▣ 819
Gelusil Antacid-Anti-gas Tablets .... ▣ 819
Maalox Antacid/Anti-Gas Tablets 889
Maalox Antacid Liquid 888
Extra Strength Maalox Antacid/Anti-Gas Liquid and Tablets 888
Mylanta Fast-Acting 1359
Mylanta Gelcaps Antacid .... ▣ 678
Fast-Acting Mylanta Liquid Antacid 1359
Mylanta Tablets .... ▣ 677
Maximum-Strength Fast-Acting Mylanta Liquid Antacid 1359
Mylanta Double Strength Tablets .... ▣ 677
Phillips' Milk of Magnesia Liquid .... ▣ 627
Rolaids Antacid Tablets .... ▣ 807
Tempo Soft Antacid .... ▣ 799

Magnesium Oxide (Absorption of itraconazole is impaired when gastric acidity is decreased; antacid should not be administered for at least two hours after itraconazole administration). Products include:
Beelith Tablets 632
Bufferin Analgesic Tablets .... ▣ 636
Arthritis Strength Bufferin Analgesic Caplets .... ▣ 637
Extra Strength Bufferin Analgesic Tablets .... ▣ 637
Caltrate PLUS .... ▣ 681
Cama Arthritis Pain Reliever .... ▣ 748
Mag-Ox 400 666
Uro-Mag 666

Metformin Hydrochloride (Potential for severe hypoglycemia). Products include:
Glucophage Tablets 754

Midazolam Hydrochloride (Co-administration with oral midazolam has resulted in elevated plasma concentration of midazolam resulting in prolonged hypnotic and sedative effects; concurrent oral use should be avoided). Products include:
Versed Injection 2324

Nicardipine Hydrochloride (Co-administration with dihydropyridine calcium channel blockers may result in edema). Products include:
Cardene Capsules 2261
Cardene I.V. 2815
Cardene SR Capsules 2264

Nifedipine (Co-administration with dihydropyridine calcium channel blockers may result in edema). Products include:
Adalat Capsules (10 mg and 20 mg) 580
Adalat CC 582
Procardia Capsules 2024
Procardia XL Extended Release Tablets 2026

(▣ Described in PDR For Nonprescription Drugs) (◉ Described in PDR For Ophthalmology)

Interactions Index

Nimodipine (Co-administration with dihydropyridine calcium channel blockers may result in edema). Products include:
- Nimotop Capsules ... 603

Nizatidine (Potential for reduced plasma levels of itraconazole; absorption of oral itraconazole is enhanced when administered with a cola beverage in patients taking acid suppressors, e.g., H_2 inhibitors). Products include:
- Axid Pulvules ... 1468

Omeprazole (Absorption of oral itraconazole is enhanced when administered with a cola beverage in patients taking acid suppressors, e.g., proton pump inhibitors). Products include:
- Prilosec Delayed-Release Capsules ... 516

Phenytoin (Potential for reduced plasma levels of itraconazole; co-administration may alter the metabolism of phenytoin). Products include:
- Dilantin Infatabs ... 1967
- Dilantin-125 Suspension ... 1969

Phenytoin Sodium (Potential for reduced plasma levels of itraconazole; co-administration may alter the metabolism of phenytoin). Products include:
- Dilantin Kapseals ... 1965

Quinidine Gluconate (Potential for tinnitus and decreased hearing when used concurrently). Products include:
- Quinaglute Dura-Tabs Tablets ... 644

Quinidine Polygalacturonate (Potential for tinnitus and decreased hearing when used concurrently). Products include:
- Cardioquin Tablets ... 2146

Quinidine Sulfate (Potential for tinnitus and decreased hearing when used concurrently). Products include:
- Quinidex Extentabs ... 2240

Ranitidine Hydrochloride (Potential for reduced plasma levels of itraconazole; absorption of oral itraconazole is enhanced when administered with a cola beverage in patients taking acid suppressors, e.g., H_2 inhibitors). Products include:
- Zantac ... 1182
- Zantac Injection ... 1180
- Zantac Syrup ... 1182

Rifampin (Potential for reduced plasma levels of itraconazole). Products include:
- Rifadin ... 1276
- Rifamate Capsules ... 1278
- Rifater ... 1280
- Rimactane Capsules ... 865

Simvastatin (Rare reports of rhabdomyolysis involving renal transplant patients on concurrent therapy with simvastatin, cyclosporine and itraconazole). Products include:
- Zocor Tablets ... 1821

Sodium Bicarbonate (Absorption of itraconazole is impaired when gastric acidity is decreased; antacid should not be administered for at least two hours after itraconazole administration). Products include:
- Alka-Seltzer Cherry Effervescent Antacid and Pain Reliever ... 609
- Alka-Seltzer Extra Strength Effervescent Antacid and Pain Reliever ... 609
- Alka-Seltzer Gold Effervescent Antacid ... 611
- Alka-Seltzer Lemon Lime Effervescent Antacid and Pain Reliever ... 609
- Alka-Seltzer Original Effervescent Antacid and Pain Reliever ... 609
- Arm & Hammer Pure Baking Soda ... 648

Colyte and Colyte-flavored ... 2540
GoLYTELY ... 694
Massengill Disposable Douches ... 780
Massengill Liquid Concentrate ... 780
NuLYTELY ... 694
Cherry Flavor NuLYTELY ... 694

Tacrolimus (Co-administration results in increased plasma concentration of tacrolimus, dosage of tacrolimus may have to be adjusted). Products include:
- Prograf ... 1028

Terfenadine (Co-administration is contraindicated; potential for serious cardiovascular adverse events, including death, cardiac dysrhythmias, ventricular tachycardia and torsade de pointes). Products include:
- Seldane Tablets ... 1284
- Seldane-D Extended-Release Tablets ... 1286

Tolazamide (Potential for severe hypoglycemia).
- No products indexed under this heading.

Tolbutamide (Potential for severe hypoglycemia).
- No products indexed under this heading.

Triazolam (Co-administration has resulted in elevated plasma concentration of triazolam resulting in prolonged hypnotic and sedative effects; concurrent use with oral triazolam is contraindicated). Products include:
- Halcion Tablets ... 2093

Warfarin Sodium (Enhanced anticoagulant effect). Products include:
- Coumadin ... 941

Food Interactions

Cola (Absorption of oral itraconazole is enhanced when administered with a cola beverage in patients with achlorhydria, such as AIDS or patients taking acid suppressors, e.g., H_2 inhibitors and proton pump inhibitors).

Food, unspecified (Presence of food increases systemic bioavailability; when taken on an empty stomach the systemic bioavailability is reduced).

SPORTSCREME EXTERNAL ANALGESIC RUB CREAM & LOTION
(Trolamine Salicylate) ... 798
None cited in PDR database.

ST. JOSEPH ADULT CHEWABLE ASPIRIN (81 MG.)
(Aspirin) ... 768
May interact with oral anticoagulants, oral hypoglycemic agents, and antigout agents. Compounds in these categories include:

Acarbose (Concurrent use is not recommended unless directed by a doctor). Products include:
- Precose ... 604

Allopurinol (Concurrent use is not recommended unless directed by a doctor). Products include:
- Zyloprim Tablets ... 1194

Antiarthritic Drugs, unspecified (Concurrent use is not recommended unless directed by a doctor).

Chlorpropamide (Concurrent use is not recommended unless directed by a doctor). Products include:
- Diabinese Tablets ... 2002

Dicumarol (Concurrent use is not recommended unless directed by a doctor).
- No products indexed under this heading.

Glimepiride (Concurrent use is not recommended unless directed by a doctor). Products include:
- Amaryl Tablets ... 1241

Glipizide (Concurrent use is not recommended unless directed by a doctor). Products include:
- Glucotrol Tablets ... 2011
- Glucotrol XL Extended Release Tablets ... 2012

Glyburide (Concurrent use is not recommended unless directed by a doctor). Products include:
- DiaBeta Tablets ... 1265
- Glynase PresTab Tablets ... 2091
- Micronase Tablets ... 2099

Metformin Hydrochloride (Concurrent use is not recommended unless directed by a doctor). Products include:
- Glucophage Tablets ... 754

Probenecid (Concurrent use is not recommended unless directed by a doctor). Products include:
- Benemid Tablets ... 1651
- ColBENEMID Tablets ... 1662

Sulfinpyrazone (Concurrent use is not recommended unless directed by a doctor). Products include:
- Anturane ... 823

Tolazamide (Concurrent use is not recommended unless directed by a doctor).
- No products indexed under this heading.

Tolbutamide (Concurrent use is not recommended unless directed by a doctor).
- No products indexed under this heading.

Warfarin Sodium (Concurrent use is not recommended unless directed by a doctor). Products include:
- Coumadin ... 941

STADOL INJECTABLE
(Butorphanol Tartrate) ... 779
See **Stadol NS Nasal Spray**

STADOL NS NASAL SPRAY
(Butorphanol Tartrate) ... 779
May interact with barbiturates, tranquilizers, central nervous system depressants, antihistamines, xanthine bronchodilators, and certain other agents. Compounds in these categories include:

Acrivastine (Potential for increased CNS depressant effect). Products include:
- Semprex-D Capsules ... 1620

Alfentanil Hydrochloride (Potential for increased CNS depressant effect). Products include:
- Alfenta Injection ... 1334

Alprazolam (Potential for increased CNS depressant effect). Products include:
- Xanax Tablets ... 2115

Aminophylline (Possibility of smaller initial dose and longer intervals between doses may be needed).
- No products indexed under this heading.

Aprobarbital (Potential for increased CNS depressant effect).
- No products indexed under this heading.

Astemizole (Potential for increased CNS depressant effect). Products include:
- Hismanal Tablets ... 1341

Azatadine Maleate (Potential for increased CNS depressant effect). Products include:
- Trinalin Repetabs Tablets ... 1373

Bromodiphenhydramine Hydrochloride (Potential for increased CNS depressant effect).
- No products indexed under this heading.

Brompheniramine Maleate (Potential for increased CNS depressant effect). Products include:
- Alka-Seltzer Plus Sinus Medicine ... 611
- Bromfed Capsules (Extended-Release) ... 1832
- Bromfed Syrup ... 712
- Bromfed Tablets ... 1832
- Bromfed-DM Cough Syrup ... 1832
- Bromfed-PD Capsules (Extended-Release) ... 1832
- Dimetane-DC Cough Syrup ... 2232
- Dimetane-DX Cough Syrup ... 2233
- Dimetapp Allergy Dye-Free Elixir ... 838
- Dimetapp Allergy Sinus Caplets ... 838
- Dimetapp Cold & Allergy Chewable Tablets ... 838
- Dimetapp Cold & Cough Liqui-Gels ... 839
- Dimetapp Cold & Fever Suspension ... 839
- Dimetapp DM Elixir ... 840
- Dimetapp Elixir ... 840
- Dimetapp Extentabs ... 841
- Dimetapp Tablets/Liqui-Gels ... 841
- Rondec Chewable Tablets ... 974
- Vicks DayQuil Allergy Relief 12-Hour Extended Release Tablets ... 733
- Vicks DayQuil Allergy Relief 4-Hour Tablets ... 733

Buprenorphine (Potential for increased CNS depressant effect). Products include:
- Buprenex Injectable ... 2170

Buspirone Hydrochloride (Potential for increased CNS depressant effect). Products include:
- BuSpar Tablets ... 738

Butabarbital (Potential for increased CNS depressant effect).
- No products indexed under this heading.

Butalbital (Potential for increased CNS depressant effect). Products include:
- Axocet Capsules ... 2469
- Esgic-plus Capsules ... 1012
- Esgic-plus Tablets ... 1012
- Fioricet Tablets ... 2386
- Fioricet with Codeine Capsules ... 2387
- Fiorinal Capsules ... 2388
- Fiorinal with Codeine Capsules ... 2390
- Fiorinal Tablets ... 2388
- Phrenilin ... 790
- Sedapap Tablets 50 mg/650 mg ... 1826

Cetirizine Hydrochloride (Potential for increased CNS depressant effect). Products include:
- Zyrtec Tablets ... 2053

Chlordiazepoxide (Potential for increased CNS depressant effect). Products include:
- Limbitrol ... 2333

Chlordiazepoxide Hydrochloride (Potential for increased CNS depressant effect). Products include:
- Librax Capsules ... 2330
- Librium Capsules ... 2331
- Librium Injectable ... 2332

Chlorpheniramine Maleate (Potential for increased CNS depressant effect). Products include:
- Alka-Seltzer Plus Cold Medicine ... 611
- Alka-Seltzer Plus Cold Medicine Liqui-Gels ... 612
- Alka-Seltzer Plus Cold & Cough Medicine ... 611
- Alka-Seltzer Plus Cold & Cough Medicine Liqui-Gels ... 612
- Alka-Seltzer Plus Flu & Body Aches Effervescent Tablets ... 612
- Allerest Maximum Strength ... 649
- Allerest Sinus Pain Formula ... 649
- Ana-Kit Anaphylaxis Emergency Treatment Kit ... 611
- Atrohist Pediatric Capsules ... 1603
- Atrohist Plus Tablets ... 1605
- BC Cold Powder Multi-Symptom Formula (Cold-Sinus-Allergy) ... 631
- Cerose DM ... 853

IMPORTANT NOTE: Always consult each drug listing in the patient's regimen for possible interactions.

Stadol — Interactions Index

Cheracol Plus Head Cold/Cough Formula .... ℞ 741
Children's TYLENOL Cold Multi-Symptom Chewable Tablets and Liquid 1559
Children's TYLENOL Cold Plus Cough Multi Symptom Chewable Tablets and Liquid 1560
Children's TYLENOL Flu Suspension Liquid 1560
Children's Vicks DayQuil Allergy Relief .... ℞ 730
Children's Vicks NyQuil Cold/Cough Relief .... ℞ 731
Chlor-Trimeton Allergy Decongestant Tablets .... ℞ 759
Chlor-Trimeton Allergy Tablets .... ℞ 758
Allergy-Sinus Comtrex Multi-Symptom Allergy-Sinus Formula Tablets and Caplets .... ℞ 639
Comtrex Multi-Symptom .... ℞ 638
Contac Continuous Action Nasal Decongestant/Antihistamine 12 Hour Capsules .... ℞ 773
Contac Maximum Strength Continuous Action Decongestant/Antihistamine 12 Hour Caplets .. ℞ 772
Contac Severe Cold and Flu Formula Caplets .... ℞ 773
Coricidin Cold + Flu Tablets .... ℞ 760
Coricidin Cough + Cold Tablets .... ℞ 760
Coricidin 'D' Decongestant Tablets .... ℞ 760
D.A. II Tablets 972
D.A. Chewable Tablets 970
Dura-Tap/PD Capsules 970
Dura-Vent/DA Tablets 972
Efidac 24 Chlorpheniramine .... ℞ 655
Extendryl 1003
Fedahist Gyrocaps 2545
Hycomine Compound Tablets 948
Kronofed-A 994
Nolamine Timed-Release Tablets 790
Novahistine Elixir .... ℞ 782
Ornade Spansule Capsules 2678
PediaCare Cough-Cold Chewable Tablets and Liquid 1569
PediaCare NightRest Cough-Cold Liquid 1569
Pediatric Vicks 44m Cough & Cold Relief .... ℞ 737
Pyrroxate Caplets .... ℞ 742
Ryna .... ℞ 804
Sinarest .... ℞ 663
Sine-Off Sinus Medicine .... ℞ 784
Singlet Tablets .... ℞ 785
Sinulin Tablets 792
Sinutab Sinus Allergy Medication, Maximum Strength Tablets and Caplets .... ℞ 823
Sudafed Cold & Allergy Tablets ..... ℞ 826
Teldrin 12 Hour Antihistamine/Nasal Decongestant Allergy Relief Capsules .... ℞ 786
TheraFlu Flu and Cold Medicine .... ℞ 750
Theraflu Maximum Strength Flu and Cold Medicine For Sore Throat .... ℞ 751
TheraFlu Flu, Cold and Cough Medicine .... ℞ 750
TheraFlu Maximum Strength Nighttime Flu, Cold & Cough Medicine .... ℞ 751
Triaminic Night Time .... ℞ 754
Triaminic Syrup .... ℞ 755
Triaminic Triaminicol Cold & Cough .... ℞ 756
Triaminicin Tablets .... ℞ 756
Tussend 1830
TYLENOL Allergy Sinus, Maximum Strength Caplets and Gelcaps 1571
TYLENOL Cold Medication, Multi-Symptom Formula Tablets and Caplets 1572
TYLENOL Cold Medication, Multi-Symptom Hot Liquid Packets 1572
Vicks 44 LiquiCaps Cough, Cold & Flu Relief .... ℞ 728
Vicks 44M Cough, Cold & Flu Relief .... ℞ 729

Chlorpheniramine Polistirex (Potential for increased CNS depressant effect). Products include:
Tussionex Pennkinetic Extended-Release Suspension 1624

Chlorpheniramine Tannate (Potential for increased CNS depressant effect). Products include:
Atrohist Pediatric Suspension 1604

Atrohist Pediatric Suspension Dye-Free 1604
Rynatan 2781
Rynatuss 2782

Chlorpromazine (Potential for increased CNS depressant effect). Products include:
Thorazine Suppositories 2701

Chlorpromazine Hydrochloride (Potential for increased CNS depressant effect). Products include:
Thorazine 2701

Chlorprothixene (Potential for increased CNS depressant effect).
No products indexed under this heading.

Chlorprothixene Hydrochloride (Potential for increased CNS depressant effect).
No products indexed under this heading.

Chlorprothixene Lactate (Potential for increased CNS depressant effect).
No products indexed under this heading.

Clemastine Fumarate (Potential for increased CNS depressant effect). Products include:
Tavist Syrup 2426
Tavist Tablets 2427
Tavist-1 12 Hour Relief Tablets .... ℞ 749
Tavist-D 12 Hour Relief Tablets .... ℞ 750

Clorazepate Dipotassium (Potential for increased CNS depressant effect). Products include:
Tranxene 459

Clozapine (Potential for increased CNS depressant effect). Products include:
Clozaril Tablets 2377

Codeine Phosphate (Potential for increased CNS depressant effect). Products include:
Brontex 2130
Dimetane-DC Cough Syrup 2232
Fioricet with Codeine Capsules 2387
Fiorinal with Codeine Capsules 2390
Nucofed 2225
Phenergan with Codeine 2883
Phenergan VC with Codeine 2888
Robitussin A-C Syrup 2248
Robitussin-DAC Syrup 2249
Ryna .... ℞ 804
Soma Compound w/Codeine Tablets 2784
Tylenol with Codeine 1592

Cyproheptadine Hydrochloride (Potential for increased CNS depressant effect). Products include:
Periactin 1767

Desflurane (Potential for increased CNS depressant effect). Products include:
Suprane (desflurane, USP) 1865

Dexchlorpheniramine Maleate (Potential for increased CNS depressant effect).
No products indexed under this heading.

Dezocine (Potential for increased CNS depressant effect). Products include:
Dalgan Injection 529

Diazepam (Potential for increased CNS depressant effect). Products include:
Dizac (diazepam injectable emulsion) CIV 1862
Valium Injectable 2336
Valium Tablets 2335

Diphenhydramine Citrate (Potential for increased CNS depressant effect). Products include:
Excedrin P.M. Analgesic/Sleeping Aid Tablets, Caplets, Liquigels 735

Diphenhydramine Hydrochloride (Potential for increased CNS depressant effect). Products include:
Actifed Allergy Daytime/Nighttime Caplets .... ℞ 808

Actifed Sinus Daytime/Nighttime Tablets and Caplets .... ℞ 809
Extra Strength Bayer PM Aspirin Plus Sleep Aid .... ℞ 617
Benadryl Allergy Chewables .... ℞ 811
Benadryl Allergy/Cold Tablets .... ℞ 811
Benadryl Allergy Decongestant Liquid Medication .... ℞ 812
Benadryl Allergy Decongestant Tablets .... ℞ 812
Benadryl Allergy Liquid Medication .... ℞ 813
Benadryl Allergy .... ℞ 811
Benadryl Allergy Sinus Headache Caplets .... ℞ 813
Benadryl Dye-Free Allergy Liquigel Softgels .... ℞ 813
Benadryl Dye-Free Allergy Liquid Medication .... ℞ 814
Benadryl Itch Relief Stick Extra Strength .... ℞ 814
Benadryl Cream .... ℞ 814
Benadryl Gel .... ℞ 815
Benadryl Spray .... ℞ 815
Benadryl Injection 1955
Contac Day & Night Cold/Flu Night Caplets .... ℞ 772
Contac Night Allergy/Sinus Caplets .... ℞ 771
Extra Strength Doan's P.M. .... ℞ 653
Excedrin P.M. Analgesic/Sleeping Aid Tablets, Caplets, Liquigels .... ℞ 643
Nytol QuickCaps Caplets .... ℞ 632
Sleepinal Night-time Sleep Aid Capsules and Softgels .... ℞ 798
TYLENOL Allergy Sinus NightTime, Maximum Strength Caplets 1571
TYLENOL Flu NightTime, Maximum Strength Gelcaps 1575
TYLENOL Flu NightTime, Maximum Strength Hot Medication Packets 1575
TYLENOL PM Pain Reliever/Sleep Aid, Extra Strength Gelcaps, Caplets, Geltabs 1576
TYLENOL Severe Allergy Medication Caplets 1571
Maximum Strength Unisom Sleepgels 1990
Unisom With Pain Relief-Nighttime Sleep Aid and Pain Reliever 1991

Diphenylpyraline Hydrochloride (Potential for increased CNS depressant effect).
No products indexed under this heading.

Droperidol (Potential for increased CNS depressant effect). Products include:
Inapsine Injection 462

Dyphylline (Possibility of smaller initial dose and longer intervals between doses may be needed). Products include:
Lufyllin & Lufyllin-400 Tablets 2778
Lufyllin-GG Elixir & Tablets 2779

Enflurane (Potential for increased CNS depressant effect).
No products indexed under this heading.

Estazolam (Potential for increased CNS depressant effect). Products include:
ProSom Tablets 457

Ethchlorvynol (Potential for increased CNS depressant effect). Products include:
Placidyl Capsules 456

Ethinamate (Potential for increased CNS depressant effect).
No products indexed under this heading.

Fentanyl (Potential for increased CNS depressant effect). Products include:
Duragesic Transdermal System 1336

Fentanyl Citrate (Potential for increased CNS depressant effect). Products include:
Sublimaze Injection 463

Fluphenazine Decanoate (Potential for increased CNS depressant effect). Products include:
Prolixin Decanoate 510

Fluphenazine Enanthate (Potential for increased CNS depressant effect). Products include:
Prolixin Enanthate 510

Fluphenazine Hydrochloride (Potential for increased CNS depressant effect). Products include:
Prolixin 510

Flurazepam Hydrochloride (Potential for increased CNS depressant effect). Products include:
Dalmane Capsules 2329

Glutethimide (Potential for increased CNS depressant effect).
No products indexed under this heading.

Haloperidol (Potential for increased CNS depressant effect). Products include:
Haldol Injection, Tablets and Concentrate 1585

Haloperidol Decanoate (Potential for increased CNS depressant effect). Products include:
Haldol Decanoate 1587

Hydrocodone Bitartrate (Potential for increased CNS depressant effect). Products include:
Codiclear DH Syrup 808
Duratuss HD Elixir 2750
Histussin D Liquid 670
Hycodan Tablets and Syrup 946
Hycomine Compound Tablets 948
Hycomine 947
Hycotuss Expectorant Syrup 950
Hydrocet Capsules 787
Lorcet 10/650 Tablets 1016
Lortab 2751
Tussend 1830
Tussend Expectorant 1831
Vicodin Tablets 1404
Vicodin ES Tablets 1405
Vicodin HP Tablets 1403
Vicodin Tuss Expectorant 1406
Zydone Capsules 967

Hydrocodone Polistirex (Potential for increased CNS depressant effect). Products include:
Tussionex Pennkinetic Extended-Release Suspension 1624

Hydroxyzine Hydrochloride (Potential for increased CNS depressant effect). Products include:
Atarax Tablets & Syrup 1992
Marax Tablets & DF Syrup 2015
Vistaril Intramuscular Solution 2042

Isoflurane (Potential for increased CNS depressant effect).
No products indexed under this heading.

Ketamine Hydrochloride (Potential for increased CNS depressant effect).
No products indexed under this heading.

Levomethadyl Acetate Hydrochloride (Potential for increased CNS depressant effect). Products include:
Orlaam Oral Solution 2361

Levorphanol Tartrate (Potential for increased CNS depressant effect). Products include:
Levo-Dromoran 2297

Loratadine (Potential for increased CNS depressant effect). Products include:
Claritin Tablets 2485
Claritin-D Tablets 2487

Lorazepam (Potential for increased CNS depressant effect). Products include:
Ativan Injection 2805
Ativan Tablets 2807

Loxapine Hydrochloride (Potential for increased CNS depressant effect). Products include:
Loxitane 1426

(℞ Described in PDR For Nonprescription Drugs)   (⊚ Described in PDR For Ophthalmology)

1009 **Interactions Index** **Stelazine**

Loxapine Succinate (Potential for increased CNS depressant effect). Products include:
- Loxitane Capsules ... 1426

Meperidine Hydrochloride (Potential for increased CNS depressant effect). Products include:
- Demerol ... 2438
- Mepergan Injection ... 2859

Mephobarbital (Potential for increased CNS depressant effect). Products include:
- Mebaral Tablets ... 2452

Meprobamate (Potential for increased CNS depressant effect). Products include:
- Miltown Tablets ... 2780
- PMB 200 and PMB 400 ... 2890

Mesoridazine Besylate (Potential for increased CNS depressant effect). Products include:
- Serentil ... 689

Methadone Hydrochloride (Potential for increased CNS depressant effect). Products include:
- Methadone Hydrochloride Oral Concentrate ... 2356
- Methadone Hydrochloride Oral Solution & Tablets ... 2357

Methdilazine Hydrochloride (Potential for increased CNS depressant effect).
- No products indexed under this heading.

Methohexital Sodium (Potential for increased CNS depressant effect).
- No products indexed under this heading.

Methotrimeprazine (Potential for increased CNS depressant effect). Products include:
- Levoprome ... 1321

Methoxyflurane (Potential for increased CNS depressant effect).
- No products indexed under this heading.

Midazolam Hydrochloride (Potential for increased CNS depressant effect). Products include:
- Versed Injection ... 2324

Molindone Hydrochloride (Potential for increased CNS depressant effect). Products include:
- Moban Tablets and Concentrate ... 1036

Morphine Sulfate (Potential for increased CNS depressant effect). Products include:
- Astramorph/PF Injection, USP (Preservative-Free) ... 526
- Duramorph Injection ... 983
- Infumorph 200 and Infumorph 500 Sterile Solutions ... 985
- Kadian Capsules ... 2948
- MS Contin Tablets ... 2149
- MSIR ... 2152
- Oramorph SR (Morphine Sulfate Sustained Release Tablets) ... 2359
- RMS Suppositories CII ... 2766
- Roxanol ... 2365

Opium Alkaloids (Potential for increased CNS depressant effect).
- No products indexed under this heading.

Oxazepam (Potential for increased CNS depressant effect). Products include:
- Serax Capsules ... 2916
- Serax Tablets ... 2916

Oxycodone Hydrochloride (Potential for increased CNS depressant effect). Products include:
- OxyContin Tablets ... 2163
- OxyIR Capsules ... 2167
- Percocet Tablets ... 955
- Percodan Tablets ... 955
- Percodan-Demi Tablets ... 956
- Roxicodone Tablets, Oral Solution & Intensol (Oxycodone) ... 2366
- Tylox Capsules ... 1593

Pentobarbital Sodium (Potential for increased CNS depressant effect). Products include:
- Nembutal Sodium Capsules ... 440
- Nembutal Sodium Solution ... 442
- Nembutal Sodium Suppositories ... 444

Perphenazine (Potential for increased CNS depressant effect). Products include:
- Etrafon ... 2495
- Triavil Tablets ... 1800
- Trilafon ... 2532

Phenobarbital (Potential for increased CNS depressant effect). Products include:
- Arco-Lase Plus Tablets ... 513
- Bellergal-S Tablets ... 2375
- Donnatal ... 2234
- Donnatal Extentabs ... 2234
- Donnatal Tablets ... 2234
- Phenobarbital Elixir and Tablets ... 1523
- Quadrinal Tablets ... 1398

Prazepam (Potential for increased CNS depressant effect).
- No products indexed under this heading.

Prochlorperazine (Potential for increased CNS depressant effect). Products include:
- Compazine ... 2644

Promethazine Hydrochloride (Potential for increased CNS depressant effect). Products include:
- Mepergan Injection ... 2859
- Phenergan with Codeine ... 2883
- Phenergan with Dextromethorphan 2885
- Phenergan Injection ... 2880
- Phenergan Suppositories ... 2882
- Phenergan Syrup ... 2881
- Phenergan Tablets ... 2882
- Phenergan VC ... 2886
- Phenergan VC with Codeine ... 2888

Propofol (Potential for increased CNS depressant effect). Products include:
- Diprivan Injectable Emulsion ... 2939

Propoxyphene Hydrochloride (Potential for increased CNS depressant effect). Products include:
- Darvon ... 1475
- Wygesic Tablets ... 2930

Propoxyphene Napsylate (Potential for increased CNS depressant effect). Products include:
- Darvon-N/Darvocet-N ... 1473

Pyrilamine Maleate (Potential for increased CNS depressant effect). Products include:
- 4-Way Fast Acting Nasal Spray (regular & mentholated) ... 644
- Maximum Strength Multi-Symptom Formula Midol ... 621
- PMS Multi-Symptom Formula Midol ... 622

Pyrilamine Tannate (Potential for increased CNS depressant effect). Products include:
- Atrohist Pediatric Suspension ... 1604
- Atrohist Pediatric Suspension Dye-Free ... 1604
- Rynatan ... 2781

Quazepam (Potential for increased CNS depressant effect). Products include:
- Doral Tablets ... 2773

Risperidone (Potential for increased CNS depressant effect). Products include:
- Risperdal Tablets ... 1348

Secobarbital Sodium (Potential for increased CNS depressant effect). Products include:
- Seconal Sodium Pulvules ... 1529

Sevoflurane (Potential for increased CNS depressant effect).
- No products indexed under this heading.

Sufentanil Citrate (Potential for increased CNS depressant effect). Products include:
- Sufenta Injection ... 1355

Temazepam (Potential for increased CNS depressant effect). Products include:
- Restoril Capsules ... 2413

Terfenadine (Potential for increased CNS depressant effect). Products include:
- Seldane Tablets ... 1284
- Seldane-D Extended-Release Tablets ... 1286

Theophylline (Possibility of smaller initial dose and longer intervals between doses may be needed). Products include:
- Marax Tablets & DF Syrup ... 2015
- Quibron ... 2227

Theophylline Anhydrous (Possibility of smaller initial dose and longer intervals between doses may be needed). Products include:
- Aerolate ... 1003
- Primatene Tablets ... 844
- Respbid Tablets ... 687
- Slo-bid Gyrocaps ... 2201
- Theo-24 Extended Release Capsules ... 2753
- Theo-Dur Extended-Release Tablets ... 1367
- Theo-X Extended-Release Tablets .. 793
- Uni-Dur Extended-Release Tablets .. 1374
- Uniphyl 400 mg and 600 mg Tablets ... 2157

Theophylline Calcium Salicylate (Possibility of smaller initial dose and longer intervals between doses may be needed). Products include:
- Quadrinal Tablets ... 1398

Theophylline Sodium Glycinate (Possibility of smaller initial dose and longer intervals between doses may be needed).
- No products indexed under this heading.

Thiamylal Sodium (Potential for increased CNS depressant effect).
- No products indexed under this heading.

Thioridazine Hydrochloride (Potential for increased CNS depressant effect). Products include:
- Mellaril ... 2398

Thiothixene (Potential for increased CNS depressant effect). Products include:
- Navane Capsules and Concentrate 2018
- Navane Intramuscular ... 2019

Triazolam (Potential for increased CNS depressant effect). Products include:
- Halcion Tablets ... 2093

Trifluoperazine Hydrochloride (Potential for increased CNS depressant effect). Products include:
- Stelazine ... 2692

Trimeprazine Tartrate (Potential for increased CNS depressant effect).
- No products indexed under this heading.

Tripelennamine Hydrochloride (Potential for increased CNS depressant effect). Products include:
- PBZ Tablets ... 863
- PBZ-SR Tablets ... 862

Triprolidine Hydrochloride (Potential for increased CNS depressant effect). Products include:
- Actifed Cold & Allergy Tablets ... 807
- Actifed Cold & Sinus Caplets and Tablets ... 808

Zolpidem Tartrate (Potential for increased CNS depressant effect). Products include:
- Ambien Tablets ... 2559

Food Interactions

Alcohol (Potential for increased CNS depressant effect).

STAR-OTIC EAR SOLUTION (Acetic Acid, Boric Acid, Burow's Solution) ... 790

None cited in PDR database.

STELAZINE CONCENTRATE (Trifluoperazine Hydrochloride) ... 2692

May interact with vasopressors, oral anticoagulants, thiazides, anticonvulsants, central nervous system depressants, and certain other agents. Compounds in these categories include:

Alfentanil Hydrochloride (Additive depressant effects). Products include:
- Alfenta Injection ... 1334

Alprazolam (Additive depressant effects). Products include:
- Xanax Tablets ... 2115

Aprobarbital (Additive depressant effects).
- No products indexed under this heading.

Bendroflumethiazide (Orthostatic hypotension that occurs with phenothiazines may be accentuated).
- No products indexed under this heading.

Buprenorphine (Additive depressant effects). Products include:
- Buprenex Injectable ... 2170

Buspirone Hydrochloride (Additive depressant effects). Products include:
- BuSpar Tablets ... 738

Butabarbital (Additive depressant effects).
- No products indexed under this heading.

Butalbital (Additive depressant effects). Products include:
- Axocet Capsules ... 2469
- Esgic-plus Capsules ... 1012
- Esgic-plus Tablets ... 1012
- Fioricet Tablets ... 2386
- Fioricet with Codeine Capsules ... 2387
- Fiorinal Capsules ... 2388
- Fiorinal with Codeine Capsules ... 2390
- Fiorinal Tablets ... 2388
- Phrenilin ... 790
- Sedapap Tablets 50 mg/650 mg .. 1826

Carbamazepine (Stelazine may lower convulsive thresholds; dosage adjustments of anticonvulsants may be necessary). Products include:
- Atretol Tablets ... 569
- Tegretol/Tegretol-XR ... 870

Chlordiazepoxide (Additive depressant effects). Products include:
- Limbitrol ... 2333

Chlordiazepoxide Hydrochloride (Additive depressant effects). Products include:
- Librax Capsules ... 2330
- Librium Capsules ... 2331
- Librium Injectable ... 2332

Chlorothiazide (Orthostatic hypotension that occurs with phenothiazines may be accentuated). Products include:
- Aldoclor Tablets ... 1638
- Diupres Tablets ... 1691
- Diuril Oral ... 1694

Chlorothiazide Sodium (Orthostatic hypotension that occurs with phenothiazines may be accentuated). Products include:
- Diuril Sodium Intravenous ... 1693

Chlorpromazine (Additive depressant effects). Products include:
- Thorazine Suppositories ... 2701

Chlorprothixene (Additive depressant effects).
- No products indexed under this heading.

IMPORTANT NOTE: Always consult each drug listing in the patient's regimen for possible interactions.

Stelazine — Interactions Index — 1010

Chlorprothixene Hydrochloride (Additive depressant effects).
- No products indexed under this heading.

Chlorprothixene Lactate (Additive depressant effects).
- No products indexed under this heading.

Clorazepate Dipotassium (Additive depressant effects). Products include:
- Tranxene ... 459

Clozapine (Additive depressant effects). Products include:
- Clozaril Tablets ... 2377

Codeine Phosphate (Additive depressant effects). Products include:
- Brontex ... 2130
- Dimetane-DC Cough Syrup ... 2232
- Fioricet with Codeine Capsules ... 2387
- Fiorinal with Codeine Capsules ... 2390
- Nucofed ... 2225
- Phenergan with Codeine ... 2883
- Phenergan VC with Codeine ... 2888
- Robitussin A-C Syrup ... 2248
- Robitussin-DAC Syrup ... 2249
- Ryna ... ▣ 804
- Soma Compound w/Codeine Tablets ... 2784
- Tylenol with Codeine ... 1592

Desflurane (Additive depressant effects). Products include:
- Suprane (desflurane, USP) ... 1865

Dezocine (Additive depressant effects). Products include:
- Dalgan Injection ... 529

Diazepam (Additive depressant effects). Products include:
- Dizac (diazepam injectable emulsion) CIV ... 1862
- Valium Injectable ... 2336
- Valium Tablets ... 2335

Dicumarol (Effect may be diminished).
- No products indexed under this heading.

Divalproex Sodium (Stelazine may lower convulsive thresholds; dosage adjustments of anticonvulsants may be necessary). Products include:
- Depakote Tablets ... 418

Dopamine Hydrochloride (May cause a paradoxical further lowering of blood pressure).
- No products indexed under this heading.

Droperidol (Additive depressant effects). Products include:
- Inapsine Injection ... 462

Enflurane (Additive depressant effects).
- No products indexed under this heading.

Epinephrine Bitartrate (Reversed epinephrine effect; may cause a paradoxical further lowering of blood pressure). Products include:
- Sensorcaine-MPF with Epinephrine Injection ... 554

Epinephrine Hydrochloride (Reversed epinephrine effect; may cause a paradoxical further lowering of blood pressure). Products include:
- Ana-Kit Anaphylaxis Emergency Treatment Kit ... 611

Estazolam (Additive depressant effects). Products include:
- ProSom Tablets ... 457

Ethchlorvynol (Additive depressant effects). Products include:
- Placidyl Capsules ... 456

Ethinamate (Additive depressant effects).
- No products indexed under this heading.

Ethosuximide (Stelazine may lower convulsive thresholds; dosage adjustments of anticonvulsants may be necessary). Products include:
- Zarontin Capsules ... 1986
- Zarontin Syrup ... 1986

Ethotoin (Stelazine may lower convulsive thresholds; dosage adjustments of anticonvulsants may be necessary). Products include:
- Peganone Tablets ... 455

Felbamate (Stelazine may lower convulsive thresholds; dosage adjustments of anticonvulsants may be necessary). Products include:
- Felbatol ... 2774

Fentanyl (Additive depressant effects). Products include:
- Duragesic Transdermal System ... 1336

Fentanyl Citrate (Additive depressant effects). Products include:
- Sublimaze Injection ... 463

Fluphenazine Decanoate (Additive depressant effects). Products include:
- Prolixin Decanoate ... 510

Fluphenazine Enanthate (Additive depressant effects). Products include:
- Prolixin Enanthate ... 510

Fluphenazine Hydrochloride (Additive depressant effects). Products include:
- Prolixin ... 510

Flurazepam Hydrochloride (Additive depressant effects). Products include:
- Dalmane Capsules ... 2329

Glutethimide (Additive depressant effects).
- No products indexed under this heading.

Guanethidine Monosulfate (Antihypertensive effects of guanethidine and related compounds may be counteracted when used concurrently). Products include:
- Esimil Tablets ... 840
- Ismelin Tablets ... 845

Haloperidol (Additive depressant effects). Products include:
- Haldol Injection, Tablets and Concentrate ... 1585

Haloperidol Decanoate (Additive depressant effects). Products include:
- Haldol Decanoate ... 1587

Hydrochlorothiazide (Orthostatic hypotension that occurs with Stelazine may be accentuated). Products include:
- Aldactazide Tablets ... 2556
- Aldoril Tablets ... 1644
- Apresazide Capsules ... 824
- Capozide Tablets ... 744
- Dyazide Capsules ... 2653
- Esidrix Tablets ... 839
- Esimil Tablets ... 840
- HydroDIURIL Tablets ... 1716
- Hydropres Tablets ... 1718
- Hyzaar Tablets ... 1720
- Inderide Tablets ... 2838
- Inderide LA Long Acting Capsules ... 2840
- Lopressor HCT Tablets ... 850
- Lotensin HCT Tablets ... 855
- Moduretic Tablets ... 1748
- Oretic Tablets ... 450
- Prinzide Tablets ... 1780
- Ser-Ap-Es Tablets ... 867
- Timolide Tablets ... 1791
- Vaseretic Tablets ... 1810
- Zestoretic Tablets ... 2968
- Ziac ... 1459

Hydrocodone Bitartrate (Additive depressant effects). Products include:
- Codiclear DH Syrup ... 808
- Duratuss HD Elixir ... 2750
- Histussin D Liquid ... 670
- Hycodan Tablets and Syrup ... 946
- Hycomine Compound Tablets ... 948
- Hycomine ... 947
- Hycotuss Expectorant Syrup ... 950
- Hydrocet Capsules ... 787
- Lorcet 10/650 Tablets ... 1016
- Lortab ... 2751
- Tussend ... 1830
- Tussend Expectorant ... 1831
- Vicodin Tablets ... 1404
- Vicodin ES Tablets ... 1405
- Vicodin HP Tablets ... 1403
- Vicodin Tuss Expectorant ... 1406
- Zydone Capsules ... 967

Hydrocodone Polistirex (Additive depressant effects). Products include:
- Tussionex Pennkinetic Extended-Release Suspension ... 1624

Hydroflumethiazide (Orthostatic hypotension that occurs with Stelazine may be accentuated). Products include:
- Diucardin Tablets ... 2824

Hydroxyzine Hydrochloride (Additive depressant effects). Products include:
- Atarax Tablets & Syrup ... 1992
- Marax Tablets & DF Syrup ... 2015
- Vistaril Intramuscular Solution ... 2042

Isoflurane (Additive depressant effects).
- No products indexed under this heading.

Ketamine Hydrochloride (Additive depressant effects).
- No products indexed under this heading.

Lamotrigine (Stelazine may lower convulsive thresholds; dosage adjustments of anticonvulsants may be necessary). Products include:
- Lamictal Tablets ... 1105

Levomethadyl Acetate Hydrochloride (Additive depressant effects). Products include:
- Orlaam Oral Solution ... 2361

Levorphanol Tartrate (Additive depressant effects). Products include:
- Levo-Dromoran ... 2297

Lorazepam (Additive depressant effects). Products include:
- Ativan Injection ... 2805
- Ativan Tablets ... 2807

Loxapine Hydrochloride (Additive depressant effects). Products include:
- Loxitane ... 1426

Loxapine Succinate (Additive depressant effects). Products include:
- Loxitane Capsules ... 1426

Meperidine Hydrochloride (Additive depressant effects). Products include:
- Demerol ... 2438
- Mepergan Injection ... 2859

Mephenytoin (Stelazine may lower convulsive thresholds; dosage adjustments of anticonvulsants may be necessary). Products include:
- Mesantoin Tablets ... 2400

Mephobarbital (Additive depressant effects). Products include:
- Mebaral Tablets ... 2452

Meprobamate (Additive depressant effects). Products include:
- Miltown Tablets ... 2780
- PMB 200 and PMB 400 ... 2890

Mesoridazine Besylate (Additive depressant effects). Products include:
- Serentil ... 689

Metaraminol Bitartrate (May cause a paradoxical further lowering of blood pressure). Products include:
- Aramine Injection ... 1649

Methadone Hydrochloride (Additive depressant effects). Products include:
- Methadone Hydrochloride Oral Concentrate ... 2356
- Methadone Hydrochloride Oral Solution & Tablets ... 2357

Methohexital Sodium (Additive depressant effects).
- No products indexed under this heading.

Methotrimeprazine (Additive depressant effects). Products include:
- Levoprome ... 1321

Methoxamine Hydrochloride (May cause a paradoxical further lowering of blood pressure). Products include:
- Vasoxyl Injection ... 1169

Methoxyflurane (Additive depressant effects).
- No products indexed under this heading.

Methsuximide (Stelazine may lower convulsive thresholds; dosage adjustments of anticonvulsants may be necessary). Products include:
- Celontin Kapseals ... 1955

Methyclothiazide (Orthostatic hypotension that occurs with Stelazine may be accentuated). Products include:
- Enduron Tablets ... 424

Metrizamide (Stelazine may lower the seizure threshold; do not use concurrently).
- No products indexed under this heading.

Midazolam Hydrochloride (Additive depressant effects). Products include:
- Versed Injection ... 2324

Molindone Hydrochloride (Additive depressant effects). Products include:
- Moban Tablets and Concentrate ... 1036

Morphine Sulfate (Additive depressant effects). Products include:
- Astramorph/PF Injection, USP (Preservative-Free) ... 526
- Duramorph Injection ... 983
- Infumorph 200 and Infumorph 500 Sterile Solutions ... 985
- Kadian Capsules ... 2948
- MS Contin Tablets ... 2149
- MSIR ... 2152
- Oramorph SR (Morphine Sulfate Sustained Release Tablets) ... 2359
- RMS Suppositories CII ... 2766
- Roxanol ... 2365

Norepinephrine Bitartrate (May cause a paradoxical further lowering of blood pressure). Products include:
- Levophed Bitartrate Injection ... 2445

Opium Alkaloids (Additive depressant effects).
- No products indexed under this heading.

Oxazepam (Additive depressant effects). Products include:
- Serax Capsules ... 2916
- Serax Tablets ... 2916

Oxycodone Hydrochloride (Additive depressant effects). Products include:
- OxyContin Tablets ... 2163
- OxyIR Capsules ... 2167
- Percocet Tablets ... 955
- Percodan Tablets ... 955
- Percodan-Demi Tablets ... 956
- Roxicodone Tablets, Oral Solution & Intensol (Oxycodone) ... 2366
- Tylox Capsules ... 1593

Paramethadione (Stelazine may lower convulsive thresholds; dosage adjustments of anticonvulsants may be necessary).
- No products indexed under this heading.

(▣ Described in PDR For Nonprescription Drugs) (◉ Described in PDR For Ophthalmology)

Pentobarbital Sodium (Additive depressant effects). Products include:
- Nembutal Sodium Capsules 440
- Nembutal Sodium Solution 442
- Nembutal Sodium Suppositories...... 444

Perphenazine (Additive depressant effects). Products include:
- Etrafon 2495
- Triavil Tablets 1800
- Trilafon 2532

Phenacemide (Stelazine may lower convulsive thresholds; dosage adjustments of anticonvulsants may be necessary). Products include:
- Phenurone Tablets 455

Phenobarbital (Additive depressant effects). Products include:
- Arco-Lase Plus Tablets 513
- Bellergal-S Tablets 2375
- Donnatal 2234
- Donnatal Extentabs....................... 2234
- Donnatal Tablets 2234
- Phenobarbital Elixir and Tablets ... 1523
- Quadrinal Tablets 1398

Phensuximide (Phenothiazines may lower convulsive thresholds; dosage adjustments of anticonvulsants may be necessary).
- No products indexed under this heading.

Phenytoin (Phenytoin toxicity may be precipitated; Stelazine may lower convulsive thresholds; dosage adjustments of anticonvulsants may be necessary). Products include:
- Dilantin Infatabs 1967
- Dilantin-125 Suspension 1969

Phenytoin Sodium (Phenytoin toxicity may be precipitated; Stelazine may lower convulsive thresholds; dosage adjustments of anticonvulsants may be necessary). Products include:
- Dilantin Kapseals 1965

Polythiazide (Orthostatic hypotension that occurs with Stelazine may be accentuated). Products include:
- Minizide Capsules 2016

Prazepam (Additive depressant effects).
- No products indexed under this heading.

Primidone (Stelazine may lower convulsive thresholds; dosage adjustments of anticonvulsants may be necessary). Products include:
- Mysoline 2860

Prochlorperazine (Additive depressant effects). Products include:
- Compazine 2644

Promethazine Hydrochloride (Additive depressant effects). Products include:
- Mepergan Injection 2859
- Phenergan with Codeine 2883
- Phenergan with Dextromethorphan 2885
- Phenergan Injection 2880
- Phenergan Suppositories 2882
- Phenergan Syrup 2881
- Phenergan Tablets 2882
- Phenergan VC 2886
- Phenergan VC with Codeine 2888

Propofol (Additive depressant effects). Products include:
- Diprivan Injectable Emulsion 2939

Propoxyphene Hydrochloride (Additive depressant effects). Products include:
- Darvon 1475
- Wygesic Tablets 2930

Propoxyphene Napsylate (Additive depressant effects). Products include:
- Darvon-N/Darvocet-N 1473

Propranolol Hydrochloride (Concomitant administration results in increased plasma levels of both drugs). Products include:
- Inderal 2834

- Inderal LA Long Acting Capsules 2836
- Inderide Tablets 2838
- Inderide LA Long Acting Capsules .. 2840

Quazepam (Additive depressant effects). Products include:
- Doral Tablets 2773

Risperidone (Additive depressant effects). Products include:
- Risperdal Tablets 1348

Secobarbital Sodium (Additive depressant effects). Products include:
- Seconal Sodium Pulvules 1529

Sevoflurane (Additive depressant effects).
- No products indexed under this heading.

Sufentanil Citrate (Additive depressant effects). Products include:
- Sufenta Injection 1355

Temazepam (Additive depressant effects). Products include:
- Restoril Capsules 2413

Thiamylal Sodium (Additive depressant effects).
- No products indexed under this heading.

Thioridazine Hydrochloride (Additive depressant effects). Products include:
- Mellaril 2398

Thiothixene (Additive depressant effects). Products include:
- Navane Capsules and Concentrate 2018
- Navane Intramuscular 2019

Triazolam (Additive depressant effects). Products include:
- Halcion Tablets 2093

Trimethadione (Stelazine may lower convulsive thresholds; dosage adjustments of anticonvulsants may be necessary).
- No products indexed under this heading.

Valproic Acid (Stelazine may lower convulsive thresholds; dosage adjustments of anticonvulsants may be necessary). Products include:
- Depakene 416

Warfarin Sodium (Effect may be diminished). Products include:
- Coumadin 941

Zolpidem Tartrate (Additive depressant effects). Products include:
- Ambien Tablets 2559

Food Interactions
Alcohol (Additive depressant effects).

STELAZINE MULTI-DOSE VIALS
(Trifluoperazine Hydrochloride) 2692
See **Stelazine Concentrate**

STELAZINE TABLETS
(Trifluoperazine Hydrochloride) 2692
See **Stelazine Concentrate**

STEPHAN BIO-NUTRITIONAL DAYTIME HYDRATING CREME
(Chamomile) 833
None cited in PDR database.

STEPHAN BIO-NUTRITIONAL EYE-FIRMING CONCENTRATE
(Chamomile) 833
None cited in PDR database.

STEPHAN BIO-NUTRITIONAL NIGHTIME MOISTURE CREME
(Moisturizing formula) 833
None cited in PDR database.

STEPHAN BIO-NUTRITIONAL REFRESHING MOISTURE GEL
(Moisturizing formula) 833
None cited in PDR database.

STEPHAN BIO-NUTRITIONAL ULTRA HYDRATING FLUID
(Moisturizing formula) 833
None cited in PDR database.

STEPHAN CLARITY
(Nutritional Supplement) 834
None cited in PDR database.

STEPHAN ELASTICITY
(Nutritional Supplement) 834
None cited in PDR database.

STEPHAN ELIXIR
(Nutritional Supplement) 834
None cited in PDR database.

STEPHAN ESSENTIAL
(Nutritional Supplement) 834
None cited in PDR database.

STEPHAN FEMININE
(Nutritional Supplement) 834
None cited in PDR database.

STEPHAN FLEXIBILITY
(Nutritional Supplement) 834
None cited in PDR database.

STEPHAN LOVPIL
(Nutritional Supplement) 834
None cited in PDR database.

STEPHAN MASCULINE
(Nutritional Supplement) 835
None cited in PDR database.

STEPHAN PROTECTOR
(Nutritional Supplement) 835
None cited in PDR database.

STEPHAN RELIEF
(Nutritional Supplement) 836
None cited in PDR database.

STEPHAN TRANQUILITY
(Nutritional Supplement) 836
None cited in PDR database.

STIMATE, (DESMOPRESSIN ACETATE) NASAL SPRAY, 1.5 MG/ML
(Desmopressin Acetate) 806
May interact with vasopressors. Compounds in this category include:

Dopamine Hydrochloride (Desmopressin has very low pressor activity, however, concurrent use with other pressor agents should be done only with careful patient monitoring).
- No products indexed under this heading.

Epinephrine Bitartrate (Desmopressin has very low pressor activity, however, concurrent use with other pressor agents should be done only with careful patient monitoring). Products include:
- Sensorcaine-MPF with Epinephrine Injection 554

Epinephrine Hydrochloride (Desmopressin has very low pressor activity, however, concurrent use with other pressor agents should be done only with careful patient monitoring). Products include:
- Ana-Kit Anaphylaxis Emergency Treatment Kit 611

Metaraminol Bitartrate (Desmopressin has very low pressor activity, however, concurrent use with other pressor agents should be done only with careful patient monitoring). Products include:
- Aramine Injection 1649

Methoxamine Hydrochloride (Desmopressin has very low pressor activity, however, concurrent use with other pressor agents should be done only with careful patient monitoring). Products include:
- Vasoxyl Injection 1169

Norepinephrine Bitartrate (Desmopressin has very low pressor activity, however, concurrent use with other pressor agents should be done only with careful patient monitoring). Products include:
- Levophed Bitartrate Injection 2445

Phenylephrine Hydrochloride (Desmopressin has very low pressor activity, however, concurrent use with other pressor agents should be done only with careful patient monitoring). Products include:
- Atrohist Plus Tablets 1605
- Cerose DM 853
- D.A. II Tablets 972
- D.A. Chewable Tablets 970
- Dura-Vent/DA Tablets 972
- Extendryl 1003
- 4-Way Fast Acting Nasal Spray (regular & mentholated) 644
- Hemorid 797
- Hycomine Compound Tablets 948
- Neo-Synephrine Hydrochloride 1% Carpuject 2455
- Neo-Synephrine Hydrochloride 1% Injection 2455
- Neo-Synephrine Hydrochloride (Ophthalmic) 2456
- Neo-Synephrine 624
- Novahistine Elixir 782
- Phenergan VC 2886
- Phenergan VC with Codeine 2888
- Preparation H 842
- Tympagesic Ear Drops 2476
- Vicks Sinex Nasal Spray and Ultra Fine Mist 738

STREPTASE FOR INFUSION
(Streptokinase)................................. 557
May interact with platelet inhibitors and anticoagulants. Compounds in these categories include:

Aspirin (Streptokinase, alone or in combination with antiplatelet and anticoagulants, may cause bleeding complications). Products include:
- Alka-Seltzer Cherry Effervescent Antacid and Pain Reliever 609
- Alka-Seltzer Extra Strength Effervescent Antacid and Pain Reliever 609
- Alka-Seltzer Lemon Lime Effervescent Antacid and Pain Reliever 609
- Alka-Seltzer Original Effervescent Antacid and Pain Reliever 609
- Alka-Seltzer Plus 611
- Alka-Seltzer Plus Sinus Medicine .. 611
- Ascriptin 650
- Arthritis Strength BC Powder......... 631
- BC Cold Powder Multi-Symptom Formula (Cold-Sinus-Allergy) 631
- BC Cold Powder Non-Drowsy Formula (Cold-Sinus) 631
- BC Powder 631
- Genuine Bayer Aspirin Tablets & Caplets 618
- Extra Strength Bayer Arthritis Pain Regimen Formula 615

IMPORTANT NOTE: Always consult each drug listing in the patient's regimen for possible interactions.

Streptase — Interactions Index

Extra Strength Bayer Aspirin Caplets & Tablets 617
Extended-Release Bayer 8-Hour Aspirin 616
Extra Strength Bayer Plus Aspirin Caplets 617
Extra Strength Bayer PM Aspirin Plus Sleep Aid 617
Aspirin Regimen Bayer 81 mg Tablets with Calcium 615
Aspirin Regimen Bayer Adult Low Strength 81 mg Tablets 613
Aspirin Regimen Bayer Children's Chewable Aspirin 616
Aspirin Regimen Bayer Regular Strength 325 mg Caplets 613
Bufferin Analgesic Tablets 636
Arthritis Strength Bufferin Analgesic Caplets 637
Extra Strength Bufferin Analgesic Tablets 637
Cama Arthritis Pain Reliever 748
Darvon Compound-65 Pulvules 1475
Easprin 1971
Ecotrin 2625
Ecotrin Enteric Coated Aspirin Maximum Strength Tablets and Caplets 775
Ecotrin Enteric Coated Aspirin Regular Strength Tablets 2625
Empirin Aspirin Tablets 818
Excedrin Extra-Strength Analgesic Tablets, Caplets, and Geltabs 734
Fiorinal Capsules 2388
Fiorinal with Codeine Capsules 2390
Fiorinal Tablets 2388
Goody's Extra Strength Headache Powders 632
Goody's Extra Strength Pain Relief Tablets 632
Halfprin Tablets 1413
Norgesic 1554
Percodan Tablets 955
Percodan-Demi Tablets 956
Robaxisal Tablets 2246
Soma Compound w/Codeine Tablets 2784
Soma Compound Tablets 2783
St. Joseph Adult Chewable Aspirin (81 mg.) 768
Talwin Compound 2466
Vanquish Analgesic Caplets 627

Azlocillin Sodium (Streptokinase, alone or in combination with antiplatelet and anticoagulants, may cause bleeding complications).
No products indexed under this heading.

Carbenicillin Indanyl Sodium (Streptokinase, alone or in combination with antiplatelet and anticoagulants, may cause bleeding complications). Products include:
Geocillin Tablets 2009

Choline Magnesium Trisalicylate (Streptokinase, alone or in combination with antiplatelet and anticoagulants, may cause bleeding complications). Products include:
Trilisate 2155

Dalteparin Sodium (Streptokinase, alone or in combination with antiplatelet and anticoagulants, may cause bleeding complications). Products include:
Fragmin Injection 2088

Diclofenac Potassium (Streptokinase, alone or in combination with antiplatelet and anticoagulants, may cause bleeding complications). Products include:
Cataflam Tablets 833

Diclofenac Sodium (Streptokinase, alone or in combination with antiplatelet and anticoagulants, may cause bleeding complications). Products include:
Voltaren Ophthalmic Sterile Ophthalmic Solution 264
Cataflam/Voltaren/Voltaren-XR 833

Dicumarol (Streptokinase, alone or in combination with antiplatelet and anticoagulants, may cause bleeding complications).
No products indexed under this heading.

Diflunisal (Streptokinase, alone or in combination with antiplatelet and anticoagulants, may cause bleeding complications). Products include:
Dolobid Tablets 1695

Dipyridamole (Streptokinase, alone or in combination with antiplatelet and anticoagulants, may cause bleeding complications). Products include:
Persantine Tablets 686

Enoxaparin (Streptokinase, alone or in combination with antiplatelet and anticoagulants, may cause bleeding complications). Products include:
Lovenox Injection 2187

Fenoprofen Calcium (Streptokinase, alone or in combination with antiplatelet and anticoagulants, may cause bleeding complications). Products include:
Nalfon 200 Pulvules & Nalfon Tablets 933

Flurbiprofen (Streptokinase, alone or in combination with antiplatelet and anticoagulants, may cause bleeding complications).
No products indexed under this heading.

Heparin Calcium (Streptokinase, alone or in combination with antiplatelet and anticoagulants, may cause bleeding complications).
No products indexed under this heading.

Heparin Sodium (Streptokinase, alone or in combination with antiplatelet and anticoagulants, may cause bleeding complications). Products include:
Heparin Lock Flush Solution 2831
Heparin Sodium Injection 2832
Heparin Sodium Vials 1486

Ibuprofen (Streptokinase, alone or in combination with antiplatelet and anticoagulants, may cause bleeding complications). Products include:
Advil Cold and Sinus Caplets and Tablets 837
Advil Ibuprofen Tablets, Caplets and Gel Caplets 836
Children's Motrin Ibuprofen Oral Suspension 1558
IBU Tablets 1389
Ibuprohm 713
Motrin IB Caplets, Tablets, and Gelcaps 802
Motrin Ibuprofen Suspension, Oral Drops, Chewable Tablets, Caplets 1563
Nuprin Ibuprofen/Analgesic Tablets & Caplets 645
Vicks DayQuil SINUS Pressure & PAIN Relief with IBUPROFEN 735

Indomethacin (Streptokinase, alone or in combination with antiplatelet and anticoagulants, may cause bleeding complications). Products include:
Indocin 1723

Indomethacin Sodium Trihydrate (Streptokinase, alone or in combination with antiplatelet and anticoagulants, may cause bleeding complications). Products include:
Indocin I.V. 1727

Ketoprofen (Streptokinase, alone or in combination with antiplatelet and anticoagulants, may cause bleeding complications). Products include:
Actron Caplets and Tablets 608
Orudis Capsules 2874

Orudis KT 842
Oruvail Capsules 2874

Magnesium Salicylate (Streptokinase, alone or in combination with antiplatelet and anticoagulants, may cause bleeding complications). Products include:
Backache Tablets 635
Doan's Extra Strength Analgesic 653
Extra Strength Doan's P.M. 653
Doan's Regular Strength Analgesic 654
Mobigesic Tablets 607

Meclofenamate Sodium (Streptokinase, alone or in combination with antiplatelet and anticoagulants, may cause bleeding complications).
No products indexed under this heading.

Mefenamic Acid (Streptokinase, alone or in combination with antiplatelet and anticoagulants, may cause bleeding complications). Products include:
Ponstel 1982

Mezlocillin Sodium (Streptokinase, alone or in combination with antiplatelet and anticoagulants, may cause bleeding complications). Products include:
Mezlin 594
Mezlin Pharmacy Bulk Package 597

Nafcillin Sodium (Streptokinase, alone or in combination with antiplatelet and anticoagulants, may cause bleeding complications).
No products indexed under this heading.

Naproxen (Streptokinase, alone or in combination with antiplatelet and anticoagulants, may cause bleeding complications). Products include:
Anaprox/Naprosyn 2277

Naproxen Sodium (Streptokinase, alone or in combination with antiplatelet and anticoagulants, may cause bleeding complications). Products include:
Aleve 2124
Anaprox/Naprosyn 2277
Naprelan Tablets 2861

Penicillin G Benzathine (Streptokinase, alone or in combination with antiplatelet and anticoagulants, may cause bleeding complications). Products include:
Bicillin C-R Injection 2810
Bicillin C-R 900/300 Injection 2812
Bicillin L-A Injection 2813

Penicillin G Procaine (Streptokinase, alone or in combination with antiplatelet and anticoagulants, may cause bleeding complications). Products include:
Bicillin C-R Injection 2810
Bicillin C-R 900/300 Injection 2812

Phenylbutazone (Streptokinase, alone or in combination with antiplatelet and anticoagulants, may cause bleeding complications).
No products indexed under this heading.

Piroxicam (Streptokinase, alone or in combination with antiplatelet and anticoagulants, may cause bleeding complications). Products include:
Feldene Capsules 2008

Salsalate (Streptokinase, alone or in combination with antiplatelet and anticoagulants, may cause bleeding complications). Products include:
Disalcid 1549
Mono-Gesic Tablets 810
Salflex Tablets 791

Sulindac (Streptokinase, alone or in combination with antiplatelet and anticoagulants, may cause bleeding complications). Products include:
Clinoril Tablets 1658

Ticarcillin Disodium (Streptokinase, alone or in combination with antiplatelet and anticoagulants, may cause bleeding complications). Products include:
Ticar for Injection 2704
Timentin for Injection 2706

Ticlopidine Hydrochloride (Streptokinase, alone or in combination with antiplatelet and anticoagulants, may cause bleeding complications). Products include:
Ticlid Tablets 2317

Tolmetin Sodium (Streptokinase, alone or in combination with antiplatelet and anticoagulants, may cause bleeding complications). Products include:
Tolectin (200, 400 and 600 mg) 1591

Warfarin Sodium (Streptokinase, alone or in combination with antiplatelet and anticoagulants, may cause bleeding complications). Products include:
Coumadin 941

STREPTOMYCIN SULFATE INJECTION
(Streptomycin Sulfate) 2031
May interact with anesthetics, muscle relaxants, diuretics, and certain other agents. Compounds in these categories include:

Alfentanil Hydrochloride (Potential for respiratory paralysis from neuromuscular blockage due to neurotoxicity, especially when given soon after the use of anesthesia). Products include:
Alfenta Injection 1334

Amiloride Hydrochloride (Interaction with furosemide is extrapolated to other diuretic where co-administration may possibly result in the potentiation of ototoxic effects). Products include:
Midamor Tablets 1746
Moduretic Tablets 1748

Atracurium Besylate (Potential for respiratory paralysis from neuromuscular blockage due to neurotoxicity, especially when given soon after the use of muscle relaxants). Products include:
Tracrium Injection 1155

Baclofen (Potential for respiratory paralysis from neuromuscular blockage due to neurotoxicity, especially when given soon after the use of muscle relaxants). Products include:
Lioresal Intrathecal 1634
Lioresal Tablets 847

Bendroflumethiazide (Interaction with furosemide is extrapolated to other diuretic where co-administration may possibly result in the potentiation of ototoxic effects).
No products indexed under this heading.

Bumetanide (Interaction with furosemide is extrapolated to other diuretic where co-administration may possibly result in the potentiation of ototoxic effects). Products include:
Bumex 2260

Carisoprodol (Potential for respiratory paralysis from neuromuscular blockage due to neurotoxicity, especially when given soon after the use of muscle relaxants). Products include:
Soma Compound w/Codeine Tablets 2784
Soma Compound Tablets 2783
Soma Tablets 2782

Cephaloridine (Concurrent and/or sequential use may increase the

(⊡ Described in PDR For Nonprescription Drugs)   (⊚ Described in PDR For Ophthalmology)

potential for increased toxicity; co-administration should be avoided).

No products indexed under this heading.

Chlorothiazide (Interaction with furosemide is extrapolated to other diuretic where co-administration may possibly result in the potentiation of ototoxic effects). Products include:

Aldoclor Tablets 1638
Diupres Tablets 1691
Diuril Oral 1694

Chlorothiazide Sodium (Interaction with furosemide is extrapolated to other diuretic where co-administration may possibly result in the potentiation of ototoxic effects). Products include:

Diuril Sodium Intravenous 1693

Chlorthalidone (Interaction with furosemide is extrapolated to other diuretic where co-administration may possibly result in the potentiation of ototoxic effects). Products include:

Combipres Tablets 682
Tenoretic Tablets 2963
Thalitone 1293

Chlorzoxazone (Potential for respiratory paralysis from neuromuscular blockage due to neurotoxicity, especially when given soon after the use of muscle relaxants). Products include:

Parafon Forte DSC Caplets 1590

Cisatracurium Besylate (Potential for respiratory paralysis from neuromuscular blockage due to neurotoxicity, especially when given soon after the use of muscle relaxants). Products include:

Nimbex Injection 1131

Colistin Sulfate (Concurrent and/or sequential use may increase the potential for increased toxicity; co-administration should be avoided). Products include:

Coly-Mycin S Otic w/Neomycin & Hydrocortisone 1965

Cyclobenzaprine Hydrochloride (Potential for respiratory paralysis from neuromuscular blockage due to neurotoxicity, especially when given soon after the use of muscle relaxants). Products include:

Flexeril Tablets 1701

Cyclosporine (Concurrent and/or sequential use may increase the potential for increased toxicity; co-administration should be avoided). Products include:

Neoral 2405
Sandimmune 2416

Dantrolene Sodium (Potential for respiratory paralysis from neuromuscular blockage due to neurotoxicity, especially when given soon after the use of muscle relaxants). Products include:

Dantrium Capsules 2131
Dantrium Intravenous 2132

Doxacurium Chloride (Potential for respiratory paralysis from neuromuscular blockage due to neurotoxicity, especially when given soon after the use of muscle relaxants). Products include:

Nuromax Injection 1136

Enflurane (Potential for respiratory paralysis from neuromuscular blockage due to neurotoxicity, especially when given soon after the use of anesthesia).

No products indexed under this heading.

Ethacrynic Acid (Co-administration results in the potentiation of ototoxic effects). Products include:

Edecrin Tablets 1698

Fentanyl Citrate (Potential for respiratory paralysis from neuromuscular blockage due to neurotoxicity, especially when given soon after the use of anesthesia). Products include:

Sublimaze Injection 463

Furosemide (Co-administration results in the potentiation of ototoxic effects). Products include:

Lasix Injection, Oral Solution and Tablets 1267

Gentamicin Sulfate (Concurrent and/or sequential use may increase the potential for increased toxicity; co-administration should be avoided). Products include:

Garamycin Cream 0.1% 2501
Garamycin Injectable 2502
Garamycin Ointment 0.1% 2501
Garamycin Ophthalmic 2501
Genoptic Sterile Ophthalmic Solution .... ◉ 241
Genoptic Sterile Ophthalmic Ointment .... ◉ 241
Gentak .... ◉ 209
Pred-G Liquifilm Sterile Ophthalmic Suspension .... ◉ 248
Pred-G S.O.P. Sterile Ophthalmic Ointment .... ◉ 249

Halothane (Potential for respiratory paralysis from neuromuscular blockage due to neurotoxicity, especially when given soon after the use of anesthesia). Products include:

Fluothane 2830

Hydrochlorothiazide (Interaction with furosemide is extrapolated to other diuretic where co-administration may possibly result in the potentiation of ototoxic effects). Products include:

Aldactazide Tablets 2556
Aldoril Tablets 1644
Apresazide Capsules 824
Capozide Tablets 744
Dyazide Capsules 2653
Esidrix Tablets 839
Esimil Tablets 840
HydroDIURIL Tablets 1716
Hydropres Tablets 1718
Hyzaar Tablets 1720
Inderide Tablets 2838
Inderide LA Long Acting Capsules .. 2840
Lopressor HCT Tablets 850
Lotensin HCT Tablets 855
Moduretic Tablets 1748
Oretic Tablets 450
Prinzide Tablets 1780
Ser-Ap-Es Tablets 867
Timolide Tablets 1791
Vaseretic Tablets 1810
Zestoretic Tablets 2968
Ziac 1459

Hydroflumethiazide (Interaction with furosemide is extrapolated to other diuretic where co-administration may possibly result in the potentiation of ototoxic effects). Products include:

Diucardin Tablets 2824

Indapamide (Interaction with furosemide is extrapolated to other diuretic where co-administration may possibly result in the potentiation of ototoxic effects).

No products indexed under this heading.

Isoflurane (Potential for respiratory paralysis from neuromuscular blockage due to neurotoxicity, especially when given soon after the use of anesthesia).

No products indexed under this heading.

Kanamycin Sulfate (Concurrent and/or sequential use may increase the potential for increased toxicity; co-administration should be avoided).

No products indexed under this heading.

Ketamine Hydrochloride (Potential for respiratory paralysis from neuromuscular blockage due to neurotoxicity, especially when given soon after the use of anesthesia).

No products indexed under this heading.

Mannitol (Co-administration results in the potentiation of ototoxic effects).

No products indexed under this heading.

Metaxalone (Potential for respiratory paralysis from neuromuscular blockage due to neurotoxicity, especially when given soon after the use of muscle relaxants). Products include:

Skelaxin Tablets 793

Methocarbamol (Potential for respiratory paralysis from neuromuscular blockage due to neurotoxicity, especially when given soon after the use of muscle relaxants). Products include:

Robaxin Injectable 2245
Robaxin Tablets 2246
Robaxisal Tablets 2246

Methohexital Sodium (Potential for respiratory paralysis from neuromuscular blockage due to neurotoxicity, especially when given soon after the use of anesthesia).

No products indexed under this heading.

Methyclothiazide (Interaction with furosemide is extrapolated to other diuretic where co-administration may possibly result in the potentiation of ototoxic effects). Products include:

Enduron Tablets 424

Metocurine Iodide (Potential for respiratory paralysis from neuromuscular blockage due to neurotoxicity, especially when given soon after the use of muscle relaxants). Products include:

Metubine Iodide Vials 932

Metolazone (Interaction with furosemide is extrapolated to other diuretic where co-administration may possibly result in the potentiation of ototoxic effects). Products include:

Mykrox Tablets 1617
Zaroxolyn Tablets 1625

Midazolam Hydrochloride (Potential for respiratory paralysis from neuromuscular blockage due to neurotoxicity, especially when given soon after the use of anesthesia). Products include:

Versed Injection 2324

Mivacurium Chloride (Potential for respiratory paralysis from neuromuscular blockage due to neurotoxicity, especially when given soon after the use of muscle relaxants). Products include:

Mivacron 1125

Neomycin Sulfate (Concurrent and/or sequential use may increase the potential for increased toxicity; co-administration should be avoided). Products include:

AK-Spore .... ◉ 205
AK-Trol Ointment & Suspension .... ◉ 205
Coly-Mycin S Otic w/Neomycin & Hydrocortisone 1965
Cortisporin Cream 1073
Cortisporin Ointment 1074
Cortisporin Ophthalmic Ointment Sterile 1074
Cortisporin Ophthalmic Suspension Sterile 1075
Cortisporin Otic Solution Sterile 1076
Cortisporin Otic Suspension Sterile 1077
Maxitrol Ophthalmic Ointment and Suspension .... ◉ 222
Mycitracin .... ▣ 803
NeoDecadron Sterile Ophthalmic Ointment 1755
NeoDecadron Sterile Ophthalmic Solution 1756
NeoDecadron Topical Cream 1757
Neosporin G.U. Irrigant Sterile 1130
Neosporin Ointment .... ▣ 821
Neosporin Plus Maximum Strength Cream .... ▣ 821
Neosporin Plus Maximum Strength Ointment .... ▣ 822
Neosporin Ophthalmic Ointment Sterile 1130
Neosporin Ophthalmic Solution Sterile 1131
Pediotic Suspension Sterile 1140
Poly-Pred Liquifilm .... ◉ 246

Neomycin, oral (Concurrent and/or sequential use may increase the potential for increased toxicity; co-administration should be avoided).

Orphenadrine Citrate (Potential for respiratory paralysis from neuromuscular blockage due to neurotoxicity, especially when given soon after the use of muscle relaxants). Products include:

Norflex 1554
Norgesic 1554

Pancuronium Bromide (Potential for respiratory paralysis from neuromuscular blockage due to neurotoxicity, especially when given soon after the use of muscle relaxants).

No products indexed under this heading.

Paromomycin Sulfate (Concurrent and/or sequential use may increase the potential for increased toxicity; co-administration should be avoided).

No products indexed under this heading.

Polymyxin B Sulfate (Concurrent and/or sequential use may increase the potential for increased toxicity; co-administration should be avoided). Products include:

AK-Spore .... ◉ 205
AK-Trol Ointment & Suspension .... ◉ 205
Betadine Brand First Aid Antibiotics & Moisturizer Ointment 2144
Cortisporin Cream 1073
Cortisporin Ointment 1074
Cortisporin Ophthalmic Ointment Sterile 1074
Cortisporin Ophthalmic Suspension Sterile 1075
Cortisporin Otic Solution Sterile 1076
Cortisporin Otic Suspension Sterile 1077
Maxitrol Ophthalmic Ointment and Suspension .... ◉ 222
Mycitracin .... ▣ 803
Neosporin G.U. Irrigant Sterile 1130
Neosporin Ointment .... ▣ 821
Neosporin Plus Maximum Strength Cream .... ▣ 821
Neosporin Plus Maximum Strength Ointment .... ▣ 822
Neosporin Ophthalmic Ointment Sterile 1130
Neosporin Ophthalmic Solution Sterile 1131
Pediotic Suspension Sterile 1140
Poly-Pred Liquifilm .... ◉ 246
Polysporin Ointment .... ▣ 822
Polysporin Ophthalmic Ointment Sterile 1140
Polysporin Powder .... ▣ 823
Polytrim Ophthalmic Solution Sterile 479
TERAK Ointment .... ◉ 210
Terramycin with Polymyxin B Sulfate Ophthalmic Ointment 2035

Polythiazide (Interaction with furosemide is extrapolated to other diuretic where co-administration may possibly result in the potentiation of ototoxic effects). Products include:

Minizide Capsules 2016

IMPORTANT NOTE: Always consult each drug listing in the patient's regimen for possible interactions.

Propofol (Potential for respiratory paralysis from neuromuscular blockage due to neurotoxicity, especially when given soon after the use of anesthesia). Products include:

Diprivan Injectable Emulsion 2939

Rocuronium Bromide (Potential for respiratory paralysis from neuromuscular blockage due to neurotoxicity, especially when given soon after the use of muscle relaxants). Products include:

Zemuron Injection 1885

Spironolactone (Interaction with furosemide is extrapolated to other diuretic where co-administration may possibly result in the potentiation of ototoxic effects). Products include:

Aldactazide Tablets 2556
Aldactone Tablets 2558

Succinylcholine Chloride (Potential for respiratory paralysis from neuromuscular blockage due to neurotoxicity, especially when given soon after the use of muscle relaxants). Products include:

Anectine 1062

Sufentanil Citrate (Potential for respiratory paralysis from neuromuscular blockage due to neurotoxicity, especially when given soon after the use of anesthesia). Products include:

Sufenta Injection 1355

Thiamylal Sodium (Potential for respiratory paralysis from neuromuscular blockage due to neurotoxicity, especially when given soon after the use of anesthesia).

No products indexed under this heading.

Tobramycin (Concurrent and/or sequential use may increase the potential for increased toxicity; co-administration should be avoided). Products include:

AKTOB .... ◉ 207
TobraDex Ophthalmic Suspension and Ointment 469
Tobrex Ophthalmic Ointment and Solution .... ◉ 226

Tobramycin Sulfate (Concurrent and/or sequential use may increase the potential for increased toxicity; co-administration should be avoided). Products include:

Nebcin Vials, Hyporets & ADD-Vantage 1518

Torsemide (Interaction with furosemide is extrapolated to other diuretic where co-administration may possibly result in the potentiation of ototoxic effects). Products include:

Demadex Tablets and Injection 691

Triamterene (Interaction with furosemide is extrapolated to other diuretic where co-administration may possibly result in the potentiation of ototoxic effects). Products include:

Dyazide Capsules 2653
Dyrenium Capsules 2655

Vecuronium Bromide (Potential for respiratory paralysis from neuromuscular blockage due to neurotoxicity, especially when given soon after the use of muscle relaxants). Products include:

Norcuron for Injection 1875

Viomycin (Concurrent and/or sequential use may increase the potential for increased toxicity; co-administration should be avoided).

STRESS GUM

(Vitamins with Minerals) .... ▣ 606
None cited in PDR database.

STRESSTABS

(Vitamin B Complex With Vitamin C) .... ▣ 685
None cited in PDR database.

STRESSTABS + IRON

(Vitamins with Iron) .... ▣ 685
None cited in PDR database.

STRESSTABS + ZINC

(Vitamins with Minerals) .... ▣ 685
None cited in PDR database.

SUBLIMAZE INJECTION

(Fentanyl Citrate) 463
May interact with barbiturates, tranquilizers, narcotic analgesics, general anesthetics, central nervous system depressants, monoamine oxidase inhibitors, and certain other agents. Compounds in these categories include:

Alfentanil Hydrochloride (Co-administration results in additive or potentiating effects). Products include:

Alfenta Injection 1334

Alprazolam (Co-administration results in additive or potentiating effects). Products include:

Xanax Tablets 2115

Aprobarbital (Co-administration results in additive or potentiating effects).

No products indexed under this heading.

Buprenorphine (Co-administration results in additive or potentiating effects). Products include:

Buprenex Injectable 2170

Buspirone Hydrochloride (Co-administration results in additive or potentiating effects). Products include:

BuSpar Tablets 738

Butabarbital (Co-administration results in additive or potentiating effects).

No products indexed under this heading.

Butalbital (Co-administration results in additive or potentiating effects). Products include:

Axocet Capsules 2469
Esgic-plus Capsules 1012
Esgic-plus Tablets 1012
Fioricet Tablets 2386
Fioricet with Codeine Capsules 2387
Fiorinal Capsules 2388
Fiorinal with Codeine Capsules 2390
Fiorinal Tablets 2388
Phrenilin 790
Sedapap Tablets 50 mg/650 mg .. 1826

Chlordiazepoxide (Co-administration results in additive or potentiating effects). Products include:

Limbitrol 2333

Chlordiazepoxide Hydrochloride (Co-administration results in additive or potentiating effects). Products include:

Librax Capsules 2330
Librium Capsules 2331
Librium Injectable 2332

Chlorpromazine (Co-administration results in additive or potentiating effects). Products include:

Thorazine Suppositories 2701

Chlorpromazine Hydrochloride (Co-administration results in additive or potentiating effects). Products include:

Thorazine 2701

Chlorprothixene (Co-administration results in additive or potentiating effects).

No products indexed under this heading.

Chlorprothixene Hydrochloride (Co-administration results in additive or potentiating effects).

No products indexed under this heading.

Chlorprothixene Lactate (Co-administration results in additive or potentiating effects).

No products indexed under this heading.

Clorazepate Dipotassium (Co-administration results in additive or potentiating effects). Products include:

Tranxene 459

Clozapine (Co-administration results in additive or potentiating effects). Products include:

Clozaril Tablets 2377

Codeine Phosphate (Co-administration results in additive or potentiating effects). Products include:

Brontex 2130
Dimetane-DC Cough Syrup 2232
Fioricet with Codeine Capsules 2387
Fiorinal with Codeine Capsules 2390
Nucofed 2225
Phenergan with Codeine 2883
Phenergan VC with Codeine 2888
Robitussin A-C Syrup 2248
Robitussin-DAC Syrup 2249
Ryna .... ▣ 804
Soma Compound w/Codeine Tablets 2784
Tylenol with Codeine 1592

Desflurane (Co-administration results in additive or potentiating effects). Products include:

Suprane (desflurane, USP) 1865

Dezocine (Co-administration results in additive or potentiating effects). Products include:

Dalgan Injection 529

Diazepam (When high dose or anesthetic dosages of fentanyl are employed, even small dosages of diazepam may cause cardiovascular depression; co-administration results in additive or potentiating effects). Products include:

Dizac (diazepam injectable emulsion) CIV 1862
Valium Injectable 2336
Valium Tablets 2335

Droperidol (Combined therapy causes a decrease in pulmonary arterial pressure; caution should be exercised if pulmonary arterial pressure measurements might determine final management of the patient). Products include:

Inapsine Injection 462

Enflurane (Co-administration results in additive or potentiating effects).

No products indexed under this heading.

Estazolam (Co-administration results in additive or potentiating effects). Products include:

ProSom Tablets 457

Ethchlorvynol (Co-administration results in additive or potentiating effects). Products include:

Placidyl Capsules 456

Ethinamate (Co-administration results in additive or potentiating effects).

No products indexed under this heading.

Fentanyl (Co-administration results in additive or potentiating effects). Products include:

Duragesic Transdermal System 1336

Fluphenazine Decanoate (Co-administration results in additive or potentiating effects). Products include:

Prolixin Decanoate 510

Fluphenazine Enanthate (Co-administration results in additive or potentiating effects). Products include:

Prolixin Enanthate 510

Fluphenazine Hydrochloride (Co-administration results in additive or potentiating effects). Products include:

Prolixin 510

Flurazepam Hydrochloride (Co-administration results in additive or potentiating effects). Products include:

Dalmane Capsules 2329

Furazolidone (Severe and unpredictable potentiation by MAO inhibitors have been reported for other narcotic analgesics; although this has not been reported with fentanyl, extreme caution should be exercised if fentanyl is administered to patients who have received MAO inhibitors within 14 days). Products include:

Furoxone 2221

Glutethimide (Co-administration results in additive or potentiating effects).

No products indexed under this heading.

Haloperidol (Co-administration results in additive or potentiating effects). Products include:

Haldol Injection, Tablets and Concentrate 1585

Haloperidol Decanoate (Co-administration results in additive or potentiating effects). Products include:

Haldol Decanoate 1587

Hydrocodone Bitartrate (Co-administration results in additive or potentiating effects). Products include:

Codiclear DH Syrup 808
Duratuss HD Elixir 2750
Histussin D Liquid 670
Hycodan Tablets and Syrup 946
Hycomine Compound Tablets 948
Hycomine 947
Hycotuss Expectorant Syrup 950
Hydrocet Capsules 787
Lorcet 10/650 Tablets 1016
Lortab 2751
Tussend 1830
Tussend Expectorant 1831
Vicodin Tablets 1404
Vicodin ES Tablets 1405
Vicodin HP Tablets 1403
Vicodin Tuss Expectorant 1406
Zydone Capsules 967

Hydrocodone Polistirex (Co-administration results in additive or potentiating effects). Products include:

Tussionex Pennkinetic Extended-Release Suspension 1624

Hydromorphone Hydrochloride (Co-administration results in additive or potentiating effects). Products include:

Dilaudid Ampules 1382
Dilaudid Cough Syrup 1383
Dilaudid-HP Injection 1384
Dilaudid-HP Lyophilized Powder 250 mg 1384
Dilaudid 1382
Dilaudid Oral Liquid 1386
Dilaudid 1382
Dilaudid Tablets - 8 mg 1386

Hydroxyzine Hydrochloride (Co-administration results in additive or potentiating effects). Products include:

Atarax Tablets & Syrup 1992
Marax Tablets & DF Syrup 2015
Vistaril Intramuscular Solution 2042

(▣ Described in PDR For Nonprescription Drugs) (◉ Described in PDR For Ophthalmology)

Isocarboxazid (Severe and unpredictable potentiation by MAO inhibitors have been reported for other narcotic analgesics; although this has not been reported with fentanyl, extreme caution should be exercised if fentanyl is administered to patients who have received MAO inhibitors within 14 days).
No products indexed under this heading.

Isoflurane (Co-administration results in additive or potentiating effects).
No products indexed under this heading.

Ketamine Hydrochloride (Co-administration results in additive or potentiating effects).
No products indexed under this heading.

Levomethadyl Acetate Hydrochloride (Co-administration results in additive or potentiating effects). Products include:
Orlaam Oral Solution 2361

Levorphanol Tartrate (Co-administration results in additive or potentiating effects). Products include:
Levo-Dromoran 2297

Lorazepam (Co-administration results in additive or potentiating effects). Products include:
Ativan Injection 2805
Ativan Tablets 2807

Loxapine Hydrochloride (Co-administration results in additive or potentiating effects). Products include:
Loxitane 1426

Loxapine Succinate (Co-administration results in additive or potentiating effects). Products include:
Loxitane Capsules 1426

Meperidine Hydrochloride (Co-administration results in additive or potentiating effects). Products include:
Demerol 2438
Mepergan Injection 2859

Mephobarbital (Co-administration results in additive or potentiating effects). Products include:
Mebaral Tablets 2452

Meprobamate (Co-administration results in additive or potentiating effects). Products include:
Miltown Tablets 2780
PMB 200 and PMB 400 2890

Mesoridazine Besylate (Co-administration results in additive or potentiating effects). Products include:
Serentil 689

Methadone Hydrochloride (Co-administration results in additive or potentiating effects). Products include:
Methadone Hydrochloride Oral Concentrate 2356
Methadone Hydrochloride Oral Solution & Tablets 2357

Methohexital Sodium (Co-administration results in additive or potentiating effects).
No products indexed under this heading.

Methotrimeprazine (Co-administration results in additive or potentiating effects). Products include:
Levoprome 1321

Methoxyflurane (Co-administration results in additive or potentiating effects).
No products indexed under this heading.

Midazolam Hydrochloride (Co-administration results in additive or potentiating effects). Products include:
Versed Injection 2324

Molindone Hydrochloride (Co-administration results in additive or potentiating effects). Products include:
Moban Tablets and Concentrate 1036

Morphine Sulfate (Co-administration results in additive or potentiating effects). Products include:
Astramorph/PF Injection, USP (Preservative-Free) 526
Duramorph Injection 983
Infumorph 200 and Infumorph 500 Sterile Solutions 985
Kadian Capsules 2948
MS Contin Tablets 2149
MSIR 2152
Oramorph SR (Morphine Sulfate Sustained Release Tablets) .. 2359
RMS Suppositories CII 2766
Roxanol 2365

Opium Alkaloids (Co-administration results in additive or potentiating effects).
No products indexed under this heading.

Oxazepam (Co-administration results in additive or potentiating effects). Products include:
Serax Capsules 2916
Serax Tablets 2916

Oxycodone Hydrochloride (Co-administration results in additive or potentiating effects). Products include:
OxyContin Tablets 2163
OxyIR Capsules 2167
Percocet Tablets 955
Percodan Tablets 955
Percodan-Demi Tablets 956
Roxicodone Tablets, Oral Solution & Intensol (Oxycodone) 2366
Tylox Capsules 1593

Pentobarbital Sodium (Co-administration results in additive or potentiating effects). Products include:
Nembutal Sodium Capsules ... 440
Nembutal Sodium Solution 442
Nembutal Sodium Suppositories 444

Perphenazine (Co-administration results in additive or potentiating effects). Products include:
Etrafon 2495
Triavil Tablets 1800
Trilafon 2532

Phenelzine Sulfate (Severe and unpredictable potentiation by MAO inhibitors have been reported for other narcotic analgesics; although this has not been reported with fentanyl, extreme caution should be exercised if fentanyl is administered to patients who have received MAO inhibitors within 14 days). Products include:
Nardil 1977

Phenobarbital (Co-administration results in additive or potentiating effects). Products include:
Arco-Lase Plus Tablets 513
Bellergal-S Tablets 2375
Donnatal 2234
Donnatal Extentabs 2234
Donnatal Tablets 2234
Phenobarbital Elixir and Tablets 1523
Quadrinal Tablets 1398

Prazepam (Co-administration results in additive or potentiating effects).
No products indexed under this heading.

Prochlorperazine (Co-administration results in additive or potentiating effects). Products include:
Compazine 2644

Promethazine Hydrochloride (Co-administration results in additive or potentiating effects). Products include:
Mepergan Injection 2859
Phenergan with Codeine 2883
Phenergan with Dextromethorphan 2885
Phenergan Injection 2880
Phenergan Suppositories 2882
Phenergan Syrup 2881
Phenergan Tablets 2882
Phenergan VC 2886
Phenergan VC with Codeine .. 2888

Propofol (Co-administration results in additive or potentiating effects). Products include:
Diprivan Injectable Emulsion .. 2939

Propoxyphene Hydrochloride (Co-administration results in additive or potentiating effects). Products include:
Darvon 1475
Wygesic Tablets 2930

Propoxyphene Napsylate (Co-administration results in additive or potentiating effects). Products include:
Darvon-N/Darvocet-N 1473

Quazepam (Co-administration results in additive or potentiating effects). Products include:
Doral Tablets 2773

Risperidone (Co-administration results in additive or potentiating effects). Products include:
Risperdal Tablets 1348

Secobarbital Sodium (Co-administration results in additive or potentiating effects). Products include:
Seconal Sodium Pulvules 1529

Selegiline Hydrochloride (Severe and unpredictable potentiation by MAO inhibitors have been reported for other narcotic analgesics; although this has not been reported with fentanyl, extreme caution should be exercised if fentanyl is administered to patients who have received MAO inhibitors within 14 days). Products include:
Eldepryl Capsules 2729

Sevoflurane (Co-administration results in additive or potentiating effects).
No products indexed under this heading.

Sufentanil Citrate (Co-administration results in additive or potentiating effects). Products include:
Sufenta Injection 1355

Temazepam (Co-administration results in additive or potentiating effects). Products include:
Restoril Capsules 2413

Thiamylal Sodium (Co-administration results in additive or potentiating effects).
No products indexed under this heading.

Thioridazine Hydrochloride (Co-administration results in additive or potentiating effects). Products include:
Mellaril 2398

Thiothixene (Co-administration results in additive or potentiating effects). Products include:
Navane Capsules and Concentrate 2018
Navane Intramuscular 2019

Tranylcypromine Sulfate (Severe and unpredictable potentiation by MAO inhibitors have been reported for other narcotic analgesics; although this has not been reported with fentanyl, extreme caution should be exercised if fentanyl is administered to patients who have received MAO inhibitors within 14 days). Products include:
Parnate Tablets 2679

Triazolam (Co-administration results in additive or potentiating effects). Products include:
Halcion Tablets 2093

Trifluoperazine Hydrochloride (Co-administration results in additive or potentiating effects). Products include:
Stelazine 2692

Zolpidem Tartrate (Co-administration results in additive or potentiating effects). Products include:
Ambien Tablets 2559

Food Interactions

Alcohol (Co-administration results in additive or potentiating effects).

SUCRETS CHILDREN'S CHERRY FLAVORED SORE THROAT LOZENGES
(Dyclonine Hydrochloride) 785
None cited in PDR database.

SUCRETS MAXIMUM STRENGTH WINTERGREEN, MAXIMUM STRENGTH VAPOR BLACK CHERRY SORE THROAT LOZENGES
(Dyclonine Hydrochloride) 785
None cited in PDR database.

SUCRETS REGULAR STRENGTH WILD CHERRY, REGULAR STRENGTH ORIGINAL MINT, REGULAR STRENGTH VAPOR LEMON SORE THROAT LOZENGES
(Dyclonine Hydrochloride) 785
None cited in PDR database.

SUCRETS 4-HOUR COUGH SUPPRESSANT
(Dextromethorphan Hydrobromide) 785
May interact with monoamine oxidase inhibitors. Compounds in this category include:

Furazolidone (Concurrent and/or sequential use is not recommended). Products include:
Furoxone 2221

Isocarboxazid (Concurrent and/or sequential use is not recommended).
No products indexed under this heading.

Phenelzine Sulfate (Concurrent and/or sequential use is not recommended). Products include:
Nardil 1977

Selegiline Hydrochloride (Concurrent and/or sequential use is not recommended). Products include:
Eldepryl Capsules 2729

Tranylcypromine Sulfate (Concurrent and/or sequential use is not recommended). Products include:
Parnate Tablets 2679

IMPORTANT NOTE: Always consult each drug listing in the patient's regimen for possible interactions.

SUDAFED CHILDREN'S COLD & COUGH LIQUID MEDICATION
(Dextromethorphan Hydrobromide, Guaifenesin, Pseudoephedrine Hydrochloride) ▣ 825
May interact with monoamine oxidase inhibitors. Compounds in this category include:

Furazolidone (Concurrent and/or sequential use is not recommended). Products include:
- Furoxone 2221

Isocarboxazid (Concurrent and/or sequential use is not recommended).
- No products indexed under this heading.

Phenelzine Sulfate (Concurrent and/or sequential use is not recommended). Products include:
- Nardil 1977

Selegiline Hydrochloride (Concurrent and/or sequential use is not recommended). Products include:
- Eldepryl Capsules 2729

Tranylcypromine Sulfate (Concurrent and/or sequential use is not recommended). Products include:
- Parnate Tablets 2679

SUDAFED CHILDREN'S NASAL DECONGESTANT LIQUID MEDICATION
(Pseudoephedrine Hydrochloride) .. ▣ 826
May interact with monoamine oxidase inhibitors. Compounds in this category include:

Furazolidone (Concurrent and/or sequential use is not recommended). Products include:
- Furoxone 2221

Isocarboxazid (Concurrent and/or sequential use is not recommended).
- No products indexed under this heading.

Phenelzine Sulfate (Concurrent and/or sequential use is not recommended). Products include:
- Nardil 1977

Selegiline Hydrochloride (Concurrent and/or sequential use is not recommended). Products include:
- Eldepryl Capsules 2729

Tranylcypromine Sulfate (Concurrent and/or sequential use is not recommended). Products include:
- Parnate Tablets 2679

SUDAFED COLD & ALLERGY TABLETS
(Chlorpheniramine Maleate, Pseudoephedrine Hydrochloride) .... ▣ 826
May interact with monoamine oxidase inhibitors, hypnotics and sedatives, tranquilizers, and certain other agents. Compounds in these categories include:

Alprazolam (May increase drowsiness effect). Products include:
- Xanax Tablets 2115

Buspirone Hydrochloride (May increase drowsiness effect). Products include:
- BuSpar Tablets 738

Chlordiazepoxide (May increase drowsiness effect). Products include:
- Limbitrol 2333

Chlordiazepoxide Hydrochloride (May increase drowsiness effect). Products include:
- Librax Capsules 2330
- Librium Capsules 2331
- Librium Injectable 2332

Chlorpromazine (May increase drowsiness effect). Products include:
- Thorazine Suppositories 2701

Chlorpromazine Hydrochloride (May increase drowsiness effect). Products include:
- Thorazine 2701

Chlorprothixene (May increase drowsiness effect).
- No products indexed under this heading.

Chlorprothixene Hydrochloride (May increase drowsiness effect).
- No products indexed under this heading.

Clorazepate Dipotassium (May increase drowsiness effect). Products include:
- Tranxene 459

Diazepam (May increase drowsiness effect). Products include:
- Dizac (diazepam injectable emulsion) CIV 1862
- Valium Injectable 2336
- Valium Tablets 2335

Droperidol (May increase drowsiness effect). Products include:
- Inapsine Injection 462

Estazolam (May increase drowsiness effect). Products include:
- ProSom Tablets 457

Ethchlorvynol (May increase drowsiness effect). Products include:
- Placidyl Capsules 456

Ethinamate (May increase drowsiness effect).
- No products indexed under this heading.

Fluphenazine Decanoate (May increase drowsiness effect). Products include:
- Prolixin Decanoate 510

Fluphenazine Enanthate (May increase drowsiness effect). Products include:
- Prolixin Enanthate 510

Fluphenazine Hydrochloride (May increase drowsiness effect). Products include:
- Prolixin 510

Flurazepam Hydrochloride (May increase drowsiness effect). Products include:
- Dalmane Capsules 2329

Furazolidone (Concurrent and/or sequential use is not recommended). Products include:
- Furoxone 2221

Glutethimide (May increase drowsiness effect).
- No products indexed under this heading.

Haloperidol (May increase drowsiness effect). Products include:
- Haldol Injection, Tablets and Concentrate 1585

Haloperidol Decanoate (May increase drowsiness effect). Products include:
- Haldol Decanoate 1587

Hydroxyzine Hydrochloride (May increase drowsiness effect). Products include:
- Atarax Tablets & Syrup 1992
- Marax Tablets & DF Syrup 2015
- Vistaril Intramuscular Solution 2042

Isocarboxazid (Concurrent and/or sequential use is not recommended).
- No products indexed under this heading.

Lorazepam (May increase drowsiness effect). Products include:
- Ativan Injection 2805
- Ativan Tablets 2807

Loxapine Hydrochloride (May increase drowsiness effect). Products include:
- Loxitane 1426

Loxapine Succinate (May increase drowsiness effect). Products include:
- Loxitane Capsules 1426

Meprobamate (May increase drowsiness effect). Products include:
- Miltown Tablets 2780
- PMB 200 and PMB 400 2890

Mesoridazine Besylate (May increase drowsiness effect). Products include:
- Serentil 689

Midazolam Hydrochloride (May increase drowsiness effect). Products include:
- Versed Injection 2324

Molindone Hydrochloride (May increase drowsiness effect). Products include:
- Moban Tablets and Concentrate 1036

Oxazepam (May increase drowsiness effect). Products include:
- Serax Capsules 2916
- Serax Tablets 2916

Perphenazine (May increase drowsiness effect). Products include:
- Etrafon 2495
- Triavil Tablets 1800
- Trilafon 2532

Phenelzine Sulfate (Concurrent and/or sequential use is not recommended). Products include:
- Nardil 1977

Prazepam (May increase drowsiness effect).
- No products indexed under this heading.

Prochlorperazine (May increase drowsiness effect). Products include:
- Compazine 2644

Promethazine Hydrochloride (May increase drowsiness effect). Products include:
- Mepergan Injection 2859
- Phenergan with Codeine 2883
- Phenergan with Dextromethorphan 2885
- Phenergan Injection 2880
- Phenergan Suppositories 2882
- Phenergan Syrup 2881
- Phenergan Tablets 2882
- Phenergan VC 2886
- Phenergan VC with Codeine 2888

Propofol (May increase drowsiness effect). Products include:
- Diprivan Injectable Emulsion 2939

Quazepam (May increase drowsiness effect). Products include:
- Doral Tablets 2773

Secobarbital Sodium (May increase drowsiness effect). Products include:
- Seconal Sodium Pulvules 1529

Selegiline Hydrochloride (Concurrent and/or sequential use is not recommended). Products include:
- Eldepryl Capsules 2729

Temazepam (May increase drowsiness effect). Products include:
- Restoril Capsules 2413

Thioridazine Hydrochloride (May increase drowsiness effect). Products include:
- Mellaril 2398

Thiothixene (May increase drowsiness effect). Products include:
- Navane Capsules and Concentrate 2018
- Navane Intramuscular 2019

Tranylcypromine Sulfate (Concurrent and/or sequential use is not recommended). Products include:
- Parnate Tablets 2679

Triazolam (May increase drowsiness effect). Products include:
- Halcion Tablets 2093

Trifluoperazine Hydrochloride (May increase drowsiness effect). Products include:
- Stelazine 2692

Zolpidem Tartrate (May increase drowsiness effect). Products include:
- Ambien Tablets 2559

Food Interactions
Alcohol (May increase drowsiness effect).

SUDAFED COLD AND COUGH LIQUID CAPS
(Acetaminophen, Dextromethorphan Hydrobromide, Guaifenesin, Pseudoephedrine Hydrochloride) .... ▣ 826
May interact with monoamine oxidase inhibitors. Compounds in this category include:

Furazolidone (Concurrent and/or sequential use is not recommended). Products include:
- Furoxone 2221

Isocarboxazid (Concurrent and/or sequential use is not recommended).
- No products indexed under this heading.

Phenelzine Sulfate (Concurrent and/or sequential use is not recommended). Products include:
- Nardil 1977

Selegiline Hydrochloride (Concurrent and/or sequential use is not recommended). Products include:
- Eldepryl Capsules 2729

Tranylcypromine Sulfate (Concurrent and/or sequential use is not recommended). Products include:
- Parnate Tablets 2679

SUDAFED NASAL DECONGESTANT TABLETS, 30 MG
(Pseudoephedrine Hydrochloride) .. ▣ 825
May interact with monoamine oxidase inhibitors. Compounds in this category include:

Furazolidone (Concurrent and/or sequential use is not recommended). Products include:
- Furoxone 2221

Isocarboxazid (Concurrent and/or sequential use is not recommended).
- No products indexed under this heading.

Phenelzine Sulfate (Concurrent and/or sequential use is not recommended). Products include:
- Nardil 1977

Selegiline Hydrochloride (Concurrent and/or sequential use is not recommended). Products include:
- Eldepryl Capsules 2729

Tranylcypromine Sulfate (Concurrent and/or sequential use is not recommended). Products include:
- Parnate Tablets 2679

SUDAFED NASAL DECONGESTANT TABLETS, 60 MG
(Pseudoephedrine Hydrochloride) .. ▣ 825
May interact with monoamine oxidase inhibitors. Compounds in this category include:

Furazolidone (Concurrent and/or sequential use is not recommended). Products include:
- Furoxone 2221

Isocarboxazid (Concurrent and/or sequential use is not recommended).
- No products indexed under this heading.

Phenelzine Sulfate (Concurrent and/or sequential use is not recommended). Products include:
- Nardil 1977

(▣ Described in PDR For Nonprescription Drugs)   (⊚ Described in PDR For Ophthalmology)

Interactions Index / Sufenta

Selegiline Hydrochloride (Concurrent and/or sequential use is not recommended). Products include:
  Eldepryl Capsules 2729
Tranylcypromine Sulfate (Concurrent and/or sequential use is not recommended). Products include:
  Parnate Tablets 2679

SUDAFED NON-DRYING SINUS LIQUID CAPS
(Pseudoephedrine Hydrochloride, Guaifenesin)................ 827
May interact with monoamine oxidase inhibitors. Compounds in this category include:

Furazolidone (Concurrent and/or sequential use is not recommended). Products include:
  Furoxone 2221
Isocarboxazid (Concurrent and/or sequential use is not recommended).
  No products indexed under this heading.
Phenelzine Sulfate (Concurrent and/or sequential use is not recommended). Products include:
  Nardil 1977
Selegiline Hydrochloride (Concurrent and/or sequential use is not recommended). Products include:
  Eldepryl Capsules 2729
Tranylcypromine Sulfate (Concurrent and/or sequential use is not recommended). Products include:
  Parnate Tablets 2679

SUDAFED PEDIATRIC NASAL DECONGESTANT LIQUID ORAL DROPS
(Pseudoephedrine Hydrochloride) .. 827
May interact with monoamine oxidase inhibitors. Compounds in this category include:

Furazolidone (Concurrent and/or sequential use is not recommended). Products include:
  Furoxone 2221
Isocarboxazid (Concurrent and/or sequential use is not recommended).
  No products indexed under this heading.
Phenelzine Sulfate (Concurrent and/or sequential use is not recommended). Products include:
  Nardil 1977
Selegiline Hydrochloride (Concurrent and/or sequential use is not recommended). Products include:
  Eldepryl Capsules 2729
Tranylcypromine Sulfate (Concurrent and/or sequential use is not recommended). Products include:
  Parnate Tablets 2679

SUDAFED SEVERE COLD FORMULA CAPLETS
(Acetaminophen, Dextromethorphan Hydrobromide, Pseudoephedrine Hydrochloride)..... 828
May interact with monoamine oxidase inhibitors. Compounds in this category include:

Furazolidone (Concurrent and/or sequential use is not recommended). Products include:
  Furoxone 2221
Isocarboxazid (Concurrent and/or sequential use is not recommended).
  No products indexed under this heading.
Phenelzine Sulfate (Concurrent and/or sequential use is not recommended). Products include:
  Nardil 1977

SUDAFED SEVERE COLD FORMULA TABLETS
(Acetaminophen, Dextromethorphan Hydrobromide, Pseudoephedrine Hydrochloride).... 828
May interact with monoamine oxidase inhibitors. Compounds in this category include:

Furazolidone (Concurrent and/or sequential use is not recommended). Products include:
  Furoxone 2221
Isocarboxazid (Concurrent and/or sequential use is not recommended).
  No products indexed under this heading.
Phenelzine Sulfate (Concurrent and/or sequential use is not recommended). Products include:
  Nardil 1977
Selegiline Hydrochloride (Concurrent and/or sequential use is not recommended). Products include:
  Eldepryl Capsules 2729
Tranylcypromine Sulfate (Concurrent and/or sequential use is not recommended). Products include:
  Parnate Tablets 2679

SUDAFED SINUS CAPLETS
(Acetaminophen, Pseudoephedrine Hydrochloride)................ 829
May interact with monoamine oxidase inhibitors. Compounds in this category include:

Furazolidone (Concurrent administration is not recommended). Products include:
  Furoxone 2221
Isocarboxazid (Concurrent administration is not recommended).
  No products indexed under this heading.
Phenelzine Sulfate (Concurrent administration is not recommended). Products include:
  Nardil 1977
Selegiline Hydrochloride (Concurrent administration is not recommended). Products include:
  Eldepryl Capsules 2729
Tranylcypromine Sulfate (Concurrent administration is not recommended). Products include:
  Parnate Tablets 2679

SUDAFED SINUS TABLETS
(Acetaminophen, Pseudoephedrine Hydrochloride)................ 829
May interact with monoamine oxidase inhibitors. Compounds in this category include:

Furazolidone (Concurrent and/or sequential use is not recommended). Products include:
  Furoxone 2221
Isocarboxazid (Concurrent and/or sequential use is not recommended).
  No products indexed under this heading.
Phenelzine Sulfate (Concurrent and/or sequential use is not recommended). Products include:
  Nardil 1977
Selegiline Hydrochloride (Concurrent and/or sequential use is not recommended). Products include:
  Eldepryl Capsules 2729
Tranylcypromine Sulfate (Concurrent and/or sequential use is not recommended). Products include:
  Parnate Tablets 2679

SUDAFED 12 HOUR CAPLETS
(Pseudoephedrine Hydrochloride) .. 824
May interact with:

Antidepressant Medications, unspecified (Effect not specified).
Antihypertensive agents, unspecified (Effect not specified).

SUFENTA INJECTION
(Sufentanil Citrate) 1355
May interact with central nervous system depressants, barbiturates, tranquilizers, narcotic analgesics, neuromuscular blocking agents, calcium channel blockers, beta blockers, benzodiazepines, and certain other agents. Compounds in these categories include:

Acebutolol Hydrochloride (The incidence and degree of bradycardia and hypotension during Sufenta-oxygen anesthesia may be greater in patients on chronic beta blocker therapy). Products include:
  Sectral Capsules 2914
Alfentanil Hydrochloride (Enhanced magnitude and duration of CNS/cardiovascular effects; respiratory depression may be enhanced). Products include:
  Alfenta Injection 1334
Alprazolam (Enhanced magnitude and duration of CNS/cardiovascular effects; respiratory depression may be enhanced; the use of benzodiazepines with Sufenta during induction may result in a decrease in mean arterial pressure and systemic vascular resistance). Products include:
  Xanax Tablets 2115
Amlodipine Besylate (The incidence and degree of bradycardia and hypotension during Sufenta-oxygen anesthesia may be greater in patients on chronic calcium channel blocker therapy). Products include:
  Lotrel Capsules 858
  Norvasc Tablets 2020
Aprobarbital (Enhanced magnitude and duration of CNS/cardiovascular effects; respiratory depression may be enhanced).
  No products indexed under this heading.
Atenolol (The incidence and degree of bradycardia and hypotension during Sufenta-oxygen anesthesia may be greater in patients on chronic beta blocker therapy). Products include:
  Tenoretic Tablets 2963
  Tenormin Tablets and I.V. Injection 2965
Atracurium Besylate (May produce bradycardia and hypotension; effect may be pronounced in the presence of calcium channel and/or beta-blockers). Products include:
  Tracrium Injection 1155
Bepridil Hydrochloride (The incidence and degree of bradycardia and hypotension during Sufenta-oxygen anesthesia may be greater in patients on chronic calcium channel blocker therapy). Products include:
  Vascor Tablets (200 and 300 mg) 1597

Betaxolol Hydrochloride (The incidence and degree of bradycardia and hypotension during Sufenta-oxygen anesthesia may be greater in patients on chronic beta blocker therapy). Products include:
  Betoptic Ophthalmic Solution....... 465
  Betoptic S Ophthalmic Suspension   467
  Kerlone Tablets 2588
Bisoprolol Fumarate (The incidence and degree of bradycardia and hypotension during Sufenta-oxygen anesthesia may be greater in patients on chronic beta blocker therapy). Products include:
  Zebeta Tablets 1457
  Ziac 1459
Buprenorphine (Enhanced magnitude and duration of CNS/cardiovascular effects; respiratory depression may be enhanced). Products include:
  Buprenex Injectable 2170
Buspirone Hydrochloride (Enhanced magnitude and duration of CNS/cardiovascular effects; respiratory depression may be enhanced). Products include:
  BuSpar Tablets 738
Butabarbital (Enhanced magnitude and duration of CNS/cardiovascular effects; respiratory depression may be enhanced).
  No products indexed under this heading.
Butalbital (Enhanced magnitude and duration of CNS/cardiovascular effects; respiratory depression may be enhanced). Products include:
  Axocet Capsules 2469
  Esgic-plus Capsules 1012
  Esgic-plus Tablets 1012
  Fioricet Tablets 2386
  Fioricet with Codeine Capsules 2387
  Fiorinal Tablets 2388
  Fiorinal with Codeine Capsules 2390
  Fiorinal Tablets 2388
  Phrenilin 790
  Sedapap Tablets 50 mg/650 mg .. 1826
Carteolol Hydrochloride (The incidence and degree of bradycardia and hypotension during Sufenta-oxygen anesthesia may be greater in patients on chronic beta blocker therapy). Products include:
  Cartrol Tablets 413
  Ocupress Ophthalmic Solution, 1% Sterile 297
Chlordiazepoxide (Enhanced magnitude and duration of CNS/cardiovascular effects; respiratory depression may be enhanced; the use of benzodiazepines with Sufenta during induction may result in a decrease in mean arterial pressure and systemic vascular resistance). Products include:
  Limbitrol 2333
Chlordiazepoxide Hydrochloride (Enhanced magnitude and duration of CNS/cardiovascular effects; respiratory depression may be enhanced; the use of benzodiazepines with Sufenta during induction may result in a decrease in mean arterial pressure and systemic vascular resistance). Products include:
  Librax Capsules 2330
  Librium Capsules 2331
  Librium Injectable 2332
Chlorpromazine (Enhanced magnitude and duration of CNS/cardiovascular effects; respiratory depression may be enhanced). Products include:
  Thorazine Suppositories 2701

IMPORTANT NOTE: Always consult each drug listing in the patient's regimen for possible interactions.

Sufenta | Interactions Index | 1018

Chlorprothixene (Enhanced magnitude and duration of CNS/cardiovascular effects; respiratory depression may be enhanced).
- No products indexed under this heading.

Chlorprothixene Hydrochloride (Enhanced magnitude and duration of CNS/cardiovascular effects; respiratory depression may be enhanced).
- No products indexed under this heading.

Chlorprothixene Lactate (Enhanced magnitude and duration of CNS/cardiovascular effects; respiratory depression may be enhanced).
- No products indexed under this heading.

Cisatracurium Besylate (May produce bradycardia and hypotension; effect may be pronounced in the presence of calcium channel and/or beta-blockers). Products include:
- Nimbex Injection 1131

Clonazepam (The use of benzodiazepines with Sufenta during induction may result in a decrease in mean arterial pressure and systemic vascular resistance). Products include:
- Klonopin Tablets 2294

Clorazepate Dipotassium (Enhanced magnitude and duration of CNS/cardiovascular effects; respiratory depression may be enhanced; the use of benzodiazepines with Sufenta during induction may result in a decrease in mean arterial pressure and systemic vascular resistance). Products include:
- Tranxene 459

Clozapine (Enhanced magnitude and duration of CNS/cardiovascular effects; respiratory depression may be enhanced). Products include:
- Clozaril Tablets 2377

Codeine Phosphate (Enhanced magnitude and duration of CNS/cardiovascular effects; respiratory depression may be enhanced). Products include:
- Brontex 2130
- Dimetane-DC Cough Syrup 2232
- Fioricet with Codeine Capsules 2387
- Fiorinal with Codeine Capsules 2390
- Nucofed 2225
- Phenergan with Codeine 2883
- Phenergan VC with Codeine 2888
- Robitussin A-C Syrup 2248
- Robitussin-DAC Syrup 2249
- Ryna .... ▣ 804
- Soma Compound w/Codeine Tablets 2784
- Tylenol with Codeine 1592

Desflurane (Enhanced magnitude and duration of CNS/cardiovascular effects; respiratory depression may be enhanced). Products include:
- Suprane (desflurane, USP) 1865

Dezocine (Enhanced magnitude and duration of CNS/cardiovascular effects; respiratory depression may be enhanced). Products include:
- Dalgan Injection 529

Diazepam (Enhanced magnitude and duration of CNS/cardiovascular effects; respiratory depression may be enhanced; the use of benzodiazepines with Sufenta during induction may result in a decrease in mean arterial pressure and systemic vascular resistance). Products include:
- Dizac (diazepam injectable emulsion) CIV 1862
- Valium Injectable 2336
- Valium Tablets 2335

Diltiazem Hydrochloride (The incidence and degree of bradycardia and hypotension during Sufenta-oxygen anesthesia may be greater in patients on chronic calcium channel blocker therapy). Products include:
- Cardizem CD Capsules 1251
- Cardizem SR Capsules 1255
- Cardizem Injectable 1253
- Cardizem Tablets 1257
- Dilacor XR Extended-release Capsules 2183
- Tiazac Capsules 1019

Doxacurium Chloride (May produce bradycardia and hypotension; effect may be pronounced in the presence of calcium channel and/or beta-blockers). Products include:
- Nuromax Injection 1136

Droperidol (Enhanced magnitude and duration of CNS/cardiovascular effects; respiratory depression may be enhanced). Products include:
- Inapsine Injection 462

Enflurane (Enhanced magnitude and duration of CNS/cardiovascular effects; respiratory depression may be enhanced).
- No products indexed under this heading.

Esmolol Hydrochloride (The incidence and degree of bradycardia and hypotension during Sufenta-oxygen anesthesia may be greater in patients on chronic beta blocker therapy). Products include:
- Brevibloc (esmolol HCl) Injection 1860

Estazolam (Enhanced magnitude and duration of CNS/cardiovascular effects; respiratory depression may be enhanced; the use of benzodiazepines with Sufenta during induction may result in a decrease in mean arterial pressure and systemic vascular resistance). Products include:
- ProSom Tablets 457

Ethchlorvynol (Enhanced magnitude and duration of CNS/cardiovascular effects; respiratory depression may be enhanced). Products include:
- Placidyl Capsules 456

Ethinamate (Enhanced magnitude and duration of CNS/cardiovascular effects; respiratory depression may be enhanced).
- No products indexed under this heading.

Felodipine (The incidence and degree of bradycardia and hypotension during Sufenta-oxygen anesthesia may be greater in patients on chronic calcium channel blocker therapy). Products include:
- Plendil Extended-Release Tablets 514

Fentanyl (Enhanced magnitude and duration of CNS/cardiovascular effects; respiratory depression may be enhanced). Products include:
- Duragesic Transdermal System 1336

Fentanyl Citrate (Enhanced magnitude and duration of CNS/cardiovascular effects; respiratory depression may be enhanced). Products include:
- Sublimaze Injection 463

Fluphenazine Decanoate (Enhanced magnitude and duration of CNS/cardiovascular effects; respiratory depression may be enhanced). Products include:
- Prolixin Decanoate 510

Fluphenazine Enanthate (Enhanced magnitude and duration of CNS/cardiovascular effects; respiratory depression may be enhanced). Products include:
- Prolixin Enanthate 510

Fluphenazine Hydrochloride (Enhanced magnitude and duration of CNS/cardiovascular effects; respiratory depression may be enhanced). Products include:
- Prolixin 510

Flurazepam Hydrochloride (Enhanced magnitude and duration of CNS/cardiovascular effects; respiratory depression may be enhanced; the use of benzodiazepines with Sufenta during induction may result in a decrease in mean arterial pressure and systemic vascular resistance). Products include:
- Dalmane Capsules 2329

Glutethimide (Enhanced magnitude and duration of CNS/cardiovascular effects; respiratory depression may be enhanced).
- No products indexed under this heading.

Halazepam (Enhanced magnitude and duration of CNS/cardiovascular effects; respiratory depression may be enhanced; the use of benzodiazepines with Sufenta during induction may result in a decrease in mean arterial pressure and systemic vascular resistance).
- No products indexed under this heading.

Haloperidol (Enhanced magnitude and duration of CNS/cardiovascular effects; respiratory depression may be enhanced). Products include:
- Haldol Injection, Tablets and Concentrate 1585

Haloperidol Decanoate (Enhanced magnitude and duration of CNS/cardiovascular effects; respiratory depression may be enhanced). Products include:
- Haldol Decanoate 1587

Hydrocodone Bitartrate (Enhanced magnitude and duration of CNS/cardiovascular effects; respiratory depression may be enhanced). Products include:
- Codiclear DH Syrup 808
- Duratuss HD Elixir 2750
- Histussin D Liquid 670
- Hycodan Tablets and Syrup 946
- Hycomine Compound Tablets 948
- Hycomine 947
- Hycotuss Expectorant Syrup 950
- Hydrocet Capsules 787
- Lorcet 10/650 Tablets 1016
- Lortab 2751
- Tussend 1830
- Tussend Expectorant 1831
- Vicodin Tablets 1404
- Vicodin ES Tablets 1405
- Vicodin HP Tablets 1403
- Vicodin Tuss Expectorant 1406
- Zydone Capsules 967

Hydrocodone Polistirex (Enhanced magnitude and duration of CNS/cardiovascular effects; respiratory depression may be enhanced). Products include:
- Tussionex Pennkinetic Extended-Release Suspension 1624

Hydromorphone Hydrochloride (Enhanced magnitude and duration of CNS/cardiovascular effects; respiratory depression may be enhanced). Products include:
- Dilaudid Ampules 1382
- Dilaudid Cough Syrup 1383
- Dilaudid-HP Injection 1384
- Dilaudid-HP Lyophilized Powder 250 mg 1384
- Dilaudid 1382
- Dilaudid Oral Liquid 1386
- Dilaudid 1382
- Dilaudid Tablets - 8 mg 1386

Hydroxyzine Hydrochloride (Enhanced magnitude and duration of CNS/cardiovascular effects; respiratory depression may be enhanced). Products include:
- Atarax Tablets & Syrup 1992
- Marax Tablets & DF Syrup 2015
- Vistaril Intramuscular Solution 2042

Isoflurane (Enhanced magnitude and duration of CNS/cardiovascular effects; respiratory depression may be enhanced).
- No products indexed under this heading.

Isradipine (The incidence and degree of bradycardia and hypotension during Sufenta-oxygen anesthesia may be greater in patients on chronic calcium channel blocker therapy). Products include:
- DynaCirc Capsules 2381
- DynaCirc CR Tablets 2383

Ketamine Hydrochloride (Enhanced magnitude and duration of CNS/cardiovascular effects; respiratory depression may be enhanced).
- No products indexed under this heading.

Labetalol Hydrochloride (The incidence and degree of bradycardia and hypotension during Sufenta-oxygen anesthesia may be greater in patients on chronic beta blocker therapy). Products include:
- Normodyne Injection 2519
- Normodyne Tablets 2522
- Trandate 1158

Levobunolol Hydrochloride (The incidence and degree of bradycardia and hypotension during Sufenta-oxygen anesthesia may be greater in patients on chronic beta blocker therapy). Products include:
- Betagan .... ⊙ 230

Levomethadyl Acetate Hydrochloride (Enhanced magnitude and duration of CNS/cardiovascular effects; respiratory depression may be enhanced). Products include:
- Orlaam Oral Solution 2361

Levorphanol Tartrate (Enhanced magnitude and duration of CNS/cardiovascular effects; respiratory depression may be enhanced). Products include:
- Levo-Dromoran 2297

Lorazepam (Enhanced magnitude and duration of CNS/cardiovascular effects; respiratory depression may be enhanced; the use of benzodiazepines with Sufenta during induction may result in a decrease in mean arterial pressure and systemic vascular resistance). Products include:
- Ativan Injection 2805
- Ativan Tablets 2807

Loxapine Hydrochloride (Enhanced magnitude and duration of CNS/cardiovascular effects; respiratory depression may be enhanced). Products include:
- Loxitane 1426

Loxapine Succinate (Enhanced magnitude and duration of CNS/cardiovascular effects; respiratory depression may be enhanced). Products include:
- Loxitane Capsules 1426

Meperidine Hydrochloride (Enhanced magnitude and duration of CNS/cardiovascular effects; respiratory depression may be enhanced). Products include:
- Demerol 2438
- Mepergan Injection 2859

(▣ Described in PDR For Nonprescription Drugs) (⊙ Described in PDR For Ophthalmology)

1019 **Interactions Index** **Sufenta**

Mephobarbital (Enhanced magnitude and duration of CNS/cardiovascular effects; respiratory depression may be enhanced). Products include:
Mebaral Tablets 2452

Meprobamate (Enhanced magnitude and duration of CNS/cardiovascular effects; respiratory depression may be enhanced). Products include:
Miltown Tablets 2780
PMB 200 and PMB 400 2890

Mesoridazine Besylate (Enhanced magnitude and duration of CNS/cardiovascular effects; respiratory depression may be enhanced). Products include:
Serentil 689

Methadone Hydrochloride (Enhanced magnitude and duration of CNS/cardiovascular effects; respiratory depression may be enhanced). Products include:
Methadone Hydrochloride Oral Concentrate 2356
Methadone Hydrochloride Oral Solution & Tablets 2357

Methohexital Sodium (Enhanced magnitude and duration of CNS/cardiovascular effects; respiratory depression may be enhanced).
No products indexed under this heading.

Methotrimeprazine (Enhanced magnitude and duration of CNS/cardiovascular effects; respiratory depression may be enhanced). Products include:
Levoprome 1321

Methoxyflurane (Enhanced magnitude and duration of CNS/cardiovascular effects; respiratory depression may be enhanced).
No products indexed under this heading.

Metipranolol Hydrochloride (The incidence and degree of bradycardia and hypotension during Sufenta-oxygen anesthesia may be greater in patients on chronic beta blocker therapy). Products include:
OptiPranolol (Metipranolol 0.3%) Sterile Ophthalmic Solution .... ◉ 256

Metocurine Iodide (May produce bradycardia and hypotension; effect may be pronounced in the presence of calcium channel and/or beta-blockers). Products include:
Metubine Iodide Vials 932

Metoprolol Succinate (The incidence and degree of bradycardia and hypotension during Sufenta-oxygen anesthesia may be greater in patients on chronic beta blocker therapy). Products include:
Toprol-XL Tablets 560

Metoprolol Tartrate (The incidence and degree of bradycardia and hypotension during Sufenta-oxygen anesthesia may be greater in patients on chronic beta blocker therapy). Products include:
Lopressor 848
Lopressor HCT Tablets 850

Midazolam Hydrochloride (Enhanced magnitude and duration of CNS/cardiovascular effects; respiratory depression may be enhanced; the use of benzodiazepines with Sufenta during induction may result in a decrease in mean arterial pressure and systemic vascular resistance). Products include:
Versed Injection 2324

Mivacurium Chloride (May produce bradycardia and hypotension; effect may be pronounced in the presence of calcium channel and/or beta-blockers). Products include:
Mivacron 1125

Molindone Hydrochloride (Enhanced magnitude and duration of CNS/cardiovascular effects; respiratory depression may be enhanced). Products include:
Moban Tablets and Concentrate 1036

Morphine Sulfate (Enhanced magnitude and duration of CNS/cardiovascular effects; respiratory depression may be enhanced). Products include:
Astramorph/PF Injection, USP (Preservative-Free) 526
Duramorph Injection 983
Infumorph 200 and Infumorph 500 Sterile Solutions 985
Kadian Capsules 2948
MS Contin Tablets 2149
MSIR 2152
Oramorph SR (Morphine Sulfate Sustained Release Tablets) 2359
RMS Suppositories CII 2766
Roxanol 2365

Nadolol (The incidence and degree of bradycardia and hypotension during Sufenta-oxygen anesthesia may be greater in patients on chronic beta blocker therapy).
No products indexed under this heading.

Nicardipine Hydrochloride (The incidence and degree of bradycardia and hypotension during Sufenta-oxygen anesthesia may be greater in patients on chronic calcium channel blocker therapy). Products include:
Cardene Capsules 2261
Cardene I.V. 2815
Cardene SR Capsules 2264

Nifedipine (The incidence and degree of bradycardia and hypotension during Sufenta-oxygen anesthesia may be greater in patients on chronic calcium channel blocker therapy). Products include:
Adalat Capsules (10 mg and 20 mg) 580
Adalat CC 582
Procardia Capsules 2024
Procardia XL Extended Release Tablets 2026

Nimodipine (The incidence and degree of bradycardia and hypotension during Sufenta-oxygen anesthesia may be greater in patients on chronic calcium channel blocker therapy). Products include:
Nimotop Capsules 603

Nisoldipine (The incidence and degree of bradycardia and hypotension during Sufenta-oxygen anesthesia may be greater in patients on chronic calcium channel blocker therapy). Products include:
Sular Tablets 2961

Nitrous Oxide (Possible cardiovascular depression).

Opium Alkaloids (Additive or potentiating effects; respiratory depression may be enhanced).
No products indexed under this heading.

Oxazepam (Enhanced magnitude and duration of CNS/cardiovascular effects; respiratory depression may be enhanced; the use of benzodiazepines with Sufenta during induction may result in a decrease in mean arterial pressure and systemic vascular resistance). Products include:
Serax Capsules 2916
Serax Tablets 2916

Oxycodone Hydrochloride (Enhanced magnitude and duration of CNS/cardiovascular effects; respiratory depression may be enhanced). Products include:
OxyContin Tablets 2163
OxyIR Capsules 2167
Percocet Tablets 955
Percodan Tablets 955
Percodan-Demi Tablets 956
Roxicodone Tablets, Oral Solution & Intensol (Oxycodone) 2366
Tylox Capsules 1593

Pancuronium Bromide (Elevated heart rate; may produce bradycardia and hypotension; effect may be pronounced in the presence of calcium channel and/or beta-blockers).
No products indexed under this heading.

Penbutolol Sulfate (The incidence and degree of bradycardia and hypotension during Sufenta-oxygen anesthesia may be greater in patients on chronic beta blocker therapy). Products include:
Levatol Tablets 2547

Pentobarbital Sodium (Enhanced magnitude and duration of CNS/cardiovascular effects; respiratory depression may be enhanced). Products include:
Nembutal Sodium Capsules 440
Nembutal Sodium Solution 442
Nembutal Sodium Suppositories 444

Perphenazine (Enhanced magnitude and duration of CNS/cardiovascular effects; respiratory depression may be enhanced). Products include:
Etrafon 2495
Triavil Tablets 1800
Trilafon 2532

Phenobarbital (Enhanced magnitude and duration of CNS/cardiovascular effects; respiratory depression may be enhanced). Products include:
Arco-Lase Plus Tablets 513
Bellergal-S Tablets 2375
Donnatal 2234
Donnatal Extentabs 2234
Donnatal Tablets 2234
Phenobarbital Elixir and Tablets 1523
Quadrinal Tablets 1398

Pindolol (The incidence and degree of bradycardia and hypotension during Sufenta-oxygen anesthesia may be greater in patients on chronic beta blocker therapy). Products include:
Visken Tablets 2428

Prazepam (Enhanced magnitude and duration of CNS/cardiovascular effects; respiratory depression may be enhanced; the use of benzodiazepines with Sufenta during induction may result in a decrease in mean arterial pressure and systemic vascular resistance).
No products indexed under this heading.

Prochlorperazine (Enhanced magnitude and duration of CNS/cardiovascular effects; respiratory depression may be enhanced). Products include:
Compazine 2644

Promethazine Hydrochloride (Enhanced magnitude and duration of CNS/cardiovascular effects; respiratory depression may be enhanced). Products include:
Mepergan Injection 2859
Phenergan with Codeine 2883
Phenergan with Dextromethorphan 2885
Phenergan Injection 2880
Phenergan Suppositories 2882
Phenergan Syrup 2881
Phenergan Tablets 2882
Phenergan VC 2886
Phenergan VC with Codeine 2888

Propofol (Enhanced magnitude and duration of CNS/cardiovascular effects; respiratory depression may be enhanced). Products include:
Diprivan Injectable Emulsion 2939

Propoxyphene Hydrochloride (Enhanced magnitude and duration of CNS/cardiovascular effects; respiratory depression may be enhanced). Products include:
Darvon 1475
Wygesic Tablets 2930

Propoxyphene Napsylate (Enhanced magnitude and duration of CNS/cardiovascular effects; respiratory depression may be enhanced). Products include:
Darvon-N/Darvocet-N 1473

Propranolol Hydrochloride (The incidence and degree of bradycardia and hypotension during Sufenta-oxygen anesthesia may be greater in patients on chronic beta blocker therapy). Products include:
Inderal 2834
Inderal LA Long Acting Capsules 2836
Inderide Tablets 2838
Inderide LA Long Acting Capsules 2840

Quazepam (Enhanced magnitude and duration of CNS/cardiovascular effects; respiratory depression may be enhanced; the use of benzodiazepines with Sufenta during induction may result in a decrease in mean arterial pressure and systemic vascular resistance). Products include:
Doral Tablets 2773

Risperidone (Enhanced magnitude and duration of CNS/cardiovascular effects; respiratory depression may be enhanced). Products include:
Risperdal Tablets 1348

Rocuronium Bromide (May produce bradycardia and hypotension; effect may be pronounced in the presence of calcium channel and/or beta-blockers). Products include:
Zemuron Injection 1885

Secobarbital Sodium (Enhanced magnitude and duration of CNS/cardiovascular effects; respiratory depression may be enhanced). Products include:
Seconal Sodium Pulvules 1529

Sevoflurane (Enhanced magnitude and duration of CNS/cardiovascular effects; respiratory depression may be enhanced).
No products indexed under this heading.

Sotalol Hydrochloride (The incidence and degree of bradycardia and hypotension during Sufenta-oxygen anesthesia may be greater in patients on chronic beta blocker therapy). Products include:
Betapace Tablets 637

Succinylcholine Chloride (May produce bradycardia and hypotension; effect may be pronounced in the presence of calcium channel and/or beta-blockers). Products include:
Anectine 1062

Temazepam (Enhanced magnitude and duration of CNS/cardiovascular effects; respiratory depression may be enhanced; the use of benzodiazepines with Sufenta during induction may result in a decrease in mean arterial pressure and systemic vascular resistance). Products include:
Restoril Capsules 2413

IMPORTANT NOTE: Always consult each drug listing in the patient's regimen for possible interactions.

Interactions Index

Sufenta

Thiamylal Sodium (Enhanced magnitude and duration of CNS/cardiovascular effects; respiratory depression may be enhanced).
No products indexed under this heading.

Thioridazine Hydrochloride (Enhanced magnitude and duration of CNS/cardiovascular effects; respiratory depression may be enhanced). Products include:
Mellaril 2398

Thiothixene (Enhanced magnitude and duration of CNS/cardiovascular effects; respiratory depression may be enhanced). Products include:
Navane Capsules and Concentrate 2018
Navane Intramuscular 2019

Timolol Maleate (The incidence and degree of bradycardia and hypotension during Sufenta-oxygen anesthesia may be greater in patients on chronic beta blocker therapy). Products include:
Blocadren Tablets 1654
Timolide Tablets 1791
Timoptic in Ocudose 1796
Timoptic Sterile Ophthalmic Solution 1794
Timoptic-XE 1798

Triazolam (Enhanced magnitude and duration of CNS/cardiovascular effects; respiratory depression may be enhanced; the use of benzodiazepines with Sufenta during induction may result in a decrease in mean arterial pressure and systemic vascular resistance). Products include:
Halcion Tablets 2093

Trifluoperazine Hydrochloride (Enhanced magnitude and duration of CNS/cardiovascular effects; respiratory depression may be enhanced). Products include:
Stelazine 2692

Vecuronium Bromide (May produce bradycardia and hypotension; effect may be pronounced in the presence of calcium channel and/or beta-blockers). Products include:
Norcuron for Injection 1875

Verapamil Hydrochloride (The incidence and degree of bradycardia and hypotension during Sufenta-oxygen anesthesia may be greater in patients on chronic calcium channel blocker therapy). Products include:
Calan SR Caplets 2571
Calan Tablets 2568
Covera-HS Tablets 2573
Isoptin Injectable 1391
Isoptin Oral Tablets 1393
Isoptin SR Tablets 1395
Verelan Capsules 1455

Zolpidem Tartrate (Enhanced magnitude and duration of CNS/cardiovascular effects; respiratory depression may be enhanced). Products include:
Ambien Tablets 2559

SULAR TABLETS
(Nisoldipine) 2961
May interact with:

Atenolol (Greater blood pressure effect of Sular with concomitant use). Products include:
Tenoretic Tablets 2963
Tenormin Tablets and I.V. Injection 2965

Cimetidine (Concomitant use increases nisoldipine AUC and Cmax by 30% to 45%). Products include:
Tagamet HB Tablets ....🅝 786
Tagamet Tablets 2694

Cimetidine Hydrochloride (Concomitant use increases nisoldipine AUC and Cmax by 30% to 45%). Products include:
Tagamet 2694

Propranolol Hydrochloride (Propranolol attenuates the heart rate increase following the administration of immediate-release nisoldipine). Products include:
Inderal 2834
Inderal LA Long Acting Capsules 2836
Inderide Tablets 2838
Inderide LA Long Acting Capsules .. 2840

Quinidine Gluconate (May decrease the bioavailability (AUC) of nisoldipine by 26%, but not the peak concentration; clinical significance is not known). Products include:
Quinaglute Dura-Tabs Tablets 644

Quinidine Polygalacturonate (May decrease the bioavailability (AUC) of nisoldipine by 26%, but not the peak concentration; clinical significance is not known). Products include:
Cardioquin Tablets 2146

Quinidine Sulfate (May decrease the bioavailability (AUC) of nisoldipine by 26%, but not the peak concentration; clinical significance is not known). Products include:
Quinidex Extentabs 2240

Ranitidine Hydrochloride (Concomitant use decreases AUC by 15%–20%). Products include:
Zantac 1182
Zantac Injection 1180
Zantac Syrup 1182

Food Interactions

Diet, high-lipid (Food with a high-fat content has a pronounced effect on the release of nisoldipine resulting in a significant increase in peak concentration (Cmax) by up to 300%; concomitant intake of high-fat meal should be avoided).

SULFACET-R LOTION
(Sodium Sulfacetamide, Sulfur) 925
None cited in PDR database.

SULFACET-R TINT FREE LOTION
(Sodium Sulfacetamide, Sulfur) 925
None cited in PDR database.

SULFAMYLON CREAM
(Mafenide Acetate) 940
None cited in PDR database.

SULTRIN TRIPLE SULFA CREAM
(Sulfathiazole, Sulfacetamide, Sulfabenzamide) 1941
None cited in PDR database.

SULTRIN TRIPLE SULFA VAGINAL TABLETS
(Sulfathiazole, Sulfacetamide, Sulfabenzamide) 1941
None cited in PDR database.

SUNKIST CHILDREN'S CHEWABLE MULTIVITAMINS - COMPLETE
(Vitamins with Minerals) ....🅝 665
None cited in PDR database.

SUNKIST CHILDREN'S CHEWABLE MULTIVITAMINS - PLUS EXTRA C
(Vitamins, Multiple) ....🅝 665
None cited in PDR database.

SUNKIST CHILDREN'S CHEWABLE MULTIVITAMINS - PLUS IRON
(Vitamins with Iron) ....🅝 665
None cited in PDR database.

SUNKIST CHILDREN'S CHEWABLE MULTIVITAMINS - REGULAR
(Vitamins, Multiple) ....🅝 664
None cited in PDR database.

SUNKIST VITAMIN C - CHEWABLE
(Vitamin C) ....🅝 666
None cited in PDR database.

SUNKIST VITAMIN C - EASY TO SWALLOW
(Vitamin C) ....🅝 666
None cited in PDR database.

SUNSOURCE ALLERGY RELIEF TABLETS
(Homeopathic Medications) ....🅝 792
None cited in PDR database.

SUNSOURCE ARTHRITIS RELIEF CREAM
(Homeopathic Medications) ....🅝 793
None cited in PDR database.

SUNSOURCE ARTHRITIS RELIEF TABLETS
(Homeopathic Medications) ....🅝 792
None cited in PDR database.

SUNSOURCE COLD RELIEF TABLETS
(Homeopathic Medications) ....🅝 792
None cited in PDR database.

SUNSOURCE FLU RELIEF TABLETS
(Homeopathic Medications) ....🅝 792
None cited in PDR database.

SUNSOURCE INSOMNIA RELIEF TABLETS
(Homeopathic Medications) ....🅝 793
May interact with hypnotics and sedatives, tranquilizers, and certain other agents. Compounds in these categories include:

Alprazolam (Concurrent use should be avoided). Products include:
Xanax Tablets 2115

Buspirone Hydrochloride (Concurrent use should be avoided). Products include:
BuSpar Tablets 738

Chlordiazepoxide (Concurrent use should be avoided). Products include:
Limbitrol 2333

Chlordiazepoxide Hydrochloride (Concurrent use should be avoided). Products include:
Librax Capsules 2330
Librium Capsules 2331
Librium Injectable 2332

Chlorpromazine (Concurrent use should be avoided). Products include:
Thorazine Suppositories 2701

Chlorpromazine Hydrochloride (Concurrent use should be avoided). Products include:
Thorazine 2701

Chlorprothixene (Concurrent use should be avoided).
No products indexed under this heading.

Chlorprothixene Hydrochloride (Concurrent use should be avoided).
No products indexed under this heading.

Clorazepate Dipotassium (Concurrent use should be avoided). Products include:
Tranxene 459

Diazepam (Concurrent use should be avoided). Products include:
Dizac (diazepam injectable emulsion) CIV 1862
Valium Injectable 2336
Valium Tablets 2335

Droperidol (Concurrent use should be avoided). Products include:
Inapsine Injection 462

Estazolam (Concurrent use should be avoided). Products include:
ProSom Tablets 457

Ethchlorvynol (Concurrent use should be avoided). Products include:
Placidyl Capsules 456

Ethinamate (Concurrent use should be avoided).
No products indexed under this heading.

Fluphenazine Decanoate (Concurrent use should be avoided). Products include:
Prolixin Decanoate 510

Fluphenazine Enanthate (Concurrent use should be avoided). Products include:
Prolixin Enanthate 510

Fluphenazine Hydrochloride (Concurrent use should be avoided). Products include:
Prolixin 510

Flurazepam Hydrochloride (Concurrent use should be avoided). Products include:
Dalmane Capsules 2329

Glutethimide (Concurrent use should be avoided).
No products indexed under this heading.

Haloperidol (Concurrent use should be avoided). Products include:
Haldol Injection, Tablets and Concentrate 1585

Haloperidol Decanoate (Concurrent use should be avoided). Products include:
Haldol Decanoate 1587

Hydroxyzine Hydrochloride (Concurrent use should be avoided). Products include:
Atarax Tablets & Syrup 1992
Marax Tablets & DF Syrup 2015
Vistaril Intramuscular Solution .. 2042

Lorazepam (Concurrent use should be avoided). Products include:
Ativan Injection 2805
Ativan Tablets 2807

Loxapine Hydrochloride (Concurrent use should be avoided). Products include:
Loxitane 1426

Loxapine Succinate (Concurrent use should be avoided). Products include:
Loxitane Capsules 1426

Meprobamate (Concurrent use should be avoided). Products include:
Miltown Tablets 2780
PMB 200 and PMB 400 2890

Mesoridazine Besylate (Concurrent use should be avoided). Products include:
Serentil 689

Midazolam Hydrochloride (Concurrent use should be avoided). Products include:
Versed Injection 2324

(🅝 Described in PDR For Nonprescription Drugs)   (Ⓞ Described in PDR For Ophthalmology)

1021 **Interactions Index** **Surmontil**

Molindone Hydrochloride (Concurrent use should be avoided). Products include:
- Moban Tablets and Concentrate 1036

Oxazepam (Concurrent use should be avoided). Products include:
- Serax Capsules 2916
- Serax Tablets 2916

Perphenazine (Concurrent use should be avoided). Products include:
- Etrafon 2495
- Triavil Tablets 1800
- Trilafon 2532

Prazepam (Concurrent use should be avoided).
- No products indexed under this heading.

Prochlorperazine (Concurrent use should be avoided). Products include:
- Compazine 2644

Promethazine Hydrochloride (Concurrent use should be avoided). Products include:
- Mepergan Injection 2859
- Phenergan with Codeine 2883
- Phenergan with Dextromethorphan 2885
- Phenergan Injection 2880
- Phenergan Suppositories 2882
- Phenergan Syrup 2881
- Phenergan Tablets 2882
- Phenergan VC 2886
- Phenergan VC with Codeine 2888

Propofol (Concurrent use should be avoided). Products include:
- Diprivan Injectable Emulsion 2939

Quazepam (Concurrent use should be avoided). Products include:
- Doral Tablets 2773

Secobarbital Sodium (Concurrent use should be avoided). Products include:
- Seconal Sodium Pulvules 1529

Temazepam (Concurrent use should be avoided). Products include:
- Restoril Capsules 2413

Thioridazine Hydrochloride (Concurrent use should be avoided). Products include:
- Mellaril 2398

Thiothixene (Concurrent use should be avoided). Products include:
- Navane Capsules and Concentrate 2018
- Navane Intramuscular 2019

Triazolam (Concurrent use should be avoided). Products include:
- Halcion Tablets 2093

Trifluoperazine Hydrochloride (Concurrent use should be avoided). Products include:
- Stelazine 2692

Zolpidem Tartrate (Concurrent use should be avoided). Products include:
- Ambien Tablets 2559

Food Interactions

Alcohol (Concurrent use should be avoided).

SUNSOURCE PSORIASIS/ECZEMA RELIEF CREAM
(Homeopathic Medications) ...... ▣ 793
None cited in PDR database.

SUNSOURCE SINUS RELIEF TABLETS
(Homeopathic Medications) ...... ▣ 793
None cited in PDR database.

SUNSOURCE SPORTS INJURY RELIEF CREAM
(Homeopathic Medications) ...... ▣ 794
None cited in PDR database.

SUPEREPA
(Docosahexaenoic Acid (DHA)) 462
None cited in PDR database.

SUPLENA SPECIALIZED LIQUID NUTRITION
(Nutritional Supplement) 2346
None cited in PDR database.

SUPPRELIN INJECTION
(Histrelin Acetate) 2230
None cited in PDR database.

SUPRANE (DESFLURANE, USP)
(Desflurane) 1865
May interact with:

Atracurium Besylate (Anesthetic concentrations of desflurane reduce the ED_{95} of atracurium by approximately 50%). Products include:
- Tracrium Injection 1155

Fentanyl (Decreases the minimum alveolar concentration (MAC) of desflurane by 50%). Products include:
- Duragesic Transdermal System...... 1336

Fentanyl Citrate (Decreases the minimum alveolar concentration (MAC) of desflurane by 50%). Products include:
- Sublimaze Injection 463

Midazolam Hydrochloride (Decreases the minimum alveolar concentration (MAC) of desflurane by 16%). Products include:
- Versed Injection 2324

Pancuronium Bromide (Anesthetic concentrations of desflurane reduce the ED_{95} of pancuronium by approximately 50%).
- No products indexed under this heading.

Succinylcholine Chloride (Anesthetic concentrations of desflurane reduce the ED_{95} of succinylcholine by approximately 30%). Products include:
- Anectine 1062

SUPRAX FOR ORAL SUSPENSION
(Cefixime) 1443
None cited in PDR database.

SUPRAX TABLETS
(Cefixime) 1443

Food Interactions

Food, unspecified (Increases time to maximal absorption approximately 0.8 hour).

SURFAK LIQUI-GELS
(Docusate Calcium) ...... ▣ 803
May interact with:

Mineral Oil (Concurrent use with oral mineral oil is not recommended unless directed by a doctor). Products include:
- Alpha Keri Moisture Rich Body Oil ▣ 635
- Anusol Hemorrhoidal Ointment...... ▣ 810
- Aquaphor Healing Ointment 636
- Aquaphor Healing Ointment, Original Formula 636
- Eucerin Original Moisturizing Creme (Unscented) 636
- Eucerin Original Moisturizing Lotion 636
- Eucerin Plus Dry Skin Care Moisturizing Lotion 636
- Eucerin Plus Moisturizing Creme 636
- Fleet Mineral Oil Enema 1001
- Hemorid ...... ▣ 797
- HypoTears Ointment ...... ◉ 262
- Keri Lotion - Original Formula ...... ▣ 644
- Kondremul ...... ▣ 656
- Lubriderm Bath and Shower Oil .... ▣ 821
- Nephrox Suspension ...... ▣ 671
- Preparation H Hemorrhoidal Ointment ...... ▣ 842
- Refresh PM Lubricant Eye Ointment ...... ◉ 252
- Replens Vaginal Moisturizer ...... ▣ 823
- Tears Renewed Ointment...... ◉ 210

SURMONTIL CAPSULES
(Trimipramine Maleate) 2917
May interact with anticholinergics, sympathomimetics, monoamine oxidase inhibitors, thyroid preparations, antidepressant drugs, phenothiazines, selective serotonin reuptake inhibitors, drugs that inhibit cytochrome p450iid6, and certain other agents. Compounds in these categories include:

Albuterol (Potentiated effects of catecholamines; careful adjustment of dosage and close supervision are required). Products include:
- Proventil Inhalation Aerosol 2524
- Ventolin Inhalation Aerosol and Refill 1170

Albuterol Sulfate (Potentiated effects of catecholamines; careful adjustment of dosage and close supervision are required). Products include:
- Airet Albuterol Sulfate Inhalation Solution 1602
- Albuterol Sulfate, USP Solution for Inhalation, Arm-a-Med 522
- Proventil Inhalation Solution 0.083% 2527
- Proventil Repetabs Tablets 2529
- Proventil Solution for Inhalation 0.5% 2525
- Proventil Syrup 2528
- Proventil Tablets 2529
- Ventolin Inhalation Solution...... 1171
- Ventolin Nebules Inhalation Solution 1172
- Ventolin Rotacaps for Inhalation...... 1173
- Ventolin Syrup 1175
- Ventolin Tablets 1176
- Volmax Extended-Release Tablets .. 1835

Amitriptyline Hydrochloride (Concurrent use with drugs that are substrate for cytochrome $P_{450}IID_6$ may make normal metabolizer resemble poor metabolizer leading to higher than expected plasma concentrations of TCA with resultant toxicity). Products include:
- Elavil 2945
- Etrafon 2495
- Limbitrol 2333
- Triavil Tablets 1800

Amoxapine (Concurrent use with drugs that are substrate for cytochrome $P_{450}IID_6$ may make normal metabolizer resemble poor metabolizer leading to higher than expected plasma concentrations of TCA with resultant toxicity). Products include:
- Asendin Tablets 1419

Atropine Sulfate (Concurrent use may result in pronounced atropinelike effects). Products include:
- Arco-Lase Plus Tablets 513
- Atrohist Plus Tablets 1605
- Donnatal 2234
- Donnatal Extentabs 2234
- Donnatal Tablets 2234
- Lomotil 2591
- Motofen Tablets 789
- Urised Tablets 2123

Belladonna Alkaloids (Concurrent use may result in pronounced atropinelike effects). Products include:
- Bellergal-S Tablets 2375
- Hyland's Bedwetting Tablets ...... ▣ 788
- Hyland's EnurAid Tablets...... ▣ 789
- Hyland's Headache Tablets ...... ▣ 790
- Hyland's Teething Tablets ...... ▣ 790
- Similasan Eye Drops # 1 ...... ▣ 769

Benztropine Mesylate (Concurrent use may result in pronounced atropinelike effects). Products include:
- Cogentin 1661

Biperiden Hydrochloride (Concurrent use may result in pronounced atropinelike effects). Products include:
- Akineton 1380

Bupropion Hydrochloride (Concurrent use with drugs that are substrate for cytochrome $P_{450}IID_6$ may make normal metabolizer resemble poor metabolizer leading to higher than expected plasma concentrations of TCA with resultant toxicity). Products include:
- Wellbutrin Tablets 1177

Chlorpromazine (Concurrent use with drugs that are substrate for cytochrome $P_{450}IID_6$ may make normal metabolizer resemble poor metabolizer leading to higher than expected plasma concentrations of TCA with resultant toxicity). Products include:
- Thorazine Suppositories 2701

Chlorpromazine Hydrochloride (Concurrent use with drugs that are substrate for cytochrome $P_{450}IID_6$ may make normal metabolizer resemble poor metabolizer leading to higher than expected plasma concentrations of TCA with resultant toxicity). Products include:
- Thorazine 2701

Cimetidine (Inhibits the elimination of tricyclic antidepressants; downward adjustment of Surmontil dosage may be required if cimetidine therapy is initiated; upward adjustment if cimetidine therapy is discontinued). Products include:
- Tagamet HB Tablets...... ▣ 786
- Tagamet Tablets 2694

Cimetidine Hydrochloride (Inhibits the elimination of tricyclic antidepressants; downward adjustment of Surmontil dosage may be required if cimetidine therapy is initiated; upward adjustment if cimetidine therapy is discontinued). Products include:
- Tagamet...... 2694

Clidinium Bromide (Concurrent use may result in pronounced atropinelike effects). Products include:
- Librax Capsules 2330

Desipramine Hydrochloride (Concurrent use with drugs that are substrate for cytochrome $P_{450}IID_6$ may make normal metabolizer resemble poor metabolizer leading to higher than expected plasma concentrations of TCA with resultant toxicity). Products include:
- Norpramin Tablets 1273

Dicyclomine Hydrochloride (Concurrent use may result in pronounced atropinelike effects). Products include:
- Bentyl 1246

Dobutamine Hydrochloride (Potentiated effects of catecholamines; careful adjustment of dosage and close supervision are required). Products include:
- Dobutrex Solution Vials...... 1480

Dopamine Hydrochloride (Potentiated effects of catecholamines; careful adjustment of dosage and close supervision are required).
- No products indexed under this heading.

IMPORTANT NOTE: Always consult each drug listing in the patient's regimen for possible interactions.

Doxepin Hydrochloride (Concurrent use with drugs that are substrate for cytochrome $P_{450}IID_6$ may make normal metabolizer resemble poor metabolizer leading to higher than expected plasma concentrations of TCA with resultant toxicity). Products include:
  Adapin Capsules 1542
  Sinequan 2028
  Zonalon Cream 1042

Ephedrine Hydrochloride (Potentiated effects of catecholamines; careful adjustment of dosage and close supervision are required). Products include:
  Primatene Tablets .... ■ 844
  Quadrinal Tablets 1398

Ephedrine Sulfate (Potentiated effects of catecholamines; careful adjustment of dosage and close supervision are required). Products include:
  Marax Tablets & DF Syrup..... 2015

Ephedrine Tannate (Potentiated effects of catecholamines; careful adjustment of dosage and close supervision are required). Products include:
  Rynatuss 2782

Epinephrine (Potentiated effects of catecholamines; careful adjustment of dosage and close supervision are required). Products include:
  EPIFRIN .... ⊚ 237
  EpiPen 808
  Marcaine with Epinephrine 2446
  Primatene Mist .... ■ 843
  Sensorcaine with Epinephrine Injection................................ 554
  Sus-Phrine Injection 1017
  Xylocaine with Epinephrine Injections................................ 562

Epinephrine Bitartrate (Potentiated effects of catecholamines; careful adjustment of dosage and close supervision are required). Products include:
  Sensorcaine-MPF with Epinephrine Injection 554

Epinephrine Hydrochloride (Potentiated effects of catecholamines; careful adjustment of dosage and close supervision are required). Products include:
  Ana-Kit Anaphylaxis Emergency Treatment Kit 611

Flecainide Acetate (Concurrent use with drugs that are substrate for cytochrome $P_{450}IID_6$ may make normal metabolizer resemble poor metabolizer leading to higher than expected plasma concentrations of TCA with resultant toxicity). Products include:
  Tambocor Tablets 1555

Fluoxetine Hydrochloride (Concurrent use with drugs that are substrate for cytochrome $P_{450}IID_6$ may make normal metabolizer resemble poor metabolizer leading to higher than expected plasma concentrations of TCA with resultant toxicity; due to variation in the extent of inhibition of $P_{450}IID_6$ and long half-life of the parent (fluoxetine) and active metabolite sufficient time must elapse, at least 5 weeks before switching to TCA). Products include:
  Prozac Pulvules & Liquid, Oral Solution 935

Fluphenazine Decanoate (Concurrent use with drugs that are substrate for cytochrome $P_{450}IID_6$ may make normal metabolizer resemble poor metabolizer leading to higher than expected plasma concentrations of TCA with resultant toxicity). Products include:
  Prolixin Decanoate 510

Fluphenazine Enanthate (Concurrent use with drugs that are substrate for cytochrome $P_{450}IID_6$ may make normal metabolizer resemble poor metabolizer leading to higher than expected plasma concentrations of TCA with resultant toxicity). Products include:
  Prolixin Enanthate 510

Fluphenazine Hydrochloride (Concurrent use with drugs that are substrate for cytochrome $P_{450}IID_6$ may make normal metabolizer resemble poor metabolizer leading to higher than expected plasma concentrations of TCA with resultant toxicity). Products include:
  Prolixin 510

Fluvoxamine Maleate (Concurrent use with drugs that are substrate for cytochrome $P_{450}IID_6$ may make normal metabolizer resemble poor metabolizer leading to higher than expected plasma concentrations of TCA with resultant toxicity; due to variation in the extent of inhibition of $P_{450}IID_6$ caution is indicated; if co-administered sufficient time must elapse). Products include:
  LUVOX Tablets 2723

Furazolidone (Potential for hyperpyretic crises, severe convulsions, and death; concurrent and/or sequential use is contraindicated). Products include:
  Furoxone 2221

Glycopyrrolate (Concurrent use may result in pronounced atropinelike effects). Products include:
  Robinul Forte Tablets............ 2247
  Robinul Injectable 2247
  Robinul Tablets..................... 2247

Guanadrel Sulfate (Trimipramine may block the antihypertensive effect). Products include:
  Hylorel Tablets 1613

Guanethidine Monosulfate (Trimipramine may block the antihypertensive effect of guanethidine or similarly acting compounds). Products include:
  Esimil Tablets 840
  Ismelin Tablets 845

Hyoscyamine (Concurrent use may result in pronounced atropinelike effects). Products include:
  Cystospaz Tablets 2123
  Urised Tablets 2123

Hyoscyamine Sulfate (Concurrent use may result in pronounced atropinelike effects). Products include:
  Arco-Lase Plus Tablets 513
  Atrohist Plus Tablets 1605
  Cystospaz-M Capsules 2123
  Donnatal 2234
  Donnatal Extentabs............... 2234
  Donnatal Tablets................... 2234
  Kutrase Capsules 2546
  Levsin/Levsinex/Levbid 2549

Imipramine Hydrochloride (Concurrent use with drugs that are substrate for cytochrome $P_{450}IID_6$ may make normal metabolizer resemble poor metabolizer leading to higher than expected plasma concentrations of TCA with resultant toxicity). Products include:
  Tofranil Ampuls 873

  Tofranil Tablets 875

Imipramine Pamoate (Concurrent use with drugs that are substrate for cytochrome $P_{450}IID_6$ may make normal metabolizer resemble poor metabolizer leading to higher than expected plasma concentrations of TCA with resultant toxicity). Products include:
  Tofranil-PM Capsules 876

Ipratropium Bromide (Concurrent use may result in pronounced atropinelike effects). Products include:
  Atrovent Inhalation Aerosol ... 674
  Atrovent Inhalation Solution .. 675
  Atrovent Nasal Spray 0.03% ... 676
  Atrovent Nasal Spray 0.06% ... 678

Isocarboxazid (Potential for hyperpyretic crises, severe convulsions, and death; concurrent and/or sequential use is contraindicated).
  No products indexed under this heading.

Isoproterenol Hydrochloride (Potentiated effects of catecholamines; careful adjustment of dosage and close supervision are required). Products include:
  Isuprel Hydrochloride Solution 2443
  Isuprel Injection 2441
  Isuprel Mistometer 2442

Isoproterenol Sulfate (Potentiated effects of catecholamines; careful adjustment of dosage and close supervision are required). Products include:
  Norisodrine with Calcium Iodide Syrup 446

Levothyroxine Sodium (Potential for cardiovascular toxicity). Products include:
  Eltroxin Tablets..................... 2214
  Levothroid Tablets 1015
  Levothyroxine Sodium, USP for Injection 546
  Levoxyl Tablets 918
  Synthroid 1410

Liothyronine Sodium (Potential for cardiovascular toxicity). Products include:
  Cytomel Tablets 2647
  Triostat Injection 2708

Liotrix (Potential for cardiovascular toxicity).
  No products indexed under this heading.

Maprotiline Hydrochloride (Concurrent use with drugs that are substrate for cytochrome $P_{450}IID_6$ may make normal metabolizer resemble poor metabolizer leading to higher than expected plasma concentrations of TCA with resultant toxicity). Products include:
  Ludiomil Tablets.................... 861

Mepenzolate Bromide (Concurrent use may result in pronounced atropinelike effects).
  No products indexed under this heading.

Mesoridazine Besylate (Concurrent use with drugs that are substrate for cytochrome $P_{450}IID_6$ may make normal metabolizer resemble poor metabolizer leading to higher than expected plasma concentrations of TCA with resultant toxicity). Products include:
  Serentil 689

Metaproterenol Sulfate (Potentiated effects of catecholamines; careful adjustment of dosage and close supervision are required). Products include:
  Alupent................................. 672

  Metaproterenol Sulfate Inhalation Solution, USP, Arm-a-Med ... 547

Metaraminol Bitartrate (Potentiated effects of catecholamines; careful adjustment of dosage and close supervision are required). Products include:
  Aramine Injection.................. 1649

Methotrimeprazine (Concurrent use with drugs that are substrate for cytochrome $P_{450}IID_6$ may make normal metabolizer resemble poor metabolizer leading to higher than expected plasma concentrations of TCA with resultant toxicity). Products include:
  Levoprome 1321

Methoxamine Hydrochloride (Potentiated effects of catecholamines; careful adjustment of dosage and close supervision are required). Products include:
  Vasoxyl Injection 1169

Nefazodone Hydrochloride (Concurrent use with drugs that are substrate for cytochrome $P_{450}IID_6$ may make normal metabolizer resemble poor metabolizer leading to higher than expected plasma concentrations of TCA with resultant toxicity). Products include:
  Serzone Tablets 776

Norepinephrine Bitartrate (Potentiated effects of catecholamines; careful adjustment of dosage and close supervision are required). Products include:
  Levophed Bitartrate Injection............ 2445

Nortriptyline Hydrochloride (Concurrent use with drugs that are substrate for cytochrome $P_{450}IID_6$ may make normal metabolizer resemble poor metabolizer leading to higher than expected plasma concentrations of TCA with resultant toxicity). Products include:
  Pamelor 2409

Oxybutynin Chloride (Concurrent use may result in pronounced atropinelike effects). Products include:
  Ditropan................................ 1267

Paroxetine Hydrochloride (Concurrent use with drugs that are substrate for cytochrome $P_{450}IID_6$ may make normal metabolizer resemble poor metabolizer leading to higher than expected plasma concentrations of TCA with resultant toxicity; due to variation in the extent of inhibition of $P_{450}IID_6$ caution is indicated; if co-administered sufficient time must elapse). Products include:
  Paxil Tablets 2681

Perphenazine (Concurrent use with drugs that are substrate for cytochrome $P_{450}IID_6$ may make normal metabolizer resemble poor metabolizer leading to higher than expected plasma concentrations of TCA with resultant toxicity). Products include:
  Etrafon.................................. 2495
  Triavil Tablets 1800
  Trilafon 2532

Phenelzine Sulfate (Potential for hyperpyretic crises, severe convulsions, and death; concurrent and/or sequential use is contraindicated). Products include:
  Nardil 1977

Phenylephrine Bitartrate (Potentiated effects of catecholamines; careful adjustment of dosage and close supervision are required).
  No products indexed under this heading.

(■ Described in PDR For Nonprescription Drugs) (⊚ Described in PDR For Ophthalmology)

Phenylephrine Hydrochloride
(Potentiated effects of catecholamines; careful adjustment of dosage and close supervision are required). Products include:

Atrohist Plus Tablets	1605
Cerose DM	◨ 853
D.A. II Tablets	972
D.A. Chewable Tablets	970
Dura-Vent/DA Tablets	972
Extendryl	1003
4-Way Fast Acting Nasal Spray (regular & mentholated)	◨ 644
Hemoril	◨ 797
Hycomine Compound Tablets	948
Neo-Synephrine Hydrochloride 1% Carpuject	2455
Neo-Synephrine Hydrochloride 1% Injection	2455
Neo-Synephrine Hydrochloride (Ophthalmic)	2456
Neo-Synephrine	◨ 624
Novahistine Elixir	◨ 782
Phenergan VC	2886
Phenergan VC with Codeine	2888
Preparation H	◨ 842
Tympagesic Ear Drops	2476
Vicks Sinex Nasal Spray and Ultra Fine Mist	◨ 738

Phenylephrine Tannate
(Potentiated effects of dosage and close supervision are required). Products include:

Atrohist Pediatric Suspension	1604
Atrohist Pediatric Suspension Dye-Free	1604
Rynatan	2781
Rynatuss	2782

Phenylpropanolamine Hydrochloride
(Potentiated effects of catecholamines; careful adjustment of dosage and close supervision are required). Products include:

Acutrim	◨ 648
Atrohist Plus Tablets	1605
BC Cold Powder Multi-Symptom Formula (Cold-Sinus-Allergy)	◨ 631
BC Cold Powder Non-Drowsy Formula (Cold-Sinus)	◨ 631
Cheracol Plus Head Cold/Cough Formula	◨ 741
Comtrex Multi-Symptom Cold Reliever Liqui-Gels	◨ 638
Comtrex Multi-Symptom Non-Drowsy Liqui-gels	◨ 640
Contac Continuous Action Nasal Decongestant/Antihistamine 12 Hour Capsules	◨ 773
Contac Maximum Strength Continuous Action Decongestant/Antihistamine 12 Hour Caplets	◨ 772
Contac Severe Cold and Flu Formula Caplets	◨ 773
Coricidin 'D' Decongestant Tablets	◨ 760
Dexatrim	◨ 795
Dexatrim Plus Vitamins Caplets	◨ 796
Dimetane-DC Cough Syrup	2232
Dimetapp Allergy Sinus Caplets	◨ 838
Dimetapp Cold & Allergy Chewable Tablets	◨ 838
Dimetapp Cold & Cough Liqui-Gels	◨ 839
Dimetapp DM Elixir	◨ 840
Dimetapp Elixir	◨ 840
Dimetapp Extentabs	◨ 841
Dimetapp Tablets/Liqui-Gels	◨ 841
Dura-Vent Tablets	971
Entex LA Tablets	972
Exgest LA Tablets	787
Hycomine	947
Nolamine Timed-Release Tablets	790
Ornade Spansule Capsules	2678
Propagest Tablets	791
Pyrroxate Caplets	◨ 742
Robitussin-CF	◨ 846
Sinulin Tablets	792
Tavist-D 12 Hour Relief Tablets	◨ 750
Teldrin 12 Hour Antihistamine/Nasal Decongestant Allergy Relief Capsules	◨ 786
Triaminic Expectorant	◨ 753
Triaminic Syrup	◨ 755
Triaminic Triaminicol Cold & Cough	◨ 756
Triaminic DM Syrup	◨ 756
Triaminicin Tablets	◨ 756

Vicks DayQuil Allergy Relief 12-Hour Extended Release Tablets	◨ 733
Vicks DayQuil Allergy Relief 4-Hour Tablets	◨ 733
Vicks DayQuil SINUS Pressure & CONGESTION Relief	◨ 734

Pirbuterol Acetate
(Potentiated effects of catecholamines; careful adjustment of dosage and close supervision are required). Products include:

Maxair Autohaler	1550
Maxair Inhaler	1552

Prochlorperazine
(Concurrent use with drugs that are substrate for cytochrome $P_{450}IID_6$ may make normal metabolizer resemble poor metabolizer leading to higher than expected plasma concentrations of TCA with resultant toxicity). Products include:

Compazine	2644

Procyclidine Hydrochloride
(Concurrent use may result in pronounced atropinelike effects). Products include:

Kemadrin Tablets	1105

Promethazine Hydrochloride
(Concurrent use with drugs that are substrate for cytochrome $P_{450}IID_6$ may make normal metabolizer resemble poor metabolizer leading to higher than expected plasma concentrations of TCA with resultant toxicity). Products include:

Mepergan Injection	2859
Phenergan with Codeine	2883
Phenergan with Dextromethorphan	2885
Phenergan Injection	2880
Phenergan Suppositories	2882
Phenergan Syrup	2881
Phenergan Tablets	2882
Phenergan VC	2886
Phenergan VC with Codeine	2888

Propafenone Hydrochloride
(Concurrent use with drugs that are substrate for cytochrome $P_{450}IID_6$ may make normal metabolizer resemble poor metabolizer leading to higher than expected plasma concentrations of TCA with resultant toxicity). Products include:

Rythmol Tablets—150mg, 225mg, 300mg	1399

Propantheline Bromide
(Concurrent use may result in pronounced atropinelike effects). Products include:

Pro-Banthine Tablets	2226

Protriptyline Hydrochloride
(Concurrent use with drugs that are substrate for cytochrome $P_{450}IID_6$ may make normal metabolizer resemble poor metabolizer leading to higher than expected plasma concentrations of TCA with resultant toxicity). Products include:

Vivactil Tablets	1820

Pseudoephedrine Hydrochloride
(Potentiated effects of catecholamines; careful adjustment of dosage and close supervision are required). Products include:

Actifed Allergy Daytime/Nighttime Caplets	◨ 808
Actifed Cold & Allergy Tablets	◨ 807
Actifed Cold & Sinus Caplets and Tablets	◨ 808
Actifed Sinus Daytime/Nighttime Tablets and Caplets	◨ 809
Advil Cold and Sinus Caplets and Tablets	◨ 837
Alka-Seltzer Plus Liqui-Gels	◨ 612
Alka-Seltzer Plus Flu & Body Aches Liqui-Gels Non-Drowsy Formula	◨ 613
Alka-Seltzer Plus Night-Time Cold Medicine Liqui-Gels	◨ 612
Allerest Maximum Strength	◨ 649
Allerest No Drowsiness	◨ 649
Allerest Sinus Pain Formula	◨ 649
Atrohist Pediatric Capsules	1603

Benadryl Allergy/Cold Tablets	◨ 811
Benadryl Allergy Decongestant Liquid Medication	◨ 812
Benadryl Allergy Decongestant Tablets	◨ 812
Benadryl Allergy Sinus Headache Caplets	◨ 813
Benylin Multisymptom	◨ 816
Bromfed Capsules (Extended-Release)	1832
Bromfed Syrup	◨ 712
Bromfed Tablets	1832
Bromfed-DM Cough Syrup	1832
Bromfed-PD Capsules (Extended-Release)	1832
Children's TYLENOL Cold Multi-Symptom Chewable Tablets and Liquid	1559
Children's TYLENOL Cold Plus Cough Multi Symptom Chewable Tablets and Liquid	1560
Children's TYLENOL Flu Suspension Liquid	1560
Children's Vicks DayQuil Allergy Relief	◨ 730
Children's Vicks NyQuil Cold/Cough Relief	◨ 731
Allergy-Sinus Comtrex Multi-Symptom Allergy-Sinus Formula Tablets and Caplets	◨ 639
Comtrex Multi-Symptom	◨ 638
Comtrex Multi-Symptom Non-Drowsy Caplets	◨ 640
Congess	1003
Contac Day Allergy/Sinus Caplets	◨ 771
Contac Day & Night	◨ 772
Contac Night Allergy/Sinus Caplets	◨ 771
Contac Severe Cold & Flu Non-Drowsy	◨ 774
Deconsal II Tablets	1605
Dimetane-DX Cough Syrup	2233
Dimetapp Cold & Fever Suspension	◨ 839
Dimetapp Decongestant Pediatric Drops	◨ 840
Dorcol Children's Cough Syrup	◨ 748
Drixoral Cough + Congestion Liquid Caps	◨ 763
Dura-Tap/PD Capsules	970
Duratuss Tablets	2750
Duratuss HD Elixir	2750
Efidac/24	◨ 655
Entex PSE Tablets	973
Fedahist Gyrocaps	2545
Guaifed	1833
Guaifed Syrup	◨ 712
Guaimax-D Tablets	809
Histussin D Liquid	670
Infants' TYLENOL Cold Decongestant & Fever-Reducer Drops	1561
Kronofed-A	994
Novahistine DMX	◨ 782
Nucofed	2225
PediaCare Cough-Cold Chewable Tablets and Liquid	1569
PediaCare Infants' Decongestant Drops	1569
PediaCare Infants' Drops Decongestant Plus Cough	1569
PediaCare NightRest Cough-Cold Liquid	1569
Pediatric Vicks 44d Cough & Head Congestion Relief	◨ 736
Pediatric Vicks 44m Cough & Cold Relief	◨ 737
Robitussin Cold & Cough Liqui-Gels	◨ 844
Robitussin Cold, Cough & Flu Liqui-Gels	◨ 844
Robitussin Maximum Strength Cough & Cold	◨ 847
Robitussin Night-Time Cold Formula	◨ 847
Robitussin Pediatric Cough & Cold Formula	◨ 848
Robitussin Pediatric Drops	◨ 849
Robitussin Severe Congestion Liqui-Gels	◨ 845
Robitussin-DAC Syrup	2249
Robitussin-PE	◨ 846
Rondec Oral Drops	974
Rondec Syrup	974
Rondec Tablet	974
Rondec Chewable Tablets	974
Rondec-TR Tablet	974
Ryna	◨ 804
Seldane-D Extended-Release Tablets	1286
Semprex-D Capsules	1620
Sinarest	◨ 663

Sine-Aid Maximum Strength Sinus Headache Gelcaps, Caplets and Tablets	1570
Sine-Off No Drowsiness Formula Caplets	◨ 784
Sine-Off Sinus Medicine	◨ 784
Singlet Tablets	◨ 785
Sinutab Non-Drying Liquid Caps	◨ 823
Sinutab Sinus Allergy Medication, Maximum Strength Tablets and Caplets	◨ 823
Sinutab Sinus Medication, Maximum Strength Without Drowsiness Formula, Tablets & Caplets	◨ 824
Sudafed Children's Cold & Cough Liquid Medication	◨ 825
Sudafed Children's Nasal Decongestant Liquid Medication	◨ 826
Sudafed Cold & Allergy Tablets	◨ 826
Sudafed Cold and Cough Liquid Caps	◨ 826
Sudafed Nasal Decongestant Tablets, 30 mg	◨ 825
Sudafed Nasal Decongestant Tablets, 60 mg	◨ 825
Sudafed Non-Drying Sinus Liquid Caps	◨ 827
Sudafed Pediatric Nasal Decongestant Liquid Oral Drops	◨ 827
Sudafed Severe Cold Formula Caplets	◨ 828
Sudafed Severe Cold Formula Tablets	◨ 828
Sudafed Sinus Caplets	◨ 829
Sudafed Sinus Tablets	◨ 829
Sudafed 12 Hour Caplets	1622
Syn-Rx Tablets	1622
Syn-Rx DM Tablets	1623
TheraFlu Flu and Cold Medicine	◨ 750
Theraflu Maximum Strength Flu and Cold Medicine For Sore Throat	◨ 751
TheraFlu Flu, Cold and Cough Medicine	◨ 750
TheraFlu Maximum Strength Nighttime Flu, Cold & Cough Medicine	◨ 751
TheraFlu Maximum Strength Non-Drowsy Formula Flu, Cold & Cough Medicine	◨ 751
TheraFlu Maximum Strength, Non-Drowsy Formula Flu, Cold and Cough Caplets	◨ 752
Theraflu Maximum Strength Sinus Non-Drowsy Formula Caplets	◨ 752
Triaminic AM Cough and Decongestant Formula	◨ 753
Triaminic AM Decongestant Formula	◨ 753
Triaminic Infant Oral Decongestant Drops	◨ 754
Triaminic Night Time	◨ 754
Triaminic Sore Throat Formula	◨ 755
Tussend	1830
Tussend Expectorant	1831
TYLENOL Allergy Sinus, Maximum Strength Caplets and Gelcaps	1571
TYLENOL Allergy Sinus NightTime, Maximum Strength Caplets	1571
TYLENOL Cold Medication, Multi-Symptom Formula Tablets and Caplets	1572
TYLENOL Cold Medication, Multi-Symptom Hot Liquid Packets	1572
TYLENOL Cold Medication, No Drowsiness Formula Caplets and Gelcaps	1572
TYLENOL Cold Severe Congestion Caplets	1573
TYLENOL Cough Medication with Decongestant, Multi Symptom	1574
TYLENOL Flu No Drowsiness Formula, Maximum Strength Gelcaps	1575
TYLENOL Flu NightTime, Maximum Strength Gelcaps	1575
TYLENOL Flu NightTime, Maximum Strength Hot Medication Packets	1575
TYLENOL Sinus, Maximum Strength Geltabs, Gelcaps, Caplets and Tablets	1576
Vicks 44 LiquiCaps Cough, Cold & Flu Relief	◨ 728
Vicks 44 LiquiCaps Non-Drowsy Cough & Cold Relief	◨ 729
Vicks 44D Cough & Head Congestion Relief	◨ 728
Vicks 44M Cough, Cold & Flu Relief	◨ 729

IMPORTANT NOTE: Always consult each drug listing in the patient's regimen for possible interactions.

- Vicks DayQuil LiquiCaps/Liquid Multi-Symptom Cold/Flu Relief .. ▣ 734
- Vicks DayQuil SINUS Pressure & PAIN Relief with IBUPROFEN ...... ▣ 735
- Vicks Nyquil Hot Therapy .... ▣ 735
- Vicks NyQuil LiquiCaps/Liquid Multi-Symptom Cold/Flu Relief, Original and Cherry Flavors .... ▣ 736

Pseudoephedrine Sulfate (Potentiated effects of catecholamines; careful adjustment of dosage and close supervision are required). Products include:

- Chlor-Trimeton Allergy Decongestant Tablets .... ▣ 759
- Claritin-D Tablets 2487
- Drixoral Cold and Allergy Sustained-Action Tablets .... ▣ 763
- Drixoral Cold and Flu Extended-Release Tablets .... ▣ 764
- Drixoral Non-Drowsy Formula Extended-Release Tablets .... ▣ 764
- Drixoral Allergy/Sinus Extended Release Tablets .... ▣ 765
- Trinalin Repetabs Tablets 1373

Quinidine Gluconate (Concurrent use with drugs that inhibit cytochrome $P_{450}IID_6$ may make normal metabolizer resemble poor metabolizer leading to higher than expected plasma concentrations of TCA with resultant toxicity). Products include:

- Quinaglute Dura-Tabs Tablets 644

Quinidine Polygalacturonate (Concurrent use with drugs that inhibit cytochrome $P_{450}IID_6$ may make normal metabolizer resemble poor metabolizer leading to higher than expected plasma concentrations of TCA with resultant toxicity). Products include:

- Cardioquin Tablets 2146

Quinidine Sulfate (Concurrent use with drugs that inhibit cytochrome $P_{450}IID_6$ may make normal metabolizer resemble poor metabolizer leading to higher than expected plasma concentrations of TCA with resultant toxicity). Products include:

- Quinidex Extentabs 2240

Salmeterol Xinafoate (Potentiated effects of catecholamines; careful adjustment of dosage and close supervision are required). Products include:

- Serevent Inhalation Aerosol 1149

Scopolamine (Concurrent use may result in pronounced atropinelike effects). Products include:

- Transderm Scōp Transdermal Therapeutic System 890

Scopolamine Hydrobromide (Concurrent use may result in pronounced atropinelike effects). Products include:

- Atrohist Plus Tablets 1605
- Donnatal 2234
- Donnatal Extentabs 2234
- Donnatal Tablets 2234

Selegiline Hydrochloride (Potential for hyperpyretic crises, severe convulsions, and death; concurrent and/or sequential use is contraindicated). Products include:

- Eldepryl Capsules 2729

Sertraline Hydrochloride (Concurrent use with drugs that are substrate for cytochrome $P_{450}IID_6$ may make normal metabolizer resemble poor metabolizer leading to higher than expected plasma concentrations of TCA with resultant toxicity; due to variation in the extent of inhibition of $P_{450}IID_6$ caution is indicated; if co-administered sufficient time must elapse). Products include:

- Zoloft Tablets 2051

Terbutaline Sulfate (Potentiated effects of catecholamines; careful adjustment of dosage and close supervision are required). Products include:

- Brethaire Inhaler 830
- Brethine Ampuls 832
- Brethine Tablets 831
- Bricanyl Subcutaneous Injection 1247
- Bricanyl Tablets 1248

Thioridazine Hydrochloride (Concurrent use with drugs that are substrate for cytochrome $P_{450}IID_6$ may make normal metabolizer resemble poor metabolizer leading to higher than expected plasma concentrations of TCA with resultant toxicity). Products include:

- Mellaril 2398

Thyroglobulin (Potential for cardiovascular toxicity).

- No products indexed under this heading.

Thyroid (Potential for cardiovascular toxicity).

- No products indexed under this heading.

Thyroxine (Potential for cardiovascular toxicity).

- No products indexed under this heading.

Thyroxine Sodium (Potential for cardiovascular toxicity).

- No products indexed under this heading.

Tranylcypromine Sulfate (Potential for hyperpyretic crises, severe convulsions, and death; concurrent and/or sequential use is contraindicated). Products include:

- Parnate Tablets 2679

Trazodone Hydrochloride (Concurrent use with drugs that are substrate for cytochrome $P_{450}IID_6$ may make normal metabolizer resemble poor metabolizer leading to higher than expected plasma concentrations of TCA with resultant toxicity). Products include:

- Desyrel and Desyrel Dividose 504

Tridihexethyl Chloride (Concurrent use may result in pronounced atropinelike effects).

- No products indexed under this heading.

Trifluoperazine Hydrochloride (Concurrent use with drugs that are substrate for cytochrome $P_{450}IID_6$ may make normal metabolizer resemble poor metabolizer leading to higher than expected plasma concentrations of TCA with resultant toxicity). Products include:

- Stelazine 2692

Trihexyphenidyl Hydrochloride (Concurrent use may result in pronounced atropinelike effects). Products include:

- Artane 1418

Venlafaxine Hydrochloride (Concurrent use with drugs that are substrate for cytochrome $P_{450}IID_6$ may make normal metabolizer resemble poor metabolizer leading to higher than expected plasma concentrations of TCA with resultant toxicity; due to variation in the extent of inhibition of $P_{450}IID_6$ caution is indicated; if co-administered sufficient time must elapse). Products include:

- Effexor 2825

Food Interactions

Alcohol (Concomitant use of alcoholic beverages and trimipramine may be associated with exaggerated effects).

SURVANTA BERACTANT INTRATRACHEAL SUSPENSION

(Beractant) 2346

None cited in PDR database.

SUS-PHRINE INJECTION

(Epinephrine) 1017

May interact with tricyclic antidepressants, cardiac glycosides, sympathomimetics, and certain other agents. Compounds in these categories include:

Albuterol (Combined effects on cardiovascular system may be deleterious). Products include:

- Proventil Inhalation Aerosol 2524
- Ventolin Inhalation Aerosol and Refill 1170

Albuterol Sulfate (Combined effects on cardiovascular system may be deleterious). Products include:

- Airet Albuterol Sulfate Inhalation Solution 1602
- Albuterol Sulfate, USP Solution for Inhalation, Arm-a-Med 522
- Proventil Inhalation Solution 0.083% 2527
- Proventil Repetabs Tablets 2529
- Proventil Solution for Inhalation 0.5% 2525
- Proventil Syrup 2528
- Proventil Tablets 2529
- Ventolin Inhalation Solution 1171
- Ventolin Nebules Inhalation Solution 1172
- Ventolin Rotacaps for Inhalation 1173
- Ventolin Syrup 1175
- Ventolin Tablets 1176
- Volmax Extended-Release Tablets .. 1835

Amitriptyline Hydrochloride (Epinephrine effects may be potentiated). Products include:

- Elavil 2945
- Etrafon 2495
- Limbitrol 2333
- Triavil Tablets 1800

Amoxapine (Epinephrine effects may be potentiated). Products include:

- Asendin Tablets 1419

Chlorpheniramine (Epinephrine effects may be potentiated).

Chlorpheniramine Maleate (Epinephrine effects may be potentiated). Products include:

- Alka-Seltzer Plus Cold Medicine .... ▣ 611
- Alka-Seltzer Plus Cold Medicine Liqui-Gels .... ▣ 612
- Alka-Seltzer Plus Cold & Cough Medicine .... ▣ 611
- Alka-Seltzer Plus Cold & Cough Medicine Liqui-Gels .... ▣ 612
- Alka-Seltzer Plus Flu & Body Aches Effervescent Tablets .... ▣ 612
- Allerest Maximum Strength .... ▣ 649
- Allerest Sinus Pain Formula .... ▣ 649
- Ana-Kit Anaphylaxis Emergency Treatment Kit 611
- Atrohist Pediatric Capsules 1603
- Atrohist Plus Tablets 1605
- BC Cold Powder Multi-Symptom Formula (Cold-Sinus-Allergy) ...... ▣ 631
- Cerose DM .... ▣ 853
- Cheracol Plus Head Cold/Cough Formula .... ▣ 741
- Children's TYLENOL Cold Multi-Symptom Chewable Tablets and Liquid 1559
- Children's TYLENOL Cold Plus Cough Multi Symptom Chewable Tablets and Liquid 1560
- Children's TYLENOL Flu Suspension Liquid 1560
- Children's Vicks DayQuil Allergy Relief .... ▣ 730
- Children's Vicks NyQuil Cold/Cough Relief .... ▣ 731
- Chlor-Trimeton Allergy Decongestant Tablets .... ▣ 759
- Chlor-Trimeton Allergy Tablets .... ▣ 758
- Allergy-Sinus Comtrex Multi-Symptom Allergy-Sinus Formula Tablets and Caplets .... ▣ 639
- Comtrex Multi-Symptom .... ▣ 638
- Contac Continuous Action Nasal Decongestant/Antihistamine 12 Hour Capsules .... ▣ 773
- Contac Maximum Strength Continuous Action Decongestant/Antihistamine 12 Hour Caplets .. ▣ 772
- Contac Severe Cold and Flu Formula Caplets .... ▣ 773
- Coricidin Cold + Flu Tablets .... ▣ 760
- Coricidin Cough + Cold Tablets .... ▣ 760
- Coricidin 'D' Decongestant Tablets .... ▣ 760
- D.A. II Tablets 972
- D.A. Chewable Tablets 970
- Dura-Tap/PD Capsules 970
- Dura-Vent/DA Tablets 972
- Efidac 24 Chlorpheniramine .... ▣ 655
- Extendryl 1003
- Fedahist Gyrocaps 2545
- Hycomine Compound Tablets 948
- Kronofed-A 994
- Nolamine Timed-Release Tablets 790
- Novahistine Elixir .... ▣ 782
- Ornade Spansule Capsules 2678
- PediaCare Cough-Cold Chewable Tablets and Liquid 1569
- PediaCare NightRest Cough-Cold Liquid 1569
- Pediatric Vicks 44m Cough & Cold Relief .... ▣ 737
- Pyrroxate Caplets .... ▣ 742
- Ryna .... ▣ 804
- Sinarest .... ▣ 663
- Sine-Off Sinus Medicine .... ▣ 784
- Singlet Tablets .... ▣ 785
- Sinulin Tablets 792
- Sinutab Sinus Allergy Medication, Maximum Strength Tablets and Caplets .... ▣ 823
- Sudafed Cold & Allergy Tablets ..... ▣ 826
- Teldrin 12 Hour Antihistamine/Nasal Decongestant Allergy Relief Capsules .... ▣ 786
- TheraFlu Flu and Cold Medicine .... ▣ 750
- Theraflu Maximum Strength Flu and Cold Medicine For Sore Throat .... ▣ 751
- TheraFlu Flu, Cold and Cough Medicine .... ▣ 750
- TheraFlu Maximum Strength Nighttime Flu, Cold & Cough Medicine .... ▣ 751
- Triaminic Night Time .... ▣ 754
- Triaminic Syrup .... ▣ 755
- Triaminic Triaminicol Cold & Cough .... ▣ 756
- Triaminicin Tablets .... ▣ 756
- Tussend 1830
- TYLENOL Allergy Sinus, Maximum Strength Caplets and Gelcaps 1571
- TYLENOL Cold Medication, Multi-Symptom Formula Tablets and Caplets 1572
- TYLENOL Cold Medication, Multi-Symptom Hot Liquid Packets 1572
- Vicks 44 LiquiCaps Cough, Cold & Flu Relief .... ▣ 728
- Vicks 44M Cough, Cold & Flu Relief .... ▣ 729

Chlorpheniramine Polistirex (Epinephrine effects may be potentiated). Products include:

- Tussionex Pennkinetic Extended-Release Suspension 1624

Chlorpheniramine Preparations (Epinephrine effects may be potentiated).

Chlorpheniramine Tannate (Epinephrine effects may be potentiated). Products include:

- Atrohist Pediatric Suspension 1604
- Atrohist Pediatric Suspension Dye-Free 1604
- Rynatan 2781
- Rynatuss 2782

Clomipramine Hydrochloride (Epinephrine effects may be potentiated). Products include:

- Anafranil Capsules 819

Desipramine Hydrochloride (Epinephrine effects may be potentiated). Products include:

- Norpramin Tablets 1273

Deslanoside (Potential for arrhythmias).

- No products indexed under this heading.

(▣ Described in PDR For Nonprescription Drugs) (⊙ Described in PDR For Ophthalmology)

1025 **Interactions Index** Sus-Phrine

Digitoxin (Potential for arrhythmias). Products include:
- Crystodigin Tablets 1472

Digoxin (Potential for arrhythmias). Products include:
- Lanoxicaps 1110
- Lanoxin Elixir Pediatric 1113
- Lanoxin Injection 1116
- Lanoxin Injection Pediatric 1119
- Lanoxin Tablets 1121

Diphenhydramine (Epinephrine effects may be potentiated).
- No products indexed under this heading.

Diphenhydramine Citrate (Epinephrine effects may be potentiated). Products include:
- Excedrin P.M. Analgesic/Sleeping Aid Tablets, Caplets, Liquigels 735

Diphenhydramine Hydrochloride (Epinephrine effects may be potentiated). Products include:
- Actifed Allergy Daytime/Nighttime Caplets 808
- Actifed Sinus Daytime/Nighttime Tablets and Caplets 809
- Extra Strength Bayer PM Aspirin Plus Sleep Aid 617
- Benadryl Allergy Chewables 811
- Benadryl Allergy/Cold Tablets 811
- Benadryl Allergy Decongestant Liquid Medication 812
- Benadryl Allergy Decongestant Tablets 812
- Benadryl Allergy Liquid Medication 813
- Benadryl Allergy 811
- Benadryl Allergy Sinus Headache Caplets 813
- Benadryl Dye-Free Allergy Liquigel Softgels 813
- Benadryl Dye-Free Allergy Liquid Medication 814
- Benadryl Itch Relief Stick Extra Strength 814
- Benadryl Cream 814
- Benadryl Gel 815
- Benadryl Spray 815
- Benadryl Injection 1955
- Contac Day & Night Cold/Flu Night Caplets 772
- Contac Night Allergy/Sinus Caplets 771
- Extra Strength Doan's P.M. 653
- Excedrin P.M. Analgesic/Sleeping Aid Tablets, Caplets, Liquigels 643
- Nytol QuickCaps Caplets 632
- Sleepinal Night-time Sleep Aid Capsules and Softgels 798
- TYLENOL Allergy Sinus NightTime, Maximum Strength Caplets 1571
- TYLENOL Flu NightTime, Maximum Strength Gelcaps 1575
- TYLENOL Flu NightTime, Maximum Strength Hot Medication Packets 1575
- TYLENOL PM Pain Reliever/Sleep Aid, Extra Strength Gelcaps, Caplets, Geltabs 1576
- TYLENOL Severe Allergy Medication Caplets 1571
- Maximum Strength Unisom Sleepgels 1990
- Unisom With Pain Relief-Nighttime Sleep Aid and Pain Reliever 1991

Dobutamine Hydrochloride (Combined effects on cardiovascular system may be deleterious). Products include:
- Dobutrex Solution Vials 1480

Dopamine Hydrochloride (Combined effects on cardiovascular system may be deleterious).
- No products indexed under this heading.

Doxepin Hydrochloride (Epinephrine effects may be potentiated). Products include:
- Adapin Capsules 1542
- Sinequan 2028
- Zonalon Cream 1042

Ephedrine Hydrochloride (Combined effects on cardiovascular system may be deleterious). Products include:
- Primatene Tablets 844
- Quadrinal Tablets 1398

Ephedrine Sulfate (Combined effects on cardiovascular system may be deleterious). Products include:
- Marax Tablets & DF Syrup 2015

Ephedrine Tannate (Combined effects on cardiovascular system may be deleterious). Products include:
- Rynatuss 2782

Epinephrine Bitartrate (Combined effects on cardiovascular system may be deleterious). Products include:
- Sensorcaine-MPF with Epinephrine Injection 554

Epinephrine Hydrochloride (Combined effects on cardiovascular system may be deleterious). Products include:
- Ana-Kit Anaphylaxis Emergency Treatment Kit 611

Imipramine Hydrochloride (Epinephrine effects may be potentiated). Products include:
- Tofranil Ampuls 873
- Tofranil Tablets 875

Imipramine Pamoate (Epinephrine effects may be potentiated). Products include:
- Tofranil-PM Capsules 876

Isoproterenol Hydrochloride (Combined effects on cardiovascular system may be deleterious). Products include:
- Isuprel Hydrochloride Solution 2443
- Isuprel Injection 2441
- Isuprel Mistometer 2442

Isoproterenol Sulfate (Combined effects on cardiovascular system may be deleterious). Products include:
- Norisodrine with Calcium Iodide Syrup 446

Maprotiline Hydrochloride (Epinephrine effects may be potentiated). Products include:
- Ludiomil Tablets 861

Metaproterenol Sulfate (Combined effects on cardiovascular system may be deleterious). Products include:
- Alupent 672
- Metaproterenol Sulfate Inhalation Solution, USP, Arm-a-Med 547

Metaraminol Bitartrate (Combined effects on cardiovascular system may be deleterious). Products include:
- Aramine Injection 1649

Norepinephrine Bitartrate (Combined effects on cardiovascular system may be deleterious). Products include:
- Levophed Bitartrate Injection 2445

Nortriptyline Hydrochloride (Epinephrine effects may be potentiated). Products include:
- Pamelor 2409

Phenylephrine Bitartrate (Combined effects on cardiovascular system may be deleterious).
- No products indexed under this heading.

Phenylephrine Hydrochloride (Combined effects on cardiovascular system may be deleterious). Products include:
- Atrohist Plus Tablets 1605
- Cerose DM 853
- D.A. II Tablets 972
- D.A. Chewable Tablets 970
- Dura-Vent/DA Tablets 972
- Extendryl 1003
- 4-Way Fast Acting Nasal Spray (regular & mentholated) 644
- Hemorid 797
- Hycomine Compound Tablets 948
- Neo-Synephrine Hydrochloride 1% Carpuject 2455
- Neo-Synephrine Hydrochloride 1% Injection 2455
- Neo-Synephrine Hydrochloride (Ophthalmic) 2456
- Neo-Synephrine 624
- Novahistine Elixir 782
- Phenergan VC 2886
- Phenergan VC with Codeine 2888
- Preparation H 842
- Tympagesic Ear Drops 2476
- Vicks Sinex Nasal Spray and Ultra Fine Mist 738

Phenylephrine Tannate (Combined effects on cardiovascular system may be deleterious). Products include:
- Atrohist Pediatric Suspension 1604
- Atrohist Pediatric Suspension Dye-Free 1604
- Rynatan 2781
- Rynatuss 2782

Phenylpropanolamine Hydrochloride (Combined effects on cardiovascular system may be deleterious). Products include:
- Acutrim 648
- Atrohist Plus Tablets 1605
- BC Cold Powder Multi-Symptom Formula (Cold-Sinus-Allergy) 631
- BC Cold Powder Non-Drowsy Formula (Cold-Sinus) 631
- Cheracol Plus Head Cold/Cough Formula 741
- Comtrex Multi-Symptom Cold Reliever Liqui-Gels 638
- Comtrex Multi-Symptom Non-Drowsy Liqui-gels 640
- Contac Continuous Action Nasal Decongestant/Antihistamine 12 Hour Capsules 773
- Contac Maximum Strength Continuous Action Decongestant/Antihistamine 12 Hour Caplets 772
- Contac Severe Cold and Flu Formula Caplets 773
- Coricidin 'D' Decongestant Tablets 760
- Dexatrim 795
- Dexatrim Plus Vitamins Caplets 796
- Dimetane-DC Cough Syrup 2232
- Dimetapp Allergy Sinus Caplets 838
- Dimetapp Cold & Allergy Chewable Tablets 838
- Dimetapp Cold & Cough Liqui-Gels 839
- Dimetapp DM Elixir 840
- Dimetapp Elixir 840
- Dimetapp Extentabs 841
- Dimetapp Tablets/Liqui-Gels 841
- Dura-Vent Tablets 971
- Entex LA Tablets 972
- Exgest LA Tablets 787
- Hycomine 947
- Nolamine Timed-Release Tablets 790
- Ornade Spansule Capsules 2678
- Propagest Tablets 791
- Pyrroxate Caplets 742
- Robitussin-CF 846
- Sinulin Tablets 792
- Tavist-D 12 Hour Relief Tablets 750
- Teldrin 12 Hour Antihistamine/Nasal Decongestant Allergy Relief Capsules 786
- Triaminic Expectorant 753
- Triaminic Syrup 755
- Triaminic Triaminicol Cold & Cough 756
- Triaminic DM Syrup 756
- Triaminicin Tablets 756
- Vicks DayQuil Allergy Relief 12-Hour Extended Release Tablets 733
- Vicks DayQuil Allergy Relief 4-Hour Tablets 733
- Vicks DayQuil SINUS Pressure & CONGESTION Relief 734

Pirbuterol Acetate (Combined effects on cardiovascular system may be deleterious). Products include:
- Maxair Autohaler 1550
- Maxair Inhaler 1552

Protriptyline Hydrochloride (Epinephrine effects may be potentiated). Products include:
- Vivactil Tablets 1820

Pseudoephedrine Hydrochloride (Combined effects on cardiovascular system may be deleterious). Products include:
- Actifed Allergy Daytime/Nighttime Caplets 808
- Actifed Cold & Allergy Tablets 807
- Actifed Cold & Sinus Caplets and Tablets 808
- Actifed Sinus Daytime/Nighttime Tablets and Caplets 809
- Advil Cold and Sinus Caplets and Tablets 837
- Alka-Seltzer Plus Liqui-Gels 612
- Alka-Seltzer Plus Flu & Body Aches Liqui-Gels Non-Drowsy Formula 613
- Alka-Seltzer Plus Night-Time Cold Medicine Liqui-Gels 612
- Allerest Maximum Strength 649
- Allerest No Drowsiness 649
- Allerest Sinus Pain Formula 649
- Atrohist Pediatric Capsules 1603
- Benadryl Allergy/Cold Tablets 811
- Benadryl Allergy Decongestant Liquid Medication 812
- Benadryl Allergy Decongestant Tablets 812
- Benadryl Allergy Sinus Headache Caplets 813
- Benylin Multisymptom 816
- Bromfed Capsules (Extended-Release) 1832
- Bromfed Syrup 712
- Bromfed Tablets 1832
- Bromfed-DM Cough Syrup 1832
- Bromfed-PD Capsules (Extended-Release) 1832
- Children's TYLENOL Cold Multi-Symptom Chewable Tablets and Liquid 1559
- Children's TYLENOL Cold Plus Cough Multi Symptom Chewable Tablets and Liquid 1560
- Children's TYLENOL Flu Suspension Liquid 1560
- Children's Vicks DayQuil Allergy Relief 730
- Children's Vicks NyQuil Cold/Cough Relief 731
- Allergy-Sinus Comtrex Multi-Symptom Allergy-Sinus Formula Tablets and Caplets 639
- Comtrex Multi-Symptom 638
- Comtrex Multi-Symptom Non-Drowsy Caplets 640
- Congess 1003
- Contac Day Allergy/Sinus Caplets 771
- Contac Day & Night 772
- Contac Night Allergy/Sinus Caplets 771
- Contac Severe Cold & Flu Non-Drowsy 774
- Deconsal II Tablets 1605
- Dimetane-DX Cough Syrup 2233
- Dimetapp Cold & Fever Suspension 839
- Dimetapp Decongestant Pediatric Drops 840
- Dorcol Children's Cough Syrup 748
- Drixoral Cough + Congestion Liquid Caps 763
- Dura-Tap/PD Capsules 970
- Duratuss Tablets 2750
- Duratuss HD Elixir 2750
- Efidac/24 655
- Entex PSE Tablets 973
- Fedahist Gyrocaps 2545
- Guaifed 1833
- Guaifed Syrup 712
- Guaimax-D Tablets 809
- Histussin D Liquid 670
- Infants' TYLENOL Cold Decongestant & Fever-Reducer Drops 1561
- Kronofed-A 994
- Novahistine DMX 782
- Nucofed 2225
- PediaCare Cough-Cold Chewable Tablets and Liquid 1569
- PediaCare Infants' Decongestant Drops 1569
- PediaCare Infants' Drops Decongestant Plus Cough 1569
- PediaCare NightRest Cough-Cold Liquid 1569

IMPORTANT NOTE: Always consult each drug listing in the patient's regimen for possible interactions.

Pediatric Vicks 44d Cough & Head Congestion Relief	736
Pediatric Vicks 44m Cough & Cold Relief	737
Robitussin Cold & Cough Liqui-Gels	844
Robitussin Cold, Cough & Flu Liqui-Gels	844
Robitussin Maximum Strength Cough & Cold	847
Robitussin Night-Time Cold Formula	847
Robitussin Pediatric Cough & Cold Formula	848
Robitussin Pediatric Drops	849
Robitussin Severe Congestion Liqui-Gels	845
Robitussin-DAC Syrup	2249
Robitussin-PE	846
Rondec Oral Drops	974
Rondec Syrup	974
Rondec Tablet	974
Rondec Chewable Tablets	974
Rondec-TR Tablet	974
Ryna	804
Seldane-D Extended-Release Tablets	1286
Semprex-D Capsules	1620
Sinarest	663
Sine-Aid Maximum Strength Sinus Headache Gelcaps, Caplets and Tablets	1570
Sine-Off No Drowsiness Formula Caplets	784
Sine-Off Sinus Medicine	784
Singlet Tablets	785
Sinutab Non-Drying Liquid Caps	823
Sinutab Sinus Allergy Medication, Maximum Strength Tablets and Caplets	823
Sinutab Sinus Medication, Maximum Strength Without Drowsiness Formula, Tablets & Caplets	824
Sudafed Children's Cold & Cough Liquid Medication	825
Sudafed Children's Nasal Decongestant Liquid Medication	826
Sudafed Cold & Allergy Tablets	826
Sudafed Cold and Cough Liquid Caps	826
Sudafed Nasal Decongestant Tablets, 30 mg	825
Sudafed Nasal Decongestant Tablets, 60 mg	825
Sudafed Non-Drying Sinus Liquid Caps	827
Sudafed Pediatric Nasal Decongestant Liquid Oral Drops	827
Sudafed Severe Cold Formula Caplets	828
Sudafed Severe Cold Formula Tablets	828
Sudafed Sinus Caplets	829
Sudafed Sinus Tablets	829
Sudafed 12 Hour Caplets	824
Syn-Rx Tablets	1622
Syn-Rx DM Tablets	1623
TheraFlu Flu and Cold Medicine	750
Theraflu Maximum Strength Flu and Cold Medicine For Sore Throat	751
TheraFlu Flu, Cold and Cough Medicine	750
TheraFlu Maximum Strength Nighttime Flu, Cold & Cough Medicine	751
TheraFlu Maximum Strength Non-Drowsy Formula Flu, Cold & Cough Medicine	751
TheraFlu Maximum Strength, Non-Drowsy Formula Flu, Cold and Cough Caplets	752
Theraflu Maximum Strength Sinus Non-Drowsy Formula Caplets	752
Triaminic AM Cough and Decongestant Formula	753
Triaminic AM Decongestant Formula	753
Triaminic Infant Oral Decongestant Drops	754
Triaminic Night Time	754
Triaminic Sore Throat Formula	755
Tussend	1830
Tussend Expectorant	1831
TYLENOL Allergy Sinus, Maximum Strength Caplets and Gelcaps	1571
TYLENOL Allergy Sinus NightTime, Maximum Strength Caplets	1571
TYLENOL Cold Medication, Multi-Symptom Formula Tablets and Caplets	1572
TYLENOL Cold Medication, Multi-Symptom Hot Liquid Packets	1572
TYLENOL Cold Medication, No Drowsiness Formula Caplets and Gelcaps	1572
TYLENOL Cold Severe Congestion Caplets	1573
TYLENOL Cough Medication with Decongestant, Multi Symptom	1574
TYLENOL Flu No Drowsiness Formula, Maximum Strength Gelcaps	1575
TYLENOL Flu NightTime, Maximum Strength Gelcaps	1575
TYLENOL Flu NightTime, Maximum Strength Hot Medication Packets	1575
TYLENOL Sinus, Maximum Strength Geltabs, Gelcaps, Caplets and Tablets	1576
Vicks 44 LiquiCaps Cough, Cold & Flu Relief	728
Vicks 44 LiquiCaps Non-Drowsy Cough & Cold Relief	729
Vicks 44D Cough & Head Congestion Relief	728
Vicks 44M Cough, Cold & Flu Relief	729
Vicks DayQuil LiquiCaps/Liquid Multi-Symptom Cold/Flu Relief	734
Vicks DayQuil SINUS Pressure & PAIN Relief with IBUPROFEN	735
Vicks Nyquil Hot Therapy	735
Vicks NyQuil LiquiCaps/Liquid Multi-Symptom Cold/Flu Relief, Original and Cherry Flavors	736

Pseudoephedrine Sulfate (Combined effects on cardiovascular system may be deleterious). Products include:

Chlor-Trimeton Allergy Decongestant Tablets	759
Claritin-D Tablets	2487
Drixoral Cold and Allergy Sustained-Action Tablets	763
Drixoral Cold and Flu Extended-Release Tablets	764
Drixoral Non-Drowsy Formula Extended-Release Tablets	764
Drixoral Allergy/Sinus Extended Release Tablets	765
Trinalin Repetabs Tablets	1373

Salmeterol Xinafoate (Combined effects on cardiovascular system may be deleterious). Products include:

Serevent Inhalation Aerosol	1149

Terbutaline Sulfate (Combined effects on cardiovascular system may be deleterious). Products include:

Brethaire Inhaler	830
Brethine Ampuls	832
Brethine Tablets	831
Bricanyl Subcutaneous Injection	1247
Bricanyl Tablets	1248

Thyroxine Sodium (Epinephrine effects may be potentiated).
No products indexed under this heading.

Trimipramine Maleate (Epinephrine effects may be potentiated). Products include:

Surmontil Capsules	2917

Tripelennamine Hydrochloride (Epinephrine effects may be potentiated). Products include:

PBZ Tablets	863
PBZ-SR Tablets	862

SYMMETREL CAPSULES
(Amantadine Hydrochloride) 965
May interact with central nervous system stimulants and certain other agents. Compounds in these categories include:

Amphetamine Resins (Co-administration with central nervous system stimulants requires careful observation).
No products indexed under this heading.

Dextroamphetamine Sulfate (Co-administration with central nervous system stimulants requires careful observation). Products include:

Adderall Tablets	2209
Dexedrine	2648
DextroStat-Dextroamphetamine Sulfate Tablets	2211

Hydrochlorothiazide (Co-administration with triamterene-hydrochlorothiazide capsules has resulted in a higher plasma amantadine concentration in a patient with Parkinsonism; it is not known which components of triamterene-hydrochlorothiazide capsules contributed this interaction). Products include:

Aldactazide Tablets	2556
Aldoril Tablets	1644
Apresazide Capsules	824
Capozide Tablets	744
Dyazide Capsules	2653
Esidrix Tablets	839
Esimil Tablets	840
HydroDIURIL Tablets	1716
Hydropres Tablets	1718
Hyzaar Tablets	1720
Inderide Tablets	2838
Inderide LA Long Acting Capsules	2840
Lopressor HCT Tablets	850
Lotensin HCT Tablets	855
Moduretic Tablets	1748
Oretic Tablets	450
Prinzide Tablets	1780
Ser-Ap-Es Tablets	867
Timolide Tablets	1791
Vaseretic Tablets	1810
Zestoretic Tablets	2968
Ziac	1459

Methamphetamine Hydrochloride (Co-administration with central nervous system stimulants requires careful observation). Products include:

Desoxyn Gradumet Tablets	422

Methylphenidate Hydrochloride (Co-administration with central nervous system stimulants requires careful observation). Products include:

Ritalin	866

Pemoline (Co-administration with central nervous system stimulants requires careful observation). Products include:

Cylert Tablets	415

Thioridazine Hydrochloride (Co-administration has been reported to worsen the tremor in elderly patients with Parkinson's disease). Products include:

Mellaril	2398

Triamterene (Co-administration with triamterene-hydrochlorothiazide capsules has resulted in a higher plasma amantadine concentration in a patient with Parkinsonism; it is not known which components of triamterene-hydrochlorothiazide capsules contributed this interaction). Products include:

Dyazide Capsules	2653
Dyrenium Capsules	2655

SYMMETREL SYRUP
(Amantadine Hydrochloride) 963
May interact with central nervous system stimulants and certain other agents. Compounds in these categories include:

Amphetamine Resins (Co-administration with central nervous system stimulants requires careful observation).
No products indexed under this heading.

Dextroamphetamine Sulfate (Co-administration with central nervous system stimulants requires careful observation). Products include:

Adderall Tablets	2209
Dexedrine	2648
DextroStat-Dextroamphetamine Sulfate Tablets	2211

Hydrochlorothiazide (Co-administration with triamterene-hydrochlorothiazide capsules has resulted in a higher plasma amantadine concentration in a patient with Parkinsonism; it is not known which components of triamterene-hydrochlorothiazide capsules contributed this interaction). Products include:

Aldactazide Tablets	2556
Aldoril Tablets	1644
Apresazide Capsules	824
Capozide Tablets	744
Dyazide Capsules	2653
Esidrix Tablets	839
Esimil Tablets	840
HydroDIURIL Tablets	1716
Hydropres Tablets	1718
Hyzaar Tablets	1720
Inderide Tablets	2838
Inderide LA Long Acting Capsules	2840
Lopressor HCT Tablets	850
Lotensin HCT Tablets	855
Moduretic Tablets	1748
Oretic Tablets	450
Prinzide Tablets	1780
Ser-Ap-Es Tablets	867
Timolide Tablets	1791
Vaseretic Tablets	1810
Zestoretic Tablets	2968
Ziac	1459

Methamphetamine Hydrochloride (Co-administration with central nervous system stimulants requires careful observation). Products include:

Desoxyn Gradumet Tablets	422

Methylphenidate Hydrochloride (Co-administration with central nervous system stimulants requires careful observation). Products include:

Ritalin	866

Pemoline (Co-administration with central nervous system stimulants requires careful observation). Products include:

Cylert Tablets	415

Thioridazine Hydrochloride (Co-administration has been reported to worsen the tremor in elderly patients with Parkinson's disease). Products include:

Mellaril	2398

Triamterene (Co-administration with triamterene-hydrochlorothiazide capsules has resulted in a higher plasma amantadine concentration in a patient with Parkinsonism; it is not known which components of triamterene-hydrochlorothiazide capsules contributed this interaction). Products include:

Dyazide Capsules	2653
Dyrenium Capsules	2655

SYNALAR CREAM 0.025%
(Fluocinolone Acetonide) 2299
None cited in PDR database.

SYNALAR TOPICAL SOLUTION 0.01%
(Fluocinolone Acetonide) 2299
None cited in PDR database.

SYNAREL NASAL SOLUTION FOR CENTRAL PRECOCIOUS PUBERTY
(Nafarelin Acetate) 2603
None cited in PDR database.

SYNAREL NASAL SOLUTION FOR ENDOMETRIOSIS
(Nafarelin Acetate) 2605
None cited in PDR database.

SYN-RX TABLETS
(Pseudoephedrine Hydrochloride, Guaifenesin) 1622
May interact with monoamine oxidase inhibitors, beta blockers, cardiac glycosides, tricyclic antidepressants, and certain other agents. Compounds in these categories include:

Acebutolol Hydrochloride (Potentiates the pressor effect). Products include:
- Sectral Capsules 2914

Amitriptyline Hydrochloride (May antagonize the effects of pseudoephedrine). Products include:
- Elavil 2945
- Etrafon 2495
- Limbitrol 2333
- Triavil Tablets 1800

Amoxapine (May antagonize the effects of pseudoephedrine). Products include:
- Asendin Tablets 1419

Atenolol (Potentiates the pressor effect). Products include:
- Tenoretic Tablets 2963
- Tenormin Tablets and I.V. Injection 2965

Betaxolol Hydrochloride (Potentiates the pressor effect). Products include:
- Betoptic Ophthalmic Solution 465
- Betoptic S Ophthalmic Suspension 467
- Kerlone Tablets 2588

Bisoprolol Fumarate (Potentiates the pressor effect). Products include:
- Zebeta Tablets 1457
- Ziac 1459

Carteolol Hydrochloride (Potentiates the pressor effect). Products include:
- Cartrol Tablets 413
- Ocupress Ophthalmic Solution, 1% Sterile .... ⊙ 297

Clomipramine Hydrochloride (May antagonize the effects of pseudoephedrine). Products include:
- Anafranil Capsules 819

Desipramine Hydrochloride (May antagonize the effects of pseudoephedrine). Products include:
- Norpramin Tablets 1273

Deslanoside (May increase the possiblity of cardiac arrhythmia). No products indexed under this heading.

Digitoxin (May increase the possiblity of cardiac arrhythmia). Products include:
- Crystodigin Tablets 1472

Digoxin (May increase the possiblity of cardiac arrhythmia). Products include:
- Lanoxicaps 1110
- Lanoxin Elixir Pediatric 1113
- Lanoxin Injection 1116
- Lanoxin Injection Pediatric 1119
- Lanoxin Tablets 1121

Doxepin Hydrochloride (May antagonize the effects of pseudoephedrine). Products include:
- Adapin Capsules 1542
- Sinequan 2028
- Zonalon Cream 1042

Esmolol Hydrochloride (Potentiates the pressor effect). Products include:
- Brevibloc (esmolol HCl) Injection 1860

Furazolidone (Concurrent and/or sequential use may lead to hypertensive crisis; co-administration is contraindicated). Products include:
- Furoxone 2221

Guanethidine Monosulfate (Reduced hypotensive effect). Products include:
- Esimil Tablets 840
- Ismelin Tablets 845

Imipramine Hydrochloride (May antagonize the effects of pseudoephedrine). Products include:
- Tofranil Ampuls 873
- Tofranil Tablets 875

Imipramine Pamoate (May antagonize the effects of pseudoephedrine). Products include:
- Tofranil-PM Capsules 876

Isocarboxazid (Concurrent and/or sequential use may lead to hypertensive crisis; co-administration is contraindicated). No products indexed under this heading.

Labetalol Hydrochloride (Potentiates the pressor effect). Products include:
- Normodyne Injection 2519
- Normodyne Tablets 2522
- Trandate 1158

Levobunolol Hydrochloride (Potentiates the pressor effect). Products include:
- Betagan .... ⊙ 230

Maprotiline Hydrochloride (May antagonize the effects of pseudoephedrine). Products include:
- Ludiomil Tablets 861

Mecamylamine Hydrochloride (Reduced hypotensive effect). Products include:
- Inversine Tablets 1729

Methyldopa (Reduced hypotensive effect). Products include:
- Aldoclor Tablets 1638
- Aldomet Oral 1640
- Aldoril Tablets 1644

Methyldopate Hydrochloride (Reduced hypotensive effect). Products include:
- Aldomet Ester HCl Injection 1642

Metipranolol Hydrochloride (Potentiates the pressor effect). Products include:
- OptiPranolol (Metipranolol 0.3%) Sterile Ophthalmic Solution .. ⊙ 256

Metoprolol Succinate (Potentiates the pressor effect). Products include:
- Toprol-XL Tablets 560

Metoprolol Tartrate (Potentiates the pressor effect). Products include:
- Lopressor 848
- Lopressor HCT Tablets 850

Nadolol (Potentiates the pressor effect). No products indexed under this heading.

Nortriptyline Hydrochloride (May antagonize the effects of pseudoephedrine). Products include:
- Pamelor 2409

Penbutolol Sulfate (Potentiates the pressor effect). Products include:
- Levatol Tablets 2547

Phenelzine Sulfate (Concurrent and/or sequential use may lead to hypertensive crisis; co-administration is contraindicated). Products include:
- Nardil 1977

Pindolol (Potentiates the pressor effect). Products include:
- Visken Tablets 2428

Propranolol Hydrochloride (Potentiates the pressor effect). Products include:
- Inderal 2834
- Inderal LA Long Acting Capsules 2836
- Inderide Tablets 2838
- Inderide LA Long Acting Capsules .. 2840

Protriptyline Hydrochloride (May antagonize the effects of pseudoephedrine). Products include:
- Vivactil Tablets 1820

Reserpine (Reduced hypotensive effect). Products include:
- Diupres Tablets 1691
- Hydropres Tablets 1718
- Ser-Ap-Es Tablets 867

Selegiline Hydrochloride (Concurrent and/or sequential use may lead to hypertensive crisis; co-administration is contraindicated). Products include:
- Eldepryl Capsules 2729

Sotalol Hydrochloride (Potentiates the pressor effect). Products include:
- Betapace Tablets 637

Timolol Hemihydrate (Potentiates the pressor effect). Products include:
- Betimol 0.25%, 0.5% .... ⊙ 259

Timolol Maleate (Potentiates the pressor effect). Products include:
- Blocadren Tablets 1654
- Timolide Tablets 1791
- Timoptic in Ocudose 1796
- Timoptic Sterile Ophthalmic Solution 1794
- Timoptic-XE 1798

Tranylcypromine Sulfate (Concurrent and/or sequential use may lead to hypertensive crisis; co-administration is contraindicated). Products include:
- Parnate Tablets 2679

Trimipramine Maleate (May antagonize the effects of pseudoephedrine). Products include:
- Surmontil Capsules 2917

SYN-RX DM TABLETS
(Guaifenesin, Pseudoephedrine Hydrochloride, Dextromethorphan Hydrobromide) 1623
May interact with monoamine oxidase inhibitors, beta blockers, veratrum alkaloids, tricyclic antidepressants, and certain other agents. Compounds in these categories include:

Acebutolol Hydrochloride (Potentiates the pressor effects of pseudoephedrine). Products include:
- Sectral Capsules 2914

Amitriptyline Hydrochloride (May antagonize the effects of pseudoephedrine). Products include:
- Elavil 2945
- Etrafon 2495
- Limbitrol 2333
- Triavil Tablets 1800

Amoxapine (May antagonize the effects of pseudoephedrine). Products include:
- Asendin Tablets 1419

Atenolol (Potentiates the pressor effects of pseudoephedrine). Products include:
- Tenoretic Tablets 2963
- Tenormin Tablets and I.V. Injection 2965

Betaxolol Hydrochloride (Potentiates the pressor effects of pseudoephedrine). Products include:
- Betoptic Ophthalmic Solution 465
- Betoptic S Ophthalmic Suspension 467
- Kerlone Tablets 2588

Bisoprolol Fumarate (Potentiates the pressor effects of pseudoephedrine). Products include:
- Zebeta Tablets 1457
- Ziac 1459

Carteolol Hydrochloride (Potentiates the pressor effects of pseudoephedrine). Products include:
- Cartrol Tablets 413
- Ocupress Ophthalmic Solution, 1% Sterile .... ⊙ 297

Clomipramine Hydrochloride (May antagonize the effects of pseudoephedrine). Products include:
- Anafranil Capsules 819

Cryptenamine Preparations (Sympathomimetic may reduce the antihypertensive effects of veratrum alkaloids).

Desipramine Hydrochloride (May antagonize the effects of pseudoephedrine). Products include:
- Norpramin Tablets 1273

Doxepin Hydrochloride (May antagonize the effects of pseudoephedrine). Products include:
- Adapin Capsules 1542
- Sinequan 2028
- Zonalon Cream 1042

Esmolol Hydrochloride (Potentiates the pressor effects of pseudoephedrine). Products include:
- Brevibloc (esmolol HCl) Injection 1860

Furazolidone (Potential for hypertensive crises; concurrent and/or sequential use is contraindicated; potentiates the pressor effects of pseudoephedrine). Products include:
- Furoxone 2221

Imipramine Hydrochloride (May antagonize the effects of pseudoephedrine). Products include:
- Tofranil Ampuls 873
- Tofranil Tablets 875

Imipramine Pamoate (May antagonize the effects of pseudoephedrine). Products include:
- Tofranil-PM Capsules 876

Isocarboxazid (Potential for hypertensive crises; concurrent and/or sequential use is contraindicated; potentiates the pressor effects of pseudoephedrine). No products indexed under this heading.

Labetalol Hydrochloride (Potentiates the pressor effects of pseudoephedrine). Products include:
- Normodyne Injection 2519
- Normodyne Tablets 2522
- Trandate 1158

Levobunolol Hydrochloride (Potentiates the pressor effects of pseudoephedrine). Products include:
- Betagan .... ⊙ 230

Maprotiline Hydrochloride (May antagonize the effects of pseudoephedrine). Products include:
- Ludiomil Tablets 861

Mecamylamine Hydrochloride (Sympathomimetic may reduce the antihypertensive effects). Products include:
- Inversine Tablets 1729

Methyldopa (Sympathomimetic may reduce the antihypertensive effects). Products include:
- Aldoclor Tablets 1638
- Aldomet Oral 1640
- Aldoril Tablets 1644

Methyldopate Hydrochloride (Sympathomimetic may reduce the antihypertensive effects). Products include:
- Aldomet Ester HCl Injection 1642

Metipranolol Hydrochloride (Potentiates the pressor effects of pseudoephedrine). Products include:
- OptiPranolol (Metipranolol 0.3%) Sterile Ophthalmic Solution .. ⊙ 256

Metoprolol Succinate (Potentiates the pressor effects of pseudoephedrine). Products include:
- Toprol-XL Tablets 560

IMPORTANT NOTE: Always consult each drug listing in the patient's regimen for possible interactions.

Syn-Rx DM **Interactions Index** 1028

Metoprolol Tartrate (Potentiates the pressor effects of pseudoephedrine). Products include:
Lopressor 848
Lopressor HCT Tablets 850
Nadolol (Potentiates the pressor effects of pseudoephedrine).
No products indexed under this heading.
Nortriptyline Hydrochloride (May antagonize the effects of pseudoephedrine). Products include:
Pamelor 2409
Penbutolol Sulfate (Potentiates the pressor effects of pseudoephedrine). Products include:
Levatol Tablets 2547
Phenelzine Sulfate (Potential for hypertensive crises; concurrent and/or sequential use is contraindicated; potentiates the pressor effects of pseudoephedrine). Products include:
Nardil 1977
Pindolol (Potentiates the pressor effects of pseudoephedrine). Products include:
Visken Tablets 2428
Propranolol Hydrochloride (Potentiates the pressor effects of pseudoephedrine). Products include:
Inderal 2834
Inderal LA Long Acting Capsules 2836
Inderide Tablets 2838
Inderide LA Long Acting Capsules 2840
Protriptyline Hydrochloride (May antagonize the effects of pseudoephedrine). Products include:
Vivactil Tablets 1820
Reserpine (Sympathomimetic may reduce the antihypertensive effects). Products include:
Diupres Tablets 1691
Hydropres Tablets 1718
Ser-Ap-Es Tablets 867
Selegiline Hydrochloride (Potential for hypertensive crises; concurrent and/or sequential use is contraindicated; potentiates the pressor effects of pseudoephedrine). Products include:
Eldepryl Capsules 2729
Sotalol Hydrochloride (Potentiates the pressor effects of pseudoephedrine). Products include:
Betapace Tablets 637
Timolol Hemihydrate (Potentiates the pressor effects of pseudoephedrine). Products include:
Betimol 0.25%, 0.5% ⊙ 259
Timolol Maleate (Potentiates the pressor effects of pseudoephedrine). Products include:
Blocadren Tablets 1654
Timolide Tablets 1791
Timoptic in Ocudose 1796
Timoptic Sterile Ophthalmic Solution 1794
Timoptic-XE 1798
Tranylcypromine Sulfate (Potential for hypertensive crises; concurrent and/or sequential use is contraindicated; potentiates the pressor effects of pseudoephedrine). Products include:
Parnate Tablets 2679
Trimipramine Maleate (May antagonize the effects of pseudoephedrine). Products include:
Surmontil Capsules 2917

SYNTHROID INJECTION
(Levothyroxine Sodium) 1410
See **Synthroid Tablets**

SYNTHROID TABLETS
(Levothyroxine Sodium) 1410
May interact with androgens, hepatic microsomal emzyme inducers, estrogens, glucocorticoids, salicylates, beta blockers, tricyclic antidepressants, sympathomimetics, xanthine bronchodilators, cardiac glycosides, insulin, oral hypoglycemic agents, oral anticoagulants, antithyroid agents, dopamine agonists, lithium preparations, sulfonylureas, thiazides, sulfonamides, cytokines, radiographic iodinated contrast media, and certain other agents. Compounds in these categories include:

Acarbose (Requirements of oral antidiabetic agents may be reduced in hypothyroid patients with diabetes and may be subsequently increased with initiation of thyroid hormone therapy). Products include:
Precose 604
Acebutolol Hydrochloride (Alters thyroid hormone or TSH levels; actions of some beta blockers may be impaired when hypothyroid patients become euthyroid). Products include:
Sectral Capsules 2914
Albuterol (Possible increased risk of coronary insufficiency in patients with coronary artery disease). Products include:
Proventil Inhalation Aerosol 2524
Ventolin Inhalation Aerosol and Refill 1170
Albuterol Sulfate (Possible increased risk of coronary insufficiency in patients with coronary artery disease). Products include:
Airet Albuterol Sulfate Inhalation Solution 1602
Albuterol Sulfate, USP Solution for Inhalation, Arm-a-Med 522
Proventil Inhalation Solution 0.083% 2527
Proventil Repetabs Tablets 2529
Proventil Solution for Inhalation 0.5% 2525
Proventil Syrup 2528
Proventil Tablets 2529
Ventolin Inhalation Solution 1171
Ventolin Nebules Inhalation Solution 1172
Ventolin Rotacaps for Inhalation 1173
Ventolin Syrup 1175
Ventolin Tablets 1176
Volmax Extended-Release Tablets 1835
Aldesleukin (Cytokines have been reported to induce both hyperthyroidism or hypothyroidism; dosage adjustment may be necessary). Products include:
Proleukin for Injection 812
Aluminum Hydroxide (Binds and decreases absorption of levothyroxine sodium from the gastrointestinal tract). Products include:
ALternaGEL Liquid 1358
Maximum Strength Ascriptin ▣ 650
Cama Arthritis Pain Reliever ▣ 748
Gaviscon Extra Strength Relief Formula Antacid Tablets ▣ 778
Gaviscon Extra Strength Relief Formula Liquid Antacid ▣ 779
Gaviscon Liquid Antacid ▣ 779
Gelusil Antacid-Anti-gas Liquid ▣ 819
Gelusil Antacid-Anti-gas Tablets ▣ 819
Maalox Antacid/Anti-Gas Tablets 889
Maalox Heartburn Relief Suspension ▣ 658
Maalox Antacid Liquid 888
Extra Strength Maalox Antacid/Anti-Gas Liquid and Tablets 888
Mylanta 1359
Tempo Soft Antacid ▣ 799
Aluminum Hydroxide Gel (Binds and decreases absorption of levothyroxine sodium from the gastrointestinal tract). Products include:
ALternaGEL Liquid ▣ 675
Aludrox Oral Suspension ▣ 850
Amphojel Suspension 2802
Amphojel Suspension without Flavor 2802
Amphojel Tablets 2802
Ascriptin ▣ 650
Gaviscon Antacid Tablets ▣ 778
Gaviscon-2 Antacid Tablets ▣ 779
Mylanta Liquid ▣ 676
Mylanta Double Strength Liquid ▣ 676
Nephrox Suspension ▣ 671
Aminoglutethimide (Alters thyroid hormone or TSH levels). Products include:
Cytadren Tablets 837
Aminophylline (Theophylline clearance may be decreased in hypothyroid patients and return toward normal when euthyroid state is achieved).
No products indexed under this heading.
p-Aminosalicylic Acid (Alters thyroid hormone or TSH levels).
No products indexed under this heading.
Amiodarone Hydrochloride (Alters thyroid hormone or TSH levels; amiodarone therapy alone can cause hypothyroidism or hyperthyroidism). Products include:
Cordarone Intravenous 2821
Cordarone Tablets 2818
Amitriptyline Hydrochloride (Concurrent use may increase the therapeutic and toxic effects of both drugs; onset of action of tricyclics may be accelerated). Products include:
Elavil 2945
Etrafon 2495
Limbitrol 2333
Triavil Tablets 1800
Amoxapine (Concurrent use may increase the therapeutic and toxic effects of both drugs; onset of action of tricyclics may be accelerated). Products include:
Asendin Tablets 1419
Asparaginase (May inhibit levothyroxine sodium binding to serum proteins or alter the concentrations of serum proteins). Products include:
Elspar 1700
Aspirin (May inhibit levothyroxine sodium binding to serum proteins or alter the concentrations of serum proteins). Products include:
Alka-Seltzer Cherry Effervescent Antacid and Pain Reliever ▣ 609
Alka-Seltzer Extra Strength Effervescent Antacid and Pain Reliever ▣ 609
Alka-Seltzer Lemon Lime Effervescent Antacid and Pain Reliever ▣ 609
Alka-Seltzer Original Effervescent Antacid and Pain Reliever ▣ 609
Alka-Seltzer Plus ▣ 611
Alka-Seltzer Plus Sinus Medicine ▣ 611
Ascriptin ▣ 650
Arthritis Strength BC Powder ▣ 631
BC Cold Powder Multi-Symptom Formula (Cold-Sinus-Allergy) ▣ 631
BC Cold Powder Non-Drowsy Formula (Cold-Sinus) ▣ 631
BC Powder ▣ 631
Genuine Bayer Aspirin Tablets & Caplets ▣ 618
Extra Strength Bayer Arthritis Pain Regimen Formula ▣ 615
Extra Strength Bayer Aspirin Caplets & Tablets ▣ 617
Extended-Release Bayer 8-Hour Aspirin ▣ 616
Extra Strength Bayer Plus Aspirin Caplets ▣ 617
Extra Strength Bayer PM Aspirin Plus Sleep Aid ▣ 617
Aspirin Regimen Bayer 81 mg Tablets with Calcium ▣ 615
Aspirin Regimen Bayer Adult Low Strength 81 mg Tablets ▣ 613
Aspirin Regimen Bayer Children's Chewable Aspirin ▣ 616
Aspirin Regimen Bayer Regular Strength 325 mg Caplets ▣ 613
Bufferin Analgesic Tablets ▣ 636
Arthritis Strength Bufferin Analgesic Caplets ▣ 637
Extra Strength Bufferin Analgesic Tablets ▣ 637
Cama Arthritis Pain Reliever ▣ 748
Darvon Compound-65 Pulvules 1475
Easprin 1971
Ecotrin 2625
Ecotrin Enteric Coated Aspirin Maximum Strength Tablets and Caplets ▣ 775
Ecotrin Enteric Coated Aspirin Regular Strength Tablets 2625
Empirin Aspirin Tablets ▣ 818
Excedrin Extra-Strength Analgesic Tablets, Caplets, and Geltabs 734
Fiorinal Capsules 2388
Fiorinal with Codeine Capsules 2390
Fiorinal Tablets 2388
Goody's Extra Strength Headache Powders ▣ 632
Goody's Extra Strength Pain Relief Tablets ▣ 632
Halfprin Tablets 1413
Norgesic 1554
Percodan Tablets 955
Percodan-Demi Tablets 956
Robaxisal Tablets 2246
Soma Compound w/Codeine Tablets 2784
Soma Compound Tablets 2783
St. Joseph Adult Chewable Aspirin (81 mg.) ▣ 768
Talwin Compound 2466
Vanquish Analgesic Caplets ▣ 627
Atenolol (Alters thyroid hormone or TSH levels; actions of some beta blockers may be impaired when hypothyroid patients become euthyroid). Products include:
Tenoretic Tablets 2963
Tenormin Tablets and I.V. Injection 2965
Bendroflumethiazide (Alters thyroid hormone or TSH levels).
No products indexed under this heading.
Betamethasone Acetate (May inhibit levothyroxine sodium binding to serum proteins or alter the concentrations of serum proteins). Products include:
Celestone Soluspan Suspension 2484
Betamethasone Sodium Phosphate (May inhibit levothyroxine sodium binding to serum proteins or alter the concentrations of serum proteins). Products include:
Celestone Soluspan Suspension 2484
Betaxolol Hydrochloride (Alters thyroid hormone or TSH levels; actions of some beta blockers may be impaired when hypothyroid patients become euthyroid). Products include:
Betoptic Ophthalmic Solution 465
Betoptic S Ophthalmic Suspension 467
Kerlone Tablets 2588
Bisoprolol Fumarate (Alters thyroid hormone or TSH levels; actions of some beta blockers may be impaired when hypothyroid patients become euthyroid). Products include:
Zebeta Tablets 1457
Ziac 1459
Bromocriptine Mesylate (Alters thyroid hormone or TSH levels). Products include:
Parlodel 2411
Carbamazepine (Alters thyroid hormone or TSH levels). Products include:
Atretol Tablets 569
Tegretol/Tegretol-XR 870
Carteolol Hydrochloride (Alters thyroid hormone or TSH levels; actions of some beta blockers may be impaired when hypothyroid patients become euthyroid). Products include:
Cartrol Tablets 413
Ocupress Ophthalmic Solution, 1% Sterile ⊙ 297

(▣ Described in PDR For Nonprescription Drugs) (⊙ Described in PDR For Ophthalmology)

Chloral Hydrate (Alters thyroid hormone or TSH levels).
No products indexed under this heading.

Chlorothiazide (Alters thyroid hormone or TSH levels). Products include:
Aldoclor Tablets 1638
Diupres Tablets 1691
Diuril Oral 1694

Chlorothiazide Sodium (Alters thyroid hormone or TSH levels). Products include:
Diuril Sodium Intravenous 1693

Chlorotrianisene (Estrogens or estrogen-containing compounds may inhibit levothyroxine sodium binding to serum proteins or alter the concentrations of serum proteins).
No products indexed under this heading.

Chlorpropamide (Alters thyroid hormone or TSH levels; requirements of oral antidiabetic agents may be reduced in hypothyroid patients with diabetes and may be subsequently increased with initiation of thyroid hormone therapy). Products include:
Diabinese Tablets 2002

Cholestyramine (Binds and decreases absorption of levothyroxine sodium from the gastrointestinal tract). Products include:
Questran 774

Choline Magnesium Trisalicylate (May inhibit levothyroxine sodium binding to serum proteins or alter the concentrations of serum proteins). Products include:
Trilisate 2155

Clofibrate (May inhibit levothyroxine sodium binding to serum proteins or alter the concentrations of serum proteins). Products include:
Atromid-S Capsules 2808

Clomipramine Hydrochloride (Concurrent use may increase the therapeutic and toxic effects of both drugs; onset of action of tricyclics may be accelerated). Products include:
Anafranil Capsules 819

Colestipol Hydrochloride (Binds and decreases absorption of levothyroxine sodium from the gastrointestinal tract). Products include:
Colestid 2073

Cortisone Acetate (May inhibit levothyroxine sodium binding to serum proteins or alter the concentrations of serum proteins). Products include:
Cortone Acetate Sterile Suspension 1663
Cortone Acetate Tablets 1664

Desipramine Hydrochloride (Concurrent use may increase the therapeutic and toxic effects of both drugs; onset of action of tricyclics may be accelerated). Products include:
Norpramin Tablets 1273

Deslanoside (Therapeutic effects of digitalis glycosides may be reduced; serum digitalis levels may be decreased in hyperthyroidism or when a hypothyroid patient becomes euthyroid).
No products indexed under this heading.

Dexamethasone (May inhibit levothyroxine sodium binding to serum proteins or alter the concentrations of serum proteins). Products include:
AK-Trol Ointment & Suspension .... ◉ 205
Decadron Elixir 1676
Decadron Tablets 1678
Decaspray Topical Aerosol 1689
Maxitrol Ophthalmic Ointment and Suspension .... ◉ 222
TobraDex Ophthalmic Suspension and Ointment 469

Dexamethasone Acetate (May inhibit levothyroxine sodium binding to serum proteins or alter the concentrations of serum proteins). Products include:
Dalalone D.P. Injectable 1009
Decadron-LA Sterile Suspension 1687

Dexamethasone Sodium Phosphate (May inhibit levothyroxine sodium binding to serum proteins or alter the concentrations of serum proteins). Products include:
Decadron Phosphate Injection 1680
Decadron Phosphate Sterile Ophthalmic Ointment 1684
Decadron Phosphate Sterile Ophthalmic Solution 1685
Decadron Phosphate Topical Cream 1686
Decadron Phosphate with Xylocaine Injection, Sterile 1683
Dexacort Phosphate in Respihaler .. 1606
Dexacort Phosphate in Turbinaire .. 1607
NeoDecadron Sterile Ophthalmic Ointment 1755
NeoDecadron Sterile Ophthalmic Solution 1756
NeoDecadron Topical Cream 1757

Diatrizoate Meglumine (Alters thyroid hormone or TSH levels).

Diatrizoate Sodium (Alters thyroid hormone or TSH levels).

Diazepam (Alters thyroid hormone or TSH levels). Products include:
Dizac (diazepam injectable emulsion) CIV 1862
Valium Injectable 2336
Valium Tablets 2335

Dicumarol (The hypoprothrombinemic effect of anticoagulants may be potentiated).
No products indexed under this heading.

Dienestrol (Estrogens or estrogen-containing compounds may inhibit levothyroxine sodium binding to serum proteins or alter the concentrations of serum proteins). Products include:
Ortho Dienestrol Cream 1922

Diethylstilbestrol (Estrogens or estrogen-containing compounds may inhibit levothyroxine sodium binding to serum proteins or alter the concentrations of serum proteins). Products include:
Diethylstilbestrol Tablets 1477

Diflunisal (May inhibit levothyroxine sodium binding to serum proteins or alter the concentrations of serum proteins). Products include:
Dolobid Tablets 1695

Digitoxin (Therapeutic effects of digitalis glycosides may be reduced; serum digitalis levels may be decreased in hyperthyroidism or when a hypothyroid patient becomes euthyroid). Products include:
Crystodigin Tablets 1472

Digoxin (Therapeutic effects of digitalis glycosides may be reduced; serum digitalis levels may be decreased in hyperthyroidism or when a hypothyroid patient becomes euthyroid). Products include:
Lanoxicaps 1110
Lanoxin Elixir Pediatric 1113
Lanoxin Injection 1116
Lanoxin Injection Pediatric 1119
Lanoxin Tablets 1121

Dobutamine Hydrochloride (Possible increased risk of coronary insufficiency in patients with coronary artery disease). Products include:
Dobutrex Solution Vials 1480

Dopamine Hydrochloride (Alters thyroid hormone or TSH levels).
No products indexed under this heading.

Doxepin Hydrochloride (Concurrent use may increase the therapeutic and toxic effects of both drugs; onset of action of tricyclics may be accelerated). Products include:
Adapin Capsules 1542
Sinequan 2028
Zonalon Cream 1042

Dyphylline (Theophylline clearance may be decreased in hypothyroid patients and return toward normal when euthyroid state is achieved). Products include:
Lufyllin & Lufyllin-400 Tablets 2778
Lufyllin-GG Elixir & Tablets 2779

Ephedrine Hydrochloride (Possible increased risk of coronary insufficiency in patients with coronary artery disease). Products include:
Primatene Tablets 844
Quadrinal Tablets 1398

Ephedrine Sulfate (Possible increased risk of coronary insufficiency in patients with coronary artery disease). Products include:
Marax Tablets & DF Syrup 2015

Ephedrine Tannate (Possible increased risk of coronary insufficiency in patients with coronary artery disease). Products include:
Rynatuss 2782

Epinephrine (Possible increased risk of coronary insufficiency in patients with coronary artery disease). Products include:
EPIFRIN .... ◉ 237
EpiPen 808
Marcaine with Epinephrine 2446
Primatene Mist 843
Sensorcaine with Epinephrine Injection 554
Sus-Phrine Injection 1017
Xylocaine with Epinephrine Injections 562

Epinephrine Bitartrate (Possible increased risk of coronary insufficiency in patients with coronary artery disease). Products include:
Sensorcaine-MPF with Epinephrine Injection 554

Epinephrine Hydrochloride (Possible increased risk of coronary insufficiency in patients with coronary artery disease). Products include:
Ana-Kit Anaphylaxis Emergency Treatment Kit 611

Esmolol Hydrochloride (Alters thyroid hormone or TSH levels; actions of some beta blockers may be impaired when hypothyroid patients become euthyroid). Products include:
Brevibloc (esmolol HCl) Injection 1860

Estradiol (Estrogens or estrogen-containing compounds may inhibit levothyroxine sodium binding to serum proteins or alter the concentrations of serum proteins). Products include:
Climara Transdermal System 640
Estrace Cream and Tablets 751
Estraderm Transdermal System 842
Estring Vaginal Ring 2086
Vivelle Transdermal System 880

Estrogens, Conjugated (Estrogens or estrogen-containing compounds may inhibit levothyroxine sodium binding to serum proteins or alter the concentrations of serum proteins). Products include:
PMB 200 and PMB 400 2890
Premarin Intravenous 2893
Premarin Tablets 2896
Premarin Vaginal Cream 2898
Premphase 2900
Prempro 2905

Estrogens, Esterified (Estrogens or estrogen-containing compounds may inhibit levothyroxine sodium binding to serum proteins or alter the concentrations of serum proteins). Products include:
ESTRATAB Tablets (0.3, 0.625, 1.25, 2.5 mg) 2715
Estratest 2718
Menest Tablets 2671

Estropipate (Estrogens or estrogen-containing compounds may inhibit levothyroxine sodium binding to serum proteins or alter the concentrations of serum proteins). Products include:
Ogen Tablets 2103
Ogen Vaginal Cream 2106
Ortho-Est 1925

Ethinyl Estradiol (Estrogens or estrogen-containing compounds may inhibit levothyroxine sodium binding to serum proteins or alter the concentrations of serum proteins). Products include:
Brevicon 2563
Demulen 2580
Desogen Tablets 1867
Levlen/Tri-Levlen 646
Lo/Ovral Tablets 2852
Lo/Ovral-28 Tablets 2857
Modicon 1928
Nordette-21 Tablets 2863
Nordette-28 Tablets 2866
Norinyl 2563
Ortho-Cept 1907
Ortho-Cyclen/Ortho-Tri-Cyclen 1914
Ortho-Novum 1928
Ortho-Cyclen/Ortho Tri-Cyclen 1914
Ovcon 765
Ovral Tablets 2877
Ovral-28 Tablets 2878
Levlen/Tri-Levlen 646
Tri-Norinyl 2607
Triphasil-21 Tablets 2919
Triphasil-28 Tablets 2924

Ethiodized Oil (Alters thyroid hormone or TSH levels).
No products indexed under this heading.

Ethionamide (Alters thyroid hormone or TSH levels). Products include:
Trecator-SC Tablets 2919

Ferrous Sulfate (Binds and decreases absorption of levothyroxine sodium from the gastrointestinal tract). Products include:
Feosol Capsules 777
Feosol Elixir 2627
Feosol Tablets 2627
Fero-Folic-500 Filmtab 433
Fero-Grad-500 Filmtab 434
Fero-Gradumet Filmtab 434
Iberet Tablets 437
Iberet-500 Liquid 438
Iberet-Folic-500 Filmtab 433
Iberet-Liquid 438
Irospan 1000
Slow Fe Tablets 889
Slow Fe with Folic Acid 890

Fludrocortisone Acetate (May inhibit levothyroxine sodium binding to serum proteins or alter the concentrations of serum proteins). Products include:
Florinef Acetate Tablets 506

IMPORTANT NOTE: Always consult each drug listing in the patient's regimen for possible interactions.

Synthroid Interactions Index 1030

Fluorouracil (May inhibit levothyroxine sodium binding to serum proteins or alter the concentrations of serum proteins). Products include:
Efudex ... 2280
Fluoroplex Topical Solution & Cream 1% ... 475
Fluorouracil Injection ... 2282

Fluoxymesterone (May inhibit levothyroxine sodium binding to serum proteins or alter the concentrations of serum proteins; alters TSH or thyroid hormone levels). Products include:
Halotestin Tablets ... 2095

Furosemide (May inhibit levothyroxine sodium binding to serum proteins or alter the concentrations of serum proteins). Products include:
Lasix Injection, Oral Solution and Tablets ... 1267

Gadopentetate Dimeglumine (Alters thyroid hormone or TSH levels).
No products indexed under this heading.

Glimepiride (Requirements of oral antidiabetic agents may be reduced in hypothyroid patients with diabetes and may be subsequently increased with initiation of thyroid hormone therapy). Products include:
Amaryl Tablets ... 1241

Glipizide (Alters thyroid hormone or TSH levels; requirements of oral antidiabetic agents may be reduced in hypothyroid patients with diabetes and may be subsequently increased with initiation of thyroid hormone therapy). Products include:
Glucotrol Tablets ... 2011
Glucotrol XL Extended Release Tablets ... 2012

Glyburide (Alters thyroid hormone or TSH levels; requirements of oral antidiabetic agents may be reduced in hypothyroid patients with diabetes and may be subsequently increased with initiation of thyroid hormone therapy). Products include:
DiaBeta Tablets ... 1265
Glynase PresTab Tablets ... 2091
Micronase Tablets ... 2099

Heparin Sodium (Alters thyroid hormone or TSH levels). Products include:
Heparin Lock Flush Solution ... 2831
Heparin Sodium Injection ... 2832
Heparin Sodium Vials ... 1486

Hydrochlorothiazide (Alters thyroid hormone or TSH levels). Products include:
Aldactazide Tablets ... 2556
Aldoril Tablets ... 1644
Apresazide Capsules ... 824
Capozide Tablets ... 744
Dyazide Capsules ... 2653
Esidrix Tablets ... 839
Esimil Tablets ... 840
HydroDIURIL Tablets ... 1716
Hydropres Tablets ... 1718
Hyzaar Tablets ... 1720
Inderide Tablets ... 2838
Inderide LA Long Acting Capsules .. 2840
Lopressor HCT Tablets ... 850
Lotensin HCT Tablets ... 855
Moduretic Tablets ... 1748
Oretic Tablets ... 450
Prinzide Tablets ... 1780
Ser-Ap-Es Tablets ... 867
Timolide Tablets ... 1791
Vaseretic Tablets ... 1810
Zestoretic Tablets ... 2968
Ziac ... 1459

Hydrocortisone (May inhibit levothyroxine sodium binding to serum proteins or alter the concentrations of serum proteins). Products include:
Anusol-HC Cream 2.5% ... 1953
Aquanil HC Lotion ... 1989
Maximum Strength Cortaid Spray ■ 800
CORTENEMA ... 2713
Cortisporin Ointment ... 1074
Cortisporin Ophthalmic Ointment Sterile ... 1074
Cortisporin Ophthalmic Suspension Sterile ... 1075
Cortisporin Otic Solution Sterile ... 1076
Cortisporin Otic Suspension Sterile 1077
Cortizone-5 ... ■ 795
Cortizone-10 ... ■ 795
Hydrocortone Tablets ... 1715
Hytone ... 922
Hytone Ointment 2 ½% ... 923
Massengill Medicated Soft Cloth Towelettes ... 2628
Pediotic Suspension Sterile ... 1140
Preparation H Hydrocortisone 1% Cream ... ■ 843
ProctoCream-HC 2.5% ... 2552
VōSoL HC Otic Solution ... 2786

Hydrocortisone Acetate (May inhibit levothyroxine sodium binding to serum proteins or alter the concentrations of serum proteins). Products include:
Analpram-HC Rectal Cream 1% and 2.5% ... 993
Anusol HC-1 Hydrocortisone Anti-Itch Ointment ... ■ 810
Anusol-HC Suppositories ... 1954
Caldecort Anti-Itch Hydrocortisone Cream ... ■ 651
Coly-Mycin S Otic w/Neomycin & Hydrocortisone ... 1965
Cortaid ... ■ 800
Cortifoam ... 2540
Cortisporin Cream ... 1073
Epifoam ... 2543
Hydrocortone Acetate Sterile Suspension ... 1712
Mantadil Cream ... 1124
Nupercainal Hydrocortisone 1% Cream ... ■ 661
Pramosone Cream, Lotion & Ointment ... 995
ProctoFoam-HC ... 2552
Terra-Cortril Ophthalmic Suspension ... 2033

Hydrocortisone Sodium Phosphate (May inhibit levothyroxine sodium binding to serum proteins or alter the concentrations of serum proteins). Products include:
Hydrocortone Phosphate Injection, Sterile ... 1713

Hydrocortisone Sodium Succinate (May inhibit levothyroxine sodium binding to serum proteins or alter the concentrations of serum proteins).
No products indexed under this heading.

Hydroflumethiazide (Alters thyroid hormone or TSH levels). Products include:
Diucardin Tablets ... 2824

Imipramine Hydrochloride (Concurrent use may increase the therapeutic and toxic effects of both drugs; onset of action of tricyclics may be accelerated). Products include:
Tofranil Ampuls ... 873
Tofranil Tablets ... 875

Imipramine Pamoate (Concurrent use may increase the therapeutic and toxic effects of both drugs; onset of action of tricyclics may be accelerated). Products include:
Tofranil-PM Capsules ... 876

Insulin, Human (Requirements of insulin may be reduced in hypothyroid patients with diabetes and may be subsequently increased with initiation of thyroid hormone therapy).
No products indexed under this heading.

Insulin, Human Isophane Suspension (Requirements of insulin may be reduced in hypothyroid patients with diabetes and may be subsequently increased with initiation of thyroid hormone therapy). Products include:
Novolin N Human Insulin 10 ml Vials ... 1846

Insulin, Human NPH (Requirements of insulin may be reduced in hypothyroid patients with diabetes and may be subsequently increased with initiation of thyroid hormone therapy). Products include:
Humulin N, 100 Units ... 1495
Novolin N PenFill 1.5 ml Cartridges Durable Insulin Delivery System ... 1849
Novolin N Prefilled Syringe Disposable Insulin Delivery System ... 1850

Insulin, Human Regular (Requirements of insulin may be reduced in hypothyroid patients with diabetes and may be subsequently increased with initiation of thyroid hormone therapy). Products include:
Humulin R, 100 Units ... 1497
Novolin R Human Insulin 10 ml Vials ... 1846
Novolin R PenFill 1.5 ml Cartridges Durable Insulin Delivery System ... 1849
Novolin R Prefilled Syringe Disposable Insulin Delivery System ... 1850
Velosulin BR Human Insulin 10 ml Vials ... 1847

Insulin, Human, Zinc Suspension (Requirements of insulin may be reduced in hypothyroid patients with diabetes and may be subsequently increased with initiation of thyroid hormone therapy). Products include:
Humulin L, 100 Units ... 1494
Humulin U, 100 Units ... 1498
Novolin L Human Insulin 10 ml Vials ... 1846

Insulin Lispro, Human (Requirements of insulin may be reduced in hypothyroid patients with diabetes and may be subsequently increased with initiation of thyroid hormone therapy). Products include:
Humalog Injection ... 1488

Insulin, NPH (Requirements of insulin may be reduced in hypothyroid patients with diabetes and may be subsequently increased with initiation of thyroid hormone therapy). Products include:
NPH, 100 Units ... 1502
Pork NPH, 100 Units ... 1506
Purified Pork NPH Isophane Insulin ... 1852

Insulin, Regular (Requirements of insulin may be reduced in hypothyroid patients with diabetes and may be subsequently increased with initiation of thyroid hormone therapy). Products include:
Regular, 100 Units ... 1503
Pork Regular, 100 Units ... 1507
Pork Regular (Concentrated), 500 Units ... 1508
Purified Pork Regular Insulin ... 1852

Insulin, Zinc Crystals (Requirements of insulin may be reduced in hypothyroid patients with diabetes and may be subsequently increased with initiation of thyroid hormone therapy). Products include:
NPH, 100 Units ... 1502

Insulin, Zinc Suspension (Requirements of insulin may be reduced in hypothyroid patients with diabetes and may be subsequently increase with initiation of thyroid hormone therapy). Products include:
Iletin I ... 1501
Lente, 100 Units ... 1501
Iletin II ... 1504
Pork Lente, 100 Units ... 1504
Purified Pork Lente Insulin ... 1852

Interferon alfa-2A, Recombinant (Cytokines have been reported to induce both hyperthyroidism or hypothyroidism; dosage adjustment may be necessary). Products include:
Roferon-A Injection ... 2308

Interferon alfa-2B, Recombinant (Cytokines have been reported to induce both hyperthyroidism or hypothyroidism; dosage adjustment may be necessary). Products include:
Intron A for Injection ... 2506

Interferon Alfa-N3 (Human Leukocyte Derived) (Cytokines have been reported to induce both hyperthyroidism or hypothyroidism; dosage adjustment may be necessary). Products include:
Alferon N Injection ... 2142

Interferon Beta-1b (Cytokines have been reported to induce both hyperthyroidism or hypothyroidism; dosage adjustment may be necessary). Products include:
Betaseron for SC Injection ... 653

Interferon Gamma-1B (Cytokines have been reported to induce both hyperthyroidism or hypothyroidism; dosage adjustment may be necessary). Products include:
Actimmune ... 1043

Iodamide Meglumine (Alters thyroid hormone or TSH levels).
No products indexed under this heading.

Iodinated Glycerol (Alters thyroid hormone or TSH levels).
No products indexed under this heading.

Iodine, radiolabeled (Uptake of radiolabeled ions may be decreased).

Iohexol (Alters thyroid hormone or TSH levels).
No products indexed under this heading.

Iopamidol (Alters thyroid hormone or TSH levels).
No products indexed under this heading.

Iothalamate Meglumine (Alters thyroid hormone or TSH levels).
No products indexed under this heading.

Iopanoic Acid (Alters thyroid hormone or TSH levels).

Ioxaglate Meglumine (Alters thyroid hormone or TSH levels).
No products indexed under this heading.

Ioxaglate Sodium (Alters thyroid hormone or TSH levels).
No products indexed under this heading.

Isoproterenol Hydrochloride (Possible increased risk of coronary insufficiency in patients with coronary artery disease). Products include:
Isuprel Hydrochloride Solution ... 2443
Isuprel Injection ... 2441
Isuprel Mistometer ... 2442

Isoproterenol Sulfate (Possible increased risk of coronary insufficiency in patients with coronary artery disease). Products include:
Norisodrine with Calcium Iodide Syrup ... 446

Ketamine Hydrochloride (Co-administration produces marked hypertension and tachycardia).
No products indexed under this heading.

(■ Described in PDR For Nonprescription Drugs) (◉ Described in PDR For Ophthalmology)

Labetalol Hydrochloride (Alters thyroid hormone or TSH levels; actions of some beta blockers may be impaired when hypothyroid patients become euthyroid). Products include:

Normodyne Injection	2519
Normodyne Tablets	2522
Trandate	1158

Levobunolol Hydrochloride (Alters thyroid hormone or TSH levels; actions of some beta blockers may be impaired when hypothyroid patients become euthyroid). Products include:

Betagan	ⓟ 230

Levodopa (Alters thyroid hormone or TSH levels). Products include:

Atamet Tablets	567
Larodopa Tablets	2296
Sinemet Tablets	959
Sinemet CR Tablets	961

Lithium Carbonate (Alters thyroid hormone or TSH levels). Products include:

Eskalith	2658
Lithium Carbonate Capsules & Tablets	2352
Lithonate/Lithotabs/Lithobid	2721

Lithium Citrate (Alters thyroid hormone or TSH levels).
No products indexed under this heading.

Lovastatin (Alters thyroid hormone or TSH levels). Products include:

Mevacor Tablets	1742

Magnesium Salicylate (May inhibit levothyroxine sodium binding to serum proteins or alter the concentrations of serum proteins). Products include:

Backache Caplets	ⓟ 635
Doan's Extra-Strength Analgesic	ⓟ 653
Extra Strength Doan's P.M.	ⓟ 653
Doan's Regular Strength Analgesic	ⓟ 654
Mobigesic Tablets	607

Maprotiline Hydrochloride (Concurrent use may increase the therapeutic and toxic effects of both drugs; onset of action of tricyclics may be acelerated; risk of cardiac arrhythmias may increase). Products include:

Ludiomil Tablets	861

Meclofenamate Sodium (Meclofenamic acid may inhibit levothyroxine sodium binding to serum proteins or alter the concentrations of serum proteins).
No products indexed under this heading.

Mefenamic Acid (May inhibit levothyroxine sodium binding to serum proteins or alter the concentrations of serum proteins). Products include:

Ponstel	1982

Mercaptopurine (Alters thyroid hormone or TSH levels). Products include:

Purinethol Tablets	1214

Metaproterenol Sulfate (Possible increased risk of coronary insufficiency in patients with coronary artery disease). Products include:

Alupent	672
Metaproterenol Sulfate Inhalation Solution, USP, Arm-a-Med	547

Metaraminol Bitartrate (Possible increased risk of coronary insufficiency in patients with coronary artery disease). Products include:

Aramine Injection	1649

Metformin Hydrochloride (Requirements of oral antidiabetic agents may be reduced in hypothyroid patients with diabetes and may be subsequently increased with initiation of thyroid hormone therapy). Products include:

Glucophage Tablets	754

Methadone Hydrochloride (May inhibit levothyroxine sodium binding to serum proteins or alter the concentrations of serum proteins). Products include:

Methadone Hydrochloride Oral Concentrate	2356
Methadone Hydrochloride Oral Solution & Tablets	2357

Methimazole (Alters thyroid hormone or TSH levels). Products include:

Tapazole Tablets	1361

Methoxamine Hydrochloride (Possible increased risk of coronary insufficiency in patients with coronary artery disease). Products include:

Vasoxyl Injection	1169

Methyclothiazide (Alters thyroid hormone or TSH levels). Products include:

Enduron Tablets	424

Methylprednisolone Acetate (May inhibit levothyroxine sodium binding to serum proteins or alter the concentrations of serum proteins).
No products indexed under this heading.

Methylprednisolone Sodium Succinate (May inhibit levothyroxine sodium binding to serum proteins or alter the concentrations of serum proteins).
No products indexed under this heading.

Methyltestosterone (May inhibit levothyroxine sodium binding to serum proteins or alter the concentrations of serum proteins; alters TSH or thyroid hormone levels). Products include:

Android Capsules, 10 mg	1297
Estratest	2718
Testred Capsules, 10 mg	1308

Metipranolol Hydrochloride (Alters thyroid hormone or TSH levels; actions of some beta blockers may be impaired when hypothyroid patients become euthyroid). Products include:

OptiPranolol (Metipranolol 0.3%) Sterile Ophthalmic Solution	ⓟ 256

Metoclopramide Hydrochloride (Alters thyroid hormone or TSH levels). Products include:

Reglan	2243

Metoprolol Succinate (Alters thyroid hormone or TSH levels; actions of some beta blockers may be impaired when hypothyroid patients become euthyroid). Products include:

Toprol-XL Tablets	560

Metoprolol Tartrate (Alters thyroid hormone or TSH levels; actions of some beta blockers may be impaired when hypothyroid patients become euthyroid). Products include:

Lopressor	848
Lopressor HCT Tablets	850

Mitotane (Alters thyroid hormone or TSH levels). Products include:

Lysodren Tablets	707

Nadolol (Alters thyroid hormone or TSH levels; actions of some beta blockers may be impaired when hypothyroid patients become euthyroid).
No products indexed under this heading.

Norepinephrine Bitartrate (Possible increased risk of coronary insufficiency in patients with coronary artery disease). Products include:

Levophed Bitartrate Injection	2445

Nortriptyline Hydrochloride (Concurrent use may increase the therapeutic and toxic effects of both drugs; onset of action of tricyclics may be accelerated). Products include:

Pamelor	2409

Octreotide Acetate (Alters thyroid hormone or TSH levels). Products include:

Sandostatin Injection	2421

Oxandrolone (May inhibit levothyroxine sodium binding to serum proteins or alter the concentrations of serum proteins; alters TSH or thyroid hormone levels). Products include:

Oxandrin	783

Oxymetholone (May inhibit levothyroxine sodium binding to serum proteins or alter the concentrations of serum proteins; alters TSH or thyroid hormone levels).
No products indexed under this heading.

Penbutolol Sulfate (Alters thyroid hormone or TSH levels; actions of some beta blockers may be impaired when hypothyroid patients become euthyroid). Products include:

Levatol Tablets	2547

Pergolide Mesylate (Alters thyroid hormone or TSH levels). Products include:

Permax Tablets	571

Perphenazine (May inhibit levothyroxine sodium binding to serum proteins or alter the concentrations of serum proteins). Products include:

Etrafon	2495
Triavil Tablets	1800
Trilafon	2532

Phenobarbital (Alters thyroid hormone or TSH levels). Products include:

Arco-Lase Plus Tablets	513
Bellergal-S Tablets	2375
Donnatal	2234
Donnatal Extentabs	2234
Donnatal Tablets	2234
Phenobarbital Elixir and Tablets	1523
Quadrinal Tablets	1398

Phenylbutazone (May inhibit levothyroxine sodium binding to serum proteins or alter the concentrations of serum proteins; alters thyroid hormone or TSH levels).
No products indexed under this heading.

Phenylephrine Bitartrate (Possible increased risk of coronary insufficiency in patients with coronary artery disease).
No products indexed under this heading.

Phenylephrine Hydrochloride (Possible increased risk of coronary insufficiency in patients with coronary artery disease). Products include:

Atrohist Plus Tablets	1605
Cerose DM	ⓟ 853
D.A. II Tablets	972
D.A. Chewable Tablets	970
Dura-Vent/DA Tablets	972
Extendryl	1003
4-Way Fast Acting Nasal Spray (regular & mentholated)	ⓟ 644
Hemorid	ⓟ 797
Hycomine Compound Tablets	948
Neo-Synephrine Hydrochloride 1% Carpuject	2455
Neo-Synephrine Hydrochloride 1% Injection	2455
Neo-Synephrine Hydrochloride (Ophthalmic)	2456
Neo-Synephrine	ⓟ 624
Novahistine Elixir	ⓟ 782
Phenergan VC	2886
Phenergan VC with Codeine	2888
Preparation H	ⓟ 842
Tympagesic Ear Drops	2476
Vicks Sinex Nasal Spray and Ultra Fine Mist	ⓟ 738

Phenylephrine Tannate (Possible increased risk of coronary insufficiency in patients with coronary artery disease). Products include:

Atrohist Pediatric Suspension	1604
Atrohist Pediatric Suspension Dye-Free	1604
Rynatan	2781
Rynatuss	2782

Phenylpropanolamine Hydrochloride (Possible increased risk of coronary insufficiency in patients with coronary artery disease). Products include:

Acutrim	ⓟ 648
Atrohist Plus Tablets	1605
BC Cold Powder Multi-Symptom Formula (Cold-Sinus-Allergy)	ⓟ 631
BC Cold Powder Non-Drowsy Formula (Cold-Sinus)	ⓟ 631
Cheracol Plus Head Cold/Cough Formula	ⓟ 741
Comtrex Multi-Symptom Cold Reliever Liqui-Gels	ⓟ 638
Comtrex Multi-Symptom Non-Drowsy Liqui-gels	ⓟ 640
Contac Continuous Action Nasal Decongestant/Antihistamine 12 Hour Capsules	ⓟ 773
Contac Maximum Strength Continuous Action Decongestant/Antihistamine 12 Hour Caplets	ⓟ 772
Contac Severe Cold and Flu Formula Caplets	ⓟ 773
Coricidin 'D' Decongestant Tablets	ⓟ 760
Dexatrim	ⓟ 795
Dexatrim Plus Vitamins Caplets	ⓟ 796
Dimetane-DC Cough Syrup	2232
Dimetapp Allergy Sinus Caplets	ⓟ 838
Dimetapp Cold & Allergy Chewable Tablets	ⓟ 838
Dimetapp Cold & Cough Liqui-Gels	ⓟ 839
Dimetapp DM Elixir	ⓟ 840
Dimetapp Elixir	ⓟ 840
Dimetapp Extentabs	ⓟ 841
Dimetapp Tablets/Liqui-Gels	ⓟ 841
Dura-Vent Tablets	971
Entex LA Tablets	972
Exgest LA Tablets	787
Hycomine	947
Nolamine Timed-Release Tablets	790
Ornade Spansule Capsules	2678
Propagest Tablets	791
Pyrroxate Caplets	ⓟ 742
Robitussin-CF	ⓟ 846
Sinulin Tablets	792
Tavist-D 12 Hour Relief Tablets	ⓟ 750
Teldrin 12 Hour Antihistamine/Nasal Decongestant Allergy Relief Capsules	ⓟ 786
Triaminic Expectorant	ⓟ 753
Triaminic Syrup	ⓟ 755
Triaminic Triaminicol Cold & Cough	ⓟ 756
Triaminic DM Syrup	ⓟ 756
Triaminicin Tablets	ⓟ 756
Vicks DayQuil Allergy Relief 12-Hour Extended Release Tablets	ⓟ 733
Vicks DayQuil Allergy Relief 4-Hour Tablets	ⓟ 733
Vicks DayQuil SINUS Pressure & CONGESTION Relief	ⓟ 734

IMPORTANT NOTE: Always consult each drug listing in the patient's regimen for possible interactions.

Synthroid — **Interactions Index** — **1032**

Phenytoin (May inhibit levothyroxine sodium binding to serum proteins or alter the concentrations of serum proteins; alters thyroid hormone or TSH levels). Products include:
Dilantin Infatabs 1967
Dilantin-125 Suspension 1969

Phenytoin Sodium (May inhibit levothyroxine sodium binding to serum proteins or alter the concentrations of serum proteins; alters thyroid hormone or TSH levels). Products include:
Dilantin Kapseals 1965

Pindolol (Alters thyroid hormone or TSH levels; actions of some beta blockers may be impaired when hypothyroid patients become euthyroid). Products include:
Visken Tablets 2428

Pirbuterol Acetate (Possible increased risk of coronary insufficiency in patients with coronary artery disease). Products include:
Maxair Autohaler 1550
Maxair Inhaler 1552

Polyestradiol Phosphate (Estrogens or estrogen-containing compounds may inhibit levothyroxine sodium binding to serum proteins or alter the concentrations of serum proteins).
No products indexed under this heading.

Polythiazide (Alters thyroid hormone or TSH levels). Products include:
Minizide Capsules 2016

Prednisolone Acetate (May inhibit levothyroxine sodium binding to serum proteins or alter the concentrations of serum proteins). Products include:
AK-CIDE .... ⊚ 203
AK-CIDE Ointment .... ⊚ 203
Blephamide Liquifilm Sterile Ophthalmic Suspension 472
Blephamide Ointment .... ⊚ 234
Econopred & Econopred Plus Ophthalmic Suspensions .... ⊚ 216
Poly-Pred Liquifilm .... ⊚ 246
Pred Forte .... ⊚ 247
Pred Mild .... ⊚ 250
Pred-G Liquifilm Sterile Ophthalmic Suspension .... ⊚ 248
Pred-G S.O.P. Sterile Ophthalmic Ointment .... ⊚ 249

Prednisolone Sodium Phosphate (May inhibit levothyroxine sodium binding to serum proteins or alter the concentrations of serum proteins). Products include:
AK-PRED .... ⊚ 204
Hydeltrasol Injection, Sterile 1708
Pediapred Oral Solution 1618

Prednisolone Tebutate (May inhibit levothyroxine sodium binding to serum proteins or alter the concentrations of serum proteins). Products include:
Hydeltra-T.B.A. Sterile Suspension 1710

Prednisone (May inhibit levothyroxine sodium binding to serum proteins or alter the concentrations of serum proteins).
No products indexed under this heading.

Propranolol Hydrochloride (Alters thyroid hormone or TSH levels; actions of some beta blockers may be impaired when hypothyroid patients become euthyroid). Products include:
Inderal 2834
Inderal LA Long Acting Capsules 2836
Inderide Tablets 2838
Inderide LA Long Acting Capsules .. 2840

Protriptyline Hydrochloride (Concurrent use may increase the therapeutic and toxic effects of both drugs; onset of action of tricyclics may be accelerated). Products include:
Vivactil Tablets 1820

Pseudoephedrine Hydrochloride (Possible increased risk of coronary insufficiency in patients with coronary artery disease). Products include:
Actifed Allergy Daytime/Nighttime Caplets .... ■ 808
Actifed Cold & Allergy Tablets .... ■ 807
Actifed Cold & Sinus Caplets and Tablets .... ■ 808
Actifed Sinus Daytime/Nighttime Tablets and Caplets .... ■ 809
Advil Cold and Sinus Caplets and Tablets .... ■ 837
Alka-Seltzer Plus Liqui-Gels .... ■ 612
Alka-Seltzer Plus Flu & Body Aches Liqui-Gels Non-Drowsy Formula .... ■ 613
Alka-Seltzer Plus Night-Time Cold Medicine Liqui-Gels .... ■ 612
Allerest Maximum Strength .... ■ 649
Allerest No Drowsiness .... ■ 649
Allerest Sinus Pain Formula .... ■ 649
Atrohist Pediatric Capsules 1603
Benadryl Allergy/Cold Tablets .... ■ 811
Benadryl Allergy Decongestant Liquid Medication .... ■ 812
Benadryl Allergy Decongestant Tablets .... ■ 812
Benadryl Allergy Sinus Headache Caplets .... ■ 813
Benylin Multisymptom .... ■ 816
Bromfed Capsules (Extended-Release) 1832
Bromfed Syrup .... ■ 712
Bromfed Tablets 1832
Bromfed-DM Cough Syrup 1832
Bromfed-PD Capsules (Extended-Release) 1832
Children's TYLENOL Cold Multi-Symptom Chewable Tablets and Liquid 1559
Children's TYLENOL Cold Plus Cough Multi Symptom Chewable Tablets and Liquid 1560
Children's TYLENOL Flu Suspension Liquid 1560
Children's Vicks DayQuil Allergy Relief .... ■ 730
Children's Vicks NyQuil Cold/Cough Relief .... ■ 731
Allergy-Sinus Comtrex Multi-Symptom Allergy-Sinus Formula Tablets and Caplets .... ■ 639
Comtrex Multi-Symptom .... ■ 638
Comtrex Multi-Symptom Non-Drowsy Caplets .... ■ 640
Congess 1003
Contac Day Allergy/Sinus Caplets ■ 771
Contac Day & Night .... ■ 772
Contac Night Allergy/Sinus Caplets .... ■ 771
Contac Severe Cold & Flu Non-Drowsy .... ■ 774
Deconsal II Tablets 1605
Dimetane-DX Cough Syrup 2233
Dimetapp Cold & Fever Suspension .... ■ 839
Dimetapp Decongestant Pediatric Drops .... ■ 840
Dorcol Children's Cough Syrup .... ■ 748
Drixoral Cough + Congestion Liquid Caps .... ■ 763
Dura-Tap/PD Capsules 970
Duratuss Tablets 2750
Duratuss HD Elixir 2750
Efidac/24 .... ■ 655
Entex PSE Tablets 973
Fedahist Gyrocaps 2545
Guaifed 1833
Guaifed Syrup .... ■ 712
Guaimax-D Tablets 809
Histussin D Liquid 670
Infants' TYLENOL Cold Decongestant & Fever-Reducer Drops 1561
Kronofed-A 994
Novahistine DMX .... ■ 782
Nucofed 2225
PediaCare Cough-Cold Chewable Tablets and Liquid 1569
PediaCare Infants' Decongestant Drops 1569
PediaCare Infants' Drops Decongestant Plus Cough 1569
PediaCare NightRest Cough-Cold Liquid 1569
Pediatric Vicks 44d Cough & Head Congestion Relief .... ■ 736
Pediatric Vicks 44m Cough & Cold Relief .... ■ 737
Robitussin Cold & Cough Liqui-Gels .... ■ 844
Robitussin Cold, Cough & Flu Liqui-Gels .... ■ 844
Robitussin Maximum Strength Cough & Cold .... ■ 847
Robitussin Night-Time Cold Formula .... ■ 847
Robitussin Pediatric Cough & Cold Formula .... ■ 848
Robitussin Pediatric Drops .... ■ 849
Robitussin Severe Congestion Liqui-Gels .... ■ 845
Robitussin-DAC Syrup 2249
Robitussin-PE .... ■ 846
Rondec Oral Drops 974
Rondec Syrup 974
Rondec Tablet 974
Rondec Chewable Tablets 974
Rondec-TR Tablet 974
Ryna .... ■ 804
Seldane-D Extended-Release Tablets 1286
Semprex-D Capsules 1620
Sinarest .... ■ 663
Sine-Aid Maximum Strength Sinus Headache Gelcaps, Caplets and Tablets 1570
Sine-Off No Drowsiness Formula Caplets .... ■ 784
Sine-Off Sinus Medicine .... ■ 784
Singlet Tablets .... ■ 785
Sinutab Non-Drying Liquid Caps .... ■ 823
Sinutab Sinus Allergy Medication, Maximum Strength Tablets and Caplets .... ■ 823
Sinutab Sinus Medication, Maximum Strength Without Drowsiness Formula, Tablets & Caplets .... ■ 824
Sudafed Children's Cold & Cough Liquid Medication .... ■ 825
Sudafed Children's Nasal Decongestant Liquid Medication .... ■ 826
Sudafed Cold & Allergy Tablets .... ■ 826
Sudafed Cold and Cough Liquid Caps .... ■ 826
Sudafed Nasal Decongestant Tablets, 30 mg .... ■ 825
Sudafed Nasal Decongestant Tablets, 60 mg .... ■ 825
Sudafed Non-Drying Sinus Liquid Caps .... ■ 827
Sudafed Pediatric Nasal Decongestant Liquid Oral Drops .... ■ 827
Sudafed Severe Cold Formula Caplets .... ■ 828
Sudafed Severe Cold Formula Tablets .... ■ 828
Sudafed Sinus Caplets .... ■ 829
Sudafed Sinus Tablets .... ■ 829
Sudafed 12 Hour Caplets .... ■ 824
Syn-Rx Tablets 1622
Syn-Rx DM Tablets 1623
TheraFlu Flu and Cold Medicine .... ■ 750
Theraflu Maximum Strength Flu and Cold Medicine For Sore Throat .... ■ 751
TheraFlu Flu, Cold and Cough Medicine .... ■ 750
TheraFlu Maximum Strength Nighttime Flu, Cold & Cough Medicine .... ■ 751
TheraFlu Maximum Strength Non-Drowsy Formula Flu, Cold & Cough Medicine .... ■ 751
TheraFlu Maximum Strength, Non-Drowsy Formula Flu, Cold and Cough Caplets .... ■ 752
Theraflu Maximum Strength Sinus Non-Drowsy Formula Caplets .... ■ 752
Triaminic AM Cough and Decongestant Formula .... ■ 753
Triaminic AM Decongestant Formula .... ■ 753
Triaminic Infant Oral Decongestant Drops .... ■ 754
Triaminic Night Time .... ■ 754
Triaminic Sore Throat Formula .... ■ 755
Tussend 1830
Tussend Expectorant 1831
TYLENOL Allergy Sinus, Maximum Strength Caplets and Gelcaps 1571
TYLENOL Allergy Sinus NightTime, Maximum Strength Caplets 1571
TYLENOL Cold Medication, Multi-Symptom Formula Tablets and Caplets 1572
TYLENOL Cold Medication, Multi-Symptom Hot Liquid Packets 1572
TYLENOL Cold Medication, No Drowsiness Formula Caplets and Gelcaps 1572
TYLENOL Cold Severe Congestion Caplets 1573
TYLENOL Cough Medication with Decongestant, Multi Symptom 1574
TYLENOL Flu No Drowsiness Formula, Maximum Strength Gelcaps 1575
TYLENOL Flu NightTime, Maximum Strength Gelcaps 1575
TYLENOL Flu NightTime, Maximum Strength Hot Medication Packets 1575
TYLENOL Sinus, Maximum Strength Geltabs, Gelcaps, Caplets and Tablets 1576
Vicks 44 LiquiCaps Cough, Cold & Flu Relief .... ■ 728
Vicks 44 LiquiCaps Non-Drowsy Cough & Cold Relief .... ■ 729
Vicks 44D Cough & Head Congestion Relief .... ■ 728
Vicks 44M Cough, Cold & Flu Relief .... ■ 729
Vicks DayQuil LiquiCaps/Liquid Multi-Symptom Cold/Flu Relief .. ■ 734
Vicks DayQuil SINUS Pressure & PAIN Relief with IBUPROFEN .... ■ 735
Vicks Nyquil Hot Therapy .... ■ 735
Vicks NyQuil LiquiCaps/Liquid Multi-Symptom Cold/Flu Relief, Original and Cherry Flavors .... ■ 736

Pseudoephedrine Sulfate (Possible increased risk of coronary insufficiency in patients with coronary artery disease). Products include:
Chlor-Trimeton Allergy Decongestant Tablets .... ■ 759
Claritin-D Tablets 2487
Drixoral Cold and Allergy Sustained-Action Tablets .... ■ 763
Drixoral Cold and Flu Extended-Release Tablets .... ■ 764
Drixoral Non-Drowsy Formula Extended-Release Tablets .... ■ 764
Drixoral Allergy/Sinus Extended Release Tablets .... ■ 765
Trinalin Repetabs Tablets 1373

Quinestrol (Estrogens or estrogen-containing compounds may inhibit levothyroxine sodium binding to serum proteins or alter the concentrations of serum proteins).
No products indexed under this heading.

Resorcinol (Alters thyroid hormone or TSH levels). Products include:
BiCozene Creme .... ■ 747

Rifampin (Alters thyroid hormone or TSH levels). Products include:
Rifadin 1276
Rifamate Capsules 1278
Rifater 1280
Rimactane Capsules 865

Salmeterol Xinafoate (Possible increased risk of coronary insufficiency in patients with coronary artery disease). Products include:
Serevent Inhalation Aerosol 1149

Salsalate (May inhibit levothyroxine sodium binding to serum proteins or alter the concentrations of serum proteins). Products include:
Disalcid 1549
Mono-Gesic Tablets 810
Salflex Tablets 791

Sodium Iodide I 123 (Uptake of radiolabeled ions may be decreased).
No products indexed under this heading.

Sodium Iodide I 131 (Uptake of radiolabeled ions may be decreased).
No products indexed under this heading.

(■ Described in PDR For Nonprescription Drugs) (⊚ Described in PDR For Ophthalmology)

Sodium Nitroprusside (Alters thyroid hormone or TSH levels).
No products indexed under this heading.

Sodium Pertechnetate (Alters thyroid hormone or TSH levels).

Sodium Polystyrene Sulfonate (Binds and decreases absorption of levothyroxine sodium from the gastrointestinal tract). Products include:
Kayexalate 2444
Sodium Polystyrene Sulfonate Suspension 2367

Somatrem (Excessive concurrent use of thyroid hormone may accelerate epiphyseal closure; untreated hypothyroidism may interfere with the growth response to somatrem). Products include:
Protropin 1053

Somatropin (Excessive concurrent use of thyroid hormone may accelerate epiphyseal closure; untreated hypothyroidism may interfere with the growth response to somatrem). Products include:
Genotropin Injection 2090
Humatrope Vials 1490
Nutropin 1049
Nutropin AQ Injection 1051

Sotalol Hydrochloride (Alters thyroid hormone or TSH levels; actions of some beta blockers may be impaired when hypothyroid patients become euthyroid). Products include:
Betapace Tablets 637

Stanozolol (May inhibit levothyroxine sodium binding to serum proteins or alter the concentrations of serum proteins; alters TSH or thyroid hormone levels). Products include:
Winstrol Tablets 2468

Sucralfate (Binds and decreases absorption of levothyroxine sodium from the gastrointestinal tract). Products include:
Carafate Suspension 1250
Carafate Tablets 1249

Sulfacytine (Alters thyroid hormone or TSH levels).

Sulfamethizole (Alters thyroid hormone or TSH levels). Products include:
Urobiotic-250 Capsules 2038

Sulfamethoxazole (Alters thyroid hormone or TSH levels). Products include:
Bactrim DS Tablets 2257
Bactrim I.V. Infusion 2255
Bactrim 2257
Gantanol Tablets 2285
Septra 1146
Septra I.V. Infusion 1142
Septra I.V. Infusion ADD-Vantage Vials 1144
Septra 1146

Sulfasalazine (Alters thyroid hormone or TSH levels). Products include:
Azulfidine 2059

Sulfinpyrazone (Alters thyroid hormone or TSH levels). Products include:
Anturane 823

Sulfisoxazole (Alters thyroid hormone or TSH levels). Products include:
Gantrisin Tablets 2286

Sulfisoxazole Diolamine (Alters thyroid hormone or TSH levels).
No products indexed under this heading.

Tamoxifen Citrate (May inhibit levothyroxine sodium binding to serum proteins or alter the concentrations of serum proteins). Products include:
Nolvadex Tablets 2957

Terbutaline Sulfate (Possible increased risk of coronary insufficiency in patients with coronary artery disease). Products include:
Brethaire Inhaler 830
Brethine Ampuls 832
Brethine Tablets 831
Bricanyl Subcutaneous Injection 1247
Bricanyl Tablets 1248

Theophylline (Theophylline clearance may be decreased in hypothyroid patients and return toward normal when euthyroid state is achieved). Products include:
Marax Tablets & DF Syrup 2015
Quibron 2227

Theophylline Anhydrous (Theophylline clearance may be decreased in hypothyroid patients and return toward normal when euthyroid state is achieved). Products include:
Aerolate 1003
Primatene Tablets 844
Respbid Tablets 687
Slo-bid Gyrocaps 2201
Theo-24 Extended Release Capsules 2753
Theo-Dur Extended-Release Tablets 1367
Theo-X Extended-Release Tablets 793
Uni-Dur Extended-Release Tablets 1374
Uniphyl 400 mg and 600 mg Tablets 2157

Theophylline Calcium Salicylate (Theophylline clearance may be decreased in hypothyroid patients and return toward normal when euthyroid state is achieved). Products include:
Quadrinal Tablets 1398

Theophylline Sodium Glycinate (Theophylline clearance may be decreased in hypothyroid patients and return toward normal when euthyroid state is achieved).
No products indexed under this heading.

Timolol Hemihydrate (Alters thyroid hormone or TSH levels; actions of some beta blockers may be impaired when hypothyroid patients become euthyroid). Products include:
Betimol 0.25%, 0.5% .... ⊙ 259

Timolol Maleate (Alters thyroid hormone or TSH levels; actions of some beta blockers may be impaired when hypothyroid patients become euthyroid). Products include:
Blocadren Tablets 1654
Timolide Tablets 1791
Timoptic in Ocudose 1796
Timoptic Sterile Ophthalmic Solution 1794
Timoptic-XE 1798

Tolazamide (Alters thyroid hormone or TSH levels; requirements of oral antidiabetic agents may be reduced in hypothyroid patients with diabetes and may be subsequently increased with initiation of thyroid hormone therapy).
No products indexed under this heading.

Tolbutamide (Alters thyroid hormone or TSH levels; requirements of oral antidiabetic agents may be reduced in hypothyroid patients with diabetes and may be subsequently increased with initiation of thyroid hormone therapy).
No products indexed under this heading.

Triamcinolone (May inhibit levothyroxine sodium binding to serum proteins or alter the concentrations of serum proteins).
No products indexed under this heading.

Triamcinolone Acetonide (May inhibit levothyroxine sodium binding to serum proteins or alter the concentrations of serum proteins). Products include:
Azmacort Oral Inhaler 2175
Nasacort AQ Nasal Spray 2191
Nasacort Nasal Inhaler 2189

Triamcinolone Diacetate (May inhibit levothyroxine sodium binding to serum proteins or alter the concentrations of serum proteins).
No products indexed under this heading.

Triamcinolone Hexacetonide (May inhibit levothyroxine sodium binding to serum proteins or alter the concentrations of serum proteins).
No products indexed under this heading.

Trimipramine Maleate (Concurrent use may increase the therapeutic and toxic effects of both drugs; onset of action of tricyclics may be accelerated). Products include:
Surmontil Capsules 2917

Tyropanoate Sodium (Alters thyroid hormone or TSH levels).
No products indexed under this heading.

Warfarin Sodium (The hypoprothrombinemic effect of anticoagulants may be potentiated). Products include:
Coumadin 941

Food Interactions

Soybean formula, children's (Binds and decreases absorption of levothyroxine sodium from the gastrointestinal tract).

SYNTOCINON INJECTION
(Oxytocin) 2425
May interact with vasopressors and certain other agents. Compounds in these categories include:

Cyclopropane (Modifies cardiovascular effects resulting in hypotension).

Dopamine Hydrochloride (Potential for severe hypertension following prophylactic administration of a vasoconstrictor in conjunction with caudal block anesthesia).
No products indexed under this heading.

Epinephrine Hydrochloride (Potential for severe hypertension following prophylactic administration of a vasoconstrictor in conjunction with caudal block anesthesia). Products include:
Ana-Kit Anaphylaxis Emergency Treatment Kit 611

Metaraminol Bitartrate (Potential for severe hypertension following prophylactic administration of a vasoconstrictor in conjunction with caudal block anesthesia). Products include:
Aramine Injection 1649

Methoxamine Hydrochloride (Potential for severe hypertension following prophylactic administration of a vasoconstrictor in conjunction with caudal block anesthesia). Products include:
Vasoxyl Injection 1169

Norepinephrine Bitartrate (Potential for severe hypertension following prophylactic administration of a vasoconstrictor in conjunction with caudal block anesthesia). Products include:
Levophed Bitartrate Injection 2445

Phenylephrine Hydrochloride (Potential for severe hypertension following prophylactic administration of a vasoconstrictor in conjunction with caudal block anesthesia). Products include:
Atrohist Plus Tablets 1605
Cerose DM 853
D.A. II Tablets 972
D.A. Chewable Tablets 970
Dura-Vent/DA Tablets 972
Extendryl 1003
4-Way Fast Acting Nasal Spray (regular & mentholated) 644
Hemorid 797
Hycomine Compound Tablets 948
Neo-Synephrine Hydrochloride 1% Carpuject 2455
Neo-Synephrine Hydrochloride 1% Injection 2455
Neo-Synephrine Hydrochloride (Ophthalmic) 2456
Neo-Synephrine 624
Novahistine Elixir 782
Phenergan VC 2886
Phenergan VC with Codeine 2888
Preparation H 842
Tympagesic Ear Drops 2476
Vicks Sinex Nasal Spray and Ultra Fine Mist 738

SYPRINE CAPSULES
(Trientine Hydrochloride) 1790
None cited in PDR database.

T-STAT 2.0% TOPICAL SOLUTION AND PADS
(Erythromycin) 2797
May interact with:

Concomitant Topical Acne Therapy (Possible cumulative irritant effect).

TAGAMET HB TABLETS
(Cimetidine) 786
May interact with dihydropyridine calcium channel blockers, xanthine bronchodilators, and certain other agents. Compounds in these categories include:

Aminophylline (Increased AUC of theophylline by 14% and peak levels by 15% when used concurrently at the maximum recommended OTC dose level; clinically significant pharmacokinetic interactions have been reported at prescription doses).
No products indexed under this heading.

Amlodipine Besylate (Clinically significant pharmacokinetic interactions have been reported with concurrent use at prescription doses of cimetidine; patients are advised to consult their physician). Products include:
Lotrel Capsules 858
Norvasc Tablets 2020

Dyphylline (Increased AUC of theophylline by 14% and peak levels by 15% when used concurrently at the maximum recommended OTC dose level; clinically significant pharmacokinetic interactions have been reported at prescription doses). Products include:
Lufyllin & Lufyllin-400 Tablets 2778
Lufyllin-GG Elixir & Tablets 2779

IMPORTANT NOTE: Always consult each drug listing in the patient's regimen for possible interactions.

Felodipine (Clinically significant pharmacokinetic interactions have been reported with concurrent use at prescription doses of cimetidine; patients are advised to consult their physician). Products include:

- Plendil Extended-Release Tablets 514

Isradipine (Clinically significant pharmacokinetic interactions have been reported with concurrent use at prescription doses of cimetidine; patients are advised to consult their physician). Products include:

- DynaCirc Capsules 2381
- DynaCirc CR Tablets 2383

Nicardipine Hydrochloride (Clinically significant pharmacokinetic interactions have been reported with concurrent use at prescription doses of cimetidine; patients are advised to consult their physician). Products include:

- Cardene Capsules 2261
- Cardene I.V. 2815
- Cardene SR Capsules 2264

Nifedipine (Clinically significant pharmacokinetic interactions have been reported with concurrent use at prescription doses of cimetidine; patients are advised to consult their physician). Products include:

- Adalat Capsules (10 mg and 20 mg) 580
- Adalat CC 582
- Procardia Capsules 2024
- Procardia XL Extended Release Tablets 2026

Nimodipine (Clinically significant pharmacokinetic interactions have been reported with concurrent use at prescription doses of cimetidine; patients are advised to consult their physician). Products include:

- Nimotop Capsules 603

Phenytoin (Clinically significant pharmacokinetic interactions have been reported with concurrent use at prescription doses of cimetidine; patients are advised to consult their physician). Products include:

- Dilantin Infatabs 1967
- Dilantin-125 Suspension 1969

Phenytoin Sodium (Clinically significant pharmacokinetic interactions have been reported with concurrent use at prescription doses of cimetidine; patients are advised to consult their physician). Products include:

- Dilantin Kapseals 1965

Theophylline (Increased AUC of theophylline by 14% and peak levels by 15% when used concurrently at the maximum recommended OTC dose level; clinically significant pharmacokinetic interactions have been reported at prescription doses). Products include:

- Marax Tablets & DF Syrup 2015
- Quibron 2227

Theophylline Anhydrous (Increased AUC of theophylline by 14% and peak levels by 15% when used concurrently at the maximum recommended OTC dose level; clinically significant pharmacokinetic interactions have been reported at prescription doses). Products include:

- Aerolate 1003
- Primatene Tablets .... ◘ 844
- Respbid Tablets 687
- Slo-bid Gyrocaps 2201
- Theo-24 Extended Release Capsules 2753
- Theo-Dur Extended-Release Tablets 1367
- Theo-X Extended-Release Tablets .. 793
- Uni-Dur Extended-Release Tablets .. 1374
- Uniphyl 400 mg and 600 mg Tablets 2157

Theophylline Calcium Salicylate (Increased AUC of theophylline by 14% and peak levels by 15% when used concurrently at the maximum recommended OTC dose level; clinically significant pharmacokinetic interactions have been reported at prescription doses). Products include:

- Quadrinal Tablets 1398

Theophylline Sodium Glycinate (Increased AUC of theophylline by 14% and peak levels by 15% when used concurrently at the maximum recommended OTC dose level; clinically significant pharmacokinetic interactions have been reported at prescription doses).

No products indexed under this heading.

Triazolam (Potential for increased AUC of triazolam by 26-28% and increased peak levels by 11-23%). Products include:

- Halcion Tablets 2093

Warfarin Sodium (Clinically significant pharmacokinetic interactions have been reported with concurrent use at prescription doses of cimetidine; patients are advised to consult their physician). Products include:

- Coumadin 941

TAGAMET INJECTION

(Cimetidine Hydrochloride) 2694

See **Tagamet Tablets**

TAGAMET LIQUID

(Cimetidine Hydrochloride) 2694

See **Tagamet Tablets**

TAGAMET TABLETS

(Cimetidine) 2694

May interact with oral anticoagulants, antacids, tricyclic antidepressants, xanthine bronchodilators, and certain other agents. Compounds in these categories include:

Aluminum Carbonate (Simultaneous administration is not recommended since antacids may interfere with the absorption of cimetidine). Products include:

- Basaljel Capsules 2810
- Basaljel Suspension 2810
- Basaljel Tablets 2810

Aluminum Hydroxide (Simultaneous administration is not recommended since antacids may interfere with the absorption of cimetidine). Products include:

- ALternaGEL Liquid 1358
- Maximum Strength Ascriptin .... ◘ 650
- Cama Arthritis Pain Reliever .... ◘ 748
- Gaviscon Extra Strength Relief Formula Antacid Tablets .... ◘ 778
- Gaviscon Extra Strength Relief Formula Liquid Antacid .... ◘ 779
- Gaviscon Liquid Antacid .... ◘ 779
- Gelusil Antacid-Anti-gas Liquid .... ◘ 819
- Gelusil Antacid-Anti-gas Tablets .... ◘ 819
- Maalox Antacid/Anti-Gas Tablets 889
- Maalox Heartburn Relief Suspension .... ◘ 658
- Maalox Antacid Liquid 888
- Extra Strength Maalox Antacid/Anti-Gas Liquid and Tablets 888
- Mylanta 1359
- Tempo Soft Antacid .... ◘ 799

Aluminum Hydroxide Gel (Simultaneous administration is not recommended since antacids may interfere with the absorption of cimetidine). Products include:

- ALternaGEL Liquid .... ◘ 675
- Aludrox Oral Suspension .... ◘ 850
- Amphojel Suspension 2802
- Amphojel Suspension without Flavor 2802
- Amphojel Tablets 2802
- Ascriptin .... ◘ 650
- Gaviscon Antacid Tablets .... ◘ 778
- Gaviscon-2 Antacid Tablets .... ◘ 779
- Mylanta Liquid .... ◘ 676
- Mylanta Double Strength Liquid .... ◘ 676
- Nephrox Suspension .... ◘ 671

Aminophylline (Reduces hepatic metabolism of theophylline resulting in delayed elimination and increased blood levels of theophylline).

No products indexed under this heading.

Amitriptyline Hydrochloride (Reduces hepatic metabolism of certain unspecified tricyclic antidepressants resulting in delayed elimination and increased blood levels of these drugs). Products include:

- Elavil 2945
- Etrafon 2495
- Limbitrol 2333
- Triavil Tablets 1800

Amoxapine (Reduces hepatic metabolism of certain unspecified tricyclic antidepressants resulting in delayed elimination and increased blood levels of these drugs). Products include:

- Asendin Tablets 1419

Chlordiazepoxide (Reduces hepatic metabolism of chlordiazepoxide resulting in delayed elimination and increased blood levels of chlordiazepoxide). Products include:

- Limbitrol 2333

Chlordiazepoxide Hydrochloride (Reduces hepatic metabolism of chlordiazepoxide resulting in delayed elimination and increased blood levels of chlordiazepoxide). Products include:

- Librax Capsules 2330
- Librium Capsules 2331
- Librium Injectable 2332

Clomipramine Hydrochloride (Reduces hepatic metabolism of certain unspecified tricyclic antidepressants resulting in delayed elimination and increased blood levels of these drugs). Products include:

- Anafranil Capsules 819

Desipramine Hydrochloride (Reduces hepatic metabolism of certain unspecified tricyclic antidepressants resulting in delayed elimination and increased blood levels of these drugs). Products include:

- Norpramin Tablets 1273

Diazepam (Reduces hepatic metabolism of diazepam resulting in delayed elimination and increased blood levels of diazepam). Products include:

- Dizac (diazepam injectable emulsion) CIV 1862
- Valium Injectable 2336
- Valium Tablets 2335

Dicumarol (Reduces hepatic metabolism of warfarin-type anticoagulants resulting in clinically significant effects; close monitoring of prothrombin time of these recommended).

No products indexed under this heading.

Doxepin Hydrochloride (Reduces hepatic metabolism of certain unspecified tricyclic antidepressants resulting in delayed elimination and increased blood levels of these drugs). Products include:

- Adapin Capsules 1542
- Sinequan 2028
- Zonalon Cream 1042

Dyphylline (Reduces hepatic metabolism of theophylline resulting in delayed elimination and increased blood levels of theophylline). Products include:

- Lufyllin & Lufyllin-400 Tablets 2778
- Lufyllin-GG Elixir & Tablets 2779

Imipramine Hydrochloride (Reduces hepatic metabolism of certain unspecified tricyclic antidepressants resulting in delayed elimination and increased blood levels of these drugs). Products include:

- Tofranil Ampuls 873
- Tofranil Tablets 875

Imipramine Pamoate (Reduces hepatic metabolism of certain unspecified tricyclic antidepressants resulting in delayed elimination and increased blood levels of these drugs). Products include:

- Tofranil-PM Capsules 876

Ketoconazole (Alteration of pH may affect absorption of ketoconazole; administer oral ketoconazole at least 2 hours before cimetidine). Products include:

- Nizoral 2% Cream 1344
- Nizoral 2% Shampoo 1344
- Nizoral Tablets 1345

Lidocaine Hydrochloride (Reduces hepatic metabolism of lidocaine resulting in delayed elimination and increased blood levels of lidocaine). Products include:

- Decadron Phosphate with Xylocaine Injection, Sterile 1683
- Unguentine Plus .... ◘ 712
- Xylocaine Injections 562

Magaldrate (Simultaneous administration is not recommended since antacids may interfere with the absorption of cimetidine).

No products indexed under this heading.

Magnesium Hydroxide (Simultaneous administration is not recommended since antacids may interfere with the absorption of cimetidine). Products include:

- Aludrox Oral Suspension .... ◘ 850
- Ascriptin .... ◘ 650
- Di-Gel Antacid/Anti-Gas .... ◘ 762
- Gelusil Antacid-Anti-gas Liquid .... ◘ 819
- Gelusil Antacid-Anti-gas Tablets .... ◘ 819
- Maalox Antacid/Anti-Gas Tablets 889
- Maalox Antacid Liquid 888
- Extra Strength Maalox Antacid/Anti-Gas Liquid and Tablets 888
- Mylanta Fast-Acting 1359
- Mylanta Gelcaps Antacid .... ◘ 678
- Fast-Acting Mylanta Liquid Antacid 1359
- Mylanta Tablets .... ◘ 677
- Maximum-Strength Fast-Acting Mylanta Liquid Antacid 1359
- Mylanta Double Strength Tablets .. ◘ 677
- Phillips' Milk of Magnesia Liquid .... ◘ 627
- Rolaids Antacid Tablets .... ◘ 807
- Tempo Soft Antacid .... ◘ 799

Magnesium Oxide (Simultaneous administration is not recommended since antacids may interfere with the absorption of cimetidine). Products include:

- Beelith Tablets 632
- Bufferin Analgesic Tablets .... ◘ 636
- Arthritis Strength Bufferin Analgesic Caplets .... ◘ 637
- Extra Strength Bufferin Analgesic Tablets .... ◘ 637
- Caltrate PLUS .... ◘ 681
- Cama Arthritis Pain Reliever .... ◘ 748
- Mag-Ox 400 666
- Uro-Mag 666

Maprotiline Hydrochloride (Reduces hepatic metabolism of certain unspecified tricyclic antidepressants resulting in delayed elimination and increased blood levels of these drugs). Products include:

- Ludiomil Tablets 861

(◘ Described in PDR For Nonprescription Drugs) (◉ Described in PDR For Ophthalmology)

Metronidazole (Reduces hepatic metabolism of metronidazole resulting in delayed elimination and increased blood levels of metronidazole). Products include:

- Flagyl 375 Capsules ... 2587
- Flagyl I.V. RTU ... 2373
- Helidac Therapy ... 2135
- MetroCream ... 1034
- MetroGel ... 1034
- MetroGel-Vaginal ... 917
- Protostat Tablets ... 1939

Metronidazole Hydrochloride (Reduces hepatic metabolism of metronidazole resulting in delayed elimination and increased blood levels of metronidazole). Products include:

- Flagyl I.V. ... 2373

Nifedipine (Reduces hepatic metabolism of nifedipine resulting in delayed elimination and increased blood levels of nifedipine). Products include:

- Adalat Capsules (10 mg and 20 mg) ... 580
- Adalat CC ... 582
- Procardia Capsules ... 2024
- Procardia XL Extended Release Tablets ... 2026

Nortriptyline Hydrochloride (Reduces hepatic metabolism of certain unspecified tricyclic antidepressants resulting in delayed elimination and increased blood levels of these drugs). Products include:

- Pamelor ... 2409

Phenytoin (Reduces hepatic metabolism of phenytoin resulting in delayed elimination and increased blood levels of phenytoin). Products include:

- Dilantin Infatabs ... 1967
- Dilantin-125 Suspension ... 1969

Phenytoin Sodium (Reduces hepatic metabolism of phenytoin resulting in delayed elimination and increased blood levels of phenytoin). Products include:

- Dilantin Kapseals ... 1965

Propranolol Hydrochloride (Reduces hepatic metabolism of propranolol resulting in delayed elimination and increased blood levels of propranolol). Products include:

- Inderal ... 2834
- Inderal LA Long Acting Capsules ... 2836
- Inderide Tablets ... 2838
- Inderide LA Long Acting Capsules ... 2840

Protriptyline Hydrochloride (Reduces hepatic metabolism of certain unspecified tricyclic antidepressants resulting in delayed elimination and increased blood levels of these drugs). Products include:

- Vivactil Tablets ... 1820

Sodium Bicarbonate (Simultaneous administration is not recommended since antacids may interfere with the absorption of cimetidine). Products include:

- Alka-Seltzer Cherry Effervescent Antacid and Pain Reliever ... 609
- Alka-Seltzer Extra Strength Effervescent Antacid and Pain Reliever ... 609
- Alka-Seltzer Gold Effervescent Antacid ... 611
- Alka-Seltzer Lemon Lime Effervescent Antacid and Pain Reliever ... 609
- Alka-Seltzer Original Effervescent Antacid and Pain Reliever ... 609
- Arm & Hammer Pure Baking Soda ... 648
- Colyte and Colyte-flavored ... 2540
- GoLYTELY ... 694
- Massengill Disposable Douches ... 780
- Massengill Liquid Concentrate ... 780
- NuLYTELY ... 694
- Cherry Flavor NuLYTELY ... 694

Theophylline (Reduces hepatic metabolism of theophylline resulting in delayed elimination and increased blood levels of theophylline). Products include:

- Marax Tablets & DF Syrup ... 2015
- Quibron ... 2227

Theophylline Anhydrous (Reduces hepatic metabolism of theophylline resulting in delayed elimination and increased blood levels of theophylline). Products include:

- Aerolate ... 1003
- Primatene Tablets ... 844
- Respbid Tablets ... 687
- Slo-bid Gyrocaps ... 2201
- Theo-24 Extended Release Capsules ... 2753
- Theo-Dur Extended-Release Tablets ... 1367
- Theo-X Extended-Release Tablets ... 793
- Uni-Dur Extended-Release Tablets ... 1374
- Uniphyl 400 mg and 600 mg Tablets ... 2157

Theophylline Calcium Salicylate (Reduces hepatic metabolism of theophylline resulting in delayed elimination and increased blood levels of theophylline). Products include:

- Quadrinal Tablets ... 1398

Theophylline Sodium Glycinate (Reduces hepatic metabolism of theophylline resulting in delayed elimination and increased blood levels of theophylline).

- No products indexed under this heading.

Trimipramine Maleate (Reduces hepatic metabolism of certain unspecified tricyclic antidepressants resulting in delayed elimination and increased blood levels of these drugs). Products include:

- Surmontil Capsules ... 2917

Warfarin Sodium (Reduces hepatic metabolism of warfarin-type anticoagulants resulting in clinically significant effects; close monitoring of prothrombin time is recommended). Products include:

- Coumadin ... 941

TALACEN CAPLETS

(Pentazocine Hydrochloride) ... 2464

May interact with narcotic analgesics, central nervous system depressants, and certain other agents. Compounds in these categories include:

Alfentanil Hydrochloride (Potential for withdrawal symptoms; additive CNS depressant effects). Products include:

- Alfenta Injection ... 1334

Alprazolam (Additive CNS depressant effects). Products include:

- Xanax Tablets ... 2115

Aprobarbital (Additive CNS depressant effects).

- No products indexed under this heading.

Buprenorphine (Potential for withdrawal symptoms; additive CNS depressant effects). Products include:

- Buprenex Injectable ... 2170

Buspirone Hydrochloride (Additive CNS depressant effects). Products include:

- BuSpar Tablets ... 738

Butabarbital (Additive CNS depressant effects).

- No products indexed under this heading.

Butalbital (Additive CNS depressant effects). Products include:

- Axocet Capsules ... 2469
- Esgic-plus Capsules ... 1012
- Esgic-plus Tablets ... 1012
- Fioricet Tablets ... 2386
- Fioricet with Codeine Capsules ... 2387
- Fiorinal Capsules ... 2388
- Fiorinal with Codeine Capsules ... 2390
- Fiorinal Tablets ... 2388
- Phrenilin ... 790
- Sedapap Tablets 50 mg/650 mg ... 1826

Chlordiazepoxide (Additive CNS depressant effects). Products include:

- Limbitrol ... 2333

Chlordiazepoxide Hydrochloride (Additive CNS depressant effects). Products include:

- Librax Capsules ... 2330
- Librium Capsules ... 2331
- Librium Injectable ... 2332

Chlorpromazine (Additive CNS depressant effects). Products include:

- Thorazine Suppositories ... 2701

Chlorprothixene (Additive CNS depressant effects).

- No products indexed under this heading.

Chlorprothixene Hydrochloride (Additive CNS depressant effects).

- No products indexed under this heading.

Chlorprothixene Lactate (Potential for withdrawal symptoms; additive CNS depressant effects).

- No products indexed under this heading.

Clorazepate Dipotassium (Additive CNS depressant effects). Products include:

- Tranxene ... 459

Clozapine (Potential for withdrawal symptoms; additive CNS depressant effects). Products include:

- Clozaril Tablets ... 2377

Codeine Phosphate (Potential for withdrawal symptoms; additive CNS depressant effects). Products include:

- Brontex ... 2130
- Dimetane-DC Cough Syrup ... 2232
- Fioricet with Codeine Capsules ... 2387
- Fiorinal with Codeine Capsules ... 2390
- Nucofed ... 2225
- Phenergan with Codeine ... 2883
- Phenergan VC with Codeine ... 2888
- Robitussin A-C Syrup ... 2248
- Robitussin-DAC Syrup ... 2249
- Ryna ... 804
- Soma Compound w/Codeine Tablets ... 2784
- Tylenol with Codeine ... 1592

Desflurane (Potential for withdrawal symptoms; additive CNS depressant effects). Products include:

- Suprane (desflurane, USP) ... 1865

Dezocine (Potential for withdrawal symptoms). Products include:

- Dalgan Injection ... 529

Diazepam (Additive CNS depressant effects). Products include:

- Dizac (diazepam injectable emulsion) CIV ... 1862
- Valium Injectable ... 2336
- Valium Tablets ... 2335

Diphenoxylate Hydrochloride (Potential for withdrawal symptoms). Products include:

- Lomotil ... 2591

Droperidol (Additive CNS depressant effects). Products include:

- Inapsine Injection ... 462

Enflurane (Additive CNS depressant effects).

- No products indexed under this heading.

Estazolam (Potential for withdrawal symptoms; additive CNS depressant effects). Products include:

- ProSom Tablets ... 457

Ethchlorvynol (Additive CNS depressant effects). Products include:

- Placidyl Capsules ... 456

Ethinamate (Additive CNS depressant effects).

- No products indexed under this heading.

Fentanyl (Potential for withdrawal symptoms). Products include:

- Duragesic Transdermal System ... 1336

Fentanyl Citrate (Potential for withdrawal symptoms; additive CNS depressant effects). Products include:

- Sublimaze Injection ... 463

Fluphenazine Decanoate (Additive CNS depressant effects). Products include:

- Prolixin Decanoate ... 510

Fluphenazine Enanthate (Additive CNS depressant effects). Products include:

- Prolixin Enanthate ... 510

Fluphenazine Hydrochloride (Additive CNS depressant effects). Products include:

- Prolixin ... 510

Flurazepam Hydrochloride (Additive CNS depressant effects). Products include:

- Dalmane Capsules ... 2329

Glutethimide (Additive CNS depressant effects).

- No products indexed under this heading.

Haloperidol (Additive CNS depressant effects). Products include:

- Haldol Injection, Tablets and Concentrate ... 1585

Haloperidol Decanoate (Additive CNS depressant effects). Products include:

- Haldol Decanoate ... 1587

Hydrocodone Bitartrate (Potential for withdrawal symptoms; additive CNS depressant effects). Products include:

- Codiclear DH Syrup ... 808
- Duratuss HD Elixir ... 2750
- Histussin D Liquid ... 670
- Hycodan Tablets and Syrup ... 946
- Hycomine Compound Tablets ... 948
- Hycomine ... 947
- Hycotuss Expectorant Syrup ... 950
- Hydrocet Capsules ... 787
- Lorcet 10/650 Tablets ... 1016
- Lortab ... 2751
- Tussend ... 1830
- Tussend Expectorant ... 1831
- Vicodin Tablets ... 1404
- Vicodin ES Tablets ... 1405
- Vicodin HP Tablets ... 1403
- Vicodin Tuss Expectorant ... 1406
- Zydone Capsules ... 967

Hydrocodone Polistirex (Potential for withdrawal symptoms; additive CNS depressant effects). Products include:

- Tussionex Pennkinetic Extended-Release Suspension ... 1624

Hydromorphone Hydrochloride (Potential for withdrawal symptoms; additive CNS depressant effects). Products include:

- Dilaudid Ampules ... 1382
- Dilaudid Cough Syrup ... 1383
- Dilaudid-HP Injection ... 1384
- Dilaudid-HP Lyophilized Powder 250 mg ... 1384
- Dilaudid ... 1382
- Dilaudid Oral Liquid ... 1386
- Dilaudid ... 1382
- Dilaudid Tablets - 8 mg ... 1386

Hydroxyzine Hydrochloride (Additive CNS depressant effects). Products include:

- Atarax Tablets & Syrup ... 1992
- Marax Tablets & DF Syrup ... 2015
- Vistaril Intramuscular Solution ... 2042

IMPORTANT NOTE: Always consult each drug listing in the patient's regimen for possible interactions.

Interactions Index

Talacen

Isoflurane (Additive CNS depressant effects).
No products indexed under this heading.

Ketamine Hydrochloride (Additive CNS depressant effects).
No products indexed under this heading.

Levomethadyl Acetate Hydrochloride (Potential for withdrawal symptoms; additive CNS depressant effects). Products include:
- Orlaam Oral Solution 2361

Levorphanol Tartrate (Potential for withdrawal symptoms; additive CNS depressant effects). Products include:
- Levo-Dromoran 2297

Lorazepam (Additive CNS depressant effects). Products include:
- Ativan Injection 2805
- Ativan Tablets 2807

Loxapine Hydrochloride (Additive CNS depressant effects). Products include:
- Loxitane 1426

Loxapine Succinate (Additive CNS depressant effects). Products include:
- Loxitane Capsules 1426

Meperidine Hydrochloride (Potential for withdrawal symptoms; additive CNS depressant effects). Products include:
- Demerol 2438
- Mepergan Injection 2859

Mephobarbital (Additive CNS depressant effects). Products include:
- Mebaral Tablets 2452

Meprobamate (Additive CNS depressant effects). Products include:
- Miltown Tablets 2780
- PMB 200 and PMB 400 2890

Mesoridazine Besylate (Additive CNS depressant effects). Products include:
- Serentil 689

Methadone Hydrochloride (Potential for withdrawal symptoms; additive CNS depressant effects). Products include:
- Methadone Hydrochloride Oral Concentrate 2356
- Methadone Hydrochloride Oral Solution & Tablets 2357

Methohexital Sodium (Additive CNS depressant effects).
No products indexed under this heading.

Methotrimeprazine (Potential for withdrawal symptoms; additive CNS depressant effects). Products include:
- Levoprome 1321

Methoxyflurane (Additive CNS depressant effects).
No products indexed under this heading.

Midazolam Hydrochloride (Additive CNS depressant effects). Products include:
- Versed Injection 2324

Molindone Hydrochloride (Additive CNS depressant effects). Products include:
- Moban Tablets and Concentrate ... 1036

Morphine Sulfate (Potential for withdrawal symptoms; additive CNS depressant effects). Products include:
- Astramorph/PF Injection, USP (Preservative-Free) 526
- Duramorph Injection 983
- Infumorph 200 and Infumorph 500 Sterile Solutions 985
- Kadian Capsules 2948
- MS Contin Tablets 2149
- MSIR 2152
- Oramorph SR (Morphine Sulfate Sustained Release Tablets) .. 2359
- RMS Suppositories CII 2766
- Roxanol 2365

Opium Alkaloids (Potential for withdrawal symptoms; additive CNS depressant effects).
No products indexed under this heading.

Oxazepam (Additive CNS depressant effects). Products include:
- Serax Capsules 2916
- Serax Tablets 2916

Oxycodone Hydrochloride (Potential for withdrawal symptoms; additive CNS depressant effects). Products include:
- OxyContin Tablets 2163
- OxyIR Capsules 2167
- Percocet Tablets 955
- Percodan Tablets 955
- Percodan-Demi Tablets 956
- Roxicodone Tablets, Oral Solution & Intensol (Oxycodone) 2366
- Tylox Capsules 1593

Paregoric (Potential for withdrawal symptoms).
No products indexed under this heading.

Pentobarbital Sodium (Additive CNS depressant effects). Products include:
- Nembutal Sodium Capsules 440
- Nembutal Sodium Solution 442
- Nembutal Sodium Suppositories ... 444

Perphenazine (Additive CNS depressant effects). Products include:
- Etrafon 2495
- Triavil Tablets 1800
- Trilafon 2532

Phenobarbital (Additive CNS depressant effects). Products include:
- Arco-Lase Plus Tablets 513
- Bellergal-S Tablets 2375
- Donnatal 2234
- Donnatal Extentabs 2234
- Donnatal Tablets 2234
- Phenobarbital Elixir and Tablets ... 1523
- Quadrinal Tablets 1398

Prazepam (Additive CNS depressant effects).
No products indexed under this heading.

Prochlorperazine (Additive CNS depressant effects). Products include:
- Compazine 2644

Promethazine Hydrochloride (Potential for withdrawal symptoms; additive CNS depressant effects). Products include:
- Mepergan Injection 2859
- Phenergan with Codeine 2883
- Phenergan with Dextromethorphan ... 2885
- Phenergan Injection 2880
- Phenergan Suppositories 2882
- Phenergan Syrup 2881
- Phenergan Tablets 2882
- Phenergan VC 2886
- Phenergan VC with Codeine .. 2888

Propofol (Additive CNS depressant effects). Products include:
- Diprivan Injectable Emulsion .. 2939

Propoxyphene Hydrochloride (Potential for withdrawal symptoms; additive CNS depressant effects). Products include:
- Darvon 1475
- Wygesic Tablets 2930

Propoxyphene Napsylate (Potential for withdrawal symptoms; additive CNS depressant effects). Products include:
- Darvon-N/Darvocet-N 1473

Quazepam (Additive CNS depressant effects). Products include:
- Doral Tablets 2773

Risperidone (Potential for withdrawal symptoms; additive CNS depressant effects). Products include:
- Risperdal Tablets 1348

Secobarbital Sodium (Potential for withdrawal symptoms; additive CNS depressant effects). Products include:
- Seconal Sodium Pulvules 1529

Sevoflurane (Potential for withdrawal symptoms; additive CNS depressant effects).
No products indexed under this heading.

Sufentanil Citrate (Potential for withdrawal symptoms; additive CNS depressant effects). Products include:
- Sufenta Injection 1355

Temazepam (Potential for withdrawal symptoms; additive CNS depressant effects). Products include:
- Restoril Capsules 2413

Thiamylal Sodium (Potential for withdrawal symptoms; additive CNS depressant effects).
No products indexed under this heading.

Thioridazine Hydrochloride (Potential for withdrawal symptoms; additive CNS depressant effects). Products include:
- Mellaril 2398

Thiothixene (Potential for withdrawal symptoms; additive CNS depressant effects). Products include:
- Navane Capsules and Concentrate ... 2018
- Navane Intramuscular 2019

Triazolam (Potential for withdrawal symptoms; additive CNS depressant effects). Products include:
- Halcion Tablets 2093

Trifluoperazine Hydrochloride (Potential for withdrawal symptoms; additive CNS depressant effects). Products include:
- Stelazine 2692

Zolpidem Tartrate (Potential for withdrawal symptoms; additive CNS depressant effects). Products include:
- Ambien Tablets 2559

Food Interactions

Alcohol (Potential for increased CNS depressant effects).

TALWIN AMPULS
(Pentazocine Lactate) 2465
May interact with narcotic analgesics, general anesthetics, preanesthetic medications, central nervous system depressants, and certain other agents. Compounds in these categories include:

Alfentanil Hydrochloride (Potential for withdrawal symptoms; may produce additive CNS depression). Products include:
- Alfenta Injection 1334

Alprazolam (May produce additive CNS depression). Products include:
- Xanax Tablets 2115

Aprobarbital (May produce additive CNS depression).
No products indexed under this heading.

Buprenorphine (Potential for withdrawal symptoms; may produce additive CNS depression). Products include:
- Buprenex Injectable 2170

Buspirone Hydrochloride (May produce additive CNS depression). Products include:
- BuSpar Tablets 738

Butabarbital (May produce additive CNS depression).
No products indexed under this heading.

Butalbital (May produce additive CNS depression). Products include:
- Axocet Capsules 2469
- Esgic-plus Capsules 1012
- Esgic-plus Tablets 1012
- Fioricet Tablets 2386
- Fioricet with Codeine Capsules ... 2387
- Fiorinal Capsules 2388
- Fiorinal with Codeine Capsules ... 2390
- Fiorinal Tablets 2388
- Phrenilin 790
- Sedapap Tablets 50 mg/650 mg .. 1826

Chlordiazepoxide (May produce additive CNS depression). Products include:
- Limbitrol 2333

Chlordiazepoxide Hydrochloride (May produce additive CNS depression). Products include:
- Librax Capsules 2330
- Librium Capsules 2331
- Librium Injectable 2332

Chlorpromazine (May produce additive CNS depression). Products include:
- Thorazine Suppositories 2701

Chlorprothixene (May produce additive CNS depression).
No products indexed under this heading.

Chlorprothixene Hydrochloride (May produce additive CNS depression).
No products indexed under this heading.

Chlorprothixene Lactate (Potential for withdrawal symptoms; may produce additive CNS depression).
No products indexed under this heading.

Clorazepate Dipotassium (May produce additive CNS depression). Products include:
- Tranxene 459

Clozapine (Potential for withdrawal symptoms; may produce additive CNS depression). Products include:
- Clozaril Tablets 2377

Codeine Phosphate (Potential for withdrawal symptoms; may produce additive CNS depression). Products include:
- Brontex 2130
- Dimetane-DC Cough Syrup .. 2232
- Fioricet with Codeine Capsules ... 2387
- Fiorinal with Codeine Capsules ... 2390
- Nucofed 2225
- Phenergan with Codeine 2883
- Phenergan VC with Codeine . 2888
- Robitussin A-C Syrup 2248
- Robitussin-DAC Syrup 2249
- Ryna 804
- Soma Compound w/Codeine Tablets 2784
- Tylenol with Codeine 1592

Desflurane (Potential for withdrawal symptoms; may produce additive CNS depression). Products include:
- Suprane (desflurane, USP) .. 1865

Dezocine (Potential for withdrawal symptoms). Products include:
- Dalgan Injection 529

Diazepam (May produce additive CNS depressant effects). Products include:
- Dizac (diazepam injectable emulsion) CIV 1862
- Valium Injectable 2336
- Valium Tablets 2335

(Described in PDR For Nonprescription Drugs)   (Described in PDR For Ophthalmology)

Droperidol (May produce additive CNS depressant effects). Products include:
- Inapsine Injection ... 462

Enflurane (May produce additive CNS depressant effects).
- No products indexed under this heading.

Estazolam (Potential for withdrawal symptoms; may produce additive CNS depression). Products include:
- ProSom Tablets ... 457

Ethchlorvynol (May produce additive CNS depression). Products include:
- Placidyl Capsules ... 456

Ethinamate (May produce additive CNS depression).
- No products indexed under this heading.

Fentanyl (Potential for withdrawal symptoms). Products include:
- Duragesic Transdermal System ... 1336

Fentanyl Citrate (Potential for withdrawal symptoms; may produce additive CNS depressant effects). Products include:
- Sublimaze Injection ... 463

Fluphenazine Decanoate (May produce additive CNS depression). Products include:
- Prolixin Decanoate ... 510

Fluphenazine Enanthate (May produce additive CNS depression). Products include:
- Prolixin Enanthate ... 510

Fluphenazine Hydrochloride (May produce additive CNS depression). Products include:
- Prolixin ... 510

Flurazepam Hydrochloride (May produce additive CNS depression). Products include:
- Dalmane Capsules ... 2329

Glutethimide (May produce additive CNS depression).
- No products indexed under this heading.

Haloperidol (May produce additive CNS depression). Products include:
- Haldol Injection, Tablets and Concentrate ... 1585

Haloperidol Decanoate (May produce additive CNS depression). Products include:
- Haldol Decanoate ... 1587

Hydrocodone Bitartrate (Potential for withdrawal symptoms; may produce additive CNS depression). Products include:
- Codiclear DH Syrup ... 808
- Duratuss HD Elixir ... 2750
- Histussin D Liquid ... 670
- Hycodan Tablets and Syrup ... 946
- Hycomine Compound Tablets ... 948
- Hycomine ... 947
- Hycotuss Expectorant Syrup ... 950
- Hydrocet Capsules ... 787
- Lorcet 10/650 Tablets ... 1016
- Lortab ... 2751
- Tussend ... 1830
- Tussend Expectorant ... 1831
- Vicodin Tablets ... 1404
- Vicodin ES Tablets ... 1405
- Vicodin HP Tablets ... 1403
- Vicodin Tuss Expectorant ... 1406
- Zydone Capsules ... 967

Hydrocodone Polistirex (Potential for withdrawal symptoms; may produce additive CNS depression). Products include:
- Tussionex Pennkinetic Extended-Release Suspension ... 1624

Hydromorphone Hydrochloride (Potential for withdrawal symptoms; may produce additive CNS depression). Products include:
- Dilaudid Ampules ... 1382
- Dilaudid Cough Syrup ... 1383
- Dilaudid-HP Injection ... 1384
- Dilaudid-HP Lyophilized Powder 250 mg ... 1384
- Dilaudid ... 1382
- Dilaudid Oral Liquid ... 1386
- Dilaudid ... 1382
- Dilaudid Tablets - 8 mg ... 1386

Hydroxyzine Hydrochloride (May produce additive CNS depressant effects). Products include:
- Atarax Tablets & Syrup ... 1992
- Marax Tablets & DF Syrup ... 2015
- Vistaril Intramuscular Solution ... 2042

Isoflurane (May produce additive CNS depressant effects).
- No products indexed under this heading.

Ketamine Hydrochloride (May produce additive CNS depressant effects).
- No products indexed under this heading.

Levomethadyl Acetate Hydrochloride (Potential for withdrawal symptoms; may produce additive CNS depression). Products include:
- Orlaam Oral Solution ... 2361

Levorphanol Tartrate (Potential for withdrawal symptoms; may produce additive CNS depression). Products include:
- Levo-Dromoran ... 2297

Lorazepam (May produce additive CNS depressant effects). Products include:
- Ativan Injection ... 2805
- Ativan Tablets ... 2807

Loxapine Hydrochloride (May produce additive CNS depression). Products include:
- Loxitane ... 1426

Loxapine Succinate (May produce additive CNS depression). Products include:
- Loxitane Capsules ... 1426

Meperidine Hydrochloride (Potential for withdrawal symptoms; may produce additive CNS depressant effects). Products include:
- Demerol ... 2438
- Mepergan Injection ... 2859

Mephobarbital (May produce additive CNS depression). Products include:
- Mebaral Tablets ... 2452

Meprobamate (May produce additive CNS depression). Products include:
- Miltown Tablets ... 2780
- PMB 200 and PMB 400 ... 2890

Mesoridazine Besylate (May produce additive CNS depression). Products include:
- Serentil ... 689

Methadone Hydrochloride (Potential for withdrawal symptoms; may produce additive CNS depression). Products include:
- Methadone Hydrochloride Oral Concentrate ... 2356
- Methadone Hydrochloride Oral Solution & Tablets ... 2357

Methohexital Sodium (May produce additive CNS depressant effects).
- No products indexed under this heading.

Methotrimeprazine (Potential for withdrawal symptoms; may produce additive CNS depression). Products include:
- Levoprome ... 1321

Methoxyflurane (Potential for withdrawal symptoms; may produce additive CNS depression).
- No products indexed under this heading.

Midazolam Hydrochloride (May produce additive CNS depression). Products include:
- Versed Injection ... 2324

Molindone Hydrochloride (May produce additive CNS depression). Products include:
- Moban Tablets and Concentrate ... 1036

Morphine Sulfate (Potential for withdrawal symptoms; may produce additive CNS depressant effects). Products include:
- Astramorph/PF Injection, USP (Preservative-Free) ... 526
- Duramorph Injection ... 983
- Infumorph 200 and Infumorph 500 Sterile Solutions ... 985
- Kadian Capsules ... 2948
- MS Contin Tablets ... 2149
- MSIR ... 2152
- Oramorph SR (Morphine Sulfate Sustained Release Tablets) ... 2359
- RMS Suppositories CII ... 2766
- Roxanol ... 2365

Opium Alkaloids (Potential for withdrawal symptoms; may produce additive CNS depressant effects).
- No products indexed under this heading.

Oxazepam (May produce additive CNS depression). Products include:
- Serax Capsules ... 2916
- Serax Tablets ... 2916

Oxycodone Hydrochloride (Potential for withdrawal symptoms; may produce additive CNS depression). Products include:
- OxyContin Tablets ... 2163
- OxyIR Capsules ... 2167
- Percocet Tablets ... 955
- Percodan Tablets ... 955
- Percodan-Demi Tablets ... 956
- Roxicodone Tablets, Oral Solution & Intensol (Oxycodone) ... 2366
- Tylox Capsules ... 1593

Pentobarbital Sodium (Potential for withdrawal symptoms; may produce additive CNS depression). Products include:
- Nembutal Sodium Capsules ... 440
- Nembutal Sodium Solution ... 442
- Nembutal Sodium Suppositories ... 444

Perphenazine (May produce additive CNS depression). Products include:
- Etrafon ... 2495
- Triavil Tablets ... 1800
- Trilafon ... 2532

Phenobarbital (May produce additive CNS depression). Products include:
- Arco-Lase Plus Tablets ... 513
- Bellergal-S Tablets ... 2375
- Donnatal ... 2234
- Donnatal Extentabs ... 2234
- Donnatal Tablets ... 2234
- Phenobarbital Elixir and Tablets ... 1523
- Quadrinal Tablets ... 1398

Prazepam (May produce additive CNS depression).
- No products indexed under this heading.

Prochlorperazine (May produce additive CNS depression). Products include:
- Compazine ... 2644

Promethazine Hydrochloride (May produce additive CNS depressant effects). Products include:
- Mepergan Injection ... 2859
- Phenergan with Codeine ... 2883
- Phenergan with Dextromethorphan ... 2885
- Phenergan Injection ... 2880
- Phenergan Suppositories ... 2882
- Phenergan Syrup ... 2881
- Phenergan Tablets ... 2882
- Phenergan VC ... 2886
- Phenergan VC with Codeine ... 2888

Propofol (May produce additive CNS depressant effects). Products include:
- Diprivan Injectable Emulsion ... 2939

Propoxyphene Hydrochloride (Potential for withdrawal symptoms; may produce additive CNS depressant effects). Products include:
- Darvon ... 1475
- Wygesic Tablets ... 2930

Propoxyphene Napsylate (Potential for withdrawal symptoms; may produce additive CNS depressant effects). Products include:
- Darvon-N/Darvocet-N ... 1473

Risperidone (Potential for withdrawal symptoms; may produce additive CNS depression). Products include:
- Risperdal Tablets ... 1348

Secobarbital Sodium (May produce additive CNS depressant effects). Products include:
- Seconal Sodium Pulvules ... 1529

Sevoflurane (Potential for withdrawal symptoms; may produce additive CNS depression).
- No products indexed under this heading.

Sufentanil Citrate (Potential for withdrawal symptoms; may produce additive CNS depressant effects). Products include:
- Sufenta Injection ... 1355

Temazepam (May produce additive CNS depressant effects). Products include:
- Restoril Capsules ... 2413

Thiamylal Sodium (Potential for withdrawal symptoms; may produce additive CNS depressant effects).
- No products indexed under this heading.

Thioridazine Hydrochloride (May produce additive CNS depressant effects). Products include:
- Mellaril ... 2398

Thiothixene (May produce additive CNS depressant effects). Products include:
- Navane Capsules and Concentrate 2018
- Navane Intramuscular ... 2019

Triazolam (May produce additive CNS depressant effects). Products include:
- Halcion Tablets ... 2093

Trifluoperazine Hydrochloride (May produce additive CNS depressant effects). Products include:
- Stelazine ... 2692

Zolpidem Tartrate (Potential for withdrawal symptoms; may produce additive CNS depression). Products include:
- Ambien Tablets ... 2559

Food Interactions

Alcohol (Potential for increased CNS depressant effects).

TALWIN CARPUJECT

(Pentazocine Lactate) ... 2465

See Talwin Ampuls

TALWIN COMPOUND

(Pentazocine Hydrochloride, Aspirin) 2466

May interact with narcotic analgesics, oral anticoagulants, and certain other agents. Compounds in these categories include:

Alfentanil Hydrochloride (Potential for withdrawal symptoms). Products include:
- Alfenta Injection ... 1334

Buprenorphine (Potential for withdrawal symptoms). Products include:
- Buprenex Injectable ... 2170

Codeine Phosphate (Potential for withdrawal symptoms). Products include:
- Brontex ... 2130
- Dimetane-DC Cough Syrup ... 2232

IMPORTANT NOTE: Always consult each drug listing in the patient's regimen for possible interactions.

Talwin Compound **Interactions Index** **1038**

Fioricet with Codeine Capsules 2387
Fiorinal with Codeine Capsules 2390
Nucofed 2225
Phenergan with Codeine 2883
Phenergan VC with Codeine 2888
Robitussin A-C Syrup 2248
Robitussin-DAC Syrup 2249
Ryna .... ▣ 804
Soma Compound w/Codeine Tablets 2784
Tylenol with Codeine 1592

Dezocine (Potential for withdrawal symptoms). Products include:
Dalgan Injection 529

Dicumarol (Effects of aspirin may be deleterious in conjunction with anticoagulant therapy).
No products indexed under this heading.

Fentanyl (Potential for withdrawal symptoms). Products include:
Duragesic Transdermal System 1336

Fentanyl Citrate (Potential for withdrawal symptoms). Products include:
Sublimaze Injection 463

Hydrocodone Bitartrate (Potential for withdrawal symptoms). Products include:
Codiclear DH Syrup 808
Duratuss HD Elixir 2750
Histussin D Liquid 670
Hycodan Tablets and Syrup 946
Hycomine Compound Tablets 948
Hycomine 947
Hycotuss Expectorant Syrup 950
Hydrocet Capsules 787
Lorcet 10/650 Tablets 1016
Lortab 2751
Tussend 1830
Tussend Expectorant 1831
Vicodin Tablets 1404
Vicodin ES Tablets 1405
Vicodin HP Tablets 1403
Vicodin Tuss Expectorant 1406
Zydone Capsules 967

Hydrocodone Polistirex (Potential for withdrawal symptoms). Products include:
Tussionex Pennkinetic Extended-Release Suspension 1624

Hydromorphone Hydrochloride (Potential for withdrawal symptoms). Products include:
Dilaudid Ampules 1382
Dilaudid Cough Syrup 1383
Dilaudid-HP Injection 1384
Dilaudid-HP Lyophilized Powder 250 mg 1384
Dilaudid 1382
Dilaudid Oral Liquid 1386
Dilaudid 1382
Dilaudid Tablets - 8 mg 1386

Levorphanol Tartrate (Potential for withdrawal symptoms). Products include:
Levo-Dromoran 2297

Meperidine Hydrochloride (Potential for withdrawal symptoms). Products include:
Demerol 2438
Mepergan Injection 2859

Methadone Hydrochloride (Potential for withdrawal symptoms). Products include:
Methadone Hydrochloride Oral Concentrate 2356
Methadone Hydrochloride Oral Solution & Tablets 2357

Morphine Sulfate (Potential for withdrawal symptoms). Products include:
Astramorph/PF Injection, USP (Preservative-Free) 526
Duramorph Injection 983
Infumorph 200 and Infumorph 500 Sterile Solutions 985
Kadian Capsules 2948
MS Contin Tablets 2149
MSIR 2152
Oramorph SR (Morphine Sulfate Sustained Release Tablets) 2359
RMS Suppositories CII 2766
Roxanol 2365

Opium Alkaloids (Potential for withdrawal symptoms).
No products indexed under this heading.

Oxycodone Hydrochloride (Potential for withdrawal symptoms). Products include:
OxyContin Tablets 2163
OxyIR Capsules 2167
Percocet Tablets 955
Percodan Tablets 955
Percodan-Demi Tablets 956
Roxicodone Tablets, Oral Solution & Intensol (Oxycodone) 2366
Tylox Capsules 1593

Propoxyphene Hydrochloride (Potential for withdrawal symptoms). Products include:
Darvon 1475
Wygesic Tablets 2930

Propoxyphene Napsylate (Potential for withdrawal symptoms). Products include:
Darvon-N/Darvocet-N 1473

Sufentanil Citrate (Potential for withdrawal symptoms). Products include:
Sufenta Injection 1355

Warfarin Sodium (Effects of aspirin may be deleterious in conjunction with anticoagulant therapy). Products include:
Coumadin 941

Food Interactions

Alcohol (Potential for increased CNS depressant effects).

TALWIN INJECTION
(Pentazocine Lactate) 2465
See **Talwin Ampuls**

TALWIN NX TABLETS
(Pentazocine Hydrochloride, Naloxone Hydrochloride) 2467
May interact with central nervous system depressants, narcotic analgesics, and certain other agents. Compounds in these categories include:

Alfentanil Hydrochloride (Pentozacine is a mild narcotic antagonist and concurrent use may lead to withdrawal symptoms). Products include:
Alfenta Injection 1334

Alprazolam (Potential for additive CNS depressant properties). Products include:
Xanax Tablets 2115

Aprobarbital (Potential for additive CNS depressant properties).
No products indexed under this heading.

Buprenorphine (Pentozacine is a mild narcotic antagonist and concurrent use may lead to withdrawal symptoms). Products include:
Buprenex Injectable 2170

Buspirone Hydrochloride (Potential for additive CNS depressant properties). Products include:
BuSpar Tablets 738

Butabarbital (Potential for additive CNS depressant properties).
No products indexed under this heading.

Butalbital (Potential for additive CNS depressant properties). Products include:
Axocet Capsules 2469
Esgic-plus Capsules 1012
Esgic-plus Tablets 1012
Fioricet Tablets 2386
Fioricet with Codeine Capsules 2387
Fiorinal Capsules 2388
Fiorinal with Codeine Capsules 2390
Fiorinal Tablets 2388
Phrenilin 790
Sedapap Tablets 50 mg/650 mg 1826

Chlordiazepoxide (Potential for additive CNS depressant properties). Products include:
Limbitrol 2333

Chlordiazepoxide Hydrochloride (Potential for additive CNS depressant properties). Products include:
Librax Capsules 2330
Librium Capsules 2331
Librium Injectable 2332

Chlorpromazine (Potential for additive CNS depressant properties). Products include:
Thorazine Suppositories 2701

Chlorpromazine Hydrochloride (Potential for additive CNS depressant properties). Products include:
Thorazine 2701

Chlorprothixene (Potential for additive CNS depressant properties).
No products indexed under this heading.

Chlorprothixene Hydrochloride (Potential for additive CNS depressant properties).
No products indexed under this heading.

Chlorprothixene Lactate (Potential for additive CNS depressant properties).
No products indexed under this heading.

Clorazepate Dipotassium (Potential for additive CNS depressant properties). Products include:
Tranxene 459

Clozapine (Potential for additive CNS depressant properties). Products include:
Clozaril Tablets 2377

Codeine Phosphate (Pentozacine is a mild narcotic antagonist and concurrent use may lead to withdrawal symptoms). Products include:
Brontex 2130
Dimetane-DC Cough Syrup 2232
Fioricet with Codeine Capsules 2387
Fiorinal with Codeine Capsules 2390
Nucofed 2225
Phenergan with Codeine 2883
Phenergan VC with Codeine 2888
Robitussin A-C Syrup 2248
Robitussin-DAC Syrup 2249
Ryna .... ▣ 804
Soma Compound w/Codeine Tablets 2784
Tylenol with Codeine 1592

Desflurane (Potential for additive CNS depressant properties). Products include:
Suprane (desflurane, USP) 1865

Dezocine (Pentozacine is a mild narcotic antagonist and concurrent use may lead to withdrawal symptoms). Products include:
Dalgan Injection 529

Diazepam (Potential for additive CNS depressant properties). Products include:
Dizac (diazepam injectable emulsion) CIV 1862
Valium Injectable 2336
Valium Tablets 2335

Droperidol (Potential for additive CNS depressant properties). Products include:
Inapsine Injection 462

Enflurane (Potential for additive CNS depressant properties).
No products indexed under this heading.

Estazolam (Potential for additive CNS depressant properties). Products include:
ProSom Tablets 457

Ethchlorvynol (Potential for additive CNS depressant properties). Products include:
Placidyl Capsules 456

Ethinamate (Potential for additive CNS depressant properties).
No products indexed under this heading.

Fentanyl (Pentozacine is a mild narcotic antagonist and concurrent use may lead to withdrawal symptoms). Products include:
Duragesic Transdermal System 1336

Fentanyl Citrate (Pentozacine is a mild narcotic antagonist and concurrent use may lead to withdrawal symptoms). Products include:
Sublimaze Injection 463

Fluphenazine Decanoate (Potential for additive CNS depressant properties). Products include:
Prolixin Decanoate 510

Fluphenazine Enanthate (Potential for additive CNS depressant properties). Products include:
Prolixin Enanthate 510

Fluphenazine Hydrochloride (Potential for additive CNS depressant properties). Products include:
Prolixin 510

Flurazepam Hydrochloride (Potential for additive CNS depressant properties). Products include:
Dalmane Capsules 2329

Glutethimide (Potential for additive CNS depressant properties).
No products indexed under this heading.

Haloperidol (Potential for additive CNS depressant properties). Products include:
Haldol Injection, Tablets and Concentrate 1585

Haloperidol Decanoate (Potential for additive CNS depressant properties). Products include:
Haldol Decanoate 1587

Hydrocodone Bitartrate (Pentozacine is a mild narcotic antagonist and concurrent use may lead to withdrawal symptoms). Products include:
Codiclear DH Syrup 808
Duratuss HD Elixir 2750
Histussin D Liquid 670
Hycodan Tablets and Syrup 946
Hycomine Compound Tablets 948
Hycomine 947
Hycotuss Expectorant Syrup 950
Hydrocet Capsules 787
Lorcet 10/650 Tablets 1016
Lortab 2751
Tussend 1830
Tussend Expectorant 1831
Vicodin Tablets 1404
Vicodin ES Tablets 1405
Vicodin HP Tablets 1403
Vicodin Tuss Expectorant 1406
Zydone Capsules 967

Hydrocodone Polistirex (Pentozacine is a mild narcotic antagonist and concurrent use may lead to withdrawal symptoms). Products include:
Tussionex Pennkinetic Extended-Release Suspension 1624

Hydromorphone Hydrochloride (Pentozacine is a mild narcotic antagonist and concurrent use may lead to withdrawal symptoms). Products include:
Dilaudid Ampules 1382
Dilaudid Cough Syrup 1383
Dilaudid-HP Injection 1384
Dilaudid-HP Lyophilized Powder 250 mg 1384
Dilaudid 1382
Dilaudid Oral Liquid 1386
Dilaudid 1382
Dilaudid Tablets - 8 mg 1386

(▣ Described in PDR For Nonprescription Drugs) (◉ Described in PDR For Ophthalmology)

1039 **Interactions Index** **Tambocor**

Hydroxyzine Hydrochloride (Potential for additive CNS depressant properties). Products include:
- Atarax Tablets & Syrup 1992
- Marax Tablets & DF Syrup 2015
- Vistaril Intramuscular Solution 2042

Isoflurane (Potential for additive CNS depressant properties).
- No products indexed under this heading.

Ketamine Hydrochloride (Potential for additive CNS depressant properties).
- No products indexed under this heading.

Levomethadyl Acetate Hydrochloride (Potential for additive CNS depressant properties). Products include:
- Orlaam Oral Solution 2361

Levorphanol Tartrate (Pentozacine is a mild narcotic antagonist and concurrent use may lead to withdrawal symptoms). Products include:
- Levo-Dromoran 2297

Lorazepam (Potential for additive CNS depressant properties). Products include:
- Ativan Injection 2805
- Ativan Tablets 2807

Loxapine Hydrochloride (Potential for additive CNS depressant properties). Products include:
- Loxitane 1426

Loxapine Succinate (Potential for additive CNS depressant properties). Products include:
- Loxitane Capsules 1426

Meperidine Hydrochloride (Pentozacine is a mild narcotic antagonist and concurrent use may lead to withdrawal symptoms). Products include:
- Demerol 2438
- Mepergan Injection 2859

Mephobarbital (Potential for additive CNS depressant properties). Products include:
- Mebaral Tablets 2452

Meprobamate (Potential for additive CNS depressant properties). Products include:
- Miltown Tablets 2780
- PMB 200 and PMB 400 2890

Mesoridazine Besylate (Potential for additive CNS depressant properties). Products include:
- Serentil 689

Methadone Hydrochloride (Pentozacine is a mild narcotic antagonist and concurrent use may lead to withdrawal symptoms). Products include:
- Methadone Hydrochloride Oral Concentrate 2356
- Methadone Hydrochloride Oral Solution & Tablets 2357

Methohexital Sodium (Potential for additive CNS depressant properties).
- No products indexed under this heading.

Methotrimeprazine (Potential for additive CNS depressant properties). Products include:
- Levoprome 1321

Methoxyflurane (Potential for additive CNS depressant properties).
- No products indexed under this heading.

Midazolam Hydrochloride (Potential for additive CNS depressant properties). Products include:
- Versed Injection 2324

Molindone Hydrochloride (Potential for additive CNS depressant properties). Products include:
- Moban Tablets and Concentrate 1036

Morphine Sulfate (Pentozacine is a mild narcotic antagonist and concurrent use may lead to withdrawal symptoms). Products include:
- Astramorph/PF Injection, USP (Preservative-Free) 526
- Duramorph Injection 983
- Infumorph 200 and Infumorph 500 Sterile Solutions 985
- Kadian Capsules 2948
- MS Contin Tablets 2149
- MSIR 2152
- Oramorph SR (Morphine Sulfate Sustained Release Tablets) 2359
- RMS Suppositories CII 2766
- Roxanol 2365

Opium Alkaloids (Pentozacine is a mild narcotic antagonist and concurrent use may lead to withdrawal symptoms).
- No products indexed under this heading.

Oxazepam (Potential for additive CNS depressant properties). Products include:
- Serax Capsules 2916
- Serax Tablets 2916

Oxycodone Hydrochloride (Pentozacine is a mild narcotic antagonist and concurrent use may lead to withdrawal symptoms). Products include:
- OxyContin Tablets 2163
- OxyIR Capsules 2167
- Percocet Tablets 955
- Percodan Tablets 955
- Percodan-Demi Tablets 956
- Roxicodone Tablets, Oral Solution & Intensol (Oxycodone) 2366
- Tylox Capsules 1593

Pentobarbital Sodium (Potential for additive CNS depressant properties). Products include:
- Nembutal Sodium Capsules 440
- Nembutal Sodium Solution 442
- Nembutal Sodium Suppositories 444

Perphenazine (Potential for additive CNS depressant properties). Products include:
- Etrafon 2495
- Triavil Tablets 1800
- Trilafon 2532

Phenobarbital (Potential for additive CNS depressant properties). Products include:
- Arco-Lase Plus Tablets 513
- Bellergal-S Tablets 2375
- Donnatal 2234
- Donnatal Extentabs 2234
- Donnatal Tablets 2234
- Phenobarbital Elixir and Tablets 1523
- Quadrinal Tablets 1398

Prazepam (Potential for additive CNS depressant properties).
- No products indexed under this heading.

Prochlorperazine (Potential for additive CNS depressant properties). Products include:
- Compazine 2644

Promethazine Hydrochloride (Potential for additive CNS depressant properties). Products include:
- Mepergan Injection 2859
- Phenergan with Codeine 2883
- Phenergan with Dextromethorphan 2885
- Phenergan Injection 2880
- Phenergan Suppositories 2882
- Phenergan Syrup 2881
- Phenergan Tablets 2882
- Phenergan VC 2886
- Phenergan VC with Codeine 2888

Propofol (Potential for additive CNS depressant properties). Products include:
- Diprivan Injectable Emulsion 2939

Propoxyphene Hydrochloride (Pentozacine is a mild narcotic antagonist and concurrent use may lead to withdrawal symptoms). Products include:
- Darvon 1475
- Wygesic Tablets 2930

Propoxyphene Napsylate (Pentozacine is a mild narcotic antagonist and concurrent use may lead to withdrawal symptoms). Products include:
- Darvon-N/Darvocet-N 1473

Quazepam (Potential for additive CNS depressant properties). Products include:
- Doral Tablets 2773

Risperidone (Potential for additive CNS depressant properties). Products include:
- Risperdal Tablets 1348

Secobarbital Sodium (Potential for additive CNS depressant properties). Products include:
- Seconal Sodium Pulvules 1529

Sevoflurane (Potential for additive CNS depressant properties).
- No products indexed under this heading.

Sufentanil Citrate (Pentozacine is a mild narcotic antagonist and concurrent use may lead to withdrawal symptoms). Products include:
- Sufenta Injection 1355

Temazepam (Potential for additive CNS depressant properties). Products include:
- Restoril Capsules 2413

Thiamylal Sodium (Potential for additive CNS depressant properties).
- No products indexed under this heading.

Thioridazine Hydrochloride (Potential for additive CNS depressant properties). Products include:
- Mellaril 2398

Thiothixene (Potential for additive CNS depressant properties). Products include:
- Navane Capsules and Concentrate 2018
- Navane Intramuscular 2019

Triazolam (Potential for additive CNS depressant properties). Products include:
- Halcion Tablets 2093

Trifluoperazine Hydrochloride (Potential for additive CNS depressant properties). Products include:
- Stelazine 2692

Zolpidem Tartrate (Potential for additive CNS depressant properties). Products include:
- Ambien Tablets 2559

Food Interactions

Alcohol (May increase CNS depression).

TAMBOCOR TABLETS

(Flecainide Acetate) 1555

May interact with beta blockers and certain other agents. Compounds in these categories include:

Acebutolol Hydrochloride (Possibility of additive negative inotropic effects). Products include:
- Sectral Capsules 2914

Amiodarone Hydrochloride (Increases plasma levels by two-fold or more; reduction of flecainide dose by 50% is recommended). Products include:
- Cordarone Intravenous 2821
- Cordarone Tablets 2818

Atenolol (Possibility of additive negative inotropic effects). Products include:
- Tenoretic Tablets 2963
- Tenormin Tablets and I.V. Injection 2965

Betaxolol Hydrochloride (Possibility of additive negative inotropic effects). Products include:
- Betoptic Ophthalmic Solution 465
- Betoptic S Ophthalmic Suspension 467
- Kerlone Tablets 2588

Bisoprolol Fumarate (Possibility of additive negative inotropic effects). Products include:
- Zebeta Tablets 1457
- Ziac 1459

Carbamazepine (A 30% increase in the rate of flecainide elimination). Products include:
- Atretol Tablets 569
- Tegretol/Tegretol-XR 870

Carteolol Hydrochloride (Possibility of additive negative inotropic effects). Products include:
- Cartrol Tablets 413
- Ocupress Ophthalmic Solution, 1% Sterile .... ◉ 297

Cimetidine (Increases flecainide plasma levels and half-life). Products include:
- Tagamet HB Tablets .... ▣ 786
- Tagamet Tablets 2694

Cimetidine Hydrochloride (Increases flecainide plasma levels and half-life). Products include:
- Tagamet 2694

Digoxin (Concurrent administration increases plasma digoxin levels by a 13% +/− 19%). Products include:
- Lanoxicaps 1110
- Lanoxin Elixir Pediatric 1113
- Lanoxin Injection 1116
- Lanoxin Injection Pediatric 1119
- Lanoxin Tablets 1121

Disopyramide Phosphate (Concurrent administration is not recommended due to negative inotropic properties). Products include:
- Norpace 2596

Esmolol Hydrochloride (Possibility of additive negative inotropic effects). Products include:
- Brevibloc (esmolol HCl) Injection 1860

Labetalol Hydrochloride (Possibility of additive negative inotropic effects). Products include:
- Normodyne Injection 2519
- Normodyne Tablets 2522
- Trandate 1158

Levobunolol Hydrochloride (Possibility of additive negative inotropic effects). Products include:
- Betagan .... ◉ 230

Metipranolol Hydrochloride (Possibility of additive negative inotropic effects). Products include:
- OptiPranolol (Metipranolol 0.3%) Sterile Ophthalmic Solution .... ◉ 256

Metoprolol Succinate (Possibility of additive negative inotropic effects). Products include:
- Toprol-XL Tablets 560

Metoprolol Tartrate (Possibility of additive negative inotropic effects). Products include:
- Lopressor 848
- Lopressor HCT Tablets 850

Nadolol (Possibility of additive negative inotropic effects).
- No products indexed under this heading.

Penbutolol Sulfate (Possibility of additive negative inotropic effects). Products include:
- Levatol Tablets 2547

Phenobarbital (A 30% increase in the rate of flecainide elimination). Products include:
- Arco-Lase Plus Tablets 513
- Bellergal-S Tablets 2375
- Donnatal 2234
- Donnatal Extentabs 2234
- Donnatal Tablets 2234
- Phenobarbital Elixir and Tablets 1523
- Quadrinal Tablets 1398

Phenytoin (A 30% increase in the rate of flecainide elimination). Products include:
- Dilantin Infatabs 1967
- Dilantin-125 Suspension 1969

IMPORTANT NOTE: Always consult each drug listing in the patient's regimen for possible interactions.

Tambocor **Interactions Index** **1040**

Phenytoin Sodium (A 30% increase in the rate of flecainide elimination). Products include:
Dilantin Kapseals ... 1965

Pindolol (Possibility of additive negative inotropic effects). Products include:
Visken Tablets ... 2428

Propranolol Hydrochloride (Increases plasma flecainide levels by 20% and propranolol levels were increased by 30%; additive negative inotropic effects). Products include:
Inderal ... 2834
Inderal LA Long Acting Capsules ... 2836
Inderide Tablets ... 2838
Inderide LA Long Acting Capsules ... 2840

Sotalol Hydrochloride (Possibility of additive negative inotropic effects). Products include:
Betapace Tablets ... 637

Timolol Hemihydrate (Possibility of additive negative inotropic effects). Products include:
Betimol 0.25%, 0.5% ... ⊙ 259

Timolol Maleate (Possibility of additive negative inotropic effects). Products include:
Blocadren Tablets ... 1654
Timolide Tablets ... 1791
Timoptic in Ocudose ... 1796
Timoptic Sterile Ophthalmic Solution ... 1794
Timoptic-XE ... 1798

Verapamil Hydrochloride (Concurrent administration is not recommended due to negative inotropic properties). Products include:
Calan SR Caplets ... 2571
Calan Tablets ... 2568
Covera-HS Tablets ... 2573
Isoptin Injectable ... 1391
Isoptin Oral Tablets ... 1393
Isoptin SR Tablets ... 1395
Verelan Capsules ... 1455

TANAC MEDICATED GEL
(Dyclonine Hydrochloride, Allantoin) ... ▣ 669
None cited in PDR database.

TANAC NO STING LIQUID
(Benzocaine, Benzalkonium Chloride) ... ▣ 669
None cited in PDR database.

TAO CAPSULES
(Troleandomycin) ... 2033
May interact with antimigraine drugs, xanthine bronchodilators, and certain other agents. Compounds in these categories include:

Aminophylline (Elevated serum concentrations of theophylline).
No products indexed under this heading.

Dihydroergotamine Mesylate (May induce ischemic reactions). Products include:
D.H.E. 45 Injection ... 2381

Dyphylline (Elevated serum concentrations of theophylline). Products include:
Lufyllin & Lufyllin-400 Tablets ... 2778
Lufyllin-GG Elixir & Tablets ... 2779

Ergotamine Tartrate (May induce ischemic reactions). Products include:
Bellergal-S Tablets ... 2375
Cafergot ... 2376
Ergomar Tablets ... 1543
Wigraine Tablets ... 1884

Metoclopramide Hydrochloride (May induce ischemic reactions). Products include:
Reglan ... 2243

Theophylline (Elevated serum concentrations of theophylline). Products include:
Marax Tablets & DF Syrup ... 2015
Quibron ... 2227

Theophylline Anhydrous (Elevated serum concentrations of theophylline). Products include:
Aerolate ... 1003
Primatene Tablets ... ▣ 844
Respbid Tablets ... 687
Slo-bid Gyrocaps ... 2201
Theo-24 Extended Release Capsules ... 2753
Theo-Dur Extended-Release Tablets ... 1367
Theo-X Extended-Release Tablets ... 793
Uni-Dur Extended-Release Tablets ... 1374
Uniphyl 400 mg and 600 mg Tablets ... 2157

Theophylline Calcium Salicylate (Elevated serum concentrations of theophylline). Products include:
Quadrinal Tablets ... 1398

Theophylline Sodium Glycinate (Elevated serum concentrations of theophylline).
No products indexed under this heading.

TAPAZOLE TABLETS
(Methimazole) ... 1361
May interact with anticoagulants. Compounds in this category include:

Dalteparin Sodium (Activity of anticoagulant may be potentiated). Products include:
Fragmin Injection ... 2088

Dicumarol (Activity of anticoagulant may be potentiated).
No products indexed under this heading.

Enoxaparin (Activity of anticoagulant may be potentiated). Products include:
Lovenox Injection ... 2187

Heparin Calcium (Activity of anticoagulant may be potentiated).
No products indexed under this heading.

Heparin Sodium (Activity of anticoagulant may be potentiated). Products include:
Heparin Lock Flush Solution ... 2831
Heparin Sodium Injection ... 2832
Heparin Sodium Vials ... 1486

Warfarin Sodium (Activity of anticoagulant may be potentiated). Products include:
Coumadin ... 941

TAVIST SYRUP
(Clemastine Fumarate) ... 2426
May interact with central nervous system depressants, hypnotics and sedatives, tranquilizers, monoamine oxidase inhibitors, and certain other agents. Compounds in these categories include:

Alfentanil Hydrochloride (Additive effects). Products include:
Alfenta Injection ... 1334

Alprazolam (Additive effects). Products include:
Xanax Tablets ... 2115

Aprobarbital (Additive effects).
No products indexed under this heading.

Buprenorphine (Additive effects). Products include:
Buprenex Injectable ... 2170

Buspirone Hydrochloride (Additive effects). Products include:
BuSpar Tablets ... 738

Butabarbital (Additive effects).
No products indexed under this heading.

Butalbital (Additive effects). Products include:
Axocet Capsules ... 2469
Esgic-plus Capsules ... 1012
Esgic-plus Tablets ... 1012
Fioricet Tablets ... 2386
Fioricet with Codeine Capsules ... 2387
Fiorinal Capsules ... 2388
Fiorinal with Codeine Capsules ... 2390
Fiorinal Tablets ... 2388
Phrenilin ... 790
Sedapap Tablets 50 mg/650 mg ... 1826

Chlordiazepoxide (Additive effects). Products include:
Limbitrol ... 2333

Chlordiazepoxide Hydrochloride (Additive effects). Products include:
Librax Capsules ... 2330
Librium Capsules ... 2331
Librium Injectable ... 2332

Chlorpromazine (Additive effects). Products include:
Thorazine Suppositories ... 2701

Chlorprothixene (Additive effects).
No products indexed under this heading.

Chlorprothixene Hydrochloride (Additive effects).
No products indexed under this heading.

Chlorprothixene Lactate (Additive effects).
No products indexed under this heading.

Clorazepate Dipotassium (Additive effects). Products include:
Tranxene ... 459

Clozapine (Additive effects). Products include:
Clozaril Tablets ... 2377

Codeine Phosphate (Additive effects). Products include:
Brontex ... 2130
Dimetane-DC Cough Syrup ... 2232
Fioricet with Codeine Capsules ... 2387
Fiorinal with Codeine Capsules ... 2390
Nucofed ... 2225
Phenergan with Codeine ... 2883
Phenergan VC with Codeine ... 2888
Robitussin A-C Syrup ... 2248
Robitussin-DAC Syrup ... 2249
Ryna ... ▣ 804
Soma Compound w/Codeine Tablets ... 2784
Tylenol with Codeine ... 1592

Desflurane (Additive effects). Products include:
Suprane (desflurane, USP) ... 1865

Dezocine (Additive effects). Products include:
Dalgan Injection ... 529

Diazepam (Additive effects). Products include:
Dizac (diazepam injectable emulsion) CIV ... 1862
Valium Injectable ... 2336
Valium Tablets ... 2335

Droperidol (Additive effects). Products include:
Inapsine Injection ... 462

Enflurane (Additive effects).
No products indexed under this heading.

Estazolam (Additive effects). Products include:
ProSom Tablets ... 457

Ethchlorvynol (Additive effects). Products include:
Placidyl Capsules ... 456

Ethinamate (Additive effects).
No products indexed under this heading.

Fentanyl (Additive effects). Products include:
Duragesic Transdermal System ... 1336

Fentanyl Citrate (Additive effects). Products include:
Sublimaze Injection ... 463

Fluphenazine Decanoate (Additive effects). Products include:
Prolixin Decanoate ... 510

Fluphenazine Enanthate (Additive effects). Products include:
Prolixin Enanthate ... 510

Fluphenazine Hydrochloride (Additive effects). Products include:
Prolixin ... 510

Flurazepam Hydrochloride (Additive effects). Products include:
Dalmane Capsules ... 2329

Furazolidone (Prolongs anticholinergic effects of Tavist). Products include:
Furoxone ... 2221

Glutethimide (Additive effects).
No products indexed under this heading.

Haloperidol (Additive effects). Products include:
Haldol Injection, Tablets and Concentrate ... 1585

Haloperidol Decanoate (Additive effects). Products include:
Haldol Decanoate ... 1587

Hydrocodone Bitartrate (Additive effects). Products include:
Codiclear DH Syrup ... 808
Duratuss HD Elixir ... 2750
Histussin D Liquid ... 670
Hycodan Tablets and Syrup ... 946
Hycomine Compound Tablets ... 948
Hycomine ... 947
Hycotuss Expectorant Syrup ... 950
Hydrocet Capsules ... 787
Lorcet 10/650 Tablets ... 1016
Lortab ... 2751
Tussend ... 1830
Tussend Expectorant ... 1831
Vicodin Tablets ... 1404
Vicodin ES Tablets ... 1405
Vicodin HP Tablets ... 1403
Vicodin Tuss Expectorant ... 1406
Zydone Capsules ... 967

Hydrocodone Polistirex (Additive effects). Products include:
Tussionex Pennkinetic Extended-Release Suspension ... 1624

Hydroxyzine Hydrochloride (Additive effects). Products include:
Atarax Tablets & Syrup ... 1992
Marax Tablets & DF Syrup ... 2015
Vistaril Intramuscular Solution ... 2042

Isocarboxazid (Prolongs anticholinergic effects of Tavist).
No products indexed under this heading.

Isoflurane (Additive effects).
No products indexed under this heading.

Ketamine Hydrochloride (Additive effects).
No products indexed under this heading.

Levomethadyl Acetate Hydrochloride (Additive effects). Products include:
Orlaam Oral Solution ... 2361

Levorphanol Tartrate (Additive effects). Products include:
Levo-Dromoran ... 2297

Lorazepam (Additive effects). Products include:
Ativan Injection ... 2805
Ativan Tablets ... 2807

Loxapine Hydrochloride (Additive effects). Products include:
Loxitane ... 1426

Loxapine Succinate (Additive effects). Products include:
Loxitane Capsules ... 1426

Meperidine Hydrochloride (Additive effects). Products include:
Demerol ... 2438
Mepergan Injection ... 2859

Mephobarbital (Additive effects). Products include:
Mebaral Tablets ... 2452

Meprobamate (Additive effects). Products include:
Miltown Tablets ... 2780
PMB 200 and PMB 400 ... 2890

Mesoridazine Besylate (Additive effects). Products include:
Serentil ... 689

(▣ Described in PDR For Nonprescription Drugs) (⊙ Described in PDR For Ophthalmology)

Methadone Hydrochloride (Additive effects). Products include:
- Methadone Hydrochloride Oral Concentrate 2356
- Methadone Hydrochloride Oral Solution & Tablets 2357

Methohexital Sodium (Additive effects).
- No products indexed under this heading.

Methotrimeprazine (Additive effects). Products include:
- Levoprome 1321

Methoxyflurane (Additive effects).
- No products indexed under this heading.

Midazolam Hydrochloride (Additive effects). Products include:
- Versed Injection 2324

Molindone Hydrochloride (Additive effects). Products include:
- Moban Tablets and Concentrate 1036

Morphine Sulfate (Additive effects). Products include:
- Astramorph/PF Injection, USP (Preservative-Free) 526
- Duramorph Injection 983
- Infumorph 200 and Infumorph 500 Sterile Solutions 985
- Kadian Capsules 2948
- MS Contin Tablets 2149
- MSIR 2152
- Oramorph SR (Morphine Sulfate Sustained Release Tablets) 2359
- RMS Suppositories CII 2766
- Roxanol 2365

Opium Alkaloids (Additive effects).
- No products indexed under this heading.

Oxazepam (Additive effects). Products include:
- Serax Capsules 2916
- Serax Tablets 2916

Oxycodone Hydrochloride (Additive effects). Products include:
- OxyContin Tablets 2163
- OxyIR Capsules 2167
- Percocet Tablets 955
- Percodan Tablets 955
- Percodan-Demi Tablets 956
- Roxicodone Tablets, Oral Solution & Intensol (Oxycodone) 2366
- Tylox Capsules 1593

Pentobarbital Sodium (Additive effects). Products include:
- Nembutal Sodium Capsules 440
- Nembutal Sodium Solution 442
- Nembutal Sodium Suppositories 444

Perphenazine (Additive effects). Products include:
- Etrafon 2495
- Triavil Tablets 1800
- Trilafon 2532

Phenelzine Sulfate (Prolongs anticholinergic effects of Tavist). Products include:
- Nardil 1977

Phenobarbital (Additive effects). Products include:
- Arco-Lase Plus Tablets 513
- Bellergal-S Tablets 2375
- Donnatal 2234
- Donnatal Extentabs 2234
- Donnatal Tablets 2234
- Phenobarbital Elixir and Tablets 1523
- Quadrinal Tablets 1398

Prazepam (Additive effects).
- No products indexed under this heading.

Prochlorperazine (Additive effects). Products include:
- Compazine 2644

Promethazine Hydrochloride (Additive effects). Products include:
- Mepergan Injection 2859
- Phenergan with Codeine 2883
- Phenergan with Dextromethorphan 2885
- Phenergan Injection 2880
- Phenergan Suppositories 2882
- Phenergan Syrup 2881
- Phenergan Tablets 2882
- Phenergan VC 2886
- Phenergan VC with Codeine 2888

Propofol (Additive effects). Products include:
- Diprivan Injectable Emulsion 2939

Propoxyphene Hydrochloride (Additive effects). Products include:
- Darvon 1475
- Wygesic Tablets 2930

Propoxyphene Napsylate (Additive effects). Products include:
- Darvon-N/Darvocet-N 1473

Quazepam (Additive effects). Products include:
- Doral Tablets 2773

Risperidone (Additive effects). Products include:
- Risperdal Tablets 1348

Secobarbital Sodium (Additive effects). Products include:
- Seconal Sodium Pulvules 1529

Selegiline Hydrochloride (Prolongs anticholinergic effects of Tavist). Products include:
- Eldepryl Capsules 2729

Sevoflurane (Additive effects).
- No products indexed under this heading.

Sufentanil Citrate (Additive effects). Products include:
- Sufenta Injection 1355

Temazepam (Additive effects). Products include:
- Restoril Capsules 2413

Thiamylal Sodium (Additive effects).
- No products indexed under this heading.

Thioridazine Hydrochloride (Additive effects). Products include:
- Mellaril 2398

Thiothixene (Additive effects). Products include:
- Navane Capsules and Concentrate 2018
- Navane Intramuscular 2019

Tranylcypromine Sulfate (Prolongs anticholinergic effects of Tavist). Products include:
- Parnate Tablets 2679

Triazolam (Additive effects). Products include:
- Halcion Tablets 2093

Trifluoperazine Hydrochloride (Additive effects). Products include:
- Stelazine 2692

Zolpidem Tartrate (Additive effects). Products include:
- Ambien Tablets 2559

Food Interactions

Alcohol (Additive effects).

TAVIST TABLETS
(Clemastine Fumarate) 2427
May interact with monoamine oxidase inhibitors, central nervous system depressants, hypnotics and sedatives, tranquilizers, and certain other agents. Compounds in these categories include:

Alfentanil Hydrochloride (Additive effects). Products include:
- Alfenta Injection 1334

Alprazolam (Additive effects). Products include:
- Xanax Tablets 2115

Aprobarbital (Additive effects).
- No products indexed under this heading.

Buprenorphine (Additive effects). Products include:
- Buprenex Injectable 2170

Buspirone Hydrochloride (Additive effects). Products include:
- BuSpar Tablets 738

Butabarbital (Additive effects).
- No products indexed under this heading.

Butalbital (Additive effects). Products include:
- Axocet Capsules 2469
- Esgic-plus Capsules 1012
- Esgic-plus Tablets 1012
- Fioricet Tablets 2386
- Fioricet with Codeine Capsules 2387
- Fiorinal Capsules 2388
- Fiorinal with Codeine Capsules 2390
- Fiorinal Tablets 2388
- Phrenilin 790
- Sedapap Tablets 50 mg/650 mg 1826

Chlordiazepoxide (Additive effects). Products include:
- Limbitrol 2333

Chlordiazepoxide Hydrochloride (Additive effects). Products include:
- Librax Capsules 2330
- Librium Capsules 2331
- Librium Injectable 2332

Chlorpromazine (Additive effects). Products include:
- Thorazine Suppositories 2701

Chlorprothixene (Additive effects).
- No products indexed under this heading.

Chlorprothixene Hydrochloride (Additive effects).
- No products indexed under this heading.

Chlorprothixene Lactate (Additive effects).
- No products indexed under this heading.

Clorazepate Dipotassium (Additive effects). Products include:
- Tranxene 459

Clozapine (Additive effects). Products include:
- Clozaril Tablets 2377

Codeine Phosphate (Additive effects). Products include:
- Brontex 2130
- Dimetane-DC Cough Syrup 2232
- Fioricet with Codeine Capsules 2387
- Fiorinal with Codeine Capsules 2390
- Nucofed 2225
- Phenergan with Codeine 2883
- Phenergan VC with Codeine 2888
- Robitussin A-C Syrup 2248
- Robitussin-DAC Syrup 2249
- Ryna 804
- Soma Compound w/Codeine Tablets 2784
- Tylenol with Codeine 1592

Desflurane (Additive effects). Products include:
- Suprane (desflurane, USP) 1865

Dezocine (Additive effects). Products include:
- Dalgan Injection 529

Diazepam (Additive effects). Products include:
- Dizac (diazepam injectable emulsion) CIV 1862
- Valium Injectable 2336
- Valium Tablets 2335

Droperidol (Additive effects). Products include:
- Inapsine Injection 462

Enflurane (Additive effects).
- No products indexed under this heading.

Estazolam (Additive effects). Products include:
- ProSom Tablets 457

Ethchlorvynol (Additive effects). Products include:
- Placidyl Capsules 456

Ethinamate (Additive effects).
- No products indexed under this heading.

Fentanyl (Additive effects). Products include:
- Duragesic Transdermal System 1336

Fentanyl Citrate (Additive effects). Products include:
- Sublimaze Injection 463

Fluphenazine Decanoate (Additive effects). Products include:
- Prolixin Decanoate 510

Fluphenazine Enanthate (Additive effects). Products include:
- Prolixin Enanthate 510

Fluphenazine Hydrochloride (Additive effects). Products include:
- Prolixin 510

Flurazepam Hydrochloride (Additive effects). Products include:
- Dalmane Capsules 2329

Furazolidone (Prolongs anticholinergic effects of Tavist; concurrent use is contraindicated). Products include:
- Furoxone 2221

Glutethimide (Additive effects).
- No products indexed under this heading.

Haloperidol (Additive effects). Products include:
- Haldol Injection, Tablets and Concentrate 1585

Haloperidol Decanoate (Additive effects). Products include:
- Haldol Decanoate 1587

Hydrocodone Bitartrate (Additive effects). Products include:
- Codiclear DH Syrup 808
- Duratuss HD Elixir 2750
- Histussin D Liquid 670
- Hycodan Tablets and Syrup 946
- Hycomine Compound Tablets 948
- Hycomine 947
- Hycotuss Expectorant Syrup 950
- Hydrocet Capsules 787
- Lorcet 10/650 Tablets 1016
- Lortab 2751
- Tussend 1830
- Tussend Expectorant 1831
- Vicodin Tablets 1404
- Vicodin ES Tablets 1405
- Vicodin HP Tablets 1403
- Vicodin Tuss Expectorant 1406
- Zydone Capsules 967

Hydrocodone Polistirex (Additive effects). Products include:
- Tussionex Pennkinetic Extended-Release Suspension 1624

Hydroxyzine Hydrochloride (Additive effects). Products include:
- Atarax Tablets & Syrup 1992
- Marax Tablets & DF Syrup 2015
- Vistaril Intramuscular Solution 2042

Isocarboxazid (Prolongs anticholinergic effects of Tavist; concurrent use is contraindicated).
- No products indexed under this heading.

Isoflurane (Additive effects).
- No products indexed under this heading.

Ketamine Hydrochloride (Additive effects).
- No products indexed under this heading.

Levomethadyl Acetate Hydrochloride (Additive effects). Products include:
- Orlaam Oral Solution 2361

Levorphanol Tartrate (Additive effects). Products include:
- Levo-Dromoran 2297

Lorazepam (Additive effects). Products include:
- Ativan Injection 2805
- Ativan Tablets 2807

Loxapine Hydrochloride (Additive effects). Products include:
- Loxitane 1426

Loxapine Succinate (Additive effects). Products include:
- Loxitane Capsules 1426

IMPORTANT NOTE: Always consult each drug listing in the patient's regimen for possible interactions.

Tavist Tablets / Interactions Index

Meperidine Hydrochloride (Additive effects). Products include:
- Demerol ... 2438
- Mepergan Injection ... 2859

Mephobarbital (Additive effects). Products include:
- Mebaral Tablets ... 2452

Meprobamate (Additive effects). Products include:
- Miltown Tablets ... 2780
- PMB 200 and PMB 400 ... 2890

Mesoridazine Besylate (Additive effects). Products include:
- Serentil ... 689

Methadone Hydrochloride (Additive effects). Products include:
- Methadone Hydrochloride Oral Concentrate ... 2356
- Methadone Hydrochloride Oral Solution & Tablets ... 2357

Methohexital Sodium (Additive effects).
No products indexed under this heading.

Methotrimeprazine (Additive effects). Products include:
- Levoprome ... 1321

Methoxyflurane (Additive effects).
No products indexed under this heading.

Midazolam Hydrochloride (Additive effects). Products include:
- Versed Injection ... 2324

Molindone Hydrochloride (Additive effects). Products include:
- Moban Tablets and Concentrate ... 1036

Morphine Sulfate (Additive effects). Products include:
- Astramorph/PF Injection, USP (Preservative-Free) ... 526
- Duramorph Injection ... 983
- Infumorph 200 and Infumorph 500 Sterile Solutions ... 985
- Kadian Capsules ... 2948
- MS Contin Tablets ... 2149
- MSIR ... 2152
- Oramorph SR (Morphine Sulfate Sustained Release Tablets) ... 2359
- RMS Suppositories CII ... 2766
- Roxanol ... 2365

Opium Alkaloids (Additive effects).
No products indexed under this heading.

Oxazepam (Additive effects). Products include:
- Serax Capsules ... 2916
- Serax Tablets ... 2916

Oxycodone Hydrochloride (Additive effects). Products include:
- OxyContin Tablets ... 2163
- OxyIR Capsules ... 2167
- Percocet Tablets ... 955
- Percodan Tablets ... 955
- Percodan-Demi Tablets ... 956
- Roxicodone Tablets, Oral Solution & Intensol (Oxycodone) ... 2366
- Tylox Capsules ... 1593

Pentobarbital Sodium (Additive effects). Products include:
- Nembutal Sodium Capsules ... 440
- Nembutal Sodium Solution ... 442
- Nembutal Sodium Suppositories ... 444

Perphenazine (Additive effects). Products include:
- Etrafon ... 2495
- Triavil Tablets ... 1800
- Trilafon ... 2532

Phenelzine Sulfate (Prolongs anticholinergic effects of Tavist; concurrent use is contraindicated). Products include:
- Nardil ... 1977

Phenobarbital (Additive effects). Products include:
- Arco-Lase Plus Tablets ... 513
- Bellergal-S Tablets ... 2375
- Donnatal ... 2234
- Donnatal Extentabs ... 2234
- Donnatal Tablets ... 2234
- Phenobarbital Elixir and Tablets ... 1523
- Quadrinal Tablets ... 1398

Prazepam (Additive effects).
No products indexed under this heading.

Prochlorperazine (Additive effects). Products include:
- Compazine ... 2644

Promethazine Hydrochloride (Additive effects). Products include:
- Mepergan Injection ... 2859
- Phenergan with Codeine ... 2883
- Phenergan with Dextromethorphan ... 2885
- Phenergan Injection ... 2880
- Phenergan Suppositories ... 2882
- Phenergan Syrup ... 2881
- Phenergan Tablets ... 2882
- Phenergan VC ... 2886
- Phenergan VC with Codeine ... 2888

Propofol (Additive effects). Products include:
- Diprivan Injectable Emulsion ... 2939

Propoxyphene Hydrochloride (Additive effects). Products include:
- Darvon ... 1475
- Wygesic Tablets ... 2930

Propoxyphene Napsylate (Additive effects). Products include:
- Darvon-N/Darvocet-N ... 1473

Quazepam (Additive effects). Products include:
- Doral Tablets ... 2773

Risperidone (Additive effects). Products include:
- Risperdal Tablets ... 1348

Secobarbital Sodium (Additive effects). Products include:
- Seconal Sodium Pulvules ... 1529

Selegiline Hydrochloride (Prolongs anticholinergic effects of Tavist; concurrent use is contraindicated). Products include:
- Eldepryl Capsules ... 2729

Sevoflurane (Additive effects).
No products indexed under this heading.

Sufentanil Citrate (Additive effects). Products include:
- Sufenta Injection ... 1355

Temazepam (Additive effects). Products include:
- Restoril Capsules ... 2413

Thiamylal Sodium (Additive effects).
No products indexed under this heading.

Thioridazine Hydrochloride (Additive effects). Products include:
- Mellaril ... 2398

Thiothixene (Additive effects). Products include:
- Navane Capsules and Concentrate ... 2018
- Navane Intramuscular ... 2019

Tranylcypromine Sulfate (Prolongs anticholinergic effects of Tavist; concurrent use is contraindicated). Products include:
- Parnate Tablets ... 2679

Triazolam (Additive effects). Products include:
- Halcion Tablets ... 2093

Trifluoperazine Hydrochloride (Additive effects). Products include:
- Stelazine ... 2692

Zolpidem Tartrate (Additive effects). Products include:
- Ambien Tablets ... 2559

Food Interactions

Alcohol (Additive effects).

TAVIST-1 12 HOUR RELIEF TABLETS
(Clemastine Fumarate) ... ⊞ 749
May interact with hypnotics and sedatives, tranquilizers, and certain other agents. Compounds in these categories include:

Alprazolam (May increase drowsiness effect). Products include:
- Xanax Tablets ... 2115

Buspirone Hydrochloride (May increase drowsiness effect). Products include:
- BuSpar Tablets ... 738

Chlordiazepoxide (May increase drowsiness effect). Products include:
- Limbitrol ... 2333

Chlordiazepoxide Hydrochloride (May increase drowsiness effect). Products include:
- Librax Capsules ... 2330
- Librium Capsules ... 2331
- Librium Injectable ... 2332

Chlorpromazine (May increase drowsiness effect). Products include:
- Thorazine Suppositories ... 2701

Chlorpromazine Hydrochloride (May increase drowsiness effect). Products include:
- Thorazine ... 2701

Chlorprothixene (May increase drowsiness effect).
No products indexed under this heading.

Chlorprothixene Hydrochloride (May increase drowsiness effect).
No products indexed under this heading.

Clorazepate Dipotassium (May increase drowsiness effect). Products include:
- Tranxene ... 459

Diazepam (May increase drowsiness effect). Products include:
- Dizac (diazepam injectable emulsion) CIV ... 1862
- Valium Injectable ... 2336
- Valium Tablets ... 2335

Droperidol (May increase drowsiness effect). Products include:
- Inapsine Injection ... 462

Estazolam (May increase drowsiness effect). Products include:
- ProSom Tablets ... 457

Ethchlorvynol (May increase drowsiness effect). Products include:
- Placidyl Capsules ... 456

Ethinamate (May increase drowsiness effect).
No products indexed under this heading.

Fluphenazine Decanoate (May increase drowsiness effect). Products include:
- Prolixin Decanoate ... 510

Fluphenazine Enanthate (May increase drowsiness effect). Products include:
- Prolixin Enanthate ... 510

Fluphenazine Hydrochloride (May increase drowsiness effect). Products include:
- Prolixin ... 510

Flurazepam Hydrochloride (May increase drowsiness effect). Products include:
- Dalmane Capsules ... 2329

Glutethimide (May increase drowsiness effect).
No products indexed under this heading.

Haloperidol (May increase drowsiness effect). Products include:
- Haldol Injection, Tablets and Concentrate ... 1585

Haloperidol Decanoate (May increase drowsiness effect). Products include:
- Haldol Decanoate ... 1587

Hydroxyzine Hydrochloride (May increase drowsiness effect). Products include:
- Atarax Tablets & Syrup ... 1992
- Marax Tablets & DF Syrup ... 2015
- Vistaril Intramuscular Solution ... 2042

Lorazepam (May increase drowsiness effect). Products include:
- Ativan Injection ... 2805
- Ativan Tablets ... 2807

Loxapine Hydrochloride (May increase drowsiness effect). Products include:
- Loxitane ... 1426

Loxapine Succinate (May increase drowsiness effect). Products include:
- Loxitane Capsules ... 1426

Meprobamate (May increase drowsiness effect). Products include:
- Miltown Tablets ... 2780
- PMB 200 and PMB 400 ... 2890

Mesoridazine Besylate (May increase drowsiness effect). Products include:
- Serentil ... 689

Midazolam Hydrochloride (May increase drowsiness effect). Products include:
- Versed Injection ... 2324

Molindone Hydrochloride (May increase drowsiness effect). Products include:
- Moban Tablets and Concentrate ... 1036

Oxazepam (May increase drowsiness effect). Products include:
- Serax Capsules ... 2916
- Serax Tablets ... 2916

Perphenazine (May increase drowsiness effect). Products include:
- Etrafon ... 2495
- Triavil Tablets ... 1800
- Trilafon ... 2532

Prazepam (May increase drowsiness effect).
No products indexed under this heading.

Prochlorperazine (May increase drowsiness effect). Products include:
- Compazine ... 2644

Promethazine Hydrochloride (May increase drowsiness effect). Products include:
- Mepergan Injection ... 2859
- Phenergan with Codeine ... 2883
- Phenergan with Dextromethorphan ... 2885
- Phenergan Injection ... 2880
- Phenergan Suppositories ... 2882
- Phenergan Syrup ... 2881
- Phenergan Tablets ... 2882
- Phenergan VC ... 2886
- Phenergan VC with Codeine ... 2888

Propofol (May increase drowsiness effect). Products include:
- Diprivan Injectable Emulsion ... 2939

Quazepam (May increase drowsiness effect). Products include:
- Doral Tablets ... 2773

Secobarbital Sodium (May increase drowsiness effect). Products include:
- Seconal Sodium Pulvules ... 1529

Temazepam (May increase drowsiness effect). Products include:
- Restoril Capsules ... 2413

Thioridazine Hydrochloride (May increase drowsiness effect). Products include:
- Mellaril ... 2398

Thiothixene (May increase drowsiness effect). Products include:
- Navane Capsules and Concentrate ... 2018
- Navane Intramuscular ... 2019

Triazolam (May increase drowsiness effect). Products include:
- Halcion Tablets ... 2093

(⊞ Described in PDR For Nonprescription Drugs) (◎ Described in PDR For Ophthalmology)

Trifluoperazine Hydrochloride (May increase drowsiness effect). Products include:
- Stelazine 2692

Zolpidem Tartrate (May increase drowsiness effect). Products include:
- Ambien Tablets 2559

Food Interactions
Alcohol (May increase drowsiness effect).

TAVIST-D 12 HOUR RELIEF TABLETS
(Clemastine Fumarate, Phenylpropanolamine Hydrochloride) ..... ⊕ 750

May interact with hypnotics and sedatives, tranquilizers, antidepressant drugs, antihypertensives, and certain other agents. Compounds in these categories include:

Acebutolol Hydrochloride (Effect of concurrent use not specified). Products include:
- Sectral Capsules 2914

Alprazolam (Increases drowsiness effect). Products include:
- Xanax Tablets 2115

Amitriptyline Hydrochloride (Effect of concurrent use not specified). Products include:
- Elavil 2945
- Etrafon 2495
- Limbitrol 2333
- Triavil Tablets 1800

Amlodipine Besylate (Effect of concurrent use not specified). Products include:
- Lotrel Capsules 858
- Norvasc Tablets 2020

Amoxapine (Effect of concurrent use not specified). Products include:
- Asendin Tablets 1419

Atenolol (Effect of concurrent use not specified). Products include:
- Tenoretic Tablets 2963
- Tenormin Tablets and I.V. Injection 2965

Benazepril Hydrochloride (Effect of concurrent use not specified). Products include:
- Lotensin Tablets 852
- Lotensin HCT Tablets 855
- Lotrel Capsules 858

Bendroflumethiazide (Effect of concurrent use not specified).
No products indexed under this heading.

Betaxolol Hydrochloride (Effect of concurrent use not specified). Products include:
- Betoptic Ophthalmic Solution 465
- Betoptic S Ophthalmic Suspension 467
- Kerlone Tablets 2588

Bisoprolol Fumarate (Effect of concurrent use not specified). Products include:
- Zebeta Tablets 1457
- Ziac 1459

Bupropion Hydrochloride (Effect of concurrent use not specified). Products include:
- Wellbutrin Tablets 1177

Buspirone Hydrochloride (Increases drowsiness effect). Products include:
- BuSpar Tablets 738

Captopril (Effect of concurrent use not specified). Products include:
- Capoten Tablets 740
- Capozide Tablets 744

Carteolol Hydrochloride (Effect of concurrent use not specified). Products include:
- Cartrol Tablets 413
- Ocupress Ophthalmic Solution, 1% Sterile ..... ⊕ 297

Chlordiazepoxide (Increases drowsiness effect). Products include:
- Limbitrol 2333

Chlordiazepoxide Hydrochloride (Increases drowsiness effect). Products include:
- Librax Capsules 2330
- Librium Capsules 2331
- Librium Injectable 2332

Chlorothiazide (Effect of concurrent use not specified). Products include:
- Aldoclor Tablets 1638
- Diupres Tablets 1691
- Diuril Oral 1694

Chlorothiazide Sodium (Effect of concurrent use not specified). Products include:
- Diuril Sodium Intravenous 1693

Chlorpromazine (Increases drowsiness effect). Products include:
- Thorazine Suppositories 2701

Chlorpromazine Hydrochloride (Increases drowsiness effect). Products include:
- Thorazine 2701

Chlorprothixene (Increases drowsiness effect).
No products indexed under this heading.

Chlorprothixene Hydrochloride (Increases drowsiness effect).
No products indexed under this heading.

Chlorthalidone (Effect of concurrent use not specified). Products include:
- Combipres Tablets 682
- Tenoretic Tablets 2963
- Thalitone 1293

Clonidine (Effect of concurrent use not specified). Products include:
- Catapres-TTS 680

Clonidine Hydrochloride (Effect of concurrent use not specified). Products include:
- Catapres Tablets 679
- Combipres Tablets 682

Clorazepate Dipotassium (Increases drowsiness effect). Products include:
- Tranxene 459

Deserpidine (Effect of concurrent use not specified).
No products indexed under this heading.

Desipramine Hydrochloride (Effect of concurrent use not specified). Products include:
- Norpramin Tablets 1273

Diazepam (Increases drowsiness effect). Products include:
- Dizac (diazepam injectable emulsion) CIV 1862
- Valium Injectable 2336
- Valium Tablets 2335

Diazoxide (Effect of concurrent use not specified). Products include:
- Hyperstat I.V. Injection 2504
- Proglycem 575

Diltiazem Hydrochloride (Effect of concurrent use not specified). Products include:
- Cardizem CD Capsules 1251
- Cardizem SR Capsules 1255
- Cardizem Injectable 1253
- Cardizem Tablets 1257
- Dilacor XR Extended-release Capsules 2183
- Tiazac Capsules 1019

Doxazosin Mesylate (Effect of concurrent use not specified). Products include:
- Cardura Tablets 1993

Doxepin Hydrochloride (Effect of concurrent use not specified). Products include:
- Adapin Capsules 1542

- Sinequan 2028
- Zonalon Cream 1042

Droperidol (Increases drowsiness effect). Products include:
- Inapsine Injection 462

Enalapril Maleate (Effect of concurrent use not specified). Products include:
- Vaseretic Tablets 1810
- Vasotec Tablets 1816

Enalaprilat (Effect of concurrent use not specified). Products include:
- Vasotec I.V. 1814

Esmolol Hydrochloride (Effect of concurrent use not specified). Products include:
- Brevibloc (esmolol HCl) Injection 1860

Estazolam (Increases drowsiness effect). Products include:
- ProSom Tablets 457

Ethchlorvynol (Increases drowsiness effect). Products include:
- Placidyl Capsules 456

Ethinamate (Increases drowsiness effect).
No products indexed under this heading.

Felodipine (Effect of concurrent use not specified). Products include:
- Plendil Extended-Release Tablets 514

Fluoxetine Hydrochloride (Effect of concurrent use not specified). Products include:
- Prozac Pulvules & Liquid, Oral Solution 935

Fluphenazine Decanoate (Increases drowsiness effect). Products include:
- Prolixin Decanoate 510

Fluphenazine Enanthate (Increases drowsiness effect). Products include:
- Prolixin Enanthate 510

Fluphenazine Hydrochloride (Increases drowsiness effect). Products include:
- Prolixin 510

Flurazepam Hydrochloride (Increases drowsiness effect). Products include:
- Dalmane Capsules 2329

Fosinopril Sodium (Effect of concurrent use not specified). Products include:
- Monopril Tablets 762

Furosemide (Effect of concurrent use not specified). Products include:
- Lasix Injection, Oral Solution and Tablets 1267

Glutethimide (Increases drowsiness effect).
No products indexed under this heading.

Guanabenz Acetate (Effect of concurrent use not specified).
No products indexed under this heading.

Guanethidine Monosulfate (Effect of concurrent use not specified). Products include:
- Esimil Tablets 840
- Ismelin Tablets 845

Haloperidol (Increases drowsiness effect). Products include:
- Haldol Injection, Tablets and Concentrate 1585

Haloperidol Decanoate (Increases drowsiness effect). Products include:
- Haldol Decanoate 1587

Hydralazine Hydrochloride (Effect of concurrent use not specified). Products include:
- Apresazide Capsules 824
- Apresoline Hydrochloride Tablets 826
- Hydralazine Hydrochloride Injection USP 2712

- Ser-Ap-Es Tablets 867

Hydrochlorothiazide (Effect of concurrent use not specified). Products include:
- Aldactazide Tablets 2556
- Aldoril Tablets 1644
- Apresazide Capsules 824
- Capozide Tablets 744
- Dyazide Capsules 2653
- Esidrix Tablets 839
- Esimil Tablets 840
- HydroDIURIL Tablets 1716
- Hydropres Tablets 1718
- Hyzaar Tablets 1720
- Inderide Tablets 2838
- Inderide LA Long Acting Capsules 2840
- Lopressor HCT Tablets 850
- Lotensin HCT Tablets 855
- Moduretic Tablets 1748
- Oretic Tablets 450
- Prinzide Tablets 1780
- Ser-Ap-Es Tablets 867
- Timolide Tablets 1791
- Vaseretic Tablets 1810
- Zestoretic Tablets 2968
- Ziac 1459

Hydroflumethiazide (Effect of concurrent use not specified). Products include:
- Diucardin Tablets 2824

Hydroxyzine Hydrochloride (Increases drowsiness effect). Products include:
- Atarax Tablets & Syrup 1992
- Marax Tablets & DF Syrup 2015
- Vistaril Intramuscular Solution 2042

Imipramine Hydrochloride (Effect of concurrent use not specified). Products include:
- Tofranil Ampuls 873
- Tofranil Tablets 875

Imipramine Pamoate (Effect of concurrent use not specified). Products include:
- Tofranil-PM Capsules 876

Indapamide (Effect of concurrent use not specified).
No products indexed under this heading.

Isocarboxazid (Effect of concurrent use not specified).
No products indexed under this heading.

Isradipine (Effect of concurrent use not specified). Products include:
- DynaCirc Capsules 2381
- DynaCirc CR Tablets 2383

Labetalol Hydrochloride (Effect of concurrent use not specified). Products include:
- Normodyne Injection 2519
- Normodyne Tablets 2522
- Trandate 1158

Lisinopril (Effect of concurrent use not specified). Products include:
- Prinivil Tablets 1776
- Prinzide Tablets 1780
- Zestoretic Tablets 2968
- Zestril Tablets 2972

Lorazepam (Increases drowsiness effect). Products include:
- Ativan Injection 2805
- Ativan Tablets 2807

Losartan Potassium (Effect of concurrent use not specified). Products include:
- Cozaar Tablets 1668
- Hyzaar Tablets 1720

Loxapine Hydrochloride (Increases drowsiness effect). Products include:
- Loxitane 1426

Loxapine Succinate (Increases drowsiness effect). Products include:
- Loxitane Capsules 1426

Maprotiline Hydrochloride (Effect of concurrent use not specified). Products include:
- Ludiomil Tablets 861

IMPORTANT NOTE: Always consult each drug listing in the patient's regimen for possible interactions.

Mecamylamine Hydrochloride (Effect of concurrent use not specified). Products include:
Inversine Tablets ... 1729
Meprobamate (Increases drowsiness effect). Products include:
Miltown Tablets ... 2780
PMB 200 and PMB 400 ... 2890
Mesoridazine Besylate (Increases drowsiness effect). Products include:
Serentil ... 689
Methyclothiazide (Effect of concurrent use not specified). Products include:
Enduron Tablets ... 424
Methyldopa (Effect of concurrent use not specified). Products include:
Aldoclor Tablets ... 1638
Aldomet Oral ... 1640
Aldoril Tablets ... 1644
Methyldopate Hydrochloride (Effect of concurrent use not specified). Products include:
Aldomet Ester HCl Injection ... 1642
Metolazone (Effect of concurrent use not specified). Products include:
Mykrox Tablets ... 1617
Zaroxolyn Tablets ... 1625
Metoprolol Succinate (Effect of concurrent use not specified). Products include:
Toprol-XL Tablets ... 560
Metoprolol Tartrate (Effect of concurrent use not specified). Products include:
Lopressor ... 848
Lopressor HCT Tablets ... 850
Metyrosine (Effect of concurrent use not specified). Products include:
Demser Capsules ... 1690
Midazolam Hydrochloride (Increases drowsiness effect). Products include:
Versed Injection ... 2324
Minoxidil (Effect of concurrent use not specified).
No products indexed under this heading.
Moexipril Hydrochloride (Effect of concurrent use not specified). Products include:
Univasc Tablets ... 2553
Molindone Hydrochloride (Increases drowsiness effect). Products include:
Moban Tablets and Concentrate ... 1036
Nadolol (Effect of concurrent use not specified).
No products indexed under this heading.
Nefazodone Hydrochloride (Effect of concurrent use not specified). Products include:
Serzone Tablets ... 776
Nicardipine Hydrochloride (Effect of concurrent use not specified). Products include:
Cardene Capsules ... 2261
Cardene I.V. ... 2815
Cardene SR Capsules ... 2264
Nifedipine (Effect of concurrent use not specified). Products include:
Adalat Capsules (10 mg and 20 mg) ... 580
Adalat CC ... 582
Procardia Capsules ... 2024
Procardia XL Extended Release Tablets ... 2026
Nisoldipine (Effect of concurrent use not specified). Products include:
Sular Tablets ... 2961
Nitroglycerin (Effect of concurrent use not specified). Products include:
Deponit NTG Transdermal Delivery System ... 2541
Nitro-Bid IV ... 1270
Nitro-Bid Ointment ... 1272
Nitro-Dur (nitroglycerin) Transdermal Infusion System ... 1365
Nitrolingual Spray ... 2193
Nitrostat Tablets ... 1981
Transderm-Nitro Transdermal Therapeutic System ... 878
Nortriptyline Hydrochloride (Effect of concurrent use not specified). Products include:
Pamelor ... 2409
Oxazepam (Increases drowsiness effect). Products include:
Serax Capsules ... 2916
Serax Tablets ... 2916
Paroxetine Hydrochloride (Effect of concurrent use not specified). Products include:
Paxil Tablets ... 2681
Penbutolol Sulfate (Effect of concurrent use not specified). Products include:
Levatol Tablets ... 2547
Perphenazine (Increases drowsiness effect). Products include:
Etrafon ... 2495
Triavil Tablets ... 1800
Trilafon ... 2532
Phenelzine Sulfate (Effect of concurrent use not specified). Products include:
Nardil ... 1977
Phenoxybenzamine Hydrochloride (Effect of concurrent use not specified). Products include:
Dibenzyline Capsules ... 2650
Phentolamine Mesylate (Effect of concurrent use not specified). Products include:
Regitine Vials ... 864
Phenylephrine Hydrochloride (Effect of concurrent use not specified). Products include:
Atrohist Plus Tablets ... 1605
Cerose DM ... ▣ 853
D.A. II Tablets ... 972
D.A. Chewable Tablets ... 970
Dura-Vent/DA Tablets ... 972
Extendryl ... 1003
4-Way Fast Acting Nasal Spray (regular & mentholated) ... ▣ 644
Hemorid ... ▣ 797
Hycomine Compound Tablets ... 948
Neo-Synephrine Hydrochloride 1% Carpuject ... 2455
Neo-Synephrine Hydrochloride 1% Injection ... 2455
Neo-Synephrine Hydrochloride (Ophthalmic) ... 2456
Neo-Synephrine ... ▣ 624
Novahistine Elixir ... ▣ 782
Phenergan VC ... 2886
Phenergan VC with Codeine ... 2888
Preparation H ... ▣ 842
Tympagesic Ear Drops ... 2476
Vicks Sinex Nasal Spray and Ultra Fine Mist ... ▣ 738
Pindolol (Effect of concurrent use not specified). Products include:
Visken Tablets ... 2428
Polythiazide (Effect of concurrent use not specified). Products include:
Minizide Capsules ... 2016
Prazepam (Increases drowsiness effect).
No products indexed under this heading.
Prazosin Hydrochloride (Effect of concurrent use not specified). Products include:
Minipress Capsules ... 2015
Minizide Capsules ... 2016
Prochlorperazine (Increases drowsiness effect). Products include:
Compazine ... 2644
Promethazine Hydrochloride (Increases drowsiness effect). Products include:
Mepergan Injection ... 2859
Phenergan with Codeine ... 2883
Phenergan with Dextromethorphan ... 2885
Phenergan Injection ... 2880
Phenergan Suppositories ... 2882
Phenergan Syrup ... 2881
Phenergan Tablets ... 2882
Phenergan VC ... 2886
Phenergan VC with Codeine ... 2888
Propofol (Increases drowsiness effect). Products include:
Diprivan Injectable Emulsion ... 2939
Propranolol Hydrochloride (Effect of concurrent use not specified). Products include:
Inderal ... 2834
Inderal LA Long Acting Capsules ... 2836
Inderide Tablets ... 2838
Inderide LA Long Acting Capsules .. 2840
Protriptyline Hydrochloride (Effect of concurrent use not specified). Products include:
Vivactil Tablets ... 1820
Pseudoephedrine Hydrochloride (Effect of concurrent use not specified). Products include:
Actifed Allergy Daytime/Nighttime Caplets ... ▣ 808
Actifed Cold & Allergy Tablets ... ▣ 807
Actifed Cold & Sinus Caplets and Tablets ... ▣ 808
Actifed Sinus Daytime/Nighttime Tablets and Caplets ... ▣ 809
Advil Cold and Sinus Caplets and Tablets ... ▣ 837
Alka-Seltzer Plus Liqui-Gels ... ▣ 612
Alka-Seltzer Plus Flu & Body Aches Liqui-Gels Non-Drowsy Formula ... ▣ 613
Alka-Seltzer Plus Night-Time Cold Medicine Liqui-Gels ... ▣ 612
Allerest Maximum Strength ... ▣ 649
Allerest No Drowsiness ... ▣ 649
Allerest Sinus Pain Formula ... ▣ 649
Atrohist Pediatric Capsules ... 1603
Benadryl Allergy/Cold Tablets ... ▣ 811
Benadryl Allergy Decongestant Liquid Medication ... ▣ 812
Benadryl Allergy Decongestant Tablets ... ▣ 812
Benadryl Allergy Sinus Headache Caplets ... ▣ 813
Benylin Multisymptom ... ▣ 816
Bromfed Capsules (Extended-Release) ... 1832
Bromfed Syrup ... ▣ 712
Bromfed Tablets ... 1832
Bromfed-DM Cough Syrup ... 1832
Bromfed-PD Capsules (Extended-Release) ... 1832
Children's TYLENOL Cold Multi-Symptom Chewable Tablets and Liquid ... 1559
Children's TYLENOL Cold Plus Cough Multi Symptom Chewable Tablets and Liquid ... 1560
Children's TYLENOL Flu Suspension Liquid ... 1560
Children's Vicks DayQuil Allergy Relief ... ▣ 730
Children's Vicks NyQuil Cold/Cough Relief ... ▣ 731
Allergy-Sinus Comtrex Multi-Symptom Allergy-Sinus Formula Tablets and Caplets ... ▣ 639
Comtrex Multi-Symptom ... ▣ 638
Comtrex Multi-Symptom Non-Drowsy Caplets ... ▣ 640
Congess ... 1003
Contac Day Allergy/Sinus Caplets ▣ 771
Contac Day & Night ... ▣ 772
Contac Night Allergy/Sinus Caplets ... ▣ 771
Contac Severe Cold & Flu Non-Drowsy ... ▣ 774
Deconsal II Tablets ... 1605
Dimetane-DX Cough Syrup ... 2233
Dimetapp Cold & Fever Suspension ... ▣ 839
Dimetapp Decongestant Pediatric Drops ... ▣ 840
Dorcol Children's Cough Syrup ... ▣ 748
Drixoral Cough + Congestion Liquid Caps ... ▣ 763
Dura-Tap/PD Capsules ... 970
Duratuss Tablets ... 2750
Duratuss HD Elixir ... 2750
Efidac/24 ... ▣ 655
Entex PSE Tablets ... 973
Fedahist Gyrocaps ... 2545
Guaifed ... 1833
Guaifed Syrup ... ▣ 712
Guaimax-D Tablets ... 809
Histussin D Liquid ... 670
Infants' TYLENOL Cold Decongestant & Fever-Reducer Drops ... 1561
Kronofed-A ... 994
Novahistine DMX ... ▣ 782
Nucofed ... 2225
PediaCare Cough-Cold Chewable Tablets and Liquid ... 1569
PediaCare Infants' Decongestant Drops ... 1569
PediaCare Infants' Drops Decongestant Plus Cough ... 1569
PediaCare NightRest Cough-Cold Liquid ... 1569
Pediatric Vicks 44d Cough & Head Congestion Relief ... ▣ 736
Pediatric Vicks 44m Cough & Cold Relief ... ▣ 737
Robitussin Cold & Cough Liqui-Gels ... ▣ 844
Robitussin Cold, Cough & Flu Liqui-Gels ... ▣ 844
Robitussin Maximum Strength Cough & Cold ... ▣ 847
Robitussin Night-Time Cold Formula ... ▣ 847
Robitussin Pediatric Cough & Cold Formula ... ▣ 848
Robitussin Pediatric Drops ... ▣ 849
Robitussin Severe Congestion Liqui-Gels ... ▣ 845
Robitussin-DAC Syrup ... 2249
Robitussin-PE ... ▣ 846
Rondec Oral Drops ... 974
Rondec Syrup ... 974
Rondec Tablet ... 974
Rondec Chewable Tablets ... 974
Rondec-TR Tablet ... 974
Ryna ... ▣ 804
Seldane-D Extended-Release Tablets ... 1286
Semprex-D Capsules ... 1620
Sinarest ... ▣ 663
Sine-Aid Maximum Strength Sinus Headache Gelcaps, Caplets and Tablets ... 1570
Sine-Off No Drowsiness Formula Caplets ... ▣ 784
Sine-Off Sinus Medicine ... ▣ 784
Singlet Tablets ... ▣ 785
Sinutab Non-Drying Liquid Caps ... ▣ 823
Sinutab Sinus Allergy Medication, Maximum Strength Tablets and Caplets ... ▣ 823
Sinutab Sinus Medication, Maximum Strength Without Drowsiness Formula, Tablets & Caplets ... ▣ 824
Sudafed Children's Cold & Cough Liquid Medication ... ▣ 825
Sudafed Children's Nasal Decongestant Liquid Medication ... ▣ 826
Sudafed Cold & Allergy Tablets ... ▣ 826
Sudafed Cold and Cough Liquid Caps ... ▣ 826
Sudafed Nasal Decongestant Tablets, 30 mg ... ▣ 825
Sudafed Nasal Decongestant Tablets, 60 mg ... ▣ 825
Sudafed Non-Drying Sinus Liquid Caps ... ▣ 827
Sudafed Pediatric Nasal Decongestant Liquid Oral Drops ... ▣ 827
Sudafed Severe Cold Formula Caplets ... ▣ 828
Sudafed Severe Cold Formula Tablets ... ▣ 828
Sudafed Sinus Caplets ... ▣ 829
Sudafed Sinus Tablets ... ▣ 829
Sudafed 12 Hour Caplets ... ▣ 824
Syn-Rx Tablets ... 1622
Syn-Rx DM Tablets ... 1623
TheraFlu Flu and Cold Medicine ... ▣ 750
Theraflu Maximum Strength Flu and Cold Medicine For Sore Throat ... ▣ 751
TheraFlu Flu, Cold and Cough Medicine ... ▣ 750
TheraFlu Maximum Strength Nighttime Flu, Cold & Cough Medicine ... ▣ 751
TheraFlu Maximum Strength Non-Drowsy Formula Flu, Cold & Cough Medicine ... ▣ 751
TheraFlu Maximum Strength, Non-Drowsy Formula Flu, Cold and Cough Caplets ... ▣ 752
Theraflu Maximum Strength Sinus Non-Drowsy Formula Caplets ... ▣ 752
Triaminic AM Cough and Decongestant Formula ... ▣ 753

(▣ Described in PDR For Nonprescription Drugs) (◉ Described in PDR For Ophthalmology)

Triaminic AM Decongestant Formula ▣ 753
Triaminic Infant Oral Decongestant Drops ▣ 754
Triaminic Night Time ▣ 754
Triaminic Sore Throat Formula ▣ 755
Tussend 1830
Tussend Expectorant 1831
TYLENOL Allergy Sinus, Maximum Strength Caplets and Gelcaps 1571
TYLENOL Allergy Sinus NightTime, Maximum Strength Caplets 1571
TYLENOL Cold Medication, Multi-Symptom Formula Tablets and Caplets 1572
TYLENOL Cold Medication, Multi-Symptom Hot Liquid Packets 1572
TYLENOL Cold Medication, No Drowsiness Formula Caplets and Gelcaps 1572
TYLENOL Cold Severe Congestion Caplets 1573
TYLENOL Cough Medication with Decongestant, Multi Symptom 1574
TYLENOL Flu No Drowsiness Formula, Maximum Strength Gelcaps 1575
TYLENOL Flu NightTime, Maximum Strength Gelcaps 1575
TYLENOL Flu NightTime, Maximum Strength Hot Medication Packets 1575
TYLENOL Sinus, Maximum Strength Geltabs, Gelcaps, Caplets and Tablets 1576
Vicks 44 LiquiCaps Cough, Cold & Flu Relief ▣ 728
Vicks 44 LiquiCaps Non-Drowsy Cough & Cold Relief ▣ 729
Vicks 44D Cough & Head Congestion Relief ▣ 728
Vicks 44M Cough, Cold & Flu Relief ▣ 729
Vicks DayQuil LiquiCaps/Liquid Multi-Symptom Cold/Flu Relief ▣ 734
Vicks DayQuil SINUS Pressure & PAIN Relief with IBUPROFEN ▣ 735
Vicks Nyquil Hot Therapy ▣ 735
Vicks NyQuil LiquiCaps/Liquid Multi-Symptom Cold/Flu Relief, Original and Cherry Flavors ▣ 736

Pseudoephedrine Sulfate (Effect of concurrent use not specified). Products include:
Chlor-Trimeton Allergy Decongestant Tablets ▣ 759
Claritin-D Tablets 2487
Drixoral Cold and Allergy Sustained-Action Tablets ▣ 763
Drixoral Cold and Flu Extended-Release Tablets ▣ 764
Drixoral Non-Drowsy Formula Extended-Release Tablets ▣ 764
Drixoral Allergy/Sinus Extended Release Tablets ▣ 765
Trinalin Repetabs Tablets 1373

Quazepam (Increases drowsiness effect). Products include:
Doral Tablets 2773

Quinapril Hydrochloride (Effect of concurrent use not specified). Products include:
Accupril Tablets 1950

Ramipril (Effect of concurrent use not specified). Products include:
Altace Capsules 1238

Rauwolfia Serpentina (Effect of concurrent use not specified).
No products indexed under this heading.

Rescinnamine (Effect of concurrent use not specified).
No products indexed under this heading.

Reserpine (Effect of concurrent use not specified). Products include:
Diupres Tablets 1691
Hydropres Tablets 1718
Ser-Ap-Es Tablets 867

Secobarbital Sodium (Increases drowsiness effect). Products include:
Seconal Sodium Pulvules 1529

Sertraline Hydrochloride (Effect of concurrent use not specified). Products include:
Zoloft Tablets 2051

Sodium Nitroprusside (Effect of concurrent use not specified).
No products indexed under this heading.

Sotalol Hydrochloride (Effect of concurrent use not specified). Products include:
Betapace Tablets 637

Spirapril Hydrochloride (Effect of concurrent use not specified).
No products indexed under this heading.

Temazepam (Increases drowsiness effect). Products include:
Restoril Capsules 2413

Terazosin Hydrochloride (Effect of concurrent use not specified). Products include:
Hytrin Capsules 434

Thioridazine Hydrochloride (Increases drowsiness effect). Products include:
Mellaril 2398

Thiothixene (Increases drowsiness effect). Products include:
Navane Capsules and Concentrate 2018
Navane Intramuscular 2019

Timolol Maleate (Effect of concurrent use not specified). Products include:
Blocadren Tablets 1654
Timolide Tablets 1791
Timoptic in Ocudose 1796
Timoptic Sterile Ophthalmic Solution 1794
Timoptic-XE 1798

Torsemide (Effect of concurrent use not specified). Products include:
Demadex Tablets and Injection 691

Tranylcypromine Sulfate (Effect of concurrent use not specified). Products include:
Parnate Tablets 2679

Trazodone Hydrochloride (Effect of concurrent use not specified). Products include:
Desyrel and Desyrel Dividose 504

Triazolam (Increases drowsiness effect). Products include:
Halcion Tablets 2093

Trifluoperazine Hydrochloride (Increases drowsiness effect). Products include:
Stelazine 2692

Trimethaphan Camsylate (Effect of concurrent use not specified).
No products indexed under this heading.

Trimipramine Maleate (Effect of concurrent use not specified). Products include:
Surmontil Capsules 2917

Venlafaxine Hydrochloride (Effect of concurrent use not specified). Products include:
Effexor 2825

Verapamil Hydrochloride (Effect of concurrent use not specified). Products include:
Calan SR Caplets 2571
Calan Tablets 2568
Covera-HS Tablets 2573
Isoptin Injectable 1391
Isoptin Oral Tablets 1393
Isoptin SR Tablets 1395
Verelan Capsules 1455

Zolpidem Tartrate (Increases drowsiness effect). Products include:
Ambien Tablets 2559

Food Interactions

Alcohol (Increases drowsiness effect).

TAXOL INJECTION

(Paclitaxel) 723

May interact with erythromycin, quinidine, and certain other agents. Compounds in these categories include:

Cyclosporine (The metabolism of paclitaxel is catalyzed by cytochrome P450 isoenzymes; based on *in vitro* studies, cyclosporine inhibits the metabolism of paclitaxel to 6-alpha-hydroxypaclitaxel, but the concentrations used exceeded those found *in vivo* following normal therapeutic doses). Products include:
Neoral 2405
Sandimmune 2416

Dexamethasone (The metabolism of paclitaxel is catalyzed by cytochrome P450 isoenzymes; based on *in vitro* studies, dexamethasone inhibits the metabolism of paclitaxel to 6-alpha-hydroxypaclitaxel, but the concentrations used exceeded those found *in vivo* following normal therapeutic doses). Products include:
AK-Trol Ointment & Suspension ◉ 205
Decadron Elixir 1676
Decadron Tablets 1678
Decaspray Topical Aerosol 1689
Maxitrol Ophthalmic Ointment and Suspension ◉ 222
TobraDex Ophthalmic Suspension and Ointment 469

Dexamethasone Acetate (The metabolism of paclitaxel is catalyzed by cytochrome P450 isoenzymes; based on *in vitro* studies, dexamethasone inhibits the metabolism of paclitaxel to 6-alpha-hydroxypaclitaxel, but the concentrations used exceeded those found *in vivo* following normal therapeutic doses). Products include:
Dalalone D.P. Injectable 1009
Decadron-LA Sterile Suspension 1687

Dexamethasone Sodium Phosphate (The metabolism of paclitaxel is catalyzed by cytochrome P450 isoenzymes; based on *in vitro* studies, dexamethasone inhibits the metabolism of paclitaxel to 6-alpha-hydroxypaclitaxel, but the concentrations used exceeded those found *in vivo* following normal therapeutic doses). Products include:
Decadron Phosphate Injection 1680
Decadron Phosphate Sterile Ophthalmic Ointment 1684
Decadron Phosphate Sterile Ophthalmic Solution 1685
Decadron Phosphate Topical Cream 1686
Decadron Phosphate with Xylocaine Injection, Sterile 1683
Dexacort Phosphate in Respihaler 1606
Dexacort Phosphate in Turbinaire 1607
NeoDecadron Sterile Ophthalmic Ointment 1755
NeoDecadron Sterile Ophthalmic Solution 1756
NeoDecadron Topical Cream 1757

Diazepam (The metabolism of paclitaxel is catalyzed by cytochrome P450 isoenzymes; based on *in vitro* studies, diazepam inhibits the metabolism of paclitaxel to 6-alpha-hydroxypaclitaxel, but the concentrations used exceeded those found *in vivo* following normal therapeutic doses). Products include:
Dizac (diazepam injectable emulsion) CIV 1862
Valium Injectable 2336
Valium Tablets 2335

Erythromycin (The metabolism of paclitaxel is catalyzed by cytochrome P450 isoenzymes; based on *in vitro* studies, erythromycin inhibits the metabolism of paclitaxel to 6-alpha-hydroxypaclitaxel). Products include:
A/T/S 2% Acne Topical Gel 1244
A/T/S 2% Acne Topical Solution 1244
Benzamycin Topical Gel 919
E-Mycin Tablets 1388
Emgel 2% Topical Gel 1081
ERYC 1972
Erycette (erythromycin 2%) Topical Solution 1943
Ery-Tab Tablets 426
Erythromycin Base Filmtab 430
Erythromycin Delayed-Release Capsules, USP 431
Ilotycin Ophthalmic Ointment 928
PCE Dispertab Tablets 453
T-Stat 2.0% Topical Solution and Pads 2797
THERAMYCIN Z 2% Solution 1629

Erythromycin Estolate (The metabolism of paclitaxel is catalyzed by cytochrome P450 isoenzymes; based on *in vitro* studies, erythromycin inhibits the metabolism of paclitaxel to 6-alpha-hydroxypaclitaxel). Products include:
Ilosone 927

Erythromycin Ethylsuccinate (The metabolism of paclitaxel is catalyzed by cytochrome P450 isoenzymes; based on *in vitro* studies, erythromycin inhibits the metabolism of paclitaxel to 6-alpha-hydroxypaclitaxel). Products include:
E.E.S. 427
EryPed 425
Pediazole Suspension 2340

Erythromycin Gluceptate (The metabolism of paclitaxel is catalyzed by cytochrome P450 isoenzymes; based on *in vitro* studies, erythromycin inhibits the metabolism of paclitaxel to 6-alpha-hydroxypaclitaxel). Products include:
Ilotycin Gluceptate, IV, Vials 929

Erythromycin Stearate (The metabolism of paclitaxel is catalyzed by cytochrome P450 isoenzymes; based on *in vitro* studies, erythromycin inhibits the metabolism of paclitaxel to 6-alpha-hydroxypaclitaxel). Products include:
Erythrocin Stearate Filmtab 429

Ethinyl Estradiol (The metabolism of paclitaxel is catalyzed by cytochrome P450 isoenzymes; based on *in vitro* studies, 17-alpha ethinyl estradiol inhibits the metabolism of paclitaxel to 6-alpha-hydroxypaclitaxel). Products include:
Brevicon 2563
Demulen 2580
Desogen Tablets 1867
Levlen/Tri-Levlen 646
Lo/Ovral Tablets 2852
Lo/Ovral-28 Tablets 2857
Modicon 1928
Nordette-21 Tablets 2863
Nordette-28 Tablets 2866
Norinyl 2563
Ortho-Cept 1907
Ortho-Cyclen/Ortho-Tri-Cyclen 1914
Ortho-Novum 1928
Ortho-Cyclen/Ortho Tri-Cyclen 1914
Ovcon 765
Ovral Tablets 2877
Ovral-28 Tablets 2878
Levlen/Tri-Levlen 646
Tri-Norinyl 2607
Triphasil-21 Tablets 2919
Triphasil-28 Tablets 2924

Etoposide (The metabolism of paclitaxel is catalyzed by cytochrome P450 isoenzymes; based on *in vitro* studies, etoposide inhibits the metabolism of paclitaxel to 6-alpha-hydroxypaclitaxel, but the concentrations used exceeded those found *in vivo* following normal therapeutic doses). Products include:
Etoposide Injection 539
VePesid Capsules and Injection 727

IMPORTANT NOTE: Always consult each drug listing in the patient's regimen for possible interactions.

Taxol / Interactions Index

Etoposide Phosphate (The metabolism of paclitaxel is catalyzed by cytochrome P450 isoenzymes; based on *in vitro* studies, etoposide inhibits the metabolism of paclitaxel to 6-alpha-hydroxypaclitaxel, but the concentrations used exceeded those found *in vivo* following normal therapeutic doses). Products include:
Etopophos for Injection 701

Etretinate (The metabolism of paclitaxel is catalyzed by cytochrome P450 isoenzymes; based on *in vitro* studies, retinoic acid inhibits the metabolism of paclitaxel to 6-alpha-hydroxypaclitaxel). Products include:
Tegison Capsules 2314

Isotretinoin (The metabolism of paclitaxel is catalyzed by cytochrome P450 isoenzymes; based on *in vitro* studies, retinoic acid inhibits the metabolism of paclitaxel to 6-alpha-hydroxypaclitaxel). Products include:
Accutane Capsules 2252

Ketoconazole (The metabolism of paclitaxel is catalyzed by cytochrome P450 isoenzymes; based on *in vitro* studies, ketoconazole inhibits the metabolism of paclitaxel to 6-alpha-hydroxypaclitaxel, but the concentrations used exceeded those found *in vivo* following normal therapeutic doses). Products include:
Nizoral 2% Cream 1344
Nizoral 2% Shampoo 1344
Nizoral Tablets 1345

Quercetin (The metabolism of paclitaxel is catalyzed by cytochrome P450 isoenzymes; based on *in vitro* studies, quercetin, a specific inhibitor of CYP2C8, inhibits the metabolism of paclitaxel to 6-alpha-hydroxypaclitaxel).
No products indexed under this heading.

Quinidine Gluconate (The metabolism of paclitaxel is catalyzed by cytochrome P450 isoenzymes; based on *in vitro* studies, quinidine inhibits the metabolism of paclitaxel to 6-alpha-hydroxypaclitaxel, but the concentrations used exceeded those found *in vivo* following normal therapeutic doses). Products include:
Quinaglute Dura-Tabs Tablets 644

Quinidine Polygalacturonate (The metabolism of paclitaxel is catalyzed by cytochrome P450 isoenzymes; based on *in vitro* studies, quinidine inhibits the metabolism of paclitaxel to 6-alpha-hydroxypaclitaxel, but the concentrations used exceeded those found *in vivo* following normal therapeutic doses). Products include:
Cardioquin Tablets 2146

Quinidine Sulfate (The metabolism of paclitaxel is catalyzed by cytochrome P450 isoenzymes; based on *in vitro* studies, quinidine inhibits the metabolism of paclitaxel to 6-alpha-hydroxypaclitaxel, but the concentrations used exceeded those found *in vivo* following normal therapeutic doses). Products include:
Quinidex Extentabs 2240

Teniposide (The metabolism of paclitaxel is catalyzed by cytochrome P450 isoenzymes; based on *in vitro* studies, teniposide inhibits the metabolism of paclitaxel to 6-alpha-hydroxypaclitaxel, but the concentrations used exceeded those found *in vivo* following normal therapeutic doses). Products include:
Vumon for Injection 729

Testosterone (The metabolism of paclitaxel is catalyzed by cytochrome P450 isoenzymes; based on *in vitro* studies, testosterone inhibits the metabolism of paclitaxel to 6-alpha-hydroxpaclitaxel). Products include:
Androderm Testosterone Transdermal System 2634
Testoderm Testosterone Transdermal System 486

Tretinoin (The metabolism of paclitaxel is catalyzed by cytochrome P450 isoenzymes; based on *in vitro* studies, retinoic acid inhibits the metabolism of paclitaxel to 6-alpha-hydroxypaclitaxel). Products include:
Renova (tretinoin emollient cream) 0.05% 1945
Retin-A (tretinoin) Cream/Gel/Liquid 1947
Vesanoid Capsules 2327

Verapamil Hydrochloride (The metabolism of paclitaxel is catalyzed by cytochrome P450 isoenzymes; based on *in vitro* studies, verapamil inhibits the metabolism of paclitaxel to 6-alpha-hydroxypaclitaxel, but the concentrations used exceeded those found *in vivo* following normal therapeutic doses). Products include:
Calan SR Caplets 2571
Calan Tablets 2568
Covera-HS Tablets 2573
Isoptin Injectable 1391
Isoptin Oral Tablets 1393
Isoptin SR Tablets 1395
Verelan Capsules 1455

Vincristine Sulfate (The metabolism of paclitaxel is catalyzed by cytochrome P450 isoenzymes; based on *in vitro* studies, vincristine inhibits the metabolism of paclitaxel to 6-alpha-hydroxypaclitaxel, but the concentrations used exceeded those found *in vivo* following normal therapeutic doses). Products include:
Oncovin Solution Vials & Hyporets 1521

TAXOTERE FOR INJECTION CONCENTRATE
(Docetaxel) 2204
May interact with erythromycin and certain other agents. Compounds in these categories include:

Cyclosporine (*In vitro* studies have shown that the metabolism of docetaxel may be modified by co-administration of compounds that induce, inhibit, or are metabolized by cytochrome P450 3A4, such as cyclosporine). Products include:
Neoral 2405
Sandimmune 2416

Erythromycin (*In vitro* studies have shown that the metabolism of docetaxel may be modified by co-administration of compounds that induce, inhibit, or are metabolized by cytochrome P450 3A4, such as erythromycin). Products include:
A/T/S 2% Acne Topical Gel 1244
A/T/S 2% Acne Topical Solution 1244
Benzamycin Topical Gel 919
E-Mycin Tablets 1388
Emgel 2% Topical Gel 1081
ERYC 1972
Erycette (erythromycin 2%) Topical Solution 1943
Ery-Tab Tablets 426
Erythromycin Base Filmtab 430
Erythromycin Delayed-Release Capsules, USP 431
Ilotycin Ophthalmic Ointment 928
PCE Dispertab Tablets 453
T-Stat 2.0% Topical Solution and Pads 2797
THERAMYCIN Z 2% Solution 1629

Erythromycin Estolate (*In vitro* studies have shown that the metabolism of docetaxel may be modified by co-administration of compounds that induce, inhibit, or are metabolized by cytochrome P450 3A4, such as erythromycin). Products include:
Ilosone 927

Erythromycin Ethylsuccinate (*In vitro* studies have shown that the metabolism of docetaxel may be modified by co-administration of compounds that induce, inhibit, or are metabolized by cytochrome P450 3A4, such as erythromycin). Products include:
E.E.S. 427
EryPed 425
Pediazole Suspension 2340

Erythromycin Gluceptate (*In vitro* studies have shown that the metabolism of docetaxel may be modified by co-administration of compounds that induce, inhibit, or are metabolized by cytochrome P450 3A4, such as erythromycin). Products include:
Ilotycin Gluceptate, IV, Vials 929

Erythromycin Stearate (*In vitro* studies have shown that the metabolism of docetaxel may be modified by co-administration of compounds that induce, inhibit, or are metabolized by cytochrome P450 3A4, such as erythromycin). Products include:
Erythrocin Stearate Filmtab 429

Ketoconazole (*In vitro* studies have shown that the metabolism of docetaxel may be modified by co-administration of compounds that induce, inhibit, or are metabolized by cytochrome P450 3A4, such as ketoconazole). Products include:
Nizoral 2% Cream 1344
Nizoral 2% Shampoo 1344
Nizoral Tablets 1345

Terfenadine (*In vitro* studies have shown that the metabolism of docetaxel may be modified by co-administration of compounds that induce, inhibit, or are metabolized by cytochrome P450 3A4, such as terfenadine). Products include:
Seldane Tablets 1284
Seldane-D Extended-Release Tablets 1286

Troleandomycin (*In vitro* studies have shown that the metabolism of docetaxel may be modified by co-administration of compounds that induce, inhibit, or are metabolized by cytochrome P450 3A4, such as troleandomycin). Products include:
Tao Capsules 2033

TAZICEF FOR INJECTION
(Ceftazidime) 2697
May interact with aminoglycosides and certain other agents. Compounds in these categories include:

Amikacin Sulfate (Concomitant administration may result in nephrotoxicity). Products include:
Amikacin Sulfate Injection, USP 523
Amikacin Sulfate Injection, USP 981
Amikin Injectable 502

Chloramphenicol (Chloramphenicol in combination with cephalosporins, including ceftazidime, has been shown to be antagonistic *in vitro*; due to possibility of antagonism *in vivo*, this combination should be avoided). Products include:
Chloromycetin Ophthalmic Ointment, 1% ...... ◎ 298
Chloromycetin Ophthalmic Solution ...... ◎ 299
Chloroptic S.O.P. ...... ◎ 236
Chloroptic Sterile Ophthalmic Solution ...... ◎ 236

Chloramphenicol Palmitate (Chloramphenicol in combination with cephalosporins, including ceftazidime, has been shown to be antagonistic *in vitro*; due to possibility of antagonism *in vivo*, this combination should be avoided).
No products indexed under this heading.

Chloramphenicol Sodium Succinate (Chloramphenicol in combination with cephalosporins, including ceftazidime, has been shown to be antagonistic *in vitro*; due to possibility of antagonism *in vivo*, this combination should be avoided). Products include:
Chloromycetin Sodium Succinate 1960

Furosemide (Concomitant administration may result in nephrotoxicity). Products include:
Lasix Injection, Oral Solution and Tablets 1267

Gentamicin Sulfate (Concomitant administration may result in nephrotoxicity). Products include:
Garamycin Cream 0.1% 2501
Garamycin Injectable 2502
Garamycin Ointment 0.1% 2501
Garamycin Ophthalmic 2501
Genoptic Sterile Ophthalmic Solution ...... ◎ 241
Genoptic Sterile Ophthalmic Ointment ...... ◎ 241
Gentak ...... ◎ 209
Pred-G Liquifilm Sterile Ophthalmic Suspension ...... ◎ 248
Pred-G S.O.P. Sterile Ophthalmic Ointment ...... ◎ 249

Kanamycin Sulfate (Concomitant administration may result in nephrotoxicity).
No products indexed under this heading.

Streptomycin Sulfate (Concomitant administration may result in nephrotoxicity). Products include:
Streptomycin Sulfate Injection 2031

Tobramycin (Concomitant administration may result in nephrotoxicity). Products include:
AKTOB ...... ◎ 207
TobraDex Ophthalmic Suspension and Ointment 469
Tobrex Ophthalmic Ointment and Solution ...... ◎ 226

Tobramycin Sulfate (Concomitant administration may result in nephrotoxicity). Products include:
Nebcin Vials, Hyporets & ADD-Vantage 1518

TAZIDIME VIALS, FASPAK & ADD-VANTAGE
(Ceftazidime) 1531
May interact with aminoglycosides and certain other agents. Compounds in these categories include:

Amikacin Sulfate (Potential for nephrotoxicity and ototoxicity; monitor renal function). Products include:
Amikacin Sulfate Injection, USP 523
Amikacin Sulfate Injection, USP 981
Amikin Injectable 502

Chloramphenicol Sodium Succinate (Chloramphenicol has been shown to be antagonistic to beta-lactam antibiotics, including ceftazidime, based on *in vitro* studies and time to kill curves with enteric gram-negative bacilli; this combination therapy should be avoided). Products include:
Chloromycetin Sodium Succinate 1960

(⊞ Described in PDR For Nonprescription Drugs)   (◎ Described in PDR For Ophthalmology)

Interactions Index — Tegretol/Tegretol-XR

Furosemide (Potential for nephrotoxicity with potent diuretics, such as furosemide). Products include:
- Lasix Injection, Oral Solution and Tablets ... 1267

Gentamicin Sulfate (Potential for nephrotoxicity and ototoxicity; monitor renal function). Products include:
- Garamycin Cream 0.1% ... 2501
- Garamycin Injectable ... 2502
- Garamycin Ointment 0.1% ... 2501
- Garamycin Ophthalmic ... 2501
- Genoptic Sterile Ophthalmic Solution ... 241
- Genoptic Sterile Ophthalmic Ointment ... 241
- Gentak ... 209
- Pred-G Liquifilm Sterile Ophthalmic Suspension ... 248
- Pred-G S.O.P. Sterile Ophthalmic Ointment ... 249

Kanamycin Sulfate (Potential for nephrotoxicity and ototoxicity; monitor renal function).
- No products indexed under this heading.

Streptomycin Sulfate (Potential for nephrotoxicity and ototoxicity; monitor renal function). Products include:
- Streptomycin Sulfate Injection ... 2031

Tobramycin (Potential for nephrotoxicity and ototoxicity; monitor renal function). Products include:
- AKTOB ... 207
- TobraDex Ophthalmic Suspension and Ointment ... 469
- Tobrex Ophthalmic Ointment and Solution ... 226

Tobramycin Sulfate (Potential for nephrotoxicity and ototoxicity; monitor renal function). Products include:
- Nebcin Vials, Hyporets & ADD-Vantage ... 1518

TEARS NATURALE II LUBRICANT EYE DROPS
(Dextran 70, Hydroxypropyl Methylcellulose) ... 469
None cited in PDR database.

TEARS NATURALE FREE LUBRICANT EYE DROPS
(Dextran 70, Hydroxypropyl Methylcellulose) ... 469
None cited in PDR database.

TEARS RENEWED OINTMENT
(Petrolatum, White) ... 210
None cited in PDR database.

TECHNI-CARE SURGICAL SCRUB AND WOUND CLEANSER
(Chloroxylenol) ... 647
None cited in PDR database.

TEGISON CAPSULES
(Etretinate) ... 2314
May interact with:

Vitamin A (Additive toxic effects). Products include:
- Aquasol A Vitamin A Capsules, USP ... 525
- Aquasol A Parenteral ... 526
- Breath + Plus ... 603
- Materna Tablets ... 1427
- Megadose ... 513
- One-A-Day Antioxidant Plus ... 625

Food Interactions
Dairy products (Increases absorption of etretinate).
Diet, high-lipid (Increases absorption of etretinate).

TEGREEN 97 CAPSULES
(Homeopathic Medications) ... 2985
None cited in PDR database.

TEGRETOL CHEWABLE TABLETS
(Carbamazepine) ... 870
See **Tegretol-XR Tablets**

TEGRETOL SUSPENSION
(Carbamazepine) ... 870
See **Tegretol-XR Tablets**

TEGRETOL TABLETS
(Carbamazepine) ... 870
See **Tegretol-XR Tablets**

TEGRETOL-XR TABLETS
(Carbamazepine) ... 870
May interact with macrolide antibiotics, erythromycin, anticonvulsants, xanthine bronchodilators, oral contraceptives, antipsychotic agents, oral anticoagulants, lithium preparations, and certain other agents. Compounds in these categories include:

Acetaminophen (Carbamazepine induces CYP activity with the potential for decreased acetaminophen levels). Products include:
- Actifed Cold & Sinus Caplets and Tablets ... 808
- Actifed Sinus Daytime/Nighttime Tablets and Caplets ... 809
- Alka-Seltzer Fast Relief Caplets ... 610
- Alka-Seltzer Plus Liqui-Gels ... 612
- Alka-Seltzer Plus Flu & Body Aches Effervescent Tablets ... 612
- Alka-Seltzer Plus Flu & Body Aches Liqui-Gels Non-Drowsy Formula ... 613
- Alka-Seltzer Plus Night-Time Cold Medicine Liqui-Gels ... 612
- Allerest No Drowsiness ... 649
- Allerest Sinus Pain Formula ... 649
- Axocet Capsules ... 2469
- Benadryl Allergy/Cold Tablets ... 811
- Benadryl Allergy Sinus Headache Caplets ... 813
- Children's TYLENOL acetaminophen Chewable Tablets, Elixir, Suspension Liquid, and Suspension Drops ... 1559
- Children's TYLENOL Cold Multi-Symptom Chewable Tablets and Liquid ... 1559
- Children's TYLENOL Cold Plus Cough Multi Symptom Chewable Tablets and Liquid ... 1560
- Children's TYLENOL Flu Suspension Liquid ... 1560
- Allergy-Sinus Comtrex Multi-Symptom Allergy-Sinus Formula Tablets and Caplets ... 639
- Comtrex Multi-Symptom ... 638
- Comtrex Non-Drowsy ... 640
- Contac Day Allergy/Sinus Caplets ... 771
- Contac Day & Night ... 772
- Contac Night Allergy/Sinus Caplets ... 771
- Contac Severe Cold and Flu Formula Caplets ... 773
- Contac Severe Cold & Flu Non-Drowsy ... 774
- Coricidin Cold + Flu Tablets ... 760
- Coricidin 'D' Decongestant Tablets ... 760
- DHCplus Capsules ... 2148
- Darvon-N/Darvocet-N ... 1473
- Dimetapp Allergy Sinus Caplets ... 838
- Dimetapp Cold & Fever Suspension ... 839
- Drixoral Cold and Flu Extended-Release Tablets ... 764
- Drixoral Cough + Sore Throat Liquid Caps ... 763
- Drixoral Allergy/Sinus Extended Release Tablets ... 765
- Esgic-plus Capsules ... 1012
- Esgic-plus Tablets ... 1012
- Aspirin Free Excedrin Analgesic Caplets and Geltabs ... 734
- Excedrin Extra-Strength Analgesic Tablets, Caplets, and Geltabs ... 734
- Excedrin P.M. Analgesic/Sleeping Aid Tablets, Caplets, Liquigels ... 735
- Fioricet Tablets ... 2386
- Fioricet with Codeine Capsules ... 2387
- Goody's Extra Strength Headache Powders ... 632
- Goody's Extra Strength Pain Relief Tablets ... 632
- Hycomine Compound Tablets ... 948
- Hydrocet Capsules ... 787
- Infants' TYLENOL acetaminophen Suspension Drops ... 1559
- Infants' TYLENOL Cold Decongestant & Fever-Reducer Drops ... 1561
- Junior Strength TYLENOL acetaminophen Coated Caplets and Chewable Tablets ... 1562
- Lorcet 10/650 Tablets ... 1016
- Lortab ... 2751
- Lurline PMS Tablets ... 1000
- Maximum Strength Multi-Symptom Formula Midol ... 621
- PMS Multi-Symptom Formula Midol ... 622
- Maximum Strength Midol Teen Multi-Symptom Formula ... 621
- Midrin Capsules ... 788
- Panodol Tablets and Caplets ... 783
- Children's Panadol Chewable Tablets, Liquid, Infant's Drops ... 783
- Percocet Tablets ... 955
- Percogesic Analgesic Tablets ... 727
- Phrenilin ... 790
- Pyrroxate Caplets ... 742
- Robitussin Cold, Cough & Flu Liqui-Gels ... 844
- Robitussin Night-Time Cold Formula ... 847
- Sedapap Tablets 50 mg/650 mg ... 1826
- Sinarest ... 663
- Sine-Aid Maximum Strength Sinus Headache Gelcaps, Caplets and Tablets ... 1570
- Sine-Off No Drowsiness Formula Caplets ... 784
- Sine-Off Sinus Medicine ... 784
- Singlet Tablets ... 785
- Sinulin Tablets ... 792
- Sinutab Sinus Allergy Medication, Maximum Strength Tablets and Caplets ... 823
- Sinutab Sinus Medication, Maximum Strength Without Drowsiness Formula, Tablets & Caplets ... 824
- Sudafed Cold and Cough Liquid Caps ... 826
- Sudafed Severe Cold Formula Caplets ... 828
- Sudafed Severe Cold Formula Tablets ... 828
- Sudafed Sinus Caplets ... 829
- Sudafed Sinus Tablets ... 829
- Talacen Caplets ... 2464
- TheraFlu Flu and Cold Medicine ... 750
- Theraflu Maximum Strength Flu and Cold Medicine For Sore Throat ... 751
- TheraFlu Flu, Cold and Cough Medicine ... 750
- TheraFlu Maximum Strength Nighttime Flu, Cold & Cough Medicine ... 751
- TheraFlu Maximum Strength Non-Drowsy Formula Flu, Cold & Cough Medicine ... 751
- TheraFlu Maximum Strength, Non-Drowsy Formula Flu, Cold and Cough Caplets ... 752
- Theraflu Maximum Strength Sinus Non-Drowsy Formula Caplets ... 752
- Triaminic Sore Throat Formula ... 755
- Triaminicin Tablets ... 756
- TYLENOL acetaminophen Extended Relief Caplets ... 1570
- TYLENOL acetaminophen, Extra Strength Adult Liquid Pain Reliever ... 1570
- TYLENOL acetaminophen, Extra Strength Gelcaps, Geltabs, Caplets, Tablets ... 1570
- TYLENOL acetaminophen, Regular Strength Caplets and Tablets ... 1570
- TYLENOL Allergy Sinus, Maximum Strength Caplets and Gelcaps ... 1571
- TYLENOL Allergy Sinus NightTime, Maximum Strength Caplets ... 1571
- TYLENOL Cold Medication, Multi-Symptom Formula Tablets and Caplets ... 1572
- TYLENOL Cold Medication, Multi-Symptom Hot Liquid Packets ... 1572
- TYLENOL Cold Medication, No Drowsiness Formula Caplets and Gelcaps ... 1572
- TYLENOL Cold Severe Congestion Caplets ... 1573
- TYLENOL Cough Medication, Multi Symptom ... 1574
- TYLENOL Cough Medication with Decongestant, Multi Symptom ... 1574
- TYLENOL Flu No Drowsiness Formula, Maximum Strength Gelcaps ... 1575
- TYLENOL Flu NightTime, Maximum Strength Gelcaps ... 1575
- TYLENOL Flu NightTime, Maximum Strength Hot Medication Packets ... 1575
- TYLENOL Headache Plus Pain Reliever with Antacid, Extra Strength Caplets ... 705
- TYLENOL PM Pain Reliever/Sleep Aid, Extra Strength Gelcaps, Caplets, Geltabs ... 1576
- TYLENOL Severe Allergy Medication Caplets ... 1571
- TYLENOL Sinus, Maximum Strength Geltabs, Gelcaps, Caplets and Tablets ... 1576
- Tylenol with Codeine ... 1592
- Tylox Capsules ... 1593
- Unisom With Pain Relief-Nighttime Sleep Aid and Pain Reliever ... 1991
- Vanquish Analgesic Caplets ... 627
- Vicks 44 LiquiCaps Cough, Cold & Flu Relief ... 728
- Vicks 44M Cough, Cold & Flu Relief ... 729
- Vicks DayQuil LiquiCaps/Liquid Multi-Symptom Cold/Flu Relief ... 734
- Vicks Nyquil Hot Therapy ... 735
- Vicks NyQuil LiquiCaps/Liquid Multi-Symptom Cold/Flu Relief, Original and Cherry Flavors ... 736
- Vicodin Tablets ... 1404
- Vicodin ES Tablets ... 1405
- Vicodin HP Tablets ... 1403
- Wygesic Tablets ... 2930
- Zydone Capsules ... 967

Alprazolam (Carbamazepine induces CYP activity with the potential for decreased alprazolam levels). Products include:
- Xanax ... 2115

Aminophylline (Theophylline, a CYP3A4 inducer, can increase carbamazepine metabolism resulting in the potential for decreased plasma carbamazepine levels; potential for decreased theophylline levels).
- No products indexed under this heading.

Azithromycin (Macrolide antibiotic, a CYP3A4 inhibitor, inhibits carbamazepine metabolism resulting in the potential for increased plasma carbamazepine levels). Products include:
- Zithromax ... 2043
- Zithromax Tablets ... 2046

Chlorpromazine (Co-administration has resulted in isolated cases of neuroleptic malignant syndrome). Products include:
- Thorazine Suppositories ... 2701

Chlorpromazine Hydrochloride (Co-administration has resulted in isolated cases of neuroleptic malignant syndrome). Products include:
- Thorazine ... 2701

Chlorprothixene (Co-administration has resulted in isolated cases of neuroleptic malignant syndrome).
- No products indexed under this heading.

Chlorprothixene Hydrochloride (Co-administration has resulted in isolated cases of neuroleptic malignant syndrome).
- No products indexed under this heading.

Cimetidine (Cimetidine, a CYP3A4 inhibitor, inhibits carbamazepine metabolism resulting in the potential for increased plasma carbamazepine levels). Products include:
- Tagamet HB Tablets ... 786
- Tagamet Tablets ... 2694

IMPORTANT NOTE: Always consult each drug listing in the patient's regimen for possible interactions.

Tegretol/Tegretol-XR — Interactions Index

Cimetidine Hydrochloride (Cimetidine, a CYP3A4 inhibitor, inhibits carbamazepine metabolism resulting in the potential for increased plasma carbamazepine levels). Products include:
- Tagamet ... 2694

Cisplatin (Cisplatin, a CYP3A4 inducer, can increase carbamazepine metabolism resulting in the potential for decreased plasma carbamazepine levels). Products include:
- Platinol for Injection ... 717
- Platinol-AQ Injection ... 719

Clarithromycin (Macrolide antibiotic, a CYP3A4 inhibitor, inhibits carbamazepine metabolism resulting in the potential for increased plasma carbamazepine levels). Products include:
- Biaxin ... 406

Clomipramine Hydrochloride (Potential for increased clomipramine levels). Products include:
- Anafranil Capsules ... 819

Clonazepam (Carbamazepine induces CYP activity with the potential for decreased clonazepam levels; combination therapy has resulted in alterations of thyroid function). Products include:
- Klonopin Tablets ... 2294

Clozapine (Carbamazepine induces CYP activity with the potential for decreased clozapine levels; co-administration has resulted in isolated cases of neuroleptic malignant syndrome). Products include:
- Clozaril Tablets ... 2377

Danazol (Danazol, a CYP3A4 inhibitor, inhibits carbamazepine metabolism resulting in the potential for increased plasma carbamazepine levels). Products include:
- Danocrine Capsules ... 2437

Desogestrel (Carbamazepine induces CYP activity with the potential for decreased oral contraceptive levels; breakthrough bleeding and reliability of oral contraceptive may be adversely affected). Products include:
- Desogen Tablets ... 1867
- Ortho-Cept ... 1907

Dicumarol (Carbamazepine induces CYP activity with the potential for decreased oral anticoagulant levels).
- No products indexed under this heading.

Diltiazem Hydrochloride (Diltiazem, a CYP3A4 inhibitor, inhibits carbamazepine metabolism resulting in the potential for increased plasma carbamazepine levels). Products include:
- Cardizem CD Capsules ... 1251
- Cardizem SR Capsules ... 1255
- Cardizem Injectable ... 1253
- Cardizem Tablets ... 1257
- Dilacor XR Extended-release Capsules ... 2183
- Tiazac Capsules ... 1019

Dirithromycin (Macrolide antibiotic, a CYP3A4 inhibitor, inhibits carbamazepine metabolism resulting in the potential for increased plasma carbamazepine levels). Products include:
- Dynabac ... 668

Divalproex Sodium (Valproate, a CYP3A4 inhibitor, inhibits carbamazepine metabolism resulting in the potential for increased plasma carbamazepine and 10,11-epoxide levels; combination therapy has resulted in alterations of thyroid function and decreased valproate levels). Products include:
- Depakote Tablets ... 418

Doxorubicin Hydrochloride (Doxorubicin, a CYP3A4 inducer, can increase carbamazepine metabolism resulting in the potential for decreased plasma carbamazepine levels). Products include:
- Adriamycin PFS ... 2056
- Adriamycin RDF ... 2056
- Doxil ... 2613
- Doxorubicin Astra ... 531
- Rubex for Injection ... 721

Doxycycline Calcium (Carbamazepine induces CYP activity with the potential for decreased doxycycline levels). Products include:
- Vibramycin Calcium Oral Suspension Syrup ... 2038

Doxycycline Hyclate (Carbamazepine induces CYP activity with the potential for decreased doxycycline levels). Products include:
- Doryx Capsules ... 1970
- Vibramycin Hyclate Capsules ... 2038
- Vibramycin Hyclate Intravenous ... 2040
- Vibra-Tabs Film Coated Tablets ... 2038

Doxycycline Monohydrate (Carbamazepine induces CYP activity with the potential for decreased doxycycline levels). Products include:
- Monodox Capsules ... 1858
- Vibramycin Monohydrate for Oral Suspension ... 2038

Dyphylline (Theophylline, a CYP3A4 inducer, can increase carbamazepine metabolism resulting in the potential for decreased plasma carbamazepine levels; potential for decreased theophylline levels). Products include:
- Lufyllin & Lufyllin-400 Tablets ... 2778
- Lufyllin-GG Elixir & Tablets ... 2779

Erythromycin (Erythromycin, a CYP3A4 inhibitor, inhibits carbamazepine metabolism resulting in the potential for increased plasma carbamazepine levels). Products include:
- A/T/S 2% Acne Topical Gel ... 1244
- A/T/S 2% Acne Topical Solution ... 1244
- Benzamycin Topical Gel ... 919
- E-Mycin Tablets ... 1388
- Emgel 2% Topical Gel ... 1081
- ERYC ... 1972
- Erycette (erythromycin 2%) Topical Solution ... 1943
- Ery-Tab Tablets ... 426
- Erythromycin Base Filmtab ... 430
- Erythromycin Delayed-Release Capsules, USP ... 431
- Ilotycin Ophthalmic Ointment ... 928
- PCE Dispertab Tablets ... 453
- T-Stat 2.0% Topical Solution and Pads ... 2797
- THERAMYCIN Z 2% Solution ... 1629

Erythromycin Estolate (Erythromycin, a CYP3A4 inhibitor, inhibits carbamazepine metabolism resulting in the potential for increased plasma carbamazepine levels). Products include:
- Ilosone ... 927

Erythromycin Ethylsuccinate (Erythromycin, a CYP3A4 inhibitor, inhibits carbamazepine metabolism resulting in the potential for increased plasma carbamazepine levels). Products include:
- E.E.S. ... 427
- EryPed ... 425
- Pediazole Suspension ... 2340

Erythromycin Glucepate (Erythromycin, a CYP3A4 inhibitor, inhibits carbamazepine metabolism resulting in the potential for increased plasma carbamazepine levels). Products include:
- Ilotycin Glucepate, IV, Vials ... 929

Erythromycin Stearate (Erythromycin, a CYP3A4 inhibitor, inhibits carbamazepine metabolism resulting in the potential for increased plasma carbamazepine levels). Products include:
- Erythrocin Stearate Filmtab ... 429

Ethinyl Estradiol (Carbamazepine induces CYP activity with the potential for decreased oral contraceptive levels; breakthrough bleeding and reliability of oral contraceptive may be adversely affected). Products include:
- Brevicon ... 2563
- Demulen ... 2580
- Desogen Tablets ... 1867
- Levlen/Tri-Levlen ... 646
- Lo/Ovral Tablets ... 2852
- Lo/Ovral-28 Tablets ... 2857
- Modicon ... 1928
- Nordette-21 Tablets ... 2863
- Nordette-28 Tablets ... 2866
- Norinyl ... 2563
- Ortho-Cept ... 1907
- Ortho-Cyclen/Ortho-Tri-Cyclen ... 1914
- Ortho-Novum ... 1928
- Ortho-Cyclen/Ortho-Tri-Cyclen ... 1914
- Ovcon ... 765
- Ovral Tablets ... 2877
- Ovral-28 Tablets ... 2878
- Levlen/Tri-Levlen ... 646
- Tri-Norinyl ... 2607
- Triphasil-21 Tablets ... 2919
- Triphasil-28 Tablets ... 2924

Ethosuximide (Carbamazepine induces CYP activity with the potential for decreased ethosuximide levels; combination therapy has resulted in alterations of thyroid function). Products include:
- Zarontin Capsules ... 1986
- Zarontin Syrup ... 1986

Ethotoin (Combination therapy has resulted in alterations of thyroid function). Products include:
- Peganone Tablets ... 455

Ethynodiol Diacetate (Carbamazepine induces CYP activity with the potential for decreased oral contraceptive levels; breakthrough bleeding and reliability of oral contraceptive may be adversely affected). Products include:
- Demulen ... 2580

Felbamate (Felbamate, a CYP3A4 inducer, can increase carbamazepine metabolism resulting in the potential for decreased plasma carbamazepine levels and increased 10,11-epoxide levels; combination therapy has resulted in alterations of thyroid function). Products include:
- Felbatol ... 2774

Fluoxetine Hydrochloride (Fluoxetine, a CYP3A4 inhibitor, inhibits carbamazepine metabolism resulting in the potential for increased plasma carbamazepine levels). Products include:
- Prozac Pulvules & Liquid, Oral Solution ... 935

Fluphenazine Decanoate (Co-administration has resulted in isolated cases of neuroleptic malignant syndrome). Products include:
- Prolixin Decanoate ... 510

Fluphenazine Enanthate (Co-administration has resulted in isolated cases of neuroleptic malignant syndrome). Products include:
- Prolixin Enanthate ... 510

Fluphenazine Hydrochloride (Co-administration has resulted in isolated cases of neuroleptic malignant syndrome). Products include:
- Prolixin ... 510

Haloperidol (Carbamazepine induces CYP activity with the potential for decreased haloperidol levels; co-administration has resulted in isolated cases of neuroleptic malignant syndrome). Products include:
- Haldol Injection, Tablets and Concentrate ... 1585

Haloperidol Decanoate (Carbamazepine induces CYP activity with the potential for decreased haloperidol levels; co-administration has resulted in isolated cases of neuroleptic malignant syndrome). Products include:
- Haldol Decanoate ... 1587

Isoniazid (Isoniazid, a CYP3A4 inhibitor, inhibits carbamazepine metabolism resulting in the potential for increased plasma carbamazepine levels). Products include:
- Nydrazid Injection ... 509
- Rifamate Capsules ... 1278
- Rifater ... 1280

Itraconazole (Itraconazole, a CYP3A4 inhibitor, inhibits carbamazepine metabolism resulting in the potential for increased plasma carbamazepine levels). Products include:
- Sporanox Capsules ... 1352

Ketoconazole (Ketoconazole, a CYP3A4 inhibitor, inhibits carbamazepine metabolism resulting in the potential for increased plasma carbamazepine levels). Products include:
- Nizoral 2% Cream ... 1344
- Nizoral 2% Shampoo ... 1344
- Nizoral Tablets ... 1345

Lamotrigine (Combination therapy has resulted in alterations of thyroid function). Products include:
- Lamictal Tablets ... 1105

Levonorgestrel (Carbamazepine induces CYP activity with the potential for decreased oral contraceptive levels; breakthrough bleeding and reliability of oral contraceptive may be adversely affected). Products include:
- Levlen/Tri-Levlen ... 646
- Nordette-21 Tablets ... 2863
- Nordette-28 Tablets ... 2866
- Norplant System ... 2868
- Levlen/Tri-Levlen ... 646
- Triphasil-21 Tablets ... 2919
- Triphasil-28 Tablets ... 2924

Lithium Carbonate (Co-administration may increase the risk of neurotoxic side effects; co-administration with psychotropic drugs has resulted in isolated cases of neuroleptic malignant syndrome). Products include:
- Eskalith ... 2658
- Lithium Carbonate Capsules & Tablets ... 2352
- Lithonate/Lithotabs/Lithobid ... 2721

Lithium Citrate (Co-administration may increase the risk of neurotoxic side effects; co-administration with psychotropic drugs has resulted in isolated cases of neuroleptic malignant syndrome).
- No products indexed under this heading.

Loxapine Hydrochloride (Co-administration has resulted in isolated cases of neuroleptic malignant syndrome). Products include:
- Loxitane ... 1426

(⊞ Described in PDR For Nonprescription Drugs) (⊚ Described in PDR For Ophthalmology)

Loxapine Succinate (Co-administration has resulted in isolated cases of neuroleptic malignant syndrome). Products include:
  Loxitane Capsules 1426
Mephenytoin (Combination therapy has resulted in alterations of thyroid function). Products include:
  Mesantoin Tablets 2400
Mesoridazine Besylate (Co-administration has resulted in isolated cases of neuroleptic malignant syndrome). Products include:
  Serentil 689
Mestranol (Carbamazepine induces CYP activity with the potential for decreased oral contraceptive levels; breakthrough bleeding and reliability of oral contraceptive may be adversely affected). Products include:
  Norinyl 2563
  Ortho-Novum 1928
Methotrimeprazine (Co-administration has resulted in isolated cases of neuroleptic malignant syndrome). Products include:
  Levoprome 1321
Methsuximide (Carbamazepine induces CYP activity with the potential for decreased methsuximide levels; combination therapy has resulted in alterations of thyroid function). Products include:
  Celontin Kapseals 1955
Molindone Hydrochloride (Co-administration has resulted in isolated cases of neuroleptic malignant syndrome). Products include:
  Moban Tablets and Concentrate ... 1036
Niacinamide (Niacinamide, a CYP3A4 inhibitor, inhibits carbamazepine metabolism resulting in the potential for increased plasma carbamazepine levels). Products include:
  Mega-B 513
Nicotinamide (Nicotinamide, a CYP3A4 inhibitor, inhibits carbamazepine metabolism resulting in the potential for increased plasma carbamazepine levels).
  No products indexed under this heading.
Norethindrone (Carbamazepine induces CYP activity with the potential for decreased oral contraceptive levels; breakthrough bleeding and reliability of oral contraceptive may be adversely affected). Products include:
  Brevicon 2563
  Micronor Tablets 1903
  Modicon 1928
  Norinyl 2563
  Nor-Q D Tablets 2598
  Ortho-Novum 1928
  Ovcon 765
  Tri-Norinyl 2607
Norethynodrel (Carbamazepine induces CYP activity with the potential for decreased oral contraceptive levels; breakthrough bleeding and reliability of oral contraceptive may be adversely affected).
  No products indexed under this heading.
Norgestimate (Carbamazepine induces CYP activity with the potential for decreased oral contraceptive levels; breakthrough bleeding and reliability of oral contraceptive may be adversely affected). Products include:
  Ortho-Cyclen/Ortho-Tri-Cyclen 1914
  Ortho-Cyclen/Ortho-Tri-Cyclen 1914

Norgestrel (Carbamazepine induces CYP activity with the potential for decreased oral contraceptive levels; breakthrough bleeding and reliability of oral contraceptive may be adversely affected). Products include:
  Lo/Ovral Tablets 2852
  Lo/Ovral-28 Tablets 2857
  Ovral Tablets 2877
  Ovral-28 Tablets 2878
  Ovrette Tablets 2878
Paramethadione (Combination therapy has resulted in alterations of thyroid function).
  No products indexed under this heading.
Perphenazine (Co-administration has resulted in isolated cases of neuroleptic malignant syndrome). Products include:
  Etrafon 2495
  Triavil Tablets 1800
  Trilafon 2532
Phenacemide (Combination therapy has resulted in alterations of thyroid function). Products include:
  Phenurone Tablets 455
Phenobarbital (Phenobarbital, a CYP3A4 inducer, can increase carbamazepine metabolism resulting in the potential for decreased plasma carbamazepine levels; combination therapy has resulted in alterations of thyroid function). Products include:
  Arco-Lase Plus Tablets 513
  Bellergal-S Tablets 2375
  Donnatal 2234
  Donnatal Extentabs 2234
  Donnatal Tablets 2234
  Phenobarbital Elixir and Tablets 1523
  Quadrinal Tablets 1398
Phensuximide (Carbamazepine induces CYP activity with the potential for decreased phensuximide levels; combination therapy has resulted in alterations of thyroid function).
  No products indexed under this heading.
Phenytoin (Phenytoin, a CYP3A4 inducer, can increase carbamazepine metabolism resulting in the potential for decreased plasma carbamazepine levels; combination therapy has resulted in alterations of thyroid function and increased or decreased phenytoin levels). Products include:
  Dilantin Infatabs 1967
  Dilantin-125 Suspension 1969
Phenytoin Sodium (Phenytoin, a CYP3A4 inducer, can increase carbamazepine metabolism resulting in the potential for decreased plasma carbamazepine levels; combination therapy has resulted in alterations of thyroid function and increased or decreased phenytoin levels). Products include:
  Dilantin Kapseals 1965
Pimozide (Co-administration has resulted in isolated cases of neuroleptic malignant syndrome). Products include:
  Orap Tablets 1037
Primidone (Primidone, a CYP3A4 inducer, can increase carbamazepine metabolism resulting in the potential for decreased plasma carbamazepine levels; combination therapy has resulted in alterations of thyroid function and increased primidone levels). Products include:
  Mysoline 2860
Prochlorperazine (Co-administration has resulted in isolated cases of neuroleptic malignant syndrome). Products include:
  Compazine 2644

Promethazine Hydrochloride (Co-administration has resulted in isolated cases of neuroleptic malignant syndrome). Products include:
  Mepergan Injection 2859
  Phenergan with Codeine 2883
  Phenergan with Dextromethorphan 2885
  Phenergan Injection 2880
  Phenergan Suppositories 2882
  Phenergan Syrup 2881
  Phenergan Tablets 2882
  Phenergan VC 2886
  Phenergan VC with Codeine 2888
Propoxyphene Hydrochloride (Propoxyphene, a CYP3A4 inhibitor, inhibits carbamazepine metabolism resulting in the potential for increased plasma carbamazepine levels). Products include:
  Darvon 1475
  Wygesic Tablets 2930
Propoxyphene Napsylate (Propoxyphene, a CYP3A4 inhibitor, inhibits carbamazepine metabolism resulting in the potential for increased plasma carbamazepine levels). Products include:
  Darvon-N/Darvocet-N 1473
Rifampin (Rifampin, a CYP3A4 inducer, can increase carbamazepine metabolism resulting in the potential for decreased plasma carbamazepine levels). Products include:
  Rifadin 1276
  Rifamate Capsules 1278
  Rifater 1280
  Rimactane Capsules 865
Risperidone (Co-administration has resulted in isolated cases of neuroleptic malignant syndrome). Products include:
  Risperdal Tablets 1348
Terfenadine (Terfenadine, a CYP3A4 inhibitor, inhibits carbamazepine metabolism resulting in the potential for increased plasma carbamazepine levels). Products include:
  Seldane Tablets 1284
  Seldane-D Extended-Release Tablets 1286
Theophylline (Theophylline, a CYP3A4 inducer, can increase carbamazepine metabolism resulting in the potential for decreased plasma carbamazepine levels; potential for decreased theophylline levels). Products include:
  Marax Tablets & DF Syrup 2015
  Quibron 2227
Theophylline Anhydrous (Theophylline, a CYP3A4 inducer, can increase carbamazepine metabolism resulting in the potential for decreased plasma carbamazepine levels; potential for decreased theophylline levels). Products include:
  Aerolate 1003
  Primatene Tablets 844
  Respbid Tablets 687
  Slo-bid Gyrocaps 2201
  Theo-24 Extended Release Capsules 2753
  Theo-Dur Extended-Release Tablets 1367
  Theo-X Extended-Release Tablets 793
  Uni-Dur Extended-Release Tablets 1374
  Uniphyl 400 mg and 600 mg Tablets 2157
Theophylline Calcium Salicylate (Theophylline, a CYP3A4 inducer, can increase carbamazepine metabolism resulting in the potential for decreased plasma carbamazepine levels; potential for decreased theophylline levels). Products include:
  Quadrinal Tablets 1398

Theophylline Sodium Glycinate (Theophylline, a CYP3A4 inducer, can increase carbamazepine metabolism resulting in the potential for decreased plasma carbamazepine levels; potential for decreased theophylline levels).
  No products indexed under this heading.
Thioridazine Hydrochloride (Co-administration has resulted in isolated cases of neuroleptic malignant syndrome). Products include:
  Mellaril 2398
Thiothixene (Co-administration has resulted in isolated cases of neuroleptic malignant syndrome). Products include:
  Navane Capsules and Concentrate 2018
  Navane Intramuscular 2019
Trifluoperazine Hydrochloride (Co-administration has resulted in isolated cases of neuroleptic malignant syndrome). Products include:
  Stelazine 2692
Trimethadione (Combination therapy has resulted in alterations of thyroid function).
  No products indexed under this heading.
Troleandomycin (Macrolide antibiotic, a CYP3A4 inhibitor, inhibits carbamazepine metabolism resulting in the potential for increased plasma carbamazepine levels). Products include:
  Tao Capsules 2033
Valproic Acid (Valproate, a CYP3A4 inhibitor, inhibits carbamazepine metabolism resulting in the potential for increased plasma carbamazepine and 10,11-epoxide levels; combination therapy has resulted in alterations of thyroid function and decreased valproate levels). Products include:
  Depakene 416
Verapamil Hydrochloride (Verapamil, a CYP3A4 inhibitor, inhibits carbamazepine metabolism resulting in the potential for increased plasma carbamazepine levels). Products include:
  Calan SR Caplets 2571
  Calan Tablets 2568
  Covera-HS Tablets 2573
  Isoptin Injectable 1391
  Isoptin Oral Tablets 1393
  Isoptin SR Tablets 1395
  Verelan Capsules 1455
Warfarin Sodium (Carbamazepine induces CYP activity with the potential for decreased oral anticoagulant levels). Products include:
  Coumadin 941

TEGRIN DANDRUFF SHAMPOO
(Coal Tar) 634
None cited in PDR database.

TEGRIN SKIN CREAM & TEGRIN MEDICATED SOAP
(Coal Tar) 634
None cited in PDR database.

TELDRIN 12 HOUR ANTIHISTAMINE/NASAL DECONGESTANT ALLERGY RELIEF CAPSULES
(Chlorpheniramine Maleate, Phenylpropanolamine Hydrochloride) 786
May interact with hypnotics and sedatives, tranquilizers, monoamine oxidase inhibitors, and certain other

IMPORTANT NOTE: Always consult each drug listing in the patient's regimen for possible interactions.

agents. Compounds in these categories include:

Alprazolam (May increase drowsiness effect; consult your doctor). Products include:
Xanax Tablets 2115
Buspirone Hydrochloride (May increase drowsiness effect; consult your doctor). Products include:
BuSpar Tablets 738
Chlordiazepoxide (May increase drowsiness effect; consult your doctor). Products include:
Limbitrol 2333
Chlordiazepoxide Hydrochloride (May increase drowsiness effect; consult your doctor). Products include:
Librax Capsules 2330
Librium Capsules 2331
Librium Injectable 2332
Chlorpromazine (May increase drowsiness effect; consult your doctor). Products include:
Thorazine Suppositories 2701
Chlorpromazine Hydrochloride (May increase drowsiness effect; consult your doctor). Products include:
Thorazine 2701
Chlorprothixene (May increase drowsiness effect; consult your doctor).
No products indexed under this heading.
Chlorprothixene Hydrochloride (May increase drowsiness effect; consult your doctor).
No products indexed under this heading.
Clorazepate Dipotassium (May increase drowsiness effect; consult your doctor). Products include:
Tranxene 459
Diazepam (May increase drowsiness effect; consult your doctor). Products include:
Dizac (diazepam injectable emulsion) CIV 1862
Valium Injectable 2336
Valium Tablets 2335
Droperidol (May increase drowsiness effect; consult your doctor). Products include:
Inapsine Injection 462
Estazolam (May increase drowsiness effect; consult your doctor). Products include:
ProSom Tablets 457
Ethchlorvynol (May increase drowsiness effect; consult your doctor). Products include:
Placidyl Capsules 456
Ethinamate (May increase drowsiness effect; consult your doctor).
No products indexed under this heading.
Fluphenazine Decanoate (May increase drowsiness effect; consult your doctor). Products include:
Prolixin Decanoate 510
Fluphenazine Enanthate (May increase drowsiness effect; consult your doctor). Products include:
Prolixin Enanthate 510
Fluphenazine Hydrochloride (May increase drowsiness effect; consult your doctor). Products include:
Prolixin 510
Flurazepam Hydrochloride (May increase drowsiness effect; consult your doctor). Products include:
Dalmane Capsules 2329
Furazolidone (Concurrent and/or sequential use is not recommended). Products include:
Furoxone 2221
Glutethimide (May increase drowsiness effect; consult your doctor).
No products indexed under this heading.
Haloperidol (May increase drowsiness effect; consult your doctor). Products include:
Haldol Injection, Tablets and Concentrate 1585
Haloperidol Decanoate (May increase drowsiness effect; consult your doctor). Products include:
Haldol Decanoate 1587
Hydroxyzine Hydrochloride (May increase drowsiness effect; consult your doctor). Products include:
Atarax Tablets & Syrup 1992
Marax Tablets & DF Syrup 2015
Vistaril Intramuscular Solution 2042
Isocarboxazid (Concurrent and/or sequential use is not recommended).
No products indexed under this heading.
Lorazepam (May increase drowsiness effect; consult your doctor). Products include:
Ativan Injection 2805
Ativan Tablets 2807
Loxapine Hydrochloride (May increase drowsiness effect; consult your doctor). Products include:
Loxitane 1426
Loxapine Succinate (May increase drowsiness effect; consult your doctor). Products include:
Loxitane Capsules 1426
Meprobamate (May increase drowsiness effect; consult your doctor). Products include:
Miltown Tablets 2780
PMB 200 and PMB 400 2890
Mesoridazine Besylate (May increase drowsiness effect; consult your doctor). Products include:
Serentil 689
Midazolam Hydrochloride (May increase drowsiness effect; consult your doctor). Products include:
Versed Injection 2324
Molindone Hydrochloride (May increase drowsiness effect; consult your doctor). Products include:
Moban Tablets and Concentrate 1036
Oxazepam (May increase drowsiness effect; consult your doctor). Products include:
Serax Capsules 2916
Serax Tablets 2916
Perphenazine (May increase drowsiness effect; consult your doctor). Products include:
Etrafon 2495
Triavil Tablets 1800
Trilafon 2532
Phenelzine Sulfate (Concurrent and/or sequential use is not recommended). Products include:
Nardil 1977
Prazepam (May increase drowsiness effect; consult your doctor).
No products indexed under this heading.
Prochlorperazine (May increase drowsiness effect; consult your doctor). Products include:
Compazine 2644
Promethazine Hydrochloride (May increase drowsiness effect; consult your doctor). Products include:
Mepergan Injection 2859
Phenergan with Codeine 2883
Phenergan with Dextromethorphan 2885
Phenergan Injection 2880
Phenergan Suppositories 2882
Phenergan Syrup 2881
Phenergan Tablets 2882
Phenergan VC 2886
Phenergan VC with Codeine 2888
Propofol (May increase drowsiness effect; consult your doctor). Products include:
Diprivan Injectable Emulsion 2939
Quazepam (May increase drowsiness effect; consult your doctor). Products include:
Doral Tablets 2773
Secobarbital Sodium (May increase drowsiness effect; consult your doctor). Products include:
Seconal Sodium Pulvules 1529
Selegiline Hydrochloride (Concurrent and/or sequential use is not recommended). Products include:
Eldepryl Capsules 2729
Temazepam (May increase drowsiness effect; consult your doctor). Products include:
Restoril Capsules 2413
Thioridazine Hydrochloride (May increase drowsiness effect; consult your doctor). Products include:
Mellaril 2398
Thiothixene (May increase drowsiness effect; consult your doctor). Products include:
Navane Capsules and Concentrate 2018
Navane Intramuscular 2019
Tranylcypromine Sulfate (Concurrent and/or sequential use is not recommended). Products include:
Parnate Tablets 2679
Triazolam (May increase drowsiness effect; consult your doctor). Products include:
Halcion Tablets 2093
Trifluoperazine Hydrochloride (May increase drowsiness effect; consult your doctor). Products include:
Stelazine 2692
Zolpidem Tartrate (May increase drowsiness effect; consult your doctor). Products include:
Ambien Tablets 2559

Food Interactions

Alcohol (May increase drowsiness effect; avoid concurrent use).

TEMOVATE CREAM
(Clobetasol Propionate) 1152
None cited in PDR database.

TEMOVATE E EMOLLIENT
(Clobetasol Propionate) 1154
None cited in PDR database.

TEMOVATE GEL
(Clobetasol Propionate) 1153
None cited in PDR database.

TEMOVATE OINTMENT
(Clobetasol Propionate) 1152
None cited in PDR database.

TEMOVATE SCALP APPLICATION
(Clobetasol Propionate) 1153
None cited in PDR database.

TEMPO SOFT ANTACID
(Calcium Carbonate, Aluminum Hydroxide, Magnesium Hydroxide, Simethicone) .... ▣ 799
May interact with:

Drugs, Oral, unspecified (Antacids may interact with certain unspecified drugs).

TENEX TABLETS
(Guanfacine Hydrochloride) 2249
May interact with central nervous system depressants and certain other agents. Compounds in these categories include:

Alfentanil Hydrochloride (Potential for increased sedation). Products include:
Alfenta Injection 1334
Alprazolam (Potential for increased sedation). Products include:
Xanax Tablets 2115
Aprobarbital (Potential for increased sedation).
No products indexed under this heading.
Buprenorphine (Potential for increased sedation). Products include:
Buprenex Injectable 2170
Buspirone Hydrochloride (Potential for increased sedation). Products include:
BuSpar Tablets 738
Butabarbital (Potential for increased sedation).
No products indexed under this heading.
Butalbital (Potential for increased sedation). Products include:
Axocet Capsules 2469
Esgic-plus Capsules 1012
Esgic-plus Tablets 1012
Fioricet Tablets 2386
Fioricet with Codeine Capsules 2387
Fiorinal Capsules 2388
Fiorinal with Codeine Capsules 2390
Fiorinal Tablets 2388
Phrenilin 790
Sedapap Tablets 50 mg/650 mg .. 1826
Chlordiazepoxide (Potential for increased sedation). Products include:
Limbitrol 2333
Chlordiazepoxide Hydrochloride (Potential for increased sedation). Products include:
Librax Capsules 2330
Librium Capsules 2331
Librium Injectable 2332
Chlorpromazine (Potential for increased sedation). Products include:
Thorazine Suppositories 2701
Chlorprothixene (Potential for increased sedation).
No products indexed under this heading.
Chlorprothixene Hydrochloride (Potential for increased sedation).
No products indexed under this heading.
Chlorprothixene Lactate (Potential for increased sedation).
No products indexed under this heading.
Clorazepate Dipotassium (Potential for increased sedation). Products include:
Tranxene 459
Clozapine (Potential for increased sedation). Products include:
Clozaril Tablets 2377
Codeine Phosphate (Potential for increased sedation). Products include:
Brontex 2130
Dimetane-DC Cough Syrup 2232
Fioricet with Codeine Capsules 2387
Fiorinal with Codeine Capsules 2390
Nucofed 2225
Phenergan with Codeine 2883
Phenergan VC with Codeine 2888
Robitussin A-C Syrup 2248
Robitussin-DAC Syrup 2249
Ryna .... ▣ 804
Soma Compound w/Codeine Tablets 2784
Tylenol with Codeine 1592

1051 Interactions Index Tenoretic

Desflurane (Potential for increased sedation). Products include:
Suprane (desflurane, USP) ... 1865
Dezocine (Potential for increased sedation). Products include:
Dalgan Injection ... 529
Diazepam (Potential for increased sedation). Products include:
Dizac (diazepam injectable emulsion) CIV ... 1862
Valium Injectable ... 2336
Valium Tablets ... 2335
Droperidol (Potential for increased sedation). Products include:
Inapsine Injection ... 462
Enflurane (Potential for increased sedation).
No products indexed under this heading.
Estazolam (Potential for increased sedation). Products include:
ProSom Tablets ... 457
Ethchlorvynol (Potential for increased sedation). Products include:
Placidyl Capsules ... 456
Ethinamate (Potential for increased sedation).
No products indexed under this heading.
Fentanyl (Potential for increased sedation). Products include:
Duragesic Transdermal System ... 1336
Fentanyl Citrate (Potential for increased sedation). Products include:
Sublimaze Injection ... 463
Fluphenazine Decanoate (Potential for increased sedation). Products include:
Prolixin Decanoate ... 510
Fluphenazine Enanthate (Potential for increased sedation). Products include:
Prolixin Enanthate ... 510
Fluphenazine Hydrochloride (Potential for increased sedation). Products include:
Prolixin ... 510
Flurazepam Hydrochloride (Potential for increased sedation). Products include:
Dalmane Capsules ... 2329
Glutethimide (Potential for increased sedation).
No products indexed under this heading.
Haloperidol (Potential for increased sedation). Products include:
Haldol Injection, Tablets and Concentrate ... 1585
Haloperidol Decanoate (Potential for increased sedation). Products include:
Haldol Decanoate ... 1587
Hydrocodone Bitartrate (Potential for increased sedation). Products include:
Codiclear DH Syrup ... 808
Duratuss HD Elixir ... 2750
Histussin D Liquid ... 670
Hycodan Tablets and Syrup ... 946
Hycomine Compound Tablets ... 948
Hycomine ... 947
Hycotuss Expectorant Syrup ... 950
Hydrocet Capsules ... 787
Lorcet 10/650 Tablets ... 1016
Lortab ... 2751
Tussend ... 1830
Tussend Expectorant ... 1831
Vicodin Tablets ... 1404
Vicodin ES Tablets ... 1405
Vicodin HP Tablets ... 1403
Vicodin Tuss Expectorant ... 1406
Zydone Capsules ... 967
Hydrocodone Polistirex (Potential for increased sedation). Products include:
Tussionex Pennkinetic Extended-Release Suspension ... 1624
Hydroxyzine Hydrochloride (Potential for increased sedation). Products include:
Atarax Tablets & Syrup ... 1992
Marax Tablets & DF Syrup ... 2015
Vistaril Intramuscular Solution ... 2042
Isoflurane (Potential for increased sedation).
No products indexed under this heading.
Ketamine Hydrochloride (Potential for increased sedation).
No products indexed under this heading.
Levomethadyl Acetate Hydrochloride (Potential for increased sedation). Products include:
Orlaam Oral Solution ... 2361
Levorphanol Tartrate (Potential for increased sedation). Products include:
Levo-Dromoran ... 2297
Lorazepam (Potential for increased sedation). Products include:
Ativan Injection ... 2805
Ativan Tablets ... 2807
Loxapine Hydrochloride (Potential for increased sedation). Products include:
Loxitane ... 1426
Loxapine Succinate (Potential for increased sedation). Products include:
Loxitane Capsules ... 1426
Meperidine Hydrochloride (Potential for increased sedation). Products include:
Demerol ... 2438
Mepergan Injection ... 2859
Mephobarbital (Potential for increased sedation). Products include:
Mebaral Tablets ... 2452
Meprobamate (Potential for increased sedation). Products include:
Miltown Tablets ... 2780
PMB 200 and PMB 400 ... 2890
Mesoridazine Besylate (Potential for increased sedation). Products include:
Serentil ... 689
Methadone Hydrochloride (Potential for increased sedation). Products include:
Methadone Hydrochloride Oral Concentrate ... 2356
Methadone Hydrochloride Oral Solution & Tablets ... 2357
Methohexital Sodium (Potential for increased sedation).
No products indexed under this heading.
Methotrimeprazine (Potential for increased sedation). Products include:
Levoprome ... 1321
Methoxyflurane (Potential for increased sedation).
No products indexed under this heading.
Midazolam Hydrochloride (Potential for increased sedation). Products include:
Versed Injection ... 2324
Molindone Hydrochloride (Potential for increased sedation). Products include:
Moban Tablets and Concentrate ... 1036
Morphine Sulfate (Potential for increased sedation). Products include:
Astramorph/PF Injection, USP (Preservative-Free) ... 526
Duramorph Injection ... 983
Infumorph 200 and Infumorph 500 Sterile Solutions ... 985
Kadian Capsules ... 2948
MS Contin Tablets ... 2149
MSIR ... 2152
Oramorph SR (Morphine Sulfate Sustained Release Tablets) ... 2359
RMS Suppositories CII ... 2766
Roxanol ... 2365
Opium Alkaloids (Potential for increased sedation).
No products indexed under this heading.
Oxazepam (Potential for increased sedation). Products include:
Serax Capsules ... 2916
Serax Tablets ... 2916
Oxycodone Hydrochloride (Potential for increased sedation). Products include:
OxyContin Tablets ... 2163
OxyIR Capsules ... 2167
Percocet Tablets ... 955
Percodan Tablets ... 955
Percodan-Demi Tablets ... 956
Roxicodone Tablets, Oral Solution & Intensol (Oxycodone) ... 2366
Tylox Capsules ... 1593
Pentobarbital Sodium (Potential for increased sedation). Products include:
Nembutal Sodium Capsules ... 440
Nembutal Sodium Solution ... 442
Nembutal Sodium Suppositories ... 444
Perphenazine (Potential for increased sedation). Products include:
Etrafon ... 2495
Triavil Tablets ... 1800
Trilafon ... 2532
Phenobarbital (Potential for increased sedation; concurrent administration may result in significant reductions in elimination half-life and plasma concentration). Products include:
Arco-Lase Plus Tablets ... 513
Bellergal-S Tablets ... 2375
Donnatal ... 2234
Donnatal Extentabs ... 2234
Donnatal Tablets ... 2234
Phenobarbital Elixir and Tablets ... 1523
Quadrinal Tablets ... 1398
Phenytoin (Concurrent administration may result in significant reductions in elimination half-life and plasma concentration). Products include:
Dilantin Infatabs ... 1967
Dilantin-125 Suspension ... 1969
Phenytoin Sodium (Concurrent administration may result in significant reductions in elimination half-life and plasma concentration). Products include:
Dilantin Kapseals ... 1965
Prazepam (Potential for increased sedation).
No products indexed under this heading.
Prochlorperazine (Potential for increased sedation). Products include:
Compazine ... 2644
Promethazine Hydrochloride (Potential for increased sedation). Products include:
Mepergan Injection ... 2859
Phenergan with Codeine ... 2883
Phenergan with Dextromethorphan ... 2885
Phenergan Injection ... 2880
Phenergan Suppositories ... 2882
Phenergan Syrup ... 2881
Phenergan Tablets ... 2882
Phenergan VC ... 2886
Phenergan VC with Codeine ... 2888
Propofol (Potential for increased sedation). Products include:
Diprivan Injectable Emulsion ... 2939
Propoxyphene Hydrochloride (Potential for increased sedation). Products include:
Darvon ... 1475
Wygesic Tablets ... 2930
Propoxyphene Napsylate (Potential for increased sedation). Products include:
Darvon-N/Darvocet-N ... 1473
Quazepam (Potential for increased sedation). Products include:
Doral Tablets ... 2773
Risperidone (Potential for increased sedation). Products include:
Risperdal Tablets ... 1348
Secobarbital Sodium (Potential for increased sedation). Products include:
Seconal Sodium Pulvules ... 1529
Sevoflurane (Potential for increased sedation).
No products indexed under this heading.
Sufentanil Citrate (Potential for increased sedation). Products include:
Sufenta Injection ... 1355
Temazepam (Potential for increased sedation). Products include:
Restoril Capsules ... 2413
Thiamylal Sodium (Potential for increased sedation).
No products indexed under this heading.
Thioridazine Hydrochloride (Potential for increased sedation). Products include:
Mellaril ... 2398
Thiothixene (Potential for increased sedation). Products include:
Navane Capsules and Concentrate 2018
Navane Intramuscular ... 2019
Triazolam (Potential for increased sedation). Products include:
Halcion Tablets ... 2093
Trifluoperazine Hydrochloride (Potential for increased sedation). Products include:
Stelazine ... 2692
Zolpidem Tartrate (Potential for increased sedation). Products include:
Ambien Tablets ... 2559

TENORETIC TABLETS
(Atenolol, Chlorthalidone) ... 2963
May interact with antihypertensives, catecholamine depleting drugs, calcium channel blockers, lithium preparations, insulin, corticosteroids, cardiac glycosides, and certain other agents. Compounds in these categories include:

Acebutolol Hydrochloride (Concurrent administration may potentiate the action of other antihypertensive agent). Products include:
Sectral Capsules ... 2914
Amlodipine Besylate (Calcium channel blockers may have an additive effect when given with Tenoretic; potential for bradycardia and heart block). Products include:
Lotrel Capsules ... 858
Norvasc Tablets ... 2020
Benazepril Hydrochloride (Concurrent administration may potentiate the action of other antihypertensive agent). Products include:
Lotensin Tablets ... 852
Lotensin HCT Tablets ... 855
Lotrel Capsules ... 858
Bendroflumethiazide (Concurrent administration may potentiate the action of other antihypertensive agent).
No products indexed under this heading.

IMPORTANT NOTE: Always consult each drug listing in the patient's regimen for possible interactions.

Tenoretic — Interactions Index

Bepridil Hydrochloride (Calcium channel blockers may have an additive effect when given with Tenoretic; potential for bradycardia and heart block). Products include:
- Vascor Tablets (200 and 300 mg) ... 1597

Betamethasone Acetate (Potential for hypokalemia). Products include:
- Celestone Soluspan Suspension ... 2484

Betamethasone Sodium Phosphate (Potential for hypokalemia). Products include:
- Celestone Soluspan Suspension ... 2484

Betaxolol Hydrochloride (Concurrent administration may potentiate the action of other antihypertensive agent). Products include:
- Betoptic Ophthalmic Solution ... 465
- Betoptic S Ophthalmic Suspension ... 467
- Kerlone Tablets ... 2588

Bisoprolol Fumarate (Concurrent administration may potentiate the action of other antihypertensive agent). Products include:
- Zebeta Tablets ... 1457
- Ziac ... 1459

Captopril (Concurrent administration may potentiate the action of other antihypertensive agent). Products include:
- Capoten Tablets ... 740
- Capozide Tablets ... 744

Carteolol Hydrochloride (Concurrent administration may potentiate the action of other antihypertensive agent). Products include:
- Cartrol Tablets ... 413
- Ocupress Ophthalmic Solution, 1% Sterile ... ⊙ 297

Chlorothiazide (Concurrent administration may potentiate the action of other antihypertensive agent). Products include:
- Aldoclor Tablets ... 1638
- Diupres Tablets ... 1691
- Diuril Oral ... 1694

Chlorothiazide Sodium (Concurrent administration may potentiate the action of other antihypertensive agent). Products include:
- Diuril Sodium Intravenous ... 1693

Clonidine (Potential for exacerbation of rebound hypertension; Tenoretic should be discontinued several days before the gradual withdrawal of clonidine). Products include:
- Catapres-TTS ... 680

Clonidine Hydrochloride (Potential for exacerbation of rebound hypertension; Tenoretic should be discontinued several days before the gradual withdrawal of clonidine). Products include:
- Catapres Tablets ... 679
- Combipres Tablets ... 682

Cortisone Acetate (Potential for hypokalemia). Products include:
- Cortone Acetate Sterile Suspension ... 1663
- Cortone Acetate Tablets ... 1664

Deserpidine (Potential for hypotension and/or marked bradycardia which may produce vertigo, syncope or postural hypotension).
- No products indexed under this heading.

Deslanoside (Hypokalemia induced by Tenoretic therapy can sensitize or exaggerate the response of the heart to the toxic effects of digitalis).
- No products indexed under this heading.

Dexamethasone (Potential for hypokalemia). Products include:
- AK-Trol Ointment & Suspension ... ⊙ 205
- Decadron Elixir ... 1676
- Decadron Tablets ... 1678
- Decaspray Topical Aerosol ... 1689
- Maxitrol Ophthalmic Ointment and Suspension ... ⊙ 222
- TobraDex Ophthalmic Suspension and Ointment ... 469

Dexamethasone Acetate (Potential for hypokalemia). Products include:
- Dalalone D.P. Injectable ... 1009
- Decadron-LA Sterile Suspension ... 1687

Dexamethasone Sodium Phosphate (Potential for hypokalemia). Products include:
- Decadron Phosphate Injection ... 1680
- Decadron Phosphate Sterile Ophthalmic Ointment ... 1684
- Decadron Phosphate Sterile Ophthalmic Solution ... 1685
- Decadron Phosphate Topical Cream ... 1686
- Decadron Phosphate with Xylocaine Injection, Sterile ... 1683
- Dexacort Phosphate in Respihaler ... 1606
- Dexacort Phosphate in Turbinaire ... 1607
- NeoDecadron Sterile Ophthalmic Ointment ... 1755
- NeoDecadron Sterile Ophthalmic Solution ... 1756
- NeoDecadron Topical Cream ... 1757

Diazoxide (Concurrent administration may potentiate the action of other antihypertensive agent). Products include:
- Hyperstat I.V. Injection ... 2504
- Proglycem ... 575

Digitoxin (Hypokalemia induced by Tenoretic therapy can sensitize or exaggerate the response of the heart to the toxic effects of digitalis). Products include:
- Crystodigin Tablets ... 1472

Digoxin (Hypokalemia induced by Tenoretic therapy can sensitize or exaggerate the response of the heart to the toxic effects of digitalis). Products include:
- Lanoxicaps ... 1110
- Lanoxin Elixir Pediatric ... 1113
- Lanoxin Injection ... 1116
- Lanoxin Injection Pediatric ... 1119
- Lanoxin Tablets ... 1121

Diltiazem Hydrochloride (Calcium channel blockers may have an additive effect when given with Tenoretic; potential for bradycardia and heart block). Products include:
- Cardizem CD Capsules ... 1251
- Cardizem SR Capsules ... 1255
- Cardizem Injectable ... 1253
- Cardizem Tablets ... 1257
- Dilacor XR Extended-release Capsules ... 2183
- Tiazac Capsules ... 1019

Doxazosin Mesylate (Concurrent administration may potentiate the action of other antihypertensive agent). Products include:
- Cardura Tablets ... 1993

Enalapril Maleate (Concurrent administration may potentiate the action of other antihypertensive agent). Products include:
- Vaseretic Tablets ... 1810
- Vasotec Tablets ... 1816

Enalaprilat (Concurrent administration may potentiate the action of other antihypertensive agent). Products include:
- Vasotec I.V. ... 1814

Epinephrine (Patients with a history of anaphylactic reaction may be unresponsive to the usual dose of epinephrine). Products include:
- EPIFRIN ... ⊙ 237
- EpiPen ... 808
- Marcaine with Epinephrine ... 2446
- Primatene Mist ... ⊡ 843
- Sensorcaine with Epinephrine Injection ... 554
- Sus-Phrine Injection ... 1017
- Xylocaine with Epinephrine Injections ... 562

Epinephrine Hydrochloride (Patients with a history of anaphylactic reaction may be unresponsive to the usual dose of epinephrine). Products include:
- Ana-Kit Anaphylaxis Emergency Treatment Kit ... 611

Esmolol Hydrochloride (Concurrent administration may potentiate the action of other antihypertensive agent). Products include:
- Brevibloc (esmolol HCl) Injection ... 1860

Felodipine (Calcium channel blockers may have an additive effect when given with Tenoretic; potential for bradycardia and heart block). Products include:
- Plendil Extended-Release Tablets ... 514

Fludrocortisone Acetate (Potential for hypokalemia). Products include:
- Florinef Acetate Tablets ... 506

Fosinopril Sodium (Concurrent administration may potentiate the action of other antihypertensive agent). Products include:
- Monopril Tablets ... 762

Furosemide (Concurrent administration may potentiate the action of other antihypertensive agent). Products include:
- Lasix Injection, Oral Solution and Tablets ... 1267

Guanabenz Acetate (Concurrent administration may potentiate the action of other antihypertensive agent).
- No products indexed under this heading.

Guanethidine Monosulfate (Potential for hypotension and/or marked bradycardia which may produce vertigo, syncope or postural hypotension). Products include:
- Esimil Tablets ... 840
- Ismelin Tablets ... 845

Hydralazine Hydrochloride (Concurrent administration may potentiate the action of other antihypertensive agent). Products include:
- Apresazide Capsules ... 824
- Apresoline Hydrochloride Tablets ... 826
- Hydralazine Hydrochloride Injection USP ... 2712
- Ser-Ap-Es Tablets ... 867

Hydrochlorothiazide (Concurrent administration may potentiate the action of other antihypertensive agent). Products include:
- Aldactazide Tablets ... 2556
- Aldoril Tablets ... 1644
- Apresazide Capsules ... 824
- Capozide Tablets ... 744
- Dyazide Capsules ... 2653
- Esidrix Tablets ... 839
- Esimil Tablets ... 840
- HydroDIURIL Tablets ... 1716
- Hydropres Tablets ... 1718
- Hyzaar Tablets ... 1720
- Inderide Tablets ... 2838
- Inderide LA Long Acting Capsules ... 2840
- Lopressor HCT Tablets ... 850
- Lotensin HCT Tablets ... 855
- Moduretic Tablets ... 1748
- Oretic Tablets ... 450
- Prinzide Tablets ... 1780
- Ser-Ap-Es Tablets ... 867
- Timolide Tablets ... 1791
- Vaseretic Tablets ... 1810
- Zestoretic Tablets ... 2968
- Ziac ... 1459

Hydrocortisone (Potential for hypokalemia). Products include:
- Anusol-HC Cream 2.5% ... 1953
- Aquanil HC Lotion ... 1989
- Maximum Strength Cortaid Spray ... ⊡ 800
- CORTENEMA ... 2713
- Cortisporin Ointment ... 1074
- Cortisporin Ophthalmic Ointment Sterile ... 1074
- Cortisporin Ophthalmic Suspension Sterile ... 1075
- Cortisporin Otic Solution Sterile ... 1076
- Cortisporin Otic Suspension Sterile ... 1077
- Cortizone-5 ... ⊡ 795
- Cortizone-10 ... ⊡ 795
- Hydrocortone Tablets ... 1715
- Hytone ... 922
- Hytone Ointment 2 ½ % ... 923
- Massengill Medicated Soft Cloth Towelettes ... 2628
- Pediotic Suspension Sterile ... 1140
- Preparation H Hydrocortisone 1% Cream ... ⊡ 843
- ProctoCream-HC 2.5% ... 2552
- VōSoL HC Otic Solution ... 2786

Hydrocortisone Acetate (Potential for hypokalemia). Products include:
- Analpram-HC Rectal Cream 1% and 2.5% ... 993
- Anusol HC-1 Hydrocortisone Anti-Itch Ointment ... ⊡ 810
- Anusol-HC Suppositories ... 1954
- Caldecort Anti-Itch Hydrocortisone Cream ... ⊡ 651
- Coly-Mycin S Otic w/Neomycin & Hydrocortisone ... ⊡ 1965
- Cortaid ... ⊡ 800
- Cortifoam ... 2540
- Cortisporin Cream ... 1073
- Epifoam ... 2543
- Hydrocortone Acetate Sterile Suspension ... 1712
- Mantadil Cream ... 1124
- Nupercainal Hydrocortisone 1% Cream ... ⊡ 661
- Pramosone Cream, Lotion & Ointment ... 995
- ProctoFoam-HC ... 2552
- Terra-Cortril Ophthalmic Suspension ... 2033

Hydrocortisone Sodium Phosphate (Potential for hypokalemia). Products include:
- Hydrocortone Phosphate Injection, Sterile ... 1713

Hydrocortisone Sodium Succinate (Potential for hypokalemia).
- No products indexed under this heading.

Hydroflumethiazide (Concurrent administration may potentiate the action of other antihypertensive agent). Products include:
- Diucardin Tablets ... 2824

Indapamide (Concurrent administration may potentiate the action of other antihypertensive agent).
- No products indexed under this heading.

Insulin, Human (Insulin requirements in diabetic patients may be altered).
- No products indexed under this heading.

Insulin, Human Isophane Suspension (Insulin requirements in diabetic patients may be altered). Products include:
- Novolin N Human Insulin 10 ml Vials ... 1846

Insulin, Human NPH (Insulin requirements in diabetic patients may be altered). Products include:
- Humulin N, 100 Units ... 1495
- Novolin N PenFill 1.5 ml Cartridges Durable Insulin Delivery System ... 1849
- Novolin N Prefilled Syringe Disposable Insulin Delivery System ... 1850

Insulin, Human Regular (Insulin requirements in diabetic patients may be altered). Products include:
- Humulin R, 100 Units ... 1497
- Novolin R Human Insulin 10 ml Vials ... 1846
- Novolin R PenFill 1.5 ml Cartridges Durable Insulin Delivery System ... 1849
- Novolin R Prefilled Syringe Disposable Insulin Delivery System ... 1850
- Velosulin BR Human Insulin 10 ml Vials ... 1847

(⊡ Described in PDR For Nonprescription Drugs)   (⊙ Described in PDR For Ophthalmology)

1053 **Interactions Index** **Tenoretic**

Insulin, Human, Zinc Suspension (Insulin requirements in diabetic patients may be altered). Products include:
- Humulin L, 100 Units 1494
- Humulin U, 100 Units 1498
- Novolin L Human Insulin 10 ml Vials 1846

Insulin Lispro, Human (Insulin requirements in diabetic patients may be altered). Products include:
- Humalog Injection 1488

Insulin, NPH (Insulin requirements in diabetic patients may be altered). Products include:
- NPH, 100 Units 1502
- Pork NPH, 100 Units 1506
- Purified Pork NPH Isophane Insulin 1852

Insulin, Regular (Insulin requirements in diabetic patients may be altered). Products include:
- Regular, 100 Units 1503
- Pork Regular, 100 Units 1507
- Pork Regular (Concentrated), 500 Units 1508
- Purified Pork Regular Insulin 1852

Insulin, Zinc Crystals (Insulin requirements in diabetic patients may be altered). Products include:
- NPH, 100 Units 1502

Insulin, Zinc Suspension (Insulin requirements in diabetic patients may be altered). Products include:
- Iletin I 1501
- Lente, 100 Units 1501
- Iletin II 1504
- Pork Lente, 100 Units 1504
- Purified Pork Lente Insulin 1852

Isradipine (Calcium channel blockers may have an additive effect when given with Tenoretic; potential for bradycardia and heart block). Products include:
- DynaCirc Capsules 2381
- DynaCirc CR Tablets 2383

Labetalol Hydrochloride (Concurrent administration may potentiate the action of other antihypertensive agent). Products include:
- Normodyne Injection 2519
- Normodyne Tablets 2522
- Trandate 1158

Lisinopril (Concurrent administration may potentiate the action of other antihypertensive agent). Products include:
- Prinivil Tablets 1776
- Prinzide Tablets 1780
- Zestoretic Tablets 2968
- Zestril Tablets 2972

Lithium Carbonate (Reduced renal clearance; lithium toxicity). Products include:
- Eskalith 2658
- Lithium Carbonate Capsules & Tablets 2352
- Lithonate/Lithotabs/Lithobid 2721

Lithium Citrate (Reduced renal clearance; lithium toxicity).
- No products indexed under this heading.

Losartan Potassium (Calcium channel blockers may have an additive effect when given with Tenoretic; potential for bradycardia and heart block). Products include:
- Cozaar Tablets 1668
- Hyzaar Tablets 1720

Mecamylamine Hydrochloride (Concurrent administration may potentiate the action of other antihypertensive agent). Products include:
- Inversine Tablets 1729

Methyclothiazide (Concurrent administration may potentiate the action of other antihypertensive agent). Products include:
- Enduron Tablets 424

Methyldopa (Concurrent administration may potentiate the action of other antihypertensive agent). Products include:
- Aldoclor Tablets 1638
- Aldomet Oral 1640
- Aldoril Tablets 1644

Methyldopate Hydrochloride (Concurrent administration may potentiate the action of other antihypertensive agent). Products include:
- Aldomet Ester HCl Injection 1642

Methylprednisolone Acetate (Potential for hypokalemia).
- No products indexed under this heading.

Methylprednisolone Sodium Succinate (Potential for hypokalemia).
- No products indexed under this heading.

Metolazone (Concurrent administration may potentiate the action of other antihypertensive agent). Products include:
- Mykrox Tablets 1617
- Zaroxolyn Tablets 1625

Metoprolol Succinate (Concurrent administration may potentiate the action of other antihypertensive agent). Products include:
- Toprol-XL Tablets 560

Metoprolol Tartrate (Concurrent administration may potentiate the action of other antihypertensive agent). Products include:
- Lopressor 848
- Lopressor HCT Tablets 850

Metyrosine (Concurrent administration may potentiate the action of other antihypertensive agent). Products include:
- Demser Capsules 1690

Minoxidil (Concurrent administration may potentiate the action of other antihypertensive agent).
- No products indexed under this heading.

Moexipril Hydrochloride (Calcium channel blockers may have an additive effect when given with Tenoretic; potential for bradycardia and heart block). Products include:
- Univasc Tablets 2553

Nadolol (Concurrent administration may potentiate the action of other antihypertensive agent).
- No products indexed under this heading.

Nicardipine Hydrochloride (Calcium channel blockers may have an additive effect when given with Tenoretic; potential for bradycardia and heart block). Products include:
- Cardene Capsules 2261
- Cardene I.V. 2815
- Cardene SR Capsules 2264

Nifedipine (Calcium channel blockers may have an additive effect when given with Tenoretic; potential for bradycardia and heart block). Products include:
- Adalat Capsules (10 mg and 20 mg) 580
- Adalat CC 582
- Procardia Capsules 2024
- Procardia XL Extended Release Tablets 2026

Nimodipine (Calcium channel blockers may have an additive effect when given with Tenoretic; potential for bradycardia and heart block). Products include:
- Nimotop Capsules 603

Nisoldipine (Calcium channel blockers may have an additive effect when given with Tenoretic; potential for bradycardia and heart block). Products include:
- Sular Tablets 2961

Nitroglycerin (Concurrent administration may potentiate the action of other antihypertensive agent). Products include:
- Deponit NTG Transdermal Delivery System 2541
- Nitro-Bid IV 1270
- Nitro-Bid Ointment 1272
- Nitro-Dur (nitroglycerin) Transdermal Infusion System 1365
- Nitrolingual Spray 2193
- Nitrostat Tablets 1981
- Transderm-Nitro Transdermal Therapeutic System 878

Norepinephrine Bitartrate (Decreased arterial responsiveness to norepinephrine). Products include:
- Levophed Bitartrate Injection 2445

Penbutolol Sulfate (Concurrent administration may potentiate the action of other antihypertensive agent). Products include:
- Levatol Tablets 2547

Phenoxybenzamine Hydrochloride (Concurrent administration may potentiate the action of other antihypertensive agent). Products include:
- Dibenzyline Capsules 2650

Phentolamine Mesylate (Concurrent administration may potentiate the action of other antihypertensive agent). Products include:
- Regitine Vials 864

Pindolol (Concurrent administration may potentiate the action of other antihypertensive agent). Products include:
- Visken Tablets 2428

Polythiazide (Concurrent administration may potentiate the action of other antihypertensive agent). Products include:
- Minizide Capsules 2016

Prazosin Hydrochloride (Concurrent administration may potentiate the action of other antihypertensive agent). Products include:
- Minipress Capsules 2015
- Minizide Capsules 2016

Prednisolone Acetate (Potential for hypokalemia). Products include:
- AK-CIDE .... ◎ 203
- AK-CIDE Ointment .... ◎ 203
- Blephamide Liquifilm Sterile Ophthalmic Suspension 472
- Blephamide Ointment .... ◎ 234
- Econopred & Econopred Plus Ophthalmic Suspensions .... ◎ 216
- Poly-Pred Liquifilm .... ◎ 246
- Pred Forte .... ◎ 247
- Pred Mild .... ◎ 250
- Pred-G Liquifilm Sterile Ophthalmic Suspension .... ◎ 248
- Pred-G S.O.P. Sterile Ophthalmic Ointment .... ◎ 249

Prednisolone Sodium Phosphate (Potential for hypokalemia). Products include:
- AK-PRED .... ◎ 204
- Hydeltrasol Injection, Sterile 1708
- Pediapred Oral Solution 1618

Prednisolone Tebutate (Potential for hypokalemia). Products include:
- Hydeltra-T.B.A. Sterile Suspension 1710

Prednisone (Potential for hypokalemia).
- No products indexed under this heading.

Propranolol Hydrochloride (Concurrent administration may potentiate the action of other antihypertensive agent). Products include:
- Inderal 2834
- Inderal LA Long Acting Capsules 2836
- Inderide Tablets 2838
- Inderide LA Long Acting Capsules .. 2840

Quinapril Hydrochloride (Concurrent administration may potentiate the action of other antihypertensive agent). Products include:
- Accupril Tablets 1950

Ramipril (Concurrent administration may potentiate the action of other antihypertensive agent). Products include:
- Altace Capsules 1238

Rauwolfia Serpentina (Potential for hypotension and/or marked bradycardia which may produce vertigo, syncope or postural hypotension).
- No products indexed under this heading.

Rescinnamine (Potential for hypotension and/or marked bradycardia which may produce vertigo, syncope or postural hypotension).
- No products indexed under this heading.

Reserpine (Potential for hypotension and/or marked bradycardia which may produce vertigo, syncope or postural hypotension). Products include:
- Diupres Tablets 1691
- Hydropres Tablets 1718
- Ser-Ap-Es Tablets 867

Sodium Nitroprusside (Concurrent administration may potentiate the action of other antihypertensive agent).
- No products indexed under this heading.

Sotalol Hydrochloride (Concurrent administration may potentiate the action of other antihypertensive agent). Products include:
- Betapace Tablets 637

Spirapril Hydrochloride (Calcium channel blockers may have an additive effect when given with Tenoretic; potential for bradycardia and heart block).
- No products indexed under this heading.

Terazosin Hydrochloride (Concurrent administration may potentiate the action of other antihypertensive agent). Products include:
- Hytrin Capsules 434

Timolol Maleate (Concurrent administration may potentiate the action of other antihypertensive agent). Products include:
- Blocadren Tablets 1654
- Timolide Tablets 1791
- Timoptic in Ocudose 1796
- Timoptic Sterile Ophthalmic Solution 1794
- Timoptic-XE 1798

Torsemide (Calcium channel blockers may have an additive effect when given with Tenoretic; potential for bradycardia and heart block). Products include:
- Demadex Tablets and Injection 691

Triamcinolone (Potential for hypokalemia).
- No products indexed under this heading.

Triamcinolone Acetonide (Potential for hypokalemia). Products include:
- Azmacort Oral Inhaler 2175
- Nasacort AQ Nasal Spray 2191
- Nasacort Nasal Inhaler 2189

IMPORTANT NOTE: Always consult each drug listing in the patient's regimen for possible interactions.

Tenoretic — Interactions Index — 1054

Triamcinolone Diacetate (Potential for hypokalemia).
  No products indexed under this heading.
Triamcinolone Hexacetonide (Potential for hypokalemia).
  No products indexed under this heading.
Trimethaphan Camsylate (Concurrent administration may potentiate the action of other antihypertensive agent).
  No products indexed under this heading.
Tubocurarine Chloride (Increased responsiveness to tubocurarine).
  No products indexed under this heading.
Verapamil Hydrochloride (Calcium channel blockers may have an additive effect when given with Tenoretic; potential for bradycardia and heart block). Products include:
  Calan SR Caplets 2571
  Calan Tablets 2568
  Covera-HS Tablets 2573
  Isoptin Injectable 1391
  Isoptin Oral Tablets 1393
  Isoptin SR Tablets 1395
  Verelan Capsules 1455

TENORMIN TABLETS AND I.V. INJECTION
(Atenolol) 2965
May interact with catecholamine depleting drugs, calcium channel blockers, and certain other agents. Compounds in these categories include:

Amlodipine Besylate (Coadministration may result in bradycardia and heart block; potential for an additive effect). Products include:
  Lotrel Capsules 858
  Norvasc Tablets 2020
Bepridil Hydrochloride (Coadministration may result in bradycardia and heart block; potential for an additive effect). Products include:
  Vascor Tablets (200 and 300 mg) .. 1597
Clonidine (Beta blockers may exacerbate the rebound hypertension which can follow the withdrawal of clonidine). Products include:
  Catapres-TTS 680
Clonidine Hydrochloride (Beta blockers may exacerbate the rebound hypertension which can follow the withdrawal of clonidine). Products include:
  Catapres Tablets 679
  Combipres Tablets 682
Deserpidine (Potential for additive effect; hypotension and/or marked bradycardia which may produce vertigo, syncope or postural hypotension).
  No products indexed under this heading.
Diltiazem Hydrochloride (Coadministration may result in bradycardia and heart block; potential for an additive effect). Products include:
  Cardizem CD Capsules 1251
  Cardizem SR Capsules 1255
  Cardizem Injectable 1253
  Cardizem Tablets 1257
  Dilacor XR Extended-release Capsules 2183
  Tiazac Capsules 1019
Epinephrine Hydrochloride (Potential for unresponsiveness to the usual dose of epinephrine to treat allergic reaction). Products include:
  Ana-Kit Anaphylaxis Emergency Treatment Kit .... ■ 611

Felodipine (Coadministration may result in bradycardia and heart block; potential for an additive effect). Products include:
  Plendil Extended-Release Tablets 514
Guanethidine Monosulfate (Potential for additive effect; hypotension and/or marked bradycardia which may produce vertigo, syncope or postural hypotension). Products include:
  Esimil Tablets 840
  Ismelin Tablets 845
Isradipine (Coadministration may result in bradycardia and heart block; potential for an additive effect). Products include:
  DynaCirc Capsules 2381
  DynaCirc CR Tablets 2383
Nicardipine Hydrochloride (Coadministration may result in bradycardia and heart block; potential for an additive effect). Products include:
  Cardene Capsules 2261
  Cardene I.V. 2815
  Cardene SR Capsules 2264
Nifedipine (Coadministration may result in bradycardia and heart block; potential for an additive effect). Products include:
  Adalat Capsules (10 mg and 20 mg) 580
  Adalat CC 582
  Procardia Capsules 2024
  Procardia XL Extended Release Tablets 2026
Nimodipine (Coadministration may result in bradycardia and heart block; potential for an additive effect). Products include:
  Nimotop Capsules 603
Nisoldipine (Coadministration may result in bradycardia and heart block; potential for an additive effect). Products include:
  Sular Tablets 2961
Rauwolfia Serpentina (Potential for additive effect; hypotension and/or marked bradycardia which may produce vertigo, syncope or postural hypotension).
  No products indexed under this heading.
Rescinnamine (Potential for additive effect; hypotension and/or marked bradycardia which may produce vertigo, syncope or postural hypotension).
  No products indexed under this heading.
Reserpine (Potential for additive effect; hypotension and/or marked bradycardia which may produce vertigo, syncope or postural hypotension). Products include:
  Diupres Tablets 1691
  Hydropres Tablets 1718
  Ser-Ap-Es Tablets 867
Verapamil Hydrochloride (Coadministration may result in bradycardia and heart block; potential for an additive effect). Products include:
  Calan SR Caplets 2571
  Calan Tablets 2568
  Covera-HS Tablets 2573
  Isoptin Injectable 1391
  Isoptin Oral Tablets 1393
  Isoptin SR Tablets 1395
  Verelan Capsules 1455

TENSILON INJECTABLE
(Edrophonium Chloride) 1307
None cited in PDR database.

TERAK OINTMENT
(Oxytetracycline Hydrochloride, Polymyxin B Sulfate) .... ◎ 210
None cited in PDR database.

TERAZOL 3 VAGINAL CREAM
(Terconazole) 1941
None cited in PDR database.

TERAZOL 3 VAGINAL SUPPOSITORIES
(Terconazole) 1942
None cited in PDR database.

TERAZOL 7 VAGINAL CREAM
(Terconazole) 1943
None cited in PDR database.

TERRA-CORTRIL OPHTHALMIC SUSPENSION
(Oxytetracycline Hydrochloride, Hydrocortisone Acetate) 2033
None cited in PDR database.

TERRAMYCIN INTRAMUSCULAR SOLUTION
(Oxytetracycline) 2034
May interact with anticoagulants, penicillins, and certain other agents. Compounds in these categories include:

Amoxicillin Trihydrate (Interference with penicillin's bactericidal action). Products include:
  Amoxil 2631
  Augmentin 2637
  Augmentin Tablets 2640
Ampicillin (Interference with penicillin's bactericidal action). Products include:
  Omnipen Capsules 2872
  Omnipen for Oral Suspension 2873
Ampicillin Sodium (Interference with penicillin's bactericidal action). Products include:
  Unasyn 2035
Ampicillin Trihydrate (Interference with penicillin's bacterial action).
  No products indexed under this heading.
Azlocillin Sodium (Interference with penicillin's bactericidal action).
  No products indexed under this heading.
Bacampicillin Hydrochloride (Interference with penicillin's bactericidal action). Products include:
  Spectrobid Tablets 2030
Carbenicillin Disodium (Interference with penicillin's bactericidal action).
  No products indexed under this heading.
Carbenicillin Indanyl Sodium (Interference with penicillin's bactericidal action). Products include:
  Geocillin Tablets 2009
Dalteparin Sodium (Depressed plasma prothrombin activity; downward adjustment of anticoagulant dosage may be necessary). Products include:
  Fragmin Injection 2088
Dicloxacillin Sodium (Interference with penicillin's bactericidal action).
  No products indexed under this heading.
Dicumarol (Depressed plasma prothrombin activity; downward adjustment of anticoagulant dosage may be necessary).
  No products indexed under this heading.

Enoxaparin (Depressed plasma prothrombin activity; downward adjustment of anticoagulant dosage may be necessary). Products include:
  Lovenox Injection 2187
Heparin Calcium (Depressed plasma prothrombin activity; downward adjustment of anticoagulant dosage may be necessary).
  No products indexed under this heading.
Heparin Sodium (Depressed plasma prothrombin activity; downward adjustment of anticoagulant dosage may be necessary). Products include:
  Heparin Lock Flush Solution 2831
  Heparin Sodium Injection 2832
  Heparin Sodium Vials 1486
Mezlocillin Sodium (Interference with penicillin's bactericidal action). Products include:
  Mezlin 594
  Mezlin Pharmacy Bulk Package 597
Nafcillin Sodium (Interference with penicillin's bactericidal action).
  No products indexed under this heading.
Penicillin G Benzathine (Interference with penicillin's bactericidal action). Products include:
  Bicillin C-R Injection 2810
  Bicillin C-R 900/300 Injection 2812
  Bicillin L-A Injection 2813
Penicillin G Potassium (Interference with penicillin's bactericidal action). Products include:
  Pfizerpen for Injection 2022
Penicillin G Procaine (Interference with penicillin's bactericidal action). Products include:
  Bicillin C-R Injection 2810
  Bicillin C-R 900/300 Injection 2812
Penicillin G Sodium (Interference with penicillin's bactericidal action).
  No products indexed under this heading.
Penicillin V Potassium (Interference with penicillin's bactericidal action). Products include:
  Pen•Vee K 2879
Ticarcillin Disodium (Interference with penicillin's bactericidal action). Products include:
  Ticar for Injection 2704
  Timentin for Injection 2706
Warfarin Sodium (Depressed plasma prothrombin activity; downward adjustment of anticoagulant dosage may be necessary). Products include:
  Coumadin 941

TERRAMYCIN WITH POLYMYXIN B SULFATE OPHTHALMIC OINTMENT
(Oxytetracycline Hydrochloride, Polymyxin B Sulfate) 2035
None cited in PDR database.

TESLAC TABLETS
(Testolactone) 727
May interact with oral anticoagulants. Compounds in this category include:

Dicumarol (Increased effects of oral anticoagulant).
  No products indexed under this heading.
Warfarin Sodium (Increased effects of oral anticoagulant). Products include:
  Coumadin 941

TESSALON PERLES
(Benzonatate) 1018
None cited in PDR database.

(■ Described in PDR For Nonprescription Drugs)   (◎ Described in PDR For Ophthalmology)

1055 Interactions Index Thalitone

TESTODERM TESTOSTERONE TRANSDERMAL SYSTEM
(Testosterone) 486
May interact with oral anticoagulants, insulin, and certain other agents. Compounds in these categories include:

Dicumarol (Potential for decreased requirements of oral anticoagulants).
No products indexed under this heading.

Insulin, Human (Possible decrease in insulin requirements).
No products indexed under this heading.

Insulin, Human Isophane Suspension (Possible decrease in insulin requirements). Products include:
Novolin N Human Insulin 10 ml Vials 1846

Insulin, Human NPH (Possible decrease in insulin requirements). Products include:
Humulin N, 100 Units 1495
Novolin N PenFill 1.5 ml Cartridges Durable Insulin Delivery System 1849
Novolin N Prefilled Syringe Disposable Insulin Delivery System 1850

Insulin, Human Regular (Possible decrease in insulin requirements). Products include:
Humulin R, 100 Units 1497
Novolin R Human Insulin 10 ml Vials 1846
Novolin R PenFill 1.5 ml Cartridges Durable Insulin Delivery System 1849
Novolin R Prefilled Syringe Disposable Insulin Delivery System 1850
Velosulin BR Human Insulin 10 ml Vials 1847

Insulin, Human, Zinc Suspension (Possible decrease in insulin requirements). Products include:
Humulin L, 100 Units 1494
Humulin U, 100 Units 1498
Novolin L Human Insulin 10 ml Vials 1846

Insulin Lispro, Human (Possible decrease in insulin requirements). Products include:
Humalog Injection 1488

Insulin, NPH (Possible decrease in insulin requirements). Products include:
NPH, 100 Units 1502
Pork NPH, 100 Units 1506
Purified Pork NPH Isophane Insulin 1852

Insulin, Regular (Possible decrease in insulin requirements). Products include:
Regular, 100 Units 1503
Pork Regular, 100 Units 1507
Pork Regular (Concentrated), 500 Units 1508
Purified Pork Regular Insulin 1852

Insulin, Zinc Crystals (Possible decrease in insulin requirements). Products include:
NPH, 100 Units 1502

Insulin, Zinc Suspension (Possible decrease in insulin requirements). Products include:
Iletin I 1501
Lente, 100 Units 1501
Iletin II 1504
Pork Lente, 100 Units 1504
Purified Pork Lente Insulin 1852

Oxyphenbutazone (Concurrent administration may result in elevated serum levels of oxyphenbutazone).

Warfarin Sodium (Potential for decreased requirements of oral anticoagulants). Products include:
Coumadin 941

TESTRED CAPSULES, 10 MG
(Methyltestosterone) 1308
May interact with oral anticoagulants, insulin, and certain other agents. Compounds in these categories include:

Dicumarol (Decreased need for anticoagulants).
No products indexed under this heading.

Insulin, Human (Possibly decreased insulin requirements).
No products indexed under this heading.

Insulin, Human Isophane Suspension (Possibly decreased insulin requirements). Products include:
Novolin N Human Insulin 10 ml Vials 1846

Insulin, Human NPH (Possibly decreased insulin requirements). Products include:
Humulin N, 100 Units 1495
Novolin N PenFill 1.5 ml Cartridges Durable Insulin Delivery System 1849
Novolin N Prefilled Syringe Disposable Insulin Delivery System 1850

Insulin, Human Regular (Possibly decreased insulin requirements). Products include:
Humulin R, 100 Units 1497
Novolin R Human Insulin 10 ml Vials 1846
Novolin R PenFill 1.5 ml Cartridges Durable Insulin Delivery System 1849
Novolin R Prefilled Syringe Disposable Insulin Delivery System 1850
Velosulin BR Human Insulin 10 ml Vials 1847

Insulin, Human, Zinc Suspension (Possibly decreased insulin requirements). Products include:
Humulin L, 100 Units 1494
Humulin U, 100 Units 1498
Novolin L Human Insulin 10 ml Vials 1846

Insulin Lispro, Human (Possibly decreased insulin requirements). Products include:
Humalog Injection 1488

Insulin, NPH (Possibly decreased insulin requirements). Products include:
NPH, 100 Units 1502
Pork NPH, 100 Units 1506
Purified Pork NPH Isophane Insulin 1852

Insulin, Regular (Possibly decreased insulin requirements). Products include:
Regular, 100 Units 1503
Pork Regular, 100 Units 1507
Pork Regular (Concentrated), 500 Units 1508
Purified Pork Regular Insulin 1852

Insulin, Zinc Crystals (Possibly decreased insulin requirements). Products include:
NPH, 100 Units 1502

Insulin, Zinc Suspension (Possibly decreased insulin requirements). Products include:
Iletin I 1501
Lente, 100 Units 1501
Iletin II 1504
Pork Lente, 100 Units 1504
Purified Pork Lente Insulin 1852

Oxyphenbutazone (Elevated serum levels of oxyphenbutazone).

Warfarin Sodium (Decreased need for anticoagulants). Products include:
Coumadin 941

TETANUS & DIPHTHERIA TOXOIDS ADSORBED PUROGENATED
(Tetanus & Diphtheria Toxoids Adsorbed) 1446
None cited in PDR database.

TETANUS TOXOID ADSORBED PUROGENATED
(Tetanus Toxoid, Adsorbed) 1447
May interact with immunosuppressive agents and certain other agents. Compounds in these categories include:

Azathioprine (Concurrent use should be avoided). Products include:
Azathioprine Tablets 2349
Imuran 1103

Cyclosporine (Concurrent use should be avoided). Products include:
Neoral 2405
Sandimmune 2416

Immune Globulin (Human) (Concurrent use should be avoided).
No products indexed under this heading.

Immune Globulin Intravenous (Human) (Concurrent use should be avoided).

Muromonab-CD3 (Concurrent use should be avoided). Products include:
Orthoclone OKT3 Sterile Solution .. 1892

Mycophenolate Mofetil (Concurrent use should be avoided). Products include:
CellCept Capsules 2265

Tacrolimus (Concurrent use should be avoided). Products include:
Prograf 1028

TETRAMUNE
(Diphtheria & Tetanus Toxoids and Pertussis with Hemophilus B Conjugate Vaccine) 1449
May interact with immunosuppressive agents, anticoagulants, and certain other agents. Compounds in these categories include:

Azathioprine (Reduces the response to active immunization procedures). Products include:
Azathioprine Tablets 2349
Imuran 1103

Cyclosporine (Reduces the response to active immunization procedures). Products include:
Neoral 2405
Sandimmune 2416

Dalteparin Sodium (Caution should be exercised if children are on anticoagulant therapy and are given IM injection of Tetramune). Products include:
Fragmin Injection 2088

Dicumarol (Caution should be exercised if children are on anticoagulant therapy and are given IM injection of Tetramune).
No products indexed under this heading.

Enoxaparin (Caution should be exercised if children are on anticoagulant therapy and are given IM injection of Tetramune). Products include:
Lovenox Injection 2187

Heparin Calcium (Caution should be exercised if children are on anticoagulant therapy and are given IM injection of Tetramune).
No products indexed under this heading.

Heparin Sodium (Caution should be exercised if children are on anticoagulant therapy and are given IM injection of Tetramune). Products include:
Heparin Lock Flush Solution 2831
Heparin Sodium Injection 2832
Heparin Sodium Vials 1486

Immune Globulin (Human) (Reduces the response to active immunization procedures).
No products indexed under this heading.

Immune Globulin Intravenous (Human) (Reduces the response to active immunization procedures).

Influenza Virus Vaccine (Potential for increased febrile reactions; influenza virus vaccine should not be administered within 3 days of immunization with a pertussis-containing vaccine). Products include:
Fluvirin (Influenza Virus Vaccine) 1608
Influenza Virus Vaccine, Trivalent, Types A and B (chromatograph- and filter-purified subviron antigen) FluShield, 1996-1997 Formula 2842

Muromonab-CD3 (Reduces the response to active immunization procedures). Products include:
Orthoclone OKT3 Sterile Solution .. 1892

Mycophenolate Mofetil (Reduces the response to active immunization procedures). Products include:
CellCept Capsules 2265

Tacrolimus (Reduces the response to active immunization procedures). Products include:
Prograf 1028

Warfarin Sodium (Caution should be exercised if children are on anticoagulant therapy and are given IM injection of Tetramune). Products include:
Coumadin 941

THALITONE
(Chlorthalidone) 1293
May interact with antihypertensives, insulin, oral hypoglycemic agents, lithium preparations, barbiturates, narcotic analgesics, and certain other agents. Compounds in these categories include:

Acarbose (Increase in serum glucose level; higher dosage of oral hypoglycemic agents may be necessary). Products include:
Precose 604

Acebutolol Hydrochloride (Chlorthalidone may add to or potentiate the action of other antihypertensive drugs). Products include:
Sectral Capsules 2914

Alfentanil Hydrochloride (Aggravates orthostatic hypotension). Products include:
Alfenta Injection 1334

Amlodipine Besylate (Chlorthalidone may add to or potentiate the action of other antihypertensive drugs). Products include:
Lotrel Capsules 858
Norvasc Tablets 2020

Aprobarbital (Aggravates orthostatic hypotension).
No products indexed under this heading.

Atenolol (Chlorthalidone may add to or potentiate the action of other antihypertensive drugs). Products include:
Tenoretic Tablets 2963
Tenormin Tablets and I.V. Injection 2965

IMPORTANT NOTE: Always consult each drug listing in the patient's regimen for possible interactions.

Thalitone — Interactions Index — 1056

Benazepril Hydrochloride (Chlorthalidone may add to or potentiate the action of other antihypertensive drugs. Products include:
- Lotensin Tablets ... 852
- Lotensin HCT Tablets ... 855
- Lotrel Capsules ... 858

Bendroflumethiazide (Chlorthalidone may add to or potentiate the action of other antihypertensive drugs).
- No products indexed under this heading.

Betaxolol Hydrochloride (Chlorthalidone may add to or potentiate the action of other antihypertensive drugs). Products include:
- Betoptic Ophthalmic Solution ... 465
- Betoptic S Ophthalmic Suspension ... 467
- Kerlone Tablets ... 2588

Bisoprolol Fumarate (Chlorthalidone may add to or potentiate the action of other antihypertensive drugs). Products include:
- Zebeta Tablets ... 1457
- Ziac ... 1459

Buprenorphine (Aggravates orthostatic hypotension). Products include:
- Buprenex Injectable ... 2170

Butabarbital (Aggravates orthostatic hypotension). Products include:
- No products indexed under this heading.

Butalbital (Aggravates orthostatic hypotension). Products include:
- Axocet Capsules ... 2469
- Esgic-plus Capsules ... 1012
- Esgic-plus Tablets ... 1012
- Fioricet Tablets ... 2386
- Fioricet with Codeine Capsules ... 2387
- Fiorinal Capsules ... 2388
- Fiorinal with Codeine Capsules ... 2390
- Fiorinal Tablets ... 2388
- Phrenilin ... 790
- Sedapap Tablets 50 mg/650 mg .. 1826

Captopril (Chlorthalidone may add to or potentiate the action of other antihypertensive drugs). Products include:
- Capoten Tablets ... 740
- Capozide Tablets ... 744

Carteolol Hydrochloride (Chlorthalidone may add to or potentiate the action of other antihypertensive drugs). Products include:
- Cartrol Tablets ... 413
- Ocupress Ophthalmic Solution, 1% Sterile ... ⊙ 297

Chlorothiazide (Chlorthalidone may add to or potentiate the action of other antihypertensive drugs). Products include:
- Aldoclor Tablets ... 1638
- Diupres Tablets ... 1691
- Diuril Oral ... 1694

Chlorothiazide Sodium (Chlorthalidone may add to or potentiate the action of other antihypertensive drugs). Products include:
- Diuril Sodium Intravenous ... 1693

Chlorpropamide (Increase in serum glucose level; higher dosage of oral hypoglycemic agents may be necessary). Products include:
- Diabinese Tablets ... 2002

Clonidine (Chlorthalidone may add to or potentiate the action of other antihypertensive drugs). Products include:
- Catapres-TTS ... 680

Clonidine Hydrochloride (Chlorthalidone may add to or potentiate the action of other antihypertensive drugs). Products include:
- Catapres Tablets ... 679
- Combipres Tablets ... 682

Codeine Phosphate (Aggravates orthostatic hypotension). Products include:
- Brontex ... 2130
- Dimetane-DC Cough Syrup ... 2232
- Fioricet with Codeine Capsules ... 2387
- Fiorinal with Codeine Capsules ... 2390
- Nucofed ... 2225
- Phenergan with Codeine ... 2883
- Phenergan VC with Codeine ... 2888
- Robitussin A-C Syrup ... 2248
- Robitussin-DAC Syrup ... 2249
- Ryna ... ⊡ 804
- Soma Compound w/Codeine Tablets ... 2784
- Tylenol with Codeine ... 1592

Deserpidine (Chlorthalidone may add to or potentiate the action of other antihypertensive drugs).
- No products indexed under this heading.

Dezocine (Aggravates orthostatic hypotension). Products include:
- Dalgan Injection ... 529

Diazoxide (Chlorthalidone may add to or potentiate the action of other antihypertensive drugs). Products include:
- Hyperstat I.V. Injection ... 2504
- Proglycem ... 575

Diltiazem Hydrochloride (Chlorthalidone may add to or potentiate the action of other antihypertensive drugs). Products include:
- Cardizem CD Capsules ... 1251
- Cardizem SR Capsules ... 1255
- Cardizem Injectable ... 1253
- Cardizem Tablets ... 1257
- Dilacor XR Extended-release Capsules ... 2183
- Tiazac Capsules ... 1019

Doxazosin Mesylate (Chlorthalidone may add to or potentiate the action of other antihypertensive drugs). Products include:
- Cardura Tablets ... 1993

Enalapril Maleate (Chlorthalidone may add to or potentiate the action of other antihypertensive drugs). Products include:
- Vaseretic Tablets ... 1810
- Vasotec Tablets ... 1816

Enalaprilat (Chlorthalidone may add to or potentiate the action of other antihypertensive drugs). Products include:
- Vasotec I.V. ... 1814

Esmolol Hydrochloride (Chlorthalidone may add to or potentiate the action of other antihypertensive drugs). Products include:
- Brevibloc (esmolol HCl) Injection ... 1860

Felodipine (Chlorthalidone may add to or potentiate the action of other antihypertensive drugs). Products include:
- Plendil Extended-Release Tablets ... 514

Fentanyl (Aggravates orthostatic hypotension). Products include:
- Duragesic Transdermal System ... 1336

Fentanyl Citrate (Aggravates orthostatic hypotension). Products include:
- Sublimaze Injection ... 463

Fosinopril Sodium (Chlorthalidone may add to or potentiate the action of other antihypertensive drugs). Products include:
- Monopril Tablets ... 762

Furosemide (Chlorthalidone may add to or potentiate the action of other antihypertensive drugs). Products include:
- Lasix Injection, Oral Solution and Tablets ... 1267

Glimepiride (Increase in serum glucose level; higher dosage of oral hypoglycemic agents may be necessary). Products include:
- Amaryl Tablets ... 1241

Glipizide (Increase in serum glucose level; higher dosage of oral hypoglycemic agents may be necessary). Products include:
- Glucotrol Tablets ... 2011
- Glucotrol XL Extended Release Tablets ... 2012

Glyburide (Increase in serum glucose level; higher dosage of oral hypoglycemic agents may be necessary). Products include:
- DiaBeta Tablets ... 1265
- Glynase PresTab Tablets ... 2091
- Micronase Tablets ... 2099

Guanabenz Acetate (Chlorthalidone may add to or potentiate the action of other antihypertensive drugs).
- No products indexed under this heading.

Guanethidine Monosulfate (Chlorthalidone may add to or potentiate the action of other antihypertensive drugs). Products include:
- Esimil Tablets ... 840
- Ismelin Tablets ... 845

Hydralazine Hydrochloride (Chlorthalidone may add to or potentiate the action of other antihypertensive drugs). Products include:
- Apresazide Capsules ... 824
- Apresoline Hydrochloride Tablets .. 826
- Hydralazine Hydrochloride Injection USP ... 2712
- Ser-Ap-Es Tablets ... 867

Hydrochlorothiazide (Chlorthalidone may add to or potentiate the action of other antihypertensive drugs). Products include:
- Aldactazide Tablets ... 2556
- Aldoril Tablets ... 1644
- Apresazide Capsules ... 824
- Capozide Tablets ... 744
- Dyazide Capsules ... 2653
- Esidrix Tablets ... 839
- Esimil Tablets ... 840
- HydroDIURIL Tablets ... 1716
- Hydropres Tablets ... 1718
- Hyzaar Tablets ... 1720
- Inderide Tablets ... 2838
- Inderide LA Long Acting Capsules .. 2840
- Lopressor HCT Tablets ... 850
- Lotensin HCT Tablets ... 855
- Moduretic Tablets ... 1748
- Oretic Tablets ... 450
- Prinzide Tablets ... 1780
- Ser-Ap-Es Tablets ... 867
- Timolide Tablets ... 1791
- Vaseretic Tablets ... 1810
- Zestoretic Tablets ... 2968
- Ziac ... 1459

Hydrocodone Bitartrate (Aggravates orthostatic hypotension). Products include:
- Codiclear DH Syrup ... 808
- Duratuss HD Elixir ... 2750
- Histussin D Liquid ... 670
- Hycodan Tablets and Syrup ... 946
- Hycomine Compound Tablets ... 948
- Hycomine ... 947
- Hycotuss Expectorant Syrup ... 950
- Hydrocet Capsules ... 787
- Lorcet 10/650 Tablets ... 1016
- Lortab ... 2751
- Tussend ... 1830
- Tussend Expectorant ... 1831
- Vicodin Tablets ... 1404
- Vicodin ES Tablets ... 1405
- Vicodin HP Tablets ... 1403
- Vicodin Tuss Expectorant ... 1406
- Zydone Capsules ... 967

Hydrocodone Polistirex (Aggravates orthostatic hypotension). Products include:
- Tussionex Pennkinetic Extended-Release Suspension ... 1624

Hydroflumethiazide (Chlorthalidone may add to or potentiate the action of other antihypertensive drugs). Products include:
- Diucardin Tablets ... 2824

Hydromorphone Hydrochloride (Aggravates orthostatic hypotension). Products include:
- Dilaudid Ampules ... 1382
- Dilaudid Cough Syrup ... 1383
- Dilaudid-HP Injection ... 1384
- Dilaudid-HP Lyophilized Powder 250 mg ... 1384
- Dilaudid ... 1382
- Dilaudid Oral Liquid ... 1386
- Dilaudid ... 1382
- Dilaudid Tablets - 8 mg ... 1386

Indapamide (Chlorthalidone may add to or potentiate the action of other antihypertensive drugs).
- No products indexed under this heading.

Insulin, Human (Increase in serum glucose level; insulin requirements in diabetic patients may be increased, decreased or unchanged).
- No products indexed under this heading.

Insulin, Human Isophane Suspension (Increase in serum glucose level; insulin requirements in diabetic patients may be increased, decreased or unchanged). Products include:
- Novolin N Human Insulin 10 ml Vials ... 1846

Insulin, Human NPH (Increase in serum glucose level; insulin requirements in diabetic patients may be increased, decreased or unchanged). Products include:
- Humulin N, 100 Units ... 1495
- Novolin N PenFill 1.5 ml Cartridges Durable Insulin Delivery System ... 1849
- Novolin N Prefilled Syringe Disposable Insulin Delivery System .. 1850

Insulin, Human Regular (Increase in serum glucose level; insulin requirements in diabetic patients may be increased, decreased or unchanged). Products include:
- Humulin R, 100 Units ... 1497
- Novolin R Human Insulin 10 ml Vials ... 1846
- Novolin R PenFill 1.5 ml Cartridges Durable Insulin Delivery System ... 1849
- Novolin R Prefilled Syringe Disposable Insulin Delivery System .. 1850
- Velosulin BR Human Insulin 10 ml Vials ... 1847

Insulin, Human, Zinc Suspension (Increase in serum glucose level; insulin requirements in diabetic patients may be increased, decreased or unchanged). Products include:
- Humulin L, 100 Units ... 1494
- Humulin U, 100 Units ... 1498
- Novolin L Human Insulin 10 ml Vials ... 1846

Insulin Lispro, Human (Increase in serum glucose level; insulin requirements in diabetic patients may be increased, decreased or unchanged). Products include:
- Humalog Injection ... 1488

Insulin, NPH (Increase in serum glucose level; insulin requirements in diabetic patients may be increased, decreased or unchanged). Products include:
- NPH, 100 Units ... 1502
- Pork NPH, 100 Units ... 1506
- Purified Pork NPH Isophane Insulin ... 1852

Insulin, Regular (Increase in serum glucose level; insulin requirements in diabetic patients may be increased, decreased or unchanged). Products include:
- Regular, 100 Units ... 1503
- Pork Regular, 100 Units ... 1507
- Pork Regular (Concentrated), 500 Units ... 1508
- Purified Pork Regular Insulin ... 1852

(⊡ Described in PDR For Nonprescription Drugs)   (⊙ Described in PDR For Ophthalmology)

Insulin, Zinc Crystals (Increase in serum glucose level; insulin requirements in diabetic patients may be increased, decreased or unchanged). Products include:
NPH, 100 Units 1502

Insulin, Zinc Suspension (Increase in serum glucose level; insulin requirements in diabetic patients may be increased, decreased or unchanged). Products include:
Iletin I 1501
Lente, 100 Units 1501
Iletin II 1504
Pork Lente, 100 Units 1504
Purified Pork Lente Insulin .. 1852

Isradipine (Chlorthalidone may add to or potentiate the action of other antihypertensive drugs). Products include:
DynaCirc Capsules 2381
DynaCirc CR Tablets 2383

Labetalol Hydrochloride (Chlorthalidone may add to or potentiate the action of other antihypertensive drugs). Products include:
Normodyne Injection 2519
Normodyne Tablets 2522
Trandate 1158

Levorphanol Tartrate (Aggravates orthostatic hypotension). Products include:
Levo-Dromoran 2297

Lisinopril (Chlorthalidone may add to or potentiate the action of other antihypertensive drugs). Products include:
Prinivil Tablets 1776
Prinzide Tablets 1780
Zestoretic Tablets 2968
Zestril Tablets 2972

Lithium Carbonate (Reduced lithium renal clearance and increased risk of lithium toxicity). Products include:
Eskalith 2658
Lithium Carbonate Capsules & Tablets 2352
Lithonate/Lithotabs/Lithobid .. 2721

Lithium Citrate (Reduced lithium renal clearance and increased risk of lithium toxicity).
No products indexed under this heading.

Losartan Potassium (Chlorthalidone may add to or potentiate the action of other antihypertensive drugs). Products include:
Cozaar Tablets 1668
Hyzaar Tablets 1720

Mecamylamine Hydrochloride (Chlorthalidone may add to or potentiate the action of other antihypertensive drugs). Products include:
Inversine Tablets 1729

Meperidine Hydrochloride (Aggravates orthostatic hypotension). Products include:
Demerol 2438
Mepergan Injection 2859

Mephobarbital (Aggravates orthostatic hypotension). Products include:
Mebaral Tablets 2452

Metformin Hydrochloride (Increase in serum glucose level; higher dosage of oral hypoglycemic agents may be necessary). Products include:
Glucophage Tablets 754

Methadone Hydrochloride (Aggravates orthostatic hypotension). Products include:
Methadone Hydrochloride Oral Concentrate 2356
Methadone Hydrochloride Oral Solution & Tablets 2357

Methyclothiazide (Chlorthalidone may add to or potentiate the action of other antihypertensive drugs). Products include:
Enduron Tablets 424

Methyldopa (Chlorthalidone may add to or potentiate the action of other antihypertensive drugs). Products include:
Aldoclor Tablets 1638
Aldomet Oral 1640
Aldoril Tablets 1644

Methyldopate Hydrochloride (Chlorthalidone may add to or potentiate the action of other antihypertensive drugs). Products include:
Aldomet Ester HCl Injection .. 1642

Metolazone (Chlorthalidone may add to or potentiate the action of other antihypertensive drugs). Products include:
Mykrox Tablets 1617
Zaroxolyn Tablets 1625

Metoprolol Succinate (Chlorthalidone may add to or potentiate the action of other antihypertensive drugs). Products include:
Toprol-XL Tablets 560

Metoprolol Tartrate (Chlorthalidone may add to or potentiate the action of other antihypertensive drugs). Products include:
Lopressor 848
Lopressor HCT Tablets 850

Metyrosine (Chlorthalidone may add to or potentiate the action of other antihypertensive drugs). Products include:
Demser Capsules 1690

Minoxidil (Chlorthalidone may add to or potentiate the action of other antihypertensive drugs).
No products indexed under this heading.

Moexipril Hydrochloride (Chlorthalidone may add to or potentiate the action of other antihypertensive drugs). Products include:
Univasc Tablets 2553

Morphine Sulfate (Aggravates orthostatic hypotension). Products include:
Astramorph/PF Injection, USP (Preservative-Free) 526
Duramorph Injection 983
Infumorph 200 and Infumorph 500 Sterile Solutions 985
Kadian Capsules 2948
MS Contin Tablets 2149
MSIR 2152
Oramorph SR (Morphine Sulfate Sustained Release Tablets) .. 2359
RMS Suppositories CII 2766
Roxanol 2365

Nadolol (Chlorthalidone may add to or potentiate the action of other antihypertensive drugs).
No products indexed under this heading.

Nicardipine Hydrochloride (Chlorthalidone may add to or potentiate the action of other antihypertensive drugs). Products include:
Cardene Capsules 2261
Cardene I.V. 2815
Cardene SR Capsules 2264

Nifedipine (Chlorthalidone may add to or potentiate the action of other antihypertensive drugs). Products include:
Adalat Capsules (10 mg and 20 mg) 580
Adalat CC 582
Procardia Capsules 2024
Procardia XL Extended Release Tablets 2026

Nisoldipine (Chlorthalidone may add to or potentiate the action of other antihypertensive drugs). Products include:
Sular Tablets 2961

Nitroglycerin (Chlorthalidone may add to or potentiate the action of other antihypertensive drugs). Products include:
Deponit NTG Transdermal Delivery System 2541
Nitro-Bid IV 1270
Nitro-Bid Ointment 1272
Nitro-Dur (nitroglycerin) Transdermal Infusion System 1365
Nitrolingual Spray 2193
Nitrostat Tablets 1981
Transderm-Nitro Transdermal Therapeutic System 878

Norepinephrine Bitartrate (Decreased arterial responsiveness). Products include:
Levophed Bitartrate Injection .. 2445

Opium Alkaloids (Aggravates orthostatic hypotension).
No products indexed under this heading.

Oxycodone Hydrochloride (Aggravates orthostatic hypotension). Products include:
OxyContin Tablets 2163
OxyIR Capsules 2167
Percocet Tablets 955
Percodan Tablets 955
Percodan-Demi Tablets 956
Roxicodone Tablets, Oral Solution & Intensol (Oxycodone) ... 2366
Tylox Capsules 1593

Penbutolol Sulfate (Chlorthalidone may add to or potentiate the action of other antihypertensive drugs). Products include:
Levatol Tablets 2547

Pentobarbital Sodium (Aggravates orthostatic hypotension). Products include:
Nembutal Sodium Capsules ... 440
Nembutal Sodium Solution ... 442
Nembutal Sodium Suppositories .. 444

Phenobarbital (Aggravates orthostatic hypotension). Products include:
Arco-Lase Plus Tablets 513
Bellergal-S Tablets 2375
Donnatal 2234
Donnatal Extentabs 2234
Donnatal Tablets 2234
Phenobarbital Elixir and Tablets .. 1523
Quadrinal Tablets 1398

Phenoxybenzamine Hydrochloride (Chlorthalidone may add to or potentiate the action of other antihypertensive drugs). Products include:
Dibenzyline Capsules 2650

Phentolamine Mesylate (Chlorthalidone may add to or potentiate the action of other antihypertensive drugs). Products include:
Regitine Vials 864

Pindolol (Chlorthalidone may add to or potentiate the action of other antihypertensive drugs). Products include:
Visken Tablets 2428

Polythiazide (Chlorthalidone may add to or potentiate the action of other antihypertensive drugs). Products include:
Minizide Capsules 2016

Prazosin Hydrochloride (Chlorthalidone may add to or potentiate the action of other antihypertensive drugs). Products include:
Minipress Capsules 2015
Minizide Capsules 2016

Propoxyphene Hydrochloride (Aggravates orthostatic hypotension). Products include:
Darvon 1475

Wygesic Tablets 2930

Propoxyphene Napsylate (Aggravates orthostatic hypotension). Products include:
Darvon-N/Darvocet-N 1473

Propranolol Hydrochloride (Chlorthalidone may add to or potentiate the action of other antihypertensive drugs). Products include:
Inderal 2834
Inderal LA Long Acting Capsules .. 2836
Inderide Tablets 2838
Inderide LA Long Acting Capsules .. 2840

Quinapril Hydrochloride (Chlorthalidone may add to or potentiate the action of other antihypertensive drugs). Products include:
Accupril Tablets 1950

Ramipril (Chlorthalidone may add to or potentiate the action of other antihypertensive drugs). Products include:
Altace Capsules 1238

Rauwolfia Serpentina (Chlorthalidone may add to or potentiate the action of other antihypertensive drugs).
No products indexed under this heading.

Rescinnamine (Chlorthalidone may add to or potentiate the action of other antihypertensive drugs).
No products indexed under this heading.

Reserpine (Chlorthalidone may add to or potentiate the action of other antihypertensive drugs). Products include:
Diupres Tablets 1691
Hydropres Tablets 1718
Ser-Ap-Es Tablets 867

Secobarbital Sodium (Aggravates orthostatic hypotension). Products include:
Seconal Sodium Pulvules 1529

Sodium Nitroprusside (Chlorthalidone may add to or potentiate the action of other antihypertensive drugs).
No products indexed under this heading.

Sotalol Hydrochloride (Chlorthalidone may add to or potentiate the action of other antihypertensive drugs). Products include:
Betapace Tablets 637

Spirapril Hydrochloride (Chlorthalidone may add to or potentiate the action of other antihypertensive drugs).
No products indexed under this heading.

Sufentanil Citrate (Aggravates orthostatic hypotension). Products include:
Sufenta Injection 1355

Terazosin Hydrochloride (Chlorthalidone may add to or potentiate the action of other antihypertensive drugs). Products include:
Hytrin Capsules 434

Thiamylal Sodium (Aggravates orthostatic hypotension).
No products indexed under this heading.

Timolol Maleate (Chlorthalidone may add to or potentiate the action of other antihypertensive drugs). Products include:
Blocadren Tablets 1654
Timolide Tablets 1791
Timoptic in Ocudose 1796
Timoptic Sterile Ophthalmic Solution 1794
Timoptic-XE 1798

IMPORTANT NOTE: Always consult each drug listing in the patient's regimen for possible interactions.

Thalitone Interactions Index 1058

Tolazamide (Increase in serum glucose level; higher dosage of oral hypoglycemic agents may be necessary).
No products indexed under this heading.
Tolbutamide (Increase in serum glucose level; higher dosage of oral hypoglycemic agents may be necessary).
No products indexed under this heading.
Torsemide (Chlorthalidone may add to or potentiate the action of other antihypertensive drugs). Products include:
Demadex Tablets and Injection 691
Trimethaphan Camsylate (Chlorthalidone may add to or potentiate the action of other antihypertensive drugs).
No products indexed under this heading.
Tubocurarine Chloride (Increased responsiveness to tubocurarine).
No products indexed under this heading.
Verapamil Hydrochloride (Chlorthalidone may add to or potentiate the action of other antihypertensive drugs). Products include:
Calan SR Caplets 2571
Calan Tablets 2568
Covera-HS Tablets 2573
Isoptin Injectable 1391
Isoptin Oral Tablets 1393
Isoptin SR Tablets 1395
Verelan Capsules 1455

Food Interactions

Alcohol (Aggravates orthostatic hypotension).

THEO-24 EXTENDED RELEASE CAPSULES

(Theophylline Anhydrous) 2753
May interact with erythromycin, lithium preparations, and certain other agents. Compounds in these categories include:

Adenosine (Theophylline blocks adenosine receptors; higher doses of adenosine may be required to achieve desired effect). Products include:
Adenocard Injection 1021
Adenoscan 1022
Allopurinol (Decreases theophylline clearance of allopurinol doses greater than or equal to 600 mg/day). Products include:
Zyloprim Tablets 1194
Aminoglutethimide (Increases theophylline clearance by induction of microsomal enzyme). Products include:
Cytadren Tablets 837
Carbamazepine (Increases theophylline clearance by induction of microsomal enzyme). Products include:
Atretol Tablets 569
Tegretol/Tegretol-XR 870
Cimetidine (Decreases theophylline clearance by inhibiting cytochrome P450 1A2). Products include:
Tagamet HB Tablets .... ▣ 786
Tagamet Tablets 2694
Cimetidine Hydrochloride (Decreases theophylline clearance by inhibiting cytochrome P450 1A2). Products include:
Tagamet 2694
Ciprofloxacin (Decreases theophylline clearance by inhibiting cytochrome P450 1A2). Products include:
Cipro I.V. 587
Cipro I.V. Pharmacy Bulk Package .. 590
Ciprofloxacin Hydrochloride (Decreases theophylline clearance by inhibiting cytochrome P450 1A2). Products include:
Ciloxan Ophthalmic Solution 468
Cipro Tablets 584
Clarithromycin (Decreases theophylline clearance by inhibiting cytochrome P450 3A3). Products include:
Biaxin 406
Diazepam (Benzodiazepines increase CNS concentrations of adenosine, a potent CNS depressant, while theophylline blocks adenosine receptors; larger diazepam doses may be required to produce desired level of sedation; discontinuation of theophylline without reduction of diazepam dose may result in respiratory depression). Products include:
Dizac (diazepam injectable emulsion) CIV 1862
Valium Injectable 2336
Valium Tablets 2335
Disulfiram (Decreases theophylline clearance by inhibiting hydroxylation and demethylation). Products include:
Antabuse Tablets 2802
Enoxacin (Decreases theophylline clearance by inhibiting cytochrome P450 1A2). Products include:
Penetrex Tablets 2196
Ephedrine Hydrochloride (Coadministration results in synergistic CNS effects resulting in increased frequency of nausea, nervousness, and insomnia). Products include:
Primatene Tablets .... ▣ 844
Quadrinal Tablets 1398
Ephedrine Sulfate (Co-administration results in synergistic CNS effects resulting in increased frequency of nausea, nervousness, and insomnia). Products include:
Marax Tablets & DF Syrup 2015
Ephedrine Tannate (Co-administration results in synergistic CNS effects resulting in increased frequency of nausea, nervousness, and insomnia). Products include:
Rynatuss 2782
Erythromycin (Erythromycin metabolite decreases theophylline clearance by inhibiting cytochrome P450 3A3; decreased erythromycin steady-state serum concentrations). Products include:
A/T/S 2% Acne Topical Gel 1244
A/T/S 2% Acne Topical Solution 1244
Benzamycin Topical Gel 919
E-Mycin Tablets 1388
Emgel 2% Topical Gel 1081
ERYC 1972
Erycette (erythromycin 2%) Topical Solution 1943
Ery-Tab Tablets 426
Erythromycin Base Filmtab 430
Erythromycin Delayed-Release Capsules, USP 431
Ilotycin Ophthalmic Ointment 928
PCE Dispertab Tablets 453
T-Stat 2.0% Topical Solution and Pads 2797
THERAMYCIN Z 2% Solution 1629
Erythromycin Estolate (Erythromycin metabolite decreases theophylline clearance by inhibiting cytochrome P450 3A3; decreased erythromycin steady-state serum concentrations). Products include:
Ilosone 927
Erythromycin Ethylsuccinate (Erythromycin metabolite decreases theophylline clearance by inhibiting cytochrome P450 3A3; decreased erythromycin steady-state serum concentrations). Products include:
E.E.S. 427
EryPed 425
Pediazole Suspension 2340
Erythromycin Gluceptate (Erythromycin metabolite decreases theophylline clearance by inhibiting cytochrome P450 3A3; decreased erythromycin steady-state serum concentrations). Products include:
Ilotycin Gluceptate, IV, Vials 929
Erythromycin Stearate (Erythromycin metabolite decreases theophylline clearance by inhibiting cytochrome P450 3A3; decreased erythromycin steady-state serum concentrations). Products include:
Erythrocin Stearate Filmtab 429
Ethinyl Estradiol (Estrogen containing oral contraceptives decreases theophylline clearance in dose dependent fashion). Products include:
Brevicon 2563
Demulen 2580
Desogen Tablets 1867
Levlen/Tri-Levlen 646
Lo/Ovral Tablets 2852
Lo/Ovral-28 Tablets 2857
Modicon 1928
Nordette-21 Tablets 2863
Nordette-28 Tablets 2866
Norinyl 2563
Ortho-Cept 1907
Ortho-Cyclen/Ortho-Tri-Cyclen 1914
Ortho-Novum 1928
Ortho-Cyclen/Ortho Tri-Cyclen 1914
Ovcon 765
Ovral Tablets 2877
Ovral-28 Tablets 2878
Levlen/Tri-Levlen 646
Tri-Norinyl 2607
Triphasil-21 Tablets 2919
Triphasil-28 Tablets 2924
Flurazepam Hydrochloride (Benzodiazepines increase CNS concentrations of adenosine, a potent CNS depressant, while theophylline blocks adenosine receptors; larger flurazepam doses may be required to produce desired level of sedation; discontinuation of theophylline without reduction of flurazepam dose may result in respiratory depression). Products include:
Dalmane Capsules 2329
Fluvoxamine Maleate (Decreases theophylline clearance by inhibiting cytochrome P450 1A2). Products include:
LUVOX Tablets 2723
Halothane (Halothane sensitizes the myocardium to catecholamines; theophylline increases release of endogenous catecholamines resulting in increased risk of ventricular arrhythmias). Products include:
Fluothane 2830
Interferon alfa-2A, Recombinant (Decreases theophylline clearance). Products include:
Roferon-A Injection 2308
Isoproterenol Hydrochloride (Co-administration with intravenous isoproterenol decreases theophylline clearance). Products include:
Isuprel Hydrochloride Solution 2443
Isuprel Injection 2441
Isuprel Mistometer 2442
Ketamine Hydrochloride (May lower theophylline seizure threshold).
No products indexed under this heading.
Lithium Carbonate (Theophylline increases renal lithium clearance; increase in lithium dose may be required to achieve a therapeutic serum concentration). Products include:
Eskalith 2658
Lithium Carbonate Capsules & Tablets 2352
Lithonate/Lithotabs/Lithobid 2721
Lithium Citrate (Theophylline increases renal lithium clearance; increase in lithium dose may be required to achieve a therapeutic serum concentration).
No products indexed under this heading.
Lorazepam (Benzodiazepines increase CNS concentrations of adenosine, a potent CNS depressant, while theophylline blocks adenosine receptors; larger lorazepam doses may be required to produce desired level of sedation; discontinuation of theophylline without reduction of lorazepam dose may result in respiratory depression). Products include:
Ativan Injection 2805
Ativan Tablets 2807
Mestranol (Estrogen containing oral contraceptives decreases theophylline clearance in dose dependent fashion). Products include:
Norinyl 2563
Ortho-Novum 1928
Methotrexate Sodium (Decreases theophylline clearance). Products include:
Methotrexate Sodium Tablets, Injection, for Injection and LPF Injection 1322
Mexiletine Hydrochloride (Decreases theophylline clearance by inhibiting hydroxylation and demethylation). Products include:
Mexitil Capsules 684
Midazolam Hydrochloride (Benzodiazepines increase CNS concentrations of adenosine, a potent CNS depressant, while theophylline blocks adenosine receptors; larger midazolam doses may be required to produce desired level of sedation; discontination of theophylline without reduction of midazolam dose may result in respiratory depression). Products include:
Versed Injection 2324
Moricizine Hydrochloride (Increases theophylline clearance). Products include:
Ethmozine Tablets 2217
Pancuronium Bromide (Theophylline may antagonize non-depolarizing neuromuscular blocking effects, possibly due to phosphodiesterase inhibition; larger pancuronium doses may be required to achieve neuromuscular blockade).
No products indexed under this heading.
Pentoxifylline (Decreases theophylline clearance). Products include:
Trental Tablets 1291
Phenobarbital (Increases theophylline clearance by induction of microsomal enzyme). Products include:
Arco-Lase Plus Tablets 513
Bellergal-S Tablets 2375
Donnatal 2234
Donnatal Extentabs 2234
Donnatal Tablets 2234
Phenobarbital Elixir and Tablets 1523
Quadrinal Tablets 1398

(▣ Described in PDR For Nonprescription Drugs) (⊚ Described in PDR For Ophthalmology)

Phenytoin (Phenytoin increases theophylline clearance by increasing microsomal enzyme activity; theophylline decreases phenytoin absorption). Products include:
Dilantin Infatabs ... 1967
Dilantin-125 Suspension ... 1969

Phenytoin Sodium (Phenytoin increases theophylline clearance by increasing microsomal enzyme activity; theophylline decreases phenytoin absorption). Products include:
Dilantin Kapseals ... 1965

Propafenone Hydrochloride (Decreases theophylline clearance). Products include:
Rythmol Tablets–150mg, 225mg, 300mg ... 1399

Propranolol Hydrochloride (Decreases theophylline clearance by inhibiting cytochrome P450 1A2). Products include:
Inderal ... 2834
Inderal LA Long Acting Capsules ... 2836
Inderide Tablets ... 2838
Inderide LA Long Acting Capsules ... 2840

Rifampin (Increases theophylline clearance by increasing cytochrome P450 1A2 and 3A3 activity). Products include:
Rifadin ... 1276
Rifamate Capsules ... 1278
Rifater ... 1280
Rimactane Capsules ... 865

Sulfinpyrazone (Increases theophylline clearance by increasing demethylation and hydroxylation; decreases renal clearance of theophylline). Products include:
Anturane ... 823

Tacrine Hydrochloride (Decreases theophylline clearance by inhibiting cytochrome P450 1A2 and also increases renal clearance of theophylline). Products include:
Cognex Capsules ... 1961

Thiabendazole (Decreases theophylline clearance). Products include:
Mintezol ... 1747

Ticlopidine Hydrochloride (Decreases theophylline clearance). Products include:
Ticlid Tablets ... 2317

Troleandomycin (Decreases theophylline clearance by inhibiting cytochrome P450 3A3). Products include:
Tao Capsules ... 2033

Verapamil Hydrochloride (Decreases theophylline clearance by inhibiting hydroxylation and demethylation). Products include:
Calan SR Caplets ... 2571
Calan Tablets ... 2568
Covera-HS Tablets ... 2573
Isoptin Injectable ... 1391
Isoptin Oral Tablets ... 1393
Isoptin SR Tablets ... 1395
Verelan Capsules ... 1455

Food Interactions

Alcohol (Concurrent use with a single dose of alcohol (3 mL/kg of whiskey) decreases theophylline clearance for up to 24 hours).

Diet, high-lipid (Taking Theo-24 one hour before a high-fat-content meal may result in a significant increase in peak serum level and the extent of absorption of theophylline).

Food, charcoal-broiled (Theophylline clearance is increased and half-life decreased by daily consumption of charcoal-broiled beef).

Food, unspecified (Theophylline clearance is increased and half-life decreased by low carbohydrate/high protein diets and parenteral nutrition; a high carbohydrate/low protein diet can decrease the clearance and prolong the half-life of theophylline).

THEO-DUR EXTENDED-RELEASE TABLETS

(Theophylline Anhydrous) ... 1367

May interact with erythromycin, lithium preparations, and certain other agents. Compounds in these categories include:

Adenosine (Theophylline blocks adenosine receptors; higher doses of adenosine may be required to achieve desired effect). Products include:
Adenocard Injection ... 1021
Adenoscan ... 1022

Allopurinol (Decreases theophylline clearance at allopurinol doses greater than or equal to 600 mg/day). Products include:
Zyloprim Tablets ... 1194

Aminoglutethimide (Increases theophylline clearance by induction of microsomal enzyme). Products include:
Cytadren Tablets ... 837

Carbamazepine (Increases theophylline clearance by induction of microsomal enzyme). Products include:
Atretol Tablets ... 569
Tegretol/Tegretol-XR ... 870

Cimetidine (Decreases theophylline clearance by inhibiting cytochrome P450 1A2). Products include:
Tagamet HB Tablets ... 786
Tagamet Tablets ... 2694

Cimetidine Hydrochloride (Decreases theophylline clearance by inhibiting cytochrome P450 1A2). Products include:
Tagamet ... 2694

Ciprofloxacin (Decreases theophylline clearance by inhibiting cytochrome P450 1A2). Products include:
Cipro I.V. ... 587
Cipro I.V. Pharmacy Bulk Package ... 590

Ciprofloxacin Hydrochloride (Decreases theophylline clearance by inhibiting cytochrome P450 1A2). Products include:
Ciloxan Ophthalmic Solution ... 468
Cipro Tablets ... 584

Clarithromycin (Decreases theophylline clearance by inhibiting cytochrome P450 3A3). Products include:
Biaxin ... 406

Diazepam (Benzodiazepines increase CNS concentrations of adenosine, a potent CNS depressant, while theophylline blocks adenosine receptors; larger diazepam doses may be required to produce desired level of sedation; discontinuation of theophylline without reduction of diazepam dose may result in respiratory depression). Products include:
Dizac (diazepam injectable emulsion) CIV ... 1862
Valium Injectable ... 2336
Valium Tablets ... 2335

Disulfiram (Decreases theophylline clearance by inhibiting hydroxylation and demethylation). Products include:
Antabuse Tablets ... 2802

Enoxacin (Decreases theophylline clearance by inhibiting cytochrome P450 1A2). Products include:
Penetrex Tablets ... 2196

Ephedrine Hydrochloride (Co-administration results in synergistic CNS effects resulting in increased frequency of nausea, nervousness, and insomnia). Products include:
Primatene Tablets ... 844
Quadrinal Tablets ... 1398

Ephedrine Sulfate (Co-administration results in synergistic CNS effects resulting in increased frequency of nausea, nervousness, and insomnia). Products include:
Marax Tablets & DF Syrup ... 2015

Ephedrine Tannate (Co-administration results in synergistic CNS effects resulting in increased frequency of nausea, nervousness, and insomnia). Products include:
Rynatuss ... 2782

Erythromycin (Erythromycin metabolite decreases theophylline clearance by inhibiting cytochrome P450 3A3; decreased erythromycin steady-state serum concentrations). Products include:
A/T/S 2% Acne Topical Gel ... 1244
A/T/S 2% Acne Topical Solution ... 1244
Benzamycin Topical Gel ... 919
E-Mycin Tablets ... 1388
Emgel 2% Topical Gel ... 1081
ERYC ... 1972
Erycette (erythromycin 2%) Topical Solution ... 1943
Ery-Tab Tablets ... 426
Erythromycin Base Filmtab ... 430
Erythromycin Delayed-Release Capsules, USP ... 431
Ilotycin Ophthalmic Ointment ... 928
PCE Dispertab Tablets ... 453
T-Stat 2.0% Topical Solution and Pads ... 2797
THERAMYCIN Z 2% Solution ... 1629

Erythromycin Estolate (Erythromycin metabolite decreases theophylline clearance by inhibiting cytochrome P450 3A3; decreased erythromycin steady-state serum concentrations). Products include:
Ilosone ... 927

Erythromycin Ethylsuccinate (Erythromycin metabolite decreases theophylline clearance by inhibiting cytochrome P450 3A3; decreased erythromycin steady-state serum concentrations). Products include:
E.E.S. ... 427
EryPed ... 425
Pediazole Suspension ... 2340

Erythromycin Gluceptate (Erythromycin metabolite decreases theophylline clearance by inhibiting cytochrome P450 3A3; decreased erythromycin steady-state serum concentrations). Products include:
Ilotycin Gluceptate, IV, Vials ... 929

Erythromycin Stearate (Erythromycin metabolite decreases theophylline clearance by inhibiting cytochrome P450 3A3; decreased erythromycin steady-state serum concentrations). Products include:
Erythrocin Stearate Filmtab ... 429

Ethinyl Estradiol (Estrogen-containing oral contraceptives decrease theophylline clearance in dose dependent fashion). Products include:
Brevicon ... 2563
Demulen ... 2580
Desogen Tablets ... 1867
Levlen/Tri-Levlen ... 646
Lo/Ovral Tablets ... 2852
Lo/Ovral-28 Tablets ... 2857
Modicon ... 1928
Nordette-21 Tablets ... 2863
Nordette-28 Tablets ... 2866
Norinyl ... 2563
Ortho-Cept ... 1907
Ortho-Cyclen/Ortho-Tri-Cyclen ... 1914
Ortho-Novum ... 1928
Ortho-Cyclen/Ortho Tri-Cyclen ... 1914
Ovcon ... 765
Ovral Tablets ... 2877
Ovral-28 Tablets ... 2878
Levlen/Tri-Levlen ... 646
Tri-Norinyl ... 2607
Triphasil-21 Tablets ... 2919
Triphasil-28 Tablets ... 2924

Flurazepam Hydrochloride (Benzodiazepines increase CNS concentrations of adenosine, a potent CNS depressant, while theophylline blocks adenosine receptors; larger flurazepam doses may be required to produce desired level of sedation; discontinuation of theophylline without reduction of flurazepam dose may result in respiratory depression). Products include:
Dalmane Capsules ... 2329

Fluvoxamine Maleate (Decreases theophylline clearance by inhibiting cytochrome P450 1A2). Products include:
LUVOX Tablets ... 2723

Fosphenytoin Sodium (Phenytoin increases theophylline clearance by increasing microsomal enzyme activity; theophylline decreases phenytoin absorption). Products include:
Cerebyx Injection ... 1956

Halothane (Halothane sensitizes the myocardium to catecholamines; theophylline increases release of endogenous catecholamines resulting in increased risk of ventricular arrhythmias). Products include:
Fluothane ... 2830

Interferon alfa-2A, Recombinant (Decreases theophylline clearance). Products include:
Roferon-A Injection ... 2308

Isoproterenol Hydrochloride (Co-administration with intravenous isoproterenol decreases theophylline clearance). Products include:
Isuprel Hydrochloride Solution ... 2443
Isuprel Injection ... 2441
Isuprel Mistometer ... 2442

Ketamine Hydrochloride (May lower theophylline seizure threshold).
No products indexed under this heading.

Lithium Carbonate (Theophylline increases renal lithium clearance; increase in lithium dose may be required to achieve a therapeutic serum concentration). Products include:
Eskalith ... 2658
Lithium Carbonate Capsules & Tablets ... 2352
Lithonate/Lithotabs/Lithobid ... 2721

Lithium Citrate (Theophylline increases renal lithium clearance; increase in lithium dose may be required to achieve a therapeutic serum concentration).
No products indexed under this heading.

Lomefloxacin Hydrochloride (Co-administration with some quinolones has increased the plasma levels of theophylline by affecting the rate of theophylline clearance). Products include:
Maxaquin Tablets ... 2593

Lorazepam (Benzodiazepines increase CNS concentrations of adenosine, a potent CNS depressant, while theophylline blocks adenosine receptors; larger lorazepam doses may be required to produce desired level of sedation; discontinuation of theophylline without reduction of lorazepam dose may result in respiratory depression). Products include:
Ativan Injection ... 2805
Ativan Tablets ... 2807

IMPORTANT NOTE: Always consult each drug listing in the patient's regimen for possible interactions.

Theo-Dur Extended-Release — Interactions Index

Mestranol (Estrogen-containing oral contraceptives decreases theophylline clearance in dose dependent fashion). Products include:
- Norinyl 2563
- Ortho-Novum 1928

Methotrexate Sodium (Decreases theophylline clearance. Products include:
- Methotrexate Sodium Tablets, Injection, for Injection and LPF Injection 1322

Mexiletine Hydrochloride (Decreases theophylline clearance by inhibiting hydroxylation and demethylation). Products include:
- Mexitil Capsules 684

Midazolam Hydrochloride (Benzodiazepines increase CNS concentrations of adenosine, a potent CNS depressant, while theophylline blocks adenosine receptors; larger midazolam doses may be required to produce desired level of sedation; discontinuation of theophylline without reduction of midazolam dose may result in respiratory depression). Products include:
- Versed Injection 2324

Moricizine Hydrochloride (Increases theophylline clearance). Products include:
- Ethmozine Tablets 2217

Norfloxacin (Co-administration with some quinolones has increased the plasma levels of theophylline by affecting the rate of theophylline clearance). Products include:
- Chibroxin Sterile Ophthalmic Solution 1657
- Noroxin Tablets 1758
- Noroxin Tablets 2222

Ofloxacin (Co-administration with some quinolones has increased the plasma levels of theophylline by affecting the rate of theophylline clearance). Products include:
- Floxin I.V. 1580
- Floxin Tablets (200 mg, 300 mg, 400 mg) 1577
- Ocuflox Ophthalmic Solution 478
- Ocuflox .... ⊚ 242

Pancuronium Bromide (Theophylline may antagonize non-depolarizing neuromuscular blocking effects; possibly due to phosphodiesterase inhibition; larger pancuronium doses may be required to achieve neuromuscular blockade).
No products indexed under this heading.

Pentoxifylline (Decreases theophylline clearance). Products include:
- Trental Tablets 1291

Phenobarbital (Increases theophylline clearance by induction of microsomal enzyme). Products include:
- Arco-Lase Plus Tablets 513
- Bellergal-S Tablets 2375
- Donnatal 2234
- Donnatal Extentabs 2234
- Donnatal Tablets 2234
- Phenobarbital Elixir and Tablets 1523
- Quadrinal Tablets 1398

Phenytoin (Phenytoin increases theophylline clearance by increasing microsomal enzyme activity; theophylline decreases phenytoin absorption). Products include:
- Dilantin Infatabs 1967
- Dilantin-125 Suspension 1969

Phenytoin Sodium (Phenytoin increases theophylline clearance by increasing microsomal enzyme activity; theophylline decreases phenytoin absorption). Products include:
- Dilantin Kapseals 1965

Propafenone Hydrochloride (Decreases theophylline clearance). Products include:
- Rythmol Tablets—150mg, 225mg, 300mg. 1399

Propranolol Hydrochloride (Decreases theophylline clearance by inhibiting cytochrome P450 1A2). Products include:
- Inderal 2834
- Inderal LA Long Acting Capsules 2836
- Inderide Tablets 2838
- Inderide LA Long Acting Capsules 2840

Rifampin (Increases theophylline clearance by increasing cytochrome P450 1A2 and 3A3 activity). Products include:
- Rifadin 1276
- Rifamate Capsules 1278
- Rifater 1280
- Rimactane Capsules 865

Sucralfate (Reduces absorption of theophylline). Products include:
- Carafate Suspension 1250
- Carafate Tablets 1249

Sulfinpyrazone (Increases theophylline clearance by increasing demethylation and hydroxylation; decreases renal clearance of theophylline). Products include:
- Anturane 823

Tacrine Hydrochloride (Decreases theophylline clearance by inhibiting cytochrome P450 1A2 and also increases renal clearance of theophylline). Products include:
- Cognex Capsules 1961

Thiabendazole (Decreases theophylline clearance). Products include:
- Mintezol 1747

Ticlopidine Hydrochloride (Decreases theophylline clearance). Products include:
- Ticlid Tablets 2317

Troleandomycin (Decreases theophylline clearance by inhibiting cytochrome P450 3A3). Products include:
- Tao Capsules 2033

Verapamil Hydrochloride (Decreases theophylline clearance by inhibiting hydroxylation and demethylation). Products include:
- Calan SR Caplets 2571
- Calan Tablets 2568
- Covera-HS Tablets 2573
- Isoptin Injectable 1391
- Isoptin Oral Tablets 1393
- Isoptin SR Tablets 1395
- Verelan Capsules 1455

Food Interactions

Alcohol (Concurrent use with a single dose of alcohol (3 mL/kg of whiskey) decreases theophylline clearance for up to 24 hours).

Food, unspecified (Available data suggests that co-administration with food may influence the absorption characteristics of controlled-release theophylline formulations).

THEO-X EXTENDED-RELEASE TABLETS
(Theophylline Anhydrous) 793
May interact with macrolide antibiotics, oral contraceptives, sympathomimetic bronchodilators, and certain other agents. Compounds in these categories include:

Albuterol (Potential for toxic synergism). Products include:
- Proventil Inhalation Aerosol 2524
- Ventolin Inhalation Aerosol and Refill 1170

Albuterol Sulfate (Potential for toxic synergism). Products include:
- Airet Albuterol Sulfate Inhalation Solution 1602
- Albuterol Sulfate, USP Solution for Inhalation, Arm-a-Med 522
- Proventil Inhalation Solution 0.083% 2527
- Proventil Repetabs Tablets 2529
- Proventil Solution for Inhalation 0.5% 2525
- Proventil Syrup 2528
- Proventil Tablets 2529
- Ventolin Inhalation Solution 1171
- Ventolin Nebules Inhalation Solution 1172
- Ventolin Rotacaps for Inhalation 1173
- Ventolin Syrup 1175
- Ventolin Tablets 1176
- Volmax Extended-Release Tablets 1835

Allopurinol (Increased theophylline levels at high dose of allopurinol). Products include:
- Zyloprim Tablets 1194

Azithromycin (Increases serum theophylline levels). Products include:
- Zithromax 2043
- Zithromax Tablets 2046

Bitolterol Mesylate (Potential for toxic synergism). Products include:
- Tornalate Solution for Inhalation, 0.2% 976
- Tornalate Metered Dose Inhaler 978

Cimetidine (Increases serum theophylline levels). Products include:
- Tagamet HB Tablets .... ▣ 786
- Tagamet Tablets 2694

Cimetidine Hydrochloride (Increases serum theophylline levels). Products include:
- Tagamet 2694

Ciprofloxacin (Increases serum theophylline levels). Products include:
- Cipro I.V. 587
- Cipro I.V. Pharmacy Bulk Package 590

Ciprofloxacin Hydrochloride (Increases serum theophylline levels). Products include:
- Ciloxan Ophthalmic Solution 468
- Cipro Tablets 584

Clarithromycin (Increases serum theophylline levels). Products include:
- Biaxin 406

Desogestrel (Increases serum theophylline levels). Products include:
- Desogen Tablets 1867
- Ortho-Cept 1907

Dirithromycin (Increases serum theophylline levels). Products include:
- Dynabac 668

Ephedrine Hydrochloride (Potential for toxic synergism). Products include:
- Primatene Tablets .... ▣ 844
- Quadrinal Tablets 1398

Ephedrine Sulfate (Potential for toxic synergism). Products include:
- Marax Tablets & DF Syrup 2015

Ephedrine Tannate (Potential for toxic synergism). Products include:
- Rynatuss 2782

Epinephrine (Potential for toxic synergism). Products include:
- EPIFRIN .... ⊚ 237
- EpiPen 808
- Marcaine with Epinephrine 2446
- Primatene Mist .... ▣ 843
- Sensorcaine with Epinephrine Injection 554
- Sus-Phrine Injection 1017
- Xylocaine with Epinephrine Injections 562

Epinephrine Hydrochloride (Potential for toxic synergism). Products include:
- Ana-Kit Anaphylaxis Emergency Treatment Kit 611

Erythromycin (Increases serum theophylline levels). Products include:
- A/T/S 2% Acne Topical Gel 1244
- A/T/S 2% Acne Topical Solution 1244
- Benzamycin Topical Gel 919
- E-Mycin Tablets 1388
- Emgel 2% Topical Gel 1081
- ERYC 1972
- Erycette (erythromycin 2%) Topical Solution 1943
- Ery-Tab Tablets 426
- Erythromycin Base Filmtab 430
- Erythromycin Delayed-Release Capsules, USP 431
- Ilotycin Ophthalmic Ointment 928
- PCE Dispertab Tablets 453
- T-Stat 2.0% Topical Solution and Pads 2797
- THERAMYCIN Z 2% Solution 1629

Erythromycin Estolate (Increases serum theophylline levels). Products include:
- Ilosone 927

Erythromycin Ethylsuccinate (Increases serum theophylline levels). Products include:
- E.E.S. 427
- EryPed 425
- Pediazole Suspension 2340

Erythromycin Glucoptate (Increases serum theophylline levels). Products include:
- Ilotycin Glucoptate, IV, Vials 929

Erythromycin Stearate (Increases serum theophylline levels). Products include:
- Erythrocin Stearate Filmtab 429

Ethinyl Estradiol (Increases serum theophylline levels). Products include:
- Brevicon 2563
- Demulen 2580
- Desogen Tablets 1867
- Levlen/Tri-Levlen 646
- Lo/Ovral Tablets 2852
- Lo/Ovral-28 Tablets 2857
- Modicon 1928
- Nordette-21 Tablets 2863
- Nordette-28 Tablets 2866
- Norinyl 2563
- Ortho-Cept 1907
- Ortho-Cyclen/Ortho-Tri-Cyclen 1914
- Ortho-Novum 1928
- Ortho-Cyclen/Ortho Tri-Cyclen 1914
- Ovcon 765
- Ovral Tablets 2877
- Ovral-28 Tablets 2878
- Levlen/Tri-Levlen 646
- Tri-Norinyl 2607
- Triphasil-21 Tablets 2919
- Triphasil-28 Tablets 2924

Ethylnorepinephrine Hydrochloride (Potential for toxic synergism).
No products indexed under this heading.

Ethynodiol Diacetate (Increases serum theophylline levels). Products include:
- Demulen 2580

Isoetharine (Potential for toxic synergism). Products include:
- Bronkometer Aerosol 2432
- Bronkosol Solution 2432
- Isoetharine Inhalation Solution, USP, Arm-a-Med 545

Isoproterenol Hydrochloride (Potential for toxic synergism). Products include:
- Isuprel Hydrochloride Solution 2443
- Isuprel Injection 2441
- Isuprel Mistometer 2442

Isoproterenol Sulfate (Potential for toxic synergism). Products include:
- Norisodrine with Calcium Iodide Syrup 446

(▣ Described in PDR For Nonprescription Drugs)   (⊚ Described in PDR For Ophthalmology)

Interactions Index

Levonorgestrel (Increases serum theophylline levels). Products include:
- Levlen/Tri-Levlen 646
- Nordette-21 Tablets 2863
- Nordette-28 Tablets 2866
- Norplant System 2868
- Levlen/Tri-Levlen 646
- Triphasil-21 Tablets 2919
- Triphasil-28 Tablets 2924

Lithium Carbonate (Increased renal excretion of lithium). Products include:
- Eskalith 2658
- Lithium Carbonate Capsules & Tablets 2352
- Lithonate/Lithotabs/Lithobid 2721

Mestranol (Increases serum theophylline levels). Products include:
- Norinyl 2563
- Ortho-Novum 1928

Metaproterenol Sulfate (Potential for toxic synergism). Products include:
- Alupent 672
- Metaproterenol Sulfate Inhalation Solution, USP, Arm-a-Med 547

Norethindrone (Increases serum theophylline levels). Products include:
- Brevicon 2563
- Micronor Tablets 1903
- Modicon 1928
- Norinyl 2563
- Nor-Q D Tablets 2598
- Ortho-Novum 1928
- Ovcon 765
- Tri-Norinyl 2607

Norethynodrel (Increases serum theophylline levels).
- No products indexed under this heading.

Norgestimate (Increases serum theophylline levels). Products include:
- Ortho-Cyclen/Ortho Tri-Cyclen 1914
- Ortho-Cyclen/Ortho Tri-Cyclen 1914

Norgestrel (Increases serum theophylline levels). Products include:
- Lo/Ovral Tablets 2852
- Lo/Ovral-28 Tablets 2857
- Ovral Tablets 2877
- Ovral-28 Tablets 2878
- Ovrette Tablets 2878

Phenytoin (Decreased theophylline and phenytoin levels). Products include:
- Dilantin Infatabs 1967
- Dilantin-125 Suspension 1969

Phenytoin Sodium (Decreased theophylline and phenytoin levels). Products include:
- Dilantin Kapseals 1965

Pirbuterol Acetate (Potential for toxic synergism). Products include:
- Maxair Autohaler 1550
- Maxair Inhaler 1552

Propranolol Hydrochloride (Increases serum theophylline levels). Products include:
- Inderal 2834
- Inderal LA Long Acting Capsules 2836
- Inderide Tablets 2838
- Inderide LA Long Acting Capsules 2840

Rifampin (Decreased serum theophylline levels). Products include:
- Rifadin 1276
- Rifamate Capsules 1278
- Rifater 1280
- Rimactane Capsules 865

Salmeterol Xinafoate (Potential for toxic synergism). Products include:
- Serevent Inhalation Aerosol 1149

Terbutaline Sulfate (Potential for toxic synergism). Products include:
- Brethaire Inhaler 830
- Brethine Ampuls 832
- Brethine Tablets 831
- Bricanyl Subcutaneous Injection 1247
- Bricanyl Tablets 1248

Troleandomycin (Increases serum theophylline levels). Products include:
- Tao Capsules 2033

Food Interactions

Diet, high-lipid (May result in a somewhat higher C_{max} and delayed T_{max}, and a somewhat greater extent of absorption when compared to taking in the fasting state).

THERACYS BCG LIVE (INTRAVESICAL)

(BCG, Live (Intravesical)) 911
May interact with immunosuppressive agents and certain other agents. Compounds in these categories include:

Azathioprine (May impair the response to TheraCys or increase the risk of osteomyelitis or disseminated BCG infection). Products include:
- Azathioprine Tablets 2349
- Imuran 1103

Bone Marrow Depressants, unspecified (May impair the response to TheraCys or increase the risk of osteomyelitis or disseminated BCG infection).

Cyclosporine (May impair the response to TheraCys or increase the risk of osteomyelitis or disseminated BCG infection). Products include:
- Neoral 2405
- Sandimmune 2416

Immune Globulin (Human) (May impair the response to TheraCys or increase the risk of osteomyelitis or disseminated BCG infection).
- No products indexed under this heading.

Immune Globulin Intravenous (Human) (May impair the response to TheraCys or increase the risk of osteomyelitis or disseminated BCG infection).

Muromonab-CD3 (May impair the response to TheraCys or increase the risk of osteomyelitis or disseminated BCG infection). Products include:
- Orthoclone OKT3 Sterile Solution 1892

Mycophenolate Mofetil (May impair the response to TheraCys or increase the risk of osteomyelitis or disseminated BCG infection). Products include:
- CellCept Capsules 2265

Tacrolimus (May impair the response to TheraCys or increase the risk of osteomyelitis or disseminated BCG infection). Products include:
- Prograf 1028

THERAFLU FLU AND COLD MEDICINE

(Acetaminophen, Chlorpheniramine Maleate, Pseudoephedrine Hydrochloride) 750
May interact with hypnotics and sedatives, tranquilizers, monoamine oxidase inhibitors, and certain other agents. Compounds in these categories include:

Alprazolam (May increase drowsiness effect). Products include:
- Xanax Tablets 2115

Buspirone Hydrochloride (May increase drowsiness effect). Products include:
- BuSpar Tablets 738

Chlordiazepoxide (May increase drowsiness effect). Products include:
- Limbitrol 2333

Chlordiazepoxide Hydrochloride (May increase drowsiness effect). Products include:
- Librax Capsules 2330
- Librium Capsules 2331
- Librium Injectable 2332

Chlorpromazine (May increase drowsiness effect). Products include:
- Thorazine Suppositories 2701

Chlorpromazine Hydrochloride (May increase drowsiness effect). Products include:
- Thorazine 2701

Chlorprothixene (May increase drowsiness effect).
- No products indexed under this heading.

Chlorprothixene Hydrochloride (May increase drowsiness effect).
- No products indexed under this heading.

Clorazepate Dipotassium (May increase drowsiness effect). Products include:
- Tranxene 459

Diazepam (May increase drowsiness effect). Products include:
- Dizac (diazepam injectable emulsion) CIV 1862
- Valium Injectable 2336
- Valium Tablets 2335

Droperidol (May increase drowsiness effect). Products include:
- Inapsine Injection 462

Estazolam (May increase drowsiness effect). Products include:
- ProSom Tablets 457

Ethchlorvynol (May increase drowsiness effect). Products include:
- Placidyl Capsules 456

Ethinamate (May increase drowsiness effect).
- No products indexed under this heading.

Fluphenazine Decanoate (May increase drowsiness effect). Products include:
- Prolixin Decanoate 510

Fluphenazine Enanthate (May increase drowsiness effect). Products include:
- Prolixin Enanthate 510

Fluphenazine Hydrochloride (May increase drowsiness effect). Products include:
- Prolixin 510

Flurazepam Hydrochloride (May increase drowsiness effect). Products include:
- Dalmane Capsules 2329

Furazolidone (Concurrent and/or sequential use is not recommended). Products include:
- Furoxone 2221

Glutethimide (May increase drowsiness effect).
- No products indexed under this heading.

Haloperidol (May increase drowsiness effect). Products include:
- Haldol Injection, Tablets and Concentrate 1585

Haloperidol Decanoate (May increase drowsiness effect). Products include:
- Haldol Decanoate 1587

Hydroxyzine Hydrochloride (May increase drowsiness effect). Products include:
- Atarax Tablets & Syrup 1992
- Marax Tablets & DF Syrup 2015
- Vistaril Intramuscular Solution 2042

Isocarboxazid (Concurrent and/or sequential use is not recommended).
- No products indexed under this heading.

Lorazepam (May increase drowsiness effect). Products include:
- Ativan Injection 2805
- Ativan Tablets 2807

Loxapine Hydrochloride (May increase drowsiness effect). Products include:
- Loxitane 1426

Loxapine Succinate (May increase drowsiness effect). Products include:
- Loxitane Capsules 1426

Meprobamate (May increase drowsiness effect). Products include:
- Miltown Tablets 2780
- PMB 200 and PMB 400 2890

Mesoridazine Besylate (May increase drowsiness effect). Products include:
- Serentil 689

Midazolam Hydrochloride (May increase drowsiness effect). Products include:
- Versed Injection 2324

Molindone Hydrochloride (May increase drowsiness effect). Products include:
- Moban Tablets and Concentrate 1036

Oxazepam (May increase drowsiness effect). Products include:
- Serax Capsules 2916
- Serax Tablets 2916

Perphenazine (May increase drowsiness effect). Products include:
- Etrafon 2495
- Triavil Tablets 1800
- Trilafon 2532

Phenelzine Sulfate (Concurrent and/or sequential use is not recommended). Products include:
- Nardil 1977

Prazepam (May increase drowsiness effect).
- No products indexed under this heading.

Prochlorperazine (May increase drowsiness effect). Products include:
- Compazine 2644

Promethazine Hydrochloride (May increase drowsiness effect). Products include:
- Mepergan Injection 2859
- Phenergan with Codeine 2883
- Phenergan with Dextromethorphan 2885
- Phenergan Injection 2880
- Phenergan Suppositories 2882
- Phenergan Syrup 2881
- Phenergan Tablets 2882
- Phenergan VC 2886
- Phenergan VC with Codeine 2888

Propofol (May increase drowsiness effect). Products include:
- Diprivan Injectable Emulsion 2939

Quazepam (May increase drowsiness effect). Products include:
- Doral Tablets 2773

Secobarbital Sodium (May increase drowsiness effect). Products include:
- Seconal Sodium Pulvules 1529

Selegiline Hydrochloride (Concurrent and/or sequential use is not recommended). Products include:
- Eldepryl Capsules 2729

Temazepam (May increase drowsiness effect). Products include:
- Restoril Capsules 2413

Thioridazine Hydrochloride (May increase drowsiness effect). Products include:
- Mellaril 2398

Thiothixene (May increase drowsiness effect). Products include:
- Navane Capsules and Concentrate 2018
- Navane Intramuscular 2019

IMPORTANT NOTE: Always consult each drug listing in the patient's regimen for possible interactions.

TheraFlu

Tranylcypromine Sulfate (Concurrent and/or sequential use is not recommended). Products include:
- Parnate Tablets 2679

Triazolam (May increase drowsiness effect). Products include:
- Halcion Tablets 2093

Trifluoperazine Hydrochloride (May increase drowsiness effect). Products include:
- Stelazine 2692

Zolpidem Tartrate (May increase drowsiness effect). Products include:
- Ambien Tablets 2559

Food Interactions
Alcohol (May increase drowsiness effect).

THERAFLU MAXIMUM STRENGTH FLU AND COLD MEDICINE FOR SORE THROAT
(Acetaminophen, Chlorpheniramine Maleate, Pseudoephedrine Hydrochloride) .... ▣ 751

May interact with monoamine oxidase inhibitors, hypnotics and sedatives, tranquilizers, and certain other agents. Compounds in these categories include:

Alprazolam (May increase drowsiness effect). Products include:
- Xanax Tablets 2115

Buspirone Hydrochloride (May increase drowsiness effect). Products include:
- BuSpar Tablets 738

Chlordiazepoxide (May increase drowsiness effect). Products include:
- Limbitrol 2333

Chlordiazepoxide Hydrochloride (May increase drowsiness effect). Products include:
- Librax Capsules 2330
- Librium Capsules 2331
- Librium Injectable 2332

Chlorpromazine (May increase drowsiness effect). Products include:
- Thorazine Suppositories 2701

Chlorpromazine Hydrochloride (May increase drowsiness effect). Products include:
- Thorazine 2701

Chlorprothixene (May increase drowsiness effect).
No products indexed under this heading.

Chlorprothixene Hydrochloride (May increase drowsiness effect).
No products indexed under this heading.

Clorazepate Dipotassium (May increase drowsiness effect). Products include:
- Tranxene 459

Diazepam (May increase drowsiness effect). Products include:
- Dizac (diazepam injectable emulsion) CIV 1862
- Valium Injectable 2336
- Valium Tablets 2335

Droperidol (May increase drowsiness effect). Products include:
- Inapsine Injection 462

Estazolam (May increase drowsiness effect). Products include:
- ProSom Tablets 457

Ethchlorvynol (May increase drowsiness effect). Products include:
- Placidyl Capsules 456

Ethinamate (May increase drowsiness effect).
No products indexed under this heading.

Fluphenazine Decanoate (May increase drowsiness effect). Products include:
- Prolixin Decanoate 510

Fluphenazine Enanthate (May increase drowsiness effect). Products include:
- Prolixin Enanthate 510

Fluphenazine Hydrochloride (May increase drowsiness effect). Products include:
- Prolixin 510

Flurazepam Hydrochloride (May increase drowsiness effect). Products include:
- Dalmane Capsules 2329

Furazolidone (Concurrent and/or sequential use is not recommended). Products include:
- Furoxone 2221

Glutethimide (May increase drowsiness effect).
No products indexed under this heading.

Haloperidol (May increase drowsiness effect). Products include:
- Haldol Injection, Tablets and Concentrate 1585

Haloperidol Decanoate (May increase drowsiness effect). Products include:
- Haldol Decanoate 1587

Hydroxyzine Hydrochloride (May increase drowsiness effect). Products include:
- Atarax Tablets & Syrup 1992
- Marax Tablets & DF Syrup 2015
- Vistaril Intramuscular Solution 2042

Isocarboxazid (Concurrent and/or sequential use is not recommended).
No products indexed under this heading.

Lorazepam (May increase drowsiness effect). Products include:
- Ativan Injection 2805
- Ativan Tablets 2807

Loxapine Hydrochloride (May increase drowsiness effect). Products include:
- Loxitane 1426

Loxapine Succinate (May increase drowsiness effect). Products include:
- Loxitane Capsules 1426

Meprobamate (May increase drowsiness effect). Products include:
- Miltown Tablets 2780
- PMB 200 and PMB 400 2890

Mesoridazine Besylate (May increase drowsiness effect). Products include:
- Serentil 689

Midazolam Hydrochloride (May increase drowsiness effect). Products include:
- Versed Injection 2324

Molindone Hydrochloride (May increase drowsiness effect). Products include:
- Moban Tablets and Concentrate 1036

Oxazepam (May increase drowsiness effect). Products include:
- Serax Capsules 2916
- Serax Tablets 2916

Perphenazine (May increase drowsiness effect). Products include:
- Etrafon 2495
- Triavil Tablets 1800
- Trilafon 2532

Phenelzine Sulfate (Concurrent and/or sequential use is not recommended). Products include:
- Nardil 1977

Prazepam (May increase drowsiness effect).
No products indexed under this heading.

Prochlorperazine (May increase drowsiness effect). Products include:
- Compazine 2644

Promethazine Hydrochloride (May increase drowsiness effect). Products include:
- Meperjan Injection 2859
- Phenergan with Codeine 2883
- Phenergan with Dextromethorphan 2885
- Phenergan Injection 2880
- Phenergan Suppositories 2882
- Phenergan Syrup 2881
- Phenergan Tablets 2882
- Phenergan VC 2886
- Phenergan VC with Codeine 2888

Propofol (May increase drowsiness effect). Products include:
- Diprivan Injectable Emulsion 2939

Quazepam (May increase drowsiness effect). Products include:
- Doral Tablets 2773

Secobarbital Sodium (May increase drowsiness effect). Products include:
- Seconal Sodium Pulvules 1529

Selegiline Hydrochloride (Concurrent and/or sequential use is not recommended). Products include:
- Eldepryl Capsules 2729

Temazepam (May increase drowsiness effect). Products include:
- Restoril Capsules 2413

Thioridazine Hydrochloride (May increase drowsiness effect). Products include:
- Mellaril 2398

Thiothixene (May increase drowsiness effect). Products include:
- Navane Capsules and Concentrate 2018
- Navane Intramuscular 2019

Tranylcypromine Sulfate (Concurrent and/or sequential use is not recommended). Products include:
- Parnate Tablets 2679

Triazolam (May increase drowsiness effect). Products include:
- Halcion Tablets 2093

Trifluoperazine Hydrochloride (May increase drowsiness effect). Products include:
- Stelazine 2692

Zolpidem Tartrate (May increase drowsiness effect). Products include:
- Ambien Tablets 2559

Food Interactions
Alcohol (May increase drowsiness effect).

THERAFLU FLU, COLD AND COUGH MEDICINE
(Acetaminophen, Pseudoephedrine Hydrochloride, Chlorpheniramine Maleate, Dextromethorphan Hydrobromide) .... ▣ 750
See TheraFlu Flu and Cold Medicine

THERAFLU MAXIMUM STRENGTH NIGHTTIME FLU, COLD & COUGH MEDICINE
(Acetaminophen, Dextromethorphan Hydrobromide, Pseudoephedrine Hydrochloride, Chlorpheniramine Maleate) .... ▣ 751

May interact with hypnotics and sedatives, tranquilizers, monoamine oxidase inhibitors, and certain other agents. Compounds in these categories include:

Alprazolam (May increase drowsiness effect). Products include:
- Xanax Tablets 2115

Buspirone Hydrochloride (May increase drowsiness effect). Products include:
- BuSpar Tablets 738

Chlordiazepoxide (May increase drowsiness effect). Products include:
- Limbitrol 2333

Chlordiazepoxide Hydrochloride (May increase drowsiness effect). Products include:
- Librax Capsules 2330
- Librium Capsules 2331
- Librium Injectable 2332

Chlorpromazine (May increase drowsiness effect). Products include:
- Thorazine Suppositories 2701

Chlorpromazine Hydrochloride (May increase drowsiness effect). Products include:
- Thorazine 2701

Chlorprothixene (May increase drowsiness effect).
No products indexed under this heading.

Chlorprothixene Hydrochloride (May increase drowsiness effect).
No products indexed under this heading.

Clorazepate Dipotassium (May increase drowsiness effect). Products include:
- Tranxene 459

Diazepam (May increase drowsiness effect). Products include:
- Dizac (diazepam injectable emulsion) CIV 1862
- Valium Injectable 2336
- Valium Tablets 2335

Droperidol (May increase drowsiness effect). Products include:
- Inapsine Injection 462

Estazolam (May increase drowsiness effect). Products include:
- ProSom Tablets 457

Ethchlorvynol (May increase drowsiness effect). Products include:
- Placidyl Capsules 456

Ethinamate (May increase drowsiness effect).
No products indexed under this heading.

Fluphenazine Decanoate (May increase drowsiness effect). Products include:
- Prolixin Decanoate 510

Fluphenazine Enanthate (May increase drowsiness effect). Products include:
- Prolixin Enanthate 510

Fluphenazine Hydrochloride (May increase drowsiness effect). Products include:
- Prolixin 510

Flurazepam Hydrochloride (May increase drowsiness effect). Products include:
- Dalmane Capsules 2329

Furazolidone (Concurrent and/or sequential use is not recommended). Products include:
- Furoxone 2221

Glutethimide (May increase drowsiness effect).
No products indexed under this heading.

Haloperidol (May increase drowsiness effect). Products include:
- Haldol Injection, Tablets and Concentrate 1585

Haloperidol Decanoate (May increase drowsiness effect). Products include:
- Haldol Decanoate 1587

Hydroxyzine Hydrochloride (May increase drowsiness effect). Products include:
- Atarax Tablets & Syrup 1992
- Marax Tablets & DF Syrup 2015
- Vistaril Intramuscular Solution 2042

(▣ Described in PDR For Nonprescription Drugs)   (⊙ Described in PDR For Ophthalmology)

Interactions Index — Thorazine

Isocarboxazid (Concurrent and/or sequential use is not recommended).
  No products indexed under this heading.
Lorazepam (May increase drowsiness effect). Products include:
  Ativan Injection 2805
  Ativan Tablets 2807
Loxapine Hydrochloride (May increase drowsiness effect). Products include:
  Loxitane 1426
Loxapine Succinate (May increase drowsiness effect). Products include:
  Loxitane Capsules 1426
Meprobamate (May increase drowsiness effect). Products include:
  Miltown Tablets 2780
  PMB 200 and PMB 400 2890
Mesoridazine Besylate (May increase drowsiness effect). Products include:
  Serentil 689
Midazolam Hydrochloride (May increase drowsiness effect). Products include:
  Versed Injection 2324
Molindone Hydrochloride (May increase drowsiness effect). Products include:
  Moban Tablets and Concentrate ... 1036
Oxazepam (May increase drowsiness effect). Products include:
  Serax Capsules 2916
  Serax Tablets 2916
Perphenazine (May increase drowsiness effect). Products include:
  Etrafon 2495
  Triavil Tablets 1800
  Trilafon 2532
Phenelzine Sulfate (Concurrent and/or sequential use is not recommended). Products include:
  Nardil 1977
Prazepam (May increase drowsiness effect). Products include:
  No products indexed under this heading.
Prochlorperazine (May increase drowsiness effect). Products include:
  Compazine 2644
Promethazine Hydrochloride (May increase drowsiness effect). Products include:
  Mepergan Injection 2859
  Phenergan with Codeine 2883
  Phenergan with Dextromethorphan 2885
  Phenergan Injection 2880
  Phenergan Suppositories 2882
  Phenergan Syrup 2881
  Phenergan Tablets 2882
  Phenergan VC 2886
  Phenergan VC with Codeine 2888
Propofol (May increase drowsiness effect). Products include:
  Diprivan Injectable Emulsion 2939
Quazepam (May increase drowsiness effect). Products include:
  Doral Tablets 2773
Secobarbital Sodium (May increase drowsiness effect). Products include:
  Seconal Sodium Pulvules 1529
Selegiline Hydrochloride (Concurrent and/or sequential use is not recommended). Products include:
  Eldepryl Capsules 2729
Temazepam (May increase drowsiness effect). Products include:
  Restoril Capsules 2413
Thioridazine Hydrochloride (May increase drowsiness effect). Products include:
  Mellaril 2398

Thiothixene (May increase drowsiness effect). Products include:
  Navane Capsules and Concentrate 2018
  Navane Intramuscular 2019
Tranylcypromine Sulfate (Concurrent and/or sequential use is not recommended). Products include:
  Parnate Tablets 2679
Triazolam (May increase drowsiness effect). Products include:
  Halcion Tablets 2093
Trifluoperazine Hydrochloride (May increase drowsiness effect). Products include:
  Stelazine 2692
Zolpidem Tartrate (May increase drowsiness effect). Products include:
  Ambien Tablets 2559

Food Interactions

Alcohol (May increase drowsiness effect).

THERAFLU MAXIMUM STRENGTH NON-DROWSY FORMULA FLU, COLD & COUGH MEDICINE
(Acetaminophen, Dextromethorphan Hydrobromide, Pseudoephedrine Hydrochloride) 751
May interact with monoamine oxidase inhibitors. Compounds in this category include:

Furazolidone (Concurrent and/or sequential use is not recommended). Products include:
  Furoxone 2221
Isocarboxazid (Concurrent and/or sequential use is not recommended).
  No products indexed under this heading.
Phenelzine Sulfate (Concurrent and/or sequential use is not recommended). Products include:
  Nardil 1977
Selegiline Hydrochloride (Concurrent and/or sequential use is not recommended). Products include:
  Eldepryl Capsules 2729
Tranylcypromine Sulfate (Concurrent and/or sequential use is not recommended). Products include:
  Parnate Tablets 2679

THERAFLU MAXIMUM STRENGTH, NON-DROWSY FORMULA FLU, COLD AND COUGH CAPLETS
(Acetaminophen, Dextromethorphan Hydrobromide, Pseudoephedrine Hydrochloride) 752
May interact with monoamine oxidase inhibitors. Compounds in this category include:

Furazolidone (Concurrent and/or sequential use is not recommended). Products include:
  Furoxone 2221
Isocarboxazid (Concurrent and/or sequential use is not recommended).
  No products indexed under this heading.
Phenelzine Sulfate (Concurrent and/or sequential use is not recommended). Products include:
  Nardil 1977
Selegiline Hydrochloride (Concurrent and/or sequential use is not recommended). Products include:
  Eldepryl Capsules 2729
Tranylcypromine Sulfate (Concurrent and/or sequential use is not recommended). Products include:
  Parnate Tablets 2679

THERAFLU MAXIMUM STRENGTH SINUS NON-DROWSY FORMULA CAPLETS
(Acetaminophen, Pseudoephedrine Hydrochloride) 752
May interact with monoamine oxidase inhibitors. Compounds in this category include:

Furazolidone (Concurrent and/or sequential use is not recommended). Products include:
  Furoxone 2221
Isocarboxazid (Concurrent and/or sequential use is not recommended).
  No products indexed under this heading.
Phenelzine Sulfate (Concurrent and/or sequential use is not recommended). Products include:
  Nardil 1977
Selegiline Hydrochloride (Concurrent and/or sequential use is not recommended). Products include:
  Eldepryl Capsules 2729
Tranylcypromine Sulfate (Concurrent and/or sequential use is not recommended). Products include:
  Parnate Tablets 2679

THERA-GESIC
(Methyl Salicylate, Menthol) 1830
None cited in PDR database.

THERAGRAN TABLETS
(Vitamin B Complex With Vitamin C, Vitamins with Minerals) 709
None cited in PDR database.

THERAGRAN-M TABLETS
(Vitamins with Minerals) 709
None cited in PDR database.

THERAMYCIN Z 2% SOLUTION
(Erythromycin) 1629
None cited in PDR database.

THERAPEUTIC MINERAL ICE, PAIN RELIEVING GEL
(Menthol) 645
None cited in PDR database.

THERATEARS ATF FORMULA
(Carboxymethylcellulose Sodium) .. 201
None cited in PDR database.

THIOGUANINE TABLETS, TABLOID BRAND
(Thioguanine) 1225
May interact with cytotoxic drugs and certain other agents. Compounds in these categories include:

Bleomycin Sulfate (Combination therapy may produce hepatic disease). Products include:
  Blenoxane 697
Busulfan (Potential for esophageal varices associated with abnormal liver function tests). Products include:
  Myleran Tablets 1209
Daunorubicin Hydrochloride (Combination therapy may produce hepatic disease). Products include:
  Cerubidine for Injection 634
Doxorubicin Hydrochloride (Combination therapy may produce hepatic disease). Products include:
  Adriamycin PFS 2056
  Adriamycin RDF 2056
  Doxil 2613
  Doxorubicin Astra 531
  Rubex for Injection 721

Fluorouracil (Combination therapy may produce hepatic disease). Products include:
  Efudex 2280
  Fluoroplex Topical Solution & Cream 1% 475
  Fluorouracil Injection 2282
Hydroxyurea (Combination therapy may produce hepatic disease). Products include:
  Hydrea Capsules 705
Mercaptopurine (Complete cross-resistance). Products include:
  Purinethol Tablets 1214
Methotrexate Sodium (Combination therapy may produce hepatic disease). Products include:
  Methotrexate Sodium Tablets, Injection, for Injection and LPF Injection 1322
Mitotane (Combination therapy may produce hepatic disease). Products include:
  Lysodren Tablets 707
Mitoxantrone Hydrochloride (Combination therapy may produce hepatic disease). Products include:
  Novantrone for Injection 1327
Procarbazine Hydrochloride (Combination therapy may produce hepatic disease). Products include:
  Matulane Capsules 2300
Tamoxifen Citrate (Combination therapy may produce hepatic disease). Products include:
  Nolvadex Tablets 2957
Vincristine Sulfate (Combination therapy may produce hepatic disease). Products include:
  Oncovin Solution Vials & Hyporets 1521

THIOPLEX (THIOTEPA FOR INJECTION)
(Thiotepa) 1329
May interact with nitrogen-mustard-type alkylating agents and certain other agents. Compounds in these categories include:

Bone Marrow Depressants, unspecified (Avoid concurrent use).
Chlorambucil (Intensified toxicity). Products include:
  Leukeran Tablets 1205
Cyclophosphamide (Intensified toxicity). Products include:
  Cytoxan 700
Estramustine Phosphate Sodium (Intensified toxicity). Products include:
  Emcyt Capsules 2085
Mechlorethamine Hydrochloride (Intensified toxicity). Products include:
  Mustargen 1752
Melphalan (Intensified toxicity). Products include:
  Alkeran Tablets 1198
Succinylcholine Chloride (Prolonged apnea after succinylcholine administration to patients receiving thiotepa and other cancer drugs). Products include:
  Anectine 1062

THORAZINE AMPULS
(Chlorpromazine Hydrochloride) 2701
See **Thorazine Concentrate**

THORAZINE CONCENTRATE
(Chlorpromazine Hydrochloride) 2701
May interact with central nervous system depressants, oral anticoagulants, anticonvulsants, thiazides, and

---
IMPORTANT NOTE: Always consult each drug listing in the patient's regimen for possible interactions.

Thorazine Interactions Index 1064

certain other agents. Compounds in these categories include:

Alfentanil Hydrochloride (Prolonged and intensified action of CNS depressants). Products include:
- Alfenta Injection ... 1334

Alprazolam (Prolonged and intensified action of CNS depressants). Products include:
- Xanax Tablets ... 2115

Aprobarbital (Prolonged and intensified action of CNS depressants).
- No products indexed under this heading.

Atropine Sulfate (Use with caution). Products include:
- Arco-Lase Plus Tablets ... 513
- Atrohist Plus Tablets ... 1605
- Donnatal ... 2234
- Donnatal Extentabs ... 2234
- Donnatal Tablets ... 2234
- Lomotil ... 2591
- Motofen Tablets ... 789
- Urised Tablets ... 2123

Bendroflumethiazide (Orthostatic hypotension that may occur with chlorpromazine may be accentuated).
- No products indexed under this heading.

Buprenorphine (Prolonged and intensified action of CNS depressants). Products include:
- Buprenex Injectable ... 2170

Buspirone Hydrochloride (Prolonged and intensified action of CNS depressants). Products include:
- BuSpar Tablets ... 738

Butabarbital (Prolonged and intensified action of CNS depressants).
- No products indexed under this heading.

Butalbital (Prolonged and intensified action of CNS depressants). Products include:
- Axocet Capsules ... 2469
- Esgic-plus Capsules ... 1012
- Esgic-plus Tablets ... 1012
- Fioricet Tablets ... 2386
- Fioricet with Codeine Capsules ... 2387
- Fiorinal Capsules ... 2388
- Fiorinal with Codeine Capsules ... 2390
- Fiorinal Tablets ... 2388
- Phrenilin ... 790
- Sedapap Tablets 50 mg/650 mg ... 1826

Carbamazepine (Chlorpromazine may lower convulsive threshold; dosage adjustments of anticonvulsants may be necessary). Products include:
- Atretol Tablets ... 569
- Tegretol/Tegretol-XR ... 870

Carmustine (BCNU) (Antiemetic action of chlorpromazine may obscure vomiting as a sign of toxicity). Products include:
- BiCNU ... 696

Chlordiazepoxide (Prolonged and intensified action of CNS depressants). Products include:
- Limbitrol ... 2333

Chlordiazepoxide Hydrochloride (Prolonged and intensified action of CNS depressants). Products include:
- Librax Capsules ... 2330
- Librium Capsules ... 2331
- Librium Injectable ... 2332

Chlorothiazide (Orthostatic hypotension that may occur with chlorpromazine may be accentuated). Products include:
- Aldoclor Tablets ... 1638
- Diupres Tablets ... 1691
- Diuril Oral ... 1694

Chlorothiazide Sodium (Orthostatic hypotension that may occur with chlorpromazine may be accentuated). Products include:
- Diuril Sodium Intravenous ... 1693

Chlorprothixene (Prolonged and intensified action of CNS depressants).
- No products indexed under this heading.

Chlorprothixene Hydrochloride (Prolonged and intensified action of CNS depressants).
- No products indexed under this heading.

Chlorprothixene Lactate (Prolonged and intensified action of CNS depressants).
- No products indexed under this heading.

Clorazepate Dipotassium (Prolonged and intensified action of CNS depressants). Products include:
- Tranxene ... 459

Clozapine (Prolonged and intensified action of CNS depressants). Products include:
- Clozaril Tablets ... 2377

Codeine Phosphate (Prolonged and intensified action of CNS depressants). Products include:
- Brontex ... 2130
- Dimetane-DC Cough Syrup ... 2232
- Fioricet with Codeine Capsules ... 2387
- Fiorinal with Codeine Capsules ... 2390
- Nucofed ... 2225
- Phenergan with Codeine ... 2883
- Phenergan VC with Codeine ... 2888
- Robitussin A-C Syrup ... 2248
- Robitussin-DAC Syrup ... 2249
- Ryna ... ▣ 804
- Soma Compound w/Codeine Tablets ... 2784
- Tylenol with Codeine ... 1592

Desflurane (Prolonged and intensified action of CNS depressants). Products include:
- Suprane (desflurane, USP) ... 1865

Dezocine (Prolonged and intensified action of CNS depressants). Products include:
- Dalgan Injection ... 529

Diazepam (Prolonged and intensified action of CNS depressants). Products include:
- Dizac (diazepam injectable emulsion) CIV ... 1862
- Valium Injectable ... 2336
- Valium Tablets ... 2335

Dicumarol (Chlorpromazine diminishes the effects of oral anticoagulants).
- No products indexed under this heading.

Divalproex Sodium (Chlorpromazine may lower convulsive threshold; dosage adjustments of anticonvulsants may be necessary). Products include:
- Depakote Tablets ... 418

Droperidol (Prolonged and intensified action of CNS depressants). Products include:
- Inapsine Injection ... 462

Enflurane (Prolonged and intensified action of CNS depressants).
- No products indexed under this heading.

Estazolam (Prolonged and intensified action of CNS depressants). Products include:
- ProSom Tablets ... 457

Estramustine Phosphate Sodium (Antiemetic action of chlorpromazine may obscure vomiting as a sign of toxicity). Products include:
- Emcyt Capsules ... 2085

Ethchlorvynol (Prolonged and intensified action of CNS depressants). Products include:
- Placidyl Capsules ... 456

Ethinamate (Prolonged and intensified action of CNS depressants).
- No products indexed under this heading.

Ethosuximide (Chlorpromazine may lower convulsive threshold; dosage adjustments of anticonvulsants may be necessary). Products include:
- Zarontin Capsules ... 1986
- Zarontin Syrup ... 1986

Ethotoin (Chlorpromazine may lower convulsive threshold; dosage adjustments of anticonvulsants may be necessary). Products include:
- Peganone Tablets ... 455

Felbamate (Chlorpromazine may lower convulsive threshold; dosage adjustments of anticonvulsants may be necessary). Products include:
- Felbatol ... 2774

Fentanyl (Prolonged and intensified action of CNS depressants). Products include:
- Duragesic Transdermal System ... 1336

Fentanyl Citrate (Prolonged and intensified action of CNS depressants). Products include:
- Sublimaze Injection ... 463

Fluphenazine Decanoate (Prolonged and intensified action of CNS depressants). Products include:
- Prolixin Decanoate ... 510

Fluphenazine Enanthate (Prolonged and intesnified action of CNS depressants). Products include:
- Prolixin Enanthate ... 510

Fluphenazine Hydrochloride (Prolonged and intensified action of CNS depressants). Products include:
- Prolixin ... 510

Flurazepam Hydrochloride (Prolonged and intensified action of CNS depressants). Products include:
- Dalmane Capsules ... 2329

Glutethimide (Prolonged and intensified action of CNS depressants).
- No products indexed under this heading.

Guanethidine Monosulfate (Antihypertensive effect of guanethidine and related compounds may be counteracted). Products include:
- Esimil Tablets ... 840
- Ismelin Tablets ... 845

Haloperidol (Prolonged and intensified action of CNS depressants). Products include:
- Haldol Injection, Tablets and Concentrate ... 1585

Haloperidol Decanoate (Prolonged and intensified action of CNS depressants). Products include:
- Haldol Decanoate ... 1587

Hydrochlorothiazide (Orthostatic hypotension that may occur with chlorpromazine may be accentuated). Products include:
- Aldactazide Tablets ... 2556
- Aldoril Tablets ... 1644
- Apresazide Capsules ... 824
- Capozide Tablets ... 744
- Dyazide Capsules ... 2653
- Esidrix Tablets ... 839
- Esimil Tablets ... 840
- HydroDIURIL Tablets ... 1716
- Hydropres Tablets ... 1718
- Hyzaar Tablets ... 1720
- Inderide Tablets ... 2838
- Inderide LA Long Acting Capsules ... 2840
- Lopressor HCT Tablets ... 850
- Lotensin HCT Tablets ... 855
- Moduretic Tablets ... 1748
- Oretic Tablets ... 450
- Prinzide Tablets ... 1780
- Ser-Ap-Es Tablets ... 867
- Timolide Tablets ... 1791
- Vaseretic Tablets ... 1810
- Zestoretic Tablets ... 2968
- Ziac ... 1459

Hydrocodone Bitartrate (Prolonged and intensified action of CNS depressants). Products include:
- Codiclear DH Syrup ... 808
- Duratuss HD Elixir ... 2750
- Histussin D Liquid ... 670
- Hycodan Tablets and Syrup ... 946
- Hycomine Compound Tablets ... 948
- Hycomine ... 947
- Hycotuss Expectorant Syrup ... 950
- Hydrocet Capsules ... 787
- Lorcet 10/650 Tablets ... 1016
- Lortab ... 2751
- Tussend ... 1830
- Tussend Expectorant ... 1831
- Vicodin Tablets ... 1404
- Vicodin ES Tablets ... 1405
- Vicodin HP Tablets ... 1403
- Vicodin Tuss Expectorant ... 1406
- Zydone Capsules ... 967

Hydrocodone Polistirex (Prolonged and intensified action of CNS depressants). Products include:
- Tussionex Pennkinetic Extended-Release Suspension ... 1624

Hydroflumethiazide (Orthostatic hypotension that may occur with chlorpromazine may be accentuated). Products include:
- Diucardin Tablets ... 2824

Hydroxyurea (Antiemetic action of chlorpromazine may obscure vomiting as a sign of toxicity). Products include:
- Hydrea Capsules ... 705

Hydroxyzine Hydrochloride (Prolonged and intensified action of CNS depressants). Products include:
- Atarax Tablets & Syrup ... 1992
- Marax Tablets & DF Syrup ... 2015
- Vistaril Intramuscular Solution ... 2042

Isoflurane (Prolonged and intensified action of CNS depressants).
- No products indexed under this heading.

Ketamine Hydrochloride (Prolonged and intensified action of CNS depressants).
- No products indexed under this heading.

Lamotrigine (Chlorpromazine may lower convulsive threshold; dosage adjustments of anticonvulsants may be necessary). Products include:
- Lamictal Tablets ... 1105

Levomethadyl Acetate Hydrochloride (Prolonged and intensified action of CNS depressants). Products include:
- Orlaam Oral Solution ... 2361

Levorphanol Tartrate (Prolonged and intensified action of CNS depressants). Products include:
- Levo-Dromoran ... 2297

Lorazepam (Prolonged and intensified action of CNS depressants). Products include:
- Ativan Injection ... 2805
- Ativan Tablets ... 2807

Loxapine Hydrochloride (Prolonged and intensified action of CNS depressants). Products include:
- Loxitane ... 1426

Loxapine Succinate (Prolonged and intensified action of CNS depressants). Products include:
- Loxitane Capsules ... 1426

Mechlorethamine Hydrochloride (Antiemetic action of chlorpromazine may obscure vomiting as a sign of toxicity). Products include:
- Mustargen ... 1752

(▣ Described in PDR For Nonprescription Drugs) (◉ Described in PDR For Ophthalmology)

Melphalan (Antiemetic action of chlorpromazine may obscure vomiting as a sign of toxicity). Products include:
Alkeran Tablets.................. 1198

Meperidine Hydrochloride (Prolonged and intensified action of CNS depressants). Products include:
Demerol 2438
Mepergan Injection 2859

Mephenytoin (Chlorpromazine may lower convulsive threshold; dosage adjustments of anticonvulsants may be necessary). Products include:
Mesantoin Tablets 2400

Mephobarbital (Prolonged and intensified action of CNS depressants). Products include:
Mebaral Tablets 2452

Meprobamate (Prolonged and intensified action of CNS depressants). Products include:
Miltown Tablets 2780
PMB 200 and PMB 400 2890

Mesoridazine Besylate (Prolonged and intensified action of CNS depressants). Products include:
Serentil 689

Methadone Hydrochloride (Prolonged and intensified action of CNS depressants). Products include:
Methadone Hydrochloride Oral Concentrate 2356
Methadone Hydrochloride Oral Solution & Tablets 2357

Methohexital Sodium (Prolonged and intensified action of CNS depressants).
No products indexed under this heading.

Methotrimeprazine (Prolonged and intensified action of CNS depressants). Products include:
Levoprome 1321

Methoxyflurane (Prolonged and intensified action of CNS depressants).
No products indexed under this heading.

Methsuximide (Chlorpromazine may lower convulsive threshold; dosage adjustments of anticonvulsants may be necessary). Products include:
Celontin Kapseals 1955

Methyclothiazide (Orthostatic hypotension that may occur with chlorpromazine may be accentuated). Products include:
Enduron Tablets 424

Metrizamide (Chlorpromazine may lower convulsive threshold; avoid concurrent use).

Midazolam Hydrochloride (Prolonged and intensified action of CNS depressants). Products include:
Versed Injection 2324

Molindone Hydrochloride (Prolonged and intensified action of CNS depressants). Products include:
Moban Tablets and Concentrate 1036

Morphine Sulfate (Prolonged and intensified action of CNS depressants). Products include:
Astramorph/PF Injection, USP (Preservative-Free) 526
Duramorph Injection 983
Infumorph 200 and Infumorph 500 Sterile Solutions 985
Kadian Capsules 2948
MS Contin Tablets 2149
MSIR 2152
Oramorph SR (Morphine Sulfate Sustained Release Tablets) 2359
RMS Suppositories CII 2766
Roxanol 2365

Opium Alkaloids (Prolonged and intensified action of CNS depressants).
No products indexed under this heading.

Oxazepam (Prolonged and intensified action of CNS depressants). Products include:
Serax Capsules 2916
Serax Tablets 2916

Oxycodone Hydrochloride (Prolonged and intensified action of CNS depressants). Products include:
OxyContin Tablets 2163
OxyIR Capsules 2167
Percocet Tablets 955
Percodan Tablets 955
Percodan-Demi Tablets 956
Roxicodone Tablets, Oral Solution & Intensol (Oxycodone) 2366
Tylox Capsules 1593

Paramethadione (Chlorpromazine may lower convulsive threshold; dosage adjustments of anticonvulsants may be necessary).
No products indexed under this heading.

Pentobarbital Sodium (Prolonged and intensified action of CNS depressants). Products include:
Nembutal Sodium Capsules 440
Nembutal Sodium Solution 442
Nembutal Sodium Suppositories 444

Perphenazine (Prolonged and intensified action of CNS depressants). Products include:
Etrafon 2495
Triavil Tablets 1800
Trilafon 2532

Phenacemide (Chlorpromazine may lower convulsive threshold; dosage adjustments of anticonvulsants may be necessary). Products include:
Phenurone Tablets 455

Phenobarbital (Chlorpromazine may lower convulsive threshold and does not potentiate anticonvulsant action of barbiturates). Products include:
Arco-Lase Plus Tablets 513
Bellergal-S Tablets 2375
Donnatal 2234
Donnatal Extentabs 2234
Donnatal Tablets 2234
Phenobarbital Elixir and Tablets 1523
Quadrinal Tablets 1398

Phensuximide (Chlorpromazine may lower convulsive threshold; dosage adjustments of anticonvulsants may be necessary).
No products indexed under this heading.

Phenytoin (Chlorpromazine may interfere with the metabolism of phenytoin and thus precipitate phenytoin toxicity). Products include:
Dilantin Infatabs 1967
Dilantin-125 Suspension ... 1969

Phenytoin Sodium (Chlorpromazine may interfere with the metabolism of phenytoin and thus precipitate phenytoin toxicity). Products include:
Dilantin Kapseals 1965

Polythiazide (Orthostatic hypotension that may occur with chlorpromazine may be accentuated). Products include:
Minizide Capsules 2016

Prazepam (Prolonged and intensified action of CNS depressants).
No products indexed under this heading.

Primidone (Chlorpromazine may lower convulsive threshold; dosage adjustments of anticonvulsants may be necessary). Products include:
Mysoline............................. 2860

Prochlorperazine (Prolonged and intensified action of CNS depressants). Products include:
Compazine 2644

Promethazine Hydrochloride (Prolonged and intensified action of CNS depressants). Products include:
Mepergan Injection 2859
Phenergan with Codeine ... 2883
Phenergan with Dextromethorphan ... 2885
Phenergan Injection 2880
Phenergan Suppositories .. 2882
Phenergan Syrup 2881
Phenergan Tablets 2882
Phenergan VC 2886
Phenergan VC with Codeine 2888

Propofol (Prolonged and intensified action of CNS depressants). Products include:
Diprivan Injectable Emulsion 2939

Propoxyphene Hydrochloride (Prolonged and intensified action of CNS depressants). Products include:
Darvon 1475
Wygesic Tablets 2930

Propoxyphene Napsylate (Prolonged and intensified action of CNS depressants). Products include:
Darvon-N/Darvocet-N 1473

Propranolol Hydrochloride (Concomitant administration results in increased plasma levels of both drugs). Products include:
Inderal 2834
Inderal LA Long Acting Capsules .. 2836
Inderide Tablets 2838
Inderide LA Long Acting Capsules .. 2840

Risperidone (Prolonged and intensified action of CNS depressants). Products include:
Risperdal Tablets 1348

Secobarbital Sodium (Prolonged and intensified action of CNS depressants). Products include:
Seconal Sodium Pulvules ... 1529

Sevoflurane (Prolonged and intensified action of CNS depressants).
No products indexed under this heading.

Sufentanil Citrate (Prolonged and intensified action of CNS depressants). Products include:
Sufenta Injection 1355

Temazepam (Prolonged and intensified action of CNS depressants). Products include:
Restoril Capsules 2413

Thiamylal Sodium (Prolonged and intensified action of CNS depressants).
No products indexed under this heading.

Thioridazine Hydrochloride (Prolonged and intensified action of CNS depressants). Products include:
Mellaril 2398

Thiothixene (Prolonged and intensified action of CNS depressants). Products include:
Navane Capsules and Concentrate 2018
Navane Intramuscular 2019

Triazolam (Prolonged and intensified action of CNS depressants). Products include:
Halcion Tablets 2093

Trifluoperazine Hydrochloride (Prolonged and intensified action of CNS depressants). Products include:
Stelazine 2692

Trimethadione (Chlorpromazine may lower convulsive threshold; dosage adjustments of anticonvulsants may be necessary).
No products indexed under this heading.

Valproic Acid (Chlorpromazine may lower convulsive threshold; dosage adjustments of anticonvulsants may be necessary). Products include:
Depakene 416

Warfarin Sodium (Chlorpromazine diminishes the effects of oral anticoagulants). Products include:
Coumadin 941

Zolpidem Tartrate (Prolonged and intensified action of CNS depressants). Products include:
Ambien Tablets 2559

THORAZINE MULTI-DOSE VIALS
(Chlorpromazine Hydrochloride) 2701
See **Thorazine Concentrate**

THORAZINE SPANSULE CAPSULES
(Chlorpromazine Hydrochloride) 2701
See **Thorazine Concentrate**

THORAZINE SUPPOSITORIES
(Chlorpromazine) 2701
See **Thorazine Concentrate**

THORAZINE SYRUP
(Chlorpromazine Hydrochloride) 2701
See **Thorazine Concentrate**

THORAZINE TABLETS
(Chlorpromazine Hydrochloride) 2701
See **Thorazine Concentrate**

THROMBATE III ANTITHROMBIN III (HUMAN)
(Antithrombin III) 631
May interact with:

Heparin Calcium (The anticoagulant effect of heparin is enhanced by concurrent treatment with antithrombin III; reduced dosage of heparin may be required).
No products indexed under this heading.

Heparin Sodium (The anticoagulant effect of heparin is enhanced by concurrent treatment with antithrombin III; reduced dosage of heparin may be required). Products include:
Heparin Lock Flush Solution 2831
Heparin Sodium Injection .. 2832
Heparin Sodium Vials 1486

THYREL TRH
(Protirelin) 2992
May interact with thyroid preparations, glucocorticoids, and certain other agents. Compounds in these categories include:

Aspirin (Inhibits the TSH response to protirelin when aspirin is given at 2 to 3 g/day). Products include:
Alka-Seltzer Cherry Effervescent Antacid and Pain Reliever 609
Alka-Seltzer Extra Strength Effervescent Antacid and Pain Reliever 609
Alka-Seltzer Lemon Lime Effervescent Antacid and Pain Reliever 609
Alka-Seltzer Original Effervescent Antacid and Pain Reliever 609
Alka-Seltzer Plus 611
Alka-Seltzer Plus Sinus Medicine .. 611
Ascriptin 650
Arthritis Strength BC Powder 631
BC Cold Powder Multi-Symptom Formula (Cold-Sinus-Allergy) 631
BC Cold Powder Non-Drowsy Formula (Cold-Sinus) 631
BC Powder 631
Genuine Bayer Aspirin Tablets & Caplets 618

IMPORTANT NOTE: Always consult each drug listing in the patient's regimen for possible interactions.

THYREL TRH — Interactions Index

Extra Strength Bayer Arthritis Pain Regimen Formula .... ▣ 615
Extra Strength Bayer Aspirin Caplets & Tablets .... ▣ 617
Extended-Release Bayer 8-Hour Aspirin .... ▣ 616
Extra Strength Bayer Plus Aspirin Caplets .... ▣ 617
Extra Strength Bayer PM Aspirin Plus Sleep Aid .... ▣ 617
Aspirin Regimen Bayer 81 mg Tablets with Calcium .... ▣ 615
Aspirin Regimen Bayer Adult Low Strength 81 mg Tablets .... ▣ 613
Aspirin Regimen Bayer Children's Chewable Aspirin .... ▣ 616
Aspirin Regimen Bayer Regular Strength 325 mg Caplets .... ▣ 613
Bufferin Analgesic Tablets .... ▣ 636
Arthritis Strength Bufferin Analgesic Caplets .... ▣ 637
Extra Strength Bufferin Analgesic Tablets .... ▣ 637
Cama Arthritis Pain Reliever 748
Darvon Compound-65 Pulvules 1475
Easprin 1971
Ecotrin 2625
Ecotrin Enteric Coated Aspirin Maximum Strength Tablets and Caplets .... ▣ 775
Ecotrin Enteric Coated Aspirin Regular Strength Tablets 2625
Empirin Aspirin Tablets .... ▣ 818
Excedrin Extra-Strength Analgesic Tablets, Caplets, and Geltabs 734
Fiorinal Capsules 2388
Fiorinal with Codeine Capsules 2390
Fiorinal Tablets 2388
Goody's Extra Strength Headache Powders .... ▣ 632
Goody's Extra Strength Pain Relief Tablets .... ▣ 632
Halfprin Tablets 1413
Norgesic 1554
Percodan Tablets 955
Percodan-Demi Tablets 956
Robaxisal Tablets 2246
Soma Compound w/Codeine Tablets 2784
Soma Compound Tablets 2783
St. Joseph Adult Chewable Aspirin (81 mg.) .... ▣ 768
Talwin Compound 2466
Vanquish Analgesic Caplets .... ▣ 627

Betamethasone Acetate (Pharmacologic doses of steroids reduce the TSH response). Products include:
Celestone Soluspan Suspension 2484

Betamethasone Sodium Phosphate (Pharmacologic doses of steroids reduce the TSH response). Products include:
Celestone Soluspan Suspension 2484

Cortisone Acetate (Pharmacologic doses of steroids reduce the TSH response). Products include:
Cortone Acetate Sterile Suspension 1663
Cortone Acetate Tablets 1664

Dexamethasone (Pharmacologic doses of steroids reduce the TSH response). Products include:
AK-Trol Ointment & Suspension .... ⊙ 205
Decadron Elixir 1676
Decadron Tablets 1678
Decaspray Topical Aerosol 1689
Maxitrol Ophthalmic Ointment and Suspension .... ⊙ 222
TobraDex Ophthalmic Suspension and Ointment 469

Dexamethasone Acetate (Pharmacologic doses of steroids reduce the TSH response). Products include:
Dalalone D.P. Injectable 1009
Decadron-LA Sterile Suspension 1687

Dexamethasone Sodium Phosphate (Pharmacologic doses of steroids reduce the TSH response). Products include:
Decadron Phosphate Injection 1680
Decadron Phosphate Sterile Ophthalmic Ointment 1684
Decadron Phosphate Sterile Ophthalmic Solution 1685
Decadron Phosphate Topical Cream 1686
Decadron Phosphate with Xylocaine Injection, Sterile 1683
Dexacort Phosphate in Respihaler 1606
Dexacort Phosphate in Turbinaire 1607
NeoDecadron Sterile Ophthalmic Ointment 1755
NeoDecadron Sterile Ophthalmic Solution 1756
NeoDecadron Topical Cream 1757

Fludrocortisone Acetate (Pharmacologic doses of steroids reduce the TSH response). Products include:
Florinef Acetate Tablets 506

Hydrocortisone (Pharmacologic doses of steroids reduce the TSH response). Products include:
Anusol-HC Cream 2.5% 1953
Aquanil HC Lotion 1989
Maximum Strength Cortaid Spray .... ▣ 800
CORTENEMA 2713
Cortisporin Ointment 1074
Cortisporin Ophthalmic Ointment Sterile 1074
Cortisporin Ophthalmic Suspension Sterile 1075
Cortisporin Otic Solution Sterile 1076
Cortisporin Otic Suspension Sterile 1077
Cortizone-5 .... ▣ 795
Cortizone-10 .... ▣ 795
Hydrocortone Tablets 1715
Hytone 922
Hytone Ointment 2 ½ % 923
Massengill Medicated Soft Cloth Towelettes 2628
Pediotic Suspension Sterile 1140
Preparation H Hydrocortisone 1% Cream .... ▣ 843
ProctoCream-HC 2.5% 2552
VōSoL HC Otic Solution 2786

Hydrocortisone Acetate (Pharmacologic doses of steroids reduce the TSH response). Products include:
Analpram-HC Rectal Cream 1% and 2.5% 993
Anusol HC-1 Hydrocortisone Anti-Itch Ointment .... ▣ 810
Anusol-HC Suppositories 1954
Caldecort Anti-Itch Hydrocortisone Cream .... ▣ 651
Coly-Mycin S Otic w/Neomycin & Hydrocortisone 1965
Cortaid .... ▣ 800
Cortifoam 2540
Cortisporin Cream 1073
Epifoam 2543
Hydrocortone Acetate Sterile Suspension 1712
Mantadil Cream 1124
Nupercainal Hydrocortisone 1% Cream .... ▣ 661
Pramosone Cream, Lotion & Ointment 995
ProctoFoam-HC 2552
Terra-Cortril Ophthalmic Suspension 2033

Hydrocortisone Sodium Phosphate (Pharmacologic doses of steroids reduce the TSH response). Products include:
Hydrocortone Phosphate Injection, Sterile 1713

Hydrocortisone Sodium Succinate (Pharmacologic doses of steroids reduce the TSH response).
No products indexed under this heading.

Levodopa (Chronic administration of levodopa inhibits the TSH response). Products include:
Atamet Tablets 567
Larodopa Tablets 2296
Sinemet Tablets 959
Sinemet CR Tablets 961

Levothyroxine Sodium (Thyroid hormones reduce the TSH response). Products include:
Eltroxin Tablets 2214
Levothroid Tablets 1015
Levothyroxine Sodium, USP for Injection 546
Levoxyl Tablets 918
Synthroid 1410

Liothyronine Sodium (Thyroid hormones reduce the TSH response). Products include:
Cytomel Tablets 2647
Triostat Injection 2708

Liotrix (Thyroid hormones reduce the TSH response).
No products indexed under this heading.

Methylprednisolone Acetate (Pharmacologic doses of steroids reduce the TSH response).
No products indexed under this heading.

Methylprednisolone Sodium Succinate (Pharmacologic doses of steroids reduce the TSH response).
No products indexed under this heading.

Prednisolone Acetate (Pharmacologic doses of steroids reduce the TSH response). Products include:
AK-CIDE .... ⊙ 203
AK-CIDE Ointment .... ⊙ 203
Blephamide Liquifilm Sterile Ophthalmic Suspension 472
Blephamide Ointment .... ⊙ 234
Econopred & Econopred Plus Ophthalmic Suspensions .... ⊙ 216
Poly-Pred Liquifilm .... ⊙ 246
Pred Forte .... ⊙ 247
Pred Mild .... ⊙ 250
Pred-G Liquifilm Sterile Ophthalmic Suspension .... ⊙ 248
Pred-G S.O.P. Sterile Ophthalmic Ointment .... ⊙ 249

Prednisolone Sodium Phosphate (Pharmacologic doses of steroids reduce the TSH response). Products include:
AK-PRED .... ⊙ 204
Hydeltrasol Injection, Sterile 1708
Pediapred Oral Solution 1618

Prednisolone Tebutate (Pharmacologic doses of steroids reduce the TSH response). Products include:
Hydeltra-T.B.A. Sterile Suspension 1710

Prednisone (Pharmacologic doses of steroids reduce the TSH response).
No products indexed under this heading.

Thyroglobulin (Thyroid hormones reduce the TSH response).
No products indexed under this heading.

Thyroid (Thyroid hormones reduce the TSH response).
No products indexed under this heading.

Thyroxine (Thyroid hormones reduce the TSH response).
No products indexed under this heading.

Thyroxine Sodium (Thyroid hormones reduce the TSH response).
No products indexed under this heading.

Triamcinolone (Pharmacologic doses of steroids reduce the TSH response).
No products indexed under this heading.

Triamcinolone Acetonide (Pharmacologic doses of steroids reduce the TSH response). Products include:
Azmacort Oral Inhaler 2175
Nasacort AQ Nasal Spray 2191
Nasacort Nasal Inhaler 2189

Triamcinolone Diacetate (Pharmacologic doses of steroids reduce the TSH response).
No products indexed under this heading.

Triamcinolone Hexacetonide (Pharmacologic doses of steroids reduce the TSH response).
No products indexed under this heading.

THYRO-BLOCK TABLETS
(Potassium Iodide) 2785
None cited in PDR database.

TIAZAC CAPSULES
(Diltiazem Hydrochloride) 1019
May interact with beta blockers, cardiac glycosides, anesthetics, and certain other agents. Compounds in these categories include:

Acebutolol Hydrochloride (Concomitant use may result in additive effects on cardiac conduction). Products include:
Sectral Capsules 2914

Alfentanil Hydrochloride (Depression of cardiac contractility, conductivity, automaticity, and vasodilation associated with anesthetic may be potentiated). Products include:
Alfenta Injection 1334

Atenolol (Concomitant use may result in additive effects on cardiac conduction). Products include:
Tenoretic Tablets 2963
Tenormin Tablets and I.V. Injection 2965

Betaxolol Hydrochloride (Concomitant use may result in additive effects on cardiac conduction). Products include:
Betoptic Ophthalmic Solution 465
Betoptic S Ophthalmic Suspension 467
Kerlone Tablets 2588

Bisoprolol Fumarate (Concomitant use may result in additive effects on cardiac conduction). Products include:
Zebeta Tablets 1457
Ziac 1459

Carbamazepine (Concomitant use may result in elevated serum levels of carbamazepine (40% to 72% increase), resulting in toxicity). Products include:
Atretol Tablets 569
Tegretol/Tegretol-XR 870

Carteolol Hydrochloride (Concomitant use may result in additive effects on cardiac conduction). Products include:
Cartrol Tablets 413
Ocupress Ophthalmic Solution, 1% Sterile .... ⊙ 297

Cimetidine (Potential for significant increase in peak plasma levels (58%) and AUC (53%); an adjustment of diltiazem dosage may be warranted). Products include:
Tagamet HB Tablets .... ▣ 786
Tagamet Tablets 2694

Cimetidine Hydrochloride (Potential for significant increase in peak plasma levels (58%) and AUC (53%); an adjustment of diltiazem dosage may be warranted). Products include:
Tagamet 2694

Cyclosporine (A pharmacokinetic interaction between diltiazem and cyclosporine has been observed in renal and cardiac transplant patients requiring a reduction of cyclosporine dose). Products include:
Neoral 2405
Sandimmune 2416

Deslanoside (Concomitant use may result in additive effects on cardiac conduction; possible increase in digitalis plasma levels).
No products indexed under this heading.

Digitoxin (Concomitant use may result in additive effects on cardiac conduction; possible increase in digitalis plasma levels). Products include:
Crystodigin Tablets 1472

(▣ Described in PDR For Nonprescription Drugs)   (⊙ Described in PDR For Ophthalmology)

Digoxin (Concomitant use may result in additive effects on cardiac conduction; possible increase in digitalis plasma levels). Products include:
- Lanoxicaps 1110
- Lanoxin Elixir Pediatric 1113
- Lanoxin Injection 1116
- Lanoxin Injection Pediatric 1119
- Lanoxin Tablets 1121

Drugs which undergo biotransformation by cytochrome P-450 mixed function oxidase (Co-administration with other agents which follow the same route of biotransformation as diltiazem may result in the competitive inhibition of metabolism).

Enflurane (Depression of cardiac contractility, conductivity, automaticity, and vasodilation associated with anesthetic may be potentiated).
- No products indexed under this heading.

Esmolol Hydrochloride (Concomitant use may result in additive effects on cardiac conduction). Products include:
- Brevibloc (esmolol HCl) Injection 1860

Fentanyl Citrate (Depression of cardiac contractility, conductivity, automaticity, and vasodilation associated with anesthetic may be potentiated). Products include:
- Sublimaze Injection 463

Halothane (Depression of cardiac contractility, conductivity, automaticity, and vasodilation associated with anesthetic may be potentiated). Products include:
- Fluothane 2830

Isoflurane (Depression of cardiac contractility, conductivity, automaticity, and vasodilation associated with anesthetic may be potentiated).
- No products indexed under this heading.

Ketamine Hydrochloride (Depression of cardiac contractility, conductivity, automaticity, and vasodilation associated with anesthetic may be potentiated).
- No products indexed under this heading.

Labetalol Hydrochloride (Concomitant use may result in additive effects on cardiac conduction). Products include:
- Normodyne Injection 2519
- Normodyne Tablets 2522
- Trandate 1158

Levobunolol Hydrochloride (Concomitant use may result in additive effects on cardiac conduction). Products include:
- Betagan .... ⊙ 230

Methohexital Sodium (Depression of cardiac contractility, conductivity, automaticity, and vasodilation associated with anesthetic may be potentiated).
- No products indexed under this heading.

Metipranolol Hydrochloride (Concomitant use may result in additive effects on cardiac conduction). Products include:
- OptiPranolol (Metipranolol 0.3%) Sterile Ophthalmic Solution .... ⊙ 256

Metoprolol Succinate (Concomitant use may result in additive effects on cardiac conduction). Products include:
- Toprol-XL Tablets 560

Metoprolol Tartrate (Concomitant use may result in additive effects on cardiac conduction). Products include:
- Lopressor 848
- Lopressor HCT Tablets 850

Midazolam Hydrochloride (Depression of cardiac contractility, conductivity, automaticity, and vasodilation associated with anesthetic may be potentiated). Products include:
- Versed Injection 2324

Nadolol (Concomitant use may result in additive effects on cardiac conduction).
- No products indexed under this heading.

Penbutolol Sulfate (Concomitant use may result in additive effects on cardiac conduction). Products include:
- Levatol Tablets 2547

Pindolol (Concomitant use may result in additive effects on cardiac conduction). Products include:
- Visken Tablets 2428

Propofol (Depression of cardiac contractility, conductivity, automaticity, and vasodilation associated with anesthetic may be potentiated). Products include:
- Diprivan Injectable Emulsion 2939

Propranolol Hydrochloride (May result in increased levels and bioavailability of propranolol; concomitant use may result in additive effects on cardiac conduction). Products include:
- Inderal 2834
- Inderal LA Long Acting Capsules 2836
- Inderide Tablets 2838
- Inderide LA Long Acting Capsules 2840

Ranitidine Hydrochloride (Produces smaller, nonsignificant increase in diltiazem plasma levels). Products include:
- Zantac 1182
- Zantac Injection 1180
- Zantac Syrup 1182

Sotalol Hydrochloride (Concomitant use may result in additive effects on cardiac conduction). Products include:
- Betapace Tablets 637

Sufentanil Citrate (Depression of cardiac contractility, conductivity, automaticity, and vasodilation associated with anesthetic may be potentiated). Products include:
- Sufenta Injection 1355

Thiamylal Sodium (Depression of cardiac contractility, conductivity, automaticity, and vasodilation associated with anesthetic may be potentiated).
- No products indexed under this heading.

Timolol Hemihydrate (Concomitant use may result in additive effects on cardiac conduction). Products include:
- Betimol 0.25%, 0.5% .... ⊙ 259

Timolol Maleate (Concomitant use may result in additive effects on cardiac conduction). Products include:
- Blocadren Tablets 1654
- Timolide Tablets 1791
- Timoptic in Ocudose 1796
- Timoptic Sterile Ophthalmic Solution 1794
- Timoptic-XE 1798

Food Interactions

Food, unspecified (When Tiazac was co-administered with high fat content breakfast the t_{max} occurred slightly earlier, however, the extent of diltiazem absorption was not affected).

TICAR FOR INJECTION
(Ticarcillin Disodium) 2704

May interact with:

Probenecid (Concurrent administration prolongs serum levels of ticarcillin). Products include:
- Benemid Tablets 1651
- ColBENEMID Tablets 1662

TICE BCG, USP
(BCG Vaccine) 1881

May interact with immunosuppressive agents and certain other agents. Compounds in these categories include:

Antimicrobial therapy, unspecified (May interfere with the effectiveness of TICE BCG therapy).

Azathioprine (May interfere with development of immune response). Products include:
- Azathioprine Tablets 2349
- Imuran 1103

Cyclosporine (May interfere with development of immune response). Products include:
- Neoral 2405
- Sandimmune 2416

Immune Globulin (Human) (May interfere with development of immune response).
- No products indexed under this heading.

Muromonab-CD3 (May interfere with development of immune response). Products include:
- Orthoclone OKT3 Sterile Solution 1892

Mycophenolate Mofetil (May interfere with development of immune response). Products include:
- CellCept Capsules 2265

Tacrolimus (May interfere with development of immune response). Products include:
- Prograf 1028

TICLID TABLETS
(Ticlopidine Hydrochloride) 2317

May interact with xanthine bronchodilators, antacids, non-steroidal anti-inflammatory agents, anticoagulants, and certain other agents. Compounds in these categories include:

Aluminum Carbonate (18% decrease in plasma levels of ticlopidine when administered after antacids). Products include:
- Basaljel Capsules 2810
- Basaljel Suspension 2810
- Basaljel Tablets 2810

Aluminum Hydroxide (18% decrease in plasma levels of ticlopidine when administered after antacids). Products include:
- ALternaGEL Liquid 1358
- Maximum Strength Ascriptin .... ▣ 650
- Cama Arthritis Pain Reliever .... ▣ 748
- Gaviscon Extra Strength Relief Formula Antacid Tablets .... ▣ 778
- Gaviscon Extra Strength Relief Formula Liquid Antacid .... ▣ 779
- Gaviscon Liquid Antacid .... ▣ 779
- Gelusil Antacid-Anti-gas Liquid .... ▣ 819
- Gelusil Antacid-Anti-gas Tablets .... ▣ 819
- Maalox Antacid/Anti-Gas Tablets 889
- Maalox Heartburn Relief Suspension .... ▣ 658
- Maalox Antacid Liquid 888
- Extra Strength Maalox Antacid/Anti-Gas Liquid and Tablets 888
- Mylanta 1359
- Tempo Soft Antacid .... ▣ 799

Aluminum Hydroxide Gel (18% decrease in plasma levels of ticlopidine when administered after antacids). Products include:
- ALternaGEL Liquid .... ▣ 675
- Aludrox Oral Suspension .... ▣ 850
- Amphojel Suspension 2802
- Amphojel Suspension without Flavor 2802
- Amphojel Tablets 2802
- Ascriptin .... ▣ 650
- Gaviscon Antacid Tablets .... ▣ 778
- Gaviscon-2 Antacid Tablets .... ▣ 779
- Mylanta Liquid .... ▣ 676
- Mylanta Double Strength Liquid .... ▣ 676
- Nephrox Suspension .... ▣ 671

Aminophylline (Co-administration may result in significant increase in the theophylline elimination half-life and a comparable reduction in total plasma clearance of theophylline).
- No products indexed under this heading.

Aspirin (Ticlopidine potentiates the effect of aspirin on collagen-induced platelet aggregation; concurrent use is not recommended). Products include:
- Alka-Seltzer Cherry Effervescent Antacid and Pain Reliever .... ▣ 609
- Alka-Seltzer Extra Strength Effervescent Antacid and Pain Reliever .... ▣ 609
- Alka-Seltzer Lemon Lime Effervescent Antacid and Pain Reliever .... ▣ 609
- Alka-Seltzer Original Effervescent Antacid and Pain Reliever .... ▣ 609
- Alka-Seltzer Plus .... ▣ 611
- Alka-Seltzer Plus Sinus Medicine .... ▣ 611
- Ascriptin .... ▣ 650
- Arthritis Strength BC Powder .... ▣ 631
- BC Cold Powder Multi-Symptom Formula (Cold-Sinus-Allergy) .... ▣ 631
- BC Cold Powder Non-Drowsy Formula (Cold-Sinus) .... ▣ 631
- BC Powder .... ▣ 631
- Genuine Bayer Aspirin Tablets & Caplets .... ▣ 618
- Extra Strength Bayer Arthritis Pain Regimen Formula .... ▣ 615
- Extra Strength Bayer Aspirin Caplets & Tablets .... ▣ 617
- Extended-Release Bayer 8-Hour Aspirin .... ▣ 616
- Extra Strength Bayer Plus Aspirin Caplets .... ▣ 617
- Extra Strength Bayer PM Aspirin Plus Sleep Aid .... ▣ 617
- Aspirin Regimen Bayer 81 mg Tablets with Calcium .... ▣ 615
- Aspirin Regimen Bayer Adult Low Strength 81 mg Tablets .... ▣ 613
- Aspirin Regimen Bayer Children's Chewable Aspirin .... ▣ 616
- Aspirin Regimen Bayer Regular Strength 325 mg Caplets .... ▣ 613
- Bufferin Analgesic Tablets .... ▣ 636
- Arthritis Strength Bufferin Analgesic Caplets .... ▣ 637
- Extra Strength Bufferin Analgesic Tablets .... ▣ 637
- Cama Arthritis Pain Reliever .... ▣ 748
- Darvon Compound-65 Pulvules 1475
- Easprin 1971
- Ecotrin 2625
- Ecotrin Enteric Coated Aspirin Maximum Strength Tablets and Caplets .... ▣ 775
- Ecotrin Enteric Coated Aspirin Regular Strength Tablets 2625
- Empirin Aspirin Tablets .... ▣ 818
- Excedrin Extra-Strength Analgesic Tablets, Caplets, and Geltabs 734
- Fiorinal Capsules 2388
- Fiorinal with Codeine Capsules 2390
- Fiorinal Tablets 2388
- Goody's Extra Strength Headache Powders .... ▣ 632
- Goody's Extra Strength Pain Relief Tablets .... ▣ 632
- Halfprin Tablets 1413
- Norgesic 1554
- Percodan Tablets 955
- Percodan-Demi Tablets 956
- Robaxisal Tablets 2246
- Soma Compound w/Codeine Tablets 2784
- Soma Compound Tablets 2783
- St. Joseph Adult Chewable Aspirin (81 mg.) .... ▣ 768
- Talwin Compound 2466
- Vanquish Analgesic Caplets .... ▣ 627

IMPORTANT NOTE: Always consult each drug listing in the patient's regimen for possible interactions.

Cimetidine (Chronic administration of cimetidine reduces the clearance of a single dose of ticlopidine by 50%). Products include:
- Tagamet HB Tablets ▣ 786
- Tagamet Tablets 2694

Cimetidine Hydrochloride (Chronic administration of cimetidine reduces the clearance of a single dose of ticlopidine by 50%). Products include:
- Tagamet 2694

Dalteparin Sodium (The tolerance and safety of co-administration has not been established; anticoagulant should be discontinued prior to Ticlid administration). Products include:
- Fragmin Injection 2088

Diclofenac Potassium (Ticlopidine potentiates the effect of NSAIDS on platelet aggregation). Products include:
- Cataflam Tablets 833

Diclofenac Sodium (Ticlopidine potentiates the effect of NSAIDS on platelet aggregation). Products include:
- Voltaren Ophthalmic Sterile Ophthalmic Solution ◉ 264
- Cataflam/Voltaren/Voltaren-XR 833

Dicumarol (The tolerance and safety of co-administration has not been established; anticoagulant should be discontinued prior to Ticlid administration).
- No products indexed under this heading.

Digoxin (Co-administration resulted in slight decrease in digoxin plasma levels. Little or no change in efficacy of digoxin). Products include:
- Lanoxicaps 1110
- Lanoxin Elixir Pediatric 1113
- Lanoxin Injection 1116
- Lanoxin Injection Pediatric 1119
- Lanoxin Tablets 1121

Dyphylline (Co-administration may result in significant increase in the theophylline elimination half-life and a comparable reduction in total plasma clearance of theophylline). Products include:
- Lufyllin & Lufyllin-400 Tablets 2778
- Lufyllin-GG Elixir & Tablets 2779

Enoxaparin (The tolerance and safety of co-administration has not been established; anticoagulant should be discontinued prior to Ticlid administration). Products include:
- Lovenox Injection 2187

Etodolac (Ticlopidine potentiates the effect of NSAIDS on platelet aggregation). Products include:
- Lodine Capsules and Tablets 2849

Fenoprofen Calcium (Ticlopidine potentiates the effect of NSAIDS on platelet aggregation). Products include:
- Nalfon 200 Pulvules & Nalfon Tablets 933

Flurbiprofen (Ticlopidine potentiates the effect of NSAIDS on platelet aggregation).
- No products indexed under this heading.

Fosphenytoin Sodium (Co-administration has resulted in several cases of elevated phenytoin plasma levels with associated somnolence and lethargy; caution is advised). Products include:
- Cerebyx Injection 1956

Heparin Calcium (The tolerance and safety of co-administration has not been established; anticoagulant should be discontinued prior to Ticlid administration).
- No products indexed under this heading.

Heparin Sodium (The tolerance and safety of co-administration has not been established; anticoagulant should be discontinued prior to Ticlid administration). Products include:
- Heparin Lock Flush Solution 2831
- Heparin Sodium Injection 2832
- Heparin Sodium Vials 1486

Ibuprofen (Ticlopidine potentiates the effect of NSAIDS on platelet aggregation). Products include:
- Advil Cold and Sinus Caplets and Tablets ▣ 837
- Advil Ibuprofen Tablets, Caplets and Gel Caplets ▣ 836
- Children's Motrin Ibuprofen Oral Suspension 1558
- IBU Tablets 1389
- Ibuprohm ▣ 713
- Motrin IB Caplets, Tablets, and Gelcaps ▣ 802
- Motrin Ibuprofen Suspension, Oral Drops, Chewable Tablets, Caplets 1563
- Nuprin Ibuprofen/Analgesic Tablets & Caplets ▣ 645
- Vicks DayQuil SINUS Pressure & PAIN Relief with IBUPROFEN ▣ 735

Indomethacin (Ticlopidine potentiates the effect of NSAIDS on platelet aggregation). Products include:
- Indocin 1723

Indomethacin Sodium Trihydrate (Ticlopidine potentiates the effect of NSAIDS on platelet aggregation). Products include:
- Indocin I.V. 1727

Ketoprofen (Ticlopidine potentiates the effect of NSAIDS on platelet aggregation). Products include:
- Actron Caplets and Tablets ▣ 608
- Orudis Capsules 2874
- Orudis KT ▣ 842
- Oruvail Capsules 2874

Ketorolac Tromethamine (Ticlopidine potentiates the effect of NSAIDS on platelet aggregation). Products include:
- Acular Sterile Ophthalmic Solution 470
- Toradol 2319

Magaldrate (18% decrease in plasma levels of ticlopidine when administered after antacids).
- No products indexed under this heading.

Magnesium Hydroxide (18% decrease in plasma levels of ticlopidine when administered after antacids). Products include:
- Aludrox Oral Suspension ▣ 850
- Ascriptin ▣ 650
- Di-Gel Antacid/Anti-Gas ▣ 762
- Gelusil Antacid-Anti-gas Liquid ▣ 819
- Gelusil Antacid-Anti-gas Tablets ▣ 819
- Maalox Antacid/Anti-Gas Tablets 889
- Maalox Antacid Liquid 888
- Extra Strength Maalox Antacid/Anti-Gas Liquid and Tablets 888
- Mylanta Fast-Acting 1359
- Mylanta Gelcaps Antacid ▣ 678
- Fast-Acting Mylanta Liquid Antacid 1359
- Mylanta Tablets ▣ 677
- Maximum-Strength Fast-Acting Mylanta Liquid Antacid 1359
- Mylanta Double Strength Tablets ▣ 677
- Phillips' Milk of Magnesia Liquid ▣ 627
- Rolaids Antacid Tablets ▣ 807
- Tempo Soft Antacid ▣ 799

Magnesium Oxide (18% decrease in plasma levels of ticlopidine when administered after antacids). Products include:
- Beelith Tablets 632
- Bufferin Analgesic Tablets ▣ 636
- Arthritis Strength Bufferin Analgesic Caplets ▣ 637
- Extra Strength Bufferin Analgesic Tablets ▣ 637
- Caltrate PLUS ▣ 681
- Cama Arthritis Pain Reliever ▣ 748
- Mag-Ox 400 666
- Uro-Mag 666

Meclofenamate Sodium (Ticlopidine potentiates the effect of NSAIDS on platelet aggregation).
- No products indexed under this heading.

Mefenamic Acid (Ticlopidine potentiates the effect of NSAIDS on platelet aggregation). Products include:
- Ponstel 1982

Nabumetone (Ticlopidine potentiates the effect of NSAIDS on platelet aggregation). Products include:
- Relafen Tablets 2688

Naproxen (Ticlopidine potentiates the effect of NSAIDS on platelet aggregation). Products include:
- Anaprox/Naprosyn 2277

Naproxen Sodium (Ticlopidine potentiates the effect of NSAIDS on platelet aggregation). Products include:
- Aleve 2124
- Anaprox/Naprosyn 2277
- Naprelan Tablets 2861

Oxaprozin (Ticlopidine potentiates the effect of NSAIDS on platelet aggregation). Products include:
- Daypro Caplets 2578

Phenylbutazone (Ticlopidine potentiates the effect of NSAIDS on platelet aggregation).
- No products indexed under this heading.

Phenytoin (Co-administration has resulted in several cases of elevated phenytoin plasma levels with associated somnolence and lethargy; caution is advised). Products include:
- Dilantin Infatabs 1967
- Dilantin-125 Suspension 1969

Phenytoin Sodium (Co-administration has resulted in several cases of elevated phenytoin plasma levels with associated somnolence and lethargy; caution is advised). Products include:
- Dilantin Kapseals 1965

Piroxicam (Ticlopidine potentiates the effect of NSAIDS on platelet aggregation). Products include:
- Feldene Capsules 2008

Propranolol Hydrochloride (Exercise caution if co-administered; *in vitro* studies indicate no alteration of plasma protein binding of propranolol). Products include:
- Inderal 2834
- Inderal LA Long Acting Capsules 2836
- Inderide Tablets 2838
- Inderide LA Long Acting Capsules 2840

Sulindac (Ticlopidine potentiates the effect of NSAIDS on platelet aggregation). Products include:
- Clinoril Tablets 1658

Theophylline (Co-administration may result in significant increase in the theophylline elimination half-life and a comparable reduction in total plasma clearance of theophylline). Products include:
- Marax Tablets & DF Syrup 2015
- Quibron 2227

Theophylline Anhydrous (Co-administration may result in significant increase in the theophylline elimination half-life and a comparable reduction in total plasma clearance of theophylline). Products include:
- Aerolate 1003
- Primatene Tablets ▣ 844
- Respbid Tablets 687
- Slo-bid Gyrocaps 2201
- Theo-24 Extended Release Capsules 2753
- Theo-Dur Extended-Release Tablets 1367
- Theo-X Extended-Release Tablets 793
- Uni-Dur Extended-Release Tablets 1374
- Uniphyl 400 mg and 600 mg Tablets 2157

Theophylline Calcium Salicylate (Co-administration may result in significant increase in the theophylline elimination half-life and a comparable reduction in total plasma clearance of theophylline). Products include:
- Quadrinal Tablets 1398

Theophylline Sodium Glycinate (Co-administration may result in significant increase in the theophylline elimination half-life and a comparable reduction in total plasma clearance of theophylline).
- No products indexed under this heading.

Tolmetin Sodium (Ticlopidine potentiates the effect of NSAIDS on platelet aggregation). Products include:
- Tolectin (200, 400 and 600 mg) 1591

Warfarin Sodium (The tolerance and safety of co-administration has not been established; anticoagulant should be discontinued prior to Ticlid administration). Products include:
- Coumadin 941

Food Interactions

Meal, unspecified (Administration after meals results in a 20% increase in the AUC of ticlopidine).

TIGAN CAPSULES

(Trimethobenzamide Hydrochloride) 2231

May interact with phenothiazines, barbiturates, belladona products, and certain other agents. Compounds in these categories include:

Aprobarbital (Exercise caution in recent recipients of barbiturates).
- No products indexed under this heading.

Atropine Sulfate (Exercise caution in recent recipients of belladonna derivatives). Products include:
- Arco-Lase Plus Tablets 513
- Atrohist Plus Tablets 1605
- Donnatal 2234
- Donnatal Extentabs 2234
- Donnatal Tablets 2234
- Lomotil 2591
- Motofen Tablets 789
- Urised Tablets 2123

Belladonna Alkaloids (Exercise caution in recent recipients of belladonna derivatives). Products include:
- Bellergal-S Tablets 2375
- Hyland's Bedwetting Tablets ▣ 788
- Hyland's EnurAid Tablets ▣ 789
- Hyland's Headache Tablets ▣ 790
- Hyland's Teething Tablets ▣ 790
- Similasan Eye Drops #1 ▣ 769

Butabarbital (Exercise caution in recent recipients of barbiturates).
- No products indexed under this heading.

Butalbital (Exercise caution in recent recipients of barbiturates). Products include:
- Axocet Capsules 2469
- Esgic-plus Capsules 1012
- Esgic-plus Tablets 1012
- Fioricet Tablets 2386
- Fioricet with Codeine Capsules 2387
- Fiorinal Capsules 2388
- Fiorinal with Codeine Capsules 2390
- Fiorinal Tablets 2388
- Phrenilin 790
- Sedapap Tablets 50 mg/650 mg 1826

(▣ Described in PDR For Nonprescription Drugs) (◉ Described in PDR For Ophthalmology)

Interactions Index

Chlorpromazine (Exercise caution in recent recipients of phenothiazines). Products include:
Thorazine Suppositories 2701

Chlorpromazine Hydrochloride (Exercise caution in recent recipients of phenothiazines). Products include:
Thorazine 2701

Fluphenazine Decanoate (Exercise caution in recent recipients of phenothiazines). Products include:
Prolixin Decanoate 510

Fluphenazine Enanthate (Exercise caution in recent recipients of phenothiazines). Products include:
Prolixin Enanthate 510

Fluphenazine Hydrochloride (Exercise caution in recent recipients of phenothiazines). Products include:
Prolixin 510

Hyoscyamine (Exercise caution in recent recipients of belladonna derivatives). Products include:
Cystospaz Tablets 2123
Urised Tablets 2123

Hyoscyamine Sulfate (Exercise caution in recent recipients of belladonna derivatives). Products include:
Arco-Lase Plus Tablets 513
Atrohist Plus Tablets 1605
Cystospaz-M Capsules 2123
Donnatal 2234
Donnatal Extentabs 2234
Donnatal Tablets 2234
Kutrase Capsules 2546
Levsin/Levsinex/Levbid 2549

Mephobarbital (Exercise caution in recent recipients of barbiturates). Products include:
Mebaral Tablets 2452

Mesoridazine Besylate (Exercise caution in recent recipients of phenothiazines). Products include:
Serentil 689

Methotrimeprazine (Exercise caution in recent recipients of phenothiazines). Products include:
Levoprome 1321

Pentobarbital Sodium (Exercise caution in recent recipients of barbiturates). Products include:
Nembutal Sodium Capsules 440
Nembutal Sodium Solution 442
Nembutal Sodium Suppositories 444

Perphenazine (Exercise caution in recent recipients of phenothiazines). Products include:
Etrafon 2495
Triavil Tablets 1800
Trilafon 2532

Phenobarbital (Exercise caution in recent recipients of barbiturates). Products include:
Arco-Lase Plus Tablets 513
Bellergal-S Tablets 2375
Donnatal 2234
Donnatal Extentabs 2234
Donnatal Tablets 2234
Phenobarbital Elixir and Tablets .. 1523
Quadrinal Tablets 1398

Prochlorperazine (Exercise caution in recent recipients of phenothiazines). Products include:
Compazine 2644

Promethazine Hydrochloride (Exercise caution in recent recipients of phenothiazines). Products include:
Mepergan Injection 2859
Phenergan with Codeine 2883
Phenergan with Dextromethorphan 2885
Phenergan Injection 2880
Phenergan Suppositories 2882
Phenergan Syrup 2881
Phenergan Tablets 2882
Phenergan VC 2886
Phenergan VC with Codeine 2888

Scopolamine (Exercise caution in recent recipients of belladonna derivatives). Products include:
Transderm Scōp Transdermal Therapeutic System 890

Scopolamine Hydrobromide (Exercise caution in recent recipients of belladonna derivatives). Products include:
Atrohist Plus Tablets 1605
Donnatal 2234
Donnatal Extentabs 2234
Donnatal Tablets 2234

Secobarbital Sodium (Exercise caution in recent recipients of barbiturates). Products include:
Seconal Sodium Pulvules 1529

Thiamylal Sodium (Exercise caution in recent recipients of barbiturates).
No products indexed under this heading.

Thioridazine Hydrochloride (Exercise caution in recent recipients of phenothiazines). Products include:
Mellaril 2398

Trifluoperazine Hydrochloride (Exercise caution in recent recipients of phenothiazines). Products include:
Stelazine 2692

Food Interactions

Alcohol (May result in an adverse drug interaction).

TIGAN INJECTABLE
(Trimethobenzamide Hydrochloride) 2231
See **Tigan Capsules**

TIGAN SUPPOSITORIES
(Trimethobenzamide Hydrochloride) 2231
See **Tigan Capsules**

TILADE INHALER
(Nedocromil Sodium) 2207
None cited in PDR database.

TIMENTIN FOR INJECTION
(Ticarcillin Disodium, Clavulanate Potassium) 2706
May interact with:

Probenecid (Increases serum concentration and prolongs half-life of ticarcillin). Products include:
Benemid Tablets 1651
ColBENEMID Tablets 1662

TIMOLIDE TABLETS
(Timolol Maleate, Hydrochlorothiazide) 1791
May interact with insulin, corticosteroids, antihypertensives, catecholamine depleting drugs, non-steroidal anti-inflammatory agents, lithium preparations, cardiac glycosides, and certain other agents. Compounds in these categories include:

Acebutolol Hydrochloride (Potentiated). Products include:
Sectral Capsules 2914

ACTH (Hypokalemia).
No products indexed under this heading.

Amlodipine Besylate (Potentiated). Products include:
Lotrel Capsules 858
Norvasc Tablets 2020

Atenolol (Potentiated). Products include:
Tenoretic Tablets 2963
Tenormin Tablets and I.V. Injection 2965

Benazepril Hydrochloride (Potentiated). Products include:
Lotensin Tablets 852
Lotensin HCT Tablets 855
Lotrel Capsules 858

Bendroflumethiazide (Potentiated).
No products indexed under this heading.

Betamethasone Acetate (Hypokalemia). Products include:
Celestone Soluspan Suspension 2484

Betamethasone Sodium Phosphate (Hypokalemia). Products include:
Celestone Soluspan Suspension 2484

Betaxolol Hydrochloride (Potentiated). Products include:
Betoptic Ophthalmic Solution 465
Betoptic S Ophthalmic Suspension 467
Kerlone Tablets 2588

Bisoprolol Fumarate (Potentiated). Products include:
Zebeta Tablets 1457
Ziac 1459

Captopril (Potentiated). Products include:
Capoten Tablets 740
Capozide Tablets 744

Carteolol Hydrochloride (Potentiated). Products include:
Cartrol Tablets 413
Ocupress Ophthalmic Solution, 1% Sterile .... Ⓡ 297

Chlorothiazide (Potentiated). Products include:
Aldoclor Tablets 1638
Diupres Tablets 1691
Diuril Oral 1694

Chlorothiazide Sodium (Potentiated). Products include:
Diuril Sodium Intravenous 1693

Chlorthalidone (Potentiated). Products include:
Combipres Tablets 682
Tenoretic Tablets 2963
Thalitone 1293

Cholestyramine (Cholestyramine resin has potential of binding hydrochlorothiazide and reducing its absorption from the GI tract by up to 85%). Products include:
Questran 774

Clonidine (Potentiated). Products include:
Catapres-TTS 680

Clonidine Hydrochloride (Potentiated). Products include:
Catapres Tablets 679
Combipres Tablets 682

Colestipol Hydrochloride (Colestipol resin has potential of binding hydrochlorothiazide and reducing its absorption from the GI tract by up to 43%). Products include:
Colestid 2073

Cortisone Acetate (Hypokalemia). Products include:
Cortone Acetate Sterile Suspension 1663
Cortone Acetate Tablets 1664

Deslanoside (Hypokalemia can lead to increased cardiac toxicity of digitalis).
No products indexed under this heading.

Dexamethasone (Hypokalemia). Products include:
AK-Trol Ointment & Suspension .... Ⓡ 205
Decadron Elixir 1676
Decadron Tablets 1678
Decaspray Topical Aerosol 1689
Maxitrol Ophthalmic Ointment and Suspension .... Ⓡ 222
TobraDex Ophthalmic Suspension and Ointment 469

Dexamethasone Acetate (Hypokalemia). Products include:
Dalalone D.P. Injectable 1009
Decadron-LA Sterile Suspension 1687

Dexamethasone Sodium Phosphate (Hypokalemia). Products include:
Decadron Phosphate Injection 1680
Decadron Phosphate Sterile Ophthalmic Ointment 1684
Decadron Phosphate Sterile Ophthalmic Solution 1685
Decadron Phosphate Topical Cream 1686
Decadron Phosphate with Xylocaine Injection, Sterile 1683
Dexacort Phosphate in Respihaler .. 1606
Dexacort Phosphate in Turbinaire .. 1607
NeoDecadron Sterile Ophthalmic Ointment 1755
NeoDecadron Sterile Ophthalmic Solution 1756
NeoDecadron Topical Cream 1757

Diazoxide (Potentiated). Products include:
Hyperstat I.V. Injection 2504
Proglycem 575

Diclofenac Potassium (Reduced diuretic, natriuretic, and antihypertensive effects of Timolide). Products include:
Cataflam Tablets 833

Diclofenac Sodium (Reduced diuretic, natriuretic, and antihypertensive effects of Timolide). Products include:
Voltaren Ophthalmic Sterile Ophthalmic Solution .... Ⓡ 264
Cataflam/Voltaren/Voltaren-XR 833

Digitoxin (Hypokalemia can lead to increased cardiac toxicity of digitalis). Products include:
Crystodigin Tablets 1472

Digoxin (Hypokalemia can lead to increased cardiac toxicity of digitalis). Products include:
Lanoxicaps 1110
Lanoxin Elixir Pediatric 1113
Lanoxin Injection 1116
Lanoxin Injection Pediatric 1119
Lanoxin Tablets 1121

Diltiazem Hydrochloride (Left ventricular failure and AV conduction disturbances). Products include:
Cardizem CD Capsules 1251
Cardizem SR Capsules 1255
Cardizem Injectable 1253
Cardizem Tablets 1257
Dilacor XR Extended-release Capsules 2183
Tiazac Capsules 1019

Doxazosin Mesylate (Potentiated). Products include:
Cardura Tablets 1993

Enalapril Maleate (Potentiated). Products include:
Vaseretic Tablets 1810
Vasotec Tablets 1816

Enalaprilat (Potentiated). Products include:
Vasotec I.V. 1814

Esmolol Hydrochloride (Potentiated). Products include:
Brevibloc (esmolol HCl) Injection 1860

Etodolac (Reduced diuretic, natriuretic, and antihypertensive effects of Timolide). Products include:
Lodine Capsules and Tablets 2849

Felodipine (Potentiated). Products include:
Plendil Extended-Release Tablets 514

Fenoprofen Calcium (Reduced diuretic, natriuretic, and antihypertensive effects of Timolide). Products include:
Nalfon 200 Pulvules & Nalfon Tablets 933

Fludrocortisone Acetate (Hypokalemia). Products include:
Florinef Acetate Tablets 506

Flurbiprofen (Reduced diuretic, natriuretic, and antihypertensive effects of Timolide).
No products indexed under this heading.

IMPORTANT NOTE: Always consult each drug listing in the patient's regimen for possible interactions.

Timolide / Interactions Index

Fosinopril Sodium (Potentiated). Products include:
- Monopril Tablets ... 762

Furosemide (Potentiated). Products include:
- Lasix Injection, Oral Solution and Tablets ... 1267

Guanabenz Acetate (Potentiated).
- No products indexed under this heading.

Guanethidine Monosulfate (Potentiated). Products include:
- Esimil Tablets ... 840
- Ismelin Tablets ... 845

Hydralazine Hydrochloride (Potentiated). Products include:
- Apresazide Capsules ... 824
- Apresoline Hydrochloride Tablets ... 826
- Hydralazine Hydrochloride Injection USP ... 2712
- Ser-Ap-Es Tablets ... 867

Hydrocortisone (Hypokalemia). Products include:
- Anusol-HC Cream 2.5% ... 1953
- Aquanil HC Lotion ... 1989
- Maximum Strength Cortaid Spray ... 800
- CORTENEMA ... 2713
- Cortisporin Ointment ... 1074
- Cortisporin Ophthalmic Ointment Sterile ... 1074
- Cortisporin Ophthalmic Suspension Sterile ... 1075
- Cortisporin Otic Solution Sterile ... 1076
- Cortisporin Otic Suspension Sterile ... 1077
- Cortizone-5 ... 795
- Cortizone-10 ... 795
- Hydrocortone Tablets ... 1715
- Hytone ... 922
- Hytone Ointment 2 ½% ... 923
- Massengill Medicated Soft Cloth Towelettes ... 2628
- Pediotic Suspension Sterile ... 1140
- Preparation H Hydrocortisone 1% Cream ... 843
- ProctoCream-HC 2.5% ... 2552
- VōSoL HC Otic Solution ... 2786

Hydrocortisone Acetate (Hypokalemia). Products include:
- Analpram-HC Rectal Cream 1% and 2.5% ... 993
- Anusol HC-1 Hydrocortisone Anti-Itch Ointment ... 810
- Anusol-HC Suppositories ... 1954
- Caldecort Anti-Itch Hydrocortisone Cream ... 651
- Coly-Mycin S Otic w/Neomycin & Hydrocortisone ... 1965
- Cortaid ... 800
- Cortifoam ... 2540
- Cortisporin Cream ... 1073
- Epifoam ... 2543
- Hydrocortone Acetate Sterile Suspension ... 1712
- Mantadil Cream ... 1124
- Nupercainal Hydrocortisone 1% Cream ... 661
- Pramosone Cream, Lotion & Ointment ... 995
- ProctoFoam-HC ... 2552
- Terra-Cortril Ophthalmic Suspension ... 2033

Hydrocortisone Sodium Phosphate (Hypokalemia). Products include:
- Hydrocortone Phosphate Injection, Sterile ... 1713

Hydrocortisone Sodium Succinate (Hypokalemia).
- No products indexed under this heading.

Hydroflumethiazide (Potentiated). Products include:
- Diucardin Tablets ... 2824

Ibuprofen (Reduced diuretic, natriuretic, and antihypertensive effects of Timolide). Products include:
- Advil Cold and Sinus Caplets and Tablets ... 837
- Advil Ibuprofen Tablets, Caplets and Gel Caplets ... 836
- Children's Motrin Ibuprofen Oral Suspension ... 1558
- IBU Tablets ... 1389
- Ibuprohm ... 713
- Motrin IB Caplets, Tablets, and Gelcaps ... 802
- Motrin Ibuprofen Suspension, Oral Drops, Chewable Tablets, Caplets ... 1563
- Nuprin Ibuprofen/Analgesic Tablets & Caplets ... 645
- Vicks DayQuil SINUS Pressure & PAIN Relief with IBUPROFEN ... 735

Indapamide (Potentiated).
- No products indexed under this heading.

Indomethacin (Reduced diuretic, natriuretic, and antihypertensive effects of Timolide). Products include:
- Indocin ... 1723

Indomethacin Sodium Trihydrate (Reduced diuretic, natriuretic, and antihypertensive effects of Timolide). Products include:
- Indocin I.V. ... 1727

Insulin, Human (Insulin requirements may be altered).
- No products indexed under this heading.

Insulin, Human Isophane Suspension (Insulin requirements may be altered). Products include:
- Novolin N Human Insulin 10 ml Vials ... 1846

Insulin, Human NPH (Insulin requirements may be altered). Products include:
- Humulin N, 100 Units ... 1495
- Novolin N PenFill 1.5 ml Cartridges Durable Insulin Delivery System ... 1849
- Novolin N Prefilled Syringe Disposable Insulin Delivery System ... 1850

Insulin, Human Regular (Insulin requirements may be altered). Products include:
- Humulin R, 100 Units ... 1497
- Novolin R Human Insulin 10 ml Vials ... 1846
- Novolin R PenFill 1.5 ml Cartridges Durable Insulin Delivery System ... 1849
- Novolin R Prefilled Syringe Disposable Insulin Delivery System ... 1850
- Velosulin BR Human Insulin 10 ml Vials ... 1847

Insulin, Human, Zinc Suspension (Insulin requirements may be altered). Products include:
- Humulin L, 100 Units ... 1494
- Humulin U, 100 Units ... 1498
- Novolin L Human Insulin 10 ml Vials ... 1846

Insulin Lispro, Human (Insulin requirements may be altered). Products include:
- Humalog Injection ... 1488

Insulin, NPH (Insulin requirements may be altered). Products include:
- NPH, 100 Units ... 1502
- Pork NPH, 100 Units ... 1506
- Purified Pork NPH Isophane Insulin ... 1852

Insulin, Regular (Insulin requirements may be altered). Products include:
- Regular, 100 Units ... 1503
- Pork Regular, 100 Units ... 1507
- Pork Regular (Concentrated), 500 Units ... 1508
- Purified Pork Regular Insulin ... 1852

Insulin, Zinc Crystals (Insulin requirements may be altered). Products include:
- NPH, 100 Units ... 1502

Insulin, Zinc Suspension (Insulin requirements may be altered). Products include:
- Iletin I ... 1501
- Lente, 100 Units ... 1501
- Iletin II ... 1504
- Pork Lente, 100 Units ... 1504
- Purified Pork Lente Insulin ... 1852

Isradipine (Potentiated). Products include:
- DynaCirc Capsules ... 2381
- DynaCirc CR Tablets ... 2383

Ketoprofen (Reduced diuretic, natriuretic, and antihypertensive effects of Timolide). Products include:
- Actron Caplets and Tablets ... 608
- Orudis Capsules ... 2874
- Orudis KT ... 842
- Oruvail Capsules ... 2874

Ketorolac Tromethamine (Reduced diuretic, natriuretic, and antihypertensive effects of Timolide). Products include:
- Acular Sterile Ophthalmic Solution ... 470
- Toradol ... 2319

Labetalol Hydrochloride (Potentiated). Products include:
- Normodyne Injection ... 2519
- Normodyne Tablets ... 2522
- Trandate ... 1158

Lisinopril (Potentiated). Products include:
- Prinivil Tablets ... 1776
- Prinzide Tablets ... 1780
- Zestoretic Tablets ... 2968
- Zestril Tablets ... 2972

Lithium Carbonate (High risk of lithium toxicity). Products include:
- Eskalith ... 2658
- Lithium Carbonate Capsules & Tablets ... 2352
- Lithonate/Lithotabs/Lithobid ... 2721

Lithium Citrate (High risk of lithium toxicity).
- No products indexed under this heading.

Losartan Potassium (Potentiated). Products include:
- Cozaar Tablets ... 1668
- Hyzaar Tablets ... 1720

Mecamylamine Hydrochloride (Potentiated). Products include:
- Inversine Tablets ... 1729

Meclofenamate Sodium (Reduced diuretic, natriuretic, and antihypertensive effects of Timolide).
- No products indexed under this heading.

Mefenamic Acid (Reduced diuretic, natriuretic, and antihypertensive effects of Timolide). Products include:
- Ponstel ... 1982

Methyclothiazide (Potentiated). Products include:
- Enduron Tablets ... 424

Methyldopa (Potentiated). Products include:
- Aldoclor Tablets ... 1638
- Aldomet Oral ... 1640
- Aldoril Tablets ... 1644

Methyldopate Hydrochloride (Potentiated). Products include:
- Aldomet Ester HCl Injection ... 1642

Methylprednisolone (Hypokalemia).
- No products indexed under this heading.

Methylprednisolone Acetate (Hypokalemia).
- No products indexed under this heading.

Methylprednisolone Sodium Succinate (Hypokalemia).
- No products indexed under this heading.

Metolazone (Potentiated). Products include:
- Mykrox Tablets ... 1617
- Zaroxolyn Tablets ... 1625

Metoprolol Succinate (Potentiated). Products include:
- Toprol-XL Tablets ... 560

Metoprolol Tartrate (Potentiated). Products include:
- Lopressor ... 848

- Lopressor HCT Tablets ... 850

Metyrosine (Potentiated). Products include:
- Demser Capsules ... 1690

Minoxidil (Potentiated).
- No products indexed under this heading.

Moexipril Hydrochloride (Potentiated). Products include:
- Univasc Tablets ... 2553

Nabumetone (Reduced diuretic, natriuretic, and antihypertensive effects of Timolide). Products include:
- Relafen Tablets ... 2688

Nadolol (Potentiated).
- No products indexed under this heading.

Naproxen (Reduced diuretic, natriuretic, and antihypertensive effects of Timolide). Products include:
- Anaprox/Naprosyn ... 2277

Naproxen Sodium (Reduced diuretic, natriuretic, and antihypertensive effects of Timolide). Products include:
- Aleve ... 2124
- Anaprox/Naprosyn ... 2277
- Naprelan Tablets ... 2861

Nicardipine Hydrochloride (Potentiated). Products include:
- Cardene Capsules ... 2261
- Cardene I.V. ... 2815
- Cardene SR Capsules ... 2264

Nifedipine (Potentiated). Products include:
- Adalat Capsules (10 mg and 20 mg) ... 580
- Adalat CC ... 582
- Procardia Capsules ... 2024
- Procardia XL Extended Release Tablets ... 2026

Nisoldipine (Potentiated). Products include:
- Sular Tablets ... 2961

Nitroglycerin (Potentiated). Products include:
- Deponit NTG Transdermal Delivery System ... 2541
- Nitro-Bid IV ... 1270
- Nitro-Bid Ointment ... 1272
- Nitro-Dur (nitroglycerin) Transdermal Infusion System ... 1365
- Nitrolingual Spray ... 2193
- Nitrostat Tablets ... 1981
- Transderm-Nitro Transdermal Therapeutic System ... 878

Norepinephrine Bitartrate (Decreased arterial responsiveness to norepinephrine). Products include:
- Levophed Bitartrate Injection ... 2445

Oxaprozin (Reduced diuretic, natriuretic, and antihypertensive effects of Timolide). Products include:
- Daypro Caplets ... 2578

Penbutolol Sulfate (Potentiated). Products include:
- Levatol Tablets ... 2547

Phenoxybenzamine Hydrochloride (Potentiated). Products include:
- Dibenzyline Capsules ... 2650

Phentolamine Mesylate (Potentiated). Products include:
- Regitine Vials ... 864

Phenylbutazone (Reduced diuretic, natriuretic, and antihypertensive effects of Timolide).
- No products indexed under this heading.

Pindolol (Potentiated). Products include:
- Visken Tablets ... 2428

Piroxicam (Reduced diuretic, natriuretic, and antihypertensive effects of Timolide). Products include:
- Feldene Capsules ... 2008

Polythiazide (Potentiated). Products include:
- Minizide Capsules ... 2016

(▣ Described in PDR For Nonprescription Drugs)   (⊙ Described in PDR For Ophthalmology)

Interactions Index — Timoptic in Ocudose

Prazosin Hydrochloride (Potentiated). Products include:
- Minipress Capsules 2015
- Minizide Capsules 2016

Prednisolone Acetate (Hypokalemia). Products include:
- AK-CIDE .... ⓡ 203
- AK-CIDE Ointment .... ⓡ 203
- Blephamide Liquifilm Sterile Ophthalmic Suspension 472
- Blephamide Ointment .... ⓡ 234
- Econopred & Econopred Plus Ophthalmic Suspensions .... ⓡ 216
- Poly-Pred Liquifilm .... ⓡ 246
- Pred Forte .... ⓡ 247
- Pred Mild .... ⓡ 250
- Pred-G Liquifilm Sterile Ophthalmic Suspension .... ⓡ 248
- Pred-G S.O.P. Sterile Ophthalmic Ointment .... ⓡ 249

Prednisolone Sodium Phosphate (Hypokalemia). Products include:
- AK-PRED .... ⓡ 204
- Hydeltrasol Injection, Sterile ... 1708
- Pediapred Oral Solution 1618

Prednisolone Tebutate (Hypokalemia). Products include:
- Hydeltra-T.B.A. Sterile Suspension 1710

Prednisone (Hypokalemia).
No products indexed under this heading.

Propranolol Hydrochloride (Potentiated). Products include:
- Inderal 2834
- Inderal LA Long Acting Capsules ... 2836
- Inderide Tablets 2838
- Inderide LA Long Acting Capsules .. 2840

Quinapril Hydrochloride (Potentiated). Products include:
- Accupril Tablets 1950

Ramipril (Potentiated). Products include:
- Altace Capsules 1238

Rauwolfia Serpentina (Potentiated; hypotension; marked bradycardia).
No products indexed under this heading.

Rescinnamine (Potentiated; hypotension; marked bradycardia).
No products indexed under this heading.

Reserpine (Potentiated; hypotension; marked bradycardia). Products include:
- Diupres Tablets 1691
- Hydropres Tablets 1718
- Ser-Ap-Es Tablets 867

Sodium Nitroprusside (Potentiated).
No products indexed under this heading.

Sotalol Hydrochloride (Potentiated). Products include:
- Betapace Tablets 637

Spirapril Hydrochloride (Potentiated).
No products indexed under this heading.

Sulindac (Reduced diuretic, natriuretic, and antihypertensive effects of Timolide). Products include:
- Clinoril Tablets 1658

Terazosin Hydrochloride (Potentiation of other antihypertensives). Products include:
- Hytrin Capsules 434

Tolmetin Sodium (Reduced diuretic, natriuretic, and antihypertensive effects of Timolide). Products include:
- Tolectin (200, 400 and 600 mg) .. 1591

Torsemide (Potentiated). Products include:
- Demadex Tablets and Injection .. 691

Triamcinolone (Hypokalemia).
No products indexed under this heading.

Triamcinolone Acetonide (Hypokalemia). Products include:
- Azmacort Oral Inhaler 2175
- Nasacort AQ Nasal Spray 2191
- Nasacort Nasal Inhaler 2189

Triamcinolone Diacetate (Hypokalemia).
No products indexed under this heading.

Triamcinolone Hexacetonide (Hypokalemia).
No products indexed under this heading.

Trimethaphan Camsylate (Potentiated).
No products indexed under this heading.

Tubocurarine Chloride (Increased responsiveness to tubocurarine).
No products indexed under this heading.

Verapamil Hydrochloride (Left ventricular failure and AV conduction disturbances). Products include:
- Calan SR Caplets 2571
- Calan Tablets 2568
- Covera-HS Tablets 2573
- Isoptin Injectable 1391
- Isoptin Oral Tablets 1393
- Isoptin SR Tablets 1395
- Verelan Capsules 1455

TIMOPTIC IN OCUDOSE
(Timolol Maleate) 1796

May interact with beta blockers, calcium channel blockers, catecholamine depleting drugs, cardiac glycosides, insulin, oral hypoglycemic agents, and certain other agents. Compounds in these categories include:

Acarbose (Beta blocking agents, usually systemic, may mask the sign and symptoms of acute hypoglycemia). Products include:
- Precose 604

Acebutolol Hydrochloride (Concurrent use with systemic beta blocker may have additive effects of beta blockade, both systemic and on intraocular pressure). Products include:
- Sectral Capsules 2914

Amlodipine Besylate (Possible atrioventricular conduction disturbances, left ventricular failure, or hypotension when used concurrently). Products include:
- Lotrel Capsules 858
- Norvasc Tablets 2020

Atenolol (Concurrent use with systemic beta blocker may have additive effects of beta blockade, both systemic and on intraocular pressure). Products include:
- Tenoretic Tablets 2963
- Tenormin Tablets and I.V. Injection 2965

Bepridil Hydrochloride (Possible atrioventricular conduction disturbances, left ventricular failure, or hypotension when used concurrently). Products include:
- Vascor Tablets (200 and 300 mg) 1597

Betaxolol Hydrochloride (Concurrent use with systemic beta blocker may have additive effects of beta blockade, both systemic and on intraocular pressure; concurrent use of two ophthalmic beta blockers is not recommended). Products include:
- Betoptic Ophthalmic Solution .. 465
- Betoptic S Ophthalmic Suspension 467
- Kerlone Tablets 2588

Bisoprolol Fumarate (Concurrent use with systemic beta blocker may have additive effects of beta blockade, both systemic and on intraocular pressure). Products include:
- Zebeta Tablets 1457
- Ziac 1459

Carteolol Hydrochloride (Concurrent use with systemic beta blocker may have additive effects of beta blockade, both systemic and on intraocular pressure; concurrent use of two ophthalmic beta blockers is not recommended). Products include:
- Cartrol Tablets 413
- Ocupress Ophthalmic Solution, 1% Sterile .... ⓡ 297

Chlorpropamide (Beta blocking agents, usually systemic, may mask the sign and symptoms of acute hypoglycemia). Products include:
- Diabinese Tablets 2002

Deserpidine (Possible additive effects and the production of hypotension and/or bradycardia).
No products indexed under this heading.

Deslanoside (Co-administration with digitalis and calcium antagonists may have additive effects in prolonging atrioventricular conduction time).
No products indexed under this heading.

Digitoxin (Co-administration with digitalis and calcium antagonists may have additive effects in prolonging atrioventricular conduction time). Products include:
- Crystodigin Tablets 1472

Digoxin (Co-administration with digitalis and calcium antagonists may have additive effects in prolonging atrioventricular conduction time). Products include:
- Lanoxicaps 1110
- Lanoxin Elixir Pediatric 1113
- Lanoxin Injection 1116
- Lanoxin Injection Pediatric 1119
- Lanoxin Tablets 1121

Diltiazem Hydrochloride (Possible atrioventricular conduction disturbances, left ventricular failure, or hypotension when used concurrently). Products include:
- Cardizem CD Capsules 1251
- Cardizem SR Capsules 1255
- Cardizem Injectable 1253
- Cardizem Tablets 1257
- Dilacor XR Extended-release Capsules 2183
- Tiazac Capsules 1019

Epinephrine (Patients with a history of atopy or anaphylactic reactions to a variety of allergens may be unresponsive to the usual dose of injectable epinephrine used to treat allergic reactions). Products include:
- EPIFRIN .... ⓡ 237
- EpiPen 808
- Marcaine with Epinephrine 2446
- Primatene Mist .... ⓡ 843
- Sensorcaine with Epinephrine Injection 554
- Sus-Phrine Injection 1017
- Xylocaine with Epinephrine Injections 562

Epinephrine Bitartrate (Patients with a history of atopy or anaphylactic reactions to a variety of allergens may be unresponsive to the usual dose of injectable epinephrine used to treat allergic reactions). Products include:
- Sensorcaine-MPF with Epinephrine Injection 554

Esmolol Hydrochloride (Concurrent use with systemic beta blocker may have additive effects of beta blockade, both systemic and on intraocular pressure). Products include:
- Brevibloc (esmolol HCl) Injection .. 1860

Felodipine (Possible atrioventricular conduction disturbances, left ventricular failure, or hypotension when used concurrently). Products include:
- Plendil Extended-Release Tablets .. 514

Glimepiride (Beta blocking agents, usually systemic, may mask the sign and symptoms of acute hypoglycemia). Products include:
- Amaryl Tablets 1241

Glipizide (Beta blocking agents, usually systemic, may mask the sign and symptoms of acute hypoglycemia). Products include:
- Glucotrol Tablets 2011
- Glucotrol XL Extended Release Tablets 2012

Glyburide (Beta blocking agents, usually systemic, may mask the sign and symptoms of acute hypoglycemia). Products include:
- DiaBeta Tablets 1265
- Glynase PresTab Tablets 2091
- Micronase Tablets 2099

Guanethidine Monosulfate (Possible additive effects and the production of hypotension and/or bradycardia). Products include:
- Esimil Tablets 840
- Ismelin Tablets 845

Insulin, Human (Beta blocking agents, usually systemic, may mask the sign and symptoms of acute hypoglycemia).
No products indexed under this heading.

Insulin, Human Isophane Suspension (Beta blocking agents, usually systemic, may mask the sign and symptoms of acute hypoglycemia). Products include:
- Novolin N Human Insulin 10 ml Vials 1846

Insulin, Human NPH (Beta blocking agents, usually systemic, may mask the sign and symptoms of acute hypoglycemia). Products include:
- Humulin N, 100 Units 1495
- Novolin N PenFill 1.5 ml Cartridges Durable Insulin Delivery System 1849
- Novolin N Prefilled Syringe Disposable Insulin Delivery System .. 1850

Insulin, Human Regular (Beta blocking agents, usually systemic, may mask the sign and symptoms of acute hypoglycemia). Products include:
- Humulin R, 100 Units 1497
- Novolin R Human Insulin 10 ml Vials 1846
- Novolin R PenFill 1.5 ml Cartridges Durable Insulin Delivery System 1849
- Novolin R Prefilled Syringe Disposable Insulin Delivery System .. 1850
- Velosulin BR Human Insulin 10 ml Vials 1847

Insulin, Human, Zinc Suspension (Beta blocking agents, usually systemic, may mask the sign and symptoms of acute hypoglycemia). Products include:
- Humulin L, 100 Units 1494
- Humulin U, 100 Units 1498
- Novolin L Human Insulin 10 ml Vials 1846

IMPORTANT NOTE: Always consult each drug listing in the patient's regimen for possible interactions.

Timoptic in Ocudose — Interactions Index — 1072

Insulin Lispro, Human (Beta blocking agents, usually systemic, may mask the sign and symptoms of acute hypoglycemia). Products include:
- Humalog Injection 1488

Insulin, NPH (Beta blocking agents, usually systemic, may mask the sign and symptoms of acute hypoglycemia). Products include:
- NPH, 100 Units 1502
- Pork NPH, 100 Units 1506
- Purified Pork NPH Isophane Insulin 1852

Insulin, Regular (Beta blocking agents, usually systemic, may mask the sign and symptoms of acute hypoglycemia). Products include:
- Regular, 100 Units 1503
- Pork Regular, 100 Units 1507
- Pork Regular (Concentrated), 500 Units 1508
- Purified Pork Regular Insulin 1852

Insulin, Zinc Crystals (Beta blocking agents, usually systemic, may mask the sign and symptoms of acute hypoglycemia). Products include:
- NPH, 100 Units 1502

Insulin, Zinc Suspension (Beta blocking agents, usually systemic, may mask the sign and symptoms of acute hypoglycemia). Products include:
- Iletin I 1501
- Lente, 100 Units 1501
- Iletin II 1504
- Pork Lente, 100 Units 1504
- Purified Pork Lente Insulin 1852

Isradipine (Possible atrioventricular conduction disturbances, left ventricular failure, or hypotension when used concurrently). Products include:
- DynaCirc Capsules 2381
- DynaCirc CR Tablets 2383

Labetalol Hydrochloride (Concurrent use with systemic beta blocker may have additive effects of beta blockade, both systemic and on intraocular pressure). Products include:
- Normodyne Injection 2519
- Normodyne Tablets 2522
- Trandate 1158

Levobunolol Hydrochloride (Concurrent use of two ophthalmic beta blockers is not recommended). Products include:
- Betagan .... ⊙ 230

Metformin Hydrochloride (Beta blocking agents, usually systemic, may mask the sign and symptoms of acute hypoglycemia). Products include:
- Glucophage Tablets 754

Metipranolol Hydrochloride (Concurrent use of two ophthalmic beta blockers is not recommended). Products include:
- OptiPranolol (Metipranolol 0.3%) Sterile Ophthalmic Solution .... ⊙ 256

Metoprolol Succinate (Concurrent use with systemic beta blocker may have additive effects of beta blockade, both systemic and on intraocular pressure). Products include:
- Toprol-XL Tablets 560

Metoprolol Tartrate (Concurrent use with systemic beta blocker may have additive effects of beta blockade, both systemic and on intraocular pressure). Products include:
- Lopressor 848
- Lopressor HCT Tablets 850

Nadolol (Concurrent use with systemic beta blocker may have additive effects of beta blockade, both systemic and on intraocular pressure).
- No products indexed under this heading.

Nicardipine Hydrochloride (Possible atrioventricular conduction disturbances, left ventricular failure, or hypotension when used concurrently). Products include:
- Cardene Capsules 2261
- Cardene I.V. 2815
- Cardene SR Capsules 2264

Nifedipine (Possible atrioventricular conduction disturbances, left ventricular failure, or hypotension when used concurrently). Products include:
- Adalat Capsules (10 mg and 20 mg) 580
- Adalat CC 582
- Procardia Capsules 2024
- Procardia XL Extended Release Tablets 2026

Nimodipine (Possible atrioventricular conduction disturbances, left ventricular failure, or hypotension when used concurrently). Products include:
- Nimotop Capsules 603

Nisoldipine (Possible atrioventricular conduction disturbances, left ventricular failure, or hypotension when used concurrently). Products include:
- Sular Tablets 2961

Penbutolol Sulfate (Concurrent use with systemic beta blocker may have additive effects of beta blockade, both systemic and on intraocular pressure). Products include:
- Levatol Tablets 2547

Pindolol (Concurrent use with systemic beta blocker may have additive effects of beta blockade, both systemic and on intraocular pressure). Products include:
- Visken Tablets 2428

Propranolol Hydrochloride (Concurrent use with systemic beta blocker may have additive effects of beta blockade, both systemic and on intraocular pressure). Products include:
- Inderal 2834
- Inderal LA Long Acting Capsules 2836
- Inderide Tablets 2838
- Inderide LA Long Acting Capsules .. 2840

Rauwolfia Serpentina (Possible additive effects and the production of hypotension and/or bradycardia).
- No products indexed under this heading.

Rescinnamine (Possible additive effects and the production of hypotension and/or bradycardia).
- No products indexed under this heading.

Reserpine (Possible additive effects and the production of hypotension and/or bradycardia). Products include:
- Diupres Tablets 1691
- Hydropres Tablets 1718
- Ser-Ap-Es Tablets 867

Sotalol Hydrochloride (Concurrent use with systemic beta blocker may have additive effects of beta blockade, both systemic and on intraocular pressure). Products include:
- Betapace Tablets 637

Timolol Hemihydrate (Concurrent use with systemic beta blocker may have additive effects of beta blockade, both systemic and on intraocular pressure). Products include:
- Betimol 0.25%, 0.5% .... ⊙ 259

Tolazamide (Beta blocking agents, usually systemic, may mask the sign and symptoms of acute hypoglycemia).
- No products indexed under this heading.

Tolbutamide (Beta blocking agents, usually systemic, may mask the sign and symptoms of acute hypoglycemia).
- No products indexed under this heading.

Verapamil Hydrochloride (Possible atrioventricular conduction disturbances, left ventricular failure, or hypotension when used concurrently). Products include:
- Calan SR Caplets 2571
- Calan Tablets 2568
- Covera-HS Tablets 2573
- Isoptin Injectable 1391
- Isoptin Oral Tablets 1393
- Isoptin SR Tablets 1395
- Verelan Capsules 1455

TIMOPTIC STERILE OPHTHALMIC SOLUTION
(Timolol Maleate) 1794

May interact with general anesthetics, beta blockers, catecholamine depleting drugs, calcium channel blockers, cardiac glycosides, and certain other agents. Compounds in these categories include:

Acebutolol Hydrochloride (Concurrent use with systemic beta blocker may have additive effects of beta blockade, both systemic and on intraocular pressure). Products include:
- Sectral Capsules 2914

Amlodipine Besylate (Possible atrioventricular conduction disturbances, left ventricular failure, or hypotension when used concurrently). Products include:
- Lotrel Capsules 858
- Norvasc Tablets 2020

Atenolol (Concurrent use with systemic beta blocker may have additive effects of beta blockade, both systemic and on intraocular pressure). Products include:
- Tenoretic Tablets 2963
- Tenormin Tablets and I.V. Injection 2965

Bepridil Hydrochloride (Possible atrioventricular conduction disturbances, left ventricular failure, or hypotension when used concurrently). Products include:
- Vascor Tablets (200 and 300 mg) 1597

Betaxolol Hydrochloride (Concurrent use with systemic beta blocker may have additive effects of beta blockade, both systemic and on intraocular pressure; concurrent use of two ophthalmic beta blockers is not recommended). Products include:
- Betoptic Ophthalmic Solution 465
- Betoptic S Ophthalmic Suspension 467
- Kerlone Tablets 2588

Bisoprolol Fumarate (Concurrent use with systemic beta blocker may have additive effects of beta blockade, both systemic and on intraocular pressure). Products include:
- Zebeta Tablets 1457
- Ziac 1459

Carteolol Hydrochloride (Concurrent use with systemic beta blocker may have additive effects of beta blockade, both systemic and on intraocular pressure; concurrent use of two ophthalmic beta blockers is not recommended). Products include:
- Cartrol Tablets 413
- Ocupress Ophthalmic Solution, 1% Sterile .... ⊙ 297

Chlorpropamide (Beta blocking agents, usually systemic, may mask the sign and symptoms of acute hypoglycemia). Products include:
- Diabinese Tablets 2002

Deserpidine (Possible additive effects and the production of hypotension and/or bradycardia).
- No products indexed under this heading.

Deslanoside (Co-administration with digitalis and calcium antagonists may have additive effects in prolonging atrioventricular conduction time).
- No products indexed under this heading.

Digitoxin (Co-administration with digitalis and calcium antagonists may have additive effects in prolonging atrioventricular conduction time). Products include:
- Crystodigin Tablets 1472

Digoxin (Co-administration with digitalis and calcium antagonists may have additive effects in prolonging atrioventricular conduction time). Products include:
- Lanoxicaps 1110
- Lanoxin Elixir Pediatric 1113
- Lanoxin Injection 1116
- Lanoxin Injection Pediatric 1119
- Lanoxin Tablets 1121

Diltiazem Hydrochloride (Possible atrioventricular conduction disturbances, left ventricular failure, or hypotension when used concurrently). Products include:
- Cardizem CD Capsules 1251
- Cardizem SR Capsules 1255
- Cardizem Injectable 1253
- Cardizem Tablets 1257
- Dilacor XR Extended-release Capsules 2183
- Tiazac Capsules 1019

Epinephrine (Patients with a history of atopy or anaphylactic reactions to a variety of allergens may be unresponsive to the usual dose of injectable epinephrine used to treat allergic reactions). Products include:
- EPIFRIN .... ⊙ 237
- EpiPen 808
- Marcaine with Epinephrine 2446
- Primatene Mist .... ▣ 843
- Sensorcaine with Epinephrine Injection 554
- Sus-Phrine Injection 1017
- Xylocaine with Epinephrine Injections 562

Epinephrine Bitartrate (Patients with a history of atopy or anaphylactic reactions to a variety of allergens may be unresponsive to the usual dose of injectable epinephrine used to treat allergic reactions). Products include:
- Sensorcaine-MPF with Epinephrine Injection 554

Esmolol Hydrochloride (Concurrent use with systemic beta blocker may have additive effects of beta blockade, both systemic and on intraocular pressure). Products include:
- Brevibloc (esmolol HCl) Injection 1860

Felodipine (Possible atrioventricular conduction disturbances, left ventricular failure, or hypotension when used concurrently). Products include:
Plendil Extended-Release Tablets.... 514

Glipizide (Beta blocking agents, usually systemic, may mask the sign and symptoms of acute hypoglycemia). Products include:
Glucotrol Tablets 2011
Glucotrol XL Extended Release Tablets 2012

Glyburide (Beta blocking agents, usually systemic, may mask the sign and symptoms of acute hypoglycemia). Products include:
DiaBeta Tablets 1265
Glynase PresTab Tablets 2091
Micronase Tablets 2099

Guanethidine Monosulfate (Possible additive effects and the production of hypotension and/or bradycardia). Products include:
Esimil Tablets 840
Ismelin Tablets 845

Insulin, Human (Beta blocking agents, usually systemic, may mask the sign and symptoms of acute hypoglycemia).
No products indexed under this heading.

Insulin, Human Isophane Suspension (Beta blocking agents, usually systemic, may mask the sign and symptoms of acute hypoglycemia). Products include:
Novolin N Human Insulin 10 ml Vials 1846

Insulin, Human NPH (Beta blocking agents, usually systemic, may mask the sign and symptoms of acute hypoglycemia). Products include:
Humulin N, 100 Units 1495
Novolin N PenFill 1.5 ml Cartridges Durable Insulin Delivery System 1849
Novolin N Prefilled Syringe Disposable Insulin Delivery System 1850

Insulin, Human Regular (Beta blocking agents, usually systemic, may mask the sign and symptoms of acute hypoglycemia). Products include:
Humulin R, 100 Units 1497
Novolin R Human Insulin 10 ml Vials 1846
Novolin R PenFill 1.5 ml Cartridges Durable Insulin Delivery System 1849
Novolin R Prefilled Syringe Disposable Insulin Delivery System 1850
Velosulin BR Human Insulin 10 ml Vials 1847

Insulin, Human, Zinc Suspension (Beta blocking agents, usually systemic, may mask the sign and symptoms of acute hypoglycemia). Products include:
Humulin L, 100 Units 1494
Humulin U, 100 Units 1498
Novolin L Human Insulin 10 ml Vials 1846

Insulin, NPH (Beta blocking agents, usually systemic, may mask the sign and symptoms of acute hypoglycemia). Products include:
NPH, 100 Units 1502
Pork NPH, 100 Units 1506
Purified Pork NPH Isophane Insulin 1852

Insulin, Regular (Beta blocking agents, usually systemic, may mask the sign and symptoms of acute hypoglycemia). Products include:
Regular, 100 Units 1503
Pork Regular, 100 Units 1507
Pork Regular (Concentrated), 500 Units 1508
Purified Pork Regular Insulin 1852

Insulin, Zinc Crystals (Beta blocking agents, usually systemic, may mask the sign and symptoms of acute hypoglycemia). Products include:
NPH, 100 Units 1502

Insulin, Zinc Suspension (Beta blocking agents, usually systemic, may mask the sign and symptoms of acute hypoglycemia). Products include:
Iletin I 1501
Lente, 100 Units 1501
Iletin II 1504
Pork Lente, 100 Units 1504
Purified Pork Lente Insulin 1852

Isradipine (Possible atrioventricular conduction disturbances, left ventricular failure, or hypotension when used concurrently). Products include:
DynaCirc Capsules 2381
DynaCirc CR Tablets 2383

Labetalol Hydrochloride (Concurrent use with systemic beta blocker may have additive effects of beta blockade, both systemic and on intraocular pressure). Products include:
Normodyne Injection 2519
Normodyne Tablets 2522
Trandate 1158

Levobunolol Hydrochloride (Concurrent use of two ophthalmic beta blockers is not recommended). Products include:
Betagan .... ⊚ 230

Metipranolol Hydrochloride (Concurrent use of two ophthalmic beta blockers is not recommended). Products include:
OptiPranolol (Metipranolol 0.3%) Sterile Ophthalmic Solution......... ⊚ 256

Metoprolol Succinate (Concurrent use with systemic beta blocker may have additive effects of beta blockade, both systemic and on intraocular pressure). Products include:
Toprol-XL Tablets 560

Metoprolol Tartrate (Concurrent use with systemic beta blocker may have additive effects of beta blockade, both systemic and on intraocular pressure). Products include:
Lopressor 848
Lopressor HCT Tablets 850

Nadolol (Concurrent use with systemic beta blocker may have additive effects of beta blockade, both systemic and on intraocular pressure).
No products indexed under this heading.

Nicardipine Hydrochloride (Possible atrioventricular conduction disturbances, left ventricular failure, or hypotension when used concurrently). Products include:
Cardene Capsules 2261
Cardene I.V. 2815
Cardene SR Capsules 2264

Nifedipine (Possible atrioventricular conduction disturbances, left ventricular failure, or hypotension when used concurrently). Products include:
Adalat Capsules (10 mg and 20 mg) 580
Adalat CC 582
Procardia Capsules 2024
Procardia XL Extended Release Tablets 2026

Nimodipine (Possible atrioventricular conduction disturbances, left ventricular failure, or hypotension when used concurrently). Products include:
Nimotop Capsules 603

Nisoldipine (Possible atrioventricular conduction disturbances, left ventricular failure, or hypotension when used concurrently). Products include:
Sular Tablets 2961

Penbutolol Sulfate (Concurrent use with systemic beta blocker may have additive effects of beta blockade, both systemic and on intraocular pressure). Products include:
Levatol Tablets 2547

Pindolol (Concurrent use with systemic beta blocker may have additive effects of beta blockade, both systemic and on intraocular pressure). Products include:
Visken Tablets 2428

Propranolol Hydrochloride (Concurrent use with systemic beta blocker may have additive effects of beta blockade, both systemic and on intraocular pressure). Products include:
Inderal 2834
Inderal LA Long Acting Capsules 2836
Inderide Tablets 2838
Inderide LA Long Acting Capsules .. 2840

Rauwolfia Serpentina (Possible additive effects and the production of hypotension and/or bradycardia).
No products indexed under this heading.

Rescinnamine (Possible additive effects and the production of hypotension and/or bradycardia).
No products indexed under this heading.

Reserpine (Possible additive effects and the production of hypotension and/or bradycardia). Products include:
Diupres Tablets 1691
Hydropres Tablets 1718
Ser-Ap-Es Tablets 867

Sotalol Hydrochloride (Concurrent use with systemic beta blocker may have additive effects of beta blockade, both systemic and on intraocular pressure). Products include:
Betapace Tablets 637

Timolol Hemihydrate (Concurrent use with systemic beta blocker may have additive effects of beta blockade, both systemic and on intraocular pressure). Products include:
Betimol 0.25%, 0.5% .... ⊚ 259

Tolazamide (Beta blocking agents, usually systemic, may mask the sign and symptoms of acute hypoglycemia).
No products indexed under this heading.

Tolbutamide (Beta blocking agents, usually systemic, may mask the sign and symptoms of acute hypoglycemia).
No products indexed under this heading.

Verapamil Hydrochloride (Possible atrioventricular conduction disturbances, left ventricular failure, or hypotension when used concurrently). Products include:
Calan SR Caplets 2571
Calan Tablets 2568
Covera-HS Tablets 2573
Isoptin Injectable 1391
Isoptin Oral Tablets 1393
Isoptin SR Tablets 1395
Verelan Capsules 1455

TIMOPTIC-XE
(Timolol Maleate) 1798
May interact with beta blockers, calcium channel blockers, catecholamine depleting drugs, cardiac glycosides, insulin, oral hypoglycemic agents, and certain other agents. Compounds in these categories include:

Acarbose (Beta blocking agents, usually systemic, may mask the sign and symptoms of acute hypoglycemia). Products include:
Precose 604

Acebutolol Hydrochloride (Concurrent use with systemic beta blocker may have additive effects of beta blockade, both systemic and on intraocular pressure). Products include:
Sectral Capsules 2914

Amlodipine Besylate (Possible atrioventricular conduction disturbances, left ventricular failure, or hypotension when used concurrently). Products include:
Lotrel Capsules 858
Norvasc Tablets 2020

Atenolol (Concurrent use with systemic beta blocker may have additive effects of beta blockade, both systemic and on intraocular pressure). Products include:
Tenoretic Tablets 2963
Tenormin Tablets and I.V. Injection 2965

Bepridil Hydrochloride (Possible atrioventricular conduction disturbances, left ventricular failure, or hypotension when used concurrently). Products include:
Vascor Tablets (200 and 300 mg) 1597

Betaxolol Hydrochloride (Concurrent use with systemic beta blocker may have additive effects of beta blockade, both systemic and on intraocular pressure; concurrent use of two ophthalmic beta blockers is not recommended). Products include:
Betoptic Ophthalmic Solution 465
Betoptic S Ophthalmic Suspension ... 467
Kerlone Tablets 2588

Bisoprolol Fumarate (Concurrent use with systemic beta blocker may have additive effects of beta blockade, both systemic and on intraocular pressure). Products include:
Zebeta Tablets 1457
Ziac 1459

Carteolol Hydrochloride (Concurrent use with systemic beta blocker may have additive effects of beta blockade, both systemic and on intraocular pressure; concurrent use of two ophthalmic beta blockers is not recommended). Products include:
Cartrol Tablets 413
Ocupress Ophthalmic Solution, 1% Sterile .... ⊚ 297

Chlorpropamide (Beta blocking agents, usually systemic, may mask the sign and symptoms of acute hypoglycemia). Products include:
Diabinese Tablets 2002

Deserpidine (Possible additive effects and the production of hypotension and/or bradycardia).
No products indexed under this heading.

Deslanoside (Co-administration with digitalis and calcium antagonists may have additive effects in prolonging atrioventricular conduction time).
No products indexed under this heading.

Digitoxin (Co-administration with digitalis and calcium antagonists may have additive effects in prolonging atrioventricular conduction time). Products include:
Crystodigin Tablets 1472

IMPORTANT NOTE: Always consult each drug listing in the patient's regimen for possible interactions.

Digoxin (Co-administration with digitalis and calcium antagonists may have additive effects in prolonging atrioventricular conduction time). Products include:
Lanoxicaps 1110
Lanoxin Elixir Pediatric 1113
Lanoxin Injection 1116
Lanoxin Injection Pediatric... 1119
Lanoxin Tablets 1121

Diltiazem Hydrochloride (Possible atrioventricular conduction disturbances, left ventricular failure, or hypotension when used concurrently). Products include:
Cardizem CD Capsules 1251
Cardizem SR Capsules 1255
Cardizem Injectable 1253
Cardizem Tablets 1257
Dilacor XR Extended-release Capsules 2183
Tiazac Capsules 1019

Epinephrine (Patients with a history of atopy or anaphylactic reactions to a variety of allergens may be unresponsive to the usual dose of injectable epinephrine used to treat allergic reactions. Products include:
EPIFRIN .... ⊙ 237
EpiPen 808
Marcaine with Epinephrine ... 2446
Primatene Mist .... ▣ 843
Sensorcaine with Epinephrine Injection 554
Sus-Phrine Injection 1017
Xylocaine with Epinephrine Injections 562

Epinephrine Bitartrate (Patients with a history of atopy or anaphylactic reactions to a variety of allergens may be unresponsive to the usual dose of injectable epinephrine used to treat allergic reactions). Products include:
Sensorcaine-MPF with Epinephrine Injection 554

Esmolol Hydrochloride (Concurrent use with systemic beta blocker may have additive effects of beta blockade, both systemic and on intraocular pressure). Products include:
Brevibloc (esmolol HCl) Injection 1860

Felodipine (Possible atrioventricular conduction disturbances, left ventricular failure, or hypotension when used concurrently). Products include:
Plendil Extended-Release Tablets..... 514

Glimepiride (Beta blocking agents, usually systemic, may mask the sign and symptoms of acute hypoglycemia). Products include:
Amaryl Tablets 1241

Glipizide (Beta blocking agents, usually systemic, may mask the sign and symptoms of acute hypoglycemia). Products include:
Glucotrol Tablets 2011
Glucotrol XL Extended Release Tablets 2012

Glyburide (Beta blocking agents, usually systemic, may mask the sign and symptoms of acute hypoglycemia). Products include:
DiaBeta Tablets 1265
Glynase PresTab Tablets 2091
Micronase Tablets 2099

Guanethidine Monosulfate (Possible additive effects and the production of hypotension and/or bradycardia). Products include:
Esimil Tablets 840
Ismelin Tablets 845

Insulin, Human (Beta blocking agents, usually systemic, may mask the sign and symptoms of acute hypoglycemia).
No products indexed under this heading.

Insulin, Human Isophane Suspension (Beta blocking agents, usually systemic, may mask the sign and symptoms of acute hypoglycemia). Products include:
Novolin N Human Insulin 10 ml Vials 1846

Insulin, Human NPH (Beta blocking agents, usually systemic, may mask the sign and symptoms of acute hypoglycemia). Products include:
Humulin N, 100 Units 1495
Novolin N PenFill 1.5 ml Cartridges Durable Insulin Delivery System 1849
Novolin N Prefilled Syringe Disposable Insulin Delivery System 1850

Insulin, Human Regular (Beta blocking agents, usually systemic, may mask the sign and symptoms of acute hypoglycemia). Products include:
Humulin R, 100 Units 1497
Novolin R Human Insulin 10 ml Vials 1846
Novolin R PenFill 1.5 ml Cartridges Durable Insulin Delivery System 1849
Novolin R Prefilled Syringe Disposable Insulin Delivery System 1850
Velosulin BR Human Insulin 10 ml Vials 1847

Insulin, Human, Zinc Suspension (Beta blocking agents, usually systemic, may mask the sign and symptoms of acute hypoglycemia). Products include:
Humulin L, 100 Units 1494
Humulin U, 100 Units 1498
Novolin L Human Insulin 10 ml Vials 1846

Insulin Lispro, Human (Beta blocking agents, usually systemic, may mask the sign and symptoms of acute hypoglycemia). Products include:
Humalog Injection 1488

Insulin, NPH (Beta blocking agents, usually systemic, may mask the sign and symptoms of acute hypoglycemia). Products include:
NPH, 100 Units 1502
Pork NPH, 100 Units............ 1506
Purified Pork NPH Isophane Insulin 1852

Insulin, Regular (Beta blocking agents, usually systemic, may mask the sign and symptoms of acute hypoglycemia). Products include:
Regular, 100 Units 1503
Pork Regular, 100 Units 1507
Pork Regular (Concentrated), 500 Units 1508
Purified Pork Regular Insulin 1852

Insulin, Zinc Crystals (Beta blocking agents, usually systemic, may mask the sign and symptoms of acute hypoglycemia). Products include:
NPH, 100 Units 1502

Insulin, Zinc Suspension (Beta blocking agents, usually systemic, may mask the sign and symptoms of acute hypoglycemia). Products include:
Iletin I 1501
Lente, 100 Units 1501
Iletin II 1504
Pork Lente, 100 Units 1504
Purified Pork Lente Insulin 1852

Isradipine (Possible atrioventricular conduction disturbances, left ventricular failure, or hypotension when used concurrently). Products include:
DynaCirc Capsules 2381
DynaCirc CR Tablets 2383

Labetalol Hydrochloride (Concurrent use with systemic beta blocker may have additive effects of beta blockade, both systemic and on intraocular pressure). Products include:
Normodyne Injection 2519
Normodyne Tablets 2522
Trandate 1158

Levobunolol Hydrochloride (Concurrent use of two ophthalmic beta blockers is not recommended). Products include:
Betagan .... ⊙ 230

Metformin Hydrochloride (Beta blocking agents, usually systemic, may mask the sign and symptoms of acute hypoglycemia). Products include:
Glucophage Tablets 754

Metipranolol Hydrochloride (Concurrent use of two ophthalmic beta blockers is not recommended). Products include:
OptiPranolol (Metipranolol 0.3%) Sterile Ophthalmic Solution.......... ⊙ 256

Metoprolol Succinate (Concurrent use with systemic beta blocker may have additive effects of beta blockade, both systemic and on intraocular pressure). Products include:
Toprol-XL Tablets 560

Metoprolol Tartrate (Concurrent use with systemic beta blocker may have additive effects of beta blockade, both systemic and on intraocular pressure). Products include:
Lopressor 848
Lopressor HCT Tablets 850

Nadolol (Concurrent use with systemic beta blocker may have additive effects of beta blockade, both systemic and on intraocular pressure).
No products indexed under this heading.

Nicardipine Hydrochloride (Possible atrioventricular conduction disturbances, left ventricular failure, or hypotension when used concurrently). Products include:
Cardene Capsules 2261
Cardene I.V. 2815
Cardene SR Capsules.......... 2264

Nifedipine (Possible atrioventricular conduction disturbances, left ventricular failure, or hypotension when used concurrently). Products include:
Adalat Capsules (10 mg and 20 mg) 580
Adalat CC 582
Procardia Capsules.............. 2024
Procardia XL Extended Release Tablets 2026

Nimodipine (Possible atrioventricular conduction disturbances, left ventricular failure, or hypotension when used concurrently). Products include:
Nimotop Capsules 603

Nisoldipine (Possible atrioventricular conduction disturbances, left ventricular failure, or hypotension when used concurrently). Products include:
Sular Tablets 2961

Penbutolol Sulfate (Concurrent use with systemic beta blocker may have additive effects of beta blockade, both systemic and on intraocular pressure). Products include:
Levatol Tablets 2547

Pindolol (Concurrent use with systemic beta blocker may have additive effects of beta blockade, both systemic and on intraocular pressure). Products include:
Visken Tablets 2428

Propranolol Hydrochloride (Concurrent use with systemic beta blocker may have additive effects of beta blockade, both systemic and on intraocular pressure). Products include:
Inderal 2834
Inderal LA Long Acting Capsules 2836
Inderide Tablets 2838
Inderide LA Long Acting Capsules .. 2840

Rauwolfia Serpentina (Possible additive effects and the production of hypotension and/or bradycardia).
No products indexed under this heading.

Rescinnamine (Possible additive effects and the production of hypotension and/or bradycardia).
No products indexed under this heading.

Reserpine (Possible additive effects and the production of hypotension and/or bradycardia). Products include:
Diupres Tablets 1691
Hydropres Tablets................ 1718
Ser-Ap-Es Tablets 867

Sotalol Hydrochloride (Concurrent use with systemic beta blocker may have additive effects of beta blockade, both systemic and on intraocular pressure). Products include:
Betapace Tablets 637

Timolol Hemihydrate (Concurrent use with systemic beta blocker may have additive effects of beta blockade, both systemic and on intraocular pressure). Products include:
Betimol 0.25%, 0.5% .... ⊙ 259

Tolazamide (Beta blocking agents, usually systemic, may mask the sign and symptoms of acute hypoglycemia).
No products indexed under this heading.

Tolbutamide (Beta blocking agents, usually systemic, may mask the sign and symptoms of acute hypoglycemia).
No products indexed under this heading.

Verapamil Hydrochloride (Possible atrioventricular conduction disturbances, left ventricular failure, or hypotension when used concurrently). Products include:
Calan SR Caplets 2571
Calan Tablets 2568
Covera-HS Tablets 2573
Isoptin Injectable 1391
Isoptin Oral Tablets 1393
Isoptin SR Tablets 1395
Verelan Capsules 1455

TING ANTIFUNGAL CREAM
(Tolnaftate)........................... ▣ 666
None cited in PDR database.

TING ANTIFUNGAL SPRAY LIQUID
(Tolnaftate) .... ▣ 666
None cited in PDR database.

TING ANTIFUNGAL SPRAY POWDER
(Miconazole Nitrate) .... ▣ 666
None cited in PDR database.

TITRALAC ANTACID REGULAR
(Calcium Carbonate) .... ▣ 686

(▣ Described in PDR For Nonprescription Drugs)   (⊙ Described in PDR For Ophthalmology)

May interact with:

Prescription Drugs, unspecified (Antacids may interact with certain unspecified prescription drugs; consult your physician).

TITRALAC ANTACID EXTRA STRENGTH
(Calcium Carbonate) 686
See **Titralac Antacid Regular**

TITRALAC PLUS LIQUID
(Calcium Carbonate, Simethicone).. 687
See **Titralac Plus Tablets**

TITRALAC PLUS TABLETS
(Calcium Carbonate, Simethicone).. 687
May interact with:

Prescription Drugs, unspecified (Antacids may interact with certain unspecified prescription drugs; consult your physician).

TOBRADEX OPHTHALMIC SUSPENSION AND OINTMENT
(Dexamethasone, Tobramycin) 469
May interact with aminoglycosides. Compounds in this category include:

Amikacin Sulfate (Monitor the total serum concentration if administered with systemic aminoglycoside). Products include:
- Amikacin Sulfate Injection, USP 523
- Amikacin Sulfate Injection, USP 981
- Amikin Injectable 502

Gentamicin Sulfate (Monitor the total serum concentration if administered with systemic aminoglycoside). Products include:
- Garamycin Cream 0.1% 2501
- Garamycin Injectable 2502
- Garamycin Ointment 0.1% 2501
- Garamycin Ophthalmic 2501
- Genoptic Sterile Ophthalmic Solution 241
- Genoptic Sterile Ophthalmic Ointment 241
- Gentak 209
- Pred-G Liquifilm Sterile Ophthalmic Suspension 248
- Pred-G S.O.P. Sterile Ophthalmic Ointment 249

Kanamycin Sulfate (Monitor the total serum concentration if administered with systemic aminoglycoside).
- No products indexed under this heading.

Streptomycin Sulfate (Monitor the total serum concentration if administered with systemic aminoglycoside). Products include:
- Streptomycin Sulfate Injection 2031

Tobramycin Sulfate (Monitor the total serum concentration if administered with systemic aminoglycoside). Products include:
- Nebcin Vials, Hyporets & ADD-Vantage 1518

TOBREX OPHTHALMIC OINTMENT AND SOLUTION
(Tobramycin) 226
May interact with aminoglycosides. Compounds in this category include:

Amikacin Sulfate (If topical ocular tobramycin is administered concomitantly with systemic aminoglycosides, care should be taken to monitor the total serum concentration). Products include:
- Amikacin Sulfate Injection, USP 523
- Amikacin Sulfate Injection, USP 981
- Amikin Injectable 502

Gentamicin Sulfate (If topical ocular tobramycin is administered concomitantly with systemic aminoglycosides, care should be taken to monitor the total serum concentration). Products include:
- Garamycin Cream 0.1% 2501
- Garamycin Injectable 2502
- Garamycin Ointment 0.1% 2501
- Garamycin Ophthalmic 2501
- Genoptic Sterile Ophthalmic Solution 241
- Genoptic Sterile Ophthalmic Ointment 241
- Gentak 209
- Pred-G Liquifilm Sterile Ophthalmic Suspension 248
- Pred-G S.O.P. Sterile Ophthalmic Ointment 249

Kanamycin Sulfate (If topical ocular tobramycin is administered concomitantly with systemic aminoglycosides, care should be taken to monitor the total serum concentration).
- No products indexed under this heading.

Streptomycin Sulfate (If topical ocular tobramycin is administered concomitantly with systemic aminoglycosides, care should be taken to monitor the total serum concentration). Products include:
- Streptomycin Sulfate Injection 2031

TOFRANIL AMPULS
(Imipramine Hydrochloride) 873
May interact with central nervous system depressants, anticholinergics, sympathomimetics, barbiturates, monoamine oxidase inhibitors, thyroid preparations, drugs that inhibit cytochrome p450iid6, antidepressant drugs, phenothiazines, selective serotonin reuptake inhibitors, and certain other agents. Compounds in these categories include:

Albuterol (Avoid concurrent use since tricyclic antidepressants can potentiate the effects of catecholamines). Products include:
- Proventil Inhalation Aerosol 2524
- Ventolin Inhalation Aerosol and Refill 1170

Albuterol Sulfate (Avoid concurrent use since tricyclic antidepressants can potentiate the effects of catecholamines). Products include:
- Airet Albuterol Sulfate Inhalation Solution 1602
- Albuterol Sulfate, USP Solution for Inhalation, Arm-a-Med 522
- Proventil Inhalation Solution 0.083% 2527
- Proventil Repetabs Tablets 2529
- Proventil Solution for Inhalation 0.5% 2525
- Proventil Syrup 2528
- Proventil Tablets 2529
- Ventolin Inhalation Solution 1171
- Ventolin Nebules Inhalation Solution 1172
- Ventolin Rotacaps for Inhalation 1173
- Ventolin Syrup 1175
- Ventolin Tablets 1176
- Volmax Extended-Release Tablets .. 1835

Alfentanil Hydrochloride (Imipramine may potentiate the effects of CNS depressant drugs). Products include:
- Alfenta Injection 1334

Alprazolam (Imipramine may potentiate the effects of CNS depressant drugs). Products include:
- Xanax Tablets 2115

Amitriptyline Hydrochloride (Concurrent use with drugs that are substrate for cytochrome $P_{450}IID_6$ may make normal metabolizer resemble poor metabolizer leading to higher than expected plasma concentrations of TCA with resultant toxicity). Products include:
- Elavil 2945
- Etrafon 2495
- Limbitrol 2333
- Triavil Tablets 1800

Amoxapine (Concurrent use with drugs that are substrate for cytochrome $P_{450}IID_6$ may make normal metabolizer resemble poor metabolizer leading to higher than expected plasma concentrations of TCA with resultant toxicity). Products include:
- Asendin Tablets 1419

Aprobarbital (The plasma concentration of imipramine may decrease when the drug is given with barbiturates, a hepatic enzyme inducer; dosage of imipramine may need to be adjusted; imipramine may potentiate the effects of CNS depressant drugs).
- No products indexed under this heading.

Atropine Sulfate (Concurrent use may result in pronounced atropine-like effects e.g., paralytic ileus). Products include:
- Arco-Lase Plus Tablets 513
- Atrohist Plus Tablets 1605
- Donnatal 2234
- Donnatal Extentabs 2234
- Donnatal Tablets 2234
- Lomotil 2591
- Motofen Tablets 789
- Urised Tablets 2123

Belladonna Alkaloids (Concurrent use may result in pronounced atropine-like effects e.g., paralytic ileus). Products include:
- Bellergal-S Tablets 2375
- Hyland's Bedwetting Tablets 788
- Hyland's EnurAid Tablets 789
- Hyland's Headache Tablets 790
- Hyland's Teething Tablets 790
- Similasan Eye Drops #1 769

Benztropine Mesylate (Concurrent use may result in pronounced atropine-like effects e.g., paralytic ileus). Products include:
- Cogentin 1661

Biperiden Hydrochloride (Concurrent use may result in pronounced atropine-like effects e.g., paralytic ileus). Products include:
- Akineton 1380

Buprenorphine (Imipramine may potentiate the effects of CNS depressant drugs). Products include:
- Buprenex Injectable 2170

Bupropion Hydrochloride (Concurrent use with drugs that are substrate for cytochrome $P_{450}IID_6$ may make normal metabolizer resemble poor metabolizer leading to higher than expected plasma concentrations of TCA with resultant toxicity). Products include:
- Wellbutrin Tablets 1177

Buspirone Hydrochloride (Imipramine may potentiate the effects of CNS depressant drugs). Products include:
- BuSpar Tablets 738

Butabarbital (The plasma concentration of imipramine may decrease when the drug is given with barbiturates, a hepatic enzyme inducer; dosage of imipramine may need to be adjusted; imipramine may potentiate the effects of CNS depressant drugs).
- No products indexed under this heading.

Butalbital (The plasma concentration of imipramine may decrease when the drug is given with barbiturates, a hepatic enzyme inducer; dosage of imipramine may need to be adjusted; imipramine may potentiate the effects of CNS depressant drugs). Products include:
- Axocet Capsules 2469
- Esgic-plus Capsules 1012
- Esgic-plus Tablets 1012
- Fioricet Tablets 2386
- Fioricet with Codeine Capsules 2387
- Fiorinal Capsules 2388
- Fiorinal with Codeine Capsules 2390
- Fiorinal Tablets 2388
- Phrenilin 790
- Sedapap Tablets 50 mg/650 mg .. 1826

Chlordiazepoxide (Imipramine may potentiate the effects of CNS depressant drugs). Products include:
- Limbitrol 2333

Chlordiazepoxide Hydrochloride (Imipramine may potentiate the effects of CNS depressant drugs). Products include:
- Librax Capsules 2330
- Librium Capsules 2331
- Librium Injectable 2332

Chlorpromazine (Concurrent use with drugs that are substrate for cytochrome $P_{450}IID_6$ may make normal metabolizer resemble poor metabolizer leading to higher than expected plasma concentrations of TCA with resultant toxicity; imipramine may potentiate the effects of CNS depressant drugs). Products include:
- Thorazine Suppositories 2701

Chlorpromazine Hydrochloride (Concurrent use with drugs that are substrate for cytochrome $P_{450}IID_6$ may make normal metabolizer resemble poor metabolizer leading to higher than expected plasma concentrations of TCA with resultant toxicity; imipramine may potentiate the effects of CNS depressant drugs). Products include:
- Thorazine 2701

Chlorprothixene (Imipramine may potentiate the effects of CNS depressant drugs).
- No products indexed under this heading.

Chlorprothixene Hydrochloride (Imipramine may potentiate the effects of CNS depressant drugs).
- No products indexed under this heading.

Chlorprothixene Lactate (Imipramine may potentiate the effects of CNS depressant drugs).
- No products indexed under this heading.

Cimetidine (The plasma concentration of imipramine may increase when the drug is given with cimetidine, a hepatic enzyme inhibitor; dosage of imipramine may need to be adjusted). Products include:
- Tagamet HB Tablets 786
- Tagamet Tablets 2694

Cimetidine Hydrochloride (The plasma concentration of imipramine may increase when the drug is given with cimetidine, a hepatic enzyme inhibitor; dosage of imipramine may need to be adjusted). Products include:
- Tagamet 2694

Clidinium Bromide (Concurrent use may result in pronounced atropine-like effects e.g., paralytic ileus). Products include:
- Librax Capsules 2330

IMPORTANT NOTE: Always consult each drug listing in the patient's regimen for possible interactions.

Tofranil — Interactions Index

Clonidine (Imipramine may block the antihypertensive effect). Products include:
Catapres-TTS 680

Clonidine Hydrochloride (Imipramine may block the antihypertensive effect). Products include:
Catapres Tablets 679
Combipres Tablets 682

Clorazepate Dipotassium (Imipramine may potentiate the effects of CNS depressant drugs). Products include:
Tranxene 459

Clozapine (Imipramine may potentiate the effects of CNS depressant drugs). Products include:
Clozaril Tablets 2377

Codeine Phosphate (Imipramine may potentiate the effects of CNS depressant drugs). Products include:
Brontex 2130
Dimetane-DC Cough Syrup 2232
Fioricet with Codeine Capsules 2387
Fiorinal with Codeine Capsules 2390
Nucofed 2225
Phenergan with Codeine 2883
Phenergan VC with Codeine 2888
Robitussin A-C Syrup 2248
Robitussin-DAC Syrup 2249
Ryna 804
Soma Compound w/Codeine Tablets 2784
Tylenol with Codeine 1592

Desflurane (Imipramine may potentiate the effects of CNS depressant drugs). Products include:
Suprane (desflurane, USP) 1865

Desipramine Hydrochloride (Concurrent use with drugs that are substrate for cytochrome $P_{450}IID_6$ may make normal metabolizer resemble poor metabolizer leading to higher than expected plasma concentrations of TCA with resultant toxicity). Products include:
Norpramin Tablets 1273

Dezocine (Imipramine may potentiate the effects of CNS depressant drugs). Products include:
Dalgan Injection 529

Diazepam (Imipramine may potentiate the effects of CNS depressant drugs). Products include:
Dizac (diazepam injectable emulsion) CIV 1862
Valium Injectable 2336
Valium Tablets 2335

Dicyclomine Hydrochloride (Concurrent use may result in pronounced atropine-like effects e.g., paralytic ileus). Products include:
Bentyl 1246

Dobutamine Hydrochloride (Avoid concurrent use since tricyclic antidepressants can potentiate the effects of catecholamines). Products include:
Dobutrex Solution Vials 1480

Dopamine Hydrochloride (Avoid concurrent use since tricyclic antidepressants can potentiate the effects of catecholamines).
No products indexed under this heading.

Doxepin Hydrochloride (Concurrent use with drugs that are substrate for cytochrome $P_{450}IID_6$ may make normal metabolizer resemble poor metabolizer leading to higher than expected plasma concentrations of TCA with resultant toxicity). Products include:
Adapin Capsules 1542
Sinequan 2028
Zonalon Cream 1042

Droperidol (Imipramine may potentiate the effects of CNS depressant drugs). Products include:
Inapsine Injection 462

Enflurane (Imipramine may potentiate the effects of CNS depressant drugs).
No products indexed under this heading.

Ephedrine Hydrochloride (Avoid concurrent use since tricyclic antidepressants can potentiate the effects of catecholamines). Products include:
Primatene Tablets 844
Quadrinal Tablets 1398

Ephedrine Sulfate (Avoid concurrent use since tricyclic antidepressants can potentiate the effects of catecholamines). Products include:
Marax Tablets & DF Syrup 2015

Ephedrine Tannate (Avoid concurrent use since tricyclic antidepressants can potentiate the effects of catecholamines). Products include:
Rynatuss 2782

Epinephrine (Avoid concurrent use since tricyclic antidepressants can potentiate the effects of catecholamines). Products include:
EPIFRIN 237
EpiPen 808
Marcaine with Epinephrine 2446
Primatene Mist 843
Sensorcaine with Epinephrine Injection 554
Sus-Phrine Injection 1017
Xylocaine with Epinephrine Injections 562

Epinephrine Bitartrate (Avoid concurrent use since tricyclic antidepressants can potentiate the effects of catecholamines). Products include:
Sensorcaine-MPF with Epinephrine Injection 554

Epinephrine Hydrochloride (Avoid concurrent use since tricyclic antidepressants can potentiate the effects of catecholamines). Products include:
Ana-Kit Anaphylaxis Emergency Treatment Kit 611

Estazolam (Imipramine may potentiate the effects of CNS depressant drugs). Products include:
ProSom Tablets 457

Ethchlorvynol (Imipramine may potentiate the effects of CNS depressant drugs). Products include:
Placidyl Capsules 456

Ethinamate (Imipramine may potentiate the effects of CNS depressant drugs).
No products indexed under this heading.

Fentanyl (Imipramine may potentiate the effects of CNS depressant drugs). Products include:
Duragesic Transdermal System 1336

Fentanyl Citrate (Imipramine may potentiate the effects of CNS depressant drugs). Products include:
Sublimaze Injection 463

Flecainide Acetate (Concurrent use with drugs that are substrate for cytochrome $P_{450}IID_6$ may make normal metabolizer resemble poor metabolizer leading to higher than expected plasma concentrations of TCA with resultant toxicity). Products include:
Tambocor Tablets 1555

Fluoxetine Hydrochloride (Concurrent use with drugs that are substrate for cytochrome $P_{450}IID_6$ may make normal metabolizer resemble poor metabolizer leading to higher than expected plasma concentrations of TCA with resultant toxicity; due to variation in the extent of inhibition of $P_{450}IID_6$ and long half-life of the parent (fluoxetine) and active must sufficient time must elapse, at least 5 weeks before switching to TCA). Products include:
Prozac Pulvules & Liquid, Oral Solution 935

Fluphenazine Decanoate (Concurrent use with drugs that are substrate for cytochrome $P_{450}IID_6$ may make normal metabolizer resemble poor metabolizer leading to higher than expected plasma concentrations of TCA with resultant toxicity; imipramine may potentiate the effects of CNS depressant drugs). Products include:
Prolixin Decanoate 510

Fluphenazine Enanthate (Concurrent use with drugs that are substrate for cytochrome $P_{450}IID_6$ may make normal metabolizer resemble poor metabolizer leading to higher than expected plasma concentrations of TCA with resultant toxicity; imipramine may potentiate the effects of CNS depressant drugs). Products include:
Prolixin Enanthate 510

Fluphenazine Hydrochloride (Concurrent use with drugs that are substrate for cytochrome $P_{450}IID_6$ may make normal metabolizer resemble poor metabolizer leading to higher than expected plasma concentrations of TCA with resultant toxicity; imipramine may potentiate the effects of CNS depressant drugs). Products include:
Prolixin 510

Flurazepam Hydrochloride (Imipramine may potentiate the effects of CNS depressant drugs). Products include:
Dalmane Capsules 2329

Fluvoxamine Maleate (Concurrent use with drugs that are substrate for cytochrome $P_{450}IID_6$ may make normal metabolizer resemble poor metabolizer leading to higher than expected plasma concentrations of TCA with resultant toxicity; due to variation in the extent of inhibition of $P_{450}IID_6$ caution is indicated if co-administered sufficient time must elapse). Products include:
LUVOX Tablets 2723

Furazolidone (Potential for hyperpyretic crises, severe convulsions, and deaths; concurrent and/or sequential use is contraindicated). Products include:
Furoxone 2221

Glutethimide (Imipramine may potentiate the effects of CNS depressant drugs).
No products indexed under this heading.

Glycopyrrolate (Concurrent use may result in pronounced atropine-like effects e.g., paralytic ileus). Products include:
Robinul Forte Tablets 2247
Robinul Injectable 2247
Robinul Tablets 2247

Guanadrel Sulfate (Imipramine may block the antihypertensive effect). Products include:
Hylorel Tablets 1613

Guanethidine Monosulfate (Imipramine may block the antihypertensive effect of guanethidine or similarly acting compounds). Products include:
Esimil Tablets 840
Ismelin Tablets 845

Haloperidol (Imipramine may potentiate the effects of CNS depressant drugs). Products include:
Haldol Injection, Tablets and Concentrate 1585

Haloperidol Decanoate (Imipramine may potentiate the effects of CNS depressant drugs). Products include:
Haldol Decanoate 1587

Hydrocodone Bitartrate (Imipramine may potentiate the effects of CNS depressant drugs). Products include:
Codiclear DH Syrup 808
Duratuss HD Elixir 2750
Histussin D Liquid 670
Hycodan Tablets and Syrup 946
Hycomine Compound Tablets 948
Hycomine 947
Hycotuss Expectorant Syrup 950
Hydrocet Capsules 787
Lorcet 10/650 Tablets 1016
Lortab 2751
Tussend 1830
Tussend Expectorant 1831
Vicodin Tablets 1404
Vicodin ES Tablets 1405
Vicodin HP Tablets 1403
Vicodin Tuss Expectorant 1406
Zydone Capsules 967

Hydrocodone Polistirex (Imipramine may potentiate the effects of CNS depressant drugs). Products include:
Tussionex Pennkinetic Extended-Release Suspension 1624

Hydroxyzine Hydrochloride (Imipramine may potentiate the effects of CNS depressant drugs). Products include:
Atarax Tablets & Syrup 1992
Marax Tablets & DF Syrup 2015
Vistaril Intramuscular Solution 2042

Hyoscyamine (Concurrent use may result in pronounced atropine-like effects e.g., paralytic ileus). Products include:
Cystospaz Tablets 2123
Urised Tablets 2123

Hyoscyamine Sulfate (Concurrent use may result in pronounced atropine-like effects e.g., paralytic ileus). Products include:
Arco-Lase Plus Tablets 513
Atrohist Plus Tablets 1605
Cystospaz-M Capsules 2123
Donnatal 2234
Donnatal Extentabs 2234
Donnatal Tablets 2234
Kutrase Capsules 2546
Levsin/Levsinex/Levbid 2549

Imipramine Pamoate (Concurrent use with drugs that are substrate for cytochrome $P_{450}IID_6$ may make normal metabolizer resemble poor metabolizer leading to higher than expected plasma concentrations of TCA with resultant toxicity). Products include:
Tofranil-PM Capsules 876

Ipratropium Bromide (Concurrent use may result in pronounced atropine-like effects e.g., paralytic ileus). Products include:
Atrovent Inhalation Aerosol 674
Atrovent Inhalation Solution 675
Atrovent Nasal Spray 0.03% 676
Atrovent Nasal Spray 0.06% 678

Isocarboxazid (Potential for hyperpyretic crises; severe convulsions, and deaths; concurrent and/or sequential use is contraindicated).
No products indexed under this heading.

(▣ Described in PDR For Nonprescription Drugs)   (⊙ Described in PDR For Ophthalmology)

1077 **Interactions Index** **Tofranil**

Isoflurane (Imipramine may potentiate the effects of CNS depressant drugs).
No products indexed under this heading.

Isoproterenol Hydrochloride (Avoid concurrent use since tricyclic antidepressants can potentiate the effects of catecholamines). Products include:
Isuprel Hydrochloride Solution 2443
Isuprel Injection 2441
Isuprel Mistometer 2442

Isoproterenol Sulfate (Avoid concurrent use since tricyclic antidepressants can potentiate the effects of catecholamines). Products include:
Norisodrine with Calcium Iodide Syrup 446

Ketamine Hydrochloride (Imipramine may potentiate the effects of CNS depressant drugs).
No products indexed under this heading.

Levomethadyl Acetate Hydrochloride (Imipramine may potentiate the effects of CNS depressant drugs). Products include:
Orlaam Oral Solution 2361

Levorphanol Tartrate (Imipramine may potentiate the effects of CNS depressant drugs). Products include:
Levo-Dromoran 2297

Levothyroxine Sodium (Co-administration may produce cardiovascular toxicity). Products include:
Eltroxin Tablets 2214
Levothroid Tablets 1015
Levothyroxine Sodium, USP for Injection 546
Levoxyl Tablets 918
Synthroid 1410

Liothyronine Sodium (Co-administration may produce cardiovascular toxicity). Products include:
Cytomel Tablets 2647
Triostat Injection 2708

Liotrix (Co-administration may produce cardiovascular toxicity).
No products indexed under this heading.

Lorazepam (Imipramine may potentiate the effects of CNS depressant drugs). Products include:
Ativan Injection 2805
Ativan Tablets 2807

Loxapine Hydrochloride (Imipramine may potentiate the effects of CNS depressant drugs). Products include:
Loxitane 1426

Loxapine Succinate (Imipramine may potentiate the effects of CNS depressant drugs). Products include:
Loxitane Capsules 1426

Maprotiline Hydrochloride (Concurrent use with drugs that are substrate for cytochrome $P_{450}IID_6$ may make normal metabolizer resemble poor metabolizer leading to higher than expected plasma concentrations of TCA with resultant toxicity). Products include:
Ludiomil Tablets 861

Mepenzolate Bromide (Concurrent use may result in pronounced atropine-like effects e.g., paralytic ileus).
No products indexed under this heading.

Meperidine Hydrochloride (Imipramine may potentiate the effects of CNS depressant drugs). Products include:
Demerol 2438
Mepergan Injection 2859

Mephobarbital (The plasma concentration of imipramine may decrease when the drug is given with barbiturates, a hepatic enzyme inducer; dosage of imipramine may need to be adjusted; imipramine may potentiate the effects of CNS depressant drugs). Products include:
Mebaral Tablets 2452

Meprobamate (Imipramine may potentiate the effects of CNS depressant drugs). Products include:
Miltown Tablets 2780
PMB 200 and PMB 400 2890

Mesoridazine Besylate (Concurrent use with drugs that are substrate for cytochrome $P_{450}IID_6$ may make normal metabolizer resemble poor metabolizer leading to higher than expected plasma concentrations of TCA with resultant toxicity; imipramine may potentiate the effects of CNS depressant drugs). Products include:
Serentil 689

Metaproterenol Sulfate (Avoid concurrent use since tricyclic antidepressants can potentiate the effects of catecholamines). Products include:
Alupent 672
Metaproterenol Sulfate Inhalation Solution, USP, Arm-a-Med 547

Metaraminol Bitartrate (Avoid concurrent use since tricyclic antidepressants can potentiate the effects of catecholamines). Products include:
Aramine Injection 1649

Methadone Hydrochloride (Imipramine may potentiate the effects of CNS depressant drugs). Products include:
Methadone Hydrochloride Oral Concentrate 2356
Methadone Hydrochloride Oral Solution & Tablets 2357

Methohexital Sodium (Imipramine may potentiate the effects of CNS depressant drugs).
No products indexed under this heading.

Methotrimeprazine (Concurrent use with drugs that are substrate for cytochrome $P_{450}IID_6$ may make normal metabolizer resemble poor metabolizer leading to higher than expected plasma concentrations of TCA with resultant toxicity; imipramine may potentiate the effects of CNS depressant drugs). Products include:
Levoprome 1321

Methoxamine Hydrochloride (Avoid concurrent use since tricyclic antidepressants can potentiate the effects of catecholamines). Products include:
Vasoxyl Injection 1169

Methoxyflurane (Imipramine may potentiate the effects of CNS depressant drugs).
No products indexed under this heading.

Methylphenidate Hydrochloride (May inhibit the metabolism of imipramine; downward dosage adjustments of imipramine may be required when given concomitantly). Products include:
Ritalin 866

Midazolam Hydrochloride (Imipramine may potentiate the effects of CNS depressant drugs). Products include:
Versed Injection 2324

Molindone Hydrochloride (Imipramine may potentiate the effects of CNS depressant drugs). Products include:
Moban Tablets and Concentrate 1036

Morphine Sulfate (Imipramine may potentiate the effects of CNS depressant drugs). Products include:
Astramorph/PF Injection, USP (Preservative-Free) 526
Duramorph Injection 983
Infumorph 200 and Infumorph 500 Sterile Solutions 985
Kadian Capsules 2948
MS Contin Tablets 2149
MSIR 2152
Oramorph SR (Morphine Sulfate Sustained Release Tablets) 2359
RMS Suppositories CII 2766
Roxanol 2365

Nefazodone Hydrochloride (Concurrent use with drugs that are substrate for cytochrome $P_{450}IID_6$ may make normal metabolizer resemble poor metabolizer leading to higher than expected plasma concentrations of TCA with resultant toxicity). Products include:
Serzone Tablets 776

Norepinephrine Bitartrate (Avoid concurrent use since tricyclic antidepressants can potentiate the effects of catecholamines). Products include:
Levophed Bitartrate Injection 2445

Nortriptyline Hydrochloride (Concurrent use with drugs that are substrate for cytochrome $P_{450}IID_6$ may make normal metabolizer resemble poor metabolizer leading to higher than expected plasma concentrations of TCA with resultant toxicity). Products include:
Pamelor 2409

Opium Alkaloids (Imipramine may potentiate the effects of CNS depressant drugs).
No products indexed under this heading.

Oxazepam (Imipramine may potentiate the effects of CNS depressant drugs). Products include:
Serax Capsules 2916
Serax Tablets 2916

Oxybutynin Chloride (Concurrent use may result in pronounced atropine-like effects e.g., paralytic ileus). Products include:
Ditropan 1267

Oxycodone Hydrochloride (Imipramine may potentiate the effects of CNS depressant drugs). Products include:
OxyContin Tablets 2163
OxyIR Capsules 2167
Percocet Tablets 955
Percodan Tablets 955
Percodan-Demi Tablets 956
Roxicodone Tablets, Oral Solution & Intensol (Oxycodone) 2366
Tylox Capsules 1593

Paroxetine Hydrochloride (Concurrent use with drugs that are substrate for cytochrome $P_{450}IID_6$ may make normal metabolizer resemble poor metabolizer leading to higher than expected plasma concentrations of TCA with resultant toxicity; due to variation in the extent of inhibition of $P_{450}IID_6$ caution is indicated if co-administered sufficient time must elapse). Products include:
Paxil Tablets 2681

Pentobarbital Sodium (The plasma concentration of imipramine may decrease when the drug is given with barbiturates, a hepatic enzyme inducer; dosage of imipramine may need to be adjusted; imipramine may potentiate the effects of CNS depressant drugs). Products include:
Nembutal Sodium Capsules 440
Nembutal Sodium Solution 442
Nembutal Sodium Suppositories 444

Perphenazine (Concurrent use with drugs that are substrate for cytochrome $P_{450}IID_6$ may make normal metabolizer resemble poor metabolizer leading to higher than expected plasma concentrations of TCA with resultant toxicity; imipramine may potentiate the effects of CNS depressant drugs). Products include:
Etrafon 2495
Triavil Tablets 1800
Trilafon 2532

Phenelzine Sulfate (Potential for hyperpyretic crises, severe convulsions, and deaths; concurrent and/or sequential use is contraindicated). Products include:
Nardil 1977

Phenobarbital (The plasma concentration of imipramine may decrease when the drug is given with barbiturates, a hepatic enzyme inducer; dosage of imipramine may need to be adjusted; imipramine may potentiate the effects of CNS depressant drugs). Products include:
Arco-Lase Plus Tablets 513
Bellergal-S Tablets 2375
Donnatal 2234
Donnatal Extentabs 2234
Donnatal Tablets 2234
Phenobarbital Elixir and Tablets 1523
Quadrinal Tablets 1398

Phenylephrine Bitartrate (Avoid concurrent use since tricyclic antidepressants can potentiate the effects of catecholamines).
No products indexed under this heading.

Phenylephrine Hydrochloride (Avoid concurrent use since tricyclic antidepressants can potentiate the effects of catecholamines). Products include:
Atrohist Plus Tablets 1605
Cerose DM 853
D.A. II Tablets 972
D.A. Chewable Tablets 970
Dura-Vent/DA Tablets 972
Extendryl 1003
4-Way Fast Acting Nasal Spray (regular & mentholated) 644
Hemorid 797
Hycomine Compound Tablets 948
Neo-Synephrine Hydrochloride 1% Carpuject 2455
Neo-Synephrine Hydrochloride 1% Injection 2455
Neo-Synephrine Hydrochloride (Ophthalmic) 2456
Neo-Synephrine 624
Novahistine Elixir 782
Phenergan VC 2886
Phenergan VC with Codeine 2888
Preparation H 842
Tympagesic Ear Drops 2476
Vicks Sinex Nasal Spray and Ultra Fine Mist 738

Phenylephrine Tannate (Avoid concurrent use since tricyclic antidepressants can potentiate the effects of catecholamines). Products include:
Atrohist Pediatric Suspension 1604
Atrohist Pediatric Suspension Dye-Free 1604
Rynatan 2781
Rynatuss 2782

IMPORTANT NOTE: Always consult each drug listing in the patient's regimen for possible interactions.

Phenylpropanolamine Hydrochloride (Avoid concurrent use since tricyclic antidepressants can potentiate the effects of catecholamines). Products include:

Acutrim	⊞ 648
Atrohist Plus Tablets	1605
BC Cold Powder Multi-Symptom Formula (Cold-Sinus-Allergy)	⊞ 631
BC Cold Powder Non-Drowsy Formula (Cold-Sinus)	⊞ 631
Cheracol Plus Head Cold/Cough Formula	⊞ 741
Comtrex Multi-Symptom Cold Reliever Liqui-Gels	⊞ 638
Comtrex Multi-Symptom Non-Drowsy Liqui-gels	⊞ 640
Contac Continuous Action Nasal Decongestant/Antihistamine 12 Hour Capsules	⊞ 773
Contac Maximum Strength Continuous Action Decongestant/Antihistamine 12 Hour Caplets	⊞ 772
Contac Severe Cold and Flu Formula Caplets	⊞ 773
Coricidin 'D' Decongestant Tablets	⊞ 760
Dexatrim	⊞ 795
Dexatrim Plus Vitamins Caplets	⊞ 796
Dimetane-DC Cough Syrup	2232
Dimetapp Allergy Sinus Caplets	⊞ 838
Dimetapp Cold & Allergy Chewable Tablets	⊞ 838
Dimetapp Cold & Cough Liqui-Gels	⊞ 839
Dimetapp DM Elixir	⊞ 840
Dimetapp Elixir	⊞ 840
Dimetapp Extentabs	⊞ 841
Dimetapp Tablets/Liqui-Gels	⊞ 841
Dura-Vent Tablets	971
Entex LA Tablets	972
Exgest LA Tablets	787
Hycomine	947
Nolamine Timed-Release Tablets	790
Ornade Spansule Capsules	2678
Propagest Tablets	791
Pyrroxate Caplets	⊞ 742
Robitussin-CF	⊞ 846
Sinulin Tablets	792
Tavist-D 12 Hour Relief Tablets	⊞ 786
Teldrin 12 Hour Antihistamine/Nasal Decongestant Allergy Relief Capsules	⊞ 786
Triaminic Expectorant	⊞ 753
Triaminic Syrup	⊞ 755
Triaminic Triaminicol Cold & Cough	⊞ 756
Triaminic DM Syrup	⊞ 756
Triaminicin Tablets	⊞ 756
Vicks DayQuil Allergy Relief 12-Hour Extended Release Tablets	⊞ 733
Vicks DayQuil Allergy Relief 4-Hour Tablets	⊞ 733
Vicks DayQuil SINUS Pressure & CONGESTION Relief	⊞ 734

Phenytoin (The plasma concentration of imipramine may decrease when the drug is given with phenytoin, a hepatic enzyme inducer; dosage of imipramine may need to be adjusted). Products include:

Dilantin Infatabs	1967
Dilantin-125 Suspension	1969

Phenytoin Sodium (The plasma concentration of imipramine may decrease when the drug is given with phenytoin, a hepatic enzyme inducer; dosage of imipramine may need to be adjusted). Products include:

Dilantin Kapseals	1965

Pirbuterol Acetate (Avoid concurrent use since tricyclic antidepressants can potentiate the effects of catecholamines). Products include:

Maxair Autohaler	1550
Maxair Inhaler	1552

Prazepam (Imipramine may potentiate the effects of CNS depressant drugs).
No products indexed under this heading.

Prochlorperazine (Concurrent use with drugs that are substrate for cytochrome $P_{450}IID_6$ may make normal metabolizer resemble poor metabolizer leading to higher than expected plasma concentrations of TCA with resultant toxicity; imipramine may potentiate the effects of CNS depressant drugs). Products include:

Compazine	2644

Procyclidine Hydrochloride (Concurrent use may result in pronounced atropine-like effects e.g., paralytic ileus). Products include:

Kemadrin Tablets	1105

Promethazine Hydrochloride (Concurrent use with drugs that are substrate for cytochrome $P_{450}IID_6$ may make normal metabolizer resemble poor metabolizer leading to higher than expected plasma concentrations of TCA with resultant toxicity; imipramine may potentiate the effects of CNS depressant drugs). Products include:

Mepergan Injection	2859
Phenergan with Codeine	2883
Phenergan with Dextromethorphan	2885
Phenergan Injection	2880
Phenergan Suppositories	2882
Phenergan Syrup	2881
Phenergan Tablets	2882
Phenergan VC	2886
Phenergan VC with Codeine	2888

Propafenone Hydrochloride (Concurrent use with drugs that are substrate for cytochrome $P_{450}IID_6$ may make normal metabolizer resemble poor metabolizer leading to higher than expected plasma concentrations of TCA with resultant toxicity). Products include:

Rythmol Tablets–150mg, 225mg, 300mg	1399

Propantheline Bromide (Concurrent use may result in pronounced atropine-like effects e.g., paralytic ileus). Products include:

Pro-Banthine Tablets	2226

Propofol (Imipramine may potentiate the effects of CNS depressant drugs). Products include:

Diprivan Injectable Emulsion	2939

Propoxyphene Hydrochloride (Imipramine may potentiate the effects of CNS depressant drugs). Products include:

Darvon	1475
Wygesic Tablets	2930

Propoxyphene Napsylate (Imipramine may potentiate the effects of CNS depressant drugs). Products include:

Darvon-N/Darvocet-N	1473

Protriptyline Hydrochloride (Concurrent use with drugs that are substrate for cytochrome $P_{450}IID_6$ may make normal metabolizer resemble poor metabolizer leading to higher than expected plasma concentrations of TCA with resultant toxicity). Products include:

Vivactil Tablets	1820

Pseudoephedrine Hydrochloride (Avoid concurrent use since tricyclic antidepressants can potentiate the effects of catecholamines). Products include:

Actifed Allergy Daytime/Nighttime Caplets	⊞ 808
Actifed Cold & Allergy Tablets	⊞ 807
Actifed Cold & Sinus Caplets and Tablets	⊞ 808
Actifed Sinus Daytime/Nighttime Tablets and Caplets	⊞ 809
Advil Cold and Sinus Caplets and Tablets	⊞ 837
Alka-Seltzer Plus Liqui-Gels	⊞ 612
Alka-Seltzer Plus Flu & Body Aches Liqui-Gels Non-Drowsy Formula	⊞ 613
Alka-Seltzer Plus Night-Time Cold Medicine Liqui-Gels	⊞ 612
Allerest Maximum Strength	⊞ 649
Allerest No Drowsiness	⊞ 649
Allerest Sinus Pain Formula	⊞ 649
Atrohist Pediatric Capsules	1603
Benadryl Allergy/Cold Tablets	⊞ 811
Benadryl Allergy Decongestant Liquid Medication	⊞ 812
Benadryl Allergy Decongestant Tablets	⊞ 812
Benadryl Allergy Sinus Headache Caplets	⊞ 813
Benylin Multisymptom	⊞ 816
Bromfed Capsules (Extended-Release)	1832
Bromfed Syrup	⊞ 712
Bromfed Tablets	1832
Bromfed-DM Cough Syrup	1832
Bromfed-PD Capsules (Extended-Release)	1832
Children's TYLENOL Cold Multi-Symptom Chewable Tablets and Liquid	1559
Children's TYLENOL Cold Plus Cough Multi Symptom Chewable Tablets and Liquid	1560
Children's TYLENOL Flu Suspension Liquid	1560
Children's Vicks DayQuil Allergy Relief	⊞ 730
Children's Vicks NyQuil Cold/Cough Relief	⊞ 731
Allergy-Sinus Comtrex Multi-Symptom Allergy-Sinus Formula Tablets and Caplets	⊞ 639
Comtrex Multi-Symptom	⊞ 638
Comtrex Multi-Symptom Non-Drowsy Caplets	⊞ 640
Congess	1003
Contac Day Allergy/Sinus Caplets	⊞ 771
Contac Day & Night	⊞ 772
Contac Night Allergy/Sinus Caplets	⊞ 771
Contac Severe Cold & Flu Non-Drowsy	⊞ 774
Deconsal II Tablets	1605
Dimetane-DX Cough Syrup	2233
Dimetapp Cold & Fever Suspension	⊞ 839
Dimetapp Decongestant Pediatric Drops	⊞ 840
Dorcol Children's Cough Syrup	⊞ 748
Drixoral Cough + Congestion Liquid Caps	⊞ 763
Dura-Tap/PD Capsules	970
Duratuss Tablets	2750
Duratuss HD Elixir	2750
Efidac/24	⊞ 655
Entex PSE Tablets	973
Fedahist Gyrocaps	2545
Guaifed	1833
Guaifed Syrup	⊞ 712
Guaimax-D Tablets	809
Histussin D Liquid	670
Infants' TYLENOL Cold Decongestant & Fever-Reducer Drops	1561
Kronofed-A	994
Novahistine DMX	⊞ 782
Nucofed	2225
PediaCare Cough-Cold Chewable Tablets and Liquid	1569
PediaCare Infants' Decongestant Drops	1569
PediaCare Infants' Drops Decongestant Plus Cough	1569
PediaCare NightRest Cough-Cold Liquid	1569
Pediatric Vicks 44d Cough & Head Congestion Relief	⊞ 736
Pediatric Vicks 44m Cough & Cold Relief	⊞ 737
Robitussin Cold & Cough Liqui-Gels	⊞ 844
Robitussin Cold, Cough & Flu Liqui-Gels	⊞ 844
Robitussin Maximum Strength Cough & Cold	⊞ 847
Robitussin Night-Time Cold Formula	⊞ 847
Robitussin Pediatric Cough & Cold Formula	⊞ 848
Robitussin Pediatric Drops	⊞ 849
Robitussin Severe Congestion Liqui-Gels	⊞ 845
Robitussin-DAC Syrup	2249
Robitussin-PE	⊞ 846
Rondec Oral Drops	974
Rondec Syrup	974
Rondec Tablet	974
Rondec Chewable Tablets	974
Rondec-TR Tablet	974
Ryna	⊞ 804
Seldane-D Extended-Release Tablets	1286
Semprex-D Capsules	1620
Sinarest	⊞ 663
Sine-Aid Maximum Strength Sinus Headache Gelcaps, Caplets and Tablets	1570
Sine-Off No Drowsiness Formula Caplets	⊞ 784
Sine-Off Sinus Medicine	⊞ 784
Singlet Tablets	⊞ 785
Sinutab Non-Drying Liquid Caps	⊞ 823
Sinutab Sinus Allergy Medication, Maximum Strength Tablets and Caplets	⊞ 823
Sinutab Sinus Medication, Maximum Strength Without Drowsiness Formula, Tablets & Caplets	⊞ 824
Sudafed Children's Cold & Cough Liquid Medication	⊞ 825
Sudafed Children's Nasal Decongestant Liquid Medication	⊞ 826
Sudafed Cold & Allergy Tablets	⊞ 826
Sudafed Cold and Cough Liquid Caps	⊞ 826
Sudafed Nasal Decongestant Tablets, 30 mg	⊞ 825
Sudafed Nasal Decongestant Tablets, 60 mg	⊞ 825
Sudafed Non-Drying Sinus Liquid Caps	⊞ 827
Sudafed Pediatric Nasal Decongestant Liquid Oral Drops	⊞ 827
Sudafed Severe Cold Formula Caplets	⊞ 828
Sudafed Severe Cold Formula Tablets	⊞ 828
Sudafed Sinus Caplets	⊞ 829
Sudafed Sinus Tablets	⊞ 829
Sudafed 12 Hour Caplets	⊞ 824
Syn-Rx Tablets	1622
Syn-Rx DM Tablets	1623
TheraFlu Flu and Cold Medicine	⊞ 750
TheraFlu Maximum Strength Flu and Cold Medicine For Sore Throat	⊞ 751
TheraFlu Flu, Cold and Cough Medicine	⊞ 750
TheraFlu Maximum Strength Nighttime Flu, Cold & Cough Medicine	⊞ 751
TheraFlu Maximum Strength Non-Drowsy Formula Flu, Cold & Cough Medicine	⊞ 751
TheraFlu Maximum Strength, Non-Drowsy Formula Flu, Cold and Cough Caplets	⊞ 752
Theraflu Maximum Strength Sinus Non-Drowsy Formula Caplets	⊞ 752
Triaminic AM Cough and Decongestant Formula	⊞ 753
Triaminic AM Decongestant Formula	⊞ 753
Triaminic Infant Oral Decongestant Drops	⊞ 754
Triaminic Night Time	⊞ 754
Triaminic Sore Throat Formula	⊞ 755
Tussend	1830
Tussend Expectorant	1831
TYLENOL Allergy Sinus, Maximum Strength Caplets and Gelcaps	1571
TYLENOL Allergy Sinus NightTime, Maximum Strength Caplets	1571
TYLENOL Cold Medication, Multi-Symptom Formula Tablets and Caplets	1572
TYLENOL Cold Medication, Multi-Symptom Hot Liquid Packets	1572
TYLENOL Cold Medication, No Drowsiness Formula Caplets and Gelcaps	1572
TYLENOL Cold Severe Congestion Caplets	1573
TYLENOL Cough Medication with Decongestant, Multi Symptom	1574
TYLENOL Flu No Drowsiness Formula, Maximum Strength Gelcaps	1575
TYLENOL Flu NightTime, Maximum Strength Gelcaps	1575
TYLENOL Flu Maximum Strength Hot Medication Packets	1575

(⊞ Described in PDR For Nonprescription Drugs) (⊙ Described in PDR For Ophthalmology)

TYLENOL Sinus, Maximum Strength Geltabs, Gelcaps, Caplets and Tablets 1576
Vicks 44 LiquiCaps Cough, Cold & Flu Relief 728
Vicks 44 LiquiCaps Non-Drowsy Cough & Cold Relief 729
Vicks 44D Cough & Head Congestion Relief 728
Vicks 44M Cough, Cold & Flu Relief 729
Vicks DayQuil LiquiCaps/Liquid Multi-Symptom Cold/Flu Relief .. 734
Vicks DayQuil SINUS Pressure & PAIN Relief with IBUPROFEN 735
Vicks Nyquil Hot Therapy 735
Vicks NyQuil LiquiCaps/Liquid Multi-Symptom Cold/Flu Relief, Original and Cherry Flavors 736

Pseudoephedrine Sulfate (Avoid concurrent use since tricyclic antidepressants can potentiate the effects of catecholamines). Products include:
Chlor-Trimeton Allergy Decongestant Tablets 759
Claritin-D Tablets 2487
Drixoral Cold and Allergy Sustained-Action Tablets 763
Drixoral Cold and Flu Extended-Release Tablets 764
Drixoral Non-Drowsy Formula Extended-Release Tablets 764
Drixoral Allergy/Sinus Extended Release Tablets 765
Trinalin Repetabs Tablets 1373

Quazepam (Imipramine may potentiate the effects of CNS depressant drugs). Products include:
Doral Tablets 2773

Quinidine Gluconate (Concurrent use with drugs that inhibit cytochrome $P_{450}IID_6$ may make normal metabolizer resemble poor metabolizer leading to higher than expected plasma concentrations of TCA with resultant toxicity). Products include:
Quinaglute Dura-Tabs Tablets 644

Quinidine Polygalacturonate (Concurrent use with drugs that inhibit cytochrome $P_{450}IID_6$ may make normal metabolizer resemble poor metabolizer leading to higher than expected plasma concentrations of TCA with resultant toxicity). Products include:
Cardioquin Tablets 2146

Quinidine Sulfate (Concurrent use with drugs that inhibit cytochrome $P_{450}IID_6$ may make normal metabolizer resemble poor metabolizer leading to higher than expected plasma concentrations of TCA with resultant toxicity). Products include:
Quinidex Extentabs 2240

Risperidone (Imipramine may potentiate the effects of CNS depressant drugs). Products include:
Risperdal Tablets 1348

Salmeterol Xinafoate (Avoid concurrent use since tricyclic antidepressants can potentiate the effects of catecholamines). Products include:
Serevent Inhalation Aerosol 1149

Scopolamine (Concurrent use may result in pronounced atropine-like effects e.g., paralytic ileus). Products include:
Transderm Scōp Transdermal Therapeutic System 890

Scopolamine Hydrobromide (Concurrent use may result in pronounced atropine-like effects e.g., paralytic ileus). Products include:
Atrohist Plus Tablets 1605
Donnatal 2234
Donnatal Extentabs 2234
Donnatal Tablets 2234

Secobarbital Sodium (The plasma concentration of imipramine may decrease when the drug is given with barbiturates, a hepatic enzyme inducer; dosage of imipramine may need to be adjusted; imipramine may potentiate the effects of CNS depressant drugs). Products include:
Seconal Sodium Pulvules 1529

Selegiline Hydrochloride (Potential for hyperpyretic crises, severe convulsions, and deaths; concurrent and/or sequential use is contraindicated). Products include:
Eldepryl Capsules 2729

Sertraline Hydrochloride (Concurrent use with drugs that are substrate for cytochrome $P_{450}IID_6$ may make normal metabolizer resemble poor metabolizer leading to higher than expected plasma concentrations of TCA with resultant toxicity; due to variation in the extent of inhibition of $P_{450}IID_6$ caution is indicated if co-administered sufficient time must elapse). Products include:
Zoloft Tablets 2051

Sevoflurane (Imipramine may potentiate the effects of CNS depressant drugs).
No products indexed under this heading.

Sufentanil Citrate (Imipramine may potentiate the effects of CNS depressant drugs). Products include:
Sufenta Injection 1355

Temazepam (Imipramine may potentiate the effects of CNS depressant drugs). Products include:
Restoril Capsules 2413

Terbutaline Sulfate (Avoid concurrent use since tricyclic antidepressants can potentiate the effects of catecholamines). Products include:
Brethaire Inhaler 830
Brethine Ampuls 832
Brethine Tablets 831
Bricanyl Subcutaneous Injection 1247
Bricanyl Tablets 1248

Thiamylal Sodium (The plasma concentration of imipramine may decrease when the drug is given with barbiturates, a hepatic enzyme inducer; dosage of imipramine may need to be adjusted; imipramine may potentiate the effects of CNS depressant drugs).
No products indexed under this heading.

Thioridazine Hydrochloride (Concurrent use with drugs that are substrate for cytochrome $P_{450}IID_6$ may make normal metabolizer resemble poor metabolizer leading to higher than expected plasma concentrations of TCA with resultant toxicity; imipramine may potentiate the effects of CNS depressant drugs). Products include:
Mellaril 2398

Thiothixene (Imipramine may potentiate the effects of CNS depressant drugs). Products include:
Navane Capsules and Concentrate 2018
Navane Intramuscular 2019

Thyroglobulin (Co-administration may produce cardiovascular toxicity).
No products indexed under this heading.

Thyroid (Co-administration may produce cardiovascular toxicity).
No products indexed under this heading.

Thyroxine (Co-administration may produce cardiovascular toxicity).
No products indexed under this heading.

Thyroxine Sodium (Co-administration may produce cardiovascular toxicity).
No products indexed under this heading.

Tranylcypromine Sulfate (Potential for hyperpyretic crises, severe convulsions, and deaths; concurrent and/or sequential use is contraindicated). Products include:
Parnate Tablets 2679

Trazodone Hydrochloride (Concurrent use with drugs that are substrate for cytochrome $P_{450}IID_6$ may make normal metabolizer resemble poor metabolizer leading to higher than expected plasma concentrations of TCA with resultant toxicity). Products include:
Desyrel and Desyrel Dividose 504

Triazolam (Imipramine may potentiate the effects of CNS depressant drugs). Products include:
Halcion Tablets 2093

Tridihexethyl Chloride (Concurrent use may result in pronounced atropine-like effects e.g., paralytic ileus).
No products indexed under this heading.

Trifluoperazine Hydrochloride (Concurrent use with drugs that are substrate for cytochrome $P_{450}IID_6$ may make normal metabolizer resemble poor metabolizer leading to higher than expected plasma concentrations of TCA with resultant toxicity; imipramine may potentiate the effects of CNS depressant drugs). Products include:
Stelazine 2692

Trihexyphenidyl Hydrochloride (Concurrent use may result in pronounced atropine-like effects e.g., paralytic ileus). Products include:
Artane 1418

Trimipramine Maleate (Concurrent use with drugs that are substrate for cytochrome $P_{450}IID_6$ may make normal metabolizer resemble poor metabolizer leading to higher than expected plasma concentrations of TCA with resultant toxicity). Products include:
Surmontil Capsules 2917

Venlafaxine Hydrochloride (Concurrent use with drugs that are substrate for cytochrome $P_{450}IID_6$ may make normal metabolizer resemble poor metabolizer leading to higher than expected plasma concentrations of TCA with resultant toxicity; due to variation in the extent of inhibition of $P_{450}IID_6$ caution is indicated if co-administered sufficient time must elapse). Products include:
Effexor 2825

Zolpidem Tartrate (Imipramine may potentiate the effects of CNS depressant drugs). Products include:
Ambien Tablets 2559

Food Interactions

Alcohol (Imipramine may enhance the CNS depressant effects of alcohol).

TOFRANIL TABLETS

(Imipramine Hydrochloride) 875
May interact with central nervous system depressants, anticholinergics, sympathomimetics, barbiturates, monoamine oxidase inhibitors, thyroid preparations, antidepressant drugs, phenothiazines, quinidine, and certain other agents. Compounds in these categories include:

Albuterol (Tricyclic antidepressants can potentiate the effects of sympathomimetics). Products include:
Proventil Inhalation Aerosol 2524
Ventolin Inhalation Aerosol and Refill 1170

Albuterol Sulfate (Tricyclic antidepressants can potentiate the effects of sympathomimetics). Products include:
Airet Albuterol Sulfate Inhalation Solution 1602
Albuterol Sulfate, USP Solution for Inhalation, Arm-a-Med 522
Proventil Inhalation Solution 0.083% 2527
Proventil Repetabs Tablets 2529
Proventil Solution for Inhalation 0.5% 2525
Proventil Syrup 2528
Proventil Tablets 2529
Ventolin Inhalation Solution 1171
Ventolin Nebules Inhalation Solution 1172
Ventolin Rotacaps for Inhalation 1173
Ventolin Syrup 1175
Ventolin Tablets 1176
Volmax Extended-Release Tablets .. 1835

Alfentanil Hydrochloride (Imipramine may potentiate the effects of CNS depressant drugs). Products include:
Alfenta Injection 1334

Alprazolam (Imipramine may potentiate the effects of CNS depressant drugs). Products include:
Xanax Tablets 2115

Amitriptyline Hydrochloride (May inhibit the activity of cytochrome P450 2D6 isoenzyme and are substrates for P450 2D6 and may make normal metabolizers resemble poor metabolizers resulting in higher than expected plasma levels of tricyclic antidepressants). Products include:
Elavil 2945
Etrafon 2495
Limbitrol 2333
Triavil Tablets 1800

Amoxapine (May inhibit the activity of cytochrome P450 2D6 isoenzyme and are substrates for P450 2D6 and may make normal metabolizers resemble poor metabolizers resulting in higher than expected plasma levels of tricyclic antidepressants). Products include:
Asendin Tablets 1419

Aprobarbital (Co-administration with hepatic enzyme inducers, such as barbiturates, may decrease imipramine plasma concentrations; imipramine may potentiate the effects of CNS depressant drugs).
No products indexed under this heading.

Atropine Sulfate (Co-administration may result in increased atropine-like effects such as paralytic ileus). Products include:
Arco-Lase Plus Tablets 513
Atrohist Plus Tablets 1605
Donnatal 2234
Donnatal Extentabs 2234
Donnatal Tablets 2234
Lomotil 2591
Motofen Tablets 789
Urised Tablets 2123

Belladonna Alkaloids (Co-administration may result in increased atropine-like effects such as paralytic ileus). Products include:
Bellergal-S Tablets 2375
Hyland's Bedwetting Tablets 788
Hyland's EnurAid Tablets 789
Hyland's Headache Tablets 790
Hyland's Teething Tablets 790
Similasan Eye Drops #1 769

IMPORTANT NOTE: Always consult each drug listing in the patient's regimen for possible interactions.

Benztropine Mesylate (Co-administration may result in increased atropine-like effects such as paralytic ileus). Products include:
Cogentin 1661

Biperiden Hydrochloride (Co-administration may result in increased atropine-like effects such as paralytic ileus). Products include:
Akineton 1380

Buprenorphine (Imipramine may potentiate the effects of CNS depressant drugs). Products include:
Buprenex Injectable 2170

Bupropion Hydrochloride (May inhibit the activity of cytochrome P450 2D6 isoenzyme and are substrates for P450 2D6 and may make normal metabolizers resemble poor metabolizers resulting in higher than expected plasma levels of tricyclic antidepressants). Products include:
Wellbutrin Tablets 1177

Buspirone Hydrochloride (Imipramine may potentiate the effects of CNS depressant drugs). Products include:
BuSpar Tablets 738

Butabarbital (Co-administration with hepatic enzyme inducers, such as barbiturates, may decrease imipramine plasma concentrations; imipramine may potentiate the effects of CNS depressant drugs).
No products indexed under this heading.

Butalbital (Co-administration with hepatic enzyme inducers, such as barbiturates, may decrease imipramine plasma concentrations; imipramine may potentiate the effects of CNS depressant drugs). Products include:
Axocet Capsules 2469
Esgic-plus Capsules 1012
Esgic-plus Tablets 1012
Fioricet Tablets 2386
Fioricet with Codeine Capsules 2387
Fiorinal Capsules 2388
Fiorinal with Codeine Capsules 2390
Fiorinal Tablets 2388
Phrenilin 790
Sedapap Tablets 50 mg/650 mg .. 1826

Chlordiazepoxide (Imipramine may potentiate the effects of CNS depressant drugs). Products include:
Limbitrol 2333

Chlordiazepoxide Hydrochloride (Imipramine may potentiate the effects of CNS depressant drugs). Products include:
Librax Capsules 2330
Librium Capsules 2331
Librium Injectable 2332

Chlorpromazine (May inhibit the activity of cytochrome P450 2D6 isoenzyme and are substrates for P450 2D6 and may make normal metabolizers resemble poor metabolizers resulting in higher than expected plasma levels of tricyclic antidepressants). Products include:
Thorazine Suppositories 2701

Chlorpromazine Hydrochloride (May inhibit the activity of cytochrome P450 2D6 isoenzyme and are substrates for P450 2D6 and may make normal metabolizers resemble poor metabolizers resulting in higher than expected plasma levels of tricyclic antidepressants). Products include:
Thorazine 2701

Chlorprothixene (Imipramine may potentiate the effects of CNS depressant drugs).
No products indexed under this heading.

Chlorprothixene Hydrochloride (Imipramine may potentiate the effects of CNS depressant drugs).
No products indexed under this heading.

Chlorprothixene Lactate (Imipramine may potentiate the effects of CNS depressant drugs).
No products indexed under this heading.

Cimetidine (Co-administration with hepatic enzyme inhibitors, such as cimetidine, may increase imipramine plasma concentrations). Products include:
Tagamet HB Tablets .... ▣ 786
Tagamet Tablets 2694

Cimetidine Hydrochloride (Co-administration with hepatic enzyme inhibitors, such as cimetidine, may increase imipramine plasma concentrations). Products include:
Tagamet 2694

Clidinium Bromide (Co-administration may result in increased atropine-like effects such as paralytic ileus). Products include:
Librax Capsules 2330

Clonidine (Imipramine may block the pharmacological effects). Products include:
Catapres-TTS 680

Clonidine Hydrochloride (Imipramine may block the pharmacological effects). Products include:
Catapres Tablets 679
Combipres Tablets 682

Clorazepate Dipotassium (Imipramine may potentiate the effects of CNS depressant drugs). Products include:
Tranxene 459

Clozapine (Imipramine may potentiate the effects of CNS depressant drugs). Products include:
Clozaril Tablets 2377

Codeine Phosphate (Imipramine may potentiate the effects of CNS depressant drugs). Products include:
Brontex 2130
Dimetane-DC Cough Syrup 2232
Fioricet with Codeine Capsules 2387
Fiorinal with Codeine Capsules 2390
Nucofed 2225
Phenergan with Codeine 2883
Phenergan VC with Codeine 2888
Robitussin A-C Syrup 2248
Robitussin-DAC Syrup 2249
Ryna .... ▣ 804
Soma Compound w/Codeine Tablets 2784
Tylenol with Codeine 1592

Desflurane (Imipramine may potentiate the effects of CNS depressant drugs). Products include:
Suprane (desflurane, USP) 1865

Desipramine Hydrochloride (May inhibit the activity of cytochrome P450 2D6 isoenzyme and are substrates for P450 2D6 and may make normal metabolizers resemble poor metabolizers resulting in higher than expected plasma levels of tricyclic antidepressants). Products include:
Norpramin Tablets 1273

Dezocine (Imipramine may potentiate the effects of CNS depressant drugs). Products include:
Dalgan Injection 529

Diazepam (Imipramine may potentiate the effects of CNS depressant drugs). Products include:
Dizac (diazepam injectable emulsion) CIV 1862
Valium Injectable 2336
Valium Tablets 2335

Dicyclomine Hydrochloride (Co-administration may result in increased atropine-like effects such as paralytic ileus). Products include:
Bentyl 1246

Dobutamine Hydrochloride (Tricyclic antidepressants can potentiate the effects of sympathomimetics). Products include:
Dobutrex Solution Vials 1480

Dopamine Hydrochloride (Tricyclic antidepressants can potentiate the effects of sympathomimetics).
No products indexed under this heading.

Doxepin Hydrochloride (May inhibit the activity of cytochrome P450 2D6 isoenzyme and are substrates for P450 2D6 and may make normal metabolizers resemble poor metabolizers resulting in higher than expected plasma levels of tricyclic antidepressants). Products include:
Adapin Capsules 1542
Sinequan 2028
Zonalon Cream 1042

Droperidol (Imipramine may potentiate the effects of CNS depressant drugs). Products include:
Inapsine Injection 462

Enflurane (Imipramine may potentiate the effects of CNS depressant drugs).
No products indexed under this heading.

Ephedrine Hydrochloride (Tricyclic antidepressants can potentiate the effects of sympathomimetics). Products include:
Primatene Tablets .... ▣ 844
Quadrinal Tablets 1398

Ephedrine Sulfate (Tricyclic antidepressants can potentiate the effects of sympathomimetics). Products include:
Marax Tablets & DF Syrup 2015

Ephedrine Tannate (Tricyclic antidepressants can potentiate the effects of sympathomimetics). Products include:
Rynatuss 2782

Epinephrine (Tricyclic antidepressants can potentiate the effects of sympathomimetics). Products include:
EPIFRIN .... ◉ 237
EpiPen 808
Marcaine with Epinephrine 2446
Primatene Mist .... ▣ 843
Sensorcaine with Epinephrine Injection 554
Sus-Phrine Injection 1017
Xylocaine with Epinephrine Injections 562

Epinephrine Bitartrate (Tricyclic antidepressants can potentiate the effects of sympathomimetics). Products include:
Sensorcaine-MPF with Epinephrine Injection 554

Epinephrine Hydrochloride (Tricyclic antidepressants can potentiate the effects of sympathomimetics). Products include:
Ana-Kit Anaphylaxis Emergency Treatment Kit 611

Estazolam (Imipramine may potentiate the effects of CNS depressant drugs). Products include:
ProSom Tablets 457

Ethchlorvynol (Imipramine may potentiate the effects of CNS depressant drugs). Products include:
Placidyl Capsules 456

Ethinamate (Imipramine may potentiate the effects of CNS depressant drugs).
No products indexed under this heading.

Fentanyl (Imipramine may potentiate the effects of CNS depressant drugs). Products include:
Duragesic Transdermal System 1336

Fentanyl Citrate (Imipramine may potentiate the effects of CNS depressant drugs). Products include:
Sublimaze Injection 463

Flecainide Acetate (May inhibit the activity of cytochrome P450 2D6 isoenzyme and are substrates for P450 2D6 and may make normal metabolizers resemble poor metabolizers resulting in higher than expected plasma levels of tricyclic antidepressants). Products include:
Tambocor Tablets 1555

Fluoxetine Hydrochloride (Co-administration with hepatic enzyme inhibitors, such as fluoxetine, may increase imipramine plasma concentrations; due to long half-life of fluoxetine, at least 5 weeks should elapse before initiating TCA treatment in a patient being withdrawn from fluoxetine). Products include:
Prozac Pulvules & Liquid, Oral Solution 935

Fluphenazine Decanoate (May inhibit the activity of cytochrome P450 2D6 isoenzyme and are substrates for P450 2D6 and may make normal metabolizers resemble poor metabolizers resulting in higher than expected plasma levels of tricyclic antidepressants). Products include:
Prolixin Decanoate 510

Fluphenazine Enanthate (May inhibit the activity of cytochrome P450 2D6 isoenzyme and are substrates for P450 2D6 and may make normal metabolizers resemble poor metabolizers resulting in higher than expected plasma levels of tricyclic antidepressants). Products include:
Prolixin Enanthate 510

Fluphenazine Hydrochloride (May inhibit the activity of cytochrome P450 2D6 isoenzyme and are substrates for P450 2D6 and may make normal metabolizers resemble poor metabolizers resulting in higher than expected plasma levels of tricyclic antidepressants). Products include:
Prolixin 510

Flurazepam Hydrochloride (Imipramine may potentiate the effects of CNS depressant drugs). Products include:
Dalmane Capsules 2329

Fosphenytoin Sodium (Co-administration with hepatic enzyme inducers, such as phenytoin, may decrease imipramine plasma concentrations). Products include:
Cerebyx Injection 1956

Furazolidone (Co-administration of tricyclic antidepressants and MAO inhibitor has produced hyperpyretic crises, severe convulsions, and deaths; concurrent and/or sequential use is contraindicated). Products include:
Furoxone 2221

Glutethimide (Imipramine may potentiate the effects of CNS depressant drugs).
No products indexed under this heading.

(▣ Described in PDR For Nonprescription Drugs) (◉ Described in PDR For Ophthalmology)

Glycopyrrolate (Co-administration may result in increased atropine-like effects such as paralytic ileus). Products include:
- Robinul Forte Tablets 2247
- Robinul Injectable 2247
- Robinul Tablets 2247

Guanadrel Sulfate (Imipramine may block the pharmacological effects). Products include:
- Hylorel Tablets 1613

Guanethidine Monosulfate (Imipramine may block the pharmacological effects). Products include:
- Esimil Tablets 840
- Ismelin Tablets 845

Haloperidol (Imipramine may potentiate the effects of CNS depressant drugs). Products include:
- Haldol Injection, Tablets and Concentrate 1585

Haloperidol Decanoate (Imipramine may potentiate the effects of CNS depressant drugs). Products include:
- Haldol Decanoate 1587

Hydrocodone Bitartrate (Imipramine may potentiate the effects of CNS depressant drugs). Products include:
- Codiclear DH Syrup 808
- Duratuss HD Elixir 2750
- Histussin D Liquid 670
- Hycodan Tablets and Syrup 946
- Hycomine Compound Tablets 948
- Hycomine 947
- Hycotuss Expectorant Syrup 950
- Hydrocet Capsules 787
- Lorcet 10/650 Tablets 1016
- Lortab 2751
- Tussend 1830
- Tussend Expectorant 1831
- Vicodin Tablets 1404
- Vicodin ES Tablets 1405
- Vicodin HP Tablets 1403
- Vicodin Tuss Expectorant 1406
- Zydone Capsules 967

Hydrocodone Polistirex (Imipramine may potentiate the effects of CNS depressant drugs). Products include:
- Tussionex Pennkinetic Extended-Release Suspension 1624

Hydromorphone Hydrochloride (Imipramine may potentiate the effects of CNS depressant drugs). Products include:
- Dilaudid Ampules 1382
- Dilaudid Cough Syrup 1383
- Dilaudid-HP Injection 1384
- Dilaudid-HP Lyophilized Powder 250 mg 1384
- Dilaudid 1382
- Dilaudid Oral Liquid 1386
- Dilaudid 1382
- Dilaudid Tablets - 8 mg 1386

Hydroxyzine Hydrochloride (Imipramine may potentiate the effects of CNS depressant drugs). Products include:
- Atarax Tablets & Syrup 1992
- Marax Tablets & DF Syrup 2015
- Vistaril Intramuscular Solution 2042

Hyoscyamine (Co-administration may result in increased atropine-like effects such as paralytic ileus). Products include:
- Cystospaz Tablets 2123
- Urised Tablets 2123

Hyoscyamine Sulfate (Co-administration may result in increased atropine-like effects such as paralytic ileus). Products include:
- Arco-Lase Plus Tablets 513
- Atrohist Plus Tablets 1605
- Cystospaz-M Capsules 2123
- Donnatal 2234
- Donnatal Extentabs 2234
- Donnatal Tablets 2234
- Kutrase Capsules 2546
- Levsin/Levsinex/Levbid 2549

Imipramine Pamoate (May inhibit the activity of cytochrome P450 2D6 isoenzyme and are substrates for P450 2D6 and may make normal metabolizers resemble poor metabolizers resulting in higher than expected plasma levels of tricyclic antidepressants). Products include:
- Tofranil-PM Capsules 876

Ipratropium Bromide (Co-administration may result in increased atropine-like effects such as paralytic ileus). Products include:
- Atrovent Inhalation Aerosol 674
- Atrovent Inhalation Solution 675
- Atrovent Nasal Spray 0.03% 676
- Atrovent Nasal Spray 0.06% 678

Isocarboxazid (Co-administration of tricyclic antidepressants and MAO inhibitor has produced hyperpyretic crises, severe convulsions, and deaths; concurrent and/or sequential use is contraindicated).
No products indexed under this heading.

Isoflurane (Imipramine may potentiate the effects of CNS depressant drugs).
No products indexed under this heading.

Isoproterenol Hydrochloride (Tricyclic antidepressants can potentiate the effects of sympathomimetics). Products include:
- Isuprel Hydrochloride Solution 2443
- Isuprel Injection 2441
- Isuprel Mistometer 2442

Isoproterenol Sulfate (Tricyclic antidepressants can potentiate the effects of sympathomimetics). Products include:
- Norisodrine with Calcium Iodide Syrup 446

Ketamine Hydrochloride (Imipramine may potentiate the effects of CNS depressant drugs).
No products indexed under this heading.

Levomethadyl Acetate Hydrochloride (Imipramine may potentiate the effects of CNS depressant drugs). Products include:
- Orlaam Oral Solution 2361

Levorphanol Tartrate (Imipramine may potentiate the effects of CNS depressant drugs). Products include:
- Levo-Dromoran 2297

Levothyroxine Sodium (Possibility of cardiovascular toxicity). Products include:
- Eltroxin Tablets 2214
- Levothroid Tablets 1015
- Levothyroxine Sodium, USP for Injection 546
- Levoxyl Tablets 918
- Synthroid 1410

Liothyronine Sodium (Possibility of cardiovascular toxicity). Products include:
- Cytomel Tablets 2647
- Triostat Injection 2708

Liotrix (Possibility of cardiovascular toxicity).
No products indexed under this heading.

Lorazepam (Imipramine may potentiate the effects of CNS depressant drugs). Products include:
- Ativan Injection 2805
- Ativan Tablets 2807

Loxapine Hydrochloride (Imipramine may potentiate the effects of CNS depressant drugs). Products include:
- Loxitane 1426

Loxapine Succinate (Imipramine may potentiate the effects of CNS depressant drugs). Products include:
- Loxitane Capsules 1426

Maprotiline Hydrochloride (May inhibit the activity of cytochrome P450 2D6 isoenzyme and are substrates for P450 2D6 and may make normal metabolizers resemble poor metabolizers resulting in higher than expected plasma levels of tricyclic antidepressants). Products include:
- Ludiomil Tablets 861

Mepenzolate Bromide (Co-administration may result in increased atropine-like effects such as paralytic ileus).
No products indexed under this heading.

Meperidine Hydrochloride (Imipramine may potentiate the effects of CNS depressant drugs). Products include:
- Demerol 2438
- Mepergan Injection 2859

Mephobarbital (Co-administration with hepatic enzyme inducers, such as barbiturates, may decrease imipramine plasma concentrations; imipramine may potentiate the effects of CNS depressant drugs). Products include:
- Mebaral Tablets 2452

Meprobamate (Imipramine may potentiate the effects of CNS depressant drugs). Products include:
- Miltown Tablets 2780
- PMB 200 and PMB 400 2890

Mesoridazine Besylate (May inhibit the activity of cytochrome P450 2D6 isoenzyme and are substrates for P450 2D6 and may make normal metabolizers resemble poor metabolizers resulting in higher than expected plasma levels of tricyclic antidepressants). Products include:
- Serentil 689

Metaproterenol Sulfate (Tricyclic antidepressants can potentiate the effects of sympathomimetics). Products include:
- Alupent 672
- Metaproterenol Sulfate Inhalation Solution, USP, Arm-a-Med 547

Metaraminol Bitartrate (Tricyclic antidepressants can potentiate the effects of sympathomimetics). Products include:
- Aramine Injection 1649

Methadone Hydrochloride (Imipramine may potentiate the effects of CNS depressant drugs). Products include:
- Methadone Hydrochloride Oral Concentrate 2356
- Methadone Hydrochloride Oral Solution & Tablets 2357

Methohexital Sodium (Imipramine may potentiate the effects of CNS depressant drugs).
No products indexed under this heading.

Methotrimeprazine (May inhibit the activity of cytochrome P450 2D6 isoenzyme and are substrates for P450 2D6 and may make normal metabolizers resemble poor metabolizers resulting in higher than expected plasma levels of tricyclic antidepressants). Products include:
- Levoprome 1321

Methoxamine Hydrochloride (Tricyclic antidepressants can potentiate the effects of sympathomimetics). Products include:
- Vasoxyl Injection 1169

Methoxyflurane (Imipramine may potentiate the effects of CNS depressant drugs).
No products indexed under this heading.

Methylphenidate Hydrochloride (Co-administration results in Inhibition of imipramine metabolism; downward dosage adjustment of imipramine may be necessary). Products include:
- Ritalin 866

Midazolam Hydrochloride (Imipramine may potentiate the effects of CNS depressant drugs). Products include:
- Versed Injection 2324

Mirtazapine (May inhibit the activity of cytochrome P450 2D6 isoenzyme and are substrates for P450 2D6 and may make normal metabolizers resemble poor metabolizers resulting in higher than expected plasma levels of tricyclic antidepressants). Products include:
- Remeron Tablets 1878

Molindone Hydrochloride (Imipramine may potentiate the effects of CNS depressant drugs). Products include:
- Moban Tablets and Concentrate 1036

Morphine Sulfate (Imipramine may potentiate the effects of CNS depressant drugs). Products include:
- Astramorph/PF Injection, USP (Preservative-Free) 526
- Duramorph Injection 983
- Infumorph 200 and Infumorph 500 Sterile Solutions 985
- Kadian Capsules 2948
- MS Contin Tablets 2149
- MSIR 2152
- Oramorph SR (Morphine Sulfate Sustained Release Tablets) 2359
- RMS Suppositories CII 2766
- Roxanol 2365

Nefazodone Hydrochloride (May inhibit the activity of cytochrome P450 2D6 isoenzyme and are substrates for P450 2D6 and may make normal metabolizers resemble poor metabolizers resulting in higher than expected plasma levels of tricyclic antidepressants). Products include:
- Serzone Tablets 776

Norepinephrine Bitartrate (Tricyclic antidepressants can potentiate the effects of sympathomimetics). Products include:
- Levophed Bitartrate Injection 2445

Nortriptyline Hydrochloride (May inhibit the activity of cytochrome P450 2D6 isoenzyme and are substrates for P450 2D6 and may make normal metabolizers resemble poor metabolizers resulting in higher than expected plasma levels of tricyclic antidepressants). Products include:
- Pamelor 2409

Opium Alkaloids (Imipramine may potentiate the effects of CNS depressant drugs).
No products indexed under this heading.

Oxazepam (Imipramine may potentiate the effects of CNS depressant drugs). Products include:
- Serax Capsules 2916
- Serax Tablets 2916

Oxybutynin Chloride (Co-administration may result in increased atropine-like effects such as paralytic ileus). Products include:
- Ditropan 1267

IMPORTANT NOTE: Always consult each drug listing in the patient's regimen for possible interactions.

Oxycodone Hydrochloride (Imipramine may potentiate the effects of CNS depressant drugs). Products include:

- OxyContin Tablets ... 2163
- OxyIR Capsules ... 2167
- Percocet Tablets ... 955
- Percodan Tablets ... 955
- Percodan-Demi Tablets ... 956
- Roxicodone Tablets, Oral Solution & Intensol (Oxycodone) ... 2366
- Tylox Capsules ... 1593

Paroxetine Hydrochloride (Selective serotonin reuptake inhibitors, such as sertraline, may have variable extent of inhibition of P450 2D6; potential for higher than expected plasma levels of tricyclic antidepressants). Products include:

- Paxil Tablets ... 2681

Pentobarbital Sodium (Co-administration with hepatic enzyme inducers, such as barbiturates, may decrease imipramine plasma concentrations; imipramine may potentiate the effects of CNS depressant drugs). Products include:

- Nembutal Sodium Capsules ... 440
- Nembutal Sodium Solution ... 442
- Nembutal Sodium Suppositories ... 444

Perphenazine (May inhibit the activity of cytochrome P450 2D6 isoenzyme and are substrates for P450 2D6 and may make normal metabolizers resemble poor metabolizers resulting in higher than expected plasma levels of tricyclic antidepressants). Products include:

- Etrafon ... 2495
- Triavil Tablets ... 1800
- Trilafon ... 2532

Phenelzine Sulfate (Co-administration of tricyclic antidepressants and MAO inhibitor has produced hyperpyretic crises, severe convulsions, and deaths; concurrent and/or sequential use is contraindicated). Products include:

- Nardil ... 1977

Phenobarbital (Co-administration with hepatic enzyme inducers, such as barbiturates, may decrease imipramine plasma concentrations; imipramine may potentiate the effects of CNS depressant drugs). Products include:

- Arco-Lase Plus Tablets ... 513
- Bellergal-S Tablets ... 2375
- Donnatal ... 2234
- Donnatal Extentabs ... 2234
- Donnatal Tablets ... 2234
- Phenobarbital Elixir and Tablets ... 1523
- Quadrinal Tablets ... 1398

Phenylephrine Bitartrate (Tricyclic antidepressants can potentiate the effects of sympathomimetics).

No products indexed under this heading.

Phenylephrine Hydrochloride (Tricyclic antidepressants can potentiate the effects of sympathomimetics). Products include:

- Atrohist Plus Tablets ... 1605
- Cerose DM ... ▣ 853
- D.A. II Tablets ... 972
- D.A. Chewable Tablets ... 970
- Dura-Vent/DA Tablets ... 972
- Extendryl ... 1003
- 4-Way Fast Acting Nasal Spray (regular & mentholated) ... ▣ 644
- Hemorid ... ▣ 797
- Hycomine Compound Tablets ... 948
- Neo-Synephrine Hydrochloride 1% Carpuject ... 2455
- Neo-Synephrine Hydrochloride 1% Injection ... 2455
- Neo-Synephrine Hydrochloride (Ophthalmic) ... 2456
- Neo-Synephrine ... ▣ 624
- Novahistine Elixir ... ▣ 782
- Phenergan VC ... 2886
- Phenergan VC with Codeine ... 2888
- Preparation H ... ▣ 842
- Tympagesic Ear Drops ... 2476
- Vicks Sinex Nasal Spray and Ultra Fine Mist ... ▣ 738

Phenylephrine Tannate (Tricyclic antidepressants can potentiate the effects of sympathomimetics). Products include:

- Atrohist Pediatric Suspension ... 1604
- Atrohist Pediatric Suspension Dye-Free ... 1604
- Rynatan ... 2781
- Rynatuss ... 2782

Phenylpropanolamine Hydrochloride (Tricyclic antidepressants can potentiate the effects of sympathomimetics). Products include:

- Acutrim ... ▣ 648
- Atrohist Plus Tablets ... 1605
- BC Cold Powder Multi-Symptom Formula (Cold-Sinus-Allergy) ... ▣ 631
- BC Cold Powder Non-Drowsy Formula (Cold-Sinus) ... ▣ 631
- Cheracol Plus Head Cold/Cough Formula ... ▣ 741
- Comtrex Multi-Symptom Cold Reliever Liqui-Gels ... ▣ 638
- Comtrex Multi-Symptom Non-Drowsy Liqui-gels ... ▣ 640
- Contac Continuous Action Nasal Decongestant/Antihistamine 12 Hour Capsules ... ▣ 773
- Contac Maximum Strength Continuous Action Decongestant/Antihistamine 12 Hour Caplets ... ▣ 772
- Contac Severe Cold and Flu Formula Caplets ... ▣ 773
- Coricidin 'D' Decongestant Tablets ... ▣ 760
- Dexatrim ... ▣ 795
- Dexatrim Plus Vitamins Caplets ... ▣ 796
- Dimetane-DC Cough Syrup ... 2232
- Dimetapp Allergy Sinus Caplets ... ▣ 838
- Dimetapp Cold & Allergy Chewable Tablets ... ▣ 838
- Dimetapp Cold & Cough Liqui-Gels ... ▣ 839
- Dimetapp DM Elixir ... ▣ 840
- Dimetapp Elixir ... ▣ 840
- Dimetapp Extentabs ... ▣ 841
- Dimetapp Tablets/Liqui-Gels ... ▣ 841
- Dura-Vent Tablets ... 971
- Entex LA Tablets ... 972
- Exgest LA Tablets ... 787
- Hycomine ... 947
- Nolamine Timed-Release Tablets ... 790
- Ornade Spansule Capsules ... 2678
- Propagest Tablets ... 791
- Pyrroxate Caplets ... ▣ 742
- Robitussin-CF ... ▣ 846
- Sinulin Tablets ... 792
- Tavist-D 12 Hour Relief Tablets ... ▣ 750
- Teldrin 12 Hour Antihistamine/Nasal Decongestant Allergy Relief Capsules ... ▣ 786
- Triaminic Expectorant ... ▣ 753
- Triaminic Syrup ... ▣ 755
- Triaminic Triaminicol Cold & Cough ... ▣ 756
- Triaminic DM Syrup ... ▣ 756
- Triaminicin Tablets ... ▣ 756
- Vicks DayQuil Allergy Relief 12-Hour Extended Release Tablets ... ▣ 733
- Vicks DayQuil Allergy Relief 4-Hour Tablets ... ▣ 733
- Vicks DayQuil SINUS Pressure & CONGESTION Relief ... ▣ 734

Phenytoin (Co-administration with hepatic enzyme inducers, such as phenytoin, may decrease imipramine plasma concentrations). Products include:

- Dilantin Infatabs ... 1967
- Dilantin-125 Suspension ... 1969

Phenytoin Sodium (Co-administration with hepatic enzyme inducers, such as phenytoin, may decrease imipramine plasma concentrations). Products include:

- Dilantin Kapseals ... 1965

Pirbuterol Acetate (Tricyclic antidepressants can potentiate the effects of sympathomimetics). Products include:

- Maxair Autohaler ... 1550
- Maxair Inhaler ... 1552

Prazepam (Imipramine may potentiate the effects of CNS depressant drugs).

No products indexed under this heading.

Prochlorperazine (May inhibit the activity of cytochrome P450 2D6 isoenzyme and are substrates for P450 2D6 and may make normal metabolizers resemble poor metabolizers resulting in higher than expected plasma levels of tricyclic antidepressants). Products include:

- Compazine ... 2644

Procyclidine Hydrochloride (Co-administration may result in increased atropine-like effects such as paralytic ileus). Products include:

- Kemadrin Tablets ... 1105

Promethazine Hydrochloride (May inhibit the activity of cytochrome P450 2D6 isoenzyme and are substrates for P450 2D6 and may make normal metabolizers resemble poor metabolizers resulting in higher than expected plasma levels of tricyclic antidepressants). Products include:

- Mepergan Injection ... 2859
- Phenergan with Codeine ... 2883
- Phenergan with Dextromethorphan ... 2885
- Phenergan Injection ... 2880
- Phenergan Suppositories ... 2882
- Phenergan Syrup ... 2881
- Phenergan Tablets ... 2882
- Phenergan VC ... 2886
- Phenergan VC with Codeine ... 2888

Propafenone Hydrochloride (May inhibit the activity of cytochrome P450 2D6 isoenzyme and are substrates for P450 2D6 and may make normal metabolizers resemble poor metabolizers resulting in higher than expected plasma levels of tricyclic antidepressants). Products include:

- Rythmol Tablets–150mg, 225mg, 300mg ... 1399

Propantheline Bromide (Co-administration may result in increased atropine-like effects such as paralytic ileus). Products include:

- Pro-Banthine Tablets ... 2226

Propofol (Imipramine may potentiate the effects of CNS depressant drugs). Products include:

- Diprivan Injectable Emulsion ... 2939

Propoxyphene Hydrochloride (Imipramine may potentiate the effects of CNS depressant drugs). Products include:

- Darvon ... 1475
- Wygesic Tablets ... 2930

Propoxyphene Napsylate (Imipramine may potentiate the effects of CNS depressant drugs). Products include:

- Darvon-N/Darvocet-N ... 1473

Protriptyline Hydrochloride (May inhibit the activity of cytochrome P450 2D6 isoenzyme and are substrates for P450 2D6 and may make normal metabolizers resemble poor metabolizers resulting in higher than expected plasma levels of tricyclic antidepressants). Products include:

- Vivactil Tablets ... 1820

Pseudoephedrine Hydrochloride (Tricyclic antidepressants can potentiate the effects of sympathomimetics). Products include:

- Actifed Allergy Daytime/Nighttime Caplets ... ▣ 808
- Actifed Cold & Allergy Tablets ... ▣ 807
- Actifed Cold & Sinus Caplets and Tablets ... ▣ 808
- Actifed Sinus Daytime/Nighttime Tablets and Caplets ... ▣ 809
- Advil Cold and Sinus Caplets and Tablets ... ▣ 837
- Alka-Seltzer Plus Liqui-Gels ... ▣ 612
- Alka-Seltzer Plus Flu & Body Aches Liqui-Gels Non-Drowsy Formula ... ▣ 613
- Alka-Seltzer Plus Night-Time Cold Medicine Liqui-Gels ... ▣ 612
- Allerest Maximum Strength ... ▣ 649
- Allerest No Drowsiness ... ▣ 649
- Allerest Sinus Pain Formula ... ▣ 649
- Atrohist Pediatric Capsules ... 1603
- Benadryl Allergy/Cold Tablets ... ▣ 811
- Benadryl Allergy Decongestant Liquid Medication ... ▣ 812
- Benadryl Allergy Decongestant Tablets ... ▣ 812
- Benadryl Allergy Sinus Headache Caplets ... ▣ 813
- Benylin Multisymptom ... ▣ 816
- Bromfed Capsules (Extended-Release) ... 1832
- Bromfed Syrup ... ▣ 712
- Bromfed Tablets ... 1832
- Bromfed-DM Cough Syrup ... 1832
- Bromfed-PD Capsules (Extended-Release) ... 1832
- Children's TYLENOL Cold Multi-Symptom Chewable Tablets and Liquid ... 1559
- Children's TYLENOL Cold Plus Cough Multi Symptom Chewable Tablets and Liquid ... 1560
- Children's TYLENOL Flu Suspension Liquid ... 1560
- Children's Vicks DayQuil Allergy Relief ... ▣ 730
- Children's Vicks NyQuil Cold/Cough Relief ... ▣ 731
- Allergy-Sinus Comtrex Multi-Symptom Allergy-Sinus Formula Tablets and Caplets ... ▣ 639
- Comtrex Multi-Symptom ... ▣ 638
- Comtrex Multi-Symptom Non-Drowsy Caplets ... ▣ 640
- Congess ... 1003
- Contac Day Allergy/Sinus Caplets ... ▣ 771
- Contac Day & Night ... ▣ 772
- Contac Night Allergy/Sinus Caplets ... ▣ 771
- Contac Severe Cold & Flu Non-Drowsy ... ▣ 774
- Deconsal II Tablets ... 1605
- Dimetane-DX Cough Syrup ... 2233
- Dimetapp Cold & Fever Suspension ... ▣ 839
- Dimetapp Decongestant Pediatric Drops ... ▣ 840
- Dorcol Children's Cough Syrup ... ▣ 748
- Drixoral Cough + Congestion Liquid Caps ... ▣ 763
- Dura-Tap/PD Capsules ... 970
- Duratuss Tablets ... 2750
- Duratuss HD Elixir ... 2750
- Efidac/24 ... ▣ 655
- Entex PSE Tablets ... 973
- Fedahist Gyrocaps ... 2545
- Guaifed ... 1833
- Guaifed Syrup ... ▣ 712
- Guaimax-D Tablets ... 809
- Histussin D Liquid ... 670
- Infants' TYLENOL Cold Decongestant & Fever-Reducer Drops ... 1561
- Kronofed-A ... 994
- Novahistine DMX ... ▣ 782
- Nucofed ... 2225
- PediaCare Cough-Cold Chewable Tablets and Liquid ... 1569
- PediaCare Infants' Decongestant Drops ... 1569
- PediaCare Infants' Drops Decongestant Plus Cough ... 1569
- PediaCare NightRest Cough-Cold Liquid ... 1569
- Pediatric Vicks 44d Cough & Head Congestion Relief ... ▣ 736
- Pediatric Vicks 44m Cough & Cold Relief ... ▣ 737
- Robitussin Cold & Cough Liqui-Gels ... ▣ 844
- Robitussin Cold, Cough & Flu Liqui-Gels ... ▣ 844
- Robitussin Maximum Strength Cough & Cold ... ▣ 847
- Robitussin Night-Time Cold Formula ... ▣ 847
- Robitussin Pediatric Cough & Cold Formula ... ▣ 848
- Robitussin Pediatric Drops ... ▣ 849
- Robitussin Severe Congestion Liqui-Gels ... ▣ 845

(▣ Described in PDR For Nonprescription Drugs)

(◉ Described in PDR For Ophthalmology)

Interactions Index

Tofranil-PM

Entry	Page
Robitussin-DAC Syrup	2249
Robitussin-PE	846
Rondec Oral Drops	974
Rondec Syrup	974
Rondec Tablet	974
Rondec Chewable Tablets	974
Rondec-TR Tablet	974
Ryna	804
Seldane-D Extended-Release Tablets	1286
Semprex-D Capsules	1620
Sinarest	663
Sine-Aid Maximum Strength Sinus Headache Gelcaps, Caplets and Tablets	1570
Sine-Off No Drowsiness Formula Caplets	784
Sine-Off Sinus Medicine	784
Singlet Tablets	785
Sinutab Non-Drying Liquid Caps	823
Sinutab Sinus Allergy Medication, Maximum Strength Tablets and Caplets	823
Sinutab Sinus Medication, Maximum Strength Without Drowsiness Formula, Tablets & Caplets	824
Sudafed Children's Cold & Cough Liquid Medication	825
Sudafed Children's Nasal Decongestant Liquid Medication	826
Sudafed Cold & Allergy Tablets	826
Sudafed Cold and Cough Liquid Caps	826
Sudafed Nasal Decongestant Tablets, 30 mg	825
Sudafed Nasal Decongestant Tablets, 60 mg	825
Sudafed Non-Drying Sinus Liquid Caps	827
Sudafed Pediatric Nasal Decongestant Liquid Oral Drops	827
Sudafed Severe Cold Formula Caplets	828
Sudafed Severe Cold Formula Tablets	828
Sudafed Sinus Caplets	829
Sudafed Sinus Tablets	829
Sudafed 12 Hour Caplets	824
Syn-Rx Tablets	1622
Syn-Rx DM Tablets	1623
TheraFlu Flu and Cold Medicine	750
Theraflu Maximum Strength Flu and Cold Medicine For Sore Throat	751
TheraFlu Flu, Cold and Cough Medicine	750
TheraFlu Maximum Strength Nighttime Flu, Cold & Cough Medicine	751
TheraFlu Maximum Strength Non-Drowsy Formula Flu, Cold & Cough Medicine	751
TheraFlu Maximum Strength, Non-Drowsy Formula Flu, Cold and Cough Caplets	752
Theraflu Maximum Strength Sinus Non-Drowsy Formula Caplets	752
Triaminic AM Cough and Decongestant Formula	753
Triaminic AM Decongestant Formula	753
Triaminic Infant Oral Decongestant Drops	754
Triaminic Night Time	754
Triaminic Sore Throat Formula	755
Tussend	1830
Tussend Expectorant	1831
TYLENOL Allergy Sinus, Maximum Strength Caplets and Gelcaps	1571
TYLENOL Allergy Sinus NightTime, Maximum Strength Caplets	1571
TYLENOL Cold Medication, Multi-Symptom Formula Tablets and Caplets	1572
TYLENOL Cold Medication, Multi-Symptom Hot Liquid Packets	1572
TYLENOL Cold Medication, No Drowsiness Formula Caplets and Gelcaps	1572
TYLENOL Cold Severe Congestion Caplets	1573
TYLENOL Cough Medication with Decongestant, Multi Symptom	1574
TYLENOL Flu No Drowsiness Formula, Maximum Strength Gelcaps	1575
TYLENOL Flu NightTime, Maximum Strength Gelcaps	1575
TYLENOL Flu NightTime, Maximum Strength Hot Medication Packets	1575
TYLENOL Sinus, Maximum Strength Geltabs, Gelcaps, Caplets and Tablets	1576
Vicks 44 LiquiCaps Cough, Cold & Flu Relief	728
Vicks 44 LiquiCaps Non-Drowsy Cough & Cold Relief	729
Vicks 44D Cough & Head Congestion Relief	728
Vicks 44M Cough, Cold & Flu Relief	729
Vicks DayQuil LiquiCaps/Liquid Multi-Symptom Cold/Flu Relief	734
Vicks DayQuil SINUS Pressure & PAIN Relief with IBUPROFEN	735
Vicks Nyquil Hot Therapy	735
Vicks NyQuil LiquiCaps/Liquid Multi-Symptom Cold/Flu Relief, Original and Cherry Flavors	736

Pseudoephedrine Sulfate (Tricyclic antidepressants can potentiate the effects of sympathomimetics). Products include:

Chlor-Trimeton Allergy Decongestant Tablets	759
Claritin-D Tablets	2487
Drixoral Cold and Allergy Sustained-Action Tablets	763
Drixoral Cold and Flu Extended-Release Tablets	764
Drixoral Non-Drowsy Formula Extended-Release Tablets	764
Drixoral Allergy/Sinus Extended Release Tablets	765
Trinalin Repetabs Tablets	1373

Quazepam (Imipramine may potentiate the effects of CNS depressant drugs). Products include:

Doral Tablets	2773

Quinidine Gluconate (May inhibit the activity of cytochrome P450 2D6 isoenzyme and may make normal metabolizers resemble poor metabolizers resulting in higher than expected plasma levels of tricyclic antidepressants). Products include:

Quinaglute Dura-Tabs Tablets	644

Quinidine Polygalacturonate (May inhibit the activity of cytochrome P450 2D6 isoenzyme and may make normal metabolizers resemble poor metabolizers resulting in higher than expected plasma levels of tricyclic antidepressants). Products include:

Cardioquin Tablets	2146

Quinidine Sulfate (May inhibit the activity of cytochrome P450 2D6 isoenzyme and may make normal metabolizers resemble poor metabolizers resulting in higher than expected plasma levels of tricyclic antidepressants). Products include:

Quinidex Extentabs	2240

Risperidone (Imipramine may potentiate the effects of CNS depressant drugs). Products include:

Risperdal Tablets	1348

Salmeterol Xinafoate (Tricyclic antidepressants can potentiate the effects of sympathomimetics). Products include:

Serevent Inhalation Aerosol	1149

Scopolamine (Co-administration may result in increased atropine-like effects such as paralytic ileus). Products include:

Transderm Scōp Transdermal Therapeutic System	890

Scopolamine Hydrobromide (Co-administration may result in increased atropine-like effects such as paralytic ileus). Products include:

Atrohist Plus Tablets	1605
Donnatal	2234
Donnatal Extentabs	2234
Donnatal Tablets	2234

Secobarbital Sodium (Co-administration with hepatic enzyme inducers, such as barbiturates, may decrease imipramine plasma concentrations; imipramine may potentiate the effects of CNS depressant drugs). Products include:

Seconal Sodium Pulvules	1529

Selegiline Hydrochloride (Co-administration of tricyclic antidepressants and MAO inhibitor has produced hyperpyretic crises, severe convulsions, and deaths; concurrent and/or sequential use is contraindicated). Products include:

Eldepryl Capsules	2729

Sertraline Hydrochloride (Selective serotonin reuptake inhibitors, such as sertraline, may have variable extent of inhibition of P450 2D6; potential for higher than expected plasma levels of tricyclic antidepressants). Products include:

Zoloft Tablets	2051

Sevoflurane (Imipramine may potentiate the effects of CNS depressant drugs).

No products indexed under this heading.

Sufentanil Citrate (Imipramine may potentiate the effects of CNS depressant drugs). Products include:

Sufenta Injection	1355

Temazepam (Imipramine may potentiate the effects of CNS depressant drugs). Products include:

Restoril Capsules	2413

Terbutaline Sulfate (Tricyclic antidepressants can potentiate the effects of sympathomimetics). Products include:

Brethaire Inhaler	830
Brethine Ampuls	832
Brethine Tablets	831
Bricanyl Subcutaneous Injection	1247
Bricanyl Tablets	1248

Thiamylal Sodium (Co-administration with hepatic enzyme inducers, such as barbiturates, may decrease imipramine plasma concentrations; imipramine may potentiate the effects of CNS depressant drugs).

No products indexed under this heading.

Thioridazine Hydrochloride (May inhibit the activity of cytochrome P450 2D6 isoenzyme and are substrates for P450 2D6 and may make normal metabolizers resemble poor metabolizers resulting in higher than expected plasma levels of tricyclic antidepressants). Products include:

Mellaril	2398

Thiothixene (Imipramine may potentiate the effects of CNS depressant drugs). Products include:

Navane Capsules and Concentrate	2018
Navane Intramuscular	2019

Thyroglobulin (Possibility of cardiovascular toxicity).

No products indexed under this heading.

Thyroid (Possibility of cardiovascular toxicity).

No products indexed under this heading.

Thyroxine (Possibility of cardiovascular toxicity).

No products indexed under this heading.

Thyroxine Sodium (Possibility of cardiovascular toxicity).

No products indexed under this heading.

Tranylcypromine Sulfate (Co-administration of tricyclic antidepressants and MAO inhibitor has produced hyperpyretic crises, severe convulsions, and deaths; concurrent and/or sequential use is contraindicated). Products include:

Parnate Tablets	2679

Trazodone Hydrochloride (May inhibit the activity of cytochrome P450 2D6 isoenzyme and are substrates for P450 2D6 and may make normal metabolizers resemble poor metabolizers resulting in higher than expected plasma levels of tricyclic antidepressants). Products include:

Desyrel and Desyrel Dividose	504

Triazolam (Imipramine may potentiate the effects of CNS depressant drugs). Products include:

Halcion Tablets	2093

Tridihexethyl Chloride (Co-administration may result in increased atropine-like effects such as paralytic ileus).

No products indexed under this heading.

Trifluoperazine Hydrochloride (May inhibit the activity of cytochrome P450 2D6 isoenzyme and are substrates for P450 2D6 and may make normal metabolizers resemble poor metabolizers resulting in higher than expected plasma levels of tricyclic antidepressants). Products include:

Stelazine	2692

Trihexyphenidyl Hydrochloride (Co-administration may result in increased atropine-like effects such as paralytic ileus). Products include:

Artane	1418

Trimipramine Maleate (May inhibit the activity of cytochrome P450 2D6 isoenzyme and are substrates for P450 2D6 and may make normal metabolizers resemble poor metabolizers resulting in higher than expected plasma levels of tricyclic antidepressants). Products include:

Surmontil Capsules	2917

Venlafaxine Hydrochloride (May inhibit the activity of cytochrome P450 2D6 isoenzyme and are substrates for P450 2D6 and may make normal metabolizers resemble poor metabolizers resulting in higher than expected plasma levels of tricyclic antidepressants). Products include:

Effexor	2825

Zolpidem Tartrate (Imipramine may potentiate the effects of CNS depressant drugs). Products include:

Ambien Tablets	2559

Food Interactions

Alcohol (Imipramine may enhance the CNS depressant effect of alcohol).

TOFRANIL-PM CAPSULES

(Imipramine Pamoate) 876

May interact with central nervous system depressants, anticholinergics, sympathomimetics, barbiturates, monoamine oxidase inhibitors, thyroid preparations, antidepressant drugs, phenothiazines, quinidine, and certain other agents. Compounds in these categories include:

Albuterol (Tricyclic antidepressants can potentiate the effects of sympathomimetics). Products include:

Proventil Inhalation Aerosol	2524

IMPORTANT NOTE: Always consult each drug listing in the patient's regimen for possible interactions.

Tofranil-PM — Interactions Index

Ventolin Inhalation Aerosol and Refill 1170

Albuterol Sulfate (Tricyclic antidepressants can potentiate the effects of sympathomimetics). Products include:
- Airet Albuterol Sulfate Inhalation Solution 1602
- Albuterol Sulfate, USP Solution for Inhalation, Arm-a-Med 522
- Proventil Inhalation Solution 0.083% 2527
- Proventil Repetabs Tablets 2529
- Proventil Solution for Inhalation 0.5% 2525
- Proventil Syrup 2528
- Proventil Tablets 2529
- Ventolin Inhalation Solution 1171
- Ventolin Nebules Inhalation Solution 1172
- Ventolin Rotacaps for Inhalation 1173
- Ventolin Syrup 1175
- Ventolin Tablets 1176
- Volmax Extended-Release Tablets .. 1835

Alfentanil Hydrochloride (Imipramine may potentiate the effects of CNS depressant drugs). Products include:
- Alfenta Injection 1334

Alprazolam (Imipramine may potentiate the effects of CNS depressant drugs). Products include:
- Xanax Tablets 2115

Amitriptyline Hydrochloride (May inhibit the activity of cytochrome P450 2D6 isoenzyme and are substrates for P450 2D6 and may make normal metabolizers resemble poor metabolizers resulting in higher than expected plasma levels of tricyclic antidepressants). Products include:
- Elavil 2945
- Etrafon 2495
- Limbitrol 2333
- Triavil Tablets 1800

Amoxapine (May inhibit the activity of cytochrome P450 2D6 isoenzyme and are substrates for P450 2D6 and may make normal metabolizers resemble poor metabolizers resulting in higher than expected plasma levels of tricyclic antidepressants). Products include:
- Asendin Tablets 1419

Aprobarbital (Co-administration with hepatic enzyme inducers, such as barbiturates, may decrease imipramine plasma concentrations; imipramine may potentiate the effects of CNS depressant drugs).
No products indexed under this heading.

Atropine Sulfate (Co-administration may result in increased atropine-like effects such as paralytic ileus). Products include:
- Arco-Lase Plus Tablets 513
- Atrohist Plus Tablets 1605
- Donnatal 2234
- Donnatal Extentabs 2234
- Donnatal Tablets 2234
- Lomotil 2591
- Motofen Tablets 789
- Urised Tablets 2123

Belladonna Alkaloids (Co-administration may result in increased atropine-like effects such as paralytic ileus). Products include:
- Bellergal-S Tablets 2375
- Hyland's Bedwetting Tablets .... ▣ 788
- Hyland's EnurAid Tablets .... ▣ 789
- Hyland's Headache Tablets .... ▣ 790
- Hyland's Teething Tablets .... ▣ 790
- Similasan Eye Drops # 1 .... ▣ 769

Benztropine Mesylate (Co-administration may result in increased atropine-like effects such as paralytic ileus). Products include:
- Cogentin 1661

Biperiden Hydrochloride (Co-administration may result in increased atropine-like effects such as paralytic ileus). Products include:
- Akineton 1380

Buprenorphine (Imipramine may potentiate the effects of CNS depressant drugs). Products include:
- Buprenex Injectable 2170

Bupropion Hydrochloride (May inhibit the activity of cytochrome P450 2D6 isoenzyme and are substrates for P450 2D6 and may make normal metabolizers resemble poor metabolizers resulting in higher than expected plasma levels of tricyclic antidepressants). Products include:
- Wellbutrin Tablets 1177

Buspirone Hydrochloride (Imipramine may potentiate the effects of CNS depressant drugs). Products include:
- BuSpar Tablets 738

Butabarbital (Co-administration with hepatic enzyme inducers, such as barbiturates, may decrease imipramine plasma concentrations; imipramine may potentiate the effects of CNS depressant drugs).
No products indexed under this heading.

Butalbital (Co-administration with hepatic enzyme inducers, such as barbiturates, may decrease imipramine plasma concentrations; imipramine may potentiate the effects of CNS depressant drugs). Products include:
- Axocet Capsules 2469
- Esgic-plus Capsules 1012
- Esgic-plus Tablets 1012
- Fioricet Tablets 2386
- Fioricet with Codeine Capsules 2387
- Fiorinal Capsules 2388
- Fiorinal with Codeine Capsules 2390
- Fiorinal Tablets 2388
- Phrenilin 790
- Sedapap Tablets 50 mg/650 mg .. 1826

Chlordiazepoxide (Imipramine may potentiate the effects of CNS depressant drugs). Products include:
- Limbitrol 2333

Chlordiazepoxide Hydrochloride (Imipramine may potentiate the effects of CNS depressant drugs). Products include:
- Librax Capsules 2330
- Librium Capsules 2331
- Librium Injectable 2332

Chlorpromazine (May inhibit the activity of cytochrome P450 2D6 isoenzyme and are substrates for P450 2D6 and may make normal metabolizers resemble poor metabolizers resulting in higher than expected plasma levels of tricyclic antidepressants). Products include:
- Thorazine Suppositories 2701

Chlorpromazine Hydrochloride (May inhibit the activity of cytochrome P450 2D6 isoenzyme and are substrates for P450 2D6 and may make normal metabolizers resemble poor metabolizers resulting in higher than expected plasma levels of tricyclic antidepressants). Products include:
- Thorazine 2701

Chlorprothixene (Imipramine may potentiate the effects of CNS depressant drugs).
No products indexed under this heading.

Chlorprothixene Hydrochloride (Imipramine may potentiate the effects of CNS depressant drugs).
No products indexed under this heading.

Chlorprothixene Lactate (Imipramine may potentiate the effects of CNS depressant drugs).
No products indexed under this heading.

Cimetidine (Co-administration with hepatic enzyme inhibitors, such as cimetidine, may increase imipramine plasma concentrations. Products include:
- Tagamet HB Tablets .... ▣ 786
- Tagamet Tablets 2694

Cimetidine Hydrochloride (Co-administration with hepatic enzyme inhibitors, such as cimetidine, may increase imipramine plasma concentrations). Products include:
- Tagamet 2694

Clidinium Bromide (Co-administration may result in increased atropine-like effects such as paralytic ileus). Products include:
- Librax Capsules 2330

Clonidine (Imipramine may block the pharmacological effects). Products include:
- Catapres-TTS 680

Clonidine Hydrochloride (Imipramine may block the pharmacological effects). Products include:
- Catapres Tablets 679
- Combipres Tablets 682

Clorazepate Dipotassium (Imipramine may potentiate the effects of CNS depressant drugs). Products include:
- Tranxene 459

Clozapine (Imipramine may potentiate the effects of CNS depressant drugs). Products include:
- Clozaril Tablets 2377

Codeine Phosphate (Imipramine may potentiate the effects of CNS depressant drugs). Products include:
- Brontex 2130
- Dimetane-DC Cough Syrup 2232
- Fioricet with Codeine Capsules 2387
- Fiorinal with Codeine Capsules 2390
- Nucofed 2225
- Phenergan with Codeine 2883
- Phenergan VC with Codeine 2888
- Robitussin A-C Syrup 2248
- Robitussin-DAC Syrup 2249
- Ryna .... ▣ 804
- Soma Compound w/Codeine Tablets 2784
- Tylenol with Codeine 1592

Desflurane (Imipramine may potentiate the effects of CNS depressant drugs). Products include:
- Suprane (desflurane, USP) 1865

Desipramine Hydrochloride (May inhibit the activity of cytochrome P450 2D6 isoenzyme and are substrates for P450 2D6 and may make normal metabolizers resemble poor metabolizers resulting in higher than expected plasma levels of tricyclic antidepressants). Products include:
- Norpramin Tablets 1273

Dezocine (Imipramine may potentiate the effects of CNS depressant drugs). Products include:
- Dalgan Injection 529

Diazepam (Imipramine may potentiate the effects of CNS depressant drugs). Products include:
- Dizac (diazepam injectable emulsion) CIV 1862
- Valium Injectable 2336
- Valium Tablets 2335

Dicyclomine Hydrochloride (Co-administration may result in increased atropine-like effects such as paralytic ileus). Products include:
- Bentyl 1246

Dobutamine Hydrochloride (Tricyclic antidepressants can potentiate the effects of sympathomimetics). Products include:
- Dobutrex Solution Vials 1480

Dopamine Hydrochloride (Tricyclic antidepressants can potentiate the effects of sympathomimetics).
No products indexed under this heading.

Doxepin Hydrochloride (May inhibit the activity of cytochrome P450 2D6 isoenzyme and are substrates for P450 2D6 and may make normal metabolizers resemble poor metabolizers resulting in higher than expected plasma levels of tricyclic antidepressants). Products include:
- Adapin Capsules 1542
- Sinequan 2028
- Zonalon Cream 1042

Droperidol (Imipramine may potentiate the effects of CNS depressant drugs). Products include:
- Inapsine Injection 462

Enflurane (Imipramine may potentiate the effects of CNS depressant drugs).
No products indexed under this heading.

Ephedrine Hydrochloride (Tricyclic antidepressants can potentiate the effects of sympathomimetics). Products include:
- Primatene Tablets .... ▣ 844
- Quadrinal Tablets 1398

Ephedrine Sulfate (Tricyclic antidepressants can potentiate the effects of sympathomimetics). Products include:
- Marax Tablets & DF Syrup 2015

Ephedrine Tannate (Tricyclic antidepressants can potentiate the effects of sympathomimetics). Products include:
- Rynatuss 2782

Epinephrine (Tricyclic antidepressants can potentiate the effects of sympathomimetics). Products include:
- EPIFRIN .... ◉ 237
- EpiPen 808
- Marcaine with Epinephrine 2446
- Primatene Mist .... ▣ 843
- Sensorcaine with Epinephrine Injection 554
- Sus-Phrine Injection 1017
- Xylocaine with Epinephrine Injections 562

Epinephrine Bitartrate (Tricyclic antidepressants can potentiate the effects of sympathomimetics). Products include:
- Sensorcaine-MPF with Epinephrine Injection 554

Epinephrine Hydrochloride (Tricyclic antidepressants can potentiate the effects of sympathomimetics). Products include:
- Ana-Kit Anaphylaxis Emergency Treatment Kit 611

Estazolam (Imipramine may potentiate the effects of CNS depressant drugs). Products include:
- ProSom Tablets 457

Ethchlorvynol (Imipramine may potentiate the effects of CNS depressant drugs). Products include:
- Placidyl Capsules 456

Ethinamate (Imipramine may potentiate the effects of CNS depressant drugs).
No products indexed under this heading.

Fentanyl (Imipramine may potentiate the effects of CNS depressant drugs). Products include:
- Duragesic Transdermal System 1336

(▣ Described in PDR For Nonprescription Drugs)   (◉ Described in PDR For Ophthalmology)

Interactions Index

Fentanyl Citrate (Imipramine may potentiate the effects of CNS depressant drugs). Products include:
Sublimaze Injection 463

Flecainide Acetate (May inhibit the activity of cytochrome P450 2D6 isoenzyme and are substrates for P450 2D6 and may make normal metabolizers resemble poor metabolizers resulting in higher than expected plasma levels of tricyclic antidepressants). Products include:
Tambocor Tablets 1555

Fluoxetine Hydrochloride (Co-administration with hepatic enzyme inhibitors, such as fluoxetine, may increase imipramine plasma concentrations; due to long half-life of fluoxetine, at least 5 weeks should elapse before initiating TCA treatment in a patient being withdrawn from fluoxetine). Products include:
Prozac Pulvules & Liquid, Oral Solution 935

Fluphenazine Decanoate (May inhibit the activity of cytochrome P450 2D6 isoenzyme and are substrates for P450 2D6 and may make normal metabolizers resemble poor metabolizers resulting in higher than expected plasma levels of tricyclic antidepressants). Products include:
Prolixin Decanoate 510

Fluphenazine Enanthate (May inhibit the activity of cytochrome P450 2D6 isoenzyme and are substrates for P450 2D6 and may make normal metabolizers resemble poor metabolizers resulting in higher than expected plasma levels of tricyclic antidepressants). Products include:
Prolixin Enanthate 510

Fluphenazine Hydrochloride (May inhibit the activity of cytochrome P450 2D6 isoenzyme and are substrates for P450 2D6 and may make normal metabolizers resemble poor metabolizers resulting in higher than expected plasma levels of tricyclic antidepressants). Products include:
Prolixin 510

Flurazepam Hydrochloride (Imipramine may potentiate the effects of CNS depressant drugs). Products include:
Dalmane Capsules 2329

Fosphenytoin Sodium (Co-administration with hepatic enzyme inducers, such as phenytoin, may decrease imipramine plasma concentrations). Products include:
Cerebyx Injection 1956

Furazolidone (Co-administration of tricyclic antidepressants and MAO inhibitor has produced hyperpyretic crises, severe convulsions, and deaths; concurrent and/or sequential use is contraindicated). Products include:
Furoxone 2221

Glutethimide (Imipramine may potentiate the effects of CNS depressant drugs).
No products indexed under this heading.

Glycopyrrolate (Co-administration may result in increased atropine-like effects such as paralytic ileus). Products include:
Robinul Forte Tablets 2247
Robinul Injectable 2247
Robinul Tablets 2247

Guanadrel Sulfate (Imipramine may block the pharmacological effects). Products include:
Hylorel Tablets 1613

Guanethidine Monosulfate (Imipramine may block the pharmacological effects). Products include:
Esimil Tablets 840
Ismelin Tablets 845

Haloperidol (Imipramine may potentiate the effects of CNS depressant drugs). Products include:
Haldol Injection, Tablets and Concentrate 1585

Haloperidol Decanoate (Imipramine may potentiate the effects of CNS depressant drugs). Products include:
Haldol Decanoate 1587

Hydrocodone Bitartrate (Imipramine may potentiate the effects of CNS depressant drugs). Products include:
Codiclear DH Syrup 808
Duratuss HD Elixir 2750
Histussin D Liquid 670
Hycodan Tablets and Syrup 946
Hycomine Compound Tablets 948
Hycomine 947
Hycotuss Expectorant Syrup 950
Hydrocet Capsules 787
Lorcet 10/650 Tablets 1016
Lortab 2751
Tussend 1830
Tussend Expectorant 1831
Vicodin Tablets 1404
Vicodin ES Tablets 1405
Vicodin HP Tablets 1403
Vicodin Tuss Expectorant 1406
Zydone Capsules 967

Hydrocodone Polistirex (Imipramine may potentiate the effects of CNS depressant drugs). Products include:
Tussionex Pennkinetic Extended-Release Suspension 1624

Hydromorphone Hydrochloride (Imipramine may potentiate the effects of CNS depressant drugs). Products include:
Dilaudid Ampules 1382
Dilaudid Cough Syrup 1383
Dilaudid-HP Injection 1384
Dilaudid-HP Lyophilized Powder 250 mg 1384
Dilaudid 1382
Dilaudid Oral Liquid 1386
Dilaudid 1382
Dilaudid Tablets - 8 mg 1386

Hydroxyzine Hydrochloride (Imipramine may potentiate the effects of CNS depressant drugs). Products include:
Atarax Tablets & Syrup 1992
Marax Tablets & DF Syrup 2015
Vistaril Intramuscular Solution ... 2042

Hyoscyamine (Co-administration may result in increased atropine-like effects such as paralytic ileus). Products include:
Cystospaz Tablets 2123
Urised Tablets 2123

Hyoscyamine Sulfate (Co-administration may result in increased atropine-like effects such as paralytic ileus). Products include:
Arco-Lase Plus Tablets 513
Atrohist Plus Tablets 1605
Cystospaz-M Capsules 2123
Donnatal 2234
Donnatal Extentabs 2234
Donnatal Tablets 2234
Kutrase Capsules 2546
Levsin/Levsinex/Levbid 2549

Imipramine Hydrochloride (May inhibit the activity of cytochrome P450 2D6 isoenzyme and are substrates for P450 2D6 and may make normal metabolizers resemble poor metabolizers resulting in higher than expected plasma levels of tricyclic antidepressants). Products include:
Tofranil Ampuls 873
Tofranil Tablets 875

Ipratropium Bromide (Co-administration may result in increased atropine-like effects such as paralytic ileus). Products include:
Atrovent Inhalation Aerosol 674
Atrovent Inhalation Solution 675
Atrovent Nasal Spray 0.03% 676
Atrovent Nasal Spray 0.06% 678

Isocarboxazid (Co-administration of tricyclic antidepressants and MAO inhibitor has produced hyperpyretic crises, severe convulsions, and deaths; concurrent and/or sequential use is contraindicated).
No products indexed under this heading.

Isoflurane (Imipramine may potentiate the effects of CNS depressant drugs).
No products indexed under this heading.

Isoproterenol Hydrochloride (Tricyclic antidepressants can potentiate the effects of sympathomimetics). Products include:
Isuprel Hydrochloride Solution ... 2443
Isuprel Injection 2441
Isuprel Mistometer 2442

Isoproterenol Sulfate (Tricyclic antidepressants can potentiate the effects of sympathomimetics). Products include:
Norisodrine with Calcium Iodide Syrup 446

Ketamine Hydrochloride (Imipramine may potentiate the effects of CNS depressant drugs).
No products indexed under this heading.

Levomethadyl Acetate Hydrochloride (Imipramine may potentiate the effects of CNS depressant drugs). Products include:
Orlaam Oral Solution 2361

Levorphanol Tartrate (Imipramine may potentiate the effects of CNS depressant drugs). Products include:
Levo-Dromoran 2297

Levothyroxine Sodium (Possibility of cardiovascular toxicity). Products include:
Eltroxin Tablets 2214
Levothroid Tablets 1015
Levothyroxine Sodium, USP for Injection 546
Levoxyl Tablets 918
Synthroid 1410

Liothyronine Sodium (Possibility of cardiovascular toxicity). Products include:
Cytomel Tablets 2647
Triostat Injection 2708

Liotrix (Possibility of cardiovascular toxicity).
No products indexed under this heading.

Lorazepam (Imipramine may potentiate the effects of CNS depressant drugs). Products include:
Ativan Injection 2805
Ativan Tablets 2807

Loxapine Hydrochloride (Imipramine may potentiate the effects of CNS depressant drugs). Products include:
Loxitane 1426

Loxapine Succinate (Imipramine may potentiate the effects of CNS depressant drugs). Products include:
Loxitane Capsules 1426

Maprotiline Hydrochloride (May inhibit the activity of cytochrome P450 2D6 isoenzyme and are substrates for P450 2D6 and may make normal metabolizers resemble poor metabolizers resulting in higher than expected plasma levels of tricyclic antidepressants). Products include:
Ludiomil Tablets 861

Mepenzolate Bromide (Co-administration may result in increased atropine-like effects such as paralytic ileus).
No products indexed under this heading.

Meperidine Hydrochloride (Imipramine may potentiate the effects of CNS depressant drugs). Products include:
Demerol 2438
Mepergan Injection 2859

Mephobarbital (Co-administration with hepatic enzyme inducers, such as barbiturates, may decrease imipramine plasma concentrations; imipramine may potentiate the effects of CNS depressant drugs). Products include:
Mebaral Tablets 2452

Meprobamate (Imipramine may potentiate the effects of CNS depressant drugs). Products include:
Miltown Tablets 2780
PMB 200 and PMB 400 2890

Mesoridazine Besylate (May inhibit the activity of cytochrome P450 2D6 isoenzyme and are substrates for P450 2D6 and may make normal metabolizers resemble poor metabolizers resulting in higher than expected plasma levels of tricyclic antidepressants). Products include:
Serentil 689

Metaproterenol Sulfate (Tricyclic antidepressants can potentiate the effects of sympathomimetics). Products include:
Alupent 672
Metaproterenol Sulfate Inhalation Solution, USP, Arm-a-Med 547

Metaraminol Bitartrate (Tricyclic antidepressants can potentiate the effects of sympathomimetics). Products include:
Aramine Injection 1649

Methadone Hydrochloride (Imipramine may potentiate the effects of CNS depressant drugs). Products include:
Methadone Hydrochloride Oral Concentrate 2356
Methadone Hydrochloride Oral Solution & Tablets 2357

Methohexital Sodium (Imipramine may potentiate the effects of CNS depressant drugs).
No products indexed under this heading.

Methotrimeprazine (May inhibit the activity of cytochrome P450 2D6 isoenzyme and are substrates for P450 2D6 and may make normal metabolizers resemble poor metabolizers resulting in higher than expected plasma levels of tricyclic antidepressants). Products include:
Levoprome 1321

Methoxamine Hydrochloride (Tricyclic antidepressants can potentiate the effects of sympathomimetics). Products include:
Vasoxyl Injection 1169

IMPORTANT NOTE: Always consult each drug listing in the patient's regimen for possible interactions.

Tofranil-PM — Interactions Index — 1086

Methoxyflurane (Imipramine may potentiate the effects of CNS depressant drugs).
No products indexed under this heading.

Methylphenidate Hydrochloride (Co-administration results in Inhibition of imipramine metabolism; downward dosage adjustment of imipramine may be necessary). Products include:
Ritalin 866

Midazolam Hydrochloride (Imipramine may potentiate the effects of CNS depressant drugs). Products include:
Versed Injection 2324

Mirtazapine (May inhibit the activity of cytochrome P450 2D6 isoenzyme and are substrates for P450 2D6 and may make normal metabolizers resemble poor metabolizers resulting in higher than expected plasma levels of tricyclic antidepressants). Products include:
Remeron Tablets 1878

Molindone Hydrochloride (Imipramine may potentiate the effects of CNS depressant drugs). Products include:
Moban Tablets and Concentrate 1036

Morphine Sulfate (Imipramine may potentiate the effects of CNS depressant drugs). Products include:
Astramorph/PF Injection, USP (Preservative-Free) 526
Duramorph Injection 983
Infumorph 200 and Infumorph 500 Sterile Solutions 985
Kadian Capsules 2948
MS Contin Tablets 2149
MSIR 2152
Oramorph SR (Morphine Sulfate Sustained Release Tablets) 2359
RMS Suppositories CII 2766
Roxanol 2365

Nefazodone Hydrochloride (May inhibit the activity of cytochrome P450 2D6 isoenzyme and are substrates for P450 2D6 and may make normal metabolizers resemble poor metabolizers resulting in higher than expected plasma levels of tricyclic antidepressants). Products include:
Serzone Tablets 776

Norepinephrine Bitartrate (Tricyclic antidepressants can potentiate the effects of sympathomimetics). Products include:
Levophed Bitartrate Injection 2445

Nortriptyline Hydrochloride (May inhibit the activity of cytochrome P450 2D6 isoenzyme and are substrates for P450 2D6 and may make normal metabolizers resemble poor metabolizers resulting in higher than expected plasma levels of tricyclic antidepressants). Products include:
Pamelor 2409

Opium Alkaloids (Imipramine may potentiate the effects of CNS depressant drugs).
No products indexed under this heading.

Oxazepam (Imipramine may potentiate the effects of CNS depressant drugs). Products include:
Serax Capsules 2916
Serax Tablets 2916

Oxybutynin Chloride (Co-administration may result in increased atropine-like effects such as paralytic ileus). Products include:
Ditropan 1267

Oxycodone Hydrochloride (Imipramine may potentiate the effects of CNS depressant drugs). Products include:
OxyContin Tablets 2163
OxyIR Capsules 2167
Percocet Tablets 955
Percodan Tablets 955
Percodan-Demi Tablets 956
Roxicodone Tablets, Oral Solution & Intensol (Oxycodone) 2366
Tylox Capsules 1593

Paroxetine Hydrochloride (Selective serotonin reuptake inhibitors, such as paroxetine may have variable extent of inhibition of P450 2D6; potential for higher than expected plasma levels of tricyclic antidepressants). Products include:
Paxil Tablets 2681

Pentobarbital Sodium (Co-administration with hepatic enzyme inducers, such as barbiturates, may decrease imipramine plasma concentrations; imipramine may potentiate the effects of CNS depressant drugs). Products include:
Nembutal Sodium Capsules 440
Nembutal Sodium Solution 442
Nembutal Sodium Suppositories 444

Perphenazine (May inhibit the activity of cytochrome P450 2D6 isoenzyme and are substrates for P450 2D6 and may make normal metabolizers resemble poor metabolizers resulting in higher than expected plasma levels of tricyclic antidepressants). Products include:
Etrafon 2495
Triavil Tablets 1800
Trilafon 2532

Phenelzine Sulfate (Co-administration of tricyclic antidepressants and MAO inhibitor has produced hyperpyretic crises, severe convulsions, and deaths; concurrent and/or sequential use is contraindicated). Products include:
Nardil 1977

Phenobarbital (Co-administration with hepatic enzyme inducers, such as barbiturates, may decrease imipramine plasma concentrations; imipramine may potentiate the effects of CNS depressant drugs). Products include:
Arco-Lase Plus Tablets 513
Bellergal-S Tablets 2375
Donnatal 2234
Donnatal Extentabs 2234
Donnatal Tablets 2234
Phenobarbital Elixir and Tablets 1523
Quadrinal Tablets 1398

Phenylephrine Bitartrate (Tricyclic antidepressants can potentiate the effects of sympathomimetics).
No products indexed under this heading.

Phenylephrine Hydrochloride (Tricyclic antidepressants can potentiate the effects of sympathomimetics). Products include:
Atrohist Plus Tablets 1605
Cerose DM ..... ▣ 853
D.A. II Tablets 972
D.A. Chewable Tablets 970
Dura-Vent/DA Tablets 972
Extendryl 1003
4-Way Fast Acting Nasal Spray (regular & mentholated) ..... ▣ 644
Hemorid ..... ▣ 797
Hycomine Compound Tablets 948
Neo-Synephrine Hydrochloride 1% Carpuject 2455
Neo-Synephrine Hydrochloride 1% Injection 2455
Neo-Synephrine Hydrochloride (Ophthalmic) 2456
Neo-Synephrine ..... ▣ 624
Novahistine Elixir ..... ▣ 782
Phenergan VC 2886
Phenergan VC with Codeine 2888
Preparation H ..... ▣ 842
Tympagesic Ear Drops 2476
Vicks Sinex Nasal Spray and Ultra Fine Mist ..... ▣ 738

Phenylephrine Tannate (Tricyclic antidepressants can potentiate the effects of sympathomimetics). Products include:
Atrohist Pediatric Suspension 1604
Atrohist Pediatric Suspension Dye-Free 1604
Rynatan 2781
Rynatuss 2782

Phenylpropanolamine Hydrochloride (Tricyclic antidepressants can potentiate the effects of sympathomimetics). Products include:
Acutrim ..... ▣ 648
Atrohist Plus Tablets 1605
BC Cold Powder Multi-Symptom Formula (Cold-Sinus-Allergy) ..... ▣ 631
BC Cold Powder Non-Drowsy Formula (Cold-Sinus) ..... ▣ 631
Cheracol Plus Head Cold/Cough Formula ..... ▣ 741
Comtrex Multi-Symptom Cold Reliever Liqui-Gels ..... ▣ 638
Comtrex Multi-Symptom Non-Drowsy Liqui-gels ..... ▣ 640
Contac Continuous Action Nasal Decongestant/Antihistamine 12 Hour Capsules ..... ▣ 773
Contac Maximum Strength Continuous Action Decongestant/Antihistamine 12 Hour Caplets ..... ▣ 772
Contac Severe Cold and Flu Formula Caplets ..... ▣ 773
Coricidin 'D' Decongestant Tablets ..... ▣ 760
Dexatrim ..... ▣ 795
Dexatrim Plus Vitamins Caplets ..... ▣ 796
Dimetane-DC Cough Syrup 2232
Dimetapp Allergy Sinus Caplets ..... ▣ 838
Dimetapp Cold & Allergy Chewable Tablets ..... ▣ 838
Dimetapp Cold & Cough Liqui-Gels ..... ▣ 839
Dimetapp DM Elixir ..... ▣ 840
Dimetapp Elixir ..... ▣ 840
Dimetapp Extentabs ..... ▣ 841
Dimetapp Tablets/Liqui-Gels ..... ▣ 841
Dura-Vent Tablets 971
Entex LA Tablets 972
Exgest LA Tablets 787
Hycomine 947
Nolamine Timed-Release Tablets 790
Ornade Spansule Capsules 2678
Propagest Tablets 791
Pyrroxate Caplets ..... ▣ 742
Robitussin-CF ..... ▣ 846
Sinulin Tablets 792
Tavist-D 12 Hour Relief Tablets ..... ▣ 750
Teldrin 12 Hour Antihistamine/Nasal Decongestant Allergy Relief Capsules ..... ▣ 786
Triaminic Expectorant ..... ▣ 753
Triaminic Syrup ..... ▣ 755
Triaminic Triaminicol Cold & Cough ..... ▣ 756
Triaminic DM Syrup ..... ▣ 756
Triaminicin Tablets ..... ▣ 756
Vicks DayQuil Allergy Relief 12-Hour Extended Release Tablets ..... ▣ 733
Vicks DayQuil Allergy Relief 4-Hour Tablets ..... ▣ 733
Vicks DayQuil SINUS Pressure & CONGESTION Relief ..... ▣ 734

Phenytoin (Co-administration with hepatic enzyme inducers, such as phenytoin, may decrease imipramine plasma concentrations). Products include:
Dilantin Infatabs 1967
Dilantin-125 Suspension 1969

Phenytoin Sodium (Co-administration with hepatic enzyme inducers, such as phenytoin, may decrease imipramine plasma concentrations). Products include:
Dilantin Kapseals 1965

Pirbuterol Acetate (Tricyclic antidepressants can potentiate the effects of sympathomimetics). Products include:
Maxair Autohaler 1550
Maxair Inhaler 1552

Prazepam (Imipramine may potentiate the effects of CNS depressant drugs).
No products indexed under this heading.

Prochlorperazine (May inhibit the activity of cytochrome P450 2D6 isoenzyme and are substrates for P450 2D6 and may make normal metabolizers resemble poor metabolizers resulting in higher than expected plasma levels of tricyclic antidepressants). Products include:
Compazine 2644

Procyclidine Hydrochloride (Co-administration may result in increased atropine-like effects such as paralytic ileus). Products include:
Kemadrin Tablets 1105

Promethazine Hydrochloride (May inhibit the activity of cytochrome P450 2D6 isoenzyme and are substrates for P450 2D6 and may make normal metabolizers resemble poor metabolizers resulting in higher than expected plasma levels of tricyclic antidepressants). Products include:
Mepergan Injection 2859
Phenergan with Codeine 2883
Phenergan with Dextromethorphan 2885
Phenergan Injection 2880
Phenergan Suppositories 2882
Phenergan Syrup 2881
Phenergan Tablets 2882
Phenergan VC 2886
Phenergan VC with Codeine 2888

Propafenone Hydrochloride (May inhibit the activity of cytochrome P450 2D6 isoenzyme and are substrates for P450 2D6 and may make normal metabolizers resemble poor metabolizers resulting in higher than expected plasma levels of tricyclic antidepressants). Products include:
Rythmol Tablets–150mg, 225mg, 300mg 1399

Propantheline Bromide (Co-administration may result in increased atropine-like effects such as paralytic ileus). Products include:
Pro-Banthine Tablets 2226

Propofol (Imipramine may potentiate the effects of CNS depressant drugs). Products include:
Diprivan Injectable Emulsion 2939

Propoxyphene Hydrochloride (Imipramine may potentiate the effects of CNS depressant drugs). Products include:
Darvon 1475
Wygesic Tablets 2930

Propoxyphene Napsylate (Imipramine may potentiate the effects of CNS depressant drugs). Products include:
Darvon-N/Darvocet-N 1473

Protriptyline Hydrochloride (May inhibit the activity of cytochrome P450 2D6 isoenzyme and are substrates for P450 2D6 and may make normal metabolizers resemble poor metabolizers resulting in higher than expected plasma levels of tricyclic antidepressants). Products include:
Vivactil Tablets 1820

Pseudoephedrine Hydrochloride (Tricyclic antidepressants can potentiate the effects of sympathomimetics). Products include:
Actifed Allergy Daytime/Nighttime Caplets ..... ▣ 808
Actifed Cold & Allergy Tablets ..... ▣ 807
Actifed Cold & Sinus Caplets and Tablets ..... ▣ 808
Actifed Sinus Daytime/Nighttime Tablets and Caplets ..... ▣ 809

(▣ Described in PDR For Nonprescription Drugs) (◉ Described in PDR For Ophthalmology)

Advil Cold and Sinus Caplets and Tablets .... ℞ 837	Robitussin Severe Congestion Liqui-Gels .... ℞ 845	TYLENOL Flu NightTime, Maximum Strength Gelcaps 1575	Donnatal Tablets 2234
Alka-Seltzer Plus Liqui-Gels .... ℞ 612	Robitussin-DAC Syrup 2249	TYLENOL Flu NightTime, Maximum Strength Hot Medication Packets 1575	**Secobarbital Sodium** (Co-administration with hepatic enzyme inducers, such as barbiturates, may decrease imipramine plasma concentrations; imipramine may potentiate the effects of CNS depressant drugs). Products include:
Alka-Seltzer Plus Flu & Body Aches Liqui-Gels Non-Drowsy Formula .... ℞ 613	Robitussin-PE .... ℞ 846
	Rondec Oral Drops 974
Alka-Seltzer Plus Night-Time Cold Medicine Liqui-Gels .... ℞ 612	Rondec Syrup 974	TYLENOL Sinus, Maximum Strength Geltabs, Gelcaps, Caplets and Tablets 1576
	Rondec Tablet 974
Allerest Maximum Strength........... ℞ 649	Rondec Chewable Tablets 974
Allerest No Drowsiness .... ℞ 649	Rondec-TR Tablet 974	Vicks 44 LiquiCaps Cough, Cold & Flu Relief .... ℞ 728
Allerest Sinus Pain Formula .... ℞ 649	Ryna 804	Seconal Sodium Pulvules 1529
Atrohist Pediatric Capsules............... 1603	Seldane-D Extended-Release Tablets 1286	Vicks 44 LiquiCaps Non-Drowsy Cough & Cold Relief .... ℞ 729	**Selegiline Hydrochloride** (Co-administration of tricyclic antidepressants and MAO inhibitor has produced hyperpyretic crises, severe convulsions, and deaths; concurrent and/or sequential use is contraindicated). Products include:
Benadryl Allergy/Cold Tablets ..... ℞ 811
Benadryl Allergy Decongestant Liquid Medication .... ℞ 812	Semprex-D Capsules 1620	Vicks 44D Cough & Head Congestion Relief .... ℞ 728
	Sinarest .... ℞ 663
Benadryl Allergy Decongestant Tablets .... ℞ 812	Sine-Aid Maximum Strength Sinus Headache Gelcaps, Caplets and Tablets 1570	Vicks 44M Cough, Cold & Flu Relief .... ℞ 729
	Vicks DayQuil LiquiCaps/Liquid Multi-Symptom Cold/Flu Relief ℞ 734
Benadryl Allergy Sinus Headache Caplets .... ℞ 813	Sine-Off No Drowsiness Formula Caplets .... ℞ 784		Eldepryl Capsules 2729
	Vicks DayQuil SINUS Pressure & PAIN Relief with IBUPROFEN 735	**Sertraline Hydrochloride** (Selective serotonin reuptake inhibitors, such as sertraline, may have variable extent of inhibition of P450 2D6; potential for higher than expected plasma levels of tricyclic antidepressants). Products include:
Benylin Multisymptom .... ℞ 816	Sine-Off Sinus Medicine .... ℞ 784
Bromfed Capsules (Extended-Release) 1832	Singlet Tablets .... ℞ 785	Vicks Nyquil Hot Therapy 735
	Sinutab Non-Drying Liquid Caps ... ℞ 823	Vicks NyQuil LiquiCaps/Liquid Multi-Symptom Cold/Flu Relief, Original and Cherry Flavors........... ℞ 736
Bromfed Syrup .... ℞ 712	Sinutab Sinus Allergy Medication, Maximum Strength Tablets and Caplets .... ℞ 823
Bromfed Tablets 1832
Bromfed-DM Cough Syrup 1832		**Pseudoephedrine Sulfate** (Tricyclic antidepressants can potentiate the effects of sympathomimetics). Products include:	Zoloft Tablets 2051
Bromfed-PD Capsules (Extended-Release) 1832	Sinutab Sinus Medication, Maximum Strength Without Drowsiness Formula, Tablets & Caplets .... ℞ 824	**Sevoflurane** (Imipramine may potentiate the effects of CNS depressant drugs).
Children's TYLENOL Cold Multi-Symptom Chewable Tablets and Liquid 1559		Chlor-Trimeton Allergy Decongestant Tablets .... ℞ 759
	Claritin-D Tablets 2487	No products indexed under this heading.
	Sudafed Children's Cold & Cough Liquid Medication .... ℞ 825
Children's TYLENOL Cold Plus Cough Multi Symptom Chewable Tablets and Liquid................... 1560		Drixoral Cold and Allergy Sustained-Action Tablets .... ℞ 763	**Sufentanil Citrate** (Imipramine may potentiate the effects of CNS depressant drugs). Products include:
	Sudafed Children's Nasal Decongestant Liquid Medication .... ℞ 826	Drixoral Cold and Flu Extended-Release Tablets .... ℞ 764
	Sudafed Cold & Allergy Tablets...... ℞ 826
Children's TYLENOL Flu Suspension Liquid 1560	Sudafed Cold and Cough Liquid Caps .... ℞ 826	Drixoral Non-Drowsy Formula Extended-Release Tablets .... ℞ 764	Sufenta Injection 1355
Children's Vicks DayQuil Allergy Relief .... ℞ 730			**Temazepam** (Imipramine may potentiate the effects of CNS depressant drugs). Products include:
	Sudafed Nasal Decongestant Tablets, 30 mg. .... ℞ 825	Drixoral Allergy/Sinus Extended Release Tablets .... ℞ 765
Children's Vicks NyQuil Cold/Cough Relief .... ℞ 731		Trinalin Repetabs Tablets 1373
	Sudafed Nasal Decongestant Tablets, 60 mg. .... ℞ 825	**Quazepam** (Imipramine may potentiate the effects of CNS depressant drugs). Products include:	Restoril Capsules........................ 2413
Allergy-Sinus Comtrex Multi-Symptom Allergy-Sinus Formula Tablets and Caplets .... ℞ 639			**Terbutaline Sulfate** (Tricyclic antidepressants can potentiate the effects of sympathomimetics). Products include:
	Sudafed Non-Drying Sinus Liquid Caps .... ℞ 827	Doral Tablets 2773
Comtrex Multi-Symptom................... ℞ 638
Comtrex Multi-Symptom Non-Drowsy Caplets .... ℞ 640	Sudafed Pediatric Nasal Decongestant Liquid Oral Drops .... ℞ 827	**Quinidine Gluconate** (May inhibit the activity of cytochrome P450 2D6 isoenzyme and may make normal metabolizers resemble poor metabolizers resulting in higher than expected plasma levels of tricyclic antidepressants). Products include:
	Brethaire Inhaler 830
Congess 1003	Sudafed Severe Cold Formula Caplets .... ℞ 828	Brethine Ampuls 832
Contac Day Allergy/Sinus Caplets ℞ 771		Brethine Tablets 831
Contac Day & Night .... ℞ 772	Sudafed Severe Cold Formula Tablets .... ℞ 828	Bricanyl Subcutaneous Injection ... 1247
Contac Night Allergy/Sinus Caplets .... ℞ 771		Bricanyl Tablets 1248
	Sudafed Sinus Caplets .... ℞ 829	Quinaglute Dura-Tabs Tablets 644	**Thiamylal Sodium** (Co-administration with hepatic enzyme inducers, such as barbiturates, may decrease imipramine plasma concentrations; imipramine may potentiate the effects of CNS depressant drugs).
Contac Severe Cold & Flu Non-Drowsy .... ℞ 774	Sudafed Sinus Tablets .... ℞ 829
	Sudafed 12 Hour Caplets .... ℞ 824	**Quinidine Polygalacturonate** (May inhibit the activity of cytochrome P450 2D6 isoenzyme and may make normal metabolizers resemble poor metabolizers resulting in higher than expected plasma levels of tricyclic antidepressants). Products include:
Deconsal II Tablets 1605	Syn-Rx Tablets 1622
Dimetane-DX Cough Syrup 2233	Syn-Rx DM Tablets 1623
Dimetapp Cold & Fever Suspension .... ℞ 839	TheraFlu Flu and Cold Medicine ..... ℞ 750
	Theraflu Maximum Strength Flu and Cold Medicine For Sore Throat .... ℞ 751		No products indexed under this heading.
Dimetapp Decongestant Pediatric Drops .... ℞ 840		Cardioquin Tablets 2146
		Thioridazine Hydrochloride (May inhibit the activity of cytochrome P450 2D6 isoenzyme and are substrates for P450 2D6 and may make normal metabolizers resemble poor metabolizers resulting in higher than expected plasma levels of tricyclic antidepressants). Products include:
Dorcol Children's Cough Syrup ...... ℞ 748	TheraFlu Flu, Cold and Cough Medicine .... ℞ 750	**Quinidine Sulfate** (May inhibit the activity of cytochrome P450 2D6 isoenzyme and may make normal metabolizers resemble poor metabolizers resulting in higher than expected plasma levels of tricyclic antidepressants). Products include:
Drixoral Cough + Congestion Liquid Caps .... ℞ 763	
	TheraFlu Maximum Strength Nighttime Flu, Cold & Cough Medicine .... ℞ 751
Dura-Tap/PD Capsules 970
Duratuss Tablets 2750	
Duratuss HD Elixir 2750	TheraFlu Maximum Strength Non-Drowsy Formula Flu, Cold & Cough Medicine .... ℞ 751	Quinidex Extentabs....................... 2240
Efidac/24 .... ℞ 655		**Risperidone** (Imipramine may potentiate the effects of CNS depressant drugs). Products include:	Mellaril 2398
Entex PSE Tablets 973	
Fedahist Gyrocaps 2545	TheraFlu Maximum Strength, Non-Drowsy Formula Flu, Cold and Cough Caplets .... ℞ 752		**Thiothixene** (Imipramine may potentiate the effects of CNS depressant drugs). Products include:
Guaifed 1833		Risperdal Tablets 1348
Guaifed Syrup .... ℞ 712	Theraflu Maximum Strength Sinus Non-Drowsy Formula Caplets ... ℞ 752	**Salmeterol Xinafoate** (Tricyclic antidepressants can potentiate the effects of sympathomimetics). Products include:
Guaimax-D Tablets 809		Navane Capsules and Concentrate 2018
Histussin D Liquid 670	Triaminic AM Cough and Decongestant Formula .... ℞ 753		Navane Intramuscular 2019
Infants' TYLENOL Cold Decongestant & Fever-Reducer Drops 1561		Serevent Inhalation Aerosol............... 1149	**Thyroglobulin** (Possibility of cardiovascular toxicity).
	Triaminic AM Decongestant Formula .... ℞ 753	**Scopolamine** (Co-administration may result in increased atropine-like effects such as paralytic ileus). Products include:
Kronofed-A 994			No products indexed under this heading.
Novahistine DMX .... ℞ 782	Triaminic Infant Oral Decongestant Drops .... ℞ 754
Nucofed 2225		Transderm Scōp Transdermal Therapeutic System 890	**Thyroid** (Possibility of cardiovascular toxicity).
PediaCare Cough-Cold Chewable Tablets and Liquid..................... 1569	Triaminic Night Time .... ℞ 754
	Triaminic Sore Throat Formula ..... ℞ 755	**Scopolamine Hydrobromide** (Co-administration may result in increased atropine-like effects such as paralytic ileus). Products include:	No products indexed under this heading.
PediaCare Infants' Decongestant Drops 1569	Tussend 1830
	Tussend Expectorant 1831		**Thyroxine** (Possibility of cardiovascular toxicity).
PediaCare Infants' Drops Decongestant Plus Cough 1569	TYLENOL Allergy Sinus, Maximum Strength Caplets and Gelcaps ... 1571
		Atrohist Plus Tablets 1605	No products indexed under this heading.
PediaCare NightRest Cough-Cold Liquid 1569	TYLENOL Allergy Sinus NightTime, Maximum Strength Caplets........... 1571	Donnatal 2234
		Donnatal Extentabs 2234	**Thyroxine Sodium** (Possibility of cardiovascular toxicity).
Pediatric Vicks 44d Cough & Head Congestion Relief .... ℞ 736	TYLENOL Cold Medication, Multi-Symptom Formula Tablets and Caplets 1572	
			No products indexed under this heading.
Pediatric Vicks 44m Cough & Cold Relief .... ℞ 737	TYLENOL Cold Medication, Multi-Symptom Hot Liquid Packets 1572
Robitussin Cold & Cough Liqui-Gels .... ℞ 844	
	TYLENOL Cold Medication, No Drowsiness Formula Caplets and Gelcaps 1572
Robitussin Cold, Cough & Flu Liqui-Gels .... ℞ 844
Robitussin Maximum Strength Cough & Cold .... ℞ 847	TYLENOL Cold Severe Congestion Caplets 1573
Robitussin Night-Time Cold Formula .... ℞ 847	TYLENOL Cough Medication with Decongestant, Multi Symptom 1574
Robitussin Pediatric Cough & Cold Formula .... ℞ 848	TYLENOL Flu No Drowsiness Formula, Maximum Strength Gelcaps 1575
Robitussin Pediatric Drops .... ℞ 849

IMPORTANT NOTE: Always consult each drug listing in the patient's regimen for possible interactions.

Tranylcypromine Sulfate (Co-administration of tricyclic antidepressants and MAO inhibitor has produced hyperpyretic crises, severe convulsions, and deaths; concurrent and/or sequential use is contraindicated). Products include:
- Parnate Tablets 2679

Trazodone Hydrochloride (May inhibit the activity of cytochrome P450 2D6 isoenzyme and are substrates for P450 2D6 and may make normal metabolizers resemble poor metabolizers resulting in higher than expected plasma levels of tricyclic antidepressants). Products include:
- Desyrel and Desyrel Dividose 504

Triazolam (Imipramine may potentiate the effects of CNS depressant drugs). Products include:
- Halcion Tablets 2093

Tridihexethyl Chloride (Co-administration may result in increased atropine-like effects such as paralytic ileus).
- No products indexed under this heading.

Trifluoperazine Hydrochloride (May inhibit the activity of cytochrome P450 2D6 isoenzyme and are substrates for P450 2D6 and may make normal metabolizers resemble poor metabolizers resulting in higher than expected plasma levels of tricyclic antidepressants). Products include:
- Stelazine 2692

Trihexyphenidyl Hydrochloride (Co-administration may result in increased atropine-like effects such as paralytic ileus). Products include:
- Artane 1418

Trimipramine Maleate (May inhibit the activity of cytochrome P450 2D6 isoenzyme and are substrates for P450 2D6 and may make normal metabolizers resemble poor metabolizers resulting in higher than expected plasma levels of tricyclic antidepressants). Products include:
- Surmontil Capsules 2917

Venlafaxine Hydrochloride (May inhibit the activity of cytochrome P450 2D6 isoenzyme and are substrates for P450 2D6 and may make normal metabolizers resemble poor metabolizers resulting in higher than expected plasma levels of tricyclic antidepressants). Products include:
- Effexor 2825

Zolpidem Tartrate (Imipramine may potentiate the effects of CNS depressant drugs). Products include:
- Ambien Tablets 2559

Food Interactions

Alcohol (Imipramine may enhance the CNS depressant effects of alcohol).

TOLECTIN (200, 400 AND 600 MG)
(Tolmetin Sodium) 1591
May interact with oral anticoagulants and certain other agents. Compounds in these categories include:

Dicumarol (Increased prothrombin time and bleeding).
- No products indexed under this heading.

Methotrexate Sodium (Reduced tubular secretion of methotrexate in an animal model). Products include:
- Methotrexate Sodium Tablets, Injection, for Injection and LPF Injection 1322

Warfarin Sodium (Increased prothrombin time and bleeding). Products include:
- Coumadin 941

Food Interactions

Dairy products (Decreases total tolmetin bioavailability by 16%).

Meal, unspecified (Decreases total tolmetin bioavailability by 16%; reduces peak plasma concentrations by 50%).

TONOCARD TABLETS
(Tocainide Hydrochloride) 519
May interact with:

Lidocaine Hydrochloride (Co-administration of these pharmacodynamically similar agents may cause an increased incidence of adverse reactions, including CNS adverse reactions such as seizures). Products include:
- Decadron Phosphate with Xylocaine Injection, Sterile 1683
- Unguentine Plus .... ▣ 712
- Xylocaine Injections 562

Metoprolol Succinate (Co-administration has produced additive effects on wedge pressure and cardiac index). Products include:
- Toprol-XL Tablets 560

Metoprolol Tartrate (Co-administration has produced additive effects on wedge pressure and cardiac index). Products include:
- Lopressor 848
- Lopressor HCT Tablets 850

TOPICORT EMOLLIENT CREAM 0.25%
(Desoximetasone) 1289
None cited in PDR database.

TOPICORT GEL 0.05%
(Desoximetasone) 1290
None cited in PDR database.

TOPICORT LP EMOLLIENT CREAM 0.05%
(Desoximetasone) 1289
None cited in PDR database.

TOPICORT OINTMENT 0.25%
(Desoximetasone) 1291
None cited in PDR database.

TOPROL-XL TABLETS
(Metoprolol Succinate) 560
May interact with catecholamine depleting drugs, cardiac glycosides, and certain other agents. Compounds in these categories include:

Deserpidine (Potential for additive effect; hypotension or marked bradycardia).
- No products indexed under this heading.

Deslanoside (Metoprolol should be used cautiously in patients with hypertension and angina who have congestive heart failure and are on digitalis and diuretics since both digitalis and metoprolol slow AV conduction).
- No products indexed under this heading.

Digitoxin (Metoprolol should be used cautiously in patients with hypertension and angina who have congestive heart failure and are on digitalis and diuretics since both digitalis and metoprolol slow AV conduction). Products include:
- Crystodigin Tablets 1472

Digoxin (Metoprolol should be used cautiously in patients with hypertension and angina who have congestive heart failure and are on digitalis and diuretics since both digitalis and metoprolol slow AV conduction). Products include:
- Lanoxicaps 1110
- Lanoxin Elixir Pediatric 1113
- Lanoxin Injection 1116
- Lanoxin Injection Pediatric 1119
- Lanoxin Tablets 1121

Epinephrine Hydrochloride (Potential unresponsiveness to the usual dose of epinephrine to treat allergic reactions in certain patients). Products include:
- Ana-Kit Anaphylaxis Emergency Treatment Kit 611

Guanethidine Monosulfate (Potential for additive effect; hypotension or marked bradycardia). Products include:
- Esimil Tablets 840
- Ismelin Tablets 845

Rauwolfia Serpentina (Potential for additive effect; hypotension or marked bradycardia).
- No products indexed under this heading.

Rescinnamine (Potential for additive effect; hypotension or marked bradycardia).
- No products indexed under this heading.

Reserpine (Potential for additive effect; hypotension or marked bradycardia). Products include:
- Diupres Tablets 1691
- Hydropres Tablets 1718
- Ser-Ap-Es Tablets 867

TORADOL IM INJECTION, IV INJECTION
(Ketorolac Tromethamine) 2319
See **Toradol Tablets**

TORADOL TABLETS
(Ketorolac Tromethamine) 2319
May interact with non-steroidal anti-inflammatory agents, lithium preparations, ACE inhibitors, nondepolarizing neuromuscular blocking agents, salicylates, and certain other agents. Compounds in these categories include:

Alprazolam (Concurrent use may produce hallucinations). Products include:
- Xanax Tablets 2115

Aspirin (Concurrent use is contraindicated because of the cumulative risk of inducing serious NSAID-related side effects). Products include:
- Alka-Seltzer Cherry Effervescent Antacid and Pain Reliever .... ▣ 609
- Alka-Seltzer Extra Strength Effervescent Antacid and Pain Reliever .... ▣ 609
- Alka-Seltzer Lemon Lime Effervescent Antacid and Pain Reliever .... ▣ 609
- Alka-Seltzer Original Effervescent Antacid and Pain Reliever .... ▣ 609
- Alka-Seltzer Plus .... ▣ 611
- Alka-Seltzer Plus Sinus Medicine .... ▣ 611
- Ascriptin .... ▣ 650
- Arthritis Strength BC Powder .... ▣ 631
- BC Cold Powder Multi-Symptom Formula (Cold-Sinus-Allergy) .... ▣ 631
- BC Cold Powder Non-Drowsy Formula (Cold-Sinus) .... ▣ 631
- BC Powder .... ▣ 631
- Genuine Bayer Aspirin Tablets & Caplets .... ▣ 618
- Extra Strength Bayer Arthritis Pain Regimen Formula .... ▣ 615
- Extra Strength Bayer Aspirin Caplets & Tablets .... ▣ 617
- Extended-Release Bayer 8-Hour Aspirin .... ▣ 616
- Extra Strength Bayer Plus Aspirin Caplets .... ▣ 617
- Extra Strength Bayer PM Aspirin Plus Sleep Aid .... ▣ 617
- Aspirin Regimen Bayer 81 mg Tablets with Calcium .... ▣ 615
- Aspirin Regimen Bayer Adult Low Strength 81 mg Tablets .... ▣ 613
- Aspirin Regimen Bayer Children's Chewable Aspirin .... ▣ 616
- Aspirin Regimen Bayer Regular Strength 325 mg Caplets .... ▣ 613
- Bufferin Analgesic Tablets .... ▣ 636
- Arthritis Strength Bufferin Analgesic Caplets .... ▣ 637
- Extra Strength Bufferin Analgesic Tablets .... ▣ 637
- Cama Arthritis Pain Reliever .... ▣ 748
- Darvon Compound-65 Pulvules 1475
- Easprin 1971
- Ecotrin 2625
- Ecotrin Enteric Coated Aspirin Maximum Strength Tablets and Caplets .... ▣ 775
- Ecotrin Enteric Coated Aspirin Regular Strength Tablets 2625
- Empirin Aspirin Tablets .... ▣ 818
- Excedrin Extra-Strength Analgesic Tablets, Caplets, and Geltabs 734
- Fiorinal Capsules 2388
- Fiorinal with Codeine Capsules 2390
- Fiorinal Tablets 2388
- Goody's Extra Strength Headache Powders .... ▣ 632
- Goody's Extra Strength Pain Relief Tablets .... ▣ 632
- Halfprin Tablets 1413
- Norgesic 1554
- Percodan Tablets 955
- Percodan-Demi Tablets 956
- Robaxisal Tablets 2246
- Soma Compound w/Codeine Tablets 2784
- Soma Compound Tablets 2783
- St. Joseph Adult Chewable Aspirin (81 mg.) .... ▣ 768
- Talwin Compound 2466
- Vanquish Analgesic Caplets .... ▣ 627

Atracurium Besylate (Concurrent use with parenteral form of Toradol has resulted in apnea). Products include:
- Tracrium Injection 1155

Benazepril Hydrochloride (Concomitant use may increase the risk of renal impairment, particularly in volume-depleted patients). Products include:
- Lotensin Tablets 852
- Lotensin HCT Tablets 855
- Lotrel Capsules 858

Captopril (Concomitant use may increase the risk of renal impairment, particularly in volume-depleted patients). Products include:
- Capoten Tablets 740
- Capozide Tablets 744

Carbamazepine (Concomitant use has resulted in sporadic cases of seizures). Products include:
- Atretol Tablets 569
- Tegretol/Tegretol-XR 870

Choline Magnesium Trisalicylate (*In Vitro* studies indicate that, at therapeutic concentrations of salicylates, the binding of ketorolac was reduced from approximately 99.2% to 97.5%, representing a potential 2-fold increase in unbound ketorolac plasma levels). Products include:
- Trilisate 2155

Cisatracurium Besylate (Concurrent use with parenteral form of Toradol has resulted in apnea). Products include:
- Nimbex Injection 1131

Diclofenac Potassium (Concurrent use is contraindicated because of the cumulative risk of inducing serious NSAID-related side effects). Products include:
- Cataflam Tablets 833

(▣ Described in PDR For Nonprescription Drugs) (◉ Described in PDR For Ophthalmology)

Diclofenac Sodium (Concurrent use is contraindicated because of the cumulative risk of inducing serious NSAID-related side effects). Products include:
- Voltaren Ophthalmic Sterile Ophthalmic Solution .... ◉ 264
- Cataflam/Voltaren/Voltaren-XR 833

Diflunisal (*In Vitro* studies indicate that, at therapeutic concentrations of salicylates, the binding of ketorolac was reduced from approximately 99.2% to 97.5%, representing a potential 2-fold increase in unbound ketorolac plasma levels). Products include:
- Dolobid Tablets........ 1695

Enalapril Maleate (Concomitant use may increase the risk of renal impairment, particularly in volume-depleted patients). Products include:
- Vaseretic Tablets........ 1810
- Vasotec Tablets........ 1816

Enalaprilat (Concomitant use may increase the risk of renal impairment, particularly in volume-depleted patients). Products include:
- Vasotec I.V........ 1814

Etodolac (Concurrent use is contraindicated because of the cumulative risk of inducing serious NSAID-related side effects). Products include:
- Lodine Capsules and Tablets 2849

Fenoprofen Calcium (Concurrent use is contraindicated because of the cumulative risk of inducing serious NSAID-related side effects). Products include:
- Nalfon 200 Pulvules & Nalfon Tablets........ 933

Fluoxetine Hydrochloride (Concurrent use may produce hallucinations). Products include:
- Prozac Pulvules & Liquid, Oral Solution........ 935

Flurbiprofen (Concurrent use is contraindicated because of the cumulative risk of inducing serious NSAID-related side effects).
- No products indexed under this heading.

Fosinopril Sodium (Concomitant use may increase the risk of renal impairment, particularly in volume-depleted patients). Products include:
- Monopril Tablets........ 762

Furosemide (Potential for reduced diuretic response in normovolemic healthy subjects by 20%). Products include:
- Lasix Injection, Oral Solution and Tablets........ 1267

Heparin Sodium (Co-administration results in mean template bleeding time of 6.4 minutes compared to 6.0 minutes, however extreme caution and close monitoring is recommended). Products include:
- Heparin Lock Flush Solution........ 2831
- Heparin Sodium Injection........ 2832
- Heparin Sodium Vials........ 1486

Ibuprofen (Concurrent use is contraindicated because of the cumulative risk of inducing serious NSAID-related side effects). Products include:
- Advil Cold and Sinus Caplets and Tablets........ 837
- Advil Ibuprofen Tablets, Caplets and Gel Caplets........ 836
- Children's Motrin Ibuprofen Oral Suspension........ 1558
- IBU Tablets........ 1389
- Ibuprohm........ 713
- Motrin IB Caplets, Tablets, and Gelcaps........ 802
- Motrin Ibuprofen Suspension, Oral Drops, Chewable Tablets, Caplets........ 1563
- Nuprin Ibuprofen/Analgesic Tablets & Caplets........ 645
- Vicks DayQuil SINUS Pressure & PAIN Relief with IBUPROFEN........ 735

Indomethacin (Concurrent use is contraindicated because of the cumulative risk of inducing serious NSAID-related side effects). Products include:
- Indocin........ 1723

Indomethacin Sodium Trihydrate (Concurrent use is contraindicated because of the cumulative risk of inducing serious NSAID-related side effects). Products include:
- Indocin I.V........ 1727

Ketoprofen (Concurrent use is contraindicated because of the cumulative risk of inducing serious NSAID-related side effects). Products include:
- Actron Caplets and Tablets........ 608
- Orudis Capsules........ 2874
- Orudis KT........ 842
- Oruvail Capsules........ 2874

Lisinopril (Concomitant use may increase the risk of renal impairment, particularly in volume-depleted patients). Products include:
- Prinivil Tablets........ 1776
- Prinzide Tablets........ 1780
- Zestoretic Tablets........ 2968
- Zestril Tablets........ 2972

Lithium Carbonate (Co-administration can result in inhibition of renal lithium clearance leading to an increase in plasma lithium concentrations). Products include:
- Eskalith........ 2658
- Lithium Carbonate Capsules & Tablets........ 2352
- Lithonate/Lithotabs/Lithobid........ 2721

Lithium Citrate (Co-administration can result in inhibition of renal lithium clearance leading to an increase in plasma lithium concentrations).
- No products indexed under this heading.

Magnesium Salicylate (*In Vitro* studies indicate that, at therapeutic concentrations of salicylates, the binding of ketorolac was reduced from approximately 99.2% to 97.5%, representing a potential 2-fold increase in unbound ketorolac plasma levels). Products include:
- Backache Caplets........ 635
- Doan's Extra-Strength Analgesic........ 653
- Extra Strength Doan's P.M........ 653
- Doan's Regular Strength Analgesic........ 654
- Mobigesic Tablets........ 607

Meclofenamate Sodium (Concurrent use is contraindicated because of the cumulative risk of inducing serious NSAID-related side effects).
- No products indexed under this heading.

Mefenamic Acid (Concurrent use is contraindicated because of the cumulative risk of inducing serious NSAID-related side effects). Products include:
- Ponstel........ 1982

Methotrexate Sodium (Co-administration may result in reduced clearance of methotrexate thereby enhancing the toxicity). Products include:
- Methotrexate Sodium Tablets, Injection, for Injection and LPF Injection........ 1322

Metocurine Iodide (Concurrent use with parenteral form of Toradol has resulted in apnea). Products include:
- Metubine Iodide Vials........ 932

Mivacurium Chloride (Concurrent use with parenteral form of Toradol has resulted in apnea). Products include:
- Mivacron........ 1125

Moexipril Hydrochloride (Concomitant use may increase the risk of renal impairment, particularly in volume-depleted patients). Products include:
- Univasc Tablets........ 2553

Nabumetone (Concurrent use is contraindicated because of the cumulative risk of inducing serious NSAID-related side effects). Products include:
- Relafen Tablets........ 2688

Naproxen (Concurrent use is contraindicated because of the cumulative risk of inducing serious NSAID-related side effects). Products include:
- Anaprox/Naprosyn........ 2277

Naproxen Sodium (Concurrent use is contraindicated because of the cumulative risk of inducing serious NSAID-related side effects). Products include:
- Aleve........ 2124
- Anaprox/Naprosyn........ 2277
- Naprelan Tablets........ 2861

Oxaprozin (Concurrent use is contraindicated because of the cumulative risk of inducing serious NSAID-related side effects). Products include:
- Daypro Caplets........ 2578

Pancuronium Bromide (Concurrent use with parenteral form of Toradol has resulted in apnea).
- No products indexed under this heading.

Phenylbutazone (Concurrent use is contraindicated because of the cumulative risk of inducing serious NSAID-related side effects).
- No products indexed under this heading.

Phenytoin (Concomitant use has resulted in sporadic cases of seizures). Products include:
- Dilantin Infatabs........ 1967
- Dilantin-125 Suspension........ 1969

Phenytoin Sodium (Concomitant use has resulted in sporadic cases of seizures). Products include:
- Dilantin Kapseals........ 1965

Piroxicam (Concurrent use is contraindicated because of the cumulative risk of inducing serious NSAID-related side effects). Products include:
- Feldene Capsules........ 2008

Probenecid (Co-administration of oral ketorolac and probenecid has resulted in decreased clearance of ketorolac and a significant increase in plasma levels, AUC increased by three-fold, and terminal half-life increased by two-fold; concomitant use is contraindicated). Products include:
- Benemid Tablets........ 1651
- ColBENEMID Tablets........ 1662

Quinapril Hydrochloride (Concomitant use may increase the risk of renal impairment, particularly in volume-depleted patients). Products include:
- Accupril Tablets........ 1950

Ramipril (Concomitant use may increase the risk of renal impairment, particularly in volume-depleted patients). Products include:
- Altace Capsules........ 1238

Rocuronium Bromide (Concurrent use with parenteral form of Toradol has resulted in apnea). Products include:
- Zemuron Injection........ 1885

Salsalate (*In Vitro* studies indicate that, at therapeutic concentrations of salicylates, the binding of ketorolac was reduced from approximately 99.2% to 97.5%, representing a potential 2-fold increase in unbound ketorolac plasma levels). Products include:
- Disalcid........ 1549
- Mono-Gesic Tablets........ 810
- Salflex Tablets........ 791

Spirapril Hydrochloride (Concomitant use may increase the risk of renal impairment, particularly in volume-depleted patients).
- No products indexed under this heading.

Sulindac (Concurrent use is contraindicated because of the cumulative risk of inducing serious NSAID-related side effects). Products include:
- Clinoril Tablets........ 1658

Thiothixene (Concurrent use may produce hallucinations). Products include:
- Navane Capsules and Concentrate 2018
- Navane Intramuscular........ 2019

Thiothixene Hydrochloride (Concurrent use may produce hallucinations).
- No products indexed under this heading.

Tolmetin Sodium (Concurrent use is contraindicated because of the cumulative risk of inducing serious NSAID-related side effects). Products include:
- Tolectin (200, 400 and 600 mg) .. 1591

Trandolapril (Concomitant use may increase the risk of renal impairment, particularly in volume-depleted patients). Products include:
- Mavik Tablets........ 1407

Vecuronium Bromide (Concurrent use with parenteral form of Toradol has resulted in apnea). Products include:
- Norcuron for Injection........ 1875

Warfarin Sodium (*In Vitro* binding of warfarin to plasma proteins is slightly reduced by ketorolac; extreme caution and close monitoring is recommended). Products include:
- Coumadin........ 941

Food Interactions

Diet, high-lipid (Oral administration of Toradol after a high-fat meal resulted in decreased peak and delayed time-to-peak concentrations of Toradol by about 1 hour).

TORECAN INJECTION

(Thiethylperazine Malate)........2367

May interact with central nervous system depressants, narcotic analgesics, barbiturates, general anesthetics, and certain other agents. Compounds in these categories include:

Alfentanil Hydrochloride (Phenothiazines are capable of potentiating CNS depressants). Products include:
- Alfenta Injection........ 1334

Alprazolam (Phenothiazines are capable of potentiating CNS depressants). Products include:
- Xanax Tablets........ 2115

Aprobarbital (Phenothiazines are capable of potentiating CNS depressants).
- No products indexed under this heading.

IMPORTANT NOTE: Always consult each drug listing in the patient's regimen for possible interactions.

Torecan / Interactions Index

Atropine Sulfate (Phenothiazines are capable of potentiating atropine). Products include:
- Arco-Lase Plus Tablets ... 513
- Atrohist Plus Tablets ... 1605
- Donnatal ... 2234
- Donnatal Extentabs ... 2234
- Donnatal Tablets ... 2234
- Lomotil ... 2591
- Motofen Tablets ... 789
- Urised Tablets ... 2123

Buprenorphine (Phenothiazines are capable of potentiating CNS depressants). Products include:
- Buprenex Injectable ... 2170

Buspirone Hydrochloride (Phenothiazines are capable of potentiating CNS depressants). Products include:
- BuSpar Tablets ... 738

Butabarbital (Phenothiazines are capable of potentiating CNS depressants).
- No products indexed under this heading.

Butalbital (Phenothiazines are capable of potentiating CNS depressants). Products include:
- Axocet Capsules ... 2469
- Esgic-plus Capsules ... 1012
- Esgic-plus Tablets ... 1012
- Fioricet Tablets ... 2386
- Fioricet with Codeine Capsules ... 2387
- Fiorinal Capsules ... 2388
- Fiorinal with Codeine Capsules ... 2390
- Fiorinal Tablets ... 2388
- Phrenilin ... 790
- Sedapap Tablets 50 mg/650 mg .. 1826

Chlordiazepoxide (Phenothiazines are capable of potentiating CNS depressants). Products include:
- Limbitrol ... 2333

Chlordiazepoxide Hydrochloride (Phenothiazines are capable of potentiating CNS depressants). Products include:
- Librax Capsules ... 2330
- Librium Capsules ... 2331
- Librium Injectable ... 2332

Chlorpromazine (Phenothiazines are capable of potentiating CNS depressants). Products include:
- Thorazine Suppositories ... 2701

Chlorpromazine Hydrochloride (Phenothiazines are capable of potentiating CNS depressants). Products include:
- Thorazine ... 2701

Chlorprothixene (Phenothiazines are capable of potentiating CNS depressants).
- No products indexed under this heading.

Chlorprothixene Hydrochloride (Phenothiazines are capable of potentiating CNS depressants).
- No products indexed under this heading.

Chlorprothixene Lactate (Phenothiazines are capable of potentiating CNS depressants).
- No products indexed under this heading.

Clorazepate Dipotassium (Phenothiazines are capable of potentiating CNS depressants). Products include:
- Tranxene ... 459

Clozapine (Phenothiazines are capable of potentiating CNS depressants). Products include:
- Clozaril Tablets ... 2377

Codeine Phosphate (Phenothiazines are capable of potentiating CNS depressants). Products include:
- Brontex ... 2130
- Dimetane-DC Cough Syrup ... 2232
- Fioricet with Codeine Capsules ... 2387
- Fiorinal with Codeine Capsules ... 2390
- Nucofed ... 2225
- Phenergan with Codeine ... 2883
- Phenergan VC with Codeine ... 2888
- Robitussin A-C Syrup ... 2248
- Robitussin-DAC Syrup ... 2249
- Ryna ... 804
- Soma Compound w/Codeine Tablets ... 2784
- Tylenol with Codeine ... 1592

Desflurane (Phenothiazines are capable of potentiating CNS depressants). Products include:
- Suprane (desflurane, USP) ... 1865

Dezocine (Phenothiazines are capable of potentiating CNS depressants). Products include:
- Dalgan Injection ... 529

Diazepam (Phenothiazines are capable of potentiating CNS depressants). Products include:
- Dizac (diazepam injectable emulsion) CIV ... 1862
- Valium Injectable ... 2336
- Valium Tablets ... 2335

Droperidol (Phenothiazines are capable of potentiating CNS depressants). Products include:
- Inapsine Injection ... 462

Enflurane (Phenothiazines are capable of potentiating CNS depressants).
- No products indexed under this heading.

Estazolam (Phenothiazines are capable of potentiating CNS depressants). Products include:
- ProSom Tablets ... 457

Ethchlorvynol (Phenothiazines are capable of potentiating CNS depressants). Products include:
- Placidyl Capsules ... 456

Ethinamate (Phenothiazines are capable of potentiating CNS depressants).
- No products indexed under this heading.

Fentanyl (Phenothiazines are capable of potentiating CNS depressants). Products include:
- Duragesic Transdermal System ... 1336

Fentanyl Citrate (Phenothiazines are capable of potentiating CNS depressants). Products include:
- Sublimaze Injection ... 463

Fluphenazine Decanoate (Phenothiazines are capable of potentiating CNS depressants). Products include:
- Prolixin Decanoate ... 510

Fluphenazine Enanthate (Phenothiazines are capable of potentiating CNS depressants). Products include:
- Prolixin Enanthate ... 510

Fluphenazine Hydrochloride (Phenothiazines are capable of potentiating CNS depressants). Products include:
- Prolixin ... 510

Flurazepam Hydrochloride (Phenothiazines are capable of potentiating CNS depressants). Products include:
- Dalmane Capsules ... 2329

Glutethimide (Phenothiazines are capable of potentiating CNS depressants).
- No products indexed under this heading.

Haloperidol (Phenothiazines are capable of potentiating CNS depressants). Products include:
- Haldol Injection, Tablets and Concentrate ... 1585

Haloperidol Decanoate (Phenothiazines are capable of potentiating CNS depressants). Products include:
- Haldol Decanoate ... 1587

Hydrocodone Bitartrate (Phenothiazines are capable of potentiating CNS depressants). Products include:
- Codiclear DH Syrup ... 808
- Duratuss HD Elixir ... 2750
- Histussin D Liquid ... 670
- Hycodan Tablets and Syrup ... 946
- Hycomine Compound Tablets ... 948
- Hycomine ... 947
- Hycotuss Expectorant Syrup ... 950
- Hydrocet Capsules ... 787
- Lorcet 10/650 Tablets ... 1016
- Lortab ... 2751
- Tussend ... 1830
- Tussend Expectorant ... 1831
- Vicodin Tablets ... 1404
- Vicodin ES Tablets ... 1405
- Vicodin HP Tablets ... 1403
- Vicodin Tuss Expectorant ... 1406
- Zydone Capsules ... 967

Hydrocodone Polistirex (Phenothiazines are capable of potentiating CNS depressants). Products include:
- Tussionex Pennkinetic Extended-Release Suspension ... 1624

Hydromorphone Hydrochloride (Phenothiazines are capable of potentiating CNS depressants). Products include:
- Dilaudid Ampules ... 1382
- Dilaudid Cough Syrup ... 1383
- Dilaudid-HP Injection ... 1384
- Dilaudid-HP Lyophilized Powder 250 mg ... 1384
- Dilaudid ... 1382
- Dilaudid Oral Liquid ... 1386
- Dilaudid ... 1382
- Dilaudid Tablets - 8 mg ... 1386

Hydroxyzine Hydrochloride (Phenothiazines are capable of potentiating CNS depressants). Products include:
- Atarax Tablets & Syrup ... 1992
- Marax Tablets & DF Syrup ... 2015
- Vistaril Intramuscular Solution ... 2042

Isoflurane (Phenothiazines are capable of potentiating CNS depressants).
- No products indexed under this heading.

Ketamine Hydrochloride (Phenothiazines are capable of potentiating CNS depressants).
- No products indexed under this heading.

Levomethadyl Acetate Hydrochloride (Phenothiazines are capable of potentiating CNS depressants). Products include:
- Orlaam Oral Solution ... 2361

Levorphanol Tartrate (Phenothiazines are capable of potentiating CNS depressants). Products include:
- Levo-Dromoran ... 2297

Lorazepam (Phenothiazines are capable of potentiating CNS depressants). Products include:
- Ativan Injection ... 2805
- Ativan Tablets ... 2807

Loxapine Hydrochloride (Phenothiazines are capable of potentiating CNS depressants). Products include:
- Loxitane ... 1426

Loxapine Succinate (Phenothiazines are capable of potentiating CNS depressants). Products include:
- Loxitane Capsules ... 1426

Meperidine Hydrochloride (Phenothiazines are capable of potentiating CNS depressants). Products include:
- Demerol ... 2438
- Mepergan Injection ... 2859

Mephobarbital (Phenothiazines are capable of potentiating CNS depressants). Products include:
- Mebaral Tablets ... 2452

Meprobamate (Phenothiazines are capable of potentiating CNS depressants). Products include:
- Miltown Tablets ... 2780
- PMB 200 and PMB 400 ... 2890

Mesoridazine Besylate (Phenothiazines are capable of potentiating CNS depressants). Products include:
- Serentil ... 689

Methadone Hydrochloride (Phenothiazines are capable of potentiating CNS depressants). Products include:
- Methadone Hydrochloride Oral Concentrate ... 2356
- Methadone Hydrochloride Oral Solution & Tablets ... 2357

Methohexital Sodium (Phenothiazines are capable of potentiating CNS depressants).
- No products indexed under this heading.

Methotrimeprazine (Phenothiazines are capable of potentiating CNS depressants). Products include:
- Levoprome ... 1321

Methoxyflurane (Phenothiazines are capable of potentiating CNS depressants).
- No products indexed under this heading.

Midazolam Hydrochloride (Phenothiazines are capable of potentiating CNS depressants). Products include:
- Versed Injection ... 2324

Molindone Hydrochloride (Phenothiazines are capable of potentiating CNS depressants). Products include:
- Moban Tablets and Concentrate ... 1036

Morphine Sulfate (Phenothiazines are capable of potentiating CNS depressants). Products include:
- Astramorph/PF Injection, USP (Preservative-Free) ... 526
- Duramorph Injection ... 983
- Infumorph 200 and Infumorph 500 Sterile Solutions ... 985
- Kadian Capsules ... 2948
- MS Contin Tablets ... 2149
- MSIR ... 2152
- Oramorph SR (Morphine Sulfate Sustained Release Tablets) ... 2359
- RMS Suppositories CII ... 2766
- Roxanol ... 2365

Opium Alkaloids (Phenothiazines are capable of potentiating CNS depressants).
- No products indexed under this heading.

Oxazepam (Phenothiazines are capable of potentiating CNS depressants). Products include:
- Serax Capsules ... 2916
- Serax Tablets ... 2916

Oxycodone Hydrochloride (Phenothiazines are capable of potentiating CNS depressants). Products include:
- OxyContin Tablets ... 2163
- OxyIR Capsules ... 2167
- Percocet Tablets ... 955
- Percodan Tablets ... 955
- Percodan-Demi Tablets ... 956
- Roxicodone Tablets, Oral Solution & Intensol (Oxycodone) ... 2366
- Tylox Capsules ... 1593

Pentobarbital Sodium (Phenothiazines are capable of potentiating CNS depressants). Products include:
- Nembutal Sodium Capsules ... 440
- Nembutal Sodium Solution ... 442
- Nembutal Sodium Suppositories ... 444

Perphenazine (Phenothiazines are capable of potentiating CNS depressants). Products include:
- Etrafon ... 2495
- Triavil Tablets ... 1800
- Trilafon ... 2532

Phenobarbital (Phenothiazines are capable of potentiating CNS depressants). Products include:
- Arco-Lase Plus Tablets ... 513
- Bellergal-S Tablets ... 2375

(■ Described in PDR For Nonprescription Drugs) (◎ Described in PDR For Ophthalmology)

1091 **Interactions Index** **Tornalate Metered Dose**

Donnatal ... 2234
Donnatal Extentabs ... 2234
Donnatal Tablets ... 2234
Phenobarbital Elixir and Tablets ... 1523
Quadrinal Tablets ... 1398

Prazepam (Phenothiazines are capable of potentiating CNS depressants).
No products indexed under this heading.

Prochlorperazine (Phenothiazines are capable of potentiating CNS depressants). Products include:
Compazine ... 2644

Promethazine Hydrochloride (Phenothiazines are capable of potentiating CNS depressants). Products include:
Mepergan Injection ... 2859
Phenergan with Codeine ... 2883
Phenergan with Dextromethorphan ... 2885
Phenergan Injection ... 2880
Phenergan Suppositories ... 2882
Phenergan Syrup ... 2881
Phenergan Tablets ... 2882
Phenergan VC ... 2886
Phenergan VC with Codeine ... 2888

Propofol (Phenothiazines are capable of potentiating CNS depressants). Products include:
Diprivan Injectable Emulsion ... 2939

Propoxyphene Hydrochloride (Phenothiazines are capable of potentiating CNS depressants). Products include:
Darvon ... 1475
Wygesic Tablets ... 2930

Propoxyphene Napsylate (Phenothiazines are capable of potentiating CNS depressants). Products include:
Darvon-N/Darvocet-N ... 1473

Quazepam (Phenothiazines are capable of potentiating CNS depressants). Products include:
Doral Tablets ... 2773

Risperidone (Phenothiazines are capable of potentiating CNS depressants). Products include:
Risperdal Tablets ... 1348

Secobarbital Sodium (Phenothiazines are capable of potentiating CNS depressants). Products include:
Seconal Sodium Pulvules ... 1529

Sevoflurane (Phenothiazines are capable of potentiating CNS depressants).
No products indexed under this heading.

Sufentanil Citrate (Phenothiazines are capable of potentiating CNS depressants). Products include:
Sufenta Injection ... 1355

Temazepam (Phenothiazines are capable of potentiating CNS depressants). Products include:
Restoril Capsules ... 2413

Thiamylal Sodium (Phenothiazines are capable of potentiating CNS depressants).
No products indexed under this heading.

Thioridazine Hydrochloride (Phenothiazines are capable of potentiating CNS depressants). Products include:
Mellaril ... 2398

Thiothixene (Phenothiazines are capable of potentiating CNS depressants). Products include:
Navane Capsules and Concentrate ... 2018
Navane Intramuscular ... 2019

Triazolam (Phenothiazines are capable of potentiating CNS depressants). Products include:
Halcion Tablets ... 2093

Trifluoperazine Hydrochloride (Phenothiazines are capable of potentiating CNS depressants). Products include:
Stelazine ... 2692

Zolpidem Tartrate (Phenothiazines are capable of potentiating CNS depressants). Products include:
Ambien Tablets ... 2559

Food Interactions

Alcohol (Phenothiazines are capable of potentiating CNS depressants).

TORECAN TABLETS
(Thiethylperazine Maleate) ... 2367
See **Torecan Injection**

TORNALATE SOLUTION FOR INHALATION, 0.2%
(Bitolterol Mesylate) ... 976
May interact with sympathomimetic bronchodilators, monoamine oxidase inhibitors, and tricyclic antidepressants. Compounds in these categories include:

Albuterol (Potential for additive effects). Products include:
Proventil Inhalation Aerosol ... 2524
Ventolin Inhalation Aerosol and Refill ... 1170

Albuterol Sulfate (Potential for additive effects). Products include:
Airet Albuterol Sulfate Inhalation Solution ... 1602
Albuterol Sulfate, USP Solution for Inhalation, Arm-a-Med ... 522
Proventil Inhalation Solution 0.083% ... 2527
Proventil Repetabs Tablets ... 2529
Proventil Solution for Inhalation 0.5% ... 2525
Proventil Syrup ... 2528
Proventil Tablets ... 2529
Ventolin Inhalation Solution ... 1171
Ventolin Nebules Inhalation Solution ... 1172
Ventolin Rotacaps for Inhalation ... 1173
Ventolin Syrup ... 1175
Ventolin Tablets ... 1176
Volmax Extended-Release Tablets ... 1835

Amitriptyline Hydrochloride (Action of bitolterol on the vascular system may be potentiated). Products include:
Elavil ... 2945
Etrafon ... 2495
Limbitrol ... 2333
Triavil Tablets ... 1800

Amoxapine (Action of bitolterol on the vascular system may be potentiated). Products include:
Asendin Tablets ... 1419

Clomipramine Hydrochloride (Action of bitolterol on the vascular system may be potentiated). Products include:
Anafranil Capsules ... 819

Desipramine Hydrochloride (Action of bitolterol on the vascular system may be potentiated). Products include:
Norpramin Tablets ... 1273

Doxepin Hydrochloride (Action of bitolterol on the vascular system may be potentiated). Products include:
Adapin Capsules ... 1542
Sinequan ... 2028
Zonalon Cream ... 1042

Ephedrine Hydrochloride (Potential for additive effects). Products include:
Primatene Tablets ... 844
Quadrinal Tablets ... 1398

Ephedrine Sulfate (Potential for additive effects). Products include:
Marax Tablets & DF Syrup ... 2015

Ephedrine Tannate (Potential for additive effects). Products include:
Rynatuss ... 2782

Epinephrine (Potential for additive effects). Products include:
EPIFRIN ... ⊙ 237
EpiPen ... 808
Marcaine with Epinephrine ... 2446
Primatene Mist ... 843
Sensorcaine with Epinephrine Injection ... 554
Sus-Phrine Injection ... 1017
Xylocaine with Epinephrine Injections ... 562

Epinephrine Hydrochloride (Potential for additive effects). Products include:
Ana-Kit Anaphylaxis Emergency Treatment Kit ... 611

Ethylnorepinephrine Hydrochloride (Potential for additive effects).
No products indexed under this heading.

Furazolidone (Action of bitolterol on the vascular system may be potentiated). Products include:
Furoxone ... 2221

Imipramine Hydrochloride (Action of bitolterol on the vascular system may be potentiated). Products include:
Tofranil Ampuls ... 873
Tofranil Tablets ... 875

Imipramine Pamoate (Action of bitolterol on the vascular system may be potentiated). Products include:
Tofranil-PM Capsules ... 876

Isocarboxazid (Action of bitolterol on the vascular system may be potentiated).
No products indexed under this heading.

Isoetharine (Potential for additive effects). Products include:
Bronkometer Aerosol ... 2432
Bronkosol Solution ... 2432
Isoetharine Inhalation Solution, USP, Arm-a-Med ... 545

Isoproterenol Hydrochloride (Potential for additive effects). Products include:
Isuprel Hydrochloride Solution ... 2443
Isuprel Injection ... 2441
Isuprel Mistometer ... 2442

Isoproterenol Sulfate (Potential for additive effects). Products include:
Norisodrine with Calcium Iodide Syrup ... 446

Maprotiline Hydrochloride (Action of bitolterol on the vascular system may be potentiated). Products include:
Ludiomil Tablets ... 861

Metaproterenol Sulfate (Potential for additive effects). Products include:
Alupent ... 672
Metaproterenol Sulfate Inhalation Solution, USP, Arm-a-Med ... 547

Nortriptyline Hydrochloride (Action of bitolterol on the vascular system may be potentiated). Products include:
Pamelor ... 2409

Phenelzine Sulfate (Action of bitolterol on the vascular system may be potentiated). Products include:
Nardil ... 1977

Pirbuterol Acetate (Potential for additive effects). Products include:
Maxair Autohaler ... 1550
Maxair Inhaler ... 1552

Protriptyline Hydrochloride (Action of bitolterol on the vascular system may be potentiated). Products include:
Vivactil Tablets ... 1820

Salmeterol Xinafoate (Potential for additive effects). Products include:
Serevent Inhalation Aerosol ... 1149

Selegiline Hydrochloride (Action of bitolterol on the vascular system may be potentiated). Products include:
Eldepryl Capsules ... 2729

Terbutaline Sulfate (Potential for additive effects). Products include:
Brethaire Inhaler ... 830
Brethine Ampuls ... 832
Brethine Tablets ... 831
Bricanyl Subcutaneous Injection ... 1247
Bricanyl Tablets ... 1248

Tranylcypromine Sulfate (Action of bitolterol on the vascular system may be potentiated). Products include:
Parnate Tablets ... 2679

Trimipramine Maleate (Action of bitolterol on the vascular system may be potentiated). Products include:
Surmontil Capsules ... 2917

TORNALATE METERED DOSE INHALER
(Bitolterol Mesylate) ... 978
May interact with sympathomimetic aerosol bronchodilators and sympathomimetic bronchodilators. Compounds in these categories include:

Albuterol (Concurrent use should be avoided to prevent deleterious cardiovascular effects). Products include:
Proventil Inhalation Aerosol ... 2524
Ventolin Inhalation Aerosol and Refill ... 1170

Albuterol Sulfate (Concurrent use should be avoided to prevent deleterious cardiovascular effects). Products include:
Airet Albuterol Sulfate Inhalation Solution ... 1602
Albuterol Sulfate, USP Solution for Inhalation, Arm-a-Med ... 522
Proventil Inhalation Solution 0.083% ... 2527
Proventil Repetabs Tablets ... 2529
Proventil Solution for Inhalation 0.5% ... 2525
Proventil Syrup ... 2528
Proventil Tablets ... 2529
Ventolin Inhalation Solution ... 1171
Ventolin Nebules Inhalation Solution ... 1172
Ventolin Rotacaps for Inhalation ... 1173
Ventolin Syrup ... 1175
Ventolin Tablets ... 1176
Volmax Extended-Release Tablets ... 1835

Ephedrine Hydrochloride (Concurrent use should be avoided to prevent deleterious cardiovascular effects). Products include:
Primatene Tablets ... 844
Quadrinal Tablets ... 1398

Ephedrine Sulfate (Concurrent use should be avoided to prevent deleterious cardiovascular effects). Products include:
Marax Tablets & DF Syrup ... 2015

Ephedrine Tannate (Concurrent use should be avoided to prevent deleterious cardiovascular effects). Products include:
Rynatuss ... 2782

Epinephrine (Concurrent use should be avoided to prevent deleterious cardiovascular effects). Products include:
EPIFRIN ... ⊙ 237
EpiPen ... 808
Marcaine with Epinephrine ... 2446
Primatene Mist ... 843
Sensorcaine with Epinephrine Injection ... 554
Sus-Phrine Injection ... 1017

IMPORTANT NOTE: Always consult each drug listing in the patient's regimen for possible interactions.

Xylocaine with Epinephrine Injections 562

Epinephrine Hydrochloride (Concurrent use should be avoided to prevent deleterious cardiovascular effects). Products include:

Ana-Kit Anaphylaxis Emergency Treatment Kit 611

Ethylnorepinephrine Hydrochloride (Concurrent use should be avoided to prevent deleterious cardiovascular effects).

No products indexed under this heading.

Isoetharine (Concurrent use should be avoided to prevent deleterious cardiovascular effects). Products include:

Bronkometer Aerosol 2432
Bronkosol Solution 2432
Isoetharine Inhalation Solution, USP, Arm-a-Med 545

Isoproterenol Hydrochloride (Concurrent use should be avoided to prevent deleterious cardiovascular effects). Products include:

Isuprel Hydrochloride Solution 2443
Isuprel Injection 2441
Isuprel Mistometer 2442

Isoproterenol Sulfate (Concurrent use should be avoided to prevent deleterious cardiovascular effects). Products include:

Norisodrine with Calcium Iodide Syrup 446

Metaproterenol Sulfate (Concurrent use should be avoided to prevent deleterious cardiovascular effects). Products include:

Alupent 672
Metaproterenol Sulfate Inhalation Solution, USP, Arm-a-Med 547

Pirbuterol Acetate (Concurrent use should be avoided to prevent deleterious cardiovascular effects). Products include:

Maxair Autohaler 1550
Maxair Inhaler 1552

Salmeterol Xinafoate (Concurrent use should be avoided to prevent deleterious cardiovascular effects). Products include:

Serevent Inhalation Aerosol 1149

Terbutaline Sulfate (Concurrent use should be avoided to prevent deleterious cardiovascular effects). Products include:

Brethaire Inhaler 830
Brethine Ampuls 832
Brethine Tablets 831
Bricanyl Subcutaneous Injection 1247
Bricanyl Tablets 1248

TRACRIUM INJECTION

(Atracurium Besylate) 1155

May interact with aminoglycosides, muscle relaxants, and certain other agents. Compounds in these categories include:

Amikacin Sulfate (Enhances neuromuscular blocking action of Tracrium). Products include:

Amikacin Sulfate Injection, USP 523
Amikacin Sulfate Injection, USP 981
Amikin Injectable 502

Baclofen (Synergistic or antagonist effect). Products include:

Lioresal Intrathecal 1634
Lioresal Tablets 847

Carisoprodol (Synergistic or antagonist effect). Products include:

Soma Compound w/Codeine Tablets 2784
Soma Compound Tablets 2783
Soma Tablets 2782

Chlorzoxazone (Synergistic or antagonist effect). Products include:

Parafon Forte DSC Caplets 1590

Cisatracurium Besylate (Synergistic or antagonist effect). Products include:

Nimbex Injection 1131

Cyclobenzaprine Hydrochloride (Synergistic or antagonist effect). Products include:

Flexeril Tablets 1701

Dantrolene Sodium (Synergistic or antagonist effect). Products include:

Dantrium Capsules 2131
Dantrium Intravenous 2132

Doxacurium Chloride (Synergistic or antagonist effect). Products include:

Nuromax Injection 1136

Enflurane (Enhances neuromuscular blocking action of Tracrium).

No products indexed under this heading.

Gentamicin Sulfate (Enhances neuromuscular blocking action of Tracrium). Products include:

Garamycin Cream 0.1% 2501
Garamycin Injectable 2502
Garamycin Ointment 0.1% 2501
Garamycin Ophthalmic 2501
Genoptic Sterile Ophthalmic Solution .... ◉ 241
Genoptic Sterile Ophthalmic Ointment .... ◉ 241
Gentak .... ◉ 209
Pred-G Liquifilm Sterile Ophthalmic Suspension .... ◉ 248
Pred-G S.O.P. Sterile Ophthalmic Ointment .... ◉ 249

Halothane (Enhances neuromuscular blocking action of Tracrium). Products include:

Fluothane 2830

Isoflurane (Enhances neuromuscular blocking action of Tracrium).

No products indexed under this heading.

Kanamycin Sulfate (Enhances neuromuscular blocking action of Tracrium).

No products indexed under this heading.

Lithium Carbonate (Enhances neuromuscular blocking action of Tracrium). Products include:

Eskalith 2658
Lithium Carbonate Capsules & Tablets 2352
Lithonate/Lithotabs/Lithobid 2721

Lithium Citrate (Enhances neuromuscular blocking action of Tracrium).

No products indexed under this heading.

Magnesium Salts (Enhances neuromuscular blocking action of Tracrium).

Metaxalone (Synergistic or antagonist effect). Products include:

Skelaxin Tablets 793

Methocarbamol (Synergistic or antagonist effect). Products include:

Robaxin Injectable 2245
Robaxin Tablets 2246
Robaxisal Tablets 2246

Metocurine Iodide (Synergistic or antagonist effect). Products include:

Metubine Iodide Vials 932

Orphenadrine Citrate (Synergistic or antagonist effect). Products include:

Norflex 1554
Norgesic 1554

Pancuronium Bromide (Synergistic or antagonist effect).

No products indexed under this heading.

Polymyxin Preparations (Enhances neuromuscular blocking action of Tracrium).

Procainamide (Enhances neuromuscular blocking action of Tracrium).

Quinidine Gluconate (Enhances neuromuscular blocking action of Tracrium). Products include:

Quinaglute Dura-Tabs Tablets 644

Quinidine Polygalacturonate (Enhances neuromuscular blocking action of Tracrium). Products include:

Cardioquin Tablets 2146

Quinidine Sulfate (Enhances neuromuscular blocking action of Tracrium). Products include:

Quinidex Extentabs 2240

Rocuronium Bromide (Synergistic or antagonist effect). Products include:

Zemuron Injection 1885

Streptomycin Sulfate (Enhances neuromuscular blocking action of Tracrium). Products include:

Streptomycin Sulfate Injection 2031

Succinylcholine Chloride (Prior administration quickens the onset and may increase the depth of neuromuscular block induced by atracurium). Products include:

Anectine 1062

Tobramycin (Enhances neuromuscular blocking action of Tracrium). Products include:

AKTOB .... ◉ 207
TobraDex Ophthalmic Suspension and Ointment 469
Tobrex Ophthalmic Ointment and Solution .... ◉ 226

Tobramycin Sulfate (Enhances neuromuscular blocking action of Tracrium). Products include:

Nebcin Vials, Hyporets & ADD-Vantage 1518

Vecuronium Bromide (Synergistic or antagonist effect). Products include:

Norcuron for Injection 1875

TRANCOPAL CAPLETS

(Chlormezanone) 2468

May interact with central nervous system depressants and certain other agents. Compounds in these categories include:

Alfentanil Hydrochloride (Possible additive effects). Products include:

Alfenta Injection 1334

Alprazolam (Possible additive effects). Products include:

Xanax Tablets 2115

Aprobarbital (Possible additive effects).

No products indexed under this heading.

Buprenorphine (Possible additive effects). Products include:

Buprenex Injectable 2170

Buspirone Hydrochloride (Possible additive effects). Products include:

BuSpar Tablets 738

Butabarbital (Possible additive effects).

No products indexed under this heading.

Butalbital (Possible additive effects). Products include:

Axocet Capsules 2469
Esgic-plus Capsules 1012
Esgic-plus Tablets 1012
Fioricet Tablets 2386
Fioricet with Codeine Capsules 2387
Fiorinal Capsules 2388
Fiorinal with Codeine Capsules 2390
Fiorinal Tablets 2388
Phrenilin 790
Sedapap Tablets 50 mg/650 mg 1826

Chlordiazepoxide (Possible additive effects). Products include:

Limbitrol 2333

Chlordiazepoxide Hydrochloride (Possible additive effects). Products include:

Librax Capsules 2330
Librium Capsules 2331
Librium Injectable 2332

Chlorpromazine (Possible additive effects). Products include:

Thorazine Suppositories 2701

Chlorprothixene (Possible additive effects).

No products indexed under this heading.

Chlorprothixene Hydrochloride (Possible additive effects).

No products indexed under this heading.

Chlorprothixene Lactate (Possible additive effects).

No products indexed under this heading.

Clorazepate Dipotassium (Possible additive effects). Products include:

Tranxene 459

Clozapine (Possible additive effects). Products include:

Clozaril Tablets 2377

Codeine Phosphate (Possible additive effects). Products include:

Brontex 2130
Dimetane-DC Cough Syrup 2232
Fioricet with Codeine Capsules 2387
Fiorinal with Codeine Capsules 2390
Nucofed 2225
Phenergan with Codeine 2883
Phenergan VC with Codeine 2888
Robitussin A-C Syrup 2248
Robitussin-DAC Syrup 2249
Ryna .... ▣ 804
Soma Compound w/Codeine Tablets 2784
Tylenol with Codeine 1592

Desflurane (Possible additive effects). Products include:

Suprane (desflurane, USP) 1865

Dezocine (Possible additive effects). Products include:

Dalgan Injection 529

Diazepam (Possible additive effects). Products include:

Dizac (diazepam injectable emulsion) CIV 1862
Valium Injectable 2336
Valium Tablets 2335

Droperidol (Possible additive effects). Products include:

Inapsine Injection 462

Enflurane (Possible additive effects).

No products indexed under this heading.

Estazolam (Possible additive effects). Products include:

ProSom Tablets 457

Ethchlorvynol (Possible additive effects). Products include:

Placidyl Capsules 456

Ethinamate (Possible additive effects).

No products indexed under this heading.

Fentanyl (Possible additive effects). Products include:

Duragesic Transdermal System 1336

Fentanyl Citrate (Possible additive effects). Products include:

Sublimaze Injection 463

Fluphenazine Decanoate (Possible additive effects). Products include:

Prolixin Decanoate 510

Fluphenazine Enanthate (Possible additive effects). Products include:

Prolixin Enanthate 510

(▣ Described in PDR For Nonprescription Drugs) (◉ Described in PDR For Ophthalmology)

1093 **Interactions Index** **Trandate**

Fluphenazine Hydrochloride (Possible additive effects). Products include:

Prolixin ... 510

Flurazepam Hydrochloride (Possible additive effects). Products include:

Dalmane Capsules ... 2329

Glutethimide (Possible additive effects).

No products indexed under this heading.

Haloperidol (Possible additive effects). Products include:

Haldol Injection, Tablets and Concentrate ... 1585

Haloperidol Decanoate (Possible additive effects). Products include:

Haldol Decanoate ... 1587

Hydrocodone Bitartrate (Possible additive effects). Products include:

Codiclear DH Syrup ... 808
Duratuss HD Elixir ... 2750
Histussin D Liquid ... 670
Hycodan Tablets and Syrup ... 946
Hycomine Compound Tablets ... 948
Hycomine ... 947
Hycotuss Expectorant Syrup ... 950
Hydrocet Capsules ... 787
Lorcet 10/650 Tablets ... 1016
Lortab ... 2751
Tussend ... 1830
Tussend Expectorant ... 1831
Vicodin Tablets ... 1404
Vicodin ES Tablets ... 1405
Vicodin HP Tablets ... 1403
Vicodin Tuss Expectorant ... 1406
Zydone Capsules ... 967

Hydrocodone Polistirex (Possible additive effects). Products include:

Tussionex Pennkinetic Extended-Release Suspension ... 1624

Hydroxyzine Hydrochloride (Possible additive effects). Products include:

Atarax Tablets & Syrup ... 1992
Marax Tablets & DF Syrup ... 2015
Vistaril Intramuscular Solution ... 2042

Isoflurane (Possible additive effects).

No products indexed under this heading.

Ketamine Hydrochloride (Possible additive effects).

No products indexed under this heading.

Levomethadyl Acetate Hydrochloride (Possible additive effects). Products include:

Orlaam Oral Solution ... 2361

Levorphanol Tartrate (Possible additive effects). Products include:

Levo-Dromoran ... 2297

Lorazepam (Possible additive effects). Products include:

Ativan Injection ... 2805
Ativan Tablets ... 2807

Loxapine Hydrochloride (Possible additive effects). Products include:

Loxitane ... 1426

Loxapine Succinate (Possible additive effects). Products include:

Loxitane Capsules ... 1426

Meperidine Hydrochloride (Possible additive effects). Products include:

Demerol ... 2438
Mepergan Injection ... 2859

Mephobarbital (Possible additive effects). Products include:

Mebaral Tablets ... 2452

Meprobamate (Possible additive effects). Products include:

Miltown Tablets ... 2780
PMB 200 and PMB 400 ... 2890

Mesoridazine Besylate (Possible additive effects). Products include:

Serentil ... 689

Methadone Hydrochloride (Possible additive effects). Products include:

Methadone Hydrochloride Oral Concentrate ... 2356
Methadone Hydrochloride Oral Solution & Tablets ... 2357

Methohexital Sodium (Possible additive effects).

No products indexed under this heading.

Methotrimeprazine (Possible additive effects). Products include:

Levoprome ... 1321

Methoxyflurane (Possible additive effects).

No products indexed under this heading.

Midazolam Hydrochloride (Possible additive effects). Products include:

Versed Injection ... 2324

Molindone Hydrochloride (Possible additive effects). Products include:

Moban Tablets and Concentrate ... 1036

Morphine Sulfate (Possible additive effects). Products include:

Astramorph/PF Injection, USP (Preservative-Free) ... 526
Duramorph Injection ... 983
Infumorph 200 and Infumorph 500 Sterile Solutions ... 985
Kadian Capsules ... 2948
MS Contin Tablets ... 2149
MSIR ... 2152
Oramorph SR (Morphine Sulfate Sustained Release Tablets) ... 2359
RMS Suppositories CII ... 2766
Roxanol ... 2365

Opium Alkaloids (Possible additive effects).

No products indexed under this heading.

Oxazepam (Possible additive effects). Products include:

Serax Capsules ... 2916
Serax Tablets ... 2916

Oxycodone Hydrochloride (Possible additive effects). Products include:

OxyContin Tablets ... 2163
OxyIR Capsules ... 2167
Percocet Tablets ... 955
Percodan Tablets ... 955
Percodan-Demi Tablets ... 956
Roxicodone Tablets, Oral Solution & Intensol (Oxycodone) ... 2366
Tylox Capsules ... 1593

Pentobarbital Sodium (Possible additive effects). Products include:

Nembutal Sodium Capsules ... 440
Nembutal Sodium Solution ... 442
Nembutal Sodium Suppositories ... 444

Perphenazine (Possible additive effects). Products include:

Etrafon ... 2495
Triavil Tablets ... 1800
Trilafon ... 2532

Phenobarbital (Possible additive effects). Products include:

Arco-Lase Plus Tablets ... 513
Bellergal-S Tablets ... 2375
Donnatal ... 2234
Donnatal Extentabs ... 2234
Donnatal Tablets ... 2234
Phenobarbital Elixir and Tablets ... 1523
Quadrinal Tablets ... 1398

Prazepam (Possible additive effects).

No products indexed under this heading.

Prochlorperazine (Possible additive effects). Products include:

Compazine ... 2644

Promethazine Hydrochloride (Possible additive effects). Products include:

Mepergan Injection ... 2859
Phenergan with Codeine ... 2883
Phenergan with Dextromethorphan 2885
Phenergan Injection ... 2880
Phenergan Suppositories ... 2882
Phenergan Syrup ... 2881
Phenergan Tablets ... 2882
Phenergan VC ... 2886
Phenergan VC with Codeine ... 2888

Propofol (Possible additive effects). Products include:

Diprivan Injectable Emulsion ... 2939

Propoxyphene Hydrochloride (Possible additive effects). Products include:

Darvon ... 1475
Wygesic Tablets ... 2930

Propoxyphene Napsylate (Possible additive effects). Products include:

Darvon-N/Darvocet-N ... 1473

Quazepam (Possible additive effects). Products include:

Doral Tablets ... 2773

Risperidone (Possible additive effects). Products include:

Risperdal Tablets ... 1348

Secobarbital Sodium (Possible additive effects). Products include:

Seconal Sodium Pulvules ... 1529

Sevoflurane (Possible additive effects).

No products indexed under this heading.

Sufentanil Citrate (Possible additive effects). Products include:

Sufenta Injection ... 1355

Temazepam (Possible additive effects). Products include:

Restoril Capsules ... 2413

Thiamylal Sodium (Possible additive effects).

No products indexed under this heading.

Thioridazine Hydrochloride (Possible additive effects). Products include:

Mellaril ... 2398

Thiothixene (Possible additive effects). Products include:

Navane Capsules and Concentrate 2018
Navane Intramuscular ... 2019

Triazolam (Possible additive effects). Products include:

Halcion Tablets ... 2093

Trifluoperazine Hydrochloride (Possible additive effects). Products include:

Stelazine ... 2692

Zolpidem Tartrate (Possible additive effects). Products include:

Ambien Tablets ... 2559

Food Interactions

Alcohol (Possible additive effects).

TRANDATE INJECTION

(Labetalol Hydrochloride) ... 1158
See **Trandate Tablets**

TRANDATE TABLETS

(Labetalol Hydrochloride) ... 1158
May interact with tricyclic antidepressants, $beta_2$ agonists, insulin, oral hypoglycemic agents, and certain other agents. Compounds in these categories include:

Acarbose (Beta-blockade may prevent the appearance of premonitory signs and symptoms of acute hypoglycemia; reduces the release of insulin in response to hyperglycemia). Products include:

Precose ... 604

Albuterol (Beta-blocker can blunt the bronchodilator effect of beta-receptor agonists in patients with bronchospasm; greater than normal anti-asthmatic dose of beta-agonist may be required). Products include:

Proventil Inhalation Aerosol ... 2524
Ventolin Inhalation Aerosol and Refill ... 1170

Albuterol Sulfate (Beta-blocker can blunt the bronchodilator effect of beta-receptor agonists in patients with bronchospasm; greater than normal anti-asthmatic dose of beta-agonist may be required). Products include:

Airet Albuterol Sulfate Inhalation Solution ... 1602
Albuterol Sulfate, USP Solution for Inhalation, Arm-a-Med ... 522
Proventil Inhalation Solution 0.083% ... 2527
Proventil Repetabs Tablets ... 2529
Proventil Solution for Inhalation 0.5% ... 2525
Proventil Syrup ... 2528
Proventil Tablets ... 2529
Ventolin Inhalation Solution ... 1171
Ventolin Nebules Inhalation Solution ... 1172
Ventolin Rotacaps for Inhalation ... 1173
Ventolin Syrup ... 1175
Ventolin Tablets ... 1176
Volmax Extended-Release Tablets .. 1835

Amitriptyline Hydrochloride (Potential for increase in tremors). Products include:

Elavil ... 2945
Etrafon ... 2495
Limbitrol ... 2333
Triavil Tablets ... 1800

Amoxapine (Potential for increase in tremors). Products include:

Asendin Tablets ... 1419

Bitolterol Mesylate (Beta-blocker can blunt the bronchodilator effect of beta-receptor agonists in patients with bronchospasm; greater than normal anti-asthmatic dose of beta-agonist may be required). Products include:

Tornalate Solution for Inhalation, 0.2% ... 976
Tornalate Metered Dose Inhaler ... 978

Chlorpropamide (Beta-blockade may prevent the appearance of premonitory signs and symptoms of acute hypoglycemia; reduces the release of insulin in response to hyperglycemia). Products include:

Diabinese Tablets ... 2002

Cimetidine (Increases bioavailability of oral labetalol). Products include:

Tagamet HB Tablets ... 786
Tagamet Tablets ... 2694

Cimetidine Hydrochloride (Increases bioavailability of oral labetalol). Products include:

Tagamet ... 2694

Clomipramine Hydrochloride (Potential for increase in tremors). Products include:

Anafranil Capsules ... 819

Desipramine Hydrochloride (Potential for increase in tremors). Products include:

Norpramin Tablets ... 1273

Doxepin Hydrochloride (Potential for increase in tremors). Products include:

Adapin Capsules ... 1542
Sinequan ... 2028
Zonalon Cream ... 1042

IMPORTANT NOTE: Always consult each drug listing in the patient's regimen for possible interactions.

Trandate

Ephedrine Hydrochloride (Beta-blocker can blunt the bronchodilator effect of beta-agonists in patients with bronchospasm; greater than normal anti-asthmatic dose of beta-agonist may be required). Products include:
Primatene Tablets ◨ 844
Quadrinal Tablets 1398

Ephedrine Sulfate (Beta-blocker can blunt the bronchodilator effect of beta-receptor agonists in patients with bronchospasm; greater than normal anti-asthmatic dose of beta-agonist may be required). Products include:
Marax Tablets & DF Syrup 2015

Ephedrine Tannate (Beta-blocker can blunt the bronchodilator effect of beta-receptor agonists in patients with bronchospasm; greater than normal anti-asthmatic dose of beta-agonist may be required). Products include:
Rynatuss 2782

Epinephrine (Beta-blocker can blunt the bronchodilator effect of beta-receptor agonists in patients with bronchospasm; greater than normal anti-asthmatic dose of beta-agonist may be required). Products include:
EPIFRIN ⊙ 237
EpiPen 808
Marcaine with Epinephrine 2446
Primatene Mist ◨ 843
Sensorcaine with Epinephrine Injection 554
Sus-Phrine Injection 1017
Xylocaine with Epinephrine Injections 562

Epinephrine Hydrochloride (Beta-blocker can blunt the bronchodilator effect of beta-receptor agonists in patients with bronchospasm; greater than normal anti-asthmatic dose of beta-agonist may be required). Products include:
Ana-Kit Anaphylaxis Emergency Treatment Kit 611

Ethylnorepinephrine Hydrochloride (Beta-blocker can blunt the bronchodilator effect of beta-receptor agonists in patients with bronchospasm; greater than normal anti-asthmatic dose of beta-agonist may be required).
No products indexed under this heading.

Glimepiride (Beta-blockade may prevent the appearance of premonitory signs and symptoms of acute hypoglycemia; reduces the release of insulin in response to hyperglycemia). Products include:
Amaryl Tablets 1241

Glipizide (Beta-blockade may prevent the appearance of premonitory signs and symptoms of acute hypoglycemia; reduces the release of insulin in response to hyperglycemia). Products include:
Glucotrol Tablets 2011
Glucotrol XL Extended Release Tablets 2012

Glyburide (Beta-blockade may prevent the appearance of premonitory signs and symptoms of acute hypoglycemia; reduces the release of insulin in response to hyperglycemia). Products include:
DiaBeta Tablets 1265
Glynase PresTab Tablets 2091
Micronase Tablets 2099

Halothane (Synergism has been reported between labetalol I.V. and halothane anesthesia; potential increased hypotensive effect, reduction in cardiac output and increased central venous pressure). Products include:
Fluothane 2830

Imipramine Hydrochloride (Potential for increase in tremors). Products include:
Tofranil Ampuls 873
Tofranil Tablets 875

Imipramine Pamoate (Potential for increase in tremors). Products include:
Tofranil-PM Capsules 876

Insulin, Human (Beta-blockade may prevent the appearance of premonitory signs and symptoms of acute hypoglycemia; reduces the release of insulin in response to hyperglycemia).
No products indexed under this heading.

Insulin, Human Isophane Suspension (Beta-blockade may prevent the appearance of premonitory signs and symptoms of acute hypoglycemia; reduces the release of insulin in response to hyperglycemia). Products include:
Novolin N Human Insulin 10 ml Vials 1846

Insulin, Human NPH (Beta-blockade may prevent the appearance of premonitory signs and symptoms of acute hypoglycemia; reduces the release of insulin in response to hyperglycemia). Products include:
Humulin N, 100 Units 1495
Novolin N PenFill 1.5 ml Cartridges Durable Insulin Delivery System 1849
Novolin N Prefilled Syringe Disposable Insulin Delivery System 1850

Insulin, Human Regular (Beta-blockade may prevent the appearance of premonitory signs and symptoms of acute hypoglycemia; reduces the release of insulin in response to hyperglycemia). Products include:
Humulin R, 100 Units 1497
Novolin R Human Insulin 10 ml Vials 1846
Novolin R PenFill 1.5 ml Cartridges Durable Insulin Delivery System 1849
Novolin R Prefilled Syringe Disposable Insulin Delivery System 1850
Velosulin BR Human Insulin 10 ml Vials 1847

Insulin, Human, Zinc Suspension (Beta-blockade may prevent the appearance of premonitory signs and symptoms of acute hypoglycemia; reduces the release of insulin in response to hyperglycemia). Products include:
Humulin L, 100 Units 1494
Humulin U, 100 Units 1498
Novolin L Human Insulin 10 ml Vials 1846

Insulin Lispro, Human (Beta-blockade may prevent the appearance of premonitory signs and symptoms of acute hypoglycemia; reduces the release of insulin in response to hyperglycemia). Products include:
Humalog Injection 1488

Insulin, NPH (Beta-blockade may prevent the appearance of premonitory signs and symptoms of acute hypoglycemia; reduces the release of insulin in response to hyperglycemia). Products include:
NPH, 100 Units 1502
Pork NPH, 100 Units 1506
Purified Pork NPH Isophane Insulin 1852

Interactions Index

Insulin, Regular (Beta-blockade may prevent the appearance of premonitory signs and symptoms of acute hypoglycemia; reduces the release of insulin in response to hyperglycemia). Products include:
Regular, 100 Units 1503
Pork Regular, 100 Units 1507
Pork Regular (Concentrated), 500 Units 1508
Purified Pork Regular Insulin 1852

Insulin, Zinc Crystals (Beta-blockade may prevent the appearance of premonitory signs and symptoms of acute hypoglycemia; reduces the release of insulin in response to hyperglycemia). Products include:
NPH, 100 Units 1502

Insulin, Zinc Suspension (Beta-blockade may prevent the appearance of premonitory signs and symptoms of acute hypoglycemia; reduces the release of insulin in response to hyperglycemia). Products include:
Iletin I 1501
Lente, 100 Units 1501
Iletin II 1504
Pork Lente, 100 Units 1504
Purified Pork Lente Insulin 1852

Isoetharine (Beta-blocker can blunt the bronchodilator effect of beta-receptor agonists in patients with bronchospasm; greater than normal anti-asthmatic dose of beta-agonist may be required). Products include:
Bronkometer Aerosol 2432
Bronkosol Solution 2432
Isoetharine Inhalation Solution, USP, Arm-a-Med 545

Isoproterenol Hydrochloride (Beta-blocker can blunt the bronchodilator effect of beta-receptor agonists in patients with bronchospasm; greater than normal anti-asthmatic dose of beta-agonist may be required). Products include:
Isuprel Hydrochloride Solution 2443
Isuprel Injection 2441
Isuprel Mistometer 2442

Isoproterenol Sulfate (Beta-blocker can blunt the bronchodilator effect of beta-receptor agonists in patients with bronchospasm; greater than normal anti-asthmatic dose of beta-agonist may be required). Products include:
Norisodrine with Calcium Iodide Syrup 446

Maprotiline Hydrochloride (Potential for increase in tremors). Products include:
Ludiomil Tablets 861

Metaproterenol Sulfate (Beta-blocker can blunt the bronchodilator effect of beta-receptor agonists in patients with bronchospasm; greater than normal anti-asthmatic dose of beta-agonist may be required). Products include:
Alupent 672
Metaproterenol Sulfate Inhalation Solution, USP, Arm-a-Med 547

Metformin Hydrochloride (Beta-blockade may prevent the appearance of premonitory signs and symptoms of acute hypoglycemia; reduces the release of insulin in response to hyperglycemia). Products include:
Glucophage Tablets 754

Nitroglycerin (Potential for additional antihypertensive effect). Products include:
Deponit NTG Transdermal Delivery System 2541
Nitro-Bid IV 1270
Nitro-Bid Ointment 1272
Nitro-Dur (nitroglycerin) Transdermal Infusion System 1365
Nitrolingual Spray 2193

1094

Nitrostat Tablets 1981
Transderm-Nitro Transdermal Therapeutic System 878

Nortriptyline Hydrochloride (Potential for increase in tremors). Products include:
Pamelor 2409

Pirbuterol Acetate (Beta-blocker can blunt the bronchodilator effect of beta-receptor agonists in patients with bronchospasm; greater than normal anti-asthmatic dose of beta-agonist may be required). Products include:
Maxair Autohaler 1550
Maxair Inhaler 1552

Protriptyline Hydrochloride (Potential for increase in tremors). Products include:
Vivactil Tablets 1820

Salmeterol Xinafoate (Beta-blocker can blunt the bronchodilator effect of beta-receptor agonists in patients with bronchospasm; greater than normal anti-asthmatic dose of beta-agonist may be required). Products include:
Serevent Inhalation Aerosol 1149

Terbutaline Sulfate (Beta-blocker can blunt the bronchodilator effect of beta-receptor agonists in patients with bronchospasm; greater than normal anti-asthmatic dose of beta-agonist may be required). Products include:
Brethaire Inhaler 830
Brethine Ampuls 832
Brethine Tablets 831
Bricanyl Subcutaneous Injection 1247
Bricanyl Tablets 1248

Tolazamide (Beta-blockade may prevent the appearance of premonitory signs and symptoms of acute hypoglycemia; reduces the release of insulin in response to hyperglycemia).
No products indexed under this heading.

Tolbutamide (Beta-blockade may prevent the appearance of premonitory signs and symptoms of acute hypoglycemia; reduces the release of insulin in response to hyperglycemia).
No products indexed under this heading.

Trimipramine Maleate (Potential for increase in tremors). Products include:
Surmontil Capsules 2917

Verapamil Hydrochloride (Care should be taken if co-administered; effects of concomitant use not specified). Products include:
Calan SR Caplets 2571
Calan Tablets 2568
Covera-HS Tablets 2573
Isoptin Injectable 1391
Isoptin Oral Tablets 1393
Isoptin SR Tablets 1395
Verelan Capsules 1455

Food Interactions

Food, unspecified (The absolute bioavailability of labetalol is increased when administered with food).

TRANSDERM SCŌP TRANSDERMAL THERAPEUTIC SYSTEM

(Scopolamine) 890
May interact with anticholinergics, belladona products, antihistamines, tricyclic antidepressants, and certain other agents. Compounds in these categories include:

Acrivastine (Effect unspecified). Products include:
Semprex-D Capsules 1620

(◨ Described in PDR For Nonprescription Drugs)   (⊙ Described in PDR For Ophthalmology)

Amitriptyline Hydrochloride (Effect unspecified). Products include:
- Elavil ... 2945
- Etrafon ... 2495
- Limbitrol ... 2333
- Triavil Tablets ... 1800

Amoxapine (Effect unspecified). Products include:
- Asendin Tablets ... 1419

Astemizole (Effect unspecified). Products include:
- Hismanal Tablets ... 1341

Atropine Sulfate (Effect unspecified). Products include:
- Arco-Lase Plus Tablets ... 513
- Atrohist Plus Tablets ... 1605
- Donnatal ... 2234
- Donnatal Extentabs ... 2234
- Donnatal Tablets ... 2234
- Lomotil ... 2591
- Motofen Tablets ... 789
- Urised Tablets ... 2123

Azatadine Maleate (Effect unspecified). Products include:
- Trinalin Repetabs Tablets ... 1373

Benztropine Mesylate (Effect unspecified). Products include:
- Cogentin ... 1661

Biperiden Hydrochloride (Effect unspecified). Products include:
- Akineton ... 1380

Bromodiphenhydramine Hydrochloride (Effect unspecified).
- No products indexed under this heading.

Brompheniramine Maleate (Effect unspecified). Products include:
- Alka-Seltzer Plus Sinus Medicine ... 611
- Bromfed Capsules (Extended-Release) ... 1832
- Bromfed Syrup ... 712
- Bromfed Tablets ... 1832
- Bromfed-DM Cough Syrup ... 1832
- Bromfed-PD Capsules (Extended-Release) ... 1832
- Dimetane-DC Cough Syrup ... 2232
- Dimetane-DX Cough Syrup ... 2233
- Dimetapp Allergy Dye-Free Elixir ... 838
- Dimetapp Allergy Sinus Caplets ... 838
- Dimetapp Cold & Allergy Chewable Tablets ... 838
- Dimetapp Cold & Cough Liqui-Gels ... 839
- Dimetapp Cold & Fever Suspension ... 839
- Dimetapp DM Elixir ... 840
- Dimetapp Elixir ... 840
- Dimetapp Extentabs ... 841
- Dimetapp Tablets/Liqui-Gels ... 841
- Rondec Chewable Tablets ... 974
- Vicks DayQuil Allergy Relief 12-Hour Extended Release Tablets ... 733
- Vicks DayQuil Allergy Relief 4-Hour Tablets ... 733

Cetirizine Hydrochloride (Effect unspecified). Products include:
- Zyrtec Tablets ... 2053

Chlorpheniramine Maleate (Effect unspecified). Products include:
- Alka-Seltzer Plus Cold Medicine ... 611
- Alka-Seltzer Plus Cold Medicine Liqui-Gels ... 612
- Alka-Seltzer Plus Cold & Cough Medicine ... 611
- Alka-Seltzer Plus Cold & Cough Medicine Liqui-Gels ... 612
- Alka-Seltzer Plus Flu & Body Aches Effervescent Tablets ... 612
- Allerest Maximum Strength ... 649
- Allerest Sinus Pain Formula ... 649
- Ana-Kit Anaphylaxis Emergency Treatment Kit ... 611
- Atrohist Pediatric Capsules ... 1603
- Atrohist Plus Tablets ... 1605
- BC Cold Powder Multi-Symptom Formula (Cold-Sinus-Allergy) ... 631
- Cerose DM ... 853
- Cheracol Plus Head Cold/Cough Formula ... 741
- Children's TYLENOL Cold Multi-Symptom Chewable Tablets and Liquid ... 1559
- Children's TYLENOL Cold Plus Cough Multi Symptom Chewable Tablets and Liquid ... 1560
- Children's TYLENOL Flu Suspension Liquid ... 1560
- Children's Vicks DayQuil Allergy Relief ... 730
- Children's Vicks NyQuil Cold/Cough Relief ... 731
- Chlor-Trimeton Allergy Decongestant Tablets ... 759
- Chlor-Trimeton Allergy Tablets ... 758
- Allergy-Sinus Comtrex Multi-Symptom Allergy-Sinus Formula Tablets and Caplets ... 639
- Comtrex Multi-Symptom ... 638
- Contac Continuous Action Nasal Decongestant/Antihistamine 12 Hour Capsules ... 773
- Contac Maximum Strength Continuous Action Decongestant/Antihistamine 12 Hour Caplets ... 772
- Contac Severe Cold and Flu Formula Caplets ... 773
- Coricidin Cold + Flu Tablets ... 760
- Coricidin Cough + Cold Tablets ... 760
- Coricidin 'D' Decongestant Tablets ... 760
- D.A. II Tablets ... 972
- D.A. Chewable Tablets ... 970
- Dura-Tap/PD Capsules ... 970
- Dura-Vent/DA Tablets ... 972
- Efidac 24 Chlorpheniramine ... 655
- Extendryl ... 1003
- Fedahist Gyrocaps ... 2545
- Hycomine Compound Tablets ... 948
- Kronofed-A ... 994
- Nolamine Timed-Release Tablets ... 790
- Novahistine Elixir ... 782
- Ornade Spansule Capsules ... 2678
- PediaCare Cough-Cold Chewable Tablets and Liquid ... 1569
- PediaCare NightRest Cough-Cold Liquid ... 1569
- Pediatric Vicks 44m Cough & Cold Relief ... 737
- Pyrroxate Caplets ... 742
- Ryna ... 804
- Sinarest ... 663
- Sine-Off Sinus Medicine ... 784
- Singlet Tablets ... 785
- Sinulin Tablets ... 792
- Sinutab Sinus Allergy Medication, Maximum Strength Tablets and Caplets ... 823
- Sudafed Cold & Allergy Tablets ... 826
- Teldrin 12 Hour Antihistamine/Nasal Decongestant Allergy Relief Capsules ... 786
- TheraFlu Flu and Cold Medicine ... 750
- Theraflu Maximum Strength Flu and Cold Medicine For Sore Throat ... 751
- TheraFlu Flu, Cold and Cough Medicine ... 750
- TheraFlu Maximum Strength Nighttime Flu, Cold & Cough Medicine ... 751
- Triaminic Night Time ... 754
- Triaminic Syrup ... 755
- Triaminic Triaminicol Cold & Cough ... 756
- Triaminicin Tablets ... 756
- Tussend ... 1830
- TYLENOL Allergy Sinus, Maximum Strength Caplets and Gelcaps ... 1571
- TYLENOL Cold Medication, Multi-Symptom Formula Tablets and Caplets ... 1572
- TYLENOL Cold Medication, Multi-Symptom Hot Liquid Packets ... 1572
- Vicks 44 LiquiCaps Cough, Cold & Flu Relief ... 728
- Vicks 44M Cough, Cold & Flu Relief ... 729

Chlorpheniramine Polistirex (Effect unspecified). Products include:
- Tussionex Pennkinetic Extended-Release Suspension ... 1624

Chlorpheniramine Tannate (Effect unspecified). Products include:
- Atrohist Pediatric Suspension ... 1604
- Atrohist Pediatric Suspension Dye-Free ... 1604
- Rynatan ... 2781
- Rynatuss ... 2782

Clemastine Fumarate (Effect unspecified). Products include:
- Tavist Syrup ... 2426
- Tavist Tablets ... 2427
- Tavist-1 12 Hour Relief Tablets ... 749
- Tavist-D 12 Hour Relief Tablets ... 750

Clidinium Bromide (Effect unspecified). Products include:
- Librax Capsules ... 2330

Clomipramine Hydrochloride (Effect unspecified). Products include:
- Anafranil Capsules ... 819

Cyproheptadine Hydrochloride (Effect unspecified). Products include:
- Periactin ... 1767

Desipramine Hydrochloride (Effect unspecified). Products include:
- Norpramin Tablets ... 1273

Dexchlorpheniramine Maleate (Effect unspecified).
- No products indexed under this heading.

Dicyclomine Hydrochloride (Effect unspecified). Products include:
- Bentyl ... 1246

Diphenhydramine Citrate (Effect unspecified). Products include:
- Excedrin P.M. Analgesic/Sleeping Aid Tablets, Caplets, Liquigels ... 735

Diphenylpyraline Hydrochloride (Effect unspecified).
- No products indexed under this heading.

Doxepin Hydrochloride (Effect unspecified). Products include:
- Adapin Capsules ... 1542
- Sinequan ... 2028
- Zonalon Cream ... 1042

Glycopyrrolate (Effect unspecified). Products include:
- Robinul Forte Tablets ... 2247
- Robinul Injectable ... 2247
- Robinul Tablets ... 2247

Hyoscyamine (Effect unspecified). Products include:
- Cystospaz Tablets ... 2123
- Urised Tablets ... 2123

Hyoscyamine Sulfate (Effect unspecified). Products include:
- Arco-Lase Plus Tablets ... 513
- Atrohist Plus Tablets ... 1605
- Cystospaz-M Capsules ... 2123
- Donnatal ... 2234
- Donnatal Extentabs ... 2234
- Donnatal Tablets ... 2234
- Kutrase Capsules ... 2546
- Levsin/Levsinex/Levbid ... 2549

Imipramine Hydrochloride (Effect unspecified). Products include:
- Tofranil Ampuls ... 873
- Tofranil Tablets ... 875

Imipramine Pamoate (Effect unspecified). Products include:
- Tofranil-PM Capsules ... 876

Ipratropium Bromide (Effect unspecified). Products include:
- Atrovent Inhalation Aerosol ... 674
- Atrovent Inhalation Solution ... 675
- Atrovent Nasal Spray 0.03% ... 676
- Atrovent Nasal Spray 0.06% ... 678

Loratadine (Effect unspecified). Products include:
- Claritin Tablets ... 2485
- Claritin-D Tablets ... 2487

Maprotiline Hydrochloride (Effect unspecified). Products include:
- Ludiomil Tablets ... 861

Meclizine Hydrochloride (Effect unspecified). Products include:
- Antivert, Antivert/25 Tablets, & Antivert/50 Tablets ... 1992
- Bonine Tablets ... 1990
- Dramamine II Tablets ... 801

Mepenzolate Bromide (Effect unspecified).
- No products indexed under this heading.

Methdilazine Hydrochloride (Effect unspecified).
- No products indexed under this heading.

Nortriptyline Hydrochloride (Effect unspecified). Products include:
- Pamelor ... 2409

Oxybutynin Chloride (Effect unspecified). Products include:
- Ditropan ... 1267

Procyclidine Hydrochloride (Effect unspecified). Products include:
- Kemadrin Tablets ... 1105

Promethazine Hydrochloride (Effect unspecified). Products include:
- Mepergan Injection ... 2859
- Phenergan with Codeine ... 2883
- Phenergan with Dextromethorphan ... 2885
- Phenergan Injection ... 2880
- Phenergan Suppositories ... 2882
- Phenergan Syrup ... 2881
- Phenergan Tablets ... 2882
- Phenergan VC ... 2886
- Phenergan VC with Codeine ... 2888

Propantheline Bromide (Effect unspecified). Products include:
- Pro-Banthine Tablets ... 2226

Protriptyline Hydrochloride (Effect unspecified). Products include:
- Vivactil Tablets ... 1820

Pyrilamine Maleate (Effect unspecified). Products include:
- 4-Way Fast Acting Nasal Spray (regular & mentholated) ... 644
- Maximum Strength Multi-Symptom Formula Midol ... 621
- PMS Multi-Symptom Formula Midol ... 622

Pyrilamine Tannate (Effect unspecified). Products include:
- Atrohist Pediatric Suspension ... 1604
- Atrohist Pediatric Suspension Dye-Free ... 1604
- Rynatan ... 2781

Terfenadine (Effect unspecified). Products include:
- Seldane Tablets ... 1284
- Seldane-D Extended-Release Tablets ... 1286

Tridihexethyl Chloride (Effect unspecified).
- No products indexed under this heading.

Trihexyphenidyl Hydrochloride (Effect unspecified). Products include:
- Artane ... 1418

Trimeprazine Tartrate (Effect unspecified).
- No products indexed under this heading.

Trimipramine Maleate (Effect unspecified). Products include:
- Surmontil Capsules ... 2917

Tripelennamine Hydrochloride (Effect unspecified). Products include:
- PBZ Tablets ... 863
- PBZ-SR Tablets ... 862

Triprolidine Hydrochloride (Effect unspecified). Products include:
- Actifed Cold & Allergy Tablets ... 807
- Actifed Cold & Sinus Caplets and Tablets ... 808

Food Interactions

Alcohol (Effect unspecified).

IMPORTANT NOTE: Always consult each drug listing in the patient's regimen for possible interactions.

Transderm-Nitro / Interactions Index

TRANSDERM-NITRO TRANSDERMAL THERAPEUTIC SYSTEM
(Nitroglycerin) 878
May interact with calcium channel blockers, vasodilators, and certain other agents. Compounds in these categories include:

Amlodipine Besylate (Potential for marked symptomatic hypotension). Products include:
- Lotrel Capsules 858
- Norvasc Tablets 2020

Bepridil Hydrochloride (Potential for marked symptomatic hypotension). Products include:
- Vascor Tablets (200 and 300 mg) 1597

Diazoxide (Additive vasodilating effects). Products include:
- Hyperstat I.V. Injection 2504
- Proglycem 575

Diltiazem Hydrochloride (Potential for marked symptomatic hypotension). Products include:
- Cardizem CD Capsules 1251
- Cardizem SR Capsules 1255
- Cardizem Injectable 1253
- Cardizem Tablets 1257
- Dilacor XR Extended-release Capsules 2183
- Tiazac Capsules 1019

Epoprostenol Sodium (Additive vasodilating effects). Products include:
- Flolan for Injection 1085

Felodipine (Potential for marked symptomatic hypotension). Products include:
- Plendil Extended-Release Tablets 514

Hydralazine Hydrochloride (Additive vasodilating effects). Products include:
- Apresazide Capsules 824
- Apresoline Hydrochloride Tablets .. 826
- Hydralazine Hydrochloride Injection USP 2712
- Ser-Ap-Es Tablets 867

Isradipine (Potential for marked symptomatic hypotension). Products include:
- DynaCirc Capsules 2381
- DynaCirc CR Tablets 2383

Minoxidil (Additive vasodilating effects).
- No products indexed under this heading.

Nicardipine Hydrochloride (Potential for marked symptomatic hypotension). Products include:
- Cardene Capsules 2261
- Cardene I.V. 2815
- Cardene SR Capsules 2264

Nifedipine (Potential for marked symptomatic hypotension). Products include:
- Adalat Capsules (10 mg and 20 mg) 580
- Adalat CC 582
- Procardia Capsules 2024
- Procardia XL Extended Release Tablets 2026

Nimodipine (Potential for marked symptomatic hypotension). Products include:
- Nimotop Capsules 603

Nisoldipine (Potential for marked symptomatic hypotension). Products include:
- Sular Tablets 2961

Verapamil Hydrochloride (Potential for marked symptomatic hypotension). Products include:
- Calan SR Caplets 2571
- Calan Tablets 2568
- Covera-HS Tablets 2573
- Isoptin Injectable 1391
- Isoptin Oral Tablets 1393
- Isoptin SR Tablets 1395
- Verelan Capsules 1455

Food Interactions
Alcohol (Additive vasodilating effects).

TRANXENE T-TAB TABLETS
(Clorazepate Dipotassium) 459
May interact with central nervous system depressants, barbiturates, narcotic analgesics, phenothiazines, antidepressant drugs, monoamine oxidase inhibitors, hypnotics and sedatives, and certain other agents. Compounds in these categories include:

Alfentanil Hydrochloride (Actions of benzodiazepines may be potentiated). Products include:
- Alfenta Injection 1334

Alprazolam (Actions of benzodiazepines may be potentiated). Products include:
- Xanax Tablets 2115

Amitriptyline Hydrochloride (Actions of benzodiazepines may be potentiated). Products include:
- Elavil 2945
- Etrafon 2495
- Limbitrol 2333
- Triavil Tablets 1800

Amoxapine (Actions of benzodiazepines may be potentiated). Products include:
- Asendin Tablets 1419

Aprobarbital (Actions of benzodiazepines may be potentiated).
- No products indexed under this heading.

Buprenorphine (Actions of benzodiazepines may be potentiated). Products include:
- Buprenex Injectable 2170

Bupropion Hydrochloride (Actions of benzodiazepines may be potentiated). Products include:
- Wellbutrin Tablets 1177

Buspirone Hydrochloride (Actions of benzodiazepines may be potentiated). Products include:
- BuSpar Tablets 738

Butabarbital (Actions of benzodiazepines may be potentiated).
- No products indexed under this heading.

Butalbital (Actions of benzodiazepines may be potentiated). Products include:
- Axocet Capsules 2469
- Esgic-plus Capsules 1012
- Esgic-plus Tablets 1012
- Fioricet Tablets 2386
- Fioricet with Codeine Capsules .. 2387
- Fiorinal Capsules 2388
- Fiorinal with Codeine Capsules .. 2390
- Fiorinal Tablets 2388
- Phrenilin 790
- Sedapap Tablets 50 mg/650 mg .. 1826

Chlordiazepoxide (Actions of benzodiazepines may be potentiated). Products include:
- Limbitrol 2333

Chlordiazepoxide Hydrochloride (Actions of benzodiazepines may be potentiated). Products include:
- Librax Capsules 2330
- Librium Capsules 2331
- Librium Injectable 2332

Chlorpromazine (Actions of benzodiazepines may be potentiated). Products include:
- Thorazine Suppositories 2701

Chlorpromazine Hydrochloride (Actions of benzodiazepines may be potentiated). Products include:
- Thorazine 2701

Chlorprothixene (Actions of benzodiazepines may be potentiated).
- No products indexed under this heading.

Chlorprothixene Hydrochloride (Actions of benzodiazepines may be potentiated).
- No products indexed under this heading.

Chlorprothixene Lactate (Actions of benzodiazepines may be potentiated).
- No products indexed under this heading.

Clozapine (Actions of benzodiazepines may be potentiated). Products include:
- Clozaril Tablets 2377

Codeine Phosphate (Actions of benzodiazepines may be potentiated). Products include:
- Brontex 2130
- Dimetane-DC Cough Syrup 2232
- Fioricet with Codeine Capsules .. 2387
- Fiorinal with Codeine Capsules .. 2390
- Nucofed 2225
- Phenergan with Codeine 2883
- Phenergan VC with Codeine 2888
- Robitussin A-C Syrup 2248
- Robitussin-DAC Syrup 2249
- Ryna .... ⓝ 804
- Soma Compound w/Codeine Tablets 2784
- Tylenol with Codeine 1592

Desflurane (Actions of benzodiazepines may be potentiated). Products include:
- Suprane (desflurane, USP) 1865

Desipramine Hydrochloride (Actions of benzodiazepines may be potentiated). Products include:
- Norpramin Tablets 1273

Dezocine (Actions of benzodiazepines may be potentiated). Products include:
- Dalgan Injection 529

Diazepam (Actions of benzodiazepines may be potentiated). Products include:
- Dizac (diazepam injectable emulsion) CIV 1862
- Valium Injectable 2336
- Valium Tablets 2335

Doxepin Hydrochloride (Actions of benzodiazepines may be potentiated). Products include:
- Adapin Capsules 1542
- Sinequan 2028
- Zonalon Cream 1042

Droperidol (Actions of benzodiazepines may be potentiated). Products include:
- Inapsine Injection 462

Enflurane (Actions of benzodiazepines may be potentiated).
- No products indexed under this heading.

Estazolam (Actions of benzodiazepines may be potentiated; increased sedation with concurrent use). Products include:
- ProSom Tablets 457

Ethchlorvynol (Actions of benzodiazepines may be potentiated; increased sedation with concurrent use). Products include:
- Placidyl Capsules 456

Ethinamate (Actions of benzodiazepines may be potentiated; increased sedation with concurrent use).
- No products indexed under this heading.

Fentanyl (Actions of benzodiazepines may be potentiated). Products include:
- Duragesic Transdermal System 1336

Fentanyl Citrate (Actions of benzodiazepines may be potentiated). Products include:
- Sublimaze Injection 463

Fluoxetine Hydrochloride (Actions of benzodiazepines may be potentiated). Products include:
- Prozac Pulvules & Liquid, Oral Solution 935

Fluphenazine Decanoate (Actions of benzodiazepines may be potentiated). Products include:
- Prolixin Decanoate 510

Fluphenazine Enanthate (Actions of benzodiazepines may be potentiated). Products include:
- Prolixin Enanthate 510

Fluphenazine Hydrochloride (Actions of benzodiazepines may be potentiated). Products include:
- Prolixin 510

Flurazepam Hydrochloride (Actions of benzodiazepines may be potentiated; increased sedation with concurrent use). Products include:
- Dalmane Capsules 2329

Furazolidone (Actions of benzodiazepines may be potentiated). Products include:
- Furoxone 2221

Glutethimide (Actions of benzodiazepines may be potentiated; increased sedation with concurrent use).
- No products indexed under this heading.

Haloperidol (Actions of benzodiazepines may be potentiated). Products include:
- Haldol Injection, Tablets and Concentrate 1585

Haloperidol Decanoate (Actions of benzodiazepines may be potentiated). Products include:
- Haldol Decanoate 1587

Hydrocodone Bitartrate (Actions of benzodiazepines may be potentiated). Products include:
- Codiclear DH Syrup 808
- Duratuss HD Elixir 2750
- Histussin D Liquid 670
- Hycodan Tablets and Syrup 946
- Hycomine Compound Tablets 948
- Hycomine 947
- Hycotuss Expectorant Syrup 950
- Hydrocet Capsules 787
- Lorcet 10/650 Tablets 1016
- Lortab 2751
- Tussend 1830
- Tussend Expectorant 1831
- Vicodin Tablets 1404
- Vicodin ES Tablets 1405
- Vicodin HP Tablets 1403
- Vicodin Tuss Expectorant 1406
- Zydone Capsules 967

Hydrocodone Polistirex (Actions of benzodiazepines may be potentiated). Products include:
- Tussionex Pennkinetic Extended-Release Suspension 1624

Hydromorphone Hydrochloride (Actions of benzodiazepines may be potentiated). Products include:
- Dilaudid Ampules 1382
- Dilaudid Cough Syrup 1383
- Dilaudid-HP Injection 1384
- Dilaudid-HP Lyophilized Powder 250 mg 1384
- Dilaudid 1382
- Dilaudid Oral Liquid 1386
- Dilaudid 1382
- Dilaudid Tablets - 8 mg 1386

Hydroxyzine Hydrochloride (Actions of benzodiazepines may be potentiated). Products include:
- Atarax Tablets & Syrup 1992
- Marax Tablets & DF Syrup 2015
- Vistaril Intramuscular Solution 2042

Imipramine Hydrochloride (Actions of benzodiazepines may be potentiated). Products include:
- Tofranil Ampuls 873
- Tofranil Tablets 875

(ⓝ Described in PDR For Nonprescription Drugs)   (ⓞ Described in PDR For Ophthalmology)

1097 **Interactions Index** **Trecator-SC**

Imipramine Pamoate (Actions of benzodiazepines may be potentiated). Products include:

Tofranil-PM Capsules 876

Isocarboxazid (Actions of benzodiazepines may be potentiated).

No products indexed under this heading.

Isoflurane (Actions of benzodiazepines may be potentiated).

No products indexed under this heading.

Ketamine Hydrochloride (Actions of benzodiazepines may be potentiated).

No products indexed under this heading.

Levomethadyl Acetate Hydrochloride (Actions of benzodiazepines may be potentiated). Products include:

Orlaam Oral Solution 2361

Levorphanol Tartrate (Actions of benzodiazepines may be potentiated). Products include:

Levo-Dromoran 2297

Lorazepam (Actions of benzodiazepines may be potentiated; increased sedation with concurrent use). Products include:

Ativan Injection 2805
Ativan Tablets 2807

Loxapine Hydrochloride (Actions of benzodiazepines may be potentiated). Products include:

Loxitane 1426

Loxapine Succinate (Actions of benzodiazepines may be potentiated). Products include:

Loxitane Capsules 1426

Maprotiline Hydrochloride (Actions of benzodiazepines may be potentiated). Products include:

Ludiomil Tablets 861

Meperidine Hydrochloride (Actions of benzodiazepines may be potentiated). Products include:

Demerol 2438
Mepergan Injection 2859

Mephobarbital (Actions of benzodiazepines may be potentiated). Products include:

Mebaral Tablets 2452

Meprobamate (Actions of benzodiazepines may be potentiated). Products include:

Miltown Tablets 2780
PMB 200 and PMB 400 2890

Mesoridazine Besylate (Actions of benzodiazepines may be potentiated). Products include:

Serentil 689

Methadone Hydrochloride (Actions of benzodiazepines may be potentiated). Products include:

Methadone Hydrochloride Oral Concentrate 2356
Methadone Hydrochloride Oral Solution & Tablets 2357

Methohexital Sodium (Actions of benzodiazepines may be potentiated).

No products indexed under this heading.

Methotrimeprazine (Actions of benzodiazepines may be potentiated). Products include:

Levoprome 1321

Methoxyflurane (Actions of benzodiazepines may be potentiated).

No products indexed under this heading.

Midazolam Hydrochloride (Actions of benzodiazepines may be potentiated; increased sedation with concurrent use). Products include:

Versed Injection 2324

Molindone Hydrochloride (Actions of benzodiazepines may be potentiated). Products include:

Moban Tablets and Concentrate 1036

Morphine Sulfate (Actions of benzodiazepines may be potentiated). Products include:

Astramorph/PF Injection, USP (Preservative-Free) 526
Duramorph Injection 983
Infumorph 200 and Infumorph 500 Sterile Solutions 985
Kadian Capsules 2948
MS Contin Tablets 2149
MSIR 2152
Oramorph SR (Morphine Sulfate Sustained Release Tablets) 2359
RMS Suppositories CII 2766
Roxanol 2365

Nefazodone Hydrochloride (Actions of benzodiazepines may be potentiated). Products include:

Serzone Tablets 776

Nortriptyline Hydrochloride (Actions of benzodiazepines may be potentiated). Products include:

Pamelor 2409

Opium Alkaloids (Actions of benzodiazepines may be potentiated).

No products indexed under this heading.

Oxazepam (Actions of benzodiazepines may be potentiated). Products include:

Serax Capsules 2916
Serax Tablets 2916

Oxycodone Hydrochloride (Actions of benzodiazepines may be potentiated). Products include:

OxyContin Tablets 2163
OxyIR Capsules 2167
Percocet Tablets 955
Percodan Tablets 955
Percodan-Demi Tablets 956
Roxicodone Tablets, Oral Solution & Intensol (Oxycodone) 2366
Tylox Capsules 1593

Paroxetine Hydrochloride (Actions of benzodiazepines may be potentiated). Products include:

Paxil Tablets 2681

Pentobarbital Sodium (Actions of benzodiazepines may be potentiated). Products include:

Nembutal Sodium Capsules 440
Nembutal Sodium Solution 442
Nembutal Sodium Suppositories 444

Perphenazine (Actions of benzodiazepines may be potentiated). Products include:

Etrafon 2495
Triavil Tablets 1800
Trilafon 2532

Phenelzine Sulfate (Actions of benzodiazepines may be potentiated). Products include:

Nardil 1977

Phenobarbital (Actions of benzodiazepines may be potentiated). Products include:

Arco-Lase Plus Tablets 513
Bellergal-S Tablets 2375
Donnatal 2234
Donnatal Extentabs 2234
Donnatal Tablets 2234
Phenobarbital Elixir and Tablets 1523
Quadrinal Tablets 1398

Prazepam (Actions of benzodiazepines may be potentiated).

No products indexed under this heading.

Prochlorperazine (Actions of benzodiazepines may be potentiated). Products include:

Compazine 2644

Promethazine Hydrochloride (Actions of benzodiazepines may be potentiated). Products include:

Mepergan Injection 2859
Phenergan with Codeine 2883
Phenergan with Dextromethorphan 2885
Phenergan Injection 2880
Phenergan Suppositories 2882
Phenergan Syrup 2881
Phenergan Tablets 2882
Phenergan VC 2886
Phenergan VC with Codeine 2888

Propofol (Actions of benzodiazepines may be potentiated; increased sedation with concurrent use). Products include:

Diprivan Injectable Emulsion 2939

Propoxyphene Hydrochloride (Actions of benzodiazepines may be potentiated). Products include:

Darvon 1475
Wygesic Tablets 2930

Propoxyphene Napsylate (Actions of benzodiazepines may be potentiated). Products include:

Darvon-N/Darvocet-N 1473

Protriptyline Hydrochloride (Actions of benzodiazepines may be potentiated). Products include:

Vivactil Tablets 1820

Quazepam (Actions of benzodiazepines may be potentiated; increased sedation with concurrent use). Products include:

Doral Tablets 2773

Risperidone (Actions of benzodiazepines may be potentiated). Products include:

Risperdal Tablets 1348

Secobarbital Sodium (Actions of benzodiazepines may be potentiated; increased sedation with concurrent use). Products include:

Seconal Sodium Pulvules 1529

Selegiline Hydrochloride (Actions of benzodiazepines may be potentiated). Products include:

Eldepryl Capsules 2729

Sertraline Hydrochloride (Actions of benzodiazepines may be potentiated). Products include:

Zoloft Tablets 2051

Sevoflurane (Actions of benzodiazepines may be potentiated).

No products indexed under this heading.

Sufentanil Citrate (Actions of benzodiazepines may be potentiated). Products include:

Sufenta Injection 1355

Temazepam (Actions of benzodiazepines may be potentiated; increased sedation with concurrent use). Products include:

Restoril Capsules 2413

Thiamylal Sodium (Actions of benzodiazepines may be potentiated).

No products indexed under this heading.

Thioridazine Hydrochloride (Actions of benzodiazepines may be potentiated). Products include:

Mellaril 2398

Thiothixene (Actions of benzodiazepines may be potentiated). Products include:

Navane Capsules and Concentrate 2018
Navane Intramuscular 2019

Tranylcypromine Sulfate (Actions of benzodiazepines may be potentiated). Products include:

Parnate Tablets 2679

Trazodone Hydrochloride (Actions of benzodiazepines may be potentiated). Products include:

Desyrel and Desyrel Dividose 504

Triazolam (Actions of benzodiazepines may be potentiated; increased sedation with concurrent use). Products include:

Halcion Tablets 2093

Trifluoperazine Hydrochloride (Actions of benzodiazepines may be potentiated). Products include:

Stelazine 2692

Trimipramine Maleate (Actions of benzodiazepines may be potentiated). Products include:

Surmontil Capsules 2917

Venlafaxine Hydrochloride (Actions of benzodiazepines may be potentiated). Products include:

Effexor 2825

Zolpidem Tartrate (Actions of benzodiazepines may be potentiated; increased sedation with concurrent use). Products include:

Ambien Tablets 2559

Food Interactions

Alcohol (Actions of benzodiazepines may be potentiated; prolonged sleeping time).

TRANXENE-SD HALF STRENGTH TABLETS
(Clorazepate Dipotassium) 459
See **Tranxene T-TAB Tablets**

TRANXENE-SD TABLETS
(Clorazepate Dipotassium) 459
See **Tranxene T-TAB Tablets**

TRASYLOL
(Aprotinin) 607
May interact with fibrinolytic agents and certain other agents. Compounds in these categories include:

Alteplase, Recombinant (Aprotinin may inhibit the effects of fibrinolytic agents). Products include:

Activase 1045

Anistreplase (Aprotinin may inhibit the effects of fibrinolytic agents). Products include:

Eminase 2215

Captopril (Aprotinin may block the acute hypotensive effects of captopril). Products include:

Capoten Tablets 740
Capozide Tablets 744

Heparin Calcium (Aprotinin, in the presence of heparin, has been found to prolong the activated clotting time (ACT) as measured by surface activation methods).

No products indexed under this heading.

Heparin Sodium (Aprotinin, in the presence of heparin, has been found to prolong the activated clotting time (ACT) as measured by surface activation methods). Products include:

Heparin Lock Flush Solution 2831
Heparin Sodium Injection 2832
Heparin Sodium Vials 1486

Streptokinase (Aprotinin may inhibit the effects of fibrinolytic agents). Products include:

Streptase for Infusion 557

Urokinase (Aprotinin may inhibit the effects of fibrinolytic agents). Products include:

Abbokinase 403
Abbokinase Open-Cath 405

TRAUMEEL INJECTION SOLUTION
(Homeopathic Medications) 1237
None cited in PDR database.

TRECATOR-SC TABLETS
(Ethionamide) 2919
May interact with antituberculosis drugs. Compounds in this category include:

Aminosalicylic Acid (Ethionamide may intensify the adverse effects of other antituberculosis

IMPORTANT NOTE: Always consult each drug listing in the patient's regimen for possible interactions.

Trecator-SC **Interactions Index** **1098**

drugs administered concurrently). Products include:
- PASER Granules 1333

p-Aminosalicylic Acid (Convulsions have been reported with concurrent use).
- No products indexed under this heading.

Cycloserine (Ethionamide may intensify the adverse effects of other antituberculosis drugs administered concurrently). Products include:
- Seromycin Capsules 975

Ethambutol Hydrochloride (Ethionamide may intensify the adverse effects of other antituberculosis drugs administered concurrently). Products include:
- Myambutol Tablets 1432

Isoniazid (Ethionamide may intensify the adverse effects of other antituberculosis drugs administered concurrently). Products include:
- Nydrazid Injection 509
- Rifamate Capsules 1278
- Rifater 1280

Pyrazinamide (Ethionamide may intensify the adverse effects of other antituberculosis drugs administered concurrently). Products include:
- Pyrazinamide Tablets 1442
- Rifater 1280

Rifampin (Ethionamide may intensify the adverse effects of other antituberculosis drugs administered concurrently). Products include:
- Rifadin 1276
- Rifamate Capsules 1278
- Rifater 1280
- Rimactane Capsules 865

TRENTAL TABLETS

(Pentoxifylline) 1291

May interact with anticoagulants, platelet inhibitors, xanthine bronchodilators, and certain other agents. Compounds in these categories include:

Aminophylline (Concomitant administration leads to increased theophylline levels and theophylline toxicity).
- No products indexed under this heading.

Aspirin (Potential for bleeding and/or prolonged prothrombin time in patients treated with Trental with or without platelet aggregation inhibitors). Products include:
- Alka-Seltzer Cherry Effervescent Antacid and Pain Reliever .... ■ 609
- Alka-Seltzer Extra Strength Effervescent Antacid and Pain Reliever .... ■ 609
- Alka-Seltzer Lemon Lime Effervescent Antacid and Pain Reliever .... ■ 609
- Alka-Seltzer Original Effervescent Antacid and Pain Reliever .... ■ 609
- Alka-Seltzer Plus .... ■ 611
- Alka-Seltzer Plus Sinus Medicine .. ■ 611
- Ascriptin .... ■ 650
- Arthritis Strength BC Powder .... ■ 631
- BC Cold Powder Multi-Symptom Formula (Cold-Sinus-Allergy) .... ■ 631
- BC Cold Powder Non-Drowsy Formula (Cold-Sinus) .... ■ 631
- BC Powder .... ■ 631
- Genuine Bayer Aspirin Tablets & Caplets .... ■ 618
- Extra Strength Bayer Arthritis Pain Regimen Formula .... ■ 615
- Extra Strength Bayer Aspirin Caplets & Tablets .... ■ 617
- Extended-Release Bayer 8-Hour Aspirin .... ■ 616
- Extra Strength Bayer Plus Aspirin Caplets .... ■ 617
- Extra Strength Bayer PM Aspirin Plus Sleep Aid .... ■ 617
- Aspirin Regimen Bayer 81 mg Tablets with Calcium .... ■ 615
- Aspirin Regimen Bayer Adult Low Strength 81 mg Tablets .... ■ 613
- Aspirin Regimen Bayer Children's Chewable Aspirin .... ■ 616
- Aspirin Regimen Bayer Regular Strength 325 mg Caplets .... ■ 613
- Bufferin Analgesic Tablets .... ■ 636
- Arthritis Strength Bufferin Analgesic Caplets .... ■ 637
- Extra Strength Bufferin Analgesic Tablets .... ■ 637
- Cama Arthritis Pain Reliever .... ■ 748
- Darvon Compound-65 Pulvules 1475
- Easprin 1971
- Ecotrin 2625
- Ecotrin Enteric Coated Aspirin Maximum Strength Tablets and Caplets .... ■ 775
- Ecotrin Enteric Coated Aspirin Regular Strength Tablets 2625
- Empirin Aspirin Tablets .... ■ 818
- Excedrin Extra-Strength Analgesic Tablets, Caplets, and Geltabs 734
- Fiorinal Capsules 2388
- Fiorinal with Codeine Capsules 2390
- Fiorinal Tablets 2388
- Goody's Extra Strength Headache Powders .... ■ 632
- Goody's Extra Strength Pain Relief Tablets .... ■ 632
- Halfprin Tablets 1413
- Norgesic 1554
- Percodan Tablets 955
- Percodan-Demi Tablets 956
- Robaxisal Tablets 2246
- Soma Compound w/Codeine Tablets 2784
- Soma Compound Tablets 2783
- St. Joseph Adult Chewable Aspirin (81 mg.) .... ■ 768
- Talwin Compound 2466
- Vanquish Analgesic Caplets .... ■ 627

Azlocillin Sodium (Potential for bleeding and/or prolonged prothrombin time in patients treated with Trental with or without platelet aggregation inhibitors).
- No products indexed under this heading.

Carbenicillin Indanyl Sodium (Potential for bleeding and/or prolonged prothrombin time in patients treated with Trental with or without platelet aggregation inhibitors). Products include:
- Geocillin Tablets 2009

Choline Magnesium Trisalicylate (Potential for bleeding and/or prolonged prothrombin time in patients treated with Trental with or without platelet aggregation inhibitors). Products include:
- Trilisate 2155

Dalteparin Sodium (Potential for bleeding and/or prolonged prothrombin time in patients treated with Trental with or without platelet aggregation inhibitors). Products include:
- Fragmin Injection 2088

Diclofenac Potassium (Potential for bleeding and/or prolonged prothrombin time in patients treated with Trental with or without platelet aggregation inhibitors). Products include:
- Cataflam Tablets 833

Diclofenac Sodium (Potential for bleeding and/or prolonged prothrombin time in patients treated with Trental with or without platelet aggregation inhibitors). Products include:
- Voltaren Ophthalmic Sterile Ophthalmic Solution .... ◉ 264
- Cataflam/Voltaren/Voltaren-XR 833

Dicumarol (Potential for bleeding and/or prolonged prothrombin time in patients treated with Trental with or without platelet aggregation inhibitors).
- No products indexed under this heading.

Diflunisal (Potential for bleeding and/or prolonged prothrombin time in patients treated with Trental with or without platelet aggregation inhibitors). Products include:
- Dolobid Tablets 1695

Dipyridamole (Potential for bleeding and/or prolonged prothrombin time in patients treated with Trental with or without platelet aggregation inhibitors). Products include:
- Persantine Tablets 686

Dyphylline (Concomitant administration leads to increased theophylline levels and theophylline toxicity). Products include:
- Lufyllin & Lufyllin-400 Tablets 2778
- Lufyllin-GG Elixir & Tablets 2779

Enoxaparin (Potential for bleeding and/or prolonged prothrombin time in patients treated with Trental with or without platelet aggregation inhibitors). Products include:
- Lovenox Injection 2187

Fenoprofen Calcium (Potential for bleeding and/or prolonged prothrombin time in patients treated with Trental with or without platelet aggregation inhibitors). Products include:
- Nalfon 200 Pulvules & Nalfon Tablets 933

Flurbiprofen (Potential for bleeding and/or prolonged prothrombin time in patients treated with Trental with or without platelet aggregation inhibitors).
- No products indexed under this heading.

Heparin Calcium (Potential for bleeding and/or prolonged prothrombin time in patients treated with Trental with or without platelet aggregation inhibitors).
- No products indexed under this heading.

Heparin Sodium (Potential for bleeding and/or prolonged prothrombin time in patients treated with Trental with or without platelet aggregation inhibitors). Products include:
- Heparin Lock Flush Solution 2831
- Heparin Sodium Injection 2832
- Heparin Sodium Vials 1486

Ibuprofen (Potential for bleeding and/or prolonged prothrombin time in patients treated with Trental with or without platelet aggregation inhibitors). Products include:
- Advil Cold and Sinus Caplets and Tablets .... ■ 837
- Advil Ibuprofen Tablets, Caplets and Gel Caplets .... ■ 836
- Children's Motrin Ibuprofen Oral Suspension 1558
- IBU Tablets 1389
- Ibuprohm .... ■ 713
- Motrin IB Caplets, Tablets, and Gelcaps .... ■ 802
- Motrin Ibuprofen Suspension, Oral Drops, Chewable Tablets, Caplets 1563
- Nuprin Ibuprofen/Analgesic Tablets & Caplets .... ■ 645
- Vicks DayQuil SINUS Pressure & PAIN Relief with IBUPROFEN .... ■ 735

Indomethacin (Potential for bleeding and/or prolonged prothrombin time in patients treated with Trental with or without platelet aggregation inhibitors). Products include:
- Indocin 1723

Indomethacin Sodium Trihydrate (Potential for bleeding and/or prolonged prothrombin time in patients treated with Trental with or without platelet aggregation inhibitors). Products include:
- Indocin I.V. 1727

Ketoprofen (Potential for bleeding and/or prolonged prothrombin time in patients treated with Trental with or without platelet aggregation inhibitors). Products include:
- Actron Caplets and Tablets .... ■ 608
- Orudis Capsules 2874
- Orudis KT .... ■ 842
- Oruvail Capsules 2874

Magnesium Salicylate (Potential for bleeding and/or prolonged prothrombin time in patients treated with Trental with or without platelet aggregation inhibitors). Products include:
- Backache Caplets .... ■ 635
- Doan's Extra-Strength Analgesic .... ■ 653
- Extra Strength Doan's P.M. .... ■ 653
- Doan's Regular Strength Analgesic .... ■ 654
- Mobigesic Tablets .... ■ 607

Meclofenamate Sodium (Potential for bleeding and/or prolonged prothrombin time in patients treated with Trental with or without platelet aggregation inhibitors).
- No products indexed under this heading.

Mefenamic Acid (Potential for bleeding and/or prolonged prothrombin time in patients treated with Trental with or without platelet aggregation inhibitors). Products include:
- Ponstel 1982

Mezlocillin Sodium (Potential for bleeding and/or prolonged prothrombin time in patients treated with Trental with or without platelet aggregation inhibitors). Products include:
- Mezlin 594
- Mezlin Pharmacy Bulk Package 597

Nafcillin Sodium (Potential for bleeding and/or prolonged prothrombin time in patients treated with Trental with or without platelet aggregation inhibitors).
- No products indexed under this heading.

Naproxen (Potential for bleeding and/or prolonged prothrombin time in patients treated with Trental with or without platelet aggregation inhibitors). Products include:
- Anaprox/Naprosyn 2277

Naproxen Sodium (Potential for bleeding and/or prolonged prothrombin time in patients treated with Trental with or without platelet aggregation inhibitors). Products include:
- Aleve 2124
- Anaprox/Naprosyn 2277
- Naprelan Tablets 2861

Penicillin G Benzathine (Potential for bleeding and/or prolonged prothrombin time in patients treated with Trental with or without platelet aggregation inhibitors). Products include:
- Bicillin C-R Injection 2810
- Bicillin C-R 900/300 Injection 2812
- Bicillin L-A Injection 2813

Penicillin G Procaine (Potential for bleeding and/or prolonged prothrombin time in patients treated with Trental with or without platelet aggregation inhibitors). Products include:
- Bicillin C-R Injection 2810
- Bicillin C-R 900/300 Injection 2812

Phenylbutazone (Potential for bleeding and/or prolonged prothrombin time in patients treated with Trental with or without platelet aggregation inhibitors).
- No products indexed under this heading.

(■ Described in PDR For Nonprescription Drugs) (◉ Described in PDR For Ophthalmology)

Piroxicam (Potential for bleeding and/or prolonged prothrombin time in patients treated with Trental with or without platelet aggregation inhibitors). Products include:
   Feldene Capsules 2008

Salsalate (Potential for bleeding and/or prolonged prothrombin time in patients treated with Trental with or without platelet aggregation inhibitors). Products include:
   Disalcid 1549
   Mono-Gesic Tablets 810
   Salflex Tablets 791

Sulindac (Potential for bleeding and/or prolonged prothrombin time in patients treated with Trental with or without platelet aggregation inhibitors). Products include:
   Clinoril Tablets 1658

Theophylline (Concomitant administration leads to increased theophylline levels and theophylline toxicity). Products include:
   Marax Tablets & DF Syrup 2015
   Quibron 2227

Theophylline Anhydrous (Concomitant administration leads to increased theophylline levels and theophylline toxicity). Products include:
   Aerolate 1003
   Primatene Tablets 844
   Respbid Tablets 687
   Slo-bid Gyrocaps 2201
   Theo-24 Extended Release Capsules 2753
   Theo-Dur Extended-Release Tablets 1367
   Theo-X Extended-Release Tablets .. 793
   Uni-Dur Extended-Release Tablets .. 1374
   Uniphyl 400 mg and 600 mg Tablets 2157

Theophylline Calcium Salicylate (Concomitant administration leads to increased theophylline levels and theophylline toxicity). Products include:
   Quadrinal Tablets 1398

Theophylline Sodium Glycinate (Concomitant administration leads to increased theophylline levels and theophylline toxicity).
   No products indexed under this heading.

Ticarcillin Disodium (Potential for bleeding and/or prolonged prothrombin time in patients treated with Trental with or without platelet aggregation inhibitors). Products include:
   Ticar for Injection 2704
   Timentin for Injection 2706

Ticlopidine Hydrochloride (Potential for bleeding and/or prolonged prothrombin time in patients treated with Trental with or without platelet aggregation inhibitors). Products include:
   Ticlid Tablets 2317

Tolmetin Sodium (Potential for bleeding and/or prolonged prothrombin time in patients treated with Trental with or without platelet aggregation inhibitors). Products include:
   Tolectin (200, 400 and 600 mg) .. 1591

Warfarin Sodium (Potential for bleeding and/or prolonged prothrombin time in patients treated with Trental with or without platelet aggregation inhibitors; frequent monitoring of prothrombin time is recommended). Products include:
   Coumadin 941

Food Interactions
Food, unspecified (Delays absorption but does not affect total absorption).

TRIAMINIC AM COUGH AND DECONGESTANT FORMULA
(Dextromethorphan Hydrobromide, Pseudoephedrine Hydrochloride) 753
May interact with monoamine oxidase inhibitors. Compounds in this category include:

Furazolidone (Concurrent and/or sequential use is not recommended). Products include:
   Furoxone 2221

Isocarboxazid (Concurrent and/or sequential use is not recommended).
   No products indexed under this heading.

Phenelzine Sulfate (Concurrent and/or sequential use is not recommended). Products include:
   Nardil 1977

Selegiline Hydrochloride (Concurrent and/or sequential use is not recommended). Products include:
   Eldepryl Capsules 2729

Tranylcypromine Sulfate (Concurrent and/or sequential use is not recommended). Products include:
   Parnate Tablets 2679

TRIAMINIC AM DECONGESTANT FORMULA
(Pseudoephedrine Hydrochloride) .. 753
May interact with monoamine oxidase inhibitors. Compounds in this category include:

Furazolidone (Concurrent and/or sequential use is not recommended). Products include:
   Furoxone 2221

Isocarboxazid (Concurrent and/or sequential use is not recommended).
   No products indexed under this heading.

Phenelzine Sulfate (Concurrent and/or sequential use is not recommended). Products include:
   Nardil 1977

Selegiline Hydrochloride (Concurrent and/or sequential use is not recommended). Products include:
   Eldepryl Capsules 2729

Tranylcypromine Sulfate (Concurrent and/or sequential use is not recommended). Products include:
   Parnate Tablets 2679

TRIAMINIC EXPECTORANT
(Phenylpropanolamine Hydrochloride, Guaifenesin) 753
May interact with monoamine oxidase inhibitors. Compounds in this category include:

Furazolidone (Concurrent and/or sequential use is not recommended). Products include:
   Furoxone 2221

Isocarboxazid (Concurrent and/or sequential use is not recommended).
   No products indexed under this heading.

Phenelzine Sulfate (Concurrent and/or sequential use is not recommended). Products include:
   Nardil 1977

Selegiline Hydrochloride (Concurrent and/or sequential use is not recommended). Products include:
   Eldepryl Capsules 2729

Tranylcypromine Sulfate (Concurrent and/or sequential use is not recommended). Products include:
   Parnate Tablets 2679

TRIAMINIC INFANT ORAL DECONGESTANT DROPS
(Pseudoephedrine Hydrochloride) .. 754
May interact with monoamine oxidase inhibitors. Compounds in this category include:

Furazolidone (Concurrent and/or sequential use is not recommended). Products include:
   Furoxone 2221

Isocarboxazid (Concurrent and/or sequential use is not recommended).
   No products indexed under this heading.

Phenelzine Sulfate (Concurrent and/or sequential use is not recommended). Products include:
   Nardil 1977

Selegiline Hydrochloride (Concurrent and/or sequential use is not recommended). Products include:
   Eldepryl Capsules 2729

Tranylcypromine Sulfate (Concurrent and/or sequential use is not recommended). Products include:
   Parnate Tablets 2679

TRIAMINIC NIGHT TIME
(Chlorpheniramine Maleate, Dextromethorphan Hydrobromide, Pseudoephedrine Hydrochloride) 754
May interact with hypnotics and sedatives, tranquilizers, monoamine oxidase inhibitors, and certain other agents. Compounds in these categories include:

Alprazolam (May increase drowsiness effect). Products include:
   Xanax Tablets 2115

Buspirone Hydrochloride (May increase drowsiness effect). Products include:
   BuSpar Tablets 738

Chlordiazepoxide (May increase drowsiness effect). Products include:
   Limbitrol 2333

Chlordiazepoxide Hydrochloride (May increase drowsiness effect). Products include:
   Librax Capsules 2330
   Librium Capsules 2331
   Librium Injectable 2332

Chlorpromazine (May increase drowsiness effect). Products include:
   Thorazine Suppositories 2701

Chlorpromazine Hydrochloride (May increase drowsiness effect). Products include:
   Thorazine 2701

Chlorprothixene (May increase drowsiness effect).
   No products indexed under this heading.

Chlorprothixene Hydrochloride (May increase drowsiness effect).
   No products indexed under this heading.

Clorazepate Dipotassium (May increase drowsiness effect). Products include:
   Tranxene 459

Diazepam (May increase drowsiness effect). Products include:
   Dizac (diazepam injectable emulsion) CIV 1862
   Valium Injectable 2336
   Valium Tablets 2335

Droperidol (May increase drowsiness effect). Products include:
   Inapsine Injection 462

Estazolam (May increase drowsiness effect). Products include:
   ProSom Tablets 457

Ethchlorvynol (May increase drowsiness effect). Products include:
   Placidyl Capsules 456

Ethinamate (May increase drowsiness effect).
   No products indexed under this heading.

Fluphenazine Decanoate (May increase drowsiness effect). Products include:
   Prolixin Decanoate 510

Fluphenazine Enanthate (May increase drowsiness effect). Products include:
   Prolixin Enanthate 510

Fluphenazine Hydrochloride (May increase drowsiness effect). Products include:
   Prolixin 510

Flurazepam Hydrochloride (May increase drowsiness effect). Products include:
   Dalmane Capsules 2329

Furazolidone (Concurrent and/or sequential use is not recommended). Products include:
   Furoxone 2221

Glutethimide (May increase drowsiness effect).
   No products indexed under this heading.

Haloperidol (May increase drowsiness effect). Products include:
   Haldol Injection, Tablets and Concentrate 1585

Haloperidol Decanoate (May increase drowsiness effect). Products include:
   Haldol Decanoate 1587

Hydroxyzine Hydrochloride (May increase drowsiness effect). Products include:
   Atarax Tablets & Syrup 1992
   Marax Tablets & DF Syrup 2015
   Vistaril Intramuscular Solution ... 2042

Isocarboxazid (Concurrent and/or sequential use is not recommended).
   No products indexed under this heading.

Lorazepam (May increase drowsiness effect). Products include:
   Ativan Injection 2805
   Ativan Tablets 2807

Loxapine Hydrochloride (May increase drowsiness effect). Products include:
   Loxitane 1426

Loxapine Succinate (May increase drowsiness effect). Products include:
   Loxitane Capsules 1426

Meprobamate (May increase drowsiness effect). Products include:
   Miltown Tablets 2780
   PMB 200 and PMB 400 2890

Mesoridazine Besylate (May increase drowsiness effect). Products include:
   Serentil 689

Midazolam Hydrochloride (May increase drowsiness effect). Products include:
   Versed Injection 2324

Molindone Hydrochloride (May increase drowsiness effect). Products include:
   Moban Tablets and Concentrate 1036

Oxazepam (May increase drowsiness effect). Products include:
   Serax Capsules 2916
   Serax Tablets 2916

Perphenazine (May increase drowsiness effect). Products include:
   Etrafon 2495
   Triavil Tablets 1800
   Trilafon 2532

Phenelzine Sulfate (Concurrent and/or sequential use is not recommended). Products include:
   Nardil 1977

IMPORTANT NOTE: Always consult each drug listing in the patient's regimen for possible interactions.

Triaminic Night Time / Interactions Index

Prazepam (May increase drowsiness effect).
　No products indexed under this heading.

Prochlorperazine (May increase drowsiness effect). Products include:
　Compazine 2644

Promethazine Hydrochloride (May increase drowsiness effect). Products include:
　Mepergan Injection 2859
　Phenergan with Codeine 2883
　Phenergan with Dextromethorphan 2885
　Phenergan Injection 2880
　Phenergan Suppositories 2882
　Phenergan Syrup 2881
　Phenergan Tablets 2882
　Phenergan VC 2886
　Phenergan VC with Codeine 2888

Propofol (May increase drowsiness effect). Products include:
　Diprivan Injectable Emulsion 2939

Quazepam (May increase drowsiness effect). Products include:
　Doral Tablets 2773

Secobarbital Sodium (May increase drowsiness effect). Products include:
　Seconal Sodium Pulvules 1529

Selegiline Hydrochloride (Concurrent and/or sequential use is not recommended). Products include:
　Eldepryl Capsules 2729

Temazepam (May increase drowsiness effect). Products include:
　Restoril Capsules 2413

Thioridazine Hydrochloride (May increase drowsiness effect). Products include:
　Mellaril 2398

Thiothixene (May increase drowsiness effect). Products include:
　Navane Capsules and Concentrate 2018
　Navane Intramuscular 2019

Tranylcypromine Sulfate (Concurrent and/or sequential use is not recommended). Products include:
　Parnate Tablets 2679

Triazolam (May increase drowsiness effect). Products include:
　Halcion Tablets 2093

Trifluoperazine Hydrochloride (May increase drowsiness effect). Products include:
　Stelazine 2692

Zolpidem Tartrate (May increase drowsiness effect). Products include:
　Ambien Tablets 2559

Food Interactions
Alcohol (May increase drowsiness effect).

TRIAMINIC SORE THROAT FORMULA
(Acetaminophen, Dextromethorphan Hydrobromide, Pseudoephedrine Hydrochloride) .... ⊞ 755
May interact with monoamine oxidase inhibitors. Compounds in this category include:

Furazolidone (Concurrent and/or sequential use is not recommended). Products include:
　Furoxone 2221

Isocarboxazid (Concurrent and/or sequential use is not recommended).
　No products indexed under this heading.

Phenelzine Sulfate (Concurrent and/or sequential use is not recommended). Products include:
　Nardil 1977

Selegiline Hydrochloride (Concurrent and/or sequential use is not recommended). Products include:
　Eldepryl Capsules 2729

Tranylcypromine Sulfate (Concurrent and/or sequential use is not recommended). Products include:
　Parnate Tablets 2679

TRIAMINIC SYRUP
(Phenylpropanolamine Hydrochloride, Chlorpheniramine Maleate) .... ⊞ 755
May interact with hypnotics and sedatives, tranquilizers, monoamine oxidase inhibitors, and certain other agents. Compounds in these categories include:

Alprazolam (May increase drowsiness). Products include:
　Xanax Tablets 2115

Buspirone Hydrochloride (May increase drowsiness). Products include:
　BuSpar Tablets 738

Chlordiazepoxide (May increase drowsiness). Products include:
　Limbitrol 2333

Chlordiazepoxide Hydrochloride (May increase drowsiness). Products include:
　Librax Capsules 2330
　Librium Capsules 2331
　Librium Injectable 2332

Chlorpromazine (May increase drowsiness). Products include:
　Thorazine Suppositories 2701

Chlorpromazine Hydrochloride (May increase drowsiness). Products include:
　Thorazine 2701

Chlorprothixene (May increase drowsiness).
　No products indexed under this heading.

Chlorprothixene Hydrochloride (May increase drowsiness).
　No products indexed under this heading.

Clorazepate Dipotassium (May increase drowsiness). Products include:
　Tranxene 459

Diazepam (May increase drowsiness). Products include:
　Dizac (diazepam injectable emulsion) CIV 1862
　Valium Injectable 2336
　Valium Tablets 2335

Droperidol (May increase drowsiness). Products include:
　Inapsine Injection 462

Estazolam (May increase drowsiness). Products include:
　ProSom Tablets 457

Ethchlorvynol (May increase drowsiness). Products include:
　Placidyl Capsules 456

Ethinamate (May increase drowsiness).
　No products indexed under this heading.

Fluphenazine Decanoate (May increase drowsiness). Products include:
　Prolixin Decanoate 510

Fluphenazine Enanthate (May increase drowsiness). Products include:
　Prolixin Enanthate 510

Fluphenazine Hydrochloride (May increase drowsiness). Products include:
　Prolixin 510

Flurazepam Hydrochloride (May increase drowsiness). Products include:
　Dalmane Capsules 2329

Furazolidone (Concurrent and/or sequential use is not recommended). Products include:
　Furoxone 2221

Glutethimide (May increase drowsiness).
　No products indexed under this heading.

Haloperidol (May increase drowsiness). Products include:
　Haldol Injection, Tablets and Concentrate 1585

Haloperidol Decanoate (May increase drowsiness). Products include:
　Haldol Decanoate 1587

Hydroxyzine Hydrochloride (May increase drowsiness). Products include:
　Atarax Tablets & Syrup 1992
　Marax Tablets & DF Syrup 2015
　Vistaril Intramuscular Solution ... 2042

Isocarboxazid (Concurrent and/or sequential use is not recommended).
　No products indexed under this heading.

Lorazepam (May increase drowsiness). Products include:
　Ativan Injection 2805
　Ativan Tablets 2807

Loxapine Hydrochloride (May increase drowsiness). Products include:
　Loxitane 1426

Loxapine Succinate (May increase drowsiness). Products include:
　Loxitane Capsules 1426

Meprobamate (May increase drowsiness). Products include:
　Miltown Tablets 2780
　PMB 200 and PMB 400 2890

Mesoridazine Besylate (May increase drowsiness). Products include:
　Serentil 689

Midazolam Hydrochloride (May increase drowsiness). Products include:
　Versed Injection 2324

Molindone Hydrochloride (May increase drowsiness). Products include:
　Moban Tablets and Concentrate ... 1036

Oxazepam (May increase drowsiness). Products include:
　Serax Capsules 2916
　Serax Tablets 2916

Perphenazine (May increase drowsiness). Products include:
　Etrafon 2495
　Triavil Tablets 1800
　Trilafon 2532

Phenelzine Sulfate (Concurrent and/or sequential use is not recommended). Products include:
　Nardil 1977

Prazepam (May increase drowsiness).
　No products indexed under this heading.

Prochlorperazine (May increase drowsiness). Products include:
　Compazine 2644

Promethazine Hydrochloride (May increase drowsiness). Products include:
　Mepergan Injection 2859
　Phenergan with Codeine 2883
　Phenergan with Dextromethorphan 2885
　Phenergan Injection 2880
　Phenergan Suppositories 2882
　Phenergan Syrup 2881
　Phenergan Tablets 2882
　Phenergan VC 2886
　Phenergan VC with Codeine 2888

Propofol (May increase drowsiness). Products include:
　Diprivan Injectable Emulsion 2939

Quazepam (May increase drowsiness). Products include:
　Doral Tablets 2773

Secobarbital Sodium (May increase drowsiness). Products include:
　Seconal Sodium Pulvules 1529

Selegiline Hydrochloride (Concurrent and/or sequential use is not recommended). Products include:
　Eldepryl Capsules 2729

Temazepam (May increase drowsiness). Products include:
　Restoril Capsules 2413

Thioridazine Hydrochloride (May increase drowsiness). Products include:
　Mellaril 2398

Thiothixene (May increase drowsiness). Products include:
　Navane Capsules and Concentrate 2018
　Navane Intramuscular 2019

Tranylcypromine Sulfate (Concurrent and/or sequential use is not recommended). Products include:
　Parnate Tablets 2679

Triazolam (May increase drowsiness). Products include:
　Halcion Tablets 2093

Trifluoperazine Hydrochloride (May increase drowsiness). Products include:
　Stelazine 2692

Zolpidem Tartrate (May increase drowsiness). Products include:
　Ambien Tablets 2559

Food Interactions
Alcohol (May increase drowsiness effect).

TRIAMINIC TRIAMINICOL COLD & COUGH
(Phenylpropanolamine Hydrochloride, Chlorpheniramine Maleate, Dextromethorphan Hydrobromide) .... ⊞ 756
May interact with hypnotics and sedatives, tranquilizers, monoamine oxidase inhibitors, and certain other agents. Compounds in these categories include:

Alprazolam (May increase drowsiness effect). Products include:
　Xanax Tablets 2115

Buspirone Hydrochloride (May increase drowsiness effect). Products include:
　BuSpar Tablets 738

Chlordiazepoxide (May increase drowsiness effect). Products include:
　Limbitrol 2333

Chlordiazepoxide Hydrochloride (May increase drowsiness effect). Products include:
　Librax Capsules 2330
　Librium Capsules 2331
　Librium Injectable 2332

Chlorpromazine (May increase drowsiness effect). Products include:
　Thorazine Suppositories 2701

Chlorpromazine Hydrochloride (May increase drowsiness effect). Products include:
　Thorazine 2701

Chlorprothixene (May increase drowsiness effect).
　No products indexed under this heading.

Chlorprothixene Hydrochloride (May increase drowsiness effect).
　No products indexed under this heading.

Clorazepate Dipotassium (May increase drowsiness effect). Products include:
　Tranxene 459

Diazepam (May increase drowsiness effect). Products include:
　Dizac (diazepam injectable emulsion) CIV 1862

(⊞ Described in PDR For Nonprescription Drugs)　　　　　　　　　　　　(⊙ Described in PDR For Ophthalmology)

Valium Injectable 2336
Valium Tablets 2335
Droperidol (May increase drowsiness effect). Products include:
Inapsine Injection 462
Estazolam (May increase drowsiness effect). Products include:
ProSom Tablets 457
Ethchlorvynol (May increase drowsiness effect). Products include:
Placidyl Capsules 456
Ethinamate (May increase drowsiness effect).
No products indexed under this heading.
Fluphenazine Decanoate (May increase drowsiness effect). Products include:
Prolixin Decanoate 510
Fluphenazine Enanthate (May increase drowsiness effect). Products include:
Prolixin Enanthate 510
Fluphenazine Hydrochloride (May increase drowsiness effect). Products include:
Prolixin 510
Flurazepam Hydrochloride (May increase drowsiness effect). Products include:
Dalmane Capsules 2329
Furazolidone (Concurrent and/or sequential use is not recommended). Products include:
Furoxone 2221
Glutethimide (May increase drowsiness effect).
No products indexed under this heading.
Haloperidol (May increase drowsiness effect). Products include:
Haldol Injection, Tablets and Concentrate 1585
Haloperidol Decanoate (May increase drowsiness effect). Products include:
Haldol Decanoate 1587
Hydroxyzine Hydrochloride (May increase drowsiness effect). Products include:
Atarax Tablets & Syrup 1992
Marax Tablets & DF Syrup 2015
Vistaril Intramuscular Solution ... 2042
Isocarboxazid (Concurrent and/or sequential use is not recommended).
No products indexed under this heading.
Lorazepam (May increase drowsiness effect). Products include:
Ativan Injection 2805
Ativan Tablets 2807
Loxapine Hydrochloride (May increase drowsiness effect). Products include:
Loxitane 1426
Loxapine Succinate (May increase drowsiness effect). Products include:
Loxitane Capsules 1426
Meprobamate (May increase drowsiness effect). Products include:
Miltown Tablets 2780
PMB 200 and PMB 400 2890
Mesoridazine Besylate (May increase drowsiness effect). Products include:
Serentil 689
Midazolam Hydrochloride (May increase drowsiness effect). Products include:
Versed Injection 2324
Molindone Hydrochloride (May increase drowsiness effect). Products include:
Moban Tablets and Concentrate 1036

Oxazepam (May increase drowsiness effect). Products include:
Serax Capsules 2916
Serax Tablets 2916
Perphenazine (May increase drowsiness effect). Products include:
Etrafon 2495
Triavil Tablets 1800
Trilafon 2532
Phenelzine Sulfate (Concurrent and/or sequential use is not recommended). Products include:
Nardil 1977
Prazepam (May increase drowsiness effect).
No products indexed under this heading.
Prochlorperazine (May increase drowsiness effect). Products include:
Compazine 2644
Promethazine Hydrochloride (May increase drowsiness effect). Products include:
Mepergan Injection 2859
Phenergan with Codeine 2883
Phenergan with Dextromethorphan 2885
Phenergan Injection 2880
Phenergan Suppositories 2882
Phenergan Syrup 2881
Phenergan Tablets 2882
Phenergan VC 2886
Phenergan VC with Codeine 2888
Propofol (May increase drowsiness effect). Products include:
Diprivan Injectable Emulsion 2939
Quazepam (May increase drowsiness effect). Products include:
Doral Tablets 2773
Secobarbital Sodium (May increase drowsiness effect). Products include:
Seconal Sodium Pulvules 1529
Selegiline Hydrochloride (Concurrent and/or sequential use is not recommended). Products include:
Eldepryl Capsules 2729
Temazepam (May increase drowsiness effect). Products include:
Restoril Capsules 2413
Thioridazine Hydrochloride (May increase drowsiness effect). Products include:
Mellaril 2398
Thiothixene (May increase drowsiness effect). Products include:
Navane Capsules and Concentrate 2018
Navane Intramuscular 2019
Tranylcypromine Sulfate (Concurrent and/or sequential use is not recommended). Products include:
Parnate Tablets 2679
Triazolam (May increase drowsiness effect). Products include:
Halcion Tablets 2093
Trifluoperazine Hydrochloride (May increase drowsiness effect). Products include:
Stelazine 2692
Zolpidem Tartrate (May increase drowsiness effect). Products include:
Ambien Tablets 2559

Food Interactions
Alcohol (May increase drowsiness effect).

TRIAMINIC DM SYRUP
(Phenylpropanolamine Hydrochloride, Dextromethorphan Hydrobromide) 756
May interact with monoamine oxidase inhibitors. Compounds in this category include:

Furazolidone (Concurrent and/or sequential use is not recommended). Products include:
Furoxone 2221

Isocarboxazid (Concurrent and/or sequential use is not recommended).
No products indexed under this heading.
Phenelzine Sulfate (Concurrent and/or sequential use is not recommended). Products include:
Nardil 1977
Selegiline Hydrochloride (Concurrent and/or sequential use is not recommended). Products include:
Eldepryl Capsules 2729
Tranylcypromine Sulfate (Concurrent and/or sequential use is not recommended). Products include:
Parnate Tablets 2679

TRIAMINICIN TABLETS
(Acetaminophen, Chlorpheniramine Maleate, Phenylpropanolamine Hydrochloride) 756
May interact with tranquilizers, hypnotics and sedatives, monoamine oxidase inhibitors, and certain other agents. Compounds in these categories include:

Alprazolam (May increase drowsiness effect). Products include:
Xanax Tablets 2115
Buspirone Hydrochloride (May increase drowsiness effect). Products include:
BuSpar Tablets 738
Chlordiazepoxide (May increase drowsiness effect). Products include:
Limbitrol 2333
Chlordiazepoxide Hydrochloride (May increase drowsiness effect). Products include:
Librax Capsules 2330
Librium Capsules 2331
Librium Injectable 2332
Chlorpromazine (May increase drowsiness effect). Products include:
Thorazine Suppositories 2701
Chlorpromazine Hydrochloride (May increase drowsiness effect). Products include:
Thorazine 2701
Chlorprothixene (May increase drowsiness effect).
No products indexed under this heading.
Chlorprothixene Hydrochloride (May increase drowsiness effect).
No products indexed under this heading.
Clorazepate Dipotassium (May increase drowsiness effect). Products include:
Tranxene 459
Diazepam (May increase drowsiness effect). Products include:
Dizac (diazepam injectable emulsion) CIV 1862
Valium Injectable 2336
Valium Tablets 2335
Droperidol (May increase drowsiness effect). Products include:
Inapsine Injection 462
Estazolam (May increase drowsiness effect). Products include:
ProSom Tablets 457
Ethchlorvynol (May increase drowsiness effect). Products include:
Placidyl Capsules 456
Ethinamate (May increase drowsiness effect).
No products indexed under this heading.
Fluphenazine Decanoate (May increase drowsiness effect). Products include:
Prolixin Decanoate 510
Fluphenazine Enanthate (May increase drowsiness effect). Products include:
Prolixin Enanthate 510

Fluphenazine Hydrochloride (May increase drowsiness effect). Products include:
Prolixin 510
Flurazepam Hydrochloride (May increase drowsiness effect). Products include:
Dalmane Capsules 2329
Furazolidone (Concurrent and/or sequential use is not recommended). Products include:
Furoxone 2221
Glutethimide (May increase drowsiness effect).
No products indexed under this heading.
Haloperidol (May increase drowsiness effect). Products include:
Haldol Injection, Tablets and Concentrate 1585
Haloperidol Decanoate (May increase drowsiness effect). Products include:
Haldol Decanoate 1587
Hydroxyzine Hydrochloride (May increase drowsiness effect). Products include:
Atarax Tablets & Syrup 1992
Marax Tablets & DF Syrup 2015
Vistaril Intramuscular Solution ... 2042
Isocarboxazid (Concurrent and/or sequential use is not recommended).
No products indexed under this heading.
Lorazepam (May increase drowsiness effect). Products include:
Ativan Injection 2805
Ativan Tablets 2807
Loxapine Hydrochloride (May increase drowsiness effect). Products include:
Loxitane 1426
Loxapine Succinate (May increase drowsiness effect). Products include:
Loxitane Capsules 1426
Meprobamate (May increase drowsiness effect). Products include:
Miltown Tablets 2780
PMB 200 and PMB 400 2890
Mesoridazine Besylate (May increase drowsiness effect). Products include:
Serentil 689
Midazolam Hydrochloride (May increase drowsiness effect). Products include:
Versed Injection 2324
Molindone Hydrochloride (May increase drowsiness effect). Products include:
Moban Tablets and Concentrate 1036
Oxazepam (May increase drowsiness effect). Products include:
Serax Capsules 2916
Serax Tablets 2916
Perphenazine (May increase drowsiness effect). Products include:
Etrafon 2495
Triavil Tablets 1800
Trilafon 2532
Phenelzine Sulfate (Concurrent and/or sequential use is not recommended). Products include:
Nardil 1977
Prazepam (May increase drowsiness effect).
No products indexed under this heading.
Prochlorperazine (May increase drowsiness effect). Products include:
Compazine 2644
Promethazine Hydrochloride (May increase drowsiness effect). Products include:
Mepergan Injection 2859
Phenergan with Codeine 2883
Phenergan with Dextromethorphan 2885

IMPORTANT NOTE: Always consult each drug listing in the patient's regimen for possible interactions.

Triaminicin | Interactions Index | 1102

Phenergan Injection 2880
Phenergan Suppositories 2882
Phenergan Syrup 2881
Phenergan Tablets 2882
Phenergan VC 2886
Phenergan VC with Codeine 2888

Propofol (May increase drowsiness effect). Products include:
Diprivan Injectable Emulsion 2939

Quazepam (May increase drowsiness effect). Products include:
Doral Tablets 2773

Secobarbital Sodium (May increase drowsiness effect). Products include:
Seconal Sodium Pulvules 1529

Selegiline Hydrochloride (Concurrent and/or sequential use is not recommended). Products include:
Eldepryl Capsules 2729

Temazepam (May increase drowsiness effect). Products include:
Restoril Capsules 2413

Thioridazine Hydrochloride (May increase drowsiness effect). Products include:
Mellaril 2398

Thiothixene (May increase drowsiness effect). Products include:
Navane Capsules and Concentrate 2018
Navane Intramuscular 2019

Tranylcypromine Sulfate (Concurrent and/or sequential use is not recommended). Products include:
Parnate Tablets 2679

Triazolam (May increase drowsiness effect). Products include:
Halcion Tablets 2093

Trifluoperazine Hydrochloride (May increase drowsiness effect). Products include:
Stelazine 2692

Zolpidem Tartrate (May increase drowsiness effect). Products include:
Ambien Tablets 2559

Food Interactions

Alcohol (May increase drowsiness effect).

TRIAVIL TABLETS
(Perphenazine, Amitriptyline Hydrochloride) 1800

May interact with thyroid preparations, antihistamines, monoamine oxidase inhibitors, peripheral adrenergic blockers, anticonvulsants, central nervous system depressants, anticholinergics, sympathomimetics, antipsychotic agents, barbiturates, and certain other agents. Compounds in these categories include:

Acrivastine (Potentiated). Products include:
Semprex-D Capsules 1620

Albuterol (Close supervision and careful dosage adjustment required). Products include:
Proventil Inhalation Aerosol 2524
Ventolin Inhalation Aerosol and Refill 1170

Albuterol Sulfate (Close supervision and careful dosage adjustment required). Products include:
Airet Albuterol Sulfate Inhalation Solution 1602
Albuterol Sulfate, USP Solution for Inhalation, Arm-a-Med 522
Proventil Inhalation Solution 0.083% 2527
Proventil Repetabs Tablets 2529
Proventil Solution for Inhalation 0.5% 2525
Proventil Syrup 2528
Proventil Tablets 2529
Ventolin Inhalation Solution 1171
Ventolin Nebules Inhalation Solution 1172
Ventolin Rotacaps for Inhalation 1173
Ventolin Syrup 1175
Ventolin Tablets 1176
Volmax Extended-Release Tablets 1835

Alfentanil Hydrochloride (Potentiated). Products include:
Alfenta Injection 1334

Alprazolam (Potentiated). Products include:
Xanax Tablets 2115

Aprobarbital (Potentiated).
No products indexed under this heading.

Astemizole (Potentiated). Products include:
Hismanal Tablets 1341

Atropine Sulfate (Potentiated; hyperpyrexia; paralytic ileus). Products include:
Arco-Lase Plus Tablets 513
Atrohist Plus Tablets 1605
Donnatal 2234
Donnatal Extentabs 2234
Donnatal Tablets 2234
Lomotil 2591
Motofen Tablets 789
Urised Tablets 2123

Azatadine Maleate (Potentiated). Products include:
Trinalin Repetabs Tablets 1373

Belladonna Alkaloids (Hyperpyrexia; paralytic ileus). Products include:
Bellergal-S Tablets 2375
Hyland's Bedwetting Tablets ▣ 788
Hyland's EnurAid Tablets ▣ 789
Hyland's Headache Tablets ▣ 790
Hyland's Teething Tablets ▣ 790
Similasan Eye Drops #1 ▣ 769

Benztropine Mesylate (Hyperpyrexia; paralytic ileus). Products include:
Cogentin 1661

Biperiden Hydrochloride (Hyperpyrexia; paralytic ileus). Products include:
Akineton 1380

Bromodiphenhydramine Hydrochloride (Potentiated).
No products indexed under this heading.

Brompheniramine Maleate (Potentiated). Products include:
Alka-Seltzer Plus Sinus Medicine ▣ 611
Bromfed Capsules (Extended-Release) 1832
Bromfed Syrup ▣ 712
Bromfed Tablets 1832
Bromfed-DM Cough Syrup 1832
Bromfed-PD Capsules (Extended-Release) 1832
Dimetane-DC Cough Syrup 2232
Dimetane-DX Cough Syrup 2233
Dimetapp Allergy Dye-Free Elixir ▣ 838
Dimetapp Allergy Sinus Caplets ▣ 838
Dimetapp Cold & Allergy Chewable Tablets ▣ 838
Dimetapp Cold & Cough Liqui-Gels ▣ 839
Dimetapp Cold & Fever Suspension ▣ 839
Dimetapp DM Elixir ▣ 840
Dimetapp Elixir ▣ 840
Dimetapp Extentabs ▣ 841
Dimetapp Tablets/Liqui-Gels ▣ 841
Rondec Chewable Tablets 974
Vicks DayQuil Allergy Relief 12-Hour Extended Release Tablets ▣ 733
Vicks DayQuil Allergy Relief 4-Hour Tablets ▣ 733

Buprenorphine (Potentiated). Products include:
Buprenex Injectable 2170

Buspirone Hydrochloride (Potentiated). Products include:
BuSpar Tablets 738

Butabarbital (Potentiated).
No products indexed under this heading.

Butalbital (Potentiated). Products include:
Axocet Capsules 2469
Esgic-plus Capsules 1012
Esgic-plus Tablets 1012
Fioricet Tablets 2386
Fioricet with Codeine Capsules 2387
Fiorinal Capsules 2388
Fiorinal with Codeine Capsules 2390
Fiorinal Tablets 2388
Phrenilin 790
Sedapap Tablets 50 mg/650 mg 1826

Carbamazepine (Increased anticonvulsant dosage may be necessary). Products include:
Atretol Tablets 569
Tegretol/Tegretol-XR 870

Cetirizine Hydrochloride (Potentiated). Products include:
Zyrtec Tablets 2053

Chlordiazepoxide (Potentiated). Products include:
Limbitrol 2333

Chlordiazepoxide Hydrochloride (Potentiated). Products include:
Librax Capsules 2330
Librium Capsules 2331
Librium Injectable 2332

Chlorpheniramine Maleate (Potentiated). Products include:
Alka-Seltzer Plus Cold Medicine ▣ 611
Alka-Seltzer Plus Cold Medicine Liqui-Gels ▣ 612
Alka-Seltzer Plus Cold & Cough Medicine ▣ 611
Alka-Seltzer Plus Cold & Cough Medicine Liqui-Gels ▣ 612
Alka-Seltzer Plus Flu & Body Aches Effervescent Tablets ▣ 612
Allerest Maximum Strength ▣ 649
Allerest Sinus Pain Formula ▣ 649
Ana-Kit Anaphylaxis Emergency Treatment Kit 611
Atrohist Pediatric Capsules 1603
Atrohist Plus Tablets 1605
BC Cold Powder Multi-Symptom Formula (Cold-Sinus-Allergy) ▣ 631
Cerose DM ▣ 853
Cheracol Plus Head Cold/Cough Formula ▣ 741
Children's TYLENOL Cold Multi-Symptom Chewable Tablets and Liquid 1559
Children's TYLENOL Cold Plus Cough Multi Symptom Chewable Tablets and Liquid 1560
Children's TYLENOL Flu Suspension Liquid 1560
Children's Vicks DayQuil Allergy Relief ▣ 730
Children's Vicks NyQuil Cold/Cough Relief ▣ 731
Chlor-Trimeton Allergy Decongestant Tablets ▣ 759
Chlor-Trimeton Allergy Tablets ▣ 758
Allergy-Sinus Comtrex Multi-Symptom Allergy-Sinus Formula Tablets and Caplets ▣ 639
Comtrex Multi-Symptom ▣ 638
Contac Continuous Action Nasal Decongestant/Antihistamine 12 Hour Capsules ▣ 773
Contac Maximum Strength Continuous Action Decongestant/Antihistamine 12 Hour Caplets ▣ 772
Contac Severe Cold and Flu Formula Caplets ▣ 773
Coricidin Cold + Flu Tablets ▣ 760
Coricidin Cough + Cold Tablets ▣ 760
Coricidin 'D' Decongestant Tablets ▣ 760
D.A. II Tablets 972
D.A. Chewable Tablets 970
Dura-Tap/PD Capsules 970
Dura-Vent/DA Tablets 972
Efidac 24 Chlorpheniramine ▣ 655
Extendryl 1003
Fedahist Gyrocaps 2545
Hycomine Compound Tablets 948
Kronofed-A 994
Nolamine Timed-Release Tablets 790
Novahistine Elixir ▣ 782
Ornade Spansule Capsules 2678
PediaCare Cough-Cold Chewable Tablets and Liquid 1569
PediaCare NightRest Cough-Cold Liquid 1569
Pediatric Vicks 44m Cough & Cold Relief ▣ 737
Pyrroxate Caplets ▣ 742
Ryna ▣ 804
Sinarest ▣ 663
Sine-Off Sinus Medicine ▣ 784
Singlet Tablets ▣ 785
Sinulin Tablets 792
Sinutab Sinus Allergy Medication, Maximum Strength Tablets and Caplets ▣ 823
Sudafed Cold & Allergy Tablets ▣ 826
Teldrin 12 Hour Antihistamine/Nasal Decongestant Allergy Relief Capsules ▣ 786
TheraFlu Flu and Cold Medicine ▣ 750
Theraflu Maximum Strength Flu and Cold Medicine For Sore Throat ▣ 751
TheraFlu Flu, Cold and Cough Medicine ▣ 750
TheraFlu Maximum Strength Nighttime Flu, Cold & Cough Medicine ▣ 751
Triaminic Night Time ▣ 754
Triaminic Syrup ▣ 755
Triaminic Triaminicol Cold & Cough ▣ 756
Triaminicin Tablets ▣ 756
Tussend 1830
TYLENOL Allergy Sinus, Maximum Strength Caplets and Gelcaps 1571
TYLENOL Cold Medication, Multi-Symptom Formula Tablets and Caplets 1572
TYLENOL Cold Medication, Multi-Symptom Hot Liquid Packets 1572
Vicks 44 LiquiCaps Cough, Cold & Flu Relief ▣ 728
Vicks 44M Cough, Cold & Flu Relief ▣ 729

Chlorpheniramine Polistirex (Potentiated). Products include:
Tussionex Pennkinetic Extended-Release Suspension 1624

Chlorpheniramine Tannate (Potentiated). Products include:
Atrohist Pediatric Suspension 1604
Atrohist Pediatric Suspension Dye-Free 1604
Rynatan 2781
Rynatuss 2782

Chlorpromazine (Potentiated; hyperpyrexia). Products include:
Thorazine Suppositories 2701

Chlorprothixene (Potentiated; hyperpyrexia).
No products indexed under this heading.

Chlorprothixene Hydrochloride (Potentiated; hyperpyrexia).
No products indexed under this heading.

Chlorprothixene Lactate (Potentiated).
No products indexed under this heading.

Cimetidine (Increased frequency and severity of side effects). Products include:
Tagamet HB Tablets ▣ 786
Tagamet Tablets 2694

Cimetidine Hydrochloride (Increased frequency and severity of side effects). Products include:
Tagamet 2694

Clemastine Fumarate (Potentiated). Products include:
Tavist Syrup 2426
Tavist Tablets 2427
Tavist-1 12 Hour Relief Tablets ▣ 749
Tavist-D 12 Hour Relief Tablets ▣ 750

Clidinium Bromide (Hyperpyrexia; paralytic ileus). Products include:
Librax Capsules 2330

Clorazepate Dipotassium (Potentiated). Products include:
Tranxene 459

Clozapine (Potentiated; hyperpyrexia). Products include:
Clozaril Tablets 2377

Codeine Phosphate (Potentiated). Products include:
Brontex 2130
Dimetane-DC Cough Syrup 2232
Fioricet with Codeine Capsules 2387
Fiorinal with Codeine Capsules 2390
Nucofed 2225
Phenergan with Codeine 2883
Phenergan VC with Codeine 2888
Robitussin A-C Syrup 2248

(▣ Described in PDR For Nonprescription Drugs) (◉ Described in PDR For Ophthalmology)

Robitussin-DAC Syrup 2249
Ryna 804
Soma Compound w/Codeine Tablets 2784
Tylenol with Codeine 1592

Cyproheptadine Hydrochloride (Potentiated). Products include:
Periactin 1767

Deserpidine (Antihypertensive effect of deserpidine blocked).
No products indexed under this heading.

Desflurane (Potentiated). Products include:
Suprane (desflurane, USP) 1865

Dexchlorpheniramine Maleate (Potentiated).
No products indexed under this heading.

Dezocine (Potentiated). Products include:
Dalgan Injection 529

Diazepam (Potentiated). Products include:
Dizac (diazepam injectable emulsion) CIV 1862
Valium Injectable 2336
Valium Tablets 2335

Dicyclomine Hydrochloride (Hyperpyrexia; paralytic ileus). Products include:
Bentyl 1246

Diphenhydramine Citrate (Potentiated). Products include:
Excedrin P.M. Analgesic/Sleeping Aid Tablets, Caplets, Liquigels 735

Diphenhydramine Hydrochloride (Potentiated). Products include:
Actifed Allergy Daytime/Nighttime Caplets 808
Actifed Sinus Daytime/Nighttime Tablets and Caplets 809
Extra Strength Bayer PM Aspirin Plus Sleep Aid 617
Benadryl Allergy Chewables 811
Benadryl Allergy/Cold Tablets 811
Benadryl Allergy Decongestant Liquid Medication 812
Benadryl Allergy Decongestant Tablets 812
Benadryl Allergy Liquid Medication 813
Benadryl Allergy 811
Benadryl Allergy Sinus Headache Caplets 813
Benadryl Dye-Free Allergy Liquigel Softgels 813
Benadryl Dye-Free Allergy Liquid Medication 814
Benadryl Itch Relief Stick Extra Strength 814
Benadryl Cream 814
Benadryl Gel 815
Benadryl Spray 815
Benadryl Injection 1955
Contac Day & Night Cold/Flu Night Caplets 772
Contac Night Allergy/Sinus Caplets 771
Extra Strength Doan's P.M. 653
Excedrin P.M. Analgesic/Sleeping Aid Tablets, Caplets, Liquigels 643
Nytol QuickCaps Caplets 632
Sleepinal Night-time Sleep Aid Capsules and Softgels 798
TYLENOL Allergy Sinus NightTime, Maximum Strength Caplets 1571
TYLENOL Flu NightTime, Maximum Strength Gelcaps 1575
TYLENOL Flu NightTime, Maximum Strength Hot Medication Packets 1575
TYLENOL PM Pain Reliever/Sleep Aid, Extra Strength Gelcaps, Caplets, Geltabs 1576
TYLENOL Severe Allergy Medication Caplets 1571
Maximum Strength Unisom Sleepgels 1990
Unisom With Pain Relief-Nighttime Sleep Aid and Pain Reliever 1991

Diphenylpyraline Hydrochloride (Potentiated).
No products indexed under this heading.

Disulfiram (Delirium). Products include:
Antabuse Tablets 2802

Divalproex Sodium (Increased anticonvulsant dosage may be necessary). Products include:
Depakote Tablets 418

Dobutamine Hydrochloride (Close supervision and careful dosage adjustment required). Products include:
Dobutrex Solution Vials 1480

Dopamine Hydrochloride (Close supervision and careful dosage adjustment required).
No products indexed under this heading.

Droperidol (Potentiated). Products include:
Inapsine Injection 462

Enflurane (Potentiated).
No products indexed under this heading.

Ephedrine (Close supervision and careful dosage adjustment required).

Ephedrine Hydrochloride (Close supervision and careful dosage adjustment required). Products include:
Primatene Tablets 844
Quadrinal Tablets 1398

Ephedrine Sulfate (Close supervision and careful dosage adjustment required). Products include:
Marax Tablets & DF Syrup 2015

Ephedrine Tannate (Close supervision and careful dosage adjustment required). Products include:
Rynatuss 2782

Epinephrine (Close supervision and careful dosage adjustment required). Products include:
EPIFRIN 237
EpiPen 808
Marcaine with Epinephrine 2446
Primatene Mist 843
Sensorcaine with Epinephrine Injection 554
Sus-Phrine Injection 1017
Xylocaine with Epinephrine Injections 562

Epinephrine Bitartrate (Close supervision and careful dosage adjustment required). Products include:
Sensorcaine-MPF with Epinephrine Injection 554

Epinephrine Hydrochloride (Close supervision and careful dosage adjustment required). Products include:
Ana-Kit Anaphylaxis Emergency Treatment Kit 611

Estazolam (Potentiated). Products include:
ProSom Tablets 457

Ethchlorvynol (Potentiated; transient delirium). Products include:
Placidyl Capsules 456

Ethinamate (Potentiated).
No products indexed under this heading.

Ethopropazine Hydrochloride (Hyperpyrexia; paralytic ileus).

Ethosuximide (Increased anticonvulsant dosage may be necessary). Products include:
Zarontin Capsules 1986
Zarontin Syrup 1986

Ethotoin (Increased anticonvulsant dosage may be necessary). Products include:
Peganone Tablets 455

Felbamate (Increased anticonvulsant dosage may be necessary). Products include:
Felbatol 2774

Fentanyl (Potentiated). Products include:
Duragesic Transdermal System 1336

Fentanyl Citrate (Potentiated). Products include:
Sublimaze Injection 463

Fluphenazine Decanoate (Potentiated; hyperpyrexia). Products include:
Prolixin Decanoate 510

Fluphenazine Enanthate (Potentiated; hyperpyrexia). Products include:
Prolixin Enanthate 510

Fluphenazine Hydrochloride (Potentiated; hyperpyrexia). Products include:
Prolixin 510

Flurazepam Hydrochloride (Potentiated). Products include:
Dalmane Capsules 2329

Furazolidone (Concomitant administration is contraindicated; hyperpyretic crises and severe convulsions have occurred). Products include:
Furoxone 2221

Glutethimide (Potentiated).
No products indexed under this heading.

Glycopyrrolate (Hyperpyrexia; paralytic ileus). Products include:
Robinul Forte Tablets 2247
Robinul Injectable 2247
Robinul Tablets 2247

Guanethidine Monosulfate (Antihypertensive effect of guanethidine). Products include:
Esimil Tablets 840
Ismelin Tablets 845

Haloperidol (Potentiated; hyperpyrexia). Products include:
Haldol Injection, Tablets and Concentrate 1585

Haloperidol Decanoate (Potentiated; hyperpyrexia). Products include:
Haldol Decanoate 1587

Hydrocodone Bitartrate (Potentiated). Products include:
Codiclear DH Syrup 808
Duratuss HD Elixir 2750
Histussin D Liquid 670
Hycodan Tablets and Syrup 946
Hycomine Compound Tablets 948
Hycomine 947
Hycotuss Expectorant Syrup 950
Hydrocet Capsules 787
Lorcet 10/650 Tablets 1016
Lortab 2751
Tussend 1830
Tussend Expectorant 1831
Vicodin Tablets 1404
Vicodin ES Tablets 1405
Vicodin HP Tablets 1403
Vicodin Tuss Expectorant 1406
Zydone Capsules 967

Hydrocodone Polistirex (Potentiated). Products include:
Tussionex Pennkinetic Extended-Release Suspension 1624

Hydroxyzine Hydrochloride (Potentiated). Products include:
Atarax Tablets & Syrup 1992
Marax Tablets & DF Syrup 2015
Vistaril Intramuscular Solution 2042

Hyoscyamine (Hyperpyrexia; paralytic ileus). Products include:
Cystospaz Tablets 2123
Urised Tablets 2123

Hyoscyamine Sulfate (Hyperpyrexia; paralytic ileus). Products include:
Arco-Lase Plus Tablets 513
Atrohist Plus Tablets 1605
Cystospaz-M Capsules 2123
Donnatal 2234
Donnatal Extentabs 2234
Donnatal Tablets 2234
Kutrase Capsules 2546

Levsin/Levsinex/Levbid 2549

Ipratropium Bromide (Hyperpyrexia; paralytic ileus). Products include:
Atrovent Inhalation Aerosol 674
Atrovent Inhalation Solution 675
Atrovent Nasal Spray 0.03% 676
Atrovent Nasal Spray 0.06% 678

Isocarboxazid (Concomitant administration is contraindicated; hyperpyretic crises and severe convulsions have occurred).
No products indexed under this heading.

Isoflurane (Potentiated; contraindication).
No products indexed under this heading.

Isoproterenol Hydrochloride (Close supervision and careful dosage adjustment required). Products include:
Isuprel Hydrochloride Solution ... 2443
Isuprel Injection 2441
Isuprel Mistometer 2442

Isoproterenol Sulfate (Close supervision and careful dosage adjustment required). Products include:
Norisodrine with Calcium Iodide Syrup 446

Ketamine Hydrochloride (Potentiated).
No products indexed under this heading.

Lamotrigine (Increased anticonvulsant dosage may be necessary). Products include:
Lamictal Tablets 1105

Levomethadyl Acetate Hydrochloride (Potentiated). Products include:
Orlaam Oral Solution 2361

Levorphanol Tartrate (Potentiated). Products include:
Levo-Dromoran 2297

Levothyroxine Sodium (Close supervision is indicated). Products include:
Eltroxin Tablets 2214
Levothroid Tablets 1015
Levothyroxine Sodium, USP for Injection 546
Levoxyl Tablets 918
Synthroid 1410

Liothyronine Sodium (Close supervision is indicated). Products include:
Cytomel Tablets 2647
Triostat Injection 2708

Lithium Carbonate (Hyperpyrexia). Products include:
Eskalith 2658
Lithium Carbonate Capsules & Tablets 2352
Lithonate/Lithotabs/Lithobid 2721

Lithium Citrate (Hyperpyrexia).
No products indexed under this heading.

Loratadine (Potentiated). Products include:
Claritin Tablets 2485
Claritin-D Tablets 2487

Lorazepam (Potentiated; contraindication). Products include:
Ativan Injection 2805
Ativan Tablets 2807

Loxapine Hydrochloride (Potentiated; hyperpyrexia). Products include:
Loxitane 1426

Loxapine Succinate (Potentiated). Products include:
Loxitane Capsules 1426

Mepenzolate Bromide (Hyperpyrexia; paralytic ileus).
No products indexed under this heading.

IMPORTANT NOTE: Always consult each drug listing in the patient's regimen for possible interactions.

Triavil **Interactions Index** 1104

Meperidine Hydrochloride (Potentiated). Products include:
Demerol 2438
Mepergan Injection 2859
Mephenytoin (Increased anticonvulsant dosage may be necessary). Products include:
Mesantoin Tablets 2400
Mephobarbital (Potentiated). Products include:
Mebaral Tablets 2452
Meprobamate (Potentiated). Products include:
Miltown Tablets 2780
PMB 200 and PMB 400 2890
Mesoridazine Besylate (Potentiated; hyperpyrexia; contraindication). Products include:
Serentil 689
Metaproterenol Sulfate (Close supervision and careful dosage adjustment required). Products include:
Alupent 672
Metaproterenol Sulfate Inhalation Solution, USP, Arm-a-Med 547
Metaraminol Bitartrate (Close supervision and careful dosage adjustment required). Products include:
Aramine Injection 1649
Methadone Hydrochloride (Potentiated). Products include:
Methadone Hydrochloride Oral Concentrate 2356
Methadone Hydrochloride Oral Solution & Tablets 2357
Methdilazine Hydrochloride (Potentiated).
No products indexed under this heading.
Methohexital Sodium (Potentiated).
No products indexed under this heading.
Methotrimeprazine (Potentiated). Products include:
Levoprome 1321
Methoxamine Hydrochloride (Close supervision and careful dosage adjustment required). Products include:
Vasoxyl Injection 1169
Methoxyflurane (Potentiated).
No products indexed under this heading.
Methsuximide (Increased anticonvulsant dosage may be necessary). Products include:
Celontin Kapseals 1955
Midazolam Hydrochloride (Potentiated). Products include:
Versed Injection 2324
Molindone Hydrochloride (Potentiated; hyperpyrexia). Products include:
Moban Tablets and Concentrate 1036
Morphine Sulfate (Potentiated). Products include:
Astramorph/PF Injection, USP (Preservative-Free) 526
Duramorph Injection 983
Infumorph 200 and Infumorph 500 Sterile Solutions 985
Kadian Capsules 2948
MS Contin Tablets 2149
MSIR 2152
Oramorph SR (Morphine Sulfate Sustained Release Tablets) 2359
RMS Suppositories CII 2766
Roxanol 2365
Norepinephrine Bitartrate (Close supervision and careful dosage adjustment required). Products include:
Levophed Bitartrate Injection 2445
Opium Alkaloids (Potentiated).
No products indexed under this heading.
Oxazepam (Potentiated). Products include:
Serax Capsules 2916
Serax Tablets 2916
Oxybutynin Chloride (Hyperpyrexia; paralytic ileus). Products include:
Ditropan 1267
Oxycodone Hydrochloride (Potentiated). Products include:
OxyContin Tablets 2163
OxyIR Capsules 2167
Percocet Tablets 955
Percodan Tablets 955
Percodan-Demi Tablets 956
Roxicodone Tablets, Oral Solution & Intensol (Oxycodone) 2366
Tylox Capsules 1593
Paramethadione (Increased anticonvulsant dosage may be necessary).
No products indexed under this heading.
Pentobarbital Sodium (Potentiated). Products include:
Nembutal Sodium Capsules 440
Nembutal Sodium Solution 442
Nembutal Sodium Suppositories 444
Phenacemide (Increased anticonvulsant dosage may be necessary). Products include:
Phenurone Tablets 455
Phenelzine Sulfate (Concomitant administration is contraindicated; hyperpyretic crises and severe convulsions have occurred). Products include:
Nardil 1977
Phenobarbital (Potentiated; increased anticonvulsant dosage may be necessary). Products include:
Arco-Lase Plus Tablets 513
Bellergal-S Tablets 2375
Donnatal 2234
Donnatal Extentabs 2234
Donnatal Tablets 2234
Phenobarbital Elixir and Tablets 1523
Quadrinal Tablets 1398
Phensuximide (Increased anticonvulsant dosage may be necessary).
No products indexed under this heading.
Phenylephrine Bitartrate (Close supervision and careful dosage adjustment required).
No products indexed under this heading.
Phenylephrine Hydrochloride (Close supervision and careful dosage adjustment required). Products include:
Atrohist Plus Tablets 1605
Cerose DM .... ▣ 853
D.A. II Tablets 972
D.A. Chewable Tablets 970
Dura-Vent/DA Tablets 972
Extendryl 1003
4-Way Fast Acting Nasal Spray (regular & mentholated) .... ▣ 644
Hemorid .... ▣ 797
Hycomine Compound Tablets 948
Neo-Synephrine Hydrochloride 1% Carpuject 2455
Neo-Synephrine Hydrochloride 1% Injection 2455
Neo-Synephrine Hydrochloride (Ophthalmic) 2456
Neo-Synephrine .... ▣ 624
Novahistine Elixir .... ▣ 782
Phenergan VC 2886
Phenergan VC with Codeine 2888
Preparation H .... ▣ 842
Tympagesic Ear Drops 2476
Vicks Sinex Nasal Spray and Ultra Fine Mist .... ▣ 738
Phenylephrine Tannate (Close supervision and careful dosage adjustment required). Products include:
Atrohist Pediatric Suspension 1604
Atrohist Pediatric Suspension Dye-Free 1604
Rynatan 2781
Rynatuss 2782
Phenylpropanolamine Hydrochloride (Close supervision and careful dosage adjustment required). Products include:
Acutrim .... ▣ 648
Atrohist Plus Tablets 1605
BC Cold Powder Multi-Symptom Formula (Cold-Sinus-Allergy) .... ▣ 631
BC Cold Powder Non-Drowsy Formula (Cold-Sinus) .... ▣ 631
Cheracol Plus Head Cold/Cough Formula .... ▣ 741
Comtrex Multi-Symptom Cold Reliever Liqui-Gels .... ▣ 638
Comtrex Multi-Symptom Non-Drowsy Liqui-gels .... ▣ 640
Contac Continuous Action Nasal Decongestant/Antihistamine 12 Hour Capsules .... ▣ 773
Contac Maximum Strength Continuous Action Decongestant/Antihistamine 12 Hour Caplets .... ▣ 772
Contac Severe Cold and Flu Formula Caplets .... ▣ 773
Coricidin 'D' Decongestant Tablets .... ▣ 760
Dexatrim .... ▣ 795
Dexatrim Plus Vitamins Caplets .... ▣ 796
Dimetane-DC Cough Syrup 2232
Dimetapp Allergy Sinus Caplets .... ▣ 838
Dimetapp Cold & Allergy Chewable Tablets .... ▣ 838
Dimetapp Cold & Cough Liqui-Gels .... ▣ 839
Dimetapp DM Elixir .... ▣ 840
Dimetapp Elixir .... ▣ 840
Dimetapp Extentabs .... ▣ 841
Dimetapp Tablets/Liqui-Gels .... ▣ 841
Dura-Vent Tablets 971
Entex LA Tablets 972
Exgest LA Tablets 787
Hycomine 947
Nolamine Timed-Release Tablets 790
Ornade Spansule Capsules 2678
Propagest Tablets 791
Pyrroxate Caplets .... ▣ 742
Robitussin-CF .... ▣ 846
Sinulin Tablets 792
Tavist-D 12 Hour Relief Tablets .... ▣ 750
Teldrin 12 Hour Antihistamine/Nasal Decongestant Allergy Relief Capsules .... ▣ 786
Triaminic Expectorant .... ▣ 753
Triaminic Syrup .... ▣ 755
Triaminic Triaminicol Cold & Cough .... ▣ 756
Triaminic DM Syrup .... ▣ 756
Triaminicin Tablets .... ▣ 756
Vicks DayQuil Allergy Relief 12-Hour Extended Release Tablets .... ▣ 733
Vicks DayQuil Allergy Relief 4-Hour Tablets .... ▣ 733
Vicks DayQuil SINUS Pressure & CONGESTION Relief .... ▣ 734
Phenytoin (Increased anticonvulsant dosage may be necessary). Products include:
Dilantin Infatabs 1967
Dilantin-125 Suspension 1969
Phenytoin Sodium (Increased anticonvulsant dosage may be necessary). Products include:
Dilantin Kapseals 1965
Pimozide (Hyperpyrexia). Products include:
Orap Tablets 1037
Pirbuterol Acetate (Close supervision and careful dosage adjustment required). Products include:
Maxair Autohaler 1550
Maxair Inhaler 1552
Prazepam (Potentiated).
No products indexed under this heading.
Prazosin Hydrochloride (Antihypertensive effect of prazosin blocked). Products include:
Minipress Capsules 2015
Minizide Capsules 2016
Primidone (Increased anticonvulsant dosage may be necessary). Products include:
Mysoline 2860
Prochlorperazine (Potentiated; hyperpyrexia). Products include:
Compazine 2644
Procyclidine Hydrochloride (Hyperpyrexia; paralytic ileus). Products include:
Kemadrin Tablets 1105
Promethazine Hydrochloride (Potentiated; hyperpyrexia). Products include:
Mepergan Injection 2859
Phenergan with Codeine 2883
Phenergan with Dextromethorphan 2885
Phenergan Injection 2880
Phenergan Suppositories 2882
Phenergan Syrup 2881
Phenergan Tablets 2882
Phenergan VC 2886
Phenergan VC with Codeine 2888
Propantheline Bromide (Hyperpyrexia; paralytic ileus). Products include:
Pro-Banthine Tablets 2226
Propofol (Potentiated). Products include:
Diprivan Injectable Emulsion 2939
Propoxyphene Hydrochloride (Potentiated). Products include:
Darvon 1475
Wygesic Tablets 2930
Propoxyphene Napsylate (Potentiated). Products include:
Darvon-N/Darvocet-N 1473
Pseudoephedrine Hydrochloride (Close supervision and careful dosage adjustment required). Products include:
Actifed Allergy Daytime/Nighttime Caplets .... ▣ 808
Actifed Cold & Allergy Tablets .... ▣ 807
Actifed Cold & Sinus Caplets and Tablets .... ▣ 808
Actifed Sinus Daytime/Nighttime Tablets and Caplets .... ▣ 809
Advil Cold and Sinus Caplets and Tablets .... ▣ 837
Alka-Seltzer Plus Liqui-Gels .... ▣ 612
Alka-Seltzer Plus Flu & Body Aches Liqui-Gels Non-Drowsy Formula .... ▣ 613
Alka-Seltzer Plus Night-Time Cold Medicine Liqui-Gels .... ▣ 612
Allerest Maximum Strength .... ▣ 649
Allerest No Drowsiness .... ▣ 649
Allerest Sinus Pain Formula .... ▣ 649
Atrohist Pediatric Capsules 1603
Benadryl Allergy/Cold Tablets .... ▣ 811
Benadryl Allergy Decongestant Liquid Medication .... ▣ 812
Benadryl Allergy Decongestant Tablets .... ▣ 812
Benadryl Allergy Sinus Headache Caplets .... ▣ 813
Benylin Multisymptom .... ▣ 816
Bromfed Capsules (Extended-Release) 1832
Bromfed Syrup .... ▣ 712
Bromfed Tablets 1832
Bromfed-DM Cough Syrup 1832
Bromfed-PD Capsules (Extended-Release) 1832
Children's TYLENOL Cold Multi-Symptom Chewable Tablets and Liquid 1559
Children's TYLENOL Cold Plus Cough Multi Symptom Chewable Tablets and Liquid 1560
Children's TYLENOL Flu Suspension Liquid 1560
Children's Vicks DayQuil Allergy Relief .... ▣ 730
Children's Vicks NyQuil Cold/Cough Relief .... ▣ 731
Allergy-Sinus Comtrex Multi-Symptom Allergy-Sinus Formula Tablets and Caplets .... ▣ 639
Comtrex Multi-Symptom .... ▣ 638
Comtrex Multi-Symptom Non-Drowsy Caplets .... ▣ 640
Congess 1003
Contac Day Allergy/Sinus Caplets ▣ 771
Contac Day & Night .... ▣ 772
Contac Night Allergy/Sinus Caplets .... ▣ 771
Contac Severe Cold & Flu Non-Drowsy .... ▣ 774
Deconsal II Tablets 1605

(▣ Described in PDR For Nonprescription Drugs) (⊙ Described in PDR For Ophthalmology)

1105 **Interactions Index** **Tri-Immunol**

Dimetane-DX Cough Syrup 2233
Dimetapp Cold & Fever Suspension 839
Dimetapp Decongestant Pediatric Drops 840
Dorcol Children's Cough Syrup 748
Drixoral Cough + Congestion Liquid Caps 763
Dura-Tap/PD Capsules 970
Duratuss Tablets 2750
Duratuss HD Elixir 2750
Efidac/24 655
Entex PSE Tablets 973
Fedahist Gyrocaps 2545
Guaifed 1833
Guaifed Syrup 712
Guaimax-D Tablets 809
Histussin D Liquid 670
Infants' TYLENOL Cold Decongestant & Fever-Reducer Drops 1561
Kronofed-A 994
Novahistine DMX 782
Nucofed 2225
PediaCare Cough-Cold Chewable Tablets and Liquid 1569
PediaCare Infants' Decongestant Drops 1569
PediaCare Infants' Drops Decongestant Plus Cough 1569
PediaCare NightRest Cough-Cold Liquid 1569
Pediatric Vicks 44d Cough & Head Congestion Relief 736
Pediatric Vicks 44m Cough & Cold Relief 737
Robitussin Cold & Cough Liqui-Gels 844
Robitussin Cold, Cough & Flu Liqui-Gels 844
Robitussin Maximum Strength Cough & Cold 847
Robitussin Night-Time Cold Formula 847
Robitussin Pediatric Cough & Cold Formula 848
Robitussin Pediatric Drops 849
Robitussin Severe Congestion Liqui-Gels 845
Robitussin-DAC Syrup 2249
Robitussin-PE 846
Rondec Oral Drops 974
Rondec Syrup 974
Rondec Tablet 974
Rondec Chewable Tablets 974
Rondec-TR Tablet 974
Ryna 804
Seldane-D Extended-Release Tablets 1286
Semprex-D Capsules 1620
Sinarest 663
Sine-Aid Maximum Strength Sinus Headache Gelcaps, Caplets and Tablets 1570
Sine-Off No Drowsiness Formula Caplets 784
Sine-Off Sinus Medicine 784
Singlet Tablets 785
Sinutab Non-Drying Liquid Caps 823
Sinutab Sinus Allergy Medication, Maximum Strength Tablets and Caplets 823
Sinutab Sinus Medication, Maximum Strength Without Drowsiness Formula, Tablets & Caplets 824
Sudafed Children's Cold & Cough Liquid Medication 825
Sudafed Children's Nasal Decongestant Liquid Medication 826
Sudafed Cold & Allergy Tablets 826
Sudafed Cold and Cough Liquid Caps 826
Sudafed Nasal Decongestant Tablets, 30 mg 825
Sudafed Nasal Decongestant Tablets, 60 mg 825
Sudafed Non-Drying Sinus Liquid Caps 827
Sudafed Pediatric Nasal Decongestant Liquid Oral Drops 827
Sudafed Severe Cold Formula Caplets 828
Sudafed Severe Cold Formula Tablets 828
Sudafed Sinus Caplets 829
Sudafed Sinus Tablets 829
Sudafed 12 Hour Caplets 824
Syn-Rx Tablets 1622
Syn-Rx DM Tablets 1623
TheraFlu Flu and Cold Medicine 750
Theraflu Maximum Strength Flu and Cold Medicine For Sore Throat 751
TheraFlu Flu, Cold and Cough Medicine 750
TheraFlu Maximum Strength Nighttime Flu, Cold & Cough Medicine 751
TheraFlu Maximum Strength Non-Drowsy Formula Flu, Cold & Cough Medicine 751
TheraFlu Maximum Strength, Non-Drowsy Formula Flu, Cold and Cough Caplets 752
Theraflu Maximum Strength Sinus Non-Drowsy Formula Caplets 752
Triaminic AM Cough and Decongestant Formula 753
Triaminic AM Decongestant Formula 753
Triaminic Infant Oral Decongestant Drops 754
Triaminic Night Time 754
Triaminic Sore Throat Formula 755
Tussend 1830
Tussend Expectorant 1831
TYLENOL Allergy Sinus, Maximum Strength Caplets and Gelcaps 1571
TYLENOL Allergy Sinus NightTime, Maximum Strength Caplets 1571
TYLENOL Cold Medication, Multi-Symptom Formula Tablets and Caplets 1572
TYLENOL Cold Medication, Multi-Symptom Hot Liquid Packets 1572
TYLENOL Cold Medication, No Drowsiness Formula Caplets and Gelcaps 1572
TYLENOL Cold Severe Congestion Caplets 1573
TYLENOL Cough Medication with Decongestant, Multi Symptom 1574
TYLENOL Flu No Drowsiness Formula, Maximum Strength Gelcaps 1575
TYLENOL Flu NightTime, Maximum Strength Gelcaps 1575
TYLENOL Flu NightTime, Maximum Strength Hot Medication Packets 1575
TYLENOL Sinus, Maximum Strength Geltabs, Gelcaps, Caplets and Tablets 1576
Vicks 44 LiquiCaps Cough, Cold & Flu Relief 728
Vicks 44 LiquiCaps Non-Drowsy Cough & Cold Relief 729
Vicks 44D Cough & Head Congestion Relief 728
Vicks 44M Cough, Cold & Flu Relief 729
Vicks DayQuil LiquiCaps/Liquid Multi-Symptom Cold/Flu Relief 734
Vicks DayQuil SINUS Pressure & PAIN Relief with IBUPROFEN 735
Vicks Nyquil Hot Therapy 735
Vicks NyQuil LiquiCaps/Liquid Multi-Symptom Cold/Flu Relief, Original and Cherry Flavors 736

Pseudoephedrine Sulfate (Close supervision and careful dosage adjustment required). Products include:
Chlor-Trimeton Allergy Decongestant Tablets 759
Claritin-D Tablets 2487
Drixoral Cold and Allergy Sustained-Action Tablets 763
Drixoral Cold and Flu Extended-Release Tablets 764
Drixoral Non-Drowsy Formula Extended-Release Tablets 764
Drixoral Allergy/Sinus Extended Release Tablets 765
Trinalin Repetabs Tablets 1373

Pyrilamine Maleate (Potentiated). Products include:
4-Way Fast Acting Nasal Spray (regular & mentholated) 644
Maximum Strength Multi-Symptom Formula Midol 621
PMS Multi-Symptom Formula Midol 622

Pyrilamine Tannate (Potentiated). Products include:
Atrohist Pediatric Suspension 1604
Atrohist Pediatric Suspension Dye-Free 1604
Rynatan 2781

Quazepam (Potentiated). Products include:
Doral Tablets 2773

Rauwolfia Serpentina (Antihypertensive effect of rauwolfia serpentina blocked).
No products indexed under this heading.

Rescinnamine (Antihypertensive effect of rescinnamine blocked).
No products indexed under this heading.

Reserpine (Antihypertensive effect of reserpine blocked). Products include:
Diupres Tablets 1691
Hydropres Tablets 1718
Ser-Ap-Es Tablets 867

Risperidone (Potentiated). Products include:
Risperdal Tablets 1348

Salmeterol Xinafoate (Close supervision and careful dosage adjustment required). Products include:
Serevent Inhalation Aerosol 1149

Scopolamine (Hyperpyrexia; paralytic ileus). Products include:
Transderm Scōp Transdermal Therapeutic System 890

Scopolamine Hydrobromide (Hyperpyrexia; paralytic ileus). Products include:
Atrohist Plus Tablets 1605
Donnatal 2234
Donnatal Extentabs 2234
Donnatal Tablets 2234

Secobarbital Sodium (Potentiated). Products include:
Seconal Sodium Pulvules 1529

Selegiline Hydrochloride (Concomitant administration is contraindicated; hyperpyretic crises and severe convulsions have occurred). Products include:
Eldepryl Capsules 2729

Sevoflurane (Potentiated).
No products indexed under this heading.

Sufentanil Citrate (Potentiated). Products include:
Sufenta Injection 1355

Temazepam (Potentiated). Products include:
Restoril Capsules 2413

Terazosin Hydrochloride (Antihypertensive effect of terazosin blocked). Products include:
Hytrin Capsules 434

Terbutaline Sulfate (Close supervision and careful dosage adjustment required). Products include:
Brethaire Inhaler 830
Brethine Ampuls 832
Brethine Tablets 831
Bricanyl Subcutaneous Injection 1247
Bricanyl Tablets 1248

Terfenadine (Potentiated). Products include:
Seldane Tablets 1284
Seldane-D Extended-Release Tablets 1286

Thiamylal Sodium (Potentiated).
No products indexed under this heading.

Thioridazine Hydrochloride (Potentiated; hyperpyrexia). Products include:
Mellaril 2398

Thiothixene (Potentiated; hyperpyrexia). Products include:
Navane Capsules and Concentrate 2018
Navane Intramuscular 2019

Thyroid (Close supervision is indicated).
No products indexed under this heading.

Thyroxine (Close supervision is indicated).
No products indexed under this heading.

Thyroxine Sodium (Close supervision is indicated).
No products indexed under this heading.

Tranylcypromine Sulfate (Concomitant administration is contraindicated; hyperpyretic crises and severe convulsions have occurred). Products include:
Parnate Tablets 2679

Triazolam (Potentiated). Products include:
Halcion Tablets 2093

Tridihexethyl Chloride (Hyperpyrexia; paralytic ileus).
No products indexed under this heading.

Trifluoperazine Hydrochloride (Potentiated; hyperpyrexia). Products include:
Stelazine 2692

Trihexyphenidyl Hydrochloride (Hyperpyrexia; paralytic ileus). Products include:
Artane 1418

Trimeprazine Tartrate (Potentiated).
No products indexed under this heading.

Trimethadione (Increased anticonvulsant dosage may be necessary).
No products indexed under this heading.

Tripelennamine Hydrochloride (Potentiated). Products include:
PBZ Tablets 863
PBZ-SR Tablets 862

Triprolidine Hydrochloride (Potentiated). Products include:
Actifed Cold & Allergy Tablets 807
Actifed Cold & Sinus Caplets and Tablets 808

Valproic Acid (Increased anticonvulsant dosage may be necessary). Products include:
Depakene 416

Zolpidem Tartrate (Potentiated). Products include:
Ambien Tablets 2559

Food Interactions
Alcohol (Potentiated; contraindication).

TRIAZ 6% AND 10% GELS AND 10% CLEANSER
(Benzoyl Peroxide) 1629
None cited in PDR database.

TRIDESILON CREAM 0.05%
(Desonide) 609
None cited in PDR database.

TRIDESILON OINTMENT 0.05%
(Desonide) 610
None cited in PDR database.

TRI-IMMUNOL ADSORBED
(Diphtheria & Tetanus Toxoids and Pertussis Vaccine Adsorbed) 1452
May interact with corticosteroids, antineoplastics, and cytotoxic drugs. Compounds in these categories include:

Altretamine (Aberrant responses to active immunization procedures). Products include:
Hexalen Capsules 2760

Anastrozole (Aberrant responses to active immunization procedures). Products include:
Arimidex Tablets 2932

IMPORTANT NOTE: Always consult each drug listing in the patient's regimen for possible interactions.

Tri-Immunol | Interactions Index | 1106

Asparaginase (Aberrant responses to active immunization procedures). Products include:
Elspar ... 1700

Betamethasone Acetate (Aberrant responses to active immunization procedures). Products include:
Celestone Soluspan Suspension ... 2484

Betamethasone Sodium Phosphate (Aberrant responses to active immunization procedures). Products include:
Celestone Soluspan Suspension ... 2484

Bicalutamide (Aberrant responses to active immunization procedures). Products include:
Casodex Tablets ... 2934

Bleomycin Sulfate (Aberrant responses to active immunization procedures). Products include:
Blenoxane ... 697

Busulfan (Aberrant responses to active immunization procedures). Products include:
Myleran Tablets ... 1209

Carboplatin (Aberrant responses to active immunization procedures). Products include:
Paraplatin for Injection ... 713

Carmustine (BCNU) (Aberrant responses to active immunization procedures). Products include:
BiCNU ... 696

Chlorambucil (Aberrant responses to active immunization procedures). Products include:
Leukeran Tablets ... 1205

Cisplatin (Aberrant responses to active immunization procedures). Products include:
Platinol for Injection ... 717
Platinol-AQ Injection ... 719

Cortisone Acetate (Aberrant responses to active immunization procedures). Products include:
Cortone Acetate Sterile Suspension ... 1663
Cortone Acetate Tablets ... 1664

Cyclophosphamide (Aberrant responses to active immunization procedures). Products include:
Cytoxan ... 700

Dacarbazine (Aberrant responses to active immunization procedures). Products include:
DTIC-Dome ... 593

Daunorubicin Citrate (Aberrant responses to active immunization procedures). Products include:
DaunoXome ... 1842

Daunorubicin Hydrochloride (Aberrant responses to active immunization procedures). Products include:
Cerubidine for Injection ... 634

Dexamethasone (Aberrant responses to active immunization procedures). Products include:
AK-Trol Ointment & Suspension ... ◉ 205
Decadron Elixir ... 1676
Decadron Tablets ... 1678
Decaspray Topical Aerosol ... 1689
Maxitrol Ophthalmic Ointment and Suspension ... ◉ 222
TobraDex Ophthalmic Suspension and Ointment ... 469

Dexamethasone Acetate (Aberrant responses to active immunization procedures). Products include:
Dalalone D.P. Injectable ... 1009
Decadron-LA Sterile Suspension ... 1687

Dexamethasone Sodium Phosphate (Aberrant responses to active immunization procedures). Products include:
Decadron Phosphate Injection ... 1680
Decadron Phosphate Sterile Ophthalmic Ointment ... 1684
Decadron Phosphate Sterile Ophthalmic Solution ... 1685
Decadron Phosphate Topical Cream ... 1686
Decadron Phosphate with Xylocaine Injection, Sterile ... 1683
Dexacort Phosphate in Respihaler .. 1606
Dexacort Phosphate in Turbinaire .. 1607
NeoDecadron Sterile Ophthalmic Ointment ... 1755
NeoDecadron Sterile Ophthalmic Solution ... 1756
NeoDecadron Topical Cream ... 1757

Docetaxel (Aberrant responses to active immunization procedures). Products include:
Taxotere for Injection Concentrate 2204

Doxorubicin Hydrochloride (Aberrant responses to active immunization procedures). Products include:
Adriamycin PFS ... 2056
Adriamycin RDF ... 2056
Doxil ... 2613
Doxorubicin Astra ... 531
Rubex for Injection ... 721

Estramustine Phosphate Sodium (Aberrant responses to active immunization procedures). Products include:
Emcyt Capsules ... 2085

Etoposide (Aberrant responses to active immunization procedures). Products include:
Etoposide Injection ... 539
VePesid Capsules and Injection ... 727

Floxuridine (Aberrant responses to active immunization procedures). Products include:
Sterile FUDR ... 2284

Fludrocortisone Acetate (Aberrant responses to active immunization procedures). Products include:
Florinef Acetate Tablets ... 506

Fluorouracil (Aberrant responses to active immunization procedures). Products include:
Efudex ... 2280
Fluoroplex Topical Solution & Cream 1% ... 475
Fluorouracil Injection ... 2282

Flutamide (Abberrant responses to active immunization procedures). Products include:
Eulexin Capsules ... 2498

Gemcitabine Hydrochloride (Aberrant responses to active immunization procedures). Products include:
Gemzar for Injection ... 1482

Hydrocortisone (Aberrant responses to active immunization procedures). Products include:
Anusol-HC Cream 2.5% ... 1953
Aquanil HC Lotion ... 1989
Maximum Strength Cortaid Spray ▣ 800
CORTENEMA ... 2713
Cortisporin Ointment ... 1074
Cortisporin Ophthalmic Ointment Sterile ... 1074
Cortisporin Ophthalmic Suspension Sterile ... 1075
Cortisporin Otic Solution Sterile ... 1076
Cortisporin Otic Suspension Sterile 1077
Cortizone-5 ... ▣ 795
Cortizone-10 ... ▣ 795
Hydrocortone Tablets ... 1715
Hytone ... 922
Hytone Ointment 2 ½% ... 923
Massengill Medicated Soft Cloth Towelettes ... 2628
Pediotic Suspension Sterile ... 1140
Preparation H Hydrocortisone 1% Cream ... ▣ 843
ProctoCream-HC 2.5% ... 2552
VõSoL HC Otic Solution ... 2786

Hydrocortisone Acetate (Aberrant responses to active immunization procedures). Products include:
Analpram-HC Rectal Cream 1% and 2.5% ... 993
Anusol HC-1 Hydrocortisone Anti-Itch Ointment ... ▣ 810
Anusol-HC Suppositories ... 1954
Caldecort Anti-Itch Hydrocortisone Cream ... ▣ 651
Coly-Mycin S Otic w/Neomycin & Hydrocortisone ... 1965
Cortaid ... ▣ 800
Cortifoam ... 2540
Cortisporin Cream ... 1073
Epifoam ... 2543
Hydrocortone Acetate Sterile Suspension ... 1712
Mantadil Cream ... 1124
Nupercainal Hydrocortisone 1% Cream ... ▣ 661
Pramosone Cream, Lotion & Ointment ... 995
ProctoFoam-HC ... 2552
Terra-Cortril Ophthalmic Suspension ... 2033

Hydrocortisone Sodium Phosphate (Aberrant responses to active immunization procedures). Products include:
Hydrocortone Phosphate Injection, Sterile ... 1713

Hydrocortisone Sodium Succinate (Aberrant responses to active immunization procedures).
No products indexed under this heading.

Hydroxyurea (Aberrant responses to active immunization procedures). Products include:
Hydrea Capsules ... 705

Idarubicin Hydrochloride (Aberrant responses to active immunization procedures). Products include:
Idamycin Injection ... 2096

Ifosfamide (Aberrant responses to active immunization procedures). Products include:
IFEX ... 706

Interferon alfa-2A, Recombinant (Aberrant responses to active immunization procedures). Products include:
Roferon-A Injection ... 2308

Interferon alfa-2B, Recombinant (Aberrant responses to active immunization procedures). Products include:
Intron A for Injection ... 2506

Irinotecan Hydrochloride (Aberrant responses to active immunization procedures).
No products indexed under this heading.

Levamisole Hydrochloride (Aberrant responses to active immunization procedures). Products include:
Ergamisol Tablets ... 1340

Lomustine (CCNU) (Aberrant responses to active immunization procedures). Products include:
CeeNU Capsules ... 699

Mechlorethamine Hydrochloride (Aberrant responses to active immunization procedures). Products include:
Mustargen ... 1752

Megestrol Acetate (Aberrant responses to active immunization procedures). Products include:
Megace Oral Suspension ... 708
Megace Tablets ... 710

Melphalan (Aberrant responses to active immunization procedures). Products include:
Alkeran Tablets ... 1198

Mercaptopurine (Aberrant responses to active immunization procedures). Products include:
Purinethol Tablets ... 1214

Methotrexate Sodium (Aberrant responses to active immunization procedures). Products include:
Methotrexate Sodium Tablets, Injection, for Injection and LPF Injection ... 1322

Methylprednisolone Acetate (Aberrant responses to active immunization procedures).
No products indexed under this heading.

Methylprednisolone Sodium Succinate (Aberrant responses to active immunization procedures).
No products indexed under this heading.

Mitomycin (Mitomycin-C) (Aberrant responses to active immunization procedures). Products include:
Mutamycin for Injection ... 712

Mitotane (Aberrant responses to active immunization procedures). Products include:
Lysodren Tablets ... 707

Mitoxantrone Hydrochloride (Aberrant responses to active immunization procedures). Products include:
Novantrone for Injection ... 1327

Paclitaxel (Aberrant responses to active immunization procedures). Products include:
Taxol Injection ... 723

Prednisolone Acetate (Aberrant responses to active immunization procedures). Products include:
AK-CIDE ... ◉ 203
AK-CIDE Ointment ... ◉ 203
Blephamide Liquifilm Sterile Ophthalmic Suspension ... 472
Blephamide Ointment ... ◉ 234
Econopred & Econopred Plus Ophthalmic Suspensions ... ◉ 216
Poly-Pred Liquifilm ... ◉ 246
Pred Forte ... ◉ 247
Pred Mild ... ◉ 250
Pred-G Liquifilm Sterile Ophthalmic Suspension ... ◉ 248
Pred-G S.O.P. Sterile Ophthalmic Ointment ... ◉ 249

Prednisolone Sodium Phosphate (Aberrant responses to active immunization procedures). Products include:
AK-PRED ... ◉ 204
Hydeltrasol Injection, Sterile ... 1708
Pediapred Oral Solution ... 1618

Prednisolone Tebutate (Aberrant responses to active immunization procedures). Products include:
Hydeltra-T.B.A. Sterile Suspension 1710

Prednisone (Aberrant responses to active immunization procedures).
No products indexed under this heading.

Procarbazine Hydrochloride (Aberrant responses to active immunization procedures). Products include:
Matulane Capsules ... 2300

Streptozocin (Aberrant responses to active immunization procedures). Products include:
Zanosar Sterile Powder ... 2119

Tamoxifen Citrate (Aberrant responses to active immunization procedures). Products include:
Nolvadex Tablets ... 2957

Teniposide (Aberrant responses to active immunization procedures). Products include:
Vumon for Injection ... 729

Thioguanine (Aberrant responses to active immunization procedures). Products include:
Thioguanine Tablets, Tabloid Brand ... 1225

Thiotepa (Aberrant responses to active immunization procedures). Products include:
Thioplex (Thiotepa For Injection) ... 1329

Topotecan Hydrochloride (Aberrant responses to active immunization procedures). Products include:
Hycamtin for Injection ... 2665

(▣ Described in PDR For Nonprescription Drugs) (◉ Described in PDR For Ophthalmology)

Interactions Index

Triamcinolone (Aberrant responses to active immunization procedures).
   No products indexed under this heading.

Triamcinolone Acetonide (Aberrant responses to active immunization procedures). Products include:
- Azmacort Oral Inhaler 2175
- Nasacort AQ Nasal Spray 2191
- Nasacort Nasal Inhaler 2189

Triamcinolone Diacetate (Aberrant responses to active immunization procedures).
   No products indexed under this heading.

Triamcinolone Hexacetonide (Aberrant responses to active immunization procedures).
   No products indexed under this heading.

Vincristine Sulfate (Aberrant responses to active immunization procedures). Products include:
- Oncovin Solution Vials & Hyporets ... 1521

Vinorelbine Tartrate (Aberrant responses to active immunization procedures). Products include:
- Navelbine Injection 1212

TRILAFON CONCENTRATE
(Perphenazine) 2532
May interact with central nervous system depressants, anticonvulsants, and certain other agents. Compounds in these categories include:

Alfentanil Hydrochloride (Potentiation of both drugs). Products include:
- Alfenta Injection 1334

Alprazolam (Potentiation of both drugs). Products include:
- Xanax Tablets 2115

Aprobarbital (Potentiation of both drugs).
   No products indexed under this heading.

Atropine Sulfate (Additive anticholinergic effects). Products include:
- Arco-Lase Plus Tablets 513
- Atrohist Plus Tablets 1605
- Donnatal 2234
- Donnatal Extentabs 2234
- Donnatal Tablets 2234
- Lomotil 2591
- Motofen Tablets 789
- Urised Tablets 2123

Buprenorphine (Potentiation of both drugs). Products include:
- Buprenex Injectable 2170

Buspirone Hydrochloride (Potentiation of both drugs). Products include:
- BuSpar Tablets 738

Butabarbital (Potentiation of both drugs).
   No products indexed under this heading.

Butalbital (Potentiation of both drugs). Products include:
- Axocet Capsules 2469
- Esgic-plus Capsules 1012
- Esgic-plus Tablets 1012
- Fioricet Tablets 2386
- Fioricet with Codeine Capsules ... 2387
- Fiorinal Capsules 2388
- Fiorinal with Codeine Capsules .. 2390
- Fiorinal Tablets 2388
- Phrenilin 790
- Sedapap Tablets 50 mg/650 mg .. 1826

Carbamazepine (Increased dosage of anticonvulsant may be required). Products include:
- Atretol Tablets 569
- Tegretol/Tegretol-XR 870

Chlordiazepoxide (Potentiation of both drugs). Products include:
- Limbitrol 2333

Chlordiazepoxide Hydrochloride (Potentiation of both drugs). Products include:
- Librax Capsules 2330
- Librium Capsules 2331
- Librium Injectable 2332

Chlorpromazine (Potentiation of both drugs). Products include:
- Thorazine Suppositories 2701

Chlorprothixene (Potentiation of both drugs).
   No products indexed under this heading.

Chlorprothixene Hydrochloride (Potentiation of both drugs).
   No products indexed under this heading.

Chlorprothixene Lactate (Potentiation of both drugs).
   No products indexed under this heading.

Clorazepate Dipotassium (Potentiation of both drugs). Products include:
- Tranxene 459

Clozapine (Potentiation of both drugs). Products include:
- Clozaril Tablets 2377

Codeine Phosphate (Potentiation of both drugs). Products include:
- Brontex 2130
- Dimetane-DC Cough Syrup 2232
- Fioricet with Codeine Capsules ... 2387
- Fiorinal with Codeine Capsules .. 2390
- Nucofed 2225
- Phenergan with Codeine 2883
- Phenergan VC with Codeine 2888
- Robitussin A-C Syrup 2248
- Robitussin-DAC Syrup 2249
- Ryna 804
- Soma Compound w/Codeine Tablets 2784
- Tylenol with Codeine 1592

Desflurane (Potentiation of both drugs). Products include:
- Suprane (desflurane, USP) 1865

Dezocine (Potentiation of both drugs). Products include:
- Dalgan Injection 529

Diazepam (Potentiation of both drugs). Products include:
- Dizac (diazepam injectable emulsion) CIV 1862
- Valium Injectable 2336
- Valium Tablets 2335

Divalproex Sodium (Increased dosage of anticonvulsant may be required). Products include:
- Depakote Tablets 418

Droperidol (Potentiation of both drugs). Products include:
- Inapsine Injection 462

Enflurane (Potentiation of both drugs).
   No products indexed under this heading.

Epinephrine (Action of epinephrine blocked and partially reversed). Products include:
- EPIFRIN 237
- EpiPen 808
- Marcaine with Epinephrine 2446
- Primatene Mist 843
- Sensorcaine with Epinephrine Injection 554
- Sus-Phrine Injection 1017
- Xylocaine with Epinephrine Injections 562

Epinephrine Bitartrate (Action of epinephrine blocked and partially reversed). Products include:
- Sensorcaine-MPF with Epinephrine Injection 554

Estazolam (Potentiation of both drugs). Products include:
- ProSom Tablets 457

Ethchlorvynol (Potentiation of both drugs). Products include:
- Placidyl Capsules 456

Ethinamate (Potentiation of both drugs).
   No products indexed under this heading.

Ethosuximide (Increased dosage of anticonvulsant may be required). Products include:
- Zarontin Capsules 1986
- Zarontin Syrup 1986

Ethotoin (Increased dosage of anticonvulsant may be required). Products include:
- Peganone Tablets 455

Felbamate (Increased dosage of anticonvulsant may be required). Products include:
- Felbatol 2774

Fentanyl (Potentiation of both drugs). Products include:
- Duragesic Transdermal System ... 1336

Fentanyl Citrate (Potentiation of both drugs). Products include:
- Sublimaze Injection 463

Fluphenazine Decanoate (Potentiation of both drugs). Products include:
- Prolixin Decanoate 510

Fluphenazine Enanthate (Potentiation of both drugs). Products include:
- Prolixin Enanthate 510

Fluphenazine Hydrochloride (Potentiation of both drugs). Products include:
- Prolixin 510

Flurazepam Hydrochloride (Potentiation of both drugs). Products include:
- Dalmane Capsules 2329

Glutethimide (Potentiation of both drugs).
   No products indexed under this heading.

Haloperidol (Potentiation of both drugs). Products include:
- Haldol Injection, Tablets and Concentrate 1585

Haloperidol Decanoate (Potentiation of both drugs). Products include:
- Haldol Decanoate 1587

Hydrocodone Bitartrate (Potentiation of both drugs). Products include:
- Codiclear DH Syrup 808
- Duratuss HD Elixir 2750
- Histussin D Liquid 670
- Hycodan Tablets and Syrup ... 946
- Hycomine Compound Tablets ... 948
- Hycomine 947
- Hycotuss Expectorant Syrup ... 950
- Hydrocet Capsules 787
- Lorcet 10/650 Tablets 1016
- Lortab 2751
- Tussend 1830
- Tussend Expectorant 1831
- Vicodin Tablets 1404
- Vicodin ES Tablets 1405
- Vicodin HP Tablets 1403
- Vicodin Tuss Expectorant 1406
- Zydone Capsules 967

Hydrocodone Polistirex (Potentiation of both drugs). Products include:
- Tussionex Pennkinetic Extended-Release Suspension 1624

Hydroxyzine Hydrochloride (Potentiation of both drugs). Products include:
- Atarax Tablets & Syrup 1992
- Marax Tablets & DF Syrup 2015
- Vistaril Intramuscular Solution ... 2042

Isoflurane (Potentiation of both drugs).
   No products indexed under this heading.

Ketamine Hydrochloride (Potentiation of both drugs).
   No products indexed under this heading.

Lamotrigine (Increased dosage of anticonvulsant may be required). Products include:
- Lamictal Tablets 1105

Levomethadyl Acetate Hydrochloride (Potentiation of both drugs). Products include:
- Orlaam Oral Solution 2361

Levorphanol Tartrate (Potentiation of both drugs). Products include:
- Levo-Dromoran 2297

Lorazepam (Potentiation of both drugs). Products include:
- Ativan Injection 2805
- Ativan Tablets 2807

Loxapine Hydrochloride (Potentiation of both drugs). Products include:
- Loxitane 1426

Loxapine Succinate (Potentiation of both drugs). Products include:
- Loxitane Capsules 1426

Meperidine Hydrochloride (Potentiation of both drugs). Products include:
- Demerol 2438
- Mepergan Injection 2859

Mephenytoin (Increased dosage of anticonvulsant may be required). Products include:
- Mesantoin Tablets 2400

Mephobarbital (Potentiation of both drugs). Products include:
- Mebaral Tablets 2452

Meprobamate (Potentiation of both drugs). Products include:
- Miltown Tablets 2780
- PMB 200 and PMB 400 2890

Mesoridazine Besylate (Potentiation of both drugs). Products include:
- Serentil 689

Methadone Hydrochloride (Potentiation of both drugs). Products include:
- Methadone Hydrochloride Oral Concentrate 2356
- Methadone Hydrochloride Oral Solution & Tablets 2357

Methohexital Sodium (Potentiation of both drugs).
   No products indexed under this heading.

Methotrimeprazine (Potentiation of both drugs). Products include:
- Levoprome 1321

Methoxyflurane (Potentiation of both drugs).
   No products indexed under this heading.

Methsuximide (Increased dosage of anticonvulsant may be required). Products include:
- Celontin Kapseals 1955

Midazolam Hydrochloride (Potentiation of both drugs). Products include:
- Versed Injection 2324

Molindone Hydrochloride (Potentiation of both drugs). Products include:
- Moban Tablets and Concentrate ... 1036

Morphine Sulfate (Potentiation of both drugs). Products include:
- Astramorph/PF Injection, USP (Preservative-Free) 526
- Duramorph Injection 983
- Infumorph 200 and Infumorph 500 Sterile Solutions 985
- Kadian Capsules 2948
- MS Contin Tablets 2149
- MSIR 2152
- Oramorph SR (Morphine Sulfate Sustained Release Tablets) ... 2359
- RMS Suppositories CII 2766
- Roxanol 2365

IMPORTANT NOTE: Always consult each drug listing in the patient's regimen for possible interactions.

Trilafon / Interactions Index

Opium Alkaloids (Potentiation of both drugs).
    No products indexed under this heading.

Oxazepam (Potentiation of both drugs). Products include:
- Serax Capsules ... 2916
- Serax Tablets ... 2916

Oxycodone Hydrochloride (Potentiation of both drugs). Products include:
- OxyContin Tablets ... 2163
- OxyIR Capsules ... 2167
- Percocet Tablets ... 955
- Percodan Tablets ... 955
- Percodan-Demi Tablets ... 956
- Roxicodone Tablets, Oral Solution & Intensol (Oxycodone) ... 2366
- Tylox Capsules ... 1593

Paramethadione (Increased dosage of anticonvulsant may be required).
    No products indexed under this heading.

Pentobarbital Sodium (Potentiation of both drugs). Products include:
- Nembutal Sodium Capsules ... 440
- Nembutal Sodium Solution ... 442
- Nembutal Sodium Suppositories ... 444

Phenacemide (Increased dosage of anticonvulsant may be required). Products include:
- Phenurone Tablets ... 455

Phenobarbital (Increased dosage of anticonvulsant may be required; potentiation of both drugs). Products include:
- Arco-Lase Plus Tablets ... 513
- Bellergal-S Tablets ... 2375
- Donnatal ... 2234
- Donnatal Extentabs ... 2234
- Donnatal ... 2234
- Phenobarbital Elixir and Tablets ... 1523
- Quadrinal Tablets ... 1398

Phensuximide (Increased dosage of anticonvulsant may be required).
    No products indexed under this heading.

Phenytoin (Increased dosage of anticonvulsant may be required). Products include:
- Dilantin Infatabs ... 1967
- Dilantin-125 Suspension ... 1969

Phenytoin Sodium (Increased dosage of anticonvulsant may be required). Products include:
- Dilantin Kapseals ... 1965

Prazepam (Potentiation of both drugs).
    No products indexed under this heading.

Primidone (Increased dosage of anticonvulsant may be required). Products include:
- Mysoline ... 2860

Prochlorperazine (Potentiation of both drugs). Products include:
- Compazine ... 2644

Promethazine Hydrochloride (Potentiation of both drugs). Products include:
- Mepergan Injection ... 2859
- Phenergan with Codeine ... 2883
- Phenergan with Dextromethorphan ... 2885
- Phenergan Injection ... 2880
- Phenergan Suppositories ... 2882
- Phenergan Syrup ... 2881
- Phenergan Tablets ... 2882
- Phenergan VC ... 2886
- Phenergan VC with Codeine ... 2888

Propofol (Potentiation of both drugs). Products include:
- Diprivan Injectable Emulsion ... 2939

Propoxyphene Hydrochloride (Potentiation of both drugs). Products include:
- Darvon ... 1475
- Wygesic Tablets ... 2930

Propoxyphene Napsylate (Potentiation of both drugs). Products include:
- Darvon-N/Darvocet-N ... 1473

Quazepam (Potentiation of both drugs). Products include:
- Doral Tablets ... 2773

Risperidone (Potentiation of both drugs). Products include:
- Risperdal Tablets ... 1348

Secobarbital Sodium (Potentiation of both drugs). Products include:
- Seconal Sodium Pulvules ... 1529

Sevoflurane (Potentiation of both drugs).
    No products indexed under this heading.

Sufentanil Citrate (Potentiation of both drugs). Products include:
- Sufenta Injection ... 1355

Temazepam (Potentiation of both drugs). Products include:
- Restoril Capsules ... 2413

Thiamylal Sodium (Potentiation of both drugs).
    No products indexed under this heading.

Thioridazine Hydrochloride (Potentiation of both drugs). Products include:
- Mellaril ... 2398

Thiothixene (Potentiation of both drugs). Products include:
- Navane Capsules and Concentrate ... 2018
- Navane Intramuscular ... 2019

Triazolam (Potentiation of both drugs). Products include:
- Halcion Tablets ... 2093

Trifluoperazine Hydrochloride (Potentiation of both drugs). Products include:
- Stelazine ... 2692

Trimethadione (Increased dosage of anticonvulsant may be required).
    No products indexed under this heading.

Valproic Acid (Increased dosage of anticonvulsant may be required). Products include:
- Depakene ... 416

Zolpidem Tartrate (Potentiation of both drugs). Products include:
- Ambien Tablets ... 2559

Food Interactions

Alcohol (Additive effects; hypotension).

TRILAFON INJECTION
(Perphenazine) ... 2532
See **Trilafon Concentrate**

TRILAFON TABLETS
(Perphenazine) ... 2532
See **Trilafon Concentrate**

TRI-LEVLEN 21 TABLETS
(Levonorgestrel, Ethinyl Estradiol) ... 646
See **Levlen 21 Tablets**

TRI-LEVLEN 28 TABLETS
(Levonorgestrel, Ethinyl Estradiol) ... 646
See **Levlen 21 Tablets**

TRILISATE LIQUID
(Choline Magnesium Trisalicylate) ... 2155
May interact with corticosteroids, oral anticoagulants, oral hypoglycemic agents, insulin, carbonic anhydrase inhibitors, and certain other agents. Compounds in these categories include:

Acarbose (Enhanced hypoglycemic effect). Products include:
- Precose ... 604

Acetazolamide (Competition for protein binding sites). Products include:
- Diamox Sequels (Sustained Release) ... ⓞ 318
- Diamox Tablets ... ⓞ 317

Allopurinol (Decreased efficacy of uricosuric agents). Products include:
- Zyloprim Tablets ... 1194

Betamethasone Acetate (Reduces plasma salicylate levels by increasing renal elimination). Products include:
- Celestone Soluspan Suspension ... 2484

Betamethasone Sodium Phosphate (Reduces plasma salicylate levels by increasing renal elimination). Products include:
- Celestone Soluspan Suspension ... 2484

Chlorpropamide (Enhanced hypoglycemic effect). Products include:
- Diabinese Tablets ... 2002

Cortisone Acetate (Reduces plasma salicylate levels by increasing renal elimination). Products include:
- Cortone Acetate Sterile Suspension ... 1663
- Cortone Acetate Tablets ... 1664

Dexamethasone (Reduces plasma salicylate levels by increasing renal elimination). Products include:
- AK-Trol Ointment & Suspension ... ⓞ 205
- Decadron Elixir ... 1676
- Decadron Tablets ... 1678
- Decaspray Topical Aerosol ... 1689
- Maxitrol Ophthalmic Ointment and Suspension ... ⓞ 222
- TobraDex Ophthalmic Suspension and Ointment ... 469

Dexamethasone Acetate (Reduces plasma salicylate levels by increasing renal elimination). Products include:
- Dalalone D.P. Injectable ... 1009
- Decadron-LA Sterile Suspension ... 1687

Dexamethasone Sodium Phosphate (Reduces plasma salicylate levels by increasing renal elimination). Products include:
- Decadron Phosphate Injection ... 1680
- Decadron Phosphate Sterile Ophthalmic Ointment ... 1684
- Decadron Phosphate Sterile Ophthalmic Solution ... 1685
- Decadron Phosphate Topical Cream ... 1686
- Decadron Phosphate with Xylocaine Injection, Sterile ... 1683
- Dexacort Phosphate in Respihaler ... 1606
- Dexacort Phosphate in Turbinaire ... 1607
- NeoDecadron Sterile Ophthalmic Ointment ... 1755
- NeoDecadron Sterile Ophthalmic Solution ... 1756
- NeoDecadron Topical Cream ... 1757

Dichlorphenamide (Competition for protein binding sites). Products include:
- Daranide Tablets ... 1676

Dicumarol (Potential exists for increased levels of unbound anticoagulant with the concurrent use).
    No products indexed under this heading.

Divalproex Sodium (Competition for protein binding sites). Products include:
- Depakote Tablets ... 418

Dorzolamide Hydrochloride (Competition for protein binding sites). Products include:
- Trusopt Sterile Ophthalmic Solution ... 1803

Fludrocortisone Acetate (Reduces plasma salicylate levels by increasing renal elimination). Products include:
- Florinef Acetate Tablets ... 506

Glimepiride (Enhanced hypoglycemic effect). Products include:
- Amaryl Tablets ... 1241

Glipizide (Enhanced hypoglycemic effect). Products include:
- Glucotrol Tablets ... 2011
- Glucotrol XL Extended Release Tablets ... 2012

Glyburide (Enhanced hypoglycemic effect). Products include:
- DiaBeta Tablets ... 1265
- Glynase PresTab Tablets ... 2091
- Micronase Tablets ... 2099

Heparin Calcium (Use cautiously).
    No products indexed under this heading.

Heparin Sodium (Use cautiously). Products include:
- Heparin Lock Flush Solution ... 2831
- Heparin Sodium Injection ... 2832
- Heparin Sodium Vials ... 1486

Hydrocortisone (Reduces plasma salicylate levels by increasing renal elimination). Products include:
- Anusol-HC Cream 2.5% ... 1953
- Aquanil HC Lotion ... 1989
- Maximum Strength Cortaid Spray ... ⓝ 800
- CORTENEMA ... 2713
- Cortisporin Ointment ... 1074
- Cortisporin Ophthalmic Ointment Sterile ... 1074
- Cortisporin Ophthalmic Suspension Sterile ... 1075
- Cortisporin Otic Solution Sterile ... 1076
- Cortisporin Otic Suspension Sterile ... 1077
- Cortizone-5 ... ⓝ 795
- Cortizone-10 ... ⓝ 795
- Hydrocortone Tablets ... 1715
- Hytone ... 922
- Hytone Ointment 2 ½% ... 923
- Massengill Medicated Soft Cloth Towelettes ... 2628
- Pediotic Suspension Sterile ... 1140
- Preparation H Hydrocortisone 1% Cream ... ⓝ 843
- ProctoCream-HC 2.5% ... 2552
- VōSoL HC Otic Solution ... 2786

Hydrocortisone Acetate (Reduces plasma salicylate levels by increasing renal elimination). Products include:
- Analpram-HC Rectal Cream 1% and 2.5% ... 993
- Anusol HC-1 Hydrocortisone Anti-Itch Ointment ... ⓝ 810
- Anusol-HC Suppositories ... 1954
- Caldecort Anti-Itch Hydrocortisone Cream ... ⓝ 651
- Coly-Mycin S Otic w/Neomycin & Hydrocortisone ... 1965
- Cortaid ... ⓝ 800
- Cortifoam ... 2540
- Cortisporin Cream ... 1073
- Epifoam ... 2543
- Hydrocortone Acetate Sterile Suspension ... 1712
- Mantadil Cream ... 1124
- Nupercainal Hydrocortisone 1% Cream ... ⓝ 661
- Pramosone Cream, Lotion & Ointment ... 995
- ProctoFoam-HC ... 2552
- Terra-Cortril Ophthalmic Suspension ... 2033

Hydrocortisone Sodium Phosphate (Reduces plasma salicylate levels by increasing renal elimination). Products include:
- Hydrocortone Phosphate Injection, Sterile ... 1713

Hydrocortisone Sodium Succinate (Reduces plasma salicylate levels by increasing renal elimination).
    No products indexed under this heading.

Insulin, Human (Insulin-treated diabetics on high doses of salicylates should be monitored for enhanced hypoglycemic response).
    No products indexed under this heading.

(ⓝ Described in PDR For Nonprescription Drugs)   (ⓞ Described in PDR For Ophthalmology)

Insulin, Human Isophane Suspension (Insulin-treated diabetics on high doses of salicylates should be monitored for enhanced hypoglycemic response). Products include:
- Novolin N Human Insulin 10 ml Vials ... 1846

Insulin, Human NPH (Insulin-treated diabetics on high doses of salicylates should be monitored for enhanced hypoglycemic response). Products include:
- Humulin N, 100 Units ... 1495
- Novolin N PenFill 1.5 ml Cartridges Durable Insulin Delivery System ... 1849
- Novolin N Prefilled Syringe Disposable Insulin Delivery System ... 1850

Insulin, Human Regular (Insulin-treated diabetics on high doses of salicylates should be monitored for enhanced hypoglycemic response). Products include:
- Humulin R, 100 Units ... 1497
- Novolin R Human Insulin 10 ml Vials ... 1846
- Novolin R PenFill 1.5 ml Cartridges Durable Insulin Delivery System ... 1849
- Novolin R Prefilled Syringe Disposable Insulin Delivery System ... 1850
- Velosulin BR Human Insulin 10 ml Vials ... 1847

Insulin, Human, Zinc Suspension (Insulin-treated diabetics on high doses of salicylates should be monitored for enhanced hypoglycemic response). Products include:
- Humulin L, 100 Units ... 1494
- Humulin U, 100 Units ... 1498
- Novolin L Human Insulin 10 ml Vials ... 1846

Insulin Lispro, Human (Insulin-treated diabetics on high doses of salicylates should be monitored for enhanced hypoglycemic response). Products include:
- Humalog Injection ... 1488

Insulin, NPH (Insulin-treated diabetics on high doses of salicylates should be monitored for enhanced hypoglycemic response). Products include:
- NPH, 100 Units ... 1502
- Pork NPH, 100 Units ... 1506
- Purified Pork NPH Isophane Insulin ... 1852

Insulin, Regular (Insulin-treated diabetics on high doses of salicylates should be monitored for enhanced hypoglycemic response). Products include:
- Regular, 100 Units ... 1503
- Pork Regular, 100 Units ... 1507
- Pork Regular (Concentrated), 500 Units ... 1508
- Purified Pork Regular Insulin ... 1852

Insulin, Zinc Crystals (Insulin-treated diabetics on high doses of salicylates should be monitored for enhanced hypoglycemic response). Products include:
- NPH, 100 Units ... 1502

Insulin, Zinc Suspension (Insulin-treated diabetics on high doses of salicylates should be monitored for enhanced hypoglycemic response). Products include:
- Iletin I ... 1501
- Lente, 100 Units ... 1501
- Iletin II ... 1504
- Pork Lente, 100 Units ... 1504
- Purified Pork Lente Insulin ... 1852

Metformin Hydrochloride (Enhanced hypoglycemic effect). Products include:
- Glucophage Tablets ... 754

Methazolamide (Competition for protein binding sites). Products include:
- GlaucTabs ... ◉ 209
- Neptazane Tablets ... ◉ 320

Methotrexate Sodium (Increased methotrexate effects). Products include:
- Methotrexate Sodium Tablets, Injection, for Injection and LPF Injection ... 1322

Methylprednisolone (Increased risk of gastrointestinal ulceration).
No products indexed under this heading.

Methylprednisolone Acetate (Reduces plasma salicylate levels by increasing renal elimination).
No products indexed under this heading.

Methylprednisolone Sodium Succinate (Reduces plasma salicylate levels by increasing renal elimination).
No products indexed under this heading.

Phenylbutazone (Increased risk of gastrointestinal ulceration).
No products indexed under this heading.

Phenytoin (Competition for protein binding sites). Products include:
- Dilantin Infatabs ... 1967
- Dilantin-125 Suspension ... 1969

Phenytoin Sodium (Competition for protein binding sites). Products include:
- Dilantin Kapseals ... 1965

Prednisolone Acetate (Reduces plasma salicylate levels by increasing renal elimination). Products include:
- AK-CIDE ... ◉ 203
- AK-CIDE Ointment ... ◉ 203
- Blephamide Liquifilm Sterile Ophthalmic Suspension ... 472
- Blephamide Ointment ... ◉ 234
- Econopred & Econopred Plus Ophthalmic Suspensions ... ◉ 216
- Poly-Pred Liquifilm ... ◉ 246
- Pred Forte ... ◉ 247
- Pred Mild ... ◉ 250
- Pred-G Liquifilm Sterile Ophthalmic Suspension ... ◉ 248
- Pred-G S.O.P. Sterile Ophthalmic Ointment ... ◉ 249

Prednisolone Sodium Phosphate (Reduces plasma salicylate levels by increasing renal elimination). Products include:
- AK-PRED ... ◉ 204
- Hydeltrasol Injection, Sterile ... 1708
- Pediapred Oral Solution ... 1618

Prednisolone Tebutate (Reduces plasma salicylate levels by increasing renal elimination). Products include:
- Hydeltra-T.B.A. Sterile Suspension 1710

Prednisone (Reduces plasma salicylate levels by increasing renal elimination).
No products indexed under this heading.

Probenecid (Decreased efficacy of uricosuric agents). Products include:
- Benemid Tablets ... 1651
- ColBENEMID Tablets ... 1662

Sulfinpyrazone (Decreased efficacy of uricosuric agents). Products include:
- Anturane ... 823

Tolazamide (Enhanced hypoglycemic effect).
No products indexed under this heading.

Tolbutamide (Enhanced hypoglycemic effect).
No products indexed under this heading.

Triamcinolone (Reduces plasma salicylate levels by increasing renal elimination).
No products indexed under this heading.

Triamcinolone Acetonide (Reduces plasma salicylate levels by increasing renal elimination). Products include:
- Azmacort Oral Inhaler ... 2175
- Nasacort AQ Nasal Spray ... 2191
- Nasacort Nasal Inhaler ... 2189

Triamcinolone Diacetate (Reduces plasma salicylate levels by increasing renal elimination).
No products indexed under this heading.

Triamcinolone Hexacetonide (Reduces plasma salicylate levels by increasing renal elimination).
No products indexed under this heading.

Valproic Acid (Competition for protein binding sites). Products include:
- Depakene ... 416

Warfarin Sodium (Potential exists for increased levels of unbound anticoagulant with the concurrent use). Products include:
- Coumadin ... 941

Food Interactions

Alcohol (Increased risk of gastrointestinal ulceration).

Food that lowers urinary pH (Decreases urinary salicylate excretion and increases plasma salicylate levels).

Food that raises urinary pH (Enhances renal salicylate clearance and diminishes plasma salicylate concentration).

TRILISATE TABLETS
(Choline Magnesium Trisalicylate) 2155
See **Trilisate Liquid**

TRIMPEX TABLETS
(Trimethoprim) 2323
May interact with:

Phenytoin (Possible excessive phenytoin effect). Products include:
- Dilantin Infatabs ... 1967
- Dilantin-125 Suspension ... 1969

Phenytoin Sodium (Possible excessive phenytoin effect). Products include:
- Dilantin Kapseals ... 1965

TRINALIN REPETABS TABLETS
(Azatadine Maleate, Pseudoephedrine Sulfate) 1373
May interact with monoamine oxidase inhibitors, tricyclic antidepressants, barbiturates, central nervous system depressants, veratrum alkaloids, antacids, oral anticoagulants, beta blockers, and certain other agents. Compounds in these categories include:

Acebutolol Hydrochloride (Effect not specified). Products include:
- Sectral Capsules ... 2914

Alfentanil Hydrochloride (Additive effect). Products include:
- Alfenta Injection ... 1334

Alprazolam (Additive effect). Products include:
- Xanax Tablets ... 2115

Aluminum Carbonate (Increased rate of absorption of pseudoephedrine). Products include:
- Basaljel Capsules ... 2810
- Basaljel Suspension ... 2810
- Basaljel Tablets ... 2810

Aluminum Hydroxide (Increased rate of absorption of pseudoephedrine). Products include:
- ALternaGEL Liquid ... 1358
- Maximum Strength Ascriptin ... ▣ 650
- Cama Arthritis Pain Reliever ... ▣ 748
- Gaviscon Extra Strength Relief Formula Antacid Tablets ... ▣ 778
- Gaviscon Extra Strength Relief Formula Liquid Antacid ... ▣ 779
- Gaviscon Liquid Antacid ... ▣ 779
- Gelusil Antacid-Anti-gas Liquid ... ▣ 819
- Gelusil Antacid-Anti-gas Tablets ... ▣ 819
- Maalox Antacid/Anti-Gas Tablets ... 889
- Maalox Heartburn Relief Suspension ... ▣ 658
- Maalox Antacid Liquid ... 888
- Extra Strength Maalox Antacid/Anti-Gas Liquid and Tablets ... 888
- Mylanta ... 1359
- Tempo Soft Antacid ... ▣ 799

Aluminum Hydroxide Gel (Increased rate of absorption of pseudoephedrine). Products include:
- ALternaGEL Liquid ... ▣ 675
- Aludrox Oral Suspension ... ▣ 850
- Amphojel Suspension ... 2802
- Amphojel Suspension without Flavor ... 2802
- Amphojel Tablets ... 2802
- Ascriptin ... ▣ 650
- Gaviscon Antacid Tablets ... ▣ 778
- Gaviscon-2 Antacid Tablets ... ▣ 779
- Mylanta Liquid ... ▣ 676
- Mylanta Double Strength Liquid ... ▣ 676
- Nephrox Suspension ... ▣ 671

Amitriptyline Hydrochloride (Additive effect). Products include:
- Elavil ... 2945
- Etrafon ... 2495
- Limbitrol ... 2333
- Triavil Tablets ... 1800

Amoxapine (Additive effect). Products include:
- Asendin Tablets ... 1419

Aprobarbital (Additive effect).
No products indexed under this heading.

Atenolol (Effect not specified). Products include:
- Tenoretic Tablets ... 2963
- Tenormin Tablets and I.V. Injection 2965

Betaxolol Hydrochloride (Effect not specified). Products include:
- Betoptic Ophthalmic Solution ... 465
- Betoptic S Ophthalmic Suspension 467
- Kerlone Tablets ... 2588

Bisoprolol Fumarate (Effect not specified). Products include:
- Zebeta Tablets ... 1457
- Ziac ... 1459

Buprenorphine (Additive effect). Products include:
- Buprenex Injectable ... 2170

Buspirone Hydrochloride (Additive effect). Products include:
- BuSpar Tablets ... 738

Butabarbital (Additive effect).
No products indexed under this heading.

Butalbital (Additive effect). Products include:
- Axocet Capsules ... 2469
- Esgic-plus Capsules ... 1012
- Esgic-plus Tablets ... 1012
- Fioricet Tablets ... 2386
- Fioricet with Codeine Capsules ... 2387
- Fiorinal Capsules ... 2388
- Fiorinal with Codeine Capsules ... 2390
- Fiorinal Tablets ... 2388
- Phrenilin ... 790
- Sedapap Tablets 50 mg/650 mg .. 1826

Carteolol Hydrochloride (Effect not specified). Products include:
- Cartrol Tablets ... 413
- Ocupress Ophthalmic Solution, 1% Sterile ... ◉ 297

Chlordiazepoxide (Additive effect). Products include:
- Limbitrol ... 2333

Chlordiazepoxide Hydrochloride (Additive effect). Products include:
- Librax Capsules ... 2330
- Librium Capsules ... 2331
- Librium Injectable ... 2332

Chlorpromazine (Additive effect). Products include:
- Thorazine Suppositories ... 2701

IMPORTANT NOTE: Always consult each drug listing in the patient's regimen for possible interactions.

Trinalin **Interactions Index** **1110**

Chlorprothixene (Additive effect).
- No products indexed under this heading.

Chlorprothixene Hydrochloride (Additive effect).
- No products indexed under this heading.

Chlorprothixene Lactate (Additive effect).
- No products indexed under this heading.

Clomipramine Hydrochloride (Additive effect). Products include:
- Anafranil Capsules 819

Clorazepate Dipotassium (Additive effect). Products include:
- Tranxene 459

Clozapine (Additive effect). Products include:
- Clozaril Tablets 2377

Codeine Phosphate (Additive effect). Products include:
- Brontex 2130
- Dimetane-DC Cough Syrup 2232
- Fioricet with Codeine Capsules 2387
- Fiorinal with Codeine Capsules 2390
- Nucofed 2225
- Phenergan with Codeine 2883
- Phenergan VC with Codeine 2888
- Robitussin A-C Syrup 2248
- Robitussin-DAC Syrup 2249
- Ryna .... ■ 804
- Soma Compound w/Codeine Tablets 2784
- Tylenol with Codeine 1592

Cryptenamine Preparations (Antihypertensive effects of veratrum alkaloids reduced).

Desflurane (Additive effect). Products include:
- Suprane (desflurane, USP) 1865

Desipramine Hydrochloride (Additive effect). Products include:
- Norpramin Tablets 1273

Deslanoside (Increased ectopic pacemaker activity).
- No products indexed under this heading.

Dezocine (Additive effect). Products include:
- Dalgan Injection 529

Diazepam (Additive effect). Products include:
- Dizac (diazepam injectable emulsion) CIV 1862
- Valium Injectable 2336
- Valium Tablets 2335

Dicumarol (Action of oral anticoagulants inhibited).
- No products indexed under this heading.

Digitoxin (Increased ectopic pacemaker activity). Products include:
- Crystodigin Tablets 1472

Digoxin (Increased ectopic pacemaker activity). Products include:
- Lanoxicaps 1110
- Lanoxin Elixir Pediatric 1113
- Lanoxin Injection 1116
- Lanoxin Injection Pediatric 1119
- Lanoxin Tablets 1121

Doxepin Hydrochloride (Additive effect). Products include:
- Adapin Capsules 1542
- Sinequan 2028
- Zonalon Cream 1042

Droperidol (Additive effect). Products include:
- Inapsine Injection 462

Enflurane (Additive effect).
- No products indexed under this heading.

Esmolol Hydrochloride (Effect not specified). Products include:
- Brevibloc (esmolol HCl) Injection 1860

Estazolam (Additive effect). Products include:
- ProSom Tablets 457

Ethchlorvynol (Additive effect). Products include:
- Placidyl Capsules 456

Ethinamate (Additive effect).
- No products indexed under this heading.

Fentanyl (Additive effect). Products include:
- Duragesic Transdermal System 1336

Fentanyl Citrate (Additive effect). Products include:
- Sublimaze Injection 463

Fluphenazine Decanoate (Additive effect). Products include:
- Prolixin Decanoate 510

Fluphenazine Enanthate (Additive effect). Products include:
- Prolixin Enanthate 510

Fluphenazine Hydrochloride (Additive effect). Products include:
- Prolixin 510

Flurazepam Hydrochloride (Additive effect). Products include:
- Dalmane Capsules 2329

Furazolidone (Hypertensive crisis; effects of antihistamines prolonged and intensified; concurrent use is contraindicated). Products include:
- Furoxone 2221

Glutethimide (Additive effect).
- No products indexed under this heading.

Haloperidol (Additive effect). Products include:
- Haldol Injection, Tablets and Concentrate 1585

Haloperidol Decanoate (Additive effect). Products include:
- Haldol Decanoate 1587

Hydrocodone Bitartrate (Additive effect). Products include:
- Codiclear DH Syrup 808
- Duratuss HD Elixir 2750
- Histussin D Liquid 670
- Hycodan Tablets and Syrup 946
- Hycomine Compound Tablets 948
- Hycomine 947
- Hycotuss Expectorant Syrup 950
- Hydrocet Capsules 787
- Lorcet 10/650 Tablets 1016
- Lortab 2751
- Tussend 1830
- Tussend Expectorant 1831
- Vicodin Tablets 1404
- Vicodin ES Tablets 1405
- Vicodin HP Tablets 1403
- Vicodin Tuss Expectorant 1406
- Zydone Capsules 967

Hydrocodone Polistirex (Additive effect). Products include:
- Tussionex Pennkinetic Extended-Release Suspension 1624

Hydroxyzine Hydrochloride (Additive effect). Products include:
- Atarax Tablets & Syrup 1992
- Marax Tablets & DF Syrup 2015
- Vistaril Intramuscular Solution 2042

Imipramine Hydrochloride (Additive effect). Products include:
- Tofranil Ampuls 873
- Tofranil Tablets 875

Imipramine Pamoate (Additive effect). Products include:
- Tofranil-PM Capsules 876

Isocarboxazid (Hypertensive crisis; effects of antihistamines prolonged and intensified; concurrent use is contraindicated).
- No products indexed under this heading.

Isoflurane (Additive effect).
- No products indexed under this heading.

Kaolin (Decreased rate of absorption of pseudoephedrine).
- No products indexed under this heading.

Ketamine Hydrochloride (Additive effect).
- No products indexed under this heading.

Labetalol Hydrochloride (Effect not specified). Products include:
- Normodyne Injection 2519
- Normodyne Tablets 2522
- Trandate 1158

Levobunolol Hydrochloride (Effect not specified). Products include:
- Betagan .... ◉ 230

Levomethadyl Acetate Hydrochloride (Additive effect). Products include:
- Orlaam Oral Solution 2361

Levorphanol Tartrate (Additive effect). Products include:
- Levo-Dromoran 2297

Lorazepam (Additive effect). Products include:
- Ativan Injection 2805
- Ativan Tablets 2807

Loxapine Hydrochloride (Additive effect). Products include:
- Loxitane 1426

Loxapine Succinate (Additive effect). Products include:
- Loxitane Capsules 1426

Magaldrate (Increased rate of absorption of pseudoephedrine).
- No products indexed under this heading.

Magnesium Hydroxide (Increased rate of absorption of pseudoephedrine). Products include:
- Aludrox Oral Suspension .... ■ 850
- Ascriptin .... ■ 650
- Di-Gel Antacid/Anti-Gas .... ■ 762
- Gelusil Antacid-Anti-gas Liquid .... ■ 819
- Gelusil Antacid-Anti-gas Tablets .... ■ 819
- Maalox Antacid/Anti-Gas Tablets 889
- Maalox Antacid Liquid 888
- Extra Strength Maalox Antacid/Anti-Gas Liquid and Tablets 888
- Mylanta Fast-Acting 1359
- Mylanta Gelcaps Antacid .... ■ 678
- Fast-Acting Mylanta Liquid Antacid 1359
- Mylanta Tablets .... ■ 677
- Maximum-Strength Fast-Acting Mylanta Liquid Antacid 1359
- Mylanta Double Strength Tablets .... ■ 677
- Phillips' Milk of Magnesia Liquid .... ■ 627
- Rolaids Antacid Tablets .... ■ 807
- Tempo Soft Antacid .... ■ 799

Magnesium Oxide (Increased rate of absorption of pseudoephedrine). Products include:
- Beelith Tablets 632
- Bufferin Analgesic Tablets .... ■ 636
- Arthritis Strength Bufferin Analgesic Caplets .... ■ 637
- Extra Strength Bufferin Analgesic Tablets .... ■ 637
- Caltrate PLUS .... ■ 681
- Cama Arthritis Pain Reliever .... ■ 748
- Mag-Ox 400 666
- Uro-Mag 666

Maprotiline Hydrochloride (Additive effect). Products include:
- Ludiomil Tablets 861

Mecamylamine Hydrochloride (Antihypertensive effects of mecamylamine reduced). Products include:
- Inversine Tablets 1729

Meperidine Hydrochloride (Additive effect). Products include:
- Demerol 2438
- Mepergan Injection 2859

Mephobarbital (Additive effect). Products include:
- Mebaral Tablets 2452

Meprobamate (Additive effect). Products include:
- Miltown Tablets 2780
- PMB 200 and PMB 400 2890

Mesoridazine Besylate (Additive effect). Products include:
- Serentil 689

Methadone Hydrochloride (Additive effect). Products include:
- Methadone Hydrochloride Oral Concentrate 2356
- Methadone Hydrochloride Oral Solution & Tablets 2357

Methohexital Sodium (Additive effect).
- No products indexed under this heading.

Methotrimeprazine (Additive effect). Products include:
- Levoprome 1321

Methoxyflurane (Additive effect).
- No products indexed under this heading.

Methyldopa (Antihypertensive effects of methyldopa reduced). Products include:
- Aldoclor Tablets 1638
- Aldomet Oral 1640
- Aldoril Tablets 1644

Methyldopate Hydrochloride (Antihypertensive effects of methyldopa reduced). Products include:
- Aldomet Ester HCl Injection 1642

Metipranolol Hydrochloride (Effect not specified). Products include:
- OptiPranolol (Metipranolol 0.3%) Sterile Ophthalmic Solution .... ◉ 256

Metoprolol Succinate (Effect not specified). Products include:
- Toprol-XL Tablets 560

Metoprolol Tartrate (Effect not specified). Products include:
- Lopressor 848
- Lopressor HCT Tablets 850

Midazolam Hydrochloride (Additive effect). Products include:
- Versed Injection 2324

Molindone Hydrochloride (Additive effect). Products include:
- Moban Tablets and Concentrate 1036

Morphine Sulfate (Additive effect). Products include:
- Astramorph/PF Injection, USP (Preservative-Free) 526
- Duramorph Injection 983
- Infumorph 200 and Infumorph 500 Sterile Solutions 985
- Kadian Capsules 2948
- MS Contin Tablets 2149
- MSIR 2152
- Oramorph SR (Morphine Sulfate Sustained Release Tablets) 2359
- RMS Suppositories CII 2766
- Roxanol 2365

Nadolol (Effect not specified).
- No products indexed under this heading.

Nortriptyline Hydrochloride (Additive effect). Products include:
- Pamelor 2409

Opium Alkaloids (Additive effect).
- No products indexed under this heading.

Oxazepam (Additive effect). Products include:
- Serax Capsules 2916
- Serax Tablets 2916

Oxycodone Hydrochloride (Additive effect). Products include:
- OxyContin Tablets 2163
- OxyIR Capsules 2167
- Percocet Tablets 955
- Percodan Tablets 955
- Percodan-Demi Tablets 956
- Roxicodone Tablets, Oral Solution & Intensol (Oxycodone) 2366
- Tylox Capsules 1593

Penbutolol Sulfate (Effect not specified). Products include:
- Levatol Tablets 2547

Pentobarbital Sodium (Additive effect). Products include:
- Nembutal Sodium Capsules 440
- Nembutal Sodium Solution 442
- Nembutal Sodium Suppositories 444

(■ Described in PDR For Nonprescription Drugs) (◉ Described in PDR For Ophthalmology)

Perphenazine (Additive effect). Products include:
Etrafon ... 2495
Triavil Tablets ... 1800
Trilafon ... 2532

Phenelzine Sulfate (Hypertensive crisis; effects of antihistamines prolonged and intensified; concurrent use is contraindicated). Products include:
Nardil ... 1977

Phenobarbital (Additive effect). Products include:
Arco-Lase Plus Tablets ... 513
Bellergal-S Tablets ... 2375
Donnatal ... 2234
Donnatal Extentabs ... 2234
Donnatal Tablets ... 2234
Phenobarbital Elixir and Tablets ... 1523
Quadrinal Tablets ... 1398

Pindolol (Effect not specified). Products include:
Visken Tablets ... 2428

Prazepam (Additive effect).
No products indexed under this heading.

Prochlorperazine (Additive effect). Products include:
Compazine ... 2644

Promethazine Hydrochloride (Additive effect). Products include:
Mepergan Injection ... 2859
Phenergan with Codeine ... 2883
Phenergan with Dextromethorphan ... 2885
Phenergan Injection ... 2880
Phenergan Suppositories ... 2882
Phenergan Syrup ... 2881
Phenergan Tablets ... 2882
Phenergan VC ... 2886
Phenergan VC with Codeine ... 2888

Propofol (Additive effect). Products include:
Diprivan Injectable Emulsion ... 2939

Propoxyphene Hydrochloride (Additive effect). Products include:
Darvon ... 1475
Wygesic Tablets ... 2930

Propoxyphene Napsylate (Additive effect). Products include:
Darvon-N/Darvocet-N ... 1473

Propranolol Hydrochloride (Effect not specified). Products include:
Inderal ... 2834
Inderal LA Long Acting Capsules ... 2836
Inderide Tablets ... 2838
Inderide LA Long Acting Capsules ... 2840

Protriptyline Hydrochloride (Additive effect). Products include:
Vivactil Tablets ... 1820

Quazepam (Additive effect). Products include:
Doral Tablets ... 2773

Reserpine (Antihypertensive effects of reserpine reduced). Products include:
Diupres Tablets ... 1691
Hydropres Tablets ... 1718
Ser-Ap-Es Tablets ... 867

Risperidone (Additive effect). Products include:
Risperdal Tablets ... 1348

Secobarbital Sodium (Additive effect). Products include:
Seconal Sodium Pulvules ... 1529

Selegiline Hydrochloride (Hypertensive crisis; effects of antihistamines prolonged and intensified; concurrent use is contraindicated). Products include:
Eldepryl Capsules ... 2729

Sevoflurane (Additive effect).
No products indexed under this heading.

Sotalol Hydrochloride (Effect not specified). Products include:
Betapace Tablets ... 637

Sufentanil Citrate (Additive effect). Products include:
Sufenta Injection ... 1355

Temazepam (Additive effect). Products include:
Restoril Capsules ... 2413

Thiamylal Sodium (Additive effect).
No products indexed under this heading.

Thioridazine Hydrochloride (Additive effect). Products include:
Mellaril ... 2398

Thiothixene (Additive effect). Products include:
Navane Capsules and Concentrate ... 2018
Navane Intramuscular ... 2019

Timolol Hemihydrate (Effect not specified). Products include:
Betimol 0.25%, 0.5% ... ⊙ 259

Timolol Maleate (Effect not specified). Products include:
Blocadren Tablets ... 1654
Timolide Tablets ... 1791
Timoptic in Ocudose ... 1796
Timoptic Sterile Ophthalmic Solution ... 1794
Timoptic-XE ... 1798

Tranylcypromine Sulfate (Hypertensive crisis; effects of antihistamines prolonged and intensified; concurrent use is contraindicated). Products include:
Parnate Tablets ... 2679

Triazolam (Additive effect). Products include:
Halcion Tablets ... 2093

Trifluoperazine Hydrochloride (Additive effect). Products include:
Stelazine ... 2692

Trimipramine Maleate (Additive effect). Products include:
Surmontil Capsules ... 2917

Warfarin Sodium (Action of oral anticoagulants inhibited). Products include:
Coumadin ... 941

Zolpidem Tartrate (Additive effect). Products include:
Ambien Tablets ... 2559

Food Interactions

Alcohol (Additive effect).

TRI-NORINYL 21-DAY TABLETS
(Norethindrone, Ethinyl Estradiol) ... 2607
May interact with barbiturates, phenothiazines, and certain other agents. Compounds in these categories include:

Ampicillin (Potential for reduced efficacy and increased incidence of breakthrough bleeding and menstrual irregularities with concomitant use). Products include:
Omnipen Capsules ... 2872
Omnipen for Oral Suspension ... 2873

Ampicillin Sodium (Potential for reduced efficacy and increased incidence of breakthrough bleeding and menstrual irregularities with concomitant use). Products include:
Unasyn ... 2035

Aprobarbital (Potential for reduced efficacy and increased incidence of breakthrough bleeding and menstrual irregularities with concomitant use).
No products indexed under this heading.

Butabarbital (Potential for reduced efficacy and increased incidence of breakthrough bleeding and menstrual irregularities with concomitant use).
No products indexed under this heading.

Butalbital (Potential for reduced efficacy and increased incidence of breakthrough bleeding and menstrual irregularities with concomitant use). Products include:
Axocet Capsules ... 2469
Esgic-plus Capsules ... 1012
Esgic-plus Tablets ... 1012
Fioricet Tablets ... 2386
Fioricet with Codeine Capsules ... 2387
Fiorinal Capsules ... 2388
Fiorinal with Codeine Capsules ... 2390
Fiorinal Tablets ... 2388
Phrenilin ... 790
Sedapap Tablets 50 mg/650 mg ... 1826

Demeclocycline Hydrochloride (Potential for reduced efficacy and increased incidence of breakthrough bleeding and menstrual irregularities with concomitant use). Products include:
Declomycin Tablets ... 1421

Doxycycline Calcium (Potential for reduced efficacy and increased incidence of breakthrough bleeding and menstrual irregularities with concomitant use). Products include:
Vibramycin Calcium Oral Suspension Syrup ... 2038

Doxycycline Hyclate (Potential for reduced efficacy and increased incidence of breakthrough bleeding and menstrual irregularities with concomitant use). Products include:
Doryx Capsules ... 1970
Vibramycin Hyclate Capsules ... 2038
Vibramycin Hyclate Intravenous ... 2040
Vibra-Tabs Film Coated Tablets ... 2038

Doxycycline Monohydrate (Potential for reduced efficacy and increased incidence of breakthrough bleeding and menstrual irregularities with concomitant use). Products include:
Monodox Capsules ... 1858
Vibramycin Monohydrate for Oral Suspension ... 2038

Fosphenytoin Sodium (Potential for reduced efficacy and increased incidence of breakthrough bleeding and menstrual irregularities with concomitant use). Products include:
Cerebyx Injection ... 1956

Griseofulvin (Potential for reduced efficacy and increased incidence of breakthrough bleeding and menstrual irregularities with concomitant use). Products include:
Fulvicin P/G Tablets ... 2499
Fulvicin P/G 165 & 330 Tablets ... 2500
Grifulvin V (griseofulvin tablets) Microsize (griseofulvin oral suspension) Microsize ... 1944
Gris-PEG Tablets, 125 mg & 250 mg ... 476

Mephobarbital (Potential for reduced efficacy and increased incidence of breakthrough bleeding and menstrual irregularities with concomitant use). Products include:
Mebaral Tablets ... 2452

Methacycline Hydrochloride (Potential for reduced efficacy and increased incidence of breakthrough bleeding and menstrual irregularities with concomitant use).
No products indexed under this heading.

Minocycline Hydrochloride (Potential for reduced efficacy and increased incidence of breakthrough bleeding and menstrual irregularities with concomitant use). Products include:
DYNACIN Capsules ... 1627
Minocin Intravenous ... 1428
Minocin Oral Suspension ... 1431
Minocin Pellet-Filled Capsules ... 1429

Oxytetracycline Hydrochloride (Potential for reduced efficacy and increased incidence of breakthrough bleeding and menstrual irregularities with concomitant use). Products include:
TERAK Ointment ... ⊙ 210
Terra-Cortril Ophthalmic Suspension ... 2033
Terramycin with Polymyxin B Sulfate Ophthalmic Ointment ... 2035
Urobiotic-250 Capsules ... 2038

Pentobarbital Sodium (Potential for reduced efficacy and increased incidence of breakthrough bleeding and menstrual irregularities with concomitant use). Products include:
Nembutal Sodium Capsules ... 440
Nembutal Sodium Solution ... 442
Nembutal Sodium Suppositories ... 444

Phenobarbital (Potential for reduced efficacy and increased incidence of breakthrough bleeding and menstrual irregularities with concomitant use). Products include:
Arco-Lase Plus Tablets ... 513
Bellergal-S Tablets ... 2375
Donnatal ... 2234
Donnatal Extentabs ... 2234
Donnatal Tablets ... 2234
Phenobarbital Elixir and Tablets ... 1523
Quadrinal Tablets ... 1398

Phenylbutazone (Potential for reduced efficacy and increased incidence of breakthrough bleeding and menstrual irregularities with concomitant use).
No products indexed under this heading.

Phenytoin (Potential for reduced efficacy and increased incidence of breakthrough bleeding and menstrual irregularities with concomitant use). Products include:
Dilantin Infatabs ... 1967
Dilantin-125 Suspension ... 1969

Phenytoin Sodium (Potential for reduced efficacy and increased incidence of breakthrough bleeding and menstrual irregularities with concomitant use). Products include:
Dilantin Kapseals ... 1965

Rifampin (Co-administration has been associated with reduced efficacy and increased incidence of breakthrough bleeding and menstrual irregularities). Products include:
Rifadin ... 1276
Rifamate Capsules ... 1278
Rifater ... 1280
Rimactane Capsules ... 865

Secobarbital Sodium (Potential for reduced efficacy and increased incidence of breakthrough bleeding and menstrual irregularities with concomitant use). Products include:
Seconal Sodium Pulvules ... 1529

Tetracycline Hydrochloride (Potential for reduced efficacy and increased incidence of breakthrough bleeding and menstrual irregularities with concomitant use). Products include:
Achromycin V Capsules ... 1417
Helidac Therapy ... 2135

Thiamylal Sodium (Potential for reduced efficacy and increased incidence of breakthrough bleeding and menstrual irregularities with concomitant use).
No products indexed under this heading.

TRI-NORINYL 28-DAY TABLETS
(Norethindrone, Ethinyl Estradiol) ... 335
See **Tri-Norinyl 21-Day Tablets**

IMPORTANT NOTE: Always consult each drug listing in the patient's regimen for possible interactions.

TRINSICON CAPSULES
(Vitamins with Iron) 2759
None cited in PDR database.

TRIOSTAT INJECTION
(Liothyronine Sodium) 2708
May interact with oral anticoagulants, insulin, oral hypoglycemic agents, estrogens, oral contraceptives, tricyclic antidepressants, cardiac glycosides, vasopressors, and certain other agents. Compounds in these categories include:

Acarbose (Potential for increased oral hypoglycemic requirements). Products include:
Precose 604

Amitriptyline Hydrochloride (Increased receptor sensitivity and enhanced antidepressant activity). Products include:
Elavil 2945
Etrafon 2495
Limbitrol 2333
Triavil Tablets 1800

Amoxapine (Increased receptor sensitivity and enhanced antidepressant activity). Products include:
Asendin Tablets 1419

Chlorotrianisene (Increases serum thyroxine-binding globulin).
No products indexed under this heading.

Chlorpropamide (Potential for increased oral hypoglycemic requirements). Products include:
Diabinese Tablets 2002

Clomipramine Hydrochloride (Increased receptor sensitivity and enhanced antidepressant activity). Products include:
Anafranil Capsules 819

Desipramine Hydrochloride (Increased receptor sensitivity and enhanced antidepressant activity). Products include:
Norpramin Tablets 1273

Deslanoside (Toxic effects of digitalis potentiated).
No products indexed under this heading.

Desogestrel (Increases serum thyroxine-binding globulin). Products include:
Desogen Tablets 1867
Ortho-Cept 1907

Dicumarol (Increased catabolism of vitamin K-dependent clotting factors).
No products indexed under this heading.

Dienestrol (Increases serum thyroxine-binding globulin). Products include:
Ortho Dienestrol Cream 1922

Diethylstilbestrol (Increases serum thyroxine-binding globulin). Products include:
Diethylstilbestrol Tablets 1477

Digitoxin (Toxic effects of digitalis potentiated). Products include:
Crystodigin Tablets 1472

Digoxin (Toxic effects of digitalis potentiated). Products include:
Lanoxicaps 1110
Lanoxin Elixir Pediatric 1113
Lanoxin Injection 1116
Lanoxin Injection Pediatric 1119
Lanoxin Tablets 1121

Dopamine Hydrochloride (Increased adrenergic effect).
No products indexed under this heading.

Doxepin Hydrochloride (Increased receptor sensitivity and enhanced antidepressant activity). Products include:
Adapin Capsules 1542
Sinequan 2028
Zonalon Cream 1042

Epinephrine Bitartrate (Increased adrenergic effect). Products include:
Sensorcaine-MPF with Epinephrine Injection 554

Epinephrine Hydrochloride (Increased adrenergic effect). Products include:
Ana-Kit Anaphylaxis Emergency Treatment Kit 611

Estradiol (Increases serum thyroxine-binding globulin). Products include:
Climara Transdermal System 640
Estrace Cream and Tablets 751
Estraderm Transdermal System 842
Estring Vaginal Ring 2086
Vivelle Transdermal System 880

Estrogens, Conjugated (Increases serum thyroxine-binding globulin). Products include:
PMB 200 and PMB 400 2890
Premarin Intravenous 2893
Premarin Tablets 2896
Premarin Vaginal Cream 2898
Premphase 2900
Prempro 2905

Estrogens, Esterified (Increases serum thyroxine-binding globulin). Products include:
ESTRATAB Tablets (0.3, 0.625, 1.25, 2.5 mg) 2715
Estratest 2718
Menest Tablets 2671

Estropipate (Increases serum thyroxine-binding globulin). Products include:
Ogen Tablets 2103
Ogen Vaginal Cream 2106
Ortho-Est 1925

Ethinyl Estradiol (Increases serum thyroxine-binding globulin). Products include:
Brevicon 2563
Demulen 2580
Desogen Tablets 1867
Levlen/Tri-Levlen 646
Lo/Ovral Tablets 2852
Lo/Ovral-28 Tablets 2857
Modicon 1928
Nordette-21 Tablets 2863
Nordette-28 Tablets 2866
Norinyl 2563
Ortho-Cept 1907
Ortho-Cyclen/Ortho-Tri-Cyclen 1914
Ortho-Novum 1928
Ortho-Cyclen/Ortho Tri-Cyclen 1914
Ovcon 765
Ovral Tablets 2877
Ovral-28 Tablets 2878
Levlen/Tri-Levlen 646
Tri-Norinyl 2607
Triphasil-21 Tablets 2919
Triphasil-28 Tablets 2924

Ethynodiol Diacetate (Increases serum thyroxine-binding globulin). Products include:
Demulen 2580

Glimepiride (Potential for increased oral hypoglycemic requirements). Products include:
Amaryl Tablets 1241

Glipizide (Potential for increased oral hypoglycemic requirements). Products include:
Glucotrol Tablets 2011
Glucotrol XL Extended Release Tablets 2012

Glyburide (Potential for increased oral hypoglycemic requirements). Products include:
DiaBeta Tablets 1265
Glynase PresTab Tablets 2091
Micronase Tablets 2099

Imipramine Hydrochloride (Increased receptor sensitivity and enhanced antidepressant activity). Products include:
Tofranil Ampuls 873
Tofranil Tablets 875

Imipramine Pamoate (Increased receptor sensitivity and enhanced antidepressant activity). Products include:
Tofranil-PM Capsules 876

Insulin, Human (Potential for increased insulin requirements).
No products indexed under this heading.

Insulin, Human Isophane Suspension (Potential for increased insulin requirements). Products include:
Novolin N Human Insulin 10 ml Vials 1846

Insulin, Human NPH (Potential for increased insulin requirements). Products include:
Humulin N, 100 Units 1495
Novolin N PenFill 1.5 ml Cartridges Durable Insulin Delivery System 1849
Novolin N Prefilled Syringe Disposable Insulin Delivery System 1850

Insulin, Human Regular (Potential for increased insulin requirements). Products include:
Humulin R, 100 Units 1497
Novolin R Human Insulin 10 ml Vials 1846
Novolin R PenFill 1.5 ml Cartridges Durable Insulin Delivery System 1849
Novolin R Prefilled Syringe Disposable Insulin Delivery System 1850
Velosulin BR Human Insulin 10 ml Vials 1847

Insulin, Human, Zinc Suspension (Potential for increased insulin requirements). Products include:
Humulin L, 100 Units 1494
Humulin U, 100 Units 1498
Novolin L Human Insulin 10 ml Vials 1846

Insulin Lispro, Human (Potential for increased insulin requirements). Products include:
Humalog Injection 1488

Insulin, NPH (Potential for increased insulin requirements). Products include:
NPH, 100 Units 1502
Pork NPH, 100 Units 1506
Purified Pork NPH Isophane Insulin 1852

Insulin, Regular (Potential for increased insulin requirements). Products include:
Regular, 100 Units 1503
Pork Regular, 100 Units 1507
Pork Regular (Concentrated), 500 Units 1508
Purified Pork Regular Insulin 1852

Insulin, Zinc Crystals (Potential for increased insulin requirements). Products include:
NPH, 100 Units 1502

Insulin, Zinc Suspension (Potential for increased insulin requirements). Products include:
Iletin I 1501
Lente, 100 Units 1501
Iletin II 1504
Pork Lente, 100 Units 1504
Purified Pork Lente Insulin 1852

Ketamine Hydrochloride (Potential for hypertension and tachycardia).
No products indexed under this heading.

Levonorgestrel (Increases serum thyroxine-binding globulin). Products include:
Levlen/Tri-Levlen 646
Nordette-21 Tablets 2863
Nordette-28 Tablets 2866
Norplant System 2868
Levlen/Tri-Levlen 646
Triphasil-21 Tablets 2919
Triphasil-28 Tablets 2924

Maprotiline Hydrochloride (Increased receptor sensitivity and enhanced antidepressant activity). Products include:
Ludiomil Tablets 861

Mestranol (Increases serum thyroxine-binding globulin). Products include:
Norinyl 2563
Ortho-Novum 1928

Metaraminol Bitartrate (Increased adrenergic effect). Products include:
Aramine Injection 1649

Metformin Hydrochloride (Potential for increased oral hypoglycemic requirements). Products include:
Glucophage Tablets 754

Methoxamine Hydrochloride (Increased adrenergic effect). Products include:
Vasoxyl Injection 1169

Norepinephrine Bitartrate (Increased adrenergic effect). Products include:
Levophed Bitartrate Injection 2445

Norethindrone (Increases serum thyroxine-binding globulin). Products include:
Brevicon 2563
Micronor Tablets 1903
Modicon 1928
Norinyl 2563
Nor-Q D Tablets 2598
Ortho-Novum 1928
Ovcon 765
Tri-Norinyl 2607

Norethynodrel (Increases serum thyroxine-binding globulin).
No products indexed under this heading.

Norgestimate (Increases serum thyroxine-binding globulin). Products include:
Ortho-Cyclen/Ortho-Tri-Cyclen 1914
Ortho-Cyclen/Ortho Tri-Cyclen 1914

Norgestrel (Increases serum thyroxine-binding globulin). Products include:
Lo/Ovral Tablets 2852
Lo/Ovral-28 Tablets 2857
Ovral Tablets 2877
Ovral-28 Tablets 2878
Ovrette Tablets 2878

Nortriptyline Hydrochloride (Increased receptor sensitivity and enhanced antidepressant activity). Products include:
Pamelor 2409

Phenylephrine Hydrochloride (Increased adrenergic effect). Products include:
Atrohist Plus Tablets 1605
Cerose DM .... ⊡ 853
D.A. II Tablets 972
D.A. Chewable Tablets 970
Dura-Vent/DA Tablets 972
Extendryl 1003
4-Way Fast Acting Nasal Spray (regular & mentholated) .... ⊡ 644
Hemorid .... ⊡ 797
Hycomine Compound Tablets 948
Neo-Synephrine Hydrochloride 1% Carpuject 2455
Neo-Synephrine Hydrochloride 1% Injection 2455
Neo-Synephrine Hydrochloride (Ophthalmic) 2456
Neo-Synephrine .... ⊡ 624
Novahistine Elixir .... ⊡ 782
Phenergan VC 2886
Phenergan VC with Codeine 2888
Preparation H .... ⊡ 842
Tympagesic Ear Drops 2476
Vicks Sinex Nasal Spray and Ultra Fine Mist .... ⊡ 738

Polyestradiol Phosphate (Increases serum thyroxine-binding globulin).
No products indexed under this heading.

(⊡ Described in PDR For Nonprescription Drugs) (⊙ Described in PDR For Ophthalmology)

1113 Interactions Index Tripedia

Protriptyline Hydrochloride (Increased receptor sensitivity and enhanced antidepressant activity). Products include:
Vivactil Tablets 1820
Quinestrol (Increases serum thyroxine-binding globulin).
No products indexed under this heading.
Tolazamide (Potential for increased oral hypoglycemic requirements).
No products indexed under this heading.
Tolbutamide (Potential for increased oral hypoglycemic requirements).
No products indexed under this heading.
Trimipramine Maleate (Increased receptor sensitivity and enhanced antidepressant activity). Products include:
Surmontil Capsules 2917
Warfarin Sodium (Increased catabolism of vitamin K-dependent clotting factors). Products include:
Coumadin 941

TRIPEDIA
(Diphtheria & Tetanus Toxoids w/Pertussis Vaccine Combined, Aluminum Potassium Sulfate Adsorbed) **908**
May interact with anticoagulants, alkylating agents, cytotoxic drugs, corticosteroids, and immunosuppressive agents. Compounds in these categories include:

Azathioprine (An adequate immunologic response may not be obtained if used concurrently). Products include:
Azathioprine Tablets 2349
Imuran 1103
Betamethasone Acetate (Corticosteroids, used in greater than physiologic doses, may reduce the immune response to vaccine). Products include:
Celestone Soluspan Suspension 2484
Betamethasone Sodium Phosphate (Corticosteroids, used in greater than physiologic doses, may reduce the immune response to vaccine). Products include:
Celestone Soluspan Suspension 2484
Bleomycin Sulfate (May reduce the immune response to vaccine). Products include:
Blenoxane 697
Busulfan (May reduce the immune response to vaccine). Products include:
Myleran Tablets 1209
Carmustine (BCNU) (May reduce the immune response to vaccine). Products include:
BiCNU 696
Chlorambucil (May reduce the immune response to vaccine). Products include:
Leukeran Tablets 1205
Cortisone Acetate (Corticosteroids, used in greater than physiologic doses, may reduce the immune response to vaccine). Products include:
Cortone Acetate Sterile Suspension 1663
Cortone Acetate Tablets 1664
Cyclophosphamide (May reduce the immune response to vaccine). Products include:
Cytoxan 700
Cyclosporine (An adequate immunologic response may not be obtained if used concurrently). Products include:
Neoral 2405
Sandimmune 2416
Cytarabine (May reduce the immune response to vaccine). Products include:
Cytosar-U Sterile Powder 2077
Dacarbazine (May reduce the immune response to vaccine). Products include:
DTIC-Dome 593
Dalteparin Sodium (Concurrent use requires caution). Products include:
Fragmin Injection 2088
Daunorubicin Hydrochloride (May reduce the immune response to vaccine). Products include:
Cerubidine for Injection 634
Dexamethasone (Corticosteroids, used in greater than physiologic doses, may reduce the immune response to vaccine). Products include:
AK-Trol Ointment & Suspension .... ⊙ 205
Decadron Elixir 1676
Decadron Tablets 1678
Decaspray Topical Aerosol 1689
Maxitrol Ophthalmic Ointment and Suspension .... ⊙ 222
TobraDex Ophthalmic Suspension and Ointment 469
Dexamethasone Acetate (Corticosteroids, used in greater than physiologic doses, may reduce the immune response to vaccine). Products include:
Dalalone D.P. Injectable 1009
Decadron-LA Sterile Suspension 1687
Dexamethasone Sodium Phosphate (Corticosteroids, used in greater than physiologic doses, may reduce the immune response to vaccine). Products include:
Decadron Phosphate Injection 1680
Decadron Phosphate Sterile Ophthalmic Ointment 1684
Decadron Phosphate Sterile Ophthalmic Solution 1685
Decadron Phosphate Topical Cream 1686
Decadron Phosphate with Xylocaine Injection, Sterile 1683
Dexacort Phosphate in Respihaler .. 1606
Dexacort Phosphate in Turbinaire .. 1607
NeoDecadron Sterile Ophthalmic Ointment 1755
NeoDecadron Sterile Ophthalmic Solution 1756
NeoDecadron Topical Cream 1757
Dicumarol (Concurrent use requires caution).
No products indexed under this heading.
Doxorubicin Hydrochloride (May reduce the immune response to vaccine). Products include:
Adriamycin PFS 2056
Adriamycin RDF 2056
Doxil 2613
Doxorubicin Astra 531
Rubex for Injection 721
Enoxaparin (Concurrent use requires caution). Products include:
Lovenox Injection 2187
Floxuridine (May reduce the immune response to vaccine). Products include:
Sterile FUDR 2284
Fludarabine Phosphate (May reduce the immune response to vaccine). Products include:
Fludara for Injection 658
Fludrocortisone Acetate (Corticosteroids, used in greater than physiologic doses, may reduce the immune response to vaccine). Products include:
Florinef Acetate Tablets 506
Fluorouracil (May reduce the immune response to vaccine). Products include:
Efudex 2280
Fluoroplex Topical Solution & Cream 1% 475
Fluorouracil Injection 2282
Heparin Calcium (Concurrent use requires caution).
No products indexed under this heading.
Heparin Sodium (Concurrent use requires caution). Products include:
Heparin Lock Flush Solution 2831
Heparin Sodium Injection 2832
Heparin Sodium Vials 1486
Hydrocortisone (Corticosteroids, used in greater than physiologic doses, may reduce the immune response to vaccine). Products include:
Anusol-HC Cream 2.5% 1953
Aquanil HC Lotion 1989
Maximum Strength Cortaid Spray ▣ 800
CORTENEMA 2713
Cortisporin Ointment 1074
Cortisporin Ophthalmic Ointment Sterile 1074
Cortisporin Ophthalmic Suspension Sterile 1075
Cortisporin Otic Solution Sterile 1076
Cortisporin Otic Suspension Sterile 1077
Cortizone-5 .... ▣ 795
Cortizone-10 .... ▣ 795
Hydrocortone Tablets 1715
Hytone 922
Hytone Ointment 2 ½% 923
Massengill Medicated Soft Cloth Towelettes 2628
Pediotic Suspension Sterile 1140
Preparation H Hydrocortisone 1% Cream .... ▣ 843
ProctoCream-HC 2.5% 2552
VōSoL HC Otic Solution 2786
Hydrocortisone Acetate (Corticosteroids, used in greater than physiologic doses, may reduce the immune response to vaccine). Products include:
Analpram-HC Rectal Cream 1% and 2.5% 993
Anusol HC-1 Hydrocortisone Anti-Itch Ointment .... ▣ 810
Anusol-HC Suppositories 1954
Caldecort Anti-Itch Hydrocortisone Cream .... ▣ 651
Coly-Mycin S Otic w/Neomycin & Hydrocortisone 1965
Cortaid .... ▣ 800
Cortifoam 2540
Cortisporin Cream 1073
Epifoam 2543
Hydrocortone Acetate Sterile Suspension 1712
Mantadil Cream 1124
Nupercainal Hydrocortisone 1% Cream .... ▣ 661
Pramosone Cream, Lotion & Ointment 995
ProctoFoam-HC 2552
Terra-Cortril Ophthalmic Suspension 2033
Hydrocortisone Sodium Phosphate (Corticosteroids, used in greater than physiologic doses, may reduce the immune response to vaccine). Products include:
Hydrocortone Phosphate Injection, Sterile 1713
Hydrocortisone Sodium Succinate (Corticosteroids, used in greater than physiologic doses, may reduce the immune response to vaccine).
No products indexed under this heading.
Hydroxyurea (May reduce the immune response to vaccine). Products include:
Hydrea Capsules 705
Immune Globulin (Human) (An adequate immunologic response may not be obtained if used concurrently).
No products indexed under this heading.
Immune Globulin Intravenous (Human) (An adequate immunologic response may not be obtained if used concurrently).
Influenza Virus Vaccine (Influenza Virus Vaccine should not be given within three days of the administration of Tripedia). Products include:
Fluvirin (Influenza Virus Vaccine) 1608
Influenza Virus Vaccine, Trivalent, Types A and B (chromatograph- and filter-purified subviron antigen) FluShield, 1996-1997 Formula 2842
Lomustine (CCNU) (May reduce the immune response to vaccine). Products include:
CeeNU Capsules 699
Mechlorethamine Hydrochloride (May reduce the immune response to vaccine). Products include:
Mustargen 1752
Melphalan (May reduce the immune response to vaccine). Products include:
Alkeran Tablets 1198
Methotrexate Sodium (May reduce the immune response to vaccine). Products include:
Methotrexate Sodium Tablets, Injection, for Injection and LPF Injection 1322
Methylprednisolone Acetate (Corticosteroids, used in greater than physiologic doses, may reduce the immune response to vaccine).
No products indexed under this heading.
Methylprednisolone Sodium Succinate (Corticosteroids, used in greater than physiologic doses, may reduce the immune response to vaccine).
No products indexed under this heading.
Mitotane (May reduce the immune response to vaccine). Products include:
Lysodren Tablets 707
Mitoxantrone Hydrochloride (May reduce the immune response to vaccine). Products include:
Novantrone for Injection 1327
Muromonab-CD3 (An adequate immunologic response may not be obtained if used concurrently). Products include:
Orthoclone OKT3 Sterile Solution .. 1892
Mycophenolate Mofetil (An adequate immunologic response may not be obtained if used concurrently). Products include:
CellCept Capsules 2265
Prednisolone Acetate (Corticosteroids, used in greater than physiologic doses, may reduce the immune response to vaccine). Products include:
AK-CIDE .... ⊙ 203
AK-CIDE Ointment .... ⊙ 203
Blephamide Liquifilm Sterile Ophthalmic Suspension 472
Blephamide Ointment .... ⊙ 234
Econopred & Econopred Plus Ophthalmic Suspensions .... ⊙ 216
Poly-Pred Liquifilm .... ⊙ 246
Pred Forte .... ⊙ 247

IMPORTANT NOTE: Always consult each drug listing in the patient's regimen for possible interactions.

Tripedia Interactions Index 1114

Pred Mild ⊙ 250
Pred-G Liquifilm Sterile Ophthalmic Suspension ⊙ 248
Pred-G S.O.P. Sterile Ophthalmic Ointment ⊙ 249

Prednisolone Sodium Phosphate (Corticosteroids, used in greater than physiologic doses, may reduce the immune response to vaccine). Products include:
AK-PRED ⊙ 204
Hydeltrasol Injection, Sterile 1708
Pediapred Oral Solution 1618

Prednisolone Tebutate (Corticosteroids, used in greater than physiologic doses, may reduce the immune response to vaccine). Products include:
Hydeltra-T.B.A. Sterile Suspension 1710

Prednisone (Corticosteroids, used in greater than physiologic doses, may reduce the immune response to vaccine).
No products indexed under this heading.

Procarbazine Hydrochloride (May reduce the immune response to vaccine). Products include:
Matulane Capsules 2300

Tacrolimus (An adequate immunologic response may not be obtained if used concurrently). Products include:
Prograf 1028

Tamoxifen Citrate (May reduce the immune response to vaccine). Products include:
Nolvadex Tablets 2957

Thioguanine (May reduce the immune response to vaccine). Products include:
Thioguanine Tablets, Tabloid Brand 1225

Thiotepa (May reduce the immune response to vaccine). Products include:
Thioplex (Thiotepa For Injection) 1329

Triamcinolone (Corticosteroids, used in greater than physiologic doses, may reduce the immune response to vaccine).
No products indexed under this heading.

Triamcinolone Acetonide (Corticosteroids, used in greater than physiologic doses, may reduce the immune response to vaccine). Products include:
Azmacort Oral Inhaler 2175
Nasacort AQ Nasal Spray 2191
Nasacort Nasal Inhaler 2189

Triamcinolone Diacetate (Corticosteroids, used in greater than physiologic doses, may reduce the immune response to vaccine).
No products indexed under this heading.

Triamcinolone Hexacetonide (Corticosteroids, used in greater than physiologic doses, may reduce the immune response to vaccine).
No products indexed under this heading.

Vincristine Sulfate (May reduce the immune response to vaccine). Products include:
Oncovin Solution Vials & Hyporets 1521

Warfarin Sodium (Concurrent use requires caution). Products include:
Coumadin 941

TRIPHASIL-21 TABLETS
(Levonorgestrel, Ethinyl Estradiol) 2919
May interact with barbiturates and certain other agents. Compounds in these categories include:

Ampicillin Sodium (Reduced efficacy; increased incidence of breakthrough bleeding). Products include:
Unasyn 2035

Aprobarbital (Reduced efficacy; increased incidence of breakthrough bleeding).
No products indexed under this heading.

Butabarbital (Reduced efficacy; increased incidence of breakthrough bleeding).
No products indexed under this heading.

Butalbital (Reduced efficacy; increased incidence of breakthrough bleeding). Products include:
Axocet Capsules 2469
Esgic-plus Capsules 1012
Esgic-plus Tablets 1012
Fioricet Tablets 2386
Fioricet with Codeine Capsules 2387
Fiorinal Capsules 2388
Fiorinal with Codeine Capsules 2390
Fiorinal Tablets 2388
Phrenilin 790
Sedapap Tablets 50 mg/650 mg 1826

Mephobarbital (Reduced efficacy; increased incidence of breakthrough bleeding). Products include:
Mebaral Tablets 2452

Oxytetracycline (Reduced efficacy; increased incidence of breakthrough bleeding). Products include:
Terramycin Intramuscular Solution 2034

Oxytetracycline Hydrochloride (Reduced efficacy; increased incidence of breakthrough bleeding). Products include:
TERAK Ointment ⊙ 210
Terra-Cortril Ophthalmic Suspension 2033
Terramycin with Polymyxin B Sulfate Ophthalmic Ointment 2035
Urobiotic-250 Capsules 2038

Pentobarbital Sodium (Reduced efficacy; increased incidence of breakthroughbleeding). Products include:
Nembutal Sodium Capsules 440
Nembutal Sodium Solution 442
Nembutal Sodium Suppositories 444

Phenobarbital (Reduced efficacy; increased incidence of breakthrough bleeding). Products include:
Arco-Lase Plus Tablets 513
Bellergal-S Tablets 2375
Donnatal 2234
Donnatal Extentabs 2234
Donnatal Tablets 2234
Phenobarbital Elixir and Tablets 1523
Quadrinal Tablets 1398

Phenylbutazone (Reduced efficacy; increased incidence of breakthrough bleeding).
No products indexed under this heading.

Phenytoin Sodium (Reduced efficacy; increased incidence of breakthrough bleeding). Products include:
Dilantin Kapseals 1965

Rifampin (Reduced efficacy; increased incidence of breakthrough bleeding). Products include:
Rifadin 1276
Rifamate Capsules 1278
Rifater 1280
Rimactane Capsules 865

Secobarbital Sodium (Reduced efficacy; increased incidence of breakthrough bleeding). Products include:
Seconal Sodium Pulvules 1529

Tetracycline Hydrochloride (Reduced efficacy; increased incidence of breakthrough bleeding). Products include:
Achromycin V Capsules 1417
Helidac Therapy 2135

Thiamylal Sodium (Reduced efficacy; increased incidence of breakthrough bleeding).
No products indexed under this heading.

TRIPHASIL-28 TABLETS
(Levonorgestrel, Ethinyl Estradiol) 2924
See **Triphasil-21 Tablets**

TRI-VI-FLOR DROPS
(Vitamins with Fluoride) 1601
None cited in PDR database.

TRISORALEN TABLETS
(Trioxsalen) 1309

Food Interactions
Food, furocoumarin-containing (Potential for severe reactions).

TRONOLANE ANESTHETIC CREAM FOR HEMORRHOIDS
(Pramoxine Hydrochloride) ▣ 746
None cited in PDR database.

TRONOLANE HEMORRHOIDAL SUPPOSITORIES
(Fat, Hard, Zinc Oxide) ▣ 747
None cited in PDR database.

TRUSOPT STERILE OPHTHALMIC SOLUTION
(Dorzolamide Hydrochloride) 1803
May interact with carbonic anhydrase inhibitors and certain other agents. Compounds in these categories include:

Acetazolamide (Potential for an additive effect on the known systemic effects of carbonic anhydrase inhibition in patients receiving a systemic carbonic anhydrase inhibitor and Trusopt). Products include:
Diamox Sequels (Sustained Release) ⊙ 318
Diamox Tablets ⊙ 317

Acetazolamide Sodium (Potential for an additive effect on the known systemic effects of carbonic anhydrase inhibition in patients receiving a systemic carbonic anhydrase inhibitor and Trusopt). Products include:
Diamox Intravenous ⊙ 317

Aspirin (Potential for acid-base and electrolyte disturbances with concomitant use; these disturbances have been reported with oral agent and have not been reported during clinical trials with Trusopt). Products include:
Alka-Seltzer Cherry Effervescent Antacid and Pain Reliever ▣ 609
Alka-Seltzer Extra Strength Effervescent Antacid and Pain Reliever ▣ 609
Alka-Seltzer Lemon Lime Effervescent Antacid and Pain Reliever ▣ 609
Alka-Seltzer Original Effervescent Antacid and Pain Reliever ▣ 609
Alka-Seltzer Plus ▣ 611
Alka-Seltzer Plus Sinus Medicine ▣ 611
Ascriptin ▣ 650
Arthritis Strength BC Powder ▣ 631
BC Cold Powder Multi-Symptom Formula (Cold-Sinus-Allergy) ▣ 631
BC Cold Powder Non-Drowsy Formula (Cold-Sinus) ▣ 631
BC Powder ▣ 631
Genuine Bayer Aspirin Tablets & Caplets ▣ 618
Extra Strength Bayer Arthritis Pain Regimen Formula ▣ 615
Extra Strength Bayer Aspirin Caplets & Tablets ▣ 617
Extended-Release Bayer 8-Hour Aspirin ▣ 616
Extra Strength Bayer Plus Aspirin Caplets ▣ 617
Extra Strength Bayer PM Aspirin Plus Sleep Aid ▣ 617
Aspirin Regimen Bayer 81 mg Tablets with Calcium ▣ 615
Aspirin Regimen Bayer Adult Low Strength 81 mg Tablets ▣ 613
Aspirin Regimen Bayer Children's Chewable Aspirin ▣ 616
Aspirin Regimen Bayer Regular Strength 325 mg Caplets ▣ 613
Bufferin Analgesic Tablets ▣ 636
Arthritis Strength Bufferin Analgesic Caplets ▣ 637
Extra Strength Bufferin Analgesic Tablets ▣ 637
Cama Arthritis Pain Reliever ▣ 748
Darvon Compound-65 Pulvules 1475
Easprin 1971
Ecotrin 2625
Ecotrin Enteric Coated Aspirin Maximum Strength Tablets and Caplets ▣ 775
Ecotrin Enteric Coated Aspirin Regular Strength Tablets 2625
Empirin Aspirin Tablets ▣ 818
Excedrin Extra-Strength Analgesic Tablets, Caplets, and Geltabs 734
Fiorinal Capsules 2388
Fiorinal with Codeine Capsules 2390
Fiorinal Tablets 2388
Goody's Extra Strength Headache Powders ▣ 632
Goody's Extra Strength Pain Relief Tablets ▣ 632
Halfprin Tablets 1413
Norgesic 1554
Percodan Tablets 955
Percodan-Demi Tablets 956
Robaxisal Tablets 2246
Soma Compound w/Codeine Tablets 2784
Soma Compound Tablets 2783
St. Joseph Adult Chewable Aspirin (81 mg.) ▣ 768
Talwin Compound 2466
Vanquish Analgesic Caplets ▣ 627

Dichlorphenamide (Potential for an additive effect on the known systemic effects of carbonic anhydrase inhibition in patients receiving a systemic carbonic anhydrase inhibitor and Trusopt). Products include:
Daranide Tablets 1676

Methazolamide (Potential for an additive effect on the known systemic effects of carbonic anhydrase inhibition in patients receiving a systemic carbonic anhydrase inhibitor and Trusopt). Products include:
GlaucTabs ⊙ 209
Neptazane Tablets ⊙ 320

T.R.U.E. TEST
(Allergens) 1162
None cited in PDR database.

TUBERCULIN, OLD, TINE TEST
(Tuberculin, Old) 2994
May interact with corticosteroids and immunosuppressive agents. Compounds in these categories include:

Azathioprine (Reactivity to the test may be suppressed). Products include:
Azathioprine Tablets 2349
Imuran 1103

Betamethasone Acetate (Reactivity to the test may be suppressed). Products include:
Celestone Soluspan Suspension 2484

Betamethasone Sodium Phosphate (Reactivity to the test may be suppressed). Products include:
Celestone Soluspan Suspension 2484

(▣ Described in PDR For Nonprescription Drugs) (⊙ Described in PDR For Ophthalmology)

Cortisone Acetate (Reactivity to the test may be suppressed). Products include:
  Cortone Acetate Sterile Suspension ... 1663
  Cortone Acetate Tablets ... 1664

Cyclosporine (Reactivity to the test may be suppressed). Products include:
  Neoral ... 2405
  Sandimmune ... 2416

Desoximetasone (Reactivity to the test may be suppressed). Products include:
  Topicort Emollient Cream 0.25% ... 1289
  Topicort Gel 0.05% ... 1290
  Topicort LP Emollient Cream 0.05% ... 1289
  Topicort Ointment 0.25% ... 1291

Dexamethasone Acetate (Reactivity to the test may be suppressed). Products include:
  Dalalone D.P. Injectable ... 1009
  Decadron-LA Sterile Suspension ... 1687

Dexamethasone Sodium Phosphate (Reactivity to the test may be suppressed). Products include:
  Decadron Phosphate Injection ... 1680
  Decadron Phosphate Sterile Ophthalmic Ointment ... 1684
  Decadron Phosphate Sterile Ophthalmic Solution ... 1685
  Decadron Phosphate Topical Cream ... 1686
  Decadron Phosphate with Xylocaine Injection, Sterile ... 1683
  Dexacort Phosphate in Respihaler .. 1606
  Dexacort Phosphate in Turbinaire .. 1607
  NeoDecadron Sterile Ophthalmic Ointment ... 1755
  NeoDecadron Sterile Ophthalmic Solution ... 1756
  NeoDecadron Topical Cream ... 1757

Fludrocortisone Acetate (Reactivity to the test may be suppressed). Products include:
  Florinef Acetate Tablets ... 506

Hydrocortisone (Reactivity to the test may be suppressed). Products include:
  Anusol-HC Cream 2.5% ... 1953
  Aquanil HC Lotion ... 1989
  Maximum Strength Cortaid Spray ... 800
  CORTENEMA ... 2713
  Cortisporin Ointment ... 1074
  Cortisporin Ophthalmic Ointment Sterile ... 1074
  Cortisporin Ophthalmic Suspension Sterile ... 1075
  Cortisporin Otic Solution Sterile ... 1076
  Cortisporin Otic Suspension Sterile 1077
  Cortizone-5 ... 795
  Cortizone-10 ... 795
  Hydrocortone Tablets ... 1715
  Hytone ... 922
  Hytone Ointment 2 ½% ... 923
  Massengill Medicated Soft Cloth Towelettes ... 2628
  Pediotic Suspension Sterile ... 1140
  Preparation H Hydrocortisone 1% Cream ... 843
  ProctoCream-HC 2.5% ... 2552
  VōSoL HC Otic Solution ... 2786

Hydrocortisone Acetate (Reactivity to the test may be suppressed). Products include:
  Analpram-HC Rectal Cream 1% and 2.5% ... 993
  Anusol HC-1 Hydrocortisone Anti-Itch Ointment ... 810
  Anusol-HC Suppositories ... 1954
  Caldecort Anti-Itch Hydrocortisone Cream ... 651
  Coly-Mycin S Otic w/Neomycin & Hydrocortisone ... 1965
  Cortaid ... 800
  Cortifoam ... 2540
  Cortisporin Cream ... 1073
  Epifoam ... 2543
  Hydrocortone Acetate Sterile Suspension ... 1712
  Mantadil Cream ... 1124
  Nupercainal Hydrocortisone 1% Cream ... 661
  Pramosone Cream, Lotion & Ointment ... 995

ProctoFoam-HC ... 2552
Terra-Cortril Ophthalmic Suspension ... 2033

Hydrocortisone Sodium Phosphate (Reactivity to the test may be suppressed). Products include:
  Hydrocortone Phosphate Injection, Sterile ... 1713

Hydrocortisone Sodium Succinate (Reactivity to the test may be suppressed).
  No products indexed under this heading.

Immune Globulin (Human) (Reactivity to the test may be suppressed).
  No products indexed under this heading.

Immune Globulin Intravenous (Human) (Reactivity to the test may be suppressed).
  No products indexed under this heading.

Methylprednisolone Acetate (Reactivity to the test may be suppressed).
  No products indexed under this heading.

Methylprednisolone Sodium Succinate (Reactivity to the test may be suppressed).
  No products indexed under this heading.

Muromonab-CD3 (Reactivity to the test may be suppressed). Products include:
  Orthoclone OKT3 Sterile Solution .. 1892

Mycophenolate Mofetil (Reactivity to the test may be suppressed). Products include:
  CellCept Capsules ... 2265

Prednisolone Acetate (Reactivity to the test may be suppressed). Products include:
  AK-CIDE ... 203
  AK-CIDE Ointment ... 203
  Blephamide Liquifilm Sterile Ophthalmic Suspension ... 472
  Blephamide Ointment ... 234
  Econopred & Econopred Plus Ophthalmic Suspensions ... 216
  Poly-Pred Liquifilm ... 246
  Pred Forte ... 247
  Pred Mild ... 250
  Pred-G Liquifilm Sterile Ophthalmic Suspension ... 248
  Pred-G S.O.P. Sterile Ophthalmic Ointment ... 249

Prednisolone Sodium Phosphate (Reactivity to the test may be suppressed). Products include:
  AK-PRED ... 204
  Hydeltrasol Injection, Sterile ... 1708
  Pediapred Oral Solution ... 1618

Prednisolone Tebutate (Reactivity to the test may be suppressed). Products include:
  Hydeltra-T.B.A. Sterile Suspension 1710

Prednisone (Reactivity to the test may be suppressed).
  No products indexed under this heading.

Tacrolimus (Reactivity to the test may be suppressed). Products include:
  Prograf ... 1028

Triamcinolone (Reactivity to the test may be suppressed).
  No products indexed under this heading.

Triamcinolone Acetonide (Reactivity to the test may be suppressed). Products include:
  Azmacort Oral Inhaler ... 2175
  Nasacort AQ Nasal Spray ... 2191
  Nasacort Nasal Inhaler ... 2189

Triamcinolone Diacetate (Reactivity to the test may be suppressed).
  No products indexed under this heading.

Triamcinolone Hexacetonide (Reactivity to the test may be suppressed).
  No products indexed under this heading.

TUBERSOL (TUBERCULIN PURIFIED PROTEIN DERIVATIVE (MANTOUX))
(Tuberculin, Purified Protein Derivative For Mantoux Test) ... 2988
May interact with corticosteroids, immunosuppressive agents, and certain other agents. Compounds in these categories include:

Azathioprine (Reactivity to the test may be suppressed or depressed). Products include:
  Azathioprine Tablets ... 2349
  Imuran ... 1103

Betamethasone Acetate (Reactivity to the test may be suppressed or depressed). Products include:
  Celestone Soluspan Suspension ... 2484

Betamethasone Sodium Phosphate (Reactivity to the test may be suppressed or depressed). Products include:
  Celestone Soluspan Suspension ... 2484

Cortisone Acetate (Reactivity to the test may be suppressed). Products include:
  Cortone Acetate Sterile Suspension ... 1663
  Cortone Acetate Tablets ... 1664

Cyclosporine (Reactivity to the test may be suppressed or depressed). Products include:
  Neoral ... 2405
  Sandimmune ... 2416

Dexamethasone (Reactivity to the test may be suppressed or depressed). Products include:
  AK-Trol Ointment & Suspension ... 205
  Decadron Elixir ... 1676
  Decadron Tablets ... 1678
  Decaspray Topical Aerosol ... 1689
  Maxitrol Ophthalmic Ointment and Suspension ... 222
  TobraDex Ophthalmic Suspension and Ointment ... 469

Dexamethasone Acetate (Reactivity to the test may be suppressed or depressed). Products include:
  Dalalone D.P. Injectable ... 1009
  Decadron-LA Sterile Suspension ... 1687

Dexamethasone Sodium Phosphate (Reactivity to the test may be suppressed or depressed). Products include:
  Decadron Phosphate Injection ... 1680
  Decadron Phosphate Sterile Ophthalmic Ointment ... 1684
  Decadron Phosphate Sterile Ophthalmic Solution ... 1685
  Decadron Phosphate Topical Cream ... 1686
  Decadron Phosphate with Xylocaine Injection, Sterile ... 1683
  Dexacort Phosphate in Respihaler .. 1606
  Dexacort Phosphate in Turbinaire .. 1607
  NeoDecadron Sterile Ophthalmic Ointment ... 1755
  NeoDecadron Sterile Ophthalmic Solution ... 1756
  NeoDecadron Topical Cream ... 1757

Fludrocortisone Acetate (Reactivity to the test may be suppressed or depressed). Products include:
  Florinef Acetate Tablets ... 506

Hydrocortisone (Reactivity to the test may be suppressed or depressed). Products include:
  Anusol-HC Cream 2.5% ... 1953
  Aquanil HC Lotion ... 1989
  Maximum Strength Cortaid Spray ... 800
  CORTENEMA ... 2713
  Cortisporin Ointment ... 1074
  Cortisporin Ophthalmic Ointment Sterile ... 1074
  Cortisporin Ophthalmic Suspension Sterile ... 1075

Cortisporin Otic Solution Sterile ... 1076
Cortisporin Otic Suspension Sterile 1077
Cortizone-5 ... 795
Cortizone-10 ... 795
Hydrocortone Tablets ... 1715
Hytone ... 922
Hytone Ointment 2 ½% ... 923
Massengill Medicated Soft Cloth Towelettes ... 2628
Pediotic Suspension Sterile ... 1140
Preparation H Hydrocortisone 1% Cream ... 843
ProctoCream-HC 2.5% ... 2552
VōSoL HC Otic Solution ... 2786

Hydrocortisone Acetate (Reactivity to the test may be suppressed or depressed). Products include:
  Analpram-HC Rectal Cream 1% and 2.5% ... 993
  Anusol HC-1 Hydrocortisone Anti-Itch Ointment ... 810
  Anusol-HC Suppositories ... 1954
  Caldecort Anti-Itch Hydrocortisone Cream ... 651
  Coly-Mycin S Otic w/Neomycin & Hydrocortisone ... 1965
  Cortaid ... 800
  Cortifoam ... 2540
  Cortisporin Cream ... 1073
  Epifoam ... 2543
  Hydrocortone Acetate Sterile Suspension ... 1712
  Mantadil Cream ... 1124
  Nupercainal Hydrocortisone 1% Cream ... 661
  Pramosone Cream, Lotion & Ointment ... 995
  ProctoFoam-HC ... 2552
  Terra-Cortril Ophthalmic Suspension ... 2033

Hydrocortisone Sodium Phosphate (Reactivity to the test may be suppressed or depressed). Products include:
  Hydrocortone Phosphate Injection, Sterile ... 1713

Hydrocortisone Sodium Succinate (Reactivity to the test may be suppressed or depressed).
  No products indexed under this heading.

Immune Globulin (Human) (Reactivity to the test may be suppressed or depressed).
  No products indexed under this heading.

Measles, Mumps & Rubella Virus Vaccine Live (Reactivity to the test may be temporarily depressed). Products include:
  M-M-R II ... 1730

Methylprednisolone Acetate (Reactivity to the test may be suppressed or depressed).
  No products indexed under this heading.

Methylprednisolone Sodium Succinate (Reactivity to the test may be suppressed or depressed).
  No products indexed under this heading.

Muromonab-CD3 (Reactivity to the test may be suppressed or depressed). Products include:
  Orthoclone OKT3 Sterile Solution .. 1892

Mycophenolate Mofetil (Reactivity to the test may be suppressed or depressed). Products include:
  CellCept Capsules ... 2265

Prednisolone Acetate (Reactivity to the test may be suppressed or depressed). Products include:
  AK-CIDE ... 203
  AK-CIDE Ointment ... 203
  Blephamide Liquifilm Sterile Ophthalmic Suspension ... 472
  Blephamide Ointment ... 234
  Econopred & Econopred Plus Ophthalmic Suspensions ... 216
  Poly-Pred Liquifilm ... 246
  Pred Forte ... 247
  Pred Mild ... 250
  Pred-G Liquifilm Sterile Ophthalmic Suspension ... 248

IMPORTANT NOTE: Always consult each drug listing in the patient's regimen for possible interactions.

Tubersol

Pred-G S.O.P. Sterile Ophthalmic
Ointment .... ⓞ 249

Prednisolone Sodium Phosphate (Reactivity to the test may be suppressed or depressed). Products include:
AK-PRED .... ⓞ 204
Hydeltrasol Injection, Sterile 1708
Pediapred Oral Solution 1618

Prednisolone Tebutate (Reactivity to the test may be suppressed or depressed). Products include:
Hydeltra-T.B.A. Sterile Suspension 1710

Prednisone (Reactivity to the test may be suppressed or depressed).
No products indexed under this heading.

Tacrolimus (Reactivity to the test may be suppressed or depressed). Products include:
Prograf 1028

Triamcinolone (Reactivity to the test may be suppressed or depressed).
No products indexed under this heading.

Triamcinolone Acetonide (Reactivity to the test may be suppressed or depressed). Products include:
Azmacort Oral Inhaler 2175
Nasacort AQ Nasal Spray 2191
Nasacort Nasal Inhaler 2189

Triamcinolone Diacetate (Reactivity to the test may be suppressed or depressed).
No products indexed under this heading.

Triamcinolone Hexacetonide (Reactivity to the test may be suppressed or depressed).
No products indexed under this heading.

TUCKS CLEAR HEMORRHOIDAL GEL
(Witch Hazel, Glycerin) .... ▣ 829
None cited in PDR database.

TUCKS PREMOISTENED HEMORRHOIDAL/VAGINAL PADS
(Witch Hazel) .... ▣ 830
None cited in PDR database.

TUCKS TAKE-ALONGS
(Witch Hazel) .... ▣ 830
None cited in PDR database.

TUMS ANTACID/CALCIUM SUPPLEMENT TABLETS
(Calcium Carbonate) .... ▣ 787
May interact with:

Drugs, Oral, unspecified (Antacids may interact with certain unspecified prescription drugs).

TUMS ANTI-GAS/ANTACID FORMULA TABLETS, ASSORTED FRUIT
(Calcium Carbonate, Simethicone) ▣ 788
May interact with:

Prescription Drugs, unspecified (Antacids may interact with certain unspecified prescription drugs; consult your doctor).

TUMS E-X ANTACID/CALCIUM SUPPLEMENT TABLETS
(Calcium Carbonate) .... ▣ 787
See **Tums Antacid/Calcium Supplement Tablets**

TUMS 500 CALCIUM SUPPLEMENT
(Calcium Carbonate) .... ▣ 788
None cited in PDR database.

TUMS ULTRA ANTACID/CALCIUM SUPPLEMENT TABLETS
(Calcium Carbonate) .... ▣ 787
See **Tums Antacid/Calcium Supplement Tablets**

TUSSEND
(Hydrocodone Bitartrate, Pseudoephedrine Hydrochloride, Chlorpheniramine Maleate) 1830
May interact with narcotic analgesics, antipsychotic agents, tranquilizers, central nervous system depressants, tricyclic antidepressants, monoamine oxidase inhibitors, beta blockers, veratrum alkaloids, anticholinergics, cardiac glycosides, and certain other agents. Compounds in these categories include:

Acebutolol Hydrochloride (Potentiates the sympathomimetic effects of pseudoephedrine; hypertensive crises can occur with concurrent use). Products include:
Sectral Capsules 2914

Alfentanil Hydrochloride (Concomitant use may exhibit additive CNS depression). Products include:
Alfenta Injection 1334

Alprazolam (Concomitant use may exhibit additive CNS depression). Products include:
Xanax Tablets 2115

Amitriptyline Hydrochloride (Concomitant use may increase the effects of either the antidepressant or hydrocodone; may antagonize the effects of pseudoephedrine). Products include:
Elavil 2945
Etrafon 2495
Limbitrol 2333
Triavil Tablets 1800

Amoxapine (Concomitant use may increase the effects of either the antidepressant or hydrocodone; may antagonize the effects of pseudoephedrine). Products include:
Asendin Tablets 1419

Aprobarbital (Concomitant use may exhibit additive CNS depression).
No products indexed under this heading.

Atenolol (Potentiates the sympathomimetic effects of pseudoephedrine; hypertensive crises can occur with concurrent use). Products include:
Tenoretic Tablets 2963
Tenormin Tablets and I.V. Injection 2965

Atropine Sulfate (Concurrent use of anticholinergics and hydrocodone may produce paralytic ileus). Products include:
Arco-Lase Plus Tablets 513
Atrohist Plus Tablets 1605
Donnatal 2234
Donnatal Extentabs 2234
Donnatal Tablets 2234
Lomotil 2591
Motofen Tablets 789
Urised Tablets 2123

Belladonna Alkaloids (Concurrent use of anticholinergics and hydrocodone may produce paralytic ileus). Products include:
Bellergal-S Tablets 2375
Hyland's Bedwetting Tablets .... ▣ 788
Hyland's EnurAid Tablets .... ▣ 789
Hyland's Headache Tablets .... ▣ 790
Hyland's Teething Tablets .... ▣ 790
Similasan Eye Drops # 1 .... ▣ 769

Benztropine Mesylate (Concurrent use of anticholinergics and hydrocodone may produce paralytic ileus). Products include:
Cogentin 1661

Betaxolol Hydrochloride (Potentiates the sympathomimetic effects of pseudoephedrine; hypertensive crises can occur with concurrent use). Products include:
Betoptic Ophthalmic Solution 465
Betoptic S Ophthalmic Suspension 467
Kerlone Tablets 2588

Biperiden Hydrochloride (Concurrent use of anticholinergics and hydrocodone may produce paralytic ileus). Products include:
Akineton 1380

Bisoprolol Fumarate (Potentiates the sympathomimetic effects of pseudoephedrine; hypertensive crises can occur with concurrent use). Products include:
Zebeta Tablets 1457
Ziac 1459

Buprenorphine (Concomitant use may exhibit additive CNS depression). Products include:
Buprenex Injectable 2170

Buspirone Hydrochloride (Concomitant use may exhibit additive CNS depression). Products include:
BuSpar Tablets 738

Butabarbital (Concomitant use may exhibit additive CNS depression).
No products indexed under this heading.

Butalbital (Concomitant use may exhibit additive CNS depression). Products include:
Axocet Capsules 2469
Esgic-plus Capsules 1012
Esgic-plus Tablets 1012
Fioricet Tablets 2386
Fioricet with Codeine Capsules ... 2387
Fiorinal Capsules 2388
Fiorinal with Codeine Capsules ... 2390
Fiorinal Tablets 2388
Phrenilin 790
Sedapap Tablets 50 mg/650 mg .. 1826

Carteolol Hydrochloride (Potentiates the sympathomimetic effects of pseudoephedrine; hypertensive crises can occur with concurrent use). Products include:
Cartrol Tablets 413
Ocupress Ophthalmic Solution, 1 % Sterile .... ⓞ 297

Chlordiazepoxide (Concomitant use may exhibit additive CNS depression). Products include:
Limbitrol 2333

Chlordiazepoxide Hydrochloride (Concomitant use may exhibit additive CNS depression). Products include:
Librax Capsules 2330
Librium Capsules 2331
Librium Injectable 2332

Chlorpromazine (Concomitant use may exhibit additive CNS depression). Products include:
Thorazine Suppositories 2701

Chlorpromazine Hydrochloride (Concomitant use may exhibit additive CNS depression). Products include:
Thorazine 2701

Chlorprothixene (Concomitant use may exhibit additive CNS depression).
No products indexed under this heading.

Chlorprothixene Hydrochloride (Concomitant use may exhibit additive CNS depression).
No products indexed under this heading.

Chlorprothixene Lactate (Concomitant use may exhibit additive CNS depression).
No products indexed under this heading.

Clidinium Bromide (Concurrent use of anticholinergics and hydrocodone may produce paralytic ileus). Products include:
Librax Capsules 2330

Clomipramine Hydrochloride (Concomitant use may increase the effects of either the antidepressant or hydrocodone; may antagonize the effects of pseudoephedrine). Products include:
Anafranil Capsules 819

Clorazepate Dipotassium (Concomitant use may exhibit additive CNS depression). Products include:
Tranxene 459

Clozapine (Concomitant use may exhibit additive CNS depression). Products include:
Clozaril Tablets 2377

Codeine Phosphate (Concomitant use may exhibit additive CNS depression). Products include:
Brontex 2130
Dimetane-DC Cough Syrup 2232
Fioricet with Codeine Capsules ... 2387
Fiorinal with Codeine Capsules ... 2390
Nucofed 2225
Phenergan with Codeine 2883
Phenergan VC with Codeine 2888
Robitussin A-C Syrup 2248
Robitussin-DAC Syrup 2249
Ryna .... ▣ 804
Soma Compound w/Codeine Tablets 2784
Tylenol with Codeine 1592

Cryptenamine Preparations (Sympathomimetic may reduce the antihypertensive effects of veratrum alkaloids).

Desflurane (Concomitant use may exhibit additive CNS depression). Products include:
Suprane (desflurane, USP) 1865

Desipramine Hydrochloride (Concomitant use may increase the effects of either the antidepressant or hydrocodone; may antagonize the effects of pseudoephedrine). Products include:
Norpramin Tablets 1273

Deslanoside (Concurrent use of digitalis glycoside may increase the possibility of cardiac arrhythmias).
No products indexed under this heading.

Dezocine (Concomitant use may exhibit additive CNS depression). Products include:
Dalgan Injection 529

Diazepam (Concomitant use may exhibit additive CNS depression). Products include:
Dizac (diazepam injectable emulsion) CIV 1862
Valium Injectable 2336
Valium Tablets 2335

Dicyclomine Hydrochloride (Concurrent use of anticholinergics and hydrocodone may produce paralytic ileus). Products include:
Bentyl 1246

Digitoxin (Concurrent use of digitalis glycoside may increase the possibility of cardiac arrhythmias). Products include:
Crystodigin Tablets 1472

Digoxin (Concurrent use of digitalis glycoside may increase the possibility of cardiac arrhythmias). Products include:
Lanoxicaps 1110
Lanoxin Elixir Pediatric 1113
Lanoxin Injection 1116
Lanoxin Injection Pediatric 1119
Lanoxin Tablets 1121

Doxepin Hydrochloride (Concomitant use may increase the effects of either the antidepressant or hydrocodone; may antagonize the effects of pseudoephedrine). Products include:
- Adapin Capsules 1542
- Sinequan 2028
- Zonalon Cream 1042

Droperidol (Concomitant use may exhibit additive CNS depression). Products include:
- Inapsine Injection 462

Enflurane (Concomitant use may exhibit additive CNS depression).
No products indexed under this heading.

Esmolol Hydrochloride (Potentiates the sympathomimetic effects of pseudoephedrine; hypertensive crises can occur with concurrent use). Products include:
- Brevibloc (esmolol HCl) Injection 1860

Estazolam (Concomitant use may exhibit additive CNS depression). Products include:
- ProSom Tablets 457

Ethchlorvynol (Concomitant use may exhibit additive CNS depression). Products include:
- Placidyl Capsules 456

Ethinamate (Concomitant use may exhibit additive CNS depression).
No products indexed under this heading.

Fentanyl (Concomitant use may exhibit additive CNS depression). Products include:
- Duragesic Transdermal System 1336

Fentanyl Citrate (Concomitant use may exhibit additive CNS depression). Products include:
- Sublimaze Injection 463

Fluphenazine Decanoate (Concomitant use may exhibit additive CNS depression). Products include:
- Prolixin Decanoate 510

Fluphenazine Enanthate (Concomitant use may exhibit additive CNS depression). Products include:
- Prolixin Enanthate 510

Fluphenazine Hydrochloride (Concomitant use may exhibit additive CNS depression). Products include:
- Prolixin 510

Flurazepam Hydrochloride (Concomitant use may exhibit additive CNS depression). Products include:
- Dalmane Capsules 2329

Furazolidone (Potentiates the sympathomimetic effects of pseudoephedrine and may result in hypertensive crisis; concurrent use is contraindicated). Products include:
- Furoxone 2221

Glutethimide (Concomitant use may exhibit additive CNS depression).
No products indexed under this heading.

Glycopyrrolate (Concurrent use of anticholinergics and hydrocodone may produce paralytic ileus). Products include:
- Robinul Forte Tablets 2247
- Robinul Injectable 2247
- Robinul Tablets 2247

Guanethidine Monosulfate (Sympathomimetic may reduce the antihypertensive effects). Products include:
- Esimil Tablets 840
- Ismelin Tablets 845

Haloperidol (Concomitant use may exhibit additive CNS depression). Products include:
- Haldol Injection, Tablets and Concentrate 1585

Haloperidol Decanoate (Concomitant use may exhibit additive CNS depression). Products include:
- Haldol Decanoate 1587

Hydrocodone Polistirex (Concomitant use may exhibit additive CNS depression). Products include:
- Tussionex Pennkinetic Extended-Release Suspension 1624

Hydromorphone Hydrochloride (Concomitant use may exhibit additive CNS depression). Products include:
- Dilaudid Ampules 1382
- Dilaudid Cough Syrup 1383
- Dilaudid-HP Injection 1384
- Dilaudid-HP Lyophilized Powder 250 mg 1384
- Dilaudid 1382
- Dilaudid Oral Liquid 1386
- Dilaudid 1382
- Dilaudid Tablets - 8 mg. 1386

Hydroxyzine Hydrochloride (Concomitant use may exhibit additive CNS depression). Products include:
- Atarax Tablets & Syrup 1992
- Marax Tablets & DF Syrup ... 2015
- Vistaril Intramuscular Solution 2042

Hyoscyamine (Concurrent use of anticholinergics and hydrocodone may produce paralytic ileus). Products include:
- Cystospaz Tablets 2123
- Urised Tablets 2123

Hyoscyamine Sulfate (Concurrent use of anticholinergics and hydrocodone may produce paralytic ileus). Products include:
- Arco-Lase Plus Tablets 513
- Atrohist Plus Tablets 1605
- Cystospaz-M Capsules 2123
- Donnatal 2234
- Donnatal Extentabs 2234
- Donnatal Tablets 2234
- Kutrase Capsules 2546
- Levsin/Levsinex/Levbid 2549

Imipramine Hydrochloride (Concomitant use may increase the effects of either the antidepressant or hydrocodone; may antagonize the effects of pseudoephedrine). Products include:
- Tofranil Ampuls 873
- Tofranil Tablets 875

Imipramine Pamoate (Concomitant use may increase the effects of either the antidepressant or hydrocodone; may antagonize the effects of pseudoephedrine). Products include:
- Tofranil-PM Capsules 876

Indomethacin (Hypertensive crises can occur with concurrent use). Products include:
- Indocin 1723

Indomethacin Sodium Trihydrate (Hypertensive crises can occur with concurrent use). Products include:
- Indocin I.V. 1727

Ipratropium Bromide (Concurrent use of anticholinergics and hydrocodone may produce paralytic ileus). Products include:
- Atrovent Inhalation Aerosol .. 674
- Atrovent Inhalation Solution . 675
- Atrovent Nasal Spray 0.03% . 676
- Atrovent Nasal Spray 0.06% . 678

Isocarboxazid (Potentiates the sympathomimetic effects of pseudoephedrine and may result in hypertensive crisis; concurrent use is contraindicated).
No products indexed under this heading.

Isoflurane (Concomitant use may exhibit additive CNS depression).
No products indexed under this heading.

Ketamine Hydrochloride (Concomitant use may exhibit additive CNS depression).
No products indexed under this heading.

Labetalol Hydrochloride (Potentiates the sympathomimetic effects of pseudoephedrine; hypertensive crises can occur with concurrent use). Products include:
- Normodyne Injection 2519
- Normodyne Tablets 2522
- Trandate 1158

Levobunolol Hydrochloride (Potentiates the sympathomimetic effects of pseudoephedrine; hypertensive crises can occur with concurrent use). Products include:
- Betagan .... ⓟ 230

Levomethadyl Acetate Hydrochloride (Concomitant use may exhibit additive CNS depression). Products include:
- Orlaam Oral Solution 2361

Levorphanol Tartrate (Concomitant use may exhibit additive CNS depression). Products include:
- Levo-Dromoran 2297

Lithium Carbonate (Concomitant use may exhibit additive CNS depression). Products include:
- Eskalith 2658
- Lithium Carbonate Capsules & Tablets 2352
- Lithonate/Lithotabs/Lithobid . 2721

Lithium Citrate (Concomitant use may exhibit additive CNS depression).
No products indexed under this heading.

Lorazepam (Concomitant use may exhibit additive CNS depression). Products include:
- Ativan Injection 2805
- Ativan Tablets 2807

Loxapine Hydrochloride (Concomitant use may exhibit additive CNS depression). Products include:
- Loxitane 1426

Loxapine Succinate (Concomitant use may exhibit additive CNS depression). Products include:
- Loxitane Capsules 1426

Maprotiline Hydrochloride (Concomitant use may increase the effects of either the antidepressant or hydrocodone; may antagonize the effects of pseudoephedrine). Products include:
- Ludiomil Tablets 861

Mecamylamine Hydrochloride (Sympathomimetic may reduce the antihypertensive effects). Products include:
- Inversine Tablets 1729

Mepenzolate Bromide (Concurrent use of anticholinergics and hydrocodone may produce paralytic ileus).
No products indexed under this heading.

Meperidine Hydrochloride (Concomitant use may exhibit additive CNS depression). Products include:
- Demerol 2438
- Mepergan Injection 2859

Mephobarbital (Concomitant use may exhibit additive CNS depression). Products include:
- Mebaral Tablets 2452

Meprobamate (Concomitant use may exhibit additive CNS depression). Products include:
- Miltown Tablets 2780
- PMB 200 and PMB 400 2890

Mesoridazine Besylate (Concomitant use may exhibit additive CNS depression). Products include:
- Serentil 689

Methadone Hydrochloride (Concomitant use may exhibit additive CNS depression). Products include:
- Methadone Hydrochloride Oral Concentrate 2356
- Methadone Hydrochloride Oral Solution & Tablets 2357

Methohexital Sodium (Concomitant use may exhibit additive CNS depression).
No products indexed under this heading.

Methotrimeprazine (Concomitant use may exhibit additive CNS depression). Products include:
- Levoprome 1321

Methoxyflurane (Concomitant use may exhibit additive CNS depression).
No products indexed under this heading.

Methyldopa (Sympathomimetic may reduce the antihypertensive effects; hypertensive crises can occur with concurrent use). Products include:
- Aldoclor Tablets 1638
- Aldomet Oral 1640
- Aldoril Tablets 1644

Methyldopate Hydrochloride (Sympathomimetic may reduce the antihypertensive effects; hypertensive crises can occur with concurrent use). Products include:
- Aldomet Ester HCl Injection . 1642

Metipranolol Hydrochloride (Potentiates the sympathomimetic effects of pseudoephedrine; hypertensive crises can occur with concurrent use). Products include:
- OptiPranolol (Metipranolol 0.3%) Sterile Ophthalmic Solution .... ⓟ 256

Metoprolol Succinate (Potentiates the sympathomimetic effects of pseudoephedrine; hypertensive crises can occur with concurrent use). Products include:
- Toprol-XL Tablets 560

Metoprolol Tartrate (Potentiates the sympathomimetic effects of pseudoephedrine; hypertensive crises can occur with concurrent use). Products include:
- Lopressor 848
- Lopressor HCT Tablets 850

Midazolam Hydrochloride (Concomitant use may exhibit additive CNS depression). Products include:
- Versed Injection 2324

Molindone Hydrochloride (Concomitant use may exhibit additive CNS depression). Products include:
- Moban Tablets and Concentrate 1036

Morphine Sulfate (Concomitant use may exhibit additive CNS depression). Products include:
- Astramorph/PF Injection, USP (Preservative-Free) 526
- Duramorph Injection 983
- Infumorph 200 and Infumorph 500 Sterile Solutions 985
- Kadian Capsules 2948
- MS Contin Tablets 2149
- MSIR 2152
- Oramorph SR (Morphine Sulfate Sustained Release Tablets) 2359
- RMS Suppositories CII 2766
- Roxanol 2365

IMPORTANT NOTE: Always consult each drug listing in the patient's regimen for possible interactions.

Nadolol (Potentiates the sympathomimetic effects of pseudoephedrine; hypertensive crises can occur with concurrent use).
No products indexed under this heading.

Nortriptyline Hydrochloride (Concomitant use may increase the effects of either the antidepressant or hydrocodone; may antagonize the effects of pseudoephedrine). Products include:
Pamelor 2409

Opium Alkaloids (Concomitant use may exhibit additive CNS depression).
No products indexed under this heading.

Oxazepam (Concomitant use may exhibit additive CNS depression). Products include:
Serax Capsules 2916
Serax Tablets 2916

Oxybutynin Chloride (Concurrent use of anticholinergics and hydrocodone may produce paralytic ileus). Products include:
Ditropan 1267

Oxycodone Hydrochloride (Concomitant use may exhibit additive CNS depression). Products include:
OxyContin Tablets 2163
OxyIR Capsules 2167
Percocet Tablets 955
Percodan Tablets 955
Percodan-Demi Tablets 956
Roxicodone Tablets, Oral Solution & Intensol (Oxycodone) 2366
Tylox Capsules 1593

Penbutolol Sulfate (Potentiates the sympathomimetic effects of pseudoephedrine; hypertensive crises can occur with concurrent use). Products include:
Levatol Tablets 2547

Pentobarbital Sodium (Concomitant use may exhibit additive CNS depression). Products include:
Nembutal Sodium Capsules 440
Nembutal Sodium Solution 442
Nembutal Sodium Suppositories 444

Perphenazine (Concomitant use may exhibit additive CNS depression). Products include:
Etrafon 2495
Triavil Tablets 1800
Trilafon 2532

Phenelzine Sulfate (Potentiates the sympathomimetic effects of pseudoephedrine and may result in hypertensive crisis; concurrent use is contraindicated). Products include:
Nardil 1977

Phenobarbital (Concomitant use may exhibit additive CNS depression). Products include:
Arco-Lase Plus Tablets 513
Bellergal-S Tablets 2375
Donnatal 2234
Donnatal Extentabs 2234
Donnatal Tablets 2234
Phenobarbital Elixir and Tablets 1523
Quadrinal Tablets 1398

Pimozide (Concomitant use may exhibit additive CNS depression). Products include:
Orap Tablets 1037

Pindolol (Potentiates the sympathomimetic effects of pseudoephedrine; hypertensive crises can occur with concurrent use). Products include:
Visken Tablets 2428

Prazepam (Concomitant use may exhibit additive CNS depression).
No products indexed under this heading.

Prochlorperazine (Concomitant use may exhibit additive CNS depression). Products include:
Compazine 2644

Procyclidine Hydrochloride (Concurrent use of anticholinergics and hydrocodone may produce paralytic ileus). Products include:
Kemadrin Tablets 1105

Promethazine Hydrochloride (Concomitant use may exhibit additive CNS depression). Products include:
Mepergan Injection 2859
Phenergan with Codeine 2883
Phenergan with Dextromethorphan 2885
Phenergan Injection 2880
Phenergan Suppositories 2882
Phenergan Syrup 2881
Phenergan Tablets 2882
Phenergan VC 2886
Phenergan VC with Codeine 2888

Propantheline Bromide (Concurrent use of anticholinergics and hydrocodone may produce paralytic ileus). Products include:
Pro-Banthine Tablets 2226

Propofol (Concomitant use may exhibit additive CNS depression). Products include:
Diprivan Injectable Emulsion 2939

Propoxyphene Hydrochloride (Concomitant use may exhibit additive CNS depression). Products include:
Darvon 1475
Wygesic Tablets 2930

Propoxyphene Napsylate (Concomitant use may exhibit additive CNS depression). Products include:
Darvon-N/Darvocet-N 1473

Propranolol Hydrochloride (Potentiates the sympathomimetic effects of pseudoephedrine; hypertensive crises can occur with concurrent use). Products include:
Inderal 2834
Inderal LA Long Acting Capsules 2836
Inderide Tablets 2838
Inderide LA Long Acting Capsules .. 2840

Protriptyline Hydrochloride (Concomitant use may increase the effects of either the antidepressant or hydrocodone; may antagonize the effects of pseudoephedrine). Products include:
Vivactil Tablets 1820

Quazepam (Concomitant use may exhibit additive CNS depression). Products include:
Doral Tablets 2773

Reserpine (Sympathomimetic may reduce the antihypertensive effects). Products include:
Diupres Tablets 1691
Hydropres Tablets 1718
Ser-Ap-Es Tablets 867

Risperidone (Concomitant use may exhibit additive CNS depression). Products include:
Risperdal Tablets 1348

Scopolamine (Concurrent use of anticholinergics and hydrocodone may produce paralytic ileus). Products include:
Transderm Scōp Transdermal Therapeutic System 890

Scopolamine Hydrobromide (Concurrent use of anticholinergics and hydrocodone may produce paralytic ileus). Products include:
Atrohist Plus Tablets 1605
Donnatal 2234
Donnatal Extentabs 2234
Donnatal Tablets 2234

Secobarbital Sodium (Concomitant use may exhibit additive CNS depression). Products include:
Seconal Sodium Pulvules 1529

Selegiline Hydrochloride (Potentiates the sympathomimetic effects of pseudoephedrine and may result in hypertensive crisis; concurrent use is contraindicated). Products include:
Eldepryl Capsules 2729

Sevoflurane (Concomitant use may exhibit additive CNS depression).
No products indexed under this heading.

Sotalol Hydrochloride (Potentiates the sympathomimetic effects of pseudoephedrine; hypertensive crises can occur with concurrent use). Products include:
Betapace Tablets 637

Sufentanil Citrate (Concomitant use may exhibit additive CNS depression). Products include:
Sufenta Injection 1355

Temazepam (Concomitant use may exhibit additive CNS depression). Products include:
Restoril Capsules 2413

Thiamylal Sodium (Concomitant use may exhibit additive CNS depression).
No products indexed under this heading.

Thioridazine Hydrochloride (Concomitant use may exhibit additive CNS depression). Products include:
Mellaril 2398

Thiothixene (Concomitant use may exhibit additive CNS depression). Products include:
Navane Capsules and Concentrate 2018
Navane Intramuscular 2019

Timolol Hemihydrate (Potentiates the sympathomimetic effects of pseudoephedrine; hypertensive crises can occur with concurrent use). Products include:
Betimol 0.25%, 0.5% .... ◉ 259

Timolol Maleate (Potentiates the sympathomimetic effects of pseudoephedrine; hypertensive crises can occur with concurrent use). Products include:
Blocadren Tablets 1654
Timolide Tablets 1791
Timoptic in Ocudose 1796
Timoptic Sterile Ophthalmic Solution 1794
Timoptic-XE 1798

Tranylcypromine Sulfate (Potentiates the sympathomimetic effects of pseudoephedrine and may result in hypertensive crisis; concurrent use is contraindicated). Products include:
Parnate Tablets 2679

Triazolam (Concomitant use may exhibit additive CNS depression). Products include:
Halcion Tablets 2093

Tridihexethyl Chloride (Concurrent use of anticholinergics and hydrocodone may produce paralytic ileus).
No products indexed under this heading.

Trifluoperazine Hydrochloride (Concomitant use may exhibit additive CNS depression). Products include:
Stelazine 2692

Trihexyphenidyl Hydrochloride (Concurrent use of anticholinergics and hydrocodone may produce paralytic ileus). Products include:
Artane 1418

Trimipramine Maleate (Concomitant use may increase the effects of either the antidepressant or hydrocodone; may antagonize the effects of pseudoephedrine). Products include:
Surmontil Capsules 2917

Zolpidem Tartrate (Concomitant use may exhibit additive CNS depression). Products include:
Ambien Tablets 2559

Food Interactions

Alcohol (Concomitant use may exhibit additive CNS depression).

TUSSEND EXPECTORANT
(Hydrocodone Bitartrate, Pseudoephedrine Hydrochloride, Guaifenesin) 1831
May interact with narcotic analgesics, general anesthetics, tranquilizers, hypnotics and sedatives, tricyclic antidepressants, central nervous system depressants, monoamine oxidase inhibitors, beta blockers, veratrum alkaloids, and certain other agents. Compounds in these categories include:

Acebutolol Hydrochloride (Potentiates the sympathomimetic effects of pseudoephedrine). Products include:
Sectral Capsules 2914

Alfentanil Hydrochloride (Hydrocodone may potentiate CNS depressant effects). Products include:
Alfenta Injection 1334

Alprazolam (Hydrocodone may potentiate CNS depressant effects). Products include:
Xanax Tablets 2115

Amitriptyline Hydrochloride (Hydrocodone may potentiate CNS depressant effects). Products include:
Elavil 2945
Etrafon 2495
Limbitrol 2333
Triavil Tablets 1800

Amoxapine (Hydrocodone may potentiate CNS depressant effects). Products include:
Asendin Tablets 1419

Aprobarbital (Hydrocodone may potentiate CNS depressant effects).
No products indexed under this heading.

Atenolol (Potentiates the sympathomimetic effects of pseudoephedrine). Products include:
Tenoretic Tablets 2963
Tenormin Tablets and I.V. Injection 2965

Betaxolol Hydrochloride (Potentiates the sympathomimetic effects of pseudoephedrine). Products include:
Betoptic Ophthalmic Solution 465
Betoptic S Ophthalmic Suspension 467
Kerlone Tablets 2588

Bisoprolol Fumarate (Potentiates the sympathomimetic effects of pseudoephedrine). Products include:
Zebeta Tablets 1457
Ziac 1459

Buprenorphine (Hydrocodone may potentiate CNS depressant effects). Products include:
Buprenex Injectable 2170

Buspirone Hydrochloride (Hydrocodone may potentiate CNS depressant effects). Products include:
BuSpar Tablets 738

Butabarbital (Hydrocodone may potentiate CNS depressant effects).
No products indexed under this heading.

(▣ Described in PDR For Nonprescription Drugs) (◉ Described in PDR For Ophthalmology)

Butalbital (Hydrocodone may potentiate CNS depressant effects). Products include:
Axocet Capsules ... 2469
Esgic-plus Capsules ... 1012
Esgic-plus Tablets ... 1012
Fioricet Tablets ... 2386
Fioricet with Codeine Capsules ... 2387
Fiorinal Capsules ... 2388
Fiorinal with Codeine Capsules ... 2390
Fiorinal Tablets ... 2388
Phrenilin ... 790
Sedapap Tablets 50 mg/650 mg .. 1826

Carteolol Hydrochloride (Potentiates the sympathomimetic effects of pseudoephedrine). Products include:
Cartrol Tablets ... 413
Ocupress Ophthalmic Solution, 1% Sterile ... ⊙ 297

Chlordiazepoxide (Hydrocodone may potentiate CNS depressant effects). Products include:
Limbitrol ... 2333

Chlordiazepoxide Hydrochloride (Hydrocodone may potentiate CNS depressant effects). Products include:
Librax Capsules ... 2330
Librium Capsules ... 2331
Librium Injectable ... 2332

Chlorpromazine (Hydrocodone may potentiate CNS depressant effects). Products include:
Thorazine Suppositories ... 2701

Chlorpromazine Hydrochloride (Hydrocodone may potentiate CNS depressant effects). Products include:
Thorazine ... 2701

Chlorprothixene (Hydrocodone may potentiate CNS depressant effects).
No products indexed under this heading.

Chlorprothixene Hydrochloride (Hydrocodone may potentiate CNS depressant effects).
No products indexed under this heading.

Chlorprothixene Lactate (Hydrocodone may potentiate CNS depressant effects).
No products indexed under this heading.

Clomipramine Hydrochloride (Hydrocodone may potentiate CNS depressant effects). Products include:
Anafranil Capsules ... 819

Clorazepate Dipotassium (Hydrocodone may potentiate CNS depressant effects). Products include:
Tranxene ... 459

Clozapine (Hydrocodone may potentiate CNS depressant effects). Products include:
Clozaril Tablets ... 2377

Codeine Phosphate (Hydrocodone may potentiate CNS depressant effects). Products include:
Brontex ... 2130
Dimetane-DC Cough Syrup ... 2232
Fioricet with Codeine Capsules ... 2387
Fiorinal with Codeine Capsules ... 2390
Nucofed ... 2225
Phenergan with Codeine ... 2883
Phenergan VC with Codeine ... 2888
Robitussin A-C Syrup ... 2248
Robitussin-DAC Syrup ... 2249
Ryna ... ⊞ 804
Soma Compound w/Codeine Tablets ... 2784
Tylenol with Codeine ... 1592

Cryptenamine Preparations (Sympathomimetic may reduce the antihypertensive effects of veratrum alkaloids).

Desflurane (Hydrocodone may potentiate CNS depressant effects). Products include:
Suprane (desflurane, USP) ... 1865

Desipramine Hydrochloride (Hydrocodone may potentiate CNS depressant effects). Products include:
Norpramin Tablets ... 1273

Dezocine (Hydrocodone may potentiate CNS depressant effects). Products include:
Dalgan Injection ... 529

Diazepam (Hydrocodone may potentiate CNS depressant effects). Products include:
Dizac (diazepam injectable emulsion) CIV ... 1862
Valium Injectable ... 2336
Valium Tablets ... 2335

Doxepin Hydrochloride (Hydrocodone may potentiate CNS depressant effects). Products include:
Adapin Capsules ... 1542
Sinequan ... 2028
Zonalon Cream ... 1042

Droperidol (Hydrocodone may potentiate CNS depressant effects). Products include:
Inapsine Injection ... 462

Enflurane (Hydrocodone may potentiate CNS depressant effects).
No products indexed under this heading.

Esmolol Hydrochloride (Potentiates the sympathomimetic effects of pseudoephedrine). Products include:
Brevibloc (esmolol HCl) Injection ... 1860

Estazolam (Hydrocodone may potentiate CNS depressant effects). Products include:
ProSom Tablets ... 457

Ethchlorvynol (Hydrocodone may potentiate CNS depressant effects). Products include:
Placidyl Capsules ... 456

Ethinamate (Hydrocodone may potentiate CNS depressant effects).
No products indexed under this heading.

Fentanyl (Hydrocodone may potentiate CNS depressant effects). Products include:
Duragesic Transdermal System ... 1336

Fentanyl Citrate (Hydrocodone may potentiate CNS depressant effects). Products include:
Sublimaze Injection ... 463

Fluphenazine Decanoate (Hydrocodone may potentiate CNS depressant effects). Products include:
Prolixin Decanoate ... 510

Fluphenazine Enanthate (Hydrocodone may potentiate CNS depressant effects). Products include:
Prolixin Enanthate ... 510

Fluphenazine Hydrochloride (Hydrocodone may potentiate CNS depressant effects). Products include:
Prolixin ... 510

Flurazepam Hydrochloride (Hydrocodone may potentiate CNS depressant effects). Products include:
Dalmane Capsules ... 2329

Furazolidone (Potentiates the sympathomimetic effects of pseudoephedrine; hydrocodone may potentiate CNS depressant effects; concurrent use is contraindicated). Products include:
Furoxone ... 2221

Glutethimide (Hydrocodone may potentiate CNS depressant effects).
No products indexed under this heading.

Haloperidol (Hydrocodone may potentiate CNS depressant effects). Products include:
Haldol Injection, Tablets and Concentrate ... 1585

Haloperidol Decanoate (Hydrocodone may potentiate CNS depressant effects). Products include:
Haldol Decanoate ... 1587

Hydrocodone Polistirex (Hydrocodone may potentiate CNS depressant effects). Products include:
Tussionex Pennkinetic Extended-Release Suspension ... 1624

Hydromorphone Hydrochloride (Hydrocodone may potentiate CNS depressant effects). Products include:
Dilaudid Ampules ... 1382
Dilaudid Cough Syrup ... 1383
Dilaudid-HP Injection ... 1384
Dilaudid-HP Lyophilized Powder 250 mg ... 1384
Dilaudid ... 1382
Dilaudid Oral Liquid ... 1386
Dilaudid ... 1382
Dilaudid Tablets - 8 mg ... 1386

Hydroxyzine Hydrochloride (Hydrocodone may potentiate CNS depressant effects). Products include:
Atarax Tablets & Syrup ... 1992
Marax Tablets & DF Syrup ... 2015
Vistaril Intramuscular Solution ... 2042

Imipramine Hydrochloride (Hydrocodone may potentiate CNS depressant effects). Products include:
Tofranil Ampuls ... 873
Tofranil Tablets ... 875

Imipramine Pamoate (Hydrocodone may potentiate CNS depressant effects). Products include:
Tofranil-PM Capsules ... 876

Isocarboxazid (Potentiates the sympathomimetic effects of pseudoephedrine; hydrocodone may potentiate CNS depressant effects; concurrent use is contraindicated).
No products indexed under this heading.

Isoflurane (Hydrocodone may potentiate CNS depressant effects).
No products indexed under this heading.

Ketamine Hydrochloride (Hydrocodone may potentiate CNS depressant effects).
No products indexed under this heading.

Labetalol Hydrochloride (Potentiates the sympathomimetic effects of pseudoephedrine). Products include:
Normodyne Injection ... 2519
Normodyne Tablets ... 2522
Trandate ... 1158

Levobunolol Hydrochloride (Potentiates the sympathomimetic effects of pseudoephedrine). Products include:
Betagan ... ⊙ 230

Levomethadyl Acetate Hydrochloride (Hydrocodone may potentiate CNS depressant effects). Products include:
Orlaam Oral Solution ... 2361

Levorphanol Tartrate (Hydrocodone may potentiate CNS depressant effects). Products include:
Levo-Dromoran ... 2297

Lorazepam (Hydrocodone may potentiate CNS depressant effects). Products include:
Ativan Injection ... 2805
Ativan Tablets ... 2807

Loxapine Hydrochloride (Hydrocodone may potentiate CNS depressant effects). Products include:
Loxitane ... 1426

Loxapine Succinate (Hydrocodone may potentiate CNS depressant effects). Products include:
Loxitane Capsules ... 1426

Maprotiline Hydrochloride (Hydrocodone may potentiate CNS depressant effects). Products include:
Ludiomil Tablets ... 861

Mecamylamine Hydrochloride (Sympathomimetic may reduce the antihypertensive effects). Products include:
Inversine Tablets ... 1729

Meperidine Hydrochloride (Hydrocodone may potentiate CNS depressant effects). Products include:
Demerol ... 2438
Mepergan Injection ... 2859

Mephobarbital (Hydrocodone may potentiate CNS depressant effects). Products include:
Mebaral Tablets ... 2452

Meprobamate (Hydrocodone may potentiate CNS depressant effects). Products include:
Miltown Tablets ... 2780
PMB 200 and PMB 400 ... 2890

Mesoridazine Besylate (Hydrocodone may potentiate CNS depressant effects). Products include:
Serentil ... 689

Methadone Hydrochloride (Hydrocodone may potentiate CNS depressant effects). Products include:
Methadone Hydrochloride Oral Concentrate ... 2356
Methadone Hydrochloride Oral Solution & Tablets ... 2357

Methohexital Sodium (Hydrocodone may potentiate CNS depressant effects).
No products indexed under this heading.

Methotrimeprazine (Hydrocodone may potentiate CNS depressant effects). Products include:
Levoprome ... 1321

Methoxyflurane (Hydrocodone may potentiate CNS depressant effects).
No products indexed under this heading.

Methyldopa (Sympathomimetic may reduce the antihypertensive effects). Products include:
Aldoclor Tablets ... 1638
Aldomet Oral ... 1640
Aldoril Tablets ... 1644

Methyldopate Hydrochloride (Sympathomimetic may reduce the antihypertensive effects). Products include:
Aldomet Ester HCl Injection ... 1642

Metipranolol Hydrochloride (Potentiates the sympathomimetic effects of pseudoephedrine). Products include:
OptiPranolol (Metipranolol 0.3%) Sterile Ophthalmic Solution ... ⊙ 256

Metoprolol Succinate (Potentiates the sympathomimetic effects of pseudoephedrine). Products include:
Toprol-XL Tablets ... 560

Metoprolol Tartrate (Potentiates the sympathomimetic effects of pseudoephedrine). Products include:
Lopressor ... 848
Lopressor HCT Tablets ... 850

Midazolam Hydrochloride (Hydrocodone may potentiate CNS depressant effects). Products include:
Versed Injection ... 2324

Molindone Hydrochloride (Hydrocodone may potentiate CNS depressant effects). Products include:
Moban Tablets and Concentrate ... 1036

IMPORTANT NOTE: Always consult each drug listing in the patient's regimen for possible interactions.

Tussend Expectorant / Interactions Index

Morphine Sulfate (Hydrocodone may potentiate CNS depressant effects). Products include:
- Astramorph/PF Injection, USP (Preservative-Free) ... 526
- Duramorph Injection ... 983
- Infumorph 200 and Infumorph 500 Sterile Solutions ... 985
- Kadian Capsules ... 2948
- MS Contin Tablets ... 2149
- MSIR ... 2152
- Oramorph SR (Morphine Sulfate Sustained Release Tablets) ... 2359
- RMS Suppositories CII ... 2766
- Roxanol ... 2365

Nadolol (Potentiates the sympathomimetic effects of pseudoephedrine).
- No products indexed under this heading.

Nortriptyline Hydrochloride (Hydrocodone may potentiate CNS depressant effects). Products include:
- Pamelor ... 2409

Opium Alkaloids (Hydrocodone may potentiate CNS depressant effects).
- No products indexed under this heading.

Oxazepam (Hydrocodone may potentiate CNS depressant effects). Products include:
- Serax Capsules ... 2916
- Serax Tablets ... 2916

Oxycodone Hydrochloride (Hydrocodone may potentiate CNS depressant effects). Products include:
- OxyContin Tablets ... 2163
- OxyIR Capsules ... 2167
- Percocet Tablets ... 955
- Percodan Tablets ... 955
- Percodan-Demi Tablets ... 956
- Roxicodone Tablets, Oral Solution & Intensol (Oxycodone) ... 2366
- Tylox Capsules ... 1593

Penbutolol Sulfate (Potentiates the sympathomimetic effects of pseudoephedrine). Products include:
- Levatol Tablets ... 2547

Pentobarbital Sodium (Hydrocodone may potentiate CNS depressant effects). Products include:
- Nembutal Sodium Capsules ... 440
- Nembutal Sodium Solution ... 442
- Nembutal Sodium Suppositories ... 444

Perphenazine (Hydrocodone may potentiate CNS depressant effects). Products include:
- Etrafon ... 2495
- Triavil Tablets ... 1800
- Trilafon ... 2532

Phenelzine Sulfate (Potentiates the sympathomimetic effects of pseudoephedrine; hydrocodone may potentiate CNS depressant effects; concurrent use is contraindicated). Products include:
- Nardil ... 1977

Phenobarbital (Hydrocodone may potentiate CNS depressant effects). Products include:
- Arco-Lase Plus Tablets ... 513
- Bellergal-S Tablets ... 2375
- Donnatal ... 2234
- Donnatal Extentabs ... 2234
- Donnatal Tablets ... 2234
- Phenobarbital Elixir and Tablets ... 1523
- Quadrinal Tablets ... 1398

Pindolol (Potentiates the sympathomimetic effects of pseudoephedrine). Products include:
- Visken Tablets ... 2428

Prazepam (Hydrocodone may potentiate CNS depressant effects).
- No products indexed under this heading.

Prochlorperazine (Hydrocodone may potentiate CNS depressant effects). Products include:
- Compazine ... 2644

Promethazine Hydrochloride (Hydrocodone may potentiate CNS depressant effects). Products include:
- Mepergan Injection ... 2859
- Phenergan with Codeine ... 2883
- Phenergan with Dextromethorphan ... 2885
- Phenergan Injection ... 2880
- Phenergan Suppositories ... 2882
- Phenergan Syrup ... 2881
- Phenergan Tablets ... 2882
- Phenergan VC ... 2886
- Phenergan VC with Codeine ... 2888

Propofol (Hydrocodone may potentiate CNS depressant effects). Products include:
- Diprivan Injectable Emulsion ... 2939

Propoxyphene Hydrochloride (Hydrocodone may potentiate CNS depressant effects). Products include:
- Darvon ... 1475
- Wygesic Tablets ... 2930

Propoxyphene Napsylate (Hydrocodone may potentiate CNS depressant effects). Products include:
- Darvon-N/Darvocet-N ... 1473

Propranolol Hydrochloride (Potentiates the sympathomimetic effects of pseudoephedrine). Products include:
- Inderal ... 2834
- Inderal LA Long Acting Capsules ... 2836
- Inderide Tablets ... 2838
- Inderide LA Long Acting Capsules ... 2840

Protriptyline Hydrochloride (Hydrocodone may potentiate CNS depressant effects). Products include:
- Vivactil Tablets ... 1820

Quazepam (Hydrocodone may potentiate CNS depressant effects). Products include:
- Doral Tablets ... 2773

Reserpine (Sympathomimetic may reduce the antihypertensive effects). Products include:
- Diupres Tablets ... 1691
- Hydropres Tablets ... 1718
- Ser-Ap-Es Tablets ... 867

Risperidone (Hydrocodone may potentiate CNS depressant effects). Products include:
- Risperdal Tablets ... 1348

Secobarbital Sodium (Hydrocodone may potentiate CNS depressant effects). Products include:
- Seconal Sodium Pulvules ... 1529

Selegiline Hydrochloride (Potentiates the sympathomimetic effects of pseudoephedrine; hydrocodone may potentiate CNS depressant effects; concurrent use is contraindicated). Products include:
- Eldepryl Capsules ... 2729

Sevoflurane (Hydrocodone may potentiate CNS depressant effects).
- No products indexed under this heading.

Sotalol Hydrochloride (Potentiates the sympathomimetic effects of pseudoephedrine). Products include:
- Betapace Tablets ... 637

Sufentanil Citrate (Hydrocodone may potentiate CNS depressant effects). Products include:
- Sufenta Injection ... 1355

Temazepam (Hydrocodone may potentiate CNS depressant effects). Products include:
- Restoril Capsules ... 2413

Thiamylal Sodium (Hydrocodone may potentiate CNS depressant effects).
- No products indexed under this heading.

Thioridazine Hydrochloride (Hydrocodone may potentiate CNS depressant effects). Products include:
- Mellaril ... 2398

Thiothixene (Hydrocodone may potentiate CNS depressant effects). Products include:
- Navane Capsules and Concentrate ... 2018
- Navane Intramuscular ... 2019

Timolol Hemihydrate (Potentiates the sympathomimetic effects of pseudoephedrine). Products include:
- Betimol 0.25%, 0.5% ... ⊙ 259

Timolol Maleate (Potentiates the sympathomimetic effects of pseudoephedrine). Products include:
- Blocadren Tablets ... 1654
- Timolide Tablets ... 1791
- Timoptic in Ocudose ... 1796
- Timoptic Sterile Ophthalmic Solution ... 1794
- Timoptic-XE ... 1798

Tranylcypromine Sulfate (Potentiates the sympathomimetic effects of pseudoephedrine; hydrocodone may potentiate CNS depressant effects; concurrent use is contraindicated). Products include:
- Parnate Tablets ... 2679

Triazolam (Hydrocodone may potentiate CNS depressant effects). Products include:
- Halcion Tablets ... 2093

Trifluoperazine Hydrochloride (Hydrocodone may potentiate CNS depressant effects). Products include:
- Stelazine ... 2692

Trimipramine Maleate (Hydrocodone may potentiate CNS depressant effects). Products include:
- Surmontil Capsules ... 2917

Zolpidem Tartrate (Hydrocodone may potentiate CNS depressant effects). Products include:
- Ambien Tablets ... 2559

Food Interactions

Alcohol (Hydrocodone may potentiate CNS depressant effects).

TUSSIONEX PENNKINETIC EXTENDED-RELEASE SUSPENSION
(Hydrocodone Polistirex, Chlorpheniramine Polistirex) ... 1624

May interact with central nervous system depressants, antihistamines, monoamine oxidase inhibitors, tricyclic antidepressants, anticholinergics, narcotic analgesics, antipsychotic agents, tranquilizers, and certain other agents. Compounds in these categories include:

Acrivastine (Additive CNS depression). Products include:
- Semprex-D Capsules ... 1620

Alfentanil Hydrochloride (Additive CNS depression). Products include:
- Alfenta Injection ... 1334

Alprazolam (Additive CNS depression). Products include:
- Xanax Tablets ... 2115

Amitriptyline Hydrochloride (Effect of either agent may be increased). Products include:
- Elavil ... 2945
- Etrafon ... 2495
- Limbitrol ... 2333
- Triavil Tablets ... 1800

Amoxapine (Effect of either agent may be increased). Products include:
- Asendin Tablets ... 1419

Aprobarbital (Additive CNS depression).
- No products indexed under this heading.

Astemizole (Additive CNS depression). Products include:
- Hismanal Tablets ... 1341

Atropine Sulfate (Concurrent use may produce paralytic ileus). Products include:
- Arco-Lase Plus Tablets ... 513
- Atrohist Plus Tablets ... 1605
- Donnatal ... 2234
- Donnatal Extentabs ... 2234
- Donnatal Tablets ... 2234
- Lomotil ... 2591
- Motofen Tablets ... 789
- Urised Tablets ... 2123

Azatadine Maleate (Additive CNS depression). Products include:
- Trinalin Repetabs Tablets ... 1373

Belladonna Alkaloids (Concurrent use may produce paralytic ileus). Products include:
- Bellergal-S Tablets ... 2375
- Hyland's Bedwetting Tablets ... ✪ 788
- Hyland's EnurAid Tablets ... ✪ 789
- Hyland's Headache Tablets ... ✪ 790
- Hyland's Teething Tablets ... ✪ 790
- Similasan Eye Drops # 1 ... ✪ 769

Benztropine Mesylate (Concurrent use may produce paralytic ileus). Products include:
- Cogentin ... 1661

Biperiden Hydrochloride (Concurrent use may produce paralytic ileus). Products include:
- Akineton ... 1380

Bromodiphenhydramine Hydrochloride (Additive CNS depression).
- No products indexed under this heading.

Brompheniramine Maleate (Additive CNS depression). Products include:
- Alka-Seltzer Plus Sinus Medicine ... 611
- Bromfed Capsules (Extended-Release) ... 1832
- Bromfed Syrup ... ✪ 712
- Bromfed Tablets ... 1832
- Bromfed-DM Cough Syrup ... 1832
- Bromfed-PD Capsules (Extended-Release) ... 1832
- Dimetane-DC Cough Syrup ... 2232
- Dimetane-DX Cough Syrup ... 2233
- Dimetapp Allergy Dye-Free Elixir ... ✪ 838
- Dimetapp Allergy Sinus Caplets ... 838
- Dimetapp Cold & Allergy Chewable Tablets ... ✪ 838
- Dimetapp Cold & Cough Liqui-Gels ... ✪ 839
- Dimetapp Cold & Fever Suspension ... ✪ 839
- Dimetapp DM Elixir ... 840
- Dimetapp Elixir ... ✪ 840
- Dimetapp Extentabs ... ✪ 841
- Dimetapp Tablets/Liqui-Gels ... ✪ 841
- Rondec Chewable Tablets ... 974
- Vicks DayQuil Allergy Relief 12-Hour Extended Release Tablets ... ✪ 733
- Vicks DayQuil Allergy Relief 4-Hour Tablets ... ✪ 733

Buprenorphine (Additive CNS depression). Products include:
- Buprenex Injectable ... 2170

Buspirone Hydrochloride (Additive CNS depression). Products include:
- BuSpar Tablets ... 738

Butabarbital (Additive CNS depression).
- No products indexed under this heading.

Butalbital (Additive CNS depression). Products include:
- Axocet Capsules ... 2469
- Esgic-plus Capsules ... 1012
- Esgic-plus Tablets ... 1012
- Fioricet Tablets ... 2386
- Fioricet with Codeine Capsules ... 2387
- Fiorinal Capsules ... 2388
- Fiorinal with Codeine Capsules ... 2390
- Fiorinal Tablets ... 2388
- Phrenilin ... 790
- Sedapap Tablets 50 mg/650 mg ... 1826

(✪ Described in PDR For Nonprescription Drugs) (⊙ Described in PDR For Ophthalmology)

Cetirizine Hydrochloride (Additive CNS depression). Products include:
Zyrtec Tablets 2053

Chlordiazepoxide (Additive CNS depression). Products include:
Limbitrol 2333

Chlordiazepoxide Hydrochloride (Additive CNS depression). Products include:
- Librax Capsules 2330
- Librium Capsules 2331
- Librium Injectable 2332

Chlorpheniramine Maleate (Additive CNS depression). Products include:
- Alka-Seltzer Plus Cold Medicine ...... ▣ 611
- Alka-Seltzer Plus Cold Medicine Liqui-Gels .... ▣ 612
- Alka-Seltzer Plus Cold & Cough Medicine .... ▣ 611
- Alka-Seltzer Plus Cold & Cough Medicine Liqui-Gels .... ▣ 612
- Alka-Seltzer Plus Flu & Body Aches Effervescent Tablets .... ▣ 612
- Allerest Maximum Strength............ ▣ 649
- Allerest Sinus Pain Formula .... ▣ 649
- Ana-Kit Anaphylaxis Emergency Treatment Kit 611
- Atrohist Pediatric Capsules 1603
- Atrohist Plus Tablets 1605
- BC Cold Powder Multi-Symptom Formula (Cold-Sinus-Allergy) ...... ▣ 631
- Cerose DM 853
- Cheracol Plus Head Cold/Cough Formula .... ▣ 741
- Children's TYLENOL Cold Multi-Symptom Chewable Tablets and Liquid 1559
- Children's TYLENOL Cold Plus Cough Multi Symptom Chewable Tablets and Liquid 1560
- Children's TYLENOL Flu Suspension Liquid 1560
- Children's Vicks DayQuil Allergy Relief .... ▣ 730
- Children's Vicks NyQuil Cold/Cough Relief .... ▣ 731
- Chlor-Trimeton Allergy Decongestant Tablets .... ▣ 759
- Chlor-Trimeton Allergy Tablets ...... ▣ 758
- Allergy-Sinus Comtrex Multi-Symptom Allergy-Sinus Formula Tablets and Caplets .... ▣ 639
- Comtrex Multi-Symptom............... ▣ 638
- Contac Continuous Action Nasal Decongestant/Antihistamine 12 Hour Capsules .... ▣ 773
- Contac Maximum Strength Continuous Action Decongestant/Antihistamine 12 Hour Capsules .. ▣ 772
- Contac Severe Cold and Flu Formula Caplets .... ▣ 773
- Coricidin Cold + Flu Tablets .... ▣ 760
- Coricidin Cough + Cold Tablets ..... ▣ 760
- Coricidin 'D' Decongestant Tablets .... ▣ 760
- D.A. II Tablets 972
- D.A. Chewable Tablets 970
- Dura-Tap/PD Capsules 970
- Dura-Vent/DA Tablets 972
- Efidac 24 Chlorpheniramine .... ▣ 655
- Extendryl 1003
- Fedahist Gyrocaps 2545
- Hycomine Compound Tablets 948
- Kronofed-A 994
- Nolamine Timed-Release Tablets ... 790
- Novahistine Elixir .... ▣ 782
- Ornade Spansule Capsules 2678
- PediaCare Cough-Cold Chewable Tablets and Liquid 1569
- PediaCare NightRest Cough-Cold Liquid 1569
- Pediatric Vicks 44m Cough & Cold Relief .... ▣ 737
- Pyrroxate Caplets .... ▣ 742
- Ryna .... ▣ 804
- Sinarest .... ▣ 663
- Sine-Off Sinus Medicine .... ▣ 784
- Singlet Tablets .... ▣ 785
- Sinulin Tablets 792
- Sinutab Sinus Allergy Medication, Maximum Strength Tablets and Caplets .... ▣ 823
- Sudafed Cold & Allergy Tablets...... ▣ 826
- Teldrin 12 Hour Antihistamine/Nasal Decongestant Allergy Relief Capsules .... ▣ 786
- TheraFlu Flu and Cold Medicine ..... ▣ 750
- TheraFlu Maximum Strength Flu and Cold Medicine For Sore Throat .... ▣ 751
- TheraFlu Flu, Cold and Cough Medicine .... ▣ 750
- TheraFlu Maximum Strength Nighttime Flu, Cold & Cough Medicine .... ▣ 751
- Triaminic Night Time .... ▣ 754
- Triaminic Syrup .... ▣ 755
- Triaminic Triaminicol Cold & Cough .... ▣ 756
- Triaminicin Tablets .... ▣ 756
- Tussend 1830
- TYLENOL Allergy Sinus, Maximum Strength Caplets and Gelcaps ... 1571
- TYLENOL Cold Medication, Multi-Symptom Formula Tablets and Caplets 1572
- TYLENOL Cold Medication, Multi-Symptom Hot Liquid Packets 1572
- Vicks 44 LiquiCaps Cough, Cold & Flu Relief .... ▣ 728
- Vicks 44M Cough, Cold & Flu Relief .... ▣ 729

Chlorpheniramine Tannate (Additive CNS depression). Products include:
- Atrohist Pediatric Suspension 1604
- Atrohist Pediatric Suspension Dye-Free 1604
- Rynatan 2781
- Rynatuss 2782

Chlorpromazine (Additive CNS depression). Products include:
Thorazine Suppositories 2701

Chlorpromazine Hydrochloride (Additive CNS depression). Products include:
Thorazine 2701

Chlorprothixene (Additive CNS depression).
No products indexed under this heading.

Chlorprothixene Hydrochloride (Additive CNS depression).
No products indexed under this heading.

Chlorprothixene Lactate (Additive CNS depression).
No products indexed under this heading.

Clemastine Fumarate (Additive CNS depression). Products include:
- Tavist Syrup 2426
- Tavist Tablets 2427
- Tavist-1 12 Hour Relief Tablets .... ▣ 749
- Tavist-D 12 Hour Relief Tablets.... ▣ 750

Clidinium Bromide (Concurrent use may produce paralytic ileus). Products include:
Librax Capsules 2330

Clomipramine Hydrochloride (Effect of either agent may be increased). Products include:
Anafranil Capsules 819

Clorazepate Dipotassium (Additive CNS depression). Products include:
Tranxene 459

Clozapine (Additive CNS depression). Products include:
Clozaril Tablets 2377

Codeine Phosphate (Additive CNS depression). Products include:
- Brontex 2130
- Dimetane-DC Cough Syrup 2232
- Fioricet with Codeine Capsules 2387
- Fiorinal with Codeine Capsules 2390
- Nucofed 2225
- Phenergan with Codeine 2883
- Phenergan VC with Codeine 2888
- Robitussin A-C Syrup 2248
- Robitussin-DAC Syrup 2249
- Ryna .... ▣ 804
- Soma Compound w/Codeine Tablets 2784
- Tylenol with Codeine 1592

Cyproheptadine Hydrochloride (Additive CNS depression). Products include:
Periactin 1767

Desflurane (Additive CNS depression). Products include:
Suprane (desflurane, USP) 1865

Desipramine Hydrochloride (Effect of either agent may be increased). Products include:
Norpramin Tablets 1273

Dexchlorpheniramine Maleate (Additive CNS depression).
No products indexed under this heading.

Dezocine (Additive CNS depression). Products include:
Dalgan Injection 529

Diazepam (Additive CNS depression). Products include:
- Dizac (diazepam injectable emulsion) CIV 1862
- Valium Injectable 2336
- Valium Tablets 2335

Dicyclomine Hydrochloride (Concurrent use may produce paralytic ileus). Products include:
Bentyl 1246

Diphenhydramine Citrate (Additive CNS depression). Products include:
Excedrin P.M. Analgesic/Sleeping Aid Tablets, Caplets, Liquigels ... 735

Diphenhydramine Hydrochloride (Additive CNS depression). Products include:
- Actifed Allergy Daytime/Nighttime Caplets .... ▣ 808
- Actifed Sinus Daytime/Nighttime Tablets and Caplets .... ▣ 809
- Extra Strength Bayer PM Aspirin Plus Sleep Aid .... ▣ 617
- Benadryl Allergy Chewables .... ▣ 811
- Benadryl Allergy/Cold Tablets ..... ▣ 811
- Benadryl Allergy Decongestant Liquid Medication .... ▣ 812
- Benadryl Allergy Decongestant Tablets .... ▣ 812
- Benadryl Allergy Liquid Medication .... ▣ 813
- Benadryl Allergy .... ▣ 811
- Benadryl Allergy Sinus Headache Caplets .... ▣ 813
- Benadryl Dye-Free Allergy Liquigel Softgels .... ▣ 813
- Benadryl Dye-Free Allergy Liquid Medication .... ▣ 814
- Benadryl Itch Relief Stick Extra Strength .... ▣ 814
- Benadryl Cream .... ▣ 814
- Benadryl Gel .... ▣ 815
- Benadryl Spray .... ▣ 815
- Benadryl Injection 1955
- Contac Day & Night Cold/Flu Night Caplets .... ▣ 772
- Contac Night Allergy/Sinus Caplets .... ▣ 771
- Extra Strength Doan's P.M. .... ▣ 653
- Excedrin P.M. Analgesic/Sleeping Aid Tablets, Caplets, Liquigels .... ▣ 643
- Nytol QuickCaps Caplets .... ▣ 632
- Sleepinal Night-time Sleep Aid Capsules and Softgels .... ▣ 798
- TYLENOL Allergy Sinus NightTime, Maximum Strength Caplets 1571
- TYLENOL Flu NightTime, Maximum Strength Gelcaps 1575
- TYLENOL Flu NightTime, Maximum Strength Hot Medication Packets 1575
- TYLENOL PM Pain Reliever/Sleep Aid, Extra Strength Gelcaps, Caplets, Geltabs 1576
- TYLENOL Severe Allergy Medication Caplets 1571
- Maximum Strength Unisom Sleepgels 1990
- Unisom With Pain Relief-Nighttime Sleep Aid and Pain Reliever....... 1991

Diphenylpyraline Hydrochloride (Additive CNS depression).
No products indexed under this heading.

Doxepin Hydrochloride (Effect of either agent may be increased). Products include:
- Adapin Capsules 1542
- Sinequan 2028
- Zonalon Cream 1042

Droperidol (Additive CNS depression). Products include:
Inapsine Injection 462

Enflurane (Additive CNS depression).
No products indexed under this heading.

Estazolam (Additive CNS depression). Products include:
ProSom Tablets 457

Ethchlorvynol (Additive CNS depression). Products include:
Placidyl Capsules 456

Ethinamate (Additive CNS depression).
No products indexed under this heading.

Fentanyl (Additive CNS depression). Products include:
Duragesic Transdermal System ... 1336

Fentanyl Citrate (Additive CNS depression). Products include:
Sublimaze Injection 463

Fluphenazine Decanoate (Additive CNS depression). Products include:
Prolixin Decanoate 510

Fluphenazine Enanthate (Additive CNS depression). Products include:
Prolixin Enanthate 510

Fluphenazine Hydrochloride (Additive CNS depression). Products include:
Prolixin 510

Flurazepam Hydrochloride (Additive CNS depression). Products include:
Dalmane Capsules 2329

Furazolidone (Effect of either agent may be increased). Products include:
Furoxone 2221

Glutethimide (Additive CNS depression).
No products indexed under this heading.

Glycopyrrolate (Concurrent use may produce paralytic ileus). Products include:
- Robinul Forte Tablets 2247
- Robinul Injectable 2247
- Robinul Tablets 2247

Haloperidol (Additive CNS depression). Products include:
Haldol Injection, Tablets and Concentrate 1585

Haloperidol Decanoate (Additive CNS depression). Products include:
Haldol Decanoate 1587

Hydrocodone Bitartrate (Additive CNS depression). Products include:
- Codiclear DH Syrup 808
- Duratuss HD Elixir 2750
- Histussin D Liquid 670
- Hycodan Tablets and Syrup 946
- Hycomine Compound Tablets 948
- Hycomine 947
- Hycotuss Expectorant Syrup 950
- Hydrocet Capsules 787
- Lorcet 10/650 Tablets 1016
- Lortab 2751
- Tussend 1830
- Tussend Expectorant 1831
- Vicodin Tablets 1404
- Vicodin ES Tablets 1405
- Vicodin HP Tablets 1403
- Vicodin Tuss Expectorant 1406
- Zydone Capsules 967

Hydromorphone Hydrochloride (Additive CNS depression). Products include:
- Dilaudid Ampules 1382
- Dilaudid Cough Syrup 1383
- Dilaudid-HP Injection 1384
- Dilaudid-HP Lyophilized Powder 250 mg 1384
- Dilaudid 1382
- Dilaudid Oral Liquid 1386

IMPORTANT NOTE: Always consult each drug listing in the patient's regimen for possible interactions.

Tussionex — **Interactions Index** — **1122**

Dilaudid 1382
Dilaudid Tablets - 8 mg 1386

Hydroxyzine Hydrochloride (Additive CNS depression). Products include:
Atarax Tablets & Syrup 1992
Marax Tablets & DF Syrup 2015
Vistaril Intramuscular Solution 2042

Hyoscyamine (Concurrent use may produce paralytic ileus). Products include:
Cystospaz Tablets 2123
Urised Tablets 2123

Hyoscyamine Sulfate (Concurrent use may produce paralytic ileus). Products include:
Arco-Lase Plus Tablets 513
Atrohist Plus Tablets 1605
Cystospaz-M Capsules 2123
Donnatal 2234
Donnatal Extentabs 2234
Donnatal Tablets 2234
Kutrase Capsules 2546
Levsin/Levsinex/Levbid 2549

Imipramine Hydrochloride (Effect of either agent may be increased). Products include:
Tofranil Ampuls 873
Tofranil Tablets 875

Imipramine Pamoate (Effect of either agent may be increased). Products include:
Tofranil-PM Capsules 876

Ipratropium Bromide (Concurrent use may produce paralytic ileus). Products include:
Atrovent Inhalation Aerosol 674
Atrovent Inhalation Solution 675
Atrovent Nasal Spray 0.03% 676
Atrovent Nasal Spray 0.06% 678

Isocarboxazid (Effect of either agent may be increased).
No products indexed under this heading.

Isoflurane (Additive CNS depression).
No products indexed under this heading.

Ketamine Hydrochloride (Additive CNS depression).
No products indexed under this heading.

Levomethadyl Acetate Hydrochloride (Additive CNS depression). Products include:
Orlaam Oral Solution 2361

Levorphanol Tartrate (Additive CNS depression). Products include:
Levo-Dromoran 2297

Lithium Carbonate (Additive CNS depression). Products include:
Eskalith 2658
Lithium Carbonate Capsules & Tablets 2352
Lithonate/Lithotabs/Lithobid 2721

Lithium Citrate (Additive CNS depression).
No products indexed under this heading.

Loratadine (Additive CNS depression). Products include:
Claritin Tablets 2485
Claritin-D Tablets 2487

Lorazepam (Additive CNS depression). Products include:
Ativan Injection 2805
Ativan Tablets 2807

Loxapine Hydrochloride (Additive CNS depression). Products include:
Loxitane 1426

Loxapine Succinate (Additive CNS depression). Products include:
Loxitane Capsules 1426

Maprotiline Hydrochloride (Effect of either agent may be increased). Products include:
Ludiomil Tablets 861

Mepenzolate Bromide (Concurrent use may produce paralytic ileus).
No products indexed under this heading.

Meperidine Hydrochloride (Additive CNS depression). Products include:
Demerol 2438
Mepergan Injection 2859

Mephobarbital (Additive CNS depression). Products include:
Mebaral Tablets 2452

Meprobamate (Additive CNS depression). Products include:
Miltown Tablets 2780
PMB 200 and PMB 400 2890

Mesoridazine Besylate (Additive CNS depression). Products include:
Serentil 689

Methadone Hydrochloride (Additive CNS depression). Products include:
Methadone Hydrochloride Oral Concentrate 2356
Methadone Hydrochloride Oral Solution & Tablets 2357

Methdilazine Hydrochloride (Additive CNS depression).
No products indexed under this heading.

Methohexital Sodium (Additive CNS depression).
No products indexed under this heading.

Methotrimeprazine (Additive CNS depression). Products include:
Levoprome 1321

Methoxyflurane (Additive CNS depression).
No products indexed under this heading.

Midazolam Hydrochloride (Additive CNS depression). Products include:
Versed Injection 2324

Molindone Hydrochloride (Additive CNS depression). Products include:
Moban Tablets and Concentrate 1036

Morphine Sulfate (Additive CNS depression). Products include:
Astramorph/PF Injection, USP (Preservative-Free) 526
Duramorph Injection 983
Infumorph 200 and Infumorph 500 Sterile Solutions 985
Kadian Capsules 2948
MS Contin Tablets 2149
MSIR 2152
Oramorph SR (Morphine Sulfate Sustained Release Tablets) 2359
RMS Suppositories CII 2766
Roxanol 2365

Nortriptyline Hydrochloride (Effect of either agent may be increased). Products include:
Pamelor 2409

Opium Alkaloids (Additive CNS depression).
No products indexed under this heading.

Oxazepam (Additive CNS depression). Products include:
Serax Capsules 2916
Serax Tablets 2916

Oxybutynin Chloride (Concurrent use may produce paralytic ileus). Products include:
Ditropan 1267

Oxycodone Hydrochloride (Additive CNS depression). Products include:
OxyContin Tablets 2163
OxyIR Capsules 2167
Percocet Tablets 955
Percodan Tablets 955
Percodan-Demi Tablets 956
Roxicodone Tablets, Oral Solution & Intensol (Oxycodone) 2366

Tylox Capsules 1593

Pentobarbital Sodium (Additive CNS depression). Products include:
Nembutal Sodium Capsules 440
Nembutal Sodium Solution 442
Nembutal Sodium Suppositories 444

Perphenazine (Additive CNS depression). Products include:
Etrafon 2495
Triavil Tablets 1800
Trilafon 2532

Phenelzine Sulfate (Effect of either agent may be increased). Products include:
Nardil 1977

Phenobarbital (Additive CNS depression). Products include:
Arco-Lase Plus Tablets 513
Bellergal-S Tablets 2375
Donnatal 2234
Donnatal Extentabs 2234
Donnatal Tablets 2234
Phenobarbital Elixir and Tablets 1523
Quadrinal Tablets 1398

Pimozide (Additive CNS depression). Products include:
Orap Tablets 1037

Prazepam (Additive CNS depression).
No products indexed under this heading.

Prochlorperazine (Additive CNS depression). Products include:
Compazine 2644

Procyclidine Hydrochloride (Concurrent use may produce paralytic ileus). Products include:
Kemadrin Tablets 1105

Promethazine Hydrochloride (Additive CNS depression). Products include:
Mepergan Injection 2859
Phenergan with Codeine 2883
Phenergan with Dextromethorphan 2885
Phenergan Injection 2880
Phenergan Suppositories 2882
Phenergan Syrup 2881
Phenergan Tablets 2882
Phenergan VC 2886
Phenergan VC with Codeine 2888

Propantheline Bromide (Concurrent use may produce paralytic ileus). Products include:
Pro-Banthine Tablets 2226

Propofol (Additive CNS depression). Products include:
Diprivan Injectable Emulsion 2939

Propoxyphene Hydrochloride (Additive CNS depression). Products include:
Darvon 1475
Wygesic Tablets 2930

Propoxyphene Napsylate (Additive CNS depression). Products include:
Darvon-N/Darvocet-N 1473

Protriptyline Hydrochloride (Effect of either agent may be increased). Products include:
Vivactil Tablets 1820

Pyrilamine Maleate (Additive CNS depression). Products include:
4-Way Fast Acting Nasal Spray (regular & mentholated) ■ 644
Maximum Strength Multi-Symptom Formula Midol ■ 621
PMS Multi-Symptom Formula Midol ■ 622

Pyrilamine Tannate (Additive CNS depression). Products include:
Atrohist Pediatric Suspension 1604
Atrohist Pediatric Suspension Dye-Free 1604
Rynatan 2781

Quazepam (Additive CNS depression). Products include:
Doral Tablets 2773

Risperidone (Additive CNS depression). Products include:
Risperdal Tablets 1348

Scopolamine (Concurrent use may produce paralytic ileus). Products include:
Transderm Scōp Transdermal Therapeutic System 890

Scopolamine Hydrobromide (Concurrent use may produce paralytic ileus). Products include:
Atrohist Plus Tablets 1605
Donnatal 2234
Donnatal Extentabs 2234
Donnatal Tablets 2234

Secobarbital Sodium (Additive CNS depression). Products include:
Seconal Sodium Pulvules 1529

Selegiline Hydrochloride (Effect of either agent may be increased). Products include:
Eldepryl Capsules 2729

Sevoflurane (Additive CNS depression).
No products indexed under this heading.

Sufentanil Citrate (Additive CNS depression). Products include:
Sufenta Injection 1355

Temazepam (Additive CNS depression). Products include:
Restoril Capsules 2413

Terfenadine (Additive CNS depression). Products include:
Seldane Tablets 1284
Seldane-D Extended-Release Tablets 1286

Thiamylal Sodium (Additive CNS depression).
No products indexed under this heading.

Thioridazine Hydrochloride (Additive CNS depression). Products include:
Mellaril 2398

Thiothixene (Additive CNS depression). Products include:
Navane Capsules and Concentrate 2018
Navane Intramuscular 2019

Tranylcypromine Sulfate (Effect of either agent may be increased). Products include:
Parnate Tablets 2679

Triazolam (Additive CNS depression). Products include:
Halcion Tablets 2093

Tridihexethyl Chloride (Concurrent use may produce paralytic ileus).
No products indexed under this heading.

Trifluoperazine Hydrochloride (Additive CNS depression). Products include:
Stelazine 2692

Trihexyphenidyl Hydrochloride (Concurrent use may produce paralytic ileus). Products include:
Artane 1418

Trimeprazine Tartrate (Additive CNS depression).
No products indexed under this heading.

Trimipramine Maleate (Effect of either agent may be increased). Products include:
Surmontil Capsules 2917

Tripelennamine Hydrochloride (Additive CNS depression). Products include:
PBZ Tablets 863
PBZ-SR Tablets 862

Triprolidine Hydrochloride (Additive CNS depression). Products include:
Actifed Cold & Allergy Tablets ■ 807
Actifed Cold & Sinus Caplets and Tablets ■ 808

Zolpidem Tartrate (Additive CNS depression). Products include:
Ambien Tablets 2559

(■ Described in PDR For Nonprescription Drugs) (◉ Described in PDR For Ophthalmology)

Food Interactions
Alcohol (Additive CNS depression).

TUSSI-ORGANIDIN DM NR LIQUID AND DM-S NR LIQUID
(Guaifenesin, Dextromethorphan Hydrobromide) 2786
May interact with monoamine oxidase inhibitors, central nervous system depressants, antihistamines, psychotropics, and certain other agents. Compounds in these categories include:

Acrivastine (Potential for additive CNS depressant effects). Products include:
- Semprex-D Capsules 1620

Alfentanil Hydrochloride (Potential for additive CNS depressant effects). Products include:
- Alfenta Injection 1334

Alprazolam (Potential for additive CNS depressant effects). Products include:
- Xanax Tablets 2115

Amitriptyline Hydrochloride (Potential for additive CNS depressant effects). Products include:
- Elavil 2945
- Etrafon 2495
- Limbitrol 2333
- Triavil Tablets 1800

Amoxapine (Potential for additive CNS depressant effects). Products include:
- Asendin Tablets 1419

Aprobarbital (Potential for additive CNS depressant effects).
No products indexed under this heading.

Astemizole (Potential for additive CNS depressant effects). Products include:
- Hismanal Tablets 1341

Azatadine Maleate (Potential for additive CNS depressant effects). Products include:
- Trinalin Repetabs Tablets 1373

Bromodiphenhydramine Hydrochloride (Potential for additive CNS depressant effects).
No products indexed under this heading.

Brompheniramine Maleate (Potential for additive CNS depressant effects). Products include:
- Alka-Seltzer Plus Sinus Medicine .. ⊞ 611
- Bromfed Capsules (Extended-Release) 1832
- Bromfed Syrup .... ⊞ 712
- Bromfed Tablets 1832
- Bromfed-DM Cough Syrup 1832
- Bromfed-PD Capsules (Extended-Release) 1832
- Dimetane-DC Cough Syrup 2232
- Dimetane-DX Cough Syrup 2233
- Dimetapp Allergy Dye-Free Elixir ... ⊞ 838
- Dimetapp Allergy Sinus Caplets .. ⊞ 838
- Dimetapp Cold & Allergy Chewable Tablets .... ⊞ 838
- Dimetapp Cold & Cough Liqui-Gels .... ⊞ 839
- Dimetapp Cold & Fever Suspension .... ⊞ 839
- Dimetapp DM Elixir .... ⊞ 840
- Dimetapp Elixir .... ⊞ 840
- Dimetapp Extentabs .... ⊞ 841
- Dimetapp Tablets/Liqui-Gels .... ⊞ 841
- Rondec Chewable Tablets 974
- Vicks DayQuil Allergy Relief 12-Hour Extended Release Tablets .. ⊞ 733
- Vicks DayQuil Allergy Relief 4-Hour Tablets .... ⊞ 733

Buprenorphine (Potential for additive CNS depressant effects). Products include:
- Buprenex Injectable 2170

Buspirone Hydrochloride (Potential for additive CNS depressant effects). Products include:
- BuSpar Tablets 738

Butabarbital (Potential for additive CNS depressant effects).
No products indexed under this heading.

Butalbital (Potential for additive CNS depressant effects). Products include:
- Axocet Capsules 2469
- Esgic-plus Capsules 1012
- Esgic-plus Tablets 1012
- Fioricet Tablets 2386
- Fioricet with Codeine Capsules .. 2387
- Fiorinal Capsules 2388
- Fiorinal with Codeine Capsules .. 2390
- Fiorinal Tablets 2388
- Phrenilin 790
- Sedapap Tablets 50 mg/650 mg .. 1826

Cetirizine Hydrochloride (Potential for additive CNS depressant effects). Products include:
- Zyrtec Tablets 2053

Chlordiazepoxide (Potential for additive CNS depressant effects). Products include:
- Limbitrol 2333

Chlordiazepoxide Hydrochloride (Potential for additive CNS depressant effects). Products include:
- Librax Capsules 2330
- Librium Capsules 2331
- Librium Injectable 2332

Chlorpheniramine Maleate (Potential for additive CNS depressant effects). Products include:
- Alka-Seltzer Plus Cold Medicine .. ⊞ 611
- Alka-Seltzer Plus Cold Medicine Liqui-Gels .... ⊞ 612
- Alka-Seltzer Plus Cold & Cough Medicine .... ⊞ 611
- Alka-Seltzer Plus Cold & Cough Medicine Liqui-Gels .... ⊞ 612
- Alka-Seltzer Plus Cold Flu & Body Aches Effervescent Tablets ...... ⊞ 612
- Allerest Maximum Strength 649
- Allerest Sinus Pain Formula 649
- Ana-Kit Anaphylaxis Emergency Treatment Kit 611
- Atrohist Pediatric Capsules 1603
- Atrohist Plus Tablets 1605
- BC Cold Powder Multi-Symptom Formula (Cold-Sinus-Allergy) ..... ⊞ 631
- Cerose DM 853
- Cheracol Plus Head Cold/Cough Formula .... ⊞ 741
- Children's TYLENOL Cold Multi-Symptom Chewable Tablets and Liquid 1559
- Children's TYLENOL Cold Plus Cough Multi Symptom Chewable Tablets and Liquid 1560
- Children's TYLENOL Flu Suspension Liquid 1560
- Children's Vicks DayQuil Allergy Relief .... ⊞ 730
- Children's Vicks NyQuil Cold/Cough Relief .... ⊞ 731
- Chlor-Trimeton Allergy Decongestant Tablets .... ⊞ 759
- Chlor-Trimeton Allergy Tablets ... ⊞ 758
- Comtrex Allergy-Sinus Multi-Symptom Allergy-Sinus Formula Tablets and Caplets .... ⊞ 639
- Comtrex Multi-Symptom .... ⊞ 638
- Contac Continuous Action Nasal Decongestant/Antihistamine 12 Hour Capsules .... ⊞ 773
- Contac Maximum Strength Continuous Action Decongestant/Antihistamine 12 Hour Caplets .... ⊞ 772
- Contac Severe Cold and Flu Formula Caplets .... ⊞ 773
- Coricidin Cold + Flu Tablets 760
- Coricidin Cough + Cold Tablets .. 760
- Coricidin 'D' Decongestant Tablets 760
- D.A. II Tablets 972
- D.A. Chewable Tablets 970
- Dura-Tap/PD Capsules 970
- Dura-Vent/DA Tablets 972
- Efidac 24 Chlorpheniramine 655
- Extendryl 1003
- Fedahist Gyrocaps 2545

- Hycomine Compound Tablets 948
- Kronofed-A 994
- Nolamine Timed-Release Tablets .. 790
- Novahistine Elixir .... ⊞ 782
- Ornade Spansule Capsules 2678
- PediaCare Cough-Cold Chewable Tablets and Liquid 1569
- PediaCare NightRest Cough-Cold Liquid 1569
- Pediatric Vicks 44m Cough & Cold Relief .... ⊞ 737
- Pyrroxate Caplets .... ⊞ 742
- Ryna .... ⊞ 804
- Sinarest .... ⊞ 663
- Sine-Off Sinus Medicine .... ⊞ 784
- Singlet Tablets .... ⊞ 785
- Sinulin Tablets 792
- Sinutab Sinus Allergy Medication, Maximum Strength Tablets and Caplets .... ⊞ 823
- Sudafed Cold & Allergy Tablets .. ⊞ 826
- Teldrin 12 Hour Antihistamine/Nasal Decongestant Allergy Relief Capsules .... ⊞ 786
- TheraFlu Flu and Cold Medicine .. ⊞ 750
- Theraflu Maximum Strength Flu and Cold Medicine For Sore Throat .... ⊞ 751
- TheraFlu Flu, Cold and Cough Medicine .... ⊞ 750
- TheraFlu Maximum Strength Nighttime Flu, Cold and Cough Medicine .... ⊞ 751
- Triaminic Night Time .... ⊞ 754
- Triaminic Syrup .... ⊞ 755
- Triaminic Triaminicol Cold & Cough .... ⊞ 756
- Triaminicin Tablets .... ⊞ 756
- Tussend 1830
- TYLENOL Allergy Sinus, Maximum Strength Caplets and Gelcaps .. 1571
- TYLENOL Cold Medication, Multi-Symptom Formula Tablets and Caplets 1572
- TYLENOL Cold Medication, Multi-Symptom Hot Liquid Packets 1572
- Vicks 44 LiquiCaps Cough, Cold & Flu Relief .... ⊞ 728
- Vicks 44M Cough, Cold & Flu Relief .... ⊞ 729

Chlorpheniramine Polistirex (Potential for additive CNS depressant effects). Products include:
- Tussionex Pennkinetic Extended-Release Suspension 1624

Chlorpheniramine Tannate (Potential for additive CNS depressant effects). Products include:
- Atrohist Pediatric Suspension 1604
- Atrohist Pediatric Suspension Dye-Free 1604
- Rynatan 2781
- Rynatuss 2782

Chlorpromazine (Potential for additive CNS depressant effects). Products include:
- Thorazine Suppositories 2701

Chlorpromazine Hydrochloride (Potential for additive CNS depressant effects). Products include:
- Thorazine 2701

Chlorprothixene (Potential for additive CNS depressant effects).
No products indexed under this heading.

Chlorprothixene Hydrochloride (Potential for additive CNS depressant effects).
No products indexed under this heading.

Chlorprothixene Lactate (Potential for additive CNS depressant effects).
No products indexed under this heading.

Clemastine Fumarate (Potential for additive CNS depressant effects). Products include:
- Tavist Syrup 2426
- Tavist Tablets 2427
- Tavist-1 12 Hour Relief Tablets ... ⊞ 749
- Tavist-D 12 Hour Relief Tablets .. ⊞ 750

Clorazepate Dipotassium (Potential for additive CNS depressant effects). Products include:
- Tranxene 459

Clozapine (Potential for additive CNS depressant effects). Products include:
- Clozaril Tablets 2377

Codeine Phosphate (Potential for additive CNS depressant effects). Products include:
- Brontex 2130
- Dimetane-DC Cough Syrup 2232
- Fioricet with Codeine Capsules .. 2387
- Fiorinal with Codeine Capsules .. 2390
- Nucofed 2225
- Phenergan with Codeine 2883
- Phenergan VC with Codeine 2888
- Robitussin A-C Syrup 2248
- Robitussin-DAC Syrup 2249
- Ryna .... ⊞ 804
- Soma Compound w/Codeine Tablets 2784
- Tylenol with Codeine 1592

Cyproheptadine Hydrochloride (Potential for additive CNS depressant effects). Products include:
- Periactin 1767

Desflurane (Potential for additive CNS depressant effects). Products include:
- Suprane (desflurane, USP) 1865

Desipramine Hydrochloride (Potential for additive CNS depressant effects). Products include:
- Norpramin Tablets 1273

Dexchlorpheniramine Maleate (Potential for additive CNS depressant effects).
No products indexed under this heading.

Dezocine (Potential for additive CNS depressant effects). Products include:
- Dalgan Injection 529

Diazepam (Potential for additive CNS depressant effects). Products include:
- Dizac (diazepam injectable emulsion) CIV 1862
- Valium Injectable 2336
- Valium Tablets 2335

Diphenhydramine Citrate (Potential for additive CNS depressant effects). Products include:
- Excedrin P.M. Analgesic/Sleeping Aid Tablets, Caplets, Liquigels 735

Diphenhydramine Hydrochloride (Potential for additive CNS depressant effects). Products include:
- Actifed Allergy Daytime/Nighttime Caplets .... ⊞ 808
- Actifed Sinus Daytime/Nighttime Tablets and Caplets .... ⊞ 809
- Extra Strength Bayer PM Aspirin Plus Sleep Aid .... ⊞ 617
- Benadryl Allergy Chewables .... ⊞ 811
- Benadryl Allergy/Cold Tablets .... ⊞ 811
- Benadryl Allergy Decongestant Liquid Medication .... ⊞ 812
- Benadryl Allergy Decongestant Tablets .... ⊞ 812
- Benadryl Allergy Liquid Medication .... ⊞ 813
- Benadryl Allergy .... ⊞ 811
- Benadryl Allergy Sinus Headache Caplets .... ⊞ 813
- Benadryl Dye-Free Allergy Liqui-gel Softgels .... ⊞ 813
- Benadryl Dye-Free Allergy Liquid Medication .... ⊞ 814
- Benadryl Itch Relief Stick Extra Strength .... ⊞ 814
- Benadryl Cream .... ⊞ 814
- Benadryl Gel .... ⊞ 815
- Benadryl Spray .... ⊞ 815
- Benadryl Injection 1955
- Contac Day & Night Cold/Flu Night Caplets .... ⊞ 772
- Contac Night Allergy/Sinus Caplets .... ⊞ 771
- Extra Strength Doan's P.M. .... ⊞ 653
- Excedrin P.M. Analgesic/Sleeping Aid Tablets, Caplets, Liquigels ... ⊞ 643
- Nytol QuickCaps Caplets .... ⊞ 632
- Sleepinal Night-time Sleep Aid Capsules and Softgels .... ⊞ 798

IMPORTANT NOTE: Always consult each drug listing in the patient's regimen for possible interactions.

TYLENOL Allergy Sinus NightTime, Maximum Strength Caplets 1571
TYLENOL Flu NightTime, Maximum Strength Gelcaps 1575
TYLENOL Flu NightTime, Maximum Strength Hot Medication Packets 1575
TYLENOL PM Pain Reliever/Sleep Aid, Extra Strength Gelcaps, Caplets, Geltabs 1576
TYLENOL Severe Allergy Medication Caplets 1571
Maximum Strength Unisom Sleep-gels 1990
Unisom With Pain Relief-Nighttime Sleep Aid and Pain Reliever 1991

Diphenylpyraline Hydrochloride (Potential for additive CNS depressant effects).
No products indexed under this heading.

Doxepin Hydrochloride (Potential for additive CNS depressant effects). Products include:
Adapin Capsules 1542
Sinequan 2028
Zonalon Cream 1042

Droperidol (Potential for additive CNS depressant effects). Products include:
Inapsine Injection 462

Enflurane (Potential for additive CNS depressant effects).
No products indexed under this heading.

Estazolam (Potential for additive CNS depressant effects). Products include:
ProSom Tablets 457

Ethchlorvynol (Potential for additive CNS depressant effects). Products include:
Placidyl Capsules 456

Ethinamate (Potential for additive CNS depressant effects).
No products indexed under this heading.

Fentanyl (Potential for additive CNS depressant effects). Products include:
Duragesic Transdermal System 1336

Fentanyl Citrate (Potential for additive CNS depressant effects). Products include:
Sublimaze Injection 463

Fluphenazine Decanoate (Potential for additive CNS depressant effects). Products include:
Prolixin Decanoate 510

Fluphenazine Enanthate (Potential for additive CNS depressant effects). Products include:
Prolixin Enanthate 510

Fluphenazine Hydrochloride (Potential for additive CNS depressant effects). Products include:
Prolixin 510

Flurazepam Hydrochloride (Potential for additive CNS depressant effects). Products include:
Dalmane Capsules 2329

Furazolidone (Coadministration may result in serious toxicity; concurrent use is contraindicated. Products include:
Furoxone 2221

Glutethimide (Potential for additive CNS depressant effects).
No products indexed under this heading.

Haloperidol (Potential for additive CNS depressant effects). Products include:
Haldol Injection, Tablets and Concentrate 1585

Haloperidol Decanoate (Potential for additive CNS depressant effects). Products include:
Haldol Decanoate 1587

Hydrocodone Bitartrate (Potential for additive CNS depressant effects). Products include:
Codiclear DH Syrup 808
Duratuss HD Elixir 2750
Histussin D Liquid 670
Hycodan Tablets and Syrup 946
Hycomine Compound Tablets 948
Hycomine 947
Hycotuss Expectorant Syrup 950
Hydrocet Capsules 787
Lorcet 10/650 Tablets 1016
Lortab 2751
Tussend 1830
Tussend Expectorant 1831
Vicodin Tablets 1404
Vicodin ES Tablets 1405
Vicodin HP Tablets 1403
Vicodin Tuss Expectorant 1406
Zydone Capsules 967

Hydrocodone Polistirex (Potential for additive CNS depressant effects). Products include:
Tussionex Pennkinetic Extended-Release Suspension 1624

Hydromorphone Hydrochloride (Potential for additive CNS depressant effects). Products include:
Dilaudid Ampules 1382
Dilaudid Cough Syrup 1383
Dilaudid-HP Injection 1384
Dilaudid-HP Lyophilized Powder 250 mg 1384
Dilaudid 1382
Dilaudid Oral Liquid 1386
Dilaudid 1382
Dilaudid Tablets - 8 mg 1386

Hydroxyzine Hydrochloride (Potential for additive CNS depressant effects). Products include:
Atarax Tablets & Syrup 1992
Marax Tablets & DF Syrup 2015
Vistaril Intramuscular Solution 2042

Imipramine Hydrochloride (Potential for additive CNS depressant effects). Products include:
Tofranil Ampuls 873
Tofranil Tablets 875

Imipramine Pamoate (Potential for additive CNS depressant effects). Products include:
Tofranil-PM Capsules 876

Isocarboxazid (Coadministration may result in serious toxicity; concurrent use is contraindicated; potential for additive CNS depressant effects).
No products indexed under this heading.

Isoflurane (Potential for additive CNS depressant effects).
No products indexed under this heading.

Ketamine Hydrochloride (Potential for additive CNS depressant effects).
No products indexed under this heading.

Levomethadyl Acetate Hydrochloride (Potential for additive CNS depressant effects). Products include:
Orlaam Oral Solution 2361

Levorphanol Tartrate (Potential for additive CNS depressant effects). Products include:
Levo-Dromoran 2297

Lithium Carbonate (Potential for additive CNS depressant effects). Products include:
Eskalith 2658
Lithium Carbonate Capsules & Tablets 2352
Lithonate/Lithotabs/Lithobid 2721

Lithium Citrate (Potential for additive CNS depressant effects).
No products indexed under this heading.

Loratadine (Potential for additive CNS depressant effects). Products include:
Claritin Tablets 2485
Claritin-D Tablets 2487

Lorazepam (Potential for additive CNS depressant effects). Products include:
Ativan Injection 2805
Ativan Tablets 2807

Loxapine Hydrochloride (Potential for additive CNS depressant effects). Products include:
Loxitane 1426

Loxapine Succinate (Potential for additive CNS depressant effects). Products include:
Loxitane Capsules 1426

Maprotiline Hydrochloride (Potential for additive CNS depressant effects). Products include:
Ludiomil Tablets 861

Meperidine Hydrochloride (Potential for additive CNS depressant effects). Products include:
Demerol 2438
Mepergan Injection 2859

Mephobarbital (Potential for additive CNS depressant effects). Products include:
Mebaral Tablets 2452

Meprobamate (Potential for additive CNS depressant effects). Products include:
Miltown Tablets 2780
PMB 200 and PMB 400 2890

Mesoridazine Besylate (Potential for additive CNS depressant effects). Products include:
Serentil 689

Methadone Hydrochloride (Potential for additive CNS depressant effects). Products include:
Methadone Hydrochloride Oral Concentrate 2356
Methadone Hydrochloride Oral Solution & Tablets 2357

Methdilazine Hydrochloride (Potential for additive CNS depressant effects).
No products indexed under this heading.

Methohexital Sodium (Potential for additive CNS depressant effects).
No products indexed under this heading.

Methotrimeprazine (Potential for additive CNS depressant effects). Products include:
Levoprome 1321

Methoxyflurane (Potential for additive CNS depressant effects).
No products indexed under this heading.

Midazolam Hydrochloride (Potential for additive CNS depressant effects). Products include:
Versed Injection 2324

Mirtazapine (Potential for additive CNS depressant effects). Products include:
Remeron Tablets 1878

Molindone Hydrochloride (Potential for additive CNS depressant effects). Products include:
Moban Tablets and Concentrate 1036

Morphine Sulfate (Potential for additive CNS depressant effects). Products include:
Astramorph/PF Injection, USP (Preservative-Free) 526
Duramorph Injection 983
Infumorph 200 and Infumorph 500 Sterile Solutions 985
Kadian Capsules 2948
MS Contin Tablets 2149
MSIR 2152
Oramorph SR (Morphine Sulfate Sustained Release Tablets) 2359

RMS Suppositories CII 2766
Roxanol 2365

Nortriptyline Hydrochloride (Potential for additive CNS depressant effects). Products include:
Pamelor 2409

Opium Alkaloids (Potential for additive CNS depressant effects).
No products indexed under this heading.

Oxazepam (Potential for additive CNS depressant effects). Products include:
Serax Capsules 2916
Serax Tablets 2916

Oxycodone Hydrochloride (Potential for additive CNS depressant effects). Products include:
OxyContin Tablets 2163
OxyIR Capsules 2167
Percocet Tablets 955
Percodan Tablets 955
Percodan-Demi Tablets 956
Roxicodone Tablets, Oral Solution & Intensol (Oxycodone) 2366
Tylox Capsules 1593

Pentobarbital Sodium (Potential for additive CNS depressant effects). Products include:
Nembutal Sodium Capsules 440
Nembutal Sodium Solution 442
Nembutal Sodium Suppositories 444

Perphenazine (Potential for additive CNS depressant effects). Products include:
Etrafon 2495
Triavil Tablets 1800
Trilafon 2532

Phenelzine Sulfate (Coadministration may result in serious toxicity; concurrent use is contraindicated; potential for additive CNS depressant effects). Products include:
Nardil 1977

Phenobarbital (Potential for additive CNS depressant effects). Products include:
Arco-Lase Plus Tablets 513
Bellergal-S Tablets 2375
Donnatal 2234
Donnatal Extentabs 2234
Donnatal Tablets 2234
Phenobarbital Elixir and Tablets 1523
Quadrinal Tablets 1398

Prazepam (Potential for additive CNS depressant effects).
No products indexed under this heading.

Prochlorperazine (Potential for additive CNS depressant effects). Products include:
Compazine 2644

Promethazine Hydrochloride (Potential for additive CNS depressant effects). Products include:
Mepergan Injection 2859
Phenergan with Codeine 2883
Phenergan with Dextromethorphan 2885
Phenergan Injection 2880
Phenergan Suppositories 2882
Phenergan Syrup 2881
Phenergan Tablets 2882
Phenergan VC 2886
Phenergan VC with Codeine 2888

Propofol (Potential for additive CNS depressant effects). Products include:
Diprivan Injectable Emulsion 2939

Propoxyphene Hydrochloride (Potential for additive CNS depressant effects). Products include:
Darvon 1475
Wygesic Tablets 2930

Propoxyphene Napsylate (Potential for additive CNS depressant effects). Products include:
Darvon-N/Darvocet-N 1473

Protriptyline Hydrochloride (Potential for additive CNS depressant effects). Products include:
Vivactil Tablets 1820

Pyrilamine Maleate (Potential for additive CNS depressant effects). Products include:
   4-Way Fast Acting Nasal Spray (regular & mentholated) 644
   Maximum Strength Multi-Symptom Formula Midol 621
   PMS Multi-Symptom Formula Midol 622

Pyrilamine Tannate (Potential for additive CNS depressant effects). Products include:
   Atrohist Pediatric Suspension 1604
   Atrohist Pediatric Suspension Dye-Free 1604
   Rynatan 2781

Quazepam (Potential for additive CNS depressant effects). Products include:
   Doral Tablets 2773

Risperidone (Potential for additive CNS depressant effects). Products include:
   Risperdal Tablets 1348

Secobarbital Sodium (Potential for additive CNS depressant effects). Products include:
   Seconal Sodium Pulvules 1529

Selegiline Hydrochloride (Coadministration may result in serious toxicity; concurrent use is contraindicated). Products include:
   Eldepryl Capsules 2729

Sevoflurane (Potential for additive CNS depressant effects).
   No products indexed under this heading.

Sufentanil Citrate (Potential for additive CNS depressant effects). Products include:
   Sufenta Injection 1355

Temazepam (Potential for additive CNS depressant effects). Products include:
   Restoril Capsules 2413

Terfenadine (Potential for additive CNS depressant effects). Products include:
   Seldane Tablets 1284
   Seldane-D Extended-Release Tablets 1286

Thiamylal Sodium (Potential for additive CNS depressant effects).
   No products indexed under this heading.

Thioridazine Hydrochloride (Potential for additive CNS depressant effects). Products include:
   Mellaril 2398

Thiothixene (Potential for additive CNS depressant effects). Products include:
   Navane Capsules and Concentrate 2018
   Navane Intramuscular 2019

Tranylcypromine Sulfate (Coadministration may result in serious toxicity; concurrent use is contraindicated; potential for additive CNS depressant effects). Products include:
   Parnate Tablets 2679

Triazolam (Potential for additive CNS depressant effects). Products include:
   Halcion Tablets 2093

Trifluoperazine Hydrochloride (Potential for additive CNS depressant effects). Products include:
   Stelazine 2692

Trimeprazine Tartrate (Potential for additive CNS depressant effects).
   No products indexed under this heading.

Trimipramine Maleate (Potential for additive CNS depressant effects). Products include:
   Surmontil Capsules 2917

Tripelennamine Hydrochloride (Potential for additive CNS depressant effects). Products include:
   PBZ Tablets 863
   PBZ-SR Tablets 862

Triprolidine Hydrochloride (Potential for additive CNS depressant effects). Products include:
   Actifed Cold & Allergy Tablets 807
   Actifed Cold & Sinus Caplets and Tablets 808

Zolpidem Tartrate (Potential for additive CNS depressant effects). Products include:
   Ambien Tablets 2559

Food Interactions
Alcohol (Potential for additive CNS depressant effects).

TYLENOL ACETAMINOPHEN EXTENDED RELIEF CAPLETS
(Acetaminophen) 1570
   See **TYLENOL acetaminophen, Regular Strength Caplets and Tablets**

TYLENOL ACETAMINOPHEN, EXTRA STRENGTH ADULT LIQUID PAIN RELIEVER
(Acetaminophen) 1570
   See **TYLENOL acetaminophen, Regular Strength Caplets and Tablets**

TYLENOL ACETAMINOPHEN, EXTRA STRENGTH GELCAPS, GELTABS, CAPLETS, TABLETS
(Acetaminophen) 1570
   See **TYLENOL acetaminophen, Regular Strength Caplets and Tablets**

TYLENOL ACETAMINOPHEN, REGULAR STRENGTH CAPLETS AND TABLETS
(Acetaminophen) 1570

Food Interactions
Alcohol (Concurrent use may increase drowsiness effect; chronic heavy alcohol abusers, 3 or more drinks per day, may be at increased risk of liver toxicity from excessive acetaminophen use).

TYLENOL ALLERGY SINUS, MAXIMUM STRENGTH CAPLETS AND GELCAPS
(Acetaminophen, Chlorpheniramine Maleate, Pseudoephedrine Hydrochloride) 1571
   See **TYLENOL Allergy Sinus Night-Time, Maximum Strength Caplets**

TYLENOL ALLERGY SINUS NIGHTTIME, MAXIMUM STRENGTH CAPLETS
(Acetaminophen, Pseudoephedrine Hydrochloride, Diphenhydramine Hydrochloride) 1571
May interact with monoamine oxidase inhibitors, hypnotics and sedatives, tranquilizers, and certain other agents. Compounds in these categories include:

Alprazolam (Concurrent use may increase drowsiness effect). Products include:
   Xanax Tablets 2115

Buspirone Hydrochloride (Concurrent use may increase drowsiness effect). Products include:
   BuSpar Tablets 738

Chlordiazepoxide (Concurrent use may increase drowsiness effect). Products include:
   Limbitrol 2333

Chlordiazepoxide Hydrochloride (Concurrent use may increase drowsiness effect). Products include:
   Librax Capsules 2330
   Librium Capsules 2331
   Librium Injectable 2332

Chlorpromazine (Concurrent use may increase drowsiness effect). Products include:
   Thorazine Suppositories 2701

Chlorpromazine Hydrochloride (Concurrent use may increase drowsiness effect). Products include:
   Thorazine 2701

Chlorprothixene (Concurrent use may increase drowsiness effect).
   No products indexed under this heading.

Chlorprothixene Hydrochloride (Concurrent use may increase drowsiness effect).
   No products indexed under this heading.

Clorazepate Dipotassium (Concurrent use may increase drowsiness effect). Products include:
   Tranxene 459

Diazepam (Concurrent use may increase drowsiness effect). Products include:
   Dizac (diazepam injectable emulsion) CIV 1862
   Valium Injectable 2336
   Valium Tablets 2335

Droperidol (Concurrent use may increase drowsiness effect). Products include:
   Inapsine Injection 462

Estazolam (Concurrent use may increase drowsiness effect). Products include:
   ProSom Tablets 457

Ethchlorvynol (Concurrent use may increase drowsiness effect). Products include:
   Placidyl Capsules 456

Ethinamate (Concurrent use may increase drowsiness effect).
   No products indexed under this heading.

Fluphenazine Decanoate (Concurrent use may increase drowsiness effect). Products include:
   Prolixin Decanoate 510

Fluphenazine Enanthate (Concurrent use may increase drowsiness effect). Products include:
   Prolixin Enanthate 510

Fluphenazine Hydrochloride (Concurrent use may increase drowsiness effect). Products include:
   Prolixin 510

Flurazepam Hydrochloride (Concurrent use may increase drowsiness effect). Products include:
   Dalmane Capsules 2329

Furazolidone (Concurrent and/or sequential use with MAO inhibitors is not recommended). Products include:
   Furoxone 2221

Glutethimide (Concurrent use may increase drowsiness effect).
   No products indexed under this heading.

Haloperidol (Concurrent use may increase drowsiness effect). Products include:
   Haldol Injection, Tablets and Concentrate 1585

Haloperidol Decanoate (Concurrent use may increase drowsiness effect). Products include:
   Haldol Decanoate 1587

Hydroxyzine Hydrochloride (Concurrent use may increase drowsiness effect). Products include:
   Atarax Tablets & Syrup 1992
   Marax Tablets & DF Syrup 2015
   Vistaril Intramuscular Solution 2042

Isocarboxazid (Concurrent and/or sequential use with MAO inhibitors is not recommended).
   No products indexed under this heading.

Lorazepam (Concurrent use may increase drowsiness effect). Products include:
   Ativan Injection 2805
   Ativan Tablets 2807

Loxapine Hydrochloride (Concurrent use may increase drowsiness effect). Products include:
   Loxitane 1426

Loxapine Succinate (Concurrent use may increase drowsiness effect). Products include:
   Loxitane Capsules 1426

Meprobamate (Concurrent use may increase drowsiness effect). Products include:
   Miltown Tablets 2780
   PMB 200 and PMB 400 2890

Mesoridazine Besylate (Concurrent use may increase drowsiness effect). Products include:
   Serentil 689

Midazolam Hydrochloride (Concurrent use may increase drowsiness effect). Products include:
   Versed Injection 2324

Molindone Hydrochloride (Concurrent use may increase drowsiness effect). Products include:
   Moban Tablets and Concentrate ... 1036

Oxazepam (Concurrent use may increase drowsiness effect). Products include:
   Serax Capsules 2916
   Serax Tablets 2916

Perphenazine (Concurrent use may increase drowsiness effect). Products include:
   Etrafon 2495
   Triavil Tablets 1800
   Trilafon 2532

Phenelzine Sulfate (Concurrent and/or sequential use with MAO inhibitors is not recommended). Products include:
   Nardil 1977

Prazepam (Concurrent use may increase drowsiness effect).
   No products indexed under this heading.

Prochlorperazine (Concurrent use may increase drowsiness effect). Products include:
   Compazine 2644

Promethazine Hydrochloride (Concurrent use may increase drowsiness effect). Products include:
   Mepergan Injection 2859
   Phenergan with Codeine 2883
   Phenergan with Dextromethorphan 2885
   Phenergan Injection 2880
   Phenergan Suppositories 2882
   Phenergan Syrup 2881
   Phenergan Tablets 2882
   Phenergan VC 2886
   Phenergan VC with Codeine 2888

Propofol (Concurrent use may increase drowsiness effect). Products include:
   Diprivan Injectable Emulsion 2939

Quazepam (Concurrent use may increase drowsiness effect). Products include:
   Doral Tablets 2773

IMPORTANT NOTE: Always consult each drug listing in the patient's regimen for possible interactions.

Tylenol Allergy Sinus

Secobarbital Sodium (Concurrent use may increase drowsiness effect). Products include:
Seconal Sodium Pulvules 1529
Selegiline Hydrochloride (Concurrent and/or sequential use with MAO inhibitors is not recommended). Products include:
Eldepryl Capsules 2729
Temazepam (Concurrent use may increase drowsiness effect). Products include:
Restoril Capsules 2413
Thioridazine Hydrochloride (Concurrent use may increase drowsiness effect). Products include:
Mellaril 2398
Thiothixene (Concurrent use may increase drowsiness effect). Products include:
Navane Capsules and Concentrate 2018
Navane Intramuscular 2019
Tranylcypromine Sulfate (Concurrent and/or sequential use with MAO inhibitors is not recommended). Products include:
Parnate Tablets 2679
Triazolam (Concurrent use may increase drowsiness effect). Products include:
Halcion Tablets 2093
Trifluoperazine Hydrochloride (Concurrent use may increase drowsiness effect). Products include:
Stelazine 2692
Zolpidem Tartrate (Concurrent use may increase drowsiness effect). Products include:
Ambien Tablets 2559

Food Interactions

Alcohol (Concurrent use may increase drowsiness effect; chronic heavy alcohol abusers, 3 or more drinks per day, may be at increased risk of liver toxicity from excessive acetaminophen use).

TYLENOL COLD MEDICATION, MULTI-SYMPTOM FORMULA TABLETS AND CAPLETS

(Acetaminophen, Chlorpheniramine Maleate, Pseudoephedrine Hydrochloride, Dextromethorphan Hydrobromide) 1572
May interact with hypnotics and sedatives, tranquilizers, monoamine oxidase inhibitors, and certain other agents. Compounds in these categories include:

Alprazolam (Concurrent use may increase drowsiness effect). Products include:
Xanax Tablets 2115
Buspirone Hydrochloride (Concurrent use may increase drowsiness effect). Products include:
BuSpar Tablets 738
Chlordiazepoxide (Concurrent use may increase drowsiness effect). Products include:
Limbitrol 2333
Chlordiazepoxide Hydrochloride (Concurrent use may increase drowsiness effect). Products include:
Librax Capsules 2330
Librium Capsules 2331
Librium Injectable 2332
Chlorpromazine (Concurrent use may increase drowsiness effect). Products include:
Thorazine Suppositories 2701
Chlorpromazine Hydrochloride (Concurrent use may increase drowsiness effect). Products include:
Thorazine 2701

Chlorprothixene (Concurrent use may increase drowsiness effect).
No products indexed under this heading.
Chlorprothixene Hydrochloride (Concurrent use may increase drowsiness effect).
No products indexed under this heading.
Clorazepate Dipotassium (Concurrent use may increase drowsiness effect). Products include:
Tranxene 459
Diazepam (Concurrent use may increase drowsiness effect). Products include:
Dizac (diazepam injectable emulsion) CIV 1862
Valium Injectable 2336
Valium Tablets 2335
Droperidol (Concurrent use may increase drowsiness effect). Products include:
Inapsine Injection 462
Estazolam (Concurrent use may increase drowsiness effect). Products include:
ProSom Tablets 457
Ethchlorvynol (Concurrent use may increase drowsiness effect). Products include:
Placidyl Capsules 456
Ethinamate (Concurrent use may increase drowsiness effect).
No products indexed under this heading.
Fluphenazine Decanoate (Concurrent use may increase drowsiness effect). Products include:
Prolixin Decanoate 510
Fluphenazine Enanthate (Concurrent use may increase drowsiness effect). Products include:
Prolixin Enanthate 510
Fluphenazine Hydrochloride (Concurrent use may increase drowsiness effect). Products include:
Prolixin 510
Flurazepam Hydrochloride (Concurrent use may increase drowsiness effect). Products include:
Dalmane Capsules 2329
Furazolidone (Concurrent and/or sequential use with MAO inhibitors is not recommended). Products include:
Furoxone 2221
Glutethimide (Concurrent use may increase drowsiness effect).
No products indexed under this heading.
Haloperidol (Concurrent use may increase drowsiness effect). Products include:
Haldol Injection, Tablets and Concentrate 1585
Haloperidol Decanoate (Concurrent use may increase drowsiness effect). Products include:
Haldol Decanoate 1587
Hydroxyzine Hydrochloride (Concurrent use may increase drowsiness effect). Products include:
Atarax Tablets & Syrup 1992
Marax Tablets & DF Syrup 2015
Vistaril Intramuscular Solution 2042
Isocarboxazid (Concurrent and/or sequential use with MAO inhibitors is not recommended).
No products indexed under this heading.
Lorazepam (Concurrent use may increase drowsiness effect). Products include:
Ativan Injection 2805
Ativan Tablets 2807

Interactions Index

Loxapine Hydrochloride (Concurrent use may increase drowsiness effect). Products include:
Loxitane 1426
Loxapine Succinate (Concurrent use may increase drowsiness effect). Products include:
Loxitane Capsules 1426
Meprobamate (Concurrent use may increase drowsiness effect). Products include:
Miltown Tablets 2780
PMB 200 and PMB 400 2890
Mesoridazine Besylate (Concurrent use may increase drowsiness effect). Products include:
Serentil 689
Midazolam Hydrochloride (Concurrent use may increase drowsiness effect). Products include:
Versed Injection 2324
Molindone Hydrochloride (Concurrent use may increase drowsiness effect). Products include:
Moban Tablets and Concentrate 1036
Oxazepam (Concurrent use may increase drowsiness effect). Products include:
Serax Capsules 2916
Serax Tablets 2916
Perphenazine (Concurrent use may increase drowsiness effect). Products include:
Etrafon 2495
Triavil Tablets 1800
Trilafon 2532
Phenelzine Sulfate (Concurrent and/or sequential use with MAO inhibitors is not recommended). Products include:
Nardil 1977
Prazepam (Concurrent use may increase drowsiness effect).
No products indexed under this heading.
Prochlorperazine (Concurrent use may increase drowsiness effect). Products include:
Compazine 2644
Promethazine Hydrochloride (Concurrent use may increase drowsiness effect). Products include:
Meperigan Injection 2859
Phenergan with Codeine 2883
Phenergan with Dextromethorphan 2885
Phenergan Injection 2880
Phenergan Suppositories 2882
Phenergan Syrup 2881
Phenergan Tablets 2882
Phenergan VC 2886
Phenergan VC with Codeine 2888
Propofol (Concurrent use may increase drowsiness effect). Products include:
Diprivan Injectable Emulsion 2939
Quazepam (Concurrent use may increase drowsiness effect). Products include:
Doral Tablets 2773
Secobarbital Sodium (Concurrent use may increase drowsiness effect). Products include:
Seconal Sodium Pulvules 1529
Selegiline Hydrochloride (Concurrent and/or sequential use with MAO inhibitors is not recommended). Products include:
Eldepryl Capsules 2729
Temazepam (Concurrent use may increase drowsiness effect). Products include:
Restoril Capsules 2413
Thioridazine Hydrochloride (Concurrent use may increase drowsiness effect). Products include:
Mellaril 2398

Thiothixene (Concurrent use may increase drowsiness effect). Products include:
Navane Capsules and Concentrate 2018
Navane Intramuscular 2019
Tranylcypromine Sulfate (Concurrent and/or sequential use with MAO inhibitors is not recommended). Products include:
Parnate Tablets 2679
Triazolam (Concurrent use may increase drowsiness effect). Products include:
Halcion Tablets 2093
Trifluoperazine Hydrochloride (Concurrent use may increase drowsiness effect). Products include:
Stelazine 2692
Zolpidem Tartrate (Concurrent use may increase drowsiness effect). Products include:
Ambien Tablets 2559

Food Interactions

Alcohol (Concurrent use may increase drowsiness effect; chronic heavy alcohol abusers, 3 or more drinks per day, may be at increased risk of liver toxicity from excessive acetaminophen use).

TYLENOL COLD MEDICATION, MULTI-SYMPTOM HOT LIQUID PACKETS

(Acetaminophen, Chlorpheniramine Maleate, Pseudoephedrine Hydrochloride, Dextromethorphan Hydrobromide) 1572
See TYLENOL Cold Medication, Multi-Symptom Formula Tablets and Caplets

TYLENOL COLD MEDICATION, NO DROWSINESS FORMULA CAPLETS AND GELCAPS

(Acetaminophen, Pseudoephedrine Hydrochloride, Dextromethorphan Hydrobromide) 1572
See TYLENOL Cold Medication, Multi-Symptom Formula Tablets and Caplets

TYLENOL COLD SEVERE CONGESTION CAPLETS

(Acetaminophen, Dextromethorphan Hydrobromide, Guaifenesin, Pseudoephedrine Hydrochloride) 1573
May interact with monoamine oxidase inhibitors and certain other agents. Compounds in these categories include:

Furazolidone (Concurrent and/or sequential use is not recommended). Products include:
Furoxone 2221
Isocarboxazid (Concurrent and/or sequential use is not recommended).
No products indexed under this heading.
Phenelzine Sulfate (Concurrent and/or sequential use is not recommended). Products include:
Nardil 1977
Selegiline Hydrochloride (Concurrent and/or sequential use is not recommended). Products include:
Eldepryl Capsules 2729
Tranylcypromine Sulfate (Concurrent and/or sequential use is not recommended). Products include:
Parnate Tablets 2679

Food Interactions

Alcohol (Chronic heavy alcohol abusers, 3 or more drinks per day, may be at increased risk of liver toxicity from acetaminophen use).

(■ Described in PDR For Nonprescription Drugs)   (⊙ Described in PDR For Ophthalmology)

TYLENOL COUGH MEDICATION, MULTI SYMPTOM
(Dextromethorphan Hydrobromide, Acetaminophen) 1574
See TYLENOL Cough Medication with Decongestant, Multi Symptom

TYLENOL COUGH MEDICATION WITH DECONGESTANT, MULTI SYMPTOM
(Dextromethorphan Hydrobromide, Acetaminophen, Pseudoephedrine Hydrochloride) 1574
May interact with monoamine oxidase inhibitors and certain other agents. Compounds in these categories include:

Furazolidone (Concurrent and/or sequential use is not recommended). Products include:
Furoxone 2221

Isocarboxazid (Concurrent and/or sequential use is not recommended).
No products indexed under this heading.

Phenelzine Sulfate (Concurrent and/or sequential use is not recommended). Products include:
Nardil 1977

Selegiline Hydrochloride (Concurrent and/or sequential use is not recommended). Products include:
Eldepryl Capsules 2729

Tranylcypromine Sulfate (Concurrent and/or sequential use is not recommended). Products include:
Parnate Tablets 2679

Food Interactions
Alcohol (Chronic heavy alcohol abusers, 3 or more drinks per day, may be at increased risk of liver toxicity from acetaminophen use).

TYLENOL FLU NO DROWSINESS FORMULA, MAXIMUM STRENGTH GELCAPS
(Acetaminophen, Dextromethorphan Hydrobromide, Pseudoephedrine Hydrochloride) 1575
See TYLENOL Flu NightTime, Maximum Strength Hot Medication Packets

TYLENOL FLU NIGHTTIME, MAXIMUM STRENGTH GELCAPS
(Acetaminophen, Pseudoephedrine Hydrochloride, Diphenhydramine Hydrochloride) 1575
See TYLENOL Flu NightTime, Maximum Strength Hot Medication Packets

TYLENOL FLU NIGHTTIME, MAXIMUM STRENGTH HOT MEDICATION PACKETS
(Acetaminophen, Diphenhydramine Hydrochloride, Pseudoephedrine Hydrochloride) 1575
May interact with monoamine oxidase inhibitors, hypnotics and sedatives, tranquilizers, and certain other agents. Compounds in these categories include:

Alprazolam (Concurrent use may increase drowsiness effect). Products include:
Xanax Tablets 2115

Buspirone Hydrochloride (Concurrent use may increase drowsiness effect). Products include:
BuSpar Tablets 738

Chlordiazepoxide (Concurrent use may increase drowsiness effect). Products include:
Limbitrol 2333

Chlordiazepoxide Hydrochloride (Concurrent use may increase drowsiness effect). Products include:
Librax Capsules 2330
Librium Capsules 2331
Librium Injectable 2332

Chlorpromazine (Concurrent use may increase drowsiness effect). Products include:
Thorazine Suppositories 2701

Chlorpromazine Hydrochloride (Concurrent use may increase drowsiness effect). Products include:
Thorazine 2701

Chlorprothixene (Concurrent use may increase drowsiness effect).
No products indexed under this heading.

Chlorprothixene Hydrochloride (Concurrent use may increase drowsiness effect).
No products indexed under this heading.

Clorazepate Dipotassium (Concurrent use may increase drowsiness effect). Products include:
Tranxene 459

Diazepam (Concurrent use may increase drowsiness effect). Products include:
Dizac (diazepam injectable emulsion) CIV 1862
Valium Injectable 2336
Valium Tablets 2335

Droperidol (Concurrent use may increase drowsiness effect). Products include:
Inapsine Injection 462

Estazolam (Concurrent use may increase drowsiness effect). Products include:
ProSom Tablets 457

Ethchlorvynol (Concurrent use may increase drowsiness effect). Products include:
Placidyl Capsules 456

Ethinamate (Concurrent use may increase drowsiness effect).
No products indexed under this heading.

Fluphenazine Decanoate (Concurrent use may increase drowsiness effect). Products include:
Prolixin Decanoate 510

Fluphenazine Enanthate (Concurrent use may increase drowsiness effect). Products include:
Prolixin Enanthate 510

Fluphenazine Hydrochloride (Concurrent use may increase drowsiness effect). Products include:
Prolixin 510

Flurazepam Hydrochloride (Concurrent use may increase drowsiness effect). Products include:
Dalmane Capsules 2329

Furazolidone (Concurrent and/or sequential use with MAO inhibitors is not recommended). Products include:
Furoxone 2221

Glutethimide (Concurrent use may increase drowsiness effect).
No products indexed under this heading.

Haloperidol (Concurrent use may increase drowsiness effect). Products include:
Haldol Injection, Tablets and Concentrate 1585

Haloperidol Decanoate (Concurrent use may increase drowsiness effect). Products include:
Haldol Decanoate 1587

Hydroxyzine Hydrochloride (Concurrent use may increase drowsiness effect). Products include:
Atarax Tablets & Syrup 1992
Marax Tablets & DF Syrup ... 2015
Vistaril Intramuscular Solution 2042

Isocarboxazid (Concurrent and/or sequential use with MAO inhibitors is not recommended).
No products indexed under this heading.

Lorazepam (Concurrent use may increase drowsiness effect). Products include:
Ativan Injection 2805
Ativan Tablets 2807

Loxapine Hydrochloride (Concurrent use may increase drowsiness effect). Products include:
Loxitane 1426

Loxapine Succinate (Concurrent use may increase drowsiness effect). Products include:
Loxitane Capsules 1426

Meprobamate (Concurrent use may increase drowsiness effect). Products include:
Miltown Tablets 2780
PMB 200 and PMB 400 2890

Mesoridazine Besylate (Concurrent use may increase drowsiness effect). Products include:
Serentil 689

Midazolam Hydrochloride (Concurrent use may increase drowsiness effect). Products include:
Versed Injection 2324

Molindone Hydrochloride (Concurrent use may increase drowsiness effect). Products include:
Moban Tablets and Concentrate 1036

Oxazepam (Concurrent use may increase drowsiness effect). Products include:
Serax Capsules 2916
Serax Tablets 2916

Perphenazine (Concurrent use may increase drowsiness effect). Products include:
Etrafon 2495
Triavil Tablets 1800
Trilafon 2532

Phenelzine Sulfate (Concurrent and/or sequential use with MAO inhibitors is not recommended). Products include:
Nardil 1977

Prazepam (Concurrent use may increase drowsiness effect).
No products indexed under this heading.

Prochlorperazine (Concurrent use may increase drowsiness effect). Products include:
Compazine 2644

Promethazine Hydrochloride (Concurrent use may increase drowsiness effect). Products include:
Mepergan Injection 2859
Phenergan with Codeine 2883
Phenergan with Dextromethorphan 2885
Phenergan Injection 2880
Phenergan Suppositories ... 2882
Phenergan Syrup 2881
Phenergan Tablets 2882
Phenergan VC 2886
Phenergan VC with Codeine 2888

Propofol (Concurrent use may increase drowsiness effect). Products include:
Diprivan Injectable Emulsion 2939

Quazepam (Concurrent use may increase drowsiness effect). Products include:
Doral Tablets 2773

Secobarbital Sodium (Concurrent use may increase drowsiness effect). Products include:
Seconal Sodium Pulvules ... 1529

Selegiline Hydrochloride (Concurrent and/or sequential use with MAO inhibitors is not recommended). Products include:
Eldepryl Capsules 2729

Temazepam (Concurrent use may increase drowsiness effect). Products include:
Restoril Capsules 2413

Thioridazine Hydrochloride (Concurrent use may increase drowsiness effect). Products include:
Mellaril 2398

Thiothixene (Concurrent use may increase drowsiness effect). Products include:
Navane Capsules and Concentrate ... 2018
Navane Intramuscular 2019

Tranylcypromine Sulfate (Concurrent and/or sequential use with MAO inhibitors is not recommended). Products include:
Parnate Tablets 2679

Triazolam (Concurrent use may increase drowsiness effect). Products include:
Halcion Tablets 2093

Trifluoperazine Hydrochloride (Concurrent use may increase drowsiness effect). Products include:
Stelazine 2692

Zolpidem Tartrate (Concurrent use may increase drowsiness effect). Products include:
Ambien Tablets 2559

Food Interactions
Alcohol (Concurrent use may increase drowsiness effect; chronic heavy alcohol abusers, 3 or more drinks per day, may be at increased risk of liver toxicity from excessive acetaminophen use).

TYLENOL HEADACHE PLUS PAIN RELIEVER WITH ANTACID, EXTRA STRENGTH CAPLETS
(Acetaminophen, Calcium Carbonate) 705
May interact with:

Prescription Drugs, unspecified (Antacid present in this product may interact with certain unspecified prescription drugs).

Food Interactions
Alcohol (Chronic heavy alcohol abusers, 3 or more drinks per day, may be at increased risk of liver toxicity from acetaminophen use).

TYLENOL PM PAIN RELIEVER/SLEEP AID, EXTRA STRENGTH GELCAPS, CAPLETS, GELTABS
(Acetaminophen, Diphenhydramine Hydrochloride) 1576
May interact with hypnotics and sedatives, tranquilizers, and certain other agents. Compounds in these categories include:

Alprazolam (Tylenol PM causes drowsiness; concurrent use may increase the drowsiness effect). Products include:
Xanax Tablets 2115

Buspirone Hydrochloride (Tylenol PM causes drowsiness; concurrent use may increase the drowsiness effect). Products include:
BuSpar Tablets 738

IMPORTANT NOTE: Always consult each drug listing in the patient's regimen for possible interactions.

Tylenol PM Extra | Interactions Index

Chlordiazepoxide (Tylenol PM causes drowsiness; concurrent use may increase the drowsiness effect). Products include:
Limbitrol 2333

Chlordiazepoxide Hydrochloride (Tylenol PM causes drowsiness; concurrent use may increase the drowsiness effect). Products include:
Librax Capsules 2330
Librium Capsules 2331
Librium Injectable 2332

Chlorpromazine (Tylenol PM causes drowsiness; concurrent use may increase the drowsiness effect). Products include:
Thorazine Suppositories 2701

Chlorpromazine Hydrochloride (Tylenol PM causes drowsiness; concurrent use may increase the drowsiness effect). Products include:
Thorazine 2701

Chlorprothixene (Tylenol PM causes drowsiness; concurrent use may increase the drowsiness effect).
No products indexed under this heading.

Chlorprothixene Hydrochloride (Tylenol PM causes drowsiness; concurrent use may increase the drowsiness effect).
No products indexed under this heading.

Clorazepate Dipotassium (Tylenol PM causes drowsiness; concurrent use may increase the drowsiness effect). Products include:
Tranxene 459

Diazepam (Tylenol PM causes drowsiness; concurrent use may increase the drowsiness effect). Products include:
Dizac (diazepam injectable emulsion) CIV 1862
Valium Injectable 2336
Valium Tablets 2335

Droperidol (Tylenol PM causes drowsiness; concurrent use may increase the drowsiness effect). Products include:
Inapsine Injection 462

Estazolam (Tylenol PM causes drowsiness; concurrent use may increase the drowsiness effect). Products include:
ProSom Tablets 457

Ethchlorvynol (Tylenol PM causes drowsiness; concurrent use may increase the drowsiness effect). Products include:
Placidyl Capsules 456

Ethinamate (Tylenol PM causes drowsiness; concurrent use may increase the drowsiness effect).
No products indexed under this heading.

Fluphenazine Decanoate (Tylenol PM causes drowsiness; concurrent use may increase the drowsiness effect). Products include:
Prolixin Decanoate 510

Fluphenazine Enanthate (Tylenol PM causes drowsiness; concurrent use may increase the drowsiness effect). Products include:
Prolixin Enanthate 510

Fluphenazine Hydrochloride (Tylenol PM causes drowsiness; concurrent use may increase the drowsiness effect). Products include:
Prolixin 510

Flurazepam Hydrochloride (Tylenol PM causes drowsiness; concurrent use may increase the drowsiness effect). Products include:
Dalmane Capsules 2329

Glutethimide (Tylenol PM causes drowsiness; concurrent use may increase the drowsiness effect).
No products indexed under this heading.

Haloperidol (Tylenol PM causes drowsiness; concurrent use may increase the drowsiness effect). Products include:
Haldol Injection, Tablets and Concentrate 1585

Haloperidol Decanoate (Tylenol PM causes drowsiness; concurrent use may increase the drowsiness effect). Products include:
Haldol Decanoate 1587

Hydroxyzine Hydrochloride (Tylenol PM causes drowsiness; concurrent use may increase the drowsiness effect). Products include:
Atarax Tablets & Syrup 1992
Marax Tablets & DF Syrup 2015
Vistaril Intramuscular Solution ... 2042

Lorazepam (Tylenol PM causes drowsiness; concurrent use may increase the drowsiness effect). Products include:
Ativan Injection 2805
Ativan Tablets 2807

Loxapine Hydrochloride (Tylenol PM causes drowsiness; concurrent use may increase the drowsiness effect). Products include:
Loxitane 1426

Loxapine Succinate (Tylenol PM causes drowsiness; concurrent use may increase the drowsiness effect). Products include:
Loxitane Capsules 1426

Meprobamate (Tylenol PM causes drowsiness; concurrent use may increase the drowsiness effect). Products include:
Miltown Tablets 2780
PMB 200 and PMB 400 2890

Mesoridazine Besylate (Tylenol PM causes drowsiness; concurrent use may increase the drowsiness effect). Products include:
Serentil 689

Midazolam Hydrochloride (Tylenol PM causes drowsiness; concurrent use may increase the drowsiness effect). Products include:
Versed Injection 2324

Molindone Hydrochloride (Tylenol PM causes drowsiness; concurrent use may increase the drowsiness effect). Products include:
Moban Tablets and Concentrate ... 1036

Oxazepam (Tylenol PM causes drowsiness; concurrent use may increase the drowsiness effect). Products include:
Serax Capsules 2916
Serax Tablets 2916

Perphenazine (Tylenol PM causes drowsiness; concurrent use may increase the drowsiness effect). Products include:
Etrafon 2495
Triavil Tablets 1800
Trilafon 2532

Prazepam (Tylenol PM causes drowsiness; concurrent use may increase the drowsiness effect).
No products indexed under this heading.

Prochlorperazine (Tylenol PM causes drowsiness; concurrent use may increase the drowsiness effect). Products include:
Compazine 2644

Promethazine Hydrochloride (Tylenol PM causes drowsiness; concurrent use may increase the drowsiness effect). Products include:
Mepergan Injection 2859
Phenergan with Codeine 2883
Phenergan with Dextromethorphan ... 2885
Phenergan Injection 2880
Phenergan Suppositories 2882
Phenergan Syrup 2881
Phenergan Tablets 2882
Phenergan VC 2886
Phenergan VC with Codeine ... 2888

Propofol (Tylenol PM causes drowsiness; concurrent use may increase the drowsiness effect). Products include:
Diprivan Injectable Emulsion ... 2939

Quazepam (Tylenol PM causes drowsiness; concurrent use may increase the drowsiness effect). Products include:
Doral Tablets 2773

Secobarbital Sodium (Tylenol PM causes drowsiness; concurrent use may increase the drowsiness effect). Products include:
Seconal Sodium Pulvules 1529

Temazepam (Tylenol PM causes drowsiness; concurrent use may increase the drowsiness effect). Products include:
Restoril Capsules 2413

Thioridazine Hydrochloride (Tylenol PM causes drowsiness; concurrent use may increase the drowsiness effect). Products include:
Mellaril 2398

Thiothixene (Tylenol PM causes drowsiness; concurrent use may increase the drowsiness effect). Products include:
Navane Capsules and Concentrate ... 2018
Navane Intramuscular 2019

Triazolam (Tylenol PM causes drowsiness; concurrent use may increase the drowsiness effect). Products include:
Halcion Tablets 2093

Trifluoperazine Hydrochloride (Tylenol PM causes drowsiness; concurrent use may increase the drowsiness effect). Products include:
Stelazine 2692

Zolpidem Tartrate (Tylenol PM causes drowsiness; concurrent use may increase the drowsiness effect). Products include:
Ambien Tablets 2559

Food Interactions

Alcohol (Avoid concurrent use; chronic heavy alcohol abusers, 3 or more drinks per day, may be at increased risk of liver toxicity from acetaminophen use).

TYLENOL SEVERE ALLERGY MEDICATION CAPLETS
(Acetaminophen, Chlorpheniramine Maleate, Pseudoephedrine Hydrochloride) 1571
See TYLENOL Allergy Sinus Night-Time, Maximum Strength Caplets

TYLENOL SINUS, MAXIMUM STRENGTH GELTABS, GELCAPS, CAPLETS AND TABLETS
(Acetaminophen, Pseudoephedrine Hydrochloride) 1576
May interact with monoamine oxidase inhibitors, and sedatives, tranquilizers, and certain other agents. Compounds in these categories include:

Furazolidone (Concurrent and/or sequential use with monoamine oxidase inhibitors is not recommended). Products include:
Furoxone 2221

Isocarboxazid (Concurrent and/or sequential use with monoamine oxidase inhibitors is not recommended).
No products indexed under this heading.

Phenelzine Sulfate (Concurrent and/or sequential use with monoamine oxidase inhibitors is not recommended). Products include:
Nardil 1977

Selegiline Hydrochloride (Concurrent and/or sequential use with monoamine oxidase inhibitors is not recommended). Products include:
Eldepryl Capsules 2729

Tranylcypromine Sulfate (Concurrent and/or sequential use with monoamine oxidase inhibitors is not recommended). Products include:
Parnate Tablets 2679

Food Interactions

Alcohol (Chronic heavy alcohol abusers, 3 or more drinks per day, may be at increased risk of liver toxicity from acetaminophen use).

TYLENOL WITH CODEINE ELIXIR
(Acetaminophen, Codeine Phosphate) 1592
May interact with central nervous system depressants, anticholinergics, antipsychotic agents, narcotic analgesics, and certain other agents. Compounds in these categories include:

Alfentanil Hydrochloride (Additive CNS depression). Products include:
Alfenta Injection 1334

Alprazolam (Additive CNS depression). Products include:
Xanax Tablets 2115

Aprobarbital (Additive CNS depression).
No products indexed under this heading.

Atropine Sulfate (May produce paralytic ileus). Products include:
Arco-Lase Plus Tablets 513
Atrohist Plus Tablets 1605
Donnatal 2234
Donnatal Extentabs 2234
Donnatal Tablets 2234
Lomotil 2591
Motofen Tablets 789
Urised Tablets 2123

Belladonna Alkaloids (May produce paralytic ileus). Products include:
Bellergal-S Tablets 2375
Hyland's Bedwetting Tablets ... 788
Hyland's EnurAid Tablets 789
Hyland's Headache Tablets 790
Hyland's Teething Tablets 790
Similasan Eye Drops #1 769

Benztropine Mesylate (May produce paralytic ileus). Products include:
Cogentin 1661

Biperiden Hydrochloride (May produce paralytic ileus). Products include:
Akineton 1380

Buprenorphine (Additive CNS depression). Products include:
Buprenex Injectable 2170

Buspirone Hydrochloride (Additive CNS depression). Products include:
BuSpar Tablets 738

Butabarbital (Additive CNS depression).
No products indexed under this heading.

(◫ Described in PDR For Nonprescription Drugs)   (◉ Described in PDR For Ophthalmology)

1129 Interactions Index Tylenol with Codeine

Butalbital (Additive CNS depression). Products include:
- Axocet Capsules ... 2469
- Esgic-plus Capsules ... 1012
- Esgic-plus Tablets ... 1012
- Fioricet Tablets ... 2386
- Fioricet with Codeine Capsules ... 2387
- Fiorinal Capsules ... 2388
- Fiorinal with Codeine Capsules ... 2390
- Fiorinal Tablets ... 2388
- Phrenilin ... 790
- Sedapap Tablets 50 mg/650 mg ... 1826

Chlordiazepoxide (Additive CNS depression). Products include:
- Limbitrol ... 2333

Chlordiazepoxide Hydrochloride (Additive CNS depression). Products include:
- Librax Capsules ... 2330
- Librium Capsules ... 2331
- Librium Injectable ... 2332

Chlorpromazine (Additive CNS depression). Products include:
- Thorazine Suppositories ... 2701

Chlorprothixene (Additive CNS depression).
- No products indexed under this heading.

Chlorprothixene Hydrochloride (Additive CNS depression).
- No products indexed under this heading.

Chlorprothixene Lactate (Additive CNS depression).
- No products indexed under this heading.

Clidinium Bromide (May produce paralytic ileus). Products include:
- Librax Capsules ... 2330

Clorazepate Dipotassium (Additive CNS depression). Products include:
- Tranxene ... 459

Clozapine (Additive CNS depression). Products include:
- Clozaril Tablets ... 2377

Desflurane (Additive CNS depression). Products include:
- Suprane (desflurane, USP) ... 1865

Dezocine (Additive CNS depression). Products include:
- Dalgan Injection ... 529

Diazepam (Additive CNS depression). Products include:
- Dizac (diazepam injectable emulsion) CIV ... 1862
- Valium Injectable ... 2336
- Valium Tablets ... 2335

Dicyclomine Hydrochloride (May produce paralytic ileus). Products include:
- Bentyl ... 1246

Droperidol (Additive CNS depression). Products include:
- Inapsine Injection ... 462

Enflurane (Additive CNS depression).
- No products indexed under this heading.

Estazolam (Additive CNS depression). Products include:
- ProSom Tablets ... 457

Ethchlorvynol (Additive CNS depression). Products include:
- Placidyl Capsules ... 456

Ethinamate (Additive CNS depression).
- No products indexed under this heading.

Ethopropazine Hydrochloride (May produce paralytic ileus).

Fentanyl (Additive CNS depression). Products include:
- Duragesic Transdermal System ... 1336

Fentanyl Citrate (Additive CNS depression). Products include:
- Sublimaze Injection ... 463

Fluphenazine Decanoate (Additive CNS depression). Products include:
- Prolixin Decanoate ... 510

Fluphenazine Enanthate (Additive CNS depression). Products include:
- Prolixin Enanthate ... 510

Fluphenazine Hydrochloride (Additive CNS depression). Products include:
- Prolixin ... 510

Flurazepam Hydrochloride (Additive CNS depression). Products include:
- Dalmane Capsules ... 2329

Glutethimide (Additive CNS depression).
- No products indexed under this heading.

Glycopyrrolate (May produce paralytic ileus). Products include:
- Robinul Forte Tablets ... 2247
- Robinul Injectable ... 2247
- Robinul Tablets ... 2247

Haloperidol (Additive CNS depression). Products include:
- Haldol Injection, Tablets and Concentrate ... 1585

Haloperidol Decanoate (Additive CNS depression). Products include:
- Haldol Decanoate ... 1587

Hydrocodone Bitartrate (Additive CNS depression). Products include:
- Codiclear DH Syrup ... 808
- Duratuss HD Elixir ... 2750
- Histussin D Liquid ... 670
- Hycodan Tablets and Syrup ... 946
- Hycomine Compound Tablets ... 948
- Hycomine ... 947
- Hycotuss Expectorant Syrup ... 950
- Hydrocet Capsules ... 787
- Lorcet 10/650 Tablets ... 1016
- Lortab ... 2751
- Tussend ... 1830
- Tussend Expectorant ... 1831
- Vicodin Tablets ... 1404
- Vicodin ES Tablets ... 1405
- Vicodin HP Tablets ... 1403
- Vicodin Tuss Expectorant ... 1406
- Zydone Capsules ... 967

Hydrocodone Polistirex (Additive CNS depression). Products include:
- Tussionex Pennkinetic Extended-Release Suspension ... 1624

Hydromorphone Hydrochloride (Additive CNS depression). Products include:
- Dilaudid Ampules ... 1382
- Dilaudid Cough Syrup ... 1383
- Dilaudid-HP Injection ... 1384
- Dilaudid-HP Lyophilized Powder 250 mg ... 1384
- Dilaudid ... 1382
- Dilaudid Oral Liquid ... 1386
- Dilaudid ... 1382
- Dilaudid Tablets - 8 mg ... 1386

Hydroxyzine Hydrochloride (Additive CNS depression). Products include:
- Atarax Tablets & Syrup ... 1992
- Marax Tablets & DF Syrup ... 2015
- Vistaril Intramuscular Solution ... 2042

Hyoscyamine (May produce paralytic ileus). Products include:
- Cystospaz Tablets ... 2123
- Urised Tablets ... 2123

Hyoscyamine Sulfate (May produce paralytic ileus). Products include:
- Arco-Lase Plus Tablets ... 513
- Atrohist Plus Tablets ... 1605
- Cystospaz-M Capsules ... 2123
- Donnatal ... 2234
- Donnatal Extentabs ... 2234
- Donnatal Tablets ... 2234
- Kutrase Capsules ... 2546
- Levsin/Levsinex/Levbid ... 2549

Ipratropium Bromide (May produce paralytic ileus). Products include:
- Atrovent Inhalation Aerosol ... 674
- Atrovent Inhalation Solution ... 675
- Atrovent Nasal Spray 0.03% ... 676
- Atrovent Nasal Spray 0.06% ... 678

Isoflurane (Additive CNS depression).
- No products indexed under this heading.

Ketamine Hydrochloride (Additive CNS depression).
- No products indexed under this heading.

Levomethadyl Acetate Hydrochloride (Additive CNS depression). Products include:
- Orlaam Oral Solution ... 2361

Levorphanol Tartrate (Additive CNS depression). Products include:
- Levo-Dromoran ... 2297

Lithium Carbonate (Additive CNS depression). Products include:
- Eskalith ... 2658
- Lithium Carbonate Capsules & Tablets ... 2352
- Lithonate/Lithotabs/Lithobid ... 2721

Lithium Citrate (Additive CNS depression).
- No products indexed under this heading.

Lorazepam (Additive CNS depression). Products include:
- Ativan Injection ... 2805
- Ativan Tablets ... 2807

Loxapine Hydrochloride (Additive CNS depression). Products include:
- Loxitane ... 1426

Loxapine Succinate (Additive CNS depression). Products include:
- Loxitane Capsules ... 1426

Maprotiline Hydrochloride (May result in increased effects). Products include:
- Ludiomil Tablets ... 861

Mepenzolate Bromide (May produce paralytic ileus).
- No products indexed under this heading.

Meperidine Hydrochloride (Additive CNS depression). Products include:
- Demerol ... 2438
- Mepergan Injection ... 2859

Mephobarbital (Additive CNS depression). Products include:
- Mebaral Tablets ... 2452

Meprobamate (Additive CNS depression). Products include:
- Miltown Tablets ... 2780
- PMB 200 and PMB 400 ... 2890

Mesoridazine Besylate (Additive CNS depression). Products include:
- Serentil ... 689

Methadone Hydrochloride (Additive CNS depression). Products include:
- Methadone Hydrochloride Oral Concentrate ... 2356
- Methadone Hydrochloride Oral Solution & Tablets ... 2357

Methohexital Sodium (Additive CNS depression).
- No products indexed under this heading.

Methotrimeprazine (Additive CNS depression). Products include:
- Levoprome ... 1321

Methoxyflurane (Additive CNS depression).
- No products indexed under this heading.

Midazolam Hydrochloride (Additive CNS depression). Products include:
- Versed Injection ... 2324

Molindone Hydrochloride (Additive CNS depression). Products include:
- Moban Tablets and Concentrate ... 1036

Morphine Sulfate (Additive CNS depression). Products include:
- Astramorph/PF Injection, USP (Preservative-Free) ... 526
- Duramorph Injection ... 983
- Infumorph 200 and Infumorph 500 Sterile Solutions ... 985
- Kadian Capsules ... 2948
- MS Contin Tablets ... 2149
- MSIR ... 2152
- Oramorph SR (Morphine Sulfate Sustained Release Tablets) ... 2359
- RMS Suppositories CII ... 2766
- Roxanol ... 2365

Opium Alkaloids (Additive CNS depression).
- No products indexed under this heading.

Oxazepam (Additive CNS depression). Products include:
- Serax Capsules ... 2916
- Serax Tablets ... 2916

Oxybutynin Chloride (May produce paralytic ileus). Products include:
- Ditropan ... 1267

Oxycodone Hydrochloride (Additive CNS depression). Products include:
- OxyContin Tablets ... 2163
- OxyIR Capsules ... 2167
- Percocet Tablets ... 955
- Percodan Tablets ... 955
- Percodan-Demi Tablets ... 956
- Roxicodone Tablets, Oral Solution & Intensol (Oxycodone) ... 2366
- Tylox Capsules ... 1593

Oxyphenonium Bromide (May produce paralytic ileus).

Pentobarbital Sodium (Additive CNS depression). Products include:
- Nembutal Sodium Capsules ... 440
- Nembutal Sodium Solution ... 442
- Nembutal Sodium Suppositories ... 444

Perphenazine (Additive CNS depression). Products include:
- Etrafon ... 2495
- Triavil Tablets ... 1800
- Trilafon ... 2532

Phenobarbital (Additive CNS depression). Products include:
- Arco-Lase Plus Tablets ... 513
- Bellergal-S Tablets ... 2375
- Donnatal ... 2234
- Donnatal Extentabs ... 2234
- Donnatal Tablets ... 2234
- Phenobarbital Elixir and Tablets ... 1523
- Quadrinal Tablets ... 1398

Pimozide (Additive CNS depression). Products include:
- Orap Tablets ... 1037

Prazepam (Additive CNS depression).
- No products indexed under this heading.

Prochlorperazine (Additive CNS depression). Products include:
- Compazine ... 2644

Procyclidine Hydrochloride (May produce paralytic ileus). Products include:
- Kemadrin Tablets ... 1105

Promethazine Hydrochloride (Additive CNS depression). Products include:
- Mepergan Injection ... 2859
- Phenergan with Codeine ... 2883
- Phenergan with Dextromethorphan ... 2885
- Phenergan Injection ... 2880
- Phenergan Suppositories ... 2882
- Phenergan Syrup ... 2881
- Phenergan Tablets ... 2882
- Phenergan VC ... 2886
- Phenergan VC with Codeine ... 2888

Propantheline Bromide (May produce paralytic ileus). Products include:
- Pro-Banthine Tablets ... 2226

IMPORTANT NOTE: Always consult each drug listing in the patient's regimen for possible interactions.

Tylenol with Codeine / Interactions Index

Propofol (Additive CNS depression). Products include:
- Diprivan Injectable Emulsion 2939

Propoxyphene Hydrochloride (Additive CNS depression). Products include:
- Darvon 1475
- Wygesic Tablets 2930

Propoxyphene Napsylate (Additive CNS depression). Products include:
- Darvon-N/Darvocet-N 1473

Quazepam (Additive CNS depression). Products include:
- Doral Tablets 2773

Risperidone (Additive CNS depression). Products include:
- Risperdal Tablets 1348

Scopolamine (May produce paralytic ileus). Products include:
- Transderm Scōp Transdermal Therapeutic System 890

Scopolamine Hydrobromide (May produce paralytic ileus). Products include:
- Atrohist Plus Tablets 1605
- Donnatal 2234
- Donnatal Extentabs 2234
- Donnatal Tablets 2234

Secobarbital Sodium (Additive CNS depression). Products include:
- Seconal Sodium Pulvules 1529

Sevoflurane (Additive CNS depression).
- No products indexed under this heading.

Sufentanil Citrate (Additive CNS depression). Products include:
- Sufenta Injection 1355

Temazepam (Additive CNS depression). Products include:
- Restoril Capsules 2413

Thiamylal Sodium (Additive CNS depression).
- No products indexed under this heading.

Thioridazine Hydrochloride (Additive CNS depression). Products include:
- Mellaril 2398

Thiothixene (Additive CNS depression). Products include:
- Navane Capsules and Concentrate 2018
- Navane Intramuscular 2019

Triazolam (Additive CNS depression). Products include:
- Halcion Tablets 2093

Tridihexethyl Chloride (May produce paralytic ileus).
- No products indexed under this heading.

Trifluoperazine Hydrochloride (Additive CNS depression). Products include:
- Stelazine 2692

Trihexyphenidyl Hydrochloride (May produce paralytic ileus). Products include:
- Artane 1418

Zolpidem Tartrate (Additive CNS depression). Products include:
- Ambien Tablets 2559

Food Interactions
Alcohol (Additive CNS depression).

TYLENOL WITH CODEINE PHOSPHATE TABLETS
(Acetaminophen, Codeine Phosphate) 1592
See Tylenol with Codeine Elixir

TYLOX CAPSULES
(Oxycodone Hydrochloride, Acetaminophen) 1593
May interact with anticholinergics, central nervous system depressants, antipsychotic agents, narcotic analgesics, phenothiazines, general anesthetics, hypnotics and sedatives, tranquilizers, and certain other agents. Compounds in these categories include:

Alfentanil Hydrochloride (Additive CNS depression). Products include:
- Alfenta Injection 1334

Alprazolam (Additive CNS depression). Products include:
- Xanax Tablets 2115

Aprobarbital (Additive CNS depression).
- No products indexed under this heading.

Atropine Sulfate (May produce paralytic ileus). Products include:
- Arco-Lase Plus Tablets 513
- Atrohist Plus Tablets 1605
- Donnatal 2234
- Donnatal Extentabs 2234
- Donnatal Tablets 2234
- Lomotil 2591
- Motofen Tablets 789
- Urised Tablets 2123

Belladonna Alkaloids (May produce paralytic ileus). Products include:
- Bellergal-S Tablets 2375
- Hyland's Bedwetting Tablets 788
- Hyland's EnurAid Tablets 789
- Hyland's Headache Tablets 790
- Hyland's Teething Tablets 790
- Similasan Eye Drops #1 769

Benztropine Mesylate (May produce paralytic ileus). Products include:
- Cogentin 1661

Biperiden Hydrochloride (May produce paralytic ileus). Products include:
- Akineton 1380

Buprenorphine (Additive CNS depression). Products include:
- Buprenex Injectable 2170

Buspirone Hydrochloride (Additive CNS depression). Products include:
- BuSpar Tablets 738

Butabarbital (Additive CNS depression).
- No products indexed under this heading.

Butalbital (Additive CNS depression). Products include:
- Axocet Capsules 2469
- Esgic-plus Capsules 1012
- Esgic-plus Tablets 1012
- Fioricet Tablets 2386
- Fioricet with Codeine Capsules 2387
- Fiorinal Capsules 2388
- Fiorinal with Codeine Capsules 2390
- Fiorinal Tablets 2388
- Phrenilin 790
- Sedapap Tablets 50 mg/650 mg 1826

Chlordiazepoxide (Additive CNS depression). Products include:
- Limbitrol 2333

Chlordiazepoxide Hydrochloride (Additive CNS depression). Products include:
- Librax Capsules 2330
- Librium Capsules 2331
- Librium Injectable 2332

Chlorpromazine (Additive CNS depression). Products include:
- Thorazine Suppositories 2701

Chlorprothixene (Additive CNS depression).
- No products indexed under this heading.

Chlorprothixene Hydrochloride (Additive CNS depression).
- No products indexed under this heading.

Chlorprothixene Lactate (Additive CNS depression).
- No products indexed under this heading.

Clidinium Bromide (May produce paralytic ileus). Products include:
- Librax Capsules 2330

Clorazepate Dipotassium (Additive CNS depression). Products include:
- Tranxene 459

Clozapine (Additive CNS depression). Products include:
- Clozaril Tablets 2377

Codeine Phosphate (Additive CNS depression). Products include:
- Brontex 2130
- Dimetane-DC Cough Syrup 2232
- Fioricet with Codeine Capsules 2387
- Fiorinal with Codeine Capsules 2390
- Nucofed 2225
- Phenergan with Codeine 2883
- Phenergan VC with Codeine 2888
- Robitussin A-C Syrup 2248
- Robitussin-DAC Syrup 2249
- Ryna 804
- Soma Compound w/Codeine Tablets 2784
- Tylenol with Codeine 1592

Desflurane (Additive CNS depression). Products include:
- Suprane (desflurane, USP) 1865

Dezocine (Additive CNS depression). Products include:
- Dalgan Injection 529

Diazepam (Additive CNS depression). Products include:
- Dizac (diazepam injectable emulsion) CIV 1862
- Valium Injectable 2336
- Valium Tablets 2335

Dicyclomine Hydrochloride (May produce paralytic ileus). Products include:
- Bentyl 1246

Droperidol (Additive CNS depression). Products include:
- Inapsine Injection 462

Enflurane (Additive CNS depression).
- No products indexed under this heading.

Estazolam (Additive CNS depression). Products include:
- ProSom Tablets 457

Ethchlorvynol (Additive CNS depression). Products include:
- Placidyl Capsules 456

Ethinamate (Additive CNS depression).
- No products indexed under this heading.

Fentanyl (Additive CNS depression). Products include:
- Duragesic Transdermal System 1336

Fentanyl Citrate (Additive CNS depression). Products include:
- Sublimaze Injection 463

Fluphenazine Decanoate (Additive CNS depression). Products include:
- Prolixin Decanoate 510

Fluphenazine Enanthate (Additive CNS depression). Products include:
- Prolixin Enanthate 510

Fluphenazine Hydrochloride (Additive CNS depression). Products include:
- Prolixin 510

Flurazepam Hydrochloride (Additive CNS depression). Products include:
- Dalmane Capsules 2329

Glutethimide (Additive CNS depression).
- No products indexed under this heading.

Glycopyrrolate (May produce paralytic ileus). Products include:
- Robinul Forte Tablets 2247
- Robinul Injectable 2247
- Robinul Tablets 2247

Haloperidol (Additive CNS depression). Products include:
- Haldol Injection, Tablets and Concentrate 1585

Haloperidol Decanoate (Additive CNS depression). Products include:
- Haldol Decanoate 1587

Hydrocodone Bitartrate (Additive CNS depression). Products include:
- Codiclear DH Syrup 808
- Duratuss HD Elixir 2750
- Histussin D Liquid 670
- Hycodan Tablets and Syrup 946
- Hycomine Compound Tablets 948
- Hycomine 947
- Hycotuss Expectorant Syrup 950
- Hydrocet Capsules 787
- Lorcet 10/650 Tablets 1016
- Lortab 2751
- Tussend 1830
- Tussend Expectorant 1831
- Vicodin Tablets 1404
- Vicodin ES Tablets 1405
- Vicodin HP Tablets 1403
- Vicodin Tuss Expectorant 1406
- Zydone Capsules 967

Hydrocodone Polistirex (Additive CNS depression). Products include:
- Tussionex Pennkinetic Extended-Release Suspension 1624

Hydromorphone Hydrochloride (Additive CNS depression). Products include:
- Dilaudid Ampules 1382
- Dilaudid Cough Syrup 1383
- Dilaudid-HP Injection 1384
- Dilaudid-HP Lyophilized Powder 250 mg 1384
- Dilaudid 1382
- Dilaudid Oral Liquid 1386
- Dilaudid 1382
- Dilaudid Tablets - 8 mg 1386

Hydroxyzine Hydrochloride (Additive CNS depression). Products include:
- Atarax Tablets & Syrup 1992
- Marax Tablets & DF Syrup 2015
- Vistaril Intramuscular Solution 2042

Hyoscyamine (May produce paralytic ileus). Products include:
- Cystospaz Tablets 2123
- Urised Tablets 2123

Hyoscyamine Sulfate (May produce paralytic ileus). Products include:
- Arco-Lase Plus Tablets 513
- Atrohist Plus Tablets 1605
- Cystospaz-M Capsules 2123
- Donnatal 2234
- Donnatal Extentabs 2234
- Donnatal Tablets 2234
- Kutrase Capsules 2546
- Levsin/Levsinex/Levbid 2549

Ipratropium Bromide (May produce paralytic ileus). Products include:
- Atrovent Inhalation Aerosol 674
- Atrovent Inhalation Solution 675
- Atrovent Nasal Spray 0.03% 676
- Atrovent Nasal Spray 0.06% 678

Isoflurane (Additive CNS depression).
- No products indexed under this heading.

Ketamine Hydrochloride (Additive CNS depression).
- No products indexed under this heading.

Levomethadyl Acetate Hydrochloride (Additive CNS depression). Products include:
- Orlaam Oral Solution 2361

Levorphanol Tartrate (Additive CNS depression). Products include:
- Levo-Dromoran 2297

Lithium Carbonate (Additive CNS depression). Products include:
- Eskalith 2658
- Lithium Carbonate Capsules & Tablets 2352
- Lithonate/Lithotabs/Lithobid 2721

(■ Described in PDR For Nonprescription Drugs)   (⊙ Described in PDR For Ophthalmology)

Lithium Citrate (Additive CNS depression).
No products indexed under this heading.

Lorazepam (Additive CNS depression). Products include:
Ativan Injection 2805
Ativan Tablets 2807

Loxapine Hydrochloride (Additive CNS depression). Products include:
Loxitane 1426

Loxapine Succinate (Additive CNS depression). Products include:
Loxitane Capsules 1426

Mepenzolate Bromide (May produce paralytic ileus).
No products indexed under this heading.

Meperidine Hydrochloride (Additive CNS depression). Products include:
Demerol 2438
Mepergan Injection 2859

Mephobarbital (Additive CNS depression). Products include:
Mebaral Tablets 2452

Meprobamate (Additive CNS depression). Products include:
Miltown Tablets 2780
PMB 200 and PMB 400 2890

Mesoridazine Besylate (Additive CNS depression). Products include:
Serentil 689

Methadone Hydrochloride (Additive CNS depression). Products include:
Methadone Hydrochloride Oral Concentrate 2356
Methadone Hydrochloride Oral Solution & Tablets 2357

Methohexital Sodium (Additive CNS depression).
No products indexed under this heading.

Methotrimeprazine (Additive CNS depression). Products include:
Levoprome 1321

Methoxyflurane (Additive CNS depression).
No products indexed under this heading.

Midazolam Hydrochloride (Additive CNS depression). Products include:
Versed Injection 2324

Molindone Hydrochloride (Additive CNS depression). Products include:
Moban Tablets and Concentrate 1036

Morphine Sulfate (Additive CNS depression). Products include:
Astramorph/PF Injection, USP (Preservative-Free) 526
Duramorph Injection 983
Infumorph 200 and Infumorph 500 Sterile Solutions 985
Kadian Capsules 2948
MS Contin Tablets 2149
MSIR 2152
Oramorph SR (Morphine Sulfate Sustained Release Tablets) 2359
RMS Suppositories CII 2766
Roxanol 2365

Opium Alkaloids (Additive CNS depression).
No products indexed under this heading.

Oxazepam (Additive CNS depression). Products include:
Serax Capsules 2916
Serax Tablets 2916

Oxybutynin Chloride (May produce paralytic ileus). Products include:
Ditropan 1267

Pentobarbital Sodium (Additive CNS depression). Products include:
Nembutal Sodium Capsules 440
Nembutal Sodium Solution 442
Nembutal Sodium Suppositories 444

Perphenazine (Additive CNS depression). Products include:
Etrafon 2495
Triavil Tablets 1800
Trilafon 2532

Phenobarbital (Additive CNS depression). Products include:
Arco-Lase Plus Tablets 513
Bellergal-S Tablets 2375
Donnatal 2234
Donnatal Extentabs 2234
Donnatal Tablets 2234
Phenobarbital Elixir and Tablets 1523
Quadrinal Tablets 1398

Pimozide (Additive CNS depression). Products include:
Orap Tablets 1037

Prazepam (Additive CNS depression).
No products indexed under this heading.

Prochlorperazine (Additive CNS depression). Products include:
Compazine 2644

Procyclidine Hydrochloride (May produce paralytic ileus). Products include:
Kemadrin Tablets 1105

Promethazine Hydrochloride (Additive CNS depression). Products include:
Mepergan Injection 2859
Phenergan with Codeine 2883
Phenergan with Dextromethorphan 2885
Phenergan Injection 2880
Phenergan Suppositories 2882
Phenergan Syrup 2881
Phenergan Tablets 2882
Phenergan VC 2886
Phenergan VC with Codeine 2888

Propantheline Bromide (May produce paralytic ileus). Products include:
Pro-Banthine Tablets 2226

Propofol (Additive CNS depression). Products include:
Diprivan Injectable Emulsion 2939

Propoxyphene Hydrochloride (Additive CNS depression). Products include:
Darvon 1475
Wygesic Tablets 2930

Propoxyphene Napsylate (Additive CNS depression). Products include:
Darvon-N/Darvocet-N 1473

Quazepam (Additive CNS depression). Products include:
Doral Tablets 2773

Risperidone (Additive CNS depression). Products include:
Risperdal Tablets 1348

Scopolamine (May produce paralytic ileus). Products include:
Transderm Scōp Transdermal Therapeutic System 890

Scopolamine Hydrobromide (May produce paralytic ileus). Products include:
Atrohist Plus Tablets 1605
Donnatal 2234
Donnatal Extentabs 2234
Donnatal Tablets 2234

Secobarbital Sodium (Additive CNS depression). Products include:
Seconal Sodium Pulvules 1529

Sevoflurane (Additive CNS depression).
No products indexed under this heading.

Sufentanil Citrate (Additive CNS depression). Products include:
Sufenta Injection 1355

Temazepam (Additive CNS depression). Products include:
Restoril Capsules 2413

Thiamylal Sodium (Additive CNS depression).
No products indexed under this heading.

Thioridazine Hydrochloride (Additive CNS depression). Products include:
Mellaril 2398

Thiothixene (Additive CNS depression). Products include:
Navane Capsules and Concentrate 2018
Navane Intramuscular 2019

Triazolam (Additive CNS depression). Products include:
Halcion Tablets 2093

Tridihexethyl Chloride (May produce paralytic ileus).
No products indexed under this heading.

Trifluoperazine Hydrochloride (Additive CNS depression). Products include:
Stelazine 2692

Trihexyphenidyl Hydrochloride (May produce paralytic ileus). Products include:
Artane 1418

Zolpidem Tartrate (Additive CNS depression). Products include:
Ambien Tablets 2559

Food Interactions

Alcohol (Additive CNS depression).

TYMPAGESIC EAR DROPS
(Antipyrine, Benzocaine, Phenylephrine Hydrochloride) 2476
None cited in PDR database.

TYPHIM VI
(Typhoid Vi Polysaccharide Vaccine) 914
May interact with anticoagulants, alkylating agents, corticosteroids, and immunosuppressive agents. Compounds in these categories include:

Azathioprine (The expected immune response may not be obtained in individuals whose immune system has been compromised by treatment with corticosteroids). Products include:
Azathioprine Tablets 2349
Imuran 1103

Betamethasone Acetate (The expected immune response may not be obtained in individuals whose immune system has been compromised by treatment with corticosteroids). Products include:
Celestone Soluspan Suspension 2484

Betamethasone Sodium Phosphate (The expected immune response may not be obtained in individuals whose immune system has been compromised by treatment with corticosteroids). Products include:
Celestone Soluspan Suspension 2484

Busulfan (The expected immune response may not be obtained in individuals whose immune system has been compromised by treatment with alkylating drugs). Products include:
Myleran Tablets 1209

Carmustine (BCNU) (The expected immune response may not be obtained in individuals whose immune system has been compromised by treatment with alkylating drugs). Products include:
BiCNU 696

Chlorambucil (The expected immune response may not be obtained in individuals whose immune system has been compromised by treatment with alkylating drugs). Products include:
Leukeran Tablets 1205

Cortisone Acetate (The expected immune response may not be obtained in individuals whose immune system has been compromised by treatment with corticosteroids). Products include:
Cortone Acetate Sterile Suspension 1663
Cortone Acetate Tablets 1664

Cyclophosphamide (The expected immune response may not be obtained in individuals whose immune system has been compromised by treatment with alkylating drugs). Products include:
Cytoxan 700

Cyclosporine (The expected immune response may not be obtained in individuals whose immune system has been compromised by treatment with corticosteroids). Products include:
Neoral 2405
Sandimmune 2416

Dacarbazine (The expected immune response may not be obtained in individuals whose immune system has been compromised by treatment with alkylating drugs). Products include:
DTIC-Dome 593

Dalteparin Sodium (Typhim VI should be given with caution to individuals on anticoagulant therapy). Products include:
Fragmin Injection 2088

Dexamethasone (The expected immune response may not be obtained in individuals whose immune system has been compromised by treatment with corticosteroids). Products include:
AK-Trol Ointment & Suspension .... ⓢ 205
Decadron Elixir 1676
Decadron Tablets 1678
Decaspray Topical Aerosol 1689
Maxitrol Ophthalmic Ointment and Suspension .... ⓢ 222
TobraDex Ophthalmic Suspension and Ointment 469

Dexamethasone Acetate (The expected immune response may not be obtained in individuals whose immune system has been compromised by treatment with corticosteroids). Products include:
Dalalone D.P. Injectable 1009
Decadron-LA Sterile Suspension 1687

Dexamethasone Sodium Phosphate (The expected immune response may not be obtained in individuals whose immune system has been compromised by treatment with corticosteroids). Products include:
Decadron Phosphate Injection ... 1680
Decadron Phosphate Sterile Ophthalmic Ointment 1684
Decadron Phosphate Sterile Ophthalmic Solution 1685
Decadron Phosphate Topical Cream 1686
Decadron Phosphate with Xylocaine Injection, Sterile 1683
Dexacort Phosphate in Respihaler .. 1606
Dexacort Phosphate in Turbinaire .. 1607
NeoDecadron Sterile Ophthalmic Ointment 1755
NeoDecadron Sterile Ophthalmic Solution 1756
NeoDecadron Topical Cream 1757

IMPORTANT NOTE: Always consult each drug listing in the patient's regimen for possible interactions.

Typhim VI / Interactions Index

Dicumarol (Typhim VI should be given with caution to individuals on anticoagulant therapy).
    No products indexed under this heading.

Enoxaparin (Typhim VI should be given with caution to individuals on anticoagulant therapy). Products include:
    Lovenox Injection 2187

Fludrocortisone Acetate (The expected immune response may not be obtained in individuals whose immune system has been compromised by treatment with corticosteroids). Products include:
    Florinef Acetate Tablets 506

Heparin Calcium (Typhim VI should be given with caution to individuals on anticoagulant therapy).
    No products indexed under this heading.

Heparin Sodium (Typhim VI should be given with caution to individuals on anticoagulant therapy). Products include:
    Heparin Lock Flush Solution 2831
    Heparin Sodium Injection 2832
    Heparin Sodium Vials 1486

Hydrocortisone (The expected immune response may not be obtained in individuals whose immune system has been compromised by treatment with corticosteroids). Products include:
    Anusol-HC Cream 2.5% 1953
    Aquanil HC Lotion 1989
    Maximum Strength Cortaid Spray ■□ 800
    CORTENEMA 2713
    Cortisporin Ointment 1074
    Cortisporin Ophthalmic Ointment Sterile 1074
    Cortisporin Ophthalmic Suspension Sterile 1075
    Cortisporin Otic Solution Sterile 1076
    Cortisporin Otic Suspension Sterile 1077
    Cortizone-5 .... ■□ 795
    Cortizone-10 .... ■□ 795
    Hydrocortone Tablets 1715
    Hytone 922
    Hytone Ointment 2 ½ % 923
    Massengill Medicated Soft Cloth Towelettes 2628
    Pediotic Suspension Sterile 1140
    Preparation H Hydrocortisone 1% Cream .... ■□ 843
    ProctoCream-HC 2.5% 2552
    VōSoL HC Otic Solution 2786

Hydrocortisone Acetate (The expected immune response may not be obtained in individuals whose immune system has been compromised by treatment with corticosteroids). Products include:
    Analpram-HC Rectal Cream 1% and 2.5% 993
    Anusol HC-1 Hydrocortisone Anti-Itch Ointment .... ■□ 810
    Anusol-HC Suppositories 1954
    Caldecort Anti-Itch Hydrocortisone Cream .... ■□ 651
    Coly-Mycin S Otic w/Neomycin & Hydrocortisone 1965
    Cortaid .... ■□ 800
    Cortifoam 2540
    Cortisporin Cream 1073
    Epifoam 2543
    Hydrocortone Acetate Sterile Suspension 1712
    Mantadil Cream 1124
    Nupercainal Hydrocortisone 1% Cream .... ■□ 661
    Pramosone Cream, Lotion & Ointment 995
    ProctoFoam-HC 2552
    Terra-Cortril Ophthalmic Suspension 2033

Hydrocortisone Sodium Phosphate (The expected immune response may not be obtained in individuals whose immune system has been compromised by treatment with corticosteroids). Products include:
    Hydrocortone Phosphate Injection, Sterile 1713

Hydrocortisone Sodium Succinate (The expected immune response may not be obtained in individuals whose immune system has been compromised by treatment with corticosteroids).
    No products indexed under this heading.

Immune Globulin (Human) (The expected immune response may not be obtained in individuals whose immune system has been compromised by treatment with corticosteroids).
    No products indexed under this heading.

Lomustine (CCNU) (The expected immune response may not be obtained in individuals whose immune system has been compromised by treatment with alkylating drugs). Products include:
    CeeNU Capsules 699

Mechlorethamine Hydrochloride (The expected immune response may not be obtained in individuals whose immune system has been compromised by treatment with alkylating drugs). Products include:
    Mustargen 1752

Melphalan (The expected immune response may not be obtained in individuals whose immune system has been compromised by treatment with alkylating drugs). Products include:
    Alkeran Tablets 1198

Methylprednisolone Acetate (The expected immune response may not be obtained in individuals whose immune system has been compromised by treatment with corticosteroids).
    No products indexed under this heading.

Methylprednisolone Sodium Succinate (The expected immune response may not be obtained in individuals whose immune system has been compromised by treatment with corticosteroids).
    No products indexed under this heading.

Muromonab-CD3 (The expected immune response may not be obtained in individuals whose immune system has been compromised by treatment with corticosteroids). Products include:
    Orthoclone OKT3 Sterile Solution .. 1892

Mycophenolate Mofetil (The expected immune response may not be obtained in individuals whose immune system has been compromised by treatment with corticosteroids). Products include:
    CellCept Capsules 2265

Prednisolone Acetate (The expected immune response may not be obtained in individuals whose immune system has been compromised by treatment with corticosteroids). Products include:
    AK-CIDE .... ⊚ 203
    AK-CIDE Ointment .... ⊚ 203
    Blephamide Liquifilm Sterile Ophthalmic Suspension 472
    Blephamide Ointment .... ⊚ 234
    Econopred & Econopred Plus Ophthalmic Suspensions .... ⊚ 216
    Poly-Pred Liquifilm .... ⊚ 246
    Pred Forte .... ⊚ 247
    Pred Mild .... ⊚ 250
    Pred-G Liquifilm Sterile Ophthalmic Suspension .... ⊚ 248
    Pred-G S.O.P. Sterile Ophthalmic Ointment .... ⊚ 249

Prednisolone Sodium Phosphate (The expected immune response may not be obtained in individuals whose immune system has been compromised by treatment with corticosteroids). Products include:
    AK-PRED .... ⊚ 204
    Hydeltrasol Injection, Sterile 1708
    Pediapred Oral Solution 1618

Prednisolone Tebutate (The expected immune response may not be obtained in individuals whose immune system has been compromised by treatment with corticosteroids). Products include:
    Hydeltra-T.B.A. Sterile Suspension 1710

Prednisone (The expected immune response may not be obtained in individuals whose immune system has been compromised by treatment with corticosteroids).
    No products indexed under this heading.

Tacrolimus (The expected immune response may not be obtained in individuals whose immune system has been compromised by treatment with corticosteroids). Products include:
    Prograf 1028

Thiotepa (The expected immune response may not be obtained in individuals whose immune system has been compromised by treatment with alkylating drugs). Products include:
    Thioplex (Thiotepa For Injection) 1329

Triamcinolone (The expected immune response may not be obtained in individuals whose immune system has been compromised by treatment with corticosteroids).
    No products indexed under this heading.

Triamcinolone Acetonide (The expected immune response may not be obtained in individuals whose immune system has been compromised by treatment with corticosteroids). Products include:
    Azmacort Oral Inhaler 2175
    Nasacort AQ Nasal Spray 2191
    Nasacort Nasal Inhaler 2189

Triamcinolone Diacetate (The expected immune response may not be obtained in individuals whose immune system has been compromised by treatment with corticosteroids).
    No products indexed under this heading.

Triamcinolone Hexacetonide (The expected immune response may not be obtained in individuals whose immune system has been compromised by treatment with corticosteroids).
    No products indexed under this heading.

Warfarin Sodium (Typhim VI should be given with caution to individuals on anticoagulant therapy). Products include:
    Coumadin 941

TYPHOID VACCINE
(Typhoid Vaccine) 2929
None cited in PDR database.

ULTRAM TABLETS (50 MG)
(Tramadol Hydrochloride) 1594
May interact with central nervous system depressants, tricyclic antidepressants, selective serotonin reuptake inhibitors, monoamine oxidase inhibitors, drugs which lower seizure threshold, quinidine, and certain other agents. Compounds in these categories include:

Alfentanil Hydrochloride (Ultram should be used with caution and in reduced dosages when administered with CNS depressants). Products include:
    Alfenta Injection 1334

Alprazolam (Co-administration with tramadol may enhance the seizure risk). Products include:
    Xanax Tablets 2115

Amitriptyline Hydrochloride (Co-administration with tramadol may enhance the seizure risk). Products include:
    Elavil 2945
    Etrafon 2495
    Limbitrol 2333
    Triavil Tablets 1800

Amoxapine (Co-administration with tramadol may enhance the seizure risk). Products include:
    Asendin Tablets 1419

Aprobarbital (Ultram should be used with caution and in reduced dosages when administered with CNS depressants).
    No products indexed under this heading.

Buprenorphine (Ultram should be used with caution and in reduced dosages when administered with CNS depressants). Products include:
    Buprenex Injectable 2170

Buspirone Hydrochloride (Ultram should be used with caution and in reduced dosages when administered with CNS depressants). Products include:
    BuSpar Tablets 738

Butabarbital (Ultram should be used with caution and in reduced dosages when administered with CNS depressants).
    No products indexed under this heading.

Butalbital (Ultram should be used with caution and in reduced dosages when administered with CNS depressants). Products include:
    Axocet Capsules 2469
    Esgic-plus Capsules 1012
    Esgic-plus Tablets 1012
    Fioricet Tablets 2386
    Fioricet with Codeine Capsules 2387
    Fiorinal Capsules 2388
    Fiorinal with Codeine Capsules 2390
    Fiorinal Tablets 2388
    Phrenilin 790
    Sedapap Tablets 50 mg/650 mg .. 1826

Carbamazepine (Co-administration causes a significant increase in tramadol metabolism, presumably through metabolic induction by carbamazepine; patients receiving chronic carbamazepine doses may require higher, up to twice the recommended, doses of tramadol). Products include:
    Atretol Tablets 569
    Tegretol/Tegretol-XR 870

Chlordiazepoxide (Co-administration with tramadol may enhance the seizure risk). Products include:
    Limbitrol 2333

Chlordiazepoxide Hydrochloride (Co-administration with tramadol may enhance the seizure risk). Products include:
    Librax Capsules 2330
    Librium Capsules 2331

(■□ Described in PDR For Nonprescription Drugs)   (⊚ Described in PDR For Ophthalmology)

Interactions Index

Chlorpromazine (Co-administration with tramadol may enhance the seizure risk). Products include:
  Librium Injectable 2332
  Thorazine Suppositories 2701

Chlorpromazine Hydrochloride (Co-administration with tramadol may enhance the seizure risk). Products include:
  Thorazine 2701

Chlorprothixene (Ultram should be used with caution and in reduced dosages when administered with CNS depressants).
  No products indexed under this heading.

Chlorprothixene Hydrochloride (Ultram should be used with caution and in reduced dosages when administered with CNS depressants).
  No products indexed under this heading.

Chlorprothixene Lactate (Ultram should be used with caution and in reduced dosages when administered with CNS depressants).
  No products indexed under this heading.

Clomipramine Hydrochloride (Co-administration with tramadol may enhance the seizure risk). Products include:
  Anafranil Capsules 819

Clorazepate Dipotassium (Ultram should be used with caution and in reduced dosages when administered with CNS depressants). Products include:
  Tranxene 459

Clozapine (Ultram should be used with caution and in reduced dosages when administered with CNS depressants). Products include:
  Clozaril Tablets 2377

Codeine Phosphate (Ultram should be used with caution and in reduced dosages when administered with CNS depressants). Products include:
  Brontex 2130
  Dimetane-DC Cough Syrup 2232
  Fioricet with Codeine Capsules . 2387
  Fiorinal with Codeine Capsules . 2390
  Nucofed 2225
  Phenergan with Codeine 2883
  Phenergan VC with Codeine 2888
  Robitussin A-C Syrup 2248
  Robitussin-DAC Syrup 2249
  Ryna 804
  Soma Compound w/Codeine Tablets 2784
  Tylenol with Codeine 1592

Cyclobenzaprine Hydrochloride (Co-administration with tramadol may enhance the seizure risk). Products include:
  Flexeril Tablets 1701

Desflurane (Ultram should be used with caution and in reduced dosages when administered with CNS depressants). Products include:
  Suprane (desflurane, USP) 1865

Desipramine Hydrochloride (Co-administration with tramadol may enhance the seizure risk). Products include:
  Norpramin Tablets 1273

Dezocine (Ultram should be used with caution and in reduced dosages when administered with CNS depressants). Products include:
  Dalgan Injection 529

Diazepam (Co-administration with tramadol may enhance the seizure risk). Products include:
  Dizac (diazepam injectable emulsion) CIV 1862
  Valium Injectable 2336
  Valium Tablets 2335

Digoxin (Rare reports of digoxin toxicity). Products include:
  Lanoxicaps 1110
  Lanoxin Elixir Pediatric 1113
  Lanoxin Injection 1116
  Lanoxin Injection Pediatric 1119
  Lanoxin Tablets 1121

Doxepin Hydrochloride (Co-administration with tramadol may enhance the seizure risk). Products include:
  Adapin Capsules 1542
  Sinequan 2028
  Zonalon Cream 1042

Droperidol (Ultram should be used with caution and in reduced dosages when administered with CNS depressants). Products include:
  Inapsine Injection 462

Enflurane (Ultram should be used with caution and in reduced dosages when administered with CNS depressants).
  No products indexed under this heading.

Estazolam (Ultram should be used with caution and in reduced dosages when administered with CNS depressants). Products include:
  ProSom Tablets 457

Ethchlorvynol (Ultram should be used with caution and in reduced dosages when administered with CNS depressants). Products include:
  Placidyl Capsules 456

Ethinamate (Ultram should be used with caution and in reduced dosages when administered with CNS depressants).
  No products indexed under this heading.

Fentanyl (Ultram should be used with caution and in reduced dosages when administered with CNS depressants). Products include:
  Duragesic Transdermal System . 1336

Fentanyl Citrate (Ultram should be used with caution and in reduced dosages when administered with CNS depressants). Products include:
  Sublimaze Injection 463

Fluoxetine Hydrochloride (Co-administration with tramadol may enhance the seizure risk). Products include:
  Prozac Pulvules y Liquid, Oral Solution 935

Fluphenazine Decanoate (Co-administration with tramadol may enhance the seizure risk). Products include:
  Prolixin Decanoate 510

Fluphenazine Enanthate (Co-administration with tramadol may enhance the seizure risk). Products include:
  Prolixin Enanthate 510

Fluphenazine Hydrochloride (Co-administration with tramadol may enhance the seizure risk). Products include:
  Prolixin 510

Flurazepam Hydrochloride (Ultram should be used with caution and in reduced dosages when administered with CNS depressants). Products include:
  Dalmane Capsules 2329

Fluvoxamine Maleate (Co-administration with tramadol may enhance the seizure risk). Products include:
  LUVOX Tablets 2723

Furazolidone (Co-administration with tramadol may enhance the seizure risk; due to interference with detoxification mechanisms, concurrent use should be undertaken with great caution). Products include:
  Furoxone 2221

Glutethimide (Ultram should be used with caution and in reduced dosages when administered with CNS depressants).
  No products indexed under this heading.

Haloperidol (Co-administration with tramadol may enhance the seizure risk). Products include:
  Haldol Injection, Tablets and Concentrate 1585

Haloperidol Decanoate (Co-administration with tramadol may enhance the seizure risk). Products include:
  Haldol Decanoate 1587

Hydrocodone Bitartrate (Ultram should be used with caution and in reduced dosages when administered with CNS depressants). Products include:
  Codiclear DH Syrup 808
  Duratuss HD Elixir 2750
  Histussin D Liquid 670
  Hycodan Tablets and Syrup 946
  Hycomine Compound Tablets .. 948
  Hycomine 947
  Hycotuss Expectorant Syrup 950
  Hydrocet Capsules 787
  Lorcet 10/650 Tablets 1016
  Lortab 2751
  Tussend 1830
  Tussend Expectorant 1831
  Vicodin Tablets 1404
  Vicodin ES Tablets 1405
  Vicodin HP Tablets 1403
  Vicodin Tuss Expectorant 1406
  Zydone Capsules 967

Hydrocodone Polistirex (Ultram should be used with caution and in reduced dosages when administered with CNS depressants). Products include:
  Tussionex Pennkinetic Extended-Release Suspension 1624

Hydroxyzine Hydrochloride (Ultram should be used with caution and in reduced dosages when administered with CNS depressants). Products include:
  Atarax Tablets & Syrup 1992
  Marax Tablets & DF Syrup 2015
  Vistaril Intramuscular Solution .. 2042

Imipramine Hydrochloride (Co-administration with tramadol may enhance the seizure risk). Products include:
  Tofranil Ampuls 873
  Tofranil Tablets 875

Imipramine Pamoate (Co-administration with tramadol may enhance the seizure risk). Products include:
  Tofranil-PM Capsules 876

Isocarboxazid (Co-administration with tramadol may enhance the seizure risk; due to interference with detoxification mechanisms, concurrent use should be undertaken with great caution).
  No products indexed under this heading.

Isoflurane (Ultram should be used with caution and in reduced dosages when administered with CNS depressants).
  No products indexed under this heading.

Ketamine Hydrochloride (Ultram should be used with caution and in reduced dosages when administered with CNS depressants).
  No products indexed under this heading.

Levomethadyl Acetate Hydrochloride (Ultram should be used with caution and in reduced dosages when administered with CNS depressants). Products include:
  Orlaam Oral Solution 2361

Levorphanol Tartrate (Ultram should be used with caution and in reduced dosages when administered with CNS depressants). Products include:
  Levo-Dromoran 2297

Lorazepam (Co-administration with tramadol may enhance the seizure risk). Products include:
  Ativan Injection 2805
  Ativan Tablets 2807

Loxapine Hydrochloride (Ultram should be used with caution and in reduced dosages when administered with CNS depressants). Products include:
  Loxitane 1426

Loxapine Succinate (Ultram should be used with caution and in reduced dosages when administered with CNS depressants). Products include:
  Loxitane Capsules 1426

Maprotiline Hydrochloride (Co-administration with tramadol may enhance the seizure risk). Products include:
  Ludiomil Tablets 861

Meperidine Hydrochloride (Ultram should be used with caution and in reduced dosages when administered with CNS depressants). Products include:
  Demerol 2438
  Mepergan Injection 2859

Mephobarbital (Ultram should be used with caution and in reduced dosages when administered with CNS depressants). Products include:
  Mebaral Tablets 2452

Meprobamate (Ultram should be used with caution and in reduced dosages when administered with CNS depressants). Products include:
  Miltown Tablets 2780
  PMB 200 and PMB 400 2890

Mesoridazine Besylate (Co-administration with tramadol may enhance the seizure risk). Products include:
  Serentil 689

Methadone Hydrochloride (Ultram should be used with caution and in reduced dosages when administered with CNS depressants). Products include:
  Methadone Hydrochloride Oral Concentrate 2356
  Methadone Hydrochloride Oral Solution & Tablets 2357

Methohexital Sodium (Ultram should be used with caution and in reduced dosages when administered with CNS depressants).
  No products indexed under this heading.

Methotrimeprazine (Ultram should be used with caution and in reduced dosages when administered with CNS depressants). Products include:
  Levoprome 1321

Methoxyflurane (Ultram should be used with caution and in reduced dosages when administered with CNS depressants).
  No products indexed under this heading.

IMPORTANT NOTE: Always consult each drug listing in the patient's regimen for possible interactions.

Ultram — Interactions Index

Midazolam Hydrochloride (Ultram should be used with caution and in reduced dosages when administered with CNS depressants). Products include:
- Versed Injection 2324

Molindone Hydrochloride (Ultram should be used with caution and in reduced dosages when administered with CNS depressants). Products include:
- Moban Tablets and Concentrate 1036

Morphine Sulfate (Ultram should be used with caution and in reduced dosages when administered with CNS depressants). Products include:
- Astramorph/PF Injection, USP (Preservative-Free) 526
- Duramorph Injection 983
- Infumorph 200 and Infumorph 500 Sterile Solutions 985
- Kadian Capsules 2948
- MS Contin Tablets 2149
- MSIR 2152
- Oramorph SR (Morphine Sulfate Sustained Release Tablets) 2359
- RMS Suppositories CII 2766
- Roxanol 2365

Nortriptyline Hydrochloride (Co-administration with tramadol may enhance the seizure risk). Products include:
- Pamelor 2409

Opium Alkaloids (Ultram should be used with caution and in reduced dosages when administered with CNS depressants).
- No products indexed under this heading.

Oxazepam (Co-administration with tramadol may enhance the seizure risk). Products include:
- Serax Capsules 2916
- Serax Tablets 2916

Oxycodone Hydrochloride (Ultram should be used with caution and in reduced dosages when administered with CNS depressants). Products include:
- OxyContin Tablets 2163
- OxyIR Capsules 2167
- Percocet Tablets 955
- Percodan Tablets 955
- Percodan-Demi Tablets 956
- Roxicodone Tablets, Oral Solution & Intensol (Oxycodone) 2366
- Tylox Capsules 1593

Paroxetine Hydrochloride (Co-administration with tramadol may enhance the seizure risk). Products include:
- Paxil Tablets 2681

Pentobarbital Sodium (Ultram should be used with caution and in reduced dosages when administered with CNS depressants). Products include:
- Nembutal Sodium Capsules 440
- Nembutal Sodium Solution 442
- Nembutal Sodium Suppositories 444

Perphenazine (Co-administration with tramadol may enhance the seizure risk). Products include:
- Etrafon 2495
- Triavil Tablets 1800
- Trilafon 2532

Phenelzine Sulfate (Co-administration with tramadol may enhance the seizure risk; due to interference with detoxification mechanisms, concurrent use should be undertaken with great caution). Products include:
- Nardil 1977

Phenobarbital (Ultram should be used with caution and in reduced dosages when administered with CNS depressants). Products include:
- Arco-Lase Plus Tablets 513
- Bellergal-S Tablets 2375
- Donnatal 2234
- Donnatal Extentabs 2234
- Donnatal Tablets 2234
- Phenobarbital Elixir and Tablets 1523
- Quadrinal Tablets 1398

Prazepam (Co-administration with tramadol may enhance the seizure risk).
- No products indexed under this heading.

Prochlorperazine (Co-administration with tramadol may enhance the seizure risk). Products include:
- Compazine 2644

Promethazine Hydrochloride (Co-administration with tramadol may enhance the seizure risk). Products include:
- Mepergan Injection 2859
- Phenergan with Codeine 2883
- Phenergan with Dextromethorphan 2885
- Phenergan Injection 2880
- Phenergan Suppositories 2882
- Phenergan Syrup 2881
- Phenergan Tablets 2882
- Phenergan VC 2886
- Phenergan VC with Codeine 2888

Propofol (Ultram should be used with caution and in reduced dosages when administered with CNS depressants). Products include:
- Diprivan Injectable Emulsion 2939

Propoxyphene Hydrochloride (Ultram should be used with caution and in reduced dosages when administered with CNS depressants). Products include:
- Darvon 1475
- Wygesic Tablets 2930

Propoxyphene Napsylate (Ultram should be used with caution and in reduced dosages when administered with CNS depressants). Products include:
- Darvon-N/Darvocet-N 1473

Protriptyline Hydrochloride (Co-administration with tramadol may enhance the seizure risk). Products include:
- Vivactil Tablets 1820

Quazepam (Ultram should be used with caution and in reduced dosages when administered with CNS depressants). Products include:
- Doral Tablets 2773

Quinidine Gluconate (Co-administration results in increased concentrations of tramadol and reduced concentrations of M1 (o-desmethyltramadol); clinical consequences of this interaction are not known). Products include:
- Quinaglute Dura-Tabs Tablets 644

Quinidine Polygalacturonate (Co-administration results in increased concentrations of tramadol and reduced concentrations of M1 (o-desmethyltramadol); clinical consequences of this interaction are not known). Products include:
- Cardioquin Tablets 2146

Quinidine Sulfate (Co-administration results in increased concentrations of tramadol and reduced concentrations of M1 (o-desmethyltramadol); clinical consequences of this interaction are not known). Products include:
- Quinidex Extentabs 2240

Risperidone (Ultram should be used with caution and in reduced dosages when administered with CNS depressants). Products include:
- Risperdal Tablets 1348

Secobarbital Sodium (Ultram should be used with caution and in reduced dosages when administered with CNS depressants). Products include:
- Seconal Sodium Pulvules 1529

Selegiline Hydrochloride (Co-administration with tramadol may enhance the seizure risk; due to interference with detoxification mechanisms, concurrent use should be undertaken with great caution). Products include:
- Eldepryl Capsules 2729

Sertraline Hydrochloride (Co-administration with tramadol may enhance the seizure risk). Products include:
- Zoloft Tablets 2051

Sevoflurane (Ultram should be used with caution and in reduced dosages when administered with CNS depressants).
- No products indexed under this heading.

Sufentanil Citrate (Ultram should be used with caution and in reduced dosages when administered with CNS depressants). Products include:
- Sufenta Injection 1355

Temazepam (Ultram should be used with caution and in reduced dosages when administered with CNS depressants). Products include:
- Restoril Capsules 2413

Thiamylal Sodium (Ultram should be used with caution and in reduced dosages when administered with CNS depressants).
- No products indexed under this heading.

Thioridazine Hydrochloride (Co-administration with tramadol may enhance the seizure risk). Products include:
- Mellaril 2398

Thiothixene (Ultram should be used with caution and in reduced dosages when administered with CNS depressants). Products include:
- Navane Capsules and Concentrate 2018
- Navane Intramuscular 2019

Tranylcypromine Sulfate (Co-administration with tramadol may enhance the seizure risk; due to interference with detoxification mechanisms, concurrent use should be undertaken with great caution). Products include:
- Parnate Tablets 2679

Trazodone Hydrochloride (Co-administration with tramadol may enhance the seizure risk). Products include:
- Desyrel and Desyrel Dividose 504

Triazolam (Ultram should be used with caution and in reduced dosages when administered with CNS depressants). Products include:
- Halcion Tablets 2093

Trifluoperazine Hydrochloride (Co-administration with tramadol may enhance the seizure risk). Products include:
- Stelazine 2692

Trimipramine Maleate (Co-administration with tramadol may enhance the seizure risk). Products include:
- Surmontil Capsules 2917

Venlafaxine Hydrochloride (Co-administration with tramadol may enhance the seizure risk). Products include:
- Effexor 2825

Warfarin Sodium (Rare reports of alteration of warfarin effect, including elevation of prothrombin times). Products include:
- Coumadin 941

Zolpidem Tartrate (Ultram should be used with caution and in reduced dosages when administered with CNS depressants). Products include:
- Ambien Tablets 2559

Food Interactions
Alcohol (Concurrent use should be avoided).

ULTRASE CAPSULES
(Pancrelipase) 2476

Food Interactions
Food having a pH greater than 5.5 (Can dissolve the protective coating resulting in early release of enzymes, irritation of oral mucosa, and/or loss of enzyme activity).

ULTRASE MT CAPSULES
(Pancrelipase) 2477

Food Interactions
Food having a pH greater than 5.5 (Can dissolve the protective enteric shell).

ULTRAVATE CREAM 0.05%
(Halobetasol Propionate) 2797
None cited in PDR database.

ULTRAVATE OINTMENT 0.05%
(Halobetasol Propionate) 2798
None cited in PDR database.

UNASYN
(Ampicillin Sodium, Sulbactam Sodium) 2035
May interact with aminoglycosides and certain other agents. Compounds in these categories include:

Allopurinol (Increased incidence of rash). Products include:
- Zyloprim Tablets 1194

Amikacin Sulfate (In vitro inactivation of aminoglycosides when reconstituted with Unasyn). Products include:
- Amikacin Sulfate Injection, USP 523
- Amikacin Sulfate Injection, USP 981
- Amikin Injectable 502

Gentamicin Sulfate (In vitro inactivation of aminoglycosides when reconstituted with Unasyn). Products include:
- Garamycin Cream 0.1% 2501
- Garamycin Injectable 2502
- Garamycin Ointment 0.1% 2501
- Garamycin Ophthalmic 2501
- Genoptic Sterile Ophthalmic Solution .... ⊙ 241
- Genoptic Sterile Ophthalmic Ointment .... ⊙ 241
- Gentak .... ⊙ 209
- Pred-G Liquifilm Sterile Ophthalmic Suspension .... ⊙ 248
- Pred-G S.O.P. Sterile Ophthalmic Ointment .... ⊙ 249

Kanamycin Sulfate (In vitro inactivation of aminoglycosides when reconstituted with Unasyn).
- No products indexed under this heading.

Probenecid (Increased and prolonged blood levels of ampicillin and sulbactam). Products include:
- Benemid Tablets 1651
- ColBENEMID Tablets 1662

Streptomycin Sulfate (In vitro inactivation of aminoglycosides when reconstituted with Unasyn). Products include:
- Streptomycin Sulfate Injection 2031

(▣ Described in PDR For Nonprescription Drugs)   (⊙ Described in PDR For Ophthalmology)

Tobramycin Sulfate (In vitro inactivation of aminoglycosides when reconstituted with Unasyn). Products include:
   Nebcin Vials, Hyporets & ADD-Vantage 1518

UNGUENTINE PLUS
(Lidocaine Hydrochloride, Phenol) .. 712
None cited in PDR database.

UNI-DUR EXTENDED-RELEASE TABLETS
(Theophylline Anhydrous) 1374
May interact with erythromycin, lithium preparations, and certain other agents. Compounds in these categories include:

Adenosine (Theophylline blocks adenosine receptors; higher doses of adenosine may be required to achieve desired effect). Products include:
   Adenocard Injection 1021
   Adenoscan 1022

Allopurinol (Decreases theophylline clearance at allopurinol doses greater than or equal to 600 mg/day). Products include:
   Zyloprim Tablets 1194

Aminoglutethimide (Increases theophylline clearance by induction of microsomal enzyme). Products include:
   Cytadren Tablets 837

Carbamazepine (Increases theophylline clearance by induction of microsomal enzyme). Products include:
   Atretol Tablets 569
   Tegretol/Tegretol-XR 870

Cimetidine (Decreases theophylline clearance by inhibiting cytochrome P450 1A2). Products include:
   Tagamet HB Tablets 786
   Tagamet Tablets 2694

Cimetidine Hydrochloride (Decreases theophylline clearance by inhibiting cytochrome P450 1A2). Products include:
   Tagamet 2694

Ciprofloxacin (Decreases theophylline clearance by inhibiting cytochrome P450 1A2). Products include:
   Cipro I.V. 587
   Cipro I.V. Pharmacy Bulk Package .. 590

Ciprofloxacin Hydrochloride (Decreases theophylline clearance by inhibiting cytochrome P450 1A2). Products include:
   Ciloxan Ophthalmic Solution 468
   Cipro Tablets 584

Clarithromycin (Decreases theophylline clearance by inhibiting cytochrome P450 3A3). Products include:
   Biaxin 406

Diazepam (Benzodiazepines increase CNS concentrations of adenosine, a potent CNS depressant, while theophylline blocks adenosine receptors; larger diazepam doses may be required to produce desired level of sedation; discontinuation of theophylline without reduction of diazepam dose may result in respiratory depression). Products include:
   Dizac (diazepam injectable emulsion) CIV 1862
   Valium Injectable 2336
   Valium Tablets 2335

Disulfiram (Decreases theophylline clearance by inhibiting hydroxylation and demethylation). Products include:
   Antabuse Tablets 2802

Enoxacin (Decreases theophylline clearance by inhibiting cytochrome P450 1A2). Products include:
   Penetrex Tablets 2196

Ephedrine Hydrochloride (Co-administration results in synergistic CNS effects resulting in increased frequency of nausea, nervousness, and insomnia). Products include:
   Primatene Tablets 844
   Quadrinal Tablets 1398

Ephedrine Sulfate (Co-administration results in synergistic CNS effects resulting in increased frequency of nausea, nervousness, and insomnia). Products include:
   Marax Tablets & DF Syrup 2015

Ephedrine Tannate (Co-administration results in synergistic CNS effects resulting in increased frequency of nausea, nervousness, and insomnia). Products include:
   Rynatuss 2782

Erythromycin (Erythromycin metabolite decreases theophylline clearance by inhibiting cytochrome P450 3A3; decreased erythromycin steady-state serum concentrations). Products include:
   A/T/S 2% Acne Topical Gel 1244
   A/T/S 2% Acne Topical Solution 1244
   Benzamycin Topical Gel 919
   E-Mycin Tablets 1388
   Emgel 2% Topical Gel 1081
   ERYC 1972
   Erycette (erythromycin 2%) Topical Solution 1943
   Ery-Tab Tablets 426
   Erythromycin Base Filmtab 430
   Erythromycin Delayed-Release Capsules, USP 431
   Ilotycin Ophthalmic Ointment 928
   PCE Dispertab Tablets 453
   T-Stat 2.0% Topical Solution and Pads 2797
   THERAMYCIN Z 2% Solution 1629

Erythromycin Estolate (Erythromycin metabolite decreases theophylline clearance by inhibiting cytochrome P450 3A3; decreased erythromycin steady-state serum concentrations). Products include:
   Ilosone 927

Erythromycin Ethylsuccinate (Erythromycin metabolite decreases theophylline clearance by inhibiting cytochrome P450 3A3; decreased erythromycin steady-state serum concentrations). Products include:
   E.E.S. 427
   EryPed 425
   Pediazole Suspension 2340

Erythromycin Gluceptate (Erythromycin metabolite decreases theophylline clearance by inhibiting cytochrome P450 3A3; decreased erythromycin steady-state serum concentrations). Products include:
   Ilotycin Gluceptate, IV, Vials 929

Erythromycin Stearate (Erythromycin metabolite decreases theophylline clearance by inhibiting cytochrome P450 3A3; decreased erythromycin steady-state serum concentrations). Products include:
   Erythrocin Stearate Filmtab 429

Ethinyl Estradiol (Estrogen-containing oral contraceptives decrease theophylline clearance in dose-dependent fashion). Products include:
   Brevicon 2563
   Demulen 2580
   Desogen Tablets 1867

   Levlen/Tri-Levlen 646
   Lo/Ovral Tablets 2852
   Lo/Ovral-28 Tablets 2857
   Modicon 1928
   Nordette-21 Tablets 2863
   Nordette-28 Tablets 2866
   Norinyl 2563
   Ortho-Cept 1907
   Ortho-Cyclen/Ortho-Tri-Cyclen 1914
   Ortho-Novum 1928
   Ortho-Cyclen/Ortho Tri-Cyclen 1914
   Ovcon 765
   Ovral Tablets 2877
   Ovral-28 Tablets 2878
   Levlen/Tri-Levlen 646
   Tri-Norinyl 2607
   Triphasil-21 Tablets 2919
   Triphasil-28 Tablets 2924

Flurazepam Hydrochloride (Benzodiazepines increase CNS concentrations of adenosine, a potent CNS depressant, while theophylline blocks adenosine receptors; larger flurazepam doses may be required to produce desired level of sedation; discontinuation of theophylline without reduction of flurazepam dose may result in respiratory depression). Products include:
   Dalmane Capsules 2329

Fluvoxamine Maleate (Decreases theophylline clearance by inhibiting cytochrome P450 1A2). Products include:
   LUVOX Tablets 2723

Fosphenytoin Sodium (Phenytoin increases theophylline clearance by increasing microsomal enzyme activity; theophylline decreases phenytoin absorption). Products include:
   Cerebyx Injection 1956

Halothane (Halothane sensitizes the myocardium to catecholamines; theophylline increases release of endogenous catecholamines resulting in increased risk of ventricular arrhythmias). Products include:
   Fluothane 2830

Interferon alfa-2A, Recombinant (Decreases theophylline clearance). Products include:
   Roferon-A Injection 2308

Isoproterenol Hydrochloride (Co-administration with intravenous isoproterenol decreases theophylline clearance). Products include:
   Isuprel Hydrochloride Solution 2443
   Isuprel Injection 2441
   Isuprel Mistometer 2442

Ketamine Hydrochloride (May lower theophylline seizure threshold).
   No products indexed under this heading.

Lithium Carbonate (Theophylline increases renal lithium clearance; increase in lithium dose may be required to achieve a therapeutic serum concentration). Products include:
   Eskalith 2658
   Lithium Carbonate Capsules & Tablets 2352
   Lithonate/Lithotabs/Lithobid 2721

Lithium Citrate (Theophylline increases renal lithium clearance; increase in lithium dose may be required to achieve a therapeutic serum concentration).
   No products indexed under this heading.

Lomefloxacin Hydrochloride (Co-administration with some quinolones has increased the plasma levels of theophylline by affecting the rate of theophylline clearance). Products include:
   Maxaquin Tablets 2593

Lorazepam (Benzodiazepines increase CNS concentrations of adenosine, a potent CNS depressant, while theophylline blocks adenosine receptors; larger lorazepam doses may be required to produce desired level of sedation; discontinuation of theophylline without reduction of lorazepam dose may result in respiratory depression). Products include:
   Ativan Injection 2805
   Ativan Tablets 2807

Mestranol (Estrogen-containing oral contraceptives decrease theophylline clearance in dose-dependent fashion). Products include:
   Norinyl 2563
   Ortho-Novum 1928

Methotrexate Sodium (Decreases theophylline clearance). Products include:
   Methotrexate Sodium Tablets, Injection, for Injection and LPF Injection 1322

Mexiletine Hydrochloride (Decreases theophylline clearance by inhibiting hydroxylation and demethylation). Products include:
   Mexitil Capsules 684

Midazolam Hydrochloride (Benzodiazepines increase CNS concentrations of adenosine, a potent CNS depressant, while theophylline blocks adenosine receptors; larger midazolam doses may be required to produce desired level of sedation; discontinuation of theophylline without reduction of midazolam dose may result in respiratory depression). Products include:
   Versed Injection 2324

Moricizine Hydrochloride (Increases theophylline clearance). Products include:
   Ethmozine Tablets 2217

Norfloxacin (Co-administration with some quinolones has increased the plasma levels of theophylline by affecting the rate of theophylline clearance). Products include:
   Chibroxin Sterile Ophthalmic Solution 1657
   Noroxin Tablets 1758
   Noroxin Tablets 2222

Ofloxacin (Co-administration with some quinolones has increased the plasma levels of theophylline by affecting the rate of theophylline clearance). Products include:
   Floxin I.V. 1580
   Floxin Tablets (200 mg, 300 mg, 400 mg) 1577
   Ocuflox Ophthalmic Solution 478
   Ocuflox 242

Pancuronium Bromide (Theophylline may antagonize non-depolarizing neuromuscular blocking effects; possibly due to phosphodiesterase inhibition; larger pancuronium doses may be required to achieve neuromuscular blockade).
   No products indexed under this heading.

Pentoxifylline (Decreases theophylline clearance). Products include:
   Trental Tablets 1291

Phenobarbital (Increases theophylline clearance by induction of microsomal enzyme). Products include:
   Arco-Lase Plus Tablets 513
   Bellergal-S Tablets 2375
   Donnatal 2234
   Donnatal Extentabs 2234
   Donnatal Tablets 2234
   Phenobarbital Elixir and Tablets 1523
   Quadrinal Tablets 1398

IMPORTANT NOTE: Always consult each drug listing in the patient's regimen for possible interactions.

Uni-Dur

Phenytoin (Phenytoin increases theophylline clearance by increasing microsomal enzyme activity; theophylline decreases phenytoin absorption). Products include:
- Dilantin Infatabs 1967
- Dilantin-125 Suspension 1969

Phenytoin Sodium (Phenytoin increases theophylline clearance by increasing microsomal enzyme activity; theophylline decreases phenytoin absorption). Products include:
- Dilantin Kapseals 1965

Propafenone Hydrochloride (Decreases theophylline clearance). Products include:
- Rythmol Tablets–150mg, 225mg, 300mg. 1399

Propranolol Hydrochloride (Decreases theophylline clearance by inhibiting cytochrome P450 1A2). Products include:
- Inderal 2834
- Inderal LA Long Acting Capsules ... 2836
- Inderide Tablets 2838
- Inderide LA Long Acting Capsules .. 2840

Rifampin (Increases theophylline clearance by increasing cytochrome P450 1A2 and 3A3 activity). Products include:
- Rifadin 1276
- Rifamate Capsules 1278
- Rifater 1280
- Rimactane Capsules 865

Sucralfate (Reduces absorption of theophylline). Products include:
- Carafate Suspension 1250
- Carafate Tablets 1249

Sulfinpyrazone (Increases theophylline clearance by increasing demethylation and hydroxylation; decreases renal clearance of theophylline). Products include:
- Anturane 823

Tacrine Hydrochloride (Decreases theophylline clearance by inhibiting cytochrome P450 1A2 and also increases renal clearance of theophylline). Products include:
- Cognex Capsules 1961

Thiabendazole (Decreases theophylline clearance). Products include:
- Mintezol 1747

Ticlopidine Hydrochloride (Decreases theophylline clearance). Products include:
- Ticlid Tablets 2317

Troleandomycin (Decreases theophylline clearance by inhibiting cytochrome P450 3A3). Products include:
- Tao Capsules 2033

Verapamil Hydrochloride (Decreases theophylline clearance by inhibiting hydroxylation and demethylation). Products include:
- Calan SR Caplets 2571
- Calan Tablets 2568
- Covera-HS Tablets 2573
- Isoptin Injectable 1391
- Isoptin Oral Tablets 1393
- Isoptin SR Tablets 1395
- Verelan Capsules 1455

Food Interactions

Alcohol (Concurrent use with a single dose of alcohol (3mL/kg of whiskey) decreases theophylline clearance for up to 24 hours).

Diet, high-lipid (Co-administration with a high-fat breakfast delays the time to peak concentration, however, the extent of theophylline absorption is similar when administered fasting or immediately after a high-fat breakfast).

UNIFIBER
(Cellulose) 1845
None cited in PDR database.

UNIPHYL 400 MG AND 600 MG TABLETS
(Theophylline Anhydrous) 2157
May interact with erythromycin, lithium preparations, and certain other agents. Compounds in these categories include:

Adenosine (Theophylline blocks adenosine receptors; higher doses of adenosine may be required to achieve desired effect). Products include:
- Adenocard Injection 1021
- Adenoscan 1022

Allopurinol (Decreases theophylline clearance at allopurinol doses greater than or equal to 600 mg/day). Products include:
- Zyloprim Tablets 1194

Aminoglutethimide (Increases theophylline clearance by induction of microsomal enzyme). Products include:
- Cytadren Tablets 837

Carbamazepine (Increases theophylline clearance by induction of microsomal enzyme). Products include:
- Atretol Tablets 569
- Tegretol/Tegretol-XR 870

Cimetidine (Decreases theophylline clearance by inhibiting cytochrome P450 1A2). Products include:
- Tagamet HB Tablets .... ▣ 786
- Tagamet Tablets 2694

Cimetidine Hydrochloride (Decreases theophylline clearance by inhibiting cytochrome P450 1A2). Products include:
- Tagamet 2694

Ciprofloxacin (Decreases theophylline clearance by inhibiting cytochrome P450 1A2). Products include:
- Cipro I.V. 587
- Cipro I.V. Pharmacy Bulk Package .. 590

Ciprofloxacin Hydrochloride (Decreases theophylline clearance by inhibiting cytochrome P450 1A2). Products include:
- Ciloxan Ophthalmic Solution 468
- Cipro Tablets 584

Clarithromycin (Decreases theophylline clearance by inhibiting cytochrome P450 3A3). Products include:
- Biaxin 406

Diazepam (Benzodiazepines increase CNS concentrations of adenosine, a potent CNS depressant, while theophylline blocks adenosine receptors; larger diazepam doses may be required to produce desired level of sedation; discontinuation of theophylline without reduction of diazepam dose may result in respiratory depression). Products include:
- Dizac (diazepam injectable emulsion) CIV 1862
- Valium Injectable 2336
- Valium Tablets 2335

Disulfiram (Decreases theophylline clearance by inhibiting hydroxylation and demethylation). Products include:
- Antabuse Tablets 2802

Enoxacin (Decreases theophylline clearance by inhibiting cytochrome P450 1A2). Products include:
- Penetrex Tablets 2196

Ephedrine Hydrochloride (Co-administration results in synergistic CNS effects resulting in increased frequency of nausea, nervousness, and insomnia). Products include:
- Primatene Tablets .... ▣ 844
- Quadrinal Tablets 1398

Ephedrine Sulfate (Co-administration results in synergistic CNS effects resulting in increased frequency of nausea, nervousness, and insomnia). Products include:
- Marax Tablets & DF Syrup 2015

Ephedrine Tannate (Co-administration results in synergistic CNS effects resulting in increased frequency of nausea, nervousness, and insomnia). Products include:
- Rynatuss 2782

Erythromycin (Erythromycin metabolite decreases theophylline clearance by inhibiting cytochrome P450 3A3; decreased erythromycin steady-state serum concentrations). Products include:
- A/T/S 2% Acne Topical Gel 1244
- A/T/S 2% Acne Topical Solution ... 1244
- Benzamycin Topical Gel 919
- E-Mycin Tablets 1388
- Emgel 2% Topical Gel 1081
- ERYC 1972
- Erycette (erythromycin 2%) Topical Solution 1943
- Ery-Tab Tablets 426
- Erythromycin Base Filmtab 430
- Erythromycin Delayed-Release Capsules, USP 431
- Ilotycin Ophthalmic Ointment 928
- PCE Dispertab Tablets 453
- T-Stat 2.0% Topical Solution and Pads 2797
- THERAMYCIN Z 2% Solution 1629

Erythromycin Estolate (Erythromycin metabolite decreases theophylline clearance by inhibiting cytochrome P450 3A3; decreased erythromycin steady-state serum concentrations). Products include:
- Ilosone 927

Erythromycin Ethylsuccinate (Erythromycin metabolite decreases theophylline clearance by inhibiting cytochrome P450 3A3; decreased erythromycin steady-state serum concentrations). Products include:
- E.E.S. 427
- EryPed 425
- Pediazole Suspension 2340

Erythromycin Glucepate (Erythromycin metabolite decreases theophylline clearance by inhibiting cytochrome P450 3A3; decreased erythromycin steady-state serum concentrations). Products include:
- Ilotycin Glucepate, IV, Vials 929

Erythromycin Stearate (Erythromycin metabolite decreases theophylline clearance by inhibiting cytochrome P450 3A3; decreased erythromycin steady-state serum concentrations). Products include:
- Erythrocin Stearate Filmtab 429

Ethinyl Estradiol (Estrogen containing oral contraceptives decreases theophylline clearance in dose-dependent fashion). Products include:
- Brevicon 2563
- Demulen 2580
- Desogen Tablets 1867
- Levlen/Tri-Levlen 646
- Lo/Ovral Tablets 2852
- Lo/Ovral-28 Tablets 2857
- Modicon 1928
- Nordette Tablets 2863
- Nordette-28 Tablets 2866
- Norinyl 2563
- Ortho-Cept 1907
- Ortho-Novum 1928
- Ortho-Cyclen/Ortho-Tri-Cyclen 1914
- Ortho-Novum 1928
- Ortho-Cyclen/Ortho-Tri-Cyclen 1914
- Ovcon 765
- Ovral Tablets 2877
- Ovral-28 Tablets 2878
- Levlen/Tri-Levlen 646
- Tri-Norinyl 2607
- Triphasil-21 Tablets 2919
- Triphasil-28 Tablets 2924

Flurazepam Hydrochloride (Benzodiazepines increase CNS concentrations of adenosine, a potent CNS depressant, while theophylline blocks adenosine receptors; larger flurazepam doses may be required to produce desired level of sedation; discontinuation of theophylline without reduction of flurazepam dose may result in respiratory depression). Products include:
- Dalmane Capsules 2329

Fluvoxamine Maleate (Decreases theophylline clearance by inhibiting cytochrome P450 1A2). Products include:
- LUVOX Tablets 2723

Halothane (Halothane sensitizes the myocardium to catecholamines; theophylline increases release of endogenous catecholamines resulting in increased risk of ventricular arrhythmias). Products include:
- Fluothane 2830

Interferon alfa-2A, Recombinant (Decreases theophylline clearance). Products include:
- Roferon-A Injection 2308

Isoproterenol Hydrochloride (Co-administration with intravenous isoproterenol decreases theophylline clearance). Products include:
- Isuprel Hydrochloride Solution 2443
- Isuprel Injection 2441
- Isuprel Mistometer 2442

Ketamine Hydrochloride (May lower theophylline seizure threshold).
No products indexed under this heading.

Lithium Carbonate (Theophylline increases renal lithium clearance; increase in lithium dose may be required to achieve a therapeutic serum concentration). Products include:
- Eskalith 2658
- Lithium Carbonate Capsules & Tablets 2352
- Lithonate/Lithotabs/Lithobid 2721

Lithium Citrate (Theophylline increases renal lithium clearance; increase in lithium dose may be required to achieve a therapeutic serum concentration).
No products indexed under this heading.

Lorazepam (Benzodiazepines increase CNS concentrations of adenosine, a potent CNS depressant, while theophylline blocks adenosine receptors; larger lorazepam doses may be required to produce desired level of sedation; discontinuation of theophylline without reduction of lorazepam dose may result in respiratory depression). Products include:
- Ativan Injection 2805
- Ativan Tablets 2807

Mestranol (Estrogen containing oral contraceptives decreases theophylline clearance in dose-dependent fashion). Products include:
- Norinyl 2563
- Ortho-Novum 1928

Methotrexate Sodium (Decreases theophylline clearance). Products include:
- Methotrexate Sodium Tablets, Injection, for Injection and LPF Injection 1322

Mexiletine Hydrochloride (Decreases theophylline clearance by inhibiting hydroxylation and demethylation). Products include:
Mexitil Capsules ... 684

Midazolam Hydrochloride (Benzodiazepines increase CNS concentrations of adenosine, a potent CNS depressant, while theophylline blocks adenosine receptors; larger midazolam doses may be required to produce desired level of sedation; discontinuation of theophylline without reduction of midazolam dose may result in respiratory depression). Products include:
Versed Injection ... 2324

Moricizine Hydrochloride (Increases theophylline clearance). Products include:
Ethmozine Tablets ... 2217

Pancuronium Bromide (Theophylline may antagonize nondepolarizing neuromusular blocking effects; possibly due to phosphodiesterase inhibition; larger pancuronium doses may be required to achieve neuromuscular blockade).
No products indexed under this heading.

Pentoxifylline (Decreases theophylline clearance). Products include:
Trental Tablets ... 1291

Phenobarbital (Increases theophylline clearance by induction of microsomal enzyme). Products include:
Arco-Lase Plus Tablets ... 513
Bellergal-S Tablets ... 2375
Donnatal ... 2234
Donnatal Extentabs ... 2234
Donnatal Tablets ... 2234
Phenobarbital Elixir and Tablets ... 1523
Quadrinal Tablets ... 1398

Phenytoin (Phenytoin increases theophylline clearance by increasing microsomal enzyme activity; theophylline decreases phenytoin absorption). Products include:
Dilantin Infatabs ... 1967
Dilantin-125 Suspension ... 1969

Phenytoin Sodium (Phenytoin increases theophylline clearance by increasing microsomal enzyme activity; theophylline decreases phenytoin absorption). Products include:
Dilantin Kapseals ... 1965

Propafenone Hydrochloride (Decreases theophylline clearance). Products include:
Rythmol Tablets–150mg, 225mg, 300mg ... 1399

Propranolol Hydrochloride (Decreases theophylline clearance by inhibiting cytochrome P450 1A2). Products include:
Inderal ... 2834
Inderal LA Long Acting Capsules ... 2836
Inderide Tablets ... 2838
Inderide LA Long Acting Capsules .. 2840

Rifampin (Increases theophylline clearance by increasing cytochrome P450 1A2 and 3A3 activity). Products include:
Rifadin ... 1276
Rifamate Capsules ... 1278
Rifater ... 1280
Rimactane Capsules ... 865

Sulfinpyrazone (Increases theophylline clearance by increasing demethylation and hydroxylation; decreases renal clearance of theophylline). Products include:
Anturane ... 823

Tacrine Hydrochloride (Decreases theophylline clearance by inhibiting cytochrome P450 1A2 and also increases renal clearance of theophylline). Products include:
Cognex Capsules ... 1961

Thiabendazole (Decreases theophylline clearance). Products include:
Mintezol ... 1747

Ticlopidine Hydrochloride (Decreases theophylline clearance). Products include:
Ticlid Tablets ... 2317

Troleandomycin (Decreases theophylline clearance by inhibiting cytochrome P450 3A3). Products include:
Tao Capsules ... 2033

Verapamil Hydrochloride (Decreases theophylline clearance by inhibiting hydroxylation and demethylation). Products include:
Calan SR Caplets ... 2571
Calan Tablets ... 2568
Covera-HS Tablets ... 2573
Isoptin Injectable ... 1391
Isoptin Oral Tablets ... 1393
Isoptin SR Tablets ... 1395
Verelan Capsules ... 1455

Food Interactions

Alcohol (Concurrent use with a single dose of alcohol (3 mL/kg of whiskey) decreases theophylline clearance for up to 24 hours).

Diet, high-lipid (Co-administration with a standardized high-fat meal results in increased peak plasma concentration and bioavailability; however, a precipitous increase in the rate and extent of absorption was not evident; the dosing should be ideally administered consistently either with or without food).

UNIQUE E VITAMIN E CAPSULES

(Vitamin E) ... 1236
None cited in PDR database.

MAXIMUM STRENGTH UNISOM SLEEPGELS

(Diphenhydramine Hydrochloride) ... 1990
May interact with monoamine oxidase inhibitors, central nervous system depressants, hypnotics and sedatives, tranquilizers, and certain other agents. Compounds in these categories include:

Alfentanil Hydrochloride (Heightens the CNS depressant effect). Products include:
Alfenta Injection ... 1334

Alprazolam (Heightens the CNS depressant effect). Products include:
Xanax Tablets ... 2115

Aprobarbital (Heightens the CNS depressant effect).
No products indexed under this heading.

Buprenorphine (Heightens the CNS depressant effect). Products include:
Buprenex Injectable ... 2170

Buspirone Hydrochloride (Heightens the CNS depressant effect). Products include:
BuSpar Tablets ... 738

Butabarbital (Heightens the CNS depressant effect).
No products indexed under this heading.

Butalbital (Heightens the CNS depressant effect). Products include:
Axocet Capsules ... 2469
Esgic-plus Capsules ... 1012
Esgic-plus Tablets ... 1012
Fioricet Tablets ... 2386
Fioricet with Codeine Capsules ... 2387
Fiorinal Capsules ... 2388
Fiorinal with Codeine Capsules ... 2390
Fiorinal Tablets ... 2388
Phrenilin ... 790
Sedapap Tablets 50 mg/650 mg .. 1826

Chlordiazepoxide (Heightens the CNS depressant effect). Products include:
Limbitrol ... 2333

Chlordiazepoxide Hydrochloride (Heightens the CNS depressant effect). Products include:
Librax Capsules ... 2330
Librium Capsules ... 2331
Librium Injectable ... 2332

Chlorpromazine (Heightens the CNS depressant effect). Products include:
Thorazine Suppositories ... 2701

Chlorpromazine Hydrochloride (Heightens the CNS depressant effect). Products include:
Thorazine ... 2701

Chlorprothixene (Heightens the CNS depressant effect).
No products indexed under this heading.

Chlorprothixene Hydrochloride (Heightens the CNS depressant effect).
No products indexed under this heading.

Chlorprothixene Lactate (Heightens the CNS depressant effect).
No products indexed under this heading.

Clorazepate Dipotassium (Heightens the CNS depressant effect). Products include:
Tranxene ... 459

Clozapine (Heightens the CNS depressant effect). Products include:
Clozaril Tablets ... 2377

Codeine Phosphate (Heightens the CNS depressant effect). Products include:
Brontex ... 2130
Dimetane-DC Cough Syrup ... 2232
Fioricet with Codeine Capsules ... 2387
Fiorinal with Codeine Capsules ... 2390
Nucofed ... 2225
Phenergan with Codeine ... 2883
Phenergan VC with Codeine ... 2888
Robitussin A-C Syrup ... 2248
Robitussin-DAC Syrup ... 2249
Ryna ... 804
Soma Compound w/Codeine Tablets ... 2784
Tylenol with Codeine ... 1592

Desflurane (Heightens the CNS depressant effect). Products include:
Suprane (desflurane, USP) ... 1865

Dezocine (Heightens the CNS depressant effect). Products include:
Dalgan Injection ... 529

Diazepam (Heightens the CNS depressant effect). Products include:
Dizac (diazepam injectable emulsion) CIV ... 1862
Valium Injectable ... 2336
Valium Tablets ... 2335

Droperidol (Heightens the CNS depressant effect). Products include:
Inapsine Injection ... 462

Enflurane (Heightens the CNS depressant effect).
No products indexed under this heading.

Estazolam (Heightens the CNS depressant effect). Products include:
ProSom Tablets ... 457

Ethchlorvynol (Heightens the CNS depressant effect). Products include:
Placidyl Capsules ... 456

Ethinamate (Heightens the CNS depressant effect).
No products indexed under this heading.

Fentanyl (Heightens the CNS depressant effect). Products include:
Duragesic Transdermal System ... 1336

Fentanyl Citrate (Heightens the CNS depressant effect). Products include:
Sublimaze Injection ... 463

Fluphenazine Decanoate (Heightens the CNS depressant effect). Products include:
Prolixin Decanoate ... 510

Fluphenazine Enanthate (Heightens the CNS depressant effect). Products include:
Prolixin Enanthate ... 510

Fluphenazine Hydrochloride (Heightens the CNS depressant effect). Products include:
Prolixin ... 510

Flurazepam Hydrochloride (Heightens the CNS depressant effect). Products include:
Dalmane Capsules ... 2329

Furazolidone (Prolongs and intensifies the anticholinergic effects of antihistamines). Products include:
Furoxone ... 2221

Glutethimide (Heightens the CNS depressant effect).
No products indexed under this heading.

Haloperidol (Heightens the CNS depressant effect). Products include:
Haldol Injection, Tablets and Concentrate ... 1585

Haloperidol Decanoate (Heightens the CNS depressant effect). Products include:
Haldol Decanoate ... 1587

Hydrocodone Bitartrate (Heightens the CNS depressant effect). Products include:
Codiclear DH Syrup ... 808
Duratuss HD Elixir ... 2750
Histussin D Liquid ... 670
Hycodan Tablets and Syrup ... 946
Hycomine Compound Tablets ... 948
Hycomine ... 947
Hycotuss Expectorant Syrup ... 950
Hydrocet Capsules ... 787
Lorcet 10/650 Tablets ... 1016
Lortab ... 2751
Tussend ... 1830
Tussend Expectorant ... 1831
Vicodin Tablets ... 1404
Vicodin ES Tablets ... 1405
Vicodin HP Tablets ... 1403
Vicodin Tuss Expectorant ... 1406
Zydone Capsules ... 967

Hydrocodone Polistirex (Heightens the CNS depressant effect). Products include:
Tussionex Pennkinetic Extended-Release Suspension ... 1624

Hydroxyzine Hydrochloride (Heightens the CNS depressant effect). Products include:
Atarax Tablets & Syrup ... 1992
Marax Tablets & DF Syrup ... 2015
Vistaril Intramuscular Solution ... 2042

Isocarboxazid (Prolongs and intensifies the anticholinergic effects of antihistamines).
No products indexed under this heading.

Isoflurane (Heightens the CNS depressant effect).
No products indexed under this heading.

Ketamine Hydrochloride (Heightens the CNS depressant effect).
No products indexed under this heading.

Levomethadyl Acetate Hydrochloride (Heightens the CNS depressant effect). Products include:
Orlaam Oral Solution ... 2361

Levorphanol Tartrate (Heightens the CNS depressant effect). Products include:
Levo-Dromoran ... 2297

IMPORTANT NOTE: Always consult each drug listing in the patient's regimen for possible interactions.

Unisom sleepgels — Interactions Index

Lorazepam (Heightens the CNS depressant effect). Products include:
- Ativan Injection 2805
- Ativan Tablets 2807

Loxapine Hydrochloride (Heightens the CNS depressant effect). Products include:
- Loxitane 1426

Loxapine Succinate (Heightens the CNS depressant effect). Products include:
- Loxitane Capsules 1426

Meperidine Hydrochloride (Heightens the CNS depressant effect). Products include:
- Demerol 2438
- Mepergan Injection 2859

Mephobarbital (Heightens the CNS depressant effect). Products include:
- Mebaral Tablets 2452

Meprobamate (Heightens the CNS depressant effect). Products include:
- Miltown Tablets 2780
- PMB 200 and PMB 400 2890

Mesoridazine Besylate (Heightens the CNS depressant effect). Products include:
- Serentil 689

Methadone Hydrochloride (Heightens the CNS depressant effect). Products include:
- Methadone Hydrochloride Oral Concentrate 2356
- Methadone Hydrochloride Oral Solution & Tablets 2357

Methohexital Sodium (Heightens the CNS depressant effect).
- No products indexed under this heading.

Methotrimeprazine (Heightens the CNS depressant effect). Products include:
- Levoprome 1321

Methoxyflurane (Heightens the CNS depressant effect).
- No products indexed under this heading.

Midazolam Hydrochloride (Heightens the CNS depressant effect). Products include:
- Versed Injection 2324

Molindone Hydrochloride (Heightens the CNS depressant effect). Products include:
- Moban Tablets and Concentrate 1036

Morphine Sulfate (Heightens the CNS depressant effect). Products include:
- Astramorph/PF Injection, USP (Preservative-Free) 526
- Duramorph Injection 983
- Infumorph 200 and Infumorph 500 Sterile Solutions 985
- Kadian Capsules 2948
- MS Contin Tablets 2149
- MSIR 2152
- Oramorph SR (Morphine Sulfate Sustained Release Tablets) 2359
- RMS Suppositories CII 2766
- Roxanol 2365

Opium Alkaloids (Heightens the CNS depressant effect).
- No products indexed under this heading.

Oxazepam (Heightens the CNS depressant effect). Products include:
- Serax Capsules 2916
- Serax Tablets 2916

Oxycodone Hydrochloride (Heightens the CNS depressant effect). Products include:
- OxyContin Tablets 2163
- OxyIR Capsules 2167
- Percocet Tablets 955
- Percodan Tablets 955
- Percodan-Demi Tablets 956
- Roxicodone Tablets, Oral Solution & Intensol (Oxycodone) 2366
- Tylox Capsules 1593

Pentobarbital Sodium (Heightens the CNS depressant effect). Products include:
- Nembutal Sodium Capsules 440
- Nembutal Sodium Solution 442
- Nembutal Sodium Suppositories 444

Perphenazine (Heightens the CNS depressant effect). Products include:
- Etrafon 2495
- Triavil Tablets 1800
- Trilafon 2532

Phenelzine Sulfate (Prolongs and intensifies the anticholinergic effects of antihistamines). Products include:
- Nardil 1977

Phenobarbital (Heightens the CNS depressant effect). Products include:
- Arco-Lase Plus Tablets 513
- Bellergal-S Tablets 2375
- Donnatal 2234
- Donnatal Extentabs 2234
- Donnatal Tablets 2234
- Phenobarbital Elixir and Tablets .. 1523
- Quadrinal Tablets 1398

Prazepam (Heightens the CNS depressant effect).
- No products indexed under this heading.

Prochlorperazine (Heightens the CNS depressant effect). Products include:
- Compazine 2644

Promethazine Hydrochloride (Heightens the CNS depressant effect). Products include:
- Mepergan Injection 2859
- Phenergan with Codeine 2883
- Phenergan with Dextromethorphan ... 2885
- Phenergan Injection 2880
- Phenergan Suppositories 2882
- Phenergan Syrup 2881
- Phenergan Tablets 2882
- Phenergan VC 2886
- Phenergan VC with Codeine 2888

Propofol (Heightens the CNS depressant effect). Products include:
- Diprivan Injectable Emulsion 2939

Propoxyphene Hydrochloride (Heightens the CNS depressant effect). Products include:
- Darvon 1475
- Wygesic Tablets 2930

Propoxyphene Napsylate (Heightens the CNS depressant effect). Products include:
- Darvon-N/Darvocet-N 1473

Quazepam (Heightens the CNS depressant effect). Products include:
- Doral Tablets 2773

Risperidone (Heightens the CNS depressant effect). Products include:
- Risperdal Tablets 1348

Secobarbital Sodium (Heightens the CNS depressant effect). Products include:
- Seconal Sodium Pulvules 1529

Selegiline Hydrochloride (Prolongs and intensifies the anticholinergic effects of antihistamines). Products include:
- Eldepryl Capsules 2729

Sevoflurane (Heightens the CNS depressant effect).
- No products indexed under this heading.

Sufentanil Citrate (Heightens the CNS depressant effect). Products include:
- Sufenta Injection 1355

Temazepam (Heightens the CNS depressant effect). Products include:
- Restoril Capsules 2413

Thiamylal Sodium (Heightens the CNS depressant effect).
- No products indexed under this heading.

Thioridazine Hydrochloride (Heightens the CNS depressant effect). Products include:
- Mellaril 2398

Thiothixene (Heightens the CNS depressant effect). Products include:
- Navane Capsules and Concentrate ... 2018
- Navane Intramuscular 2019

Tranylcypromine Sulfate (Prolongs and intensifies the anticholinergic effects of antihistamines). Products include:
- Parnate Tablets 2679

Triazolam (Heightens the CNS depressant effect). Products include:
- Halcion Tablets 2093

Trifluoperazine Hydrochloride (Heightens the CNS depressant effect). Products include:
- Stelazine 2692

Zolpidem Tartrate (Heightens the CNS depressant effect). Products include:
- Ambien Tablets 2559

Food Interactions
Alcohol (Heightens the CNS depressant effect).

UNISOM NIGHTTIME SLEEP AID
(Doxylamine Succinate) 1990

Food Interactions
Alcohol (Use Unisom cautiously).

UNISOM WITH PAIN RELIEF-NIGHTTIME SLEEP AID AND PAIN RELIEVER
(Diphenhydramine Hydrochloride, Acetaminophen) 1991
May interact with monoamine oxidase inhibitors, central nervous system depressants, and certain other agents. Compounds in these categories include:

Alfentanil Hydrochloride (Heightened CNS depressant effect of antihistamines). Products include:
- Alfenta Injection 1334

Alprazolam (Heightened CNS depressant effect of antihistamines). Products include:
- Xanax Tablets 2115

Aprobarbital (Heightened CNS depressant effect of antihistamines).
- No products indexed under this heading.

Buprenorphine (Heightened CNS depressant effect of antihistamines). Products include:
- Buprenex Injectable 2170

Buspirone Hydrochloride (Heightened CNS depressant effect of antihistamines). Products include:
- BuSpar Tablets 738

Butabarbital (Heightened CNS depressant effect of antihistamines).
- No products indexed under this heading.

Butalbital (Heightened CNS depressant effect of antihistamines). Products include:
- Axocet Capsules 2469
- Esgic-plus Capsules 1012
- Esgic-plus Tablets 1012
- Fioricet Tablets 2386
- Fioricet with Codeine Capsules 2387
- Fiorinal Capsules 2388
- Fiorinal with Codeine Capsules 2390
- Fiorinal Tablets 2388
- Phrenilin 790
- Sedapap Tablets 50 mg/650 mg 1826

Chlordiazepoxide (Heightened CNS depressant effect of antihistamines). Products include:
- Limbitrol 2333

Chlordiazepoxide Hydrochloride (Heightened CNS depressant effect of antihistamines). Products include:
- Librax Capsules 2330

- Librium Capsules 2331
- Librium Injectable 2332

Chlorpromazine (Heightened CNS depressant effect of antihistamines). Products include:
- Thorazine Suppositories 2701

Chlorpromazine Hydrochloride (Heightened CNS depressant effect of antihistamines). Products include:
- Thorazine 2701

Chlorprothixene (Heightened CNS depressant effect of antihistamines).
- No products indexed under this heading.

Chlorprothixene Hydrochloride (Heightened CNS depressant effect of antihistamines).
- No products indexed under this heading.

Chlorprothixene Lactate (Heightened CNS depressant effect of antihistamines).
- No products indexed under this heading.

Clorazepate Dipotassium (Heightened CNS depressant effect of antihistamines). Products include:
- Tranxene 459

Clozapine (Heightened CNS depressant effect of antihistamines). Products include:
- Clozaril Tablets 2377

Codeine Phosphate (Heightened CNS depressant effect of antihistamines). Products include:
- Brontex 2130
- Dimetane-DC Cough Syrup 2232
- Fioricet with Codeine Capsules 2387
- Fiorinal with Codeine Capsules 2390
- Nucofed 2225
- Phenergan with Codeine 2883
- Phenergan VC with Codeine 2888
- Robitussin A-C Syrup 2248
- Robitussin-DAC Syrup 2249
- Ryna 804
- Soma Compound w/Codeine Tablets ... 2784
- Tylenol with Codeine 1592

Desflurane (Heightened CNS depressant effect of antihistamines). Products include:
- Suprane (desflurane, USP) 1865

Dezocine (Heightened CNS depressant effect of antihistamines). Products include:
- Dalgan Injection 529

Diazepam (Heightened CNS depressant effect of antihistamines). Products include:
- Dizac (diazepam injectable emulsion) CIV 1862
- Valium Injectable 2336
- Valium Tablets 2335

Droperidol (Heightened CNS depressant effect of antihistamines). Products include:
- Inapsine Injection 462

Enflurane (Heightened CNS depressant effect of antihistamines).
- No products indexed under this heading.

Estazolam (Heightened CNS depressant effect of antihistamines). Products include:
- ProSom Tablets 457

Ethchlorvynol (Heightened CNS depressant effect of antihistamines). Products include:
- Placidyl Capsules 456

Ethinamate (Heightened CNS depressant effect of antihistamines).
- No products indexed under this heading.

Fentanyl (Heightened CNS depressant effect of antihistamines). Products include:
- Duragesic Transdermal System 1336

(⬛ Described in PDR For Nonprescription Drugs) (⊙ Described in PDR For Ophthalmology)

Fentanyl Citrate (Heightened CNS depressant effect of antihistamines). Products include:
Sublimaze Injection 463

Fluphenazine Decanoate (Heightened CNS depressant effect of antihistamines). Products include:
Prolixin Decanoate 510

Fluphenazine Enanthate (Heightened CNS depressant effect of antihistamines). Products include:
Prolixin Enanthate 510

Fluphenazine Hydrochloride (Heightened CNS depressant effect of antihistamines). Products include:
Prolixin 510

Flurazepam Hydrochloride (Heightened CNS depressant effect of antihistamines). Products include:
Dalmane Capsules 2329

Furazolidone (Prolonged and intensified anticholinergic effects of antihistamines). Products include:
Furoxone 2221

Glutethimide (Heightened CNS depressant effect of antihistamines).
No products indexed under this heading.

Haloperidol (Heightened CNS depressant effect of antihistamines). Products include:
Haldol Injection, Tablets and Concentrate 1585

Haloperidol Decanoate (Heightened CNS depressant effect of antihistamines). Products include:
Haldol Decanoate 1587

Hydrocodone Bitartrate (Heightened CNS depressant effect of antihistamines). Products include:
Codiclear DH Syrup 808
Duratuss HD Elixir 2750
Histussin D Liquid 670
Hycodan Tablets and Syrup 946
Hycomine Compound Tablets ... 948
Hycomine 947
Hycotuss Expectorant Syrup 950
Hydrocet Capsules 787
Lorcet 10/650 Tablets 1016
Lortab 2751
Tussend 1830
Tussend Expectorant 1831
Vicodin Tablets 1404
Vicodin ES Tablets 1405
Vicodin HP Tablets 1403
Vicodin Tuss Expectorant 1406
Zydone Capsules 967

Hydrocodone Polistirex (Heightened CNS depressant effect of antihistamines). Products include:
Tussionex Pennkinetic Extended-Release Suspension 1624

Hydroxyzine Hydrochloride (Heightened CNS depressant effect of antihistamines). Products include:
Atarax Tablets & Syrup 1992
Marax Tablets & DF Syrup 2015
Vistaril Intramuscular Solution .. 2042

Isocarboxazid (Prolonged and intensified anticholinergic effects of antihistamines).
No products indexed under this heading.

Isoflurane (Heightened CNS depressant effect of antihistamines).
No products indexed under this heading.

Ketamine Hydrochloride (Heightened CNS depressant effect of antihistamines).
No products indexed under this heading.

Levomethadyl Acetate Hydrochloride (Heightened CNS depressant effect of antihistamines). Products include:
Orlaam Oral Solution 2361

Levorphanol Tartrate (Heightened CNS depressant effect of antihistamines). Products include:
Levo-Dromoran 2297

Lorazepam (Heightened CNS depressant effect of antihistamines). Products include:
Ativan Injection 2805
Ativan Tablets 2807

Loxapine Hydrochloride (Heightened CNS depressant effect of antihistamines). Products include:
Loxitane 1426

Loxapine Succinate (Heightened CNS depressant effect of antihistamines). Products include:
Loxitane Capsules 1426

Meperidine Hydrochloride (Heightened CNS depressant effect of antihistamines). Products include:
Demerol 2438
Mepergan Injection 2859

Mephobarbital (Heightened CNS depressant effect of antihistamines). Products include:
Mebaral Tablets 2452

Meprobamate (Heightened CNS depressant effect of antihistamines). Products include:
Miltown Tablets 2780
PMB 200 and PMB 400 2890

Mesoridazine Besylate (Heightened CNS depressant effect of antihistamines). Products include:
Serentil 689

Methadone Hydrochloride (Heightened CNS depressant effect of antihistamines). Products include:
Methadone Hydrochloride Oral Concentrate 2356
Methadone Hydrochloride Oral Solution & Tablets 2357

Methohexital Sodium (Heightened CNS depressant effect of antihistamines).
No products indexed under this heading.

Methotrimeprazine (Heightened CNS depressant effect of antihistamines). Products include:
Levoprome 1321

Methoxyflurane (Heightened CNS depressant effect of antihistamines).
No products indexed under this heading.

Midazolam Hydrochloride (Heightened CNS depressant effect of antihistamines). Products include:
Versed Injection 2324

Molindone Hydrochloride (Heightened CNS depressant effect of antihistamines). Products include:
Moban Tablets and Concentrate 1036

Morphine Sulfate (Heightened CNS depressant effect of antihistamines). Products include:
Astramorph/PF Injection, USP (Preservative-Free) 526
Duramorph Injection 983
Infumorph 200 and Infumorph 500 Sterile Solutions 985
Kadian Capsules 2948
MS Contin Tablets 2149
MSIR 2152
Oramorph SR (Morphine Sulfate Sustained Release Tablets) .. 2359
RMS Suppositories CII 2766
Roxanol 2365

Opium Alkaloids (Heightened CNS depressant effect of antihistamines).
No products indexed under this heading.

Oxazepam (Heightened CNS depressant effect of antihistamines). Products include:
Serax Capsules 2916
Serax Tablets 2916

Oxycodone Hydrochloride (Heightened CNS depressant effect of antihistamines). Products include:
OxyContin Tablets 2163
OxyIR Capsules 2167
Percocet Tablets 955
Percodan Tablets 955
Percodan-Demi Tablets 956
Roxicodone Tablets, Oral Solution & Intensol (Oxycodone) ... 2366
Tylox Capsules 1593

Pentobarbital Sodium (Heightened CNS depressant effect of antihistamines). Products include:
Nembutal Sodium Capsules 440
Nembutal Sodium Solution 442
Nembutal Sodium Suppositories ... 444

Perphenazine (Heightened CNS depressant effect of antihistamines). Products include:
Etrafon 2495
Triavil Tablets 1800
Trilafon 2532

Phenelzine Sulfate (Prolonged and intensified anticholinergic effects of antihistamines). Products include:
Nardil 1977

Phenobarbital (Heightened CNS depressant effect of antihistamines). Products include:
Arco-Lase Plus Tablets 513
Bellergal-S Tablets 2375
Donnatal 2234
Donnatal Extentabs 2234
Donnatal Tablets 2234
Phenobarbital Elixir and Tablets ... 1523
Quadrinal Tablets 1398

Prazepam (Heightened CNS depressant effect of antihistamines).
No products indexed under this heading.

Prochlorperazine (Heightened CNS depressant effect of antihistamines). Products include:
Compazine 2644

Promethazine Hydrochloride (Heightened CNS depressant effect of antihistamines). Products include:
Mepergan Injection 2859
Phenergan with Codeine 2883
Phenergan with Dextromethorphan ... 2885
Phenergan Injection 2880
Phenergan Suppositories 2882
Phenergan Syrup 2881
Phenergan Tablets 2882
Phenergan VC 2886
Phenergan VC with Codeine .. 2888

Propofol (Heightened CNS depressant effect of antihistamines). Products include:
Diprivan Injectable Emulsion . 2939

Propoxyphene Hydrochloride (Heightened CNS depressant effect of antihistamines). Products include:
Darvon 1475
Wygesic Tablets 2930

Propoxyphene Napsylate (Heightened CNS depressant effect of antihistamines). Products include:
Darvon-N/Darvocet-N 1473

Quazepam (Heightened CNS depressant effect of antihistamines). Products include:
Doral Tablets 2773

Risperidone (Heightened CNS depressant effect of antihistamines). Products include:
Risperdal Tablets 1348

Secobarbital Sodium (Heightened CNS depressant effect of antihistamines). Products include:
Seconal Sodium Pulvules 1529

Selegiline Hydrochloride (Prolonged and intensified anticholinergic effects of antihistamines). Products include:
Eldepryl Capsules 2729

Sevoflurane (Heightened CNS depressant effect of antihistamines).
No products indexed under this heading.

Sufentanil Citrate (Heightened CNS depressant effect of antihistamines). Products include:
Sufenta Injection 1355

Temazepam (Heightened CNS depressant effect of antihistamines). Products include:
Restoril Capsules 2413

Thiamylal Sodium (Heightened CNS depressant effect of antihistamines).
No products indexed under this heading.

Thioridazine Hydrochloride (Heightened CNS depressant effect of antihistamines). Products include:
Mellaril 2398

Thiothixene (Heightened CNS depressant effect of antihistamines). Products include:
Navane Capsules and Concentrate ... 2018
Navane Intramuscular 2019

Tranylcypromine Sulfate (Prolonged and intensified anticholinergic effects of antihistamines). Products include:
Parnate Tablets 2679

Triazolam (Heightened CNS depressant effect of antihistamines). Products include:
Halcion Tablets 2093

Trifluoperazine Hydrochloride (Heightened CNS depressant effect of antihistamines). Products include:
Stelazine 2692

Zolpidem Tartrate (Heightened CNS depressant effect of antihistamines). Products include:
Ambien Tablets 2559

Food Interactions

Alcohol (Heightened CNS depressant effect of antihistamines).

UNIVASC TABLETS
(Moexipril Hydrochloride) 2553
May interact with diuretics, potassium sparing diuretics, potassium preparations, lithium preparations, and certain other agents. Compounds in these categories include:

Amiloride Hydrochloride (ACE inhibitors can increase the risk of hyperkalemia with concomitant use). Products include:
Midamor Tablets 1746
Moduretic Tablets 1748

Bendroflumethiazide (Excessive reduction in blood pressure may occur in patients on diuretic therapy when ACE inhibitors are started).
No products indexed under this heading.

Bumetanide (Excessive reduction in blood pressure may occur in patients on diuretic therapy when ACE inhibitors are started). Products include:
Bumex 2260

Chlorothiazide (Excessive reduction in blood pressure may occur in patients on diuretic therapy when ACE inhibitors are started). Products include:
Aldoclor Tablets 1638
Diupres Tablets 1691
Diuril Oral 1694

Chlorothiazide Sodium (Excessive reduction in blood pressure may occur in patients on diuretic therapy when ACE inhibitors are started). Products include:
Diuril Sodium Intravenous 1693

IMPORTANT NOTE: Always consult each drug listing in the patient's regimen for possible interactions.

Chlorthalidone (Excessive reduction in blood pressure may occur in patients on diuretic therapy when ACE inhibitors are started). Products include:

- Combipres Tablets 682
- Tenoretic Tablets 2963
- Thalitone 1293

Ethacrynic Acid (Excessive reduction in blood pressure may occur in patients on diuretic therapy when ACE inhibitors are started). Products include:

- Edecrin Tablets 1698

Furosemide (Excessive reduction in blood pressure may occur in patients on diuretic therapy when ACE inhibitors are started). Products include:

- Lasix Injection, Oral Solution and Tablets 1267

Hydrochlorothiazide (Excessive reduction in blood pressure may occur in patients on diuretic therapy when ACE inhibitors are started). Products include:

- Aldactazide Tablets 2556
- Aldoril Tablets 1644
- Apresazide Capsules 824
- Capozide Tablets 744
- Dyazide Capsules 2653
- Esidrix Tablets 839
- Esimil Tablets 840
- HydroDIURIL Tablets 1716
- Hydropres Tablets 1718
- Hyzaar Tablets 1720
- Inderide Tablets 2838
- Inderide LA Long Acting Capsules .. 2840
- Lopressor HCT Tablets 850
- Lotensin HCT Tablets 855
- Moduretic Tablets 1748
- Oretic Tablets 450
- Prinzide Tablets 1780
- Ser-Ap-Es Tablets 867
- Timolide Tablets 1791
- Vaseretic Tablets 1810
- Zestoretic Tablets 2968
- Ziac 1459

Hydroflumethiazide (Excessive reduction in blood pressure may occur in patients on diuretic therapy when ACE inhibitors are started). Products include:

- Diucardin Tablets 2824

Indapamide (Excessive reduction in blood pressure may occur in patients on diuretic therapy when ACE inhibitors are started).

No products indexed under this heading.

Lithium Carbonate (Potential for increased serum lithium levels and risk of lithium toxicity). Products include:

- Eskalith 2658
- Lithium Carbonate Capsules & Tablets 2352
- Lithonate/Lithotabs/Lithobid 2721

Lithium Citrate (Potential for increased serum lithium levels and risk of lithium toxicity).

No products indexed under this heading.

Methyclothiazide (Excessive reduction in blood pressure may occur in patients on diuretic therapy when ACE inhibitors are started). Products include:

- Enduron Tablets 424

Metolazone (Excessive reduction in blood pressure may occur in patients on diuretic therapy when ACE inhibitors are started). Products include:

- Mykrox Tablets 1617
- Zaroxolyn Tablets 1625

Polythiazide (Excessive reduction in blood pressure may occur in patients on diuretic therapy when ACE inhibitors are started). Products include:

- Minizide Capsules 2016

Potassium Acid Phosphate (ACE inhibitors can increase the risk of hyperkalemia with concomitant use). Products include:

- K-Phos Original Formula 'Sodium Free' Tablets 633

Potassium Bicarbonate (ACE inhibitors can increase the risk of hyperkalemia with concomitant use). Products include:

- Alka-Seltzer Gold Effervescent Antacid .... ▣ 611

Potassium Chloride (ACE inhibitors can increase the risk of hyperkalemia with concomitant use). Products include:

- Chlor-3 Condiment 1003
- Colyte and Colyte-flavored 2540
- GoLYTELY 694
- K-Dur Microburst Release System (potassium chloride, USP) E.R. Tablets 1364
- K-Lor Powder Packets 438
- K-Norm Capsules 1615
- K-Tab Filmtab 439
- Micro-K 2237
- Micro-K LS Packets 2238
- NuLYTELY 694
- Cherry Flavor NuLYTELY 694
- Rum-K Syrup 1004
- Slow-K Extended-Release Tablets 869

Potassium Citrate (ACE inhibitors can increase the risk of hyperkalemia with concomitant use). Products include:

- Polycitra Syrup 574
- Polycitra-K Crystals 574
- Polycitra-K Oral Solution 575
- Polycitra-LC 574
- Urocit-K Tablets 1828

Potassium Gluconate (ACE inhibitors can increase the risk of hyperkalemia with concomitant use).

No products indexed under this heading.

Potassium Phosphate, Dibasic (ACE inhibitors can increase the risk of hyperkalemia with concomitant use).

No products indexed under this heading.

Potassium Phosphate, Monobasic (ACE inhibitors can increase the risk of hyperkalemia with concomitant use). Products include:

- K-Phos Neutral Tablets 633
- K-Phos Original Formula 'Sodium Free' Tablets 633

Spironolactone (ACE inhibitors can increase the risk of hyperkalemia with concomitant use). Products include:

- Aldactazide Tablets 2556
- Aldactone Tablets 2558

Torsemide (Excessive reduction in blood pressure may occur in patients on diuretic therapy when ACE inhibitors are started). Products include:

- Demadex Tablets and Injection 691

Triamterene (ACE inhibitors can increase the risk of hyperkalemia with concomitant use). Products include:

- Dyazide Capsules 2653
- Dyrenium Capsules 2655

Food Interactions

Food, unspecified (Food reduces C_{max} and AUC by about 70% and 40% respectively after ingestion of a low-fat breakfast or by 80% and 50% respectively after the ingestion of high-fat breakfast).

URECHOLINE INJECTION

(Bethanechol Chloride) 1804

See **Urecholine Tablets**

URECHOLINE TABLETS

(Bethanechol Chloride) 1804

May interact with ganglionic blocking agents. Compounds in this category include:

Mecamylamine Hydrochloride (Critical fall in blood pressure). Products include:

- Inversine Tablets 1729

Trimethaphan Camsylate (Critical fall in blood pressure).

No products indexed under this heading.

URISED TABLETS

(Atropine Sulfate, Hyoscyamine, Methenamine, Phenyl Salicylate) 2123

May interact with sulfonamides, urinary alkalizing agents, and certain other agents. Compounds in these categories include:

Potassium Citrate (Methenamine has therapeutic activity in acidic urine; concurrent use with drugs which produce an alkaline urine should be restricted). Products include:

- Polycitra Syrup 574
- Polycitra-K Crystals 574
- Polycitra-K Oral Solution 575
- Polycitra-LC 574
- Urocit-K Tablets 1828

Sodium Citrate (Methenamine has therapeutic activity in acidic urine; concurrent use with drugs which produce an alkaline urine should be restricted). Products include:

- Bicitra 573
- Polycitra 574
- Salix SST Lozenges Saliva Stimulant .... ▣ 757

Sulfamethizole (Mutual antagonism; concurrent use should be avoided since insoluble precipitate may form in the urine). Products include:

- Urobiotic-250 Capsules 2038

Sulfamethoxazole (Mutual antagonism; concurrent use should be avoided since insoluble precipitate may form in the urine). Products include:

- Bactrim DS Tablets 2257
- Bactrim I.V. Infusion 2255
- Bactrim 2257
- Gantanol Tablets 2285
- Septra 1146
- Septra I.V. Infusion 1142
- Septra I.V. Infusion ADD-Vantage Vials 1144
- Septra 1146

Sulfasalazine (Mutual antagonism; concurrent use should be avoided since insoluble precipitate may form in the urine). Products include:

- Azulfidine 2059

Sulfinpyrazone (Mutual antagonism; concurrent use should be avoided since insoluble precipitate may form in the urine). Products include:

- Anturane 823

Sulfisoxazole (Mutual antagonism; concurrent use should be avoided since insoluble precipitate may form in the urine). Products include:

- Gantrisin Tablets 2286

Sulfisoxazole Diolamine (Mutual antagonism; concurrent use should be avoided since insoluble precipitate may form in the urine).

No products indexed under this heading.

Food Interactions

Food that raises urinary pH (Methenamine has therapeutic activity in acidic urine; concurrent use with foods which produce an alkaline urine should be restricted).

URISPAS TABLETS

(Flavoxate Hydrochloride) 2710

None cited in PDR database.

UROBIOTIC-250 CAPSULES

(Oxytetracycline Hydrochloride, Sulfamethizole, Phenazopyridine Hydrochloride) 2038

May interact with:

Aluminum Hydroxide (Decreases absorption of Urobiotic). Products include:

- ALternaGEL Liquid 1358
- Maximum Strength Ascriptin .... ▣ 650
- Cama Arthritis Pain Reliever .... ▣ 748
- Gaviscon Extra Strength Relief Formula Antacid Tablets .... ▣ 778
- Gaviscon Extra Strength Relief Formula Liquid Antacid .... ▣ 779
- Gaviscon Liquid Antacid .... ▣ 779
- Gelusil Antacid-Anti-gas Liquid .... ▣ 819
- Gelusil Antacid-Anti-gas Tablets .... ▣ 819
- Maalox Antacid/Anti-Gas Tablets 889
- Maalox Heartburn Relief Suspension .... ▣ 658
- Maalox Antacid Liquid 888
- Extra Strength Maalox Antacid/Anti-Gas Liquid and Tablets 888
- Mylanta 1359
- Tempo Soft Antacid .... ▣ 799

Aluminum Hydroxide Gel (Decreases absorption of Urobiotic). Products include:

- ALternaGEL Liquid .... ▣ 675
- Aludrox Oral Suspension .... ▣ 850
- Amphojel Suspension 2802
- Amphojel Suspension without Flavor 2802
- Amphojel Tablets 2802
- Ascriptin .... ▣ 650
- Gaviscon Antacid Tablets .... ▣ 778
- Gaviscon-2 Antacid Tablets .... ▣ 779
- Mylanta Liquid .... ▣ 676
- Mylanta Double Strength Liquid .... ▣ 676
- Nephrox Suspension .... ▣ 671

UROCIT-K TABLETS

(Potassium Citrate) 1828

May interact with anticholinergics and potassium sparing diuretics. Compounds in these categories include:

Amiloride Hydrochloride (Coadministration can produce severe hyperkalemia; concurrent use should be avoided). Products include:

- Midamor Tablets 1746
- Moduretic Tablets 1748

Atropine Sulfate (Co-administration with drugs that slow gastrointestinal transit time, such as anticholinergics, can be expected to increase the gastrointestinal irritation produced by potassium salts; concurrent use is contraindicated). Products include:

- Arco-Lase Plus Tablets 513
- Atrohist Plus Tablets 1605
- Donnatal 2234
- Donnatal Extentabs 2234
- Donnatal Tablets 2234
- Lomotil 2591
- Motofen Tablets 789
- Urised Tablets 2123

Belladonna Alkaloids (Co-administration with drugs that slow gastrointestinal transit time, such as anticholinergics, can be expected to increase the gastrointestinal irritation produced by potassium salts; concurrent use is contraindicated). Products include:

- Bellergal-S Tablets 2375
- Hyland's Bedwetting Tablets .... ▣ 788

(▣ Described in PDR For Nonprescription Drugs) (◉ Described in PDR For Ophthalmology)

Hyland's EnurAid Tablets ... 789
Hyland's Headache Tablets ... 790
Hyland's Teething Tablets ... 790
Similasan Eye Drops #1 ... 769

Benztropine Mesylate (Co-administration with drugs that slow gastrointestinal transit time, such as anticholinergics, can be expected to increase the gastrointestinal irritation produced by potassium salts; concurrent use is contraindicated). Products include:

Cogentin ... 1661

Biperiden Hydrochloride (Co-administration with drugs that slow gastrointestinal transit time, such as anticholinergics, can be expected to increase the gastrointestinal irritation produced by potassium salts; concurrent use is contraindicated). Products include:

Akineton ... 1380

Clidinium Bromide (Co-administration with drugs that slow gastrointestinal transit time, such as anticholinergics, can be expected to increase the gastrointestinal irritation produced by potassium salts; concurrent use is contraindicated). Products include:

Librax Capsules ... 2330

Dicyclomine Hydrochloride (Co-administration with drugs that slow gastrointestinal transit time, such as anticholinergics, can be expected to increase the gastrointestinal irritation produced by potassium salts; concurrent use is contraindicated). Products include:

Bentyl ... 1246

Glycopyrrolate (Co-administration with drugs that slow gastrointestinal transit time, such as anticholinergics, can be expected to increase the gastrointestinal irritation produced by potassium salts; concurrent use is contraindicated). Products include:

Robinul Forte Tablets ... 2247
Robinul Injectable ... 2247
Robinul Tablets ... 2247

Hyoscyamine (Co-administration with drugs that slow gastrointestinal transit time, such as anticholinergics, can be expected to increase the gastrointestinal irritation produced by potassium salts; concurrent use is contraindicated). Products include:

Cystospaz Tablets ... 2123
Urised Tablets ... 2123

Hyoscyamine Sulfate (Co-administration with drugs that slow gastrointestinal transit time, such as anticholinergics, can be expected to increase the gastrointestinal irritation produced by potassium salts; concurrent use is contraindicated). Products include:

Arco-Lase Plus Tablets ... 513
Atrohist Plus Tablets ... 1605
Cystospaz-M Capsules ... 2123
Donnatal ... 2234
Donnatal Extentabs ... 2234
Donnatal Tablets ... 2234
Kutrase Capsules ... 2546
Levsin/Levsinex/Levbid ... 2549

Ipratropium Bromide (Co-administration with drugs that slow gastrointestinal transit time, such as anticholinergics, can be expected to increase the gastrointestinal irritation produced by potassium salts; concurrent use is contraindicated). Products include:

Atrovent Inhalation Aerosol ... 674
Atrovent Inhalation Solution ... 675
Atrovent Nasal Spray 0.03% ... 676
Atrovent Nasal Spray 0.06% ... 678

Mepenzolate Bromide (Co-administration with drugs that slow gastrointestinal transit time, such as anticholinergics, can be expected to increase the gastrointestinal irritation produced by potassium salts; concurrent use is contraindicated).

No products indexed under this heading.

Oxybutynin Chloride (Co-administration with drugs that slow gastrointestinal transit time, such as anticholinergics, can be expected to increase the gastrointestinal irritation produced by potassium salts; concurrent use is contraindicated). Products include:

Ditropan ... 1267

Procyclidine Hydrochloride (Co-administration with drugs that slow gastrointestinal transit time, such as anticholinergics, can be expected to increase the gastrointestinal irritation produced by potassium salts; concurrent use is contraindicated). Products include:

Kemadrin Tablets ... 1105

Propantheline Bromide (Co-administration with drugs that slow gastrointestinal transit time, such as anticholinergics, can be expected to increase the gastrointestinal irritation produced by potassium salts; concurrent use is contraindicated). Products include:

Pro-Banthine Tablets ... 2226

Scopolamine (Co-administration with drugs that slow gastrointestinal transit time, such as anticholinergics, can be expected to increase the gastrointestinal irritation produced by potassium salts; concurrent use is contraindicated). Products include:

Transderm Scōp Transdermal Therapeutic System ... 890

Scopolamine Hydrobromide (Co-administration with drugs that slow gastrointestinal transit time, such as anticholinergics, can be expected to increase the gastrointestinal irritation produced by potassium salts; concurrent use is contraindicated). Products include:

Atrohist Plus Tablets ... 1605
Donnatal ... 2234
Donnatal Extentabs ... 2234
Donnatal Tablets ... 2234

Spironolactone (Co-administration can produce severe hyperkalemia; concurrent use should be avoided). Products include:

Aldactazide Tablets ... 2556
Aldactone Tablets ... 2558

Triamterene (Co-administration can produce severe hyperkalemia; concurrent use should be avoided). Products include:

Dyazide Capsules ... 2653
Dyrenium Capsules ... 2655

Tridihexethyl Chloride (Co-administration with drugs that slow gastrointestinal transit time, such as anticholinergics, can be expected to increase the gastrointestinal irritation produced by potassium salts; concurrent use is contraindicated).

No products indexed under this heading.

Trihexyphenidyl Hydrochloride (Co-administration with drugs that slow gastrointestinal transit time, such as anticholinergics, can be expected to increase the gastrointestinal irritation produced by potassium salts; concurrent use is contraindicated). Products include:

Artane ... 1418

URO-MAG
(Magnesium Oxide) ... 666
None cited in PDR database.

UROQID-ACID NO. 2 TABLETS
(Methenamine Mandelate, Sodium Acid Phosphate) ... 633
May interact with:

Acetazolamide (Reduces the effectiveness of methenamine by causing urine to become alkaline). Products include:

Diamox Sequels (Sustained Release) ... 318
Diamox Tablets ... 317

ACTH (Concurrent use with sodium phosphate may result in hypernatremia).

No products indexed under this heading.

Aluminum Carbonate (Reduces the effectiveness of methenamine by causing urine to become alkaline). Products include:

Basaljel Capsules ... 2810
Basaljel Suspension ... 2810
Basaljel Tablets ... 2810

Aluminum Hydroxide (Reduces the effectiveness of methenamine by causing urine to become alkaline). Products include:

ALternaGEL Liquid ... 1358
Maximum Strength Ascriptin ... 650
Cama Arthritis Pain Reliever ... 748
Gaviscon Extra Strength Relief Formula Antacid Tablets ... 778
Gaviscon Extra Strength Relief Formula Liquid Antacid ... 779
Gaviscon Liquid Antacid ... 779
Gelusil Antacid-Anti-gas Liquid ... 819
Gelusil Antacid-Anti-gas Tablets ... 819
Maalox Antacid/Anti-Gas Tablets ... 889
Maalox Heartburn Relief Suspension ... 658
Maalox Antacid Liquid ... 888
Extra Strength Maalox Antacid/Anti-Gas Liquid and Tablets ... 888
Mylanta ... 1359
Tempo Soft Antacid ... 799

Aluminum Hydroxide Gel (Reduces the effectiveness of methenamine by causing urine to become alkaline). Products include:

ALternaGEL Liquid ... 675
Aludrox Oral Suspension ... 850
Amphojel Suspension ... 2802
Amphojel Suspension without Flavor ... 2802
Amphojel Tablets ... 2802
Ascriptin ... 650
Gaviscon Antacid Tablets ... 778
Gaviscon-2 Antacid Tablets ... 779
Mylanta Liquid ... 676
Mylanta Double Strength Liquid ... 676
Nephrox Suspension ... 671

Aspirin (Concurrent use may lead to increased serum salicylate levels since excretion of salicylates is reduced in acidic urine). Products include:

Alka-Seltzer Cherry Effervescent Antacid and Pain Reliever ... 609
Alka-Seltzer Extra Strength Effervescent Antacid and Pain Reliever ... 609
Alka-Seltzer Lemon Lime Effervescent Antacid and Pain Reliever ... 609
Alka-Seltzer Original Effervescent Antacid and Pain Reliever ... 611
Alka-Seltzer Plus ... 611
Alka-Seltzer Plus Sinus Medicine ... 611
Ascriptin ... 650
Arthritis Strength BC Powder ... 631
BC Cold Powder Multi-Symptom Formula (Cold-Sinus-Allergy) ... 631
BC Cold Powder Non-Drowsy Formula (Cold-Sinus) ... 631
BC Powder ... 631
Genuine Bayer Aspirin Tablets & Caplets ... 618
Extra Strength Bayer Arthritis Pain Regimen Formula ... 615

Extra Strength Bayer Aspirin Caplets & Tablets ... 617
Extended-Release Bayer 8-Hour Aspirin ... 616
Extra Strength Bayer Plus Aspirin Caplets ... 617
Extra Strength Bayer PM Aspirin Plus Sleep Aid ... 617
Aspirin Regimen Bayer 81 mg Tablets with Calcium ... 615
Aspirin Regimen Bayer Adult Low Strength 81 mg Tablets ... 613
Aspirin Regimen Bayer Children's Chewable Aspirin ... 616
Aspirin Regimen Bayer Regular Strength 325 mg Caplets ... 613
Bufferin Analgesic Tablets ... 636
Arthritis Strength Bufferin Analgesic Caplets ... 637
Extra Strength Bufferin Analgesic Tablets ... 637
Cama Arthritis Pain Reliever ... 748
Darvon Compound-65 Pulvules ... 1475
Easprin ... 1971
Ecotrin ... 2625
Ecotrin Enteric Coated Aspirin Maximum Strength Tablets and Caplets ... 775
Ecotrin Enteric Coated Aspirin Regular Strength Tablets ... 2625
Empirin Aspirin Tablets ... 818
Excedrin Extra-Strength Analgesic Tablets, Caplets, and Geltabs ... 734
Fiorinal Capsules ... 2388
Fiorinal with Codeine Capsules ... 2390
Fiorinal Tablets ... 2388
Goody's Extra Strength Headache Powders ... 632
Goody's Extra Strength Pain Relief Tablets ... 632
Halfprin Tablets ... 1413
Norgesic ... 1554
Percodan Tablets ... 955
Percodan-Demi Tablets ... 956
Robaxisal Tablets ... 2246
Soma Compound w/Codeine Tablets ... 2784
Soma Compound Tablets ... 2783
St. Joseph Adult Chewable Aspirin (81 mg.) ... 768
Talwin Compound ... 2466
Vanquish Analgesic Caplets ... 627

Bendroflumethiazide (Reduces the effectiveness of methenamine by causing urine to become alkaline).

No products indexed under this heading.

Betamethasone Acetate (Concurrent use with sodium phosphate may result in hypernatremia). Products include:

Celestone Soluspan Suspension ... 2484

Betamethasone Sodium Phosphate (Concurrent use with sodium phosphate may result in hypernatremia). Products include:

Celestone Soluspan Suspension ... 2484

Chlorothiazide (Reduces the effectiveness of methenamine by causing urine to become alkaline). Products include:

Aldoclor Tablets ... 1638
Diupres Tablets ... 1691
Diuril Oral ... 1694

Chlorothiazide Sodium (Reduces the effectiveness of methenamine by causing urine to become alkaline). Products include:

Diuril Sodium Intravenous ... 1693

Choline Magnesium Trisalicylate (Concurrent use may lead to increased serum salicylate levels since excretion of salicylates is reduced in acidic urine). Products include:

Trilisate ... 2155

Cortisone Acetate (Concurrent use with sodium phosphate may result in hypernatremia). Products include:

Cortone Acetate Sterile Suspension ... 1663
Cortone Acetate Tablets ... 1664

IMPORTANT NOTE: Always consult each drug listing in the patient's regimen for possible interactions.

Uroqid-Acid Interactions Index 1142

Deserpidine (Concurrent use with sodium phosphate may result in hypernatremia).
No products indexed under this heading.

Desoxycorticosterone Acetate (Concurrent use with sodium phosphate may result in hypernatremia).

Desoxycorticosterone Pivalate (Concurrent use with sodium phosphate may result in hypernatremia).

Dexamethasone (Concurrent use with sodium phosphate may result in hypernatremia). Products include:
- AK-Trol Ointment & Suspension ◉ 205
- Decadron Elixir 1676
- Decadron Tablets 1678
- Decaspray Topical Aerosol 1689
- Maxitrol Ophthalmic Ointment and Suspension ◉ 222
- TobraDex Ophthalmic Suspension and Ointment 469

Dexamethasone Acetate (Concurrent use with sodium phosphate may result in hypernatremia). Products include:
- Dalalone D.P. Injectable 1009
- Decadron-LA Sterile Suspension 1687

Dexamethasone Sodium Phosphate (Concurrent use with sodium phosphate may result in hypernatremia). Products include:
- Decadron Phosphate Injection 1680
- Decadron Phosphate Sterile Ophthalmic Ointment 1684
- Decadron Phosphate Sterile Ophthalmic Solution 1685
- Decadron Phosphate Topical Cream 1686
- Decadron Phosphate with Xylocaine Injection, Sterile 1683
- Dexacort Phosphate in Respihaler 1606
- Dexacort Phosphate in Turbinaire 1607
- NeoDecadron Sterile Ophthalmic Ointment 1755
- NeoDecadron Sterile Ophthalmic Solution 1756
- NeoDecadron Topical Cream 1757

Diazoxide (Concurrant use with sodium phosphate may result in hypernatremia). Products include:
- Hyperstat I.V. Injection 2504
- Proglycem 575

Dichlorphenamide (Reduces the effectiveness of methenamine by causing urine to become alkaline). Products include:
- Daranide Tablets 1676

Diflunisal (Concurrent use may lead to increased serum salicylate levels since excretion of salicylates is reduced in acidic urine). Products include:
- Dolobid Tablets 1695

Fludrocortisone Acetate (Concurrent use with sodium phosphate may result in hypernatremia). Products include:
- Florinef Acetate Tablets 506

Guanethidine Monosulfate (Concurrent use with sodium phosphate may result in hypernatremia). Products include:
- Esimil Tablets 840
- Ismelin Tablets 845

Hydralazine Hydrochloride (Concurrent use with sodium phosphate may result in hypernatremia). Products include:
- Apresazide Capsules 824
- Apresoline Hydrochloride Tablets 826
- Hydralazine Hydrochloride Injection USP 2712
- Ser-Ap-Es Tablets 867

Hydrochlorothiazide (Reduces the effectiveness of methenamine by causing urine to become alkaline). Products include:
- Aldactazide Tablets 2556
- Aldoril Tablets 1644
- Apresazide Capsules 824
- Capozide Tablets 744
- Dyazide Capsules 2653
- Esidrix Tablets 839
- Esimil Tablets 840
- HydroDIURIL Tablets 1716
- Hydropres Tablets 1718
- Hyzaar Tablets 1720
- Inderide Tablets 2838
- Inderide LA Long Acting Capsules 2840
- Lopressor HCT Tablets 850
- Lotensin HCT Tablets 855
- Moduretic Tablets 1748
- Oretic Tablets 450
- Prinzide Tablets 1780
- Ser-Ap-Es Tablets 867
- Timolide Tablets 1791
- Vaseretic Tablets 1810
- Zestoretic Tablets 2968
- Ziac 1459

Hydrocortisone (Concurrent use with sodium phosphate may result in hypernatremia). Products include:
- Anusol-HC Cream 2.5% 1953
- Aquanil HC Lotion 1989
- Maximum Strength Cortaid Spray ▣ 800
- CORTENEMA 2713
- Cortisporin Ointment 1074
- Cortisporin Ophthalmic Ointment Sterile 1074
- Cortisporin Ophthalmic Suspension Sterile 1075
- Cortisporin Otic Solution Sterile 1076
- Cortisporin Otic Suspension Sterile 1077
- Cortizone-5 ▣ 795
- Cortizone-10 ▣ 795
- Hydrocortone Tablets 1715
- Hytone 922
- Hytone Ointment 2 ½% 923
- Massengill Medicated Soft Cloth Towelettes 2628
- Pediotic Suspension Sterile 1140
- Preparation H Hydrocortisone 1% Cream ▣ 843
- ProctoCream-HC 2.5% 2552
- VōSoL HC Otic Solution 2786

Hydrocortisone Acetate (Concurrent use with sodium phosphate may result in hypernatremia). Products include:
- Analpram-HC Rectal Cream 1% and 2.5% 993
- Anusol HC-1 Hydrocortisone Anti-Itch Ointment ▣ 810
- Anusol-HC Suppositories 1954
- Caldecort Anti-Itch Hydrocortisone Cream ▣ 651
- Coly-Mycin S Otic w/Neomycin & Hydrocortisone 1965
- Cortaid ▣ 800
- Cortifoam 2540
- Cortisporin Cream 1073
- Epifoam 2543
- Hydrocortone Acetate Sterile Suspension 1712
- Mantadil Cream 1124
- Nupercainal Hydrocortisone 1% Cream ▣ 661
- Pramosone Cream, Lotion & Ointment 995
- ProctoFoam-HC 2552
- Terra-Cortril Ophthalmic Suspension 2033

Hydrocortisone Sodium Phosphate (Concurrent use with sodium phosphate may result in hypernatremia). Products include:
- Hydrocortone Phosphate Injection, Sterile 1713

Hydrocortisone Sodium Succinate (Concurrent use with sodium phosphate may result in hypernatremia).
No products indexed under this heading.

Hydroflumethiazide (Reduces the effectiveness of methenamine by causing urine to become alkaline). Products include:
- Diucardin Tablets 2824

Magaldrate (Reduces the effectiveness of methenamine by causing urine to become alkaline).
No products indexed under this heading.

Magnesium Hydroxide (Reduces the effectiveness of methenamine by causing urine to become alkaline). Products include:
- Aludrox Oral Suspension ▣ 850
- Ascriptin ▣ 650
- Di-Gel Antacid/Anti-Gas ▣ 762
- Gelusil Antacid-Anti-gas Liquid ▣ 819
- Gelusil Antacid-Anti-gas Tablets ▣ 819
- Maalox Antacid/Anti-Gas Tablets 889
- Maalox Antacid Liquid 888
- Extra Strength Maalox Antacid/Anti-Gas Liquid and Tablets 888
- Mylanta Fast-Acting 1359
- Mylanta Gelcaps Antacid ▣ 678
- Fast-Acting Mylanta Liquid Antacid 1359
- Mylanta Tablets ▣ 677
- Maximum-Strength Fast-Acting Mylanta Liquid Antacid 1359
- Mylanta Double Strength Tablets ▣ 677
- Phillips' Milk of Magnesia Liquid ▣ 627
- Rolaids Antacid Tablets ▣ 807
- Tempo Soft Antacid ▣ 799

Magnesium Oxide (Reduces the effectiveness of methenamine by causing urine to become alkaline). Products include:
- Beelith Tablets 632
- Bufferin Analgesic Tablets ▣ 636
- Arthritis Strength Bufferin Analgesic Caplets ▣ 637
- Extra Strength Bufferin Analgesic Tablets ▣ 637
- Caltrate PLUS ▣ 681
- Cama Arthritis Pain Reliever ▣ 748
- Mag-Ox 400 666
- Uro-Mag 666

Magnesium Salicylate (Concurrent use may lead to increased serum salicylate levels since excretion of salicylates is reduced in acidic urine). Products include:
- Backache Caplets ▣ 635
- Doan's Extra-Strength Analgesic ▣ 653
- Extra Strength Doan's P.M. ▣ 653
- Doan's Regular Strength Analgesic ▣ 654
- Mobigesic Tablets ▣ 607

Methazolamide (Reduces the effectiveness of methenamine by causing urine to become alkaline). Products include:
- GlaucTabs ◉ 209
- Neptazane Tablets ◉ 320

Methyclothiazide (Reduces the effectiveness of methenamine by causing urine to become alkaline). Products include:
- Enduron Tablets 424

Methyldopa (Concurrent use with sodium phosphate may result in hypernatremia). Products include:
- Aldoclor Tablets 1638
- Aldomet Oral 1640
- Aldoril Tablets 1644

Methylprednisolone Acetate (Concurrent use with sodium phosphate may result in hypernatremia).
No products indexed under this heading.

Methylprednisolone Sodium Succinate (Concurrent use with sodium phosphate may result in hypernatremia).
No products indexed under this heading.

Polythiazide (Reduces the effectiveness of methenamine by causing urine to become alkaline). Products include:
- Minizide Capsules 2016

Potassium Citrate (Reduces the effectiveness of methenamine by causing urine to become alkaline). Products include:
- Polycitra Syrup 574
- Polycitra-K Crystals 574
- Polycitra-K Oral Solution 575
- Polycitra-LC 574
- Urocit-K Tablets 1828

Prednisolone Acetate (Concurrent use with sodium phosphate may result in hypernatremia). Products include:
- AK-CIDE ◉ 203
- AK-CIDE Ointment ◉ 203
- Blephamide Liquifilm Sterile Ophthalmic Suspension 472
- Blephamide Ointment ◉ 234
- Econopred & Econopred Plus Ophthalmic Suspensions ◉ 216
- Poly-Pred Liquifilm ◉ 246
- Pred Forte ◉ 247
- Pred Mild ◉ 250
- Pred-G Liquifilm Sterile Ophthalmic Suspension ◉ 248
- Pred-G S.O.P. Sterile Ophthalmic Ointment ◉ 249

Prednisolone Sodium Phosphate (Concurrent use with sodium phosphate may result in hypernatremia). Products include:
- AK-PRED ◉ 204
- Hydeltrasol Injection, Sterile 1708
- Pediapred Oral Solution 1618

Prednisolone Tebutate (Concurrent use with sodium phosphate may result in hypernatremia). Products include:
- Hydeltra-T.B.A. Sterile Suspension 1710

Prednisone (Concurrent use with sodium phosphate may result in hypernatremia).
No products indexed under this heading.

Rauwolfia Serpentina (Concurrent use with sodium phosphate may result in hypernatremia).
No products indexed under this heading.

Rescinnamine (Concurrent use with sodium phosphate may result in hypernatremia).
No products indexed under this heading.

Reserpine (Concurrent use with sodium phosphate may result in hypernatremia). Products include:
- Diupres Tablets 1691
- Hydropres Tablets 1718
- Ser-Ap-Es Tablets 867

Salsalate (Concurrent use may lead to increased serum salicylate levels since excretion of salicylates is reduced in acidic urine). Products include:
- Disalcid 1549
- Mono-Gesic Tablets 810
- Salflex Tablets 791

Sodium Bicarbonate (Reduces the effectiveness of methenamine by causing urine to become alkaline). Products include:
- Alka-Seltzer Cherry Effervescent Antacid and Pain Reliever ▣ 609
- Alka-Seltzer Extra Strength Effervescent Antacid and Pain Reliever ▣ 609
- Alka-Seltzer Gold Effervescent Antacid ▣ 611
- Alka-Seltzer Lemon Lime Effervescent Antacid and Pain Reliever ▣ 609
- Alka-Seltzer Original Effervescent Antacid and Pain Reliever ▣ 609
- Arm & Hammer Pure Baking Soda ▣ 648
- Colyte and Colyte-flavored 2540
- GoLYTELY 694
- Massengill Disposable Douches ▣ 780
- Massengill Liquid Concentrate ▣ 780
- NuLYTELY 694
- Cherry Flavor NuLYTELY 694

Sodium Citrate (Reduces the effectiveness of methenamine by causing urine to become alkaline). Products include:
- Bicitra 573
- Polycitra 574
- Salix SST Lozenges Saliva Stimulant ▣ 757

(▣ Described in PDR For Nonprescription Drugs) (◉ Described in PDR For Ophthalmology)

Sulfamethizole (Concurrent use with sulfamethizole and formaldehyde forms an insoluble precipitate in acid urine and increases the risk of crystaluria). Products include:
Urobiotic-250 Capsules 2038

Triamcinolone (Concurrent use with sodium phosphate may result in hypernatremia).
No products indexed under this heading.

Triamcinolone Acetonide (Concurrent use with sodium phosphate may result in hypernatremia). Products include:
Azmacort Oral Inhaler 2175
Nasacort AQ Nasal Spray 2191
Nasacort Nasal Inhaler 2189

Triamcinolone Diacetate (Concurrent use with sodium phosphate may result in hypernatremia).
No products indexed under this heading.

Triamcinolone Hexacetonide (Concurrent use with sodium phosphate may result in hypernatremia).
No products indexed under this heading.

VAGISTAT-1
(Tioconazole) 783
May interact with:

Rubber or latex products (The Vagistat ointment base may interact with rubber or latex products, such as condoms or vaginal contraceptive diaphragms; therefore, use of such products within 72 hours following treatment is not recommended).

VALIUM INJECTABLE
(Diazepam) 2336
May interact with central nervous system depressants, barbiturates, narcotic analgesics, phenothiazines, monoamine oxidase inhibitors, antidepressant drugs, and certain other agents. Compounds in these categories include:

Alfentanil Hydrochloride (Concomitant use increases central nervous system depression with increased risk of apnea; dosage of narcotic analgesics should be reduced by at least one-third). Products include:
Alfenta Injection 1334

Alprazolam (Concomitant use increases central nervous system depression with increased risk of apnea). Products include:
Xanax Tablets 2115

Amitriptyline Hydrochloride (May potentiate the actions of diazepam). Products include:
Elavil 2945
Etrafon 2495
Limbitrol 2333
Triavil Tablets 1800

Amoxapine (May potentiate the actions of diazepam). Products include:
Asendin Tablets 1419

Aprobarbital (Concomitant use increases central nervous system depression with increased risk of apnea).
No products indexed under this heading.

Buprenorphine (Concomitant use increases central nervous system depression with increased risk of apnea; dosage of narcotic analgesics should be reduced by at least one-third). Products include:
Buprenex Injectable 2170

Bupropion Hydrochloride (May potentiate the actions of diazepam). Products include:
Wellbutrin Tablets 1177

Buspirone Hydrochloride (Concomitant use increases central nervous system depression with increased risk of apnea). Products include:
BuSpar Tablets 738

Butabarbital (Concomitant use increases central nervous system depression with increased risk of apnea).
No products indexed under this heading.

Butalbital (Concomitant use increases central nervous system depression with increased risk of apnea). Products include:
Axocet Capsules 2469
Esgic-plus Capsules 1012
Esgic-plus Tablets 1012
Fioricet Tablets 2386
Fioricet with Codeine Capsules 2387
Fiorinal Capsules 2388
Fiorinal with Codeine Capsules ... 2390
Fiorinal Tablets 2388
Phrenilin 790
Sedapap Tablets 50 mg/650 mg .. 1826

Chlordiazepoxide (Concomitant use increases central nervous system depression with increased risk of apnea). Products include:
Limbitrol 2333

Chlordiazepoxide Hydrochloride (Concomitant use increases central nervous system depression with increased risk of apnea). Products include:
Librax Capsules 2330
Librium Capsules 2331
Librium Injectable 2332

Chlorpromazine (May potentiate the actions of diazepam). Products include:
Thorazine Suppositories 2701

Chlorpromazine Hydrochloride (May potentiate the actions of diazepam). Products include:
Thorazine 2701

Chlorprothixene (Concomitant use increases central nervous system depression with increased risk of apnea).
No products indexed under this heading.

Chlorprothixene Hydrochloride (Concomitant use increases central nervous system depression with increased risk of apnea).
No products indexed under this heading.

Chlorprothixene Lactate (Concomitant use increases central nervous system depression with increased risk of apnea).
No products indexed under this heading.

Cimetidine (Co-administration delays diazepam clearance; clinical significance of this interaction is unclear). Products include:
Tagamet HB Tablets 786
Tagamet Tablets 2694

Cimetidine Hydrochloride (Co-administration delays diazepam clearance; clinical significance of this interaction is unclear). Products include:
Tagamet................................... 2694

Clonazepam (May potentiate the CNS depression caused by diazepam). Products include:
Klonopin Tablets 2294

Clorazepate Dipotassium (Concomitant use increases central nervous system depression with increased risk of apnea). Products include:
Tranxene 459

Clozapine (Concomitant use increases central nervous system depression with increased risk of apnea). Products include:
Clozaril Tablets 2377

Codeine Phosphate (Concomitant use increases central nervous system depression with increased risk of apnea; dosage of narcotic analgesics should be reduced by at least one-third). Products include:
Brontex 2130
Dimetane-DC Cough Syrup 2232
Fioricet with Codeine Capsules ... 2387
Fiorinal with Codeine Capsules ... 2390
Nucofed 2225
Phenergan with Codeine 2883
Phenergan VC with Codeine ... 2888
Robitussin A-C Syrup 2248
Robitussin-DAC Syrup 2249
Ryna 804
Soma Compound w/Codeine Tablets 2784
Tylenol with Codeine 1592

Desflurane (Concomitant use increases central nervous system depression with increased risk of apnea). Products include:
Suprane (desflurane, USP) 1865

Desipramine Hydrochloride (May potentiate the actions of diazepam). Products include:
Norpramin Tablets 1273

Dezocine (Concomitant use increases central nervous system depression with increased risk of apnea; dosage of narcotic analgesics should be reduced by at least one-third). Products include:
Dalgan Injection 529

Doxepin Hydrochloride (May potentiate the actions of diazepam). Products include:
Adapin Capsules 1542
Sinequan 2028
Zonalon Cream 1042

Droperidol (Concomitant use increases central nervous system depression with increased risk of apnea). Products include:
Inapsine Injection 462

Enflurane (Concomitant use increases central nervous system depression with increased risk of apnea).
No products indexed under this heading.

Estazolam (Concomitant use increases central nervous system depression with increased risk of apnea). Products include:
ProSom Tablets 457

Ethchlorvynol (Concomitant use increases central nervous system depression with increased risk of apnea). Products include:
Placidyl Capsules 456

Ethinamate (Concomitant use increases central nervous system depression with increased risk of apnea).
No products indexed under this heading.

Fentanyl (Concomitant use increases central nervous system depression with increased risk of apnea; dosage of narcotic analgesics should be reduced by at least one-third). Products include:
Duragesic Transdermal System 1336

Fentanyl Citrate (Concomitant use increases central nervous system depression with increased risk of apnea; dosage of narcotic analgesics should be reduced by at least one-third). Products include:
Sublimaze Injection 463

Fluoxetine Hydrochloride (May potentiate the actions of diazepam). Products include:
Prozac Pulvules & Liquid, Oral Solution 935

Fluphenazine Decanoate (May potentiate the actions of diazepam). Products include:
Prolixin Decanoate 510

Fluphenazine Enanthate (May potentiate the actions of diazepam). Products include:
Prolixin Enanthate 510

Fluphenazine Hydrochloride (May potentiate the actions of diazepam). Products include:
Prolixin 510

Flurazepam Hydrochloride (Concomitant use increases central nervous system depression with increased risk of apnea). Products include:
Dalmane Capsules 2329

Furazolidone (May potentiate the actions of diazepam). Products include:
Furoxone 2221

Glutethimide (Concomitant use increases central nervous system depression with increased risk of apnea).
No products indexed under this heading.

Haloperidol (Concomitant use increases central nervous system depression with increased risk of apnea). Products include:
Haldol Injection, Tablets and Concentrate 1585

Haloperidol Decanoate (Concomitant use increases central nervous system depression with increased risk of apnea). Products include:
Haldol Decanoate.................... 1587

Hydrocodone Bitartrate (Concomitant use increases central nervous system depression with increased risk of apnea; dosage of narcotic analgesics should be reduced by at least one-third). Products include:
Codiclear DH Syrup 808
Duratuss HD Elixir 2750
Histussin D Liquid 670
Hycodan Tablets and Syrup 946
Hycomine Compound Tablets .. 948
Hycomine 947
Hycotuss Expectorant Syrup ... 950
Hydrocet Capsules 787
Lorcet 10/650 Tablets 1016
Lortab 2751
Tussend 1830
Tussend Expectorant 1831
Vicodin Tablets 1404
Vicodin ES Tablets 1405
Vicodin HP Tablets 1403
Vicodin Tuss Expectorant 1406
Zydone Capsules 967

Hydrocodone Polistirex (Concomitant use increases central nervous system depression with increased risk of apnea; dosage of narcotic analgesics should be reduced by at least one-third). Products include:
Tussionex Pennkinetic Extended-Release Suspension 1624

IMPORTANT NOTE: Always consult each drug listing in the patient's regimen for possible interactions.

Valium Injectable — Interactions Index

Hydromorphone Hydrochloride (Concomitant use increases central nervous system depression with increased risk of apnea; dosage of narcotic analgesics should be reduced by at least one-third). Products include:
- Dilaudid Ampules 1382
- Dilaudid Cough Syrup 1383
- Dilaudid-HP Injection 1384
- Dilaudid-HP Lyophilized Powder 250 mg 1384
- Dilaudid 1382
- Dilaudid Oral Liquid 1386
- Dilaudid 1382
- Dilaudid Tablets - 8 mg 1386

Hydroxyzine Hydrochloride (Concomitant use increases central nervous system depression with increased risk of apnea). Products include:
- Atarax Tablets & Syrup 1992
- Marax Tablets & DF Syrup 2015
- Vistaril Intramuscular Solution 2042

Imipramine Hydrochloride (May potentiate the actions of diazepam). Products include:
- Tofranil Ampuls 873
- Tofranil Tablets 875

Imipramine Pamoate (May potentiate the actions of diazepam). Products include:
- Tofranil-PM Capsules 876

Isocarboxazid (May potentiate the actions of diazepam).
No products indexed under this heading.

Isoflurane (Concomitant use increases central nervous system depression with increased risk of apnea).
No products indexed under this heading.

Ketamine Hydrochloride (Concomitant use increases central nervous system depression with increased risk of apnea).
No products indexed under this heading.

Levomethadyl Acetate Hydrochloride (Concomitant use increases central nervous system depression with increased risk of apnea). Products include:
- Orlaam Oral Solution 2361

Levorphanol Tartrate (Concomitant use increases central nervous system depression with increased risk of apnea; dosage of narcotic analgesics should be reduced by at least one-third). Products include:
- Levo-Dromoran 2297

Lorazepam (Concomitant use increases central nervous system depression with increased risk of apnea). Products include:
- Ativan Injection 2805
- Ativan Tablets 2807

Loxapine Hydrochloride (Concomitant use increases central nervous system depression with increased risk of apnea). Products include:
- Loxitane 1426

Loxapine Succinate (Concomitant use increases central nervous system depression with increased risk of apnea). Products include:
- Loxitane Capsules 1426

Maprotiline Hydrochloride (May potentiate the actions of diazepam). Products include:
- Ludiomil Tablets 861

Meperidine Hydrochloride (Concomitant use increases central nervous system depression with increased risk of apnea; dosage of narcotic analgesics should be reduced by at least one-third). Products include:
- Demerol 2438
- Mepergan Injection 2859

Mephobarbital (Concomitant use increases central nervous system depression with increased risk of apnea). Products include:
- Mebaral Tablets 2452

Meprobamate (Concomitant use increases central nervous system depression with increased risk of apnea). Products include:
- Miltown Tablets 2780
- PMB 200 and PMB 400 2890

Mesoridazine Besylate (May potentiate the actions of diazepam). Products include:
- Serentil 689

Methadone Hydrochloride (Concomitant use increases central nervous system depression with increased risk of apnea; dosage of narcotic analgesics should be reduced by at least one-third). Products include:
- Methadone Hydrochloride Oral Concentrate 2356
- Methadone Hydrochloride Oral Solution & Tablets 2357

Methohexital Sodium (Concomitant use increases central nervous system depression with increased risk of apnea).
No products indexed under this heading.

Methotrimeprazine (May potentiate the actions of diazepam). Products include:
- Levoprome 1321

Methoxyflurane (Concomitant use increases central nervous system depression with increased risk of apnea).
No products indexed under this heading.

Midazolam Hydrochloride (Concomitant use increases central nervous system depression with increased risk of apnea). Products include:
- Versed Injection 2324

Molindone Hydrochloride (Concomitant use increases central nervous system depression with increased risk of apnea). Products include:
- Moban Tablets and Concentrate 1036

Morphine Sulfate (Concomitant use increases central nervous system depression with increased risk of apnea; dosage of narcotic analgesics should be reduced by at least one-third). Products include:
- Astramorph/PF Injection, USP (Preservative-Free) 526
- Duramorph Injection 983
- Infumorph 200 and Infumorph 500 Sterile Solutions 985
- Kadian Capsules 2948
- MS Contin Tablets 2149
- MSIR 2152
- Oramorph SR (Morphine Sulfate Sustained Release Tablets) 2359
- RMS Suppositories CII 2766
- Roxanol 2365

Nefazodone Hydrochloride (May potentiate the actions of diazepam). Products include:
- Serzone Tablets 776

Nortriptyline Hydrochloride (May potentiate the actions of diazepam). Products include:
- Pamelor 2409

Opium Alkaloids (Concomitant use increases central nervous system depression with increased risk of apnea; dosage of narcotic analgesics should be reduced by at least one-third).
No products indexed under this heading.

Oxazepam (Concomitant use increases central nervous system depression with increased risk of apnea). Products include:
- Serax Capsules 2916
- Serax Tablets 2916

Oxycodone Hydrochloride (Concomitant use increases central nervous system depression with increased risk of apnea; dosage of narcotic analgesics should be reduced by at least one-third). Products include:
- OxyContin Tablets 2163
- OxyIR Capsules 2167
- Percocet Tablets 955
- Percodan Tablets 955
- Percodan-Demi Tablets 956
- Roxicodone Tablets, Oral Solution & Intensol (Oxycodone) 2366
- Tylox Capsules 1593

Paroxetine Hydrochloride (May potentiate the actions of diazepam). Products include:
- Paxil Tablets 2681

Pentobarbital Sodium (Concomitant use increases central nervous system depression with increased risk of apnea). Products include:
- Nembutal Sodium Capsules 440
- Nembutal Sodium Solution 442
- Nembutal Sodium Suppositories 444

Perphenazine (May potentiate the actions of diazepam). Products include:
- Etrafon 2495
- Triavil Tablets 1800
- Trilafon 2532

Phenelzine Sulfate (May potentiate the actions of diazepam). Products include:
- Nardil 1977

Phenobarbital (Concomitant use increases central nervous system depression with increased risk of apnea). Products include:
- Arco-Lase Plus Tablets 513
- Bellergal-S Tablets 2375
- Donnatal 2234
- Donnatal Extentabs 2234
- Donnatal Tablets 2234
- Phenobarbital Elixir and Tablets 1523
- Quadrinal Tablets 1398

Prazepam (Concomitant use increases central nervous system depression with increased risk of apnea).
No products indexed under this heading.

Prochlorperazine (May potentiate the actions of diazepam). Products include:
- Compazine 2644

Promethazine Hydrochloride (May potentiate the actions of diazepam). Products include:
- Mepergan Injection 2859
- Phenergan with Codeine 2883
- Phenergan with Dextromethorphan 2885
- Phenergan Injection 2880
- Phenergan Suppositories 2882
- Phenergan Syrup 2881
- Phenergan Tablets 2882
- Phenergan VC 2886
- Phenergan VC with Codeine 2888

Propofol (Concomitant use increases central nervous system depression with increased risk of apnea). Products include:
- Diprivan Injectable Emulsion 2939

Propoxyphene Hydrochloride (Concomitant use increases central nervous system depression with increased risk of apnea; dosage of narcotic analgesics should be reduced by at least one-third). Products include:
- Darvon 1475
- Wygesic Tablets 2930

Propoxyphene Napsylate (Concomitant use increases central nervous system depression with increased risk of apnea; dosage of narcotic analgesics should be reduced by at least one-third). Products include:
- Darvon-N/Darvocet-N 1473

Protriptyline Hydrochloride (May potentiate the actions of diazepam). Products include:
- Vivactil Tablets 1820

Quazepam (Concomitant use increases central nervous system depression with increased risk of apnea). Products include:
- Doral Tablets 2773

Risperidone (Concomitant use increases central nervous system depression with increased risk of apnea). Products include:
- Risperdal Tablets 1348

Secobarbital Sodium (Concomitant use increases central nervous system depression with increased risk of apnea). Products include:
- Seconal Sodium Pulvules 1529

Selegiline Hydrochloride (May potentiate the actions of diazepam). Products include:
- Eldepryl Capsules 2729

Sertraline Hydrochloride (May potentiate the actions of diazepam). Products include:
- Zoloft Tablets 2051

Sevoflurane (Concomitant use increases central nervous system depression with increased risk of apnea).
No products indexed under this heading.

Sufentanil Citrate (Concomitant use increases central nervous system depression with increased risk of apnea; dosage of narcotic analgesics should be reduced by at least one-third). Products include:
- Sufenta Injection 1355

Temazepam (Concomitant use increases central nervous system depression with increased risk of apnea). Products include:
- Restoril Capsules 2413

Thiamylal Sodium (Concomitant use increases central nervous system depression with increased risk of apnea).
No products indexed under this heading.

Thioridazine Hydrochloride (May potentiate the actions of diazepam). Products include:
- Mellaril 2398

Thiothixene (Concomitant use increases central nervous system depression with increased risk of apnea). Products include:
- Navane Capsules and Concentrate 2018
- Navane Intramuscular 2019

Tranylcypromine Sulfate (May potentiate the actions of diazepam). Products include:
- Parnate Tablets 2679

Trazodone Hydrochloride (May potentiate the actions of diazepam). Products include:
- Desyrel and Desyrel Dividose 504

(■ Described in PDR For Nonprescription Drugs)   (◉ Described in PDR For Ophthalmology)

Triazolam (Concomitant use increases central nervous system depression with increased risk of apnea). Products include:
Halcion Tablets 2093
Trifluoperazine Hydrochloride (May potentiate the actions of diazepam). Products include:
Stelazine 2692
Trimipramine Maleate (May potentiate the actions of diazepam). Products include:
Surmontil Capsules 2917
Venlafaxine Hydrochloride (May potentiate the actions of diazepam). Products include:
Effexor 2825
Zolpidem Tartrate (Concomitant use increases central nervous system depression with increased risk of apnea). Products include:
Ambien Tablets 2559

Food Interactions

Alcohol (Concomitant use increases central nervous system depression with increased risk of apnea; injectable diazepam should not be administered in acute alcoholic intoxication.)

VALIUM TABLETS
(Diazepam) 2335
May interact with central nervous system depressants, phenothiazines, narcotic analgesics, barbiturates, monoamine oxidase inhibitors, antidepressant drugs, anticonvulsants, and certain other agents. Compounds in these categories include:

Alfentanil Hydrochloride (May potentiate the actions of diazepam). Products include:
Alfenta Injection 1334
Alprazolam (May potentiate the actions of diazepam). Products include:
Xanax Tablets 2115
Amitriptyline Hydrochloride (May potentiate the actions of diazepam). Products include:
Elavil 2945
Etrafon 2495
Limbitrol 2333
Triavil Tablets 1800
Amoxapine (May potentiate the actions of diazepam). Products include:
Asendin Tablets 1419
Aprobarbital (May potentiate the actions of diazepam).
No products indexed under this heading.
Buprenorphine (May potentiate the actions of diazepam). Products include:
Buprenex Injectable 2170
Bupropion Hydrochloride (May potentiate the actions of diazepam). Products include:
Wellbutrin Tablets 1177
Buspirone Hydrochloride (May potentiate the actions of diazepam). Products include:
BuSpar Tablets 738
Butabarbital (May potentiate the actions of diazepam).
No products indexed under this heading.
Butalbital (May potentiate the actions of diazepam). Products include:
Axocet Capsules 2469
Esgic-plus Capsules 1012
Esgic-plus Tablets 1012
Fioricet Tablets 2386
Fioricet with Codeine Capsules ... 2387
Fiorinal Capsules 2388
Fiorinal with Codeine Capsules ... 2390

Fiorinal Tablets 2388
Phrenilin 790
Sedapap Tablets 50 mg/650 mg .. 1826
Carbamazepine (Co-administration of diazepam as an adjunct in treating convulsive disorders results in possibility of an increase in the frequency and/or severity of grand mal seizures which may require an increase in the dosage of standard anticonvulsant agent). Products include:
Atretol Tablets 569
Tegretol/Tegretol-XR 870
Chlordiazepoxide (May potentiate the actions of diazepam). Products include:
Limbitrol 2333
Chlordiazepoxide Hydrochloride (May potentiate the actions of diazepam). Products include:
Librax Capsules 2330
Librium Capsules 2331
Librium Injectable 2332
Chlorpromazine (May potentiate the actions of diazepam). Products include:
Thorazine Suppositories 2701
Chlorpromazine Hydrochloride (May potentiate the actions of diazepam). Products include:
Thorazine 2701
Chlorprothixene (May potentiate the actions of diazepam).
No products indexed under this heading.
Chlorprothixene Hydrochloride (May potentiate the actions of diazepam).
No products indexed under this heading.
Chlorprothixene Lactate (May potentiate the actions of diazepam).
No products indexed under this heading.
Cimetidine (Co-administration delays diazepam clearance; clinical significance of this interaction is unclear). Products include:
Tagamet HB Tablets 786
Tagamet Tablets 2694
Cimetidine Hydrochloride (Co-administration delays diazepam clearance; clinical significance of this interaction is unclear). Products include:
Tagamet 2694
Clonazepam (Co-administration of diazepam as an adjunct in treating convulsive disorders results in possibility of an increase in the frequency and/or severity of grand mal seizures which may require an increase in the dosage of standard anticonvulsant agent; may potentiate the CNS depression caused by diazepam). Products include:
Klonopin Tablets 2294
Clorazepate Dipotassium (May potentiate the actions of diazepam). Products include:
Tranxene 459
Clozapine (May potentiate the actions of diazepam). Products include:
Clozaril Tablets 2377
Codeine Phosphate (May potentiate the actions of diazepam). Products include:
Brontex 2130
Dimetane-DC Cough Syrup 2232
Fioricet with Codeine Capsules ... 2387
Fiorinal with Codeine Capsules ... 2390
Nucofed 2225
Phenergan with Codeine 2883
Phenergan VC with Codeine 2888
Robitussin A-C Syrup 2248
Robitussin-DAC Syrup 2249
Ryna 804

Soma Compound w/Codeine Tablets 2784
Tylenol with Codeine 1592
Desflurane (May potentiate the actions of diazepam). Products include:
Suprane (desflurane, USP) 1865
Desipramine Hydrochloride (May potentiate the actions of diazepam). Products include:
Norpramin Tablets 1273
Dezocine (May potentiate the actions of diazepam). Products include:
Dalgan Injection 529
Divalproex Sodium (Co-administration of diazepam as an adjunct in treating convulsive disorders results in possibility of an increase in the frequency and/or severity of grand mal seizures which may require an increase in the dosage of standard anticonvulsant agent). Products include:
Depakote Tablets 418
Doxepin Hydrochloride (May potentiate the actions of diazepam). Products include:
Adapin Capsules 1542
Sinequan 2028
Zonalon Cream 1042
Droperidol (May potentiate the actions of diazepam). Products include:
Inapsine Injection 462
Enflurane (May potentiate the actions of diazepam).
No products indexed under this heading.
Estazolam (May potentiate the actions of diazepam). Products include:
ProSom Tablets 457
Ethchlorvynol (May potentiate the actions of diazepam). Products include:
Placidyl Capsules 456
Ethinamate (May potentiate the actions of diazepam).
No products indexed under this heading.
Ethosuximide (Co-administration of diazepam as an adjunct in treating convulsive disorders results in possibility of an increase in the frequency and/or severity of grand mal seizures which may require an increase in the dosage of standard anticonvulsant agent). Products include:
Zarontin Capsules 1986
Zarontin Syrup 1986
Ethotoin (Co-administration of diazepam as an adjunct in treating convulsive disorders results in possibility of an increase in the frequency and/or severity of grand mal seizures which may require an increase in the dosage of standard anticonvulsant agent). Products include:
Peganone Tablets 455
Felbamate (Co-administration of diazepam as an adjunct in treating convulsive disorders results in possibility of an increase in the frequency and/or severity of grand mal seizures which may require an increase in the dosage of standard anticonvulsant agent). Products include:
Felbatol 2774
Fentanyl (May potentiate the actions of diazepam). Products include:
Duragesic Transdermal System ... 1336
Fentanyl Citrate (May potentiate the actions of diazepam). Products include:
Sublimaze Injection 463

Fluoxetine Hydrochloride (May potentiate the actions of diazepam). Products include:
Prozac Pulvules & Liquid, Oral Solution 935
Fluphenazine Decanoate (May potentiate the actions of diazepam). Products include:
Prolixin Decanoate 510
Fluphenazine Enanthate (May potentiate the actions of diazepam). Products include:
Prolixin Enanthate 510
Fluphenazine Hydrochloride (May potentiate the actions of diazepam). Products include:
Prolixin 510
Flurazepam Hydrochloride (May potentiate the actions of diazepam). Products include:
Dalmane Capsules 2329
Furazolidone (May potentiate the actions of diazepam). Products include:
Furoxone 2221
Glutethimide (May potentiate the actions of diazepam).
No products indexed under this heading.
Haloperidol (May potentiate the actions of diazepam). Products include:
Haldol Injection, Tablets and Concentrate 1585
Haloperidol Decanoate (May potentiate the actions of diazepam). Products include:
Haldol Decanoate 1587
Hydrocodone Bitartrate (May potentiate the actions of diazepam). Products include:
Codiclear DH Syrup 808
Duratuss HD Elixir 2750
Histussin D Liquid 670
Hycodan Tablets and Syrup 946
Hycomine Compound Tablets 948
Hycomine 947
Hycotuss Expectorant Syrup 950
Hydrocet Capsules 787
Lorcet 10/650 Tablets 1016
Lortab 2751
Tussend 1830
Tussend Expectorant 1831
Vicodin Tablets 1404
Vicodin ES Tablets 1405
Vicodin HP Tablets 1403
Vicodin Tuss Expectorant 1406
Zydone Capsules 967
Hydrocodone Polistirex (May potentiate the actions of diazepam). Products include:
Tussionex Pennkinetic Extended-Release Suspension 1624
Hydromorphone Hydrochloride (May potentiate the actions of diazepam). Products include:
Dilaudid Ampules 1382
Dilaudid Cough Syrup 1383
Dilaudid-HP Injection 1384
Dilaudid-HP Lyophilized Powder 250 mg 1384
Dilaudid 1382
Dilaudid Oral Liquid 1386
Dilaudid 1382
Dilaudid Tablets - 8 mg 1386
Hydroxyzine Hydrochloride (May potentiate the actions of diazepam). Products include:
Atarax Tablets & Syrup 1992
Marax Tablets & DF Syrup 2015
Vistaril Intramuscular Solution 2042
Imipramine Hydrochloride (May potentiate the actions of diazepam). Products include:
Tofranil Ampuls 873
Tofranil Tablets 875
Imipramine Pamoate (May potentiate the actions of diazepam). Products include:
Tofranil-PM Capsules 876

IMPORTANT NOTE: Always consult each drug listing in the patient's regimen for possible interactions.

Valium Tablets — Interactions Index

Isocarboxazid (May potentiate the actions of diazepam).
No products indexed under this heading.

Isoflurane (May potentiate the actions of diazepam).
No products indexed under this heading.

Ketamine Hydrochloride (May potentiate the actions of diazepam).
No products indexed under this heading.

Lamotrigine (Co-administration of diazepam as an adjunct in treating convulsive disorders results in possibility of an increase in the frequency and/or severity of grand mal seizures which may require an increase in the dosage of standard anticonvulsant agent). Products include:
Lamictal Tablets 1105

Levomethadyl Acetate Hydrochloride (May potentiate the actions of diazepam). Products include:
Orlaam Oral Solution 2361

Levorphanol Tartrate (May potentiate the actions of diazepam). Products include:
Levo-Dromoran 2297

Lorazepam (May potentiate the actions of diazepam). Products include:
Ativan Injection 2805
Ativan Tablets 2807

Loxapine Hydrochloride (May potentiate the actions of diazepam). Products include:
Loxitane 1426

Loxapine Succinate (May potentiate the actions of diazepam). Products include:
Loxitane Capsules 1426

Maprotiline Hydrochloride (May potentiate the actions of diazepam). Products include:
Ludiomil Tablets 861

Meperidine Hydrochloride (May potentiate the actions of diazepam). Products include:
Demerol 2438
Mepergan Injection 2859

Mephenytoin (Co-administration of diazepam as an adjunct in treating convulsive disorders results in possibility of an increase in the frequency and/or severity of grand mal seizures which may require an increase in the dosage of standard anticonvulsant agent). Products include:
Mesantoin Tablets 2400

Mephobarbital (May potentiate the actions of diazepam). Products include:
Mebaral Tablets 2452

Meprobamate (May potentiate the actions of diazepam). Products include:
Miltown Tablets 2780
PMB 200 and PMB 400 2890

Mesoridazine Besylate (May potentiate the actions of diazepam). Products include:
Serentil 689

Methadone Hydrochloride (May potentiate the actions of diazepam). Products include:
Methadone Hydrochloride Oral Concentrate 2356
Methadone Hydrochloride Oral Solution & Tablets 2357

Methohexital Sodium (May potentiate the actions of diazepam).
No products indexed under this heading.

Methotrimeprazine (May potentiate the actions of diazepam). Products include:
Levoprome 1321

Methoxyflurane (May potentiate the actions of diazepam).
No products indexed under this heading.

Methsuximide (Co-administration of diazepam as an adjunct in treating convulsive disorders results in possibility of an increase in the frequency and/or severity of grand mal seizures which may require an increase in the dosage of standard anticonvulsant agent). Products include:
Celontin Kapseals 1955

Midazolam Hydrochloride (May potentiate the actions of diazepam). Products include:
Versed Injection 2324

Molindone Hydrochloride (May potentiate the actions of diazepam). Products include:
Moban Tablets and Concentrate 1036

Morphine Sulfate (May potentiate the actions of diazepam). Products include:
Astramorph/PF Injection, USP (Preservative-Free) 526
Duramorph Injection 983
Infumorph 200 and Infumorph 500 Sterile Solutions 985
Kadian Capsules 2948
MS Contin Tablets 2149
MSIR 2152
Oramorph SR (Morphine Sulfate Sustained Release Tablets) 2359
RMS Suppositories CII 2766
Roxanol 2365

Nefazodone Hydrochloride (May potentiate the actions of diazepam). Products include:
Serzone Tablets 776

Nortriptyline Hydrochloride (May potentiate the actions of diazepam). Products include:
Pamelor 2409

Opium Alkaloids (May potentiate the actions of diazepam).
No products indexed under this heading.

Oxazepam (May potentiate the actions of diazepam). Products include:
Serax Capsules 2916
Serax Tablets 2916

Oxycodone Hydrochloride (May potentiate the actions of diazepam). Products include:
OxyContin Tablets 2163
OxyIR Capsules 2167
Percocet Tablets 955
Percodan Tablets 955
Percodan-Demi Tablets 956
Roxicodone Tablets, Oral Solution & Intensol (Oxycodone) 2366
Tylox Capsules 1593

Paramethadione (Co-administration of diazepam as an adjunct in treating convulsive disorders results in possibility of an increase in the frequency and/or severity of grand mal seizures which may require an increase in the dosage of standard anticonvulsant agent).
No products indexed under this heading.

Paroxetine Hydrochloride (May potentiate the actions of diazepam). Products include:
Paxil Tablets 2681

Pentobarbital Sodium (May potentiate the actions of diazepam). Products include:
Nembutal Sodium Capsules 440
Nembutal Sodium Solution 442
Nembutal Sodium Suppositories 444

Perphenazine (May potentiate the actions of diazepam). Products include:
Etrafon 2495
Triavil Tablets 1800
Trilafon 2532

Phenacemide (Co-administration of diazepam as an adjunct in treating convulsive disorders results in possibility of an increase in the frequency and/or severity of grand mal seizures which may require an increase in the dosage of standard anticonvulsant agent). Products include:
Phenurone Tablets 455

Phenelzine Sulfate (May potentiate the actions of diazepam). Products include:
Nardil 1977

Phenobarbital (Co-administration of diazepam as an adjunct in treating convulsive disorders results in possibility of an increase in the frequency and/or severity of grand mal seizures which may require an increase in the dosage of standard anticonvulsant agent; may potentiate the CNS depression caused by diazepam). Products include:
Arco-Lase Plus Tablets 513
Bellergal-S Tablets 2375
Donnatal 2234
Donnatal Extentabs 2234
Donnatal Tablets 2234
Phenobarbital Elixir and Tablets 1523
Quadrinal Tablets 1398

Phensuximide (Co-administration of diazepam as an adjunct in treating convulsive disorders results in possibility of an increase in the frequency and/or severity of grand mal seizures which may require an increase in the dosage of standard anticonvulsant agent).
No products indexed under this heading.

Phenytoin (Co-administration of diazepam as an adjunct in treating convulsive disorders results in possibility of an increase in the frequency and/or severity of grand mal seizures which may require an increase in the dosage of standard anticonvulsant agent). Products include:
Dilantin Infatabs 1967
Dilantin-125 Suspension 1969

Phenytoin Sodium (Co-administration of diazepam as an adjunct in treating convulsive disorders results in possibility of an increase in the frequency and/or severity of grand mal seizures which may require an increase in the dosage of standard anticonvulsant agent). Products include:
Dilantin Kapseals 1965

Prazepam (May potentiate the actions of diazepam).
No products indexed under this heading.

Primidone (Co-administration of diazepam as an adjunct in treating convulsive disorders results in possibility of an increase in the frequency and/or severity of grand mal seizures which may require an increase in the dosage of standard anticonvulsant agent). Products include:
Mysoline 2860

Prochlorperazine (May potentiate the actions of diazepam). Products include:
Compazine 2644

Promethazine Hydrochloride (May potentiate the actions of diazepam). Products include:
Mepergan Injection 2859

Phenergan with Codeine 2883
Phenergan with Dextromethorphan 2885
Phenergan Injection 2880
Phenergan Suppositories 2882
Phenergan Syrup 2881
Phenergan Tablets 2882
Phenergan VC 2886
Phenergan VC with Codeine 2888

Propofol (May potentiate the actions of diazepam). Products include:
Diprivan Injectable Emulsion 2939

Propoxyphene Hydrochloride (May potentiate the actions of diazepam). Products include:
Darvon 1475
Wygesic Tablets 2930

Propoxyphene Napsylate (May potentiate the actions of diazepam). Products include:
Darvon-N/Darvocet-N 1473

Protriptyline Hydrochloride (May potentiate the actions of diazepam). Products include:
Vivactil Tablets 1820

Quazepam (May potentiate the actions of diazepam). Products include:
Doral Tablets 2773

Risperidone (May potentiate the actions of diazepam). Products include:
Risperdal Tablets 1348

Secobarbital Sodium (May potentiate the actions of diazepam). Products include:
Seconal Sodium Pulvules 1529

Selegiline Hydrochloride (May potentiate the actions of diazepam). Products include:
Eldepryl Capsules 2729

Sertraline Hydrochloride (May potentiate the actions of diazepam). Products include:
Zoloft Tablets 2051

Sevoflurane (May potentiate the actions of diazepam).
No products indexed under this heading.

Sufentanil Citrate (May potentiate the actions of diazepam). Products include:
Sufenta Injection 1355

Temazepam (May potentiate the actions of diazepam). Products include:
Restoril Capsules 2413

Thiamylal Sodium (May potentiate the actions of diazepam).
No products indexed under this heading.

Thioridazine Hydrochloride (May potentiate the actions of diazepam). Products include:
Mellaril 2398

Thiothixene (May potentiate the actions of diazepam). Products include:
Navane Capsules and Concentrate 2018
Navane Intramuscular 2019

Tranylcypromine Sulfate (May potentiate the actions of diazepam). Products include:
Parnate Tablets 2679

Trazodone Hydrochloride (May potentiate the actions of diazepam). Products include:
Desyrel and Desyrel Dividose 504

Triazolam (May potentiate the actions of diazepam). Products include:
Halcion Tablets 2093

Trifluoperazine Hydrochloride (May potentiate the actions of diazepam). Products include:
Stelazine 2692

(▣ Described in PDR For Nonprescription Drugs)   (◉ Described in PDR For Ophthalmology)

Trimethadione (Co-administration of diazepam as an adjunct in treating convulsive disorders results in possibility of an increase in the frequency and/or severity of grand mal seizures which may require an increase in the dosage of standard anticonvulsant agent).
 No products indexed under this heading.

Trimipramine Maleate (May potentiate the actions of diazepam). Products include:
 Surmontil Capsules 2917

Valproic Acid (Co-administration of diazepam as an adjunct in treating convulsive disorders results in possibility of an increase in the frequency and/or severity of grand mal seizures which may require an increase in the dosage of standard anticonvulsant agent). Products include:
 Depakene 416

Venlafaxine Hydrochloride (May potentiate the actions of diazepam). Products include:
 Effexor 2825

Zolpidem Tartrate (May potentiate the actions of diazepam). Products include:
 Ambien Tablets 2559

Food Interactions
Alcohol (May potentiate the actions of diazepam).

VALTREX CAPLETS
(Valacyclovir Hydrochloride) 1167
May interact with:

Cimetidine (Co-administration reduces the rate but not the extent of conversion of valacyclovir to acyclovir; additive increase in acyclovir AUC and C_{max}). Products include:
 Tagamet HB Tablets .... ⊙ 786
 Tagamet Tablets 2694

Cimetidine Hydrochloride (Co-administration reduces the rate but not the extent of conversion of valacyclovir to acyclovir; additive increase in acyclovir AUC and C_{max}). Products include:
 Tagamet 2694

Probenecid (Co-administration reduces the rate but not the extent of conversion of valacyclovir to acyclovir; additive increase in acyclovir AUC and C_{max}). Products include:
 Benemid Tablets 1651
 ColBENEMID Tablets 1662

VANCENASE AQ NASAL SPRAY 0.042%
(Beclomethasone Dipropionate) 2535
None cited in PDR database.

VANCENASE AQ DOUBLE STRENGTH NASAL SPRAY 0.084%
(Beclomethasone Dipropionate) 2536
None cited in PDR database.

VANCENASE POCKETHALER NASAL INHALER
(Beclomethasone Dipropionate) 2534
May interact with:

Prednisone (Increased likelihood of HPA suppression).
 No products indexed under this heading.

VANCERIL INHALER
(Beclomethasone Dipropionate) 2538
None cited in PDR database.

VANCOCIN HCL, ORAL SOLUTION & PULVULES
(Vancomycin Hydrochloride) 1536
May interact with aminoglycosides and ototoxic drugs. Compounds in these categories include:

Amikacin Sulfate (Concurrent use may result in increased ototoxicity and/or nephrotoxicity). Products include:
 Amikacin Sulfate Injection, USP 523
 Amikacin Sulfate Injection, USP 981
 Amikin Injectable 502

Cisplatin (Concurrent use may result in increased ototoxicity and/or nephrotoxicity). Products include:
 Platinol for Injection 717
 Platinol-AQ Injection 719

Gentamicin Sulfate (Concurrent use may result in increased ototoxicity and/or nephrotoxicity). Products include:
 Garamycin Cream 0.1% 2501
 Garamycin Injectable 2502
 Garamycin Ointment 0.1% 2501
 Garamycin Ophthalmic 2501
 Genoptic Sterile Ophthalmic Solution .... ⊙ 241
 Genoptic Sterile Ophthalmic Ointment .... ⊙ 241
 Gentak .... ⊙ 209
 Pred-G Liquifilm Sterile Ophthalmic Suspension .... ⊙ 248
 Pred-G S.O.P. Sterile Ophthalmic Ointment .... ⊙ 249

Kanamycin Sulfate (Concurrent use may result in increased ototoxicity and/or nephrotoxicity).
 No products indexed under this heading.

Streptomycin Sulfate (Concurrent use may result in increased ototoxicity and/or nephrotoxicity). Products include:
 Streptomycin Sulfate Injection 2031

Tobramycin Sulfate (Concurrent use may result in increased ototoxicity and/or nephrotoxicity). Products include:
 Nebcin Vials, Hyporets & ADD-Vantage 1518

VANCOCIN HCL, VIALS & ADD-VANTAGE
(Vancomycin Hydrochloride) 1534
May interact with aminoglycosides, anesthetics, and certain other agents. Compounds in these categories include:

Alfentanil Hydrochloride (Co-administration with anesthetic agents has been associated with erythema and histamine-like flushing in children). Products include:
 Alfenta Injection 1334

Amikacin Sulfate (Concurrent and/or sequential use may result in increased potential for neurotoxicity and/or nephrotoxicity). Products include:
 Amikacin Sulfate Injection, USP 523
 Amikacin Sulfate Injection, USP 981
 Amikin Injectable 502

Amphotericin B (Concurrent and/or sequential use may result in increased potential for neurotoxicity and/or nephrotoxicity). Products include:
 Abelcet Injection 1540
 Fungizone Intravenous 507
 Fungizone Oral Suspension 704

Bacitracin Zinc (Concurrent and/or sequential use may result in increased potential for neurotoxicity and/or nephrotoxicity). Products include:
 AK-Spore Ointment .... ⊙ 205
 Betadine Brand First Aid Antibiotics & Moisturizer Ointment 2144
 Cortisporin Ointment 1074
 Cortisporin Ophthalmic Ointment Sterile 1074
 Mycitracin .... ⊙ 803
 Neosporin Ointment .... ⊙ 821
 Neosporin Plus Maximum Strength Ointment .... ⊙ 822
 Neosporin Ophthalmic Ointment Sterile 1130
 Polysporin Ointment .... ⊙ 822
 Polysporin Ophthalmic Ointment Sterile 1140
 Polysporin Powder .... ⊙ 823

Cisplatin (Concurrent and/or sequential use may result in increased potential for neurotoxicity and/or nephrotoxicity). Products include:
 Platinol for Injection 717
 Platinol-AQ Injection 719

Colistin Sulfate (Concurrent and/or sequential use may result in increased potential for neurotoxicity and/or nephrotoxicity). Products include:
 Coly-Mycin S Otic w/Neomycin & Hydrocortisone 1965

Enflurane (Co-administration with anesthetic agents has been associated with erythema and histamine-like flushing in children).
 No products indexed under this heading.

Fentanyl Citrate (Co-administration with anesthetic agents has been associated with erythema and histamine-like flushing in children). Products include:
 Sublimaze Injection 463

Gentamicin Sulfate (Concurrent and/or sequential use may result in increased potential for neurotoxicity and/or nephrotoxicity). Products include:
 Garamycin Cream 0.1% 2501
 Garamycin Injectable 2502
 Garamycin Ointment 0.1% 2501
 Garamycin Ophthalmic 2501
 Genoptic Sterile Ophthalmic Solution .... ⊙ 241
 Genoptic Sterile Ophthalmic Ointment .... ⊙ 241
 Gentak .... ⊙ 209
 Pred-G Liquifilm Sterile Ophthalmic Suspension .... ⊙ 248
 Pred-G S.O.P. Sterile Ophthalmic Ointment .... ⊙ 249

Halothane (Co-administration with anesthetic agents has been associated with erythema and histamine-like flushing in children). Products include:
 Fluothane 2830

Isoflurane (Co-administration with anesthetic agents has been associated with erythema and histamine-like flushing in children).
 No products indexed under this heading.

Kanamycin Sulfate (Concurrent and/or sequential use may result in increased potential for neurotoxicity and/or nephrotoxicity).
 No products indexed under this heading.

Ketamine Hydrochloride (Co-administration with anesthetic agents has been associated with erythema and histamine-like flushing in children).
 No products indexed under this heading.

Methohexital Sodium (Co-administration with anesthetic agents has been associated with erythema and histamine-like flushing in children).
 No products indexed under this heading.

Midazolam Hydrochloride (Co-administration with anesthetic agents has been associated with erythema and histamine-like flushing in children). Products include:
 Versed Injection 2324

Polymyxin B Sulfate (Concurrent and/or sequential use may result in increased potential for neurotoxicity and/or nephrotoxicity). Products include:
 AK-Spore .... ⊙ 205
 AK-Trol Ointment & Suspension ... ⊙ 205
 Betadine Brand First Aid Antibiotics & Moisturizer Ointment 2144
 Cortisporin Cream 1073
 Cortisporin Ointment 1074
 Cortisporin Ophthalmic Ointment Sterile 1074
 Cortisporin Ophthalmic Suspension Sterile 1075
 Cortisporin Otic Solution Sterile 1076
 Cortisporin Otic Suspension Sterile ... 1077
 Maxitrol Ophthalmic Ointment and Suspension .... ⊙ 222
 Mycitracin .... ⊙ 803
 Neosporin G.U. Irrigant Sterile 1130
 Neosporin Ointment .... ⊙ 821
 Neosporin Plus Maximum Strength Cream .... ⊙ 821
 Neosporin Plus Maximum Strength Ointment .... ⊙ 822
 Neosporin Ophthalmic Ointment Sterile 1130
 Neosporin Ophthalmic Solution Sterile 1131
 Pediotic Suspension Sterile 1140
 Poly-Pred Liquifilm .... ⊙ 246
 Polysporin Ointment .... ⊙ 822
 Polysporin Ophthalmic Ointment Sterile 1140
 Polysporin Powder .... ⊙ 823
 Polytrim Ophthalmic Solution Sterile 479
 TERAK Ointment .... ⊙ 210
 Terramycin with Polymyxin B Sulfate Ophthalmic Ointment 2035

Propofol (Co-administration with anesthetic agents has been associated with erythema and histamine-like flushing in children). Products include:
 Diprivan Injectable Emulsion ... 2939

Streptomycin Sulfate (Concurrent and/or sequential use may result in increased potential for neurotoxicity and/or nephrotoxicity). Products include:
 Streptomycin Sulfate Injection 2031

Sufentanil Citrate (Co-administration with anesthetic agents has been associated with erythema and histamine-like flushing in children). Products include:
 Sufenta Injection 1355

Thiamylal Sodium (Co-administration with anesthetic agents has been associated with erythema and histamine-like flushing in children).
 No products indexed under this heading.

Tobramycin (Concurrent and/or sequential use may result in increased potential for neurotoxicity and/or nephrotoxicity). Products include:
 AKTOB .... ⊙ 207
 TobraDex Ophthalmic Suspension and Ointment 469
 Tobrex Ophthalmic Ointment and Solution .... ⊙ 226

Tobramycin Sulfate (Concurrent and/or sequential use may result in increased potential for neurotoxicity and/or nephrotoxicity). Products include:
 Nebcin Vials, Hyporets & ADD-Vantage 1518

Viomycin (Concurrent and/or sequential use may result in increased potential for neurotoxicity and/or nephrotoxicity).

IMPORTANT NOTE: Always consult each drug listing in the patient's regimen for possible interactions.

VANQUISH ANALGESIC CAPLETS
(Acetaminophen, Aspirin, Caffeine, Aluminum Hydroxide Gel, Magnesium Hydroxide) ◘ 627
May interact with oral anticoagulants and certain other agents. Compounds in these categories include:

Antiarthritic Drugs, unspecified (Effect not specified).

Antidiabetic Drugs, unspecified (Effect not specified).

Antigout Drugs, unspecified (Effect not specified).

Dicumarol (Concurrent use requires caution).
No products indexed under this heading.

Warfarin Sodium (Concurrent use requires caution). Products include:
Coumadin ... 941

VANTIN FOR ORAL SUSPENSION AND VANTIN TABLETS
(Cefpodoxime Proxetil) ... 2112
May interact with antacids, histamine H_2-receptor antagonists, anticholinergics, and certain other agents. Compounds in these categories include:

Aluminum Carbonate (High doses of antacids reduces peak plasma levels by 24% and the extent of absorption by 27%; the rate of absorption is not altered). Products include:
Basaljel Capsules ... 2810
Basaljel Suspension ... 2810
Basaljel Tablets ... 2810

Aluminum Hydroxide (High doses of antacids reduces peak plasma levels by 24% and the extent of absorption by 27%; the rate of absorption is not altered). Products include:
ALternaGEL Liquid ... 1358
Maximum Strength Ascriptin ... ◘ 650
Cama Arthritis Pain Reliever ... ◘ 748
Gaviscon Extra Strength Relief Formula Antacid Tablets ... ◘ 778
Gaviscon Extra Strength Relief Formula Liquid Antacid ... ◘ 779
Gaviscon Liquid Antacid ... ◘ 779
Gelusil Antacid-Anti-gas Liquid ... ◘ 819
Gelusil Antacid-Anti-gas Tablets ... ◘ 819
Maalox Antacid/Anti-Gas Tablets ... 889
Maalox Heartburn Relief Suspension ... ◘ 658
Maalox Antacid Liquid ... 888
Extra Strength Maalox Antacid/Anti-Gas Liquid and Tablets ... 888
Mylanta ... 1359
Tempo Soft Antacid ... ◘ 799

Aluminum Hydroxide Gel (High doses of antacids reduces peak plasma levels by 24% and the extent of absorption by 27%; the rate of absorption is not altered). Products include:
ALternaGEL Liquid ... ◘ 675
Aludrox Oral Suspension ... ◘ 850
Amphojel Suspension ... 2802
Amphojel Suspension without Flavor ... 2802
Amphojel Tablets ... 2802
Ascriptin ... ◘ 650
Gaviscon Antacid Tablets ... ◘ 778
Gaviscon-2 Antacid Tablets ... ◘ 779
Mylanta Liquid ... ◘ 676
Mylanta Double Strength Liquid ... ◘ 676
Nephrox Suspension ... ◘ 671

Atropine Sulfate (Oral anti-cholinergics delay peak plasma levels but do not affect the extent of absorption). Products include:
Arco-Lase Plus Tablets ... 513
Atrohist Plus Tablets ... 1605
Donnatal ... 2234
Donnatal Extentabs ... 2234
Donnatal Tablets ... 2234
Lomotil ... 2591
Motofen Tablets ... 789
Urised Tablets ... 2123

Belladonna Alkaloids (Oral anti-cholinergics delay peak plasma levels but do not affect the extent of absorption). Products include:
Bellergal-S Tablets ... 2375
Hyland's Bedwetting Tablets ... ◘ 788
Hyland's EnurAid Tablets ... ◘ 789
Hyland's Headache Tablets ... ◘ 790
Hyland's Teething Tablets ... ◘ 790
Similasan Eye Drops #1 ... ◘ 769

Benztropine Mesylate (Oral anti-cholinergics delay peak plasma levels but do not affect the extent of absorption). Products include:
Cogentin ... 1661

Biperiden Hydrochloride (Oral anti-cholinergics delay peak plasma levels but do not affect the extent of absorption). Products include:
Akineton ... 1380

Cimetidine (High doses of H_2 blockers reduces peak plasma levels by 42% and the extent of absorption by 32%; the rate of absorption is not altered). Products include:
Tagamet HB Tablets ... ◘ 786
Tagamet Tablets ... 2694

Cimetidine Hydrochloride (High doses of H_2 blockers reduces peak plasma levels by 42% and the extent of absorption by 32%; the rate of absorption is not altered). Products include:
Tagamet ... 2694

Clidinium Bromide (Oral anti-cholinergics delay peak plasma levels but do not affect the extent of absorption). Products include:
Librax Capsules ... 2330

Dicyclomine Hydrochloride (Oral anti-cholinergics delay peak plasma levels but do not affect the extent of absorption). Products include:
Bentyl ... 1246

Famotidine (High doses of H_2 blockers reduces peak plasma levels by 42% and the extent of absorption by 32%; the rate of absorption is not altered). Products include:
Pepcid AC Acid Controller ... 1360
Pepcid Injection ... 1765
Pepcid ... 1763

Glycopyrrolate (Oral anti-cholinergics delay peak plasma levels but do not affect the extent of absorption). Products include:
Robinul Forte Tablets ... 2247
Robinul Injectable ... 2247
Robinul Tablets ... 2247

Hyoscyamine (Oral anti-cholinergics delay peak plasma levels but do not affect the extent of absorption). Products include:
Cystospaz Tablets ... 2123
Urised Tablets ... 2123

Hyoscyamine Sulfate (Oral anti-cholinergics delay peak plasma levels but do not affect the extent of absorption). Products include:
Arco-Lase Plus Tablets ... 513
Atrohist Plus Tablets ... 1605
Cystospaz-M Capsules ... 2123
Donnatal ... 2234
Donnatal Extentabs ... 2234
Donnatal Tablets ... 2234
Kutrase Capsules ... 2546
Levsin/Levsinex/Levbid ... 2549

Ipratropium Bromide (Oral anti-cholinergics delay peak plasma levels but do not affect the extent of absorption). Products include:
Atrovent Inhalation Aerosol ... 674
Atrovent Inhalation Solution ... 675
Atrovent Nasal Spray 0.03% ... 676
Atrovent Nasal Spray 0.06% ... 678

Magaldrate (High doses of antacids reduces peak plasma levels by 24% and the extent of absorption by 27%; the rate of absorption is not altered).
No products indexed under this heading.

Magnesium Hydroxide (High doses of antacids reduces peak plasma levels by 24% and the extent of absorption by 27%; the rate of absorption is not altered). Products include:
Aludrox Oral Suspension ... ◘ 850
Ascriptin ... ◘ 650
Di-Gel Antacid/Anti-Gas ... ◘ 762
Gelusil Antacid-Anti-gas Liquid ... ◘ 819
Gelusil Antacid-Anti-gas Tablets ... ◘ 819
Maalox Antacid/Anti-Gas Tablets ... 889
Maalox Antacid Liquid ... 888
Extra Strength Maalox Antacid/Anti-Gas Liquid and Tablets ... 888
Mylanta Fast-Acting ... 1359
Mylanta Gelcaps Antacid ... ◘ 678
Fast-Acting Mylanta Liquid Antacid 1359
Mylanta Tablets ... ◘ 677
Maximum-Strength Fast-Acting Mylanta Liquid Antacid ... 1359
Mylanta Double Strength Tablets ... ◘ 677
Phillips' Milk of Magnesia Liquid ... ◘ 627
Rolaids Antacid Tablets ... ◘ 807
Tempo Soft Antacid ... ◘ 799

Magnesium Oxide (High doses of antacids reduces peak plasma levels by 24% and the extent of absorption by 27%; the rate of absorption is not altered). Products include:
Beelith Tablets ... 632
Bufferin Analgesic Tablets ... ◘ 636
Arthritis Strength Bufferin Analgesic Caplets ... ◘ 637
Extra Strength Bufferin Analgesic Tablets ... ◘ 637
Caltrate PLUS ... ◘ 681
Cama Arthritis Pain Reliever ... ◘ 748
Mag-Ox 400 ... 666
Uro-Mag ... 666

Mepenzolate Bromide (Oral anti-cholinergics delay peak plasma levels but do not affect the extent of absorption).
No products indexed under this heading.

Nephrotoxic Drugs (Close monitoring of renal function is required when co-administered with compounds of known nephrotoxicity potential).

Nizatidine (High doses of H_2 blockers reduces peak plasma levels by 42% and the extent of absorption by 32%; the rate of absorption is not altered). Products include:
Axid Pulvules ... 1468

Oxybutynin Chloride (Oral anti-cholinergics delay peak plasma levels but do not affect the extent of absorption). Products include:
Ditropan ... 1267

Probenecid (Renal excretion of cefpodoxime is inhibited by probenecid and resulting in an approximately 31% increase in AUC and 20% increase in peak plasma levels). Products include:
Benemid Tablets ... 1651
ColBENEMID Tablets ... 1662

Procyclidine Hydrochloride (Oral anti-cholinergics delay peak plasma levels but do not affect the extent of absorption). Products include:
Kemadrin Tablets ... 1105

Propantheline Bromide (Oral anti-cholinergics delay peak plasma levels but do not affect the extent of absorption). Products include:
Pro-Banthine Tablets ... 2226

Ranitidine Hydrochloride (High doses of H_2 blockers reduces peak plasma levels by 42% and the extent of absorption by 32%; the rate of absorption is not altered). Products include:
Zantac ... 1182
Zantac Injection ... 1180
Zantac Syrup ... 1182

Scopolamine (Oral anti-cholinergics delay peak plasma levels but do not affect the extent of absorption). Products include:
Transderm Scōp Transdermal Therapeutic System ... 890

Scopolamine Hydrobromide (Oral anti-cholinergics delay peak plasma levels but do not affect the extent of absorption). Products include:
Atrohist Plus Tablets ... 1605
Donnatal ... 2234
Donnatal Extentabs ... 2234
Donnatal Tablets ... 2234

Sodium Bicarbonate (High doses of antacids reduces peak plasma levels by 24% and the extent of absorption by 27%; the rate of absorption is not altered). Products include:
Alka-Seltzer Cherry Effervescent Antacid and Pain Reliever ... ◘ 609
Alka-Seltzer Extra Strength Effervescent Antacid and Pain Reliever ... ◘ 609
Alka-Seltzer Gold Effervescent Antacid ... ◘ 611
Alka-Seltzer Lemon Lime Effervescent Antacid and Pain Reliever ... ◘ 609
Alka-Seltzer Original Effervescent Antacid and Pain Reliever ... ◘ 609
Arm & Hammer Pure Baking Soda ... ◘ 648
Colyte and Colyte-flavored ... 2540
GoLYTELY ... 694
Massengill Disposable Douches ... ◘ 780
Massengill Liquid Concentrate ... ◘ 780
NuLYTELY ... 694
Cherry Flavor NuLYTELY ... 694

Tridihexethyl Chloride (Oral anti-cholinergics delay peak plasma levels but do not affect the extent of absorption).
No products indexed under this heading.

Trihexyphenidyl Hydrochloride (Oral anti-cholinergics delay peak plasma levels but do not affect the extent of absorption). Products include:
Artane ... 1418

Food Interactions

Food, unspecified (The extent of absorption and the mean peak plasma concentration increased when film-coated tablets were administered with food).

VAQTA
(Hepatitis A Vaccine, Inactivated) ... 1805
None cited in PDR database.

VARIVAX
(Varicella Virus Vaccine Live) ... 1807
May interact with salicylates and certain other agents. Compounds in these categories include:

Aspirin (Vaccine recipients should avoid use of salicylates for 6 weeks after vaccination with Varivax because of the potential for Reye's syndrome). Products include:
Alka-Seltzer Cherry Effervescent Antacid and Pain Reliever ... ◘ 609
Alka-Seltzer Extra Strength Effervescent Antacid and Pain Reliever ... ◘ 609
Alka-Seltzer Lemon Lime Effervescent Antacid and Pain Reliever ... ◘ 609

(◘ Described in PDR For Nonprescription Drugs) (◉ Described in PDR For Ophthalmology)

1149 **Interactions Index** **Varivax**

Alka-Seltzer Original Effervescent Antacid and Pain Reliever ▣ 609
Alka-Seltzer Plus ▣ 611
Alka-Seltzer Plus Sinus Medicine ▣ 611
Ascriptin ▣ 650
Arthritis Strength BC Powder ▣ 631
BC Cold Powder Multi-Symptom Formula (Cold-Sinus-Allergy) ▣ 631
BC Cold Powder Non-Drowsy Formula (Cold-Sinus) ▣ 631
BC Powder ▣ 631
Genuine Bayer Aspirin Tablets & Caplets ▣ 618
Extra Strength Bayer Arthritis Pain Regimen Formula ▣ 615
Extra Strength Bayer Aspirin Caplets & Tablets ▣ 617
Extended-Release Bayer 8-Hour Aspirin ▣ 616
Extra Strength Bayer Plus Aspirin Caplets ▣ 617
Extra Strength Bayer PM Aspirin Plus Sleep Aid ▣ 617
Aspirin Regimen Bayer 81 mg Tablets with Calcium ▣ 615
Aspirin Regimen Bayer Adult Low Strength 81 mg Tablets ▣ 613
Aspirin Regimen Bayer Children's Chewable Aspirin ▣ 616
Aspirin Regimen Bayer Regular Strength 325 mg Caplets ▣ 613
Bufferin Analgesic Tablets ▣ 636
Arthritis Strength Bufferin Analgesic Caplets ▣ 637
Extra Strength Bufferin Analgesic Tablets ▣ 637
Cama Arthritis Pain Reliever ▣ 748
Darvon Compound-65 Pulvules 1475
Easprin 1971
Ecotrin 2625
Ecotrin Enteric Coated Aspirin Maximum Strength Tablets and Caplets ▣ 775
Ecotrin Enteric Coated Aspirin Regular Strength Tablets 2625
Empirin Aspirin Tablets ▣ 818
Excedrin Extra-Strength Analgesic Tablets, Caplets, and Geltabs 734
Fiorinal Capsules 2388
Fiorinal with Codeine Capsules 2390
Fiorinal Tablets 2388
Goody's Extra Strength Headache Powders ▣ 632
Goody's Extra Strength Pain Relief Tablets ▣ 632
Halfprin Tablets 1413
Norgesic 1554
Percodan Tablets 955
Percodan-Demi Tablets 956
Robaxisal Tablets 2246
Soma Compound w/Codeine Tablets 2784
Soma Compound Tablets 2783
St. Joseph Adult Chewable Aspirin (81 mg.) ▣ 768
Talwin Compound 2466
Vanquish Analgesic Caplets ▣ 627

Azathioprine (Concurrent use in individuals who are on immunosuppressant drugs are more susceptible to infections; co-administration is contraindicated). Products include:
Azathioprine Tablets 2349
Imuran 1103

Betamethasone Acetate (Co-administration in individuals on immunosuppressant doses of corticosteroids can result in more extensive vaccine-associated rash or disseminated disease). Products include:
Celestone Soluspan Suspension 2484

Betamethasone Sodium Phosphate (Co-administration in individuals on immunosuppressant doses of corticosteroids can result in more extensive vaccine-associated rash or disseminated disease). Products include:
Celestone Soluspan Suspension 2484

Choline Magnesium Trisalicylate (Vaccine recipients should avoid use of salicylates for 6 weeks after vaccination with Varivax because of the potential for Reye's syndrome). Products include:
Trilisate 2155

Cortisone Acetate (Co-administration in individuals on immunosuppressant doses of corticosteroids can result in more extensive vaccine-associated rash or disseminated disease). Products include:
Cortone Acetate Sterile Suspension 1663
Cortone Acetate Tablets 1664

Cyclosporine (Concurrent use in individuals who are on immunosuppressant drugs are more susceptible to infections; co-administration is contraindicated). Products include:
Neoral 2405
Sandimmune 2416

Dexamethasone (Co-administration in individuals on immunosuppressant doses of corticosteroids can result in more extensive vaccine-associated rash or disseminated disease). Products include:
AK-Trol Ointment & Suspension ⊙ 205
Decadron Elixir 1676
Decadron Tablets 1678
Decaspray Topical Aerosol 1689
Maxitrol Ophthalmic Ointment and Suspension ⊙ 222
TobraDex Ophthalmic Suspension and Ointment 469

Dexamethasone Acetate (Co-administration in individuals on immunosuppressant doses of corticosteroids can result in more extensive vaccine-associated rash or disseminated disease). Products include:
Dalalone D.P. Injectable 1009
Decadron-LA Sterile Suspension 1687

Dexamethasone Sodium Phosphate (Co-administration in individuals on immunosuppressant doses of corticosteroids can result in more extensive vaccine-associated rash or disseminated disease). Products include:
Decadron Phosphate Injection 1680
Decadron Phosphate Sterile Ophthalmic Ointment 1684
Decadron Phosphate Sterile Ophthalmic Solution 1685
Decadron Phosphate Topical Cream 1686
Decadron Phosphate with Xylocaine Injection, Sterile 1683
Dexacort Phosphate in Respihaler 1606
Dexacort Phosphate in Turbinaire 1607
NeoDecadron Sterile Ophthalmic Ointment 1755
NeoDecadron Sterile Ophthalmic Solution 1756
NeoDecadron Topical Cream 1757

Diflunisal (Vaccine recipients should avoid use of salicylates for 6 weeks after vaccination with Varivax because of the potential for Reye's syndrome). Products include:
Dolobid Tablets 1695

Fludrocortisone Acetate (Co-administration in individuals on immunosuppressant doses of corticosteroids can result in more extensive vaccine-associated rash or disseminated disease). Products include:
Florinef Acetate Tablets 506

Globulin, Immune (Human) (Vaccination should be deferred for at least 5 months following immune globulin administration; following administration of Varivax, immune globulin should not be given for 2 months). Products include:
Gamimune N, 5% Immune Globulin Intravenous (Human), 5% 612
Gamimune N, 10% Immune Globulin Intravenous (Human), 10% 615
Gammagard S/D, Immune Globulin, Intravenous (Human) 577
Gammar-P I.V., Immune Globulin Intravenous (Human) 798
MICRhoGAM $Rh_0(D)$ Immune Globulin (Human) 1902
RhoGAM $Rh_0(D)$ Immune Globulin (Human) 1902
Sandoglobulin I.V. 2419

Hydrocortisone (Co-administration in individuals on immunosuppressant doses of corticosteroids can result in more extensive vaccine-associated rash or disseminated disease). Products include:
Anusol-HC Cream 2.5% 1953
Aquanil HC Lotion 1989
Maximum Strength Cortaid Spray ▣ 800
CORTENEMA 2713
Cortisporin Ointment 1074
Cortisporin Ophthalmic Ointment Sterile 1074
Cortisporin Ophthalmic Suspension Sterile 1075
Cortisporin Otic Solution Sterile 1076
Cortisporin Otic Suspension Sterile 1077
Cortizone-5 ▣ 795
Cortizone-10 ▣ 795
Hydrocortone Tablets 1715
Hytone 922
Hytone Ointment 2 ½% 923
Massengill Medicated Soft Cloth Towelettes 2628
Pediotic Suspension Sterile 1140
Preparation H Hydrocortisone 1% Cream ▣ 843
ProctoCream-HC 2.5% 2552
VōSoL HC Otic Solution 2786

Hydrocortisone Acetate (Co-administration in individuals on immunosuppressant doses of corticosteroids can result in more extensive vaccine-associated rash or disseminated disease). Products include:
Analpram-HC Rectal Cream 1% and 2.5% 993
Anusol HC-1 Hydrocortisone Anti-Itch Ointment ▣ 810
Anusol-HC Suppositories 1954
Caldecort Anti-Itch Hydrocortisone Cream ▣ 651
Coly-Mycin S Otic w/Neomycin & Hydrocortisone 1965
Cortaid ▣ 800
Cortifoam 2540
Cortisporin Cream 1073
Epifoam 2543
Hydrocortone Acetate Sterile Suspension 1712
Mantadil Cream 1124
Nupercainal Hydrocortisone 1% Cream ▣ 661
Pramosone Cream, Lotion & Ointment 995
ProctoFoam-HC 2552
Terra-Cortril Ophthalmic Suspension 2033

Hydrocortisone Sodium Phosphate (Co-administration in individuals on immunosuppressant doses of corticosteroids can result in more extensive vaccine-associated rash or disseminated disease). Products include:
Hydrocortone Phosphate Injection, Sterile 1713

Hydrocortisone Sodium Succinate (Co-administration in individuals on immunosuppressant doses of corticosteroids can result in more extensive vaccine-associated rash or disseminated disease).
No products indexed under this heading.

Magnesium Salicylate (Vaccine recipients should avoid use of salicylates for 6 weeks after vaccination with Varivax because of the potential for Reye's syndrome). Products include:
Backache Caplets ▣ 635
Doan's Extra-Strength Analgesic ▣ 653
Extra Strength Doan's P.M. ▣ 653
Doan's Regular Strength Analgesic ▣ 654
Mobigesic Tablets ▣ 607

Methylprednisolone Acetate (Co-administration in individuals on immunosuppressant doses of corticosteroids can result in more extensive vaccine-associated rash or disseminated disease).
No products indexed under this heading.

Methylprednisolone Sodium Succinate (Co-administration in individuals on immunosuppressant doses of corticosteroids can result in more extensive vaccine-associated rash or disseminated disease).
No products indexed under this heading.

Muromonab-CD3 (Concurrent use in individuals who are on immunosuppressant drugs are more susceptible to infections; co-administration is contraindicated). Products include:
Orthoclone OKT3 Sterile Solution 1892

Mycophenolate Mofetil (Concurrent use in individuals who are on immunosuppressant drugs are more susceptible to infections; co-administration is contraindicated). Products include:
CellCept Capsules 2265

Prednisolone Acetate (Co-administration in individuals on immunosuppressant doses of corticosteroids can result in more extensive vaccine-associated rash or disseminated disease). Products include:
AK-CIDE ⊙ 203
AK-CIDE Ointment ⊙ 203
Blephamide Liquifilm Sterile Ophthalmic Suspension 472
Blephamide Ointment ⊙ 234
Econopred & Econopred Plus Ophthalmic Suspensions ⊙ 216
Poly-Pred Liquifilm ⊙ 246
Pred Forte ⊙ 247
Pred Mild ⊙ 250
Pred-G Liquifilm Sterile Ophthalmic Suspension ⊙ 248
Pred-G S.O.P. Sterile Ophthalmic Ointment ⊙ 249

Prednisolone Sodium Phosphate (Co-administration in individuals on immunosuppressant doses of corticosteroids can result in more extensive vaccine-associated rash or disseminated disease). Products include:
AK-PRED ⊙ 204
Hydeltrasol Injection, Sterile 1708
Pediapred Oral Solution 1618

Prednisolone Tebutate (Co-administration in individuals on immunosuppressant doses of corticosteroids can result in more extensive vaccine-associated rash or disseminated disease). Products include:
Hydeltra-T.B.A. Sterile Suspension 1710

Prednisone (Co-administration in individuals on immunosuppressant doses of corticosteroids can result in more extensive vaccine-associated rash or disseminated disease).
No products indexed under this heading.

Salsalate (Vaccine recipients should avoid use of salicylates for 6 weeks after vaccination with Varivax because of the potential for Reye's syndrome). Products include:
Disalcid 1549
Mono-Gesic Tablets 810
Salflex Tablets 791

Tacrolimus (Concurrent use in individuals who are on immunosuppressant drugs are more susceptible to infections; co-administration is contraindicated). Products include:
Prograf 1028

IMPORTANT NOTE: Always consult each drug listing in the patient's regimen for possible interactions.

Varivax — Interactions Index

Triamcinolone (Co-administration in individuals on immunosuppressant doses of corticosteroids can result in more extensive vaccine-associated rash or disseminated disease).
No products indexed under this heading.

Triamcinolone Acetonide (Co-administration in individuals on immunosuppressant doses of corticosteroids can result in more extensive vaccine-associated rash or disseminated disease). Products include:
Azmacort Oral Inhaler 2175
Nasacort AQ Nasal Spray 2191
Nasacort Nasal Inhaler 2189

Triamcinolone Diacetate (Co-administration in individuals on immunosuppressant doses of corticosteroids can result in more extensive vaccine-associated rash or disseminated disease).
No products indexed under this heading.

Triamcinolone Hexacetonide (Co-administration in individuals on immunosuppressant doses of corticosteroids can result in more extensive vaccine-associated rash or disseminated disease).
No products indexed under this heading.

VASCOR TABLETS (200 AND 300 MG)
(Bepridil Hydrochloride) 1597
May interact with type 1 antiarrhythmic drugs, tricyclic antidepressants, cardiac glycosides, beta blockers, and certain other agents. Compounds in these categories include:

Acebutolol Hydrochloride (Available data are not sufficient to predict the effects of concomitant medication on patients with impaired ventricular function or cardiac conduction abnormalities). Products include:
Sectral Capsules 2914

Amitriptyline Hydrochloride (Potential for exaggeration of the QT interval prolongation). Products include:
Elavil 2945
Etrafon 2495
Limbitrol 2333
Triavil Tablets 1800

Amoxapine (Potential for exaggeration of the QT interval prolongation). Products include:
Asendin Tablets 1419

Atenolol (Available data are not sufficient to predict the effects of concomitant medication on patients with impaired ventricular function or cardiac conduction abnormalities). Products include:
Tenoretic Tablets 2963
Tenormin Tablets and I.V. Injection 2965

Betaxolol Hydrochloride (Available data are not sufficient to predict the effects of concomitant medication on patients with impaired ventricular function or cardiac conduction abnormalities). Products include:
Betoptic Ophthalmic Solution 465
Betoptic S Ophthalmic Suspension 467
Kerlone Tablets 2588

Bisoprolol Fumarate (Available data are not sufficient to predict the effects of concomitant medication on patients with impaired ventricular function or cardiac conduction abnormalities). Products include:
Zebeta Tablets 1457
Ziac 1459

Carteolol Hydrochloride (Available data are not sufficient to predict the effects of concomitant medication on patients with impaired ventricular function or cardiac conduction abnormalities). Products include:
Cartrol Tablets 413
Ocupress Ophthalmic Solution, 1% Sterile .... ◉ 297

Clomipramine Hydrochloride (Potential for exaggeration of the QT interval prolongation). Products include:
Anafranil Capsules 819

Desipramine Hydrochloride (Potential for exaggeration of the QT interval prolongation). Products include:
Norpramin Tablets 1273

Deslanoside (Cardiac glycosides could exaggerate the depression of AV nodal conduction).
No products indexed under this heading.

Digitoxin (Cardiac glycosides could exaggerate the depression of AV nodal conduction). Products include:
Crystodigin Tablets 1472

Digoxin (May be associated with modest increases in steady-state serum digoxin concentrations; cardiac glycosides could exaggerate the depression of AV nodal conduction). Products include:
Lanoxicaps 1110
Lanoxin Elixir Pediatric 1113
Lanoxin Injection 1116
Lanoxin Injection Pediatric 1119
Lanoxin Tablets 1121

Disopyramide Phosphate (Potential for exaggeration of the QT interval prolongation). Products include:
Norpace 2596

Doxepin Hydrochloride (Potential for exaggeration of the QT interval prolongation). Products include:
Adapin Capsules 1542
Sinequan 2028
Zonalon Cream 1042

Esmolol Hydrochloride (Available data are not sufficient to predict the effects of concomitant medication on patients with impaired ventricular function or cardiac conduction abnormalities). Products include:
Brevibloc (esmolol HCl) Injection ... 1860

Imipramine Hydrochloride (Potential for exaggeration of the QT interval prolongation). Products include:
Tofranil Ampuls 873
Tofranil Tablets 875

Imipramine Pamoate (Potential for exaggeration of the QT interval prolongation). Products include:
Tofranil-PM Capsules 876

Labetalol Hydrochloride (Available data are not sufficient to predict the effects of concomitant medication on patients with impaired ventricular function or cardiac conduction abnormalities). Products include:
Normodyne Injection 2519
Normodyne Tablets 2522
Trandate 1158

Levobunolol Hydrochloride (Available data are not sufficient to predict the effects of concomitant medication on patients with impaired ventricular function or cardiac conduction abnormalities). Products include:
Betagan .... ◉ 230

Maprotiline Hydrochloride (Potential for exaggeration of the QT interval prolongation). Products include:
Ludiomil Tablets 861

Metipranolol Hydrochloride (Available data are not sufficient to predict the effects of concomitant medication on patients with impaired ventricular function or cardiac conduction abnormalities). Products include:
OptiPranolol (Metipranolol 0.3%) Sterile Ophthalmic Solution .... ◉ 256

Metoprolol Succinate (Available data are not sufficient to predict the effects of concomitant medication on patients with impaired ventricular function or cardiac conduction abnormalities). Products include:
Toprol-XL Tablets 560

Metoprolol Tartrate (Available data are not sufficient to predict the effects of concomitant medication on patients with impaired ventricular function or cardiac conduction abnormalities). Products include:
Lopressor 848
Lopressor HCT Tablets 850

Moricizine Hydrochloride (Potential for exaggeration of the QT interval prolongation). Products include:
Ethmozine Tablets 2217

Nadolol (Available data are not sufficient to predict the effects of concomitant medication on patients with impaired ventricular function or cardiac conduction abnormalities).
No products indexed under this heading.

Nortriptyline Hydrochloride (Potential for exaggeration of the QT interval prolongation). Products include:
Pamelor 2409

Penbutolol Sulfate (Available data are not sufficient to predict the effects of concomitant medication on patients with impaired ventricular function or cardiac conduction abnormalities). Products include:
Levatol Tablets 2547

Pindolol (Available data are not sufficient to predict the effects of concomitant medication on patients with impaired ventricular function or cardiac conduction abnormalities). Products include:
Visken Tablets 2428

Procainamide Hydrochloride (Potential for exaggeration of the QT interval prolongation). Products include:
Procanbid Extended-Release Tablets 1983

Propafenone Hydrochloride (Potential for exaggeration of the QT interval prolongation). Products include:
Rythmol Tablets–150mg, 225mg, 300mg 1399

Propranolol Hydrochloride (Available data are not sufficient to predict the effects of concomitant medication on patients with impaired ventricular function or cardiac conduction abnormalities). Products include:
Inderal 2834
Inderal LA Long Acting Capsules 2836
Inderide Tablets 2838
Inderide LA Long Acting Capsules 2840

Protriptyline Hydrochloride (Potential for exaggeration of the QT interval prolongation). Products include:
Vivactil Tablets 1820

Quinidine Gluconate (Potential for exaggeration of the QT interval prolongation). Products include:
Quinaglute Dura-Tabs Tablets ... 644

Quinidine Polygalacturonate (Potential for exaggeration of the QT interval prolongation). Products include:
Cardioquin Tablets 2146

Quinidine Sulfate (Potential for exaggeration of the QT interval prolongation). Products include:
Quinidex Extentabs 2240

Sotalol Hydrochloride (Available data are not sufficient to predict the effects of concomitant medication on patients with impaired ventricular function or cardiac conduction abnormalities). Products include:
Betapace Tablets 637

Timolol Hemihydrate (Available data are not sufficient to predict the effects of concomitant medication on patients with impaired ventricular function or cardiac conduction abnormalities). Products include:
Betimol 0.25%, 0.5% .... ◉ 259

Timolol Maleate (Available data are not sufficient to predict the effects of concomitant medication on patients with impaired ventricular function or cardiac conduction abnormalities). Products include:
Blocadren Tablets 1654
Timolide Tablets 1791
Timoptic in Ocudose 1796
Timoptic Sterile Ophthalmic Solution 1794
Timoptic-XE 1798

Trimipramine Maleate (Potential for exaggeration of the QT interval prolongation). Products include:
Surmontil Capsules 2917

Food Interactions
Meal, unspecified (May result in a clinically insignificant delay in time to peak concentration, but neither peak plasma levels nor the extent of absorption was changed).

VASERETIC TABLETS
(Enalapril Maleate, Hydrochlorothiazide) 1810
May interact with insulin, potassium preparations, diuretics, potassium sparing diuretics, barbiturates, narcotic analgesics, oral hypoglycemic agents, antihypertensives, corticosteroids, nondepolarizing neuromuscular blocking agents, lithium preparations, non-steroidal anti-inflammatory agents, cardiac glycosides, and certain other agents. Compounds in these categories include:

Acarbose (Dosage adjustment of hypoglycemic may be required). Products include:
Precose 604

Acebutolol Hydrochloride (Additive effect or potentiation). Products include:
Sectral Capsules 2914

ACTH (Intensified electrolyte depletion, particularly hypokalemia).
No products indexed under this heading.

Alfentanil Hydrochloride (Potentiation of orthostatic hypotension may occur). Products include:
Alfenta Injection 1334

Amiloride Hydrochloride (Significant increases in serum potassium; excessive hypotension). Products include:
Midamor Tablets 1746
Moduretic Tablets 1748

(◨ Described in PDR For Nonprescription Drugs)   (◉ Described in PDR For Ophthalmology)

1151 **Interactions Index** **Vaseretic**

Amlodipine Besylate (Additive effect or potentiation). Products include:
Lotrel Capsules ... 858
Norvasc Tablets ... 2020

Aprobarbital (Potentiation of orthostatic hypotension may occur).
No products indexed under this heading.

Atenolol (Additive effect or potentiation). Products include:
Tenoretic Tablets ... 2963
Tenormin Tablets and I.V. Injection 2965

Atracurium Besylate (Increased responsiveness to muscle relaxant). Products include:
Tracrium Injection ... 1155

Benazepril Hydrochloride (Additive effect or potentiation). Products include:
Lotensin Tablets ... 852
Lotensin HCT Tablets ... 855
Lotrel Capsules ... 858

Bendroflumethiazide (Additive effect or potentiation; excessive hypotension).
No products indexed under this heading.

Betamethasone Acetate (Intensified electrolyte depletion, particularly hypokalemia). Products include:
Celestone Soluspan Suspension ... 2484

Betamethasone Sodium Phosphate (Intensified electrolyte depletion, particularly hypokalemia). Products include:
Celestone Soluspan Suspension ... 2484

Betaxolol Hydrochloride (Additive effect or potentiation). Products include:
Betoptic Ophthalmic Solution... 465
Betoptic S Ophthalmic Suspension 467
Kerlone Tablets ... 2588

Bisoprolol Fumarate (Additive effect or potentiation). Products include:
Zebeta Tablets ... 1457
Ziac ... 1459

Bumetanide (Excessive hypotension). Products include:
Bumex ... 2260

Buprenorphine (Potentiation of orthostatic hypotension may occur). Products include:
Buprenex Injectable ... 2170

Butabarbital (Potentiation of orthostatic hypotension may occur).
No products indexed under this heading.

Butalbital (Potentiation of orthostatic hypotension may occur). Products include:
Axocet Capsules ... 2469
Esgic-plus Capsules ... 1012
Esgic-plus Tablets ... 1012
Fioricet Tablets ... 2386
Fioricet with Codeine Capsules ... 2387
Fiorinal Capsules ... 2388
Fiorinal with Codeine Capsules ... 2390
Fiorinal Tablets ... 2388
Phrenilin ... 790
Sedapap Tablets 50 mg/650 mg .. 1826

Captopril (Additive effect or potentiation). Products include:
Capoten Tablets ... 740
Capozide Tablets ... 744

Carteolol Hydrochloride (Additive effect or potentiation). Products include:
Cartrol Tablets ... 413
Ocupress Ophthalmic Solution, 1% Sterile... ◉ 297

Chlorothiazide (Additive effect or potentiation; excessive hypotension). Products include:
Aldoclor Tablets ... 1638
Diupres Tablets ... 1691
Diuril Oral ... 1694

Chlorothiazide Sodium (Additive effect or potentiation; excessive hypotension). Products include:
Diuril Sodium Intravenous ... 1693

Chlorpropamide (Dosage adjustment of hypoglycemic may be required). Products include:
Diabinese Tablets ... 2002

Chlorthalidone (Additive effect or potentiation; significant increases in serum potassium; excessive hypotension). Products include:
Combipres Tablets ... 682
Tenoretic Tablets ... 2963
Thalitone ... 1293

Cholestyramine (Binds the hydrochlorothiazide and reduces its absorption from gastrointestinal tract by up to 85%). Products include:
Questran ... 774

Cisatracurium Besylate (Increased responsiveness to muscle relaxant). Products include:
Nimbex Injection ... 1131

Clonidine (Additive effect or potentiation). Products include:
Catapres-TTS... 680

Clonidine Hydrochloride (Additive effect or potentiation). Products include:
Catapres Tablets ... 679
Combipres Tablets ... 682

Codeine Phosphate (Potentiation of orthostatic hypotension may occur). Products include:
Brontex ... 2130
Dimetane-DC Cough Syrup ... 2232
Fioricet with Codeine Capsules ... 2387
Fiorinal with Codeine Capsules ... 2390
Nucofed ... 2225
Phenergan with Codeine ... 2883
Phenergan VC with Codeine ... 2888
Robitussin A-C Syrup ... 2248
Robitussin-DAC Syrup ... 2249
Ryna ... 804
Soma Compound w/Codeine Tablets ... 2784
Tylenol with Codeine ... 1592

Colestipol Hydrochloride (Binds the hydrochlorothiazide and reduces its absorption from gastrointestinal tract by up to 43%). Products include:
Colestid ... 2073

Cortisone Acetate (Intensified electrolyte depletion, particularly hypokalemia). Products include:
Cortone Acetate Sterile Suspension ... 1663
Cortone Acetate Tablets ... 1664

Deserpidine (Additive effect or potentiation).
No products indexed under this heading.

Deslanoside (Hypokalemia produced by hydrochlorothiazide may exaggerate the response of the heart to the digitalis toxicity).
No products indexed under this heading.

Dexamethasone (Intensified electrolyte depletion, particularly hypokalemia). Products include:
AK-Trol Ointment & Suspension .... ◉ 205
Decadron Elixir ... 1676
Decadron Tablets... 1678
Decaspray Topical Aerosol ... 1689
Maxitrol Ophthalmic Ointment and Suspension ... ◉ 222
TobraDex Ophthalmic Suspension and Ointment... 469

Dexamethasone Acetate (Intensified electrolyte depletion, particularly hypokalemia). Products include:
Dalalone D.P. Injectable ... 1009
Decadron-LA Sterile Suspension... 1687

Dexamethasone Sodium Phosphate (Intensified electrolyte depletion, particularly hypokalemia). Products include:
Decadron Phosphate Injection ... 1680
Decadron Phosphate Sterile Ophthalmic Ointment ... 1684
Decadron Phosphate Sterile Ophthalmic Solution ... 1685
Decadron Phosphate Topical Cream ... 1686
Decadron Phosphate with Xylocaine Injection, Sterile ... 1683
Dexacort Phosphate in Respihaler .. 1606
Dexacort Phosphate in Turbinaire .. 1607
NeoDecadron Sterile Ophthalmic Ointment ... 1755
NeoDecadron Sterile Ophthalmic Solution ... 1756
NeoDecadron Topical Cream ... 1757

Dezocine (Potentiation of orthostatic hypotension may occur). Products include:
Dalgan Injection ... 529

Diazoxide (Additive effect or potentiation). Products include:
Hyperstat I.V. Injection ... 2504
Proglycem... 575

Diclofenac Potassium (Reduced diuretic, natriuretic, and antihypertensive effects of Vaseretic). Products include:
Cataflam Tablets ... 833

Diclofenac Sodium (Reduced diuretic, natriuretic, and antihypertensive effects of Vaseretic). Products include:
Voltaren Ophthalmic Sterile Ophthalmic Solution ... ◉ 264
Cataflam/Voltaren/Voltaren-XR ... 833

Digitoxin (Hypokalemia produced by hydrochlorothiazide may exaggerate the response of the heart to the digitalis toxicity). Products include:
Crystodigin Tablets... 1472

Digoxin (Hypokalemia produced by hydrochlorothiazide may exaggerate the response of the heart to the digitalis toxicity). Products include:
Lanoxicaps ... 1110
Lanoxin Elixir Pediatric ... 1113
Lanoxin Injection ... 1116
Lanoxin Injection Pediatric... 1119
Lanoxin Tablets ... 1121

Diltiazem Hydrochloride (Additive effect or potentiation). Products include:
Cardizem CD Capsules ... 1251
Cardizem SR Capsules ... 1255
Cardizem Injectable ... 1253
Cardizem Tablets... 1257
Dilacor XR Extended-release Capsules ... 2183
Tiazac Capsules ... 1019

Doxazosin Mesylate (Additive effect or potentiation). Products include:
Cardura Tablets ... 1993

Enalaprilat (Additive effect or potentiation). Products include:
Vasotec I.V... 1814

Esmolol Hydrochloride (Additive effect or potentiation). Products include:
Brevibloc (esmolol HCl) Injection 1860

Ethacrynic Acid (Excessive hypotension). Products include:
Edecrin Tablets... 1698

Etodolac (Reduced diuretic, natriuretic, and antihypertensive effects of Vaseretic). Products include:
Lodine Capsules and Tablets ... 2849

Felodipine (Additive effect or potentiation). Products include:
Plendil Extended-Release Tablets.... 514

Fenoprofen Calcium (Reduced diuretic, natriuretic, and antihypertensive effects of Vaseretic). Products include:
Nalfon 200 Pulvules & Nalfon Tablets ... 933

Fentanyl (Potentiation of orthostatic hypotension may occur). Products include:
Duragesic Transdermal System... 1336

Fentanyl Citrate (Potentiation of orthostatic hypotension may occur). Products include:
Sublimaze Injection... 463

Fludrocortisone Acetate (Intensified electrolyte depletion, particularly hypokalemia). Products include:
Florinef Acetate Tablets ... 506

Flurbiprofen (Reduced diuretic, natriuretic, and antihypertensive effects of Vaseretic).
No products indexed under this heading.

Fosinopril Sodium (Additive effect or potentiation). Products include:
Monopril Tablets ... 762

Furosemide (Additive effect or potentiation; excessive hypotension). Products include:
Lasix Injection, Oral Solution and Tablets ... 1267

Glimepiride (Dosage adjustment of hypoglycemic may be required). Products include:
Amaryl Tablets ... 1241

Glipizide (Dosage adjustment of hypoglycemic may be required). Products include:
Glucotrol Tablets ... 2011
Glucotrol XL Extended Release Tablets ... 2012

Glyburide (Dosage adjustment of hypoglycemic may be required). Products include:
DiaBeta Tablets ... 1265
Glynase PresTab Tablets ... 2091
Micronase Tablets ... 2099

Guanabenz Acetate (Additive effect or potentiation).
No products indexed under this heading.

Guanethidine Monosulfate (Additive effect or potentiation). Products include:
Esimil Tablets ... 840
Ismelin Tablets ... 845

Hydralazine Hydrochloride (Additive effect or potentiation). Products include:
Apresazide Capsules ... 824
Apresoline Hydrochloride Tablets .. 826
Hydralazine Hydrochloride Injection USP... 2712
Ser-Ap-Es Tablets ... 867

Hydrocodone Bitartrate (Potentiation of orthostatic hypotension may occur). Products include:
Codiclear DH Syrup ... 808
Duratuss HD Elixir... 2750
Histussin D Liquid ... 670
Hycodan Tablets and Syrup ... 946
Hycomine Compound Tablets ... 948
Hycomine ... 947
Hycotuss Expectorant Syrup ... 950
Hydrocet Capsules ... 787
Lorcet 10/650 Tablets ... 1016
Lortab... 2751
Tussend... 1830
Tussend Expectorant ... 1831
Vicodin Tablets... 1404
Vicodin ES Tablets ... 1405
Vicodin HP Tablets ... 1403
Vicodin Tuss Expectorant ... 1406
Zydone Capsules ... 967

Hydrocodone Polistirex (Potentiation of orthostatic hypotension may occur). Products include:
Tussionex Pennkinetic Extended-Release Suspension ... 1624

IMPORTANT NOTE: Always consult each drug listing in the patient's regimen for possible interactions.

Vaseretic **Interactions Index** **1152**

Hydrocortisone (Intensified electrolyte depletion, particularly hypokalemia). Products include:
- Anusol-HC Cream 2.5% 1953
- Aquanil HC Lotion 1989
- Maximum Strength Cortaid Spray ■ 800
- CORTENEMA 2713
- Cortisporin Ointment 1074
- Cortisporin Ophthalmic Ointment Sterile 1074
- Cortisporin Ophthalmic Suspension Sterile 1075
- Cortisporin Otic Solution Sterile 1076
- Cortisporin Otic Suspension Sterile 1077
- Cortizone-5 .... ■ 795
- Cortizone-10 .... ■ 795
- Hydrocortone Tablets 1715
- Hytone 922
- Hytone Ointment 2 ½% 923
- Massengill Medicated Soft Cloth Towelettes 2628
- Pediotic Suspension Sterile 1140
- Preparation H Hydrocortisone 1% Cream .... ■ 843
- ProctoCream-HC 2.5% 2552
- VōSoL HC Otic Solution 2786

Hydrocortisone Acetate (Intensified electrolyte depletion, particularly hypokalemia). Products include:
- Analpram-HC Rectal Cream 1% and 2.5% 993
- Anusol HC-1 Hydrocortisone Anti-Itch Ointment .... ■ 810
- Anusol-HC Suppositories 1954
- Caldecort Anti-Itch Hydrocortisone Cream .... ■ 651
- Coly-Mycin S Otic w/Neomycin & Hydrocortisone 1965
- Cortaid .... ■ 800
- Cortifoam 2540
- Cortisporin Cream 1073
- Epifoam 2543
- Hydrocortone Acetate Sterile Suspension 1712
- Mantadil Cream 1124
- Nupercainal Hydrocortisone 1% Cream .... ■ 661
- Pramosone Cream, Lotion & Ointment 995
- ProctoFoam-HC 2552
- Terra-Cortril Ophthalmic Suspension 2033

Hydrocortisone Sodium Phosphate (Intensified electrolyte depletion, particularly hypokalemia). Products include:
- Hydrocortone Phosphate Injection, Sterile 1713

Hydrocortisone Sodium Succinate (Intensified electrolyte depletion, particularly hypokalemia).
- No products indexed under this heading.

Hydroflumethiazide (Additive effect or potentiation; excessive hypotension). Products include:
- Diucardin Tablets 2824

Hydromorphone Hydrochloride (Potentiation of orthostatic hypotension may occur). Products include:
- Dilaudid Ampules 1382
- Dilaudid Cough Syrup 1383
- Dilaudid-HP Injection 1384
- Dilaudid-HP Lyophilized Powder 250 mg 1384
- Dilaudid 1382
- Dilaudid Oral Liquid 1386
- Dilaudid 1382
- Dilaudid Tablets - 8 mg 1386

Ibuprofen (Reduced diuretic, natriuretic, and antihypertensive effects of Vaseretic). Products include:
- Advil Cold and Sinus Caplets and Tablets .... ■ 837
- Advil Ibuprofen Tablets, Caplets and Gel Caplets .... ■ 836
- Children's Motrin Ibuprofen Oral Suspension 1558
- IBU Tablets 1389
- Ibuprohm .... ■ 713
- Motrin IB Caplets, Tablets, and Gelcaps .... ■ 802
- Motrin Ibuprofen Suspension, Oral Drops, Chewable Tablets, Caplets 1563
- Nuprin Ibuprofen/Analgesic Tablets & Caplets .... ■ 645
- Vicks DayQuil SINUS Pressure & PAIN Relief with IBUPROFEN .... ■ 735

Indapamide (Additive effect or potentiation; excessive hypotension).
- No products indexed under this heading.

Indomethacin (Reduced diuretic, natriuretic, and antihypertensive effects of Vaseretic). Products include:
- Indocin 1723

Indomethacin Sodium Trihydrate (Reduced diuretic, natriuretic, and antihypertensive effects of Vaseretic). Products include:
- Indocin I.V. 1727

Insulin, Human (Dosage adjustments of insulin may be required).
- No products indexed under this heading.

Insulin, Human Isophane Suspension (Dosage adjustments of insulin may be required). Products include:
- Novolin N Human Insulin 10 ml Vials 1846

Insulin, Human NPH (Dosage adjustments of insulin may be required). Products include:
- Humulin N, 100 Units 1495
- Novolin N PenFill 1.5 ml Cartridges Durable Insulin Delivery System 1849
- Novolin N Prefilled Syringe Disposable Insulin Delivery System 1850

Insulin, Human Regular (Dosage adjustments of insulin may be required). Products include:
- Humulin R, 100 Units 1497
- Novolin R Human Insulin 10 ml Vials 1846
- Novolin R PenFill 1.5 ml Cartridges Durable Insulin Delivery System 1849
- Novolin R Prefilled Syringe Disposable Insulin Delivery System 1850
- Velosulin BR Human Insulin 10 ml Vials 1847

Insulin, Human, Zinc Suspension (Dosage adjustments of insulin may be required). Products include:
- Humulin L, 100 Units 1494
- Humulin U, 100 Units 1498
- Novolin L Human Insulin 10 ml Vials 1846

Insulin Lispro, Human (Dosage adjustments of insulin may be required). Products include:
- Humalog Injection 1488

Insulin, NPH (Dosage adjustments of insulin may be required). Products include:
- NPH, 100 Units 1502
- Pork NPH, 100 Units 1506
- Purified Pork NPH Isophane Insulin 1852

Insulin, Regular (Dosage adjustments of insulin may be required). Products include:
- Regular, 100 Units 1503
- Pork Regular, 100 Units 1507
- Pork Regular (Concentrated), 500 Units 1508
- Purified Pork Regular Insulin 1852

Insulin, Zinc Crystals (Dosage adjustments of insulin may be required). Products include:
- NPH, 100 Units 1502

Insulin, Zinc Suspension (Dosage adjustments of insulin may be required). Products include:
- Iletin I 1501
- Lente, 100 Units 1501
- Iletin II 1504
- Pork Lente, 100 Units 1504
- Purified Pork Lente Insulin 1852

Isradipine (Additive effect or potentiation). Products include:
- DynaCirc Capsules 2381
- DynaCirc CR Tablets 2383

Ketoprofen (Reduced diuretic, natriuretic, and antihypertensive effects of Vaseretic). Products include:
- Actron Caplets and Tablets .... ■ 608
- Orudis Capsules 2874
- Orudis KT .... ■ 842
- Oruvail Capsules 2874

Ketorolac Tromethamine (Reduced diuretic, natriuretic, and antihypertensive effects of Vaseretic). Products include:
- Acular Sterile Ophthalmic Solution 470
- Toradol 2319

Labetalol Hydrochloride (Additive effect or potentiation). Products include:
- Normodyne Injection 2519
- Normodyne Tablets 2522
- Trandate 1158

Levorphanol Tartrate (Potentiation of orthostatic hypotension may occur). Products include:
- Levo-Dromoran 2297

Lisinopril (Additive effect or potentiation). Products include:
- Prinivil Tablets 1776
- Prinzide Tablets 1780
- Zestoretic Tablets 2968
- Zestril Tablets 2972

Lithium Carbonate (High risk of lithium toxicity; frequent monitoring of lithium serum levels is recommended). Products include:
- Eskalith 2658
- Lithium Carbonate Capsules & Tablets 2352
- Lithonate/Lithotabs/Lithobid 2721

Lithium Citrate (High risk of lithium toxicity; frequent monitoring of lithium serum levels is recommended).
- No products indexed under this heading.

Losartan Potassium (Additive effect or potentiation). Products include:
- Cozaar Tablets 1668
- Hyzaar Tablets 1720

Mecamylamine Hydrochloride (Additive effect or potentiation). Products include:
- Inversine Tablets 1729

Meclofenamate Sodium (Reduced diuretic, natriuretic, and antihypertensive effects of Vaseretic).
- No products indexed under this heading.

Mefenamic Acid (Reduced diuretic, natriuretic, and antihypertensive effects of Vaseretic). Products include:
- Ponstel 1982

Meperidine Hydrochloride (Potentiation of orthostatic hypotension may occur). Products include:
- Demerol 2438
- Mepergan Injection 2859

Mephobarbital (Potentiation of orthostatic hypotension may occur). Products include:
- Mebaral Tablets 2452

Metformin Hydrochloride (Dosage adjustment of hypoglycemic may be required). Products include:
- Glucophage Tablets 754

Methadone Hydrochloride (Potentiation of orthostatic hypotension may occur). Products include:
- Methadone Hydrochloride Oral Concentrate 2356
- Methadone Hydrochloride Oral Solution & Tablets 2357

Methyclothiazide (Additive effect or potentiation; excessive hypotension). Products include:
- Enduron Tablets 424

Methyldopa (Additive effect or potentiation). Products include:
- Aldoclor Tablets 1638
- Aldomet Oral 1640
- Aldoril Tablets 1644

Methyldopate Hydrochloride (Additive effect or potentiation). Products include:
- Aldomet Ester HCI Injection 1642

Methylprednisolone Acetate (Intensified electrolyte depletion, particularly hypokalemia).
- No products indexed under this heading.

Methylprednisolone Sodium Succinate (Intensified electrolyte depletion, particularly hypokalemia).
- No products indexed under this heading.

Metocurine Iodide (Increased responsiveness to muscle relaxant). Products include:
- Metubine Iodide Vials 932

Metolazone (Additive effect or potentiation; excessive hypotension). Products include:
- Mykrox Tablets 1617
- Zaroxolyn Tablets 1625

Metoprolol Succinate (Additive effect or potentiation). Products include:
- Toprol-XL Tablets 560

Metoprolol Tartrate (Additive effect or potentiation). Products include:
- Lopressor 848
- Lopressor HCT Tablets 850

Metyrosine (Additive effect or potentiation). Products include:
- Demser Capsules 1690

Minoxidil (Additive effect or potentiation).
- No products indexed under this heading.

Mivacurium Chloride (Increased responsiveness to muscle relaxant). Products include:
- Mivacron 1125

Moexipril Hydrochloride (Additive effect or potentiation). Products include:
- Univasc Tablets 2553

Morphine Sulfate (Potentiation of orthostatic hypotension may occur). Products include:
- Astramorph/PF Injection, USP (Preservative-Free) 526
- Duramorph Injection 983
- Infumorph 200 and Infumorph 500 Sterile Solutions 985
- Kadian Capsules 2948
- MS Contin Tablets 2149
- MSIR 2152
- Oramorph SR (Morphine Sulfate Sustained Release Tablets) 2359
- RMS Suppositories CII 2766
- Roxanol 2365

Nabumetone (Reduced diuretic, natriuretic, and antihypertensive effects of Vaseretic). Products include:
- Relafen Tablets 2688

Nadolol (Additive effect or potentiation).
- No products indexed under this heading.

Naproxen (Reduced diuretic, natriuretic, and antihypertensive effects of Vaseretic). Products include:
- Anaprox/Naprosyn 2277

Naproxen Sodium (Reduced diuretic, natriuretic, and antihypertensive effects of Vaseretic). Products include:
- Aleve 2124
- Anaprox/Naprosyn 2277
- Naprelan Tablets 2861

(■ Described in PDR For Nonprescription Drugs) (⊙ Described in PDR For Ophthalmology)

Nicardipine Hydrochloride (Additive effect or potentiation). Products include:
Cardene Capsules 2261
Cardene I.V. 2815
Cardene SR Capsules 2264

Nifedipine (Additive effect or potentiation). Products include:
Adalat Capsules (10 mg and 20 mg) 580
Adalat CC 582
Procardia Capsules 2024
Procardia XL Extended Release Tablets 2026

Nisoldipine (Additive effect or potentiation). Products include:
Sular Tablets 2961

Nitroglycerin (Additive effect or potentiation). Products include:
Deponit NTG Transdermal Delivery System 2541
Nitro-Bid IV 1270
Nitro-Bid Ointment 1272
Nitro-Dur (nitroglycerin) Transdermal Infusion System 1365
Nitrolingual Spray 2193
Nitrostat Tablets 1981
Transderm-Nitro Transdermal Therapeutic System 878

Norepinephrine Bitartrate (Decreased reponse to pressor amines). Products include:
Levophed Bitartrate Injection 2445

Opium Alkaloids (Potentiation of orthostatic hypotension may occur). No products indexed under this heading.

Oxaprozin (Reduced diuretic, natriuretic, and antihypertensive effects of Vaseretic). Products include:
Daypro Caplets 2578

Oxycodone Hydrochloride (Potentiation of orthostatic hypotension may occur). Products include:
OxyContin Tablets 2163
OxyIR Capsules 2167
Percocet Tablets 955
Percodan Tablets 955
Percodan-Demi Tablets 956
Roxicodone Tablets, Oral Solution & Intensol (Oxycodone) 2366
Tylox Capsules 1593

Pancuronium Bromide (Increased responsiveness to muscle relaxant).
No products indexed under this heading.

Penbutolol Sulfate (Additive effect or potentiation). Products include:
Levatol Tablets 2547

Pentobarbital Sodium (Potentiation of orthostatic hypotension may occur). Products include:
Nembutal Sodium Capsules ... 440
Nembutal Sodium Solution 442
Nembutal Sodium Suppositories 444

Phenobarbital (Potentiation of orthostatic hypotension may occur). Products include:
Arco-Lase Plus Tablets 513
Bellergal-S Tablets 2375
Donnatal 2234
Donnatal Extentabs 2234
Donnatal Tablets 2234
Phenobarbital Elixir and Tablets 1523
Quadrinal Tablets 1398

Phenoxybenzamine Hydrochloride (Additive effect or potentiation). Products include:
Dibenzyline Capsules 2650

Phentolamine Mesylate (Additive effect or potentiation). Products include:
Regitine Vials 864

Phenylbutazone (Reduced diuretic, natriuretic, and antihypertensive effects of Vaseretic).
No products indexed under this heading.

Pindolol (Additive effect or potentiation). Products include:
Visken Tablets 2428

Piroxicam (Reduced diuretic, natriuretic, and antihypertensive effects of Vaseretic). Products include:
Feldene Capsules 2008

Polythiazide (Additive effect or potentiation; excessive hypotension). Products include:
Minizide Capsules 2016

Potassium Acid Phosphate (Significant increases in serum potassium). Products include:
K-Phos Original Formula 'Sodium Free' Tablets 633

Potassium Bicarbonate (Significant increases in serum potassium). Products include:
Alka-Seltzer Gold Effervescent Antacid .... ⊕ 611

Potassium Chloride (Significant increases in serum potassium). Products include:
Chlor-3 Condiment 1003
Colyte and Colyte-flavored 2540
GoLYTELY 694
K-Dur Microburst Release System (potassium chloride, USP) E.R. Tablets 1364
K-Lor Powder Packets 438
K-Norm Capsules 1615
K-Tab Filmtab 439
Micro-K 2237
Micro-K LS Packets 2238
NuLYTELY 694
Cherry Flavor NuLYTELY 694
Rum-K Syrup 1004
Slow-K Extended-Release Tablets 869

Potassium Citrate (Significant increases in serum potassium). Products include:
Polycitra Syrup 574
Polycitra-K Crystals 574
Polycitra-K Oral Solution 575
Polycitra-LC 574
Urocit-K Tablets 1828

Potassium Gluconate (Significant increases in serum potassium).
No products indexed under this heading.

Potassium Phosphate, Dibasic (Significant increases in serum potassium).
No products indexed under this heading.

Potassium Phosphate, Monobasic (Significant increases in serum potassium). Products include:
K-Phos Neutral Tablets 633
K-Phos Original Formula 'Sodium Free' Tablets 633

Prazosin Hydrochloride (Additive effect or potentiation). Products include:
Minipress Capsules 2015
Minizide Capsules 2016

Prednisolone Acetate (Intensified electrolyte depletion, particularly hypokalemia). Products include:
AK-CIDE .... ⊕ 203
AK-CIDE Ointment .... ⊕ 203
Blephamide Liquifilm Sterile Ophthalmic Suspension 472
Blephamide Ointment .... ⊕ 234
Econopred & Econopred Plus Ophthalmic Suspensions ..... ⊕ 216
Poly-Pred Liquifilm .... ⊕ 246
Pred Forte .... ⊕ 247
Pred Mild .... ⊕ 250
Pred-G Liquifilm Sterile Ophthalmic Suspension .... ⊕ 248
Pred-G S.O.P. Sterile Ophthalmic Ointment .... ⊕ 249

Prednisolone Sodium Phosphate (Intensified electrolyte depletion, particularly hypokalemia). Products include:
AK-PRED .... ⊕ 204
Hydeltrasol Injection, Sterile 1708
Pediapred Oral Solution 1618

Prednisolone Tebutate (Intensified electrolyte depletion, particularly hypokalemia). Products include:
Hydeltra-T.B.A. Sterile Suspension 1710

Prednisone (Intensified electrolyte depletion, particularly hypokalemia).
No products indexed under this heading.

Propoxyphene Hydrochloride (Potentiation of orthostatic hypotension may occur). Products include:
Darvon 1475
Wygesic Tablets 2930

Propoxyphene Napsylate (Potentiation of orthostatic hypotension may occur). Products include:
Darvon-N/Darvocet-N 1473

Propranolol Hydrochloride (Additive effect or potentiation). Products include:
Inderal 2834
Inderal LA Long Acting Capsules 2836
Inderide Tablets 2838
Inderide LA Long Acting Capsules 2840

Quinapril Hydrochloride (Additive effect or potentiation). Products include:
Accupril Tablets 1950

Ramipril (Additive effect or potentiation). Products include:
Altace Capsules 1238

Rauwolfia Serpentina (Additive effect or potentiation).
No products indexed under this heading.

Rescinnamine (Additive effect or potentiation).
No products indexed under this heading.

Reserpine (Additive effect or potentiation). Products include:
Diupres Tablets 1691
Hydropres Tablets 1718
Ser-Ap-Es Tablets 867

Rocuronium Bromide (Increased responsiveness to muscle relaxant). Products include:
Zemuron Injection 1885

Secobarbital Sodium (Potentiation of orthostatic hypotension may occur). Products include:
Seconal Sodium Pulvules 1529

Sodium Nitroprusside (Additive effect or potentiation).
No products indexed under this heading.

Sotalol Hydrochloride (Additive effect or potentiation). Products include:
Betapace Tablets 637

Spirapril Hydrochloride (Additive effect or potentiation).
No products indexed under this heading.

Spironolactone (Significant increases in serum potassium; excessive hypotension). Products include:
Aldactazide Tablets 2556
Aldactone Tablets 2558

Sufentanil Citrate (Potentiation of orthostatic hypotension may occur). Products include:
Sufenta Injection 1355

Sulindac (Reduced diuretic, natriuretic, and antihypertensive effects of Vaseretic). Products include:
Clinoril Tablets 1658

Terazosin Hydrochloride (Additive effect or potentiation). Products include:
Hytrin Capsules 434

Thiamylal Sodium (Potentiation of orthostatic hypotension may occur).
No products indexed under this heading.

Timolol Maleate (Additive effect or potentiation). Products include:
Blocadren Tablets 1654
Timolide Tablets 1791
Timoptic in Ocudose 1796
Timoptic Sterile Ophthalmic Solution 1794
Timoptic-XE 1798

Tolazamide (Dosage adjustment of hypoglycemic may be required).
No products indexed under this heading.

Tolbutamide (Dosage adjustment of hypoglycemic may be required).
No products indexed under this heading.

Tolmetin Sodium (Reduced diuretic, natriuretic, and antihypertensive effects of Vaseretic). Products include:
Tolectin (200, 400 and 600 mg) .. 1591

Torsemide (Additive effect or potentiation). Products include:
Demadex Tablets and Injection 691

Triamcinolone (Intensified electrolyte depletion, particularly hypokalemia).
No products indexed under this heading.

Triamcinolone Acetonide (Intensified electrolyte depletion, particularly hypokalemia). Products include:
Azmacort Oral Inhaler 2175
Nasacort AQ Nasal Spray 2191
Nasacort Nasal Inhaler 2189

Triamcinolone Diacetate (Intensified electrolyte depletion, particularly hypokalemia).
No products indexed under this heading.

Triamcinolone Hexacetonide (Intensified electrolyte depletion, particularly hypokalemia).
No products indexed under this heading.

Triamterene (Significant increases potentiation; excessive hypotension). Products include:
Dyazide Capsules 2653
Dyrenium Capsules 2655

Trimethaphan Camsylate (Additive effect or potentiation).
No products indexed under this heading.

Vecuronium Bromide (Increased responsiveness to muscle relaxant). Products include:
Norcuron for Injection 1875

Verapamil Hydrochloride (Additive effect or potentiation). Products include:
Calan SR Caplets 2571
Calan Tablets 2568
Covera-HS Tablets 2573
Isoptin Injectable 1391
Isoptin Oral Tablets 1393
Isoptin SR Tablets 1395
Verelan Capsules 1455

Food Interactions

Alcohol (Potentiation of orthostatic hypotension may occur).

VASOCON-A
(Antazoline Phosphate, Naphazoline Hydrochloride) .... ⊕ 263
None cited in PDR database.

VASOTEC I.V.
(Enalaprilat) 1814
May interact with diuretics, potassium sparing diuretics, potassium preparations, lithium preparations, and certain other agents. Compounds in these categories include:

Amiloride Hydrochloride (Potential for excessive hypotension and significant hyperkalemia). Products include:

IMPORTANT NOTE: Always consult each drug listing in the patient's regimen for possible interactions.

Vasotec I.V.

Midamor Tablets 1746
Moduretic Tablets 1748

Bendroflumethiazide (Potential for excessive hypotension).
No products indexed under this heading.

Bumetanide (Potential for excessive hypotension). Products include:
Bumex 2260

Chlorothiazide (Potential for excessive hypotension). Products include:
Aldoclor Tablets 1638
Diupres Tablets 1691
Diuril Oral 1694

Chlorothiazide Sodium (Potential for excessive hypotension). Products include:
Diuril Sodium Intravenous 1693

Chlorthalidone (Potential for excessive hypotension). Products include:
Combipres Tablets 682
Tenoretic Tablets 2963
Thalitone 1293

Ethacrynic Acid (Potential for excessive hypotension). Products include:
Edecrin Tablets 1698

Furosemide (Potential for excessive hypotension). Products include:
Lasix Injection, Oral Solution and Tablets 1267

Hydrochlorothiazide (Potential for excessive hypotension). Products include:
Aldactazide Tablets 2556
Aldoril Tablets 1644
Apresazide Capsules 824
Capozide Tablets 744
Dyazide Capsules 2653
Esidrix Tablets 839
Esimil Tablets 840
HydroDIURIL Tablets 1716
Hydropres Tablets 1718
Hyzaar Tablets 1720
Inderide Tablets 2838
Inderide LA Long Acting Capsules .. 2840
Lopressor HCT Tablets 850
Lotensin HCT Tablets 855
Moduretic Tablets 1748
Oretic Tablets 450
Prinzide Tablets 1780
Ser-Ap-Es Tablets 867
Timolide Tablets 1791
Vaseretic Tablets 1810
Zestoretic Tablets 2968
Ziac 1459

Hydroflumethiazide (Potential for excessive hypotension). Products include:
Diucardin Tablets 2824

Indapamide (Potential for excessive hypotension).
No products indexed under this heading.

Lithium Carbonate (Potential for reversible lithium toxicity; monitor lithium levels frequently). Products include:
Eskalith 2658
Lithium Carbonate Capsules & Tablets 2352
Lithonate/Lithotabs/Lithobid .. 2721

Lithium Citrate (Potential for reversible lithium toxicity; monitor lithium levels frequently).
No products indexed under this heading.

Methyclothiazide (Potential for excessive hypotension). Products include:
Enduron Tablets 424

Metolazone (Potential for excessive hypotension). Products include:
Mykrox Tablets 1617
Zaroxolyn Tablets 1625

Polythiazide (Potential for excessive hypotension). Products include:
Minizide Capsules 2016

Interactions Index

Potassium Acid Phosphate (Potential for significant hyperkalemia). Products include:
K-Phos Original Formula 'Sodium Free' Tablets 633

Potassium Bicarbonate (Potential for significant hyperkalemia). Products include:
Alka-Seltzer Gold Effervescent Antacid 611

Potassium Chloride (Potential for significant hyperkalemia). Products include:
Chlor-3 Condiment 1003
Colyte and Colyte-flavored ... 2540
GoLYTELY 694
K-Dur Microburst Release System (potassium chloride, USP) E.R. Tablets 1364
K-Lor Powder Packets 438
K-Norm Capsules 1615
K-Tab Filmtab 439
Micro-K 2237
Micro-K LS Packets 2238
NuLYTELY 694
Cherry Flavor NuLYTELY 694
Rum-K Syrup 1004
Slow-K Extended-Release Tablets .. 869

Potassium Citrate (Potential for significant hyperkalemia). Products include:
Polycitra Syrup 574
Polycitra-K Crystals 574
Polycitra-K Oral Solution 575
Polycitra-LC 574
Urocit-K Tablets 1828

Potassium Gluconate (Potential for significant hyperkalemia).
No products indexed under this heading.

Potassium Phosphate, Dibasic (Potential for significant hyperkalemia).
No products indexed under this heading.

Potassium Phosphate, Monobasic (Potential for significant hyperkalemia). Products include:
K-Phos Neutral Tablets 633
K-Phos Original Formula 'Sodium Free' Tablets 633

Spironolactone (Potential for excessive hypotension and significant hyperkalemia). Products include:
Aldactazide Tablets 2556
Aldactone Tablets 2558

Torsemide (Potential for excessive hypotension). Products include:
Demadex Tablets and Injection .. 691

Triamterene (Potential for excessive hypotension and significant hyperkalemia). Products include:
Dyazide Capsules 2653
Dyrenium Capsules 2655

VASOTEC TABLETS
(Enalapril Maleate) 1816

May interact with diuretics, thiazides, potassium preparations, lithium preparations, potassium sparing diuretics, and certain other agents. Compounds in these categories include:

Amiloride Hydrochloride (Significant increases in serum potassium; excessive hypotension). Products include:
Midamor Tablets 1746
Moduretic Tablets 1748

Bendroflumethiazide (Attenuated potassium loss; excessive hypotension).
No products indexed under this heading.

Bumetanide (Excessive hypotension). Products include:
Bumex 2260

Chlorothiazide (Attenuated potassium loss; excessive hypotension). Products include:
Aldoclor Tablets 1638
Diupres Tablets 1691
Diuril Oral 1694

Chlorothiazide Sodium (Attenuated potassium loss; excessive hypotension). Products include:
Diuril Sodium Intravenous 1693

Chlorthalidone (Significant increases in serum potassium; excessive hypotension). Products include:
Combipres Tablets 682
Tenoretic Tablets 2963
Thalitone 1293

Ethacrynic Acid (Excessive hypotension). Products include:
Edecrin Tablets 1698

Furosemide (Excessive hypotension). Products include:
Lasix Injection, Oral Solution and Tablets 1267

Hydrochlorothiazide (Attenuated potassium loss; excessive hypotension). Products include:
Aldactazide Tablets 2556
Aldoril Tablets 1644
Apresazide Capsules 824
Capozide Tablets 744
Dyazide Capsules 2653
Esidrix Tablets 839
Esimil Tablets 840
HydroDIURIL Tablets 1716
Hydropres Tablets 1718
Hyzaar Tablets 1720
Inderide Tablets 2838
Inderide LA Long Acting Capsules .. 2840
Lopressor HCT Tablets 850
Lotensin HCT Tablets 855
Moduretic Tablets 1748
Oretic Tablets 450
Prinzide Tablets 1780
Ser-Ap-Es Tablets 867
Timolide Tablets 1791
Vaseretic Tablets 1810
Zestoretic Tablets 2968
Ziac 1459

Hydroflumethiazide (Attenuated potassium loss; excessive hypotension). Products include:
Diucardin Tablets 2824

Indapamide (Excessive hypotension).
No products indexed under this heading.

Lithium Carbonate (Potential for reversible lithium toxicity; frequent monitoring of serum lithium levels is recommended). Products include:
Eskalith 2658
Lithium Carbonate Capsules & Tablets 2352
Lithonate/Lithotabs/Lithobid .. 2721

Lithium Citrate (Potential for reversible lithium toxicity; frequent monitoring of serum lithium levels is recommended).
No products indexed under this heading.

Methyclothiazide (Attenuated potassium loss; excessive hypotension). Products include:
Enduron Tablets 424

Metolazone (Excessive hypotension). Products include:
Mykrox Tablets 1617
Zaroxolyn Tablets 1625

Polythiazide (Attenuated potassium loss; excessive hypotension). Products include:
Minizide Capsules 2016

Potassium Acid Phosphate (Significant increases in serum potassium). Products include:
K-Phos Original Formula 'Sodium Free' Tablets 633

Potassium Bicarbonate (Significant increases in serum potassium). Products include:
Alka-Seltzer Gold Effervescent Antacid 611

Potassium Chloride (Significant increases in serum potassium). Products include:
Chlor-3 Condiment 1003
Colyte and Colyte-flavored ... 2540
GoLYTELY 694
K-Dur Microburst Release System (potassium chloride, USP) E.R. Tablets 1364
K-Lor Powder Packets 438
K-Norm Capsules 1615
K-Tab Filmtab 439
Micro-K 2237
Micro-K LS Packets 2238
NuLYTELY 694
Cherry Flavor NuLYTELY 694
Rum-K Syrup 1004
Slow-K Extended-Release Tablets .. 869

Potassium Citrate (Significant increases in serum potassium). Products include:
Polycitra Syrup 574
Polycitra-K Crystals 574
Polycitra-K Oral Solution 575
Polycitra-LC 574
Urocit-K Tablets 1828

Potassium Gluconate (Significant increases in serum potassium).
No products indexed under this heading.

Potassium Phosphate, Dibasic (Significant increases in serum potassium).
No products indexed under this heading.

Potassium Phosphate, Monobasic (Significant increases in serum potassium). Products include:
K-Phos Neutral Tablets 633
K-Phos Original Formula 'Sodium Free' Tablets 633

Spironolactone (Significant increases in serum potassium; excessive hypotension). Products include:
Aldactazide Tablets 2556
Aldactone Tablets 2558

Torsemide (Excessive hypotension). Products include:
Demadex Tablets and Injection .. 691

Triamterene (Significant increases in serum potassium; excessive hypotension). Products include:
Dyazide Capsules 2653
Dyrenium Capsules 2655

VASOXYL INJECTION
(Methoxamine Hydrochloride) .. 1169

May interact with monoamine oxidase inhibitors, tricyclic antidepressants, and certain other agents. Compounds in these categories include:

Amitriptyline Hydrochloride (Potentiation of pressor effect). Products include:
Elavil 2945
Etrafon 2495
Limbitrol 2333
Triavil Tablets 1800

Amoxapine (Potentiation of pressor effect). Products include:
Asendin Tablets 1419

Clomipramine Hydrochloride (Potentiation of pressor effect). Products include:
Anafranil Capsules 819

Desipramine Hydrochloride (Potentiation of pressor effect). Products include:
Norpramin Tablets 1273

Doxepin Hydrochloride (Potentiation of pressor effect). Products include:
Adapin Capsules 1542
Sinequan 2028
Zonalon Cream 1042

(■ Described in PDR For Nonprescription Drugs)   (⊙ Described in PDR For Ophthalmology)

Ergonovine Maleate (Potentiation of pressor effect).
  No products indexed under this heading.
Ergot Alkaloids (Hydrogenated) (Potentiation of pressor effect).
Ergotamine Tartrate (Potentiation of pressor effect). Products include:
  Bellergal-S Tablets 2375
  Cafergot 2376
  Ergomar Tablets 1543
  Wigraine Tablets 1884
Furazolidone (Potentiation of pressor effect). Products include:
  Furoxone 2221
Imipramine Hydrochloride (Potentiation of pressor effect). Products include:
  Tofranil Ampuls 873
  Tofranil Tablets 875
Imipramine Pamoate (Potentiation of pressor effect). Products include:
  Tofranil-PM Capsules 876
Isocarboxazid (Potentiation of pressor effect).
  No products indexed under this heading.
Maprotiline Hydrochloride (Potentiation of pressor effect). Products include:
  Ludiomil Tablets 861
Methylergonovine Maleate (Potentiation of pressor effect). Products include:
  Methergine 2401
Nortriptyline Hydrochloride (Potentiation of pressor effect). Products include:
  Pamelor 2409
Phenelzine Sulfate (Potentiation of pressor effect). Products include:
  Nardil 1977
Protriptyline Hydrochloride (Potentiation of pressor effect). Products include:
  Vivactil Tablets 1820
Selegiline Hydrochloride (Potentiation of pressor effect). Products include:
  Eldepryl Capsules 2729
Tranylcypromine Sulfate (Potentiation of pressor effect). Products include:
  Parnate Tablets 2679
Trimipramine Maleate (Potentiation of pressor effect). Products include:
  Surmontil Capsules 2917
Vasopressin (Potentiation of pressor effect).
  No products indexed under this heading.

VELBAN VIALS
(Vinblastine Sulfate) 1537
May interact with:
Itraconazole (Co-administration with drugs that inhibit metabolism via cytochrome P450 3A, such as itraconazole, may cause an earlier onset and/or an increased severity of side effects). Products include:
  Sporanox Capsules 1352
Ketoconazole (Co-administration with drugs that inhibit metabolism via cytochrome P450 3A, such as ketoconazole, may cause an earlier onset and/or an increased severity of side effects). Products include:
  Nizoral 2% Cream 1344
  Nizoral 2% Shampoo 1344
  Nizoral Tablets 1345

Mitomycin (Mitomycin-C) (Acute shortness of breath; severe bronchospasm). Products include:
  Mutamycin for Injection 712
Phenytoin (Reduced blood levels of phenytoin and increased seizure activity). Products include:
  Dilantin Infatabs 1967
  Dilantin-125 Suspension 1969
Phenytoin Sodium (Reduced blood levels of phenytoin and increased seizure activity). Products include:
  Dilantin Kapseals 1965

VELOSULIN BR HUMAN INSULIN 10 ML VIALS
(Insulin, Human Regular) 1847
None cited in PDR database.

VENOLAX
(Vitamin B$_6$, Vitamin C) 686
None cited in PDR database.

VENTOLIN INHALATION AEROSOL AND REFILL
(Albuterol) 1170
May interact with sympathomimetic bronchodilators, monoamine oxidase inhibitors, tricyclic antidepressants, beta blockers, and certain other agents. Compounds in these categories include:

Acebutolol Hydrochloride (Beta receptor blocking agents and albuterol inhibit effect of each other). Products include:
  Sectral Capsules 2914
Amitriptyline Hydrochloride (Action of albuterol on vascular system may be potentiated). Products include:
  Elavil 2945
  Etrafon 2495
  Limbitrol 2333
  Triavil Tablets 1800
Amoxapine (Action of albuterol on vascular system may be potentiated). Products include:
  Asendin Tablets 1419
Atenolol (Beta receptor blocking agents and albuterol inhibit effect of each other). Products include:
  Tenoretic Tablets 2963
  Tenormin Tablets and I.V. Injection 2965
Betaxolol Hydrochloride (Beta receptor blocking agents and albuterol inhibit effect of each other). Products include:
  Betoptic Ophthalmic Solution 465
  Betoptic S Ophthalmic Suspension 467
  Kerlone Tablets 2588
Bisoprolol Fumarate (Beta receptor blocking agents and albuterol inhibit effect of each other). Products include:
  Zebeta Tablets 1457
  Ziac 1459
Bitolterol Mesylate (Sympathomimetic aerosol bronchodilators should not be used concomitantly with albuterol, may have additive effects). Products include:
  Tornalate Solution for Inhalation, 0.2% 976
  Tornalate Metered Dose Inhaler 978
Carteolol Hydrochloride (Beta receptor blocking agents and albuterol inhibit effect of each other). Products include:
  Cartrol Tablets 413
  Ocupress Ophthalmic Solution, 1% Sterile 297
Clomipramine Hydrochloride (Action of albuterol on vascular system may be potentiated). Products include:
  Anafranil Capsules 819

Desipramine Hydrochloride (Action of albuterol on vascular system may be potentiated). Products include:
  Norpramin Tablets 1273
Doxepin Hydrochloride (Action of albuterol on vascular system may be potentiated). Products include:
  Adapin Capsules 1542
  Sinequan 2028
  Zonalon Cream 1042
Ephedrine Hydrochloride (Sympathomimetic aerosol bronchodilators should not be used concomitantly with albuterol, may have additive effects). Products include:
  Primatene Tablets 844
  Quadrinal Tablets 1398
Ephedrine Sulfate (Sympathomimetic aerosol bronchodilators should not be used concomitantly with albuterol, may have additive effects). Products include:
  Marax Tablets & DF Syrup 2015
Ephedrine Tannate (Sympathomimetic aerosol bronchodilators should not be used concomitantly with albuterol, may have additive effects). Products include:
  Rynatuss 2782
Epinephrine (Sympathomimetic aerosol bronchodilators should not be used concomitantly with albuterol, may have additive effects). Products include:
  EPIFRIN 237
  EpiPen 808
  Marcaine with Epinephrine 2446
  Primatene Mist 843
  Sensorcaine with Epinephrine Injection 554
  Sus-Phrine Injection 1017
  Xylocaine with Epinephrine Injections 562
Epinephrine Hydrochloride (Sympathomimetic aerosol bronchodilators should not be used concomitantly with albuterol, may have additive effects). Products include:
  Ana-Kit Anaphylaxis Emergency Treatment Kit 611
Esmolol Hydrochloride (Beta receptor blocking agents and albuterol inhibit effect of each other). Products include:
  Brevibloc (esmolol HCl) Injection 1860
Ethylnorepinephrine Hydrochloride (Sympathomimetic aerosol bronchodilators should not be used concomitantly with albuterol, may have additive effects).
  No products indexed under this heading.
Furazolidone (Action of albuterol on vascular system may be potentiated). Products include:
  Furoxone 2221
Imipramine Hydrochloride (Action of albuterol on vascular system may be potentiated). Products include:
  Tofranil Ampuls 873
  Tofranil Tablets 875
Imipramine Pamoate (Action of albuterol on vascular system may be potentiated). Products include:
  Tofranil-PM Capsules 876
Isocarboxazid (Action of albuterol on vascular system may be potentiated).
  No products indexed under this heading.
Isoetharine (Sympathomimetic aerosol bronchodilators should not be used concomitantly with albuterol, may have additive effects). Products include:
  Bronkometer Aerosol 2432
  Bronkosol Solution 2432

Isoetharine Inhalation Solution, USP, Arm-a-Med 545
Isoproterenol Hydrochloride (Sympathomimetic aerosol bronchodilators should not be used concomitantly with albuterol, may have additive effects). Products include:
  Isuprel Hydrochloride Solution 2443
  Isuprel Injection 2441
  Isuprel Mistometer 2442
Isoproterenol Sulfate (Sympathomimetic aerosol bronchodilators should not be used concomitantly with albuterol, may have additive effects). Products include:
  Norisodrine with Calcium Iodide Syrup 446
Labetalol Hydrochloride (Beta receptor blocking agents and albuterol inhibit effect of each other). Products include:
  Normodyne Injection 2519
  Normodyne Tablets 2522
  Trandate 1158
Levobunolol Hydrochloride (Beta receptor blocking agents and albuterol inhibit effect of each other). Products include:
  Betagan 230
Maprotiline Hydrochloride (Action of albuterol on vascular system may be potentiated). Products include:
  Ludiomil Tablets 861
Metaproterenol Sulfate (Sympathomimetic aerosol bronchodilators should not be used concomitantly with albuterol, may have additive effects). Products include:
  Alupent 672
  Metaproterenol Sulfate Inhalation Solution, USP, Arm-a-Med 547
Metipranolol Hydrochloride (Beta receptor blocking agents and albuterol inhibit effect of each other). Products include:
  OptiPranolol (Metipranolol 0.3%) Sterile Ophthalmic Solution ... 256
Metoprolol Succinate (Beta receptor blocking agents and albuterol inhibit effect of each other). Products include:
  Toprol-XL Tablets 560
Metoprolol Tartrate (Beta receptor blocking agents and albuterol inhibit effect of each other). Products include:
  Lopressor 848
  Lopressor HCT Tablets 850
Nadolol (Beta receptor blocking agents and albuterol inhibit effect of each other).
  No products indexed under this heading.
Nortriptyline Hydrochloride (Action of albuterol on vascular system may be potentiated). Products include:
  Pamelor 2409
Penbutolol Sulfate (Beta receptor blocking agents and albuterol inhibit effect of each other). Products include:
  Levatol Tablets 2547
Phenelzine Sulfate (Action of albuterol on vascular system may be potentiated). Products include:
  Nardil 1977
Pindolol (Beta receptor blocking agents and albuterol inhibit effect of each other). Products include:
  Visken Tablets 2428
Pirbuterol Acetate (Sympathomimetic aerosol bronchodilators should not be used concomitantly with albuterol, may have additive effects). Products include:
  Maxair Autohaler 1550
  Maxair Inhaler 1552

IMPORTANT NOTE: Always consult each drug listing in the patient's regimen for possible interactions.

Ventolin Inhalation Aerosol **Interactions Index** **1156**

Propranolol Hydrochloride (Beta-receptor blocking agents and albuterol inhibit effect of each other). Products include:
Inderal 2834
Inderal LA Long Acting Capsules 2836
Inderide Tablets 2838
Inderide LA Long Acting Capsules .. 2840

Protriptyline Hydrochloride (Action of albuterol on vascular system may be potentiated). Products include:
Vivactil Tablets 1820

Salmeterol Xinafoate (Sympathomimetic aerosol bronchodilators should not be used concomitantly with albuterol, may have additive effects). Products include:
Serevent Inhalation Aerosol 1149

Selegiline Hydrochloride (Action of albuterol on vascular system may be potentiated). Products include:
Eldepryl Capsules 2729

Sotalol Hydrochloride (Beta receptor blocking agents and albuterol inhibit effect of each other). Products include:
Betapace Tablets 637

Terbutaline Sulfate (Sympathomimetic aerosol bronchodilators should not be used concomitantly with albuterol, may have additive effects). Products include:
Brethaire Inhaler 830
Brethine Ampuls 832
Brethine Tablets 831
Bricanyl Subcutaneous Injection 1247
Bricanyl Tablets 1248

Timolol Hemihydrate (Beta receptor blocking agents and albuterol inhibit effect of each other). Products include:
Betimol 0.25%, 0.5% .... ⊙ 259

Timolol Maleate (Beta receptor blocking agents and albuterol inhibit effect of each other). Products include:
Blocadren Tablets 1654
Timolide Tablets 1791
Timoptic in Ocudose 1796
Timoptic Sterile Ophthalmic Solution 1794
Timoptic-XE 1798

Tranylcypromine Sulfate (Action of albuterol on vascular system may be potentiated). Products include:
Parnate Tablets 2679

Trimipramine Maleate (Action of albuterol on vascular system may be potentiated). Products include:
Surmontil Capsules 2917

VENTOLIN INHALATION SOLUTION
(Albuterol Sulfate) 1171
May interact with sympathomimetics, monoamine oxidase inhibitors, beta blockers, and tricyclic antidepressants. Compounds in these categories include:

Acebutolol Hydrochloride (Beta-receptor blocking agents and albuterol inhibit effect of each other). Products include:
Sectral Capsules 2914

Amitriptyline Hydrochloride (Action of albuterol on the vascular system may be potentiated). Products include:
Elavil 2945
Etrafon 2495
Limbitrol 2333
Triavil Tablets 1800

Amoxapine (Action of albuterol on the vascular system may be potentiated). Products include:
Asendin Tablets 1419

Atenolol (Beta-receptor blocking agents and albuterol inhibit effect of each other). Products include:
Tenoretic Tablets 2963
Tenormin Tablets and I.V. Injection 2965

Betaxolol Hydrochloride (Beta-receptor blocking agents and albuterol inhibit effect of each other). Products include:
Betoptic Ophthalmic Solution 465
Betoptic S Ophthalmic Suspension 467
Kerlone Tablets 2588

Bisoprolol Fumarate (Beta-receptor blocking agents and albuterol inhibit effect of each other). Products include:
Zebeta Tablets 1457
Ziac 1459

Carteolol Hydrochloride (Beta-receptor blocking agents and albuterol inhibit effect of each other). Products include:
Cartrol Tablets 413
Ocupress Ophthalmic Solution, 1% Sterile .... ⊙ 297

Clomipramine Hydrochloride (Action of albuterol on the vascular system may be potentiated). Products include:
Anafranil Capsules 819

Desipramine Hydrochloride (Action of albuterol on the vascular system may be potentiated). Products include:
Norpramin Tablets 1273

Doxepin Hydrochloride (Action of albuterol on the vascular system may be potentiated). Products include:
Adapin Capsules 1542
Sinequan 2028
Zonalon Cream 1042

Ephedrine Hydrochloride (Concomitant use of albuterol with oral sympathomimetic agents is not recommended due to potential for cardiovascular toxicity). Products include:
Primatene Tablets .... ▣ 844
Quadrinal Tablets 1398

Ephedrine Sulfate (Concomitant use of albuterol with oral sympathomimetic agents is not recommended due to potential for cardiovascular toxicity). Products include:
Marax Tablets & DF Syrup 2015

Ephedrine Tannate (Concomitant use of albuterol with oral sympathomimetic agents is not recommended due to potential for cardiovascular toxicity). Products include:
Rynatuss 2782

Esmolol Hydrochloride (Beta-receptor blocking agents and albuterol inhibit effect of each other). Products include:
Brevibloc (esmolol HCl) Injection 1860

Furazolidone (Action of albuterol on the vascular system may be potentiated). Products include:
Furoxone 2221

Imipramine Hydrochloride (Action of albuterol on the vascular system may be potentiated). Products include:
Tofranil Ampuls 873
Tofranil Tablets 875

Imipramine Pamoate (Action of albuterol on the vascular system may be potentiated). Products include:
Tofranil-PM Capsules 876

Isocarboxazid (Action of albuterol on the vascular system may be potentiated).
No products indexed under this heading.

Labetalol Hydrochloride (Beta-receptor blocking agents and albuterol inhibit effect of each other). Products include:
Normodyne Injection 2519
Normodyne Tablets 2522
Trandate 1158

Levobunolol Hydrochloride (Beta-receptor blocking agents and albuterol inhibit effect of each other). Products include:
Betagan .... ⊙ 230

Maprotiline Hydrochloride (Action of albuterol on the vascular system may be potentiated). Products include:
Ludiomil Tablets 861

Metaproterenol Sulfate (Concomitant use of albuterol with oral sympathomimetic agents is not recommended due to potential for cardiovascular toxicity). Products include:
Alupent 672
Metaproterenol Sulfate Inhalation Solution, USP, Arm-a-Med 547

Metipranolol Hydrochloride (Beta-receptor blocking agents and albuterol inhibit effect of each other). Products include:
OptiPranolol (Metipranolol 0.3%) Sterile Ophthalmic Solution .... ⊙ 256

Metoprolol Succinate (Beta-receptor blocking agents and albuterol inhibit effect of each other). Products include:
Toprol-XL Tablets 560

Metoprolol Tartrate (Beta-receptor blocking agents and albuterol inhibit effect of each other). Products include:
Lopressor 848
Lopressor HCT Tablets 850

Nadolol (Beta-receptor blocking agents and albuterol inhibit effect of each other).
No products indexed under this heading.

Norepinephrine Bitartrate (Concomitant use of albuterol with oral sympathomimetic agents is not recommended due to potential for cardiovascular toxicity). Products include:
Levophed Bitartrate Injection 2445

Nortriptyline Hydrochloride (Action of albuterol on the vascular system may be potentiated). Products include:
Pamelor 2409

Penbutolol Sulfate (Beta-receptor blocking agents and albuterol inhibit effect of each other). Products include:
Levatol Tablets 2547

Phenelzine Sulfate (Action of albuterol on the vascular system may be potentiated). Products include:
Nardil 1977

Phenylephrine Bitartrate (Concomitant use of albuterol with oral sympathomimetic agents is not recommended due to potential for cardiovascular toxicity).
No products indexed under this heading.

Phenylephrine Hydrochloride (Concomitant use of albuterol with oral sympathomimetic agents is not recommended due to potential for cardiovascular toxicity). Products include:
Atrohist Plus Tablets 1605
Cerose DM .... ▣ 853
D.A. II Tablets 972
D.A. Chewable Tablets 970
Dura-Vent/DA Tablets 972
Extendryl 1003
4-Way Fast Acting Nasal Spray (regular & mentholated) .... ▣ 644
Hemorid .... ▣ 797
Hycomine Compound Tablets 948
Neo-Synephrine Hydrochloride 1% Carpuject 2455
Neo-Synephrine Hydrochloride 1% Injection 2455
Neo-Synephrine Hydrochloride (Ophthalmic) 2456
Neo-Synephrine .... ▣ 624
Novahistine Elixir .... ▣ 782
Phenergan VC 2886
Phenergan VC with Codeine 2888
Preparation H .... ▣ 842
Tympagesic Ear Drops 2476
Vicks Sinex Nasal Spray and Ultra Fine Mist .... ▣ 738

Phenylephrine Tannate (Concomitant use of albuterol with oral sympathomimetic agents is not recommended due to potential for cardiovascular toxicity). Products include:
Atrohist Pediatric Suspension 1604
Atrohist Pediatric Suspension Dye-Free 1604
Rynatan 2781
Rynatuss 2782

Phenylpropanolamine Hydrochloride (Concomitant use of albuterol with oral sympathomimetic agents is not recommended due to potential for cardiovascular toxicity). Products include:
Acutrim .... ▣ 648
Atrohist Plus Tablets 1605
BC Cold Powder Multi-Symptom Formula (Cold-Sinus-Allergy) .... ▣ 631
BC Cold Powder Non-Drowsy Formula (Cold-Sinus) .... ▣ 631
Cheracol Plus Head Cold/Cough Formula .... ▣ 741
Comtrex Multi-Symptom Cold Reliever Liqui-Gels .... ▣ 638
Comtrex Multi-Symptom Non-Drowsy Liqui-gels .... ▣ 640
Contac Continuous Action Nasal Decongestant/Antihistamine 12 Hour Capsules .... ▣ 773
Contac Maximum Strength Continuous Action Decongestant/Antihistamine 12 Hour Caplets .. ▣ 772
Contac Severe Cold and Flu Formula Caplets .... ▣ 773
Coricidin 'D' Decongestant Tablets .... ▣ 760
Dexatrim .... ▣ 795
Dexatrim Plus Vitamins Caplets .... ▣ 796
Dimetane-DC Cough Syrup 2232
Dimetapp Allergy Sinus Caplets .... ▣ 838
Dimetapp Cold & Allergy Chewable Tablets .... ▣ 838
Dimetapp Cold & Cough Liqui-Gels .... ▣ 839
Dimetapp DM Elixir .... ▣ 840
Dimetapp Elixir .... ▣ 840
Dimetapp Extentabs .... ▣ 841
Dimetapp Tablets/Liqui-Gels .... ▣ 841
Dura-Vent Tablets 971
Entex LA Tablets 972
Exgest LA Tablets 787
Hycomine 947
Nolamine Timed-Release Tablets 790
Ornade Spansule Capsules 2678
Propagest Tablets 791
Pyrroxate Caplets .... ▣ 742
Robitussin-CF .... ▣ 846
Sinulin Tablets 792
Tavist-D 12 Hour Relief Tablets .... ▣ 750
Teldrin 12 Hour Antihistamine/Nasal Decongestant Allergy Relief Capsules .... ▣ 786
Triaminic Expectorant .... ▣ 753
Triaminic Syrup .... ▣ 755
Triaminic Triaminicol Cold & Cough .... ▣ 756
Triaminic DM Syrup .... ▣ 756
Triaminicin Tablets .... ▣ 756
Vicks DayQuil Allergy Relief 12-Hour Extended Release Tablets .... ▣ 733
Vicks DayQuil Allergy Relief 4-Hour Tablets .... ▣ 733
Vicks DayQuil SINUS Pressure & CONGESTION Relief .... ▣ 734

(▣ Described in PDR For Nonprescription Drugs) (⊙ Described in PDR For Ophthalmology)

1157 **Interactions Index** **Ventolin Nebules**

Pindolol (Beta-receptor blocking agents and albuterol inhibit effect of each other). Products include:
Visken Tablets 2428

Pirbuterol Acetate (Concomitant use of albuterol with oral sympathomimetic agents is not recommended due to potential for cardiovascular toxicity). Products include:
Maxair Autohaler 1550
Maxair Inhaler 1552

Propranolol Hydrochloride (Beta-receptor blocking agents and albuterol inhibit effect of each other). Products include:
Inderal 2834
Inderal LA Long Acting Capsules 2836
Inderide Tablets 2838
Inderide LA Long Acting Capsules 2840

Protriptyline Hydrochloride (Action of albuterol on the vascular system may be potentiated). Products include:
Vivactil Tablets 1820

Pseudoephedrine Hydrochloride (Concomitant use of albuterol with oral sympathomimetic agents is not recommended due to potential for cardiovascular toxicity). Products include:
Actifed Allergy Daytime/Nighttime Caplets 808
Actifed Cold & Allergy Tablets 807
Actifed Cold & Sinus Caplets and Tablets 808
Actifed Sinus Daytime/Nighttime Tablets and Caplets 809
Advil Cold and Sinus Caplets and Tablets 837
Alka-Seltzer Plus Liqui-Gels 612
Alka-Seltzer Plus Flu & Body Aches Liqui-Gels Non-Drowsy Formula 613
Alka-Seltzer Plus Night-Time Cold Medicine Liqui-Gels 612
Allerest Maximum Strength 649
Allerest No Drowsiness 649
Allerest Sinus Pain Formula 649
Atrohist Pediatric Capsules 1603
Benadryl Allergy/Cold Tablets 811
Benadryl Allergy Decongestant Liquid Medication 812
Benadryl Allergy Decongestant Tablets 812
Benadryl Allergy Sinus Headache Caplets 813
Benylin Multisymptom 816
Bromfed Capsules (Extended-Release) 1832
Bromfed Syrup 712
Bromfed Tablets 1832
Bromfed-DM Cough Syrup 1832
Bromfed-PD Capsules (Extended-Release) 1832
Children's TYLENOL Cold Multi-Symptom Chewable Tablets and Liquid 1559
Children's TYLENOL Cold Plus Cough Multi Symptom Chewable Tablets and Liquid 1560
Children's TYLENOL Flu Suspension Liquid 1560
Children's Vicks DayQuil Allergy Relief 730
Children's Vicks NyQuil Cold/Cough Relief 731
Allergy-Sinus Comtrex Multi-Symptom Allergy-Sinus Formula Tablets and Caplets 639
Comtrex Multi-Symptom 638
Comtrex Multi-Symptom Non-Drowsy Caplets 640
Congess 1003
Contac Day Allergy/Sinus Caplets 771
Contac Day & Night 772
Contac Night Allergy/Sinus Caplets 771
Contac Severe Cold & Flu Non-Drowsy 774
Deconsal II Tablets 1605
Dimetane-DX Cough Syrup 2233
Dimetapp Cold & Fever Suspension 839
Dimetapp Decongestant Pediatric Drops 840
Dorcol Children's Cough Syrup 748
Drixoral Cough + Congestion Liquid Caps 763
Dura-Tap/PD Capsules 970
Duratuss Tablets 2750
Duratuss HD Elixir 2750
Efidac/24 655
Entex PSE Tablets 973
Fedahist Gyrocaps 2545
Guaifed 1833
Guaifed Syrup 712
Guaimax-D Tablets 809
Histussin D Liquid 670
Infants' TYLENOL Cold Decongestant & Fever-Reducer Drops 1561
Kronofed-A 994
Novahistine DMX 782
Nucofed 2225
PediaCare Cough-Cold Chewable Tablets and Liquid 1569
PediaCare Infants' Decongestant Drops 1569
PediaCare Infants' Drops Decongestant Plus Cough 1569
PediaCare NightRest Cough-Cold Liquid 1569
Pediatric Vicks 44d Cough & Head Congestion Relief 736
Pediatric Vicks 44m Cough & Cold Relief 737
Robitussin Cold & Cough Liqui-Gels 844
Robitussin Cold, Cough & Flu Liqui-Gels 844
Robitussin Maximum Strength Cough & Cold 847
Robitussin Night-Time Cold Formula 847
Robitussin Pediatric Cough & Cold Formula 848
Robitussin Pediatric Drops 849
Robitussin Severe Congestion Liqui-Gels 845
Robitussin-DAC Syrup 2249
Robitussin-PE 846
Rondec Oral Drops 974
Rondec Syrup 974
Rondec Tablet 974
Rondec Chewable Tablets 974
Rondec-TR Tablet 974
Ryna 804
Seldane-D Extended-Release Tablets 1286
Semprex-D Capsules 1620
Sinarest 663
Sine-Aid Maximum Strength Sinus Headache Gelcaps, Caplets and Tablets 1570
Sine-Off No Drowsiness Formula Caplets 784
Sine-Off Sinus Medicine 784
Singlet Tablets 785
Sinutab Non-Drying Liquid Caps 823
Sinutab Sinus Allergy Medication, Maximum Strength Tablets and Caplets 823
Sinutab Sinus Medication, Maximum Strength Without Drowsiness Formula, Tablets & Caplets 824
Sudafed Children's Cold & Cough Liquid Medication 825
Sudafed Children's Nasal Decongestant Liquid Medication 826
Sudafed Cold & Allergy Tablets 826
Sudafed Cold and Cough Liquid Caps 826
Sudafed Nasal Decongestant Tablets, 30 mg 825
Sudafed Nasal Decongestant Tablets, 60 mg 825
Sudafed Non-Drying Sinus Liquid Caps 827
Sudafed Pediatric Nasal Decongestant Liquid Oral Drops 827
Sudafed Severe Cold Formula Caplets 828
Sudafed Severe Cold Formula Tablets 828
Sudafed Sinus Caplets 829
Sudafed Sinus Tablets 829
Sudafed 12 Hour Caplets 824
Syn-Rx Tablets 1622
Syn-Rx DM Tablets 1623
TheraFlu Flu and Cold Medicine 750
Theraflu Maximum Strength Flu and Cold Medicine For Sore Throat 751
TheraFlu Flu, Cold and Cough Medicine 750
TheraFlu Maximum Strength Nighttime Flu, Cold & Cough Medicine 751
TheraFlu Maximum Strength Non-Drowsy Formula Flu, Cold & Cough Medicine 751
TheraFlu Maximum Strength, Non-Drowsy Formula Flu, Cold and Cough Caplets 752
Theraflu Maximum Strength Sinus Non-Drowsy Formula Caplets 752
Triaminic AM Cough and Decongestant Formula 753
Triaminic AM Decongestant Formula 753
Triaminic Infant Oral Decongestant Drops 754
Triaminic Night Time 754
Triaminic Sore Throat Formula 755
Tussend 1830
Tussend Expectorant 1831
TYLENOL Allergy Sinus, Maximum Strength Caplets and Gelcaps 1571
TYLENOL Allergy Sinus NightTime, Maximum Strength Caplets 1571
TYLENOL Cold Medication, Multi-Symptom Formula Tablets and Caplets 1572
TYLENOL Cold Medication, Multi-Symptom Hot Liquid Packets 1572
TYLENOL Cold Medication, No Drowsiness Formula Caplets and Gelcaps 1572
TYLENOL Cold Severe Congestion Caplets 1573
TYLENOL Cough Medication with Decongestant, Multi Symptom 1574
TYLENOL Flu No Drowsiness Formula, Maximum Strength Gelcaps 1575
TYLENOL Flu NightTime, Maximum Strength Gelcaps 1575
TYLENOL Flu NightTime, Maximum Strength Hot Medication Packets 1575
TYLENOL Sinus, Maximum Strength Geltabs, Gelcaps, Caplets and Tablets 1576
Vicks 44 LiquiCaps Cough, Cold & Flu Relief 728
Vicks 44 LiquiCaps Non-Drowsy Cough & Cold Relief 729
Vicks 44D Cough & Head Congestion Relief 728
Vicks 44M Cough, Cold & Flu Relief 729
Vicks DayQuil LiquiCaps/Liquid Multi-Symptom Cold/Flu Relief 734
Vicks DayQuil SINUS Pressure & PAIN Relief with IBUPROFEN 735
Vicks Nyquil Hot Therapy 735
Vicks NyQuil LiquiCaps/Liquid Multi-Symptom Cold/Flu Relief, Original and Cherry Flavors 736

Pseudoephedrine Sulfate (Concomitant use of albuterol with oral sympathomimetic agents is not recommended due to potential for cardiovascular toxicity). Products include:
Chlor-Trimeton Allergy Decongestant Tablets 759
Claritin-D Tablets 2487
Drixoral Cold and Allergy Sustained-Action Tablets 763
Drixoral Cold and Flu Extended-Release Tablets 764
Drixoral Non-Drowsy Formula Extended-Release Tablets 764
Drixoral Allergy/Sinus Extended Release Tablets 765
Trinalin Repetabs Tablets 1373

Salmeterol Xinafoate (Concomitant use of albuterol with oral sympathomimetic agents is not recommended due to potential for cardiovascular toxicity). Products include:
Serevent Inhalation Aerosol 1149

Selegiline Hydrochloride (Action of albuterol on the vascular system may be potentiated). Products include:
Eldepryl Capsules 2729

Sotalol Hydrochloride (Beta-receptor blocking agents and albuterol inhibit effect of each other). Products include:
Betapace Tablets 637

Terbutaline Sulfate (Concomitant use of albuterol with oral sympathomimetic agents is not recommended due to potential for cardiovascular toxicity). Products include:
Brethaire Inhaler 830
Brethine Ampuls 832
Brethine Tablets 831
Bricanyl Subcutaneous Injection 1247
Bricanyl Tablets 1248

Timolol Hemihydrate (Beta-receptor blocking agents and albuterol inhibit effect of each other). Products include:
Betimol 0.25%, 0.5% ⊙ 259

Timolol Maleate (Beta-receptor blocking agents and albuterol inhibit effect of each other). Products include:
Blocadren Tablets 1654
Timolide Tablets 1791
Timoptic in Ocudose 1796
Timoptic Sterile Ophthalmic Solution 1794
Timoptic-XE 1798

Tranylcypromine Sulfate (Action of albuterol on the vascular system may be potentiated). Products include:
Parnate Tablets 2679

Trimipramine Maleate (Action of albuterol on the vascular system may be potentiated). Products include:
Surmontil Capsules 2917

VENTOLIN NEBULES INHALATION SOLUTION
(Albuterol Sulfate) 1172
May interact with sympathomimetic bronchodilators, monoamine oxidase inhibitors, beta blockers, and tricyclic antidepressants. Compounds in these categories include:

Acebutolol Hydrochloride (Beta-receptor blocking agents and albuterol inhibit effect of each other). Products include:
Sectral Capsules 2914

Amitriptyline Hydrochloride (Action of albuterol on the vascular system may be potentiated). Products include:
Elavil 2945
Etrafon 2495
Limbitrol 2333
Triavil Tablets 1800

Amoxapine (Action of albuterol on the vascular system may be potentiated). Products include:
Asendin Tablets 1419

Atenolol (Beta-receptor blocking agents and albuterol inhibit effect of each other). Products include:
Tenoretic Tablets 2963
Tenormin Tablets and I.V. Injection 2965

Betaxolol Hydrochloride (Beta-receptor blocking agents and albuterol inhibit effect of each other). Products include:
Betoptic Ophthalmic Solution 465
Betoptic S Ophthalmic Suspension 467
Kerlone Tablets 2588

Bisoprolol Fumarate (Beta-receptor blocking agents and albuterol inhibit effect of each other). Products include:
Zebeta Tablets 1457
Ziac 1459

IMPORTANT NOTE: Always consult each drug listing in the patient's regimen for possible interactions.

Ventolin Nebules

Bitolterol Mesylate (Concomitant use with other sympathomimetic aerosol bronchodilators is not recommended). Products include:
- Tornalate Solution for Inhalation, 0.2% 976
- Tornalate Metered Dose Inhaler 978

Carteolol Hydrochloride (Beta-receptor blocking agents and albuterol inhibit effect of each other). Products include:
- Cartrol Tablets 413
- Ocupress Ophthalmic Solution, 1% Sterile............ ⊚ 297

Clomipramine Hydrochloride (Action of albuterol on the vascular system may be potentiated). Products include:
- Anafranil Capsules 819

Desipramine Hydrochloride (Action of albuterol on the vascular system may be potentiated). Products include:
- Norpramin Tablets 1273

Doxepin Hydrochloride (Action of albuterol on the vascular system may be potentiated). Products include:
- Adapin Capsules 1542
- Sinequan 2028
- Zonalon Cream 1042

Ephedrine Hydrochloride (Concomitant use with other sympathomimetic aerosol bronchodilators is not recommended). Products include:
- Primatene Tablets .... ✦ 844
- Quadrinal Tablets 1398

Ephedrine Sulfate (Concomitant use with other sympathomimetic aerosol bronchodilators is not recommended). Products include:
- Marax Tablets & DF Syrup............ 2015

Ephedrine Tannate (Concomitant use with other sympathomimetic aerosol bronchodilators is not recommended). Products include:
- Rynatuss 2782

Epinephrine (Concomitant use with other sympathomimetic aerosol bronchodilators is not recommended). Products include:
- EPIFRIN .... ⊚ 237
- EpiPen 808
- Marcaine with Epinephrine 2446
- Primatene Mist .... ✦ 843
- Sensorcaine with Epinephrine Injection 554
- Sus-Phrine Injection 1017
- Xylocaine with Epinephrine Injections 562

Epinephrine Hydrochloride (Concomitant use with other sympathomimetic aerosol bronchodilators is not recommended). Products include:
- Ana-Kit Anaphylaxis Emergency Treatment Kit 611

Esmolol Hydrochloride (Beta-receptor blocking agents and albuterol inhibit effect of each other). Products include:
- Brevibloc (esmolol HCl) Injection 1860

Ethylnorepinephrine Hydrochloride (Concomitant use with other sympathomimetic aerosol bronchodilators is not recommended).
- No products indexed under this heading.

Furazolidone (Action of albuterol on the vascular system may be potentiated). Products include:
- Furoxone 2221

Imipramine Hydrochloride (Action of albuterol on the vascular system may be potentiated). Products include:
- Tofranil Ampuls 873

Interactions Index

- Tofranil Tablets 875

Imipramine Pamoate (Action of albuterol on the vascular system may be potentiated). Products include:
- Tofranil-PM Capsules 876

Isocarboxazid (Action of albuterol on the vascular system may be potentiated).
- No products indexed under this heading.

Isoetharine (Concomitant use with other sympathomimetic aerosol bronchodilators is not recommended). Products include:
- Bronkometer Aerosol............ 2432
- Bronkosol Solution 2432
- Isoetharine Inhalation Solution, USP, Arm-a-Med............ 545

Isoproterenol Hydrochloride (Concomitant use with other sympathomimetic aerosol bronchodilators is not recommended). Products include:
- Isuprel Hydrochloride Solution 2443
- Isuprel Injection 2441
- Isuprel Mistometer 2442

Isoproterenol Sulfate (Concomitant use with other sympathomimetic aerosol bronchodilators is not recommended). Products include:
- Norisodrine with Calcium Iodide Syrup............ 446

Labetalol Hydrochloride (Beta-receptor blocking agents and albuterol inhibit effect of each other). Products include:
- Normodyne Injection 2519
- Normodyne Tablets 2522
- Trandate 1158

Levobunolol Hydrochloride (Beta-receptor blocking agents and albuterol inhibit effect of each other). Products include:
- Betagan .... ⊚ 230

Maprotiline Hydrochloride (Action of albuterol on the vascular system may be potentiated). Products include:
- Ludiomil Tablets............ 861

Metaproterenol Sulfate (Concomitant use with other sympathomimetic aerosol bronchodilators is not recommended). Products include:
- Alupent 672
- Metaproterenol Sulfate Inhalation Solution, USP, Arm-a-Med 547

Metipranolol Hydrochloride (Beta-receptor blocking agents and albuterol inhibit effect of each other). Products include:
- OptiPranolol (Metipranolol 0.3%) Sterile Ophthalmic Solution.......... ⊚ 256

Metoprolol Succinate (Beta-receptor blocking agents and albuterol inhibit effect of each other). Products include:
- Toprol-XL Tablets 560

Metoprolol Tartrate (Beta-receptor blocking agents and albuterol inhibit effect of each other). Products include:
- Lopressor 848
- Lopressor HCT Tablets 850

Nadolol (Beta-receptor blocking agents and albuterol inhibit effect of each other).
- No products indexed under this heading.

Nortriptyline Hydrochloride (Action of albuterol on the vascular system may be potentiated). Products include:
- Pamelor 2409

Penbutolol Sulfate (Beta-receptor blocking agents and albuterol inhibit effect of each other). Products include:
- Levatol Tablets 2547

Phenelzine Sulfate (Action of albuterol on the vascular system may be potentiated). Products include:
- Nardil 1977

Pindolol (Beta-receptor blocking agents and albuterol inhibit effect of each other). Products include:
- Visken Tablets............ 2428

Pirbuterol Acetate (Concomitant use with other sympathomimetic aerosol bronchodilators is not recommended). Products include:
- Maxair Autohaler 1550
- Maxair Inhaler 1552

Propranolol Hydrochloride (Beta-receptor blocking agents and albuterol inhibit effect of each other). Products include:
- Inderal 2834
- Inderal LA Long Acting Capsules 2836
- Inderide Tablets 2838
- Inderide LA Long Acting Capsules 2840

Protriptyline Hydrochloride (Action of albuterol on the vascular system may be potentiated). Products include:
- Vivactil Tablets 1820

Salmeterol Xinafoate (Concomitant use with other sympathomimetic aerosol bronchodilators is not recommended). Products include:
- Serevent Inhalation Aerosol............ 1149

Selegiline Hydrochloride (Action of albuterol on the vascular system may be potentiated). Products include:
- Eldepryl Capsules 2729

Sotalol Hydrochloride (Beta-receptor blocking agents and albuterol inhibit effect of each other). Products include:
- Betapace Tablets 637

Terbutaline Sulfate (Concomitant use with other sympathomimetic aerosol bronchodilators is not recommended). Products include:
- Brethaire Inhaler 830
- Brethine Ampuls 832
- Brethine Tablets 831
- Bricanyl Subcutaneous Injection 1247
- Bricanyl Tablets 1248

Timolol Hemihydrate (Beta-receptor blocking agents and albuterol inhibit effect of each other). Products include:
- Betimol 0.25%, 0.5% .... ⊚ 259

Timolol Maleate (Beta-receptor blocking agents and albuterol inhibit effect of each other). Products include:
- Blocadren Tablets 1654
- Timolide Tablets 1791
- Timoptic in Ocudose 1796
- Timoptic Sterile Ophthalmic Solution............ 1794
- Timoptic-XE 1798

Tranylcypromine Sulfate (Action of albuterol on the vascular system may be potentiated). Products include:
- Parnate Tablets 2679

Trimipramine Maleate (Action of albuterol on the vascular system may be potentiated). Products include:
- Surmontil Capsules............ 2917

VENTOLIN ROTACAPS FOR INHALATION

(Albuterol Sulfate) 1173
May interact with sympathomimetic bronchodilators, monoamine oxidase inhibitors, beta blockers, and tricyclic antidepressants. Compounds in these categories include:

Acebutolol Hydrochloride (Beta-receptor blocking agents and albuterol inhibit effect of each other). Products include:
- Sectral Capsules 2914

Amitriptyline Hydrochloride (Action of albuterol on the vascular system may be potentiated). Products include:
- Elavil 2945
- Etrafon 2495
- Limbitrol 2333
- Triavil Tablets 1800

Amoxapine (Action of albuterol on the vascular system may be potentiated). Products include:
- Asendin Tablets 1419

Atenolol (Beta-receptor blocking agents and albuterol inhibit effect of each other). Products include:
- Tenoretic Tablets............ 2963
- Tenormin Tablets and I.V. Injection 2965

Betaxolol Hydrochloride (Beta-receptor blocking agents and albuterol inhibit effect of each other). Products include:
- Betoptic Ophthalmic Solution............ 465
- Betoptic S Ophthalmic Suspension 467
- Kerlone Tablets 2588

Bisoprolol Fumarate (Beta-receptor blocking agents and albuterol inhibit effect of each other). Products include:
- Zebeta Tablets 1457
- Ziac 1459

Bitolterol Mesylate (Concomitant use with other sympathomimetic aerosol bronchodilators is not recommended). Products include:
- Tornalate Solution for Inhalation, 0.2% 976
- Tornalate Metered Dose Inhaler 978

Carteolol Hydrochloride (Beta-receptor blocking agents and albuterol inhibit effect of each other). Products include:
- Cartrol Tablets 413
- Ocupress Ophthalmic Solution, 1% Sterile............ ⊚ 297

Clomipramine Hydrochloride (Action of albuterol on the vascular system may be potentiated). Products include:
- Anafranil Capsules 819

Desipramine Hydrochloride (Action of albuterol on the vascular system may be potentiated). Products include:
- Norpramin Tablets 1273

Doxepin Hydrochloriae (Action of albuterol on the vascular system may be potentiated). Products include:
- Adapin Capsules 1542
- Sinequan 2028
- Zonalon Cream 1042

Ephedrine Hydrochloride (Concomitant use with other sympathomimetic aerosol bronchodilators is not recommended). Products include:
- Primatene Tablets .... ✦ 844
- Quadrinal Tablets 1398

Ephedrine Sulfate (Concomitant use with other sympathomimetic aerosol bronchodilators is not recommended). Products include:
- Marax Tablets & DF Syrup............ 2015

Ephedrine Tannate (Concomitant use with other sympathomimetic aerosol bronchodilators is not recommended). Products include:
- Rynatuss 2782

(✦ Described in PDR For Nonprescription Drugs)   (⊚ Described in PDR For Ophthalmology)

Epinephrine (Concomitant use with other sympathomimetic aerosol bronchodilators is not recommended). Products include:

EPIFRIN	ⓟ 237
EpiPen	808
Marcaine with Epinephrine	2446
Primatene Mist	ⓟ 843
Sensorcaine with Epinephrine Injection	554
Sus-Phrine Injection	1017
Xylocaine with Epinephrine Injections	562

Epinephrine Hydrochloride (Concomitant use with other sympathomimetic aerosol bronchodilators is not recommended). Products include:

Ana-Kit Anaphylaxis Emergency Treatment Kit	611

Esmolol Hydrochloride (Beta-receptor blocking agents and albuterol inhibit effect of each other). Products include:

Brevibloc (esmolol HCl) Injection	1860

Ethylnorepinephrine Hydrochloride (Concomitant use with other sympathomimetic aerosol bronchodilators is not recommended).
No products indexed under this heading.

Furazolidone (Action of albuterol on the vascular system may be potentiated). Products include:

Furoxone	2221

Imipramine Hydrochloride (Action of albuterol on the vascular system may be potentiated). Products include:

Tofranil Ampuls	873
Tofranil Tablets	875

Imipramine Pamoate (Action of albuterol on the vascular system may be potentiated). Products include:

Tofranil-PM Capsules	876

Isocarboxazid (Action of albuterol on the vascular system may be potentiated).
No products indexed under this heading.

Isoetharine (Concomitant use with other sympathomimetic aerosol bronchodilators is not recommended). Products include:

Bronkometer Aerosol	2432
Bronkosol Solution	2432
Isoetharine Inhalation Solution, USP, Arm-a-Med	545

Isoproterenol Hydrochloride (Concomitant use with other sympathomimetic aerosol bronchodilators is not recommended). Products include:

Isuprel Hydrochloride Solution	2443
Isuprel Injection	2441
Isuprel Mistometer	2442

Isoproterenol Sulfate (Concomitant use with other sympathomimetic aerosol bronchodilators is not recommended). Products include:

Norisodrine with Calcium Iodide Syrup	446

Labetalol Hydrochloride (Beta-receptor blocking agents and albuterol inhibit effect of each other). Products include:

Normodyne Injection	2519
Normodyne Tablets	2522
Trandate	1158

Levobunolol Hydrochloride (Beta-receptor blocking agents and albuterol inhibit effect of each other). Products include:

Betagan	ⓟ 230

Maprotiline Hydrochloride (Action of albuterol on the vascular system may be potentiated). Products include:

Ludiomil Tablets	861

Metaproterenol Sulfate (Concomitant use with other sympathomimetic aerosol bronchodilators is not recommended). Products include:

Alupent	672
Metaproterenol Sulfate Inhalation Solution, USP, Arm-a-Med	547

Metipranolol Hydrochloride (Beta-receptor blocking agents and albuterol inhibit effect of each other). Products include:

OptiPranolol (Metipranolol 0.3%) Sterile Ophthalmic Solution	ⓟ 256

Metoprolol Succinate (Beta-receptor blocking agents and albuterol inhibit effect of each other). Products include:

Toprol-XL Tablets	560

Metoprolol Tartrate (Beta-receptor blocking agents and albuterol inhibit effect of each other). Products include:

Lopressor	848
Lopressor HCT Tablets	850

Nadolol (Beta-receptor blocking agents and albuterol inhibit effect of each other).
No products indexed under this heading.

Nortriptyline Hydrochloride (Action of albuterol on the vascular system may be potentiated). Products include:

Pamelor	2409

Penbutolol Sulfate (Beta-receptor blocking agents and albuterol inhibit effect of each other). Products include:

Levatol Tablets	2547

Phenelzine Sulfate (Action of albuterol on the vascular system may be potentiated). Products include:

Nardil	1977

Pindolol (Beta-receptor blocking agents and albuterol inhibit effect of each other). Products include:

Visken Tablets	2428

Pirbuterol Acetate (Concomitant use with other sympathomimetic aerosol bronchodilators is not recommended). Products include:

Maxair Autohaler	1550
Maxair Inhaler	1552

Propranolol Hydrochloride (Beta-receptor blocking agents and albuterol inhibit effect of each other). Products include:

Inderal	2834
Inderal LA Long Acting Capsules	2836
Inderide Tablets	2838
Inderide LA Long Acting Capsules	2840

Protriptyline Hydrochloride (Action of albuterol on the vascular system may be potentiated). Products include:

Vivactil Tablets	1820

Salmeterol Xinafoate (Concomitant use with other sympathomimetic aerosol bronchodilators is not recommended). Products include:

Serevent Inhalation Aerosol	1149

Selegiline Hydrochloride (Action of albuterol on the vascular system may be potentiated). Products include:

Eldepryl Capsules	2729

Sotalol Hydrochloride (Beta-receptor blocking agents and albuterol inhibit effect of each other). Products include:

Betapace Tablets	637

Terbutaline Sulfate (Concomitant use with other sympathomimetic aerosol bronchodilators is not recommended). Products include:

Brethaire Inhaler	830
Brethine Ampuls	832
Brethine Tablets	831
Bricanyl Subcutaneous Injection	1247
Bricanyl Tablets	1248

Timolol Hemihydrate (Beta-receptor blocking agents and albuterol inhibit effect of each other). Products include:

Betimol 0.25%, 0.5%	ⓟ 259

Timolol Maleate (Beta-receptor blocking agents and albuterol inhibit effect of each other). Products include:

Blocadren Tablets	1654
Timolide Tablets	1791
Timoptic in Ocudose	1796
Timoptic Sterile Ophthalmic Solution	1794
Timoptic-XE	1798

Tranylcypromine Sulfate (Action of albuterol on the vascular system may be potentiated). Products include:

Parnate Tablets	2679

Trimipramine Maleate (Action of albuterol on the vascular system may be potentiated). Products include:

Surmontil Capsules	2917

VENTOLIN SYRUP

(Albuterol Sulfate) 1175

May interact with monoamine oxidase inhibitors, beta blockers, tricyclic antidepressants, oral sympathomimetics, drugs which lower serum potassium (selected), and certain other agents. Compounds in these categories include:

Acebutolol Hydrochloride (Beta receptor blocking agents and albuterol inhibit effect of each other). Products include:

Sectral Capsules	2914

Amitriptyline Hydrochloride (Action of albuterol on vascular system may be potentiated). Products include:

Elavil	2945
Etrafon	2495
Limbitrol	2333
Triavil Tablets	1800

Amoxapine (Action of albuterol on vascular system may be potentiated). Products include:

Asendin Tablets	1419

Atenolol (Beta receptor blocking agents and albuterol inhibit effect of each other). Products include:

Tenoretic Tablets	2963
Tenormin Tablets and I.V. Injection	2965

Bendroflumethiazide (Potential for additive hypokalemic effect with concurrent use).
No products indexed under this heading.

Betamethasone Acetate (Potential for additive hypokalemic effect with concurrent use). Products include:

Celestone Soluspan Suspension	2484

Betamethasone Sodium Phosphate (Potential for additive hypokalemic effect with concurrent use). Products include:

Celestone Soluspan Suspension	2484

Betaxolol Hydrochloride (Beta receptor blocking agents and albuterol inhibit effect of each other). Products include:

Betoptic Ophthalmic Solution	465
Betoptic S Ophthalmic Suspension	467
Kerlone Tablets	2588

Bisoprolol Fumarate (Beta receptor blocking agents and albuterol inhibit effect of each other). Products include:

Zebeta Tablets	1457
Ziac	1459

Carteolol Hydrochloride (Beta receptor blocking agents and albuterol inhibit effect of each other). Products include:

Cartrol Tablets	413
Ocupress Ophthalmic Solution, 1% Sterile	ⓟ 297

Chlorothiazide (Potential for additive hypokalemic effect with concurrent use). Products include:

Aldoclor Tablets	1638
Diupres Tablets	1691
Diuril Oral	1694

Chlorothiazide Sodium (Potential for additive hypokalemic effect with concurrent use). Products include:

Diuril Sodium Intravenous	1693

Clomipramine Hydrochloride (Action of albuterol on vascular system may be potentiated). Products include:

Anafranil Capsules	819

Cortisone Acetate (Potential for additive hypokalemic effect with concurrent use). Products include:

Cortone Acetate Sterile Suspension	1663
Cortone Acetate Tablets	1664

Desipramine Hydrochloride (Action of albuterol on vascular system may be potentiated). Products include:

Norpramin Tablets	1273

Dexamethasone (Potential for additive hypokalemic effect with concurrent use). Products include:

AK-Trol Ointment & Suspension	ⓟ 205
Decadron Elixir	1676
Decadron Tablets	1678
Decaspray Topical Aerosol	1689
Maxitrol Ophthalmic Ointment and Suspension	ⓟ 222
TobraDex Ophthalmic Suspension and Ointment	469

Dexamethasone Acetate (Potential for additive hypokalemic effect with concurrent use). Products include:

Dalalone D.P. Injectable	1009
Decadron-LA Sterile Suspension	1687

Dexamethasone Sodium Phosphate (Potential for additive hypokalemic effect with concurrent use). Products include:

Decadron Phosphate Injection	1680
Decadron Phosphate Sterile Ophthalmic Ointment	1684
Decadron Phosphate Sterile Ophthalmic Solution	1685
Decadron Phosphate Topical Cream	1686
Decadron Phosphate with Xylocaine Injection, Sterile	1683
Dexacort Phosphate in Respihaler	1606
Dexacort Phosphate in Turbinaire	1607
NeoDecadron Sterile Ophthalmic Ointment	1755
NeoDecadron Sterile Ophthalmic Solution	1756
NeoDecadron Topical Cream	1757

Digoxin (Decreased serum digoxin levels (16%-22%); the clinical significance of these findings for patients with COPD who are concurrently taking these on a chronic basis is unclear). Products include:

Lanoxicaps	1110
Lanoxin Elixir Pediatric	1113
Lanoxin Injection	1116
Lanoxin Injection Pediatric	1119
Lanoxin Tablets	1121

Doxepin Hydrochloride (Action of albuterol on vascular system may be potentiated). Products include:

Adapin Capsules	1542

IMPORTANT NOTE: Always consult each drug listing in the patient's regimen for possible interactions.

Ventolin Syrup — Interactions Index — 1160

Sinequan ... 2028
Zonalon Cream ... 1042

Ephedrine Hydrochloride (Concomitant use of albuterol with oral sympathomimetic agents is not recommended due to the potential for cardiovascular toxicity). Products include:
Primatene Tablets ... ▣ 844
Quadrinal Tablets ... 1398

Ephedrine Sulfate (Concomitant use of albuterol with oral sympathomimetic agents is not recommended due to the potential for cardiovascular toxicity). Products include:
Marax Tablets & DF Syrup ... 2015

Ephedrine Tannate (Concomitant use of albuterol with oral sympathomimetic agents is not recommended due to the potential for cardiovascular toxicity). Products include:
Rynatuss ... 2782

Esmolol Hydrochloride (Beta receptor blocking agents and albuterol inhibit effect of each other). Products include:
Brevibloc (esmolol HCl) Injection ... 1860

Furazolidone (Action of albuterol on vascular system may be potentiated). Products include:
Furoxone ... 2221

Hydrochlorothiazide (Potential for additive hypokalemic effect with concurrent use). Products include:
Aldactazide Tablets ... 2556
Aldoril Tablets ... 1644
Apresazide Capsules ... 824
Capozide Tablets ... 744
Dyazide Capsules ... 2653
Esidrix Tablets ... 839
Esimil Tablets ... 840
HydroDIURIL Tablets ... 1716
Hydropres Tablets ... 1718
Hyzaar Tablets ... 1720
Inderide Tablets ... 2838
Inderide LA Long Acting Capsules ... 2840
Lopressor HCT Tablets ... 850
Lotensin HCT Tablets ... 855
Moduretic Tablets ... 1748
Oretic Tablets ... 450
Prinzide Tablets ... 1780
Ser-Ap-Es Tablets ... 867
Timolide Tablets ... 1791
Vaseretic Tablets ... 1810
Zestoretic Tablets ... 2968
Ziac ... 1459

Hydrocortisone (Potential for additive hypokalemic effect with concurrent use). Products include:
Anusol-HC Cream 2.5% ... 1953
Aquanil HC Lotion ... 1989
Maximum Strength Cortaid Spray ▣ 800
CORTENEMA ... 2713
Cortisporin Ointment ... 1074
Cortisporin Ophthalmic Ointment Sterile ... 1074
Cortisporin Ophthalmic Suspension Sterile ... 1075
Cortisporin Otic Solution Sterile ... 1076
Cortisporin Otic Suspension Sterile 1077
Cortizone-5 ... ▣ 795
Cortizone-10 ... ▣ 795
Hydrocortone Tablets ... 1715
Hytone ... 922
Hytone Ointment 2 ½% ... 923
Massengill Medicated Soft Cloth Towelettes ... 2628
Pediotic Suspension Sterile ... 1140
Preparation H Hydrocortisone 1% Cream ... ▣ 843
ProctoCream-HC 2.5% ... 2552
VōSoL HC Otic Solution ... 2786

Hydrocortisone Acetate (Potential for additive hypokalemic effect with concurrent use). Products include:
Analpram-HC Rectal Cream 1% and 2.5% ... 993
Anusol HC-1 Hydrocortisone Anti-Itch Ointment ... ▣ 810
Anusol-HC Suppositories ... 1954
Caldecort Anti-Itch Hydrocortisone Cream ... ▣ 651
Coly-Mycin S Otic w/Neomycin & Hydrocortisone ... 1965
Cortaid ... ▣ 800
Cortifoam ... 2540
Cortisporin Cream ... 1073
Epifoam ... 2543
Hydrocortone Acetate Sterile Suspension ... 1712
Mantadil Cream ... 1124
Nupercainal Hydrocortisone 1% Cream ... ▣ 661
Pramosone Cream, Lotion & Ointment ... 995
ProctoFoam-HC ... 2552
Terra-Cortril Ophthalmic Suspension ... 2033

Hydrocortisone Sodium Phosphate (Potential for additive hypokalemic effect with concurrent use). Products include:
Hydrocortone Phosphate Injection, Sterile ... 1713

Hydrocortisone Sodium Succinate (Potential for additive hypokalemic effect with concurrent use).
No products indexed under this heading.

Hydroflumethiazide (Potential for additive hypokalemic effect with concurrent use). Products include:
Diucardin Tablets ... 2824

Imipramine Hydrochloride (Action of albuterol on vascular system may be potentiated). Products include:
Tofranil Ampuls ... 873
Tofranil Tablets ... 875

Imipramine Pamoate (Action of albuterol on vascular system may be potentiated). Products include:
Tofranil-PM Capsules ... 876

Isocarboxazid (Action of albuterol on vascular system may be potentiated).
No products indexed under this heading.

Labetalol Hydrochloride (Beta receptor blocking agents and albuterol inhibit effect of each other). Products include:
Normodyne Injection ... 2519
Normodyne Tablets ... 2522
Trandate ... 1158

Levobunolol Hydrochloride (Beta receptor blocking agents and albuterol inhibit effect of each other). Products include:
Betagan ... ⊙ 230

Maprotiline Hydrochloride (Action of albuterol on vascular system may be potentiated). Products include:
Ludiomil Tablets ... 861

Metaproterenol Sulfate (Concomitant use of albuterol with oral sympathomimetic agents is not recommended due to the potential for cardiovascular toxicity). Products include:
Alupent ... 672
Metaproterenol Sulfate Inhalation Solution, USP, Arm-a-Med ... 547

Methyclothiazide (Potential for additive hypokalemic effect with concurrent use). Products include:
Enduron Tablets ... 424

Methylprednisolone Acetate (Potential for additive hypokalemic effect with concurrent use).
No products indexed under this heading.

Methylprednisolone Sodium Succinate (Potential for additive hypokalemic effect with concurrent use).
No products indexed under this heading.

Metipranolol Hydrochloride (Beta receptor blocking agents and albuterol inhibit effect of each other). Products include:
OptiPranolol (Metipranolol 0.3%) Sterile Ophthalmic Solution ... ⊙ 256

Metoprolol Succinate (Beta receptor blocking agents and albuterol inhibit effect of each other). Products include:
Toprol-XL Tablets ... 560

Metoprolol Tartrate (Beta receptor blocking agents and albuterol inhibit effect of each other). Products include:
Lopressor ... 848
Lopressor HCT Tablets ... 850

Nadolol (Beta receptor blocking agents and albuterol inhibit effect of each other).
No products indexed under this heading.

Nortriptyline Hydrochloride (Action of albuterol on vascular system may be potentiated). Products include:
Pamelor ... 2409

Penbutolol Sulfate (Beta receptor blocking agents and albuterol inhibit effect of each other). Products include:
Levatol Tablets ... 2547

Phenelzine Sulfate (Action of albuterol on vascular system may be potentiated). Products include:
Nardil ... 1977

Phenylephrine Hydrochloride (Concomitant use of albuterol with oral sympathomimetic agents is not recommended due to the potential for cardiovascular toxicity). Products include:
Atrohist Plus Tablets ... 1605
Cerose DM ... ▣ 853
D.A. II Tablets ... 972
D.A. Chewable Tablets ... 970
Dura-Vent/DA Tablets ... 972
Extendryl ... 1003
4-Way Fast Acting Nasal Spray (regular & mentholated) ... ▣ 644
Hemorid ... ▣ 797
Hycomine Compound Tablets ... 948
Neo-Synephrine Hydrochloride 1% Carpuject ... 2455
Neo-Synephrine Hydrochloride 1% Injection ... 2455
Neo-Synephrine Hydrochloride (Ophthalmic) ... 2456
Neo-Synephrine ... ▣ 624
Novahistine Elixir ... ▣ 782
Phenergan VC ... 2886
Phenergan VC with Codeine ... 2888
Preparation H ... ▣ 842
Tympagesic Ear Drops ... 2476
Vicks Sinex Nasal Spray and Ultra Fine Mist ... ▣ 738

Phenylephrine Tannate (Concomitant use of albuterol with oral sympathomimetic agents is not recommended due to the potential for cardiovascular toxicity). Products include:
Atrohist Pediatric Suspension ... 1604
Atrohist Pediatric Suspension Dye-Free ... 1604
Rynatan ... 2781
Rynatuss ... 2782

Phenylpropanolamine Hydrochloride (Concomitant use of albuterol with oral sympathomimetic agents is not recommended due to the potential for cardiovascular toxicity). Products include:
Acutrim ... ▣ 648
Atrohist Plus Tablets ... 1605
BC Cold Powder Multi-Symptom Formula (Cold-Sinus-Allergy) ... ▣ 631
BC Cold Powder Non-Drowsy Formula (Cold-Sinus) ... ▣ 631
Cheracol Plus Head Cold/Cough Formula ... ▣ 741
Comtrex Multi-Symptom Cold Reliever Liqui-Gels ... ▣ 638
Comtrex Multi-Symptom Non-Drowsy Liqui-gels ... ▣ 640
Contac Continuous Action Nasal Decongestant/Antihistamine 12 Hour Capsules ... ▣ 773
Contac Maximum Strength Continuous Action Decongestant/Antihistamine 12 Hour Caplets ... ▣ 772
Contac Severe Cold and Flu Formula Caplets ... ▣ 773
Coricidin 'D' Decongestant Tablets ... ▣ 760
Dexatrim ... ▣ 795
Dexatrim Plus Vitamins Caplets ... ▣ 796
Dimetane-DC Cough Syrup ... 2232
Dimetapp Allergy Sinus Caplets ... ▣ 838
Dimetapp Cold & Allergy Chewable Tablets ... ▣ 838
Dimetapp Cold & Cough Liqui-Gels ... ▣ 839
Dimetapp DM Elixir ... ▣ 840
Dimetapp Elixir ... ▣ 840
Dimetapp Extentabs ... ▣ 841
Dimetapp Tablets/Liqui-Gels ... ▣ 841
Dura-Vent Tablets ... 971
Entex LA Tablets ... 972
Exgest LA Tablets ... 787
Hycomine ... 947
Nolamine Timed-Release Tablets ... 790
Ornade Spansule Capsules ... 2678
Propagest Tablets ... 791
Pyrroxate Caplets ... ▣ 742
Robitussin-CF ... ▣ 846
Sinulin Tablets ... 792
Tavist-D 12 Hour Relief Tablets ... ▣ 750
Teldrin 12 Hour Antihistamine/Nasal Decongestant Allergy Relief Capsules ... ▣ 786
Triaminic Expectorant ... ▣ 753
Triaminic Syrup ... ▣ 755
Triaminic Triaminicol Cold & Cough ... ▣ 756
Triaminic DM Syrup ... ▣ 756
Triaminicin Tablets ... ▣ 756
Vicks DayQuil Allergy Relief 12-Hour Extended Release Tablets ... ▣ 733
Vicks DayQuil Allergy Relief 4-Hour Tablets ... ▣ 733
Vicks DayQuil SINUS Pressure & CONGESTION Relief ... ▣ 734

Pindolol (Beta receptor blocking agents and albuterol inhibit effect of each other). Products include:
Visken Tablets ... 2428

Polythiazide (Potential for additive hypokalemic effect with concurrent use). Products include:
Minizide Capsules ... 2016

Prednisolone Acetate (Potential for additive hypokalemic effect with concurrent use). Products include:
AK-CIDE ... ⊙ 203
AK-CIDE Ointment ... ⊙ 203
Blephamide Liquifilm Sterile Ophthalmic Suspension ... 472
Blephamide Ointment ... ⊙ 234
Econopred & Econopred Plus Ophthalmic Suspensions ... ⊙ 216
Poly-Pred Liquifilm ... ⊙ 246
Pred Forte ... ⊙ 247
Pred Mild ... ⊙ 250
Pred-G Liquifilm Sterile Ophthalmic Suspension ... ⊙ 248
Pred-G S.O.P. Sterile Ophthalmic Ointment ... ⊙ 249

Prednisolone Sodium Phosphate (Potential for additive hypokalemic effect with concurrent use). Products include:
AK-PRED ... ⊙ 204
Hydeltrasol Injection, Sterile ... 1708
Pediapred Oral Solution ... 1618

Prednisolone Tebutate (Potential for additive hypokalemic effect with concurrent use). Products include:
Hydeltra-T.B.A. Sterile Suspension 1710

Prednisone (Potential for additive hypokalemic effect with concurrent use).
No products indexed under this heading.

(▣ Described in PDR For Nonprescription Drugs) (⊙ Described in PDR For Ophthalmology)

Propranolol Hydrochloride (Beta receptor blocking agents and albuterol inhibit effect of each other). Products include:

Inderal	2834
Inderal LA Long Acting Capsules	2836
Inderide Tablets	2838
Inderide LA Long Acting Capsules	2840

Protriptyline Hydrochloride (Action of albuterol on vascular system may be potentiated). Products include:

Vivactil Tablets	1820

Pseudoephedrine Hydrochloride (Concomitant use of albuterol with oral sympathomimetic agents is not recommended due to the potential for cardiovascular toxicity). Products include:

Actifed Allergy Daytime/Nighttime Caplets	808
Actifed Cold & Allergy Tablets	807
Actifed Cold & Sinus Caplets and Tablets	808
Actifed Sinus Daytime/Nighttime Tablets and Caplets	809
Advil Cold and Sinus Caplets and Tablets	837
Alka-Seltzer Plus Liqui-Gels	612
Alka-Seltzer Plus Flu & Body Aches Liqui-Gels Non-Drowsy Formula	613
Alka-Seltzer Plus Night-Time Cold Medicine Liqui-Gels	612
Allerest Maximum Strength	649
Allerest No Drowsiness	649
Allerest Sinus Pain Formula	649
Atrohist Pediatric Capsules	1603
Benadryl Allergy/Cold Tablets	811
Benadryl Allergy Decongestant Liquid Medication	812
Benadryl Allergy Decongestant Tablets	812
Benadryl Allergy Sinus Headache Caplets	813
Benylin Multisymptom	816
Bromfed Capsules (Extended-Release)	1832
Bromfed Syrup	712
Bromfed Tablets	1832
Bromfed-DM Cough Syrup	1832
Bromfed-PD Capsules (Extended-Release)	1832
Children's TYLENOL Cold Multi-Symptom Chewable Tablets and Liquid	1559
Children's TYLENOL Cold Plus Cough Multi Symptom Chewable Tablets and Liquid	1560
Children's TYLENOL Flu Suspension Liquid	1560
Children's Vicks DayQuil Allergy Relief	730
Children's Vicks NyQuil Cold/Cough Relief	731
Allergy-Sinus Comtrex Multi-Symptom Allergy-Sinus Formula Tablets and Caplets	639
Comtrex Multi-Symptom	638
Comtrex Multi-Symptom Non-Drowsy Caplets	640
Congess	1003
Contac Day Allergy/Sinus Caplets	771
Contac Day & Night	772
Contac Night Allergy/Sinus Caplets	771
Contac Severe Cold & Flu Non-Drowsy	774
Deconsal II Tablets	1605
Dimetane-DX Cough Syrup	2233
Dimetapp Cold & Fever Suspension	839
Dimetapp Decongestant Pediatric Drops	840
Dorcol Children's Cough Syrup	748
Drixoral Cough + Congestion Liquid Caps	763
Dura-Tap/PD Capsules	970
Duratuss Tablets	2750
Duratuss HD Elixir	2750
Efidac/24	655
Entex PSE Tablets	973
Fedahist Gyrocaps	2545
Guaifed	1833
Guaifed Syrup	712
Guaimax-D Tablets	809
Histussin D Liquid	670
Infants' TYLENOL Cold Decongestant & Fever-Reducer Drops	1561
Kronofed-A	994
Novahistine DMX	782
Nucofed	2225
PediaCare Cough-Cold Chewable Tablets and Liquid	1569
PediaCare Infants' Decongestant Drops	1569
PediaCare Infants' Drops Decongestant Plus Cough	1569
PediaCare NightRest Cough-Cold Liquid	1569
Pediatric Vicks 44d Cough & Head Congestion Relief	736
Pediatric Vicks 44m Cough & Cold Relief	737
Robitussin Cold & Cough Liqui-Gels	844
Robitussin Cold, Cough & Flu Liqui-Gels	844
Robitussin Maximum Strength Cough & Cold	847
Robitussin Night-Time Cold Formula	847
Robitussin Pediatric Cough & Cold Formula	848
Robitussin Pediatric Drops	849
Robitussin Severe Congestion Liqui-Gels	845
Robitussin-DAC Syrup	2249
Robitussin-PE	846
Rondec Oral Drops	974
Rondec Syrup	974
Rondec Tablet	974
Rondec Chewable Tablets	974
Rondec-TR Tablet	974
Ryna	804
Seldane-D Extended-Release Tablets	1286
Semprex-D Capsules	1620
Sinarest	663
Sine-Aid Maximum Strength Sinus Headache Gelcaps, Caplets and Tablets	1570
Sine-Off No Drowsiness Formula Caplets	784
Sine-Off Sinus Medicine	784
Singlet Tablets	785
Sinutab Non-Drying Liquid Caps	823
Sinutab Sinus Allergy Medication, Maximum Strength Tablets and Caplets	823
Sinutab Sinus Medication, Maximum Strength Without Drowsiness Formula, Tablets & Caplets	824
Sudafed Children's Cold & Cough Liquid Medication	825
Sudafed Children's Nasal Decongestant Liquid Medication	826
Sudafed Cold & Allergy Tablets	826
Sudafed Cold and Cough Liquid Caps	826
Sudafed Nasal Decongestant Tablets, 30 mg	825
Sudafed Nasal Decongestant Tablets, 60 mg	825
Sudafed Non-Drying Sinus Liquid Caps	827
Sudafed Pediatric Nasal Decongestant Liquid Oral Drops	827
Sudafed Severe Cold Formula Caplets	828
Sudafed Severe Cold Formula Tablets	828
Sudafed Sinus Caplets	829
Sudafed Sinus Tablets	829
Sudafed 12 Hour Caplets	824
Syn-Rx Tablets	1622
Syn-Rx DM Tablets	1623
TheraFlu Flu and Cold Medicine	750
Theraflu Maximum Strength Flu and Cold Medicine For Sore Throat	751
TheraFlu Flu, Cold and Cough Medicine	750
TheraFlu Maximum Strength Nighttime Flu, Cold & Cough Medicine	751
TheraFlu Maximum Strength Non-Drowsy Formula Flu, Cold & Cough Medicine	751
TheraFlu Maximum Strength, Non-Drowsy Formula Flu, Cold and Cough Caplets	752
Theraflu Maximum Strength Sinus Non-Drowsy Formula Caplets	752
Triaminic AM Cough and Decongestant Formula	753
Triaminic AM Decongestant Formula	753
Triaminic Infant Oral Decongestant Drops	754
Triaminic Night Time	754
Triaminic Sore Throat Formula	755
Tussend	1830
Tussend Expectorant	1831
TYLENOL Allergy Sinus, Maximum Strength Caplets and Gelcaps	1571
TYLENOL Allergy Sinus NightTime, Maximum Strength Caplets	1571
TYLENOL Cold Medication, Multi-Symptom Formula Tablets and Caplets	1572
TYLENOL Cold Medication, Multi-Symptom Hot Liquid Packets	1572
TYLENOL Cold Medication, No Drowsiness Formula Caplets and Gelcaps	1572
TYLENOL Cold Severe Congestion Caplets	1573
TYLENOL Cough Medication with Decongestant, Multi Symptom	1574
TYLENOL Flu No Drowsiness Formula, Maximum Strength Gelcaps	1575
TYLENOL Flu NightTime, Maximum Strength Gelcaps	1575
TYLENOL Flu NightTime, Maximum Strength Hot Medication Packets	1575
TYLENOL Sinus, Maximum Strength Geltabs, Gelcaps, Caplets and Tablets	1576
Vicks 44 LiquiCaps Cough, Cold & Flu Relief	728
Vicks 44 LiquiCaps Non-Drowsy Cough & Cold Relief	729
Vicks 44D Cough & Head Congestion Relief	728
Vicks 44M Cough, Cold & Flu Relief	729
Vicks DayQuil LiquiCaps/Liquid Multi-Symptom Cold/Flu Relief	734
Vicks DayQuil SINUS Pressure & PAIN Relief with IBUPROFEN	735
Vicks Nyquil Hot Therapy	735
Vicks NyQuil LiquiCaps/Liquid Multi-Symptom Cold/Flu Relief, Original and Cherry Flavors	736

Pseudoephedrine Sulfate (Concomitant use of albuterol with oral sympathomimetic agents is not recommended due to the potential for cardiovascular toxicity). Products include:

Chlor-Trimeton Allergy Decongestant Tablets	759
Claritin-D Tablets	2487
Drixoral Cold and Allergy Sustained-Action Tablets	763
Drixoral Cold and Flu Extended-Release Tablets	764
Drixoral Non-Drowsy Formula Extended-Release Tablets	764
Drixoral Allergy/Sinus Extended Release Tablets	765
Trinalin Repetabs Tablets	1373

Selegiline Hydrochloride (Action of albuterol on vascular system may be potentiated). Products include:

Eldepryl Capsules	2729

Sotalol Hydrochloride (Beta receptor blocking agents and albuterol inhibit effect of each other). Products include:

Betapace Tablets	637

Terbutaline Sulfate (Concomitant use of albuterol with oral sympathomimetic agents is not recommended due to the potential for cardiovascular toxicity). Products include:

Brethaire Inhaler	830
Brethine Ampuls	832
Brethine Tablets	831
Bricanyl Subcutaneous Injection	1247
Bricanyl Tablets	1248

Timolol Hemihydrate (Beta receptor blocking agents and albuterol inhibit effect of each other). Products include:

Betimol 0.25%, 0.5%	259

Timolol Maleate (Beta receptor blocking agents and albuterol inhibit effect of each other). Products include:

Blocadren Tablets	1654
Timolide Tablets	1791
Timoptic in Ocudose	1796
Timoptic Sterile Ophthalmic Solution	1794
Timoptic-XE	1798

Tranylcypromine Sulfate (Action of albuterol on vascular system may be potentiated). Products include:

Parnate Tablets	2679

Triamcinolone (Potential for additive hypokalemic effect with concurrent use).

No products indexed under this heading.

Triamcinolone Acetonide (Potential for additive hypokalemic effect with concurrent use). Products include:

Azmacort Oral Inhaler	2175
Nasacort AQ Nasal Spray	2191
Nasacort Nasal Inhaler	2189

Triamcinolone Diacetate (Potential for additive hypokalemic effect with concurrent use).

No products indexed under this heading.

Triamcinolone Hexacetonide (Potential for additive hypokalemic effect with concurrent use).

No products indexed under this heading.

Trimipramine Maleate (Action of albuterol on vascular system may be potentiated). Products include:

Surmontil Capsules	2917

VENTOLIN TABLETS (Albuterol Sulfate) ... 1176

May interact with sympathomimetics, monoamine oxidase inhibitors, beta blockers, and tricyclic antidepressants. Compounds in these categories include:

Acebutolol Hydrochloride (Beta-receptor blocking agents and albuterol inhibit effect of each other). Products include:

Sectral Capsules	2914

Amitriptyline Hydrochloride (Action of albuterol on the vascular system may be potentiated). Products include:

Elavil	2945
Etrafon	2495
Limbitrol	2333
Triavil Tablets	1800

Amoxapine (Action of albuterol on the vascular system may be potentiated). Products include:

Asendin Tablets	1419

Atenolol (Beta-receptor blocking agents and albuterol inhibit effect of each other). Products include:

Tenoretic Tablets	2963
Tenormin Tablets and I.V. Injection	2965

Betaxolol Hydrochloride (Beta-receptor blocking agents and albuterol inhibit effect of each other). Products include:

Betoptic Ophthalmic Solution	465
Betoptic S Ophthalmic Suspension	467
Kerlone Tablets	2588

Bisoprolol Fumarate (Beta-receptor blocking agents and albuterol inhibit effect of each other). Products include:

Zebeta Tablets	1457
Ziac	1459

Carteolol Hydrochloride (Beta-receptor blocking agents and albuterol inhibit effect of each other). Products include:

Cartrol Tablets	413
Ocupress Ophthalmic Solution, 1% Sterile	297

IMPORTANT NOTE: Always consult each drug listing in the patient's regimen for possible interactions.

Ventolin Tablets | Interactions Index | 1162

Clomipramine Hydrochloride (Action of albuterol on the vascular system may be potentiated). Products include:
- Anafranil Capsules ... 819

Desipramine Hydrochloride (Action of albuterol on the vascular system may be potentiated). Products include:
- Norpramin Tablets ... 1273

Dobutamine Hydrochloride (Concomitant use of albuterol with oral sympathomimetic agents is not recommended due to potential for cardiovascular toxicity). Products include:
- Dobutrex Solution Vials ... 1480

Dopamine Hydrochloride (Concomitant use of albuterol with oral sympathomimetic agents is not recommended due to potential for cardiovascular toxicity).
- No products indexed under this heading.

Doxepin Hydrochloride (Action of albuterol on the vascular system may be potentiated). Products include:
- Adapin Capsules ... 1542
- Sinequan ... 2028
- Zonalon Cream ... 1042

Ephedrine Hydrochloride (Concomitant use of albuterol with oral sympathomimetic agents is not recommended due to potential for cardiovascular toxicity). Products include:
- Primatene Tablets ... ▣ 844
- Quadrinal Tablets ... 1398

Ephedrine Sulfate (Concomitant use of albuterol with oral sympathomimetic agents is not recommended due to potential for cardiovascular toxicity). Products include:
- Marax Tablets & DF Syrup ... 2015

Ephedrine Tannate (Concomitant use of albuterol with oral sympathomimetic agents is not recommended due to potential for cardiovascular toxicity). Products include:
- Rynatuss ... 2782

Esmolol Hydrochloride (Beta-receptor blocking agents and albuterol inhibit effect of each other). Products include:
- Brevibloc (esmolol HCl) Injection ... 1860

Furazolidone (Action of albuterol on the vascular system may be potentiated). Products include:
- Furoxone ... 2221

Imipramine Hydrochloride (Action of albuterol on the vascular system may be potentiated). Products include:
- Tofranil Ampuls ... 873
- Tofranil Tablets ... 875

Imipramine Pamoate (Action of albuterol on the vascular system may be potentiated). Products include:
- Tofranil-PM Capsules ... 876

Isocarboxazid (Action of albuterol on the vascular system may be potentiated).
- No products indexed under this heading.

Labetalol Hydrochloride (Beta-receptor blocking agents and albuterol inhibit effect of each other). Products include:
- Normodyne Injection ... 2519
- Normodyne Tablets ... 2522
- Trandate ... 1158

Levobunolol Hydrochloride (Beta-receptor blocking agents and albuterol inhibit effect of each other). Products include:
- Betagan ... ⊙ 230

Maprotiline Hydrochloride (Action of albuterol on the vascular system may be potentiated). Products include:
- Ludiomil Tablets ... 861

Metaproterenol Sulfate (Concomitant use of albuterol with oral sympathomimetic agents is not recommended due to potential for cardiovascular toxicity). Products include:
- Alupent ... 672
- Metaproterenol Sulfate Inhalation Solution, USP, Arm-a-Med ... 547

Metaraminol Bitartrate (Concomitant use of albuterol with oral sympathomimetic agents is not recommended due to potential for cardiovascular toxicity). Products include:
- Aramine Injection ... 1649

Metipranolol Hydrochloride (Beta-receptor blocking agents and albuterol inhibit effect of each other). Products include:
- OptiPranolol (Metipranolol 0.3%) Sterile Ophthalmic Solution ... ⊙ 256

Metoprolol Succinate (Beta-receptor blocking agents and albuterol inhibit effect of each other). Products include:
- Toprol-XL Tablets ... 560

Metoprolol Tartrate (Beta-receptor blocking agents and albuterol inhibit effect of each other). Products include:
- Lopressor ... 848
- Lopressor HCT Tablets ... 850

Nadolol (Beta-receptor blocking agents and albuterol inhibit effect of each other).
- No products indexed under this heading.

Nortriptyline Hydrochloride (Action of albuterol on the vascular system may be potentiated). Products include:
- Pamelor ... 2409

Penbutolol Sulfate (Beta-receptor blocking agents and albuterol inhibit effect of each other). Products include:
- Levatol Tablets ... 2547

Phenelzine Sulfate (Action of albuterol on the vascular system may be potentiated). Products include:
- Nardil ... 1977

Phenylephrine Bitartrate (Concomitant use of albuterol with oral sympathomimetic agents is not recommended due to potential for cardiovascular toxicity).
- No products indexed under this heading.

Phenylephrine Hydrochloride (Concomitant use of albuterol with oral sympathomimetic agents is not recommended due to potential for cardiovascular toxicity). Products include:
- Atrohist Plus Tablets ... 1605
- Cerose DM ... ▣ 853
- D.A. II Tablets ... 972
- D.A. Chewable Tablets ... 970
- Dura-Vent/DA Tablets ... 972
- Extendryl ... 1003
- 4-Way Fast Acting Nasal Spray (regular & mentholated) ... ▣ 644
- Hemorid ... ▣ 797
- Hycomine Compound Tablets ... 948
- Neo-Synephrine Hydrochloride 1% Carpuject ... 2455
- Neo-Synephrine Hydrochloride 1% Injection ... 2455
- Neo-Synephrine Hydrochloride (Ophthalmic) ... 2456
- Neo-Synephrine ... ▣ 624
- Novahistine Elixir ... ▣ 782
- Phenergan VC ... 2886
- Phenergan VC with Codeine ... 2888
- Preparation H ... ▣ 842
- Tympagesic Ear Drops ... 2476
- Vicks Sinex Nasal Spray and Ultra Fine Mist ... ▣ 738

Phenylephrine Tannate (Concomitant use of albuterol with oral sympathomimetic agents is not recommended due to potential for cardiovascular toxicity). Products include:
- Atrohist Pediatric Suspension ... 1604
- Atrohist Pediatric Suspension Dye-Free ... 1604
- Rynatan ... 2781
- Rynatuss ... 2782

Phenylpropanolamine Hydrochloride (Concomitant use of albuterol with oral sympathomimetic agents is not recommended due to potential for cardiovascular toxicity). Products include:
- Acutrim ... ▣ 648
- Atrohist Plus Tablets ... 1605
- BC Cold Powder Multi-Symptom Formula (Cold-Sinus-Allergy) ... ▣ 631
- BC Cold Powder Non-Drowsy Formula (Cold-Sinus) ... ▣ 631
- Cheracol Plus Head Cold/Cough Formula ... ▣ 741
- Comtrex Multi-Symptom Cold Reliever Liqui-Gels ... ▣ 638
- Comtrex Multi-Symptom Non-Drowsy Liqui-gels ... ▣ 640
- Contac Continuous Action Nasal Decongestant/Antihistamine 12 Hour Capsules ... ▣ 773
- Contac Maximum Strength Continuous Action Decongestant/Antihistamine 12 Hour Caplets ... ▣ 772
- Contac Severe Cold and Flu Formula Caplets ... ▣ 773
- Coricidin 'D' Decongestant Tablets ... ▣ 760
- Dexatrim ... ▣ 795
- Dexatrim Plus Vitamins Caplets ... ▣ 796
- Dimetane-DC Cough Syrup ... 2232
- Dimetapp Allergy Sinus Caplets ... ▣ 838
- Dimetapp Cold & Allergy Chewable Tablets ... ▣ 838
- Dimetapp Cold & Cough Liqui-Gels ... ▣ 839
- Dimetapp DM Elixir ... ▣ 840
- Dimetapp Elixir ... ▣ 840
- Dimetapp Extentabs ... ▣ 841
- Dimetapp Tablets/Liqui-Gels ... ▣ 841
- Dura-Vent Tablets ... 971
- Entex LA Tablets ... 972
- Exgest LA Tablets ... 787
- Hycomine ... 947
- Nolamine Timed-Release Tablets ... 790
- Ornade Spansule Capsules ... 2678
- Propagest Tablets ... 791
- Pyrroxate Caplets ... ▣ 742
- Robitussin-CF ... ▣ 846
- Sinulin Tablets ... 792
- Tavist-D 12 Hour Relief Tablets ... ▣ 750
- Teldrin 12 Hour Antihistamine/Nasal Decongestant Allergy Relief Capsules ... ▣ 786
- Triaminic Expectorant ... ▣ 753
- Triaminic Syrup ... ▣ 755
- Triaminic Triaminicol Cold & Cough ... ▣ 756
- Triaminic DM Syrup ... ▣ 756
- Triaminicin Tablets ... ▣ 756
- Vicks DayQuil Allergy Relief 12-Hour Extended Release Tablets ... ▣ 733
- Vicks DayQuil Allergy Relief 4-Hour Tablets ... ▣ 733
- Vicks DayQuil SINUS Pressure & CONGESTION Relief ... ▣ 734

Pindolol (Beta-receptor blocking agents and albuterol inhibit effect of each other). Products include:
- Visken Tablets ... 2428

Pirbuterol Acetate (Concomitant use of albuterol with oral sympathomimetic agents is not recommended due to potential for cardiovascular toxicity). Products include:
- Maxair Autohaler ... 1550
- Maxair Inhaler ... 1552

Propranolol Hydrochloride (Beta-receptor blocking agents and albuterol inhibit effect of each other). Products include:
- Inderal ... 2834
- Inderal LA Long Acting Capsules ... 2836
- Inderide Tablets ... 2838
- Inderide LA Long Acting Capsules ... 2840

Protriptyline Hydrochloride (Action of albuterol on the vascular system may be potentiated). Products include:
- Vivactil Tablets ... 1820

Pseudoephedrine Hydrochloride (Concomitant use of albuterol with oral sympathomimetic agents is not recommended due to potential for cardiovascular toxicity). Products include:
- Actifed Allergy Daytime/Nighttime Caplets ... ▣ 808
- Actifed Cold & Allergy Tablets ... ▣ 807
- Actifed Cold & Sinus Caplets and Tablets ... ▣ 808
- Actifed Sinus Daytime/Nighttime Tablets and Caplets ... ▣ 809
- Advil Cold and Sinus Caplets and Tablets ... ▣ 837
- Alka-Seltzer Plus Liqui-Gels ... ▣ 612
- Alka-Seltzer Plus Flu & Body Aches Liqui-Gels Non-Drowsy Formula ... ▣ 613
- Alka-Seltzer Plus Night-Time Cold Medicine Liqui-Gels ... ▣ 612
- Allerest Maximum Strength ... ▣ 649
- Allerest No Drowsiness ... ▣ 649
- Allerest Sinus Pain Formula ... ▣ 649
- Atrohist Pediatric Capsules ... 1603
- Benadryl Allergy/Cold Tablets ... ▣ 811
- Benadryl Allergy Decongestant Liquid Medication ... ▣ 812
- Benadryl Allergy Decongestant Tablets ... ▣ 812
- Benadryl Allergy Sinus Headache Caplets ... ▣ 813
- Benylin Multisymptom ... ▣ 816
- Bromfed Capsules (Extended-Release) ... 1832
- Bromfed Syrup ... ▣ 712
- Bromfed Tablets ... 1832
- Bromfed-DM Cough Syrup ... 1832
- Bromfed-PD Capsules (Extended-Release) ... 1832
- Children's TYLENOL Cold Multi-Symptom Chewable Tablets and Liquid ... 1559
- Children's TYLENOL Cold Plus Cough Multi Symptom Chewable Tablets and Liquid ... 1560
- Children's TYLENOL Flu Suspension Liquid ... 1560
- Children's Vicks DayQuil Allergy Relief ... ▣ 730
- Children's Vicks NyQuil Cold/Cough Relief ... ▣ 731
- Allergy-Sinus Comtrex Multi-Symptom Allergy-Sinus Formula Tablets and Caplets ... ▣ 639
- Comtrex Multi-Symptom ... ▣ 638
- Comtrex Multi-Symptom Non-Drowsy Caplets ... ▣ 640
- Congess ... 1003
- Contac Day Allergy/Sinus Caplets ... ▣ 771
- Contac Day & Night ... ▣ 772
- Contac Night Allergy/Sinus Caplets ... ▣ 771
- Contac Severe Cold & Flu Non-Drowsy ... ▣ 774
- Deconsal II Tablets ... 1605
- Dimetane-DX Cough Syrup ... 2233
- Dimetapp Cold & Fever Suspension ... ▣ 839
- Dimetapp Decongestant Pediatric Drops ... ▣ 840
- Dorcol Children's Cough Syrup ... ▣ 748
- Drixoral Cough + Congestion Liquid Caps ... ▣ 763
- Dura-Tap/PD Capsules ... 970
- Duratuss Tablets ... 2750
- Duratuss HD Elixir ... 2750
- Efidac/24 ... ▣ 655
- Entex PSE Tablets ... 973
- Fedahist Gyrocaps ... 2545
- Guaifed ... 1833
- Guaifed Syrup ... ▣ 712
- Guaimax-D Tablets ... 809
- Histussin D Liquid ... 670
- Infants' TYLENOL Cold Decongestant & Fever-Reducer Drops ... 1561
- Kronofed-A ... 994
- Novahistine DMX ... ▣ 782
- Nucofed ... 2225
- PediaCare Cough-Cold Chewable Tablets and Liquid ... 1569

(▣ Described in PDR For Nonprescription Drugs) (⊙ Described in PDR For Ophthalmology)

PediaCare Infants' Decongestant Drops ... 1569
PediaCare Infants' Drops Decongestant Plus Cough ... 1569
PediaCare NightRest Cough-Cold Liquid ... 1569
Pediatric Vicks 44d Cough & Head Congestion Relief ... 736
Pediatric Vicks 44m Cough & Cold Relief ... 737
Robitussin Cold & Cough Liqui-Gels ... 844
Robitussin Cold, Cough & Flu Liqui-Gels ... 844
Robitussin Maximum Strength Cough & Cold ... 847
Robitussin Night-Time Cold Formula ... 847
Robitussin Pediatric Cough & Cold Formula ... 848
Robitussin Pediatric Drops ... 849
Robitussin Severe Congestion Liqui-Gels ... 845
Robitussin-DAC Syrup ... 2249
Robitussin-PE ... 846
Rondec Oral Drops ... 974
Rondec Syrup ... 974
Rondec Tablet ... 974
Rondec Chewable Tablets ... 974
Rondec-TR Tablet ... 974
Ryna ... 804
Seldane-D Extended-Release Tablets ... 1286
Semprex-D Capsules ... 1620
Sinarest ... 663
Sine-Aid Maximum Strength Sinus Headache Gelcaps, Caplets and Tablets ... 1570
Sine-Off No Drowsiness Formula Caplets ... 784
Sine-Off Sinus Medicine ... 784
Singlet Tablets ... 785
Sinutab Non-Drying Liquid Caps ... 823
Sinutab Sinus Allergy Medication, Maximum Strength Tablets and Caplets ... 823
Sinutab Sinus Medication, Maximum Strength Without Drowsiness Formula, Tablets & Caplets ... 824
Sudafed Children's Cold & Cough Liquid Medication ... 825
Sudafed Children's Nasal Decongestant Liquid Medication ... 826
Sudafed Cold & Allergy Tablets ... 826
Sudafed Cold and Cough Liquid Caps ... 826
Sudafed Nasal Decongestant Tablets, 30 mg ... 825
Sudafed Nasal Decongestant Tablets, 60 mg ... 825
Sudafed Non-Drying Sinus Liquid Caps ... 827
Sudafed Pediatric Nasal Decongestant Liquid Oral Drops ... 827
Sudafed Severe Cold Formula Caplets ... 828
Sudafed Severe Cold Formula Tablets ... 828
Sudafed Sinus Caplets ... 829
Sudafed Sinus Tablets ... 829
Sudafed 12 Hour Caplets ... 824
Syn-Rx Tablets ... 1622
Syn-Rx DM Tablets ... 1623
TheraFlu Flu and Cold Medicine ... 750
Theraflu Maximum Strength Flu and Cold Medicine For Sore Throat ... 751
TheraFlu Flu, Cold and Cough Medicine ... 750
TheraFlu Maximum Strength Nighttime Flu, Cold & Cough Medicine ... 751
TheraFlu Maximum Strength Non-Drowsy Formula Flu, Cold & Cough Medicine ... 751
TheraFlu Maximum Strength, Non-Drowsy Formula Flu, Cold and Cough Caplets ... 752
Theraflu Maximum Strength Sinus Non-Drowsy Formula Caplets ... 752
Triaminic AM Cough and Decongestant Formula ... 753
Triaminic AM Decongestant Formula ... 753
Triaminic Infant Oral Decongestant Drops ... 754
Triaminic Night Time ... 754
Triaminic Sore Throat Formula ... 755
Tussend ... 1830

Tussend Expectorant ... 1831
TYLENOL Allergy Sinus, Maximum Strength Caplets and Gelcaps ... 1571
TYLENOL Allergy Sinus NightTime, Maximum Strength Caplets ... 1571
TYLENOL Cold Medication, Multi-Symptom Formula Tablets and Caplets ... 1572
TYLENOL Cold Medication, Multi-Symptom Hot Liquid Packets ... 1572
TYLENOL Cold Medication, No Drowsiness Formula Caplets and Gelcaps ... 1572
TYLENOL Cold Severe Congestion Caplets ... 1573
TYLENOL Cough Medication with Decongestant, Multi Symptom ... 1574
TYLENOL Flu No Drowsiness Formula, Maximum Strength Gelcaps ... 1575
TYLENOL Flu NightTime, Maximum Strength Gelcaps ... 1575
TYLENOL Flu NightTime, Maximum Strength Hot Medication Packets ... 1575
TYLENOL Sinus, Maximum Strength Geltabs, Gelcaps, Caplets and Tablets ... 1576
Vicks 44 LiquiCaps Cough, Cold & Flu Relief ... 728
Vicks 44 LiquiCaps Non-Drowsy Cough & Cold Relief ... 729
Vicks 44D Cough & Head Congestion Relief ... 728
Vicks 44M Cough, Cold & Flu Relief ... 729
Vicks DayQuil LiquiCaps/Liquid Multi-Symptom Cold/Flu Relief .. 734
Vicks DayQuil SINUS Pressure & PAIN Relief with IBUPROFEN ... 735
Vicks Nyquil Hot Therapy ... 735
Vicks NyQuil LiquiCaps/Liquid Multi-Symptom Cold/Flu Relief, Original and Cherry Flavors ... 736

Pseudoephedrine Sulfate (Concomitant use of albuterol with oral sympathomimetic agents is not recommended due to potential for cardiovascular toxicity). Products include:
Chlor-Trimeton Allergy Decongestant Tablets ... 759
Claritin-D Tablets ... 2487
Drixoral Cold and Allergy Sustained-Action Tablets ... 763
Drixoral Cold and Flu Extended-Release Tablets ... 764
Drixoral Non-Drowsy Formula Extended-Release Tablets ... 764
Drixoral Allergy/Sinus Extended Release Tablets ... 765
Trinalin Repetabs Tablets ... 1373

Salmeterol Xinafoate (Concomitant use of albuterol with oral sympathomimetic agents is not recommended due to potential for cardiovascular toxicity). Products include:
Serevent Inhalation Aerosol ... 1149

Selegiline Hydrochloride (Action of albuterol on the vascular system may be potentiated). Products include:
Eldepryl Capsules ... 2729

Sotalol Hydrochloride (Beta-receptor blocking agents and albuterol inhibit effect of each other). Products include:
Betapace Tablets ... 637

Terbutaline Sulfate (Concomitant use of albuterol with oral sympathomimetic agents is not recommended due to potential for cardiovascular toxicity). Products include:
Brethaire Inhaler ... 830
Brethine Ampuls ... 832
Brethine Tablets ... 831
Bricanyl Subcutaneous Injection ... 1247
Bricanyl Tablets ... 1248

Timolol Hemihydrate (Beta-receptor blocking agents and albuterol inhibit effect of each other). Products include:
Betimol 0.25%, 0.5% ... 259

Timolol Maleate (Beta-receptor blocking agents and albuterol inhibit effect of each other). Products include:
Blocadren Tablets ... 1654
Timolide Tablets ... 1791
Timoptic in Ocudose ... 1796
Timoptic Sterile Ophthalmic Solution ... 1794
Timoptic-XE ... 1798

Tranylcypromine Sulfate (Action of albuterol on the vascular system may be potentiated). Products include:
Parnate Tablets ... 2679

Trimipramine Maleate (Action of albuterol on the vascular system may be potentiated). Products include:
Surmontil Capsules ... 2917

VEPESID CAPSULES AND INJECTION
(Etoposide) ... 727
None cited in PDR database.

VERELAN CAPSULES
(Verapamil Hydrochloride) ... 1455
May interact with antihypertensives, ACE inhibitors, beta blockers, cardiac glycosides, quinidine, lithium preparations, inhalant anesthetics, neuromuscular blocking agents, and certain other agents. Compounds in these categories include:

Acebutolol Hydrochloride (Concomitant therapy may result in additive negative effects on heart rate, AV conduction, and/or cardiac contractility; excessive bradycardia and AV block has been reported with concurrent use in hypertensive patients; possible additive effect on blood pressure). Products include:
Sectral Capsules ... 2914

Amlodipine Besylate (Co-administration with oral antihypertensive agents will usually have an additive effect on lowering blood pressure). Products include:
Lotrel Capsules ... 858
Norvasc Tablets ... 2020

Atenolol (Concomitant therapy may result in additive negative effects on heart rate, AV conduction, and/or cardiac contractility; excessive bradycardia and AV block has been reported with concurrent use in hypertensive patients; possible additive effect on blood pressure). Products include:
Tenoretic Tablets ... 2963
Tenormin Tablets and I.V. Injection ... 2965

Atracurium Besylate (Verapamil may potentiate the activity of neuromuscular blocking drugs). Products include:
Tracrium Injection ... 1155

Benazepril Hydrochloride (Co-administration with oral antihypertensive agents will usually have an additive effect on lowering blood pressure). Products include:
Lotensin Tablets ... 852
Lotensin HCT Tablets ... 855
Lotrel Capsules ... 858

Bendroflumethiazide (Co-administration with oral antihypertensive agents will usually have an additive effect on lowering blood pressure).
No products indexed under this heading.

Betaxolol Hydrochloride (Concomitant therapy may result in additive negative effects on heart rate, AV conduction, and/or cardiac contractility; excessive bradycardia and AV block has been reported with concurrent use in hypertensive patients; possible additive effect on blood pressure). Products include:
Betoptic Ophthalmic Solution ... 465
Betoptic S Ophthalmic Suspension ... 467
Kerlone Tablets ... 2588

Bisoprolol Fumarate (Concomitant therapy may result in additive negative effects on heart rate, AV conduction, and/or cardiac contractility; excessive bradycardia and AV block has been reported with concurrent use in hypertensive patients; possible additive effect on blood pressure). Products include:
Zebeta Tablets ... 1457
Ziac ... 1459

Captopril (Co-administration with oral antihypertensive agents will usually have an additive effect on lowering blood pressure). Products include:
Capoten Tablets ... 740
Capozide Tablets ... 744

Carbamazepine (Verapamil therapy may increase carbamazepine concentrations during combined therapy resulting in side effects such as diplopia, headache, ataxia, or dizziness). Products include:
Atretol Tablets ... 569
Tegretol/Tegretol-XR ... 870

Carteolol Hydrochloride (Concomitant therapy may result in additive negative effects on heart rate, AV conduction, and/or cardiac contractility; excessive bradycardia and AV block has been reported with concurrent use in hypertensive patients; possible additive effect on blood pressure). Products include:
Cartrol Tablets ... 413
Ocupress Ophthalmic Solution, 1% Sterile ... 297

Chlorothiazide (Co-administration with oral antihypertensive agents will usually have an additive effect on lowering blood pressure). Products include:
Aldoclor Tablets ... 1638
Diupres Tablets ... 1691
Diuril Oral ... 1694

Chlorothiazide Sodium (Co-administration with oral antihypertensive agents will usually have an additive effect on lowering blood pressure). Products include:
Diuril Sodium Intravenous ... 1693

Chlorthalidone (Co-administration with oral antihypertensive agents will usually have an additive effect on lowering blood pressure). Products include:
Combipres Tablets ... 682
Tenoretic Tablets ... 2963
Thalitone ... 1293

Cimetidine (Variable results on verapamil clearance acute studies, either reduced or unchanged). Products include:
Tagamet HB Tablets ... 786
Tagamet Tablets ... 2694

Cimetidine Hydrochloride (Variable results on verapamil clearance acute studies, either reduced or unchanged). Products include:
Tagamet ... 2694

Cisatracurium Besylate (Verapamil may potentiate the activity of neuromuscular blocking drugs). Products include:
Nimbex Injection ... 1131

IMPORTANT NOTE: Always consult each drug listing in the patient's regimen for possible interactions.

Clonidine (Co-administration with oral antihypertensive agents will usually have an additive effect on lowering blood pressure). Products include:

- Catapres-TTS ... 680

Clonidine Hydrochloride (Co-administration with oral antihypertensive agents will usually have an additive effect on lowering blood pressure). Products include:

- Catapres Tablets ... 679
- Combipres Tablets ... 682

Cyclosporine (Verapamil therapy may increase serum levels of cyclosporine). Products include:

- Neoral ... 2405
- Sandimmune ... 2416

Deserpidine (Co-administration with oral antihypertensive agents will usually have an additive effect on lowering blood pressure).

No products indexed under this heading.

Desflurane (Potential for excessive cardiovascular depression based on animal studies). Products include:

- Suprane (desflurane, USP) ... 1865

Deslanoside (Chronic verapamil treatment can increase serum digoxin levels by 50% to 70% resulting in digitalis toxicity; influence on digoxin kinetics is magnified in hepatic cirrhosis patients).

No products indexed under this heading.

Diazoxide (Co-administration with oral antihypertensive agents will usually have an additive effect on lowering blood pressure). Products include:

- Hyperstat I.V. Injection ... 2504
- Proglycem ... 575

Digitoxin (Chronic verapamil treatment can increase serum digoxin levels by 50% to 70% resulting in digitalis toxicity; influence on digoxin kinetics is magnified in hepatic cirrhosis patients). Products include:

- Crystodigin Tablets ... 1472

Digoxin (Chronic verapamil treatment can increase serum digoxin levels by 50% to 70% resulting in digitalis toxicity; influence on digoxin kinetics is magnified in hepatic cirrhosis patients). Products include:

- Lanoxicaps ... 1110
- Lanoxin Elixir Pediatric ... 1113
- Lanoxin Injection ... 1116
- Lanoxin Injection Pediatric ... 1119
- Lanoxin Tablets ... 1121

Diltiazem Hydrochloride (Co-administration with oral antihypertensive agents will usually have an additive effect on lowering blood pressure). Products include:

- Cardizem CD Capsules ... 1251
- Cardizem SR Capsules ... 1255
- Cardizem Injectable ... 1253
- Cardizem Tablets ... 1257
- Dilacor XR Extended-release Capsules ... 2183
- Tiazac Capsules ... 1019

Disopyramide Phosphate (Disopyramide should not be administered within 48 hours before or 24 hours after verapamil administration). Products include:

- Norpace ... 2596

Doxacurium Chloride (Verapamil may potentiate the activity of neuromuscular blocking drugs). Products include:

- Nuromax Injection ... 1136

Doxazosin Mesylate (Concomitant use of agents that attenuate alpha-adrenergic function, such as doxazosin, may result in excessive reduction in blood pressure). Products include:

- Cardura Tablets ... 1993

Enalapril Maleate (Co-administration with oral antihypertensive agents will usually have an additive effect on lowering blood pressure). Products include:

- Vaseretic Tablets ... 1810
- Vasotec Tablets ... 1816

Enalaprilat (Co-administration with oral antihypertensive agents will usually have an additive effect on lowering blood pressure). Products include:

- Vasotec I.V. ... 1814

Enflurane (Potential for excessive cardiovascular depression based on animal studies).

No products indexed under this heading.

Esmolol Hydrochloride (Concomitant therapy may result in additive negative effects on heart rate, AV conduction, and/or cardiac contractility; excessive bradycardia and AV block has been reported with concurrent use in hypertensive patients; possible additive effect on blood pressure). Products include:

- Brevibloc (esmolol HCl) Injection ... 1860

Felodipine (Co-administration with oral antihypertensive agents will usually have an additive effect on lowering blood pressure). Products include:

- Plendil Extended-Release Tablets ... 514

Flecainide Acetate (Co-administration may have additive effects on myocardial contractility, AV conduction, and repolarization). Products include:

- Tambocor Tablets ... 1555

Fosinopril Sodium (Co-administration with oral antihypertensive agents will usually have an additive effect on lowering blood pressure). Products include:

- Monopril Tablets ... 762

Furosemide (Co-administration with oral antihypertensive agents will usually have an additive effect on lowering blood pressure). Products include:

- Lasix Injection, Oral Solution and Tablets ... 1267

Guanabenz Acetate (Co-administration with oral antihypertensive agents will usually have an additive effect on lowering blood pressure).

No products indexed under this heading.

Guanethidine Monosulfate (Co-administration with oral antihypertensive agents will usually have an additive effect on lowering blood pressure). Products include:

- Esimil Tablets ... 840
- Ismelin Tablets ... 845

Halothane (Potential for excessive cardiovascular depression based on animal studies). Products include:

- Fluothane ... 2830

Hydralazine Hydrochloride (Co-administration with oral antihypertensive agents will usually have an additive effect on lowering blood pressure). Products include:

- Apresazide Capsules ... 824
- Apresoline Hydrochloride Tablets ... 826
- Hydralazine Hydrochloride Injection USP ... 2712
- Ser-Ap-Es Tablets ... 867

Hydrochlorothiazide (Co-administration with oral antihypertensive agents will usually have an additive effect on lowering blood pressure). Products include:

- Aldactazide Tablets ... 2556
- Aldoril Tablets ... 1644
- Apresazide Capsules ... 824
- Capozide Tablets ... 744
- Dyazide Capsules ... 2653
- Esidrix Tablets ... 839
- Esimil Tablets ... 840
- HydroDIURIL Tablets ... 1716
- Hydropres Tablets ... 1718
- Hyzaar Tablets ... 1720
- Inderide Tablets ... 2838
- Inderide LA Long Acting Capsules ... 2840
- Lopressor HCT Tablets ... 850
- Lotensin HCT Tablets ... 855
- Moduretic Tablets ... 1748
- Oretic Tablets ... 450
- Prinzide Tablets ... 1780
- Ser-Ap-Es Tablets ... 867
- Timolide Tablets ... 1791
- Vaseretic Tablets ... 1810
- Zestoretic Tablets ... 2968
- Ziac ... 1459

Hydroflumethiazide (Co-administration with oral antihypertensive agents will usually have an additive effect on lowering blood pressure). Products include:

- Diucardin Tablets ... 2824

Indapamide (Co-administration with oral antihypertensive agents will usually have an additive effect on lowering blood pressure).

No products indexed under this heading.

Isoflurane (Potential for excessive cardiovascular depression based on animal studies).

No products indexed under this heading.

Isradipine (Co-administration with oral antihypertensive agents will usually have an additive effect on lowering blood pressure). Products include:

- DynaCirc Capsules ... 2381
- DynaCirc CR Tablets ... 2383

Labetalol Hydrochloride (Concomitant therapy may result in additive negative effects on heart rate, AV conduction, and/or cardiac contractility; excessive bradycardia and AV block has been reported with concurrent use in hypertensive patients; possible additive effect on blood pressure). Products include:

- Normodyne Injection ... 2519
- Normodyne Tablets ... 2522
- Trandate ... 1158

Levobunolol Hydrochloride (Concomitant therapy may result in additive negative effects on heart rate, AV conduction, and/or cardiac contractility; excessive bradycardia and AV block has been reported with concurrent use in hypertensive patients; possible additive effect on blood pressure). Products include:

- Betagan ... ⊙ 230

Lisinopril (Co-administration with oral antihypertensive agents will usually have an additive effect on lowering blood pressure). Products include:

- Prinivil Tablets ... 1776
- Prinzide Tablets ... 1780
- Zestoretic Tablets ... 2968
- Zestril Tablets ... 2972

Lithium Carbonate (Combined therapy of oral verapamil and lithium may result in a lowering of serum lithium levels in patients on receiving chronic stable oral lithium; potential for increased sensitivity to the effect of lithium). Products include:

- Eskalith ... 2658
- Lithium Carbonate Capsules & Tablets ... 2352
- Lithonate/Lithotabs/Lithobid ... 2721

Lithium Citrate (Combined therapy of oral verapamil and lithium may result in a lowering of serum lithium levels in patients on receiving chronic stable oral lithium; potential for increased sensitivity to the effect of lithium).

No products indexed under this heading.

Losartan Potassium (Co-administration with oral antihypertensive agents will usually have an additive effect on lowering blood pressure). Products include:

- Cozaar Tablets ... 1668
- Hyzaar Tablets ... 1720

Mecamylamine Hydrochloride (Co-administration with oral antihypertensive agents will usually have an additive effect on lowering blood pressure). Products include:

- Inversine Tablets ... 1729

Methoxyflurane (Potential for excessive cardiovascular depression based on animal studies).

No products indexed under this heading.

Methyclothiazide (Co-administration with oral antihypertensive agents will usually have an additive effect on lowering blood pressure). Products include:

- Enduron Tablets ... 424

Methyldopa (Co-administration with oral antihypertensive agents will usually have an additive effect on lowering blood pressure). Products include:

- Aldoclor Tablets ... 1638
- Aldomet Oral ... 1640
- Aldoril Tablets ... 1644

Methyldopate Hydrochloride (Co-administration with oral antihypertensive agents will usually have an additive effect on lowering blood pressure). Products include:

- Aldomet Ester HCl Injection ... 1642

Metipranolol Hydrochloride (Concomitant therapy may result in additive negative effects on heart rate, AV conduction, and/or cardiac contractility; excessive bradycardia and AV block has been reported with concurrent use in hypertensive patients; possible additive effect on blood pressure). Products include:

- OptiPranolol (Metipranolol 0.3%) Sterile Ophthalmic Solution ... ⊙ 256

Metocurine Iodide (Verapamil may potentiate the activity of neuromuscular blocking drugs). Products include:

- Metubine Iodide Vials ... 932

Metolazone (Co-administration with oral antihypertensive agents will usually have an additive effect on lowering blood pressure). Products include:

- Mykrox Tablets ... 1617
- Zaroxolyn Tablets ... 1625

Metoprolol Succinate (Co-administration has resulted in a decrease in metoprolol clearance; concomitant therapy may result in additive negative effects on heart rate, AV conduction, and/or cardiac contractility; excessive bradycardia and AV block has been reported with concurrent use in hypertensive patients). Products include:

- Toprol-XL Tablets ... 560

(▣ Described in PDR For Nonprescription Drugs) (⊙ Described in PDR For Ophthalmology)

Metoprolol Tartrate (Co-administration has resulted in a decrease in metoprolol clearance; concomitant therapy may result in additive negative effects on heart rate, AV conduction, and/or cardiac contractility; excessive bradycardia and AV block has been reported with concurrent use in hypertensive patients). Products include:
- Lopressor 848
- Lopressor HCT Tablets 850

Metyrosine (Co-administration with oral antihypertensive agents will usually have an additive effect on lowering blood pressure). Products include:
- Demser Capsules 1690

Minoxidil (Co-administration with oral antihypertensive agents will usually have an additive effect on lowering blood pressure).
No products indexed under this heading.

Mivacurium Chloride (Verapamil may potentiate the activity of neuromuscular blocking drugs). Products include:
- Mivacron 1125

Moexipril Hydrochloride (Co-administration with oral antihypertensive agents will usually have an additive effect on lowering blood pressure). Products include:
- Univasc Tablets 2553

Nadolol (Concomitant therapy may result in additive negative effects on heart rate, AV conduction, and/or cardiac contractility; excessive bradycardia and AV block has been reported with concurrent use in hypertensive patients; possible additive effect on blood pressure).
No products indexed under this heading.

Nicardipine Hydrochloride (Co-administration with oral antihypertensive agents will usually have an additive effect on lowering blood pressure). Products include:
- Cardene Capsules 2261
- Cardene I.V. 2815
- Cardene SR Capsules 2264

Nifedipine (Co-administration with oral antihypertensive agents will usually have an additive effect on lowering blood pressure). Products include:
- Adalat Capsules (10 mg and 20 mg) 580
- Adalat CC 582
- Procardia Capsules 2024
- Procardia XL Extended Release Tablets 2026

Nisoldipine (Co-administration with oral antihypertensive agents will usually have an additive effect on lowering blood pressure). Products include:
- Sular Tablets 2961

Nitroglycerin (Co-administration with oral antihypertensive agents will usually have an additive effect on lowering blood pressure). Products include:
- Deponit NTG Transdermal Delivery System 2541
- Nitro-Bid IV 1270
- Nitro-Bid Ointment 1272
- Nitro-Dur (nitroglycerin) Transdermal Infusion System 1365
- Nitrolingual Spray 2193
- Nitrostat Tablets 1981
- Transderm-Nitro Transdermal Therapeutic System 878

Pancuronium Bromide (Verapamil may potentiate the activity of neuromuscular blocking drugs).
No products indexed under this heading.

Penbutolol Sulfate (Concomitant therapy may result in additive negative effects on heart rate, AV conduction, and/or cardiac contractility; excessive bradycardia and AV block has been reported with concurrent use in hypertensive patients; possible additive effect on blood pressure). Products include:
- Levatol Tablets 2547

Phenobarbital (Combined therapy with phenobarbital may increase verapamil clearance). Products include:
- Arco-Lase Plus Tablets 513
- Bellergal-S Tablets 2375
- Donnatal 2234
- Donnatal Extentabs 2234
- Donnatal Tablets 2234
- Phenobarbital Elixir and Tablets 1523
- Quadrinal Tablets 1398

Phenoxybenzamine Hydrochloride (Co-administration with oral antihypertensive agents will usually have an additive effect on lowering blood pressure). Products include:
- Dibenzyline Capsules 2650

Phentolamine Mesylate (Co-administration with oral antihypertensive agents will usually have an additive effect on lowering blood pressure). Products include:
- Regitine Vials 864

Pindolol (Concomitant therapy may result in additive negative effects on heart rate, AV conduction, and/or cardiac contractility; excessive bradycardia and AV block has been reported with concurrent use in hypertensive patients; possible additive effect on blood pressure). Products include:
- Visken Tablets 2428

Polythiazide (Co-administration with oral antihypertensive agents will usually have an additive effect on lowering blood pressure). Products include:
- Minizide Capsules 2016

Prazosin Hydrochloride (Concomitant use of agents that attenuate alpha-adrenergic function, such as prazosin, has resulted in excessive reduction in blood pressure). Products include:
- Minipress Capsules 2015
- Minizide Capsules 2016

Propranolol Hydrochloride (Concomitant therapy may result in additive negative effects on heart rate, AV conduction, and/or cardiac contractility; excessive bradycardia and AV block has been reported with concurrent use in hypertensive patients; possible additive effect on blood pressure). Products include:
- Inderal 2834
- Inderal LA Long Acting Capsules 2836
- Inderide Tablets 2838
- Inderide LA Long Acting Capsules .. 2840

Quinapril Hydrochloride (Co-administration with oral antihypertensive agents will usually have an additive effect on lowering blood pressure). Products include:
- Accupril Tablets 1950

Quinidine Gluconate (In a small number of patients with hypertrophic cardiomyopathy, co-administration has resulted in significant hypotension; combined use in these patients should probably be avoided). Products include:
- Quinaglute Dura-Tabs Tablets 644

Quinidine Polygalacturonate (In a small number of patients with hypertrophic cardiomyopathy, co-administration has resulted in significant hypotension; combined use in these patients should probably be avoided). Products include:
- Cardioquin Tablets 2146

Quinidine Sulfate (In a small number of patients with hypertrophic cardiomyopathy, co-administration has resulted in significant hypotension; combined use in these patients should probably be avoided). Products include:
- Quinidex Extentabs 2240

Ramipril (Co-administration with oral antihypertensive agents will usually have an additive effect on lowering blood pressure). Products include:
- Altace Capsules 1238

Rauwolfia Serpentina (Co-administration with oral antihypertensive agents will usually have an additive effect on lowering blood pressure).
No products indexed under this heading.

Rescinnamine (Co-administration with oral antihypertensive agents will usually have an additive effect on lowering blood pressure).
No products indexed under this heading.

Reserpine (Co-administration with oral antihypertensive agents will usually have an additive effect on lowering blood pressure). Products include:
- Diupres Tablets 1691
- Hydropres Tablets 1718
- Ser-Ap-Es Tablets 867

Rifampin (Combined therapy with rifampin may markedly reduce oral verapamil bioavailability). Products include:
- Rifadin 1276
- Rifamate Capsules 1278
- Rifater 1280
- Rimactane Capsules 865

Rocuronium Bromide (Verapamil may potentiate the activity of neuromuscular blocking drugs). Products include:
- Zemuron Injection 1885

Sodium Nitroprusside (Co-administration with oral antihypertensive agents will usually have an additive effect on lowering blood pressure).
No products indexed under this heading.

Sotalol Hydrochloride (Concomitant therapy may result in additive negative effects on heart rate, AV conduction, and/or cardiac contractility; excessive bradycardia and AV block has been reported with concurrent use in hypertensive patients; possible additive effect on blood pressure). Products include:
- Betapace Tablets 637

Spirapril Hydrochloride (Co-administration with oral antihypertensive agents will usually have an additive effect on lowering blood pressure).
No products indexed under this heading.

Succinylcholine Chloride (Verapamil may potentiate the activity of neuromuscular blocking drugs). Products include:
- Anectine 1062

Terazosin Hydrochloride (Concomitant use of agents that attenuate alpha-adrenergic function, such as terazosin, may result in excessive reduction in blood pressure). Products include:
- Hytrin Capsules 434

Timolol Hemihydrate (Co-administration of oral verapamil and timolol eye drops has resulted in asymptomatic bradycardia with a wandering atrial pacemaker). Products include:
- Betimol 0.25%, 0.5% 259

Timolol Maleate (Co-administration of oral verapamil and timolol eye drops has resulted in asymptomatic bradycardia with a wandering atrial pacemaker; concomitant therapy may result in additive negative effects on heart rate, AV conduction, and/or cardiac contractility; excessive bradycardia and AV block has been reported with concurrent use in hypertensive patients). Products include:
- Blocadren Tablets 1654
- Timolide Tablets 1791
- Timoptic in Ocudose 1796
- Timoptic Sterile Ophthalmic Solution 1794
- Timoptic-XE 1798

Torsemide (Co-administration with oral antihypertensive agents will usually have an additive effect on lowering blood pressure). Products include:
- Demadex Tablets and Injection 691

Trandolapril (Co-administration with oral antihypertensive agents will usually have an additive effect on lowering blood pressure). Products include:
- Mavik Tablets 1407

Trimethaphan Camsylate (Co-administration with oral antihypertensive agents will usually have an additive effect on lowering blood pressure).
No products indexed under this heading.

Tubocurarine Chloride (Verapamil may potentiate the activity of neuromuscular blocking drugs).
No products indexed under this heading.

Vecuronium Bromide (Verapamil may potentiate the activity of neuromuscular blocking drugs). Products include:
- Norcuron for Injection 1875

Food Interactions

Alcohol (Verapamil has been found to significantly inhibit ethanol elimination resulting in elevated blood ethanol concentration that may prolong the intoxicating effects of alcohol).

VERMOX CHEWABLE TABLETS
(Mebendazole) 1357
May interact with:

Cimetidine (Inhibits mebendazole metabolism and may result in an increase in plasma concentrations of mebendazole). Products include:
- Tagamet HB Tablets 786
- Tagamet Tablets 2694

Cimetidine Hydrochloride (Inhibits mebendazole metabolism and may result in an increase in plasma concentrations of mebendazole). Products include:
- Tagamet 2694

IMPORTANT NOTE: Always consult each drug listing in the patient's regimen for possible interactions.

Versed — Interactions Index

VERSED INJECTION 2324
(Midazolam Hydrochloride)
May interact with central nervous system depressants, barbiturates, narcotic analgesics, erythromycin, and certain other agents. Compounds in these categories include:

Alfentanil Hydrochloride (The sedative effect of intravenous midazolam is accentuated by narcotics; narcotic premedications also depress the ventilatory response to carbon dioxide stimulation). Products include:
Alfenta Injection 1334

Alprazolam (Concomitant use may increase the risk of underventilation or apnea and may contribute to profound and/or prolonged drug effect). Products include:
Xanax Tablets 2115

Aprobarbital (Concomitant use may increase the risk of underventilation or apnea and may contribute to profound and/or prolonged drug effect).
No products indexed under this heading.

Buprenorphine (The sedative effect of intravenous midazolam is accentuated by narcotics; narcotic premedications also depress the ventilatory response to carbon dioxide stimulation). Products include:
Buprenex Injectable 2170

Buspirone Hydrochloride (Concomitant use may increase the risk of underventilation or apnea and may contribute to profound and/or prolonged drug effect). Products include:
BuSpar Tablets 738

Butabarbital (Concomitant use may increase the risk of underventilation or apnea and may contribute to profound and/or prolonged drug effect).
No products indexed under this heading.

Butalbital (Concomitant use may increase the risk of underventilation or apnea and may contribute to profound and/or prolonged drug effect). Products include:
Axocet Capsules 2469
Esgic-plus Capsules 1012
Esgic-plus Tablets 1012
Fioricet Tablets 2386
Fioricet with Codeine Capsules 2387
Fiorinal Capsules 2388
Fiorinal with Codeine Capsules 2390
Fiorinal Tablets 2388
Phrenilin 790
Sedapap Tablets 50 mg/650 mg .. 1826

Chlordiazepoxide (Concomitant use may increase the risk of underventilation or apnea and may contribute to profound and/or prolonged drug effect). Products include:
Limbitrol 2333

Chlordiazepoxide Hydrochloride (Concomitant use may increase the risk of underventilation or apnea and may contribute to profound and/or prolonged drug effect). Products include:
Librax Capsules 2330
Librium Capsules 2331
Librium Injectable 2332

Chlorpromazine (Concomitant use may increase the risk of underventilation or apnea and may contribute to profound and/or prolonged drug effect). Products include:
Thorazine Suppositories 2701

Chlorpromazine Hydrochloride (Concomitant use may increase the risk of underventilation or apnea and may contribute to profound and/or prolonged drug effect). Products include:
Thorazine 2701

Chlorprothixene (Concomitant use may increase the risk of underventilation or apnea and may contribute to profound and/or prolonged drug effect).
No products indexed under this heading.

Chlorprothixene Hydrochloride (Concomitant use may increase the risk of underventilation or apnea and may contribute to profound and/or prolonged drug effect).
No products indexed under this heading.

Chlorprothixene Lactate (Concomitant use may increase the risk of underventilation or apnea and may contribute to profound and/or prolonged drug effect).
No products indexed under this heading.

Cimetidine (Co-administration may result in delayed clearance of midazolam; clinical significance of this interaction is unclear). Products include:
Tagamet HB Tablets .... ▣ 786
Tagamet Tablets 2694

Cimetidine Hydrochloride (Co-administration may result in delayed clearance of midazolam; clinical significance of this interaction is unclear). Products include:
Tagamet 2694

Clorazepate Dipotassium (Concomitant use may increase the risk of underventilation or apnea and may contribute to profound and/or prolonged drug effect). Products include:
Tranxene 459

Clozapine (Concomitant use may increase the risk of underventilation or apnea and may contribute to profound and/or prolonged drug effect). Products include:
Clozaril Tablets 2377

Codeine Phosphate (The sedative effect of intravenous midazolam is accentuated by narcotics; narcotic premedications also depress the ventilatory response to carbon dioxide stimulation). Products include:
Brontex 2130
Dimetane-DC Cough Syrup 2232
Fioricet with Codeine Capsules 2387
Fiorinal with Codeine Capsules 2390
Nucofed 2225
Phenergan with Codeine 2883
Phenergan VC with Codeine 2888
Robitussin A-C Syrup 2248
Robitussin-DAC Syrup 2249
Ryna .... ▣ 804
Soma Compound w/Codeine Tablets 2784
Tylenol with Codeine 1592

Desflurane (Concomitant use may increase the risk of underventilation or apnea and may contribute to profound and/or prolonged drug effect). Products include:
Suprane (desflurane, USP) 1865

Dezocine (The sedative effect of intravenous midazolam is accentuated by narcotics; narcotic premedications also depress the ventilatory response to carbon dioxide stimulation). Products include:
Dalgan Injection 529

Diazepam (Concomitant use may increase the risk of underventilation or apnea and may contribute to profound and/or prolonged drug effect). Products include:
Dizac (diazepam injectable emulsion) CIV 1862
Valium Injectable 2336
Valium Tablets 2335

Droperidol (Concomitant use may increase the risk of underventilation or apnea and may contribute to profound and/or prolonged drug effect). Products include:
Inapsine Injection 462

Enflurane (Concomitant use may increase the risk of underventilation or apnea and may contribute to profound and/or prolonged drug effect).
No products indexed under this heading.

Erythromycin (Co-administration may result in a decrease in the plasma clearance of midazolam). Products include:
A/T/S 2% Acne Topical Gel 1244
A/T/S 2% Acne Topical Solution 1244
Benzamycin Topical Gel 919
E-Mycin Tablets 1388
Emgel 2% Topical Gel 1081
ERYC 1972
Erycette (erythromycin 2%) Topical Solution 1943
Ery-Tab Tablets 426
Erythromycin Base Filmtab 430
Erythromycin Delayed-Release Capsules, USP 431
Ilotycin Ophthalmic Ointment 928
PCE Dispertab Tablets 453
T-Stat 2.0% Topical Solution and Pads 2797
THERAMYCIN Z 2% Solution 1629

Erythromycin Estolate (Co-administration may result in a decrease in the plasma clearance of midazolam). Products include:
Ilosone 927

Erythromycin Ethylsuccinate (Co-administration may result in a decrease in the plasma clearance of midazolam). Products include:
E.E.S. 427
EryPed 425
Pediazole Suspension 2340

Erythromycin Glucepate (Co-administration may result in a decrease in the plasma clearance of midazolam). Products include:
Ilotycin Glucepate, IV, Vials 929

Erythromycin Stearate (Co-administration may result in a decrease in the plasma clearance of midazolam). Products include:
Erythrocin Stearate Filmtab 429

Estazolam (Concomitant use may increase the risk of underventilation or apnea and may contribute to profound and/or prolonged drug effect). Products include:
ProSom Tablets 457

Etchlorvynol (Concomitant use may increase the risk of underventilation or apnea and may contribute to profound and/or prolonged drug effect). Products include:
Placidyl Capsules 456

Ethinamate (Concomitant use may increase the risk of underventilation or apnea and may contribute to profound and/or prolonged drug effect).
No products indexed under this heading.

Fentanyl (The sedative effect of intravenous midazolam is accentuated by narcotics; narcotic premedications also depress the ventilatory response to carbon dioxide stimulation). Products include:
Duragesic Transdermal System 1336

Fentanyl Citrate (The sedative effect of intravenous midazolam is accentuated by narcotics; narcotic premedications also depress the ventilatory response to carbon dioxide stimulation). Products include:
Sublimaze Injection 463

Fluphenazine Decanoate (Concomitant use may increase the risk of underventilation or apnea and may contribute to profound and/or prolonged drug effect). Products include:
Prolixin Decanoate 510

Fluphenazine Enanthate (Concomitant use may increase the risk of underventilation or apnea and may contribute to profound and/or prolonged drug effect). Products include:
Prolixin Enanthate 510

Fluphenazine Hydrochloride (Concomitant use may increase the risk of underventilation or apnea and may contribute to profound and/or prolonged drug effect). Products include:
Prolixin 510

Flurazepam Hydrochloride (Concomitant use may increase the risk of underventilation or apnea and may contribute to profound and/or prolonged drug effect). Products include:
Dalmane Capsules 2329

Glutethimide (Concomitant use may increase the risk of underventilation or apnea and may contribute to profound and/or prolonged drug effect).
No products indexed under this heading.

Haloperidol (Concomitant use may increase the risk of underventilation or apnea and may contribute to profound and/or prolonged drug effect). Products include:
Haldol Injection, Tablets and Concentrate 1585

Haloperidol Decanoate (Concomitant use may increase the risk of underventilation or apnea and may contribute to profound and/or prolonged drug effect). Products include:
Haldol Decanoate 1587

Halothane (The intravenous administration of midazolam decreases the minimum alveolar concentration of halothane required for general anesthesia). Products include:
Fluothane 2830

Hydrocodone Bitartrate (The sedative effect of intravenous midazolam is accentuated by narcotics; narcotic premedications also depress the ventilatory response to carbon dioxide stimulation). Products include:
Codiclear DH Syrup 808
Duratuss HD Elixir 2750
Histussin D Liquid 670
Hycodan Tablets and Syrup 946
Hycomine Compound Tablets 948
Hycomine 947
Hycotuss Expectorant Syrup 950
Hydrocet Capsules 787
Lorcet 10/650 Tablets 1016
Lortab 2751
Tussend 1830
Tussend Expectorant 1831
Vicodin Tablets 1404
Vicodin ES Tablets 1405
Vicodin HP Tablets 1403
Vicodin Tuss Expectorant 1406
Zydone Capsules 967

(▣ Described in PDR For Nonprescription Drugs)   (⊙ Described in PDR For Ophthalmology)

Interactions Index — Versed

Hydrocodone Polistirex (The sedative effect of intravenous midazolam is accentuated by narcotics; narcotic premedications also depress the ventilatory response to carbon dioxide stimulation). Products include:
- Tussionex Pennkinetic Extended-Release Suspension 1624

Hydromorphone Hydrochloride (The sedative effect of intravenous midazolam is accentuated by narcotics; narcotic premedications also depress the ventilatory response to carbon dioxide stimulation). Products include:
- Dilaudid Ampules 1382
- Dilaudid Cough Syrup 1383
- Dilaudid-HP Injection 1384
- Dilaudid-HP Lyophilized Powder 250 mg 1384
- Dilaudid 1382
- Dilaudid Oral Liquid 1386
- Dilaudid 1382
- Dilaudid Tablets - 8 mg 1386

Hydroxyzine Hydrochloride (Concomitant use may increase the risk of underventilation or apnea and may contribute to profound and/or prolonged drug effect). Products include:
- Atarax Tablets & Syrup 1992
- Marax Tablets & DF Syrup 2015
- Vistaril Intramuscular Solution 2042

Isoflurane (Concomitant use may increase the risk of underventilation or apnea and may contribute to profound and/or prolonged drug effect).
- No products indexed under this heading.

Ketamine Hydrochloride (Concomitant use may increase the risk of underventilation or apnea and may contribute to profound and/or prolonged drug effect).
- No products indexed under this heading.

Levomethadyl Acetate Hydrochloride (Concomitant use may increase the risk of underventilation or apnea and may contribute to profound and/or prolonged drug effect). Products include:
- Orlaam Oral Solution 2361

Levorphanol Tartrate (The sedative effect of intravenous midazolam is accentuated by narcotics; narcotic premedications also depress the ventilatory response to carbon dioxide stimulation). Products include:
- Levo-Dromoran 2297

Lorazepam (Concomitant use may increase the risk of underventilation or apnea and may contribute to profound and/or prolonged drug effect). Products include:
- Ativan Injection 2805
- Ativan Tablets 2807

Loxapine Hydrochloride (Concomitant use may increase the risk of underventilation or apnea and may contribute to profound and/or prolonged drug effect). Products include:
- Loxitane 1426

Loxapine Succinate (Concomitant use may increase the risk of underventilation or apnea and may contribute to profound and/or prolonged drug effect). Products include:
- Loxitane Capsules 1426

Meperidine Hydrochloride (The sedative effect of intravenous midazolam is accentuated by narcotics; narcotic premedications also depress the ventilatory response to carbon dioxide stimulation). Products include:
- Demerol 2438
- Mepergan Injection 2859

Mephobarbital (Concomitant use may increase the risk of underventilation or apnea and may contribute to profound and/or prolonged drug effect). Products include:
- Mebaral Tablets 2452

Meprobamate (Concomitant use may increase the risk of underventilation or apnea and may contribute to profound and/or prolonged drug effect). Products include:
- Miltown Tablets 2780
- PMB 200 and PMB 400 2890

Mesoridazine Besylate (Concomitant use may increase the risk of underventilation or apnea and may contribute to profound and/or prolonged drug effect). Products include:
- Serentil 689

Methadone Hydrochloride (The sedative effect of intravenous midazolam is accentuated by narcotics; narcotic premedications also depress the ventilatory response to carbon dioxide stimulation). Products include:
- Methadone Hydrochloride Oral Concentrate 2356
- Methadone Hydrochloride Oral Solution & Tablets 2357

Methohexital Sodium (Concomitant use may increase the risk of underventilation or apnea and may contribute to profound and/or prolonged drug effect).
- No products indexed under this heading.

Methotrimeprazine (Concomitant use may increase the risk of underventilation or apnea and may contribute to profound and/or prolonged drug effect). Products include:
- Levoprome 1321

Methoxyflurane (Concomitant use may increase the risk of underventilation or apnea and may contribute to profound and/or prolonged drug effect).
- No products indexed under this heading.

Molindone Hydrochloride (Concomitant use may increase the risk of underventilation or apnea and may contribute to profound and/or prolonged drug effect). Products include:
- Moban Tablets and Concentrate 1036

Morphine Sulfate (The sedative effect of intravenous midazolam is accentuated by narcotics; narcotic premedications also depress the ventilatory response to carbon dioxide stimulation). Products include:
- Astramorph/PF Injection, USP (Preservative-Free) 526
- Duramorph Injection 983
- Infumorph 200 and Infumorph 500 Sterile Solutions 985
- Kadian Capsules 2948
- MS Contin Tablets 2149
- MSIR 2152
- Oramorph SR (Morphine Sulfate Sustained Release Tablets) 2359
- RMS Suppositories CII 2766
- Roxanol 2365

Opium Alkaloids (The sedative effect of intravenous midazolam is accentuated by narcotics; narcotic premedications also depress the ventilatory response to carbon dioxide stimulation).
- No products indexed under this heading.

Oxazepam (Concomitant use may increase the risk of underventilation or apnea and may contribute to profound and/or prolonged drug effect). Products include:
- Serax Capsules 2916
- Serax Tablets 2916

Oxycodone Hydrochloride (The sedative effect of intravenous midazolam is accentuated by narcotics; narcotic premedications also depress the ventilatory response to carbon dioxide stimulation). Products include:
- OxyContin Tablets 2163
- OxyIR Capsules 2167
- Percocet Tablets 955
- Percodan Tablets 955
- Percodan-Demi Tablets 956
- Roxicodone Tablets, Oral Solution & Intensol (Oxycodone) 2366
- Tylox Capsules 1593

Pentobarbital Sodium (Concomitant use may increase the risk of underventilation or apnea and may contribute to profound and/or prolonged drug effect). Products include:
- Nembutal Sodium Capsules 440
- Nembutal Sodium Solution 442
- Nembutal Sodium Suppositories 444

Perphenazine (Concomitant use may increase the risk of underventilation or apnea and may contribute to profound and/or prolonged drug effect). Products include:
- Etrafon 2495
- Triavil Tablets 1800
- Trilafon 2532

Phenobarbital (Concomitant use may increase the risk of underventilation or apnea and may contribute to profound and/or prolonged drug effect). Products include:
- Arco-Lase Plus Tablets 513
- Bellergal-S Tablets 2375
- Donnatal 2234
- Donnatal Extentabs 2234
- Donnatal Tablets 2234
- Phenobarbital Elixir and Tablets 1523
- Quadrinal Tablets 1398

Prazepam (Concomitant use may increase the risk of underventilation or apnea and may contribute to profound and/or prolonged drug effect).
- No products indexed under this heading.

Prochlorperazine (Concomitant use may increase the risk of underventilation or apnea and may contribute to profound and/or prolonged drug effect). Products include:
- Compazine 2644

Promethazine Hydrochloride (Concomitant use may increase the risk of underventilation or apnea and may contribute to profound and/or prolonged drug effect). Products include:
- Mepergan Injection 2859
- Phenergan with Codeine 2883
- Phenergan with Dextromethorphan 2885
- Phenergan Injection 2880
- Phenergan Suppositories 2882
- Phenergan Syrup 2881
- Phenergan Tablets 2882
- Phenergan VC 2886
- Phenergan VC with Codeine 2888

Propofol (Concomitant use may increase the risk of underventilation or apnea and may contribute to profound and/or prolonged drug effect). Products include:
- Diprivan Injectable Emulsion 2939

Propoxyphene Hydrochloride (The sedative effect of intravenous midazolam is accentuated by narcotics; narcotic premedications also depress the ventilatory response to carbon dioxide stimulation). Products include:
- Darvon 1475
- Wygesic Tablets 2930

Propoxyphene Napsylate (The sedative effect of intravenous midazolam is accentuated by narcotics; narcotic premedications also depress the ventilatory response to carbon dioxide stimulation). Products include:
- Darvon-N/Darvocet-N 1473

Quazepam (Concomitant use may increase the risk of underventilation or apnea and may contribute to profound and/or prolonged drug effect). Products include:
- Doral Tablets 2773

Risperidone (Concomitant use may increase the risk of underventilation or apnea and may contribute to profound and/or prolonged drug effect). Products include:
- Risperdal Tablets 1348

Secobarbital Sodium (Concomitant use may increase the risk of underventilation or apnea and may contribute to profound and/or prolonged drug effect). Products include:
- Seconal Sodium Pulvules 1529

Sevoflurane (Concomitant use may increase the risk of underventilation or apnea and may contribute to profound and/or prolonged drug effect).
- No products indexed under this heading.

Sufentanil Citrate (The sedative effect of intravenous midazolam is accentuated by narcotics; narcotic premedications also depress the ventilatory response to carbon dioxide stimulation). Products include:
- Sufenta Injection 1355

Temazepam (Concomitant use may increase the risk of underventilation or apnea and may contribute to profound and/or prolonged drug effect). Products include:
- Restoril Capsules 2413

Thiamylal Sodium (Concomitant use may increase the risk of underventilation or apnea and may contribute to profound and/or prolonged drug effect).
- No products indexed under this heading.

Thioridazine Hydrochloride (Concomitant use may increase the risk of underventilation or apnea and may contribute to profound and/or prolonged drug effect). Products include:
- Mellaril 2398

Thiothixene (Concomitant use may increase the risk of underventilation or apnea and may contribute to profound and/or prolonged drug effect). Products include:
- Navane Capsules and Concentrate 2018
- Navane Intramuscular 2019

IMPORTANT NOTE: Always consult each drug listing in the patient's regimen for possible interactions.

Triazolam (Concomitant use may increase the risk of underventilation or apnea and may contribute to profound and/or prolonged drug effect). Products include:
- Halcion Tablets 2093

Trifluoperazine Hydrochloride (Concomitant use may increase the risk of underventilation or apnea and may contribute to profound and/or prolonged drug effect). Products include:
- Stelazine 2692

Zolpidem Tartrate (Concomitant use may increase the risk of underventilation or apnea and may contribute to profound and/or prolonged drug effect). Products include:
- Ambien Tablets 2559

Food Interactions

Alcohol (Concomitant use may increase the risk of underventilation or apnea and may contribute to profound and/or prolonged drug effect).

VESANOID CAPSULES

(Tretinoin) 2327

May interact with glucocorticoids, erythromycin, and certain other agents. Compounds in these categories include:

Betamethasone Acetate (Potential for alteration of pharmacokinetic parameters in patients on concomitant drugs that are inducers of hepatic CYP enzymes). Products include:
- Celestone Soluspan Suspension 2484

Betamethasone Sodium Phosphate (Potential for alteration of pharmacokinetic parameters in patients on concomitant drugs that are inducers of hepatic CYP enzymes). Products include:
- Celestone Soluspan Suspension 2484

Cimetidine (Potential for alteration of pharmacokinetic parameters in patients on concomitant drugs that inhibit hepatic CYP enzymes). Products include:
- Tagamet HB Tablets .... ⊡ 786
- Tagamet Tablets 2694

Cimetidine Hydrochloride (Potential for alteration of pharmacokinetic parameters in patients on concomitant drugs that inhibit hepatic CYP enzymes). Products include:
- Tagamet 2694

Cortisone Acetate (Potential for alteration of pharmacokinetic parameters in patients on concomitant drugs that are inducers of hepatic CYP enzymes). Products include:
- Cortone Acetate Sterile Suspension 1663
- Cortone Acetate Tablets 1664

Cyclosporine (Potential for alteration of pharmacokinetic parameters in patients on concomitant drugs that inhibit hepatic CYP enzymes). Products include:
- Neoral 2405
- Sandimmune 2416

Dexamethasone (Potential for alteration of pharmacokinetic parameters in patients on concomitant drugs that are inducers of hepatic CYP enzymes). Products include:
- AK-Trol Ointment & Suspension .... ⊙ 205
- Decadron Elixir 1676
- Decadron Tablets 1678
- Decaspray Topical Aerosol 1689
- Maxitrol Ophthalmic Ointment and Suspension .... ⊙ 222
- TobraDex Ophthalmic Suspension and Ointment 469

Dexamethasone Acetate (Potential for alteration of pharmacokinetic parameters in patients on concomitant drugs that are inducers of hepatic CYP enzymes). Products include:
- Dalalone D.P. Injectable 1009
- Decadron-LA Sterile Suspension 1687

Dexamethasone Sodium Phosphate (Potential for alteration of pharmacokinetic parameters in patients on concomitant drugs that are inducers of hepatic CYP enzymes). Products include:
- Decadron Phosphate Injection 1680
- Decadron Phosphate Sterile Ophthalmic Ointment 1684
- Decadron Phosphate Sterile Ophthalmic Solution 1685
- Decadron Phosphate Topical Cream 1686
- Decadron Phosphate with Xylocaine Injection, Sterile 1683
- Dexacort Phosphate in Respihaler 1606
- Dexacort Phosphate in Turbinaire 1607
- NeoDecadron Sterile Ophthalmic Ointment 1755
- NeoDecadron Sterile Ophthalmic Solution 1756
- NeoDecadron Topical Cream 1757

Diltiazem Hydrochloride (Potential for alteration of pharmacokinetic parameters in patients on concomitant drugs that inhibit hepatic CYP enzymes). Products include:
- Cardizem CD Capsules 1251
- Cardizem SR Capsules 1255
- Cardizem Injectable 1253
- Cardizem Tablets 1257
- Dilacor XR Extended-release Capsules 2183
- Tiazac Capsules 1019

Erythromycin (Potential for alteration of pharmacokinetic parameters in patients on concomitant drugs that inhibit hepatic CYP enzymes). Products include:
- A/T/S 2% Acne Topical Gel 1244
- A/T/S 2% Acne Topical Solution 1244
- Benzamycin Topical Gel 919
- E-Mycin Tablets 1388
- Emgel 2% Topical Gel 1081
- ERYC 1972
- Erycette (erythromycin 2%) Topical Solution 1943
- Ery-Tab Tablets 426
- Erythromycin Base Filmtab 430
- Erythromycin Delayed-Release Capsules, USP 431
- Ilotycin Ophthalmic Ointment 928
- PCE Dispertab Tablets 453
- T-Stat 2.0% Topical Solution and Pads 2797
- THERAMYCIN Z 2% Solution 1629

Erythromycin Estolate (Potential for alteration of pharmacokinetic parameters in patients on concomitant drugs that inhibit hepatic CYP enzymes). Products include:
- Ilosone 927

Erythromycin Ethylsuccinate (Potential for alteration of pharmacokinetic parameters in patients on concomitant drugs that inhibit hepatic CYP enzymes). Products include:
- E.E.S. 427
- EryPed 425
- Pediazole Suspension 2340

Erythromycin Gluceptate (Potential for alteration of pharmacokinetic parameters in patients on concomitant drugs that inhibit hepatic CYP enzymes). Products include:
- Ilotycin Gluceptate, IV, Vials 929

Erythromycin Stearate (Potential for alteration of pharmacokinetic parameters in patients on concomitant drugs that inhibit hepatic CYP enzymes). Products include:
- Erythrocin Stearate Filmtab 429

Fludrocortisone Acetate (Potential for alteration of pharmacokinetic parameters in patients on concomitant drugs that are inducers of hepatic CYP enzymes). Products include:
- Florinef Acetate Tablets 506

Hydrocortisone (Potential for alteration of pharmacokinetic parameters in patients on concomitant drugs that are inducers of hepatic CYP enzymes). Products include:
- Anusol-HC Cream 2.5% 1953
- Aquanil HC Lotion 1989
- Maximum Strength Cortaid Spray .... ⊡ 800
- CORTENEMA 2713
- Cortisporin Ointment 1074
- Cortisporin Ophthalmic Ointment Sterile 1074
- Cortisporin Ophthalmic Suspension Sterile 1075
- Cortisporin Otic Solution Sterile 1076
- Cortisporin Otic Suspension Sterile 1077
- Cortizone-5 .... ⊡ 795
- Cortizone-10 .... ⊡ 795
- Hydrocortone Tablets 1715
- Hytone 922
- Hytone Ointment 2 ½% 923
- Massengill Medicated Soft Cloth Towelettes 2628
- Pediotic Suspension Sterile 1140
- Preparation H Hydrocortisone 1% Cream .... ⊡ 843
- ProctoCream-HC 2.5% 2552
- VōSoL HC Otic Solution 2786

Hydrocortisone Acetate (Potential for alteration of pharmacokinetic parameters in patients on concomitant drugs that are inducers of hepatic CYP enzymes). Products include:
- Analpram-HC Rectal Cream 1% and 2.5% 993
- Anusol HC-1 Hydrocortisone Anti-Itch Ointment .... ⊡ 810
- Anusol-HC Suppositories 1954
- Caldecort Anti-Itch Hydrocortisone Cream .... ⊡ 651
- Coly-Mycin S Otic w/Neomycin & Hydrocortisone 1965
- Cortaid .... ⊡ 800
- Cortifoam 2540
- Cortisporin Cream 1073
- Epifoam 2543
- Hydrocortone Acetate Sterile Suspension 1712
- Mantadil Cream 1124
- Nupercainal Hydrocortisone 1% Cream .... ⊡ 661
- Pramosone Cream, Lotion & Ointment 995
- ProctoFoam-HC 2552
- Terra-Cortril Ophthalmic Suspension 2033

Hydrocortisone Sodium Phosphate (Potential for alteration of pharmacokinetic parameters in patients on concomitant drugs that are inducers of hepatic CYP enzymes). Products include:
- Hydrocortone Phosphate Injection, Sterile 1713

Hydrocortisone Sodium Succinate (Potential for alteration of pharmacokinetic parameters in patients on concomitant drugs that are inducers of hepatic CYP enzymes).
- No products indexed under this heading.

Ketoconazole (Potential for alteration of pharmacokinetic parameters in patients on concomitant drugs that inhibit hepatic CYP enzymes). Products include:
- Nizoral 2% Cream 1344
- Nizoral 2% Shampoo 1344
- Nizoral Tablets 1345

Methylprednisolone Acetate (Potential for alteration of pharmacokinetic parameters in patients on concomitant drugs that are inducers of hepatic CYP enzymes).
- No products indexed under this heading.

Methylprednisolone Sodium Succinate (Potential for alteration of pharmacokinetic parameters in patients on concomitant drugs that are inducers of hepatic CYP enzymes).
- No products indexed under this heading.

Pentobarbital Sodium (Potential for alteration of pharmacokinetic parameters in patients on concomitant drugs that are inducers of hepatic CYP enzymes). Products include:
- Nembutal Sodium Capsules 440
- Nembutal Sodium Solution 442
- Nembutal Sodium Suppositories 444

Phenobarbital (Potential for alteration of pharmacokinetic parameters in patients on concomitant drugs that are inducers of hepatic CYP enzymes). Products include:
- Arco-Lase Plus Tablets 513
- Bellergal-S Tablets 2375
- Donnatal 2234
- Donnatal Extentabs 2234
- Donnatal Tablets 2234
- Phenobarbital Elixir and Tablets 1523
- Quadrinal Tablets 1398

Prednisolone Acetate (Potential for alteration of pharmacokinetic parameters in patients on concomitant drugs that are inducers of hepatic CYP enzymes). Products include:
- AK-CIDE .... ⊙ 203
- AK-CIDE Ointment .... ⊙ 203
- Blephamide Liquifilm Sterile Ophthalmic Suspension 472
- Blephamide Ointment .... ⊙ 234
- Econopred & Econopred Plus Ophthalmic Suspensions .... ⊙ 216
- Poly-Pred Liquifilm .... ⊙ 246
- Pred Forte .... ⊙ 247
- Pred Mild .... ⊙ 250
- Pred-G Liquifilm Sterile Ophthalmic Suspension .... ⊙ 248
- Pred-G S.O.P. Sterile Ophthalmic Ointment .... ⊙ 249

Prednisolone Sodium Phosphate (Potential for alteration of pharmacokinetic parameters in patients on concomitant drugs that are inducers of hepatic CYP enzymes). Products include:
- AK-PRED .... ⊙ 204
- Hydeltrasol Injection, Sterile 1708
- Pediapred Oral Solution 1618

Prednisolone Tebutate (Potential for alteration of pharmacokinetic parameters in patients on concomitant drugs that are inducers of hepatic CYP enzymes). Products include:
- Hydeltra-T.B.A. Sterile Suspension 1710

Prednisone (Potential for alteration of pharmacokinetic parameters in patients on concomitant drugs that are inducers of hepatic CYP enzymes).
- No products indexed under this heading.

Rifampin (Potential for alteration of pharmacokinetic parameters in patients on concomitant drugs that are inducers of hepatic CYP enzymes). Products include:
- Rifadin 1276
- Rifamate Capsules 1278
- Rifater 1280
- Rimactane Capsules 865

Triamcinolone (Potential for alteration of pharmacokinetic parameters in patients on concomitant drugs that are inducers of hepatic CYP enzymes).
- No products indexed under this heading.

(⊡ Described in PDR For Nonprescription Drugs) (⊙ Described in PDR For Ophthalmology)

Triamcinolone Acetonide (Potential for alteration of pharmacokinetic parameters in patients on concomitant drugs that are inducers of hepatic CYP enzymes). Products include:
- Azmacort Oral Inhaler 2175
- Nasacort AQ Nasal Spray 2191
- Nasacort Nasal Inhaler 2189

Triamcinolone Diacetate (Potential for alteration of pharmacokinetic parameters in patients on concomitant drugs that are inducers of hepatic CYP enzymes).
- No products indexed under this heading.

Triamcinolone Hexacetonide (Potential for alteration of pharmacokinetic parameters in patients on concomitant drugs that are inducers of hepatic CYP enzymes).
- No products indexed under this heading.

Verapamil Hydrochloride (Potential for alteration of pharmacokinetic parameters in patients on concomitant drugs that inhibit hepatic CYP enzymes). Products include:
- Calan SR Caplets 2571
- Calan Tablets 2568
- Covera-HS Tablets 2573
- Isoptin Injectable 1391
- Isoptin Oral Tablets 1393
- Isoptin SR Tablets 1395
- Verelan Capsules 1455

Food Interactions

Food, unspecified (The absorption of retinoids as a class has been shown to be enhanced when taken with food).

VEXOL 1% OPHTHALMIC SUSPENSION

(Rimexolone) .... ⊙ 227

None cited in PDR database.

VIBRAMYCIN CALCIUM ORAL SUSPENSION SYRUP

(Doxycycline Calcium) 2038

See **Vibramycin Hyclate Capsules**

VIBRAMYCIN HYCLATE CAPSULES

(Doxycycline Hyclate) 2038

May interact with oral anticoagulants, penicillins, antacids containing aluminium, calcium and magnesium, barbiturates, oral contraceptives, and certain other agents. Compounds in these categories include:

Aluminum Carbonate (Concomitant therapy may impair oral absorption of tetracycline). Products include:
- Basaljel Capsules 2810
- Basaljel Suspension 2810
- Basaljel Tablets 2810

Aluminum Hydroxide (Concomitant therapy may impair oral absorption of tetracycline). Products include:
- ALternaGEL Liquid 1358
- Maximum Strength Ascriptin 650
- Cama Arthritis Pain Reliever 748
- Gaviscon Extra Strength Relief Formula Antacid Tablets 778
- Gaviscon Extra Strength Relief Formula Liquid Antacid 779
- Gaviscon Liquid Antacid 779
- Gelusil Antacid-Anti-gas Liquid 819
- Gelusil Antacid-Anti-gas Tablets 819
- Maalox Antacid/Anti-Gas Tablets 889
- Maalox Heartburn Relief Suspension 658
- Maalox Antacid Liquid 888
- Extra Strength Maalox Antacid/Anti-Gas Liquid and Tablets 888
- Mylanta 1359
- Tempo Soft Antacid 799

Aluminum Hydroxide Gel (Concomitant therapy may impair oral absorption of tetracycline). Products include:
- ALternaGEL Liquid 675
- Aludrox Oral Suspension 850
- Amphojel Suspension 2802
- Amphojel Suspension without Flavor 2802
- Amphojel Tablets 2802
- Ascriptin 650
- Gaviscon Antacid Tablets 778
- Gaviscon-2 Antacid Tablets 779
- Mylanta Liquid 676
- Mylanta Double Strength Liquid 676
- Nephrox Suspension 671

Amoxicillin Trihydrate (Bacteriostatic drugs may interfere with bactericidal action of penicillin). Products include:
- Amoxil 2631
- Augmentin 2637
- Augmentin Tablets 2640

Ampicillin Sodium (Bacteriostatic drugs may interfere with bactericidal action of penicillin). Products include:
- Unasyn 2035

Aprobarbital (Decreases the half-life of doxycycline).
- No products indexed under this heading.

Azlocillin Sodium (Bacteriostatic drugs may interfere with bactericidal action of penicillin).
- No products indexed under this heading.

Bacampicillin Hydrochloride (Bacteriostatic drugs may interfere with bactericidal action of penicillin). Products include:
- Spectrobid Tablets 2030

Bismuth Subsalicylate (Absorption of tetracyclines is impaired by bismuth subsalicylate). Products include:
- Helidac Therapy 2135
- Pepto-Bismol Original Liquid, Original and Cherry Tablets and Easy-To-Swallow Caplets 2126
- Pepto-Bismol Maximum Strength Liquid 2126

Butabarbital (Decreases the half-life of doxycycline).
- No products indexed under this heading.

Butalbital (Decreases the half-life of doxycycline). Products include:
- Axocet Capsules 2469
- Esgic-plus Capsules 1012
- Esgic-plus Tablets 1012
- Fioricet Tablets 2386
- Fioricet with Codeine Capsules 2387
- Fiorinal Capsules 2388
- Fiorinal with Codeine Capsules 2390
- Fiorinal Tablets 2388
- Phrenilin 790
- Sedapap Tablets 50 mg/650 mg 1826

Carbamazepine (Decreases the half-life of doxycycline). Products include:
- Atretol Tablets 569
- Tegretol/Tegretol-XR 870

Carbenicillin Disodium (Bacteriostatic drugs may interfere with bactericidal action of penicillin).
- No products indexed under this heading.

Carbenicillin Indanyl Sodium (Bacteriostatic drugs may interfere with bactericidal action of penicillin). Products include:
- Geocillin Tablets 2009

Desogestrel (Concurrent use may render oral contraceptive less effective). Products include:
- Desogen Tablets 1867
- Ortho-Cept 1907

Dicloxacillin Sodium (Bacteriostatic drugs may interfere with bactericidal action of penicillin).
- No products indexed under this heading.

Dicumarol (Depressed plasma prothrombin activity; may require downward adjustment of the anticoagulant dosage).
- No products indexed under this heading.

Ethinyl Estradiol (Concurrent use may render oral contraceptive less effective). Products include:
- Brevicon 2563
- Demulen 2580
- Desogen Tablets 1867
- Levlen/Tri-Levlen 646
- Lo/Ovral Tablets 2852
- Lo/Ovral-28 Tablets 2857
- Modicon 1928
- Nordette-21 Tablets 2863
- Nordette-28 Tablets 2866
- Norinyl 2563
- Ortho-Cept 1907
- Ortho-Cyclen/Ortho-Tri-Cyclen 1914
- Ortho-Novum 1928
- Ortho-Cyclen/Ortho Tri-Cyclen 1914
- Ovcon 765
- Ovral Tablets 2877
- Ovral-28 Tablets 2878
- Levlen/Tri-Levlen 646
- Tri-Norinyl 2607
- Triphasil-21 Tablets 2919
- Triphasil-28 Tablets 2924

Ethynodiol Diacetate (Concurrent use may render oral contraceptive less effective). Products include:
- Demulen 2580

Levonorgestrel (Concurrent use may render oral contraceptive less effective). Products include:
- Levlen/Tri-Levlen 646
- Nordette-21 Tablets 2863
- Nordette-28 Tablets 2866
- Norplant System 2868
- Levlen/Tri-Levlen 646
- Triphasil-21 Tablets 2919
- Triphasil-28 Tablets 2924

Magaldrate (Concomitant therapy may impair oral absorption of tetracycline).
- No products indexed under this heading.

Magnesium Hydroxide (Concomitant therapy may impair oral absorption of tetracycline). Products include:
- Aludrox Oral Suspension 850
- Ascriptin 650
- Di-Gel Antacid/Anti-Gas 762
- Gelusil Antacid-Anti-gas Liquid 819
- Gelusil Antacid-Anti-gas Tablets 819
- Maalox Antacid/Anti-Gas Tablets 889
- Maalox Antacid Liquid 888
- Extra Strength Maalox Antacid/Anti-Gas Liquid and Tablets 888
- Mylanta Fast-Acting 1359
- Mylanta Gelcaps Antacid 678
- Fast-Acting Mylanta Liquid Antacid 1359
- Mylanta Tablets 677
- Maximum-Strength Fast-Acting Mylanta Liquid Antacid 1359
- Mylanta Double Strength Tablets 677
- Phillips' Milk of Magnesia Liquid 627
- Rolaids Antacid Tablets 807
- Tempo Soft Antacid 799

Magnesium Oxide (Concomitant therapy may impair oral absorption of tetracycline). Products include:
- Beelith Tablets 632
- Bufferin Analgesic Tablets 636
- Arthritis Strength Bufferin Analgesic Caplets 637
- Extra Strength Bufferin Analgesic Tablets 637
- Caltrate PLUS 681
- Cama Arthritis Pain Reliever 748
- Mag-Ox 400 666
- Uro-Mag 666

Mephobarbital (Decreases the half-life of doxycycline). Products include:
- Mebaral Tablets 2452

Mestranol (Concurrent use may render oral contraceptive less effective). Products include:
- Norinyl 2563
- Ortho-Novum 1928

Methoxyflurane (Potential for fatal renal toxicity).
- No products indexed under this heading.

Mezlocillin Sodium (Bacteriostatic drugs may interfere with bactericidal action of penicillin). Products include:
- Mezlin 594
- Mezlin Pharmacy Bulk Package 597

Nafcillin Sodium (Bacteriostatic drugs may interfere with bactericidal action of penicillin).
- No products indexed under this heading.

Norethindrone (Concurrent use may render oral contraceptive less effective). Products include:
- Brevicon 2563
- Micronor Tablets 1903
- Modicon 1928
- Norinyl 2563
- Nor-Q D Tablets 2598
- Ortho-Novum 1928
- Ovcon 765
- Tri-Norinyl 2607

Norethynodrel (Concurrent use may render oral contraceptive less effective).
- No products indexed under this heading.

Norgestimate (Concurrent use may render oral contraceptive less effective). Products include:
- Ortho-Cyclen/Ortho-Tri-Cyclen 1914
- Ortho-Cyclen/Ortho Tri-Cyclen 1914

Norgestrel (Concurrent use may render oral contraceptive less effective). Products include:
- Lo/Ovral Tablets 2852
- Lo/Ovral-28 Tablets 2857
- Ovral Tablets 2877
- Ovral-28 Tablets 2878
- Ovrette Tablets 2878

Penicillin G Benzathine (Bacteriostatic drugs may interfere with bactericidal action of penicillin). Products include:
- Bicillin C-R Injection 2810
- Bicillin C-R 900/300 Injection 2812
- Bicillin L-A Injection 2813

Penicillin G Potassium (Bacteriostatic drugs may interfere with bactericidal action of penicillin). Products include:
- Pfizerpen for Injection 2022

Penicillin G Procaine (Bacteriostatic drugs may interfere with bactericidal action of penicillin). Products include:
- Bicillin C-R Injection 2810
- Bicillin C-R 900/300 Injection 2812

Penicillin G Sodium (Bacteriostatic drugs may interfere with bactericidal action of penicillin).
- No products indexed under this heading.

Penicillin V Potassium (Bacteriostatic drugs may interfere with bactericidal action of penicillin). Products include:
- Pen•Vee K 2879

Pentobarbital Sodium (Decreases the half-life of doxycycline). Products include:
- Nembutal Sodium Capsules 440
- Nembutal Sodium Solution 442
- Nembutal Sodium Suppositories 444

Phenobarbital (Decreases the half-life of doxycycline). Products include:
- Arco-Lase Plus Tablets 513
- Bellergal-S Tablets 2375
- Donnatal 2234
- Donnatal Extentabs 2234

IMPORTANT NOTE: Always consult each drug listing in the patient's regimen for possible interactions.

Vibramycin

Donnatal Tablets 2234
Phenobarbital Elixir and Tablets 1523
Quadrinal Tablets 1398

Phenytoin (Decreases the half-life of doxycycline). Products include:
Dilantin Infatabs 1967
Dilantin-125 Suspension 1969

Phenytoin Sodium (Decreases the half-life of doxycycline). Products include:
Dilantin Kapseals 1965

Secobarbital Sodium (Decreases the half-life of doxycycline). Products include:
Seconal Sodium Pulvules 1529

Thiamylal Sodium (Decreases the half-life of doxycycline).
No products indexed under this heading.

Ticarcillin Disodium (Bacteriostatic drugs may interfere with bactericidal action of penicillin). Products include:
Ticar for Injection 2704
Timentin for Injection 2706

Warfarin Sodium (Depressed plasma prothrombin activity; may require downward adjustment of the anticoagulant dosage). Products include:
Coumadin 941

Food Interactions

Dairy products (Absorption of doxycycline is not markedly influenced by simultaneous ingestion of milk).

Food, unspecified (Absorption of doxycycline is not markedly influenced by simultaneous ingestion of food).

VIBRAMYCIN HYCLATE INTRAVENOUS

(Doxycycline Hyclate) 2040
May interact with anticoagulants and penicillins. Compounds in these categories include:

Amoxicillin Trihydrate (Interference with bactericidal action of penicillin). Products include:
Amoxil 2631
Augmentin 2637
Augmentin Tablets 2640

Ampicillin Sodium (Interference with bactericidal action of penicillin). Products include:
Unasyn 2035

Azlocillin Sodium (Interference with bactericidal action of penicillin).
No products indexed under this heading.

Bacampicillin Hydrochloride (Interference with bactericidal action of penicillin). Products include:
Spectrobid Tablets 2030

Carbenicillin Disodium (Interference with bactericidal action of penicillin).
No products indexed under this heading.

Carbenicillin Indanyl Sodium (Interference with bactericidal action of penicillin). Products include:
Geocillin Tablets 2009

Dalteparin Sodium (Depressed plasma prothrombin activity; downward adjustment of anticoagulant dosage may be necessary). Products include:
Fragmin Injection 2088

Dicloxacillin Sodium (Interference with bactericidal action of penicillin).
No products indexed under this heading.

Dicumarol (Depressed plasma prothrombin activity; downward adjustment of anticoagulant dosage may be necessary).
No products indexed under this heading.

Enoxaparin (Depressed plasma prothrombin activity; downward adjustment of anticoagulant dosage may be necessary). Products include:
Lovenox Injection 2187

Heparin Calcium (Depressed plasma prothrombin activity; downward adjustment of anticoagulant dosage may be necessary).
No products indexed under this heading.

Heparin Sodium (Depressed plasma prothrombin activity; downward adjustment of anticoagulant dosage may be necessary). Products include:
Heparin Lock Flush Solution 2831
Heparin Sodium Injection 2832
Heparin Sodium Vials 1486

Mezlocillin Sodium (Interference with bactericidal action of penicillin). Products include:
Mezlin 594
Mezlin Pharmacy Bulk Package 597

Nafcillin Sodium (Interference with bactericidal action of penicillin).
No products indexed under this heading.

Penicillin G Benzathine (Interference with bactericidal action of penicillin). Products include:
Bicillin C-R Injection 2810
Bicillin C-R 900/300 Injection 2812
Bicillin L-A Injection 2813

Penicillin G Potassium (Interference with bactericidal action of penicillin). Products include:
Pfizerpen for Injection 2022

Penicillin G Procaine (Interference with bactericidal action of penicillin). Products include:
Bicillin C-R Injection 2810
Bicillin C-R 900/300 Injection 2812

Penicillin G Sodium (Interference with bactericidal action of penicillin).
No products indexed under this heading.

Penicillin V Potassium (Interference with bactericidal action of penicillin). Products include:
Pen·Vee K 2879

Ticarcillin Disodium (Interference with bactericidal action of penicillin). Products include:
Ticar for Injection 2704
Timentin for Injection 2706

Warfarin Sodium (Depressed plasma prothrombin activity; downward adjustment of anticoagulant dosage may be necessary). Products include:
Coumadin 941

VIBRAMYCIN MONOHYDRATE FOR ORAL SUSPENSION

(Doxycycline Monohydrate) 2038
See Vibramycin Hyclate Capsules

VIBRA-TABS FILM COATED TABLETS

(Doxycycline Hyclate) 2038
See Vibramycin Hyclate Capsules

VICKS 44 COUGH RELIEF

(Dextromethorphan Hydrobromide) 728
May interact with monoamine oxidase inhibitors. Compounds in this category include:

Furazolidone (Concurrent or sequential use not recommended). Products include:
Furoxone 2221

Isocarboxazid (Concurrent or sequential use not recommended).
No products indexed under this heading.

Phenelzine Sulfate (Concurrent or sequential use not recommended). Products include:
Nardil 1977

Selegiline Hydrochloride (Concurrent or sequential use not recommended). Products include:
Eldepryl Capsules 2729

Tranylcypromine Sulfate (Concurrent or sequential use not recommended). Products include:
Parnate Tablets 2679

VICKS 44 LIQUICAPS COUGH, COLD & FLU RELIEF

(Dextromethorphan Hydrobromide, Pseudoephedrine Hydrochloride, Chlorpheniramine Maleate, Acetaminophen) 728
May interact with monoamine oxidase inhibitors, hypnotics and sedatives, tranquilizers, and certain other agents. Compounds in these categories include:

Alprazolam (May increase the drowsiness effect). Products include:
Xanax Tablets 2115

Buspirone Hydrochloride (May increase the drowsiness effect). Products include:
BuSpar Tablets 738

Chlordiazepoxide (May increase the drowsiness effect). Products include:
Limbitrol 2333

Chlordiazepoxide Hydrochloride (May increase the drowsiness effect). Products include:
Librax Capsules 2330
Librium Capsules 2331
Librium Injectable 2332

Chlorpromazine (May increase the drowsiness effect). Products include:
Thorazine Suppositories 2701

Chlorpromazine Hydrochloride (May increase the drowsiness effect). Products include:
Thorazine 2701

Chlorprothixene (May increase the drowsiness effect).
No products indexed under this heading.

Chlorprothixene Hydrochloride (May increase the drowsiness effect).
No products indexed under this heading.

Clorazepate Dipotassium (May increase the drowsiness effect). Products include:
Tranxene 459

Diazepam (May increase the drowsiness effect). Products include:
Dizac (diazepam injectable emulsion) CIV 1862
Valium Injectable 2336
Valium Tablets 2335

Droperidol (May increase the drowsiness effect). Products include:
Inapsine Injection 462

Estazolam (May increase the drowsiness effect). Products include:
ProSom Tablets 457

Ethchlorvynol (May increase the drowsiness effect). Products include:
Placidyl Capsules 456

Ethinamate (May increase the drowsiness effect).
No products indexed under this heading.

Fluphenazine Decanoate (May increase the drowsiness effect). Products include:
Prolixin Decanoate 510

Fluphenazine Enanthate (May increase the drowsiness effect). Products include:
Prolixin Enanthate 510

Fluphenazine Hydrochloride (May increase the drowsiness effect). Products include:
Prolixin 510

Flurazepam Hydrochloride (May increase the drowsiness effect). Products include:
Dalmane Capsules 2329

Furazolidone (Concomitant and/or sequential use not recommended). Products include:
Furoxone 2221

Glutethimide (May increase the drowsiness effect).
No products indexed under this heading.

Haloperidol (May increase the drowsiness effect). Products include:
Haldol Injection, Tablets and Concentrate 1585

Haloperidol Decanoate (May increase the drowsiness effect). Products include:
Haldol Decanoate 1587

Hydroxyzine Hydrochloride (May increase the drowsiness effect). Products include:
Atarax Tablets & Syrup 1992
Marax Tablets & DF Syrup 2015
Vistaril Intramuscular Solution 2042

Isocarboxazid (Concomitant and/or sequential use not recommended).
No products indexed under this heading.

Lorazepam (May increase the drowsiness effect). Products include:
Ativan Injection 2805
Ativan Tablets 2807

Loxapine Hydrochloride (May increase the drowsiness effect). Products include:
Loxitane 1426

Loxapine Succinate (May increase the drowsiness effect). Products include:
Loxitane Capsules 1426

Meprobamate (May increase the drowsiness effect). Products include:
Miltown Tablets 2780
PMB 200 and PMB 400 2890

Mesoridazine Besylate (May increase the drowsiness effect). Products include:
Serentil 689

Midazolam Hydrochloride (May increase the drowsiness effect). Products include:
Versed Injection 2324

Molindone Hydrochloride (May increase the drowsiness effect). Products include:
Moban Tablets and Concentrate 1036

Oxazepam (May increase the drowsiness effect). Products include:
Serax Capsules 2916
Serax Tablets 2916

Perphenazine (May increase the drowsiness effect). Products include:
Etrafon 2495
Triavil Tablets 1800
Trilafon 2532

(Described in PDR For Nonprescription Drugs)   (Described in PDR For Ophthalmology)

Phenelzine Sulfate (Concomitant and/or sequential use not recommended). Products include:
- Nardil 1977

Prazepam (May increase the drowsiness effect).
- No products indexed under this heading.

Prochlorperazine (May increase the drowsiness effect). Products include:
- Compazine 2644

Promethazine Hydrochloride (May increase the drowsiness effect). Products include:
- Mepergan Injection 2859
- Phenergan with Codeine 2883
- Phenergan with Dextromethorphan ... 2885
- Phenergan Injection 2880
- Phenergan Suppositories 2882
- Phenergan Syrup 2881
- Phenergan Tablets 2882
- Phenergan VC 2886
- Phenergan VC with Codeine .. 2888

Propofol (May increase the drowsiness effect). Products include:
- Diprivan Injectable Emulsion .. 2939

Quazepam (May increase the drowsiness effect). Products include:
- Doral Tablets 2773

Secobarbital Sodium (May increase the drowsiness effect). Products include:
- Seconal Sodium Pulvules 1529

Selegiline Hydrochloride (Concomitant and/or sequential use not recommended). Products include:
- Eldepryl Capsules 2729

Temazepam (May increase the drowsiness effect). Products include:
- Restoril Capsules 2413

Thioridazine Hydrochloride (May increase the drowsiness effect). Products include:
- Mellaril 2398

Thiothixene (May increase the drowsiness effect). Products include:
- Navane Capsules and Concentrate ... 2018
- Navane Intramuscular 2019

Tranylcypromine Sulfate (Concomitant and/or sequential use not recommended). Products include:
- Parnate Tablets 2679

Triazolam (May increase the drowsiness effect). Products include:
- Halcion Tablets 2093

Trifluoperazine Hydrochloride (May increase the drowsiness effect). Products include:
- Stelazine 2692

Zolpidem Tartrate (May increase the drowsiness effect). Products include:
- Ambien Tablets 2559

Food Interactions

Alcohol (May increase the drowsiness effect).

VICKS 44 LIQUICAPS NON-DROWSY COUGH & COLD RELIEF
(Dextromethorphan Hydrobromide, Pseudoephedrine Hydrochloride) 729
May interact with monoamine oxidase inhibitors. Compounds in this category include:

Furazolidone (Concurrent and/or sequential use is not recommended). Products include:
- Furoxone 2221

Isocarboxazid (Concurrent and/or sequential use is not recommended).
- No products indexed under this heading.

Phenelzine Sulfate (Concurrent and/or sequential use is not recommended). Products include:
- Nardil 1977

Selegiline Hydrochloride (Concurrent and/or sequential use is not recommended). Products include:
- Eldepryl Capsules 2729

Tranylcypromine Sulfate (Concurrent and/or sequential use is not recommended). Products include:
- Parnate Tablets 2679

VICKS 44D COUGH & HEAD CONGESTION RELIEF
(Dextromethorphan Hydrobromide, Pseudoephedrine Hydrochloride) 728
May interact with monoamine oxidase inhibitors. Compounds in this category include:

Furazolidone (Concurrent and/or sequential use is not recommended). Products include:
- Furoxone 2221

Isocarboxazid (Concurrent and/or sequential use is not recommended).
- No products indexed under this heading.

Phenelzine Sulfate (Concurrent and/or sequential use is not recommended). Products include:
- Nardil 1977

Selegiline Hydrochloride (Concurrent and/or sequential use is not recommended). Products include:
- Eldepryl Capsules 2729

Tranylcypromine Sulfate (Concurrent and/or sequential use is not recommended). Products include:
- Parnate Tablets 2679

VICKS 44E COUGH & CHEST CONGESTION RELIEF
(Dextromethorphan Hydrobromide, Guaifenesin) 729
May interact with monoamine oxidase inhibitors. Compounds in this category include:

Furazolidone (Concurrent and/or sequential use is not recommended). Products include:
- Furoxone 2221

Isocarboxazid (Concurrent and/or sequential use is not recommended).
- No products indexed under this heading.

Phenelzine Sulfate (Concurrent and/or sequential use is not recommended). Products include:
- Nardil 1977

Selegiline Hydrochloride (Concurrent and/or sequential use is not recommended). Products include:
- Eldepryl Capsules 2729

Tranylcypromine Sulfate (Concurrent and/or sequential use is not recommended). Products include:
- Parnate Tablets 2679

VICKS 44M COUGH, COLD & FLU RELIEF
(Acetaminophen, Dextromethorphan Hydrobromide, Chlorpheniramine Maleate, Pseudoephedrine Hydrochloride) 729
May interact with hypnotics and sedatives, tranquilizers, monoamine oxidase inhibitors, and certain other agents. Compounds in these categories include:

Alprazolam (May increase drowsiness effect). Products include:
- Xanax Tablets 2115

Buspirone Hydrochloride (May increase drowsiness effect). Products include:
- BuSpar Tablets 738

Chlordiazepoxide (May increase drowsiness effect). Products include:
- Limbitrol 2333

Chlordiazepoxide Hydrochloride (May increase drowsiness effect). Products include:
- Librax Capsules 2330
- Librium Capsules 2331
- Librium Injectable 2332

Chlorpromazine (May increase drowsiness effect). Products include:
- Thorazine Suppositories 2701

Chlorpromazine Hydrochloride (May increase drowsiness effect). Products include:
- Thorazine 2701

Chlorprothixene (May increase drowsiness effect).
- No products indexed under this heading.

Chlorprothixene Hydrochloride (May increase drowsiness effect).
- No products indexed under this heading.

Clorazepate Dipotassium (May increase drowsiness effect). Products include:
- Tranxene 459

Diazepam (May increase drowsiness effect). Products include:
- Dizac (diazepam injectable emulsion) CIV 1862
- Valium Injectable 2336
- Valium Tablets 2335

Droperidol (May increase drowsiness effect). Products include:
- Inapsine Injection 462

Estazolam (May increase drowsiness effect). Products include:
- ProSom Tablets 457

Ethchlorvynol (May increase drowsiness effect). Products include:
- Placidyl Capsules 456

Ethinamate (May increase drowsiness effect).
- No products indexed under this heading.

Fluphenazine Decanoate (May increase drowsiness effect). Products include:
- Prolixin Decanoate 510

Fluphenazine Enanthate (May increase drowsiness effect). Products include:
- Prolixin Enanthate 510

Fluphenazine Hydrochloride (May increase drowsiness effect). Products include:
- Prolixin 510

Flurazepam Hydrochloride (May increase drowsiness effect). Products include:
- Dalmane Capsules 2329

Furazolidone (Concurrent and/or sequential use is not recommended). Products include:
- Furoxone 2221

Glutethimide (May increase drowsiness effect).
- No products indexed under this heading.

Haloperidol (May increase drowsiness effect). Products include:
- Haldol Injection, Tablets and Concentrate 1585

Haloperidol Decanoate (May increase drowsiness effect). Products include:
- Haldol Decanoate 1587

Hydroxyzine Hydrochloride (May increase drowsiness effect). Products include:
- Atarax Tablets & Syrup 1992

- Marax Tablets & DF Syrup 2015
- Vistaril Intramuscular Solution ... 2042

Isocarboxazid (Concurrent and/or sequential use is not recommended).
- No products indexed under this heading.

Lorazepam (May increase drowsiness effect). Products include:
- Ativan Injection 2805
- Ativan Tablets 2807

Loxapine Hydrochloride (May increase drowsiness effect). Products include:
- Loxitane 1426

Loxapine Succinate (May increase drowsiness effect). Products include:
- Loxitane Capsules 1426

Meprobamate (May increase drowsiness effect). Products include:
- Miltown Tablets 2780
- PMB 200 and PMB 400 2890

Mesoridazine Besylate (May increase drowsiness effect). Products include:
- Serentil 689

Midazolam Hydrochloride (May increase drowsiness effect). Products include:
- Versed Injection 2324

Molindone Hydrochloride (May increase drowsiness effect). Products include:
- Moban Tablets and Concentrate ... 1036

Oxazepam (May increase drowsiness effect). Products include:
- Serax Capsules 2916
- Serax Tablets 2916

Perphenazine (May increase drowsiness effect). Products include:
- Etrafon 2495
- Triavil Tablets 1800
- Trilafon 2532

Phenelzine Sulfate (Concurrent and/or sequential use is not recommended). Products include:
- Nardil 1977

Prazepam (May increase drowsiness effect).
- No products indexed under this heading.

Prochlorperazine (May increase drowsiness effect). Products include:
- Compazine 2644

Promethazine Hydrochloride (May increase drowsiness effect). Products include:
- Mepergan Injection 2859
- Phenergan with Codeine 2883
- Phenergan with Dextromethorphan ... 2885
- Phenergan Injection 2880
- Phenergan Suppositories 2882
- Phenergan Syrup 2881
- Phenergan Tablets 2882
- Phenergan VC 2886
- Phenergan VC with Codeine .. 2888

Propofol (May increase drowsiness effect). Products include:
- Diprivan Injectable Emulsion .. 2939

Quazepam (May increase drowsiness effect). Products include:
- Doral Tablets 2773

Secobarbital Sodium (May increase drowsiness effect). Products include:
- Seconal Sodium Pulvules 1529

Selegiline Hydrochloride (Concurrent and/or sequential use is not recommended). Products include:
- Eldepryl Capsules 2729

Temazepam (May increase drowsiness effect). Products include:
- Restoril Capsules 2413

Thioridazine Hydrochloride (May increase drowsiness effect). Products include:
- Mellaril 2398

IMPORTANT NOTE: Always consult each drug listing in the patient's regimen for possible interactions.

Vicks 44M

Thiothixene (May increase drowsiness effect). Products include:
- Navane Capsules and Concentrate ... 2018
- Navane Intramuscular ... 2019

Tranylcypromine Sulfate (Concurrent and/or sequential use is not recommended). Products include:
- Parnate Tablets ... 2679

Triazolam (May increase drowsiness effect). Products include:
- Halcion Tablets ... 2093

Trifluoperazine Hydrochloride (May increase drowsiness effect). Products include:
- Stelazine ... 2692

Zolpidem Tartrate (May increase drowsiness effect). Products include:
- Ambien Tablets ... 2559

Food Interactions
Alcohol (May increase drowsiness effect).

VICKS CHLORASEPTIC COUGH & THROAT DROPS, MENTHOL, CHERRY AND HONEY LEMON FLAVORS
(Menthol) ... 732
None cited in PDR database.

VICKS CHLORASEPTIC SORE THROAT LOZENGES, MENTHOL AND CHERRY FLAVORS
(Benzocaine, Menthol) ... 732
None cited in PDR database.

VICKS CHLORASPETIC SORE THROAT SPRAY, GARGLE AND MOUTH RINSE, MENTHOL AND CHERRY FLAVORS
(Phenol) ... 732
None cited in PDR database.

VICKS COUGH DROPS, MENTHOL AND CHERRY FLAVORS
(Menthol) ... 732
None cited in PDR database.

VICKS DAYQUIL ALLERGY RELIEF 12-HOUR EXTENDED RELEASE TABLETS
(Phenylpropanolamine Hydrochloride, Brompheniramine Maleate) ... 733
May interact with monoamine oxidase inhibitors and certain other agents. Compounds in these categories include:

Furazolidone (Concurrent use is not recommended). Products include:
- Furoxone ... 2221

Isocarboxazid (Concurrent use is not recommended).
No products indexed under this heading.

Phenelzine Sulfate (Concurrent use is not recommended). Products include:
- Nardil ... 1977

Selegiline Hydrochloride (Concurrent use is not recommended). Products include:
- Eldepryl Capsules ... 2729

Tranylcypromine Sulfate (Concurrent use is not recommended). Products include:
- Parnate Tablets ... 2679

Food Interactions
Alcohol (Avoid concurrent use).

VICKS DAYQUIL ALLERGY RELIEF 4-HOUR TABLETS
(Phenylpropanolamine Hydrochloride, Brompheniramine Maleate) ... 733
May interact with monoamine oxidase inhibitors, hypnotics and sedatives, tranquilizers, and certain other agents. Compounds in these categories include:

Alprazolam (May increase drowsiness effect). Products include:
- Xanax Tablets ... 2115

Buspirone Hydrochloride (May increase drowsiness effect). Products include:
- BuSpar Tablets ... 738

Chlordiazepoxide (May increase drowsiness effect). Products include:
- Limbitrol ... 2333

Chlordiazepoxide Hydrochloride (May increase drowsiness effect). Products include:
- Librax Capsules ... 2330
- Librium Capsules ... 2331
- Librium Injectable ... 2332

Chlorpromazine (May increase drowsiness effect). Products include:
- Thorazine Suppositories ... 2701

Chlorpromazine Hydrochloride (May increase drowsiness effect). Products include:
- Thorazine ... 2701

Chlorprothixene (May increase drowsiness effect).
No products indexed under this heading.

Chlorprothixene Hydrochloride (May increase drowsiness effect).
No products indexed under this heading.

Clorazepate Dipotassium (May increase drowsiness effect). Products include:
- Tranxene ... 459

Diazepam (May increase drowsiness effect). Products include:
- Dizac (diazepam injectable emulsion) CIV ... 1862
- Valium Injectable ... 2336
- Valium Tablets ... 2335

Droperidol (May increase drowsiness effect). Products include:
- Inapsine Injection ... 462

Estazolam (May increase drowsiness effect). Products include:
- ProSom Tablets ... 457

Ethchlorvynol (May increase drowsiness effect). Products include:
- Placidyl Capsules ... 456

Ethinamate (May increase drowsiness effect).
No products indexed under this heading.

Fluphenazine Decanoate (May increase drowsiness effect). Products include:
- Prolixin Decanoate ... 510

Fluphenazine Enanthate (May increase drowsiness effect). Products include:
- Prolixin Enanthate ... 510

Fluphenazine Hydrochloride (May increase drowsiness effect). Products include:
- Prolixin ... 510

Flurazepam Hydrochloride (May increase drowsiness effect). Products include:
- Dalmane Capsules ... 2329

Furazolidone (Concurrent and/or sequential use is not recommended). Products include:
- Furoxone ... 2221

Glutethimide (May increase drowsiness effect).
No products indexed under this heading.

Interactions Index

Haloperidol (May increase drowsiness effect). Products include:
- Haldol Injection, Tablets and Concentrate ... 1585

Haloperidol Decanoate (May increase drowsiness effect). Products include:
- Haldol Decanoate ... 1587

Hydroxyzine Hydrochloride (May increase drowsiness effect). Products include:
- Atarax Tablets & Syrup ... 1992
- Marax Tablets & DF Syrup ... 2015
- Vistaril Intramuscular Solution ... 2042

Isocarboxazid (Concurrent and/or sequential use is not recommended).
No products indexed under this heading.

Lorazepam (May increase drowsiness effect). Products include:
- Ativan Injection ... 2805
- Ativan Tablets ... 2807

Loxapine Hydrochloride (May increase drowsiness effect). Products include:
- Loxitane ... 1426

Loxapine Succinate (May increase drowsiness effect). Products include:
- Loxitane Capsules ... 1426

Meprobamate (May increase drowsiness effect). Products include:
- Miltown Tablets ... 2780
- PMB 200 and PMB 400 ... 2890

Mesoridazine Besylate (May increase drowsiness effect). Products include:
- Serentil ... 689

Midazolam Hydrochloride (May increase drowsiness effect). Products include:
- Versed Injection ... 2324

Molindone Hydrochloride (May increase drowsiness effect). Products include:
- Moban Tablets and Concentrate ... 1036

Oxazepam (May increase drowsiness effect). Products include:
- Serax Capsules ... 2916
- Serax Tablets ... 2916

Perphenazine (May increase drowsiness effect). Products include:
- Etrafon ... 2495
- Triavil Tablets ... 1800
- Trilafon ... 2532

Phenelzine Sulfate (Concurrent and/or sequential use is not recommended). Products include:
- Nardil ... 1977

Prazepam (May increase drowsiness effect).
No products indexed under this heading.

Prochlorperazine (May increase drowsiness effect). Products include:
- Compazine ... 2644

Promethazine Hydrochloride (May increase drowsiness effect). Products include:
- Mepergan Injection ... 2859
- Phenergan with Codeine ... 2883
- Phenergan with Dextromethorphan ... 2885
- Phenergan Injection ... 2880
- Phenergan Suppositories ... 2882
- Phenergan Syrup ... 2881
- Phenergan Tablets ... 2882
- Phenergan VC ... 2886
- Phenergan VC with Codeine ... 2888

Propofol (May increase drowsiness effect). Products include:
- Diprivan Injectable Emulsion ... 2939

Quazepam (May increase drowsiness effect). Products include:
- Doral Tablets ... 2773

Secobarbital Sodium (May increase drowsiness effect). Products include:
- Seconal Sodium Pulvules ... 1529

Selegiline Hydrochloride (Concurrent and/or sequential use is not recommended). Products include:
- Eldepryl Capsules ... 2729

Temazepam (May increase drowsiness effect). Products include:
- Restoril Capsules ... 2413

Thioridazine Hydrochloride (May increase drowsiness effect). Products include:
- Mellaril ... 2398

Thiothixene (May increase drowsiness effect). Products include:
- Navane Capsules and Concentrate ... 2018
- Navane Intramuscular ... 2019

Tranylcypromine Sulfate (Concurrent and/or sequential use is not recommended). Products include:
- Parnate Tablets ... 2679

Triazolam (May increase drowsiness effect). Products include:
- Halcion Tablets ... 2093

Trifluoperazine Hydrochloride (May increase drowsiness effect). Products include:
- Stelazine ... 2692

Zolpidem Tartrate (May increase drowsiness effect). Products include:
- Ambien Tablets ... 2559

Food Interactions
Alcohol (May increase drowsiness effect).

VICKS DAYQUIL LIQUICAPS/LIQUID MULTI-SYMPTOM COLD/FLU RELIEF
(Acetaminophen, Dextromethorphan Hydrobromide, Pseudoephedrine Hydrochloride, Guaifenesin) ... 734
May interact with monoamine oxidase inhibitors. Compounds in this category include:

Furazolidone (Concurrent and/or sequential use is not recommended). Products include:
- Furoxone ... 2221

Isocarboxazid (Concurrent and/or sequential use is not recommended).
No products indexed under this heading.

Phenelzine Sulfate (Concurrent and/or sequential use is not recommended). Products include:
- Nardil ... 1977

Selegiline Hydrochloride (Concurrent and/or sequential use is not recommended). Products include:
- Eldepryl Capsules ... 2729

Tranylcypromine Sulfate (Concurrent and/or sequential use is not recommended). Products include:
- Parnate Tablets ... 2679

VICKS DAYQUIL SINUS PRESSURE & CONGESTION RELIEF
(Guaifenesin, Phenylpropanolamine Hydrochloride) ... 734
May interact with monoamine oxidase inhibitors. Compounds in this category include:

Furazolidone (Concurrent and/or sequential use is not recommended). Products include:
- Furoxone ... 2221

Isocarboxazid (Concurrent and/or sequential use is not recommended).
No products indexed under this heading.

Phenelzine Sulfate (Concurrent and/or sequential use is not recommended). Products include:
- Nardil ... 1977

(■ Described in PDR For Nonprescription Drugs) (◉ Described in PDR For Ophthalmology)

Selegiline Hydrochloride (Concurrent and/or sequential use is not recommended). Products include:
  Eldepryl Capsules 2729
Tranylcypromine Sulfate (Concurrent and/or sequential use is not recommended). Products include:
  Parnate Tablets 2679

VICKS DAYQUIL SINUS PRESSURE & PAIN RELIEF WITH IBUPROFEN
(Ibuprofen, Pseudoephedrine Hydrochloride) 735
May interact with monoamine oxidase inhibitors. Compounds in this category include:

Furazolidone (Concurrent and/or sequential use is not recommended. Products include:
  Furoxone 2221
Isocarboxazid (Concurrent and/or sequential use is not recommended).
  No products indexed under this heading.
Phenelzine Sulfate (Concurrent and/or sequential use is not recommended). Products include:
  Nardil 1977
Selegiline Hydrochloride (Concurrent and/or sequential use is not recommended). Products include:
  Eldepryl Capsules 2729
Tranylcypromine Sulfate (Concurrent and/or sequential use is not recommended). Products include:
  Parnate Tablets 2679

VICKS NYQUIL HOT THERAPY
(Acetaminophen, Pseudoephedrine Hydrochloride, Dextromethorphan Hydrobromide, Doxylamine Succinate) 735
May interact with hypnotics and sedatives, tranquilizers, monoamine oxidase inhibitors, and certain other agents. Compounds in these categories include:

Alprazolam (May increase the drowsiness effect). Products include:
  Xanax Tablets 2115
Buspirone Hydrochloride (May increase the drowsiness effect). Products include:
  BuSpar Tablets 738
Chlordiazepoxide (May increase the drowsiness effect). Products include:
  Limbitrol 2333
Chlordiazepoxide Hydrochloride (May increase the drowsiness effect). Products include:
  Librax Capsules 2330
  Librium Capsules 2331
  Librium Injectable 2332
Chlorpromazine (May increase the drowsiness effect). Products include:
  Thorazine Suppositories 2701
Chlorpromazine Hydrochloride (May increase the drowsiness effect). Products include:
  Thorazine 2701
Chlorprothixene (May increase the drowsiness effect).
  No products indexed under this heading.
Chlorprothixene Hydrochloride (May increase the drowsiness effect).
  No products indexed under this heading.

Clorazepate Dipotassium (May increase the drowsiness effect). Products include:
  Tranxene 459
Diazepam (May increase the drowsiness effect). Products include:
  Dizac (diazepam injectable emulsion) CIV 1862
  Valium Injectable 2336
  Valium Tablets 2335
Droperidol (May increase the drowsiness effect). Products include:
  Inapsine Injection 462
Estazolam (May increase the drowsiness effect). Products include:
  ProSom Tablets 457
Ethchlorvynol (May increase the drowsiness effect). Products include:
  Placidyl Capsules 456
Ethinamate (May increase the drowsiness effect).
  No products indexed under this heading.
Fluphenazine Decanoate (May increase the drowsiness effect). Products include:
  Prolixin Decanoate 510
Fluphenazine Enanthate (May increase the drowsiness effect). Products include:
  Prolixin Enanthate 510
Fluphenazine Hydrochloride (May increase the drowsiness effect). Products include:
  Prolixin 510
Flurazepam Hydrochloride (May increase the drowsiness effect). Products include:
  Dalmane Capsules 2329
Furazolidone (Concurrent and/or sequential use is not recommended. Products include:
  Furoxone 2221
Glutethimide (May increase the drowsiness effect).
  No products indexed under this heading.
Haloperidol (May increase the drowsiness effect). Products include:
  Haldol Injection, Tablets and Concentrate 1585
Haloperidol Decanoate (May increase the drowsiness effect). Products include:
  Haldol Decanoate 1587
Hydroxyzine Hydrochloride (May increase the drowsiness effect). Products include:
  Atarax Tablets & Syrup 1992
  Marax Tablets & DF Syrup 2015
  Vistaril Intramuscular Solution 2042
Isocarboxazid (Concurrent and/or sequential use is not recommended).
  No products indexed under this heading.
Lorazepam (May increase the drowsiness effect). Products include:
  Ativan Injection 2805
  Ativan Tablets 2807
Loxapine Hydrochloride (May increase the drowsiness effect). Products include:
  Loxitane 1426
Loxapine Succinate (May increase the drowsiness effect). Products include:
  Loxitane Capsules 1426
Meprobamate (May increase the drowsiness effect). Products include:
  Miltown Tablets 2780
  PMB 200 and PMB 400 2890
Mesoridazine Besylate (May increase the drowsiness effect). Products include:
  Serentil 689

Midazolam Hydrochloride (May increase the drowsiness effect). Products include:
  Versed Injection 2324
Molindone Hydrochloride (May increase the drowsiness effect). Products include:
  Moban Tablets and Concentrate 1036
Oxazepam (May increase the drowsiness effect). Products include:
  Serax Capsules 2916
  Serax Tablets 2916
Perphenazine (May increase the drowsiness effect). Products include:
  Etrafon 2495
  Triavil Tablets 1800
  Trilafon 2532
Phenelzine Sulfate (Concurrent and/or sequential use is not recommended). Products include:
  Nardil 1977
Prazepam (May increase the drowsiness effect).
  No products indexed under this heading.
Prochlorperazine (May increase the drowsiness effect). Products include:
  Compazine 2644
Promethazine Hydrochloride (May increase the drowsiness effect). Products include:
  Mepergan Injection 2859
  Phenergan with Codeine 2883
  Phenergan with Dextromethorphan 2885
  Phenergan Injection 2880
  Phenergan Suppositories 2882
  Phenergan Syrup 2881
  Phenergan Tablets 2882
  Phenergan VC 2886
  Phenergan VC with Codeine 2888
Propofol (May increase the drowsiness effect). Products include:
  Diprivan Injectable Emulsion 2939
Quazepam (May increase the drowsiness effect). Products include:
  Doral Tablets 2773
Secobarbital Sodium (May increase the drowsiness effect). Products include:
  Seconal Sodium Pulvules 1529
Selegiline Hydrochloride (Concurrent and/or sequential use is not recommended). Products include:
  Eldepryl Capsules 2729
Temazepam (May increase the drowsiness effect). Products include:
  Restoril Capsules 2413
Thioridazine Hydrochloride (May increase the drowsiness effect). Products include:
  Mellaril 2398
Thiothixene (May increase the drowsiness effect). Products include:
  Navane Capsules and Concentrate .. 2018
  Navane Intramuscular 2019
Tranylcypromine Sulfate (Concurrent and/or sequential use is not recommended). Products include:
  Parnate Tablets 2679
Triazolam (May increase the drowsiness effect). Products include:
  Halcion Tablets 2093
Trifluoperazine Hydrochloride (May increase the drowsiness effect). Products include:
  Stelazine 2692
Zolpidem Tartrate (May increase the drowsiness effect). Products include:
  Ambien Tablets 2559

Food Interactions
Alcohol (May increase drowsiness effect).

VICKS NYQUIL LIQUICAPS/LIQUID MULTI-SYMPTOM COLD/FLU RELIEF, ORIGINAL AND CHERRY FLAVORS
(Acetaminophen, Pseudoephedrine Hydrochloride, Dextromethorphan Hydrobromide, Doxylamine Succinate) 736
May interact with hypnotics and sedatives, tranquilizers, monoamine oxidase inhibitors, and certain other agents. Compounds in these categories include:

Alprazolam (May increase drowsiness effect). Products include:
  Xanax Tablets 2115
Buspirone Hydrochloride (May increase drowsiness effect). Products include:
  BuSpar Tablets 738
Chlordiazepoxide (May increase drowsiness effect). Products include:
  Limbitrol 2333
Chlordiazepoxide Hydrochloride (May increase drowsiness effect). Products include:
  Librax Capsules 2330
  Librium Capsules 2331
  Librium Injectable 2332
Chlorpromazine (May increase drowsiness effect). Products include:
  Thorazine Suppositories 2701
Chlorpromazine Hydrochloride (May increase drowsiness effect). Products include:
  Thorazine 2701
Chlorprothixene (May increase drowsiness effect).
  No products indexed under this heading.
Chlorprothixene Hydrochloride (May increase drowsiness effect).
  No products indexed under this heading.
Clorazepate Dipotassium (May increase drowsiness effect). Products include:
  Tranxene 459
Diazepam (May increase drowsiness effect). Products include:
  Dizac (diazepam injectable emulsion) CIV 1862
  Valium Injectable 2336
  Valium Tablets 2335
Droperidol (May increase drowsiness effect). Products include:
  Inapsine Injection 462
Estazolam (May increase drowsiness effect). Products include:
  ProSom Tablets 457
Ethchlorvynol (May increase drowsiness effect). Products include:
  Placidyl Capsules 456
Ethinamate (May increase drowsiness effect).
  No products indexed under this heading.
Fluphenazine Decanoate (May increase drowsiness effect). Products include:
  Prolixin Decanoate 510
Fluphenazine Enanthate (May increase drowsiness effect). Products include:
  Prolixin Enanthate 510
Fluphenazine Hydrochloride (May increase drowsiness effect). Products include:
  Prolixin 510
Flurazepam Hydrochloride (May increase drowsiness effect). Products include:
  Dalmane Capsules 2329

IMPORTANT NOTE: Always consult each drug listing in the patient's regimen for possible interactions.

Vicks NyQuil LiquiCaps **Interactions Index** **1174**

Furazolidone (Concurrent and/or sequential use is not recommended). Products include:
- Furoxone 2221

Glutethimide (May increase drowsiness effect).
- No products indexed under this heading.

Haloperidol (May increase drowsiness effect). Products include:
- Haldol Injection, Tablets and Concentrate 1585

Haloperidol Decanoate (May increase drowsiness effect). Products include:
- Haldol Decanoate 1587

Hydroxyzine Hydrochloride (May increase drowsiness effect). Products include:
- Atarax Tablets & Syrup 1992
- Marax Tablets & DF Syrup 2015
- Vistaril Intramuscular Solution 2042

Isocarboxazid (Concurrent and/or sequential use is not recommended).
- No products indexed under this heading.

Lorazepam (May increase drowsiness effect). Products include:
- Ativan Injection 2805
- Ativan Tablets 2807

Loxapine Hydrochloride (May increase drowsiness effect). Products include:
- Loxitane 1426

Loxapine Succinate (May increase drowsiness effect). Products include:
- Loxitane Capsules 1426

Meprobamate (May increase drowsiness effect). Products include:
- Miltown Tablets 2780
- PMB 200 and PMB 400 2890

Mesoridazine Besylate (May increase drowsiness effect). Products include:
- Serentil 689

Midazolam Hydrochloride (May increase drowsiness effect). Products include:
- Versed Injection 2324

Molindone Hydrochloride (May increase drowsiness effect). Products include:
- Moban Tablets and Concentrate 1036

Oxazepam (May increase drowsiness effect). Products include:
- Serax Capsules 2916
- Serax Tablets 2916

Perphenazine (May increase drowsiness effect). Products include:
- Etrafon 2495
- Triavil Tablets 1800
- Trilafon 2532

Phenelzine Sulfate (Concurrent and/or sequential use is not recommended). Products include:
- Nardil 1977

Prazepam (May increase drowsiness effect).
- No products indexed under this heading.

Prochlorperazine (May increase drowsiness effect). Products include:
- Compazine 2644

Promethazine Hydrochloride (May increase drowsiness effect). Products include:
- Mepergan Injection 2859
- Phenergan with Codeine 2883
- Phenergan with Dextromethorphan 2885
- Phenergan Injection 2880
- Phenergan Suppositories 2882
- Phenergan Syrup 2881
- Phenergan Tablets 2882
- Phenergan VC 2886
- Phenergan VC with Codeine 2888

Propofol (May increase drowsiness effect). Products include:
- Diprivan Injectable Emulsion 2939

Quazepam (May increase drowsiness effect). Products include:
- Doral Tablets 2773

Secobarbital Sodium (May increase drowsiness effect). Products include:
- Seconal Sodium Pulvules 1529

Selegiline Hydrochloride (Concurrent and/or sequential use is not recommended). Products include:
- Eldepryl Capsules 2729

Temazepam (May increase drowsiness effect). Products include:
- Restoril Capsules 2413

Thioridazine Hydrochloride (May increase drowsiness effect). Products include:
- Mellaril 2398

Thiothixene (May increase drowsiness effect). Products include:
- Navane Capsules and Concentrate 2018
- Navane Intramuscular 2019

Tranylcypromine Sulfate (Concurrent and/or sequential use is not recommended). Products include:
- Parnate Tablets 2679

Triazolam (May increase drowsiness effect). Products include:
- Halcion Tablets 2093

Trifluoperazine Hydrochloride (May increase drowsiness effect). Products include:
- Stelazine 2692

Zolpidem Tartrate (May increase drowsiness effect). Products include:
- Ambien Tablets 2559

Food Interactions

Alcohol (May increase drowsiness effect).

VICKS SINEX 12-HOUR NASAL DECONGESTANT SPRAY AND ULTRA FINE MIST
(Oxymetazoline Hydrochloride) .... ■ 738
None cited in PDR database.

VICKS SINEX NASAL SPRAY AND ULTRA FINE MIST
(Phenylephrine Hydrochloride) .... ■ 738
None cited in PDR database.

VICKS VAPOR INHALER
(Desoxyephedrine-Levo) .... ■ 738
None cited in PDR database.

VICKS VAPORUB CREAM
(Menthol, Camphor, Eucalyptus, Oil of) .... ■ 739
None cited in PDR database.

VICKS VAPORUB OINTMENT
(Menthol, Camphor, Eucalyptus, Oil of) .... ■ 739
None cited in PDR database.

VICKS VAPOSTEAM
(Camphor, Eucalyptus, Oil of, Menthol) .... ■ 739
None cited in PDR database.

VICODIN TABLETS
(Hydrocodone Bitartrate, Acetaminophen) 1404
May interact with tricyclic antidepressants, monoamine oxidase inhibitors, anticholinergics, antipsychotic agents, tranquilizers, central nervous system depressants, narcotic analgesics, and certain other agents. Compounds in these categories include:

Alfentanil Hydrochloride (May exhibit an additive CNS depression; the dose of one or both agents should be reduced). Products include:
- Alfenta Injection 1334

Alprazolam (May exhibit an additive CNS depression; the dose of one or both agents should be reduced). Products include:
- Xanax Tablets 2115

Amitriptyline Hydrochloride (Co-administration may increase the effect of either drug). Products include:
- Elavil 2945
- Etrafon 2495
- Limbitrol 2333
- Triavil Tablets 1800

Amoxapine (Co-administration may increase the effect of either drug). Products include:
- Asendin Tablets 1419

Aprobarbital (May exhibit an additive CNS depression; the dose of one or both agents should be reduced).
- No products indexed under this heading.

Atropine Sulfate (Potential for paralytic ileus). Products include:
- Arco-Lase Plus Tablets 513
- Atrohist Plus Tablets 1605
- Donnatal 2234
- Donnatal Extentabs 2234
- Donnatal Tablets 2234
- Lomotil 2591
- Motofen Tablets 789
- Urised Tablets 2123

Belladonna Alkaloids (Potential for paralytic ileus). Products include:
- Bellergal-S Tablets 2375
- Hyland's Bedwetting Tablets .... ■ 788
- Hyland's EnurAid Tablets .... ■ 789
- Hyland's Headache Tablets .... ■ 790
- Hyland's Teething Tablets .... ■ 790
- Similasan Eye Drops #1 .... ■ 769

Benztropine Mesylate (Potential for paralytic ileus). Products include:
- Cogentin 1661

Biperiden Hydrochloride (Potential for paralytic ileus). Products include:
- Akineton 1380

Buprenorphine (May exhibit an additive CNS depression; the dose of one or both agents should be reduced). Products include:
- Buprenex Injectable 2170

Buspirone Hydrochloride (May exhibit an additive CNS depression; the dose of one or both agents should be reduced). Products include:
- BuSpar Tablets 738

Butabarbital (May exhibit an additive CNS depression; the dose of one or both agents should be reduced).
- No products indexed under this heading.

Butalbital (May exhibit an additive CNS depression; the dose of one or both agents should be reduced). Products include:
- Axocet Capsules 2469
- Esgic-plus Capsules 1012
- Esgic-plus Tablets 1012
- Fioricet Tablets 2386
- Fioricet with Codeine Capsules 2387
- Fiorinal Capsules 2388
- Fiorinal with Codeine Capsules 2390
- Fiorinal Tablets 2388
- Phrenilin 790
- Sedapap Tablets 50 mg/650 mg .. 1826

Chlordiazepoxide (May exhibit an additive CNS depression; the dose of one or both agents should be reduced). Products include:
- Limbitrol 2333

Chlordiazepoxide Hydrochloride (May exhibit an additive CNS depression; the dose of one or both agents should be reduced). Products include:
- Librax Capsules 2330
- Librium Capsules 2331
- Librium Injectable 2332

Chlorpromazine (May exhibit an additive CNS depression; the dose of one or both agents should be reduced). Products include:
- Thorazine Suppositories 2701

Chlorpromazine Hydrochloride (May exhibit an additive CNS depression; the dose of one or both agents should be reduced). Products include:
- Thorazine 2701

Chlorprothixene (May exhibit an additive CNS depression; the dose of one or both agents should be reduced).
- No products indexed under this heading.

Chlorprothixene Hydrochloride (May exhibit an additive CNS depression; the dose of one or both agents should be reduced).
- No products indexed under this heading.

Chlorprothixene Lactate (May exhibit an additive CNS depression; the dose of one or both agents should be reduced).
- No products indexed under this heading.

Clidinium Bromide (Potential for paralytic ileus). Products include:
- Librax Capsules 2330

Clomipramine Hydrochloride (Co-administration may increase the effect of either drug). Products include:
- Anafranil Capsules 819

Clorazepate Dipotassium (May exhibit an additive CNS depression; the dose of one or both agents should be reduced). Products include:
- Tranxene 459

Clozapine (May exhibit an additive CNS depression; the dose of one or both agents should be reduced). Products include:
- Clozaril Tablets 2377

Codeine Phosphate (May exhibit an additive CNS depression; the dose of one or both agents should be reduced). Products include:
- Brontex 2130
- Dimetane-DC Cough Syrup 2232
- Fioricet with Codeine Capsules 2387
- Fiorinal with Codeine Capsules 2390
- Nucofed 2225
- Phenergan with Codeine 2883
- Phenergan VC with Codeine 2888
- Robitussin A-C Syrup 2248
- Robitussin-DAC Syrup 2249
- Ryna .... ■ 804
- Soma Compound w/Codeine Tablets 2784
- Tylenol with Codeine 1592

Desflurane (May exhibit an additive CNS depression; the dose of one or both agents should be reduced). Products include:
- Suprane (desflurane, USP) 1865

Desipramine Hydrochloride (Co-administration may increase the effect of either drug). Products include:
- Norpramin Tablets 1273

Dezocine (May exhibit an additive CNS depression; the dose of one or both agents should be reduced). Products include:
- Dalgan Injection 529

Interactions Index

Diazepam (May exhibit an additive CNS depression; the dose of one or both agents should be reduced. Products include:
- Dizac (diazepam injectable emulsion) CIV 1862
- Valium Injectable 2336
- Valium Tablets 2335

Dicyclomine Hydrochloride (Potential for paralytic ileus). Products include:
- Bentyl 1246

Doxepin Hydrochloride (Co-administration may increase the effect of either drug). Products include:
- Adapin Capsules 1542
- Sinequan 2028
- Zonalon Cream 1042

Droperidol (May exhibit an additive CNS depression; the dose of one or both agents should be reduced). Products include:
- Inapsine Injection 462

Enflurane (May exhibit an additive CNS depression; the dose of one or both agents should be reduced).
- No products indexed under this heading.

Estazolam (May exhibit an additive CNS depression; the dose of one or both agents should be reduced). Products include:
- ProSom Tablets 457

Ethchlorvynol (May exhibit an additive CNS depression; the dose of one or both agents should be reduced). Products include:
- Placidyl Capsules 456

Ethinamate (May exhibit an additive CNS depression; the dose of one or both agents should be reduced).
- No products indexed under this heading.

Fentanyl (May exhibit an additive CNS depression; the dose of one or both agents should be reduced). Products include:
- Duragesic Transdermal System........ 1336

Fentanyl Citrate (May exhibit an additive CNS depression; the dose of one or both agents should be reduced). Products include:
- Sublimaze Injection 463

Fluphenazine Decanoate (May exhibit an additive CNS depression; the dose of one or both agents should be reduced). Products include:
- Prolixin Decanoate 510

Fluphenazine Enanthate (May exhibit an additive CNS depression; the dose of one or both agents should be reduced). Products include:
- Prolixin Enanthate 510

Fluphenazine Hydrochloride (May exhibit an additive CNS depression; the dose of one or both agents should be reduced). Products include:
- Prolixin 510

Flurazepam Hydrochloride (May exhibit an additive CNS depression; the dose of one or both agents should be reduced). Products include:
- Dalmane Capsules 2329

Furazolidone (Co-administration may increase the effect of either drug). Products include:
- Furoxone 2221

Glutethimide (May exhibit an additive CNS depression; the dose of one or both agents should be reduced).
- No products indexed under this heading.

Glycopyrrolate (Potential for paralytic ileus). Products include:
- Robinul Forte Tablets 2247
- Robinul Injectable 2247
- Robinul Tablets 2247

Haloperidol (May exhibit an additive CNS depression; the dose of one or both agents should be reduced). Products include:
- Haldol Injection, Tablets and Concentrate 1585

Haloperidol Decanoate (May exhibit an additive CNS depression; the dose of one or both agents should be reduced). Products include:
- Haldol Decanoate 1587

Hydrocodone Polistirex (May exhibit an additive CNS depression; the dose of one or both agents should be reduced). Products include:
- Tussionex Pennkinetic Extended-Release Suspension 1624

Hydromorphone Hydrochloride (May exhibit an additive CNS depression; the dose of one or both agents should be reduced). Products include:
- Dilaudid Ampules 1382
- Dilaudid Cough Syrup 1383
- Dilaudid-HP Injection 1384
- Dilaudid-HP Lyophilized Powder 250 mg 1384
- Dilaudid 1382
- Dilaudid Oral Liquid 1386
- Dilaudid 1382
- Dilaudid Tablets - 8 mg. 1386

Hydroxyzine Hydrochloride (May exhibit an additive CNS depression; the dose of one or both agents should be reduced). Products include:
- Atarax Tablets & Syrup. 1992
- Marax Tablets & DF Syrup... 2015
- Vistaril Intramuscular Solution... 2042

Hyoscyamine (Potential for paralytic ileus). Products include:
- Cystospaz Tablets 2123
- Urised Tablets 2123

Hyoscyamine Sulfate (Potential for paralytic ileus). Products include:
- Arco-Lase Plus Tablets 513
- Atrohist Plus Tablets 1605
- Cystospaz-M Capsules 2123
- Donnatal 2234
- Donnatal Extentabs 2234
- Donnatal Tablets 2234
- Kutrase Capsules 2546
- Levsin/Levsinex/Levbid 2549

Imipramine Hydrochloride (Co-administration may increase the effect of either drug). Products include:
- Tofranil Ampuls 873
- Tofranil Tablets 875

Imipramine Pamoate (Co-administration may increase the effect of either drug). Products include:
- Tofranil-PM Capsules 876

Ipratropium Bromide (Potential for paralytic ileus). Products include:
- Atrovent Inhalation Aerosol ... 674
- Atrovent Inhalation Solution ... 675
- Atrovent Nasal Spray 0.03% ... 676
- Atrovent Nasal Spray 0.06% ... 678

Isocarboxazid (Co-administration may increase the effect of either drug).
- No products indexed under this heading.

Isoflurane (May exhibit an additive CNS depression; the dose of one or both agents should be reduced).
- No products indexed under this heading.

Ketamine Hydrochloride (May exhibit an additive CNS depression; the dose of one or both agents should be reduced).
- No products indexed under this heading.

Levomethadyl Acetate Hydrochloride (May exhibit an additive CNS depression; the dose of one or both agents should be reduced). Products include:
- Orlaam Oral Solution 2361

Levorphanol Tartrate (May exhibit an additive CNS depression; the dose of one or both agents should be reduced). Products include:
- Levo-Dromoran 2297

Lithium Carbonate (May exhibit an additive CNS depression; the dose of one or both agents should be reduced). Products include:
- Eskalith 2658
- Lithium Carbonate Capsules & Tablets 2352
- Lithonate/Lithotabs/Lithobid ... 2721

Lithium Citrate (May exhibit an additive CNS depression; the dose of one or both agents should be reduced).
- No products indexed under this heading.

Lorazepam (May exhibit an additive CNS depression; the dose of one or both agents should be reduced). Products include:
- Ativan Injection 2805
- Ativan Tablets 2807

Loxapine Hydrochloride (May exhibit an additive CNS depression; the dose of one or both agents should be reduced). Products include:
- Loxitane 1426

Loxapine Succinate (May exhibit an additive CNS depression; the dose of one or both agents should be reduced). Products include:
- Loxitane Capsules 1426

Maprotiline Hydrochloride (Co-administration may increase the effect of either drug). Products include:
- Ludiomil Tablets 861

Mepenzolate Bromide (Potential for paralytic ileus).
- No products indexed under this heading.

Meperidine Hydrochloride (May exhibit an additive CNS depression; the dose of one or both agents should be reduced). Products include:
- Demerol 2438
- Mepergan Injection 2859

Mephobarbital (May exhibit an additive CNS depression; the dose of one or both agents should be reduced). Products include:
- Mebaral Tablets 2452

Meprobamate (May exhibit an additive CNS depression; the dose of one or both agents should be reduced). Products include:
- Miltown Tablets 2780
- PMB 200 and PMB 400 2890

Mesoridazine Besylate (May exhibit an additive CNS depression; the dose of one or both agents should be reduced). Products include:
- Serentil 689

Methadone Hydrochloride (May exhibit an additive CNS depression; the dose of one or both agents should be reduced). Products include:
- Methadone Hydrochloride Oral Concentrate 2356
- Methadone Hydrochloride Oral Solution & Tablets 2357

Methohexital Sodium (May exhibit an additive CNS depression; the dose of one or both agents should be reduced).
- No products indexed under this heading.

Methotrimeprazine (May exhibit an additive CNS depression; the dose of one or both agents should be reduced). Products include:
- Levoprome 1321

Methoxyflurane (May exhibit an additive CNS depression; the dose of one or both agents should be reduced).
- No products indexed under this heading.

Midazolam Hydrochloride (May exhibit an additive CNS depression; the dose of one or both agents should be reduced). Products include:
- Versed Injection 2324

Molindone Hydrochloride (May exhibit an additive CNS depression; the dose of one or both agents should be reduced). Products include:
- Moban Tablets and Concentrate 1036

Morphine Sulfate (May exhibit an additive CNS depression; the dose of one or both agents should be reduced). Products include:
- Astramorph/PF Injection, USP (Preservative-Free) 526
- Duramorph Injection 983
- Infumorph 200 and Infumorph 500 Sterile Solutions 985
- Kadian Capsules 2948
- MS Contin Tablets 2149
- MSIR 2152
- Oramorph SR (Morphine Sulfate Sustained Release Tablets) ... 2359
- RMS Suppositories CII 2766
- Roxanol 2365

Nortriptyline Hydrochloride (Co-administration may increase the effect of either drug). Products include:
- Pamelor 2409

Opium Alkaloids (May exhibit an additive CNS depression; the dose of one or both agents should be reduced).
- No products indexed under this heading.

Oxazepam (May exhibit an additive CNS depression; the dose of one or both agents should be reduced). Products include:
- Serax Capsules 2916
- Serax Tablets 2916

Oxybutynin Chloride (Potential for paralytic ileus). Products include:
- Ditropan 1267

Oxycodone Hydrochloride (May exhibit an additive CNS depression; the dose of one or both agents should be reduced). Products include:
- OxyContin Tablets 2163
- OxyIR Capsules 2167
- Percocet Tablets 955
- Percodan Tablets 955
- Percodan-Demi Tablets 956
- Roxicodone Tablets, Oral Solution & Intensol (Oxycodone) ... 2366
- Tylox Capsules 1593

Pentobarbital Sodium (May exhibit an additive CNS depression; the dose of one or both agents should be reduced). Products include:
- Nembutal Sodium Capsules ... 440
- Nembutal Sodium Solution ... 442
- Nembutal Sodium Suppositories ... 444

IMPORTANT NOTE: Always consult each drug listing in the patient's regimen for possible interactions.

Perphenazine (May exhibit an additive CNS depression; the dose of one or both agents should be reduced). Products include:
Etrafon 2495
Triavil Tablets 1800
Trilafon 2532

Phenelzine Sulfate (Co-administration may increase the effect of either drug). Products include:
Nardil 1977

Phenobarbital (May exhibit an additive CNS depression; the dose of one or both agents should be reduced). Products include:
Arco-Lase Plus Tablets 513
Bellergal-S Tablets 2375
Donnatal 2234
Donnatal Extentabs 2234
Donnatal Tablets 2234
Phenobarbital Elixir and Tablets ... 1523
Quadrinal Tablets 1398

Pimozide (May exhibit an additive CNS depression; the dose of one or both agents should be reduced). Products include:
Orap Tablets 1037

Prazepam (May exhibit an additive CNS depression; the dose of one or both agents should be reduced).
No products indexed under this heading.

Prochlorperazine (May exhibit an additive CNS depression; the dose of one or both agents should be reduced). Products include:
Compazine 2644

Procyclidine Hydrochloride (Potential for paralytic ileus). Products include:
Kemadrin Tablets 1105

Promethazine Hydrochloride (May exhibit an additive CNS depression; the dose of one or both agents should be reduced). Products include:
Mepergan Injection 2859
Phenergan with Codeine 2883
Phenergan with Dextromethorphan .. 2885
Phenergan Injection 2880
Phenergan Suppositories 2882
Phenergan Syrup 2881
Phenergan Tablets 2882
Phenergan VC 2886
Phenergan VC with Codeine 2888

Propantheline Bromide (Potential for paralytic ileus). Products include:
Pro-Banthine Tablets 2226

Propofol (May exhibit an additive CNS depression; the dose of one or both agents should be reduced). Products include:
Diprivan Injectable Emulsion 2939

Propoxyphene Hydrochloride (May exhibit an additive CNS depression; the dose of one or both agents should be reduced). Products include:
Darvon 1475
Wygesic Tablets 2930

Propoxyphene Napsylate (May exhibit an additive CNS depression; the dose of one or both agents should be reduced). Products include:
Darvon-N/Darvocet-N 1473

Protriptyline Hydrochloride (Co-administration may increase the effect of either drug). Products include:
Vivactil Tablets 1820

Quazepam (May exhibit an additive CNS depression; the dose of one or both agents should be reduced). Products include:
Doral Tablets 2773

Risperidone (May exhibit an additive CNS depression; the dose of one or both agents should be reduced). Products include:
Risperdal Tablets 1348

Scopolamine (Potential for paralytic ileus). Products include:
Transderm Scōp Transdermal Therapeutic System 890

Scopolamine Hydrobromide (Potential for paralytic ileus). Products include:
Atrohist Plus Tablets 1605
Donnatal 2234
Donnatal Extentabs 2234
Donnatal Tablets 2234

Secobarbital Sodium (May exhibit an additive CNS depression; the dose of one or both agents should be reduced). Products include:
Seconal Sodium Pulvules 1529

Selegiline Hydrochloride (Co-administration may increase the effect of either drug). Products include:
Eldepryl Capsules 2729

Sevoflurane (May exhibit an additive CNS depression; the dose of one or both agents should be reduced).
No products indexed under this heading.

Sufentanil Citrate (May exhibit an additive CNS depression; the dose of one or both agents should be reduced). Products include:
Sufenta Injection 1355

Temazepam (May exhibit an additive CNS depression; the dose of one or both agents should be reduced). Products include:
Restoril Capsules 2413

Thiamylal Sodium (May exhibit an additive CNS depression; the dose of one or both agents should be reduced).
No products indexed under this heading.

Thioridazine Hydrochloride (May exhibit an additive CNS depression; the dose of one or both agents should be reduced). Products include:
Mellaril 2398

Thiothixene (May exhibit an additive CNS depression; the dose of one or both agents should be reduced). Products include:
Navane Capsules and Concentrate .. 2018
Navane Intramuscular 2019

Tranylcypromine Sulfate (Co-administration may increase the effect of either drug). Products include:
Parnate Tablets 2679

Triazolam (May exhibit an additive CNS depression; the dose of one or both agents should be reduced). Products include:
Halcion Tablets 2093

Tridihexethyl Chloride (Potential for paralytic ileus).
No products indexed under this heading.

Trifluoperazine Hydrochloride (May exhibit an additive CNS depression; the dose of one or both agents should be reduced). Products include:
Stelazine 2692

Trihexyphenidyl Hydrochloride (Potential for paralytic ileus). Products include:
Artane 1418

Trimipramine Maleate (Co-administration may increase the effect of either drug). Products include:
Surmontil Capsules 2917

Zolpidem Tartrate (May exhibit an additive CNS depression; the dose of one or both agents should be reduced). Products include:
Ambien Tablets 2559

Food Interactions
Alcohol (May exhibit an additive CNS depression).

VICODIN ES TABLETS
(Hydrocodone Bitartrate, Acetaminophen).................1405
May interact with central nervous system depressants, narcotic analgesics, psychotropics, tranquilizers, monoamine oxidase inhibitors, tricyclic antidepressants, anticholinergics, and certain other agents. Compounds in these categories include:

Alfentanil Hydrochloride (Additive CNS depression; the dose of one or both agents should be reduced). Products include:
Alfenta Injection 1334

Alprazolam (Additive CNS depression; the dose of one or both agents should be reduced). Products include:
Xanax Tablets 2115

Amitriptyline Hydrochloride (Additive CNS depression; the dose of one or both agents should be reduced; increased effect of either hydrocodone or antidepressant). Products include:
Elavil 2945
Etrafon 2495
Limbitrol 2333
Triavil Tablets 1800

Amoxapine (Additive CNS depression; the dose of one or both agents should be reduced; increased effect of either hydrocodone or antidepressant). Products include:
Asendin Tablets 1419

Aprobarbital (Additive CNS depression; the dose of one or both agents should be reduced).
No products indexed under this heading.

Atropine Sulfate (May produce paralytic ileus). Products include:
Arco-Lase Plus Tablets 513
Atrohist Plus Tablets 1605
Donnatal 2234
Donnatal Extentabs 2234
Donnatal Tablets 2234
Lomotil 2591
Motofen Tablets 789
Urised Tablets 2123

Belladonna Alkaloids (May produce paralytic ileus). Products include:
Bellergal-S Tablets 2375
Hyland's Bedwetting Tablets .....◨ 788
Hyland's EnurAid Tablets..........◨ 789
Hyland's Headache Tablets ......◨ 790
Hyland's Teething Tablets ....◨ 790
Similasan Eye Drops # 1 ....◨ 769

Benztropine Mesylate (May produce paralytic ileus). Products include:
Cogentin 1661

Biperiden Hydrochloride (May produce paralytic ileus). Products include:
Akineton 1380

Buprenorphine (Additive CNS depression; the dose of one or both agents should be reduced). Products include:
Buprenex Injectable 2170

Buspirone Hydrochloride (Additive CNS depression; the dose of one or both agents should be reduced). Products include:
BuSpar Tablets 738

Butabarbital (Additive CNS depression; the dose of one or both agents should be reduced).
No products indexed under this heading.

Butalbital (Additive CNS depression; the dose of one or both agents should be reduced). Products include:
Axocet Capsules 2469
Esgic-plus Capsules 1012
Esgic-plus Tablets 1012
Fioricet Tablets 2386
Fioricet with Codeine Capsules .. 2387
Fiorinal Capsules 2388
Fiorinal with Codeine Capsules .. 2390
Fiorinal Tablets 2388
Phrenilin 790
Sedapap Tablets 50 mg/650 mg .. 1826

Chlordiazepoxide (Additive CNS depression; the dose of one or both agents should be reduced). Products include:
Limbitrol 2333

Chlordiazepoxide Hydrochloride (Additive CNS depression; the dose of one or both agents should be reduced). Products include:
Librax Capsules 2330
Librium Capsules 2331
Librium Injectable 2332

Chlorpromazine (Additive CNS depression; the dose of one or both agents should be reduced). Products include:
Thorazine Suppositories 2701

Chlorprothixene (Additive CNS depression; the dose of one or both agents should be reduced).
No products indexed under this heading.

Chlorprothixene Hydrochloride (Additive CNS depression; the dose of one or both agents should be reduced).
No products indexed under this heading.

Chlorprothixene Lactate (Additive CNS depression; the dose of one or both agents should be reduced).
No products indexed under this heading.

Clidinium Bromide (May produce paralytic ileus). Products include:
Librax Capsules 2330

Clomipramine Hydrochloride (Additive CNS depression; the dose of one or both agents should be reduced; increased effect of either hydrocodone or antidepressant). Products include:
Anafranil Capsules 819

Clorazepate Dipotassium (Additive CNS depression; the dose of one or both agents should be reduced). Products include:
Tranxene 459

Clozapine (Additive CNS depression; the dose of one or both agents should be reduced). Products include:
Clozaril Tablets 2377

Codeine Phosphate (Additive CNS depression; the dose of one or both agents should be reduced). Products include:
Brontex 2130
Dimetane-DC Cough Syrup 2232
Fioricet with Codeine Capsules .. 2387
Fiorinal with Codeine Capsules .. 2390
Nucofed 2225
Phenergan with Codeine 2883
Phenergan VC with Codeine ... 2888
Robitussin A-C Syrup 2248
Robitussin-DAC Syrup 2249
Ryna ....◨ 804
Soma Compound w/Codeine Tablets 2784
Tylenol with Codeine 1592

(◨ Described in PDR For Nonprescription Drugs)   (◉ Described in PDR For Ophthalmology)

1177 **Interactions Index** **Vicodin ES**

Desflurane (Additive CNS depression; the dose of one or both agents should be reduced). Products include:
Suprane (desflurane, USP) 1865
Desipramine Hydrochloride (Additive CNS depression; the dose of one or both agents should be reduced; increased effect of either hydrocodone or antidepressant). Products include:
Norpramin Tablets 1273
Dezocine (Additive CNS depression; the dose of one or both agents should be reduced). Products include:
Dalgan Injection 529
Diazepam (Additive CNS depression; the dose of one or both agents should be reduced). Products include:
Dizac (diazepam injectable emulsion) CIV 1862
Valium Injectable 2336
Valium Tablets 2335
Dicyclomine Hydrochloride (May produce paralytic ileus). Products include:
Bentyl 1246
Doxepin Hydrochloride (Additive CNS depression; the dose of one or both agents should be reduced; increased effect of either hydrocodone or antidepressant). Products include:
Adapin Capsules 1542
Sinequan 2028
Zonalon Cream 1042
Droperidol (Additive CNS depression; the dose of one or both agents should be reduced). Products include:
Inapsine Injection 462
Enflurane (Additive CNS depression; the dose of one or both agents should be reduced).
No products indexed under this heading.
Estazolam (Additive CNS depression; the dose of one or both agents should be reduced). Products include:
ProSom Tablets 457
Ethchlorvynol (Additive CNS depression; the dose of one or both agents should be reduced). Products include:
Placidyl Capsules 456
Ethinamate (Additive CNS depression; the dose of one or both agents should be reduced).
No products indexed under this heading.
Fentanyl (Additive CNS depression; the dose of one or both agents should be reduced). Products include:
Duragesic Transdermal System 1336
Fentanyl Citrate (Additive CNS depression; the dose of one or both agents should be reduced). Products include:
Sublimaze Injection 463
Fluphenazine Decanoate (Additive CNS depression; the dose of one or both agents should be reduced). Products include:
Prolixin Decanoate 510
Fluphenazine Enanthate (Additive CNS depression; the dose of one or both agents should be reduced). Products include:
Prolixin Enanthate 510
Fluphenazine Hydrochloride (Additive CNS depression; the dose of one or both agents should be reduced). Products include:
Prolixin 510
Flurazepam Hydrochloride (Additive CNS depression; the dose of one or both agents should be reduced). Products include:
Dalmane Capsules 2329
Furazolidone (Additive CNS depression; the dose of one or both agents should be reduced; increased effect of either hydrocodone or MAO inhibitor). Products include:
Furoxone 2221
Glutethimide (Additive CNS depression; the dose of one or both agents should be reduced).
No products indexed under this heading.
Glycopyrrolate (May produce paralytic ileus). Products include:
Robinul Forte Tablets 2247
Robinul Injectable 2247
Robinul Tablets 2247
Haloperidol (Additive CNS depression; the dose of one or both agents should be reduced). Products include:
Haldol Injection, Tablets and Concentrate 1585
Haloperidol Decanoate (Additive CNS depression; the dose of one or both agents should be reduced). Products include:
Haldol Decanoate 1587
Hydrocodone Polistirex (Additive CNS depression; the dose of one or both agents should be reduced). Products include:
Tussionex Pennkinetic Extended-Release Suspension 1624
Hydromorphone Hydrochloride (Additive CNS depression; the dose of one or both agents should be reduced). Products include:
Dilaudid Ampules 1382
Dilaudid Cough Syrup 1383
Dilaudid-HP Injection 1384
Dilaudid-HP Lyophilized Powder 250 mg 1384
Dilaudid 1382
Dilaudid Oral Liquid 1386
Dilaudid 1382
Dilaudid Tablets - 8 mg 1386
Hydroxyzine Hydrochloride (Additive CNS depression; the dose of one or both agents should be reduced). Products include:
Atarax Tablets & Syrup 1992
Marax Tablets & DF Syrup 2015
Vistaril Intramuscular Solution 2042
Hyoscyamine (May produce paralytic ileus). Products include:
Cystospaz Tablets 2123
Urised Tablets 2123
Hyoscyamine Sulfate (May produce paralytic ileus). Products include:
Arco-Lase Plus Tablets 513
Atrohist Plus Tablets 1605
Cystospaz-M Capsules 2123
Donnatal 2234
Donnatal Extentabs 2234
Donnatal Tablets 2234
Kutrase Capsules 2546
Levsin/Levsinex/Levbid 2549
Imipramine Hydrochloride (Additive CNS depression; the dose of one or both agents should be reduced; increased effect of either hydrocodone or antidepressant). Products include:
Tofranil Ampuls 873
Tofranil Tablets 875
Imipramine Pamoate (Additive CNS depression; the dose of one or both agents should be reduced; increased effect of either hydrocodone or antidepressant). Products include:
Tofranil-PM Capsules 876
Ipratropium Bromide (May produce paralytic ileus). Products include:
Atrovent Inhalation Aerosol 674
Atrovent Inhalation Solution 675
Atrovent Nasal Spray 0.03% 676
Atrovent Nasal Spray 0.06% 678
Isocarboxazid (Additive CNS depression; the dose of one or both agents should be reduced; increased effect of either hydrocodone or MAO inhibitor).
No products indexed under this heading.
Isoflurane (Additive CNS depression; the dose of one or both agents should be reduced).
No products indexed under this heading.
Ketamine Hydrochloride (Additive CNS depression; the dose of one or both agents should be reduced).
No products indexed under this heading.
Levomethadyl Acetate Hydrochloride (Additive CNS depression; the dose of one or both agents should be reduced). Products include:
Orlaam Oral Solution 2361
Levorphanol Tartrate (Additive CNS depression; the dose of one or both agents should be reduced). Products include:
Levo-Dromoran 2297
Lithium Carbonate (Additive CNS depression; the dose of one or both agents should be reduced). Products include:
Eskalith 2658
Lithium Carbonate Capsules & Tablets 2352
Lithonate/Lithotabs/Lithobid 2721
Lithium Citrate (Additive CNS depression; the dose of one or both agents should be reduced).
No products indexed under this heading.
Lorazepam (Additive CNS depression; the dose of one or both agents should be reduced). Products include:
Ativan Injection 2805
Ativan Tablets 2807
Loxapine Hydrochloride (Additive CNS depression; the dose of one or both agents should be reduced). Products include:
Loxitane 1426
Loxapine Succinate (Additive CNS depression; the dose of one or both agents should be reduced). Products include:
Loxitane Capsules 1426
Maprotiline Hydrochloride (Additive CNS depression; the dose of one or both agents should be reduced; increased effect of either hydrocodone or antidepressant). Products include:
Ludiomil Tablets 861
Mepenzolate Bromide (May produce paralytic ileus).
No products indexed under this heading.
Meperidine Hydrochloride (Additive CNS depression; the dose of one or both agents should be reduced). Products include:
Demerol 2438
Mepergan Injection 2859
Mephobarbital (Additive CNS depression; the dose of one or both agents should be reduced). Products include:
Mebaral Tablets 2452
Meprobamate (Additive CNS depression; the dose of one or both agents should be reduced). Products include:
Miltown Tablets 2780
PMB 200 and PMB 400 2890
Mesoridazine Besylate (Additive CNS depression; the dose of one or both agents should be reduced). Products include:
Serentil 689
Methadone Hydrochloride (Additive CNS depression; the dose of one or both agents should be reduced). Products include:
Methadone Hydrochloride Oral Concentrate 2356
Methadone Hydrochloride Oral Solution & Tablets 2357
Methohexital Sodium (Additive CNS depression; the dose of one or both agents should be reduced).
No products indexed under this heading.
Methotrimeprazine (Additive CNS depression; the dose of one or both agents should be reduced). Products include:
Levoprome 1321
Methoxyflurane (Additive CNS depression; the dose of one or both agents should be reduced).
No products indexed under this heading.
Midazolam Hydrochloride (Additive CNS depression; the dose of one or both agents should be reduced). Products include:
Versed Injection 2324
Molindone Hydrochloride (Additive CNS depression; the dose of one or both agents should be reduced). Products include:
Moban Tablets and Concentrate 1036
Morphine Sulfate (Additive CNS depression; the dose of one or both agents should be reduced). Products include:
Astramorph/PF Injection, USP (Preservative-Free) 526
Duramorph Injection 983
Infumorph 200 and Infumorph 500 Sterile Solutions 985
Kadian Capsules 2948
MS Contin Tablets 2149
MSIR 2152
Oramorph SR (Morphine Sulfate Sustained Release Tablets) 2359
RMS Suppositories CII 2766
Roxanol 2365
Nortriptyline Hydrochloride (Additive CNS depression; the dose of one or both agents should be reduced; increased effect of either hydrocodone or antidepressant). Products include:
Pamelor 2409
Opium Alkaloids (Additive CNS depression; the dose of one or both agents should be reduced).
No products indexed under this heading.
Oxazepam (Additive CNS depression; the dose of one or both agents should be reduced). Products include:
Serax Capsules 2916
Serax Tablets 2916
Oxybutynin Chloride (May produce paralytic ileus). Products include:
Ditropan 1267
Oxycodone Hydrochloride (Additive CNS depression; the dose of one or both agents should be reduced). Products include:
OxyContin Tablets 2163
OxyIR Capsules 2167
Percocet Tablets 955
Percodan Tablets 955

IMPORTANT NOTE: Always consult each drug listing in the patient's regimen for possible interactions.

Vicodin ES **Interactions Index** **1178**

Percodan-Demi Tablets 956
Roxicodone Tablets, Oral Solution & Intensol (Oxycodone) 2366
Tylox Capsules 1593

Pentobarbital Sodium (Additive CNS depression; the dose of one or both agents should be reduced). Products include:
Nembutal Sodium Capsules 440
Nembutal Sodium Solution 442
Nembutal Sodium Suppositories 444

Perphenazine (Additive CNS depression; the dose of one or both agents should be reduced). Products include:
Etrafon 2495
Triavil Tablets 1800
Trilafon 2532

Phenelzine Sulfate (Additive CNS depression; the dose of one or both agents should be reduced; increased effect of either hydrocodone or MAO inhibitor). Products include:
Nardil 1977

Phenobarbital (Additive CNS depression; the dose of one or both agents should be reduced). Products include:
Arco-Lase Plus Tablets 513
Bellergal-S Tablets 2375
Donnatal 2234
Donnatal Extentabs 2234
Donnatal Tablets 2234
Phenobarbital Elixir and Tablets 1523
Quadrinal Tablets 1398

Prazepam (Additive CNS depression; the dose of one or both agents should be reduced).
No products indexed under this heading.

Prochlorperazine (Additive CNS depression; the dose of one or both agents should be reduced). Products include:
Compazine 2644

Procyclidine Hydrochloride (May produce paralytic ileus). Products include:
Kemadrin Tablets 1105

Promethazine Hydrochloride (Additive CNS depression; the dose of one or both agents should be reduced). Products include:
Mepergan Injection 2859
Phenergan with Codeine 2883
Phenergan with Dextromethorphan 2885
Phenergan Injection 2880
Phenergan Suppositories 2882
Phenergan Syrup 2881
Phenergan Tablets 2882
Phenergan VC 2886
Phenergan VC with Codeine 2888

Propantheline Bromide (May produce paralytic ileus). Products include:
Pro-Banthine Tablets 2226

Propofol (Additive CNS depression; the dose of one or both agents should be reduced). Products include:
Diprivan Injectable Emulsion 2939

Propoxyphene Hydrochloride (Additive CNS depression; the dose of one or both agents should be reduced). Products include:
Darvon 1475
Wygesic Tablets 2930

Propoxyphene Napsylate (Additive CNS depression; the dose of one or both agents should be reduced). Products include:
Darvon-N/Darvocet-N 1473

Protriptyline Hydrochloride (Additive CNS depression; the dose of one or both agents should be reduced; increased effect of either hydrocodone or antidepressant). Products include:
Vivactil Tablets 1820

Quazepam (Additive CNS depression; the dose of one or both agents should be reduced). Products include:
Doral Tablets 2773

Risperidone (Additive CNS depression; the dose of one or both agents should be reduced). Products include:
Risperdal Tablets 1348

Scopolamine (May produce paralytic ileus). Products include:
Transderm Scōp Transdermal Therapeutic System 890

Scopolamine Hydrobromide (May produce paralytic ileus). Products include:
Atrohist Plus Tablets 1605
Donnatal 2234
Donnatal Extentabs 2234
Donnatal Tablets 2234

Secobarbital Sodium (Additive CNS depression; the dose of one or both agents should be reduced). Products include:
Seconal Sodium Pulvules 1529

Selegiline Hydrochloride (Additive CNS depression; the dose of one or both agents should be reduced; increased effect of either hydrocodone or MAO inhibitor). Products include:
Eldepryl Capsules 2729

Sevoflurane (Additive CNS depression; the dose of one or both agents should be reduced).
No products indexed under this heading.

Sufentanil Citrate (Additive CNS depression; the dose of one or both agents should be reduced). Products include:
Sufenta Injection 1355

Temazepam (Additive CNS depression; the dose of one or both agents should be reduced). Products include:
Restoril Capsules 2413

Thiamylal Sodium (Additive CNS depression; the dose of one or both agents should be reduced).
No products indexed under this heading.

Thioridazine Hydrochloride (Additive CNS depression; the dose of one or both agents sjould be reduced). Products include:
Mellaril 2398

Thiothixene (Additive CNS depression; the dose of one or both agents should be reduced). Products include:
Navane Capsules and Concentrate 2018
Navane Intramuscular 2019

Tranylcypromine Sulfate (Additive CNS depression; the dose of one or both agents should be reduced; increased effect of either hydrocodone or MAO inhibitor). Products include:
Parnate Tablets 2679

Triazolam (Additive CNS depression; the dose of one or both agents should be reduced). Products include:
Halcion Tablets 2093

Tridihexethyl Chloride (May produce paralytic ileus).
No products indexed under this heading.

Trifluoperazine Hydrochloride (Additive CNS depression; the dose of one or both agents should be reduced). Products include:
Stelazine 2692

Trihexyphenidyl Hydrochloride (May produce paralytic ileus). Products include:
Artane 1418

Trimipramine Maleate (Additive CNS depression; the dose of one or both agents should be reduced; increased effect of either hydrocodone or antidepressant). Products include:
Surmontil Capsules 2917

Zolpidem Tartrate (Additive CNS depression; the dose of one or both agents should be reduced). Products include:
Ambien Tablets 2559

Food Interactions

Alcohol (Additive CNS depression).

VICODIN HP TABLETS

(Hydrocodone Bitartrate, Acetaminophen) 1403

May interact with antihistamines, tranquilizers, narcotic analgesics, central nervous system depressants, monoamine oxidase inhibitors, tricyclic antidepressants, and certain other agents. Compounds in these categories include:

Acrivastine (Co-administration may result in an additive CNS depression). Products include:
Semprex-D Capsules 1620

Alfentanil Hydrochloride (Co-administration may result in an additive CNS depression). Products include:
Alfenta Injection 1334

Alprazolam (Co-administration may result in an additive CNS depression). Products include:
Xanax Tablets 2115

Amitriptyline Hydrochloride (Co-administration with an MAO inhibitor may increase the effect of either hydrocodone or the tricyclic antidepressant). Products include:
Elavil 2945
Etrafon 2495
Limbitrol 2333
Triavil Tablets 1800

Amoxapine (Co-administration with an MAO inhibitor may increase the effect of either hydrocodone or the tricyclic antidepressant). Products include:
Asendin Tablets 1419

Aprobarbital (Co-administration may result in an additive CNS depression).
No products indexed under this heading.

Astemizole (Co-administration may result in an additive CNS depression). Products include:
Hismanal Tablets 1341

Azatadine Maleate (Co-administration may result in an additive CNS depression). Products include:
Trinalin Repetabs Tablets 1373

Bromodiphenhydramine Hydrochloride (Co-administration may result in an additive CNS depression).
No products indexed under this heading.

Brompheniramine Maleate (Co-administration may result in an additive CNS depression). Products include:
Alka-Seltzer Plus Sinus Medicine .. ■ 611
Bromfed Capsules (Extended-Release) 1832
Bromfed Syrup .... ■ 712
Bromfed Tablets 1832
Bromfed-DM Cough Syrup 1832
Bromfed-PD Capsules (Extended-Release) 1832
Dimetane-DC Cough Syrup 2232
Dimetane-DX Cough Syrup 2233
Dimetapp Allergy Dye-Free Elixir .... ■ 838
Dimetapp Allergy Sinus Caplets .... ■ 838
Dimetapp Cold & Allergy Chewable Tablets .... ■ 838
Dimetapp Cold & Cough Liqui-Gels .... ■ 839
Dimetapp Cold & Fever Suspension .... ■ 839
Dimetapp DM Elixir .... ■ 840
Dimetapp Elixir .... ■ 840
Dimetapp Extentabs .... ■ 841
Dimetapp Tablets/Liqui-Gels .... ■ 841
Rondec Chewable Tablets 974
Vicks DayQuil Allergy Relief 12-Hour Extended Release Tablets .. ■ 733
Vicks DayQuil Allergy Relief 4-Hour Tablets .... ■ 733

Buprenorphine (Co-administration may result in an additive CNS depression). Products include:
Buprenex Injectable 2170

Buspirone Hydrochloride (Co-administration may result in an additive CNS depression). Products include:
BuSpar Tablets 738

Butabarbital (Co-administration may result in an additive CNS depression).
No products indexed under this heading.

Butalbital (Co-administration may result in an additive CNS depression). Products include:
Axocet Capsules 2469
Esgic-plus Capsules 1012
Esgic-plus Tablets 1012
Fioricet Tablets 2386
Fioricet with Codeine Capsules 2387
Fiorinal Capsules 2388
Fiorinal with Codeine Capsules 2390
Fiorinal Tablets 2388
Phrenilin 790
Sedapap Tablets 50 mg/650 mg .. 1826

Cetirizine Hydrochloride (Co-administration may result in an additive CNS depression). Products include:
Zyrtec Tablets 2053

Chlordiazepoxide (Co-administration may result in an additive CNS depression). Products include:
Limbitrol 2333

Chlordiazepoxide Hydrochloride (Co-administration may result in an additive CNS depression). Products include:
Librax Capsules 2330
Librium Capsules 2331
Librium Injectable 2332

Chlorpheniramine Maleate (Co-administration may result in an additive CNS depression). Products include:
Alka-Seltzer Plus Cold Medicine .... ■ 611
Alka-Seltzer Plus Cold Medicine Liqui-Gels .... ■ 612
Alka-Seltzer Plus Cold & Cough Medicine .... ■ 611
Alka-Seltzer Plus Cold & Cough Medicine Liqui-Gels .... ■ 612
Alka-Seltzer Plus Flu & Body Aches Effervescent Tablets .... ■ 612
Allerest Maximum Strength .... ■ 649
Allerest Sinus Pain Formula .... ■ 649
Ana-Kit Anaphylaxis Emergency Treatment Kit 611
Atrohist Pediatric Capsules 1603
Atrohist Plus Tablets 1605
BC Cold Powder Multi-Symptom Formula (Cold-Sinus-Allergy) .... ■ 631
Cerose DM .... ■ 853
Cheracol Plus Head Cold/Cough Formula .... ■ 741
Children's TYLENOL Cold Multi-Symptom Chewable Tablets and Liquid 1559
Children's TYLENOL Cold Plus Cough Multi Symptom Chewable Tablets and Liquid 1560
Children's TYLENOL Flu Suspension Liquid 1560
Children's Vicks DayQuil Allergy Relief .... ■ 730

(■ Described in PDR For Nonprescription Drugs) (◉ Described in PDR For Ophthalmology)

Interactions Index — Vicodin HP

Children's Vicks NyQuil Cold/Cough Relief ... 731
Chlor-Trimeton Allergy Decongestant Tablets ... 759
Chlor-Trimeton Allergy Tablets ... 758
Allergy-Sinus Comtrex Multi-Symptom Allergy-Sinus Formula Tablets and Caplets ... 639
Comtrex Multi-Symptom ... 638
Contac Continuous Action Nasal Decongestant/Antihistamine 12 Hour Capsules ... 773
Contac Maximum Strength Continuous Action Decongestant/Antihistamine 12 Hour Caplets ... 772
Contac Severe Cold and Flu Formula Caplets ... 773
Coricidin Cold + Flu Tablets ... 760
Coricidin Cough + Cold Tablets ... 760
Coricidin 'D' Decongestant Tablets ... 760
D.A. II Tablets ... 972
D.A. Chewable Tablets ... 970
Dura-Tap/PD Capsules ... 970
Dura-Vent/DA Tablets ... 972
Efidac 24 Chlorpheniramine ... 655
Extendryl ... 1003
Fedahist Gyrocaps ... 2545
Hycomine Compound Tablets ... 948
Kronofed-A ... 994
Nolamine Timed-Release Tablets ... 790
Novahistine Elixir ... 782
Ornade Spansule Capsules ... 2678
PediaCare Cough-Cold Chewable Tablets and Liquid ... 1569
PediaCare NightRest Cough-Cold Liquid ... 1569
Pediatric Vicks 44m Cough & Cold Relief ... 737
Pyrroxate Caplets ... 742
Ryna ... 804
Sinarest ... 663
Sine-Off Sinus Medicine ... 784
Singlet Tablets ... 785
Sinulin Tablets ... 792
Sinutab Sinus Allergy Medication, Maximum Strength Tablets and Caplets ... 823
Sudafed Cold & Allergy Tablets ... 826
Teldrin 12 Hour Antihistamine/Nasal Decongestant Allergy Relief Capsules ... 786
TheraFlu Flu and Cold Medicine ... 750
Theraflu Maximum Strength Flu and Cold Medicine For Sore Throat ... 751
TheraFlu Flu, Cold and Cough Medicine ... 750
TheraFlu Maximum Strength Nighttime Flu, Cold & Cough Medicine ... 751
Triaminic Night Time ... 754
Triaminic Syrup ... 755
Triaminic Triaminicol Cold & Cough ... 756
Triaminicin Tablets ... 756
Tussend ... 1830
TYLENOL Allergy Sinus, Maximum Strength Caplets and Gelcaps ... 1571
TYLENOL Cold Medication, Multi-Symptom Formula Tablets and Caplets ... 1572
TYLENOL Cold Medication, Multi-Symptom Hot Liquid Packets ... 1572
Vicks 44 LiquiCaps Cough, Cold & Flu Relief ... 728
Vicks 44M Cough, Cold & Flu Relief ... 729

Chlorpheniramine Polistirex (Co-administration may result in an additive CNS depression). Products include:
Tussionex Pennkinetic Extended-Release Suspension ... 1624

Chlorpheniramine Tannate (Co-administration may result in an additive CNS depression). Products include:
Atrohist Pediatric Suspension ... 1604
Atrohist Pediatric Suspension Dye-Free ... 1604
Rynatan ... 2781
Rynatuss ... 2782

Chlorpromazine (Co-administration may result in an additive CNS depression). Products include:
Thorazine Suppositories ... 2701

Chlorpromazine Hydrochloride (Co-administration may result in an additive CNS depression). Products include:
Thorazine ... 2701

Chlorprothixene (Co-administration may result in an additive CNS depression).
No products indexed under this heading.

Chlorprothixene Hydrochloride (Co-administration may result in an additive CNS depression).
No products indexed under this heading.

Chlorprothixene Lactate (Co-administration may result in an additive CNS depression).
No products indexed under this heading.

Clemastine Fumarate (Co-administration may result in an additive CNS depression). Products include:
Tavist Syrup ... 2426
Tavist Tablets ... 2427
Tavist-1 12 Hour Relief Tablets ... 749
Tavist-D 12 Hour Relief Tablets ... 750

Clomipramine Hydrochloride (Co-administration with an MAO inhibitor may increase the effect of either hydrocodone or the tricyclic antidepressant). Products include:
Anafranil Capsules ... 819

Clorazepate Dipotassium (Co-administration may result in an additive CNS depression). Products include:
Tranxene ... 459

Clozapine (Co-administration may result in an additive CNS depression). Products include:
Clozaril Tablets ... 2377

Codeine Phosphate (Co-administration may result in an additive CNS depression). Products include:
Brontex ... 2130
Dimetane-DC Cough Syrup ... 2232
Fioricet with Codeine Capsules ... 2387
Fiorinal with Codeine Capsules ... 2390
Nucofed ... 2225
Phenergan with Codeine ... 2883
Phenergan VC with Codeine ... 2888
Robitussin A-C Syrup ... 2248
Robitussin-DAC Syrup ... 2249
Ryna ... 804
Soma Compound w/Codeine Tablets ... 2784
Tylenol with Codeine ... 1592

Cyproheptadine Hydrochloride (Co-administration may result in an additive CNS depression). Products include:
Periactin ... 1767

Desflurane (Co-administration may result in an additive CNS depression). Products include:
Suprane (desflurane, USP) ... 1865

Desipramine Hydrochloride (Co-administration with an MAO inhibitor may increase the effect of either hydrocodone or the tricyclic antidepressant). Products include:
Norpramin Tablets ... 1273

Dexchlorpheniramine Maleate (Co-administration may result in an additive CNS depression).
No products indexed under this heading.

Dezocine (Co-administration may result in an additive CNS depression). Products include:
Dalgan Injection ... 529

Diazepam (Co-administration may result in an additive CNS depression). Products include:
Dizac (diazepam injectable emulsion) CIV ... 1862
Valium Injectable ... 2336
Valium Tablets ... 2335

Diphenhydramine Citrate (Co-administration may result in an additive CNS depression). Products include:
Excedrin P.M. Analgesic/Sleeping Aid Tablets, Caplets, Liquigels ... 735

Diphenhydramine Hydrochloride (Co-administration may result in an additive CNS depression). Products include:
Actifed Allergy Daytime/Nighttime Caplets ... 808
Actifed Sinus Daytime/Nighttime Tablets and Caplets ... 809
Extra Strength Bayer PM Aspirin Plus Sleep Aid ... 617
Benadryl Allergy Chewables ... 811
Benadryl Allergy/Cold Tablets ... 811
Benadryl Allergy Decongestant Liquid Medication ... 812
Benadryl Allergy Decongestant Tablets ... 812
Benadryl Allergy Liquid Medication ... 813
Benadryl Allergy ... 811
Benadryl Allergy Sinus Headache Caplets ... 813
Benadryl Dye-Free Allergy Liquigel Softgels ... 813
Benadryl Dye-Free Allergy Liquid Medication ... 814
Benadryl Itch Relief Stick Extra Strength ... 814
Benadryl Cream ... 814
Benadryl Gel ... 815
Benadryl Spray ... 815
Benadryl Injection ... 1955
Contac Day & Night Cold/Flu Night Caplets ... 772
Contac Night Allergy/Sinus Caplets ... 771
Extra Strength Doan's P.M. ... 653
Excedrin P.M. Analgesic/Sleeping Aid Tablets, Caplets, Liquigels ... 643
Nytol QuickCaps Caplets ... 632
Sleepinal Night-time Sleep Aid Capsules and Softgels ... 798
TYLENOL Allergy Sinus NightTime, Maximum Strength Caplets ... 1571
TYLENOL Flu NightTime, Maximum Strength Gelcaps ... 1575
TYLENOL Flu NightTime, Maximum Strength Hot Medication Packets ... 1575
TYLENOL PM Pain Reliever/Sleep Aid, Extra Strength Gelcaps, Caplets, Geltabs ... 1576
TYLENOL Severe Allergy Medication Caplets ... 1571
Maximum Strength Unisom Sleepgels ... 1990
Unisom With Pain Relief-Nighttime Sleep Aid and Pain Reliever ... 1991

Diphenylpyraline Hydrochloride (Co-administration may result in an additive CNS depression).
No products indexed under this heading.

Doxepin Hydrochloride (Co-administration with an MAO inhibitor may increase the effect of either hydrocodone or the tricyclic antidepressant). Products include:
Adapin Capsules ... 1542
Sinequan ... 2028
Zonalon Cream ... 1042

Droperidol (Co-administration may result in an additive CNS depression). Products include:
Inapsine Injection ... 462

Enflurane (Co-administration may result in an additive CNS depression).
No products indexed under this heading.

Estazolam (Co-administration may result in an additive CNS depression). Products include:
ProSom Tablets ... 457

Ethchlorvynol (Co-administration may result in an additive CNS depression). Products include:
Placidyl Capsules ... 456

Ethinamate (Co-administration may result in an additive CNS depression).
No products indexed under this heading.

Fentanyl (Co-administration may result in an additive CNS depression). Products include:
Duragesic Transdermal System ... 1336

Fentanyl Citrate (Co-administration may result in an additive CNS depression). Products include:
Sublimaze Injection ... 463

Fluphenazine Decanoate (Co-administration may result in an additive CNS depression). Products include:
Prolixin Decanoate ... 510

Fluphenazine Enanthate (Co-administration may result in an additive CNS depression). Products include:
Prolixin Enanthate ... 510

Fluphenazine Hydrochloride (Co-administration may result in an additive CNS depression). Products include:
Prolixin ... 510

Flurazepam Hydrochloride (Co-administration may result in an additive CNS depression). Products include:
Dalmane Capsules ... 2329

Furazolidone (Co-administration with an MAO inhibitor may increase the effect of either hydrocodone or the MAO inhibitor). Products include:
Furoxone ... 2221

Glutethimide (Co-administration may result in an additive CNS depression).
No products indexed under this heading.

Haloperidol (Co-administration may result in an additive CNS depression). Products include:
Haldol Injection, Tablets and Concentrate ... 1585

Haloperidol Decanoate (Co-administration may result in an additive CNS depression). Products include:
Haldol Decanoate ... 1587

Hydrocodone Polistirex (Co-administration may result in an additive CNS depression). Products include:
Tussionex Pennkinetic Extended-Release Suspension ... 1624

Hydromorphone Hydrochloride (Co-administration may result in an additive CNS depression). Products include:
Dilaudid Ampules ... 1382
Dilaudid Cough Syrup ... 1383
Dilaudid-HP Injection ... 1384
Dilaudid-HP Lyophilized Powder 250 mg ... 1384
Dilaudid ... 1382
Dilaudid Oral Liquid ... 1386
Dilaudid ... 1382
Dilaudid Tablets - 8 mg ... 1386

Hydroxyzine Hydrochloride (Co-administration may result in an additive CNS depression). Products include:
Atarax Tablets & Syrup ... 1992
Marax Tablets & DF Syrup ... 2015
Vistaril Intramuscular Solution ... 2042

Imipramine Hydrochloride (Co-administration with an MAO inhibitor may increase the effect of either hydrocodone or the tricyclic antidepressant). Products include:
Tofranil Ampuls ... 873
Tofranil Tablets ... 875

IMPORTANT NOTE: Always consult each drug listing in the patient's regimen for possible interactions.

Vicodin HP — Interactions Index

Imipramine Pamoate (Co-administration with an MAO inhibitor may increase the effect of either hydrocodone or the tricyclic antidepressant). Products include:
- Tofranil-PM Capsules 876

Isocarboxazid (Co-administration with an MAO inhibitor may increase the effect of either hydrocodone or the MAO inhibitor).
- No products indexed under this heading.

Isoflurane (Co-administration may result in an additive CNS depression).
- No products indexed under this heading.

Ketamine Hydrochloride (Co-administration may result in an additive CNS depression).
- No products indexed under this heading.

Levomethadyl Acetate Hydrochloride (Co-administration may result in an additive CNS depression). Products include:
- Orlaam Oral Solution 2361

Levorphanol Tartrate (Co-administration may result in an additive CNS depression). Products include:
- Levo-Dromoran 2297

Loratadine (Co-administration may result in an additive CNS depression). Products include:
- Claritin Tablets 2485
- Claritin-D Tablets 2487

Lorazepam (Co-administration may result in an additive CNS depression). Products include:
- Ativan Injection 2805
- Ativan Tablets 2807

Loxapine Hydrochloride (Co-administration may result in an additive CNS depression). Products include:
- Loxitane 1426

Loxapine Succinate (Co-administration may result in an additive CNS depression). Products include:
- Loxitane Capsules 1426

Maprotiline Hydrochloride (Co-administration with an MAO inhibitor may increase the effect of either hydrocodone or the tricyclic antidepressant). Products include:
- Ludiomil Tablets 861

Meperidine Hydrochloride (Co-administration may result in an additive CNS depression). Products include:
- Demerol 2438
- Mepergan Injection 2859

Mephobarbital (Co-administration may result in an additive CNS depression). Products include:
- Mebaral Tablets 2452

Meprobamate (Co-administration may result in an additive CNS depression). Products include:
- Miltown Tablets 2780
- PMB 200 and PMB 400 2890

Mesoridazine Besylate (Co-administration may result in an additive CNS depression). Products include:
- Serentil 689

Methadone Hydrochloride (Co-administration may result in an additive CNS depression). Products include:
- Methadone Hydrochloride Oral Concentrate 2356
- Methadone Hydrochloride Oral Solution & Tablets 2357

Methdilazine Hydrochloride (Co-administration may result in an additive CNS depression).
- No products indexed under this heading.

Methohexital Sodium (Co-administration may result in an additive CNS depression).
- No products indexed under this heading.

Methotrimeprazine (Co-administration may result in an additive CNS depression). Products include:
- Levoprome 1321

Methoxyflurane (Co-administration may result in an additive CNS depression).
- No products indexed under this heading.

Midazolam Hydrochloride (Co-administration may result in an additive CNS depression). Products include:
- Versed Injection 2324

Molindone Hydrochloride (Co-administration may result in an additive CNS depression). Products include:
- Moban Tablets and Concentrate 1036

Morphine Sulfate (Co-administration may result in an additive CNS depression). Products include:
- Astramorph/PF Injection, USP (Preservative-Free) 526
- Duramorph Injection 983
- Infumorph 200 and Infumorph 500 Sterile Solutions 985
- Kadian Capsules 2948
- MS Contin Tablets 2149
- MSIR 2152
- Oramorph SR (Morphine Sulfate Sustained Release Tablets) 2359
- RMS Suppositories CII 2766
- Roxanol 2365

Nortriptyline Hydrochloride (Co-administration with an MAO inhibitor may increase the effect of either hydrocodone or the tricyclic antidepressant). Products include:
- Pamelor 2409

Opium Alkaloids (Co-administration may result in an additive CNS depression).
- No products indexed under this heading.

Oxazepam (Co-administration may result in an additive CNS depression). Products include:
- Serax Capsules 2916
- Serax Tablets 2916

Oxycodone Hydrochloride (Co-administration may result in an additive CNS depression). Products include:
- OxyContin Tablets 2163
- OxyIR Capsules 2167
- Percocet Tablets 955
- Percodan Tablets 955
- Percodan-Demi Tablets 956
- Roxicodone Tablets, Oral Solution & Intensol (Oxycodone) 2366
- Tylox Capsules 1593

Pentobarbital Sodium (Co-administration may result in an additive CNS depression). Products include:
- Nembutal Sodium Capsules 440
- Nembutal Sodium Solution 442
- Nembutal Sodium Suppositories 444

Perphenazine (Co-administration may result in an additive CNS depression). Products include:
- Etrafon 2495
- Triavil Tablets 1800
- Trilafon 2532

Phenelzine Sulfate (Co-administration with an MAO inhibitor may increase the effect of either hydrocodone or the MAO inhibitor). Products include:
- Nardil 1977

Phenobarbital (Co-administration may result in an additive CNS depression). Products include:
- Arco-Lase Plus Tablets 513
- Bellergal-S Tablets 2375
- Donnatal 2234
- Donnatal Extentabs 2234
- Donnatal Tablets 2234
- Phenobarbital Elixir and Tablets 1523
- Quadrinal Tablets 1398

Prazepam (Co-administration may result in an additive CNS depression).
- No products indexed under this heading.

Prochlorperazine (Co-administration may result in an additive CNS depression). Products include:
- Compazine 2644

Promethazine Hydrochloride (Co-administration may result in an additive CNS depression). Products include:
- Mepergan Injection 2859
- Phenergan with Codeine 2883
- Phenergan with Dextromethorphan 2885
- Phenergan Injection 2880
- Phenergan Suppositories 2882
- Phenergan Syrup 2881
- Phenergan Tablets 2882
- Phenergan VC 2886
- Phenergan VC with Codeine 2888

Propofol (Co-administration may result in an additive CNS depression). Products include:
- Diprivan Injectable Emulsion 2939

Propoxyphene Hydrochloride (Co-administration may result in an additive CNS depression). Products include:
- Darvon 1475
- Wygesic Tablets 2930

Propoxyphene Napsylate (Co-administration may result in an additive CNS depression). Products include:
- Darvon-N/Darvocet-N 1473

Protriptyline Hydrochloride (Co-administration with an MAO inhibitor may increase the effect of either hydrocodone or the tricyclic antidepressant). Products include:
- Vivactil Tablets 1820

Pyrilamine Maleate (Co-administration may result in an additive CNS depression). Products include:
- 4-Way Fast Acting Nasal Spray (regular & mentholated) 644
- Maximum Strength Multi-Symptom Formula Midol 621
- PMS Multi-Symptom Formula Midol 622

Pyrilamine Tannate (Co-administration may result in an additive CNS depression). Products include:
- Atrohist Pediatric Suspension 1604
- Atrohist Pediatric Suspension Dye-Free 1604
- Rynatan 2781

Quazepam (Co-administration may result in an additive CNS depression). Products include:
- Doral Tablets 2773

Risperidone (Co-administration may result in an additive CNS depression). Products include:
- Risperdal Tablets 1348

Secobarbital Sodium (Co-administration may result in an additive CNS depression). Products include:
- Seconal Sodium Pulvules 1529

Selegiline Hydrochloride (Co-administration with an MAO inhibitor may increase the effect of either hydrocodone or the MAO inhibitor). Products include:
- Eldepryl Capsules 2729

Sevoflurane (Co-administration may result in an additive CNS depression).
- No products indexed under this heading.

Sufentanil Citrate (Co-administration may result in an additive CNS depression). Products include:
- Sufenta Injection 1355

Temazepam (Co-administration may result in an additive CNS depression). Products include:
- Restoril Capsules 2413

Terfenadine (Co-administration may result in an additive CNS depression). Products include:
- Seldane Tablets 1284
- Seldane-D Extended-Release Tablets 1286

Thiamylal Sodium (Co-administration may result in an additive CNS depression).
- No products indexed under this heading.

Thioridazine Hydrochloride (Co-administration may result in an additive CNS depression). Products include:
- Mellaril 2398

Thiothixene (Co-administration may result in an additive CNS depression). Products include:
- Navane Capsules and Concentrate 2018
- Navane Intramuscular 2019

Tranylcypromine Sulfate (Co-administration with an MAO inhibitor may increase the effect of either hydrocodone or the MAO inhibitor). Products include:
- Parnate Tablets 2679

Triazolam (Co-administration may result in an additive CNS depression). Products include:
- Halcion Tablets 2093

Trifluoperazine Hydrochloride (Co-administration may result in an additive CNS depression). Products include:
- Stelazine 2692

Trimeprazine Tartrate (Co-administration may result in an additive CNS depression).
- No products indexed under this heading.

Trimipramine Maleate (Co-administration with an MAO inhibitor may increase the effect of either hydrocodone or the tricyclic antidepressant). Products include:
- Surmontil Capsules 2917

Tripelennamine Hydrochloride (Co-administration may result in an additive CNS depression). Products include:
- PBZ Tablets 863
- PBZ-SR Tablets 862

Triprolidine Hydrochloride (Co-administration may result in an additive CNS depression). Products include:
- Actifed Cold & Allergy Tablets 807
- Actifed Cold & Sinus Caplets and Tablets 808

Zolpidem Tartrate (Co-administration may result in an additive CNS depression). Products include:
- Ambien Tablets 2559

Food Interactions

Alcohol (Concurrent use results in an additive CNS depression).

VICODIN TUSS EXPECTORANT
(Hydrocodone Bitartrate, Guaifenesin) 1406

May interact with central nervous system depressants, phenothiazines, narcotic analgesics, general anes-

(Described in PDR For Nonprescription Drugs)   (Described in PDR For Ophthalmology)

thetics, tranquilizers, hypnotics and sedatives, and certain other agents. Compounds in these categories include:

Alfentanil Hydrochloride (Co-administration may exhibit an additive CNS depression; the dose of one or both agents should be reduced). Products include:
- Alfenta Injection 1334

Alprazolam (Co-administration may exhibit an additive CNS depression; the dose of one or both agents should be reduced). Products include:
- Xanax Tablets 2115

Aprobarbital (Co-administration may exhibit an additive CNS depression; the dose of one or both agents should be reduced).
No products indexed under this heading.

Buprenorphine (Co-administration may exhibit an additive CNS depression; the dose of one or both agents should be reduced). Products include:
- Buprenex Injectable 2170

Buspirone Hydrochloride (Co-administration may exhibit an additive CNS depression; the dose of one or both agents should be reduced). Products include:
- BuSpar Tablets 738

Butabarbital (Co-administration may exhibit an additive CNS depression; the dose of one or both agents should be reduced).
No products indexed under this heading.

Butalbital (Co-administration may exhibit an additive CNS depression; the dose of one or both agents should be reduced). Products include:
- Axocet Capsules 2469
- Esgic-plus Capsules 1012
- Esgic-plus Tablets 1012
- Fioricet Tablets 2386
- Fioricet with Codeine Capsules 2387
- Fiorinal Capsules 2388
- Fiorinal with Codeine Capsules 2390
- Fiorinal Tablets 2388
- Phrenilin 790
- Sedapap Tablets 50 mg/650 mg .. 1826

Chlordiazepoxide (Co-administration may exhibit an additive CNS depression; the dose of one or both agents should be reduced). Products include:
- Limbitrol 2333

Chlordiazepoxide Hydrochloride (Co-administration may exhibit an additive CNS depression; the dose of one or both agents should be reduced). Products include:
- Librax Capsules 2330
- Librium Capsules 2331
- Librium Injectable 2332

Chlorpromazine (Co-administration may exhibit an additive CNS depression; the dose of one or both agents should be reduced). Products include:
- Thorazine Suppositories 2701

Chlorpromazine Hydrochloride (Co-administration may exhibit an additive CNS depression; the dose of one or both agents should be reduced). Products include:
- Thorazine 2701

Chlorprothixene (Co-administration may exhibit an additive CNS depression; the dose of one or both agents should be reduced).
No products indexed under this heading.

Chlorprothixene Hydrochloride (Co-administration may exhibit an additive CNS depression; the dose of one or both agents should be reduced).
No products indexed under this heading.

Chlorprothixene Lactate (Co-administration may exhibit an additive CNS depression; the dose of one or both agents should be reduced).
No products indexed under this heading.

Clorazepate Dipotassium (Co-administration may exhibit an additive CNS depression; the dose of one or both agents should be reduced). Products include:
- Tranxene 459

Clozapine (Co-administration may exhibit an additive CNS depression; the dose of one or both agents should be reduced). Products include:
- Clozaril Tablets 2377

Codeine Phosphate (Co-administration may exhibit an additive CNS depression; the dose of one or both agents should be reduced). Products include:
- Brontex 2130
- Dimetane-DC Cough Syrup 2232
- Fioricet with Codeine Capsules 2387
- Fiorinal with Codeine Capsules 2390
- Nucofed 2225
- Phenergan with Codeine 2883
- Phenergan VC with Codeine 2888
- Robitussin A-C Syrup 2248
- Robitussin-DAC Syrup 2249
- Ryna 804
- Soma Compound w/Codeine Tablets 2784
- Tylenol with Codeine 1592

Desflurane (Co-administration may exhibit an additive CNS depression; the dose of one or both agents should be reduced). Products include:
- Suprane (desflurane, USP) 1865

Dezocine (Co-administration may exhibit an additive CNS depression; the dose of one or both agents should be reduced). Products include:
- Dalgan Injection 529

Diazepam (Co-administration may exhibit an additive CNS depression; the dose of one or both agents should be reduced). Products include:
- Dizac (diazepam injectable emulsion) CIV 1862
- Valium Injectable 2336
- Valium Tablets 2335

Droperidol (Co-administration may exhibit an additive CNS depression; the dose of one or both agents should be reduced). Products include:
- Inapsine Injection 462

Enflurane (Co-administration may exhibit an additive CNS depression; the dose of one or both agents should be reduced).
No products indexed under this heading.

Estazolam (Co-administration may exhibit an additive CNS depression; the dose of one or both agents should be reduced). Products include:
- ProSom Tablets 457

Ethchlorvynol (Co-administration may exhibit an additive CNS depression; the dose of one or both agents should be reduced). Products include:
- Placidyl Capsules 456

Ethinamate (Co-administration may exhibit an additive CNS depression; the dose of one or both agents should be reduced).
No products indexed under this heading.

Fentanyl (Co-administration may exhibit an additive CNS depression; the dose of one or both agents should be reduced). Products include:
- Duragesic Transdermal System 1336

Fentanyl Citrate (Co-administration may exhibit an additive CNS depression; the dose of one or both agents should be reduced). Products include:
- Sublimaze Injection 463

Fluphenazine Decanoate (Co-administration may exhibit an additive CNS depression; the dose of one or both agents should be reduced). Products include:
- Prolixin Decanoate 510

Fluphenazine Enanthate (Co-administration may exhibit an additive CNS depression; the dose of one or both agents should be reduced). Products include:
- Prolixin Enanthate 510

Fluphenazine Hydrochloride (Co-administration may exhibit an additive CNS depression; the dose of one or both agents should be reduced). Products include:
- Prolixin 510

Flurazepam Hydrochloride (Co-administration may exhibit an additive CNS depression; the dose of one or both agents should be reduced). Products include:
- Dalmane Capsules 2329

Glutethimide (Co-administration may exhibit an additive CNS depression; the dose of one or both agents should be reduced).
No products indexed under this heading.

Haloperidol (Co-administration may exhibit an additive CNS depression; the dose of one or both agents should be reduced). Products include:
- Haldol Injection, Tablets and Concentrate 1585

Haloperidol Decanoate (Co-administration may exhibit an additive CNS depression; the dose of one or both agents should be reduced). Products include:
- Haldol Decanoate 1587

Hydrocodone Polistirex (Co-administration may exhibit an additive CNS depression; the dose of one or both agents should be reduced). Products include:
- Tussionex Pennkinetic Extended-Release Suspension 1624

Hydromorphone Hydrochloride (Co-administration may exhibit an additive CNS depression; the dose of one or both agents should be reduced). Products include:
- Dilaudid Ampules 1382
- Dilaudid Cough Syrup 1383
- Dilaudid-HP Injection 1384
- Dilaudid-HP Lyophilized Powder 250 mg 1384
- Dilaudid 1382
- Dilaudid Oral Liquid 1386
- Dilaudid 1382
- Dilaudid Tablets - 8 mg 1386

Hydroxyzine Hydrochloride (Co-administration may exhibit an additive CNS depression; the dose of one or both agents should be reduced). Products include:
- Atarax Tablets & Syrup 1992
- Marax Tablets & DF Syrup 2015
- Vistaril Intramuscular Solution 2042

Isoflurane (Co-administration may exhibit an additive CNS depression; the dose of one or both agents should be reduced).
No products indexed under this heading.

Ketamine Hydrochloride (Co-administration may exhibit an additive CNS depression; the dose of one or both agents should be reduced).
No products indexed under this heading.

Levomethadyl Acetate Hydrochloride (Co-administration may exhibit an additive CNS depression; the dose of one or both agents should be reduced). Products include:
- Orlaam Oral Solution 2361

Levorphanol Tartrate (Co-administration may exhibit an additive CNS depression; the dose of one or both agents should be reduced). Products include:
- Levo-Dromoran 2297

Lorazepam (Co-administration may exhibit an additive CNS depression; the dose of one or both agents should be reduced). Products include:
- Ativan Injection 2805
- Ativan Tablets 2807

Loxapine Hydrochloride (Co-administration may exhibit an additive CNS depression; the dose of one or both agents should be reduced). Products include:
- Loxitane 1426

Loxapine Succinate (Co-administration may exhibit an additive CNS depression; the dose of one or both agents should be reduced). Products include:
- Loxitane Capsules 1426

Meperidine Hydrochloride (Co-administration may exhibit an additive CNS depression; the dose of one or both agents should be reduced). Products include:
- Demerol 2438
- Mepergan Injection 2859

Mephobarbital (Co-administration may exhibit an additive CNS depression; the dose of one or both agents should be reduced). Products include:
- Mebaral Tablets 2452

Meprobamate (Co-administration may exhibit an additive CNS depression; the dose of one or both agents should be reduced). Products include:
- Miltown Tablets 2780
- PMB 200 and PMB 400 2890

Mesoridazine Besylate (Co-administration may exhibit an additive CNS depression; the dose of one or both agents should be reduced). Products include:
- Serentil 689

Methadone Hydrochloride (Co-administration may exhibit an additive CNS depression; the dose of one or both agents should be reduced). Products include:
- Methadone Hydrochloride Oral Concentrate 2356
- Methadone Hydrochloride Oral Solution & Tablets 2357

Methohexital Sodium (Co-administration may exhibit an additive CNS depression; the dose of one or both agents should be reduced).
No products indexed under this heading.

IMPORTANT NOTE: Always consult each drug listing in the patient's regimen for possible interactions.

Methotrimeprazine (Co-administration may exhibit an additive CNS depression; the dose of one or both agents should be reduced). Products include:

Levoprome ... 1321

Methoxyflurane (Co-administration may exhibit an additive CNS depression; the dose of one or both agents should be reduced).

No products indexed under this heading.

Midazolam Hydrochloride (Co-administration may exhibit an additive CNS depression; the dose of one or both agents should be reduced). Products include:

Versed Injection ... 2324

Molindone Hydrochloride (Co-administration may exhibit an additive CNS depression; the dose of one or both agents should be reduced). Products include:

Moban Tablets and Concentrate ... 1036

Morphine Sulfate (Co-administration may exhibit an additive CNS depression; the dose of one or both agents should be reduced). Products include:

Astramorph/PF Injection, USP (Preservative-Free) ... 526
Duramorph Injection ... 983
Infumorph 200 and Infumorph 500 Sterile Solutions ... 985
Kadian Capsules ... 2948
MS Contin Tablets ... 2149
MSIR ... 2152
Oramorph SR (Morphine Sulfate Sustained Release Tablets) ... 2359
RMS Suppositories CII ... 2766
Roxanol ... 2365

Opium Alkaloids (Co-administration may exhibit an additive CNS depression; the dose of one or both agents should be reduced).

No products indexed under this heading.

Oxazepam (Co-administration may exhibit an additive CNS depression; the dose of one or both agents should be reduced). Products include:

Serax Capsules ... 2916
Serax Tablets ... 2916

Oxycodone Hydrochloride (Co-administration may exhibit an additive CNS depression; the dose of one or both agents should be reduced). Products include:

OxyContin Tablets ... 2163
OxyIR Capsules ... 2167
Percocet Tablets ... 955
Percodan Tablets ... 955
Percodan-Demi Tablets ... 956
Roxicodone Tablets, Oral Solution & Intensol (Oxycodone) ... 2366
Tylox Capsules ... 1593

Pentobarbital Sodium (Co-administration may exhibit an additive CNS depression; the dose of one or both agents should be reduced). Products include:

Nembutal Sodium Capsules ... 440
Nembutal Sodium Solution ... 442
Nembutal Sodium Suppositories ... 444

Perphenazine (Co-administration may exhibit an additive CNS depression; the dose of one or both agents should be reduced). Products include:

Etrafon ... 2495
Triavil Tablets ... 1800
Trilafon ... 2532

Phenobarbital (Co-administration may exhibit an additive CNS depression; the dose of one or both agents should be reduced). Products include:

Arco-Lase Plus Tablets ... 513
Bellergal-S Tablets ... 2375
Donnatal ... 2234
Donnatal Extentabs ... 2234
Donnatal Tablets ... 2234
Phenobarbital Elixir and Tablets ... 1523
Quadrinal Tablets ... 1398

Prazepam (Co-administration may exhibit an additive CNS depression; the dose of one or both agents should be reduced).

No products indexed under this heading.

Prochlorperazine (Co-administration may exhibit an additive CNS depression; the dose of one or both agents should be reduced). Products include:

Compazine ... 2644

Promethazine Hydrochloride (Co-administration may exhibit an additive CNS depression; the dose of one or both agents should be reduced). Products include:

Mepergan Injection ... 2859
Phenergan with Codeine ... 2883
Phenergan with Dextromethorphan 2885
Phenergan Injection ... 2880
Phenergan Suppositories ... 2882
Phenergan Syrup ... 2881
Phenergan Tablets ... 2882
Phenergan VC ... 2886
Phenergan VC with Codeine ... 2888

Propofol (Co-administration may exhibit an additive CNS depression; the dose of one or both agents should be reduced). Products include:

Diprivan Injectable Emulsion ... 2939

Propoxyphene Hydrochloride (Co-administration may exhibit an additive CNS depression; the dose of one or both agents should be reduced). Products include:

Darvon ... 1475
Wygesic Tablets ... 2930

Propoxyphene Napsylate (Co-administration may exhibit an additive CNS depression; the dose of one or both agents should be reduced). Products include:

Darvon-N/Darvocet-N ... 1473

Quazepam (Co-administration may exhibit an additive CNS depression; the dose of one or both agents should be reduced). Products include:

Doral Tablets ... 2773

Risperidone (Co-administration may exhibit an additive CNS depression; the dose of one or both agents should be reduced). Products include:

Risperdal Tablets ... 1348

Secobarbital Sodium (Co-administration may exhibit an additive CNS depression; the dose of one or both agents should be reduced). Products include:

Seconal Sodium Pulvules ... 1529

Sevoflurane (Co-administration may exhibit an additive CNS depression; the dose of one or both agents should be reduced).

No products indexed under this heading.

Sufentanil Citrate (Co-administration may exhibit an additive CNS depression; the dose of one or both agents should be reduced). Products include:

Sufenta Injection ... 1355

Temazepam (Co-administration may exhibit an additive CNS depression; the dose of one or both agents should be reduced). Products include:

Restoril Capsules ... 2413

Thiamylal Sodium (Co-administration may exhibit an additive CNS depression; the dose of one or both agents should be reduced).

No products indexed under this heading.

Thioridazine Hydrochloride (Co-administration may exhibit an additive CNS depression; the dose of one or both agents should be reduced). Products include:

Mellaril ... 2398

Thiothixene (Co-administration may exhibit an additive CNS depression; the dose of one or both agents should be reduced). Products include:

Navane Capsules and Concentrate 2018
Navane Intramuscular ... 2019

Triazolam (Co-administration may exhibit an additive CNS depression; the dose of one or both agents should be reduced). Products include:

Halcion Tablets ... 2093

Trifluoperazine Hydrochloride (Co-administration may exhibit an additive CNS depression; the dose of one or both agents should be reduced). Products include:

Stelazine ... 2692

Zolpidem Tartrate (Co-administration may exhibit an additive CNS depression; the dose of one or both agents should be reduced). Products include:

Ambien Tablets ... 2559

Food Interactions

Alcohol (Co-administration may exhibit an additive CNS depression).

VICON FORTE CAPSULES

(Vitamins with Minerals) ... 2760
None cited in PDR database.

VIDEX TABLETS, POWDER FOR ORAL SOLUTION, & PEDIATRIC POWDER FOR ORAL SOLUTION

(Didanosine) ... 2980
May interact with drugs that are known to cause peripheral neuropathy and pancreatitis (selected), tetracyclines, antacids containing aluminium, calcium and magnesium, and certain other agents. Compounds in these categories include:

Altretamine (Increased risk of toxicity due to peripheral neuropathy and pancreatitis). Products include:

Hexalen Capsules ... 2760

Aluminum Carbonate (Co-administration of these antacids with Videx chewable/dispersible buffered tablets or pediatric powder for oral solution may potentiate adverse effects associated with the antacid component). Products include:

Basaljel Capsules ... 2810
Basaljel Suspension ... 2810
Basaljel Tablets ... 2810

Aluminum Hydroxide (Co-administration of these antacids with Videx chewable/dispersible buffered tablets or pediatric powder for oral solution may potentiate adverse effects associated with the antacid component). Products include:

ALternaGEL Liquid ... 1358
Maximum Strength Ascriptin ... ▣ 650
Cama Arthritis Pain Reliever ... ▣ 748
Gaviscon Extra Strength Relief Formula Antacid Tablets ... ▣ 778
Gaviscon Extra Strength Relief Formula Liquid Antacid ... ▣ 779
Gaviscon Liquid Antacid ... ▣ 779
Gelusil Antacid-Anti-gas Liquid ... ▣ 819
Gelusil Antacid-Anti-gas Tablets ... ▣ 819
Maalox Antacid/Anti-Gas Tablets ... 889
Maalox Heartburn Relief Suspension ... ▣ 658
Maalox Antacid Liquid ... 888
Extra Strength Maalox Antacid/Anti-Gas Liquid and Tablets ... 888
Mylanta ... 1359
Tempo Soft Antacid ... ▣ 799

Aluminum Hydroxide Gel (Co-administration of these antacids with Videx chewable/dispersible buffered tablets or pediatric powder for oral solution may potentiate adverse effects associated with the antacid component). Products include:

ALternaGEL Liquid ... ▣ 675
Aludrox Oral Suspension ... ▣ 850
Amphojel Suspension ... 2802
Amphojel Suspension without Flavor ... 2802
Amphojel Tablets ... 2802
Ascriptin ... ▣ 650
Gaviscon Antacid Tablets ... ▣ 778
Gaviscon-2 Antacid Tablets ... ▣ 779
Mylanta Liquid ... ▣ 676
Mylanta Double Strength Liquid ... ▣ 676
Nephrox Suspension ... ▣ 671

Auranofin (Increased risk of toxicity due to peripheral neuropathy and pancreatitis). Products include:

Ridaura Capsules ... 2691

Carboplatin (Increased risk of toxicity due to peripheral neuropathy and pancreatitis). Products include:

Paraplatin for Injection ... 713

Chloramphenicol (Increased risk of toxicity due to peripheral neuropathy and pancreatitis). Products include:

Chloromycetin Ophthalmic Ointment, 1% ... ◉ 298
Chloromycetin Ophthalmic Solution ... ◉ 299
Chloroptic S.O.P. ... ◉ 236
Chloroptic Sterile Ophthalmic Solution ... ◉ 236

Chloramphenicol Palmitate (Increased risk of toxicity due to peripheral neuropathy and pancreatitis).

No products indexed under this heading.

Chloramphenicol Sodium Succinate (Increased risk of toxicity due to peripheral neuropathy and pancreatitis). Products include:

Chloromycetin Sodium Succinate ... 1960

Ciprofloxacin (Potential for decreased plasma concentrations of some quinolone antibiotics). Products include:

Cipro I.V. ... 587
Cipro I.V. Pharmacy Bulk Package ... 590

Ciprofloxacin Hydrochloride (Plasma concentrations of some oral quinolone antibiotics are decreased when administered with antacids used in conjunction with Videx; doses of quinolones should not be administered within 2 hours of taking Videx). Products include:

Ciloxan Ophthalmic Solution ... 468
Cipro Tablets ... 584

Cisplatin (Increased risk of toxicity due to peripheral neuropathy and pancreatitis). Products include:

Platinol for Injection ... 717
Platinol-AQ Injection ... 719

Dapsone (Drugs whose oral absorption can be affected by the level of acidity in the stomach, e.g., dapsone, should be administered at least 2 hours prior to dosing with Videx; potential for increased risk of toxicity due to peripheral neuropathy and pancreatitis). Products include:

Dapsone Tablets USP ... 1331

(▣ Described in PDR For Nonprescription Drugs) (◉ Described in PDR For Ophthalmology)

1183 **Interactions Index** **Viramune**

Demeclocycline Hydrochloride (Due to the magnesium and/or aluminum component of antacids present in Videx, concurrent use with any oral form of tetracycline should be avoided). Products include:
Declomycin Tablets 1421

Disulfiram (Increased risk of toxicity due to peripheral neuropathy and pancreatitis). Products include:
Antabuse Tablets 2802

Doxycycline Calcium (Due to the magnesium and/or aluminum component of antacids present in Videx, concurrent use with any oral form of tetracycline should be avoided). Products include:
Vibramycin Calcium Oral Suspension Syrup 2038

Doxycycline Hyclate (Due to the magnesium and/or aluminum component of antacids present in Videx, concurrent use with any oral form of tetracycline should be avoided). Products include:
Doryx Capsules 1970
Vibramycin Hyclate Capsules 2038
Vibramycin Hyclate Intravenous 2040
Vibra-Tabs Film Coated Tablets 2038

Doxycycline Monohydrate (Due to the magnesium and/or aluminum component of antacids present in Videx, concurrent use with any oral form of tetracycline should be avoided). Products include:
Monodox Capsules 1858
Vibramycin Monohydrate for Oral Suspension 2038

Enoxacin (Plasma concentrations of some oral quinolone antibiotics are decreased when administered with antacids used in conjunction with Videx; doses of quinolones should not be administered within 2 hours of taking Videx). Products include:
Penetrex Tablets 2196

Ethionamide (Increased risk of toxicity due to peripheral neuropathy and pancreatitis). Products include:
Trecator-SC Tablets 2919

Fosphenytoin Sodium (Increased risk of toxicity due to peripheral neuropathy and pancreatitis). Products include:
Cerebyx Injection 1956

Glutethimide (Increased risk of toxicity due to peripheral neuropathy and pancreatitis).
No products indexed under this heading.

Gold Sodium Thiomalate (Increased risk of toxicity due to peripheral neuropathy and pancreatitis). Products include:
Myochrysine Injection 1754

Hydralazine Hydrochloride (Increased risk of toxicity due to peripheral neuropathy and pancreatitis). Products include:
Apresazide Capsules 824
Apresoline Hydrochloride Tablets 826
Hydralazine Hydrochloride Injection USP 2712
Ser-Ap-Es Tablets 867

Iodoquinol (Increased risk of toxicity due to peripheral neuropathy and pancreatitis). Products include:
Yodoxin Tablets 1235

Isoniazid (Increased risk of toxicity due to peripheral neuropathy and pancreatitis). Products include:
Nydrazid Injection 509
Rifamate Capsules 1278
Rifater 1280

Ketoconazole (Drugs whose oral absorption can be affected by the level of acidity in the stomach, e.g., ketoconazole, should be administered at least 2 hours prior to dosing with Videx). Products include:
Nizoral 2% Cream 1344
Nizoral 2% Shampoo 1344
Nizoral Tablets 1345

Leuprolide Acetate (Increased risk of toxicity due to peripheral neuropathy and pancreatitis). Products include:
Lupron Depot 3.75 mg 2739
Lupron Depot 7.5 mg 2741
Lupron Depot - 3 Month 22.5 mg 2743
Lupron Depot-PED 7.5 mg, 11.25 mg and 15 mg 2744
Lupron Injection 2736
Lupron Injection Pediatric 2737

Lomefloxacin Hydrochloride (Plasma concentrations of some oral quinolone antibiotics are decreased when administered with antacids used in conjunction with Videx; doses of quinolones should not be administered within 2 hours of taking Videx). Products include:
Maxaquin Tablets 2593

Magaldrate (Co-administration of these antacids with Videx chewable/dispersible buffered tablets or pediatric powder for oral solution may potentiate adverse effects associated with the antacid component).
No products indexed under this heading.

Magnesium Hydroxide (Co-administration of these antacids with Videx chewable/dispersible buffered tablets or pediatric powder for oral solution may potentiate adverse effects associated with the antacid component). Products include:
Aludrox Oral Suspension .... ▣ 850
Ascriptin .... ▣ 650
Di-Gel Antacid/Anti-Gas .... ▣ 762
Gelusil Antacid-Anti-gas Liquid .... ▣ 819
Gelusil Antacid-Anti-gas Tablets .... ▣ 819
Maalox Antacid/Anti-Gas Tablets 889
Maalox Antacid Liquid 888
Extra Strength Maalox Antacid/Anti-Gas Liquid and Tablets 888
Mylanta Fast-Acting 1359
Mylanta Gelcaps Antacid .... ▣ 678
Fast-Acting Mylanta Liquid Antacid 1359
Mylanta Tablets .... ▣ 677
Maximum-Strength Fast-Acting Mylanta Liquid Antacid 1359
Mylanta Double Strength Tablets .... ▣ 677
Phillips' Milk of Magnesia Liquid .... ▣ 627
Rolaids Antacid Tablets .... ▣ 807
Tempo Soft Antacid .... ▣ 799

Magnesium Oxide (Co-administration of these antacids with Videx chewable/dispersible buffered tablets or pediatric powder for oral solution may potentiate adverse effects associated with the antacid component). Products include:
Beelith Tablets 632
Bufferin Analgesic Tablets .... ▣ 636
Arthritis Strength Bufferin Analgesic Caplets .... ▣ 637
Extra Strength Bufferin Analgesic Tablets .... ▣ 637
Caltrate PLUS .... ▣ 681
Cama Arthritis Pain Reliever .... ▣ 748
Mag-Ox 400 666
Uro-Mag 666

Methacycline Hydrochloride (Due to the magnesium and/or aluminum component of antacids present in Videx, concurrent use with any oral form of tetracycline should be avoided).
No products indexed under this heading.

Metronidazole (Increased risk of toxicity due to peripheral neuropathy and pancreatitis). Products include:
Flagyl 375 Capsules 2587
Flagyl I.V. RTU 2373
Helidac Therapy 2135
MetroCream 1034
MetroGel 1034
MetroGel-Vaginal 917
Protostat Tablets 1939

Minocycline Hydrochloride (Due to the magnesium and/or aluminum component of antacids present in Videx, concurrent use with any oral form of tetracycline should be avoided). Products include:
DYNACIN Capsules 1627
Minocin Intravenous 1428
Minocin Oral Suspension 1431
Minocin Pellet-Filled Capsules 1429

Nitrofurantoin (Increased risk of toxicity due to peripheral neuropathy and pancreatitis). Products include:
Macrodantin Capsules 2140

Norfloxacin (Plasma concentrations of some oral quinolone antibiotics are decreased when administered with antacids used in conjunction with Videx; doses of quinolones should not be administered within 2 hours of taking Videx). Products include:
Chibroxin Sterile Ophthalmic Solution 1657
Noroxin Tablets 1758
Noroxin Tablets 2222

Ofloxacin (Plasma concentrations of some oral quinolone antibiotics are decreased when administered with antacids used in conjunction with Videx; doses of quinolones should not be administered within 2 hours of taking Videx). Products include:
Floxin I.V. 1580
Floxin Tablets (200 mg, 300 mg, 400 mg) 1577
Ocuflox Ophthalmic Solution 478
Ocuflox .... ◎ 242

Oxytetracycline Hydrochloride (Due to the magnesium and/or aluminum component of antacids present in Videx, concurrent use with any oral form of tetracycline should be avoided). Products include:
TERAK Ointment .... ◎ 210
Terra-Cortril Ophthalmic Suspension 2033
Terramycin with Polymyxin B Sulfate Ophthalmic Ointment 2035
Urobiotic-250 Capsules 2038

Pentamidine Isethionate (Increased risk of toxicity due to peripheral neuropathy and pancreatitis).
No products indexed under this heading.

Phenytoin (Increased risk of toxicity due to peripheral neuropathy and pancreatitis). Products include:
Dilantin Infatabs 1967
Dilantin-125 Suspension 1969

Phenytoin Sodium (Increased risk of toxicity due to peripheral neuropathy and pancreatitis). Products include:
Dilantin Kapseals 1965

Ribavirin (Increased risk of toxicity due to peripheral neuropathy and pancreatitis). Products include:
Virazole 1310

Sulfamethoxazole (Increased risk of toxicity due to peripheral neuropathy and pancreatitis). Products include:
Bactrim DS Tablets 2257
Bactrim I.V. Infusion 2255
Bactrim 2257
Gantanol Tablets 2285
Septra 1146
Septra I.V. Infusion 1142
Septra I.V. Infusion ADD-Vantage Vials 1144
Septra 1146

Tetracycline Hydrochloride (Due to the magnesium and/or aluminum component of antacids present in Videx, concurrent use with any oral form of tetracycline should be avoided). Products include:
Achromycin V Capsules 1417
Helidac Therapy 2135

Vincristine Sulfate (Increased risk of toxicity due to peripheral neuropathy and pancreatitis). Products include:
Oncovin Solution Vials & Hyporets 1521

Food Interactions

Food, unspecified (Reduces the absorption of Videx by 50%; administer Videx on an empty stomach).

VIOKASE POWDER
(Pancrelipase) 2251
None cited in PDR database.

VIOKASE TABLETS
(Pancrelipase) 2251
None cited in PDR database.

VIQUIN FORTE 4% CREAM
(Hydroquinone, Dioxybenzone, Oxybenzone, Padimate O (Octyl Dimethyl Paba)) 1299
None cited in PDR database.

VIRA-A OPHTHALMIC OINTMENT, 3%
(Vidarabine) .... ◎ 299
None cited in PDR database.

VIRAMUNE TABLETS
(Nevirapine) 2368
May interact with oral contraceptives, macrolide antibiotics, protease inhibitors, and certain other agents. Compounds in these categories include:

Azithromycin (Co-administration with macrolides has resulted in elevated steady-state nevirapine trough plasma concentrations). Products include:
Zithromax 2043
Zithromax Tablets 2046

Cimetidine (Co-administration has resulted in elevated steady-state nevirapine trough plasma concentrations). Products include:
Tagamet HB Tablets .... ▣ 786
Tagamet Tablets 2694

Cimetidine Hydrochloride (Co-administration has resulted in elevated steady-state nevirapine trough plasma concentrations). Products include:
Tagamet 2694

Clarithromycin (Co-administration with macrolides has resulted in elevated steady-state nevirapine trough plasma concentrations). Products include:
Biaxin 406

Desogestrel (Nevirapine may decrease plasma concentrations of oral contraceptives and other hormonal contraceptives; concurrent use is not recommended). Products include:
Desogen Tablets 1867
Ortho-Cept 1907

Dirithromycin (Co-administration with macrolides has resulted in elevated steady-state nevirapine trough plasma concentrations). Products include:
Dynabac 668

IMPORTANT NOTE: Always consult each drug listing in the patient's regimen for possible interactions.

Viramune | Interactions Index | 1184

Erythromycin (Co-administration with macrolides has resulted in elevated steady-state nevirapine trough plasma concentrations). Products include:

A/T/S 2% Acne Topical Gel	1244
A/T/S 2% Acne Topical Solution	1244
Benzamycin Topical Gel	919
E-Mycin Tablets	1388
Emgel 2% Topical Gel	1081
ERYC	1972
Erycette (erythromycin 2%) Topical Solution	1943
Ery-Tab Tablets	426
Erythromycin Base Filmtab	430
Erythromycin Delayed-Release Capsules, USP	431
Ilotycin Ophthalmic Ointment	928
PCE Dispertab Tablets	453
T-Stat 2.0% Topical Solution and Pads	2797
THERAMYCIN Z 2% Solution	1629

Erythromycin Estolate (Co-administration with macrolides has resulted in elevated steady-state nevirapine trough plasma concentrations). Products include:

Ilosone	927

Erythromycin Ethylsuccinate (Co-administration with macrolides has resulted in elevated steady-state nevirapine trough plasma concentrations). Products include:

E.E.S.	427
EryPed	425
Pediazole Suspension	2340

Erythromycin Gluceptate (Co-administration with macrolides has resulted in elevated steady-state nevirapine trough plasma concentrations). Products include:

Ilotycin Gluceptate, IV, Vials	929

Erythromycin Stearate (Co-administration with macrolides has resulted in elevated steady-state nevirapine trough plasma concentrations). Products include:

Erythrocin Stearate Filmtab	429

Ethinyl Estradiol (Nevirapine may decrease plasma concentrations of oral contraceptives and other hormonal contraceptives; concurrent use is not recommended). Products include:

Brevicon	2563
Demulen	2580
Desogen Tablets	1867
Levlen/Tri-Levlen	646
Lo/Ovral Tablets	2852
Lo/Ovral-28 Tablets	2857
Modicon	1928
Nordette-21 Tablets	2863
Nordette-28 Tablets	2866
Norinyl	2563
Ortho-Cept	1907
Ortho-Cyclen/Ortho-Tri-Cyclen	1914
Ortho-Novum	1928
Ortho-Cyclen/Ortho-Tri-Cyclen	1914
Ovcon	765
Ovral Tablets	2877
Ovral-28 Tablets	2878
Levlen/Tri-Levlen	646
Tri-Norinyl	2607
Triphasil-21 Tablets	2919
Triphasil-28 Tablets	2924

Ethynodiol Diacetate (Nevirapine may decrease plasma concentrations of oral contraceptives and other hormonal contraceptives; concurrent use is not recommended). Products include:

Demulen	2580

Indinavir Sulfate (Nevirapine may decrease plasma concentrations of protease inhibitors; concurrent use is not recommended). Products include:

Crixivan Capsules	1670

Ketoconazole (*In vitro* studies indicates that ketoconazole significantly inhibited the formation of nevirapine hydroxylated metabolites; *in vivo* studies revealed no evidence of significant inhibitory effects). Products include:

Nizoral 2% Cream	1344
Nizoral 2% Shampoo	1344
Nizoral Tablets	1345

Levonorgestrel (Nevirapine may decrease plasma concentrations of oral contraceptives and other hormonal contraceptives; concurrent use is not recommended). Products include:

Levlen/Tri-Levlen	646
Nordette-21 Tablets	2863
Nordette-28 Tablets	2866
Norplant System	2868
Levlen/Tri-Levlen	646
Triphasil-21 Tablets	2919
Triphasil-28 Tablets	2924

Mestranol (Nevirapine may decrease plasma concentrations of oral contraceptives and other hormonal contraceptives; concurrent use is not recommended). Products include:

Norinyl	2563
Ortho-Novum	1928

Norethindrone (Nevirapine may decrease plasma concentrations of oral contraceptives and other hormonal contraceptives; concurrent use is not recommended). Products include:

Brevicon	2563
Micronor Tablets	1903
Modicon	1928
Norinyl	2563
Nor-Q D Tablets	2598
Ortho-Novum	1928
Ovcon	765
Tri-Norinyl	2607

Norethynodrel (Nevirapine may decrease plasma concentrations of oral contraceptives and other hormonal contraceptives; concurrent use is not recommended).

No products indexed under this heading.

Norgestimate (Nevirapine may decrease plasma concentrations of oral contraceptives and other hormonal contraceptives; concurrent use is not recommended). Products include:

Ortho-Cyclen/Ortho-Tri-Cyclen	1914
Ortho-Cyclen/Ortho Tri-Cyclen	1914

Norgestrel (Nevirapine may decrease plasma concentrations of oral contraceptives and other hormonal contraceptives; concurrent use is not recommended). Products include:

Lo/Ovral Tablets	2852
Lo/Ovral-28 Tablets	2857
Ovral Tablets	2877
Ovral-28 Tablets	2878
Ovrette Tablets	2878

Rifabutin (Co-administration with known inducers of CYP3A has resulted in reduced steady-state nevirapine trough plasma concentrations). Products include:

Mycobutin Capsules	2101

Rifampin (Co-administration with known inducers of CYP3A has resulted in reduced steady-state nevirapine trough plasma concentrations). Products include:

Rifadin	1276
Rifamate Capsules	1278
Rifater	1280
Rimactane Capsules	865

Ritonavir (Nevirapine may decrease plasma concentrations of protease inhibitors; concurrent use is not recommended). Products include:

Norvir	447

Saquinavir Mesylate (Nevirapine may decrease plasma concentrations of protease inhibitors; concurrent use is not recommended). Products include:

Invirase Capsules	2291

Troleandomycin (Co-administration with macrolides has resulted in elevated steady-state nevirapine trough plasma concentrations). Products include:

Tao Capsules	2033

Zidovudine (Co-administration with ddI on a background of zidovudine (ZDV) therapy, has produced a significant decline of 32% in ZDV AUC and a non-significant decline of 27% in ZDV C_{max}). Products include:

Retrovir Capsules	1216
Retrovir I.V. Infusion	1221
Retrovir Syrup	1216

VIRAZOLE
(Ribavirin) 1310
None cited in PDR database.

VIROPTIC OPHTHALMIC SOLUTION, 1% STERILE
(Trifluridine) 1177
None cited in PDR database.

VISINE A.C. SEASONAL RELIEF FROM POLLEN AND DUST
(Tetrahydrozoline Hydrochloride, Zinc Sulfate) .... ⊚ 301
None cited in PDR database.

VISINE L.R. EYE DROPS
(Oxymetazoline Hydrochloride) .... ⊚ 301
None cited in PDR database.

VISINE MOISTURIZING EYE DROPS
(Tetrahydrozoline Hydrochloride, Polyethylene Glycol) .... ⊚ 301
None cited in PDR database.

VISINE ORIGINAL EYE DROPS
(Tetrahydrozoline Hydrochloride) .. ⊚ 301
None cited in PDR database.

VISKEN TABLETS
(Pindolol) 2428
May interact with general anesthetics, insulin, oral hypoglycemic agents, catecholamine depleting drugs, beta₂ agonists, and certain other agents. Compounds in these categories include:

Acarbose (Beta-blockade reduces the release of insulin in response to hyperglycemia; adjust the dose of antidiabetic drugs). Products include:

Precose	604

Albuterol (Beta-blockade may block bronchodilation produced by exogenous catecholamine stimulation of beta₂ receptors). Products include:

Proventil Inhalation Aerosol	2524
Ventolin Inhalation Aerosol and Refill	1170

Albuterol Sulfate (Beta-blockade may block bronchodilation produced by exogenous catecholamine stimulation of beta₂ receptors). Products include:

Airet Albuterol Sulfate Inhalation Solution	1602
Albuterol Sulfate, USP Solution for Inhalation, Arm-a-Med	522
Proventil Inhalation Solution 0.083%	2527
Proventil Repetabs Tablets	2529
Proventil Solution for Inhalation 0.5%	2525
Proventil Syrup	2528
Proventil Tablets	2529
Ventolin Inhalation Solution	1171
Ventolin Nebules Inhalation Solution	1172
Ventolin Rotacaps for Inhalation	1173
Ventolin Syrup	1175
Ventolin Tablets	1176
Volmax Extended-Release Tablets	1835

Bitolterol Mesylate (Beta-blockade may block bronchodilation produced by exogenous catecholamine stimulation of beta₂ receptors). Products include:

Tornalate Solution for Inhalation, 0.2%	976
Tornalate Metered Dose Inhaler	978

Chlorpropamide (Beta-blockade reduces the release of insulin in response to hyperglycemia; adjust the dose of antidiabetic drugs). Products include:

Diabinese Tablets	2002

Deserpidine (Potential for additive effect; observe patients for evidence of hypotension, and/or bradycardia, vertigo, syncope, or postural hypotension).

No products indexed under this heading.

Enflurane (Risks of general anesthesia increased).

No products indexed under this heading.

Ephedrine Hydrochloride (Beta-blockade may block bronchodilation produced by exogenous catecholamine stimulation of beta₂ receptors). Products include:

Primatene Tablets	▣ 844
Quadrinal Tablets	1398

Ephedrine Sulfate (Beta-blockade may block bronchodilation produced by exogenous catecholamine stimulation of beta₂ receptors). Products include:

Marax Tablets & DF Syrup	2015

Ephedrine Tannate (Beta-blockade may block bronchodilation produced by exogenous catecholamine stimulation of beta₂ receptors). Products include:

Rynatuss	2782

Epinephrine (Patients with a history of severe anaphylactic reaction may be unresponsive to the usual dose of epinephrine used to treat allergy; Beta-blockade may block bronchodilation produced by exogenous catecholamine stimulation of beta₂ receptors). Products include:

EPIFRIN	⊚ 237
EpiPen	808
Marcaine with Epinephrine	2446
Primatene Mist	▣ 843
Sensorcaine with Epinephrine Injection	554
Sus-Phrine Injection	1017
Xylocaine with Epinephrine Injections	562

Epinephrine Hydrochloride (Patients with a history of severe anaphylactic reaction may be unresponsive to the usual dose of epinephrine used to treat allergy; Beta-blockade may block bronchodilation produced by exogenous catecholamine stimulation of beta₂ receptors). Products include:

Ana-Kit Anaphylaxis Emergency Treatment Kit	611

Ethylnorepinephrine Hydrochloride (Beta-blockade may block bronchodilation produced by exogenous catecholamine stimulation of beta₂ receptors).

No products indexed under this heading.

(▣ Described in PDR For Nonprescription Drugs)   (⊚ Described in PDR For Ophthalmology)

1185 Interactions Index Vistaril

Glimepiride (Beta-blockade reduces the release of insulin in response to hyperglycemia; adjust the dose of antidiabetic drugs). Products include:
Amaryl Tablets 1241
Glipizide (Beta-blockade reduces the release of insulin in response to hyperglycemia; adjust the dose of antidiabetic drugs). Products include:
Glucotrol Tablets 2011
Glucotrol XL Extended Release Tablets 2012
Glyburide (Beta-blockade reduces the release of insulin in response to hyperglycemia; adjust the dose of antidiabetic drugs). Products include:
DiaBeta Tablets 1265
Glynase PresTab Tablets 2091
Micronase Tablets 2099
Guanethidine Monosulfate (Potential for additive effect; observe patients for evidence of hypotension, and/or bradycardia, vertigo, syncope or postural hypotension). Products include:
Esimil Tablets 840
Ismelin Tablets 845
Insulin, Human (Beta-blockade reduces the release of insulin in response to hyperglycemia; adjust the dose of antidiabetic drugs).
No products indexed under this heading.
Insulin, Human Isophane Suspension (Beta-blockade reduces the release of insulin in response to hyperglycemia; adjust the dose of antidiabetic drugs). Products include:
Novolin N Human Insulin 10 ml Vials 1846
Insulin, Human NPH (Beta-blockade reduces the release of insulin in response to hyperglycemia; adjust the dose of antidiabetic drugs). Products include:
Humulin N, 100 Units 1495
Novolin N PenFill 1.5 ml Cartridges Durable Insulin Delivery System 1849
Novolin N Prefilled Syringe Disposable Insulin Delivery System 1850
Insulin, Human Regular (Beta-blockade reduces the release of insulin in response to hyperglycemia; adjust the dose of antidiabetic drugs). Products include:
Humulin R, 100 Units 1497
Novolin R Human Insulin 10 ml Vials 1846
Novolin R PenFill 1.5 ml Cartridges Durable Insulin Delivery System 1849
Novolin R Prefilled Syringe Disposable Insulin Delivery System 1850
Velosulin BR Human Insulin 10 ml Vials 1847
Insulin, Human, Zinc Suspension (Beta-blockade reduces the release of insulin in response to hyperglycemia; adjust the dose of antidiabetic drugs). Products include:
Humulin L, 100 Units 1494
Humulin U, 100 Units 1498
Novolin L Human Insulin 10 ml Vials 1846
Insulin Lispro, Human (Beta-blockade reduces the release of insulin in response to hyperglycemia; adjust the dose of antidiabetic drugs). Products include:
Humalog Injection 1488
Insulin, NPH (Beta-blockade reduces the release of insulin in response to hyperglycemia; adjust the dose of antidiabetic drugs). Products include:
NPH, 100 Units 1502
Pork NPH, 100 Units 1506
Purified Pork NPH Isophane Insulin 1852
Insulin, Regular (Beta-blockade reduces the release of insulin in response to hyperglycemia; adjust the dose of antidiabetic drugs). Products include:
Regular, 100 Units 1503
Pork Regular, 100 Units 1507
Pork Regular (Concentrated), 500 Units 1508
Purified Pork Regular Insulin 1852
Insulin, Zinc Crystals (Beta-blockade reduces the release of insulin in response to hyperglycemia; adjust the dose of antidiabetic drugs). Products include:
NPH, 100 Units 1502
Insulin, Zinc Suspension (Beta-blockade reduces the release of insulin in response to hyperglycemia; adjust the dose of antidiabetic drugs). Products include:
Iletin I 1501
Lente, 100 Units 1501
Iletin II 1504
Pork Lente, 100 Units 1504
Purified Pork Lente Insulin 1852
Isoetharine (Beta-blockade may block bronchodilation produced by exogenous catecholamine stimulation of $beta_2$ receptors). Products include:
Bronkometer Aerosol 2432
Bronkosol Solution 2432
Isoetharine Inhalation Solution, USP, Arm-a-Med 545
Isoflurane (Risks of general anesthesia increased).
No products indexed under this heading.
Isoproterenol Hydrochloride (Beta-blockade may block bronchodilation produced by exogenous catecholamine stimulation of $beta_2$ receptors). Products include:
Isuprel Hydrochloride Solution 2443
Isuprel Injection 2441
Isuprel Mistometer 2442
Isoproterenol Sulfate (Beta-blockade may block bronchodilation produced by exogenous catecholamine stimulation of $beta_2$ receptors). Products include:
Norisodrine with Calcium Iodide Syrup 446
Ketamine Hydrochloride (Risks of general anesthesia increased).
No products indexed under this heading.
Metaproterenol Sulfate (Beta-blockade may block bronchodilation produced by exogenous catecholamine stimulation of $beta_2$ receptors). Products include:
Alupent 672
Metaproterenol Sulfate Inhalation Solution, USP, Arm-a-Med 547
Metformin Hydrochloride (Beta-blockade reduces the release of insulin in response to hyperglycemia; adjust the dose of antidiabetic drugs). Products include:
Glucophage Tablets 754
Methohexital Sodium (Risks of general anesthesia increased).
No products indexed under this heading.
Methoxyflurane (Risks of general anesthesia increased).
No products indexed under this heading.
Pirbuterol Acetate (Beta-blockade may block bronchodilation produced by exogenous catecholamine stimulation of $beta_2$ receptors). Products include:
Maxair Autohaler 1550
Maxair Inhaler 1552
Propofol (Risks of general anesthesia increased). Products include:
Diprivan Injectable Emulsion 2939
Rauwolfia Serpentina (Potential for additive effect; observe patients for evidence of hypotension, and/or bradycardia, vertigo, syncope, or postural hypotension).
No products indexed under this heading.
Rescinnamine (Potential for additive effect; observe patients for evidence of hypotension, and/or bradycardia, vertigo, syncope, or postural hypotension).
No products indexed under this heading.
Reserpine (Potential for additive effect; observe patients for evidence of hypotension, and/or bradycardia, vertigo, syncope, or postural hypotension). Products include:
Diupres Tablets 1691
Hydropres Tablets 1718
Ser-Ap-Es Tablets 867
Salmeterol Xinafoate (Beta-blockade may block bronchodilation produced by exogenous catecholamine stimulation of $beta_2$ receptors). Products include:
Serevent Inhalation Aerosol 1149
Sevoflurane (Risks of general anesthesia increased).
No products indexed under this heading.
Terbutaline Sulfate (Beta-blockade may block bronchodilation produced by exogenous catecholamine stimulation of $beta_2$ receptors). Products include:
Brethaire Inhaler 830
Brethine Ampuls 832
Brethine Tablets 831
Bricanyl Subcutaneous Injection 1247
Bricanyl Tablets 1248
Thioridazine Hydrochloride (Increased serum levels of both drugs). Products include:
Mellaril 2398
Tolazamide (Beta-blockade reduces the release of insulin in response to hyperglycemia; adjust the dose of antidiabetic drugs).
No products indexed under this heading.
Tolbutamide (Beta-blockade reduces the release of insulin in response to hyperglycemia; adjust the dose of antidiabetic drugs).
No products indexed under this heading.

VISTARIL CAPSULES
(Hydroxyzine Pamoate) 2042
May interact with barbiturates, narcotic analgesics, central nervous system depressants, and certain other agents. Compounds in these categories include:

Alfentanil Hydrochloride (Potential for increased CNS depression when used concurrently). Products include:
Alfenta Injection 1334
Alprazolam (Potential for increased CNS depression when used concurrently). Products include:
Xanax Tablets 2115
Aprobarbital (Potential for increased CNS depression when used concurrently).
No products indexed under this heading.
Buprenorphine (Potential for increased CNS depression when used concurrently). Products include:
Buprenex Injectable 2170
Buspirone Hydrochloride (Potential for increased CNS depression when used concurrently). Products include:
BuSpar Tablets 738
Butabarbital (Potential for increased CNS depression when used concurrently).
No products indexed under this heading.
Butalbital (Potential for increased CNS depression when used concurrently). Products include:
Axocet Capsules 2469
Esgic-plus Capsules 1012
Esgic-plus Tablets 1012
Fioricet Tablets 2386
Fioricet with Codeine Capsules 2387
Fiorinal Capsules 2388
Fiorinal with Codeine Capsules 2390
Fiorinal Tablets 2388
Phrenilin 790
Sedapap Tablets 50 mg/650 mg 1826
Chlordiazepoxide (Potential for increased CNS depression when used concurrently). Products include:
Limbitrol 2333
Chlordiazepoxide Hydrochloride (Potential for increased CNS depression when used concurrently). Products include:
Librax Capsules 2330
Librium Capsules 2331
Librium Injectable 2332
Chlorpromazine (Potential for increased CNS depression when used concurrently). Products include:
Thorazine Suppositories 2701
Chlorpromazine Hydrochloride (Potential for increased CNS depression when used concurrently). Products include:
Thorazine 2701
Chlorprothixene (Potential for increased CNS depression when used concurrently).
No products indexed under this heading.
Chlorprothixene Hydrochloride (Potential for increased CNS depression when used concurrently).
No products indexed under this heading.
Chlorprothixene Lactate (Potential for increased CNS depression when used concurrently).
No products indexed under this heading.
Clorazepate Dipotassium (Potential for increased CNS depression when used concurrently). Products include:
Tranxene 459
Clozapine (Potential for increased CNS depression when used concurrently). Products include:
Clozaril Tablets 2377
Codeine Phosphate (Potential for increased CNS depression when used concurrently). Products include:
Brontex 2130
Dimetane-DC Cough Syrup 2232
Fioricet with Codeine Capsules 2387
Fiorinal with Codeine Capsules 2390
Nucofed 2225
Phenergan with Codeine 2883
Phenergan VC with Codeine 2888
Robitussin A-C Syrup 2248

IMPORTANT NOTE: Always consult each drug listing in the patient's regimen for possible interactions.

Vistaril

Robitussin-DAC Syrup 2249
Ryna .... ▣ 804
Soma Compound w/Codeine Tablets 2784
Tylenol with Codeine 1592

Desflurane (Potential for increased CNS depression when used concurrently). Products include:
Suprane (desflurane, USP) 1865

Dezocine (Potential for increased CNS depression when used concurrently). Products include:
Dalgan Injection 529

Diazepam (Potential for increased CNS depression when used concurrently). Products include:
Dizac (diazepam injectable emulsion) CIV 1862
Valium Injectable 2336
Valium Tablets 2335

Droperidol (Potential for increased CNS depression when used concurrently). Products include:
Inapsine Injection 462

Enflurane (Potential for increased CNS depression when used concurrently).
No products indexed under this heading.

Estazolam (Potential for increased CNS depression when used concurrently). Products include:
ProSom Tablets 457

Ethchlorvynol (Potential for increased CNS depression when used concurrently). Products include:
Placidyl Capsules 456

Ethinamate (Potential for increased CNS depression when used concurrently).
No products indexed under this heading.

Fentanyl (Potential for increased CNS depression when used concurrently). Products include:
Duragesic Transdermal System 1336

Fentanyl Citrate (Potential for increased CNS depression when used concurrently). Products include:
Sublimaze Injection 463

Fluphenazine Decanoate (Potential for increased CNS depression when used concurrently). Products include:
Prolixin Decanoate 510

Fluphenazine Enanthate (Potential for increased CNS depression when used concurrently). Products include:
Prolixin Enanthate 510

Fluphenazine Hydrochloride (Potential for increased CNS depression when used concurrently). Products include:
Prolixin 510

Flurazepam Hydrochloride (Potential for increased CNS depression when used concurrently). Products include:
Dalmane Capsules 2329

Glutethimide (Potential for increased CNS depression when used concurrently).
No products indexed under this heading.

Haloperidol (Potential for increased CNS depression when used concurrently). Products include:
Haldol Injection, Tablets and Concentrate 1585

Haloperidol Decanoate (Potential for increased CNS depression when used concurrently). Products include:
Haldol Decanoate 1587

Hydrocodone Bitartrate (Potential for increased CNS depression when used concurrently). Products include:
Codiclear DH Syrup 808
Duratuss HD Elixir 2750
Histussin D Liquid 670
Hycodan Tablets and Syrup 946
Hycomine Compound Tablets ... 948
Hycomine 947
Hycotuss Expectorant Syrup 950
Hydrocet Capsules 787
Lorcet 10/650 Tablets 1016
Lortab 2751
Tussend 1830
Tussend Expectorant 1831
Vicodin Tablets 1404
Vicodin ES Tablets 1405
Vicodin HP Tablets 1403
Vicodin Tuss Expectorant 1406
Zydone Capsules 967

Hydrocodone Polistirex (Potential for increased CNS depression when used concurrently). Products include:
Tussionex Pennkinetic Extended-Release Suspension 1624

Hydromorphone Hydrochloride (Potential for increased CNS depression when used concurrently). Products include:
Dilaudid Ampules 1382
Dilaudid Cough Syrup 1383
Dilaudid-HP Injection 1384
Dilaudid-HP Lyophilized Powder 250 mg 1384
Dilaudid 1382
Dilaudid Oral Liquid 1386
Dilaudid 1382
Dilaudid Tablets - 8 mg 1386

Hydroxyzine Hydrochloride (Potential for increased CNS depression when used concurrently). Products include:
Atarax Tablets & Syrup 1992
Marax Tablets & DF Syrup 2015
Vistaril Intramuscular Solution 2042

Isoflurane (Potential for increased CNS depression when used concurrently).
No products indexed under this heading.

Ketamine Hydrochloride (Potential for increased CNS depression when used concurrently).
No products indexed under this heading.

Levomethadyl Acetate Hydrochloride (Potential for increased CNS depression when used concurrently). Products include:
Orlaam Oral Solution 2361

Levorphanol Tartrate (Potential for increased CNS depression when used concurrently). Products include:
Levo-Dromoran 2297

Lorazepam (Potential for increased CNS depression when used concurrently). Products include:
Ativan Injection 2805
Ativan Tablets 2807

Loxapine Hydrochloride (Potential for increased CNS depression when used concurrently). Products include:
Loxitane 1426

Loxapine Succinate (Potential for increased CNS depression when used concurrently). Products include:
Loxitane Capsules 1426

Meperidine Hydrochloride (Potential for increased CNS depression when used concurrently). Products include:
Demerol 2438
Mepergan Injection 2859

Interactions Index

Mephobarbital (Potential for increased CNS depression when used concurrently). Products include:
Mebaral Tablets 2452

Meprobamate (Potential for increased CNS depression when used concurrently). Products include:
Miltown Tablets 2780
PMB 200 and PMB 400 2890

Mesoridazine Besylate (Potential for increased CNS depression when used concurrently). Products include:
Serentil 689

Methadone Hydrochloride (Potential for increased CNS depression when used concurrently). Products include:
Methadone Hydrochloride Oral Concentrate 2356
Methadone Hydrochloride Oral Solution & Tablets 2357

Methohexital Sodium (Potential for increased CNS depression when used concurrently).
No products indexed under this heading.

Methotrimeprazine (Potential for increased CNS depression when used concurrently). Products include:
Levoprome 1321

Methoxyflurane (Potential for increased CNS depression when used concurrently).
No products indexed under this heading.

Midazolam Hydrochloride (Potential for increased CNS depression when used concurrently). Products include:
Versed Injection 2324

Molindone Hydrochloride (Potential for increased CNS depression when used concurrently). Products include:
Moban Tablets and Concentrate 1036

Morphine Sulfate (Potential for increased CNS depression when used concurrently). Products include:
Astramorph/PF Injection, USP (Preservative-Free) 526
Duramorph Injection 983
Infumorph 200 and Infumorph 500 Sterile Solutions 985
Kadian Capsules 2948
MS Contin Tablets 2149
MSIR 2152
Oramorph SR (Morphine Sulfate Sustained Release Tablets) 2359
RMS Suppositories CII 2766
Roxanol 2365

Opium Alkaloids (Potential for increased CNS depression when used concurrently).
No products indexed under this heading.

Oxazepam (Potential for increased CNS depression when used concurrently). Products include:
Serax Capsules 2916
Serax Tablets 2916

Oxycodone Hydrochloride (Potential for increased CNS depression when used concurrently). Products include:
OxyContin Tablets 2163
OxyIR Capsules 2167
Percocet Tablets 955
Percodan Tablets 955
Percodan-Demi Tablets 956
Roxicodone Tablets, Oral Solution & Intensol (Oxycodone) 2366
Tylox Capsules 1593

Pentobarbital Sodium (Potential for increased CNS depression when used concurrently). Products include:
Nembutal Sodium Capsules 440

Nembutal Sodium Solution 442
Nembutal Sodium Suppositories 444

Perphenazine (Potential for increased CNS depression when used concurrently). Products include:
Etrafon 2495
Triavil Tablets 1800
Trilafon 2532

Phenobarbital (Potential for increased CNS depression when used concurrently). Products include:
Arco-Lase Plus Tablets 513
Bellergal-S Tablets 2375
Donnatal 2234
Donnatal Extentabs 2234
Donnatal Tablets 2234
Phenobarbital Elixir and Tablets 1523
Quadrinal Tablets 1398

Prazepam (Potential for increased CNS depression when used concurrently).
No products indexed under this heading.

Prochlorperazine (Potential for increased CNS depression when used concurrently). Products include:
Compazine 2644

Promethazine Hydrochloride (Potential for increased CNS depression when used concurrently). Products include:
Mepergan Injection 2859
Phenergan with Codeine 2883
Phenergan with Dextromethorphan 2885
Phenergan Injection 2880
Phenergan Suppositories 2882
Phenergan Syrup 2881
Phenergan Tablets 2882
Phenergan VC 2886
Phenergan VC with Codeine 2888

Propofol (Potential for increased CNS depression when used concurrently). Products include:
Diprivan Injectable Emulsion 2939

Propoxyphene Hydrochloride (Potential for increased CNS depression when used concurrently). Products include:
Darvon 1475
Wygesic Tablets 2930

Propoxyphene Napsylate (Potential for increased CNS depression when used concurrently). Products include:
Darvon-N/Darvocet-N 1473

Quazepam (Potential for increased CNS depression when used concurrently). Products include:
Doral Tablets 2773

Risperidone (Potential for increased CNS depression when used concurrently). Products include:
Risperdal Tablets 1348

Secobarbital Sodium (Potential for increased CNS depression when used concurrently). Products include:
Seconal Sodium Pulvules 1529

Sevoflurane (Potential for increased CNS depression when used concurrently).
No products indexed under this heading.

Sufentanil Citrate (Potential for increased CNS depression when used concurrently). Products include:
Sufenta Injection 1355

Temazepam (Potential for increased CNS depression when used concurrently). Products include:
Restoril Capsules 2413

Thiamylal Sodium (Potential for increased CNS depression when used concurrently).
No products indexed under this heading.

(▣ Described in PDR For Nonprescription Drugs)   (⊙ Described in PDR For Ophthalmology)

1187 Interactions Index Vistaril Intramuscular

Thioridazine Hydrochloride (Potential for increased CNS depression when used concurrently). Products include:

Mellaril 2398

Thiothixene (Potential for increased CNS depression when used concurrently). Products include:

Navane Capsules and Concentrate 2018
Navane Intramuscular 2019

Triazolam (Potential for increased CNS depression when used concurrently). Products include:

Halcion Tablets 2093

Trifluoperazine Hydrochloride (Potential for increased CNS depression when used concurrently). Products include:

Stelazine 2692

Zolpidem Tartrate (Potential for increased CNS depression when used concurrently). Products include:

Ambien Tablets 2559

Food Interactions

Alcohol (Increased effect of alcohol).

VISTARIL INTRAMUSCULAR SOLUTION

(Hydroxyzine Hydrochloride) 2042

May interact with central nervous system depressants, narcotic analgesics, barbiturates, and certain other agents. Compounds in these categories include:

Alfentanil Hydrochloride (May be potentiated; dosage should be decreased by up to 50%; rare potential for cardiac arrest and death). Products include:

Alfenta Injection 1334

Alprazolam (May be potentiated; dosage should be decreased by up to 50%; rare potential for cardiac arrest and death). Products include:

Xanax Tablets 2115

Aprobarbital (May be potentiated; dosage should be decreased by up to 50%; rare potential for cardiac arrest and death).

No products indexed under this heading.

Buprenorphine (May be potentiated; dosage should be decreased by up to 50%; rare potential for cardiac arrest and death). Products include:

Buprenex Injectable 2170

Buspirone Hydrochloride (May be potentiated; dosage should be decreased by up to 50%; rare potential for cardiac arrest and death). Products include:

BuSpar Tablets 738

Butabarbital (May be potentiated; dosage should be decreased by up to 50%; rare potential for cardiac arrest and death).

No products indexed under this heading.

Butalbital (May be potentiated; dosage should be decreased by up to 50%; rare potential for cardiac arrest and death). Products include:

Axocet Capsules 2469
Esgic-plus Capsules 1012
Esgic-plus Tablets 1012
Fioricet Tablets 2386
Fioricet with Codeine Capsules 2387
Fiorinal Capsules 2388
Fiorinal with Codeine Capsules 2390
Fiorinal Tablets 2388
Phrenilin 790
Sedapap Tablets 50 mg/650 mg .. 1826

Chlordiazepoxide (May be potentiated; dosage should be decreased by up to 50%; rare potential for cardiac arrest and death). Products include:

Limbitrol 2333

Chlordiazepoxide Hydrochloride (May be potentiated; dosage should be decreased by up to 50%; rare potential for cardiac arrest and death). Products include:

Librax Capsules 2330
Librium Capsules 2331
Librium Injectable 2332

Chlorpromazine (May be potentiated; dosage should be decreased by up to 50%; rare potential for cardiac arrest and death). Products include:

Thorazine Suppositories 2701

Chlorprothixene (May be potentiated; dosage should be decreased by up to 50%; rare potential for cardiac arrest and death).

No products indexed under this heading.

Chlorprothixene Hydrochloride (May be potentiated; dosage should be decreased by up to 50%; rare potential for cardiac arrest and death).

No products indexed under this heading.

Chlorprothixene Lactate (May be potentiated; dosage should be decreased by up to 50%; rare potential for cardiac arrest and death).

No products indexed under this heading.

Clorazepate Dipotassium (May be potentiated; dosage should be decreased by up to 50%; rare potential for cardiac arrest and death). Products include:

Tranxene 459

Clozapine (May be potentiated; dosage should be decreased by up to 50%; rare potential for cardiac arrest and death). Products include:

Clozaril Tablets 2377

Codeine Phosphate (May be potentiated; dosage should be decreased by up to 50%; rare potential for cardiac arrest and death). Products include:

Brontex 2130
Dimetane-DC Cough Syrup 2232
Fioricet with Codeine Capsules 2387
Fiorinal with Codeine Capsules 2390
Nucofed 2225
Phenergan with Codeine 2883
Phenergan VC with Codeine 2888
Robitussin A-C Syrup 2248
Robitussin-DAC Syrup 2249
Ryna 804
Soma Compound w/Codeine Tablets 2784
Tylenol with Codeine 1592

Desflurane (May be potentiated; dosage should be decreased by up to 50%; rare potential for cardiac arrest and death). Products include:

Suprane (desflurane, USP) 1865

Dezocine (May be potentiated; dosage should be decreased by up to 50%; rare potential for cardiac arrest and death). Products include:

Dalgan Injection 529

Diazepam (May be potentiated; dosage should be decreased by up to 50%; rare potential for cardiac arrest and death). Products include:

Dizac (diazepam injectable emulsion) CIV 1862
Valium Injectable 2336
Valium Tablets 2335

Droperidol (May be potentiated; dosage should be decreased by up to 50%; rare potential for cardiac arrest and death). Products include:

Inapsine Injection 462

Enflurane (May be potentiated; dosage should be decreased by up to 50%; rare potential for cardiac arrest and death).

No products indexed under this heading.

Estazolam (May be potentiated; dosage should be decreased by up to 50%; rare potential for cardiac arrest and death). Products include:

ProSom Tablets 457

Ethchlorvynol (May be potentiated; dosage should be decreased by up to 50%; rare potential for cardiac arrest and death). Products include:

Placidyl Capsules 456

Ethinamate (May be potentiated; dosage should be decreased by up to 50%; rare potential for cardiac arrest and death).

No products indexed under this heading.

Fentanyl (May be potentiated; dosage should be decreased by up to 50%; rare potential for cardiac arrest and death). Products include:

Duragesic Transdermal System 1336

Fentanyl Citrate (May be potentiated; dosage should be decreased by up to 50%; rare potential for cardiac arrest and death). Products include:

Sublimaze Injection 463

Fluphenazine Decanoate (May be potentiated; dosage should be decreased by up to 50%; rare potential for cardiac arrest and death). Products include:

Prolixin Decanoate 510

Fluphenazine Enanthate (May be potentiated; dosage should be decreased by up to 50%; rare potential for cardiac arrest and death). Products include:

Prolixin Enanthate 510

Fluphenazine Hydrochloride (May be potentiated; dosage should be decreased by up to 50%; rare potential for cardiac arrest and death). Products include:

Prolixin 510

Flurazepam Hydrochloride (May be potentiated; dosage should be decreased by up to 50%; rare potential for cardiac arrest and death). Products include:

Dalmane Capsules 2329

Glutethimide (May be potentiated; dosage should be decreased by up to 50%; rare potential for cardiac arrest and death).

No products indexed under this heading.

Haloperidol (May be potentiated; dosage should be decreased by up to 50%; rare potential for cardiac arrest and death). Products include:

Haldol Injection, Tablets and Concentrate 1585

Haloperidol Decanoate (May be potentiated; dosage should be decreased by up to 50%; rare potential for cardiac arrest and death). Products include:

Haldol Decanoate 1587

Hydrocodone Bitartrate (May be potentiated; dosage should be decreased by up to 50%; rare potential for cardiac arrest and death). Products include:

Codiclear DH Syrup 808
Duratuss HD Elixir 2750
Histussin D Liquid 670
Hycodan Tablets and Syrup 946
Hycomine Compound Tablets 948
Hycomine 947
Hycotuss Expectorant Syrup 950
Hydrocet Capsules 787
Lorcet 10/650 Tablets 1016
Lortab 2751
Tussend 1830
Tussend Expectorant 1831
Vicodin Tablets 1404
Vicodin ES Tablets 1405
Vicodin HP Tablets 1403
Vicodin Tuss Expectorant 1406
Zydone Capsules 967

Hydrocodone Polistirex (May be potentiated; dosage should be decreased by up to 50%; rare potential for cardiac arrest and death). Products include:

Tussionex Pennkinetic Extended-Release Suspension 1624

Hydromorphone Hydrochloride (May be potentiated; dosage should be decreased by up to 50%; rare potential for cardiac arrest and death). Products include:

Dilaudid Ampules 1382
Dilaudid Cough Syrup 1383
Dilaudid-HP Injection 1384
Dilaudid-HP Lyophilized Powder 250 mg 1384
Dilaudid 1382
Dilaudid Oral Liquid 1386
Dilaudid 1382
Dilaudid Tablets - 8 mg 1386

Isoflurane (May be potentiated; dosage should be decreased by up to 50%; rare potential for cardiac arrest and death).

No products indexed under this heading.

Ketamine Hydrochloride (May be potentiated; dosage should be decreased by up to 50%; rare potential for cardiac arrest and death).

No products indexed under this heading.

Levomethadyl Acetate Hydrochloride (May be potentiated; dosage should be decreased by up to 50%; rare potential for cardiac arrest and death). Products include:

Orlaam Oral Solution 2361

Levorphanol Tartrate (May be potentiated; dosage should be decreased by up to 50%; rare potential for cardiac arrest and death). Products include:

Levo-Dromoran 2297

Lorazepam (May be potentiated; dosage should be decreased by up to 50%; rare potential for cardiac arrest and death). Products include:

Ativan Injection 2805
Ativan Tablets 2807

Loxapine Hydrochloride (May be potentiated; dosage should be decreased by up to 50%; rare potential for cardiac arrest and death). Products include:

Loxitane 1426

Loxapine Succinate (May be potentiated; dosage should be decreased by up to 50%; rare potential for cardiac arrest and death). Products include:

Loxitane Capsules 1426

Meperidine Hydrochloride (May be potentiated; dosage should be decreased by up to 50%; rare potential for cardiac arrest and death). Products include:

Demerol 2438
Mepergan Injection 2859

Mephobarbital (May be potentiated; dosage should be decreased by up to 50%; rare potential for cardiac arrest and death). Products include:

Mebaral Tablets 2452

Meprobamate (May be potentiated; dosage should be decreased by up to 50%; rare potential for cardiac arrest and death). Products include:

Miltown Tablets 2780
PMB 200 and PMB 400 2890

IMPORTANT NOTE: Always consult each drug listing in the patient's regimen for possible interactions.

Vistaril Intramuscular / Interactions Index

Mesoridazine Besylate (May be potentiated; dosage should be decreased by up to 50%; rare potential for cardiac arrest and death). Products include:
- Serentil 689

Methadone Hydrochloride (May be potentiated; dosage should be decreased by up to 50%; rare potential for cardiac arrest and death). Products include:
- Methadone Hydrochloride Oral Concentrate 2356
- Methadone Hydrochloride Oral Solution & Tablets 2357

Methohexital Sodium (May be potentiated; dosage should be decreased by up to 50%; rare potential for cardiac arrest and death).
- No products indexed under this heading.

Methotrimeprazine (May be potentiated; dosage should be decreased by up to 50%; rare potential for cardiac arrest and death). Products include:
- Levoprome 1321

Methoxyflurane (May be potentiated; dosage should be decreased by up to 50%; rare potential for cardiac arrest and death).
- No products indexed under this heading.

Midazolam Hydrochloride (May be potentiated; dosage should be decreased by up to 50%; rare potential for cardiac arrest and death). Products include:
- Versed Injection 2324

Molindone Hydrochloride (May be potentiated; dosage should be decreased by up to 50%; rare potential for cardiac arrest and death). Products include:
- Moban Tablets and Concentrate 1036

Morphine Sulfate (May be potentiated; dosage should be decreased by up to 50%; rare potential for cardiac arrest and death). Products include:
- Astramorph/PF Injection, USP (Preservative-Free) 526
- Duramorph Injection 983
- Infumorph 200 and Infumorph 500 Sterile Solutions 985
- Kadian Capsules 2948
- MS Contin Tablets 2149
- MSIR 2152
- Oramorph SR (Morphine Sulfate Sustained Release Tablets) 2359
- RMS Suppositories CII 2766
- Roxanol 2365

Opium Alkaloids (May be potentiated; dosage should be decreased by up to 50%; rare potential for cardiac arrest and death).
- No products indexed under this heading.

Oxazepam (May be potentiated; dosage should be decreased by up to 50%; rare potential for cardiac arrest and death). Products include:
- Serax Capsules 2916
- Serax Tablets 2916

Oxycodone Hydrochloride (May be potentiated; dosage should be decreased by up to 50%; rare potential for cardiac arrest and death). Products include:
- OxyContin Tablets 2163
- OxyIR Capsules 2167
- Percocet Tablets 955
- Percodan Tablets 955
- Percodan-Demi Tablets 956
- Roxicodone Tablets, Oral Solution & Intensol (Oxycodone) 2366
- Tylox Capsules 1593

Pentobarbital Sodium (May be potentiated; dosage should be decreased by up to 50%; rare potential for cardiac arrest and death). Products include:
- Nembutal Sodium Capsules 440
- Nembutal Sodium Solution 442
- Nembutal Sodium Suppositories 444

Perphenazine (May be potentiated; dosage should be decreased by up to 50%; rare potential for cardiac arrest and death). Products include:
- Etrafon 2495
- Triavil Tablets 1800
- Trilafon 2532

Phenobarbital (May be potentiated; dosage should be decreased by up to 50%; rare potential for cardiac arrest and death). Products include:
- Arco-Lase Plus Tablets 513
- Bellergal-S Tablets 2375
- Donnatal 2234
- Donnatal Extentabs 2234
- Donnatal Tablets 2234
- Phenobarbital Elixir and Tablets 1523
- Quadrinal Tablets 1398

Prazepam (May be potentiated; dosage should be decreased by up to 50%; rare potential for cardiac arrest and death).
- No products indexed under this heading.

Prochlorperazine (May be potentiated; dosage should be decreased by up to 50%; rare potential for cardiac arrest and death). Products include:
- Compazine 2644

Promethazine Hydrochloride (May be potentiated; dosage should be decreased by up to 50%; rare potential for cardiac arrest and death). Products include:
- Mepergan Injection 2859
- Phenergan with Codeine 2883
- Phenergan with Dextromethorphan 2885
- Phenergan Injection 2880
- Phenergan Suppositories 2882
- Phenergan Syrup 2881
- Phenergan Tablets 2882
- Phenergan VC 2886
- Phenergan VC with Codeine 2888

Propofol (May be potentiated; dosage should be decreased by up to 50%; rare potential for cardiac arrest and death). Products include:
- Diprivan Injectable Emulsion 2939

Propoxyphene Hydrochloride (May be potentiated; dosage should be decreased by up to 50%; rare potential for cardiac arrest and death). Products include:
- Darvon 1475
- Wygesic Tablets 2930

Propoxyphene Napsylate (May be potentiated; dosage should be decreased by up to 50%; rare potential for cardiac arrest and death). Products include:
- Darvon-N/Darvocet-N 1473

Quazepam (May be potentiated; dosage should be decreased by up to 50%; rare potential for cardiac arrest and death). Products include:
- Doral Tablets 2773

Risperidone (May be potentiated; dosage should be decreased by up to 50%; rare potential for cardiac arrest and death). Products include:
- Risperdal Tablets 1348

Secobarbital Sodium (May be potentiated; dosage should be decreased by up to 50%; rare potential for cardiac arrest and death). Products include:
- Seconal Sodium Pulvules 1529

Sevoflurane (May be potentiated; dosage should be decreased by up to 50%; rare potential for cardiac arrest and death).
- No products indexed under this heading.

Sufentanil Citrate (May be potentiated; dosage should be decreased by up to 50%; rare potential for cardiac arrest and death). Products include:
- Sufenta Injection 1355

Temazepam (May be potentiated; dosage should be decreased by up to 50%; rare potential for cardiac arrest and death). Products include:
- Restoril Capsules 2413

Thiamylal Sodium (May be potentiated; dosage should be decreased by up to 50%; rare potential for cardiac arrest and death).
- No products indexed under this heading.

Thioridazine Hydrochloride (May be potentiated; dosage should be decreased by up to 50%; rare potential for cardiac arrest and death). Products include:
- Mellaril 2398

Thiothixene (May be potentiated; dosage should be decreased by up to 50%; rare potential for cardiac arrest and death). Products include:
- Navane Capsules and Concentrate 2018
- Navane Intramuscular 2019

Triazolam (May be potentiated; dosage should be decreased by up to 50%; rare potential for cardiac arrest and death). Products include:
- Halcion Tablets 2093

Trifluoperazine Hydrochloride (May be potentiated; dosage should be decreased by up to 50%; rare potential for cardiac arrest and death). Products include:
- Stelazine 2692

Zolpidem Tartrate (May be potentiated; dosage should be decreased by up to 50%; rare potential for cardiac arrest and death). Products include:
- Ambien Tablets 2559

Food Interactions

Alcohol (May be potentiated).

VISTARIL ORAL SUSPENSION
(Hydroxyzine Pamoate) 2042
See **Vistaril Capsules**

VISTIDE INJECTION
(Cidofovir) 1057
May interact with aminoglycosides, ACE inhibitors, barbiturates, benzodiazepines, non-steroidal anti-inflammatory agents, xanthine bronchodilators, and certain other agents. Compounds in these categories include:

Acetaminophen (Probenecid must be used with each cidofovir infusion; probenecid is known to interact with the metabolism or renal tubular excretion of acetaminophen; concomitant use should be carefully assessed). Products include:
- Actifed Cold & Sinus Caplets and Tablets 808
- Actifed Sinus Daytime/Nighttime Tablets and Caplets 809
- Alka-Seltzer Fast Relief Caplets 610
- Alka-Seltzer Plus Liqui-Gels 612
- Alka-Seltzer Plus Flu & Body Aches Effervescent Tablets 612
- Alka-Seltzer Plus Flu & Body Aches Liqui-Gels Non-Drowsy Formula 613
- Alka-Seltzer Plus Night-Time Cold Medicine Liqui-Gels 612
- Allerest No Drowsiness 649
- Allerest Sinus Pain Formula 649
- Axocet Capsules 2469
- Benadryl Allergy/Cold Tablets 811
- Benadryl Allergy Sinus Headache Caplets 813
- Children's TYLENOL acetaminophen Chewable Tablets, Elixir, Suspension Liquid, and Suspension Drops 1559
- Children's TYLENOL Cold Multi-Symptom Chewable Tablets and Liquid 1559
- Children's TYLENOL Cold Plus Cough Multi Symptom Chewable Tablets and Liquid 1560
- Children's TYLENOL Flu Suspension Liquid 1560
- Allergy-Sinus Comtrex Multi-Symptom Allergy-Sinus Formula Tablets and Caplets 639
- Comtrex Multi-Symptom 638
- Comtrex Non-Drowsy 640
- Contac Day Allergy/Sinus Caplets 771
- Contac Day & Night 772
- Contac Night Allergy/Sinus Caplets 771
- Contac Severe Cold and Flu Formula Caplets 773
- Contac Severe Cold & Flu Non-Drowsy 774
- Coricidin Cold + Flu Tablets 760
- Coricidin 'D' Decongestant Tablets 760
- DHCplus Capsules 2148
- Darvon-N/Darvocet-N 1473
- Dimetapp Allergy Sinus Caplets 838
- Dimetapp Cold & Fever Suspension 839
- Drixoral Cold and Flu Extended-Release Tablets 764
- Drixoral Cough + Sore Throat Liquid Caps 763
- Drixoral Allergy/Sinus Extended Release Tablets 765
- Esgic-plus Capsules 1012
- Esgic-plus Tablets 1012
- Aspirin Free Excedrin Analgesic Caplets and Geltabs 734
- Excedrin Extra-Strength Analgesic Tablets, Caplets, and Geltabs 734
- Excedrin P.M. Analgesic/Sleeping Aid Tablets, Caplets, Liquigels 735
- Fioricet Tablets 2386
- Fioricet with Codeine Capsules 2387
- Goody's Extra Strength Headache Powders 632
- Goody's Extra Strength Pain Relief Tablets 632
- Hycomine Compound Tablets 948
- Hydrocet Capsules 787
- Infants' TYLENOL acetaminophen Suspension Drops 1559
- Infants' TYLENOL Cold Decongestant & Fever-Reducer Drops 1561
- Junior Strength TYLENOL acetaminophen Coated Caplets and Chewable Tablets 1562
- Lorcet 10/650 Tablets 1016
- Lortab 2751
- Lurline PMS Tablets 1000
- Maximum Strength Multi-Symptom Formula Midol 621
- PMS Multi-Symptom Formula Midol 622
- Maximum Strength Midol Teen Multi-Symptom Formula 621
- Midrin Capsules 788
- Panodol Tablets and Caplets 783
- Children's Panadol Chewable Tablets, Liquid, Infant's Drops 783
- Percocet Tablets 955
- Percogesic Analgesic Tablets 727
- Phrenilin 790
- Pyrroxate Caplets 742
- Robitussin Cold, Cough & Flu Liqui-Gels 844
- Robitussin Night-Time Cold Formula 847
- Sedapap Tablets 50 mg/650 mg 1826
- Sinarest 663
- Sine-Aid Maximum Strength Sinus Headache Gelcaps, Caplets and Tablets 1570
- Sine-Off No Drowsiness Formula Caplets 784
- Sine-Off Sinus Medicine 784
- Singlet Tablets 785
- Sinulin Tablets 792

(▣ Described in PDR For Nonprescription Drugs) (⊙ Described in PDR For Ophthalmology)

1189 **Interactions Index** **Vistide**

Sinutab Sinus Allergy Medication, Maximum Strength Tablets and Caplets 823
Sinutab Sinus Medication, Maximum Strength Without Drowsiness Formula, Tablets & Caplets 824
Sudafed Cold and Cough Liquid Caps 826
Sudafed Severe Cold Formula Caplets 828
Sudafed Severe Cold Formula Tablets 828
Sudafed Sinus Caplets 829
Sudafed Sinus Tablets 829
Talacen Caplets 2464
TheraFlu Flu and Cold Medicine 750
Theraflu Maximum Strength Flu and Cold Medicine For Sore Throat 751
TheraFlu Flu, Cold and Cough Medicine 750
TheraFlu Maximum Strength Nighttime Flu, Cold & Cough Medicine 751
TheraFlu Maximum Strength Non-Drowsy Formula Flu, Cold & Cough Medicine 751
TheraFlu Maximum Strength, Non-Drowsy Formula Flu, Cold and Cough Caplets 752
Theraflu Maximum Strength Sinus Non-Drowsy Formula Caplets 752
Triaminic Sore Throat Formula 755
Triaminicin Tablets 756
TYLENOL acetaminophen Extended Relief Caplets 1570
TYLENOL acetaminophen, Extra Strength Adult Liquid Pain Reliever 1570
TYLENOL acetaminophen, Extra Strength Gelcaps, Geltabs, Caplets, Tablets 1570
TYLENOL acetaminophen, Regular Strength Caplets and Tablets 1570
TYLENOL Allergy Sinus, Maximum Strength Caplets and Gelcaps 1571
TYLENOL Allergy Sinus NightTime, Maximum Strength Caplets 1571
TYLENOL Cold Medication, Multi-Symptom Formula Tablets and Caplets 1572
TYLENOL Cold Medication, Multi-Symptom Hot Liquid Packets 1572
TYLENOL Cold Medication, No Drowsiness Formula Caplets and Gelcaps 1572
TYLENOL Cold Severe Congestion Caplets 1573
TYLENOL Cough Medication, Multi Symptom 1574
TYLENOL Cough Medication with Decongestant, Multi Symptom 1574
TYLENOL Flu No Drowsiness Formula, Maximum Strength Gelcaps 1575
TYLENOL Flu NightTime, Maximum Strength Gelcaps 1575
TYLENOL Flu NightTime, Maximum Strength Hot Medication Packets 1575
TYLENOL Headache Plus Pain Reliever with Antacid, Extra Strength Caplets 705
TYLENOL PM Pain Reliever/Sleep Aid, Extra Strength Gelcaps, Caplets, Geltabs 1576
TYLENOL Severe Allergy Medication Caplets 1571
TYLENOL Sinus, Maximum Strength Geltabs, Gelcaps, Caplets and Tablets 1576
Tylenol with Codeine 1592
Tylox Capsules 1593
Unisom With Pain Relief-Nighttime Sleep Aid and Pain Reliever 1991
Vanquish Analgesic Caplets 627
Vicks 44 LiquiCaps Cough, Cold & Flu Relief 728
Vicks 44M Cough, Cold & Flu Relief 729
Vicks DayQuil LiquiCaps/Liquid Multi-Symptom Cold/Flu Relief 734
Vicks Nyquil Hot Therapy 735
Vicks NyQuil LiquiCaps/Liquid Multi-Symptom Cold/Flu Relief, Original and Cherry Flavors 736
Vicodin Tablets 1404
Vicodin ES Tablets 1405
Vicodin HP Tablets 1403
Wygesic Tablets 2930
Zydone Capsules 967

Acyclovir (Probenecid must be used with each cidofovir infusion; probenecid is known to interact with the metabolism or renal tubular excretion of acyclovir; concomitant use should be carefully assessed). Products include:
Zovirax Capsules 1187
Zovirax Ointment 5% 1190
Zovirax 1187

Acyclovir Sodium (Probenecid must be used with each cidofovir infusion; probenecid is known to interact with the metabolism or renal tubular excretion of acyclovir; concomitant use should be carefully assessed). Products include:
Zovirax Sterile Powder 1191

Alprazolam (Probenecid must be used with each cidofovir infusion; probenecid is known to interact with the metabolism or renal tubular excretion of benzodiazepines; concomitant use should be carefully assessed). Products include:
Xanax Tablets 2115

Amikacin Sulfate (Renal impairment is the major toxicity of cidofovir; co-administration with potential nephrotoxic agents should be avoided). Products include:
Amikacin Sulfate Injection, USP 523
Amikacin Sulfate Injection, USP 981
Amikin Injectable 502

Aminophylline (Probenecid must be used with each cidofovir infusion; probenecid is known to interact with the metabolism or renal tubular excretion of theophylline; concomitant use should be carefully assessed).
No products indexed under this heading.

Amphotericin B (Renal impairment is the major toxicity of cidofovir; co-administration with potential nephrotoxic agents should be avoided). Products include:
Abelcet Injection 1540
Fungizone Intravenous 507
Fungizone Oral Suspension 704

Aprobarbital (Probenecid must be used with each cidofovir infusion; probenecid is known to interact with the metabolism or renal tubular excretion of barbiturates; concomitant use should be carefully assessed).
No products indexed under this heading.

Benazepril Hydrochloride (Probenecid must be used with each cidofovir infusion; probenecid is known to interact with the metabolism or renal tubular excretion of ACE inhibitors; concomitant use should be carefully assessed). Products include:
Lotensin Tablets 852
Lotensin HCT Tablets 855
Lotrel Capsules 858

Bumetanide (Probenecid must be used with each cidofovir infusion; probenecid is known to interact with the metabolism or renal tubular excretion of bumetanide; concomitant use should be carefully assessed). Products include:
Bumex 2260

Butabarbital (Probenecid must be used with each cidofovir infusion; probenecid is known to interact with the metabolism or renal tubular excretion of barbiturates; concomitant use should be carefully assessed).
No products indexed under this heading.

Butalbital (Probenecid must be used with each cidofovir infusion; probenecid is known to interact with the metabolism or renal tubular excretion of barbiturates; concomitant use should be carefully assessed). Products include:
Axocet Capsules 2469
Esgic-plus Capsules 1012
Esgic-plus Tablets 1012
Fioricet Tablets 2386
Fioricet with Codeine Capsules 2387
Fiorinal Capsules 2388
Fiorinal with Codeine Capsules 2390
Fiorinal Tablets 2388
Phrenilin 790
Sedapap Tablets 50 mg/650 mg 1826

Captopril (Probenecid must be used with each cidofovir infusion; probenecid is known to interact with the metabolism or renal tubular excretion of ACE inhibitors; concomitant use should be carefully assessed). Products include:
Capoten Tablets 740
Capozide Tablets 744

Chlordiazepoxide (Probenecid must be used with each cidofovir infusion; probenecid is known to interact with the metabolism or renal tubular excretion of benzodiazepines; concomitant use should be carefully assessed). Products include:
Limbitrol 2333

Chlordiazepoxide Hydrochloride (Probenecid must be used with each cidofovir infusion; probenecid is known to interact with the metabolism or renal tubular excretion of benzodiazepines; concomitant use should be carefully assessed). Products include:
Librax Capsules 2330
Librium Capsules 2331
Librium Injectable 2332

Clofibrate (Probenecid must be used with each cidofovir infusion; probenecid is known to interact with the metabolism or renal tubular excretion of clofibrate; concomitant use should be carefully assessed). Products include:
Atromid-S Capsules 2808

Clonazepam (Probenecid must be used with each cidofovir infusion; probenecid is known to interact with the metabolism or renal tubular excretion of benzodiazepines; concomitant use should be carefully assessed). Products include:
Klonopin Tablets 2294

Clorazepate Dipotassium (Probenecid must be used with each cidofovir infusion; probenecid is known to interact with the metabolism or renal tubular excretion of benzodiazepines; concomitant use should be carefully assessed). Products include:
Tranxene 459

Diazepam (Probenecid must be used with each cidofovir infusion; probenecid is known to interact with the metabolism or renal tubular excretion of benzodiazepines; concomitant use should be carefully assessed). Products include:
Dizac (diazepam injectable emulsion) CIV 1862
Valium Injectable 2336
Valium Tablets 2335

Diclofenac Potassium (Probenecid must be used with each cidofovir infusion; probenecid is known to interact with the metabolism or renal tubular excretion of non-steroidal anti-inflammatory agents; concomitant use should be carefully assessed). Products include:
Cataflam Tablets 833

Diclofenac Sodium (Probenecid must be used with each cidofovir infusion; probenecid is known to interact with the metabolism or renal tubular excretion of non-steroidal anti-inflammatory agents; concomitant use should be carefully assessed). Products include:
Voltaren Ophthalmic Sterile Ophthalmic Solution .... ⊙ 264
Cataflam/Voltaren/Voltaren-XR 833

Dyphylline (Probenecid must be used with each cidofovir infusion; probenecid is known to interact with the metabolism or renal tubular excretion of theophylline; concomitant use should be carefully assessed). Products include:
Lufyllin & Lufyllin-400 Tablets 2778
Lufyllin-GG Elixir & Tablets 2779

Enalapril Maleate (Probenecid must be used with each cidofovir infusion; probenecid is known to interact with the metabolism or renal tubular excretion of ACE inhibitors; concomitant use should be carefully assessed). Products include:
Vaseretic Tablets 1810
Vasotec Tablets 1816

Enalaprilat (Probenecid must be used with each cidofovir infusion; probenecid is known to interact with the metabolism or renal tubular excretion of ACE inhibitors; concomitant use should be carefully assessed). Products include:
Vasotec I.V. 1814

Estazolam (Probenecid must be used with each cidofovir infusion; probenecid is known to interact with the metabolism or renal tubular excretion of benzodiazepines; concomitant use should be carefully assessed). Products include:
ProSom Tablets 457

Etodolac (Probenecid must be used with each cidofovir infusion; probenecid is known to interact with the metabolism or renal tubular excretion of non-steroidal anti-inflammatory agents; concomitant use should be carefully assessed). Products include:
Lodine Capsules and Tablets 2849

Famotidine (Probenecid must be used with each cidofovir infusion; probenecid is known to interact with the metabolism or renal tubular excretion of famotidine; concomitant use should be carefully assessed). Products include:
Pepcid AC Acid Controller 1360
Pepcid Injection 1765
Pepcid 1763

Fenoprofen Calcium (Probenecid must be used with each cidofovir infusion; probenecid is known to interact with the metabolism or renal tubular excretion of non-steroidal anti-inflammatory agents; concomitant use should be carefully assessed). Products include:
Nalfon 200 Pulvules & Nalfon Tablets 933

IMPORTANT NOTE: Always consult each drug listing in the patient's regimen for possible interactions.

Flurazepam Hydrochloride (Probenecid must be used with each cidofovir infusion; probenecid is known to interact with the metabolism or renal tubular excretion of benzodiazepines; concomitant use should be carefully assessed). Products include:
Dalmane Capsules 2329

Flurbiprofen (Probenecid must be used with each cidofovir infusion; probenecid is known to interact with the metabolism or renal tubular excretion of non–steroidal anti-inflammatory agents; concomitant use should be carefully assessed).
No products indexed under this heading.

Foscarnet Sodium (Renal impairment is the major toxicity of cidofovir; co-administration with potential nephrotoxic agents should be avoided). Products include:
Foscavir Injection 541

Fosinopril Sodium (Probenecid must be used with each cidofovir infusion; probenecid is known to interact with the metabolism or renal tubular excretion of ACE inhibitors; concomitant use should be carefully assessed). Products include:
Monopril Tablets 762

Furosemide (Probenecid must be used with each cidofovir infusion; probenecid is known to interact with the metabolism or renal tubular excretion of furosemide; concomitant use should be carefully assessed). Products include:
Lasix Injection, Oral Solution and Tablets 1267

Gentamicin Sulfate (Renal impairment is the major toxicity of cidofovir; co-administration with potential nephrotoxic agents should be avoided). Products include:
Garamycin Cream 0.1 % 2501
Garamycin Injectable 2502
Garamycin Ointment 0.1 % 2501
Garamycin Ophthalmic 2501
Genoptic Sterile Ophthalmic Solution .... ⊙ 241
Genoptic Sterile Ophthalmic Ointment .... ⊙ 241
Gentak .... ⊙ 209
Pred-G Liquifilm Sterile Ophthalmic Suspension .... ⊙ 248
Pred-G S.O.P. Sterile Ophthalmic Ointment .... ⊙ 249

Halazepam (Probenecid must be used with each cidofovir infusion; probenecid is known to interact with the metabolism or renal tubular excretion of benzodiazepines; concomitant use should be carefully assessed).
No products indexed under this heading.

Ibuprofen (Probenecid must be used with each cidofovir infusion; probenecid is known to interact with the metabolism or renal tubular excretion of non–steroidal anti-inflammatory agents; concomitant use should be carefully assessed). Products include:
Advil Cold and Sinus Caplets and Tablets .... ▣ 837
Advil Ibuprofen Tablets, Caplets and Gel Caplets .... ▣ 836
Children's Motrin Ibuprofen Oral Suspension 1558
IBU Tablets 1389
Ibuprohm 713
Motrin IB Caplets, Tablets, and Gelcaps .... ▣ 802
Motrin Ibuprofen Suspension, Oral Drops, Chewable Tablets, Caplets 1563
Nuprin Ibuprofen/Analgesic Tablets & Caplets .... ▣ 645
Vicks DayQuil SINUS Pressure & PAIN Relief with IBUPROFEN ...... ▣ 735

Indomethacin (Probenecid must be used with each cidofovir infusion; probenecid is known to interact with the metabolism or renal tubular excretion of non–steroidal anti-inflammatory agents; concomitant use should be carefully assessed). Products include:
Indocin 1723

Indomethacin Sodium Trihydrate (Probenecid must be used with each cidofovir infusion; probenecid is known to interact with the metabolism or renal tubular excretion of non–steroidal anti-inflammatory agents; concomitant use should be carefully assessed). Products include:
Indocin I.V. 1727

Kanamycin Sulfate (Renal impairment is the major toxicity of cidofovir; co-administration with potential nephrotoxic agents should be avoided).
No products indexed under this heading.

Ketoprofen (Probenecid must be used with each cidofovir infusion; probenecid is known to interact with the metabolism or renal tubular excretion of non–steroidal anti-inflammatory agents; concomitant use should be carefully assessed). Products include:
Actron Caplets and Tablets .... ▣ 608
Orudis Capsules 2874
Orudis KT .... ▣ 842
Oruvail Capsules 2874

Ketorolac Tromethamine (Probenecid must be used with each cidofovir infusion; probenecid is known to interact with the metabolism or renal tubular excretion of non–steroidal anti-inflammatory agents; concomitant use should be carefully assessed). Products include:
Acular Sterile Ophthalmic Solution   470
Toradol 2319

Lisinopril (Probenecid must be used with each cidofovir infusion; probenecid is known to interact with the metabolism or renal tubular excretion of ACE inhibitors; concomitant use should be carefully assessed). Products include:
Prinivil Tablets 1776
Prinzide Tablets 1780
Zestoretic Tablets 2968
Zestril Tablets 2972

Lorazepam (Probenecid must be used with each cidofovir infusion; probenecid is known to interact with the metabolism or renal tubular excretion of benzodiazepines; concomitant use should be carefully assessed). Products include:
Ativan Injection 2805
Ativan Tablets 2807

Meclofenamate Sodium (Probenecid must be used with each cidofovir infusion; probenecid is known to interact with the metabolism or renal tubular excretion of non–steroidal anti-inflammatory agents; concomitant use should be carefully assessed).
No products indexed under this heading.

Mefenamic Acid (Probenecid must be used with each cidofovir infusion; probenecid is known to interact with the metabolism or renal tubular excretion of non–steroidal anti-inflammatory agents; concomitant use should be carefully assessed). Products include:
Ponstel 1982

Mephobarbital (Probenecid must be used with each cidofovir infusion; probenecid is known to interact with the metabolism or renal tubular excretion of barbiturates; concomitant use should be carefully assessed). Products include:
Mebaral Tablets 2452

Methotrexate Sodium (Probenecid must be used with each cidofovir infusion; probenecid is known to interact with the metabolism or renal tubular excretion of methotrexate; concomitant use should be carefully assessed). Products include:
Methotrexate Sodium Tablets, Injection; for Injection and LPF Injection 1322

Midazolam Hydrochloride (Probenecid must be used with each cidofovir infusion; probenecid is known to interact with the metabolism or renal tubular excretion of benzodiazepines; concomitant use should be carefully assessed). Products include:
Versed Injection 2324

Moexipril Hydrochloride (Probenecid must be used with each cidofovir infusion; probenecid is known to interact with the metabolism or renal tubular excretion of ACE inhibitors; concomitant use should be carefully assessed). Products include:
Univasc Tablets 2553

Nabumetone (Probenecid must be used with each cidofovir infusion; probenecid is known to interact with the metabolism or renal tubular excretion of non–steroidal anti-inflammatory agents; concomitant use should be carefully assessed). Products include:
Relafen Tablets 2688

Naproxen (Probenecid must be used with each cidofovir infusion; probenecid is known to interact with the metabolism or renal tubular excretion of non–steroidal anti-inflammatory agents; concomitant use should be carefully assessed). Products include:
Anaprox/Naprosyn 2277

Naproxen Sodium (Probenecid must be used with each cidofovir infusion; probenecid is known to interact with the metabolism or renal tubular excretion of non–steroidal anti-inflammatory agents; concomitant use should be carefully assessed). Products include:
Aleve 2124
Anaprox/Naprosyn 2277
Naprelan Tablets 2861

Oxaprozin (Probenecid must be used with each cidofovir infusion; probenecid is known to interact with the metabolism or renal tubular excretion of non–steroidal anti-inflammatory agents; concomitant use should be carefully assessed). Products include:
Daypro Caplets 2578

Oxazepam (Probenecid must be used with each cidofovir infusion; probenecid is known to interact with the metabolism or renal tubular excretion of benzodiazepines; concomitant use should be carefully assessed). Products include:
Serax Capsules 2916
Serax Tablets 2916

Pentamidine Isethionate (Renal impairment is the major toxicity of cidofovir; co-administration with potential nephrotoxic agents, such as intravenous pentamidine, should be avoided).
No products indexed under this heading.

Pentobarbital Sodium (Probenecid must be used with each cidofovir infusion; probenecid is known to interact with the metabolism or renal tubular excretion of barbiturates; concomitant use should be carefully assessed). Products include:
Nembutal Sodium Capsules 440
Nembutal Sodium Solution 442
Nembutal Sodium Suppositories 444

Phenobarbital (Probenecid must be used with each cidofovir infusion; probenecid is known to interact with the metabolism or renal tubular excretion of barbiturates; concomitant use should be carefully assessed). Products include:
Arco-Lase Plus Tablets 513
Bellergal-S Tablets 2375
Donnatal 2234
Donnatal Extentabs 2234
Donnatal Tablets 2234
Phenobarbital Elixir and Tablets 1523
Quadrinal Tablets 1398

Phenylbutazone (Probenecid must be used with each cidofovir infusion; probenecid is known to interact with the metabolism or renal tubular excretion of non–steroidal anti-inflammatory agents; concomitant use should be carefully assessed).
No products indexed under this heading.

Piroxicam (Probenecid must be used with each cidofovir infusion; probenecid is known to interact with the metabolism or renal tubular excretion of non–steroidal anti-inflammatory agents; concomitant use should be carefully assessed). Products include:
Feldene Capsules 2008

Prazepam (Probenecid must be used with each cidofovir infusion; probenecid is known to interact with the metabolism or renal tubular excretion of benzodiazepines; concomitant use should be carefully assessed).
No products indexed under this heading.

Quazepam (Probenecid must be used with each cidofovir infusion; probenecid is known to interact with the metabolism or renal tubular excretion of benzodiazepines; concomitant use should be carefully assessed). Products include:
Doral Tablets 2773

Quinapril Hydrochloride (Probenecid must be used with each cidofovir infusion; probenecid is known to interact with the metabolism or renal tubular excretion of ACE inhibitors; concomitant use should be carefully assessed). Products include:
Accupril Tablets 1950

(▣ Described in PDR For Nonprescription Drugs)   (⊙ Described in PDR For Ophthalmology)

Ramipril (Probenecid must be used with each cidofovir infusion; probenecid is known to interact with the metabolism or renal tubular excretion of ACE inhibitors; concomitant use should be carefully assessed). Products include:
- Altace Capsules ... 1238

Secobarbital Sodium (Probenecid must be used with each cidofovir infusion; probenecid is known to interact with the metabolism or renal tubular excretion of barbiturates; concomitant use should be carefully assessed). Products include:
- Seconal Sodium Pulvules ... 1529

Spirapril Hydrochloride (Probenecid must be used with each cidofovir infusion; probenecid is known to interact with the metabolism or renal tubular excretion of ACE inhibitors; concomitant use should be carefully assessed).
- No products indexed under this heading.

Streptomycin Sulfate (Renal impairment is the major toxicity of cidofovir; co-administration with potential nephrotoxic agents should be avoided). Products include:
- Streptomycin Sulfate Injection ... 2031

Sulindac (Probenecid must be used with each cidofovir infusion; probenecid is known to interact with the metabolism or renal tubular excretion of non–steroidal anti-inflammatory agents; concomitant use should be carefully assessed). Products include:
- Clinoril Tablets ... 1658

Temazepam (Probenecid must be used with each cidofovir infusion; probenecid is known to interact with the metabolism or renal tubular excretion of benzodiazepines; concomitant use should be carefully assessed). Products include:
- Restoril Capsules ... 2413

Theophylline (Probenecid must be used with each cidofovir infusion; probenecid is known to interact with the metabolism or renal tubular excretion of theophylline; concomitant use should be carefully assessed). Products include:
- Marax Tablets & DF Syrup ... 2015
- Quibron ... 2227

Theophylline Anhydrous (Probenecid must be used with each cidofovir infusion; probenecid is known to interact with the metabolism or renal tubular excretion of theophylline; concomitant use should be carefully assessed). Products include:
- Aerolate ... 1003
- Primatene Tablets ... ▣ 844
- Respbid Tablets ... 687
- Slo-bid Gyrocaps ... 2201
- Theo-24 Extended Release Capsules ... 2753
- Theo-Dur Extended-Release Tablets ... 1367
- Theo-X Extended-Release Tablets .. 793
- Uni-Dur Extended-Release Tablets .. 1374
- Uniphyl 400 mg and 600 mg Tablets ... 2157

Theophylline Calcium Salicylate (Probenecid must be used with each cidofovir infusion; probenecid is known to interact with the metabolism or renal tubular excretion of theophylline; concomitant use should be carefully assessed). Products include:
- Quadrinal Tablets ... 1398

Theophylline Sodium Glycinate (Probenecid must be used with each cidofovir infusion; probenecid is known to interact with the metabolism or renal tubular excretion of theophylline; concomitant use should be carefully assessed).
- No products indexed under this heading.

Thiamylal Sodium (Probenecid must be used with each cidofovir infusion; probenecid is known to interact with the metabolism or renal tubular excretion of barbiturates; concomitant use should be carefully assessed).
- No products indexed under this heading.

Tobramycin (Renal impairment is the major toxicity of cidofovir; co-administration with potential nephrotoxic agents should be avoided). Products include:
- AKTOB ... ⊙ 207
- TobraDex Ophthalmic Suspension and Ointment ... 469
- Tobrex Ophthalmic Ointment and Solution ... ⊙ 226

Tobramycin Sulfate (Renal impairment is the major toxicity of cidofovir; co-administration with potential nephrotoxic agents should be avoided). Products include:
- Nebcin Vials, Hyporets & ADD-Vantage ... 1518

Tolmetin Sodium (Probenecid must be used with each cidofovir infusion; probenecid is known to interact with the metabolism or renal tubular excretion of non–steroidal anti-inflammatory agents; concomitant use should be carefully assessed). Products include:
- Tolectin (200, 400 and 600 mg) .. 1591

Trandolapril (Probenecid must be used with each cidofovir infusion; probenecid is known to interact with the metabolism or renal tubular excretion of ACE inhibitors; concomitant use should be carefully assessed). Products include:
- Mavik Tablets ... 1407

Triazolam (Probenecid must be used with each cidofovir infusion; probenecid is known to interact with the metabolism or renal tubular excretion of benzodiazepines; concomitant use should be carefully assessed). Products include:
- Halcion Tablets ... 2093

Zidovudine (Probenecid must be used with each cidofovir infusion; probenecid is known to interact with the metabolism or renal tubular excretion of zidovudine; concomitant use should be carefully assessed). Products include:
- Retrovir Capsules ... 1216
- Retrovir I.V. Infusion ... 1221
- Retrovir Syrup ... 1216

VITAL HIGH NITROGEN NUTRITIONALLY COMPLETE PARTIALLY HYDROLYZED DIET

(Nutritional Supplement) ... 2348
None cited in PDR database.

VITRON-C TABLETS

(Ferrous Fumarate, Vitamin C) ... ▣ 667
May interact with tetracyclines. Compounds in this category include:

Demeclocycline Hydrochloride (Oral iron products interfere with absorption of oral tetracycline antibiotics; should not be taken within 2 hours of each other). Products include:
- Declomycin Tablets ... 1421

Doxycycline Calcium (Oral iron products interfere with absorption of oral tetracycline antibiotics; should not be taken within 2 hours of each other). Products include:
- Vibramycin Calcium Oral Suspension Syrup ... 2038

Doxycycline Hyclate (Oral iron products interfere with absorption of oral tetracycline antibiotics; should not be taken within 2 hours of each other). Products include:
- Doryx Capsules ... 1970
- Vibramycin Hyclate Capsules ... 2038
- Vibramycin Hyclate Intravenous ... 2040
- Vibra-Tabs Film Coated Tablets ... 2038

Doxycycline Monohydrate (Oral iron products interfere with absorption of oral tetracycline antibiotics; should not be taken within 2 hours of each other). Products include:
- Monodox Capsules ... 1858
- Vibramycin Monohydrate for Oral Suspension ... 2038

Methacycline Hydrochloride (Oral iron products interfere with absorption of oral tetracycline antibiotics; should not be taken within 2 hours of each other).
- No products indexed under this heading.

Minocycline Hydrochloride (Oral iron products interfere with absorption of oral tetracycline antibiotics; should not be taken within 2 hours of each other). Products include:
- DYNACIN Capsules ... 1627
- Minocin Intravenous ... 1428
- Minocin Oral Suspension ... 1431
- Minocin Pellet-Filled Capsules ... 1429

Oxytetracycline Hydrochloride (Oral iron products interfere with absorption of oral tetracycline antibiotics; should not be taken within 2 hours of each other). Products include:
- TERAK Ointment ... ⊙ 210
- Terra-Cortril Ophthalmic Suspension ... 2033
- Terramycin with Polymyxin B Sulfate Ophthalmic Ointment ... 2035
- Urobiotic-250 Capsules ... 2038

Tetracycline Hydrochloride (Oral iron products interfere with absorption of oral tetracycline antibiotics; should not be taken within 2 hours of each other). Products include:
- Achromycin V Capsules ... 1417
- Helidac Therapy ... 2135

VIVA-DROPS

(Polysorbate 80) ... ⊙ 326
None cited in PDR database.

VIVACTIL TABLETS

(Protriptyline Hydrochloride) ... 1820
May interact with barbiturates, central nervous system depressants, anticholinergics, phenothiazines, quinidine, antidepressant drugs, selective serotonin reuptake inhibitors, monoamine oxidase inhibitors, sympathomimetics, thyroid preparations, and certain other agents. Compounds in these categories include:

Albuterol (Effects of concurrent use not specified; careful adjustment of dosage and close supervision are required). Products include:
- Proventil Inhalation Aerosol ... 2524
- Ventolin Inhalation Aerosol and Refill ... 1170

Albuterol Sulfate (Effects of concurrent use not specified; careful adjustment of dosage and close supervision are required). Products include:
- Airet Albuterol Sulfate Inhalation Solution ... 1602
- Albuterol Sulfate, USP Solution for Inhalation, Arm-a-Med ... 522
- Proventil Inhalation Solution 0.083% ... 2527
- Proventil Repetabs Tablets ... 2529
- Proventil Solution for Inhalation 0.5% ... 2525
- Proventil Syrup ... 2528
- Proventil Tablets ... 2529
- Ventolin Inhalation Solution ... 1171
- Ventolin Nebules Inhalation Solution ... 1172
- Ventolin Rotacaps for Inhalation ... 1173
- Ventolin Syrup ... 1175
- Ventolin Tablets ... 1176
- Volmax Extended-Release Tablets .. 1835

Alfentanil Hydrochloride (Co-administration results in enhanced response to CNS depressants). Products include:
- Alfenta Injection ... 1334

Alprazolam (Co-administration results in enhanced response to CNS depressants). Products include:
- Xanax Tablets ... 2115

Amitriptyline Hydrochloride (Co-administration with cytochrome P4502D6 inhibitors, such as antidepressants, may make normal metabolizer resemble poor metabolizer leading to higher than expected plasma concentration of TCA with resultant toxicity; lower than usual doses of either drug may be required). Products include:
- Elavil ... 2945
- Etrafon ... 2495
- Limbitrol ... 2333
- Triavil Tablets ... 1800

Amoxapine (Co-administration with cytochrome P4502D6 inhibitors, such as antidepressants, may make normal metabolizer resemble poor metabolizer leading to higher than expected plasma concentration of TCA with resultant toxicity; lower than usual doses of either drug may be required). Products include:
- Asendin Tablets ... 1419

Aprobarbital (Co-administration results in enhanced response to CNS depressants).
- No products indexed under this heading.

Atropine Sulfate (Co-administration may result in hyperpyrexia, particularly during hot weather). Products include:
- Arco-Lase Plus Tablets ... 513
- Atrohist Plus Tablets ... 1605
- Donnatal ... 2234
- Donnatal Extentabs ... 2234
- Donnatal Tablets ... 2234
- Lomotil ... 2591
- Motofen Tablets ... 789
- Urised Tablets ... 2123

Belladonna Alkaloids (Co-administration may result in hyperpyrexia, particularly during hot weather). Products include:
- Bellergal-S Tablets ... 2375
- Hyland's Bedwetting Tablets ... ▣ 788
- Hyland's EnurAid Tablets ... ▣ 789
- Hyland's Headache Tablets ... ▣ 790
- Hyland's Teething Tablets ... ▣ 790
- Similasan Eye Drops #1 ... ▣ 769

Benztropine Mesylate (Co-administration may result in hyperpyrexia, particularly during hot weather). Products include:
- Cogentin ... 1661

IMPORTANT NOTE: Always consult each drug listing in the patient's regimen for possible interactions.

Vivactil **Interactions Index** **1192**

Biperiden Hydrochloride (Co-administration may result in hyperpyrexia, particularly during hot weather). Products include:

Akineton 1380

Buprenorphine (Co-administration results in enhanced response to CNS depressants). Products include:

Buprenex Injectable 2170

Bupropion Hydrochloride (Co-administration with cytochrome P4502D6 inhibitors, such as antidepressants, may make normal metabolizer resemble poor metabolizer leading to higher than expected plasma concentration of TCA with resultant toxicity; lower than usual doses of either drug may be required). Products include:

Wellbutrin Tablets 1177

Buspirone Hydrochloride (Co-administration results in enhanced response to CNS depressants). Products include:

BuSpar Tablets 738

Butabarbital (Co-administration results in enhanced response to CNS depressants).

No products indexed under this heading.

Butalbital (Co-administration results in enhanced response to CNS depressants). Products include:

Axocet Capsules 2469
Esgic-plus Capsules 1012
Esgic-plus Tablets 1012
Fioricet Tablets 2386
Fioricet with Codeine Capsules 2387
Fiorinal Capsules 2388
Fiorinal with Codeine Capsules 2390
Fiorinal Tablets 2388
Phrenilin 790
Sedapap Tablets 50 mg/650 mg .. 1826

Chlordiazepoxide (Co-administration results in enhanced response to CNS depressants). Products include:

Limbitrol 2333

Chlordiazepoxide Hydrochloride (Co-administration results in enhanced response to CNS depressants). Products include:

Librax Capsules 2330
Librium Capsules 2331
Librium Injectable 2332

Chlorpromazine (Co-administration with cytochrome P4502D6 inhibitors, such as phenothiazines, may make normal metabolizer resemble poor metabolizer leading to higher than expected plasma concentration of TCA with resultant toxicity; lower than usual doses of either drug may be required; co-administration results in enhanced response to CNS depressants). Products include:

Thorazine Suppositories 2701

Chlorpromazine Hydrochloride (Co-administration with cytochrome P4502D6 inhibitors, such as phenothiazines, may make normal metabolizer resemble poor metabolizer leading to higher than expected plasma concentration of TCA with resultant toxicity; lower than usual doses of either drug may be required; co-administration results in enhanced response to CNS depressants). Products include:

Thorazine 2701

Chlorprothixene (Co-administration results in enhanced response to CNS depressants).

No products indexed under this heading.

Chlorprothixene Hydrochloride (Co-administration results in enhanced response to CNS depressants).

No products indexed under this heading.

Chlorprothixene Lactate (Co-administration results in enhanced response to CNS depressants).

No products indexed under this heading.

Cimetidine (Co-administration has been reported to reduce hepatic metabolism of certain tricyclic antidepressants, thereby delaying elimination and increasing steady-state concentrations of TCA resulting in the frequency and severity of side effects, particularly anticholinergic). Products include:

Tagamet HB Tablets .... ◙ 786
Tagamet Tablets 2694

Cimetidine Hydrochloride (Co-administration has been reported to reduce hepatic metabolism of certain tricyclic antidepressants, thereby delaying elimination and increasing steady-state concentrations of TCA resulting in the frequency and severity of side effects, particularly anticholinergic). Products include:

Tagamet 2694

Clidinium Bromide (Co-administration may result in hyperpyrexia, particularly during hot weather). Products include:

Librax Capsules 2330

Clorazepate Dipotassium (Co-administration results in enhanced response to CNS depressants). Products include:

Tranxene 459

Clozapine (Co-administration results in enhanced response to CNS depressants). Products include:

Clozaril Tablets 2377

Codeine Phosphate (Co-administration results in enhanced response to CNS depressants). Products include:

Brontex 2130
Dimetane-DC Cough Syrup 2232
Fioricet with Codeine Capsules 2387
Fiorinal with Codeine Capsules 2390
Nucofed 2225
Phenergan with Codeine 2883
Phenergan VC with Codeine 2888
Robitussin A-C Syrup 2248
Robitussin-DAC Syrup 2249
Ryna .... ◙ 804
Soma Compound w/Codeine Tablets 2784
Tylenol with Codeine 1592

Desflurane (Co-administration results in enhanced response to CNS depressants). Products include:

Suprane (desflurane, USP) 1865

Desipramine Hydrochloride (Co-administration with cytochrome P4502D6 inhibitors, such as antidepressants, may make normal metabolizer resemble poor metabolizer leading to higher than expected plasma concentration of TCA with resultant toxicity; lower than usual doses of either drug may be required). Products include:

Norpramin Tablets 1273

Dezocine (Co-administration results in enhanced response to CNS depressants). Products include:

Dalgan Injection 529

Diazepam (Co-administration results in enhanced response to CNS depressants). Products include:

Dizac (diazepam injectable emulsion) CIV 1862
Valium Injectable 2336
Valium Tablets 2335

Dicyclomine Hydrochloride (Co-administration may result in hyperpyrexia, particularly during hot weather). Products include:

Bentyl 1246

Dobutamine Hydrochloride (Effects of concurrent use not specified; careful adjustment of dosage and close supervision are required). Products include:

Dobutrex Solution Vials 1480

Dopamine Hydrochloride (Effects of concurrent use not specified; careful adjustment of dosage and close supervision are required).

No products indexed under this heading.

Doxepin Hydrochloride (Co-administration with cytochrome P4502D6 inhibitors, such as antidepressants, may make normal metabolizer resemble poor metabolizer leading to higher than expected plasma concentration of TCA with resultant toxicity; lower than usual doses of either drug may be required). Products include:

Adapin Capsules 1542
Sinequan 2028
Zonalon Cream 1042

Droperidol (Co-administration results in enhanced response to CNS depressants). Products include:

Inapsine Injection 462

Enflurane (Co-administration results in enhanced response to CNS depressants).

No products indexed under this heading.

Ephedrine Hydrochloride (Effects of concurrent use not specified; careful adjustment of dosage and close supervision are required). Products include:

Primatene Tablets .... ◙ 844
Quadrinal Tablets 1398

Ephedrine Sulfate (Effects of concurrent use not specified; careful adjustment of dosage and close supervision are required). Products include:

Marax Tablets & DF Syrup 2015

Ephedrine Tannate (Effects of concurrent use not specified; careful adjustment of dosage and close supervision are required). Products include:

Rynatuss 2782

Epinephrine (Effects of concurrent use not specified; careful adjustment of dosage and close supervision are required). Products include:

EPIFRIN .... ⊙ 237
EpiPen 808
Marcaine with Epinephrine 2446
Primatene Mist .... ◙ 843
Sensorcaine with Epinephrine Injection 554
Sus-Phrine Injection 1017
Xylocaine with Epinephrine Injections 562

Epinephrine Bitartrate (Effects of concurrent use not specified; careful adjustment of dosage and close supervision are required). Products include:

Sensorcaine-MPF with Epinephrine Injection 554

Epinephrine Hydrochloride (Effects of concurrent use not specified; careful adjustment of dosage and close supervision are required). Products include:

Ana-Kit Anaphylaxis Emergency Treatment Kit 611

Estazolam (Co-administration results in enhanced response to CNS depressants). Products include:

ProSom Tablets 457

Ethchlorvynol (Co-administration results in enhanced response to CNS depressants). Products include:

Placidyl Capsules 456

Ethinamate (Co-administration results in enhanced response to CNS depressants).

No products indexed under this heading.

Fentanyl (Co-administration results in enhanced response to CNS depressants). Products include:

Duragesic Transdermal System 1336

Fentanyl Citrate (Co-administration results in enhanced response to CNS depressants). Products include:

Sublimaze Injection 463

Flecainide Acetate (Co-administration with cytochrome P4502D6 inhibitors, such as flecainide, may make normal metabolizer resemble poor metabolizer leading to higher than expected plasma concentration of TCA with resultant toxicity; lower than usual doses of either drug may be required). Products include:

Tambocor Tablets 1555

Fluoxetine Hydrochloride (Co-administration with cytochrome P4502D6 inhibitors, such as antidepressants, may make normal metabolizer resemble poor metabolizer leading to higher than expected plasma concentration of TCA with resultant toxicity; due to variation in the extent of inhibition P4502D6 and long half-life of fluoxetine, sufficient time, at least 5 weeks, should elapse in switching to TCA). Products include:

Prozac Pulvules & Liquid, Oral Solution 935

Fluphenazine Decanoate (Co-administration with cytochrome P4502D6 inhibitors, such as phenothiazines, may make normal metabolizer resemble poor metabolizer leading to higher than expected plasma concentration of TCA with resultant toxicity; lower than usual doses of either drug may be required; co-administration results in enhanced response to CNS depressants). Products include:

Prolixin Decanoate 510

Fluphenazine Enanthate (Co-administration with cytochrome P4502D6 inhibitors, such as phenothiazines, may make normal metabolizer resemble poor metabolizer leading to higher than expected plasma concentration of TCA with resultant toxicity; lower than usual doses of either drug may be required; co-administration results in enhanced response to CNS depressants). Products include:

Prolixin Enanthate 510

Fluphenazine Hydrochloride (Co-administration with cytochrome P4502D6 inhibitors, such as phenothiazines, may make normal metabolizer resemble poor metabolizer leading to higher than expected plasma concentration of TCA with resultant toxicity; lower than usual doses of either drug may be required; co-administration results in enhanced response to CNS depressants). Products include:

Prolixin 510

Flurazepam Hydrochloride (Co-administration results in enhanced response to CNS depressants). Products include:

Dalmane Capsules 2329

(◙ Described in PDR For Nonprescription Drugs) (⊙ Described in PDR For Ophthalmology)

Fluvoxamine Maleate (Co-administration with cytochrome P4502D6 inhibitors, such as antidepressants, may make normal metabolizer resemble poor metabolizer leading to higher than expected plasma concentration of TCA with resultant toxicity; due to variation in the extent of inhibition P4502D6, sufficient time should elapse in switching from one class to the other). Products include:
LUVOX Tablets ... 2723
Furazolidone (Co-administration of tricyclic antidepressants and MAO inhibitors has resulted in hyperpyretic crises, severe convulsion, and deaths; concurrent and/or sequential use is contraindicated). Products include:
Furoxone ... 2221
Glutethimide (Co-administration results in enhanced response to CNS depressants).
No products indexed under this heading.
Glycopyrrolate (Co-administration may result in hyperpyrexia, particularly during hot weather). Products include:
Robinul Forte Tablets ... 2247
Robinul Injectable ... 2247
Robinul Tablets ... 2247
Guanadrel Sulfate (Protriptyline may block the antihypertensive action). Products include:
Hylorel Tablets ... 1613
Guanethidine Monosulfate (Protriptyline may block the antihypertensive action of guanethidine). Products include:
Esimil Tablets ... 840
Ismelin Tablets ... 845
Haloperidol (Co-administration results in enhanced response to CNS depressants). Products include:
Haldol Injection, Tablets and Concentrate ... 1585
Haloperidol Decanoate (Co-administration results in enhanced response to CNS depressants). Products include:
Haldol Decanoate ... 1587
Hydrocodone Bitartrate (Co-administration results in enhanced response to CNS depressants). Products include:
Codiclear DH Syrup ... 808
Duratuss HD Elixir ... 2750
Histussin D Liquid ... 670
Hycodan Tablets and Syrup ... 946
Hycomine Compound Tablets ... 948
Hycomine ... 947
Hycotuss Expectorant Syrup ... 950
Hydrocet Capsules ... 787
Lorcet 10/650 Tablets ... 1016
Lortab ... 2751
Tussend ... 1830
Tussend Expectorant ... 1831
Vicodin Tablets ... 1404
Vicodin ES Tablets ... 1405
Vicodin HP Tablets ... 1403
Vicodin Tuss Expectorant ... 1406
Zydone Capsules ... 967
Hydrocodone Polistirex (Co-administration results in enhanced response to CNS depressants). Products include:
Tussionex Pennkinetic Extended-Release Suspension ... 1624
Hydromorphone Hydrochloride (Co-administration results in enhanced response to CNS depressants). Products include:
Dilaudid Ampules ... 1382
Dilaudid Cough Syrup ... 1383
Dilaudid-HP Injection ... 1384
Dilaudid-HP Lyophilized Powder 250 mg ... 1384
Dilaudid ... 1382
Dilaudid Oral Liquid ... 1386
Dilaudid ... 1382
Dilaudid Tablets - 8 mg ... 1386
Hydroxyzine Hydrochloride (Co-administration results in enhanced response to CNS depressants). Products include:
Atarax Tablets & Syrup ... 1992
Marax Tablets & DF Syrup ... 2015
Vistaril Intramuscular Solution ... 2042
Hyoscyamine (Co-administration may result in hyperpyrexia, particularly during hot weather). Products include:
Cystospaz Tablets ... 2123
Urised Tablets ... 2123
Hyoscyamine Sulfate (Co-administration may result in hyperpyrexia, particularly during hot weather). Products include:
Arco-Lase Plus Tablets ... 513
Atrohist Plus Tablets ... 1605
Cystospaz-M Capsules ... 2123
Donnatal ... 2234
Donnatal Extentabs ... 2234
Donnatal Tablets ... 2234
Kutrase Capsules ... 2546
Levsin/Levsinex/Levbid ... 2549
Imipramine Hydrochloride (Co-administration with cytochrome P4502D6 inhibitors, such as antidepressants, may make normal metabolizer resemble poor metabolizer leading to higher than expected plasma concentration of TCA with resultant toxicity; lower than usual doses of either drug may be required). Products include:
Tofranil Ampuls ... 873
Tofranil Tablets ... 875
Imipramine Pamoate (Co-administration with cytochrome P4502D6 inhibitors, such as antidepressants, may make normal metabolizer resemble poor metabolizer leading to higher than expected plasma concentration of TCA with resultant toxicity; lower than usual doses of either drug may be required). Products include:
Tofranil-PM Capsules ... 876
Ipratropium Bromide (Co-administration may result in hyperpyrexia, particularly during hot weather). Products include:
Atrovent Inhalation Aerosol ... 674
Atrovent Inhalation Solution ... 675
Atrovent Nasal Spray 0.03% ... 676
Atrovent Nasal Spray 0.06% ... 678
Isocarboxazid (Co-administration of tricyclic antidepressants and MAO inhibitors has resulted in hyperpyretic crises, severe convulsion, and deaths; concurrent and/or sequential use is contraindicated).
No products indexed under this heading.
Isoflurane (Co-administration results in enhanced response to CNS depressants).
No products indexed under this heading.
Isoproterenol Hydrochloride (Effects of concurrent use not specified; careful adjustment of dosage and close supervision are required). Products include:
Isuprel Hydrochloride Solution ... 2443
Isuprel Injection ... 2441
Isuprel Mistometer ... 2442
Isoproterenol Sulfate (Effects of concurrent use not specified; careful adjustment of dosage and close supervision are required). Products include:
Norisodrine with Calcium Iodide Syrup ... 446
Ketamine Hydrochloride (Co-administration results in enhanced response to CNS depressants).
No products indexed under this heading.
Levomethadyl Acetate Hydrochloride (Co-administration results in enhanced response to CNS depressants). Products include:
Orlaam Oral Solution ... 2361
Levorphanol Tartrate (Co-administration results in enhanced response to CNS depressants). Products include:
Levo-Dromoran ... 2297
Levothyroxine Sodium (On rare occasions, concurrent use may result in arrhythmias). Products include:
Eltroxin Tablets ... 2214
Levothroid Tablets ... 1015
Levothyroxine Sodium, USP for Injection ... 546
Levoxyl Tablets ... 918
Synthroid ... 1410
Liothyronine Sodium (On rare occasions, concurrent use may result in arrhythmias). Products include:
Cytomel Tablets ... 2647
Triostat Injection ... 2708
Liotrix (On rare occasions, concurrent use may result in arrhythmias).
No products indexed under this heading.
Lorazepam (Co-administration results in enhanced response to CNS depressants). Products include:
Ativan Injection ... 2805
Ativan Tablets ... 2807
Loxapine Hydrochloride (Co-administration results in enhanced response to CNS depressants). Products include:
Loxitane ... 1426
Loxapine Succinate (Co-administration results in enhanced response to CNS depressants). Products include:
Loxitane Capsules ... 1426
Maprotiline Hydrochloride (Co-administration with cytochrome P4502D6 inhibitors, such as antidepressants, may make normal metabolizer resemble poor metabolizer leading to higher than expected plasma concentration of TCA with resultant toxicity; lower than usual doses of either drug may be required). Products include:
Ludiomil Tablets ... 861
Mepenzolate Bromide (Co-administration may result in hyperpyrexia, particularly during hot weather).
No products indexed under this heading.
Meperidine Hydrochloride (Co-administration results in enhanced response to CNS depressants). Products include:
Demerol ... 2438
Mepergan Injection ... 2859
Mephobarbital (Co-administration results in enhanced response to CNS depressants). Products include:
Mebaral Tablets ... 2452
Meprobamate (Co-administration results in enhanced response to CNS depressants). Products include:
Miltown Tablets ... 2780
PMB 200 and PMB 400 ... 2890
Mesoridazine Besylate (Co-administration with cytochrome P4502D6 inhibitors, such as phenothiazines, may make normal metabolizer resemble poor metabolizer leading to higher than expected plasma concentration of TCA with resultant toxicity; lower than usual doses of either drug may be required; co-administration results in enhanced response to CNS depressants). Products include:
Serentil ... 689
Metaproterenol Sulfate (Effects of concurrent use not specified; careful adjustment of dosage and close supervision are required). Products include:
Alupent ... 672
Metaproterenol Sulfate Inhalation Solution, USP, Arm-a-Med ... 547
Metaraminol Bitartrate (Effects of concurrent use not specified; careful adjustment of dosage and close supervision are required). Products include:
Aramine Injection ... 1649
Methadone Hydrochloride (Co-administration results in enhanced response to CNS depressants). Products include:
Methadone Hydrochloride Oral Concentrate ... 2356
Methadone Hydrochloride Oral Solution & Tablets ... 2357
Methohexital Sodium (Co-administration results in enhanced response to CNS depressants).
No products indexed under this heading.
Methotrimeprazine (Co-administration with cytochrome P4502D6 inhibitors, such as phenothiazines, may make normal metabolizer resemble poor metabolizer leading to higher than expected plasma concentration of TCA with resultant toxicity; lower than usual doses of either drug may be required; co-administration results in enhanced response to CNS depressants). Products include:
Levoprome ... 1321
Methoxamine Hydrochloride (Effects of concurrent use not specified; careful adjustment of dosage and close supervision are required). Products include:
Vasoxyl Injection ... 1169
Methoxyflurane (Co-administration results in enhanced response to CNS depressants).
No products indexed under this heading.
Midazolam Hydrochloride (Co-administration results in enhanced response to CNS depressants). Products include:
Versed Injection ... 2324
Mirtazapine (Co-administration with cytochrome P4502D6 inhibitors, such as antidepressants, may make normal metabolizer resemble poor metabolizer leading to higher than expected plasma concentration of TCA with resultant toxicity; lower than usual doses of either drug may be required). Products include:
Remeron Tablets ... 1878
Molindone Hydrochloride (Co-administration results in enhanced response to CNS depressants). Products include:
Moban Tablets and Concentrate ... 1036

IMPORTANT NOTE: Always consult each drug listing in the patient's regimen for possible interactions.

Morphine Sulfate (Co-administration results in enhanced response to CNS depressants). Products include:
- Astramorph/PF Injection, USP (Preservative-Free) ... 526
- Duramorph Injection ... 983
- Infumorph 200 and Infumorph 500 Sterile Solutions ... 985
- Kadian Capsules ... 2948
- MS Contin Tablets ... 2149
- MSIR ... 2152
- Oramorph SR (Morphine Sulfate Sustained Release Tablets) ... 2359
- RMS Suppositories CII ... 2766
- Roxanol ... 2365

Nefazodone Hydrochloride (Co-administration with cytochrome P4502D6 inhibitors, such as antidepressants, may make normal metabolizer resemble poor metabolizer leading to higher than expected plasma concentration of TCA with resultant toxicity; lower than usual doses of either drug may be required). Products include:
- Serzone Tablets ... 776

Norepinephrine Bitartrate (Effects of concurrent use not specified; careful adjustment of dosage and close supervision are required). Products include:
- Levophed Bitartrate Injection ... 2445

Nortriptyline Hydrochloride (Co-administration with cytochrome P4502D6 inhibitors, such as antidepressants, may make normal metabolizer resemble poor metabolizer leading to higher than expected plasma concentration of TCA with resultant toxicity; lower than usual doses of either drug may be required). Products include:
- Pamelor ... 2409

Opium Alkaloids (Co-administration results in enhanced response to CNS depressants).
- No products indexed under this heading.

Oxazepam (Co-administration results in enhanced response to CNS depressants). Products include:
- Serax Capsules ... 2916
- Serax Tablets ... 2916

Oxybutynin Chloride (Co-administration may result in hyperpyrexia, particularly during hot weather). Products include:
- Ditropan ... 1267

Oxycodone Hydrochloride (Co-administration results in enhanced response to CNS depressants). Products include:
- OxyContin Tablets ... 2163
- OxyIR Capsules ... 2167
- Percocet Tablets ... 955
- Percodan Tablets ... 955
- Percodan-Demi Tablets ... 956
- Roxicodone Tablets, Oral Solution & Intensol (Oxycodone) ... 2366
- Tylox Capsules ... 1593

Paroxetine Hydrochloride (Co-administration with cytochrome P4502D6 inhibitors, such as antidepressants, may make normal metabolizer resemble poor metabolizer leading to higher than expected plasma concentration of TCA with resultant toxicity; due to variation in the extent of inhibition P4502D6, sufficient time should elapse in switching from one class to the other). Products include:
- Paxil Tablets ... 2681

Pentobarbital Sodium (Co-administration results in enhanced response to CNS depressants). Products include:
- Nembutal Sodium Capsules ... 440
- Nembutal Sodium Solution ... 442
- Nembutal Sodium Suppositories ... 444

Perphenazine (Co-administration with cytochrome P4502D6 inhibitors, such as phenothiazines, may make normal metabolizer resemble poor metabolizer leading to higher than expected plasma concentration of TCA with resultant toxicity; lower than usual doses of either drug may be required; co-administration results in enhanced response to CNS depressants). Products include:
- Etrafon ... 2495
- Triavil Tablets ... 1800
- Trilafon ... 2532

Phenelzine Sulfate (Co-administration of tricyclic antidepressants and MAO inhibitors has resulted in hyperpyretic crises, severe convulsion, and deaths; concurrent and/or sequential use is contraindicated). Products include:
- Nardil ... 1977

Phenobarbital (Co-administration results in enhanced response to CNS depressants). Products include:
- Arco-Lase Plus Tablets ... 513
- Bellergal-S Tablets ... 2375
- Donnatal ... 2234
- Donnatal Extentabs ... 2234
- Donnatal Tablets ... 2234
- Phenobarbital Elixir and Tablets ... 1523
- Quadrinal Tablets ... 1398

Phenylephrine Bitartrate (Effects of concurrent use not specified; careful adjustment of dosage and close supervision are required).
- No products indexed under this heading.

Phenylephrine Hydrochloride (Effects of concurrent use not specified; careful adjustment of dosage and close supervision are required). Products include:
- Atrohist Plus Tablets ... 1605
- Cerose DM ... ▣ 853
- D.A. II Tablets ... 972
- D.A. Chewable Tablets ... 970
- Dura-Vent/DA Tablets ... 972
- Extendryl ... 1003
- 4-Way Fast Acting Nasal Spray (regular & mentholated) ... ▣ 644
- Hemorid ... ▣ 797
- Hycomine Compound Tablets ... 948
- Neo-Synephrine Hydrochloride 1% Carpuject ... 2455
- Neo-Synephrine Hydrochloride 1% Injection ... 2455
- Neo-Synephrine Hydrochloride (Ophthalmic) ... 2456
- Neo-Synephrine ... ▣ 624
- Novahistine Elixir ... ▣ 782
- Phenergan VC ... 2886
- Phenergan VC with Codeine ... 2888
- Preparation H ... ▣ 842
- Tympagesic Ear Drops ... 2476
- Vicks Sinex Nasal Spray and Ultra Fine Mist ... ▣ 738

Phenylephrine Tannate (Effects of concurrent use not specified; careful adjustment of dosage and close supervision are required). Products include:
- Atrohist Pediatric Suspension ... 1604
- Atrohist Pediatric Suspension Dye-Free ... 1604
- Rynatan ... 2781
- Rynatuss ... 2782

Phenylpropanolamine Hydrochloride (Effects of concurrent use not specified; careful adjustment of dosage and close supervision are required). Products include:
- Acutrim ... ▣ 648
- Atrohist Plus Tablets ... 1605
- BC Cold Powder Multi-Symptom Formula (Cold-Sinus-Allergy) ... ▣ 631
- BC Cold Powder Non-Drowsy Formula (Cold-Sinus) ... ▣ 631
- Cheracol Plus Head Cold/Cough Formula ... ▣ 741
- Comtrex Multi-Symptom Cold Reliever Liqui-Gels ... ▣ 638
- Comtrex Multi-Symptom Non-Drowsy Liqui-gels ... ▣ 640
- Contac Continuous Action Nasal Decongestant/Antihistamine 12 Hour Capsules ... ▣ 773
- Contac Maximum Strength Continuous Action Decongestant/Antihistamine 12 Hour Caplets ... ▣ 772
- Contac Severe Cold and Flu Formula Caplets ... ▣ 773
- Coricidin 'D' Decongestant Tablets ... ▣ 760
- Dexatrim ... ▣ 795
- Dexatrim Plus Vitamins Caplets ... ▣ 796
- Dimetane-DC Cough Syrup ... 2232
- Dimetapp Allergy Sinus Caplets ... ▣ 838
- Dimetapp Cold & Allergy Chewable Tablets ... ▣ 838
- Dimetapp Cold & Cough Liqui-Gels ... ▣ 839
- Dimetapp DM Elixir ... ▣ 840
- Dimetapp Elixir ... ▣ 840
- Dimetapp Extentabs ... ▣ 841
- Dimetapp Tablets/Liqui-Gels ... ▣ 841
- Dura-Vent Tablets ... 971
- Entex LA Tablets ... 972
- Exgest LA Tablets ... 787
- Hycomine ... 947
- Nolamine Timed-Release Tablets ... 790
- Ornade Spansule Capsules ... 2678
- Propagest Tablets ... 791
- Pyrroxate Caplets ... ▣ 742
- Robitussin-CF ... ▣ 846
- Sinulin Tablets ... 792
- Tavist-D 12 Hour Relief Tablets ... ▣ 750
- Teldrin 12 Hour Antihistamine/Nasal Decongestant Allergy Relief Capsules ... ▣ 786
- Triaminic Expectorant ... ▣ 753
- Triaminic Syrup ... ▣ 755
- Triaminic Triaminicol Cold & Cough ... ▣ 756
- Triaminic DM Syrup ... ▣ 756
- Triaminicin Tablets ... ▣ 756
- Vicks DayQuil Allergy Relief 12-Hour Extended Release Tablets ... ▣ 733
- Vicks DayQuil Allergy Relief 4-Hour Tablets ... ▣ 733
- Vicks DayQuil SINUS Pressure & CONGESTION Relief ... ▣ 734

Pirbuterol Acetate (Effects of concurrent use not specified; careful adjustment of dosage and close supervision are required). Products include:
- Maxair Autohaler ... 1550
- Maxair Inhaler ... 1552

Prazepam (Co-administration results in enhanced response to CNS depressants).
- No products indexed under this heading.

Prochlorperazine (Co-administration with cytochrome P4502D6 inhibitors, such as phenothiazines, may make normal metabolizer resemble poor metabolizer leading to higher than expected plasma concentration of TCA with resultant toxicity; lower than usual doses of either drug may be required; co-administration results in enhanced response to CNS depressants). Products include:
- Compazine ... 2644

Procyclidine Hydrochloride (Co-administration may result in hyperpyrexia, particularly during hot weather). Products include:
- Kemadrin Tablets ... 1105

Promethazine Hydrochloride (Co-administration with cytochrome P4502D6 inhibitors, such as phenothiazines, may make normal metabolizer resemble poor metabolizer leading to higher than expected plasma concentration of TCA with resultant toxicity; lower than usual doses of either drug may be required; co-administration results in enhanced response to CNS depressants). Products include:
- Mepergan Injection ... 2859
- Phenergan with Codeine ... 2883
- Phenergan with Dextromethorphan ... 2885
- Phenergan Injection ... 2880
- Phenergan Suppositories ... 2882
- Phenergan Syrup ... 2881
- Phenergan Tablets ... 2882
- Phenergan VC ... 2886
- Phenergan VC with Codeine ... 2888

Propafenone Hydrochloride (Co-administration with cytochrome P4502D6 inhibitors, such as propafenone, may make normal metabolizer resemble poor metabolizer leading to higher than expected plasma concentration of TCA with resultant toxicity; lower than usual doses of either drug may be required). Products include:
- Rythmol Tablets–150mg, 225mg, 300mg ... 1399

Propantheline Bromide (Co-administration may result in hyperpyrexia, particularly during hot weather). Products include:
- Pro-Banthine Tablets ... 2226

Propofol (Co-administration results in enhanced response to CNS depressants). Products include:
- Diprivan Injectable Emulsion ... 2939

Propoxyphene Hydrochloride (Co-administration results in enhanced response to CNS depressants). Products include:
- Darvon ... 1475
- Wygesic Tablets ... 2930

Propoxyphene Napsylate (Co-administration results in enhanced response to CNS depressants). Products include:
- Darvon-N/Darvocet-N ... 1473

Pseudoephedrine Hydrochloride (Effects of concurrent use not specified; careful adjustment of dosage and close supervision are required). Products include:
- Actifed Allergy Daytime/Nighttime Caplets ... ▣ 808
- Actifed Cold & Allergy Tablets ... ▣ 807
- Actifed Cold & Sinus Caplets and Tablets ... ▣ 808
- Actifed Sinus Daytime/Nighttime Tablets and Caplets ... ▣ 809
- Advil Cold and Sinus Caplets and Tablets ... ▣ 837
- Alka-Seltzer Plus Liqui-Gels ... ▣ 612
- Alka-Seltzer Plus Flu & Body Aches Liqui-Gels Non-Drowsy Formula ... ▣ 613
- Alka-Seltzer Plus Night-Time Cold Medicine Liqui-Gels ... ▣ 612
- Allerest Maximum Strength ... ▣ 649
- Allerest No Drowsiness ... ▣ 649
- Allerest Sinus Pain Formula ... ▣ 649
- Atrohist Pediatric Capsules ... 1603
- Benadryl Allergy/Cold Tablets ... ▣ 811
- Benadryl Allergy Decongestant Liquid Medication ... ▣ 812
- Benadryl Allergy Decongestant Tablets ... ▣ 812
- Benadryl Allergy Sinus Headache Caplets ... ▣ 813
- Benylin Multisymptom ... ▣ 816
- Bromfed Capsules (Extended-Release) ... 1832
- Bromfed Syrup ... ▣ 712
- Bromfed Tablets ... 1832
- Bromfed-DM Cough Syrup ... 1832
- Bromfed-PD Capsules (Extended-Release) ... 1832
- Children's TYLENOL Cold Multi-Symptom Chewable Tablets and Liquid ... 1559
- Children's TYLENOL Cold Plus Cough Multi Symptom Chewable Tablets and Liquid ... 1560
- Children's TYLENOL Flu Suspension Liquid ... 1560
- Children's Vicks DayQuil Allergy Relief ... ▣ 730
- Children's Vicks NyQuil Cold/Cough Relief ... ▣ 731
- Allergy-Sinus Comtrex Multi-Symptom Allergy-Sinus Formula Tablets and Caplets ... ▣ 639
- Comtrex Multi-Symptom ... ▣ 638
- Comtrex Multi-Symptom Non-Drowsy Caplets ... ▣ 640
- Congess ... 1003
- Contac Day Allergy/Sinus Caplets ... ▣ 771
- Contac Day & Night ... ▣ 772

(▣ Described in PDR For Nonprescription Drugs) (⊙ Described in PDR For Ophthalmology)

Contac Night Allergy/Sinus Caplets ... 771
Contac Severe Cold & Flu Non-Drowsy ... 774
Deconsal II Tablets ... 1605
Dimetane-DX Cough Syrup ... 2233
Dimetapp Cold & Fever Suspension ... 839
Dimetapp Decongestant Pediatric Drops ... 840
Dorcol Children's Cough Syrup ... 748
Drixoral Cough + Congestion Liquid Caps ... 763
Dura-Tap/PD Capsules ... 970
Duratuss Tablets ... 2750
Duratuss HD Elixir ... 2750
Efidac/24 ... 655
Entex PSE Tablets ... 973
Fedahist Gyrocaps ... 2545
Guaifed ... 1833
Guaifed Syrup ... 712
Guaimax-D Tablets ... 809
Histussin D Liquid ... 670
Infants' TYLENOL Cold Decongestant & Fever-Reducer Drops ... 1561
Kronofed-A ... 994
Novahistine DMX ... 782
Nucofed ... 2225
PediaCare Cough-Cold Chewable Tablets and Liquid ... 1569
PediaCare Infants' Decongestant Drops ... 1569
PediaCare Infants' Drops Decongestant Plus Cough ... 1569
PediaCare NightRest Cough-Cold Liquid ... 1569
Pediatric Vicks 44d Cough & Head Congestion Relief ... 736
Pediatric Vicks 44m Cough & Cold Relief ... 737
Robitussin Cold & Cough Liqui-Gels ... 844
Robitussin Cold, Cough & Flu Liqui-Gels ... 844
Robitussin Maximum Strength Cough & Cold ... 847
Robitussin Night-Time Cold Formula ... 847
Robitussin Pediatric Cough & Cold Formula ... 848
Robitussin Pediatric Drops ... 849
Robitussin Severe Congestion Liqui-Gels ... 845
Robitussin-DAC Syrup ... 2249
Robitussin-PE ... 846
Rondec Oral Drops ... 974
Rondec Syrup ... 974
Rondec Tablet ... 974
Rondec Chewable Tablets ... 974
Rondec-TR Tablet ... 974
Ryna ... 804
Seldane-D Extended-Release Tablets ... 1286
Semprex-D Capsules ... 1620
Sinarest ... 663
Sine-Aid Maximum Strength Sinus Headache Gelcaps, Caplets and Tablets ... 1570
Sine-Off No Drowsiness Formula Caplets ... 784
Sine-Off Sinus Medicine ... 784
Singlet Tablets ... 785
Sinutab Non-Drying Liquid Caps ... 823
Sinutab Sinus Allergy Medication, Maximum Strength Tablets and Caplets ... 823
Sinutab Sinus Medication, Maximum Strength Without Drowsiness Formula, Tablets & Caplets ... 824
Sudafed Children's Cold & Cough Liquid Medication ... 825
Sudafed Children's Nasal Decongestant Liquid Medication ... 826
Sudafed Cold & Allergy Tablets ... 826
Sudafed Cold and Cough Liquid Caps ... 826
Sudafed Nasal Decongestant Tablets, 30 mg ... 825
Sudafed Nasal Decongestant Tablets, 60 mg ... 825
Sudafed Non-Drying Sinus Liquid Caps ... 827
Sudafed Pediatric Nasal Decongestant Liquid Oral Drops ... 827
Sudafed Severe Cold Formula Caplets ... 828
Sudafed Severe Cold Formula Tablets ... 828
Sudafed Sinus Caplets ... 829
Sudafed Sinus Tablets ... 829
Sudafed 12 Hour Caplets ... 824
Syn-Rx Tablets ... 1622
Syn-Rx DM Tablets ... 1623
TheraFlu Flu and Cold Medicine ... 750
Theraflu Maximum Strength Flu and Cold Medicine For Sore Throat ... 751
TheraFlu Flu, Cold and Cough Medicine ... 750
TheraFlu Maximum Strength Nighttime Flu, Cold & Cough Medicine ... 751
TheraFlu Maximum Strength Non-Drowsy Formula Flu, Cold & Cough Medicine ... 751
TheraFlu Maximum Strength, Non-Drowsy Formula Flu, Cold and Cough Caplets ... 752
Theraflu Maximum Strength Sinus Non-Drowsy Formula Caplets ... 752
Triaminic AM Cough and Decongestant Formula ... 753
Triaminic AM Decongestant Formula ... 753
Triaminic Infant Oral Decongestant Drops ... 754
Triaminic Night Time ... 754
Triaminic Sore Throat Formula ... 755
Tussend ... 1830
Tussend Expectorant ... 1831
TYLENOL Allergy Sinus, Maximum Strength Caplets and Gelcaps ... 1571
TYLENOL Allergy Sinus NightTime, Maximum Strength Caplets ... 1571
TYLENOL Cold Medication, Multi-Symptom Formula Tablets and Caplets ... 1572
TYLENOL Cold Medication, Multi-Symptom Hot Liquid Packets ... 1572
TYLENOL Cold Medication, No Drowsiness Formula Caplets and Gelcaps ... 1572
TYLENOL Cold Severe Congestion Caplets ... 1573
TYLENOL Cough Medication with Decongestant, Multi Symptom ... 1574
TYLENOL Flu No Drowsiness Formula, Maximum Strength Gelcaps ... 1575
TYLENOL Flu NightTime, Maximum Strength Gelcaps ... 1575
TYLENOL Flu NightTime, Maximum Strength Hot Medication Packets ... 1575
TYLENOL Sinus, Maximum Strength Geltabs, Gelcaps, Caplets and Tablets ... 1576
Vicks 44 LiquiCaps Cough, Cold & Flu Relief ... 728
Vicks 44 LiquiCaps Non-Drowsy Cough & Cold Relief ... 729
Vicks 44D Cough & Head Congestion Relief ... 728
Vicks 44M Cough, Cold & Flu Relief ... 729
Vicks DayQuil LiquiCaps/Liquid Multi-Symptom Cold/Flu Relief ... 734
Vicks DayQuil SINUS Pressure & PAIN Relief with IBUPROFEN ... 735
Vicks Nyquil Hot Therapy ... 735
Vicks NyQuil LiquiCaps/Liquid Multi-Symptom Cold/Flu Relief, Original and Cherry Flavors ... 736

Pseudoephedrine Sulfate (Effects of concurrent use not specified; careful adjustment of dosage and close supervision are required). Products include:
Chlor-Trimeton Allergy Decongestant Tablets ... 759
Claritin-D Tablets ... 2487
Drixoral Cold and Allergy Sustained-Action Tablets ... 763
Drixoral Cold and Flu Extended-Release Tablets ... 764
Drixoral Non-Drowsy Formula Extended-Release Tablets ... 764
Drixoral Allergy/Sinus Extended Release Tablets ... 765
Trinalin Repetabs Tablets ... 1373

Quazepam (Co-administration results in enhanced response to CNS depressants). Products include:
Doral Tablets ... 2773

Quinidine Gluconate (Co-administration with cytochrome P4502D6 inhibitors, such as quinidine, may make normal metabolizer resemble poor metabolizer leading to higher than expected plasma concentration of TCA with resultant toxicity; lower than usual doses of either drug may be required). Products include:
Quinaglute Dura-Tabs Tablets ... 644

Quinidine Polygalacturonate (Co-administration with cytochrome P4502D6 inhibitors, such as quinidine, may make normal metabolizer resemble poor metabolizer leading to higher than expected plasma concentration of TCA with resultant toxicity; lower than usual doses of either drug may be required). Products include:
Cardioquin Tablets ... 2146

Quinidine Sulfate (Co-administration with cytochrome P4502D6 inhibitors, such as quinidine, may make normal metabolizer resemble poor metabolizer leading to higher than expected plasma concentration of TCA with resultant toxicity; lower than usual doses of either drug may be required). Products include:
Quinidex Extentabs ... 2240

Risperidone (Co-administration results in enhanced response to CNS depressants). Products include:
Risperdal Tablets ... 1348

Salmeterol Xinafoate (Effects of concurrent use not specified; careful adjustment of dosage and close supervision are required). Products include:
Serevent Inhalation Aerosol ... 1149

Scopolamine (Co-administration may result in hyperpyrexia, particularly during hot weather). Products include:
Transderm Scōp Transdermal Therapeutic System ... 890

Scopolamine Hydrobromide (Co-administration may result in hyperpyrexia, particularly during hot weather). Products include:
Atrohist Plus Tablets ... 1605
Donnatal ... 2234
Donnatal Extentabs ... 2234
Donnatal Tablets ... 2234

Secobarbital Sodium (Co-administration results in enhanced response to CNS depressants). Products include:
Seconal Sodium Pulvules ... 1529

Selegiline Hydrochloride (Co-administration of tricyclic antidepressants and MAO inhibitors has resulted in hyperpyretic crises, severe convulsion, and deaths; concurrent and/or sequential use is contraindicated). Products include:
Eldepryl Capsules ... 2729

Sertraline Hydrochloride (Co-administration with cytochrome P4502D6 inhibitors, such as antidepressants, may make normal metabolizer resemble poor metabolizer leading to higher than expected plasma concentration of TCA with resultant toxicity; due to variation in the extent of inhibition P4502D6, sufficient time should elapse in switching from one class to the other). Products include:
Zoloft Tablets ... 2051

Sevoflurane (Co-administration results in enhanced response to CNS depressants).
No products indexed under this heading.

Sufentanil Citrate (Co-administration results in enhanced response to CNS depressants). Products include:
Sufenta Injection ... 1355

Temazepam (Co-administration results in enhanced response to CNS depressants). Products include:
Restoril Capsules ... 2413

Terbutaline Sulfate (Effects of concurrent use not specified; careful adjustment of dosage and close supervision are required). Products include:
Brethaire Inhaler ... 830
Brethine Ampuls ... 832
Brethine Tablets ... 831
Bricanyl Subcutaneous Injection ... 1247
Bricanyl Tablets ... 1248

Thiamylal Sodium (Co-administration results in enhanced response to CNS depressants).
No products indexed under this heading.

Thioridazine Hydrochloride (Co-administration with cytochrome P4502D6 inhibitors, such as phenothiazines, may make normal metabolizer resemble poor metabolizer leading to higher than expected plasma concentration of TCA with resultant toxicity; lower than usual doses of either drug may be required; co-administration results in enhanced response to CNS depressants). Products include:
Mellaril ... 2398

Thiothixene (Co-administration results in enhanced response to CNS depressants). Products include:
Navane Capsules and Concentrate 2018
Navane Intramuscular ... 2019

Thyroglobulin (On rare occasions, concurrent use may result in arrhythmias).
No products indexed under this heading.

Thyroid (On rare occasions, concurrent use may result in arrhythmias).
No products indexed under this heading.

Thyroxine (On rare occasions, concurrent use may result in arrhythmias).
No products indexed under this heading.

Thyroxine Sodium (On rare occasions, concurrent use may result in arrhythmias).
No products indexed under this heading.

Tranylcypromine Sulfate (Co-administration of tricyclic antidepressants and MAO inhibitors has resulted in hyperpyretic crises, severe convulsion, and deaths; concurrent and/or sequential use is contraindicated). Products include:
Parnate Tablets ... 2679

Trazodone Hydrochloride (Co-administration with cytochrome P4502D6 inhibitors, such as antidepressants, may make normal metabolizer resemble poor metabolizer leading to higher than expected plasma concentration of TCA with resultant toxicity; lower than usual doses of either drug may be required). Products include:
Desyrel and Desyrel Dividose ... 504

Triazolam (Co-administration results in enhanced response to CNS depressants). Products include:
Halcion Tablets ... 2093

IMPORTANT NOTE: Always consult each drug listing in the patient's regimen for possible interactions.

Vivactil — Interactions Index

Tridihexethyl Chloride (Co-administration may result in hyperpyrexia, particularly during hot weather).
    No products indexed under this heading.

Trifluoperazine Hydrochloride (Co-administration with cytochrome P4502D6 inhibitors, such as phenothiazines, may make normal metabolizer resemble poor metabolizer leading to higher than expected plasma concentration of TCA with resultant toxicity; lower than usual doses of either drug may be required; co-administration results in enhanced response to CNS depressants). Products include:
    Stelazine 2692

Trihexyphenidyl Hydrochloride (Co-administration may result in hyperpyrexia, particularly during hot weather). Products include:
    Artane 1418

Trimipramine Maleate (Co-administration with cytochrome P4502D6 inhibitors, such as antidepressants, may make normal metabolizer resemble poor metabolizer leading to higher than expected plasma concentration of TCA with resultant toxicity; lower than usual doses of either drug may be required). Products include:
    Surmontil Capsules 2917

Venlafaxine Hydrochloride (Co-administration with cytochrome P4502D6 inhibitors, such as antidepressants, may make normal metabolizer resemble poor metabolizer leading to higher than expected plasma concentration of TCA with resultant toxicity; due to variation in the extent of inhibition P4502D6, sufficient time should elapse in switching from one class to the other). Products include:
    Effexor 2825

Zolpidem Tartrate (Co-administration results in enhanced response to CNS depressants). Products include:
    Ambien Tablets 2559

Food Interactions

Alcohol (Co-administration results in enhanced response to alcohol).

VIVELLE TRANSDERMAL SYSTEM

(Estradiol) 880
May interact with progestins. Compounds in this category include:

Desogestrel (Potential for adverse effects on carbohydrate and lipid metabolism). Products include:
    Desogen Tablets 1867
    Ortho-Cept 1907

Medroxyprogesterone Acetate (Potential for adverse effects on carbohydrate and lipid metabolism). Products include:
    Amen Tablets 785
    Cycrin Tablets 991
    Depo-Provera Contraceptive Injection 2079
    Depo-Provera Sterile Aqueous Suspension 2083
    Premphase 2900
    Prempro 2905
    Provera Tablets 2110

Megestrol Acetate (Potential for adverse effects on carbohydrate and lipid metabolism). Products include:
    Megace Oral Suspension 708
    Megace Tablets 710

Norgestimate (Potential for adverse effects on carbohydrate and lipid metabolism). Products include:
    Ortho-Cyclen/Ortho-Tri-Cyclen 1914
    Ortho-Cyclen/Ortho-Tri-Cyclen 1914

VIVOTIF BERNA

(Typhoid Vaccine Live Oral Ty21a) .. 660
May interact with:

Antibiotics, unspecified (The vaccine should not be administered to individuals receiving unspecified antibiotics and other antibacterial drugs including sulfonamides since these agents may interfere with protective immune response).

VOLMAX EXTENDED-RELEASE TABLETS

(Albuterol Sulfate) 1835
May interact with sympathomimetics, monoamine oxidase inhibitors, tricyclic antidepressants, beta blockers, and certain other agents. Compounds in these categories include:

Acebutolol Hydrochloride (Effect of each other inhibited). Products include:
    Sectral Capsules 2914

Albuterol (Potential for deleterious cardiovascular effects with other oral sympathomimetic agents). Products include:
    Proventil Inhalation Aerosol ... 2524
    Ventolin Inhalation Aerosol and Refill 1170

Amitriptyline Hydrochloride (Action of albuterol on the vascular system may be potentiated). Products include:
    Elavil 2945
    Etrafon 2495
    Limbitrol 2333
    Triavil Tablets 1800

Amoxapine (Action of albuterol on the vascular system may be potentiated). Products include:
    Asendin Tablets 1419

Atenolol (Effect of each other inhibited). Products include:
    Tenoretic Tablets 2963
    Tenormin Tablets and I.V. Injection 2965

Betaxolol Hydrochloride (Effect of each other inhibited). Products include:
    Betoptic Ophthalmic Solution 465
    Betoptic S Ophthalmic Suspension 467
    Kerlone Tablets 2588

Bisoprolol Fumarate (Effect of each other inhibited). Products include:
    Zebeta Tablets 1457
    Ziac 1459

Carteolol Hydrochloride (Effect of each other inhibited). Products include:
    Cartrol Tablets 413
    Ocupress Ophthalmic Solution, 1% Sterile .... ⊙ 297

Clomipramine Hydrochloride (Action of albuterol on the vascular system may be potentiated). Products include:
    Anafranil Capsules 819

Desipramine Hydrochloride (Action of albuterol on the vascular system may be potentiated). Products include:
    Norpramin Tablets 1273

Dobutamine Hydrochloride (Potential for deleterious cardiovascular effects with other oral sympathomimetic agents). Products include:
    Dobutrex Solution Vials 1480

Dopamine Hydrochloride (Potential for deleterious cardiovascular effects with other oral sympathomimetic agents).
    No products indexed under this heading.

Doxepin Hydrochloride (Action of albuterol on the vascular system may be potentiated). Products include:
    Adapin Capsules 1542
    Sinequan 2028
    Zonalon Cream 1042

Ephedrine Hydrochloride (Potential for deleterious cardiovascular effects with other oral sympathomimetic agents). Products include:
    Primatene Tablets .... ▣ 844
    Quadrinal Tablets 1398

Ephedrine Sulfate (Potential for deleterious cardiovascular effects with other oral sympathomimetic agents). Products include:
    Marax Tablets & DF Syrup ... 2015

Ephedrine Tannate (Potential for deleterious cardiovascular effects with other oral sympathomimetic agents). Products include:
    Rynatuss 2782

Epinephrine (Potential for deleterious cardiovascular effects with other oral sympathomimetic agents). Products include:
    EPIFRIN .... ⊙ 237
    EpiPen 808
    Marcaine with Epinephrine .. 2446
    Primatene Mist .... ▣ 843
    Sensorcaine with Epinephrine Injection 554
    Sus-Phrine Injection 1017
    Xylocaine with Epinephrine Injections 562

Epinephrine Bitartrate (Potential for deleterious cardiovascular effects with other oral sympathomimetic agents). Products include:
    Sensorcaine-MPF with Epinephrine Injection 554

Epinephrine Hydrochloride (Potential for deleterious cardiovascular effects with other oral sympathomimetic agents). Products include:
    Ana-Kit Anaphylaxis Emergency Treatment Kit 611

Esmolol Hydrochloride (Effect of each other inhibited). Products include:
    Brevibloc (esmolol HCl) Injection 1860

Furazolidone (Action of albuterol on the vascular system may be potentiated). Products include:
    Furoxone 2221

Imipramine Hydrochloride (Action of albuterol on the vascular system may be potentiated). Products include:
    Tofranil Ampuls 873
    Tofranil Tablets 875

Imipramine Pamoate (Action of albuterol on the vascular system may be potentiated). Products include:
    Tofranil-PM Capsules 876

Isocarboxazid (Action of albuterol on the vascular system may be potentiated).
    No products indexed under this heading.

Isoproterenol Hydrochloride (Potential for deleterious cardiovascular effects with other oral sympathomimetic agents). Products include:
    Isuprel Hydrochloride Solution 2443
    Isuprel Injection 2441
    Isuprel Mistometer 2442

Isoproterenol Sulfate (Potential for deleterious cardiovascular effects with other oral sympathomimetic agents). Products include:
    Norisodrine with Calcium Iodide Syrup 446

Labetalol Hydrochloride (Effect of each other inhibited). Products include:
    Normodyne Injection 2519
    Normodyne Tablets 2522
    Trandate 1158

Levobunolol Hydrochloride (Effect of each other inhibited). Products include:
    Betagan .... ⊙ 230

Maprotiline Hydrochloride (Action of albuterol on the vascular system may be potentiated). Products include:
    Ludiomil Tablets 861

Metaproterenol Sulfate (Potential for deleterious cardiovascular effects with other oral sympathomimetic agents). Products include:
    Alupent 672
    Metaproterenol Sulfate Inhalation Solution, USP, Arm-a-Med ... 547

Metaraminol Bitartrate (Potential for deleterious cardiovascular effects with other oral sympathomimetic agents). Products include:
    Aramine Injection 1649

Methoxamine Hydrochloride (Potential for deleterious cardiovascular effects with other oral sympathomimetic agents). Products include:
    Vasoxyl Injection 1169

Metipranolol Hydrochloride (Effect of each other inhibited). Products include:
    OptiPranolol (Metipranolol 0.3%) Sterile Ophthalmic Solution .... ⊙ 256

Metoprolol Succinate (Effect of each other inhibited). Products include:
    Toprol-XL Tablets 560

Metoprolol Tartrate (Effect of each other inhibited). Products include:
    Lopressor 848
    Lopressor HCT Tablets 850

Nadolol (Effect of each other inhibited).
    No products indexed under this heading.

Norepinephrine Bitartrate (Potential for deleterious cardiovascular effects with other oral sympathomimetic agents). Products include:
    Levophed Bitartrate Injection 2445

Nortriptyline Hydrochloride (Action of albuterol on the vascular system may be potentiated). Products include:
    Pamelor 2409

Penbutolol Sulfate (Effect of each other inhibited). Products include:
    Levatol Tablets 2547

Phenelzine Sulfate (Action of albuterol on the vascular system may be potentiated). Products include:
    Nardil 1977

Phenylephrine Bitartrate (Potential for deleterious cardiovascular effects with other oral sympathomimetic agents).
    No products indexed under this heading.

Phenylephrine Hydrochloride (Potential for deleterious cardiovascular effects with other oral sympathomimetic agents). Products include:
    Atrohist Plus Tablets 1605

(▣ Described in PDR For Nonprescription Drugs)   (⊙ Described in PDR For Ophthalmology)

Cerose DM 853
D.A. II Tablets 972
D.A. Chewable Tablets 970
Dura-Vent/DA Tablets 972
Extendryl 1003
4-Way Fast Acting Nasal Spray (regular & mentholated) 644
Hemorid 797
Hycomine Compound Tablets 948
Neo-Synephrine Hydrochloride 1% Carpuject 2455
Neo-Synephrine Hydrochloride 1% Injection 2455
Neo-Synephrine Hydrochloride (Ophthalmic) 2456
Neo-Synephrine 624
Novahistine Elixir 782
Phenergan VC 2886
Phenergan VC with Codeine 2888
Preparation H 842
Tympagesic Ear Drops 2476
Vicks Sinex Nasal Spray and Ultra Fine Mist 738

Phenylephrine Tannate (Potential for deleterious cardiovascular effects with other oral sympathomimetic agents). Products include:
Atrohist Pediatric Suspension 1604
Atrohist Pediatric Suspension Dye-Free 1604
Rynatan 2781
Rynatuss 2782

Phenylpropanolamine Hydrochloride (Potential for deleterious cardiovascular effects with other oral sympathomimetic agents). Products include:
Acutrim 648
Atrohist Plus Tablets 1605
BC Cold Powder Multi-Symptom Formula (Cold-Sinus-Allergy) 631
BC Cold Powder Non-Drowsy Formula (Cold-Sinus) 631
Cheracol Plus Head Cold/Cough Formula 741
Comtrex Multi-Symptom Cold Reliever Liqui-Gels 638
Comtrex Multi-Symptom Non-Drowsy Liqui-gels 640
Contac Continuous Action Nasal Decongestant/Antihistamine 12 Hour Capsules 773
Contac Maximum Strength Continuous Action Decongestant/Antihistamine 12 Hour Caplets 772
Contac Severe Cold and Flu Formula Caplets 773
Coricidin 'D' Decongestant Tablets 760
Dexatrim 795
Dexatrim Plus Vitamins Caplets 796
Dimetane-DC Cough Syrup 2232
Dimetapp Allergy Sinus Caplets 838
Dimetapp Cold & Allergy Chewable Tablets 838
Dimetapp Cold & Cough Liqui-Gels 839
Dimetapp DM Elixir 840
Dimetapp Elixir 840
Dimetapp Extentabs 841
Dimetapp Tablets/Liqui-Gels 841
Dura-Vent Tablets 971
Entex LA Tablets 972
Exgest LA Tablets 787
Hycomine 947
Nolamine Timed-Release Tablets 790
Ornade Spansule Capsules 2678
Propagest Tablets 791
Pyrroxate Caplets 742
Robitussin-CF 846
Sinulin Tablets 792
Tavist-D 12 Hour Relief Tablets 750
Teldrin 12 Hour Antihistamine/Nasal Decongestant Allergy Relief Capsules 786
Triaminic Expectorant 753
Triaminic Syrup 755
Triaminic Triaminicol Cold & Cough 756
Triaminic DM Syrup 756
Triaminicin Tablets 756
Vicks DayQuil Allergy Relief 12-Hour Extended Release Tablets 733
Vicks DayQuil Allergy Relief 4-Hour Tablets 733
Vicks DayQuil SINUS Pressure & CONGESTION Relief 734

Pindolol (Effect of each other inhibited). Products include:
Visken Tablets 2428

Pirbuterol Acetate (Potential for deleterious cardiovascular effects with other oral sympathomimetic agents). Products include:
Maxair Autohaler 1550
Maxair Inhaler 1552

Propranolol Hydrochloride (Effect of each other inhibited). Products include:
Inderal 2834
Inderal LA Long Acting Capsules 2836
Inderide Tablets 2838
Inderide LA Long Acting Capsules 2840

Protriptyline Hydrochloride (Action of albuterol on the vascular system may be potentiated). Products include:
Vivactil Tablets 1820

Pseudoephedrine Hydrochloride (Potential for deleterious cardiovascular effects with other oral sympathomimetic agents). Products include:
Actifed Allergy Daytime/Nighttime Caplets 808
Actifed Cold & Allergy Tablets 807
Actifed Cold & Sinus Caplets and Tablets 808
Actifed Sinus Daytime/Nighttime Tablets and Caplets 809
Advil Cold and Sinus Caplets and Tablets 837
Alka-Seltzer Plus Liqui-Gels 612
Alka-Seltzer Plus Flu & Body Aches Liqui-Gels Non-Drowsy Formula 613
Alka-Seltzer Plus Night-Time Cold Medicine Liqui-Gels 612
Allerest Maximum Strength 649
Allerest No Drowsiness 649
Allerest Sinus Pain Formula 649
Atrohist Pediatric Capsules 1603
Benadryl Allergy/Cold Tablets 811
Benadryl Allergy Decongestant Liquid Medication 812
Benadryl Allergy Decongestant Tablets 812
Benadryl Allergy Sinus Headache Caplets 813
Benylin Multisymptom 816
Bromfed Capsules (Extended-Release) 1832
Bromfed Syrup 712
Bromfed Tablets 1832
Bromfed-DM Cough Syrup 1832
Bromfed-PD Capsules (Extended-Release) 1832
Children's TYLENOL Cold Multi-Symptom Chewable Tablets and Liquid 1559
Children's TYLENOL Cold Plus Cough Multi Symptom Chewable Tablets and Liquid 1560
Children's TYLENOL Flu Suspension Liquid 1560
Children's Vicks DayQuil Allergy Relief 730
Children's Vicks NyQuil Cold/Cough Relief 731
Allergy-Sinus Comtrex Multi-Symptom Allergy-Sinus Formula Tablets and Caplets 639
Comtrex Multi-Symptom 638
Comtrex Multi-Symptom Non-Drowsy Caplets 640
Congess 1003
Contac Day Allergy/Sinus Caplets 771
Contac Day & Night 772
Contac Night Allergy/Sinus Caplets 771
Contac Severe Cold & Flu Non-Drowsy 774
Deconsal II Tablets 1605
Dimetane-DX Cough Syrup 2233
Dimetapp Cold & Fever Suspension 839
Dimetapp Decongestant Pediatric Drops 840
Dorcol Children's Cough Syrup 748
Drixoral Cough + Congestion Liquid Caps 763
Dura-Tap/PD Capsules 970
Duratuss Tablets 2750
Duratuss HD Elixir 2750
Efidac/24 655
Entex PSE Tablets 973
Fedahist Gyrocaps 2545
Guaifed 1833
Guaifed Syrup 712
Guaimax-D Tablets 809
Histussin D Liquid 670
Infants' TYLENOL Cold Decongestant & Fever-Reducer Drops 1561
Kronofed-A 994
Novahistine DMX 782
Nucofed 2225
PediaCare Cough-Cold Chewable Tablets and Liquid 1569
PediaCare Infants' Decongestant Drops 1569
PediaCare Infants' Drops Decongestant Plus Cough 1569
PediaCare NightRest Cough-Cold Liquid 1569
Pediatric Vicks 44d Cough & Head Congestion Relief 736
Pediatric Vicks 44m Cough & Cold Relief 737
Robitussin Cold & Cough Liqui-Gels 844
Robitussin Cold, Cough & Flu Liqui-Gels 844
Robitussin Maximum Strength Cough & Cold 847
Robitussin Night-Time Cold Formula 847
Robitussin Pediatric Cough & Cold Formula 848
Robitussin Pediatric Drops 849
Robitussin Severe Congestion Liqui-Gels 845
Robitussin-DAC Syrup 2249
Robitussin-PE 846
Rondec Oral Drops 974
Rondec Syrup 974
Rondec Tablet 974
Rondec Chewable Tablets 974
Rondec-TR Tablet 974
Ryna 804
Seldane-D Extended-Release Tablets 1286
Semprex-D Capsules 1620
Sinarest 663
Sine-Aid Maximum Strength Sinus Headache Gelcaps, Caplets and Tablets 1570
Sine-Off No Drowsiness Formula Caplets 784
Sine-Off Sinus Medicine 784
Singlet Tablets 785
Sinutab Non-Drying Liquid Caps 823
Sinutab Sinus Allergy Medication, Maximum Strength Tablets and Caplets 823
Sinutab Sinus Medication, Maximum Strength Without Drowsiness Formula, Tablets & Caplets 824
Sudafed Children's Cold & Cough Liquid Medication 825
Sudafed Children's Nasal Decongestant Liquid Medication 826
Sudafed Cold & Allergy Tablets 826
Sudafed Cold and Cough Liquid Caps 826
Sudafed Nasal Decongestant Tablets, 30 mg 825
Sudafed Nasal Decongestant Tablets, 60 mg 825
Sudafed Non-Drying Sinus Liquid Caps 827
Sudafed Pediatric Nasal Decongestant Liquid Oral Drops 827
Sudafed Severe Cold Formula Caplets 828
Sudafed Severe Cold Formula Tablets 828
Sudafed Sinus Caplets 829
Sudafed Sinus Tablets 829
Sudafed 12 Hour Caplets 824
Syn-Rx Tablets 1622
Syn-Rx DM Tablets 1623
TheraFlu Flu and Cold Medicine 750
Theraflu Maximum Strength Flu and Cold Medicine For Sore Throat 751
TheraFlu Flu, Cold and Cough Medicine 750
TheraFlu Maximum Strength Nighttime Flu, Cold & Cough Medicine 751
TheraFlu Maximum Strength Non-Drowsy Formula Flu, Cold & Cough Medicine 751
TheraFlu Maximum Strength, Non-Drowsy Formula Flu, Cold and Cough Caplets 752
Theraflu Maximum Strength Sinus Non-Drowsy Formula Caplets 752
Triaminic AM Cough and Decongestant Formula 753
Triaminic AM Decongestant Formula 753
Triaminic Infant Oral Decongestant Drops 754
Triaminic Night Time 754
Triaminic Sore Throat Formula 755
Tussend 1830
Tussend Expectorant 1831
TYLENOL Allergy Sinus, Maximum Strength Caplets and Gelcaps 1571
TYLENOL Allergy Sinus NightTime, Maximum Strength Caplets 1571
TYLENOL Cold Medication, Multi-Symptom Formula Tablets and Caplets 1572
TYLENOL Cold Medication, Multi-Symptom Hot Liquid Packets 1572
TYLENOL Cold Medication, No Drowsiness Formula Caplets and Gelcaps 1572
TYLENOL Cold Severe Congestion Caplets 1573
TYLENOL Cough Medication with Decongestant, Multi Symptom 1574
TYLENOL Flu No Drowsiness Formula, Maximum Strength Gelcaps 1575
TYLENOL Flu NightTime, Maximum Strength Gelcaps 1575
TYLENOL Flu NightTime, Maximum Strength Hot Medication Packets 1575
TYLENOL Sinus, Maximum Strength Geltabs, Gelcaps, Caplets and Tablets 1576
Vicks 44 LiquiCaps Cough, Cold & Flu Relief 728
Vicks 44 LiquiCaps Non-Drowsy Cough & Cold Relief 729
Vicks 44D Cough & Head Congestion Relief 728
Vicks 44M Cough, Cold & Flu Relief 729
Vicks DayQuil LiquiCaps/Liquid Multi-Symptom Cold/Flu Relief 734
Vicks DayQuil SINUS Pressure & PAIN Relief with IBUPROFEN 735
Vicks Nyquil Hot Therapy 735
Vicks NyQuil LiquiCaps/Liquid Multi-Symptom Cold/Flu Relief, Original and Cherry Flavors 736

Pseudoephedrine Sulfate (Potential for deleterious cardiovascular effects with other oral sympathomimetic agents). Products include:
Chlor-Trimeton Allergy Decongestant Tablets 759
Claritin-D Tablets 2487
Drixoral Cold and Allergy Sustained-Action Tablets 763
Drixoral Cold and Flu Extended-Release Tablets 764
Drixoral Non-Drowsy Formula Extended-Release Tablets 764
Drixoral Allergy/Sinus Extended Release Tablets 765
Trinalin Repetabs Tablets 1373

Salmeterol Xinafoate (Potential for deleterious cardiovascular effects with other oral sympathomimetic agents). Products include:
Serevent Inhalation Aerosol 1149

Selegiline Hydrochloride (Action of albuterol on the vascular system may be potentiated). Products include:
Eldepryl Capsules 2729

Sotalol Hydrochloride (Effect of each other inhibited). Products include:
Betapace Tablets 637

Terbutaline Sulfate (Potential for deleterious cardiovascular effects with other oral sympathomimetic agents). Products include:
Brethaire Inhaler 830
Brethine Ampuls 832
Brethine Tablets 831
Bricanyl Subcutaneous Injection 1247
Bricanyl Tablets 1248

IMPORTANT NOTE: Always consult each drug listing in the patient's regimen for possible interactions.

Timolol Hemihydrate (Effect of each other inhibited). Products include:

Betimol 0.25%, 0.5% .... ⊙ 259

Timolol Maleate (Effect of each other inhibited). Products include:

Blocadren Tablets 1654
Timolide Tablets 1791
Timoptic in Ocudose 1796
Timoptic Sterile Ophthalmic Solution 1794
Timoptic-XE 1798

Tranylcypromine Sulfate (Action of albuterol on the vascular system may be potentiated). Products include:

Parnate Tablets 2679

Trimipramine Maleate (Action of albuterol on the vascular system may be potentiated). Products include:

Surmontil Capsules 2917

Food Interactions

Food, unspecified (Food may decrease the rate of absorption without altering the extent of bioavailability).

VOLTAREN OPHTHALMIC STERILE OPHTHALMIC SOLUTION

(Diclofenac Sodium) .... ⊙ 264
None cited in PDR database.

VOLTAREN TABLETS

(Diclofenac Sodium) 833
May interact with oral anticoagulants, oral hypoglycemic agents, diuretics, lithium preparations, potassium sparing diuretics, insulin, and certain other agents. Compounds in these categories include:

Acarbose (Both hypo- and hyperglycemic effects have been reported rarely; possibility exists that diclofenac may alter diabetic patient's response to oral hypoglycemic agents). Products include:

Precose 604

Amiloride Hydrochloride (Concomitant treatment may be associated with hyperkalemia). Products include:

Midamor Tablets 1746
Moduretic Tablets 1748

Aspirin (Co-administration is not recommended because diclofenac is displaced from its binding sites resulting in lower peak plasma concentrations, peak plasma levels and AUC values). Products include:

Alka-Seltzer Cherry Effervescent Antacid and Pain Reliever .... ▣ 609
Alka-Seltzer Extra Strength Effervescent Antacid and Pain Reliever .... ▣ 609
Alka-Seltzer Lemon Lime Effervescent Antacid and Pain Reliever .... ▣ 609
Alka-Seltzer Original Effervescent Antacid and Pain Reliever .... ▣ 609
Alka-Seltzer Plus .... ▣ 611
Alka-Seltzer Plus Sinus Medicine .. ▣ 611
Ascriptin .... ▣ 650
Arthritis Strength BC Powder .... ▣ 631
BC Cold Powder Multi-Symptom Formula (Cold-Sinus-Allergy) .... ▣ 631
BC Cold Powder Non-Drowsy Formula (Cold-Sinus) .... ▣ 631
BC Powder .... ▣ 631
Genuine Bayer Aspirin Tablets & Caplets .... ▣ 618
Extra Strength Bayer Arthritis Pain Regimen Formula .... ▣ 615
Extra Strength Bayer Aspirin Caplets & Tablets .... ▣ 617
Extended-Release Bayer 8-Hour Aspirin .... ▣ 616
Extra Strength Bayer Plus Aspirin Caplets .... ▣ 617
Extra Strength Bayer PM Aspirin Plus Sleep Aid .... ▣ 617
Aspirin Regimen Bayer 81 mg Tablets with Calcium .... ▣ 615
Aspirin Regimen Bayer Adult Low Strength 81 mg Tablets .... ▣ 613
Aspirin Regimen Bayer Children's Chewable Aspirin .... ▣ 616
Aspirin Regimen Bayer Regular Strength 325 mg Caplets .... ▣ 613
Bufferin Analgesic Tablets .... ▣ 636
Arthritis Strength Bufferin Analgesic Caplets .... ▣ 637
Extra Strength Bufferin Analgesic Tablets .... ▣ 637
Cama Arthritis Pain Reliever .... ▣ 748
Darvon Compound-65 Pulvules 1475
Easprin 1971
Ecotrin 2625
Ecotrin Enteric Coated Aspirin Maximum Strength Tablets and Caplets .... ▣ 775
Ecotrin Enteric Coated Aspirin Regular Strength Tablets 2625
Empirin Aspirin Tablets .... ▣ 818
Excedrin Extra-Strength Analgesic Tablets, Caplets, and Geltabs 734
Fiorinal Capsules 2388
Fiorinal with Codeine Capsules 2390
Fiorinal Tablets 2388
Goody's Extra Strength Headache Powders .... ▣ 632
Goody's Extra Strength Pain Relief Tablets .... ▣ 632
Halfprin Tablets 1413
Norgesic 1554
Percodan Tablets 955
Percodan-Demi Tablets 956
Robaxisal Tablets 2246
Soma Compound w/Codeine Tablets 2784
Soma Compound Tablets 2783
St. Joseph Adult Chewable Aspirin (81 mg.) .... ▣ 768
Talwin Compound 2466
Vanquish Analgesic Caplets .... ▣ 627

Bendroflumethiazide (Diclofenac can inhibit the activity of diuretics).

No products indexed under this heading.

Bumetanide (Diclofenac can inhibit the activity of diuretics). Products include:

Bumex 2260

Chlorothiazide (Diclofenac can inhibit the activity of diuretics). Products include:

Aldoclor Tablets 1638
Diupres Tablets 1691
Diuril Oral 1694

Chlorothiazide Sodium (Diclofenac can inhibit the activity of diuretics). Products include:

Diuril Sodium Intravenous 1693

Chlorpropamide (Both hypo- and hyperglycemic effects have been reported rarely; possibility exists that diclofenac may alter diabetic patient's response to oral hypoglycemic agents). Products include:

Diabinese Tablets 2002

Chlorthalidone (Diclofenac can inhibit the activity of diuretics). Products include:

Combipres Tablets 682
Tenoretic Tablets 2963
Thalitone 1293

Cyclosporine (Co-administration may increase cyclosporine's nephrotoxicity since diclofenac may affect renal prostaglandins). Products include:

Neoral 2405
Sandimmune 2416

Dicumarol (While studies have not shown interactions with oral anticoagulants, concurrent therapy requires close monitoring of patients for potential modification in anticoagulant dosage).

No products indexed under this heading.

Digoxin (Co-administration may increase serum digoxin concentrations resulting in digoxin toxicity since diclofenac may affect renal prostaglandins). Products include:

Lanoxicaps 1110
Lanoxin Elixir Pediatric 1113
Lanoxin Injection 1116
Lanoxin Injection Pediatric 1119
Lanoxin Tablets 1121

Ethacrynic Acid (Diclofenac can inhibit the activity of diuretics). Products include:

Edecrin Tablets 1698

Furosemide (Diclofenac can inhibit the activity of diuretics). Products include:

Lasix Injection, Oral Solution and Tablets 1267

Glimepiride (Both hypo- and hyperglycemic effects have been reported rarely; possibility exists that diclofenac may alter diabetic patient's response to oral hypoglycemic agents). Products include:

Amaryl Tablets 1241

Glipizide (Both hypo- and hyperglycemic effects have been reported rarely; possibility exists that diclofenac may alter diabetic patient's response to oral hypoglycemic agents). Products include:

Glucotrol Tablets 2011
Glucotrol XL Extended Release Tablets 2012

Glyburide (Both hypo- and hyperglycemic effects have been reported rarely; possibility exists that diclofenac may alter diabetic patient's response to oral hypoglycemic agents). Products include:

DiaBeta Tablets 1265
Glynase PresTab Tablets 2091
Micronase Tablets 2099

Hydrochlorothiazide (Diclofenac can inhibit the activity of diuretics). Products include:

Aldactazide Tablets 2556
Aldoril Tablets 1644
Apresazide Capsules 824
Capozide Tablets 744
Dyazide Capsules 2653
Esidrix Tablets 839
Esimil Tablets 840
HydroDIURIL Tablets 1716
Hydropres Tablets 1718
Hyzaar Tablets 1720
Inderide Tablets 2838
Inderide LA Long Acting Capsules .. 2840
Lopressor HCT Tablets 850
Lotensin HCT Tablets 855
Moduretic Tablets 1748
Oretic Tablets 450
Prinzide Tablets 1780
Ser-Ap-Es Tablets 867
Timolide Tablets 1791
Vaseretic Tablets 1810
Zestoretic Tablets 2968
Ziac 1459

Hydroflumethiazide (Diclofenac can inhibit the activity of diuretics). Products include:

Diucardin Tablets 2824

Indapamide (Diclofenac can inhibit the activity of diuretics).

No products indexed under this heading.

Insulin, Human (Both hypo- and hyperglycemic effects have been reported rarely; possibility exists that diclofenac may alter diabetic patient's response to insulin).

No products indexed under this heading.

Insulin, Human Isophane Suspension (Both hypo- and hyperglycemic effects have been reported rarely; possibility exists that diclofenac may alter diabetic patient's response to insulin). Products include:

Novolin N Human Insulin 10 ml Vials 1846

Insulin, Human NPH (Both hypo- and hyperglycemic effects have been reported rarely; possibility exists that diclofenac may alter diabetic patient's response to insulin). Products include:

Humulin N, 100 Units 1495
Novolin N PenFill 1.5 ml Cartridges Durable Insulin Delivery System 1849
Novolin N Prefilled Syringe Disposable Insulin Delivery System 1850

Insulin, Human Regular (Both hypo- and hyperglycemic effects have been reported rarely; possibility exists that diclofenac may alter diabetic patient's response to insulin). Products include:

Humulin R, 100 Units 1497
Novolin R Human Insulin 10 ml Vials 1846
Novolin R PenFill 1.5 ml Cartridges Durable Insulin Delivery System 1849
Novolin R Prefilled Syringe Disposable Insulin Delivery System 1850
Velosulin BR Human Insulin 10 ml Vials 1847

Insulin, Human, Zinc Suspension (Both hypo- and hyperglycemic effects have been reported rarely; possibility exists that diclofenac may alter diabetic patient's response to insulin). Products include:

Humulin L, 100 Units 1494
Humulin U, 100 Units 1498
Novolin L Human Insulin 10 ml Vials 1846

Insulin Lispro, Human (Both hypo- and hyperglycemic effects have been reported rarely; possibility exists that diclofenac may alter diabetic patient's response to insulin). Products include:

Humalog Injection 1488

Insulin, NPH (Both hypo- and hyperglycemic effects have been reported rarely; possibility exists that diclofenac may alter diabetic patient's response to insulin). Products include:

NPH, 100 Units 1502
Pork NPH, 100 Units 1506
Purified Pork NPH Isophane Insulin 1852

Insulin, Regular (Both hypo- and hyperglycemic effects have been reported rarely; possibility exists that diclofenac may alter diabetic patient's response to insulin). Products include:

Regular, 100 Units 1503
Pork Regular, 100 Units 1507
Pork Regular (Concentrated), 500 Units 1508
Purified Pork Regular Insulin 1852

Insulin, Zinc Crystals (Both hypo- and hyperglycemic effects have been reported rarely; possibility exists that diclofenac may alter diabetic patient's response to insulin). Products include:

NPH, 100 Units 1502

Insulin, Zinc Suspension (Both hypo- and hyperglycemic effects have been reported rarely; possibility exists that diclofenac may alter diabetic patient's response to insulin). Products include:

Iletin I 1501
Lente, 100 Units 1501
Iletin II 1504

(▣ Described in PDR For Nonprescription Drugs) (⊙ Described in PDR For Ophthalmology)

Interactions Index / Wellbutrin

Pork Lente, 100 Units.................... 1504
Purified Pork Lente Insulin 1852

Lithium Carbonate (Decreased lithium renal clearance resulting in increased lithium plasma levels; potential for lithium toxicity). Products include:
Eskalith 2658
Lithium Carbonate Capsules & Tablets 2352
Lithonate/Lithotabs/Lithobid 2721

Lithium Citrate (Decreased lithium renal clearance resulting in increased lithium plasma levels; potential for lithium toxicity).
No products indexed under this heading.

Metformin Hydrochloride (Both hypo- and hyperglycemic effects have been reported rarely; possibility exists that diclofenac may alter diabetic patient's response to oral hypoglycemic agents). Products include:
Glucophage Tablets 754

Methotrexate Sodium (Co-administration may increase serum methotrexate concentrations resulting in methotrexate toxicity since diclofenac may affect renal prostaglandins). Products include:
Methotrexate Sodium Tablets, Injection, for Injection and LPF Injection 1322

Methyclothiazide (Diclofenac can inhibit the activity of diuretics). Products include:
Enduron Tablets 424

Metolazone (Diclofenac can inhibit the activity of diuretics). Products include:
Mykrox Tablets 1617
Zaroxolyn Tablets 1625

Phenobarbital (Potential for phenobarbital toxicity in patients on chronic phenobarbital treatment following the initiation of diclofenac therapy). Products include:
Arco-Lase Plus Tablets 513
Bellergal-S Tablets 2375
Donnatal 2234
Donnatal Extentabs 2234
Donnatal Tablets 2234
Phenobarbital Elixir and Tablets 1523
Quadrinal Tablets 1398

Polythiazide (Diclofenac can inhibit the activity of diuretics). Products include:
Minizide Capsules 2016

Spironolactone (Concomitant treatment may be associated with hyperkalemia). Products include:
Aldactazide Tablets 2556
Aldactone Tablets 2558

Tolazamide (Both hypo- and hyperglycemic effects have been reported rarely; possibility exists that diclofenac may alter diabetic patient's response to oral hypoglycemic agents).
No products indexed under this heading.

Tolbutamide (Both hypo- and hyperglycemic effects have been reported rarely; possibility exists that diclofenac may alter diabetic patient's response to oral hypoglycemic agents).
No products indexed under this heading.

Torsemide (Diclofenac can inhibit the activity of diuretics). Products include:
Demadex Tablets and Injection 691

Triamterene (Concomitant treatment may be associated with hyperkalemia). Products include:
Dyazide Capsules 2653
Dyrenium Capsules 2655

Warfarin Sodium (While studies have not shown interactions with oral anticoagulants, concurrent therapy requires close monitoring of patients for potential modification in anticoagulant dosage). Products include:
Coumadin 941

Food Interactions

Food, unspecified (Food significantly alters the absorption pattern of extended-release dosage form as indicated by delay of 1 to 2 hours in T_{max} and a two-fold increase in C_{max} values; food also delays the onset of absorption of delayed-release and immediate-release formulations).

VOLTAREN-XR TABLETS
(Diclofenac Sodium) 833
See **Voltaren Tablets**

VōSOL HC OTIC SOLUTION
(Acetic Acid, Hydrocortisone) 2786
None cited in PDR database.

VōSOL OTIC SOLUTION
(Acetic Acid) 2786
None cited in PDR database.

VUMON FOR INJECTION
(Teniposide) 729
May interact with:

Methotrexate Sodium (Co-administration slightly increases methotrexate clearance; an increase in intracellular levels of methotrexate has been observed *in vitro* in the presence of teniposide). Products include:
Methotrexate Sodium Tablets, Injection, for Injection and LPF Injection 1322

Sodium Salicylate (Possible potentiation of drug toxicity due to small decrease in protein binding causing substantial increase in free teniposide).
No products indexed under this heading.

Sulfamethizole (Possible potentiation of drug toxicity due to small decrease in protein binding causing substantial increase in free teniposide). Products include:
Urobiotic-250 Capsules 2038

Tolbutamide (Possible potentiation of drug toxicity due to small decrease in protein binding causing substantial increase in free teniposide).
No products indexed under this heading.

WART-OFF WART REMOVER
(Salicylic Acid) 720
None cited in PDR database.

WELLBUTRIN TABLETS
(Bupropion Hydrochloride) 1177
May interact with drugs affecting hepatic drug metabolizing enzyme systems, monoamine oxidase inhibitors, drugs which lower seizure threshold, and certain other agents. Compounds in these categories include:

Alprazolam (Concurrent therapy should be undertaken with extreme caution). Products include:
Xanax Tablets 2115

Amitriptyline Hydrochloride (Concurrent therapy should be undertaken with extreme caution). Products include:
Elavil 2945
Etrafon 2495
Limbitrol 2333
Triavil Tablets 1800

Amoxapine (Concurrent therapy should be undertaken with extreme caution). Products include:
Asendin Tablets 1419

Carbamazepine (Concurrent therapy may affect metabolism of bupropion). Products include:
Atretol Tablets 569
Tegretol/Tegretol-XR 870

Chlordiazepoxide (Concurrent therapy should be undertaken with extreme caution). Products include:
Limbitrol 2333

Chlordiazepoxide Hydrochloride (Concurrent therapy should be undertaken with extreme caution). Products include:
Librax Capsules 2330
Librium Capsules 2331
Librium Injectable 2332

Chlorpromazine (Concurrent therapy should be undertaken with extreme caution). Products include:
Thorazine Suppositories 2701

Cimetidine (Concurrent therapy may affect metabolism of bupropion). Products include:
Tagamet HB Tablets 786
Tagamet Tablets 2694

Cimetidine Hydrochloride (Concurrent therapy may affect metabolism of bupropion). Products include:
Tagamet 2694

Desipramine Hydrochloride (Concurrent therapy should be undertaken with extreme caution). Products include:
Norpramin Tablets 1273

Diazepam (Concurrent therapy should be undertaken with extreme caution). Products include:
Dizac (diazepam injectable emulsion) CIV 1862
Valium Injectable 2336
Valium Tablets 2335

Doxepin Hydrochloride (Concurrent therapy should be undertaken with extreme caution). Products include:
Adapin Capsules 1542
Sinequan 2028
Zonalon Cream 1042

Fluoxetine Hydrochloride (Concurrent therapy should be undertaken with extreme caution). Products include:
Prozac Pulvules & Liquid, Oral Solution 935

Fluphenazine Decanoate (Concurrent therapy should be undertaken with extreme caution). Products include:
Prolixin Decanoate 510

Fluphenazine Enanthate (Concurrent therapy should be undertaken with extreme caution). Products include:
Prolixin Enanthate 510

Fluphenazine Hydrochloride (Concurrent therapy should be undertaken with extreme caution). Products include:
Prolixin 510

Furazolidone (Concurrent administration is contraindicated). Products include:
Furoxone 2221

Haloperidol (Concurrent therapy should be undertaken with extreme caution). Products include:
Haldol Injection, Tablets and Concentrate 1585

Haloperidol Decanoate (Concurrent therapy should be undertaken with extreme caution). Products include:
Haldol Decanoate 1587

Imipramine Hydrochloride (Concurrent therapy should be undertaken with extreme caution). Products include:
Tofranil Ampuls 873
Tofranil Tablets 875

Imipramine Pamoate (Concurrent therapy should be undertaken with extreme caution). Products include:
Tofranil-PM Capsules 876

Isocarboxazid (Concurrent administration is contraindicated).
No products indexed under this heading.

Levodopa (Potential for higher incidence of adverse experiences). Products include:
Atamet Tablets 567
Larodopa Tablets 2296
Sinemet Tablets 959
Sinemet CR Tablets 961

Lorazepam (Concurrent therapy should be undertaken with extreme caution). Products include:
Ativan Injection 2805
Ativan Tablets 2807

Maprotiline Hydrochloride (Concurrent therapy should be undertaken with extreme caution). Products include:
Ludiomil Tablets 861

Mesoridazine Besylate (Concurrent therapy should be undertaken with extreme caution). Products include:
Serentil 689

Nortriptyline Hydrochloride (Concurrent therapy should be undertaken with extreme caution). Products include:
Pamelor 2409

Oxazepam (Concurrent therapy should be undertaken with extreme caution). Products include:
Serax Capsules 2916
Serax Tablets 2916

Perphenazine (Concurrent therapy should be undertaken with extreme caution). Products include:
Etrafon 2495
Triavil Tablets 1800
Trilafon 2532

Phenelzine Sulfate (Concurrent administration is contraindicated). Products include:
Nardil 1977

Phenobarbital (Concurrent therapy may affect metabolism of bupropion). Products include:
Arco-Lase Plus Tablets 513
Bellergal-S Tablets 2375
Donnatal 2234
Donnatal Extentabs 2234
Donnatal Tablets 2234
Phenobarbital Elixir and Tablets ... 1523
Quadrinal Tablets 1398

Phenytoin (Concurrent therapy may affect metabolism of bupropion). Products include:
Dilantin Infatabs 1967
Dilantin-125 Suspension 1969

Phenytoin Sodium (Concurrent therapy may affect metabolism of bupropion). Products include:
Dilantin Kapseals 1965

Prazepam (Concurrent therapy should be undertaken with extreme caution).
No products indexed under this heading.

Prochlorperazine (Concurrent therapy should be undertaken with extreme caution). Products include:
Compazine 2644

IMPORTANT NOTE: Always consult each drug listing in the patient's regimen for possible interactions.

Wellbutrin / Interactions Index

Promethazine Hydrochloride (Concurrent therapy should be undertaken with extreme caution). Products include:
- Mepergan Injection ... 2859
- Phenergan with Codeine ... 2883
- Phenergan with Dextromethorphan ... 2885
- Phenergan Injection ... 2880
- Phenergan Suppositories ... 2882
- Phenergan Syrup ... 2881
- Phenergan Tablets ... 2882
- Phenergan VC ... 2886
- Phenergan VC with Codeine ... 2888

Protriptyline Hydrochloride (Concurrent therapy should be undertaken with extreme caution). Products include:
- Vivactil Tablets ... 1820

Selegiline Hydrochloride (Concurrent administration is contraindicated). Products include:
- Eldepryl Capsules ... 2729

Thioridazine Hydrochloride (Concurrent therapy should be undertaken with extreme caution). Products include:
- Mellaril ... 2398

Tranylcypromine Sulfate (Concurrent administration is contraindicated). Products include:
- Parnate Tablets ... 2679

Trazodone Hydrochloride (Concurrent therapy should be undertaken with extreme caution). Products include:
- Desyrel and Desyrel Dividose ... 504

Trifluoperazine Hydrochloride (Concurrent therapy should be undertaken with extreme caution). Products include:
- Stelazine ... 2692

Trimipramine Maleate (Concurrent therapy should be undertaken with extreme caution). Products include:
- Surmontil Capsules ... 2917

Food Interactions
Alcohol (Concurrent alcohol consumption should be avoided or minimized).

WESTCORT CREAM 0.2%
(Hydrocortisone Valerate) ... 2799
None cited in PDR database.

WESTCORT OINTMENT 0.2%
(Hydrocortisone Valerate) ... 2800
None cited in PDR database.

WIGRAINE TABLETS
(Ergotamine Tartrate, Caffeine) ... 1884
None cited in PDR database.

WINRGY
(Nutritional Beverage) ... ◼ 836
May interact with:

Aluminum Carbonate (Concomitant use with aluminum-containing antacids should be avoided). Products include:
- Basaljel Capsules ... 2810
- Basaljel Suspension ... 2810
- Basaljel Tablets ... 2810

Aluminum Hydroxide (Concomitant use with aluminum-containing antacids should be avoided). Products include:
- ALternaGEL Liquid ... 1358
- Maximum Strength Ascriptin ... ◼ 650
- Cama Arthritis Pain Reliever ... ◼ 748
- Gaviscon Extra Strength Relief Formula Antacid Tablets ... ◼ 778
- Gaviscon Extra Strength Relief Formula Liquid Antacid ... ◼ 779
- Gaviscon Liquid Antacid ... ◼ 779
- Gelusil Antacid-Anti-gas Liquid ... ◼ 819
- Gelusil Antacid-Anti-gas Tablets ... ◼ 819
- Maalox Antacid/Anti-Gas Tablets ... 889
- Maalox Heartburn Relief Suspension ... ◼ 658
- Maalox Antacid Liquid ... 888
- Extra Strength Maalox Antacid/Anti-Gas Liquid and Tablets ... 888
- Mylanta ... 1359
- Tempo Soft Antacid ... ◼ 799

Aluminum Hydroxide Gel (Concomitant use with aluminum-containing antacids should be avoided). Products include:
- ALternaGEL Liquid ... ◼ 675
- Aludrox Oral Suspension ... ◼ 850
- Amphojel Suspension ... 2802
- Amphojel Suspension without Flavor ... 2802
- Amphojel Tablets ... 2802
- Ascriptin ... ◼ 650
- Gaviscon Antacid Tablets ... ◼ 778
- Gaviscon-2 Antacid Tablets ... ◼ 779
- Mylanta Liquid ... ◼ 676
- Mylanta Double Strength Liquid ... ◼ 676
- Nephrox Suspension ... ◼ 671

WINRHO SD
(Rh₀(D) Immune Globulin (Human)) ... 1839
None cited in PDR database.

WINRHO SD
(Rh₀(D) Immune Globulin (Human)) ... 1840
None cited in PDR database.

WINSTROL TABLETS
(Stanozolol) ... 2468
May interact with oral anticoagulants. Compounds in this category include:

Dicumarol (Increased sensitivity to anticoagulants).
No products indexed under this heading.

Warfarin Sodium (Increased sensitivity to anticoagulants). Products include:
- Coumadin ... 941

WYANOIDS RELIEF FACTOR HEMORRHOIDAL SUPPOSITORIES
(Liver, Desiccated, Shark Liver Oil) ... ◼ 856
None cited in PDR database.

WYGESIC TABLETS
(Propoxyphene Hydrochloride, Acetaminophen) ... 2930
May interact with central nervous system depressants, antidepressant drugs, oral anticoagulants, anticonvulsants, tranquilizers, and certain other agents. Compounds in these categories include:

Alfentanil Hydrochloride (Additive effects). Products include:
- Alfenta Injection ... 1334

Alprazolam (Additive effects). Products include:
- Xanax Tablets ... 2115

Amitriptyline Hydrochloride (Propoxyphene may slow the metabolism of antidepressants). Products include:
- Elavil ... 2945
- Etrafon ... 2495
- Limbitrol ... 2333
- Triavil Tablets ... 1800

Amoxapine (Propoxyphene may slow the metabolism of antidepressants). Products include:
- Asendin Tablets ... 1419

Aprobarbital (Additive effects).
No products indexed under this heading.

Buprenorphine (Additive effects). Products include:
- Buprenex Injectable ... 2170

Bupropion Hydrochloride (Propoxyphene may slow the metabolism of antidepressants). Products include:
- Wellbutrin Tablets ... 1177

Buspirone Hydrochloride (Additive effects). Products include:
- BuSpar Tablets ... 738

Butabarbital (Additive effects).
No products indexed under this heading.

Butalbital (Additive effects). Products include:
- Axocet Capsules ... 2469
- Esgic-plus Capsules ... 1012
- Esgic-plus Tablets ... 1012
- Fioricet Tablets ... 2386
- Fioricet with Codeine Capsules ... 2387
- Fiorinal Capsules ... 2388
- Fiorinal with Codeine Capsules ... 2390
- Fiorinal Tablets ... 2388
- Phrenilin ... 790
- Sedapap Tablets 50 mg/650 mg ... 1826

Carbamazepine (Propoxyphene may slow the metabolism of anticonvulsants). Products include:
- Atretol Tablets ... 569
- Tegretol/Tegretol-XR ... 870

Chlordiazepoxide (Additive effects). Products include:
- Limbitrol ... 2333

Chlordiazepoxide Hydrochloride (Additive effects). Products include:
- Librax Capsules ... 2330
- Librium Capsules ... 2331
- Librium Injectable ... 2332

Chlorpromazine (Additive effects). Products include:
- Thorazine Suppositories ... 2701

Chlorprothixene (Additive effects).
No products indexed under this heading.

Chlorprothixene Hydrochloride (Additive effects).
No products indexed under this heading.

Chlorprothixene Lactate (Additive effects).
No products indexed under this heading.

Clorazepate Dipotassium (Additive effects). Products include:
- Tranxene ... 459

Clozapine (Additive effects). Products include:
- Clozaril Tablets ... 2377

Codeine Phosphate (Additive effects). Products include:
- Brontex ... 2130
- Dimetane-DC Cough Syrup ... 2232
- Fioricet with Codeine Capsules ... 2387
- Fiorinal with Codeine Capsules ... 2390
- Nucofed ... 2225
- Phenergan with Codeine ... 2883
- Phenergan VC with Codeine ... 2888
- Robitussin A-C Syrup ... 2248
- Robitussin-DAC Syrup ... 2249
- Ryna ... ◼ 804
- Soma Compound w/Codeine Tablets ... 2784
- Tylenol with Codeine ... 1592

Desflurane (Additive effects). Products include:
- Suprane (desflurane, USP) ... 1865

Desipramine Hydrochloride (Propoxyphene may slow the metabolism of antidepressants). Products include:
- Norpramin Tablets ... 1273

Dezocine (Additive effects). Products include:
- Dalgan Injection ... 529

Diazepam (Additive effects). Products include:
- Dizac (diazepam injectable emulsion) CIV ... 1862
- Valium Injectable ... 2336
- Valium Tablets ... 2335

Dicumarol (Propoxyphene may slow the metabolism of warfarin-like drug).
No products indexed under this heading.

Divalproex Sodium (Propoxyphene may slow the metabolism of anticonvulsants). Products include:
- Depakote Tablets ... 418

Doxepin Hydrochloride (Propoxyphene may slow the metabolism of antidepressants). Products include:
- Adapin Capsules ... 1542
- Sinequan ... 2028
- Zonalon Cream ... 1042

Droperidol (Additive effects). Products include:
- Inapsine Injection ... 462

Enflurane (Additive effects).
No products indexed under this heading.

Estazolam (Additive effects). Products include:
- ProSom Tablets ... 457

Ethchlorvynol (Additive effects). Products include:
- Placidyl Capsules ... 456

Ethinamate (Additive effects).
No products indexed under this heading.

Ethosuximide (Propoxyphene may slow the metabolism of anticonvulsants). Products include:
- Zarontin Capsules ... 1986
- Zarontin Syrup ... 1986

Ethotoin (Propoxyphene may slow the metabolism of anticonvulsants). Products include:
- Peganone Tablets ... 455

Felbamate (Propoxyphene may slow the metabolism of anticonvulsants). Products include:
- Felbatol ... 2774

Fentanyl (Additive effects). Products include:
- Duragesic Transdermal System ... 1336

Fentanyl Citrate (Additive effects). Products include:
- Sublimaze Injection ... 463

Fluoxetine Hydrochloride (Propoxyphene may slow the metabolism of antidepressants). Products include:
- Prozac Pulvules & Liquid, Oral Solution ... 935

Fluphenazine Decanoate (Additive effects). Products include:
- Prolixin Decanoate ... 510

Fluphenazine Enanthate (Additive effects). Products include:
- Prolixin Enanthate ... 510

Fluphenazine Hydrochloride (Additive effects). Products include:
- Prolixin ... 510

Flurazepam Hydrochloride (Additive effects). Products include:
- Dalmane Capsules ... 2329

Glutethimide (Additive effects).
No products indexed under this heading.

Haloperidol (Additive effects). Products include:
- Haldol Injection, Tablets and Concentrate ... 1585

Haloperidol Decanoate (Additive effects). Products include:
- Haldol Decanoate ... 1587

Hydrocodone Bitartrate (Additive effects). Products include:
- Codiclear DH Syrup ... 808
- Duratuss HD Elixir ... 2750
- Histussin D Liquid ... 670
- Hycodan Tablets and Syrup ... 946
- Hycomine Compound Tablets ... 948
- Hycomine ... 947
- Hycotuss Expectorant Syrup ... 950
- Hydrocet Capsules ... 787
- Lorcet 10/650 Tablets ... 1016
- Lortab ... 2751
- Tussend ... 1830
- Tussend Expectorant ... 1831
- Vicodin Tablets ... 1404
- Vicodin ES Tablets ... 1405
- Vicodin HP Tablets ... 1403

(◼ Described in PDR For Nonprescription Drugs)   (⊙ Described in PDR For Ophthalmology)

Interactions Index / Xanax

Vicodin Tuss Expectorant	1406
Zydone Capsules	967

Hydrocodone Polistirex (Additive effects). Products include:
Tussionex Pennkinetic Extended-Release Suspension	1624

Hydroxyzine Hydrochloride (Additive effects). Products include:
Atarax Tablets & Syrup	1992
Marax Tablets & DF Syrup	2015
Vistaril Intramuscular Solution	2042

Imipramine Hydrochloride (Propoxyphene may slow the metabolism of antidepressants). Products include:
Tofranil Ampuls	873
Tofranil Tablets	875

Imipramine Pamoate (Propoxyphene may slow the metabolism of antidepressants). Products include:
Tofranil-PM Capsules	876

Isocarboxazid (Propoxyphene may slow the metabolism of antidepressants).
No products indexed under this heading.

Isoflurane (Additive effects).
No products indexed under this heading.

Ketamine Hydrochloride (Additive effects).
No products indexed under this heading.

Lamotrigine (Propoxyphene may slow the metabolism of anticonvulsants). Products include:
Lamictal Tablets	1105

Levomethadyl Acetate Hydrochloride (Additive effects). Products include:
Orlaam Oral Solution	2361

Levorphanol Tartrate (Additive effects). Products include:
Levo-Dromoran	2297

Lorazepam (Additive effects). Products include:
Ativan Injection	2805
Ativan Tablets	2807

Loxapine Hydrochloride (Additive effects). Products include:
Loxitane	1426

Loxapine Succinate (Additive effects). Products include:
Loxitane Capsules	1426

Maprotiline Hydrochloride (Propoxyphene may slow the metabolism of antidepressants). Products include:
Ludiomil Tablets	861

Meperidine Hydrochloride (Additive effects). Products include:
Demerol	2438
Mepergan Injection	2859

Mephenytoin (Propoxyphene may slow the metabolism of anticonvulsants). Products include:
Mesantoin Tablets	2400

Mephobarbital (Additive effects). Products include:
Mebaral Tablets	2452

Meprobamate (Additive effects). Products include:
Miltown Tablets	2780
PMB 200 and PMB 400	2890

Mesoridazine Besylate (Additive effects). Products include:
Serentil	689

Methadone Hydrochloride (Additive effects). Products include:
Methadone Hydrochloride Oral Concentrate	2356
Methadone Hydrochloride Oral Solution & Tablets	2357

Methohexital Sodium (Additive effects).
No products indexed under this heading.

Methotrimeprazine (Additive effects). Products include:
Levoprome	1321

Methoxyflurane (Additive effects).
No products indexed under this heading.

Methsuximide (Propoxyphene may slow the metabolism of anticonvulsants). Products include:
Celontin Kapseals	1955

Midazolam Hydrochloride (Additive effects). Products include:
Versed Injection	2324

Molindone Hydrochloride (Additive effects). Products include:
Moban Tablets and Concentrate	1036

Morphine Sulfate (Additive effects). Products include:
Astramorph/PF Injection, USP (Preservative-Free)	526
Duramorph Injection	983
Infumorph 200 and Infumorph 500 Sterile Solutions	985
Kadian Capsules	2948
MS Contin Tablets	2149
MSIR	2152
Oramorph SR (Morphine Sulfate Sustained Release Tablets)	2359
RMS Suppositories CII	2766
Roxanol	2365

Nefazodone Hydrochloride (Propoxyphene may slow the metabolism of antidepressants). Products include:
Serzone Tablets	776

Nortriptyline Hydrochloride (Propoxyphene may slow the metabolism of antidepressants). Products include:
Pamelor	2409

Opium Alkaloids (Additive effects).
No products indexed under this heading.

Oxazepam (Additive effects). Products include:
Serax Capsules	2916
Serax Tablets	2916

Oxycodone Hydrochloride (Additive effects). Products include:
OxyContin Tablets	2163
OxyIR Capsules	2167
Percocet Tablets	955
Percodan Tablets	955
Percodan-Demi Tablets	956
Roxicodone Tablets, Oral Solution & Intensol (Oxycodone)	2366
Tylox Capsules	1593

Paramethadione (Propoxyphene may slow the metabolism of anticonvulsants).
No products indexed under this heading.

Paroxetine Hydrochloride (Propoxyphene may slow the metabolism of antidepressants). Products include:
Paxil Tablets	2681

Pentobarbital Sodium (Additive effects). Products include:
Nembutal Sodium Capsules	440
Nembutal Sodium Solution	442
Nembutal Sodium Suppositories	444

Perphenazine (Additive effects). Products include:
Etrafon	2495
Triavil Tablets	1800
Trilafon	2532

Phenacemide (Propoxyphene may slow the metabolism of anticonvulsants). Products include:
Phenurone Tablets	455

Phenelzine Sulfate (Propoxyphene may slow the metabolism of antidepressants). Products include:
Nardil	1977

Phenobarbital (Additive effects; propoxyphene may slow the metabolism of anticonvulsants). Products include:
Arco-Lase Plus Tablets	513
Bellergal-S Tablets	2375
Donnatal	2234
Donnatal Extentabs	2234
Donnatal Tablets	2234
Phenobarbital Elixir and Tablets	1523
Quadrinal Tablets	1398

Phensuximide (Propoxyphene may slow the metabolism of anticonvulsants).
No products indexed under this heading.

Phenytoin (Propoxyphene may slow the metabolism of anticonvulsants). Products include:
Dilantin Infatabs	1967
Dilantin-125 Suspension	1969

Phenytoin Sodium (Propoxyphene may slow the metabolism of anticonvulsants). Products include:
Dilantin Kapseals	1965

Prazepam (Additive effects).
No products indexed under this heading.

Primidone (Propoxyphene may slow the metabolism of anticonvulsants). Products include:
Mysoline	2860

Prochlorperazine (Additive effects). Products include:
Compazine	2644

Promethazine Hydrochloride (Additive effects). Products include:
Mepergan Injection	2859
Phenergan with Codeine	2883
Phenergan with Dextromethorphan	2885
Phenergan Injection	2880
Phenergan Suppositories	2882
Phenergan Syrup	2881
Phenergan Tablets	2882
Phenergan VC	2886
Phenergan VC with Codeine	2888

Propofol (Additive effects). Products include:
Diprivan Injectable Emulsion	2939

Propoxyphene Napsylate (Additive effects). Products include:
Darvon-N/Darvocet-N	1473

Protriptyline Hydrochloride (Propoxyphene may slow the metabolism of antidepressants). Products include:
Vivactil Tablets	1820

Quazepam (Additive effects). Products include:
Doral Tablets	2773

Risperidone (Additive effects). Products include:
Risperdal Tablets	1348

Secobarbital Sodium (Additive effects). Products include:
Seconal Sodium Pulvules	1529

Sertraline Hydrochloride (Propoxyphene may slow the metabolism of antidepressants). Products include:
Zoloft Tablets	2051

Sevoflurane (Additive effects).
No products indexed under this heading.

Sufentanil Citrate (Additive effects). Products include:
Sufenta Injection	1355

Temazepam (Additive effects). Products include:
Restoril Capsules	2413

Thiamylal Sodium (Additive effects).
No products indexed under this heading.

Thioridazine Hydrochloride (Additive effects). Products include:
Mellaril	2398

Thiothixene (Additive effects). Products include:
Navane Capsules and Concentrate	2018
Navane Intramuscular	2019

Tranylcypromine Sulfate (Propoxyphene may slow the metabolism of antidepressants). Products include:
Parnate Tablets	2679

Trazodone Hydrochloride (Propoxyphene may slow the metabolism of antidepressants). Products include:
Desyrel and Desyrel Dividose	504

Triazolam (Additive effects). Products include:
Halcion Tablets	2093

Trifluoperazine Hydrochloride (Additive effects). Products include:
Stelazine	2692

Trimethadione (Propoxyphene may slow the metabolism of anticonvulsants).
No products indexed under this heading.

Trimipramine Maleate (Propoxyphene may slow the metabolism of antidepressants). Products include:
Surmontil Capsules	2917

Valproic Acid (Propoxyphene may slow the metabolism of anticonvulsants). Products include:
Depakene	416

Venlafaxine Hydrochloride (Propoxyphene may slow the metabolism of antidepressants). Products include:
Effexor	2825

Warfarin Sodium (Propoxyphene may slow the metabolism of warfarin-like drug). Products include:
Coumadin	941

Zolpidem Tartrate (Additive effects). Products include:
Ambien Tablets	2559

Food Interactions
Alcohol (Additive effects).

XALATAN
(Latanoprost) ... ⊙ 304

May interact with:

Thimerosal (*In vitro* studies have shown that precipitation occurs when eye drops containing thiomersal are mixed with Xalatan; administer with an interval of at least five minutes between applications).
No products indexed under this heading.

XANAX TABLETS
(Alprazolam) ... 2115

May interact with central nervous system depressants, anticonvulsants, antihistamines, oral contraceptives, and certain other agents. Compounds in these categories include:

Acrivastine (Additive CNS depressant effects). Products include:
Semprex-D Capsules	1620

Alfentanil Hydrochloride (Additive CNS depressant effects). Products include:
Alfenta Injection	1334

Amiodarone Hydrochloride (Possible interaction based on data from *in vitro* studies of other benzodiazepines suggests a possible interaction when co-administered; concurrent use requires caution). Products include:
Cordarone Intravenous	2821
Cordarone Tablets	2818

IMPORTANT NOTE: Always consult each drug listing in the patient's regimen for possible interactions.

Xanax — Interactions Index

Aprobarbital (Additive CNS depressant effects).
No products indexed under this heading.

Astemizole (Additive CNS depressant effects). Products include:
Hismanal Tablets ... 1341

Azatadine Maleate (Additive CNS depressant effects). Products include:
Trinalin Repetabs Tablets ... 1373

Bromodiphenhydramine Hydrochloride (Additive CNS depressant effects).
No products indexed under this heading.

Brompheniramine Maleate (Additive CNS depressant effects). Products include:
Alka-Seltzer Plus Sinus Medicine .. ◨ 611
Bromfed Capsules (Extended-Release) ... 1832
Bromfed Syrup ... ◨ 712
Bromfed Tablets ... 1832
Bromfed-DM Cough Syrup ... 1832
Bromfed-PD Capsules (Extended-Release) ... 1832
Dimetane-DC Cough Syrup ... 2232
Dimetane-DX Cough Syrup ... 2233
Dimetapp Allergy Dye-Free Elixir ... ◨ 838
Dimetapp Allergy Sinus Caplets ... ◨ 838
Dimetapp Cold & Allergy Chewable Tablets ... ◨ 838
Dimetapp Cold & Cough Liqui-Gels ... ◨ 839
Dimetapp Cold & Fever Suspension ... ◨ 839
Dimetapp DM Elixir ... ◨ 840
Dimetapp Elixir ... ◨ 840
Dimetapp Extentabs ... ◨ 841
Dimetapp Tablets/Liqui-Gels ... ◨ 841
Rondec Chewable Tablets ... 974
Vicks DayQuil Allergy Relief 12-Hour Extended Release Tablets. ◨ 733
Vicks DayQuil Allergy Relief 4-Hour Tablets ... ◨ 733

Buprenorphine (Additive CNS depressant effects). Products include:
Buprenex Injectable ... 2170

Buspirone Hydrochloride (Additive CNS depressant effects). Products include:
BuSpar Tablets ... 738

Butabarbital (Additive CNS depressant effects).
No products indexed under this heading.

Butalbital (Additive CNS depressant effects). Products include:
Axocet Capsules ... 2469
Esgic-plus Capsules ... 1012
Esgic-plus Tablets ... 1012
Fioricet Tablets ... 2386
Fioricet with Codeine Capsules ... 2387
Fiorinal Capsules ... 2388
Fiorinal with Codeine Capsules ... 2390
Fiorinal Tablets ... 2388
Phrenilin ... 790
Sedapap Tablets 50 mg/650 mg .. 1826

Carbamazepine (Additive CNS depressant effects). Products include:
Atretol Tablets ... 569
Tegretol/Tegretol-XR ... 870

Cetirizine Hydrochloride (Additive CNS depressant effects). Products include:
Zyrtec Tablets ... 2053

Chlordiazepoxide (Additive CNS depressant effects). Products include:
Limbitrol ... 2333

Chlordiazepoxide Hydrochloride (Additive CNS depressant effects). Products include:
Librax Capsules ... 2330
Librium Capsules ... 2331
Librium Injectable ... 2332

Chlorpheniramine Maleate (Additive CNS depressant effects). Products include:
Alka-Seltzer Plus Cold Medicine ... ◨ 611
Alka-Seltzer Plus Cold Medicine Liqui-Gels ... ◨ 612
Alka-Seltzer Plus Cold & Cough Medicine ... ◨ 611
Alka-Seltzer Plus Cold & Cough Medicine Liqui-Gels ... ◨ 612
Alka-Seltzer Plus Flu & Body Aches Effervescent Tablets ... ◨ 612
Allerest Maximum Strength ... ◨ 649
Allerest Sinus Pain Formula ... ◨ 649
Ana-Kit Anaphylaxis Emergency Treatment Kit ... 611
Atrohist Pediatric Capsules ... 1603
Atrohist Plus Tablets ... 1605
BC Cold Powder Multi-Symptom Formula (Cold-Sinus-Allergy) ... ◨ 631
Cerose DM ... ◨ 853
Ceracol Plus Head Cold/Cough Formula ... ◨ 741
Children's TYLENOL Cold Multi-Symptom Chewable Tablets and Liquid ... 1559
Children's TYLENOL Cold Plus Cough Multi Symptom Chewable Tablets and Liquid ... 1560
Children's TYLENOL Flu Suspension Liquid ... 1560
Children's Vicks DayQuil Allergy Relief ... ◨ 730
Children's Vicks NyQuil Cold/Cough Relief ... ◨ 731
Chlor-Trimeton Allergy Decongestant Tablets ... 759
Chlor-Trimeton Allergy Tablets ... 758
Allergy-Sinus Comtrex Multi-Symptom Allergy-Sinus Formula Tablets and Caplets ... ◨ 639
Comtrex Multi-Symptom ... ◨ 638
Contac Continuous Action Nasal Decongestant/Antihistamine 12 Hour Capsules ... ◨ 773
Contac Maximum Strength Continuous Action Decongestant/Antihistamine 12 Hour Caplets. ◨ 772
Contac Severe Cold and Flu Formula Caplets ... ◨ 773
Coricidin Cold + Flu Tablets ... ◨ 760
Coricidin Cough + Cold Tablets ... ◨ 760
Coricidin 'D' Decongestant Tablets ... ◨ 760
D.A. II Tablets ... 972
D.A. Chewable Tablets ... 970
Dura-Tap/PD Capsules ... 970
Dura-Vent/DA Tablets ... 972
Efidac 24 Chlorpheniramine ... ◨ 655
Extendryl ... 1003
Fedahist Gyrocaps ... 2545
Hycomine Compound Tablets ... 948
Kronofed-A ... 994
Nolamine Timed-Release Tablets ... 790
Novahistine Elixir ... ◨ 782
Ornade Spansule Capsules ... 2678
PediaCare Cough-Cold Chewable Tablets and Liquid ... 1569
PediaCare NightRest Cough-Cold Liquid ... 1569
Pediatric Vicks 44m Cough & Cold Relief ... ◨ 737
Pyrroxate Caplets ... 742
Ryna ... ◨ 804
Sinarest ... ◨ 663
Sine-Off Sinus Medicine ... ◨ 784
Singlet Tablets ... ◨ 785
Sinulin Tablets ... 792
Sinutab Sinus Allergy Medication, Maximum Strength Tablets and Caplets ... ◨ 823
Sudafed Cold & Allergy Tablets ... ◨ 826
Teldrin 12 Hour Antihistamine/Nasal Decongestant Allergy Relief Capsules ... ◨ 786
TheraFlu Flu and Cold Medicine ... ◨ 750
Theraflu Maximum Strength Flu and Cold Medicine For Sore Throat ... ◨ 751
TheraFlu Flu, Cold and Cough Medicine ... ◨ 750
TheraFlu Maximum Strength Nighttime Flu, Cold & Cough Medicine ... ◨ 751
Triaminic Night Time ... ◨ 754
Triaminic Syrup ... ◨ 755
Triaminic Triaminicol Cold & Cough ... ◨ 756
Triaminicin Tablets ... ◨ 756
Tussend ... 1830

TYLENOL Allergy Sinus, Maximum Strength Caplets and Gelcaps ... 1571
TYLENOL Cold Medication, Multi-Symptom Formula Tablets and Caplets ... 1572
TYLENOL Cold Medication, Multi-Symptom Hot Liquid Packets ... 1572
Vicks 44 LiquiCaps Cough, Cold & Flu Relief ... ◨ 728
Vicks 44M Cough, Cold & Flu Relief ... ◨ 729

Chlorpheniramine Polistirex (Additive CNS depressant effects). Products include:
Tussionex Pennkinetic Extended-Release Suspension ... 1624

Chlorpheniramine Tannate (Additive CNS depressant effects). Products include:
Atrohist Pediatric Suspension ... 1604
Atrohist Pediatric Suspension Dye-Free ... 1604
Rynatan ... 2781
Rynatuss ... 2782

Chlorpromazine (Additive CNS depressant effects). Products include:
Thorazine Suppositories ... 2701

Chlorpromazine Hydrochloride (Additive CNS depressant effects). Products include:
Thorazine ... 2701

Chlorprothixene (Additive CNS depressant effects).
No products indexed under this heading.

Chlorprothixene Hydrochloride (Additive CNS depressant effects).
No products indexed under this heading.

Chlorprothixene Lactate (Additive CNS depressant effects).
No products indexed under this heading.

Cimetidine (Co-administration of cimetidine has increased the maximum plasma concentration of alprazolam by 86%, decreased clearance by 42%, and increased half-life by 16%). Products include:
Tagamet HB Tablets ... ◨ 786
Tagamet Tablets ... 2694

Cimetidine Hydrochloride (Co-administration of cimetidine has increased the maximum plasma concentration of alprazolam by 86%, decreased clearance by 42%, and increased half-life by 16%). Products include:
Tagamet ... 2694

Clarithromycin (Possible interaction based on the clinical studies involving other benzodiazepines metabolized similarly as alprazolam; co-administration requires caution). Products include:
Biaxin ... 406

Clemastine Fumarate (Additive CNS depressant effects). Products include:
Tavist Syrup ... 2426
Tavist Tablets ... 2427
Tavist-1 12 Hour Relief Tablets ... ◨ 749
Tavist-D 12 Hour Relief Tablets ... ◨ 750

Clorazepate Dipotassium (Additive CNS depressant effects). Products include:
Tranxene ... 459

Clozapine (Additive CNS depressant effects). Products include:
Clozaril Tablets ... 2377

Codeine Phosphate (Additive CNS depressant effects). Products include:
Brontex ... 2130
Dimetane-DC Cough Syrup ... 2232
Fioricet with Codeine Capsules ... 2387
Fiorinal with Codeine Capsules ... 2390
Nucofed ... 2225
Phenergan with Codeine ... 2883
Phenergan VC with Codeine ... 2888

Robitussin A-C Syrup ... 2248
Robitussin-DAC Syrup ... 2249
Ryna ... ◨ 804
Soma Compound w/Codeine Tablets ... 2784
Tylenol with Codeine ... 1592

Cyclosporine (Possible interaction based on the data from in vitro studies of other benzodiazepines suggests a possible interaction when co-administered; concurrent use requires caution). Products include:
Neoral ... 2405
Sandimmune ... 2416

Cyproheptadine Hydrochloride (Additive CNS depressant effects). Products include:
Periactin ... 1767

Desflurane (Additive CNS depressant effects). Products include:
Suprane (desflurane, USP) ... 1865

Desipramine Hydrochloride (Increased steady state-plasma concentrations of desipramine by 20%). Products include:
Norpramin Tablets ... 1273

Desogestrel (Co-administration of oral contraceptives has increased the maximum plasma concentration of alprazolam by 18%, decreased clearance by 2%, and increased half-life by 29%). Products include:
Desogen Tablets ... 1867
Ortho-Cept ... 1907

Dexchlorpheniramine Maleate (Additive CNS depressant effects).
No products indexed under this heading.

Dezocine (Additive CNS depressant effects). Products include:
Dalgan Injection ... 529

Diazepam (Additive CNS depressant effects). Products include:
Dizac (diazepam injectable emulsion) CIV ... 1862
Valium Injectable ... 2336
Valium Tablets ... 2335

Diltiazem Hydrochloride (Possible interaction based on the clinical studies involving other benzodiazepines metabolized similarly as alprazolam; co-administration requires caution). Products include:
Cardizem CD Capsules ... 1251
Cardizem SR Capsules ... 1255
Cardizem Injectable ... 1253
Cardizem Tablets ... 1257
Dilacor XR Extended-release Capsules ... 2183
Tiazac Capsules ... 1019

Diphenhydramine Citrate (Additive CNS depressant effects). Products include:
Excedrin P.M. Analgesic/Sleeping Aid Tablets, Caplets, Liquigels ... 735

Diphenhydramine Hydrochloride (Additive CNS depressant effects). Products include:
Actifed Allergy Daytime/Nighttime Caplets ... ◨ 808
Actifed Sinus Daytime/Nighttime Tablets and Caplets ... ◨ 809
Extra Strength Bayer PM Aspirin Plus Sleep Aid ... ◨ 617
Benadryl Allergy Chewables ... ◨ 811
Benadryl Allergy/Cold Tablets ... ◨ 811
Benadryl Allergy Decongestant Liquid Medication ... ◨ 812
Benadryl Allergy Decongestant Tablets ... ◨ 812
Benadryl Allergy Liquid Medication ... ◨ 813
Benadryl Allergy ... ◨ 811
Benadryl Allergy Sinus Headache Caplets ... ◨ 813
Benadryl Dye-Free Allergy Liquigel Softgels ... ◨ 813
Benadryl Dye-Free Allergy Liquid Medication ... ◨ 814
Benadryl Itch Relief Stick Extra Strength ... ◨ 814
Benadryl Cream ... ◨ 814
Benadryl Gel ... ◨ 815

(◨ Described in PDR For Nonprescription Drugs)   (⊙ Described in PDR For Ophthalmology)

Benadryl Spray 815
Benadryl Injection 1955
Contac Day & Night Cold/Flu Night Caplets 772
Contac Night Allergy/Sinus Caplets 771
Extra Strength Doan's P.M. 653
Excedrin P.M. Analgesic/Sleeping Aid Tablets, Caplets, Liquigels 643
Nytol QuickCaps Caplets 632
Sleepinal Night-time Sleep Aid Capsules and Softgels 798
TYLENOL Allergy Sinus NightTime, Maximum Strength Caplets 1571
TYLENOL Flu NightTime, Maximum Strength Gelcaps 1575
TYLENOL Flu NightTime, Maximum Strength Hot Medication Packets 1575
TYLENOL PM Pain Reliever/Sleep Aid, Extra Strength Gelcaps, Caplets, Geltabs 1576
TYLENOL Severe Allergy Medication Caplets 1571
Maximum Strength Unisom Sleepgels 1990
Unisom With Pain Relief-Nighttime Sleep Aid and Pain Reliever 1991

Diphenylpyraline Hydrochloride (Additive CNS depressant effects).
No products indexed under this heading.

Divalproex Sodium (Additive CNS depressant effects). Products include:
Depakote Tablets 418

Droperidol (Additive CNS depressant effects). Products include:
Inapsine Injection 462

Enflurane (Additive CNS depressant effects).
No products indexed under this heading.

Ergotamine Tartrate (Possible interaction based on the data from *in vitro* studies of other benzodiazepines suggests a possible interaction when co-administered; concurrent use requires caution). Products include:
Bellergal-S Tablets 2375
Cafergot 2376
Ergomar Tablets 1543
Wigraine Tablets 1884

Erythromycin (Possible interaction based on the clinical studies involving other benzodiazepines metabolized similarly as alprazolam; co-administration requires caution). Products include:
A/T/S 2% Acne Topical Gel 1244
A/T/S 2% Acne Topical Solution 1244
Benzamycin Topical Gel 919
E-Mycin Tablets 1388
Emgel 2% Topical Gel 1081
ERYC 1972
Erycette (erythromycin 2%) Topical Solution 1943
Ery-Tab Tablets 426
Erythromycin Base Filmtab 430
Erythromycin Delayed-Release Capsules, USP 431
Ilotycin Ophthalmic Ointment 928
PCE Dispertab Tablets 453
T-Stat 2.0% Topical Solution and Pads 2797
THERAMYCIN Z 2% Solution 1629

Erythromycin Estolate (Possible interaction based on the clinical studies involving other benzodiazepines metabolized similarly as alprazolam; co-administration requires caution). Products include:
Ilosone 927

Erythromycin Ethylsuccinate (Possible interaction based on the clinical studies involving other benzodiazepines metabolized similarly as alprazolam; co-administration requires caution). Products include:
E.E.S. 427
EryPed 425
Pediazole Suspension 2340

Erythromycin Gluceptate (Possible interaction based on the clinical studies involving other benzodiazepines metabolized similarly as alprazolam; co-administration requires caution). Products include:
Ilotycin Gluceptate, IV, Vials 929

Erythromycin Stearate (Possible interaction based on the clinical studies involving other benzodiazepines metabolized similarly as alprazolam; co-administration requires caution). Products include:
Erythrocin Stearate Filmtab 429

Estazolam (Additive CNS depressant effects). Products include:
ProSom Tablets 457

Ethchlorvynol (Additive CNS depressant effects). Products include:
Placidyl Capsules 456

Ethinamate (Additive CNS depressant effects).
No products indexed under this heading.

Ethinyl Estradiol (Co-administration of oral contraceptives has increased the maximum plasma concentration of alprazolam by 18%, decreased clearance by 2%, and increased half-life by 29%). Products include:
Brevicon 2563
Demulen 2580
Desogen Tablets 1867
Levlen/Tri-Levlen 646
Lo/Ovral Tablets 2852
Lo/Ovral-28 Tablets 2857
Modicon 1928
Nordette-21 Tablets 2863
Nordette-28 Tablets 2866
Norinyl 2563
Ortho-Cept 1907
Ortho-Cyclen/Ortho-Tri-Cyclen 1914
Ortho-Novum 1928
Ortho-Cyclen/Ortho Tri-Cyclen 1914
Ovcon 765
Ovral Tablets 2877
Ovral-28 Tablets 2878
Levlen/Tri-Levlen 646
Tri-Norinyl 2607
Triphasil-21 Tablets 2919
Triphasil-28 Tablets 2924

Ethosuximide (Additive CNS depressant effects). Products include:
Zarontin Capsules 1986
Zarontin Syrup 1986

Ethotoin (Additive CNS depressant effects). Products include:
Peganone Tablets 455

Ethynodiol Diacetate (Co-administration of oral contraceptives has increased the maximum plasma concentration of alprazolam by 18%, decreased clearance by 2%, and increased half-life by 29%). Products include:
Demulen 2580

Felbamate (Additive CNS depressant effects). Products include:
Felbatol 2774

Fentanyl (Additive CNS depressant effects). Products include:
Duragesic Transdermal System 1336

Fentanyl Citrate (Additive CNS depressant effects). Products include:
Sublimaze Injection 463

Fluconazole (Other azole-type antifungal agents should be considered potent CYP 3A inhibitors and they may have an effect on alprozolam clearance; co-administration is not recommended). Products include:
Diflucan Tablets, Injection, and Oral Suspension 2003

Fluoxetine Hydrochloride (Co-administration of fluoxetine has increased the maximum plasma concentration of alprazolam by 46%, decreased clearance by 21%, increased half-life by 17%, and decreased measured psychomotor performance). Products include:
Prozac Pulvules & Liquid, Oral Solution 935

Fluphenazine Decanoate (Additive CNS depressant effects). Products include:
Prolixin Decanoate 510

Fluphenazine Enanthate (Additive CNS depressant effects). Products include:
Prolixin Enanthate 510

Fluphenazine Hydrochloride (Additive CNS depressant effects). Products include:
Prolixin 510

Flurazepam Hydrochloride (Additive CNS depressant effects). Products include:
Dalmane Capsules 2329

Fluvoxamine Maleate (Co-administration of fluvoxamine approximately doubled the maximum plasma concentration of alprazolam, decreased clearance by 49%, increased half-life by 71%, and decreased measured psychomotor performance). Products include:
LUVOX Tablets 2723

Fosphenytoin Sodium (Additive CNS depressant effects). Products include:
Cerebyx Injection 1956

Glutethimide (Additive CNS depressant effects).
No products indexed under this heading.

Haloperidol (Additive CNS depressant effects). Products include:
Haldol Injection, Tablets and Concentrate 1585

Haloperidol Decanoate (Additive CNS depressant effects). Products include:
Haldol Decanoate 1587

Hydrocodone Bitartrate (Additive CNS depressant effects). Products include:
Codiclear DH Syrup 808
Duratuss HD Elixir 2750
Histussin D Liquid 670
Hycodan Tablets and Syrup 946
Hycomine Compound Tablets 948
Hycomine 947
Hycotuss Expectorant Syrup 950
Hydrocet Capsules 787
Lorcet 10/650 Tablets 1016
Lortab 2751
Tussend 1830
Tussend Expectorant 1831
Vicodin Tablets 1404
Vicodin ES Tablets 1405
Vicodin HP Tablets 1403
Vicodin Tuss Expectorant 1406
Zydone Capsules 967

Hydrocodone Polistirex (Additive CNS depressant effects). Products include:
Tussionex Pennkinetic Extended-Release Suspension 1624

Hydromorphone Hydrochloride (Additive CNS depressant effects). Products include:
Dilaudid Ampules 1382
Dilaudid Cough Syrup 1383
Dilaudid-HP Injection 1384
Dilaudid-HP Lyophilized Powder 250 mg 1384
Dilaudid 1382
Dilaudid Oral Liquid 1386
Dilaudid 1382
Dilaudid Tablets - 8 mg 1386

Hydroxyzine Hydrochloride (Additive CNS depressant effects). Products include:
Atarax Tablets & Syrup 1992
Marax Tablets & DF Syrup 2015
Vistaril Intramuscular Solution 2042

Imipramine Hydrochloride (Increased steady state-plasma concentrations of imipramine by 31%). Products include:
Tofranil Ampuls 873
Tofranil Tablets 875

Imipramine Pamoate (Increased steady state-plasma concentrations of imipramine by 31%). Products include:
Tofranil-PM Capsules 876

Isoflurane (Additive CNS depressant effects).
No products indexed under this heading.

Isoniazid (Possible interaction based on the clinical studies involving other benzodiazepines metabolized similarly as alprazolam; co-administration requires caution). Products include:
Nydrazid Injection 509
Rifamate Capsules 1278
Rifater 1280

Itraconazole (Co-administration with drugs that inhibit metabolism via cytochrome P450 3A, such as itraconazole, may have profound effect on the clearance of alprazolam; concurrent use is contraindicated). Products include:
Sporanox Capsules 1352

Ketamine Hydrochloride (Additive CNS depressant effects).
No products indexed under this heading.

Ketoconazole (Co-administration with drugs that inhibit metabolism via cytochrome P450 3A, such as ketoconazole, may have profound effect on the clearance of alprozolam; concurrent use is contraindicated). Products include:
Nizoral 2% Cream 1344
Nizoral 2% Shampoo 1344
Nizoral Tablets 1345

Lamotrigine (Additive CNS depressant effects). Products include:
Lamictal Tablets 1105

Levomethadyl Acetate Hydrochloride (Additive CNS depressant effects). Products include:
Orlaam Oral Solution 2361

Levonorgestrel (Co-administration of oral contraceptives has increased the maximum plasma concentration of alprazolam by 18%, decreased clearance by 2%, and increased half-life by 29%). Products include:
Levlen/Tri-Levlen 646
Nordette-21 Tablets 2863
Nordette-28 Tablets 2866
Norplant System 2868
Levlen/Tri-Levlen 646
Triphasil-21 Tablets 2919
Triphasil-28 Tablets 2924

Levorphanol Tartrate (Additive CNS depressant effects). Products include:
Levo-Dromoran 2297

Loratadine (Additive CNS depressant effects). Products include:
Claritin Tablets 2485
Claritin-D Tablets 2487

Lorazepam (Additive CNS depressant effects). Products include:
Ativan Injection 2805
Ativan Tablets 2807

Loxapine Hydrochloride (Additive CNS depressant effects). Products include:
Loxitane 1426

IMPORTANT NOTE: Always consult each drug listing in the patient's regimen for possible interactions.

Xanax / Interactions Index

Loxapine Succinate (Additive CNS depressant effects). Products include:
- Loxitane Capsules 1426

Meperidine Hydrochloride (Additive CNS depressant effects). Products include:
- Demerol 2438
- Mepergan Injection 2859

Mephenytoin (Additive CNS depressant effects). Products include:
- Mesantoin Tablets 2400

Mephobarbital (Additive CNS depressant effects). Products include:
- Mebaral Tablets 2452

Meprobamate (Additive CNS depressant effects). Products include:
- Miltown Tablets 2780
- PMB 200 and PMB 400 2890

Mesoridazine Besylate (Additive CNS depressant effects). Products include:
- Serentil 689

Mestranol (Co-administration of oral contraceptives has increased the maximum plasma concentration of alprazolam by 18%, decreased clearance by 2%, and increased half-life by 29%). Products include:
- Norinyl 2563
- Ortho-Novum 1928

Methadone Hydrochloride (Additive CNS depressant effects). Products include:
- Methadone Hydrochloride Oral Concentrate 2356
- Methadone Hydrochloride Oral Solution & Tablets 2357

Methdilazine Hydrochloride (Additive CNS depressant effects).
No products indexed under this heading.

Methohexital Sodium (Additive CNS depressant effects).
No products indexed under this heading.

Methotrimeprazine (Additive CNS depressant effects). Products include:
- Levoprome 1321

Methoxyflurane (Additive CNS depressant effects).
No products indexed under this heading.

Methsuximide (Additive CNS depressant effects). Products include:
- Celontin Kapseals 1955

Midazolam Hydrochloride (Additive CNS depressant effects). Products include:
- Versed Injection 2324

Molindone Hydrochloride (Additive CNS depressant effects). Products include:
- Moban Tablets and Concentrate 1036

Morphine Sulfate (Additive CNS depressant effects). Products include:
- Astramorph/PF Injection, USP (Preservative-Free) 526
- Duramorph Injection 983
- Infumorph 200 and Infumorph 500 Sterile Solutions 985
- Kadian Capsules 2948
- MS Contin Tablets 2149
- MSIR 2152
- Oramorph SR (Morphine Sulfate Sustained Release Tablets) 2359
- RMS Suppositories CII 2766
- Roxanol 2365

Nefazodone Hydrochloride (Co-administration has resulted in increased alprazolam concentration two-fold). Products include:
- Serzone Tablets 776

Nicardipine Hydrochloride (Possible interaction based on the data from *in vitro* studies of other benzodiazepines suggests a possible interaction when co-administered; concurrent use requires caution). Products include:
- Cardene Capsules 2261
- Cardene I.V. 2815
- Cardene SR Capsules 2264

Nifedipine (Possible interaction based on the data from *in vitro* studies of other benzodiazepines suggests a possible interaction when co-administered; concurrent use requires caution). Products include:
- Adalat Capsules (10 mg and 20 mg) 580
- Adalat CC 582
- Procardia Capsules 2024
- Procardia XL Extended Release Tablets 2026

Norethindrone (Co-administration of oral contraceptives has increased the maximum plasma concentration of alprazolam by 18%, decreased clearance by 2%, and increased half-life by 29%). Products include:
- Brevicon 2563
- Micronor Tablets 1903
- Modicon 1928
- Norinyl 2563
- Nor-Q D Tablets 2598
- Ortho-Novum 1928
- Ovcon 765
- Tri-Norinyl 2607

Norethynodrel (Co-administration of oral contraceptives has increased the maximum plasma concentration of alprazolam by 18%, decreased clearance by 2%, and increased half-life by 29%).
No products indexed under this heading.

Norgestimate (Co-administration of oral contraceptives has increased the maximum plasma concentration of alprazolam by 18%, decreased clearance by 2%, and increased half-life by 29%). Products include:
- Ortho-Cyclen/Ortho-Tri-Cyclen 1914
- Ortho-Cyclen/Ortho-Tri-Cyclen 1914

Norgestrel (Co-administration of oral contraceptives has increased the maximum plasma concentration of alprazolam by 18%, decreased clearance by 2%, and increased half-life by 29%). Products include:
- Lo/Ovral Tablets 2852
- Lo/Ovral-28 Tablets 2857
- Ovral Tablets 2877
- Ovral-28 Tablets 2878
- Ovrette Tablets 2878

Opium Alkaloids (Additive CNS depressant effects).
No products indexed under this heading.

Oxazepam (Additive CNS depressant effects). Products include:
- Serax Capsules 2916
- Serax Tablets 2916

Oxycodone Hydrochloride (Additive CNS depressant effects). Products include:
- OxyContin Tablets 2163
- OxyIR Capsules 2167
- Percocet Tablets 955
- Percodan Tablets 955
- Percodan-Demi Tablets 956
- Roxicodone Tablets, Oral Solution & Intensol (Oxycodone) 2366
- Tylox Capsules 1593

Paramethadione (Additive CNS depressant effects).
No products indexed under this heading.

Paroxetine Hydrochloride (Possible interaction based on the data from *in vitro* studies suggest a possible interaction when co-administered; concurrent use requires caution). Products include:
- Paxil Tablets 2681

Pentobarbital Sodium (Additive CNS depressant effects). Products include:
- Nembutal Sodium Capsules 440
- Nembutal Sodium Solution 442
- Nembutal Sodium Suppositories 444

Perphenazine (Additive CNS depressant effects). Products include:
- Etrafon 2495
- Triavil Tablets 1800
- Trilafon 2532

Phenacemide (Additive CNS depressant effects). Products include:
- Phenurone Tablets 455

Phenobarbital (Additive CNS depressant effects). Products include:
- Arco-Lase Plus Tablets 513
- Bellergal-S Tablets 2375
- Donnatal 2234
- Donnatal Extentabs 2234
- Donnatal Tablets 2234
- Phenobarbital Elixir and Tablets 1523
- Quadrinal Tablets 1398

Phensuximide (Additive CNS depressant effects).
No products indexed under this heading.

Phenytoin (Additive CNS depressant effects). Products include:
- Dilantin Infatabs 1967
- Dilantin-125 Suspension 1969

Phenytoin Sodium (Additive CNS depressant effects). Products include:
- Dilantin Kapseals 1965

Prazepam (Additive CNS depressant effects).
No products indexed under this heading.

Primidone (Additive CNS depressant effects). Products include:
- Mysoline 2860

Prochlorperazine (Additive CNS depressant effects). Products include:
- Compazine 2644

Promethazine Hydrochloride (Additive CNS depressant effects). Products include:
- Mepergan Injection 2859
- Phenergan with Codeine 2883
- Phenergan with Dextromethorphan 2885
- Phenergan Injection 2880
- Phenergan Suppositories 2882
- Phenergan Syrup 2881
- Phenergan Tablets 2882
- Phenergan VC 2886
- Phenergan VC with Codeine 2888

Propofol (Additive CNS depressant effects). Products include:
- Diprivan Injectable Emulsion 2939

Propoxyphene Hydrochloride (Co-administration of propoxyphene has decreased the maximum concentration of alprazolam by 6%, decreased clearance by 38%, and increased half-life by 16%). Products include:
- Darvon 1475
- Wygesic Tablets 2930

Propoxyphene Napsylate (Co-administration of propoxyphene has decreased the maximum plasma concentration of alprazolam by 6%, decreased clearance by 38%, and increased half-life by 16%). Products include:
- Darvon-N/Darvocet-N 1473

Pyrilamine Maleate (Additive CNS depressant effects). Products include:
- 4-Way Fast Acting Nasal Spray (regular & mentholated) .... ◼ 644

- Maximum Strength Multi-Symptom Formula Midol .... ◼ 621
- PMS Multi-Symptom Formula Midol .... ◼ 622

Pyrilamine Tannate (Additive CNS depressant effects). Products include:
- Atrohist Pediatric Suspension 1604
- Atrohist Pediatric Suspension Dye-Free 1604
- Rynatan 2781

Quazepam (Additive CNS depressant effects). Products include:
- Doral Tablets 2773

Risperidone (Additive CNS depressant effects). Products include:
- Risperdal Tablets 1348

Secobarbital Sodium (Additive CNS depressant effects). Products include:
- Seconal Sodium Pulvules 1529

Sertraline Hydrochloride (Possible interaction based on the data from *in vitro* studies suggests a possible interaction when co-administered; concurrent use requires caution). Products include:
- Zoloft Tablets 2051

Sevoflurane (Additive CNS depressant effects).
No products indexed under this heading.

Sufentanil Citrate (Additive CNS depressant effects). Products include:
- Sufenta Injection 1355

Temazepam (Additive CNS depressant effects). Products include:
- Restoril Capsules 2413

Terfenadine (Additive CNS depressant effects). Products include:
- Seldane Tablets 1284
- Seldane-D Extended-Release Tablets 1286

Thiamylal Sodium (Additive CNS depressant effects).
No products indexed under this heading.

Thioridazine Hydrochloride (Additive CNS depressant effects). Products include:
- Mellaril 2398

Thiothixene (Additive CNS depressant effects). Products include:
- Navane Capsules and Concentrate 2018
- Navane Intramuscular 2019

Triazolam (Additive CNS depressant effects). Products include:
- Halcion Tablets 2093

Trifluoperazine Hydrochloride (Additive CNS depressant effects). Products include:
- Stelazine 2692

Trimeprazine Tartrate (Additive CNS depressant effects).
No products indexed under this heading.

Trimethadione (Additive CNS depressant effects).
No products indexed under this heading.

Tripelennamine Hydrochloride (Additive CNS depressant effects). Products include:
- PBZ Tablets 863
- PBZ-SR Tablets 862

Triprolidine Hydrochloride (Additive CNS depressant effects). Products include:
- Actifed Cold & Allergy Tablets .... ◼ 807
- Actifed Cold & Sinus Caplets and Tablets .... ◼ 808

Valproic Acid (Additive CNS depressant effects). Products include:
- Depakene 416

Zolpidem Tartrate (Additive CNS depressant effects). Products include:
- Ambien Tablets 2559

(◼ Described in PDR For Nonprescription Drugs)   (◉ Described in PDR For Ophthalmology)

Food Interactions

Alcohol (Additive CNS depressant effects).

Grapefruit Juice (Possible interaction based on the clinical studies involving other benzodiazepines metabolized by similarly as alprazolam; co-administration requires caution).

XERAC AC SOLUTION
(Aluminum Chloride)..................1990
None cited in PDR database.

XYLOCAINE INJECTIONS
(Lidocaine Hydrochloride) 562
See **Xylocaine with Epinephrine Injections**

XYLOCAINE WITH EPINEPHRINE INJECTIONS
(Lidocaine Hydrochloride, Epinephrine) 562
May interact with monoamine oxidase inhibitors, tricyclic antidepressants, phenothiazines, butyrophenones, and certain other agents. Compounds in these categories include:

Amitriptyline Hydrochloride (Potential for severe, prolonged hypertension). Products include:
  Elavil 2945
  Etrafon 2495
  Limbitrol 2333
  Triavil Tablets 1800

Amoxapine (Potential for severe, prolonged hypertension). Products include:
  Asendin Tablets 1419

Chlorpromazine (Reduces or reverses the pressor effect of epinephrine). Products include:
  Thorazine Suppositories 2701

Clomipramine Hydrochloride (Potential for severe, prolonged hypertension). Products include:
  Anafranil Capsules 819

Desipramine Hydrochloride (Potential for severe, prolonged hypertension). Products include:
  Norpramin Tablets 1273

Doxepin Hydrochloride (Potential for severe, prolonged hypertension). Products include:
  Adapin Capsules 1542
  Sinequan 2028
  Zonalon Cream 1042

Ergonovine Maleate (Potential for severe, persistent hypertension or cerebrovascular accidents).
  No products indexed under this heading.

Fluphenazine Decanoate (Reduces or reverses the pressor effect of epinephrine). Products include:
  Prolixin Decanoate 510

Fluphenazine Enanthate (Reduces or reverses the pressor effect of epinephrine). Products include:
  Prolixin Enanthate 510

Fluphenazine Hydrochloride (Reduces or reverses the pressor effect of epinephrine). Products include:
  Prolixin 510

Furazolidone (Potential for severe, prolonged hypertension). Products include:
  Furoxone 2221

Haloperidol (Reduces or reverses the pressor effect of epinephrine). Products include:
  Haldol Injection, Tablets and Concentrate 1585

Haloperidol Decanoate (Reduces or reverses the pressor effect of epinephrine). Products include:
  Haldol Decanoate 1587

Imipramine Hydrochloride (Potential for severe, prolonged hypertension). Products include:
  Tofranil Ampuls 873
  Tofranil Tablets 875

Imipramine Pamoate (Potential for severe, prolonged hypertension). Products include:
  Tofranil-PM Capsules 876

Isocarboxazid (Potential for severe, prolonged hypertension).
  No products indexed under this heading.

Maprotiline Hydrochloride (Potential for severe, prolonged hypertension). Products include:
  Ludiomil Tablets 861

Mesoridazine Besylate (Reduces or reverses the pressor effect of epinephrine). Products include:
  Serentil 689

Methotrimeprazine (Reduces or reverses the pressor effect of epinephrine). Products include:
  Levoprome 1321

Methylergonovine Maleate (Potential for severe, persistent hypertension or cerebrovascular accidents). Products include:
  Methergine 2401

Nortriptyline Hydrochloride (Potential for severe, prolonged hypertension). Products include:
  Pamelor 2409

Perphenazine (Reduces or reverses the pressor effect of epinephrine). Products include:
  Etrafon 2495
  Triavil Tablets 1800
  Trilafon 2532

Phenelzine Sulfate (Potential for severe, prolonged hypertension). Products include:
  Nardil 1977

Prochlorperazine (Reduces or reverses the pressor effect of epinephrine). Products include:
  Compazine 2644

Promethazine Hydrochloride (Reduces or reverses the pressor effect of epinephrine). Products include:
  Mepergan Injection 2859
  Phenergan with Codeine 2883
  Phenergan with Dextromethorphan 2885
  Phenergan Injection 2880
  Phenergan Suppositories 2882
  Phenergan Syrup 2881
  Phenergan Tablets 2882
  Phenergan VC 2886
  Phenergan VC with Codeine 2888

Protriptyline Hydrochloride (Potential for severe, prolonged hypertension). Products include:
  Vivactil Tablets 1820

Selegiline Hydrochloride (Potential for severe, prolonged hypertension). Products include:
  Eldepryl Capsules 2729

Thioridazine Hydrochloride (Reduces or reverses the pressor effect of epinephrine). Products include:
  Mellaril 2398

Tranylcypromine Sulfate (Potential for severe, prolonged hypertension). Products include:
  Parnate Tablets 2679

Trifluoperazine Hydrochloride (Reduces or reverses the pressor effect of epinephrine). Products include:
  Stelazine 2692

Trimipramine Maleate (Potential for severe, prolonged hypertension). Products include:
  Surmontil Capsules 2917

XYLOCAINE 2.5% OINTMENT
(Lidocaine) 608
None cited in PDR database.

YOCON TABLETS
(Yohimbine Hydrochloride) 1235
May interact with antidepressant drugs. Compounds in this category include:

Amitriptyline Hydrochloride (Should not be used together). Products include:
  Elavil 2945
  Etrafon 2495
  Limbitrol 2333
  Triavil Tablets 1800

Amoxapine (Should not be used together). Products include:
  Asendin Tablets 1419

Bupropion Hydrochloride (Should not be used together). Products include:
  Wellbutrin Tablets 1177

Clomipramine Hydrochloride (Should not be used together). Products include:
  Anafranil Capsules 819

Desipramine Hydrochloride (Should not be used together). Products include:
  Norpramin Tablets 1273

Doxepin Hydrochloride (Should not be used together). Products include:
  Adapin Capsules 1542
  Sinequan 2028
  Zonalon Cream 1042

Fluoxetine Hydrochloride (Should not be used together). Products include:
  Prozac Pulvules & Liquid, Oral Solution 935

Imipramine Hydrochloride (Should not be used together). Products include:
  Tofranil Ampuls 873
  Tofranil Tablets 875

Imipramine Pamoate (Should not be used together). Products include:
  Tofranil-PM Capsules 876

Isocarboxazid (Should not be used together).
  No products indexed under this heading.

Maprotiline Hydrochloride (Should not be used together). Products include:
  Ludiomil Tablets 861

Nefazodone Hydrochloride (Should not be used together). Products include:
  Serzone Tablets 776

Nortriptyline Hydrochloride (Should not be used together). Products include:
  Pamelor 2409

Paroxetine Hydrochloride (Should not be used together). Products include:
  Paxil Tablets 2681

Phenelzine Sulfate (Should not be used together). Products include:
  Nardil 1977

Protriptyline Hydrochloride (Should not be used together). Products include:
  Vivactil Tablets 1820

Sertraline Hydrochloride (Should not be used together). Products include:
  Zoloft Tablets 2051

Tranylcypromine Sulfate (Should not be used together). Products include:
  Parnate Tablets 2679

Trazodone Hydrochloride (Should not be used together). Products include:
  Desyrel and Desyrel Dividose 504

Trimipramine Maleate (Should not be used together). Products include:
  Surmontil Capsules 2917

Venlafaxine Hydrochloride (Should not be used together). Products include:
  Effexor 2825

YODOXIN TABLETS
(Iodoquinol) 1235
None cited in PDR database.

YOHIMEX TABLETS
(Yohimbine Hydrochloride) 1414
May interact with antidepressant drugs, antipsychotic agents, and certain other agents. Compounds in these categories include:

Amitriptyline Hydrochloride (Do not use concomitantly). Products include:
  Elavil 2945
  Etrafon 2495
  Limbitrol 2333
  Triavil Tablets 1800

Amoxapine (Do not use concomitantly). Products include:
  Asendin Tablets 1419

Bupropion Hydrochloride (Do not use concomitantly). Products include:
  Wellbutrin Tablets 1177

Chlorpromazine (Do not use concomitantly). Products include:
  Thorazine Suppositories 2701

Chlorprothixene (Do not use concomitantly).
  No products indexed under this heading.

Chlorprothixene Hydrochloride (Do not use concomitantly).
  No products indexed under this heading.

Clomipramine Hydrochloride (Do not use concomitantly). Products include:
  Anafranil Capsules 819

Clozapine (Do not use concomitantly). Products include:
  Clozaril Tablets 2377

Desipramine Hydrochloride (Do not use concomitantly). Products include:
  Norpramin Tablets 1273

Doxepin Hydrochloride (Do not use concomitantly). Products include:
  Adapin Capsules 1542
  Sinequan 2028
  Zonalon Cream 1042

Fluoxetine Hydrochloride (Do not use concomitantly). Products include:
  Prozac Pulvules & Liquid, Oral Solution 935

Fluphenazine Decanoate (Do not use concomitantly). Products include:
  Prolixin Decanoate 510

Fluphenazine Enanthate (Do not use concomitantly). Products include:
  Prolixin Enanthate 510

Fluphenazine Hydrochloride (Do not use concomitantly). Products include:
  Prolixin 510

Haloperidol (Do not use concomitantly). Products include:
  Haldol Injection, Tablets and Concentrate 1585

IMPORTANT NOTE: Always consult each drug listing in the patient's regimen for possible interactions.

Yohimex

Interactions Index

Haloperidol Decanoate (Do not use concomitantly). Products include:
Haldol Decanoate 1587

Imipramine Hydrochloride (Do not use concomitantly). Products include:
Tofranil Ampuls 873
Tofranil Tablets 875

Imipramine Pamoate (Do not use concomitantly). Products include:
Tofranil-PM Capsules 876

Isocarboxazid (Do not use concomitantly).
No products indexed under this heading.

Lithium Carbonate (Do not use concomitantly). Products include:
Eskalith 2658
Lithium Carbonate Capsules & Tablets 2352
Lithonate/Lithotabs/Lithobid 2721

Lithium Citrate (Do not use concomitantly).
No products indexed under this heading.

Loxapine Hydrochloride (Do not use concomitantly). Products include:
Loxitane 1426

Loxapine Succinate (Do not use concomitantly). Products include:
Loxitane Capsules 1426

Maprotiline Hydrochloride (Do not use concomitantly). Products include:
Ludiomil Tablets 861

Mesoridazine Besylate (Do not use concomitantly). Products include:
Serentil 689

Molindone Hydrochloride (Do not use concomitantly). Products include:
Moban Tablets and Concentrate 1036

Nefazodone Hydrochloride (Do not use concomitantly). Products include:
Serzone Tablets 776

Nortriptyline Hydrochloride (Do not use concomitantly). Products include:
Pamelor 2409

Paroxetine Hydrochloride (Do not use concomitantly). Products include:
Paxil Tablets 2681

Perphenazine (Do not use concomitantly). Products include:
Etrafon 2495
Triavil Tablets 1800
Trilafon 2532

Phenelzine Sulfate (Do not use concomitantly). Products include:
Nardil 1977

Pimozide (Do not use concomitantly). Products include:
Orap Tablets 1037

Prochlorperazine (Do not use concomitantly). Products include:
Compazine 2644

Promethazine Hydrochloride (Do not use concomitantly). Products include:
Mepergan Injection 2859
Phenergan with Codeine 2883
Phenergan with Dextromethorphan .. 2885
Phenergan Injection 2880
Phenergan Suppositories 2882
Phenergan Syrup 2881
Phenergan Tablets 2882
Phenergan VC 2886
Phenergan VC with Codeine 2888

Protriptyline Hydrochloride (Do not use concomitantly). Products include:
Vivactil Tablets 1820

Risperidone (Do not use concomitantly). Products include:
Risperdal Tablets 1348

Sertraline Hydrochloride (Do not use concomitantly). Products include:
Zoloft Tablets 2051

Thioridazine Hydrochloride (Do not use concomitantly). Products include:
Mellaril 2398

Thiothixene (Do not use concomitantly). Products include:
Navane Capsules and Concentrate . 2018
Navane Intramuscular 2019

Tranylcypromine Sulfate (Do not use concomitantly). Products include:
Parnate Tablets 2679

Trazodone Hydrochloride (Do not use concomitantly). Products include:
Desyrel and Desyrel Dividose 504

Trifluoperazine Hydrochloride (Do not use concomitantly). Products include:
Stelazine 2692

Trimipramine Maleate (Do not use concomitantly). Products include:
Surmontil Capsules 2917

Venlafaxine Hydrochloride (Do not use concomitantly). Products include:
Effexor 2825

YUTOPAR INTRAVENOUS INJECTION
(Ritodrine Hydrochloride) 566
May interact with corticosteroids, general anesthetics, anticholinergics, sympathomimetics, beta blockers, and certain other agents. Compounds in these categories include:

Acebutolol Hydrochloride (Inhibition of Yutopar's action). Products include:
Sectral Capsules 2914

Albuterol (Possible additive effects). Products include:
Proventil Inhalation Aerosol 2524
Ventolin Inhalation Aerosol and Refill 1170

Albuterol Sulfate (Possible additive effects). Products include:
Airet Albuterol Sulfate Inhalation Solution 1602
Albuterol Sulfate, USP Solution for Inhalation, Arm-a-Med 522
Proventil Inhalation Solution 0.083% 2527
Proventil Repetabs Tablets 2529
Proventil Solution for Inhalation 0.5% 2525
Proventil Syrup 2528
Proventil Tablets 2529
Ventolin Inhalation Solution 1171
Ventolin Nebules Inhalation Solution 1172
Ventolin Rotacaps for Inhalation .. 1173
Ventolin Syrup 1175
Ventolin Tablets 1176
Volmax Extended-Release Tablets .. 1835

Atenolol (Inhibition of Yutopar's action). Products include:
Tenoretic Tablets 2963
Tenormin Tablets and I.V. Injection 2965

Atropine Sulfate (Systemic hypertension exaggerated). Products include:
Arco-Lase Plus Tablets 513
Atrohist Plus Tablets 1605
Donnatal 2234
Donnatal Extentabs 2234
Donnatal Tablets 2234
Lomotil 2591
Motofen Tablets 789
Urised Tablets 2123

Belladonna Alkaloids (Systemic hypertension exaggerated). Products include:
Bellergal-S Tablets 2375
Hyland's Bedwetting Tablets ...... ◨ 788
Hyland's EnurAid Tablets .... ◨ 789
Hyland's Headache Tablets .... ◨ 790
Hyland's Teething Tablets .... ◨ 790
Similasan Eye Drops #1 .... ◨ 769

Benztropine Mesylate (Systemic hypertension exaggerated). Products include:
Cogentin 1661

Betamethasone Acetate (Increased risk of pulmonary edema with concomitant use). Products include:
Celestone Soluspan Suspension ... 2484

Betamethasone Sodium Phosphate (Increased risk of pulmonary edema with concomitant use). Products include:
Celestone Soluspan Suspension ... 2484

Betaxolol Hydrochloride (Inhibition of Yutopar's action). Products include:
Betoptic Ophthalmic Solution 465
Betoptic S Ophthalmic Suspension . 467
Kerlone Tablets 2588

Biperiden Hydrochloride (Systemic hypertension exaggerated). Products include:
Akineton 1380

Bisoprolol Fumarate (Inhibition of Yutopar's action). Products include:
Zebeta Tablets 1457
Ziac 1459

Carteolol Hydrochloride (Inhibition of Yutopar's action). Products include:
Cartrol Tablets 413
Ocupress Ophthalmic Solution, 1% Sterile .... ⊚ 297

Clidinium Bromide (Systemic hypertension exaggerated). Products include:
Librax Capsules 2330

Cortisone Acetate (Increased risk of pulmonary edema with concomitant use). Products include:
Cortone Acetate Sterile Suspension 1663
Cortone Acetate Tablets 1664

Dexamethasone (Increased risk of pulmonary edema with concomitant use). Products include:
AK-Trol Ointment & Suspension ... ⊚ 205
Decadron Elixir 1676
Decadron Tablets 1678
Decaspray Topical Aerosol 1689
Maxitrol Ophthalmic Ointment and Suspension .... ⊚ 222
TobraDex Ophthalmic Suspension and Ointment 469

Dexamethasone Acetate (Increased risk of pulmonary edema with concomitant use). Products include:
Dalalone D.P. Injectable 1009
Decadron-LA Sterile Suspension ... 1687

Dexamethasone Sodium Phosphate (Increased risk of pulmonary edema with concomitant use). Products include:
Decadron Phosphate Injection 1680
Decadron Phosphate Sterile Ophthalmic Ointment 1684
Decadron Phosphate Sterile Ophthalmic Solution 1685
Decadron Phosphate Topical Cream 1686
Decadron Phosphate with Xylocaine Injection, Sterile 1683
Dexacort Phosphate in Respihaler . 1606
Dexacort Phosphate in Turbinaire . 1607
NeoDecadron Sterile Ophthalmic Ointment 1755
NeoDecadron Sterile Ophthalmic Solution 1756
NeoDecadron Topical Cream 1757

Diazoxide (Potentiates Yutopar's cardiovascular effects, particularly cardiac arrhythmia or hypotension). Products include:
Hyperstat I.V. Injection 2504
Proglycem 575

Dicyclomine Hydrochloride (Systemic hypertension exaggerated). Products include:
Bentyl 1246

Dobutamine Hydrochloride (Possible additive effects). Products include:
Dobutrex Solution Vials 1480

Dopamine Hydrochloride (Possible additive effects).
No products indexed under this heading.

Enflurane (Potentiates Yutopar's cardiovascular effects, particularly cardiac arrhythmia or hypotension).
No products indexed under this heading.

Ephedrine Hydrochloride (Possible additive effects). Products include:
Primatene Tablets .... ◨ 844
Quadrinal Tablets 1398

Ephedrine Sulfate (Possible additive effects). Products include:
Marax Tablets & DF Syrup 2015

Ephedrine Tannate (Possible additive effects). Products include:
Rynatuss 2782

Epinephrine (Possible additive effects). Products include:
EPIFRIN .... ⊚ 237
EpiPen 808
Marcaine with Epinephrine 2446
Primatene Mist .... ◨ 843
Sensorcaine with Epinephrine Injection 554
Sus-Phrine Injection 1017
Xylocaine with Epinephrine Injections 562

Epinephrine Bitartrate (Possible additive effects). Products include:
Sensorcaine-MPF with Epinephrine Injection 554

Epinephrine Hydrochloride (Possible additive effects). Products include:
Ana-Kit Anaphylaxis Emergency Treatment Kit 611

Esmolol Hydrochloride (Inhibition of Yutopar's action). Products include:
Brevibloc (esmolol HCI) Injection .. 1860

Fludrocortisone Acetate (Increased risk of pulmonary edema with concomitant use). Products include:
Florinef Acetate Tablets 506

Glycopyrrolate (Systemic hypertension exaggerated). Products include:
Robinul Forte Tablets 2247
Robinul Injectable 2247
Robinul Tablets 2247

Hydrocortisone (Increased risk of pulmonary edema with concomitant use). Products include:
Anusol-HC Cream 2.5% 1953
Aquanil HC Lotion 1989
Maximum Strength Cortaid Spray . ◨ 800
CORTENEMA 2713
Cortisporin Ointment 1074
Cortisporin Ophthalmic Ointment Sterile 1074
Cortisporin Ophthalmic Suspension Sterile 1075
Cortisporin Otic Solution Sterile ... 1076
Cortisporin Otic Suspension Sterile . 1077
Cortizone-5 .... ◨ 795
Cortizone-10 .... ◨ 795
Hydrocortone Tablets 1715
Hytone 922
Hytone Ointment 2 ½% 923
Massengill Medicated Soft Cloth Towelettes 2628
Pediotic Suspension Sterile 1140

(◨ Described in PDR For Nonprescription Drugs)   (⊚ Described in PDR For Ophthalmology)

1207 Interactions Index Yutopar

Preparation H Hydrocortisone 1% Cream ▣ 843
ProctoCream-HC 2.5% 2552
VōSoL HC Otic Solution 2786

Hydrocortisone Acetate (Increased risk of pulmonary edema with concomitant use). Products include:
Analpram-HC Rectal Cream 1% and 2.5% 993
Anusol HC-1 Hydrocortisone Anti-Itch Ointment ▣ 810
Anusol-HC Suppositories 1954
Caldecort Anti-Itch Hydrocortisone Cream ▣ 651
Coly-Mycin S Otic w/Neomycin & Hydrocortisone 1965
Cortaid ▣ 800
Cortifoam 2540
Cortisporin Cream 1073
Epifoam 2543
Hydrocortone Acetate Sterile Suspension 1712
Mantadil Cream 1124
Nupercainal Hydrocortisone 1% Cream ▣ 661
Pramosone Cream, Lotion & Ointment 995
ProctoFoam-HC 2552
Terra-Cortril Ophthalmic Suspension 2033

Hydrocortisone Sodium Phosphate (Increased risk of pulmonary edema with concomitant use). Products include:
Hydrocortone Phosphate Injection, Sterile 1713

Hydrocortisone Sodium Succinate (Increased risk of pulmonary edema with concomitant use).
No products indexed under this heading.

Hyoscyamine (Systemic hypertension exaggerated). Products include:
Cystospaz Tablets 2123
Urised Tablets 2123

Hyoscyamine Sulfate (Systemic hypertension exaggerated). Products include:
Arco-Lase Plus Tablets 513
Atrohist Plus Tablets 1605
Cystospaz-M Capsules 2123
Donnatal 2234
Donnatal Extentabs 2234
Donnatal Tablets 2234
Kutrase Capsules 2546
Levsin/Levsinex/Levbid 2549

Ipratropium Bromide (Systemic hypertension exaggerated). Products include:
Atrovent Inhalation Aerosol 674
Atrovent Inhalation Solution 675
Atrovent Nasal Spray 0.03% 676
Atrovent Nasal Spray 0.06% 678

Isoflurane (Potentiates Yutopar's cardiovascular effects, particularly cardiac arrhythmia or hypotension).
No products indexed under this heading.

Isoproterenol Hydrochloride (Possible additive effects). Products include:
Isuprel Hydrochloride Solution 2443
Isuprel Injection 2441
Isuprel Mistometer 2442

Isoproterenol Sulfate (Possible additive effects). Products include:
Norisodrine with Calcium Iodide Syrup 446

Labetalol Hydrochloride (Inhibition of Yutopar's action). Products include:
Normodyne Injection 2519
Normodyne Tablets 2522
Trandate 1158

Levobunolol Hydrochloride (Inhibition of Yutopar's action). Products include:
Betagan ◉ 230

Magnesium Sulfate (Potentiates Yutopar's cardiovascular effects, particularly cardiac arrhythmia or hypotension hypotension).
No products indexed under this heading.

Mepenzolate Bromide (Systemic hypertension exaggerated).
No products indexed under this heading.

Meperidine Hydrochloride (Potentiates Yutopar's cardiovascular effects, particularly cardiac arrhythmia or hypotension). Products include:
Demerol 2438
Mepergan Injection 2859

Metaproterenol Sulfate (Possible additive effects). Products include:
Alupent 672
Metaproterenol Sulfate Inhalation Solution, USP, Arm-a-Med 547

Metaraminol Bitartrate (Possible additive effects). Products include:
Aramine Injection 1649

Methohexital Sodium (Potentiates Yutopar's cardiovascular effects, particularly cardiac arrhythmia or hypotension).
No products indexed under this heading.

Methoxamine Hydrochloride (Possible additive effects). Products include:
Vasoxyl Injection 1169

Methoxyflurane (Potentiates Yutopar's cardiovascular effects, particularly cardiac arrhythmia or hypotension).
No products indexed under this heading.

Methylprednisolone Acetate (Increased risk of pulmonary edema with concomitant use).
No products indexed under this heading.

Methylprednisolone Sodium Succinate (Increased risk of pulmonary edema with concomitant use).
No products indexed under this heading.

Metipranolol Hydrochloride (Inhibition of Yutopar's action). Products include:
OptiPranolol (Metipranolol 0.3%) Sterile Ophthalmic Solution ◉ 256

Metoprolol Succinate (Inhibition of Yutopar's action). Products include:
Toprol-XL Tablets 560

Metoprolol Tartrate (Inhibition of Yutopar's action). Products include:
Lopressor 848
Lopressor HCT Tablets 850

Nadolol (Inhibition of Yutopar's action).
No products indexed under this heading.

Norepinephrine Bitartrate (Possible additive effects). Products include:
Levophed Bitartrate Injection 2445

Oxybutynin Chloride (Systemic hypertension exaggerated). Products include:
Ditropan 1267

Penbutolol Sulfate (Inhibition of Yutopar's action). Products include:
Levatol Tablets 2547

Phenylephrine Bitartrate (Possible additive effects).
No products indexed under this heading.

Phenylephrine Hydrochloride (Possible additive effects). Products include:
Atrohist Plus Tablets 1605
Cerose DM ▣ 853
D.A. II Tablets 972
D.A. Chewable Tablets 970
Dura-Vent/DA Tablets 972
Extendryl 1003
4-Way Fast Acting Nasal Spray (regular & mentholated) ▣ 644
Hemorid ▣ 797
Hycomine Compound Tablets 948
Neo-Synephrine Hydrochloride 1% Carpuject 2455
Neo-Synephrine Hydrochloride 1% Injection 2455
Neo-Synephrine Hydrochloride (Ophthalmic) 2456
Neo-Synephrine ▣ 624
Novahistine Elixir ▣ 782
Phenergan VC 2886
Phenergan VC with Codeine 2888
Preparation H ▣ 842
Tympagesic Ear Drops 2476
Vicks Sinex Nasal Spray and Ultra Fine Mist ▣ 738

Phenylephrine Tannate (Possible additive effects). Products include:
Atrohist Pediatric Suspension 1604
Atrohist Pediatric Suspension Dye-Free 1604
Rynatan 2781
Rynatuss 2782

Phenylpropanolamine Hydrochloride (Possible additive effects). Products include:
Acutrim ▣ 648
Atrohist Plus Tablets 1605
BC Cold Powder Multi-Symptom Formula (Cold-Sinus-Allergy) ▣ 631
BC Cold Powder Non-Drowsy Formula (Cold-Sinus) ▣ 631
Cheracol Plus Head Cold/Cough Formula ▣ 741
Comtrex Multi-Symptom Cold Reliever Liqui-Gels ▣ 638
Comtrex Multi-Symptom Non-Drowsy Liqui-gels ▣ 640
Contac Continuous Action Nasal Decongestant/Antihistamine 12 Hour Capsules ▣ 773
Contac Maximum Strength Continuous Action Decongestant/Antihistamine 12 Hour Caplets ▣ 772
Contac Severe Cold and Flu Formula Caplets ▣ 773
Coricidin 'D' Decongestant Tablets ▣ 760
Dexatrim ▣ 795
Dexatrim Plus Vitamins Caplets ▣ 796
Dimetane-DC Cough Syrup 2232
Dimetapp Allergy Sinus Caplets ▣ 838
Dimetapp Cold & Allergy Chewable Tablets ▣ 838
Dimetapp Cold & Cough Liqui-Gels ▣ 839
Dimetapp DM Elixir ▣ 840
Dimetapp Elixir ▣ 840
Dimetapp Extentabs ▣ 841
Dimetapp Tablets/Liqui-Gels ▣ 841
Dura-Vent Tablets 971
Entex LA Tablets 972
Exgest LA Tablets 787
Hycomine 947
Nolamine Timed-Release Tablets 790
Ornade Spansule Capsules 2678
Propagest Tablets 791
Pyrroxate Caplets ▣ 742
Robitussin-CF ▣ 846
Sinulin Tablets 792
Tavist-D 12 Hour Relief Tablets ▣ 750
Teldrin 12 Hour Antihistamine/Nasal Decongestant Allergy Relief Capsules ▣ 786
Triaminic Expectorant ▣ 753
Triaminic Syrup ▣ 755
Triaminic Triaminicol Cold & Cough ▣ 756
Triaminic DM Syrup ▣ 756
Triaminicin Tablets ▣ 756
Vicks DayQuil Allergy Relief 12-Hour Extended Release Tablets ▣ 733
Vicks DayQuil Allergy Relief 4-Hour Tablets ▣ 733
Vicks DayQuil SINUS Pressure & CONGESTION Relief ▣ 734

Pindolol (Inhibition of Yutopar's action). Products include:
Visken Tablets 2428

Pirbuterol Acetate (Possible additive effects). Products include:
Maxair Autohaler 1550
Maxair Inhaler 1552

Prednisolone Acetate (Increased risk of pulmonary edema with concomitant use). Products include:
AK-CIDE ◉ 203
AK-CIDE Ointment ◉ 203
Blephamide Liquifilm Sterile Ophthalmic Suspension 472
Blephamide Ointment ◉ 234
Econopred & Econopred Plus Ophthalmic Suspensions ◉ 216
Poly-Pred Liquifilm ◉ 246
Pred Forte ◉ 247
Pred Mild ◉ 250
Pred-G Liquifilm Sterile Ophthalmic Suspension ◉ 248
Pred-G S.O.P. Sterile Ophthalmic Ointment ◉ 249

Prednisolone Sodium Phosphate (Increased risk of pulmonary edema with concomitant use). Products include:
AK-PRED ◉ 204
Hydeltrasol Injection, Sterile 1708
Pediapred Oral Solution 1618

Prednisolone Tebutate (Increased risk of pulmonary edema with concomitant use). Products include:
Hydeltra-T.B.A. Sterile Suspension 1710

Prednisone (Increased risk of pulmonary edema with concomitant use).
No products indexed under this heading.

Procyclidine Hydrochloride (Systemic hypertension exaggerated). Products include:
Kemadrin Tablets 1105

Propantheline Bromide (Systemic hypertension exaggerated). Products include:
Pro-Banthine Tablets 2226

Propofol (Potentiates Yutopar's cardiovascular effects, particularly cardiac arrhythmia or hypotension). Products include:
Diprivan Injectable Emulsion 2939

Propranolol Hydrochloride (Inhibition of Yutopar's action). Products include:
Inderal 2834
Inderal LA Long Acting Capsules 2836
Inderide Tablets 2838
Inderide LA Long Acting Capsules 2840

Pseudoephedrine Hydrochloride (Possible additive effects). Products include:
Actifed Allergy Daytime/Nighttime Caplets ▣ 808
Actifed Cold & Allergy Tablets ▣ 807
Actifed Cold & Sinus Caplets and Tablets ▣ 808
Actifed Sinus Daytime/Nighttime Tablets and Caplets ▣ 809
Advil Cold and Sinus Caplets and Tablets ▣ 837
Alka-Seltzer Plus Liqui-Gels ▣ 612
Alka-Seltzer Plus Flu & Body Aches Liqui-Gels Non-Drowsy Formula ▣ 613
Alka-Seltzer Plus Night-Time Cold Medicine Liqui-Gels ▣ 612
Allerest Maximum Strength ▣ 649
Allerest No Drowsiness ▣ 649
Allerest Sinus Pain Formula ▣ 649
Atrohist Pediatric Capsules 1603
Benadryl Allergy/Cold Tablets ▣ 811
Benadryl Allergy Decongestant Liquid Medication ▣ 812
Benadryl Allergy Decongestant Tablets ▣ 812
Benadryl Allergy Sinus Headache Caplets ▣ 813
Benylin Multisymptom ▣ 816
Bromfed Capsules (Extended-Release) 1832
Bromfed Syrup ▣ 712

IMPORTANT NOTE: Always consult each drug listing in the patient's regimen for possible interactions.

Yutopar   Interactions Index   1208

Bromfed Tablets 1832	Sinutab Sinus Allergy Medication, Maximum Strength Tablets and Caplets .... ▫ 823	Vicks NyQuil LiquiCaps/Liquid Multi-Symptom Cold/Flu Relief, Original and Cherry Flavors. ▫ 736
Bromfed-DM Cough Syrup 1832		
Bromfed-PD Capsules (Extended-Release) 1832	Sinutab Sinus Medication, Maximum Strength Without Drowsiness Formula, Tablets & Caplets .... ▫ 824	**Pseudoephedrine Sulfate** (Possible additive effects). Products include:
Children's TYLENOL Cold Multi-Symptom Chewable Tablets and Liquid 1559		Chlor-Trimeton Allergy Decongestant Tablets .... ▫ 759
	Sudafed Children's Cold & Cough Liquid Medication .... ▫ 825	Claritin-D Tablets 2487
Children's TYLENOL Cold Plus Cough Multi Symptom Chewable Tablets and Liquid 1560	Sudafed Children's Nasal Decongestant Liquid Medication .... ▫ 826	Drixoral Cold and Allergy Sustained-Action Tablets .... ▫ 763
Children's TYLENOL Flu Suspension Liquid 1560	Sudafed Cold & Allergy Tablets .... ▫ 826	Drixoral Cold and Flu Extended-Release Tablets .... ▫ 764
Children's Vicks DayQuil Allergy Relief .... ▫ 730	Sudafed Cold and Cough Liquid Caps .... ▫ 826	Drixoral Non-Drowsy Formula Extended-Release Tablets .... ▫ 764
Children's Vicks NyQuil Cold/Cough Relief .... ▫ 731	Sudafed Nasal Decongestant Tablets, 30 mg .... ▫ 825	Drixoral Allergy/Sinus Extended Release Tablets .... ▫ 765
Allergy-Sinus Comtrex Multi-Symptom Allergy-Sinus Formula Tablets and Caplets .... ▫ 639	Sudafed Nasal Decongestant Tablets, 60 mg .... ▫ 825	Trinalin Repetabs Tablets 1373
	Sudafed Non-Drying Sinus Liquid Caps .... ▫ 827	**Salmeterol Xinafoate** (Possible additive effects). Products include:
Comtrex Multi-Symptom .... ▫ 638	Sudafed Pediatric Nasal Decongestant Liquid Oral Drops .... ▫ 827	Serevent Inhalation Aerosol 1149
Comtrex Multi-Symptom Non-Drowsy Caplets .... ▫ 640	Sudafed Severe Cold Formula Caplets .... ▫ 828	**Scopolamine** (Systemic hypertension exaggerated). Products include:
Congess 1003	Sudafed Severe Cold Formula Tablets .... ▫ 828	Transderm Scōp Transdermal Therapeutic System 890
Contac Day Allergy/Sinus Caplets 771	Sudafed Sinus Caplets .... ▫ 829	**Scopolamine Hydrobromide** (Systemic hypertension exaggerated). Products include:
Contac Day & Night 772	Sudafed Sinus Tablets .... ▫ 829	
Contac Night Allergy/Sinus Caplets 771	Sudafed 12 Hour Caplets .... ▫ 824	Atrohist Plus Tablets 1605
Contac Severe Cold & Flu Non-Drowsy 774	Syn-Rx Tablets 1622	Donnatal 2234
Deconsal II Tablets 1605	Syn-Rx DM Tablets 1623	Donnatal Extentabs 2234
Dimetane-DX Cough Syrup 2233	TheraFlu Flu and Cold Medicine 750	Donnatal Tablets 2234
Dimetapp Cold & Fever Suspension .... ▫ 839	Theraflu Maximum Strength Flu and Cold Medicine for Sore Throat 751	**Sevoflurane** (Potentiates Yutopar's cardiovascular effects, particularly cardiac arrhythymia or hypotension).
Dimetapp Decongestant Pediatric Drops .... ▫ 840	TheraFlu Flu, Cold and Cough Medicine .... ▫ 750	No products indexed under this heading.
Dorcol Children's Cough Syrup .... ▫ 748	TheraFlu Maximum Strength Nighttime Flu, Cold & Cough Medicine .... ▫ 751	**Sotalol Hydrochloride** (Inhibition of Yutopar's action). Products include:
Drixoral Cough + Congestion Liquid Caps .... ▫ 763	TheraFlu Maximum Strength Non-Drowsy Formula Flu, Cold & Cough Medicine .... ▫ 751	Betapace Tablets 637
Dura-Tap/PD Capsules 970		**Terbutaline Sulfate** (Possible additive effects). Products include:
Duratuss Tablets 2750	TheraFlu Maximum Strength, Non-Drowsy Formula Flu, Cold and Cough Caplets 752	Brethaire Inhaler 830
Duratuss HD Elixir 2750		Brethine Ampuls 832
Efidac/24 .... ▫ 655	Theraflu Maximum Strength Sinus Non-Drowsy Formula Caplets 752	Brethine Tablets 831
Entex PSE Tablets 973		Bricanyl Subcutaneous Injection 1247
Fedahist Gyrocaps 2545	Triaminic AM Cough and Decongestant Formula 753	Bricanyl Tablets 1248
Guaifed 1833	Triaminic AM Decongestant Formula 753	**Timolol Hemihydrate** (Inhibition of Yutopar's action). Products include:
Guaifed Syrup .... ▫ 712	Triaminic Infant Oral Decongestant Drops 754	
Guaimax-D Tablets 809	Triaminic Night Time 754	Betimol 0.25%, 0.5% .... ⊙ 259
Histussin D Liquid 670	Triaminic Sore Throat Formula 755	**Timolol Maleate** (Inhibition of Yutopar's action). Products include:
Infants' TYLENOL Cold Decongestant & Fever-Reducer Drops 1561	Tussend 1830	Blocadren Tablets 1654
	Tussend Expectorant 1831	Timolide Tablets 1791
Kronofed-A 994	TYLENOL Allergy Sinus, Maximum Strength Caplets and Gelcaps 1571	Timoptic in Ocudose 1796
Novahistine DMX .... ▫ 782		Timoptic Sterile Ophthalmic Solution 1794
Nucofed 2225	TYLENOL Allergy Sinus NightTime, Maximum Strength Caplets 1571	Timoptic-XE 1798
PediaCare Cough-Cold Chewable Tablets and Liquid 1569	TYLENOL Cold Medication, Multi-Symptom Formula Tablets and Caplets 1572	**Triamcinolone** (Increased risk of pulmonary edema with concomitant use).
PediaCare Infants' Decongestant Drops 1569	TYLENOL Cold Medication, Multi-Symptom Hot Liquid Packets 1572	No products indexed under this heading.
PediaCare Infants' Drops Decongestant Plus Cough 1569	TYLENOL Cold Medication, No Drowsiness Formula Caplets and Gelcaps 1572	**Triamcinolone Acetonide** (Increased risk of pulmonary edema with concomitant use). Products include:
PediaCare NightRest Cough-Cold Liquid 1569	TYLENOL Cold Severe Congestion Caplets 1573	Azmacort Oral Inhaler 2175
Pediatric Vicks 44d Cough & Head Congestion Relief .... ▫ 736	TYLENOL Cough Medication with Decongestant, Multi Symptom 1574	Nasacort AQ Nasal Spray 2191
Pediatric Vicks 44m Cough & Cold Relief .... ▫ 737	TYLENOL Flu No Drowsiness Formula, Maximum Strength Gelcaps 1575	Nasacort Nasal Inhaler 2189
Robitussin Cold & Cough Liqui-Gels .... ▫ 844		**Triamcinolone Diacetate** (Increased risk of pulmonary edema with concomitant use).
Robitussin Cold, Cough & Flu Liqui-Gels .... ▫ 844	TYLENOL Flu NightTime, Maximum Strength Gelcaps 1575	No products indexed under this heading.
Robitussin Maximum Strength Cough & Cold .... ▫ 847	TYLENOL Flu NightTime, Maximum Strength Hot Medication Packets 1575	**Triamcinolone Hexacetonide** (Increased risk of pulmonary edema with concomitant use).
Robitussin Night-Time Cold Formula .... ▫ 847	TYLENOL Sinus, Maximum Strength Geltabs, Gelcaps, Caplets and Tablets 1576	No products indexed under this heading.
Robitussin Pediatric Cough & Cold Formula .... ▫ 848		**Tridihexethyl Chloride** (Systemic hypertension exaggerated).
Robitussin Pediatric Drops .... ▫ 849	Vicks 44 LiquiCaps Cough, Cold & Flu Relief .... ▫ 728	No products indexed under this heading.
Robitussin Severe Congestion Liqui-Gels .... ▫ 845	Vicks 44 LiquiCaps Non-Drowsy Cough & Cold Relief .... ▫ 729	**Trihexyphenidyl Hydrochloride** (Systemic hypertension exaggerated). Products include:
Robitussin-DAC Syrup 2249	Vicks 44D Cough & Head Congestion Relief .... ▫ 728	
Robitussin-PE .... ▫ 846	Vicks 44M Cough, Cold & Flu Relief .... ▫ 729	Artane 1418
Rondec Oral Drops 974	Vicks DayQuil LiquiCaps/Liquid Multi-Symptom Cold/Flu Relief .... ▫ 734	
Rondec Syrup 974		
Rondec Tablet 974	Vicks DayQuil SINUS Pressure & PAIN Relief with IBUPROFEN .... ▫ 735	
Rondec Chewable Tablets 974		
Rondec-TR Tablet 974	Vicks Nyquil Hot Therapy .... ▫ 735	
Ryna .... ▫ 804		
Seldane-D Extended-Release Tablets 1286		
Semprex-D Capsules 1620		
Sinarest 663		
Sine-Aid Maximum Strength Sinus Headache Gelcaps, Caplets and Tablets 1570		
Sine-Off No Drowsiness Formula Caplets .... ▫ 784		
Sine-Off Sinus Medicine .... ▫ 784		
Singlet Tablets 785		
Sinutab Non-Drying Liquid Caps .... ▫ 823		

ZANOSAR STERILE POWDER
(Streptozocin) 2119
May interact with:

Nephrotoxic Drugs (Concomitant or combination use should be avoided).

ZANTAC 150 EFFERDOSE GRANULES
(Ranitidine Hydrochloride) 1182
See **Zantac 150 Tablets**

ZANTAC 150 EFFERDOSE TABLETS
(Ranitidine Hydrochloride) 1182
See **Zantac 150 Tablets**

ZANTAC 150 GELDOSE CAPSULES
(Ranitidine Hydrochloride) 1182
See **Zantac 150 Tablets**

ZANTAC 300 GELDOSE CAPSULES
(Ranitidine Hydrochloride) 1182
See **Zantac 150 Tablets**

ZANTAC 150 TABLETS
(Ranitidine Hydrochloride) 1182
May interact with:

Warfarin Sodium (Potential for increased or decreased prothrombin time; doses of ranitidine up to 400 mg per day had no effect on prothrombin time or warfarin clearance). Products include:
Coumadin 941

ZANTAC 300 TABLETS
(Ranitidine Hydrochloride) 1182
See **Zantac 150 Tablets**

ZANTAC INJECTION
(Ranitidine Hydrochloride) 1180
May interact with:

Warfarin Sodium (Potential for increased or decreased prothrombin time; doses of ranitidine up to 400 mg per day had no effect on prothrombin time or warfarin clearance). Products include:
Coumadin 941

ZANTAC INJECTION PREMIXED
(Ranitidine Hydrochloride) 1180
See **Zantac Injection**

ZANTAC SYRUP
(Ranitidine Hydrochloride) 1182
See **Zantac 150 Tablets**

ZARONTIN CAPSULES
(Ethosuximide) 1986
May interact with:

Divalproex Sodium (Valproic acid may increase or decrease ethosuximide levels). Products include:
Depakote Tablets 418

Phenytoin (Ethosuximide may elevate phenytoin serum levels). Products include:
Dilantin Infatabs 1967
Dilantin-125 Suspension 1969

Phenytoin Sodium (Ethosuximide may elevate phenytoin serum levels). Products include:
Dilantin Kapseals 1965

Valproic Acid (Valproic acid may increase or decrease ethosuximide levels). Products include:
Depakene 416

(▫ Described in PDR For Nonprescription Drugs)   (⊙ Described in PDR For Ophthalmology)

1209 Interactions Index Zaroxolyn

ZARONTIN SYRUP
(Ethosuximide) 1986
May interact with:

Divalproex Sodium (Valproic acid may increase or decrease ethosuximide levels). Products include:
Depakote Tablets 418

Phenytoin (Ethosuximide may elevate phenytoin serum levels). Products include:
Dilantin Infatabs 1967
Dilantin-125 Suspension 1969

Phenytoin Sodium (Ethosuximide may elevate phenytoin serum levels). Products include:
Dilantin Kapseals 1965

Valproic Acid (Valproic acid may increase or decrease ethosuximide levels). Products include:
Depakene 416

ZAROXOLYN TABLETS
(Metolazone) 1625
May interact with loop diuretics, antihypertensives, barbiturates, narcotic analgesics, cardiac glycosides, corticosteroids, lithium preparations, salicylates, non-steroidal anti-inflammatory agents, oral hypoglycemic agents, insulin, and certain other agents. Compounds in these categories include:

Acarbose (Blood glucose concentration may be raised). Products include:
Precose 604

Acebutolol Hydrochloride (Excessive hypotension may result especially during initial therapy). Products include:
Sectral Capsules 2914

ACTH (May increase the risk of hypokalemia and increase salt and water retention).
No products indexed under this heading.

Alfentanil Hydrochloride (Hypotensive effect may be potentiated). Products include:
Alfenta Injection 1334

Amlodipine Besylate (Excessive hypotension may result especially during initial therapy). Products include:
Lotrel Capsules 858
Norvasc Tablets 2020

Aprobarbital (Hypotensive effect may be potentiated).
No products indexed under this heading.

Aspirin (Increases the antihypertensive effect). Products include:
Alka-Seltzer Cherry Effervescent Antacid and Pain Reliever 609
Alka-Seltzer Extra Strength Effervescent Antacid and Pain Reliever 609
Alka-Seltzer Lemon Lime Effervescent Antacid and Pain Reliever 609
Alka-Seltzer Original Effervescent Antacid and Pain Reliever 609
Alka-Seltzer Plus 611
Alka-Seltzer Plus Sinus Medicine .. 611
Ascriptin 650
Arthritis Strength BC Powder 631
BC Cold Powder Multi-Symptom Formula (Cold-Sinus-Allergy) 631
BC Cold Powder Non-Drowsy Formula (Cold-Sinus) 631
BC Powder 631
Genuine Bayer Aspirin Tablets & Caplets 618
Extra Strength Bayer Arthritis Pain Regimen Formula 615
Extra Strength Bayer Aspirin Caplets & Tablets 617
Extended-Release Bayer 8-Hour Aspirin 616
Extra Strength Bayer Plus Aspirin Caplets 617
Extra Strength Bayer PM Aspirin Plus Sleep Aid 617
Aspirin Regimen Bayer 81 mg Tablets with Calcium 615
Aspirin Regimen Bayer Adult Low Strength 81 mg Tablets 613
Aspirin Regimen Bayer Children's Chewable Aspirin 616
Aspirin Regimen Bayer Regular Strength 325 mg Caplets 613
Bufferin Analgesic Tablets 636
Arthritis Strength Bufferin Analgesic Caplets 637
Extra Strength Bufferin Analgesic Tablets 637
Cama Arthritis Pain Reliever 748
Darvon Compound-65 Pulvules 1475
Easprin 1971
Ecotrin 2625
Ecotrin Enteric Coated Aspirin Maximum Strength Tablets and Caplets 775
Ecotrin Enteric Coated Aspirin Regular Strength Tablets 2625
Empirin Aspirin Tablets 818
Excedrin Extra-Strength Analgesic Tablets, Caplets, and Geltabs 734
Fiorinal Capsules 2388
Fiorinal with Codeine Capsules 2390
Fiorinal Tablets 2388
Goody's Extra Strength Headache Powders 632
Goody's Extra Strength Pain Relief Tablets 632
Halfprin Tablets 1413
Norgesic 1554
Percodan Tablets 955
Percodan-Demi Tablets 956
Robaxisal Tablets 2246
Soma Compound w/Codeine Tablets 2784
Soma Compound Tablets 2783
St. Joseph Adult Chewable Aspirin (81 mg.) 768
Talwin Compound 2466
Vanquish Analgesic Caplets 627

Atenolol (Excessive hypotension may result especially during initial therapy). Products include:
Tenoretic Tablets 2963
Tenormin Tablets and I.V. Injection 2965

Benazepril Hydrochloride (Excessive hypotension may result especially during initial therapy). Products include:
Lotensin Tablets 852
Lotensin HCT Tablets 855
Lotrel Capsules 858

Bendroflumethiazide (Excessive hypotension may result especially during initial therapy).
No products indexed under this heading.

Betamethasone Acetate (May increase the risk of hypokalemia and increase salt and water retention). Products include:
Celestone Soluspan Suspension 2484

Betamethasone Sodium Phosphate (May increase the risk of hypokalemia and increase salt and water retention). Products include:
Celestone Soluspan Suspension 2484

Betaxolol Hydrochloride (Excessive hypotension may result especially during initial therapy). Products include:
Betoptic Ophthalmic Solution 465
Betoptic S Ophthalmic Suspension 467
Kerlone Tablets 2588

Bisoprolol Fumarate (Excessive hypotension may result especially during initial therapy). Products include:
Zebeta Tablets 1457
Ziac 1459

Bumetanide (May result in large or prolonged losses of fluids and electrolytes). Products include:
Bumex 2260

Buprenorphine (Hypotensive effect may be potentiated). Products include:
Buprenex Injectable 2170

Butabarbital (Hypotensive effect may be potentiated).
No products indexed under this heading.

Butalbital (Hypotensive effect may be potentiated). Products include:
Axocet Capsules 2469
Esgic-plus Capsules 1012
Esgic-plus Tablets 1012
Fioricet Tablets 2386
Fioricet with Codeine Capsules 2387
Fiorinal Capsules 2388
Fiorinal with Codeine Capsules 2390
Fiorinal Tablets 2388
Phrenilin 790
Sedapap Tablets 50 mg/650 mg .. 1826

Captopril (Excessive hypotension may result especially during initial therapy). Products include:
Capoten Tablets 740
Capozide Tablets 744

Carteolol Hydrochloride (Excessive hypotension may result especially during initial therapy). Products include:
Cartrol Tablets 413
Ocupress Ophthalmic Solution, 1% Sterile .... ⊙ 297

Chlorothiazide (Excessive hypotension may result especially during initial therapy). Products include:
Aldoclor Tablets 1638
Diupres Tablets 1691
Diuril Oral 1694

Chlorothiazide Sodium (Excessive hypotension may result especially during initial therapy). Products include:
Diuril Sodium Intravenous 1693

Chlorpropamide (Blood glucose concentration may be raised). Products include:
Diabinese Tablets 2002

Chlorthalidone (Excessive hypotension may result especially during initial therapy). Products include:
Combipres Tablets 682
Tenoretic Tablets 2963
Thalitone 1293

Choline Magnesium Trisalicylate (Increases the antihypertensive effect). Products include:
Trilisate 2155

Clonidine (Excessive hypotension may result especially during initial therapy). Products include:
Catapres-TTS 680

Clonidine Hydrochloride (Excessive hypotension may result especially during initial therapy). Products include:
Catapres Tablets 679
Combipres Tablets 682

Codeine Phosphate (Hypotensive effect may be potentiated). Products include:
Brontex 2130
Dimetane-DC Cough Syrup 2232
Fioricet with Codeine Capsules 2387
Fiorinal with Codeine Capsules 2390
Nucofed 2225
Phenergan with Codeine 2883
Phenergan VC with Codeine 2888
Robitussin A-C Syrup 2248
Robitussin-DAC Syrup 2249
Ryna 804
Soma Compound w/Codeine Tablets 2784
Tylenol with Codeine 1592

Cortisone Acetate (May increase the risk of hypokalemia and increase salt and water retention). Products include:
Cortone Acetate Sterile Suspension 1663
Cortone Acetate Tablets 1664

Deserpidine (Excessive hypotension may result especially during initial therapy).
No products indexed under this heading.

Deslanoside (Hypokalemia induced by diuretic may increase the sensitivity of the myocardium to digitalis therapy).
No products indexed under this heading.

Dexamethasone (May increase the risk of hypokalemia and increase salt and water retention). Products include:
AK-Trol Ointment & Suspension .... ⊙ 205
Decadron Elixir 1676
Decadron Tablets 1678
Decaspray Topical Aerosol 1689
Maxitrol Ophthalmic Ointment and Suspension .... ⊙ 222
TobraDex Ophthalmic Suspension and Ointment 469

Dexamethasone Acetate (May increase the risk of hypokalemia and increase salt and water retention). Products include:
Dalalone D.P. Injectable 1009
Decadron-LA Sterile Suspension 1687

Dexamethasone Sodium Phosphate (May increase the risk of hypokalemia and increase salt and water retention). Products include:
Decadron Phosphate Injection 1680
Decadron Phosphate Sterile Ophthalmic Ointment 1684
Decadron Phosphate Sterile Ophthalmic Solution 1685
Decadron Phosphate Topical Cream 1686
Decadron Phosphate with Xylocaine Injection, Sterile 1683
Dexacort Phosphate in Respihaler .. 1606
Dexacort Phosphate in Turbinaire .. 1607
NeoDecadron Sterile Ophthalmic Ointment 1755
NeoDecadron Sterile Ophthalmic Solution 1756
NeoDecadron Topical Cream 1757

Dezocine (Hypotensive effect may be potentiated). Products include:
Dalgan Injection 529

Diazoxide (Excessive hypotension may result especially during initial therapy). Products include:
Hyperstat I.V. Injection 2504
Proglycem 575

Diclofenac Potassium (Increases the antihypertensive effect). Products include:
Cataflam Tablets 833

Diclofenac Sodium (Increases the antihypertensive effect). Products include:
Voltaren Ophthalmic Sterile Ophthalmic Solution .... ⊙ 264
Cataflam/Voltaren/Voltaren-XR 833

Dicumarol (May affect the hypoprothrombinemic response to anticoagulants; dosage adjustments may be necessary).
No products indexed under this heading.

Diflunisal (Increases the antihypertensive effect). Products include:
Dolobid Tablets 1695

Digitoxin (Hypokalemia induced by diuretic may increase the sensitivity of the myocardium to digitalis therapy). Products include:
Crystodigin Tablets 1472

Digoxin (Hypokalemia induced by diuretic may increase the sensitivity of the myocardium to digitalis therapy). Products include:
Lanoxicaps 1110
Lanoxin Elixir Pediatric 1113
Lanoxin Injection 1116
Lanoxin Injection Pediatric 1119
Lanoxin Tablets 1121

Diltiazem Hydrochloride (Excessive hypotension may result especially during initial therapy). Products include:
Cardizem CD Capsules 1251
Cardizem SR Capsules 1255

IMPORTANT NOTE: Always consult each drug listing in the patient's regimen for possible interactions.

Zaroxolyn — Interactions Index — 1210

Cardizem Injectable 1253
Cardizem Tablets 1257
Dilacor XR Extended-release Capsules 2183
Tiazac Capsules 1019

Doxazosin Mesylate (Excessive hypotension may result especially during initial therapy). Products include:
Cardura Tablets 1993

Enalapril Maleate (Excessive hypotension may result especially during initial therapy). Products include:
Vaseretic Tablets 1810
Vasotec Tablets 1816

Enalaprilat (Excessive hypotension may result especially during initial therapy). Products include:
Vasotec I.V. 1814

Esmolol Hydrochloride (Excessive hypotension may result especially during initial therapy). Products include:
Brevibloc (esmolol HCl) Injection 1860

Ethacrynic Acid (May result in large or prolonged losses of fluids and electrolytes). Products include:
Edecrin Tablets 1698

Etodolac (Increases the antihypertensive effect). Products include:
Lodine Capsules and Tablets 2849

Felodipine (Excessive hypotension may result especially during initial therapy). Products include:
Plendil Extended-Release Tablets 514

Fenoprofen Calcium (Increases the antihypertensive effect). Products include:
Nalfon 200 Pulvules & Nalfon Tablets 933

Fentanyl (Hypotensive effect may be potentiated). Products include:
Duragesic Transdermal System 1336

Fentanyl Citrate (Hypotensive effect may be potentiated). Products include:
Sublimaze Injection 463

Fludrocortisone Acetate (May increase the risk of hypokalemia and increase salt and water retention). Products include:
Florinef Acetate Tablets 506

Flurbiprofen (Increases the antihypertensive effect).
No products indexed under this heading.

Fosinopril Sodium (Excessive hypotension may result especially during initial therapy). Products include:
Monopril Tablets 762

Furosemide (May result in large or prolonged losses of fluids and electrolytes; excessive hypotension may result especially during initial therapy). Products include:
Lasix Injection, Oral Solution and Tablets 1267

Glimepiride (Blood glucose concentration may be raised). Products include:
Amaryl Tablets 1241

Glipizide (Blood glucose concentration may be raised). Products include:
Glucotrol Tablets 2011
Glucotrol XL Extended Release Tablets 2012

Glyburide (Blood glucose concentration may be raised). Products include:
DiaBeta Tablets 1265
Glynase PresTab Tablets 2091
Micronase Tablets 2099

Guanabenz Acetate (Excessive hypotension may result especially during initial therapy).
No products indexed under this heading.

Guanethidine Monosulfate (Excessive hypotension may result especially during initial therapy). Products include:
Esimil Tablets 840
Ismelin Tablets 845

Hydralazine Hydrochloride (Excessive hypotension may result especially during initial therapy). Products include:
Apresazide Capsules 824
Apresoline Hydrochloride Tablets .. 826
Hydralazine Hydrochloride Injection USP 2712
Ser-Ap-Es Tablets 867

Hydrochlorothiazide (Excessive hypotension may result especially during initial therapy). Products include:
Aldactazide Tablets 2556
Aldoril Tablets 1644
Apresazide Capsules 824
Capozide Tablets 744
Dyazide Capsules 2653
Esidrix Tablets 839
Esimil Tablets 840
HydroDIURIL Tablets 1716
Hydropres Tablets 1718
Hyzaar Tablets 1720
Inderide Tablets 2838
Inderide LA Long Acting Capsules . 2840
Lopressor HCT Tablets 850
Lotensin HCT Tablets 855
Moduretic Tablets 1748
Oretic Tablets 450
Prinzide Tablets 1780
Ser-Ap-Es Tablets 867
Timolide Tablets 1791
Vaseretic Tablets 1810
Zestoretic Tablets 2968
Ziac 1459

Hydrocodone Bitartrate (Hypotensive effect may be potentiated). Products include:
Codiclear DH Syrup 808
Duratuss HD Elixir 2750
Histussin D Liquid 670
Hycodan Tablets and Syrup 946
Hycomine Compound Tablets 948
Hycomine 947
Hycotuss Expectorant Syrup 950
Hydrocet Capsules 787
Lorcet 10/650 Tablets 1016
Lortab 2751
Tussend 1830
Tussend Expectorant 1831
Vicodin Tablets 1404
Vicodin ES Tablets 1405
Vicodin HP Tablets 1403
Vicodin Tuss Expectorant 1406
Zydone Capsules 967

Hydrocodone Polistirex (Hypotensive effect may be potentiated). Products include:
Tussionex Pennkinetic Extended-Release Suspension 1624

Hydrocortisone (May increase the risk of hypokalemia and increase salt and water retention). Products include:
Anusol-HC Cream 2.5% 1953
Aquanil HC Lotion 1989
Maximum Strength Cortaid Spray 800
CORTENEMA 2713
Cortisporin Ointment 1074
Cortisporin Ophthalmic Ointment Sterile 1074
Cortisporin Ophthalmic Suspension Sterile 1075
Cortisporin Otic Solution Sterile 1076
Cortisporin Otic Suspension Sterile 1077
Cortizone-5 795
Cortizone-10 795
Hydrocortone Tablets 1715
Hytone 922
Hytone Ointment 2½% 923
Massengill Medicated Soft Cloth Towelettes 2628
Pediotic Suspension Sterile 1140
Preparation H Hydrocortisone 1% Cream 843

ProctoCream-HC 2.5% 2552
VōSoL HC Otic Solution 2786

Hydrocortisone Acetate (May increase the risk of hypokalemia and increase salt and water retention). Products include:
Analpram-HC Rectal Cream 1% and 2.5% 993
Anusol HC-1 Hydrocortisone Anti-Itch Ointment 810
Anusol-HC Suppositories 1954
Caldecort Anti-Itch Hydrocortisone Cream 651
Coly-Mycin S Otic w/Neomycin & Hydrocortisone 1965
Cortaid 800
Cortifoam 2540
Cortisporin Cream 1073
Epifoam 2543
Hydrocortone Acetate Sterile Suspension 1712
Mantadil Cream 1124
Nupercainal Hydrocortisone 1% Cream 661
Pramosone Cream, Lotion & Ointment 995
ProctoFoam-HC 2552
Terra-Cortril Ophthalmic Suspension 2033

Hydrocortisone Sodium Phosphate (May increase the risk of hypokalemia and increase salt and water retention). Products include:
Hydrocortone Phosphate Injection, Sterile 1713

Hydrocortisone Sodium Succinate (May increase the risk of hypokalemia and increase salt and water retention).
No products indexed under this heading.

Hydroflumethiazide (Excessive hypotension may result especially during initial therapy). Products include:
Diucardin Tablets 2824

Hydromorphone Hydrochloride (Hypotensive effect may be potentiated). Products include:
Dilaudid Ampules 1382
Dilaudid Cough Syrup 1383
Dilaudid-HP Injection 1384
Dilaudid-HP Lyophilized Powder 250 mg 1384
Dilaudid 1382
Dilaudid Oral Liquid 1386
Dilaudid 1382
Dilaudid Tablets - 8 mg 1386

Ibuprofen (Increases the antihypertensive effect). Products include:
Advil Cold and Sinus Caplets and Tablets 837
Advil Ibuprofen Tablets, Caplets and Gel Caplets 836
Children's Motrin Ibuprofen Oral Suspension 1558
IBU Tablets 1389
Ibuprohm 713
Motrin IB Caplets, Tablets, and Gelcaps 802
Motrin Ibuprofen Suspension, Oral Drops, Chewable Tablets, Caplets 1563
Nuprin Ibuprofen/Analgesic Tablets & Caplets 645
Vicks DayQuil SINUS Pressure & PAIN Relief with IBUPROFEN 735

Indapamide (Excessive hypotension may result especially during initial therapy).
No products indexed under this heading.

Indomethacin (Increases the antihypertensive effect). Products include:
Indocin 1723

Indomethacin Sodium Trihydrate (Increases the antihypertensive effect). Products include:
Indocin I.V. 1727

Insulin, Human (Blood glucose concentration may be raised).
No products indexed under this heading.

Insulin, Human Isophane Suspension (Blood glucose concentration may be raised). Products include:
Novolin N Human Insulin 10 ml Vials 1846

Insulin, Human NPH (Blood glucose concentration may be raised). Products include:
Humulin N, 100 Units 1495
Novolin N PenFill 1.5 ml Cartridges Durable Insulin Delivery System 1849
Novolin N Prefilled Syringe Disposable Insulin Delivery System 1850

Insulin, Human Regular (Blood glucose concentration may be raised). Products include:
Humulin R, 100 Units 1497
Novolin R Human Insulin 10 ml Vials 1846
Novolin R PenFill 1.5 ml Cartridges Durable Insulin Delivery System 1849
Novolin R Prefilled Syringe Disposable Insulin Delivery System 1850
Velosulin BR Human Insulin 10 ml Vials 1847

Insulin, Human, Zinc Suspension (Blood glucose concentration may be raised). Products include:
Humulin L, 100 Units 1494
Humulin U, 100 Units 1498
Novolin L Human Insulin 10 ml Vials 1846

Insulin Lispro, Human (Blood glucose concentration may be raised). Products include:
Humalog Injection 1488

Insulin, NPH (Blood glucose concentration may be raised). Products include:
NPH, 100 Units 1502
Pork NPH, 100 Units 1506
Purified Pork NPH Isophane Insulin 1852

Insulin, Regular (Blood glucose concentration may be raised). Products include:
Regular, 100 Units 1503
Pork Regular, 100 Units 1507
Pork Regular (Concentrated), 500 Units 1508
Purified Pork Regular Insulin 1852

Insulin, Zinc Crystals (Blood glucose concentration may be raised). Products include:
NPH, 100 Units 1502

Insulin, Zinc Suspension (Blood glucose concentration may be raised). Products include:
Iletin I 1501
Lente, 100 Units 1501
Iletin II 1504
Pork Lente, 100 Units 1504
Purified Pork Lente Insulin 1852

Isradipine (Excessive hypotension may result especially during initial therapy). Products include:
DynaCirc Capsules 2381
DynaCirc CR Tablets 2383

Ketoprofen (Increases the antihypertensive effect). Products include:
Actron Caplets and Tablets 608
Orudis Capsules 2874
Orudis KT 842
Oruvail Capsules 2874

Ketorolac Tromethamine (Increases the antihypertensive effect). Products include:
Acular Sterile Ophthalmic Solution 470
Toradol 2319

Labetalol Hydrochloride (Excessive hypotension may result especially during initial therapy). Products include:
Normodyne Injection 2519
Normodyne Tablets 2522
Trandate 1158

(■ Described in PDR For Nonprescription Drugs) (◎ Described in PDR For Ophthalmology)

1211 Interactions Index Zaroxolyn

Levorphanol Tartrate (Hypotensive effect may be potentiated). Products include:
Levo-Dromoran ... 2297

Lisinopril (Excessive hypotension may result especially during initial therapy). Products include:
Prinivil Tablets ... 1776
Prinzide Tablets ... 1780
Zestoretic Tablets ... 2968
Zestril Tablets ... 2972

Lithium Carbonate (Serum lithium levels may increase). Products include:
Eskalith ... 2658
Lithium Carbonate Capsules & Tablets ... 2352
Lithonate/Lithotabs/Lithobid ... 2721

Lithium Citrate (Serum lithium levels may increase).
No products indexed under this heading.

Losartan Potassium (Excessive hypotension may result especially during initial therapy). Products include:
Cozaar Tablets ... 1668
Hyzaar Tablets ... 1720

Magnesium Salicylate (Increases the antihypertensive effect). Products include:
Backache Caplets ... ■D 635
Doan's Extra-Strength Analgesic ... ■D 653
Extra Strength Doan's P.M. ... ■D 653
Doan's Regular Strength Analgesic ... ■D 654
Mobigesic Tablets ... ■D 607

Mecamylamine Hydrochloride (Excessive hypotension may result especially during initial therapy). Products include:
Inversine Tablets ... 1729

Meclofenamate Sodium (Increases the antihypertensive effect).
No products indexed under this heading.

Mefenamic Acid (Increases the antihypertensive effect). Products include:
Ponstel ... 1982

Meperidine Hydrochloride (Hypotensive effect may be potentiated). Products include:
Demerol ... 2438
Mepergan Injection ... 2859

Mephobarbital (Hypotensive effect may be potentiated). Products include:
Mebaral Tablets ... 2452

Metformin Hydrochloride (Blood glucose concentration may be raised). Products include:
Glucophage Tablets ... 754

Methadone Hydrochloride (Hypotensive effect may be potentiated). Products include:
Methadone Hydrochloride Oral Concentrate ... 2356
Methadone Hydrochloride Oral Solution & Tablets ... 2357

Methenamine (Efficacy of methenamine may be decreased). Products include:
Urised Tablets ... 2123

Methenamine Hippurate (Efficacy of methenamine may be decreased).
No products indexed under this heading.

Methenamine Mandelate (Efficacy of methenamine may be decreased). Products include:
Uroqid-Acid No. 2 Tablets ... 633

Methyclothiazide (Excessive hypotension may result especially during initial therapy). Products include:
Enduron Tablets ... 424

Methyldopa (Excessive hypotension may result especially during initial therapy). Products include:
Aldoclor Tablets ... 1638
Aldomet Oral ... 1640
Aldoril Tablets ... 1644

Methyldopate Hydrochloride (Excessive hypotension may result especially during initial therapy). Products include:
Aldomet Ester HCl Injection ... 1642

Methylprednisolone Acetate (May increase the risk of hypokalemia and increase salt and water retention).
No products indexed under this heading.

Methylprednisolone Sodium Succinate (May increase the risk of hypokalemia and increase salt and water retention).
No products indexed under this heading.

Metoprolol Succinate (Excessive hypotension may result especially during initial therapy). Products include:
Toprol-XL Tablets ... 560

Metoprolol Tartrate (Excessive hypotension may result especially during initial therapy). Products include:
Lopressor ... 848
Lopressor HCT Tablets ... 850

Metyrosine (Excessive hypotension may result especially during initial therapy). Products include:
Demser Capsules ... 1690

Minoxidil (Excessive hypotension may result especially during initial therapy).
No products indexed under this heading.

Moexipril Hydrochloride (Excessive hypotension may result especially during initial therapy). Products include:
Univasc Tablets ... 2553

Morphine Sulfate (Hypotensive effect may be potentiated). Products include:
Astramorph/PF Injection, USP (Preservative-Free) ... 526
Duramorph Injection ... 983
Infumorph 200 and Infumorph 500 Sterile Solutions ... 985
Kadian Capsules ... 2948
MS Contin Tablets ... 2149
MSIR ... 2152
Oramorph SR (Morphine Sulfate Sustained Release Tablets) ... 2359
RMS Suppositories CII ... 2766
Roxanol ... 2365

Nabumetone (Increases the antihypertensive effect). Products include:
Relafen Tablets ... 2688

Nadolol (Excessive hypotension may result especially during initial therapy).
No products indexed under this heading.

Naproxen (Increases the antihypertensive effect). Products include:
Anaprox/Naprosyn ... 2277

Naproxen Sodium (Increases the antihypertensive effect). Products include:
Aleve ... 2124
Anaprox/Naprosyn ... 2277
Naprelan Tablets ... 2861

Nicardipine Hydrochloride (Excessive hypotension may result especially during initial therapy). Products include:
Cardene Capsules ... 2261
Cardene I.V. ... 2815
Cardene SR Capsules ... 2264

Nifedipine (Excessive hypotension may result especially during initial therapy). Products include:
Adalat Capsules (10 mg and 20 mg) ... 580
Adalat CC ... 582
Procardia Capsules ... 2024
Procardia XL Extended Release Tablets ... 2026

Nisoldipine (Excessive hypotension may result especially during initial therapy). Products include:
Sular Tablets ... 2961

Nitroglycerin (Excessive hypotension may result especially during initial therapy). Products include:
Deponit NTG Transdermal Delivery System ... 2541
Nitro-Bid IV ... 1270
Nitro-Bid Ointment ... 1272
Nitro-Dur (nitroglycerin) Transdermal Infusion System ... 1365
Nitrolingual Spray ... 2193
Nitrostat Tablets ... 1981
Transderm-Nitro Transdermal Therapeutic System ... 878

Norepinephrine Bitartrate (Arterial responsiveness to norepinephrine may be decreased). Products include:
Levophed Bitartrate Injection ... 2445

Opium Alkaloids (Hypotensive effect may be potentiated).
No products indexed under this heading.

Oxaprozin (Increases the antihypertensive effect). Products include:
Daypro Caplets ... 2578

Oxycodone Hydrochloride (Hypotensive effect may be potentiated). Products include:
OxyContin Tablets ... 2163
OxyIR Capsules ... 2167
Percocet Tablets ... 955
Percodan Tablets ... 955
Percodan-Demi Tablets ... 956
Roxicodone Tablets, Oral Solution & Intensol (Oxycodone) ... 2366
Tylox Capsules ... 1593

Penbutolol Sulfate (Excessive hypotension may result especially during initial therapy). Products include:
Levatol Tablets ... 2547

Pentobarbital Sodium (Hypotensive effect may be potentiated). Products include:
Nembutal Sodium Capsules ... 440
Nembutal Sodium Solution ... 442
Nembutal Sodium Suppositories ... 444

Phenobarbital (Hypotensive effect may be potentiated). Products include:
Arco-Lase Plus Tablets ... 513
Bellergal-S Tablets ... 2375
Donnatal ... 2234
Donnatal Extentabs ... 2234
Donnatal Tablets ... 2234
Phenobarbital Elixir and Tablets ... 1523
Quadrinal Tablets ... 1398

Phenoxybenzamine Hydrochloride (Excessive hypotension may result especially during initial therapy). Products include:
Dibenzyline Capsules ... 2650

Phentolamine Mesylate (Excessive hypotension may result especially during initial therapy). Products include:
Regitine Vials ... 864

Phenylbutazone (Increases the antihypertensive effect).
No products indexed under this heading.

Pindolol (Excessive hypotension may result especially during initial therapy). Products include:
Visken Tablets ... 2428

Piroxicam (Increases the antihypertensive effect). Products include:
Feldene Capsules ... 2008

Polythiazide (Excessive hypotension may result especially during initial therapy). Products include:
Minizide Capsules ... 2016

Prazosin Hydrochloride (Excessive hypotension may result especially during initial therapy). Products include:
Minipress Capsules ... 2015
Minizide Capsules ... 2016

Prednisolone Acetate (May increase the risk of hypokalemia and increase salt and water retention). Products include:
AK-CIDE ... ⊛ 203
AK-CIDE Ointment ... ⊛ 203
Blephamide Liquifilm Sterile Ophthalmic Suspension ... 472
Blephamide Ointment ... ⊛ 234
Econopred & Econopred Plus Ophthalmic Suspensions ... ⊛ 216
Poly-Pred Liquifilm ... ⊛ 246
Pred Forte ... ⊛ 247
Pred Mild ... ⊛ 250
Pred-G Liquifilm Sterile Ophthalmic Suspension ... ⊛ 248
Pred-G S.O.P. Sterile Ophthalmic Ointment ... ⊛ 249

Prednisolone Sodium Phosphate (May increase the risk of hypokalemia and increase salt and water retention). Products include:
AK-PRED ... ⊛ 204
Hydeltrasol Injection, Sterile ... 1708
Pediapred Oral Solution ... 1618

Prednisolone Tebutate (May increase the risk of hypokalemia and increase salt and water retention). Products include:
Hydeltra-T.B.A. Sterile Suspension 1710

Prednisone (May increase the risk of hypokalemia and increase salt and water retention).
No products indexed under this heading.

Propoxyphene Hydrochloride (Hypotensive effect may be potentiated). Products include:
Darvon ... 1475
Wygesic Tablets ... 2930

Propoxyphene Napsylate (Hypotensive effect may be potentiated). Products include:
Darvon-N/Darvocet-N ... 1473

Propranolol Hydrochloride (Excessive hypotension may result especially during initial therapy). Products include:
Inderal ... 2834
Inderal LA Long Acting Capsules ... 2836
Inderide Tablets ... 2838
Inderide LA Long Acting Capsules ... 2840

Quinapril Hydrochloride (Excessive hypotension may result especially during initial therapy). Products include:
Accupril Tablets ... 1950

Ramipril (Excessive hypotension may result especially during initial therapy). Products include:
Altace Capsules ... 1238

Rauwolfia Serpentina (Excessive hypotension may result especially during initial therapy).
No products indexed under this heading.

Rescinnamine (Excessive hypotension may result especially during initial therapy).
No products indexed under this heading.

Reserpine (Excessive hypotension may result especially during initial therapy). Products include:
Diupres Tablets ... 1691
Hydropres Tablets ... 1718
Ser-Ap-Es Tablets ... 867

Salsalate (Increases the antihypertensive effect). Products include:
Disalcid ... 1549

IMPORTANT NOTE: Always consult each drug listing in the patient's regimen for possible interactions.

Zaroxolyn / Interactions Index

Mono-Gesic Tablets 810
Salflex Tablets 791

Secobarbital Sodium (Hypotensive effect may be potentiated). Products include:
Seconal Sodium Pulvules 1529

Sodium Nitroprusside (Excessive hypotension may result especially during initial therapy).
No products indexed under this heading.

Sotalol Hydrochloride (Excessive hypotension may result especially during initial therapy). Products include:
Betapace Tablets 637

Spirapril Hydrochloride (Excessive hypotension may result especially during initial therapy).
No products indexed under this heading.

Sufentanil Citrate (Hypotensive effect may be potentiated). Products include:
Sufenta Injection 1355

Sulindac (Increases the antihypertensive effect). Products include:
Clinoril Tablets 1658

Terazosin Hydrochloride (Excessive hypotension may result especially during initial therapy). Products include:
Hytrin Capsules 434

Thiamylal Sodium (Hypotensive effect may be potentiated).
No products indexed under this heading.

Timolol Maleate (Excessive hypotension may result especially during initial therapy). Products include:
Blocadren Tablets 1654
Timolide Tablets 1791
Timoptic in Ocudose 1796
Timoptic Sterile Ophthalmic Solution 1794
Timoptic-XE 1798

Tolazamide (Blood glucose concentration may be raised).
No products indexed under this heading.

Tolbutamide (Blood glucose concentration may be raised).
No products indexed under this heading.

Tolmetin Sodium (Increases the antihypertensive effect). Products include:
Tolectin (200, 400 and 600 mg) .. 1591

Torsemide (Excessive hypotension may result especially during initial therapy). Products include:
Demadex Tablets and Injection 691

Triamcinolone (May increase the risk of hypokalemia and increase salt and water retention).
No products indexed under this heading.

Triamcinolone Acetonide (May increase the risk of hypokalemia and increase salt and water retention). Products include:
Azmacort Oral Inhaler 2175
Nasacort AQ Nasal Spray 2191
Nasacort Nasal Inhaler 2189

Triamcinolone Diacetate (May increase the risk of hypokalemia and increase salt and water retention).
No products indexed under this heading.

Triamcinolone Hexacetonide (May increase the risk of hypokalemia and increase salt and water retention).
No products indexed under this heading.

Trimethaphan Camsylate (Excessive hypotension may result especially during initial therapy).
No products indexed under this heading.

Tubocurarine Chloride (Neuromuscular blocking effects of curariform drugs may be enhanced).
No products indexed under this heading.

Verapamil Hydrochloride (Excessive hypotension may result especially during initial therapy). Products include:
Calan SR Caplets 2571
Calan Tablets 2568
Covera-HS Tablets 2573
Isoptin Injectable 1391
Isoptin Oral Tablets 1393
Isoptin SR Tablets 1395
Verelan Capsules 1455

Warfarin Sodium (May affect the hypoprothrombinemic response to anticoagulants; dosage adjustments may be necessary). Products include:
Coumadin 941

Food Interactions

Alcohol (Hypotensive effect may be potentiated).

ZEBETA TABLETS

(Bisoprolol Fumarate) 1457
May interact with beta blockers, catecholamine depleting drugs, oral hypoglycemic agents, and insulin. Compounds in these categories include:

Acarbose (Possible masking of some of the manifestations of hypoglycemia). Products include:
Precose 604

Acebutolol Hydrochloride (Zebeta should not be combined with other beta-blocking drugs). Products include:
Sectral Capsules 2914

Atenolol (Zebeta should not be combined with other beta-blocking drugs). Products include:
Tenoretic Tablets 2963
Tenormin Tablets and I.V. Injection 2965

Betaxolol Hydrochloride (Zebeta should not be combined with other beta-blocking drugs). Products include:
Betoptic Ophthalmic Solution 465
Betoptic S Ophthalmic Suspension .. 467
Kerlone Tablets 2588

Carteolol Hydrochloride (Zebeta should not be combined with other beta-blocking drugs). Products include:
Cartrol Tablets 413
Ocupress Ophthalmic Solution, 1% Sterile .... ⊚ 297

Chlorpropamide (Possible masking of some of the manifestations of hypoglycemia). Products include:
Diabinese Tablets 2002

Clonidine (In patients receiving concurrent clonidine, Zebeta should be discontinued for several days before the withdrawal of clonidine). Products include:
Catapres-TTS 680

Clonidine Hydrochloride (In patients receiving concurrent clonidine, Zebeta should be discontinued for several days before the withdrawal of clonidine). Products include:
Catapres Tablets 679
Combipres Tablets 682

Cyclopropane (Care should be taken when anesthetic agents which depress myocardial function are used with Zebeta).

Deserpidine (Potential for added beta-adrenergic blocking action of Zebeta resulting in excessive reduction of sympathetic activity).
No products indexed under this heading.

Diltiazem Hydrochloride (Potential for additional myocardial depression and/or inhibition of AV conduction). Products include:
Cardizem CD Capsules 1251
Cardizem SR Capsules 1255
Cardizem Injectable 1253
Cardizem Tablets 1257
Dilacor XR Extended-release Capsules 2183
Tiazac Capsules 1019

Disopyramide Phosphate (Potential for additional myocardial depression and/or inhibition of AV conduction). Products include:
Norpace 2596

Epinephrine (Patients with a history of anaphylactic reactions to a variety of allergens may be unresponsive to the usual dose of epinephrine used to treat allergic reactions). Products include:
EPIFRIN .... ⊚ 237
EpiPen 808
Marcaine with Epinephrine 2446
Primatene Mist .... ▣ 843
Sensorcaine with Epinephrine Injection 554
Sus-Phrine Injection 1017
Xylocaine with Epinephrine Injections 562

Epinephrine Bitartrate (Patients with a history of anaphylactic reactions to a variety of allergens may be unresponsive to the usual dose of epinephrine used to treat allergic reactions). Products include:
Sensorcaine-MPF with Epinephrine Injection 554

Esmolol Hydrochloride (Zebeta should not be combined with other beta-blocking drugs). Products include:
Brevibloc (esmolol HCl) Injection 1860

Ether (Care should be taken when anesthetic agents which depress myocardial function are used with Zebeta).
No products indexed under this heading.

Glimepiride (Possible masking of some of the manifestations of hypoglycemia). Products include:
Amaryl Tablets 1241

Glipizide (Possible masking of some of the manifestations of hypoglycemia). Products include:
Glucotrol Tablets 2011
Glucotrol XL Extended Release Tablets 2012

Glyburide (Possible masking of some of the manifestations of hypoglycemia). Products include:
DiaBeta Tablets 1265
Glynase PresTab Tablets 2091
Micronase Tablets 2099

Guanethidine Monosulfate (Potential for added beta-adrenergic blocking action of Zebeta resulting in excessive reduction of sympathetic activity). Products include:
Esimil Tablets 840
Ismelin Tablets 845

Insulin, Human (Possible masking of some of the manifestations of hypoglycemia).
No products indexed under this heading.

Insulin, Human Isophane Suspension (Possible masking of some of the manifestations of hypoglycemia). Products include:
Novolin N Human Insulin 10 ml Vials 1846

Insulin, Human NPH (Possible masking of some of the manifestations of hypoglycemia). Products include:
Humulin N, 100 Units 1495
Novolin N PenFill 1.5 ml Cartridges Durable Insulin Delivery System 1849
Novolin N Prefilled Syringe Disposable Insulin Delivery System ... 1850

Insulin, Human Regular (Possible masking of some of the manifestations of hypoglycemia). Products include:
Humulin R, 100 Units 1497
Novolin R Human Insulin 10 ml Vials 1846
Novolin R PenFill 1.5 ml Cartridges Durable Insulin Delivery System 1849
Novolin R Prefilled Syringe Disposable Insulin Delivery System ... 1850
Velosulin BR Human Insulin 10 ml Vials 1847

Insulin, Human, Zinc Suspension (Possible masking of some of the manifestations of hypoglycemia). Products include:
Humulin L, 100 Units 1494
Humulin U, 100 Units 1498
Novolin L Human Insulin 10 ml Vials 1846

Insulin Lispro, Human (Possible masking of some of the manifestations of hypoglycemia). Products include:
Humalog Injection 1488

Insulin, NPH (Possible masking of some of the manifestations of hypoglycemia). Products include:
NPH, 100 Units 1502
Pork NPH, 100 Units 1506
Purified Pork NPH Isophane Insulin 1852

Insulin, Regular (Possible masking of some of the manifestations of hypoglycemia). Products include:
Regular, 100 Units 1503
Pork Regular, 100 Units 1507
Pork Regular (Concentrated), 500 Units 1508
Purified Pork Regular Insulin 1852

Insulin, Zinc Crystals (Possible masking of some of the manifestations of hypoglycemia). Products include:
NPH, 100 Units 1502

Insulin, Zinc Suspension (Possible masking of some of the manifestations of hypoglycemia). Products include:
Iletin I 1501
Lente, 100 Units 1501
Iletin II 1504
Pork Lente, 100 Units 1504
Purified Pork Lente Insulin 1852

Labetalol Hydrochloride (Zebeta should not be combined with other beta-blocking drugs). Products include:
Normodyne Injection 2519
Normodyne Tablets 2522
Trandate 1158

Levobunolol Hydrochloride (Zebeta should not be combined with other beta-blocking drugs). Products include:
Betagan .... ⊚ 230

Metformin Hydrochloride (Possible masking of some of the manifestations of hypoglycemia). Products include:
Glucophage Tablets 754

Metipranolol Hydrochloride (Zebeta should not be combined with other beta-blocking drugs). Products include:
OptiPranolol (Metipranolol 0.3%) Sterile Ophthalmic Solution .... ⊚ 256

(▣ Described in PDR For Nonprescription Drugs)   (⊚ Described in PDR For Ophthalmology)

Interactions Index

Metoprolol Succinate (Zebeta should not be combined with other beta-blocking drugs). Products include:
- Toprol-XL Tablets 560

Metoprolol Tartrate (Zebeta should not be combined with other beta-blocking drugs). Products include:
- Lopressor 848
- Lopressor HCT Tablets 850

Nadolol (Zebeta should not be combined with other beta-blocking drugs).
- No products indexed under this heading.

Penbutolol Sulfate (Zebeta should not be combined with other beta-blocking drugs). Products include:
- Levatol Tablets 2547

Pindolol (Zebeta should not be combined with other beta-blocking drugs). Products include:
- Visken Tablets 2428

Propranolol Hydrochloride (Zebeta should not be combined with other beta-blocking drugs). Products include:
- Inderal 2834
- Inderal LA Long Acting Capsules 2836
- Inderide Tablets 2838
- Inderide LA Long Acting Capsules 2840

Rauwolfia Serpentina (Potential for added beta-adrenergic blocking action of Zebeta resulting in excessive reduction of sympathetic activity).
- No products indexed under this heading.

Rescinnamine (Potential for added beta-adrenergic blocking action of Zebeta resulting in excessive reduction of sympathetic activity).
- No products indexed under this heading.

Reserpine (Potential for added beta-adrenergic blocking action of Zebeta resulting in excessive reduction of sympathetic activity). Products include:
- Diupres Tablets 1691
- Hydropres Tablets 1718
- Ser-Ap-Es Tablets 867

Rifampin (Concurrent use increases the metabolic clearance of Zebeta, resulting in shortened elimination half-life of Zebeta). Products include:
- Rifadin 1276
- Rifamate Capsules 1278
- Rifater 1280
- Rimactane Capsules 865

Sotalol Hydrochloride (Zebeta should not be combined with other beta-blocking drugs). Products include:
- Betapace Tablets 637

Timolol Hemihydrate (Zebeta should not be combined with other beta-blocking drugs). Products include:
- Betimol 0.25%, 0.5% .... ⓐ 259

Timolol Maleate (Zebeta should not be combined with other beta-blocking drugs). Products include:
- Blocadren Tablets 1654
- Timolide Tablets 1791
- Timoptic in Ocudose 1796
- Timoptic Sterile Ophthalmic Solution 1794
- Timoptic-XE 1798

Tolazamide (Possible masking of some of the manifestations of hypoglycemia).
- No products indexed under this heading.

Tolbutamide (Possible masking of some of the manifestations of hypoglycemia).
- No products indexed under this heading.

Verapamil Hydrochloride (Potential for additional myocardial depression and/or inhibition of AV conduction). Products include:
- Calan SR Caplets 2571
- Calan Tablets 2568
- Covera-HS Tablets 2573
- Isoptin Injectable 1391
- Isoptin Oral Tablets 1393
- Isoptin SR Tablets 1395
- Verelan Capsules 1455

ZEMURON INJECTION
(Rocuronium Bromide) 1885
May interact with aminoglycosides, tetracyclines, anticonvulsants, inhalant anesthetics, and certain other agents. Compounds in these categories include:

Amikacin Sulfate (Possible prolongation of neuromuscular blockade). Products include:
- Amikacin Sulfate Injection, USP 523
- Amikacin Sulfate Injection, USP 981
- Amikin Injectable 502

Bacitracin (Possible prolongation of neuromuscular blockade).
- No products indexed under this heading.

Carbamazepine (Potential for apparent resistance to the effects of rocuronium in the form of diminished magnitude of neuromuscular blockade). Products include:
- Atretol Tablets 569
- Tegretol/Tegretol-XR 870

Colistimethate Sodium (Possible prolongation of neuromuscular blockade).
- No products indexed under this heading.

Colistin Sulfate (Possible prolongation of neuromuscular blockade). Products include:
- Coly-Mycin S Otic w/Neomycin & Hydrocortisone 1965

Demeclocycline Hydrochloride (Possible prolongation of neuromuscular blockade). Products include:
- Declomycin Tablets 1421

Desflurane (Possible enhanced activity of neuromuscular blocking agent). Products include:
- Suprane (desflurane, USP) 1865

Divalproex Sodium (Potential for apparent resistance to the effects of rocuronium in the form of diminished magnitude of neuromuscular blockade). Products include:
- Depakote Tablets 418

Doxycycline Calcium (Possible prolongation of neuromuscular blockade). Products include:
- Vibramycin Calcium Oral Suspension Syrup 2038

Doxycycline Hyclate (Possible prolongation of neuromuscular blockade). Products include:
- Doryx Capsules 1970
- Vibramycin Hyclate Capsules 2038
- Vibramycin Hyclate Intravenous 2040
- Vibra-Tabs Film Coated Tablets 2038

Doxycycline Monohydrate (Possible prolongation of neuromuscular blockade). Products include:
- Monodox Capsules 1858
- Vibramycin Monohydrate for Oral Suspension 2038

Enflurane (Possible enhanced activity of neuromuscular blocking agent; may prolong the duration of action).
- No products indexed under this heading.

Ethosuximide (Potential for apparent resistance to the effects of rocuronium in the form of diminished magnitude of neuromuscular blockade). Products include:
- Zarontin Capsules 1986
- Zarontin Syrup 1986

Ethotoin (Potential for apparent resistance to the effects of rocuronium in the form of diminished magnitude of neuromuscular blockade). Products include:
- Peganone Tablets 455

Felbamate (Potential for apparent resistance to the effects of rocuronium in the form of diminished magnitude of neuromuscular blockade). Products include:
- Felbatol 2774

Gentamicin Sulfate (Possible prolongation of neuromuscular blockade). Products include:
- Garamycin Cream 0.1% 2501
- Garamycin Injectable 2502
- Garamycin Ointment 0.1% 2501
- Garamycin Ophthalmic 2501
- Genoptic Sterile Ophthalmic Solution .... ⓐ 241
- Genoptic Sterile Ophthalmic Ointment .... ⓐ 241
- Gentak .... ⓐ 209
- Pred-G Liquifilm Sterile Ophthalmic Suspension .... ⓐ 248
- Pred-G S.O.P. Sterile Ophthalmic Ointment .... ⓐ 249

Halothane (Possible enhanced activity of neuromuscular blocking agent). Products include:
- Fluothane 2830

Isoflurane (Possible enhanced activity of neuromuscular blocking agent; may prolong the duration of action).
- No products indexed under this heading.

Kanamycin Sulfate (Possible prolongation of neuromuscular blockade).
- No products indexed under this heading.

Lamotrigine (Potential for apparent resistance to the effects of rocuronium in the form of diminished magnitude of neuromuscular blockade). Products include:
- Lamictal Tablets 1105

Lithium Carbonate (May increase the duration of neuromuscular block). Products include:
- Eskalith 2658
- Lithium Carbonate Capsules & Tablets 2352
- Lithonate/Lithotabs/Lithobid 2721

Lithium Citrate (May increase the duration of neuromuscular block).
- No products indexed under this heading.

Magnesium Sulfate Injection (May enhance the neuromuscular blockade).

Mephenytoin (Potential for apparent resistance to the effects of rocuronium in the form of diminished magnitude of neuromuscular blockade). Products include:
- Mesantoin Tablets 2400

Methacycline Hydrochloride (Possible prolongation of neuromuscular blockade).
- No products indexed under this heading.

Methoxyflurane (Possible enhanced activity of neuromuscular blocking agent).
- No products indexed under this heading.

Methsuximide (Potential for apparent resistance to the effects of rocuronium in the form of diminished magnitude of neuromuscular blockade). Products include:
- Celontin Kapseals 1955

Minocycline Hydrochloride (Possible prolongation of neuromuscular blockade). Products include:
- DYNACIN Capsules 1627
- Minocin Intravenous 1428
- Minocin Oral Suspension 1431
- Minocin Pellet-Filled Capsules 1429

Oxytetracycline Hydrochloride (Possible prolongation of neuromuscular blockade). Products include:
- TERAK Ointment .... ⓐ 210
- Terra-Cortril Ophthalmic Suspension 2033
- Terramycin with Polymyxin B Sulfate Ophthalmic Ointment 2035
- Urobiotic-250 Capsules 2038

Paramethadione (Potential for apparent resistance to the effects of rocuronium in the form of diminished magnitude of neuromuscular blockade).
- No products indexed under this heading.

Phenacemide (Potential for apparent resistance to the effects of rocuronium in the form of diminished magnitude of neuromuscular blockade). Products include:
- Phenurone Tablets 455

Phenobarbital (Potential for apparent resistance to the effects of rocuronium in the form of diminished magnitude of neuromuscular blockade). Products include:
- Arco-Lase Plus Tablets 513
- Bellergal-S Tablets 2375
- Donnatal 2234
- Donnatal Extentabs 2234
- Donnatal Tablets 2234
- Phenobarbital Elixir and Tablets 1523
- Quadrinal Tablets 1398

Phensuximide (Potential for apparent resistance to the effects of rocuronium in the form of diminished magnitude of neuromuscular blockade).
- No products indexed under this heading.

Phenytoin (Potential for apparent resistance to the effects of rocuronium in the form of diminished magnitude of neuromuscular blockade). Products include:
- Dilantin Infatabs 1967
- Dilantin-125 Suspension 1969

Phenytoin Sodium (Potential for apparent resistance to the effects of rocuronium in the form of diminished magnitude of neuromuscular blockade). Products include:
- Dilantin Kapseals 1965

Polymyxin B Sulfate (Possible prolongation of neuromuscular blockade). Products include:
- AK-Spore .... ⓐ 205
- AK-Trol Ointment & Suspension .... ⓐ 205
- Betadine Brand First Aid Antibiotics & Moisturizer Ointment 2144
- Cortisporin Cream 1073
- Cortisporin Ointment 1074
- Cortisporin Ophthalmic Ointment Sterile 1074
- Cortisporin Ophthalmic Suspension Sterile 1075
- Cortisporin Otic Solution Sterile 1076
- Cortisporin Otic Suspension Sterile 1077
- Maxitrol Ophthalmic Ointment and Suspension .... ⓐ 222
- Mycitracin .... ⓐ 803
- Neosporin G.U. Irrigant Sterile 1130
- Neosporin Ointment .... ⓐ 821
- Neosporin Plus Maximum Strength Cream 1130
- Neosporin Plus Maximum Strength Ointment .... ⓐ 822
- Neosporin Ophthalmic Ointment Sterile 1130

IMPORTANT NOTE: Always consult each drug listing in the patient's regimen for possible interactions.

Zemuron Interactions Index 1214

Neosporin Ophthalmic Solution Sterile ... 1131
Pediotic Suspension Sterile ... 1140
Poly-Pred Liquifilm ... ◉ 246
Polysporin Ointment ... ▣ 822
Polysporin Ophthalmic Ointment Sterile ... 1140
Polysporin Powder ... ▣ 823
Polytrim Ophthalmic Solution Sterile ... 479
TERAK Ointment ... ◉ 210
Terramycin with Polymyxin B Sulfate Ophthalmic Ointment ... 2035

Primidone (Potential for apparent resistance to the effects of rocuronium in the form of diminished magnitude of neuromuscular blockade). Products include:
Mysoline ... 2860

Procainamide Hydrochloride (May increase the duration of neuromuscular block). Products include:
Procanbid Extended-Release Tablets ... 1983

Quinidine Gluconate (Possible recurrent paralysis; increased duration of neuromuscular block). Products include:
Quinaglute Dura-Tabs Tablets ... 644

Quinidine Polygalacturonate (Possible recurrent paralysis; increased duration of neuromuscular block). Products include:
Cardioquin Tablets ... 2146

Quinidine Sulfate (Possible recurrent paralysis; increased duration of neuromuscular block). Products include:
Quinidex Extentabs ... 2240

Streptomycin Sulfate (Possible prolongation of neuromuscular blockade). Products include:
Streptomycin Sulfate Injection ... 2031

Succinylcholine Chloride (Rocuronium should not be given until recovery from succinylcholine has been observed). Products include:
Anectine ... 1062

Tetracycline Hydrochloride (Possible prolongation of neuromuscular blockade). Products include:
Achromycin V Capsules ... 1417
Helidac Therapy ... 2135

Tobramycin (Possible prolongation of neuromuscular blockade). Products include:
AKTOB ... ◉ 207
TobraDex Ophthalmic Suspension and Ointment ... 469
Tobrex Ophthalmic Ointment and Solution ... ◉ 226

Tobramycin Sulfate (Possible prolongation of neuromuscular blockade). Products include:
Nebcin Vials, Hyporets & ADD-Vantage ... 1518

Trimethadione (Potential for apparent resistance to the effects of rocuronium in the form of diminished magnitude of neuromuscular blockade).
No products indexed under this heading.

Valproic Acid (Potential for apparent resistance to the effects of rocuronium in the form of diminished magnitude of neuromuscular blockade). Products include:
Depakene ... 416

Vancomycin Hydrochloride (Possible prolongation of neuromuscular blockade). Products include:
Vancocin HCl, Oral Solution & Pulvules ... 1536
Vancocin HCl, Vials & ADD-Vantage ... 1534

ADVANCED FORMULA ZENATE TABLETS
(Vitamins with Minerals) ... 2728
None cited in PDR database.

ZERIT CAPSULES
(Stavudine) ... 731
May interact with drugs that may exacerbate peripheral neuropathy (selected). Compounds in this category include:

Carboplatin (Concurrent use may exacerbate peripheral neuropathy). Products include:
Paraplatin for Injection ... 713

Didanosine (Concurrent use may exacerbate peripheral neuropathy). Products include:
Videx Tablets, Powder for Oral Solution, & Pediatric Powder for Oral Solution ... 2980

Isoniazid (Concurrent use may exacerbate peripheral neuropathy). Products include:
Nydrazid Injection ... 509
Rifamate Capsules ... 1278
Rifater ... 1280

Paclitaxel (Concurrent use may exacerbate peripheral neuropathy). Products include:
Taxol Injection ... 723

Zalcitabine (Concurrent use may exacerbate peripheral neuropathy). Products include:
Hivid Tablets ... 2287

Food Interactions

Meal, unspecified (Co-administration with food decreases C_{max} by approximately 45%, however, the systemic availability (AUC) is unchanged; Zerit capsules can be taken without regard to meals).

ZESTORETIC TABLETS
(Lisinopril, Hydrochlorothiazide) ... 2968
May interact with diuretics, non-steroidal anti-inflammatory agents, potassium sparing diuretics, potassium preparations, barbiturates, narcotic analgesics, oral hypoglycemic agents, insulin, antihypertensives, corticosteroids, lithium preparations, nondepolarizing neuromuscular blocking agents, and certain other agents. Compounds in these categories include:

Acarbose (Dosage adjustment of the antidiabetic may be required). Products include:
Precose ... 604

Acebutolol Hydrochloride (Additive effects). Products include:
Sectral Capsules ... 2914

ACTH (Intensifies electrolyte depletion).
No products indexed under this heading.

Alfentanil Hydrochloride (Potentiates orthostatic hypotension). Products include:
Alfenta Injection ... 1334

Amiloride Hydrochloride (Additive antihypertensive effects; potential for hyperkalemia). Products include:
Midamor Tablets ... 1746
Moduretic Tablets ... 1748

Amlodipine Besylate (Additive effects). Products include:
Lotrel Capsules ... 858
Norvasc Tablets ... 2020

Aprobarbital (Potentiates orthostatic hypotension).
No products indexed under this heading.

Atenolol (Additive effects). Products include:
Tenoretic Tablets ... 2963
Tenormin Tablets and I.V. Injection 2965

Atracurium Besylate (Possible increased responsiveness to the muscle relaxant). Products include:
Tracrium Injection ... 1155

Benazepril Hydrochloride (Additive effects). Products include:
Lotensin Tablets ... 852
Lotensin HCT Tablets ... 855
Lotrel Capsules ... 858

Bendroflumethiazide (Additive effects).
No products indexed under this heading.

Betamethasone Acetate (Intensifies electrolyte depletion). Products include:
Celestone Soluspan Suspension ... 2484

Betamethasone Sodium Phosphate (Intensifies electrolyte depletion). Products include:
Celestone Soluspan Suspension ... 2484

Betaxolol Hydrochloride (Additive effects). Products include:
Betoptic Ophthalmic Solution ... 465
Betoptic S Ophthalmic Suspension 467
Kerlone Tablets ... 2588

Bisoprolol Fumarate (Additive effects). Products include:
Zebeta Tablets ... 1457
Ziac ... 1459

Bumetanide (Additive effects). Products include:
Bumex ... 2260

Buprenorphine (Potentiates orthostatic hypotension). Products include:
Buprenex Injectable ... 2170

Butabarbital (Potentiates orthostatic hypotension).
No products indexed under this heading.

Butalbital (Potentiates orthostatic hypotension). Products include:
Axocet Capsules ... 2469
Esgic-plus Capsules ... 1012
Esgic-plus Tablets ... 1012
Fioricet Tablets ... 2386
Fioricet with Codeine Capsules ... 2387
Fiorinal Capsules ... 2388
Fiorinal with Codeine Capsules ... 2390
Fiorinal Tablets ... 2388
Phrenilin ... 790
Sedapap Tablets 50 mg/650 mg .. 1826

Captopril (Additive effects). Products include:
Capoten Tablets ... 740
Capozide Tablets ... 744

Carteolol Hydrochloride (Additive effects). Products include:
Cartrol Tablets ... 413
Ocupress Ophthalmic Solution, 1% Sterile ... ◉ 297

Chlorothiazide (Additive effects). Products include:
Aldoclor Tablets ... 1638
Diupres Tablets ... 1691
Diuril Oral ... 1694

Chlorothiazide Sodium (Additive effects). Products include:
Diuril Sodium Intravenous ... 1693

Chlorpropamide (Dosage adjustment of the antidiabetic may be required). Products include:
Diabinese Tablets ... 2002

Chlorthalidone (Additive effects). Products include:
Combipres Tablets ... 682
Tenoretic Tablets ... 2963
Thalitone ... 1293

Cholestyramine (Absorption of hydrochlorothiazide is impaired in the presence of anionic exchange resins, such as cholestyramine; binds hydrochlorothiazide and reduces its absorption from the GI tract by up to 85%). Products include:
Questran ... 774

Cisatracurium Besylate (Possible increased responsiveness to the muscle relaxant). Products include:
Nimbex Injection ... 1131

Clonidine (Additive effects). Products include:
Catapres-TTS ... 680

Clonidine Hydrochloride (Additive effects). Products include:
Catapres Tablets ... 679
Combipres Tablets ... 682

Codeine Phosphate (Potentiates orthostatic hypotension). Products include:
Brontex ... 2130
Dimetane-DC Cough Syrup ... 2232
Fioricet with Codeine Capsules ... 2387
Fiorinal with Codeine Capsules ... 2390
Nucofed ... 2225
Phenergan with Codeine ... 2883
Phenergan VC with Codeine ... 2888
Robitussin A-C Syrup ... 2248
Robitussin-DAC Syrup ... 2249
Ryna ... ▣ 804
Soma Compound w/Codeine Tablets ... 2784
Tylenol with Codeine ... 1592

Colestipol Hydrochloride (Absorption of hydrochlorothiazide is impaired in the presence of anionic exchange resins, such as colestipol; binds hydrochlorothiazide and reduces its absorption from the GI tract by up to 43%). Products include:
Colestid ... 2073

Cortisone Acetate (Intensifies electrolyte depletion). Products include:
Cortone Acetate Sterile Suspension ... 1663
Cortone Acetate Tablets ... 1664

Deserpidine (Additive effects).
No products indexed under this heading.

Dexamethasone (Intensifies electrolyte depletion). Products include:
AK-Trol Ointment & Suspension ... ◉ 205
Decadron Elixir ... 1676
Decadron Tablets ... 1678
Decaspray Topical Aerosol ... 1689
Maxitrol Ophthalmic Ointment and Suspension ... ◉ 222
TobraDex Ophthalmic Suspension and Ointment ... 469

Dexamethasone Acetate (Intensifies electrolyte depletion). Products include:
Dalalone D.P. Injectable ... 1009
Decadron-LA Sterile Suspension ... 1687

Dexamethasone Sodium Phosphate (Intensifies electrolyte depletion). Products include:
Decadron Phosphate Injection ... 1680
Decadron Phosphate Sterile Ophthalmic Ointment ... 1684
Decadron Phosphate Sterile Ophthalmic Solution ... 1685
Decadron Phosphate Topical Cream ... 1686
Decadron Phosphate with Xylocaine Injection, Sterile ... 1683
Dexacort Phosphate in Respihaler .. 1606
Dexacort Phosphate in Turbinaire .. 1607
NeoDecadron Sterile Ophthalmic Ointment ... 1755
NeoDecadron Sterile Ophthalmic Solution ... 1756
NeoDecadron Topical Cream ... 1757

Dezocine (Potentiates orthostatic hypotension). Products include:
Dalgan Injection ... 529

Diazoxide (Additive effects). Products include:
Hyperstat I.V. Injection ... 2504
Proglycem ... 575

Diclofenac Potassium (Reduces antihypertensive effects). Products include:
Cataflam Tablets ... 833

(▣ Described in PDR For Nonprescription Drugs) (◉ Described in PDR For Ophthalmology)

Interactions Index

Diclofenac Sodium (Reduces antihypertensive effects). Products include:
- Voltaren Ophthalmic Sterile Ophthalmic Solution ... 264
- Cataflam/Voltaren/Voltaren-XR ... 833

Diltiazem Hydrochloride (Additive effects). Products include:
- Cardizem CD Capsules ... 1251
- Cardizem SR Capsules ... 1255
- Cardizem Injectable ... 1253
- Cardizem Tablets ... 1257
- Dilacor XR Extended-release Capsules ... 2183
- Tiazac Capsules ... 1019

Doxazosin Mesylate (Additive effects). Products include:
- Cardura Tablets ... 1993

Enalapril Maleate (Additive effects). Products include:
- Vaseretic Tablets ... 1810
- Vasotec Tablets ... 1816

Enalaprilat (Additive effects). Products include:
- Vasotec I.V. ... 1814

Esmolol Hydrochloride (Additive effects). Products include:
- Brevibloc (esmolol HCl) Injection ... 1860

Ethacrynic Acid (Additive effects). Products include:
- Edecrin Tablets ... 1698

Etodolac (Reduces antihypertensive effects). Products include:
- Lodine Capsules and Tablets ... 2849

Felodipine (Additive effects). Products include:
- Plendil Extended-Release Tablets ... 514

Fenoprofen Calcium (Reduces antihypertensive effects). Products include:
- Nalfon 200 Pulvules & Nalfon Tablets ... 933

Fentanyl (Potentiates orthostatic hypotension). Products include:
- Duragesic Transdermal System ... 1336

Fentanyl Citrate (Potentiates orthostatic hypotension). Products include:
- Sublimaze Injection ... 463

Fludrocortisone Acetate (Intensifies electrolyte depletion). Products include:
- Florinef Acetate Tablets ... 506

Flurbiprofen (Reduces antihypertensive effects).
- No products indexed under this heading.

Fosinopril Sodium (Additive effects). Products include:
- Monopril Tablets ... 762

Furosemide (Additive effects). Products include:
- Lasix Injection, Oral Solution and Tablets ... 1267

Glimepiride (Dosage adjustment of the antidiabetic may be required). Products include:
- Amaryl Tablets ... 1241

Glipizide (Dosage adjustment of the antidiabetic may be required). Products include:
- Glucotrol Tablets ... 2011
- Glucotrol XL Extended Release Tablets ... 2012

Glyburide (Dosage adjustment of the antidiabetic may be required). Products include:
- DiaBeta Tablets ... 1265
- Glynase PresTab Tablets ... 2091
- Micronase Tablets ... 2099

Guanabenz Acetate (Additive effects).
- No products indexed under this heading.

Guanethidine Monosulfate (Additive effects). Products include:
- Esimil Tablets ... 840
- Ismelin Tablets ... 845

Hydralazine Hydrochloride (Additive effects). Products include:
- Apresazide Capsules ... 824
- Apresoline Hydrochloride Tablets ... 826
- Hydralazine Hydrochloride Injection USP ... 2712
- Ser-Ap-Es Tablets ... 867

Hydrocodone Bitartrate (Potentiates orthostatic hypotension). Products include:
- Codiclear DH Syrup ... 808
- Duratuss HD Elixir ... 2750
- Histussin D Liquid ... 670
- Hycodan Tablets and Syrup ... 946
- Hycomine Compound Tablets ... 948
- Hycomine ... 947
- Hycotuss Expectorant Syrup ... 950
- Hydrocet Capsules ... 787
- Lorcet 10/650 Tablets ... 1016
- Lortab ... 2751
- Tussend ... 1830
- Tussend Expectorant ... 1831
- Vicodin Tablets ... 1404
- Vicodin ES Tablets ... 1405
- Vicodin HP Tablets ... 1403
- Vicodin Tuss Expectorant ... 1406
- Zydone Capsules ... 967

Hydrocodone Polistirex (Potentiates orthostatic hypotension). Products include:
- Tussionex Pennkinetic Extended-Release Suspension ... 1624

Hydrocortisone (Intensifies electrolyte depletion). Products include:
- Anusol-HC Cream 2.5% ... 1953
- Aquanil HC Lotion ... 1989
- Maximum Strength Cortaid Spray ... 800
- CORTENEMA ... 2713
- Cortisporin Ointment ... 1074
- Cortisporin Ophthalmic Ointment Sterile ... 1074
- Cortisporin Ophthalmic Suspension Sterile ... 1075
- Cortisporin Otic Solution Sterile ... 1076
- Cortisporin Otic Suspension Sterile ... 1077
- Cortizone-5 ... 795
- Cortizone-10 ... 795
- Hydrocortone Tablets ... 1715
- Hytone ... 922
- Hytone Ointment 2 ½% ... 923
- Massengill Medicated Soft Cloth Towelettes ... 2628
- Pediotic Suspension Sterile ... 1140
- Preparation H Hydrocortisone 1% Cream ... 843
- ProctoCream-HC 2.5% ... 2552
- VōSoL HC Otic Solution ... 2786

Hydrocortisone Acetate (Intensifies electrolyte depletion). Products include:
- Analpram-HC Rectal Cream 1% and 2.5% ... 993
- Anusol HC-1 Hydrocortisone Anti-Itch Ointment ... 810
- Anusol-HC Suppositories ... 1954
- Caldecort Anti-Itch Hydrocortisone Cream ... 651
- Coly-Mycin S Otic w/Neomycin & Hydrocortisone ... 1965
- Cortaid ... 800
- Cortifoam ... 2540
- Cortisporin Cream ... 1073
- Epifoam ... 2543
- Hydrocortone Acetate Sterile Suspension ... 1712
- Mantadil Cream ... 1124
- Nupercainal Hydrocortisone 1% Cream ... 661
- Pramosone Cream, Lotion & Ointment ... 995
- ProctoFoam-HC ... 2552
- Terra-Cortril Ophthalmic Suspension ... 2033

Hydrocortisone Sodium Phosphate (Intensifies electrolyte depletion). Products include:
- Hydrocortone Phosphate Injection, Sterile ... 1713

Hydrocortisone Sodium Succinate (Intensifies electrolyte depletion).
- No products indexed under this heading.

Hydroflumethiazide (Additive effects). Products include:
- Diucardin Tablets ... 2824

Hydromorphone Hydrochloride (Potentiates orthostatic hypotension). Products include:
- Dilaudid Ampules ... 1382
- Dilaudid Cough Syrup ... 1383
- Dilaudid-HP Injection ... 1384
- Dilaudid-HP Lyophilized Powder 250 mg ... 1384
- Dilaudid ... 1382
- Dilaudid Oral Liquid ... 1386
- Dilaudid ... 1382
- Dilaudid Tablets - 8 mg ... 1386

Ibuprofen (Reduces antihypertensive effects). Products include:
- Advil Cold and Sinus Caplets and Tablets ... 837
- Advil Ibuprofen Tablets, Caplets and Gel Caplets ... 836
- Children's Motrin Ibuprofen Oral Suspension ... 1558
- IBU Tablets ... 1389
- Ibuprohm ... 713
- Motrin IB Caplets, Tablets, and Gelcaps ... 802
- Motrin Ibuprofen Suspension, Oral Drops, Chewable Tablets, Caplets ... 1563
- Nuprin Ibuprofen/Analgesic Tablets & Caplets ... 645
- Vicks DayQuil SINUS Pressure & PAIN Relief with IBUPROFEN ... 735

Indapamide (Additive effects).
- No products indexed under this heading.

Indomethacin (Reduces antihypertensive effects). Products include:
- Indocin ... 1723

Indomethacin Sodium Trihydrate (Reduces antihypertensive effects). Products include:
- Indocin I.V. ... 1727

Insulin, Human (Dosage adjustment of the antidiabetic may be required).
- No products indexed under this heading.

Insulin, Human Isophane Suspension (Dosage adjustment of the antidiabetic may be required). Products include:
- Novolin N Human Insulin 10 ml Vials ... 1846

Insulin, Human NPH (Dosage adjustment of the antidiabetic may be required). Products include:
- Humulin N, 100 Units ... 1495
- Novolin N PenFill 1.5 ml Cartridges Durable Insulin Delivery System ... 1849
- Novolin N Prefilled Syringe Disposable Insulin Delivery System ... 1850

Insulin, Human Regular (Dosage adjustment of the antidiabetic may be required). Products include:
- Humulin R, 100 Units ... 1497
- Novolin R Human Insulin 10 ml Vials ... 1846
- Novolin R PenFill 1.5 ml Cartridges Durable Insulin Delivery System ... 1849
- Novolin R Prefilled Syringe Disposable Insulin Delivery System ... 1850
- Velosulin BR Human Insulin 10 ml Vials ... 1847

Insulin, Human, Zinc Suspension (Dosage adjustment of the antidiabetic may be required). Products include:
- Humulin L, 100 Units ... 1494
- Humulin L, 100 Units ... 1498
- Novolin L Human Insulin 10 ml Vials ... 1846

Insulin Lispro, Human (Dosage adjustment of the antidiabetic may be required). Products include:
- Humalog Injection ... 1488

Insulin, NPH (Dosage adjustment of the antidiabetic may be required). Products include:
- NPH, 100 Units ... 1502
- Pork NPH, 100 Units ... 1506
- Purified Pork NPH Isophane Insulin ... 1852

Insulin, Regular (Dosage adjustment of the antidiabetic may be required). Products include:
- Regular, 100 Units ... 1503
- Pork Regular, 100 Units ... 1507
- Pork Regular (Concentrated), 500 Units ... 1508
- Purified Pork Regular Insulin ... 1852

Insulin, Zinc Crystals (Dosage adjustment of the antidiabetic may be required). Products include:
- NPH, 100 Units ... 1502

Insulin, Zinc Suspension (Dosage adjustment of the antidiabetic may be required). Products include:
- Iletin I ... 1501
- Lente, 100 Units ... 1501
- Iletin II ... 1504
- Pork Lente, 100 Units ... 1504
- Purified Pork Lente Insulin ... 1852

Isradipine (Additive effects). Products include:
- DynaCirc Capsules ... 2381
- DynaCirc CR Tablets ... 2383

Ketoprofen (Reduces antihypertensive effects). Products include:
- Actron Caplets and Tablets ... 608
- Orudis Capsules ... 2874
- Orudis KT ... 842
- Oruvail Capsules ... 2874

Ketorolac Tromethamine (Reduces antihypertensive effects). Products include:
- Acular Sterile Ophthalmic Solution ... 470
- Toradol ... 2319

Labetalol Hydrochloride (Additive effects). Products include:
- Normodyne Injection ... 2519
- Normodyne Tablets ... 2522
- Trandate ... 1158

Levorphanol Tartrate (Potentiates orthostatic hypotension). Products include:
- Levo-Dromoran ... 2297

Lithium Carbonate (Reduced renal clearance of lithium resulting in lithium toxicity). Products include:
- Eskalith ... 2658
- Lithium Carbonate Capsules & Tablets ... 2352
- Lithonate/Lithotabs/Lithobid ... 2721

Lithium Citrate (Reduced renal clearance of lithium resulting in lithium toxicity).
- No products indexed under this heading.

Losartan Potassium (Additive effects). Products include:
- Cozaar Tablets ... 1668
- Hyzaar Tablets ... 1720

Mecamylamine Hydrochloride (Additive effects). Products include:
- Inversine Tablets ... 1729

Meclofenamate Sodium (Reduces antihypertensive effects).
- No products indexed under this heading.

Mefenamic Acid (Reduces antihypertensive effects). Products include:
- Ponstel ... 1982

Meperidine Hydrochloride (Potentiates orthostatic hypotension). Products include:
- Demerol ... 2438
- Mepergan Injection ... 2859

Mephobarbital (Potentiates orthostatic hypotension). Products include:
- Mebaral Tablets ... 2452

Metformin Hydrochloride (Dosage adjustment of the antidiabetic may be required). Products include:
- Glucophage Tablets ... 754

IMPORTANT NOTE: Always consult each drug listing in the patient's regimen for possible interactions.

Zestoretic | Interactions Index | 1216

Methadone Hydrochloride (Potentiates orthostatic hypotension). Products include:
- Methadone Hydrochloride Oral Concentrate 2356
- Methadone Hydrochloride Oral Solution & Tablets 2357

Methyclothiazide (Additive effects). Products include:
- Enduron Tablets 424

Methyldopa (Additive effects). Products include:
- Aldoclor Tablets 1638
- Aldomet Oral 1640
- Aldoril Tablets 1644

Methyldopate Hydrochloride (Additive effects). Products include:
- Aldomet Ester HCl Injection 1642

Methylprednisolone Acetate (Intensifies electrolyte depletion).
- No products indexed under this heading.

Methylprednisolone Sodium Succinate (Intensifies electrolyte depletion).
- No products indexed under this heading.

Metocurine Iodide (Possible increased responsiveness to the muscle relaxant). Products include:
- Metubine Iodide Vials 932

Metolazone (Additive effects). Products include:
- Mykrox Tablets 1617
- Zaroxolyn Tablets 1625

Metoprolol Succinate (Additive effects). Products include:
- Toprol-XL Tablets 560

Metoprolol Tartrate (Additive effects). Products include:
- Lopressor 848
- Lopressor HCT Tablets 850

Metyrosine (Additive effects). Products include:
- Demser Capsules 1690

Minoxidil (Additive effects).
- No products indexed under this heading.

Mivacurium Chloride (Possible increased responsiveness to the muscle relaxant). Products include:
- Mivacron 1125

Moexipril Hydrochloride (Additive effects). Products include:
- Univasc Tablets 2553

Morphine Sulfate (Potentiates orthostatic hypotension). Products include:
- Astramorph/PF Injection, USP (Preservative-Free) 526
- Duramorph Injection 983
- Infumorph 200 and Infumorph 500 Sterile Solutions 985
- Kadian Capsules 2948
- MS Contin Tablets 2149
- MSIR 2152
- Oramorph SR (Morphine Sulfate Sustained Release Tablets) 2359
- RMS Suppositories CII 2766
- Roxanol 2365

Nabumetone (Reduces antihypertensive effects). Products include:
- Relafen Tablets 2688

Nadolol (Additive effects).
- No products indexed under this heading.

Naproxen (Reduces antihypertensive effects). Products include:
- Anaprox/Naprosyn 2277

Naproxen Sodium (Reduces antihypertensive effects). Products include:
- Aleve 2124
- Anaprox/Naprosyn 2277
- Naprelan Tablets 2861

Nicardipine Hydrochloride (Additive effects). Products include:
- Cardene Capsules 2261
- Cardene I.V. 2815
- Cardene SR Capsules 2264

Nifedipine (Additive effects). Products include:
- Adalat Capsules (10 mg and 20 mg) 580
- Adalat CC 582
- Procardia Capsules 2024
- Procardia XL Extended Release Tablets 2026

Nisoldipine (Additive effects). Products include:
- Sular Tablets 2961

Nitroglycerin (Additive effects). Products include:
- Deponit NTG Transdermal Delivery System 2541
- Nitro-Bid IV 1270
- Nitro-Bid Ointment 1272
- Nitro-Dur (nitroglycerin) Transdermal Infusion System 1365
- Nitrolingual Spray 2193
- Nitrostat Tablets 1981
- Transderm-Nitro Transdermal Therapeutic System 878

Norepinephrine Bitartrate (Possible decreased response to pressor amines). Products include:
- Levophed Bitartrate Injection 2445

Opium Alkaloids (Potentiates orthostatic hypotension).
- No products indexed under this heading.

Oxaprozin (Reduces antihypertensive effects). Products include:
- Daypro Caplets 2578

Oxycodone Hydrochloride (Potentiates orthostatic hypotension). Products include:
- OxyContin Tablets 2163
- OxyIR Capsules 2167
- Percocet Tablets 955
- Percodan Tablets 955
- Percodan-Demi Tablets 956
- Roxicodone Tablets, Oral Solution & Intensol (Oxycodone) 2366
- Tylox Capsules 1593

Pancuronium Bromide (Possible increased responsiveness to the muscle relaxant).
- No products indexed under this heading.

Penbutolol Sulfate (Additive effects). Products include:
- Levatol Tablets 2547

Pentobarbital Sodium (Potentiates orthostatic hypotension). Products include:
- Nembutal Sodium Capsules 440
- Nembutal Sodium Solution 442
- Nembutal Sodium Suppositories 444

Phenobarbital (Potentiates orthostatic hypotension). Products include:
- Arco-Lase Plus Tablets 513
- Bellergal-S Tablets 2375
- Donnatal 2234
- Donnatal Extentabs 2234
- Donnatal Tablets 2234
- Phenobarbital Elixir and Tablets 1523
- Quadrinal Tablets 1398

Phenoxybenzamine Hydrochloride (Additive effects). Products include:
- Dibenzyline Capsules 2650

Phentolamine Mesylate (Additive effects). Products include:
- Regitine Vials 864

Phenylbutazone (Reduces antihypertensive effects).
- No products indexed under this heading.

Pindolol (Additive effects). Products include:
- Visken Tablets 2428

Piroxicam (Reduces antihypertensive effects). Products include:
- Feldene Capsules 2008

Polythiazide (Additive effects). Products include:
- Minizide Capsules 2016

Potassium Acid Phosphate (Potential for hyperkalemia). Products include:
- K-Phos Original Formula 'Sodium Free' Tablets 633

Potassium Bicarbonate (Potential for hyperkalemia). Products include:
- Alka-Seltzer Gold Effervescent Antacid .... ▣ 611

Potassium Chloride (Potential for hyperkalemia). Products include:
- Chlor-3 Condiment 1003
- Colyte and Colyte-flavored 2540
- GoLYTELY 694
- K-Dur Microburst Release System (potassium chloride, USP) E.R. Tablets 1364
- K-Lor Powder Packets 438
- K-Norm Capsules 1615
- K-Tab Filmtab 439
- Micro-K 2237
- Micro-K LS Packets 2238
- NuLYTELY 694
- Cherry Flavor NuLYTELY 694
- Rum-K Syrup 1004
- Slow-K Extended-Release Tablets 869

Potassium Citrate (Potential for hyperkalemia). Products include:
- Polycitra Syrup 574
- Polycitra-K Crystals 574
- Polycitra-K Oral Solution 575
- Polycitra-LC 574
- Urocit-K Tablets 1828

Potassium Gluconate (Potential for hyperkalemia).
- No products indexed under this heading.

Potassium Phosphate, Dibasic (Potential for hyperkalemia).
- No products indexed under this heading.

Potassium Phosphate, Monobasic (Potential for hyperkalemia). Products include:
- K-Phos Neutral Tablets 633
- K-Phos Original Formula 'Sodium Free' Tablets 633

Prazosin Hydrochloride (Additive effects). Products include:
- Minipress Capsules 2015
- Minizide Capsules 2016

Prednisolone Acetate (Intensifies electrolyte depletion). Products include:
- AK-CIDE .... ◉ 203
- AK-CIDE Ointment .... ◉ 203
- Blephamide Liquifilm Sterile Ophthalmic Suspension 472
- Blephamide Ointment .... ◉ 234
- Econopred & Econopred Plus Ophthalmic Suspensions .... ◉ 216
- Poly-Pred Liquifilm .... ◉ 246
- Pred Forte .... ◉ 247
- Pred Mild .... ◉ 250
- Pred-G Liquifilm Sterile Ophthalmic Suspension .... ◉ 248
- Pred-G S.O.P. Sterile Ophthalmic Ointment .... ◉ 249

Prednisolone Sodium Phosphate (Intensifies electrolyte depletion). Products include:
- AK-PRED .... ◉ 204
- Hydeltrasol Injection, Sterile 1708
- Pediapred Oral Solution 1618

Prednisolone Tebutate (Intensifies electrolyte depletion). Products include:
- Hydeltra-T.B.A. Sterile Suspension 1710

Prednisone (Intensifies electrolyte depletion).
- No products indexed under this heading.

Propoxyphene Hydrochloride (Potentiates orthostatic hypotension). Products include:
- Darvon 1475
- Wygesic Tablets 2930

Propoxyphene Napsylate (Potentiates orthostatic hypotension). Products include:
- Darvon-N/Darvocet-N 1473

Propranolol Hydrochloride (Additive effects). Products include:
- Inderal 2834
- Inderal LA Long Acting Capsules 2836
- Inderide Tablets 2838
- Inderide LA Long Acting Capsules 2840

Quinapril Hydrochloride (Additive effects). Products include:
- Accupril Tablets 1950

Ramipril (Additive effects). Products include:
- Altace Capsules 1238

Rauwolfia Serpentina (Additive effects).
- No products indexed under this heading.

Rescinnamine (Additive effects).
- No products indexed under this heading.

Reserpine (Additive effects). Products include:
- Diupres Tablets 1691
- Hydropres Tablets 1718
- Ser-Ap-Es Tablets 867

Rocuronium Bromide (Possible increased responsiveness to the muscle relaxant). Products include:
- Zemuron Injection 1885

Secobarbital Sodium (Potentiates orthostatic hypotension). Products include:
- Seconal Sodium Pulvules 1529

Sodium Nitroprusside (Additive effects).
- No products indexed under this heading.

Sotalol Hydrochloride (Additive effects). Products include:
- Betapace Tablets 637

Spirapril Hydrochloride (Additive effects).
- No products indexed under this heading.

Spironolactone (Additive antihypertensive effects; potential for hyperkalemia). Products include:
- Aldactazide Tablets 2556
- Aldactone Tablets 2558

Sufentanil Citrate (Potentiates orthostatic hypotension). Products include:
- Sufenta Injection 1355

Sulindac (Reduces antihypertensive effects). Products include:
- Clinoril Tablets 1658

Terazosin Hydrochloride (Additive effects). Products include:
- Hytrin Capsules 434

Thiamylal Sodium (Potentiates orthostatic hypotension).
- No products indexed under this heading.

Timolol Maleate (Additive effects). Products include:
- Blocadren Tablets 1654
- Timolide Tablets 1791
- Timoptic in Ocudose 1796
- Timoptic Sterile Ophthalmic Solution 1794
- Timoptic-XE 1798

Tolazamide (Dosage adjustment of the antidiabetic may be required).
- No products indexed under this heading.

Tolbutamide (Dosage adjustment of the antidiabetic may be required).
- No products indexed under this heading.

Tolmetin Sodium (Reduces antihypertensive effects). Products include:
- Tolectin (200, 400 and 600 mg) .. 1591

Torsemide (Additive effects). Products include:
- Demadex Tablets and Injection 691

(▣ Described in PDR For Nonprescription Drugs) (◉ Described in PDR For Ophthalmology)

1217 **Interactions Index** **Ziac**

Triamcinolone (Intensifies electrolyte depletion).
No products indexed under this heading.

Triamcinolone Acetonide (Intensifies electrolyte depletion). Products include:
Azmacort Oral Inhaler 2175
Nasacort AQ Nasal Spray 2191
Nasacort Nasal Inhaler 2189

Triamcinolone Diacetate (Intensifies electrolyte depletion).
No products indexed under this heading.

Triamcinolone Hexacetonide (Intensifies electrolyte depletion).
No products indexed under this heading.

Triamterene (Additive antihypertensive effects; potential for hyperkalemia). Products include:
Dyazide Capsules 2653
Dyrenium Capsules 2655

Trimethaphan Camsylate (Additive effects).
No products indexed under this heading.

Tubocurarine Chloride (Possible increased responsiveness to the muscle relaxant).
No products indexed under this heading.

Vecuronium Bromide (Possible increased responsiveness to the muscle relaxant). Products include:
Norcuron for Injection 1875

Verapamil Hydrochloride (Additive effects). Products include:
Calan SR Caplets 2571
Calan Tablets 2568
Covera-HS Tablets 2573
Isoptin Injectable 1391
Isoptin Oral Tablets 1393
Isoptin SR Tablets 1395
Verelan Capsules 1455

Food Interactions

Alcohol (Potentiates orthostatic hypotension).

ZESTRIL TABLETS

(Lisinopril) 2972

May interact with diuretics, potassium sparing diuretics, potassium preparations, thiazides, lithium preparations, and certain other agents. Compounds in these categories include:

Amiloride Hydrochloride (Potential for significant hyperkalemia; possibility of excessive reduction in blood pressure). Products include:
Midamor Tablets 1746
Moduretic Tablets 1748

Bendroflumethiazide (Thiazide-induced potassium loss attenuated; possibility of excessive reduction in blood pressure).
No products indexed under this heading.

Bumetanide (Possibility of excessive reduction in blood pressure). Products include:
Bumex 2260

Chlorothiazide (Thiazide-induced potassium loss attenuated; possibility of excessive reduction in blood pressure). Products include:
Aldoclor Tablets 1638
Diupres Tablets 1691
Diuril Oral 1694

Chlorothiazide Sodium (Thiazide-induced potassium loss attenuated; possibility of excessive reduction in blood pressure). Products include:
Diuril Sodium Intravenous 1693

Chlorthalidone (Possibility of excessive reduction in blood pressure). Products include:
Combipres Tablets 682
Tenoretic Tablets 2963
Thalitone 1293

Ethacrynic Acid (Possibility of excessive reduction in blood pressure). Products include:
Edecrin Tablets 1698

Furosemide (Possibility of excessive reduction in blood pressure). Products include:
Lasix Injection, Oral Solution and Tablets 1267

Hydrochlorothiazide (Thiazide-induced potassium loss attenuated; possibility of excessive reduction in blood pressure). Products include:
Aldactazide Tablets 2556
Aldoril Tablets 1644
Apresazide Capsules 824
Capozide Tablets 744
Dyazide Capsules 2653
Esidrix Tablets 839
Esimil Tablets 840
HydroDIURIL Tablets 1716
Hydropres Tablets 1718
Hyzaar Tablets 1720
Inderide Tablets 2838
Inderide LA Long Acting Capsules .. 2840
Lopressor HCT Tablets 850
Lotensin HCT Tablets 855
Moduretic Tablets 1748
Oretic Tablets 450
Prinzide Tablets 1780
Ser-Ap-Es Tablets 867
Timolide Tablets 1791
Vaseretic Tablets 1810
Zestoretic Tablets 2968
Ziac 1459

Hydroflumethiazide (Thiazide-induced potassium loss attenuated; possibility of excessive reduction in blood pressure). Products include:
Diucardin Tablets 2824

Indapamide (Possibility of excessive reduction in blood pressure).
No products indexed under this heading.

Indomethacin (Reduces antihypertensive effect). Products include:
Indocin 1723

Indomethacin Sodium Trihydrate (Reduces antihypertensive effect). Products include:
Indocin I.V. 1727

Lithium Carbonate (Possibility of lithium toxicity—serum lithium levels should be monitored frequently). Products include:
Eskalith 2658
Lithium Carbonate Capsules & Tablets 2352
Lithonate/Lithotabs/Lithobid 2721

Lithium Citrate (Possibility of lithium toxicity—serum lithium levels should be monitored frequently).
No products indexed under this heading.

Methyclothiazide (Thiazide-induced potassium loss attenuated; possibility of excessive reduction in blood pressure). Products include:
Enduron Tablets 424

Metolazone (Possibility of excessive reduction in blood pressure). Products include:
Mykrox Tablets 1617
Zaroxolyn Tablets 1625

Polythiazide (Thiazide-induced potassium loss attenuated; possibility of excessive reduction in blood pressure). Products include:
Minizide Capsules 2016

Potassium Acid Phosphate (Potential for significant hyperkalemia). Products include:
K-Phos Original Formula 'Sodium Free' Tablets 633

Potassium Bicarbonate (Potential for significant hyperkalemia). Products include:
Alka-Seltzer Gold Effervescent Antacid 611

Potassium Chloride (Potential for significant hyperkalemia). Products include:
Chlor-3 Condiment 1003
Colyte and Colyte-flavored 2540
GoLYTELY 694
K-Dur Microburst Release System (potassium chloride, USP) E.R. Tablets 1364
K-Lor Powder Packets 438
K-Norm Capsules 1615
K-Tab Filmtab 439
Micro-K 2237
Micro-K LS Packets 2238
NuLYTELY 694
Cherry Flavor NuLYTELY 694
Rum-K Syrup 1004
Slow-K Extended-Release Tablets 869

Potassium Citrate (Potential for significant hyperkalemia). Products include:
Polycitra Syrup 574
Polycitra-K Crystals 574
Polycitra-K Oral Solution 575
Polycitra-LC 574
Urocit-K Tablets 1828

Potassium Gluconate (Potential for significant hyperkalemia).
No products indexed under this heading.

Potassium Phosphate, Dibasic (Potential for significant hyperkalemia).
No products indexed under this heading.

Potassium Phosphate, Monobasic (Potential for significant hyperkalemia). Products include:
K-Phos Neutral Tablets 633
K-Phos Original Formula 'Sodium Free' Tablets 633

Spironolactone (Potential for significant hyperkalemia; possibility of excessive reduction in blood pressure). Products include:
Aldactazide Tablets 2556
Aldactone Tablets 2558

Torsemide (Possibility of excessive reduction in blood pressure). Products include:
Demadex Tablets and Injection 691

Triamterene (Potential for significant hyperkalemia; possibility of excessive reduction in blood pressure). Products include:
Dyazide Capsules 2653
Dyrenium Capsules 2655

ZIAC

(Bisoprolol Fumarate, Hydrochlorothiazide) 1459

May interact with insulin, oral hypoglycemic agents, antihypertensives, catecholamine depleting drugs, barbiturates, narcotic analgesics, corticosteroids, nondepolarizing neuromuscular blocking agents, lithium preparations, non-steroidal anti-inflammatory agents, and certain other agents. Compounds in these categories include:

Acarbose (Beta blockers may mask some of the manifestations of hypoglycemia, particularly tachycardia; dosage adjustment of the antidiabetic drug may be required). Products include:
Precose 604

Acebutolol Hydrochloride (Ziac may potentiate the action of other antihypertensive agents used concomitantly). Products include:
Sectral Capsules 2914

ACTH (Intensifies electrolyte depletion, particularly hypokalemia).
No products indexed under this heading.

Alfentanil Hydrochloride (Potentiation of orthostatic hypotension may occur when thiazide diuretics are used with narcotics). Products include:
Alfenta Injection 1334

Amlodipine Besylate (Ziac may potentiate the action of other antihypertensive agents used concomitantly). Products include:
Lotrel Capsules 858
Norvasc Tablets 2020

Aprobarbital (Potentiation of orthostatic hypotension may occur when thiazide diuretics are used with barbiturates).
No products indexed under this heading.

Atenolol (Ziac may potentiate the action of other antihypertensive agents used concomitantly). Products include:
Tenoretic Tablets 2963
Tenormin Tablets and I.V. Injection 2965

Atracurium Besylate (Possible increased responsiveness to the muscle relaxant). Products include:
Tracrium Injection 1155

Benazepril Hydrochloride (Ziac may potentiate the action of other antihypertensive agents used concomitantly). Products include:
Lotensin Tablets 852
Lotensin HCT Tablets 855
Lotrel Capsules 858

Bendroflumethiazide (Ziac may potentiate the action of other antihypertensive agents used concomitantly).
No products indexed under this heading.

Betamethasone Acetate (Intensifies electrolyte depletion, particularly hypokalemia). Products include:
Celestone Soluspan Suspension 2484

Betamethasone Sodium Phosphate (Intensifies electrolyte depletion, particularly hypokalemia). Products include:
Celestone Soluspan Suspension 2484

Betaxolol Hydrochloride (Ziac may potentiate the action of other antihypertensive agents used concomitantly). Products include:
Betoptic Ophthalmic Solution 465
Betoptic S Ophthalmic Suspension 467
Kerlone Tablets 2588

Buprenorphine (Potentiation of orthostatic hypotension may occur when thiazide diuretics are used with narcotics). Products include:
Buprenex Injectable 2170

Butabarbital (Potentiation of orthostatic hypotension may occur when thiazide diuretics are used with barbiturates).
No products indexed under this heading.

Butalbital (Potentiation of orthostatic hypotension may occur when thiazide diuretics are used with barbiturates). Products include:
Axocet Capsules 2469
Esgic-plus Capsules 1012
Esgic-plus Tablets 1012
Fioricet Tablets 2386
Fioricet with Codeine Capsules 2387
Fiorinal Capsules 2388
Fiorinal with Codeine Capsules 2390
Fiorinal Tablets 2388
Phrenilin 790
Sedapap Tablets 50 mg/650 mg .. 1826

IMPORTANT NOTE: Always consult each drug listing in the patient's regimen for possible interactions.

Captopril (Ziac may potentiate the action of other antihypertensive agents used concomitantly). Products include:
- Capoten Tablets 740
- Capozide Tablets 744

Carteolol Hydrochloride (Ziac may potentiate the action of other antihypertensive agents used concomitantly). Products include:
- Cartrol Tablets 413
- Ocupress Ophthalmic Solution, 1% Sterile .... ◉ 297

Chlorothiazide (Ziac may potentiate the action of other antihypertensive agents used concomitantly). Products include:
- Aldoclor Tablets 1638
- Diupres Tablets 1691
- Diuril Oral 1694

Chlorothiazide Sodium (Ziac may potentiate the action of other antihypertensive agents used concomitantly). Products include:
- Diuril Sodium Intravenous 1693

Chlorpropamide (Beta blockers may mask some of the manifestations of hypoglycemia, particularly tachycardia; dosage adjustment of the antidiabetic drug may be required). Products include:
- Diabinese Tablets 2002

Chlorthalidone (Ziac may potentiate the action of other antihypertensive agents used concomitantly). Products include:
- Combipres Tablets 682
- Tenoretic Tablets 2963
- Thalitone 1293

Cholestyramine (Binds the hydrochlorothiazide and reduces its absorption in the GI tract by up to 85%). Products include:
- Questran 774

Cisatracurium Besylate (Possible increased responsiveness to the muscle relaxant). Products include:
- Nimbex Injection 1131

Clonidine (Ziac may potentiate the action of other antihypertensive agents used concomitantly). Products include:
- Catapres-TTS 680

Clonidine Hydrochloride (Ziac may potentiate the action of other antihypertensive agents used concomitantly). Products include:
- Catapres Tablets 679
- Combipres Tablets 682

Codeine Phosphate (Potentiation of orthostatic hypotension may occur when thiazide diuretics are used with narcotics). Products include:
- Brontex 2130
- Dimetane-DC Cough Syrup 2232
- Fioricet with Codeine Capsules 2387
- Fiorinal with Codeine Capsules 2390
- Nucofed 2225
- Phenergan with Codeine 2883
- Phenergan VC with Codeine 2888
- Robitussin A-C Syrup 2248
- Robitussin-DAC Syrup 2249
- Ryna .... ▣ 804
- Soma Compound w/Codeine Tablets 2784
- Tylenol with Codeine 1592

Colestipol Hydrochloride (Binds the hydrochlorothiazide and reduces its absorption in the GI tract by up to 43%). Products include:
- Colestid 2073

Cortisone Acetate (Intensifies electrolyte depletion, particularly hypokalemia). Products include:
- Cortone Acetate Sterile Suspension 1663
- Cortone Acetate Tablets 1664

Cyclopropane (Use with caution when administered with anesthetic agent that depresses myocardial function).

Deserpidine (Concomitant use may produce excessive reduction of sympathetic activity).
- No products indexed under this heading.

Dexamethasone (Intensifies electrolyte depletion, particularly hypokalemia). Products include:
- AK-Trol Ointment & Suspension .... ◉ 205
- Decadron Elixir 1676
- Decadron Tablets 1678
- Decaspray Topical Aerosol 1689
- Maxitrol Ophthalmic Ointment and Suspension .... ◉ 222
- TobraDex Ophthalmic Suspension and Ointment 469

Dexamethasone Acetate (Intensifies electrolyte depletion, particularly hypokalemia). Products include:
- Dalalone D.P. Injectable 1009
- Decadron-LA Sterile Suspension 1687

Dexamethasone Sodium Phosphate (Intensifies electrolyte depletion, particularly hypokalemia). Products include:
- Decadron Phosphate Injection 1680
- Decadron Phosphate Sterile Ophthalmic Ointment 1684
- Decadron Phosphate Sterile Ophthalmic Solution 1685
- Decadron Phosphate Topical Cream 1686
- Decadron Phosphate with Xylocaine Injection, Sterile 1683
- Dexacort Phosphate in Respihaler 1606
- Dexacort Phosphate in Turbinaire 1607
- NeoDecadron Sterile Ophthalmic Ointment 1755
- NeoDecadron Sterile Ophthalmic Solution 1756
- NeoDecadron Topical Cream 1757

Dezocine (Potentiation of orthostatic hypotension may occur when thiazide diuretics are used with narcotics). Products include:
- Dalgan Injection 529

Diazoxide (Ziac may potentiate the action of other antihypertensive agents used concomitantly). Products include:
- Hyperstat I.V. Injection 2504
- Proglycem 575

Diclofenac Potassium (Reduces the diuretic, natriuretic, and antihypertensive effects of thiazides). Products include:
- Cataflam Tablets 833

Diclofenac Sodium (Reduces the diuretic, natriuretic, and antihypertensive effects of thiazides). Products include:
- Voltaren Ophthalmic Sterile Ophthalmic Solution .... ◉ 264
- Cataflam/Voltaren/Voltaren-XR 833

Diltiazem Hydrochloride (Ziac should be used with caution when myocardial depressants or inhibitors of AV conduction are used concurrently). Products include:
- Cardizem CD Capsules 1251
- Cardizem SR Capsules 1255
- Cardizem Injectable 1253
- Cardizem Tablets 1257
- Dilacor XR Extended-release Capsules 2183
- Tiazac Capsules 1019

Disopyramide Phosphate (Ziac should be used with caution when myocardial depressants or inhibitors of AV conduction are used concurrently). Products include:
- Norpace 2596

Doxazosin Mesylate (Ziac may potentiate the action of other antihypertensive agents used concomitantly). Products include:
- Cardura Tablets 1993

Enalapril Maleate (Ziac may potentiate the action of other antihypertensive agents used concomitantly). Products include:
- Vaseretic Tablets 1810
- Vasotec Tablets 1816

Enalaprilat (Ziac may potentiate the action of other antihypertensive agents used concomitantly). Products include:
- Vasotec I.V. 1814

Epinephrine Hydrochloride (Patients with history of severe anaphylactic reaction to variety of allergens may be unresponsive to the usual doses of epinephrine used to treat allergic reactions). Products include:
- Ana-Kit Anaphylaxis Emergency Treatment Kit 611

Esmolol Hydrochloride (Ziac may potentiate the action of other antihypertensive agents used concomitantly). Products include:
- Brevibloc (esmolol HCl) Injection 1860

Ether (Use with caution when administered with anesthetic agent that depresses myocardial function).

Etodolac (Reduces the diuretic, natriuretic, and antihypertensive effects of thiazides). Products include:
- Lodine Capsules and Tablets 2849

Felodipine (Ziac may potentiate the action of other antihypertensive agents used concomitantly). Products include:
- Plendil Extended-Release Tablets 514

Fenoprofen Calcium (Reduces the diuretic, natriuretic, and antihypertensive effects of thiazides). Products include:
- Nalfon 200 Pulvules & Nalfon Tablets 933

Fentanyl (Potentiation of orthostatic hypotension may occur when thiazide diuretics are used with narcotics). Products include:
- Duragesic Transdermal System 1336

Fentanyl Citrate (Potentiation of orthostatic hypotension may occur when thiazide diuretics are used with narcotics). Products include:
- Sublimaze Injection 463

Fludrocortisone Acetate (Intensifies electrolyte depletion, particularly hypokalemia). Products include:
- Florinef Acetate Tablets 506

Flurbiprofen (Reduces the diuretic, natriuretic, and antihypertensive effects of thiazides).
- No products indexed under this heading.

Fosinopril Sodium (Ziac may potentiate the action of other antihypertensive agents used concomitantly). Products include:
- Monopril Tablets 762

Furosemide (Ziac may potentiate the action of other antihypertensive agents used concomitantly). Products include:
- Lasix Injection, Oral Solution and Tablets 1267

Glimepiride (Beta blockers may mask some of the manifestations of hypoglycemia, particularly tachycardia; dosage adjustment of the antidiabetic drug may be required). Products include:
- Amaryl Tablets 1241

Glipizide (Beta blockers may mask some of the manifestations of hypoglycemia, particularly tachycardia; dosage adjustment of the antidiabetic drug may be required). Products include:
- Glucotrol Tablets 2011
- Glucotrol XL Extended Release Tablets 2012

Glyburide (Beta blockers may mask some of the manifestations of hypoglycemia, particularly tachycardia; dosage adjustment of the antidiabetic drug may be required). Products include:
- DiaBeta Tablets 1265
- Glynase PresTab Tablets 2091
- Micronase Tablets 2099

Guanabenz Acetate (Ziac may potentiate the action of other antihypertensive agents used concomitantly).
- No products indexed under this heading.

Guanethidine Monosulfate (Concomitant use may produce excessive reduction of sympathetic activity). Products include:
- Esimil Tablets 840
- Ismelin Tablets 845

Hydralazine Hydrochloride (Ziac may potentiate the action of other antihypertensive agents used concomitantly). Products include:
- Apresazide Capsules 824
- Apresoline Hydrochloride Tablets 826
- Hydralazine Hydrochloride Injection USP 2712
- Ser-Ap-Es Tablets 867

Hydrocodone Bitartrate (Potentiation of orthostatic hypotension may occur when thiazide diuretics are used with narcotics). Products include:
- Codiclear DH Syrup 808
- Duratuss HD Elixir 2750
- Histussin D Liquid 670
- Hycodan Tablets and Syrup 946
- Hycomine Compound Tablets 948
- Hycomine 947
- Hycotuss Expectorant Syrup 950
- Hydrocet Capsules 787
- Lorcet 10/650 Tablets 1016
- Lortab 2751
- Tussend 1830
- Tussend Expectorant 1831
- Vicodin Tablets 1404
- Vicodin ES Tablets 1405
- Vicodin HP Tablets 1403
- Vicodin Tuss Expectorant 1406
- Zydone Capsules 967

Hydrocodone Polistirex (Potentiation of orthostatic hypotension may occur when thiazide diuretics are used with narcotics). Products include:
- Tussionex Pennkinetic Extended-Release Suspension 1624

Hydrocortisone (Intensifies electrolyte depletion, particularly hypokalemia). Products include:
- Anusol-HC Cream 2.5% 1953
- Aquanil HC Lotion 1989
- Maximum Strength Cortaid Spray .... ▣ 800
- CORTENEMA 2713
- Cortisporin Ointment 1074
- Cortisporin Ophthalmic Ointment Sterile 1074
- Cortisporin Ophthalmic Suspension Sterile 1075
- Cortisporin Otic Solution Sterile 1076
- Cortisporin Otic Suspension Sterile 1077
- Cortizone-5 .... ▣ 795
- Cortizone-10 .... ▣ 795
- Hydrocortone Tablets 1715
- Hytone 922
- Hytone Ointment 2 ½% 923
- Massengill Medicated Soft Cloth Towelettes 2628
- Pediotic Suspension Sterile 1140
- Preparation H Hydrocortisone 1% Cream .... ▣ 843
- ProctoCream-HC 2.5% 2552
- VōSoL HC Otic Solution 2786

(▣ Described in PDR For Nonprescription Drugs) (◉ Described in PDR For Ophthalmology)

Interactions Index

Hydrocortisone Acetate (Intensifies electrolyte depletion, particularly hypokalemia). Products include:
   Analpram-HC Rectal Cream 1% and 2.5% 993
   Anusol HC-1 Hydrocortisone Anti-Itch Ointment 810
   Anusol-HC Suppositories 1954
   Caldecort Anti-Itch Hydrocortisone Cream 651
   Coly-Mycin S Otic w/Neomycin & Hydrocortisone 1965
   Cortaid 800
   Cortifoam 2540
   Cortisporin Cream 1073
   Epifoam 2543
   Hydrocortone Acetate Sterile Suspension 1712
   Mantadil Cream 1124
   Nupercainal Hydrocortisone 1% Cream 661
   Pramosone Cream, Lotion & Ointment 995
   ProctoFoam-HC 2552
   Terra-Cortril Ophthalmic Suspension 2033

Hydrocortisone Sodium Phosphate (Intensifies electrolyte depletion, particularly hypokalemia). Products include:
   Hydrocortone Phosphate Injection, Sterile 1713

Hydrocortisone Sodium Succinate (Intensifies electrolyte depletion, particularly hypokalemia).
   No products indexed under this heading.

Hydroflumethiazide (Ziac may potentiate the action of other antihypertensive agents used concomitantly). Products include:
   Diucardin Tablets 2824

Hydromorphone Hydrochloride (Potentiation of orthostatic hypotension may occur when thiazide diuretics are used with narcotics). Products include:
   Dilaudid Ampules 1382
   Dilaudid Cough Syrup 1383
   Dilaudid-HP Injection 1384
   Dilaudid-HP Lyophilized Powder 250 mg 1384
   Dilaudid 1382
   Dilaudid Oral Liquid 1386
   Dilaudid 1382
   Dilaudid Tablets - 8 mg 1386

Ibuprofen (Reduces the diuretic, natriuretic, and antihypertensive effects of thiazides). Products include:
   Advil Cold and Sinus Caplets and Tablets 837
   Advil Ibuprofen Tablets, Caplets and Gel Caplets 836
   Children's Motrin Ibuprofen Oral Suspension 1558
   IBU Tablets 1389
   Ibuprohm 713
   Motrin IB Caplets, Tablets, and Gelcaps 802
   Motrin Ibuprofen Suspension, Oral Drops, Chewable Tablets, Caplets 1563
   Nuprin Ibuprofen/Analgesic Tablets & Caplets 645
   Vicks DayQuil SINUS Pressure & PAIN Relief with IBUPROFEN 735

Indapamide (Ziac may potentiate the action of other antihypertensive agents used concomitantly).
   No products indexed under this heading.

Indomethacin (Reduces the diuretic, natriuretic, and antihypertensive effects of thiazides). Products include:
   Indocin 1723

Indomethacin Sodium Trihydrate (Reduces the diuretic, natriuretic, and antihypertensive effects of thiazides). Products include:
   Indocin I.V. 1727

Insulin, Human (Beta blockers may mask some of the manifestations of hypoglycemia, particularly tachycardia; dosage adjustment of the antidiabetic drug may be required).
   No products indexed under this heading.

Insulin, Human Isophane Suspension (Beta blockers may mask some of the manifestations of hypoglycemia, particularly tachycardia; dosage adjustment of the antidiabetic drug may be required). Products include:
   Novolin N Human Insulin 10 ml Vials 1846

Insulin, Human NPH (Beta blockers may mask some of the manifestations of hypoglycemia, particularly tachycardia; dosage adjustment of the antidiabetic drug may be required). Products include:
   Humulin N, 100 Units 1495
   Novolin N PenFill 1.5 ml Cartridges Durable Insulin Delivery System 1849
   Novolin N Prefilled Syringe Disposable Insulin Delivery System 1850

Insulin, Human Regular (Beta blockers may mask some of the manifestations of hypoglycemia, particularly tachycardia; dosage adjustment of the antidiabetic drug may be required). Products include:
   Humulin R, 100 Units 1497
   Novolin R Human Insulin 10 ml Vials 1846
   Novolin R PenFill 1.5 ml Cartridges Durable Insulin Delivery System 1849
   Novolin R Prefilled Syringe Disposable Insulin Delivery System 1850
   Velosulin BR Human Insulin 10 ml Vials 1847

Insulin, Human, Zinc Suspension (Beta blockers may mask some of the manifestations of hypoglycemia, particularly tachycardia; dosage adjustment of the antidiabetic drug may be required). Products include:
   Humulin L, 100 Units 1494
   Humulin U, 100 Units 1498
   Novolin L Human Insulin 10 ml Vials 1846

Insulin Lispro, Human (Beta blockers may mask some of the manifestations of hypoglycemia, particularly tachycardia; dosage adjustment of the antidiabetic drug may be required). Products include:
   Humalog Injection 1488

Insulin, NPH (Beta blockers may mask some of the manifestations of hypoglycemia, particularly tachycardia; dosage adjustment of the antidiabetic drug may be required). Products include:
   NPH, 100 Units 1502
   Pork NPH, 100 Units 1506
   Purified Pork NPH Isophane Insulin 1852

Insulin, Regular (Beta blockers may mask some of the manifestations of hypoglycemia, particularly tachycardia; dosage adjustment of the antidiabetic drug may be required). Products include:
   Regular, 100 Units 1503
   Pork Regular, 100 Units 1507
   Pork Regular (Concentrated), 500 Units 1508
   Purified Pork Regular Insulin 1852

Insulin, Zinc Crystals (Beta blockers may mask some of the manifestations of hypoglycemia, particularly tachycardia; dosage adjustment of the antidiabetic drug may be required). Products include:
   NPH, 100 Units 1502

Insulin, Zinc Suspension (Beta blockers may mask some of the manifestations of hypoglycemia, particularly tachycardia; dosage adjustment of the antidiabetic drug may be required). Products include:
   Iletin I 1501
   Lente, 100 Units 1501
   Iletin II 1504
   Pork Lente, 100 Units 1504
   Purified Pork Lente Insulin 1852

Isradipine (Ziac may potentiate the action of other antihypertensive agents used concomitantly). Products include:
   DynaCirc Capsules 2381
   DynaCirc CR Tablets 2383

Ketoprofen (Reduces the diuretic, natriuretic, and antihypertensive effects of thiazides). Products include:
   Actron Caplets and Tablets 608
   Orudis Capsules 2874
   Orudis KT 842
   Oruvail Capsules 2874

Ketorolac Tromethamine (Reduces the diuretic, natriuretic, and antihypertensive effects of thiazides). Products include:
   Acular Sterile Ophthalmic Solution 470
   Toradol 2319

Labetalol Hydrochloride (Ziac may potentiate the action of other antihypertensive agents used concomitantly). Products include:
   Normodyne Injection 2519
   Normodyne Tablets 2522
   Trandate 1158

Levorphanol Tartrate (Potentiation of orthostatic hypotension may occur when thiazide diuretics are used with narcotics). Products include:
   Levo-Dromoran 2297

Lisinopril (Ziac may potentiate the action of other antihypertensive agents used concomitantly). Products include:
   Prinivil Tablets 1776
   Prinzide Tablets 1780
   Zestoretic Tablets 2968
   Zestril Tablets 2972

Lithium Carbonate (Reduced renal clearance of lithium and increased risk of lithium toxicity). Products include:
   Eskalith 2658
   Lithium Carbonate Capsules & Tablets 2352
   Lithonate/Lithotabs/Lithobid 2721

Lithium Citrate (Reduced renal clearance of lithium and increased risk of lithium toxicity).
   No products indexed under this heading.

Losartan Potassium (Ziac may potentiate the action of other antihypertensive agents used concomitantly). Products include:
   Cozaar Tablets 1668
   Hyzaar Tablets 1720

Mecamylamine Hydrochloride (Ziac may potentiate the action of other antihypertensive agents used concomitantly). Products include:
   Inversine Tablets 1729

Meclofenamate Sodium (Reduces the diuretic, natriuretic, and antihypertensive effects of thiazides).
   No products indexed under this heading.

Mefenamic Acid (Reduces the diuretic, natriuretic, and antihypertensive effects of thiazides). Products include:
   Ponstel 1982

Meperidine Hydrochloride (Potentiation of orthostatic hypotension may occur when thiazide diuretics are used with narcotics). Products include:
   Demerol 2438
   Mepergan Injection 2859

Mephobarbital (Potentiation of orthostatic hypotension may occur when thiazide diuretics are used with barbiturates). Products include:
   Mebaral Tablets 2452

Metformin Hydrochloride (Beta blockers may mask some of the manifestations of hypoglycemia, particularly tachycardia; dosage adjustment of the antidiabetic drug may be required). Products include:
   Glucophage Tablets 754

Methadone Hydrochloride (Potentiation of orthostatic hypotension may occur when thiazide diuretics are used with narcotics). Products include:
   Methadone Hydrochloride Oral Concentrate 2356
   Methadone Hydrochloride Oral Solution & Tablets 2357

Methyclothiazide (Ziac may potentiate the action of other antihypertensive agents used concomitantly). Products include:
   Enduron Tablets 424

Methyldopa (Ziac may potentiate the action of other antihypertensive agents used concomitantly). Products include:
   Aldoclor Tablets 1638
   Aldomet Oral 1640
   Aldoril Tablets 1644

Methyldopate Hydrochloride (Ziac may potentiate the action of other antihypertensive agents used concomitantly). Products include:
   Aldomet Ester HCl Injection 1642

Methylprednisolone Acetate (Intensifies electrolyte depletion, particularly hypokalemia).
   No products indexed under this heading.

Methylprednisolone Sodium Succinate (Intensifies electrolyte depletion, particularly hypokalemia).
   No products indexed under this heading.

Metocurine Iodide (Possible increased responsiveness to the muscle relaxant). Products include:
   Metubine Iodide Vials 932

Metolazone (Ziac may potentiate the action of other antihypertensive agents used concomitantly). Products include:
   Mykrox Tablets 1617
   Zaroxolyn Tablets 1625

Metoprolol Succinate (Ziac may potentiate the action of other antihypertensive agents used concomitantly). Products include:
   Toprol-XL Tablets 560

Metoprolol Tartrate (Ziac may potentiate the action of other antihypertensive agents used concomitantly). Products include:
   Lopressor 848
   Lopressor HCT Tablets 850

Metyrosine (Ziac may potentiate the action of other antihypertensive agents used concomitantly). Products include:
   Demser Capsules 1690

Minoxidil (Ziac may potentiate the action of other antihypertensive agents used concomitantly).
   No products indexed under this heading.

IMPORTANT NOTE: Always consult each drug listing in the patient's regimen for possible interactions.

Ziac **Interactions Index** 1220

Mivacurium Chloride (Possible increased responsiveness to the muscle relaxant). Products include:
Mivacron 1125

Moexipril Hydrochloride (Ziac may potentiate the action of other antihypertensive agents used concomitantly). Products include:
Univasc Tablets 2553

Morphine Sulfate (Potentiation of orthostatic hypotension may occur when thiazide diuretics are used with narcotics). Products include:
Astramorph/PF Injection, USP (Preservative-Free) 526
Duramorph Injection 983
Infumorph 200 and Infumorph 500 Sterile Solutions 985
Kadian Capsules 2948
MS Contin Tablets 2149
MSIR 2152
Oramorph SR (Morphine Sulfate Sustained Release Tablets) 2359
RMS Suppositories CII 2766
Roxanol 2365

Nabumetone (Reduces the diuretic, natriuretic, and antihypertensive effects of thiazides). Products include:
Relafen Tablets 2688

Nadolol (Ziac may potentiate the action of other antihypertensive agents used concomitantly).
No products indexed under this heading.

Naproxen (Reduces the diuretic, natriuretic, and antihypertensive effects of thiazides). Products include:
Anaprox/Naprosyn 2277

Naproxen Sodium (Reduces the diuretic, natriuretic, and antihypertensive effects of thiazides). Products include:
Aleve 2124
Anaprox/Naprosyn 2277
Naprelan Tablets 2861

Nicardipine Hydrochloride (Ziac may potentiate the action of other antihypertensive agents used concomitantly). Products include:
Cardene Capsules 2261
Cardene I.V. 2815
Cardene SR Capsules 2264

Nifedipine (Ziac may potentiate the action of other antihypertensive agents used concomitantly). Products include:
Adalat Capsules (10 mg and 20 mg) 580
Adalat CC 582
Procardia Capsules 2024
Procardia XL Extended Release Tablets 2026

Nisoldipine (Ziac may potentiate the action of other antihypertensive agents used concomitantly). Products include:
Sular Tablets 2961

Nitroglycerin (Ziac may potentiate the action of other antihypertensive agents used concomitantly). Products include:
Deponit NTG Transdermal Delivery System 2541
Nitro-Bid IV 1270
Nitro-Bid Ointment 1272
Nitro-Dur (nitroglycerin) Transdermal Infusion System 1365
Nitrolingual Spray 2193
Nitrostat Tablets 1981
Transderm-Nitro Transdermal Therapeutic System 878

Norepinephrine Bitartrate (Possible decreased response to pressor amines). Products include:
Levophed Bitartrate Injection 2445

Norepinephrine Hydrochloride (Possible decreased response to pressor amines).
No products indexed under this heading.

Opium Alkaloids (Potentiation of orthostatic hypotension may occur when thiazide diuretics are used with narcotics).
No products indexed under this heading.

Oxaprozin (Reduces the diuretic, natriuretic, and antihypertensive effects of thiazides). Products include:
Daypro Caplets 2578

Oxycodone Hydrochloride (Potentiation of orthostatic hypotension may occur when thiazide diuretics are used with narcotics). Products include:
OxyContin Tablets 2163
OxyIR Capsules 2167
Percocet Tablets 955
Percodan Tablets 955
Percodan-Demi Tablets 956
Roxicodone Tablets, Oral Solution & Intensol (Oxycodone) 2366
Tylox Capsules 1593

Pancuronium Bromide (Possible increased responsiveness to the muscle relaxant).
No products indexed under this heading.

Penbutolol Sulfate (Ziac may potentiate the action of other antihypertensive agents used concomitantly). Products include:
Levatol Tablets 2547

Pentobarbital Sodium (Potentiation of orthostatic hypotension may occur when thiazide diuretics are used with barbiturates). Products include:
Nembutal Sodium Capsules 440
Nembutal Sodium Solution 442
Nembutal Sodium Suppositories 444

Phenobarbital (Potentiation of orthostatic hypotension may occur when thiazide diuretics are used with barbiturates). Products include:
Arco-Lase Plus Tablets 513
Bellergal-S Tablets 2375
Donnatal 2234
Donnatal Extentabs 2234
Donnatal Tablets 2234
Phenobarbital Elixir and Tablets 1523
Quadrinal Tablets 1398

Phenoxybenzamine Hydrochloride (Ziac may potentiate the action of other antihypertensive agents used concomitantly). Products include:
Dibenzyline Capsules 2650

Phentolamine Mesylate (Ziac may potentiate the action of other antihypertensive agents used concomitantly). Products include:
Regitine Vials 864

Phenylbutazone (Reduces the diuretic, natriuretic, and antihypertensive effects of thiazides).
No products indexed under this heading.

Pindolol (Ziac may potentiate the action of other antihypertensive agents used concomitantly). Products include:
Visken Tablets 2428

Piroxicam (Reduces the diuretic, natriuretic, and antihypertensive effects of thiazides). Products include:
Feldene Capsules 2008

Polythiazide (Ziac may potentiate the action of other antihypertensive agents used concomitantly). Products include:
Minizide Capsules 2016

Prazosin Hydrochloride (Ziac may potentiate the action of other antihypertensive agents used concomitantly). Products include:
Minipress Capsules 2015
Minizide Capsules 2016

Prednisolone Acetate (Intensifies electrolyte depletion, particularly hypokalemia). Products include:
AK-CIDE .... ◉ 203
AK-CIDE Ointment .... ◉ 203
Blephamide Liquifilm Sterile Ophthalmic Suspension 472
Blephamide Ointment .... ◉ 234
Econopred & Econopred Plus Ophthalmic Suspensions .... ◉ 216
Poly-Pred Liquifilm .... ◉ 246
Pred Forte .... ◉ 247
Pred Mild .... ◉ 250
Pred-G Liquifilm Sterile Ophthalmic Suspension .... ◉ 248
Pred-G S.O.P. Sterile Ophthalmic Ointment .... ◉ 249

Prednisolone Sodium Phosphate (Intensifies electrolyte depletion, particularly hypokalemia). Products include:
AK-PRED .... ◉ 204
Hydeltrasol Injection, Sterile 1708
Pediapred Oral Solution 1618

Prednisolone Tebutate (Intensifies electrolyte depletion, particularly hypokalemia). Products include:
Hydeltra-T.B.A. Sterile Suspension 1710

Prednisone (Intensifies electrolyte depletion, particularly hypokalemia).
No products indexed under this heading.

Propoxyphene Hydrochloride (Potentiation of orthostatic hypotension may occur when thiazide diuretics are used with narcotics). Products include:
Darvon 1475
Wygesic Tablets 2930

Propoxyphene Napsylate (Potentiation of orthostatic hypotension may occur when thiazide diuretics are used with narcotics). Products include:
Darvon-N/Darvocet-N 1473

Propranolol Hydrochloride (Ziac may potentiate the action of other antihypertensive agents used concomitantly). Products include:
Inderal 2834
Inderal LA Long Acting Capsules 2836
Inderide Tablets 2838
Inderide LA Long Acting Capsules 2840

Quinapril Hydrochloride (Ziac may potentiate the action of other antihypertensive agents used concomitantly). Products include:
Accupril Tablets 1950

Ramipril (Ziac may potentiate the action of other antihypertensive agents used concomitantly). Products include:
Altace Capsules 1238

Rauwolfia Serpentina (Concomitant use may produce excessive reduction of sympathetic activity).
No products indexed under this heading.

Rescinnamine (Concomitant use may produce excessive reduction of sympathetic activity).
No products indexed under this heading.

Reserpine (Concomitant use may produce excessive reduction of sympathetic activity). Products include:
Diupres Tablets 1691
Hydropres Tablets 1718
Ser-Ap-Es Tablets 867

Rifampin (Increases the metabolic clearance of bisoprolol fumarate and shortening its elimination half-life). Products include:
Rifadin 1276
Rifamate Capsules 1278
Rifater 1280
Rimactane Capsules 865

Rocuronium Bromide (Possible increased responsiveness to the muscle relaxant). Products include:
Zemuron Injection 1885

Secobarbital Sodium (Potentiation of orthostatic hypotension may occur when thiazide diuretics are used with barbiturates). Products include:
Seconal Sodium Pulvules 1529

Sodium Nitroprusside (Ziac may potentiate the action of other antihypertensive agents used concomitantly).
No products indexed under this heading.

Sotalol Hydrochloride (Ziac may potentiate the action of other antihypertensive agents used concomitantly). Products include:
Betapace Tablets 637

Spirapril Hydrochloride (Ziac may potentiate the action of other antihypertensive agents used concomitantly).
No products indexed under this heading.

Sufentanil Citrate (Potentiation of orthostatic hypotension may occur when thiazide diuretics are used with narcotics). Products include:
Sufenta Injection 1355

Sulindac (Reduces the diuretic, natriuretic, and antihypertensive effects of thiazides). Products include:
Clinoril Tablets 1658

Terazosin Hydrochloride (Ziac may potentiate the action of other antihypertensive agents used concomitantly). Products include:
Hytrin Capsules 434

Thiamylal Sodium (Potentiation of orthostatic hypotension may occur when thiazide diuretics are used with barbiturates).
No products indexed under this heading.

Timolol Maleate (Ziac may potentiate the action of other antihypertensive agents used concomitantly). Products include:
Blocadren Tablets 1654
Timolide Tablets 1791
Timoptic in Ocudose 1796
Timoptic Sterile Ophthalmic Solution 1794
Timoptic-XE 1798

Tolazamide (Beta blockers may mask some of the manifestations of hypoglycemia, particularly tachycardia; dosage adjustment of the antidiabetic drug may be required).
No products indexed under this heading.

Tolbutamide (Beta blockers may mask some of the manifestations of hypoglycemia, particularly tachycardia; dosage adjustment of the antidiabetic drug may be required).
No products indexed under this heading.

Tolmetin Sodium (Reduces the diuretic, natriuretic, and antihypertensive effects of thiazides). Products include:
Tolectin (200, 400 and 600 mg) 1591

Torsemide (Ziac may potentiate the action of other antihypertensive agents used concomitantly). Products include:
Demadex Tablets and Injection 691

Triamcinolone (Intensifies electrolyte depletion, particularly hypokalemia).
No products indexed under this heading.

(▣ Described in PDR For Nonprescription Drugs) (◉ Described in PDR For Ophthalmology)

Interactions Index — Zinecard

Triamcinolone Acetonide (Intensifies electrolyte depletion, particularly hypokalemia). Products include:
  Azmacort Oral Inhaler 2175
  Nasacort AQ Nasal Spray 2191
  Nasacort Nasal Inhaler 2189

Triamcinolone Diacetate (Intensifies electrolyte depletion, particularly hypokalemia).
  No products indexed under this heading.

Triamcinolone Hexacetonide (Intensifies electrolyte depletion, particularly hypokalemia).
  No products indexed under this heading.

Trichloroethylene (Use with caution when administered with anesthetic agent that depresses myocardial function).
  No products indexed under this heading.

Trimethaphan Camsylate (Ziac may potentiate the action of other antihypertensive agents used concomitantly).
  No products indexed under this heading.

Tubocurarine Chloride (Possible increased responsiveness to the muscle relaxant).
  No products indexed under this heading.

Vecuronium Bromide (Possible increased responsiveness to the muscle relaxant). Products include:
  Norcuron for Injection 1875

Verapamil Hydrochloride (Ziac should be used with caution when myocardial depressants or inhibitors of AV conduction are used concurrently). Products include:
  Calan SR Caplets 2571
  Calan Tablets 2568
  Covera-HS Tablets 2573
  Isoptin Injectable 1391
  Isoptin Oral Tablets 1393
  Isoptin SR Tablets 1395
  Verelan Capsules 1455

Food Interactions

Alcohol (Potentiation of orthostatic hypotension may occur when thiazide diuretics are used with alcohol).

ZILACTIN MEDICATED GEL
(Benzyl Alcohol) .... ⓔ 856
None cited in PDR database.

ZILACTIN-B MEDICATED GEL WITH BENZOCAINE
(Benzocaine) .... ⓔ 856
None cited in PDR database.

ZILACTIN-L LIQUID
(Lidocaine) .... ⓔ 856
None cited in PDR database.

ZINACEF
(Cefuroxime Sodium) 1184
May interact with aminoglycosides and certain other agents. Compounds in these categories include:

Amikacin Sulfate (Concomitant administration may produce nephrotoxicity). Products include:
  Amikacin Sulfate Injection, USP ... 523
  Amikacin Sulfate Injection, USP ... 981
  Amikin Injectable 502

Gentamicin Sulfate (Concomitant administration may produce nephrotoxicity). Products include:
  Garamycin Cream 0.1% 2501
  Garamycin Injectable 2502
  Garamycin Ointment 0.1% 2501
  Garamycin Ophthalmic 2501
  Genoptic Sterile Ophthalmic Solution .... ⓔ 241
  Genoptic Sterile Ophthalmic Ointment .... ⓔ 241
  Gentak .... ⓔ 209
  Pred-G Liquifilm Sterile Ophthalmic Suspension .... ⓔ 248
  Pred-G S.O.P. Sterile Ophthalmic Ointment .... ⓔ 249

Kanamycin Sulfate (Concomitant administration may produce nephrotoxicity).
  No products indexed under this heading.

Probenecid (Concurrent administration of probenecid decreases renal clearance and increases peak serum levels of cefuroxime). Products include:
  Benemid Tablets 1651
  ColBENEMID Tablets 1662

Streptomycin Sulfate (Concomitant administration may produce nephrotoxicity). Products include:
  Streptomycin Sulfate Injection .. 2031

Tobramycin Sulfate (Concomitant administration may produce nephrotoxicity). Products include:
  Nebcin Vials, Hyporets & ADD-Vantage 1518

ZINECARD INJECTION
(Dexrazoxane) 2120
May interact with antineoplastics and certain other agents. Compounds in these categories include:

Altretamine (Dexrazoxane may add to the myelosuppression caused by chemotherapeutic agents). Products include:
  Hexalen Capsules 2760

Anastrozole (Dexrazoxane may add to the myelosuppression caused by chemotherapeutic agents). Products include:
  Arimidex Tablets 2932

Asparaginase (Dexrazoxane may add to the myelosuppression caused by chemotherapeutic agents). Products include:
  Elspar 1700

Bicalutamide (Dexrazoxane may add to the myelosuppression caused by chemotherapeutic agents). Products include:
  Casodex Tablets 2934

Bleomycin Sulfate (Dexrazoxane may add to the myelosuppression caused by chemotherapeutic agents). Products include:
  Blenoxane 697

Busulfan (Dexrazoxane may add to the myelosuppression caused by chemotherapeutic agents). Products include:
  Myleran Tablets 1209

Carboplatin (Dexrazoxane may add to the myelosuppression caused by chemotherapeutic agents). Products include:
  Paraplatin for Injection 713

Carmustine (BCNU) (Dexrazoxane may add to the myelosuppression caused by chemotherapeutic agents). Products include:
  BiCNU 696

Chlorambucil (Dexrazoxane may add to the myelosuppression caused by chemotherapeutic agents). Products include:
  Leukeran Tablets 1205

Cisplatin (Dexrazoxane may add to the myelosuppression caused by chemotherapeutic agents). Products include:
  Platinol for Injection 717
  Platinol-AQ Injection 719

Cyclophosphamide (Use of dexrazoxane concurrently with the initiation of fluorouracil, doxorubicin and cyclophosphamide (FAC) therapy may interfere with the antitumor efficacy of the regimen). Products include:
  Cytoxan 700

Dacarbazine (Dexrazoxane may add to the myelosuppression caused by chemotherapeutic agents). Products include:
  DTIC-Dome 593

Daunorubicin Citrate (Use of dexrazoxane concurrently with the initiation of fluorouracil, doxorubicin and cyclophosphamide (FAC) therapy may interfere with the antitumor efficacy of the regimen). Products include:
  DaunoXome 1842

Daunorubicin Hydrochloride (Dexrazoxane may add to the myelosuppression caused by chemotherapeutic agents). Products include:
  Cerubidine for Injection 634

Docetaxel (Dexrazoxane may add to the myelosuppression caused by chemotherapeutic agents). Products include:
  Taxotere for Injection Concentrate ... 2204

Doxorubicin Hydrochloride (Use of dexrazoxane concurrently with the initiation of fluorouracil, doxorubicin and cyclophosphamide (FAC) therapy may interfere with the antitumor efficacy of the regimen). Products include:
  Adriamycin PFS 2056
  Adriamycin RDF 2056
  Doxil 2613
  Doxorubicin Astra 531
  Rubex for Injection 721

Estramustine Phosphate Sodium (Dexrazoxane may add to the myelosuppression caused by chemotherapeutic agents). Products include:
  Emcyt Capsules 2085

Etoposide (Dexrazoxane may add to the myelosuppression caused by chemotherapeutic agents). Products include:
  Etoposide Injection 539
  VePesid Capsules and Injection ... 727

Floxuridine (Dexrazoxane may add to the myelosuppression caused by chemotherapeutic agents). Products include:
  Sterile FUDR 2284

Fluorouracil (Use of dexrazoxane concurrently with the initiation of fluorouracil, doxorubicin and cyclophosphamide (FAC) therapy may interfere with the antitumor efficacy of the regimen). Products include:
  Efudex 2280
  Fluoroplex Topical Solution & Cream 1% 475
  Fluorouracil Injection 2282

Flutamide (Dexrazoxane may add to the myelosuppression caused by chemotherapeutic agents). Products include:
  Eulexin Capsules 2498

Gemcitabine Hydrochloride (Dexrazoxane may add to the myelosuppression caused by chemotherapeutic agents). Products include:
  Gemzar for Injection 1482

Hydroxyurea (Dexrazoxane may add to the myelosuppression caused by chemotherapeutic agents). Products include:
  Hydrea Capsules 705

Idarubicin Hydrochloride (Dexrazoxane may add to the myelosuppression caused by chemotherapeutic agents). Products include:
  Idamycin Injection 2096

Ifosfamide (Dexrazoxane may add to the myelosuppression caused by chemotherapeutic agents). Products include:
  IFEX 706

Interferon alfa-2A, Recombinant (Dexrazoxane may add to the myelosuppression caused by chemotherapeutic agents). Products include:
  Roferon-A Injection 2308

Interferon alfa-2B, Recombinant (Dexrazoxane may add to the myelosuppression caused by chemotherapeutic agents). Products include:
  Intron A for Injection 2506

Irinotecan Hydrochloride (Dexrazoxane may add to the myelosuppression caused by chemotherapeutic agents).
  No products indexed under this heading.

Levamisole Hydrochloride (Dexrazoxane may add to the myelosuppression caused by chemotherapeutic agents). Products include:
  Ergamisol Tablets 1340

Lomustine (CCNU) (Dexrazoxane may add to the myelosuppression caused by chemotherapeutic agents). Products include:
  CeeNU Capsules 699

Mechlorethamine Hydrochloride (Dexrazoxane may add to the myelosuppression caused by chemotherapeutic agents). Products include:
  Mustargen 1752

Megestrol Acetate (Dexrazoxane may add to the myelosuppression caused by chemotherapeutic agents). Products include:
  Megace Oral Suspension 708
  Megace Tablets 710

Melphalan (Dexrazoxane may add to the myelosuppression caused by chemotherapeutic agents). Products include:
  Alkeran Tablets 1198

Mercaptopurine (Dexrazoxane may add to the myelosuppression caused by chemotherapeutic agents). Products include:
  Purinethol Tablets 1214

Methotrexate Sodium (Dexrazoxane may add to the myelosuppression caused by chemotherapeutic agents). Products include:
  Methotrexate Sodium Tablets, Injection, for Injection and LPF Injection 1322

Mitomycin (Mitomycin-C) (Dexrazoxane may add to the myelosuppression caused by chemotherapeutic agents). Products include:
  Mutamycin for Injection 712

Mitotane (Dexrazoxane may add to the myelosuppression caused by chemotherapeutic agents). Products include:
  Lysodren Tablets 707

Mitoxantrone Hydrochloride (Dexrazoxane may add to the myelosuppression caused by chemotherapeutic agents). Products include:
  Novantrone for Injection 1327

Paclitaxel (Dexrazoxane may add to the myelosuppression caused by chemotherapeutic agents). Products include:
  Taxol Injection 723

IMPORTANT NOTE: Always consult each drug listing in the patient's regimen for possible interactions.

Zinecard   Interactions Index   1222

Procarbazine Hydrochloride (Dexrazoxane may add to the myelosuppression caused by chemotherapeutic agents). Products include:
Matulane Capsules 2300

Streptozocin (Dexrazoxane may add to the myelosuppression caused by chemotherapeutic agents). Products include:
Zanosar Sterile Powder 2119

Tamoxifen Citrate (Dexrazoxane may add to the myelosuppression caused by chemotherapeutic agents). Products include:
Nolvadex Tablets 2957

Teniposide (Dexrazoxane may add to the myelosuppression caused by chemotherapeutic agents). Products include:
Vumon for Injection 729

Thioguanine (Dexrazoxane may add to the myelosuppression caused by chemotherapeutic agents). Products include:
Thioguanine Tablets, Tabloid Brand 1225

Thiotepa (Dexrazoxane may add to the myelosuppression caused by chemotherapeutic agents). Products include:
Thioplex (Thiotepa For Injection) 1329

Topotecan Hydrochloride (Dexrazoxane may add to the myelosuppression caused by chemotherapeutic agents). Products include:
Hycamtin for Injection 2665

Vincristine Sulfate (Dexrazoxane may add to the myelosuppression caused by chemotherapeutic agents). Products include:
Oncovin Solution Vials & Hyporets   1521

Vinorelbine Tartrate (Dexrazoxane may add to the myelosuppression caused by chemotherapeutic agents). Products include:
Navelbine Injection 1212

ZITHROMAX CAPSULES
(Azithromycin) 2043
May interact with antacids containing aluminium, calcium and magnesium, xanthine bronchodilators, oral anticoagulants, and certain other agents. Compounds in these categories include:

Aluminum Carbonate (Aluminum- and magnesium-containing antacids reduce the peak serum levels (rate) but not the AUC (extent) of azithromycin absorption; simultaneous administration should be avoided). Products include:
Basaljel Capsules 2810
Basaljel Suspension 2810
Basaljel Tablets 2810

Aluminum Hydroxide (Aluminum- and magnesium-containing antacids reduce the peak serum levels (rate) but not the AUC (extent) of azithromycin absorption; simultaneous administration should be avoided). Products include:
ALternaGEL Liquid 1358
Maximum Strength Ascriptin .... ⊡ 650
Cama Arthritis Pain Reliever .... ⊡ 748
Gaviscon Extra Strength Relief Formula Antacid Tablets............ ⊡ 778
Gaviscon Extra Strength Relief Formula Liquid Antacid .... ⊡ 779
Gaviscon Liquid Antacid .... ⊡ 779
Gelusil Antacid-Anti-gas Liquid .... ⊡ 819
Gelusil Antacid-Anti-gas Tablets .... ⊡ 819
Maalox Antacid/Anti-Gas Tablets ... 889
Maalox Heartburn Relief Suspension .... ⊡ 658
Maalox Antacid Liquid 888

Extra Strength Maalox Antacid/ Anti-Gas Liquid and Tablets 888
Mylanta 1359
Tempo Soft Antacid .... ⊡ 799

Aluminum Hydroxide Gel (Aluminum- and magnesium-containing antacids reduce the peak serum levels (rate) but not the AUC (extent) of azithromycin absorption; simultaneous administration should be avoided). Products include:
ALternaGEL Liquid .... ⊡ 675
Aludrox Oral Suspension .... ⊡ 850
Amphojel Suspension 2802
Amphojel Suspension without Flavor 2802
Amphojel Tablets 2802
Ascriptin .... ⊡ 650
Gaviscon Antacid Tablets .... ⊡ 778
Gaviscon-2 Antacid Tablets .... ⊡ 779
Mylanta Liquid .... ⊡ 676
Mylanta Double Strength Liquid ... ⊡ 676
Nephrox Suspension .... ⊡ 671

Aminophylline (Careful monitoring of plasma theophylline levels in patient receiving azithromycin and theophylline concurrently is recommended; possible increases in serum concentrations of theophylline).
No products indexed under this heading.

Carbamazepine (Caution is advised since co-administration of drugs metabolized by cytochrome P450 system and macrolide antibiotics is associated with elevation in carbamazepine serum levels). Products include:
Atretol Tablets 569
Tegretol/Tegretol-XR 870

Cyclosporine (Caution is advised since co-administration of drugs metabolized by cytochrome P450 system and macrolide antibiotics is associated with elevation in cyclosporine serum levels). Products include:
Neoral 2405
Sandimmune 2416

Dicumarol (Concurrent use of macrolides and warfarin in clinical practice has been associated with increased anticoagulant effects).
No products indexed under this heading.

Digoxin (Caution is advised since macrolide antibiotics elevate digoxin serum levels). Products include:
Lanoxicaps 1110
Lanoxin Elixir Pediatric 1113
Lanoxin Injection 1116
Lanoxin Injection Pediatric............ 1119
Lanoxin Tablets 1121

Dihydroergotamine Mesylate (Caution is advised since macrolide antibiotics and ergotamine co-administration is associated with acute ergot toxicity). Products include:
D.H.E. 45 Injection 2381

Dyphylline (Careful monitoring of plasma theophylline levels in patient receiving azithromycin and theophylline concurrently is recommended; possible increases in serum concentrations of theophylline). Products include:
Lufyllin & Lufyllin-400 Tablets 2778
Lufyllin-GG Elixir & Tablets 2779

Ergotamine Tartrate (Caution is advised since macrolide antibiotics and ergotamine co-administration is associated with acute ergot toxicity). Products include:
Bellergal-S Tablets 2375
Cafergot 2376
Ergomar Tablets 1543
Wigraine Tablets 1884

Hexobarbital (Caution is advised since co-administration of drugs

metabolized by cytochrome P450 system and macrolide antibiotics is associated with elevation in hexobarbital serum levels).
No products indexed under this heading.

Magaldrate (Aluminum- and magnesium-containing antacids reduce the peak serum levels (rate) but not the AUC (extent) of azithromycin absorption; simultaneous administration should be avoided).
No products indexed under this heading.

Magnesium Hydroxide (Aluminum- and magnesium-containing antacids reduce the peak serum levels (rate) but not the AUC (extent) of azithromycin absorption; simultaneous administration should be avoided). Products include:
Aludrox Oral Suspension .... ⊡ 850
Ascriptin .... ⊡ 650
Di-Gel Antacid/Anti-Gas .... ⊡ 762
Gelusil Antacid-Anti-gas Liquid .... ⊡ 819
Gelusil Antacid-Anti-gas Tablets .... ⊡ 819
Maalox Antacid/Anti-Gas Tablets ... 889
Maalox Antacid Liquid 888
Extra Strength Maalox Antacid/ Anti-Gas Liquid and Tablets 888
Mylanta Fast-Acting 1359
Mylanta Gelcaps Antacid .... ⊡ 678
Fast-Acting Mylanta Liquid Antacid 1359
Mylanta Tablets .... ⊡ 677
Maximum-Strength Fast-Acting Mylanta Liquid Antacid 1359
Mylanta Double Strength Tablets .. ⊡ 677
Phillips' Milk of Magnesia Liquid ... ⊡ 627
Rolaids Antacid Tablets .... ⊡ 807
Tempo Soft Antacid .... ⊡ 799

Magnesium Oxide (Aluminum- and magnesium-containing antacids reduce the peak serum levels (rate) but not the AUC (extent) of azithromycin absorption; simultaneous administration should be avoided). Products include:
Beelith Tablets 632
Bufferin Analgesic Tablets............. ⊡ 636
Arthritis Strength Bufferin Analgesic Caplets .... ⊡ 637
Extra Strength Bufferin Analgesic Tablets .... ⊡ 637
Caltrate PLUS .... ⊡ 681
Cama Arthritis Pain Reliever .... ⊡ 748
Mag-Ox 400 666
Uro-Mag 666

Phenytoin (Caution is advised since co-administration of drugs metabolized by cytochrome P450 system and macrolide antibiotics is associated with elevation in phenytoin serum levels). Products include:
Dilantin Infatabs 1967
Dilantin-125 Suspension 1969

Phenytoin Sodium (Caution is advised since co-administration of drugs metabolized by cytochrome P450 system and macrolide antibiotics is associated with elevation in phenytoin serum levels). Products include:
Dilantin Kapseals 1965

Terfenadine (Caution is advised since co-administration of drugs metabolized by cytochrome P450 system and macrolide antibiotics is associated with elevation in terfenadine serum levels). Products include:
Seldane Tablets 1284
Seldane-D Extended-Release Tablets 1286

Theophylline (Careful monitoring of plasma theophylline levels in patient receiving azithromycin and theophylline concurrently is recommended; possible increases in serum concentrations of theophylline). Products include:
Marax Tablets & DF Syrup............. 2015

Quibron 2227

Theophylline Anhydrous (Careful monitoring of plasma theophylline levels in patient receiving azithromycin and theophylline concurrently is recommended; possible increases in serum concentrations of theophylline). Products include:
Aerolate 1003
Primatene Tablets .... ⊡ 844
Respbid Tablets 687
Slo-bid Gyrocaps 2201
Theo-24 Extended Release Capsules 2753
Theo-Dur Extended-Release Tablets 1367
Theo-X Extended-Release Tablets .. 793
Uni-Dur Extended-Release Tablets . 1374
Uniphyl 400 mg and 600 mg Tablets 2157

Theophylline Calcium Salicylate (Careful monitoring of plasma theophylline levels in patient receiving azithromycin and theophylline concurrently is recommended; possible increases in serum concentrations of theophylline). Products include:
Quadrinal Tablets 1398

Theophylline Sodium Glycinate (Careful monitoring of plasma theophylline levels in patient receiving azithromycin and theophylline concurrently is recommended; possible increases in serum concentrations of theophylline).
No products indexed under this heading.

Triazolam (Caution is advised since macrolide antibiotics decrease the clearance of triazolam and thereby increasing the pharmacologic effect of triazolam). Products include:
Halcion Tablets 2093

Warfarin Sodium (Concurrent use of macrolides and warfarin in clinical practice has been associated with increased anticoagulant effects). Products include:
Coumadin 941

Food Interactions
Food, unspecified (Zithromax should not be taken with food; reduces the rate of absorption (Cmax) of azithromycin capsules by 52% and the extent of absorption (AUC) by 43%; when oral suspension of azithromycin was administered with food the Cmax increased by 56% and the AUC was unchanged).

ZITHROMAX FOR ORAL SUSPENSION
(Azithromycin) 2043
See **Zithromax Capsules**

ZITHROMAX TABLETS
(Azithromycin) 2046
See **Zithromax Capsules**

ZOCOR TABLETS
(Simvastatin) 1821
May interact with fibrates, erythromycin, and certain other agents. Compounds in these categories include:

Clofibrate (Potential for myopathy and rhabdomyolysis; combined therapy with fibrates should be avoided). Products include:
Atromid-S Capsules 2808

(⊡ Described in PDR For Nonprescription Drugs)   (⊙ Described in PDR For Ophthalmology)

Interactions Index — Zoladex

Cyclosporine (Co-administration has been associated with rhabdomyolysis in cardiac transplant patients; concurrent use has resulted in muscle weakness accompanied by marked elevation of creatine phosphokinase in a renal transplant patient following initiation of itraconazole therapy). Products include:
- Neoral 2405
- Sandimmune 2416

Digoxin (Slight elevation in digoxin plasma levels). Products include:
- Lanoxicaps 1110
- Lanoxin Elixir Pediatric 1113
- Lanoxin Injection 1116
- Lanoxin Injection Pediatric 1119
- Lanoxin Tablets 1121

Erythromycin (Co-administration may produce rhabdomyolysis in seriously ill patients). Products include:
- A/T/S 2% Acne Topical Gel 1244
- A/T/S 2% Acne Topical Solution 1244
- Benzamycin Topical Gel 919
- E-Mycin Tablets 1388
- Emgel 2% Topical Gel 1081
- ERYC 1972
- Erycette (erythromycin 2%) Topical Solution 1943
- Ery-Tab Tablets 426
- Erythromycin Base Filmtab 430
- Erythromycin Delayed-Release Capsules, USP 431
- Ilotycin Ophthalmic Ointment 928
- PCE Dispertab Tablets 453
- T-Stat 2.0% Topical Solution and Pads 2797
- THERAMYCIN Z 2% Solution 1629

Erythromycin Estolate (Co-administration may produce rhabdomyolysis in seriously ill patients). Products include:
- Ilosone 927

Erythromycin Ethylsuccinate (Co-administration may produce rhabdomyolysis in seriously ill patients). Products include:
- E.E.S. 427
- EryPed 425
- Pediazole Suspension 2340

Erythromycin Gluceptate (Co-administration may produce rhabdomyolysis in seriously ill patients). Products include:
- Ilotycin Gluceptate, IV, Vials 929

Erythromycin Stearate (Co-administration may produce rhabdomyolysis in seriously ill patients). Products include:
- Erythrocin Stearate Filmtab 429

Gemfibrozil (Potential for myopathy and rhabdomyolysis; combined therapy with fibrates should be avoided). Products include:
- Lopid Tablets 1974

Itraconazole (Concurrent use has resulted in muscle weakness accompanied by marked elevation of creatine phosphokinase in a renal transplant patient on cyclosporine and simvastatin following initiation of itraconazole therapy). Products include:
- Sporanox Capsules 1352

Muromonab-CD3 (Concomitant administration may produce rhabdomyolysis). Products include:
- Orthoclone OKT3 Sterile Solution 1892

Niacin (Co-administration with lipid-lowering doses (greater than or equal to 1 g/day) has been associated with rhabdomyolysis). Products include:
- Kyo-Chrome 680
- Nicotinex Elixir 671
- Slo-Niacin Tablets 2767

Propranolol Hydrochloride (Significant decreases in mean C_{max}, but no change in AUC). Products include:
- Inderal 2834
- Inderal LA Long Acting Capsules 2836
- Inderide Tablets 2838
- Inderide LA Long Acting Capsules 2840

Warfarin Sodium (Slightly enhanced anticoagulant effect). Products include:
- Coumadin 941

ZOFRAN INJECTION
(Ondansetron Hydrochloride) 1227
May interact with quinidine and certain other agents. Compounds in these categories include:

Cimetidine (Co-administration with inhibitors of cytochrome P450, such as cimetidine may change the clearance and, hence, the half-life of ondansetron; based on the limited data, no dosage adjustment is recommended for patients on concomitant therapy). Products include:
- Tagamet HB Tablets 786
- Tagamet Tablets 2694

Cimetidine Hydrochloride (Co-administration with inhibitors of cytochrome P450, such as cimetidine may change the clearance and, hence, the half-life of ondansetron; based on the limited data, no dosage adjustment is recommended for patients on concomitant therapy). Products include:
- Tagamet 2694

Fosphenytoin Sodium (Co-administration with inducers of cytochrome P450, such as phenytoin, may change the clearance and, hence, the half-life of ondansetron; based on the limited data, no dosage adjustment is recommended for patients on concomitant therapy). Products include:
- Cerebyx Injection 1956

Phenobarbital (Co-administration with inducers of cytochrome P450, such as phenobarbital, may change the clearance and, hence, the half-life of ondansetron; based on the limited data, no dosage adjustment is recommended for patients on concomitant therapy). Products include:
- Arco-Lase Plus Tablets 513
- Bellergal-S Tablets 2375
- Donnatal 2234
- Donnatal Extentabs 2234
- Donnatal Tablets 2234
- Phenobarbital Elixir and Tablets 1523
- Quadrinal Tablets 1398

Phenytoin (Co-administration with inducers of cytochrome P450, such as phenytoin, may change the clearance and, hence, the half-life of ondansetron; based on the limited data, no dosage adjustment is recommended for patients on concomitant therapy). Products include:
- Dilantin Infatabs 1967
- Dilantin-125 Suspension 1969

Phenytoin Sodium (Co-administration with inducers of cytochrome P450, such as phenytoin, may change the clearance and, hence, the half-life of ondansetron; based on the limited data, no dosage adjustment is recommended for patients on concomitant therapy). Products include:
- Dilantin Kapseals 1965

Quinidine Gluconate (Co-administration with inhibitors of cytochrome P450, such as quinidine, may change the clearance and, hence, the half-life of ondansetron; based on the limited data, no dosage adjustment is recommended for patients on concomitant therapy). Products include:
- Quinaglute Dura-Tabs Tablets 644

Quinidine Polygalacturonate (Co-administration with inhibitors of cytochrome P450, such as quinidine, may change the clearance and, hence, the half-life of ondansetron; based on the limited data, no dosage adjustment is recommended for patients on concomitant therapy). Products include:
- Cardioquin Tablets 2146

Quinidine Sulfate (Co-administration with inhibitors of cytochrome P450, such as quinidine, may change the clearance and, hence, the half-life of ondansetron; based on the limited data, no dosage adjustment is recommended for patients on concomitant therapy). Products include:
- Quinidex Extentabs 2240

Rifampin (Co-administration with inducers of cytochrome P450, such as rifampin, may change the clearance and, hence, the half-life of ondansetron; based on the limited data, no dosage adjustment is recommended for patients on concomitant therapy). Products include:
- Rifadin 1276
- Rifamate Capsules 1278
- Rifater 1280
- Rimactane Capsules 865

ZOFRAN INJECTION PREMIXED
(Ondansetron Hydrochloride) 1227
See Zofran Injection

ZOFRAN TABLETS
(Ondansetron Hydrochloride) 1231
May interact with quinidine and certain other agents. Compounds in these categories include:

Cimetidine (Co-administration with inhibitors of cytochrome P450, such as quinidine, may change the clearance and, hence, the half-life of ondansetron; based on the limited data, no dosage adjustment is recommended for patients on concomitant therapy). Products include:
- Tagamet HB Tablets 786
- Tagamet Tablets 2694

Cimetidine Hydrochloride (Co-administration with inhibitors of cytochrome P450, such as quinidine, may change the clearance and, hence, the half-life of ondansetron; based on the limited data, no dosage adjustment is recommended for patients on concomitant therapy). Products include:
- Tagamet 2694

Fosphenytoin Sodium (Co-administration with inducers of cytochrome P450, such as phenytoin, may change the clearance and, hence, the half-life of ondansetron; based on the limited data, no dosage adjustment is recommended for patients on concomitant therapy). Products include:
- Cerebyx Injection 1956

Phenobarbital (Co-administration with inducers of cytochrome P450, such as phenobarbital, may change the clearance and, hence, the half-life of ondansetron; based on the limited data, no dosage adjustment is recommended for patients on concomitant therapy). Products include:
- Arco-Lase Plus Tablets 513
- Bellergal-S Tablets 2375
- Donnatal 2234
- Donnatal Extentabs 2234
- Donnatal Tablets 2234
- Phenobarbital Elixir and Tablets 1523
- Quadrinal Tablets 1398

Phenytoin (Co-administration with inducers of cytochrome P450, such as phenytoin, may change the clearance and, hence, the half-life of ondansetron; based on the limited data, no dosage adjustment is recommended for patients on concomitant therapy). Products include:
- Dilantin Infatabs 1967
- Dilantin-125 Suspension 1969

Phenytoin Sodium (Co-administration with inducers of cytochrome P450, such as phenytoin, may change the clearance and, hence, the half-life of ondansetron; based on the limited data, no dosage adjustment is recommended for patients on concomitant therapy). Products include:
- Dilantin Kapseals 1965

Quinidine Gluconate (Co-administration with inhibitors of cytochrome P450, such as quinidine, may change the clearance and, hence, the half-life of ondansetron; based on the limited data, no dosage adjustment is recommended for patients on concomitant therapy). Products include:
- Quinaglute Dura-Tabs Tablets 644

Quinidine Polygalacturonate (Co-administration with inhibitors of cytochrome P450, such as quinidine, may change the clearance and, hence, the half-life of ondansetron; based on the limited data, no dosage adjustment is recommended for patients on concomitant therapy). Products include:
- Cardioquin Tablets 2146

Quinidine Sulfate (Co-administration with inhibitors of cytochrome P450, such as quinidine, may change the clearance and, hence, the half-life of ondansetron; based on the limited data, no dosage adjustment is recommended for patients on concomitant therapy). Products include:
- Quinidex Extentabs 2240

Rifampin (Co-administration with inducers of cytochrome P450, such as rifampin, may change the clearance and, hence, the half-life of ondansetron; based on the limited data, no dosage adjustment is recommended for patients on concomitant therapy). Products include:
- Rifadin 1276
- Rifamate Capsules 1278
- Rifater 1280
- Rimactane Capsules 865

Food Interactions
Food, unspecified (Increases significantly (about 17%) the extent of absorption of ondansetron).

ZOLADEX
(Goserelin Acetate) 2976
None cited in PDR database.

IMPORTANT NOTE: Always consult each drug listing in the patient's regimen for possible interactions.

ZOLADEX 3-MONTH
(Goserelin Acetate) **2978**
None cited in PDR database.

ZOLOFT TABLETS
(Sertraline Hydrochloride) **2051**
May interact with oral anticoagulants, antidepressant drugs, lithium preparations, monoamine oxidase inhibitors, highly protein bound drugs (selected), tricyclic antidepressants, and certain other agents. Compounds in these categories include:

Amiodarone Hydrochloride (Co-administration with another drug which is tightly bound to protein may cause a shift in plasma concentrations resulting in an adverse effect). Products include:
Cordarone Intravenous **2821**
Cordarone Tablets **2818**

Amitriptyline Hydrochloride (Concurrent use of drugs that inhibit the biochemical activity of $P_{450}IID_6$, such as tricyclic antidepressants, may increase plasma concentrations of co-administered drugs that are metabolized by $P_{450}IID_6$; changes in the dosage may be required; the duration of an appropriate washout period which should intervene before switching has not been established). Products include:
Elavil **2945**
Etrafon **2495**
Limbitrol **2333**
Triavil Tablets **1800**

Amoxapine (Concurrent use of drugs that inhibit the biochemical activity of $P_{450}IID_6$, such as tricyclic antidepressants, may increase plasma concentrations of co-administered drugs that are metabolized by $P_{450}IID_6$; changes in the dosage may be required; the duration of an appropriate washout period which should intervene before switching has not been established). Products include:
Asendin Tablets **1419**

Astemizole (Sertraline has been shown to have some inhibition of P4503A4 *in vitro*, astemizole is metabolized by P4503A4 isoenzyme and inhibition of this enzyme system may result in increased serum levels of astemizole; co-administration requires caution). Products include:
Hismanal Tablets **1341**

Atovaquone (Co-administration with another drug which is tightly bound to protein may cause a shift in plasma concentrations resulting in an adverse effect). Products include:
Mepron Suspension **1206**

Cefonicid Sodium (Co-administration with another drug which is tightly bound to protein may cause a shift in plasma concentrations resulting in an adverse effect). Products include:
Monocid Injection **2674**

Chlordiazepoxide (Co-administration with another drug which is tightly bound to protein may cause a shift in plasma concentrations resulting in an adverse effect). Products include:
Limbitrol **2333**

Chlordiazepoxide Hydrochloride (Co-administration with another drug which is tightly bound to protein may cause a shift in plasma concentrations resulting in an adverse effect). Products include:
Librax Capsules **2330**
Librium Capsules **2331**
Librium Injectable **2332**

Chlorpromazine (Co-administration with another drug which is tightly bound to protein may cause a shift in plasma concentrations resulting in an adverse effect). Products include:
Thorazine Suppositories **2701**

Chlorpromazine Hydrochloride (Co-administration with another drug which is tightly bound to protein may cause a shift in plasma concentrations resulting in an adverse effect). Products include:
Thorazine **2701**

Cimetidine (Potential for increase in Zoloft mean AUC (50%), C_{max} (24%) and half-life (26%); clinical significance is unknown). Products include:
Tagamet HB Tablets .... ▣ **786**
Tagamet Tablets **2694**

Cimetidine Hydrochloride (Potential for increase in Zoloft mean AUC (50%), C_{max} (24%) and half-life (26%); clinical significance is unknown). Products include:
Tagamet **2694**

Cisapride (Sertraline has been shown to have some inhibition of P4503A4 *in vitro*, cisapride is metabolized by P4503A4 isoenzyme and inhibition of this enzyme system may result in increased serum levels of cisapride; co-administration requires caution). Products include:
Propulsid **1346**

Clomipramine Hydrochloride (Concurrent use of drugs that inhibit the biochemical activity of $P_{450}IID_6$, such as tricyclic antidepressants, may increase plasma concentrations of co-administered drugs that are metabolized by $P_{450}IID_6$; changes in the dosage may be required; the duration of an appropriate washout period which should intervene before switching has not been established). Products include:
Anafranil Capsules **819**

Clozapine (Co-administration with another drug which is tightly bound to protein may cause a shift in plasma concentrations resulting in an adverse effect). Products include:
Clozaril Tablets **2377**

CNS-Active Drugs, unspecified (Caution is advised if Zoloft is co-administered with other CNS active drugs).

Cyclosporine (Co-administration with another drug which is tightly bound to protein may cause a shift in plasma concentrations resulting in an adverse effect). Products include:
Neoral **2405**
Sandimmune **2416**

Desipramine Hydrochloride (Concurrent use of drugs that inhibit the biochemical activity of $P_{450}IID_6$, such as tricyclic antidepressants, may increase plasma concentrations of co-administered drugs that are metabolized by $P_{450}IID_6$; changes in the dosage may be required; the duration of an appropriate washout period which should intervene before switching has not been established). Products include:
Norpramin Tablets **1273**

Diazepam (Co-administration with intravenous diazepam has resulted in decrease in relative to baseline diazepam clearance and increase in T_{max} for desmethyldiazepam; the clinical significance is unknown). Products include:
Dizac (diazepam injectable emulsion) CIV **1862**
Valium Injectable **2336**
Valium Tablets **2335**

Diclofenac Potassium (Co-administration with another drug which is tightly bound to protein may cause a shift in plasma concentrations resulting in an adverse effect). Products include:
Cataflam Tablets **833**

Diclofenac Sodium (Co-administration with another drug which is tightly bound to protein may cause a shift in plasma concentrations resulting in an adverse effect). Products include:
Voltaren Ophthalmic Sterile Ophthalmic Solution .... ⊙ **264**
Cataflam/Voltaren/Voltaren-XR **833**

Dicumarol (May cause a shift in plasma concentrations potentially resulting in an adverse effect; prothrombin time should be carefully monitored when Zoloft therapy is initiated or stopped).
No products indexed under this heading.

Digitoxin (May cause shift in plasma concentrations potentially resulting in an adverse effect; in clinical trials, during co-administration, there was no change in serum digoxin levels or plasma digitalis glycoside clearance). Products include:
Crystodigin Tablets **1472**

Digoxin (May cause a shift in plasma concentrations potentially resulting in an adverse effect; in clinical trials, during co-administration, there was no change in serum digoxin levels or digoxin clearance). Products include:
Lanoxicaps **1110**
Lanoxin Elixir Pediatric **1113**
Lanoxin Injection **1116**
Lanoxin Injection Pediatric **1119**
Lanoxin Tablets **1121**

Dipyridamole (Co-administration with another drug which is tightly bound to protein may cause a shift in plasma concentrations resulting in an adverse effect). Products include:
Persantine Tablets **686**

Doxepin Hydrochloride (Concurrent use of drugs that inhibit the biochemical activity of $P_{450}IID_6$, such as tricyclic antidepressants, may increase plasma concentrations of co-administered drugs that are metabolized by $P_{450}IID_6$; changes in the dosage may be required; the duration of an appropriate washout period which should intervene before switching has not been established). Products include:
Adapin Capsules **1542**
Sinequan **2028**
Zonalon Cream **1042**

Fenoprofen Calcium (Co-administration with another drug which is tightly bound to protein may cause a shift in plasma concentrations resulting in an adverse effect). Products include:
Nalfon 200 Pulvules & Nalfon Tablets **933**

Flecainide Acetate (Concurrent use of drugs that inhibit the biochemical activity of $P_{450}IID_6$, such as flecainide, may increase plasma concentrations of co-administered drugs that are metabolized by $P_{450}IID_6$; changes in the dosage may be required). Products include:
Tambocor Tablets **1555**

Fluoxetine Hydrochloride (Concurrent use of drugs that inhibit the biochemical activity of $P_{450}IID_6$, such as SSRIs, may increase plasma concentrations of co-administered drugs that are metabolized by $P_{450}IID_6$; changes in the dosage may be required; the duration of an appropriate washout period which should intervene before switching has not been established). Products include:
Prozac Pulvules & Liquid, Oral Solution **935**

Flurazepam Hydrochloride (Co-administration with another drug which is tightly bound to protein may cause a shift in plasma concentrations resulting in an adverse effect). Products include:
Dalmane Capsules **2329**

Flurbiprofen (Co-administration with another drug which is tightly bound to protein may cause a shift in plasma concentrations resulting in an adverse effect).
No products indexed under this heading.

Fluvoxamine Maleate (Concurrent use of drugs that inhibit the biochemical activity of $P_{450}IID_6$, such as SSRIs, may increase plasma concentrations of co-administered drugs that are metabolized by $P_{450}IID_6$; changes in the dosage may be required; the duration of an appropriate washout period which should intervene before switching has not been established). Products include:
LUVOX Tablets **2723**

Furazolidone (Co-administration has resulted in serious, sometimes fatal, reactions including hyperthermia, rigidity, myoclonus, autonomic instability, extreme agitation progressing to delirium and coma; concurrent and/or sequential use is contraindicated). Products include:
Furoxone **2221**

Glipizide (Co-administration with another drug which is tightly bound to protein may cause a shift in plasma concentrations resulting in an adverse effect). Products include:
Glucotrol Tablets **2011**
Glucotrol XL Extended Release Tablets **2012**

Ibuprofen (Co-administration with another drug which is tightly bound to protein may cause a shift in plasma concentrations resulting in an adverse effect). Products include:
Advil Cold and Sinus Caplets and Tablets .... ▣ **837**
Advil Ibuprofen Tablets, Caplets and Gel Caplets .... ▣ **836**
Children's Motrin Ibuprofen Oral Suspension **1558**
IBU Tablets **1389**
Ibuprohm .... ▣ **713**
Motrin IB Caplets, Tablets, and Gelcaps .... ▣ **802**
Motrin Ibuprofen Suspension, Oral Drops, Chewable Tablets, Caplets **1563**
Nuprin Ibuprofen/Analgesic Tablets & Caplets .... ▣ **645**
Vicks DayQuil SINUS Pressure & PAIN Relief with IBUPROFEN ...... ▣ **735**

(▣ Described in PDR For Nonprescription Drugs) (⊙ Described in PDR For Ophthalmology)

Imipramine Hydrochloride (Concurrent use of drugs that inhibit the biochemical activity of $P_{450}IID_6$, such as tricyclic antidepressants, may increase plasma concentrations of co-administered drugs that are metabolized by $P_{450}IID_6$; changes in the dosage may be required; the duration of an appropriate washout period which should intervene before switching has not been established). Products include:
- Tofranil Ampuls 873
- Tofranil Tablets 875

Imipramine Pamoate (Concurrent use of drugs that inhibit the biochemical activity of $P_{450}IID_6$, such as tricyclic antidepressants, may increase plasma concentrations of co-administered drugs that are metabolized by $P_{450}IID_6$; changes in the dosage may be required; the duration of an appropriate washout period which should intervene before switching has not been established). Products include:
- Tofranil-PM Capsules 876

Indomethacin (Co-administration with another drug which is tightly bound to protein may cause a shift in plasma concentrations resulting in an adverse effect). Products include:
- Indocin 1723

Indomethacin Sodium Trihydrate (Co-administration with another drug which is tightly bound to protein may cause a shift in plasma concentrations resulting in an adverse effect). Products include:
- Indocin I.V. 1727

Isocarboxazid (Co-administration has resulted in serious, sometimes fatal, reactions including hyperthermia, rigidity, myoclonus, autonomic instability, extreme agitation progressing to delirium and coma; concurrent and/or sequential use is contraindicated).
- No products indexed under this heading.

Ketoprofen (Co-administration with another drug which is tightly bound to protein may cause a shift in plasma concentrations resulting in an adverse effect). Products include:
- Actron Caplets and Tablets 608
- Orudis Capsules 2874
- Orudis KT 842
- Oruvail Capsules 2874

Ketorolac Tromethamine (Co-administration with another drug which is tightly bound to protein may cause a shift in plasma concentrations resulting in an adverse effect). Products include:
- Acular Sterile Ophthalmic Solution 470
- Toradol 2319

Lithium Carbonate (No significant alteration in plasma lithium levels or renal clearance, nonetheless, plasma lithium levels should be monitored). Products include:
- Eskalith 2658
- Lithium Carbonate Capsules & Tablets 2352
- Lithonate/Lithotabs/Lithobid 2721

Lithium Citrate (No significant alteration in plasma lithium levels or renal clearance, nonetheless, plasma lithium levels should be monitored).
- No products indexed under this heading.

Maprotiline Hydrochloride (Concurrent use of drugs that inhibit the biochemical activity of $P_{450}IID_6$, such as tricyclic antidepressants, may increase plasma concentrations of co-administered drugs that are metabolized by $P_{450}IID_6$; changes in the dosage may be required; the duration of an appropriate washout period which should intervene before switching has not been established). Products include:
- Ludiomil Tablets 861

Meclofenamate Sodium (Co-administration with another drug which is tightly bound to protein may cause a shift in plasma concentrations resulting in an adverse effect).
- No products indexed under this heading.

Mefenamic Acid (Co-administration with another drug which is tightly bound to protein may cause a shift in plasma concentrations resulting in an adverse effect). Products include:
- Ponstel 1982

Midazolam Hydrochloride (Co-administration with another drug which is tightly bound to protein may cause a shift in plasma concentrations resulting in an adverse effect). Products include:
- Versed Injection 2324

Naproxen (Co-administration with another drug which is tightly bound to protein may cause a shift in plasma concentrations resulting in an adverse effect). Products include:
- Anaprox/Naprosyn 2277

Naproxen Sodium (Co-administration with another drug which is tightly bound to protein may cause a shift in plasma concentrations resulting in an adverse effect). Products include:
- Aleve 2124
- Anaprox/Naprosyn 2277
- Naprelan Tablets 2861

Nefazodone Hydrochloride (Care and prudent medical judgment should be exercised regarding the optimal timing of switching from another antidepressant to Zoloft; the duration of an appropriate washout period which should intervene before switching has not been established). Products include:
- Serzone Tablets 776

Nortriptyline Hydrochloride (Concurrent use of drugs that inhibit the biochemical activity of $P_{450}IID_6$, such as tricyclic antidepressants, may increase plasma concentrations of co-administered drugs that are metabolized by $P_{450}IID_6$; changes in the dosage may be required; the duration of an appropriate washout period which should intervene before switching has not been established). Products include:
- Pamelor 2409

Oxaprozin (Co-administration with another drug which is tightly bound to protein may cause a shift in plasma concentrations resulting in an adverse effect). Products include:
- Daypro Caplets 2578

Oxazepam (Co-administration with another drug which is tightly bound to protein may cause a shift in plasma concentrations resulting in an adverse effect). Products include:
- Serax Capsules 2916
- Serax Tablets 2916

Paroxetine Hydrochloride (Concurrent use of drugs that inhibit the biochemical activity of $P_{450}IID_6$, such as SSRIs, may increase plasma concentrations of co-administered drugs that are metabolized by $P_{450}IID_6$; changes in the dosage may be required; the duration of an appropriate washout period which should intervene before switching has not been established). Products include:
- Paxil Tablets 2681

Phenelzine Sulfate (Co-administration has resulted in serious, sometimes fatal, reactions including hyperthermia, rigidity, myoclonus, autonomic instability, extreme agitation progressing to delirium and coma; concurrent and/or sequential use is contraindicated). Products include:
- Nardil 1977

Phenylbutazone (Co-administration with another drug which is tightly bound to protein may cause a shift in plasma concentrations resulting in an adverse effect).
- No products indexed under this heading.

Piroxicam (Co-administration with another drug which is tightly bound to protein may cause a shift in plasma concentrations resulting in an adverse effect). Products include:
- Feldene Capsules 2008

Propafenone Hydrochloride (Concurrent use of drugs that inhibit the biochemical activity of $P_{450}IID_6$, such as propafenone, may increase plasma concentrations of co-administered drugs that are metabolized by $P_{450}IID_6$; changes in the dosage may be required). Products include:
- Rythmol Tablets–150mg, 225mg, 300mg 1399

Propranolol Hydrochloride (Co-administration with another drug which is tightly bound to protein may cause a shift in plasma concentrations resulting in an adverse effect). Products include:
- Inderal 2834
- Inderal LA Long Acting Capsules 2836
- Inderide Tablets 2838
- Inderide LA Long Acting Capsules 2840

Protriptyline Hydrochloride (Concurrent use of drugs that inhibit the biochemical activity of $P_{450}IID_6$, such as tricyclic antidepressants, may increase plasma concentrations of co-administered drugs that are metabolized by $P_{450}IID_6$; changes in the dosage may be required; the duration of an appropriate washout period which should intervene before switching has not been established). Products include:
- Vivactil Tablets 1820

Selegiline Hydrochloride (Co-administration has resulted in serious, sometimes fatal, reactions including hyperthermia, rigidity, myoclonus, autonomic instability, extreme agitation progressing to delirium and coma; concurrent and/or sequential use is contraindicated). Products include:
- Eldepryl Capsules 2729

Sulindac (Co-administration with another drug which is tightly bound to protein may cause a shift in plasma concentrations resulting in an adverse effect). Products include:
- Clinoril Tablets 1658

Temazepam (Co-administration with another drug which is tightly bound to protein may cause a shift in plasma concentrations resulting in an adverse effect). Products include:
- Restoril Capsules 2413

Terfenadine (Sertraline has been shown to have some inhibition of P4503A4 *in vitro*, terfenadine is metabolized by P4503A4 isoenzyme and inhibition of this enzyme system may result in increased serum levels of terfenadine; co-administration requires caution). Products include:
- Seldane Tablets 1284
- Seldane-D Extended-Release Tablets 1286

Tolbutamide (A statistically significant decrease in tolbutamide clearance due to a change in the metabolism of the drug).
- No products indexed under this heading.

Tolmetin Sodium (Co-administration with another drug which is tightly bound to protein may cause a shift in plasma concentrations resulting in an adverse effect). Products include:
- Tolectin (200, 400 and 600 mg) 1591

Tranylcypromine Sulfate (Co-administration has resulted in serious, sometimes fatal, reactions including hyperthermia, rigidity, myoclonus, autonomic instability, extreme agitation progressing to delirium and coma; concurrent and/or sequential use is contraindicated). Products include:
- Parnate Tablets 2679

Trimipramine Maleate (Concurrent use of drugs that inhibit the biochemical activity of $P_{450}IID_6$, such as tricyclic antidepressants, may increase plasma concentrations of co-administered drugs that are metabolized by $P_{450}IID_6$; changes in the dosage may be required; the duration of an appropriate washout period which should intervene before switching has not been established). Products include:
- Surmontil Capsules 2917

Venlafaxine Hydrochloride (Concurrent use of drugs that inhibit the biochemical activity of $P_{450}IID_6$, such as SSRIs, may increase plasma concentrations of co-administered drugs that are metabolized by $P_{450}IID_6$; changes in the dosage may be required; the duration of an appropriate washout period which should intervene before switching has not been established). Products include:
- Effexor 2825

Warfarin Sodium (May cause a shift in plasma concentrations potentially resulting in an adverse effect; prothrombin time should be carefully monitored when Zoloft therapy is initiated or stopped). Products include:
- Coumadin 941

Food Interactions

Alcohol (Concomitant use of Zoloft and alcohol in depressed patient is not recommended).

Food, unspecified (AUC was slightly increased when drug was administered with food but the C_{max} was 25% greater).

ZONALON CREAM
(Doxepin Hydrochloride) 1042
May interact with monoamine oxidase inhibitors, antidepressant

---

IMPORTANT NOTE: Always consult each drug listing in the patient's regimen for possible interactions.

drugs, phenothiazines, and certain other agents. Compounds in these categories include:

Amitriptyline Hydrochloride (Concomitant use of doxepin, a tricyclic antidepressant, with other drugs metabolized by cytochrome $P_{450}IID_6$ may require lower than usual doses prescribed for either drug). Products include:

Elavil	2945
Etrafon	2495
Limbitrol	2333
Triavil Tablets	1800

Amoxapine (Concomitant use of doxepin, a tricyclic antidepressant, with other drugs metabolized by cytochrome $P_{450}IID_6$ may require lower than usual doses prescribed for either drug). Products include:

Asendin Tablets	1419

Bupropion Hydrochloride (Concomitant use of doxepin, a tricyclic antidepressant, with other drugs metabolized by cytochrome $P_{450}IID_6$ may require lower than usual doses prescribed for either drug). Products include:

Wellbutrin Tablets	1177

Carbamazepine (Concomitant use of doxepin, a tricyclic antidepressant, with other drugs metabolized by cytochrome $P_{450}IID_6$ may require lower than usual doses prescribed for either drug). Products include:

Atretol Tablets	569
Tegretol/Tegretol-XR	870

Chlorpromazine (Concomitant use of doxepin, a tricyclic antidepressant, with other drugs metabolized by cytochrome $P_{450}IID_6$ may require lower than usual doses prescribed for either drug). Products include:

Thorazine Suppositories	2701

Chlorpromazine Hydrochloride (Concomitant use of doxepin, a tricyclic antidepressant, with other drugs metabolized by cytochrome $P_{450}IID_6$ may require lower than usual doses prescribed for either drug). Products include:

Thorazine	2701

Cimetidine (Potential for clinically significant fluctuations in steady-state serum concentrations). Products include:

Tagamet HB Tablets	▣ 786
Tagamet Tablets	2694

Cimetidine Hydrochloride (Potential for clinically significant fluctuations in steady-state serum concentrations). Products include:

Tagamet	2694

Desipramine Hydrochloride (Concomitant use of doxepin, a tricyclic antidepressant, with other drugs metabolized by cytochrome $P_{450}IID_6$ may require lower than usual doses prescribed for either drug). Products include:

Norpramin Tablets	1273

Flecainide Acetate (Concomitant use of doxepin, a tricyclic antidepressant, with other drugs metabolized by cytochrome $P_{450}IID_6$ may require lower than usual doses prescribed for either drug). Products include:

Tambocor Tablets	1555

Fluoxetine Hydrochloride (Concomitant use of doxepin, a tricyclic antidepressant, with other drugs metabolized by cytochrome $P_{450}IID_6$ may require lower than usual doses prescribed for either drug). Products include:

Prozac Pulvules & Liquid, Oral Solution	935

Fluphenazine Decanoate (Concomitant use of doxepin, a tricyclic antidepressant, with other drugs metabolized by cytochrome $P_{450}IID_6$ may require lower than usual doses prescribed for either drug). Products include:

Prolixin Decanoate	510

Fluphenazine Enanthate (Concomitant use of doxepin, a tricyclic antidepressant, with other drugs metabolized by cytochrome $P_{450}IID_6$ may require lower than usual doses prescribed for either drug). Products include:

Prolixin Enanthate	510

Fluphenazine Hydrochloride (Concomitant use of doxepin, a tricyclic antidepressant, with other drugs metabolized by cytochrome $P_{450}IID_6$ may require lower than usual doses prescribed for either drug). Products include:

Prolixin	510

Furazolidone (Potential for serious side effects and fatality have been reported with orally administered drugs; plasma levels of doxepin obtained with topical administered doxepin are similar to systemic therapy; concurrent and/or sequential therapy is not recommended). Products include:

Furoxone	2221

Imipramine Hydrochloride (Concomitant use of doxepin, a tricyclic antidepressant, with other drugs metabolized by cytochrome $P_{450}IID_6$ may require lower than usual doses prescribed for either drug). Products include:

Tofranil Ampuls	873
Tofranil Tablets	875

Imipramine Pamoate (Concomitant use of doxepin, a tricyclic antidepressant, with other drugs metabolized by cytochrome $P_{450}IID_6$ may require lower than usual doses prescribed for either drug). Products include:

Tofranil-PM Capsules	876

Isocarboxazid (Potential for serious side effects and fatality have been reported with orally administered drugs; plasma levels of doxepin obtained with topical administered doxepin are similar to systemic therapy; concurrent and/or sequential therapy is not recommended; concomitant use of doxepin, a tricyclic antidepressant, with other drugs metabolized by cytochrome $P,450 IID,6$ may require lower than usual doses prescribed for either drug).
No products indexed under this heading.

Maprotiline Hydrochloride (Concomitant use of doxepin, a tricyclic antidepressant, with other drugs metabolized by cytochrome $P_{450}IID_6$ may require lower than usual doses prescribed for either drug). Products include:

Ludiomil Tablets	861

Mesoridazine Besylate (Concomitant use of doxepin, a tricyclic antidepressant, with other drugs metabolized by cytochrome $P_{450}IID_6$ may require lower than usual doses prescribed for either drug). Products include:

Serentil	689

Methotrimeprazine (Concomitant use of doxepin, a tricyclic antidepressant, with other drugs metabolized by cytochrome $P_{450}IID_6$ may require lower than usual doses prescribed for either drug). Products include:

Levoprome	1321

Nefazodone Hydrochloride (Concomitant use of doxepin, a tricyclic antidepressant, with other drugs metabolized by cytochrome $P_{450}IID_6$ may require lower than usual doses prescribed for either drug). Products include:

Serzone Tablets	776

Nortriptyline Hydrochloride (Concomitant use of doxepin, a tricyclic antidepressant, with other drugs metabolized by cytochrome $P_{450}IID_6$ may require lower than usual doses prescribed for either drug). Products include:

Pamelor	2409

Paroxetine Hydrochloride (Concomitant use of doxepin, a tricyclic antidepressant, with other drugs metabolized by cytochrome $P_{450}IID_6$ may require lower than usual doses prescribed for either drug). Products include:

Paxil Tablets	2681

Perphenazine (Concomitant use of doxepin, a tricyclic antidepressant, with other drugs metabolized by cytochrome $P_{450}IID_6$ may require lower than usual doses prescribed for either drug). Products include:

Etrafon	2495
Triavil Tablets	1800
Trilafon	2532

Phenelzine Sulfate (Potential for serious side effects and fatality have been reported with orally administered drugs; plasma levels of doxepin obtained with topical administered doxepin are similar to systemic therapy; concurrent and/or sequential therapy is not recommended; concomitant use of doxepin, a tricyclic antidepressant, with other drugs metabolized by cytochrome $P,450 IID,6$ may require lower than usual doses prescribed for either drug). Products include:

Nardil	1977

Prochlorperazine (Concomitant use of doxepin, a tricyclic antidepressant, with other drugs metabolized by cytochrome $P_{450}IID_6$ may require lower than usual doses prescribed for either drug). Products include:

Compazine	2644

Promethazine Hydrochloride (Concomitant use of doxepin, a tricyclic antidepressant, with other drugs metabolized by cytochrome $P_{450}IID_6$ may require lower than usual doses prescribed for either drug). Products include:

Mepergan Injection	2859
Phenergan with Codeine	2883
Phenergan with Dextromethorphan	2885
Phenergan Injection	2880
Phenergan Suppositories	2882
Phenergan Syrup	2881
Phenergan Tablets	2882
Phenergan VC	2886
Phenergan VC with Codeine	2888

Propafenone Hydrochloride (Concomitant use of doxepin, a tricyclic antidepressant, with other drugs metabolized by cytochrome $P_{450}IID_6$ may require lower than usual doses prescribed for either drug). Products include:

Rythmol Tablets–150mg, 225mg, 300mg	1399

Protriptyline Hydrochloride (Concomitant use of doxepin, a tricyclic antidepressant, with other drugs metabolized by cytochrome $P_{450}IID_6$ may require lower than usual doses prescribed for either drug). Products include:

Vivactil Tablets	1820

Quinidine Gluconate (Concomitant use of doxepin, a tricyclic antidepressant, with quinidine which inhibits cytochrome $P_{450}IID_6$ should be approached with caution). Products include:

Quinaglute Dura-Tabs Tablets	644

Quinidine Polygalacturonate (Concomitant use of doxepin, a tricyclic antidepressant, with quinidine which inhibits cytochrome $P_{450}IID_6$ should be approached with caution). Products include:

Cardioquin Tablets	2146

Quinidine Sulfate (Concomitant use of doxepin, a tricyclic antidepressant, with quinidine which inhibits cytochrome $P_{450}IID_6$ should be approached with caution). Products include:

Quinidex Extentabs	2240

Selegiline Hydrochloride (Potential for serious side effects and fatality have been reported with orally administered drugs; plasma levels of doxepin obtained with topical administered doxepin are similar to systemic therapy; concurrent and/or sequential therapy is not recommended). Products include:

Eldepryl Capsules	2729

Sertraline Hydrochloride (Concomitant use of doxepin, a tricyclic antidepressant, with other drugs metabolized by cytochrome $P_{450}IID_6$ may require lower than usual doses prescribed for either drug). Products include:

Zoloft Tablets	2051

Thioridazine Hydrochloride (Concomitant use of doxepin, a tricyclic antidepressant, with other drugs metabolized by cytochrome $P_{450}IID_6$ may require lower than usual doses prescribed for either drug). Products include:

Mellaril	2398

Tranylcypromine Sulfate (Potential for serious side effects and fatality have been reported with orally administered drugs; plasma levels of doxepin obtained with topical administered doxepin are similar to systemic therapy; concurrent and/or sequential therapy is not recommended; concomitant use of doxepin, a tricyclic antidepressant, with other drugs metabolized by cytochrome $P,450 IID,6$ may require lower than usual doses prescribed for either drug). Products include:

Parnate Tablets	2679

Trazodone Hydrochloride (Concomitant use of doxepin, a tricyclic antidepressant, with other drugs metabolized by cytochrome $P_{450}IID_6$ may require lower than usual doses prescribed for either drug). Products include:

Desyrel and Desyrel Dividose	504

(▣ Described in PDR For Nonprescription Drugs)   (⊙ Described in PDR For Ophthalmology)

Trifluoperazine Hydrochloride (Concomitant use of doxepin, a tricyclic antidepressant, with other drugs metabolized by cytochrome $P_{450}IID_6$ may require lower than usual doses prescribed for either drug). Products include:
Stelazine 2692

Trimipramine Maleate (Concomitant use of doxepin, a tricyclic antidepressant, with other drugs metabolized by cytochrome $P_{450}IID_6$ may require lower than usual doses prescribed for either drug). Products include:
Surmontil Capsules 2917

Venlafaxine Hydrochloride (Concomitant use of doxepin, a tricyclic antidepressant, with other drugs metabolized by cytochrome $P_{450}IID_6$ may require lower than usual doses prescribed for either drug). Products include:
Effexor 2825

Food Interactions
Alcohol (Alcohol ingestion may exacerbate the potential sedative effects of Zonalon Cream).

ZOSTRIX CREAM
(Capsaicin) 1043
None cited in PDR database.

ZOSTRIX-HP CREAM
(Capsaicin) 1043
None cited in PDR database.

ZOSYN
(Piperacillin Sodium, Tazobactam Sodium) 1463
May interact with aminoglycosides, anticoagulants, nondepolarizing neuromuscular blocking agents, and certain other agents. Compounds in these categories include:

Amikacin Sulfate (The mixing of Zosyn with an aminoglycoside *in vitro* can result in substantial inactivation due to penicillin-aminoglycoside complex; this complex is microbiologically inactive and of unknown toxicity). Products include:
Amikacin Sulfate Injection, USP 523
Amikacin Sulfate Injection, USP 981
Amikin Injectable 502

Atracurium Besylate (Due to similar mechanism of action as vecuronium, it is expected that the neuromuscular blockade produced by other non-depolarizing muscle relaxants could be prolonged in the presence of piperacillin). Products include:
Tracrium Injection 1155

Cisatracurium Besylate (Due to similar mechanism of action as vecuronium, it is expected that the neuromuscular blockade produced by other non-depolarizing muscle relaxants could be prolonged in the presence of piperacillin). Products include:
Nimbex Injection 1131

Dalteparin Sodium (Coagulation parameters should be tested more frequently and monitored regularly during simultaneous administration; effect of concurrent use is not specified). Products include:
Fragmin Injection 2088

Dicumarol (Coagulation parameters should be tested more frequently and monitored regularly during simultaneous administration; effect of concurrent use is not specified).
No products indexed under this heading.

Enoxaparin (Coagulation parameters should be tested more frequently and monitored regularly during simultaneous administration; effect of concurrent use is not specified). Products include:
Lovenox Injection 2187

Gentamicin Sulfate (The mixing of Zosyn with an aminoglycoside *in vitro* can result in substantial inactivation due to penicillin-aminoglycoside complex; this complex is microbiologically inactive and of unknown toxicity). Products include:
Garamycin Cream 0.1% 2501
Garamycin Injectable 2502
Garamycin Ointment 0.1% 2501
Garamycin Ophthalmic 2501
Genoptic Sterile Ophthalmic Solution .... ◎ 241
Genoptic Sterile Ophthalmic Ointment .... ◎ 241
Gentak .... ◎ 209
Pred-G Liquifilm Sterile Ophthalmic Suspension .... ◎ 248
Pred-G S.O.P. Sterile Ophthalmic Ointment .... ◎ 249

Heparin Calcium (Coagulation parameters should be tested more frequently and monitored regularly during simultaneous administration; effect of concurrent use is not specified).
No products indexed under this heading.

Heparin Sodium (Coagulation parameters should be tested more frequently and monitored regularly during simultaneous administration; effect of concurrent use is not specified). Products include:
Heparin Lock Flush Solution 2831
Heparin Sodium Injection 2832
Heparin Sodium Vials 1486

Kanamycin Sulfate (The mixing of Zosyn with an aminoglycoside *in vitro* can result in substantial inactivation due to penicillin-aminoglycoside complex; this complex is microbiologically inactive and of unknown toxicity).
No products indexed under this heading.

Metocurine Iodide (Due to similar mechanism of action as vecuronium, it is expected that the neuromuscular blockade produced by other non-depolarizing muscle relaxants could be prolonged in the presence of piperacillin). Products include:
Metubine Iodide Vials 932

Mivacurium Chloride (Due to similar mechanism of action as vecuronium, it is expected that the neuromuscular blockade produced by other non-depolarizing muscle relaxants could be prolonged in the presence of piperacillin). Products include:
Mivacron 1125

Pancuronium Bromide (Due to similar mechanism of action as vecuronium, it is expected that the neuromuscular blockade produced by other non-depolarizing muscle relaxants could be prolonged in the presence of piperacillin).
No products indexed under this heading.

Probenecid (Concomitant administration prolongs half-life of piperacillin by 21% and of tazobactam by 71%). Products include:
Benemid Tablets 1651
ColBENEMID Tablets 1662

Rocuronium Bromide (Due to similar mechanism of action as vecuronium, it is expected that the neuromuscular blockade produced by other non-depolarizing muscle relaxants could be prolonged in the presence of piperacillin). Products include:
Zemuron Injection 1885

Streptomycin Sulfate (The mixing of Zosyn with an aminoglycoside *in vitro* can result in substantial inactivation due to penicillin-aminoglycoside complex; this complex is microbiologically inactive and of unknown toxicity). Products include:
Streptomycin Sulfate Injection 2031

Tobramycin (The mixing of Zosyn with an aminoglycoside *in vitro* can result in substantial inactivation due to penicillin-aminoglycoside complex; this complex is microbiologically inactive and of unknown toxicity). Products include:
AKTOB .... ◎ 207
TobraDex Ophthalmic Suspension and Ointment 469
Tobrex Ophthalmic Ointment and Solution .... ◎ 226

Tobramycin Sulfate (Co-administration has resulted in the alteration of tobramycin pharmacokinetics which may be due to *in vitro* and *in vivo* inactivation of tobramycin). Products include:
Nebcin Vials, Hyporets & ADD-Vantage 1518

Vecuronium Bromide (Co-administration of piperacillin and vecuronium has been implicated in the prolongation of the neuromuscular blockade). Products include:
Norcuron for Injection 1875

Warfarin Sodium (Coagulation parameters should be tested more frequently and monitored regularly during simultaneous administration; effect of concurrent use is not specified). Products include:
Coumadin 941

ZOVIRAX CAPSULES
(Acyclovir) 1187
May interact with:

Nephrotoxic Drugs (Increased risk of renal dysfunction).

Probenecid (Increases mean half-life and the AUC when co-administered with intravenous acyclovir). Products include:
Benemid Tablets 1651
ColBENEMID Tablets 1662

ZOVIRAX OINTMENT 5%
(Acyclovir) 1190
None cited in PDR database.

ZOVIRAX STERILE POWDER
(Acyclovir Sodium) 1191
May interact with cytotoxic drugs and certain other agents. Compounds in these categories include:

Bleomycin Sulfate (Use with caution in patients who have manifested prior neurologic reactions to cytotoxic drugs). Products include:
Blenoxane 697

Daunorubicin Hydrochloride (Use with caution in patients who have manifested prior neurologic reactions to cytotoxic drugs). Products include:
Cerubidine for Injection 634

Doxorubicin Hydrochloride (Use with caution in patients who have manifested prior neurologic reactions to cytotoxic drugs). Products include:
Adriamycin PFS 2056
Adriamycin RDF 2056
Doxil 2613
Doxorubicin Astra 531
Rubex for Injection 721

Fluorouracil (Use with caution in patients who have manifested prior neurologic reactions to cytotoxic drugs). Products include:
Efudex 2280
Fluoroplex Topical Solution & Cream 1% 475
Fluorouracil Injection 2282

Hydroxyurea (Use with caution in patients who have manifested prior neurologic reactions to cytotoxic drugs). Products include:
Hydrea Capsules 705

Interferon alfa-2A, Recombinant (Concomitant administration requires caution). Products include:
Roferon-A Injection 2308

Interferon alfa-2B, Recombinant (Concomitant administration requires caution). Products include:
Intron A for Injection 2506

Methotrexate Sodium (Use with caution in patients who have manifested prior neurologic reactions to cytotoxic drugs; use with caution in patients receiving intrathecal methotrexate). Products include:
Methotrexate Sodium Tablets, Injection, for Injection and LPF Injection 1322

Mitotane (Use with caution in patients who have manifested prior neurologic reactions to cytotoxic drugs). Products include:
Lysodren Tablets 707

Mitoxantrone Hydrochloride (Use with caution in patients who have manifested prior neurologic reactions to cytotoxic drugs). Products include:
Novantrone for Injection 1327

Probenecid (Increases mean half-life of Zovirax). Products include:
Benemid Tablets 1651
ColBENEMID Tablets 1662

Procarbazine Hydrochloride (Use with caution in patients who have manifested prior neurologic reactions to cytotoxic drugs). Products include:
Matulane Capsules 2300

Tamoxifen Citrate (Use with caution in patients who have manifested prior neurologic reactions to cytotoxic drugs). Products include:
Nolvadex Tablets 2957

Vincristine Sulfate (Use with caution in patients who have manifested prior neurologic reactions to cytotoxic drugs). Products include:
Oncovin Solution Vials & Hyporets 1521

ZOVIRAX SUSPENSION
(Acyclovir) 1187
See Zovirax Capsules

ZOVIRAX TABLETS
(Acyclovir) 1187
See Zovirax Capsules

IMPORTANT NOTE: Always consult each drug listing in the patient's regimen for possible interactions.

ZYDONE CAPSULES
(Hydrocodone Bitartrate, Acetaminophen) 967
May interact with narcotic analgesics, antipsychotic agents, tranquilizers, central nervous system depressants, monoamine oxidase inhibitors, tricyclic antidepressants, anticholinergics, phenothiazines, and certain other agents. Compounds in these categories include:

Alfentanil Hydrochloride (Additive CNS depression). Products include:
Alfenta Injection 1334

Alprazolam (Additive CNS depression). Products include:
Xanax Tablets 2115

Amitriptyline Hydrochloride (Increased effect of either drug). Products include:
Elavil 2945
Etrafon 2495
Limbitrol 2333
Triavil Tablets 1800

Amoxapine (Increased effect of either drug). Products include:
Asendin Tablets 1419

Aprobarbital (Additive CNS depression).
No products indexed under this heading.

Atropine Sulfate (May produce paralytic). Products include:
Arco-Lase Plus Tablets 513
Atrohist Plus Tablets 1605
Donnatal 2234
Donnatal Extentabs 2234
Donnatal Tablets 2234
Lomotil 2591
Motofen Tablets 789
Urised Tablets 2123

Belladonna Alkaloids (May produce paralytic ileus). Products include:
Bellergal-S Tablets 2375
Hyland's Bedwetting Tablets ▣ 788
Hyland's EnurAid Tablets ...... ▣ 789
Hyland's Headache Tablets .... ▣ 790
Hyland's Teething Tablets ..... ▣ 790
Similasan Eye Drops #1 .... ▣ 769

Benztropine Mesylate (May produce paralytic ileus). Products include:
Cogentin 1661

Biperiden Hydrochloride (May produce paralytic ileus). Products include:
Akineton 1380

Buprenorphine (Additive CNS depression). Products include:
Buprenex Injectable 2170

Buspirone Hydrochloride (Additive CNS depression). Products include:
BuSpar Tablets 738

Butabarbital (Additive CNS depression).
No products indexed under this heading.

Butalbital (Additive CNS depression). Products include:
Axocet Capsules 2469
Esgic-plus Capsules 1012
Esgic-plus Tablets 1012
Fioricet Tablets 2386
Fioricet with Codeine Capsules 2387
Fiorinal Capsules 2388
Fiorinal with Codeine Capsules 2390
Fiorinal Tablets 2388
Phrenilin 790
Sedapap Tablets 50 mg/650 mg .. 1826

Chlordiazepoxide (Additive CNS depression). Products include:
Limbitrol 2333

Chlordiazepoxide Hydrochloride (Additive CNS depression). Products include:
Librax Capsules 2330
Librium Capsules 2331
Librium Injectable 2332

Chlorpromazine (Reduction or increase in amount of narcotic needed for pain relief; additive CNS depression). Products include:
Thorazine Suppositories 2701

Chlorpromazine Hydrochloride (Reduction or increase in amount of narcotic needed for pain relief; additive CNS depression). Products include:
Thorazine 2701

Chlorprothixene (Additive CNS depression).
No products indexed under this heading.

Chlorprothixene Hydrochloride (Additive CNS depression).
No products indexed under this heading.

Chlorprothixene Lactate (Additive CNS depression).
No products indexed under this heading.

Clidinium Bromide (May produce paralytic ileus). Products include:
Librax Capsules 2330

Clomipramine Hydrochloride (Increased effect of either drug). Products include:
Anafranil Capsules 819

Clorazepate Dipotassium (Additive CNS depression). Products include:
Tranxene 459

Clozapine (Additive CNS depression). Products include:
Clozaril Tablets 2377

Codeine Phosphate (Additive CNS depression). Products include:
Brontex 2130
Dimetane-DC Cough Syrup 2232
Fioricet with Codeine Capsules 2387
Fiorinal with Codeine Capsules 2390
Nucofed 2225
Phenergan with Codeine 2883
Phenergan VC with Codeine . 2888
Robitussin A-C Syrup 2248
Robitussin-DAC Syrup 2249
Ryna .... ▣ 804
Soma Compound w/Codeine Tablets 2784
Tylenol with Codeine 1592

Desflurane (Additive CNS depression). Products include:
Suprane (desflurane, USP) 1865

Desipramine Hydrochloride (Increased effect of either drug). Products include:
Norpramin Tablets 1273

Dezocine (Additive CNS depression). Products include:
Dalgan Injection 529

Diazepam (Additive CNS depression). Products include:
Dizac (diazepam injectable emulsion) CIV 1862
Valium Injectable 2336
Valium Tablets 2335

Dicyclomine Hydrochloride (May produce paralytic ileus). Products include:
Bentyl 1246

Doxepin Hydrochloride (Increased effect of either drug). Products include:
Adapin Capsules 1542
Sinequan 2028
Zonalon Cream 1042

Droperidol (Additive CNS depression). Products include:
Inapsine Injection 462

Enflurane (Additive CNS depression).
No products indexed under this heading.

Estazolam (Additive CNS depression). Products include:
ProSom Tablets 457

Ethchlorvynol (Additive CNS depression). Products include:
Placidyl Capsules 456

Ethinamate (Additive CNS depression).
No products indexed under this heading.

Fentanyl (Additive CNS depression). Products include:
Duragesic Transdermal System 1336

Fentanyl Citrate (Additive CNS depression). Products include:
Sublimaze Injection 463

Fluphenazine Decanoate (Reduction or increase in amount of narcotic needed for pain relief; additive CNS depression). Products include:
Prolixin Decanoate 510

Fluphenazine Enanthate (Reduction or increase in amount of narcotic needed for pain relief; additive CNS depression). Products include:
Prolixin Enanthate 510

Fluphenazine Hydrochloride (Reduction or increase in amount of narcotic needed for pain relief; additive CNS depression). Products include:
Prolixin 510

Flurazepam Hydrochloride (Additive CNS depression). Products include:
Dalmane Capsules 2329

Furazolidone (Increased effect of either drug). Products include:
Furoxone 2221

Glutethimide (Additive CNS depression).
No products indexed under this heading.

Glycopyrrolate (May produce paralytic ileus). Products include:
Robinul Forte Tablets 2247
Robinul Injectable 2247
Robinul Tablets 2247

Haloperidol (Additive CNS depression). Products include:
Haldol Injection, Tablets and Concentrate 1585

Haloperidol Decanoate (Additive CNS depression). Products include:
Haldol Decanoate 1587

Hydrocodone Polistirex (Additive CNS depression). Products include:
Tussionex Pennkinetic Extended-Release Suspension 1624

Hydromorphone Hydrochloride (Additive CNS depression). Products include:
Dilaudid Ampules 1382
Dilaudid Cough Syrup 1383
Dilaudid-HP Injection 1384
Dilaudid-HP Lyophilized Powder 250 mg 1384
Dilaudid 1382
Dilaudid Oral Liquid 1386
Dilaudid 1382
Dilaudid Tablets - 8 mg. 1386

Hydroxyzine Hydrochloride (Additive CNS depression). Products include:
Atarax Tablets & Syrup 1992
Marax Tablets & DF Syrup 2015
Vistaril Intramuscular Solution 2042

Hyoscyamine (May produce paralytic ileus). Products include:
Cystospaz Tablets 2123
Urised Tablets 2123

Hyoscyamine Sulfate (May produce paralytic ileus). Products include:
Arco-Lase Plus Tablets 513
Atrohist Plus Tablets 1605
Cystospaz-M Capsules 2123
Donnatal 2234
Donnatal Extentabs 2234
Donnatal Tablets 2234
Kutrase Capsules 2546

Levsin/Levsinex/Levbid 2549

Imipramine Hydrochloride (Increased effect of either drug). Products include:
Tofranil Ampuls 873
Tofranil Tablets 875

Imipramine Pamoate (Increased effect of either drug). Products include:
Tofranil-PM Capsules 876

Ipratropium Bromide (May produce paralytic ileus). Products include:
Atrovent Inhalation Aerosol 674
Atrovent Inhalation Solution 675
Atrovent Nasal Spray 0.03% 676
Atrovent Nasal Spray 0.06% 678

Isocarboxazid (Increased effect of either drug).
No products indexed under this heading.

Isoflurane (Additive CNS depression).
No products indexed under this heading.

Ketamine Hydrochloride (Additive CNS depression).
No products indexed under this heading.

Levomethadyl Acetate Hydrochloride (Additive CNS depression). Products include:
Orlaam Oral Solution 2361

Levorphanol Tartrate (Additive CNS depression). Products include:
Levo-Dromoran 2297

Lithium Carbonate (Additive CNS depression). Products include:
Eskalith 2658
Lithium Carbonate Capsules & Tablets 2352
Lithonate/Lithotabs/Lithobid .. 2721

Lithium Citrate (Additive CNS depression).
No products indexed under this heading.

Lorazepam (Additive CNS depression). Products include:
Ativan Injection 2805
Ativan Tablets 2807

Loxapine Hydrochloride (Additive CNS depression). Products include:
Loxitane 1426

Loxapine Succinate (Additive CNS depression). Products include:
Loxitane Capsules 1426

Maprotiline Hydrochloride (Increased effect of either drug). Products include:
Ludiomil Tablets 861

Mepenzolate Bromide (May produce paralytic ileus).
No products indexed under this heading.

Meperidine Hydrochloride (Additive CNS depression). Products include:
Demerol 2438
Mepergan Injection 2859

Mephobarbital (Additive CNS depression). Products include:
Mebaral Tablets 2452

Meprobamate (Additive CNS depression). Products include:
Miltown Tablets 2780
PMB 200 and PMB 400 2890

Mesoridazine Besylate (Reduction or increase in amount of narcotic needed for pain relief; additive CNS depression). Products include:
Serentil 689

Methadone Hydrochloride (Additive CNS depression). Products include:
Methadone Hydrochloride Oral Concentrate 2356
Methadone Hydrochloride Oral Solution & Tablets 2357

(▣ Described in PDR For Nonprescription Drugs)   (⊚ Described in PDR For Ophthalmology)

Methohexital Sodium (Additive CNS depression).
No products indexed under this heading.

Methotrimeprazine (Reduction or increase in amount of narcotic needed for pain relief; additive CNS depression). Products include:
Levoprome 1321

Methoxyflurane (Additive CNS depression).
No products indexed under this heading.

Midazolam Hydrochloride (Additive CNS depression). Products include:
Versed Injection 2324

Molindone Hydrochloride (Additive CNS depression). Products include:
Moban Tablets and Concentrate 1036

Morphine Sulfate (Additive CNS depression). Products include:
Astramorph/PF Injection, USP (Preservative-Free) 526
Duramorph Injection 983
Infumorph 200 and Infumorph 500 Sterile Solutions............... 985
Kadian Capsules........................ 2948
MS Contin Tablets..................... 2149
MSIR 2152
Oramorph SR (Morphine Sulfate Sustained Release Tablets) 2359
RMS Suppositories CII 2766
Roxanol 2365

Nortriptyline Hydrochloride (Increased effect of either drug). Products include:
Pamelor 2409

Opium Alkaloids (Additive CNS depression).
No products indexed under this heading.

Oxazepam (Additive CNS depression). Products include:
Serax Capsules 2916
Serax Tablets 2916

Oxybutynin Chloride (May produce paralytic ileus). Products include:
Ditropan 1267

Oxycodone Hydrochloride (Additive CNS depression). Products include:
OxyContin Tablets 2163
OxyIR Capsules 2167
Percocet Tablets 955
Percodan Tablets 955
Percodan-Demi Tablets 956
Roxicodone Tablets, Oral Solution & Intensol (Oxycodone) 2366
Tylox Capsules 1593

Pentobarbital Sodium (Additive CNS depression). Products include:
Nembutal Sodium Capsules 440
Nembutal Sodium Solution 442
Nembutal Sodium Suppositories...... 444

Perphenazine (Reduction or increase in amount of narcotic needed for pain relief; additive CNS depression). Products include:
Etrafon 2495
Triavil Tablets 1800
Trilafon 2532

Phenelzine Sulfate (Increased effect of either drug). Products include:
Nardil 1977

Phenobarbital (Additive CNS depression). Products include:
Arco-Lase Plus Tablets 513
Bellergal-S Tablets 2375
Donnatal 2234
Donnatal Extentabs 2234
Donnatal Tablets 2234
Phenobarbital Elixir and Tablets .. 1523
Quadrinal Tablets 1398

Pimozide (Additive CNS depression). Products include:
Orap Tablets 1037

Prazepam (Additive CNS depression).
No products indexed under this heading.

Prochlorperazine (Reduction or increase in amount of narcotic needed for pain relief; additive CNS depression). Products include:
Compazine 2644

Procyclidine Hydrochloride (May produce paralytic ileus). Products include:
Kemadrin Tablets 1105

Promethazine Hydrochloride (Reduction or increase in amount of narcotic needed for pain relief; additive CNS depression). Products include:
Mepergan Injection 2859
Phenergan with Codeine 2883
Phenergan with Dextromethorphan 2885
Phenergan Injection 2880
Phenergan Suppositories 2882
Phenergan Syrup 2881
Phenergan Tablets 2882
Phenergan VC 2886
Phenergan VC with Codeine ... 2888

Propantheline Bromide (May produce paralytic ileus). Products include:
Pro-Banthine Tablets 2226

Propofol (Additive CNS depression). Products include:
Diprivan Injectable Emulsion .. 2939

Propoxyphene Hydrochloride (Additive CNS depression). Products include:
Darvon 1475
Wygesic Tablets 2930

Propoxyphene Napsylate (Additive CNS depression). Products include:
Darvon-N/Darvocet-N 1473

Protriptyline Hydrochloride (Increased effect of either drug). Products include:
Vivactil Tablets 1820

Quazepam (Additive CNS depression). Products include:
Doral Tablets 2773

Risperidone (Additive CNS depression). Products include:
Risperdal Tablets 1348

Scopolamine (May produce paralytic ileus). Products include:
Transderm Scōp Transdermal Therapeutic System 890

Scopolamine Hydrobromide (May produce paralytic ileus). Products include:
Atrohist Plus Tablets 1605
Donnatal 2234
Donnatal Extentabs 2234
Donnatal Tablets 2234

Secobarbital Sodium (Additive CNS depression). Products include:
Seconal Sodium Pulvules 1529

Selegiline Hydrochloride (Increased effect of either drug). Products include:
Eldepryl Capsules 2729

Sevoflurane (Additive CNS depression).
No products indexed under this heading.

Sufentanil Citrate (Additive CNS depression). Products include:
Sufenta Injection 1355

Temazepam (Additive CNS depression). Products include:
Restoril Capsules 2413

Thiamylal Sodium (Additive CNS depression).
No products indexed under this heading.

Thioridazine Hydrochloride (Reduction or increase in amount of narcotic needed for pain relief; additive CNS depression). Products include:
Mellaril 2398

Thiothixene (Additive CNS depression). Products include:
Navane Capsules and Concentrate 2018
Navane Intramuscular 2019

Tranylcypromine Sulfate (Increased effect of either drug). Products include:
Parnate Tablets 2679

Triazolam (Additive CNS depression). Products include:
Halcion Tablets 2093

Tridihexethyl Chloride (May produce paralytic ileus).
No products indexed under this heading.

Trifluoperazine Hydrochloride (Additive CNS depression). Products include:
Stelazine 2692

Trihexyphenidyl Hydrochloride (May produce paralytic ileus). Products include:
Artane...................................... 1418

Trimipramine Maleate (Increased effect of either drug). Products include:
Surmontil Capsules 2917

Zolpidem Tartrate (Additive CNS depression). Products include:
Ambien Tablets........................ 2559

Food Interactions
Alcohol (Additive CNS depression).

ZYLOPRIM TABLETS
(Allopurinol) 1194
May interact with antigout agents, thiazides, and certain other agents. Compounds in these categories include:

Amoxicillin Trihydrate (Increased frequency of skin rash). Products include:
Amoxil 2631
Augmentin 2637
Augmentin Tablets 2640

Ampicillin Sodium (Increased frequency of skin rash). Products include:
Unasyn 2035

Azathioprine (Enhanced therapeutic response). Products include:
Azathioprine Tablets 2349
Imuran 1103

Bendroflumethiazide (May enhance allopurinol toxicity).
No products indexed under this heading.

Chlorothiazide (May enhance allopurinol toxicity). Products include:
Aldoclor Tablets 1638
Diupres Tablets 1691
Diuril Oral 1694

Chlorothiazide Sodium (May enhance allopurinol toxicity). Products include:
Diuril Sodium Intravenous 1693

Chlorpropamide (Prolonged half-life). Products include:
Diabinese Tablets 2002

Cyclophosphamide (Enhanced bone marrow suppression). Products include:
Cytoxan 700

Cyclosporine (Rare reports indicate that cyclosporine levels may be increased during concomitant treatment with allopurinol). Products include:
Neoral 2405

Sandimmune 2416

Dicumarol (Prolonged half-life).
No products indexed under this heading.

Hydrochlorothiazide (May enhance allopurinol toxicity). Products include:
Aldactazide Tablets 2556
Aldoril Tablets 1644
Apresazide Capsules 824
Capozide Tablets 744
Dyazide Capsules 2653
Esidrix Tablets 839
Esimil Tablets 840
HydroDIURIL Tablets 1716
Hydropres Tablets 1718
Hyzaar Tablets 1720
Inderide Tablets 2838
Inderide LA Long Acting Capsules .. 2840
Lopressor HCT Tablets 850
Lotensin HCT Tablets 855
Moduretic Tablets 1748
Oretic Tablets 450
Prinzide Tablets 1780
Ser-Ap-Es Tablets 867
Timolide Tablets 1791
Vaseretic Tablets 1810
Zestoretic Tablets 2968
Ziac 1459

Hydroflumethiazide (May enhance allopurinol toxicity). Products include:
Diucardin Tablets 2824

Mercaptopurine (Enhanced therapeutic response). Products include:
Purinethol Tablets 1214

Methyclothiazide (May enhance allopurinol toxicity). Products include:
Enduron Tablets 424

Polythiazide (May enhance allopurinol toxicity). Products include:
Minizide Capsules 2016

Probenecid (Decreased excretion of oxypurines and increased excretion of urinary uric acid). Products include:
Benemid Tablets 1651
ColBENEMID Tablets 1662

Sulfinpyrazone (Decreased excretion of oxypurines and increased excretion of urinary uric acid). Products include:
Anturane 823

Tolbutamide (Metabolism of tolbutamide may be affected).
No products indexed under this heading.

ZYMASE CAPSULES
(Pancrelipase) 1889
None cited in PDR database.

ZYRTEC TABLETS
(Cetirizine Hydrochloride) 2053
May interact with central nervous system depressants, xanthine bronchodilators, and certain other agents. Compounds in these categories include:

Alfentanil Hydrochloride (Concurrent use may result in additional impairment of CNS performance and reduction in mental alertness). Products include:
Alfenta Injection 1334

Alprazolam (Concurrent use may result in additional impairment of CNS performance and reduction in mental alertness). Products include:
Xanax Tablets 2115

Aminophylline (Small decrease in the clearance of cetirizine caused by a larger dose, e.g., 400 mg dose of theophylline).
No products indexed under this heading.

IMPORTANT NOTE: Always consult each drug listing in the patient's regimen for possible interactions.

Aprobarbital (Concurrent use may result in additional impairment of CNS performance and reduction in mental alertness).
    No products indexed under this heading.

Buprenorphine (Concurrent use may result in additional impairment of CNS performance and reduction in mental alertness). Products include:
    Buprenex Injectable 2170

Buspirone Hydrochloride (Concurrent use may result in additional impairment of CNS performance and reduction in mental alertness). Products include:
    BuSpar Tablets 738

Butabarbital (Concurrent use may result in additional impairment of CNS performance and reduction in mental alertness).
    No products indexed under this heading.

Butalbital (Concurrent use may result in additional impairment of CNS performance and reduction in mental alertness). Products include:
    Axocet Capsules 2469
    Esgic-plus Capsules 1012
    Esgic-plus Tablets 1012
    Fioricet Tablets 2386
    Fioricet with Codeine Capsules ... 2387
    Fiorinal Capsules 2388
    Fiorinal with Codeine Capsules ... 2390
    Fiorinal Tablets 2388
    Phrenilin 790
    Sedapap Tablets 50 mg/650 mg .. 1826

Chlordiazepoxide (Concurrent use may result in additional impairment of CNS performance and reduction in mental alertness). Products include:
    Limbitrol 2333

Chlordiazepoxide Hydrochloride (Concurrent use may result in additional impairment of CNS performance and reduction in mental alertness). Products include:
    Librax Capsules 2330
    Librium Capsules 2331
    Librium Injectable 2332

Chlorpromazine (Concurrent use may result in additional impairment of CNS performance and reduction in mental alertness). Products include:
    Thorazine Suppositories 2701

Chlorpromazine Hydrochloride (Concurrent use may result in additional impairment of CNS performance and reduction in mental alertness). Products include:
    Thorazine 2701

Chlorprothixene (Concurrent use may result in additional impairment of CNS performance and reduction in mental alertness).
    No products indexed under this heading.

Chlorprothixene Hydrochloride (Concurrent use may result in additional impairment of CNS performance and reduction in mental alertness).
    No products indexed under this heading.

Chlorprothixene Lactate (Concurrent use may result in additional impairment of CNS performance and reduction in mental alertness).
    No products indexed under this heading.

Clorazepate Dipotassium (Concurrent use may result in additional impairment of CNS performance and reduction in mental alertness). Products include:
    Tranxene 459

Clozapine (Concurrent use may result in additional impairment of CNS performance and reduction in mental alertness). Products include:
    Clozaril Tablets 2377

Codeine Phosphate (Concurrent use may result in additional impairment of CNS performance and reduction in mental alertness). Products include:
    Brontex 2130
    Dimetane-DC Cough Syrup 2232
    Fioricet with Codeine Capsules .. 2387
    Fiorinal with Codeine Capsules .. 2390
    Nucofed 2225
    Phenergan with Codeine 2883
    Phenergan VC with Codeine 2888
    Robitussin A-C Syrup 2248
    Robitussin-DAC Syrup 2249
    Ryna .... ▣ 804
    Soma Compound w/Codeine Tablets 2784
    Tylenol with Codeine 1592

Desflurane (Concurrent use may result in additional impairment of CNS performance and reduction in mental alertness). Products include:
    Suprane (desflurane, USP) 1865

Dezocine (Concurrent use may result in additional impairment of CNS performance and reduction in mental alertness). Products include:
    Dalgan Injection 529

Diazepam (Concurrent use may result in additional impairment of CNS performance and reduction in mental alertness). Products include:
    Dizac (diazepam injectable emulsion) CIV 1862
    Valium Injectable 2336
    Valium Tablets 2335

Droperidol (Concurrent use may result in additional impairment of CNS performance and reduction in mental alertness). Products include:
    Inapsine Injection 462

Dyphylline (Small decrease in the clearance of cetirizine caused by a larger dose, e.g., 400 mg dose of theophylline). Products include:
    Lufyllin & Lufyllin-400 Tablets ... 2778
    Lufyllin-GG Elixir & Tablets 2779

Enflurane (Concurrent use may result in additional impairment of CNS performance and reduction in mental alertness).
    No products indexed under this heading.

Estazolam (Concurrent use may result in additional impairment of CNS performance and reduction in mental alertness). Products include:
    ProSom Tablets 457

Ethchlorvynol (Concurrent use may result in additional impairment of CNS performance and reduction in mental alertness). Products include:
    Placidyl Capsules 456

Ethinamate (Concurrent use may result in additional impairment of CNS performance and reduction in mental alertness).
    No products indexed under this heading.

Fentanyl (Concurrent use may result in additional impairment of CNS performance and reduction in mental alertness). Products include:
    Duragesic Transdermal System ... 1336

Fentanyl Citrate (Concurrent use may result in additional impairment of CNS performance and reduction in mental alertness). Products include:
    Sublimaze Injection 463

Fluphenazine Decanoate (Concurrent use may result in additional impairment of CNS performance and reduction in mental alertness). Products include:
    Prolixin Decanoate 510

Fluphenazine Enanthate (Concurrent use may result in additional impairment of CNS performance and reduction in mental alertness). Products include:
    Prolixin Enanthate 510

Fluphenazine Hydrochloride (Concurrent use may result in additional impairment of CNS performance and reduction in mental alertness). Products include:
    Prolixin 510

Flurazepam Hydrochloride (Concurrent use may result in additional impairment of CNS performance and reduction in mental alertness). Products include:
    Dalmane Capsules 2329

Glutethimide (Concurrent use may result in additional impairment of CNS performance and reduction in mental alertness).
    No products indexed under this heading.

Haloperidol (Concurrent use may result in additional impairment of CNS performance and reduction in mental alertness). Products include:
    Haldol Injection, Tablets and Concentrate 1585

Haloperidol Decanoate (Concurrent use may result in additional impairment of CNS performance and reduction in mental alertness). Products include:
    Haldol Decanoate 1587

Hydrocodone Bitartrate (Concurrent use may result in additional impairment of CNS performance and reduction in mental alertness). Products include:
    Codiclear DH Syrup 808
    Duratuss HD Elixir 2750
    Histussin D Liquid 670
    Hycodan Tablets and Syrup 946
    Hycomine Compound Tablets ... 948
    Hycomine 947
    Hycotuss Expectorant Syrup 950
    Hydrocet Capsules 787
    Lorcet 10/650 Tablets 1016
    Lortab 2751
    Tussend 1830
    Tussend Expectorant 1831
    Vicodin Tablets 1404
    Vicodin ES Tablets 1405
    Vicodin HP Tablets 1403
    Vicodin Tuss Expectorant 1406
    Zydone Capsules 967

Hydrocodone Polistirex (Concurrent use may result in additional impairment of CNS performance and reduction in mental alertness). Products include:
    Tussionex Pennkinetic Extended-Release Suspension 1624

Hydroxyzine Hydrochloride (Concurrent use may result in additional impairment of CNS performance and reduction in mental alertness). Products include:
    Atarax Tablets & Syrup 1992
    Marax Tablets & DF Syrup 2015
    Vistaril Intramuscular Solution ... 2042

Isoflurane (Concurrent use may result in additional impairment of CNS performance and reduction in mental alertness).
    No products indexed under this heading.

Ketamine Hydrochloride (Concurrent use may result in additional impairment of CNS performance and reduction in mental alertness).
    No products indexed under this heading.

Levomethadyl Acetate Hydrochloride (Concurrent use may result in additional impairment of CNS performance and reduction in mental alertness). Products include:
    Orlaam Oral Solution 2361

Levorphanol Tartrate (Concurrent use may result in additional impairment of CNS performance and reduction in mental alertness). Products include:
    Levo-Dromoran 2297

Lorazepam (Concurrent use may result in additional impairment of CNS performance and reduction in mental alertness). Products include:
    Ativan Injection 2805
    Ativan Tablets 2807

Loxapine Hydrochloride (Concurrent use may result in additional impairment of CNS performance and reduction in mental alertness). Products include:
    Loxitane 1426

Loxapine Succinate (Concurrent use may result in additional impairment of CNS performance and reduction in mental alertness). Products include:
    Loxitane Capsules 1426

Meperidine Hydrochloride (Concurrent use may result in additional impairment of CNS performance and reduction in mental alertness). Products include:
    Demerol 2438
    Mepergan Injection 2859

Mephobarbital (Concurrent use may result in additional impairment of CNS performance and reduction in mental alertness). Products include:
    Mebaral Tablets 2452

Meprobamate (Concurrent use may result in additional impairment of CNS performance and reduction in mental alertness). Products include:
    Miltown Tablets 2780
    PMB 200 and PMB 400 2890

Mesoridazine Besylate (Concurrent use may result in additional impairment of CNS performance and reduction in mental alertness). Products include:
    Serentil 689

Methadone Hydrochloride (Concurrent use may result in additional impairment of CNS performance and reduction in mental alertness). Products include:
    Methadone Hydrochloride Oral Concentrate 2356
    Methadone Hydrochloride Oral Solution & Tablets 2357

Methohexital Sodium (Concurrent use may result in additional impairment of CNS performance and reduction in mental alertness).
    No products indexed under this heading.

Methotrimeprazine (Concurrent use may result in additional impairment of CNS performance and reduction in mental alertness). Products include:
    Levoprome 1321

(▣ Described in PDR For Nonprescription Drugs) (◉ Described in PDR For Ophthalmology)

Interactions Index

Methoxyflurane (Concurrent use may result in additional impairment of CNS performance and reduction in mental alertness).
No products indexed under this heading.

Midazolam Hydrochloride (Concurrent use may result in additional impairment of CNS performance and reduction in mental alertness). Products include:
Versed Injection 2324

Molindone Hydrochloride (Concurrent use may result in additional impairment of CNS performance and reduction in mental alertness). Products include:
Moban Tablets and Concentrate 1036

Morphine Sulfate (Concurrent use may result in additional impairment of CNS performance and reduction in mental alertness). Products include:
Astramorph/PF Injection, USP (Preservative-Free) 526
Duramorph Injection 983
Infumorph 200 and Infumorph 500 Sterile Solutions 985
Kadian Capsules 2948
MS Contin Tablets 2149
MSIR 2152
Oramorph SR (Morphine Sulfate Sustained Release Tablets) 2359
RMS Suppositories CII 2766
Roxanol 2365

Opium Alkaloids (Concurrent use may result in additional impairment of CNS performance and reduction in mental alertness).
No products indexed under this heading.

Oxazepam (Concurrent use may result in additional impairment of CNS performance and reduction in mental alertness). Products include:
Serax Capsules 2916
Serax Tablets 2916

Oxycodone Hydrochloride (Concurrent use may result in additional impairment of CNS performance and reduction in mental alertness). Products include:
OxyContin Tablets 2163
OxyIR Capsules 2167
Percocet Tablets 955
Percodan Tablets 955
Percodan-Demi Tablets 956
Roxicodone Tablets, Oral Solution & Intensol (Oxycodone) 2366
Tylox Capsules 1593

Pentobarbital Sodium (Concurrent use may result in additional impairment of CNS performance and reduction in mental alertness). Products include:
Nembutal Sodium Capsules 440
Nembutal Sodium Solution 442
Nembutal Sodium Suppositories 444

Perphenazine (Concurrent use may result in additional impairment of CNS performance and reduction in mental alertness). Products include:
Etrafon 2495
Triavil Tablets 1800
Trilafon 2532

Phenobarbital (Concurrent use may result in additional impairment of CNS performance and reduction in mental alertness). Products include:
Arco-Lase Plus Tablets 513
Bellergal-S Tablets 2375
Donnatal 2234
Donnatal Extentabs 2234
Donnatal Tablets 2234
Phenobarbital Elixir and Tablets 1523
Quadrinal Tablets 1398

Prazepam (Concurrent use may result in additional impairment of CNS performance and reduction in mental alertness).
No products indexed under this heading.

Prochlorperazine (Concurrent use may result in additional impairment of CNS performance and reduction in mental alertness). Products include:
Compazine 2644

Promethazine Hydrochloride (Concurrent use may result in additional impairment of CNS performance and reduction in mental alertness). Products include:
Mepergan Injection 2859
Phenergan with Codeine 2883
Phenergan with Dextromethorphan ... 2885
Phenergan Injection 2880
Phenergan Suppositories 2882
Phenergan Syrup 2881
Phenergan Tablets 2882
Phenergan VC 2886
Phenergan VC with Codeine 2888

Propofol (Concurrent use may result in additional impairment of CNS performance and reduction in mental alertness). Products include:
Diprivan Injectable Emulsion 2939

Propoxyphene Hydrochloride (Concurrent use may result in additional impairment of CNS performance and reduction in mental alertness). Products include:
Darvon 1475
Wygesic Tablets 2930

Propoxyphene Napsylate (Concurrent use may result in additional impairment of CNS performance and reduction in mental alertness). Products include:
Darvon-N/Darvocet-N 1473

Quazepam (Concurrent use may result in additional impairment of CNS performance and reduction in mental alertness). Products include:
Doral Tablets 2773

Risperidone (Concurrent use may result in additional impairment of CNS performance and reduction in mental alertness). Products include:
Risperdal Tablets 1348

Secobarbital Sodium (Concurrent use may result in additional impairment of CNS performance and reduction in mental alertness). Products include:
Seconal Sodium Pulvules 1529

Sevoflurane (Concurrent use may result in additional impairment of CNS performance and reduction in mental alertness).
No products indexed under this heading.

Sufentanil Citrate (Concurrent use may result in additional impairment of CNS performance and reduction in mental alertness). Products include:
Sufenta Injection 1355

Temazepam (Concurrent use may result in additional impairment of CNS performance and reduction in mental alertness). Products include:
Restoril Capsules 2413

Theophylline (Small decrease in the clearance of cetirizine caused by a larger dose, e.g., 400 mg dose of theophylline). Products include:
Marax Tablets & DF Syrup 2015
Quibron 2227

Theophylline Anhydrous (Small decrease in the clearance of cetirizine caused by a larger dose, e.g., 400 mg dose of theophylline). Products include:
Aerolate 1003
Primatene Tablets 844
Respbid Tablets 687
Slo-bid Gyrocaps 2201
Theo-24 Extended Release Capsules 2753
Theo-Dur Extended-Release Tablets 1367
Theo-X Extended-Release Tablets .. 793
Uni-Dur Extended-Release Tablets .. 1374
Uniphyl 400 mg and 600 mg Tablets 2157

Theophylline Calcium Salicylate (Small decrease in the clearance of cetirizine caused by a larger dose, e.g., 400 mg dose of theophylline). Products include:
Quadrinal Tablets 1398

Theophylline Sodium Glycinate (Small decrease in the clearance of cetirizine caused by a larger dose, e.g., 400 mg dose of theophylline).
No products indexed under this heading.

Thiamylal Sodium (Concurrent use may result in additional impairment of CNS performance and reduction in mental alertness).
No products indexed under this heading.

Thioridazine Hydrochloride (Concurrent use may result in additional impairment of CNS performance and reduction in mental alertness). Products include:
Mellaril 2398

Thiothixene (Concurrent use may result in additional impairment of CNS performance and reduction in mental alertness). Products include:
Navane Capsules and Concentrate 2018
Navane Intramuscular 2019

Triazolam (Concurrent use may result in additional impairment of CNS performance and reduction in mental alertness). Products include:
Halcion Tablets 2093

Trifluoperazine Hydrochloride (Concurrent use may result in additional impairment of CNS performance and reduction in mental alertness). Products include:
Stelazine 2692

Zolpidem Tartrate (Concurrent use may result in additional impairment of CNS performance and reduction in mental alertness). Products include:
Ambien Tablets 2559

Food Interactions

Alcohol (Concurrent use may result in additional impairment of CNS performance and reduction in mental alertness).

Food, unspecified (Food has no effect on the extent of cetirizine absorption, but T_{max} may be delayed and C_{max} may be decreased in the presence of food).

IMPORTANT NOTE: Always consult each drug listing in the patient's regimen for possible interactions.

SECTION 2

FOOD INTERACTIONS CROSS-REFERENCE

In this section, drug/food and drug/alcohol interactions listed in the preceding index are cross-referenced by dietary item. Under each entry is an alphabetical list, by brand name, of drugs said to interact with the item. A brief description of the interaction follows each brand, along with the page number of the underlying text. Page numbers refer to the 1997 editions of PDR and PDR For Ophthalmology and the 1996 edition of PDR For Nonprescription Drugs, which is published later each year. A key to the symbols denoting the companion volumes appears in the bottom margin.

Entries in this section are limited to drug/food and drug/alcohol interactions cited in official prescribing information as published by PDR.

Alcohol

Actifed Allergy Daytime/Nighttime Caplets (May increase drowsiness effect) 808
Actifed Cold & Allergy Tablets (May increase drowsiness effect) 807
Actifed Cold & Sinus Caplets and Tablets (May increase drowsiness effect) 808
Actifed Sinus Daytime/Nighttime Tablets and Caplets (May increase drowsiness effect) 809
Actron Caplets and Tablets (Patients consuming 3 or more alcohol-containing drinks per day should consult their physician for advice on when and how they should take Actron) 608
Adapin Capsules (Doxepin may potentiate the CNS depressant effects of alcohol) 1542
Adipex-P Tablets and Capsules (May result in adverse drug interaction) 1035
Aldoclor Tablets (Aggravates orthostatic hypotension) 1638
Aldoril Tablets (Aggravates orthostatic hypotension) 1644
Aleve (Concurrent use should be undertaken with the physician's consultation) 2124
Alka-Seltzer Plus Cold & Cough Medicine (May increase drowsiness effect) 611
Alka-Seltzer Plus Flu & Body Aches Effervescent Tablets (May increase drowsiness effect) 612
Alka-Seltzer Plus Night-Time Cold Medicine Liqui-Gels (May increase drowsiness effect) 612

Allerest Maximum Strength (May increase drowsiness) 649
Ambien Tablets (Co-administration produces additive effects on psychomotor performance) 2559
Anafranil Capsules (Co-administration may exaggerate patient's response to alcohol) 819
Antabuse Tablets (Antabuse plus alcohol, even small amounts, produces flushing, throbbing in head and neck, respiratory difficulty, headache and other serious reactions including convulsions and death; concurrent use is contraindicated) 2802
Antivert, Antivert/25 Tablets, & Antivert/50 Tablets (Concurrent use should be avoided) 1992
Apresazide Capsules (May potentiate orthostatic hypotension) 824
Asendin Tablets (Enhanced response to alcohol) 1419
Astramorph/PF Injection, USP (Preservative-Free) (Potentiation of depressant effects of morphine) 526
Atarax Tablets & Syrup (Increased effect of alcohol) 1992
Ativan Injection (Additive CNS depressant effects) 2805
Ativan Tablets (Diminished tolerance for alcohol when used concurrently; potential for increased CNS-depressant effects) 2807
Atrohist Pediatric Capsules (Potential for additive effects) 1603
Atrohist Pediatric Suspension (Potential for additive central nervous system effects) 1604

Atrohist Pediatric Suspension Dye-Free (Potential for additive central nervous system effects) 1604
Atrohist Plus Tablets (Possible additive drowsiness effects) 1605
Axocet Capsules (Concurrent use may cause increased CNS depression) 2469
BC Cold Powder Multi-Symptom Formula (Cold-Sinus-Allergy) (Concurrent use not recommended; consult your doctor) 631
Extra Strength Bayer PM Aspirin Plus Sleep Aid (Avoid concurrent use) 617
Bellergal-S Tablets (Combined use may result in a potentiation of the depressant action) 2375
Benadryl Allergy Chewables (May increase drowsiness effect) 811
Benadryl Allergy/Cold Tablets (May increase drowsiness effect) 811
Benadryl Allergy Decongestant Liquid Medication (May increase drowsiness effect; avoid concurrent use) 812
Benadryl Allergy Decongestant Tablets (Increases the drowsiness effect; avoid concomitant use) 812
Benadryl Allergy Liquid Medication (Increases drowsiness effect) 813
Benadryl Allergy Kapseals (May increase drowsiness effect) 811
Benadryl Allergy Sinus Headache Caplets (May increase drowsiness effect) 813
Benadryl Dye-Free Allergy Liqui-gel Softgels (May increase the drowsiness effect) 813

Benadryl Dye-Free Allergy Liquid Medication (May increase the drowsiness effect) 814
Benadryl Parenteral (Additive effects) 1955
Bonine Tablets (May increase drowsiness effect) 1990
Bromfed Capsules (Extended-Release) (Additive effects) 1832
Bromfed Syrup (May increase drowsiness effect) 712
Bromfed-DM Cough Syrup (Potential for additive effects) 1832
Brontex Tablets (Potential for greater sedation) 2130
Buprenex Injectable (Increased CNS depression) 2170
BuSpar Tablets (Concomitant use should be avoided) 738
Butisol Sodium Elixir & Tablets (Concurrent use may produce additive CNS depressant effects) 2768
Capozide Tablets (Potentation of orthostatic hypotension) 744
Catapres Tablets (Clonidine may potentiate the CNS-depressive effects) 679
Catapres-TTS (Clonidine may potentiate the CNS-depressive effects) 680
Cefobid Intravenous/Intramuscular (When ingested within 72 hours, flushing, sweating, headache, and tachycardia have been reported) 1996
Cefobid Pharmacy Bulk Package - Not for Direct Infusion (A disulfiram-like reaction characterized by flushing, sweating, headache, and tachycardia has been reported when alcohol was ingested within

(■ Described in PDR For Nonprescription Drugs)   (◉ Described in PDR For Ophthalmology)

Alcohol **Food Interactions Cross-Reference** 1234

72 hours after Cefobid administration) ... 1999
Cefotan for Injection (When ingested within 72 hours after Cefotan administration may cause disulfiram-like reactions, including flushing, headache, sweating and tachycardia) ... 2936
Cerebyx Injection (Acute alcohol intake may increase plasma phenytoin concentration; chronic alcohol abuse may decrease plasma phenytoin concentration) 1956
Cerose DM (May increase drowsiness effect) ... ▣ 853
Children's Vicks DayQuil Allergy Relief (May increase drowsiness effect) ... ▣ 730
Children's Vicks NyQuil Cold/Cough Relief (May increase drowsiness effect) ... ▣ 731
Chlor-Trimeton Allergy Decongestant Tablets (May increase drowsiness effect) ... ▣ 759
Chlor-Trimeton Allergy Tablets (Do not use concomitantly) ... ▣ 758
Cholestin Capsules (Concurrent use in patients consuming more than 3 drinks per day is not recommended) ... 2985
Clozaril Tablets (Caution is advised with concomitant use) ... 2377
Codiclear DH Syrup (Additive CNS depression) ... 808
Combipres Tablets (Orthostatic hypotension produced by chlorthalidone may be aggravated by alcohol; potential for enhanced CNS-depressive effects) ... 682
Compazine Tablets (Phenothiazines may intensify or prolong the action of other central nervous system depressants) ... 2644
Allergy-Sinus Comtrex Multi-Symptom Allergy-Sinus Formula Tablets and Caplets (Increases drowsiness effect) ... ▣ 639
Comtrex Multi-Symptom Cold Reliever Tablets and Caplets (May increase drowsiness effect) ... ▣ 638
Contac Continuous Action Nasal Decongestant/Antihistamine 12 Hour Capsules (May increase drowsiness effect; concurrent use should be avoided) ... ▣ 773
Contac Day & Night Cold/Flu Night Caplets (Increases drowsiness effect) ... ▣ 772
Contac Maximum Strength Continuous Action Decongestant/Antihistamine 12 Hour Caplets (May increase drowsiness effect; concurrent use should be avoided) ... ▣ 772
Contac Night Allergy/Sinus Caplets (May increase the drowsiness effect; avoid concurrent use) ... ▣ 771
Contac Severe Cold and Flu Formula Caplets (May increase drowsiness effect; concurrent use should be avoided) ... ▣ 773
Coricidin 'D' Decongestant Tablets (May increase drowsiness effect) ... ▣ 760
Coumadin Tablets (Decreased or increased prothrombin time response) ... 941
Covera-HS Tablets (Verapamil may increase blood alcohol concentrations and prolong its effect) ... 2573
Cytadren Tablets (Effects of alcohol potentiated) ... 837
D.A. Chewable Tablets (Potential for additive effects) ... 970
DHCplus Capsules (Potential for additive CNS depression) ... 2148
Dalgan Injection (Concomitant administration may have an additive effect) ... 529
Dalmane Capsules (Additive effects; potential for continuation of interaction after discontinuance of flurazepam) ... 2329
Darvocet-N 50 Tablets (Additive CNS depression) ... 1473
Darvon Compound-65 Pulvules (The CNS-depressant effect of propoxyphene is additive with that of other CNS depressants) ... 1475
Demerol Tablets (Concurrent use may result in respiratory depression, hypotension, and profound sedation or coma) ... 2438
Demser Capsules (Additive sedative effects) ... 1690
Depakene Capsules (Depakene may potentiate CNS depressant activity) ... 416
Depakote Tablets (Co-administration may result in additive CNS depression) ... 418
Deponit NTG Transdermal Delivery System (Additive vasodilating effects) ... 2541
Desyrel and Desyrel Dividose (Enhanced response to alcohol) .. 504
DiaBeta Tablets (Potential for hypoglycemia) ... 1265
Diabinese Tablets (In some patients disulfiram-like reaction may be produced by the ingestion of alcohol) ... 2002
Dilantin Infatabs (Acute alcohol intake increases serum phenytoin levels; chronic alcohol intake decreases serum phenytoin levels) ... 1967
Dilantin Kapseals (Acute alcohol intake increases serum phenytoin levels; chronic alcohol intake decreases serum phenytoin levels) ... 1965
Dilantin-125 Suspension (Acute alcohol intake increases serum phenytoin levels; chronic alcohol intake decreases serum phenytoin levels) ... 1969
Dilatrate-SR Capsules (Alcohol has been found to exhibit additive vasodilating effects) ... 2542
Dilaudid Ampules (Additive CNS depression) ... 1382
Dilaudid Cough Syrup (Additive CNS depression) ... 1383
Dilaudid-HP Injection (Additive depressant effects) ... 1384
Dilaudid Oral Liquid (May exhibit an additive CNS depression) ... 1386
Dimetane-DC Cough Syrup (Antihistamines have additive effects with alcohol) ... 2232
Dimetane-DX Cough Syrup (Additive effect) ... 2233
Dimetapp Allergy Dye-Free Elixir (May increase drowsiness effect) ... ▣ 838
Dimetapp Allergy Sinus Caplets (May increase drowsiness effect) ... ▣ 838
Dimetapp Cold & Cough Liqui-Gels (May increase drowsiness effect) ... ▣ 839
Dimetapp Cold & Fever Suspension (May increase drowsiness effect) ... ▣ 839
Dimetapp DM Elixir (Increases drowsiness effect; avoid concurrent use) ... ▣ 840
Dimetapp Elixir (May increase drowsiness effect) ... ▣ 840
Dimetapp Extentabs (May increase drowsiness effect) ... ▣ 841
Dimetapp Liqui-Gels (Increases drowsiness effect; avoid concurrent use) ... ▣ 841
Ditropan Tablets (Enhances the drowsiness effect) ... 1267
Diucardin Tablets (Thiazide-induced orthostatic hypotension may be potentiated) 2824
Diupres Tablets (Orthostatic hypotension may be aggravated) 1691
Diuril Oral Suspension (Potentiation of orthostatic hypotension may occur) ... 1694
Diuril Sodium Intravenous (Potentiation of orthostatic hypotension may occur) ... 1693
Dizac (diazepam injectable emulsion) CIV (Potentiates the action of diazepam; concomitant use increases depression with increased risk of apnea) ... 1862
Extra Strength Doan's P.M. (Avoid concomitant use) ... ▣ 653
Doral Tablets (Additive CNS depressant effects) ... 2773
Dramamine Tablets (May increase drowsiness effect) ... ▣ 801
Dramamine II Tablets (May increase drowsiness effect) ... ▣ 801
Drixoral Cold and Allergy Sustained-Action Tablets (May increase drowsiness effect) ... ▣ 763
Drixoral Cold and Flu Extended-Release Tablets (May increase drowsiness effect) ... ▣ 764
Drixoral Allergy/Sinus Extended Release Tablets (May increase the drowsiness effect) ... ▣ 765
Duragesic Transdermal System (May produce additive depressant effects) ... 1336
Duramorph Injection (Potentiation of depressant effect) ... 983
Dura-Tap/PD Capsules (Potential for additive effects) ... 970
Dura-Vent/DA Tablets (Potential for additive effects) ... 972
Duratuss HD Elixir (Potentiation of central nervous system effects) .. 2750
Easprin (Alcohol has a synergistic effect with aspirin in causing gastrointestinal bleeding) ... 1971
Effexor (Concurrent use should be avoided) ... 2825
Efidac 24 Chlorpheniramine (May increase drowsiness effect) ... ▣ 655
Elavil Injection (Co-administration results in enhanced response to alcohol) ... 2945
Enduron Tablets (Potentiates orthostatic hypotension) ... 424
Ergamisol Tablets (May result in ANTABUSE-like side effects) ... 1340
Esgic-plus Tablets (May exhibit additive CNS depressant effects) 1012
Esidrix Tablets (May potentiate orthostatic hypotension) ... 839
Esimil Tablets (Orthostatic hypotension aggravated) ... 840
Etrafon Tablets (2-25) (Amitriptyline may enhance the response to alcohol; potential for additive effects and hypotension; concurrent use should be avoided) ... 2495
Aspirin Free Excedrin Analgesic Caplets and Geltabs (Concurrent use should be undertaken with the physician's consultation) ... 734
Aspirin Free Excedrin Analgesic Caplets and Geltabs (Concurrent use should be undertaken with the physician's consultation) ... 734
Excedrin P.M. Analgesic/Sleeping Aid Tablets, Caplets, Liquigels (Concurrent use is not recommended; chronic users of alcohol, 3 or more drinks per day should consult their physician for advice before taking this product) ... 735
Fastin Capsules (Concomitant use may result in adverse drug interaction) ... 2662
Fedahist Gyrocaps (May have an additive CNS depressant effect) .. 2545
Fioricet Tablets (Additive CNS depressant effects) ... 2386
Fioricet with Codeine Capsules (Increased CNS depression) ... 2387
Fiorinal Capsules (Increased CNS depression) ... 2388
Fiorinal with Codeine Capsules (Increased CNS depression) ... 2390
Flagyl 375 Capsules (Alcohol should not be consumed during metronidazole therapy and for at least three days afterward because abdominal cramps, nausea, vomiting, headaches, and flushing may occur) ... 2587
Flagyl I.V. (Potential for abdominal cramps, nausea, vomiting, and headaches, and flushing) ... 2373
Flexeril Tablets (Concurrent use results in enhanced effects) ... 1701
Fulvicin P/G Tablets (Potentiation of effects of alcohol) ... 2499
Fulvicin P/G 165 & 330 Tablets (Potentiation of effects of alcohol) ... 2500
Furoxone Liquid (Possible disulfiram-like reaction may occur; alcohol intake should be avoided during or within four days after Furoxone therapy) ... 2221
Glucophage Tablets (Alcohol potentiates the effect of metfomrin on lactate metabolism; patients should be warned against excessive alcohol intake, acute or chronic) ... 754
Glucotrol Tablets (Co-administration with alcohol may result in hypoglycemia) ... 2011
Glucotrol XL Extended Release Tablets (Co-administration with alcohol may result in hypoglycemia) ... 2012
Gris-PEG Tablets, 125 mg & 250 mg (Griseofulvin potentiates the effects of alcohol, producing tachycardia and flushing) ... 476
Halcion Tablets (Additive CNS depressant effects) ... 2093
Haldol Decanoate 50 (50 mg/mL) Injection (CNS depressant potentiated) ... 1587
Haldol Injection, Tablets and Concentrate (CNS depressant potentiated) ... 1585
Helidac Therapy (Concurrent use has resulted in abdominal cramps, nausea, vomiting, headaches, and flushing; avoid alcoholic beverages concurrently and/or at least 1 day afterward) 2135
Histussin D Liquid (Co-administration may produce additive CNS depressant effects) 670
Humalog Injection (Co-administration with drugs with hypoglycemic activity may result in decreased insulin requirements) ... 1488
Hycodan Tablets and Syrup (Exhibits an additive CNS depression) ... 946
Hycomine Compound Tablets (Exhibits an additive CNS depression) ... 948
Hycotuss Expectorant Syrup (Exhibits an additive CNS depression) ... 950
Hydrocet Capsules (Additive CNS depression) ... 787
HydroDIURIL Tablets (Potentiation of orthostatic hypotension) ... 1716
Hydropres Tablets (Potentiation of orthostatic hypotension) ... 1718
Hylorel Tablets (Exaggerates postural hypotension) ... 1613
Hyzaar Tablets (Potentiation of orthostatic hypotension) ... 1720
Imdur (Additive vasodilating effects) ... 1362
Inderal Injectable (Slows the rate of absorption of propranolol) ... 2834
Inderal LA Long Acting Capsules (Absorption rate of propranolol slowed) ... 2836
Inderide Tablets (Slows the rate of absorption of propranolol) ... 2838
Inderide LA Long Acting Capsules (May aggravate orthostatic hypotension) ... 2840
Infumorph 200 and Infumorph 500 Sterile Solutions (Potentiates CNS depressant effects) ... 985
Inversine Tablets (Potentiation of Inversine) ... 1729
Ionamin Capsules (Possibility of adverse interactions) ... 1615
Ismelin Tablets (Aggravates orthostatic hypotensive effects) .. 845
Ismo Tablets (Additive vasodilating effects) ... 2844
Isordil Sublingual Tablets (Alcohol exhibits additive vasodilating effects) ... 2845
Isordil Tembids Capsules (Alcohol exhibits additive vasodilating effects) ... 2847
Isordil Titradose Tablets (Alcohol exhibits additive vasodilating effects) ... 2848
Kadian Capsules (Co-administration may increase the risk of respiratory depression, hypotension and profound sedation and coma) ... 2948
Klonopin Tablets (Potentiates CNS-depressant action) ... 2294

(▣ Described in PDR For Nonprescription Drugs) (◉ Described in PDR For Ophthalmology)

Lasix Injection, Oral Solution and Tablets (Orthostatic hypotension may be aggravated by alcohol) 1267
Levatol Tablets (Concurrent use increases the number of errors in the eye-hand psychomotor function test) 2547
Levo-Dromoran Injectable (Concurrent use may result in additive central nervous system depressant effects, including respiratory depression, hypotension, profound sedation and coma) 2297
Levoprome (Potentiation of CNS depression) 1321
Librax Capsules (Co-administration may produce additive CNS depressant effects) 2330
Librium Capsules (Potential for additive effects) 2331
Librium Injectable (Additive effect) 2332
Limbitrol Tablets (Concurrent use may produce additive effects resulting in harmful level of sedation and CNS depression) 2333
Lioresal Intrathecal (CNS depressant effect of Lioresal Intrathecal may be additive to those of alcohol) 1634
Lioresal Tablets (Additive depressant effect) 847
Lomotil Liquid (Potentiation of alcohol) 2591
Lopressor HCT Tablets (Orthostatic hypotension may be potentiated) 850
Lorcet 10/650 Tablets (Potential for additive CNS depression) 1016
Lortab 10/500 Tablets (Co-administration may exhibit additive CNS depression; concurrent use should be avoided) 2751
Lotensin HCT Tablets (Thiazide-induced orthostatic hypotension potentiated by alcohol) 855
Ludiomil Tablets (Enhanced response to central nervous system depressants) 861
LUVOX Tablets (Concurrent use should be avoided) 2723
MS Contin Tablets (Respiratory depression, hypotension and profound sedation or coma may result) 2149
MSIR Oral Solution (Additive depressant effects; potential for respiratory depression, hypotension and profound sedation or coma) 2152
Mandol Vials, Faspak & ADD-Vantage (Concurrent ingestion of ethanol may result in nausea, vomiting, vasomotor instability with hypotension and peripheral vasodilation) 1516
Marax Tablets & DF Syrup (Potentiated) 2015
Marinol (Dronabinol) Capsules (Co-administration results in additive drowsiness and CNS depression) 2353
Matulane Capsules (Concurrent use may result in disulfiram-like reaction) 2300
Mellaril Concentrate (Concurrent use results in the potentiation of CNS depression) 2398
Mepergan Injection (Respiratory depression, hypotension, profound sedation or coma) 2859
Mesantoin Tablets (Co-administration may result in possible additive effects; acute alcohol intoxication may increase the anticonvulsant effect; chronic alcohol abuse may decrease anticonvulsant effect) .. 2400
Methadone Hydrochloride Oral Concentrate (Potential for respiratory depression, hypotension, and profound sedation or coma; use caution and reduced dosage in patients who are concurrently receiving these drugs) 2356
Methadone Hydrochloride Oral Solution & Tablets (Respiratory depression, hypotension, and profound sedation or coma may result) 2357
MetroGel-Vaginal (Possibility of a disulfiram-like reaction) 917
Mevacor Tablets (Lovastatin should be used with caution in patients who have consumed a substantial quantity of alcohol and have a past history of liver disease; active liver disease and unexplained elevation in transaminase are contraindications to the use of lovastatin) 1742
Maximum Strength Multi-Symptom Formula Midol (May increase drowsiness) .... ▣ 621
PMS Multi-Symptom Formula Midol (May increase drowsiness) .... ▣ 622
Miltown Tablets (Additive effects) .. 2780
Minizide Capsules (Concurrent use may aggravate orthostatic hypotension) 2016
Mobigesic Tablets (Avoid concurrent use; may cause drowsiness) .... ▣ 607
Moduretic Tablets (Potentiation of orthostatic hypotension) 1748
Monoket Tablets (Additive vasodilating effects) 2550
Motofen Tablets (Effects potentiated) 789
Mykrox Tablets (Potentiates orthostatic hypotensive effects) .. 1617
Nardil (Concurrent use should be avoided) 1977
Navane Capsules and Concentrate (Possible additive effects which may include hypotension) 2018
Navane Intramuscular (Possible additive effects which may include hypotension) 2019
Nitro-Bid Ointment (Exhibits additive vasodilating effects) 1272
Nitro-Dur (nitroglycerin) Transdermal Infusion System (Enhances sensitivity to the hypotensive effects) 1365
Nitrolingual Spray (Enhanced sensitivity to hypotensive effects) 2193
Nitrostat Tablets (Concomitant use may cause hypotension) 1981
Nizoral Tablets (Potential for disulfiram-like reaction to alcohol resulting in flushing, rash, peripheral edema, nausea and headache) 1345
Nolahist Tablets (Increased drowsiness) 790
Norpramin Tablets (Concurrent use results in exaggerated response to alcohol; alcohol induces liver enzyme activity and thereby reduces tricyclic antidepressant plasma levels) 1273
Novahistine Elixir (May increase the drowsiness effect; avoid concurrent use) .... ▣ 782
Nubain Injection (Additive CNS depression) 952
Nucofed Syrup and Capsules (May increase the depressant effects of codeine) 2225
Numorphan Injection (Additive CNS depression) 953
Numorphan Suppositories (Additive CNS depression) 953
Nydrazid Injection (Daily ingestion of alcohol may be associated with a higher incidence of isoniazid hepatitis) 509
Maximum Strength Nytol Caplets (When consuming alcohol, use Nytol with caution) .... ▣ 632
Nytol QuickCaps Caplets (Heightens depressant effect) .. ▣ 632
Oramorph SR (Morphine Sulfate Sustained Release Tablets) (CNS depressant effects are potentiated) 2359
Orap Tablets (CNS depression potentiated) 1037
Oretic Tablets (May aggravate orthostatic hypotension) 450
Orlaam Oral Solution (Potential for serious side effects, including respiratory depression, hypotension, profound sedation and coma, if used concurrently) .. 2361
Ornade Spansule Capsules (Concurrent use results in potentiation of CNS depressant effects) 2678
Orudis KT (Patients consuming three or more alcohol-containing drinks should consult doctor for advice on when and how they should take Orudis KT) .... ▣ 842
OxyContin Tablets (Concurrent use with the usual dose of OxyContin may result in respiratory depression, profound sedation or coma) 2163
OxyIR Capsules (Concomitant use may exhibit an additive CNS depression) 2167
PBZ Tablets (CNS effects may be additive) 863
PBZ-SR Tablets (CNS effects may be additive) 862
Pamelor Capsules (Excessive consumption of alcohol with nortriptyline may have a potentiating effect and exaggerated response to alcohol) 2409
Parafon Forte DSC Caplets (May produce additive effect) 1590
Parlodel Capsules (Alcohol may potentiate the side effects of bromocriptine) 2411
Parnate Tablets (Concurrent use is contraindicated; a marked potentiating effect on alcohol has been reported) 2679
Paxil Tablets (Concurrent use should be avoided) 2681
Pediatric Vicks 44m Cough & Cold Relief (May increase drowsiness effect) .... ▣ 737
Percocet Tablets (Additive CNS depression) 955
Percodan Tablets (Additive CNS depression) 955
Percodan-Demi Tablets (CNS depressant effects of Percodan-Demi may be additive) 956
Percogesic Analgesic Tablets (May increase the drowsiness effect) .... ▣ 727
Periactin Syrup (Additive effects).... 1767
Phenergan with Codeine (Additive sedative effects) 2883
Phenergan with Dextromethorphan (Additive sedative effects) 2885
Phenergan Injection (Additive sedative effects) 2880
Phenergan Suppositories (Additive sedative effects) 2882
Phenergan Syrup Fortis (Additive sedative effects) 2881
Phenergan VC (Additive sedative effects) 2886
Phenergan VC with Codeine (Additive sedative effects) 2888
Phenobarbital Elixir and Tablets (Additive depressant effects) 1523
Phrenilin Forte Capsules (Potential for increased CNS depression) 790
PMB 200 and PMB 400 (Additive effects) 2890
Pondimin Tablets (Possible additive effects of CNS depressants; avoid alcoholic beverages) 2239
Prinzide Tablets (Potentiates orthostatic hypotension) 1780
Procanbid Extended-Release Tablets (Alcohol consumption tends to decrease the half-life of procainamide in the blood through induction of its acetylation to NAPA) 1983
Prolixin Decanoate (Potentiation of the effect of alcohol may occur) .. 510
Propulsid Tablets (Sedative effects of alcohol may be accelerated) 1346
ProSom Tablets (Co-administration results in increased CNS depression) 457
Protostat Tablets (Abdominal cramps, nausea, vomiting, headache, and flushing may occur; alcohol should not be consumed during and for at least one day after therapy) 1939
Prozac Pulvules & Liquid, Oral Solution (Concurrent use with CNS active agents, such as alcohol, requires caution) 935
Pyrroxate Caplets (Concurrent use not recommended) .... ▣ 742
Quadrinal Tablets (Co-administration of phenobarbital with alcohol results in increased effects of either agent) 1398
RMS Suppositories CII (Additive CNS depressant effect) 2766
Reglan Injectable (Increased rate and/or extent of absorption from the small bowel; additive sedative effects) 2243
Remeron Tablets (Co-administration has shown to result in an additive impairment of cognitive and motor skills) 1878
Restoril Capsules (Additive effects) 2413
Rifamate Capsules (Daily ingestion of alcohol may be associated with a higher incidence of isoniazid hepatitis) 1278
Rifater (Daily ingestion of alcohol may be associated with higher incidence of isoniazid hepatitis) .. 1280
Rilutek Tablets (Alcohol may increase the risk of hepatotoxicity; patients on riluzole should be discouraged from drinking excessive amounts of alcohol) 2198
Risperdal Tablets (Effects not specified; concurrent use should be avoided) 1348
Robaxin Injectable (Increased depressant effect) 2245
Robaxin Tablets (Increased CNS depressant effect) 2246
Robaxisal Tablets (Increased depressant effect) 2246
Robitussin Night-Time Cold Formula (May increase drowsiness effect) .... ▣ 847
Romazicon (Concurrent use should be avoided) 2311
Rondec Oral Drops (Enhanced effects of alcohol) 974
Rondec Chewable Tablets (Concomitant use of antihistamines with alcohol may have an additive effect) 974
Roxanol (Morphine Sulfate Concentrated Oral Solution) (Respiratory depression, hypotension, and profound sedation or coma may result; depressant effects of morphine may be enhanced) 2365
Roxicodone Tablets, Oral Solution & Intensol (Oxycodone) (Possible additive CNS depression) 2366
Ryna-C Liquid (May increase drowsiness effect) .... ▣ 804
Rynatan-S Pediatric Suspension (Antihistamines cause drowsiness and co-administration may increase drowsiness effect) 2781
Rynatuss Pediatric Suspension (Antihistamines cause drowsiness and co-administration may increase drowsiness effect) 2782
Seconal Sodium Pulvules (Concomitant use may produce additive CNS-depressant effects) 1529
Sedapap Tablets 50 mg/650 mg (Additive CNS depression) 1826
Semprex-D Capsules (Co-administration may result in additional reduction in alertness and impairment of CNS performance and should be avoided) 1620
Ser-Ap-Es Tablets (Thiazide-induced orthostatic hypotension may be potentiated) 867
Serax Capsules (Effects may be additive) 2916
Serentil Ampuls (Potentiation of central nervous system depressant) 689
Seromycin Capsules (Concurrent use increases the possibility and risk of epileptic episodes) 975
Serzone Tablets (Concomitant use should be avoided) 776
Sinarest Tablets (May increase drowsiness effect) .... ▣ 663

Sine-Aid Maximum Strength Sinus Headache Gelcaps, Caplets and Tablets (Chronic heavy alcohol abusers, 3 or more drinks per day, may be at increased risk of liver toxicity from acetaminophen use) 1570
Sine-Off Sinus Medicine (May increase drowsiness effect) .... ▣ 784
Sinequan Capsules (Doxepin may enhance the response to alcohol) 2028
Singlet Tablets (May increase drowsiness effect) .... ▣ 785
Sinulin Tablets (Increased drowsiness) 792
Sinutab Sinus Allergy Medication, Maximum Strength Tablets and Caplets (May increase drowsiness effect) .... ▣ 823
Sleepinal Night-time Sleep Aid Capsules and Softgels (Avoid alcoholic beverages) .... ▣ 798
Soma Compound w/Codeine Tablets (Additive effects including gastrointestinal bleeding) 2784
Soma Compound Tablets (Additive effects including enhanced aspirin-induced fecal blood loss) 2783
Soma Tablets (Carisoprodol causes drowsiness and co-administration may increase drowsiness effect) 2782
Sorbitrate Chewable Tablets (Enhances sensitivity to hypotensive activity of nitrates) .. 2959
Stadol NS Nasal Spray (Potential for increased CNS depressant effect) 779
Stelazine Concentrate (Additive depressant effects) 2692
Sublimaze Injection (Co-administration results in additive or potentiating effects) .. 463
Sudafed Cold & Allergy Tablets (May increase drowsiness effect) .... ▣ 826
Sunsource Insomnia Relief Tablets (Concurrent use should be avoided) .... ▣ 793
Surmontil Capsules (Concomitant use of alcoholic beverages and trimipramine may be associated with exaggerated effects) 2917
Talacen Caplets (Potential for increased CNS depressant effects) 2464
Talwin Ampuls (Potential for increased CNS depressant effects) 2465
Talwin Compound (Potential for increased CNS depressant effects) 2466
Talwin Nx Tablets (May increase CNS depression) 2467
Tavist Syrup (Additive effects) 2426
Tavist Tablets (Additive effects) 2427
Tavist-1 12 Hour Relief Tablets (May increase drowsiness effect) .... ▣ 749
Tavist-D 12 Hour Relief Tablets (Increases drowsiness effect) .... ▣ 750
Teldrin 12 Hour Antihistamine/Nasal Decongestant Allergy Relief Capsules (May increase drowsiness effect; avoid concurrent use) .... ▣ 786
Thalitone (Aggravates orthostatic hypotension) 1293
Theo-24 Extended Release Capsules (Concurrent use with a single dose of alcohol (3 mL/kg of whiskey) decreases theophylline clearance for up to 24 hours) 2753
Theo-Dur Extended-Release Tablets (Concurrent use with a single dose of alcohol (3 mL/kg of whiskey) decreases theophylline clearance for up to 24 hours) 1367
TheraFlu Flu and Cold Medicine (May increase drowsiness effect.) .... ▣ 750
Theraflu Maximum Strength Flu and Cold Medicine For Sore Throat (May increase drowsiness effect) .... ▣ 751
TheraFlu Maximum Strength Nighttime Flu, Cold & Cough Medicine (May increase drowsiness effect.) .... ▣ 751
Tigan Capsules (May result in an adverse drug interaction) 2231
Tofranil Ampuls (Imipramine may enhance the CNS depressant effects of alcohol) 873
Tofranil Tablets (Imipramine may enhance the CNS depressant effect of alcohol) 875
Tofranil-PM Capsules (Imipramine may enhance the CNS depressant effects of alcohol) 876
Torecan Injection (Phenothiazines are capable of potentiating CNS depressants) 2367
Trancopal Caplets (Possible additive effects) 2468
Transderm Scōp Transdermal Therapeutic System (Effect unspecified) 890
Transderm-Nitro Transdermal Therapeutic System (Additive vasodilating effects) 878
Tranxene T-TAB Tablets (Actions of benzodiazepines may be potentiated; prolonged sleeping time) 459
Triaminic Night Time (May increase drowsiness effect) .... ▣ 754
Triaminic Syrup (May increase drowsiness effect) .... ▣ 755
Triaminic Triaminicol Cold & Cough (May increase drowsiness effect) .... ▣ 756
Triaminicin Tablets (May increase drowsiness effect) .... ▣ 756
Triavil Tablets (Potentiated; contraindication) 1800
Trilafon Concentrate (Additive effects; hypotension) 2532
Trilisate Liquid (Increased risk of gastrointestinal ulceration) 2155
Trinalin Repetabs Tablets (Additive effect) 1373
Tussend (Concomitant use may exhibit additive CNS depression) 1830
Tussend Expectorant (Hydrocodone may potentiate CNS depressant effects) 1831
Tussionex Pennkinetic Extended-Release Suspension (Additive CNS depression) 1624
Tussi-Organidin DM NR Liquid and DM-S NR Liquid (Potential for additive CNS depressant effects) 2786
TYLENOL acetaminophen, Regular Strength Caplets and Tablets (Concurrent use may increase drowsiness effect; chronic heavy alcohol abusers, 3 or more drinks per day, may be at increased risk of liver toxicity from excessive acetaminophen use) 1570
TYLENOL Allergy Sinus NightTime, Maximum Strength Caplets (Concurrent use may increase drowsiness effect; chronic heavy alcohol abusers, 3 or more drinks per day, may be at increased risk of liver toxicity from excessive acetaminophen use) 1571
TYLENOL Cold Medication, Multi-Symptom Formula Tablets and Caplets (Concurrent use may increase drowsiness effect; chronic heavy alcohol abusers, 3 or more drinks per day, may be at increased risk of liver toxicity from excessive acetaminophen use) 1572
TYLENOL Cold Severe Congestion Caplets (Chronic heavy alcohol abusers, 3 or more drinks per day, may be at increased risk of liver toxicity from acetaminophen use) 1573
TYLENOL Cough Medication with Decongestant, Multi Symptom (Chronic heavy alcohol abusers, 3 or more drinks per day, may be at increased risk of liver toxicity from acetaminophen use) 1574
TYLENOL Flu NightTime, Maximum Strength Hot Medication Packets (Concurrent use may increase drowsiness effect; chronic heavy alcohol abusers, 3 or more drinks per day, may be at increased risk of liver toxicity from excessive acetaminophen use) 1575
TYLENOL Headache Plus Pain Reliever with Antacid, Extra Strength Caplets (Chronic heavy alcohol abusers, 3 or more drinks per day, may be at increased risk of liver toxicity from acetaminophen use) .... ▣ 705
TYLENOL PM Pain Reliever/Sleep Aid, Extra Strength Gelcaps, Caplets, Geltabs (Avoid concurrent use; chronic heavy alcohol abusers, 3 or more drinks per day, may be at increased risk of liver toxicity from acetaminophen use) 1576
TYLENOL Sinus, Maximum Strength Geltabs, Gelcaps, Caplets and Tablets (Chronic heavy alcohol abusers, 3 or more drinks per day, may be at increased risk of liver toxicity from acetaminophen use) 1576
Tylenol with Codeine Elixir (Additive CNS depression) 1592
Tylox Capsules (Additive CNS depression) 1593
Ultram Tablets (50 mg) (Concurrent use should be avoided) 1594
Uni-Dur Extended-Release Tablets (Concurrent use with a single dose of alcohol (3mL/kg of whiskey) decreases theophylline clearance for up to 24 hours) 1374
Uniphyl 400 mg and 600 mg Tablets (Concurrent use with a single dose of alcohol (3 mL/kg of whiskey) decreases theophylline clearance for up to 24 hours) 2157
Maximum Strength Unisom Sleepgels (Heightens the CNS depressant effect) 1990
Unisom Nighttime Sleep Aid (Use Unisom cautiously) 1990
Unisom With Pain Relief-Nighttime Sleep Aid and Pain Reliever (Heightened CNS depressant effect of antihistamines) 1991
Valium Injectable (Concomitant use increases central nervous system depression with increased risk of apnea: injectable diazepam should not be administered in acute alcoholic intoxication) 2336
Valium Tablets (May potentiate the actions of diazepam) 2335
Vaseretic Tablets (Potentiation of orthostatic hypotension may occur) 1810
Verelan Capsules (Verapamil has been found to significantly inhibit ethanol elimination resulting in elevated blood ethanol concentration that may prolong the intoxicating effects of alcohol) 1455
Versed Injection (Concomitant use may increase the risk of underventilation or apnea and may contribute to profound and/or prolonged drug effect) 2324
Vicks 44 LiquiCaps Cough, Cold & Flu Relief (May increase the drowsiness effect) .... ▣ 728
Vicks 44M Cough, Cold & Flu Relief (May increase drowsiness effect) .... ▣ 729
Vicks DayQuil Allergy Relief 12-Hour Extended Release Tablets (Avoid concurrent use) ▣ 733
Vicks DayQuil Allergy Relief 4-Hour Tablets (May increase drowsiness effect) .... ▣ 733
Vicks Nyquil Hot Therapy (May increase drowsiness effect) .... ▣ 735
Vicks NyQuil LiquiCaps/Liquid Multi-Symptom Cold/Flu Relief, Original and Cherry Flavors (May increase drowsiness effect) .... ▣ 736
Vicodin Tablets (May exhibit an additive CNS depression) 1404
Vicodin ES Tablets (Additive CNS depression) 1405
Vicodin HP Tablets (Concurrent use results in an additive CNS depression) 1403
Vicodin Tuss Expectorant (Co-administration may exhibit an additive CNS depression) 1406
Vistaril Capsules (Increased effect of alcohol) 2042
Vistaril Intramuscular Solution (May be potentiated) 2042
Vivactil Tablets (Co-administration results in enhanced response to alcohol) 1820
Wellbutrin Tablets (Concurrent alcohol consumption should be avoided or minimized) 1177
Wygesic Tablets (Additive effects) .. 2930
Xanax Tablets (Additive CNS depressant effects) 2115
Zaroxolyn Tablets (Hypotensive effect may be potentiated) 1625
Zestoretic Tablets (Potentiates orthostatic hypotension) 2968
Ziac (Potentiation of orthostatic hypotension may occur when thiazide diuretics are used with alcohol) 1459
Zoloft Tablets (Concomitant use of Zoloft and alcohol in depressed patient is not recommended) 2051
Zonalon Cream (Alcohol ingestion may exacerbate the potential sedative effects of Zonalon Cream) 1042
Zydone Capsules (Additive CNS depression) 967
Zyrtec Tablets (Concurrent use may result in additional impairment of CNS performance and reduction in mental alertness) 2053

Anchovies

Parnate Tablets (Potential for hypertensive crisis; concurrent use is contraindicated) 2679

Avocados

Parnate Tablets (Potential for hypertensive crisis; concurrent use is contraindicated) 2679

Bananas

Matulane Capsules (Procarbazine exhibits some monoamine oxidase inhibitory activity; concurrent use should be avoided) 2300
Parnate Tablets (Potential for hypertensive crisis; concurrent use is contraindicated) 2679

Beans, broad

Furoxone Liquid (Concurrent and/or sequential intake must be avoided) 2221
Nardil (Concurrent and/or sequential intake must be avoided) 1977
Parnate Tablets (Potential for hypertensive crisis; concurrent use is contraindicated) 2679

Beans, Fava

Nardil (Concurrent and/or sequential intake must be avoided) 1977
Parnate Tablets (Potential for hypertensive crisis; concurrent use is contraindicated) 2679

Beer, alcohol-free

Nardil (Concurrent and/or sequential intake must be avoided) 1977
Parnate Tablets (Potential for hypertensive crisis; concurrent use is contraindicated) 2679

Beer, reduced-alcohol (see also under Alcohol)

Nardil (Concurrent and/or sequential intake must be avoided) 1977

Beer, unspecified (see also under Alcohol)

Furoxone Liquid (Concurrent and/or sequential intake must be avoided) 2221

(▣ Described in PDR For Nonprescription Drugs) (◉ Described in PDR For Ophthalmology)

Food Interactions Cross-Reference / Food that lowers urinary pH

Nardil (Concurrent and/or sequential intake must be avoided) 1977
Parnate Tablets (Potential for hypertensive crisis; concurrent use is contraindicated) 2679

Beverages, alcoholic
(see under Alcohol; Beer, unspecified; Wine products; Wine, Chianti; Wine, unspecified)

Beverages, caffeine-containing
BioLean Free (Concurrent caffeine intake should be minimized) 831
Fosamax Tablets (Concomitant administration of alendronate with coffee reduces bioavailability by approximately 60%) 1703
Maximum Strength Multi-Symptom Formula Midol (Concomitant use may cause nervousness, irritability, sleeplessness, and occasionally, rapid heartbeat) .. 621
Nardil (Excessive caffeine intake should be avoided) 1977
No Doz Maximum Strength Caplets (May cause sleeplessness, irritability, nervousness and rapid heart beat) 644
Parnate Tablets (Potential for hypertensive crisis; concurrent use is contraindicated) 2679
Penetrex Tablets (Enoxacin causes a dose-related increase in the mean elimination half-life of caffeine leading to caffeine-related adverse effects; consumption of caffeine-containing products should be avoided) 2196
Respbid Tablets (Avoid large quantities; increased side effects) 687

Bologna, Lebanon
Nardil (Concurrent and/or sequential intake must be avoided) 1977

Broccoli
(see under Diet high in vitamin K)

Carrots
(see under Food, furocoumarin-containing)

Celery
(see under Food, furocoumarin-containing)

Caviar
Parnate Tablets (Potential for hypertensive crisis; concurrent use is contraindicated) 2679

Cheese, aged
Matulane Capsules (Procarbazine exhibits some monoamine oxidase inhibitory activity; concurrent use should be avoided) 2300
Nardil (Concurrent and/or sequential intake must be avoided) 1977
Parnate Tablets (Potential for hypertensive crisis; concurrent use is contraindicated) 2679

Cheese, strong, unpasteurized
Furoxone Liquid (Concurrent and/or sequential intake must be avoided) 2221
Parnate Tablets (Potential for hypertensive crisis; concurrent use is contraindicated) 2679

Cheese, unspecified
Nardil (Concurrent and/or sequential intake must be avoided) 1977
Parnate Tablets (Potential for hypertensive crisis; concurrent use is contraindicated) 2679
Rifater (Isoniazid has some MAO inhibiting activity, an interaction with tyramine-containing food may occur) 1280

Chocolate
Nardil (Concurrent and/or sequential intake must be avoided) 1977
Parnate Tablets (Potential for hypertensive crisis; concurrent use is contraindicated) 2679
Penetrex Tablets (Enoxacin causes a dose-related increase in the mean elimination half-life of caffeine leading to caffeine-related adverse effects; consumption of caffeine-containing products should be avoided) 2196
Respbid Tablets (Eating large quantity of chocolate increases theophylline side effects) 687

Coffee
(see under Beverages, caffeine-containing)

Cola
Penetrex Tablets (Enoxacin causes a dose-related increase in the mean elimination half-life of caffeine leading to caffeine-related adverse effects; consumption of caffeine-containing products should be avoided) 2196
Respbid Tablets (Drinking large quantity of cola increases theophylline side effects) 687
Sporanox Capsules (Absorption of oral itraconazole is enhanced when administered with a cola beverage in patients with achlorhydria, such as AIDS or patients taking acid suppressors, e.g., H_2 inhibitors and proton pump inhibitors) 1352

Cream, sour
Parnate Tablets (Potential for hypertensive crisis; concurrent use is contraindicated) 2679

Dairy products
Accutane Capsules (Increases oral absorption of isotretinoin) 2252
Achromycin V Capsules (Interfers with absorption of oral forms of tetracycline) 1417
Correctol Laxative Tablets & Caplets (Concurrent use within one hour after taking milk is not recommended) 761
Declomycin Tablets (Interferes with absorption) 1421
Emcyt Capsules (Calcium-rich foods may impair the absorption of estramustine) 2085
Fero-Folic-500 Filmtab (Ingestion of milk inhibits iron absorption) .. 433
Fleet Prep Kits (Concurrent use within one-hour should be avoided) 1002
Helidac Therapy (Impairs absorption of tetracyclines) 2135
Luride Drops 50 ml (Incompatibility of fluoride with dairy) 891
Luride Lozi-Tabs Tablets (Incompatibility of fluoride with dairy foods results in the formation of poorly absorbed calcium fluoride) 892
Minocin Pellet-Filled Capsules (The peak plasma concentrations were slightly decreased (11.2%) and delayed by 1 hour) 1429
Nalfon 200 Pulvules & Nalfon Tablets (Peak blood levels are delayed and diminished) 933
Noroxin Tablets (Avoid simultaneous ingestion; administer norfloxacin at least one hour before or two hours after milk ingestion) 1758
Noroxin Tablets (Avoid simultaneous ingestion; administer norfloxacin at least one hour before or two hours after milk ingestion) 2222
Relafen Tablets (Potential for more rapid absorption, however, the total amount of GMNA in the plasma is unchanged) 2688
Tegison Capsules (Increases absorption of etretinate) 2314
Tolectin (200, 400 and 600 mg) (Decreases total tolmetin bioavailability by 16%) 1591
Vibramycin Hyclate Capsules (Absorption of doxycycline is not markedly influenced by simultaneous ingestion of milk) 2038

Diet high in protein
Atamet Tablets (Levodopa competes with certain amino acids, the absorption of levodopa may be impaired in some patients on a high protein diet) 567
Sinemet Tablets (Levodopa competes with certain amino acids, the absorption of levodopa may be impaired in some patients on a high protein diet) 959

Diet high in vitamin K
Coumadin Tablets (Decreased prothrombin time) 941

Diet, high-lipid
Accupril Tablets (Rate and extent of Quinapril absorption are diminished moderately) 1950
Adalat CC (High fat meal increases peak plasma nifedipine concentrations by 60%, a prolongation in the time to peak concentration, but no significant change in the AUC; administer on an empty stomach) 582
Albenza Tablets (Oral bioavailability appears to be enhanced when albendazole is co-administered with a fatty meal) 2629
Cardene SR Capsules (Results in lower C_{max} and AUC; higher trough levels) 2264
Dilacor XR Extended-release Capsules (Simultaneous administration of Dilacor XR with a high-fat breakfast has a modest effect on diltiazem bioavailability) 2183
Glucotrol XL Extended Release Tablets (Administration of Glucotrol XL immediately before a high-fat breakfast resulted in a 40% increase in the glipizide mean Cmax value; the effect on the AUC was not significant) 2012
Mycobutin Capsules (High-fat meals slow the rate without influencing the extent of absorption from the capsule dosage form) 2101
Neoral Soft Gelatin Capsules for Microemulsion (A high fat meal consumed within one-half hour before Neoral administration decreased the AUC by 13% and C_{max} by 33%) 2405
Respbid Tablets (Reduced plasma concentration levels; delay in time of peak plasma levels) 687
Rilutek Tablets (Co-administration with high-fat meal decreases absorption, reduces AUC by about 20% and peak blood levels by about 45%) 2198
Salagen Tablets (Decrease in the rate of absorption of pilocarpine when taken with high fat meal) 1546
Slo-bid Gyrocaps (Decreases the rate of absorption, but with no significant difference in the extent of absorption) 2201
Sular Tablets (Food with a high-fat content has a pronounced effect on the release of nisoldipine resulting in a significant increase in peak concentration (Cax by 33%) 2961
Tegison Capsules (Increases absorption of etretinate) 2314
Theo-24 Extended Release Capsules (Taking Theo-24 one hour before a high-fat-content meal may result in a significant increase in peak serum level and the extent of absorption of theophylline) 2753
Theo-X Extended-Release Tablets (May result in a somewhat higher C_{max} and delayed T_{max}, and a somewhat greater extent of absorption when compared to taking in the fasting state) 793
Theo-X Extended-Release Tablets (May result in a somewhat higher C_{max} and delayed T_{max}, and a somewhat greater extent of absorption when compared to taking in the fasting state) 793
Uni-Dur Extended-Release Tablets (Co-administration with a high-fat breakfast delays the time to peak concentration, however, the extent of theophylline absorption is similar when administered fasting or immediately after a high-fat breakfast) 1374
Uniphyl 400 mg and 600 mg Tablets (Co-administration with a standardized high-fat meal results in increased peak plasma concentration and bioavailability; however, a precipitous increase in the rate and extent of absorption was not evident; the dosing should be ideally administered consistently either with or without food) 2157

Diet, potassium-rich
Aldactone Tablets (Concurrent use with diet rich in potassium should not ordinarily be given with spironolactone since this may result in hyperkalemia) 2558
Midamor Tablets (Potential for rapid increases in serum potassium levels) 1746
Moduretic Tablets (Potential for rapid increases in serum potassium levels) 1748

Eggs
Fero-Folic-500 Filmtab (Ingestion of eggs inhibits iron absorption) .. 433

Figs
(see under Food, furocoumarin-containing)

Figs, canned
Parnate Tablets (Potential for hypertensive crisis; concurrent use is contraindicated) 2679

Fish, smoked
Nardil (Concurrent and/or sequential intake must be avoided) 1977

Fish, tropical
Rifater (Isoniazid may inhibit diamine oxidase, causing exaggerated response (headache, sweating, palpitations, flushing, hypotension) to food containing histamine) 1280

Food having a pH greater than 5.5
CREON 5 Capsules (Can dissolve the protective coating resulting in early release of enzymes, irritation of oral mucosa, and/or loss of enzyme activity) 2714
Ultrase Capsules (Can dissolve the protective coating resulting in early release of enzymes, irritation of oral mucosa, and/or loss of enzyme activity) 2476
Ultrase MT Capsules (Can dissolve the protective enteric shell) 2477

Food that lowers urinary pH
Disalcid Capsules (Co-administration with food that lowers urine pH will decrease renal clearance and urinary excretion of salicylic acid, thus increase plasma levels) 1549
Mono-Gesic Tablets (Decreases urinary excretion and increases plasma levels) 810
Trilisate Liquid (Decreases urinary salicylate excretion and increases plasma levels) 2155

(■ Described in PDR For Nonprescription Drugs) (◎ Described in PDR For Ophthalmology)

Food Interactions Cross-Reference

Food that raises urinary pH

- Disalcid Capsules (Co-administration with food that raises urine pH will increase renal clearance and urinary excretion of salicylic acid, thus lowering plasma levels) ... 1549
- Mono-Gesic Tablets (Increases renal clearance and urinary excretion of salicylic acid) ... 810
- Trilisate Liquid (Enhances renal salicylate clearance and diminishes plasma salicylate concentration) ... 2155
- Urised Tablets (Methenamine has therapeutic activity in acidic urine; concurrent use with foods which produce an alkaline urine should be restricted) ... 2123

Food with high concentration of dopamine

- Nardil (Concurrent and/or sequential intake must be avoided) ... 1977

Food with high concentration of tyramine

- Furoxone Liquid (Concurrent and/or sequential intake must be avoided) ... 2221
- Matulane Capsules (Procarbazine exhibits some monoamine oxidase inhibitory activity; concurrent use should be avoided) ... 2300
- Nardil (Concurrent and/or sequential intake must be avoided) ... 1977
- Parnate Tablets (Potential for hypertensive crisis; concurrent use is contraindicated) ... 2679
- Rifater (Isoniazid has some MAO inhibiting activity, an interaction with tyramine-containing food may occur) ... 1280

Food, caffeine containing

- DHCplus Capsules (Concomitant use may result in caffeine accumulation when DHC Plus is consumed with caffeine-containing foods) ... 2148
- Maximum Strength Multi-Symptom Formula Midol (Concomitant use may cause nervousness, irritability, sleeplessness, and occasionally, rapid heartbeat) ... 621
- No Doz Maximum Strength Caplets (May cause sleeplessness, irritability, nervousness and rapid heart beat) ... 644

Food, calcium-rich

- Emcyt Capsules (Calcium-rich foods may impair the absorption of estramustine) ... 2085

Food, charcoal-broiled

- Rilutek Tablets (Potential inducers of CYP1A2, such as charcoal-broiled food, could increase the rate of riluzole elimination) ... 2198
- Theo-24 Extended Release Capsules (Theophylline clearance is increased and half-life decreased by daily consumption of charcoal-broiled beef) ... 2753

Food, furocoumarin-containing

- Trisoralen Tablets (Potential for severe reactions) ... 1309

Food, unspecified

- Accutane Capsules (Increases oral absorption of isotretinoin) ... 2252
- Achromycin V Capsules (Interferes with absorption of oral forms of tetracycline) ... 1417
- Altace Capsules (The rate of absorption is reduced, not the extent of absorption) ... 1238
- Apresazide Capsules (Enhances gastrointestinal absorption of hydrochlorothiazide) ... 824
- Apresoline Hydrochloride Tablets (Administration of hydralazine with food results in higher plasma levels) ... 826
- Biaxin Filmtab (Food slightly delays both the onset of absorption and the formation of the active metabolite, but does not affect the extent of bioavailability; Biaxin may be administered without regard to food) ... 406
- BuSpar Tablets (Food may decrease presystemic clearance of buspirone) ... 738
- Calan SR Caplets (Produces decreased bioavailability (AUC) but a narrower peak-to-trough ratio) ... 2571
- Capoten Tablets (Reduces absorption by about 30 to 40%; should be given one hour before meals) ... 740
- Capozide Tablets (Reduces captopril's absorption by about 30% to 40%; should be given one hour before meals) ... 744
- Cardioquin Tablets (Food delays absorption, but not the extent) ... 2146
- Cardura Tablets (Reduction of 18% in mean maximum plasma concentration and 12% in the AUC occurred when Cardura was administered with food; neither of these differences were statistically or clinically significant) ... 1993
- Cedax Capsules (Food delays the time of C_{max}, decreases the C_{max}, and the extent of absorption (AUC); cefibuten oral suspension should be taken at least 2 hours before meal or at least 1 hour after meal) ... 2480
- Ceftin Tablets (Absorption is greater when taken after food) ... 1067
- CellCept Capsules (Decreased Cmax of mycophenolate mofetil by 40% in the presence of food; no effect on the extent of absorption) ... 2265
- Cipro Tablets (Delays the absorption of the drug resulting in peak concentrations that are closer to 2 hours after dosing) ... 584
- Clinoril Tablets (The peak plasma concentrations of biologically active sulfide metabolite is delayed slightly in the presence of food) ... 1658
- Cognex Capsules (Food reduces tacrine bioavailability by approximately 30% to 40%; no effect if tacrine is administered at least one hour before meals) ... 1961
- Crixivan Capsules (Co-administration with a meal high in calories, fat, and protein has resulted in a 77% C_{max}; administer without food 1 hour before or 2 hours after a meal) ... 1670
- Cytotec (Diminishes maximum plasma concentrations) ... 2576
- Daypro Caplets (Reduces the rate of absorption of oxaprozin, but the extent of absorption is unchanged) ... 2578
- Declomycin Tablets (Interferes with absorption) ... 1421
- Demadex Tablets and Injection (Simultaneous food intake delays the time to C_{max} by about 30 minutes, but overall bioavailability (AUC) and diuretic activity are unchanged) ... 691
- Desyrel and Desyrel Dividose (Total drug absorption may be up to 20% higher when the drug is taken with food rather than on an empty stomach; the risk of dizziness, lightheadedness may increase under fasting conditions) ... 504
- Dyclone 0.5% and 1% Topical Solutions, USP (Topical anesthesia may impair swallowing and thus enhance the danger of aspiration; food should not be ingested for 60 minutes) ... 535
- Dynabac (Slight increase in the absorption of erythromycylamine when dirithromycin tablets were administered after food; significant decrease in C_{max} (33%) and AUC (31%) occurs when administered one hour before food; administer with food or within an hour of having eaten) ... 668
- DYNACIN Capsules (The peak plasma concentrations were slightly decreased and delayed by one hour when administered with a meal which included dairy products; extent of absorption was not noticeably influenced) ... 1627
- DynaCirc Capsules (Coadministration significantly increases the time to peak by about an hour with no effect on AUC) ... 2381
- DynaCirc CR Tablets (Food has been shown to decrease the extent of bioavailability of DynaCirc CR by up to 25%) ... 2383
- EC-Naprosyn Delayed-Release Tablets (The presence of food prolonged the time the EC-Naprosyn remained in the stomach, time to first detectable serum naproxen levels, and time to maximal naproxen levels (T_{max}), but did not affect peak naproxen levels (C_{max})) ... 2277
- Eldepryl Capsules (The bioavailability of selegiline is increased 3 to 4 fold when it is taken with food) ... 2729
- Epivir Tablets (Food slows the absorption; no significant difference in systemic exposure AUC (infinity) in the fed and fasted states) ... 1200
- Erythromycin Delayed-Release Capsules, USP (Lowers the blood levels of systemically available erythromycin) ... 431
- Esimil Tablets (Enhances gastrointestinal absorption of hydrochlorothiazide) ... 840
- Floxin Tablets (200 mg, 300 mg, 400 mg) (Food does not affect the C_{max} and AUC_{∞} of the drug, but T_{max} is prolonged) ... 1577
- Glucophage Tablets (Food decreases the extent and slightly delays the absorption of metformin) ... 754
- Glucotrol Tablets (Delays absorption by 40 minutes; administer 30 minutes prior to meals) ... 2011
- GoLYTELY (For best results, no solid food should be consumed during 3 to 4 hour period before drinking solution) ... 694
- Hivid Tablets (The absorption rate of a 15 mg oral dose of zalactabine was reduced when administered with food) ... 2287
- Hytrin Capsules (Delays the time to peak concentration by about 40 minutes; minimal effect on the extent of absorption) ... 434
- IBU Tablets (Food affects the rate but not the extent of absorption) ... 1389
- Imdur (May decrease the rate (increase in T_{max}) but not the extent (AUC) of absorption) ... 1362
- Imitrex Tablets (Delays the T_{max} slightly by about 0.5 hour with no significant effect on the bioavailability) ... 1099
- Invirase Capsules (Saquinavir 24-AUC and Cmax following a high-caloric meal is on average two times higher than a lower calorie, lower fat meal; patients should be advised to take saquinavir within 2 hours after a full meal) ... 2291
- Isoptin SR Tablets (Produces decreased bioavailability (AUC) but a narrower peak to trough ratio) ... 1395
- Kadian Capsules (Concurrent administration of food slows the rate of absorption; the extent of absorption is not affected) ... 2948
- Kytril Tablets (When oral granisetron was administered with food, AUC was decreased by 5% and Cmax increased by 30% in non-fasted individuals) ... 2669
- Lamisil Tablets (Co-administration has resulted in an increase in the AUC of terbinafine of less than 20%) ... 2394
- Lodine Capsules and Tablets (Reduces the peak concentration reached by approximately one-half and increases the time-to-peak concentration by 1.4 to 3.8 hours) ... 2849
- Lorabid Suspension and Pulvules (Delays the peak plasma concentration with no change in the total absorption) ... 1513
- Macrobid Capsules (Increases bioavailability by approximately 40%) ... 2138
- Macrodantin Capsules (Increases bioavailability of Macrodantin) ... 2140
- Mavik Tablets (Slows absorption of trandolapril but does not affect AUC or C_{max}) ... 1407
- Maxaquin Tablets (The rate of drug absorption may be delayed by 41%, however, the drug can be taken without regard to meal) ... 2593
- Mepron Suspension (Food enhances absorption by approximately two-fold) ... 1206
- Methotrexate Sodium Tablets, Injection, for Injection and LPF Injection (Delays absorption and reduces peak concentration) ... 1322
- Monopril Tablets (Rate of absorption may be slowed by the presence of food in the GI tract; the extent of absorption is not affected) ... 762
- Motrin Ibuprofen Suspension, Oral Drops, Chewable Tablets, Caplets (Food affects the rate but not the extent of absorption; T_{max} is delayed by approximately 30 to 60 minutes and peak levels are reduced by approximately 30 to 50%) ... 1563
- Naprelan Tablets (Food causes a slight decrease in the rate of naproxen absorption following Naprelan administration) ... 2861
- Neoral Soft Gelatin Capsules for Microemulsion (Administration of food with Neoral decreases the AUC and C_{max}) ... 2405
- Noroxin Tablets (Co-administration may decrease the absorption of norfloxacin; administer at least one hour before or two hours after a meal) ... 1758
- Noroxin Tablets (Co-administration may decrease the absorption of norfloxacin; administer at least one hour before or two hours after a meal) ... 2222
- NuLYTELY (Solid food should not be given for at least two hours before the solution is given) ... 694
- Orudis Capsules (Slows rate of absorption resulting in delayed and reduced peak concentrations) ... 2874
- Pepcid Oral Suspension (Bioavailability may be slightly increased by antacids) ... 1763
- Premphase (Administration with a high-fat breakfast decreased total estrone C_{max} and increased total equilin C_{max} compared to fasting state, no other effect on rate or extent of absorption; administration with food doubles MPA C_{max} and increases MPA AUC) ... 2900
- Prempro (Administration with food decreased C_{max} of total estrone compared to fasting state, no other effect on rate or extent of absorption; administration with food doubles MPA C_{max} and increases MPA AUC) ... 2905
- Prevacid Delayed-Release Capsules (Cmax and AUC are diminished by about 50% if the drug is given 30 minutes after food as opposed to the fasting condition; Prevacid should be taken before eating) ... 2746
- Procardia XL Extended Release Tablets (Presence of food

(■ Described in PDR For Nonprescription Drugs)   (◎ Described in PDR For Ophthalmology)

slightly alters the early rate of drug absorption) 2026
Prozac Pulvules & Liquid, Oral Solution (May delay absorption of fluoxetine inconsequentially) 935
Quibron-T/SR Tablets (Food ingestion may influence the absorption characteristics of some or all theophylline controlled-release products) 2227
Quinaglute Dura-Tabs Tablets (Increases absorption of quinidine in both rate (27%) and extent (17%)) 644
Quinidex Extentabs (Peak serum quinidine levels obtained from immediate-release quinidine sulfate are known to be delayed by nearly an hour without change in total absorption when these products are taken with food) 2240
Relafen Tablets (Potential for more rapid absorption, however, the total amount of GMNA in the plasma is unchanged) 2688
Remeron Tablets (The presence of food in the stomach has a minimal effect on both the rate and extent of absorption and does not require a dosage adjustment) 1878
Retrovir Capsules (Administration of Retrovir Capsules with food decreased peak plasma concentrations by greater than 50%, however, bioavailability as determined by AUC may not be affected) 1216
Rythmol Tablets–150mg, 225mg, 300mg (Increased peak blood level and bioavailability in a single dose study) 1399
Salflex Tablets (Slows the absorption) 791
Sectral Capsules (Slightly decreases absorption and peak concentration) 2914
Ser-Ap-Es Tablets (Gastrointestinal absorption of hydrochlorothiazide is enhanced when administered with food) 867
Serzone Tablets (Food delays the absorption of nefazodone and decreases the bioavailability by approximately 20%) 776
Sinemet CR Tablets (Increases the extent of availability and peak concentrations of levodopa) 961
Sporanox Capsules (Presence of food increases systemic bioavailability; when taken on an empty stomach the systemic bioavailability is reduced) 1352
Suprax Tablets (Increases time to maximal absorption approximately 0.8 hour) 1443
Theo-24 Extended Release Capsules (Theophylline clearance is increased and half-life decreased by low carbohydrate/high protein diets and parenteral nutrition; a high carbohydrate/low protein diet can decrease the clearance and prolong the half-life of theophylline) 2753
Theo-Dur Extended-Release Tablets (Available data suggests that co-administration with food may influence the absorption characteristics of controlled-release theophylline formulations) 1367
Tiazac Capsules (When Tiazac was co-administered with high fat content breakfast the t_{max} occurred slightly earlier, however, the extent of diltiazem absorption was not affected) 1019
Trandate Tablets (The absolute bioavailability of labetalol is increased when administered with food) 1158
Trental Tablets (Delays absorption but does not affect total absorption) 1291
Univasc Tablets (Food reduces C_{max} and AUC by about 70% and 40% respectively after ingestion of a low-fat breakfast or by 80% and 50%

respectively after the ingestion of high-fat breakfast) 2553
Vantin for Oral Suspension and Vantin Tablets (The extent of absorption and the mean peak plasma concentration increased when film-coated tablets were administered with food) 2112
Vesanoid Capsules (The absorption of retinoids as a class has been shown to be enhanced when taken with food) 2327
Vibramycin Hyclate Capsules (Absorption of doxycycline is not markedly influenced by simultaneous ingestion of food) .. 2038
Videx Tablets, Powder for Oral Solution, & Pediatric Powder for Oral Solution (Reduces the absorption of Videx by 50%; administer Videx on an empty stomach) 2980
Videx Tablets, Powder for Oral Solution, & Pediatric Powder for Oral Solution (Reduces the absorption of Videx by 50%; administer Videx on an empty stomach) 2980
Volmax Extended-Release Tablets (Food may decrease the rate of absorption without altering the extent of bioavailability) 1835
Voltaren Tablets (Food significantly alters the absorption pattern of extended-release dosage form as indicated by delay of 1 to 2 hours in T_{max} and a two-fold increase in C_{max} values; food also delays the onset of absorption of delayed-release and immediate-release formulations) 833
Zithromax Capsules (Zithromax should not be taken with food; reduces the rate of absorption (Cmax) of azithromycin capsules by 52% and the extent of absorption (AUC) by 43%; when oral suspension of azithromycin was administered with food the Cmax increased by 56% and the AUC was unchanged) 2043
Zofran Tablets (Increases significantly (about 17%) the extent of absorption of ondansetron) 1231
Zoloft Tablets (AUC was slightly increased when drug was administered with food but the C_{max} was 25% greater) 2051
Zyrtec Tablets (Food has no effect on the extent of cetirizine absorption, but T_{max} may be delayed and C_{max} may be decreased in the presence of food) 2053

Fruit juices, unspecified
Adderall Tablets (Lowers absorption of amphetamines, blood levels and efficacy) 2209
Dexedrine Spansule Capsules (Lowers absorption of amphetamines) 2648
DextroStat-Dextroamphetamine Sulfate Tablets (Lowers absorption of amphetamines by acting as gastrointestinal acidifying agent) 2211

Grapefruit
Neoral Soft Gelatin Capsules for Microemulsion (Affects the metabolism of cyclosporine and should be avoided) 2405

Grapefruit Juice
Crixivan Capsules (Potential for decrease in indinavir AUC) 1670
Neoral Soft Gelatin Capsules for Microemulsion (Affects the metabolism of cyclosporine and should be avoided) 2405
Xanax Tablets (Possible interaction based on the clinical studies involving other benzodiazepines metabolized by similarly as alprazolam; co-administration requires caution) 2115

Grapefruit juice, doubly concentrated
Plendil Extended-Release Tablets (Increases bioavailability more than two-fold) 514

Herring, pickled
Furoxone Liquid (Concurrent and/or sequential intake must be avoided) 2221
Nardil (Concurrent and/or sequential intake must be avoided) 1977
Parnate Tablets (Potential for hypertensive crisis; concurrent use is contraindicated) 2679

Limes
(see under Food, furocoumarin-containing)

Liqueurs
(see also under Alcohol)
Parnate Tablets (Potential for hypertensive crisis; concurrent use is contraindicated) 2679

Liver
Nardil (Concurrent and/or sequential intake must be avoided) 1977
Parnate Tablets (Potential for hypertensive crisis; concurrent use is contraindicated) 2679

Liver, chicken
Furoxone Liquid (Concurrent and/or sequential intake must be avoided) 2221

Meal with dairy products
Minocin Pellet-Filled Capsules (The peak plasma concentrations were slightly decreased (11.2%) and delayed by 1 hour) 1429

Meal, high in bran fiber
Lanoxicaps (Reduces the amount of digoxin from an oral dose) 1110
Lanoxin Elixir Pediatric (The amount of digoxin from an oral dose may be reduced) 1113
Lanoxin Tablets (The amount of digoxin from an oral dose may be reduced) 1121

Meal, unspecified
Amaryl Tablets (When glimepiride is given with meals the mean T_{max} is slightly increased (12%) and mean C_{max} and AUC are slightly decreased) 1241
Ambien Tablets (Mean AUC and C_{max} decreased by 15% and 25% respectively, while T_{max} was prolonged by 60%; for faster sleep onset, Ambien should not be administered with or immediately after meal) 2559
Betapace Tablets (Reduces oral absorption by 20%) 637
Claritin Tablets (Food increases the AUC by approximately 73%, the time to peak plasma concentration is delayed by one-hour; Claritin should be administered on an empty stomach) 2485
Claritin-D Tablets (Food increases the AUC of loratadine by approximately 40% and of decarboethoxyloratadine by approximately 15%; the time of peak plasma concentration (T_{max}) of loratadine and decarboethoxyloratadine was delayed by 1 hour with meal) 2487
Cozaar Tablets (Meal slows absorption and decreases C_{max} but has minor effects on losartan AUC or on the AUC of the metabolite) 1668
Cytovene Capsules (Meal containing 46.5% fat increases the steady-state AUC of oral Cytovene by 22% +/- 22% and significant prolongation of time T_{max} and a higher C_{max}) 2270
Depen Titratable Tablets (Potential for reduced absorption and the

likelihood of inactivation by metal binding in the GI tract; Depen should be given on an empty stomach) 2770
ERYC (Optimum blood levels are obtained on a fasting stomach; administration is preferable one-half hour pre- or two hours post-meal) 1972
Ethmozine Tablets (Administration 30 minutes after a meal delays the rate of absorption but the extent of absorption is not altered) 2217
Famvir Tablets (Penciclovir C_{max} decreased approximately 50% and T_{max} was delayed by 1.5 hours when a capsule formulation of famciclovir was administered with food; there is no effect on the extent of availability (AUC) of penciclovir).. 2660
Fosamax Tablets (Standardized breakfast decreases bioavailability by approximately 40% when alendronate is administered either 0.5 or 1 hour before breakfast) 1703
Hismanal Tablets (Reduces the absorption by 60%; patients should be instructed to take Hismanal on an empty stomach, e.g. at least 2 hours after a meal) 1341
Hyzaar Tablets (Meal slows absorption and decreases C_{max} but has minor effects on losartan AUC or on the AUC of the metabolite) 1720
Lanoxicaps (The rate of absorption is slowed) 1110
Lanoxin Elixir Pediatric (Slows the rate of absorption) 1113
Lanoxin Tablets (Slows the rate of absorption) 1121
Lescol Capsules (Administration of fluvastatin with the evening meal results in a two-fold decrease in C_{max} and more than two-fold increase in t_{max} as compared to patients receiving the drug 4 hours after evening meal) 2395
Mevacor Tablets (When lovastatin was given under fasting conditions, plasma concentrations of total inhibitors were on average about two-thirds those found when lovastatin was administered immediately after a standard meal) 1742
Nalfon 200 Pulvules & Nalfon Tablets (Peak blood levels are delayed and diminished) 933
Nimotop Capsules (Administration of nimodipine capsules following a standard breakfast resulted in 68% lower peak plasma concentration and 38% lower bioavailability) 603
Norvir Capsules (Relative to fasting conditions, the extent of absorption of ritonavir from capsule formulation was 15% higher when administered with a meal; decreased peak ritonavir concentrations when oral solution was given under non-fasting condition) 447
PCE Dispertab Tablets (Optimal blood levels are obtained when PCE is given in the fasting state) 453
Prograf (The presence of food reduces the absorption of tacrolimus (decrease in AUC and C_{max}, and increase in T_{max}) 1028
Ticlid Tablets (Administration after meals results in a 20% increase in the AUC of ticlopidine) 2317
Tolectin (200, 400 and 600 mg) (Decreases total tolmetin bioavailability by 16%; reduces peak plasma concentrations by 50%) 1591
Vascor Tablets (200 and 300 mg) (May result in a clinically insignificant delay in time to peak concentration, but neither peak plasma levels nor the extent of absorption was changed) 1597

Meal, unspecified

Zerit Capsules (Co-administration with food decreases C_{max} by approximately 45%, however, the systemic availability (AUC) is unchanged; Zerit capsules can be taken without regard to meals).................. 731

Meat extracts
Nardil (Concurrent and/or sequential intake must be avoided).................. 1977
Parnate Tablets (Potential for hypertensive crisis; concurrent use is contraindicated).................. 2679

Meat prepared with tenderizers
Parnate Tablets (Potential for hypertensive crisis; concurrent use is contraindicated).................. 2679

Meat, unspecified
Nardil (Concurrent and/or sequential intake must be avoided).................. 1977

Milk
(see under Dairy products)

Milk products
(see under Dairy products)

Milk, low fat
Dyazide Capsules (Concurrent use of low-salt milk with triamterene may result in hyperkalemia, especially in patients with renal insufficiency).................. 2653

Milk, low salt
Dyrenium Capsules (Co-administration may promote serum potassium accumulation and possibly resulting in hyperkalemia).................. 2655

Mustard
(see under Food, furocoumarin-containing)

Orange Juice
Fosamax Tablets (Concomitant administration of alendronate with orange juice reduces bioavailability by approximately 60%).................. 1703

Parsley
(see under Food, furocoumarin-containing)

Parsnips
(see under Food, furocoumarin-containing)

Pepperoni
Nardil (Concurrent and/or sequential intake must be avoided).................. 1977

Raisins
Parnate Tablets (Potential for hypertensive crisis; concurrent use is contraindicated).................. 2679

Salami, hard
Nardil (Concurrent and/or sequential intake must be avoided).................. 1977

Salami, Genoa
Nardil (Concurrent and/or sequential intake must be avoided).................. 1977

Salt substitutes, potassium-containing
Altace Capsules (Increases risk of hyperkalemia).................. 1238

Sauerkraut
Nardil (Concurrent and/or sequential intake must be avoided).................. 1977
Parnate Tablets (Potential for hypertensive crisis; concurrent use is contraindicated).................. 2679

Sausage, dry
Nardil (Concurrent and/or sequential intake must be avoided).................. 1977

Sherry
Parnate Tablets (Potential for hypertensive crisis; concurrent use is contraindicated).................. 2679

Skipjack fish
Rifater (Isoniazid may inhibit diamine oxidase, causing exaggerated response (headache, sweating, palpitations, flushing, hypotension) to food containing histamine).................. 1280

Soy sauce
Parnate Tablets (Potential for hypertensive crisis; concurrent use is contraindicated).................. 2679

Soybean formula, children's
Synthroid Tablets (Binds and decreases absorption of levothyroxine sodium from the gastrointestinal tract).................. 1410

Tea
(see under Beverages, caffeine-containing)

Tonic water
Hismanal Tablets (May elevate plasma levels of astemizole and desmethyastemizole; potential for insignificant prolongation of the QT interval).................. 1341

Tuna fish
Rifater (Isoniazid may inhibit diamine oxidase, causing exaggerated response (headache, sweating, palpitations, flushing, hypotension) to food containing histamine).................. 1280

Vegetables, green leafy
Coumadin Tablets (Large amounts of green leafy vegetables may affect Coumadin therapy).................. 941

Wine products
(see also under Alcohol)
Nardil (Concurrent and/or sequential intake must be avoided).................. 1977

Wine, unspecified
(see also under Alcohol)
Furoxone Liquid (Concurrent and/or sequential intake must be avoided).................. 2221
Matulane Capsules (Procarbazine exhibits some monoamine oxidase inhibitory activity; concurrent use should be avoided).................. 2300
Nardil (Concurrent and/or sequential intake must be avoided).................. 1977

Wine, Chianti
(see also under Alcohol)
Parnate Tablets (Potential for hypertensive crisis; concurrent use is contraindicated).................. 2679

Wine, red
Rifater (Isoniazid has some MAO inhibiting activity, an interaction with tyramine-containing food may occur).................. 1280

Yeast extract
Furoxone Liquid (Concurrent and/or sequential intake must be avoided).................. 2221
Nardil (Concurrent and/or sequential intake must be avoided).................. 1977
Parnate Tablets (Potential for hypertensive crisis; concurrent use is contraindicated).................. 2679

Yeast, brewer's
Nardil (Concurrent and/or sequential intake must be avoided).................. 1977

Yogurt
Matulane Capsules (Procarbazine exhibits some monoamine oxidase inhibitory activity; concurrent use should be avoided).................. 2300
Nardil (Concurrent and/or sequential intake must be avoided).................. 1977
Parnate Tablets (Potential for hypertensive crisis; concurrent use is contraindicated).................. 2679

SECTION 3

SIDE EFFECTS INDEX

Presented in this section is an alphabetical list of every side effect reported in the "Adverse Reactions" section of the product descriptions in PDR and its companion volumes. Under each side effect is an alphabetical list of brands associated with the reaction.

If noted in the underlying text, incidence is shown in parentheses immediately after the brand name. Products reporting an incidence rate of 3% or more are marked with a ▲ symbol at their left. Because incidence data are sometimes drawn from controlled clinical trials, the rates seen in actual clinical practice may vary from those found in the published reports.

This index lists only side effects noted in official prescribing information as published by PDR. To alert you to the full range of possibilities, the entries include adverse effects shared by an entire class of drugs, but not necessarily reported for the specific drug in question. The index is restricted to reactions that may be expected to occur at recommended dosages in the general patient population. Precautions to be taken under special circumstances are not listed, nor are the effects of overdosage.

The page numbers shown for the products refer to the 1997 editions of PDR and PDR For Ophthalmology, and the 1996 edition of PDR For Nonprescription Drugs, which is published later in the year. A key to the symbols denoting the companion volumes appears in the bottom margin.

A

A-V block
- Adenocard Injection 1021
- Atretol Tablets 569
- Blocadren Tablets (Less than 1%) 1654
- Brethaire Inhaler 830
- Calan SR Caplets (0.8% to 1.2%) 2571
- Calan Tablets (0.8% to 1.2%) 2568
- Cardene I.V. (Rare) 2815
- ▲ Cardizem SR Capsules (0.6% to 7.6%) 1255
- Cardizem Tablets (Less than 1%) 1257
- Cartrol Tablets 413
- Catapres Tablets (Rare) 679
- Catapres-TTS 680
- Cognex Capsules (Rare) 1961
- Combipres Tablets (Rare) 682
- Cordarone Intravenous 2821
- Corvert Injection (1.5%) 2075
- Covera-HS Tablets (0.8% to 2%) 2573
- Dilacor XR Extended-release Capsules 2183
- Diprivan Injectable Emulsion (Less than 1%) 2939
- Ethmozine Tablets 2217
- Inderide Tablets 2838
- Inderide LA Long Acting Capsules 2840
- Isoptin Injectable (Rare) 1391
- Isoptin Oral Tablets (0.8 to 1.2%) 1393
- Isoptin SR Tablets (0.8% to 1.2%) 1395
- Kerlone Tablets 2588
- Kytril Injection (Rare) 2667
- Lanoxicaps 1110
- Lanoxin Elixir Pediatric (Common) 1113
- Lanoxin Injection 1116
- ▲ Lanoxin Injection Pediatric (Among most common) 1119
- Lanoxin Tablets 1121
- Levatol Tablets 2547
- LUVOX Tablets (Rare) 2723
- Mexitil Capsules (Less than 1% or about 2 in 1,000) 684
- Nipent for Injection (Less than 3%) 2733
- Normodyne Tablets 2522
- Norpace (Less than 1%) 2596
- Pepcid Injection (Infrequent) 1765
- Pepcid (Infrequent) 1763
- Permax Tablets (Infrequent) 571
- Prostigmin Injectable 1305
- Prostigmin Tablets 1306
- ReoPro Vials (1.3%) 1526
- Risperdal Tablets (Infrequent) 1348
- Salagen Tablets (Rare) 1546
- Sectral Capsules 2914
- Serzone Tablets (Rare) 776
- Tagamet (Rare) 2694
- Tambocor Tablets 1555
- Taxol Injection 723
- Tegretol/Tegretol-XR 870
- Timolide Tablets 1791
- Tonocard Tablets (Less than 1%) 519
- Verelan Capsules (0.8 to 1.2%) 1455
- Zantac (Rare) 1182
- Zantac Injection (Rare) 1180
- Zantac Syrup (Rare) 1182

A-V block, first-degree
- Adenocard Injection 1021
- Adenoscan (2.9% to 3%) 1022
- Calan SR Caplets (1.2%) 2571
- Calan Tablets (1.2%) 2568
- Cardizem CD Capsules (2.4% to 3.3%) 1251
- ▲ Cardizem SR Capsules (1.8% to 7.6%) 1255
- Cardizem Injectable (Less than 1%) 1253
- Cardizem Tablets (Less than 1%) 1257
- Covera-HS Tablets (1.2% to 1.7%) 2573
- Dilacor XR Extended-release Capsules (Infrequent) 2183
- Effexor (Rare) 2825
- Foscavir Injection (Between 1% and 5%) 541
- Isoptin Oral Tablets (1.2%) 1393
- Isoptin SR Tablets (1.2%) 1395
- Mavik Tablets (0.3% to 1.0%) 1407
- Prozac Pulvules & Liquid, Oral Solution (Rare) 935
- ▲ Rythmol Tablets–150mg, 225mg, 300mg (0.8 to 4.5%) 1399
- Sular Tablets (Less than or equal to 1%) 2961
- Verelan Capsules (1.2%) 1455

A-V block, intensification of
- Blocadren Tablets 1654
- Cartrol Tablets 413
- Inderal 2834
- Inderal LA Long Acting Capsules 2836
- Inderide Tablets 2838
- Inderide LA Long Acting Capsules 2840
- Levatol Tablets 2547
- Lopressor HCT Tablets 850
- Sectral Capsules 2914
- Tenoretic Tablets 2963
- Toprol-XL Tablets 560
- Trandate Tablets 1158
- Visken Tablets 2428

A-V block, second-degree
- Adenocard Injection 1021
- Adenoscan (2.6% to 3%) 1022
- Blocadren Tablets (Less than 1%) 1654
- Calan SR Caplets (0.8%) 2571
- Calan Tablets (0.8%) 2568
- Cardizem CD Capsules (Less than 1%) 1251
- Cardizem SR Capsules (0.6%) 1255
- Cardizem Injectable (Less than 1%) 1253
- Cardizem Tablets (Less than 1%) 1257
- Covera-HS Tablets (0.8% to 2%) 2573
- Cozaar Tablets (Less than 1%) 1668
- Hyzaar Tablets 1720
- Isoptin Oral Tablets (0.8%) 1393
- Isoptin SR Tablets (0.8%) 1395
- Rythmol Tablets–150mg, 225mg, 300mg (1.2%) 1399
- Tambocor Tablets (Less than 1%) 1555
- Tiazac Capsules (Less than 1%) 1019
- Verelan Capsules (0.8% to 1.2%) 1455

A-V block, third-degree
- Adenocard Injection 1021
- Adenoscan (0.8%; less than 1%) 1022
- Blocadren Tablets (Less than 1%) 1654
- Calan SR Caplets (0.8%) 2571
- Calan Tablets (0.8%) 2568
- Cardizem CD Capsules (Less than 1%) 1251
- Cardizem SR Capsules (Less than 1%) 1255
- Cardizem Injectable 1253
- Cardizem Tablets (Less than 1%) 1257
- Covera-HS Tablets (0.8% to 2%) 2573
- Isoptin Oral Tablets (0.8%) 1393
- Isoptin SR Tablets (0.8%) 1395
- Tambocor Tablets (Less than 1%) 1555
- Tiazac Capsules (Less than 1%) 1019
- Verelan Capsules (0.8% to 1.2%) 1455

A-V conduction, prolongation
- Isoptin Injectable 1391
- Sensorcaine 554

A-V conduction changes, unspecified
- Elavil 2945
- Nimotop Capsules 603

A-V shunt, thrombosis of (see under Thrombosis of vascular access)

Abdominal adhesion
- ParaGard T 380A Intrauterine Copper Contraceptive 1936

(⊡ Described in PDR For Nonprescription Drugs)   Incidence data in parenthesis; ▲ 3% or more   (⊚ Described in PDR For Ophthalmology)

Abdominal bloating
Side Effects Index
1242

Abdominal bloating

AeroBid Inhaler System (Less than 1%) 1004
Aerobid-M Inhaler System (Less than 1%) 1004
Asacol Delayed-Release Tablets 2129
Atromid-S Capsules 2808
Brevicon 2563
Climara Transdermal System 640
▲ Clomid (5.5%) 1262
Colestid (Less frequent) 2073
▲ Colyte and Colyte-flavored (Among most frequent) 2540
▲ Creon (Among most frequent) 2714
Demulen 2580
DiaBeta Tablets (1.8%) 1265
Estraderm Transdermal System 842
ESTRATAB Tablets (0.3, 0.625, 1.25, 2.5 mg) 2715
Estratest 2718
▲ Glucophage Tablets (Among most common) 754
Glynase PresTab Tablets (1.8%) 2091
▲ GoLYTELY (Up to 50%) 694
Hivid Tablets (Less than 1%) 2287
Humegon for Injection 1873
Levlen/Tri-Levlen 646
Metrodin (urofollitropin for injection) 2616
Midamor Tablets (Less than or equal to 1%) 1746
Moduretic Tablets (Less than or equal to 1%) 1748
Motrin Ibuprofen Suspension, Oral Drops, Chewable Tablets, Caplets (1% to less than 3%) 1563
Mycelex-G 500 mg Vaginal Tablets (Rare) 602
Mykrox Tablets (Less than 2%) 1617
Norinyl 2563
Noroxin Tablets (Less frequent) 1758
Noroxin Tablets (Less frequent) 2222
▲ Norpace (3 to 9%) 2596
Nor-Q D Tablets 2598
Norvir (Less than 2%) 447
▲ NuLYTELY (Up to 50% of patients) 694
▲ Cherry Flavor NuLYTELY (Among most common) 694
Ogen Tablets 2103
Ogen Vaginal Cream 2106
Pergonal (menotropins for injection, USP) 2618
PMB 200 and PMB 400 2890
Premarin Intravenous 2893
Premarin Tablets 2896
Premarin Vaginal Cream 2898
Premphase 2900
Prempro 2905
Prilosec Delayed-Release Capsules (Less than 1%) 516
Roferon-A Injection (Infrequent) 2308
▲ THROMBATE III Antithrombin III (Human) (1 of 17) 631
Ticlid Tablets (0.5% to 1.0%) 2317
Toradol (Greater than 1%) 2319
Trental Tablets (0.6%) 1291
Levlen/Tri-Levlen 646
Tri-Norinyl 2607
Vivelle Transdermal System 880
Zaroxolyn Tablets 1625

Abdominal discomfort (see also under Distress, gastrointestinal; Distress, abdominal)

Aquasol A Vitamin A Capsules, USP 525
Aquasol A Parenteral 526
Biaxin (2%) 406
Brevibloc (esmolol HCl) Injection (Less than 1%) 1860
BuSpar Tablets (2%) 738
Carafate Tablets (Less than 0.5%) 1249
Children's Motrin Ibuprofen Oral Suspension 1558
Cipro I.V. (1.7%) 587
Cipro Tablets (0.3% to 1%) 584
▲ Clomid (5.5%) 1262
▲ Clozaril Tablets (4%) 2377
Colestid (Less frequent) 2073
CordyMax Cs-4 Capsules (One case) 2985
Correctol Laxative Tablets & Caplets ■ 761
Crystodigin Tablets 1472
Cytoxan (Less frequent) 700
Dalgan Injection (Less than 1%) 529
Desferal Vials 838
Dulcolax 883
DynaCirc CR Tablets (1.3% to 5.1%) 2383
▲ E.E.S. (Most frequent) 427
▲ E-Mycin Tablets (One of the two most frequent) 1388
▲ EryPed 200 & EryPed 400 Granules (Most frequent) 425
Feldene Capsules (Greater than 1%) 2008
Flagyl I.V. 2373
Fleet Bisacodyl Enema 1000
Fleet Prep Kits 1002
Hyperstat I.V. Injection 2504
Imodium Capsules 1343
K-Dur Microburst Release System (potassium chloride, USP) E.R. Tablets 1364
Lomotil 2591
Mykrox Tablets (Less than 2%) 1617
▲ Neoral (Up to 7%) 2405
Papaverine Hydrochloride Vials and Ampoules 1523
Parlodel 2411
Pepcid Injection (Infrequent) 1765
Pepcid (Infrequent) 1763
▲ Rowasa (8.10%) 2727
▲ Sandimmune (Less than 1 to 7%) 2416
▲ Serophene (clomiphene citrate tablets, USP) (Approximately 1 in 15 patients) 2621
▲ Slow-K Extended-Release Tablets (Among most common) 869
Tonocard Tablets (Less than 1%) 519
Trental Tablets 1291
Urocit-K Tablets (Some patients) 1828
▲ Visken Tablets (4%) 2428

Abdominal distention

Aldoclor Tablets 1638
Aldomet Ester HCl Injection 1642
Aldomet Oral 1640
Aldoril Tablets 1644
Cataflam Tablets (1% to 3%) 833
Celestone Soluspan Suspension 2484
▲ CellCept Capsules (More than or equal to 3%) 2265
Claritin-D Tablets (Less frequent) 2487
▲ Clomid (5.5%) 1262
Clozaril Tablets (Less than 1%) 2377
CORTENEMA 2713
Cortone Acetate Sterile Suspension 1663
Cortone Acetate Tablets 1664
Crixivan Capsules (Less than 2%) 1670
Cytovene (1% or less) 2270
Dalalone D.P. Injectable 1009
Decadron Elixir 1676
Decadron Phosphate Injection 1680
Decadron Phosphate with Xylocaine Injection, Sterile 1683
Decadron Tablets 1678
Decadron-LA Sterile Suspension 1687
Dexacort Phosphate in Respihaler 1606
Dexacort Phosphate in Turbinaire 1607
Duragesic Transdermal System (Less than 1%) 1336
DynaCirc CR Tablets (1.2%) 2383
Effexor (Infrequent) 2825
Ensure Plus High Calorie Complete Nutrition 2338
Estring Vaginal Ring (At least 1 report) 2086
Florinef Acetate Tablets 506
Fosamax Tablets (1.0%) 1703
Humegon for Injection 1873
Hydeltrasol Injection, Sterile 1708
Hydeltra-T.B.A. Sterile Suspension 1710
Hydrocortone Acetate Sterile Suspension 1712
Hydrocortone Phosphate Injection, Sterile 1713
Hydrocortone Tablets 1715
Imodium Capsules 1343
Indocin I.V. (1% to 3%) 1727
Intron A for Injection (Less than 5%) 2506
Lamictal Tablets (Rare) 1105
▲ Leukine (4%) 1317
Lupron Depot - 3 Month 22.5 mg (Less than 5%) 2743
Mavik Tablets (0.3% to 1.0%) 1407
Merrem I.V. (0.1% to 1.0%) 2952
▲ Metrodin (urofollitropin for injection) (Approximately 20%) 2616
Monopril Tablets (0.2% to 1.0%) 762
Naprelan Tablets (Less than 1%) 2861
NuLYTELY 694
▲ Cherry Flavor NuLYTELY (Among most common) 694
Osmolite HN High Nitrogen Isotonic Liquid Nutrition 2339
Pediapred Oral Solution 1618
Pentasa (Less than 1%) 1275
Pergonal (menotropins for injection, USP) 2618
Permax Tablets (Infrequent) 571
Prelone Syrup 1834
▲ Prograf (Greater than 3%) 1028
Prozac Pulvules & Liquid, Oral Solution (Rare) 935
Remeron Tablets (Infrequent) 1878
Rilutek Tablets (Infrequent) 2198
Risperdal Tablets (Rare) 1348
▲ Sandostatin Injection (Less than 10%) 2421
Serophene (clomiphene citrate tablets, USP) 2621
Serzone Tablets (Infrequent) 776
▲ Taxotere for Injection Concentrate (6%) 2204
Unasyn (Less than 1%) 2035
▲ Vesanoid Capsules (11%) 2327
Cataflam/Voltaren/Voltaren-XR (1% to 3%) 833
Zoloft Tablets (Rare) 2051
Zyrtec Tablets (Less than 2%) 2053

Abdominal mass

Demulen 2580
Estratest 2718

Abdominal pain/cramps

▲ Abelcet Injection (3% to 5%) 1540
Accupril Tablets (1.0%) 1950
Accutane Capsules 2252
▲ Actigall Capsules (43.2%) 818
▲ Actimmune (8%) 1043
Adalat CC (Less than 1.0%) 582
▲ AeroBid Inhaler System (3% to 9%) 1004
▲ Aerobid-M Inhaler System (3% to 9%) 1004
▲ Albenza Tablets (Up to 6.0%) 2629
Aldactazide Tablets 2556
Aldactone Tablets 2558
Aldoclor Tablets 1638
Aldoril Tablets 1644
Altace Capsules (Less than 1%) 1238
Ambien Tablets (2%) 2559
Amicar Syrup, Tablets, and Injection 1312
Aminohippurate Sodium Injection 1646
▲ Anafranil Capsules (11% to 13%) 819
▲ Anaprox/Naprosyn (3% to 9%) 2277
Ancef Injection 2632
Ancobon Capsules 2254
Apresazide Capsules 824
Aralen Hydrochloride Injection 2430
Aralen Phosphate Tablets 2431
▲ Aredia for Injection (Up to at least 15%) 827
▲ Arimidex Tablets (5.7% to 6.9%) 2932
▲ Asacol Delayed-Release Tablets (18%) 2129
Asendin Tablets (Less than 1%) 1419
Atamet Tablets 567
Atretol Tablets 569
▲ Avonex (9%) 662
▲ Axid Pulvules (7.5%) 1468
▲ Axocet Capsules (Among most frequent) 2469
Azactam for Injection (Less than 1%) 736
Azathioprine Tablets (Rare) 2349
Azulfidine (Rare) 2059
Bactrim DS Tablets 2257
Bactrim I.V. Infusion 2255
Bactrim 2257
Bentyl 1246
Betapace Tablets (Less than 1% to 3%) 637
▲ Betaseron for SC Injection (32%) 653
Biaxin (2% to 3%) 406
Blocadren Tablets 1654
Brevicon 2563
Bumex (0.2%) 2260
Capoten Tablets (About 0.5 to 2%) 740
Capozide Tablets (0.5 to 2%) 744
Carbastat Intraocular Solution ⊙ 260
Cardene I.V. (0.7%) 2815
Cardura Tablets (2.4%) 1993
Carnitor Tablets and Solution 2624
Cartrol Tablets (1.3%) 413
▲ Casodex Tablets (8%) 2934
▲ Cataflam Tablets (3% to 9%) 833
Catapres Tablets (Rare) 679
Cedax (1% to 2%) 2480
Cefotan 2936
Ceftin (0.1% to 1%) 1067
Cefzil Tablets and Oral Suspension (1%) 747
▲ CellCept Capsules (24.7% to 27.6%; 11.9% to 12.1%) 2265
Celontin Kapseals (Frequent) 1955
Ceptaz (One in 416 patients) 1070
Ceredase 1055
Cervidil (Less than 1%) 1008
▲ Chemet Capsules (5.2% to 15.7%) 666
Cipro I.V. (1% or less) 587
Cipro I.V. Pharmacy Bulk Package (Less than 1%) 590
Cipro Tablets (1.7%) 584
Claritin-D Tablets (Less frequent) 2487
Cleocin Phosphate Injection 2068
Cleocin T Topical 2072
Climara Transdermal System 640
Cleocin Vaginal Cream (Less than 1% to 2%) 2070
▲ Clinoril Tablets (10%) 1658
Clomid 1262
▲ Cognex Capsules (8%) 1961
ColBENEMID Tablets 1662
Colestid (Less frequent) 2073
Colyte and Colyte-flavored 2540
Cordarone Tablets (1 to 3%) 2818
Correctol Laxative Tablets & Caplets ■ 761
Cosmegen Injection 1666
Coumadin (Infrequent) 941
Cozaar Tablets (1% or greater) 1668
▲ Creon (Among most frequent) 2714
▲ Crixivan Capsules (8.7%) 1670
Crystodigin Tablets 1472
Cytosar-U Sterile Powder (Less frequent) 2077
▲ Cytotec (13% to 20%) 2576
▲ Cytovene (17%) 2270
Cytoxan (Less frequent) 700
DDAVP Injection (Infrequent) 2178
DDAVP Injection 15 mcg/mL (Infrequent) 2179
DDAVP (2%) 2180
DDAVP Tablets 2182
Dalgan Injection (Less than 1%) 529
Dalmane Capsules (Rare) 2329
Dantrium Capsules (Less frequent) 2131
Dapsone Tablets USP 1331
Darvon-N/Darvocet-N 1473
Darvon 1475
Darvon-N Suspension & Tablets 1473
▲ DaunoXome (3% to 20%) 1842
Daypro Caplets (1% to 3%) 2578
Demser Capsules (Infrequent) 1690
Demulen 2580
Depakene 416
▲ Depakote Tablets (9%) 418
▲ Depo-Provera Contraceptive Injection (More than 5%) 2079
Desmopressin Acetate Injection (Infrequent) 996
Desmopressin Acetate Rhinal Tube (2%) 997
Desogen Tablets 1867
Diethylstilbestrol Tablets 1477
▲ Diflucan Tablets, Injection, and Oral Suspension (1.7% to 6%) 2003
Dilacor XR Extended-release Capsules (1.0%) 2183
Dilaudid-HP Injection (Less frequent) 1384
Dilaudid-HP Lyophilized Powder 250 mg (Less frequent) 1384
▲ Dipentum Capsules (10.1%) 2084
Diprivan Injectable Emulsion (Less than 1%) 2939
Disalcid 1549
Diucardin Tablets 2824
Diuril Sodium Intravenous 1693
Doral Tablets 2773
Doxil (1% to 5%) 2613
DUPHALAC Solution 2714
▲ Duragesic Transdermal System (3% to 10%) 1336
Duricef Capsules, Tablets, and Oral Suspension 750
Dyazide Capsules 2653
▲ Dynabac (9.7%) 668
▲ E.E.S. (Most frequent) 427
▲ E-Mycin Tablets (One of the most frequent) 1388
▲ EC-Naprosyn Delayed-Release Tablets (3% to 9%) 2277
Edecrin 1698
▲ Effexor (2.2% to 8.0%) 2825
▲ Eldepryl Capsules (4 of 49 patients) 2729
Elspar 1700
Enduron Tablets 424
Engerix-B Unit-Dose Vials (Less than 1%) 2656

(■ Described in PDR For Nonprescription Drugs) Incidence data in parenthesis; ▲ 3% or more (⊙ Described in PDR For Ophthalmology)

Side Effects Index — Abdominal pain/cramps

Ensure Plus High Calorie Complete Nutrition ... 2338
▲ Epivir (6% to 9%) ... 1200
▲ Ergamisol Tablets (2% to 5%) ... 1340
▲ ERYC (Among most frequent) ... 1972
▲ EryPed (Among most frequent) ... 425
▲ Ery-Tab Tablets (Among most frequent) ... 426
▲ Erythrocin Stearate Filmtab (Among most frequent) ... 429
▲ Erythromycin Base Filmtab (Among most frequent) ... 430
▲ Erythromycin Delayed-Release Capsules, USP (Among most frequent) ... 431
▲ Esgic-plus Capsules (Among most frequent) ... 1012
▲ Esgic-plus Tablets (Among most frequent) ... 1012
Esidrix Tablets ... 839
Esimil Tablets ... 840
Eskalith ... 2658
Estrace Cream and Tablets ... 751
Estraderm Transdermal System ... 842
ESTRATAB (0.3, 0.625, 1.25, 2.5 mg) ... 2715
Estratest ... 2718
▲ Estring Vaginal Ring (4%) ... 2086
Ethiodol Injection ... 2472
▲ Ethmozine Tablets (2% to 5%) ... 2217
Etopophos for Injection (Infrequent) ... 701
Etoposide Injection (Infrequent) ... 539
▲ Famvir Tablets (1.1% to 3.9%) ... 2660
Fansidar Tablets ... 2281
▲ Felbatol (5.3%) ... 2774
Feldene Capsules (Greater than 1%) ... 2008
▲ Fioricet Tablets (Among most frequent) ... 2386
Fioricet with Codeine Capsules (Frequent) ... 2387
▲ Fiorinal with Codeine Capsules (3.7%) ... 2390
Flagyl 375 Capsules ... 2587
Fleet Bisacodyl Enema ... 1000
Fleet Prep Kits ... 1002
▲ Flolan for Injection (5% to 27%) ... 1085
Floxin I.V. (1% to 3%) ... 1580
Floxin Tablets (200 mg, 300 mg, 400 mg) (1% to 3%) ... 1577
Flumadine Tablets & Syrup (1.4%) ... 1013
Fortaz (1 in 416) ... 1092
▲ Fosamax Tablets (6.6%) ... 1703
▲ Foscavir Injection (5% or greater) ... 541
Sterile FUDR ... 2284
▲ Fungizone Intravenous (Among most common) ... 507
Gamimune N, 5% Immune Globulin Intravenous (Human), 5% ... 612
Gamimune N, 10% Immune Globulin Intravenous (Human), 10% ... 615
Gammar-P I.V., Immune Globulin Intravenous (Human) ... 798
Gantanol Tablets ... 2285
Gantrisin ... 2286
Gastrocrom Capsules (2 of 87 patients) ... 1611
Gastrocrom Oral Concentrate (2 of 87 patients) ... 1611
Geocillin Tablets ... 2009
GoLYTELY (Infrequent) ... 694
▲ Habitrol Nicotine Transdermal System (3% to 9% of patients) ... 884
Halcion Tablets (0.9% to 0.5%) ... 2093
Havrix (Less than 1%) ... 2663
▲ Helidac Therapy (3.0%) ... 2135
Hismanal Tablets (1.4%) ... 1341
Hivid Tablets (Less than 1% to 3.0%) ... 2287
Humegon for Injection ... 1873
Humorsol Sterile Ophthalmic Solution (Rare) ... 1707
▲ Hycamtin for Injection (Less than 1% to 33%) ... 2665
HydroDIURIL Tablets ... 1716
Hylorel Tablets (1.7%) ... 1613
Hytrin Capsules (At least 1%) ... 434
Hyzaar Tablets (1.2%) ... 1720
IBU Tablets (Greater than 1%) ... 1389
▲ Idamycin Injection (73%) ... 2096
▲ Ilosone (One of the two most frequent) ... 927
Imdur (Less than or equal to 5%) ... 1362
Imodium Capsules ... 1343
▲ Imovax Rabies Vaccine (About 20%) ... 899
Imuran (Rare) ... 1103
Inderal ... 2834

Inderal LA Long Acting Capsules ... 2836
Inderide Tablets ... 2838
Inderide LA Long Acting Capsules ... 2840
Indocin (Greater than 1%) ... 1723
INFeD (Iron Dextran Injection, USP) ... 2478
Inocor Lactate Injection (0.4%) ... 2439
▲ Intron A for Injection (1% to 21%) ... 2506
Invirase Capsules (Rare) ... 2291
IOPIDINE Sterile Ophthalmic Solution ... ⊙ 218
Isopto Carbachol Ophthalmic Solution ... ⊙ 221
Ismo Tablets (Fewer than 1%) ... 2844
▲ JE-VAX (Approximately 10%) ... 904
K-Dur Microburst Release System (potassium chloride, USP) E.R. Tablets ... 1364
▲ K-Lor Powder Packets (Among most common) ... 438
▲ K-Norm Capsules (Among most common) ... 1615
Kadian Capsules (Less than 3%) ... 2948
Keflex Pulvules & Oral Suspension ... 930
Keftab Tablets ... 931
Ku-Zyme HP Capsules ... 2547
▲ Kytril Tablets (6%) ... 2669
▲ Lamictal Tablets (5.2%) ... 1105
Lamisil Tablets (2.4%) ... 2394
▲ Lamprene Capsules (40-50%) ... 846
Lanoxicaps (Very rare) ... 1110
Lanoxin Elixir Pediatric (Very rare) ... 1113
Lanoxin Injection (Very rare) ... 1116
Lanoxin Injection Pediatric (Very rare) ... 1119
Lanoxin Tablets (Very rare) ... 1121
▲ Lariam Tablets (Among most frequent) ... 2295
Larodopa Tablets (Relatively frequent) ... 2296
Lasix Injection, Oral Solution and Tablets ... 1267
▲ Lescol Capsules (4.9%) ... 2395
Leukine (38%) ... 1317
▲ Leustatin (6%) ... 1889
Levlen/Tri-Levlen ... 646
Levo-Dromoran ... 2297
Lioresal Intrathecal (1% or more) ... 1634
Lioresal Tablets (Rare) ... 847
Lithonate/Lithotabs/Lithobid ... 2721
▲ Lodine Capsules and Tablets (3% to 9%) ... 2849
Lo/Ovral Tablets ... 2852
Lo/Ovral-28 Tablets ... 2857
▲ Lopid Tablets (9.8%) ... 1974
Lopressor (Less than 1%) ... 848
Lorabid Suspension and Pulvules (1.4%) ... 1513
Lotensin HCT Tablets (0.3% to 1.0%) ... 855
Lotrel Capsules ... 858
Ludiomil Tablets (Rare) ... 861
LUVOX Tablets ... 2723
MS Contin Tablets (Less frequent) ... 2149
MSIR (Infrequent) ... 2152
Macrobid Capsules (Less than 1%) ... 2138
Macrodantin Capsules (Less common) ... 2140
Marax Tablets & DF Syrup (Frequent, on empty stomach) ... 2015
▲ Marinol (Dronabinol) Capsules (3% to 10%) ... 2353
Massengill Disposable Douche ... 2627
Massengill Medicated Disposable Douche ... 2628
Matulane Capsules ... 2300
Mavik Tablets (0.3% to 1.0%) ... 1407
Maxair Autohaler ... 1550
Maxair Inhaler (Less than 1%) ... 1552
Maxaquin Tablets (Less than 1%) ... 2593
Megace Oral Suspension (1% to 3%) ... 708
Menest Tablets ... 2671
▲ Mepron Suspension (4% to 10%) ... 1206
Merrem I.V. (0.1% to 1.0%) ... 2952
Mestinon Injectable ... 1300
Mestinon ... 1300
Methadone Hydrochloride Oral Concentrate ... 2356
▲ Metrodin (urofollitropin for injection) (Approximately 20%) ... 2616
MetroGel-Vaginal (Equal to or less than 3.4%) ... 917
▲ Mevacor Tablets (2.0% to 5.7%) ... 1742
Mexitil Capsules (1.2%) ... 684
Miacalcin Injection ... 2402
Miacalcin Nasal Spray (1% to 3%) ... 2403
Micro-K ... 2237

Micro-K LS Packets (Among most common) ... 2238
Micronor Tablets (Rare) ... 1903
▲ Midamor Tablets (Between 1% and 3%) ... 1746
Minipress Capsules (Less than 1%) ... 2015
Minizide Capsules (Rare) ... 2016
MIOSTAT Intraocular Solution ... ⊙ 222
Modicon ... 1928
Moduretic Tablets (Greater than 1%, less than 3%) ... 1748
Monoket Tablets (Up to 2%) ... 2550
Monopril Tablets (0.2% to 1.0% or more) ... 762
Motrin Ibuprofen Suspension, Oral Drops, Chewable Tablets, Caplets (1% to less than 3%) ... 1563
Myambutol Tablets ... 1432
Mycelex-G 500 mg Vaginal Tablets (Rare) ... 602
▲ Mycobutin Capsules (4%) ... 2101
Mykrox Tablets (Less than 2%) ... 1617
Myochrysine Injection ... 1754
Nalfon 200 Pulvules & Nalfon Tablets (2%) ... 933
▲ Naprelan Tablets (3% to 9%) ... 2861
Anaprox/Naprosyn (3% to 9%) ... 2277
NegGram ... 2453
Neupogen for Injection (Infrequent) ... 495
Neurontin Capsules (More than 1%) ... 1978
Nicotrol NS Nicotine Nasal Spray (3%) ... 1565
▲ Nipent for Injection (4% to 16%) ... 2733
Nizoral Tablets (1.2%) ... 1345
Nolvadex Tablets (1%) ... 2957
Nordette-21 Tablets ... 2863
Nordette-28 Tablets ... 2866
Norinyl ... 2563
Normodyne Tablets ... 2522
Noroxin Tablets (0.3% to 1.6%) ... 1758
Noroxin Tablets (0.3% to 1.6%) ... 2222
▲ Norpace (3 to 9%) ... 2596
Norpramin Tablets ... 1273
Nor-Q D Tablets ... 2598
Norvasc Tablets (1.6%) ... 2020
▲ Norvir (3.4% to 7.0%) ... 447
▲ Novantrone for Injection (9 to 15%) ... 1327
Nubain Injection (1% or less) ... 952
NuLYTELY (Less frequent) ... 694
Cherry Flavor NuLYTELY (Less frequent) ... 694
Ogen Tablets ... 2103
Ogen Vaginal Cream ... 2106
▲ Oncaspar (Greater than 1% but less than 5%) ... 2194
Oncovin Solution Vials & Hyporets ... 1521
Oramorph SR (Morphine Sulfate Sustained Release Tablets) (Less frequent) ... 2359
▲ Orlaam Oral Solution (3% to 9%) ... 2361
Ornade Spansule Capsules ... 2678
Ortho-Cept ... 1907
Ortho-Cyclen/Ortho-Tri-Cyclen ... 1914
Ortho Dienestrol Cream ... 1922
Ortho-Est ... 1925
Ortho-Novum ... 1928
Ortho-Cyclen/Ortho Tri-Cyclen ... 1914
Orthoclone OKT3 Sterile Solution ... 1892
▲ Orudis Capsules (3% to 9%) ... 2874
▲ Oruvail Capsules (3% to 9%) ... 2874
Osmolite HN High Nitrogen Isotonic Liquid Nutrition ... 2339
Ovcon ... 765
Ovral Tablets ... 2877
Ovral-28 Tablets ... 2878
Ovrette Tablets ... 2878
OxyContin Tablets (Between 1% and 5%) ... 2163
▲ PCE Dispertab Tablets (Among most frequent) ... 453
Pamelor ... 2409
ParaGard T 380A Intrauterine Copper Contraceptive ... 1936
▲ Parlodel (3% to 9%) ... 2411
Parnate Tablets ... 2679
▲ PASER Granules (Among most common) ... 1333
▲ Paxil Tablets (4%) ... 2681
▲ Pediazole Suspension (Among most frequent) ... 2340
Penetrex Tablets (Less than 1% to 2%) ... 2196
Pentasa (1.1% to 1.7%) ... 1275
Peptavlon ... 2997
Pergonal (menotropins for injection, USP) ... 2618
Peri-Colace Capsules and Syrup ... 2226

▲ Permax Tablets (5.8%) ... 571
▲ Phrenilin (Among most frequent) ... 790
Plaquenil Sulfate Tablets ... 2459
Plendil Extended-Release Tablets (0.5% to 1.5%) ... 514
PMB 200 and PMB 400 ... 2890
Pondimin Tablets ... 2239
Ponstel ... 1982
▲ Pravachol Tablets (2.0% to 5.4%) ... 770
▲ Precose (21%) ... 604
Premarin Intravenous ... 2893
Premarin Tablets ... 2896
Premarin Vaginal Cream ... 2898
Premphase ... 2900
Prempro ... 2905
Prevacid Delayed-Release Capsules (1.8%) ... 2746
▲ Prilosec Delayed-Release Capsules (2.4% to 5.2%) ... 516
Primaxin I.M. ... 1770
Primaxin I.V. (Less than 0.2%) ... 1772
▲ Prinivil Tablets (0.3% to 4.0%) ... 1776
Prinzide Tablets (0.3 to 1%) ... 1780
▲ Procanbid Extended-Release Tablets (3% to 4%) ... 1983
Procardia Capsules (2% or less) ... 2024
Procardia XL Extended Release Tablets (Less than 3%) ... 2026
Proglycem (Frequent) ... 575
▲ Prograf (26% to 59%) ... 1028
▲ Proleukin for Injection (15%) ... 812
▲ Propulsid (10.2%) ... 1346
ProSom Tablets (1%) ... 457
Prostep (nicotine transdermal system) (1% to 3% of patients) ... 1439
▲ Prostigmin Injectable (Most common) ... 1305
Prostigmin Tablets ... 1306
Protostat Tablets (Occasional) ... 1939
▲ Prozac Pulvules & Liquid, Oral Solution (3.4%) ... 935
Pulmozyme Inhalation ... 1054
Questran (Less frequent) ... 774
▲ Rabies Vaccine, Imovax Rabies I.D. (About 20%) ... 901
Recombivax HB (Less than 1%) ... 1787
▲ Redux Capsules (6.7%) ... 2911
▲ Relafen Tablets (12%) ... 2688
Remeron Tablets (Frequent) ... 1878
RespiGam ... 1631
▲ Retrovir Capsules (3.2%) ... 1216
▲ Retrovir I.V. Infusion (4%) ... 1221
▲ Retrovir Syrup (3.2%) ... 1216
▲ ReVia Tablets (More than 10%) ... 957
Revex (nalmefene hydrochloride injection) ... 1863
▲ Ridaura Capsules (14%) ... 2691
Rifadin (Some patients) ... 1276
Rifater ... 1280
▲ Rilutek Tablets (6.8% to 7.8%) ... 2198
Rimactane Capsules ... 865
Risperdal Tablets (1% to 4%) ... 1348
Ritalin ... 866
Rocephin Injectable Vials, ADD-Vantage, Galaxy Container (Rare) ... 2305
▲ Roferon-A Injection (15%) ... 2308
▲ Rowasa (3.0 to 8.10%) ... 2727
Rythmol Tablets–150mg, 225mg, 300mg (0.8 to 1.9%) ... 1399
▲ Salagen Tablets (4%) ... 1546
Salflex Tablets ... 791
Sansert Tablets ... 2424
Sectral Capsules (Up to 2%) ... 2914
▲ Sedapap Tablets 50 mg/650 mg (Among the most frequent) ... 1826
Septra ... 1146
Septra I.V. Infusion ... 1142
Septra I.V. Infusion ADD-Vantage Vials ... 1144
Septra ... 1146
Ser-Ap-Es Tablets ... 867
Serevent Inhalation Aerosol (1% to 3%) ... 1149
Serophene (clomiphene citrate tablets, USP) ... 2621
Serzone Tablets ... 776
Sinemet Tablets ... 959
Sinemet CR Tablets ... 961
Solganal Suspension (Rare) ... 2530
Sporanox Capsules (1.4% to 1.5%) ... 1352
Stimate, (desmopressin acetate) Nasal Spray, 1.5 mg/mL (Infrequent) ... 806
▲ Supprelin Injection (1% to 12%) ... 2230
▲ Suprax (3%) ... 1443
Surmontil Capsules ... 2917
Talwin Injection (Rare) ... 2465
▲ Tambocor Tablets (3.3%) ... 1555
Tao Capsules (Most frequent) ... 2033

(▣ Described in PDR For Nonprescription Drugs) Incidence data in parenthesis; ▲ 3% or more (⊙ Described in PDR For Ophthalmology)

Abdominal pain/cramps — Side Effects Index — 1244

Taxotere for Injection Concentrate 2204
Tazicef for Injection (Less than 2%; 1 in 416 patients) 2697
Tazidime Vials, Faspak & ADD-Vantage (1 in 416) 1531
▲ Tegison Capsules (25-50%) 2314
Tegretol/Tegretol-XR 870
Tenex Tablets (3% or less) 2249
Tensilon Injectable 1307
▲ Terazol 3 Vaginal Cream (3.4%) 1941
▲ TheraCys BCG Live (Intravesical) (2.7% to 6.3%) 911
Thioplex (Thiotepa For Injection) 1329
▲ TICE BCG, USP (1.5% to 4.0%) 1881
Tilade Inhaler (1.2%) 2207
Tofranil Ampuls 873
Tofranil Tablets 875
Tofranil-PM Capsules 876
▲ Tolectin (200, 400 and 600 mg) (3 to 9%) 1591
Tonocard Tablets (Less than 1%) 519
Levlen/Tri-Levlen 646
Trinalin Repetabs Tablets 1373
Tri-Norinyl 2607
Triphasil-21 Tablets (Occasional) 2919
Triphasil-28 Tablets 2924
Tylenol with Codeine 1592
Typhim Vi 914
Ultram Tablets (50 mg) (1% to less than 5%) 1594
Ultrase Capsules 2476
▲ Ultrase MT Capsules (5.7%) 2477
Univasc Tablets (Less than 1%) 2553
Urecholine 1804
Valtrex Caplets (2% to 3%) 1167
Vancocin HCl, Vials & ADD-Vantage 1534
Vantin for Oral Suspension and Vantin Tablets (Less than 1% to 1.6%) 2112
Vaqta (1.1% to 1.6%) 1805
Varivax (Greater than or equal to 1%) 1807
▲ Vascor Tablets (200 and 300 mg) (3.02%) 1597
Vaseretic Tablets (0.5% to 2.0%) 1810
Vasotec I.V. 1814
Vasotec Tablets (1.6%) 1816
Velban Vials 1537
VePesid Capsules and Injection (Infrequent; up to 2%) 727
Vermox Chewable Tablets 1357
▲ Vesanoid Capsules (31%) 2327
▲ Videx Tablets, Powder for Oral Solution, & Pediatric Powder for Oral Solution (7% to 35%) 2980
Viramune Tablets (1%) 2368
▲ Vistide Injection (17%) 1057
Vivactil Tablets 1820
Vivelle Transdermal System 880
Vivotif Berna 660
▲ Cataflam/Voltaren/Voltaren-XR (3% to 9%) 833
Wygesic Tablets 2930
Yodoxin Tablets 1235
Zantac 1182
Zantac Injection 1180
Zantac Syrup 1182
Zarontin Capsules (Frequent) 1986
Zarontin Syrup (Frequent) 1986
Zaroxolyn Tablets 1625
Zebeta Tablets 1457
▲ Zerit Capsules (4% to 34%) 731
Zestoretic Tablets (0.3 to 1.0%) 2968
Zestril Tablets (0.3% to 2.2%) 2972
Ziac 1459
Zinacef 1184
▲ Zithromax (2% to 5%) 2043
▲ Zithromax Tablets (3% to 5%) 2046
▲ Zocor Tablets (3.2%) 1821
Zofran Injection (2%) 1227
Zofran Tablets (1% to 3%) 1231
▲ Zoladex (7%) 2976
Zoladex 3-month (1% to 5%) 2978
Zoloft Tablets (2.4%) 2051
Zosyn (1.3%) 1463
Zovirax Capsules (0.6%) 1187
Zovirax Sterile Powder (Less than 1%) 1191
Zovirax (0.6%) 1187
Zyloprim Tablets (Less than 1%) 1194
Zyrtec Tablets (Less than 2%) 2053

Abdominal symptom complex, acute

Clomid (Fewer than 1%) 1262
Permax Tablets (Rare) 571
Questran (One patient) 774
Remeron Tablets (Frequent) 1878

Abortion

Amen Tablets 785
Effexor (Rare) 2825
Imitrex Tablets (Rare) 1099
Methotrexate Sodium Tablets, Injection, for Injection and LPF Injection 1322
Metrodin (urofollitropin for injection) (3 reported) 2616
Paxil Tablets (Infrequent) 2681
Permax Tablets (Infrequent) 571
Prozac Pulvules & Liquid, Oral Solution (Rare) 935

Abortion, septic

ParaGard T 380A Intrauterine Copper Contraceptive 1936

Abortion, spontaneous

Accutane Capsules 2252
Depo-Provera Sterile Aqueous Suspension 2083
Lupron Depot-PED 7.5 mg, 11.25 mg and 15 mg (Possible) 2744
Nolvadex Tablets (A small number of reports) 2957
ParaGard T 380A Intrauterine Copper Contraceptive 1936
▲ Parlodel (11.4%) 2411
Redux Capsules (Rare) 2911
Syntocinon Injection 2425
Vermox Chewable Tablets 1357

Abscess

Ambien Tablets (Rare) 2559
Aramine Injection 1649
Avonex 662
Betaseron for SC Injection 653
Capastat Sulfate Injection 968
Celestone Soluspan Suspension 2484
Cortone Acetate Sterile Suspension 1663
Cytovene (1% or less) 2270
Dalalone D.P. Injectable 1009
Decadron Phosphate Injection 1680
Decadron Phosphate with Xylocaine Injection, Sterile 1683
Decadron-LA Sterile Suspension 1687
Depo-Provera Sterile Aqueous Suspension (A few instances) 2083
Diphtheria and Tetanus Toxoids and Pertussis Vaccine Adsorbed 2650
Doxil (Less than 1%) 2613
Foscavir Injection (Between 1% and 5%) 541
Sterile FUDR 2284
Hydeltrasol Injection, Sterile 1708
Hydeltra-T.B.A. Sterile Suspension 1710
Hydrocortone Acetate Sterile Suspension 1712
Hydrocortone Phosphate Injection, Sterile 1713
INFeD (Iron Dextran Injection, USP) 2478
Intron A for Injection (Less than 5%) 2506
Invirase Capsules (Less than 2%) 2291
Lamictal Tablets (Rare) 1105
▲ Lupron Depot-PED 7.5 mg, 11.25 mg and 15 mg (5%) 2744
Naprelan Tablets (Less than 1%) 2861
▲ Neoral (4.4%) 2405
Nipent for Injection (2%) 2733
Paxil Tablets (Rare) 2681
Permax Tablets (Infrequent) 571
▲ Prograf (Greater than 3%) 1028
Rilutek Tablets (Infrequent) 2198
▲ Sandimmune (4.4 to 5.3%) 2416
TICE BCG, USP (1.8%) 1881
Videx Tablets, Powder for Oral Solution, & Pediatric Powder for Oral Solution (Less than 1%) 2980

Abscess at injection site

Ceredase 1055
Cleocin Phosphate Injection 2068
Cytovene-IV (1% or less) 2270
Lupron Depot 3.75 mg 2739
Lupron Depot 7.5 mg 2741
Lupron Depot - 3 Month 22.5 mg 2743
Lupron Injection Pediatric 2737
MSTA Mumps Skin Test Antigen 2988
PedvaxHIB 1761

Abscess, periesophageal

Ethamolin Injection (0.1 to 0.4%) 2544

Abscess, periodontal

Avonex 662
Betaseron for SC Injection 653
Depakote Tablets (1% to 5%) 418
Hivid Tablets (Less than 1%) 2287
Naprelan Tablets (Less than 1%) 2861
Norvir (Less than 2%) 447
Permax Tablets (Infrequent) 571
Serzone Tablets (Infrequent) 776

Abscess, tubo-ovarian

ParaGard T 380A Intrauterine Copper Contraceptive 1936

Abuse

Astramorph/PF Injection, USP (Preservative-Free) 526
Cafergot 2376
Fioricet with Codeine Capsules 2387
Fiorinal with Codeine Capsules 2390
Miltown Tablets 2780
Prozac Pulvules & Liquid, Oral Solution 935

Accommodation, impaired

AK-CIDE (Occasional) ⊙ 203
AK-CIDE Ointment (Occasional) ⊙ 203
Amaryl Tablets 1241
Ambien Tablets (Rare) 2559
Anafranil Capsules (Infrequent) 819
Aralen Hydrochloride Injection 2430
Aralen Phosphate Tablets 2431
Asendin Tablets (Less than 1%) 1419
Atrovent Inhalation Aerosol (About 1 in 100) 674
Blephamide Liquifilm Sterile Ophthalmic Suspension 472
Blephamide Ointment (Occasional) ⊙ 234
Clomid 1262
Crixivan Capsules (Less than 2%) 1670
DiaBeta Tablets 1265
Econopred & Econopred Plus Ophthalmic Suspensions (Occasional) ⊙ 216
▲ Effexor (5.6% to 9.1%) 2825
Elavil 2945
Etrafon 2495
FML Forte Liquifilm (Occasional) ⊙ 237
FML Liquifilm (Occasional) ⊙ 238
FML S.O.P. (Occasional) ⊙ 239
Glynase PresTab Tablets 2091
Lamictal Tablets (Infrequent) 1105
Limbitrol 2333
Lioresal Intrathecal (1% or more) 1634
Ludiomil Tablets (Rare) 861
LUVOX Tablets (Infrequent) 2723
Micronase Tablets 2099
Neurontin Capsules (Rare) 1978
Norpramin Tablets 1273
Norvasc Tablets (Less than or equal to 0.1%) 2020
▲ Orap Tablets (4 of 20 patients) 1037
Pamelor 2409
Paxil Tablets (Infrequent) 2681
Plaquenil Sulfate Tablets 2459
PMB 200 and PMB 400 2890
Pred Forte (Occasional) ⊙ 247
Pred Mild (Occasional) ⊙ 250
Protopam Chloride for Injection 2909
Redux Capsules (Rare) 2911
Remeron Tablets (Infrequent) 1878
Risperdal Tablets (Infrequent) 1348
Ritalin 866
Serzone Tablets (Infrequent) 776
Surmontil Capsules 2917
Tofranil Ampuls 873
Tofranil Tablets (Rare) 875
Tofranil-PM Capsules 876
Transderm Scōp Transdermal Therapeutic System 890
Triavil Tablets 1800
Urispas Tablets 2710
Vivactil Tablets 1820
Zantac (Rare) 1182
Zantac Injection (Rare) 1180
Zantac Syrup (Rare) 1182
Zofran Injection 1227
Zoloft Tablets (Infrequent) 2051
Zyrtec Tablets (Less than 2%) 2053

Accommodation, paresis

Tripedia 908

Accommodation, spasm

Pilagan ⊙ 245
Tensilon Injectable 1307

Aches

Asacol Delayed-Release Tablets 2129
Cartrol Tablets 413
Cipro I.V. (1% or less) 587
Cipro I.V. Pharmacy Bulk Package (Less than 1%) 590
Cipro Tablets (Less than 1%) 584
Cytotec (Infrequent) 2576
Eldepryl Capsules (1 of 49 patients) 2729
Gammar-P I.V., Immune Globulin Intravenous (Human) 798
Humegon for Injection 1873
Humorsol Sterile Ophthalmic Solution 1707
Hydropres Tablets 1718
Inderal 2834
Inderal LA Long Acting Capsules 2836
Inderide Tablets 2838
Inderide LA Long Acting Capsules 2840
Kerlone Tablets 2588
Levatol Tablets 2547
Lysodren Tablets (Infrequent) 707
Methadone Hydrochloride Oral Concentrate 2356
Midamor Tablets (Less than or equal to 1%) 1746
Normodyne Tablets 2522
Orlaam Oral Solution 2361
Orthoclone OKT3 Sterile Solution 1892
Pergonal (menotropins for injection, USP) 2618
Recombivax HB (Less than 1%) 1787
Sectral Capsules 2914
Tenoretic Tablets 2963
Tenormin Tablets and I.V. Injection 2965
Teslac Tablets 727
Timoptic in Ocudose 1796
Timoptic Sterile Ophthalmic Solution 1794
Timoptic-XE 1798
Toprol-XL Tablets 560
Trandate Tablets 1158
Trilafon 2532
Visken Tablets 2428
Ziac 1459

Aches, joints (see under Arthralgia)

Acid-base disturbances

Demadex Tablets and Injection 691

Acidosis

Abbokinase 403
Abbokinase Open-Cath 405
▲ Abelcet Injection (3%) 1540
Achromycin V Capsules 1417
▲ CellCept Capsules (More than or equal to 3%) 2265
Cipro I.V. (1% or less) 587
Cipro I.V. Pharmacy Bulk Package (Less than 1%) 590
Cipro Tablets (Less than 1%) 584
Cytovene-IV (Two or more reports) 2270
Dyazide Capsules 2653
Fleet Enema 1001
Floxin I.V. 1580
Floxin Tablets (200 mg, 300 mg, 400 mg) 1577
Foscavir Injection (Between 1% and 5%) 541
IBU Tablets (Less than 1%) 1389
IFEX (Rare) 706
Indocin I.V. (Less than 3%) 1727
Kerlone Tablets (Less than 2%) 2588
Maxaquin Tablets 2593
Minocin Intravenous 1428
Minocin Oral Suspension 1431
Minocin Pellet-Filled Capsules 1429
Motrin Ibuprofen Suspension, Oral Drops, Chewable Tablets, Caplets (Less than 1%) 1563
Permax Tablets (Rare) 571
Proglycem (Infrequent) 575
▲ Prograf (Greater than 3%) 1028
▲ Proleukin for Injection (16%) 812
Sulfamylon Cream 940
▲ Vesanoid Capsules (3%) 2327
Videx Tablets, Powder for Oral Solution, & Pediatric Powder for Oral Solution (Less than 1%) 2980

Acidosis, hypochloremic metabolic

Neoral (Occasional) 2405
Sandimmune (Occasional) 2416

Acidosis, metabolic

Cerebyx Injection (Infrequent) 1956
Daranide Tablets 1676
Diamox Intravenous (Occasional) ⊙ 317
Diamox Sequels (Sustained Release) ⊙ 318
Diamox Tablets (Occasional) ⊙ 317
Diprivan Injectable Emulsion (Less than 1%) 2939
Etopophos for Injection 701
Etoposide Injection 539

(Described in PDR For Nonprescription Drugs) Incidence data in parenthesis; ▲ 3% or more (⊙ Described in PDR For Ophthalmology)

Side Effects Index

Fludara for Injection ... 658
GlaucTabs ... ⊚ 209
Hespan Injection ... 945
▲ IFEX (31%) ... 706
Nardil (Less frequent) ... 1977
NegGram (Rare) ... 2453
Neptazane Tablets ... ⊚ 320
Nydrazid Injection ... 509
Oncaspar ... 2194
Rifamate Capsules ... 1278
Rifater ... 1280
Sensorcaine ... 554
VePesid Capsules and Injection ... 727
Vistide Injection (Less than 1%) ... 1057

Acidosis, renal tubular
Abelcet Injection ... 1540
▲ Fungizone Intravenous (Among most common) ... 507
IFEX (1 episode) ... 706
Zanosar Sterile Powder ... 2119

Acidosis, respiratory
▲ Diprivan Injectable Emulsion (3% to 10%) ... 2939
Rilutek Tablets (Infrequent) ... 2198

Acne
(see under Acneiform eruptions)

Acne fulminaris
Accutane Capsules ... 2252

Acne vulgaris
Hyland's ClearAc ... ⊞ 789

Acne, cystic, flare-up
Parnate Tablets ... 2679

Acne, transient exacerbation of
Accutane Capsules ... 2252
Oxandrin ... 783

Acneiform eruptions
Aclovate (Infrequent) ... 1061
AeroBid Inhaler System (1% to 3%) ... 1004
Aerobid-M Inhaler System (1% to 3%) ... 1004
Ambien Tablets (Rare) ... 2559
Amen Tablets (Few cases) ... 785
Anafranil Capsules (Up to 2%) ... 819
Analpram-HC Rectal Cream 1% and 2.5% ... 993
Androderm Testosterone Transdermal System (Less than 1%) ... 2634
▲ Android Capsules, 10 mg (Among most common) ... 1297
Antabuse Tablets (Small number of patients) ... 2802
Anusol-HC Cream 2.5% (Infrequent to frequent) ... 1953
Asacol Delayed-Release Tablets (1% to 2%) ... 2129
Brevicon ... 2563
BuSpar Tablets (Rare) ... 738
▲ CellCept Capsules (9.7% to 10.1%) ... 2265
Claritin-D Tablets (Less frequent) ... 2487
Clomid ... 1262
Cognex Capsules (Infrequent) ... 1961
Cordran Lotion (Infrequent) ... 1854
Cordran Tape (Infrequent) ... 1855
Cormax Ointment (Infrequent) ... 1856
Cormax Scalp Application (Infrequent) ... 1857
Cortifoam ... 2540
Cortisporin Cream ... 1073
Cortisporin Ointment ... 1074
Cortisporin Otic Solution Sterile ... 1076
Cortisporin Otic Suspension Sterile ... 1077
Cosmegen Injection ... 1666
Cutivate Cream ... 1078
Cutivate Ointment (Infrequent to more frequent) ... 1078
Cycrin Tablets (A few cases) ... 991
Cytovene (1% or less) ... 2270
Danocrine Capsules ... 2437
Dantrium Capsules (Less frequent) ... 2131
Decadron Phosphate Topical Cream ... 1686
Decaspray Topical Aerosol ... 1689
Demulen ... 2580
Depo-Provera Contraceptive Injection (1% to 5%) ... 2079
Depo-Provera Sterile Aqueous Suspension ... 2083
Dermatop Emollient Cream 0.1% (Infrequent to frequent) ... 1264
Desogen Tablets ... 1867

DesOwen Cream, Ointment and Lotion (Infrequent) ... 1032
Diprolene AF Cream 0.05% (Infrequent) ... 2489
Diprolene Gel 0.05% (Infrequent) ... 2490
Diprolene Lotion 0.05% (1%) ... 2491
Diprolene Ointment 0.05% (Infrequent) ... 2491
Effexor (Infrequent) ... 2825
Elocon Cream 0.1% (Infrequent) ... 2492
Elocon Lotion 0.1% (Infrequent) ... 2493
Elocon Ointment 0.1% (Infrequent) ... 2494
Epifoam (Infrequent) ... 2543
Eskalith ... 2658
Estratest ... 2718
▲ Felbatol (3.4%) ... 2774
Florinef Acetate Tablets ... 506
Florone/Florone E ... 921
Foscavir Injection (Less than 1%) ... 541
Halog (Infrequent) ... 2795
Halotestin Tablets ... 2095
Hivid Tablets (Less than 1%) ... 2287
Hytone ... 922
Hytone Ointment 2 ½% ... 923
Imdur (Less than or equal to 5%) ... 1362
Intron A for Injection (Less than 5%) ... 2506
Invirase Capsules (Less than 2%) ... 2291
Lamictal Tablets (1.3%) ... 1105
Lamprene Capsules (Less than 1%) ... 846
Levlen/Tri-Levlen ... 646
Lidex (Infrequent) ... 2299
Lithonate/Lithotabs/Lithobid ... 2721
Lotrisone Cream (Infrequent) ... 2515
Lupron Depot-PED 7.5 mg, 11.25 mg and 15 mg (2%) ... 2744
Lupron Injection Pediatric ... 2737
LUVOX Tablets (Infrequent) ... 2723
Mantadil Cream ... 1124
Methotrexate Sodium Tablets, Injection, for Injection and LPF Injection ... 1322
Micronor Tablets ... 1903
Modicon ... 1928
Naprelan Tablets (Less than 1%) ... 2861
NeoDecadron Topical Cream ... 1757
Neoral (1% to 2%) ... 2405
Neurontin Capsules (More than 1%) ... 1978
▲ Nicotrol NS Nicotine Nasal Spray (3%) ... 1565
Nimotop Capsules (Up to 1.4%) ... 603
Nipent for Injection (Less than 3%) ... 2733
Norinyl ... 2563
Norisodrine with Calcium Iodide Syrup ... 446
Norplant System ... 2868
Nor-Q D Tablets ... 2598
Norvir (Less than 2%) ... 447
Ortho-Cept ... 1907
Ortho-Cyclen/Ortho-Tri-Cyclen ... 1914
Ortho-Novum ... 1928
Ortho-Cyclen/Ortho Tri-Cyclen ... 1914
Ovcon ... 765
Oxandrin ... 783
Pandel Cream, 0.1% ... 2475
Paxil Tablets (Infrequent) ... 2681
Pediotic Suspension Sterile ... 1140
Pentasa (0.2%) ... 1275
Pentaspan Injection ... 954
Pepcid Injection (Infrequent) ... 1765
Pepcid (Infrequent) ... 1763
Permax Tablets (Infrequent) ... 571
Pramosone Cream, Lotion & Ointment ... 995
Premphase ... 2900
Prempro ... 2905
Prevacid Delayed-Release Capsules (Less than 1%) ... 2746
ProctoCream-HC 2.5% (Infrequent to frequent) ... 2552
ProctoFoam-HC ... 2552
ProSom Tablets (Rare) ... 457
Provera Tablets (A few cases) ... 2110
Prozac Pulvules & Liquid, Oral Solution (2%) ... 935
Psorcon Cream 0.05% (Infrequent) ... 924
Psorcon Ointment 0.05% ... 923
Pyrazinamide Tablets (Rare) ... 1442
Relafen Tablets (Less than 1%) ... 2688
Retrovir Capsules ... 1216
Retrovir I.V. Infusion ... 1221
Retrovir Syrup ... 1216
ReVia Tablets (Less than 1%) ... 957
Rifater (Rare) ... 1280
Risperdal Tablets (Infrequent) ... 1348
Rowasa (1.2%) ... 2727

▲ Sandimmune (1 to 6%) ... 2416
Serzone Tablets (Infrequent) ... 776
Sular Tablets (Less than or equal to 1%) ... 2961
▲ Supprelin Injection (3% to 10%) ... 2230
Synalar (Infrequent) ... 2299
▲ Synarel Nasal Solution for Central Precocious Puberty (10%) ... 2603
▲ Synarel Nasal Solution for Endometriosis (13% of patients) ... 2605
Temovate Cream ... 1152
Temovate E Emollient (Infrequent) ... 1154
Temovate Gel (Infrequent) ... 1153
Temovate Ointment ... 1152
Temovate Scalp Application (Infrequent) ... 1153
Testoderm Testosterone Transdermal System (Four in 104 patients) ... 486
Testred Capsules, 10 mg. ... 1308
Topicort Emollient Cream 0.25% (Infrequent) ... 1289
Topicort Gel 0.05% (Infrequent) ... 1290
Topicort LP Emollient Cream 0.05% (Infrequent) ... 1289
Topicort Ointment 0.25% (Infrequent) ... 1291
Tridesilon Cream 0.05% ... 609
Tridesilon Ointment 0.05% ... 610
Levlen/Tri-Levlen ... 646
Tri-Norinyl ... 2607
Ultravate Cream 0.05% (Infrequent) ... 2797
Ultravate Ointment 0.05% (Less frequent) ... 2798
Vantin for Oral Suspension and Vantin Tablets (Less than 1%) ... 2112
Videx Tablets, Powder for Oral Solution, & Pediatric Powder for Oral Solution (Less than 1%) ... 2980
Vistide Injection ... 1057
Wellbutrin Tablets (Rare) ... 1177
Westcort Cream 0.2% (Infrequent) ... 2799
Westcort Ointment 0.2% ... 2800
Winstrol Tablets ... 2468
Yodoxin Tablets ... 1235
Zebeta Tablets ... 1457
Ziac ... 1459
▲ Zoladex (42%) ... 2976
Zoladex 3-month ... 2978
Zoloft Tablets (Infrequent) ... 2051
Zyrtec Tablets (Less than 2%) ... 2053

Acneiform reactions
Elocon Lotion 0.1% (2 in 209 patients) ... 2493
Haldol Decanoate ... 1587
Haldol Injection, Tablets and Concentrate ... 1585

Adams-Stokes syndrome
Isuprel Injection ... 2441

Adenitis
Asendin Tablets ... 1419
Clinoril Tablets ... 1658
Dolobid Tablets (Less than 1 in 100) ... 1695
Ludiomil Tablets (Isolated reports) ... 861
Norpramin Tablets (Rare) ... 1273
Pamelor (Rare) ... 2409
Pneumovax 23 (Rare) ... 1768
Pnu-Imune 23 (Rare) ... 1437
Surmontil Capsules ... 2917
Tofranil Ampuls (Rare) ... 873
Tofranil Tablets (Rare) ... 875
Tofranil-PM Capsules (Rare) ... 876
Vivactil Tablets (Rare) ... 1820

Adenoma, nephrogenic
TICE BCG, USP (Two cases) ... 1881

Adenomas, benign
Betaseron for SC Injection ... 653
Demulen ... 2580
Redux Capsules (Rare) ... 2911

Adenomas, endocrine system
Permax Tablets (Infrequent) ... 571

Adenopathy
Atretol Tablets ... 569
Miltown Tablets ... 2780
PMB 200 and PMB 400 ... 2890
Tegretol/Tegretol-XR ... 870
Tetanus Toxoid Adsorbed Purogenated ... 1447

Adenopathy, inguinal
Zovirax (0.3%) ... 1187

Adnexal enlargement
Norplant System ... 2868

Adnexal torsion, ovarian
Humegon for Injection ... 1873
Metrodin (urofollitropin for injection) ... 2616
Pergonal (menotropins for injection, USP) ... 2618
Serophene (clomiphene citrate tablets, USP) ... 2621

Adrenal insufficiency
Azmacort Oral Inhaler ... 2175
Beclovent Inhalation Aerosol and Refill ... 1063
Beconase ... 1065
Cortifoam ... 2540
Heparin Lock Flush Solution ... 2831
Heparin Sodium Injection ... 2832
Heparin Sodium Vials ... 1486
Megace Tablets (Rare) ... 710
Nasacort Nasal Inhaler ... 2189
Sporanox Capsules (Infrequent) ... 1352

Adrenergic syndrome, unspecified
Paxil Tablets (Rare) ... 2681

Adrenocortical suppression
Dermatop Emollient Cream 0.1% ... 1264
Dexacort Phosphate in Respihaler ... 1606
Dexacort Phosphate in Turbinaire ... 1607
Nasacort Nasal Inhaler ... 2189
ProctoCream-HC 2.5% ... 2552

Adrenocortical unresponsiveness, secondary
Celestone Soluspan Suspension ... 2484
CORTENEMA ... 2713
Cortone Acetate Sterile Suspension ... 1663
Cortone Acetate Tablets ... 1664
Dalalone D.P. Injectable ... 1009
Decadron Elixir ... 1676
Decadron Phosphate Injection ... 1680
Decadron Phosphate with Xylocaine Injection, Sterile ... 1683
Decadron Tablets ... 1678
Decadron-LA Sterile Suspension ... 1687
Dexacort Phosphate in Respihaler ... 1606
Dexacort Phosphate in Turbinaire ... 1607
Florinef Acetate Tablets ... 506
Hydeltrasol Injection, Sterile ... 1708
Hydeltra-T.B.A. Sterile Suspension ... 1710
Hydrocortone Acetate Sterile Suspension ... 1712
Hydrocortone Phosphate Injection, Sterile ... 1713
Hydrocortone Tablets ... 1715
Pediapred Oral Solution ... 1618
Prelone Syrup ... 1834

Afibrinogenemia
Depakene (One infant) ... 416
Depakote Tablets (One infant) ... 418
Syntocinon Injection ... 2425

Aftertaste
Antabuse Tablets (Small number of patients) ... 2802
Etopophos for Injection (Infrequent) ... 701
Etoposide Injection (Infrequent) ... 539
▲ Nasarel Nasal Solution (8% to 17%) ... 2302
Placidyl Capsules ... 456
VePesid Capsules and Injection (Infrequent) ... 727

Ageusia
▲ AeroBid Inhaler System (3% to 9%) ... 1004
▲ Aerobid-M Inhaler System (3% to 9%) ... 1004
Anafranil Capsules (Infrequent) ... 819
Beclovent Inhalation Aerosol and Refill (Rare) ... 1063
Beconase (Rare) ... 1065
Bentyl ... 1246
Betaseron for SC Injection ... 653
Capoten Tablets (Approximately 2 to 4 of 100 patients) ... 740
Capozide Tablets (Approximately 2 to 4 of 100 patients) ... 744
Cerebyx Injection (Infrequent) ... 1956
Claritin-D Tablets (Less frequent) ... 2487
Clinoril Tablets (Less than 1 in 100) ... 1658
▲ Depen Titratable Tablets (12%) ... 2770
▲ Didronel I.V. Infusion (5%) ... 1545
Donnatal ... 2234

(⊞ Described in PDR For Nonprescription Drugs)   Incidence data in parenthesis; ▲ 3% or more   (⊚ Described in PDR For Ophthalmology)

Donnatal Extentabs 2234
Donnatal Tablets 2234
Effexor (Infrequent) 2825
Elavil 2945
Flexeril Tablets (Less than 1%) 1701
Flumadine Tablets & Syrup (Less than 0.3%) 1013
Hivid Tablets (Less than 1%) 2287
Intron A for Injection (Less than 5%) 2506
Kerlone Tablets (Less than 2%) 2588
Lamictal Tablets (Rare) 1105
Lamisil Tablets (Rare) 2394
Levsin/Levsinex/Levbid 2549
Lioresal Intrathecal (1% or more) 1634
LUVOX Tablets (Infrequent) 2723
Nasalide Nasal Solution 0.025% 2301
Neptazane Tablets .... ⊙ 320
Neurontin Capsules (Infrequent) 1978
Nolvadex Tablets (Infrequent) 2957
Norvir (Less than 2%) 447
Paxil Tablets (Infrequent) 2681
Platinol for Injection 717
Platinol-AQ Injection 719
Pro-Banthine Tablets 2226
Proglycem (Frequent) 575
Prolixin 510
Prozac Pulvules & Liquid, Oral Solution (Rare) 935
Remeron Tablets (Rare) 1878
Rilutek Tablets (Rare) 2198
Robinul Forte Tablets 2247
Robinul Injectable 2247
Robinul Tablets 2247
Serzone Tablets (Rare) 776
Tapazole Tablets 1361
Tornalate Solution for Inhalation, 0.2% (Less than 1%) 976
Zyloprim Tablets (Less than 1%) 1194
Zyrtec Tablets (Less than 2%) 2053

Aggression

Ambien Tablets (Rare) 2559
Anafranil Capsules (Up to 2%) 819
Celontin Kapseals 1955
Claritin-D Tablets (Less frequent) 2487
Depakene 416
Depakote Tablets 418
Felbatol (Frequent) 2774
Floxin I.V. 1580
Floxin Tablets (200 mg, 300 mg, 400 mg) 1577
Foscavir Injection (Between 1% and 5%) 541
Halcion Tablets 2093
Imitrex Tablets (Rare) 1099
Intron A for Injection (Less than 5%) 2506
Prilosec Delayed-Release Capsules (Less than 1%) 516
Risperdal Tablets (1% to 3%) 1348
Seromycin Capsules 975
Ventolin Inhalation Aerosol and Refill (1%) 1170
Xanax Tablets (Rare) 2115
Zarontin Capsules 1986
Zarontin Syrup 1986
Zoloft Tablets (Infrequent) 2051
Zosyn (1.0% or less) 1463

Agitation

Akineton 1380
Alfenta Injection 1334
Ambien Tablets (Infrequent) 2559
Amoxil (Rare) 2631
Anafranil Capsules (Up to 3%) 819
Artane 1418
Atamet Tablets 567
Ativan Tablets (Less frequent) 2807
Atretol Tablets 569
Augmentin (Rare) 2637
Augmentin Tablets (Rare) 2640
Axocet Capsules (Infrequent) 2469
Betaseron for SC Injection 653
Bontril Slow-Release Capsules 786
Brevibloc (esmolol HCl) Injection (About 2%) 1860
Buprenex Injectable (Rare) 2170
Butisol Sodium Elixir & Tablets (Less than 1 in 100) 2768
Cardura Tablets (0.5% to 1%) 1993
Catapres Tablets (About 3 in 100 patients) 679
Catapres-TTS 680
Cedax (0.1% to 1%) 2480
▲ Cerebyx Injection (3.3%) 1956
Cipro Tablets 584
Claritin Tablets (2% or fewer patients) 2485
Claritin-D Tablets (Less frequent) 2487
▲ Clozaril Tablets (4%) 2377
▲ Cognex Capsules (7%) 1961
▲ Combipres Tablets (About 3%) 682
Compazine 2644
Crixivan Capsules (Less than 2%) 1670
Cytovene (1% or less) 2270
Demerol 2438
Depakote Tablets (1% to 5%) 418
Desyrel and Desyrel Dividose 504
Dexedrine 2648
Dilaudid-HP Injection (Less frequent) 1384
Dilaudid-HP Lyophilized Powder 250 mg (Less frequent) 1384
Dilaudid Tablets and Liquid (Less frequent) 1386
Diprivan Injectable Emulsion (Less than 1%) 2939
Donnatal (In elderly patients) 2234
Donnatal Extentabs (In elderly patients) 2234
Donnatal Tablets (In elderly patients) 2234
Doral Tablets 2773
Duragesic Transdermal System (1% or greater) 1336
▲ Effexor (2% to 4.5%) 2825
Eldepryl Capsules 2729
Elspar 1700
▲ Eminase (Less than 10%) 2215
Engerix-B Unit-Dose Vials (Less than 1%) 2656
Esgic-plus Capsules (Infrequent) 1012
Esgic-plus Tablets (Infrequent) 1012
Ethmozine Tablets (Less than 2%) 2217
Felbatol (Frequent) 2774
Fioricet Tablets (Infrequent) 2386
Fioricet with Codeine Capsules (Infrequent) 2387
Fiorinal with Codeine Capsules (Infrequent) 2390
Flexeril Tablets (Less than 1%) 1701
▲ Flolan for Injection (11%) 1085
Floxin I.V. 1580
Floxin Tablets (200 mg, 300 mg, 400 mg) 1577
Fludara for Injection 658
Flumadine Tablets & Syrup (0.3% to 1%) 1013
Foscavir Injection (Between 1% and 5%) 541
Halcion Tablets 2093
Haldol Decanoate 1587
Haldol Injection, Tablets and Concentrate 1585
Hivid Tablets (Less than 1%) 2287
Imitrex Injection (Infrequent) 1095
Imitrex Tablets (Up to 2%) 1099
Intron A for Injection (Less than 5%) 2506
Invirase Capsules (Less than 2%) 2291
Ismo Tablets (Fewer than 1%) 2844
Kadian Capsules (Less than 3%) 2948
Keflex Pulvules & Oral Suspension 930
Keftab Tablets 931
Kytril Injection (Less than 2%) 2667
Lamictal Tablets (Infrequent) 1105
Larodopa Tablets (Relatively frequent) 2296
Leukeran Tablets (Rare) 1205
Levsin/Levsinex/Levbid 2549
Lioresal Intrathecal (Up to 1.3%) 1634
Loxitane 1426
Ludiomil Tablets (2%) 861
Lufyllin & Lufyllin-400 Tablets 2778
Lufyllin-GG Elixir & Tablets 2779
LUVOX Tablets (2%) 2723
MS Contin Tablets (Less frequent) 2149
MSIR (Infrequent) 2152
Maxaquin Tablets (Less than 1%) 2593
Mebaral Tablets (Less than 1 in 100) 2452
Mellaril 2398
Mepergan Injection 2859
Merrem I.V. (0.1% to 1.0%) 2952
Methadone Hydrochloride Oral Concentrate 2356
Methadone Hydrochloride Oral Solution & Tablets 2357
Miacalcin Nasal Spray (Less than 1%) 2403
Nardil (Uncommon) 1977
Navane Capsules and Concentrate 2018
Navane Intramuscular 2019
Nembutal Sodium Capsules (Less than 1%) 440
Nembutal Sodium Solution (Less than 1%) 442
Nembutal Sodium Suppositories (Less than 1%) 444
Neurontin Capsules (Infrequent) 1978
Norflex 1554
Norgesic 1554
Norpramin Tablets 1273
Norvasc Tablets (Less than or equal to 0.1%) 2020
Norvir (Less than 2%) 447
Oramorph SR (Morphine Sulfate Sustained Release Tablets) (Less frequent) 2359
Orthoclone OKT3 Sterile Solution 1892
OxyContin Tablets (Less than 1%) 2163
Pamelor 2409
Parnate Tablets 2679
Paxil Tablets (1.1% to 5%) 2681
Penetrex Tablets (0.1% to 1%) 2196
Pepcid Injection (Infrequent) 1765
Pepcid (Infrequent) 1763
Permax Tablets (Infrequent) 571
Phenobarbital Elixir and Tablets (Less than 1 in 100 patients) 1523
Phrenilin (Infrequent) 790
Placidyl Capsules 456
Pondimin Tablets 2239
Prevacid Delayed-Release Capsules (Less than 1%) 2746
▲ Prograf (Greater than 3%) 1028
Proleukin for Injection 812
ProSom Tablets (Infrequent) 457
Prozac Pulvules & Liquid, Oral Solution (Frequent to 2%) 935
RMS Suppositories CII 2766
Recombivax HB 1787
Redux Capsules (Infrequent) 2911
Reglan 2243
Relafen Tablets (1%) 2688
Remeron Tablets (Frequent) 1878
Revex (nalmefene hydrochloride injection) (Less than 1%) 1863
Rilutek Tablets (Frequent) 2198
▲ Risperdal Tablets (22% to 26%) 1348
Roferon-A Injection 2308
▲ Romazicon (3% to 9%) 2311
Roxanol 2365
Salagen Tablets (Rare) 1546
Seconal Sodium Pulvules (Less than 1 in 100) 1529
Sedapap Tablets 50 mg/650 mg (Infrequent) 1826
Serentil 689
Serzone Tablets 776
Sinemet Tablets 959
Sinemet CR Tablets 961
Soma Compound w/Codeine Tablets (Infrequent or rare) 2784
Soma Compound Tablets (Very rare to infrequent) 2783
Soma Tablets 2782
Stadol (Less than 1%) 779
Stelazine 2692
Stimate, (desmopressin acetate) Nasal Spray, 1.5 mg/mL 806
Suprane (desflurane, USP) (Less than 1%) 1865
Surmontil Capsules 2917
Symmetrel Capsules (1% to 5%) 965
Symmetrel Syrup (1% to 5%) 963
Tagamet 2694
Tegretol/Tegretol-XR 870
Tenex Tablets (Less frequent) 2249
Thorazine 2701
Tofranil Ampuls 873
Tofranil Tablets 875
Tofranil-PM Capsules 876
Tonocard Tablets (Less than 1%) 519
Torecan 2367
Trental Tablets 1291
▲ Ultram Tablets (50 mg) (1% to 14%) 1594
Ventolin Inhalation Aerosol and Refill (1%) 1170
Versed Injection (Less than 1%) 2324
▲ Vesanoid Capsules (9%) 2327
Videx Tablets, Powder for Oral Solution, & Pediatric Powder for Oral Solution (Up to 1%) 2980
Vivactil Tablets 1820
▲ Wellbutrin Tablets (31.9%) 1177
Xanax Tablets (Rare; 2.9%) 2115
Zantac (Rare) 1182
Zantac Injection 1180
Zantac Syrup (Rare) 1182
Zithromax (1% or less) 2043
Zofran Injection (2%) 1227
▲ Zofran Tablets (6%) 1231
▲ Zoloft Tablets (5.6%) 2051
▲ Zosyn (2.1% to 7.1%) 1463
Zovirax Sterile Powder (Approximately 1%) 1191
Zyrtec Tablets (Less than 2%) 2053

Agnosia

▲ Vesanoid Capsules (3%) 2327

Agoraphobia

LUVOX Tablets (Infrequent) 2723

Agranulocytopenia

Sterile FUDR (Remote possibility) 2284

Agranulocytosis

Accupril Tablets (Rare) 1950
Adapin Capsules (Occasional) 1542
Albenza Tablets (Rare) 2629
Aldactazide Tablets (A few cases) 2556
Aldactone Tablets (A few cases) 2558
Aldoclor Tablets 1638
Aldoril Tablets 1644
Altace Capsules (Rare to more frequent) 1238
Amaryl Tablets 1241
Amicar Syrup, Tablets, and Injection 1312
Amoxil 2631
Anafranil Capsules 819
Anaprox/Naprosyn (Less than 1%) 2277
Ancobon Capsules 2254
Anturane (Rare) 823
Apresazide Capsules (Less frequent) 824
Apresoline Hydrochloride Tablets (Less frequent) 826
Asacol Delayed-Release Tablets (Rare) 2129
Asendin Tablets (Less than 1%) 1419
Atamet Tablets (Rare) 567
Atretol Tablets 569
Atrohist Plus Tablets 1605
Atromid-S Capsules 2808
Augmentin 2637
Augmentin Tablets 2640
Axocet Capsules 2469
Azulfidine (Rare) 2059
Bactrim DS Tablets (Rare) 2257
Bactrim I.V. Infusion (Rare) 2255
Bactrim (Rare) 2257
Benadryl Injection 1955
Blephamide Liquifilm Sterile Ophthalmic Suspension 472
▲ Blephamide Ointment (Among most often) .... ⊙ 234
Blocadren Tablets 1654
▲ Bromfed-DM Cough Syrup (Among most frequent) 1832
Capoten Tablets 740
Capozide Tablets 744
Cardioquin Tablets 2146
Cartrol Tablets 413
Cataflam Tablets (Rare) 833
Cedax 2480
Cefizox for Intramuscular or Intravenous Use 1025
Cefotan 2936
Ceftin 1067
Cefzil Tablets and Oral Suspension 747
Ceptaz (Very rare) 1070
Cipro I.V. 587
Cipro I.V. Pharmacy Bulk Package (Less than 1%) 590
Cipro Tablets 584
Claforan Sterile and Injection (Less than 1%) 1259
Cleocin Phosphate Injection 2068
Cleocin Vaginal Cream 2070
Clinoril Tablets (Less than 1%) 1658
Clozaril Tablets (1%; approximately 1.3%) 2377
ColBENEMID Tablets 1662
Combipres Tablets 682
Compazine 2644
Cosmegen Injection 1666
Cuprimine Capsules 1673
▲ Cytadren Tablets (4 out of 27) 837
Dapsone Tablets USP 1331
Daranide Tablets 1676
Depen Titratable Tablets 2770
DiaBeta Tablets 1265
Diabinese Tablets 2002
Diamox Intravenous .... ⊙ 317
Diamox Sequels (Sustained Release) .... ⊙ 318
Diamox Tablets .... ⊙ 317
Didronel Tablets (Rare) 2133
Diflucan Tablets, Injection, and Oral Suspension 2003
Dilantin Infatabs (Occasional) 1967
Dilantin Kapseals (Occasional) 1965
Dilantin-125 Suspension (Occasional) 1969
Dimetane-DC Cough Syrup 2232
Dimetane-DX Cough Syrup 2233
Diucardin Tablets 2824
Diupres Tablets 1691
Diuril Oral Suspension 1694

(▭ Described in PDR For Nonprescription Drugs)   Incidence data in parenthesis; ▲ 3% or more   (⊙ Described in PDR For Ophthalmology)

1247 Side Effects Index Alcohol abuse

Diuril Sodium Intravenous 1693
Diuril Tablets 1694
Dolobid Tablets (Less than 1 in 100) 1695
Duricef Capsules, Tablets, and Oral Suspension 750
Dyazide Capsules 2653
EC-Naprosyn Delayed-Release Tablets (Less than 1%) 2277
Edecrin 1698
Elavil 2945
Enduron Tablets 424
Ergamisol Tablets (One patient) 1340
Esgic-plus Capsules 1012
Esgic-plus Tablets 1012
Esidrix Tablets 839
Esimil Tablets 840
Etrafon 2495
FML-S Liquifilm ⊙ 240
Fansidar Tablets 2281
Felbatol (Rare) 2774
Fioricet Tablets 2386
Fioricet with Codeine Capsules 2387
Floxin I.V. 1580
Floxin Tablets (200 mg, 300 mg, 400 mg) 1577
Fluorouracil Injection 2282
Fortaz (Very rare) 1092
Fungizone Intravenous 507
Gantanol Tablets 2285
Gantrisin (Rare) 2286
Garamycin Injectable 2502
GlaucTabs ⊙ 209
Glucotrol Tablets 2011
Glucotrol XL Extended Release Tablets 2012
Glynase PresTab Tablets 2091
Haldol Decanoate (Rare) 1587
Haldol Injection, Tablets and Concentrate (Rare) 1585
Hydralazine Hydrochloride Injection USP (Less frequent) 2712
Hydrocet Capsules 787
HydroDIURIL Tablets 1716
Hydropres Tablets 1718
Hyzaar Tablets 1720
IBU Tablets (Less than 1%) 1389
Inderal 2834
Inderal LA Long Acting Capsules 2836
Inderide Tablets 2838
Inderide LA Long Acting Capsules 2840
Indocin Capsules (Less than 1%) 1723
Indocin I.V. (Less than 1%) 1727
Indocin (Less than 1%) 1723
Kefurox Vials, Faspak & ADD-Vantage 1509
Kerlone Tablets 2588
Larodopa Tablets (Rare) 2296
Lasix Injection, Oral Solution and Tablets (Rare) 1267
▲ Leukine (6%) 1317
Levatol Tablets 2547
Levoprome 1321
Librax Capsules (Occasional) 2330
Librium Capsules (Occasional) 2331
Librium Injectable (Occasional) 2332
Limbitrol 2333
Lodine Capsules and Tablets (Less than 1%) 2849
Lopressor (Rare) 848
Lopressor HCT Tablets 850
Lorabid Suspension and Pulvules 1513
Lortab 2751
Lotensin Tablets (Rare) 852
Lotensin HCT Tablets 855
Lotrel Capsules 858
Loxitane (Rare) 1426
Ludiomil Tablets (Isolated reports) 861
LUVOX Tablets 2723
Macrobid Capsules 2138
Macrodantin Capsules 2140
Mavik Tablets (Rare) 1407
Maxaquin Tablets 2593
Mellaril (Infrequent) 2398
Mepergan Injection (1 instance) 2859
Mesantoin Tablets 2400
Mexitil Capsules (About 1 in 1,000) 684
Micronase Tablets 2099
Miltown Tablets 2780
Minizide Capsules 2016
Moduretic Tablets 1748
Monopril Tablets 762
Motrin Ibuprofen Suspension, Oral Drops, Chewable Tablets, Caplets (Less than 1%) 1563
Mustargen (Relatively infrequent) 1752
Mykrox Tablets 1617
Mysoline Suspension 2860
Nalfon 200 Pulvules & Nalfon Tablets (Less than 1%) 933
▲ Naprelan Tablets (3% to 9%) 2861
Anaprox/Naprosyn (Less than 1%) 2277
Navane Capsules and Concentrate 2018
Navane Intramuscular 2019
Neptazane Tablets ⊙ 320
▲ Nipent for Injection (3% to 10%) 2733
Normodyne Tablets 2522
Noroxin Tablets 1758
Noroxin Tablets 2222
Norpace (Rare) 2596
Norpramin Tablets 1273
Nydrazid Injection 509
Omnipen Capsules 2872
Omnipen for Oral Suspension 2873
Oncaspar 2194
Oretic Tablets 450
Ornade Spansule Capsules 2678
Orudis Capsules (Less than 1%) 2874
Oruvail Capsules (Less than 1%) 2874
PBZ Tablets 863
PBZ-SR Tablets 862
Pamelor 2409
Parnate Tablets 2679
PASER Granules 1333
Pediazole Suspension 2340
Penetrex Tablets 2196
Pepcid Injection (Rare) 1765
Pepcid (Rare) 1763
Periactin 1767
Phenergan with Codeine (1 case) 2883
Phenergan with Dextromethorphan (1 case) 2885
Phenergan Injection 2880
Phenergan Suppositories (1 case) 2882
Phenergan Syrup (1 case) 2881
Phenergan Tablets (1 case) 2882
Phenergan VC (1 case) 2886
Phenergan VC with Codeine (1 case) 2888
Phrenilin (Infrequent) 790
Plaquenil Sulfate Tablets 2459
PMB 200 and PMB 400 2890
Ponstel (Occasional) 1982
Prilosec Delayed-Release Capsules (Rare) 516
Primaxin I.M. 1770
Primaxin I.V. 1772
Prinivil Tablets (Rare to frequent) 1776
Prinzide Tablets (Rare) 1780
Procanbid Extended-Release Tablets (Approximately 0.5%) 1983
Prolixin 510
ProSom Tablets (Rare) 457
Quinaglute Dura-Tabs Tablets 644
Quinidex Extentabs 2240
Redux Capsules 2911
Reglan (A few cases) 2243
Remeron Tablets (Three patients) 1878
Ridaura Capsules (Less than 0.1%) 2691
Rifamate Capsules 1278
Rifater 1280
Rythmol Tablets–150mg, 225mg, 300mg (Less than 1%) 1399
SSD 1402
Sectral Capsules 2914
Sedapap Tablets 50 mg/650 mg 1826
Septra 1146
Septra I.V. Infusion 1142
Septra I.V. Infusion ADD-Vantage Vials (Rare) 1144
Septra 1146
Ser-Ap-Es Tablets 867
Serax Capsules 2916
Serax Tablets 2916
Serentil 689
Silvadene Cream 1% 1288
Sinemet Tablets (Rare) 959
Sinemet CR Tablets 961
Sinequan (Occasional) 2028
Solganal Suspension (Rare) 2530
Spectrobid Tablets 2030
Stelazine 2692
Sultrin (One case) 1941
Suprax 1443
Surmontil Capsules 2917
Tagamet (Approximately 3 per 1,000,000) 2694
Talacen Caplets (Rare) 2464
Tapazole Tablets 1361
Tavist Syrup 2426
Tavist Tablets 2427
Tazicef for Injection (Very rare) 2697
Tazidime Vials, Faspak & ADD-Vantage (Very rare) 1531
Tegretol/Tegretol-XR (Very low incidence) 870
Tenoretic Tablets 2963
Tenormin Tablets and I.V. Injection 2965
Thalitone 1293
Thorazine 2701
Ticlid Tablets (Rare; 0.8%) 2317
Timolide Tablets 1791
Timoptic in Ocudose 1796
Timoptic Sterile Ophthalmic Solution 1794
Timoptic-XE 1798
Tofranil Ampuls 873
Tofranil Tablets 875
Tofranil-PM Capsules 876
Tolectin (200, 400 and 600 mg) (Less than 1%) 1591
Tonocard Tablets (Less than 1%) 519
Toprol-XL Tablets (Rare) 560
Torecan 2367
Trandate Tablets 1158
Triavil Tablets 1800
Trilafon 2532
Trinalin Repetabs Tablets 1373
Trusopt Sterile Ophthalmic Solution (Rare) 1803
Tussend 1830
Tympagesic Ear Drops 2476
Unasyn 2035
Univasc Tablets (More than 1%) 2553
Urobiotic-250 Capsules 2038
Vancocin HCl, Vials & ADD-Vantage (Rare) 1534
Vantin for Oral Suspension and Vantin Tablets 2112
Vascor Tablets (200 and 300 mg) 1597
Vaseretic Tablets (Rare; several cases) 1810
Vasotec I.V. (Several cases) 1814
Vasotec Tablets (Several cases) 1816
Vicodin HP Tablets 1403
Visken Tablets 2428
Vivactil Tablets 1820
Cataflam/Voltaren/Voltaren-XR (Rare) 833
Yutopar Intravenous Injection 566
Zantac (Rare) 1182
Zantac Injection (Rare) 1180
Zantac Syrup (Rare) 1182
Zarontin Capsules 1986
Zarontin Syrup 1986
Zaroxolyn Tablets 1625
Zebeta Tablets 1457
Zestoretic Tablets 2968
Zestril Tablets 2972
Ziac 1459
Zinacef 1184
Zyloprim Tablets (Less than 1%) 1194

Airway obstruction

Altace Capsules 1238
Ativan Injection (5 patients) 2805
Capoten Tablets 740
Capozide Tablets 744
Diprivan Injectable Emulsion (Less than 1%) 2939
Fiorinal with Codeine Capsules 2390
Floxin I.V. 1580
Floxin Tablets (200 mg, 300 mg, 400 mg) 1577
Monopril Tablets 762
Orthoclone OKT3 Sterile Solution 1892
Prinivil Tablets 1776
Prinzide Tablets 1780
Vaseretic Tablets 1810
Vasotec I.V. 1814
Vasotec Tablets 1816
Versed Injection (Less than 1%) 2324
Zestoretic Tablets 2968
Zestril Tablets 2972

Airway resistance

Demerol 2438
Isuprel Mistometer (Occasional) 2442

Akathisia

BuSpar Tablets (Infrequent) 738
Cerebyx Injection (Infrequent) 1956
▲ Clozaril Tablets (3%) 2377
Cognex Capsules (Rare) 1961
Compazine 2644
Desyrel and Desyrel Dividose 504
Effexor (Rare) 2825
Ethmozine Tablets (Less than 2%) 2217
Etrafon 2495
Feldene Capsules (Less than 1%) 2008
Haldol Decanoate (Frequent) 1587
Haldol Injection, Tablets and Concentrate 1585
Inapsine Injection 462
Lamictal Tablets (Infrequent) 1105
Lioresal Intrathecal (1% or more) 1634
Loxitane 1426
Ludiomil Tablets (Rare) 861
LUVOX Tablets (Infrequent) 2723
Mellaril 2398
Moban Tablets and Concentrate 1036
Navane Capsules and Concentrate 2018
Navane Intramuscular 2019
▲ Orap Tablets (8 of 20 patients) 1037
Paxil Tablets 2681
Permax Tablets (1.6%) 571
Prolixin 510
Prozac Pulvules & Liquid, Oral Solution (Infrequent) 935
Reglan 2243
Remeron Tablets (Rare) 1878
▲ Risperdal Tablets (17% to 34%) 1348
Serentil 689
Stelazine 2692
Torecan 2367
Triavil Tablets 1800
Trilafon 2532
Vascor Tablets (200 and 300 mg) (0.5 to 2.0%) 1597
Wellbutrin Tablets (1.5%) 1177
Xanax Tablets (1.6% to 3.0%) 2115

Akinesia

Cardura Tablets (1%) 1993
▲ Clozaril Tablets (4%) 2377
Effexor (Rare) 2825
Loxitane 1426
LUVOX Tablets (Rare) 2723
Mellaril 2398
Moban Tablets and Concentrate 1036
▲ Orap Tablets (8 of 20 patients) 1037
Parnate Tablets 2679
Paxil Tablets (Infrequent) 2681
Permax Tablets (1.1%) 571
Serentil 689
Torecan 2367
▲ Wellbutrin Tablets (8.0%) 1177

Albuminuria

Amikacin Sulfate Injection, USP 523
Amikacin Sulfate Injection, USP 981
Amikin Injectable 502
Anafranil Capsules (Rare) 819
Atretol Tablets 569
Calcijex Injection 412
▲ CellCept Capsules (More than or equal to 3%) 2265
Cerebyx Injection (Infrequent) 1956
Cipro I.V. (1% or less) 587
Cipro I.V. Pharmacy Bulk Package (Less than 1%) 590
Cipro Tablets 584
Dapsone Tablets USP 1331
Dopram Injectable 2235
Doxil (1% to 5%) 2613
Effexor (Infrequent) 2825
Eskalith 2658
Floxin I.V. 1580
Floxin Tablets (200 mg, 300 mg, 400 mg) 1577
Foscavir Injection (Between 1% and 5%) 541
Hivid Tablets (Less than 1%) 2287
Intron A for Injection (Less than 5%) 2506
Lamprene Capsules (Less than 1%) 846
Lioresal Intrathecal (1% or more) 1634
Lithium Carbonate Capsules & Tablets 2352
Lithonate/Lithotabs/Lithobid 2721
Lufyllin & Lufyllin-400 Tablets 2778
Lufyllin-GG Elixir & Tablets 2779
Lysodren Tablets (Infrequent) 707
Maxaquin Tablets 2593
Megace Oral Suspension (1% to 3%) 708
Naprelan Tablets (Less than 1%) 2861
Noroxin Tablets 1758
Noroxin Tablets 2222
Pentasa (Less than 1%) 1275
Prevacid Delayed-Release Capsules (Less than 1%) 2746
Proglycem 575
Prozac Pulvules & Liquid, Oral Solution (Rare) 935
Quadrinal Tablets 1398
Redux Capsules (Infrequent) 2911
Relafen Tablets (Less than 1%) 2688
Rocaltrol Capsules 2303
Solganal Suspension 2530
Sporanox Capsules (0.1% to 1.2%) 1352
Tegretol/Tegretol-XR 870
Uroqid-Acid No. 2 Tablets 633
Xanax Tablets (Less than 1%) 2115
Zyloprim Tablets (Less than 1%) 1194

Alcohol abuse

BuSpar Tablets (Rare) 738
Effexor (Rare) 2825

(▭ Described in PDR For Nonprescription Drugs) Incidence data in parenthesis; ▲ 3% or more (⊙ Described in PDR For Ophthalmology)

Side Effects Index

Alcohol abuse
- Paxil Tablets (Infrequent) ... 2681

Alcohol, increased sensitivity to
- Ativan Injection ... 2805
- Betaseron for SC Injection ... 653
- Catapres Tablets ... 679
- Combipres Tablets ... 682
- Effexor (Rare) ... 2825
- Lamictal Tablets (Rare) ... 1105
- Neurontin Capsules (Rare) ... 1978
- Nicotinex Elixir ... ▫ 671
- Parlodel (Less than 1%) ... 2411

Aldosterone synthesis, suppression
- Heparin Lock Flush Solution ... 2831
- Heparin Sodium Injection ... 2832
- Heparin Sodium Vials ... 1486

Alkalinuria
- Floxin I.V. (More than or equal to 1%) ... 1580
- Floxin Tablets (200 mg, 300 mg, 400 mg) (More than or equal to 1%) ... 1577

Alkalosis
- Ancef Injection ... 2632
- Bicitra ... 573
- CeeNU Capsules (Small percentage) ... 699
- Kefurox Vials, Faspak & ADD-Vantage (1 in 50) ... 1509
- Lioresal Tablets ... 847
- Naprelan Tablets (Less than 1%) .. 2861
- Netromycin Injection 100 mg/ml (15 of 1000 patients) ... 2516
- Polycitra Syrup ... 574
- Polycitra-K Crystals ... 574
- Polycitra-K Oral Solution ... 575
- Polycitra-LC ... 574
- ▲ Prograf (Greater than 3%) ... 1028
- ▲ Proleukin for Injection (4%) ... 812

Alkalosis, metabolic
- Cerebyx Injection (Infrequent) ... 1956
- Indocin I.V. (Less than 3%) ... 1727

Allergic contact dermatitis
- Aclovate (Infrequent) ... 1061
- Analpram-HC Rectal Cream 1% and 2.5% ... 993
- ▲ Androderm Testosterone Transdermal System (4%) ... 2634
- Anusol-HC Cream 2.5% (Infrequent to frequent) ... 1953
- Anusol-HC Suppositories ... 1954
- Benzac ... 1031
- ▲ Catapres-TTS (About 19 in 100).. 680
- Cerumenex Drops ... 2148
- Cordran Lotion (Infrequent) ... 1854
- Cordran Tape (Infrequent) ... 1855
- Cormax Ointment (Infrequent) ... 1856
- Cormax Scalp Application (Infrequent) ... 1857
- Cortisporin Cream ... 1073
- Cortisporin Ointment ... 1074
- Cortisporin Otic Solution Sterile ... 1076
- Cortisporin Otic Suspension Sterile ... 1077
- Cutivate Cream ... 1078
- Cutivate Ointment (Infrequent to more frequent) ... 1078
- Decadron Phosphate Topical Cream ... 1686
- Decaspray Topical Aerosol ... 1689
- Dermatop Emollient Cream 0.1% (Less than 2%) ... 1264
- DesOwen Cream, Ointment and Lotion (Less than 2%) ... 1032
- Diprolene AF Cream 0.05% (Infrequent) ... 2489
- Diprolene Gel 0.05% (Less frequent) ... 2490
- Diprolene Lotion 0.05% (Infrequent) ... 2491
- Diprolene Ointment 0.05% (Infrequent) ... 2491
- ▲ Efudex (Among most frequent) ... 2280
- Elocon Cream 0.1% (Infrequent) ... 2492
- Elocon Lotion 0.1% (Infrequent) ... 2493
- Elocon Ointment 0.1% (Infrequent) ... 2494
- Epifoam (Infrequent) ... 2543
- Florone/Florone E ... 921
- FLUORACAINE ... ⊙ 208
- Fluoroplex Topical Solution & Cream 1% ... 475
- FLURESS ... ⊙ 208
- Habitrol Nicotine Transdermal System (3 patients or 2% of patients) ... 884
- Hytone ... 922
- Hytone Ointment 2 ½% ... 923
- Locoid Cream, Ointment and Topical Solution (Infrequent) ... 994
- Mantadil Cream ... 1124
- Monistat Dual-Pak ... 1906
- NeoDecadron Topical Cream ... 1757
- Ophthetic ... ⊙ 244
- Oxistat Cream ... 1139
- Pandel Cream, 0.1% ... 2475
- Pediotic Suspension Sterile ... 1140
- Pramosone Cream, Lotion & Ointment ... 995
- ProctoCream-HC 2.5% (Infrequent to frequent) ... 2552
- Psorcon Cream 0.05% (Infrequent) ... 924
- Psorcon Ointment 0.05% ... 923
- Retin-A (tretinoin) Cream/Gel/Liquid (Rare) ... 1947
- Synalar (Infrequent) ... 2299
- Temovate Cream ... 1152
- Temovate E Emollient (Infrequent) ... 1154
- Temovate Gel (Infrequent) ... 1153
- Temovate Ointment ... 1152
- Temovate Scalp Application (Infrequent) ... 1153
- Topicort Emollient Cream 0.25% (Infrequent) ... 1289
- Topicort Gel 0.05% (Infrequent) ... 1290
- Topicort LP Emollient Cream 0.05% (Infrequent) ... 1289
- Topicort Ointment 0.25% (Infrequent) ... 1291
- TRIAZ 6% and 10% Gels and 10% Cleanser ... 1629
- Ultravate Cream 0.05% (Infrequent) ... 2797
- Ultravate Ointment 0.05% (Infrequent) ... 2798
- Westcort Cream 0.2% ... 2799
- Westcort Ointment 0.2% ... 2800

Allergic reactions
- Abbokinase ... 403
- Abbokinase Open-Cath ... 405
- Abelcet Injection ... 1540
- ▲ Actigall Capsules (5.2%) ... 818
- Activase (Very rare) ... 1045
- ▲ Acular Sterile Ophthalmic Solution (3%) ... 470
- Adapin Capsules (Occasional) ... 1542
- Adipex-P Tablets and Capsules ... 1035
- AKPRO (Infrequent) ... ⊙ 206
- Albenza Tablets (Rare) ... 2629
- Alkeran for Injection ... 1196
- Alkeran Tablets ... 1198
- Amaryl Tablets (Less than 1%) ... 1241
- Ambien Tablets (Rare to 4%) ... 2559
- Americaine Hemorrhoidal Ointment ... ▫ 649
- Amicar Syrup, Tablets, and Injection ... 1312
- Amoxil ... 2631
- ▲ Anafranil Capsules (3% to 7%) ... 819
- Ancef Injection ... 2632
- AquaMEPHYTON Injection ... 1648
- Aquasol A Parenteral (Rare) ... 526
- Aredia for Injection (One patient) ... 827
- Atromid-S Capsules ... 2808
- Atrovent Inhalation Aerosol ... 674
- Attenuvax (Rare) ... 1650
- Augmentin ... 2637
- Augmentin Tablets ... 2640
- Axocet Capsules (Infrequent) ... 2469
- Azelex ... 471
- ▲ Bactrim DS Tablets (Among most common) ... 2257
- ▲ Bactrim I.V. Infusion (Among most common) ... 2255
- ▲ Bactrim (Among most common) ... 2257
- Benemid Tablets ... 1651
- Bentyl ... 1246
- Berocca Plus Tablets (Possible) ... 2259
- Berocca Tablets ... 2259
- Betasept Surgical Scrub ... 2145
- Betimol 0.25%, 0.5% (1% to 5%) ... ⊙ 259
- Betoptic Ophthalmic Solution (Small numbers of patients) ... 465
- Betoptic S Ophthalmic Suspension ... 467
- Biavax II ... 1653
- Biaxin (Rare) ... 406
- Bicillin L-A Injection ... 2813
- Bio-Ginkgo (Rare) ... 2984
- BuSpar Tablets (Rare) ... 738
- Calcimar Injection, Synthetic (A few cases) ... 2176
- Carbocaine Injection ... 2432
- Cardene Capsules (Rare) ... 2261
- Cardene SR Capsules (Rare) ... 2264
- Cardizem SR Capsules (Infrequent) ... 1255
- Cardizem Tablets (Infrequent) ... 1257
- Cataflam Tablets ... 833
- Catapres Tablets ... 679
- ▲ Catapres-TTS (5 of 101 patients) .. 680
- Ceclor Pulvules & Suspension ... 1470
- Cedax ... 2480
- Cefol Filmtab ... 415
- Ceftin Tablets ... 1067
- CellCept Capsules ... 2265
- ▲ Ceptaz (Among most common) ... 1070
- Cetacaine Topical Anesthetic ... 812
- Chloromycetin Ophthalmic Ointment, 1% ... ⊙ 298
- Ciloxan Ophthalmic Solution (Less than 1%) ... 468
- Cipro I.V. (1% or less) ... 587
- Cipro I.V. Pharmacy Bulk Package (Less than 1%) ... 590
- Cipro Tablets ... 584
- Claritin Tablets (2% or fewer patients) ... 2485
- Clomid ... 1262
- Cogentin Injection ... 1661
- ColBENEMID Tablets ... 1662
- Colyte and Colyte-flavored ... 2540
- Compazine ... 2644
- CordyMax Cs-4 Capsules (One case) ... 2985
- Cortisporin Cream (Approximately 1%) ... 1073
- Cortisporin Ointment (Approximately 1%) ... 1074
- Cortisporin Otic Solution Sterile (0.09% to approximately 1%) ... 1076
- Cortisporin Otic Suspension Sterile (0.09% to approximately 1%) ... 1077
- Creon (Less frequent) ... 2714
- Cystospaz ... 2123
- Cytadren Tablets (Rare) ... 837
- CytoGam (Rare) ... 1630
- Cytomel Tablets (Rare) ... 2647
- DDAVP Injection (Rare) ... 2178
- DDAVP Injection 15 mcg/mL (Rare) ... 2179
- DDAVP ... 2180
- DDAVP Tablets (Rare) ... 2182
- Danocrine Capsules ... 2437
- ▲ DaunoXome (3% to 21%) ... 1842
- Depakote Tablets (1% to 5%) ... 418
- Depen Titratable Tablets ... 2770
- Depo-Provera Contraceptive Injection (Fewer than 1%) ... 2079
- Deponit NTG Transdermal Delivery System (Uncommon) ... 2541
- Desmopressin Acetate Injection (Rare) ... 996
- Desquam-E Gel (10 to 25 patients per 1,000) ... 2792
- Desquam-X Gel (10 to 25 patients per 1,000) ... 2792
- Desquam-X 10 Bar (10 to 25 patients per 1,000) ... 2792
- Desquam-X Wash (10 to 25 patients per 1,000) ... 2792
- Desyrel and Desyrel Dividose ... 504
- DiaBeta Tablets (1.5%) ... 1265
- Digibind (Rare) ... 1079
- Dilantin-125 Suspension ... 1969
- Dilaudid Tablets and Liquid ... 1386
- Diphtheria and Tetanus Toxoids and Pertussis Vaccine Adsorbed ... 2650
- Donnatal ... 2234
- Donnatal Extentabs ... 2234
- Donnatal Tablets ... 2234
- Doxil (1% to 5%) ... 2613
- Drithocreme 0.1%, 0.25%, 0.5%, 1.0% (HP) (Very few instances) .. 920
- Dritho-Scalp 0.25%, 0.5% (Very few instances) ... 921
- Duranest Injections ... 533
- Dyclone 0.5% and 1% Topical Solutions, USP ... 535
- Dynabac (0.1% to 1%) ... 668
- E.E.S. ... 427
- E-Mycin Tablets ... 1388
- Effexor (Infrequent) ... 2825
- Elspar ... 1700
- Emete-con Intramuscular/Intravenous ... 2007
- Eminase (0.2%) ... 2215
- EMLA Cream ... 536
- EPIFRIN ... ⊙ 237
- Epogen for Injection (Rare) ... 489
- Ergamisol Tablets ... 1340
- ERYC ... 1972
- EryPed 200 & EryPed 400 Granules ... 425
- Ery-Tab Tablets ... 426
- Erythrocin Stearate Filmtab ... 429
- Esgic-plus Capsules ... 1012
- Esgic-plus Tablets ... 1012
- Estrace Cream and Tablets ... 751
- Estraderm Transdermal System (Rare) ... 842
- Estring Vaginal Ring (1%) ... 2086
- Ethyol (amifostine) for Injection (Rare; less than 1%) ... 485
- Etopophos for Injection (1% to 2%) ... 701
- Etoposide Injection (1% to 2%) ... 539
- Eurax Cream & Lotion ... 2794
- FML Liquifilm ... ⊙ 238
- Felbatol (Rare) ... 2774
- Fero-Folic-500 Filmtab ... 433
- Fioricet Tablets (Infrequent) ... 2386
- Fioricet with Codeine Capsules (Infrequent) ... 2387
- Fiorinal with Codeine Capsules ... 2390
- Fluorouracil Injection ... 2282
- Fluvirin (Influenza Virus Vaccine) (Rare) ... 1608
- ▲ Fortaz (Among most common) ... 1092
- Fragmin Injection (Rare) ... 2088
- Sterile FUDR (Remote possibility) .. 2284
- Fungizone Intravenous ... 507
- Gamimune N, 5% Immune Globulin Intravenous (Human), 5% ... 612
- Gamimune N, 10% Immune Globulin Intravenous (Human), 10% ... 615
- Gammar-P I.V., Immune Globulin Intravenous (Human) ... 798
- Gantanol Tablets ... 2285
- Gantrisin ... 2286
- Garamycin Ophthalmic ... 2501
- Genoptic Sterile Ophthalmic Solution (Rare) ... ⊙ 241
- Genoptic Sterile Ophthalmic Ointment (Rare) ... ⊙ 241
- Gentak (Rare) ... ⊙ 209
- Geref (sermorelin acetate for injection) (One patient) ... 2995
- Glucagon for Injection Vials and Emergency Kit ... 1485
- Glynase PresTab Tablets (1.5%) ... 2091
- ▲ Habitrol Nicotine Transdermal System (3% to 9% of patients) .. 884
- Halcion Tablets (Rare) ... 2093
- Haldol Injection, Tablets and Concentrate ... 1585
- Halotestin Tablets ... 2095
- Hibiclens Antimicrobial Skin Cleanser ... 2947
- Hibistat (Very rare) ... 2948
- Hivid Tablets (Less than 1%) ... 2287
- Humalog Injection (Less common) .. 1488
- Humate-P, Antihemophilic Factor (Human), Dried Pasteurized (Rare) ... 801
- Humegon for Injection ... 1873
- Humulin 50/50, 100 Units (Less common to occasional) ... 1491
- Humulin 70/30, 100 Units ... 1492
- Humulin L, 100 Units ... 1494
- Hydrocet Capsules ... 787
- Hytrin Capsules (Rare) ... 434
- IBU Tablets (Less than 1%) ... 1389
- Iberet-Folic-500 Filmtab ... 433
- IFEX (Less than 1%) ... 706
- Regular, 100 Units ... 1503
- Pork Regular, 100 Units ... 1507
- Ilosone ... 927
- Ilotycin Gluceptate, IV, Vials ... 929
- Inderide Tablets ... 2838
- Influenza Virus Vaccine, Trivalent, Types A and B (chromatograph- and filter-purified subviron antigen) FluShield, 1996-1997 Formula (Rare) ... 2842
- Invirase Capsules (Less than 2%) .. 2291
- IOPIDINE Sterile Ophthalmic Solution ... ⊙ 218
- Keflex Pulvules & Oral Suspension ... 930
- Keftab Tablets ... 931
- Kefzol Vials, Faspak & ADD-Vantage ... 1511
- Kerlone Tablets (Less than 2%) ... 2588
- Koãte-HP Antihemophilic Factor (Human) ... 624
- Konsyl Powder Sugar Free Unflavored ... ▫ 680
- Kutrase Capsules ... 2546
- Kytril Injection (Rare) ... 2667
- Lamictal Tablets (Infrequent) ... 1105
- Lamisil Tablets (Rare) ... 2394
- Lescol Capsules (2.3%) ... 2395
- ▲ Leukine (12%) ... 1317
- Levsin/Levsinex/Levbid ... 2549

(▫ Described in PDR For Nonprescription Drugs)   Incidence data in parenthesis; ▲ 3% or more   (⊙ Described in PDR For Ophthalmology)

1249 Side Effects Index Alopecia

Lodine Capsules and Tablets (Less than 1%) 2849
Lorabid Suspension and Pulvules 1513
Lortab 2751
Lovenox Injection 2187
Lutrepulse for Injection 998
LUVOX Tablets (Infrequent) 2723
M-M-R II 1730
M-R-VAX II 1732
Marcaine (Rare) 2446
Marcaine Spinal (Rare) 2449
Matulane Capsules 2300
Maxaquin Tablets (Less than 1%) 2593
May-Vita Elixir 1826
Mefoxin 1734
Mefoxin Premixed Intravenous Solution 1737
▲ Mesnex Injection (17%) 711
Metamucil 2125
Metubine Iodide Vials 932
Mezlin 594
Miacalcin Injection (A few cases) 2402
Miacalcin Nasal Spray (Less than 1%; a few reports) 2403
Micronase Tablets (1.5%) 2099
Miltown Tablets 2780
Minocin Intravenous (Rare) 1428
Minocin Oral Suspension 1431
Mivacron 1125
8-MOP Capsules 1294
Monoclate-P, Factor VIII:C Pasteurized, Monoclonal Antibody Purified Antihemophilic Factor (Human) 802
Monoket Tablets (Extremely rare) 2550
Mononine, Coagulation Factor IX (Human), Monoclonal Antibody Purified 804
Mumpsvax (Extremely rare) 1751
Myochrysine Injection 1754
Naprelan Tablets (Less than 1%) 2861
Natacyn Antifungal Ophthalmic Suspension (One case) ⊙ 223
Navelbine Injection 1212
Neoral (2% or less) 2405
Neosporin G.U. Irrigant Sterile 1130
Nescaine/Nescaine MPF (Rare) 549
Neupogen for Injection 495
Neurontin Capsules (Infrequent) 1978
Nicotrol NS Nicotine Nasal Spray (Less than 1%) 1565
Niferex-PN Tablets 811
▲ Nipent for Injection (2% to 11%) 2733
Nitro-Bid IV (Uncommon) 1270
Nitro-Bid Ointment (Uncommon;) 1272
Nitro-Dur (nitroglycerin) Transdermal Infusion System (Uncommon) 1365
▲ Nizoral 2% Cream (5%) 1344
Noroxin Tablets (Less frequent) 1758
Noroxin Tablets (Less frequent) 2222
Norvir (Less than 2%) 447
Novocain Hydrochloride for Spinal Anesthesia 2457
Novolin 70/30 Prefilled Disposable Insulin Delivery System (Rare) 1850
Nubain Injection (1% or less) 952
NuLYTELY (Isolated cases) 694
Cherry Flavor NuLYTELY (Isolated cases) 694
Nutropin 1049
Nutropin AQ Injection 1051
Ocusert Pilo-20 and Pilo-40 Ocular Therapeutic Systems (Uncommon) ⊙ 252
▲ Oncaspar (Greater than 5%) 2194
Oncovin Solution Vials & Hyporets (Rare) 1521
OptiPranolol (Metipranolol 0.3%) Sterile Ophthalmic Solution (A small number of patients) ⊙ 256
Orudis Capsules (Less than 1%) 2874
Oruvail Capsules (Less than 1%) 2874
PBZ Tablets 863
PBZ-SR Tablets 862
PCE Dispertab Tablets 453
Pamelor 2409
Pancrease Capsules (Less frequent) 1589
Pancrease MT Capsules (Less frequent) 1589
ParaGard T 380A Intrauterine Copper Contraceptive 1936
▲ Paraplatin for Injection (10% to 12%) 713
Paremyd ⊙ 244
Paxil Tablets (Infrequent) 2681
Pediazole Suspension 2340
Pediotic Suspension Sterile (0.09% to approximately 1%) 1140
Peptavlon 2997
Pergonal (menotropins for injection, USP) 2618
Peridex (Rare) 2127
Periogard Oral Rinse (Rare) 892
Phenergan Injection 2880
Phenobarbital Elixir and Tablets 1523
PhosLo Tablets 695
Phrenilin (Infrequent) 790
PMB 200 and PMB 400 2890
Polysporin Ophthalmic Ointment Sterile 1140
Pontocaine Hydrochloride for Spinal Anesthesia 2460
Pred Forte ⊙ 247
Pred Mild ⊙ 250
Primaxin I.M. 1770
Pro-Banthine Tablets 2226
Procrit for Injection (Rare) 1896
Profasi (chorionic gonadotropin for injection, USP) 2620
Prolastin Alpha$_1$-Proteinase Inhibitor (Human) (Occasional) 629
Proleukin for Injection (1%) 812
Prolixin Oral Concentrate 510
PROPINE with C CAP Compliance Cap ⊙ 251
ProSom Tablets (Infrequent) 457
Prostigmin Injectable 1305
Prostigmin Tablets 1306
Protropin 1053
Prozac Pulvules & Liquid, Oral Solution (1.2% to 3%) 935
Rabies Vaccine Adsorbed 2686
Redux Capsules (Frequent) 2911
ReoPro Vials 1526
RespiGam 1631
Risperdal Tablets (Rare) 1348
Robinul Forte Tablets 2247
Robinul Injectable 2247
Robinul Tablets 2247
Rowasa 2727
SSD 1402
Sandimmune (2% or less) 2416
Sandostatin Injection (Less than 1%) 2421
Secretin-Ferring 2991
Sedapap Tablets 50 mg/650 mg (Infrequent) 1826
Selsun Rx 2.5% Selenium Sulfide Lotion, USP 2345
Sensorcaine (Rare) 554
▲ Septra (Among most common) 1146
▲ Septra I.V. Infusion (Among the most common) 1142
▲ Septra I.V. Infusion ADD-Vantage Vials (Among most common) 1144
▲ Septra (Among most common) 1146
Seromycin Capsules 975
Serzone Tablets (Infrequent) 776
Silvadene Cream 1% 1288
Sinequan (Occasional) 2028
Slo-Niacin Tablets 2767
Soma Compound w/Codeine Tablets 2784
Soma Compound Tablets 2783
Soma Tablets 2782
Sotradecol (Sodium Tetradecyl Sulfate Injection) 987
Sporanox Capsules (Infrequent) 1352
Stelazine (Occasional) 2692
Stimate, (desmopressin acetate) Nasal Spray, 1.5 mg/mL (Rare) 806
▲ Streptase for Infusion (Among most common; 1% to 4%) 557
Sultrin (Frequent) 1941
Suprax 1443
Synarel Nasal Solution for Central Precocious Puberty (2.6%) 2603
Tagamet (Rare) 2694
Talacen Caplets 2464
▲ Tazicef for Injection (Among most common) 2697
TERAK Ointment (Rare) ⊙ 210
Terra-Cortril Ophthalmic Suspension 2033
Terramycin Intramuscular Solution 2034
Terramycin with Polymyxin B Sulfate Ophthalmic Ointment (Rare) 2035
Thioplex (Thiotepa For Injection) (Rare) 1329
Thorazine (Occasional) 2701
THYREL TRH (Less frequent) 2992
Thyro-Block Tablets (A few people) 2785
Tiazac Capsules (1%) 1019
TICE BCG, USP (2.1%) 1881
Tigan 2231
Torecan 2367
Tracrium Injection 1155
Transderm-Nitro Transdermal Therapeutic System (Uncommon) 878
Trasylol (0.3%) 607
Traumeel Injection Solution (Rare) 1237
Trinsicon Capsules 2759
Triostat Injection (Rare) 2708
Tronolane Anesthetic Cream for Hemorrhoids ▣ 746
Trusopt Sterile Ophthalmic Solution 1803
Tylenol with Codeine 1592
Tylox Capsules 1593
Tympagesic Ear Drops (Infrequently) 2476
Typhim Vi (Rare) 914
Ultram Tablets (50 mg) (Less than 1%) 1594
Ultrase Capsules (Less frequent) 2476
Ultrase MT Capsules (Less frequent) 2477
Urobiotic-250 Capsules (Rare) 2038
Vantin for Oral Suspension and Vantin Tablets 2112
Varivax (Greater than or equal to 1%) 1807
VePesid Capsules and Injection (1% to 2%) 727
Versed Injection 2324
Vibramycin Hyclate Intravenous 2040
Vicodin HP Tablets 1403
Videx Tablets, Powder for Oral Solution, & Pediatric Powder for Oral Solution (1% to 2%) 2980
Vistide Injection 1057
Cataflam/Voltaren/Voltaren-XR 833
▲ Xanax Tablets (3.8%) 2115
Xylocaine Injections (Extremely rare) 562
▲ Zerit Capsules (Up to 9%) 731
Zinacef 1184
Zithromax (Rare) 2043
Zithromax Tablets (Rare) 2046
Zoladex (1% or greater) 2976
Zoladex 3-month 2978
Zosyn 1463

Allergic sensitization

▲ AK-CIDE (Most often) ⊙ 203
▲ AK-CIDE Ointment (Most often) ⊙ 203
▲ AK-Trol Ointment & Suspension (Most often) ⊙ 205
▲ Alferon N Injection (1% to 18%) 2142
▲ Blephamide Liquifilm Sterile Ophthalmic Suspension (Most often) 472
▲ Blephamide Ointment (Among most often) ⊙ 234
Cerezyme (A number of patients) 1056
Chloroptic S.O.P. ⊙ 236
Cortisporin Ophthalmic Ointment Sterile 1074
Cortisporin Ophthalmic Suspension Sterile 1075
▲ Cortisporin Otic Solution Sterile (Most often) 1076
▲ Cortisporin Otic Suspension Sterile (Most often) 1077
Desquam-E Gel (10 to 25 per 1,000) 2792
Desquam-X Gel (10 to 25 per 1,000) 2792
Desquam-X 10 Bar (10 to 25 per 1,000) 2792
Desquam-X Wash (10 to 25 per 1,000) 2792
▲ FML-S Liquifilm (Among most often) ⊙ 240
Leucovorin Calcium for Injection, Wellcovorin Brand 1203
Leucovorin Calcium for Injection 1313
Leucovorin Calcium Tablets, Wellcovorin Brand 1204
Leucovorin Calcium Tablets 1315
▲ Maxitrol Ophthalmic Ointment and Suspension (Most often) ⊙ 222
NeoDecadron Sterile Ophthalmic Ointment 1755
▲ NeoDecadron Sterile Ophthalmic Solution (Most often) 1756
Neosporin Ophthalmic Ointment Sterile 1130
Neosporin Ophthalmic Solution Sterile 1131
▲ Pediotic Suspension Sterile (Most often) 1140
▲ Poly-Pred Liquifilm (Most often) ⊙ 246
▲ Polysporin Ophthalmic Ointment Sterile (Among those occurring most often) 1140
Precare Prenatal Multi-Vitamin/Mineral 2753
▲ Pred-G Liquifilm Sterile Ophthalmic Suspension (Most often) ⊙ 248
Pred-G S.O.P. Sterile Ophthalmic Ointment ⊙ 249
Advanced Formula ZENATE Tablets 2728

Allergic vasospastic reactions

Heparin Lock Flush Solution 2831
Heparin Sodium Injection 2832

Allergy (see under Allergic reactions)

Alopecia

Accupril Tablets (0.5% to 1.0%) 1950
Adalat CC (Rare) 582
Adapin Capsules (Occasional) 1542
▲ Adriamycin PFS (Most cases) 2056
▲ Adriamycin RDF (Most cases) 2056
Albenza Tablets (Less than 1.0% to 1.6%) 2629
Aldoclor Tablets 1638
Aldoril Tablets 1644
Alkeran for Injection 1196
Alkeran Tablets 1198
Amen Tablets (Few cases) 785
Anafranil Capsules (Infrequent) 819
Anaprox/Naprosyn (Less than 1%) 2277
Aquasol A Vitamin A Capsules, USP 525
Aquasol A Parenteral 526
Aralen Phosphate Tablets 2431
Asacol Delayed-Release Tablets 2129
Asendin Tablets (Very rare) 1419
Atamet Tablets 567
Atretol Tablets 569
Atromid-S Capsules (Less frequent) 2808
Atrovent Inhalation Aerosol (Less frequent) 674
▲ Avonex (4%) 662
Azathioprine Tablets (Less than 1%) 2349
Azulfidine (Rare) 2059
Benemid Tablets 1651
Betagan ⊙ 230
Betapace Tablets (Rare) 637
▲ Betaseron for SC Injection (4%) 653
Betimol 0.25%, 0.5% ⊙ 259
Betoptic Ophthalmic Solution (Rare) 465
Betoptic S Ophthalmic Suspension (Rare) 467
Blenoxane 697
Blocadren Tablets (Less than 1%) 1654
Brevicon 2563
BuSpar Tablets (Infrequent) 738
Calan SR Caplets (1% or less) 2571
Calan Tablets (1% or less) 2568
Capoten Tablets (About 0.5 to 2%) 740
Capozide Tablets (0.5 to 2%) 744
Cardizem CD Capsules (Infrequent) 1251
Cardizem SR Capsules (Infrequent) 1255
Cardizem Injectable 1253
Cardizem Tablets (Infrequent) 1257
Cardura Tablets (Less than 0.5% of 3960 patients) 1993
Cartrol Tablets 413
Casodex Tablets (2% to 5%) 2934
Cataflam Tablets (Less than 1%) 833
Catapres Tablets (About 2 in 1,000 patients) 679
Catapres-TTS 680
CeeNU Capsules (Infrequent) 699
▲ CellCept Capsules (More than or equal to 3%) 2265
▲ Cerubidine for Injection (In most patients) 634
Claritin Tablets (Rare) 2485
Claritin-D Tablets 2487
Climara Transdermal System 640
Clinoril Tablets (Less than 1%) 1658
Clomid (Fewer than 1%) 1262
Cognex Capsules (Infrequent) 1961
ColBENEMID Tablets 1662
Combipres Tablets (About 2 in 1,000) 682
Cordarone Tablets (Less than 1%) 2818
Cormax Scalp Application (Approximately 0.3%) 1857
Cosmegen Injection 1666
Coumadin (Infrequent) 941
Covera-HS Tablets (Less than 2%) 2573

(▣ Described in PDR For Nonprescription Drugs) Incidence data in parenthesis; ▲ 3% or more (⊙ Described in PDR For Ophthalmology)

Cozaar Tablets (Less than 1%) 1668
Cuprimine Capsules (Rare) 1673
Cycrin Tablets (A few cases) 991
Cytosar-U Sterile Powder (Less frequent) 2077
Cytotec (Infrequent) 2576
Cytovene (1% or less) 2270
Cytoxan (Common) 700
DTIC-Dome 593
Danocrine Capsules 2437
▲ DaunoXome (2% to 8%) 1842
Daypro Caplets (Less than 1%) 2578
Demulen 2580
Depakene 416
▲ Depakote Tablets (1% to 7%) 418
Depen Titratable Tablets (Rare) 2770
Depo-Provera Contraceptive Injection (1% to 5%) 2079
Depo-Provera Sterile Aqueous Suspension 2083
Desogen Tablets 1867
Desyrel and Desyrel Dividose 504
Didronel Tablets 2133
Diethylstilbestrol Tablets 1477
Diflucan Tablets, Injection, and Oral Suspension 2003
Dipentum Capsules (Rare) 2084
Diupres Tablets 1691
Diuril Oral Suspension 1694
Diuril Sodium Intravenous 1693
Diuril Tablets 1694
▲ Doxil (8.9% to 9.1%) 2613
▲ Doxorubicin Astra (Most cases) 531
EC-Naprosyn Delayed-Release Tablets (Less than 1%) 2277
Effexor (Infrequent) 2825
Efudex 2280
Elavil 2945
Eldepryl Capsules 2729
Emcyt Capsules (1%) 2085
Engerix-B Unit-Dose Vials 2656
▲ Ergamisol Tablets (3% to 22%) 1340
Esimil Tablets 840
Eskalith 2658
Estrace Cream and Tablets 751
Estraderm Transdermal System 842
ESTRATAB Tablets (0.3, 0.625, 1.25, 2.5 mg) 2715
Estratest 2718
▲ Etopophos for Injection (Up to 66%) 701
▲ Etoposide Injection (Up to 66%) 539
Etrafon 2495
Felbatol 2774
Feldene Capsules (Less than 1%) 2008
Flexeril Tablets (Rare) 1701
Fludara for Injection (Up to 3%) 658
Fluorouracil Injection (Substantial number of cases) 2282
Foscavir Injection (Less than 1%) 541
Sterile FUDR 2284
Garamycin Injectable 2502
▲ Gemzar for Injection (15% to 18%) 1482
Haldol Decanoate (Isolated cases) 1587
Haldol Injection, Tablets and Concentrate (Isolated cases) 1585
Heparin Lock Flush Solution 2831
Heparin Sodium Injection 2832
Heparin Sodium Vials 1486
Hexalen Capsules (Less than 1%) 2760
Hivid Tablets (Less than 1%) 2287
▲ Hycamtin for Injection (42% to 62%) 2665
Hydrea Capsules (Very rare) 705
HydroDIURIL Tablets 1716
Hydropres Tablets 1718
Hyzaar Tablets 1720
IBU Tablets (Less than 1%) 1389
▲ Idamycin Injection (77%) 2096
▲ IFEX (83%) 706
Imuran (Less than 1%) 1103
Inderal (Rare) 2834
Inderal LA Long Acting Capsules (Rare) 2836
Inderide Tablets (Rare) 2838
Inderide LA Long Acting Capsules (Rare) 2840
Indocin Capsules (Less than 1%) 1723
Indocin I.V. (Less than 1%) 1727
Indocin (Less than 1%) 1723
▲ Intron A for Injection (Up to 38%) 2506
Ismelin Tablets 845
Isoptin Oral Tablets (Less than 1%) 1393
Isoptin SR Tablets (1% or less) 1395
Kerlone Tablets (Less than 2%) 2588
Klonopin Tablets 2294
▲ Kytril Tablets (3%) 2669
Lamictal Tablets (1.3%) 1105
Lariam Tablets (Less than 1%) 2295
Larodopa Tablets (Rare) 2296
▲ Leucovorin Calcium for Injection (5% to 43%) 1313
▲ Leukine (37% to 73%) 1317
Levatol Tablets 2547
Levlen/Tri-Levlen 646
Levothroid Tablets 1015
Limbitrol 2333
Lioresal Intrathecal (1% or more) 1634
Lithium Carbonate Capsules & Tablets 2352
Lithonate/Lithotabs/Lithobid 2721
Lodine Capsules and Tablets (Less than 1%) 2849
Lo/Ovral Tablets 2852
Lo/Ovral-28 Tablets 2857
Lopid Tablets 1974
Lopressor (Rare) 848
Lopressor HCT Tablets 850
Loxitane 1426
Ludiomil Tablets (Rare) 861
▲ Lupron Depot 3.75 mg (Among most frequent) 2739
Lupron Depot-PED 7.5 mg, 11.25 mg and 15 mg (Less than 2%) 2744
Lupron Injection (Less than 5%) 2736
Lupron Injection Pediatric (Less than 2%) 2737
LUVOX Tablets (Infrequent) 2723
Macrobid Capsules (Less than 1%) 2138
Macrodantin Capsules 2140
Matulane Capsules 2300
Maxair Autohaler 1550
Maxair Inhaler (Less than 1%) 1552
Megace Oral Suspension (1% to 3%) 708
Megace Tablets 710
Menest Tablets 2671
Mesantoin Tablets 2400
▲ Methotrexate Sodium Tablets, Injection, for Injection and LPF Injection (1% to 10%) 1322
Metrodin (urofollitropin for injection) 2616
Mevacor Tablets (0.5% to 1.0%) 1742
Mexitil Capsules (About 4 in 1,000) 684
Miacalcin Nasal Spray (Less than 1%) 2403
Midamor Tablets (Less than or equal to 1%) 1746
Minipress Capsules (Less than 1%) 2015
Minizide Capsules (Rare) 2016
Modicon 1928
Moduretic Tablets 1748
Motrin Ibuprofen Suspension, Oral Drops, Chewable Tablets, Caplets (Less than 1%) 1563
Mustargen (Infrequent) 1752
Mutamycin for Injection (Frequent) 712
Myleran Tablets (Rare) 1209
Myochrysine Injection 1754
Nalfon 200 Pulvules & Nalfon Tablets (Less than 1%) 933
Naprelan Tablets (Less than 1%) 2861
Anaprox/Naprosyn (Less than 1%) 2277
▲ Navelbine Injection (Up to 12%) 1212
▲ Neupogen for Injection (18%) 495
Neurontin Capsules (Infrequent) 1978
Nipent for Injection (Less than 3%) 2733
Nizoral 2% Shampoo (Less than 1%) 1344
Nizoral Tablets (Rare) 1345
Nolvadex Tablets (Infrequent) 2957
Nordette-21 Tablets 2863
Nordette-28 Tablets 2866
Norinyl 2563
Normodyne Tablets (Less common) 2522
Norplant System 2868
Norpramin Tablets 1273
Nor-Q D Tablets 2598
Norvasc Tablets (Less than or equal to 0.1%) 2020
▲ Novantrone for Injection (22 to 37%) 1327
Ogen Tablets 2103
Ogen Vaginal Cream 2106
Oncaspar 2194
▲ Oncovin Solution Vials & Hyporets (Most common) 1521
Ortho-Cept 1907
Ortho-Cyclen/Ortho-Tri-Cyclen 1914
Ortho Dienestrol Cream 1922
Ortho-Est 1925
Ortho-Novum 1928
Ortho-Cyclen/Ortho Tri-Cyclen 1914
Orudis Capsules (Less than 1%) 2874
Oruvail Capsules (Less than 1%) 2874
Ovcon 765
Ovral Tablets 2877
Ovral-28 Tablets 2878
Ovrette Tablets 2878
Pamelor 2409
▲ Paraplatin for Injection (2% to 50%) 713
Parlodel (Less than 1%) 2411
Paxil Tablets (Infrequent) 2681
Pentasa (Less than 1%) 1275
Pepcid Injection (Infrequent) 1765
Pepcid (Infrequent) 1763
Permax Tablets (Infrequent) 571
Plaquenil Sulfate Tablets 2459
Platinol for Injection 717
Platinol-AQ Injection 719
PMB 200 and PMB 400 2890
Pondimin Tablets 2239
Pravachol Tablets 770
Premarin Intravenous 2893
Premarin Tablets 2896
Premarin Vaginal Cream 2898
Premphase 2900
Prempro 2905
Prevacid Delayed-Release Capsules (Less than 1%) 2746
Prilosec Delayed-Release Capsules (Less than 1%) 516
Prinivil Tablets (0.3% to 1.0%) 1776
Prinzide Tablets 1780
Procardia XL Extended Release Tablets (1% or less) 2026
Proglycem 575
▲ Prograf (Greater than 3%) 1028
Proleukin for Injection (1%) 812
Provera Tablets (A few cases) 2110
Prozac Pulvules & Liquid, Oral Solution (Infrequent) 935
Quibron 2227
Redux Capsules (Frequent) 2911
Relafen Tablets (Less than 1%) 2688
Remeron Tablets (Infrequent) 1878
Respbid Tablets 687
ReVia Tablets (Less than 1%) 957
Rhinocort Nasal Inhaler (Rare) 552
Ridaura Capsules (Rare) 2691
Rilutek Tablets (Up to 1.2%) 2198
Risperdal Tablets (Infrequent) 1348
Ritalin (A few instances) 866
▲ Roferon-A Injection (17% to 22%) 2308
Rowasa (0.86%) 2727
▲ Rubex for Injection (Most cases) 721
Rythmol Tablets–150mg, 225mg, 300mg (Less than 1%) 1399
Sandostatin Injection (1% to 4%) 2421
Sectral Capsules 2914
Seldane Tablets 1284
Seldane-D Extended-Release Tablets 1286
Selsun Rx 2.5% Selenium Sulfide Lotion, USP 2345
Serophene (clomiphene citrate tablets, USP) (Less than 1 in 100 patients) 2621
Serzone Tablets (Infrequent) 776
Sinemet Tablets 959
Sinemet CR Tablets 961
Sinequan (Occasional) 2028
Slo-bid Gyrocaps 2201
Solganal Suspension 2530
Sular Tablets (Less than or equal to 1%) 2961
Supprelin Injection (1% to 3%) 2230
Surmontil Capsules 2917
Synarel Nasal Solution for Endometriosis (Some patients) 2605
Synthroid 1410
Tagamet (Very rare) 2694
Tambocor Tablets (Less than 1%) 1555
Tapazole Tablets 1361
▲ Taxol Injection (87%) 723
▲ Taxotere for Injection Concentrate (80%) 2204
▲ Tegison Capsules (Less than 75%) 2314
Tegretol/Tegretol-XR 870
Temovate Scalp Application (1 of 294 patients) 1153
Tenex Tablets (Less frequent) 2249
Tenoretic Tablets 2963
Tenormin Tablets and I.V. Injection 2965
Teslac Tablets (Rare) 727
Theo-Dur Extended-Release Tablets 1367
Theo-X Extended-Release Tablets 793
Thioplex (Thiotepa For Injection) 1329
Tiazac Capsules (Infrequent) 1019
Timolide Tablets 1791
Timoptic in Ocudose (Less frequent) 1796
Timoptic Sterile Ophthalmic Solution (Less frequent) 1794
Timoptic-XE 1798
Tofranil Ampuls 873
Tofranil Tablets 875
Tofranil-PM Capsules 876
Tonocard Tablets (Less than 1%) 519
Toprol-XL Tablets (Rare) 560
Trandate Tablets (Less common) 1158
Triavil Tablets 1800
Levlen/Tri-Levlen 646
Tri-Norinyl 2607
Triphasil-21 Tablets 2919
Triphasil-28 Tablets 2924
Uni-Dur Extended-Release Tablets 1374
Vaseretic Tablets 1810
Vasotec I.V. 1814
Vasotec Tablets (0.5% to 1.0%) 1816
▲ Velban Vials (Among most common) 1537
▲ VePesid Capsules and Injection (Up to 66%) 727
Verelan Capsules (1% or less) 1455
▲ Vesanoid Capsules (14%) 2327
▲ Videx Tablets, Powder for Oral Solution, & Pediatric Powder for Oral Solution (5%) 2980
Visken Tablets 2428
▲ Vistide Injection (25%) 1057
Vivactil Tablets 1820
Vivelle Transdermal System 880
Cataflam/Voltaren/Voltaren-XR (Less than 1%) 833
▲ Vumon for Injection (9%) 729
Wellbutrin Tablets (Infrequent) 1177
Winstrol Tablets 2468
Zantac (Rare) 1182
Zantac Injection (Rare) 1180
Zantac Syrup (Rare) 1182
Zebeta Tablets 1457
Zestoretic Tablets 2968
Zestril Tablets (0.3% to 1.0%) 2972
Ziac 1459
▲ Zinecard Injection (94% to 100%) 2120
Zocor Tablets 1821
Zoladex (1% or greater) 2976
Zoladex 3-month 2978
Zoloft Tablets (Infrequent) 2051
Zovirax 1187
Zyloprim Tablets (Less than 1%) 1194
Zyrtec Tablets (Less than 2%) 2053

Alopecia hereditaria

Androderm Testosterone Transdermal System 2634
▲ Android Capsules, 10 mg (Among most common) 1297
Estratest 2718
Halotestin Tablets 2095
Oxandrin 783
Testoderm Testosterone Transdermal System 486
Testred Capsules, 10 mg 1308

Alpha-glutamyl transferase, elevation

Eulexin Capsules 2498

Alveolar infiltrates, interstitial

Cytadren Tablets (Rare) 837

Alveolitis

Cordarone Tablets 2818
Cuprimine Capsules 1673
Prozac Pulvules & Liquid, Oral Solution (Rare) 935

Alveolitis, allergic

Cytadren Tablets (Rare) 837
Depen Titratable Tablets (Rare) 2770
Relafen Tablets (Less than 1%) 2688

Alveolitis, fibrosing

Azulfidine (Rare) 2059
Rowasa 2727
Tonocard Tablets (Less than 1%) 519

Amaurosis

Zofran Injection (One patient) 1227

Amblyopia

Accupril Tablets (0.5% to 1.0%) 1950
Adalat CC (Less than 1.0%) 582
Axid Pulvules (1.0%) 1468
Buprenex Injectable (Infrequent) 2170
Cardizem CD Capsules (Less than 1%) 1251
Cardizem SR Capsules (Less than 1%) 1255

(Described in PDR For Nonprescription Drugs) Incidence data in parenthesis; ▲ 3% or more (Described in PDR For Ophthalmology)

1251 Side Effects Index Anaphylactic reactions

Cardizem Injectable (Less than 1%) 1253
Cardizem Tablets (Less than 1%) 1257
Cataflam Tablets (Less than 1%) 833
▲ CellCept Capsules (More than or equal to 3%) 2265
Cerebyx Injection (2.2%) 1956
Cognex Capsules (Infrequent) 1961
Cytovene (1% or less) 2270
Depakote Tablets (1% to 5%) 418
Dilacor XR Extended-release Capsules (Infrequent) 2183
Diprivan Injectable Emulsion (Less than 1%) 2939
Ditropan 1267
Duragesic Transdermal System (Less than 1%) 1336
Dynabac (0.1% to 1%) 668
▲ Flolan for Injection (8%) 1085
Hytrin Capsules (0.6% to 1.3%) 434
IBU Tablets (Less than 1%) 1389
Kadian Capsules (Less than 3%) 2948
Lioresal Intrathecal (0.2% to 2.3%) 1634
Lupron Depot - 3 Month 22.5 mg (Less than 5%) 2743
▲ LUVOX Tablets (3%) 2723
Macrobid Capsules (Less than 1%) 2138
Megace Oral Suspension (1% to 3%) 708
Monoket Tablets (Fewer than 1%) 2550
Motrin Ibuprofen Suspension, Oral Drops, Chewable Tablets, Caplets (Less than 1%) 1563
▲ Neurontin Capsules (4.2%) 1978
Nipent for Injection (Less than 3%) 2733
Norvir (Less than 2%) 447
Paxil Tablets (Rare) 2681
Penetrex Tablets (0.1% to 1%) 2196
Placidyl Capsules 456
Prevacid Delayed-Release Capsules (Less than 1%) 2746
▲ Prograf (Greater than 3%) 1028
Prozac Pulvules & Liquid, Oral Solution (Infrequent to 3%) 935
Redux Capsules (Frequent) 2911
Retrovir Capsules 1216
Retrovir I.V. Infusion 1221
Retrovir Syrup 1216
Rilutek Tablets (Infrequent) 2198
▲ Salagen Tablets (4%) 1546
Sular Tablets (Less than or equal to 1%) 2961
Tiazac Capsules (Less than 1%) 1019
Vistide Injection 1057
Cataflam/Voltaren/Voltaren-XR (Less than 1%) 833
Zoladex (1% or greater) 2976
Zoladex 3-month 2978
Zyloprim Tablets (Less than 1%) 1194

Amblyopia scleritis

Naprelan Tablets (Less than 1%) 2861

Amebiasis, precipitation of latent

Dexacort Phosphate in Respihaler 1606

Amenorrhea

Aldactazide Tablets 2556
Aldactone Tablets 2558
Aldoclor Tablets 1638
Aldomet Ester HCl Injection 1642
Aldomet Oral 1640
Aldoril Tablets 1644
Alkeran for Injection 1196
Alkeran Tablets (A significant number of patients) 1198
Amen Tablets 785
Anafranil Capsules (Up to 1%) 819
▲ Android Capsules, 10 mg (Among most common) 1297
Aygestin Tablets 990
Brevicon 2563
BuSpar Tablets (Rare) 738
Compazine 2644
Cycrin Tablets 991
Cytoxan (A significant proportion of women) 700
Danocrine Capsules (Occasional) 2437
Demulen 2580
Depakene 416
Depakote Tablets 418
▲ Depo-Provera Contraceptive Injection (Up to 68%) 2079
Depo-Provera Sterile Aqueous Suspension 2083
Desogen Tablets 1867
Diethylstilbestrol Tablets 1477
Effexor (Infrequent) 2825
▲ Estratest (Among most common) 2718
Etrafon 2495
Haldol Decanoate 1587
Haldol Injection, Tablets and Concentrate 1585
Halotestin Tablets 2095
Intron A for Injection (Less than 5%) 2506
Kadian Capsules (Less than 3%) 2948
Lamictal Tablets (1.9%) 1105
Leukeran Tablets 1205
Levlen/Tri-Levlen 646
Lo/Ovral Tablets 2852
Lo/Ovral-28 Tablets 2857
Loxitane (Rare) 1426
Mellaril 2398
Menest Tablets 2671
Micronor Tablets 1903
Moban Tablets and Concentrate (Infrequent) 1036
Modicon 1928
Mustargen 1752
Navane Capsules and Concentrate 2018
Navane Intramuscular 2019
Neurontin Capsules (Infrequent) 1978
Nipent for Injection (Less than 3%) 2733
▲ Nolvadex Tablets (16.3%) 2957
Nordette-21 Tablets 2863
Nordette-28 Tablets 2866
Norinyl 2563
▲ Norplant System (9.4%) 2868
Nor-Q D Tablets 2598
Orlaam Oral Solution (Low frequency) 2361
Ortho-Cept 1907
Ortho-Cyclen/Ortho-Tri-Cyclen 1914
Ortho Dienestrol Cream 1922
Ortho-Est 1925
Ortho-Novum 1928
Ortho-Cyclen/Ortho Tri-Cyclen 1914
Ovcon 765
Ovral Tablets 2877
Ovral-28 Tablets 2878
Ovrette Tablets 2878
ParaGard T 380A Intrauterine Copper Contraceptive 1936
Paxil Tablets (Infrequent) 2681
Pentasa (Less than 1%) 1275
Permax Tablets (Rare) 571
PMB 200 and PMB 400 2890
Premarin Intravenous 2893
Premarin Vaginal Cream 2898
Premphase 2900
Prempro 2905
Prolixin Oral Concentrate 510
Provera Tablets 2110
Prozac Pulvules & Liquid, Oral Solution (Infrequent) 935
Redux Capsules (Infrequent) 2911
Reglan 2243
Remeron Tablets (Infrequent) 1878
Rilutek Tablets (Rare) 2198
Risperdal Tablets (Infrequent) 1348
Sandostatin Injection (Less than 1%) 2421
Serentil 689
Serzone Tablets (Infrequent) 776
Stelazine 2692
Testred Capsules, 10 mg 1308
Thioplex (Thiotepa For Injection) 1329
Thorazine 2701
Trilafon 2532
Levlen/Tri-Levlen 646
Tri-Norinyl 2607
Triphasil-21 Tablets 2919
Triphasil-28 Tablets 2924
Zoladex (Rare) 2976
Zoloft Tablets (Rare) 2051

Amnesia

Altace Capsules (Less than 1%) 1238
Ambien Tablets (1%) 2559
Ativan Tablets 2807
Avonex 662
Betaseron for SC Injection (2%) 653
Cardizem CD Capsules (Less than 1%) 1251
Cardizem SR Capsules (Less than 1%) 1255
Cardizem Injectable 1253
Cardizem Tablets (Less than 1%) 1257
Cardura Tablets (Less than 0.5% of 3960 patients) 1993
Cerebyx Injection (Infrequent) 1956
Claritin Tablets (2% or fewer patients) 2485
Claritin-D Tablets 2487
Clozaril Tablets (Less than 1%) 2377
Cognex Capsules (Infrequent) 1961
Cytovene (1% or less) 2270
DaunoXome (Less than or equal to 5%) 1842
Depakote Tablets (1% to 5%) 418
Didronel Tablets 2133
Doral Tablets 2773
Duragesic Transdermal System (1% or greater) 1336
Effexor 2825
Ergamisol Tablets (Up to 1%) 1340
Foscavir Injection (Between 1% and 5%) 541
Halcion Tablets 2093
Hivid Tablets (Less than 1%) 2287
▲ Intron A for Injection (Up to 14%) 2506
Invirase Capsules (Less than 2%) 2291
Kadian Capsules (Less than 3%) 2948
Kerlone Tablets (Less than 2%) 2588
Klonopin Tablets 2294
Lamictal Tablets (Frequent) 1105
Levo-Dromoran 2297
Lioresal Intrathecal (1% or more) 1634
LUVOX Tablets (Frequent) 2723
Marinol (Dronabinol) Capsules (Greater than 1%) 2353
Naprelan Tablets (Less than 1%) 2861
Neurontin Capsules (2.2%) 1978
Nicotrol NS Nicotine Nasal Spray (Less than 1%) 1565
Norvasc Tablets (Less than or equal to 0.1%) 2020
Norvir (Less than 2%) 447
Orudis Capsules (Less than 1%) 2874
Oruvail Capsules (Less than 1%) 2874
OxyContin Tablets (Less than 1%) 2163
Paxil Tablets (Frequent; 2%) 2681
Penetrex Tablets (Less than 0.1%) 2196
Permax Tablets (Frequent) 571
Prevacid Delayed-Release Capsules (Less than 1%) 2746
ProSom Tablets (Infrequent) 457
Prozac Pulvules & Liquid, Oral Solution (2%) 935
Redux Capsules (Infrequent) 2911
Remeron Tablets (Frequent) 1878
Rilutek Tablets (Infrequent) 2198
Risperdal Tablets (Infrequent) 1348
Roferon-A Injection (Less than 0.5% to less than 3%) 2308
Sandostatin Injection (Less than 1%) 2421
Serax Capsules 2916
Serax Tablets 2916
Sular Tablets (Less than or equal to 1%) 2961
Symmetrel Capsules (0.1% to 1%) 965
Symmetrel Syrup (0.1% to 1%) 963
Tambocor Tablets (Less than 1%) 1555
Tegison Capsules (Less than 1%) 2314
Tenex Tablets (3% or less) 2249
Tiazac Capsules (Less than 1%) 1019
Ultram Tablets (50 mg) (Less than 1%) 1594
Versed Injection (Less than 1%) 2324
Videx Tablets, Powder for Oral Solution, & Pediatric Powder for Oral Solution (1%) 2980
Vistide Injection 1057
Xanax Tablets 2115
Zoloft Tablets (Infrequent) 2051
Zyloprim Tablets (Less than 1%) 1194
Zyrtec Tablets (Less than 2%) 2053

Amnesia, traveler's

Halcion Tablets 2093

Amnionitis

▲ Cleocin Vaginal Cream (6%) 2070
Prepidil Gel 2108

Amputation, gangrene of the extremities-induced

Heparin Lock Flush Solution 2831
Heparin Sodium Injection 2832

Analgesia, reversal

Narcan Injection 950

Anaphylactic reactions

Acel-Imune Diphtheria and Tetanus Toxoids and Acellular Pertussis Vaccine Adsorbed (Rare) 1415
Aldoclor Tablets 1638
Aldoril Tablets 1644
Amoxil 2631
Ancef Injection 2632
Antivenin (Black Widow Spider) 1647
AquaMEPHYTON Injection 1648
Atrovent Inhalation Aerosol 674
Atrovent Nasal Spray 0.06% 678
Augmentin 2637
Augmentin Tablets 2640
Benemid Tablets 1651
Biavax II 1653
Bicillin C-R Injection 2810
Bicillin L-A Injection 2813
Brontex (Rare) 2130
Capozide Tablets 744
Cefotan 2936
Chloromycetin Sodium Succinate 1960
Cipro I.V. (1% or less) 587
Cipro I.V. Pharmacy Bulk Package (Less than 1%) 590
Cipro Tablets 584
Cortisporin Otic Solution Sterile 1076
Cytosar-U Sterile Powder (Less frequent) 2077
Cytovene-IV (Two or more reports) 2270
Cytoxan (Rare) 700
Desferal Vials 838
Diflucan Tablets, Injection, and Oral Suspension (Rare) 2003
Digibind 1079
Dilaudid Tablets and Liquid 1386
Diphtheria and Tetanus Toxoids and Pertussis Vaccine Adsorbed (Rare) 2650
Diucardin Tablets 2824
Diupres Tablets 1691
Diuril Oral Suspension 1694
Diuril Sodium Intravenous 1693
Diuril Tablets 1694
Dobutrex Solution Vials 1480
Dolobid Tablets (Less than 1 in 100) 1695
Dyclone 0.5% and 1% Topical Solutions, USP 535
Easprin 1971
Elspar 1700
Eminase (0.2%) 2215
Enduron Tablets 424
▲ Etopophos for Injection (3%) 701
Etoposide Injection (0.7% to 2%) 539
Factrel (Rare) 2996
Floxin I.V. 1580
Floxin Tablets (200 mg, 300 mg, 400 mg) 1577
Gamimune N, 5% Immune Globulin Intravenous (Human), 5% 612
Gamimune N, 10% Immune Globulin Intravenous (Human), 10% 615
Gammagard S/D, Immune Globulin, Intravenous (Human) (A remote possibility) 577
Gammar-P I.V., Immune Globulin Intravenous (Human) 798
Gastrocrom Oral Concentrate (Rare) 1611
Geocillin Tablets 2009
Heparin Lock Flush Solution 2831
Heparin Sodium Injection 2832
Hep-B-Gammagee (Rare) 1706
Hespan Injection (Rare) 945
Humalog Injection (Less common) 1488
HydroDIURIL Tablets 1716
Hydropres Tablets 1718
HyperHep Hepatitis B Immune Globulin (Human) (Rare) 619
Hyskon Hysteroscopy Fluid (Rare) 1633
Hyzaar Tablets 1720
Imogam Rabies Immune Globulin (Human) (Rare) 897
Imovax Rabies Vaccine 899
Inderide Tablets 2838
Inderide LA Long Acting Capsules 2840
INFeD (Iron Dextran Injection, USP) 2478
Isuprel Hydrochloride Solution 2443
Levatol Tablets 2547
Lupron Depot 7.5 mg (One report) 2741
Lupron Injection (One report) 2736
Lupron Injection Pediatric 2737
LUVOX Tablets 2723
M-M-R II 1730
Marcaine Spinal (Rare) 2449
Maxaquin Tablets (Occasional) 2593
Mefoxin Premixed Intravenous Solution 1737
Merrem I.V. 2952
Meruvax II 1740
Mesnex Injection 711
Mezlin 594
Mezlin Pharmacy Bulk Package 597
Mintezol 1747
Moduretic Tablets 1748
MSTA Mumps Skin Test Antigen 2988
Mykrox Tablets (rare) 1617
Nasalcrom Nasal Solution (1 in 430) 2192
Norflex (Rare) 1554

(▣ Described in PDR For Nonprescription Drugs) Incidence data in parenthesis; ▲ 3% or more (◉ Described in PDR For Ophthalmology)

Normodyne Injection 2519
Normodyne Tablets 2522
Noroxin Tablets (Occasional) 1758
Noroxin Tablets (Occasional) 2222
Nubain Injection (1% or less) 952
Omnipen Capsules 2872
▲ Oncaspar (Greater than 1% but less than 5%) 2194
Orthoclone OKT3 Sterile Solution 1892
Orudis Capsules (Less than 1%) 2874
Oruvail Capsules (Less than 1%) 2874
Parafon Forte DSC Caplets (Extremely rare) 1590
Paraplatin for Injection 713
Pergonal (menotropins for injection, USP) (Some patients) 2618
Pfizerpen for Injection (Occasional) 2022
Phenergan Injection 2880
Pipracil 1435
Platinol for Injection (Occasional) 717
Platinol-AQ Injection (Occasional) 719
Pred Mild ⊙ 250
Primaxin I.M. 1770
Primaxin I.V. 1772
Prinzide Tablets 1780
Prograf (A few patients) 1028
Protamine Sulfate Vials 1526
Rabies Vaccine, Imovax Rabies I.D. 901
RespiGam 1631
Ridaura Capsules 2691
Risperdal Tablets 1348
Robaxin Injectable 2245
Roferon-A Injection (Rare) 2308
Rowasa 2727
Sandimmune I.V. Ampuls for Infusion (Rare) 2416
Sandoglobulin I.V. 2419
Sensorcaine 554
Septra I.V. Infusion 1142
Septra I.V. Infusion ADD-Vantage Vials 1144
Soma Compound w/Codeine Tablets 2784
Spectrobid Tablets (Occasional) 2030
Stelazine 2692
Streptase for Infusion (Rare) 557
Streptomycin Sulfate Injection 2031
Syntocinon Injection 2425
Talacen Caplets (One instance) 2464
Tao Capsules 2033
Terramycin Intramuscular Solution 2034
Tetramune (Rare) 1449
Thorazine 2701
Timentin for Injection 2706
Timolide Tablets 1791
Toradol 2319
Tracrium Injection 1155
Trandate Injection 1158
Trasylol (Less than 0.5%) 607
Triavil Tablets 1800
Tri-Immunol Adsorbed (Rare) 1452
Trilafon 2532
Tripedia 908
Tympagesic Ear Drops 2476
Typhim Vi 914
Unasyn (Occasional) 2035
Vaseretic Tablets 1810
VePesid Capsules and Injection 727
Vibramycin Hyclate Intravenous 2040
Vibra-Tabs Film Coated Tablets 2038
Zaroxolyn Tablets 1625
Zestoretic Tablets 2968
Ziac 1459
Zoladex 3-month (One report) 2978
Zosyn (Occasional) 1463

Anaphylactic shock

Ambien Tablets (Rare) 2559
Aquasol A Parenteral 526
Benadryl Injection 1955
Calcimar Injection, Synthetic (A few cases) 2176
CytoGam (A possibility) 1630
Declomycin Tablets 1421
Disalcid 1549
Eminase (0,1%) 2215
Ethamolin Injection 2544
Fioricet with Codeine Capsules 2387
Fiorinal with Codeine Capsules 2390
Hep-B-Gammagee 1706
Hyperab Rabies Immune Globulin (Human) (Rare) 618
Hyper-Tet Tetanus Immune Globulin (Human) (Few isolated cases) 621
Miacalcin Injection (A few cases) 2402
Myochrysine Injection 1754
Ornade Spansule Capsules 2678
Orthoclone OKT3 Sterile Solution 1892
PBZ Tablets 863
PBZ-SR Tablets 862
Periactin 1767
Protamine Sulfate Vials 1526
Salflex Tablets 791
Sandostatin Injection (Several patients) 2421
Solganal Suspension 2530
Soma Compound w/Codeine Tablets 2784
Soma Compound Tablets 2783
Soma Tablets 2782
Sotradecol (Sodium Tetradecyl Sulfate Injection) 987
Streptase for Infusion (Very rare) 557
Tavist Syrup 2426
Tavist Tablets 2427
Tetramune (Rare) 1449
Thioplex (Thiotepa For Injection) 1329
Toradol 2319
Trasylol 607
Trinalin Repetabs Tablets 1373
Tripedia 908
Tussend 1830
Vantin for Oral Suspension and Vantin Tablets (Less than 1%) 2112
Yutopar Intravenous Injection (Infrequent) 566

Anaphylactoid reactions

Abelcet Injection 1540
Accupril Tablets 1950
Achromycin V Capsules 1417
Activase (Very rare) 1045
Altace Capsules (Less than 1%) 1238
Amen Tablets 785
Amicar Syrup, Tablets, and Injection 1312
Amoxil (occasional) 2631
Anaprox/Naprosyn (Less than 1%) 2277
Androderm Testosterone Transdermal System (Rare) 2634
Android Capsules, 10 mg (Rare) 1297
Aquasol A Parenteral (One case) 526
Attenuvax 1650
Betaseron for SC Injection 653
Biavax II 1653
Capoten Tablets 740
Capozide Tablets 744
Carbocaine Injection (Rare) 2432
Cataflam Tablets (Less than 1%) 833
Ceclor Pulvules & Suspension 1470
Celestone Soluspan Suspension (Rare) 2484
Cerubidine for Injection (Rare) 634
Chibroxin Sterile Ophthalmic Solution (With oral form) 1657
Cleocin Phosphate Injection (A few cases) 2068
Cleocin Vaginal Cream (A few cases) 2070
Compazine 2644
Cortone Acetate Sterile Suspension 1663
Cycrin Tablets 991
Dalalone D.P. Injectable 1009
Decadron Phosphate Injection 1680
Decadron Phosphate with Xylocaine Injection, Sterile 1683
Decadron-LA Sterile Suspension 1687
Depo-Provera Contraceptive Injection 2079
Depo-Provera Sterile Aqueous Suspension 2083
Deponit NTG Transdermal Delivery System 2541
Digibind 1079
Diprivan Injectable Emulsion (Less than 1%) 2939
Duranest Injections 533
EC-Naprosyn Delayed-Release Tablets (Less than 1%) 2277
Eminase (0.2%) 2215
EMLA Cream 536
Engerix-B Unit-Dose Vials 2656
Epogen for Injection 489
Estratest (Rare) 2718
Etrafon 2495
Fansidar Tablets 2281
Felbatol (Rare) 2774
Florinef Acetate Tablets 506
Floxin I.V. 1580
Floxin Tablets (200 mg, 300 mg, 400 mg) 1577
Fragmin Injection (A few cases) 2088
Fungizone Intravenous 507
Gamimune N, 5% Immune Globulin Intravenous (Human), 5% (Very rare) 612
Gamimune N, 10% Immune Globulin Intravenous (Human), 10% (Very rare) 615
Gammar-P I.V., Immune Globulin Intravenous (Human) (Very rare) 798
Garamycin Injectable 2502
Gemzar for Injection (Rare) 1482
Halotestin Tablets 2095
Havrix (Rare) 2663
Heparin Sodium Vials (Rare) 1486
Hespan Injection (Rare) 945
Hivid Tablets (One patient) 2287
Hydeltrasol Injection, Sterile 1708
Hydeltra-T.B.A. Sterile Suspension 1710
Hydrocortone Acetate Sterile Suspension 1712
Hydrocortone Phosphate Injection, Sterile 1713
Imitrex Injection (Rare) 1095
Imitrex Tablets (Rare) 1099
Imogam Rabies Immune Globulin (Human) (Rare) 897
Kytril Injection (Rare) 2667
Leucovorin Calcium for Injection 1313
Leucovorin Calcium Tablets 1315
Levoprome 1321
Lodine Capsules and Tablets (Less than 1%) 2849
Lotensin Tablets 852
Lotensin HCT Tablets (Two patients) 855
Lotrel Capsules 858
Lupron Depot 3.75 mg (Rare) 2739
Lupron Depot 7.5 mg (Rare) 2741
Lupron Depot - 3 Month 22.5 mg (Rare) 2743
Lupron Depot-PED 7.5 mg, 11.25 mg and 15 mg 2744
M-M-R II 1730
M-R-VAX II 1732
Marcaine 2446
Mavik Tablets 1407
Maxaquin Tablets 2593
Meruvax II 1740
Methotrexate Sodium Tablets, Injection, for Injection and LPF Injection 1322
Mezlin 594
Monocid Injection (Less than 1%) 2674
Monopril Tablets 762
Motrin Ibuprofen Suspension, Oral Drops, Chewable Tablets, Caplets (Less than 1%) 1563
Mumpsvax 1751
Myambutol Tablets 1432
▲ Naprelan Tablets (3% to 9%) 2861
Anaprox/Naprosyn (Less than 1%) 2277
NegGram (Occasional) 2453
Nescaine/Nescaine MPF 549
Neutrexin for Injection (One report) 2761
Nitro-Bid IV (A few reports) 1270
Nitro-Bid Ointment (A few reports) 1272
Nitro-Dur (nitroglycerin) Transdermal Infusion System (A few reports) 1365
Normodyne Injection (Rare) 2519
Normodyne Tablets (Rare) 2522
Noroxin Tablets (Occasional) 1758
Noroxin Tablets (Occasional) 2222
Novocain Hydrochloride for Spinal Anesthesia 2457
Nubain Injection (1% or less) 952
Orthoclone OKT3 Sterile Solution 1892
Pen•Vee K (Occasional) 2879
Pneumovax 23 (Rare) 1768
Pnu-Imune 23 (Rare) 1437
Premphase 2900
Prempro 2905
Prinivil Tablets (0.3% to 1.0%) 1776
Prinzide Tablets 1780
Procrit for Injection 1896
Prolixin 510
Protamine Sulfate Vials 1526
Provera Tablets 2110
Pyridium (One report) 1985
Relafen Tablets (Rarer) 2688
Sandoglobulin I.V. 2419
Sandostatin Injection (Several patients) 2421
Sensorcaine 554
Stelazine Concentrate 2692
Streptase for Infusion (Rare) 557
Testoderm Testosterone Transdermal System (Rare) 486
Testred Capsules, 10 mg (Rare) 1308
Tetanus Toxoid Adsorbed Purogenated 1447
Tolectin (200, 400 and 600 mg) (Less than 1%) 1591
Toradol 2319
Tracrium Injection 1155
Trandate (Rare) 1158
Transderm-Nitro Transdermal Therapeutic System (A few reports) 878
Trental Tablets (Rare) 1291
Ultram Tablets (50 mg) 1594
Univasc Tablets 2553
Vancocin HCl, Oral Solution & Pulvules 1536
Vancocin HCl, Vials & ADD-Vantage 1534
Vaseretic Tablets 1810
Vasotec I.V. 1814
Vasotec Tablets (0.5% to 1.0%) 1816
Versed Injection 2324
Videx Tablets, Powder for Oral Solution, & Pediatric Powder for Oral Solution (Less than 1%) 2980
Cataflam/Voltaren/Voltaren-XR (Less than 1%) 833
Xylocaine Injections (Extremely rare) 562
Zestoretic Tablets 2968
Zestril Tablets (0.3% to 1.0%) 2972

Anaphylaxis

Abbokinase (Rare) 403
Abbokinase Open-Cath (Rare) 405
Abelcet Injection (One case) 1540
Achromycin V Capsules 1417
Adriamycin PFS 2056
Adriamycin RDF 2056
Alfenta Injection 1334
Alferon N Injection 2142
Alkeran for Injection (2.4%) 1196
Alkeran Tablets (Rare) 1198
Amen Tablets 785
Amicar Syrup, Tablets, and Injection 1312
Amoxil 2631
Ancef Injection 2632
Anectine (Rare) 1062
Antivenin (Crotalidae) Polyvalent 2803
AquaMEPHYTON Injection 1648
Atrovent Inhalation Solution (A single case) 675
Attenuvax 1650
Axid Pulvules (Rare) 1468
Azactam for Injection (Less than 1%) 736
Azulfidine (Rare) 2059
Bactrim DS Tablets 2257
Bactrim I.V. Infusion 2255
Bactrim 2257
Benemid Tablets 1651
Bentyl 1246
Biavax II 1653
Biaxin (Rare) 406
Bicillin C-R Injection 2810
Bicillin C-R 900/300 Injection 2812
Blenoxane (Approximately 1%) 697
Calcimar Injection, Synthetic (One case) 2176
Cataflam Tablets (Rare) 833
Ceclor Pulvules & Suspension (Rare) 1470
Cedax 2480
Cefizox for Intramuscular or Intravenous Use (Rare) 1025
Ceftin 1067
Cefzil Tablets and Oral Suspension (Rare) 747
Ceptaz (Very rare) 1070
Chloromycetin Sodium Succinate 1960
Claforan Sterile and Injection (Less frequent) 1259
Claritin Tablets (Rare) 2485
Claritin-D Tablets 2487
Clinoril Tablets 1658
ColBENEMID Tablets 1662
Cortisporin Ophthalmic Ointment Sterile (Rare) 1074
Cortisporin Ophthalmic Suspension Sterile (Rare) 1075
Cycrin Tablets 991
CytoGam 1630
Cytosar-U Sterile Powder (One case) 2077
Cytotec (Infrequent) 2576
DDAVP Injection (Rare) 2178
DDAVP Injection 15 mcg/mL (Rare) 2179
Dantrium Capsules (Less frequent) 2131
Dantrium Intravenous (One case) 2132
Daypro Caplets (Less than 1%) 2578
Declomycin Tablets 1421
Depo-Provera Contraceptive Injection 2079

(Described in PDR For Nonprescription Drugs) Incidence data in parenthesis; ▲ 3% or more (⊙ Described in PDR For Ophthalmology)

1253 Side Effects Index Anemia

Depo-Provera Sterile Aqueous Suspension 2083
Desmopressin Acetate Injection (Rare) 996
Diamox ⊙ 317
Diflucan Tablets, Injection, and Oral Suspension (Rare) 2003
Digibind 1079
Diprivan Injectable Emulsion (Rare; less than 1%) 2939
Donnatal 2234
Donnatal Extentabs 2234
Donnatal Tablets 2234
Doryx Capsules 1970
Doxorubicin Astra 531
Duricef Capsules, Tablets, and Oral Suspension 750
Dyazide Capsules 2653
Dynabac 668
DYNACIN Capsules 1627
Dyrenium Capsules 2655
E.E.S. 427
E-Mycin Tablets 1388
Easprin 1971
Elspar 1700
Engerix-B Unit-Dose Vials 2656
Ergamisol Tablets (Less frequent) 1340
ERYC 1972
EryPed 425
Ery-Tab Tablets 426
Erythrocin Stearate Filmtab 429
Erythromycin Base Filmtab 430
Erythromycin Delayed-Release Capsules, USP 431
Ethamolin Injection (Three reports) 2544
Feldene Capsules (Less than 1%) 2008
Flexeril Tablets 1701
Fludara for Injection (Up to 1%) 658
Fluorescite ⊙ 217
Fluorouracil Injection 2282
Fluvirin (Influenza Virus Vaccine) (Rare) 1608
Fortaz (Very rare) 1092
Sterile FUDR (Remote possibility) 2284
Gamimune N, 5% Immune Globulin Intravenous (Human), 5% (Rare) 612
Gantanol Tablets 2285
Gantrisin 2286
GlaucTabs ⊙ 209
Havrix (Rare) 2663
Helidac Therapy 2135
Hep-B-Gammagee 1706
Hytrin Capsules (Rare) 434
IBU Tablets (Less than 1%) 1389
Ilosone 927
Ilotycin Gluceptate, IV, Vials 929
Imitrex Injection (Rare) 1095
Imitrex Tablets (Rare) 1099
Inapsine Injection (Less common) 462
Indocin Capsules (Less than 1%) 1723
Indocin I.V. (Less than 1%) 1727
Indocin (Less than 1%) 1723
INFeD (Iron Dextran Injection, USP) 2478
Influenza Virus Vaccine, Trivalent, Types A and B (chromatograph- and filter-purified subviron antigen) FluShield, 1996-1997 Formula (Rare) 2842
Intal Inhaler (Infrequent) 2185
Intal Nebulizer Solution (Rare) 2186
Intron A for Injection (Rare) 2506
JE-VAX (One episode) 904
Keflex Pulvules & Oral Suspension 930
Keftab Tablets 931
Kefurox Vials, Faspak & ADD-Vantage (Rare) 1509
Kefzol Vials, Faspak & ADD-Vantage 1511
Kytril Injection (Rare) 2667
Kytril Tablets (Rare) 2669
Lamisil Tablets (Rare) 2394
Lescol Capsules (Rare) 2395
Lomotil 2591
Lopid Tablets 1974
Lorabid Suspension and Pulvules (Rare) 1513
Lutrepulse for Injection 998
M-M-R II 1730
M-R-VAX II 1732
Macrobid Capsules 2138
Macrodantin Capsules 2140
Mandol Vials, Faspak & ADD-Vantage 1516
Maxaquin Tablets 2593
Mefoxin 1734
Mefoxin Premixed Intravenous Solution 1737
Meruvax II 1740
Methergine (Rare isolated reports) 2401
Mevacor Tablets (Rare) 1742
Miltown Tablets (Rare) 2780
Minocin Intravenous 1428
Minocin Oral Suspension 1431
Minocin Pellet-Filled Capsules 1429
Mintezol 1747
Monoclate-P, Factor VIII:C Pasteurized, Monoclonal Antibody Purified Antihemophilic Factor (Human) 802
Monodox Capsules 1858
Mononine, Coagulation Factor IX (Human), Monoclonal Antibody Purified 804
Motofen Tablets 789
Motrin Ibuprofen Suspension, Oral Drops, Chewable Tablets, Caplets (Less than 1%) 1563
Mumpsvax 1751
Mustargen 1752
Nalfon 200 Pulvules & Nalfon Tablets (Less than 1%) 933
Nasalcrom Nasal Solution (1 case) 2192
Navane Capsules and Concentrate (Rare) 2018
Navane Intramuscular (Rare) 2019
Navelbine Injection 1212
Neosporin Ophthalmic Ointment Sterile (Rare) 1130
Neosporin Ophthalmic Solution Sterile (Rare) 1131
Neptazane Tablets ⊙ 320
Nizoral Tablets (Rare) 1345
Omnipen Capsules 2872
Omnipen for Oral Suspension 2873
Oncaspar 2194
Oncovin Solution Vials & Hyporets (Rare) 1521
Orthoclone OKT3 Sterile Solution 1892
Orudis Capsules (Less than 1%) 2874
Oruvail Capsules (Less than 1%) 2874
PCE Dispertab Tablets 453
Pediazole Suspension 2340
Pen•Vee K (Occasional) 2879
Pepcid Injection (Infrequent) 1765
Pepcid (Infrequent) 1763
Pfizerpen for Injection (Severe & occasionally fatal. (See Warnings)) 2022
PMB 200 and PMB 400 2890
Polysporin Ophthalmic Ointment Sterile (Rare) 1140
Pontocaine Hydrochloride for Spinal Anesthesia 2460
Pravachol Tablets (Rare) 770
Premphase 2900
Prempro 2905
Pro-Banthine Tablets 2226
Prograf (A small percentage of patients) 1028
Proloprim Tablets (Rare) 1141
Prostigmin Injectable 1305
Prostigmin Tablets 1306
Protamine Sulfate Vials 1526
Proventil Syrup (Rare) 2528
Provera Tablets 2110
Recombivax HB (Less than 1%) 1787
Redux Capsules 2911
Relafen Tablets (Rarer) 2688
ReoPro Vials 1526
Retrovir Capsules (One patient) 1216
Retrovir I.V. Infusion (One patient) 1221
Retrovir Syrup (One patient) 1216
Robinul Forte Tablets 2247
Robinul Injectable 2247
Robinul Tablets 2247
Rocephin Injectable Vials, ADD-Vantage, Galaxy Container (Rare) 2305
Rubex for Injection 721
Seldane Tablets 1284
Seldane-D Extended-Release Tablets 1286
Semprex-D Capsules (Rare) 1620
Septra 1146
Septra I.V. Infusion 1142
Septra I.V. Infusion ADD-Vantage Vials 1144
Septra 1146
Sporanox Capsules (Rare) 1352
Stimate, (desmopressin acetate) Nasal Spray, 1.5 mg/mL (One patient) 806
Sublimaze Injection 463
Sufenta Injection 1355
Suprax 1443
Tagamet (Rare) 2694
Tao Capsules 2033
Taxol Injection (2%) 723
Tazicef for Injection (Very rare) 2697
Tazidime Vials, Faspak & ADD-Vantage (Very rare) 1531
Terramycin Intramuscular Solution 2034
Tetanus Toxoid Adsorbed Purogenated 1447
Tilade Inhaler (Isolated cases) 2207
Toradol 2319
Trasylol 607
Trimpex Tablets (Rare) 2323
Ultram Tablets (50 mg) (Less than 1%) 1594
Vancocin HCl, Oral Solution & Pulvules (Infrequent) 1536
Vancocin HCl, Vials & ADD-Vantage (Infrequent) 1534
Varivax 1807
Velosulin BR Human Insulin 10 ml Vials 1847
Ventolin Inhalation Aerosol and Refill 1170
Ventolin Rotacaps for Inhalation 1173
Ventolin Syrup (Rare) 1175
Vibramycin 2038
Vistide Injection 1057
Cataflam/Voltaren/Voltaren-XR (Rare) 833
Vumon for Injection 729
Zantac (Rare) 1182
Zantac Injection (Rare) 1180
Zantac Syrup (Rare) 1182
Zinacef (Rare) 1184
Zithromax (Rare) 2043
Zithromax Tablets (Rare) 2046
Zocor Tablets (Rare) 1821
Zofran Injection (Rare) 1227
Zofran Tablets (Rare) 1231
Zosyn (1.0% or less) 1463
Zovirax Capsules (Rare) 1187
Zovirax Sterile Powder (Rare) 1191
Zovirax (Rare) 1187
Zyrtec Tablets (Rare) 2053

Androgen excess, signs or symptoms of

Danocrine Capsules 2437
Lupron Depot 3.75 mg (Less than 5%) 2739

Anemia (see also under Aplastic anemia; Hypoplastic anemia; Megaloblastic anemia)

▲ Abelcet Injection (4%) 1540
Accutane Capsules (Less than 1%) 2252
Adalat Capsules (10 mg and 20 mg) (Less than 0.5%) 580
Adalat CC (Rare) 582
Alkeran for Injection 1196
Alkeran Tablets 1198
Ambien Tablets (Rare) 2559
Amikacin Sulfate Injection, USP (Rare) 523
Amikacin Sulfate Injection, USP (Rare) 981
Amikin Injectable (Rare) 502
Amoxil 2631
Anafranil Capsules (Up to 2%) 819
Ancobon Capsules 2254
Anturane (Rare) 823
▲ Aredia for Injection (Up to 29.6%) 827
Arimidex Tablets (2% to 5%) 2932
Asacol Delayed-Release Tablets 2129
Atamet Tablets (Rare) 567
Atromid-S Capsules 2808
Augmentin 2637
Augmentin Tablets 2640
▲ Avonex (8%) 662
▲ Axid Pulvules (More frequent) 1468
Azactam for Injection (Less than 1%) 736
Azulfidine 2059
Benemid Tablets 1651
BiCNU (Less frequent) 696
Capoten Tablets 740
Capozide Tablets 744
▲ Casodex Tablets (7%) 2934
Cataflam Tablets (Sometimes) 833
CeeNU Capsules 699
Cefizox for Intramuscular or Intravenous Use (Rare) 1025
▲ CellCept Capsules (25.6% to 25.8%) 2265
Cerebyx Injection (Infrequent) 1956
Cipro Tablets (Less than 0.1%) 584
Clinoril Tablets (Less than 1%) 1658
Clozaril Tablets (Less than 1%) 2377
Cognex Capsules (Infrequent) 1961
ColBENEMID Tablets 1662
Cosmegen Injection 1666
Cozaar Tablets (Less than 1%) 1668
Crixivan Capsules (Less than 2%) 1670
Cytosar-U Sterile Powder 2077
Cytotec (Infrequent) 2576
▲ Cytovene (19%) 2270
Cytoxan (Occasional) 700
DTIC-Dome 593
Dalgan Injection (Less than 1%) 529
Daypro Caplets (Less than 1%) 2578
Demser Capsules (Rare) 1690
Demulen 2580
Depakene 416
Depakote Tablets 418
Depo-Provera Contraceptive Injection (Fewer than 1%) 2079
Desyrel and Desyrel Dividose 504
Dipentum Capsules (Rare) 2084
▲ Doxil (6.5% to 19.4%) 2613
Effexor (Infrequent) 2825
Eldepryl Capsules 2729
Epivir (2% to 2.9%) 1200
Ergamisol Tablets (Up to 6%) 1340
Esimil Tablets (A few instances) 840
▲ Etopophos for Injection (Up to 72%) 701
▲ Etoposide Injection (Up to 33%) 539
▲ Eulexin Capsules (6%) 2498
Felbatol 2774
Feldene Capsules (Greater than 1%) 2008
Floxin I.V. (More than or equal to 1%) 1580
Floxin Tablets (200 mg, 300 mg, 400 mg) (More than or equal to 1%) 1577
▲ Fludara for Injection (Among most common) 658
Fluorouracil Injection 2282
▲ Foscavir Injection (5% or greater up to 33%) 541
▲ Sterile FUDR (Among more common) 2284
Ganite 2711
Garamycin Injectable 2502
Gemzar for Injection 1482
Geocillin Tablets 2009
Glucophage Tablets (Very rare) 754
Haldol Decanoate 1587
Haldol Injection, Tablets and Concentrate 1585
▲ Hivid Tablets (Less than 1% to 8.4%) 2287
▲ Hycamtin for Injection (40% to 95%) 2665
Hydrea Capsules (Less often) 705
Hyzaar Tablets 1720
Imitrex Tablets (Rare) 1099
Indocin Capsules (Less than 1%) 1723
Indocin I.V. (Less than 1%) 1727
Indocin (Less than 1%) 1723
Intal Inhaler (Rare) 2185
Intal Nebulizer Solution (Rare) 2186
▲ Intron A for Injection (Less than 5% to 22%) 2506
Invirase Capsules (Less than 2%) 2291
Ismelin Tablets 845
Kadian Capsules (Less than 3%) 2948
Kerlone Tablets (Less than 2%) 2588
Klonopin Tablets 2294
▲ Kytril Tablets (4%) 2669
Lamictal Tablets (Infrequent) 1105
Lamprene Capsules (Less than 1%) 846
Lasix Injection, Oral Solution and Tablets 1267
▲ Leustatin (Common; 37%) 1889
Lioresal Intrathecal (1% or more) 1634
Lodine Capsules and Tablets (Less than 1%) 2849
Lopid Tablets (Rare) 1974
Lupron Depot - 3 Month 22.5 mg (Less than 5%) 2743
▲ Lupron Injection (5% or more) 2736
LUVOX Tablets (Infrequent) 2723
Macrobid Capsules 2138
Macrodantin Capsules 2140
▲ Matulane Capsules (Frequent) 2300
Maxaquin Tablets (Less than or equal to 0.1%) 2593
Mefoxin 1734
Mefoxin Premixed Intravenous Solution 1737
▲ Megace Oral Suspension (Up to 5%) 708
Mellaril 2398
▲ Mepron Suspension (4% to 6%) 1206
Merrem I.V. (0.1% to 1.0%) 2952
Mesantoin Tablets (Uncommon) 2400

(▭ Described in PDR For Nonprescription Drugs) Incidence data in parenthesis; ▲ 3% or more (⊙ Described in PDR For Ophthalmology)

Anemia — Side Effects Index

Methotrexate Sodium Tablets, Injection, for Injection and LPF Injection ... 1322
Miacalcin Nasal Spray (Less than 1%) ... 2403
Monopril Tablets ... 762
▲ Mycobutin Capsules (6%) ... 2101
Myleran Tablets ... 1209
Naprelan Tablets (Less than 3%) .. 2861
▲ Navelbine Injection (1% to 77%) .. 1212
Nebcin Vials, Hyporets & ADD-Vantage ... 1518
Neoral (2% or less) ... 2405
Netromycin Injection 100 mg/ml (Fewer than 1 per 1000 patients) ... 2516
▲ Neupogen for Injection (Approximately 10%) ... 495
Neurontin Capsules (Infrequent) 1978
▲ Neutrexin for Injection (7.3%) ... 2761
Nimotop Capsules (Less than 1%) ... 603
▲ Nipent for Injection (8% to 35%) .. 2733
Nolvadex Tablets ... 2957
Norvir (Less than 2%) ... 447
Omnipen Capsules ... 2872
Omnipen for Oral Suspension ... 2873
Oncaspar ... 2194
Oncovin Solution Vials & Hyporets 1521
Orudis Capsules (Less than 1%) ... 2874
Oruvail Capsules (Less than 1%).... 2874
ParaGard T 380A Intrauterine Copper Contraceptive ... 1936
▲ Paraplatin for Injection (8% to 91%) ... 713
Parnate Tablets ... 2679
Paxil Tablets (Infrequent) ... 2681
Pentasa ... 1275
Permax Tablets (1.1%) ... 571
Platinol for Injection ... 717
Platinol-AQ Injection ... 719
Plendil Extended-Release Tablets (0.5% to 1.5%) ... 514
Pravachol Tablets ... 770
Prevacid Delayed-Release Capsules (Less than 1%) ... 2746
Prilosec Delayed-Release Capsules (Rare) ... 516
Prinivil Tablets ... 1776
Procardia Capsules (Less than 0.5%) ... 2024
▲ Prograf (4% to 47%) ... 1028
▲ Proleukin for Injection (77%) ... 812
Prozac Pulvules & Liquid, Oral Solution (Infrequent) ... 935
Purinethol Tablets (Frequent) ... 1214
Questran ... 774
Redux Capsules (Infrequent) ... 2911
Relafen Tablets (Less than 1%) 2688
Remeron Tablets (Rare) ... 1878
ReoPro Vials (1.2%) ... 1526
▲ Retrovir Capsules (1.1% to 29%) ... 1216
▲ Retrovir I.V. Infusion (1.1% to 29%) ... 1221
▲ Retrovir Syrup (1.1% to 29%)........ 1216
▲ Ridaura Capsules (3.1%) ... 2691
Rilutek Tablets (Infrequent) ... 2198
Risperdal Tablets (Infrequent) 1348
Ritalin ... 866
Rocephin Injectable Vials, ADD-Vantage, Galaxy Container (Less than 1%) ... 2305
Rythmol Tablets–150mg, 225mg, 300mg (Less than 1%) ... 1399
Sandimmune (2% or less) ... 2416
Sandostatin Injection (Less than 1%) ... 2421
Serentil ... 689
Serzone Tablets (Infrequent) ... 776
Sinemet Tablets (Rare) ... 959
Spectrobid Tablets ... 2030
Stelazine ... 2692
Sular Tablets (Less than or equal to 1%) ... 2961
Supprelin Injection (1%) ... 2230
▲ Taxol Injection (16% to 78%) ... 723
▲ Taxotere for Injection Concentrate (89.5%) ... 2204
▲ TheraCys BCG Live (Intravesical) (Up to 20.5%) ... 911
Thioguanine Tablets, Tabloid Brand ... 1225
Thioplex (Thiotepa For Injection) ... 1329
Ticar for Injection ... 2704
TICE BCG, USP (1.3%) ... 1881
Tonocard Tablets (Less than 1%) .. 519
Toradol (1% or less) ... 2319
Vaseretic Tablets ... 1810
Vasotec I.V. ... 1814
Vasotec Tablets ... 1816
Velban Vials ... 1537
▲ VePesid Capsules and Injection (Up to 33%) ... 727
Videx Tablets, Powder for Oral Solution, & Pediatric Powder for Oral Solution ... 2980
Virazole ... 1310
▲ Vistide Injection (20%) ... 1057
Cataflam/Voltaren/Voltaren-XR (Sometimes) ... 833
▲ Vumon for Injection (88%) ... 729
Wellbutrin Tablets (Rare) ... 1177
Zerit Capsules (Up to 3%) ... 731
Zestoretic Tablets ... 2968
Zoladex (Greater than 1% but less than 5%) ... 2976
Zoladex 3-month (1% to 5%) ... 2978
Zoloft Tablets (Rare) ... 2051
Zovirax Sterile Powder (Less than 1%) ... 1191
Zyloprim Tablets (Less than 1%).... 1194

Anemia, aplastic
(see under Aplastic anemia)

Anemia, dilutional
Prolastin Alpha₁-Proteinase Inhibitor (Human) ... 629

Anemia, glucose-6-phosphate dehydrogenase deficiency
Macrobid Capsules ... 2138
Macrodantin Capsules ... 2140

Anemia, Heinz-body
▲ Azulfidine (One in every 30 patients or less) ... 2059

Anemia, hemolytic, immune
Fludara for Injection ... 658
Tagamet (Extremely rare) ... 2694
Zantac (Exceedingly rare) ... 1182
Zantac Injection (Exceedingly rare) 1180
Zantac Syrup (Exceedingly rare)... 1182

Anemia, hemolytic, sideroblastic
Rifamate Capsules ... 1278

Anemia, hypochromic
▲ Casodex Tablets (7%) ... 2934
▲ CellCept Capsules (7.4% to 11.5%) ... 2265
Cerebyx Injection (Infrequent) 1956
Cytovene (1% or less) ... 2270
▲ Doxil (5.2% to 9.8%) ... 2613
Felbatol ... 2774
Foscavir Injection (Less than 1%) ... 541
Imdur (Less than or equal to 5%) .. 1362
Lovenox Injection (2%) ... 2187
Paxil Tablets (Rare) ... 2681
▲ Prograf (Greater than 3%) ... 1028
Rilutek Tablets (Rare) ... 2198
Risperdal Tablets (Infrequent) 1348

Anemia, hypoplastic
(see under Hypoplastic anemia)

Anemia, iron deficiency
▲ Casodex Tablets (7%) ... 2934
Fiorinal with Codeine Capsules 2390
Lamictal Tablets (Rare) ... 1105
Paxil Tablets (Rare) ... 2681
Prozac Pulvules & Liquid, Oral Solution (Rare) ... 935
Rilutek Tablets (Rare) ... 2198

Anemia, microangiopathic hemolytic
Mutamycin for Injection ... 712
Sandimmune (Occasional) ... 2416

Anemia, microcytic
Paxil Tablets (Rare) ... 2681

Anemia, nonhemolytic
Sinemet CR Tablets ... 961

Anemia, normochromic
▲ Fungizone Intravenous (Among most common) ... 507

Anemia, normocytic
▲ Fungizone Intravenous (Among most common) ... 507
Paxil Tablets (Rare) ... 2681
Risperdal Tablets (Rare) ... 1348

Anemia, sideroblastic
Cuprimine Capsules ... 1673
Depen Titratable Tablets ... 2770
Nydrazid Injection ... 509
Pyrazinamide Tablets (Rare) ... 1442

Rifater (Rare) ... 1280

Anencephaly
Felbatol ... 2774
Serophene (clomiphene citrate tablets, USP) ... 2621

Anesthesia, local
Zoloft Tablets (Rare) ... 2051

Anesthesia, persistent
Marcaine ... 2446

Anesthetic effect
Lithium Carbonate Capsules & Tablets ... 2352
Sensorcaine ... 554
Tonocard Tablets (Less than 1%) .. 519
Versed Injection ... 2324

Anetoderma
Cuprimine Capsules (Rare) ... 1673
Depen Titratable Tablets (Rare) ... 2770

Aneurysm
Anafranil Capsules (Rare) ... 819
Cognex Capsules (Infrequent) ... 1961
Fludara for Injection (Up to 1%) ... 658
Videx Tablets, Powder for Oral Solution, & Pediatric Powder for Oral Solution (Less than 1%)....... 2980

Anger
BuSpar Tablets (2%) ... 738
Desyrel and Desyrel Dividose (1.3% to 3.5%) ... 504
Valium Injectable ... 2336

Angiectases, cutaneous
Adalat CC (Less than 1.0%) ... 582

Angiitis
Esidrix Tablets ... 839
Esimil Tablets ... 840
Indocin Capsules (Less than 1%) ... 1723
Indocin I.V. (Less than 1%) ... 1727
Indocin (Less than 1%) ... 1723
Timolide Tablets ... 1791

Angina
Adalat Capsules (10 mg and 20 mg) (1 in 8 patients) ... 580
Ana-Kit Anaphylaxis Emergency Treatment Kit ... 611
Apresazide Capsules ... 824
Atromid-S Capsules ... 2808
Cardizem CD Capsules (Less than 1%) ... 1251
Cardizem SR Capsules (Less than 1%) ... 1255
Cardizem Tablets (Less than 1%) .. 1257
Clozaril Tablets (1%) ... 2377
Colestid (Infrequent) ... 2073
Dobutrex Solution Vials (1% to 3%) ... 1480
Ergamisol Tablets ... 1340
Esimil Tablets ... 840
▲ Fludara for Injection (Up to 6%) ... 658
Fluorouracil Injection ... 2282
Sterile FUDR (Remote possibility) ... 2284
Hyperstat I.V. Injection ... 2504
Imitrex Tablets (Rare) ... 1099
Intron A for Injection (Less than 5%) ... 2506
Ismelin Tablets ... 845
Isuprel Hydrochloride Solution 2443
Isuprel Injection ... 2441
Isuprel Mistometer ... 2442
Lupron Depot 7.5 mg (Less than 5%) ... 2741
Lupron Injection (Less than 5%) ... 2736
Mexitil Capsules (1.7% or about 3 in 1,000) ... 684
Monopril Tablets (0.2% to 1.0%).. 762
Norisodrine with Calcium Iodide Syrup ... 446
Normodyne Tablets ... 2522
OptiPranolol (Metipranolol 0.3%) Sterile Ophthalmic Solution (A small number of patients) ... ⓞ 256
Ornade Spansule Capsules ... 2678
Orthoclone OKT3 Sterile Solution .. 1892
Pravachol Tablets (0.1% to 4.0%) ... 770
Prevacid Delayed-Release Capsules (Less than 1%) ... 2746
Prilosec Delayed-Release Capsules (Less than 1%) ... 516
Primacor Injection (1.2%) ... 2461
Proleukin for Injection ... 812
Proventil Inhalation Aerosol ... 2524

Proventil Repetabs Tablets ... 2529
Proventil Syrup ... 2528
Proventil Tablets ... 2529
▲ Quinidex Extentabs (6%) ... 2240
Relafen Tablets (Less than 1%) ... 2688
Rifater ... 1280
Ritalin ... 866
▲ Rythmol Tablets–150mg, 225mg, 300mg (1.2% to 4.6%) ... 1399
Ser-Ap-Es Tablets ... 867
Sus-Phrine Injection ... 1017
Taxotere for Injection Concentrate (Rare) ... 2204
Tiazac Capsules (Less than 1%) 1019
Tonocard Tablets (Less than 1%) .. 519
Trandate ... 1158
Trental Tablets (0.3%) ... 1291
Trinalin Repetabs Tablets ... 1373
Triostat Injection (Approximately 1%) ... 2708
Univasc Tablets (Less than 1%) ... 2553
Ventolin Inhalation Aerosol and Refill ... 1170
Ventolin Rotacaps for Inhalation ... 1173
Ventolin Syrup ... 1175
Ventolin Tablets ... 1176
Volmax Extended-Release Tablets .. 1835
Zofran Injection (Rare) ... 1227
Zofran Tablets (Rare) ... 1231
Zosyn (1.0% or less) ... 1463

Angina, crescendo
Deponit NTG Transdermal Delivery System (Uncommon) ... 2541
Dilatrate-SR Capsules (Uncommon) ... 2542
Isordil Sublingual Tablets (Uncommon) ... 2845
Isordil Tembids (Uncommon) ... 2847
Isordil Titradose Tablets (Uncommon) ... 2848
Nitro-Bid IV (Uncommon) ... 1270
Nitro-Bid Ointment (Uncommon) ... 1272
Nitro-Dur (nitroglycerin) Transdermal Infusion System (Uncommon) ... 1365
Sorbitrate (Uncommon) ... 2959
Transderm-Nitro Transdermal Therapeutic System (Uncommon) ... 878

Angina, increased
▲ Cardene Capsules (5.6%) ... 2261
Deponit NTG Transdermal Delivery System (2%) ... 2541
Isordil Sublingual Tablets ... 2845
Isordil Tembids ... 2847
Isordil Titradose Tablets ... 2848
Lotrel Capsules (Rare) ... 858
Nitro-Bid IV ... 1270
Nitrostat Tablets ... 1981
Norvasc Tablets (Rare) ... 2020
Procardia Capsules (Very rare) ... 2024
Procardia XL Extended Release Tablets (1% or less) ... 2026
Transderm-Nitro Transdermal Therapeutic System (2%) ... 878
▲ Vascor Tablets (200 and 300 mg) (4.5%) ... 1597

Angina, Prinzmetal's, episodes of
Imitrex Injection ... 1095
Respbid Tablets ... 687

Angina tonsillaris
Invirase Capsules (Less than 2%) .. 2291

Angina pectoris
Accupril Tablets (Rare) ... 1950
Altace Capsules (Less than 1% to 2.9%) ... 1238
Ambien Tablets (Rare) ... 2559
Apresazide Capsules (Common) ... 824
Apresoline Hydrochloride Tablets (Common) ... 826
Betaseron for SC Injection ... 653
Brethaire Inhaler ... 830
Calan SR Caplets (1% or less) ... 2571
Calan Tablets (1% or less) ... 2568
Capoten Tablets (2 to 3 of 1000 patients) ... 740
Capozide Tablets (2 to 3 of 1000 patients) ... 744
Cardene I.V. ... 2815
Cardene SR Capsules (Rare) ... 2264
Cardura Tablets (Less than 0.5% of 3960 patients to 0.6%) ... 1993
Cartrol Tablets (Less common) ... 413
Casodex Tablets (2% to 5%) ... 2934
▲ CellCept Capsules (More than or equal to 3%) ... 2265

(🅟 Described in PDR For Nonprescription Drugs)   Incidence data in parenthesis; ▲ 3% or more   (ⓞ Described in PDR For Ophthalmology)

Side Effects Index

Cipro I.V. (1% or less) ... 587
Cipro I.V. Pharmacy Bulk Package (Less than 1%) ... 590
Cipro Tablets (Less than 1%) ... 584
Cognex Capsules (Infrequent) ... 1961
Covera-HS Tablets (2% or less) ... 2573
Cozaar Tablets (Less than 1%) ... 1668
Demulen ... 2580
Dilacor XR Extended-release Capsules ... 2183
Diupres Tablets ... 1691
Dobutrex Solution Vials (1% to 3%) ... 1480
Effexor (Infrequent) ... 2825
Eldepryl Capsules ... 2729
Esimil Tablets ... 840
▲ Flolan for Injection (19%) ... 1085
Hydralazine Hydrochloride Injection USP (Common) ... 2712
Hydropres Tablets ... 1718
Hyzaar Tablets ... 1720
Imitrex Injection ... 1095
Imitrex Tablets ... 1099
Ismelin Tablets ... 845
Isoptin Oral Tablets (Less than 1%) ... 1393
Isoptin SR Tablets (1% or less) ... 1395
Kerlone Tablets (Less than 2%) ... 2588
Kytril Tablets (Rare) ... 2669
Lamictal Tablets (Rare) ... 1105
Levlen/Tri-Levlen (Very infrequent) ... 646
Lotensin Tablets ... 852
LUVOX Tablets (Infrequent) ... 2723
Maxaquin Tablets (Less than 1%) ... 2593
Miacalcin Nasal Spray (1% to 3%) ... 2403
Midamor Tablets (Less than or equal to 1%) ... 1746
Modicon ... 1928
Moduretic Tablets (Less than or equal to 1%) ... 1748
Monopril Tablets (1.0% or more) ... 762
Naprelan Tablets (Less than 1%) ... 2861
Neurontin Capsules (Infrequent) ... 1978
Nipent for Injection (Less than 3%) ... 2733
Ortho-Cyclen/Ortho-Tri-Cyclen ... 1914
Ortho-Novum ... 1928
Ortho-Cyclen/Ortho Tri-Cyclen ... 1914
Paxil Tablets (Rare) ... 2681
Permax Tablets (Infrequent) ... 571
Persantine Tablets (Rare) ... 686
Plendil Extended-Release Tablets (0.5% to 1.5%) ... 514
Pondimin Tablets ... 2239
Prinivil Tablets (Greater than 1%) ... 1776
Prinzide Tablets ... 1780
Prozac Pulvules & Liquid, Oral Solution (Infrequent) ... 935
Redux Capsules (Frequent) ... 2911
Remeron Tablets (Infrequent) ... 1878
Rilutek Tablets (Infrequent) ... 2198
Risperdal Tablets (Rare) ... 1348
Ser-Ap-Es Tablets ... 867
Serzone Tablets (Infrequent) ... 776
Tambocor Tablets (Less than 1%) ... 1555
Timolide Tablets ... 1791
Levlen/Tri-Levlen (Very infrequent) ... 646
Vaseretic Tablets ... 1810
Vasotec I.V. ... 1814
Vasotec Tablets (1.5%) ... 1816
Verelan Capsules (1% or less) ... 1455
Videx Tablets, Powder for Oral Solution, & Pediatric Powder for Oral Solution (Less than 1%) ... 2980
Xalatan (1% to 2%) ... ⊚ 304
Zestoretic Tablets ... 2968
Zestril Tablets (Greater than 1%) ... 2972
Zoladex 3-month (1% to 5%) ... 2978

Angina pectoris, aggravation

Aldoclor Tablets ... 1638
Aldomet Ester HCl Injection ... 1642
Aldomet Oral ... 1640
Aldoril Tablets ... 1644
Blocadren Tablets (Less than 1%) ... 1654
Eldepryl Capsules ... 2729
Feldene Capsules (Less than 1%) ... 2008
Imdur (Less than or equal to 5%) ... 1362
Ismo Tablets (Fewer than 1%) ... 2844
Isordil Sublingual Tablets ... 2845
Isordil Tembids ... 2847
Isordil Titradose Tablets ... 2848
Nitro-Bid IV ... 1270
Nitrostat Tablets ... 1981
Sorbitrate ... 2959
Timoptic in Ocudose (Less frequent) ... 1796
Timoptic Sterile Ophthalmic Solution (Less frequent) ... 1794
Timoptic-XE ... 1798

Angina pectoris, exacerbation of, post-abrupt discontinuation

Cartrol Tablets ... 413
Inderal ... 2834
Inderal LA Long Acting Capsules ... 2836
Normodyne Injection ... 2519
Normodyne Tablets ... 2522
Tenoretic Tablets ... 2963
Tenormin Tablets and I.V. Injection ... 2965
Toprol-XL Tablets ... 560
Trandate ... 1158
Visken Tablets ... 2428

Angioedema
(see also under Edema, angioneurotic)

Bactrim DS Tablets ... 2257
Bactrim I.V. Infusion ... 2255
Bactrim ... 2257
Beclovent Inhalation Aerosol and Refill ... 1063
Beconase (Rare) ... 1065
Butisol Sodium Elixir & Tablets (Less than 1 in 100) ... 2768
Capoten Tablets (Approximately 1 in 1000 patients) ... 740
Capozide Tablets (Approximately 1 in 1000 patients) ... 744
Cardioquin Tablets ... 2146
Cataflam Tablets (Less than 1%) ... 833
Catapres Tablets (About 5 in 1,000 patients) ... 679
Ceptaz (Very rare) ... 1070
Chloromycetin Sodium Succinate ... 1960
Cipro I.V. (1% or less) ... 587
Cipro Tablets (Less than 1%) ... 584
Didronel Tablets ... 2133
Easprin ... 1971
Eskalith ... 2658
Feldene Capsules (Less than 1%) ... 2008
Fortaz (Very rare) ... 1092
Hep-B-Gammagee ... 1706
Indocin (Less than 1%) ... 1723
Intal Inhaler (Infrequent) ... 2185
Keflex Pulvules & Oral Suspension ... 930
Keftab Tablets ... 931
Lotrel Capsules (About 0.5%) ... 858
Macrobid Capsules ... 2138
Macrodantin Capsules ... 2140
Mebaral Tablets ... 2452
Mintezol ... 1747
Nalfon 200 Pulvules & Nalfon Tablets ... 933
Nasalcrom Nasal Solution ... 2192
NegGram ... 2453
Nembutal Sodium Capsules ... 440
Nembutal Sodium Solution ... 442
Nembutal Sodium Suppositories (Less than 1%) ... 444
Noroxin Tablets ... 1758
Noroxin Tablets ... 2222
Phenobarbital Elixir and Tablets (Less than 1 in 100 patients) ... 1523
Prinivil Tablets (0.3% to 1.0%) ... 1776
Proventil Inhalation Aerosol (Rare) ... 2524
Quinaglute Dura-Tabs Tablets ... 644
Quinidex Extentabs ... 2240
Recombivax HB (Less than 1%) ... 1787
Reglan (Rare) ... 2243
Ridaura Capsules ... 2691
Robaxisal Tablets ... 2246
Seconal Sodium Pulvules (Less than 1 in 100) ... 1529
Septra ... 1146
Septra I.V. Infusion ... 1142
Septra I.V. Infusion ADD-Vantage Vials ... 1144
Septra ... 1146
Soma Compound w/Codeine Tablets ... 2784
Soma Compound Tablets (Less common) ... 2783
Trental Tablets (Less than 1%) ... 1291
Vancenase PocketHaler Nasal Inhaler (Rare) ... 2534
Vanceril Inhaler ... 2538
Vaseretic Tablets (0.6%) ... 1810
Vasotec I.V. (0.5 to 1%) ... 1814
Vasotec Tablets ... 1816
Ventolin Inhalation Aerosol and Refill (Rare) ... 1170
Ventolin Inhalation Solution ... 1171
Ventolin Syrup ... 1175
Ventolin Tablets ... 1176
Cataflam/Voltaren/Voltaren-XR (Less than 1%) ... 833
Zestril Tablets (0.1%) ... 2972
Zithromax (1% or less; rare) ... 2043
Zithromax Tablets (1% or less) ... 2046

Angioedema, extremities

Accupril Tablets (0.1%) ... 1950
Altace Capsules ... 1238
Capoten Tablets (Approximately 1 in 1000 patients) ... 740
Capozide Tablets (Approximately 1 in 1000 patients) ... 744
Lotensin Tablets (0.5%) ... 852
Lotensin HCT Tablets (About 0.5%) ... 855
Lotrel Capsules ... 858
Monopril Tablets ... 762
Prinivil Tablets ... 1776
Prinzide Tablets (Rare) ... 1780
Univasc Tablets ... 2553
Vaseretic Tablets ... 1810
Vasotec I.V. ... 1814
Vasotec Tablets ... 1816
Zestoretic Tablets (Rare) ... 2968
Zestril Tablets ... 2972

Angioedema, eyes

Accupril Tablets ... 1950
Altace Capsules ... 1238
Capoten Tablets ... 740
Capozide Tablets ... 744
Lotensin HCT Tablets ... 855
Zestoretic Tablets ... 2968
Zestril Tablets ... 2972

Angioedema, face

Accupril Tablets (0.1%) ... 1950
Altace Capsules ... 1238
Atrovent Inhalation Aerosol ... 674
Atrovent Nasal Spray 0.06% ... 678
Capoten Tablets (Approximately 1 in 1000 patients) ... 740
Capozide Tablets (Approximately 1 in 1000 patients) ... 744
Catapres-TTS (2 of 3,539 patients) ... 680
Hyzaar Tablets (Rare) ... 1720
Lotensin Tablets (0.5%) ... 852
Lotensin HCT Tablets (0.3% to about 0.5%) ... 855
Lotrel Capsules (About 0.5%) ... 858
Monopril Tablets ... 762
Prinivil Tablets ... 1776
Prinzide Tablets (Rare) ... 1780
Univasc Tablets (Less than 0.5%) ... 2553
Vaseretic Tablets ... 1810
Vasotec I.V. ... 1814
Vasotec Tablets ... 1816
Zestoretic Tablets (Rare) ... 2968
Zestril Tablets ... 2972

Angioedema, glottis

Accupril Tablets (0.1%) ... 1950
Altace Capsules ... 1238
Capoten Tablets (Approximately 1 in 1000 patients) ... 740
Capozide Tablets (Approximately 1 in 1000 patients) ... 744
Lotensin Tablets (0.5%) ... 852
Lotensin HCT Tablets (About 0.5%) ... 855
Lotrel Capsules (About 0.5%) ... 858
Mavik Tablets (0.3% to 1.0%) ... 1407
Monopril Tablets ... 762
Prinivil Tablets ... 1776
Prinzide Tablets (Rare) ... 1780
Univasc Tablets ... 2553
Vaseretic Tablets ... 1810
Vasotec I.V. ... 1814
Vasotec Tablets ... 1816
Zestoretic Tablets (Rare) ... 2968
Zestril Tablets ... 2972

Angioedema, larynx

Accupril Tablets (0.1%) ... 1950
Altace Capsules ... 1238
Capoten Tablets (Approximately 1 in 1000 patients) ... 740
Capozide Tablets (Approximately 1 in 1000 patients) ... 744
Floxin Tablets (200 mg, 300 mg, 400 mg) ... 1577
Lotensin Tablets (0.5%) ... 852
Lotensin HCT Tablets (About 0.5%) ... 855
Monopril Tablets ... 762
Prinivil Tablets ... 1776
Prinzide Tablets (Rare) ... 1780
Univasc Tablets ... 2553
Vaseretic Tablets ... 1810
Vasotec I.V. ... 1814
Vasotec Tablets ... 1816
Zestoretic Tablets (Rare) ... 2968
Zestril Tablets ... 2972

Angioedema, lips

Accupril Tablets (0.1%) ... 1950
Altace Capsules ... 1238
Atrovent Inhalation Aerosol ... 674
Atrovent Nasal Spray 0.06% ... 678
Capoten Tablets (Approximately 1 in 1000 patients) ... 740
Capozide Tablets (Approximately 1 in 1000 patients) ... 744
Hyzaar Tablets (Rare) ... 1720
Lotensin Tablets (0.5%) ... 852
Lotensin HCT Tablets (0.3% to about 0.5%) ... 855
Lotrel Capsules ... 858
Monopril Tablets ... 762
Prinivil Tablets ... 1776
Prinzide Tablets (Rare) ... 1780
Univasc Tablets ... 2553
Vaseretic Tablets ... 1810
Vasotec I.V. ... 1814
Vasotec Tablets ... 1816
Zestoretic Tablets (Rare) ... 2968
Zestril Tablets ... 2972

Angioedema, mucous membranes of the mouth

Capozide Tablets (Approximately 1 in 1000 patients) ... 744

Angioedema, oropharyngeal

Adalat Capsules (10 mg and 20 mg) (Less than 0.5%) ... 580

Angioedema of tongue

Accupril Tablets (0.1%) ... 1950
Altace Capsules ... 1238
Atrovent Inhalation Aerosol ... 674
Atrovent Nasal Spray 0.06% ... 678
Capoten Tablets (Approximately 1 in 1000 patients) ... 740
Capozide Tablets (Approximately 1 in 1000 patients) ... 744
Catapres-TTS (One case) ... 680
Floxin I.V. ... 1580
Floxin Tablets (200 mg, 300 mg, 400 mg) ... 1577
Hyzaar Tablets (Rare) ... 1720
Lotensin Tablets (0.5%) ... 852
Lotensin HCT Tablets (About 0.5%) ... 855
Lotrel Capsules (About 0.5%) ... 858
Monopril Tablets ... 762
Prinivil Tablets ... 1776
Prinzide Tablets (Rare) ... 1780
Univasc Tablets ... 2553
Vaseretic Tablets ... 1810
Vasotec I.V. ... 1814
Vasotec Tablets ... 1816
Zestoretic Tablets (Rare) ... 2968
Zestril Tablets ... 2972

Angioma, spider

Avonex ... 662
Betaseron for SC Injection ... 653

Anhidrosis

Cogentin ... 1661
Kutrase Capsules ... 2546

Anisocoria

Anafranil Capsules (Up to 2%) ... 819
Betoptic Ophthalmic Solution (Rare) ... 465
Betoptic S Ophthalmic Suspension ... 467
Paxil Tablets (Rare) ... 2681
Redux Capsules (Rare) ... 2911

Ankylosing spondylosis

Lupron Injection ... 2736

Anorexia

Abelcet Injection ... 1540
Achromycin V Capsules (Rare) ... 1417
▲ ActHIB (2.2% to 26.1%) ... 893
▲ Actimmune (3%) ... 1043
Adapin Capsules ... 1542
Adderall Tablets ... 2209
Adriamycin PFS (Occasional) ... 2056
Adriamycin RDF (Occasional) ... 2056
Aldactazide Tablets ... 2556
Aldoclor Tablets ... 1638
Aldoril Tablets ... 1644
▲ Alferon N Injection (1% to 68%) ... 2142
Altace Capsules (Less than 1%) ... 1238
Ambien Tablets (1%) ... 2559
▲ Anafranil Capsules (12% to 22%) ... 819
Ancef Injection ... 2632
Ancobon Capsules ... 2254
Apresazide Capsules (Common) ... 824
Apresoline Hydrochloride Tablets (Common) ... 826

(⊡ Described in PDR For Nonprescription Drugs) Incidence data in parenthesis; ▲ 3% or more (⊚ Described in PDR For Ophthalmology)

Anorexia Side Effects Index 1256

Aquasol A Vitamin A Capsules, USP 525
Aquasol A Parenteral 526
Aralen Hydrochloride Injection 2430
Aralen Phosphate Tablets 2431
▲ Aredia for Injection (1% to at least 15%) 827
▲ Arimidex Tablets (6.9% to 7.7%) 2932
Asacol Delayed-Release Tablets 2129
Asendin Tablets (Very rare) 1419
Atamet Tablets (Less frequent) 567
Atretol Tablets 569
Atrohist Plus Tablets 1605
▲ Avonex (7%) 662
Axid Pulvules (1.2%) 1468
▲ Azulfidine (Approximately one-third of patients) 2059
▲ Bactrim DS Tablets (Among most common) 2257
▲ Bactrim I.V. Infusion (Among most common) 2255
▲ Bactrim (Among most common) 2257
Benadryl Injection 1955
Benemid Tablets 1651
Bentyl 1246
Blenoxane (Common) 697
Brevibloc (esmolol HCl) Injection (Less than 1%) 1860
▲ Bromfed-DM Cough Syrup (Among most frequent) 1832
Buprenex Injectable (Rare) 2170
BuSpar Tablets (Infrequent) 738
Calcijex Injection 412
Capoten Tablets (About 0.5 to 2%) 740
Capozide Tablets (0.5 to 2%) 744
Cardizem CD Capsules (Less than 1%) 1251
Cardizem SR Capsules (Less than 1%) 1255
Cardizem Injectable 1253
Cardizem Tablets (Less than 1%) 1257
Cardura Tablets (Less than 0.5% of 3960 patients) 1993
Casodex Tablets (2% to 5%) 2934
Catapres Tablets (About 1 in 100 patients) 679
Catapres-TTS 680
Cedax (0.1% to 1%) 2480
Ceftin (0.1% to 1%) 1067
▲ CellCept Capsules (More than or equal to 3%) 2265
Celontin Kapseals (Frequent) 1955
Cerebyx Injection (Infrequent) 1956
Cipro I.V. (1% or less) 587
Cipro I.V. Pharmacy Bulk Package (Less than 1%) 590
Cipro Tablets (Less than 1%) 584
Claritin Tablets (2% or fewer patients) 2485
Claritin-D Tablets (2%) 2487
Clinoril Tablets (Greater than 1%) 1658
Clozaril Tablets (1%) 2377
▲ Cognex Capsules (9%) 1961
ColBENEMID Tablets 1662
Colestid (Infrequent) 2073
Combipres Tablets (About 1%) 682
▲ Cordarone Tablets (4 to 9%) 2818
Cosmegen Injection 1666
Cozaar Tablets (Less than 1%) 1668
Crixivan Capsules (0.5% to less than 2%) 1670
Crystodigin Tablets 1472
Cuprimine Capsules 1673
Cylert Tablets 415
▲ Cytadren Tablets (1 in 8) 837
▲ Cytosar-U Sterile Powder (Among most frequent) 2077
▲ Cytovene (15%) 2270
Cytoxan 700
▲ DTIC-Dome (90% with the initial few doses) 593
Dalmane Capsules (Rare) 2329
Dantrium Capsules (Less frequent) 2131
▲ Daranide Tablets (Among the most common effects) 1676
Daraprim Tablets 1199
▲ DaunoXome (2% to 21%) 1842
Daypro Caplets (1% to 3%) 2578
Declomycin Tablets 1421
Demulen 2580
Depakene 416
Depakote Tablets (1% to 5%) 418
▲ Depen Titratable Tablets (17%) 2770
Dexedrine 2648
DextroStat-Dextroamphetamine Sulfate Tablets 2211
Diabinese Tablets (Less Than 2%) 2002
Diamox Intravenous ◉ 317
Diamox Sequels (Sustained Release) ◉ 318
Diamox Tablets ◉ 317
Dilacor XR Extended-release Capsules (Infrequent) 2183
Dilaudid-HP Injection (Less frequent) 1384
Dilaudid-HP Lyophilized Powder 250 mg (Less frequent) 1384
Dilaudid Tablets and Liquid 1386
Dimetane-DC Cough Syrup 2232
Dimetane-DX Cough Syrup 2233
Dipentum Capsules (1.3%) 2084
Diphtheria and Tetanus Toxoids and Pertussis Vaccine Adsorbed 2650
Diucardin Tablets 2824
Diupres Tablets 1691
Diuril Oral Suspension 1694
Diuril Sodium Intravenous 1693
Diuril Tablets 1694
Dolobid Tablets (Less than 1 in 100) 1695
Doral Tablets 2773
Doryx Capsules 1970
Doxil (1% to 5%) 2613
Doxorubicin Astra (Occasional) 531
▲ Duragesic Transdermal System (3% to 10%) 1336
Dynabac (0.1% to 1%) 668
DYNACIN Capsules 1627
▲ E.E.S. (Among most frequent) 427
Edecrin 1698
▲ Effexor (11% to 17.0%) 2825
Elavil 2945
Eldepryl Capsules 2729
Elspar 1700
▲ Emcyt Capsules (4%) 2085
Emete-con Intramuscular/Intravenous 2007
Enduron Tablets 424
Engerix-B Unit-Dose Vials (Less than 1%) 2656
▲ Epivir (10%) 1200
▲ Ergamisol Tablets (2% to 6%) 1340
▲ ERYC (Among most frequent) 1972
▲ EryPed (Among most frequent) 425
▲ Ery-Tab Tablets (Among most frequent) 426
▲ Erythrocin Stearate Filmtab (Among most frequent) 429
▲ Erythromycin Base Filmtab (Among most frequent) 430
▲ Erythromycin Delayed-Release Capsules, USP (Among most frequent) 431
Esidrix Tablets 839
Esimil Tablets 840
Eskalith 2658
Ethmozine Tablets (Less than 2%) 2217
▲ Etopophos for Injection (10% to 16%) 701
▲ Etoposide Injection (10% to 13%) 539
Etrafon 2495
▲ Eulexin Capsules (4%) 2498
Famvir Tablets (1.1% to 2.6%) 2660
Fedahist Gyrocaps 2545
▲ Felbatol (Among most common; 19.3% to 54.8%) 2774
Feldene Capsules (Greater than 1%) 2008
Fioricet with Codeine Capsules 2387
Fiorinal with Codeine Capsules 2390
Flagyl 375 Capsules (Sometimes) 2587
Flexeril Tablets (Less than 1%) 1701
▲ Flolan for Injection (25%) 1085
▲ Fludara for Injection (7% to 34%) 658
Flumadine Tablets & Syrup (1.6%) 1013
Fluorouracil Injection (Common) 2282
▲ Foscavir Injection (5% or greater) 541
Sterile FUDR 2284
▲ Fungizone Intravenous (Among most common) 507
Gantanol Tablets 2285
Gantrisin 2286
Gemzar for Injection (Common) 1482
Geocillin Tablets 2009
GlaucTabs ◉ 209
▲ Glucophage Tablets (Among most common) 754
Glucotrol XL Extended Release Tablets (Less than 1%) 2012
Halcion Tablets 2093
Haldol Decanoate 1587
Haldol Injection, Tablets and Concentrate 1585
▲ Havrix (1% to 10%) 2663
Helidac Therapy (1.5%) 2135
Hexalen Capsules (1%) 2760
HibTITER 1423
Hivid Tablets (Less than 1%) 2287
▲ Hycamtin for Injection (Up to 19%) 2665
Hydralazine Hydrochloride Injection USP (Common) 2712
Hydrea Capsules (Less frequent) 705
HydroDIURIL Tablets 1716
Hydropres Tablets 1718
▲ Hylorel Tablets (18.7%) 1613
Hyperstat I.V. Injection 2504
Hyzaar Tablets 1720
IFEX (Less than 1%) 706
Inderide Tablets 2838
Inderide LA Long Acting Capsules 2840
Indocin (Less than 1%) 1723
Inocor Lactate Injection (0.4%) 2439
▲ Intron A for Injection (1% to 69%) 2506
Inversine Tablets 1729
Kadian Capsules (Less than 3%) 2948
Kayexalate 2444
Kefzol Vials, Faspak & ADD-Vantage 1511
Kerlone Tablets (Less than 2%) 2588
Klonopin Tablets 2294
Lamictal Tablets (1.8%) 1105
Lamprene Capsules (Less than 1%) 846
Lanoxicaps (Common) 1110
Lanoxin Elixir Pediatric 1113
Lanoxin Injection (Common) 1116
Lanoxin Injection Pediatric 1119
Lanoxin Tablets (Common) 1121
▲ Lariam Tablets (Among most frequent) 2295
Larodopa Tablets (Relatively frequent) 2296
Lasix Injection, Oral Solution and Tablets 1267
Lescol Capsules 2395
▲ Leucovorin Calcium for Injection (1% to 22%) 1313
▲ Leukine (13% to 54%) 1317
Levlen/Tri-Levlen 646
Limbitrol 2333
Lioresal Intrathecal (Up to 0.9%) 1634
Lioresal Tablets (Rare) 847
Lithium Carbonate Capsules & Tablets 2352
Lithonate/Lithotabs/Lithobid 2721
Lodine Capsules and Tablets (Less than 1%) 2849
Lomotil 2591
Lopressor HCT Tablets (1 in 100 patients) 850
Lorabid Suspension and Pulvules (0.3% to 2.3%) 1513
Lotensin HCT Tablets (0.3% to 1.0%) 855
Lupron Depot 7.5 mg (Less than 5%) 2741
Lupron Depot - 3 Month 22.5 mg (Less than 5%) 2743
▲ Lupron Injection (5% or more) 2736
▲ LUVOX Tablets (6%) 2723
Lysodren Tablets 707
MS Contin Tablets (Less frequent) 2149
MSIR (Infrequent) 2152
▲ Macrodantin Capsules (Among most often) 2140
Marinol (Dronabinol) Capsules (Less than 1%) 2353
Maxair Autohaler 1550
Maxair Inhaler (Less than 1%) 1552
Maxaquin Tablets (Less than 1%) 2593
Mellaril 2398
▲ Mepron Suspension (7%) 1206
Merrem I.V. (0.1% to 1.0%) 2952
Methadone Hydrochloride Oral Concentrate 2356
Methadone Hydrochloride Oral Solution & Tablets 2357
Methotrexate Sodium Tablets, Injection, for Injection and LPF Injection (Less common) 1322
MetroGel-Vaginal 917
Mevacor Tablets (Rare) 1742
Miacalcin Nasal Spray (Less than 1%) 2403
▲ Midamor Tablets (3% to 8%) 1746
Minizide Capsules 2016
Minocin Intravenous 1428
Minocin Oral Suspension 1431
Minocin Pellet-Filled Capsules 1429
Mintezol 1747
Mithracin 599
Modicon 1928
▲ Moduretic Tablets (3% to 8%) 1748
Monodox Capsules 1858
Monoket Tablets (Fewer than 1%) 2550
Motofen Tablets 789
Motrin Ibuprofen Suspension, Oral Drops, Chewable Tablets, Caplets 1563
MSTA Mumps Skin Test Antigen 2988
Mustargen 1752
▲ Mutamycin for Injection (14%) 712
Myambutol Tablets 1432
Mycobutin Capsules (2%) 2101
Mykrox Tablets 1617
Myleran Tablets 1209
Myochrysine Injection 1754
Mysoline (Occasional) 2860
Nalfon 200 Pulvules & Nalfon Tablets (Less than 1%) 933
Naprelan Tablets (Less than 1%) 2861
Navane Capsules and Concentrate 2018
Navane Intramuscular 2019
▲ Navelbine Injection (Less than 20%) 1212
Neoral (2% or less) 2405
Neptazane Tablets ◉ 320
▲ Neupogen for Injection (9%) 495
Neurontin Capsules (Frequent) 1978
▲ Nipent for Injection (13% to 16%) 2733
Nizoral Tablets 1345
Nolvadex Tablets (1%) 2957
Normodyne Injection 2519
Normodyne Tablets 2522
Noroxin Tablets (Less frequent) 1758
Noroxin Tablets (Less frequent) 2222
Norpace (1 to 3%) 2596
Norpramin Tablets 1273
Norvasc Tablets (More than 0.1% to 1%) 2020
▲ Norvir (0.9% to 6.1%) 447
Novahistine Elixir ▣ 782
Nydrazid Injection 509
▲ OmniHIB (2.2% t0 15.3%) 2676
▲ Oncaspar (Greater than 1% but less than 5%) 2194
Oncovin Solution Vials & Hyporets 1521
Oramorph SR (Morphine Sulfate Sustained Release Tablets) (Less frequent) 2359
Orap Tablets 1037
Oretic Tablets 450
Ornade Spansule Capsules 2678
Ortho-Cyclen/Ortho-Tri-Cyclen 1914
Ortho-Novum 1928
Ortho-Cyclen/Ortho Tri-Cyclen 1914
Orthoclone OKT3 Sterile Solution 1892
Orudis Capsules (Greater than 1%) 2874
Oruvail Capsules (Greater than 1%) 2874
OxyContin Tablets (Between 1% and 5%) 2163
PBZ Tablets 863
PBZ-SR Tablets 862
▲ PCE Dispertab Tablets (Among most frequent) 453
Pamelor 2409
Papaverine Hydrochloride Vials and Ampoules 1523
▲ Parlodel (4%) 2411
Parnate Tablets 2679
PASER Granules (Less frequent) 1333
▲ Pediazole Suspension (Among most frequent) 2340
Penetrex Tablets (0.1% to 1%) 2196
Pentasa (Less than 1% to 1.1%) 1275
Pepcid Injection (Infrequent) 1765
Pepcid (Infrequent) 1763
Periactin 1767
▲ Permax Tablets (4.8%) 571
▲ Phenurone Tablets (5%) 455
PhosLo Tablets 695
Placidyl Capsules 456
Plaquenil Sulfate Tablets 2459
Platinol for Injection 717
Platinol-AQ Injection 719
Ponstel (Less frequent) 1982
Potaba Capsules, Envules, Powder, and Tablets (Infrequent) 1234
Pravachol Tablets (Rare) 770
Prevacid Delayed-Release Capsules (Less than 1%) 2746
Prilosec Delayed-Release Capsules (Less than 1%) 516
Prinivil Tablets (Greater than 1%) 1776
Prinzide Tablets 1780
▲ Procanbid Extended-Release Tablets (3% to 4%) 1983
Proglycem (Frequent) 575
▲ Prograf (6% to 34%) 1028
▲ Proleukin for Injection (27%) 812
Protostat Tablets 1939
Proventil Syrup (Children 2 to 6 years, 1%) 2528
▲ Prozac Pulvules & Liquid, Oral Solution (8.7% to 17%) 935
Purinethol Tablets (Uncommon) 1214
Pyrazinamide Tablets 1442

(▣ Described in PDR For Nonprescription Drugs) Incidence data in parenthesis; ▲ 3% or more (◉ Described in PDR For Ophthalmology)

Quadrinal Tablets ... 1398
Questran (Less frequent) ... 774
RMS Suppositories CII ... 2766
Relafen Tablets (1%) ... 2688
Remeron Tablets (Frequent) ... 1878
Restoril Capsules (1-2%) ... 2413
▲ Retrovir Capsules (11% to 20.1%) ... 1216
▲ Retrovir I.V. Infusion (11% to 20.1%) ... 1221
▲ Retrovir Syrup (11% to 20.1%) ... 1216
ReVia Tablets (Less than 10%) ... 957
▲ Ridaura Capsules (3 to 9%) ... 2691
Rifadin (Some patients) ... 1276
Rifamate Capsules (Some patients) ... 1278
Rifater ... 1280
▲ Rilutek Tablets (3.8% to 8.6%) ... 2198
Rimactane Capsules ... 865
Risperdal Tablets (Frequent) ... 1348
Ritalin ... 866
Rocaltrol Capsules ... 2303
▲ Roferon-A Injection (43% to 65%) ... 2308
Rondec Oral Drops ... 974
Rondec Syrup ... 974
Rondec ... 974
Roxanol ... 2365
Rubex for Injection (Occasional) ... 721
Rythmol Tablets—150mg, 225mg, 300mg (0.5 to 1.7%) ... 1399
Salagen Tablets (Less than 1%) ... 1546
Sandimmune (2% or less) ... 2416
Sectral Capsules ... 2914
▲ Seldane-D Extended-Release Tablets (3.7%) ... 1286
▲ Septra (Among most common) ... 1146
▲ Septra I.V. Infusion (Among the most common) ... 1142
▲ Septra I.V. Infusion ADD-Vantage Vials (Among most common) ... 1144
▲ Septra (Among most common) ... 1146
Ser-Ap-Es Tablets ... 867
Serentil ... 689
Serzone Tablets ... 776
Sinemet Tablets (Less frequent) ... 959
Sinemet CR Tablets (1.2%) ... 961
Sinequan ... 2028
Slo-Niacin Tablets ... 2767
Sodium Polystyrene Sulfonate Suspension ... 2367
Solganal Suspension (Rare) ... 2530
Sporanox Capsules (0.3% to 1.2%) ... 1352
▲ Stadol (3% to 9%) ... 779
Stelazine ... 2692
Sular Tablets (Less than or equal to 1%) ... 2961
Surmontil Capsules ... 2917
Symmetrel Capsules (1% to 5%) ... 965
Symmetrel Syrup (1% to 5%) ... 963
Talacen Caplets (Rare) ... 2464
Talwin Compound (Rare) ... 2466
Talwin Nx Tablets ... 2467
Tambocor Tablets (1% to less than 3%) ... 1555
Tapazole Tablets ... 1361
Tavist Syrup ... 2426
Tavist Tablets ... 2427
Tegretol/Tegretol-XR ... 870
Tenoretic Tablets ... 2963
Terramycin Intramuscular Solution ... 2034
Teslac Tablets ... 727
Tetramune (Up to 4%) ... 1449
Thalitone ... 1293
▲ TheraCys BCG Live (Intravesical) (Up to 10.7%) ... 911
Thioguanine Tablets, Tabloid Brand (Less frequent) ... 1225
Thioplex (Thiotepa For Injection) ... 1329
Tiazac Capsules (Less than 1% to 1%) ... 1019
TICE BCG, USP (2.2%) ... 1881
Ticlid Tablets (1.0%) ... 2317
Timolide Tablets ... 1791
Timoptic in Ocudose (Less frequent) ... 1796
Timoptic Sterile Ophthalmic Solution (Less frequent) ... 1794
Timoptic-XE ... 1798
Tofranil Ampuls ... 873
Tofranil Tablets ... 875
Tofranil-PM Capsules ... 876
▲ Tonocard Tablets (1.2% to 11.3%) ... 519
Toradol (1% or less) ... 2319
Torecan ... 2367
Trandate ... 1158
Trental Tablets (Less than 1%) ... 1291
Triavil Tablets ... 1800
Tri-Immunol Adsorbed ... 1452
Trilafon (Occasional) ... 2532

Levlen/Tri-Levlen ... 646
Trilisate (Less than 1%) ... 2155
Trinalin Repetabs Tablets ... 1373
▲ Tripedia (1% to 6%) ... 908
Tussend ... 1830
Ultram Tablets (50 mg) (1% to less than 5%) ... 1594
Valtrex Caplets (Less than 1% to 3%) ... 1167
▲ Vascor Tablets (200 and 300 mg) (3.02 to 6.82%) ... 1597
Vaseretic Tablets ... 1810
Vasotec I.V. ... 1814
Vasotec Tablets (0.5% to 1.0%) ... 1816
Velban Vials ... 1537
Ventolin Syrup (1% of children) ... 1175
▲ VePesid Capsules and Injection (10% to 13%) ... 727
▲ Vesanoid Capsules (17%) ... 2327
Vibramycin ... 2038
Vibramycin Hyclate Intravenous ... 2040
Vibramycin ... 2038
▲ Videx Tablets, Powder for Oral Solution, & Pediatric Powder for Oral Solution (2% to 51%) ... 2980
▲ Vistide Injection (22%) ... 1057
Vivactil Tablets ... 1820
▲ Wellbutrin Tablets (18.3%) ... 1177
Xanax Tablets ... 2115
Zarontin Capsules (Frequent) ... 1986
Zarontin Syrup (Frequent) ... 1986
Zaroxolyn Tablets ... 1625
▲ Zerit Capsules (Fewer than 1% to 22%) ... 731
Zestoretic Tablets ... 2968
Zestril Tablets (Greater than 1%) ... 2972
Ziac ... 1459
▲ Zinecard Injection (27% to 42%) ... 2120
Zithromax (1% or less) ... 2043
Zocor Tablets ... 1821
Zoladex (1% to 5%) ... 2976
Zoladex 3-month ... 2978
Zoloft Tablets (2.8%) ... 2051
Zovirax Capsules (0.3%) ... 1187
Zovirax Sterile Powder (Less than 1%) ... 1191
Zovirax (0.3%) ... 1187
Zyloprim Tablets (Less than 1%) ... 1194
Zyrtec Tablets (Less than 2%) ... 2053

Anorgasmia

Anafranil Capsules (Rare) ... 819
Depo-Provera Contraceptive Injection (1% to 5%) ... 2079
Effexor (Frequent) ... 2825
Eldepryl Capsules ... 2729
LUVOX Tablets (2%) ... 2723
Nardil (Common) ... 1977
Neurontin Capsules (Infrequent) ... 1978
▲ Paxil Tablets (2% to 10.0%) ... 2681
Risperdal Tablets (Frequent) ... 1348
Serzone Tablets (Rare) ... 776

Anosmia

▲ AeroBid Inhaler System (3% to 9%) ... 1004
▲ Aerobid-M Inhaler System (3% to 9%) ... 1004
Beclovent Inhalation Aerosol and Refill (Rare) ... 1063
Beconase (Rare) ... 1065
Cipro I.V. (1% or less) ... 587
Cipro I.V. Pharmacy Bulk Package (Less than 1%) ... 590
Cipro Tablets ... 584
Cytovene-IV (One report) ... 2270
Dexacort Phosphate in Turbinaire ... 1607
Nasalide Nasal Solution 0.025% ... 2301
Vaseretic Tablets ... 1810
Vasotec I.V. ... 1814
Vasotec Tablets (0.5% to 1.0%) ... 1816

Anotia, fetal

Accutane Capsules ... 2252

Antibodies development, persistent

Geref (sermorelin acetate for injection) (Approximately 1 in 4 patients) ... 2995
Humatrope Vials ... 1490
Protropin (A small percentage of patients) ... 1053

Anticholinergic syndrome

Anafranil Capsules (Rare) ... 819
Clozaril Tablets ... 2377
Serentil ... 689

Antidiuretic effect

Brontex ... 2130
Demerol ... 2438

Dilaudid-HP Injection (Less frequent) ... 1384
Dilaudid-HP Lyophilized Powder 250 mg (Less frequent) ... 1384
MS Contin Tablets (Less frequent) ... 2149
MSIR ... 2152
Mepergan Injection ... 2859
Methadone Hydrochloride Oral Concentrate ... 2356
Oramorph SR (Morphine Sulfate Sustained Release Tablets) (Less frequent) ... 2359
Phenergan with Codeine ... 2883
Phenergan VC with Codeine ... 2888
RMS Suppositories CII ... 2766
Risperdal Tablets (Rare) ... 1348
Yohimex Tablets ... 1414

Antimitochondrial antibodies

Normodyne Tablets (Less common) ... 2522
Trandate Tablets (Less common) ... 1158

Antithrombin, decrease

Brevicon ... 2563
Estrace Cream and Tablets ... 751
Estratest ... 2718
Norinyl ... 2563
Nor-Q D Tablets ... 2598
Oncaspar ... 2194
Ortho-Cyclen/Ortho-Tri-Cyclen ... 1914
Ortho-Cyclen/Ortho Tri-Cyclen ... 1914
Tri-Norinyl ... 2607

Anuria

Azulfidine (Rare) ... 2059
Bactrim DS Tablets ... 2257
Bactrim I.V. Infusion ... 2255
Bactrim ... 2257
Betaseron for SC Injection ... 653
Calcium Disodium Versenate Injection ... 1548
Fansidar Tablets ... 2281
Floxin I.V. ... 1580
Floxin Tablets (200 mg, 300 mg, 400 mg) ... 1577
Fungizone Intravenous ... 507
Gantanol Tablets ... 2285
Gantrisin ... 2286
LUVOX Tablets (Infrequent) ... 2723
Maxaquin Tablets (Less than 1%) ... 2593
Miltown Tablets (Rare) ... 2780
Nalfon 200 Pulvules & Nalfon Tablets (Less than 1%) ... 933
Neurontin Capsules (Infreq.) ... 1978
Orthoclone OKT3 Sterile Solution ... 1892
Pediazole Suspension ... 2340
PMB 200 and PMB 400 (Rare) ... 2890
Primaxin I.M. ... 1770
Primaxin I.V. (Less than 0.2%) ... 1772
Prinivil Tablets (0.3% to 1.0%) ... 1776
Prinzide Tablets ... 1780
▲ Proleukin for Injection (76%) ... 812
Septra ... 1146
Septra I.V. Infusion ... 1142
Septra I.V. Infusion ADD-Vantage Vials ... 1144
Septra ... 1146
Zanosar Sterile Powder ... 2119
Zestoretic Tablets ... 2968
Zestril Tablets (0.3% to 1.0%) ... 2972
Zovirax Sterile Powder (Less than 1%) ... 1191

Anuria, neonatal

Accupril Tablets ... 1950
Altace Capsules ... 1238
Capoten Tablets ... 740
Capozide Tablets ... 744
Cozaar Tablets ... 1668
Hyzaar Tablets ... 1720
Lotensin Tablets ... 852
Lotensin HCT Tablets ... 855
Lotrel Capsules ... 858
Monopril Tablets ... 762
Prinivil Tablets ... 1776
Prinzide Tablets ... 1780
Univasc Tablets ... 2553
Vaseretic Tablets ... 1810
Vasotec I.V. ... 1814
Vasotec Tablets ... 1816
Zestoretic Tablets ... 2968
Zestril Tablets ... 2972

Anxiety

▲ Acel-Imune Diphtheria and Tetanus Toxoids and Acellular Pertussis Vaccine Adsorbed (17% to 20%) ... 1415
Actigall Tablets ... 818
Adalat CC (Less than 1.0%) ... 582

AeroBid Inhaler System (1% to 3%) ... 1004
Aerobid-M Inhaler System (1% to 3%) ... 1004
Altace Capsules (Less than 1%) ... 1238
Ambien Tablets (1%) ... 2559
Amoxil (Rare) ... 2631
▲ Anafranil Capsules (2% to 9%) ... 819
Ana-Kit Anaphylaxis Emergency Treatment Kit (Common) ... 611
Androderm Testosterone Transdermal System (Less than 1%) ... 2634
▲ Android Capsules, 10 mg (Among most common) ... 1297
Apresazide Capsules (Less frequent) ... 824
Apresoline Hydrochloride Tablets (Less frequent) ... 826
Arimidex Tablets (2% to 5%) ... 2932
Asacol Delayed-Release Tablets ... 2129
Asendin Tablets (Less frequent) ... 1419
Astramorph/PF Injection, USP (Preservative-Free) ... 526
Atamet Tablets ... 567
Augmentin (Rare) ... 2637
Augmentin Tablets (Rare) ... 2640
Axid Pulvules (1.6%) ... 1468
▲ Betapace Tablets (2% to 4%) ... 637
▲ Betaseron for SC Injection (15%) ... 653
Brethine Ampuls (Less than 0.5%) ... 832
Brevibloc (esmolol HCl) Injection (Less than 1%) ... 1860
Bronkometer Aerosol ... 2432
Bronkosol Solution ... 2432
Butisol Sodium Elixir & Tablets (Less than 1 in 100) ... 2768
Carbocaine Injection ... 2432
Cardene Capsules (Rare) ... 2261
Cardene SR Capsules (Rare) ... 2264
Cardura Tablets (1.1%) ... 1993
Cartrol Tablets (Less common) ... 413
Casodex Tablets (2% to 5%) ... 2934
Cataflam Tablets (Less than 1%) ... 833
Catapres Tablets ... 679
Catapres-TTS ... 680
▲ CellCept Capsules (More than or equal to 3%) ... 2265
Cipro I.V. (1% or less) ... 587
Cipro I.V. Pharmacy Bulk Package (Less than 1%) ... 590
Claritin Tablets (2% or fewer patients) ... 2485
Claritin-D Tablets (Less frequent) ... 2487
Clomid ... 1262
Clozaril Tablets (1%) ... 2377
▲ Cognex Capsules (3%) ... 1961
Combipres Tablets ... 682
Cozaar Tablets (Less than 1%) ... 1668
Crixivan Capsules (Less than 2%) ... 1670
Cytotec (Infrequent) ... 2576
Cytovene (1% or less) ... 2270
D.A. II Tablets ... 972
D.A. Chewable Tablets ... 970
D.H.E. 45 Injection (Occasional) ... 2381
Dalgan Injection (Less than 1%) ... 529
Danocrine Capsules (Rare) ... 2437
DaunoXome (Less than or equal to 5%) ... 1842
Deconsal II Tablets ... 1605
Demser Capsules ... 1690
Desyrel and Desyrel Dividose ... 504
Dilaudid Ampules ... 1382
Dilaudid Cough Syrup ... 1383
Dilaudid ... 1382
Diphtheria and Tetanus Toxoids and Pertussis Vaccine Adsorbed ... 2650
Diprivan Injectable Emulsion (Less than 1%) ... 2939
Doral Tablets ... 2773
Doxil (Less than 1%) ... 2613
▲ Duragesic Transdermal System (3% to 10%) ... 1336
Duramorph Injection ... 983
Dura-Tap/PD Capsules ... 970
Dura-Vent/DA Tablets ... 972
Dura-Vent Tablets ... 971
Dynabac (0.1% to 1%) ... 668
▲ Effexor (2% to 11.2%) ... 2825
Elavil ... 2945
Eldepryl Capsules (1 of 49 patients) ... 2729
Emcyt Capsules (1%) ... 2085
Entex PSE Tablets ... 973
EpiPen ... 808
Ergamisol Tablets (1%) ... 1340
Estratest ... 2718
Estring Vaginal Ring (1% to 3%) ... 2086
Ethmozine Tablets (Less than 2%) ... 2217
Etrafon ... 2495
Eulexin Capsules (1%) ... 2498

Fedahist Gyrocaps 2545
▲ Felbatol (5.2% to 5.3%) 2774
Fioricet with Codeine Capsules 2387
Fiorinal with Codeine Capsules 2390
Flexeril Tablets (Less than 1%) 1701
▲ Flolan for Injection (11% to 21%) 1085
Floxin I.V. (Less than 1%) 1580
Floxin Tablets (200 mg, 300 mg, 400 mg) (Less than 1%) 1577
▲ Foscavir Injection (5% or greater) 541
Gamimune N, 5% Immune Globulin Intravenous (Human), 5% 612
Gamimune N, 10% Immune Globulin Intravenous (Human), 10% 615
Gammar-P I.V., Immune Globulin Intravenous (Human) 798
Gastrocrom Capsules (Infrequent) 1611
Gastrocrom Oral Concentrate (Less common) 1611
Glucotrol XL Extended Release Tablets (Less than 3%) 2012
Guaimax-D Tablets 809
Haldol Decanoate 1587
Haldol Injection, Tablets and Concentrate 1585
Halotestin Tablets 2095
Histussin D Liquid 670
Hivid Tablets (Less than 1%) 2287
Hycodan Tablets and Syrup 946
Hycomine Compound Tablets 948
Hycomine 947
Hycotuss Expectorant Syrup 950
Hydralazine Hydrochloride Injection USP (Less frequent) 2712
Hydrocet Capsules 787
Hyperstat I.V. Injection 2504
Hytrin Capsules (At least 1%) 434
Hyzaar Tablets 1720
Imdur (Less than or equal to 5%) 1362
Imitrex Injection (1.1%) 1095
Imitrex Tablets 1099
▲ Inapsine Injection (Among most common) 462
Indocin (Less than 1%) 1723
Infumorph 200 and Infumorph 500 Sterile Solutions 985
▲ Intron A for Injection (Up to 5%) 2506
Invirase Capsules (Less than 2%) 2291
Ismo Tablets (Fewer than 1%) 2844
Isoetharine Inhalation Solution, USP, Arm-a-Med 545
▲ Kadian Capsules (Less than 3% to 6%) 2948
Kytril Injection (Less than 2%) 2667
Kytril Tablets (2%) 2669
▲ Lamictal Tablets (3.8%) 1105
Lariam Tablets 2295
Larodopa Tablets (Relatively frequent) 2296
Lescol Capsules 2395
▲ Leukine (11%) 1317
Levbid Extended-Release Tablets 2549
Levophed Bitartrate Injection 2445
Levsin/Levsinex/Levbid 2549
Lioresal Intrathecal (0.2% to 0.9%) 1634
Lorcet 10/650 Tablets 1016
Lortab 2751
Lotensin Tablets 852
Lotrel Capsules 858
▲ Ludiomil Tablets (3%) 861
▲ Lupron Depot 3.75 mg (Among most frequent; less than 5%) 2739
Lupron Depot - 3 Month 22.5 mg (Less than 5%) 2743
Lupron Injection (Less than 5%) 2736
▲ LUVOX Tablets (5%) 2723
Marcaine 2446
Marcaine Spinal 2449
Marinol (Dronabinol) Capsules (Greater than 1%) 2353
Mavik Tablets (0.3% to 1.0%) 1407
Maxair Autohaler 1550
Maxair Inhaler (Less than 1%) 1552
Maxaquin Tablets (Less than 1%) 2593
Mebaral Tablets (Less than 1 in 100) 2452
▲ Mepron Suspension (7%) 1206
Merrem I.V. (0.1% to 1.0%) 2952
Methadone Hydrochloride Oral Concentrate 2356
Mevacor Tablets (0.5% to 1.0%) 1742
Miacalcin Nasal Spray (Less than 1%) 2403
Monoket Tablets (Fewer than 1%) 2550
Mykrox Tablets (Less than 2%) 1617
Naprelan Tablets (Less than 1%) 2861
Nardil (Less frequent) 1977
Nembutal Sodium Capsules (Less than 1%) 440
Nembutal Sodium Solution (Less than 1%) 442
Nembutal Sodium Suppositories (Less than 1%) 444
Neoral (Rare) 2405
Nescaine/Nescaine MPF 549
Neurontin Capsules (Frequent) 1978
▲ Nicotrol NS Nicotine Nasal Spray (Over 5%) 1565
▲ Nipent for Injection (3% to 10%) 2733
Noroxin Tablets (Less frequent) 1758
Noroxin Tablets (Less frequent) 2222
Norplant System 2868
Norpramin Tablets 1273
Norvasc Tablets (More than 0.1% to 1%) 2020
Norvir (Less than 2%) 447
Novahistine DMX ▣ 782
Novahistine Elixir ▣ 782
OptiPranolol (Metipranolol 0.3%) Sterile Ophthalmic Solution (A small number of patients) ◉ 256
Orlaam Oral Solution (1% to 3%) 2361
OxyContin Tablets (Between 1% and 5%) 2163
Pamelor 2409
Parlodel 2411
Parnate Tablets 2679
▲ Paxil Tablets (5% to 5.9%) 2681
Pediazole Suspension 2340
Penetrex Tablets (1%) 2196
Pentaspan Injection 954
Pepcid Injection (Infrequent) 1765
Pepcid (Infrequent) 1763
▲ Permax Tablets (6.4%) 571
Phenergan VC 2886
Phenergan VC with Codeine 2888
Phenobarbital Elixir and Tablets (Less than 1 in 100 patients) 1523
Placidyl Capsules 456
Plendil Extended-Release Tablets (0.5% to 1.5%) 514
Pondimin Tablets 2239
Pravachol Tablets 770
Prevacid Delayed-Release Capsules (Less than 1%) 2746
Prilosec Delayed-Release Capsules (Less than 1%) 516
Procardia XL Extended Release Tablets (1% or less) 2026
Proglycem 575
▲ Prograf (Greater than 3%) 1028
Propulsid (1.4%) 1346
ProSom Tablets (Frequent) 457
▲ Prozac Pulvules & Liquid, Oral Solution (5% to 14%) 935
Questran 774
Redux Capsules (Frequent) 2911
Reglan 2243
Relafen Tablets (1%) 2688
Remeron Tablets (Frequent) 1878
RespiGam 1631
Retrovir Capsules 1216
Retrovir I.V. Infusion 1221
Retrovir Syrup 1216
▲ ReVia Tablets (2% to more than 10%) 957
Rifater 1280
▲ Risperdal Tablets (12% to 20%) 1348
Roferon-A Injection (Less than 3% to 6%) 2308
▲ Romazicon (3% to 9%) 2311
Rythmol Tablets–150mg, 225mg, 300mg (0.7 to 2.0%) 1399
Salagen Tablets (Less than 1%) 1546
Sandimmune (Rare) 2416
Sandostatin Injection (Less than 1%) 2421
Seconal Sodium Pulvules (Less than 1 in 100) 1529
Sectral Capsules (Up to 2%) 2914
Seldane-D Extended-Release Tablets 1286
Sensorcaine 554
Ser-Ap-Es Tablets 867
Serzone Tablets 776
Sinemet Tablets 959
Sinemet CR Tablets 961
Stadol (1% or greater) 779
Sular Tablets (Less than or equal to 1%) 2961
▲ Supprelin Injection (3% to 10%) 2230
Surmontil Capsules 2917
Sus-Phrine Injection 1017
Symmetrel Capsules (1% to 5%) 965
Symmetrel Syrup (1% to 5%) 963
Syn-Rx Tablets 1622
Syn-Rx DM Tablets 1623
Tagamet 2694
Tambocor Tablets (1% to less than 3%) 1555
Tegison Capsules (Less than 1%) 2314
Tenex Tablets (Less frequent) 2249
Testoderm Testosterone Transdermal System 486
Testred Capsules, 10 mg 1308
THYREL TRH (Less frequent) 2992
Timoptic in Ocudose (Less frequent) 1796
Timoptic Sterile Ophthalmic Solution (Less frequent) 1794
Timoptic-XE 1798
Tofranil Ampuls 873
Tofranil Tablets 875
Tofranil-PM Capsules 876
Tonocard Tablets (1.1% to 1.5%) 519
Tornalate Solution for Inhalation, 0.2% (Less than 1%) 976
Trental Tablets (Less than 1%) 1291
Triavil Tablets 1800
Trinalin Repetabs Tablets 1373
Tripedia 908
Tussend 1830
Tussend Expectorant 1831
Tussionex Pennkinetic Extended-Release Suspension 1624
Tympagesic Ear Drops 2476
▲ Ultram Tablets (50 mg) (1% to 14%) 1594
Univasc Tablets (Less than 1%) 2553
Vantin for Oral Suspension and Vantin Tablets (Less than 1%) 2112
Vascor Tablets (200 and 300 mg) (0.5 to 2.0%) 1597
Vasoxyl Injection 1169
Versed Injection (Less than 1%) 2324
▲ Vesanoid Capsules (17%) 2327
Vicodin Tablets 1404
Vicodin ES Tablets 1405
Vicodin HP Tablets 1403
Vicodin Tuss Expectorant 1406
Videx Tablets, Powder for Oral Solution, & Pediatric Powder for Oral Solution (Up to 2%) 2980
Visken Tablets (2% or fewer patients) 2428
Vistide Injection 1057
Vivactil Tablets 1820
Cataflam/Voltaren/Voltaren-XR (Less than 1%) 833
▲ Wellbutrin Tablets (3.1%) 1177
▲ Xanax Tablets (16.6%) 2115
Xylocaine Injections 562
▲ Yutopar Intravenous Injection (5% to 6%) 566
Zebeta Tablets 1457
▲ Zerit Capsules (Fewer than 1% to 22%) 731
Ziac 1459
Zocor Tablets 1821
Zofran Injection (2%) 1227
▲ Zofran Tablets (6%) 1231
Zoladex (1% or greater but less than 5%) 2976
Zoladex 3-month 2978
Zoloft Tablets (2.6%) 2051
Zonalon Cream (Less than 1%) 1042
Zosyn (1.2% to 3.2%) 1463
Zydone Capsules 967
Zyrtec Tablets (Less than 2%) 2053

Anxiety, paradoxical

Diupres Tablets 1691
Dizac (diazepam injectable emulsion) CIV (Less frequent) 1862
Halcion Tablets 2093
Hydropres Tablets 1718
Ser-Ap-Es Tablets 867
Valium Injectable 2336
Valium Tablets 2335
Vivactil Tablets 1820

Apathy

Ambien Tablets (Rare) 2559
Anafranil Capsules (Infrequent) 819
Bactrim DS Tablets 2257
Bactrim I.V. Infusion 2255
Bactrim 2257
Betaseron for SC Injection 653
BuSpar Tablets (Infrequent) 738
Claritin-D Tablets (Less frequent) 2487
Cognex Capsules (Infrequent) 1961
Doral Tablets 2773
Effexor (Infrequent) 2825
Eldepryl Capsules 2729
Fansidar Tablets 2281
Felbatol 2774
Gantanol Tablets 2285
Gantrisin 2286
Imitrex Tablets (Rare) 1099
Intron A for Injection (Less than 5%) 2506
Kadian Capsules (Less than 3%) 2948
Lamictal Tablets (Infrequent) 1105
Lanoxicaps 1110
Lanoxin Elixir Pediatric 1113
Lanoxin Injection 1116
Lanoxin Injection Pediatric 1119
Lanoxin Tablets 1121
LUVOX Tablets (Frequent) 2723
Neurontin Capsules (Infrequent) 1978
Nicotrol NS Nicotine Nasal Spray (Under 5%) 1565
Norvasc Tablets (Less than or equal to 0.1%) 2020
Permax Tablets (Infrequent) 571
Prevacid Delayed-Release Capsules (Less than 1%) 2746
Prilosec Delayed-Release Capsules (Less than 1%) 516
ProSom Tablets (Infrequent) 457
Prozac Pulvules & Liquid, Oral Solution (Infrequent) 935
Redux Capsules (Rare) 2911
Remeron Tablets (Frequent) 1878
Rilutek Tablets (Infrequent) 2198
Risperdal Tablets (Infrequent) 1348
Roferon-A Injection (Infrequent) 2308
Septra 1146
Septra I.V. Infusion 1142
Septra I.V. Infusion ADD-Vantage Vials 1144
Septra 1146
Serzone Tablets (Infrequent) 776
Tambocor Tablets (Less than 1%) 1555
Zoloft Tablets (Infrequent) 2051

Apgar score, low

Syntocinon Injection 2425

Aphasia

Anafranil Capsules (Rare) 819
Betaseron for SC Injection 653
Cedax 2480
Cerebyx Injection (Infrequent) 1956
Cognex Capsules (Infrequent) 1961
Desyrel and Desyrel Dividose 504
Duragesic Transdermal System (Less than 1%) 1336
Effexor (Rare) 2825
Foscavir Injection (Between 1% and 5%) 541
Hivid Tablets (Less than 1%) 2287
Intron A for Injection (Less than 5%) 2506
Lamictal Tablets (Infrequent) 1105
Methotrexate Sodium Tablets, Injection, for Injection and LPF Injection 1322
Mycobutin Capsules (More than one patient) 2101
Neurontin Capsules (Infrequent) 1978
Nicotrol NS Nicotine Nasal Spray (Less than 1%) 1565
Norvir (Less than 2%) 447
Orthoclone OKT3 Sterile Solution 1892
Paxil Tablets (Rare) 2681
Remeron Tablets (Rare) 1878
Risperdal Tablets (Rare) 1348
Roferon-A Injection (Less than 0.5%) 2308
▲ Vesanoid Capsules (3%) 2327
Videx Tablets, Powder for Oral Solution, & Pediatric Powder for Oral Solution (Up to 1%) 2980
Wellbutrin Tablets (Rare) 1177

Aphonia

BuSpar Tablets (Rare) 738
Klonopin Tablets 2294
Roferon-A Injection (Less than 0.5%) 2308

Aphthous stomatitis (see under Stomatitis, ulcerative)

Aplasia, red cell

Cuprimine Capsules 1673
Depen Titratable Tablets 2770
Lamictal Tablets (One case) 1105
Ridaura Capsules (Less than 1%) 2691

Aplasia cutis, fetal

Tapazole Tablets (Rare) 1361

Aplastic anemia

Aldactazide Tablets 2556
Aldoclor Tablets 1638
Aldoril Tablets 1644
Amaryl Tablets 1241

(▣ Described in PDR For Nonprescription Drugs) Incidence data in parenthesis; ▲ 3% or more (◉ Described in PDR For Ophthalmology)

1259 **Side Effects Index** **Appetite, decreased**

Anaprox/Naprosyn (Less than 1%) 2277
Ancobon Capsules 2254
Anturane 823
Apresazide Capsules 824
Asacol Delayed-Release Tablets (Rare) 2129
Atretol Tablets 569
Azulfidine (Rare) 2059
Bactrim DS Tablets (Rare) 2257
Bactrim I.V. Infusion (Rare) 2255
Bactrim (Rare) 2257
Blephamide Liquifilm Sterile Ophthalmic Suspension 472
▲ Blephamide Ointment (Among most often) ⊙ 234
Capozide Tablets 744
Cataflam Tablets (Rare) 833
Cedax 2480
Cefizox for Intramuscular or Intravenous Use 1025
Cefotan 2936
Ceftin 1067
Cefzil Tablets and Oral Suspension 747
Ceptaz 1070
Chloromycetin Ophthalmic Ointment, 1% ⊙ 298
Chloromycetin Ophthalmic Solution ⊙ 299
Chloromycetin Sodium Succinate 1960
Chloroptic Sterile Ophthalmic Solution (Rare) ⊙ 236
Clinoril Tablets (Less than 1 in 100) 1658
Combipres Tablets 682
Compazine 2644
Cosmegen Injection 1666
Cuprimine Capsules 1673
Cylert Tablets (Isolated reports) 415
Dantrium Capsules (Less frequent) 2131
Dantrium Intravenous 2132
Dapsone Tablets USP 1331
Depen Titratable Tablets 2770
DiaBeta Tablets (Occasional) 1265
Diabinese Tablets 2002
Diamox Intravenous ⊙ 317
Diamox Sequels (Sustained Release) ⊙ 318
Diamox Tablets ⊙ 317
Diucardin Tablets 2824
Diupres Tablets 1691
Diuril Oral Suspension 1694
Diuril Sodium Intravenous 1693
Diuril Tablets 1694
Duricef Capsules, Tablets, and Oral Suspension 750
Dyazide Capsules 2653
EC-Naprosyn Delayed-Release Tablets (Less than 1%) 2277
Eminase (Less than 1%) 2215
Enduron Tablets 424
Esidrix Tablets 839
Esimil Tablets 840
FML-S Liquifilm ⊙ 240
Fansidar Tablets 2281
Felbatol (A marked increase (maybe more than 100 fold)) 2774
Feldene Capsules (Less than 1%) 2008
Floxin I.V. 1580
Floxin Tablets (200 mg, 300 mg, 400 mg) 1577
Fortaz 1092
Gantanol Tablets 2285
Gantrisin (Rare) 2286
GlaucTabs ⊙ 209
Glucotrol Tablets 2011
Glucotrol XL Extended Release Tablets 2012
Glynase PresTab Tablets 2091
▲ Hexalen Capsules (13% to 33%) 2760
HydroDIURIL Tablets 1716
Hydropres Tablets 1718
Hyzaar Tablets 1720
IBU Tablets (Less than 1%) 1389
Inderide Tablets 2838
Inderide LA Long Acting Capsules 2840
Indocin Capsules (Less than 1%) 1723
Indocin I.V. (Less than 1%) 1727
Indocin (Less than 1%) 1723
Kefurox Vials, Faspak & ADD-Vantage 1509
Lamictal Tablets 1105
Lasix Injection, Oral Solution and Tablets (Rare) 1267
Leustatin (Some reports) 1889
Lopressor HCT Tablets 850
Lorabid Suspension and Pulvules 1513
Lotensin HCT Tablets 855
LUVOX Tablets 2723
Macrobid Capsules (Rare) 2138
Macrodantin Capsules (Rare) 2140
Maxipime for Injection 758
Mellaril 2398
Mesantoin Tablets (Uncommon) 2400
Micronase Tablets 2099
Midamor Tablets (Rare) 1746
Miltown Tablets 2780
Minizide Capsules 2016
Moduretic Tablets 1748
Monopril Tablets 762
Motrin Ibuprofen Suspension, Oral Drops, Chewable Tablets, Caplets (Less than 1%) 1563
Mykrox Tablets 1617
Myochrysine Injection 1754
Nalfon 200 Pulvules & Nalfon Tablets (Less than 1%) 933
▲ Naprelan Tablets (3% to 9%) 2861
Anaprox/Naprosyn (Less than 1%) 2277
Neptazane Tablets ⊙ 320
Nipent for Injection (Less than 3%) 2733
Norflex (Very rare) 1554
Norgesic (1 case) 1554
Nydrazid Injection 509
Oretic Tablets 450
Orthoclone OKT3 Sterile Solution 1892
PBZ Tablets 863
PBZ-SR Tablets 862
Pediazole Suspension 2340
Pentasa 1275
Phenurone Tablets (2%) 455
Plaquenil Sulfate Tablets 2459
PMB 200 and PMB 400 2890
Prinzide Tablets 1780
Propulsid (Rare) 1346
Prozac Pulvules & Liquid, Oral Solution 935
Ridaura Capsules (Less than 0.1%) 2691
Rifamate Capsules 1278
Rifater (Rare) 1280
Rilutek Tablets (Rare) 2198
Roferon-A Injection (Rare) 2308
SSD 1402
Septra 1146
Septra I.V. Infusion 1142
Septra I.V. Infusion ADD-Vantage Vials (Rare) 1144
Septra 1146
Ser-Ap-Es Tablets 867
Serentil 689
Silvadene Cream 1% 1288
Solganal Suspension (Rare) 2530
Stelazine 2692
Suprax 1443
Tagamet (Very rare) 2694
Tapazole Tablets 1361
Tazicef for Injection 2697
Tazidime Vials, Faspak & ADD-Vantage 1531
Tegretol/Tegretol-XR (Very low incidence) 870
Tenoretic Tablets 2963
Thalitone 1293
Thorazine 2701
Ticlid Tablets (Rare) 2317
Timolide Tablets 1791
Torecan 2367
Trental Tablets (Rare) 1291
Trusopt Sterile Ophthalmic Solution (Rare) 1803
Urobiotic-250 Capsules 2038
Vantin for Oral Suspension and Vantin Tablets 2112
Vaseretic Tablets 1810
Cataflam/Voltaren/Voltaren-XR (Rare) 833
Zantac (Rare) 1182
Zantac Injection (Rare) 1180
Zantac Syrup (Rare) 1182
Zaroxolyn Tablets 1625
Zestoretic Tablets 2968
Zinacef 1184
Zyloprim Tablets (Less than 1%) 1194

Apnea

▲ Alfenta Injection (3% to 9%) 1334
Amikacin Sulfate Injection, USP 523
Amikacin Sulfate Injection, USP 981
Amikin Injectable 502
Anectine 1062
Bentyl 1246
Betaseron for SC Injection 653
Buprenex Injectable (Infrequent) 2170
Butisol Sodium Elixir & Tablets (Less than 1 in 100) 2768
Carbocaine Injection 2432
Cerebyx Injection (Infrequent) 1956
Demerol 2438
Desyrel and Desyrel Dividose 504
Dilaudid-HP Injection 1384
Dilaudid-HP Lyophilized Powder 250 mg 1384
Dilaudid Tablets and Liquid 1386
Diphtheria and Tetanus Toxoids and Pertussis Vaccine Adsorbed 2650
Diprivan Injectable Emulsion (1% to 3%) 2939
▲ Duragesic Transdermal System (3% to 10%) 1336
Ethmozine Tablets (Less than 2%) 2217
Etopophos for Injection (Rare) 701
Etoposide Injection (Rare) 539
▲ Exosurf Neonatal for Intratracheal Suspension (33% to 73%) 1081
Indocin I.V. (Less than 3%) 1727
Lamictal Tablets 1105
Levo-Dromoran 2297
Lioresal Intrathecal (1% or more) 1634
LUVOX Tablets (Rare) 2723
MS Contin Tablets 2149
MSIR 2152
Marcaine 2446
Mebaral Tablets (Less than 1 in 100) 2452
Merrem I.V. (1.2%) 2952
Metubine Iodide Vials 932
Motrin Ibuprofen Suspension, Oral Drops, Chewable Tablets, Caplets (Less than 1%) 1563
Nembutal Sodium Capsules (Less than 1%) 440
Nembutal Sodium Solution (Less than 1%) 442
Nembutal Sodium Suppositories (Less than 1%) 444
Nescaine/Nescaine MPF 549
Netromycin Injection 100 mg/ml 2516
Neurontin Capsules (Infrequent) 1978
Norcuron for Injection 1875
Nuromax Injection 1136
Oramorph SR (Morphine Sulfate Sustained Release Tablets) (Less frequent) 2359
Orthoclone OKT3 Sterile Solution 1892
OxyContin Tablets 2163
Permax Tablets (Infrequent) 571
Phenobarbital Elixir and Tablets (Less than 1 in 100 patients) 1523
Proleukin for Injection (1%) 812
Prozac Pulvules & Liquid, Oral Solution (Rare) 935
Pulmozyme Inhalation 1054
Redux Capsules (Rare) 2911
Rilutek Tablets (More than 2%) 2198
Risperdal Tablets 1348
Rythmol Tablets–150mg, 225mg, 300mg (Less than 1%) 1399
Seconal Sodium Pulvules (Less than 1 in 100) 1529
Sensorcaine 554
Stadol (Less than 1%) 779
▲ Sublimaze Injection (Among most common) 463
Sufenta Injection (0.3% to 1%) 1355
▲ Suprane (desflurane, USP) (3% to 15%) 1865
▲ Survanta Beractant Intratracheal Suspension (46.1 to 65.4%) 2346
Talwin Injection 2465
Tetramune (Rare) 1449
Thioplex (Thiotepa For Injection) 1329
▲ Trasylol (3%) 607
Tri-Immunol Adsorbed (Rare) 1452
VePesid Capsules and Injection (Rare) 727
▲ Versed Injection (15.4%) 2324
Videx Tablets, Powder for Oral Solution, & Pediatric Powder for Oral Solution (Less than 1%) 2980
Virazole 1310

Apnea, neonatal

Adapin Capsules (One case) 1542
Sinequan (One case) 2028
Survanta Beractant Intratracheal Suspension (Less than 1%) 2346

Appendicitis, acute

Effexor (Rare) 2825
Lopid Tablets (1.2%) 1974
Redux Capsules (Rare) 2911
Sandostatin Injection (Less than 1%) 2421

Appetite, changes

Alupent Tablets (0.4%) 672
Amen Tablets 785
Asendin Tablets (Less frequent) 1419
Ativan Tablets (Less frequent) 2807
Betapace Tablets (1% to 3%) 637
Brevicon 2563
Cataflam Tablets (Less than 1%) 833
Compazine 2644
Cortone Acetate Sterile Suspension 1663
Cortone Acetate Tablets 1664
Cycrin Tablets 991
Cytotec (Infrequent) 2576
Danocrine Capsules (Rare) 2437
Decadron Elixir 1676
Decadron Phosphate Injection 1680
Decadron Phosphate with Xylocaine Injection, Sterile 1683
Decadron Tablets 1678
Decadron-LA Sterile Suspension 1687
Demulen 2580
Depo-Provera Contraceptive Injection (Fewer than 1%) 2079
Depo-Provera Sterile Aqueous Suspension 2083
Desogen Tablets 1867
▲ Effexor (1% to 6%) 2825
Eldepryl Capsules 2729
▲ Hismanal Tablets (3.9%) 1341
Hydeltrasol Injection, Sterile 1708
Hydeltra-T.B.A. Sterile Suspension 1710
Hydrocortone Acetate Sterile Suspension 1712
Hydrocortone Phosphate Injection, Sterile 1713
Hydrocortone Tablets 1715
Klonopin Tablets 2294
Levlen/Tri-Levlen 646
Lo/Ovral Tablets 2852
Lo/Ovral-28 Tablets 2857
▲ Lupron Depot 3.75 mg (Among most frequent; less than 5%) 2739
Mexitil Capsules (2.6%) 684
Midamor Tablets (Between 1% and 3%) 1746
Modicon 1928
Moduretic Tablets (Less than or equal to 1%) 1748
Monopril Tablets (0.2% to 1.0%) 762
Navane Capsules and Concentrate 2018
Navane Intramuscular 2019
Nordette-21 Tablets 2863
Nordette-28 Tablets 2866
Norinyl 2563
Norplant System 2868
Nor-Q D Tablets 2598
Ortho-Cept 1907
Ortho-Cyclen/Ortho-Tri-Cyclen 1914
Ortho-Novum 1928
Ortho-Cyclen/Ortho Tri-Cyclen 1914
Ovcon 765
Ovral Tablets 2877
Ovral-28 Tablets 2878
Ovrette Tablets 2878
Premphase 2900
Prempro 2905
Provera Tablets 2110
Quadrinal Tablets 1398
Stelazine (Occasional) 2692
▲ Tegison Capsules (25-50%) 2314
Thorazine (Sometimes) 2701
Trilafon 2532
Levlen/Tri-Levlen 646
Tri-Norinyl 2607
Triphasil-21 Tablets 2919
Triphasil-28 Tablets 2924
Univasc Tablets (Less than 1%) 2553
▲ Videx Tablets, Powder for Oral Solution, & Pediatric Powder for Oral Solution (6%) 2980
Cataflam/Voltaren/Voltaren-XR (Less than 1%) 833
▲ Wellbutrin Tablets (3.7%) 1177

Appetite, decreased

AeroBid Inhaler System 1004
▲ Aerobid-M Inhaler System (3% to 9%) 1004
Desyrel and Desyrel Dividose (Up to 3.5%) 504
DynaCirc CR Tablets (0.5% to 1.0%) 2383
▲ Epivir (10%) 1200
Floxin I.V. (1% to 3%) 1580
Floxin Tablets (200 mg, 300 mg, 400 mg) (1% to 3%) 1577
Garamycin Injectable 2502
IBU Tablets (Greater than 1%) 1389
Imitrex Injection (Rare) 1095
Imitrex Tablets (Rare) 1099
IPOL Poliovirus Vaccine Inactivated 903
▲ Kytril Tablets (5%) 2669
▲ Leustatin (17%) 1889
MetroGel-Vaginal (Equal to or less than 2%) 917

(▣ Described in PDR For Nonprescription Drugs) Incidence data in parenthesis; ▲ 3% or more (⊙ Described in PDR For Ophthalmology)

Appetite, decreased

Oncaspar ... 2194
▲ Paxil Tablets (2.0% to 9%) ... 2681
ProSom Tablets (Infrequent) ... 457
Recombivax HB (Less to greater than 1%) ... 1787
Supprelin Injection (1% to 3%) ... 2230
Vantin for Oral Suspension and Vantin Tablets (Less than 1%) ... 2112
▲ Xanax Tablets (27.8%) ... 2115

Appetite, increased

AeroBid Inhaler System (1% to 3%) ... 1004
Aerobid-M Inhaler System (1% to 3%) ... 1004
Ambien Tablets (Rare) ... 2559
▲ Anafranil Capsules (Up to 11%) ... 819
Androderm Testosterone Transdermal System (Less than 1%) ... 2634
Arimidex Tablets (Up to 0.4%) ... 2932
Asacol Delayed-Release Tablets ... 2129
Avonex ... 662
BuSpar Tablets (Infrequent) ... 738
Cardura Tablets (Less than 0.5% of 3960 patients) ... 1993
Claritin Tablets (2% or fewer patients) ... 2485
Claritin-D Tablets (Less frequent) ... 2487
Clomid (Fewer than 1%) ... 1262
Clozaril Tablets (Less than 1%) ... 2377
Cognex Capsules (Infrequent) ... 1961
Cortifoam ... 2540
Crixivan Capsules (Less than 2%) ... 1670
Dalalone D.P. Injectable ... 1009
DaunoXome (Less than or equal to 5%) ... 1842
Depakene ... 416
▲ Depakote Tablets (6%) ... 418
Desyrel and Desyrel Dividose ... 504
Dexacort Phosphate in Respihaler ... 1606
Dexacort Phosphate in Turbinaire ... 1607
Doxil (Less than 1%) ... 2613
DynaCirc CR Tablets (0.5% to 1.0%) ... 2383
Etrafon ... 2495
Felbatol (Infrequent) ... 2774
Fioricet with Codeine Capsules ... 2387
Fiorinal with Codeine Capsules ... 2390
Intron A for Injection (Less than 5%) ... 2506
Ismo Tablets (Fewer than 1%) ... 2844
Kerlone Tablets (Less than 2%) ... 2588
Lamictal Tablets (Infrequent) ... 1105
Lupron Depot - 3 Month 22.5 mg (Less than 5%) ... 2743
LUVOX Tablets ... 2723
Maxaquin Tablets (Less than 1%) ... 2593
Megace Tablets ... 710
Miacalcin Nasal Spray (Less than 1%) ... 2403
Neurontin Capsules (1.1%) ... 1978
Nicotrol NS Nicotine Nasal Spray (Under 5%) ... 1565
Norvasc Tablets (Less than or equal to 0.1%) ... 2020
Oncaspar (Less than 1%) ... 2194
▲ Orap Tablets (1 of 20 patients) ... 1037
Orudis Capsules (Less than 1%) ... 2874
Oruvail Capsules (Less than 1%) ... 2874
OxyContin Tablets (Less than 1%) ... 2163
▲ Paxil Tablets (4%) ... 2681
Periactin ... 1767
Permax Tablets (Infrequent) ... 571
Prevacid Delayed-Release Capsules (Less than 1%) ... 2746
▲ Prograf (Greater than 3%) ... 1028
ProSom Tablets (Infrequent) ... 457
▲ Proventil Syrup (3 of 100 patients) ... 2528
Prozac Pulvules & Liquid, Oral Solution (Frequent) ... 935
Redux Capsules (Frequent) ... 2911
Relafen Tablets (1%) ... 2688
▲ Remeron Tablets (17%) ... 1878
ReVia Tablets (Less than 1%) ... 957
Rilutek Tablets (Infrequent) ... 2198
Risperdal Tablets (Infrequent) ... 1348
Salagen Tablets (Less than 1%) ... 1546
Seldane Tablets (0.5% to 0.6%) ... 1284
Seldane-D Extended-Release Tablets ... 1286
▲ Serzone Tablets (5%) ... 776
Sular Tablets (Less than or equal to 1%) ... 2961
Toradol (1% or less) ... 2319
Vascor Tablets (200 and 300 mg) (0.5 to 2.0%) ... 1597
Ventolin Syrup (3 of 100 patients) ... 1175

Videx Tablets, Powder for Oral Solution, & Pediatric Powder for Oral Solution (2%) ... 2980
▲ Xanax Tablets (32.7%) ... 2115
Zoladex (2%) ... 2976
Zoladex 3-month ... 2978
Zoloft Tablets (1.3%) ... 2051
Zyrtec Tablets (Less than 2%) ... 2053

Appetite, loss of
(see also under Anorexia)

▲ Chemet Capsules (12.0% to 20.9%) ... 666
HibTITER (23 of 1,118 vaccinations) ... 1423
Miacalcin Injection ... 2402
Varivax (Greater than or equal to 1%) ... 1807

Apprehension

Adenocard Injection (Less than 1%) ... 1021
Ana-Kit Anaphylaxis Emergency Treatment Kit ... 611
Antivenin (Crotalidae) Polyvalent ... 2803
Cardioquin Tablets ... 2146
Dalmane Capsules ... 2329
Dilaudid-HP Injection (Less frequent) ... 1384
Dilaudid-HP Lyophilized Powder 250 mg (Less frequent) ... 1384
Dilaudid Tablets and Liquid (Less frequent) ... 1386
Dopram Injectable ... 2235
Duranest Injections ... 533
Dyclone 0.5% and 1% Topical Solutions, USP ... 535
Edecrin ... 1698
EMLA Cream (Unlikely with cream) ... 536
EpiPen Jr.- Epinephrine Auto-Injector ... 808
Hyperstat I.V. Injection ... 2504
Limbitrol ... 2333
MS Contin Tablets (Less frequent) ... 2149
MSIR (Infrequent) ... 2152
Matulane Capsules ... 2300
Oramorph SR (Morphine Sulfate Sustained Release Tablets) (Less frequent) ... 2359
Quinaglute Dura-Tabs Tablets ... 644
Quinidex Extentabs ... 2240
▲ Xylocaine Injections (Among most common) ... 562

Apraxia

Anafranil Capsules (Rare) ... 819
Cognex Capsules (Rare) ... 1961
Eldepryl Capsules ... 2729
Neurontin Capsules (Rare) ... 1978

Arachnoiditis

Marcaine Spinal ... 2449
Methotrexate Sodium Tablets, Injection, for Injection and LPF Injection ... 1322
Nescaine/Nescaine MPF ... 549
Novocain Hydrochloride for Spinal Anesthesia ... 2457
Pontocaine Hydrochloride for Spinal Anesthesia ... 2460
Streptomycin Sulfate Injection ... 2031

Areflexia

Cognex Capsules (Infrequent) ... 1961
Neurontin Capsules (Frequent) ... 1978
Platinol for Injection ... 717
Platinol-AQ Injection ... 719

Argumentativeness

Versed Injection (Less than 1%) ... 2324

Arm, stiffness of

Engerix-B Unit-Dose Vials (Less than 1%) ... 2656

Arrhythmia, exacerbation of

Cordarone Tablets ... 2818
Corvert Injection ... 2075

Arrhythmias

Abbokinase (Occasional) ... 403
Abelcet Injection ... 1540
Activase ... 1045
Adenocard Injection ... 1021
Adenoscan (1%) ... 1022
Adriamycin PFS ... 2056
Adriamycin RDF ... 2056
AKPRO ... ⊚ 206
▲ Alfenta Injection (14%) ... 1334
Altace Capsules (Less than 1%) ... 1238
Ambien Tablets (Rare) ... 2559

Anafranil Capsules (Infrequent) ... 819
Ana-Kit Anaphylaxis Emergency Treatment Kit ... 611
Anectine ... 1062
Aramine Injection ... 1649
Atretol Tablets ... 569
Atromid-S Capsules ... 2808
Avonex ... 662
Betagan ... ⊚ 230
Betaseron for SC Injection ... 653
Betimol 0.25%, 0.5% ... ⊚ 259
Blocadren Tablets (Greater than 1.1%) ... 1654
▲ Bromfed-DM Cough Syrup (Among most frequent) ... 1832
Calcijex Injection ... 412
Carbocaine Injection ... 2432
Cardizem CD Capsules (Less than 1%) ... 1251
Cardizem SR Capsules (Less than 1%) ... 1255
Cardizem Injectable (1.0%) ... 1253
Cardizem Tablets (Less than 1%) ... 1257
Cardura Tablets (1%) ... 1993
Cartrol Tablets (Less common) ... 413
Catapres Tablets (Rare) ... 679
Catapres-TTS ... 680
Chemet Capsules (Up to 1.8%) ... 666
Cipro I.V. (1% or less) ... 587
Cipro I.V. Pharmacy Bulk Package (Less than 1%) ... 590
Claforan Sterile and Injection ... 1259
Claritin-D Tablets ... 2487
Clinoril Tablets (Rare) ... 1658
Clomid ... 1262
Clozaril Tablets (Several patients) ... 2377
Combipres Tablets (Rare) ... 682
Compazine ... 2644
Cordarone Tablets (1 to 3%) ... 2818
Corvert Injection (1.7%) ... 2075
Cozaar Tablets (Less than 1%) ... 1668
Cytotec (Infrequent) ... 2576
Cytovene (1% or less) ... 2270
D.A. II Tablets ... 972
D.A. Chewable Tablets ... 970
Dalgan Injection (Less than 1%) ... 529
Deconsal II Tablets ... 1605
Demadex Tablets and Injection ... 691
Desyrel and Desyrel Dividose ... 504
Dexatrim ... ⊞ 795
Dexatrim Plus Vitamins Caplets ... ⊞ 796
Dilacor XR Extended-release Capsules (Infrequent) ... 2183
Dimetane-DC Cough Syrup ... 2232
Dimetane-DX Cough Syrup ... 2233
Diprivan Injectable Emulsion (Less than 1%) ... 2939
Diupres Tablets ... 1691
Dopram Injectable ... 2235
Doxil ... 2613
Doxorubicin Astra ... 531
Duragesic Transdermal System (1% or greater) ... 1336
Dura-Tap/PD Capsules ... 970
Dura-Vent/DA Tablets ... 972
Dura-Vent Tablets ... 971
Dyazide Capsules ... 2653
E.E.S. (Occasional reports) ... 427
Effexor (Rare) ... 2825
Elavil ... 2945
Eldepryl Capsules ... 2729
▲ Eminase (38%) ... 2215
EpiPen Jr.- Epinephrine Auto-Injector ... 808
EryPed (Occasional reports) ... 425
Ery-Tab Tablets (Occasional reports) ... 426
Erythrocin Stearate Filmtab (Occasional reports) ... 429
Erythromycin Base Filmtab (Occasional reports) ... 430
Erythromycin Delayed-Release Capsules, USP (Occasional reports) ... 431
Eskalith ... 2658
Etrafon ... 2495
Fedahist Gyrocaps ... 2545
Flexeril Tablets (Less than 1%) ... 1701
▲ Flolan for Injection (27%) ... 1085
Fludara for Injection (Up to 3%) ... 658
Fluothane ... 2830
Foscavir Injection (Less than 1%) ... 541
Fungizone Intravenous ... 507
Gemzar for Injection (2%) ... 1482
Glucotrol XL Extended Release Tablets (Less than 1%) ... 2012
Haldol Decanoate ... 1587
Histussin D Liquid ... 670
Hivid Tablets (Less than 1%) ... 2287
Hydropres Tablets ... 1718
Hytrin Capsules (At least 1%) ... 434

Hyzaar Tablets ... 1720
IBU Tablets (Less than 1%) ... 1389
Idamycin Injection ... 2096
Imdur (Less than or equal to 5%) ... 1362
Imitrex Injection (Rare) ... 1095
Imitrex Tablets (Rare to infrequent) ... 1099
Indocin Capsules (Less than 1%) ... 1723
Indocin I.V. (Less than 1%) ... 1727
Indocin (Less than 1%) ... 1723
INFeD (Iron Dextran Injection, USP) ... 2478
▲ Inocor Lactate Injection (3%) ... 2439
Intron A for Injection (Less than 5%) ... 2506
Iopidine 0.5% (Less than 1%) ... ⊚ 219
Ismo Tablets (Fewer than 1%) ... 2844
Isopto Carbachol Ophthalmic Solution ... ⊚ 221
Kerlone Tablets (Less than 2%) ... 2588
Kytril Injection (Rare) ... 2667
Lanoxicaps ... 1110
Lanoxin Elixir Pediatric ... 1113
Lanoxin Injection ... 1116
Lanoxin Injection Pediatric ... 1119
Lanoxin Tablets ... 1121
Lasix Injection, Oral Solution and Tablets ... 1267
Leukine ... 1317
Levo-Dromoran ... 2297
Levophed Bitartrate Injection ... 2445
Limbitrol ... 2333
Lithium Carbonate Capsules & Tablets ... 2352
Lithonate/Lithotabs/Lithobid ... 2721
Lodine Capsules and Tablets (Less than 1%) ... 2849
Ludiomil Tablets (Rare) ... 861
Lupron Depot 7.5 mg (Less than 5%) ... 2741
Lupron Depot - 3 Month 22.5 mg (Less than 5%) ... 2743
Lupron Injection (Less than 5%) ... 2736
Marax Tablets & DF Syrup ... 2015
Maxaquin Tablets (Less than 1%) ... 2593
Mellaril ... 2398
Midamor Tablets (Less than or equal to 1%) ... 1746
Miltown Tablets ... 2780
Mivacron (Less than 1%) ... 1125
Moban Tablets and Concentrate ... 1036
Moduretic Tablets (Greater than 1%, less than 3%) ... 1748
Monoket Tablets (Fewer than 1%) ... 2550
Monopril Tablets (0.2% to 1.0%) ... 762
Motrin Ibuprofen Suspension, Oral Drops, Chewable Tablets, Caplets (Less than 1%) ... 1563
Naprelan Tablets (Less than 1%) ... 2861
Navane Capsules and Concentrate ... 2018
Navane Intramuscular ... 2019
Neo-Synephrine Hydrochloride 1% Carpuject (Rare) ... 2455
Neo-Synephrine Hydrochloride 1% Injection (Rare) ... 2455
▲ Neupogen for Injection (11 of 375 cancer patients) ... 495
Nipent for Injection (Less than 3%) ... 2733
Norisodrine with Calcium Iodide Syrup ... 446
Norpramin Tablets ... 1273
Norvasc Tablets (More than 0.1% to 1%) ... 2020
Novahistine DMX ... ⊞ 782
Novahistine Elixir ... ⊞ 782
▲ Novantrone for Injection (3 to 4%) ... 1327
Ocupress Ophthalmic Solution, 1% Sterile (Occasional) ... ⊚ 297
Orap Tablets ... 1037
Orthoclone OKT3 Sterile Solution ... 1892
Orudis Capsules (Rare) ... 2874
Oruvail Capsules (Rare) ... 2874
OSMOGLYN Oral Osmotic Agent ... ⊚ 225
PCE Dispertab Tablets (Rare) ... 453
Pamelor ... 2409
Parlodel (Less than 1%) ... 2411
Paxil Tablets (Rare) ... 2681
Pepcid Injection (Infrequent) ... 1765
Pepcid (Infrequent) ... 1763
Permax Tablets (1.1%) ... 571
Pfizerpen for Injection ... 2022
Plendil Extended-Release Tablets (0.5% to 1.5%) ... 514
PMB 200 and PMB 400 ... 2890
Prinivil Tablets (0.3% to 1.0%) ... 1776
Prinzide Tablets ... 1780
Priscoline Hydrochloride Ampuls ... 864
Procardia XL Extended Release Tablets (1% or less) ... 2026
▲ Proleukin for Injection (22%) ... 812

(⊞ Described in PDR For Nonprescription Drugs)   Incidence data in parenthesis; ▲ 3% or more   (⊚ Described in PDR For Ophthalmology)

1261 **Side Effects Index** **Arthralgia**

Prolixin 510
PROPINE with C CAP Compliance Cap ◉ 251
Propulsid (Rare) 1346
ProSom Tablets (Rare) 457
Prostigmin Injectable 1305
Prostigmin Tablets 1306
Prostin E2 Suppository 2109
Prozac Pulvules & Liquid, Oral Solution (Infrequent) 935
Quibron 2227
▲ Quinaglute Dura-Tabs Tablets (3%) 644
Redux Capsules (Infrequent) 2911
Regitine Vials 864
Relafen Tablets (Less than 1%) 2688
Revex (nalmefene hydrochloride injection) (Less than 1%) 1863
Risperdal Tablets 1348
Ritalin 866
Rocaltrol Capsules 2303
Roferon-A Injection (Less than 3%) 2308
Romazicon (Less than 1%) 2311
Rondec Oral Drops 974
Rondec Syrup 974
Rondec 974
Rubex for Injection 721
Rum-K Syrup 1004
▲ Sandostatin Injection (9%) 2421
Seldane Tablets 1284
Seldane-D Extended-Release Tablets 1286
Sensorcaine 554
Ser-Ap-Es Tablets 867
Serentil 689
Serevent Inhalation Aerosol 1149
Slo-bid Gyrocaps 2201
Sodium Polystyrene Sulfonate Suspension 2367
Stelazine 2692
Streptase for Infusion 557
Sufenta Injection (0.3% to 1%) 1355
Suprane (desflurane, USP) (Less than 1%) 1865
Surmontil Capsules 2917
Sus-Phrine Injection 1017
Syn-Rx Tablets 1622
Syn-Rx DM Tablets 1623
Syntocinon Injection 2425
Tagamet Injection (Rare) 2694
Taxol Injection (Approximately 1%) 723
Tegretol/Tegretol-XR 870
Tensilon Injectable 1307
Theo-Dur Extended-Release Tablets 1367
Tiazac Capsules (Less than 1%) 1019
Timolide Tablets (Less than 1%) 1791
Timoptic in Ocudose (Less frequent) 1796
Timoptic Sterile Ophthalmic Solution (Less frequent) 1794
Timoptic-XE 1798
Tofranil Ampuls 873
Tofranil Tablets 875
Tofranil-PM Capsules 876
▲ Trasylol (4%) 607
Trental Tablets (Rare) 1291
Triavil Tablets 1800
Trilafon 2532
Trinalin Repetabs Tablets 1373
▲ Triostat Injection (6%) 2708
Tussend 1830
Tussend Expectorant 1831
Uni-Dur Extended-Release Tablets 1374
Uniphyl 400 mg and 600 mg Tablets 2157
Univasc Tablets (Less than 1%) 2553
Vascor Tablets (200 and 300 mg) (About 2.4%) 1597
Vaseretic Tablets 1810
Vasotec Tablets (0.5% to 1.0%) 1816
Ventolin Inhalation Solution 1171
Ventolin Nebules Inhalation Solution 1172
▲ Vesanoid Capsules (23%) 2327
Videx Tablets, Powder for Oral Solution, & Pediatric Powder for Oral Solution (Less than 1% to 6%) 2980
Vivactil Tablets 1820
Vumon for Injection 729
▲ Wellbutrin Tablets (5.3%) 1177
Yutopar Intravenous Injection (1% to 2%) 566
Zantac (Rare) 1182
Zantac Injection (Rare) 1180
Zantac Syrup (Rare) 1182
Zaroxolyn Tablets 1625
Zemuron Injection (Less than 1%) 1885
Zestoretic Tablets 2968
Zestril Tablets (0.3% to 1.0%) 2972
Ziac (Up to 0.4%) 1459
Zoladex (Greater than 1% but less than 5%) 2976
Zoladex 3-month 2978
Zosyn (1.0% or less) 1463

Arrhythmias, junctional

Proleukin for Injection (1%) 812
Tornalate Solution for Inhalation, 0.2% (Less than 1%) 976

Arrhythmias, pre-existing, worsening of

Cordarone Intravenous 2821
Corvert Injection 2075
Mexitil Capsules 684
Quibron 2227
▲ Rythmol Tablets–150mg, 225mg, 300mg (4.7%) 1399
Slo-bid Gyrocaps 2201

Arrhythmias, sinus

Imitrex Injection (Infrequent) 1095

Arrhythmias, supraventricular

Ethmozine Tablets (Less than 2%) 2217
Intron A for Injection (Rare) 2506
Leukine (Occasional) 1317
▲ Primacor Injection (3.8%) 2461
▲ Proleukin for Injection (5%) 812

Arterial carbon dioxide, decrease

Sulfamylon Cream 940

Arterial insufficiency

Blocadren Tablets 1654
Inderal 2834
Inderal LA Long Acting Capsules 2836
Inderide Tablets 2838
Inderide LA Long Acting Capsules 2840
Lopressor (1%) 848
Lopressor HCT Tablets 850
Timolide Tablets 1791
Timoptic in Ocudose 1796
Timoptic Sterile Ophthalmic Solution 1794
Timoptic-XE 1798
Toprol-XL Tablets (About 1 of 100 patients) 560

Arterial occlusion

Humegon for Injection 1873
Metrodin (urofollitropin for injection) 2616
Serophene (clomiphene citrate tablets, USP) (Rare) 2621

Arteriospasm

Ceptaz 1070
Fortaz 1092

Arteritis

Ambien Tablets (Rare) 2559
Avonex 662
Pediazole Suspension 2340

Arteritis, temporal

Imitrex Tablets 1099
Orthoclone OKT3 Sterile Solution 1892

Arthralgia

Abelcet Injection 1540
▲ Accutane Capsules (Approximately 16%) 2252
Acel-Imune Diphtheria and Tetanus Toxoids and Acellular Pertussis Vaccine Adsorbed (Rare) 1415
▲ Actigall Capsules (7.7%) 818
Actimmune (2%) 1043
Adalat CC (Less than 1.0%) 582
Aldoclor Tablets 1638
Aldomet Ester HCl Injection 1642
Aldomet Oral 1640
Aldoril Tablets 1644
▲ Alferon N Injection (3% to 10%) 2142
All-Flex Arcing Spring Diaphragm (See also Ortho Diaphragm Kits) 1921
Altace Capsules (Less than 1%) 1238
▲ Ambien Tablets (4%) 2559
Amikacin Sulfate Injection, USP (Rare) 523
Amikacin Sulfate Injection, USP (Rare) 981
Amikin Injectable (Rare) 502
Anafranil Capsules (Up to 3%) 819
Antivenin (Crotalidae) Polyvalent 2803
Apresazide Capsules (Less frequent) 824
Apresoline Hydrochloride Tablets (Less frequent) 826
▲ Aredia for Injection (6.4%) 827
Arimidex Tablets (2% to 5%) 2932
▲ Asacol Delayed-Release Tablets (5%) 2129
Atretol Tablets 569
Atromid-S Capsules 2808
Augmentin 2637
Augmentin Tablets 2640
▲ Avonex (9%) 662
Azathioprine Tablets (Less than 1%) 2349
Azmacort Oral Inhaler 2175
Azulfidine (Rare) 2059
Bactrim DS Tablets 2257
Bactrim I.V. Infusion 2255
Bactrim 2257
Beconase 1065
Biavax II 1653
Bicillin C-R Injection 2810
Bicillin C-R 900/300 Injection 2812
Bicillin L-A Injection 2813
Blocadren Tablets (Less than 1%) 1654
BuSpar Tablets (Infrequent) 738
Calan SR Caplets (1% or less) 2571
Calan Tablets (1% or less) 2568
▲ Capoten Tablets (About 4 to 7 of 100 patients) 740
Capozide Tablets (Sometimes) 744
Cardene Capsules (Rare) 2261
Cardene SR Capsules (Rare) 2264
Cardioquin Tablets 2146
Cardura Tablets (1%) 1993
Cartrol Tablets (1.2%) 413
Catapres Tablets (About 6 in 1,000 patients) 679
Catapres-TTS 680
Ceclor Pulvules & Suspension 1470
Ceftin for Oral Suspension (0.1% to 1%) 1067
▲ CellCept Capsules (More than or equal to 3%) 2265
Cerebyx Injection (Infrequent) 1956
Chibroxin Sterile Ophthalmic Solution (With oral form) 1657
Cipro I.V. (1% or less) 587
Cipro I.V. Pharmacy Bulk Package (Less than 1%) 590
Cipro Tablets (Less than 1%) 584
Claritin Tablets (2% or fewer patients) 2485
Claritin-D Tablets (Less frequent) 2487
Clinoril Tablets (Less than 1 in 100) 1658
Clomid 1262
Clozaril Tablets (Less than 1%) 2377
Cognex Capsules (Frequent) 1961
Colestid 2073
Combipres Tablets (About 6 in 1,000) 682
Coumadin 941
Covera-HS Tablets (Less than 2%) 2573
Cozaar Tablets (Less than 1%) 1668
Crixivan Capsules (Less than 2%) 1670
Cuprimine Capsules 1673
CytoGam (Less than 5.0%) 1630
Cytotec (Infrequent) 2576
Danocrine Capsules 2437
▲ DaunoXome (Up to 7%) 1842
Demadex Tablets and Injection (1.8%) 691
Depakote Tablets (1% to 5%) 418
Depen Titratable Tablets 2770
Depo-Provera Contraceptive Injection (1% to 5%) 2079
DiaBeta Tablets 1265
Didronel Tablets 2133
Dilacor XR Extended-release Capsules (Infrequent; 1.4%) 2183
Dilantin Infatabs 1967
Dilantin Kapseals 1965
Dilantin-125 Suspension 1969
▲ Dipentum Capsules (4.0%) 2084
Diphtheria and Tetanus Toxoids and Pertussis Vaccine Adsorbed 2650
Dolobid Tablets (Less than 1 in 100) 1695
Doxil (Less than 1%) 2613
Duricef Capsules, Tablets, and Oral Suspension (Rare) 750
DynaCirc CR Tablets (0.5% to 1.0%) 2383
Effexor 2825
Elspar 1700
▲ Eminase (Less than 10%) 2215
Engerix-B Unit-Dose Vials (Less than 1%) 2656
▲ Epivir (5%) 1200
▲ Epogen for Injection (11%; rare) 489
▲ Ergamisol Tablets (4% to 5%) 1340
Eskalith 2658
▲ Estring Vaginal Ring (3%) 2086
Famvir Tablets (1.3% to 1.5%) 2660
Fansidar Tablets 2281
Felbatol 2774
Feldene Capsules (Occasional) 2008
Flagyl 375 Capsules 2587
▲ Flolan for Injection (6%) 1085
▲ Flovent (1% to 19%) 1089
Floxin I.V. (Less than 1%) 1580
Floxin Tablets (200 mg, 300 mg, 400 mg) (Less than 1%) 1577
Fludara for Injection (Up to 1%) 658
Foscavir Injection (Between 1% and 5%) 541
▲ Fungizone Intravenous (Among most common) 507
Furoxone 2221
Gamimune N, 5% Immune Globulin Intravenous (Human), 5% 612
Gamimune N, 10% Immune Globulin Intravenous (Human), 10% 615
Gammar-P I.V., Immune Globulin Intravenous (Human) 798
Gantanol Tablets 2285
Gantrisin 2286
Garamycin Injectable 2502
Gastrocrom Capsules (Infrequent) 1611
Gastrocrom Oral Concentrate (Less common) 1611
Glucotrol XL Extended Release Tablets (Less than 3%) 2012
Glynase PresTab Tablets 2091
▲ Habitrol Nicotine Transdermal System (3% to 9% of patients) 884
Havrix (Less than 1%) 2663
Helidac Therapy 2135
Hismanal Tablets (1.2%) 1341
Hivid Tablets (Less than 1%) 2287
Humegon for Injection 1873
Hycamtin for Injection (0.2% to 0.9%) 2665
Hydralazine Hydrochloride Injection USP (Less frequent) 2712
Hylorel Tablets (1.7%) 1613
Hyskon Hysteroscopy Fluid (Rare) 1633
Hytrin Capsules (At least 1%) 434
Hyzaar Tablets 1720
Imdur (Less than or equal to 5%) 1362
Imitrex Injection (Infrequent) 1095
▲ Imovax Rabies Vaccine (Up to 6%) 899
Imuran (Less than 1%) 1103
INFeD (Iron Dextran Injection, USP) 2478
Intal Inhaler (Infrequent) 2185
Intal Nebulizer Solution 2186
▲ Intron A for Injection (Up to 19%) 2506
Invirase Capsules (Less than 2%) 2291
Ismo Tablets (Fewer than 1%) 2844
Isoptin Oral Tablets (Less than 1%) 1393
Isoptin SR Tablets (1% or less) 1395
K-Phos Neutral Tablets 633
K-Phos Original Formula 'Sodium Free' Tablets (Less frequent) 633
Kadian Capsules (Less than 3%) 2948
Keflex Pulvules & Oral Suspension 930
Keftab Tablets 931
▲ Kerlone Tablets (3.1%) 2588
Lamictal Tablets (2.0%) 1105
▲ Lescol Capsules (4.0%) 2395
▲ Leukine (11% to 21%) 1317
▲ Leustatin (5%) 1889
Lithonate/Lithotabs/Lithobid 2721
Lopid Tablets 1974
Lotensin Tablets 852
Lotensin HCT Tablets (0.3% to more than 1%) 855
Lumitene ▭ 799
Lupron Injection (Less than 5%) 2736
LUVOX Tablets (Infrequent) 2723
M-M-R II 1730
M-R-VAX II 1732
Macrobid Capsules 2138
Macrodantin Capsules 2140
Matulane Capsules 2300
Maxaquin Tablets (Less than 1%) 2593
Meruvax II 1740
Methotrexate Sodium Tablets, Injection, for Injection and LPF Injection (Rare to less common) 1322
Metrodin (urofollitropin for injection) 2616
MetroGel-Vaginal 917
Mevacor Tablets (0.5% to 1.0%; rare) 1742
Mexitil Capsules (1.7%) 684
▲ Miacalcin Nasal Spray (3.8%) 2403
Micronase Tablets 2099

(▭ Described in PDR For Nonprescription Drugs) Incidence data in parenthesis; ▲ 3% or more (◉ Described in PDR For Ophthalmology)

Midamor Tablets (Less than or equal to 1%) 1746
Minipress Capsules 2015
Moduretic Tablets (Less than or equal to 1%) 1748
Monopril Tablets (0.2% to 1.0%) 762
Myambutol Tablets 1432
Mycobutin Capsules (Less than 1%) 2101
▲ Mykrox Tablets (3.1%) 1617
Myochrysine Injection 1754
Naprelan Tablets (Less than 3%) 2861
Nasacort Nasal Inhaler 2189
Nasalcrom Nasal Solution 2192
Navelbine Injection (Less than 5%) 1212
NegGram 2453
Neoral (Rare) 2405
Neupogen for Injection (Infrequent) 495
Neurontin Capsules (Frequent) 1978
▲ Nicotrol NS Nicotine Nasal Spray (5%) 1565
▲ Nipent for Injection (3% to 10%) 2733
Noroxin Tablets 1758
Noroxin Tablets 2222
Norvasc Tablets (More than 0.1% to 1%) 2020
Norvir (Less than 2%) 447
▲ Oncaspar (Greater than 1% but less than 5%) 2194
▲ Orlaam Oral Solution (3% to 9%) 2361
Ortho Diaphragm Kits—All-Flex Arcing Spring; Ortho Coil Spring; Ortho-White Flat Spring 1921
Ortho Diaphragm Kit 1921
Orthoclone OKT3 Sterile Solution 1892
Paxil Tablets (Frequent) 2681
Penetrex Tablets (0.1% to 1%) 2196
Pentasa (Less than 1%) 1275
Pepcid Injection (Infrequent) 1765
Pepcid (Infrequent) 1763
Pergonal (menotropins for injection, USP) 2618
Permax Tablets (1.6%) 571
Pfizerpen for Injection 2022
Phenobarbital Elixir and Tablets (Rare) 1523
Plendil Extended-Release Tablets (0.5% to 1.5%) 514
Pneumovax 23 (Rare) 1768
Pnu-Imune 23 (Rare to infrequent) 1437
Pravachol Tablets (Rare) 770
Prevacid Delayed-Release Capsules (Less than 1%) 2746
Prilosec Delayed-Release Capsules (Less than 1%) 516
Prinivil Tablets (0.3% to 1.0%) 1776
Prinzide Tablets 1780
Procanbid Extended-Release Tablets (Fairly common) 1983
Procardia XL Extended Release Tablets (Less than 3%) 2026
▲ Procrit for Injection (Rare to 11%) 1896
▲ Prograf (Greater than 3%) 1028
▲ Proleukin for Injection (6%) 812
Propulsid (1.4%) 1346
ProSom Tablets (Rare) 457
Prostigmin Injectable 1305
Prostigmin Tablets 1306
Prostin E2 Suppository 2109
Protostat Tablets 1939
Prozac Pulvules & Liquid, Oral Solution (1.2% to 3%) 935
Pyrazinamide Tablets (Frequent) 1442
Quadrinal Tablets 1398
Questran 774
Quinaglute Dura-Tabs Tablets 644
Quinidex Extentabs 2240
Rabies Vaccine Adsorbed (Less than 1%) 2686
▲ Rabies Vaccine, Imovax Rabies I.D. (Less frequent; up to 6%) 901
Recombivax HB (Less than 1%) 1787
Redux Capsules (Frequent) 2911
Remeron Tablets (Frequent) 1878
RespiGam 1631
Retrovir Capsules 1216
Retrovir I.V. Infusion 1221
Retrovir Syrup 1216
▲ ReVia Tablets (More than 10%) 957
Revex (nalmefene hydrochloride injection) 1863
Rhinocort Nasal Inhaler (Less than 1%) 552
Rifater (Frequent) 1280
Rilutek Tablets (1.6% to 5.1%) 2198
Risperdal Tablets (2% to 3%) 1348
Ritalin 866
▲ Roferon-A Injection (24% to 47%) 2308
Rowasa (2.09%) 2727
Rythmol Tablets–150mg, 225mg, 300mg (0.2 to 1.0%) 1399
Sandimmune (Rare) 2416
Sandostatin Injection (1% to 4%) 2421
Sansert Tablets 2424
Sectral Capsules 2914
Septra 1146
Septra I.V. Infusion 1142
Septra I.V. Infusion ADD-Vantage Vials 1144
Septra 1146
Ser-Ap-Es Tablets 867
Serevent Inhalation Aerosol (1% to 3%) 1149
Serzone Tablets (1%) 776
Solganal Suspension 2530
Sular Tablets (Less than or equal to 1%) 2961
▲ Supprelin Injection (3% to 10%) 2230
Synarel Nasal Solution for Endometriosis (Less than 1%) 2605
Tagamet (Rare) 2694
Tambocor Tablets (Less than 1%) 1555
Tapazole Tablets 1361
▲ Taxol Injection (8% to 60%) 723
Taxotere for Injection Concentrate 2204
▲ Tegison Capsules (50-75%) 2314
Tegretol/Tegretol-XR 870
Tenex Tablets (Less frequent) 2249
Tetramune 1449
▲ TheraCys BCG Live (Intravesical) (1.0% to 7.1%) 911
Thyro-Block Tablets (A few people) 2785
TICE BCG, USP 1881
Timentin for Injection 2706
Timolide Tablets 1791
Timoptic in Ocudose 1796
Timoptic Sterile Ophthalmic Solution 1794
Timoptic-XE 1798
▲ Tonocard Tablets (Less than 1% to 4.7%) 519
Tornalate Solution for Inhalation, 0.2% (Less than 1%) 976
Tri-Immunol Adsorbed 1452
Typhim Vi (One report) 914
Univasc Tablets (Less than 1%) 2553
Uroqid-Acid No. 2 Tablets 633
Varivax (Greater than or equal to 1%) 1807
Vaseretic Tablets (0.5% to 2.0%) 1810
Vasotec I.V. 1814
Vasotec Tablets (0.5% to 1.0%) 1816
Verelan Capsules (1% or less) 1455
Videx Tablets, Powder for Oral Solution, & Pediatric Powder for Oral Solution (Up to 2%) 2980
Viramune Tablets 2368
▲ Visken Tablets (7%) 2428
Vistide Injection 1057
Wellbutrin Tablets 1177
Xalatan ◉ 304
Zantac (Rare) 1182
Zantac Injection (Rare) 1180
Zantac Syrup (Rare) 1182
Zaroxolyn Tablets 1625
Zebeta Tablets (2.2% to 2.7%) 1457
▲ Zerit Capsules (Fewer than 1% to 19%) 731
Zestoretic Tablets 2968
Zestril Tablets (0.3% to 1.0%) 2972
Ziac 1459
Zocor Tablets 1821
Zofran Injection (2%) 1227
Zoladex (1% or greater) 2976
Zoladex 3-month 2978
Zoloft Tablets (Infrequent) 2051
Zosyn (1.0% or less) 1463
Zyloprim Tablets (Less than 1%) 1194
Zyrtec Tablets (Less than 2%) 2053

Arthralgia, migratory

Aquasol A Vitamin A Capsules, USP 525
Aquasol A Parenteral 526

Arthralgia, monoarticular

Recombivax HB (Less than 1%) 1787

Arthritis

Accutane Capsules (Less than 1%) 2252
▲ Actigall Capsules (5.8%) 818
Adalat Capsules (10 mg and 20 mg) (Less than 0.5%) 580
Adalat CC (Less than 1.0%) 582
Altace Capsules (Less than 1%) 1238
Ambien Tablets (Infrequent) 2559
Asacol Delayed-Release Tablets (1% to 2%) 2129
Atrovent Inhalation Solution (0.9%) 675
Augmentin 2637
Augmentin Tablets 2640
Avonex 662
Benemid Tablets 1651
Betaseron for SC Injection 653
Biavax II (Rare) 1653
Bumex (0.2%) 2260
Cardura Tablets (1%) 1993
Cartrol Tablets (Less common) 413
Casodex Tablets (2% to 5%) 2934
Ceclor Pulvules & Suspension 1470
Chibroxin Sterile Ophthalmic Solution (With oral form) 1657
Clinoril Tablets (Less than 1 in 100) 1658
Cognex Capsules (Frequent) 1961
ColBENEMID Tablets 1662
Colestid 2073
Cozaar Tablets (Less than 1%) 1668
Cytovene-IV (One report) 2270
Demadex Tablets and Injection 691
Didronel Tablets 2133
Dolobid Tablets (Less than 1 in 100) 1695
Effexor (Infrequent) 2825
Engerix-B Unit-Dose Vials 2656
▲ Estring Vaginal Ring (4%) 2086
Hivid Tablets (Less than 1%) 2287
Hylorel Tablets (1.7%) 1613
Hytrin Capsules (At least 1%) 434
Hyzaar Tablets 1720
▲ Imovax Rabies Vaccine (Up to 6%) 899
INFeD (Iron Dextran Injection, USP) 2478
Intron A for Injection (Less than 5%) 2506
Invirase Capsules (Less than 2%) 2291
Keflex Pulvules & Oral Suspension 930
Keftab Tablets 931
Lamictal Tablets (Rare) 1105
Lescol Capsules (Rare; 2.1%) 2395
Lotensin Tablets 852
Lotensin HCT Tablets (0.3% or more) 855
LUVOX Tablets (Infrequent) 2723
M-M-R II 1730
M-R-VAX II 1732
Meruvax II (Rare) 1740
Mevacor Tablets (Rare) 1742
Miacalcin Nasal Spray (Less than 1%) 2403
Monopril Tablets 762
Neurontin Capsules (Infrequent) 1978
Nipent for Injection (Less than 3%) 2733
Noroxin Tablets 1758
Noroxin Tablets 2222
OptiPranolol (Metipranolol 0.3%) Sterile Ophthalmic Solution (A small number of patients) ◉ 256
Orthoclone OKT3 Sterile Solution 1892
Paxil Tablets (Infrequent) 2681
Permax Tablets (Infrequent) 571
Pneumovax 23 1768
Pnu-Imune 23 (Rare) 1437
Pravachol Tablets (Rare) 770
Prevacid Delayed-Release Capsules (Less than 1%) 2746
Prinivil Tablets (0.3% to 1.0%) 1776
Prinzide Tablets 1780
Procanbid Extended-Release Tablets (Fairly common) 1983
Procardia Capsules (Less than 0.5%) 2024
Proleukin for Injection (1%) 812
ProSom Tablets (Infrequent) 457
Prostin E2 Suppository 2109
Prozac Pulvules & Liquid, Oral Solution (Infrequent) 935
Questran 774
▲ Rabies Vaccine, Imovax Rabies I.D. (Less frequent; up to 6%) 901
Recombivax HB 1787
Redux Capsules (Frequent) 2911
Remeron Tablets (Infrequent) 1878
Risperdal Tablets (Rare) 1348
Roferon-A Injection (Rare) 2308
Sandostatin Injection (Less than 1%) 2421
Serzone Tablets (Infrequent) 776
Sular Tablets (Less than or equal to 1%) 2961
▲ TheraCys BCG Live (Intravesical) (1.0% to 7.1%) 911
TICE BCG, USP (2.7%) 1881
Tilade Inhaler (Less than 1%) 2207
▲ Tonocard Tablets (4.7%) 519
Vascor Tablets (200 and 300 mg) (0.5 to 2.0%) 1597
Vaseretic Tablets 1810
Vasotec I.V. 1814
Vasotec Tablets (0.5% to 1.0%) 1816
▲ Videx Tablets, Powder for Oral Solution, & Pediatric Powder for Oral Solution (Less than 1% to 11%) 2980
▲ Wellbutrin Tablets (3.1%) 1177
Zestoretic Tablets 2968
Zestril Tablets (0.3% to 1.0%) 2972
Zocor Tablets (Rare) 1821
Zyrtec Tablets (Less than 2%) 2053

Arthritis, acute gouty, precipitation of

Benemid Tablets 1651
Pyrazinamide Tablets 1442

Arthritis, migratory

Elavil 2945

Arthropathy, Charcot-like

Celestone Soluspan Suspension 2484
Dalalone D.P. Injectable 1009
Decadron Phosphate Injection 1680
Decadron Phosphate with Xylocaine Injection, Sterile 1683
Decadron-LA Sterile Suspension 1687
Hydeltrasol Injection, Sterile 1708
Hydeltra-T.B.A. Sterile Suspension 1710
Hydrocortone Acetate Sterile Suspension 1712

Arthropathy, unspecified

Didronel Tablets 2133
Hivid Tablets (Less than 1%) 2287
Kerlone Tablets (Less than 2%) 2588
Ticlid Tablets (Rare) 2317

Arthrosis

Ambien Tablets (Rare) 2559
Anafranil Capsules (Infrequent) 819
▲ Aredia for Injection (At least 10%) 827
Betaseron for SC Injection 653
Depakote Tablets (1% to 5%) 418
Dilacor XR Extended-release Capsules (1.0%) 2183
Effexor (Infrequent) 2825
Foscavir Injection (Less than 1%) 541
Hivid Tablets (Less than 1%) 2287
Intron A for Injection (Less than 5%) 2506
LUVOX Tablets (Rare) 2723
Miacalcin Nasal Spray (1% to 3%) 2403
Norvasc Tablets (More than 0.1% to 1%) 2020
Norvir (Less than 2%) 447
Paxil Tablets (Rare) 2681
Remeron Tablets (Rare) 1878
Rilutek Tablets (Infrequent) 2198
Risperdal Tablets (Rare) 1348
Zoloft Tablets (Infrequent) 2051
Zyrtec Tablets (Less than 2%) 2053

Ascaris, appearance in mouth and nose

Mintezol 1747

Ascites

Avonex 662
Betaseron for SC Injection 653
Clomid 1262
Cosmegen Injection 1666
Doxil (Less than 1%) 2613
▲ Flolan for Injection (12%) 1085
Foscavir Injection (Less than 1%) 541
Humegon for Injection 1873
Hyskon Hysteroscopy Fluid (Rare) 1633
Inocor Lactate Injection (1 case) 2439
Intron A for Injection (Less than 5%) 2506
Invirase Capsules (Rare) 2291
Lutrepulse for Injection (Rare) 998
Metrodin (urofollitropin for injection) 2616
Oncaspar 2194
Profasi (chorionic gonadotropin for injection, USP) 2620
▲ Prograf (5% to 27%) 1028
▲ Proleukin for Injection (4%) 812
Risperdal Tablets (Rare) 1348
Serophene (clomiphene citrate tablets, USP) 2621
Taxotere for Injection Concentrate (Less frequent) 2204
▲ Vesanoid Capsules (3%) 2327

(▣ Described in PDR For Nonprescription Drugs) Incidence data in parenthesis; ▲ 3% or more (◉ Described in PDR For Ophthalmology)

Aseptic meningitis syndrome
Clinoril Tablets (Less than 1 in 100) ... 1658
CytoGam (Infrequent) ... 1630
Gamimune N, 5% Immune Globulin Intravenous (Human), 5% (Infrequent) ... 612
Gamimune N, 10% Immune Globulin Intravenous (Human), 10% (Infrequent) ... 615
Gammar-P I.V., Immune Globulin Intravenous (Human) (Infrequent) ... 798
Orthoclone OKT3 Sterile Solution ... 1892
RespiGam (Rare) ... 1631
Trimpex Tablets (Rare) ... 2323

Aseptic necrosis of femoral/humeral heads
Celestone Soluspan Suspension ... 2484
CORTENEMA ... 2713
Cortone Acetate Sterile Suspension ... 1663
Cortone Acetate Tablets ... 1664
Dalalone D.P. Injectable ... 1009
Decadron Elixir ... 1676
Decadron Phosphate Injection ... 1680
Decadron Phosphate with Xylocaine Injection, Sterile ... 1683
Decadron Tablets ... 1678
Decadron-LA Sterile Suspension ... 1687
Dexacort Phosphate in Respihaler ... 1606
Dexacort Phosphate in Turbinaire ... 1607
Florinef Acetate Tablets ... 506
Hydeltrasol Injection, Sterile ... 1708
Hydeltra-T.B.A. Sterile Suspension ... 1710
Hydrocortone Acetate Sterile Suspension ... 1712
Hydrocortone Phosphate Injection, Sterile ... 1713
Hydrocortone Tablets ... 1715
Pediapred Oral Solution ... 1618
Prelone Syrup ... 1834
Vancenase AQ Double Strength Nasal Spray 0.084% (Single cases) ... 2536

Aspermatogenesis
Velban Vials ... 1537

Asphyxia
Bentyl ... 1246
Compazine ... 2644
Navane Intramuscular ... 2019
Remeron Tablets (Rare) ... 1878
Stelazine ... 2692
Thorazine ... 2701

Aspiration
Clozaril Tablets ... 2377
Compazine ... 2644
Risperdal Tablets (Rare) ... 1348

Asterixis
Bumex (0.1%) ... 2260
Ceptaz ... 1070
Depakene ... 416
Depakote Tablets ... 418
Dilantin Infatabs (Rare) ... 1967
Dilantin Kapseals (Rare) ... 1965
Dilantin-125 Suspension (Rare) ... 1969
Fortaz ... 1092
Orthoclone OKT3 Sterile Solution ... 1892
Tazidime Vials, Faspak & ADD-Vantage ... 1531
▲ Vesanoid Capsules (3%) ... 2327

Asthenia
Accutane Capsules ... 2252
▲ Adalat Capsules (10 mg and 20 mg) (About 10% to 12%) ... 580
▲ Adalat CC (4%) ... 582
Adapin Capsules (Occasional) ... 1542
Adenoscan (Less than 1%) ... 1022
AeroBid Inhaler System (1% to 3%) ... 1004
Aerobid-M Inhaler System (1% to 3%) ... 1004
Albalon Solution with Liquifilm ... ⊙ 229
Aldactazide Tablets ... 2556
Aldoclor Tablets ... 1638
Aldomet Ester HCl Injection ... 1642
Aldomet Oral ... 1640
Aldoril Tablets ... 1644
All-Flex Arcing Spring Diaphragm (See also Ortho Diaphragm Kits) ... 1921
Altace Capsules (0.3% to 2.0%) ... 1238
Alupent Tablets (0.2%) ... 672
Amaryl Tablets (1.6%) ... 1241
Ambien Tablets (Frequent) ... 2559
Amicar Syrup, Tablets, and Injection ... 1312
Anafranil Capsules (Up to 2%) ... 819
Ana-Kit Anaphylaxis Emergency Treatment Kit (Common) ... 611
Ancobon Capsules ... 2254
Apresazide Capsules ... 824
▲ Arimidex Tablets (13.4% to 16.0%) ... 2932
Artane ... 1418
▲ Asacol Delayed-Release Tablets (7%) ... 2129
Asendin Tablets (Less frequent) ... 1419
Atamet Tablets ... 567
▲ Ativan Tablets (4.2%) ... 2807
Atromid-S Capsules (Less often) ... 2808
▲ Avonex (21%) ... 662
▲ Axid Pulvules (3.1%) ... 1468
Azactam for Injection (Less than 1%) ... 736
Bactrim DS Tablets ... 2257
Bactrim I.V. Infusion ... 2255
Bactrim ... 2257
▲ Bentyl (7%) ... 1246
Betagan ... ⊙ 230
▲ Betapace Tablets (4% to 13%) ... 637
▲ Betaseron for SC Injection (49%) ... 653
Betimol 0.25%, 0.5% (1% to 5%) ... ⊙ 259
Blocadren Tablets (0.6%) ... 1654
Brevibloc (esmolol HCl) Injection (Less than 1%) ... 1860
▲ Bromfed-DM Cough Syrup (Among most frequent) ... 1832
Bronkometer Aerosol ... 2432
Bronkosol Solution ... 2432
Brontex ... 2130
Bumex (0.2%) ... 2260
BuSpar Tablets (2%) ... 738
Cafergot ... 2376
Calcijex Injection ... 412
Capoten Tablets ... 740
Capozide Tablets ... 744
Carbocaine Injection ... 2432
▲ Cardene Capsules (4.2% to 5.8%) ... 2261
Cardene I.V. (0.7%) ... 2815
▲ Cardene SR Capsules (0.9% to 4.4%) ... 2264
▲ Cardioquin Tablets (5%) ... 2146
Cardizem CD Capsules (1.8% to 2.6%) ... 1251
▲ Cardizem SR Capsules (2.8% to 5%) ... 1255
Cardizem Injectable (Less than 1%) ... 1253
Cardizem Tablets (1.2%) ... 1257
Cardura Tablets (1%) ... 1993
▲ Cartrol Tablets (7.1%) ... 413
▲ Casodex Tablets (15%) ... 2934
▲ Catapres Tablets (About 10 in 100 patients) ... 679
Catapres-TTS ... 680
Caverject Injection (Less than 1%) ... 2064
Ceclor Pulvules & Suspension ... 1470
▲ CellCept Capsules (13.7% to 16.1%) ... 2265
▲ Cerebyx Injection (2.2% to 3.9%) ... 1956
Ceredase ... 1055
Cipro I.V. (1% or less) ... 587
Cipro I.V. Pharmacy Bulk Package (Less than 1%) ... 590
Cipro Tablets (Less than 1%) ... 584
Claritin Tablets (2% or fewer patients) ... 2485
Claritin-D Tablets (Less frequent) ... 2487
Clinoril Tablets (Less than 1 in 100) ... 1658
Clomid ... 1262
Clozaril Tablets (1%) ... 2377
Cogentin ... 1661
Cognex Capsules (2%) ... 1961
ColBENEMID Tablets ... 1662
Colestid (Infrequent) ... 2073
▲ Combipres Tablets (About 10%) ... 682
Cortone Acetate Sterile Suspension ... 1663
Cortone Acetate Tablets ... 1664
Coumadin ... 941
Cozaar Tablets (1% or greater) ... 1668
▲ Crixivan Capsules (3.6%) ... 1670
Cystospaz ... 2123
Cytotec (Infrequent) ... 2576
▲ Cytovene (6%) ... 2270
D.A. II Tablets ... 972
D.A. Chewable Tablets ... 970
DDAVP (Up to 2%) ... 2180
Dalmane Capsules ... 2329
Danocrine Capsules ... 2437
▲ Dantrium Capsules (Among most frequent) ... 2131
Dapsone Tablets USP ... 1331
Daranide Tablets ... 1676
Darvon-N/Darvocet-N ... 1473
Darvon ... 1475
Darvon-N Suspension & Tablets ... 1473
Daypro Caplets (Less than 1%) ... 2578
Decadron Elixir ... 1676
Decadron Phosphate with Xylocaine Injection, Sterile ... 1683
Deconsal II Tablets ... 1605
Demadex Tablets and Injection (2.0%) ... 691
Demerol ... 2438
Demulen ... 2580
Depakene ... 416
▲ Depakote Tablets (10% to 20%) ... 418
▲ Depo-Provera Contraceptive Injection (More than 5%) ... 2079
Desmopressin Acetate Rhinal Tube (Up to 2%) ... 997
Desyrel and Desyrel Dividose ... 504
Dilacor XR Extended-release Capsules (1.7% to 3.6%) ... 2183
Dilaudid-HP Injection (Less frequent) ... 1384
Dilaudid-HP Lyophilized Powder 250 mg (Less frequent) ... 1384
Dilaudid Tablets and Liquid (Less frequent) ... 1386
Dimetane-DC Cough Syrup ... 2232
Dimetane-DX Cough Syrup ... 2233
Diprivan Injectable Emulsion (Less than 1%) ... 2939
Ditropan ... 1267
Diucardin Tablets ... 2824
Diupres Tablets ... 1691
Diuril Oral Suspension ... 1694
Diuril Sodium Intravenous ... 1693
Diuril Tablets ... 1694
Dolobid Tablets (Less than 1 in 100) ... 1695
Donnatal ... 2234
Donnatal Extentabs ... 2234
Donnatal Tablets ... 2234
Doral Tablets ... 2773
▲ Doxil (6.5% to 9.9%) ... 2613
▲ Duragesic Transdermal System (10% or more) ... 1336
Dura-Tap/PD Capsules ... 970
Dura-Vent/DA Tablets ... 972
Dura-Vent Tablets ... 971
Dyazide Capsules ... 2653
Dynabac (2.0%) ... 668
DynaCirc Capsules (Up to 1.2%) ... 2381
Dyrenium Capsules (Rare) ... 2655
▲ Effexor (2% to 16.9%) ... 2825
Elavil ... 2945
Eldepryl Capsules ... 2729
Emete-con Intramuscular/Intravenous ... 2007
Enduron Tablets ... 424
Engerix-B Unit-Dose Vials (Less than 1%) ... 2656
Entex PSE Tablets ... 973
EpiPen ... 808
▲ Epogen for Injection (7% to 13%) ... 489
Ergamisol Tablets (10 out of 463 patients) ... 1340
Esidrix Tablets ... 839
Esimil Tablets ... 840
Eskalith ... 2658
Estrace Cream and Tablets ... 751
▲ Ethmozine Tablets (2% to 5%) ... 2217
▲ Etopophos for Injection (39%) ... 701
Etrafon ... 2495
Fansidar Tablets ... 2281
Fedahist Gyrocaps ... 2545
Felbatol (Frequent) ... 2774
Feldene Capsules (Less than 1%) ... 2008
Flagyl 375 Capsules ... 2587
Flexeril Tablets (Less than 1%) ... 1701
▲ Flolan for Injection (87%) ... 1085
Floxin I.V. (Less than 1%) ... 1580
Floxin Tablets (200 mg, 300 mg, 400 mg) (Less than 1%) ... 1577
▲ Fludara for Injection (9% to 65%) ... 658
Flumadine Tablets & Syrup (1.4%) ... 1013
▲ Foscavir Injection (5% or greater) ... 541
Sterile FUDR ... 2284
Gantanol Tablets ... 2285
Gantrisin ... 2286
Gemzar for Injection (Common) ... 1482
▲ Glucotrol XL Extended Release Tablets (10.1%) ... 2012
Guaimax-D Tablets ... 809
Halcion Tablets (Rare) ... 2093
Helidac Therapy (1.0%) ... 2135
Histussin D Liquid ... 670
Hivid Tablets (Less than 1%) ... 2287
Humatrope Vials (Infrequent) ... 1490
▲ Hycamtin for Injection (Less than 1% to 21%) ... 2665
Hydeltrasol Injection, Sterile ... 1708
HydroDIURIL Tablets ... 1716
Hydropres Tablets ... 1718
Hyperstat I.V. Injection (2%) ... 2504
▲ Hytrin Capsules (1.6% to 11.3%) ... 434
Hyzaar Tablets (1% or greater) ... 1720
Imdur (Less than or equal to 5%) ... 1362
▲ Imitrex Injection (4.9%) ... 1095
Imitrex Tablets (Less than 1% to 2%) ... 1099
Inderal ... 2834
Inderal LA Long Acting Capsules ... 2836
Inderide Tablets ... 2838
Inderide LA Long Acting Capsules ... 2840
INFeD (Iron Dextran Injection, USP) ... 2478
▲ Intron A for Injection (Less than 5% to 24%) ... 2506
Inversine Tablets ... 1729
Invirase Capsules (Rare; 1.3%) ... 2291
Iopidine 0.5% (Less than 3%) ... ⊙ 219
Ismelin Tablets ... 845
Ismo Tablets (Fewer than 1%) ... 2844
Isoetharine Inhalation Solution, USP, Arm-a-Med ... 545
Isuprel Hydrochloride Solution ... 2443
Isuprel Injection ... 2441
Isuprel Mistometer ... 2442
K-Phos Neutral Tablets ... 633
Kadian Capsules (Less than 3%) ... 2948
▲ Kerlone Tablets (7.1%) ... 2588
Kutrase Capsules ... 2546
▲ Kytril Injection (5%) ... 2667
▲ Kytril Tablets (5% to 14%) ... 2669
Lamictal Tablets (More than 1%) ... 1105
Lanoxicaps ... 1110
Lanoxin Elixir Pediatric ... 1113
Lanoxin Injection ... 1116
Lanoxin Injection Pediatric ... 1119
Lanoxin Tablets ... 1121
Lariam Tablets (Less than 1%) ... 2295
Larodopa Tablets (Relatively frequent) ... 2296
Lasix Injection, Oral Solution and Tablets ... 1267
Lescol Capsules (Rare) ... 2395
▲ Leukine (17% to 66%) ... 1317
▲ Leustatin (9%) ... 1889
Levatol Tablets (1.6%) ... 2547
Levbid Extended-Release Tablets ... 2549
Levlen/Tri-Levlen ... 646
▲ Levoprome (Among the most important) ... 1321
Levsin/Levsinex/Levbid ... 2549
Limbitrol ... 2333
Lioresal Intrathecal (Up to 2.0%) ... 1634
▲ Lioresal Tablets (5% to 15%) ... 847
Lithonate/Lithotabs/Lithobid ... 2721
Lodine Capsules and Tablets (1% to 3%) ... 2849
Lopid Tablets ... 1974
Lopressor HCT Tablets ... 850
Lotensin Tablets ... 852
Lotensin HCT Tablets (0.3% to more than 1%) ... 855
Lotrel Capsules ... 858
Loxitane ... 1426
▲ Ludiomil Tablets (4%) ... 861
▲ Lupron Depot 3.75 mg (8.4%) ... 2739
▲ Lupron Depot 7.5 mg (5.4%) ... 2741
▲ Lupron Depot - 3 Month 22.5 mg (7.4%) ... 2743
▲ Lupron Injection (5% or more) ... 2736
▲ LUVOX Tablets (14%) ... 2723
MS Contin Tablets (Less frequent) ... 2149
MSIR (Infrequent) ... 2152
Macrobid Capsules ... 2138
Macrodantin Capsules ... 2140
Marcaine ... 2446
Marcaine Spinal ... 2449
Marinol (Dronabinol) Capsules (Greater than 1%) ... 2353
Matulane Capsules ... 2300
Maxair Autohaler ... 1550
Maxair Inhaler (Less than 1%) ... 1552
Maxaquin Tablets (Less than 1%) ... 2593
▲ Megace Oral Suspension (2% to 6%) ... 708
Mepergan Injection ... 2859
▲ Mepron Suspension (8%) ... 1206
Mestinon Injectable ... 1300
Mestinon ... 1300
Methadone Hydrochloride Oral Concentrate ... 2356
Methadone Hydrochloride Oral Solution & Tablets ... 2357
Mevacor Tablets (1.2% to 1.7%; rare) ... 1742
▲ Mexitil Capsules (1.9% to 5%) ... 684
▲ Midamor Tablets (Between 1% and 3%) ... 1746

(▣ Described in PDR For Nonprescription Drugs) Incidence data in parenthesis; ▲ 3% or more (⊙ Described in PDR For Ophthalmology)

Asthenia

▲ Minipress Capsules (6.5%) ... 2015
▲ Minizide Capsules (6.5%) ... 2016
Mithracin ... 599
Modicon ... 1928
▲ Moduretic Tablets (3% to 8%) ... 1748
Monopril Tablets (0.2% to 1.4%) ... 762
Mustargen ... 1752
Mycobutin Capsules (1%) ... 2101
Mykrox Tablets (Less than 2%) ... 1617
Myleran Tablets ... 1209
Myochrysine Injection ... 1754
▲ Nalfon 200 Pulvules & Nalfon Tablets (5.4%) ... 933
Naprelan Tablets (Less than 3%) ... 2861
Nardil (Common) ... 1977
Navane Capsules and Concentrate ... 2018
Navane Intramuscular ... 2019
▲ Navelbine Injection (Up to 27%) ... 1212
NegGram ... 2453
Neoral (Rare) ... 2405
▲ Neupogen for Injection (4%) ... 495
Neurontin Capsules (Frequent) ... 1978
▲ Nipent for Injection (10% to 13%) ... 2733
Nitrolingual Spray ... 2193
Nitrostat Tablets (Occasional) ... 1981
Norflex ... 1554
Norgesic ... 1554
Norisodrine with Calcium Iodide Syrup ... 446
Normodyne Tablets (1%) ... 2522
Noroxin Tablets (Less frequent) ... 1758
Noroxin Tablets (0.3% to 1.3%) ... 2222
Norpramin Tablets ... 1273
Norvasc Tablets (Less than 1% to 2%) ... 2020
▲ Norvir (9.4% to 14.2%) ... 447
Novahistine DMX ... 782
Novahistine Elixir ... 782
Nubain Injection (1% or less) ... 952
Nucofed ... 2225
Nydrazid Injection ... 509
Ocupress Ophthalmic Solution, 1% Sterile (Occasional) ... ⊚ 297
OptiPranolol (Metipranolol 0.3%) Sterile Ophthalmic Solution (A small number of patients) ... ⊚ 256
Oramorph SR (Morphine Sulfate Sustained Release Tablets) (Less frequent) ... 2359
▲ Orap Tablets (25.0%) ... 1037
Oretic Tablets ... 450
▲ Orlaam Oral Solution (3% to 9%) ... 2361
Ornade Spansule Capsules ... 2678
Ortho-Cyclen/Ortho-Tri-Cyclen ... 1914
Ortho Diaphragm Kits—All-Flex Arcing Spring; Ortho Coil Spring; Ortho-White Flat Spring ... 1921
Ortho Diaphragm Kit-Coil Spring ... 1921
Ortho-Est ... 1925
Ortho-Novum ... 1928
Ortho-Cyclen/Ortho Tri-Cyclen ... 1914
Ortho-White Diaphragm Kit-Flat Spring (See also Ortho Diaphragm Kits) ... 1921
Orthoclone OKT3 Sterile Solution ... 1892
▲ OxyContin Tablets (6%) ... 2163
Pamelor ... 2409
▲ Paraplatin for Injection (11% to 43%) ... 713
Parlodel ... 2411
Parnate Tablets ... 2679
▲ Paxil Tablets (1.6% to 22%) ... 2681
Pediazole Suspension ... 2340
Penetrex Tablets (0.1% to 1%) ... 2196
Pentasa (Less than 1%) ... 1275
Pentaspan Injection ... 954
Pepcid Injection (Infrequent) ... 1765
Pepcid (Infrequent) ... 1763
▲ Permax Tablets (4.2%) ... 571
Phenergan with Codeine ... 2883
Phenergan VC ... 2886
Phenergan VC with Codeine ... 2888
Placidyl Capsules ... 456
Plaquenil Sulfate Tablets ... 2459
▲ Plendil Extended-Release Tablets (2.2% to 3.9%) ... 514
PMB 200 and PMB 400 ... 2890
Pneumovax 23 ... 1768
Polycitra Syrup ... 574
Polycitra-K Crystals ... 574
Polycitra-K Oral Solution ... 575
Polycitra-LC ... 574
Pondimin Tablets ... 2239
Pravachol Tablets (Rare) ... 770
Prevacid Delayed-Release Capsules (Less than 1%) ... 2746
Prilosec Delayed-Release Capsules (1.1% to 1.3%) ... 516
Primaxin I.M. ... 1770

Primaxin I.V. (Less than 0.2%) ... 1772
Prinivil Tablets (Greater than 1%) ... 1776
Prinzide Tablets (1.8%) ... 1780
Pro-Banthine Tablets ... 2226
Procanbid Extended-Release Tablets (Occasional) ... 1983
▲ Procardia Capsules (Approximately 10% to 12%) ... 2024
▲ Procardia XL Extended Release Tablets (Less than 3% to 12%) ... 2026
▲ Procrit for Injection (7% to 13%) ... 1896
Proglycem ... 575
▲ Prograf (7% to 52%) ... 1028
▲ Proleukin for Injection (53%) ... 812
▲ ProSom Tablets (11%) ... 457
Prostigmin Injectable ... 1305
Prostigmin Tablets ... 1306
Prostin E2 Suppository ... 2109
Protostat Tablets ... 1939
Proventil Repetabs Tablets (2%) ... 2529
Proventil Syrup (Less than 1 of 100 patients) ... 2528
Proventil Tablets (2%) ... 2529
▲ Prozac Pulvules & Liquid, Oral Solution (4.4% to 15%) ... 935
Pulmozyme Inhalation ... 1054
Quadrinal Tablets ... 1398
Quinaglute Dura-Tabs Tablets (2%) ... 644
▲ Quinidex Extentabs (5%) ... 2240
RMS Suppositories CII ... 2766
Recombivax HB (Equal to or greater than 1%) ... 1787
▲ Redux Capsules (15.8%) ... 2911
Regitine Vials ... 864
Relafen Tablets (1%) ... 2688
▲ Remeron Tablets (8%) ... 1878
Restoril Capsules (1-2%) ... 2413
▲ Retrovir Capsules (8.6% to 69%) ... 1216
▲ Retrovir I.V. Infusion (8.6% to 69%) ... 1221
▲ Retrovir Syrup (8.6% to 69%) ... 1216
Rifamate Capsules ... 1278
Rifater ... 1280
▲ Rilutek Tablets (14.8% to 20.1%) ... 2198
Risperdal Tablets ... 1348
Robinul Forte Tablets ... 2247
Robinul Injectable ... 2247
Robinul Tablets ... 2247
Rocaltrol Capsules ... 2303
▲ Roferon-A Injection (Less than 0.5% to 88%) ... 2308
Romazicon (1% to 3%) ... 2311
Rondec Oral Drops ... 974
Rondec Syrup ... 974
Rondec ... 974
Rowasa (0.12% to 1.2%) ... 2727
Roxanol ... 2365
Rum-K Syrup ... 1004
Rythmol Tablets–150mg, 225mg, 300mg (0.6 to 2.4%) ... 1399
▲ Salagen Tablets (6% to 12%) ... 1546
Sandimmune (Rare) ... 2416
Sandostatin Injection (1% to 4%) ... 2421
Sanorex Tablets ... 2423
Sansert Tablets ... 2424
Scleromate Injection (Rare) ... 1234
Seldane Tablets (0.6% to 0.9%) ... 1284
Seldane-D Extended-Release Tablets ... 1286
Semprex-D Capsules (2%) ... 1620
Sensorcaine ... 554
Septra ... 1146
Septra I.V. Infusion ... 1142
Septra I.V. Infusion ADD-Vantage Vials ... 1144
Septra ... 1146
Ser-Ap-Es Tablets ... 867
Serentil ... 689
▲ Serzone Tablets (11%) ... 776
Sinemet Tablets ... 959
Sinemet CR Tablets ... 961
Sinequan (Occasional) ... 2028
Solganal Suspension (Rare) ... 2530
Soma Compound w/Codeine Tablets (Very rare) ... 2784
Soma Compound Tablets (Very rare) ... 2783
Soma Tablets ... 2782
Sorbitrate ... 2959
Stadol (1% or greater) ... 779
Surmontil Capsules ... 2917
Sus-Phrine Injection ... 1017
Symmetrel Capsules (0.1% to 1%) ... 965
Symmetrel Syrup (0.1% to 1%) ... 963
Synarel Nasal Solution for Endometriosis (Less than 1%) ... 2605
Syn-Rx Tablets ... 1622
Syn-Rx DM Tablets ... 1623
Talacen Caplets (Infrequent) ... 2464

Talwin Injection (Infrequent) ... 2465
Talwin Compound (Infrequent) ... 2466
Talwin Injection (Infrequent) ... 2465
Talwin Nx Tablets (Infrequent) ... 2467
▲ Tambocor Tablets (Less than 1% to 4.9%) ... 1555
▲ Taxotere for Injection Concentrate (11.1%) ... 2204
▲ Tenex Tablets (Up to 10%) ... 2249
Tenoretic Tablets ... 2963
Tensilon Injectable ... 1307
Thalitone ... 1293
Thioplex (Thiotepa For Injection) ... 1329
▲ Tiazac Capsules (6%) ... 1019
Ticlid Tablets (0.5% to 1.0%) ... 2317
Timolide Tablets (1.9%) ... 1791
Timoptic in Ocudose (Less frequent) ... 1796
Timoptic Sterile Ophthalmic Solution (Less frequent) ... 1794
Timoptic-XE ... 1798
Tofranil Ampuls ... 873
Tofranil Tablets ... 875
Tofranil-PM Capsules ... 876
▲ Tolectin (200, 400 and 600 mg) (3 to 9%) ... 1591
Tonocard Tablets (Less than 1%) ... 519
Toradol (1% or less) ... 2319
Tornalate Solution for Inhalation, 0.2% (Less than 1%) ... 976
Trancopal Caplets ... 2468
Trandate Tablets (1%) ... 1158
Triavil Tablets ... 1800
Levlen/Tri-Levlen ... 646
Trinalin Repetabs Tablets ... 1373
Trusopt Sterile Ophthalmic Solution (Infrequent) ... 1803
Tussend ... 1830
Tussend Expectorant ... 1831
Tympagesic Ear Drops ... 2476
▲ Ultram Tablets (50 mg) (6% to 12%) ... 1594
Uroqid-Acid No. 2 Tablets ... 633
Valtrex Caplets (2% to 4%) ... 1167
Vantin for Oral Suspension and Vantin Tablets (Less than 1%) ... 2112
▲ Vaqta (3.9%) ... 1805
▲ Vascor Tablets (200 and 300 mg) (0.5 to 13.95%) ... 1597
Vaseretic Tablets (2.4%) ... 1810
Vasotec I.V. ... 1814
Vasotec Tablets (1.1% to 1.6%) ... 1816
Velban Vials ... 1537
Ventolin Syrup (Less than 1 of 100) ... 1175
Ventolin Tablets (2 of 100 patients) ... 1176
Versed Injection (Less than 1%) ... 2324
Vesanoid Capsules ... 2327
▲ Videx Tablets, Powder for Oral Solution, & Pediatric Powder for Oral Solution (4% to 41%) ... 2980
Virazole ... 1310
▲ Visken Tablets (4%) ... 2428
▲ Vistide Injection (7% to 46%) ... 1057
Vivactil Tablets ... 1820
Volmax Extended-Release Tablets ... 1835
Wygesic Tablets ... 2930
▲ Xanax Tablets (7.1%) ... 2115
Yutopar Intravenous Injection (Infrequent) ... 566
Zaroxolyn Tablets ... 1625
Zebeta Tablets (0.4% to 1.5%) ... 1457
▲ Zerit Capsules (2% to 28%) ... 731
Zestoretic Tablets (1.8%) ... 2968
Zestril Tablets (1.3% to greater than 1%) ... 2972
Ziac ... 1459
Zocor Tablets (1.6%; rare) ... 1821
Zofran Tablets (Up to 2%) ... 1231
▲ Zoladex (11%) ... 2976
Zoloft Tablets (Frequent) ... 2051
Zosyn (1.0% or less) ... 1463
Zovirax (1.2%) ... 1187
Zyloprim Tablets (Less than 1%) ... 1194
Zyrtec Tablets (Less than 2%) ... 2053

Asthma, allergic

Abelcet Injection ... 1540
Fluvirin (Influenza Virus Vaccine) (Rare) ... 1608
Influenza Virus Vaccine, Trivalent, Types A and B (chromatograph- and filter-purified subviron antigen) FluShield, 1996-1997 Formula (Rare) ... 2842

Asthma, bronchial

▲ CellCept Capsules (More than or equal to 3%) ... 2265
Cerebyx Injection (Infrequent) ... 1956

Cuprimine Capsules ... 1673
Cytovene-IV (One report) ... 2270
Depen Titratable Tablets ... 2770
Dexacort Phosphate in Turbinaire ... 1607
Doxil (Less than 1%) ... 2613
Felbatol ... 2774
Haldol Injection, Tablets and Concentrate ... 1585
Halotestin Tablets ... 2095
Kadian Capsules (Less than 3%) ... 2948
Naprelan Tablets (Less than 1%) ... 2861
Norvir (Less than 2%) ... 447
Nubain Injection (1% or less) ... 952
Permax Tablets (Infrequent) ... 571
Prevacid Delayed-Release Capsules (Less than 1%) ... 2746
Prinivil Tablets (0.3% to 1.0%) ... 1776
Prolixin ... 510
Prozac Pulvules & Liquid, Oral Solution (Infrequent) ... 935
Redux Capsules (Infrequent) ... 2911
Relafen Tablets (Less than 1%) ... 2688
Serzone Tablets (Infrequent) ... 776
Soma Compound Tablets ... 2783
Toradol ... 2319
Vaqta (Less than 1%) ... 1805
Vaseretic Tablets ... 1810
Vasotec I.V. ... 1814
Vasotec Tablets (0.5% to 1.0%) ... 1816
▲ Vesanoid Capsules (3%) ... 2327
Vistide Injection ... 1057
Zestoretic Tablets ... 2968
Zyloprim Tablets (Less than 1%) ... 1194

Asthma, worsening of

Azelex (Rare) ... 471
Sinequan (Occasional) ... 2028

Asthmatic episodes

Alupent (1% to 4%) ... 672
Betapace Tablets (1% to 2%) ... 637
Betaseron for SC Injection ... 653
Betoptic Ophthalmic Solution (Rare) ... 465
Betoptic S Ophthalmic Suspension (Rare) ... 467
Cataflam Tablets (Less than 1%) ... 833
Cognex Capsules (Infrequent) ... 1961
Compazine ... 2644
Cortisporin Otic Solution Sterile ... 1076
Depo-Provera Contraceptive Injection (Fewer than 1%) ... 2079
Dilaudid Tablets and Liquid ... 1386
Dobutrex Solution Vials ... 1480
Duragesic Transdermal System (Less than 1%) ... 1336
Easprin ... 1971
Effexor (Infrequent) ... 2825
Eldepryl Capsules ... 2729
Engerix-B Unit-Dose Vials ... 2656
Esimil Tablets ... 840
Estrace Cream and Tablets ... 751
Ethmozine Tablets (Less than 2%) ... 2217
Etrafon ... 2495
Heparin Lock Flush Solution ... 2831
Heparin Sodium Injection ... 2832
Heparin Sodium Vials (Rare) ... 1486
Imitrex Tablets (Infrequent) ... 1099
Indocin Capsules (Less than 1%) ... 1723
Indocin I.V. (Less than 1%) ... 1727
Indocin (Less than 1%) ... 1723
Iopidine 0.5% (Less than 1%) ... ⊚ 219
Ismelin Tablets ... 845
Isopto Carbachol Ophthalmic Solution ... ⊚ 221
Isuprel Hydrochloride Solution ... 2443
Kutrase Capsules ... 2546
Levoprome ... 1321
Lodine Capsules and Tablets (Less than 1%) ... 2849
Lotensin Tablets ... 852
Lupron Depot 3.75 mg (Rare) ... 2739
Lupron Depot 7.5 mg (Rare) ... 2741
Lupron Depot - 3 Month 22.5 mg (Rare) ... 2743
Lupron Depot-PED 7.5 mg, 11.25 mg and 15 mg ... 2744
LUVOX Tablets (Infrequent) ... 2723
Mellaril ... 2398
Minocin Oral Suspension ... 1431
Monoket Tablets (Fewer than 1%) ... 2550
▲ Nipent for Injection (3% to 10%) ... 2733
Paxil Tablets (Infrequent) ... 2681
Phenergan Injection ... 2880
Phenergan Tablets ... 2882
Pred Mild ... ⊚ 250
Prinzide Tablets ... 1780
▲ Prograf (Greater than 3%) ... 1028
Prolixin ... 510
ProSom Tablets (Infrequent) ... 457
Questran ... 774

(▣ Described in PDR For Nonprescription Drugs)   Incidence data in parenthesis; ▲ 3% or more   (⊚ Described in PDR For Ophthalmology)

1265 Side Effects Index Atrial tachycardia

Remeron Tablets (Infrequent) 1878
Rilutek Tablets (Infrequent) 2198
Risperdal Tablets (Rare) 1348
Robaxisal Tablets 2246
Rowasa 2727
Scleromate Injection (Rare) 1234
Sensorcaine 554
Septra I.V. Infusion 1142
Septra I.V. Infusion ADD-Vantage Vials 1144
Serentil 689
Soma Compound w/Codeine Tablets (Rare) 2784
Soma Compound Tablets (Less common) 2783
Soma Tablets 2782
Sotradecol (Sodium Tetradecyl Sulfate Injection) 987
Stelazine 2692
Streptomycin Sulfate Injection 2031
Sular Tablets (Less than or equal to 1%) 2961
Supprelin Injection (2% to 3%) 2230
Suprane (desflurane, USP) (Less than 1%) 1865
Terramycin Intramuscular Solution 2034
Thioplex (Thiotepa For Injection) 1329
Thorazine 2701
Torecan 2367
▲ Trasylol (3%) 607
Triavil Tablets 1800
Trilafon 2532
Trilisate (Rare) 2155
Urecholine 1804
▲ Videx Tablets, Powder for Oral Solution, & Pediatric Powder for Oral Solution (Up to 21%) 2980
Viokase 2251
Cataflam/Voltaren/Voltaren-XR (Less than 1%) 833
Zebeta Tablets 1457
Zemuron Injection (Less than 1%) 1885
Zerit Capsules (Fewer than 1% to 2%) 731
Zestril Tablets (0.3% to 1.0%) 2972
Ziac 1459

Asystole
Acthrel for Injection (One patient) 2990
Adenocard Injection 1021
Alfenta Injection 1334
Brevibloc (esmolol HCl) Injection (2 Patients) 1860
Cardizem SR Capsules (Infrequent) 1255
Cardizem Tablets (Infrequent) 1257
Diprivan Injectable Emulsion 2939
Isoptin Injectable (In extreme cases) 1391
Zantac Injection (Rare) 1180

Asystole, ventricular
Procanbid Extended-Release Tablets 1983

Ataxia
Adapin Capsules (Infrequent) 1542
Aldactazide Tablets 2556
Aldactone Tablets 2558
Ambien Tablets (Frequent) 2559
Anafranil Capsules (Infrequent) 819
Ancobon Capsules 2254
Asendin Tablets (Less frequent) 1419
Atamet Tablets 567
Atrohist Plus Tablets 1605
Attenuvax (Rare) 1650
Avonex (2%) 662
Azulfidine (Rare) 2059
Bactrim DS Tablets 2257
Bactrim I.V. Infusion 2255
Bactrim 2257
Bentyl 10 mg Capsules 1246
Betagan (Rare) ⊙ 230
Betapace Tablets (Rare) 637
Betaseron for SC Injection 653
▲ Bromfed-DM Cough Syrup (Among most frequent) 1832
Buprenex Injectable (Rare) 2170
BuSpar Tablets (1%) 738
Butisol Sodium Elixir & Tablets (Less than 1 in 100) 2768
Capoten Tablets 740
Capozide Tablets 744
Cardioquin Tablets (1% to 3%) 2146
Cardura Tablets (1%) 1993
CeeNU Capsules 699
Celontin Kapseals (Frequent) 1955
▲ Cerebyx Injection (4.4% to 11.1%) 1956
Chibroxin Sterile Ophthalmic Solution (With oral form) 1657
Cipro I.V. (1% or less) 587
Cipro I.V. Pharmacy Bulk Package (Less than 1%) 590
Cipro Tablets (Less than 1%) 584
Clozaril Tablets (1%) 2377
▲ Cognex Capsules (6%) 1961
▲ Cordarone Tablets (4 to 9%) 2818
Cozaar Tablets (Less than 1%) 1668
Cytovene (1% or less) 2270
Dalalone D.P. Injectable 1009
Dalmane Capsules 2329
Daranide Tablets 1676
DaunoXome (Less than or equal to 5%) 1842
Decadron-LA Sterile Suspension (Low) 1687
Demerol 2438
Depakene 416
Depakote Tablets (1% to 5%) 418
▲ Desyrel and Desyrel Dividose (1.9% to 4.9%) 504
▲ Dilantin Infatabs (Among most common) 1967
▲ Dilantin Kapseals (Among most common) 1965
▲ Dilantin-125 Suspension (Among most common) 1969
▲ Dizac (diazepam injectable emulsion) CIV (Among most common) 1862
Doral Tablets 2773
Effexor (Infrequent) 2825
Elavil 2945
Ergamisol Tablets (Up to 2%) 1340
Eskalith 2658
Ethmozine Tablets (Less than 2%) 2217
Etrafon 2495
Fansidar Tablets 2281
▲ Felbatol (3.5% to 6.5%) 2774
Flagyl 375 Capsules 2587
Flagyl I.V. 2373
Flexeril Tablets (Less than 1%) 1701
Floxin I.V. 1580
Floxin Tablets (200 mg, 300 mg, 400 mg) 1577
Flumadine Tablets & Syrup (0.3% to 1%) 1013
Foscavir Injection (Between 1% and 5%) 541
Gantanol Tablets 2285
Gantrisin 2286
Garamycin Injectable 2502
▲ Halcion Tablets (4.6%) 2093
Helidac Therapy 2135
Hexalen Capsules 2760
Hivid Tablets (Less than 1%) 2287
Hyzaar Tablets 1720
Imitrex Tablets (Infrequent) 1099
Intron A for Injection (Less than 5%) 2506
Invirase Capsules (Rare; less than 2%) 2291
Kadian Capsules (Less than 3%) 2948
Kerlone Tablets (Less than 2%) 2588
▲ Klonopin Tablets (30%) 2294
▲ Lamictal Tablets (Among most common; 10% to 28%) 1105
Larodopa Tablets (Relatively frequent) 2296
Leukeran Tablets (Rare) 1205
Levsin/Levsinex/Levbid 2549
Librax Capsules 2330
Librium Capsules (Some patients) 2331
Librium Injectable 2332
Limbitrol 2333
Lioresal Intrathecal (1% or more) 1634
Lioresal Tablets 847
Lithium Carbonate Capsules & Tablets 2352
Lithonate/Lithotabs/Lithobid 2721
Ludiomil Tablets (Rare) 861
LUVOX Tablets (Infrequent) 2723
M-M-R II (Rare) 1730
M-R-VAX II (Rare) 1732
Marinol (Dronabinol) Capsules (Greater than 1%) 2353
Matulane Capsules 2300
Maxaquin Tablets 2593
Mebaral Tablets (Less than 1 in 100) 2452
Mepergan Injection 2859
Mesantoin Tablets 2400
Methotrexate Sodium Tablets, Injection, for Injection and LPF Injection 1322
MetroGel-Vaginal 917
Miltown Tablets 2780
▲ Mysoline (Among most frequent) 2860
Nardil (Less frequent) 1977
Nembutal Sodium Capsules (Less than 1%) 440
Nembutal Sodium Solution (Less than 1%) 442
Nembutal Sodium Suppositories (Less than 1%) 444
▲ Neurontin Capsules (Among most common; 12.5%) 1978
Nipent for Injection (Less than 3%) 2733
Noroxin Tablets 1758
Noroxin Tablets 2222
Norpramin Tablets 1273
Norvasc Tablets (Less than or equal to 0.1%) 2020
Norvir (Less than 2%) 447
Oncovin Solution Vials & Hyporets 1521
PBZ-SR Tablets 862
Pamelor 2409
Parlodel 2411
Parnate Tablets 2679
Paxil Tablets (Infrequent) 2681
Pediazole Suspension 2340
Peganone Tablets (Rare) 455
Penetrex Tablets (Less than 0.1%) 2196
Permax Tablets (1.6%) 571
Phenergan Injection 2880
Phenergan Tablets 2882
Phenobarbital Elixir and Tablets (Less than 1 in 100 patients) 1523
Placidyl Capsules 456
Plaquenil Sulfate Tablets 2459
PMB 200 and PMB 400 (Rare) 2890
Pondimin Tablets 2239
Prinivil Tablets (0.3% to 1.0%) 1776
Prinzide Tablets 1780
Procardia XL Extended Release Tablets (1% or less) 2026
▲ Prograf (Greater than 3%) 1028
ProSom Tablets (Rare) 457
Protostat Tablets 1939
Prozac Pulvules & Liquid, Oral Solution (Infrequent) 935
Quinaglute Dura-Tabs Tablets 644
Quinidex Extentabs (1%) 2240
Redux Capsules (Infrequent) 2911
Remeron Tablets (Infrequent) 1878
Restoril Capsules (Less than 1%) 2413
Rifadin 1276
Rifamate Capsules 1278
Rifater 1280
Rilutek Tablets (Infrequent) 2198
Rimactane Capsules 865
▲ Risperdal Tablets (17% to 34%) 1348
Robaxin Injectable 2245
Roferon-A Injection (Less than 1%) 2308
▲ Romazicon (10%) 2311
Rythmol Tablets–150mg, 225mg, 300mg (0.3 to 1.6%) 1399
Sansert Tablets 2424
Seconal Sodium Pulvules (Less than 1 in 100) 1529
Septra 1146
Septra I.V. Infusion 1142
Septra I.V. Infusion ADD-Vantage Vials 1144
Septra 1146
Serax Capsules (Rare) 2916
Serax Tablets (Rare) 2916
Serentil 689
Serzone Tablets (2%) 776
Sinemet Tablets 959
Sinequan (Infrequent) 2028
Soma Compound w/Codeine Tablets 2784
Soma Compound Tablets (Very rare to less frequent) 2783
Soma Tablets 2782
Sular Tablets (Less than or equal to 1%) 2961
Surmontil Capsules 2917
Symmetrel Capsules (1% to 5%) 965
Symmetrel Syrup (1% to 5%) 963
Tambocor Tablets (1% to less than 3%) 1555
Taxol Injection (Rare; less than 1%) 723
Tofranil Ampuls 873
Tofranil Tablets 875
Tofranil-PM Capsules 876
▲ Tonocard Tablets (0.2% to 10.8%) 519
Tornalate Solution for Inhalation, 0.2% (Less than 1%) 976
Tranxene 459
Triavil Tablets 1800
Trilafon 2532
Tussend 1830
▲ Valium Injectable (Among most common) 2336
▲ Valium Tablets (Among most common) 2335
Varivax 1807
Vaseretic Tablets 1810
Vasotec I.V. 1814
Vasotec Tablets (0.5% to 1.0%) 1816
Versed Injection (Less than 1%) 2324
Videx Tablets, Powder for Oral Solution, & Pediatric Powder for Oral Solution (Less than 1% to 6%) 2980
Vivactil Tablets 1820
Wellbutrin Tablets (Frequent) 1177
Xanax Tablets 2115
Yohimex Tablets 1414
Zarontin Capsules 1986
Zarontin Syrup 1986
Zestoretic Tablets 2968
Zestril Tablets (0.3% to 1.0%) 2972
Zoloft Tablets (Infrequent) 2051
Zyrtec Tablets (Less than 2%) 2053

Ataxia, cerebellar
JE-VAX (One case) 904
Redux Capsules 2911

Atelectasis
Betaseron for SC Injection 653
Cerebyx Injection (Infrequent) 1956
Dalgan Injection (Less than 1%) 529
Effexor (Rare) 2825
Humegon for Injection 1873
Kadian Capsules (Less than 3%) 2948
Metrodin (urofollitropin for injection) 2616
Pergonal (menotropins for injection, USP) 2618
▲ Prograf (5% to 28%) 1028
Virazole (Infrequent) 1310
Zosyn (1.0% or less) 1463

Athetosis
Versed Injection (Less than 1%) 2324

Atrial arrhythmias
Adalat Capsules (10 mg and 20 mg) (1 in 150 patients) 580
Asendin Tablets (Very rare) 1419
Felbatol 2774
Foscavir Injection (Less than 1%) 541
Hyperstat I.V. Injection 2504
Imdur (Less than or equal to 5%) 1362
Mexitil Capsules (1 in 1,000) 684
Monopril Tablets (0.4% to 1.0%) 762
▲ Proleukin for Injection (8%) 812
Remeron Tablets (Rare) 1878
Romazicon (Less than 1%) 2311
Tornalate Solution for Inhalation, 0.2% (Less than 1%) 976
Trasylol (2%) 607

Atrial contractions, premature
Adenocard Injection 1021
Brethaire Inhaler 830
Cognex Capsules (Rare) 1961
Diprivan Injectable Emulsion (Less than 1%) 2939
Emete-con Intramuscular/Intravenous 2007
Neurontin Capsules (Rare) 1978
▲ Proleukin for Injection (4%) 812
Risperdal Tablets (Rare) 1348
Sodium Polystyrene Sulfonate Suspension 2367
Yutopar Intravenous Injection 566

Atrial flutter
Anafranil Capsules (Rare) 819
Aredia for Injection (Up to 1%) 827
Cardizem Injectable (Less than 1%) 1253
Cerebyx Injection (Infrequent) 1956
Cipro Tablets (Less than 1%) 584
Cognex Capsules (Infrequent) 1961
Ethmozine Tablets (Less than 2%) 2217
▲ ReoPro Vials (3.5%) 1526
Rythmol Tablets–150mg, 225mg, 300mg (Less than 1%) 1399
Taxotere for Injection Concentrate (Rare) 2204
Tenormin Tablets and I.V. Injection (1.6%) 2965
Theo-Dur Extended-Release Tablets 1367
▲ Trasylol (8%) 607
Uni-Dur Extended-Release Tablets 1374
Uniphyl 400 mg and 600 mg Tablets 2157

Atrial tachycardia
▲ Lanoxicaps (Among most common) 1110

(▣ Described in PDR For Nonprescription Drugs) Incidence data in parenthesis; ▲ 3% or more (⊙ Described in PDR For Ophthalmology)

Atrial tachycardia — Side Effects Index — 1266

▲ Lanoxin Elixir Pediatric (Among most common) 1113
▲ Lanoxin Injection (Among most common) 1116
▲ Lanoxin Injection Pediatric (Among most common) 1119
▲ Lanoxin Tablets (Among most common) 1121
Prinivil Tablets (0.3% to 1.0%) 1776
Prinzide Tablets 1780
Theo-Dur Extended-Release Tablets 1367
Uni-Dur Extended-Release Tablets 1374
Uniphyl 400 mg and 600 mg Tablets 2157
Vaseretic Tablets 1810
Vasotec I.V. 1814
Vasotec Tablets (0.5% to 1.0%) 1816
Zestril Tablets (0.3% to 1.0%) 2972

Atrioventricular dissociation
Calan SR Caplets (1% or less) 2571
Calan Tablets (1% or less) 2568
Covera-HS Tablets (Less than 2%) 2573
Isoptin Oral Tablets (Less than 1%) 1393
Isoptin SR Tablets (1% or less) 1395
Lanoxicaps (Common) 1110
Lanoxin Injection (Common) 1116
Lanoxin Tablets (Common) 1121
Rythmol Tablets–150mg, 225mg, 300mg (Less than 1%) 1399
Verelan Capsules (1% or less) 1455

Atrophy
Antivenin (Crotalidae) Polyvalent 2803
Cuprimine Capsules 1673
Norcuron for Injection 1875
Nydrazid Injection (Uncommon) 509

Atrophy, acute yellow
Solganal Suspension 2530

Atrophy, cutaneous
Anusol-HC Cream 2.5% (Infrequent to frequent) 1953
Celestone Soluspan Suspension 2484
▲ Cordran Lotion (More frequent) 1854
▲ Cordran Tape (More frequent) 1855
Cortone Acetate Sterile Suspension 1663
Dalalone D.P. Injectable 1009
Decadron Phosphate Injection 1680
Decadron Phosphate with Xylocaine Injection, Sterile 1683
Decadron-LA Sterile Suspension 1687
Depen Titratable Tablets (Rare) 2770
Hydeltrasol Injection, Sterile 1708
Hydeltra-T.B.A. Sterile Suspension 1710
Hydrocortone Acetate Sterile Suspension 1712
Hydrocortone Phosphate Injection, Sterile 1713
Psorcon Cream 0.05% (Infrequent) 924

Atrophy, iris
Healon GV ◉ 303

Atrophy, subcutaneous
Celestone Soluspan Suspension 2484
Cortone Acetate Sterile Suspension 1663
Dalalone D.P. Injectable 1009
Decadron Phosphate Injection 1680
Decadron Phosphate with Xylocaine Injection, Sterile 1683
Decadron-LA Sterile Suspension 1687
Diphtheria and Tetanus Toxoids and Pertussis Vaccine Adsorbed 2650
Garamycin Injectable (Rare) 2502
Hydeltrasol Injection, Sterile 1708
Hydeltra-T.B.A. Sterile Suspension 1710
Hydrocortone Acetate Sterile Suspension 1712
Hydrocortone Phosphate Injection, Sterile 1713
Lidex 2299
Synalar 2299

Atypical measles
Attenuvax 1650

Auditory acuity, decrease
▲ Capastat Sulfate Injection (Approximately 11%) 968
Desferal Vials 838

Auditory canals, small or absent, fetal
Accutane Capsules 2252

Auditory disturbances
Amikacin Sulfate Injection, USP 523
Aralen Hydrochloride Injection 2430
Aralen Phosphate Tablets 2431
Oncovin Solution Vials & Hyporets (Rare) 1521
Velban Vials (Rare) 1537
▲ Wellbutrin Tablets (5.3%) 1177

Autonomic deficit, persistent
Duranest Injections 533
Inapsine Injection (Very rare) 462
Nescaine/Nescaine MPF 549
Stelazine 2692
Symmetrel Capsules (Uncommon) 965
Symmetrel Syrup (Uncommon) 963
Torecan 2367
Xylocaine Injections (Rare) 562

Avitaminosis
Norvir (Less than 2%) 447

Awareness, altered
Diprivan Injectable Emulsion (Less than 1%) 2939
Halcion Tablets 2093
▲ Tonocard Tablets (1.5% to 11.0%) 519

Awareness, heightened
Demser Capsules 1690
Imitrex Tablets (Rare) 1099
▲ Marinol (Dronabinol) Capsules (8% to 24%) 2353

Azoospermia
ColBENEMID Tablets 1662
Cytoxan (Reported in a number of patients) 700
Matulane Capsules 2300
Mustargen 1752

Azotemia
Achromycin V Capsules 1417
Altace Capsules 1238
Amikacin Sulfate Injection, USP 523
Amikacin Sulfate Injection, USP 981
Amikin Injectable 502
Ancobon Capsules 2254
Aredia for Injection (Up to 4%) 827
Atretol Tablets 569
BiCNU 696
▲ Bumex (10.6%) 2260
Cataflam Tablets (Less than 1%) 833
CeeNU Capsules 699
Cleocin Phosphate Injection (Rare) 2068
Cleocin Vaginal Cream (Rare) 2070
Daypro Caplets 2578
Demadex Tablets and Injection 691
Diuril Sodium Intravenous 1693
Dyrenium Capsules (Rare) 2655
Effexor (Rare) 2825
Elspar (Frequent) 1700
Esidrix Tablets 839
Foscavir Injection (Less than 1%) 541
▲ Fungizone Intravenous (Among most common) 507
Glucophage Tablets 754
HydroDIURIL Tablets 1716
Hydropres Tablets 1718
Hyzaar Tablets 1720
IBU Tablets (Less than 1%) 1389
▲ Indocin I.V. (41% of infants) 1727
Lasix Injection, Oral Solution and Tablets 1267
Lotrel Capsules 858
Methotrexate Sodium Tablets, Injection, for Injection and LPF Injection 1322
Minocin Intravenous 1428
Minocin Oral Suspension 1431
Minocin Pellet-Filled Capsules 1429
Monopril Tablets 762
Motrin Ibuprofen Suspension, Oral Drops, Chewable Tablets, Caplets (Less than 1%) 1563
Mykrox Tablets 1617
Nalfon 200 Pulvules & Nalfon Tablets (Less than 1%) 933
Prinivil Tablets (0.3% to 1.0%) 1776
Prinzide Tablets 1780
Proglycem 575
Relafen Tablets (Less than 1%) 2688
Tegretol/Tegretol-XR 870
Tenoretic Tablets 2963
Toradol 2319
Vancocin HCl, Oral Solution & Pulvules 1536
Vancocin HCl, Vials & ADD-Vantage 1534
Vaseretic Tablets 1810
Vasotec I.V. 1814
Vasotec Tablets 1816
Cataflam/Voltaren/Voltaren-XR (Less than 1%) 833
Zanosar Sterile Powder 2119
Zaroxolyn Tablets 1625
Zestoretic Tablets 2968
Zestril Tablets (0.3% to 1.0%) 2972
Zyloprim Tablets (Less than 1%) 1194

ADH syndrome, inappropriate
Adapin Capsules 1542
Amaryl Tablets 1241
Asendin Tablets (Less than 1%) 1419
Atretol Tablets 569
Betaseron for SC Injection 653
Cytovene-IV (One report) 2270
Depakene 416
Depakote Tablets 418
Desyrel and Desyrel Dividose 504
DiaBeta Tablets 1265
Diabinese Tablets (Rare) 2002
Elavil 2945
Etrafon 2495
Felbatol 2774
Flexeril Tablets (Rare) 1701
Foscavir Injection (Less than 1%) 541
Glucotrol Tablets 2011
Glucotrol XL Extended Release Tablets 2012
Glynase PresTab Tablets 2091
Kadian Capsules (Less than 3%) 2948
Limbitrol 2333
Lufyllin & Lufyllin-400 Tablets 2778
Lufyllin-GG Elixir & Tablets 2779
Methadone Hydrochloride Oral Solution & Tablets 2357
Micronase Tablets 2099
Navelbine Injection (Less than 1%) 1212
Norpramin Tablets 1273
Oncovin Solution Vials & Hyporets (Rare) 1521
Oretic Tablets 450
OxyContin Tablets (Less than 1%) 2163
Pamelor 2409
Parnate Tablets 2679
Paxil Tablets 2681
Permax Tablets (Infrequent) 571
Platinol for Injection 717
Platinol-AQ Injection 719
Quadrinal Tablets 1398
Quibron 2227
Respbid Tablets 687
Roxanol 2365
Rythmol Tablets–150mg, 225mg, 300mg (Less than 1%) 1399
Sinequan 2028
Slo-bid Gyrocaps 2201
Surmontil Capsules 2917
Tegretol/Tegretol-XR 870
Theo-Dur Extended-Release Tablets 1367
Theo-X Extended-Release Tablets 793
Tofranil Ampuls 873
Tofranil Tablets 875
Tofranil-PM Capsules 876
Triavil Tablets 1800
Trilafon 2532
Uni-Dur Extended-Release Tablets 1374
Velban Vials 1537
Videx Tablets, Powder for Oral Solution, & Pediatric Powder for Oral Solution (Less than 1%) 2980
Vivactil Tablets 1820
Wellbutrin Tablets 1177

AICD discharge
Betapace Tablets (Less than 1% to 3%) 637

ANA, positive
Adalat Capsules (10 mg and 20 mg) (Less than 0.5%) 580
Adalat CC (Rare) 582
Aldoclor Tablets 1638
Aldomet Ester HCl Injection 1642
Aldomet Oral 1640
Aldoril Tablets 1644
Altace Capsules (Less than 1%) 1238
Capoten Tablets 740
Capozide Tablets 744
Depen Titratable Tablets (Certain patients) 2770
Elavil 2945
Felbatol (Rare) 2774
Feldene Capsules (Less than 1%) 2008
Lescol Capsules (Rare) 2395
Lopid Tablets 1974
Mevacor Tablets (Rare) 1742
Mexitil Capsules (About 2 in 1,000) 684
Minipress Capsules 2015
Monopril Tablets 762
Normodyne Tablets (Less common) 2522
Pravachol Tablets (Rare) 770
Prinivil Tablets (0.3% to 1.0%) 1776
Prinzide Tablets 1780
Procanbid Extended-Release Tablets 1983
Procardia Capsules (Less than 0.5%) 2024
Redux Capsules 2911
Rythmol Tablets–150mg, 225mg, 300mg (0.7%) 1399
Tenoretic Tablets 2963
Tenormin Tablets and I.V. Injection 2965
Ticlid Tablets (Rare) 2317
Tonocard Tablets (Less than 1%) 519
Trandate Tablets (Less common) 1158
Vaseretic Tablets 1810
Vasotec I.V. 1814
Vasotec Tablets (0.5% to 1.0%) 1816
Zestoretic Tablets 2968
Zestril Tablets (0.3% to 1.0%) 2972
Zocor Tablets (Rare) 1821

B

Babinski's phenomenon, bilateral
Cerebyx Injection (Infrequent) 1956
Dopram Injectable 2235
Neurontin Capsules (Infrequent) 1978

Backache
Abbokinase 403
Abbokinase Open-Cath 405
Accupril Tablets (0.5% to 1.2%) 1950
▲ Actigall Capsules (7.1%) 818
Actimmune (2%) 1043
Adenocard Injection (Less than 1%) 1021
Adenoscan (Less than 1%) 1022
Alferon N Injection (Up to 4%) 2142
▲ Ambien Tablets (3%) 2559
Amen Tablets 785
▲ Anafranil Capsules (Up to 6%) 819
▲ Aredia for Injection (At least 5%) 827
▲ Arimidex Tablets (10.6% to 10.7%) 2932
▲ Asacol Delayed-Release Tablets (7%) 2129
▲ Atrovent Inhalation Solution (3.2%) 675
Axid Pulvules (2.4%) 1468
Betapace Tablets (1% to 3%) 637
Carafate Suspension (Less than 0.5%) 1250
Carafate Tablets (Less than 0.5%) 1249
Carbocaine Injection 2432
Cardura Tablets (Less than 0.5% of 3960 patients to 1.8%) 1993
Cartrol Tablets (2.1%) 413
▲ Casodex Tablets (15%) 2934
Caverject Injection (1%) 2064
▲ CellCept Capsules (11.6% to 12.1%) 2265
Cerebyx Injection (2.2%) 1956
Ceredase 1055
▲ Chemet Capsules (5.2% to 15.7%) 666
Cipro I.V. (1% or less) 587
Cipro I.V. Pharmacy Bulk Package (Less than 1%) 590
Cipro Tablets (Less than 1%) 584
Claritin Tablets (2% or fewer patients) 2485
Claritin-D Tablets (Less frequent) 2487
Clomid 1262
Clozaril Tablets (1%) 2377
Cognex Capsules (2%) 1961
Colestid 2073
Cozaar Tablets (1.8%) 1668
Crixivan Capsules (Less than 2% to 2%) 1670
Cycrin Tablets 991
CytoGam (Less than 5.0%) 1630
Cytotec (Infrequent) 2576
Cytovene (1% or less) 2270
Danocrine Capsules 2437
Dantrium Capsules (Less frequent) 2131
▲ DaunoXome (13.8% to 16%) 1842
▲ Depakote Tablets (8%) 418
Depo-Provera Contraceptive Injection (1% to 5%) 2079
Depo-Provera Sterile Aqueous Suspension 2083
Dilacor XR Extended-release Capsules (1.7% to 2.9%) 2183
▲ Doxil (Approximately 6.8%) 2613
Duranest Injections 533

(▣ Described in PDR For Nonprescription Drugs) Incidence data in parenthesis; ▲ 3% or more (◉ Described in PDR For Ophthalmology)

Side Effects Index — Birth, premature

Entry	Page
DynaCirc CR Tablets (0.5% to 1.0%)	2383
Effexor	2825
Eldepryl Capsules (1 of 49 patients)	2729
Engerix-B Unit-Dose Vials (Less than 1%)	2656
▲ Estring Vaginal Ring (6%)	2086
Etopophos for Injection (Sometimes)	701
Etoposide Injection (Sometimes)	539
Famvir Tablets (1.5% to 1.9%)	2660
Flolan for Injection (2%)	1085
Foscavir Injection (Between 1% and 5%)	541
Gamimune N, 5% Immune Globulin Intravenous (Human), 5%	612
Gamimune N, 10% Immune Globulin Intravenous (Human), 10%	615
Gammagard S/D, Immune Globulin, Intravenous (Human) (Occasional)	577
▲ Gammar-P I.V., Immune Globulin Intravenous (Human) (3.6%)	798
▲ Habitrol Nicotine Transdermal System (3% to 9% of patients)	884
Hivid Tablets (Less than 1%)	2287
Hylorel Tablets (1.5%)	1613
Hyperstat I.V. Injection	2504
Hytrin Capsules (2.4%)	434
Hyzaar Tablets (2.1%)	1720
Imdur (Less than or equal to 5%)	1362
Imitrex Injection (Rare)	1095
INFeD (Iron Dextran Injection, USP)	2478
▲ Intron A for Injection (Up to 19%)	2506
Invirase Capsules (Less than 2%)	2291
Kadian Capsules (Less than 3%)	2948
Lamictal Tablets (More than 1%)	1105
▲ Lescol Capsules (5.7%)	2395
▲ Leukine (9%)	1317
Lioresal Intrathecal (0.7% to 2.0%)	1634
Lotensin HCT Tablets (More than 1.0%)	855
Lotrel Capsules	858
LUVOX Tablets	2723
Marcaine	2446
Marcaine Spinal	2449
Maxaquin Tablets (Less than 1%)	2593
Merrem I.V. (0.1% to 1.0%)	2952
Methotrexate Sodium Tablets, Injection, for Injection and LPF Injection	1322
▲ Miacalcin Nasal Spray (5.0%)	2403
Midamor Tablets (Less than or equal to 1%)	1746
Moduretic Tablets (Less than or equal to 1%)	1748
Monoket Tablets (Fewer than 1%)	2550
Mykrox Tablets (Less than 2%)	1617
▲ Naprelan Tablets (3% to 9%)	2861
Navelbine Injection	1212
Nescaine/Nescaine MPF	549
Neurontin Capsules (1.8%)	1978
▲ Nicotrol NS Nicotine Nasal Spray (6%)	1565
Noroxin Tablets (0.3% to 1.0%)	1758
Noroxin Tablets (0.3% to 1.0%)	2222
Norvasc Tablets (More than 0.1% to 1%)	2020
Norvir (Less than 2%)	447
Oncovin Solution Vials & Hyporets	1521
Orlaam Oral Solution (1% to 3%)	2361
ParaGard T 380A Intrauterine Copper Contraceptive	1936
▲ Paxil Tablets (3%)	2681
Penetrex Tablets (0.1% to 1%)	2196
Permax Tablets (1.6%)	571
Plendil Extended-Release Tablets (0.5% to 1.5%)	514
Premphase	2900
Prempro	2905
▲ Prepidil Gel (3.1%)	2108
Prilosec Delayed-Release Capsules (1.1%)	516
Prinivil Tablets (0.3% to greater than 1%)	1776
Prinzide Tablets (0.3% to 1%)	1780
Procardia XL Extended Release Tablets (1% or less)	2026
▲ Prograf (13% to 30%)	1028
▲ Proleukin for Injection (9%)	812
Propulsid (More than 1%)	1346
ProSom Tablets (2%)	457
Prostep (nicotine transdermal system) (1% to 3% of patients)	1439
Prostin E2 Suppository	2109
Protamine Sulfate Vials	1526
Provera Tablets	2110
Prozac Pulvules & Liquid, Oral Solution (2.0%)	935
Questran	774
Recombivax HB (Less than 1%)	1787
Redux Capsules (Frequent)	2911
Remeron Tablets (2%)	1878
Retrovir Capsules	1216
Retrovir I.V. Infusion	1221
Retrovir Syrup	1216
▲ Rilutek Tablets (1.7% to 4.1%)	2198
Risperdal Tablets (Up to 2%)	1348
▲ Roferon-A Injection (16%)	2308
Rowasa (1.35%)	2727
Sandostatin Injection (1% to 4%)	2421
Sansert Tablets	2424
Sectral Capsules (Up to 2%)	2914
Sensorcaine	554
Serevent Inhalation Aerosol (1% to 3%)	1149
Serzone Tablets	776
Sinemet CR Tablets (1.6%)	961
Taxol Injection (Rare)	723
Taxotere for Injection Concentrate	2204
Vancocin HCl, Oral Solution & Pulvules	1536
Vancocin HCl, Vials & ADD-Vantage	1534
Vaqta (1.1%)	1805
Vaseretic Tablets (0.5% to 2.0%)	1810
VePesid Capsules and Injection (Sometimes)	727
Vistide Injection	1057
Xalatan (1 to 2%)	⊙ 304
▲ Xylocaine Injections (3%)	562
Zebeta Tablets	1457
▲ Zerit Capsules (Fewer than 1% to 20%)	731
Zestoretic Tablets (0.3 to 1%)	2968
Zestril Tablets (0.3% to 1.0%)	2972
Ziac	1459
▲ Zoladex (7%)	2976
Zoladex 3-month (1% to 5%)	2978
Zoloft Tablets (1.5%)	2051
Zosyn (1.0% or less)	1463
Zyrtec Tablets (Less than 2%)	2053

Back strain
Prinzide Tablets (0.3% to 1.0%)	1780
Zestoretic Tablets (0.3% to 1.0%)	2968

Bacteremia
Ethamolin Injection	2544
Retrovir Capsules (1.6%)	1216
Retrovir I.V. Infusion (2%)	1221
Retrovir Syrup (1.6%)	1216

Bacteriuria
Primaxin I.M.	1770
Sinemet CR Tablets (1% or greater)	961

Balance, loss of
(see also under Equilibrium, dysfunction)
Adalat Capsules (10 mg and 20 mg) (2% or less)	580
Amikacin Sulfate Injection, USP	523
Amikacin Sulfate Injection, USP	981
Amikin Injectable	502
Eldepryl Capsules	2729
Rythmol Tablets–150mg, 225mg, 300mg (1.2%)	1399
Versed Injection (Less than 1%)	2324

Balanitis
Achromycin V Capsules (Rare)	1417
Betaseron for SC Injection	653
Caverject Injection (Less than 1%)	2064
Declomycin Tablets	1421
Doxil (Less than 1%)	2613
DYNACIN Capsules (Rare)	1627
Minocin Intravenous (Rare)	1428
Minocin Oral Suspension (Rare)	1431
Minocin Pellet-Filled Capsules (Rare)	1429
Stimate, (desmopressin acetate) Nasal Spray, 1.5 mg/mL	806

Balanoposthitis
Zoloft Tablets (Rare)	2051
Zosyn (1.0% or less)	1463

Baldness, male pattern
(see under Alopecia hereditaria)

Bartter's syndrome
Capastat Sulfate Injection (1 patient)	968

Basophils, increase
Dynabac (0.1% to 1%)	668
Effexor (Rare)	2825
Paxil Tablets (Rare)	2681
Primaxin I.M.	1770
Primaxin I.V.	1772
Rocephin Injectable Vials, ADD-Vantage, Galaxy Container (Rare)	2305
Unasyn	2035
Vantin for Oral Suspension and Vantin Tablets	2112
Vesanoid Capsules (Isolated cases)	2327

Behavior, hypochondriacal
Celontin Kapseals	1955

Behavior, inappropriate
Artane	1418
Ativan Injection (Occasional)	2805
Diprivan Injectable Emulsion (Less than 1%)	2939
Halcion Tablets	2093
Mellaril	2398
ProSom Tablets	457
Ritalin	866
Serentil	689
Tessalon Perles (Isolated instances)	1018
Xanax Tablets (Rare)	2115

Behavior, violent
Prozac Pulvules & Liquid, Oral Solution	935

Behavioral changes
Akineton	1380
Ambien Tablets	2559
Amoxil (Rare)	2631
Augmentin (Rare)	2637
Augmentin Tablets (Rare)	2640
Biaxin	406
Catapres Tablets	679
Catapres-TTS	680
Combipres Tablets	682
Cytotec (Infrequent)	2576
Eldepryl Capsules	2729
Gastrocrom Capsules (Infrequent)	1611
Gastrocrom Oral Concentrate (Less common)	1611
JE-VAX (One case)	904
▲ Klonopin Tablets (25%)	2294
Monopril Tablets (0.4% to 1.0%)	762
▲ Orap Tablets (27.7%)	1037
Paremyd	⊙ 244
Rifadin	1276
Rifater	1280
Timoptic in Ocudose (Less frequent)	1796
Timoptic Sterile Ophthalmic Solution (Less frequent)	1794
Timoptic-XE	1798
Torecan	2367
Uniphyl 400 mg and 600 mg Tablets	2157
Vascor Tablets (200 and 300 mg) (0.5 to 2.0%)	1597

Behavioral deterioration
Depakene	416
Depakote Tablets	418

Bell's palsy
Aldoclor Tablets	1638
Aldomet Ester HCl Injection	1642
Aldomet Oral	1640
Aldoril Tablets	1644
Avonex	662
Cognex Capsules (Rare)	1961
Cytovene-IV (One report)	2270
Engerix-B Unit-Dose Vials	2656
Flexeril Tablets (Rare)	1701
Hivid Tablets (Less than 1%)	2287
JE-VAX (One case)	904
Lescol Capsules	2395
Mevacor Tablets (0.5% to 1.0%)	1742
Permax Tablets (Rare)	571
Pravachol Tablets	770
Recombivax HB	1787
Sandostatin Injection (Less than 1%)	2421
Zocor Tablets	1821

Benzyl alcohol, sensitivity to
Amicar Syrup, Tablets, and Injection	1312
AquaMEPHYTON Injection	1648
Cleocin Phosphate Injection	2068
Cytosar-U Sterile Powder	2077
Leukine	1317
Leustatin	1889

Entry	Page
Lupron Injection	2736
Lupron Injection Pediatric	2737
Mesnex Injection	711
Mivacron Injection	1125
Nimbex Injection	1131
Nuromax Injection	1136
Nutropin	1049
Procrit for Injection	1896
Profasi (chorionic gonadotropin for injection, USP)	2620
Protropin	1053
Roferon-A Injection	2308
Septra I.V. Infusion	1142
Septra I.V. Infusion ADD-Vantage Vials	1144
Tracrium Injection	1155

Bezoar
Carafate Suspension	1250
Carafate Tablets	1249
Ecotrin	2625
Prevacid Delayed-Release Capsules (Less than 1%)	2746

Bigeminy
Diprivan Injectable Emulsion (Less than 1%)	2939
Remeron Tablets (Rare)	1878
Suprane (desflurane, USP) (Less than 1%)	1865
Taxol Injection (Approximately 1%)	723
Versed Injection (Less than 1%)	2324
Virazole (Infrequent)	1310

Bile duct "sludge," presence of metabolites
Clinoril Tablets (Rare)	1658

Biliary duct dilation
▲ Sandostatin Injection (12%)	2421

Biliary sclerosis
Sterile FUDR	2284

Biliary sludge
Rocephin Injectable Vials, ADD-Vantage, Galaxy Container (Rare)	2305
▲ Sandostatin Injection (24% to 52%)	2421

Biliary stasis
Compazine	2644
Levoprome	1321
Mellaril	2398
Serentil	689
Stelazine	2692
Torecan	2367
Triavil Tablets	1800
Trilafon	2532

Biliary tract abnormalities
▲ Sandostatin Injection (12% to 63%)	2421

Biliary tract spasm
Levo-Dromoran	2297
Mepergan Injection	2859
Methadone Hydrochloride Oral Concentrate	2356

Biliary tree, calcification
Questran (Occasional)	774

Bilirubinemia
▲ Abelcet Injection (4% to 5%)	1540
Ambien Tablets (Rare)	2559
Effexor (Rare)	2825
Hivid Tablets (Less than 1%)	2287
▲ Intron A for Injection (Less than 5%)	2506
Lamictal Tablets (Rare)	1105
▲ Oncaspar (Greater than 1% but less than 5%)	2194
Paxil Tablets (Rare)	2681
Prevacid Delayed-Release Capsules (Less than 1%)	2746
▲ Prograf (Greater than 3%)	1028
Rifater	1280

Bilirubinuria
Primaxin I.M.	1770
Primaxin I.V.	1772
Relafen Tablets (Less than 1%)	2688
Rifamate Capsules	1278
Rifater	1280

Birth, premature
Accutane Capsules	2252
Sandimmune	2416

(⊞ Described in PDR For Nonprescription Drugs)   Incidence data in parenthesis; ▲ 3% or more   (⊙ Described in PDR For Ophthalmology)

Birth defects — Side Effects Index

Birth defects
- Aygestin Tablets ... 990
- Celontin Kapseals ... 1955
- Coumadin ... 941
- Cuprimine Capsules ... 1673
- Depakene (Multiple reports) ... 416
- Depakote Tablets (Multiple reports) ... 418
- Depen Titratable Tablets ... 2770
- Dilantin Infatabs ... 1967
- Dilantin Kapseals ... 1965
- Dilantin-125 Suspension ... 1969
- Encare Vaginal Contraceptive Suppositories ... ⊡ 797
- Estraderm Transdermal System ... 842
- Humegon for Injection (1.7%) ... 1873
- Klonopin Tablets ... 2294
- Lo/Ovral Tablets ... 2852
- Lo/Ovral-28 Tablets ... 2857
- Mesantoin Tablets ... 2400
- Metrodin (urofollitropin for injection) (4 incidents) ... 2616
- Mysoline ... 2860
- Nolvadex Tablets (A small number of reports) ... 2957
- Nordette-21 Tablets ... 2863
- Nordette-28 Tablets ... 2866
- Ortho Dienestrol Cream ... 1922
- Ortho-Est ... 1925
- Ovral Tablets ... 2877
- Ovral-28 Tablets ... 2878
- Ovrette Tablets ... 2878
- ▲ Parlodel (3.3%) ... 2411
- Peganone Tablets (Multiple reports) ... 455
- Pergonal (menotropins for injection, USP) (1.7%) ... 2618
- Phenurone Tablets (Multiple reports) ... 455
- Podocon-25 ... 1949
- Premarin Intravenous ... 2893
- Premarin Vaginal Cream ... 2898
- Premphase ... 2900
- Prempro ... 2905
- Quadrinal Tablets ... 1398
- Serophene (clomiphene citrate tablets, USP) (2.5%) ... 2621
- Triphasil-21 Tablets ... 2919
- Triphasil-28 Tablets ... 2924
- Vivelle Transdermal System ... 880
- Zarontin Capsules ... 1986
- Zarontin Syrup ... 1986

Birth weight, low
- Adderall Tablets ... 2209
- Betapace Tablets ... 637
- Cytosar-U Sterile Powder (Five infants) ... 2077
- Dexedrine ... 2648
- Easprin ... 1971
- Sandimmune ... 2416
- Sectral Capsules ... 2914

Births, multiple
- ▲ Humegon for Injection (20%) ... 1873
- ▲ Metrodin (urofollitropin for injection) (18.6%) ... 2616
- ▲ Pergonal (menotropins for injection, USP) (20%) ... 2618
- Profasi (chorionic gonadotropin for injection) ... 2620
- ▲ Serophene (clomiphene citrate tablets, USP) (Less than 1% to 10%) ... 2621

Blackout spells
- Eskalith ... 2658
- Lithium Carbonate Capsules & Tablets ... 2352
- Lithonate/Lithotabs/Lithobid ... 2721
- Lupron Injection (Less than 5%) ... 2736

Bladder, dysfunction
- ▲ TheraCys BCG Live (Intravesical) (Up to 5.4%) ... 911

Bladder, irritability
- IFEX ... 706
- Oxandrin ... 783
- Winstrol Tablets ... 2468

Bladder, loss of control
- Duranest Injections ... 533
- Nescaine/Nescaine MPF ... 549
- Trilafon ... 2532
- Xylocaine Injections ... 562

Bladder, spasms
- Lasix Injection, Oral Solution and Tablets ... 1267
- Lupron Injection (Less than 5%) ... 2736

- Midamor Tablets (Less than or equal to 1%) ... 1746
- Moduretic Tablets ... 1748

Blanching
- Catapres-TTS (1 of 101 patients) ... 680
- ▲ EMLA Cream (37%) ... 536
- Iopidine 0.5% (Less than 3%) ... ⊙ 219
- Tympagesic Ear Drops ... 2476

Blebs, filtering (ocular)
- Blephamide Ointment (Increased incidence) ... ⊙ 234
- Cortisporin Ophthalmic Ointment Sterile ... 1074
- Decadron Phosphate Sterile Ophthalmic Ointment (Rare) ... 1684
- Decadron Phosphate Sterile Ophthalmic Solution (Rare) ... 1685
- FML Forte Liquifilm ... ⊙ 237
- FML Liquifilm ... ⊙ 238
- FML S.O.P. ... ⊙ 239
- Pred Forte ... ⊙ 247
- Pred Mild ... ⊙ 250

Bleeding
- Abbokinase ... 403
- Abbokinase Open-Cath ... 405
- ▲ Activase (Most common complication) ... 1045
- Adriamycin PFS ... 2056
- Adriamycin RDF ... 2056
- Alka-Seltzer ... ⊡ 609
- Alkeran for Injection ... 1196
- Alkeran Tablets ... 1198
- Amicar Syrup, Tablets, and Injection ... 1312
- Avonex ... 662
- Azathioprine Tablets (2 patients) ... 2349
- Betapace Tablets (1% to 2%) ... 637
- Betaseron for SC Injection ... 653
- BiCNU ... 696
- Cedax ... 2480
- CeeNU Capsules ... 699
- Cefizox for Intramuscular or Intravenous Use ... 1025
- Cefotan ... 2936
- Ceftin ... 1067
- Cefzil Tablets and Oral Suspension ... 747
- CellCept Capsules (More than or equal to 3%) ... 2265
- Ceptaz ... 1070
- Condylox Topical Solution (Less than 5%) ... 1853
- Coumadin ... 941
- ▲ Cytosar-U Sterile Powder (Among most frequent) ... 2077
- Cytovene (1% or less) ... 2270
- Demadex Tablets and Injection ... 691
- Depakene ... 416
- Depakote Tablets ... 418
- Depen Titratable Tablets ... 2770
- Diprivan Injectable Emulsion (Less than 1%) ... 2939
- Diupres Tablets ... 1691
- Doxil (1% to 5%) ... 2613
- Doxorubicin Astra ... 531
- Duricef Capsules, Tablets, and Oral Suspension ... 750
- Elspar ... 1700
- ▲ Eminase (14.6% to 14.8%) ... 2215
- Etopophos for Injection ... 701
- Etoposide Injection ... 539
- Felbatol ... 2774
- ▲ Flolan for Injection (19%) ... 1085
- Floxin I.V. ... 1580
- Floxin Tablets (200 mg, 300 mg, 400 mg) ... 1577
- Fludara for Injection (Up to 1%) ... 658
- Fluorouracil Injection ... 2282
- Fortaz ... 1092
- Fragmin Injection ... 2088
- Sterile FUDR ... 2284
- ▲ Gemzar for Injection (Up to 17%) ... 1482
- Halotestin Tablets ... 2095
- Heparin Lock Flush Solution ... 2831
- Heparin Sodium Injection ... 2832
- Heparin Sodium Vials ... 1486
- Hydropres Tablets ... 1718
- ▲ Idamycin Injection (63%) ... 2096
- Imuran (2 cases) ... 1103
- Lamictal Tablets (Rare) ... 1105
- Leukeran Tablets ... 1205
- ▲ Leukine (23% to 29%) ... 1317
- Lorabid Suspension and Pulvules ... 1513
- ▲ Lovenox Injection (4%) ... 2187
- Maxipime for Injection ... 758
- Motrin Ibuprofen Suspension, Oral Drops, Chewable Tablets, Caplets (Less than 1%) ... 1563
- Mustargen ... 1752

- Naprelan Tablets (Less than 1%) ... 2861
- ▲ Nipent for Injection (3% to 10%) ... 2733
- Norvir (Less than 2%) ... 447
- ▲ Novantrone for Injection (20 to 37%) ... 1327
- Oncaspar ... 2194
- ▲ Paraplatin for Injection (6% to 10%) ... 713
- PPD Tine Test ... 2993
- Priscoline Hydrochloride Ampuls ... 864
- Proglycem ... 575
- ▲ Prograf (Greater than 3%) ... 1028
- Protamine Sulfate Vials (Some patients) ... 1526
- Prozac Pulvules & Liquid, Oral Solution (Infrequent) ... 935
- Quadrinal Tablets ... 1398
- Redux Capsules (Infrequent) ... 2911
- ▲ ReoPro Vials (Most common) ... 1526
- Rilutek Tablets (Rare) ... 2198
- Risperdal Tablets (Rare) ... 1348
- Rubex for Injection ... 721
- Serzone Tablets (Rare) ... 776
- Soma Compound w/Codeine Tablets ... 2784
- Streptase for Infusion ... 557
- Suprane (desflurane, USP) (Less than 1%) ... 1865
- Suprax ... 1443
- Tapazole Tablets ... 1361
- ▲ Taxol Injection (14%) ... 723
- Tazicef for Injection ... 2697
- Tazidime Vials, Faspak & ADD-Vantage ... 1531
- Testred Capsules, 10 mg. ... 1308
- Thioplex (Thiotepa For Injection) ... 1329
- Ticlid Tablets ... 2317
- Tonocard Tablets ... 519
- Tuberculin, Old, Tine Test ... 2994
- Vantin for Oral Suspension and Vantin Tablets ... 2112
- VePesid Capsules and Injection ... 727
- ▲ Vesanoid Capsules (60%) ... 2327
- Videx Tablets, Powder for Oral Solution, & Pediatric Powder for Oral Solution (Up to 10%) ... 2980
- ▲ Vumon for Injection (5%) ... 729
- Winstrol Tablets ... 2468
- Zinacef ... 1184
- Zinecard Injection (2% to 3%) ... 2120
- Zoladex (1% or greater) ... 2976
- Zoladex 3-month ... 2978
- Zosyn (1.0% or less) ... 1463

Bleeding, at invaded sites
- Eminase ... 2215
- Streptase for Infusion ... 557

Bleeding, at site of administration
- Avonex ... 662
- Caverject Injection ... 2064
- Cerebyx Injection (Infrequent) ... 1956
- Cytovene (1% or less) ... 2270
- Doxil (Less than 1%) ... 2613
- Eminase ... 2215
- Genotropin Injection (Infrequent) ... 2090
- Intron A for Injection (Less than 5%) ... 2506
- ReoPro Vials (1 to 50 events) ... 1526
- Streptase for Infusion ... 557

Bleeding, breakthrough
- Amen Tablets ... 785
- Aygestin Tablets ... 990
- Brevicon ... 2563
- Climara Transdermal System ... 640
- Cycrin Tablets ... 991
- Demulen ... 2580
- Depo-Provera Sterile Aqueous Suspension ... 2083
- Desogen Tablets ... 1867
- Diethylstilbestrol Tablets ... 1477
- Estrace Cream and Tablets ... 751
- Estraderm Transdermal System ... 842
- ESTRATAB Tablets (0.3, 0.625, 1.25, 2.5 mg) ... 2715
- Estratest ... 2718
- Levlen/Tri-Levlen (Sometimes) ... 646
- Lo/Ovral Tablets ... 2852
- Lo/Ovral-28 Tablets ... 2857
- Megace Oral Suspension ... 708
- Megace Tablets ... 710
- Menest Tablets ... 2671
- Micronor Tablets ... 1903
- Modicon (Sometimes) ... 1928
- Nordette-21 Tablets ... 2863
- Nordette-28 Tablets ... 2866
- Norinyl ... 2563
- Nor-Q D Tablets ... 2598
- Ogen Tablets ... 2103
- Ogen Vaginal Cream ... 2106

- Ortho-Cept ... 1907
- Ortho-Cyclen/Ortho-Tri-Cyclen ... 1914
- Ortho Dienestrol Cream ... 1922
- Ortho-Est ... 1925
- Ortho-Novum (Sometimes) ... 1928
- Ortho-Cyclen/Ortho Tri-Cyclen ... 1914
- Ovcon (Sometimes) ... 765
- Ovral Tablets ... 2877
- Ovral-28 Tablets ... 2878
- Ovrette Tablets ... 2878
- PMB 200 and PMB 400 ... 2890
- Premarin Intravenous ... 2893
- Premarin Tablets ... 2896
- Premarin Vaginal Cream ... 2898
- Premphase ... 2900
- Prempro ... 2905
- Provera Tablets ... 2110
- Levlen/Tri-Levlen (Sometimes) ... 646
- Tri-Norinyl (Sometimes) ... 2607
- Triphasil-21 Tablets ... 2919
- Triphasil-28 Tablets ... 2924
- Vivelle Transdermal System ... 880

Bleeding, dental
- Accutane Capsules (Less than 1%) ... 2252
- Activase (Less than 1%) ... 1045
- Anafranil Capsules (Rare) ... 819
- Avonex ... 662
- Claritin-D Tablets (Less frequent) ... 2487
- Coumadin ... 941
- Crixivan Capsules (Less than 2%) ... 1670
- Danocrine Capsules (Rare) ... 2437
- DaunoXome (Less than or equal to 5%) ... 1842
- Effexor (Rare) ... 2825
- Eminase (1%) ... 2215
- Felbatol ... 2774
- Hivid Tablets (Less than 1%) ... 2287
- Intron A for Injection (Less than 5%) ... 2506
- Lamictal Tablets (Rare) ... 1105
- Mustargen ... 1752
- Neurontin Capsules (Infrequent) ... 1978
- Questran ... 774
- Remeron Capsules (Infrequent) ... 1878
- Retrovir Capsules ... 1216
- Retrovir I.V. Infusion ... 1221
- Retrovir Syrup ... 1216
- Rilutek Tablets (Infrequent) ... 2198
- Roferon-A Injection (Rare) ... 2308
- ▲ Tegison Capsules (1-10%) ... 2314
- Videx Tablets, Powder for Oral Solution, & Pediatric Powder for Oral Solution (Less than 1%) ... 2980

Bleeding, duodenal ulcer
- Questran ... 774

Bleeding, gastrointestinal
- Abbokinase ... 403
- Abbokinase Open-Cath ... 405
- ▲ Abelcet Injection (3%) ... 1540
- Accupril Tablets (Rare) ... 1950
- Actimmune (Rare) ... 1043
- ▲ Activase (5%) ... 1045
- Adalat CC (Less than 1.0%) ... 582
- Aldactazide Tablets ... 2556
- Aldactone Tablets ... 2558
- Anaprox/Naprosyn (Approximately 1% to 4%) ... 2277
- Ancobon Capsules ... 2254
- Androderm Testosterone Transdermal System (2%) ... 2634
- ▲ Aredia for Injection (Up to 6%) ... 827
- Regular Strength Ascriptin Tablets ... ⊡ 650
- Atamet Tablets (Rare) ... 567
- Atromid-S Capsules ... 2808
- Avonex ... 662
- Azactam for Injection (Less than 1%) ... 736
- Genuine Bayer Aspirin Tablets & Caplets ... ⊡ 618
- Aspirin Regimen Bayer Regular Strength 325 mg Caplets ... ⊡ 613
- Betaseron for SC Injection ... 653
- Bufferin Analgesic Tablets ... ⊡ 636
- Cataflam Tablets (0.6% to 4%) ... 833
- ▲ CellCept Capsules (More than or equal to 3%) ... 2265
- Cerebyx Injection (Infrequent) ... 1956
- Cipro I.V. (Less than 1%) ... 587
- Cipro I.V. Pharmacy Bulk Package (Less than 1%) ... 590
- Cipro Tablets (Less than 1%) ... 584
- Clinoril Tablets (Less than 1%) ... 1658
- Cognex Capsules (Infrequent) ... 1961
- Cortone Acetate Sterile Suspension ... 1663
- Cortone Acetate Tablets ... 1664

(⊡ Described in PDR For Nonprescription Drugs)   Incidence data in parenthesis; ▲ 3% or more   (⊙ Described in PDR For Ophthalmology)

Cytotec (Infrequent) ... 2576
Dantrium Capsules (Less frequent) 2131
DaunoXome (Less than or equal to 5%) ... 1842
Daypro Caplets (Less than 1%) ... 2578
Demadex Tablets and Injection ... 691
Dilacor XR Extended-release Capsules ... 2183
Disalcid ... 1549
Dolobid Tablets (Less than 1 in 100) ... 1695
Doxil ... 2613
Easprin ... 1971
EC-Naprosyn Delayed-Release Tablets (Approximately 1% to 4%) ... 2277
Ecotrin ... 2625
Edecrin ... 1698
Eldepryl Capsules ... 2729
Emcyt Capsules (1%) ... 2085
Eminase (2%) ... 2215
Ergamisol Tablets ... 1340
Felbatol ... 2774
Feldene Capsules (Less than 1%) .. 2008
Floxin I.V. ... 1580
Floxin Tablets (200 mg, 300 mg, 400 mg) ... 1577
▲ Fludara for Injection (3% to 13%) 658
Fluorouracil Injection ... 2282
Sterile FUDR ... 2284
Fulvicin P/G Tablets (Rare) ... 2499
Fulvicin P/G 165 & 330 Tablets (Rare) ... 2500
Glucotrol XL Extended Release Tablets (Rare) ... 2012
Halfprin Tablets ... 1413
Helidac Therapy (Less than 1%) 2135
Heparin Lock Flush Solution ... 2831
Heparin Sodium Injection ... 2832
Hivid Tablets (Less than 1%) ... 2287
IBU Tablets (Less than 1%) ... 1389
Imitrex Tablets (Rare) ... 1099
Indocin Capsules (Less than 1%).... 1723
▲ Indocin I.V. (3% to 9%) ... 1727
Indocin (Less than 1%) ... 1723
Intron A for Injection (Less than 5%) ... 2506
K-Dur Microburst Release System (potassium chloride, USP) E.R. Tablets ... 1364
K-Norm Capsules ... 1615
K-Tab Filmtab ... 439
Lamictal Tablets (Rare) ... 1105
Lamprene Capsules (Less than 1%) ... 846
Larodopa Tablets (Rare) ... 2296
▲ Leukine (11% to 27%) ... 1317
Lioresal Intrathecal (1% or more) .. 1634
Lodine Capsules and Tablets ... 2849
Lupron Injection (Less than 5%) ... 2736
LUVOX Tablets (Infrequent) ... 2723
Maxaquin Tablets (Less than 1%) .. 2593
Merrem I.V. (0.7%) ... 2952
Methotrexate Sodium Tablets, Injection, for Injection and LPF Injection ... 1322
Mexitil Capsules (About 7 in 10,000) ... 684
Micro-K ... 2237
Micro-K LS Packets ... 2238
Midamor Tablets (Less than or equal to 1%) ... 1746
Moduretic Tablets (Less than or equal to 1%) ... 1748
Motrin Ibuprofen Suspension, Oral Drops, Chewable Tablets, Caplets (Less than 1% to 4%) ... 1563
Mustargen ... 1752
Nalfon 200 Pulvules & Nalfon Tablets (Less than 1%) ... 933
Naprelan Tablets (Less than 1% to 4%) ... 2861
Anaprox/Naprosyn (Approximately 1% to 4%) ... 2277
Neoral (Rare) ... 2405
Nimotop Capsules (Less than 1%) ... 603
Norgesic (Rare) ... 1554
Norvir (Less than 2%) ... 447
▲ Novantrone for Injection (2 to 16%) ... 1327
Orthoclone OKT3 Sterile Solution .. 1892
Orudis Capsules (Less than 1%) ... 2874
Oruvail Capsules (Less than 1%) ... 2874
Parafon Forte DSC Caplets (Rare) .. 1590
Parlodel (Less than 2%) ... 2411
Pediazole Suspension ... 2340
Pentasa (Less than 1%) ... 1275
Ponstel ... 1982
Prevacid Delayed-Release Capsules (Less than 1%) ... 2746
Priscoline Hydrochloride Ampuls 864

Procardia XL Extended Release Tablets (Less than 1%) ... 2026
▲ Prograf (Greater than 3%) ... 1028
▲ Proleukin for Injection (13%) ... 812
Questran ... 774
Redux Capsules (Infrequent) ... 2911
Relafen Tablets (1%) ... 2688
ReoPro Vials (11 events) ... 1526
Ridaura Capsules (0.1 to 1%) ... 2691
Rilutek Tablets (Infrequent) ... 2198
Risperdal Tablets (Rare) ... 1348
Roferon-A Injection (Infrequent) ... 2308
SSKI Solution (Less frequent) ... 2767
Salflex Tablets ... 791
Sandimmune (Rare) ... 2416
Sandostatin Injection (Less than 1%) ... 2421
Serzone Tablets (Rare) ... 776
Sinemet Tablets (Rare) ... 959
Sinemet CR Tablets ... 961
Slow-K Extended-Release Tablets .. 869
Soma Compound Tablets ... 2783
St. Joseph Adult Chewable Aspirin (81 mg.) ... ⊡ 768
Streptase for Infusion ... 557
Sular Tablets (Less than or equal to 1%) ... 2961
Taxotere for Injection Concentrate (One patient) ... 2204
Ticlid Tablets ... 2317
Tolectin (200, 400 and 600 mg) (Less than 1%) ... 1591
Toradol ... 2319
Ultram Tablets (50 mg) (Infrequent) ... 1594
▲ Vesanoid Capsules (34%) ... 2327
Videx Tablets, Powder for Oral Solution, & Pediatric Powder for Oral Solution (Up to 2%) ... 2980
Cataflam/Voltaren/Voltaren-XR (0.6% to 4%) ... 833
Wellbutrin Tablets (Rare) ... 1177
Zylophim Tablets (Less than 1%) ... 1194

Bleeding, genitourinary tract
Abbokinase ... 403
Abbokinase Open-Cath ... 405
▲ Activase (4%) ... 1045
Eminase ... 2215
Premphase ... 2900
Prempro ... 2905
ReoPro Vials (5 to 8 events) ... 1526
Streptase for Infusion ... 557

Bleeding, gingival
(see under Bleeding, dental)

Bleeding, hemorrhoidal
Colestid (Infrequent) ... 2073
Daypro Caplets (Less than 1%) ... 2578
Questran ... 774

Bleeding, in immediate coronary catheterization
▲ Eminase (13.3%) ... 2215

Bleeding, in patients not undergoing coronary catheterization
▲ Eminase (3%) ... 2215

Bleeding, intermenstrual
Estring Vaginal Ring (At least 1 report) ... 2086
▲ Felbatol (3.4%) ... 2774
Imitrex Tablets (Infrequent) ... 1099
Levlen/Tri-Levlen ... 646
Maxaquin Tablets (Less than 1%).. 2593
Risperdal Tablets (Infrequent) ... 1348
Levlen/Tri-Levlen ... 646
Zoloft Tablets (Infrequent) ... 2051
Zyrtec Tablets (Less than 2%) ... 2053

Bleeding, internal
Abbokinase ... 403
Activase ... 1045
Eminase ... 2215
Streptase for Infusion ... 557

Bleeding, intracerebral
▲ Lopid Tablets (More common) ... 1974
Streptase for Infusion ... 557
Ticlid Tablets (Rare) ... 2317

Bleeding, intracranial
Abbokinase ... 403
Abbokinase Open-Cath ... 405
Activase (0.4% to 1.3%) ... 1045
Cardene I.V. (0.7%) ... 2815
Elspar ... 1700
Eminase (1%) ... 2215

Hespan Injection ... 945
▲ Indocin I.V. (3% to 9%) ... 1727
Neurontin Capsules (Infrequent) ... 1978
ReoPro Vials (1 to 3 events) ... 1526
▲ Survanta Beractant Intratracheal Suspension (24.1 to 48.1%) ... 2346
Videx Tablets, Powder for Oral Solution, & Pediatric Powder for Oral Solution (Less than 1%) ... 2980

Bleeding, menstrual, frequent onsets
▲ Norplant System (7.0%) ... 2868

Bleeding, menstrual, prolonged episodes
▲ Norplant System (27.6%) ... 2868

Bleeding, menstrual, scanty
▲ Norplant System (5.2%) ... 2868

Bleeding, mouth
Eminase (1%) ... 2215
Foscavir Injection (Less than 1%) .. 541
ReoPro Vials (4 events) ... 1526

Bleeding, mucosal
Effexor (Rare) ... 2825
Quadrinal Tablets ... 1398
Unasyn (Less than 1%) ... 2035
Vancenase PocketHaler Nasal Inhaler (2 per 100 patients) ... 2534

Bleeding, nasal
(see under Epistaxis)

Bleeding, nonpuncture site
▲ Eminase (10.2%) ... 2215

Bleeding, otic
ReoPro Vials (9 to 11 events) ... 1526

Bleeding, pericardial
Activase ... 1045
Eminase ... 2215

Bleeding, perioperative
Ticlid Tablets ... 2317

Bleeding, postmenopausal
Aldactazide Tablets ... 2556
Aldactone Tablets ... 2558
Avonex ... 662

Bleeding, puncture site
Capastat Sulfate Injection ... 968
▲ Eminase (Up to 5.7%) ... 2215

Bleeding, renal-pelvic
Cipro I.V. (1% or less) ... 587

Bleeding, retroperitoneal
ReoPro Vials (2 to 12 events) ... 1526
Streptase for Infusion ... 557

Bleeding, superficial
Abbokinase ... 403
Abbokinase Open-Cath ... 405
Activase ... 1045
Eminase ... 2215

Bleeding, upper GI
(see under Bleeding, gastrointestinal)

Bleeding, urethral
Caverject Injection (Less than 1%) 2064
Ceftin (0.1% to 1%) ... 1067
Cipro Tablets (Less than 1%) ... 584

Bleeding, uterine
Anafranil Capsules (Infrequent) ... 819
Climara Transdermal System ... 640
Clomid ... 1262
Cytotec ... 2576
Effexor (Infrequent) ... 2825
Estrace Cream and Tablets ... 751
Estraderm Transdermal System ... 842
Estratest ... 2718
Intron A for Injection (Less than 5%) ... 2506
Menest Tablets ... 2671
Ogen Tablets ... 2103
Ogen Vaginal Cream ... 2106
Ortho-Est ... 1925
Permax Tablets (Infrequent) ... 571
PMB 200 and PMB 400 ... 2890
Premarin Intravenous ... 2893
Premarin Tablets ... 2896
Premarin Vaginal Cream ... 2898
Premphase ... 2900

Prempro ... 2905
Prozac Pulvules & Liquid, Oral Solution (Rare) ... 935
Redux Capsules (Rare) ... 2911
Rilutek Tablets (Rare) ... 2198
Serophene (clomiphene citrate tablets, USP) (Less than 1 in 100 patients) ... 2621
Serzone Tablets (Rare) ... 776

Bleeding, uterine, irregularities
Clomid (1.3%) ... 1262
Depo-Provera Contraceptive Injection ... 2079
ESTRATAB Tablets (0.3, 0.625, 1.25, 2.5 mg) ... 2715
Estring Vaginal Ring (Uncommon) .. 2086
Lodine Capsules and Tablets (Less than 1%) ... 2849

Bleeding, vaginal
Abbokinase ... 403
Abbokinase Open-Cath ... 405
Anafranil Capsules (Infrequent) ... 819
▲ Arimidex Tablets (1.6% to 2.3%) .. 2932
Avonex ... 662
Betaseron for SC Injection ... 653
Brevicon ... 2563
Cataflam Tablets (Less than 1%) ... 833
Climara Transdermal System ... 640
Clinoril Tablets (Less than 1%) ... 1658
Cognex Capsules (Infrequent) ... 1961
Coumadin ... 941
Demulen ... 2580
Depakote Tablets (1% to 5%) ... 418
▲ Depo-Provera Contraceptive Injection (More than 5%) ... 2079
Effexor (Infrequent) ... 2825
Ergamisol Capsules (Less frequent) . 1340
Estrace Cream and Tablets ... 751
Estraderm Transdermal System ... 842
Estratest ... 2718
▲ Estring Vaginal Ring (4%) ... 2086
Felbatol ... 2774
Indocin Capsules (Less than 1%) ... 1723
Indocin I.V. (Less than 1%) ... 1727
Indocin (Less than 1%) ... 1723
Levlen/Tri-Levlen ... 646
Lo/Ovral Tablets ... 2852
Lo/Ovral-28 Tablets ... 2857
Lupron Depot-PED 7.5 mg, 11.25 mg and 15 mg (2%) ... 2744
Lupron Injection Pediatric ... 2737
LUVOX Tablets (Infrequent) ... 2723
Massengill Disposable Douche ... 2627
Micronor Tablets ... 1903
Modicon ... 1928
Neurontin Capsules (Infrequent) ... 1978
Nolvadex Tablets (Less frequent; 2%) ... 2957
Norinyl ... 2563
Nor-Q D Tablets ... 2598
Ogen Tablets ... 2103
Ogen Vaginal Cream ... 2106
Ortho-Cyclen/Ortho-Tri-Cyclen ... 1914
Ortho-Novum ... 1928
Ortho-Cyclen/Ortho Tri-Cyclen ... 1914
Ovral Tablets ... 2877
Ovral-28 Tablets ... 2878
Ovrette Tablets ... 2878
Paxil Tablets (Rare) ... 2681
Permax Tablets (Infrequent) ... 571
Premarin Tablets ... 2896
Prozac Pulvules & Liquid, Oral Solution (Rare) ... 935
Relafen Tablets (Less than 1%) ... 2688
Risperdal Tablets (Infrequent) ... 1348
Serzone Tablets (Infrequent) ... 776
Sular Tablets (Less than or equal to 1%) ... 2961
▲ Supprelin Injection (22%) ... 2230
▲ Synarel Nasal Solution for Central Precocious Puberty (8%) ... 2603
Synarel Nasal Solution for Endometriosis ... 2605
Levlen/Tri-Levlen ... 646
Tri-Norinyl ... 2607
Triphasil-21 Tablets ... 2919
Triphasil-28 Tablets ... 2924
Videx Tablets, Powder for Oral Solution, & Pediatric Powder for Oral Solution (Less than 1%) ... 2980
Vivelle Transdermal System ... 880
Cataflam/Voltaren/Voltaren-XR (Less than 1%) ... 833
Zarontin Capsules ... 1986
Zarontin Syrup ... 1986
Zoladex (1% or greater) ... 2976

Bleeding diathesis
Cipro I.V. (Rare) ... 587

(⊡ Described in PDR For Nonprescription Drugs)   Incidence data in parentheses; ▲ 3% or more   (⊙ Described in PDR For Ophthalmology)

Side Effects Index

Bleeding diathesis
- Cipro Tablets (Less than 0.1%) ... 584

Bleeding irregularities
- BuSpar Tablets (Rare) ... 738
- Climara Transdermal System ... 640
- Cycrin Tablets ... 991
- ▲ Demulen (Among most common) ... 2580
- Estrace Cream and Tablets ... 751
- Levlen/Tri-Levlen ... 646
- Modicon (Sometimes) ... 1928
- ▲ Norplant System (7.6%) ... 2868
- Ogen Tablets ... 2103
- Ortho-Est ... 1925
- Ortho-Novum (Sometimes) ... 1928
- Ovcon ... 765
- Premarin Tablets ... 2896
- Premphase ... 2900
- Prempro ... 2905
- Quadrinal Tablets ... 1398
- Levlen/Tri-Levlen ... 646

Bleeding syndrome
- Mithracin ... 599

Bleeding tendencies due to hypoprothrombinemia
- Questran (Less frequent) ... 774

Bleeding time, prolongation
- Cardizem CD Capsules (Infrequent) ... 1251
- Cardizem SR Capsules (Infrequent) ... 1255
- Cardizem Injectable ... 1253
- Cardizem Tablets (Infrequent) ... 1257
- Daypro Caplets ... 2578
- Depakene ... 416
- Easprin ... 1971
- Fiorinal with Codeine Capsules ... 2390
- Hespan Injection ... 945
- Lodine Capsules and Tablets (Less than 1%) ... 2849
- Mithracin ... 599
- Naprelan Tablets (Less than 1%) ... 2861
- Neurontin Capsules (Rare) ... 1978
- Pentaspan Injection ... 954
- Procardia Capsules (Some patients) ... 2024
- Procardia XL Extended Release Tablets (Some patients) ... 2026
- Prozac Pulvules & Liquid, Oral Solution (Rare) ... 935
- Rythmol Tablets–150mg, 225mg, 300mg (Less than 1%) ... 1399
- Tiazac Capsules (Infrequent) ... 1019
- Timentin for Injection ... 2706
- Tolectin (200, 400 and 600 mg) ... 1591
- Toradol ... 2319

Blepharitis
- Alomide Ophthalmic Solution (Less than 1%) ... 465
- Anafranil Capsules (Rare) ... 819
- Bactroban Nasal (Less than 1%) ... 2643
- Betaseron for SC Injection ... 653
- Betimol 0.25%, 0.5% (1% to 5%) ... ⊙ 259
- Cognex Capsules (Rare) ... 1961
- Effexor (Rare) ... 2825
- Invirase Capsules (Less than 2%) ... 2291
- Iopidine 0.5% (Less than 3%) ... ⊙ 219
- Kerlone Tablets (Less than 2%) ... 2588
- Norvir (Less than 2%) ... 447
- OptiPranolol (Metipranolol 0.3%) Sterile Ophthalmic Solution (A small number of patients) ... ⊙ 256
- Paxil Tablets (Rare) ... 2681
- Prozac Pulvules & Liquid, Oral Solution (Rare) ... 935
- Remeron Tablets (Rare) ... 1878
- Rilutek Tablets (Rare) ... 2198
- Risperdal Tablets (Rare) ... 1348
- Sular Tablets (Less than or equal to 1%) ... 2961
- Timoptic in Ocudose (Less frequent) ... 1796
- Timoptic Sterile Ophthalmic Solution (Less frequent) ... 1794
- Timoptic-XE ... 1798

Blepharoconjunctivitis
- ▲ Betagan (About 1 in 20 patients) ... ⊙ 230
- Iopidine 0.5% (Less than 3%) ... ⊙ 219
- Ocupress Ophthalmic Solution, 1% Sterile (Occasional) ... ⊙ 297

Blepharoptosis
(see also under Ptosis, eyelids)
- Betagan ... ⊙ 230

- Betimol 0.25%, 0.5% ... ⊙ 259

Blepharospasm
- Anafranil Capsules (Up to 2%) ... 819
- Atamet Tablets ... 567
- Claritin Tablets (2% or fewer patients) ... 2485
- Claritin-D Tablets ... 2487
- Eldepryl Capsules ... 2729
- Larodopa Tablets (Infrequent) ... 2296
- Parlodel ... 2411
- Sinemet Tablets ... 959
- Sinemet CR Tablets ... 961

Blind spot, enlargement
- Eskalith ... 2658

Blindness
- Betaseron for SC Injection ... 653
- Celestone Soluspan Suspension (Rare) ... 2484
- Cortone Acetate Sterile Suspension ... 1663
- Cytovene (1% or less) ... 2270
- Dalalone D.P. Injectable (Rare) ... 1009
- Decadron Phosphate Injection (Rare) ... 1680
- Decadron Phosphate with Xylocaine Injection, Sterile (Rare) ... 1683
- Decadron-LA Sterile Suspension (Rare) ... 1687
- Doxil (Less than 1%) ... 2613
- Eskalith ... 2658
- Foscavir Injection (Less than 1%) ... 541
- Hydeltrasol Injection, Sterile (Rare) ... 1708
- Hydeltra-T.B.A. Sterile Suspension (Rare) ... 1710
- Hydrocortone Acetate Sterile Suspension (Rare) ... 1712
- Hydrocortone Phosphate Injection, Sterile (Rare) ... 1713
- Levlen/Tri-Levlen (Rare) ... 646
- Modicon (Rare) ... 1928
- Neurontin Capsules (Rare) ... 1978
- Oncovin Solution Vials & Hyporets ... 1521
- Ortho-Cyclen/Ortho-Tri-Cyclen (Rare) ... 1914
- Ortho-Novum (Rare) ... 1928
- Ortho-Cyclen/Ortho Tri-Cyclen (Rare) ... 1914
- Orthoclone OKT3 Sterile Solution ... 1892
- Permax Tablets (Rare) ... 571
- Proleukin for Injection (Less than 1%) ... 812
- Levlen/Tri-Levlen (Rare) ... 646
- Zyrtec Tablets (Less than 2%) ... 2053

Blindness, cerebral
- Platinol for Injection (Infrequent) ... 717
- Platinol-AQ Injection (Infrequent) ... 719

Blindness, night
(see under Nyctalopia)

Blindness, sudden
- Factrel ... 2996

Blindness, transient
- Adalat Capsules (10 mg and 20 mg) (Less than 0.5%) ... 580
- Adalat CC (Rare) ... 582
- Proleukin for Injection (Less than 1%) ... 812
- THYREL TRH ... 2992

Blindness, transient cortical
- Etopophos for Injection (Infrequent) ... 701
- Etoposide Injection (Infrequent) ... 539
- Oncovin Solution Vials & Hyporets ... 1521
- Procardia Capsules (Less than 0.5%) ... 2024
- VePesid Capsules and Injection (Infrequent) ... 727

Blistering
- ▲ Androderm Testosterone Transdermal System (12%) ... 2634
- Avonex ... 662
- BuSpar Tablets (Infrequent) ... 738
- Doxorubicin Astra ... 531
- Efudex (Infrequent) ... 2280
- Lotrimin ... 2514
- Lotrisone Cream ... 2515
- Maxaquin Tablets ... 2593
- Norplant System ... 2868
- Retin-A (tretinoin) Cream/Gel/Liquid ... 1947
- Sulfamylon Cream ... 940
- Viramune Tablets ... 2368

Bloated feeling
(see under Bloating)

Bloating
- Bentyl ... 1246
- ▲ Colyte and Colyte-flavored (Among most frequent) ... 2540
- ▲ CREON 5 Capsules (Among most frequent) ... 2714
- Depo-Provera Contraceptive Injection (1% to 5%) ... 2079
- Desogen Tablets ... 1867
- Dipentum Capsules (1.5%) ... 2084
- Donnatal ... 2234
- Donnatal Extentabs ... 2234
- Donnatal Tablets ... 2234
- Estrace Cream and Tablets ... 751
- ▲ GoLYTELY (Up to 50%) ... 694
- IBU Tablets (Greater than 1%) ... 1389
- Indocin Capsules (Less than 1%) ... 1723
- Indocin I.V. (Less than 1%) ... 1727
- Indocin (Less than 1%) ... 1723
- Levsin/Levsinex/Levbid ... 2549
- ▲ Limbitrol (Among most frequent) ... 2333
- Lo/Ovral Tablets ... 2852
- Lo/Ovral-28 Tablets ... 2857
- Menest Tablets ... 2671
- Modicon ... 1928
- Nephro-Fer Rx Tablets ... 2168
- Nordette-21 Tablets ... 2863
- Nordette-28 Tablets ... 2866
- ▲ Norpace (3 to 9%) ... 2596
- Ortho-Cept ... 1907
- Ortho-Cyclen/Ortho-Tri-Cyclen ... 1914
- Ortho Dienestrol Cream ... 1922
- Ortho-Est ... 1925
- Ortho-Novum ... 1928
- Ortho-Cyclen/Ortho Tri-Cyclen ... 1914
- Ovcon ... 765
- Ovral Tablets ... 2877
- Ovral-28 Tablets ... 2878
- Ovrette Tablets ... 2878
- Premarin Vaginal Cream ... 2898
- Pro-Banthine Tablets ... 2226
- Robinul Forte Tablets ... 2247
- Robinul Injectable ... 2247
- Robinul Tablets ... 2247
- Rowasa (1.47%) ... 2727
- Triphasil-21 Tablets ... 2919
- Triphasil-28 Tablets ... 2924
- Yutopar Intravenous Injection (Infrequent) ... 566

Blood clotting, mechanisms, disorders of
- Estrace Cream and Tablets ... 751
- Ortho-Est ... 1925
- Pyrazinamide Tablets (Rare) ... 1442
- Rifater (Rare) ... 1280

Blood dyscrasias
- Anturane (Rare) ... 823
- Apresazide Capsules (Less frequent) ... 824
- Apresoline Hydrochloride Tablets (Less frequent) ... 826
- Aralen Hydrochloride Injection ... 2430
- Aralen Phosphate Tablets ... 2431
- Azulfidine ... 2059
- Bactrim DS Tablets (Rare) ... 2257
- Bactrim I.V. Infusion (Rare) ... 2255
- Bactrim (Rare) ... 2257
- Blephamide Liquifilm Sterile Ophthalmic Suspension ... 472
- ▲ Blephamide Ointment (Among most often) ... ⊙ 234
- Celontin Kapseals ... 1955
- Chloromycetin Ophthalmic Ointment, 1% ... ⊙ 298
- Chloromycetin Ophthalmic Solution ... ⊙ 299
- Chloromycetin Sodium Succinate ... 1960
- Chloroptic Sterile Ophthalmic Solution (Rare) ... ⊙ 236
- Compazine ... 2644
- Dapsone Tablets USP ... 1331
- Depo-Provera Contraceptive Injection (Fewer than 1%) ... 2079
- Diamox Intravenous ... ⊙ 317
- Diamox Sequels (Sustained Release) ... ⊙ 318
- Diamox Tablets ... ⊙ 317
- Esimil Tablets (A few instances) ... 840
- Etrafon (Less frequent) ... 2495
- Fansidar Tablets ... 2281
- Gantrisin (Rare) ... 2286
- GlaucTabs ... ⊙ 209
- Hydralazine Hydrochloride Injection USP (Less frequent) ... 2712
- Ismelin Tablets ... 845

- Lasix Injection, Oral Solution and Tablets ... 1267
- ▲ Leukine (25%) ... 1317
- Levoprome ... 1321
- Librax Capsules ... 2330
- Librium Capsules (Occasional) ... 2331
- Mesantoin Tablets ... 2400
- Mexitil Capsules ... 684
- Myochrysine Injection (Rare) ... 1754
- Neptazane Tablets ... ⊙ 320
- Phenurone Tablets (2%) ... 455
- Plaquenil Sulfate Tablets ... 2459
- Procanbid Extended-Release Tablets (Approximately 0.5%) ... 1983
- Prolixin ... 510
- Prozac Pulvules & Liquid, Oral Solution (Rare) ... 935
- Ridaura Capsules ... 2691
- SSD ... 1402
- Septra ... 1146
- Septra I.V. Infusion ... 1142
- Septra I.V. Infusion ADD-Vantage Vials (Rare) ... 1144
- Septra ... 1146
- Ser-Ap-Es Tablets ... 867
- Serax Capsules ... 2916
- Serax Tablets ... 2916
- Silvadene Cream 1% ... 1288
- Solganal Suspension (Rare) ... 2530
- Stelazine ... 2692
- Tambocor Tablets (Extremely rare) ... 1555
- Tigan ... 2231
- Tonocard Tablets ... 519
- Triavil Tablets ... 1800
- Trusopt Sterile Ophthalmic Solution (Rare) ... 1803
- Urobiotic-250 Capsules ... 2038
- Zarontin Capsules ... 1986
- Zarontin Syrup ... 1986

Blood glucose, elevation
(see under Hyperglycemia)

Blood glucose, reduction
(see under Hypoglycemia)

Blood loss, increase
(see under Bleeding)

Blood pressure, changes
- Alka-Seltzer Cherry Effervescent Antacid and Pain Reliever ... ▣ 609
- Alka-Seltzer Lemon Lime Effervescent Antacid and Pain Reliever ... ▣ 609
- Alka-Seltzer Original Effervescent Antacid and Pain Reliever ... ▣ 609
- Asendin Tablets ... 1419
- Bronkometer Aerosol ... 2432
- Bronkosol Solution ... 2432
- Bufferin Analgesic Tablets ... ▣ 636
- Cartrol Tablets ... 413
- Clozaril Tablets ... 2377
- DDAVP Injection (Infrequent) ... 2178
- DDAVP Injection 15 mcg/mL (Infrequent) ... 2179
- Dantrium Capsules (Less frequent) ... 2131
- Daypro Caplets (Less than 1%) ... 2578
- Desmopressin Acetate Injection (Infrequent) ... 996
- Desoxyn Gradumet Tablets ... 422
- Dilatrate-SR Capsules ... 2542
- Gammar-P I.V., Immune Globulin Intravenous (Human) ... 798
- Haldol Decanoate ... 1587
- Isoetharine Inhalation Solution, USP, Arm-a-Med ... 545
- Isordil Sublingual Tablets ... 2845
- Isordil Tembids ... 2847
- Isordil Titradose Tablets ... 2848
- Loxitane ... 1426
- Mellaril ... 2398
- Moban Tablets and Concentrate ... 1036
- Orap Tablets ... 1037
- Pontocaine Hydrochloride for Spinal Anesthesia ... 2460
- Premphase (Occasional) ... 2900
- Prempro (Occasional) ... 2905
- Prolixin ... 510
- RespiGam ... 1631
- Risperdal Tablets ... 1348
- Ritalin ... 866
- Sandimmune ... 2416
- Sensorcaine ... 554
- Serentil ... 689
- Stelazine ... 2692
- Tornalate Metered Dose Inhaler ... 978
- Trilafon ... 2532
- Ventolin Rotacaps for Inhalation ... 1173

(▣ Described in PDR For Nonprescription Drugs)   Incidence data in parenthesis; ▲ 3% or more   (⊙ Described in PDR For Ophthalmology)

1271 Side Effects Index Blurred vision

▲ Vumon for Injection (Approximately 5%) 729
▲ Yutopar Intravenous Injection (80% to 100%) 566
Zemuron Injection 1885

Blood pressure, elevation (see under Hypertension)

Blood pressure, reduction (see under Hypotension)

Blood urea levels, increase

Ceptaz (Occasional) 1070
Fortaz (Occasional) 1092
Inderide Tablets 2838
Normodyne Tablets (Rare) 2522
▲ Paraplatin for Injection (Up to 17%) 713
Tazidime Vials, Faspak & ADD-Vantage (Occasional) 1531

Blood urea nitrogen levels, increase (see under BUN levels, elevation)

Blurred vision

Achromycin V Capsules 1417
Adalat Capsules (10 mg and 20 mg) (2% or less) 580
Adapin Capsules 1542
Adenocard Injection (Less than 1%) 1021
Adenoscan (Less than 1%) 1022
AeroBid Inhaler System (1% to 3%) 1004
Aerobid-M Inhaler System (1% to 3%) 1004
Akineton 1380
Albalon Solution with Liquifilm ⊙ 229
Alfenta Injection (1% to 3%) 1334
▲ Alferon N Injection (3% to 6%) 2142
▲ Alomide Ophthalmic Solution (1% to 5%) 465
Alupent Tablets (0.2%) 672
Amaryl Tablets (0.4%) 1241
Ana-Kit Anaphylaxis Emergency Treatment Kit 611
Antivert, Antivert/25 Tablets, & Antivert/50 Tablets (Rare) 1992
Aralen Hydrochloride Injection 2430
Aralen Phosphate Tablets 2431
Arco-Lase Plus Tablets 513
▲ Artane (30% to 50%) 1418
Asacol Delayed-Release Tablets 2129
▲ Asendin Tablets (7%) 1419
Atamet Tablets 567
Ativan Injection (Occasional) 2805
Atretol Tablets 569
Atrohist Pediatric Capsules 1603
Atrohist Plus Tablets 1605
Atromid-S Capsules 2808
Atrovent Inhalation Aerosol (1.2%; about 1 in 100) 674
Atrovent Nasal Spray 0.03% (Less than 2%) 676
Atrovent Nasal Spray 0.06% (Less than 1%) 678
Bellergal-S Tablets (Rare) 2375
Benadryl Injection 1955
▲ Bentyl (27%) 1246
Betimol 0.25%, 0.5% (1% to 5%) ⊙ 259
Betoptic Ophthalmic Solution 465
Betoptic S Ophthalmic Suspension (Small number of patients) 467
Bonine Tablets (Rare) 1990
Bontril Slow-Release Capsules 786
Bromfed 1832
BuSpar Tablets (2%) 738
Calan SR Caplets (1% or less) 2571
Calan Tablets (1% or less) 2568
Capoten Tablets 740
Capozide Tablets 744
Carbocaine Injection 2432
Cardene Capsules (Rare) 2261
Cardene SR Capsules (Rare) 2264
Cardioquin Tablets 2146
Cartrol Tablets (Less common) 413
Cataflam Tablets (Less than 1%) 833
Catapres Tablets 679
Catapres-TTS 680
Celontin Kapseals 1955
Cipro I.V. (1% or less) 587
Cipro I.V. Pharmacy Bulk Package (Less than 1%) 590
Cipro Tablets (Less than 1%) 584
Claritin Tablets (2% or fewer patients) 2485
Claritin-D Tablets (Less frequent) 2487
Clinoril Tablets (Less than 1 in 100) 1658
Clomid (Occasional; 1.5%) 1262
Cogentin 1661
Combipres Tablets 682
Compazine 2644
Covera-HS Tablets (Less than 2%) 2573
Cozaar Tablets (Less than 1%) 1668
Crixivan Capsules (Less than 2%) 1670
Cystospaz 2123
D.A. II Tablets 972
D.A. Chewable Tablets 970
Dalgan Injection (Less than 1%) 529
Dalmane Capsules (Rare) 2329
Dapsone Tablets USP 1331
Daypro Caplets (Less than 1%) 2578
Decadron Phosphate Sterile Ophthalmic Ointment 1684
Decadron Phosphate Sterile Ophthalmic Solution 1685
Decadron Phosphate with Xylocaine Injection, Sterile 1683
Declomycin Tablets 1421
Desferal Vials 838
▲ Desyrel and Desyrel Dividose (6.3% to 14.7%) 504
DiaBeta Tablets 1265
Dilacor XR Extended-release Capsules (Infrequent) 2183
Dilaudid-HP Injection (Less frequent) 1384
Dilaudid-HP Lyophilized Powder 250 mg (Less frequent) 1384
Dilaudid Tablets and Liquid (Less frequent) 1386
Dipentum Capsules (Rare) 2084
Ditropan 1267
Diucardin Tablets 2824
Diupres Tablets 1691
Dizac (diazepam injectable emulsion) CIV (Less frequent) 1862
Dolobid Tablets (Less than 1 in 100) 1695
Donnagel Liquid and Donnagel Chewable Tablets (Rare) ⊡ 854
Donnatal 2234
Donnatal Extentabs 2234
Donnatal Tablets 2234
Duranest Injections 533
Dura-Tap/PD Capsules 970
Dura-Vent/DA Tablets 972
Dyclone 0.5% and 1% Topical Solutions, USP 535
Edecrin 1698
▲ Effexor (6%) 2825
Elavil 2945
Eldepryl Capsules 2729
Emete-con Intramuscular/Intravenous 2007
EMLA Cream (Unlikely with cream) 536
Enduron Tablets 424
Ergamisol Tablets (1% to 2%) 1340
Esimil Tablets 840
Eskalith 2658
▲ Ethmozine Tablets (2% to 5%) 2217
Etrafon 2495
FML Forte Liquifilm ⊙ 237
FML Liquifilm ⊙ 238
Fedahist Gyrocaps 2545
Feldene Capsules (Less than 1%) 2008
Flexeril Tablets (1% to 3%) 1701
Floxin I.V. 1580
Floxin Tablets (200 mg, 300 mg, 400 mg) 1577
Glucotrol XL Extended Release Tablets (Less than 3%) 2012
Glynase PresTab Tablets 2091
Haldol Decanoate 1587
Haldol Injection, Tablets and Concentrate 1585
Hivid Tablets (Less than 1%) 2287
Humorsol Sterile Ophthalmic Solution 1707
Hycomine Compound Tablets 948
Hycomine 947
Hycotuss Expectorant Syrup 950
HydroDIURIL Tablets 1716
Hydropres Tablets 1718
Hyperstat I.V. Injection 2504
Hytrin Capsules (0.6% to 1.6%) 434
Hyzaar Tablets 1720
IBU Tablets (Less than 1%) 1389
Indocin (Less than 1%) 1723
Intron A for Injection (Less than 5%) 2506
Inversine Tablets 1729
IOPIDINE Sterile Ophthalmic Solution ⊙ 218
Iopidine 0.5% (Less than 3%) ⊙ 219
Ismelin Tablets 845
Ismo Tablets (Fewer than 1%) 2844
Isoptin Oral Tablets (Less than 1%) 1393
Isoptin SR Tablets (1% or less) 1395
Kadian Capsules (Less than 3%) 2948
Kemadrin Tablets 1105
Kutrase Capsules 2546
Lacrisert Sterile Ophthalmic Insert 1730
▲ Lamictal Tablets (Among most common; 11% to 25%) 1105
Lanoxicaps 1110
Lanoxin Elixir Pediatric 1113
Lanoxin Injection 1116
Lanoxin Injection Pediatric 1119
Lanoxin Tablets 1121
Larodopa Tablets (Infrequent) 2296
Lasix Injection, Oral Solution and Tablets 1267
Levsin/Levsinex/Levbid 2549
Librax Capsules 2330
Librium Injectable (Isolated instances) 2332
▲ Limbitrol (Among most frequent) 2333
Lioresal Tablets 847
Lithium Carbonate Capsules & Tablets 2352
Lithonate/Lithotabs/Lithobid 2721
Lodine Capsules and Tablets (1% to 3%) 2849
Lopid Tablets 1974
Lopressor 848
Lopressor HCT Tablets (1 in 100 patients) 850
Loxitane 1426
▲ Ludiomil Tablets (4%) 861
Lupron Injection (Less than 5%) 2736
▲ LUVOX Tablets (3%) 2723
Lysodren Tablets (Infrequent) 707
MS Contin Tablets (Less frequent) 2149
MSIR (Infrequent) 2152
Marcaine 2446
Marcaine Spinal 2449
Mellaril 2398
Mepergan Injection (Occasional) 2859
Methotrexate Sodium Tablets, Injection, for Injection and LPF Injection 1322
Mevacor Tablets (0.9% to 1.5%) 1742
▲ Mexitil Capsules (5.7% to 7.5%) 684
Miacalcin Nasal Spray (Less than 1%) 2403
Micronase Tablets 2099
Minipress Capsules (1-4%) 2015
Minizide Capsules 2016
Minocin Intravenous 1428
Minocin Oral Suspension 1431
Minocin Pellet-Filled Capsules 1429
Mintezol 1747
Moban Tablets and Concentrate (Occasional) 1036
Moduretic Tablets 1748
Motofen Tablets (Less frequent) 789
Motrin Ibuprofen Suspension, Oral Drops, Chewable Tablets, Caplets (Less than 1%) 1563
Mutamycin for Injection 712
Nalfon 200 Pulvules & Nalfon Tablets (2.2%) 933
Nardil (Less common) 1977
Navane Capsules and Concentrate 2018
Navane Intramuscular 2019
Nescaine/Nescaine MPF 549
Netromycin Injection 100 mg/ml (Fewer than 1 of 1000 patients) 2516
Norflex 1554
Norgesic 1554
Noroxin Tablets (Less frequent) 1758
Noroxin Tablets (Less frequent) 2222
▲ Norpace (3 to 9%) 2596
Norpramin Tablets 1273
Norvir (Less than 2%) 447
Novocain Hydrochloride for Spinal Anesthesia 2457
Nubain Injection (1% or less) 952
Ocuflox Ophthalmic Solution 478
Ocupress Ophthalmic Solution, 1% Sterile (Occasional) ⊙ 297
OptiPranolol (Metipranolol 0.3%) Sterile Ophthalmic Solution (A small number of patients) ⊙ 256
Oramorph SR (Morphine Sulfate Sustained Release Tablets) (Less frequent) 2359
Orap Tablets 1037
Orlaam Oral Solution (1% to 3%) 2361
Ornade Spansule Capsules 2678
Orthoclone OKT3 Sterile Solution 1892
PBZ Tablets 863
PBZ-SR Tablets 862
Pamelor 2409
Paremyd ⊙ 244
Parnate Tablets 2679
▲ Paxil Tablets (2.0% to 7.8%) 2681
Periactin 1767
Phenergan with Codeine (Occasional) 2883
Phenergan with Dextromethorphan (Occasional) 2885
Phenergan Injection 2880
Phenergan Suppositories (Occasional) 2882
Phenergan Syrup (Occasional) 2881
Phenergan Tablets (Occasional) 2882
Phenergan VC (Occasional) 2886
Phenergan VC with Codeine (Occasional) 2888
Phospholine Iodide ⊙ 323
Pilagan ⊙ 245
Placidyl Capsules 456
Plaquenil Sulfate Tablets (Fairly common) 2459
Platinol for Injection 717
Platinol-AQ Injection 719
Pondimin Tablets 2239
Ponstel 1982
Pontocaine Hydrochloride for Spinal Anesthesia 2460
Pred Forte ⊙ 247
Prinivil Tablets (0.3% to 1.0%) 1776
Prinzide Tablets (0.3 to 1%) 1780
Pro-Banthine Tablets 2226
Procardia Capsules (2% or less) 2024
Proglycem 575
Prolixin 510
PROPINE with C CAP Compliance Cap ⊙ 251
Prostin E2 Suppository 2109
Protopam Chloride for Injection 2909
Quinaglute Dura-Tabs Tablets 644
Quinidex Extentabs 2240
Rev-Eyes Ophthalmic Eyedrops 0.5% (Less frequently) ⊙ 324
ReVia Tablets (Less than 1%) 957
Ritalin 866
Robaxin Injectable 2245
Robaxin Tablets 2246
Robaxisal Tablets 2246
Robinul Forte Tablets 2247
Robinul Injectable 2247
Robinul Tablets 2247
▲ Romazicon (1% to 9%) 2311
Rondec Chewable Tablets 974
▲ Rythmol Tablets–150mg, 225mg, 300mg (0.6 to 5.7%) 1399
Sandostatin Injection (1% to 4%) 2421
Sanorex Tablets 2423
Seldane-D Extended-Release Tablets (1.1%) 1286
Sensorcaine 554
Ser-Ap-Es Tablets 867
Serax Capsules 2916
Serax Tablets 2916
Serentil 689
Serophene (clomiphene citrate tablets, USP) (Occasionally) 2621
▲ Serzone Tablets (3% to 9%) 776
Sinemet Tablets 959
Sinemet CR Tablets 961
Sinequan 2028
Slo-Niacin Tablets 2767
Stadol (1% or greater) 779
Stelazine 2692
Sublimaze Injection 463
Surmontil Capsules 2917
Talacen Caplets (Infrequent) 2464
Talwin Injection 2465
Talwin Compound (Infrequent) 2466
Talwin Injection 2465
Talwin Nx Tablets 2467
Tambocor Tablets 1555
Tavist Syrup 2426
Tavist Tablets 2427
Tegretol/Tegretol-XR 870
Tenex Tablets (Less frequent) 2249
Thioplex (Thiotepa For Injection) 1329
Tigan 2231
Timolide Tablets 1791
Tofranil Ampuls 873
Tofranil Tablets (Rare) 875
Tofranil-PM Capsules 876
▲ Tonocard Tablets (1.3% to 10.0%) 519
Toprol-XL Tablets 560
Toradol (1% or less) 2319
Torecan 2367
Transderm Scōp Transdermal Therapeutic System 890
Tranxene (Less common) 459
Trental Tablets (Less than 1%) 1291
Triavil Tablets 1800
Trilafon (Occasional) 2532
Trinalin Repetabs Tablets 1373

(⊡ Described in PDR For Nonprescription Drugs) Incidence data in parenthesis; ▲ 3% or more (⊙ Described in PDR For Ophthalmology)

Blurred vision

Trusopt Sterile Ophthalmic Solution (Approximately 1% to 5%) ... 1803
Tussend ... 1830
Urised Tablets ... 2123
Urispas Tablets ... 2710
Valium Injectable ... 2336
Valium Tablets (Infrequent) ... 2335
Vascor Tablets (200 and 300 mg) (0.5 to 2.0%) ... 1597
Vasotec I.V. ... 1814
Vasotec Tablets (0.5% to 1.0%) ... 1816
Verelan Capsules (1% or less) ... 1455
Versed Injection (Less than 1%) ... 2324
Vexol 1% Ophthalmic Suspension (1% to 5%) ... ⊚ 227
Vicodin Tuss Expectorant ... 1406
Videx Tablets, Powder for Oral Solution, & Pediatric Powder for Oral Solution (Up to 2%) ... 2980
Vivactil Tablets ... 1820
Cataflam/Voltaren/Voltaren-XR (Less than 1%) ... 833
▲ Wellbutrin Tablets (14.6%) ... 1177
▲ Xalatan (5% to 15%) ... ⊚ 304
▲ Xanax Tablets (6.2% to 21.0%) ... 2115
▲ Xylocaine Injections (Among most common) ... 562
Zantac (Rare) ... 1182
Zantac Injection (Rare) ... 1180
Zantac Syrup (Rare) ... 1182
Zestoretic Tablets (0.3 to 1%) ... 2968
Zestril Tablets (0.3% to 1.0%) ... 2972
Ziac ... 1459
Zofran Injection ... 1227

Blurred vision, transient
(see also under Blurred vision)

Aldoclor Tablets ... 1638
Aldoril Tablets ... 1644
Apresazide Capsules ... 824
Capozide Tablets ... 744
Diucardin Tablets ... 2824
Diupres Tablets ... 1691
Diuril Oral Suspension ... 1694
Diuril Sodium Intravenous ... 1693
Diuril Tablets ... 1694
Dyazide Capsules ... 2653
Esidrix Tablets ... 839
Esimil Tablets ... 840
HydroDIURIL Tablets ... 1716
Inderide Tablets ... 2838
Inderide LA Long Acting Capsules ... 2840
Lopressor HCT Tablets ... 850
Lotensin HCT Tablets ... 855
Mykrox Tablets ... 1617
Peptavlon ... 2997
Ser-Ap-Es Tablets ... 867
Vaseretic Tablets ... 1810
Zaroxolyn Tablets ... 1625

Body odor

Carnitor Injection (Less frequent) ... 2623
Carnitor Tablets and Solution ... 2624
Crixivan Capsules (Less than 2%) ... 1670
Depo-Provera Contraceptive Injection (Fewer than 1%) ... 2079
Effexor (Rare) ... 2825
Felbatol ... 2774
Lupron Depot 3.75 mg (Less than 5%) ... 2739
Lupron Depot-PED 7.5 mg, 11.25 mg and 15 mg (Less than 2%) ... 2744
Lupron Injection Pediatric (Less than 2%) ... 2737
Retrovir Capsules ... 1216
Retrovir I.V. Infusion ... 1221
Retrovir Syrup ... 1216
Salagen Tablets (Less than 1%) ... 1546
Supprelin Injection (1% to 3%) ... 2230
▲ Synarel Nasal Solution for Central Precocious Puberty (4%) ... 2603
Wellbutrin Tablets (Rare) ... 1177

Bone density, changes

Depo-Provera Contraceptive Injection ... 2079
Proglycem Suspension ... 575
▲ Zoladex (4.3% decrease) ... 2976

Bone disorders

Accutane Capsules ... 2252
Clomid ... 1262
Effexor (Infrequent) ... 2825
Naprelan Tablets (Less than 1%) ... 2861
Proglycem Capsules ... 575
Redux Capsules (Infrequent) ... 2911
Risperdal Tablets (Rare) ... 1348
▲ Vesanoid Capsules (3%) ... 2327

Videx Tablets, Powder for Oral Solution, & Pediatric Powder for Oral Solution (Less than 1%) ... 2980

Bone fractures

Didronel Tablets ... 2133
Naprelan Tablets (Less than 1%) ... 2861

Bone marrow depression

Accupril Tablets (Rare) ... 1950
Adapin Capsules (Occasional) ... 1542
▲ Adriamycin PFS (High incidence) ... 2056
▲ Adriamycin RDF (High incidence) ... 2056
Aldoclor Tablets ... 1638
Aldomet Ester HCl Injection ... 1642
Aldomet Oral ... 1640
Aldoril Tablets ... 1644
Altace Capsules (Rare to more frequent) ... 1238
Anafranil Capsules (Rare) ... 819
Atretol Tablets ... 569
Azathioprine Tablets ... 2349
Bleph-10 Ophthalmic Solution 10% ... 472
Chloromycetin Sodium Succinate ... 1960
Chloroptic Sterile Ophthalmic Solution (Three cases) ... ⊚ 236
Clinoril Tablets (Less than 1%) ... 1658
Cuprimine Capsules ... 1673
Depen Titratable Tablets ... 2770
Diamox ... ⊚ 317
Doxil ... 2613
▲ Doxorubicin Astra (High incidence) ... 531
Elavil ... 2945
Elspar (Rare) ... 1700
FML-S Liquifilm ... ⊚ 240
Felbatol ... 2774
Feldene Capsules (Less than 1%) ... 2008
Flexeril Tablets (Rare) ... 1701
Floxin I.V. ... 1580
Floxin Tablets (200 mg, 300 mg, 400 mg) ... 1577
GlaucTabs ... ⊚ 209
Hydrea Capsules ... 705
Indocin Capsules (Less than 1%) ... 1723
Indocin I.V. (Less than 1%) ... 1727
Indocin (Less than 1%) ... 1723
Limbitrol ... 2333
Lotensin Tablets (Rare) ... 852
Lotensin HCT Tablets ... 855
Lotrel Capsules ... 858
Ludiomil Tablets (Isolated reports) ... 861
Mavik Tablets (Rare) ... 1407
Mefoxin ... 1734
Mefoxin Premixed Intravenous Solution ... 1737
Methotrexate Sodium Tablets, Injection, for Injection and LPF Injection ... 1322
Neptazane Tablets ... ⊚ 320
Norpramin Tablets ... 1273
Oncovin Solution Vials & Hyporets ... 1521
Pamelor ... 2409
Primaxin I.M. ... 1770
Primaxin I.V. ... 1772
Prinivil Tablets (Rare) ... 1776
Prinzide Tablets (Rare) ... 1780
Procanbid Extended-Release Tablets (Approximately 0.5%) ... 1983
Redux Capsules ... 2911
Rubex for Injection (A high incidence) ... 721
Sinequan (Occasional) ... 2028
Sulfamylon Cream (A single case) ... 940
Surmontil Capsules ... 2917
Tegretol/Tegretol-XR ... 870
Thioplex (Thiotepa For Injection) ... 1329
Ticlid Tablets ... 2317
Tofranil Ampuls ... 873
Tofranil Tablets ... 875
Tofranil-PM Capsules ... 876
Tonocard Tablets (Less than 1%) ... 519
Triavil Tablets ... 1800
Vaseretic Tablets (Rare) ... 1810
Vasotec I.V. (Rare) ... 1814
Vasotec Tablets (Rare) ... 1816
Vivactil Tablets ... 1820
Zestoretic Tablets (Rare) ... 2968
Zestril Tablets (Rare) ... 2972

Bone marrow dysplasia

BiCNU ... 696
CeeNU Capsules ... 699

Bone marrow fibrosis

Fludara for Injection (One patient) ... 658

Bone marrow hyperplasia

Ponstel (Occasional) ... 1982

Bone marrow hypoplasia

Capoten Tablets ... 740
Capozide Tablets ... 744
Chloromycetin Ophthalmic Ointment, 1% ... ⊚ 298
Chloromycetin Ophthalmic Solution ... ⊚ 299
Lopid Tablets (Rare) ... 1974
Zantac (Rare) ... 1182
Zantac Injection (Sometimes) ... 1180
Zantac Syrup (Rare) ... 1182

Bone marrow suppression

▲ Alkeran for Injection (Most common) ... 1196
▲ Alkeran Tablets (Most common) ... 1198
▲ BiCNU (Most common) ... 696
▲ CeeNU Capsules (Most common) ... 699
Celontin Kapseals ... 1955
▲ Cerubidine for Injection (All patients) ... 634
Chloroptic S.O.P. ... ⊚ 236
Clozaril Tablets ... 2377
Cytosar-U Sterile Powder ... 2077
Depakene ... 416
Depakote Tablets ... 418
Dilantin Infatabs ... 1967
Dilantin Kapseals ... 1965
Dilantin-125 Suspension ... 1969
Doxil ... 2613
Etopophos for Injection ... 701
Etoposide Injection ... 539
Etrafon ... 2495
Fiorinal (Single case) ... 2388
Fludara for Injection ... 658
▲ Foscavir Injection (10%) ... 541
Hycamtin for Injection ... 2665
Hydrea Capsules ... 705
Imuran (Rare) ... 1103
Leukeran Tablets (Frequent) ... 1205
Leustatin (Common) ... 1889
Neutrexin for Injection ... 2761
Paraplatin for Injection ... 713
Purinethol Tablets (Frequent) ... 1214
▲ Septra I.V. Infusion (Among most frequent) ... 1142
Taxol Injection ... 723
Taxotere for Injection Concentrate ... 2204
Thioguanine Tablets, Tabloid Brand ... 1225
VePesid Capsules and Injection ... 727
Vumon for Injection ... 729
Zarontin Capsules ... 1986
Zarontin Syrup ... 1986

Borborygmi

Peptavlon ... 2997
Urecholine ... 1804

Bowel, loss of control

Duranest Injections ... 533
Nescaine/Nescaine MPF ... 549
Xylocaine Injections ... 562

Bowel disease, inflammatory, exacerbation of

Accutane Capsules ... 2252
Asacol Delayed-Release Tablets ... 2129

Bowel frequency, increase

Esimil Tablets ... 840
Fluorouracil Injection ... 2282
Sterile FUDR ... 2284
▲ Hylorel Tablets (4.9%) ... 1613
Invirase Capsules (Less than 2%) ... 2291
Ismelin Tablets ... 845

Bowel habits, changes

▲ Seldane Tablets (4.6% to 7.6%) ... 1284
Seldane-D Extended-Release Tablets ... 1286

Bowel infarction

Activase ... 1045
Orthoclone OKT3 Sterile Solution ... 1892
Proleukin for Injection ... 812

Bowel strictures, fibrotic

Pancrease MT Capsules ... 1589

Bowel syndrome, irritable

Anafranil Capsules (Infrequent) ... 819
Neurontin Capsules (Rare) ... 1978

Bowels, perforation

Cortone Acetate Sterile Suspension ... 1663
Cortone Acetate Tablets ... 1664
Dalalone D.P. Injectable ... 1009
Decadron Elixir ... 1676
Decadron Phosphate Injection ... 1680

Decadron Phosphate with Xylocaine Injection, Sterile ... 1683
Decadron Tablets ... 1678
Decadron-LA Sterile Suspension ... 1687
Dexacort Phosphate in Respihaler ... 1606
Dexacort Phosphate in Turbinaire ... 1607
Hydeltrasol Injection, Sterile ... 1708
Hydeltra-T.B.A. Sterile Suspension ... 1710
Hydrocortone Acetate Sterile Suspension ... 1712
Hydrocortone Phosphate Injection, Sterile ... 1713
Hydrocortone Tablets ... 1715
Indocin I.V. (1% to 3%) ... 1727
Proleukin for Injection ... 812

Brachial plexus neuropathies

Tripedia ... 908

Bradycardia

Adalat CC (Less than 1.0%) ... 582
Adenoscan (Less than 1%) ... 1022
Akineton ... 1380
Aldoclor Tablets ... 1638
Aldomet Ester HCl Injection ... 1642
Aldomet Oral ... 1640
Aldoril Tablets ... 1644
▲ Alfenta Injection (14%) ... 1334
Amicar Syrup, Tablets, and Injection ... 1312
Anafranil Capsules (Infrequent) ... 819
Anectine ... 1062
Antilirium Injectable ... 1007
Betagan ... ⊚ 230
▲ Betapace Tablets (8% to 16%) ... 637
Betimol 0.25%, 0.5% ... ⊚ 259
Betoptic Ophthalmic Solution (Rare) ... 465
Betoptic S Ophthalmic Suspension (Rare) ... 467
▲ Blocadren Tablets (5% to 9.1%) ... 1654
Brevibloc (esmolol HCl) Injection (Less than 1%) ... 1860
Brontex ... 2130
Buprenex Injectable (Less than 1%) ... 2170
BuSpar Tablets (Rare) ... 738
Butisol Sodium Elixir & Tablets (Less than 1 in 100) ... 2768
Cafergot ... 2376
Calan SR Caplets (1.4%) ... 2571
Calan Tablets (1.4%) ... 2568
Carbocaine Injection ... 2432
Cardizem CD Capsules (1.7% to 3.3%) ... 1251
▲ Cardizem SR Capsules (1.5% to 6%) ... 1255
Cardizem Injectable (Less than 1%) ... 1253
Cardizem Tablets (Less than 1%) ... 1257
Cartrol Tablets ... 413
Catapres Tablets (About 5 in 1,000 patients) ... 679
Catapres-TTS ... 680
Clozaril Tablets (Less than 1%) ... 2377
Cognex Capsules (Infrequent) ... 1961
Combipres Tablets (About 5 in 1,000) ... 682
▲ Cordarone Intravenous (4.9%) ... 2821
Cordarone Tablets (Uncommon) ... 2818
Corvert Injection (1.2%) ... 2075
Covera-HS Tablets (1.4%) ... 2573
D.H.E. 45 Injection ... 2381
Decadron Phosphate with Xylocaine Injection, Sterile ... 1683
Demerol ... 2438
Desyrel and Desyrel Dividose ... 504
Dilacor XR Extended-release Capsules (1.4%) ... 2183
Dilaudid-HP Injection (Less frequent) ... 1384
Dilaudid-HP Lyophilized Powder 250 mg (Less frequent) ... 1384
Dilaudid Tablets and Liquid ... 1386
▲ Diprivan Injectable Emulsion (1% to 3%) ... 2939
Diupres Tablets ... 1691
Dizac (diazepam injectable emulsion) CIV (Less frequent) ... 1862
Duragesic Transdermal System (Less than 1%) ... 1336
Duranest Injections ... 533
Dyclone 0.5% and 1% Topical Solutions, USP ... 535
Effexor (Rare) ... 2825
EMLA Cream (Unlikely with cream) ... 536
Esimil Tablets ... 840
Eskalith ... 2658
Ethmozine Tablets (Less than 2%) ... 2217
Etrafon ... 2495
Felbatol ... 2774

(⊞ Described in PDR For Nonprescription Drugs)   Incidence data in parenthesis; ▲ 3% or more   (⊚ Described in PDR For Ophthalmology)

1273 Side Effects Index Breast enlargement

▲ Flolan for Injection (5% to 15%).... 1085
Foscavir Injection (Less than 1%) .. 541
Glucophage Tablets ... 754
Hespan Injection ... 945
Humorsol Sterile Ophthalmic Solution (Rare) ... 1707
Hydropres Tablets ... 1718
Hyperstat I.V. Injection ... 2504
Imdur (Less than or equal to 5%) .. 1362
Imitrex Injection (Infrequent) ... 1095
Imitrex Tablets (Rare) ... 1099
Inderal ... 2834
Inderal LA Long Acting Capsules ... 2836
Inderide Tablets ... 2838
Inderide LA Long Acting Capsules .. 2840
Indocin I.V. (Less than 3%) ... 1727
Intron A for Injection (Less than 5%) ... 2506
IOPIDINE Sterile Ophthalmic Solution ... ◉ 218
Ismelin Tablets ... 845
Isoptin Injectable (1.2%) ... 1391
Isoptin Oral Tablets (1.4%) ... 1393
Isoptin SR Tablets (1.4%) ... 1395
Kadian Capsules (Less than 3%) 2948
▲ Kerlone Tablets (5.8% to 8.8%) ... 2588
Lariam Tablets (Less than 1%) ... 2295
Levo-Dromoran ... 2297
Levophed Bitartrate Injection ... 2445
Lioresal Intrathecal (1% or more) .. 1634
Lithonate/Lithotabs/Lithobid ... 2721
▲ Lopressor (3%) ... 848
▲ Lopressor HCT Tablets (3 to 6 in 100 patients) ... 850
Lupron Depot - 3 Month 22.5 mg (Less than 5%) ... 2743
LUVOX Tablets (Infrequent) ... 2723
MS Contin Tablets (Less frequent) 2149
MSIR (Infrequent) ... 2152
Marcaine ... 2446
Marcaine Spinal ... 2449
Mavik Tablets (0.3% to 1.0%) ... 1407
Maxaquin Tablets (Less than 1%) .. 2593
Mebaral Tablets (Less than 1 in 100) ... 2452
Mepergan Injection ... 2859
Merrem I.V. (0.1% to 1.0%) ... 2952
Methadone Hydrochloride Oral Concentrate ... 2356
Methadone Hydrochloride Oral Solution & Tablets ... 2357
Mexitil Capsules (About 4 in 1,000) ... 684
Midamor Tablets ... 1746
Miochol-E with Iocare Steri-Tags and Miochol-E System Pak (Rare) ... ◉ 263
Mivacron (Less than 1%) ... 1125
Monoket Tablets (Fewer than 1%) 2550
Monopril Tablets (0.4% to 1.0%) .. 762
Myochrysine Injection ... 1754
Nembutal Sodium Capsules (Less than 1%) ... 440
Nembutal Sodium Solution (Less than 1%) ... 442
Nembutal Sodium Suppositories (Less than 1%) ... 444
Neo-Synephrine Hydrochloride 1% Carpuject ... 2455
Neo-Synephrine Hydrochloride 1% Injection ... 2455
Nescaine/Nescaine MPF ... 549
Neurontin Capsules (Rare) ... 1978
Nimbex Injection (0.4%) ... 1131
Nimotop Capsules (Up to 1.0%) 603
Nipent for Injection (Less than 3%) ... 2733
Normodyne Injection (Rare) ... 2519
Normodyne Tablets (Rare) ... 2522
Norvasc Tablets (More than 0.1% to 1%) ... 2020
Novocain Hydrochloride for Spinal Anesthesia ... 2457
Nubain Injection (1% or less) ... 952
Ocupress Ophthalmic Solution, 1% Sterile ... ◉ 297
OptiPranolol (Metipranolol 0.3%) Sterile Ophthalmic Solution (A small number of patients) ... ◉ 256
Oramorph SR (Morphine Sulfate Sustained Release Tablets) (Less frequent) ... 2359
Orthoclone OKT3 Sterile Solution .. 1892
ParaGard T 380A Intrauterine Copper Contraceptive ... 1936
Parlodel (Less than 1%) ... 2411
Paxil Tablets (Infrequent) ... 2681
Permax Tablets (Infrequent) ... 571
Phenergan with Codeine ... 2883
Phenergan Injection ... 2880
Phenergan Tablets ... 2882
Phenergan VC with Codeine ... 2888
Phenobarbital Elixir and Tablets (Less than 1 in 100 patients) ... 1523
Prilosec Delayed-Release Capsules (Less than 1%) ... 516
Prinivil Tablets (0.3% to 1.0%) ... 1776
Prinzide Tablets ... 1780
▲ Proleukin for Injection (7%) ... 812
Prostigmin Injectable ... 1305
Prostigmin Tablets ... 1306
Protamine Sulfate Vials ... 1526
Prozac Pulvules & Liquid, Oral Solution (Rare) ... 935
RMS Suppositories CII ... 2766
Reglan ... 2243
Remeron Tablets (Infrequent) ... 1878
▲ ReoPro Vials (5.2%) ... 1526
Revex (nalmefene hydrochloride injection) (Less than 1%) ... 1863
Rilutek Tablets (Rare) ... 2198
Risperdal Tablets ... 1348
Robaxin Injectable ... 2245
Romazicon (Less than 1%) ... 2311
Roxanol ... 2365
Rythmol Tablets–150mg, 225mg, 300mg (0.5 to 1.5%) ... 1399
Salagen Tablets (Less than 1%) ... 1546
▲ Sandostatin Injection (25%) ... 2421
Seconal Sodium Pulvules (Less than 1 in 100) ... 1529
Sectral Capsules (Up to 2%) ... 2914
Sensorcaine ... 554
Ser-Ap-Es Tablets ... 867
Solganal Suspension ... 2530
▲ Sublimaze Injection (Among most common) ... 463
▲ Sufenta Injection (3% to 9%) ... 1355
Suprane (desflurane, USP) (Greater than 1%) ... 1865
Tagamet (Rare) ... 2694
Tambocor Tablets (Less than 1%) 1555
▲ Taxol Injection (3%) ... 723
Tenex Tablets (3% or less) ... 2249
▲ Tenoretic Tablets (3%) ... 2963
▲ Tenormin Tablets and I.V. Injection (3% to 18%) ... 2965
Tensilon Injectable ... 1307
Timolide Tablets (1.2%) ... 1791
Timoptic in Ocudose (Less frequent) ... 1796
Timoptic Sterile Ophthalmic Solution (Less frequent) ... 1794
Timoptic-XE ... 1798
Tonocard Tablets (0.4% to 1.8%) 519
▲ Toprol-XL Tablets (Approximately 3 of 100 patients) ... 560
Tracrium Injection ... 1155
Trandate (Rare) ... 1158
Trilafon ... 2532
Valium Injectable ... 2336
Vancocin HCl, Vials & ADD-Vantage (Infrequent) ... 1534
Vascor Tablets (200 and 300 mg) 1597
Vaseretic Tablets ... 1810
Vasotec I.V. ... 1814
Vasotec Tablets (0.5% to 1.0%) ... 1816
Verelan Capsules (1.4%) ... 1455
Versed Injection ... 2324
Virazole (Infrequent) ... 1310
Visken Tablets (2% or fewer patients) ... 2428
Xylocaine Injections ... 562
Zantac (Rare) ... 1182
Zantac Injection (Rare) ... 1180
Zantac Syrup (Rare) ... 1182
Zebeta Tablets (0.4% to 0.5%) ... 1457
Zestril Tablets (0.3% to 1.0%) ... 2972
Ziac (0.9% to 1.1%) ... 1459
Zofran Injection (Rare) ... 1227
▲ Zofran Tablets (6%) ... 1231
Zosyn (1.0% or less) ... 1463
Zyloprim Tablets (Less than 1%).... 1194

Bradycardia, fetal
Carbocaine Injection ... 2432
Duranest Injections ... 533
Nescaine/Nescaine MPF ... 549
▲ Prepidil Gel (4.1%) ... 2108
Sensorcaine ... 554
Sufenta Injection (One case) ... 1355
Syntocinon Injection ... 2425
Vasoxyl Injection ... 1169
▲ Xylocaine Injections (20% to 30%) ... 562

Bradycardia, neonatal
Diupres Tablets ... 1691
Hydropres Tablets ... 1718
Normodyne Injection ... 2519
Normodyne Tablets (Rare) ... 2522
Syntocinon Injection ... 2425
Tenoretic Tablets ... 2963
Tenormin Tablets and I.V. Injection 2965
Trandate ... 1158

Bradycardia, paradoxical
Ismo Tablets ... 2844
Isordil Sublingual Tablets ... 2845
Isordil Tembids ... 2847
Isordil Titradose Tablets ... 2848
Nitro-Bid IV ... 1270
Nitrostat Tablets ... 1981
Sorbitrate ... 2959
Transderm-Nitro Transdermal Therapeutic System ... 878

Bradycardia, severe
Eskalith ... 2658

Bradycardia, symptomatic
Kerlone Tablets (0.8% to 1.9%) 2588

Bradycardia, transient
Calan SR Caplets ... 2571
Calan Tablets ... 2568
Covera-HS Tablets (1.4%) ... 2573
▲ Survanta Beractant Intratracheal Suspension (11.9%) ... 2346
Wigraine Tablets ... 1884

Bradycardia with nodal escape rhythms
Isoptin SR Tablets ... 1395
Verelan Capsules ... 1455

Bradykinesia
Cognex Capsules (Infrequent) ... 1961
Effexor (Rare) ... 2825
Eldepryl Capsules ... 2729
Paxil Tablets ... 2681
Reglan ... 2243
▲ Wellbutrin Tablets (8.0%) ... 1177

Bradykinetic episodes
Atamet Tablets (Less frequent) ... 567
Larodopa Tablets (Infrequent) ... 2296
Sinemet Tablets (Less frequent) ... 959
Sinemet CR Tablets ... 961

Bradylogia
Imitrex Tablets (Rare) ... 1099

Bradypnea
Alfenta Injection ... 1334
Zoloft Tablets (Rare) ... 2051

Brain syndrome, acute
Betaseron for SC Injection ... 653
Cerebyx Injection (Infrequent) ... 1956
Doxil (Less than 1%) ... 2613
Permax Tablets (Infrequent) ... 571
Prozac Pulvules & Liquid, Oral Solution (Infrequent) ... 935
Rilutek Tablets (Rare) ... 2198
Videx Tablets, Powder for Oral Solution, & Pediatric Powder for Oral Solution (Less than 1%) ... 2980
Virazole ... 1310

Brain syndrome, chronic
Betaseron for SC Injection ... 653
Prozac Pulvules & Liquid, Oral Solution (Rare) ... 935

Brain syndrome, organic, acute
Garamycin Injectable ... 2502

Breast abscess
Lamictal Tablets (Rare) ... 1105
Rilutek Tablets (Rare) ... 2198
Videx Tablets, Powder for Oral Solution, & Pediatric Powder for Oral Solution (Less than 1%) ... 2980

Breast atrophy
Paxil Tablets (Rare) ... 2681
▲ Zoladex (33%) ... 2976

Breast carcinoma
Aldactazide Tablets ... 2556
Aldactone Tablets ... 2558
Ambien Tablets (Rare) ... 2559
Betaseron for SC Injection (2%) ... 653
Climara Transdermal System (Moderate increased risk) ... 640
Clomid ... 1262
Cognex Capsules (Rare) ... 1961
Demulen ... 2580
Depo-Provera Contraceptive Injection (Fewer than 1%) ... 2079
Estratest ... 2718
Eulexin Capsules (Two reports) ... 2498
Lamictal Tablets (Rare) ... 1105
Levlen/Tri-Levlen ... 646
Naprelan Tablets (Less than 1%) .. 2861
Ogen Tablets ... 2103
Ogen Vaginal Cream ... 2106
Ortho-Cyclen/Ortho-Tri-Cyclen ... 1914
Ortho-Est ... 1925
Ortho-Cyclen/Ortho Tri-Cyclen ... 1914
Paxil Tablets (Rare) ... 2681
Permax Tablets (Infrequent) ... 571
Premphase (A moderate increased risk) ... 2900
Prempro (A moderate increased risk) ... 2905
Protostat Tablets ... 1939
Redux Capsules ... 2911
Levlen/Tri-Levlen ... 646

Breast changes, unspecified
Brevicon ... 2563
Demulen ... 2580
Desogen Tablets ... 1867
▲ Emcyt Capsules (Up to 66%) ... 2085
Lo/Ovral Tablets ... 2852
Lo/Ovral-28 Tablets ... 2857
Lupron Depot 3.75 mg (Less than 5%) ... 2739
Lupron Depot-PED 7.5 mg, 11.25 mg and 15 mg (Less than 2%).... 2744
Lupron Injection Pediatric (Less than 2%) ... 2737
Modicon ... 1928
Nordette-21 Tablets ... 2863
Nordette-28 Tablets ... 2866
Norinyl ... 2563
Nor-Q D Tablets ... 2598
Ortho-Cept ... 1907
Ortho-Cyclen/Ortho-Tri-Cyclen ... 1914
Ortho-Novum ... 1928
Ortho-Cyclen/Ortho Tri-Cyclen ... 1914
Ovral Tablets ... 2877
Ovral-28 Tablets ... 2878
Ovrette Tablets ... 2878
Proglycem ... 575
Tri-Norinyl ... 2607
Triphasil-21 Tablets ... 2919
Triphasil-28 Tablets ... 2924

Breast engorgement
Adalat CC (Less than 1.0%) ... 582
Anafranil Capsules (Rare) ... 819
Betaseron for SC Injection ... 653
Desyrel and Desyrel Dividose ... 504
Effexor (Rare) ... 2825
Estring Vaginal Ring (At least 1 report) ... 2086
Haldol Decanoate ... 1587
Haldol Injection, Tablets and Concentrate ... 1585
Mellaril ... 2398
Permax Tablets (Rare) ... 571
Remeron Tablets (Rare) ... 1878
Ser-Ap-Es Tablets ... 867
Synarel Nasal Solution for Endometriosis (Less than 1%) ... 2605
Zoladex (Greater than 1% but less than 5%) ... 2976

Breast enlargement
Adapin Capsules ... 1542
Aldoclor Tablets ... 1638
Aldomet Ester HCl Injection ... 1642
Aldomet Oral ... 1640
Aldoril Tablets ... 1644
Anafranil Capsules (Up to 2%) ... 819
Asendin Tablets (Less than 1%) ... 1419
Brevicon ... 2563
Catapres-TTS ... 680
Claritin Tablets (Rare) ... 2485
Claritin-D Tablets ... 2487
Climara Transdermal System ... 640
Demser Capsules (Infrequent) ... 1690
Demulen ... 2580
Depakene ... 416
Depakote Tablets ... 418
Desogen Tablets ... 1867
Desyrel and Desyrel Dividose ... 504
Diethylstilbestrol Tablets ... 1477
Effexor (Rare) ... 2825
Elavil ... 2945
▲ Emcyt Capsules (60%) ... 2085
Estrace Cream and Tablets ... 751
Estraderm Transdermal System ... 842
ESTRATAB Tablets (0.3, 0.625, 1.25, 2.5 mg) ... 2715
Estratest ... 2718
Estring Vaginal Ring (At least 1 report) ... 2086
Etrafon ... 2495
Flexeril Tablets (Rare) ... 1701

(▣ Described in PDR For Nonprescription Drugs) Incidence data in parenthesis; ▲ 3% or more (◉ Described in PDR For Ophthalmology)

Breast enlargement — Side Effects Index — 1274

Indocin Capsules (Less than 1%) 1723
Indocin I.V. (Less than 1%) 1727
Indocin (Less than 1%) 1723
Levlen/Tri-Levlen 646
Limbitrol 2333
Ludiomil Tablets (Isolated reports) 861
Menest Tablets 2671
Modicon 1928
Navane Capsules and Concentrate 2018
Navane Intramuscular 2019
Norinyl 2563
Norpramin Tablets 1273
Nor-Q D Tablets 2598
Ogen Tablets 2103
Ogen Vaginal Cream 2106
Ortho-Cept 1907
Ortho-Cyclen/Ortho-Tri-Cyclen 1914
Ortho Dienestrol Cream 1922
Ortho-Est 1925
Ortho-Novum 1928
Ortho-Cyclen/Ortho Tri-Cyclen 1914
Ovcon 765
Pamelor 2409
Paxil Tablets (Rare) 2681
PMB 200 and PMB 400 2890
Premarin Intravenous 2893
Premarin Tablets 2896
Premarin Vaginal Cream 2898
Premphase 2900
Prempro 2905
Prevacid Delayed-Release Capsules (Less than 1%) 2746
Proscar Tablets 1784
ProSom Tablets (Rare) 457
Prozac Pulvules & Liquid, Oral Solution (Rare) 935
Redux Capsules 2911
Remeron Tablets (Rare) 1878
Serzone Tablets (Infrequent) 776
Sinequan 2028
▲ Supprelin Injection (1% to 10%) 2230
Surmontil Capsules 2917
▲ Synarel Nasal Solution for Central Precocious Puberty (8%) 2603
Thorazine 2701
THYREL TRH (A small number of patients) 2992
Tofranil Ampuls 873
Tofranil Tablets 875
Tofranil-PM Capsules 876
Triavil Tablets 1800
Trilafon 2532
Levlen/Tri-Levlen 646
Tri-Norinyl 2607
Triphasil-21 Tablets 2919
Triphasil-28 Tablets 2924
Vivactil Tablets 1820
Vivelle Transdermal System 880
▲ Zoladex (18%) 2976
Zoloft Tablets (Rare) 2051

Breast fibroadenosis

Ambien Tablets (Rare) 2559
Anafranil Capsules (Rare) 819
Avonex 662
Kerlone Tablets (Less than 2%) 2588

Breast, fibrocystic

Avonex 662
▲ Betaseron for SC Injection (3%) 653
Clomid 1262
Levlen/Tri-Levlen 646
Modicon 1928
Ortho-Cyclen/Ortho-Tri-Cyclen 1914
Ortho-Novum 1928
Ortho-Cyclen/Ortho Tri-Cyclen 1914
Paxil Tablets (Rare) 2681
Permax Tablets (Infrequent) 571
Prozac Pulvules & Liquid, Oral Solution (Infrequent) 935
Levlen/Tri-Levlen 646

Breast lumps

Avonex 662
Depo-Provera Contraceptive Injection (Fewer than 1%) 2079
Levlen/Tri-Levlen 646
Nipent for Injection (Less than 3%) 2733
Ortho-Cyclen/Ortho-Tri-Cyclen 1914
Ortho-Est 1925
Ortho-Cyclen/Ortho Tri-Cyclen 1914
Levlen/Tri-Levlen 646

Breast milk, maternal, excreted in

AVC 1245
Achromycin V Capsules 1417
Adalat Capsules (10 mg and 20 mg) 580
Adalat CC 582
Adderall Tablets 2209
Aldactazide Tablets 2556
Aldactone Tablets 2558
Aldoclor Tablets 1638
Aldomet Ester HCl Injection 1642
Aldomet Oral 1640
Aldoril Tablets 1644
Alfenta Injection 1334
Altace Capsules 1238
Ambien Tablets 2559
Amen Tablets 785
Anafranil Capsules 819
Anaprox/Naprosyn 2277
Androderm Testosterone Transdermal System 2634
Apresoline Hydrochloride Tablets 826
Asacol Delayed-Release Tablets 2129
Asendin Tablets 1419
Astramorph/PF Injection, USP (Preservative-Free) 526
Atretol Tablets 569
Atromid-S Capsules 2808
Augmentin 2637
Augmentin Tablets 2640
Axid Pulvules 1468
Axocet Capsules 2469
Azactam for Injection 736
Azathioprine Tablets 2349
Azulfidine 2059
Bactrim DS Tablets 2257
Bactrim I.V. Infusion 2255
Bactrim 2257
Bentyl 1246
Betapace Tablets 637
Biavax II 1653
Bicillin C-R Injection 2810
Bicillin C-R 900/300 Injection 2812
Bicillin L-A Injection 2813
Biltricide Tablets 584
Blocadren Tablets 1654
Brevicon 2563
Bricanyl Subcutaneous Injection 1247
Bricanyl Tablets 1248
Brontex 2130
Butisol Sodium Elixir & Tablets 2768
Cafergot 2376
Calan SR Caplets 2571
Calan Tablets 2568
Capoten Tablets 740
Capozide Tablets 744
Cardioquin Tablets 2146
Cardizem CD Capsules 1251
Cardizem SR Capsules 1255
Cardizem Injectable 1253
Cardizem Tablets 1257
Cataflam Tablets 833
Catapres Tablets 679
Catapres-TTS 680
Ceclor Pulvules & Suspension 1470
Cefizox for Intramuscular or Intravenous Use 1025
Cefotan 2936
Ceftin 1067
CellCept Capsules 2265
Ceptaz 1070
Cerebyx Injection 1956
Ceredase 1055
Cipro I.V. 587
Cipro Tablets 584
Claforan Sterile and Injection 1259
Claritin Tablets 2485
Cleocin Phosphate Injection 2068
Clozaril Tablets 2377
Combipres Tablets 682
Compazine 2644
Cordarone Intravenous 2821
Cordarone Tablets 2818
Cortisporin Cream 1073
Cortisporin Ointment 1074
Cortisporin Otic Solution Sterile 1076
Cortisporin Otic Suspension Sterile 1077
Cortone Acetate Sterile Suspension 1663
Cortone Acetate Tablets 1664
Coumadin 941
Covera-HS Tablets 2573
Cycrin Tablets 991
Cystospaz 2123
Cytotec 2576
Cytoxan 700
Dalalone D.P. Injectable 1009
Dapsone Tablets USP 1331
Daraprim Tablets 1199
Decadron Elixir 1676
Decadron Phosphate Injection 1680
Decadron Phosphate with Xylocaine Injection, Sterile 1683
Decadron Tablets 1678
Decadron-LA Sterile Suspension 1687
Deconsal II Tablets 1605
Demerol 2438
Demulen 2580
Depakene 416
Depakote Tablets 418
Depo-Provera Sterile Aqueous Suspension 2083
Desogen Tablets 1867
Desoxyn Gradumet Tablets 422
Desyrel and Desyrel Dividose 504
Dexacort Phosphate in Respihaler 1606
Dexacort Phosphate in Turbinaire 1607
Dexedrine 2648
DextroStat-Dextroamphetamine Sulfate Tablets 2211
Diabinese Tablets 2002
Diflucan Tablets, Injection, and Oral Suspension 2003
Dilacor XR Extended-release Capsules 2183
Dilantin Infatabs 1967
Dilantin Kapseals 1965
Dilantin-125 Suspension 1969
Dilaudid-HP Injection 1384
Dilaudid-HP Lyophilized Powder 250 mg 1384
Dilaudid Tablets and Liquid 1386
Diprivan Injectable Emulsion 2939
Disalcid 1549
Diucardin Tablets 2824
Diupres Tablets 1691
Diuril Oral Suspension 1694
Diuril Sodium Intravenous 1693
Diuril Tablets 1694
Dolobid Tablets 1695
Doral Tablets 2773
Doryx Capsules 1970
Duragesic Transdermal System 1336
Duramorph Injection 983
Duratuss HD Elixir 2750
Dyazide Capsules 2653
Dyrenium Capsules 2655
E.E.S. 427
E-Mycin Tablets 1388
EC-Naprosyn Delayed-Release Tablets 2277
Elavil 2945
Eltroxin Tablets 2214
EMLA Cream 536
Enduron Tablets 424
Ergomar Tablets 1543
ERYC 1972
EryPed 200 & EryPed 400 Granules 425
Ery-Tab Tablets 426
Erythrocin Stearate Filmtab 429
Esgic-plus Capsules 1012
Esgic-plus Tablets 1012
Esidrix Tablets 839
Esimil Tablets 840
Eskalith 2658
Ethmozine Tablets 2217
Fansidar Tablets 2281
Fedahist Gyrocaps 2545
Felbatol 2774
Fioricet Tablets 2386
Fioricet with Codeine Capsules 2387
Fiorinal Capsules 2388
Fiorinal with Codeine Capsules 2390
Fiorinal Tablets 2388
Flagyl 375 Capsules 2587
Flagyl I.V. 2373
Florinef Acetate Tablets 506
Floxin I.V. 1580
Floxin Tablets (200 mg, 300 mg, 400 mg) 1577
Fluorescite ◉ 217
Fortaz 1092
Gantanol Tablets 2285
Gantrisin 2286
Glucophage Tablets 754
Halcion Tablets 2093
Haldol Decanoate 1587
Haldol Injection, Tablets and Concentrate 1585
Helidac Therapy 2135
Hydeltrasol Injection, Sterile 1708
Hydeltra-T.B.A. Sterile Suspension 1710
Hydrocet Capsules 787
Hydrocortone Acetate Sterile Suspension 1712
Hydrocortone Phosphate Injection, Sterile 1713
Hydrocortone Tablets 1715
HydroDIURIL Tablets 1716
Hydropres Tablets 1718
IFEX 706
Ilosone 927
Imitrex Injection 1095
Imitrex Tablets 1099
Imuran 1103
Inderal 2834
Inderal LA Long Acting Capsules 2836
Inderide Tablets 2838
Inderide LA Long Acting Capsules 2840
Indocin 1723
INFeD (Iron Dextran Injection, USP) 2478
Inversine Tablets 1729
Isoptin Injectable 1391
Isoptin Oral Tablets 1393
Isoptin SR Tablets 1395
Kadian Capsules 2948
Keflex Pulvules & Oral Suspension 930
Kefurox Vials, Faspak & ADD-Vantage 1509
Kefzol Vials, Faspak & ADD-Vantage 1511
Kerlone Tablets (Less than 2%) 2588
Kutrase Capsules 2546
Kwell Cream & Lotion 2172
Kwell Shampoo 2173
Lamictal Tablets 1105
Lamisil Tablets 2394
Lamprene Capsules 846
Lanoxicaps 1110
Lanoxin Injection 1116
Lanoxin Tablets 1121
Lariam Tablets 2295
Lasix Injection, Oral Solution and Tablets 1267
Lescol Capsules 2395
Levbid Extended-Release Tablets 2549
Levlen/Tri-Levlen 646
Levothroid Tablets 1015
Levoxyl Tablets 918
Levsin/Levsinex/Levbid 2549
Lindane Lotion USP 1% 481
Lindane Shampoo USP 1% 483
Lioresal Intrathecal 1634
Lithium Carbonate Capsules & Tablets 2352
Lithonate/Lithotabs/Lithobid 2721
Lomotil 2591
Lo/Ovral Tablets 2852
Lo/Ovral-28 Tablets 2857
Lopressor 848
Lopressor HCT Tablets 850
Lortab 2751
Lotensin Tablets 852
Lotensin HCT Tablets 855
Lotrel Capsules 858
Ludiomil Tablets 861
Lufyllin & Lufyllin-400 Tablets 2778
Lufyllin-GG Elixir & Tablets 2779
LUVOX Tablets 2723
MS Contin Tablets 2149
MSIR Oral Solution 2152
Macrobid Capsules 2138
Macrodantin Capsules 2140
Marinol (Dronabinol) Capsules 2353
Maxipime for Injection 758
Mefoxin 1734
Mefoxin Premixed Intravenous Solution 1737
Mepergan Injection 2859
Meruvax II 1740
Methergine 2401
Methotrexate Sodium Tablets, Injection, for Injection and LPF Injection 1322
MetroCream 1034
MetroGel 1034
Mexitil Capsules 684
Mezlin 594
Micronor Tablets 1903
Midamor Tablets 1746
Miltown Tablets 2780
Minizide Capsules 2016
Minocin Intravenous 1428
Minocin Oral Suspension 1431
Minocin Pellet-Filled Capsules 1429
Modicon 1928
Moduretic Tablets 1748
Monocid Injection 2674
Monodox Capsules 1858
Mono-Gesic Tablets 810
Monopril Tablets 762
Mykrox Tablets 1617
Myochrysine Injection 1754
Mysoline 2860
Naprelan Tablets 2861
Anaprox/Naprosyn 2277
Nembutal Sodium Solution 442
Neoral 2405
Nicotrol NS Nicotine Nasal Spray 1565
Nizoral Tablets 1345
Nordette-21 Tablets 2863
Nordette-28 Tablets 2866
Norinyl 2563
Norisodrine with Calcium Iodide Syrup 446
Normodyne Injection 2519
Normodyne Tablets 2522
Norpace 2596

(▣ Described in PDR For Nonprescription Drugs) Incidence data in parenthesis; ▲ 3% or more (◉ Described in PDR For Ophthalmology)

1275 Side Effects Index Breath, shortness

Norplant System 2868
Nor-Q D Tablets 2598
Nucofed 2225
Nydrazid Injection 509
Omnipen for Oral Suspension 2873
Oramorph SR (Morphine Sulfate Sustained Release Tablets) 2359
Oretic Tablets 450
Ortho-Cept 1907
Ortho-Cyclen/Ortho-Tri-Cyclen 1914
Ortho-Novum 1928
Ortho-Cyclen/Ortho Tri-Cyclen 1914
Ovcon 765
Ovral Tablets 2877
Ovral-28 Tablets 2878
Ovrette Tablets 2878
Oxistat 1139
OxyContin Tablets 2163
PCE Dispertab Tablets 453
Paxil Tablets 2681
Pediapred Oral Solution 1618
Pediazole Suspension 2340
Pediotic Suspension Sterile 1140
Pentasa 1275
Pepcid Injection 1765
Pepcid 1763
Persantine Tablets 686
Pfizerpen for Injection 2022
Phenergan with Codeine 2883
Phenergan VC with Codeine 2888
Phenobarbital Elixir and Tablets 1523
Phrenilin 790
PMB 200 and PMB 400 2890
Pravachol Tablets 770
Premphase 2900
Prempro 2905
Prevacid Delayed-Release Capsules 2746
Prinzide Tablets 1780
Procanbid Extended-Release Tablets 1983
Prograf 1028
Proloprim Tablets 1141
Propulsid 1346
Prostep (nicotine transdermal system) 1439
Protostat Tablets 1939
Provera Tablets 2110
Prozac Pulvules & Liquid, Oral Solution 935
Psorcon Cream 0.05% 924
Pyrazinamide Tablets 1442
Quadrinal Tablets 1398
Quibron 2227
Quinaglute Dura-Tabs Tablets 644
Quinidex Extentabs 2240
RMS Suppositories CII 2766
Reglan 2243
Retrovir I.V. Infusion 1221
Ridaura Capsules 2691
Rifamate Capsules 1278
Rifater 1280
Rimactane Capsules 865
Robaxisal Tablets 2246
Rocaltrol Capsules 2303
Rocephin Injectable Vials, ADD-Vantage, Galaxy Container 2305
Roxanol 2365
Salflex Tablets 791
Sandimmune 2416
Sansert Tablets 2424
Sectral Capsules 2914
Sedapap Tablets 50 mg/650 mg 1826
Semprex-D Capsules 1620
Septra 1146
Septra I.V. Infusion 1142
Septra I.V. Infusion ADD-Vantage Vials 1144
Septra 1146
Ser-Ap-Es Tablets 867
Slo-bid Gyrocaps 2201
Solganal Suspension 2530
Soma Compound w/Codeine Tablets 2784
Soma Compound Tablets 2783
Soma Tablets 2782
Spectrobid Tablets 2030
Sporanox Capsules 1352
Stadol 779
Stelazine 2692
Symmetrel Capsules 965
Symmetrel Syrup 963
Syn-Rx Tablets 1622
Syn-Rx DM Tablets 1623
Synthroid 1410
Syntocinon Injection 2425
Tagamet 2694
Tambocor Tablets 1555
Tapazole Tablets 1361
Tavist Syrup 2426
Tazicef for Injection 2697
Tazidime Vials, Faspak & ADD-Vantage 1531
Tegretol/Tegretol-XR 870
Tenoretic Tablets 2963
Tenormin Tablets and I.V. Injection 2965
Testoderm Testosterone Transdermal System 486
Thalitone 1293
Theo-24 Extended Release Capsules 2753
Theo-Dur Extended-Release Tablets 1367
Theo-X Extended-Release Tablets 793
Thorazine 2701
Tiazac Capsules 1019
Timolide Tablets 1791
Timoptic in Ocudose 1796
Timoptic Sterile Ophthalmic Solution 1794
Timoptic-XE 1798
Tofranil Ampuls 873
Tofranil Tablets 875
Tofranil-PM Capsules 876
Tolectin (200, 400 and 600 mg) 1591
Toprol-XL Tablets 560
Toradol 2319
Trandate 1158
Tranxene 459
Trental Tablets 1291
Levlen/Tri-Levlen 646
Trilisate 2155
Trimpex Tablets 2323
Tri-Norinyl 2607
Triostat Injection 2708
Triphasil-21 Tablets 2919
Triphasil-28 Tablets 2924
Tylenol with Codeine 1592
Ultram Tablets (50 mg) 1594
Unasyn 2035
Uni-Dur Extended-Release Tablets 1374
Uniphyl 400 mg and 600 mg Tablets 2157
Uroqid-Acid No. 2 Tablets 633
Vanceril Inhaler 2538
Vancocin HCl, Oral Solution & Pulvules 1536
Vancocin HCl, Vials & ADD-Vantage 1534
Vantin for Oral Suspension and Vantin Tablets 2112
Vascor Tablets (200 and 300 mg) 1597
Vaseretic Tablets 1810
Vasotec Tablets 1816
Verelan Capsules 1455
Versed Injection 2324
Vibramycin 2038
Vibramycin Hyclate Intravenous 2040
Vibramycin 2038
Vicodin ES Tablets 1405
Vicodin HP Tablets 1403
Viramune Tablets 2368
Visken Tablets 2428
Cataflam/Voltaren/Voltaren-XR 833
Wygesic Tablets 2930
Xanax Tablets 2115
Zantac 1182
Zantac Injection 1180
Zantac Syrup 1182
Zaroxolyn Tablets 1625
Zestoretic Tablets 2968
Ziac 1459
Zinacef 1184
Zonalon Cream 1042
Zosyn 1463
Zovirax Capsules 1187
Zovirax Sterile Powder 1191
Zovirax 1187
Zyloprim Tablets 1194
Zyrtec Tablets 2053

Breast nipple bleeding

Depo-Provera Contraceptive Injection (Fewer than 1%) 2079

Breast pain

Anafranil Capsules (Up to 1%) 819
Arimidex Tablets (2% to 5%) 2932
▲ Betaseron for SC Injection (7%) 653
Cardura Tablets (Less than 0.5% of 3960 patients) 1993
Cipro Tablets (0.3% to 1%) 584
Claritin-D Tablets 2487
Clomid (1.5%) 1262
Clozaril Tablets (Less than 1%) 2377
Cognex Capsules (Infrequent) 1961
Cytovene (1% or less) 2270
Effexor (Infrequent) 2825
Estring Vaginal Ring (1%) 2086
Humegon for Injection (Occasional) 1873
Imdur (Less than or equal to 5%) 1362
Lamictal Tablets (Infrequent) 1105
Lupron Depot 3.75 mg (Less than 5%) 2739
LUVOX Tablets (Infrequent) 2723
Paxil Tablets (Infrequent) 2681
Pentasa (Less than 1%) 1275
▲ Premphase (Approximately one-third of subjects) 2900
▲ Prempro (Approximately one-third of subjects) 2905
Prinzide Tablets 1780
Procardia XL Extended Release Tablets (1% or less) 2026
Prozac Pulvules & Liquid, Oral Solution (Infrequent) 935
Redux Capsules (Infrequent) 2911
Remeron Tablets (Infrequent) 1878
Rilutek Tablets (Rare) 2198
Sporanox Capsules (Infrequent) 1352
▲ Zoladex (7%) 2976
Zoladex 3-month (1% to 5%) 2978
Zoloft Tablets (Rare) 2051

Breast secretion

Brevicon 2563
Danocrine Capsules (Rare) 2437
Demulen 2580
Desogen Tablets 1867
Diethylstilbestrol Tablets 1477
ESTRATAB Tablets (0.3, 0.625, 1.25, 2.5 mg) 2715
Estratest 2718
Imitrex Tablets (Rare) 1099
Levlen/Tri-Levlen 646
Menest Tablets 2671
Modicon 1928
Norinyl 2563
▲ Norplant System (5% or greater) 2868
Nor-Q D Tablets 2598
Ortho-Cept 1907
Ortho-Cyclen/Ortho-Tri-Cyclen 1914
Ortho Dienestrol Cream 1922
Ortho-Novum 1928
Ortho-Cyclen/Ortho Tri-Cyclen 1914
Ovcon 765
PMB 200 and PMB 400 2890
Premarin Intravenous 2893
Premarin Vaginal Cream 2898
▲ Supprelin Injection (1% to 12%) 2230
Levlen/Tri-Levlen 646
Tri-Norinyl 2607

Breast size reduction

Danocrine Capsules 2437
Supprelin Injection (2% to 3%) 2230
▲ Synarel Nasal Solution for Endometriosis (10% of patients) 2605

Breast size, changes

Depo-Provera Contraceptive Injection (Fewer than 1%) 2079

Breast tenderness

Amen Tablets (Rare) 785
Azactam for Injection (Less than 1%) 736
Brevicon 2563
Bumex (0.1%) 2260
Climara Transdermal System 640
Cycrin Tablets (Rare) 991
▲ Demulen (Among most common) 2580
Depo-Provera Sterile Aqueous Suspension 2083
Desogen Tablets 1867
Diethylstilbestrol Tablets 1477
▲ Emcyt Capsules (66%) 2085
Estrace Cream and Tablets 751
Estraderm Transdermal System 842
ESTRATAB Tablets (0.3, 0.625, 1.25, 2.5 mg) 2715
Estratest 2718
Imitrex Tablets (Infrequent) 1099
Indocin Capsules (Less than 1%) 1723
Indocin I.V. (Less than 1%) 1727
Indocin (Less than 1%) 1723
Levlen/Tri-Levlen 646
Lo/Ovral Tablets 2852
Lo/Ovral-28 Tablets 2857
Lupron Depot 3.75 mg (Less than 5%) 2739
▲ Lupron Injection (5% or more) 2736
Menest Tablets 2671
Metrodin (urofollitropin for injection) 2616
Micronor Tablets (Less common) 1903
Modicon 1928
Norinyl 2563
Nor-Q D Tablets 2598
Ogen Tablets 2103
Ogen Vaginal Cream 2106
Ortho-Cept 1907
Ortho-Cyclen/Ortho-Tri-Cyclen 1914
Ortho Dienestrol Cream 1922
Ortho-Est 1925
Ortho-Novum 1928
Ortho-Cyclen/Ortho Tri-Cyclen 1914
Ovcon 765
Ovral Tablets 2877
Ovral-28 Tablets 2878
Ovrette Tablets 2878
PMB 200 and PMB 400 2890
Premarin Intravenous 2893
Premarin Tablets 2896
Premarin Vaginal Cream 2898
Premphase 2900
Prempro 2905
Prevacid Delayed-Release Capsules (Less than 1%) 2746
Proscar Tablets 1784
Prostin E2 Suppository 2109
Provera Tablets (Rare) 2110
Serophene (clomiphene citrate tablets, USP) (Approximately 1 in 50) 2621
Testoderm Testosterone Transdermal System (Three in 104 patients) 486
Levlen/Tri-Levlen 646
Tri-Norinyl 2607
Triphasil-21 Tablets 2919
Triphasil-28 Tablets 2924
Vivelle Transdermal System 880
Zoladex (Greater than 1% but less than 5%) 2976
Zoladex 3-month 2978

Breath, shortness

Adalat Capsules (10 mg and 20 mg) (2% or less) 580
▲ Adenocard Injection (12%) 1021
AeroBid Inhaler System (Less than 1%) 1004
Aerobid-M Inhaler System (Less than 1%) 1004
▲ Axocet Capsules (Among most frequent) 2469
▲ Bromfed-DM Cough Syrup (Among most frequent) 1832
BuSpar Tablets (Infrequent) 738
Ceftin (0.1% to 1%) 1067
Clomid 1262
Clozaril Tablets (1%) 2377
Colestid (Infrequent) 2073
Coumadin 941
Cytosar-U Sterile Powder (Less frequent) 2077
Dalmane Capsules (Rare) 2329
Demulen 2580
Desyrel and Desyrel Dividose (Less than 1% to 1.3%) 504
Dimetane-DC Cough Syrup 2232
Dimetane-DX Cough Syrup 2233
Dipentum Capsules (Rare) 2084
Dobutrex Solution Vials (1% to 3%) 1480
▲ Doxil (Approximately 6.8%) 2613
DynaCirc Capsules (0.5% to 1%) 2381
DynaCirc CR Tablets (0.5% to 1.0%) 2383
Eldepryl Capsules 2729
▲ Epogen for Injection (0.14% to 14%) 489
▲ Esgic-plus Capsules (Among most frequent) 1012
▲ Esgic-plus Tablets (Among most frequent) 1012
Estrace Cream and Tablets 751
▲ Fioricet Tablets (Among most frequent) 2386
Fioricet with Codeine Capsules (Frequent) 2387
Floxin I.V. 1580
Floxin Tablets (200 mg, 300 mg, 400 mg) 1577
Gamimune N, 5% Immune Globulin Intravenous (Human), 5% 612
Gamimune N, 10% Immune Globulin Intravenous (Human), 10% 615
Gantrisin 2286
Guaifed 1833
Hespan Injection 945
Humalog Injection (Less common) 1488
Humulin 50/50, 100 Units 1491
Humulin 70/30, 100 Units (Less common) 1492
Humulin L, 100 Units (Less common) 1494
▲ Hylorel Tablets (18.3% to 45.9%) 1613
Regular, 100 Units (Less common) 1503

(▭ Described in PDR For Nonprescription Drugs) Incidence data in parenthesis; ▲ 3% or more (◉ Described in PDR For Ophthalmology)

Breath, shortness

Pork Regular, 100 Units (Less common) ... 1507
Imitrex Injection ... 1095
Imitrex Tablets ... 1099
IOPIDINE Sterile Ophthalmic Solution ... ⊚ 218
K-Phos Neutral Tablets ... 633
K-Phos Original Formula 'Sodium Free' Tablets (Less frequent) ... 633
Klonopin Tablets ... 2294
Kytril Injection (Rare) ... 2667
Kytril Tablets (Rare) ... 2669
▲ Leustatin (7%) ... 1889
Levlen/Tri-Levlen ... 646
▲ Lopressor (3%) ... 848
Lopressor HCT Tablets ... 850
Midamor Tablets (Less than or equal to 1%) ... 1746
Modicon ... 1928
Moduretic Tablets ... 1748
▲ Navelbine Injection (3%; infrequent) ... 1212
Norpace (1 to 3%) ... 2596
Novolin 70/30 Prefilled Disposable Insulin Delivery System (Rare) ... 1850
Oncovin Solution Vials & Hyporets ... 1521
Ortho-Cyclen/Ortho-Tri-Cyclen ... 1914
Ortho-Est ... 1925
Ortho-Novum ... 1928
Ortho-Cyclen/Ortho Tri-Cyclen ... 1914
Orthoclone OKT3 Sterile Solution ... 1892
Parlodel (Less than 1%) ... 2411
Pediazole Suspension ... 2340
Peptavlon ... 2997
▲ Phrenilin (Among most frequent) ... 790
Procardia Capsules (2% or less) ... 2024
▲ Procrit for Injection (0.14% to 14%) ... 1896
Profasi (chorionic gonadotropin for injection, USP) ... 2620
Quadrinal Tablets ... 1398
Questran ... 774
Retrovir Capsules ... 1216
Retrovir I.V. Infusion ... 1221
Retrovir Syrup ... 1216
ReVia Tablets (Less than 1%) ... 957
Rifadin ... 1276
Rifater ... 1280
Sandostatin Injection (Less than 1%) ... 2421
Sansert Tablets ... 2424
▲ Sedapap Tablets 50 mg/650 mg (Among the most frequent) ... 1826
Septra (Rare) ... 1146
Septra I.V. Infusion ... 1142
Septra I.V. Infusion ADD-Vantage Vials ... 1144
Septra (Rare) ... 1146
Soma Compound Tablets ... 2783
Synarel Nasal Solution for Central Precocious Puberty (2.6%) ... 2603
▲ THROMBATE III Antithrombin III (Human) (1 of 17) ... 631
Thyro-Block Tablets (A few people) ... 2785
▲ Toprol-XL Tablets (Approximately 3 of 100 patients) ... 560
Levlen/Tri-Levlen ... 646
▲ Tylenol with Codeine (Among most frequent) ... 1592
Uroqid-Acid No. 2 Tablets ... 633
Velban Vials ... 1537
Velosulin BR Human Insulin 10 ml Vials ... 1847
Vivelle Transdermal System ... 880
Wellbutrin Tablets (Infrequent) ... 1177
Zofran Injection (Rare) ... 1227

Breathholding

▲ Suprane (desflurane, USP) (30% to 68%) ... 1865

Breathing, difficult
(see under Dyspnea)

Breathing, irregular

Dilaudid Ampules ... 1382
Dilaudid Cough Syrup ... 1383
Dilaudid-HP Injection ... 1384
Dilaudid-HP Lyophilized Powder 250 mg ... 1384
Dilaudid ... 1382
Hydrocet Capsules ... 787
Larodopa Tablets (Infrequent) ... 2296
Lortab ... 2751
Monopril Tablets (0.4% to 1.0%) ... 1928
Quadrinal Tablets ... 1398
Sinemet CR Tablets ... 961
Supprelin Injection (2% to 3%) ... 2230
Vicodin Tablets ... 1404
Vicodin ES Tablets ... 1405

Zydone Capsules ... 967

Breathing, labored
(see under Dyspnea)

Breathing, shallow
(see under Hypopnea)

Breathing, stertorous

Duragesic Transdermal System (Less than 1%) ... 1336
Neurontin Capsules (Rare) ... 1978

Bromsulphalein retention, increase
(see under BSP retention, increase)

Bronchial constriction

Vaqta (Less than 1%) ... 1805

Bronchial obstruction

Blocadren Tablets ... 1654
Timoptic in Ocudose ... 1796
Timoptic Sterile Ophthalmic Solution ... 1794
Timoptic-XE ... 1798

Bronchial secretion, decreased

Atrovent Inhalation Aerosol (About 1 in 100) ... 674

Bronchial secretions, increase

Klonopin Tablets ... 2294
Mestinon Injectable ... 1300
Mestinon ... 1300
Prostigmin Injectable ... 1305
Prostigmin Tablets ... 1306
Tensilon Injectable ... 1307

Bronchial secretions, thickening

Atrohist Plus Tablets ... 1605
▲ Benadryl Injection (Among most frequent) ... 1955
Betoptic Ophthalmic Solution (Rare) ... 465
Betoptic S Ophthalmic Suspension (Rare) ... 467
▲ Bromfed-DM Cough Syrup (Among most frequent) ... 1832
▲ Dimetane-DC Cough Syrup (Most frequent) ... 2232
▲ Dimetane-DX Cough Syrup (Among most frequent) ... 2233
Ornade Spansule Capsules ... 2678
▲ PBZ Tablets (Among most frequent) ... 863
▲ PBZ-SR Tablets (Among most frequent) ... 862
Periactin ... 1767
▲ Tavist Syrup (Among most frequent) ... 2426
▲ Tavist Tablets (Among most frequent) ... 2427
▲ Trinalin Repetabs Tablets (Among most frequent) ... 1373
Tussend ... 1830

Bronchiectasis

Pulmozyme Inhalation ... 1054
Videx Tablets, Powder for Oral Solution, & Pediatric Powder for Oral Solution (Less than 1%) ... 2980

Bronchiolitis

Cuprimine Capsules ... 1673
Haldol Decanoate ... 1587
▲ Proventil Solution for Inhalation 0.5% (1.5% to 4%) ... 2525
Solganal Suspension ... 2530
▲ Tetramune (Among most common) ... 1449

Bronchiolitis, obliterative

Depen Titratable Tablets (Rare) ... 2770
Pentasa (One case) ... 1275

Bronchitis

▲ Actigall Capsules (6.5%) ... 818
AeroBid Inhaler System (1% to 3%) ... 1004
Aerobid-M Inhaler System (1% to 3%) ... 1004
Airet Albuterol Sulfate Inhalation Solution (1.5% to 4%) ... 1602
Albuterol Sulfate, USP Solution for Inhalation, Arm-a-Med (1.5% to 4%) ... 522
Ambien Tablets (Infrequent) ... 2559
Anafranil Capsules (Infrequent) ... 819
Arimidex Tablets (2% to 5%) ... 2932

▲ Atrovent Inhalation Solution (14.6%) ... 675
Cartrol Tablets (Less common) ... 413
Casodex Tablets (2% to 5%) ... 2934
▲ CellCept Capsules (8.5% to 11.9%) ... 2265
Cerebyx Injection (Infrequent) ... 1956
Claritin Tablets (2% or fewer patients) ... 2485
Claritin-D Tablets (Less frequent) ... 2487
Clozaril Tablets (Less than 1%) ... 2377
Cognex Capsules (Frequent) ... 1961
Cozaar Tablets (Less than 1%) ... 1668
Cytotec (Infrequent) ... 2576
Dilacor XR Extended-release Capsules (Infrequent) ... 2183
Doxil (Less than 1%) ... 2613
Effexor (Frequent) ... 2825
Estring Vaginal Ring (1% to 3%) ... 2086
Flonase Nasal Spray (Less than 1%) ... 1088
Flovent (1% to 3%) ... 1089
Fludara for Injection (Up to 1%) ... 658
Foscavir Injection (Less than 1%) ... 541
Hytrin Capsules (At least 1%) ... 434
Hyzaar Tablets (1% or greater) ... 1720
Imdur (Less than or equal to 5%) ... 1362
Intron A for Injection (Less than or equal to 5%) ... 2506
Invirase Capsules (Less than 2%) ... 2291
Ismo Tablets (Fewer than 1%) ... 2844
Kerlone Tablets (Less than 2%) ... 2588
Lodine Capsules and Tablets (Less than 1%) ... 2849
Lotensin Tablets ... 852
Lotensin HCT Tablets (0.3% or more) ... 855
LUVOX Tablets (Infrequent) ... 2723
Miacalcin Nasal Spray (Less than 1%) ... 2403
Naprelan Tablets (Less than 3%) ... 2861
Nicotrol NS Nicotine Nasal Spray (Less than 1%) ... 1565
▲ Nipent for Injection (3%) ... 2733
OptiPranolol (Metipranolol 0.3%) Sterile Ophthalmic Solution (A small number of patients) ... ⊚ 256
Paxil Tablets (Infrequent) ... 2681
Permax Tablets (Infrequent) ... 571
Plendil Extended-Release Tablets (0.5% to 1.5%) ... 514
Prevacid Delayed-Release Capsules (Less than 1%) ... 2746
Prinivil Tablets (0.3% to 1.0%) ... 1776
Prinzide Tablets (0.3 to 1%) ... 1780
▲ Prograf (Greater than 3%) ... 1028
Proventil Inhalation Solution 0.083% (1.5% to 4%) ... 2527
Prozac Pulvules & Liquid, Oral Solution (Frequent) ... 935
Pulmozyme Inhalation ... 1054
▲ Redux Capsules (3.4%) ... 2911
Remeron Tablets (Infrequent) ... 1878
Ridaura Capsules (Rare) ... 2691
Rilutek Tablets (More than 2%) ... 2198
Serevent Inhalation Aerosol (1% to 3%) ... 1149
Serzone Tablets (Frequent) ... 776
Stadol (1% or greater) ... 779
Supprelin Injection (2% to 3%) ... 2230
▲ Tetramune (Among most common) ... 1449
Tilade Inhaler (1.2%) ... 2207
Vaseretic Tablets ... 1810
Vasotec I.V. ... 1814
Vasotec Tablets (0.5% to 1.0%) ... 1816
▲ Ventolin Inhalation Solution (1.5% to 4%) ... 1171
Ventolin Nebules Inhalation Solution (1.5% to 4%) ... 1172
Videx Tablets, Powder for Oral Solution, & Pediatric Powder for Oral Solution (Up to 1%) ... 2980
Vistide Injection ... 1057
Wellbutrin Tablets (Infrequent) ... 1177
Zebeta Tablets ... 1457
Zestoretic Tablets (0.3 to 1%) ... 2968
Zestril Tablets (0.3% to 1.0%) ... 2972
Ziac ... 1459
Zoladex (1% or greater) ... 2976
Zoladex 3-month ... 2978
Zyrtec Tablets (Less than 2%) ... 2053

Bronchoconstriction

Intron A for Injection (Rare) ... 2506
Platinol for Injection ... 717
Platinol-AQ Injection ... 719
Sublimaze Injection ... 463
Tensilon Injectable ... 1307
Urecholine ... 1804

Bronchoconstriction, paradoxical

Maxair Inhaler ... 1552
Metaproterenol Sulfate Inhalation Solution, USP, Arm-a-Med ... 547
Tornalate Solution for Inhalation, 0.2% ... 976
Tornalate Metered Dose Inhaler ... 978

Bronchospasm

Abbokinase ... 403
Abbokinase Open-Cath ... 405
Abelcet Injection ... 1540
Actimmune (Rare) ... 1043
Adenocard Injection ... 1021
Airet Albuterol Sulfate Inhalation Solution (Rare) ... 1602
▲ Albuterol Sulfate, USP Solution for Inhalation, Arm-a-Med (8% to 15.4%) ... 522
Alfenta Injection (0.3% to 1%) ... 1334
Alkeran for Injection (In some patients) ... 1196
Ambien Tablets (Rare) ... 2559
▲ Anafranil Capsules (2% to 7%) ... 819
Atrovent Inhalation Solution (2.3%) ... 675
Atrovent Nasal Spray 0.06% (Rare) ... 678
Axid Pulvules (Rare) ... 1468
Azactam for Injection (Less than 1%) ... 736
Beclovent Inhalation Aerosol and Refill (Rare) ... 1063
Beconase (Rare) ... 1065
Betagan ... ⊚ 230
Betimol 0.25%, 0.5% ... ⊚ 259
Betoptic Ophthalmic Solution (Rare) ... 465
Betoptic S Ophthalmic Suspension (Rare) ... 467
Blocadren Tablets (0.6%) ... 1654
Brevibloc (esmolol HCl) Injection (Less than 1%) ... 1860
Calcimar Injection, Synthetic (A few cases) ... 2176
Capoten Tablets ... 740
Capozide Tablets ... 744
Cardioquin Tablets ... 2146
Cardura Tablets (Less than 0.5% of 3960 patients) ... 1993
Cartrol Tablets (Rare) ... 413
Cataflam Tablets ... 833
Ceptaz (Very rare) ... 1070
Cipro Tablets (Less than 1%) ... 584
Claritin Tablets (2% or fewer patients) ... 2485
Claritin-D Tablets (Less frequent) ... 2487
Clinoril Tablets (Less than 1 in 100) ... 1658
Cytotec (Infrequent) ... 2576
Dilaudid-HP Injection (Less frequent) ... 1384
Dilaudid-HP Lyophilized Powder 250 mg (Less frequent) ... 1384
Dilaudid Tablets and Liquid ... 1386
Dipentum Capsules (Rare) ... 2084
Diprivan Injectable Emulsion (Rare; less than 1%) ... 2939
Disalcid ... 1549
Dobutrex Solution Vials (Occasional) ... 1480
Dolobid Tablets (Less than 1 in 100) ... 1695
Dopram Injectable ... 2235
Eminase ... 2215
EMLA Cream ... 536
Engerix-B Unit-Dose Vials ... 2656
▲ Etopophos for Injection (3%) ... 701
Etoposide Injection (0.7% to 2%) ... 539
Factrel (Rare) ... 2996
Feldene Capsules (Less than 1%) ... 2008
Flonase Nasal Spray (Rare) ... 1088
Flovent (Rare) ... 1089
Floxin I.V. ... 1580
Floxin Tablets (200 mg, 300 mg, 400 mg) ... 1577
Flumadine Tablets & Syrup (Less than 0.3%) ... 1013
Fluorescite ... ⊚ 217
Fortaz (Very rare) ... 1092
Foscavir Injection (Between 1% and 5%) ... 541
Fungizone Intravenous ... 507
Gemzar for Injection (Less than 2%) ... 1482
Haldol Decanoate ... 1587
Haldol Injection, Tablets and Concentrate ... 1585
Hespan Injection ... 945
Hismanal Tablets (Less frequent) ... 1341
IBU Tablets (Less than 1%) ... 1389

1277 **Side Effects Index** **Burning**

Imdur (Less than or equal to 5%) .. 1362
Imitrex Injection (1%) 1095
Inapsine Injection (Less common) .. 462
Inderal 2834
Inderal LA Long Acting Capsules 2836
Inderide Tablets 2838
Inderide LA Long Acting Capsules .. 2840
INFeD (Iron Dextran Injection, USP) 2478
▲ Intal Inhaler (Among most frequent) 2185
Intal Nebulizer Solution (Rare) 2186
Intron A for Injection (Less than or equal to 5%) 2506
Isoptin Injectable (Rare) 1391
Kerlone Tablets (Less than 2%) 2588
Lamictal Tablets (Rare) 1105
Lopressor HCT Tablets (Fewer than 1 in 100) 850
Lutrepulse for Injection 998
Maxaquin Tablets (Less than 1%) .. 2593
Metubine Iodide Vials 932
Miacalcin Injection (A few cases) 2402
Miacalcin Nasal Spray (1% to 3%) 2403
Miltown Tablets (Rare) 2780
Mivacron (Less than 1%) 1125
Monopril Tablets (0.2% to 1.0%) .. 762
Motrin Ibuprofen Suspension, Oral Drops, Chewable Tablets, Caplets (Less than 1%) 1563
Mykrox Tablets 1617
Navelbine Injection (Infrequent) 1212
Neurontin Capsules (Rare) 1978
Nicotrol NS Nicotine Nasal Spray (Less than 1%) 1565
Nimbex Injection (0.2%; one patient) 1131
Nipent for Injection (Less than 3%) 2733
Norcuron for Injection (Rare) 1875
Normodyne Tablets (Less common) 2522
Nubain Injection (1% or less) 952
Nuromax Injection (Less than or equal to 0.1%) 1136
Ocupress Ophthalmic Solution, 1% Sterile .... ⊙ 297
▲ Oncaspar (Less than 1% to greater than 5%) 2194
Oncovin Solution Vials & Hyporets 1521
Orthoclone OKT3 Sterile Solution .. 1892
Orudis Capsules (Less than 1%) 2874
Oruvail Capsules (Less than 1%) 2874
Paraplatin for Injection (Rare) 713
Pepcid Injection (Infrequent) 1765
Pepcid (Infrequent) 1763
PMB 200 and PMB 400 (Rare) 2890
Prinivil Tablets (0.3% to 1.0%) 1776
Prinzide Tablets 1780
Prostigmin Injectable 1305
Prostigmin Tablets 1306
Proventil Inhalation Aerosol (Rare) 2524
▲ Proventil Inhalation Solution 0.083% (8% to 15.4%) 2527
▲ Proventil Solution for Inhalation 0.5% (8% to 15.4%) 2525
Proventil Syrup (Rare) 2528
Quinaglute Dura-Tabs Tablets 644
Quinidex Extentabs 2240
Recombivax HB (Less than 1%) 1787
Reglan (A few cases) 2243
Risperdal Tablets (Infrequent) 1348
Rocephin Injectable Vials, ADD-Vantage, Galaxy Container (Rare) 2305
Roferon-A Injection (Less than 1%; rare) 2308
Salflex Tablets 791
Seldane Tablets 1284
Seldane-D Extended-Release Tablets 1286
Semprex-D Capsules (Rare) 1620
Serevent Inhalation Aerosol (Rare) 1149
Streptase for Infusion (Rare) 557
Sufenta Injection (0.3% to 1%) 1355
▲ Suprane (desflurane, USP) (3% to 10%) 1865
Tambocor Tablets (Less than 1%) 1555
Taxotere for Injection Concentrate (0.9%) 2204
Tazicef for Injection (Very rare) 2697
Tazidime Vials, Faspak & ADD-Vantage (Very rare) 1531
Tenormin Tablets and I.V. Injection (1.2%) 2965
Tessalon Perles 1018
▲ Tilade Inhaler (5.4%) 2207
Timolide Tablets (1.6%) 1791
Timoptic in Ocudose (Less frequent) 1796
Timoptic Sterile Ophthalmic Solution (Less frequent) 1794
Timoptic-XE 1798
Toprol-XL Tablets (About 1 of 100 patients) 560
Toradol 2319
Tornalate Solution for Inhalation, 0.2% (1.5%) 976
Tornalate Metered Dose Inhaler (Less than 1% to 1%) 978
Tracrium Injection 1155
Trandate Tablets (Less common) 1158
Ultram Tablets (50 mg) 1594
Univasc Tablets (Less than 1%) 2553
Vancenase PocketHaler Nasal Inhaler (Rare) 2534
Vanceril Inhaler (Rare) 2538
Vaseretic Tablets 1810
Vasotec I.V. 1814
Vasotec Tablets (0.5% to 1.0%) 1816
Velban Vials 1537
Ventolin Inhalation Aerosol and Refill (Rare) 1170
▲ Ventolin Inhalation Solution (Rare to 15.4%) 1171
▲ Ventolin Nebules Inhalation Solution (Rare to 15.4%) 1172
Ventolin Rotacaps for Inhalation (Rare to 1%) 1173
Ventolin Syrup (Rare) 1175
Ventolin Tablets (Rare) 1176
VePesid Capsules and Injection (0.7% to 2%) 727
Versed Injection (Less than 1%) 2324
Virazole (Infrequent) 1310
Volmax Extended-Release Tablets (Rare) 1835
Cataflam/Voltaren/Voltaren-XR 833
▲ Vumon for Injection (Approximately 5%) 729
Zantac (Rare) 1182
Zantac Injection 1180
Zantac Syrup (Rare) 1182
Zaroxolyn Tablets 1625
Zebeta Tablets 1457
Zemuron Injection (Less than 1%) 1885
Zestoretic Tablets 2968
Zestril Tablets (0.3% to 1.0%) 2972
Ziac (Rare) 1459
Zofran Injection (Rare) 1227
Zofran Tablets (Rare) 1231
Zoloft Tablets (Infrequent) 2051
Zosyn (1.0% or less) 1463
Zyloprim Tablets (Less than 1%) 1194
Zyrtec Tablets (Less than 2%) 2053

Bronchospasm, exacerbation of
▲ Airet Albuterol Sulfate Inhalation Solution (15.4%) 1602
Asacol Delayed-Release Tablets 2129
Brethine Ampuls 832
Brethine Tablets 831
Didronel Tablets (Rare) 2133
Nicotrol NS Nicotine Nasal Spray 1565
Serevent Inhalation Aerosol 1149

Bronchospasm, paradoxical
Albuterol Sulfate, USP Solution for Inhalation, Arm-a-Med 522
Alupent 672
Proventil Solution for Inhalation 0.5% 2525
Serevent Inhalation Aerosol 1149
Tilade Inhaler (Rare) 2207
Ventolin Inhalation Solution 1171
Ventolin Nebules Inhalation Solution 1172
Ventolin Rotacaps for Inhalation 1173

Browache
EPIFRIN .... ⊙ 237
Humorsol Sterile Ophthalmic Solution 1707
OptiPranolol (Metipranolol 0.3%) Sterile Ophthalmic Solution (A small number of patients) .... ⊙ 256
Phospholine Iodide .... ⊙ 323
▲ Rev-Eyes Ophthalmic Eyedrops 0.5% (10% to 40%) .... ⊙ 324
Vexol 1% Ophthalmic Suspension (Less than 1%) ...... ⊙ 227

Bruising
Accutane Capsules (Less than 1%) 2252
Anafranil Capsules (Rare) 819
Atretol Tablets 569
Beclovent Inhalation Aerosol and Refill 1063
BuSpar Tablets (Infrequent) 738
Calan SR Caplets (1% or less) 2571
Calan Tablets (1% or less) 2568
Cataflam Tablets (Rare) 833
Clozaril Tablets (Less than 1%) 2377
Coumadin 941
Covera-HS Tablets (Less than 2%) 2573
Depakene 416
Depakote Tablets 418
Depen Titratable Tablets 2770
▲ Emcyt Capsules (3%) 2085
Eminase 2215
Felbatol 2774
Feldene Capsules (Less than 1%) .. 2008
Florinef Acetate Tablets 506
Floxin I.V. 1580
Floxin Tablets (200 mg, 300 mg, 400 mg) 1577
Hycamtin for Injection 2665
Isoptin Oral Tablets (Less than 1%) 1393
Isoptin SR Tablets (1% or less) 1395
Maxair Autohaler (0.6%) 1550
Maxair Inhaler (Less than 1%) 1552
Nalfon 200 Pulvules & Nalfon Tablets (Less than 1%) 933
Oncaspar 2194
Plendil Extended-Release Tablets (0.5% to 1.5%) 514
Quadrinal Tablets 1398
Roferon-A Injection (Less than 4%) 2308
Rythmol Tablets–150mg, 225mg, 300mg (Less than 1%) 1399
Sandostatin Injection (1% to 4%) .. 2421
▲ Tegison Capsules (25-50%) 2314
Tegretol/Tegretol-XR 870
Tonocard Tablets 519
Verelan Capsules (1% or less) 1455
Cataflam/Voltaren/Voltaren-XR (Rare) 833

Bruxism
Atamet Tablets 567
Crixivan Capsules (Less than 2%) .. 1670
Eldepryl Capsules 2729
Larodopa Tablets (Relatively frequent) 2296
Paxil Tablets (Infrequent) 2681
Sinemet Tablets 959
Sinemet CR Tablets 961
Wellbutrin Tablets (Infrequent) 1177

Buccal-lingual-masticatory syndrome
Prozac Pulvules & Liquid, Oral Solution (One case) 935

Buccoglossal syndrome
Prozac Pulvules & Liquid, Oral Solution (Infrequent) 935

Bucking
Diprivan Injectable Emulsion (Less than 1%) 2939

Budd-Chiari syndrome
Brevicon 2563
Demulen 2580
Desogen Tablets 1867
Levlen/Tri-Levlen 646
Micronor Tablets 1903
Modicon 1928
Norinyl 2563
Nor-Q D Tablets 2598
Ortho-Cept 1907
Ortho-Cyclen/Ortho-Tri-Cyclen 1914
Ortho-Novum 1928
Ortho-Cyclen/Ortho Tri-Cyclen 1914
Ovcon 765
Levlen/Tri-Levlen 646
Tri-Norinyl 2607

Bulbus oculi, perforation
AK-CIDE .... ⊙ 203
AK-CIDE Ointment .... ⊙ 203
AK-PRED .... ⊙ 204
Blephamide Liquifilm Sterile Ophthalmic Suspension 472
Blephamide Ointment .... ⊙ 234
FML Forte Liquifilm .... ⊙ 237
FML Liquifilm .... ⊙ 238
FML S.O.P. .... ⊙ 239
FML-S Liquifilm .... ⊙ 240
Maxitrol Ophthalmic Ointment and Suspension .... ⊙ 222
Pred Forte .... ⊙ 247
Pred Mild .... ⊙ 250
TobraDex Ophthalmic Suspension and Ointment 469
Vexol 1% Ophthalmic Suspension .... ⊙ 227

Bulimia
Paxil Tablets (Rare) 2681

Bullae
▲ Androderm Testosterone Transdermal System (Less than 1% to 12%) 2634
8-MOP Capsules 1294
NegGram 2453

Bundle branch block
Anafranil Capsules (Rare) 819
Cardizem CD Capsules (Less than 1%) 1251
Cardizem SR Capsules (Less than 1%) 1255
Cardizem Injectable 1253
Cardizem Tablets (Less than 1%) .. 1257
Cerebyx Injection (Infrequent) 1956
Cognex Capsules (Rare) 1961
Corvert Injection (1.9%) 2075
Diprivan Injectable Emulsion (Less than 1%) 2939
Doxil (Less than 1%) 2613
Effexor (Rare) 2825
Imdur (Less than or equal to 5%) .. 1362
Macrobid Capsules 2138
Macrodantin Capsules 2140
Miacalcin Nasal Spray (Less than 1%) 2403
Naprelan Tablets (Less than 1%) .. 2861
Paxil Tablets (Rare) 2681
Prozac Pulvules & Liquid, Oral Solution (Rare) 935
Rilutek Tablets (Infrequent) 2198
Rythmol Tablets–150mg, 225mg, 300mg (0.3 to 1.9%) 1399
▲ Tenormin Tablets and I.V. Injection (6.6%) 2965
Tiazac Capsules (Less than 1%) 1019
Tonocard Tablets (Less than 1%) .. 519
Yutopar Intravenous Injection 566

Burning
Aclovate (Approximately 2%) 1061
▲ Acular Sterile Ophthalmic Solution (Approximately 40%) 470
Afrin .... ▣ 757
▲ Alomide Ophthalmic Solution (Among most frequent) 465
Americaine Anesthetic Lubricant 1603
Americaine Otic Topical Anesthetic Ear Drops 1603
Analpram-HC Rectal Cream 1% and 2.5% 993
Anusol Hemorrhoidal Ointment .... ▣ 810
Anusol-HC Cream 2.5% (Infrequent to frequent) 1953
Anusol-HC Suppositories 1954
▲ A/T/S 2% Acne Topical Gel (Most common) 1244
▲ A/T/S 2% Acne Topical Solution (Most common) 1244
Azelex (Approximately 1% to 5%) 471
Bactroban Nasal (2%) 2643
Bactroban Ointment (1.5%) 2642
BiCNU 696
Caladryl Cream For Kids .... ▣ 817
Capzasin-P .... ▣ 794
Catapres-TTS (3 of 101 patients) .. 680
▲ Cerebyx Injection (7 of 16 volunteers) 1956
Chloromycetin Ophthalmic Ointment, 1% (Occasional) ...... ⊙ 298
Cipro I.V. Pharmacy Bulk Package (Less than 1%) 590
▲ Condylox Topical Solution (64% to 78%) 1853
Cordran Lotion (Infrequent) 1854
Cordran Tape (Infrequent) 1855
Cormax Ointment (Infrequent) 1856
Cormax Scalp Application (Infrequent) 1857
Cortisporin Cream 1073
Cortisporin Ointment 1074
Cortisporin Otic Solution Sterile 1076
Cortisporin Otic Suspension Sterile (Rare) 1077
Cutivate Cream (0.6%) 1078
Cutivate Ointment (Less than 1%) 1078
Decadron Phosphate Injection 1680
Decadron Phosphate Topical Cream 1686
Decaspray Topical Aerosol 1689
Dermatop Emollient Cream 0.1% (Less than 1%) 1264
DesOwen Cream, Ointment and Lotion (Approximately 3%) 1032
▲ Diprolene Gel 0.05% (6%) 2490
▲ Elimite (permethrin) 5% Cream (10%) 475

(▣ Described in PDR For Nonprescription Drugs) Incidence data in parenthesis; ▲ 3% or more (⊙ Described in PDR For Ophthalmology)

Burning **Side Effects Index** 1278

Elocon Cream 0.1% (1.6%) 2492
Elocon Lotion 0.1% (4 in 209 patients) 2493
▲ Elocon Ointment 0.1% (4.8%)........ 2494
▲ Exelderm Cream 1.0% (3%)........... 2794
Exelderm Solution 1.0% (Approximately 1%)........... 2795
4-Way Fast Acting Nasal Spray (regular & mentholated)............. ▣ 644
4-Way 12 Hour Nasal Spray.......... ▣ 644
Fleet Bisacodyl Enema........... 1000
Fleet Prep Kits........... 1002
Florone/Florone E 921
Fluoroplex Topical Solution & Cream 1% 475
Garamycin Injectable 2502
Heparin Lock Flush Solution........... 2831
Heparin Sodium Injection........... 2832
Heparin Sodium Vials........... 1486
Humorsol Sterile Ophthalmic Solution 1707
Hydeltrasol Injection, Sterile........... 1708
Hydrocortone Phosphate Injection, Sterile 1713
Hytone 922
Hytone Ointment 2 ½% 923
IOPIDINE Sterile Ophthalmic Solution .... ⊙ 218
▲ Lac-Hydrin 12% Lotion (1 in 10 to 30 patients)........... 2796
Lamisil Cream 1% (0.8%) 2393
Lidex (Infrequent) 2299
Locoid Cream, Ointment and Topical Solution (Infrequent) 994
Lotrimin 2514
Lotrisone Cream (Infrequent)........... 2515
Monistat-Derm (miconazole nitrate 2%) Cream (Isolated reports) 1944
▲ Naftin Gel 1% (5.0%) 477
NeoDecadron Topical Cream 1757
Ophthetic (Occasional) .... ⊙ 244
Oxistat (1.4%) 1139
Panafil Ointment (Occasional)........... 2372
Panafil-White Ointment (Occasional)........... 2372
Pandel Cream, 0.1% 2475
Pediotic Suspension Sterile (Rare).. 1140
Phospholine Iodide .... ⊙ 323
Pramosone Cream, Lotion & Ointment 995
Pred-G Liquifilm Sterile Ophthalmic Suspension .... ⊙ 248
ProctoCream-HC 2.5% (Infrequent to frequent) 2552
Psorcon Cream 0.05% (Infrequent) 924
Psorcon Ointment 0.05% 923
▲ Renova (tretinoin emollient cream) 0.05% (Almost all subjects) 1945
▲ Rev-Eyes Ophthalmic Eyedrops 0.5% (Approximately 50%) .... ⊙ 324
Rowasa (0.61%) 2727
▲ Spectazole (econazole nitrate 1%) Cream (3%)........... 1947
Synalar (Infrequent) 2299
Temovate Cream (1%) 1152
▲ Temovate E Emollient (5%) 1154
▲ Temovate Gel (Among most frequent) 1153
Temovate Scalp Application (Infrequent) 1153
Terazol 3 Vaginal Suppositories 1942
▲ Timoptic-XE (1 in 8 patients)........... 1798
Topicort Emollient Cream 0.25% (0.8%)........... 1289
Topicort Gel 0.05% (Infrequent).... 1290
Topicort LP Emollient Cream 0.05% (Infrequent) 1289
Topicort Ointment 0.25% (Infrequent) 1291
Tridesilon Cream 0.05% (Infrequent) 609
Tridesilon Ointment 0.05% (Infrequent) 610
▲ Ultravate Cream 0.05% (4.4%) 2797
Ultravate Ointment 0.05% (1.6%) 2798
▲ Vagistat-1 (Approximately 6%) 783
▲ Viroptic Ophthalmic Solution, 1% Sterile (4.6%)........... 1177
VōSol (Occasional) 2786
Westcort Cream 0.2% (Infrequent) 2799
Westcort Ointment 0.2%........... 2800
Zantac Injection 1180
▲ Zovirax Ointment 5% (28.3%)........ 1190

Burning, at injection site

▲ Ativan Injection (17%) 2805
Attenuvax 1650
Biavax II 1653
BiCNU 696
Brevibloc (esmolol HCl) Injection (Less than 1%)........... 1860
▲ Cardizem Injectable (3.9%) 1253
Cefizox for Intramuscular or Intravenous Use (1% to 5%)........ 1025
Ceredase 1055
Cipro I.V. (1% or less)........... 587
DDAVP Injection (Occasional) 2178
Desmopressin Acetate Injection (Occasional)........... 996
▲ Diprivan Injectable Emulsion (10% to 17.6%)........... 2939
Genotropin Injection (Infrequent).... 2090
Helixate, Antihemophilic Factor (Recombinant) 799
Inocor Lactate Injection (0.2%) 2439
Intron A for Injection (Less than 5%)........... 2506
KOGENATE Antihemophilic Factor (Recombinant) 626
M-M-R II 1730
M-R-VAX II 1732
Meruvax II 1740
Monocid Injection (Less often)........... 2674
Mononine, Coagulation Factor IX (Human), Monoclonal Antibody Purified 804
Mumpsvax 1751
Timentin for Injection........... 2706
Versed Injection (Less than 1%) 2324
▲ Zofran Injection (4%) 1227

Burning, local

Aci-Jel Therapeutic Vaginal Jelly (Occasional cases) 1903
Americaine Anesthetic Lubricant 1603
▲ Androderm Testosterone Transdermal System (3%) 2634
▲ Betimol 0.25%, 0.5% (One of the two most frequent) .... ⊙ 259
▲ Chibroxin Sterile Ophthalmic Solution (One of the two most frequent) 1657
▲ Condylox Topical Solution (64% to 78%) 1853
CORTENEMA........... 2713
▲ Efudex (Among most frequent)........ 2280
▲ Elimite (permethrin) 5% Cream (10%) 475
Exact .... ▣ 722
▲ Garamycin Ophthalmic (Among most frequent) 2501
▲ Gentak (Among most frequent).... ⊙ 209
Habitrol Nicotine Transdermal System (Once in 35% of patients) 884
Loprox 1% Cream and Lotion (1 out of 514 patients)........... 1269
Mumpsvax 1751
▲ Naftin Cream 1% (6%) 477
12 Hour Nōstrilla........... ▣ 660
Otrivin........... ▣ 662
Prostep (nicotine transdermal system) (At least once in 54% of patients) 1439
Selsun Rx 2.5% Selenium Sulfide Lotion, USP........... 2345
Spectazole (econazole nitrate 1%) Cream 1947
▲ Zonalon Cream (Approximately 21%) 1042

Burning, mild

Mycelex-G 500 mg Vaginal Tablets (6 in 1,116 patients)........... 602

Burning, sexual partner

Mycelex-G 500 mg Vaginal Tablets (Rare) 602

Burning, vaginal (see under Vaginal burning)

Burning, vulvovaginal (see under Vaginal burning)

Burning sensation

AVC (Occasional)........... 1245
Accuzyme Ointment (A small percentage) 1236
Adenocard Injection (Less than 1%)........... 1021
▲ A/T/S 2% Acne Topical Solution (17 out of 90 patients)........... 1244
Benoquin Cream 20% 1298
Benzamycin Topical Gel (Occasional) 919
Chloromycetin Ophthalmic Solution .... ⊙ 299
Cormax Ointment (0.5%) 1856
▲ Cormax Scalp Application (Approximately 10%) 1857
Decadron Phosphate Sterile Ophthalmic Ointment (Rare) 1684
Decadron Phosphate Sterile Ophthalmic Solution (Rare)........... 1685
Dopram Injectable 2235
Doxil 2613
Doxorubicin Astra 531
Erycette (erythromycin 2%) Topical Solution 1943
Fleet Babylax 1000
Gamimune N, 5% Immune Globulin Intravenous (Human), 5% 612
Gamimune N, 10% Immune Globulin Intravenous (Human), 10% 615
Idamycin Injection 2096
▲ Imitrex Injection (7.5%)........... 1095
Imitrex Tablets (Frequent)........... 1099
Mutamycin for Injection 712
Pandel Cream, 0.1% (4 of 226 patients) 2475
Peptavlon 2997
Pondimin Tablets........... 2239
Quadrinal Tablets 1398
Rubex for Injection 721
SSD (Infrequent) 1402
Scleromate Injection........... 1234
Silvadene Cream 1% (Infrequent) .. 1288
▲ Sulfamylon Cream (One of two most frequent) 940
T-Stat 2.0% Topical Solution and Pads 2797
Temovate Cream (1%) 1152
Temovate Gel (1.8%) 1153
Temovate Ointment (0.5%)........... 1152
▲ Temovate Scalp Application (29 of 294 patients) 1153
THERAMYCIN Z 2% Solution........... 1629
Topicort LP Emollient Cream 0.05% (0.8%)........... 1289
T.R.U.E. Test (Common; up to 14 reports) 1162
Vagistat-1 (Less than 1%) 783
Ventolin Rotacaps for Inhalation (Less than 1%)........... 1173
Zilactin Medicated Gel........... ▣ 856

Bursitis

Betaseron for SC Injection........... 653
Cognex Capsules (Infrequent) 1961
Dilacor XR Extended-release Capsules (Infrequent) 2183
Effexor (Infrequent) 2825
Hivid Tablets (Less than 1%) 2287
Lamictal Tablets (Rare)........... 1105
LUVOX Tablets (Infrequent) 2723
Naprelan Tablets (Less than 1%) ... 2861
Neurontin Capsules (Rare) 1978
Noroxin Tablets (Less frequent) 1758
Noroxin Tablets (Less frequent) 2222
Paxil Tablets (Rare) 2681
Permax Tablets (1.6%) 571
Prozac Pulvules & Liquid, Oral Solution (Infrequent) 935
Redux Capsules (Rare) 2911
Remeron Tablets (Rare) 1878
Risperdal Tablets (Rare)........... 1348
Serzone Tablets (Infrequent) 776

BBB+ Major Axis Deviation

▲ Tenormin Tablets and I.V. Injection (6.6%) 2965

BCG infection, disseminated

TICE BCG, USP (Very rare; about 1 per 5,000,000 vaccinees) 1881

BEI, increase

Amen Tablets 785
Aygestin Tablets........... 990

BSP retention

Atromid-S Capsules 2808
Capastat Sulfate Injection 968
Sterile FUDR 2284
Hydrea Capsules 705

BSP retention, increase

Depo-Provera Sterile Aqueous Suspension........... 2083
Estratest 2718
Mithracin 599
Oxandrin 783
Rifadin 1276
Rifamate Capsules 1278
Rimactane Capsules........... 865
▲ Serophene (clomiphene citrate tablets, USP) (Approximately 10% to 20% of patients) 2621
Winstrol Tablets 2468

BUN levels, changes

Atamet Tablets 567
Celestone Soluspan Suspension 2484
CORTENEMA........... 2713
Cortifoam 2540
Cortone Acetate Sterile Suspension........... 1663
Cortone Acetate Tablets........... 1664
Dalalone D.P. Injectable 1009
Decadron Elixir 1676
Decadron Phosphate Injection 1680
Decadron Phosphate with Xylocaine Injection, Sterile........... 1683
Decadron Tablets........... 1678
Decadron-LA Sterile Suspension...... 1687
Dexacort Phosphate in Respihaler .. 1606
Dexacort Phosphate in Turbinaire .. 1607
Doral Tablets (Less than 1%) 2773
Etrafon 2495
Florinef Acetate Tablets 506
Hydeltrasol Injection, Sterile........... 1708
Intron A for Injection (Up to 2%).... 2506
Moban Tablets and Concentrate...... 1036
▲ Paraplatin for Injection (14%) 713
Pediapred Oral Solution 1618
Prelone Syrup 1834
Prolixin 510
Roferon-A Injection (Up to less than 1%)........... 2308
Sinemet Tablets 959
▲ Vasotec I.V. (About 0.2 to 20%) 1814
▲ Vasotec Tablets (About 0.2% to 20%) 1816

BUN levels, decrease

Azathioprine Tablets (Less than 1%)........... 2349
Cipro I.V. (Infrequent) 587
Cipro I.V. Pharmacy Bulk Package (Less than 1%)........... 590
Imuran (Less than 1%)........... 1103

BUN levels, elevation

Accupril Tablets (2%)........... 1950
Achromycin V Capsules 1417
Aldactone Tablets 2558
Aldoclor Tablets........... 1638
Aldomet Ester HCl Injection 1642
Aldomet Oral 1640
Aldoril Tablets........... 1644
Alka-Seltzer Cherry Effervescent Antacid and Pain Reliever (Less than 1%) .... ▣ 609
Alka-Seltzer Lemon Lime Effervescent Antacid and Pain Reliever (Less than 1%) .. ▣ 609
Alka-Seltzer Original Effervescent Antacid and Pain Reliever (Less than 1%) .. ▣ 609
Altace Capsules (0.5% to 3%)........ 1238
Ambien Tablets (Rare) 2559
Amicar Syrup, Tablets, and Injection 1312
Amikacin Sulfate Injection, USP 523
Ancef Injection 2632
Ancobon Capsules........... 2254
Asacol Delayed-Release Tablets 2129
Regular Strength Ascriptin Tablets .... ▣ 650
Atretol Tablets 569
Bactrim DS Tablets........... 2257
Bactrim I.V. Infusion........... 2255
Bactrim 2257
Genuine Bayer Aspirin Tablets & Caplets (Less than 1.0% at doses of 1000 mg/day)........... ▣ 618
Betaseron for SC Injection........... 653
▲ Biaxin (4%) 406
Blocadren Tablets 1654
Bufferin Analgesic Tablets........... ▣ 636
Calcijex Injection 412
▲ Capastat Sulfate Injection (36%)..... 968
Capoten Tablets 740
Capozide Tablets 744
Casodex Tablets (2% to 5%) 2934
Ceclor Pulvules & Suspension (Less than 1 in 500) 1470
Cedax (2% to 4%) 2480
Cefizox for Intramuscular or Intravenous Use (Occasional)........ 1025
▲ Cefobid Intravenous/Intramuscular (1 in 16) 1996
▲ Cefobid Pharmacy Bulk Package - Not for Direct Infusion (1 in 16).. 1999
Cefotan........... 2936
Ceftin 1067

(▣ Described in PDR For Nonprescription Drugs) Incidence data in parenthesis; ▲ 3% or more (⊙ Described in PDR For Ophthalmology)

Side Effects Index — Carbohydrate tolerance, decrease

Cefzil Tablets and Oral Suspension (0.1%) ... 747
Ceptaz (Occasional) ... 1070
Chibroxin Sterile Ophthalmic Solution (With oral form) ... 1657
▲ Cipro I.V. (Among most frequent) .. 587
▲ Cipro I.V. Pharmacy Bulk Package (Among most frequent) ... 590
Cipro Tablets (0.9%) ... 584
Claforan Sterile and Injection (Occasional) ... 1259
Cozaar Tablets (Less than 0.1%) .. 1668
Cytotec (Infrequent) ... 2576
Cytovene (1% or less) ... 2270
Daypro Caplets (Occasional) ... 2578
Declomycin Tablets ... 1421
Demadex Tablets and Injection ... 691
Didronel I.V. Infusion (Occasional) .. 1545
Diprivan Injectable Emulsion (Less than 1%) ... 2939
Dopram Injectable ... 2235
Doryx Capsules ... 1970
Doxil (Less than 1%) ... 2613
Duricef Capsules, Tablets, and Oral Suspension ... 750
Dyazide Capsules ... 2653
DYNACIN Capsules ... 1627
Dyrenium Capsules (Rare) ... 2655
Ecotrin ... 2625
Effexor (Rare) ... 2825
Esimil Tablets ... 840
Eulexin Capsules ... 2498
Feldene Capsules (Greater than 1%) ... 2008
Floxin I.V. (More than or equal to 1%) ... 1580
Floxin Tablets (200 mg, 300 mg, 400 mg) (More than or equal to 1%) ... 1577
Fortaz (Occasional) ... 1092
Foscavir Injection (Between 1% and 5%) ... 541
Fungizone Intravenous ... 507
▲ Ganite (About 12.5%) ... 2711
Garamycin Injectable ... 2502
▲ Gemzar for Injection (8% to 16%) 1482
Glucotrol Tablets ... 2011
Glucotrol XL Extended Release Tablets ... 2012
Halfprin Tablets (Less than %) ... 1413
Helidac Therapy ... 2135
▲ Hexalen Capsules (1% to 9%) ... 2760
Hivid Tablets (Less than 1%) ... 2287
Hydrea Capsules (Occasional) ... 705
Hyzaar Tablets (0.6%) ... 1720
IFEX ... 706
Indocin Capsules (Less than 1%) ... 1723
▲ Indocin I.V. (41% of infants) ... 1727
Indocin (Less than 1%) ... 1723
Intron A for Injection (Less than 5%) ... 2506
Ismelin Tablets ... 845
Keftab Tablets ... 931
Kefurox Vials, Faspak & ADD-Vantage ... 1509
Kefzol Vials, Faspak & ADD-Vantage ... 1511
Larodopa Tablets (Rare) ... 2296
▲ Leukine (23%) ... 1317
Lithonate/Lithotabs/Lithobid ... 2721
Lodine Capsules and Tablets (Less than 1%) ... 2849
Lorabid Suspension and Pulvules ... 1513
Lotensin Tablets (Less than 0.1%) ... 852
Lotensin HCT Tablets ... 855
Lotrel Capsules ... 858
Lupron Depot - 3 Month 22.5 mg .. 2743
Lupron Injection (Less than 5%) ... 2736
Mandol Vials, Faspak & ADD-Vantage ... 1516
Mavik Tablets (0.6% to 1.4%) ... 1407
Maxaquin Tablets ... 2593
Maxipime for Injection (0.1% to 1%) ... 758
Mefoxin ... 1734
Mefoxin Premixed Intravenous Solution ... 1737
Mepron Suspension (1%) ... 1206
Merrem I.V. (Greater than 0.2%) ... 2952
Mezlin ... 594
Mezlin Pharmacy Bulk Package ... 597
Minocin Intravenous ... 1428
Minocin Oral Suspension ... 1431
Minocin Pellet-Filled Capsules ... 1429
Mithracin ... 599
Monocid Injection (Occasional) ... 2674
Monodox Capsules ... 1858
Monopril Tablets ... 762

Motrin Ibuprofen Suspension, Oral Drops, Chewable Tablets, Caplets ... 1563
Mykrox Tablets ... 1617
Naprelan Tablets (Less than 1%) .. 2861
Nebcin Vials, Hyporets & ADD-Vantage ... 1518
Neoral ... 2405
Netromycin Injection 100 mg/ml ... 2516
▲ Nolvadex Tablets (18.1%) ... 2957
▲ Normodyne Injection (8%) ... 2519
Noroxin Tablets (Less frequent) ... 1758
Noroxin Tablets (Less frequent) ... 2222
Norpace (1%) ... 2596
▲ Orudis Capsules (3% to 9%) ... 2874
▲ Oruvail Capsules (3% to 9%) ... 2874
Parlodel ... 2411
Paxil Tablets (Rare) ... 2681
Pediazole Suspension ... 2340
Pipracil ... 1435
Platinol for Injection ... 717
Platinol-AQ Injection ... 719
Primaxin I.M. ... 1770
Primaxin I.V. ... 1772
▲ Prinivil Tablets (2.0% to 11.6%) .. 1776
Prinzide Tablets ... 1780
Procardia Capsules (Rare) ... 2024
Procardia XL Extended Release Tablets (Rare) ... 2026
▲ Prograf (8% to 30%) ... 1028
▲ Proleukin for Injection (63%) ... 812
Proloprim Tablets ... 1141
Rifadin ... 1276
Rifamate Capsules ... 1278
Rifater ... 1280
Rimactane Capsules ... 865
Rocaltrol Capsules ... 2303
Rocephin Injectable Vials, ADD-Vantage, Galaxy Container (1.2%) ... 2305
Sandimmune ... 2416
Sansert Tablets ... 2424
Septra ... 1146
Septra I.V. Infusion ... 1142
Septra I.V. Infusion ADD-Vantage Vials ... 1144
Septra ... 1146
Sinemet CR Tablets ... 961
Sular Tablets (Less than or equal to 1%) ... 2961
Suprax (Less than 2%) ... 1443
Tazicef for Injection (Occasional) ... 2697
Tazidime Vials, Faspak & ADD-Vantage (Occasional) ... 1531
▲ Tegison Capsules (1-10%) ... 2314
Tegretol/Tegretol-XR ... 870
Terramycin Intramuscular Solution 2034
Timentin for Injection ... 2706
▲ Tolectin (200, 400 and 600 mg) (1 to 3%) ... 1591
Toradol ... 2319
▲ Trandate (8 of 100 patients) ... 1158
Trilisate (Less than 1%) ... 2155
Trimpex Tablets ... 2323
Unasyn ... 2035
Univasc Tablets (Approximately 1%) ... 2553
Vancocin HCl, Oral Solution & Pulvules (Rare) ... 1536
Vancocin HCl, Vials & ADD-Vantage (Rare) ... 1534
Vantin for Oral Suspension and Vantin Tablets ... 2112
Vaseretic Tablets (About 0.6% to 20%) ... 1810
Vibramycin ... 2038
Vibramycin Hyclate Intravenous ... 2040
Vibramycin ... 2038
Zaroxolyn Tablets ... 1625
Zebeta Tablets ... 1457
Zestoretic Tablets ... 2968
Zestril Tablets (About 2.0%) ... 2972
Zinacef ... 1184
Zithromax (Less than 1%) ... 2043
Zithromax Tablets (Less than 1%) ... 2046
Zosyn ... 1463
▲ Zovirax Sterile Powder (5% to 10%) ... 1191

C

Cachexia
Cerebyx Injection (Infrequent) ... 1956
Cognex Capsules (Infrequent) ... 1961
Cytovene-IV (One report) ... 2270
Foscavir Injection (Between 1% and 5%) ... 541
Hivid Tablets (Less than 1%) ... 2287
Intron A for Injection (Less than or equal to 5%) ... 2506
Norvir (Less than 2%) ... 447

Permax Tablets (Rare) ... 571
Risperdal Tablets (Rare) ... 1348

Calcification, ectopic
Calcijex Injection ... 412
Rocaltrol Capsules ... 2303

Calcium retention
Estratest ... 2718
Halotestin Tablets ... 2095
Inderide Tablets ... 2838
Lupron Injection (Less than 5%) ... 2736
Oxandrin ... 783
Testred Capsules, 10 mg ... 1308

Calf muscles, need to flex
Imitrex Injection (Rare) ... 1095
Respbid Tablets ... 687

Cancer, breast
Estrace Cream and Tablets ... 751
Helidac Therapy (Some reports) ... 2135
Micronor Tablets ... 1903
Modicon ... 1928
Neurontin Capsules (Infrequent) ... 1978
Nor-Q D Tablets ... 2598
Ortho-Novum ... 1928
Ovcon ... 765

Cancer, cervical
Demulen ... 2580
Depo-Provera Contraceptive Injection (Fewer than 1%) ... 2079
Diethylstilbestrol Tablets ... 1477
Estratest ... 2718
Levlen/Tri-Levlen ... 646
Micronor Tablets ... 1903
Modicon ... 1928
Ortho-Cyclen/Ortho-Tri-Cyclen ... 1914
Ortho-Novum ... 1928
Ortho-Cyclen/Ortho Tri-Cyclen ... 1914
Ovcon ... 765
Permax Tablets (Infrequent) ... 571
PMB 200 and PMB 400 ... 2890
Premarin Intravenous ... 2893
Premarin Vaginal Cream ... 2898
Levlen/Tri-Levlen ... 646

Cancer, vaginal
Diethylstilbestrol Tablets ... 1477
Estratest ... 2718
Ortho-Est ... 1925
PMB 200 and PMB 400 ... 2890
Premarin Intravenous ... 2893
Premarin Vaginal Cream ... 2898
Vivelle Transdermal System ... 880

Candidiasis
▲ AeroBid Inhaler System (3% to 9%) ... 1004
▲ Aerobid-M Inhaler System (3% to 9%) ... 1004
Augmentin ... 2637
Augmentin Tablets ... 2640
Beconase Inhalation Aerosol (Rare) 1065
Ceftin for Oral Suspension (0.1% to 1%) ... 1067
CellCept Capsules (Up to 0.6%) ... 2265
Ceptaz (Fewer than 1%) ... 1070
Cipro I.V. (1% or less) ... 587
Cipro I.V. Pharmacy Bulk Package (Less than 1%) ... 590
Cipro Tablets (Less than 1%) ... 584
Doxil (23.5%) ... 2613
Flagyl I.V. ... 2373
Floxin I.V. ... 1580
Fortaz (Less than 1%) ... 1092
Helidac Therapy ... 2135
Invirase Capsules (Less than 2%) ... 2291
Macrobid Capsules ... 2138
Pipracil ... 1435
Prevacid Delayed-Release Capsules (Less than 1%) ... 2746
Primaxin I.M. ... 1770
Primaxin I.V. (Less than 0.2%) ... 1772
Suprax (Less than 2%) ... 1443
Tazicef for Injection (Less than 1%) ... 2697
Unasyn (Less than 1%) ... 2035
Vantin for Oral Suspension and Vantin Tablets (Less than 1%) ... 2112

Candidiasis, esophageal
Prilosec Delayed-Release Capsules (Less than 1%) ... 516

Candidiasis, mouth
(see under Candidiasis, oral)

Candidiasis, nasal
Nasacort Nasal Inhaler (Rare) ... 2189

Vancenase PocketHaler Nasal Inhaler (Rare) ... 2534

Candidiasis, oral
Ancef Injection ... 2632
Azmacort Oral Inhaler (A few cases) ... 2175
Ceptaz ... 1070
Cipro I.V. (1% or less) ... 587
Cipro I.V. Pharmacy Bulk Package (Less than 1%) ... 590
Cipro Tablets (Less than 1%) ... 584
Effexor (Rare) ... 2825
Flagyl 375 Capsules ... 2587
▲ Flovent (2% to 25%) ... 1089
Fortaz (Less than 1%) ... 1092
Fulvicin P/G Tablets (Occasional) .. 2499
Fulvicin P/G 165 & 330 Tablets (Occasional) ... 2500
Grifulvin V (griseofulvin tablets) Microsize (griseofulvin oral suspension) Microsize (Occasional) ... 1944
Gris-PEG Tablets, 125 mg & 250 mg (Occasional) ... 476
Helidac Therapy ... 2135
Kefzol Vials, Faspak & ADD-Vantage ... 1511
Megace Oral Suspension (1% to 3%) ... 708
▲ Prograf (Greater than 3%) ... 1028
Tazidime Vials, Faspak & ADD-Vantage (Less than 1%) ... 1531
▲ Videx Tablets, Powder for Oral Solution, & Pediatric Powder for Oral Solution (Up to 9%) ... 2980
▲ Zosyn (3.9%) ... 1463

Candidiasis, penile
Caverject Injection (Less than 1%) 2064

Candidiasis, pharynx
Azmacort Oral Inhaler (A few cases) ... 2175
Dexacort Phosphate in Respihaler .. 1606
Dexacort Phosphate in Turbinaire ... 1607
▲ Flovent (19% to 25%) ... 1089
Nasacort Nasal Inhaler (Rare) ... 2189
Vancenase PocketHaler Nasal Inhaler (Rare) ... 2534

Candidiasis, vaginal
(see under Vaginal candidiasis)

Candiduria
Cipro I.V. (1% or less) ... 587
Cipro I.V. Pharmacy Bulk Package (Less than 1%) ... 590
Cipro Tablets ... 584
Floxin Tablets (200 mg, 300 mg, 400 mg) ... 1577
Maxaquin Tablets ... 2593
Noroxin Tablets ... 1758
Noroxin Tablets ... 2222
Penetrex Tablets ... 2196
Zosyn (1.0% or less) ... 1463

Capillary fragility
AeroBid Inhaler System (1% to 3%) ... 1004
Aerobid-M Inhaler System (1% to 3%) ... 1004

Capillary leak syndrome
Leukine (Less than 1%) ... 1317
Neupogen for Injection (One event) ... 495
Orthoclone OKT3 Sterile Solution .. 1892
Proleukin for Injection ... 812
Protamine Sulfate Vials ... 1526

Carbohydrate tolerance, decrease
Brevicon ... 2563
Celestone Soluspan Suspension ... 2484
Climara Transdermal System ... 640
CORTENEMA ... 2713
Cortone Acetate Sterile Suspension ... 1663
Cortone Acetate Tablets ... 1664
Dalalone D.P. Injectable ... 1009
Decadron Elixir ... 1676
Decadron Phosphate Injection ... 1680
Decadron Phosphate with Xylocaine Injection, Sterile ... 1683
Decadron Tablets ... 1678
Decadron-LA Sterile Suspension ... 1687
Demulen ... 2580
Desogen Tablets ... 1867
Dexacort Phosphate in Respihaler .. 1606
Dexacort Phosphate in Turbinaire ... 1607
Diethylstilbestrol Tablets ... 1477
Estrace Cream and Tablets ... 751

(▥ Described in PDR For Nonprescription Drugs)   Incidence data in parentheses; ▲ 3% or more   (⊚ Described in PDR For Ophthalmology)

Carbohydrate tolerance, decrease

- Estraderm Transdermal System ... 842
- ESTRATAB Tablets (0.3, 0.625, 1.25, 2.5 mg) ... 2715
- Estratest ... 2718
- Florinef Acetate Tablets ... 506
- Hydeltrasol Injection, Sterile ... 1708
- Hydeltra-T.B.A. Sterile Suspension ... 1710
- Hydrocortone Acetate Sterile Suspension ... 1712
- Hydrocortone Phosphate Injection, Sterile ... 1713
- Hydrocortone Tablets ... 1715
- Levlen/Tri-Levlen ... 646
- Lo/Ovral Tablets ... 2852
- Lo/Ovral-28 Tablets ... 2857
- Menest Tablets ... 2671
- Modicon ... 1928
- Nordette-21 Tablets ... 2863
- Nordette-28 Tablets ... 2866
- Norinyl ... 2563
- Nor-Q D Tablets ... 2598
- Ogen Tablets ... 2103
- Ogen Vaginal Cream ... 2106
- Ortho-Cept ... 1907
- Ortho-Cyclen/Ortho-Tri-Cyclen ... 1914
- Ortho Dienestrol Cream ... 1922
- Ortho-Est ... 1925
- Ortho-Novum ... 1928
- Ortho-Cyclen/Ortho Tri-Cyclen ... 1914
- Ovcon ... 765
- Ovral Tablets ... 2877
- Ovral-28 Tablets ... 2878
- Ovrette Tablets ... 2878
- PMB 200 and PMB 400 ... 2890
- Prelone Syrup ... 1834
- Premarin Intravenous ... 2893
- Premarin Tablets ... 2896
- Premarin Vaginal Cream ... 2898
- Premphase ... 2900
- Prempro ... 2905
- Levlen/Tri-Levlen ... 646
- Tri-Norinyl ... 2607
- Triphasil-21 Tablets ... 2919
- Triphasil-28 Tablets ... 2924
- Vivelle Transdermal System ... 880

Carcinoma

- Avonex ... 662
- Azathioprine Tablets (2.8%) ... 2349
- Casodex Tablets (2% to 5%) ... 2934
- Demulen ... 2580
- Diethylstilbestrol Tablets ... 1477
- Effexor (Rare) ... 2825
- Felbatol ... 2774
- Lioresal Intrathecal (1% or more) .. 1634
- Naprelan Tablets (Less than 1%) .. 2861
- Nipent for Injection (Less than 3%) ... 2733
- Paxil Tablets (Infrequent) ... 2681
- Permax Tablets (Infrequent) ... 571
- Redux Capsules (Infrequent) ... 2911
- Rilutek Tablets (Infrequent) ... 2198
- ▲ Zerit Capsules (2% to 4%) ... 731

Carcinoma, basal cell

- Sandostatin Injection (Less than 1%) ... 2421

Carcinoma, bladder

- Clomid ... 1262
- Testoderm Testosterone Transdermal System (One in 104 patients) ... 486
- Videx Tablets, Powder for Oral Solution, & Pediatric Powder for Oral Solution (Less than 1%) ... 2980
- Zoladex 3-month (1% to 5%) ... 2978

Carcinoma, ear

- Lupron Injection (Less than 5%) 2736

Carcinoma, endometrial

- Climara Transdermal System ... 640
- Clomid ... 1262
- Demulen ... 2580
- Estrace Cream and Tablets ... 751
- Estraderm Transdermal System ... 842
- ESTRATAB Tablets (0.3, 0.625, 1.25, 2.5 mg) ... 2715
- Estratest ... 2718
- Levlen/Tri-Levlen ... 646
- Menest Tablets ... 2671
- Nolvadex Tablets ... 2957
- Ogen Tablets ... 2103
- Ogen Vaginal Cream ... 2106
- Ortho Dienestrol Cream ... 1922
- Ortho-Est ... 1925
- Premarin Intravenous ... 2893
- Premarin Tablets ... 2896
- Premarin Vaginal Cream ... 2898

- Premphase (About 2- to 12-fold or greater than in nonusers) ... 2900
- Prempro (About 2- to 12-fold or greater than in nonusers) ... 2905
- Levlen/Tri-Levlen ... 646
- Vivelle Transdermal System ... 880

Carcinoma, hepatocellular

- Androderm Testosterone Transdermal System ... 2634
- Android Capsules, 10 mg (Rare) 1297
- Brevicon (Extremely rare) ... 2563
- Clomid ... 1262
- Demulen (Rare) ... 2580
- Halotestin Tablets ... 2095
- Levlen/Tri-Levlen (Extremely rare) ... 646
- Micronor Tablets (Rare) ... 1903
- Modicon (Rare) ... 1928
- Nolvadex Tablets (3 cases) ... 2957
- Norinyl (Extremely rare) ... 2563
- Nor-Q D Tablets (Extremely rare) ... 2598
- Ortho-Cyclen/Ortho-Tri-Cyclen (Rare) ... 1914
- Ortho-Novum (Rare) ... 1928
- Ortho-Cyclen/Ortho Tri-Cyclen (Rare) ... 1914
- Testoderm Testosterone Transdermal System (Rare) ... 486
- Levlen/Tri-Levlen (Extremely rare) ... 646
- Tri-Norinyl (Extremely rare) ... 2607
- Winstrol Tablets (Rare) ... 2468

Carcinoma, ovarian

- Clomid ... 1262
- Humegon for Injection (Infrequent) ... 1873
- Metrodin (urofollitropin for injection) (Infrequent) ... 2616
- Pergonal (menotropins for injection, USP) ... 2618

Carcinoma, prostate

- Androderm Testosterone Transdermal System (Less than 1%) ... 2634
- Android Capsules, 10 mg ... 1297
- Cognex Capsules (Infrequent) ... 1961
- Halotestin Tablets ... 2095
- Paxil Tablets (Rare) ... 2681
- Rilutek Tablets (Rare) ... 2198
- Testoderm Testosterone Transdermal System ... 486
- Winstrol Tablets ... 2468

Carcinoma, renal pelvis

- Cytoxan (One case) ... 700

Carcinoma, uterine

- Nolvadex Tablets ... 2957

Carcinoma, skin

- Avonex ... 662
- Betaseron for SC Injection ... 653
- Caverject Injection (Less than 1%) ... 2064
- Cognex Capsules (Infrequent) ... 1961
- Lupron Injection (Less than 5%) ... 2736
- 8-MOP Capsules ... 1294
- Orthoclone OKT3 Sterile Solution .. 1892
- Permax Tablets (Infrequent) ... 571
- ▲ Prograf (One of the two most common forms) ... 1028
- Sandimmune ... 2416
- Videx Tablets, Powder for Oral Solution, & Pediatric Powder for Oral Solution (Less than 1%) ... 2980

Carcinoma, skin, benign

- CellCept Capsules (1.6% to 4.0%) ... 2265
- Permax Tablets (Rare) ... 571
- Virazole ... 1310

Cardiac abnormalities

- Albalon Solution with Liquifilm... ⊚ 229
- Atamet Tablets (Less frequent) ... 567
- Clozaril Tablets (1%) ... 2377
- Cordarone Tablets (Infrequent) ... 2818
- Hivid Tablets (Less than 1%) ... 2287
- Humorsol Sterile Ophthalmic Solution ... 1707
- ▲ Leukine (23%) ... 1317
- Marax Tablets & DF Syrup ... 2015
- Novantrone for Injection ... 1327
- Pergonal (menotropins for injection, USP) (One report) ... 2618
- Phospholine Iodide ... ⊚ 323
- Platinol for Injection (Infrequent) 717
- Platinol-AQ Injection (Infrequent) ... 719
- Sansert Tablets ... 2424
- Sinemet Tablets (Less frequent) ... 959
- Sinemet CR Tablets ... 961
- Tri-Immunol Absorbed ... 1452

Cardiac anomalies

- Eskalith ... 2658
- Lithium Carbonate Capsules & Tablets ... 2352
- Tetramune (Rare) ... 1449

Cardiac arrest

- ▲ Abelcet Injection (5%) ... 1540
- Activase ... 1045
- Adalat CC (Less than 1.0%) ... 582
- Adenoscan ... 1022
- AK-FLUOR Injection 10% and 25% ... ⊚ 204
- Alupent Inhalation Aerosol (Several cases) ... 672
- Anafranil Capsules (Infrequent) ... 819
- Ancobon Capsules ... 2254
- Anectine (Rare) ... 1062
- AquaMEPHYTON Injection ... 1648
- Avonex ... 662
- Betagan ... ⊚ 230
- Betaseron for SC Injection ... 653
- Betimol 0.25%, 0.5% ... ⊚ 259
- Blocadren Tablets (Less than 1%) ... 1654
- Capoten Tablets ... 740
- Capozide Tablets ... 744
- Carbocaine Injection ... 2432
- Cerebyx Injection (Infrequent) ... 1956
- Clozaril Tablets (Rare) ... 2377
- Cognex Capsules (Rare) ... 1961
- Compazine ... 2644
- Cordarone Intravenous (2.9%) ... 2821
- Cytovene-IV (Two or more reports) ... 2270
- Decadron Phosphate with Xylocaine Injection, Sterile ... 1683
- Demerol ... 2438
- Desyrel and Desyrel Dividose ... 504
- Dilaudid Ampules ... 1382
- Dilaudid-HP Injection ... 1384
- Dilaudid-HP Lyophilized Powder 250 mg ... 1384
- Dilaudid ... 1382
- Dilaudid Oral Liquid ... 1386
- Dilaudid ... 1382
- Dilaudid Tablets - 8 mg ... 1386
- Diprivan Injectable Emulsion (Rare; Less than 1%) ... 2939
- Doxil (Less than 1%) ... 2613
- Duranest Injections ... 533
- Dyclone 0.5% and 1% Topical Solutions, USP ... 535
- EMLA Cream (Unlikely with cream) ... 536
- Ethmozine Tablets (Less than 2%) ... 2217
- Etrafon ... 2495
- Felbatol ... 2774
- Floxin I.V. (Less than 1%) ... 1580
- Fluorescite ... ⊚ 217
- Fluothane ... 2830
- Foscavir Injection (Less than 1%) .. 541
- Fungizone Intravenous ... 507
- Hespan Injection ... 945
- Hismanal Tablets ... 1341
- Imitrex Injection ... 1095
- Isuprel Hydrochloride Solution (Several instances) ... 2443
- Isuprel Mistometer (Several instances) ... 2442
- K-Lor Powder Packets ... 438
- K-Norm Capsules ... 1615
- K-Tab Filmtab ... 439
- Kadian Capsules ... 2948
- Levo-Dromoran ... 2297
- Levoprome ... 1321
- MS Contin Tablets ... 2149
- MSIR ... 2152
- Marcaine ... 2446
- Marcaine Spinal ... 2449
- Mellaril (Rare) ... 2398
- Mepergan Injection ... 2859
- Merrem I.V. (0.1% to 1.0%) ... 2952
- Metaproterenol Sulfate Inhalation Solution, USP, Arm-a-Med (Several cases) ... 547
- Methadone Hydrochloride Oral Solution & Tablets ... 2357
- Micro-K ... 2237
- Micro-K LS Packets ... 2238
- Monopril Tablets ... 762
- Narcan Injection ... 950
- Navane Intramuscular ... 2019
- Nescaine/Nescaine MPF ... 549
- Nipent for Injection (Less than 3%) ... 2733
- Novocain Hydrochloride for Spinal Anesthesia ... 2457
- Nubain Injection (1% or less) ... 952
- Oramorph SR (Morphine Sulfate Sustained Release Tablets) (Less frequent) ... 2359
- Orthoclone OKT3 Sterile Solution .. 1892

- Permax Tablets (Infrequent) ... 571
- Pfizerpen for Injection ... 2022
- Pontocaine Hydrochloride for Spinal Anesthesia ... 2460
- Prinivil Tablets (0.3% to 1.0%) ... 1776
- Prinzide Tablets ... 1780
- Proleukin for Injection (Less than 1% to 2%) ... 812
- Prolixin ... 510
- Prostigmin Injectable ... 1305
- Prostigmin Tablets ... 1306
- Proventil Inhalation Aerosol ... 2524
- Prozac Pulvules & Liquid, Oral Solution ... 935
- Pulmozyme Inhalation ... 1054
- RMS Suppositories CII ... 2766
- Redux Capsules ... 2911
- Rilutek Tablets (More than 2%) ... 2198
- Roxanol ... 2365
- Rythmol Tablets – 150mg, 225mg, 300mg (Less than 1%) ... 1399
- Seldane Tablets (Rare) ... 1284
- Seldane-D Extended-Release Tablets (Rare) ... 1286
- Sensorcaine ... 554
- Serentil (Rare) ... 689
- Slow-K Extended-Release Tablets ... 869
- Stelazine ... 2692
- Sublimaze Injection ... 463
- Sufenta Injection ... 1355
- ▲ Tambocor Tablets (5.1%) ... 1555
- Tenormin Tablets and I.V. Injection (1.6%) ... 2965
- Thorazine ... 2701
- Timolide Tablets ... 1791
- Timoptic in Ocudose (Less frequent) ... 1796
- Timoptic Sterile Ophthalmic Solution (Less frequent) ... 1794
- Timoptic-XE ... 1798
- Tonocard Tablets ... 519
- Torecan (Rare) ... 2367
- Tracrium Injection ... 1155
- ▲ Trasylol (3%) ... 607
- Trilafon ... 2532
- Vancocin HCl, Vials & ADD-Vantage (Rare) ... 1534
- Vaseretic Tablets ... 1810
- Vasotec I.V. ... 1814
- Vasotec Tablets (0.5% to 1.0%) ... 1816
- ▲ Vesanoid Capsules (3%) ... 2327
- Videx Tablets, Powder for Oral Solution, & Pediatric Powder for Oral Solution (Less than 1%) ... 2980
- Virazole ... 1310
- Xylocaine Injections ... 562
- Zestoretic Tablets ... 2968
- Zestril Tablets (0.3% to 1.0%) ... 2972
- Zosyn (1.0% or less) ... 1463

Cardiac arrhythmias
(see under Arrhythmias)

Cardiac asystole
(see under Asystole)

Cardiac collapse

- BOTOX (Botulinum Toxin Type A) Purified Neurotoxin Complex (2 patients) ... 473

Cardiac death

- ▲ Ethmozine Tablets (2% to 5%) ... 2217

Cardiac dysrhythmias
(see under Arrhythmias)

Cardiac enzymes, elevation

- Cytotec (Infrequent) ... 2576

Cardiac failure

- Abelcet Injection ... 1540
- Anafranil Capsules (Rare) ... 819
- Aredia for Injection (Up to 1%) ... 827
- Betimol 0.25%, 0.5% ... ⊚ 259
- Blocadren Tablets ... 1654
- Brevibloc (esmolol HCl) Injection ... 1860
- Felbatol ... 2774
- Flumadine Tablets & Syrup (Less than 0.3%) ... 1013
- Foscavir Injection (Less than 1%) .. 541
- Fungizone Intravenous ... 507
- Hivid Tablets (Less than 1%) ... 2287
- Imdur (Less than or equal to 5%) .. 1362
- Intron A for Injection (Less than 5%) ... 2506
- Levatol Tablets ... 2547
- Maxaquin (Less than 1%) ... 2593
- Normodyne Tablets ... 2522
- Norvasc Tablets (Less than or equal to 0.1%) ... 2020

(⊞ Described in PDR For Nonprescription Drugs)   Incidence data in parenthesis; ▲ 3% or more   (⊚ Described in PDR For Ophthalmology)

Ocupress Ophthalmic Solution, 1% Sterile (In some cases) ⊚ 297	Cerebyx Injection (Infrequent) 1956	Guaimax-D Tablets 809	Betimol 0.25%, 0.5% (1% to 5%) ⊚ 259
Paraplatin for Injection 713	Cytosar-U Sterile Powder 2077	Histussin D Liquid 670	Brevicon 2563
Tenoretic Tablets 2963	Doxil (Less than 1%) 2613	INFeD (Iron Dextran Injection, USP) 2478	▲ CellCept Capsules (More than or equal to 3%) 2265
Tenormin Tablets and I.V. Injection 2965	Remeron Tablets (Rare) 1878	Lioresal Intrathecal 1634	Clomid 1262
Timolide Tablets (Less than 1%) 1791	Tonocard Tablets (Less than 1%) 519	Lutrepulse for Injection 998	Cognex Capsules (Infrequent) 1961
Timoptic in Ocudose (Less frequent) 1796	**Cardiomyopathy**	Marcaine Spinal 2449	Cytovene-IV (Two or more reports) 2270
Timoptic Sterile Ophthalmic Solution (Less frequent) 1794	Abelcet Injection 1540	Maxaquin Tablets 2593	Danocrine Capsules (Rare) 2437
Timoptic-XE 1798	Adderall Tablets (Isolated reports) 2209	NegGram 2453	Demulen 2580
Toprol-XL Tablets 560	Adriamycin PFS 2056	Nescaine/Nescaine MPF 549	Desogen Tablets 1867
Trandate 1158	Adriamycin RDF 2056	Noroxin Tablets 1758	Doral Tablets 2773
▲ Vesanoid Capsules (6%) 2327	BuSpar Tablets (Rare) 738	Noroxin Tablets 2222	Effexor (Infrequent) 2825
Visken Tablets (Some cases) 2428	Cytosar-U Sterile Powder 2077	Novahistine DMX ⊡ 782	Eflone Sterile Ophthalmic Suspension ⊚ 261
Zebeta Tablets 1457	DaunoXome 1842	Novahistine Elixir ⊡ 782	Flarex Ophthalmic Suspension ⊚ 217
Zosyn (1.0% or less) 1463	Dexedrine (Isolated reports) 2648	Orthoclone OKT3 Sterile Solution 1892	Floxin I.V. 1580
Zyrtec Tablets (Less than 2%) 2053	DextroStat-Dextroamphetamine Sulfate Tablets (Isolated reports) 2211	Seldane-D Extended-Release Tablets 1286	Floxin Tablets (200 mg, 300 mg, 400 mg) 1577
Cardiac output, decrease	Doxil (1% to 5%) 2613	Syn-Rx Tablets 1622	Haldol Decanoate 1587
Carbocaine Injection 2432	Doxorubicin Astra 531	Syn-Rx DM Tablets 1623	Haldol Injection, Tablets and Concentrate 1585
Digibind (Few instances) 1079	Foscavir Injection (Less than 1%) 541	Tegretol/Tegretol-XR 870	Hyperstat I.V. Injection 2504
Diprivan Injectable Emulsion (1% to 3%) 2939	Hivid Tablets (Less than 1%) 2287	Tessalon Perles 1018	IBU Tablets (Less than 1%) 1389
Marcaine 2446	Idamycin Injection 2096	Trinalin Repetabs Tablets 1373	ISPAN Perfluoropropane ⊚ 267
Marcaine Spinal 2449	Imitrex Tablets 1099	Tussend 1830	ISPAN Sulfur Hexafluoride ⊚ 266
Paxil Tablets (Rare) 2681	Intron A for Injection (Less than 5%) 2506	Tussend Expectorant 1831	Kerlone Tablets (Less than 2%) 2588
Protamine Sulfate Vials 1526	LUVOX Tablets (Infrequent) 2723	Valium Injectable 2336	Lescol Capsules 2395
Sensorcaine 554	Maxaquin Tablets (Less than 1%) 2593	Xylocaine Injections 562	Levlen/Tri-Levlen 646
Tensilon Injectable 1307	Megace Oral Suspension (1% to 3%) 708	**Cardiovascular depression**	Lo/Ovral Tablets 2852
Trandate 1158	Novantrone for Injection 1327	Nardil (Less frequent) 1977	Lo/Ovral-28 Tablets 2857
Cardiac rhythms, disturbances	Plaquenil Sulfate Tablets (Rare) 2459	**Cardiovascular disorders**	▲ Lopid Tablets (More common) 1974
Accupril Tablets (Rare) 1950	Redux Capsules 2911	Adapin Capsules (Occasional) 1542	Minipress Capsules (A few reports) 2015
Capoten Tablets 740	Retrovir Capsules (0.8%) 1216	Betapace Tablets (1% to 3%) 637	Minizide Capsules (Rare) 2016
Capozide Tablets 744	Retrovir I.V. Infusion (1%) 1221	● CellCept Capsules (More than or equal to 3%) 2265	Modicon 1928
Daraprim Tablets 1199	Retrovir Syrup (0.8%) 1216	▲ Cleocin Vaginal Cream (4%) 2070	Motrin Ibuprofen Suspension, Oral Drops, Chewable Tablets, Caplets (Less than 1%) 1563
Monopril Tablets (0.2% to 1.4%) 762	Roferon-A Injection (Rare) 2308	Crixivan Capsules (Less than 2%) 1670	Mylerin Tablets (Rare) 1209
Prinzide Tablets 1780	Rubex for Injection 721	Demulen 2580	Naprelan Tablets (Less than 1%) 2861
Vaseretic Tablets 1810	**Cardiopulmonary arrest**	Estrace Cream and Tablets 751	Neurontin Capsules (Infrequent) 1978
Vasotec I.V. 1814	Cipro I.V. (1% or less) 587	Larodopa Tablets 2296	Nolvadex Tablets 2957
Vasotec Tablets (0.5% to 1.0%) 1816	Cipro I.V. Pharmacy Bulk Package (Less than 1%) 590	LUVOX Tablets (Infrequent) 2723	Nordette-21 Tablets 2863
Zebeta Tablets 1457	Cipro Tablets (Less than 1%) 584	Monoket Tablets (Up to 2%) 2550	Nordette-28 Tablets 2866
Zestoretic Tablets 2968	Cleocin Phosphate Injection (Rare) 2068	Nor-Q D Tablets 2598	Norinyl 2563
Cardiac rupture	Lariam Tablets (One patient) 2295	▲ Novantrone for Injection (11 to 26%) 1327	Nor-Q D Tablets 2598
▲ Eminase (Less than 10%) 2215	Maxaquin Tablets 2593	▲ Paraplatin for Injection (6% to 23%) 713	Orap Tablets 1037
Cardiac stimulation, unspecified	Penetrex Tablets 2196	Phospholine Iodide ⊚ 323	Ortho-Cept 1907
Esgic-plus Capsules 1012	Pulmozyme Inhalation 1054	Redux Capsules (Infrequent) 2911	Ortho-Cyclen/Ortho Tri-Cyclen 1914
Esgic-plus Tablets 1012	Risperdal Tablets 1348	Salagen Tablets (Two patients) 1546	Ortho-Novum 1928
Fioricet Tablets 2386	Triostat Injection (Approximately 2%) 2708	Seldane Tablets (Rare) 1284	Ortho-Cyclen/Ortho Tri-Cyclen 1914
Fioricet with Codeine Capsules 2387	**Cardiorespiratory arrest**	Seldane-D Extended-Release Tablets (Rare) 1286	Ovcon 765
Fiorinal with Codeine Capsules 2390	Monopril Tablets (0.4% to 1.0%) 762	Sinequan (Occasional) 2028	Ovral Tablets 2877
Sensorcaine 554	Orthoclone OKT3 Sterile Solution 1892	Taxol Injection (Approximately 1%) 723	Ovral-28 Tablets 2878
Cardiac tamponade	**Cardiorespiratory collapse**	Videx Tablets, Powder for Oral Solution, & Pediatric Powder for Oral Solution (Less than 1%) 2980	Ovrette Tablets 2878
Activase 1045	Paremyd ⊚ 244	Vumon for Injection (2%) 729	Paxil Tablets (Rare) 2681
Mylerin Tablets (A small number of patients) 1209	**Cardiospasm**	**Carnitine concentrations, decreased**	Permax Tablets (Rare) 571
▲ Taxotere for Injection Concentrate (6%) 2204	Betaseron for SC Injection 653	Depakene 416	Pravachol Tablets 770
Zovirax Sterile Powder (Less than 1%) 1191	Desyrel and Desyrel Dividose 504	**Carotid sinus hypersensitivity**	Proglycem 575
Cardiac toxicity	Lodine Capsules and Tablets (Less than 1%) 2849	Aldoclor Tablets 1638	Prozac Pulvules & Liquid, Oral Solution (Rare) 935
Adriamycin PFS 2056	Naprelan Tablets (Less than 1%) 2861	Aldomet Ester HCl Injection 1642	Rilutek Tablets (Rare) 2198
Adriamycin RDF 2056	Prevacid Delayed-Release Capsules (Less than 1%) 2746	Aldomet Oral 1640	Levlen/Tri-Levlen 646
Cerubidine for Injection 634	**Cardiovascular abnormalities, fetal**	Aldoril Tablets 1644	Tri-Norinyl 2607
Cytoxan 700	Accutane Capsules 2252	**Carpal tunnel syndrome**	Triphasil-21 Tablets 2919
DaunoXome 1842	Cataflam Tablets 833	Danocrine Capsules 2437	Triphasil-28 Tablets 2924
Doxil 2613	Clinoril Tablets 1658	Humatrope Vials (Rare) 1490	Ultram Tablets (50 mg) (Infrequent) 1594
Doxorubicin Astra 531	Dolobid Tablets 1695	Intron A for Injection (Less than 5%) 2506	Zyloprim Tablets (Less than 1%) 1194
▲ Idamycin Injection (16%) 2096	Cataflam/Voltaren/Voltaren-XR 833	Megace Tablets 710	**Cataracts, posterior subcapsular**
IFEX (Less than 1%) 706	**Cardiovascular collapse**	Nutropin (Rare) 1049	AK-CIDE (Infrequent) ⊚ 203
Lanoxicaps 1110	Aralen Hydrochloride Injection 2430	Nutropin AQ Injection (Rare) 1051	AK-CIDE Ointment (Infrequent) ⊚ 203
Lanoxin Elixir Pediatric 1113	Atretol Tablets 569	Protropin (Rare) 1053	AK-PRED ⊚ 204
Lanoxin Injection 1116	Cipro I.V. (1% or less) 587	**Carpopedal spasm**	AK-Trol Ointment & Suspension ⊚ 205
Lanoxin Injection Pediatric 1119	Cipro I.V. Pharmacy Bulk Package (Less than 1%) 590	Compazine 2644	Blephamide Liquifilm Sterile Ophthalmic Suspension 472
Lanoxin Tablets 1121	Cipro Tablets 584	Stelazine 2692	Blephamide Ointment (Infrequent) ⊚ 234
Rubex for Injection 721	Claritin-D Tablets 2487	Thorazine 2701	Celestone Soluspan Suspension 2484
TheraCys BCG Live (Intravesical) (Up to 2.7%) 911	D.A. II Tablets 972	Triavil Tablets 1800	CORTENEMA 2713
TICE BCG, USP (1.9%) 1881	D.A. Chewable Tablets 970	**Catalepsy**	Cortisporin Ophthalmic Ointment Sterile 1074
Cardialgia	Deconsal II Tablets 1605	Anafranil Capsules (Rare) 819	Cortisporin Ophthalmic Suspension Sterile 1075
(see under Heartburn)	Dizac (diazepam injectable emulsion) CIV (Less frequent) 1862	**Cataplexy**	Cortone Acetate Sterile Suspension 1663
Cardiodynia	Duranest Injections 533	Clozaril Tablets 2377	Cortone Acetate Tablets 1664
(see under Heartburn)	Dura-Tap/PD Capsules 970	**Cataracts**	Dalalone D.P. Injectable 1009
Cardiogenic shock	Dura-Vent/DA Tablets 972	Accutane Capsules 2252	Decadron Elixir 1676
Accupril Tablets (Rare) 1950	Dura-Vent Tablets 971	▲ AdatoSil 5000 (Approximately 50% to 70%) ⊚ 265	Decadron Phosphate Injection 1680
Activase 1045	Dyclone 0.5% and 1% Topical Solutions, USP 535	Beclovent Inhalation Aerosol and Refill (Rare) 1063	Decadron Phosphate Sterile Ophthalmic Ointment 1684
Mexitil Capsules (1 in 1,000) 684	EMLA Cream (Unlikely with cream) 536	Beconase 1065	Decadron Phosphate Sterile Ophthalmic Solution 1685
Tenormin Tablets and I.V. Injection (0.4%) 2965	Entex PSE Tablets 973		Decadron Phosphate with Xylocaine Injection, Sterile 1683
Tonocard Tablets (Less than 1%) 519	Fedahist Gyrocaps 2545		Decadron Tablets 1678
Cardiomegaly	Floxin I.V. 1580		Decadron-LA Sterile Suspension 1606
Betaseron for SC Injection 653	Floxin Tablets (200 mg, 300 mg, 400 mg) 1577		Dexacort Phosphate in Respihaler 1606
	Glucophage Tablets 754		Dexacort Phosphate in Turbinaire 1607

(⊡ Described in PDR For Nonprescription Drugs)   Incidence data in parenthesis; ▲ 3% or more   (⊚ Described in PDR For Ophthalmology)

Cataracts, posterior subcapsular — Side Effects Index

Econopred & Econopred Plus Ophthalmic Suspensions ... ⊛ 216
FML Forte Liquifilm (Infrequent) .. ⊛ 237
FML Liquifilm ... ⊛ 238
FML S.O.P. (Infrequent) ... ⊛ 239
FML-S Liquifilm ... ⊛ 240
Florinef Acetate Tablets ... 506
HMS Liquifilm (Rare) ... ⊛ 241
Hydeltrasol Injection, Sterile ... 1708
Hydeltra-T.B.A. Sterile Suspension ... 1710
Hydrocortone Acetate Sterile Suspension ... 1712
Hydrocortone Phosphate Injection, Sterile ... 1713
Hydrocortone Tablets ... 1715
Maxitrol Ophthalmic Ointment and Suspension ... ⊛ 222
NeoDecadron Sterile Ophthalmic Ointment ... 1755
NeoDecadron Sterile Ophthalmic Solution ... 1756
Pediapred Oral Solution ... 1618
Poly-Pred Liquifilm ... ⊛ 246
Pred Forte ... ⊛ 247
Pred Mild (Infrequent) ... ⊛ 250
Pred-G Liquifilm Sterile Ophthalmic Suspension ... ⊛ 248
Pred-G S.O.P. Sterile Ophthalmic Ointment ... ⊛ 249
Prelone Syrup ... 1834
Terra-Cortril Ophthalmic Suspension ... 2033
TobraDex Ophthalmic Suspension and Ointment ... 469
Vexol 1% Ophthalmic Suspension ... ⊛ 227

Catatonia

Blocadren Tablets ... 1654
Cartrol Tablets ... 413
Compazine ... 2644
Depakote Tablets (1% to 5%) ... 418
Etrafon ... 2495
Haldol Decanoate ... 1587
Haldol Injection, Tablets and Concentrate ... 1585
Inderal ... 2834
Inderal LA Long Acting Capsules ... 2836
Inderide Tablets ... 2838
Inderide LA Long Acting Capsules .. 2840
Kerlone Tablets ... 2588
Levatol Tablets ... 2547
Levoprome ... 1321
Lopressor HCT Tablets ... 850
Normodyne Tablets ... 2522
Phenergan Injection ... 2880
Phenergan Tablets ... 2882
Prolixin ... 510
Risperdal Tablets (Infrequent) ... 1348
Sectral Capsules ... 2914
Stelazine ... 2692
Tenoretic Tablets ... 2963
Tenormin Tablets and I.V. Injection ... 2965
Thorazine (Rare) ... 2701
Timolide Tablets ... 1791
Timoptic in Ocudose ... 1796
Timoptic Sterile Ophthalmic Solution ... 1794
Timoptic-XE ... 1798
Toprol-XL Tablets ... 560
Trandate Tablets ... 1158
Triavil Tablets ... 1800
Trilafon ... 2532
Visken Tablets ... 2428
Zebeta Tablets ... 1457
Ziac ... 1459

Cauda equina syndrome

Azulfidine (Rare) ... 2059

Cellulitis

Adalat CC (Less than 1.0%) ... 582
Adriamycin PFS ... 2056
Adriamycin RDF ... 2056
Anafranil Capsules (Infrequent) ... 819
Avonex ... 662
Betaseron for SC Injection ... 653
Cognex Capsules (Infrequent) ... 1961
Cytovene (1% or less) ... 2270
Doxil (Less than 1%) ... 2613
Doxorubicin Astra ... 531
Effexor (Rare) ... 2825
Hivid Tablets (Less than 1%) ... 2287
Hyperstat I.V. Injection ... 2504
Intron A for Injection (Less than 5%) ... 2506
Naprelan Tablets (Less than 1%) .. 2861
▲ Nipent for Injection (6%) ... 2733
Norplant System (Uncommon) ... 2868
Oncovin Solution Vials & Hyporets ... 1521
Paxil Tablets (Rare) ... 2681

Permax Tablets (Infrequent) ... 571
Platinol for Injection ... 717
Platinol-AQ Injection ... 719
Prozac Pulvules & Liquid, Oral Solution (Rare) ... 935
Remeron Tablets (Rare) ... 1878
ReoPro Vials (0.3%) ... 1526
Rilutek Tablets (Infrequent) ... 2198
Rubex for Injection ... 721
Sandostatin Injection (Less than 1%) ... 2421
Serzone Tablets (Rare) ... 776
Sular Tablets (Less than or equal to 1%) ... 2961
Taxol Injection (Rare) ... 723
Velban Vials ... 1537
▲ Vesanoid Capsules (8%) ... 2327
Videx Tablets, Powder for Oral Solution, & Pediatric Powder for Oral Solution (Less than 1%) ... 2980

Cellulitis, at injection site

Cefizox for Intramuscular or Intravenous Use (1% to 5%) ... 1025
Cytosar-U Sterile Powder (Less frequent) ... 2077
INFeD (Iron Dextran Injection, USP) ... 2478
Mutamycin for Injection ... 712

Cellulitis, scrotal

Testoderm Testosterone Transdermal System (One in 104 patients) ... 486

Central retinal artery occlusion

Sus-Phrine Injection ... 1017

Cephalic flocculation, increase

Prolixin ... 510

Cephalin flocculation test, positive

Cuprimine Capsules ... 1673
Depen Titratable Tablets (Few reports) ... 2770

Cerebellar dysfunction

Cerebyx Injection (Rare) ... 1956
Cytosar-U Sterile Powder (With experimental doses) ... 2077
▲ Idamycin Injection (4%) ... 2096
Neurontin Capsules (Infrequent) ... 1978

Cerebellar malformation, fetal

Accutane Capsules ... 2252

Cerebellar syndrome, acute

Ergamisol Tablets ... 1340
Fludara for Injection (Up to 1%) ... 658
Fluorouracil Injection ... 2282
Sterile FUDR (Remote possibility) .. 2284
Lamictal Tablets (Rare) ... 1105

Cerebral abnormalities, fetal

Accutane Capsules ... 2252

Cerebral arterial insufficiency, symptoms

Atretol Tablets ... 569
Tegretol/Tegretol-XR ... 870

Cerebral arteritis

Blenoxane (Rare) ... 697
Platinol for Injection (Rare) ... 717
Platinol-AQ Injection (Rare) ... 719
Ritalin (Isolated cases) ... 866

Cerebral bleeding

(see under Cerebral hemorrhage)

Cerebral hemorrhage

Anafranil Capsules (Rare) ... 819
Ana-Kit Anaphylaxis Emergency Treatment Kit ... 611
Betaseron for SC Injection ... 653
Brevicon ... 2563
Cerebyx Injection (Infrequent) ... 1956
Demulen ... 2580
Desogen Tablets ... 1867
Imitrex Injection ... 1095
Imitrex Tablets ... 1099
Levlen/Tri-Levlen ... 646
Lo/Ovral Tablets ... 2852
Lo/Ovral-28 Tablets ... 2857
Modicon ... 1928
Nordette-21 Tablets ... 2863
Nordette-28 Tablets ... 2866
Norinyl ... 2563
Nor-Q D Tablets ... 2598
Ortho-Cept ... 1907
Ortho-Cyclen/Ortho Tri-Cyclen ... 1914

Ortho-Novum ... 1928
Ortho-Cyclen/Ortho Tri-Cyclen ... 1914
Ovcon ... 765
Ovral Tablets ... 2877
Ovral-28 Tablets ... 2878
Ovrette Tablets ... 2878
Permax Tablets (Rare) ... 571
Redux Capsules ... 2911
Rifadin ... 1276
Rilutek Tablets (Infrequent) ... 2198
Levlen/Tri-Levlen ... 646
Tri-Norinyl ... 2607
Triphasil-21 Tablets ... 2919
Triphasil-28 Tablets ... 2924
▲ Vesanoid Capsules (9%) ... 2327

Cerebral infarction

Activase ... 1045
Cerebyx Injection (Infrequent) ... 1956
Hyperstat I.V. Injection ... 2504
Monopril Tablets (0.4% to 1.0%) .. 762
Redux Capsules ... 2911
Trandate ... 1158

Cerebral ischemia

(see under Ischemia, cerebral)

Cerebral occlusion

Humegon for Injection ... 1873
Ritalin (Isolated cases) ... 866

Cerebral thrombosis

Amen Tablets ... 785
Brevicon ... 2563
Cipro I.V. (1% or less) ... 587
Cipro I.V. Pharmacy Bulk Package (Less than 1%) ... 590
Cipro Tablets (Less than 1%) ... 584
Cycrin Tablets ... 991
DDAVP Injection (Rare) ... 2178
DDAVP Injection 15 mcg/mL (Rare) ... 2179
Demulen ... 2580
Desogen Tablets ... 1867
Floxin I.V. ... 1580
Floxin Tablets (200 mg, 300 mg, 400 mg) ... 1577
Lamictal Tablets (Rare) ... 1105
Levlen/Tri-Levlen ... 646
Lo/Ovral Tablets ... 2852
Lo/Ovral-28 Tablets ... 2857
Maxaquin Tablets ... 2593
Modicon ... 1928
Nordette-21 Tablets ... 2863
Nordette-28 Tablets ... 2866
Norinyl ... 2563
Nor-Q D Tablets ... 2598
Ortho-Cept ... 1907
Ortho-Cyclen/Ortho-Tri-Cyclen ... 1914
Ortho-Novum ... 1928
Ortho-Cyclen/Ortho Tri-Cyclen ... 1914
Ovcon ... 765
Ovral Tablets ... 2877
Ovral-28 Tablets ... 2878
Ovrette Tablets ... 2878
Penetrex Tablets ... 2196
Premphase ... 2900
Prempro ... 2905
Provera Tablets ... 2110
Stimate, (desmopressin acetate) Nasal Spray, 1.5 mg/mL (Rare) .. 806
Trasylol (0.5%) ... 607
Levlen/Tri-Levlen ... 646
Tri-Norinyl ... 2607
Triphasil-21 Tablets ... 2919
Triphasil-28 Tablets ... 2924

Cerebral vascular spasm

Torecan (Occasional case) ... 2367

Cerebrospinal fluid proteins, changes

Compazine ... 2644
Etrafon ... 2495
Navane Capsules and Concentrate ... 2018
Navane Intramuscular ... 2019
Prolixin ... 510
Stelazine ... 2692
Thorazine ... 2701
Triavil Tablets ... 1800
Trilafon ... 2532

Cerebrospinal fluid rhinorrhea

Parlodel (A few cases) ... 2411

Cerebrovascular accident

Accupril Tablets (Rare) ... 1950
Betagan ... ⊛ 230

Betimol 0.25%, 0.5% ... ⊛ 259
Blenoxane (Rare) ... 697
Blocadren Tablets (Less than 1%) ... 1654
BuSpar Tablets (Rare) ... 738
Calan SR Caplets (1% or less) ... 2571
Calan Tablets (1% or less) ... 2568
Capoten Tablets ... 740
Capozide Tablets ... 744
Cardura Tablets (Less than 0.5% of 3960 patients) ... 1993
Catapres-TTS ... 680
Cognex Capsules (Infrequent) ... 1961
Covera-HS Tablets (Less than 2%) ... 2573
Cozaar Tablets (Less than 1%) ... 1668
D.H.E. 45 Injection (Extremely rare) ... 2381
Desyrel and Desyrel Dividose ... 504
Effexor (Rare) ... 2825
Emcyt Capsules (2%) ... 2085
Epogen for Injection (0.4%) ... 489
▲ Flolan for Injection (4%) ... 1085
Fludara for Injection (Up to 3%) ... 658
Gemzar for Injection (2%) ... 1482
Hyzaar Tablets ... 1720
Imitrex Injection (Rare) ... 1095
Imitrex Tablets ... 1099
Isoptin Oral Tablets (Less than 1%) ... 1393
Isoptin SR Tablets (1% or less) ... 1395
Lamictal Tablets (Rare) ... 1105
Lioresal Intrathecal (1% or more) .. 1634
Lodine Capsules and Tablets (Less than 1%) ... 2849
LUVOX Tablets (Rare) ... 2723
Miacalcin Nasal Spray (Less than 1%) ... 2403
Monopril Tablets (0.2% to 1.0%) .. 762
Motrin Ibuprofen Suspension, Oral Drops, Chewable Tablets, Caplets (Less than 1%) ... 1563
Neurontin Capsules (Rare) ... 1978
Ocupress Ophthalmic Solution, 1% Sterile ... ⊛ 297
Orthoclone OKT3 Sterile Solution .. 1892
Paraplatin for Injection ... 713
Paxil Tablets (Rare) ... 2681
Permax Tablets (Infrequent) ... 571
Platinol for Injection (Rare) ... 717
Platinol-AQ Injection (Rare) ... 719
Prevacid Delayed-Release Capsules (Less than 1%) ... 2746
Prinivil Tablets (0.3% to 1.0%) ... 1776
Prinzide Tablets ... 1780
Procrit for Injection (0.4% to 3.2%) ... 1896
Prozac Pulvules & Liquid, Oral Solution ... 935
Redux Capsules ... 2911
Serzone Tablets (Rare) ... 776
Sular Tablets (Less than or equal to 1%) ... 2961
Tenex Tablets (Rare) ... 2249
Timolide Tablets ... 1791
Timoptic in Ocudose (Less frequent) ... 1796
Timoptic Sterile Ophthalmic Solution (Less frequent) ... 1794
Timoptic-XE ... 1798
Tonocard Tablets ... 519
Trasylol (0.5%) ... 607
Vaseretic Tablets ... 1810
Vasotec I.V. ... 1814
Vasotec Tablets (0.5% to 1.0%) ... 1816
Velban Vials ... 1537
Verelan Capsules (1% or less) ... 1455
Zestoretic Tablets ... 2968
Zestril Tablets (0.3% to 1.0%) ... 2972
Zoladex (Greater than 1% but less than 5%) ... 2976
Zoladex 3-month (1% to 5%) ... 2978
Zosyn (1.0% or less) ... 1463

Cerebrovascular disorders

Aldoclor Tablets ... 1638
Aldomet Ester HCl Injection ... 1642
Aldomet Oral ... 1640
Aldoril Tablets ... 1644
Altace Capsules (Less than 1%) ... 1238
Ambien Tablets (Infrequent) ... 2559
Amen Tablets ... 785
Brevicon ... 2563
Cycrin Tablets ... 991
Demulen ... 2580
Depo-Provera Contraceptive Injection ... 2079
Depo-Provera Sterile Aqueous Suspension ... 2083
Ethmozine Tablets (Less than 2%) ... 2217
Felbatol ... 2774
Flumadine Tablets & Syrup (Less than 0.3%) ... 1013

(⊛ Described in PDR For Nonprescription Drugs)   Incidence data in parenthesis; ▲ 3% or more   (⊛ Described in PDR For Ophthalmology)

Side Effects Index

Chest pain

Foscavir Injection (Between 1% and 5%)	541
Kerlone Tablets (Less than 2%)	2588
Levlen/Tri-Levlen	646
Maxaquin Tablets (Less than 1%)	2593
Modicon	1928
Norinyl	2563
Norplant System	2868
Nor-Q D Tablets	2598
Ortho-Cyclen/Ortho-Tri-Cyclen	1914
Ortho-Novum	1928
Ortho-Cyclen/Ortho Tri-Cyclen	1914
Ovcon	765
Premphase	2900
Prempro	2905
Provera Tablets	2110
Risperdal Tablets	1348
Levlen/Tri-Levlen	646
Tri-Norinyl	2607

Cerebrovascular insufficiency
Capoten Tablets	740
Capozide Tablets	744

Cervical disorders (see under Cervical irregularities)

Cervical erosion, changes
Amen Tablets	785
Aygestin Tablets	990
Brevicon	2563
Cycrin Tablets	991
Demulen	2580
Depo-Provera Sterile Aqueous Suspension	2083
Desogen Tablets	1867
ESTRATAB Tablets (0.3, 0.625, 1.25, 2.5 mg)	2715
Estratest	2718
Levlen/Tri-Levlen	646
Lo/Ovral Tablets	2852
Lo/Ovral-28 Tablets	2857
Menest Tablets	2671
Modicon	1928
Nordette-21 Tablets	2863
Nordette-28 Tablets	2866
Norinyl	2563
Nor-Q D Tablets	2598
Ortho-Cept	1907
Ortho-Cyclen/Ortho-Tri-Cyclen	1914
Ortho-Novum	1928
Ortho-Cyclen/Ortho Tri-Cyclen	1914
Ovcon	765
Ovral Tablets	2877
Ovral-28 Tablets	2878
Ovrette Tablets	2878
ParaGard T 380A Intrauterine Copper Contraceptive	1936
PMB 200 and PMB 400	2890
Premarin Intravenous	2893
Premarin Vaginal Cream	2898
Premphase	2900
Prempro	2905
Provera Tablets	2110
Levlen/Tri-Levlen	646
Tri-Norinyl	2607
Triphasil-21 Tablets	2919
Triphasil-28 Tablets	2924

Cervical eversion, changes in
Diethylstilbestrol Tablets	1477
Ortho Dienestrol Cream	1922

Cervical irregularities
Demulen	2580
Hivid Tablets (Less than 1%)	2287
Lupron Depot-PED 7.5 mg, 11.25 mg and 15 mg (Less than 2%)	2744
Lupron Injection Pediatric (Less than 2%)	2737

Cervical secretion, changes
Amen Tablets	785
Aygestin Tablets	990
Brevicon	2563
Climara Transdermal System	640
Cycrin Tablets	991
Demulen	2580
Depo-Provera Sterile Aqueous Suspension	2083
Desogen Tablets	1867
Diethylstilbestrol Tablets	1477
Estrace Cream and Tablets	751
Estraderm Transdermal System	842
ESTRATAB Tablets (0.3, 0.625, 1.25, 2.5 mg)	2715
Estratest	2718
Levlen/Tri-Levlen	646
Lo/Ovral Tablets	2852
Lo/Ovral-28 Tablets	2857
Menest Tablets	2671
Modicon	1928
Nordette-21 Tablets	2863
Nordette-28 Tablets	2866
Norinyl	2563
Nor-Q D Tablets	2598
Ogen Tablets	2103
Ogen Vaginal Cream	2106
Ortho-Cept	1907
Ortho-Cyclen/Ortho-Tri-Cyclen	1914
Ortho Dienestrol Cream	1922
Ortho-Est	1925
Ortho-Novum	1928
Ortho-Cyclen/Ortho Tri-Cyclen	1914
Ovcon	765
Ovral Tablets	2877
Ovral-28 Tablets	2878
Ovrette Tablets	2878
PMB 200 and PMB 400	2890
Premarin Intravenous	2893
Premarin Tablets	2896
Premarin Vaginal Cream	2898
Premphase	2900
Prempro	2905
Provera Tablets	2110
Levlen/Tri-Levlen	646
Tri-Norinyl	2607
Triphasil-21 Tablets	2919
Triphasil-28 Tablets	2924
Vivelle Transdermal System	880

Cervicitis
Betaseron for SC Injection	653
▲Cleocin Vaginal Cream (16% to 33%)	2070
▲Norplant System (5% or greater)	2868

Chafing, genital
Condylox Topical Solution (Less than 5%)	1853

Change in blood glucose levels (see under Insulin reaction)

Character changes
Seromycin Capsules	975

Charcot's syndrome
Atromid-S Capsules	2808
Imdur (Less than or equal to 5%)	1362
Isoptin Oral Tablets (Less than 1%)	1393
Kerlone Tablets (Less than 2%)	2588
ReoPro Vials (0.4%)	1526
Timolide Tablets	1791
Tonocard Tablets (Less than 1%)	519

Cheek puffing
Compazine	2644
Etrafon	2495
Haldol Decanoate	1587
Haldol Injection, Tablets and Concentrate	1585
Mellaril	2398
Moban Tablets and Concentrate	1036
Navane Intramuscular	2019
Orap Tablets	1037
Phenobarbital Elixir and Tablets	1523
Prolixin	510
Stelazine	2692
Thorazine	2701

Cheilitis
▲Accutane Capsules (More than 90%)	2252
Anafranil Capsules (Rare)	819
Betaseron for SC Injection	653
Cosmegen Injection	1666
Crixivan Capsules (Less than 2%)	1670
Effexor (Rare)	2825
Invirase Capsules (Less than 2%)	2291
Norvir (Less than 2%)	447
Rilutek Tablets (Rare)	2198
▲Tegison Capsules (Less than 75%)	2314

Cheilitis, actinic
▲Tegison Capsules (Greater than 75%)	2314

Cheilosis
Cuprimine Capsules (Rare)	1673
Depen Titratable Tablets (Rare)	2770

Cheilosis, monilial
Lamprene Capsules (Less than 1%)	846

Chemosis
Alomide Ophthalmic Solution (Less than 1%)	465
Chibroxin Sterile Ophthalmic Solution	1657
▲Rev-Eyes Ophthalmic Eyedrops 0.5% (10% to 40%)	⊚ 324

Chest congestion
▲AeroBid Inhaler System (3% to 9%)	1004
▲Aerobid-M Inhaler System (3% to 9%)	1004
BuSpar Tablets (Infrequent)	738
Claritin-D Tablets (Less frequent)	2487
Cognex Capsules (Infrequent)	1961
Effexor (Infrequent)	2825
Flovent (1% to 3%)	1089
Hivid Tablets (Less than 1%)	2287
Klonopin Tablets	2294
Roferon-A Injection (Less than 3%)	2308

Chest numbness
Tessalon Perles	1018

Chest pain
Accupril Tablets (2.4%)	1950
Accutane Capsules (Less frequent)	2252
▲Actigall Capsules (3.2%)	818
Adalat CC (3% or less)	582
Adenocard Injection (Less than 1%)	1021
▲AeroBid Inhaler System (3% to 9%)	1004
▲Aerobid-M Inhaler System (3% to 9%)	1004
▲Alferon N Injection (6% to 10%)	2142
Altace Capsules (Less than 1% to 1.1%)	1238
Alupent Tablets (0.2%)	672
Ambien Tablets (1%)	2559
▲Anafranil Capsules (4% to 7%)	819
Ancobon Capsules	2254
Apresazide Capsules	824
▲Arimidex Tablets (5.0% to 7.3%)	2932
▲Asacol Delayed-Release Tablets (3%)	2129
▲Atrovent Inhalation Solution (3.2%)	675
▲Avonex (6%)	662
Axid Pulvules (2.3%)	1468
Azactam for Injection (One patient)	736
Betagan	⊚ 230
▲Betapace Tablets (4% to 16%)	637
Betimol 0.25%, 0.5%	⊚ 259
Blenoxane (Rare)	697
Blocadren Tablets (0.6%)	1654
Brevibloc (esmolol HCl) Injection (Less than 1%)	1860
Bumex (0.1%)	2260
BuSpar Tablets (Frequent)	738
Cafergot	2376
Calan SR Caplets (1% or less)	2571
Calan Tablets (1% or less)	2568
Capoten Tablets (Approximately 1 in 100 patients)	740
Capozide Tablets (Approximately 1 of 100 patients)	744
Cardene Capsules (Rare)	2261
Cardene I.V. (0.7%)	2815
Cardene SR Capsules (Rare)	2264
Cardizem Injectable (Less than 1%)	1253
Cardura Tablets (1.2% to 2%)	1993
Cartrol Tablets (2.2%)	413
▲Casodex Tablets (6%)	2934
Cataflam Tablets (Less than 1%)	833
Catapres-TTS	680
Ceftin (0.1% to 1%)	1067
▲CellCept Capsules (13.3% to 13.4%)	2265
Cipro I.V. (1% or less)	587
Cipro I.V. Pharmacy Bulk Package (Less than 1%)	590
Cipro Tablets (Less than 1%)	584
Claritin Tablets (2% or fewer patients)	2485
Claritin-D Tablets (Less frequent)	2487
Clinoril Tablets (Less than 1 in 100)	1658
Clomid	1262
Clozaril Tablets (1%)	2377
▲Cognex Capsules (4%)	1961
Colestid (Infrequent)	2073
Coumadin	941
Covera-HS Tablets (Less than 2%)	2573
Cozaar Tablets (1% or greater)	1668
Crixivan Capsules (Less than 2%)	1670
Cytosar-U Sterile Powder (Less frequent; occasional)	2077
Cytotec (Infrequent)	2576
Cytovene (1% or less)	2270
D.H.E. 45 Injection	2381
Dalgan Injection (Less than 1%)	529
Dalmane Capsules	2329
▲DaunoXome (1% to 9%)	1842
Demadex Tablets and Injection (1.2%)	691
Depakote Tablets (1% to 5%)	418
Depo-Provera Contraceptive Injection (Fewer than 1%)	2079
Desyrel and Desyrel Dividose	504
Dilacor XR Extended-release Capsules (Infrequent)	2183
Dipentum Capsules (Rare)	2084
Diprivan Injectable Emulsion (Less than 1%)	2939
Dizac (diazepam injectable emulsion) CIV	1862
Dobutrex Solution Vials (1% to 3%)	1480
Dolobid Tablets (Rare)	1695
Dopram Injectable	2235
Doxil (1% to 5%)	2613
Duragesic Transdermal System (1% or greater)	1336
▲DynaCirc Capsules (2.7% to 7%)	2381
DynaCirc CR Tablets (0.5% to 1.0%)	2383
E.E.S. (Isolated reports)	427
Effexor (2%)	2825
Emcyt Capsules (1%)	2085
▲Eminase (Less than 10%)	2215
▲Epogen for Injection (7%)	489
Ergamisol Tablets (Less than 1% to 1%)	1340
EryPed (Isolated reports)	425
Ery-Tab Tablets (Isolated reports)	426
Erythrocin Stearate Filmtab (Isolated reports)	429
Erythromycin Base Filmtab (Isolated reports)	430
Erythromycin Delayed-Release Capsules, USP (Isolated reports)	431
Esimil Tablets	840
Estrace Cream and Tablets	751
Estring Vaginal Ring (1% to 3%)	2086
▲Ethmozine Tablets (2% to 5%)	2217
Felbatol (2.6%)	2774
Fioricet with Codeine Capsules	2387
Fiorinal with Codeine Capsules	2390
Flexeril Tablets (Rare)	1701
▲Flolan for Injection (11% to 67%)	1085
Floxin I.V. (1% to 3%)	1580
Floxin Tablets (200 mg, 300 mg, 400 mg) (1% to 3%)	1577
Foscavir Injection (Between 1% and 5%)	541
Gamimune N, 5% Immune Globulin Intravenous (Human), 5%	612
Gamimune N, 10% Immune Globulin Intravenous (Human), 10%	615
Gastrocrom Oral Concentrate (Less common)	1611
Halcion Tablets	2093
Hespan Injection	945
Hivid Tablets (Less than 1%)	2287
▲Hylorel Tablets (27.9%)	1613
Hytrin Capsules (At least 1%)	434
Hyzaar Tablets	1720
Idamycin Injection	2096
Imdur (Less than or equal to 5%)	1362
Imitrex Injection	1095
Imitrex Tablets (Frequent)	1099
Indocin (Less than 1%)	1723
INFeD (Iron Dextran Injection, USP)	2478
Inocor Lactate Injection (0.2%)	2439
▲Intron A for Injection (Up to 28%)	2506
Invirase Capsules (Less than 2%)	2291
Iopidine 0.5% (Less than 1%)	⊚ 219
Ismelin Tablets	845
Isoptin Oral Tablets (Less than 1%)	1393
Isoptin SR Tablets (1% or less)	1395
Kadian Capsules (Less than 3%)	2948
▲Kerlone Tablets (2.4% to 7.1%)	2588
Lamictal Tablets (More than 1%)	1105
▲Leukine (15%)	1317
Levatol Tablets (2.4%)	2547
Levlen/Tri-Levlen	646
Lioresal Intrathecal (1% or more)	1634
Lioresal Tablets (Rare)	847
Lotensin HCT Tablets (0.3% to 1.0%)	855
Lotrel Capsules (Infrequent)	858
LUVOX Tablets	2723
Macrobid Capsules	2138
Macrodantin Capsules	2140
Mavik Tablets (0.3% to 1.0%)	1407
Maxair Autohaler (1.3%)	1550

(🅱 Described in PDR For Nonprescription Drugs) Incidence data in parenthesis; ▲ 3% or more (⊚ Described in PDR For Ophthalmology)

Maxair Inhaler (Less than 1%) 1552
Maxaquin Tablets (Less than 1%).. 2593
Megace Oral Suspension (1% to 3%) 708
Merrem I.V. (0/.1% to 1.0%) 2952
Methergine (Rare) 2401
Methotrexate Sodium Tablets, Injection, for Injection and LPF Injection (Less common) 1322
Mevacor Tablets (0.5% to 1.0%) .. 1742
▲ Mexitil Capsules (2.6% to 7.5%) .. 684
Midamor Tablets (Less than or equal to 1%) 1746
Modicon 1928
Moduretic Tablets (Less than or equal to 1%) 1748
Monoket Tablets (Less than 1% to 2%) 2550
Monopril Tablets (0.2% to 2.2%).. 762
Mycobutin Capsules (1%) 2101
Mykrox Tablets (2.7%) 1617
Naprelan Tablets (Less than 3%) .. 2861
▲ Navelbine Injection (5%) 1212
Neoral (Rare) 2405
▲ Neupogen for Injection (5%) 495
▲ Nipent for Injection (3% to 10%) .. 2733
Noroxin Tablets (Less frequent) 1758
Noroxin Tablets (Less frequent) 2222
Norpace (1 to 3%) 2596
Norvasc Tablets (More than 0.1% to 1%) 2020
Norvir (Less than 2%) 447
Novantrone for Injection 1327
Oncaspar (Less than 1%) 2194
Orap Tablets 1037
Ortho-Cyclen/Ortho-Tri-Cyclen 1914
Ortho-Est 1925
Ortho-Novum 1928
Ortho-Cyclen/Ortho Tri-Cyclen 1914
▲ Orthoclone OKT3 Sterile Solution (14%) 1892
OxyContin Tablets (Less than 1%) 2163
▲ Paxil Tablets (3%) 2681
Peganone Tablets 455
Penetrex Tablets (0.1% to 1%) 2196
Pentasa (Infrequent) 1275
Pentaspan Injection 954
▲ Permax Tablets (3.7%) 571
Plendil Extended-Release Tablets (0.5% to 1.5%) 514
Pondimin Tablets 2239
Pravachol Tablets (0.3% to 3.7%) 770
Prevacid Delayed-Release Capsules (Less than 1%) 2746
Prilosec Delayed-Release Capsules (Less than 1%) 516
Primacor Injection (1.2%) 2461
▲ Prinivil Tablets (3.4%) 1776
Prinzide Tablets (0.3 to 1%) 1780
Procardia XL Extended Release Tablets (Less than 3%) 2026
▲ Procrit for Injection (7%) 1896
Proglycem (Rare) 575
▲ Prograf (Greater than 3%) 1028
▲ Proleukin for Injection (12%) 812
Propulsid (More than 1%) 1346
ProSom Tablets (1%) 457
Prostin E2 Suppository 2109
Proventil Syrup (Less than 1 of 100 patients) 2528
Prozac Pulvules & Liquid, Oral Solution (1.3% to 3%) 935
▲ Pulmozyme Inhalation (18% to 21%) 1054
Redux Capsules (Infrequent) 2911
Retrovir Capsules 1216
Retrovir I.V. Infusion 1221
Retrovir Syrup 1216
Rifater 1280
Risperdal Tablets (2% to 3%) 1348
▲ Roferon-A Injection (4% to 11%) .. 2308
Romazicon (Less than 1%) 2311
Rowasa 2727
Rythmol Tablets–150mg, 225mg, 300mg (0.5 to 1.8%) 1399
Sandimmune (Rare) 2416
Sandostatin Injection (Less than 1%) 2421
Sansert Tablets 2424
Sectral Capsules (2%) 2914
Serzone Tablets 776
Sinemet CR Tablets (1.0%) 961
Stadol (Infrequent) 779
Stimate, (desmopressin acetate) Nasal Spray, 1.5 mg/mL 806
Sular Tablets (2%) 2961
▲ Supprelin Injection (1% to 10%) 2230
Synarel Nasal Solution for Central Precocious Puberty (2.6%) 2603
▲ Tambocor Tablets (5.4%) 1555
Taxol Injection 723
Taxotere for Injection Concentrate 2204
Tegison Capsules (Less than 1%) .. 2314
Tenex Tablets (Less frequent) 2249
▲ THROMBATE III Antithrombin III (Human) (1 of 17) 631
▲ Tilade Inhaler (4.0%) 2207
Timolide Tablets (Less than 1%) 1791
Timoptic in Ocudose (Less frequent) 1796
Timoptic Sterile Ophthalmic Solution (Less frequent) 1794
Timoptic-XE 1798
Tolectin (200, 400 and 600 mg) (1 to 3%) 1591
Tonocard Tablets (0.4% to 1.6%) 519
Toprol-XL Tablets (About 1 of 100 patients) 560
Trental Tablets (0.3%) 1291
Levlen/Tri-Levlen 646
Unasyn (Less than 1%) 2035
Univasc Tablets (More than 1%) 2553
Valium Injectable 2336
Vancocin HCl, Oral Solution & Pulvules 1536
Vancocin HCl, Vials & ADD-Vantage 1534
Vantin for Oral Suspension and Vantin Tablets (Less than 1%) 2112
Vaseretic Tablets (0.5% to 2.0%) 1810
Vasotec I.V. 1814
Vasotec Tablets (0.5% to 2.1%) 1816
Ventolin Syrup (Less than 1 of 100 patients) 1175
Verelan Capsules (1% or less) 1455
Videx Tablets, Powder for Oral Solution, & Pediatric Powder for Oral Solution (Up to 2%) 2980
Virazole 1310
▲ Visken Tablets (3%) 2428
Vistide Injection 1057
Vivelle Transdermal System 880
Cataflam/Voltaren/Voltaren-XR (Less than 1%) 833
Wellbutrin Tablets (Infrequent) 1177
Xalatan (1% to 2%) .... ⊙ 304
▲ Xanax Tablets (10.6%) 2115
Yutopar Intravenous Injection (1% to 2%) 566
Zaroxolyn Tablets 1625
Zebeta Tablets (1.1% to 1.5%) 1457
▲ Zerit Capsules (Fewer than 1% to 8%) 731
Zestoretic Tablets (0.3 to 1.0%) 2968
▲ Zestril Tablets (3.4%) 2972
Ziac (0.9% to 1.8%) 1459
Zithromax (1% or less) 2043
Zithromax Tablets (1% or less) 2046
Zofran Injection (Rare; 2%) 1227
Zofran Tablets (Rare) 1231
Zoladex (1% or greater) 2976
Zoladex 3-month 2978
Zoloft Tablets (1.0%) 2051
Zosyn (1.0% or less to 1.3%) 1463
Zovirax Sterile Powder (Less than 1%) 1191

Chest pain, substernal

Effexor (Infrequent) 2825
Felbatol (Rare) 2774
Foscavir Injection (Less than 1%) .. 541
Intron A for Injection (Less than 5%) 2506
Norvir (Less than 2%) 447
Remeron Tablets (Rare) 1878
Videx Tablets, Powder for Oral Solution, & Pediatric Powder for Oral Solution (Less than 1%) 2980
Zoloft Tablets (Rare) 2051

Chest sound, abnormalities

Imdur (Less than or equal to 5%) .. 1362
▲ Leustatin (9%) 1889
Orthoclone OKT3 Sterile Solution .. 1892
Prinivil Tablets (Greater than 1%).. 1776
Prinzide Tablets 1780
Zestoretic Tablets 2968
Zestril Tablets (Greater than 1%) .. 2972

Chest tightness

Acthrel for Injection 2990
▲ Adenocard Injection (7%) 1021
AeroBid Inhaler System (1% to 3%) 1004
Aerobid-M Inhaler System (1% to 3%) 1004
▲ Alfenta Injection (17%) 1334
Alferon N Injection 2142
Atrohist Plus Tablets 1605
Benadryl Injection 1955
Bioclate, Antihemophilic Factor (Recombinant) 797
▲ Bromfed-DM Cough Syrup (Among most frequent) 1832
Ceftin (0.1% to 1%) 1067
▲ DaunoXome (13.8% to 16%) 1842
Dimetane-DC Cough Syrup 2232
Dimetane-DX Cough Syrup 2233
Dopram Injectable 2235
▲ Doxil (Approximately 6.8%) 2613
Eskalith 2658
Furoxone (Rare) 2221
Gamimune N, 5% Immune Globulin Intravenous (Human), 5% 612
Gamimune N, 10% Immune Globulin Intravenous (Human), 10% 615
Gammar-P I.V., Immune Globulin Intravenous (Human) 798
Geref (sermorelin acetate for injection) 2995
Hivid Tablets (Less than 1%) 2287
Hyperstat I.V. Injection 2504
Hyskon Hysteroscopy Fluid (Rare).. 1633
Imitrex Injection (2.7%) 1095
Imitrex Tablets (Frequent) 1099
INFeD (Iron Dextran Injection, USP) 2478
Levlen/Tri-Levlen 646
Lithonate/Lithotabs/Lithobid 2721
Maxair Autohaler (1.3%) 1550
Modicon 1928
Monoclate-P, Factor VIII:C Pasteurized, Monoclonal Antibody Purified Antihemophilic Factor (Human) 802
Mononine, Coagulation Factor IX (Human), Monoclonal Antibody Purified 804
Nicotrol NS Nicotine Nasal Spray (Common) 1565
Ornade Spansule Capsules 2678
Ortho-Cyclen/Ortho-Tri-Cyclen 1914
Ortho-Novum 1928
Ortho-Cyclen/Ortho Tri-Cyclen 1914
Orthoclone OKT3 Sterile Solution .. 1892
PBZ Tablets 863
PBZ-SR Tablets 862
Periactin 1767
Prostin E2 Suppository 2109
Quadrinal Tablets 1398
RespiGam 1631
Rifater 1280
Sandoglobulin I.V. (Less than 1%).. 2419
Sansert Tablets 2424
▲ Sufenta Injection (3% to 9%) 1355
Tavist Syrup 2426
Tavist Tablets 2427
Taxotere for Injection Concentrate 2204
▲ THROMBATE III Antithrombin III (Human) (3 of 17) 631
THYREL TRH (Less frequent) 2992
Tornalate Metered Dose Inhaler (Less than 1%) 978
Levlen/Tri-Levlen 646
Trinalin Repetabs Tablets 1373
Tussend 1830
Tussionex Pennkinetic Extended-Release Suspension (Occasional) 1624
Yutopar Intravenous Injection (1% to 2%) 566

Chewing movements

Compazine 2644
Etrafon 2495
Haldol Decanoate 1587
Haldol Injection, Tablets and Concentrate 1585
Mellaril 2398
Moban Tablets and Concentrate 1036
Navane Capsules and Concentrate 2018
Navane Intramuscular 2019
Orap Tablets 1037
Prolixin 510
Serentil 689
Stelazine 2692
Thorazine 2701
Triavil Tablets 1800
Trilafon 2532

Chills

Abbokinase 403
Abbokinase Open-Cath 405
▲ Abelcet Injection (15% to 16%) 1540
▲ Actimmune (14%) 1043
Adalat Capsules (10 mg and 20 mg) (2% or less) 580
Adalat CC (Less than 1.0%) 582
Adapin Capsules (Occasional) 1542
Adriamycin PFS (Occasional) 2056
Adriamycin RDF (Occasional) 2056
AeroBid Inhaler System (1% to 3%) 1004
Aerobid-M Inhaler System (1% to 3%) 1004
▲ Alferon N Injection (14% to 87%) 2142
Alupent Tablets (0.2%) 672
Anafranil Capsules (Up to 2%) 819
Anaprox/Naprosyn (Less than 1%) 2277
Apresazide Capsules (Less frequent) 824
Apresoline Hydrochloride Tablets (Less frequent) 826
▲ Asacol Delayed-Release Tablets (3%) 2129
Atretol Tablets 569
▲ Avonex (21%) 662
Bactrim DS Tablets 2257
Bactrim I.V. Infusion 2255
Bactrim 2257
Benadryl Injection 1955
▲ Betaseron for SC Injection (46%) .. 653
Bicillin C-R Injection 2810
Bicillin C-R 900/300 Injection 2812
Bicillin L-A Injection 2813
Bioclate, Antihemophilic Factor (Recombinant) (Extremely rare) .. 797
Blenoxane (Frequent) 697
Buprenex Injectable (Less than 1%) 2170
Carbocaine Injection 2432
Casodex Tablets (2% to 5%) 2934
Ceftin (0.1% to 1%) 1067
▲ CellCept Capsules (More than or equal to 3%) 2265
Cerebyx Injection (Frequent) 1956
Ceredase 1055
Cerubidine for Injection (Rare) 634
▲ Chemet Capsules (5.2% to 15.7%) 666
Cipro I.V. (1% or less) 587
Cipro I.V. Pharmacy Bulk Package (Less than 1%) 590
Cipro Tablets (Less than 1%) 584
Clinoril Tablets (Less than 1 in 100) 1658
Clozaril Tablets (Less than 1%) 2377
Cognex Capsules (Frequent) 1961
Crixivan Capsules (Less than 2%).. 1670
CytoGam (Less than 5.0%) 1630
▲ Cytovene (7%) 2270
DDAVP (Up to 2%) 2180
Dalgan Injection (Less than 1%) 529
Danocrine Capsules (Rare) 2437
Dantrium Capsules (Less frequent) 2131
Depakote Tablets (1% to 5%) 418
Depen Titratable Tablets 2770
Depo-Provera Contraceptive Injection (Fewer than 1%) 2079
Desmopressin Acetate Rhinal Tube (Up to 2%) 997
Desyrel and Desyrel Dividose 504
Dilaudid-HP Injection (Less frequent) 1384
Dilaudid-HP Lyophilized Powder 250 mg (Less frequent) 1384
Dilaudid Tablets and Liquid 1386
Dipentum Capsules (Rare) 2084
Diphtheria & Tetanus Toxoids Adsorbed Purogenated (Mild) 1422
Diprivan Injectable Emulsion (Less than 1%) 2939
Dolobid Tablets (Less than 1 in 100) 1695
Doxil (1% to 5%) 2613
Doxorubicin Astra (Occasional) 531
EC-Naprosyn Delayed-Release Tablets (Less than 1%) 2277
Edecrin 1698
▲ Effexor (2.2% to 6.8%) 2825
Eldepryl Capsules 2729
Elspar 1700
Emete-con Intramuscular/Intravenous 2007
▲ Eminase (Less than 10%) 2215
Engerix-B Unit-Dose Vials (Less than 1%) 2656
▲ Epivir (10%) 1200
Ergamisol Tablets (5 patients) 1340
Ethyol (amifostine) for Injection 485
▲ Etopophos for Injection (3% to 24%) 701
Etoposide Injection (0.7% to 2%).. 539
Fansidar Tablets 2281
▲ Flolan for Injection (25%) 1085
Floxin I.V. (Less than 1%) 1580
Floxin Tablets (200 mg, 300 mg, 400 mg) (Less than 1%) 1577
▲ Fludara for Injection (11% to 19%) 658

Side Effects Index — Cholestasis, intrahepatic

▲ Fungizone Intravenous (Among most common) ... 507
▲ Gamimune N, 5% Immune Globulin Intravenous (Human), 5% (Among most common; 9 patients) ... 612
▲ Gamimune N, 10% Immune Globulin Intravenous (Human), 10% (Among most common; 9 patients) ... 615
Gammagard S/D, Immune Globulin, Intravenous (Human) (Occasional) ... 577
▲ Gammar-P I.V., Immune Globulin Intravenous (Human) (8.9%) ... 798
Gantanol Tablets ... 2285
Gantrisin ... 2286
Gemzar for Injection (Common) ... 1482
Glucotrol XL Extended Release Tablets (Less than 1%) ... 2012
Heparin Lock Flush Solution ... 2831
Heparin Sodium Injection ... 2832
▲ Heparin Sodium Vials (Among most common) ... 1486
Hespan Injection ... 945
Hivid Tablets (Less than 1%) ... 2287
Humegon for Injection ... 1873
Hydralazine Hydrochloride Injection USP (Less frequent) ... 2712
Hydrea Capsules ... 705
IBU Tablets (Less than 1%) ... 1389
Imitrex Injection (Infrequent) ... 1095
Inapsine Injection (Less common) ... 462
INFeD (Iron Dextran Injection, USP) ... 2478
▲ Intron A for Injection (Up to 54%) ... 2506
▲ JE-VAX (Approximately 10%) ... 904
Kadian Capsules (Less than 3%) ... 2948
Konÿne 80 Factor IX Complex ... 627
Lamictal Tablets (1.3%) ... 1105
▲ Lariam Tablets (Among most frequent) ... 2295
Lescol Capsules (Rare) ... 2395
▲ Leukine (19% to 25%) ... 1317
▲ Leustatin (9%) ... 1889
Levoprome (Sometimes) ... 1321
Lioresal Intrathecal (Up to 1.3%) ... 1634
Lodine Capsules and Tablets (Greater than or equal to 1%) ... 2849
Lotensin HCT Tablets (0.3% or more) ... 855
Lupron Depot 7.5 mg (Less than 5%) ... 2741
Lupron Injection (Less than 5%) ... 2736
LUVOX Tablets (2%) ... 2723
MS Contin Tablets (Less frequent) ... 2149
MSIR (Infrequent) ... 2152
Macrobid Capsules (Less than 1%) ... 2138
Macrodantin Capsules ... 2140
Marcaine ... 2446
Marinol (Dronabinol) Capsules (Less than 1%) ... 2353
Matulane Capsules ... 2300
Maxaquin Tablets (Less than 1%) ... 2593
Methadone Hydrochloride Oral Concentrate ... 2356
Methotrexate Sodium Tablets, Injection, for Injection and LPF Injection (Frequent) ... 1322
Metrodin (urofollitropin for injection) ... 2616
Mevacor Tablets (Rare) ... 1742
Miltown Tablets (Rare) ... 2780
Mintezol ... 1747
Monoclate-P, Factor VIII:C Pasteurized, Monoclonal Antibody Purified Antihemophilic Factor (Human) ... 802
Mononine, Coagulation Factor IX (Human), Monoclonal Antibody Purified ... 804
Mykrox Tablets ... 1617
▲ Naprelan Tablets (3% to 9%) ... 2861
Anaprox/Naprosyn (Less than 1%) ... 2277
Navelbine Injection ... 1212
Neurontin Capsules (Infrequent) ... 1978
▲ Nipent for Injection (11% to 19%) ... 2733
Nizoral Tablets (Less than 1%) ... 1345
Noroxin Tablets (Less frequent) ... 1758
Noroxin Tablets (Less frequent) ... 2222
Norvir (Less than 2%) ... 447
▲ Oncaspar (Greater than 5%) ... 2194
Oramorph SR (Morphine Sulfate Sustained Release Tablets) (Less frequent) ... 2359
Orlaam Oral Solution (1% to 3%) ... 2361
Ornade Spansule Capsules ... 2678

▲ Orthoclone OKT3 Sterile Solution (59%) ... 1892
Orudis Capsules (Less than 1%) ... 2874
Oruvail Capsules (Less than 1%) ... 2874
OxyContin Tablets (Between 1% and 5%) ... 2163
PBZ Tablets ... 863
PBZ-SR Tablets ... 862
Parnate Tablets ... 2679
Paxil Tablets (Frequent; 2%) ... 2681
Penetrex Tablets (0.1% to 1%) ... 2196
Pentaspan Injection ... 954
Peptavlon ... 2997
Pergonal (menotropins for injection, USP) ... 2618
Periactin ... 1767
Permax Tablets (1.1%) ... 571
Pfizerpen for Injection ... 2022
PMB 200 and PMB 400 (Rare) ... 2890
Pondimin Tablets ... 2239
Pontocaine Hydrochloride for Spinal Anesthesia ... 2460
Pravachol Tablets (Rare) ... 770
Prinivil Tablets (0.3% to 1.0%) ... 1776
Prinzide Tablets ... 1780
Priscoline Hydrochloride Ampuls ... 864
Procanbid Extended-Release Tablets (Fairly common) ... 1983
Procardia Capsules (2% or less) ... 2024
▲ Prograf (Greater than 3%) ... 1028
Prolastin Alpha₁-Proteinase Inhibitor (Human) (Occasional) ... 629
▲ Proleukin for Injection (89%) ... 812
ProSom Tablets (Infrequent) ... 457
▲ Prostin E2 Suppository (Approximately one-tenth) ... 2109
Prozac Pulvules & Liquid, Oral Solution (Frequent) ... 935
Recombivax HB (Less than 1%) ... 1787
Redux Capsules (2.9%) ... 2911
Relafen Tablets (Less than 1%) ... 2688
Remeron Tablets (Infrequent) ... 1878
Retrovir Capsules ... 1216
Retrovir I.V. Infusion ... 1221
Retrovir Syrup ... 1216
▲ ReVia Tablets (Less than 10%) ... 957
Revex (nalmefene hydrochloride injection) (1%) ... 1863
Rifadin ... 1276
Rifater ... 1280
Rilutek Tablets (Infrequent) ... 2198
Rocephin Injectable Vials, ADD-Vantage, Galaxy Container (Less than 1%) ... 2305
▲ Roferon-A Injection (41% to 64%) 2308
Rubex for Injection (Occasional) ... 721
Rythmol Tablets–150mg, 225mg, 300mg ... 1399
▲ Salagen Tablets (3% to 14%) ... 1546
Sandoglobulin I.V. (Less than 1%) ... 2419
Sensorcaine ... 554
Septra ... 1146
Septra I.V. Infusion ... 1142
Septra I.V. Infusion ADD-Vantage Vials ... 1144
Septra ... 1146
Ser-Ap-Es Tablets ... 867
Serzone Tablets (2%) ... 776
Sinequan (Occasional) ... 2028
Stimate, (desmopressin acetate) Nasal Spray, 1.5 mg/mL ... 806
Sufenta Injection (0.3% to 1%) ... 1355
Sular Tablets (Less than or equal to 1%) ... 2961
▲ Supprelin Injection (1% to 3%) ... 2230
Talacen Caplets (Rare) ... 2464
Talwin Injection (Rare) ... 2465
Talwin Compound (Rare) ... 2466
Talwin Injection (Rare) ... 2465
Talwin Nx Tablets (Rare) ... 2467
Tavist Syrup ... 2426
Tavist Tablets ... 2427
Taxol Injection (Rare) ... 723
Taxotere for Injection Concentrate ... 2204
Tegretol/Tegretol-XR ... 870
Terazol 3 Vaginal Suppositories (1.8% of 284 patients) ... 1942
Terazol 7 Vaginal Cream (0.4% of 521 patients) ... 1943
Tessalon Perles ... 1018
Tetanus & Diphtheria Toxoids Adsorbed Purogenated (Rare) ... 1446
Tetanus Toxoid Adsorbed Purogenated ... 1447
▲ TheraCys BCG Live (Intravesical) (2.6% to 33.9%) ... 911
▲ THROMBATE III Antithrombin III (Human) (2 of 17) ... 631
▲ TICE BCG, USP (3.3%) ... 1881
Ticlid Tablets ... 2317
Timentin for Injection ... 2706

Tonocard Tablets (Less than 1%) ... 519
Tornalate Solution for Inhalation, 0.2% (Less than 1%) ... 976
Trinalin Repetabs Tablets ... 1373
Tussend ... 1830
Tympagesic Ear Drops ... 2476
Unasyn (Less than 1%) ... 2035
Vancocin HCl, Oral Solution & Pulvules (Infrequent) ... 1536
Vancocin HCl, Vials & ADD-Vantage (Infrequent) ... 1534
Varivax (Greater than or equal to 1%) ... 1807
VePesid Capsules and Injection (0.7% to 2%) ... 727
Versed Injection (Less than 1%) ... 2324
▲ Videx Tablets, Powder for Oral Solution, & Pediatric Powder for Oral Solution (9% to 82%) ... 2980
▲ Vistide Injection (24%) ... 1057
▲ Vumon for Injection (Approximately 5%) ... 729
Wellbutrin Tablets (1.2%) ... 1177
WinRho SD (One report) ... 1839
WinRho SD (Less than 2%) ... 1840
Yodoxin Tablets ... 1235
Yutopar Intravenous Injection (Infrequent) ... 566
Zaroxolyn Tablets ... 1625
▲ Zerit Capsules (6% to 51%) ... 731
Zestoretic Tablets ... 2968
Zestril Tablets (0.3% to 1.0%) ... 2972
Zocor Tablets (Rare) ... 1821
Zoladex (Greater than 1% but less than 5%) ... 2976
Zoladex 3-month ... 2978
Zyloprim Tablets (Less than 1%) ... 1194

Chloasma
Anafranil Capsules (Rare) ... 819
Aygestin Tablets ... 990
Climara Transdermal System ... 640
Demulen ... 2580
Depo-Provera Contraceptive Injection (Fewer than 1%) ... 2079
Diethylstilbestrol Tablets ... 1477
Estrace Cream and Tablets ... 751
Estraderm Transdermal System ... 842
ESTRATAB Tablets (0.3, 0.625, 1.25, 2.5 mg) ... 2715
Estratest ... 2718
Lo/Ovral Tablets ... 2852
Lo/Ovral-28 Tablets ... 2857
Menest Tablets ... 2671
Nordette-21 Tablets ... 2863
Nordette-28 Tablets ... 2866
Ogen Tablets ... 2103
Ogen Vaginal Cream ... 2106
Ortho Dienestrol Cream ... 1922
Ortho-Est ... 1925
Ovral Tablets ... 2877
Ovral-28 Tablets ... 2878
Ovrette Tablets ... 2878
PMB 200 and PMB 400 ... 2890
Premarin Intravenous ... 2893
Premarin Tablets ... 2896
Premarin Vaginal Cream ... 2900
Premphase ... 2900
Prempro ... 2905
Synarel Nasal Solution for Endometriosis (Less than 1%) ... 2605
Triphasil-21 Tablets ... 2919
Triphasil-28 Tablets ... 2924
Vivelle Transdermal System ... 880

Chloride retention
Estratest ... 2718
Halotestin Tablets ... 2095
Oxandrin ... 783
Testred Capsules, 10 mg ... 1308

Choking sensation
Dantrium Intravenous ... 2132
Hyperstat I.V. Injection ... 2504
Serevent Inhalation Aerosol (Rare) ... 1149

Cholangiocarcinoma
Fioricet with Codeine Capsules ... 2387
Fiorinal with Codeine Capsules ... 2390

Cholangitis
Cytovene-IV (Two or more reports) ... 2270
Norvir (Less than 2%) ... 447
▲ Prograf (Greater than 3%) ... 1028

Cholangitis, sclerosing
Doxil (Less than 1%) ... 2613

Cholecystitis
▲ Actigall Capsules (5.2%) ... 818
Asacol Delayed-Release Tablets ... 2129

Betaseron for SC Injection ... 653
Cognex Capsules (Infrequent) ... 1961
Colestid (Rare) ... 2073
Crixivan Capsules (Less than 2%) ... 1670
Effexor (Rare) ... 2825
Foscavir Injection (Less than 1%) ... 541
Hivid Tablets (Less than 1%) ... 2287
Lopid Tablets ... 1974
LUVOX Tablets (Rare) ... 2723
Naprelan Tablets (Less than 1%) ... 2861
Permax Tablets (Rare) ... 571
Premphase ... 2900
Prempro ... 2905
Prozac Pulvules & Liquid, Oral Solution (Rare) ... 935
Remeron Tablets (Infrequent) ... 1878
Rilutek Tablets (Rare) ... 2198
Risperdal Tablets (Rare) ... 1348
Trental Tablets (Less than 1%) ... 1291
Videx Tablets, Powder for Oral Solution, & Pediatric Powder for Oral Solution (Less than 1%) ... 2980
Ziac ... 1459

Cholecystitis, acalculus
Sterile FUDR ... 2284

Cholelithiasis
Atromid-S Capsules ... 2808
Betaseron for SC Injection ... 653
Cognex Capsules (Infrequent) ... 1961
Colestid (Rare) ... 2073
Effexor (Rare) ... 2825
Fludara for Injection (Up to 3%) ... 658
Foscavir Injection (Less than 1%) ... 541
Lopid Tablets ... 1974
LUVOX Tablets (Rare) ... 2723
Miacalcin Nasal Spray (Less than 1%) ... 2403
Naprelan Tablets (Less than 1%) ... 2861
Paxil Tablets (Rare) ... 2681
Permax Tablets (Infrequent) ... 571
Premphase ... 2900
Prempro ... 2905
Prevacid Delayed-Release Capsules (Less than 1%) ... 2746
Prozac Pulvules & Liquid, Oral Solution (Rare) ... 935
Redux Capsules (Rare) ... 2911
Risperdal Tablets (Rare) ... 1348
Videx Tablets, Powder for Oral Solution, & Pediatric Powder for Oral Solution (Less than 1%) ... 2980

Cholestasis
Capoten Tablets (Rare) ... 740
Capozide Tablets (Rare) ... 744
Cefotan ... 2936
Ceftin Tablets ... 1067
Ceptaz ... 1070
Clinoril Tablets (Less than 1%) ... 1658
Clozaril Tablets ... 2377
Crixivan Capsules (Less than 2%) ... 1670
Cytovene-IV (Two or more reports) ... 2270
Desyrel and Desyrel Dividose ... 504
Diflucan Tablets, Injection, and Oral Suspension (Rare) ... 2003
Dolobid Tablets (Less than 1 in 100) ... 1695
Duricef Capsules, Tablets, and Oral Suspension ... 750
Flexeril Tablets (Less than 1%) ... 1701
Fortaz ... 1092
Keftab Tablets ... 931
Lorabid Suspension and Pulvules (Rare) ... 1513
Maxipime for Injection ... 758
Mintezol ... 1747
NegGram Tablets ... 2453
Nolvadex Tablets (Rare) ... 2957
Norvasc Tablets ... 2020
Procardia Capsules ... 2024
Procardia XL Extended Release Tablets ... 2026
Rythmol Tablets–150mg, 225mg, 300mg (0.1%) ... 1399
Suprax ... 1443
Tagamet (Rare) ... 2694
Tambocor Tablets (Rare) ... 1555
Tazicef for Injection ... 2697
Tazidime Vials, Faspak & ADD-Vantage ... 1531
Ticlid Tablets ... 2317
Vantin for Oral Suspension and Vantin Tablets ... 2112
Zinacef ... 1184
Zyrtec Tablets (Rare) ... 2053

Cholestasis, intrahepatic
Cedax ... 2480
Ceftin for Oral Suspension ... 1067

(▣ Described in PDR For Nonprescription Drugs)   Incidence data in parenthesis; ▲ 3% or more   (⊙ Described in PDR For Ophthalmology)

Side Effects Index

Cholestasis, intrahepatic
- Cuprimine Capsules (Rare) 1673
- Depen Titratable Tablets (Rare) 2770

Cholestatic hepatic injury
- Axid Pulvules (Rare) 1468
- Coumadin (Infrequent) 941

Cholesterol, systemic, microembolism
- Coumadin (Infrequent) 941

Cholinergic reactions
- Anafranil Capsules (Rare) 819
- Cognex Capsules (Rare) 1961
- Risperdal Tablets (Rare) 1348
- Tensilon Injectable 1307

Chondrodystrophy
- Prozac Pulvules & Liquid, Oral Solution (Rare) 935

Chorea
- ▲ Atamet Tablets (Among most common) 567
- Climara Transdermal System 640
- Diethylstilbestrol Tablets 1477
- Dilantin Infatabs (Rare) 1967
- Dilantin Kapseals (Rare) 1965
- Dilantin-125 Suspension (Rare) 1969
- Dilaudid-HP Injection 1384
- Dilaudid-HP Lyophilized Powder 250 mg 1384
- Eldepryl Capsules 2729
- Estrace Cream and Tablets 751
- Estraderm Transdermal System 842
- ESTRATAB Tablets (0.3, 0.625, 1.25, 2.5 mg) 2715
- Estratest 2718
- Inversine Tablets 1729
- Klonopin Tablets 2294
- Larodopa Tablets (Frequent) 2296
- Lo/Ovral Tablets 2852
- Lo/Ovral-28 Tablets 2857
- Menest Tablets 2671
- Mesantoin Tablets 2400
- Nordette-21 Tablets 2863
- Nordette-28 Tablets 2866
- Ogen Tablets 2103
- Ogen Vaginal Cream 2106
- Ortho Dienestrol Cream 1922
- Ortho-Est 1925
- Ovral Tablets 2877
- Ovral-28 Tablets 2878
- Ovrette Tablets 2878
- PMB 200 and PMB 400 2890
- Premarin Intravenous 2893
- Premarin Tablets 2896
- Premarin Vaginal Cream 2898
- Premphase 2900
- Prempro 2905
- ▲ Sinemet Tablets (Among most common) 959
- Sinemet CR Tablets 961
- Trilafon Concentrate 2532
- Triphasil-21 Tablets 2919
- Triphasil-28 Tablets 2924
- Vivelle Transdermal System 880

Choreoathetotic movements
- Aldoclor Tablets 1638
- Aldomet Ester HCl Injection 1642
- Aldomet Oral 1640
- Aldoril Tablets 1644
- Anafranil Capsules (Rare) 819
- Eskalith 2658
- Felbatol 2774
- Lamictal Tablets (Rare) 1105
- Lithium Carbonate Capsules & Tablets 2352
- Lithonate/Lithotabs/Lithobid 2721
- Loxitane 1426
- Mellaril 2398
- Neurontin Capsules (Rare) 1978
- Paxil Tablets (Rare) 2681
- Permax Tablets (Frequent) 571
- Prolixin 510
- Redux Capsules 2911
- Reglan 2243
- Risperdal Tablets (Rare) 1348
- Serentil 689
- Triavil Tablets 1800

Chorioretinitis
- Neurontin Capsules (Rare) 1978

Choroidal detachment, post-filtration procedures
- AdatoSil 5000 (Less than 2%) .... ⊚ 265
- ISPAN Perfluoropropane .... ⊚ 267
- ISPAN Sulfur Hexafluoride .... ⊚ 266

- Timoptic in Ocudose 1796
- Timoptic Sterile Ophthalmic Solution 1794
- Timoptic-XE 1798

Chromatopsia
- Anafranil Capsules (Rare) 819
- Effexor (Rare) 2825

Chromosomal abnormalities
- Clomid 1262
- Depo-Provera Contraceptive Injection 2079
- Imuran 1103
- Metrodin (urofollitropin for injection) (3 incidents) 2616
- Mustargen 1752
- Roferon-A Injection 2308

Chrysiasis
- Solganal Suspension 2530

Ciliary injection
- Isopto Carbachol Ophthalmic Solution .... ⊚ 221

Ciliary redness
- Humorsol Sterile Ophthalmic Solution 1707
- Phospholine Iodide .... ⊚ 323

Ciliary spasm
- Isopto Carbachol Ophthalmic Solution .... ⊚ 221
- Isopto Carpine Ophthalmic Solution .... ⊚ 221
- Ocusert Pilo-20 and Pilo-40 Ocular Therapeutic Systems .... ⊚ 252
- Pilopine HS Ophthalmic Gel .... ⊚ 224

Cinchonism
- Cardioquin Tablets 2146
- Quinaglute Dura-Tabs Tablets 644
- Quinidex Extentabs 2240
- Tonocard Tablets (Less than 1%) 519

Circulatory collapse
- Etrafon (Extremely rare) 2495
- Lasix Injection, Oral Solution and Tablets 1267
- Protamine Sulfate Vials 1526

Circulatory collapse, peripheral
- Eskalith 2658
- Lithium Carbonate Capsules & Tablets 2352
- Lithonate/Lithotabs/Lithobid 2721
- Phenobarbital Elixir and Tablets 1523
- Tenormin Tablets and I.V. Injection 2965

Circulatory depression
- Demerol 2438
- Dilaudid Ampules 1382
- Dilaudid-HP Injection 1384
- Dilaudid-HP Lyophilized Powder 250 mg 1384
- Dilaudid 1382
- Dilaudid Oral Liquid 1386
- Dilaudid 1382
- Dilaudid Tablets - 8 mg 1386
- MS Contin Tablets 2149
- MSIR 2152
- Mepergan Injection 2859
- OxyContin Tablets 2163
- Phenergan with Codeine 2883
- Phenergan VC with Codeine 2888
- Talwin Injection 2465

Circulatory failure
- Ambien Tablets (Rare) 2559
- Dilaudid 1382
- Lufyllin & Lufyllin-400 Tablets 2778
- Lufyllin-GG Elixir & Tablets 2779
- Metubine Iodide Vials 932
- Prevacid Delayed-Release Capsules (Less than 1%) 2746
- Quadrinal Tablets 1398
- Quibron 2227
- Respbid Tablets 687
- Slo-bid Gyrocaps 2201
- Theo-Dur Extended-Release Tablets 1367
- Theo-X Extended-Release Tablets 793
- Trasylol 607
- Trilafon (Extremely rare) 2532
- Uni-Dur Extended-Release Tablets 1374
- Zosyn (1.0% or less) 1463

Circulatory overload
- Hespan Injection 945
- Pentaspan Injection 954

Cirrhosis, hepatic
(see under Cirrhosis of liver)

Cirrhosis of liver
- Cataflam Tablets (Rare) 833
- Cordarone Tablets (Rare) 2818
- Crixivan Capsules (Less than 2%) 1670
- Lescol Capsules (Rare) 2395
- Methotrexate Sodium Tablets, Injection, for Injection and LPF Injection 1322
- Mevacor Tablets (Rare) 1742
- Papaverine Hydrochloride Vials and Ampoules (Rare) 1523
- Pravachol Tablets (Rare) 770
- Remeron Tablets (Rare) 1878
- Cataflam/Voltaren/Voltaren-XR (Rare) 833
- Zocor Tablets (Rare) 1821

Clamminess
- Avonex 662
- BuSpar Tablets (1%) 738
- Desyrel and Desyrel Dividose (Less than 1% to 1.4%) 504
- Intron A for Injection (Less than 5%) 2506
- IOPIDINE Sterile Ophthalmic Solution .... ⊚ 218
- Norvasc Tablets (Less than or equal to 0.1%) 2020
- ▲ Nubain Injection (9%) 952
- Sanorex Tablets 2423
- ▲ Stadol (3% to 9%) 779
- ▲ Tegison Capsules (1-10%) 2314
- Zoloft Tablets (Infrequent) 2051

Claudication
- Blocadren Tablets 1654
- Calan SR Caplets (1% or less) 2571
- Calan Tablets (1% or less) 2568
- Covera-HS Tablets (Less than 2%) 2573
- Isoptin Oral Tablets 1393
- Isoptin SR Tablets (1% or less) 1395
- Monopril Tablets (0.2% to 1.0%) 762
- Timolide Tablets 1791
- Timoptic in Ocudose 1796
- Timoptic Sterile Ophthalmic Solution 1794
- Timoptic-XE 1798
- Tonocard Tablets (Less than 1%) 519
- Verelan Capsules (1% or less) 1455
- Visken Tablets (2% or fewer patients) 2428
- Zebeta Tablets 1457
- Ziac 1459

Claudication, intermittent
(see under Charcot's syndrome)

Claustrophobia
- BuSpar Tablets (Rare) 738
- Roferon-A Injection (Infrequent) 2308

Cleft palate, neonatal
- Accutane Capsules 2252
- Proventil Inhalation Aerosol 2524
- Proventil Inhalation Solution 0.083% 2527
- Proventil Repetabs Tablets 2529
- Proventil Solution for Inhalation 0.5% 2525
- Proventil Syrup 2528
- Ventolin Inhalation Aerosol and Refill 1170
- Ventolin Inhalation Solution (Rare) 1171
- Ventolin Nebules Inhalation Solution (Rare) 1172
- Ventolin Rotacaps for Inhalation 1173
- Ventolin Syrup 1175
- Ventolin Tablets 1176

Climacteric, onset masked
- Cycrin Tablets 991
- Demulen 2580

Clitoral hypertrophy
- Danocrine Capsules (Rare) 2437
- Desyrel and Desyrel Dividose 504

Clitoris, enlargement
(see under Clitoromegaly)

Clitoromegaly
- ▲ Android Capsules, 10 mg (Among most common) 1297
- Depo-Provera Sterile Aqueous Suspension (Rare) 2083
- Estratest 2718
- Halotestin Tablets 2095

- Oxandrin 783
- Provera Tablets (Rare) 2110
- Testred Capsules, 10 mg 1308
- Winstrol Tablets 2468

Clonic movements of whole limbs
- Diprivan Injectable Emulsion (Less than 1%) 2939
- Eskalith 2658
- Lithium Carbonate Capsules & Tablets 2352
- Lithonate/Lithotabs/Lithobid 2721

Clonus
- Alupent Tablets (0.2%) 672
- Dopram Injectable 2235

Clostridial myonecrosis
- Sus-Phrine Injection 1017

Clotting time, prolongation
- Hespan Injection 945
- Hyskon Hysteroscopy Fluid (Rare) 1633
- Mithracin 599
- Oncaspar (Less than 1%) 2194
- Pentaspan Injection 954
- Zosyn 1463

Coagulation, dysfunction
- Abelcet Injection 1540
- Amicar Syrup, Tablets, and Injection 1312
- Avonex 662
- Bentyl Injection 1246
- Cordarone Tablets (1 to 3%) 2818
- Depakene 416
- Depakote Tablets 418
- Diprivan Injectable Emulsion (Less than 1%) 2939
- Elspar 1700
- Estratest 2718
- Felbatol 2774
- Foscavir Injection (Less than 1%) 541
- Fungizone Intravenous 507
- Hespan Injection 945
- IFEX (Less than 1%) 706
- ▲ Leukine (19%) 1317
- Lo/Ovral Tablets 2852
- Lo/Ovral-28 Tablets 2857
- Maxaquin Tablets 2593
- Mononine, Coagulation Factor IX (Human), Monoclonal Antibody Purified 804
- Nimotop Capsules (Less than 1%) 603
- Oncaspar (Less than 1%) 2194
- Orthoclone OKT3 Sterile Solution 1892
- Ovral Tablets 2877
- Ovral-28 Tablets 2878
- Ovrette Tablets 2878
- Pediazole Suspension 2340
- Pentaspan Injection 954
- PMB 200 and PMB 400 2890
- Premarin Intravenous 2893
- Premarin Tablets 2896
- Premarin Vaginal Cream 2898
- ▲ Prograf (Greater than 3%) 1028
- ▲ Proleukin for Injection (10%) 812
- Redux Capsules (Rare) 2911
- Roferon-A Injection (Less than 4%) 2308
- Tegison Capsules (Less than 1%) 2314
- TICE BCG, USP (0.3%) 1881
- Vantin for Oral Suspension and Vantin Tablets 2112

Coagulation defects, neonatal
- Dilantin Infatabs 1967
- Dilantin Kapseals 1965
- Dilantin-125 Suspension 1969

Coagulation tests, altered results
- Cycrin Tablets 991
- Depo-Provera Sterile Aqueous Suspension 2083
- Eminase 2215
- Provera Tablets 2110
- Zosyn 1463

Cochlear damage
- Amikacin Sulfate Injection, USP 523
- Amikacin Sulfate Injection, USP 981
- Nebcin Vials, Hyporets & ADD-Vantage 1518
- Streptomycin Sulfate Injection 2031
- Tripedia 908

Cochlear lesion
- Redux Capsules 2911

Cognitive dysfunction
- Ambien Tablets (Infrequent) 2559

(⊡ Described in PDR For Nonprescription Drugs)   Incidence data in parenthesis; ▲ 3% or more   (⊚ Described in PDR For Ophthalmology)

Anaprox/Naprosyn (Less than 1%) 2277
Doral Tablets 2773
EC-Naprosyn Delayed-Release Tablets (Rare) 2277
Floxin I.V. (Less than 1%) 1580
Floxin Tablets (200 mg, 300 mg, 400 mg) (Less than 1%) 1577
Methotrexate Sodium Tablets, Injection, for Injection and LPF Injection (Occasional) 1322
Anaprox/Naprosyn 2277
Orthoclone OKT3 Sterile Solution 1892
Risperdal Tablets 1348
Supprelin Injection (2% to 3%) 2230
Ultram Tablets (50 mg) (Less than 1%) 1594
▲ Xanax Tablets (28.8%) 2115

Cogwheel rigidity

BuSpar Tablets (Rare) 738
Cognex Capsules (Infrequent) 1961
Compazine 2644
Eskalith 2658
Lithonate/Lithotabs/Lithobid 2721
Paxil Tablets 2681
Prolixin 510
Reglan 2243
Stelazine 2692
Thorazine 2701

Cold, reduced tolerance

BuSpar Tablets (Rare) 738
Parlodel (Less than 1%) 2411

Coldness of extremities

▲ Blocadren Tablets (8%) 1654
Cafergot 2376
Effexor (Infrequent) 2825
Eskalith (A few reports) 2658
Helixate, Antihemophilic Factor (Recombinant) 799
Hivid Tablets (Less than 1%) 2287
Kerlone Tablets (1.9%) 2588
Lithium Carbonate Capsules & Tablets (A single report) 2352
Lithonate/Lithotabs/Lithobid 2721
Lopressor (1%) 848
Lopressor HCT Tablets 850
LUVOX Tablets (Infrequent) 2723
Mykrox Tablets (Less than 2%) 1617
Parlodel (Rare) 2411
ReVia Tablets (Less than 1%) 957
Sansert Tablets 2424
▲ Tenoretic Tablets (Up to 12%) 2963
▲ Tenormin Tablets and I.V. Injection (Up to 12%) 2965
Timolide Tablets 1791
Timoptic in Ocudose 1796
Timoptic Sterile Ophthalmic Solution 1794
Timoptic-XE 1798
Tonocard Tablets (Less than 1%) 519
Toprol-XL Tablets (About 1 of 100 patients) 560
Visken Tablets (2% or fewer patients) 2428
Zebeta Tablets 1457
Ziac 1459

Cold sensations

Buprenex Injectable (Less than 1%) 2170
Duranest Injections 533
Dyclone 0.5% and 1% Topical Solutions, USP 535
EMLA Cream (Unlikely with cream) 536
Ethyol (amifostine) for Injection 485
Imitrex Injection (1.1%) 1095
Imitrex Tablets (Rare) 1099
Monopril Tablets (0.4% to 1.0%) 762
Sanorex Tablets 2423
Versed Injection (Less than 1%) 2324
▲ Xylocaine Injections (Among most common) 562
Zofran Injection (2%) 1227

Cold sore, non-herpetic

Hivid Tablets (Less than 1%) 2287
Intron A for Injection (Less than 5%) 2506
ReVia Tablets (Less than 1%) 957
Varivax (Greater than or equal to 1%) 1807

Cold symptoms, unspecified

▲ AeroBid Inhaler System (15%) 1004
▲ Aerobid-M Inhaler System (15%) 1004
Cartrol Tablets (Less common) 413
Paxil Tablets 2681
Prinivil Tablets (1.1%) 1776
▲ ProSom Tablets (3%) 457
Sandostatin Injection (1% to 4%) 2421
Thyro-Block Tablets 2785
▲ Xalatan (Approximately 4%) ⊙ 304
Zestril Tablets (1.1%) 2972

Colds, susceptibility

Betimol 0.25%, 0.5% (1% to 5%) ⊙ 259
Diupres Tablets 1691
Hydropres Tablets 1718
Hytrin Capsules (At least 1%) 434
Lopid Tablets 1974
▲ Pravachol Tablets (Up to 7.0%) 770
Prinzide Tablets (0.3% to 1%) 1780
Rowasa (2.33%) 2727
Sinemet CR Tablets 961
Zestoretic Tablets (0.3 to 1%) 2968

Colic

Feldene Capsules (Less than 1%) 2008
Glucotrol Tablets (1 in 100) 2011
Solganal Suspension (Rare) 2530
Urecholine 1804

Colic, biliary

Kadian Capsules (Less than 3%) 2948
Questran (One patient) 774

Colitis

Aldoclor Tablets 1638
Aldomet Ester HCl Injection 1642
Aldomet Oral 1640
Aldoril Tablets 1644
Anafranil Capsules (Infrequent) 819
Anaprox/Naprosyn (Less than 1%) 2277
Ancef Injection 2632
Avonex 662
Brevicon 2563
Cataflam Tablets (Rare; less than 1%) 833
Cefotan 2936
Cefzil Tablets and Oral Suspension (Rare) 747
Ceptaz 1070
Claforan Sterile and Injection (1.4%) 1259
Cleocin Phosphate Injection 2068
Cleocin T Topical (Rare) 2072
Cleocin Vaginal Cream 2070
Clinoril Tablets (Less than 1%) 1658
Demulen 2580
Desogen Tablets 1867
Dilacor XR Extended-release Capsules 2183
Doxil (Less than 1%) 2613
EC-Naprosyn Delayed-Release Tablets (Less than 1%) 2277
Effexor (Infrequent) 2825
Fortaz 1092
Foscavir Injection (Less than 1%) 541
Furoxone 2221
Hivid Tablets (Less than 1%) 2287
Keftab Tablets 931
Kefurox Vials, Faspak & ADD-Vantage 1509
Levlen/Tri-Levlen 646
Lodine Capsules and Tablets (Less than 1%) 2849
Lopid Tablets 1974
LUVOX Tablets (Infrequent) 2723
Maxipime for Injection (0.1% to 1%) 758
Modicon 1928
Naprelan Tablets (Less than 1%) 2861
Anaprox/Naprosyn (Less than 1%) 2277
Neurontin Capsules (Rare) 1978
Norinyl 2563
Nor-Q D Tablets 2598
Norvir (Less than 2%) 447
Oncaspar 2194
Ortho-Cept 1907
Ortho-Cyclen/Ortho-Tri-Cyclen 1914
Ortho-Novum 1928
Ortho-Cyclen/Ortho Tri-Cyclen 1914
Ovcon 765
Paxil Tablets (Rare) 2681
Permax Tablets (Rare) 571
Prozac Pulvules & Liquid, Oral Solution (Rare) 935
Redux Capsules (Infrequent) 2911
Remeron Tablets (Infrequent) 1878
Rocephin Injectable Vials, ADD-Vantage, Galaxy Container (Rare) 2305
Roferon-A Injection (Infrequent) 2308
Rowasa (1.2%) 2727
Serzone Tablets (Infrequent) 776
Solganal Suspension 2530
Sular Tablets (Less than or equal to 1%) 2961
Tazicef for Injection 2697
Tazidime Vials, Faspak & ADD-Vantage 1531
Ticlid Tablets 2317
Levlen/Tri-Levlen 646
Tri-Norinyl 2607
Videx Tablets, Powder for Oral Solution, & Pediatric Powder for Oral Solution (Less than 1%) 2980
Vistide Injection 1057
Cataflam/Voltaren/Voltaren-XR (Rare; less than 1%) 833
Wellbutrin Tablets (Rare) 1177
Zinacef 1184

Colitis, ischemic

Blocadren Tablets 1654
Cartrol Tablets 413
Taxol Injection (Rare) 723
Tenoretic Tablets 2963
Tenormin Tablets and I.V. Injection 2965
Timoptic-XE 1798
Trandate Tablets 1158
Visken Tablets 2428
Zebeta Tablets 1457
Ziac 1459

Colitis, necrotizing

Adriamycin PFS 2056
Adriamycin RDF 2056
Cytosar-U Sterile Powder (With experimental doses) 2077
Doxorubicin Astra 531
Rubex for Injection 721

Colitis, pseudomembranous (see under Pseudomembranous colitis)

Colitis, ulcerative

Ancobon Capsules 2254
Indocin (Less than 1%) 1723
Orudis Capsules (Rare) 2874
Oruvail Capsules (Rare) 2874
Prevacid Delayed-Release Capsules (Less than 1%) 2746
Serzone Tablets (Rare) 776
Vantin for Oral Suspension and Vantin Tablets 2112

Colitis, ulcerative, worsening of

▲ Asacol Delayed-Release Tablets (3%) 2129
Pentasa (0.4%) 1275

Collapse

Antivenin (Crotalidae) Polyvalent 2803
Atretol Tablets 569
Clozaril Tablets (Rare) 2377
Diphtheria and Tetanus Toxoids and Pertussis Vaccine Adsorbed 2650
Fluvirin (Influenza Virus Vaccine) 1608
Mintezol 1747
Nitrolingual Spray 2193
Nitrostat Tablets 1981
Norpramin Tablets (One report) 1273
Tegretol/Tegretol-XR 870
Tofranil Tablets 875

Colon problem, unspecified

Betapace Tablets (2% to 3%) 637

Colon, cancer of

Helidac Therapy (Some reports) 2135
Protostat Tablets 1939

Colon, dilatation

Artane (Rare) 1418
Phenergan with Codeine 2883
Phenergan VC with Codeine 2888

Colon, irritable

BuSpar Tablets (Infrequent) 738
Compazine 2644
Prilosec Delayed-Release Capsules (Less than 1%) 516

Colon, motility, increase

Phenergan with Codeine 2883
Phenergan VC with Codeine 2888

Colonic strictures

Creon 2714
Ultrase Capsules 2476
Ultrase MT Capsules 2477

Color perception, disturbed

Cardioquin Tablets (Occasional) 2146
Cataflam Tablets 833
Cipro Tablets (Less than 1%) 584
IBU Tablets (Less than 1%) 1389
NegGram (Infrequent) 2453
Platinol for Injection 717
Platinol-AQ Injection 719
Quinaglute Dura-Tabs Tablets (Occasional) 644
Quinidex Extentabs (Occasional) 2240
Cataflam/Voltaren/Voltaren-XR 833

Coma

Anafranil Capsules (Infrequent) 819
Betaseron for SC Injection 653
Buprenex Injectable (Infrequent) 2170
Cataflam Tablets (Rare) 833
Cerebyx Injection (Infrequent) 1956
Cognex Capsules (Rare) 1961
Compazine 2644
Cytosar-U Sterile Powder (With experimental doses) 2077
Cytovene (1% or less) 2270
DDAVP Injection (Rare) 2178
DDAVP (Rare) 2180
Dalmane Capsules 2329
Depakene (Rare) 416
Depakote Tablets (Rare) 418
Desmopressin Acetate Injection (Rare) 996
Elavil 2945
Elspar 1700
Ergamisol Tablets 1340
Eskalith 2658
Ethmozine Tablets (Less than 2%) 2217
Felbatol 2774
Fludara for Injection 658
Foscavir Injection (Less than 1%) 541
IBU Tablets (Rare; less than 1%) 1389
IFEX (Occasional) 706
Indocin Capsules (Less than 1%) 1723
Indocin I.V. (Less than 1%) 1727
Indocin (Less than 1%) 1723
Intron A for Injection (Less than 5%) 2506
Klonopin Tablets 2294
Levbid Extended-Release Tablets 2549
Levo-Dromoran 2297
Levsin/Levsinex/Levbid 2549
Lioresal Intrathecal (Up to 1.5%) 1634
Lithium Carbonate Capsules & Tablets 2352
Lithonate/Lithotabs/Lithobid 2721
LUVOX Tablets (Rare) 2723
Matulane Capsules 2300
Maxaquin Tablets (Less than 1%) 2593
Motrin Ibuprofen Suspension, Oral Drops, Chewable Tablets, Caplets (Rare; less than 1%) 1563
Nardil (Less frequent) 1977
Oncaspar 2194
Oncovin Solution Vials & Hyporets 1521
Orthoclone OKT3 Sterile Solution 1892
Permax Tablets (Infrequent) 571
Pfizerpen for Injection 2022
PhosLo Tablets 695
Podocon-25 1949
Prograf 1028
Proleukin for Injection (1%) 812
Prozac Pulvules & Liquid, Oral Solution (Rare) 935
ReoPro Vials (0.4%) 1526
Rilutek Tablets (Infrequent) 2198
Risperdal Tablets (Rare) 1348
Roferon-A Injection (Infrequent) 2308
Rythmol Tablets–150mg, 225mg, 300mg (Less than 1%) 1399
Seromycin Capsules 975
Stimate, (desmopressin acetate) Nasal Spray, 1.5 mg/mL 806
Streptomycin Sulfate Injection (Occasional) 2031
Syntocinon Injection 2425
Tigan 2231
Tonocard Tablets (Less than 1%) 519
Triavil Tablets 1800
▲ Vesanoid Capsules (3%) 2327
Cataflam/Voltaren/Voltaren-XR (Rare) 833
Wellbutrin Tablets 1177
Zoloft Tablets (Rare) 2051
Zovirax Sterile Powder (Approximately 1%) 1191

Coma, hepatic (see under Hepatic coma)

Coma, hyperosmolar non-ketonic

Hyperstat I.V. Injection 2504
OSMOGLYN Oral Osmotic Agent ⊙ 225
Proglycem 575

(▭ Described in PDR For Nonprescription Drugs) Incidence data in parenthesis; ▲ 3% or more (⊙ Described in PDR For Ophthalmology)

Coma, hypoglycemic — Side Effects Index — 1288

Coma, hypoglycemic
Redux Capsules ... 2911
Tapazole Tablets ... 1361

Combativeness
Diprivan Injectable Emulsion (Less than 1%) ... 2939
Orthoclone OKT3 Sterile Solution .. 1892
Zosyn (1.0% or less) ... 1463

Conduct disorder
Supprelin Injection (1%) ... 2230

Conduction delay, intraventricular
▲Rythmol Tablets–150mg, 225mg, 300mg (0.2 to 4.0%) ... 1399

Conduction disturbances
Adalat Capsules (10 mg and 20 mg) (Fewer than 0.5%) ... 580
Blocadren Tablets ... 1654
Catapres-TTS ... 680
Combipres Tablets (Rare) ... 682
Desyrel and Desyrel Dividose ... 504
▲Eminase (38%) ... 2215
Ethmozine Tablets ... 2217
Etrafon ... 2495
▲Lanoxicaps (Among most common) ... 1110
▲Lanoxin Elixir Pediatric (Among most common) ... 1113
▲Lanoxin Injection (Among most common) ... 1116
▲Lanoxin Injection Pediatric (Among most common) ... 1119
▲Lanoxin Tablets (Among most common) ... 1121
LUVOX Tablets (Infrequent) ... 2723
Mexitil Capsules (2 in 1,000) ... 684
Monopril Tablets (0.4% to 1.0%) .. 762
Paxil Tablets (Infrequent) ... 2681
Procardia Capsules (Fewer than 0.5%) ... 2024
Procardia XL Extended Release Tablets (Fewer than 0.5%) ... 2026
▲Rythmol Tablets–150mg, 225mg, 300mg (0.2 to 4.0%) ... 1399
▲Sandostatin Injection (10%) ... 2421
Taxol Injection (Less than 1%) ... 723
Tonocard Tablets (Up to 1.5%) ... 519

Confusion
Actimmune (Rare) ... 1043
Adalat CC (Less than 1.0%) ... 582
Adapin Capsules (Infrequent) ... 1542
Aldactazide Tablets ... 2556
Aldactone Tablets ... 2558
Aldoclor Tablets ... 1638
Aldomet Ester HCl Injection ... 1642
Aldomet Oral ... 1640
Aldoril Tablets ... 1644
Alfenta Injection (0.3% to 1%) ... 1334
Alferon N Injection (One patient to 3%) ... 2142
Ambien Tablets (Frequent) ... 2559
Amicar Syrup, Tablets, and Injection ... 1312
Amoxil (Rare) ... 2631
Anafranil Capsules (2% to 3%) ... 819
Ancobon Capsules ... 2254
Androderm Testosterone Transdermal System (Less than 1%) ... 2634
Arimidex Tablets (2% to 5%) ... 2932
Artane ... 1418
Asacol Delayed-Release Tablets ... 2129
Asendin Tablets (Less frequent) ... 1419
Atamet Tablets ... 567
Ativan Injection (1.3%) ... 2805
Atretol Tablets ... 569
Augmentin (Rare) ... 2637
Augmentin Tablets (Rare) ... 2640
Axid Pulvules (Rare) ... 1468
Axocet Capsules (Infrequent) ... 2469
Azactam for Injection (Less than 1%) ... 736
Benadryl Injection ... 1955
Bentyl ... 1246
Betagan ... ⊙ 230
▲Betaseron for SC Injection (4%) ... 653
Biaxin ... 406
Blenoxane (Approximately 1%) ... 697
Brevibloc (esmolol HCl) Injection (About 2%) ... 1860
BuSpar Tablets (2%) ... 738
Butisol Sodium Elixir & Tablets (Less than 1 in 100) ... 2768
Calan SR Caplets (1% or less) ... 2571
Calan Tablets (1% or less) ... 2568
Capoten Tablets ... 740
Capozide Tablets ... 744
Cardene Capsules (Rare) ... 2261
Cardene I.V. (Rare) ... 2815
Cardene SR Capsules (Rare) ... 2264
Cardioquin Tablets ... 2146
Cardura Tablets (Less than 0.5% of 3960 patients) ... 1993
Casodex Tablets (2% to 5%) ... 2934
Ceclor Pulvules & Suspension (Rare) ... 1470
Cefzil Tablets and Oral Suspension (Less than 1%) ... 747
Celontin Kapseals ... 1955
Cerebyx Injection (Infrequent) ... 1956
Chibroxin Sterile Ophthalmic Solution (With oral form) ... 1657
Chloromycetin Sodium Succinate ... 1960
Cipro I.V. (1% or less) ... 587
Cipro I.V. Pharmacy Bulk Package (Less than 1%) ... 590
Cipro Tablets ... 584
Claritin Tablets (2% or fewer patients) ... 2485
Claritin-D Tablets (Less frequent) .. 2487
▲Clozaril Tablets (3%) ... 2377
Cogentin ... 1661
▲Cognex Capsules (7%) ... 1961
Covera-HS Tablets (Less than 2%) 2573
Cozaar Tablets (Less than 1%) ... 1668
Cytotec ... 2576
Cytovene (1% or less) ... 2270
Dalgan Injection (Less than 1%) ... 529
Dalmane Capsules (Rare) ... 2329
Dantrium Capsules (Less frequent) 2131
Daranide Tablets ... 1676
DaunoXome (Less than or equal to 5%) ... 1842
Daypro Caplets (1% to 3%) ... 2578
Demser Capsules ... 1690
Depakote Tablets (1% to 5%) ... 418
▲Desyrel and Desyrel Dividose (4.9% to 5.7%) ... 504
Diamox Intravenous (Occasional) ⊙ 317
Diamox Sequels (Sustained Release) (Occasional) ... ⊙ 318
Diamox Tablets (Occasional) ... ⊙ 317
Didronel Tablets ... 2133
▲Dilantin Infatabs (Among most common) ... 1967
▲Dilantin Kapseals (Among most common) ... 1965
▲Dilantin-125 Suspension (Among most common) ... 1969
Dilaudid Ampules ... 1382
Dilaudid Cough Syrup ... 1383
Dilaudid ... 1382
Diprivan Injectable Emulsion (Less than 1%) ... 2939
Diupres Tablets ... 1691
Diuril Oral Suspension ... 1694
Diuril Sodium Intravenous ... 1693
Diuril Tablets ... 1694
Dizac (diazepam injectable emulsion) CIV (Less frequent) ... 1862
Dolobid Tablets (Less than 1 in 100) ... 1695
Doral Tablets ... 2773
Doxil (Less than 1%) ... 2613
▲Duragesic Transdermal System (10% or more) ... 1336
Duranest Injections ... 533
Dyazide Capsules ... 2653
Dyclone 0.5% and 1% Topical Solutions, USP ... 535
E.E.S. (Isolated reports) ... 427
Easprin ... 1971
Edecrin ... 1698
Effexor (2%) ... 2825
Elavil ... 2945
▲Eldepryl Capsules (3 of 49 patients) ... 2729
Elspar ... 1700
EMLA Cream (Unlikely with cream) 536
Ergamisol Tablets (Less frequent) .. 1340
EryPed (Isolated reports) ... 425
Ery-Tab Tablets (Isolated reports) .. 426
Erythrocin Stearate Filmtab (Isolated reports) ... 429
Erythromycin Base Filmtab (Isolated reports) ... 430
Erythromycin Delayed-Release Capsules, USP (Isolated reports) 431
Esgic-plus Capsules (Infrequent) ... 1012
Esgic-plus Tablets (Infrequent) ... 1012
Eskalith ... 2658
Ethmozine Tablets (Less than 2%) 2217
Etrafon ... 2495
Eulexin Capsules (1%) ... 2498
Famvir Tablets (Very rare) ... 2660
Felbatol ... 2774
Feldene Capsules (Less than 1%) .. 2008
Fioricet Tablets (Infrequent) ... 2386
Fioricet with Codeine Capsules (Infrequent) ... 2387
Flagyl 375 Capsules ... 2587
Flagyl I.V. ... 2373
▲Flolan for Injection (6%) ... 1085
Floxin I.V. (Less than 1%) ... 1580
Floxin Tablets (200 mg, 300 mg, 400 mg) ... 1577
Fludara for Injection ... 658
Flumadine Tablets & Syrup (Less than 0.3%) ... 1013
Fluorouracil Injection ... 2282
▲Foscavir Injection (5% or greater) .. 541
Sterile FUDR (Remote possibility) .. 2284
Fulvicin P/G Tablets (Occasional) .. 2499
Fulvicin P/G 165 & 330 Tablets (Occasional) ... 2500
Ganite ... 2711
Garamycin Injectable ... 2502
GlaucTabs (Occasional instances) ... ⊙ 209
Glucotrol XL Extended Release Tablets (Less than 1%) ... 2012
Grifulvin V (griseofulvin tablets) Microsize (griseofulvin oral suspension) Microsize (Occasional) ... 1944
Gris-PEG Tablets, 125 mg & 250 mg (Occasional) ... 476
Halcion Tablets (0.9% to 0.5%) ... 2093
Haldol Decanoate ... 1587
Haldol Injection, Tablets and Concentrate ... 1585
Helidac Therapy ... 2135
Hivid Tablets (Less than 1%) ... 2287
HydroDIURIL Tablets ... 1716
Hydropres Tablets ... 1718
▲Hylorel Tablets (14.8%) ... 1613
Hyperstat I.V. Injection ... 2504
Hyzaar Tablets ... 1720
IBU Tablets (Less than 1%) ... 1389
▲IFEX (Among most common) ... 706
Imdur (Less than or equal to 5%) .. 1362
Imitrex Injection (Infrequent) ... 1095
Imitrex Tablets (Infrequent) ... 1099
Indocin (Less than 1%) ... 1723
▲Intron A for Injection (Up to 12%) 2506
Invirase Capsules (Rare; less than 2%) ... 2291
Ismo Tablets (Fewer than 1%) ... 2844
ISMOTIC 45% w/v Solution ... ⊙ 221
Isoptin Oral Tablets (Less than 1%) ... 1393
Isoptin SR Tablets (1% or less) ... 1395
K-Phos Neutral Tablets ... 633
K-Phos Original Formula 'Sodium Free' Tablets (Less frequent) ... 633
Kadian Capsules (Less than 3%) ... 2948
Keflex Pulvules & Oral Suspension 930
Keftab Tablets ... 931
Kerlone Tablets (Less than 2%) ... 2588
Klonopin Tablets ... 2294
Lamictal Tablets (1.8%) ... 1105
Lariam Tablets ... 2295
Larodopa Tablets (Relatively frequent) ... 2296
Leukeran Tablets (Rare) ... 1205
Levbid Extended-Release Tablets ... 2549
Levo-Dromoran ... 2297
Levsin/Levsinex/Levbid ... 2549
Librax Capsules ... 2330
Librium Capsules (Some patients) .. 2331
Librium Injectable ... 2332
Limbitrol (Less common) ... 2333
Lioresal Intrathecal (0.5% to 2.3%) ... 1634
▲Lioresal Tablets (1% to 11%) ... 847
Lithium Carbonate Capsules & Tablets ... 2352
Lithonate/Lithotabs/Lithobid ... 2721
Lodine Capsules and Tablets (Less than 1%) ... 2849
Lomotil ... 2591
Lopid Tablets ... 1974
Lopressor ... 848
Lopressor HCT Tablets ... 850
Loxitane ... 1426
Ludiomil Tablets (Rare) ... 861
Lupron Depot 3.75 mg ... 2739
LUVOX Tablets ... 2723
Macrobid Capsules (Rare) ... 2138
Macrodantin Capsules (Rare) ... 2140
Marinol (Dronabinol) Capsules (Greater than 1%) ... 2353
Matulane Capsules ... 2300
Maxair Autohaler ... 1550
Maxair Inhaler (Less than 1%) ... 1552
Maxaquin Tablets (Less than 1%) .. 2593
Mebaral Tablets (Less than 1 in 100) ... 2452
Megace Oral Suspension (1% to 3%) ... 708
Mellaril ... 2398
Merrem I.V. (0.1% to 1.0%) ... 2952
Methadone Hydrochloride Oral Solution & Tablets ... 2357
Methotrexate Sodium Tablets, Injection, for Injection and LPF Injection ... 1322
MetroGel-Vaginal ... 917
Mexitil Capsules (1.9% to 2.6%) .. 684
Midamor Tablets (Less than or equal to 1%) ... 1746
Moduretic Tablets (Less than or equal to 1%) ... 1748
Mono-Gesic Tablets ... 810
Monopril Tablets (0.2% to 1.0%) .. 762
Motofen Tablets (1 in 200 to 1 in 600) ... 789
Motrin Ibuprofen Suspension, Oral Drops, Chewable Tablets, Caplets (Less than 1%) ... 1563
Mutamycin for Injection ... 712
Myambutol Tablets ... 1432
Mycobutin Capsules (More than one patient) ... 2101
Myochrysine Injection (Rare) ... 1754
Nalfon 200 Pulvules & Nalfon Tablets (1.4%) ... 933
Naprelan Tablets (Less than 1%) .. 2861
Nebcin Vials, Hyporets & ADD-Vantage ... 1518
NegGram ... 2453
Nembutal Sodium Capsules (Less than 1%) ... 440
Nembutal Sodium Solution (Less than 1%) ... 442
Nembutal Sodium Suppositories (Less than 1%) ... 444
Neoral (2% or less) ... 2405
Neptazane Tablets (Occasional) .. ⊙ 320
Neurontin Capsules (More than 1%) ... 1978
Neutrexin for Injection (2.8%) ... 2761
▲Nicotrol NS Nicotine Nasal Spray (3%) ... 1565
Norflex (Infrequent) ... 1554
Norgesic (Infrequent) ... 1554
Noroxin Tablets ... 1758
Noroxin Tablets ... 2222
Norpramin Tablets ... 1273
Norvir (Less than 2%) ... 447
Nubain Injection (1% or less) ... 952
Oncaspar (Less than 1%) ... 2194
Oramorph SR (Morphine Sulfate Sustained Release Tablets) ... 2359
Ornade Spansule Capsules ... 2678
Orthoclone OKT3 Sterile Solution .. 1892
Orudis Capsules (Less than 1%) .. 2874
Oruvail Capsules (Less than 1%) ... 2874
OSMOGLYN Oral Osmotic Agent ⊙ 225
OxyContin Tablets (Between 1% and 5%) ... 2163
PBZ Tablets ... 863
PBZ-SR Tablets ... 862
Pamelor ... 2409
Parlodel ... 2411
Parnate Tablets ... 2679
Paxil Tablets (1%) ... 2681
Penetrex Tablets (0.1% to 1%) ... 2196
Pepcid Injection (Infrequent) ... 1765
Pepcid (Infrequent) ... 1763
Periactin ... 1767
▲Permax Tablets (11.1%) ... 571
Phenergan with Codeine (Rare) ... 2883
Phenergan with Dextromethorphan (Rare) ... 2885
Phenergan Suppositories (Rare) ... 2882
Phenergan Syrup (Rare) ... 2881
Phenergan VC (Rare) ... 2886
Phenergan VC with Codeine (Rare) 2888
Phenobarbital Elixir and Tablets (Less than 1 in 100 patients) ... 1523
PhosLo Tablets ... 695
Phrenilin ... 790
Placidyl Capsules ... 456
Polycitra Syrup ... 574
Polycitra-K Crystals ... 574
Polycitra-K Oral Solution ... 575
Polycitra-LC ... 574
Pondimin Tablets ... 2239
Prevacid Delayed-Release Capsules (Less than 1%) ... 2746
Prilosec Delayed-Release Capsules (Less than 1%) ... 516
Primaxin I.M. ... 1770
Primaxin I.V. (Less than 0.2%) ... 1772
Prinivil Tablets (0.3 to 1.0%) ... 1776
Prinzide Tablets ... 1780
Pro-Banthine Tablets ... 2226
▲Prograf (Greater than 3%) ... 1028

(▣ Described in PDR For Nonprescription Drugs) Incidence data in parenthesis; ▲ 3% or more (⊙ Described in PDR For Ophthalmology)

Side Effects Index

Congestive heart failure

Proleukin for Injection	812
ProSom Tablets (2%)	457
Protostat Tablets	1939
Prozac Pulvules & Liquid, Oral Solution (2%)	935
Quadrinal Tablets	1398
Quinaglute Dura-Tabs Tablets	644
Quinidex Extentabs	2240
Redux Capsules (Infrequent)	2911
Reglan (Less frequent)	2243
Relafen Tablets (1%)	2688
Remeron Tablets (2%)	1878
ReoPro Vials (0.6%)	1526
Restoril Capsules (2-3%)	2413
Retrovir Capsules	1216
Retrovir I.V. Infusion	1221
Retrovir Syrup	1216
ReVia Tablets (Less than 1%)	957
Revex (nalmefene hydrochloride injection) (Less than 1%)	1863
Rifadin	1276
Rifamate Capsules	1278
Rifater	1280
Rilutek Tablets (Infrequent)	2198
Rimactane Capsules	865
Risperdal Tablets (Infrequent)	1348
Robinul Forte Tablets	2247
Robinul Injectable	2247
Robinul Tablets	2247
▲ Roferon-A Injection (Less than 4% to 8%)	2308
Romazicon (Less than 1%)	2311
Roxanol	2365
Roxicodone Tablets, Oral Solution & Intensol (Oxycodone)	2366
Rythmol Tablets—150mg, 225mg, 300mg (Less than 1%)	1399
SSKI Solution (Less frequent)	2767
Salagen Tablets (Less than 1%)	1546
Sandimmune (2% or less)	2416
Seconal Sodium Pulvules (Less than 1 in 100)	1529
Sedapap Tablets 50 mg/650 mg (Infrequent)	1826
Seldane Tablets	1284
Seldane-D Extended-Release Tablets	1286
Sensorcaine	554
Serentil	689
Seromycin Capsules	975
▲ Serzone Tablets (7% to 8%)	776
Sinemet Tablets	959
▲ Sinemet CR Tablets (3.7%)	961
Sinequan (Infrequent)	2028
Soma Compound w/Codeine Tablets (Very rare)	2784
Soma Compound Tablets (Very rare)	2783
Soma Tablets	2782
▲ Stadol (3% to 9%)	779
Sular Tablets (Less than or equal to 1%)	2961
Surmontil Capsules	2917
Symmetrel Capsules (0.1% to 5%)	965
Symmetrel Syrup (0.1% to 5%)	963
Tagamet (Occasional)	2694
Talacen Caplets	2464
Talwin Injection	2465
Talwin Compound	2466
Talwin Injection	2465
Talwin Nx Tablets	2467
Tambocor Tablets (Less than 1%)	1555
Tavist Syrup	2426
Tavist Tablets	2427
Taxotere for Injection Concentrate	2204
Tegretol/Tegretol-XR	870
Tenex Tablets (3% or less)	2249
Tessalon Perles	1018
Timolide Tablets (Less than 1%)	1791
Timoptic in Ocudose (Less frequent)	1796
Timoptic Sterile Ophthalmic Solution (Less frequent)	1794
Timoptic-XE	1798
Tofranil Ampuls	873
Tofranil Tablets	875
Tofranil-PM Capsules	876
▲ Tonocard Tablets (2.1% to 11.2%)	519
Toprol-XL Tablets	560
Torecan	2367
Trancopal Caplets	2468
Transderm Scōp Transdermal Therapeutic System (Infrequent)	890
Tranxene (Less common)	459
▲ Trasylol (4%)	607
Trental Tablets (Less than 1%)	1291
Triavil Tablets	1800
Trilisate (Rare)	2155
Trinalin Repetabs Tablets	1373
Tussend	1830
Ultram Tablets (50 mg) (1% to less than 5%)	1594
Urispas Tablets	2710
Uroqid-Acid No. 2 Tablets	633
Valium Injectable	2336
Valium Tablets (Infrequent)	2335
Vaseretic Tablets	1810
Vasotec I.V.	1814
Vasotec Tablets (0.5% to 1%)	1816
Verelan Capsules (1% or less)	1455
Versed Injection (Less than 1%)	2324
▲ Vesanoid Capsules (14%)	2327
Videx Tablets, Powder for Oral Solution, & Pediatric Powder for Oral Solution (1% to 2%)	2980
Vistide Injection	1057
Vivactil Tablets	1820
▲ Wellbutrin Tablets (8.4%)	1177
▲ Xanax Tablets (9.9% to 10.4%)	2115
▲ Xylocaine Injections (Among most common)	562
Zantac (Rare)	1182
Zantac Injection (Rare)	1180
Zantac Syrup (Rare)	1182
Zerit Capsules (Fewer than 1% to 3%)	731
Zestoretic Tablets	2968
Zestril Tablets (0.3% to 1.0%)	2972
Zoloft Tablets (Frequent)	2051
Zosyn (1.0% or less)	1463
Zovirax Capsules	1187
Zovirax Sterile Powder (Approximately 1%)	1191
Zovirax	1187
Zyloprim Tablets (Less than 1%)	1194
Zyrtec Tablets (Less than 2%)	2053

Confusion, mental
(see under Confusion)

Confusion, nocturnal

Mellaril (Extremely rare)	2398
Trilafon	2532

Confusional state
(see under Confusion)

Congelation

Eldepryl Capsules	2729
Ethyl Chloride, U.S.P.	1040
Fluori-Methane	1040

Congenital anomalies

Airet Albuterol Sulfate Inhalation Solution	1602
Amen Tablets	785
Aygestin Tablets	990
Cordarone Intravenous	2821
Cytotec	2576
Cytovene-IV (Two or more reports)	2270
Depakene	416
Depakote Tablets	418
Depo-Provera Sterile Aqueous Suspension	2083
Diabinese Tablets	2002
Diethylstilbestrol Tablets	1477
Estrace Cream and Tablets	751
Estraderm Transdermal System	842
ESTRATAB Tablets (0.3, 0.625, 1.25, 2.5 mg)	2715
Halcion Tablets	2093
Havrix (Rare)	2663
Humegon for Injection	1873
Lescol Capsules (Rare)	2395
Levlen/Tri-Levlen	646
Lo/Ovral Tablets	2852
Lo/Ovral-28 Tablets	2857
Methotrexate Sodium Tablets, Injection, for Injection and LPF Injection	1322
Metrodin (urofollitropin for injection)	2616
Mevacor Tablets (Rare)	1742
Nordette-21 Tablets	2863
Nordette-28 Tablets	2866
Norplant System (Rare; less than 1%)	2868
Ogen Tablets	2103
Ogen Vaginal Cream	2106
Ortho Dienestrol Cream	1922
Ortho-Est	1925
Ovral Tablets	2877
Ovral-28 Tablets	2878
Ovrette Tablets	2878
Pergonal (menotropins for injection, USP)	2618
Permax Tablets	571
PMB 200 and PMB 400	2890
Premarin Intravenous	2893
Premarin Tablets	2896
Proventil Inhalation Aerosol	2524
Proventil Inhalation Solution 0.083%	2527
Proventil Repetabs Tablets	2529
Proventil Solution for Inhalation 0.5%	2525
Proventil Syrup	2528
Provera Tablets	2110
Redux Capsules	2911
Retrovir Capsules	1216
Retrovir I.V. Infusion	1221
Retrovir Syrup	1216
▲ Septra I.V. Infusion (4.5%)	1142
Serophene (clomiphene citrate tablets, USP)	2621
Levlen/Tri-Levlen	646
Triphasil-21 Tablets	2919
Triphasil-28 Tablets	2924
Ventolin Inhalation Aerosol and Refill	1170
Ventolin Inhalation Solution (Rare)	1171
Ventolin Nebules Inhalation Solution (Rare)	1172
Ventolin Rotacaps for Inhalation	1173
Ventolin Syrup	1175
Ventolin Tablets	1176
Vivelle Transdermal System	880
Xanax Tablets	2115

Congenital malformation

Ativan Injection	2805
Ativan Tablets	2807
Atretol Tablets	569
Cerebyx Injection	1956
Cytosar-U Sterile Powder (Two cases)	2077
Dalmane Capsules	2329
Dilantin Infatabs	1967
Dilantin Kapseals	1965
Dilantin-125 Suspension	1969
Dizac (diazepam injectable emulsion) CIV	1862
Doral Tablets	2773
Halcion Tablets	2093
Librax Capsules	2330
Librium Capsules	2331
Librium Injectable	2332
Limbitrol	2333
Miltown Tablets	2780
PMB 200 and PMB 400	2890
Pravachol Tablets (One case)	770
Premphase	2900
Prempro	2905
ProSom Tablets	457
Restoril Capsules	2413
Tegretol/Tegretol-XR	870
Tofranil Ampuls	873
Tofranil Tablets	875
Tofranil-PM Capsules	876
Tranxene	459
Valium Injectable	2336
Valium Tablets	2335
Versed Injection	2324

Congestion

Adalat Capsules (10 mg and 20 mg) (2% or less)	580
Halcion Tablets (Rare)	2093
Procardia Capsules (2% or less)	2024

Congestion, nasal
(see under Nasal congestion)

Congestive heart failure

Adalat Capsules (10 mg and 20 mg) (About 2%)	580
Adriamycin PFS	2056
Adriamycin RDF	2056
Aldoclor Tablets	1638
Aldomet Ester HCl Injection	1642
Aldomet Oral	1640
Aldoril Tablets	1644
Aminohippurate Sodium Injection	1646
Anaprox/Naprosyn (Less than 1%)	2277
Atretol Tablets	569
Betagan	⊙ 230
Betoptic Ophthalmic Solution (Rare)	465
Betoptic S Ophthalmic Suspension (Rare)	467
BuSpar Tablets (Rare)	738
Calan SR Caplets (1.8%)	2571
Calan Tablets (1.8%)	2568
Capoten Tablets (2 to 3 of 1000 patients)	740
Capozide Tablets (2 to 3 of 1000 patients)	744
Cardizem CD Capsules (Less than 1%)	1251
Cardizem SR Capsules (Less than 1%)	1255
Cardizem Injectable (Less than 1%)	1253
Cardizem Tablets (Less than 1%)	1257
Cartrol Tablets (Rare)	413
Casodex Tablets (2% to 5%)	2934
Cataflam Tablets (Less than 1%)	833
Catapres Tablets (Rare)	679
Catapres-TTS	680
Celestone Soluspan Suspension	2484
Cerebyx Injection (Infrequent)	1956
Cerubidine for Injection	634
Clinoril Tablets (Less than 1%)	1658
Clozaril Tablets	2377
Combipres Tablets (Rare)	682
Cordarone Intravenous (2.1%)	2821
Cordarone Tablets (1 to 3%)	2818
CORTENEMA	2713
Cortone Acetate Sterile Suspension	1663
Cortone Acetate Tablets	1664
Corvert Injection (0.5%)	2075
Covera-HS Tablets (1.8% to 2%)	2573
Cytoxan	700
Dalalone D.P. Injectable	1009
DaunoXome	1842
Decadron Elixir	1676
Decadron Phosphate Injection	1680
Decadron Phosphate with Xylocaine Injection, Sterile	1683
Decadron Tablets	1678
Decadron-LA Sterile Suspension	1687
Desyrel and Desyrel Dividose	504
Dexacort Phosphate in Respihaler	1606
Dexacort Phosphate in Turbinaire	1607
Digibind (Few instances)	1079
Diupres Tablets	1691
Doxil (1% to 5%)	2613
Doxorubicin Astra	531
EC-Naprosyn Delayed-Release Tablets (Less than 1%)	2277
▲ Emcyt Capsules (3%)	2085
Esimil Tablets (Occasional)	840
▲ Ethmozine Tablets (1%-5%)	2217
Feldene Capsules (Less than 1%)	2008
Florinef Acetate Tablets	506
Fludara for Injection (Up to 3%)	658
Glucophage Tablets	754
Hespan Injection	945
Hivid Tablets (Infrequent)	2287
Hydeltrasol Injection, Sterile	1708
Hydeltra-T.B.A. Sterile Suspension	1710
Hydrocortone Acetate Sterile Suspension	1712
Hydrocortone Phosphate Injection, Sterile	1713
Hydrocortone Tablets	1715
Hydropres Tablets	1718
IBU Tablets (Less than 1%)	1389
Idamycin Injection	2096
Inderal	2834
Inderal LA Long Acting Capsules	2836
Inderide Tablets	2838
Inderide LA Long Acting Capsules	2840
Indocin Capsules (Less than 1%)	1723
Indocin I.V. (Less than 1%)	1727
Indocin (Less than 1%)	1723
Ismelin Tablets	845
Isoptin Oral Tablets (1.8%)	1393
Isoptin SR Tablets (1.8%)	1395
Lodine Capsules and Tablets (Less than 1%)	2849
Lopressor (1%)	848
Lopressor HCT Tablets	850
Lupron Depot - 3 Month 22.5 mg (Less than 5%)	2743
▲ Lupron Injection (5% or more)	2736
LUVOX Tablets (Infrequent)	2723
Mexitil Capsules (Less than 1%)	684
Motrin Ibuprofen Suspension, Oral Drops, Chewable Tablets, Caplets (Less than 1%)	1563
Mutamycin for Injection (Rare)	712
▲ Naprelan Tablets (3% to 9%)	2861
Anaprox/Naprosyn (Less than 1%)	2277
Nimotop Capsules (Less than 1%)	603
Normodyne Injection	2519
Normodyne Tablets	2522
Norpace (1 to 3%)	2596
Novantrone for Injection (Up to 5%)	1327
Ocupress Ophthalmic Solution, 1% Sterile	⊙ 297
Orudis Capsules (Less than 1%)	2874
Oruvail Capsules (Less than 1%)	2874
Paxil Tablets (Rare)	2681
Pediapred Oral Solution	1618
Permax Tablets (Frequent)	571
Prelone Syrup	1834

(⊞ Described in PDR For Nonprescription Drugs)   Incidence data in parenthesis; ▲ 3% or more   (⊙ Described in PDR For Ophthalmology)

Side Effects Index

Congestive heart failure (cont.)

- Procardia Capsules (About 2%; rare, about 1 patient in 15) ... 2024
- Procardia XL Extended Release Tablets (Rare) ... 2026
- Proglycem ... 575
- Proleukin for Injection (1%) ... 812
- Retrovir Capsules (0.8%) ... 1216
- Retrovir I.V. Infusion (1%) ... 1221
- Retrovir Syrup (0.8%) ... 1216
- Rilutek Tablets (Infrequent) ... 2198
- Roferon-A Injection (Infrequent) ... 2308
- Rubex for Injection ... 721
- ▲ Rythmol Tablets—150mg, 225mg, 300mg (0.8 to 3.7%) ... 1399
- Sandostatin Injection (Less than 1%) ... 2421
- Seromycin Capsules ... 975
- Serzone Tablets (Rare) ... 776
- Sular Tablets (Less than or equal to 1%) ... 2961
- Symmetrel Capsules (0.1% to 1%) ... 965
- Symmetrel Syrup (0.1% to 1%) ... 963
- Tambocor Tablets ... 1555
- Taxol Injection ... 723
- Tegretol/Tegretol-XR ... 870
- Tenex Tablets (Rare) ... 2249
- Testoderm Testosterone Transdermal System (One in 104 patients) ... 486
- Tiazac Capsules (Less than 1%) ... 1019
- Tofranil Ampuls ... 873
- Tofranil Tablets ... 875
- Tofranil-PM Capsules ... 876
- Tolectin (200, 400 and 600 mg) (Less than 1%) ... 1591
- ▲ Tonocard Tablets (4.0%) ... 519
- Toprol-XL Tablets (About 1 of 100 patients) ... 560
- Trasylol (3%) ... 607
- Triostat Injection (Approximately 1%) ... 2708
- Vascor Tablets (200 and 300 mg) (About 1%) ... 1597
- Vasotec I.V. (1.8%) ... 1814
- Verelan Capsules (1.8%) ... 1455
- Cataflam/Voltaren/Voltaren-XR (Less than 1%) ... 833
- Zebeta Tablets ... 1457
- Ziac ... 1459
- ▲ Zoladex (5%) ... 2976
- Zoladex 3-month (1% to 5%) ... 2978

Conjunctiva, progressive pigmentation
- Serentil ... 689
- Torecan ... 2367

Conjunctiva, sensitization
- Neosporin Ophthalmic Ointment Sterile ... 1130
- Polysporin Ophthalmic Ointment Sterile ... 1140

Conjunctiva, suffusion
- BiCNU ... 696

Conjunctiva, thickening
- Humorsol Sterile Ophthalmic Solution ... 1707
- Phospholine Iodide ... ⊚ 323

Conjunctival blanching
- IOPIDINE Sterile Ophthalmic Solution (0.4%) ... ⊚ 218

Conjunctival chemosis
- Natacyn Antifungal Ophthalmic Suspension (One case) ... ⊚ 223

Conjunctival deposits
- AKPRO ... ⊚ 206
- EPIFRIN ... ⊚ 237
- PROPINE with C CAP Compliance Cap ... ⊚ 251
- Solganal Suspension ... 2530

Conjunctival epithelial defects, unspecified
- ▲ Garamycin Ophthalmic (Among most frequent) ... 2501
- ▲ Genoptic Sterile Ophthalmic Solution (Among most frequent) ... ⊚ 241
- ▲ Genoptic Sterile Ophthalmic Ointment (Among most frequent) ... ⊚ 241
- ▲ Gentak (Among most frequent) ... ⊚ 209

Conjunctival erythema
- Cortisporin Ophthalmic Ointment Sterile ... 1074
- Cortisporin Ophthalmic Suspension Sterile ... 1075
- FLURESS (Occasional) ... ⊚ 208
- Ocusert Pilo-20 and Pilo-40 Ocular Therapeutic Systems ... ⊚ 252

Conjunctival hyperemia
- AK-Spore ... ⊚ 205
- ▲ Ciloxan Ophthalmic Solution (Less than 10%) ... 468
- EPIFRIN ... ⊚ 237
- ▲ Garamycin Ophthalmic (Among most frequent) ... 2501
- ▲ Gentak (Among most frequent) ... ⊚ 209
- Natacyn Antifungal Ophthalmic Suspension (One case) ... ⊚ 223
- Ophthetic ... ⊚ 244
- Phospholine Iodide ... ⊚ 323
- Pilagan ... ⊚ 245
- Pred Forte (Occasional) ... ⊚ 247
- Pred Mild (Occasional) ... ⊚ 250
- Suprane (desflurane, USP) (Greater than 1%) ... 1865

Conjunctival injection
- Azulfidine (Rare) ... 2059
- Bactrim DS Tablets ... 2257
- Bactrim I.V. Infusion ... 2255
- Bactrim ... 2257
- ▲ Betimol 0.25%, 0.5% (More than 5%) ... ⊚ 259
- Crolom (Infrequent) ... ⊚ 254
- Diupres Tablets ... 1691
- Fansidar Tablets ... 2281
- Gantanol Tablets ... 2285
- Gantrisin ... 2286
- Hydropres Tablets ... 1718
- Isopto Carbachol Ophthalmic Solution ... ⊚ 221
- Mintezol ... 1747
- Pediazole Suspension ... 2340
- Pepcid Injection (Infrequent) ... 1765
- Pepcid (Infrequent) ... 1763
- ▲ Rev-Eyes Ophthalmic Eyedrops 0.5% (80%) ... ⊚ 324
- Septra ... 1146
- Septra I.V. Infusion ... 1142
- Septra I.V. Infusion ADD-Vantage Vials ... 1144
- Septra ... 1146
- Ser-Ap-Es Tablets ... 867
- Vira-A Ophthalmic Ointment, 3% ... ⊚ 299

Conjunctival irritation
- Efudex (Infrequent) ... 2280
- Ocusert Pilo-20 and Pilo-40 Ocular Therapeutic Systems ... ⊚ 252

Conjunctival microhemorrhage
- IOPIDINE Sterile Ophthalmic Solution ... ⊚ 218
- RespiGam (Infrequent) ... 1631

Conjunctival vascular congestion
- Isopto Carpine Ophthalmic Solution ... ⊚ 221
- Pilopine HS Ophthalmic Gel ... ⊚ 224

Conjunctivitis
- ▲ Accutane Capsules (About 2 patients in 5) ... 2252
- Adalat CC (Less than 1.0%) ... 582
- Adriamycin PFS (Rare) ... 2056
- Adriamycin RDF (Rare) ... 2056
- Ambien Tablets (Rare) ... 2559
- Anafranil Capsules (Up to 1%) ... 819
- Apresazide Capsules (Less frequent) ... 824
- Apresoline Hydrochloride Tablets (Less frequent) ... 826
- Asacol Delayed-Release Tablets (1% to 2%) ... 2129
- Atretol Tablets ... 569
- Atrovent Nasal Spray 0.03% (Less than 2%) ... 676
- Atrovent Nasal Spray 0.06% (Less than 1%) ... 678
- Avonex ... 662
- ▲ Betaseron for SC Injection (12%) ... 653
- Betimol 0.25%, 0.5% ... ⊚ 259
- Buprenex Injectable (Less than 1%) ... 2170
- BuSpar Tablets (Infrequent) ... 738
- Cardene I.V. (Rare) ... 2815
- Cardura Tablets (1%) ... 1993
- Cartrol Tablets (Less common) ... 413
- ▲ CellCept Capsules (More than or equal to 3%) ... 2265
- Cerebyx Injection (Infrequent) ... 1956
- Claritin Tablets (2% or fewer patients) ... 2485
- Claritin-D Tablets (Less frequent) ... 2487
- Clinoril Tablets (Less than 1 in 100) ... 1658
- Cognex Capsules (Frequent) ... 1961
- Cozaar Tablets (Less than 1%) ... 1668
- Cytosar-U Sterile Powder (Less frequent) ... 2077
- Cytotec (Infrequent) ... 2576
- Cytovene (1% or less) ... 2270
- DDAVP (Up to 2%) ... 2180
- DaunoXome (Less than or equal to 5%) ... 1842
- Daypro Caplets (Less than 1%) ... 2578
- Depakote Tablets (1% to 5%) ... 418
- Desmopressin Acetate Rhinal Tube (Up to 2%) ... 997
- Doxil (1% to 5%) ... 2613
- Doxorubicin Astra (Rare) ... 531
- Econopred & Econopred Plus Ophthalmic Suspensions (Occasional) ... ⊚ 216
- Effexor (Infrequent) ... 2825
- Engerix-B Unit-Dose Vials ... 2656
- Ergamisol Tablets (Less than 1% to 2%) ... 1340
- FML Forte Liquifilm (Occasional) ... ⊚ 237
- FML Liquifilm (Occasional) ... ⊚ 238
- FML S.O.P. (Occasional) ... ⊚ 239
- Felbatol ... 2774
- Floxin I.V. ... 1580
- Foscavir Injection (Between 1% and 5%) ... 541
- ▲ Garamycin Ophthalmic (Among most frequent) ... 2501
- ▲ Genoptic Sterile Ophthalmic Solution (Among most frequent) ... ⊚ 241
- ▲ Genoptic Sterile Ophthalmic Ointment (Among most frequent) ... ⊚ 241
- ▲ Gentak (Among most frequent) ... ⊚ 209
- Glucotrol XL Extended Release Tablets (Less than 1%) ... 2012
- Hismanal Tablets (1.2%) ... 1341
- Hydralazine Hydrochloride Injection USP ... 2712
- Hytrin Capsules (At least 1%) ... 434
- Hyzaar Tablets ... 1720
- IBU Tablets (Less than 1%) ... 1389
- Imdur (Less than or equal to 5%) ... 1362
- Intron A for Injection (Less than 5%) ... 2506
- Iopidine 0.5% (Less than 3%) ... ⊚ 219
- Kadian Capsules (Less than 3%) ... 2948
- Kerlone Tablets (Less than 2%) ... 2588
- Lamictal Tablets (Infrequent) ... 1105
- Lodine Capsules and Tablets (Less than 1%) ... 2849
- Lotensin HCT Tablets (0.3% or more) ... 855
- Lupron Depot 3.75 mg (Less than 5%) ... 2739
- LUVOX Tablets (Infrequent) ... 2723
- M-M-R II ... 1730
- Marinol (Dronabinol) Capsules (0.3% to 1%) ... 2353
- Maxaquin Tablets (Less than 1%) ... 2593
- Mesantoin Tablets ... 2400
- Methotrexate Sodium Tablets, Injection, for Injection and LPF Injection ... 1322
- Miacalcin Nasal Spray (1% to 3%) ... 2403
- Motrin Ibuprofen Suspension, Oral Drops, Chewable Tablets, Caplets (Less than 1%) ... 1563
- Myochrysine Injection (Rare) ... 1754
- Naprelan Tablets (Less than 1%) ... 2861
- Neoral (2% or less) ... 2405
- Neurontin Capsules (Infrequent) ... 1978
- ▲ Nipent for Injection (4%) ... 2733
- Norvasc Tablets (More than 0.1% to 1%) ... 2020
- Novantrone for Injection (Up to 5%) ... 1327
- Ocuflox Ophthalmic Solution ... 478
- OptiPranolol (Metipranolol 0.3%) Sterile Ophthalmic Solution (A small number of patients) ... ⊚ 256
- Orthoclone OKT3 Sterile Solution ... 1892
- Orudis Capsules (Less than 1%) ... 2874
- Oruvail Capsules (Less than 1%) ... 2874
- Pandel Cream, 0.1% (7 of 226 patients) ... 2475
- Paxil Tablets (Infrequent) ... 2681
- Penetrex Tablets (0.1% to 1%) ... 2196
- Pentasa (Less than 1%) ... 1275
- Permax Tablets (Infrequent) ... 571
- Pred Forte (Occasional) ... ⊚ 247
- Pred Mild (Occasional) ... ⊚ 250
- ▲ Proleukin for Injection (4%) ... 812
- Proventil Syrup (Children 2 to 6 years, 1%) ... 2528
- Prozac Pulvules & Liquid, Oral Solution (Infrequent) ... 935
- ▲ Pulmozyme Inhalation (4% to 5%) ... 1054
- Recombivax HB ... 1787
- Redux Capsules (Infrequent) ... 2911
- Remeron Tablets (Infrequent) ... 1878
- ▲ Ridaura Capsules (3 to 9%) ... 2691
- Rifadin (Occasional) ... 1276
- Rifater (Occasional) ... 1280
- Rimactane Capsules ... 865
- Robaxin Injectable ... 2245
- Robaxin Tablets ... 2246
- Rocaltrol Capsules ... 2303
- Rubex for Injection (Rare) ... 721
- Salagen Tablets (2%) ... 1546
- Sandimmune (2% or less) ... 2416
- Sectral Capsules (Up to 2%) ... 2914
- Ser-Ap-Es Tablets ... 867
- Serzone Tablets (Infrequent) ... 776
- Solganal Suspension (Rare) ... 2530
- Sular Tablets (Less than or equal to 1%) ... 2961
- Suprane (desflurane, USP) (Greater than 1%) ... 1865
- ▲ Tegison Capsules (10-25%) ... 2314
- Tegretol/Tegretol-XR ... 870
- Tenex Tablets (3% or less) ... 2249
- Thioplex (Thiotepa For Injection) ... 1329
- Timoptic in Ocudose (Less frequent) ... 1796
- Timoptic Sterile Ophthalmic Solution (Less frequent) ... 1794
- Timoptic-XE (1% to 5% of patients) ... 1798
- Trental Tablets (Less than 1%) ... 1291
- Vancenase AQ Double Strength Nasal Spray 0.084% (2%) ... 2536
- Vaseretic Tablets ... 1810
- Vasotec I.V. ... 1814
- Vasotec Tablets (0.5% to 1.0%) ... 1816
- Ventolin Syrup (1% of children) ... 1175
- Videx Tablets, Powder for Oral Solution, & Pediatric Powder for Oral Solution (Less than 1%) ... 2980
- Viramune Tablets ... 2368
- Virazole ... 1310
- Vistide Injection ... 1057
- Xalatan (Less than 1%) ... ⊚ 304
- ▲ Zerit Capsules (Fewer than 1% to 5%) ... 731
- Zithromax (1% or less) ... 2043
- Zoloft Tablets (Infrequent) ... 2051
- Zosyn (1.0% or less) ... 1463
- Zyloprim Tablets (Less than 1%) ... 1194
- Zyrtec Tablets (Less than 2%) ... 2053

Conjunctivitis, calcific
- Calcijex Injection ... 412

Conjunctivitis, exudative
- Rifamate Capsules (Occasional) ... 1278
- Rimactane Capsules ... 865

Conjunctivitis, follicular
- AKPRO (Infrequent) ... ⊚ 206
- PROPINE with C CAP Compliance Cap ... ⊚ 251

Conjunctivitis, hemorrhagic
- Anafranil Capsules (Rare) ... 819
- Cytosar-U Sterile Powder (With experimental doses) ... 2077

Conjunctivitis, mucopurulent
- Hivid Tablets (Less than 1%) ... 2287

Conjunctivitis sicca
- Orudis Capsules (Less than 1%) ... 2874
- Oruvail Capsules (Less than 1%) ... 2874

Consciousness, disorders
- ▲ Betapace Tablets (2% to 4%) ... 637
- Hexalen Capsules ... 2760
- Inapsine Injection (Very rare) ... 462
- Intron A for Injection (Less than 5%) ... 2506
- Permax Tablets ... 571
- Reglan ... 2243
- Supprelin Injection (1% to 3%) ... 2230
- Symmetrel Capsules (Uncommon) ... 965
- Symmetrel Syrup (Uncommon) ... 963

Consciousness, loss of
- Acthrel for Injection (Two patients) ... 2990
- Carbocaine Injection ... 2432
- Cipro I.V. (1% or less) ... 587

(▨ Described in PDR For Nonprescription Drugs)   Incidence data in parenthesis; ▲ 3% or more   (⊚ Described in PDR For Ophthalmology)

1291 **Side Effects Index** **Constipation**

Cipro Tablets ... 584
Decadron Phosphate with Xylocaine Injection, Sterile ... 1683
Duranest Injections ... 533
Dyclone 0.5% and 1% Topical Solutions, USP ... 535
Effexor (Rare) ... 2825
EMLA Cream (Unlikely with cream) 536
Etopophos for Injection (Sometimes; 3%) ... 701
Etoposide Injection (Sometimes) ... 539
Fioricet with Codeine Capsules ... 2387
Fiorinal with Codeine Capsules ... 2390
Floxin I.V. ... 1580
Floxin Tablets (200 mg, 300 mg, 400 mg) ... 1577
Hyperstat I.V. Injection ... 2504
Lutrepulse for Injection ... 998
Marcaine ... 2446
Marcaine Spinal ... 2449
Maxaquin Tablets ... 2593
Mexitil Capsules (Less than 1% or about 6 in 10,000) ... 684
NegGram ... 2453
Nescaine/Nescaine MPF ... 549
Noroxin Tablets ... 1758
Noroxin Tablets ... 2222
Novocain Hydrochloride for Spinal Anesthesia ... 2457
Orthoclone OKT3 Sterile Solution .. 1892
Pontocaine Hydrochloride for Spinal Anesthesia ... 2460
Prostigmin Injectable ... 1305
Prostigmin Tablets ... 1306
Sensorcaine ... 554
Stelazine ... 2692
Typhim Vi ... 914
VePesid Capsules and Injection (Sometimes) ... 727
▲ Vesanoid Capsules (3%) ... 2327
▲ Xylocaine Injections (Among most common) ... 562

Constipation

Accupril Tablets (0.5% to 1.0%) .. 1950
▲ Actigall Capsules (9.7%) ... 818
Adalat Capsules (10 mg and 20 mg) (2% or less) ... 580
▲ Adalat CC (1% to 3% or less) ... 582
Adapin Capsules ... 1542
Adderall Tablets ... 2209
Adipex-P Tablets and Capsules ... 1035
▲ AeroBid Inhaler System (1% to 3%) ... 1004
▲ Aerobid-M Inhaler System (1% to 3%) ... 1004
Akineton ... 1380
Aldoclor Tablets ... 1638
Aldomet Ester HCl Injection ... 1642
Aldomet Oral ... 1640
Aldoril Tablets ... 1644
Alferon N Injection (One patient) ... 2142
Alka-Mints Chewable Antacid ... ▣ 609
Altace Capsules (Less than 1%) ... 1238
ALternaGEL Liquid ... 1358
Ambien Tablets (Infrequent; 2%) ... 2559
Amphojel ... 2802
▲ Anafranil Capsules (22% to 47%) 819
▲ Anaprox/Naprosyn (3% to 9%) ... 2277
Apresazide Capsules (Less frequent) ... 824
Apresoline Hydrochloride Tablets (Less frequent) ... 826
▲ Aredia for Injection (Up to 18.2%) 827
▲ Arimidex Tablets (6.9% to 7.3%) .. 2932
Artane ... 1418
▲ Asacol Delayed-Release Tablets (5%) ... 2129
▲ Asendin Tablets (12%) ... 1419
Astramorph/PF Injection, USP (Preservative-Free) ... 526
Atamet Tablets ... 567
Atretol Tablets ... 569
Atrohist Plus Tablets ... 1605
Atrovent Inhalation Aerosol (Less frequent) ... 674
Atrovent Inhalation Solution (0.9%) ... 675
Atrovent Nasal Spray 0.03% ... 676
Atrovent Nasal Spray 0.06% ... 678
Avonex ... 662
Axid Pulvules (2.5%) ... 1468
Axocet Capsules (Infrequent) ... 2469
Basaljel ... 2810
Benadryl Injection ... 1955
Bentyl ... 1246
▲ Betaseron for SC Injection (24%) .. 653
Bontril Slow-Release Capsules ... 786
Brevibloc (esmolol HCl) Injection (Less than 1%) ... 1860
▲ Bromfed-DM Cough Syrup (Among most frequent) ... 1832
Brontex ... 2130
Buprenex Injectable (Less than 1%) ... 2170
BuSpar Tablets (1%) ... 738
Butisol Sodium Elixir & Tablets (Less than 1 in 100) ... 2768
▲ Calan SR Caplets (7.3%) ... 2571
▲ Calan Tablets (7.3%) ... 2568
Calcijex Injection ... 412
Capoten Tablets (About 0.5 to 2%) ... 740
Capozide Tablets (0.5 to 2%) ... 744
Carafate Suspension (2%) ... 1250
Carafate Tablets (2%) ... 1249
Cardene Capsules (0.6%) ... 2261
Cardizem CD Capsules (Less than 1%) ... 1251
Cardizem SR Capsules (1.6%) ... 1255
Cardizem Injectable (Less than 1%) ... 1253
Cardizem Tablets (Less than 1%) .. 1257
Cardura Tablets (1%) ... 1993
Cartrol Tablets (Less common) ... 413
▲ Casodex Tablets (17%) ... 2934
▲ Cataflam Tablets (3% to 9%) ... 833
▲ Catapres Tablets (About 10 in 100 patients) ... 679
Catapres-TTS (1 of 101 patients) .. 680
Cedax (0.1% to 1%) ... 2480
▲ CellCept Capsules (18.5% to 22.9%) ... 2265
Celontin Kapseals (Frequent) ... 1955
Cerebyx Injection (Frequent) ... 1956
Cipro I.V. (1% or less) ... 587
Cipro I.V. Pharmacy Bulk Package (Less than 1%) ... 590
Cipro Tablets ... 584
Claritin Tablets (2% or fewer patients) ... 2485
Claritin-D Tablets (Less frequent) .. 2487
Cleocin Vaginal Cream (Less than 1%) ... 2070
▲ Clinoril Tablets (3% to 9%) ... 1658
Clomid (Fewer than 1%) ... 1262
▲ Clozaril Tablets (More than 5 to 14%) ... 2377
Codiclear DH Syrup ... 808
Cogentin ... 1661
▲ Cognex Capsules (4%) ... 1961
Colestid ... 2073
▲ Combipres Tablets (About 10%) ... 682
Compazine ... 2644
▲ Cordarone Tablets (4 to 9%) ... 2818
▲ Covera-HS Tablets (7.2% to 11.7%) ... 2573
Cozaar Tablets (Less than 1%) ... 1668
▲ Creon (Among most frequent) ... 2714
Crixivan Capsules (Less than 2%) . 1670
Cytotec (1.1%) ... 2576
Cytovene (1% or less) ... 2270
▲ DHCplus Capsules (Among most frequent) ... 2148
Dalgan Injection (Less than 1%) ... 529
Dalmane Capsules ... 2329
Danocrine Capsules ... 2437
Dantrium Capsules (Less frequent) 2131
Daranide Tablets ... 1676
Darvon-N/Darvocet-N ... 1473
Darvon ... 1475
Darvon-N Suspension & Tablets ... 1473
▲ DaunoXome (Up to 7%) ... 1842
▲ Daypro Caplets (3% to 9%) ... 2578
Demadex Tablets and Injection (1.8%) ... 691
Demerol ... 2438
Depakene ... 416
▲ Depakote Tablets (1% to 5%) ... 418
Desoxyn Gradumet Tablets ... 422
▲ Desyrel and Desyrel Dividose (7.0% to 7.6%) ... 504
Dexedrine ... 2648
DextroStat-Dextroamphetamine Sulfate Tablets ... 2211
▲ Dilacor XR Extended-release Capsules (2.2% to 3.6%) ... 2183
Dilantin Infatabs ... 1967
Dilantin Kapseals ... 1965
Dilantin-125 Suspension ... 1969
Dilaudid Ampules ... 1382
Dilaudid Cough Syrup ... 1383
Dilaudid-HP Injection (Less frequent) ... 1384
Dilaudid-HP Lyophilized Powder 250 mg (Less frequent) ... 1384
Dilaudid ... 1382
Dilaudid Oral Liquid ... 1386
Dilaudid ... 1382
Dilaudid Tablets - 8 mg ... 1386
Dimetane-DC Cough Syrup ... 2232
Dimetane-DX Cough Syrup ... 2233
Ditropan ... 1267
Diucardin Tablets ... 2824
Diupres Tablets ... 1691
Diuril Oral Suspension ... 1694
Diuril Sodium Intravenous ... 1693
Diuril Tablets ... 1694
Dizac (diazepam injectable emulsion) CIV (Less frequent) ... 1862
Dolobid Tablets (Greater than 1 in 100) ... 1695
Donnatal ... 2234
Donnatal Extentabs ... 2234
Donnatal Tablets ... 2234
Doral Tablets ... 2773
Doxil (1% to 5%) ... 2613
▲ Duragesic Transdermal System (10% or more) ... 1336
Duramorph Injection (Frequent) ... 983
Duratuss HD Elixir ... 2750
Dyazide Capsules ... 2653
Dynabac (0.1% to 1%) ... 668
DynaCirc Capsules (0.5% to 1%) .. 2381
DynaCirc CR Tablets (1.7% to 3.8%) ... 2383
▲ EC-Naprosyn Delayed-Release Tablets (3% to 9%) ... 2277
▲ Effexor (15%) ... 2825
Elavil ... 2945
Eldepryl Capsules ... 2729
Enduron Tablets ... 424
Engerix-B Unit-Dose Vials (Less than 1%) ... 2656
Ergamisol Tablets (2% to 3%) ... 1340
Esgic-plus Capsules (Infrequent) ... 1012
Esgic-plus Tablets (Infrequent) ... 1012
Esidrix Tablets ... 839
Esimil Tablets ... 840
▲ Etopophos for Injection (Infrequent; 8%) ... 701
Etoposide Injection (Infrequent) ... 539
Etrafon ... 2495
Famvir Tablets (1.4% to 4.4%) ... 2660
Fastin Capsules ... 2662
▲ Felbatol (6.9% to 12.9%) ... 2774
Feldene Capsules (Greater than 1%) ... 2008
Feosol Caplets (Occasional) ... 2626
Feosol Capsules (Occasional) ... ▣ 777
Feosol Elixir (Occasional) ... 2627
Feosol Tablets (Occasional) ... 2627
Fioricet Tablets (Infrequent) ... 2386
Fioricet with Codeine Capsules (Infrequent) ... 2387
Fiorinal with Codeine Capsules ... 2390
Flagyl 375 Capsules ... 2587
Flagyl I.V. ... 2373
Flexeril Tablets (1% to 3%) ... 1701
▲ Flolan for Injection (6%) ... 1085
Floxin I.V. (1% to 3%) ... 1580
Floxin Tablets (200 mg, 300 mg, 400 mg) (1% to 3%) ... 1577
Fludara for Injection (1% to 3%) ... 658
Flumadine Tablets & Syrup ... 1013
▲ Fosamax Tablets (3.1%) ... 1703
Foscavir Injection (Between 1% and 5%) ... 541
Ganite ... 2711
Gastrocrom Oral Concentrate ... 1611
▲ Gemzar for Injection (10% to 31%) ... 1482
Glucotrol Tablets (1 in 100) ... 2011
Glucotrol XL Extended Release Tablets (Less than 3%) ... 2012
▲ Habitrol Nicotine Transdermal System (3% to 9% of patients) .. 884
Halcion Tablets (Rare) ... 2093
Haldol Decanoate ... 1587
Haldol Injection, Tablets and Concentrate ... 1585
Helidac Therapy (1.0%) ... 2135
▲ Histussin D Liquid (Among most frequent) ... 670
Hivid Tablets (Less than 1% to 2.5%) ... 2287
▲ Hycamtin for Injection (Less than 1% to 39%) ... 2665
Hycodan Tablets and Syrup ... 946
Hycomine ... 947
Hydralazine Hydrochloride Injection USP (Less frequent) ... 2712
Hydrea Capsules (Less frequent) ... 705
Hydrocet Capsules ... 787
HydroDIURIL Tablets ... 1716
Hydropres Tablets ... 1718
▲ Hylorel Tablets (21.0%) ... 1613
Hyperstat I.V. Injection ... 2504
Hytrin Capsules (At least 1%) ... 434
Hyzaar Tablets ... 1720
IBU Tablets (Greater than 1%) ... 1389
IFEX (Less than 1%) ... 706
Imdur (Less than or equal to 5%) .. 1362
Imitrex Tablets (Infrequent) ... 1099
Imodium Capsules ... 1343
Inderal ... 2834
Inderal LA Long Acting Capsules ... 2836
Inderide Tablets ... 2838
Inderide LA Long Acting Capsules .. 2840
Indocin Capsules (Greater than 1%) ... 1723
Indocin I.V. (1% to 3%) ... 1727
Indocin (Greater than 1%) ... 1723
Infumorph 200 and Infumorph 500 Sterile Solutions (Frequent) 985
▲ Intron A for Injection (Up to 10%) 2506
Inversine Tablets ... 1729
Invirase Capsules (Less than 2%) .. 2291
Ionamin Capsules ... 1615
Iopidine 0.5% (Less than 1%) ... ⊙ 219
▲ Isoptin Oral Tablets (7.3%) ... 1393
▲ Isoptin SR Tablets (7.3%) ... 1395
▲ Kadian Capsules (Virtually all patients) ... 2948
Kayexalate ... 2444
Kemadrin Tablets ... 1105
Kerlone Tablets (Less than 2%) ... 2588
Klonopin Tablets ... 2294
▲ Kytril Injection (3%) ... 2667
▲ Kytril Tablets (3% to 18%) ... 2669
▲ Lamictal Tablets (4.1%) ... 1105
Lamprene Capsules (Less than 1%) ... 846
Larodopa Tablets (Infrequent) ... 2296
Lasix Injection, Oral Solution and Tablets ... 1267
▲ Lescol Capsules (3.1%) ... 2395
Leucovorin Calcium for Injection (Up to 4%) ... 1313
▲ Leukine (8%) ... 1317
▲ Leustatin (9%) ... 1889
Levbid Extended-Release Tablets ... 2549
Levoprome ... 1321
Levsin/Levsinex/Levbid ... 2549
Librax Capsules (Infrequent) ... 2330
Librium Capsules (Isolated cases) .. 2331
Librium Injectable (Isolated instances) ... 2332
▲ Limbitrol (Among most frequent) ... 2333
Lioresal Intrathecal (0.2% to 5.1%) ... 1634
▲ Lioresal Tablets (2% to 6%) ... 847
Lodine Capsules and Tablets (1% to 3%) ... 2849
Lopid Tablets (1.4%) ... 1974
Lopressor (1%) ... 848
Lopressor HCT Tablets (1 in 100 patients) ... 850
Lorcet 10/650 Tablets ... 1016
Lortab ... 2751
Lotensin Tablets ... 852
Lotensin HCT Tablets (0.3% to 1.0%) ... 855
Lotrel Capsules ... 858
Loxitane ... 1426
▲ Ludiomil Tablets (6%) ... 861
▲ Lupron Injection (5% or more) ... 2736
▲ LUVOX Tablets (10%) ... 2723
▲ MS Contin Tablets (Less frequent to among most frequent) ... 2149
▲ MSIR (Among most frequent) ... 2152
Macrobid Capsules (Less than 1%) ... 2138
Matulane Capsules ... 2300
Mavik Tablets (0.3% to 1.0%) ... 1407
Maxaquin Tablets (Less than 1%) .. 2593
Mebaral Tablets (Less than 1 in 100) ... 2452
Megace Oral Suspension (1% to 3%) ... 708
Mellaril ... 2398
Mepergan Injection ... 2859
▲ Mepron Suspension (3%) ... 1206
Merrem I.V. (1.2%) ... 2952
Methadone Hydrochloride Oral Concentrate ... 2356
Methadone Hydrochloride Oral Solution & Tablets ... 2357
MetroGel-Vaginal (Equal to or less than 2%) ... 917
▲ Mevacor Tablets (2.0% to 4.9%) . 1742
▲ Mexitil Capsules (4%) ... 684
Miacalcin Nasal Spray (1% to 3%) 2403
Midamor Tablets (Between 1% and 3%) ... 1746
Minipress Capsules (1-4%) ... 2015
Minizide Capsules (Rare) ... 2016
Moban Tablets and Concentrate ... 1036
Moduretic Tablets (Less than or equal to 1%) ... 1748
Monopril Tablets (0.2% to 1.0%) .. 762

(▣ Described in PDR For Nonprescription Drugs) Incidence data in parenthesis; ▲ 3% or more (⊙ Described in PDR For Ophthalmology)

Motofen Tablets (1 in 300) 789
Motrin Ibuprofen Suspension, Oral Drops, Chewable Tablets, Caplets (1% to less than 3%) 1563
Mykrox Tablets (Less than 2%) 1617
▲ Nalfon 200 Pulvules & Nalfon Tablets (7%) 933
▲ Naprelan Tablets (3% to 9%) 2861
▲ Anaprox/Naprosyn (3% to 9%) 2277
Nardil (Common) 1977
Navane Capsules and Concentrate 2018
Navane Intramuscular 2019
▲ Navelbine Injection (Up to 29%) 1212
Nembutal Sodium Capsules (Less than 1%) 440
Nembutal Sodium Solution (Less than 1%) 442
Nembutal Sodium Suppositories (Less than 1%) 444
Neoral (Rare) 2405
Nephro-Fer Rx Tablets 2168
▲ Neupogen for Injection (5%) 495
Neurontin Capsules (1.5%) 1978
Nicotrol NS Nicotine Nasal Spray (Common) 1565
Nipent for Injection (Less than 3%) 2733
Norflex 1554
Norgesic 1554
Noroxin Tablets (0.3% to 1.0%) 1758
Noroxin Tablets (0.3% to 1.0%) 2222
▲ Norpace (11%) 2596
Norpramin Tablets 1273
Norvasc Tablets (More than 0.1% to 1%) 2020
Nucofed 2225
Oncaspar (Less than 1%) 2194
Oncovin Solution Vials & Hyporets 1521
▲ Oramorph SR (Morphine Sulfate Sustained Release Tablets) (Among most frequent) 2359
▲ Orap Tablets (4 of 20 patients) 1037
Oretic Tablets 450
▲ Orlaam Oral Solution (3% to 9%) 2361
Ornade Spansule Capsules 2678
▲ Orudis Capsules (3% to 9%) 2874
▲ Oruvail Capsules (3% to 9%) 2874
▲ OxyContin Tablets (23%) 2163
OxyIR Capsules 2167
PBZ Tablets 863
PBZ-SR Tablets 862
Pamelor 2409
Papaverine Hydrochloride Vials and Ampoules 1523
▲ Paraplatin for Injection (6%) 713
▲ Parlodel (3% to 14%) 2411
Parnate Tablets 2679
▲ Paxil Tablets (1.1% to 16%) 2681
Penetrex Tablets (0.1% to 1%) 2196
Pentasa (Less than 1%) 1275
Pepcid Injection (1.2%) 1765
Pepcid (1.2%) 1763
Percocet Tablets 955
Percodan Tablets 955
Percodan-Demi Tablets 956
Periactin 1767
▲ Permax Tablets (10.6%; frequent) 571
Phenergan with Codeine 2883
Phenergan VC with Codeine 2888
Phenobarbital Elixir and Tablets (Less than 1 in 100 patients) 1523
PhosLo Tablets 695
Phrenilin (Infrequent) 790
Plendil Extended-Release Tablets (0.3% to 1.5%) 514
Pondimin Tablets 2239
Ponstel (Less frequent) 1982
▲ Pravachol Tablets (2.4% to 4.0%) 770
Prelu-2 Timed Release Capsules 687
Prevacid Delayed-Release Capsules (Less than 1%) 2746
Prilosec Delayed-Release Capsules (1.1% to 1.5%) 516
Prinivil Tablets (0.3 to 1.0%) 1776
Prinzide Tablets (0.3% to 1%) 1780
Pro-Banthine Tablets 2226
Procardia Capsules (2% or less) 2024
▲ Procardia XL Extended Release Tablets (3.3%) 2026
▲ Prograf (19% to 24%) 1028
▲ Proleukin for Injection (5%) 812
Prolixin 510
▲ Propulsid (6.7%) 1346
ProSom Tablets (Frequent) 457
Prostep (nicotine transdermal system) (1% to 3% of patients) 1439
Protostat Tablets 1939
▲ Prozac Pulvules & Liquid, Oral Solution (4.5%) 935
▲ Questran (Most common) 774
RMS Suppositories CII 2766
Recombivax HB 1787
Redux Capsules (Frequent) 2911
▲ Relafen Tablets (3% to 9%) 2688
▲ Remeron Tablets (13%) 1878
ReoPro Vials (0.3%) 1526
▲ Retrovir Capsules (6.4%) 1216
▲ Retrovir I.V. Infusion (6.4%) 1221
▲ Retrovir Syrup (6.4%) 1216
▲ ReVia Tablets (Less than 10%) 957
Ridaura Capsules (1 to 3%) 2691
Rilutek Tablets (More than 2%) 2198
▲ Risperdal Tablets (7% to 13%) 1348
Robaxisal Tablets 2246
Robinul Forte Tablets 2247
Robinul Injectable 2247
Robinul Tablets 2247
Robitussin A-C Syrup 2248
Robitussin-DAC Syrup 2249
Rocaltrol Capsules 2303
Roferon-A Injection (Less than 3%) 2308
Rowasa (0.98%) 2727
Roxanol 2365
Roxicodone Tablets, Oral Solution & Intensol (Oxycodone) 2366
Ryna ▣ 804
▲ Rythmol Tablets–150mg, 225mg, 300mg (2.0 to 7.2%) 1399
Sandimmune (Rare) 2416
▲ Sandostatin Injection (Less than 10%) 2421
▲ Sanorex Tablets (Among most common) 2423
Sansert Tablets 2424
Seconal Sodium Pulvules (Less than 1 in 100) 1529
▲ Sectral Capsules (4%) 2914
Sedapap Tablets 50 mg/650 mg (Infrequent) 1826
Ser-Ap-Es Tablets 867
Serentil 689
▲ Serzone Tablets (10% to 17%) 776
Sinemet Tablets 959
Sinemet CR Tablets (0.2%) 961
Sinequan 2028
Sodium Polystyrene Sulfonate Suspension 2367
Soma Compound w/Codeine Tablets 2784
▲ Soma Compound Tablets (Among most common) 2783
Sporanox Capsules (Infrequent) 1352
▲ Stadol (3% to 9%) 779
Stelazine 2692
Supprelin Injection (1% to 3%) 2230
Surmontil Capsules 2917
Symmetrel Capsules (1% to 5%) 965
Symmetrel Syrup (1% to 5%) 963
Talacen Caplets (Infrequent) 2464
Talwin Injection (Infrequent) 2465
Talwin Compound (Infrequent) 2466
Talwin Injection (Infrequent) 2465
Talwin Nx Tablets 2467
▲ Tambocor Tablets (4.4%) 1555
Tavist Syrup 2426
Tavist Tablets 2427
Taxotere for Injection Concentrate 2204
Tegison Capsules (Less than 1%) 2314
Tegretol/Tegretol-XR 870
▲ Tenex Tablets (Up to 16%) 2249
Tenoretic Tablets 2963
Tessalon Perles 1018
Thalitone 1293
TheraCys BCG Live (Intravesical) (Up to 0.9%) 911
Thorazine 2701
Tiazac Capsules (Less than 1% to 2%) 1019
Timolide Tablets (Less than 1%) 1791
Tofranil Ampuls 873
Tofranil Tablets (Rare) 875
Tofranil-PM Capsules 876
Tolectin (200, 400 and 600 mg) (1 to 3%) 1591
Tonocard Tablets (Less than 1%) 519
Toprol-XL Tablets (About 1 of 100 patients) 560
Toradol (Greater than 1%) 2319
Trental Tablets (Less than 1%) 1291
Triavil Tablets 1800
Trilafon (Occasional) 2532
▲ Trilisate (Less than 20%) 2155
Trinalin Repetabs Tablets 1373
Trinsicon Capsules (Rare) 2759
Tussend 1830
Tussend Expectorant 1831
Tussionex Pennkinetic Extended-Release Suspension 1624
Tylenol with Codeine 1592
Tylox Capsules 1593
▲ Ultram Tablets (50 mg) (24% to 46%) 1594
Univasc Tablets (Less than 1%) 2553
Valium Injectable 2336
Valium Tablets (Infrequent) 2335
Valtrex Caplets (Less than 1% to 5%) 1167
Varivax (Greater than or equal to 1%) 1807
Vascor Tablets (200 and 300 mg) (0.5 to 2.84%) 1597
Vaseretic Tablets (0.5% to 2.0%) 1810
Vasotec I.V. (0.5 to 1%) 1814
Vasotec Tablets (0.5% to 1.0%) 1816
▲ Velban Vials (Among most common) 1537
VePesid Capsules and Injection (Infrequent) 727
▲ Verelan Capsules (7.3% to 7.4%) 1455
▲ Vesanoid Capsules (17%) 2327
Vicodin Tablets 1404
Vicodin ES Tablets 1405
Vicodin HP Tablets 1403
▲ Videx Tablets, Powder for Oral Solution, & Pediatric Powder for Oral Solution (Up to 12%) 2980
Vistide Injection 1057
Vivactil Tablets 1820
▲ Cataflam/Voltaren/Voltaren-XR (3% to 9%) 833
▲ Wellbutrin Tablets (26.0%) 1177
Wygesic Tablets 2930
▲ Xanax Tablets (10.4% to 26.2%) 2115
Yutopar Intravenous Injection (Infrequent) 566
Zantac 1182
Zantac Injection 1180
Zantac Syrup 1182
Zaroxolyn Tablets 1625
Zebeta Tablets 1457
▲ Zerit Capsules (Fewer than 1% to 7%) 731
Zestoretic Tablets (0.3 to 1%) 2968
Zestril Tablets (0.3% to 1.0%) 2972
Ziac 1459
Zithromax (1% or less) 2043
Zocor Tablets (2.3%) 1821
▲ Zofran Injection (11%) 1227
▲ Zofran Tablets (6% to 9%) 1231
Zoladex (1% or greater but less than 5%) 2976
Zoladex 3-month 2978
▲ Zoloft Tablets (8.4%) 2051
▲ Zosyn (7.7% to 8.4%) 1463
Zovirax (0.9%) 1187
Zydone Capsules 967
Zyrtec Tablets (Less than 2%) 2053

Constriction, pupillary (see under Miosis)

Constriction, pupils (see under Miosis)

Contact lenses, intolerance

Accutane Capsules 2252
Brevicon 2563
Climara Transdermal System 640
▲ Demulen (Among most common) 2580
Desogen Tablets 1867
Diethylstilbestrol Tablets 1477
Estrace Cream and Tablets 751
Estraderm Transdermal System 842
ESTRATAB Tablets (0.3, 0.625, 1.25, 2.5 mg) 2715
Estratest 2718
Levlen/Tri-Levlen 646
Lo/Ovral Tablets 2852
Lo/Ovral-28 Tablets 2857
Menest Tablets 2671
Modicon 1928
Nordette-21 Tablets 2863
Nordette-28 Tablets 2866
Norinyl 2563
Nor-Q D Tablets 2598
Ogen Tablets 2103
Ogen Vaginal Cream 2106
Ortho-Cept 1907
Ortho-Cyclen/Ortho-Tri-Cyclen 1914
Ortho Dienestrol Cream 1922
Ortho-Est 1925
Ortho-Novum 1928
Ortho-Cyclen/Ortho Tri-Cyclen 1914
Ovcon 765
Ovral Tablets 2877
Ovral-28 Tablets 2878
Ovrette Tablets 2878
PMB 200 and PMB 400 2890
Premarin Intravenous 2893
Premarin Tablets 2896
Premarin Vaginal Cream 2898
Premphase 2900
Prempro 2905
Levlen/Tri-Levlen 646
Tri-Norinyl 2607
Vivelle Transdermal System 880

Contact lens staining

Prodium 695
Pyridium 1985
Rifadin 1276
Rifater 1280

Convulsions

Abelcet Injection 1540
ActHIB (2 definite; 3 possible) 893
AK-FLUOR Injection 10% and 25% ⊙ 204
Aldoclor Tablets 1638
Aldoril Tablets 1644
Altace Capsules (Less than 1%) 1238
Ambien Tablets 2559
Amicar Syrup, Tablets, and Injection 1312
Amikacin Sulfate Injection, USP 523
Anafranil Capsules (Infrequent) 819
Ana-Kit Anaphylaxis Emergency Treatment Kit (Occasional) 611
Antilirium Injectable 1007
Aralen Hydrochloride Injection 2430
Astramorph/PF Injection, USP (Preservative-Free) 526
Atamet Tablets 567
Atarax Tablets & Syrup (Rare) 1992
Attenuvax (Rare) 1650
Azulfidine (Rare) 2059
Bactrim DS Tablets 2257
Bactrim I.V. Infusion 2255
Bactrim 2257
Benadryl Injection 1955
Betaseron for SC Injection (2%) 653
Biavax II (Rare) 1653
Brevibloc (esmolol HCl) Injection (Less than 1%) 1860
▲ Bromfed-DM Cough Syrup (Among most frequent) 1832
Brontex 2130
Buprenex Injectable (Rare) 2170
Carbocaine Injection 2432
Cardioquin Tablets 2146
Cataflam Tablets (Rare) 833
Cefotan 2936
Ceftin for Oral Suspension 1067
Celestone Soluspan Suspension 2484
Cerebyx Injection (Infrequent) 1956
Chibroxin Sterile Ophthalmic Solution (With oral form) 1657
Cipro I.V. Pharmacy Bulk Package (Less than 1%) 590
Cipro Tablets 584
Claritin Tablets (2% or fewer patients) 2485
Claritin-D Tablets 2487
Clinoril Tablets (Less than 1%) 1658
▲ Clozaril Tablets (3%) 2377
Cognex Capsules (Frequent) 1961
Compazine 2644
CORTENEMA 2713
Cortone Acetate Sterile Suspension 1663
Cortone Acetate Tablets 1664
Cytovene (1% or less) 2270
D.A. II Tablets 972
D.A. Chewable Tablets 970
Dalalone D.P. Injectable 1009
Danocrine Capsules (Rare) 2437
DaunoXome (Less than or equal to 5%) 1842
Decadron Elixir 1676
Decadron Phosphate Injection 1680
Decadron Phosphate with Xylocaine Injection, Sterile 1683
Decadron Tablets 1678
Decadron-LA Sterile Suspension 1687
Deconsal II Tablets 1605
Demerol 2438
Depo-Provera Contraceptive Injection (A few cases; fewer than 1%) 2079
Dexacort Phosphate in Respihaler 1606
Dexacort Phosphate in Turbinaire 1607
Dexatrim ▣ 795
Dexatrim Plus Vitamins Caplets ▣ 796
Diamox Intravenous (Occasional) ⊙ 317
Diamox Sequels (Sustained Release) ⊙ 318
Diamox Tablets (Occasional) ⊙ 317
Dimetane-DC Cough Syrup 2232
Dimetane-DX Cough Syrup 2233
Diphtheria and Tetanus Toxoids and Pertussis Vaccine Adsorbed (Infrequent) 2650

(▣ Described in PDR For Nonprescription Drugs) Incidence data in parenthesis; ▲ 3% or more (⊙ Described in PDR For Ophthalmology)

Diprivan Injectable Emulsion (Rare) 2939
Diupres Tablets 1691
Diuril Oral Suspension 1694
Diuril Sodium Intravenous 1693
Diuril Tablets 1694
Dopram Injectable 2235
Doxil (Less than 1%) 2613
Duramorph Injection (May accompany high doses) 983
Duranest Injections 533
Dura-Tap/PD Capsules 970
Dura-Vent/DA Tablets 972
Dura-Vent Tablets 971
Dyclone 0.5% and 1% Topical Solutions, USP 535
Effexor (Infrequent) 2825
EMLA Cream (Unlikely with cream) 536
Entex PSE Tablets 973
Ergamisol Tablets (Less frequent) 1340
Esgic-plus Capsules (Infrequent) 1012
Esgic-plus Tablets (Infrequent) 1012
Fansidar Tablets 2281
Fedahist Gyrocaps 2545
Fioricet Tablets (Infrequent) 2386
Flexeril Tablets (Less than 1%) 1701
▲ Flolan for Injection (4%) 1085
Florinef Acetate Tablets 506
Floxin Tablets (200 mg, 300 mg, 400 mg) 1577
Flumadine Tablets & Syrup (Less than 0.3%) 1013
Fluorescite ⊙ 217
Fungizone Intravenous 507
Gantanol Tablets 2285
Gantrisin 2286
Garamycin Injectable 2502
Gastrocrom Oral Concentrate (Less common) 1611
GlaucTabs (Occasional) ⊙ 209
Guaimax-D Tablets 809
Havrix (Rare) 2663
HibTITER 1423
Hismanal Tablets (Isolated cases) 1341
Histussin D Liquid 670
Hydeltrasol Injection, Sterile 1708
Hydeltra-T.B.A. Sterile Suspension 1710
Hydrea Capsules (Extremely rare) 705
Hydrocortone Acetate Sterile Suspension 1712
Hydrocortone Phosphate Injection, Sterile 1713
Hydrocortone Tablets 1715
HydroDIURIL Tablets 1716
Hydropres Tablets 1718
Hyperstat I.V. Injection 2504
Hyskon Hysteroscopy Fluid (Rare) 1633
Imitrex Injection (Rare) 1095
Imitrex Tablets (Rare) 1099
Indocin Capsules (Less than 1%) 1723
Indocin I.V. (Less than 1%) 1727
Indocin (Less than 1%) 1723
INFeD (Iron Dextran Injection, USP) 2478
Infumorph 200 and Infumorph 500 Sterile Solutions 985
Intron A for Injection (Less than 5%) 2506
Inversine Tablets 1729
Invirase Capsules (Rare; less than 2%) 2291
Kefzol Vials, Faspak & ADD-Vantage 1511
Kwell Cream & Lotion 2172
Kwell Shampoo (Exceedingly rare cases) 2173
▲ Lamictal Tablets (3.2%) 1105
Larodopa Tablets (Rare) 2296
Levo-Dromoran 2297
Lindane Lotion USP 1% 481
Lindane Shampoo USP 1% 483
▲ Lioresal Intrathecal (0.5% to 10.0%) 1634
Lopid Tablets 1974
Lufyllin-GG Elixir & Tablets 2779
LUVOX Tablets (Infrequent) 2723
M-M-R II (Rare) 1730
M-R-VAX II (Rare) 1732
Marcaine 2446
Marcaine Spinal 2449
Matulane Capsules 2300
Maxaquin Tablets (Less than 1%) 2593
Megace Oral Suspension (1% to 3%) 708
Methotrexate Sodium Tablets, Injection, for Injection and LPF Injection 1322
Mexitil Capsules (About 2 in 1,000) 684
Mintezol 1747
Motrin Ibuprofen Suspension, Oral Drops, Chewable Tablets, Caplets (Less than 1%) 1563
Mycobutin Capsules (More than one patient) 2101
Nardil (Less frequent) 1977
Nebcin Vials, Hyporets & ADD-Vantage 1518
NegGram (Rare) 2453
Neoral (1% to 5%) 2405
Neptazane Tablets ⊙ 320
Nescaine/Nescaine MPF 549
Netromycin Injection 100 mg/ml 2516
Neurontin Capsules (More than 1%) 1978
Neutrexin for Injection (Rare; less than 1%) 2761
Nipent for Injection (Less than 3%) 2733
Noroxin Tablets 1758
Noroxin Tablets 2222
Norvir (Less than 2%) 447
Novahistine DMX ▣ 782
Novahistine Elixir ▣ 782
Novocain Hydrochloride for Spinal Anesthesia 2457
Nydrazid Injection (Uncommon) 509
OmniHIB (Two definite and 3 possible out of 5,000 infants) 2676
▲ Oncaspar (Greater than 1% but less than 5%) 2194
Oncovin Solution Vials & Hyporets (A few patients) 1521
Ornade Spansule Capsules 2678
PBZ Tablets 863
PBZ-SR Tablets 862
Paxil Tablets (0.1%; infrequent) 2681
Pediapred Oral Solution 1618
Pediazole Suspension 2340
Penetrex Tablets (0.1% to 1%) 2196
Periactin 1767
Permax Tablets (Infrequent) 571
Pfizerpen for Injection 2022
Phenergan with Codeine 2883
Phenergan VC with Codeine 2888
Phrenilin (Infrequent) 790
Placidyl Capsules 456
Plaquenil Sulfate Tablets 2459
Pontocaine Hydrochloride for Spinal Anesthesia 2460
Prelone Syrup 1834
▲ Prograf (Greater than 3%) 1028
Propulsid (Rare) 1346
Prostigmin Injectable 1305
Prostigmin Tablets 1306
Prozac Pulvules & Liquid, Oral Solution (Infrequent) 935
Quinaglute Dura-Tabs Tablets 644
Quinidex Extentabs 2240
Redux Capsules 2911
Rifamate Capsules (Uncommon) 1278
Rifater (Uncommon) 1280
Rilutek Tablets (Infrequent) 2198
Romazicon 2311
Rondec Oral Drops 974
Rondec Syrup 974
Rondec 974
▲ Sandimmune (1 to 5%) 2416
Sandostatin Injection (Less than 1%) 2421
Sedapap Tablets 50 mg/650 mg (Infrequent) 1826
Seldane-D Extended-Release Tablets 1286
Sensorcaine (0.1%) 554
Septra 1146
Septra I.V. Infusion 1142
Septra I.V. Infusion ADD-Vantage Vials 1144
Septra 1146
Seromycin Capsules 975
Sinemet Tablets 959
Sinemet CR Tablets 961
Slo-bid Gyrocaps 2201
Stadol (Less than 1%) 779
Stelazine 2692
Supprelin Injection (2%) 2230
Symmetrel Capsules (Less than 0.1%) 965
Symmetrel Syrup (Less than 0.1%) 963
Syn-Rx Tablets 1622
Syn-Rx DM Tablets 1623
Tambocor Tablets (Less than 1%) 1555
Tavist Syrup 2426
Tavist Tablets 2427
Tazicef for Injection 2697
Tensilon Injectable 1307
Tetramune (One child) 1449
THYREL TRH (Rare) 2992
Ticar for Injection (With very high doses) 2704
Tigan 2231
Timolide Tablets 1791
Tofranil Ampuls 873
Tofranil Tablets 875
Tonocard Tablets (Less than 1%) 519
Toradol 2319
Torecan 2367
Tracrium Injection (Rare) 1155
Trental Tablets (Less than 1%) 1291
Tri-Immunol Adsorbed (1 per 1,750) 1452
Trinalin Repetabs Tablets 1373
Tussend 1830
Tussend Expectorant 1831
Ultram Tablets (50 mg) 1594
Urecholine 1804
Vantin for Oral Suspension and Vantin Tablets 2112
Velban Vials 1537
Vermox Chewable Tablets (Very rare) 1357
▲ Vesanoid Capsules (3%) 2327
Videx Tablets, Powder for Oral Solution, & Pediatric Powder for Oral Solution (2% to 4%) 2980
Virazole 1310
Vistaril Capsules (Rare) 2042
Vistaril Intramuscular Solution (Rare) 2042
Vistaril Oral Suspension (Rare) 2042
Vistide Injection 1057
Cataflam/Voltaren/Voltaren-XR (Rare) 833
▲ Xylocaine Injections (Among most common) 562
Zestoretic Tablets 2968
Zoloft Tablets (Rare) 2051
Zosyn (1.0% or less) 1463
Zovirax Sterile Powder 1191

Convulsions, clonic

Cocaine Hydrochloride Topical Solutions 529
Lufyllin & Lufyllin-400 Tablets 2778
Lufyllin-GG Elixir & Tablets 2779
M-M-R II (Rare) 1730
Quadrinal Tablets 1398
Quibron 2227
Respbid Tablets 687
Seromycin Capsules 975
Slo-bid Gyrocaps 2201
Theo-X Extended-Release Tablets 793
Uniphyl 400 mg and 600 mg Tablets (A few isolated reports) 2157

Convulsions, grand mal

Compazine 2644
Lamictal Tablets (Rare) 1105
Levoprome 1321
Norvir (Less than 2%) 447
Paxil Tablets (Rare) 2681
Redux Capsules 2911
Remeron Tablets (Rare) 1878
Stelazine 2692
Triavil Tablets 1800
Videx Tablets, Powder for Oral Solution, & Pediatric Powder for Oral Solution (Less than 1%) 2980

Convulsions, major

Seromycin Capsules 975

Convulsions, tonic generalized

Cocaine Hydrochloride Topical Solutions 529
Lufyllin & Lufyllin-400 Tablets 2778
Lufyllin-GG Elixir & Tablets 2779
Quadrinal Tablets 1398
Quibron 2227
Respbid Tablets 687
Slo-bid Gyrocaps 2201
Theo-X Extended-Release Tablets 793
Uniphyl 400 mg and 600 mg Tablets (A few isolated reports) 2157

Coombs' test, positive

Adalat CC 582
Aldoclor Tablets 1638
Aldomet Ester HCl Injection 1642
Aldomet Oral 1640
Aldoril Tablets 1644
Atamet Tablets 567
Azactam for Injection 736
Catapres Tablets 679
Ceclor Pulvules & Suspension (Less than 1 in 200) 1470
Cefizox for Intramuscular or Intravenous Use (1% to 5%) 1025
Cefobid Intravenous/Intramuscular (1 in 60) 1996
Cefobid Pharmacy Bulk Package - Not for Direct Infusion (1 in 60) 1999
Cefotan (1 in 250) 2936
Ceftin (0.1% to 1%) 1067
Cefzil Tablets and Oral Suspension 747
Ceptaz (One in 23) 1070
Claforan Sterile and Injection (Less than 1%) 1259
Combipres Tablets 682
Duricef Capsules, Tablets, and Oral Suspension 750
▲ Fortaz (1 in 23) 1092
IBU Tablets (Sometimes) 1389
Keflex Pulvules & Oral Suspension 930
Kefurox Vials, Faspak & ADD-Vantage (Less than 1 in 250) 1509
Kefzol Vials, Faspak & ADD-Vantage 1511
Larodopa Tablets 2296
Lorabid Suspension and Pulvules 1513
Mandol Vials, Faspak & ADD-Vantage 1516
▲ Maxipime for Injection (16.2%) 758
Mefoxin 1734
Mefoxin Premixed Intravenous Solution 1737
Merrem I.V. (Greater than 0.2%) 2952
Mezlin 594
Mezlin Pharmacy Bulk Package 597
Monocid Injection (Less than 1%) 2674
Motrin Ibuprofen Suspension, Oral Drops, Chewable Tablets, Caplets (Sometimes) 1563
PASER Granules 1333
Pipracil (Less frequent) 1435
Platinol for Injection 717
Platinol-AQ Injection 719
Ponstel 1982
Primaxin I.M. 1770
Primaxin I.V. 1772
Procardia Capsules 2024
Procardia XL Extended Release Tablets 2026
Rilutek Tablets (Infrequent) 2198
Roferon-A Injection (Rare) 2308
Sinemet Tablets 959
Sinemet CR Tablets 961
Suprax 1443
▲ Tazicef for Injection (1 in 23 patients) 2697
▲ Tazidime Vials, Faspak & ADD-Vantage (1 in 23) 1531
Unasyn (Some individuals) 2035
Vantin for Oral Suspension and Vantin Tablets 2112
Zinacef (Fewer than 1 in 250 patients) 1184
Zosyn 1463

Coordination, disturbed (see under Coordination, impaired)

Coordination, impaired

Anafranil Capsules (Infrequent) 819
Atretol Tablets 569
Atrovent Inhalation Aerosol (Less frequent) 674
▲ Benadryl Injection (Among most frequent) 1955
Cataflam Tablets (Rare) 833
Clozaril Tablets (Less than 1%) 2377
▲ Cordarone Tablets (4 to 9%) 2818
Dilantin Infatabs 1967
▲ Dilantin Kapseals (Among most common) 1965
Dilantin-125 Suspension 1969
Dimetane-DX Cough Syrup 2233
Duragesic Transdermal System (1% or greater) 1336
Ethmozine Tablets (Less than 2%) 2217
Foscavir Injection (Between 1% and 5%) 541
▲ Halcion Tablets (4.6%) 2093
Helidac Therapy 2135
Hivid Tablets (Less than 1%) 2287
Intron A for Injection (Less than 5%) 2506
Iopidine 0.5% (Less than 1%) ⊙ 219
Ismo Tablets (Fewer than 1%) 2844
Lioresal Intrathecal (1% or more) 1634
Lioresal Tablets 847
Lithium Carbonate Capsules & Tablets 2352
Marinol (Dronabinol) Capsules 2353
▲ Mexitil Capsules (9.4% to 10.2%) 684
Naprelan Tablets (Less than 1%) 2861
Neurontin Capsules (1.1%) 1978

(▣ Described in PDR For Nonprescription Drugs) Incidence data in parenthesis; ▲ 3% or more (⊙ Described in PDR For Ophthalmology)

Coordination, impaired

- Nicotrol NS Nicotine Nasal Spray (Under 5%) ... 1565
- Ornade Spansule Capsules ... 2678
- ▲ PBZ Tablets (Among most frequent) ... 863
- ▲ PBZ-SR Tablets (Among most frequent) ... 862
- Pamelor ... 2409
- Periactin ... 1767
- ▲ ProSom Tablets (4%) ... 457
- Remeron Tablets (Infrequent) ... 1878
- Rilutek Tablets (Infrequent) ... 2198
- Roferon-A Injection (Less than 0.5%) ... 2308
- ▲ Tavist Syrup (Among most frequent) ... 2426
- ▲ Tavist Tablets (Among most frequent) ... 2427
- Tegretol/Tegretol-XR ... 870
- Tofranil Ampuls ... 873
- Tofranil Tablets ... 875
- Tofranil-PM Capsules ... 876
- Tonocard Tablets (Up to 1.2%) ... 519
- Triavil Tablets ... 1800
- ▲ Trinalin Repetabs Tablets (Among most frequent) ... 1373
- Ultram Tablets (50 mg) (1% to less than 5%) ... 1594
- Cataflam/Voltaren/Voltaren-XR (Rare) ... 833
- ▲ Xanax Tablets (40.1%) ... 2115
- Zoloft Tablets (Infrequent) ... 2051
- Zyrtec Tablets (Less than 2%) ... 2053

Coordination, lack of
(see under Ataxia)

Coordination difficulty
(see under Coordination, impaired)

Cor pulmonale
- Pulmozyme Inhalation ... 1054

Cornea, discoloration
- Mellaril ... 2398
- Serentil ... 689
- Torecan ... 2367
- Xalatan ... ⊚ 304

Cornea, fungal infections
- AK-CIDE ... ⊚ 203
- AK-CIDE Ointment ... ⊚ 203
- AK-PRED ... ⊚ 204
- AK-Trol Ointment & Suspension .. ⊚ 205
- Blephamide Ointment ... ⊚ 234
- NeoDecadron Sterile Ophthalmic Ointment ... 1755
- NeoDecadron Sterile Ophthalmic Solution ... 1756
- Polysporin Ophthalmic Ointment Sterile ... 1140
- Pred Forte ... ⊚ 247
- Pred Mild ... ⊚ 250
- Pred-G Liquifilm Sterile Ophthalmic Suspension ... ⊚ 248
- Terra-Cortril Ophthalmic Suspension ... 2033
- TobraDex Ophthalmic Suspension and Ointment ... 469

Cornea, gray, ground-glass appearance
- FLUORACAINE ... ⊚ 208
- FLURESS (Rare) ... ⊚ 208
- Ophthetic ... ⊚ 244

Cornea, opacities
- ▲ Accutane Capsules (5 of 72 patients) ... 2252
- FLUORACAINE ... ⊚ 208
- Imitrex Injection ... 1095
- Imitrex Tablets ... 1099
- Mellaril ... 2398
- Plaquenil Sulfate Tablets ... 2459
- Serentil ... 689
- Symmetrel Capsules (0.1% to 1%) ... 965
- Symmetrel Syrup (0.1% to 1%) ... 963
- Torecan ... 2367

Cornea, white crystalline precipitates, presence of
- ▲ Ciloxan Ophthalmic Solution (Approximately 17%) ... 468

Corneal abrasion
- Alomide Ophthalmic Solution (Less than 1%) ... 465
- Ocusert Pilo-20 and Pilo-40 Ocular Therapeutic Systems ... ⊚ 252

Corneal changes
- Alomide Ophthalmic Solution (Less than 1%) ... 465
- Aralen Phosphate Tablets ... 2431
- Azulfidine (Rare) ... 2059
- Cocaine Hydrochloride Topical Solutions ... 529
- Efudex (Infrequent) ... 2280
- Neurontin Capsules (Rare) ... 1978
- Nolvadex Tablets ... 2957
- Plaquenil Sulfate Tablets ... 2459
- Prozac Pulvules & Liquid, Oral Solution (Rare) ... 935
- ▲ Tegison Capsules (10-25%) ... 2314

Corneal clouding
- Carbastat Intraocular Solution (Occasional) ... ⊚ 260
- Chemet Capsules (1.0% to 3.7%) ... 666
- Cocaine Hydrochloride Topical Solutions ... 529
- Miochol-E with Iocare Steri-Tags and Miochol-E System Pak (Infrequent) ... ⊚ 263
- MIOSTAT Intraocular Solution ... ⊚ 222

Corneal curvature, steepening
- Brevicon ... 2563
- Climara Transdermal System ... 640
- Demulen ... 2580
- Desogen Tablets ... 1867
- Diethylstilbestrol Tablets ... 1477
- Estrace Cream and Tablets ... 751
- Estraderm Transdermal System ... 842
- ESTRATAB Tablets (0.3, 0.625, 1.25, 2.5 mg) ... 2715
- Estratest ... 2718
- Levlen/Tri-Levlen ... 646
- Lo/Ovral Tablets ... 2852
- Lo/Ovral-28 Tablets ... 2857
- Menest Tablets ... 2671
- Modicon ... 1928
- Nordette-21 Tablets ... 2863
- Nordette-28 Tablets ... 2866
- Norinyl ... 2563
- Nor-Q D Tablets ... 2598
- Ogen Tablets ... 2103
- Ogen Vaginal Cream ... 2106
- Ortho-Cept ... 1907
- Ortho-Cyclen/Ortho-Tri-Cyclen ... 1914
- Ortho Dienestrol Cream ... 1922
- Ortho-Est ... 1925
- Ortho-Novum ... 1928
- Ortho-Cyclen/Ortho Tri-Cyclen ... 1914
- Ovcon ... 765
- Ovral Tablets ... 2877
- Ovral-28 Tablets ... 2878
- Ovrette Tablets ... 2878
- PMB 200 and PMB 400 ... 2890
- Premarin Intravenous ... 2893
- Premarin Tablets ... 2896
- Premarin Vaginal Cream ... 2898
- Premphase ... 2900
- Prempro ... 2905
- Levlen/Tri-Levlen ... 646
- Tri-Norinyl ... 2607
- Triphasil-21 Tablets ... 2919
- Triphasil-28 Tablets ... 2924
- Vivelle Transdermal System ... 880

Corneal decompensation
- AMVISC Plus ... ⊚ 327
- Cytovene-IV (One report) ... 2270
- Healon (Rare) ... ⊚ 302
- Healon GV ... ⊚ 303
- Miochol-E with Iocare Steri-Tags and Miochol-E System Pak (Infrequent) ... ⊚ 263
- OcuCoat ... ⊚ 321

Corneal deposits
- AKPRO ... ⊚ 206
- Compazine ... 2644
- Cordarone Tablets ... 2818
- EPIFRIN ... ⊚ 237
- Etrafon ... 2495
- Indocin (Less than 1%) ... 1723
- Levoprome ... 1321
- Plaquenil Sulfate Tablets ... 2459
- Prolixin ... 510
- PROPINE with C CAP Compliance Cap ... ⊚ 251
- Ridaura Capsules (Less than 1%) ... 2691
- Solganal Suspension ... 2530
- Stelazine ... 2692
- Thorazine ... 2701
- Trilafon ... 2532

Corneal infiltrate
- Ciloxan Ophthalmic Solution (Less than 1%) ... 468

Iopidine 0.5% (Less than 3%) ... ⊚ 219
Vexol 1% Ophthalmic Suspension (Less than 1%) ... ⊚ 227

Corneal pitting
- Cocaine Hydrochloride Topical Solutions ... 529

Corneal punctate, defects
- Symmetrel Capsules (0.1% to 1%) ... 965
- Symmetrel Syrup (0.1% to 1%) ... 963

Corneal punctate keratitis
- Betoptic Ophthalmic Solution (Rare) ... 465
- Betoptic S Ophthalmic Suspension (Small number of patients) ... 467

Corneal punctate staining
- Betoptic Ophthalmic Solution (Rare) ... 465

Corneal sensitivity, decrease
- Betagan (A small number of patients) ... ⊚ 230
- Betimol 0.25%, 0.5% ... ⊚ 259
- Betoptic Ophthalmic Solution (Rare) ... 465
- Betoptic S Ophthalmic Suspension ... 467
- Plaquenil Sulfate Tablets ... 2459
- Timoptic in Ocudose (Less frequent) ... 1796
- Timoptic Sterile Ophthalmic Solution (Less frequent) ... 1794
- Timoptic-XE ... 1798

Corneal sensitivity, unspecified
- Ocupress Ophthalmic Solution, 1% Sterile (Occasional) ... ⊚ 297

Corneal staining
- Betimol 0.25%, 0.5% (1% to 5%) ... ⊚ 259
- Ciloxan Ophthalmic Solution (Less than 1%) ... 468
- Iopidine 0.5% (Less than 3%) ... ⊚ 219
- Ocupress Ophthalmic Solution, 1% Sterile (Occasional) ... ⊚ 297
- Paremyd ... ⊚ 244
- Vexol 1% Ophthalmic Suspension (Less than 1%) ... ⊚ 227

Corneal toxicity
- Cytosar-U Sterile Powder (With experimental doses) ... 2077

Corneal ulceration
- Alomide Ophthalmic Solution (Less than 1%) ... 465
- Ambien Tablets (Rare) ... 2559
- BOTOX (Botulinum Toxin Type A) Purified Neurotoxin Complex ... 473
- Cocaine Hydrochloride Topical Solutions ... 529
- Econopred & Econopred Plus Ophthalmic Suspensions (Occasional) ... ⊚ 216
- Gentak ... ⊚ 209
- Paxil Tablets (Rare) ... 2681
- Pred Forte (Occasional) ... ⊚ 247
- Pred Mild (Occasional) ... ⊚ 250
- Vexol 1% Ophthalmic Suspension (Less than 1%) ... ⊚ 227

Coronary artery disease, aggravation
- Atretol Tablets ... 569
- Oncovin Solution Vials & Hyporets ... 1521
- Tegretol/Tegretol-XR ... 870
- Tenoretic Tablets ... 2963
- Vasotec I.V. (One case) ... 1814

Coronary artery disease, unspecified
- LUVOX Tablets (Rare) ... 2723
- Naprelan Tablets (Less than 1%) ... 2861

Coronary thrombosis
- Demulen ... 2580
- Lo/Ovral Tablets ... 2852
- Lo/Ovral-28 Tablets ... 2857
- Modicon ... 1928
- Nordette-21 Tablets ... 2863
- Nordette-28 Tablets ... 2866
- Ortho-Novum ... 1928
- Ovral Tablets ... 2877
- Ovral-28 Tablets ... 2878
- Ovrette Tablets ... 2878
- Triphasil-21 Tablets ... 2919
- Triphasil-28 Tablets ... 2924

Cortical lens opacities, scattered punctate
- Atretol Tablets ... 569
- Tegretol/Tegretol-XR ... 870

Cortical proliferation of long bones
- Aquasol A Vitamin A Capsules, USP ... 525

Coryza
- Quadrinal Tablets ... 1398

Costochondritis
- Neurontin Capsules (Rare) ... 1978

Costovertebral pain
- Benemid Tablets ... 1651
- ColBENEMID Tablets ... 1662

Cough
- ▲ Accupril Tablets (2.0% to 4.3%) .. 1950
- ▲ ActHIB (4.3% to 9.6%) ... 893
- ▲ Actigall Capsules (7.1%) ... 818
- ▲ Adalat Capsules (10 mg and 20 mg) (6%) ... 580
- Adalat CC (Less than 1.0%) ... 582
- Adenoscan (Less than 1%) ... 1022
- AeroBid Inhaler System (3% to 9%) ... 1004
- Aerobid-M Inhaler System (3% to 9%) ... 1004
- ▲ Airet Albuterol Sulfate Inhalation Solution (3.1% to 4%) ... 1602
- ▲ Albuterol Sulfate, USP Solution for Inhalation, Arm-a-Med (3.1% to 4%) ... 522
- Alferon N Injection (One patient to 1%) ... 2142
- Alkeran for Injection ... 1196
- Alkeran Tablets ... 1198
- ▲ Altace Capsules (7.6% to almost 12%) ... 1238
- Alupent (1% to 4%) ... 672
- Ambien Tablets (Infrequent) ... 2559
- ▲ Anafranil Capsules (4% to 6%) ... 819
- Antivenin (Crotalidae) Polyvalent ... 2803
- ▲ Aredia for Injection (15.9%) ... 827
- ▲ Arimidex Tablets (7.3% to 8.4%) .. 2932
- Asacol Delayed-Release Tablets (1% to 2%) ... 2129
- ▲ Atrovent Inhalation Aerosol (5.9%) ... 674
- ▲ Atrovent Inhalation Solution (4.6%) ... 675
- Atrovent Nasal Spray 0.03% (Less than 2%) ... 676
- Atrovent Nasal Spray 0.06% (Less than 1%) ... 678
- Axid Pulvules (2.0%) ... 1468
- Azmacort Oral Inhaler ... 2175
- Bactroban Nasal (2%) ... 2643
- Blocadren Tablets ... 1654
- Capoten Tablets (0.5 to 2%) ... 740
- Capozide Tablets (0.5 to 2%) ... 744
- Cardura Tablets (Less than 0.5% of 3960 patients) ... 1993
- Cartrol Tablets (Less common) ... 413
- Casodex Tablets (2% to 5%) ... 2934
- Caverject Injection (1%) ... 2064
- Ceftin for Oral Suspension (0.1% to 1%) ... 1067
- ▲ CellCept Capsules (13.3% to 15.5%) ... 2265
- Cerebyx Injection (Infrequent) ... 1956
- Chemet Capsules (0.7% to 3.7%) ... 666
- Claritin Tablets (2% or fewer patients) ... 2485
- Claritin-D Tablets (Less frequent) .. 2487
- Clozaril Tablets (Less than 1%) ... 2377
- ▲ Cognex Capsules (3%) ... 1961
- Cordarone Tablets (2% to 7%) ... 2818
- ▲ Cozaar Tablets (3.4%) ... 1668
- Crixivan Capsules (Less than 2%) .. 1670
- Cytovene (1% or less) ... 2270
- DDAVP ... 2180
- ▲ DaunoXome (2% to 26%) ... 1842
- Demadex Tablets and Injection (2.0%) ... 691
- Depakote Tablets (1% to 5%) ... 418
- Depen Titratable Tablets ... 2770
- Desmopressin Acetate Rhinal Tube ... 997
- Dexacort Phosphate in Respihaler ... 1606
- ▲ Dilacor XR Extended-release Capsules (2.2% to 3.0%) ... 2183
- Diprivan Injectable Emulsion (Less than 1%) ... 2939
- Dizac (diazepam injectable emulsion) CIV ... 1862
- Dopram Injectable ... 2235
- Doxil (Less than 1%) ... 2613
- Dynabac (1.5%) ... 668
- DynaCirc Capsules (0.5% to 1%) .. 2381
- DynaCirc CR Tablets (0.5% to 1.0%) ... 2383

1295 **Side Effects Index** **Cramping, muscular**

Effexor ... 2825
▲ Epivir (18%) ... 1200
▲ Epogen for Injection (18%) ... 489
Ergamisol Tablets (1 out of 463 patients) ... 1340
Ethmozine Tablets (Less than 2%) 2217
Etopophos for Injection (Sometimes) ... 701
Etoposide Injection (Sometimes) ... 539
▲ Felbatol (6.5%) ... 2774
▲ Flolan for Injection (38%) ... 1085
Floxin I.V. (Less than 1%) ... 1580
Floxin Tablets (200 mg, 300 mg, 400 mg) (Less than 1%) ... 1577
▲ Fludara for Injection (10% to 44%) ... 658
Flumadine Tablets & Syrup (Less than 0.3%) ... 1013
▲ Foscavir Injection (5% or greater) .. 541
Gantrisin ... 2286
Gemzar for Injection (Common) ... 1482
▲ Habitrol Nicotine Transdermal System (3% to 9% of patients) .. 884
Hespan Injection ... 945
Hivid Tablets (Less than 1%) ... 2287
▲ Hylorel Tablets (26.9%) ... 1613
Hyperstat I.V. Injection ... 2504
Hyskon Hysteroscopy Fluid (Rare) .. 1633
Hytrin Capsules (At least 1%) ... 434
Hyzaar Tablets (2.6%) ... 1720
Imdur (Less than or equal to 5%) .. 1362
Imitrex Tablets (Infrequent) ... 1099
▲ Intal Inhaler (Among most frequent) ... 2185
Intal Nebulizer Solution (Rare; occasional) ... 2186
▲ Intron A for Injection (Up to 31%) 2506
Invirase Capsules (Less than 2%) .. 2291
Kerlone Tablets (Less than 2%) ... 2588
▲ Lamictal Tablets (7.5%) ... 1105
Lescol Capsules (2.4%) ... 2395
Leukeran Tablets ... 1205
▲ Leustatin (7% to 10%) ... 1889
Levatol Tablets (2.1%) ... 2547
Livostin (Approximately 1% to 3%) ... ⊙ 262
▲ Lopid Tablets (More common) ... 1974
Lotensin Tablets (1.2%) ... 852
Lotensin HCT Tablets (2.1%) ... 855
▲ Lotrel Capsules (3.3%) ... 858
Lupron Injection (Less than 5%) ... 2736
LUVOX Tablets (Frequent) ... 2723
Macrobid Capsules (Common) ... 2138
Macrodantin Capsules (Common) .. 2140
Marinol (Dronabinol) Capsules (Less than 1%) ... 2353
Matulane Capsules ... 2300
Mavik Tablets (0.3% to 2%) ... 1407
Maxair Autohaler (1.2%) ... 1550
Maxair Inhaler (1.2%) ... 1552
Maxaquin Tablets (Less than 1%) .. 2593
Megace Oral Suspension (1% to 3%) ... 708
Methotrexate Sodium Tablets, Injection, for Injection and LPF Injection (Less common) ... 1322
Miacalcin Nasal Spray (Less than 1%) ... 2403
Midamor Tablets (Between 1% and 3%) ... 1746
Moduretic Tablets ... 1748
Monoket Tablets (Less than 1% to 4%) ... 2550
▲ Monopril Tablets (2.2% to 9.7%) .. 762
Mumpsvax ... 1751
Mykrox Tablets (Less than 2%) ... 1617
Naprelan Tablets (Less than 3%) . 2861
Nasacort AQ Nasal Spray (2.1%) .. 2191
Nasalcrom Nasal Solution ... 2192
Nasarel Nasal Solution (Greater than 1%) ... 2302
▲ Neupogen for Injection (6%) ... 495
Neurontin Capsules (1.8%) ... 1978
Nicotrol NS Nicotine Nasal Spray (Common) ... 1565
▲ Nipent for Injection (17% to 20%) ... 2733
▲ Nolvadex Tablets (3.8%) ... 2957
Norvasc Tablets (Less than or equal to 0.1%) ... 2020
Norvir (Less than 2%) ... 447
▲ Novantrone for Injection (9 to 13%) ... 1327
▲ OmniHIB (4.3% to 9.6%) ... 2676
Oncaspar (Less than 1%) ... 2194
OptiPranolol (Metipranolol 0.3%) Sterile Ophthalmic Solution (A small number of patients) ... ⊙ 256
Orlaam Oral Solution (1% to 3%) .. 2361
OxyContin Tablets (Less than 1%) 2163
Pandel Cream, 0.1% (1 of 226 patients) ... 2475
Paxil Tablets (Frequent) ... 2681
Pediazole Suspension ... 2340
Penetrex Tablets (0.1% to 1%) ... 2196
Plendil Extended-Release Tablets (0.8% to 1.7%) ... 514
Pravachol Tablets (0.1% to 2.6%) 770
Prevacid Delayed-Release Capsules (Less than 1%) ... 2746
Prilosec Delayed-Release Capsules (1.1%) ... 516
Prinivil Tablets (1% to 3.5%) ... 1776
▲ Prinzide Tablets (3.9%) ... 1780
▲ Procardia Capsules (6%) ... 2024
▲ Procardia XL Extended Release Tablets (1% or less to 6%) ... 2026
▲ Procrit for Injection (18%) ... 1896
▲ Prograf (Greater than 3%) ... 1028
Propulsid (1.5%) ... 1346
ProSom Tablets (Infrequent) ... 457
Prostin E2 Suppository ... 2109
▲ Proventil Inhalation Solution 0.083% (3.1% to 4%) ... 2527
▲ Proventil Solution for Inhalation 0.5% (3.1% to 4%) ... 2525
Proventil Syrup (Less than 1 of 100 patients) ... 2528
Prozac Pulvules & Liquid, Oral Solution (1.6% to 3%) ... 935
Pulmozyme Inhalation ... 1054
Quadrinal Tablets ... 1398
Recombivax HB (Less than 1%) ... 1787
▲ Redux Capsules (3.6%) ... 2911
Relafen Tablets (Less than 1%) ... 2688
Remeron Tablets (Frequent) ... 1878
RespiGam (Infrequent) ... 1631
Retrovir Capsules ... 1216
Retrovir I.V. Infusion ... 1221
Retrovir Syrup ... 1216
ReVia Tablets (Less than 1%) ... 957
▲ Rhinocort Nasal Inhaler (3 to 9%) .. 552
Rifater ... 1280
Rilutek Tablets (2.1% to 3.7%) ... 2198
▲ Risperdal Tablets (3%) ... 1348
▲ Roferon-A Injection (16% to 27%) 2308
Sectral Capsules (1%) ... 2914
Seldane Tablets (0.9% to 2.5%) ... 1284
Seldane-D Extended-Release Tablets (1.6%) ... 1286
Semprex-D Capsules (2%) ... 1620
Septra (Rare) ... 1146
Septra I.V. Infusion ... 1142
Septra I.V. Infusion ADD-Vantage Vials ... 1144
Septra (Rare) ... 1146
▲ Serevent Inhalation Aerosol (7%) .. 1149
▲ Serzone Tablets (3%) ... 776
Sinemet CR Tablets ... 961
Stadol (1% or greater) ... 779
Stimate, (desmopressin acetate) Nasal Spray, 1.5 mg/mL ... 806
Sular Tablets (Less than or equal to 1%) ... 2961
▲ Supprelin Injection (3% to 10%) ... 2230
▲ Suprane (desflurane, USP) (34% to 72%) ... 1865
Tegison Capsules (Less than 1%) .. 2314
TheraCys BCG Live (Intravesical) (Rare) ... 911
Tiazac Capsules (1%) ... 1019
TICE BCG, USP ... 1881
▲ Tilade Inhaler (7.0%) ... 2207
Timolide Tablets ... 1791
Timoptic in Ocudose (Less frequent) ... 1796
Timoptic Sterile Ophthalmic Solution (Less frequent) ... 1794
Timoptic-XE ... 1798
Toradol (1% or less) ... 2319
Tornalate Solution for Inhalation, 0.2% (2.5%) ... 976
▲ Tornalate Metered Dose Inhaler (4% to 4.1%) ... 978
▲ Univasc Tablets (6.1%) ... 2553
Valium Injectable ... 2336
▲ Vancenase AQ Double Strength Nasal Spray 0.084% (6%) ... 2536
Vantin for Oral Suspension and Vantin Tablets (Less than 1%) ... 2112
Vaqta (1.0%) ... 1805
Varivax (Greater than or equal to 1%) ... 1807
Vascor Tablets (200 and 300 mg) (0.5 to 2.0%) ... 1597
▲ Vaseretic Tablets (3.5%) ... 1810
Vasotec I.V. ... 1814
Vasotec Tablets (1.3% to 2.2%) ... 1816
Ventolin Inhalation Aerosol and Refill (2%) ... 1170
▲ Ventolin Inhalation Solution (3.1% to 4%) ... 1171
▲ Ventolin Nebules Inhalation Solution (3.1% to 4%) ... 1172
▲ Ventolin Rotacaps for Inhalation (2% to 5%) ... 1173
Ventolin Syrup (Less than 1 of 100 patients) ... 1175
VePesid Capsules and Injection (Sometimes) ... 727
Versed Injection (1.3%) ... 2324
▲ Videx Tablets, Powder for Oral Solution, & Pediatric Powder for Oral Solution (1% to 85%) ... 2980
Vistide Injection ... 1057
Zebeta Tablets (2.5% to 2.6%) ... 1457
▲ Zestoretic Tablets (3.9%) ... 2968
Zestril Tablets (Greater than 1% to 3.5%) ... 2972
Ziac (1.5% to 2.2%) ... 1459
Zoladex (1% or greater) ... 2976
Zoladex 3-month (1% to 5%) ... 2978
Zoloft Tablets (Infrequent) ... 2051
Zosyn (1.0% or less) ... 1463
Zyrtec Tablets (Less than 2%) ... 2053

Cough, productive

Permax Tablets (Frequent) ... 571

Cough reflex, depression

Astramorph/PF Injection, USP (Preservative-Free) ... 526
Compazine ... 2644
Duramorph Injection ... 983
Infumorph 200 and Infumorph 500 Sterile Solutions ... 985
Kadian Capsules (Less than 3%) ... 2948
Lorcet 10/650 Tablets ... 1016
Stelazine ... 2692
Thorazine ... 2701

Cramping

Adalat Capsules (10 mg and 20 mg) (2% or less) ... 580
Aldactazide Tablets ... 2556
Aldactone Tablets ... 2558
Aldoclor Tablets ... 1638
Aldoril Tablets ... 1644
Alferon N Injection (One patient) ... 2142
Aminohippurate Sodium Injection .. 1646
Capozide Tablets ... 744
Clinoril Tablets (Greater than 1%) 1658
Combipres Tablets ... 682
Coumadin (Infrequent) ... 941
Cytotec (0.6%) ... 2576
Dilaudid Tablets and Liquid ... 1386
Diucardin Tablets ... 2824
Diupres Tablets ... 1691
Diuril Oral Suspension ... 1694
Diuril Sodium Intravenous ... 1693
Diuril Tablets ... 1694
Enduron Tablets ... 424
Esidrix Tablets ... 839
Esimil Tablets ... 840
Sterile FUDR ... 2284
HydroDIURIL Tablets ... 1716
Hydropres Tablets ... 1718
Hyzaar Tablets ... 1720
Inderide Tablets ... 2838
Inderide LA Long Acting Capsules .. 2840
Lopressor HCT Tablets ... 850
Lotensin HCT Tablets ... 855
Moduretic Tablets ... 1748
Monistat Dual-Pak (2%) ... 1906
Monistat 3 Vaginal Suppositories (2%) ... 1905
Mycelex-G 500 mg Vaginal Tablets (Rare) ... 602
Neoral (Up to 2%) ... 2405
Oramorph SR (Morphine Sulfate Sustained Release Tablets) (Less frequent) ... 2359
Oretic Tablets ... 450
ParaGard T 380A Intrauterine Copper Contraceptive ... 1936
Prinzide Tablets ... 1780
Rifamate Capsules ... 1278
▲ Sandimmune (Up to 4%) ... 2416
Scleromate Injection ... 1234
Serzone Tablets ... 776
Tenoretic Tablets ... 2963
Thalitone ... 1293
▲ THROMBATE III Antithrombin III (Human) (2 of 17) ... 631
Timolide Tablets ... 1791
Vaseretic Tablets ... 1810
Zarontin Capsules (Frequent) ... 1986
Zarontin Syrup (Frequent) ... 1986
Zestoretic Tablets (0.3 to 1%) ... 2968
Ziac ... 1459

Cramping, abdominal (see under Abdominal pain/cramps)

Cramping, muscular

▲ Adalat Capsules (10 mg and 20 mg) (2% or less to 8%) ... 580
Adalat CC (Rare) ... 582
Alferon N Injection (1%) ... 2142
Apresazide Capsules (Less frequent) ... 824
Apresoline Hydrochloride Tablets (Less frequent) ... 826
Asacol Delayed-Release Tablets ... 2129
Atamet Tablets ... 567
Atromid-S Capsules (Less often) ... 2808
Brethine Ampuls (Less than 0.5%) 832
Brethine Tablets ... 831
Bricanyl Subcutaneous Injection ... 1247
Bricanyl Tablets ... 1248
Bumex (1.1%) ... 2260
BuSpar Tablets (Infrequent) ... 738
Calan SR Caplets (1% or less) ... 2571
Calan Tablets (1% or less) ... 2568
Capozide Tablets ... 744
Cardizem CD Capsules (Less than 1%) ... 1251
Cardizem SR Capsules (Less than 1%) ... 1255
Cardizem Injectable ... 1253
Cardizem Tablets (Less than 1%) .. 1257
Cardura Tablets (1%) ... 1993
Cartrol Tablets (2.6%) ... 413
Ceftin (0.1% to 1%) ... 1067
Covera-HS Tablets (Less than 2%) 2573
Cozaar Tablets (1.1%) ... 1668
Crixivan Capsules (Less than 2%) . 1670
▲ CytoGam (Less than 5.0%) ... 1630
Cytotec (Infrequent) ... 2576
Dalgan Injection (Less than 1%) ... 529
Danocrine Capsules ... 2437
Demadex Tablets and Injection ... 691
Dipentum Capsules (Rare) ... 2084
Diucardin Tablets ... 2824
Diuril Sodium Intravenous ... 1693
Dolobid Tablets (Rare) ... 1695
Dyazide Capsules ... 2653
Eldepryl Capsules ... 2729
Esidrix Tablets ... 839
Hivid Tablets (Less than 1%) ... 2287
Hydralazine Hydrochloride Injection USP (Less frequent) ... 2712
Hyzaar Tablets ... 1720
Imitrex Injection (1.1%) ... 1095
Imitrex Tablets (Infrequent) ... 1099
Invirase Capsules (Less than 2%) .. 2291
Isoptin Oral Tablets (Less than 1%) ... 1393
Isoptin SR Tablets (1% or less) ... 1395
K-Phos Neutral Tablets ... 633
K-Phos Original Formula 'Sodium Free' Tablets (Less frequent) ... 633
Kerlone Tablets (Less than 2%) ... 2588
Lasix Injection, Oral Solution and Tablets ... 1267
Lescol Capsules ... 2395
Lotrel Capsules ... 858
Mavik Tablets (0.3% to 1.0%) ... 1407
Mestinon Injectable ... 1300
Mestinon ... 1300
Mevacor Tablets (0.6% to 1.1%) .. 1742
Midamor Tablets (Between 1% and 3%) ... 1746
Moduretic Tablets (Less than or equal to 1%) ... 1748
Monoket Tablets (Fewer than 1%) 2550
Monopril Tablets (0.2% to 1.0% or more) ... 762
▲ Mykrox Tablets (5.8%) ... 1617
Nimotop Capsules (Up to 1.4%) ... 603
Normodyne Tablets (Less common) ... 2522
Norvasc Tablets (Less than 1% to 2%) ... 2020
Norvir (Less than 2%) ... 447
Oncaspar ... 2194
Parlodel (Less than 1%) ... 2411
Pepcid Injection (Infrequent) ... 1765
Pepcid (Infrequent) ... 1763
Platinol for Injection ... 717
Platinol-AQ Injection ... 719
Plendil Extended-Release Tablets (0.5% to 1.5%) ... 514
Prilosec Delayed-Release Capsules (Less than 1%) ... 516
Prinivil Tablets (Greater than 1%) .. 1776
Prinzide Tablets (2%) ... 1780
▲ Procardia Capsules (2% or less to 8%) ... 2024
▲ Procardia XL Extended Release Tablets (8%) ... 2026

(Described in PDR For Nonprescription Drugs) Incidence data in parenthesis; ▲ 3% or more (⊙ Described in PDR For Ophthalmology)

Cramping, muscular / Side Effects Index

Cramping, muscular (continued)

- Prostigmin Injectable ... 1305
- Prostigmin Tablets ... 1306
- Prostin E2 Suppository ... 2109
- ▲ Proventil (3%) ... 2529
- Rythmol Tablets–150mg, 225mg, 300mg (Less than 1%) ... 1399
- Ser-Ap-Es Tablets ... 867
- Serevent Inhalation Aerosol (1% to 3%) ... 1149
- Sinemet Tablets ... 959
- Sinemet CR Tablets (0.8%) ... 961
- ▲ Supprelin Injection (3% to 10%) ... 2230
- ▲ Tegison Capsules (25-50%) ... 2314
- Tenoretic Tablets ... 2963
- Thalitone (Common) ... 1293
- Tiazac Capsules (Less than 1%) ... 1019
- Tigan ... 2231
- Timolide Tablets ... 1791
- Tonocard Tablets (Less than 1%) ... 519
- Trandate Tablets (Less common) ... 1158
- Uroqid-Acid No. 2 Tablets ... 633
- Vaseretic Tablets (2.7%) ... 1810
- Vasotec I.V. ... 1814
- Vasotec Tablets (0.5% to 1.0%) ... 1816
- Ventolin Inhalation Aerosol and Refill (1%) ... 1170
- Ventolin Syrup (1%) ... 1175
- ▲ Ventolin Tablets (3 of 100 patients) ... 1176
- Verelan Capsules (1% or less) ... 1455
- ▲ Visken Tablets (3%) ... 2428
- Volmax Extended-Release Tablets (2.7%) ... 1835
- Xanax Tablets (2.4%) ... 2115
- Zaroxolyn Tablets ... 1625
- Zebeta Tablets ... 1457
- Zestoretic Tablets (2.0%) ... 2968
- Zestril Tablets (0.5% to greater than 1%) ... 2972
- Ziac (1.1% to 1.2%) ... 1459
- Zocor Tablets ... 1821
- Zoloft Tablets (Infrequent) ... 2051

Cramps, abdominal
(see under Abdominal pain/cramps)

Cramps, lower limbs

- Adalat CC (3% or less) ... 582
- Ambien Tablets (Infrequent) ... 2559
- Anafranil Capsules (Infrequent) ... 819
- Atretol Tablets ... 569
- Betaseron for SC Injection ... 653
- Casodex Tablets (2% to 5%) ... 2934
- Catapres Tablets (About 3 in 1,000) ... 679
- Catapres-TTS ... 680
- Caverject Injection (Less than 1%) ... 2064
- ▲ CellCept Capsules (More than or equal to 3%) ... 2265
- Cerebyx Injection (Infrequent) ... 1956
- Claritin Tablets (2% or fewer patients) ... 2485
- Claritin-D Tablets (Less frequent) ... 2487
- Combipres Tablets (About 3 in 1,000) ... 682
- Depakote Tablets (1% to 5%) ... 418
- Depo-Provera Contraceptive Injection (1% to 5%) ... 2079
- Desferal Vials ... 838
- DynaCirc Capsules (0.5% to 1%) ... 2381
- DynaCirc CR Tablets (0.5% to 1.0%) ... 2383
- ▲ Emcyt Capsules (8%) ... 2085
- Foscavir Injection (Between 1% and 5%) ... 541
- Gammagard S/D, Immune Globulin, Intravenous (Human) (Occasional) ... 577
- Glucotrol XL Extended Release Tablets (Less than 3%) ... 2012
- Hivid Tablets (Less than 1%) ... 2287
- ▲ Hylorel Tablets (21.1% to 25.6%) ... 1613
- Intron A for Injection (Less than 5%) ... 2506
- Kerlone Tablets (Less than 2%) ... 2588
- Lamictal Tablets (Rare) ... 1105
- LUVOX Tablets ... 2723
- Maxaquin Tablets (Less than 1%) ... 2593
- Methergine (Rare) ... 2401
- 8-MOP Capsules ... 1294
- Naprelan Tablets (Less than 3%) ... 2861
- Oxsoralen-Ultra Capsules ... 1302
- Pentasa (Less than 1%) ... 1275
- Procardia XL Extended Release Tablets (Less than 3%) ... 2026
- ▲ Prograf (Greater than 3%) ... 1028
- Redux Capsules (Infrequent) ... 2911
- Rilutek Tablets (Infrequent) ... 2198
- Risperdal Tablets (Rare) ... 1348
- Sansert Tablets ... 2424
- Sular Tablets (Less than or equal to 1%) ... 2961
- Tegretol/Tegretol-XR ... 870
- Tenex Tablets (3% or less) ... 2249
- Videx Tablets, Powder for Oral Solution, & Pediatric Powder for Oral Solution (Less than 1%) ... 2980
- Zoladex (2%) ... 2976
- Zoladex 3-month ... 2978
- Zyrtec Tablets (Less than 2%) ... 2053

Cramps, pelvic
- Cytotec (0.6%) ... 2576

Cranial nerve, dysfunction
- Garamycin Injectable ... 2502
- IFEX (Less frequent) ... 706
- JE-VAX (One case) ... 904
- Lescol Capsules ... 2395
- Oncovin Solution Vials & Hyporets (Rare) ... 1521
- Pravachol Tablets ... 770
- Velban Vials (Rare) ... 1537
- Zocor Tablets ... 1821

Cranial nerve deficit, fetal
- Accutane Capsules ... 2252

Cranial sensations, unspecified
- Methotrexate Sodium Tablets, Injection, for Injection and LPF Injection (Occasional) ... 1322

Craniofacial deformities
- Accupril Tablets ... 1950
- Altace Capsules ... 1238
- Capoten Tablets ... 740
- Capozide Tablets ... 744
- Cozaar Tablets ... 1668
- Hyzaar Tablets ... 1720
- Lotensin Tablets ... 852
- Lotensin HCT Tablets ... 855
- Lotrel Capsules ... 858
- Monopril Tablets ... 762
- Prinivil Tablets ... 1776
- Prinzide Tablets ... 1780
- Univasc Tablets ... 2553
- Vaseretic Tablets ... 1810
- Vasotec I.V. ... 1814
- Vasotec Tablets ... 1816
- Zestoretic Tablets ... 2968
- Zestril Tablets ... 2972

Creatinine, increase
(see under Serum creatinine, elevation)

Creatinine clearance, decrease
- Amikacin Sulfate Injection, USP ... 523
- Bumex (0.3%) ... 2260
- Cytovene (1% or less) ... 2270
- Disalcid ... 1549
- Eskalith ... 2658
- ▲ Foscavir Injection (5% or greater up to 27%) ... 541
- IBU Tablets (Less than 1%) ... 1389
- IFEX ... 706
- Kefurox Vials, Faspak & ADD-Vantage ... 1509
- Lithonate/Lithotabs/Lithobid ... 2721
- Macrobid Capsules ... 2138
- Macrodantin Capsules ... 2140
- Mandol Vials, Faspak & ADD-Vantage ... 1516
- Motrin Ibuprofen Suspension, Oral Drops, Chewable Tablets, Caplets (Less than 1%) ... 1563
- Netromycin Injection 100 mg/ml ... 2516
- Platinol for Injection ... 717
- Platinol-AQ Injection ... 719
- Proglycem ... 575
- Salflex Tablets ... 791
- ▲ Vistide Injection (8% to 53%) ... 1057
- Zinacef ... 1184

Creatine phosphokinase, increase
- Accutane Capsules (Some patients) ... 2252
- Adalat CC (Rare) ... 582
- Amicar Syrup, Tablets, and Injection ... 1312
- Atamet Tablets ... 567
- Atromid-S Capsules ... 2808
- Cardizem CD Capsules (Less than 1%) ... 1251
- Cardizem SR Capsules (Less than 1%) ... 1255
- Cardizem Injectable ... 1253
- Cardizem Tablets (Less than 1%) ... 1257
- Clozaril Tablets ... 2377
- Danocrine Capsules ... 2437
- Dynabac (1.2%) ... 668
- Felbatol (Rare) ... 2774
- Lopid Tablets ... 1974
- ▲ Mevacor Tablets (11%) ... 1742
- Nardil ... 1977
- Orap Tablets ... 1037
- Oxandrin ... 783
- Parlodel ... 2411
- Paxil Tablets (Rare) ... 2681
- Pravachol Tablets (Rare) ... 770
- Procardia Capsules (Rare) ... 2024
- Procardia XL Extended Release Tablets (Rare) ... 2026
- Prolixin ... 510
- Revex (nalmefene hydrochloride injection) (0.5%) ... 1863
- Sandostatin Injection (Less than 1%) ... 2421
- Sinemet Tablets ... 959
- Tegison Capsules ... 2314
- Tiazac Capsules (Less than 1%) ... 1019
- Winstrol Tablets (no incidence data in labeling) ... 2468
- Zocor Tablets ... 1821

Cretinism, fetal
- Tapazole Tablets ... 1361

Crohn's disease, exacerbation
- Proleukin for Injection (Two patients) ... 812

Crying
- ActHIB (Up to 1.6%) ... 893
- Ambien Tablets ... 2559
- Ativan Injection (1.3%) ... 2805
- Dalgan Injection (Less than 1%) ... 529
- Diphtheria and Tetanus Toxoids and Pertussis Vaccine Adsorbed (Infrequent) ... 2650
- Foscavir Injection (Less than 1%) ... 541
- HibTITER (38 of 1,118 vaccinations) ... 1423
- IPOL Poliovirus Vaccine Inactivated ... 903
- Nubain Injection (1% or less) ... 952
- OmniHIB (0.3% to 1.6%) ... 2676
- Recombivax HB (Greater than 1%) ... 1787
- Romazicon (1% to 3%) ... 2311
- Tetramune ... 1449
- Tri-Immunol Adsorbed ... 1452
- Tripedia ... 908

Cryptococcosis
- Cerebyx Injection (Infrequent) ... 1956
- Doxil (Less than 1%) ... 2613

Crystalluria
- Ancobon Capsules ... 2254
- Azulfidine (Rare) ... 2059
- Bactrim DS Tablets ... 2257
- Bactrim I.V. Infusion ... 2255
- Bactrim ... 2257
- Cipro I.V. (1% or less) ... 587
- Cipro I.V. Pharmacy Bulk Package (Less than 1%) ... 590
- Cipro Tablets (Rare) ... 584
- Clinoril Tablets (Less than 1 in 100) ... 1658
- Dantrium Capsules (Less frequent) ... 2131
- Demser Capsules (A few patients) ... 1690
- Diamox ... ⊙ 317
- Effexor (Rare) ... 2825
- Floxin I.V. ... 1580
- Floxin Tablets (200 mg, 300 mg, 400 mg) ... 1577
- Fludara for Injection ... 658
- GlaucTabs (Rare) ... ⊙ 209
- Maxaquin Tablets ... 2593
- Mintezol ... 1747
- Neptazane Tablets (Rare) ... ⊙ 320
- Noroxin Tablets ... 1758
- Noroxin Tablets ... 2222
- PASER Granules ... 1333
- Pediazole Suspension ... 2340
- Penetrex Tablets ... 2196
- Septra ... 1146
- Septra I.V. Infusion ... 1142
- Septra I.V. Infusion ADD-Vantage Vials ... 1144
- Septra ... 1146
- Urobiotic-250 Capsules ... 2038

Cushingoid state
(see under Cushing's syndrome)

Cushing's syndrome
- Aclovate ... 1061
- Beclovent Inhalation Aerosol and Refill ... 1063
- Beconase Inhalation Aerosol ... 1065
- Betaseron for SC Injection ... 653
- Celestone Soluspan Suspension ... 2484
- Cormax Ointment ... 1856
- Cormax Scalp Application ... 1857
- CORTENEMA ... 2713
- Cortone Acetate Sterile Suspension ... 1663
- Cortone Acetate Tablets ... 1664
- Cutivate Cream ... 1078
- Cutivate Ointment ... 1078
- ▲ Cytadren Tablets (2 out of 3) ... 837
- Dalalone D.P. Injectable ... 1009
- Decadron Elixir ... 1676
- Decadron Phosphate Injection ... 1680
- Decadron Phosphate with Xylocaine Injection, Sterile ... 1683
- Decadron Tablets ... 1678
- Decadron-LA Sterile Suspension ... 1687
- Dermatop Emollient Cream 0.1% ... 1264
- Dexacort Phosphate in Respihaler ... 1606
- Dexacort Phosphate in Turbinaire ... 1607
- Diprolene AF Cream 0.05% (Some patients) ... 2489
- Diprolene Lotion 0.05% (Some patients) ... 2491
- Diprolene Ointment 0.05% (Some patients) ... 2491
- Elocon Cream 0.1% ... 2492
- Florinef Acetate Tablets ... 506
- Hydeltrasol Injection, Sterile ... 1708
- Hydeltra-T.B.A. Sterile Suspension ... 1710
- Hydrocortone Acetate Sterile Suspension ... 1712
- Hydrocortone Phosphate Injection, Sterile ... 1713
- Hydrocortone Tablets ... 1715
- Nasalide Nasal Solution 0.025% (With excessive dose) ... 2301
- Neurontin Capsules (Rare) ... 1978
- Pediapred Oral Solution ... 1618
- Prelone Syrup ... 1834
- ProctoCream-HC 2.5% ... 2552
- Temovate Cream ... 1152
- Temovate E Emollient ... 1154
- Temovate Gel ... 1153
- Temovate Ointment ... 1152
- Temovate Scalp Application ... 1153
- Ultravate Cream 0.05% ... 2797
- Ultravate Ointment 0.05% ... 2798

Cutaneous tenderness
- 8-MOP Capsules ... 1294
- Oxsoralen-Ultra Capsules ... 1302

Cyanosis
- Abbokinase ... 403
- Abbokinase Open-Cath ... 405
- Americaine Anesthetic Lubricant ... 1603
- Americaine Otic Topical Anesthetic Ear Drops ... 1603
- Anafranil Capsules (Rare) ... 819
- Antivenin (Crotalidae) Polyvalent ... 2803
- AquaMEPHYTON Injection ... 1648
- Azulfidine (One in every 30 patients or less) ... 2059
- Betaseron for SC Injection ... 653
- Buprenex Injectable (Less than 1%) ... 2170
- Cafergot ... 2376
- Cerebyx Injection (Infrequent) ... 1956
- Chloromycetin Sodium Succinate ... 1960
- Clozaril Tablets (Less than 1%) ... 2377
- Cytovene-IV (One report) ... 2270
- Diupres Tablets ... 1691
- Effexor (Rare) ... 2825
- Etopophos for Injection (Sometimes) ... 701
- Etoposide Injection (Sometimes) ... 539
- ▲ Flolan for Injection (31%) ... 1085
- Gammar-P I.V., Immune Globulin Intravenous (Human) ... 798
- Heparin Sodium Vials ... 1486
- Hivid Tablets (Less than 1%) ... 2287
- Hydropres Tablets ... 1718
- Hyskon Hysteroscopy Fluid (Rare) ... 1633
- Imitrex Tablets ... 1099
- Intron A for Injection (Less than or equal to 5%) ... 2506
- Invirase Capsules (Less than 2%) ... 2291
- Levo-Dromoran ... 2297
- Macrobid Capsules (Rare) ... 2138
- Macrodantin Capsules (Rare) ... 2140
- Maxaquin Tablets (Less than 1%) ... 2593
- Mephyton Tablets (Rare) ... 1739
- Pediazole Suspension ... 2340
- Permax Tablets (Infrequent) ... 571
- Primaxin I.M. ... 1770
- Primaxin I.V. (Less than 0.2%) ... 1772
- RespiGam (Infrequent) ... 1631
- Rilutek Tablets (Rare) ... 2198

(℞ Described in PDR For Nonprescription Drugs) Incidence data in parenthesis; ▲ 3% or more (⊙ Described in PDR For Ophthalmology)

Side Effects Index — CNS stimulation, paradoxical

Cyanosis, hand (cont.)
- Roferon-A Injection (Less than 1%) ... 2308
- Ser-Ap-Es Tablets ... 867
- VePesid Capsules and Injection (Sometimes) ... 727
- Virazole (Infrequent) ... 1310

Cyanosis, hand
- Intron A for Injection (Less than 5%) ... 2506

Cycloplegia
- Bentyl ... 1246
- Cystospaz ... 2123
- Ditropan ... 1267
- Donnatal ... 2234
- Donnatal Extentabs ... 2234
- Donnatal Tablets ... 2234
- Kutrase Capsules ... 2546
- Levsin/Levsinex/Levbid ... 2549
- Pro-Banthine Tablets ... 2226
- Robinul Forte Tablets ... 2247
- Robinul Injectable ... 2247
- Robinul Tablets ... 2247

Cylindruria
- Cipro I.V. (1% or less) ... 587
- Cipro I.V. Pharmacy Bulk Package (Less than 1%) ... 590
- Cipro Tablets ... 584
- Floxin I.V. ... 1580
- Floxin Tablets (200 mg, 300 mg, 400 mg) ... 1577
- Garamycin Injectable ... 2502
- Nebcin Vials, Hyporets & ADD-Vantage ... 1518
- Netromycin Injection 100 mg/ml ... 2516
- Noroxin Tablets ... 1758
- Noroxin Tablets ... 2222

Cyst
- Anafranil Capsules (Infrequent) ... 819
- ▲ Betaseron for SC Injection (4%) ... 653
- ▲ CellCept Capsules (More than or equal to 3%) ... 2265
- Cognex Capsules (Infrequent) ... 1961
- Depakote Tablets (1% to 5%) ... 418
- Effexor (Infrequent) ... 2825
- LUVOX Tablets (Rare) ... 2723
- Neurontin Capsules (Infrequent) ... 1978
- Videx Tablets, Powder for Oral Solution, & Pediatric Powder for Oral Solution (Less than 1%) ... 2980

Cyst, renal
- Anafranil Capsules (Rare) ... 819
- Hivid Tablets (Less than 1%) ... 2287

Cystic masses in the pelvis
- ParaGard T 380A Intrauterine Copper Contraceptive ... 1936

Cystitis
- Ambien Tablets (Infrequent) ... 2559
- Amen Tablets ... 785
- Anafranil Capsules (Up to 2%) ... 819
- ▲ Betaseron for SC Injection (8%) ... 653
- Brevicon ... 2563
- Cognex Capsules (Infrequent) ... 1961
- Cycrin Tablets ... 991
- Demulen ... 2580
- Depo-Provera Sterile Aqueous Suspension ... 2083
- Desogen Tablets ... 1867
- Diethylstilbestrol Tablets ... 1477
- Dilacor XR Extended-release Capsules (Infrequent) ... 2183
- Doxil (Less than 1%) ... 2613
- Effexor (Infrequent) ... 2825
- ESTRATAB Tablets (0.3, 0.625, 1.25, 2.5 mg) ... 2715
- Estratest ... 2718
- Estring Vaginal Ring (1% to 3%) ... 2086
- ▲ Eulexin Capsules (16%) ... 2498
- Flagyl 375 Capsules ... 2587
- Flagyl I.V. ... 2373
- Helidac Therapy ... 2135
- IBU Tablets (Less than 1%) ... 1389
- Kerlone Tablets (Less than 2%) ... 2588
- Lamictal Tablets (Rare) ... 1105
- Lamprene Capsules (Less than 1%) ... 846
- Leukeran Tablets ... 1205
- Levlen/Tri-Levlen ... 646
- Lodine Capsules and Tablets (Less than 1%) ... 2849
- Lo/Ovral Tablets ... 2852
- Lo/Ovral-28 Tablets ... 2857
- LUVOX Tablets (Infrequent) ... 2723
- Menest Tablets ... 2671
- Methotrexate Sodium Tablets, Injection, for Injection and LPF Injection ... 1322
- MetroGel-Vaginal ... 917
- ▲ Miacalcin Nasal Spray (1% to 3%) ... 2403
- Modicon ... 1928
- Motrin Ibuprofen Suspension, Oral Drops, Chewable Tablets, Caplets (Less than 1%) ... 1563
- Nalfon 200 Pulvules & Nalfon Tablets (Less than 1%) ... 933
- Naprelan Tablets (Less than 3%) ... 2861
- Neurontin Capsules (Infrequent) ... 1978
- Nordette-21 Tablets ... 2863
- Nordette-28 Tablets ... 2866
- Norinyl ... 2563
- Nor-Q D Tablets ... 2598
- Ortho-Cept ... 1907
- Ortho-Cyclen/Ortho-Tri-Cyclen ... 1914
- Ortho Dienestrol Cream ... 1922
- Ortho-Novum ... 1928
- Ortho-Cyclen/Ortho Tri-Cyclen ... 1914
- Ovcon ... 765
- Ovral Tablets ... 2877
- Ovral-28 Tablets ... 2878
- Ovrette Tablets ... 2878
- Paxil Tablets (Infrequent) ... 2681
- Permax Tablets (Infrequent) ... 571
- PMB 200 and PMB 400 ... 2890
- Premarin Intravenous ... 2893
- Premarin Vaginal Cream ... 2898
- Premphase ... 2900
- Prempro ... 2905
- Protostat Tablets ... 1939
- Provera Tablets ... 2110
- Prozac Pulvules & Liquid, Oral Solution (Infrequent) ... 935
- Remeron Tablets (Infrequent) ... 1878
- Risperdal Tablets (Rare) ... 1348
- Serzone Tablets (Infrequent) ... 776
- ▲ TheraCys BCG Live (Intravesical) (Up to 29.5%) ... 911
- Thioplex (Thiotepa For Injection) (Rare) ... 1329
- ▲ TICE BCG, USP (5.9%) ... 1881
- Levlen/Tri-Levlen ... 646
- Tri-Norinyl ... 2607
- Triphasil-21 Tablets ... 2919
- Triphasil-28 Tablets ... 2924
- Wellbutrin Tablets (Rare) ... 1177
- Zebeta Tablets ... 1457
- Ziac ... 1459
- Zyrtec Tablets (Less than 2%) ... 2053

Cystitis, hemorrhagic
- Adriamycin PFS ... 2056
- Adriamycin RDF ... 2056
- Cipro I.V. (1% or less) ... 587
- Cipro I.V. Pharmacy Bulk Package (Less than 1%) ... 590
- Cytoxan ... 700
- Fludara for Injection (Rare) ... 658
- IFEX (Frequent) ... 706
- Lysodren Tablets (Infrequent) ... 707
- Navelbine Injection (Less than 1%) ... 1212
- Oncaspar ... 2194
- Thioplex (Thiotepa For Injection) (Rare) ... 1329

Cystitis, non-hemorrhagic
- Cytoxan ... 700

Cystitis, viral
- Retrovir Capsules (0.8%) ... 1216
- Retrovir I.V. Infusion (1%) ... 1221
- Retrovir Syrup (0.8%) ... 1216

Cystitis-like syndrome
(see under Cystitis)

Cysts, vaginal
- Depo-Provera Contraceptive Injection (Fewer than 1%) ... 2079

Cytarabine syndrome
- Cytosar-U Sterile Powder ... 2077

Cytokine Released Syndrome
- Orthoclone OKT3 Sterile Solution (Occasional) ... 1892

cAMP, elevation
- ▲ Yutopar Intravenous Injection (80% to 100%) ... 566

CHF
(see under Congestive heart failure)

CNS abnormalities, fetal
- Accutane Capsules ... 2252

- Elavil ... 2945
- Sensorcaine ... 554

CNS damage
- Tri-Immunol Adsorbed (1 per 330,000) ... 1452

CNS damage, permanent
- Syntocinon Injection ... 2425

CNS depression
- Ana-Kit Anaphylaxis Emergency Treatment Kit ... 611
- Anaprox/Naprosyn (Less than 1%) ... 2277
- Ativan Injection ... 2805
- Brontex ... 2130
- Butisol Sodium Elixir & Tablets (Less than 1 in 100) ... 2768
- Carbocaine Injection ... 2432
- Cerebyx Injection (Infrequent) ... 1956
- Cocaine Hydrochloride Topical Solutions ... 529
- D.A. II Tablets ... 972
- D.A. Chewable Tablets ... 970
- Deconsal II Tablets ... 1605
- Depakote Tablets ... 418
- Duranest Injections ... 533
- Dura-Tap/PD Capsules ... 970
- Dura-Vent/DA Tablets ... 972
- Dura-Vent Tablets ... 971
- EC-Naprosyn Delayed-Release Tablets (Less than 1%) ... 2277
- EMLA Cream (Unlikely with cream) ... 536
- Entex PSE Tablets ... 973
- Fedahist Gyrocaps ... 2545
- Guaimax-D Tablets ... 809
- Histussin D Liquid ... 670
- ▲ Klonopin Tablets (Most frequent) ... 2294
- Lamictal Tablets (Infrequent) ... 1105
- Lioresal Intrathecal ... 1634
- LUVOX Tablets (Infrequent) ... 2723
- ▲ Lysodren Tablets (40%) ... 707
- Mebaral Tablets (Less than 1 in 100) ... 2452
- Anaprox/Naprosyn (Less than 1%) ... 2277
- Nembutal Sodium Capsules (Less than 1%) ... 440
- Nembutal Sodium Solution (Less than 1%) ... 442
- Nembutal Sodium Suppositories (Less than 1%) ... 444
- Neurontin Capsules ... 1978
- Novahistine DMX ... 782
- Novahistine Elixir ... 782
- Phenergan with Codeine ... 2883
- Phenergan VC with Codeine ... 2888
- Phenobarbital Elixir and Tablets (Less than 1 in 100 patients) ... 1523
- Pontocaine Hydrochloride for Spinal Anesthesia ... 2460
- Prozac Pulvules & Liquid, Oral Solution (Rare) ... 935
- Rilutek Tablets (Rare) ... 2198
- Seconal Sodium Pulvules (Less than 1 in 100) ... 1529
- Seldane-D Extended-Release Tablets ... 1286
- Syn-Rx Tablets ... 1622
- Syn-Rx DM Tablets ... 1623
- Trinalin Repetabs Tablets ... 1373
- Tussend ... 1830
- Tussend Expectorant ... 1831
- ▲ Vesanoid Capsules (3%) ... 2327
- Videx Tablets, Powder for Oral Solution, & Pediatric Powder for Oral Solution (Less than 1%) ... 2980
- Vumon for Injection ... 729
- ▲ Xanax Tablets (13.8% to 13.9%) ... 2115
- Xylocaine Injections ... 562

CNS depression, neonatal
- Halcion Tablets ... 2093
- ProSom Tablets ... 457
- Streptomycin Sulfate Injection ... 2031
- Versed Injection ... 2324

CNS reactions
- Attenuvax ... 1650
- Azulfidine ... 2059
- Biavax II ... 1653
- BuSpar Tablets ... 738
- Chibroxin Sterile Ophthalmic Solution (With oral form) ... 1657
- ▲ Cipro I.V. Pharmacy Bulk Package (Among most frequent) ... 590
- Clozaril Tablets ... 2377
- Compazine ... 2644
- Danocrine Capsules ... 2437
- Desyrel and Desyrel Dividose ... 504

- Diupres Tablets ... 1691
- Hexalen Capsules ... 2760
- Hydrocet Capsules ... 787
- Hydropres Tablets ... 1718
- Intron A for Injection (Less than 5%) ... 2506
- Lanoxicaps (Rare) ... 1110
- Lanoxin Elixir Pediatric ... 1113
- Lanoxin Injection ... 1116
- Lanoxin Injection Pediatric ... 1119
- Lanoxin Tablets ... 1121
- Lariam Tablets ... 2295
- ▲ Leukine (11%) ... 1317
- Levsin/Levsinex/Levbid ... 2549
- Marax Tablets & DF Syrup (Rare) ... 2015
- ▲ Nipent for Injection (1% to 11%) ... 2733
- Noroxin Tablets ... 1758
- Noroxin Tablets ... 2222
- ▲ Novantrone for Injection (30 to 34%) ... 1327
- Orap Tablets ... 1037
- Orthoclone OKT3 Sterile Solution ... 1892
- Orudis Capsules (Less than 1%) ... 2874
- Oruvail Capsules (Less than 1%) ... 2874
- ▲ Paraplatin for Injection (5%) ... 713
- Paremyd (Rare) ... ⊙ 244
- Prolixin ... 510
- Rabies Vaccine, Imovax Rabies I.D. (One report) ... 901
- Roferon-A Injection (Less than 5%) ... 2308
- SSD ... 1402
- Sandostatin Injection (Less than 1%) ... 2421
- Serentil ... 689
- Silvadene Cream 1% ... 1288
- Stelazine ... 2692
- Thalitone ... 1293

CNS stimulation
- Adipex-P Tablets and Capsules ... 1035
- Brethaire Inhaler ... 830
- Carbocaine Injection ... 2432
- Chibroxin Sterile Ophthalmic Solution (With oral form) ... 1657
- ▲ Cipro I.V. (Among most frequent) ... 587
- Cipro Tablets ... 584
- Claritin-D Tablets ... 2487
- Cocaine Hydrochloride Topical Solutions ... 529
- D.A. Chewable Tablets ... 970
- Duranest Injections ... 533
- Dura-Tap/PD Capsules ... 970
- Dura-Vent Tablets ... 971
- Effexor (Infrequent) ... 2825
- EMLA Cream (Unlikely with cream) ... 536
- Floxin Tablets (200 mg, 300 mg, 400 mg) ... 1577
- Kwell Cream & Lotion ... 2172
- Kwell Shampoo ... 2173
- Kytril Injection (Less than 2%) ... 2667
- Lamictal Tablets (Rare) ... 1105
- Levo-Dromoran ... 2297
- Lindane Lotion USP 1% ... 481
- Lindane Shampoo USP 1% ... 483
- Lufyllin-GG Elixir & Tablets ... 2779
- LUVOX Tablets (2%) ... 2723
- Maxaquin Tablets ... 2593
- NegGram ... 2453
- Noroxin Tablets ... 1758
- Noroxin Tablets ... 2222
- Paxil Tablets (Frequent) ... 2681
- Penetrex Tablets ... 2196
- Pontocaine Hydrochloride for Spinal Anesthesia ... 2460
- Proventil Inhalation Aerosol ... 2524
- Proventil Repetabs Tablets ... 2529
- Proventil Syrup ... 2528
- Prozac Pulvules & Liquid, Oral Solution (Infrequent) ... 935
- Rondec Oral Drops ... 974
- Rondec Syrup ... 974
- Rondec ... 974
- Serzone Tablets ... 776
- Syn-Rx Tablets ... 1622
- Tussend ... 1830
- ▲ Ultram Tablets (50 mg) (7% to 14%) ... 1594
- Ventolin Inhalation Aerosol and Refill ... 1170
- Ventolin Rotacaps for Inhalation ... 1173
- Ventolin Syrup ... 1175
- Ventolin Tablets ... 1176
- Volmax Extended-Release Tablets ... 1835
- Xylocaine Injections ... 562

CNS stimulation, paradoxical
- Doral Tablets ... 2773
- Halcion Tablets ... 2093
- Librium Capsules ... 2331

(▭ Described in PDR For Nonprescription Drugs) Incidence data in parenthesis; ▲ 3% or more (⊙ Described in PDR For Ophthalmology)

CNS stimulation, paradoxical — Side Effects Index — 1298

Restoril Capsules (Less than 0.5%) ... 2413

CNS toxicity

Cytosar-U Sterile Powder (With experimental doses) ... 2077
Duranest Injections ... 533
▲ IFEX (12%) ... 706
Kefzol Vials, Faspak & ADD-Vantage ... 1511
Kwell Cream & Lotion ... 2172
Lindane Lotion USP 1% ... 481
Lindane Shampoo USP 1% ... 483
Marcaine Spinal ... 2449
▲ Nipent for Injection (1% to 11%) .. 2733
Parlodel ... 2411

CNS unresponsiveness, unspecified

▲ Cipro I.V. (Among most frequent) .. 587

CPK, elevation (see under Creatine phosphokinase, increase)

D

Deafness

Amicar Syrup, Tablets, and Injection ... 1312
Amikacin Sulfate Injection, USP ... 523
Amikacin Sulfate Injection, USP ... 981
Amikin Injectable ... 502
Anafranil Capsules (Infrequent) ... 819
Aralen Hydrochloride Injection (A few cases) ... 2430
Aralen Phosphate Tablets (A few cases) ... 2431
Betasept Surgical Scrub ... 2145
Betaseron for SC Injection ... 653
Cardioquin Tablets ... 2146
Cerebyx Injection (2.2%; infrequent) ... 1956
Clomid ... 1262
Cognex Capsules (Infrequent) ... 1961
Cytotec (Infrequent) ... 2576
Cytovene (1% or less) ... 2270
DaunoXome (Less than or equal to 5%) ... 1842
Depakote Tablets (1% to 5%) ... 418
Diupres Tablets ... 1691
Edecrin ... 1698
Effexor (Rare) ... 2825
Foscavir Injection (Less than 1%) .. 541
Hibiclens Antimicrobial Skin Cleanser ... 2947
Hibistat ... 2948
Hydropres Tablets ... 1718
Imitrex Tablets ... 1099
Indocin Capsules (Less than 1%) ... 1723
Indocin I.V. (Less than 1%) ... 1727
Indocin (Less than 1%) ... 1723
Kerlone Tablets (Less than 2%) ... 2588
Lamictal Tablets (Rare) ... 1105
Lodine Capsules and Tablets (Less than 1%) ... 2849
LUVOX Tablets (Infrequent) ... 2723
M-M-R II ... 1730
Naprelan Tablets (Less than 1%) .. 2861
Nebcin Vials, Hyporets & ADD-Vantage ... 1518
Nipent for Injection (Less than 3%) ... 2733
Oncovin Solution Vials & Hyporets (Rare) ... 1521
Paxil Tablets (Rare) ... 2681
Permax Tablets (Infrequent) ... 571
Platinol for Injection (Rare) ... 717
Platinol-AQ Injection (Rare to occasional) ... 719
Prevacid Delayed-Release Capsules (Less than 1%) ... 2746
Prozac Pulvules & Liquid, Oral Solution (Rare) ... 935
Quinaglute Dura-Tabs Tablets ... 644
Quinidex Extentabs ... 2240
Remeron Tablets (Infrequent) ... 1878
Rilutek Tablets (Rare) ... 2198
Salagen Tablets (Less than 1%) ... 1546
Ser-Ap-Es Tablets ... 867
Serzone Tablets (Rare) ... 776
Ultram Tablets (50 mg) (Infrequent) ... 1594
Velban Vials (Rare) ... 1537
Videx Tablets, Powder for Oral Solution, & Pediatric Powder for Oral Solution (Less than 1%) ... 2980
Zosyn (1.0% or less) ... 1463
Zyrtec Tablets (Less than 2%) ... 2053

Deafness, transient

Dynabac (A few cases) ... 668
Oncovin Solution Vials & Hyporets (Rare) ... 1521
Redux Capsules ... 2911
Remeron Tablets (Rare) ... 1878
Velban Vials (Rare) ... 1537

Death, fetal

Accupril Tablets ... 1950
Altace Capsules ... 1238
Capoten Tablets ... 740
Capozide Tablets ... 744
Cozaar Tablets ... 1668
Cytotec ... 2576
Felbatol ... 2774
Hyzaar Tablets ... 1720
Lotensin Tablets ... 852
Lotensin HCT Tablets (Several dozen cases) ... 855
Lotrel Capsules ... 858
Methotrexate Sodium Tablets, Injection, for Injection and LPF Injection ... 1322
Monopril Tablets ... 762
Nolvadex Tablets (A small number of reports) ... 2957
Podocon-25 ... 1949
Prinivil Tablets ... 1776
Prinzide Tablets ... 1780
Sensorcaine ... 554
Syntocinon Injection ... 2425
Univasc Tablets ... 2553
Vaseretic Tablets ... 1810
Vasotec I.V. ... 1814
Vasotec Tablets ... 1816
Zestoretic Tablets ... 2968
Zestril Tablets ... 2972
Zyrtec Tablets (Rare) ... 2053

Death, infants

Virazole (20 cases) ... 1310

Death, sudden

Clozaril Tablets (Rare) ... 2377
Felbatol ... 2774
Haldol Decanoate ... 1587
Imitrex Tablets ... 1099
Inapsine Injection ... 462
JE-VAX (One case) ... 904
LUVOX Tablets (Rare) ... 2723
Monopril Tablets (0.4% to 1.0%) .. 762
Neurontin Capsules (8 out of 2,203 patients) ... 1978
Norpramin Tablets (One report) ... 1273
Orap Tablets ... 1037
Prozac Pulvules & Liquid, Oral Solution ... 935
Redux Capsules ... 2911
Risperdal Tablets (Rare) ... 1348
Thorazine ... 2701
Vascor Tablets (200 and 300 mg) (1.6%) ... 1597
Vumon for Injection (One episode) ... 729

Deep tendon reflexes, loss

Oncovin Solution Vials & Hyporets ... 1521
Plaquenil Sulfate Tablets ... 2459
Velban Vials ... 1537

Defecate, desire to

Aminohippurate Sodium Injection .. 1646
Dopram Injectable ... 2235
Peptavlon ... 2997

Defecation, painful

Invirase Capsules (Less than 2%) .. 2291

Dehydration

Anafranil Capsules (Infrequent) ... 819
Avonex ... 662
Bumex (0.1%) ... 2260
Capoten Tablets ... 740
Capozide Tablets ... 744
▲ Casodex Tablets (2% to 5%) ... 2934
Cedax (0.1% to 1%) ... 2480
▲ CellCept Capsules (More than or equal to 3%) ... 2265
Cerebyx Injection (Infrequent) ... 1956
Claritin-D Tablets (Less frequent) .. 2487
Cognex Capsules (Infrequent) ... 1961
Cytotec (Rare) ... 2576
▲ DaunoXome (Less than or equal to 5%) ... 1842
Demadex Tablets and Injection ... 691
Dipentum Capsules (Rare) ... 2084
Diprivan Injectable Emulsion (Less than 1%) ... 2939
Doxil (Less than 1%) ... 2613
Dynabac (0.1% to 1%) ... 668
Eskalith ... 2658
Felbatol ... 2774
Fleet Enema ... 1001
Fludara for Injection (Up to 1%) ... 658
Foscavir Injection (Less than 1%) .. 541
Garamycin Injectable ... 2502
Glucophage Tablets ... 754
Haldol Decanoate ... 1587
Imitrex Injection (Rare) ... 1095
Intron A for Injection (Less than or equal to 5%) ... 2506
Invirase Capsules (Less than 2%) .. 2291
Klonopin Tablets ... 2294
Lasix Injection, Oral Solution and Tablets ... 1267
Leucovorin Calcium Tablets, Wellcovorin Brand ... 1204
Lioresal Intrathecal (1% or more) .. 1634
Lithium Carbonate Capsules & Tablets ... 2352
Lithonate/Lithotabs/Lithobid ... 2721
Lupron Depot - 3 Month 22.5 mg (Less than 5%) ... 2743
LUVOX Tablets (Infrequent) ... 2723
Methotrexate Sodium Tablets, Injection, for Injection and LPF Injection ... 1322
Moduretic Tablets (Less than or equal to 1%) ... 1748
Naprelan Tablets (Less than 1%) .. 2861
Norvir (Less than 2%) ... 447
OxyContin Tablets (Less than 1%) 2163
Paxil Tablets (Rare) ... 2681
Permax Tablets (Infrequent) ... 571
Prinivil Tablets (0.3% to 1.0%) ... 1776
Prinzide Tablets ... 1780
Propulsid (More than 1%) ... 1346
Prostin E2 Suppository ... 2109
Prozac Pulvules & Liquid, Oral Solution (Rare) ... 935
Redux Capsules ... 2911
Remeron Tablets (Infrequent) ... 1878
Risperdal Tablets (Rare) ... 1348
Serzone Tablets (Infrequent) ... 776
Univasc Tablets ... 2553
Vaseretic Tablets ... 1810
Vasotec Tablets ... 1816
Videx Tablets, Powder for Oral Solution, & Pediatric Powder for Oral Solution (1% to 5%) ... 2980
Vistide Injection ... 1057
Zestoretic Tablets ... 2968
Zestril Tablets (0.3% to 1.0%) ... 2972
Zoloft Tablets (Rare) ... 2051
Zyrtec Tablets (Less than 2%) ... 2053

Delirium

Amicar Syrup, Tablets, and Injection ... 1312
Anafranil Capsules (Infrequent) ... 819
Ativan Injection (1.3%) ... 2805
Betaseron for SC Injection ... 653
Catapres Tablets ... 679
Catapres-TTS ... 680
Cerebyx Injection ... 1956
Chloromycetin Sodium Succinate ... 1960
Cipro Tablets ... 584
Clozaril Tablets ... 2377
Cognex Capsules (Infrequent) ... 1961
Combipres Tablets ... 682
Dalgan Injection (Less than 1%) ... 529
Diprivan Injectable Emulsion (Less than 1%) ... 2939
Famvir Tablets (Very rare) ... 2660
Foscavir Injection (Less than 1%) .. 541
Lamictal Tablets (Rare) ... 1105
LUVOX Tablets (Infrequent) ... 2723
Merrem I.V. (0.1% to 1.0%) ... 2952
Nardil (Less frequent) ... 1977
Orthoclone OKT3 Sterile Solution .. 1892
Paxil Tablets (Rare) ... 2681
Phenobarbital Elixir and Tablets ... 1523
PhosLo Tablets ... 695
Placidyl Capsules ... 456
Prograf ... 1028
Quinaglute Dura-Tabs Tablets ... 644
Quinidex Extentabs ... 2240
Redux Capsules ... 2911
Remeron Tablets (Infrequent) ... 1878
Rilutek Tablets (Infrequent) ... 2198
Risperdal Tablets (Rare) ... 1348
Romazicon (Less than 1%) ... 2311
Wellbutrin Tablets ... 1177
Zovirax Sterile Powder ... 1191

Delivery complications, unspecified

Actron Caplets and Tablets ... ▣ 608
Advil Cold and Sinus Caplets and Tablets ... ▣ 837
Advil Ibuprofen Tablets, Caplets and Gel Caplets ... ▣ 836
Aleve ... 2124
Alka-Seltzer Cherry Effervescent Antacid and Pain Reliever ... ▣ 609
Alka-Seltzer Extra Strength Effervescent Antacid and Pain Reliever ... ▣ 609
Alka-Seltzer Lemon Lime Effervescent Antacid and Pain Reliever ... ▣ 609
Alka-Seltzer Original Effervescent Antacid and Pain Reliever ... ▣ 609
Alka-Seltzer Plus ... ▣ 611
Alka-Seltzer Plus Sinus Medicine ▣ 611
Ascriptin ... ▣ 650
BC Cold Powder Multi-Symptom Formula (Cold-Sinus-Allergy) ... ▣ 631
BC Cold Powder Non-Drowsy Formula (Cold-Sinus) ... ▣ 631
BC Powder ... ▣ 631
Genuine Bayer Aspirin Tablets & Caplets ... ▣ 618
Extra Strength Bayer Arthritis Pain Regimen Formula ... ▣ 615
Extra Strength Bayer Aspirin Caplets & Tablets ... ▣ 617
Extended-Release Bayer 8-Hour Aspirin ... ▣ 616
Extra Strength Bayer Plus Aspirin Caplets ... ▣ 617
Extra Strength Bayer PM Aspirin Plus Sleep Aid ... ▣ 617
Aspirin Regimen Bayer 81 mg Tablets with Calcium ... ▣ 615
Aspirin Regimen Bayer Adult Low Strength 81 mg Tablets ... ▣ 613
Aspirin Regimen Bayer Children's Chewable Aspirin ... ▣ 616
Aspirin Regimen Bayer Regular Strength 325 mg Caplets ... ▣ 613
Cama Arthritis Pain Reliever ... ▣ 748
Ecotrin ... 2625
Empirin Aspirin Tablets ... ▣ 818
Fiorinal with Codeine Capsules ... 2390
Goody's Extra Strength Headache Powders ... ▣ 632
Goody's Extra Strength Pain Relief Tablets ... ▣ 632
Marcaine ... 2446
Motrin IB Caplets, Tablets, and Gelcaps ... ▣ 802
Orudis KT ... ▣ 842
Sensorcaine ... 554
Soma Compound w/Codeine Tablets ... 2784
Soma Compound Tablets ... 2783
St. Joseph Adult Chewable Aspirin (81 mg.) ... ▣ 768
Vanquish Analgesic Caplets ... ▣ 627

Delusions

Ambien Tablets (Rare) ... 2559
Anafranil Capsules (Infrequent) ... 819
Artane (Rare) ... 1418
Asendin Tablets ... 1419
Atamet Tablets ... 567
Betaseron for SC Injection ... 653
Clozaril Tablets (Less than 1%) ... 2377
Dalgan Injection (Less than 1%) ... 529
Desyrel and Desyrel Dividose ... 504
Effexor (Rare) ... 2825
Elavil ... 2945
Eldepryl Capsules ... 2729
Etrafon ... 2495
Felbatol ... 2774
Flexeril Tablets (Rare) ... 1701
Halcion Tablets ... 2093
Lamictal Tablets (Rare) ... 1105
Larodopa Tablets (Relatively frequent) ... 2296
Limbitrol ... 2333
Ludiomil Tablets (Rare) ... 861
▲ Lupron Depot 3.75 mg (Among most frequent) ... 2739
Lupron Depot - 3 Month 22.5 mg (Less than 5%) ... 2743
LUVOX Tablets (Infrequent) ... 2723
Norpramin Tablets ... 1273
Nubain Injection (1% or less) ... 952
Pamelor ... 2409
Paxil Tablets (Rare) ... 2681
Permax Tablets (Infrequent) ... 571
Prozac Pulvules & Liquid, Oral Solution (Infrequent) ... 935
Remeron Tablets (Infrequent) ... 1878
Rilutek Tablets (Infrequent) ... 2198
Salagen Tablets (Rare) ... 1546
Sinemet Tablets ... 959
Sinemet CR Tablets ... 961
Stadol (Less than 1%) ... 779
Surmontil Capsules ... 2917
Tofranil Ampuls ... 873

(▣ Described in PDR For Nonprescription Drugs) Incidence data in parenthesis; ▲ 3% or more (◉ Described in PDR For Ophthalmology)

1299 Side Effects Index Depression

Tofranil Tablets 875
Tofranil-PM Capsules 876
Triavil Tablets 1800
Vivactil Tablets 1820
Wellbutrin Tablets (1.2%) 1177
Zoloft Tablets (Infrequent) 2051

Dementia

Ambien Tablets (Rare) 2559
Atamet Tablets 567
Betaseron for SC Injection 653
Effexor (Rare) 2825
Foscavir Injection (Between 1% and 5%) 541
Larodopa Tablets (Infrequent) 2296
Methotrexate Sodium Tablets, Injection, for Injection and LPF Injection 1322
Redux Capsules (Rare) 2911
Remeron Tablets (Rare) 1878
Rilutek Tablets (Rare) 2198
Sinemet Tablets 959
Sinemet CR Tablets 961
▲ Vesanoid Capsules (3%) 2327
Videx Tablets, Powder for Oral Solution, & Pediatric Powder for Oral Solution (Less than 1%) 2980
Zerit Capsules (1%) 731

Dental calculus formation, an increase in

Peridex 2127
Periogard Oral Rinse 892

Dental caries

Ambien Tablets (Rare) 2559
Anafranil Capsules (Infrequent) 819
Claritin Tablets (2% or fewer patients) 2485
DaunoXome (Less than or equal to 5%) 1842
Eskalith 2658
Lithonate/Lithotabs/Lithobid 2721
▲ LUVOX Tablets (3%) 2723
Paxil Tablets (Rare) 2681
Permax Tablets (Infrequent) 571
Questran 774
Tegison Capsules (Less than 1%) 2314

Dependence, drug

Adderall Tablets 2209
Adipex-P Tablets and Capsules 1035
Alfenta Injection 1334
Astramorph/PF Injection, USP (Preservative-Free) 526
Avonex 662
Dalmane Capsules 2329
Darvon-N/Darvocet-N 1473
Darvon 1475
Darvon-N Suspension & Tablets 1473
Demerol 2438
Dexedrine 2648
DextroStat-Dextroamphetamine Sulfate Tablets 2211
Dilaudid Ampules 1382
Dilaudid Cough Syrup 1383
Dilaudid 1382
Dilaudid Oral Liquid 1386
Dilaudid 1382
Dilaudid Tablets - 8 mg 1386
Dizac (diazepam injectable emulsion) CIV 1862
Duragesic Transdermal System 1336
Duramorph Injection 983
Esgic-plus Capsules 1012
Esgic-plus Tablets 1012
Ex-Lax Chocolated Laxative Tablets ▣ 748
Extra Gentle Ex-Lax Laxative Pills ▣ 749
Regular Strength Ex-Lax Laxative Pills ▣ 749
Ex-Lax Gentle Nature Laxative Pills ▣ 749
Fioricet Tablets 2386
Fioricet with Codeine Capsules 2387
Fiorinal Capsules 2388
Fiorinal with Codeine Capsules 2390
Fiorinal Tablets 2388
Halcion Tablets 2093
Ionamin Capsules 1615
Librium Capsules 2331
Librium Injectable 2332
Limbitrol 2333
Lioresal Intrathecal (1% or more) 1634
Lortab 2751
LUVOX Tablets (Infrequent) 2723
MS Contin Tablets 2149
MSIR 2152
Mepergan Injection 2859
Methadone Hydrochloride Oral Concentrate 2356
Methadone Hydrochloride Oral Solution & Tablets 2357
Nembutal Sodium Capsules 440
Nembutal Sodium Solution 442
Nembutal Sodium Suppositories 444
Oramorph SR (Morphine Sulfate Sustained Release Tablets) 2359
OxyIR Capsules 2167
Paxil Tablets (Rare) 2681
Percocet Tablets 955
Percodan Tablets 955
Percodan-Demi Tablets 956
Peri-Colace Capsules and Syrup 2226
Phenergan with Codeine 2883
Phenergan VC with Codeine 2888
Phenobarbital Elixir and Tablets 1523
Placidyl Capsules 456
PMB 200 and PMB 400 2890
Prelu-2 Timed Release Capsules 687
RMS Suppositories CII 2766
Redux Capsules 2911
Remeron Tablets (Rare) 1878
Restoril Capsules 2413
Ritalin 866
Roxanol 2365
Roxicodone Tablets, Oral Solution & Intensol (Oxycodone) 2366
Seconal Sodium Pulvules 1529
Stadol (Less than 1%) 779
Sublimaze Injection 463
Talwin Injection 2465
Talwin Compound 2466
Talwin Injection 2465
Talwin Nx Tablets 2467
Tranxene 459
Tylenol with Codeine 1592
Tylox Capsules 1593
Valium Injectable 2336
Valium Tablets 2335
Vicodin Tuss Expectorant 1406
Videx Tablets, Powder for Oral Solution, & Pediatric Powder for Oral Solution (Less than 1%) 2980
Wygesic Tablets 2930

Dependence, physical

Axocet Capsules 2469
Bellergal-S Tablets 2375
Brontex 2130
Butisol Sodium Elixir & Tablets 2768
Codiclear DH Syrup 808
DHCplus Capsules 2148
Demerol 2438
Dexedrine 2648
Dilaudid Tablets and Liquid 1386
Doral Tablets 2773
Duragesic Transdermal System 1336
Duramorph Injection 983
Esgic-plus Capsules 1012
Esgic-plus Tablets 1012
Fioricet Tablets 2386
Fiorinal Capsules 2388
Fiorinal with Codeine Capsules 2390
Fiorinal Tablets 2388
Hycodan Tablets and Syrup 946
Hycomine Compound Tablets 948
Hycomine 947
Hycotuss Expectorant Syrup 950
Hydrocet Capsules 787
Infumorph 200 and Infumorph 500 Sterile Solutions 985
Isordil Tembids 2847
Isordil Titradose Tablets 2848
Klonopin Tablets 2294
Levo-Dromoran 2297
Lorcet 10/650 Tablets 1016
Lortab 2751
MS Contin Tablets 2149
MSIR 2152
Marinol (Dronabinol) Capsules (Uncommon) 2353
Mebaral Tablets 2452
Methadone Hydrochloride Oral Concentrate 2356
Methadone Hydrochloride Oral Solution & Tablets 2357
Miltown Tablets 2780
Oramorph SR (Morphine Sulfate Sustained Release Tablets) 2359
OxyContin Tablets 2163
Percocet Tablets 955
Percodan Tablets 955
Phrenilin 790
ProSom Tablets 457
Quadrinal Tablets 1398
RMS Suppositories CII 2766
Roxanol 2365
Seconal Sodium Pulvules 1529
Sedapap Tablets 50 mg/650 mg 1826
Serax Capsules 2916
Serax Tablets 2916
Sorbitrate 2959
Talacen Caplets 2464
Talwin Injection 2465
Talwin Nx Tablets 2467
Tranxene 459
Tylenol with Codeine 1592
Tylox Capsules 1593
Ultram Tablets (50 mg) 1594
Versed Injection 2324
Vicodin HP Tablets 1403
Vicodin Tuss Expectorant 1406
Xanax Tablets 2115

Dependence, psychic (see under Dependence, psychological)

Dependence, psychological

Adderall Tablets 2209
Axocet Capsules 2469
Bellergal-S Tablets 2375
Brontex 2130
Butisol Sodium Elixir & Tablets 2768
Cafergot 2376
DHCplus Capsules 2148
Darvon-N/Darvocet-N 1473
Darvon 1475
Darvon-N Suspension & Tablets 1473
Demerol 2438
Desoxyn Gradumet Tablets 422
Dexedrine 2648
DextroStat-Dextroamphetamine Sulfate Tablets 2211
Dilaudid 1382
Dilaudid Oral Liquid 1386
Dilaudid 1382
Dilaudid Tablets - 8 mg 1386
Duragesic Transdermal System 1336
Duramorph Injection 983
Esgic-plus Capsules 1012
Esgic-plus Tablets 1012
Etrafon 2495
Fastin Capsules 2662
Fioricet Tablets 2386
Fiorinal Capsules 2388
Fiorinal with Codeine Capsules 2390
Fiorinal Tablets 2388
Hycodan Tablets and Syrup 946
Hycomine Compound Tablets 948
Hycomine 947
Hycotuss Expectorant Syrup 950
Hydrocet Capsules 787
Infumorph 200 and Infumorph 500 Sterile Solutions 985
Ionamin Capsules 1615
Kadian Capsules (Very rare) 2948
Klonopin Tablets 2294
Levo-Dromoran 2297
Lorcet 10/650 Tablets 1016
Lortab 2751
MS Contin Tablets (Very rare) 2149
MSIR 2152
Marinol (Dronabinol) Capsules (Uncommon) 2353
Mebaral Tablets 2452
Methadone Hydrochloride Oral Concentrate 2356
Methadone Hydrochloride Oral Solution & Tablets 2357
Miltown Tablets 2780
Nembutal Sodium Capsules 440
Nembutal Sodium Solution 442
Nembutal Sodium Suppositories 444
Oramorph SR (Morphine Sulfate Sustained Release Tablets) 2359
OxyContin Tablets 2163
OxyIR Capsules 2167
Percocet Tablets 955
Percodan Tablets 955
Phrenilin 790
Placidyl Capsules 456
ProSom Tablets 457
RMS Suppositories CII 2766
Ritalin 866
Roxanol 2365
Roxicodone Tablets, Oral Solution & Intensol (Oxycodone) 2366
Sedapap Tablets 50 mg/650 mg 1826
Serax Capsules 2916
Serax Tablets 2916
Talacen Caplets 2464
Talwin Nx Tablets 2467
Tranxene 459
Tussend 1830
Tussionex Pennkinetic Extended-Release Suspension 1624
Tylenol with Codeine 1592
Tylox Capsules 1593
Ultram Tablets (50 mg) 1594
Vicodin Tablets 1404
Vicodin ES Tablets 1405
Vicodin HP Tablets 1403
Vicodin Tuss Expectorant 1406
Zydone Capsules 967

Depersonalization

Ambien Tablets (Rare) 2559
Anafranil Capsules (2%) 819
Avonex 662
Betaseron for SC Injection 653
Biaxin 406
Buprenex Injectable (Infrequent) 2170
BuSpar Tablets (Infrequent) 738
Cardura Tablets (Less than 0.5% of 3960 patients) 1993
Cerebyx Injection (Infrequent) 1956
Cipro I.V. (1% or less) 587
Cipro I.V. Pharmacy Bulk Package (Less than 1%) 590
Cipro Tablets (Less than 1%) 584
Duragesic Transdermal System (Less than 1%) 1336
Effexor (1%) 2825
Halcion Tablets 2093
Hivid Tablets (Less than 1%) 2287
Indocin (Less than 1%) 1723
Lamictal Tablets (Infrequent) 1105
LUVOX Tablets (Infrequent) 2723
Marinol (Dronabinol) Capsules (Greater than 1%) 2353
Maxaquin Tablets (Less than 1%) 2593
Neurontin Capsules (Infrequent) 1978
Norvasc Tablets (More than 0.1% to 1%) 2020
Nubain Injection (1% or less) 952
OxyContin Tablets (Less than 1%) 2163
Paxil Tablets (Infrequent) 2681
Penetrex Tablets (0.1% to 1%) 2196
Prozac Pulvules & Liquid, Oral Solution (Infrequent) 935
Redux Capsules (Infrequent) 2911
Remeron Tablets (Infrequent) 1878
Rilutek Tablets (Infrequent) 2198
Romazicon (1% to 3%) 2311
Serzone Tablets (Infrequent) 776
Tambocor Tablets (Less than 1%) 1555
Wellbutrin Tablets (Infrequent) 1177
Xanax Tablets 2115
Zoloft Tablets (Infrequent) 2051
Zyrtec Tablets (Less than 2%) 2053

Depigmentation

Azelex (Rare) 471
Intron A for Injection (Less than 5%) 2506
Thioplex (Thiotepa For Injection) 1329

Depilation (see under Epilation)

Depression (see also under Depression, mental)

Accupril Tablets (0.5% to 1.0%) 1950
Accutane Capsules (Some patients) 2252
Actigall Capsules 818
▲ Actimmune (3%) 1043
Adalat Capsules (10 mg and 20 mg) (Less than 0.5%) 580
AeroBid Inhaler System (1% to 3%) 1004
Aerobid-M Inhaler System (1% to 3%) 1004
Aldoclor Tablets 1638
Aldomet Ester HCl Injection 1642
Aldomet Oral 1640
Aldoril Tablets 1644
Alferon N Injection (One patient to 3%) 2142
Altace Capsules (Less than 1%) 1238
Anafranil Capsules (Up to 5%) 819
Apresazide Capsules (Less frequent) 824
Apresoline Hydrochloride Tablets (Less frequent) 826
▲ Arimidex Tablets (2.4% to 5.3%) 2932
Asacol Delayed-Release Tablets 2129
Atamet Tablets 567
Ativan Injection (1.3%) 2805
Ativan Tablets (Less frequent) 2807
Atretol Tablets 569
Avonex 662
Axocet Capsules (Infrequent) 2469
Azmacort Oral Inhaler 2175
Bactrim DS Tablets 2257
Bactrim I.V. Infusion 2255
Bactrim 2257
Betagan ⊙ 230
Betimol 0.25%, 0.5% ⊙ 259
Betoptic Ophthalmic Solution (Rare) 465

Betoptic S Ophthalmic Suspension (Rare) ... 467
Blocadren Tablets ... 1654
Brevibloc (esmolol HCl) Injection (Less than 1%) ... 1860
Brevicon ... 2563
BuSpar Tablets (2%) ... 738
Capoten Tablets ... 740
Capozide Tablets ... 744
Cardene Capsules (Rare) ... 2261
Cardene SR Capsules (Rare) ... 2264
Cardioquin Tablets (Occasional) ... 2146
Cardizem SR Capsules (Less than 1%) ... 1255
Cardizem Injectable ... 1253
Cardizem Tablets (Less than 1%) .. 1257
Cardura Tablets (1%) ... 1993
Cartrol Tablets (Less common) ... 413
Casodex Tablets (2% to 5%) ... 2934
Cataflam Tablets (Less than 1%) ... 833
Celestone Soluspan Suspension ... 2484
▲ CellCept Capsules (More than or equal to 3%) ... 2265
Cerebyx Injection (Infrequent) ... 1956
Cipro I.V. (1% or less) ... 587
Cipro I.V. Pharmacy Bulk Package (Less than 1%) ... 590
Cipro Tablets (Less than 1%) ... 584
Clinoril Tablets (Less than 1%) ... 1658
Clomid (Fewer than 1%) ... 1262
Clozaril Tablets (1%) ... 2377
Cogentin ... 1661
Cozaar Tablets (Less than 1%) ... 1668
Crixivan Capsules (Less than 2%) .. 1670
Cylert Tablets ... 415
DDAVP ... 2180
Dalgan Injection (Less than 1%) ... 529
Dalmane Capsules (Rare) ... 2329
Danocrine Capsules ... 2437
Daranide Tablets ... 1676
Daraprim Tablets (Rare) ... 1199
▲ DaunoXome (3% to 7%) ... 1842
Demser Capsules ... 1690
Diethylstilbestrol Tablets ... 1477
Dilaudid-HP Injection (Less frequent) ... 1384
Dilaudid-HP Lyophilized Powder 250 mg (Less frequent) ... 1384
Dipentum Capsules (1.5%) ... 2084
Diprivan Injectable Emulsion (Less than 1%) ... 2939
Dizac (diazepam injectable emulsion) CIV (Less frequent) ... 1862
Dolobid Tablets (Less than 1 in 100) ... 1695
Doral Tablets ... 2773
Doxil (Less than 1%) ... 2613
▲ Duragesic Transdermal System (3% to 10%) ... 1336
Dynabac (0.1% to 1%) ... 668
DynaCirc Capsules (0.5% to 1%) .. 2381
DynaCirc CR Tablets (0.5% to 1.0%) ... 2383
Eldepryl Capsules ... 2729
Elspar ... 1700
Ergamisol Tablets (1% to 2%) ... 1340
Estrace Cream and Tablets ... 751
Estratest ... 2718
Estring Vaginal Ring (At least 1 report) ... 2086
Ethmozine Tablets (Less than 2%) 2217
Eulexin Capsules (1%) ... 2498
Feldene Capsules (Less than 1%) .. 2008
Fioricet Tablets (Infrequent) ... 2386
Fioricet with Codeine Capsules (Infrequent) ... 2387
Fiorinal with Codeine Capsules ... 2390
Flagyl 375 Capsules ... 2587
Flagyl I.V. ... 2373
▲ Flolan for Injection (37%) ... 1085
Floxin I.V. (Less than 1%) ... 1580
Floxin Tablets (200 mg, 300 mg, 400 mg) (Less than 1%) ... 1577
Fludara for Injection (Up to 1%) ... 658
▲ Foscavir Injection (5% or greater) .. 541
Gantanol Tablets ... 2285
Gantrisin ... 2286
Garamycin Injectable ... 2502
Gastrocrom Capsules (Infrequent) .. 1611
Gastrocrom Oral Concentrate (Less common) ... 1611
Halcion Tablets (0.9% to 0.5%) ... 2093
Haldol Decanoate ... 1587
Haldol Injection, Tablets and Concentrate ... 1585
Halotestin Tablets ... 2095
Helidac Therapy ... 2135
Hismanal Tablets (Less frequent) ... 1341
Hivid Tablets (Less than 1%; 0.4%) ... 2287
Hydralazine Hydrochloride Injection USP (Less frequent) ... 2712
Hydropres Tablets ... 1718
Hylorel Tablets (1.9%) ... 1613
Hytrin Capsules (0.3%) ... 434
Hyzaar Tablets ... 1720
IBU Tablets (Less than 1%) ... 1389
Indocin (Greater than 1%) ... 1723
▲ Intron A for Injection (2% to 40%) ... 2506
Invirase Capsules (Less than 2%) .. 2291
Isoptin Injectable ... 1391
Kadian Capsules (Less than 3%) ... 2948
Kerlone Tablets (0.8%) ... 2588
Klonopin Tablets ... 2294
Lamprene Capsules (Less than 1%) ... 846
Lariam Tablets ... 2295
Larodopa Tablets (Infrequent) ... 2296
Levatol Tablets (0.6%) ... 2547
Levo-Dromoran ... 2297
Lioresal Tablets ... 847
Lodine Capsules and Tablets (1% to 3%) ... 2849
Lomotil ... 2591
Lopid Tablets ... 1974
▲ Lopressor (5%) ... 848
▲ Lopressor HCT Tablets (5 in 100) 850
▲ Lupron Depot 3.75 mg (10.8%) ... 2739
Lupron Depot - 3 Month 22.5 mg (Less than 5%) ... 2743
Lupron Injection (Less than 5%) ... 2736
MS Contin Tablets (Less frequent) 2149
MSIR (Infrequent) ... 2152
Marcaine ... 2446
Marcaine Spinal ... 2449
Marinol (Dronabinol) Capsules (Less than 1%) ... 2353
Matulane Capsules ... 2300
Maxair Inhaler (Less than 1%) ... 1552
Maxaquin Tablets (Less than 1%) .. 2593
Mebaral Tablets ... 2452
Merrem I.V. (0.1% to 1.0%) ... 2952
Mesantoin Tablets ... 2400
Mevacor Tablets (0.5% to 1.0%) .. 1742
Mexitil Capsules (2.4%) ... 684
Miacalcin Nasal Spray (1% to 3%) 2403
Midamor Tablets (Less than or equal to 1%) ... 1746
Minipress Capsules (1-4%) ... 2015
Minizide Capsules (Rare) ... 2016
Mithracin ... 599
Moban Tablets and Concentrate (Less frequent) ... 1036
Modicon ... 1928
Moduretic Tablets (Less than or equal to 1%) ... 1748
8-MOP Capsules ... 1294
Monopril Tablets (0.4% to 1.0%) .. 762
Motofen Tablets ... 789
Mykrox Tablets (Less than 2%) ... 1617
Nalfon 200 Pulvules & Nalfon Tablets (Less than 1%) ... 933
Nasacort Nasal Inhaler ... 2189
Neoral (Rare) ... 2405
Nescaine/Nescaine MPF ... 549
Nicotrol NS Nicotine Nasal Spray (Under 5%) ... 1565
Nimotop Capsules (Up to 1.4%) ... 603
▲ Nipent for Injection (3% to 10%) .. 2733
Nolvadex Tablets (Infrequent; 1.9%) ... 2957
Norinyl ... 2563
Noroxin Tablets (Less frequent) ... 1758
Noroxin Tablets (Less frequent) ... 2222
Nor-Q D Tablets ... 2598
Norvasc Tablets (More than 0.1% to 1%) ... 2020
Norvir (Less than 2%) ... 447
Nubain Injection (1% or less) ... 952
Ocupress Ophthalmic Solution, 1% Sterile ... ◉ 297
OptiPranolol (Metipranolol 0.3%) Sterile Ophthalmic Solution (A small number of patients) ... ◉ 256
Oramorph SR (Morphine Sulfate Sustained Release Tablets) (Less frequent) ... 2359
▲ Orap Tablets (2 of 20 patients) ... 1037
Orlaam Oral Solution (1% to 3%) .. 2361
Ortho-Novum ... 1928
Orudis Capsules (Greater than 1%) ... 2874
Oruvail Capsules (Greater than 1%) ... 2874
Ovcon ... 765
Oxandrin ... 783
Oxsoralen-Ultra Capsules ... 1302
OxyContin Tablets (Less than 1%) 2163
Parlodel ... 2411
Pediazole Suspension ... 2340
Penetrex Tablets (0.1% to 1%) ... 2196
Pepcid Injection (Infrequent) ... 1765
Pepcid (Infrequent) ... 1763
▲ Permax Tablets (3.2%) ... 571
Phrenilin ... 790
Plendil Extended-Release Tablets (0.5% to 1.5%) ... 514
Pondimin Tablets ... 2239
Pregnyl for Injection ... 1878
Prelone Syrup ... 1834
Prevacid Delayed-Release Capsules (Less than 1%) ... 2746
Prilosec Delayed-Release Capsules (Less than 1%) ... 516
Prinivil Tablets (Greater than 1%) .. 1776
Prinzide Tablets (0.3% to 1%) ... 1780
Procardia Capsules (Less than 0.5%) ... 2024
Procardia XL Extended Release Tablets (1% or less) ... 2026
Profasi (chorionic gonadotropin for injection, USP) ... 2620
Protostat Tablets ... 1939
Quadrinal Tablets ... 1398
Quinaglute Dura-Tabs Tablets ... 644
Quinidex Extentabs (Occasional) ... 2240
▲ Redux Capsules (4.7%) ... 2911
Reglan (Less frequent) ... 2243
Relafen Tablets (1%) ... 2688
Remeron Tablets (Frequent) ... 1878
Retrovir Capsules ... 1216
Retrovir I.V. Infusion ... 1221
Retrovir Syrup ... 1216
Revex (nalmefene hydrochloride injection) (Less than 1%) ... 1863
▲ Rilutek Tablets (4.2% to 6.1%) ... 2198
Romazicon (1% to 3%) ... 2311
Rythmol Tablets–150mg, 225mg, 300mg (Less than 1%) ... 1399
Sandimmune (Rare) ... 2416
Sandostatin Injection (1% to 4%) .. 2421
Sanorex Tablets ... 2423
Sectral Capsules (2%) ... 2914
Sedapap Tablets 50 mg/650 mg (Infrequent) ... 1826
Seldane Tablets ... 1284
Seldane-D Extended-Release Tablets ... 1286
Sensorcaine ... 554
Septra ... 1146
Septra I.V. Infusion ... 1142
Septra I.V. Infusion ADD-Vantage Vials ... 1144
Septra ... 1146
Ser-Ap-Es Tablets ... 867
Serophene (clomiphene citrate tablets, USP) (Less than 1 in 100 patients) ... 2621
Sinemet Tablets ... 959
Sinemet CR Tablets (2.2%) ... 961
Stadol (Less than 1%) ... 779
Sular Tablets (Less than or equal to 1%) ... 2961
▲ Supprelin Injection (3% to 10%) ... 2230
Symmetrel Capsules (1% to 5%) .. 965
Symmetrel Syrup (1% to 5%) ... 963
▲ Synarel Nasal Solution for Endometriosis (3% of patients) .. 2605
Tagamet ... 2694
Talacen Caplets (Infrequent) ... 2464
Talwin Injection (Infrequent) ... 2465
Talwin Compound (Infrequent) ... 2466
Talwin Injection ... 2465
Talwin Nx Tablets ... 2467
Tambocor Tablets (1% to less than 3%) ... 1555
Tegison Capsules (Less than 1%) .. 2314
Tegretol/Tegretol-XR ... 870
Tenex Tablets (3% or less) ... 2249
▲ Tenoretic Tablets (0.6% to 12%) .. 2963
▲ Tenormin Tablets and I.V. Injection (0.6% to 12%) ... 2965
Testred Capsules, 10 mg ... 1308
Timolide Tablets ... 1791
Timoptic in Ocudose (Less frequent) ... 1796
Timoptic Sterile Ophthalmic Solution (Less frequent) ... 1794
Tolectin (200, 400 and 600 mg) (1 to 3%) ... 1591
Tonocard Tablets (Less than 1%) .. 519
▲ Toprol-XL Tablets (About 5 of 100 patients) ... 560
Toradol (1% or less) ... 2319
Trancopal Caplets ... 2468
Tranxene ... 459
Tri-Norinyl 28-Day Tablets ... 335
Valium Injectable ... 2336
Valium Tablets (Infrequent) ... 2335
Vascor Tablets (200 and 300 mg) (0.5 to 2.0%) ... 1597
Vaseretic Tablets ... 1810
Vasotec I.V. ... 1814
Vasotec Tablets (0.5% to 1%) ... 1816
Velban Vials ... 1537
▲ Vesanoid Capsules (14%) ... 2327
Vistide Injection ... 1057
Cataflam/Voltaren/Voltaren-XR (Less than 1%) ... 833
Wellbutrin Tablets (Frequent) ... 1177
Winstrol Tablets ... 2468
▲ Xanax Tablets (13.8% to 13.9%) .. 2115
Zantac (Rare) ... 1182
Zantac Injection (Rare) ... 1180
Zantac Syrup (Rare) ... 1182
Zaroxolyn Tablets ... 1625
Zestoretic Tablets (0.3 to 1%) ... 2968
Zestril Tablets (Greater than 1%) .. 2972
Zocor Tablets ... 1821
▲ Zoladex (Greater than 1% to 54%) ... 2976
Zoladex 3-month ... 2978
Zoloft Tablets (Infrequent) ... 2051
Zyloprim Tablets (Less than 1%) ... 1194
Zyrtec Tablets (Less than 2%) ... 2053

Depression, aggravation of

Halcion Tablets ... 2093
Intron A for Injection (Less than 5%) ... 2506
Lupron Depot 3.75 mg (A possibility) ... 2739
Tegretol-XR Tablets ... 870
Zoloft Tablets (Infrequent) ... 2051

Depression, circulatory

Brontex ... 2130
Kadian Capsules ... 2948
Methadone Hydrochloride Oral Solution & Tablets ... 2357
Oramorph SR (Morphine Sulfate Sustained Release Tablets) ... 2359
RMS Suppositories CII ... 2766
Roxanol ... 2365
Sublimaze Injection ... 463

Depression, mental

Adalat CC (Less than 1.0%) ... 582
Aldomet Ester HCl Injection ... 1642
Ambien Tablets (2%) ... 2559
Amen Tablets ... 785
▲ Androderm Testosterone Transdermal System (3%) ... 2634
▲ Android Capsules, 10 mg (Among most common) ... 1297
Aygestin Tablets ... 990
Azulfidine (Rare) ... 2059
Beconase ... 1065
Betapace Tablets (1% to 4%) ... 637
Betaseron for SC Injection ... 653
Blocadren Tablets ... 1654
Brevicon ... 2563
Cardizem CD Capsules (Less than 1%) ... 1251
Cartrol Tablets ... 413
Catapres Tablets (About 1 in 100 patients) ... 679
Catapres-TTS ... 680
Celontin Kapseals ... 1955
Chibroxin Sterile Ophthalmic Solution (With oral form) ... 1657
Chloromycetin Sodium Succinate ... 1960
Claritin Tablets (2% or fewer patients) ... 2485
Claritin-D Tablets (Less frequent) .. 2487
Climara Transdermal System ... 640
▲ Cognex Capsules (4%) ... 1961
Combipres Tablets (About 1%) ... 682
CORTENEMA ... 2713
Cortone Acetate Sterile Suspension ... 1663
Cortone Acetate Tablets ... 1664
Cycrin Tablets ... 991
Cytovene (1% or less) ... 2270
Dantrium Capsules (Less frequent) 2131
Daypro Caplets (1% to 3%) ... 2578
Decadron Elixir ... 1676
Decadron Phosphate Injection ... 1680
Decadron Phosphate with Xylocaine Injection, Sterile ... 1683
Decadron Tablets ... 1678
Decadron-LA Sterile Suspension ... 1687
Demulen ... 2580
Depakene ... 416
Depakote Tablets (1% to 5%) ... 418
Depo-Provera Contraceptive Injection (1% to 5%) ... 2079
Depo-Provera Sterile Aqueous Suspension ... 2083
Desmopressin Acetate Rhinal Tube 997

(▭ Described in PDR For Nonprescription Drugs) Incidence data in parenthesis; ▲ 3% or more (◉ Described in PDR For Ophthalmology)

1301 **Side Effects Index** **Dermatitis**

Desogen Tablets 1867
Dexacort Phosphate in Respihaler 1606
Dexacort Phosphate in Turbinaire 1607
Didronel Tablets 2133
Dilaudid Tablets and Liquid (Less frequent) 1386
Diupres Tablets 1691
Duranest Injections 533
Effexor (1%) 2825
Esgic-plus Capsules (Infrequent) 1012
Esgic-plus Tablets (Infrequent) 1012
Esimil Tablets 840
Estraderm Transdermal System 842
ESTRATAB Tablets (0.3, 0.625, 1.25, 2.5 mg) 2715
Estratest 2718
Fansidar Tablets 2281
▲ Felbatol (5.3%) 2774
Flexeril Tablets (Less than 1%) 1701
Florinef Acetate Tablets 506
Flumadine Tablets & Syrup (0.3% to 1%) 1013
Glucotrol XL Extended Release Tablets (Less than 3%) 2012
Hydeltrasol Injection, Sterile 1708
Hydeltra-T.B.A. Sterile Suspension 1710
Hydrocortone Acetate Sterile Suspension 1712
Hydrocortone Phosphate Injection, Sterile 1713
Hydrocortone Tablets 1715
Hydropres Tablets 1718
Hylorel Tablets (1.9%) 1613
Imdur (Less than or equal to 5%) 1362
Imitrex Injection (Rare) 1095
Imitrex Tablets (Infrequent) 1099
Inapsine Injection 462
Inderal 2834
Inderal LA Long Acting Capsules 2836
Inderide Tablets 2838
Inderide LA Long Acting Capsules 2840
Iopidine 0.5% (Less than 1%) ⊙ 219
Ismelin Tablets 845
Isoptin Injectable 1391
Kerlone Tablets 2588
▲ Lamictal Tablets (4.2%) 1105
Lescol Capsules 2395
Levatol Tablets 2547
Levlen/Tri-Levlen 646
Lioresal Intrathecal (Up to 1.6%) 1634
Lo/Ovral Tablets 2852
Lo/Ovral-28 Tablets 2857
Lopressor HCT Tablets 850
LUVOX Tablets (2%) 2723
Macrobid Capsules (Rare) 2138
Macrodantin Capsules (Rare) 2140
Maxair Autohaler 1550
Megace Oral Suspension (1% to 3%) 708
Menest Tablets 2671
Methadone Hydrochloride Oral Concentrate 2356
MetroGel-Vaginal 917
Modicon 1928
Monoket Tablets (Fewer than 1%) 2550
Motrin Ibuprofen Suspension, Oral Drops, Chewable Tablets, Caplets (Less than 1%) 1563
Naprelan Tablets (Less than 1%) 2861
Neurontin Capsules (1.8%) 1978
Nizoral Tablets (Rare) 1345
Nordette-21 Tablets 2863
Nordette-28 Tablets 2866
Norinyl 2563
Normodyne Tablets 2522
Nor-Q D Tablets 2598
Ogen Tablets 2103
Ogen Vaginal Cream 2106
Ortho-Cept 1907
Ortho-Cyclen/Ortho-Tri-Cyclen 1914
Ortho Dienestrol Cream 1922
Ortho-Est 1925
Ortho-Novum 1928
Ortho-Cyclen/Ortho Tri-Cyclen 1914
Ovral Tablets 2877
Ovral-28 Tablets 2878
Ovrette Tablets 2878
Paxil Tablets (Frequent) 2681
Pentasa (Less than 1%) 1275
PMB 200 and PMB 400 2890
Pravachol Tablets 770
Premarin Intravenous 2893
Premarin Tablets 2896
Premarin Vaginal Cream 2898
Premphase 2900
Prempro 2905
Prinivil Tablets (Greater than 1%) 1776
Procanbid Extended-Release Tablets (Occasional) 1983
▲ Prograf (Greater than 3%) 1028
Proleukin for Injection (Less than 1%) 812
Propulsid (More than 1%) 1346
ProSom Tablets (2%) 457
Provera Tablets 2110
Quadrinal Tablets 1398
Reglan (Less frequent) 2243
▲ ReVia Tablets (Less than 1% to 7%) 957
Risperdal Tablets (Infrequent) 1348
Ritalin 866
▲ Roferon-A Injection (16% to 28%) 2308
Salagen Tablets (Less than 1%) 1546
Sectral Capsules 2914
Serzone Tablets 776
Sporanox Capsules (Infrequent) 1352
Tenoretic Tablets 2963
Tenormin Tablets and I.V. Injection 2965
Testoderm Testosterone Transdermal System 486
Tiazac Capsules (Less than 1%) 1019
Tigan 2231
Timoptic in Ocudose 1796
Timoptic Sterile Ophthalmic Solution 1794
Timoptic-XE 1798
Toprol-XL Tablets 560
Trandate Tablets 1158
Trecator-SC Tablets 2919
Trental Tablets (Less than 1%) 1291
Levlen/Tri-Levlen 646
Tri-Norinyl 2607
Triphasil-21 Tablets 2919
Triphasil-28 Tablets 2924
Ultram Tablets (50 mg) (Less than 1%) 1594
Videx Tablets, Powder for Oral Solution, & Pediatric Powder for Oral Solution (1% to 5%) 2980
Visken Tablets 2428
Vivelle Transdermal System 880
Zantac (Rare) 1182
Zantac Injection (Rare) 1180
Zantac Syrup (Rare) 1182
Zarontin Capsules (Rare) 1986
Zarontin Syrup (Rare) 1986
Zaroxolyn Tablets 1625
Zebeta Tablets (Up to 0.2%) 1457
▲ Zerit Capsules (Fewer than 1% to 14%) 731
Ziac 1459
Zoladex (Greater than 1% but less than 5%) 2976
Zoladex 3-month 2978
Zosyn (1.0% or less) 1463

Depression, mood (see under Depression, mental)

Depression, psychotic

Effexor (Infrequent) 2825
▲ IFEX (Among most common) 706
Lioresal Intrathecal (1% or more) 1634
8-MOP Capsules 1294
Paxil Tablets (Rare) 2681
Remeron Tablets (Rare) 1878
Rilutek Tablets (Rare) 2198

Depression, respiratory

▲ Alfenta Injection (One of the two most common) 1334
Anectine 1062
Aralen Hydrochloride Injection 2430
Astramorph/PF Injection, USP (Preservative-Free) 526
Brontex 2130
Codiclear DH Syrup 808
Dalgan Injection (Less than 1%) 529
Demerol 2438
Dilaudid Ampules 1382
Dilaudid Cough Syrup 1383
Dilaudid-HP Injection 1384
Dilaudid-HP Lyophilized Powder 250 mg 1384
Dilaudid 1382
Dilaudid Oral Liquid 1386
Dilaudid 1382
Dilaudid Tablets - 8 mg 1386
Dizac (diazepam injectable emulsion) CIV 1862
Doral Tablets 2773
Duramorph Injection 983
Duranest Injections 533
Dyclone 0.5% and 1% Topical Solutions, USP 535
EMLA Cream (Unlikely with cream) 536
Felbatol 2774
Foscavir Injection (Less than 1%) 541
Garamycin Injectable 2502
Hycodan Tablets and Syrup 946
Hycomine Compound Tablets 948
Hycomine 947
Hycotuss Expectorant Syrup 950
Hydrocet Capsules 787
Infumorph 200 and Infumorph 500 Sterile Solutions 985
Kadian Capsules 2948
Klonopin Tablets 2294
Levo-Dromoran 2297
Lioresal Intrathecal 1634
Lorcet 10/650 Tablets 1016
Lortab 2751
MS Contin Tablets 2149
MSIR 2152
Marcaine 2446
Mepergan Injection 2859
Methadone Hydrochloride Oral Solution & Tablets 2357
Metubine Iodide Vials 932
Nardil (Less frequent) 1977
Norcuron for Injection 1875
Numorphan Injection 953
Numorphan Suppositories 953
Oramorph SR (Morphine Sulfate Sustained Release Tablets) 2359
OxyContin Tablets 2163
Percocet Tablets 955
Phenergan with Codeine 2883
Phenergan VC with Codeine 2888
Phenobarbital Elixir and Tablets 1523
ProSom Tablets 457
Prostigmin Injectable 1305
Prostigmin Tablets 1306
RMS Suppositories CII 2766
Roxanol 2365
Scleromate Injection (Rare) 1234
Sensorcaine 554
▲ Sublimaze Injection (Among most common) 463
▲ Sufenta Injection (One of the two most common) 1355
Survanta Beractant Intratracheal Suspension 2346
Talacen Caplets (Rare) 2464
Talwin Injection (Infrequent) 2465
Talwin Compound 2466
Talwin Injection (Infrequent) 2465
Talwin Nx Tablets (Rare) 2467
Tussionex Pennkinetic Extended-Release Suspension 1624
Tylenol with Codeine 1592
Tylox Capsules 1593
Valium Injectable 2336
Versed Injection 2324
Vicodin Tablets 1404
Vicodin ES Tablets 1405
Vicodin HP Tablets 1403
Vicodin Tuss Expectorant 1406
Xylocaine Injections 562
Zydone Capsules 967

Depression, respiratory, neonatal

Astramorph/PF Injection, USP (Preservative-Free) 526
Brontex 2130
Demerol 2438
Dilaudid Ampules 1382
Dilaudid Cough Syrup 1383
Dilaudid 1382
Duramorph Injection 983
Fioricet with Codeine Capsules 2387
Fiorinal with Codeine Capsules 2390
Hydrocet Capsules 787
Kadian Capsules 2948
Lortab 2751
MS Contin Tablets 2149
MSIR 2152
Mepergan Injection 2859
Methadone Hydrochloride Oral Solution & Tablets 2357
Normodyne Injection 2519
Oramorph SR (Morphine Sulfate Sustained Release Tablets) 2359
Percocet Tablets 955
Quadrinal Tablets 1398
Roxanol 2365
Streptomycin Sulfate Injection (Occasional) 2031
Tracrium Injection 1155
Trandate 1158
Tussionex Pennkinetic Extended-Release Suspension 1624
Tylenol with Codeine 1592
Tylox Capsules 1593
Vicodin Tablets 1404
Vicodin ES Tablets 1405

Depressive reactions

▲ Epivir (9%) 1200
Soma Compound w/Codeine Tablets (Infrequent or rare) 2784
Soma Compound Tablets (Infrequent or rare) 2783
Soma Tablets 2782
Xanax Tablets 2115

Dermal creases

Doxorubicin Astra (A few cases) 531

Dermatitis

Adalat Capsules (10 mg and 20 mg) (2% or less) 580
Ambien Tablets (Rare) 2559
Anafranil Capsules (Up to 2%) 819
Azelex (Less than 1%) 471
Benemid Tablets 1651
Benoquin Cream 20% 1298
Cataflam Tablets (Less than 1%) 833
Cerumenex Drops (1% of 2,700 patients) 2148
Claritin Tablets (2% or fewer patients) 2485
Claritin-D Tablets 2487
Clomid (Fewer than 1%) 1262
Clozaril Tablets (Less than 1%) 2377
Cognex Capsules (Infrequent) 1961
ColBENEMID Tablets 1662
Colestid (Rare) 2073
Colyte and Colyte-flavored (Isolated cases) 2540
Cormax Scalp Application (Approximately 0.3%) 1857
Coumadin (Infrequent) 941
Cozaar Tablets (Less than 1%) 1668
Crixivan Capsules (Less than 2%) 1670
Cytotec (Infrequent) 2576
Daraprim Tablets (Rare) 1199
Dilantin Infatabs 1967
Dilantin Kapseals (Rare) 1965
Dilantin-125 Suspension (Rare) 1969
▲ Dovonex Cream 0.005% (1% to 10%) 2792
▲ Dovonex Ointment 0.005% (1% to 10%) 2793
▲ Ergamisol Tablets (8% to 23%) 1340
Esimil Tablets 840
Estring Vaginal Ring (1% to 3%) 2086
Fedahist Gyrocaps (Very rare) 2545
Flovent (1% to 3%) 1089
Fluorouracil Injection (Substantial number of cases) 2282
Foscavir Injection (Less than 1%) 541
Sterile FUDR 2284
Glucophage Tablets 754
GoLYTELY (Isolated cases) 694
Halcion Tablets (Rare) 2093
Hibistat Germicidal Hand Rinse (Rare) 2948
Hivid Tablets (Less than 1%) 2287
Hyzaar Tablets 1720
IFEX (Less than 1%) 706
▲ Intron A for Injection (Up to 8%) 2506
Invirase Capsules (Less than 2%) 2291
Iopidine 0.5% (Less than 1%) ⊙ 219
Ismelin Tablets 845
▲ Leucovorin Calcium for Injection (1% to 25%) 1313
Lopid Tablets 1974
Lotensin Tablets 852
Lotrel Capsules 858
Loxitane 1426
Lupron Depot 7.5 mg (Less than 5%) 2741
▲ Lupron Injection (5% or more) 2736
Matulane Capsules 2300
Maxair Autohaler 1550
Maxair Inhaler (Less than 1%) 1552
Maxaquin Tablets 2593
Mellaril (Infrequent) 2398
Methotrexate Sodium Tablets, Injection, for Injection and LPF Injection (1% to 3%) 1322
Myambutol Tablets 1432
Mykrox Tablets 1617
Myochrysine Injection 1754
Norplant System 2868
Norvasc Tablets (Less than or equal to 0.1%) 2020
Novahistine Elixir (Very rare) ▣ 782
NuLYTELY (Isolated cases) 694
Cherry Flavor NuLYTELY (Isolated cases) 694
pHisoHex 2458
Phenergan Injection 2880
Phenergan Tablets 2882
Prinzide Tablets (0.3 to 1%) 1780
Procardia Capsules (2% or less) 2024
Proglycem 575
▲ Ridaura Capsules (Second most common) 2691
Salagen Tablets (Rare) 1546
Solganal Suspension 2530

(▣ Described in PDR For Nonprescription Drugs) Incidence data in parenthesis; ▲ 3% or more (⊙ Described in PDR For Ophthalmology)

Dermatitis | Side Effects Index | 1302

Talwin Injection 2465
Talwin Nx Tablets 2467
Temovate Scalp Application (1 of 294 patients) 1153
Tenex Tablets (3% or less) 2249
Thioplex (Thiotepa For Injection) 1329
Urispas Tablets 2710
Urobiotic-250 Capsules (Rare) 2038
Vaqta (Less than 1%) 1805
Varivax (Greater than or equal to 1%) 1807
Cataflam/Voltaren/Voltaren-XR (Less than 1%) 833
▲ Xanax Tablets (3.8%) 2115
Zaroxolyn Tablets 1625
Ziac 1459
Zoloft Tablets (Rare) 2051
Zyrtec Tablets (Less than 2%) 2053

Dermatitis, allergic

Antabuse Tablets (Small number of patients) 2802
Cortone Acetate Sterile Suspension 1663
Cortone Acetate Tablets 1664
Dalalone D.P. Injectable 1009
Decadron Elixir 1676
Decadron Phosphate Injection 1680
Decadron Phosphate with Xylocaine Injection, Sterile 1683
Decadron Tablets 1678
Decadron-LA Sterile Suspension 1687
Dexacort Phosphate in Respihaler 1606
Dexacort Phosphate in Turbinaire 1607
Halog (Infrequent) 2795
Hydeltrasol Injection, Sterile 1708
Hydeltra-T.B.A. Sterile Suspension 1710
Hydrocortone Acetate Sterile Suspension 1712
Hydrocortone Phosphate Injection, Sterile 1713
Hydrocortone Tablets 1715
Lidex (Infrequent) 2299
Lotrisone Cream (Infrequent) 2515
Monistat-Derm (miconazole nitrate 2%) Cream (Isolated reports) 1944
ProctoFoam-HC 2552
Serophene (clomiphene citrate tablets, USP) (Less than 1 in 100 patients) 2621
Tridesilon Cream 0.05% (Infrequent) 609
Tridesilon Ointment 0.05% (Infrequent) 610

Dermatitis, bullous

Chloroptic Sterile Ophthalmic Solution ⊙ 236
Dilantin Infatabs 1967
Dilantin Kapseals 1965
Dilantin-125 Suspension 1969
Miltown Tablets (Rare) 2780
PMB 200 and PMB 400 (Rare) 2890
Solganal Suspension (Occasional) 2530
T.R.U.E. Test 1162
Zyloprim Tablets (Less than 1%) 1194

Dermatitis, contact

Americaine Anesthetic Lubricant 1603
Americaine Otic Topical Anesthetic Ear Drops 1603
Avonex 662
Azelex (Less than 1%) 471
Bactroban Ointment (Less than 1%) 2642
BENZASHAVE Medicated Shave Cream 5% and 10% 1627
Betaseron for SC Injection 653
Capitrol Shampoo 2791
Catapres-TTS 680
Cerebyx Injection (Infrequent) 1956
Cleocin Vaginal Cream 2070
Compazine 2644
Crixivan Capsules (Less than 2%) 1670
Deponit NTG Transdermal Delivery System 2541
Dilacor XR Extended-release Capsules 2183
Effexor (Infrequent) 2825
Eldopaque/Eldoquin/Solaquin/Viquin (Occasional) 1299
Etrafon 2495
Furacin Soluble Dressing (Approximately 1%) 2220
Furacin Topical Cream (Approximately 1%) 2220
Iopidine 0.5% (Less than 1%) ⊙ 219
Lioresal Intrathecal (1% or more) 1634
Mellaril 2398
Naprelan Tablets (Less than 1%) 2861
Navane Capsules and Concentrate 2018
Navane Intramuscular 2019
Nitro-Bid IV 1270
Nitro-Bid Ointment (Uncommon) 1272
Nitro-Dur (nitroglycerin) Transdermal Infusion System (Uncommon) 1365
Nizoral 2% Cream (Rare) 1344
Norvir (Less than 2%) 447
Paxil Tablets (Rare) 2681
Prozac Pulvules & Liquid, Oral Solution (Infrequent) 935
Rhinocort Nasal Inhaler (Less than 1%) 552
Rilutek Tablets (Rare) 2198
Serentil 689
Eldopaque/Eldoquin/Solaquin/Viquin (Occasional) 1299
Thioplex (Thiotepa For Injection) 1329
Thorazine 2701
Torecan 2367
Tympagesic Ear Drops 2476
Varivax (Greater than or equal to 1%) 1807
Viquin Forte 4% Cream (Occasional) 1299

Dermatitis, eczematoid

Symmetrel Capsules (Less than 0.1%) 965
Symmetrel Syrup (Less than 0.1%) 963
Zyloprim Tablets (Less than 1%) 1194

Dermatitis, erythematous

Phenobarbital Elixir and Tablets 1523

Dermatitis, exfoliative

Abelcet Injection 1540
Accupril Tablets (Rare) 1950
Achromycin V Capsules (Uncommon) 1417
Adalat Capsules (10 mg and 20 mg) (Less than 0.5%) 580
Adalat CC (Rare) 582
Aldoclor Tablets 1638
Aldoril Tablets 1644
Aquasol A Vitamin A Capsules, USP 525
Atretol Tablets 569
Augmentin (Occasional) 2637
Augmentin Tablets (Occasional) 2640
Axid Pulvules 1468
Azactam for Injection (Less than 1%) 736
Azulfidine (Rare) 2059
Bactrim DS Tablets 2257
Bactrim I.V. Infusion 2255
Bactrim 2257
Betaseron for SC Injection 653
Bicillin C-R Injection 2810
Bicillin C-R 900/300 Injection 2812
Bicillin L-A Injection 2813
Butisol Sodium Elixir & Tablets (Less than 1 in 100) 2768
Capoten Tablets 740
Capozide Tablets 744
Cardizem CD Capsules (Infrequent) 1251
Cardizem SR Capsules (Infrequent) 1255
Cardizem Injectable 1253
Cardizem Tablets 1257
Cataflam Tablets (Rare) 833
Chibroxin Sterile Ophthalmic Solution (With oral form) 1657
Cipro I.V. (1% or less) 587
Cipro I.V. Pharmacy Bulk Package (Less than 1%) 590
Cipro Tablets 584
Clinoril Tablets 1658
Compazine 2644
Cuprimine Capsules 1673
Cytovene-IV (One report) 2270
Daypro Caplets (Less than 1%) 2578
Declomycin Tablets (Uncommon) 1421
Depen Titratable Tablets 2770
Diabinese Tablets 2002
Diflucan Tablets, Injection, and Oral Suspension (Rare) 2003
Dilantin Infatabs 1967
Dilantin Kapseals 1965
Dilantin-125 Suspension 1969
Diupres Tablets 1691
Diuril Oral Suspension 1694
Diuril Sodium Intravenous 1693
Diuril Tablets 1694
Dolobid Tablets (Less than 1 in 100) 1695
Doryx Capsules (Uncommon) 1970
Doxil (Less than 1%) 2613
Duragesic Transdermal System (Less than 1%) 1336
DYNACIN Capsules (Uncommon) 1627
Effexor (Rare) 2825
Ergamisol Tablets (Less frequent) 1340
Etrafon 2495
Fansidar Tablets 2281
Feldene Capsules (Less than 1%) 2008
Fioricet with Codeine Capsules 2387
Fiorinal with Codeine Capsules 2390
Floxin I.V. 1580
Floxin Tablets (200 mg, 300 mg, 400 mg) 1577
Gantanol Tablets 2285
Gantrisin 2286
Helidac Therapy (Rare) 2135
Hivid Tablets (Less than 1%) 2287
HydroDIURIL Tablets 1716
Hydropres Tablets 1718
Hyzaar Tablets 1720
Imitrex Tablets (Rare) 1099
Indocin Capsules (Less than 1%) 1723
Indocin I.V. (Less than 1%) 1727
Indocin (Less than 1%) 1723
Intal Inhaler (Rare) 2185
Intal Nebulizer Solution (Rare) 2186
Lasix Injection, Oral Solution and Tablets 1267
Levoprome 1321
Lopid Tablets 1974
LUVOX Tablets (Infrequent) 2723
Macrobid Capsules (Rare) 2138
Macrodantin Capsules (Rare) 2140
Maxaquin Tablets 2593
Mebaral Tablets (Less than 1 in 100) 2452
Mefoxin 1734
Mefoxin Premixed Intravenous Solution 1737
Mellaril 2398
Mesantoin Tablets (Rare) 2400
Mexitil Capsules (Rare) 684
Miltown Tablets (Rare) 2780
Minocin Intravenous (Uncommon) 1428
Minocin Oral Suspension (Uncommon) 1431
Minocin Pellet-Filled Capsules (Uncommon) 1429
Moduretic Tablets 1748
Monodox Capsules (Uncommon) 1858
Monopril Tablets 762
Motrin Ibuprofen Suspension, Oral Drops, Chewable Tablets, Caplets (Less than 1%) 1563
Myochrysine Injection 1754
Nalfon 200 Pulvules & Nalfon Tablets (Less than 1%) 933
Nasalcrom Nasal Solution (Rare) 2192
Navane Capsules and Concentrate 2018
Navane Intramuscular 2019
Nebcin Vials, Hyporets & ADD-Vantage 1518
Nembutal Sodium Capsules (Less than 1%) 440
Nembutal Sodium Solution 442
Nembutal Sodium Suppositories (Less than 1%) 444
Nitrolingual Spray 2193
Nitrostat Tablets 1981
Noroxin Tablets 1758
Noroxin Tablets 2222
Omnipen Capsules (Occasional) 2872
Omnipen for Oral Suspension (Occasional) 2873
Orudis Capsules (Less than 1%) 2874
Oruvail Capsules (Less than 1%) 2874
OxyContin Tablets (Less than 1%) 2163
PASER Granules 1333
Pediazole Suspension 2340
Pen•Vee K 2879
Pfizerpen for Injection 2022
Phenobarbital Elixir and Tablets (Less than 1 in 100 patients) 1523
Plaquenil Sulfate Tablets 2459
PMB 200 and PMB 400 (Rare) 2890
Prinzide Tablets 1780
Procardia Capsules (Less than 0.5%) 2024
Procardia XL Extended Release Tablets (Rare) 2026
▲ Proleukin for Injection (14%) 812
Prolixin 510
Proloprim Tablets (Rare) 1141
Prozac Pulvules & Liquid, Oral Solution 935
Remeron Tablets (Infrequent) 1878
Rifamate Capsules 1278
Rifater 1280
Rilutek Tablets (Up to 1.2%) 2198
Risperdal Tablets (Infrequent) 1348
Ritalin 866
SSD 1402
Seconal Sodium Pulvules (Less than 1 in 100) 1529
Septra 1146
Septra I.V. Infusion 1142
Septra I.V. Infusion ADD-Vantage Vials 1144
Septra 1146
Serentil 689
Silvadene Cream 1% 1288
Solganal Suspension (Occasional) 2530
Spectrobid Tablets (Occasional) 2030
Stelazine (Occasional) 2692
Sular Tablets (Less than or equal to 1%) 2961
Tagamet (Very rare) 2694
Tambocor Tablets (Less than 1%) 1555
Tapazole Tablets 1361
Taxol Injection (Rare) 723
Tegretol/Tegretol-XR 870
Tenex Tablets (Less frequent) 2249
Terramycin Intramuscular Solution (Uncommon) 2034
Thorazine 2701
Tiazac Capsules (Infrequent) 1019
Ticlid Tablets (Rare) 2317
Timolide Tablets 1791
Tonocard Tablets (Less than 1%) 519
Toradol 2319
Torecan 2367
Triavil Tablets 1800
Trilafon 2532
Trimpex Tablets (Rare) 2323
Unasyn (Occasional) 2035
Vancocin HCl, Oral Solution & Pulvules (Infrequent) 1536
Vancocin HCl, Vials & ADD-Vantage (Infrequent) 1534
Vantin for Oral Suspension and Vantin Tablets (Less than 1%) 2112
Vaseretic Tablets 1810
Vasotec I.V. 1814
Vasotec Tablets (0.5% to 1.0%) 1816
Vibramycin (Uncommon) 2038
Vibramycin Hyclate Intravenous (Uncommon) 2040
Vibramycin (Uncommon) 2038
Videx Tablets, Powder for Oral Solution, & Pediatric Powder for Oral Solution (Less than 1%) 2980
Cataflam/Voltaren/Voltaren-XR (Rare) 833
Wellbutrin Tablets 1177
Zebeta Tablets 1457
Zerit Capsules (Up to 1%) 731
Zestoretic Tablets 2968
Ziac (Very rare) 1459
Zyloprim Tablets (Less than 1%) 1194

Dermatitis, eyelid

OptiPranolol (Metipranolol 0.3%) Sterile Ophthalmic Solution (A small number of patients) ⊙ 256
Vantin for Oral Suspension and Vantin Tablets 2112

Dermatitis, flare-up

T.R.U.E. Test 1162

Dermatitis, fungal

▲ CellCept Capsules (More than or equal to 3%) 2265
Effexor (Rare) 2825
Lamictal Tablets (Rare) 1105
Paxil Tablets (Rare) 2681
Permax Tablets (Infrequent) 571
Prozac Pulvules & Liquid, Oral Solution (Rare) 935
Redux Capsules (Infrequent) 2911
Rilutek Tablets (Infrequent) 2198
Sular Tablets (Less than or equal to 1%) 2961
Videx Tablets, Powder for Oral Solution, & Pediatric Powder for Oral Solution (Less than 1%) 2980

Dermatitis, gold-induced

Ridaura Capsules 2691
Solganal Suspension 2530

Dermatitis, lichenoides

Betaseron for SC Injection 653
Effexor (Rare) 2825
Intron A for Injection (Less than 5%) 2506
Permax Tablets (Rare) 571
Risperdal Tablets (Rare) 1348

Dermatitis, maculopapular

Chloroptic S.O.P. ⊙ 236

(Described in PDR For Nonprescription Drugs) Incidence data in parenthesis; ▲ 3% or more (⊙ Described in PDR For Ophthalmology)

Side Effects Index — Diaphoresis

Chloroptic Sterile Ophthalmic Solution ... ⊚ 236
Solganal Suspension (Occasional) .. 2530

Dermatitis, perioral

Aclovate (Infrequent) ... 1061
Analpram-HC Rectal Cream 1% and 2.5% ... 993
Anusol-HC Cream 2.5% (Infrequent to frequent) ... 1953
Cordran Lotion (Infrequent) ... 1854
Cordran Tape (Infrequent) ... 1855
Cormax Ointment (Infrequent) ... 1856
Cormax Scalp Application (Infrequent) ... 1857
Cortisporin Cream ... 1073
Cortisporin Ointment ... 1074
Cortisporin Otic Solution Sterile ... 1076
Cortisporin Otic Suspension Sterile ... 1077
Cutivate Cream ... 1078
Cutivate Ointment (Infrequent to more frequent) ... 1078
Decadron Phosphate Topical Cream ... 1686
Decaspray Topical Aerosol ... 1689
Dermatop Emollient Cream 0.1% (Infrequent to frequent) ... 1264
DesOwen Cream, Ointment and Lotion (Infrequent) ... 1032
Diprolene AF Cream 0.05% (Infrequent) ... 2489
Diprolene Gel 0.05% (Infrequent) ... 2490
Diprolene Lotion 0.05% (Infrequent) ... 2491
Diprolene Ointment 0.05% (Infrequent) ... 2491
Elocon Cream 0.1% (Infrequent) ... 2492
Elocon Lotion 0.1% (Infrequent) ... 2493
Elocon Ointment 0.1% (Infrequent) ... 2494
Epifoam (Infrequent) ... 2543
Florone/Florone E ... 921
Halog (Infrequent) ... 2795
Hytone ... 922
Hytone Ointment 2 ½% ... 923
Lidex (Infrequent) ... 2299
Locoid Cream, Ointment and Topical Solution (Infrequent) ... 994
Lotrisone Cream (Infrequent) ... 2515
NeoDecadron Topical Cream ... 1757
Pandel Cream, 0.1% ... 2475
Pediotic Suspension Sterile ... 1140
Pramosone Cream, Lotion & Ointment ... 995
ProctoCream-HC 2.5% (Infrequent to frequent) ... 2552
ProctoFoam-HC ... 2552
Psorcon Cream 0.05% (Infrequent) ... 924
Psorcon Ointment 0.05% (Infrequent) ... 923
Synalar (Infrequent) ... 2299
Temovate Cream ... 1152
Temovate E Emollient (Infrequent) ... 1154
Temovate Gel (Infrequent) ... 1153
Temovate Ointment ... 1152
Temovate Scalp Application (Infrequent) ... 1153
Topicort Emollient Cream 0.25% (Infrequent) ... 1289
Topicort Gel 0.05% (Infrequent) ... 1290
Topicort LP Emollient Cream 0.05% (Infrequent) ... 1289
Topicort Ointment 0.25% (Infrequent) ... 1291
Tridesilon Cream 0.05% (Infrequent) ... 609
Tridesilon Ointment 0.05% (Infrequent) ... 610
Ultravate Cream 0.05% (Infrequent) ... 2797
Ultravate Ointment 0.05% (Infrequent) ... 2798
Westcort Cream 0.2% (Infrequent) ... 2799
Westcort Ointment 0.2% ... 2800

Dermatitis, photosensitive

Anaprox/Naprosyn (Less than 1%) ... 2277
▲ Cordarone Tablets (4 to 9%) ... 2818
EC-Naprosyn Delayed-Release Tablets (Less than 1%) ... 2277
Intal Inhaler (Rare) ... 2185
Intal Nebulizer Solution (Rare) ... 2186
▲ Naprelan Tablets (3% to 9%) ... 2861
Anaprox/Naprosyn (Less than 1%) ... 2277

Dermatitis, purpuric

Dilantin Infatabs ... 1967
Dilantin Kapseals ... 1965

Dilantin-125 Suspension ... 1969

Dermatitis, radiation recall

Etopophos for Injection (Single report) ... 701
Etoposide Injection (Single case) ... 539
Methotrexate Sodium Tablets, Injection, for Injection and LPF Injection ... 1322
Taxol Injection (Rare) ... 723
VePesid Capsules and Injection (Single case) ... 727

Dermatitis, vesicular bullous
(see under Dermatitis, bullous)

Dermatologic reactions, unspecified

Altace Capsules (Less than 1%) ... 1238
Ativan Tablets (Less frequent) ... 2807
Axocet Capsules (Infrequent) ... 2469
Bentyl ... 1246
Capoten Tablets ... 740
Capozide Tablets ... 744
Clinoril Tablets (Less than 1 in 100) ... 1658
Depen Titratable Tablets (Rare) ... 2770
Esgic-plus Capsules (Infrequent) ... 1012
Esgic-plus Tablets (Infrequent) ... 1012
Fioricet Tablets (Several cases) ... 2386
Fioricet with Codeine Capsules (Several cases) ... 2387
Floxin I.V. ... 1580
Floxin Tablets (200 mg, 300 mg, 400 mg) ... 1577
Hydrea Capsules (Less frequent) ... 705
▲ Idamycin Injection (46%) ... 2096
Kerlone Tablets (Less than 2%) ... 2588
Kutrase Capsules ... 2546
Levbid Extended-Release Tablets ... 2549
Levoprome ... 1321
Levsin/Levsinex/Levbid ... 2549
Metrodin (urofollitropin for injection) ... 2616
Monopril Tablets ... 762
Norflex (Rare) ... 1554
Norgesic (Rare) ... 1554
Phrenilin (Several cases) ... 790
Prinivil Tablets (0.3% to 1.0%) ... 1776
Prinzide Tablets ... 1780
Pro-Banthine Tablets ... 2226
SSD ... 1402
Sedapap Tablets 50 mg/650 mg (Several cases) ... 1826
Silvadene Cream 1% ... 1288
Vaseretic Tablets ... 1810
Vasotec I.V. ... 1814
Vasotec Tablets (0.5% to 1.0%) ... 1816
Zestoretic Tablets ... 2968
Zestril Tablets (0.3% to 1.0%) ... 2972

Dermatomyositis

Cuprimine Capsules (Rare) ... 1673
Depen Titratable Tablets (Rare) ... 2770
Pravachol Tablets (Rare) ... 770

Dermatomyositis, exacerbation of

Actimmune (Rare) ... 1043

Dermatopolymycositis

Accupril Tablets (Rare) ... 1950

Descemetitis

FLUORACAINE (Sometimes) ... ⊚ 208
FLURESS (Sometimes) ... ⊚ 208
Ophthetic ... ⊚ 244

Despondency

Hydropres Tablets ... 1718

Desquamation

Aquasol A Vitamin A Capsules, USP ... 525
Aquasol A Parenteral ... 526
A/T/S 2% Acne Topical Solution ... 1244
Cognex Capsules (Rare) ... 1961
Cytosar-U Sterile Powder (Rare) ... 2077
Doxil (Some patients) ... 2613
Erycette (erythromycin 2%) Topical Solution ... 1943
Feldene Capsules (Less than 1%) ... 2008
Fluorouracil Injection ... 2282
Hivid Tablets (Less than 1%) ... 2287
Neurontin Capsules (Rare) ... 1978
Peridex ... 2127
Periogard Oral Rinse ... 892
T-Stat 2.0% Topical Solution and Pads ... 2797
▲ Taxotere for Injection Concentrate (5.6%) ... 2204
THERAMYCIN Z 2% Solution ... 1629

Vagistat-1 (Less than 1%) ... 783

Diabetes
(see under Diabetes mellitus)

Diabetes insipidus

Sandostatin Injection (Less than 1%) ... 2421

Diabetes insipidus, nephrogenic

Betaseron for SC Injection ... 653
Declomycin Tablets ... 1421
Eskalith (Some reports) ... 2658
Foscavir Injection (Rare) ... 541
Lithonate/Lithotabs/Lithobid (Occasional) ... 2721
Zanosar Sterile Powder (Two patients) ... 2119

Diabetes mellitus

Accutane Capsules ... 2252
Anafranil Capsules (Infrequent) ... 819
Betaseron for SC Injection ... 653
Casodex Tablets (2% to 5%) ... 2934
▲ CellCept Capsules (More than or equal to 3%) ... 2265
Cognex Capsules (Infrequent) ... 1961
Doxil (Less than 1%) ... 2613
Dyazide Capsules ... 2653
Effexor (Infrequent) ... 2825
Foscavir Injection (Less than 1%) ... 541
Hivid Tablets (Less than 1%) ... 2287
Hydeltra-T.B.A. Sterile Suspension ... 1710
Kerlone Tablets (Less than 2%) ... 2588
Lupron Depot 7.5 mg (Less than 5%) ... 2741
Lupron Injection (Less than 5%) ... 2736
LUVOX Tablets (Rare) ... 2723
Macrobid Capsules ... 2138
Macrodantin Capsules ... 2140
Methotrexate Sodium Tablets, Injection, for Injection and LPF Injection ... 1322
Norvir (Less than 2%) ... 447
Paxil Tablets (Rare) ... 2681
Permax Tablets (Infrequent) ... 571
Prevacid Delayed-Release Capsules (Less than 1%) ... 2746
Prinivil Tablets (0.3% to 1.0%) ... 1776
Prinzide Tablets ... 1780
▲ Prograf (Greater than 3%) ... 1028
Pulmozyme Inhalation ... 1054
Redux Capsules (Infrequent) ... 2911
Remeron Tablets (Rare) ... 1878
Rilutek Tablets (Infrequent) ... 2198
Risperdal Tablets (Infrequent) ... 1348
Roferon-A Injection (Infrequent) ... 2308
Sular Tablets (Less than or equal to 1%) ... 2961
Videx Tablets, Powder for Oral Solution, & Pediatric Powder for Oral Solution (Rare) ... 2980
Zestoretic Tablets ... 2968
Zestril Tablets (0.3% to 1.0%) ... 2972
Zoladex 3-month (1% to 5%) ... 2978
Zyrtec Tablets (Less than 2%) ... 2053

Diabetes mellitus, increase

Hydrocortone Phosphate Injection, Sterile ... 1713

Diabetes mellitus, precipitation of latent

Apresazide Capsules ... 824
Capozide Tablets ... 744
Celestone Soluspan Suspension ... 2484
CORTENEMA ... 2713
Cortone Acetate Sterile Suspension ... 1663
Cortone Acetate Tablets ... 1664
Dalalone D.P. Injectable ... 1009
Decadron Elixir ... 1676
Decadron Phosphate Injection ... 1680
Decadron Phosphate with Xylocaine Injection, Sterile ... 1683
Decadron Tablets ... 1678
Decadron-LA Sterile Suspension ... 1687
Dexacort Phosphate in Respihaler ... 1606
Dexacort Phosphate in Turbinaire ... 1607
Esidrix Tablets ... 839
Florinef Acetate Tablets ... 506
Hydeltrasol Injection, Sterile ... 1708
Hydrocortone Acetate Sterile Suspension ... 1712
Hydrocortone Tablets ... 1715
Intron A for Injection (Less than 5%) ... 2506
Lasix Injection, Oral Solution and Tablets (Rare) ... 1267
Oretic Tablets ... 450
Orudis Capsules (Rare) ... 2874

Oruvail Capsules (Rare) ... 2874
Pediapred Oral Solution ... 1618
Prelone Syrup ... 1834
Prinzide Tablets ... 1780
Risperdal Tablets ... 1348
Tenoretic Tablets ... 2963
Vaseretic Tablets ... 1810
Zestoretic Tablets ... 2968

Dialysis encephalopathy

ALternaGEL Liquid ... 1358
Amphojel ... 2802
Basaljel ... 2810
Gelusil Antacid-Anti-gas Liquid ... ᴺᴾ 819
Gelusil Antacid-Anti-gas Tablets ... ᴺᴾ 819
Maalox Antacid/Anti-Gas Tablets ... 889
Maalox Heartburn Relief Suspension ... ᴺᴾ 658
Maalox Antacid Liquid ... 888
Extra Strength Maalox Antacid/Anti-Gas Liquid and Tablets ... 888
Mylanta ... 1359
Rolaids Antacid Tablets ... ᴺᴾ 807

Dialysis osteomalacia, results in, or worsening of

ALternaGEL Liquid ... 1358
Amphojel ... 2802
Basaljel ... 2810
Gelusil Antacid-Anti-gas Liquid ... ᴺᴾ 819
Gelusil Antacid-Anti-gas Tablets ... ᴺᴾ 819
Maalox Antacid/Anti-Gas Tablets ... 889
Maalox Heartburn Relief Suspension ... ᴺᴾ 658
Maalox Antacid Liquid ... 888
Mylanta ... 1359
Rolaids Antacid Tablets ... ᴺᴾ 807

Diaphoresis

Accupril Tablets (0.5% to 1.0%) ... 1950
Accutane Capsules (Less than 1%) ... 2252
Actigall Capsules ... 818
Adalat Capsules (10 mg and 20 mg) (2% or less) ... 580
Adalat CC (Less than 1.0%) ... 582
Adapin Capsules (Occasional) ... 1542
Adenocard Injection (Less than 1%) ... 1021
Adenoscan (Less than 1%) ... 1022
AeroBid Inhaler System (1% to 3%) ... 1004
Aerobid-M Inhaler System (1% to 3%) ... 1004
Albalon Solution with Liquifilm ... ⊚ 229
Alferon N Injection (One patient to 3%) ... 2142
Altace Capsules (Less than 1%) ... 1238
Alupent Tablets (0.2%) ... 672
Ambien Tablets (Infrequent) ... 2559
▲ Anafranil Capsules (9% to 29%) ... 819
Ana-Kit Anaphylaxis Emergency Treatment Kit ... 611
Anaprox/Naprosyn (Less than 3%) ... 2277
AquaMEPHYTON Injection ... 1648
Aredia for Injection ... 827
Arimidex Tablets (1.2% to 1.5%) ... 2932
▲ Asacol Delayed-Release Tablets (3%) ... 2129
Asendin Tablets (Less frequent) ... 1419
Atamet Tablets ... 567
Atretol Tablets ... 569
Atromid-S Capsules ... 2808
▲ Axid Pulvules (More frequent) ... 1468
Azactam for Injection (Less than 1%) ... 736
Benadryl Injection ... 1955
▲ Betapace Tablets (1% to 6%) ... 637
▲ Betaseron for SC Injection (23%) ... 653
Blocadren Tablets (Less than 1%) ... 1654
Bontril Slow-Release Capsules ... 786
Brethine Ampuls (0.0 to 2.4%) ... 832
Brethine Tablets ... 831
▲ Brevibloc (esmolol HCl) Injection (12%) ... 1860
Bricanyl Subcutaneous Injection ... 1247
Bricanyl Tablets ... 1248
Brontex ... 2130
Bumex (0.1%) ... 2260
▲ Buprenex Injectable (1-5%) ... 2170
BuSpar Tablets (1%) ... 738
Calan SR Caplets (1% or less) ... 2571
Calan Tablets (1% or less) ... 2568
Capoten Tablets ... 740
Capozide Tablets ... 744
Carbastat Intraocular Solution ... ⊚ 260
Carbocaine Injection ... 2432
Cardene I.V. (1.4%) ... 2815
Cardene SR Capsules (0.6%) ... 2264

(ᴺᴾ Described in PDR For Nonprescription Drugs)   Incidence data in parentheses; ▲ 3% or more   (⊚ Described in PDR For Ophthalmology)

Diaphoresis
Side Effects Index
1304

Cardizem Injectable (Less than 1%) 1253
Cardura Tablets (0.5% to 1.1%) 1993
Cartrol Tablets (0.7-1.0%) 413
▲ Casodex Tablets (5%) 2934
Cataflam Tablets (Less than 1%) 833
Caverject Injection (Less than 1%) 2064
Celestone Soluspan Suspension 2484
▲ CellCept Capsules (More than or equal to 3%) 2265
Cerebyx Injection (Infrequent) 1956
Cipro I.V. (1% or less) 587
Cipro I.V. Pharmacy Bulk Package (Less than 1%) 590
Claritin Tablets (2% or fewer patients) 2485
Claritin-D Tablets (Less frequent) 2487
Clinoril Tablets (Less than 1 in 100) 1658
▲ Clozaril Tablets (More than 5 to 6%) 2377
Cognex Capsules (Frequent) 1961
Compazine 2644
CORTENEMA 2713
Cortifoam 2540
Cortone Acetate Sterile Suspension 1663
Cortone Acetate Tablets 1664
Covera-HS Tablets (Less than 2%) 2573
Cozaar Tablets (Less than 1%) 1668
Crixivan Capsules (Less than 2%) 1670
Cystospaz 2123
Cytotec (Infrequent) 2576
▲ Cytovene (11%) 2270
D.H.E. 45 Injection (Occasional) 2381
Dalalone D.P. Injectable 1009
Dalgan Injection (Less than 1%) 529
Dalmane Capsules (Rare) 2329
Danocrine Capsules 2437
Dantrium Capsules (Less frequent) 2131
▲ DaunoXome (2% to 12%) 1842
Decadron Elixir 1676
Decadron Phosphate Injection 1680
Decadron Phosphate with Xylocaine Injection, Sterile 1683
Decadron Tablets 1678
Decadron-LA Sterile Suspension 1687
▲ Demerol (Among most frequent) 2438
Depo-Provera Contraceptive Injection (Fewer than 1%) 2079
Desyrel and Desyrel Dividose (Less than 1% to 1.4%) 504
Dexacort Phosphate in Respihaler 1606
Dexacort Phosphate in Turbinaire 1607
Dilacor XR Extended-release Capsules 2183
▲ Dilaudid-HP Injection (Among most frequent) 1384
▲ Dilaudid-HP Lyophilized Powder 250 mg (Among most frequent) 1384
Dilaudid Tablets and Liquid 1386
Diprivan Injectable Emulsion (Less than 1%) 2939
Dolobid Tablets (Less than 1 in 100) 1695
Dopram Injectable 2235
▲ Duragesic Transdermal System (10% or more) 1336
Dyazide Capsules 2653
Dynabac (0.1% to 1%) 668
Easprin 1971
EC-Naprosyn Delayed-Release Tablets (Less than 3%) 2277
▲ Effexor (2% to 19.3%) 2825
Elavil 2945
Eldepryl Capsules 2729
Emete-con Intramuscular/Intravenous 2007
▲ Eminase (Less than 10%) 2215
Engerix-B Unit-Dose Vials (Less than 1%) 2656
▲ Ethmozine Tablets (2% to 5%) 2217
Etopophos for Injection (Sometimes; 3%) 701
Etoposide Injection (Sometimes) 539
Etrafon 2495
Felbatol 2774
Feldene Capsules (Less than 1%) 2008
Flexeril Tablets (Less than 1%) 1701
▲ Flolan for Injection (1% to 15%) 1085
Florinef Acetate Tablets 506
Floxin I.V. (Less than 1%) 1580
Floxin Tablets (200 mg, 300 mg, 400 mg) (Less than 1%) 1577
▲ Fludara for Injection (1% to 13%) 658
Flumadine Tablets & Syrup 1013
▲ Foscavir Injection (5% or greater) 541
Gammar-P I.V., Immune Globulin Intravenous (Human) 798
Gemzar for Injection (Infrequent) 1482
Glucotrol XL Extended Release Tablets (Less than 3%) 2012
Haldol Decanoate 1587
Haldol Injection, Tablets and Concentrate 1585
Hivid Tablets (Less than 1%) 2287
Humalog Injection (Less common) 1488
Humorsol Sterile Ophthalmic Solution (Rare) 1707
Humulin 50/50, 100 Units 1491
Humulin 70/30, 100 Units 1492
Humulin L, 100 Units (Less common) 1494
Hydeltrasol Injection, Sterile 1708
Hydeltra-T.B.A. Sterile Suspension 1710
Hydrocortone Acetate Sterile Suspension 1712
Hydrocortone Phosphate Injection, Sterile 1713
Hydrocortone Tablets 1715
Hyperstat I.V. Injection 2504
Hytrin Capsules (At least 1%) 434
Hyzaar Tablets 1720
Regular, 100 Units 1503
Pork Regular, 100 Units (Less common) 1507
Imdur (Less than or equal to 5%) 1362
Imitrex Injection (1.6%) 1095
Imitrex Tablets (Infrequent) 1099
Indocin (Less than 1%) 1723
INFeD (Iron Dextran Injection, USP) 2478
▲ Intron A for Injection (1% to 21%) 2506
Invirase Capsules (Less than 2%) 2291
Isoptin Injectable 1391
Isoptin Oral Tablets (Less than 1%) 1393
Isoptin SR Tablets (1% or less) 1395
Isopto Carbachol Ophthalmic Solution ⊙ 221
Isuprel Hydrochloride Solution 2443
Isuprel Injection 2441
Isuprel Mistometer 2442
Kadian Capsules (Less than 3%) 2948
Kerlone Tablets (Less than 2%) 2588
Lamictal Tablets (Infrequent) 1105
Larodopa Tablets (Infrequent) 2296
▲ Leukine (6%) 1317
▲ Leustatin (9%) 1889
Levatol Tablets (1.6%) 2547
Levo-Dromoran 2297
Levophed Bitartrate Injection 2445
Limbitrol 2333
Lioresal Intrathecal (1% or more) 1634
Lioresal Tablets 847
Lithonate/Lithotabs/Lithobid 2721
Lodine Capsules and Tablets (Less than 1%) 2849
Lopressor HCT Tablets (1 in 100 patients) 850
Lotensin Tablets 852
Lotensin HCT Tablets (0.3% to 1.0%) 855
Loxitane 1426
Ludiomil Tablets (Rare) 861
▲ Lupron Depot 3.75 mg (72.9%) 2739
▲ Lupron Depot 7.5 mg (58.9%) 2741
▲ Lupron Depot - 3 Month 22.5 mg (58.5%) 2743
▲ LUVOX Tablets (7%) 2723
▲ MS Contin Tablets (Less frequent to among most frequent) 2149
▲ MSIR (Among most frequent) 2152
Marax Tablets & DF Syrup 2015
Marcaine (Rare) 2446
Marcaine Spinal (Rare) 2449
Marinol (Dronabinol) Capsules (Less than 1%) 2353
Matulane Capsules 2300
Maxaquin Tablets (Less than 1%) 2593
▲ Megace Oral Suspension (1% to 3%) 708
Mellaril 2398
▲ Mepergan Injection (Among most frequent) 2859
Mephyton Tablets (Rare) 1739
▲ Mepron Suspension (10%) 1206
Merrem I.V. (0.1% to 1.0%) 2952
Mestinon Injectable 1300
Mestinon 1300
Methadone Hydrochloride Oral Concentrate 2356
Methadone Hydrochloride Oral Solution & Tablets 2357
Methergine (Rare) 2401
Methotrexate Sodium Tablets, Injection, for Injection and LPF Injection (Less common) 1322
Mexitil Capsules (Less than 1% or about 6 in 1,000) 684
Minipress Capsules 2015
Minizide Capsules 2016
Miochol-E with Iocare Steri-Tags and Miochol-E System Pak (Rare) ⊙ 263
MIOSTAT Intraocular Solution ⊙ 222
Moban Tablets and Concentrate 1036
Moduretic Tablets (Less than or equal to 1%) 1748
Mono-Gesic Tablets 810
Monoket Tablets (Fewer than 1%) 2550
Monopril Tablets (0.2% to 1.0%) 762
MSTA Mumps Skin Test Antigen 2988
Myochrysine Injection 1754
▲ Nalfon 200 Pulvules & Nalfon Tablets (4.6%) 933
Naprelan Tablets (Less than 1%) 2861
Anaprox/Naprosyn (Less than 3%) 2277
Narcan Injection 950
Nardil (Less common) 1977
Navane Capsules and Concentrate 2018
Navane Intramuscular 2019
Nescaine/Nescaine MPF 549
Neurontin Capsules (Infrequent) 1978
▲ Nicotrol NS Nicotine Nasal Spray (Over 5%) 1565
Nimotop Capsules (Less than 1%) 603
▲ Nipent for Injection (8% to 10%) 2733
Nitrolingual Spray 2193
Nitrostat Tablets 1981
Norisodrine with Calcium Iodide Syrup 446
▲ Normodyne Injection (4%) 2519
Normodyne Tablets (Less than 1%) 2522
Norpramin Tablets 1273
Norvasc Tablets (More than 0.1% to 1%) 2020
Norvir (1.3% to 2.6%) 447
Novolin 70/30 Prefilled Disposable Insulin Delivery System (Rare) 1850
▲ Nubain Injection (9%) 952
Nucofed 2225
▲ Oramorph SR (Morphine Sulfate Sustained Release Tablets) (Among most frequent) 2359
Orap Tablets 1037
▲ Orlaam Oral Solution (3% to 9%) 2361
Ornade Spansule Capsules 2678
Orthoclone OKT3 Sterile Solution 1892
Orudis Capsules (Less than 1%) 2874
Oruvail Capsules (Less than 1%) 2874
▲ OxyContin Tablets (5%) 2163
Pamelor 2409
Papaverine Hydrochloride Vials and Ampoules 1523
▲ Paxil Tablets (1.0% to 19.2%) 2681
Pediapred Oral Solution 1618
Pentasa (Less than 1%) 1275
Peptavlon 2997
Periactin 1767
Permax Tablets (2.1%) 571
Phenergan with Codeine 2883
Phenergan VC with Codeine 2888
Pilopine HS Ophthalmic Gel (Occasional) ⊙ 224
Placidyl Capsules 456
Pondimin Tablets 2239
Ponstel 1982
Prelone Syrup 1834
Prinivil Tablets (0.3% to 1.0%) 1776
Prinzide Tablets (0.3% to 1%) 1780
Procardia Capsules (2% or less) 2024
Procardia XL Extended Release Tablets (1% or less) 2026
▲ Prograf (Greater than 3%) 1028
Prolixin 510
ProSom Tablets (Infrequent) 457
Prostep (nicotine transdermal system) (1% to 3% of patients) 1439
Prostigmin Injectable 1305
Prostigmin Tablets 1306
Prostin E2 Suppository 2109
Proventil Syrup (Less than 1 of 100 patients) 2528
▲ Prozac Pulvules & Liquid, Oral Solution (5% to 8.4%) 935
Quadrinal Tablets 1398
▲ RMS Suppositories CII (Among most frequent) 2766
Recombivax HB (Less than 1%) 1787
Redux Capsules (Frequent) 2911
Relafen Tablets (1% to 3%) 2688
▲ Retrovir Capsules (5%) 1216
▲ Retrovir I.V. Infusion (5%) 1221
▲ Retrovir Syrup (5%) 1216
Rifater 1280
Risperdal Tablets (Infrequent) 1348
Rocephin Injectable Vials, ADD-Vantage, Galaxy Container (Occasional) 2305
▲ Roferon-A Injection (7% to 22%) 2308
▲ Romazicon (1% to 9%) 2311
▲ Roxanol (Among most frequent) 2365
Rythmol Tablets–150mg, 225mg, 300mg (0.6 to 1.4%) 1399
▲ Salagen Tablets (29% to 68%) 1546
Sandoglobulin I.V. (Less than 1%) 2419
Sanorex Tablets 2423
Seldane Tablets 1284
Seldane-D Extended-Release Tablets 1286
Sensorcaine (Rare) 554
Serentil 689
Serzone Tablets 776
Sinemet Tablets 959
Sinemet CR Tablets 961
Sinequan (Occasional) 2028
Solganal Suspension 2530
Stadol (1% or greater) 779
Stelazine 2692
Sublimaze Injection 463
Sular Tablets (Less than or equal to 1%) 2961
▲ Supprelin Injection (1% to 10%) 2230
Surmontil Capsules 2917
Talacen Caplets 2464
Talwin Injection 2465
Talwin Compound 2466
Talwin Injection 2465
Talwin Nx Tablets 2467
Tambocor Tablets (1% to less than 3%) 1555
Tavist Syrup 2426
Tavist Tablets 2427
▲ Tegison Capsules (1-10%) 2314
Tegretol/Tegretol-XR 870
Tenex Tablets (3% or less) 2249
Tensilon Injectable 1307
Thorazine 2701
THYREL TRH (Less frequent) 2992
Timolide Tablets 1791
Timoptic in Ocudose 1796
Timoptic Sterile Ophthalmic Solution 1794
Timoptic-XE 1798
Tofranil Ampuls 873
Tofranil Tablets 875
Tofranil-PM Capsules 876
▲ Tonocard Tablets (2.3% to 5.1%) 519
Toradol (Greater than 1%) 2319
▲ Trandate (4 of 100 patients) 1158
Triavil Tablets 1800
Trilafon 2532
Trinalin Repetabs Tablets 1373
▲ Ultram Tablets (50 mg) (6% to 9%) 1594
Univasc Tablets (Less than 1%) 2553
Urecholine 1804
Vascor Tablets (200 and 300 mg) (0.5 to 2.0%) 1597
Vaseretic Tablets (0.5% to 2.0%) 1810
Vasotec I.V. 1814
Vasotec Tablets (0.5% to 1.0%) 1816
Vasoxyl Injection 1169
Velosulin BR Human Insulin 10 ml Vials 1847
Ventolin Syrup (Less than 1 of 100 patients) 1175
VePesid Capsules and Injection (Sometimes) 727
Verelan Capsules (1% or less) 1455
▲ Vesanoid Capsules (20%) 2327
▲ Videx Tablets, Powder for Oral Solution, & Pediatric Powder for Oral Solution (Up to 7%) 2980
Vistide Injection 1057
Vivactil Tablets 1820
Cataflam/Voltaren/Voltaren-XR (Less than 1%) 833
▲ Wellbutrin Tablets (22.3%) 1177
▲ Xanax Tablets (15.1%) 2115
Yocon Tablets (Common) 1235
Yutopar Intravenous Injection (Infrequent) 566
Zebeta Tablets (0.7% to 1.0%) 1457
▲ Zerit Capsules (Fewer than 1% to 19%) 731
Zestoretic Tablets (0.3 to 1%) 2968
Zestril Tablets (0.3% to 1.0%) 2972
Ziac 1459
▲ Zoladex (6% to 45%) 2976
Zoladex 3-month 2978
▲ Zoloft Tablets (8.4%) 2051
Zosyn (1.0% or less) 1463
Zovirax Sterile Powder (Less than 1%) 1191
Zyrtec Tablets (Less than 2%) 2053

(Described in PDR For Nonprescription Drugs) Incidence data in parenthesis; ▲ 3% or more (⊙ Described in PDR For Ophthalmology)

1305 Side Effects Index Diarrhea

Diaphoresis, nocturnal

Sandimmune (Rare) ... 2416

Diaphragm, paralyzed

Survanta Beractant Intratracheal Suspension ... 2346

Diarrhea

▲ Abelcet Injection (5% to 10%) ... 1540
Accupril Tablets (1.7%) ... 1950
Accutane Capsules ... 2252
▲ Acel-Imune Diphtheria and Tetanus Toxoids and Acellular Pertussis Vaccine Adsorbed (3.5%) ... 1415
Achromycin V Capsules (Rare) ... 1417
▲ ActHIB (1.5% to 9.0%) ... 893
▲ Actigall Capsules (27.1%) ... 818
▲ Actimmune (14%) ... 1043
Adalat Capsules (10 mg and 20 mg) (2% or less) ... 580
Adalat CC (Less than 1.0%) ... 582
Adapin Capsules ... 1542
Adderall Tablets ... 2209
Adipex-P Tablets and Capsules ... 1035
Adriamycin PFS (Occasional) ... 2056
Adriamycin RDF (Occasional) ... 2056
▲ AeroBid Inhaler System (10%) ... 1004
▲ Aerobid-M Inhaler System (10%) .. 1004
Aldactazide Tablets ... 2556
Aldactone Tablets ... 2558
Aldoclor Tablets ... 1638
Aldomet Ester HCl Injection ... 1642
Aldomet Oral ... 1640
Aldoril Tablets ... 1644
▲ Alferon N Injection (2% to 6%) ... 2142
Alkeran for Injection (Infrequent) ... 1196
Alkeran Tablets (Infrequent) ... 1198
All-Flex Arcing Spring Diaphragm (See also Ortho Diaphragm Kits) 1921
Altace Capsules (Less than 1% to 1.1%) ... 1238
Alupent Tablets (1.2%) ... 672
Amaryl Tablets (Less than 1%) ... 1241
Ambien Tablets (1% to 3%) ... 2559
Amicar Syrup, Tablets, and Injection ... 1312
Amoxil ... 2631
▲ Anafranil Capsules (7% to 13%) ... 819
Anaprox/Naprosyn (Less than 3%) ... 2277
Ancef Injection ... 2632
Ancobon Capsules ... 2254
Apresazide Capsules (Common) ... 824
Apresoline Hydrochloride Tablets (Common) ... 826
Aralen Hydrochloride Injection ... 2430
Aralen Phosphate Tablets ... 2431
▲ Aredia for Injection (Up to 19.2%) 827
▲ Arimidex Tablets (7.3% to 8.4%) .. 2932
▲ Asacol Delayed-Release Tablets (7%) ... 2129
Asendin Tablets (Less than 1%) ... 1419
Atamet Tablets ... 567
Atretol Tablets ... 569
Atrohist Plus Tablets ... 1605
Atromid-S Capsules ... 2808
Attenuvax (Rare) ... 1650
▲ Augmentin (9%) ... 2637
▲ Augmentin Tablets (9%) ... 2640
▲ Avonex (16%) ... 662
▲ Axid Pulvules (7.2%) ... 1468
Azactam for Injection (1 to 1.3%) .. 736
Azathioprine Tablets (Less than 1%) ... 2349
Azulfidine (Rare) ... 2059
Bactrim DS Tablets ... 2257
Bactrim I.V. Infusion ... 2255
Bactrim ... 2257
Bactroban Nasal (Less than 1%) ... 2643
Benadryl Injection ... 1955
Betagan ... ⊙ 230
▲ Betapace Tablets (2% to 7%) ... 637
▲ Betaseron for SC Injection (35%) .. 653
Betimol 0.25%, 0.5% ... ⊙ 259
Biavax II ... 1653
▲ Biaxin (3% to 6%) ... 406
Blocadren Tablets (Less than 1%) 1654
Bontril Slow-Release Capsules ... 786
▲ Bromfed-DM Cough Syrup (Among most frequent) ... 1832
Bumex (0.1%) ... 2260
Buprenex Injectable (Rare) ... 2170
BuSpar Tablets (2%) ... 738
Calan SR Caplets (1% or less) ... 2571
Calan Tablets (1% or less) ... 2568
Capoten Tablets (About 0.5 to 2%) ... 740
Capozide Tablets (0.5 to 2%) ... 744
Carafate Suspension (Less than 0.5%) ... 1250
Carafate Tablets (Less than 0.5%) 1249
▲ Cardioquin Tablets (Among most frequent; 35%) ... 2146
Cardizem CD Capsules (Less than 1%) ... 1251
Cardizem SR Capsules (Less than 1%) ... 1255
Cardizem Injectable ... 1253
Cardizem Tablets (Less than 1%) .. 1257
Cardura Tablets (2% to 2.3%) ... 1993
Carnitor Tablets and Solution ... 2624
Cartrol Tablets (2.1-4.4%) ... 413
▲ Casodex Tablets (10%) ... 2934
▲ Cataflam Tablets (3% to 9%) ... 833
Ceclor Pulvules & Suspension (1 in 70) ... 1470
▲ Cedax (3% to 4%) ... 2480
Cefizox for Intramuscular or Intravenous Use (Occasional) ... 1025
▲ Cefobid Intravenous/Intramuscular (1 in 30) ... 1996
▲ Cefobid Pharmacy Bulk Package - Not for Direct Infusion (1 in 30) .. 1999
Cefotan (1 in 80) ... 2936
▲ Ceftin (3.7% to 8.6%) ... 1067
Cefzil Tablets and Oral Suspension (2.9%) ... 747
▲ CellCept Capsules (31.0% to 36.1%; 16.4% to 18.8%) ... 2265
Celontin Kapseals (Frequent) ... 1955
Ceptaz (One in 78 patients) ... 1070
Cerebyx Injection (Infrequent) ... 1956
Ceredase ... 1055
Cerubidine for Injection (Occasional) ... 634
Cervidil (Less than 1%) ... 1008
▲ Chemet Capsules (12.0% to 20.9%) ... 666
Chloromycetin Sodium Succinate ... 1960
Chromagen Capsules ... 2470
Chromagen FA ... 2471
Chromagen Forte ... 2471
Cipro I.V. (1% or less) ... 587
▲ Cipro I.V. Pharmacy Bulk Package - (Among most frequent) ... 590
Cipro Tablets (2.3%) ... 584
Claforan Sterile and Injection (1.4%) ... 1259
Claritin Tablets (2% or fewer patients) ... 2485
Claritin-D Tablets (Less frequent) .. 2487
Cleocin Phosphate Injection ... 2068
Cleocin T Topical (Rare) ... 2072
Cleocin Vaginal Cream (Less than 1%) ... 2070
▲ Clinoril Tablets (3% to 9%) ... 1658
Clomid (Fewer than 1%) ... 1262
Clozaril Tablets (2%) ... 2377
▲ Cognex Capsules (16%) ... 1961
ColBENEMID Tablets ... 1662
Colestid (Less frequent) ... 2073
Combipres Tablets ... 682
Cordarone Intravenous (Less than 2%) ... 2821
Cosmegen Injection ... 1666
Coumadin (Infrequent) ... 941
Covera-HS Tablets (Less than 2%) 2573
Cozaar Tablets (2.4%) ... 1668
▲ Creon (Among most frequent) ... 2714
▲ Crixivan Capsules (4.6%) ... 1670
Crystodigin Tablets ... 1472
Cuprimine Capsules ... 1673
▲ Cytosar-U Sterile Powder (Among most frequent) ... 2077
▲ Cytotec (14% to 40%) ... 2576
▲ Cytovene (41%) ... 2270
Cytoxan (Less frequent) ... 700
D.H.E. 45 Injection (Occasional) ... 2381
DTIC-Dome (Rare) ... 593
Dalgan Injection (Less than 1%) ... 529
Dalmane Capsules ... 2329
▲ Dantrium Capsules (Among most frequent) ... 2131
Daraprim Tablets (Rare) ... 1199
▲ DaunoXome (4% to 34%) ... 1842
▲ Daypro Caplets (3% to 9%) ... 2578
Declomycin Tablets ... 1421
Demadex Tablets and Injection (2.0%) ... 691
▲ Demser Capsules (10%) ... 1690
Depakene ... 416
▲ Depakote Tablets (12%) ... 418
▲ Depen Titratable Tablets (17%) ... 2770
Desferal Vials ... 838
Desoxyn Gradumet Tablets ... 422
Desyrel and Desyrel Dividose (Up to 4.5%) ... 504
Dexedrine ... 2648
DextroStat-Dextroamphetamine Sulfate Tablets ... 2211
Diabinese Tablets (Less than 2%) .. 2002
Diamox Intravenous ... ⊙ 317
Diamox Sequels (Sustained Release) ... ⊙ 318
Diamox Tablets ... ⊙ 317
▲ Didronel Tablets (About 1 patient in 15; possibly 2 or 3 in 10) ... 2133
Diflucan Tablets, Injection, and Oral Suspension (1.5% to 3%) .. 2003
Dilacor XR Extended-release Capsules (2.0%) ... 2183
Dilaudid-HP Injection (Less frequent) ... 1384
Dilaudid-HP Lyophilized Powder 250 mg (Less frequent) ... 1384
Dilaudid Tablets and Liquid ... 1386
Dimetane-DC Cough Syrup ... 2232
Dimetane-DX Cough Syrup ... 2233
▲ Dipentum Capsules (11.1% to about 17%) ... 2084
Diprivan Injectable Emulsion (Less than 1%) ... 2939
Disalcid ... 1549
Diucardin Tablets ... 2824
Diupres Tablets ... 1691
Diuril Oral Suspension ... 1694
Diuril Sodium Intravenous ... 1693
Diuril Tablets ... 1694
▲ Dolobid Tablets (3% to 9%) ... 1695
Dopram Injectable ... 2235
Doral Tablets ... 2773
Doryx Capsules (Infrequent) ... 1970
▲ Doxil (5.2% to 7.8%) ... 2613
Doxorubicin Astra (Occasional) ... 531
DUPHALAC Solution ... 2714
▲ Duragesic Transdermal System (3% to 10%) ... 1336
Dura-Vent Tablets ... 971
Duricef Capsules, Tablets, and Oral Suspension ... 750
Dyazide Capsules ... 2653
▲ Dynabac (7.7%) ... 668
DYNACIN Capsules (Infrequent) ... 1627
DynaCirc Capsules (Up to 3.4%) ... 2381
DynaCirc CR Tablets (0.5% to 1.0%) ... 2383
Dyrenium Capsules (Rare) ... 2655
▲ E.E.S. (Most frequent) ... 427
E-Mycin Tablets (Infrequent) ... 1388
Easprin ... 1971
EC-Naprosyn Delayed-Release Tablets (Less than 3%) ... 2277
Edecrin ... 1698
▲ Effexor (8%) ... 2825
Elavil ... 2945
Eldepryl Capsules (1 of 49 patients) ... 2729
▲ Emcyt Capsules (12%) ... 2085
Enduron Tablets ... 424
Engerix-B Unit-Dose Vials (Less than 1%) ... 2656
Ensure Plus High Calorie Complete Nutrition ... 2338
▲ Epivir (18%) ... 1200
▲ Epogen for Injection (0.11 to 21%) ... 489
▲ Ergamisol Tablets (13% to 52%) .. 1340
▲ ERYC (Among most frequent) ... 1972
▲ EryPed (Among most frequent) ... 425
▲ Ery-Tab Tablets (Among most frequent) ... 426
▲ Erythrocin Stearate Filmtab (Among most frequent) ... 429
▲ Erythromycin Base Filmtab (Among most frequent) ... 430
▲ Erythromycin Delayed-Release Capsules, USP (Among most frequent) ... 431
Esidrix Tablets ... 839
Esimil Tablets ... 840
Eskalith ... 2658
Estring Vaginal Ring (1% to 3%) ... 2086
▲ Ethmozine Tablets (2% to 5%) ... 2217
▲ Etopophos for Injection (1% to 13%) ... 701
▲ Etoposide Injection (1% to 13%) .. 539
Etrafon ... 2495
▲ Eulexin Capsules (12% to 40%) ... 2498
▲ Famvir Tablets (4.5% to 7.7%) ... 2660
Fansidar Tablets ... 2281
Fastin Capsules ... 2662
▲ Felbatol (5.2% to 5.3%) ... 2774
Feldene Capsules (Greater than 1%) ... 2008
Feosol Caplets (Occasional) ... 2626
Feosol Capsules (Occasional) ... ▣ 777
Feosol Elixir (Occasional) ... 2627
Feosol Tablets (Occasional) ... 2627
Fioricet with Codeine Capsules ... 2387
Fiorinal with Codeine Capsules ... 2390
Flagyl 375 Capsules ... 2587
Flagyl I.V. ... 2373
Flexeril Tablets (Less than 1%) ... 1701
▲ Flolan for Injection (37%) ... 1085
Flovent (1% to 3%) ... 1089
▲ Floxin I.V. (1% to 4%) ... 1580
Floxin Tablets (200 mg, 300 mg, 400 mg) (1% to 4%) ... 1577
▲ Fludara for Injection (13% to 15%) ... 658
Flumadine Tablets & Syrup (0.3% to 1%) ... 1013
Fluorouracil Injection (Rare to common) ... 2282
Fortaz (1 in 78 patients) ... 1092
▲ Fosamax Tablets (3.1%) ... 1703
▲ Foscavir Injection (5% or greater up to 30%) ... 541
▲ Sterile FUDR (Among more common) ... 2284
Fulvicin P/G Tablets (Occasional) .. 2499
Fulvicin P/G 165 & 330 Tablets (Occasional) ... 2500
▲ Fungizone Intravenous (Among most common) ... 507
Fungizone Oral Suspension ... 704
Ganite ... 2711
Gantanol Tablets ... 2285
Gantrisin ... 2286
▲ Gastrocrom Capsules (4 of 87 patients) ... 1611
▲ Gastrocrom Oral Concentrate (4 of 87 patients) ... 1611
▲ Gemzar for Injection (19% to 31%) ... 1482
Geocillin Tablets ... 2009
GlaucTabs ... ⊙ 209
▲ Glucophage Tablets (Among most common) ... 754
Glucotrol Tablets (1 in 70) ... 2011
▲ Glucotrol XL Extended Release Tablets (5.4%) ... 2012
Grifulvin V (griseofulvin tablets) Microsize (griseofulvin oral suspension) Microsize (Occasional) ... 1944
Gris-PEG Tablets, 125 mg & 250 mg (Occasional) ... 476
Guaifed ... 1833
▲ Habitrol Nicotine Transdermal System (3% to 9% of patients) .. 884
Halcion Tablets (Rare) ... 2093
Haldol Decanoate ... 1587
Haldol Injection, Tablets and Concentrate ... 1585
Havrix (Less than 1%) ... 2663
▲ Helidac Therapy (5.1%) ... 2135
Helixate, Antihemophilic Factor (Recombinant) (One report out of 3,254 patients) ... 799
HibTITER (2 of 1,118 vaccinations) ... 1423
Hismanal Tablets (1.8%) ... 1341
Hivid Tablets (2.5%) ... 2287
Humegon for Injection ... 1873
Humorsol Sterile Ophthalmic Solution (Rare) ... 1707
▲ Hycamtin for Injection (Less than 1% to 42%) ... 2665
Hydralazine Hydrochloride Injection USP (Common) ... 2712
Hydrea Capsules (Less frequent) ... 705
HydroDIURIL Tablets ... 1716
Hydropres Tablets ... 1718
Hyperstat I.V. Injection ... 2504
Hytrin Capsules (At least 1%) ... 434
Hyzaar Tablets (1% or greater) ... 1720
IBU Tablets (Greater than 1%) ... 1389
▲ Idamycin Injection (73%) ... 2096
IFEX (Less than 1%) ... 706
Ilosone (Infrequent) ... 927
Imdur (Less than or equal to 5%) .. 1362
Imitrex Injection (Infrequent) ... 1095
Imitrex Tablets (Frequent) ... 1099
Imuran (Less than 1%) ... 1103
Inderal ... 2834
Inderal LA Long Acting Capsules ... 2836
Inderide Tablets ... 2838
Inderide LA Long Acting Capsules .. 2840
Indocin Capsules (Greater than 1%) ... 1723
Indocin I.V. (1% to 3%) ... 1727
Indocin (Greater than 1%) ... 1723
INFeD (Iron Dextran Injection, USP) ... 2478
▲ Intron A for Injection (2% to 45%) ... 2506
▲ Invirase Capsules (3.8%) ... 2291
Ionamin Capsules ... 1615
IOPIDINE Sterile Ophthalmic Solution ... ⊙ 218
Ismelin Tablets ... 845
Ismo Tablets (Fewer than 1%) ... 2844

(▣ Described in PDR For Nonprescription Drugs) Incidence data in parenthesis; ▲ 3% or more (⊙ Described in PDR For Ophthalmology)

Diarrhea
Side Effects Index

Isoptin Oral Tablets (Less than 1%) ... 1393
Isoptin SR Tablets (1% or less) ... 1395
Isopto Carbachol Ophthalmic Solution ... ⊚ 221
K-Dur Microburst Release System (potassium chloride, USP) E.R. Tablets ... 1364
▲ K-Lor Powder Packets (Among most common) ... 438
▲ K-Norm Capsules (Among most common) ... 1615
K-Phos Neutral Tablets ... 633
K-Phos Original Formula 'Sodium Free' Tablets ... 633
▲ K-Tab Filmtab (Most common) ... 439
Kadian Capsules (Less than 3%) ... 2948
Kayexalate (Occasional) ... 2444
▲ Keflex Pulvules & Oral Suspension (Most frequent) ... 930
▲ Keftab Tablets (Most frequent) ... 931
Kefurox Vials, Faspak & ADD-Vantage (1 in 220) ... 1509
Kefzol Vials, Faspak & ADD-Vantage ... 1511
Kerlone Tablets (1.9% to 2.0%) ... 2588
Klonopin Tablets ... 2294
KOGENATE Antihemophilic Factor (Recombinant) (One report) ... 626
Ku-Zyme HP Capsules ... 2547
▲ Kytril Injection (4%) ... 2667
▲ Kytril Tablets (4% to 8%) ... 2669
▲ Lamictal Tablets (6.3%) ... 1105
▲ Lamisil Tablets (5.6%) ... 2394
▲ Lamprene Capsules (40-50%) ... 846
Lanoxicaps (Less common) ... 1110
Lanoxin Elixir Pediatric (Less common) ... 1113
Lanoxin Injection (Less common) ... 1116
Lanoxin Injection Pediatric ... 1119
Lanoxin Tablets (Less common) ... 1121
▲ Lariam Tablets (Among most frequent) ... 2295
Larodopa Tablets (Infrequent) ... 2296
Lasix Injection, Oral Solution and Tablets ... 1267
▲ Lescol Capsules (9%) ... 2395
▲ Leucovorin Calcium for Injection (11% to 66%) ... 1313
Leucovorin Calcium Tablets, Wellcovorin Brand ... 1204
Leukeran Tablets (Infrequent) ... 1205
▲ Leukine (52% to 89%) ... 1317
▲ Leustatin (10%) ... 1889
▲ Levatol Tablets (3.3%) ... 2547
Levsin/Levsinex/Levbid ... 2549
Limbitrol ... 2333
Lioresal Intrathecal (Up to 2.3%) .. 1634
Lioresal Tablets (Rare) ... 847
Lithium Carbonate Capsules & Tablets ... 2352
Lithonate/Lithotabs/Lithobid ... 2721
▲ Lodine Capsules and Tablets (3% to 9%) ... 2849
▲ Lopid Tablets (7.2%) ... 1974
▲ Lopressor (5%) ... 848
Lopressor HCT Tablets (1 to 5 in 100 patients) ... 850
▲ Lorabid Suspension and Pulvules (3.6% to 5.8%) ... 1513
Lotensin HCT Tablets (0.3% to 1.0%) ... 855
Lotrel Capsules ... 858
Ludiomil Tablets (Rare) ... 861
Lufyllin & Lufyllin-400 Tablets ... 2778
Lufyllin-GG Elixir & Tablets ... 2779
Lupron Depot 7.5 mg (Less than 5%) ... 2741
Lupron Injection (Less than 5%) ... 2736
▲ LUVOX Tablets (11%) ... 2723
Lysodren Tablets (80%) ... 707
M-M-R II ... 1730
M-R-VAX II ... 1732
MS Contin Tablets (Less frequent) ... 2149
MSIR (Infrequent) ... 2152
Macrobid Capsules (Less than 1%) ... 2138
Macrodantin Capsules (Less common) ... 2140
MagTab SR Caplets ... 1844
Marinol (Dronabinol) Capsules (0.3% to 1%) ... 2353
Mavik Tablets (More than 1%) ... 1407
Maxair Autohaler (1.3%) ... 1550
Maxair Inhaler (Less than 1%) ... 1552
Maxaquin Tablets (1.4%) ... 2593
Maxipime for Injection (0.1% to 1%) ... 758
Mefoxin ... 1734
Mefoxin Premixed Intravenous Solution ... 1737

▲ Megace Oral Suspension (8% to 15%) ... 708
Mellaril ... 2398
▲ Mepron Suspension (19% to 21%) ... 1206
▲ Merrem I.V. (3.5% to 5.0%) ... 2952
Meruvax II ... 1740
▲ Mesnex Injection (83%) ... 711
Mestinon Injectable ... 1300
Mestinon ... 1300
Methadone Hydrochloride Oral Concentrate ... 2356
Methergine (Rare) ... 2401
Methotrexate Sodium Tablets, Injection, for Injection and LPF Injection (1% to 3%) ... 1322
Metrodin (urofollitropin for injection) ... 2616
MetroGel-Vaginal (Equal to or less than 2%) ... 917
▲ Mevacor Tablets (2.2% to 5.5%) ... 1742
Mexitil Capsules (5.2%) ... 684
Mezlin ... 594
Mezlin Pharmacy Bulk Package ... 597
Miacalcin Nasal Spray (1% to 3%) 2403
▲ Micro-K (Among most common) ... 2237
▲ Micro-K LS Packets (Among most common) ... 2238
▲ Midamor Tablets (3% to 8%) ... 1746
Miltown Tablets ... 2780
Minipress Capsules (1-4%) ... 2015
Minizide Capsules (Rare) ... 2016
Minocin Intravenous ... 1428
Minocin Oral Suspension ... 1431
Minocin Pellet-Filled Capsules (Infrequent) ... 1429
Mintezol ... 1747
Mithracin ... 599
Moduretic Tablets (Greater than 1%, less than 3%) ... 1748
Monocid Injection (Less than 1%) .. 2674
Monodox Capsules (Infrequent) ... 1858
Mono-Gesic Tablets ... 810
Monoket Tablets (Up to 2%) ... 2550
▲ Monopril Tablets (Less than 1% to 11.9%) ... 762
Motrin Ibuprofen Suspension, Oral Drops, Chewable Tablets, Caplets (1% to less than 3%) ... 1563
Mumpsvax ... 1751
Mustargen ... 1752
Mutamycin for Injection ... 712
▲ Mycobutin Capsules (3%) ... 2101
Mycostatin Pastilles (Occasional) ... 713
Mykrox Tablets (Less than 2%) ... 1617
Mylanta (Occasional) ... 1359
Myochrysine Injection ... 1754
Nalfon 200 Pulvules & Nalfon Tablets (1.8%) ... 933
▲ Naprelan Tablets (3% to 9%) ... 2861
Anaprox/Naprosyn (Less than 3%) ... 2277
Navane Capsules and Concentrate ... 2018
Navane Intramuscular ... 2019
▲ Navelbine Injection (Up to 13% but less than 20%) ... 1212
Nebcin Vials, Hyporets & ADD-Vantage ... 1518
NegGram ... 2453
Neoral (3% to 8%) ... 2405
Nephro-Fer Rx Tablets ... 2168
Neptazane Tablets ... ⊚ 320
Netromycin Injection 100 mg/ml (Fewer than 1 of 1000 patients) 2516
Neupogen for Injection (14%) ... 495
Neurontin Capsules (More than 1%) ... 1978
Nicotrol NS Nicotine Nasal Spray (Less than 1%) ... 1565
▲ Nimotop Capsules (Up to 4.2%) ... 603
▲ Nipent for Injection (15% to 17%) ... 2733
Nizoral Tablets (Less than 1%) ... 1345
▲ Nolvadex Tablets (11.2%) ... 2957
Normodyne Tablets (Less than 1%) ... 2522
Noroxin Tablets (0.3% to 1.0%) ... 1758
Noroxin Tablets (0.3% to 1.0%) ... 2222
Norpace (1 to 3%) ... 2596
Norpramin Tablets ... 1273
Norvasc Tablets (More than 0.1% to 1%) ... 2020
▲ Norvir (12.8% to 18.3%) ... 447
▲ Novantrone for Injection (18 to 47%) ... 1327
▲ OmniHIB (3.6% to 8.5%) ... 2676
Omnipen Capsules ... 2872
Omnipen for Oral Suspension ... 2873
▲ Oncaspar (Greater than 1% but less than 5%) ... 2194
Oncovin Solution Vials & Hyporets ... 1521

Oramorph SR (Morphine Sulfate Sustained Release Tablets) (Less frequent) ... 2359
▲ Orap Tablets (1 of 20 patients) ... 1037
Oretic Tablets ... 450
Orlaam Oral Solution (1% to 3%) ... 2361
Ornade Spansule Capsules ... 2678
Ortho Diaphragm Kits—All-Flex Arcing Spring; Ortho Coil Spring; Ortho-White Flat Spring ... 1921
Ortho Diaphragm Kit ... 1921
▲ Orthoclone OKT3 Sterile Solution (14%) ... 1892
▲ Orudis Capsules (3% to 9%) ... 2874
▲ Oruvail Capsules (3% to 9%) ... 2874
Osmolite HN High Nitrogen Isotonic Liquid Nutrition ... 2339
Ovcon ... 765
OxyContin Tablets (Between 1% and 5%) ... 2163
PBZ Tablets ... 863
PBZ-SR Tablets ... 862
▲ PCE Dispertab Tablets (Among most frequent) ... 453
Pamelor ... 2409
Papaverine Hydrochloride Vials and Ampoules ... 1523
▲ Paraplatin for Injection (6%) ... 713
Parlodel (0.4 to 3%) ... 2411
Parnate Tablets ... 2679
▲ PASER Granules (Among most common) ... 1333
▲ Paxil Tablets (1.0% to 12%) ... 2681
▲ Pediazole Suspension (Among most frequent) ... 2340
PedvaxHIB (One case) ... 1761
Peganone Tablets ... 455
▲ Pen•Vee K (Among most common) 2879
Penetrex Tablets (1% to 2%) ... 2196
▲ Pentasa (3.4% to 3.5%) ... 1275
Pentaspan Injection ... 954
Pepcid Injection (1.7%) ... 1765
Pepcid (1.7%) ... 1763
Pergonal (menotropins for injection, USP) ... 2618
Periactin ... 1767
Peri-Colace Capsules and Syrup ... 2226
▲ Permax Tablets (6.4%) ... 571
Persantine Tablets ... 686
Pipracil (2%) ... 1435
Plaquenil Sulfate Tablets ... 2459
Platinol for Injection ... 717
Platinol-AQ Injection ... 719
Plendil Extended-Release Tablets (0.5% to 1.5%) ... 514
PMB 200 and PMB 400 ... 2890
▲ Pondimin Tablets (Among most common) ... 2239
▲ Ponstel (Approximately 5%) ... 1982
▲ Pravachol Tablets (2.0% to 6.2%) ... 770
▲ Precose (33%) ... 604
Prelu-2 Timed Release Capsules ... 687
▲ Prevacid Delayed-Release Capsules (1.4% to 7.4%) ... 2746
▲ Prilosec Delayed-Release Capsules (3.0% to 3.7%) ... 516
Primaxin I.M. (0.6%) ... 1770
Primaxin I.V. (1.8%) ... 1772
Prinivil Tablets (3.7%) ... 1776
Prinzide Tablets (2.5%) ... 1780
Priscoline Hydrochloride Ampuls ... 864
Procanbid Extended-Release Tablets (Occasional) ... 1983
Procardia Capsules (2% or less) ... 2024
Procardia XL Extended Release Tablets (Less than 3%) ... 2026
▲ Procrit for Injection (0.11% to 21%) ... 1896
Proglycem (Frequent) ... 575
▲ Prograf (32% to 72%) ... 1028
▲ Proleukin for Injection (76%) ... 812
▲ Propulsid (14.2%) ... 1346
Prostigmin Injectable ... 1305
Prostigmin Tablets ... 1306
Prostin E2 Suppository (Approximately two-fifths) ... 2109
Protostat Tablets (Occasional) ... 1939
▲ Prozac Pulvules & Liquid, Oral Solution (12.3% to 18%) ... 935
Purinethol Tablets (Occasional) ... 1214
Quadrinal Tablets ... 1398
Questran (Less frequent) ... 774
Quibron ... 2227
▲ Quinaglute Dura-Tabs Tablets (24%) ... 644
▲ Quinidex Extentabs (35%) ... 2240
RMS Suppositories CII ... 2766
Recombivax HB (Equal to or greater than 1%) ... 1787
▲ Redux Capsules (17.5%) ... 2911
Regitine Vials ... 864

Reglan ... 2243
▲ Relafen Tablets (14%) ... 2688
ReoPro Vials (0.9%) ... 1526
Respbid Tablets ... 687
RespiGam (1%) ... 1631
Restoril Capsules (1-2%) ... 2413
▲ Retrovir Capsules (0.8% to 12%) ... 1216
▲ Retrovir I.V. Infusion (1% to 12%) 1221
▲ Retrovir Syrup (0.8% to 12%) ... 1216
▲ ReVia Tablets (Less than 1% to less than 10%) ... 957
Revex (nalmefene hydrochloride injection) (Less than 1%) ... 1863
▲ Ridaura Capsules (42.5%) ... 2691
Rifadin (Some patients) ... 1276
Rifamate Capsules (Some patients) ... 1278
Rifater ... 1280
▲ Rilutek Tablets (5.5% to 9.0%) ... 2198
Rimactane Capsules ... 865
Risperdal Tablets (Infrequent) ... 1348
Robaxisal Tablets ... 2246
Rocephin Injectable Vials, ADD-Vantage, Galaxy Container (2.7%) ... 2305
▲ Roferon-A Injection (34% to 42%) 2308
Rondec Oral Drops ... 974
Rondec Syrup ... 974
Rondec ... 974
Rowasa (2.09% to 3.0%) ... 2727
Rubex for Injection (Occasional) ... 721
Rum-K Syrup ... 1004
▲ Rythmol Tablets—150mg, 225mg, 300mg (0.5 to 5.7%) ... 1399
▲ SSKI Solution (Among most frequent) ... 2767
▲ Salagen Tablets (6%) ... 1546
Salflex Tablets ... 791
▲ Sandimmune (3 to 8%) ... 2416
▲ Sandostatin Injection (4% to 61%) ... 2421
Sanorex Tablets ... 2423
Sansert Tablets ... 2424
▲ Sectral Capsules (4%) ... 2914
Septra ... 1146
Septra I.V. Infusion ... 1142
Septra I.V. Infusion ADD-Vantage Vials ... 1144
Septra ... 1146
Ser-Ap-Es Tablets ... 867
Serevent Inhalation Aerosol (1% to 3%) ... 1149
Serophene (clomiphene citrate tablets, USP) ... 2621
▲ Serzone Tablets (8%) ... 776
Sinemet Tablets ... 959
Sinemet CR Tablets (1.2%) ... 961
Sinequan ... 2028
Slo-bid Gyrocaps ... 2201
▲ Slow-K Extended-Release Tablets (Among most common) ... 869
Sodium Polystyrene Sulfonate Suspension (Occasional) ... 2367
Solganal Suspension (Rare) ... 2530
Soma Compound w/Codeine Tablets ... 2784
▲ Soma Compound Tablets (Among most common) ... 2783
Spectrobid Tablets (2% to 4%) ... 2030
▲ Sporanox Capsules (0.6% to 3.3%) ... 1352
Sular Tablets (Less than or equal to 1%) ... 2961
Sulfamylon Cream ... 940
▲ Supprelin Injection (1% to 10%) ... 2230
▲ Suprax (16%) ... 1443
Surmontil Capsules ... 2917
Symmetrel Capsules (1% to 5%) ... 965
Symmetrel Syrup (1% to 5%) ... 963
Tagamet (Approximately 1 in 100) 2694
Talacen Caplets (Rare) ... 2464
Talwin Injection (Rare) ... 2465
Talwin Compound (Rare) ... 2466
Talwin Injection (Rare) ... 2465
Talwin Nx Tablets ... 2467
Tambocor Tablets (1% to less than 3%) ... 1555
Tao Capsules (Infrequent) ... 2033
Tavist Syrup ... 2426
Tavist Tablets ... 2427
▲ Taxol Injection (38%) ... 723
Taxotere for Injection Concentrate 2204
Tazicef for Injection (Less than 2%; 1 in 78 patients) ... 2697
Tazidime Vials, Faspak & ADD-Vantage (1 in 78) ... 1531
Tegison Capsules (Less than 1%) .. 2314
Tegretol/Tegretol-XR ... 870
Tenex Tablets (3% or less) ... 2249
Tenoretic Tablets (2% to 3%) ... 2963

(⊚ Described in PDR For Nonprescription Drugs)   Incidence data in parenthesis; ▲ 3% or more   (⊚ Described in PDR For Ophthalmology)

Side Effects Index

▲ Tenormin Tablets and I.V. Injection (2% to 3%) ... 2965
Tensilon Injectable ... 1307
Terramycin Intramuscular Solution ... 2034
▲ Tetramune (1% to 10%) ... 1449
Thalitone ... 1293
Theo-24 Extended Release Capsules ... 2753
Theo-Dur Extended-Release Tablets ... 1367
Theo-X Extended-Release Tablets ... 793
▲ TheraCys BCG Live (Intravesical) (Up to 6.3%) ... 911
Thyro-Block Tablets (Sometimes) ... 2785
Tiazac Capsules (Less than 1% to 2%) ... 1019
TICE BCG, USP (1.2%) ... 1881
▲ Ticlid Tablets (12.5%) ... 2317
Tigan ... 2231
Tilade Inhaler (0.9%) ... 2207
Timentin for Injection ... 2706
Timolide Tablets (Less than 1%) ... 1791
Timoptic in Ocudose (Less frequent) ... 1796
Timoptic Sterile Ophthalmic Solution (Less frequent) ... 1794
Timoptic-XE ... 1798
Tofranil Ampuls ... 873
Tofranil Tablets ... 875
Tofranil-PM Capsules ... 876
▲ Tolectin (200, 400 and 600 mg) (3 to 9%) ... 1591
▲ Tonocard Tablets (Up to 6.8%) ... 519
▲ Toprol-XL Tablets (About 5 of 100 patients) ... 560
▲ Toradol (7%) ... 2319
Trandate Tablets (Less than 1%) ... 1158
Trasylol (2%) ... 607
Trental Tablets ... 1291
Triavil Tablets ... 1800
Trilafon (Occasional) ... 2532
▲ Trilisate (Less than 20%) ... 2155
Trinalin Repetabs Tablets ... 1373
Trinsicon Capsules (Rare) ... 2759
Tripedia (Up to 3%) ... 908
Tussend ... 1830
Typhim Vi (Up to 3.1%) ... 914
▲ Ultram Tablets (50 mg) (5% to 10%) ... 1594
Ultrase Capsules ... 2476
▲ Ultrase MT Capsules (3.7%; among most frequent) ... 2477
▲ Unasyn (3%) ... 2035
Uni-Dur Extended-Release Tablets ... 1374
Uniphyl 400 mg and 600 mg Tablets ... 2157
▲ Univasc Tablets (3.1%) ... 2553
Urecholine ... 1804
Urobiotic-250 Capsules (Rare) ... 2038
Urocit-K Tablets (Some patients) ... 1828
Uroqid-Acid No. 2 Tablets ... 633
▲ Valtrex Caplets (4% to 5%) ... 1167
Vancocin HCl, Vials & ADD-Vantage ... 1534
▲ Vantin for Oral Suspension and Vantin Tablets (1.2% to 7.2%) ... 2112
Vaqta (1.0% to 2.4%) ... 1805
Varivax (Greater than or equal to 1%) ... 1807
▲ Vascor Tablets (200 and 300 mg) (6.82 to 10.87%) ... 1597
Vaseretic Tablets (2.1%) ... 1810
Vasotec I.V. ... 1814
Vasotec Tablets (1.4% to 2.1%) ... 1816
Velban Vials ... 1537
Ventolin Inhalation Aerosol and Refill (1%) ... 1170
Ventolin Rotacaps for Inhalation (Less than 1%) ... 1173
▲ VePesid Capsules and Injection (1% to 13%) ... 727
Verelan Capsules (1% or less) ... 1455
Vermox Chewable Tablets ... 1357
▲ Vesanoid Capsules (23%) ... 2327
Vibramycin (Infrequent) ... 2038
Vibramycin Hyclate Intravenous ... 2040
Vibramycin (Infrequent) ... 2038
▲ Videx Tablets, Powder for Oral Solution, & Pediatric Powder for Oral Solution (17% to 81%) ... 2980
Viokase ... 2251
Viramune Tablets (2%) ... 2368
Visken Tablets (2% or fewer patients) ... 2428
▲ Vistide Injection (7% to 27%) ... 1057
Vivactil Tablets ... 1820
Vivotif Berna ... 660
▲ Cataflam/Voltaren/Voltaren-XR (3% to 9%) ... 833
▲ Vumon for Injection (33%) ... 729
▲ Wellbutrin Tablets (6.8%) ... 1177

Wigraine Tablets ... 1884
Winstrol Tablets ... 2468
▲ Xanax Tablets (10.1% to 20.6%) ... 2115
Yodoxin Tablets ... 1235
Yutopar Intravenous Injection (Infrequent) ... 566
Zanosar Sterile Powder (Some patients) ... 2119
Zantac ... 1182
Zantac Injection ... 1180
Zantac Syrup ... 1182
Zarontin Capsules (Frequent) ... 1986
Zarontin Syrup (Frequent) ... 1986
Zaroxolyn Tablets ... 1625
▲ Zebeta Tablets (2.6% to 3.5%) ... 1457
▲ Zerit Capsules (5% to 50%) ... 731
Zestoretic Tablets (2.5%) ... 2968
▲ Zestril Tablets (3.7%) ... 2972
▲ Ziac (1.1% to 4.3%) ... 1459
Zinacef (1 in 220 patients) ... 1184
▲ Zinecard Injection (14% to 21%) ... 2120
▲ Zithromax (2% to 7%) ... 2043
▲ Zithromax Tablets (5% to 7%) ... 2046
Zocor Tablets (1.9%) ... 1821
▲ Zofran Injection (8% to 16%) ... 1227
▲ Zofran Tablets (4% to 6%) ... 1231
Zoladex (1% or greater but less than 5%) ... 2976
Zoladex 3-month (1% to 5%) ... 2978
▲ Zoloft Tablets (17.7%) ... 2051
▲ Zosyn (11.3% to 20%) ... 1463
Zovirax (0.3% to 3.2%) ... 1187
Zyloprim Tablets (Less than 1%) ... 1194
Zyrtec Tablets (Less than 2%) ... 2053

Diarrhea, bloody

Asacol Delayed-Release Tablets ... 2129
Azulfidine (Rare) ... 2059
Cataflam Tablets (Less than 1%) ... 833
Cleocin Phosphate Injection ... 2068
Cleocin T Topical (Rare) ... 2072
Norvir (Less than 2%) ... 447
Paxil Tablets (Rare) ... 2681
Pentasa (0.9%) ... 1275
Pipracil (Less frequent) ... 1435
Prozac Pulvules & Liquid, Oral Solution (Rare) ... 935
Rowasa ... 2727
Ticlid Tablets ... 2317
Vantin for Oral Suspension and Vantin Tablets ... 2112
Cataflam/Voltaren/Voltaren-XR (Less than 1%) ... 833

Digitalis toxicity

Demadex Tablets and Injection ... 691
Lanoxicaps ... 1110
Virazole ... 1310

Diplegia

Imitrex Injection (Rare) ... 1095

Diplopia

Abelcet Injection ... 1540
Adalat CC (Less than 1.0%) ... 582
Ambien Tablets (Frequent) ... 2559
Amen Tablets ... 785
Anafranil Capsules (Infrequent) ... 819
Atamet Tablets ... 567
Ativan Injection (Occasional) ... 2805
Atretol Tablets ... 569
Azactam for Injection (Less than 1%) ... 736
Benadryl Injection ... 1955
Bentyl ... 1246
Betagan ... ⊙ 230
Betaseron for SC Injection ... 653
Betimol 0.25%, 0.5% ... ⊙ 259
Blocadren Tablets ... 1654
BOTOX (Botulinum Toxin Type A Purified Neurotoxin Complex (Less than 1%) ... 473
Brevicon ... 2563
Buprenex Injectable (Less than 1%) ... 2170
Cardioquin Tablets ... 2146
Cataflam Tablets (Less than 1%) ... 833
▲ Cerebyx Injection (3.3%) ... 1956
Chibroxin Sterile Ophthalmic Solution (With oral form) ... 1657
Cipro I.V. (1% or less) ... 587
Cipro I.V. Pharmacy Bulk Package (Less than 1%) ... 590
Cipro Tablets (Less than 1%) ... 584
Clomid (1.5%) ... 1262
Cognex Capsules (Infrequent) ... 1961
Cycrin Tablets ... 991
Cytovene-IV (One report) ... 2270
Dalgan Injection (Less than 1%) ... 529
Dalmane Capsules ... 2329
Dantrium Capsules (Less frequent) ... 2131

Demulen ... 2580
Depakene ... 416
▲ Depakote Tablets (1% to 5%) ... 418
Depen Titratable Tablets ... 2770
Depo-Provera Contraceptive Injection ... 2079
Depo-Provera Sterile Aqueous Suspension ... 2083
Desyrel and Desyrel Dividose ... 504
Dilaudid-HP Injection (Less frequent) ... 1384
Dilaudid-HP Lyophilized Powder 250 mg (Less frequent) ... 1384
Dilaudid Tablets and Liquid (Less frequent) ... 1386
Diprivan Injectable Emulsion (Less than 1%) ... 2939
Dizac (diazepam injectable emulsion) CIV (Less frequent) ... 1862
Duranest Injections ... 533
Dyclone 0.5% and 1% Topical Solutions, USP ... 535
Effexor (Infrequent) ... 2825
Eldepryl Capsules ... 2729
EMLA Cream (Unlikely with cream) ... 536
Ethmozine Tablets (Less than 2%) ... 2217
▲ Felbatol (3.4% to 6.1%) ... 2774
Flexeril Tablets (Less than 1%) ... 1701
Floxin I.V. ... 1580
Floxin Tablets (200 mg, 300 mg, 400 mg) ... 1577
Foscavir Injection (Less than 1%) ... 541
Fungizone Intravenous ... 507
IBU Tablets (Less than 1%) ... 1389
Indocin (Less than 1%) ... 1723
Intron A for Injection (Less than 5%) ... 2506
Ismo Tablets (Fewer than 1%) ... 2844
Kadian Capsules (Less than 3%) ... 2948
Klonopin Tablets ... 2294
▲ Lamictal Tablets (Among most common; 24% to 49%) ... 1105
Larodopa Tablets (Infrequent) ... 2296
Levlen/Tri-Levlen (Rare) ... 646
Levo-Dromoran ... 2297
Lioresal Intrathecal (Up to 0.9%) ... 1634
Lioresal Tablets ... 847
LUVOX Tablets (Infrequent) ... 2723
Lysodren Tablets (Infrequent) ... 707
MS Contin Tablets (Less frequent) ... 2149
MSIR (Infrequent) ... 2152
Matulane Capsules ... 2300
Maxaquin Tablets ... 2593
Mesantoin Tablets ... 2400
Modicon (Rare) ... 1928
Motrin Ibuprofen Suspension, Oral Drops, Chewable Tablets, Caplets (Less than 1%) ... 1563
Mysoline (Occasional) ... 2860
Nalfon 200 Pulvules & Nalfon Tablets (Less than 1%) ... 933
Naprelan Tablets (Less than 1%) ... 2861
NegGram (Infrequent) ... 2453
▲ Neurontin Capsules (5.9%) ... 1978
Norinyl ... 2563
Noroxin Tablets ... 1758
Noroxin Tablets ... 2222
Nor-Q D Tablets ... 2598
Norvasc Tablets (More than 0.1% to 1%) ... 2020
Norvir (Less than 2%) ... 447
Novahistine Elixir ... ◨ 782
Nuromax Injection (Less than or equal to 0.1%) ... 1136
Ocupress Ophthalmic Solution, 1% Sterile ... ⊙ 297
Oramorph SR (Morphine Sulfate Sustained Release Tablets) (Less frequent) ... 2359
Ornade Spansule Capsules ... 2678
Ortho-Cyclen/Ortho-Tri-Cyclen ... 1914
Ortho-Novum (Rare) ... 1928
Ortho-Cyclen/Ortho Tri-Cyclen ... 1914
Orthoclone OKT3 Sterile Solution ... 1892
Ovcon ... 765
PBZ Tablets ... 863
PBZ-SR Tablets ... 862
Paxil Tablets (Rare) ... 2681
Peganone Tablets ... 455
Periactin ... 1767
Permax Tablets (2.1%) ... 571
Phenergan Injection ... 2880
Phenergan Tablets ... 2882
Placidyl Capsules ... 456
Premphase ... 2900
Prempro ... 2905
Prinivil Tablets (0.3% to 1.0%) ... 1776
Prinzide Tablets ... 1780
Proglycem ... 575
ProSom Tablets (Rare) ... 457
Protopam Chloride for Injection ... 2909

Provera Tablets ... 2110
Prozac Pulvules & Liquid, Oral Solution (Rare) ... 935
Quinaglute Dura-Tabs Tablets ... 644
Quinidex Extentabs ... 2240
Redux Capsules (Infrequent) ... 2911
Remeron Tablets (Rare) ... 1878
Rilutek Tablets (Rare) ... 2198
Risperdal Tablets (Rare) ... 1348
Robaxin Injectable ... 2245
Romazicon (1% to 3%) ... 2311
Rondec Oral Drops ... 974
Rondec Syrup ... 974
Rondec ... 974
Serax Capsules ... 2916
Serax Tablets ... 2916
Serophene (clomiphene citrate tablets, USP) ... 2621
Serzone Tablets (Infrequent) ... 776
Sinemet Tablets ... 959
Soma Compound w/Codeine Tablets (Very rare) ... 2784
Soma Compound Tablets (Very rare) ... 2783
Soma Tablets ... 2782
Supprelin Injection (1% to 3%) ... 2230
Talwin Injection ... 2465
Tambocor Tablets (1% to less than 3%) ... 1555
Tavist Syrup ... 2426
Tavist Tablets ... 2427
▲ Tegison Capsules (10-25%) ... 2314
Tegretol/Tegretol-XR ... 870
Tensilon Injectable ... 1307
Timolide Tablets ... 1791
Timoptic in Ocudose (Less frequent) ... 1796
Timoptic Sterile Ophthalmic Solution (Less frequent) ... 1794
Timoptic-XE ... 1798
Tonocard Tablets (Less than 1%) ... 519
Tranxene ... 459
Levlen/Tri-Levlen (Rare) ... 646
Tri-Norinyl ... 2607
Tussend ... 1830
Valium Injectable ... 2336
Valium Tablets (Infrequent) ... 2335
Versed Injection (Less than 1%) ... 2324
Videx Tablets, Powder for Oral Solution, & Pediatric Powder for Oral Solution (Less than 1%) ... 2980
Cataflam/Voltaren/Voltaren-XR (Less than 1%) ... 833
Wellbutrin Tablets (Rare) ... 1177
Xalatan (Less than 1%) ... ⊙ 304
Xanax Tablets ... 2115
▲ Xylocaine Injections (Less than 1% to among most common) ... 562
Zestoretic Tablets ... 2968
Zestril Tablets (0.3% to 1.0%) ... 2972
Zoloft Tablets (Infrequent) ... 2051

Dipsesis

Aldactone Tablets ... 2558
Alferon N Injection (1%) ... 2142
Ambien Tablets (Infrequent) ... 2559
Anafranil Capsules (Up to 2%) ... 819
Anaprox/Naprosyn (Less than 3%) ... 2277
Apresazide Capsules ... 824
Atrovent Nasal Spray 0.06% (Less than 1%) ... 678
Avonex ... 662
Betaseron for SC Injection ... 653
Capozide Tablets ... 744
Cardizem CD Capsules (Less than 1%) ... 1251
Cardizem SR Capsules (Less than 1%) ... 1255
Cardizem Injectable ... 1253
Cardizem Tablets (Less than 1%) ... 1257
Cardura Tablets (Less than 0.5% of 3960 patients) ... 1993
Ceftin (0.1% to 1%) ... 1067
Claritin Tablets (2% or fewer patients) ... 2485
Claritin-D Tablets (2%) ... 2487
CordyMax Cs-4 Capsules (Sometimes) ... 2985
Cytotec (Infrequent) ... 2576
DaunoXome (Less than or equal to 5%) ... 1842
Demadex Tablets and Injection ... 691
Depo-Provera Contraceptive Injection (Fewer than 1%) ... 2079
Dyazide Capsules ... 2653
Dynabac (0.1% to 1%) ... 668
Easprin ... 1971
EC-Naprosyn Delayed-Release Tablets (Less than 3%) ... 2277
Effexor (Infrequent) ... 2825

(◨ Described in PDR For Nonprescription Drugs)   Incidence data in parenthesis; ▲ 3% or more   (⊙ Described in PDR For Ophthalmology)

Dipsesis
Side Effects Index
1308

Emcyt Capsules (1%) 2085
Esidrix Tablets 839
Eskalith 2658
Flexeril Tablets (Less than 1%) 1701
Floxin I.V. (Less than 1%) 1580
Floxin Tablets (200 mg, 300 mg, 400 mg) (Less than 1%) 1577
Foscavir Injection (Between 1% and 5%) 541
Glucotrol XL Extended Release Tablets (Less than 1%) 2012
Imitrex Injection (Infrequent) 1095
Imitrex Tablets (Infrequent) 1099
Intron A for Injection (Less than or equal to 5%) 2506
ISMOTIC 45% w/v Solution (Very rare) .... ⊙ 221
K-Phos Neutral Tablets 633
Kerlone Tablets (Less than 2%) 2588
Lamictal Tablets (Infrequent) 1105
Lasix Injection, Oral Solution and Tablets 1267
Lithium Carbonate Capsules & Tablets 2352
Lithonate/Lithotabs/Lithobid 2721
Lodine Capsules and Tablets (Less than 1%) 2849
▲ Lupron Depot 3.75 mg (Among most frequent) 2739
Lupron Depot - 3 Month 22.5 mg (Less than 5%) 2743
LUVOX Tablets 2723
Maxaquin Tablets (Less than 1%) 2593
Miacalcin Nasal Spray (Less than 1%) 2403
Midamor Tablets (Less than or equal to 1%) 1746
Moduretic Tablets (Less than or equal to 1%) 1748
Monoket Tablets (Fewer than 1%) 2550
Naprelan Tablets (Less than 3%) 2861
Anaprox/Naprosyn (Less than 3%) 2277
Neurontin Capsules (Infrequent) 1978
Norvasc Tablets (More than 0.1% to 1%) 2020
Norvir (Less than 2%) 447
Oncaspar (Less than 1%) 2194
▲ Orap Tablets (1 of 20 patients) 1037
Oretic Tablets 450
Orudis Capsules (Less than 1%) 2874
Oruvail Capsules (Less than 1%) 2874
OxyContin Tablets (Less than 1%) 2163
Paxil Tablets (Infrequent) 2681
Pentasa (Less than 1%) 1275
Permax Tablets (Infrequent) 571
Prevacid Delayed-Release Capsules (Less than 1%) 2746
Prinzide Tablets 1780
ProSom Tablets (Infrequent) 457
Prozac Pulvules & Liquid, Oral Solution (Infrequent) 935
Redux Capsules (2.8%) 2911
Remeron Tablets (Frequent) 1878
▲ ReVia Tablets (Less than 10%) 957
Rilutek Tablets (Infrequent) 2198
Risperdal Tablets (Infrequent) 1348
Sanorex Tablets 2423
Serzone Tablets (1%) 776
Supprelin Injection (1% to 3%) 2230
▲ Tegison Capsules (50-75%) 2314
Tenoretic Tablets 2963
Thalitone (Common) 1293
Tiazac Capsules (Less than 1%) 1019
Tonocard Tablets (Less than 1%) 519
Toradol (1% or less) 2319
Trental Tablets (Less than 1%) 1291
Uroqid-Acid No. 2 Tablets 633
Vaseretic Tablets 1810
Videx Tablets, Powder for Oral Solution, & Pediatric Powder for Oral Solution (Less than 1%) 2980
Zaroxolyn Tablets 1625
Zestoretic Tablets 2968
Zoloft Tablets (1.4%) 2051
▲ Zonalon Cream (Approximately 1% to 10%) 1042
Zosyn (1.0% or less) 1463
Zovirax Sterile Powder (Less than 1%) 1191
Zyrtec Tablets (Less than 2%) 2053

Discoloration, injection site
Depo-Provera Sterile Aqueous Suspension 2083
Diprivan Injectable Emulsion (Less than 1%) 2939
▲ Navelbine Injection (Approximately one-third of patients) 1212

Discomfort, arm
▲ Adenoscan (4%) 1022
Respbid Tablets 687

Discomfort, chest
▲ Adenoscan (40%) 1022
Brethine Ampuls (1.3 to 1.5%) 832
Ceredase 1055
Helixate, Antihemophilic Factor (Recombinant) 799
Imitrex Injection (Rare; 4.5%) 1095
Imitrex Tablets (Frequent) 1099
KOGENATE Antihemophilic Factor (Recombinant) 626
Primaxin I.M. 1770
Primaxin I.V. (Less than 0.2%) 1772
Prinivil Tablets (0.3 to 1.0%) 1776
Prinzide Tablets (0.3 to 1%) 1780
Proventil (Less than 1%) 2529
Recombivax HB (Less than 1%) 1787
Timentin for Injection 2706
Tornalate Solution for Inhalation, 0.2% (Less than 1% to 1.5%) 976
Tornalate Metered Dose Inhaler (Approximately 1%; 0.5%) 978
Ventolin Tablets (Fewer than 1 of 100 patients) 1176
▲ Vesanoid Capsules (32%) 2327
Volmax Extended-Release Tablets (Less frequent) 1835
Zaroxolyn Tablets 1625
Zestoretic Tablets (0.3 to 1.0%) 2968
Zestril Tablets (0.3% to 1.0%) 2972

Discomfort, general
AVC (Occasional) 1245
Coumadin 941
EPIFRIN .... ⊙ 237
Eskalith 2658
IOPIDINE Sterile Ophthalmic Solution .... ⊙ 218
Lithium Carbonate Capsules & Tablets 2352
Lithonate/Lithotabs/Lithobid 2721
Papaverine Hydrochloride Vials and Ampoules 1523
Pilopine HS Ophthalmic Gel .... ⊙ 224
Zovirax Ointment 5% 1190

Discomfort, jaw
▲ Adenoscan (15%) 1022
Imitrex Injection (1.8%) 1095

Discomfort, local
Albalon Solution with Liquifilm .... ⊙ 229
▲ Betimol 0.25%, 0.5% (More than 5%) .... ⊙ 259
▲ Chibroxin Sterile Ophthalmic Solution (One of the two most frequent) 1657
▲ Ciloxan Ophthalmic Solution (Among most frequent) 468
Efudex (Infrequent) 2280
OptiPranolol (Metipranolol 0.3%) Sterile Ophthalmic Solution (A small number of patients) .... ⊙ 256
▲ Testoderm Testosterone Transdermal System (4%) 486

Discomfort, nasal
Imitrex Injection (2.2%) 1095
▲ Imitrex Tablets (5% to 7%) 1099

Discomfort at injection site
Azactam for Injection (2.4%) 736
Cefotan (1 in 500) 2936
Ceredase 1055
MICRhoGAM $Rh_0(D)$ Immune Globulin (Human) 1902
▲ Monocid Injection (5.7%) 2674
Oncovin Solution Vials & Hyporets 1521
PPD Tine Test 2993
▲ Rabies Vaccine Adsorbed (Approximately 65% to 70%) 2686
RhoGAM $Rh_0(D)$ Immune Globulin (Human) 1902
Tuberculin, Old, Tine Test 2994
Tubersol (Tuberculin Purified Protein Derivative (Mantoux)) 2988
WinRho SD (A small number of cases) 1839

Discontinuation syndrome
Catapres-TTS 680
Combipres Tablets (About 1%) 682

Disorientation
Actimmune (Rare) 1043
Adapin Capsules (Infrequent) 1542
Akineton 1380
Alferon N Injection (1%) 2142
Apresazide Capsules (Less frequent) 824
Apresoline Hydrochloride Tablets (Less frequent) 826
Asacol Delayed-Release Tablets 2129
Asendin Tablets (Less than 1%) 1419
Ativan Tablets (Less frequent) 2807
Bentyl 10 mg Capsules 1246
Biaxin 406
BOTOX (Botulinum Toxin Type A) Purified Neurotoxin Complex 473
Brontex 2130
Cataflam Tablets (Rare) 833
CeeNU Capsules 699
Dalmane Capsules 2329
Daranide Tablets 1676
Demerol 2438
Demser Capsules 1690
Desyrel and Desyrel Dividose (Less than 1% to 2.1%) 504
Dilaudid-HP Injection (Less frequent) 1384
Dilaudid-HP Lyophilized Powder 250 mg (Less frequent) 1384
Dilaudid Tablets and Liquid (Less frequent) 1386
Dolobid Tablets (Less than 1 in 100) 1695
Dopram Injectable 2235
Elavil 2945
Eldepryl Capsules 2729
Etrafon 2495
Famvir Tablets (Very rare) 2660
Fioricet with Codeine Capsules 2387
Fiorinal with Codeine Capsules 2390
Flexeril Tablets (Less than 1%) 1701
Floxin I.V. 1580
Floxin Tablets (200 mg, 300 mg, 400 mg) 1577
Fluorouracil Injection 2282
Sterile FUDR (Remote possibility) 2284
Halcion Tablets 2093
Hydralazine Hydrochloride Injection USP (Less frequent) 2712
Hydrea Capsules (Extremely rare) 705
IFEX (Less frequent) 706
INFeD (Iron Dextran Injection, USP) 2478
ISMOTIC 45% w/v Solution .... ⊙ 221
Levbid Extended-Release Tablets 2549
Levoprome (Sometimes) 1321
Levsin/Levsinex/Levbid 2549
Ludiomil Tablets (Rare) 861
MS Contin Tablets (Less frequent) 2149
MSIR (Infrequent) 2152
Mepergan Injection 2859
Methadone Hydrochloride Oral Concentrate 2356
Methadone Hydrochloride Oral Solution & Tablets 2357
Myambutol Tablets 1432
Nalfon 200 Pulvules & Nalfon Tablets (Less than 1%) 933
Nebcin Vials, Hyporets & ADD-Vantage 1518
Netromycin Injection 100 mg/ml (1 of 1000 patients) 2516
Norpramin Tablets 1273
Oncaspar 2194
Oramorph SR (Morphine Sulfate Sustained Release Tablets) (Less frequent) 2359
Orthoclone OKT3 Sterile Solution 1892
OSMOGLYN Oral Osmotic Agent .... ⊙ 225
Pamelor 2409
Parnate Tablets 2679
Pediazole Suspension 2340
Phenergan with Codeine 2883
Phenergan with Dextromethorphan 2885
Phenergan Suppositories 2882
Phenergan Syrup 2881
Phenergan VC 2886
Phenergan VC with Codeine 2888
RMS Suppositories CII 2766
ReVia Tablets (Less than 1%) 957
Roxanol 2365
Seldane-D Extended-Release Tablets (1.1%) 1286
Ser-Ap-Es Tablets 867
Serax Capsules 2916
Serax Tablets 2916
Seromycin Capsules 975
Sinemet CR Tablets 961
Sinequan (Infrequent) 2028
Soma Compound w/Codeine Tablets (Very rare) 2784
Soma Compound Tablets (Very rare) 2783
Soma Tablets 2782
Surmontil Capsules 2917
Tagamet 2694
Talacen Caplets 2464
Talwin Injection 2465
Talwin Compound 2466
Talwin Injection 2465
Talwin Nx Tablets 2467
Tigan 2231
Timoptic in Ocudose (Less frequent) 1796
Timoptic Sterile Ophthalmic Solution (Less frequent) 1794
Timoptic-XE 1798
Tofranil Ampuls 873
Tofranil Tablets 875
Tofranil-PM Capsules 876
▲ Tonocard Tablets (2.1% to 11.2%) 519
Transderm Scōp Transdermal Therapeutic System (Infrequent) 890
Triavil Tablets 1800
Vivactil Tablets 1820
Cataflam/Voltaren/Voltaren-XR (Rare) 833
WinRho SD (One report) 1839

Disorientation, place
Blocadren Tablets 1654
Cartrol Tablets 413
Inderal 2834
Inderal LA Long Acting Capsules 2836
Inderide Tablets 2838
Inderide LA Long Acting Capsules 2840
Kerlone Tablets 2588
Levatol Tablets 2547
Lopressor HCT Tablets 850
Normodyne Tablets 2522
Sectral Capsules 2914
Tenoretic Tablets 2963
Tenormin Tablets and I.V. Injection 2965
Timolide Tablets 1791
Timoptic in Ocudose 1796
Timoptic Sterile Ophthalmic Solution 1794
Timoptic-XE 1798
Toprol-XL Tablets 560
Trandate Tablets 1158
Visken Tablets 2428
Zebeta Tablets 1457
Ziac 1459

Disorientation, time
Blocadren Tablets 1654
Cartrol Tablets 413
Inderal 2834
Inderal LA Long Acting Capsules 2836
Inderide Tablets 2838
Inderide LA Long Acting Capsules 2840
Kerlone Tablets 2588
Levatol Tablets 2547
Lopressor HCT Tablets 850
Normodyne Tablets 2522
Sectral Capsules 2914
Tenoretic Tablets 2963
Tenormin Tablets and I.V. Injection 2965
Timolide Tablets 1791
Timoptic in Ocudose 1796
Timoptic Sterile Ophthalmic Solution 1794
Timoptic-XE 1798
Toprol-XL Tablets 560
Trandate Tablets 1158
Visken Tablets 2428
Zebeta Tablets 1457
Ziac 1459

Distention, abdominal (see under Abdominal distention)

Distress, abdominal
Ambien Tablets (Rare) 2559
Atamet Tablets 567
Atromid-S Capsules (Less frequent) 2808
Augmentin (Less frequent) 2637
Augmentin Tablets (Less frequent) 2640
Ceredase 1055
Cerezyme (One patient) 1056
Claritin-D Tablets (Less frequent) 2487
Daypro Caplets (1% to 3%) 2578
▲ Depo-Provera Contraceptive Injection (More than 5%) 2079
EryPed 200 & EryPed 400 Granules 425
Ery-Tab Tablets 426
Erythrocin Stearate Filmtab 429
Estrace Cream and Tablets 751
Factrel (Rare) 2996
Glucophage Tablets 754
Hylorel Tablets (1.7%) 1613
IBU Tablets (Greater than 1%) 1389

(▭ Described in PDR For Nonprescription Drugs) Incidence data in parenthesis; ▲ 3% or more (⊙ Described in PDR For Ophthalmology)

1309 Side Effects Index Dizziness

▲ Ilosone (One of the two most frequent) 927
Imitrex Injection (1.3%) 1095
Imitrex Tablets 1099
Indocin (Greater than 1%) 1723
▲ Invirase Capsules (Among most frequent) 2291
IOPIDINE Sterile Ophthalmic Solution ⊙ 218
▲ K-Lor Powder Packets (Among most common) 438
▲ K-Tab Filmtab (Most common) 439
Levoprome (Sometimes) 1321
▲ Methotrexate Sodium Tablets, Injection, for Injection and LPF Injection (Among most frequent) 1322
Mexitil Capsules (1.2%) 684
Motrin Ibuprofen Suspension, Oral Drops, Chewable Tablets, Caplets (1% to less than 3%) 1563
▲ Norplant System (5% or greater) 2868
▲ Persantine Tablets (6.1%) 686
Protostat Tablets 1939
Questran (Less frequent) 774
Rum-K Syrup 1004
Sanorex Tablets 2423
▲ Seldane Tablets (4.6% to 7.6%) 1284
Seldane-D Extended-Release Tablets 1286
Senna X-Prep Bowel Evacuant Liquid 1236
Sinemet Tablets 959
Talacen Caplets (Rare) 2464
Talwin Compound (Rare) 2466
Talwin Nx Tablets (Rare) 2467
THYREL TRH 2992
▲ Ultrase MT Capsules (Among most frequent) 2477
▲ Xanax Tablets (18.3%) 2115
Zantac Injection 1180

Distress, epigastric

Abelcet Injection 1540
Aerolate 1003
Amaryl Tablets (Less than 1%) 1241
Asendin Tablets (Less than 1%) 1419
Atrohist Plus Tablets 1605
▲ Benadryl Injection (Among most frequent) 1955
▲ Bromfed-DM Cough Syrup (Among most frequent) 1832
Carbastat Intraocular Solution ⊙ 260
Celontin Kapseals (Frequent) 1955
Cipro I.V. (1% or less) 587
Cipro I.V. Pharmacy Bulk Package (Less than 1%) 590
Combipres Tablets 682
Cuprimine Capsules 1673
D.H.E. 45 Injection 2381
▲ Depen Titratable Tablets (17%) 2770
DiaBeta Tablets (1.8%) 1265
Dimetane-DC Cough Syrup 2232
Dimetane-DX Cough Syrup 2233
Dipentum Capsules (Rare) 2084
Elavil 2945
Etrafon 2495
▲ Feldene Capsules (3% to 9%) 2008
Flagyl 375 Capsules 2587
Flagyl I.V. 2373
Fulvicin P/G Tablets (Occasional) 2499
Fulvicin P/G 165 & 330 Tablets (Occasional) 2500
▲ Fungizone Intravenous (Among most common) 507
Geocillin Tablets 2009
Grifulvin V (griseofulvin tablets) Microsize (griseofulvin oral suspension) Microsize (Occasional) 1944
Gris-PEG Tablets, 125 mg & 250 mg (Occasional) 476
Helidac Therapy (Sometimes) 2135
Hivid Tablets (Less than 1%) 2287
▲ IBU Tablets (3% to 9%) 1389
Inderal 2834
Inderal LA Long Acting Capsules 2836
Inderide Tablets 2838
Inderide LA Long Acting Capsules 2840
▲ Indocin (3% to 9%) 1723
Isuprel Hydrochloride Solution 2443
Isuprel Mistometer 2442
Kemadrin Tablets 1105
▲ Lamprene Capsules (40-50%) 846
Limbitrol 2333
Ludiomil Tablets (Rare) 861
Lufyllin & Lufyllin-400 Tablets 2778
Lufyllin-GG Elixir & Tablets 2779
MetroGel-Vaginal 917
▲ Mexitil Capsules (41%) 684
Micronase Tablets (1.8%) 2099
Mintezol 1747
MIOSTAT Intraocular Solution ⊙ 222
Motofen Tablets (1 in 100) 789
▲ Motrin Ibuprofen Suspension, Oral Drops, Chewable Tablets, Caplets (3% to 9%) 1563
Norisodrine with Calcium Iodide Syrup 446
Norpramin Tablets 1273
Nydrazid Injection 509
Oncaspar (Less than 1%) 2194
Ornade Spansule Capsules 2678
▲ PBZ Tablets (Among most frequent) 863
▲ PBZ-SR Tablets (Among most frequent) 862
Pamelor 2409
▲ Pen•Vee K (Among most common) 2879
Periactin 1767
Phenergan VC 2886
Phenergan VC with Codeine 2888
Pima Syrup 1004
Proloprim Tablets 1141
Protostat Tablets (Occasional) 1939
Proventil Syrup (Less than 1 of 100 patients) 2528
Quadrinal Tablets 1398
Quibron 2227
Respbid Tablets 687
Rifadin (Some patients) 1276
Rifamate Capsules (Some patients) 1278
Rifater 1280
Rimactane Capsules 865
Slo-bid Gyrocaps 2201
Soma Compound w/Codeine Tablets 2784
Soma Compound Tablets 2783
Soma Tablets 2782
Spectrobid Tablets (2%) 2030
Surmontil Capsules 2917
Tapazole Tablets 1361
▲ Tavist Syrup (Among most frequent) 2426
▲ Tavist Tablets (Among most frequent) 2427
Theo-24 Extended Release Capsules 2753
Theo-Dur Extended-Release Tablets 1367
Theo-X Extended-Release Tablets 793
▲ Ticlid Tablets (3.7%) 2317
Timentin for Injection 2706
Tofranil Ampuls 873
Tofranil Tablets 875
Tofranil-PM Capsules 876
Toprol-XL Tablets (About 1 of 100 patients) 560
▲ Toradol (13%) 2319
Triavil Tablets 1800
▲ Trilisate (Less than 20%) 2155
Trimpex Tablets 2323
▲ Trinalin Repetabs Tablets (Among most frequent) 1373
Tussend 1830
Uni-Dur Extended-Release Tablets 1374
Ventolin Syrup (Less than 1 of 100 patients) 1175
Vivactil Tablets 1820
Wigraine Tablets 1884
Yutopar Intravenous Injection (Infrequent) 566
Zarontin Capsules (Frequent) 1986
Zarontin Syrup (Frequent) 1986
Zaroxolyn Tablets 1625
Zebeta Tablets 1457
Ziac 1459

Distress, gastric (see under Distress, gastrointestinal)

Distress, gastrointestinal

AK-FLUOR Injection 10% and 25% ⊙ 204
Alferon N Injection (One patient) 2142
Alupent (1% to 4%) 672
Atretol Tablets 569
Atrovent Inhalation Aerosol (2.4%) 674
▲ Azulfidine (Approximately one-third of patients) 2059
Biltricide Tablets 584
Bumex (0.1%) 2260
BuSpar Tablets (2%) 738
Calan SR Caplets (1% or less) 2571
Calan Tablets (1% or less) 2568
Carafate Suspension (Less than 0.5%) 1250
Carafate Tablets (Less than 0.5%) 1249
Celontin Kapseals (Frequent) 1955
Claritin Tablets (2% or fewer patients) 2485
▲ Clinoril Tablets (10%) 1658
Covera-HS Tablets (Less than 2%) 2573
Cuprimine Capsules 1673
▲ Desyrel and Desyrel Dividose (3.5% to 5.7%) 504
▲ Dolobid Tablets (3% to 9%) 1695
DynaCirc Capsules (Up to 3.3%) 2381
▲ Emcyt Capsules (11%) 2085
Esimil Tablets 840
Fastin Capsules 2662
Feldene Capsules (Greater than 1%) 2008
Feosol Caplets 2626
Feosol Elixir (Occasional) 2627
Feosol Tablets (Occasional) 2627
Fioricet with Codeine Capsules 2387
Fiorinal with Codeine Capsules 2390
Flexeril Tablets (Less than 1%) 1701
Floxin I.V. (1% to 3%) 1580
Floxin Tablets (200 mg, 300 mg, 400 mg) (1% to 3%) 1577
Fluorescite ⊙ 217
Hydergine 2392
Imitrex Tablets (Frequent) 1099
▲ Imuran (Approximately 12%) 1103
ISMOTIC 45% w/v Solution (Very rare) ⊙ 221
Isoptin Injectable (0.6%) 1391
Isoptin Oral Tablets (Less than 1%) 1393
Isoptin SR Tablets (1% or less) 1395
K-Dur Microburst Release System (potassium chloride, USP) E.R. Tablets 1364
▲ K-Norm Capsules (Among most common) 1615
Kadian Capsules (Less than 3%) 2948
Larodopa Tablets 2296
Lopid Tablets 1974
Lopressor (1%) 848
Lopressor HCT Tablets (1 in 100 patients) 850
Lupron Depot - 3 Month 22.5 mg 2743
▲ Lysodren Tablets (80%) 707
Midamor Tablets (Between 1% and 3%) 1746
Minipress Capsules (Less than 1%) 2015
Minizide Capsules (Rare) 2016
Moduretic Tablets (Greater than 1%, less than 3%) 1748
Nardil (Common) 1977
Norisodrine with Calcium Iodide Syrup 446
Orap Tablets 1037
▲ Phenurone Tablets (8%) 455
Placidyl Capsules 456
Ponstel 1982
Prelu-2 Timed Release Capsules 687
Pyridium (Occasional) 1985
▲ Quinidex Extentabs (22%) 2240
Robaxisal Tablets 2246
Roferon-A Injection (Less than 1%) 2308
▲ Sandostatin Injection (4% to 61%) 2421
Scleromate Injection (Rare) 1234
Sedapap Tablets 50 mg/650 mg (Less frequent) 1826
Supprelin Injection (1% to 3%) 2230
Tegretol/Tegretol-XR 870
Timolide Tablets (Less than 1%) 1791
Timoptic in Ocudose 1796
Timoptic Sterile Ophthalmic Solution 1794
▲ Tolectin (200, 400 and 600 mg) (3 to 9%) 1591
▲ Vascor Tablets (200 and 300 mg) (4.35 to about 22%) 1597
Verelan Capsules (1% or less) 1455
Zarontin Capsules (Frequent) 1986
Zarontin Syrup (Frequent) 1986
Zebeta Tablets 1457
Ziac 1459
Zovirax 1187

Distress, precordial (see under Distress, epigastric)

Distress, stomach (see under Distress, gastrointestinal)

Distress, upper GI (see under Distress, epigastric)

Disturbances, emotional (see under Emotional disturbances)

Disturbances, gastrointestinal (see under Distress, gastrointestinal)

Disulfiram-like reactions

Amaryl Tablets 1241
DiaBeta Tablets (Very rare) 1265
Diabinese Tablets 2002
Furoxone (Rare) 2221
Glucotrol Tablets 2011
Glynase PresTab Tablets (Very rare) 2091
Micronase Tablets (Very rare) 2099

Diuresis

Axocet Capsules (Infrequent) 2469
Azulfidine (Rare) 2059
Bactrim DS Tablets (Rare) 2257
Bactrim I.V. Infusion (Rare) 2255
Bactrim (Rare) 2257
Esgic-plus Capsules (Infrequent) 1012
Esgic-plus Tablets (Infrequent) 1012
Fansidar Tablets (Rare) 2281
Fioricet Tablets (Infrequent) 2386
Fioricet with Codeine Capsules (Infrequent) 2387
Fiorinal with Codeine Capsules (Infrequent) 2390
Gantanol Tablets (Rare) 2285
Gantrisin (Rare) 2286
Lufyllin & Lufyllin-400 Tablets 2778
Lufyllin-GG Elixir & Tablets 2779
Marax Tablets & DF Syrup 2015
Pediazole Suspension (Rare) 2340
Phrenilin (Infrequent) 790
Quadrinal Tablets 1398
Questran 774
Quibron 2227
Respbid Tablets 687
Sedapap Tablets 50 mg/650 mg (Infrequent) 1826
Septra (Rare) 1146
Septra I.V. Infusion (Rare) 1142
Septra I.V. Infusion ADD-Vantage Vials (Rare) 1144
Septra (Rare) 1146
Theo-24 Extended Release Capsules 2753
Theo-Dur Extended-Release Tablets 1367
Tonocard Tablets (Less than 1%) 519
Uni-Dur Extended-Release Tablets 1374

Diuresis, potentiation of

Slo-bid Gyrocaps 2201
Theo-X Extended-Release Tablets 793
Uniphyl 400 mg and 600 mg Tablets 2157

Diverticulitis

Avonex 662
Cognex Capsules (Infrequent) 1961
Questran 774
Risperdal Tablets (Rare) 1348
Zoloft Tablets (Rare) 2051

Dizziness

▲ Accupril Tablets (3.9% to 7.7%) 1950
Accutane Capsules 2252
Achromycin V Capsules 1417
Actifed Cold & Allergy Tablets ▣ 807
Actifed Cold & Sinus Caplets and Tablets ▣ 808
Acutrim ▣ 648
▲ Adalat Capsules (10 mg and 20 mg) (About 10% to 27%) 580
▲ Adalat CC (4%) 582
Adapin Capsules (Occasional) 1542
Adderall Tablets 2209
Adenocard Injection (1%) 1021
▲ Adenoscan (12%) 1022
Adipex-P Tablets and Capsules 1035
Advil Cold and Sinus Caplets and Tablets ▣ 837
▲ AeroBid Inhaler System (3% to 9%) 1004

(▣ Described in PDR For Nonprescription Drugs) Incidence data in parenthesis; ▲ 3% or more (⊙ Described in PDR For Ophthalmology)

Dizziness — Side Effects Index

▲ Aerobid-M Inhaler System (3% to 9%)	1004	▲ Brevibloc (esmolol HCl) Injection (3% to 12%)	1860
Aerolate	1003	Brevicon	2563
▲ Airet Albuterol Sulfate Inhalation Solution (7%)	1602	Bricanyl Subcutaneous Injection (Common)	1247
Albalon Solution with Liquifilm	⊙ 229	Bricanyl Tablets (Common)	1248
Albenza Tablets (Less than 1.0% to 1.2%)	2629	Bromfed	1832
▲ Albuterol Sulfate, USP Solution for Inhalation, Arm-a-Med (7%)	522	▲ Bromfed-DM Cough Syrup (Among most frequent)	1832
Aldactazide Tablets	2556	Bromfed-PD Capsules (Extended-Release)	1832
Aldoclor Tablets	1638	Bronkometer Aerosol	2432
Aldomet Ester HCl Injection	1642	Bronkosol Solution	2432
Aldomet Oral	1640	Brontex	2130
Aldoril Tablets	1644	Arthritis Strength Bufferin Analgesic Caplets	⊡ 637
▲ Alfenta Injection (3% to 9%)	1334	Bumex (1.1%)	2260
▲ Alferon N Injection (9%)	2142	▲ Buprenex Injectable (5-10%)	2170
Alka-Seltzer Plus	⊡ 611	▲ BuSpar Tablets (12%)	738
Alka-Seltzer Plus Sinus Medicine	⊡ 611	Butisol Sodium Elixir & Tablets (Less than 1 in 100)	2768
Allerest Maximum Strength	⊡ 649	▲ Calan SR Caplets (3.3%)	2571
Allerest No Drowsiness	⊡ 649	▲ Calan Tablets (3.3%)	2568
Allerest Sinus Pain Formula	⊡ 649	Cama Arthritis Pain Reliever	⊡ 748
All-Flex Arcing Spring Diaphragm (See also Ortho Diaphragm Kits)	1921	Capoten Tablets (About 0.5 to 2%)	740
Alomide Ophthalmic Solution (Less than 1%)	465	Capozide Tablets (0.5 to 2%)	744
▲ Altace Capsules (2.2% to 4.1%)	1238	Carafate Suspension (Less than 0.5%)	1250
Alupent (1% to 4%)	672	Carafate Tablets (Less than 0.5%)	1249
Amaryl Tablets (1.7%)	1241	Carbocaine Injection	2432
Ambien Tablets (1% to 5%)	2559	▲ Cardene Capsules (4.0% to 6.9%)	2261
Amen Tablets	785	Cardene I.V. (1.4%)	2815
Amicar Syrup, Tablets, and Injection	1312	▲ Cardene SR Capsules (1.6% to 3.3%)	2264
Amikacin Sulfate Injection, USP	523	▲ Cardizem CD Capsules (3.0% to 3.5%)	1251
Amoxil (Rare)	2631	▲ Cardizem SR Capsules (3.4% to 7%)	1255
▲ Anafranil Capsules (41% to 54%)	819	Cardizem Injectable (Less than 1%)	1253
Ana-Kit Anaphylaxis Emergency Treatment Kit (Common)	611	Cardizem Tablets (1.5%)	1257
▲ Anaprox/Naprosyn (3% to 9%)	2277	▲ Cardura Tablets (Up to 23%)	1993
Apresazide Capsules (Less frequent)	824	Cartrol Tablets (Less common)	413
Apresoline Hydrochloride Tablets (Less frequent)	826	▲ Casodex Tablets (7%)	2934
AquaMEPHYTON Injection	1648	Cataflam Tablets (1% to 3%)	833
Aredia for Injection	827	▲ Catapres Tablets (About 16 in 100 patients)	679
▲ Arimidex Tablets (4.9% to 6.1%)	2932	Catapres-TTS (2 of 101 patients)	680
▲ Artane (30% to 50%)	1418	Caverject Injection (1%)	2064
▲ Asacol Delayed-Release Tablets (8%)	2129	Ceclor Pulvules & Suspension (Rare)	1470
Asendin Tablets (Less frequent)	1419	Cedax (0.1% to 1%)	2480
Atamet Tablets (Less frequent)	567	Ceftin (0.1% to 1%)	1067
Ativan Injection (Occasional)	2805	Cefzil Tablets and Oral Suspension (1%)	747
Ativan Tablets (6.9%)	2807	▲ CellCept Capsules (5.7% to 11.2%)	2265
▲ Atretol Tablets (Among most frequent)	569	Celontin Kapseals (Frequent)	1955
Atrohist Pediatric Capsules	1603	Ceptaz (Fewer than 1%)	1070
Atrohist Plus Tablets	1605	▲ Cerebyx Injection (5.0% to 31.1%)	1956
Atromid-S Capsules (Less often)	2808	Cerezyme (One patient)	1056
Atrovent Inhalation Aerosol (2.4%; about 1 in 100)	674	Cerose DM	⊡ 853
Atrovent Inhalation Solution (2.3%)	675	▲ Chemet Capsules (1.0% to 12.7%)	666
Atrovent Nasal Spray 0.03% (Less than 2%)	676	Children's TYLENOL Cold Multi-Symptom Chewable Tablets and Liquid	1559
Atrovent Nasal Spray 0.06% (Less than 1%)	678	Children's Vicks DayQuil Allergy Relief	⊡ 730
Augmentin (Rare)	2637	Children's Vicks NyQuil Cold/Cough Relief	⊡ 731
Augmentin Tablets (Rare)	2640	Chlor-Trimeton Allergy Decongestant Tablets	⊡ 759
▲ Avonex (15%)	662	Cipro I.V. (1% or less)	587
▲ Axid Pulvules (4.6%)	1468	Cipro I.V. Pharmacy Bulk Package (Less than 1%)	590
▲ Axocet Capsules (Among most frequent)	2469	Cipro Tablets (0.3% to 1%)	584
Azactam for Injection (Less than 1%)	736	Claritin Tablets (2% or fewer patients)	2485
Benadryl Allergy Decongestant Liquid Medication	⊡ 812	▲ Claritin-D Tablets (4%)	2487
Benadryl Allergy Decongestant Tablets	⊡ 812	Climara Transdermal System	640
Benadryl Allergy Sinus Headache Caplets	⊡ 813	Cleocin Vaginal Cream (Less than 1%)	2070
▲ Benadryl Injection (Among most frequent)	1955	▲ Clinoril Tablets (3% to 9%)	1658
Benemid Tablets	1651	Clomid (Fewer than 1%)	1262
▲ Bentyl (29%)	1246	▲ Clozaril Tablets (More than 5 to 19%)	2377
Benylin Multisymptom	⊡ 816	Codiclear DH Syrup	808
Betagan (Rare)	⊙ 230	▲ Cognex Capsules (12%)	1961
▲ Betapace Tablets (7% to 20%)	637	ColBENEMID Tablets	1662
▲ Betaseron for SC Injection (35%)	653	Colestid (Infrequent)	2073
Betimol 0.25%, 0.5% (1% to 5%)	⊙ 259	▲ Combipres Tablets (About 16%)	682
Betoptic Ophthalmic Solution (Rare)	465	Compazine	2644
Betoptic S Ophthalmic Suspension (Rare)	467	Allergy-Sinus Comtrex Multi-Symptom Allergy-Sinus Formula Tablets and Caplets	⊡ 639
Biavax II	1653	Condylox Topical Solution (Less than 5%)	1853
Diaxin	406		
Biltricide Tablets	584		
Blocadren Tablets (2.3%)	1654		
Bontril Slow-Release Capsules	786		
▲ Brethine Ampuls (1.3 to 10.2%)	832		

Contac Continuous Action Nasal Decongestant/Antihistamine 12 Hour Capsules	⊡ 773	Diuril Oral Suspension	1694
Contac Maximum Strength Continuous Action Decongestant/Antihistamine 12 Hour Caplets	⊡ 772	Diuril Sodium Intravenous	1693
Contac Severe Cold and Flu Formula Caplets	⊡ 773	Diuril Tablets	1694
▲ Cordarone Tablets (4 to 9%)	2818	Dolobid Tablets (Greater than 1 in 100)	1695
Coricidin Cough + Cold Tablets	⊡ 760	Donnagel Liquid and Donnagel Chewable Tablets (Rare)	⊡ 854
Coricidin 'D' Decongestant Tablets	⊡ 760	Donnatal	2234
▲ Covera-HS Tablets (3.3% to 4.7%)	2573	Donnatal Extentabs	2234
▲ Cozaar Tablets (3.5%)	1668	Donnatal Tablets	2234
Crixivan Capsules (1.0% to less than 2%)	1670	Dopram Injectable	2235
Cycrin Tablets	991	Doral Tablets (1.5%)	2773
Cylert Tablets	415	Dorcol Children's Cough Syrup	⊡ 748
Cystospaz	2123	Doxil (1% to 5%)	2613
▲ Cytadren Tablets (5%)	837	Drixoral Cold and Allergy Sustained-Action Tablets	⊡ 763
Cytosar-U Sterile Powder (Less frequent)	2077	Drixoral Cold and Flu Extended-Release Tablets	⊡ 764
Cytotec (Infrequent)	2576	Drixoral Allergy/Sinus Extended Release Tablets	⊡ 765
Cytovene (1% or less)	2270	▲ Duragesic Transdermal System (3% to 10%)	1336
D.A. II Tablets	972	Duramorph Injection	983
D.A. Chewable Tablets	970	Duranest Injections	533
DDAVP (Up to 3%)	2180	Dura-Tap/PD Capsules	970
▲ DHCplus Capsules (Among most frequent)	2148	Dura-Vent/DA Tablets	972
D.H.E. 45 Injection (Occasional)	2381	Dyazide Capsules	2653
Dalgan Injection (1 to less than 3%)	529	Dyclone 0.5% and 1% Topical Solutions, USP	535
Dalmane Capsules	2329	Dynabac (2.3%)	668
Danocrine Capsules	2437	DYNACIN Capsules	1627
▲ Dantrium Capsules (Among most frequent)	2131	▲ DynaCirc Capsules (3.4% to 8.0%)	2381
Daranide Tablets	1676	▲ DynaCirc CR Tablets (4.7% to 6.4%)	2383
▲ Darvon-N/Darvocet-N (Among most frequent)	1473	Dyrenium Capsules (Rare)	2655
▲ Darvon (Among most frequent)	1475	E.E.S. (Isolated reports)	427
▲ Darvon-N Suspension & Tablets (Among most frequent)	1473	Easprin	1971
▲ DaunoXome (Up to 8%)	1842	▲ EC-Naprosyn Delayed-Release Tablets (3% to 9%)	2277
Decadron Phosphate with Xylocaine Injection, Sterile	1683	Ecotrin	2625
Deconsal II Tablets	1605	▲ Effexor (3% to 23.9%)	2825
▲ Demadex Tablets and Injection (3.2%)	691	Efidac/24	⊡ 655
▲ Demerol (Among most frequent)	2438	Elavil	2945
Demulen	2580	▲ Eldepryl Capsules (7 of 49 patients)	2729
Depakene	416	Emete-con Intramuscular/Intravenous	2007
▲ Depakote Tablets (12%)	418	▲ Eminase (Less than 10%)	2215
Depo-Provera Contraceptive Injection (More than 5%)	2079	EMLA Cream (Unlikely with cream)	536
Depo-Provera Sterile Aqueous Suspension	2083	Enduron Tablets	424
Desmopressin Acetate Rhinal Tube (Up to 3%)	997	▲ Engerix-B Unit-Dose Vials (1% to 10%)	2656
Desogen Tablets	1867	Entex PSE Tablets	973
Desoxyn Graudumet Tablets (Rare)	422	EpiPen	808
▲ Desyrel and Desyrel Dividose (19.7% to 28.0%)	504	▲ Epivir (10%)	1200
Dexatrim	⊡ 795	Epogen for Injection (5% to 9%)	489
Dexatrim Plus Vitamins Caplets	⊡ 796	▲ Ergamisol Tablets (3% to 4%)	1340
Dexedrine	2648	EryPed (Isolated reports)	425
DextroStat-Dextroamphetamine Sulfate Tablets	2211	Ery-Tab Tablets (Isolated reports)	426
Diethylstilbestrol Tablets	1477	Erythrocin Stearate Filmtab (Isolated reports)	429
Diflucan Tablets, Injection, and Oral Suspension (1%)	2003	Erythromycin Base Filmtab (Isolated reports)	430
Dilacor XR Extended-release Capsules (Infrequent; 2.2%)	2183	Erythromycin Delayed-Release Capsules, USP (Isolated reports)	431
Dilantin Infatabs	1967	▲ Esgic-plus Capsules (Among most frequent)	1012
Dilantin Kapseals	1965	▲ Esgic-plus Tablets (Among most frequent)	1012
Dilantin-125 Suspension	1969	Esidrix Tablets	839
Dilaudid Ampules	1382	Esimil Tablets	840
Dilaudid Cough Syrup	1383	Eskalith	2658
▲ Dilaudid-HP Injection (Among most frequent)	1384	Estrace Cream and Tablets	751
▲ Dilaudid-HP Lyophilized Powder 250 mg (Among most frequent)	1384	Estraderm Transdermal System	842
Dilaudid	1382	ESTRATAB Tablets (0.3, 0.625, 1.25, 2.5 mg)	2715
Dilaudid Oral Liquid	1386	Estratest	2718
Dilaudid	1382	Estring Vaginal Ring (At least 1 report)	2086
Dilaudid Tablets - 8 mg	1386	▲ Ethmozine Tablets (11.3% to more than 20%)	2217
▲ Dimetane-DC Cough Syrup (Most frequent)	2232	Ethyol (amifostine) for Injection	485
▲ Dimetane-DX Cough Syrup (Among most frequent)	2233	▲ Etopophos for Injection (5%)	701
Dimetapp Cold & Allergy Chewable Tablets	⊡ 838	Etrafon	2495
Dimetapp Extentabs	⊡ 841	▲ Famvir Tablets (3.3% to 5.5%)	2660
Dimetapp Tablets/Liqui-Gels	⊡ 841	Fastin Capsules	2662
Dipentum Capsules (1.0%)	2084	Fedahist Gyrocaps	2545
Diprivan Injectable Emulsion (Less than 1%)	2939	▲ Felbatol (Among most common; 18.4%)	2774
Ditropan	1267	Feldene Capsules (Greater than 1%)	2008
Diucardin Tablets	2824	▲ Fioricet Tablets (Among most frequent)	2386
Diupres Tablets	1691	Fioricet with Codeine Capsules (Frequent)	2387
		▲ Fiorinal Capsules (One of the two most frequent)	2388
		Fiorinal with Codeine Capsules (2.6%)	2390

(⊡ Described in PDR For Nonprescription Drugs) Incidence data in parenthesis; ▲ 3% or more (⊙ Described in PDR For Ophthalmology)

1311 Side Effects Index Dizziness

▲ Fiorinal Tablets (One of the two most frequent) 2388
Flagyl 375 Capsules 2587
Flagyl I.V. 2373
▲ Flexeril Tablets (3% to 11%) 1701
▲ Flolan for Injection (8% to 83%) 1085
Flonase Nasal Spray (Less than 1%) 1088
Flovent (1% to 3%) 1089
▲ Floxin I.V. (1% to 5%) 1580
▲ Floxin Tablets (200 mg, 300 mg, 400 mg) (1% to 5%) 1577
Flumadine Tablets & Syrup (0.7% to 1.9%) 1013
Fortaz (Less than 1%) 1092
▲ Foscavir Injection (5% or greater) 541
Fulvicin P/G Tablets (Occasional) 2499
Fulvicin P/G 165 & 330 Tablets (Occasional) 2500
Gamimune N, 5% Immune Globulin Intravenous (Human), 5% 612
Gamimune N, 10% Immune Globulin Intravenous (Human), 10% 615
Gammar-P I.V., Immune Globulin Intravenous (Human) 798
Gantrisin (Rare) 2286
Garamycin Injectable 2502
Gastrocrom Capsules (Infrequent) 1611
Gastrocrom Oral Concentrate (Less common) 1611
Glucotrol Tablets (About 1 in 50) 2011
▲ Glucotrol XL Extended Release Tablets (6.8%) 2012
Grifulvin V (griseofulvin tablets) Microsize (griseofulvin oral suspension) Microsize (Occasional) 1944
Gris-PEG Tablets, 125 mg & 250 mg (Occasional) 476
Guaifed 1833
Guaimax-D Tablets 809
▲ Habitrol Nicotine Transdermal System (3% to 9% of patients) 884
▲ Halcion Tablets (7.8%) 2093
Havrix (Rare) 2663
Helidac Therapy (1.5%) 2135
Hexalen Capsules 2760
Helixate, Antihemophilic Factor (Recombinant) 799
Hismanal Tablets (Rare to 2.0%) 1341
Histussin D Liquid 670
Hivid Tablets (Less than 1%) 2287
Humegon for Injection 1873
Hycodan Tablets and Syrup 946
Hycomine Compound Tablets 948
Hycomine 947
Hycotuss Expectorant Syrup 950
Hydralazine Hydrochloride Injection USP (Less frequent) 2712
Hydrea Capsules (Extremely rare) 705
Hydrocet Capsules 787
HydroDIURIL Tablets 1716
Hydropres Tablets 1718
Hyperstat I.V. Injection (2%) 2504
▲ Hytrin Capsules (2.0% to 28%) 434
▲ Hyzaar Tablets (5.7%) 1720
▲ IBU Tablets (3% to 9%) 1389
IFEX (Less frequent) 706
▲ Imdur (8% to 11%) 1362
▲ Imitrex Injection (11.9%) 1095
Imitrex Tablets 1099
Imodium Capsules 1343
▲ Imovax Rabies Vaccine (About 20%) 899
Inapsine Injection (Less common) 462
Inderide Tablets 2838
Inderide LA Long Acting Capsules 2840
▲ Indocin (3% to 9%) 1723
INFeD (Iron Dextran Injection, USP) 2478
Infumorph 200 and Infumorph 500 Sterile Solutions 985
Intal Inhaler (Infrequent) 2185
Intal Nebulizer Solution 2186
▲ Intron A for Injection (7% to 24%) 2506
Inversine Tablets 1729
Iopidine 0.5% (Less than 1%) ⊙ 219
Ismelin Tablets 845
▲ Ismo Tablets (3% to 5%) 2844
ISMOTIC 45% w/v Solution (Very rare) ⊙ 221
Isoetharine Inhalation Solution, USP, Arm-a-Med 545
Isoptin Injectable (1.2%) 1391
▲ Isoptin Oral Tablets (3.3%) 1393
▲ Isoptin SR Tablets (3.3%) 1395
Isuprel Hydrochloride Solution 2443
Isuprel Injection 2441
Isuprel Mistometer 2442
▲ JE-VAX (Approximately 10%) 904
K-Phos Neutral Tablets 633
K-Phos Original Formula 'Sodium Free' Tablets (Less frequent) 633
▲ Kadian Capsules (Among frequent) 2948
Keflex Pulvules & Oral Suspension 930
Keftab Tablets 931
Kemadrin Tablets 1105
▲ Kerlone Tablets (4.5% to 14.8%) 2588
KOGENATE Antihemophilic Factor (Recombinant) 626
Kwell Cream & Lotion 2172
Kwell Shampoo 2173
▲ Kytril Tablets (3%) 2669
▲ Lamictal Tablets (Among most common; 31% to 54%) 1105
Lamprene Capsules (Less than 1%) 846
Lanoxicaps 1110
Lanoxin Elixir Pediatric 1113
Lanoxin Injection 1116
Lanoxin Injection Pediatric 1119
Lanoxin Tablets 1121
▲ Lariam Tablets (Among most frequent; less than 1%) 2295
Larodopa Tablets (Relatively frequent) 2296
Lasix Injection, Oral Solution and Tablets 1267
Lescol Capsules (2.2%) 2395
▲ Leustatin (9%) 1889
▲ Levatol Tablets (4.9%) 2547
Levbid Extended-Release Tablets 2549
Levlen/Tri-Levlen 646
Levo-Dromoran 2297
Levoprome (Sometimes) 1321
Levsin/Levsinex/Levbid 2549
▲ Limbitrol (Among most frequent) 2333
Lindane Lotion USP 1% 481
Lindane Shampoo USP 1% 483
▲ Lioresal Intrathecal (1.7% to 8.0%) 1634
▲ Lioresal Tablets (5% to 15%) 847
Lithium Carbonate Capsules & Tablets 2352
Lithonate/Lithotabs/Lithobid 2721
▲ Lodine Capsules and Tablets (3% to 9%) 2849
Lomotil 2591
Lo/Ovral Tablets 2852
Lo/Ovral-28 Tablets 2857
Lopid Tablets 1974
▲ Lopressor (10%) 848
▲ Lopressor HCT Tablets (10 in 100 patients) 850
Lorabid Suspension and Pulvules 1513
▲ Lorcet 10/650 Tablets (Among most frequent) 1016
▲ Lortab (Among most frequent) 2751
▲ Lotensin Tablets (1.5% to 3.6%) 852
▲ Lotensin HCT Tablets (3.5% to 6.3%) 855
Lotrel Capsules (1.3%) 858
Loxitane 1426
▲ Ludiomil Tablets (8%) 861
Lupron Depot 3.75 mg (Less than 5%) 2739
▲ Lupron Depot - 3 Month 22.5 mg (6.4%) 2743
▲ Lupron Injection (5% or more) 2736
▲ LUVOX Tablets (11%) 2723
▲ Lysodren Tablets (15%) 707
M-M-R II 1730
M-R-VAX II 1732
▲ MS Contin Tablets (Among most frequent) 2149
▲ MSIR (Among most frequent) 2152
Macrobid Capsules (Less than 1%) 2138
Marax Tablets & DF Syrup 2015
Marcaine (Rare) 2446
Marcaine Spinal (Rare) 2449
▲ Marinol (Dronabinol) Capsules (3% to 10%) 2353
Matulane Capsules 2300
Mavik Tablets (1.0%) 1407
Maxair Autohaler (0.6% to 1.2%) 1550
Maxair Inhaler (1.2%) 1552
Maxaquin Tablets (2.3%) 2593
Mebaral Tablets (Less than 1 in 100) 2452
Menest Tablets 2671
▲ Mepergan Injection (Among most frequent) 2859
Mephyton Tablets (Rare) 1739
▲ Mepron Suspension (3% to 8%) 1206
Merrem I.V. (0.1% to 1.0%) 2952
Meruvax II 1740
Mesantoin Tablets 2400
▲ Methadone Hydrochloride Oral Concentrate (Among most frequent) 2356
Methadone Hydrochloride Oral Solution & Tablets 2357
Methergine (Rare) 2401
Methotrexate Sodium Tablets, Injection, for Injection and LPF Injection (Frequent; 1% to 3%) 1322
MetroGel-Vaginal (Equal to or less than 2%) 917
Mevacor Tablets (0.5% to 2.0%) 1742
▲ Mexitil Capsules (18.9% to 26.4%) 684
Miacalcin Nasal Spray (1% to 3%) 2403
Micronor Tablets (Less common) 1903
Midamor Tablets (Between 1% and 3%) 1746
Midrin Capsules 788
Miltown Tablets 2780
▲ Minipress Capsules (10.3%) 2015
▲ Minizide Capsules (10.3%) 2016
Minocin Intravenous 1428
Minocin Oral Suspension 1431
Minocin Pellet-Filled Capsules 1429
Mintezol 1747
Mivacron (Less than 1%) 1125
Modicon 1928
▲ Moduretic Tablets (3% to 8%) 1748
8-MOP Capsules 1294
Monoket Tablets (Up to 4%) 2550
▲ Monopril Tablets (1.6% to 11.9%) 762
Motofen Tablets (1 in 20) 789
▲ Motrin Ibuprofen Suspension, Oral Drops, Chewable Tablets, Caplets (3% to 9%) 1563
Myambutol Tablets 1432
▲ Mykrox Tablets (10.2%) 1617
Myochrysine Injection 1754
▲ Nalfon 200 Pulvules & Nalfon Tablets (6.5%) 933
Naprelan Tablets (Less than 3%) 2861
▲ Anaprox/Naprosyn (3% to 9%) 2277
Nardil (Common) 1977
Nebcin Vials, Hyporets & ADD-Vantage 1518
NegGram 2453
Nembutal Sodium Capsules (Less than 1%) 440
Nembutal Sodium Solution (Less than 1%) 442
Nembutal Sodium Suppositories (Less than 1%) 444
Nescaine/Nescaine MPF 549
Netromycin Injection 100 mg/ml 2516
▲ Neurontin Capsules (Among most common; 17.1%) 1978
▲ Nicotrol NS Nicotine Nasal Spray (Over 5%) 1565
Nimotop Capsules (Less than 1%) 603
▲ Nipent for Injection (3% to 10%) 2733
Nitrolingual Spray (Occasional) 2193
Nizoral Tablets (Less than 1%) 1345
Nolamine Timed-Release Tablets (Occasional) 790
Nolvadex Tablets (Infrequent) 2957
Nordette-21 Tablets 2863
Nordette-28 Tablets 2866
Norflex 1554
Norgesic 1554
Norinyl 2563
Norisodrine with Calcium Iodide Syrup 446
▲ Normodyne Injection (2% to 16%) 2519
▲ Normodyne Tablets (1% to 16%) 2522
Noroxin Tablets (1.7% to 2.6%) 1758
Noroxin Tablets (1.7% to 2.6%) 2222
▲ Norpace (3 to 9%) 2596
Norplant System 2868
Norpramin Tablets 1273
Nor-Q D Tablets 2598
▲ Norvasc Tablets (0.1% to 3.4%) 2020
Norvir (2.6% to 3.3%) 447
Novahistine DMX ◘ 782
Novahistine Elixir ◘ 782
Novocain Hydrochloride for Spinal Anesthesia 2457
▲ Nubain Injection (5%) 952
Nucofed 2225
Ocuflox Ophthalmic Solution (Rare) 478
Ocupress Ophthalmic Solution, 1% Sterile (Occasional) ⊙ 297
Ogen Tablets 2103
Ogen Vaginal Cream 2106
Oncaspar (Less than 1%) 2194
Oncovin Solution Vials & Hyporets (Rare) 1521
OptiPranolol (Metipranolol 0.3%) Sterile Ophthalmic Solution (A small number of patients) ⊙ 256
▲ Oramorph SR (Morphine Sulfate Sustained Release Tablets) (Among most frequent) 2359
Orap Tablets 1037
Oretic Tablets 450
Organidin NR Tablets and Liquid (Rare) 2781
Ornade Spansule Capsules 2678
Ortho-Cept 1907
Ortho-Cyclen/Ortho-Tri-Cyclen 1914
Ortho Diaphragm Kits—All-Flex Arcing Spring; Ortho Coil Spring; Ortho-White Flat Spring 1921
Ortho Diaphragm Kit-Coil Spring 1921
Ortho Dienestrol Cream 1922
Ortho-Est 1925
Ortho-Novum 1928
Ortho-Cyclen/Ortho Tri-Cyclen 1914
Ortho-White Diaphragm Kit-Flat Spring (See also Ortho Diaphragm Kits) 1921
Orthoclone OKT3 Sterile Solution 1892
Orudis Capsules (Greater than 1%) 2874
Oruvail Capsules (Greater than 1%) 2874
Ovcon 765
Ovral Tablets 2877
Ovral-28 Tablets 2878
Ovrette Tablets 2878
Oxsoralen-Ultra Capsules 1302
▲ OxyContin Tablets (13%) 2163
▲ OxyIR Capsules (Among most frequent) 2167
▲ PBZ Tablets (Among most frequent) 863
▲ PBZ-SR Tablets (Among most frequent) 862
Pamelor 2409
Parafon Forte DSC Caplets (Occasional) 1590
▲ Parlodel (Less than 2% to 17%) 2411
Parnate Tablets 2679
▲ Paxil Tablets (6.7% to 14%) 2681
Pediatric Vicks 44d Cough & Head Congestion Relief ◘ 736
Pediatric Vicks 44m Cough & Cold Relief ◘ 737
Pediazole Suspension 2340
Peganone Tablets 455
▲ Penetrex Tablets (Less than 1% to 3%) 2196
Pentasa (Less than 1%) 1275
Pentaspan Injection 954
Pepcid Injection (1.3%) 1765
Pepcid (1.3%) 1763
Peptavlon 2997
▲ Percocet Tablets (Among most frequent) 955
▲ Percodan Tablets (Among most frequent) 955
▲ Percodan-Demi Tablets (Among most frequent) 956
Pergonal (menotropins for injection, USP) 2618
Periactin 1767
▲ Permax Tablets (19.1%) 571
▲ Persantine Tablets (13.6%) 686
Phenergan with Codeine 2883
Phenergan with Dextromethorphan 2885
Phenergan Injection 2880
Phenergan Suppositories 2882
Phenergan Syrup 2881
Phenergan Tablets 2882
Phenergan VC 2886
Phenergan VC with Codeine 2888
Phenobarbital Elixir and Tablets (Less than 1 in 100 patients) 1523
Phenurone Tablets (Less than 1%) 455
▲ Phrenilin (Among most frequent) 790
Pipracil 1435
Placidyl Capsules 456
Plaquenil Sulfate Tablets 2459
▲ Plendil Extended-Release Tablets (2.7% to 3.7%) 514
PMB 200 and PMB 400 2890
Pondimin Tablets 2239
Ponstel 1982
Pontocaine Hydrochloride for Spinal Anesthesia 2460
Pravachol Tablets (1.0% to 3.3%) 770
Prelu-2 Timed Release Capsules 687
Premarin Intravenous 2893
Premarin Tablets 2896
Premarin Vaginal Cream 2898
Premphase 2900
Prempro 2905
Prevacid Delayed-Release Capsules (Less than 1%) 2746

(◘ Described in PDR For Nonprescription Drugs) Incidence data in parenthesis; ▲ 3% or more (⊙ Described in PDR For Ophthalmology)

Dizziness Side Effects Index 1312

Prilosec Delayed-Release Capsules (1.5%) ... 516
Primaxin I.M. ... 1770
Primaxin I.V. (0.3%) ... 1772
▲ Prinivil Tablets (5.4% to 11.8%) .. 1776
▲ Prinzide Tablets (7.5%) ... 1780
Pro-Banthine Tablets ... 2226
Procanbid Extended-Release Tablets (Occasional) ... 1983
▲ Procardia Capsules (Approximately 10% to 27%; 1 in 8 patients) ... 2024
▲ Procardia XL Extended Release Tablets (4.1% to 27%) ... 2026
▲ Procrit for Injection (5% to 9%) 1896
Proglycem ... 575
▲ Prograf (Greater than 3%) ... 1028
Prolastin Alpha$_1$-Proteinase Inhibitor (Human) (0.19%) ... 629
▲ Proleukin for Injection (17%) ... 812
Prolixin ... 510
Propagest Tablets ... 791
Propulsid (More than 1%) ... 1346
▲ ProSom Tablets (7%) ... 457
Prostep (nicotine transdermal system) (1% to 3% of patients).. 1439
Prostigmin Injectable ... 1305
Prostigmin Tablets ... 1306
Prostin E2 Suppository ... 2109
Protopam Chloride for Injection ... 2909
Protostat Tablets ... 1939
Proventil Inhalation Aerosol (Less than 5%) ... 2524
▲ Proventil Inhalation Solution 0.083% (7%) ... 2527
Proventil Repetabs Tablets (2%) 2529
▲ Proventil Solution for Inhalation 0.5% (7%) ... 2525
▲ Proventil Syrup (3 of 100 patients) ... 2528
Proventil Tablets (2%) ... 2529
Provera Tablets ... 2110
▲ Prozac Pulvules & Liquid, Oral Solution (5.7% to 13%) ... 935
Pyrroxate Caplets ... ■ 742
Quadrinal Tablets ... 1398
Questran ... 774
▲ Quinaglute Dura-Tabs Tablets (3%) ... 644
▲ RMS Suppositories CII (Among most frequent) ... 2766
▲ Rabies Vaccine, Imovax Rabies I.D. (About 20%) ... 901
▲ Redux Capsules (5.5%) ... 2911
Regitine Vials ... 864
Reglan (Less frequent) ... 2243
▲ Relafen Tablets (3% to 9%) ... 2688
▲ Remeron Tablets (7%) ... 1878
ReoPro Vials (1.8%) ... 1526
RespiGam ... 1631
▲ Restoril Capsules (7%) ... 2413
▲ Retrovir Capsules (6% to 17.9%) 1216
▲ Retrovir I.V. Infusion (6% to 17.9%) ... 1221
▲ Retrovir Syrup (6% to 17.9%) ... 1216
▲ ReVia Tablets (4% to less than 10%) ... 957
▲ Revex (nalmefene hydrochloride injection) (3%) ... 1863
Rifadin ... 1276
Rifamate Capsules ... 1278
Rifater ... 1280
▲ Rilutek Tablets (5.1% to 12.7%) .. 2198
Rimactane Capsules ... 865
▲ Risperdal Tablets (4% to 7%) ... 1348
Ritalin ... 866
Robaxin Injectable ... 2245
Robaxin Tablets ... 2246
▲ Robaxisal Tablets (One in 20-25) .. 2246
Robinul Forte Tablets ... 2247
Robinul Injectable ... 2247
Robinul Tablets ... 2247
Robitussin Maximum Strength Cough & Cold ... ■ 847
Robitussin Pediatric Cough & Cold Formula ... ■ 848
Robitussin-CF ... ■ 846
Robitussin-DAC Syrup ... 2249
Robitussin-PE ... ■ 846
Rocephin Injectable Vials, ADD-Vantage, Galaxy Container (Occasional) ... 2305
▲ Roferon-A Injection (11% to 40%) 2308
▲ Romazicon (1% to 9%) ... 2311
Rondec Oral Drops ... 974
Rondec Syrup ... 974
Rondec Tablet ... 974
Rondec Chewable Tablets ... 974
Rondec-TR Tablet ... 974
Rowasa (1.84% to 3.0%) ... 2727
▲ Roxanol (Among most frequent) ... 2365
▲ Roxicodone Tablets, Oral Solution & Intensol (Oxycodone) (Among most frequent) ... 2366
Ryna ... ■ 804
Rynatan ... 2781
▲ Rythmol Tablets–150mg, 225mg, 300mg (3.6 to 15.1%) ... 1399
▲ Salagen Tablets (5% to 12%) ... 1546
Sandoglobulin I.V. (Less than 1%).. 2419
▲ Sandostatin Injection (5%) ... 2421
Sanorex Tablets ... 2423
Sansert Tablets ... 2424
Scleromate Injection (Rare) ... 1234
Seconal Sodium Pulvules (Less than 1 in 100) ... 1529
▲ Sectral Capsules (6%) ... 2914
▲ Sedapap Tablets 50 mg/650 mg (Among the most frequent) ... 1826
▲ Seldane Tablets (2.9% to 5.8%) 1284
Seldane-D Extended-Release Tablets (Rare) ... 1286
▲ Semprex-D Capsules (3%) ... 1620
Sensorcaine (Rare) ... 554
Ser-Ap-Es Tablets ... 867
Serax Capsules (In few instances) .. 2916
Serax Tablets (In few instances) ... 2916
Serentil ... 689
Serophene (clomiphene citrate tablets, USP) (Less than 1 in 100 patients) ... 2621
▲ Serzone Tablets (11% to 22%) ... 776
Sinarest ... ■ 663
Sine-Aid Maximum Strength Sinus Headache Gelcaps, Caplets and Tablets ... 1570
Sine-Off No Drowsiness Formula Caplets ... ■ 784
Sinemet Tablets (Less frequent) ... 959
Sinemet CR Tablets (2.9%) ... 961
Sinequan (Occasional) ... 2028
Sinulin Tablets ... 792
Sinutab Non-Drying Liquid Caps .. ■ 823
Skelaxin Tablets ... 793
Solganal Suspension ... 2530
Soma Compound w/Codeine Tablets ... 2784
Soma Compound Tablets (Very rare to less frequent) ... 2783
Soma Tablets ... 2782
Sorbitrate ... 2959
Sporanox Capsules (0.7% to 1.7%) ... 1352
▲ Stadol (19%) ... 779
Stelazine ... 2692
Stimate, (desmopressin acetate) Nasal Spray, 1.5 mg/mL ... 806
Sublimaze Injection ... 463
Sudafed Cold & Allergy Tablets .... ■ 826
Sudafed Nasal Decongestant Tablets, 30 mg ... ■ 825
Sudafed Nasal Decongestant Tablets, 60 mg ... ■ 825
Sudafed Sinus Caplets ... ■ 829
Sudafed Sinus Tablets ... ■ 829
Sudafed 12 Hour Caplets ... ■ 824
▲ Sular Tablets (5%) ... 2961
Supprelin Injection (1% to 3%) ... 2230
Suprane (desflurane, USP) (Less than 1%) ... 1865
Suprax (Less than 2%) ... 1443
Surmontil Capsules ... 2917
Sus-Phrine Injection ... 1017
▲ Symmetrel Capsules (5% to 10%) ... 965
▲ Symmetrel Syrup (5% to 10%) ... 963
Syn-Rx Tablets ... 1622
Syn-Rx DM Tablets ... 1623
Tagamet (Approximately 1 in 100) 2694
Talacen Caplets ... 2464
▲ Talwin Injection (Most common) ... 2465
Talwin Compound ... 2466
▲ Talwin Injection (Most common) ... 2465
Talwin Nx Tablets ... 2467
▲ Tambocor Tablets (18.9%) ... 1555
▲ Tavist Syrup (Among most frequent) ... 2426
▲ Tavist Tablets (Among most frequent) ... 2427
Tazicef for Injection (Less than 1%) ... 2697
Tazidime Vials, Faspak & ADD-Vantage (Less than 1%) ... 1531
▲ Tegison Capsules (1-10%) ... 2314
▲ Tegretol/Tegretol-XR (Among most frequent) ... 870
Teldrin 12 Hour Antihistamine/Nasal Decongestant Allergy Relief Capsules ... ■ 786
▲ Tenex Tablets (1% to 15%) ... 2249
▲ Tenoretic Tablets (4% to 13%) ... 2963
▲ Tenormin Tablets and I.V. Injection (4% to 13%) ... 2965
Tessalon Perles ... 1018
Thalitone ... 1293
TheraCys BCG Live (Intravesical) (Up to 0.9%) ... 911
TheraFlu ... ■ 750
TheraFlu Maximum Strength Nighttime Flu, Cold & Cough Medicine ... ■ 751
Thioplex (Thiotepa For Injection) 1329
Thorazine ... 2701
▲ THROMBATE III Antithrombin III (Human) (7 of 17) ... 631
▲ Tiazac Capsules (5%) ... 1019
TICE BCG, USP (2.4%) ... 1881
Ticlid Tablets (1.1%) ... 2317
Tigan ... 2231
Tilade Inhaler (0.9%) ... 2207
Timentin for Injection ... 2706
Timolide Tablets (1.2%) ... 1791
Timoptic in Ocudose (Less frequent) ... 1796
Timoptic Sterile Ophthalmic Solution (Less frequent) ... 1794
Timoptic-XE (1% to 5% of patients) ... 1798
Tofranil Ampuls ... 873
Tofranil Tablets ... 875
Tofranil-PM Capsules ... 876
▲ Tolectin (200, 400 and 600 mg) (3 to 9%) ... 1591
▲ Tonocard Tablets (8.0% to 25.3%) ... 519
▲ Toprol-XL Tablets (About 10 of 100 patients) ... 560
▲ Toradol (7%) ... 2319
Torecan (Occasional) ... 2367
▲ Tornalate Solution for Inhalation, 0.2% (4.0%) ... 976
Tornalate Metered Dose Inhaler (1.0% to 3%) ... 978
Trancopal Caplets ... 2468
▲ Trandate (9 of 100 patients; 1% to 16%) ... 1158
Transderm Scōp Transdermal Therapeutic System (Infrequent) 890
Tranxene (Less common) ... 459
Trental Tablets (1.9%) ... 1291
Triaminic Syrup ... ■ 755
Triaminic Triaminicol Cold & Cough ... ■ 756
Triaminic DM Syrup ... ■ 756
Triaminicin Tablets ... ■ 756
Triavil Tablets ... 1800
Trilafon (Rare) ... 2532
Levlen/Tri-Levlen ... 646
Trilisate (Less than 2%) ... 2155
▲ Trinalin Repetabs Tablets (Among most frequent) ... 1373
Tri-Norinyl ... 2607
Triphasil-21 Tablets ... 2919
Triphasil-28 Tablets ... 2924
Trusopt Sterile Ophthalmic Solution ... 1803
Tussend ... 1830
Tussend Expectorant ... 1831
Tussionex Pennkinetic Extended-Release Suspension ... 1624
Tussi-Organidin DM NR Liquid and DM-S NR Liquid (Rare) ... 2786
TYLENOL Cold Medication, Multi-Symptom Formula Tablets and Caplets ... 1572
TYLENOL Cold Medication, Multi-Symptom Hot Liquid Packets ... 1572
TYLENOL Cold Medication, No Drowsiness Formula Caplets and Gelcaps ... 1572
TYLENOL Cough Medication with Decongestant, Multi Symptom ... 1574
TYLENOL Flu NightTime, Maximum Strength Hot Medication Packets ... 1575
TYLENOL Sinus, Maximum Strength Geltabs, Gelcaps, Caplets and Tablets ... 1576
▲ Tylenol with Codeine (Among most frequent) ... 1592
▲ Tylox Capsules (Among most frequent) ... 1593
Tympagesic Ear Drops ... 2476
▲ Ultram Tablets (50 mg) (26% to 33%) ... 1594
▲ Univasc Tablets (4.3%) ... 2553
Urecholine ... 1804
Urised Tablets ... 2123
Uroqid-Acid No. 2 Tablets ... 633
▲ Valtrex Caplets (2% to 4%) ... 1167
Vancocin HCl, Oral Solution & Pulvules (Rare) ... 1536
Vancocin HCl, Vials & ADD-Vantage (Rare) ... 1534
Vantin for Oral Suspension and Vantin Tablets (Less than 1%) 2112
▲ Vascor Tablets (200 and 300 mg) (11.63 to 27.27%) ... 1597
▲ Vaseretic Tablets (8.6%) ... 1810
Vasotec I.V. (0.5 to 1%) ... 1814
▲ Vasotec Tablets (4.3% to 7.9%) 1816
Velban Vials ... 1537
▲ Ventolin Inhalation Aerosol and Refill (Fewer than 5 per 100 patients) ... 1170
▲ Ventolin Inhalation Solution (7%) .. 1171
▲ Ventolin Nebules Inhalation Solution (7%) ... 1172
Ventolin Rotacaps for Inhalation (Less than 1%) ... 1173
▲ Ventolin Syrup (3 of 100 patients) 1175
Ventolin Tablets (2 of 100 patients) ... 1176
▲ Verelan Capsules (3.3% to 4.2%) 1455
Versed Injection (Less than 1%) 2324
▲ Vesanoid Capsules (20%) ... 2327
Vicks 44 LiquiCaps Cough, Cold & Flu Relief ... ■ 728
Vicks 44 LiquiCaps Non-Drowsy Cough & Cold Relief ... ■ 729
Vicks 44D Cough & Head Congestion Relief ... ■ 728
Vicks 44M Cough, Cold & Flu Relief ... ■ 729
Vicks DayQuil Allergy Relief 4-Hour Tablets ... ■ 733
Vicks DayQuil LiquiCaps/Liquid Multi-Symptom Cold/Flu Relief ■ 734
Vicks DayQuil SINUS Pressure & CONGESTION Relief ... ■ 734
Vicks Nyquil Hot Therapy ... ■ 735
Vicks NyQuil LiquiCaps/Liquid Multi-Symptom Cold/Flu Relief, Original and Cherry Flavors ... ■ 736
Vicodin Tablets ... 1404
▲ Vicodin ES Tablets (Among most frequent) ... 1405
▲ Vicodin HP Tablets (Among most frequent) ... 1403
Vicodin Tuss Expectorant ... 1406
▲ Videx Tablets, Powder for Oral Solution, & Pediatric Powder for Oral Solution (1% to 7%) ... 2980
▲ Visken Tablets (9%) ... 2428
Vistide Injection ... 1057
Vivactil Tablets ... 1820
Vivelle Transdermal System ... 880
Cataflam/Voltaren/Voltaren-XR (1% to 3%) ... 833
▲ Wellbutrin Tablets (22.3%) ... 1177
▲ Wygesic Tablets (Most frequent) ... 2930
▲ Xanax Tablets (1.8% to 29.8%) 2115
▲ Xylocaine Injections (Among most common) ... 562
Yocon Tablets ... 1235
Yohimex Tablets ... 1414
Zantac (Rare) ... 1182
Zantac Injection (Rare) ... 1180
Zantac Syrup (Rare) ... 1182
Zarontin Capsules ... 1986
Zarontin Syrup ... 1986
Zaroxolyn Tablets ... 1625
▲ Zebeta Tablets (2.9% to 3.5%) ... 1457
▲ Zerit Capsules (Fewer than 1% to 9%) ... 731
▲ Zestoretic Tablets (7.5%) ... 2968
▲ Zestril Tablets (5.4% to 11.8%) ... 2972
▲ Ziac (3.2% to 5.1%) ... 1459
Zithromax (1% or less) ... 2043
Zithromax Tablets (1% or less) ... 2046
Zocor Tablets ... 1821
▲ Zofran Injection (12%) ... 1227
▲ Zofran Tablets (4% to 7%) ... 1231
▲ Zoladex (5% to 6%) ... 2976
Zoladex 3-month (1% to 5%) ... 2978
▲ Zoloft Tablets (Infrequent to 11.7) 2051
▲ Zonalon Cream (Approximately 1% to 10%) ... 1042
Zosyn (1.4%) ... 1463
Zovirax (0.3%) ... 1187
▲ Zydone Capsules (Among most frequent) ... 967
Zyloprim Tablets (Less than 1%) 1194
Zyrtec Tablets (2%) ... 2053

Down's syndrome

Pergonal (menotropins for injection, USP) ... 2618
Serophene (clomiphene citrate tablets, USP) (Six cases) ... 2621

(■ Described in PDR For Nonprescription Drugs) Incidence data in parenthesis; ▲ 3% or more (◉ Described in PDR For Ophthalmology)

1313 Side Effects Index Drowsiness

Dreaming

Dilaudid Tablets and Liquid (Less frequent) 1386
Ganite 2711
Limbitrol (Less common) 2333
MS Contin Tablets (Less frequent) 2149
MSIR (Infrequent) 2152
Nicotrol NS Nicotine Nasal Spray (Under 5%) 1565
▲Orudis Capsules (3% to 9%) 2874
▲Oruvail Capsules (3% to 9%) 2874
Tenoretic Tablets (Up to 3%) 2963
Tenormin Tablets and I.V. Injection (Up to 3%) 2965
Versed Injection (Less than 1%) 2324

Dreaming, abnormalities

Aldomet Ester HCl Injection 1642
Ambien Tablets (1%) 2559
Anafranil Capsules (Up to 3%) 819
Anaprox/Naprosyn (Less than 1%) 2277
Axid Pulvules (1.9%) 1468
Blocadren Tablets (Less than 1%) 1654
Buprenex Injectable (Less than 1%) 2170
BuSpar Tablets (Frequent) 738
Cardene Capsules (0.4%) 2261
Cardizem CD Capsules (Less than 1%) 1251
Cardizem SR Capsules (Less than 1%) 1255
Cardizem Injectable 1253
Cardizem Tablets (Less than 1%) 1257
Cartrol Tablets (Rare) 413
Catapres Tablets 679
Catapres-TTS 680
Cognex Capsules (Infrequent) 1961
Combipres Tablets 682
Cozaar Tablets (Less than 1%) 1668
Crixivan Capsules (Less than 2%) 1670
Cytovene (1% or less) 2270
Depakote Tablets (1% to 5%) 418
Desyrel and Desyrel Dividose (Less than 1% to 5.1%) 504
Dilacor XR Extended-release Capsules (1.4%) 2183
Dilaudid-HP Injection (Less frequent) 1384
Dilaudid-HP Lyophilized Powder 250 mg (Less frequent) 1384
Diprivan Injectable Emulsion (Less than 1%) 2939
Duragesic Transdermal System (1% or greater) 1336
EC-Naprosyn Delayed-Release Tablets (Less than 1%) 2277
▲Effexor (4%) 2825
Elavil 2945
▲Eldepryl Capsules (2 of 49 patients) 2729
Etrafon 2495
Feldene Capsules (Less than 1%) 2008
Flexeril Tablets (Less than 1%) 1701
Floxin I.V. (Less than 1%) 1580
Floxin Tablets (200 mg, 300 mg, 400 mg) (Less than 1%) 1577
▲Habitrol Nicotine Transdermal System (3% to 9% of patients) 884
Halcion Tablets (Rare) 2093
Hyzaar Tablets 1720
IBU Tablets (Less than 1%) 1389
Inderal 2834
Inderal LA Long Acting Capsules 2836
Inderide Tablets 2838
Intron A for Injection (Less than 5%) 2506
Invirase Capsules (Less than 2%) 2291
IOPIDINE Sterile Ophthalmic Solution ⊙ 218
Kadian Capsules (Less than 3%) 2948
Kerlone Tablets (1.0%) 2588
Lamictal Tablets (Infrequent) 1105
Levo-Dromoran 2297
Lotensin HCT Tablets (0.3% or more) 855
LUVOX Tablets 2723
Mellaril 2398
Motrin Ibuprofen Suspension, Oral Drops, Chewable Tablets, Caplets (Less than 1%) 1563
▲Naprelan Tablets (3% to 9%) 2861
Anaprox/Naprosyn (Less than 1%) 2277
Neurontin Capsules (Infrequent) 1978
Nipent for Injection (Less than 3%) 2733
Norvasc Tablets (More than 0.1% to 1%) 2020
Norvir (Less than 2%) 447
Nubain Injection (1% or less) 952
Oramorph SR (Morphine Sulfate Sustained Release Tablets) (Less frequent) 2359
Orap Tablets (2.7%) 1037
Orlaam Oral Solution (1% to 3%) 2361
OxyContin Tablets (Between 1% and 5%) 2163
▲Paxil Tablets (4%) 2681
Permax Tablets (2.7%) 571
Prilosec Delayed-Release Capsules (Less than 1%) 516
▲Prograf (Greater than 3%) 1028
Prolixin 510
ProSom Tablets (2%) 457
▲Prozac Pulvules & Liquid, Oral Solution (5%) 935
Redux Capsules (2.0%) 2911
▲Remeron Tablets (4%) 1878
ReVia Tablets (Less than 1%) 957
Rilutek Tablets (Rare) 2198
Risperdal Tablets (Frequent) 1348
Rythmol Tablets–150mg, 225mg, 300mg (Less than 1%) 1399
Salagen Tablets (Less than 1%) 1546
Sectral Capsules (2%) 2914
Serentil 689
▲Serzone Tablets (3%) 776
Sinemet CR Tablets (1.8%) 961
Stadol (Less than 1%) 779
Sular Tablets (Less than or equal to 1%) 2961
Symmetrel Capsules (1% to 5%) 965
Symmetrel Syrup (1% to 5%) 963
Talacen Caplets (Infrequent) 2464
Talwin Injection (Infrequent) 2465
Talwin Compound (Infrequent) 2466
Talwin Injection 2465
Talwin Nx Tablets 2467
Tambocor Tablets (Less than 1%) 1555
Tiazac Capsules (Less than 1%) 1019
Tonocard Tablets (Less than 1%) 519
Toradol (1% or less) 2319
Torecan 2367
Triavil Tablets 1800
Trilafon 2532
▲Visken Tablets (5%) 2428
Wellbutrin Tablets 1177
Xanax Tablets (1.8%) 2115
Zebeta Tablets (0%) 1457
Ziac 1459
Zoloft Tablets (Infrequent) 2051

Drowsiness

Accupril Tablets (0.5% to 1.0%) 1950
Accutane Capsules 2252
▲Acel-Imune Diphtheria and Tetanus Toxoids and Acellular Pertussis Vaccine Adsorbed (6% to 12%) 1415
▲ActHIB (23.5% to 63.7%) 893
Actifed Allergy Daytime/Nighttime Caplets ▣ 808
Actifed Cold & Allergy Tablets ▣ 807
Actifed Cold & Sinus Caplets and Tablets ▣ 808
Actifed Sinus Daytime/Nighttime Tablets and Caplets ▣ 809
Adalat CC (Less than 1.0%) 582
▲Adapin Capsules (Most common) 1542
Adenoscan (Less than 1%) 1022
Akineton 1380
Albalon Solution with Liquifilm ⊙ 229
Aldactazide Tablets 2556
Aldactone Tablets 2558
Alfenta Injection (1% to 3%) 1334
▲Alferon N Injection (3% to 10%) 2142
Alka-Seltzer Plus Cold Medicine ▣ 611
Alka-Seltzer Plus Cold Medicine Liqui-Gels ▣ 612
Alka-Seltzer Plus Cold & Cough Medicine ▣ 611
Alka-Seltzer Plus Cold & Cough Medicine Liqui-Gels ▣ 612
Alka-Seltzer Plus Flu & Body Aches Effervescent Tablets ▣ 612
Alka-Seltzer Plus Night-Time Cold Medicine ▣ 611
Alka-Seltzer Plus Night-Time Cold Medicine Liqui-Gels ▣ 612
Alka-Seltzer Plus Sinus Medicine ▣ 611
Allerest Maximum Strength ▣ 649
Allerest No Drowsiness ▣ 649
Allerest Sinus Pain Formula ▣ 649
Alomide Ophthalmic Solution (Less than 1%) 465
Altace Capsules (Less than 1%) 1238
Alupent Tablets (0.6%) 672
▲Ambien Tablets (2% to 8%) 2559
Amen Tablets 785
▲Anafranil Capsules (46% to 54%) 819
Ana-Kit Anaphylaxis Emergency Treatment Kit 611
▲Anaprox/Naprosyn (3% to 9%) 2277
Antabuse Tablets (Small number of patients) 2802
Antivert, Antivert/25 Tablets, & Antivert/50 Tablets 1992
Apresazide Capsules 824
▲Aredia for Injection (Up to 6%) 827
Arimidex Tablets (2% to 5%) 2932
Artane 1418
Asacol Delayed-Release Tablets 2129
▲Asendin Tablets (14%) 1419
Atamet Tablets 567
Atarax Tablets & Syrup 1992
▲Ativan Injection (6%) 2805
▲Atretol Tablets (Among most frequent) 569
Atrohist Pediatric Capsules 1603
▲Atrohist Pediatric Suspension (Among most common) 1604
▲Atrohist Pediatric Suspension Dye-Free (Among most common) 1604
Atrohist Plus Tablets 1605
Atromid-S Capsules 2808
Atrovent Inhalation Aerosol (Less frequent) 674
Axid Pulvules (1.9%) 1468
▲Axocet Capsules (Among most frequent) 2469
Azulfidine (Rare) 2059
BC Cold Powder Multi-Symptom Formula (Cold-Sinus-Allergy) ▣ 631
Bellergal-S Tablets (Rare) 2375
Benadryl Allergy Chewables ▣ 811
Benadryl Allergy/Cold Tablets ▣ 811
Benadryl Allergy Decongestant Liquid Medication ▣ 812
Benadryl Allergy Decongestant Tablets ▣ 812
Benadryl Allergy Liquid Medication ▣ 813
Benadryl Allergy ▣ 811
Benadryl Dye-Free Allergy Liqui-gel Softgels ▣ 813
Benadryl Dye-Free Allergy Liquid Medication ▣ 814
▲Benadryl Injection (Among most frequent) 1955
▲Bentyl (9%) 1246
▲Betaseron for SC Injection (6%) 653
Blocadren Tablets (Less than 1%) 1654
Bonine Tablets 1990
Brethaire Inhaler 830
▲Brethine Ampuls (9.8 to 11.7%) 832
Brethine Tablets 831
▲Brevibloc (esmolol HCl) Injection (3%) 1860
Bricanyl Subcutaneous Injection 1247
Bricanyl Tablets 1248
Bromfed Capsules (Extended-Release) 1832
Bromfed Syrup ▣ 712
Bromfed 1832
Brontex 2130
▲BuSpar Tablets (10%) 738
Butisol Sodium Elixir & Tablets (1 to 3 patients per 100) 2768
Calan SR Caplets (1% or less) 2571
Calan Tablets (1% or less) 2568
Calcijex Injection 412
Capoten Tablets 740
Capozide Tablets 744
Carafate Suspension (Less than 0.5%) 1250
Carafate Tablets (Less than 0.5%) 1249
Carbocaine Injection 2432
Cardene Capsules (1.1% to 1.4%) 2261
Cardizem CD Capsules (Less than 1%) 1251
Cardizem SR Capsules (1.3%) 1255
Cardizem Injectable 1253
Cardizem Tablets (Less than 1%) 1257
▲Cardura Tablets (3% to 5%) 1993
▲Cartrol Tablets (1%-7.4%) 413
Casodex Tablets (2% to 5%) 2934
Cataflam Tablets (Less than 1%) 833
▲Catapres Tablets (About 33 in 100 patients) 679
▲Catapres-TTS (12 of 101 patients) 680
Ceclor Pulvules & Suspension (Rare) 1470
Cedax (0.1% to 1%) 2480
Ceftin (0.1% to 1%) 1067
Cefzil Tablets and Oral Suspension (Less than 1%) 747
▲CellCept Capsules (More than or equal to 3%) 2265
Celontin Kapseals (Frequent) 1955
▲Cerebyx Injection (6.7% to 20.0%) 1956
Cerose DM ▣ 853
▲Chemet Capsules (1.0% to 12.7%) 666
Cheracol Plus Head Cold/Cough Formula ▣ 741
Children's TYLENOL Cold Multi-Symptom Chewable Tablets and Liquid 1559
Children's TYLENOL Cold Plus Cough Multi Symptom Chewable Tablets and Liquid 1560
Children's TYLENOL Flu Suspension Liquid 1560
Children's Vicks DayQuil Allergy Relief ▣ 730
Children's Vicks NyQuil Cold/Cough Relief ▣ 731
Chlor-Trimeton Allergy Decongestant Tablets ▣ 759
Chlor-Trimeton Allergy Tablets ▣ 758
Cipro I.V. (1% or less) 587
Cipro I.V. Pharmacy Bulk Package (Less than 1%) 590
Cipro Tablets (Less than 1%) 584
▲Claritin Tablets (8%) 2485
▲Claritin-D Tablets (7%) 2487
Clinoril Tablets (Less than 1%) 1658
▲Clozaril Tablets (More than 5 to 39%) 2377
Codiclear DH Syrup 808
▲Cognex Capsules (4%) 1961
▲Combipres Tablets (About 33%) 682
Compazine 2644
Allergy-Sinus Comtrex Multi-Symptom Allergy-Sinus Formula Tablets and Caplets ▣ 639
Comtrex Multi-Symptom ▣ 638
Contac Continuous Action Nasal Decongestant/Antihistamine 12 Hour Capsules ▣ 773
Contac Day & Night Cold/Flu Night Caplets ▣ 772
Contac Maximum Strength Continuous Action Decongestant/Antihistamine 12 Hour Caplets ▣ 772
Contac Night Allergy/Sinus Caplets ▣ 771
Contac Severe Cold and Flu Formula Caplets ▣ 773
Coricidin Cold + Flu Tablets ▣ 760
Coricidin Cough + Cold Tablets ▣ 760
Coricidin 'D' Decongestant Tablets ▣ 760
Covera-HS Tablets (Less than 2%) 2573
Cozaar Tablets (Less than 1%) 1668
Crixivan Capsules (1.0% to less than 2%) 1670
Cycrin Tablets 991
Cylert Tablets 415
Cystospaz 2123
▲Cytadren Tablets (1 in 3) 837
CytoGam (Infrequent) 1630
Cytosar-U Sterile Powder (With experimental doses) 2077
Cytotec (Infrequent) 2576
Cytovene (1% or less) 2270
D.A. II Tablets 972
D.A. Chewable Tablets 970
▲DHCplus Capsules (Among most frequent) 2148
Dalmane Capsules 2329
▲Dantrium Capsules (Among most frequent) 2131
▲Daranide Tablets (Among the most common effects) 1676
▲DaunoXome (Less than or equal to 5%) 1842
▲Daypro Caplets (1% to 3%) 2578
Decadron Phosphate with Xylocaine Injection, Sterile 1683
Demadex Tablets and Injection 691
▲Depakote Tablets (17% to 19%) 418
Depo-Provera Contraceptive Injection (Fewer than 1%) 2079
Depo-Provera Sterile Aqueous Suspension 2083
▲Desyrel and Desyrel Dividose (23.9% to 40.8%) 504
Diamox Intravenous (Occasional) ⊙ 317
Diamox Sequels (Sustained Release) (Occasional) ⊙ 318
Diamox Tablets (Occasional) ⊙ 317
Dibenzyline Capsules 2650
Dilacor XR Extended-release Capsules (Infrequent) 2183
Dilaudid Ampules 1382
Dilaudid Cough Syrup 1383
Dilaudid 1382
Dimetapp Allergy Dye-Free Elixir ▣ 838
Dimetapp Allergy Sinus Caplets ▣ 838

(▣ Described in PDR For Nonprescription Drugs) Incidence data in parenthesis; ▲ 3% or more (⊙ Described in PDR For Ophthalmology)

Drowsiness Side Effects Index 1314

Dimetapp Cold & Allergy Chewable Tablets ▣ 838
Dimetapp Cold & Cough Liqui-Gels ▣ 839
Dimetapp Cold & Fever Suspension ▣ 839
Dimetapp Elixir ▣ 840
Dimetapp Extentabs ▣ 841
Dimetapp Tablets/Liqui-Gels ▣ 841
Dipentum Capsules (1.8%) 2084
Diphtheria and Tetanus Toxoids and Pertussis Vaccine Adsorbed 2650
Diprivan Injectable Emulsion (Less than 1%) 2939
Ditropan 1267
Diuril Sodium Intravenous 1693
▲ Dizac (diazepam injectable emulsion) CIV (Among most common) 1862
Dolobid Tablets (Greater than 1 in 100) 1695
Donnatal (In elderly patients) 2234
Donnatal Extentabs (In elderly patients) 2234
Donnatal Tablets (In elderly patients) 2234
▲ Doral Tablets (12%) 2773
Doxil (1% to 5%) 2613
Dramamine Chewable Tablets ▣ 801
Children's Dramamine Liquid ▣ 801
Dramamine Tablets ▣ 801
Dramamine II Tablets ▣ 801
Drixoral Cold and Allergy Sustained-Action Tablets ▣ 763
Drixoral Cold and Flu Extended-Release Tablets ▣ 764
Drixoral Allergy/Sinus Extended Release Tablets ▣ 765
▲ Duragesic Transdermal System (10% or more) 1336
Duranest Injections 533
Dura-Tap/PD Capsules 970
Dura-Vent/DA Tablets 972
Duratuss HD Elixir 2750
Dyazide Capsules 2653
Dyclone 0.5% and 1% Topical Solutions, USP 535
Dynabac (0.1% to 1%) 668
DynaCirc Capsules (0.5% to 1%) 2381
DynaCirc CR Tablets (0.5% to 1.0%) 2383
Easprin 1971
▲ EC-Naprosyn Delayed-Release Tablets (3% to 9%) 2277
▲ Effexor (3% to 26.1%) 2825
Efidac 24 Chlorpheniramine ▣ 655
Elavil 2945
Eldepryl Capsules 2729
Elspar 1700
▲ Emete-con Intramuscular/Intravenous (Most common) 2007
EMLA Cream (Unlikely with cream) 536
Engerix-B Unit-Dose Vials (Less than 1%) 2656
Ergamisol Tablets (2% to 3%) 1340
▲ Esgic-plus Capsules (Among most frequent) 1012
▲ Esgic-plus Tablets (Among most frequent) 1012
Esidrix Tablets 839
Eskalith 2658
Ethmozine Tablets (Less than 2%) 2217
Ethyol (amifostine) for Injection 485
Etrafon 2495
Eulexin Capsules (1%) 2498
Extendryl 1003
Famvir Tablets (1.6% to 2.6%) 2660
Fedahist Gyrocaps 2545
▲ Felbatol (Among most common; 19.3% to 48.4%) 2774
Feldene Capsules (Greater than 1%) 2008
▲ Fioricet Tablets (Among most frequent) 2386
Fioricet with Codeine Capsules (Frequent) 2387
▲ Fiorinal Capsules (One of the two most frequent) 2388
Fiorinal with Codeine Capsules (2.4%) 2390
▲ Fiorinal Tablets (One of the two most frequent) 2388
▲ Flexeril Tablets (16% to 39%) 1701
Floxin I.V. (1% to 3%) 1580
Floxin Tablets (200 mg, 300 mg, 400 mg) (1% to 3%) 1577
Flumadine Tablets & Syrup (0.3% to 1%) 1013
Foscavir Injection (Between 1% and 5%) 541
Gamimune N, 5% Immune Globulin Intravenous (Human), 5% (Infrequent) 612
Gamimune N, 10% Immune Globulin Intravenous (Human), 10% (Infrequent) 615
Gammar-P I.V., Immune Globulin Intravenous (Human) (Infrequent) 798
▲ Gemzar for Injection (5% to 11%) 1482
GlaucTabs (Occasional instances) ◉ 209
Glucophage Tablets 754
Glucotrol Tablets (About 1 in 50) 2011
Glucotrol XL Extended Release Tablets (Less than 1%) 2012
Guaifed 1833
▲ Habitrol Nicotine Transdermal System (3% to 9% of patients) 884
▲ Halcion Tablets (14.0%) 2093
Haldol Decanoate 1587
Haldol Injection, Tablets and Concentrate 1585
Havrix (Rare) 2663
HibTITER (91 of 1,118 vaccinations) 1423
▲ Hismanal Tablets (7.1%) 1341
▲ Histussin D Liquid (Among most frequent) 670
Hivid Tablets (Less than 1%) 2287
Hycodan Tablets and Syrup 946
Hycomine Compound Tablets 948
Hycomine 947
Hycotuss Expectorant Syrup 950
Hydrea Capsules 705
Hydrocet Capsules 787
▲ Hylorel Tablets (15.3% to 44.6%) 1613
Hyperstat I.V. Injection 2504
▲ Hytrin Capsules (0.6% to 5.4%) 434
Hyzaar Tablets 1720
IBU Tablets (Less than 1%) 1389
▲ IFEX (Among most common) 706
Imdur (Less than or equal to 5%) 1362
Imitrex Injection (2.7%) 1095
Imitrex Tablets 1099
Imodium Capsules 1343
▲ Inapsine Injection (Among most common) 462
Indocin (Less than 1%) 1723
Intal Inhaler (Rare) 2185
Intal Nebulizer Solution 2186
▲ Intron A for Injection (Up to 14%) 2506
Invirase Capsules (Less than 2%) 2291
Iopidine 0.5% (Less than 1%) ◉ 219
IPOL Poliovirus Vaccine Inactivated 903
Isoptin Injectable 1391
Isoptin Oral Tablets (Less than 1%) 1393
Isoptin SR Tablets (1% or less) 1395
▲ Kadian Capsules (Among frequent) 2948
▲ Klonopin Tablets (50%) 2294
Kutrase Capsules 2546
▲ Kytril Injection (4%) 2667
Kytril Tablets (1% to 4%) 2669
▲ Lamictal Tablets (Among most common; 14.2%) 1105
Lamprene Capsules (Less than 1%) 846
Lasix Injection, Oral Solution and Tablets 1267
Levsin/Levsinex/Levbid 2549
Librax Capsules 2330
Librium Capsules (Some patients) 2331
Librium Injectable 2332
▲ Limbitrol (Among most frequent) 2333
▲ Lioresal Intrathecal (5.7% to 20.9%) 1634
▲ Lioresal Tablets (10% to 63%) 847
Lithium Carbonate Capsules & Tablets 2352
Lithonate/Lithotabs/Lithobid 2721
Livostin (Approximately 1% to 3%) ◉ 262
Lodine Capsules and Tablets (Less than 1%) 2849
Lomotil 2591
Lopid Tablets 1974
▲ Lopressor HCT Tablets (10 in 100 patients) 850
Lorabid Suspension and Pulvules (0.4% to 2.1%) 1513
Lorcet 10/650 Tablets 1016
Lortab 2751
Lotensin Tablets (1.6%) 852
Lotensin HCT Tablets (1.2%) 855
Lotrel Capsules (Up to 0.3%) 858
Loxitane 1426
▲ Ludiomil Tablets (16%) 861
Lupron Depot-PED 7.5 mg, 11.25 mg and 15 mg (Less than 2%) 2744
Lupron Injection Pediatric (Less than 2%) 2737
▲ LUVOX Tablets (22%) 2723
▲ Lysodren Tablets (25%) 707
Macrobid Capsules (Less than 1%) 2138
Marax Tablets & DF Syrup (Occasional) 2015
Marcaine 2446
Marcaine Spinal 2449
▲ Marinol (Dronabinol) Capsules (3% to 10%) 2353
Matulane Capsules 2300
Mavik Tablets (0.3% to 1.0%) 1407
Maxaquin Tablets (Less than 1%) 2593
Mebaral Tablets (1 to 3 in 100) 2452
Mellaril (Occasional) 2398
Merrem I.V. (0.1% to 1.0%) 2952
Mesantoin Tablets 2400
Methotrexate Sodium Tablets, Injection, for Injection and LPF Injection 1322
Midamor Tablets (Less than or equal to 1%) 1746
Maximum Strength Multi-Symptom Formula Midol ▣ 621
PMS Multi-Symptom Formula Midol ▣ 622
Miltown Tablets 2780
▲ Minipress Capsules (7.6%) 2015
▲ Minizide Capsules (7.6%) 2016
Mintezol 1747
Mithracin 599
▲ Moban Tablets and Concentrate (Most frequent) 1036
Mobigesic Tablets ▣ 607
Moduretic Tablets (Less than or equal to 1%) 1748
Mono-Gesic Tablets 810
Monopril Tablets (0.2% to 1.0%) 762
Motofen Tablets (1 in 25) 789
Motrin Ibuprofen Suspension, Oral Drops, Chewable Tablets, Caplets (Less than 1%) 1563
MSTA Mumps Skin Test Antigen 2988
Mutamycin for Injection 712
Mykrox Tablets 1617
Mysoline (Occasional) 2860
▲ Nalfon 200 Pulvules & Nalfon Tablets (8.5%) 933
▲ Naprelan Tablets (3% to 9%) 2861
▲ Anaprox/Naprosyn (3% to 9%) 2277
Nardil (Common) 1977
Navane Capsules and Concentrate 2018
Navane Intramuscular 2019
NegGram 2453
Nembutal Sodium Capsules (1% to 3%) 440
Nembutal Sodium Solution (1%-3%) 442
Nembutal Sodium Suppositories (1%-3%) 444
Neptazane Tablets (Occasional) ◉ 320
Nescaine/Nescaine MPF 549
▲ Neurontin Capsules (Among most common; 19.3%) 1978
▲ Nicotrol NS Nicotine Nasal Spray (Over 5%) 1565
▲ Nipent for Injection (3% to 10%) 2733
Nizoral Tablets (Less than 1%) 1345
Nolahist Tablets 790
Nolamine Timed-Release Tablets (Occasional) 790
Norflex 1554
Norgesic 1554
▲ Normodyne Injection (3%) 2519
Normodyne Tablets (Less than 1%) 2522
Noroxin Tablets (0.3% to 1.0%) 1758
Noroxin Tablets (0.3% to 1.0%) 2222
Norpramin Tablets 1273
Norvasc Tablets (1.3% to 1.6%) 2020
Norvir (2.0% to 2.6%) 447
Novahistine Elixir ▣ 782
Novocain Hydrochloride for Spinal Anesthesia 2457
Nucofed 2225
Numorphan Injection 953
Numorphan Suppositories 953
Maximum Strength Nytol Caplets ▣ 632
▲ OmniHIB (2.5% to 57.5%) 2676
Oncaspar (Less than 1%) 2194
OptiPranolol (Metipranolol 0.3%) Sterile Ophthalmic Solution (A small number of patients) ◉ 256
▲ Orap Tablets (27.7%) 1037
Oretic Tablets 450
Orlaam Oral Solution (1% to 3%) 2361
Ornade Spansule Capsules 2678
Orudis Capsules (Greater than 1%) 2874
Oruvail Capsules (Greater than 1%) 2874
▲ OxyContin Tablets (23%) 2163
▲ PBZ Tablets (Among most frequent) 863
▲ PBZ-SR Tablets (Among most frequent) 862
Pamelor 2409
Parafon Forte DSC Caplets (Occasional) 1590
▲ Parlodel (3%) 2411
Parnate Tablets 2679
▲ Paxil Tablets (1.9% to 24%) 2681
PediaCare 1569
Pediatric Vicks 44m Cough & Cold Relief ▣ 737
Pediazole Suspension 2340
▲ PedvaxHIB (Among most frequent) 1761
Penetrex Tablets (0.1% to 1%) 2196
Pentasa (Less than 1%) 1275
Pepcid Injection (Infrequent) 1765
Pepcid (Infrequent) 1763
Peptavlon 2997
Percogesic Analgesic Tablets ▣ 727
Periactin 1767
▲ Permax Tablets (10.1%) 571
Phenergan with Codeine 2883
Phenergan with Dextromethorphan 2885
Phenergan Injection 2880
Phenergan Suppositories 2882
Phenergan Syrup 2881
Phenergan Tablets 2882
Phenergan VC 2886
Phenergan VC with Codeine 2888
Phenobarbital Elixir and Tablets (1 to 3 patients per 100) 1523
▲ Phenurone Tablets (4%) 455
▲ Phrenilin (Among most frequent) 790
Plendil Extended-Release Tablets (0.5% to 1.5%) 514
PMB 200 and PMB 400 2890
▲ Pondimin Tablets (Among most common) 2239
Ponstel 1982
Pontocaine Hydrochloride for Spinal Anesthesia 2460
Premphase 2900
Prempro 2905
Prilosec Delayed-Release Capsules (Less than 1%) 516
Primaxin I.M. 1770
Primaxin I.V. (0.2%) 1772
Prinivil Tablets (0.3 to 1.0%) 1776
Prinzide Tablets (0.3% to 1%) 1780
Pro-Banthine Tablets 2226
Procardia XL Extended Release Tablets (Less than 3%) 2026
▲ Prograf (Greater than 3%) 1028
Proleukin for Injection 812
Prolixin 510
Propulsid (1% or less) 1346
▲ ProSom Tablets (42%) 457
▲ Prostep (nicotine transdermal system) (3% to 9% of patients) 1439
Prostigmin Injectable 1305
Prostigmin Tablets 1306
Protopam Chloride for Injection 2909
Proventil (Less than 1% to 2%) 2529
Provera Tablets 2110
▲ Prozac Pulvules & Liquid, Oral Solution (5% to 17%) 935
Pyrroxate Caplets ▣ 742
Questran 774
RMS Suppositories CII 2766
Recombivax HB 1787
▲ Redux Capsules (7.1%) 2911
▲ Reglan (Approximately 10%) 2243
Relafen Tablets (1% to 3%) 2688
▲ Remeron Tablets (10.4% to 54%) 1878
RespiGam (Infrequent) 1631
▲ Restoril Capsules (17%) 2413
▲ Retrovir Capsules (8%) 1216
▲ Retrovir I.V. Infusion (8%) 1221
▲ Retrovir Syrup (8%) 1216
ReVia Tablets (Less than 1% to 2%) 957
Revex (nalmefene hydrochloride injection) (Less than 1%) 1863
Rifadin 1276
Rifamate Capsules 1278
Rifater 1280
Rilutek Tablets (0.8% to 4.1%) 2198
Rimactane Capsules 865
▲ Risperdal Tablets (3% to 8%; 41%) 1348
Ritalin 866
Robaxin Injectable 2245
Robaxin Tablets 2246
Robaxisal Tablets 2246

(▣ Described in PDR For Nonprescription Drugs) Incidence data in parenthesis; ▲ 3% or more (◉ Described in PDR For Ophthalmology)

Side Effects Index — Dryness

Robinul Forte Tablets ... 2247
Robinul Injectable ... 2247
Robinul Tablets ... 2247
Robitussin Night-Time Cold Formula ... ⊡ 847
Rocaltrol Capsules ... 2303
Romazicon (Less than 1%) ... 2311
Rondec Chewable Tablets ... 974
Ryna ... ⊡ 804
▲ Rynatan (Among most common) ... 2781
▲ Rynatuss (Among most common) ... 2782
Rythmol Tablets–150mg, 225mg, 300mg (0.6 to 1.2%) ... 1399
Sandoglobulin I.V. (Infrequent) ... 2419
Sanorex Tablets ... 2423
Sansert Tablets ... 2424
Scleromate Injection (Rare) ... 1234
▲ Seconal Sodium Pulvules (Most common) ... 1529
▲ Sedapap Tablets 50 mg/650 mg (Among the most frequent) ... 1826
▲ Seldane (8.5% to 9.0%) ... 1284
▲ Seldane-D Extended-Release Tablets (7.2%) ... 1286
▲ Semprex-D Capsules (12%) ... 1620
Sensorcaine ... 554
Ser-Ap-Es Tablets ... 867
Serax Capsules ... 2916
Serax Tablets ... 2916
▲ Serentil (One of the two most prevalent) ... 689
Seromycin Capsules ... 975
▲ Serzone Tablets (16% to 28%) ... 776
Sinarest ... ⊡ 663
Sine-Off Sinus Medicine ... ⊡ 784
Sinemet Tablets ... 959
Sinemet CR Tablets ... 961
▲ Sinequan (Most common) ... 2028
Singlet Tablets ... ⊡ 785
Sinulin Tablets ... 792
Sinutab Sinus Allergy Medication, Maximum Strength Tablets and Caplets ... ⊡ 823
Skelaxin Tablets ... 793
▲ Soma Compound w/Codeine Tablets (Most frequent) ... 2784
▲ Soma Compound Tablets (Most frequent) ... 2783
Soma Tablets ... 2782
Sporanox Capsules (0.3% to 1.2%) ... 1352
▲ Stadol (43%) ... 779
Stelazine ... 2692
Stimate, (desmopressin acetate) Nasal Spray, 1.5 mg/mL ... 806
▲ Sublimaze Injection (Frequent) ... 463
Sudafed Cold & Allergy Tablets ... ⊡ 826
▲ Sufenta Injection (3% to 9%) ... 1355
Sular Tablets (Less than or equal to 1%) ... 2961
Supprelin Injection (1% to 3%) ... 2230
Surmontil Capsules ... 2917
Symmetrel Capsules (1% to 5%) ... 965
Symmetrel Syrup (1% to 5%) ... 963
Tagamet (Approximately 1 in 100) ... 2694
Tambocor Tablets (1% to less than 3%) ... 1555
Tapazole Tablets ... 1361
▲ Tavist Syrup (Among most frequent) ... 2426
▲ Tavist Tablets (Among most frequent) ... 2427
Tavist-1 12 Hour Relief Tablets ... ⊡ 749
Tavist-D 12 Hour Relief Tablets ... ⊡ 750
▲ Tegretol/Tegretol-XR (Among most frequent) ... 870
Teldrin 12 Hour Antihistamine/Nasal Decongestant Allergy Relief Capsules ... ⊡ 786
▲ Tenex Tablets (Up to 39%) ... 2249
Tenoretic Tablets (0.6% to 2%) ... 2963
Tenormin Tablets and I.V. Injection (0.6% to 2%) ... 2965
▲ Tetramune (Up to 26%) ... 1449
Thalitone (Common) ... 1293
▲ TheraFlu Flu and Cold Medicine ... ⊡ 750
Theraflu Maximum Strength Flu and Cold Medicine For Sore Throat ... ⊡ 751
TheraFlu, Cold and Cough Medicine ... ⊡ 750
TheraFlu Maximum Strength Nighttime Flu, Cold & Cough Medicine ... ⊡ 751
Thorazine ... 2701
THYREL TRH (Less frequent) ... 2992
Tiazac Capsules (Less than 1% to 2%) ... 1019
Tigan ... 2231
Timolide Tablets (Less than 1%) ... 1791

Timoptic in Ocudose (Less frequent) ... 1796
Timoptic Sterile Ophthalmic Solution (Less frequent) ... 1794
Timoptic-XE ... 1798
Tofranil Ampuls ... 873
Tofranil Tablets ... 875
Tofranil-PM Capsules ... 876
Tolectin (200, 400 and 600 mg) (1 to 3%) ... 1591
Tonocard Tablets (0.8% to 1.6%) ... 519
Toprol-XL Tablets ... 560
▲ Toradol (6%) ... 2319
Torecan (Occasional) ... 2367
Tornalate Solution for Inhalation, 0.2% (1.2%) ... 976
Trancopal Caplets ... 2468
▲ Trandate (3 of 100 patients) ... 1158
▲ Transderm Scōp Transdermal Therapeutic System (Less than one-sixth) ... 890
▲ Tranxene (Most frequent) ... 459
Trental Tablets ... 1291
Triaminic Night Time ... ⊡ 754
Triaminic Syrup ... ⊡ 755
Triaminic Triaminicol Cold & Cough ... ⊡ 756
Triaminicin Tablets ... ⊡ 756
Triavil Tablets ... 1800
Tri-Immunol Adsorbed (Rare) ... 1452
Trilafon ... 2532
Trilisate (Less than 2%) ... 2155
▲ Trinalin Repetabs Tablets (Among most frequent) ... 1373
▲ Tripedia (1% to 13%) ... 908
▲ Tussend (Most frequent) ... 1830
Tussend Expectorant ... 1831
Tussionex Pennkinetic Extended-Release Suspension ... 1624
Tussi-Organidin DM NR Liquid and DM-S NR Liquid (Rare) ... 2786
Tylenol Allergy Sinus ... 1571
TYLENOL Cold Medication, Multi-Symptom Formula Tablets and Caplets ... 1572
TYLENOL Cold Medication, Multi-Symptom Hot Liquid Packets ... 1572
TYLENOL Flu NightTime, Maximum Strength Gelcaps ... 1575
TYLENOL Flu NightTime, Maximum Strength Hot Medication Packets ... 1575
TYLENOL PM Pain Reliever/Sleep Aid, Extra Strength Gelcaps, Caplets, Geltabs ... 1576
TYLENOL Severe Allergy Medication Caplets ... 1571
▲ Ultram Tablets (50 mg) (16% to 25%) ... 1594
Univasc Tablets (Less than 1%) ... 2553
Urispas Tablets ... 2710
▲ Valium Injectable (Among most common) ... 2336
▲ Valium Tablets (Among most common) ... 2335
Vascor Tablets (200 and 300 mg) (0.5 to 6.98%) ... 1597
Vaseretic Tablets (0.5% to 2.0%) ... 1810
Vasotec I.V. ... 1814
Vasotec Tablets (0.5% to 1.0%) ... 1816
Ventolin Tablets (Fewer than 1 of 100 patients) ... 1176
Verelan Capsules (1% or less) ... 1455
Versed Injection (1.2%) ... 2324
▲ Vesanoid Capsules (3%) ... 2327
Vicks 44 LiquiCaps Cough, Cold & Flu Relief ... ⊡ 728
Vicks 44M Cough, Cold & Flu Relief ... ⊡ 729
Vicks DayQuil Allergy Relief 12-Hour Extended Release Tablets ... ⊡ 733
Vicks DayQuil Allergy Relief 4-Hour Tablets ... ⊡ 733
Vicks Nyquil Hot Therapy ... ⊡ 735
Vicks NyQuil LiquiCaps/Liquid Multi-Symptom Cold/Flu Relief, Original and Cherry Flavors ... ⊡ 736
Vicodin Tablets ... 1404
Vicodin ES Tablets ... 1405
Vicodin HP Tablets ... 1403
Vicodin Tuss Expectorant ... 1406
Vistaril Capsules ... 2042
Vistaril Intramuscular Solution ... 2042
Vistaril Oral Suspension ... 2042
Vistide Injection ... 1057
Vivactil Tablets ... 1820
Volmax Extended-Release Tablets (0.3%) ... 1835

Cataflam/Voltaren/Voltaren-XR (Less than 1%) ... 833
WinRho SD (One report) ... 1839
▲ Xanax Tablets (41% to 76.8%) ... 2115
▲ Xylocaine Injections (Among most common) ... 562
Yutopar Intravenous Injection (Infrequent) ... 566
Zantac (Rare) ... 1182
Zantac Injection ... 1180
Zantac Syrup (Rare) ... 1182
Zarontin Capsules ... 1986
Zarontin Syrup ... 1986
Zaroxolyn Tablets ... 1625
Zebeta Tablets ... 1457
Zerit Capsules (Fewer than 1% to 2%) ... 731
Zestoretic Tablets (0.3 to 1%) ... 2968
Zestril Tablets (0.3% to 1.0%) ... 2972
Ziac (0.9% to 1.1%) ... 1459
Zithromax (1% or less) ... 2043
Zithromax Tablets (1% or less) ... 2046
▲ Zofran Injection (8%) ... 1227
▲ Zofran Tablets (20%) ... 1231
Zoladex (1% or greater) ... 2976
Zoladex 3-month ... 2978
▲ Zoloft Tablets (13.4%) ... 2051
▲ Zonalon Cream (22%) ... 1042
Zovirax ... 1187
Zydone Capsules ... 967
Zyloprim Tablets (Less than 1%) ... 1194
▲ Zyrtec Tablets (11% to 14%) ... 2053

Drug administration site reactions, unspecified

Abelcet Injection ... 1540
Amicar Syrup, Tablets, and Injection ... 1312
▲ Avonex (4%) ... 662
Cardene I.V. (1.4%) ... 2815
Casodex Tablets (2% to 5%) ... 2934
▲ Ceptaz (Among most common) ... 1070
Cerebyx Injection (Frequent) ... 1956
▲ Cytovene-IV (22%) ... 2270
D.H.E. 45 Injection ... 2381
Doxil ... 2613
Duragesic Transdermal System (1% or greater) ... 1336
Engerix-B Unit-Dose Vials ... 2656
▲ Fortaz (Among most common) ... 1092
Fragmin Injection (Rare) ... 2088
▲ Imitrex Injection (58.7%) ... 1095
Intron A for Injection (Less than 5%) ... 2506
Leukine ... 1317
▲ Leustatin (9% to 19%) ... 1889
Levo-Dromoran ... 2297
Lupron Depot 3.75 mg (Less than 5%) ... 2739
▲ Lupron Depot - 3 Month 22.5 mg (13.8%) ... 2743
▲ Lupron Depot-PED 7.5 mg, 11.25 mg and 15 mg (5%) ... 2744
Lupron Injection Pediatric ... 2737
Merrem I.V. (1.1%) ... 2952
▲ Navelbine Injection (Up to 38%) ... 1212
Neupogen for Injection (Infrequent) ... 495
Nuromax Injection (Less than or equal to 0.1%) ... 1136
Oncaspar (Greater than 1% but less than 5%) ... 2194
▲ Proleukin for Injection (3%) ... 812
Retrovir I.V. Infusion (Infrequent) ... 1221
Rilutek Tablets (Infrequent) ... 2198
Rocephin Injectable Vials, ADD-Vantage, Galaxy Container (5% to 17%) ... 2305
Septra I.V. Infusion ... 1142
Septra I.V. Infusion ADD-Vantage Vials (Infrequent) ... 1144
▲ Supprelin Injection (12%) ... 2230
▲ Taxol Injection (13%) ... 723
Taxotere for Injection Concentrate ... 2204
▲ Tazicef for Injection (Among most common) ... 2697
▲ Vesanoid Capsules (17%) ... 2327
▲ Zoladex (6%) ... 2976
Zoladex 3-month ... 2978
Zosyn (0.5%) ... 1463

Drug effect, unspecified, prolonged

Diprivan Injectable Emulsion (Less than 1%) ... 2939
Mivacron (Less than 1%) ... 1125
Nuromax Injection (Less than or equal to 0.1%) ... 1136

Drug fever

Aldactazide Tablets ... 2556
Aldactone Tablets ... 2558

Aldoclor Tablets ... 1638
Aldomet Oral ... 1640
Aldoril Tablets ... 1644
Amikacin Sulfate Injection, USP (Rare) ... 523
Amikacin Sulfate Injection, USP (Rare) ... 981
Amikin Injectable (Rare) ... 502
Ancef Injection ... 2632
Asendin Tablets (Less than 1%) ... 1419
Bactrim DS Tablets ... 2257
Bactrim I.V. Infusion ... 2255
Bactrim ... 2257
Cedax ... 2480
Cefobid Intravenous/Intramuscular (1 in 260) ... 1996
Cefobid Pharmacy Bulk Package - Not for Direct Infusion (1 in 260) ... 1999
Clozaril Tablets ... 2377
Compazine ... 2644
Depen Titratable Tablets ... 2770
DynaCirc CR Tablets (0.5% to 1.0%) ... 2383
Ethmozine Tablets (Less than 2%) ... 2217
Fansidar Tablets ... 2281
Kefzol Vials, Faspak & ADD-Vantage ... 1511
Leukeran Tablets ... 1205
Ludiomil Tablets (Rare) ... 861
Macrobid Capsules ... 2138
Macrodantin Capsules ... 2140
Mandol Vials, Faspak & ADD-Vantage ... 1516
Mezlin ... 594
Mezlin Pharmacy Bulk Package ... 597
Norpramin Tablets ... 1273
Orap Tablets ... 1037
Pamelor ... 2409
Prolixin ... 510
Purinethol Tablets (Very rare) ... 1214
Septra ... 1146
Septra I.V. Infusion ... 1142
Septra I.V. Infusion ADD-Vantage Vials ... 1144
Septra ... 1146
Serentil ... 689
Stelazine ... 2692
Suprax (Less than 2%) ... 1443
Tapazole Tablets ... 1361
Taxotere for Injection Concentrate ... 2204
Ticar for Injection ... 2704
Timentin for Injection ... 2706
Tofranil Ampuls ... 873
Tofranil Tablets ... 875
Tofranil-PM Capsules ... 876
Urobiotic-250 Capsules ... 2038
Vancocin HCl, Oral Solution & Pulvules (Infrequent) ... 1536
Vancocin HCl, Vials & ADD-Vantage (Infrequent) ... 1534
Vivactil Tablets ... 1820
Zinacef (Rare) ... 1184

Drug idiosyncrasies
(see under Allergic reactions)

Dry mouth
(see under Xerostomia)

Dryness

Aclovate Cream (Approximately 2%) ... 1061
Analpram-HC Rectal Cream 1% and 2.5% ... 993
Anusol-HC Cream 2.5% (Infrequent to frequent) ... 1953
Anusol-HC Suppositories ... 1954
A/T/S 2% Acne Topical Gel (Occasional) ... 1244
A/T/S 2% Acne Topical Solution (Occasional) ... 1244
Azelex (Less than 1%) ... 471
Condylox Topical Solution (Less than 5%) ... 1853
Cordran Lotion (Infrequent) ... 1854
Cordran Tape (Infrequent) ... 1855
Cormax Ointment (Infrequent) ... 1856
Cormax Scalp Application (Infrequent) ... 1857
Cortisporin Cream ... 1073
Cortisporin Ointment ... 1074
Cortisporin Otic Solution Sterile ... 1076
Cortisporin Otic Suspension Sterile ... 1077
Cutivate Cream (1.2%) ... 1078
Cutivate Ointment (Infrequent to more frequent) ... 1078
Decadron Phosphate Topical Cream ... 1686
Decaspray Topical Aerosol ... 1689
▲ Desquam-E Gel (2 in 50 patients) ... 2792

(⊡ Described in PDR For Nonprescription Drugs)   Incidence data in parenthesis; ▲ 3% or more   (⊙ Described in PDR For Ophthalmology)

▲Desquam-X Gel (2 in 50 patients).. 2792
▲Desquam-X 10 Bar (2 in 50 patients) 2792
▲Desquam-X Wash (2 in 50 patients) 2792
Elocon Lotion 0.1% (Infrequent) 2493
Erycette (erythromycin 2%) Topical Solution 1943
Florone/Florone E 921
FLUORACAINE ⊙ 208
Lamisil Cream 1% (0.2%) 2393
Lidex (Infrequent) 2299
Locoid Cream, Ointment and Topical Solution (Infrequent) 994
Melanex Topical Solution 1842
▲Naftin Cream 1% (3%) 477
NeoDecadron Topical Cream 1757
Ophthetic ⊙ 244
Pediotic Suspension Sterile 1140
Pramosone Cream, Lotion & Ointment 995
Psorcon Cream 0.05% (Infrequent) 924
SalAc 1042
Synalar (Infrequent) 2299
T-Stat 2.0% Topical Solution and Pads 2797
Temovate Cream 1152
Temovate E Emollient (Infrequent) 1154
Temovate Gel (Infrequent) 1153
Temovate Ointment 1152
Temovate Scalp Application (Infrequent) 1153
THERAMYCIN Z 2% Solution 1629
Topicort Emollient Cream 0.25% (Infrequent) 1289
Topicort Gel 0.05% (Infrequent) 1290
Topicort LP Emollient Cream 0.05% (Infrequent) 1289
Topicort Ointment 0.25% (Infrequent) 1291
TRIAZ 6% and 10% Gels and 10% Cleanser 1629
Tridesilon Cream 0.05% (Infrequent) 609
Tridesilon Ointment 0.05% (Infrequent) 610
Westcort Cream 0.2% (Infrequent) 2799
Westcort Ointment 0.2% 2800

Dryness, mucous membrane

▲Atrohist Pediatric Suspension (Among most common) 1604
▲Atrohist Pediatric Suspension Dye-Free (Among most common) 1604
Cataflam Tablets (Less than 1%).... 833
Dolobid Tablets (Less than 1 in 100) 1695
Lomotil 2591
Mintezol Chewable Tablets 1747
Myleran Tablets (Rare) 1209
Nasacort Nasal Inhaler (Fewer than 5%) 2189
Pravachol Tablets 770
▲Rynatan (Among most common) 2781
▲Rynatuss (Among most common) .. 2782
Timolide Tablets (Less than 1%) 1791
Trinalin Repetabs Tablets 1373
▲Vesanoid Capsules (77%) 2327
Cataflam/Voltaren/Voltaren-XR (Less than 1%) 833

Dryness, nose (see under Xeromycteria)

Duodenitis

Anafranil Capsules (Infrequent) 819
Sterile FUDR 2284
Lodine Capsules and Tablets (Less than 1%) 2849
Motrin Ibuprofen Suspension, Oral Drops, Chewable Tablets, Caplets (Less than 1%) 1563
Paxil Tablets (Rare) 2681
Permax Tablets (Rare) 571
Relafen Tablets (Less than 1%) 2688
Videx Tablets, Powder for Oral Solution, & Pediatric Powder for Oral Solution (Less than 1%) 2980

Dysarthria

Ambien Tablets (Infrequent) 2559
CeeNU Capsules 699
Cerebyx Injection (2.2%; frequent) 1956
Clozaril Tablets (Less than 1%) 2377
Cognex Capsules (Infrequent) 1961
Depakene 416
Depakote Tablets (1% to 5%) 418
Dizac (diazepam injectable emulsion) CIV (Less frequent) 1862
Doral Tablets 2773
Elavil 2945
Felbatol 2774
Flexeril Tablets (Less than 1%) 1701
Halcion Tablets 2093
Imitrex Injection (Rare) 1095
Imitrex Tablets (Infrequent) 1099
Indocin Capsules (Less than 1%).... 1723
Indocin I.V. (Less than 1%) 1727
Indocin (Less than 1%) 1723
Invirase Capsules (Less than 2%) .. 2291
Klonopin Tablets 2294
Lamictal Tablets (1.0%) 1105
Levsin/Levsinex/Levbid 2549
Lioresal Tablets 847
Ludiomil Tablets (Rare) 861
Mesantoin Tablets 2400
Neurontin Capsules (2.4%) 1978
Nipent for Injection (Less than 3%) 2733
Paxil Tablets (Rare) 2681
Pondimin Tablets 2239
Prostigmin Injectable 1305
Prostigmin Tablets 1306
Prozac Pulvules & Liquid, Oral Solution (Rare) 935
Remeron Tablets (Infrequent) 1878
Rilutek Tablets (Infrequent) 2198
Risperdal Tablets (Infrequent) 1348
Roferon-A Injection (Less than 0.5%) 2308
Seromycin Capsules 975
Serzone Tablets (Infrequent) 776
Soma Compound w/Codeine Tablets (Very rare) 2784
Soma Compound Tablets (Very rare) 2783
Soma Tablets 2782
Tensilon Injectable 1307
Tonocard Tablets (Less than 1%) .. 519
Triavil Tablets 1800
Valium Injectable 2336
Valium Tablets (Infrequent) 2335
▲Vesanoid Capsules (3%) 2327
Wellbutrin Tablets (Infrequent) 1177
▲Xanax Tablets (23.3%) 2115

Dysautonomia

Lioresal Intrathecal (0.2% to 0.9%) 1634

Dyscrasias, blood (see under Blood dyscrasias)

Dysdiadochokinesia

Klonopin Tablets 2294

Dysesthesia

Cognex Capsules (Rare) 1961
Crixivan Capsules (Less than 2%).. 1670
Cytovene-IV (One report) 2270
Halcion Tablets (Rare) 2093
Hivid Tablets 2287
Imitrex Injection (Rare) 1095
Imitrex Tablets (Rare) 1099
Invirase Capsules (Less than 2%) .. 2291
Neurontin Capsules (Infrequent) 1978
Prinivil Tablets (0.3% to 1.0%) 1776
Prinzide Tablets 1780
▲Taxotere for Injection Concentrate (7% of 134 patients) 2204
Vaseretic Tablets 1810
Vasotec I.V. 1814
Vasotec Tablets (0.5% to 1.0%).... 1816
Zestril Tablets (0.3% to 1.0%) 2972

Dysesthesia, hemifacial

Prilosec Delayed-Release Capsules (Less than 1%) 516

Dysgeusia

Capoten Tablets (Approximately 2 to 4 of 100 patients) 740
Capozide Tablets (Approximately 2 to 4 of 100 patients) 744
Cardizem CD Capsules (Less than 1%) 1251
Cardizem SR Capsules (Less than 1%) 1255
Cardizem Injectable 1253
Cardizem Tablets (Less than 1%) .. 1257
Eskalith 2658
Floxin I.V. (1% to 3%) 1580
Floxin Tablets (200 mg, 300 mg, 400 mg) (1% to 3%) 1577
Havrix (Less than 1%) 2663
Lithonate/Lithotabs/Lithobid 2721
Maxaquin Tablets 2593
Mevacor Tablets (0.8%) 1742
Ridaura Capsules (1-3%) 2691
Rocephin Injectable Vials, ADD-Vantage, Galaxy Container (Less than 1%) 2305
Tiazac Capsules (Less than 1%) 1019
Trilisate (Less than 1%) 2155
Ultram Tablets (50 mg) (Less than 1%) 1594

Dyskinesia

Adderall Tablets 2209
Anafranil Capsules (Infrequent) 819
Bentyl 1246
BuSpar Tablets (Rare) 738
Cognex Capsules (Rare) 1961
Compazine 2644
Cylert Tablets 415
Dexedrine 2648
DextroStat-Dextroamphetamine Sulfate Tablets 2211
Dilantin Infatabs (Rare) 1967
Dilantin Kapseals (Rare) 1965
Dilantin-125 Suspension (Rare) 1969
▲Eldepryl Capsules (2 of 49 patients) 2729
Ethmozine Tablets (Less than 2%) 2217
Etrafon 2495
Felbatol 2774
Foscavir Injection (Less than 1%) .. 541
Haldol Decanoate 1587
Haldol Injection, Tablets and Concentrate 1585
Lamictal Tablets (Infrequent) 1105
Levo-Dromoran 2297
Levoprome 1321
Loxitane (Less frequent) 1426
LUVOX Tablets (Infrequent) 2723
MSIR (Infrequent) 2152
Orap Tablets 1037
Paxil Tablets (Rare) 2681
▲Permax Tablets (62.4%) 571
Prolixin 510
Prozac Pulvules & Liquid, Oral Solution 935
Remeron Tablets (Infrequent) 1878
Ritalin 866
▲Sinemet CR Tablets (16.5%) 961
Stelazine 2692
Triavil Tablets 1800
Trilafon 2532
Vistaril 2042
Wellbutrin Tablets (Frequent) 1177
Zoloft Tablets (Rare) 2051

Dyskinesia, orofacial

Zyrtec Tablets (Rare) 2053

Dyskinesia, tardive (see under Tardive dyskinesia)

Dyskinesia, transient

Orap Tablets 1037

Dyslexia

Redux Capsules 2911

Dysmenorrhea

▲Anafranil Capsules (10% to 12%) 819
▲Asacol Delayed-Release Tablets (3%) 2129
▲Betaseron for SC Injection (18%) .. 653
Claritin Tablets (2% or fewer patients) 2485
Claritin-D Tablets (Less frequent) .. 2487
Clozaril Tablets (Less than 1%) 2377
Cytotec (0.1%) 2576
Depakote Tablets (1% to 5%) 418
Depo-Provera Contraceptive Injection (Fewer than 1%) 2079
Diethylstilbestrol Tablets 1477
Dilacor XR Extended-release Capsules (Infrequent) 2183
Dynabac (0.1% to 1%) 668
Effexor 2825
ESTRATAB Tablets (0.3, 0.625, 1.25, 2.5 mg) 2715
Estratest 2718
Flovent (1% to 3%) 1089
Floxin I.V. (Less than 1%) 1580
Floxin Tablets (200 mg, 300 mg, 400 mg) (Less than 1%) 1577
▲Habitrol Nicotine Transdermal System (3% to 9% of patients) .. 884
Imitrex Injection (Rare) 1095
Imitrex Tablets (Infrequent) 1099
▲Lamictal Tablets (6.6%) 1105
Lo/Ovral Tablets 2852
Lo/Ovral-28 Tablets 2857
LUVOX Tablets 2723
Menest Tablets 2671
Naprelan Tablets (Less than 1%) .. 2861
Neurontin Capsules (Infrequent) 1978
▲Nicotrol NS Nicotine Nasal Spray (3%) 1565
Nordette-21 Tablets 2863
Nordette-28 Tablets 2866
Noroxin Tablets (Less frequent) 1758
Noroxin Tablets (Less frequent) 2222
Norplant System 2868
Ortho Dienestrol Cream 1922
Ovral Tablets 2877
Ovral-28 Tablets 2878
Ovrette Tablets 2878
ParaGard T 380A Intrauterine Copper Contraceptive 1936
Paxil Tablets (Infrequent) 2681
Permax Tablets (Frequent) 571
PMB 200 and PMB 400 2890
Premarin Intravenous 2893
Premarin Vaginal Cream 2898
Prostep (nicotine transdermal system) (1% to 3% of patients).. 1439
Redux Capsules (Frequent) 2911
Remeron Tablets (Infrequent) 1878
Risperdal Tablets (Infrequent) 1348
Seldane Tablets 1284
Seldane-D Extended-Release Tablets 1286
Semprex-D Capsules (2%) 1620
Serevent Inhalation Aerosol (1% to 3%) 1149
Serzone Tablets 776
▲Supprelin Injection (3% to 10%).... 2230
▲Terazol 3 Vaginal Cream (6%) 1941
Triphasil-21 Tablets 2919
Triphasil-28 Tablets 2924
Zerit Capsules (Up to 2%) 731
Zoladex (1% or greater) 2976
Zoloft Tablets (Infrequent) 2051
Zyrtec Tablets (Less than 2%) 2053

Dyspareunia

Depo-Provera Contraceptive Injection (Fewer than 1%) 2079
Flagyl 375 Capsules 2587
Flagyl I.V. 2373
Helidac Therapy 2135
MetroGel-Vaginal 917
Mycelex-G 500 mg Vaginal Tablets (1 in 149 patients) 602
ParaGard T 380A Intrauterine Copper Contraceptive 1936
Protostat Tablets 1939
Prozac Pulvules & Liquid, Oral Solution (Rare) 935
Supprelin Injection (2% to 3%) 2230
Vagistat-1 (Less than 1%) 783
Wellbutrin Tablets (Rare) 1177
▲Zoladex (14%) 2976

Dyspepsia

Abelcet Injection 1540
▲Actigall Capsules (16.8%) 818
Adalat CC (Less than 1.0%) 582
AeroBid Inhaler System (1% to 3%) 1004
Aerobid-M Inhaler System (1% to 3%) 1004
Airet Albuterol Sulfate Inhalation Solution (1% to 1.5%) 1602
Albuterol Sulfate, USP Solution for Inhalation, Arm-a-Med (1% to 1.5%) 522
▲Alferon N Injection (3%) 2142
Altace Capsules (Less than 1%) 1238
▲Ambien Tablets (5%) 2559
▲Anafranil Capsules (13% to 22%) 819
Anaprox/Naprosyn (Less than 3%) 2277
Aredia for Injection (Up to 4%) 827
▲Asacol Delayed-Release Tablets (6%) 2129
Atromid-S Capsules 2808
▲Avonex (11%) 662
▲Axid Pulvules (3.6%) 1468
▲Betapace Tablets (2% to 6%) 637
Biaxin (2%) 406
Blocadren Tablets (0.6%) 1654
Brevibloc (esmolol HCl) Injection (Less than 1%) 1860
Buprenex Injectable (Infrequent) 2170
Capoten Tablets 740
Capozide Tablets 744
Cardene Capsules (0.8% to 1.5%) 2261
Cardene I.V. (Rare) 2815
Cardizem CD Capsules (Less than 1%) 1251
Cardizem SR Capsules (1.3%) 1255
Cardizem Injectable 1253
Cardizem Tablets (Less than 1%) .. 1257
Cardura Tablets (1% to 1.7%) 1993
Cartrol Tablets (Less common) 413
Casodex Tablets (2% to 5%) 2934

1317 Side Effects Index Dysphoria

Cataflam Tablets (Common) 833
Cedax (0.1% to 2%) 2480
Ceftin (0.1% to 1%) 1067
▲CellCept Capsules (13.6% to 17.6%) 2265
Cerebyx Injection (Infrequent) 1956
Cipro I.V. 587
Cipro Tablets 584
Claritin Tablets (2% or fewer patients) 2485
▲Claritin-D Tablets (3%) 2487
▲Clinoril Tablets (3% to 9%) 1658
▲Cognex Capsules (9%) 1961
Cozaar Tablets (1.3%) 1668
Crixivan Capsules (Less than 2%) 1670
Cytotec (2.0%) 2576
Cytovene (2%) 2270
▲Daypro Caplets (3% to 9%) 2578
Demadex Tablets and Injection (1.6%) 691
▲Depakote Tablets (9% to 13%) 418
Diflucan Tablets, Injection, and Oral Suspension (1%) 2003
Dilacor XR Extended-release Capsules (1.3%) 2183
▲Dipentum Capsules (4.0%) 2084
▲Dolobid Tablets (3% to 9%) 1695
Doral Tablets (1.1%) 2773
Doxil (Less than 1%) 2613
▲Duragesic Transdermal System (3% to 10%) 1336
Duricef Capsules, Tablets, and Oral Suspension (Rare) 750
Dynabac (2.6%) 668
Easprin 1971
EC-Naprosyn Delayed-Release Tablets (Less than 3%) 2277
▲Effexor (4.5% to 5%) 2825
Engerix-B Unit-Dose Vials 2656
▲Epivir (5%) 1200
Ergamisol Tablets (Less than 1% to 1%) 1340
Estring Vaginal Ring (1% to 3%) 2086
▲Ethmozine Tablets (2% to 5%) 2217
Famvir Tablets (1.1% to 3.4%) 2660
▲Felbatol (6.5% to 12.3%) 2774
Feldene Capsules (Common) 2008
Flexeril Tablets (1 to 3%) 1701
Flolan for Injection (1%) 1085
Flovent (1% to 3%) 1089
Floxin I.V. (Less than 1%) 1580
Floxin Tablets (200 mg, 300 mg, 400 mg) (Less than 1%) 1577
Flumadine Tablets & Syrup (0.3% to 1%) 1013
▲Fosamax Tablets (3.6%) 1703
Foscavir Injection (Between 1% and 5%) 541
▲Fungizone Intravenous (Among most common) 507
Gastrocrom Oral Concentrate 1611
Glucotrol XL Extended Release Tablets (Less than 3%) 2012
▲Habitrol Nicotine Transdermal System (3% to 9% of patients) 884
Haldol Decanoate 1587
Haldol Injection, Tablets and Concentrate 1585
Helidac Therapy (Less than 1%) 2135
Hivid Tablets (Less than 1%) 2287
Hytrin Capsules (At least 1%) 434
Hyzaar Tablets 1720
Imdur (Less than or equal to 5%) 1362
▲Indocin (3% to 9%) 1723
▲Intron A for Injection (Up to 8%) 2506
Ismo Tablets (Fewer than 1%) 2844
Kadian Capsules (Less than 3%) 2948
Keflex Pulvules & Oral Suspension 930
Keftab Tablets 931
▲Kerlone Tablets (3.9% to 4.7%) 2588
▲Lamictal Tablets (5.3%) 1105
▲Lamisil Tablets (4.3%) 2394
▲Lescol Capsules (7.9%) 2395
▲Leukine (17%) 1317
Levatol Tablets (2.7%) 2547
Levo-Dromoran 2297
Lioresal Intrathecal (1% or more) 1634
▲Lodine Capsules and Tablets (10%) 2849
▲Lopid Tablets (19.6%) 1974
Lotensin HCT Tablets (0.3% to 1.0%) 855
Lotrel Capsules 858
▲LUVOX Tablets (10%) 2723
Macrobid Capsules (Less than 1%) 2138
Mavik Tablets (0.3% to 1.0%) 1407
Maxaquin Tablets (Less than 1%) 2593
Megace Oral Suspension (Up to 4%) 708
▲Mepron Suspension (5%) 1206
▲Mevacor Tablets (1.0% to 3.9%) 1742
Miacalcin Nasal Spray (1% to 3%) 2403
Midamor Tablets (Less than or equal to 1%) 1746
Moduretic Tablets 1748
Monoket Tablets (Fewer than 1%) 2550
Motrin Ibuprofen Suspension, Oral Drops, Chewable Tablets, Caplets (Common) 1563
▲Mycobutin Capsules (3%) 2101
▲Nalfon 200 Pulvules & Nalfon Tablets (10.3%) 933
▲Naprelan Tablets (14%) 2861
Anaprox/Naprosyn (Less than 3%) 2277
Neurontin Capsules (2.2%) 1978
Nicotrol NS Nicotine Nasal Spray (Common) 1565
▲Nipent for Injection (3% to 10%) 2733
▲Normodyne Injection (Up to 4%) 2519
▲Normodyne Tablets (Up to 4%) 2522
Noroxin Tablets (0.3% to 1.0%) 1758
Noroxin Tablets (0.3% to 1.0%) 2222
Norvasc Tablets (Less than 1% to 2%) 2020
▲Norvir (4.8%) 447
Nubain Injection (1% or less) 952
▲Orudis Capsules (11%) 2874
▲Oruvail Capsules (11%) 2874
OxyContin Tablets (Between 1% and 5%) 2163
▲Parlodel (4%) 2411
Paxil Tablets (2%) 2681
Penetrex Tablets (1%) 2196
Pentasa (1.6%) 1275
▲Permax Tablets (6.4%) 571
▲Plendil Extended-Release Tablets (0.5% to 3.9%) 514
Ponstel (Common) 1982
Prevacid Delayed-Release Capsules (Less than 1%) 2746
Prinivil Tablets (0.3% to 1.0%) 1776
Prinzide Tablets (1.3%) 1780
Procardia XL Extended Release Tablets (Less than 3%) 2026
▲Prograf (Greater than 3%) 1028
▲Proleukin for Injection (7%) 812
Propulsid (2.7%) 1346
ProSom Tablets (2%) 457
Prostep (nicotine transdermal system) (Less than 1% of patients) 1439
Proventil Inhalation Solution 0.083% (1% to 1.5%) 2527
Proventil Repetabs Tablets (2%) 2529
Proventil Solution for Inhalation 0.5% (1% to 1.5%) 2525
Proventil Tablets (2%) 2529
▲Prozac Pulvules & Liquid, Oral Solution (5% to 10%) 935
Recombivax HB (Less than 1%) 1787
Redux Capsules (Frequent) 2911
▲Relafen Tablets (13%) 2688
▲Retrovir Capsules (5% to 6%) 1216
▲Retrovir I.V. Infusion (5% to 6%) 1221
▲Retrovir Syrup (5% to 6%) 1216
Rhinocort Nasal Inhaler (1 to 3%) 552
▲Ridaura Capsules (3 to 9%) 2691
▲Rilutek Tablets (2.5% to 6.1%) 2198
▲Risperdal Tablets (5% to 10%) 1348
Rocephin Injectable Vials, ADD-Vantage, Galaxy Container (Rare) 2305
▲Rythmol Tablets–150mg, 225mg, 300mg (1.3 to 3.4%) 1399
▲Salagen Tablets (7%) 1546
▲Sectral Capsules (4%) 2914
Semprex-D Capsules (2%) 1620
▲Serzone Tablets (9%) 776
Sinemet CR Tablets (0.6%) 961
Stimate, (desmopressin acetate) Nasal Spray, 1.5 mg/mL 806
Sular Tablets (Less than or equal to 1%) 2961
Supprelin Injection (2% to 3%) 2230
▲Suprax (3%) 1443
Tambocor Tablets (1% to less than 3%) 1555
Tenex Tablets (3% or less) 2249
▲Tiazac Capsules (4%) 1019
▲Ticlid Tablets (7.0%) 2317
Tilade Inhaler (1.3%) 2207
Timolide Tablets (Less than 1%) 1791
Timoptic in Ocudose (Less frequent) 1796
Timoptic Sterile Ophthalmic Solution 1794
Timoptic-XE 1798
▲Tolectin (200, 400 and 600 mg) (3 to 9%) 1591
Tonocard Tablets (Less than 1%) 519
▲Toradol (12%) 2319
Tornalate Metered Dose Inhaler (0.5%) 978
Trandate (1 of 100 patients; up to 4%) 1158
Trental Tablets (2.8%) 1291
▲Ultram Tablets (50 mg) (5% to 13%) 1594
Univasc Tablets (More than 1%) 2553
▲Vascor Tablets (200 and 300 mg) (6.81 to about 22%) 1597
Vaseretic Tablets (0.5% to 2.0%) 1810
Vasotec I.V. 1814
Vasotec Tablets (0.5% to 1.0%) 1816
Ventolin Inhalation Solution (1% to 1.5%) 1171
Ventolin Nebules Inhalation Solution (1% to 1.5%) 1172
Verelan Capsules (2.5%) 1455
▲Vesanoid Capsules (14%) 2327
Videx Tablets, Powder for Oral Solution, & Pediatric Powder for Oral Solution (Less than 1%) 2980
Vistide Injection 1057
Cataflam/Voltaren/Voltaren-XR (Common) 833
▲Wellbutrin Tablets (3.1%) 1177
Zebeta Tablets 1457
▲Zerit Capsules (Fewer than 1% to 9%) 731
Zestoretic Tablets (1.3%) 2968
Zestril Tablets (0.3% to 1.0%) 2972
Ziac (0.9% to 1.2%) 1459
Zithromax (1% or less to 1%) 2043
Zithromax Tablets (1% or less to 1%) 2046
Zocor Tablets (1.1%) 1821
Zoladex (1% or greater) 2976
Zoladex 3-month 2978
▲Zoloft Tablets (6.0%) 2051
Zosyn (1.9% to 3.3%) 1463
Zyloprim Tablets (Less than 1%) 1194
Zyrtec Tablets (Less than 2%) 2053

Dysphagia

Achromycin V Capsules (Rare) 1417
Altace Capsules (Less than 1%) 1238
Ambien Tablets (Infrequent) 2559
Anafranil Capsules (Up to 2%) 819
Atamet Tablets 567
Cerebyx Injection (Infrequent) 1956
Cipro I.V. (1% or less) 587
Cipro I.V. Pharmacy Bulk Package (Less than 1%) 590
Cipro Tablets (Less than 1%) 584
Clozaril Tablets 2377
Cognex Capsules (Infrequent) 1961
Cosmegen Injection 1666
Cytotec (Infrequent) 2576
Cytovene (1% or less) 2270
DaunoXome (Less than or equal to 5%) 1842
Declomycin Tablets 1421
Doryx Capsules 1970
Doxil (1% to 5%) 2613
DYNACIN Capsules 1627
Edecrin 1698
Effexor (Frequent) 2825
Eldepryl Capsules 2729
Ethmozine Tablets (Less than 2%) 2217
Etopophos for Injection (Infrequent) 701
Etoposide Injection (Infrequent) 539
Etrafon 2495
Felbatol 2774
Fludara for Injection (Up to 1%) 658
Flumadine Tablets & Syrup 1013
Fosamax Tablets (1.0%) 1703
Foscavir Injection (Between 1% and 5%) 541
Gastrocrom Capsules (Infrequent) 1611
Gastrocrom Oral Concentrate (Less common) 1611
Helidac Therapy (Less than 1%) 2135
Hivid Tablets (Less than 1%) 2287
Imitrex Injection (1.1%) 1095
Imitrex Tablets (Infrequent) 1099
Intron A for Injection (Less than 5%) 2506
Invirase Capsules (Less than 2%) 2291
Kadian Capsules (Less than 3%) 2948
Kerlone Tablets (Less than 2%) 2588
Lamictal Tablets (Infrequent) 1105
Larodopa Tablets (Relatively frequent) 2296
▲Leukine (11%) 1317
Lioresal Intrathecal (1% or more) 1634
Ludiomil Tablets (Rare) 861
Lupron Depot-PED 7.5 mg, 11.25 mg and 15 mg (Less than 2%) 2744
Lupron Injection (Less than 5%) 2736
Lupron Injection Pediatric (Less than 2%) 2737
LUVOX Tablets (2%) 2723
Maxaquin Tablets (Less than 1%) 2593
Mexitil Capsules (About 2 in 1,000) 684
Minocin Intravenous 1428
Minocin Oral Suspension 1431
Minocin Pellet-Filled Capsules 1429
Monodox Capsules 1858
Monopril Tablets (0.2% to 1.0%) 762
Naprelan Tablets (Less than 3%) 2861
Neurontin Capsules (Rare) 1978
Nipent for Injection (Less than 3%) 2733
Noroxin Tablets 1758
Noroxin Tablets 2222
Norvasc Tablets (More than 0.1% to 1%) 2020
Norvir (Less than 2%) 447
Orap Tablets (2.7%) 1037
OxyContin Tablets (Less than 1%) 2163
Parlodel 2411
Paxil Tablets (Infrequent) 2681
Pentasa (Less than 1%) 1275
Permax Tablets (Frequent) 571
Prevacid Delayed-Release Capsules (Less than 1%) 2746
Prozac Pulvules & Liquid, Oral Solution (Infrequent) 935
Questran 774
Redux Capsules 2911
Relafen Tablets (1%) 2688
Retrovir Capsules 1216
Retrovir I.V. Infusion 1221
Retrovir Syrup 1216
Ridaura Capsules (Less than 0.1%) 2691
Rilutek Tablets (More than 2%) 2198
Risperdal Tablets (Infrequent) 1348
Salagen Tablets (2%) 1546
Serzone Tablets (Rare) 776
Sinemet Tablets 959
Sinemet CR Tablets 961
Sular Tablets (Less than or equal to 1%) 2961
Tenex Tablets (3% or less) 2249
Tensilon Injectable 1307
Terramycin Intramuscular Solution 2034
Tonocard Tablets (Less than 1%) 519
Triavil Tablets 1800
Trilafon 2532
VePesid Capsules and Injection (Infrequent) 727
Vibramycin 2038
Vibramycin Hyclate Intravenous 2040
Vibramycin 2038
Videx Tablets, Powder for Oral Solution, & Pediatric Powder for Oral Solution (Up to 1%) 2980
Vistide Injection 1057
Wellbutrin Tablets (Infrequent) 1177
Zinecard Injection (Up to 8%) 2120
Zoloft Tablets (Infrequent) 2051

Dysphasia

Ambien Tablets (Rare) 2559
Cipro I.V. (1% or less) 587
Cipro I.V. Pharmacy Bulk Package (Less than 1%) 590
Cipro Tablets 584
Floxin I.V. 1580
Floxin Tablets (200 mg, 300 mg, 400 mg) 1577
Imitrex Injection 1095
Maxaquin Tablets 2593
▲Prograf (Greater than 3%) 1028
Roferon-A Injection (Infrequent) 2308
Torecan 2367

Dysphonia

Anafranil Capsules (Infrequent) 819
Claritin Tablets (2% or fewer patients) 2485
Claritin-D Tablets (Less frequent) 2487
▲Flovent (3% to 19%) 1089
Hivid Tablets (Less than 1%) 2287
Intron A for Injection (Less than 5%) 2506
ReoPro Vials (0.3%) 1526
Romazicon (Less than 1%) 2311
Tegison Capsules (Less than 1%) 2314
Tensilon Injectable 1307
Tilade Inhaler (1.0%) 2207
Versed Injection (Less than 1%) 2324
Zoloft Tablets (Rare) 2051
Zyrtec Tablets (Less than 2%) 2053

Dysphoria

Adderall Tablets 2209
Adipex-P Tablets and Capsules 1035

(▭ Described in PDR For Nonprescription Drugs) Incidence data in parenthesis; ▲ 3% or more (◉ Described in PDR For Ophthalmology)

Dysphoria **Side Effects Index** **1318**

Aldactazide Tablets 2556
Aldoclor Tablets 1638
Aldoril Tablets 1644
Ambien Tablets 2559
Ana-Kit Anaphylaxis Emergency Treatment Kit 611
Apresazide Capsules 824
Asendin Tablets (Less frequent) 1419
Astramorph/PF Injection, USP (Preservative-Free) 526
Ativan Injection (1.3%) 2805
Benadryl Injection 1955
Bontril Slow-Release Capsules 786
▲ Bromfed-DM Cough Syrup (Among most frequent) 1832
Bronkometer Aerosol 2432
Bronkosol Solution 2432
Brontex 2130
Buprenex Injectable (Rare) 2170
BuSpar Tablets (Infrequent) 738
Capozide Tablets 744
Carbocaine Injection 2432
Catapres Tablets 679
Catapres-TTS 680
Chibroxin Sterile Ophthalmic Solution (With oral form) 1657
▲ Cipro I.V. (Among most frequent) 587
Cipro I.V. Pharmacy Bulk Package (Greater than 1%) 590
Cipro Tablets (1.1%) 584
Claritin-D Tablets 2487
▲ Clozaril Tablets (4%) 2377
Cocaine Hydrochloride Topical Solutions 529
Combipres Tablets 682
Allergy-Sinus Comtrex Multi-Symptom Allergy-Sinus Formula Tablets and Caplets ▣ 639
D.A. II Tablets 972
D.A. Chewable Tablets 970
Dalmane Capsules (Rare) 2329
Darvon-N/Darvocet-N 1473
Darvon 1475
Darvon-N Suspension & Tablets 1473
Deconsal II Tablets 1605
Demadex Tablets and Injection 691
Demerol 2438
Desoxyn Gradumet Tablets (Rare) 422
Dexedrine 2648
DextroStat-Dextroamphetamine Sulfate Tablets 2211
Dilaudid Ampules 1382
Dilaudid Cough Syrup 1383
Dilaudid-HP Injection (Less frequent) 1384
Dilaudid-HP Lyophilized Powder 250 mg (Less frequent) 1384
Dilaudid 1382
Dilaudid Oral Liquid 1386
Dilaudid 1382
Dilaudid Tablets - 8 mg 1386
Dimetane-DC Cough Syrup 2232
Dimetane-DX Cough Syrup 2233
Ditropan 1267
Diucardin Tablets 2824
Diupres Tablets 1691
Diuril Oral Suspension 1694
Diuril Sodium Intravenous 1693
Diuril Tablets 1694
Duramorph Injection 983
Duranest Injections 533
Dura-Tap/PD Capsules 970
Duratuss Tablets 2750
Dura-Vent/DA Tablets 972
Dura-Vent Tablets 971
Elavil 2945
Eldepryl Capsules 2729
Emete-con Intramuscular/Intravenous 2007
Enduron Tablets 424
Entex LA Tablets 972
EpiPen–Epinephrine Auto-Injector 808
Esidrix Tablets 839
Esimil Tablets 840
Eskalith 2658
Etrafon 2495
Exgest LA Tablets 787
Fastin Capsules 2662
Fedahist Gyrocaps 2545
Floxin I.V. 1580
Floxin Tablets (200 mg, 300 mg, 400 mg) 1577
Halcion Tablets 2093
Haldol Decanoate 1587
Haldol Injection, Tablets and Concentrate 1585
Hespan Injection 945
Histussin D Liquid 670
Hycodan Tablets and Syrup 946
Hycomine Compound Tablets 948
Hycomine 947
Hycotuss Expectorant Syrup 950
Hydrocet Capsules 787
HydroDIURIL Tablets 1716
Hydropres Tablets 1718
Hyzaar Tablets 1720
▲ Inapsine Injection (Among most common) 462
Inderide LA Long Acting Capsules 2840
Infumorph 200 and Infumorph 500 Sterile Solutions 985
Ionamin Capsules 1615
Isoetharine Inhalation Solution, USP, Arm-a-Med 545
Lamictal Tablets (Infrequent) 1105
Lariam Tablets 2295
Lasix Injection, Oral Solution and Tablets 1267
Limbitrol 2333
Lithium Carbonate Capsules & Tablets 2352
Lithonate/Lithotabs/Lithobid 2721
Lomotil 2591
Lopressor HCT Tablets 850
Lorcet 10/650 Tablets 1016
Lortab 2751
Lotensin HCT Tablets 855
Ludiomil Tablets (Rare) 861
Lufyllin & Lufyllin-400 Tablets 2778
Lufyllin-GG Elixir & Tablets 2779
▲ MS Contin Tablets (Among most frequent) 2149
▲ MSIR (Among most frequent) 2152
Marcaine 2446
Marcaine Spinal 2449
Maxaquin Tablets 2593
Mellaril (Extremely rare) 2398
Mepergan Injection 2859
Methadone Hydrochloride Oral Concentrate 2356
Methadone Hydrochloride Oral Solution & Tablets 2357
Minizide Capsules 2016
Moduretic Tablets 1748
Monoket Tablets (Fewer than 1%) 2550
Mykrox Tablets 1617
Navane Capsules and Concentrate 2018
Navane Intramuscular 2019
NegGram 2453
Neo-Synephrine Hydrochloride 1% Carpuject 2455
Neo-Synephrine Hydrochloride 1% Injection 2455
Nescaine/Nescaine MPF 549
▲ Nicotrol NS Nicotine Nasal Spray (Over 5%) 1565
Nitrolingual Spray 2193
Noroxin Tablets 1758
Noroxin Tablets 2222
Norpramin Tablets 1273
Novahistine DMX ▣ 782
Novahistine Elixir ▣ 782
Nubain Injection (1% or less) 952
Nucofed 2225
Numorphan Injection 953
Numorphan Suppositories 953
▲ Oramorph SR (Morphine Sulfate Sustained Release Tablets) (Among most frequent) 2359
Oretic Tablets 450
Orlaam Oral Solution 2361
Ornade Spansule Capsules 2678
Orudis Capsules (Rare) 2874
Oruvail Capsules (Rare) 2874
Oxsoralen-Ultra Capsules 1302
OxyIR Capsules 2167
PBZ Tablets 863
PBZ-SR Tablets 862
Pamelor 2409
Parnate Tablets 2679
Penetrex Tablets 2196
Percocet Tablets 955
Percodan Tablets 955
Percodan-Demi Tablets 956
Periactin 1767
Phenergan with Codeine 2883
Phenergan VC 2886
Phenergan VC with Codeine 2888
Phenobarbital Elixir and Tablets 1523
Pregnyl for Injection 1878
Prelu-2 Timed Release Capsules 687
Prinzide Tablets 1780
Profasi (chorionic gonadotropin for injection, USP) 2620
Prolixin 510
Proventil (Less than 1%) 2529
Quadrinal Tablets 1398
Quibron 2227
RMS Suppositories CII 2766
▲ Reglan (Approximately 10%) 2243
Respbid Tablets 687
ReVia Tablets (Less than 1%) 957
Revex (nalmefene hydrochloride injection) 1863
Romazicon (1% to 3%) 2311
Roxanol 2365
Roxicodone Tablets, Oral Solution & Intensol (Oxycodone) 2366
Sanorex Tablets 2423
Seldane-D Extended-Release Tablets (2.1%) 1286
Sensorcaine 554
Ser-Ap-Es Tablets 867
Serentil 689
Serzone Tablets 776
Slo-bid Gyrocaps 2201
Stadol (Less than 1%) 779
Surmontil Capsules 2917
Sus-Phrine Injection 1017
Syn-Rx Tablets 1622
Syn-Rx DM Tablets 1623
Tavist Syrup 2426
Tavist Tablets 2427
Tenoretic Tablets 2963
Thalitone 1293
Theo-24 Extended Release Capsules 2753
Theo-Dur Extended-Release Tablets 1367
Theo-X Extended-Release Tablets 793
Timolide Tablets 1791
Tofranil Ampuls 873
Tofranil Tablets 875
Tofranil-PM Capsules 876
Torecan (Occasional) 2367
Transderm Scōp Transdermal Therapeutic System (Infrequent) 890
Triavil Tablets 1800
Trilafon 2532
Tussend 1830
Tussend Expectorant 1831
Tussionex Pennkinetic Extended-Release Suspension 1624
Tylenol with Codeine 1592
Tylox Capsules 1593
Tympagesic Ear Drops 2476
Uni-Dur Extended-Release Tablets 1374
Uniphyl 400 mg and 600 mg Tablets 2157
Vaseretic Tablets 1810
Ventolin Tablets (Fewer than 1 of 100 patients) 1176
Versed Injection (Less than 1%) 2324
Vicodin Tablets 1404
Vicodin ES Tablets 1405
Vicodin HP Tablets 1403
Vicodin Tuss Expectorant 1406
Vivactil Tablets 1820
Volmax Extended-Release Tablets (Less frequent) 1835
Wellbutrin Tablets (Infrequent) 1177
Wygesic Tablets 2930
Xylocaine Injections 562
▲ Yutopar Intravenous Injection (5% to 6%) 566
Zaroxolyn Tablets 1625
Zebeta Tablets 1457
Zestoretic Tablets 2968
Ziac 1459
Zydone Capsules 967

Dysplasia, bone marrow (see under Bone marrow dysplasia)

Dysplasia, cervical

Anafranil Capsules (Rare) 819
Demulen 2580
Ortho-Est 1.25 Tablets 1925
Vivelle Transdermal System 880

Dyspnea

Abbokinase 403
Abbokinase Open-Cath 405
▲ Abelcet Injection (5% to 8%) 1540
Accupril Tablets (1.9%) 1950
Acel-Imune Diphtheria and Tetanus Toxoids and Acellular Pertussis Vaccine Adsorbed (Rare) 1415
Acthrel for Injection 2990
▲ Adalat Capsules (10 mg and 20 mg) (6%) 580
Adalat CC (Less than 1.0%) 582
▲ Adenocard Injection (12%) 1021
▲ Adenoscan (Approximately 28%) 1022
AeroBid Inhaler System (1% to 3%) 1004
Aerobid-M Inhaler System (1% to 3%) 1004
Airet Albuterol Sulfate Inhalation Solution (1.5%) 1602
Albuterol Sulfate, USP Solution for Inhalation, Arm-a-Med (1.5%) 522
Alkeran for Injection (In some patients) 1196
Altace Capsules (Less than 1%) 1238
Ambien Tablets (Infrequent) 2559
Amicar Syrup, Tablets, and Injection 1312
Anafranil Capsules (Up to 2%) 819
▲ Anaprox/Naprosyn (3% to 9%) 2277
Ancobon Capsules 2254
Antivenin (Crotalidae) Polyvalent 2803
Apresazide Capsules (Less frequent) 824
Apresoline Hydrochloride Tablets (Less frequent) 826
AquaMEPHYTON Injection 1648
▲ Aredia for Injection (16.4%) 827
▲ Arimidex Tablets (9.2% to 11.0%) 2932
Atamet Tablets 567
Atretol Tablets 569
▲ Atrovent Inhalation Solution (9.6%) 675
▲ Avonex (6%) 662
Azactam for Injection (One patient) 736
Bentyl 1246
Betagan ⊙ 230
▲ Betapace Tablets (5% to 21%) 637
▲ Betaseron for SC Injection (8%) 653
Betimol 0.25%, 0.5% ⊙ 259
Betoptic Ophthalmic Solution (Rare) 465
Betoptic S Ophthalmic Suspension (Rare) 467
Blenoxane 697
Blocadren Tablets (1.7%) 1654
Brethaire Inhaler 830
Brethine Ampuls (0.0 to 2.0%) 832
Brevibloc (esmolol HCl) Injection (Less than 1%) 1860
Buprenex Injectable (Less than 1%) 2170
Calan SR Caplets (1.4%) 2571
Calan Tablets (1.4%) 2568
Capoten Tablets (About 0.5 to 2%) 740
Capozide Tablets (0.5 to 2%) 744
Cardene Capsules (0.6%) 2261
Cardene I.V. (0.7%) 2815
Cardizem CD Capsules (Less than 1%) 1251
Cardizem SR Capsules (Less than 1%) 1255
Cardizem Injectable (Less than 1%) 1253
Cardizem Tablets (Less than 1%) 1257
Cardura Tablets (1% to 2.6%) 1993
Cartrol Tablets (Less common) 413
▲ Casodex Tablets (7%) 2934
Cataflam Tablets (Less than 1%) 833
Ceclor Pulvules & Suspension 1470
Cedax (0.1% to 1%) 2480
▲ CellCept Capsules (15.5% to 17.3%) 2265
Cerebyx Injection (Infrequent) 1956
Chibroxin Sterile Ophthalmic Solution (With oral form) 1657
Cipro I.V. (1% or less) 587
Cipro I.V. Pharmacy Bulk Package (Less than 1%) 590
Cipro Tablets (Less than 1%) 584
Claritin Tablets (2% or fewer patients) 2485
Claritin-D Tablets (Less frequent) 2487
Clinoril Tablets (Less than 1%) 1658
Clomid 1262
Clozaril Tablets (1%) 2377
Cognex Capsules (Frequent) 1961
▲ Cordarone Tablets (2% to 7%) 2818
Coumadin 941
Covera-HS Tablets (1.4% to 2%) 2573
Cozaar Tablets (Less than 1%) 1668
Crixivan Capsules (Less than 2%) 1670
Cytotec (Infrequent) 2576
Cytovene (1% or less) 2270
D.H.E. 45 Injection (Occasional) 2381
▲ DaunoXome (3% to 23%) 1842
Depakote Tablets (1% to 5%) 418
Depen Titratable Tablets 2770
Depo-Provera Contraceptive Injection (Fewer than 1%) 2079
Dilacor XR Extended-release Capsules (1.0% to 1.4%) 2183
Diphtheria and Tetanus Toxoids and Pertussis Vaccine Adsorbed (Rare) 2650
Diprivan Injectable Emulsion (Less than 1%) 2939
Diupres Tablets 1691
Dizac (diazepam injectable emulsion) CIV 1862

(▣ Described in PDR For Nonprescription Drugs) Incidence data in parenthesis; ▲ 3% or more (⊙ Described in PDR For Ophthalmology)

1319 **Side Effects Index** **Dystonia**

Dolobid Tablets (Rare) 1695
Dopram Injectable 2235
Doxil (1% to 5%) 2613
▲ Duragesic Transdermal System (3% to 10%) 1336
Dynabac (1.2%) 668
DynaCirc Capsules (0.5% to 3.4%) 2381
DynaCirc CR Tablets (0.5% to 1.0%) 2383
▲ EC-Naprosyn Delayed-Release Tablets (3% to 9%) 2277
Effexor (Frequent) 2825
▲ Emcyt Capsules (11%) 2085
▲ Eminase (Less than 10%) 2215
Esimil Tablets 840
▲ Ethmozine Tablets (3.8% to 5.7%) 2217
▲ Etopophos for Injection (3%) 701
Etoposide Injection (0.7% to 2%) 539
Felbatol 2774
Feldene Capsules (Less than 1%) 2008
Flexeril Tablets (Rare) 1701
▲ Flolan for Injection (2% to 90%) 1085
Floxin I.V. 1580
Floxin Tablets (200 mg, 300 mg, 400 mg) 1577
▲ Fludara for Injection (9% to 22%) 658
Flumadine Tablets & Syrup (0.3% to 1%) 1013
▲ Foscavir Injection (5% or greater) 541
Fungizone Intravenous 507
Furoxone (Rare) 2221
Gamimune N, 5% Immune Globulin Intravenous (Human), 5% 612
Gamimune N, 10% Immune Globulin Intravenous (Human), 10% 615
Ganite 2711
Gastrocrom Capsules (Infrequent) 1611
Gastrocrom Oral Concentrate (Less common) 1611
▲ Gemzar for Injection (3% to 23%) 1482
Glucotrol XL Extended Release Tablets (Less than 1%) 2012
Guaifed 1833
Havrix (Rare) 2663
Hivid Tablets (Less than 1%) 2287
Humegon for Injection 1873
Humorsol Sterile Ophthalmic Solution 1707
▲ Hycamtin for Injection (1.8% to 20%) 2665
Hydralazine Hydrochloride Injection USP (Less frequent) 2712
Hydrea Capsules (Rare) 705
Hydropres Tablets 1718
Hyperstat I.V. Injection 2504
Hyskon Hysteroscopy Fluid (Rare) 1633
▲ Hytrin Capsules (0.5% to 3.1%) 434
Hyzaar Tablets 1720
Imdur (Less than or equal to 5%) 1362
Imitrex Injection (Infrequent) 1095
Imitrex Tablets (Frequent) 1099
Indocin Capsules (Less than 1%) 1723
Indocin I.V. (Less than 1%) 1727
Indocin (Less than 1%) 1723
INFeD (Iron Dextran Injection, USP) 2478
▲ Intron A for Injection (Up to 34%) 2506
Invirase Capsules (Less than 2%) 2291
Iopidine 0.5% (Less than 1%) ⊙ 219
Ismelin Tablets 845
Isoptin Oral Tablets (1.4%) 1393
Isoptin SR Tablets (1.4%) 1395
K-Phos Neutral Tablets 633
K-Phos Original Formula 'Sodium Free' Tablets (Less frequent) 633
Kadian Capsules (Less than 3%) 2948
Kerlone Tablets (2.4%) 2588
Lamictal Tablets (1.1%) 1105
Lescol Capsules (Rare) 2395
▲ Leukine (15% to 28%) 1317
▲ Leustatin (11%) 1889
Levatol Tablets (2.1%) 2547
Lioresal Intrathecal (Up to 1.2%) 1634
Lioresal Tablets (Rare) 847
Livostin (Approximately 1% to 3%) ⊙ 262
Lodine Capsules and Tablets (Less than 1%) 2849
Lopressor (1%) 848
Lopressor HCT Tablets (1 in 100 patients) 850
Lorcet 10/650 Tablets 1016
Lortab 2751
Lotensin Tablets 852
Lotensin HCT Tablets 855
Loxitane 1426
▲ Lupron Depot 7.5 mg (5.4%) 2741
▲ Lupron Injection (5% or more) 2736
Lutrepulse for Injection 998
LUVOX Tablets (2%) 2723
Macrobid Capsules (Common) 2138
Macrodantin Capsules (Common) 2140
Mavik Tablets (0.3% to 1.0%) 1407
Maxaquin Tablets (Less than 1%) 2593
Mefoxin 1734
Mefoxin Premixed Intravenous Solution 1737
Megace Oral Suspension (1% to 3%) 708
Megace Tablets 710
Mephyton Tablets (Rare) 1739
Merrem I.V. (0.1% to 1.0%) 2952
Methergine (Rare) 2401
Methotrexate Sodium Tablets, Injection, for Injection and LPF Injection 1322
Metrodin (urofollitropin for injection) 2616
Mevacor Tablets (Rare) 1742
▲ Mexitil Capsules (3.3% to 5.7%) 684
Miacalcin Nasal Spray (Less than 1%) 2403
Midamor Tablets (Between 1% and 3%) 1746
Minipress Capsules (1-4%) 2015
Minizide Capsules 2016
Miochol-E with Iocare Steri-Tags and Miochol-E System Pak (Rare) ⊙ 263
Moduretic Tablets (Greater than 1%, less than 3%) 1748
Monoket Tablets (Fewer than 1%) 2550
Monopril Tablets (1.0% or more) 762
Motrin Ibuprofen Suspension, Oral Drops, Chewable Tablets, Caplets (Less than 1%) 1563
Mutamycin for Injection 712
Mycobutin Capsules (Less than 1%) 2101
Myochrysine Injection 1754
Nalfon 200 Pulvules & Nalfon Tablets (2.8%) 933
▲ Naprelan Tablets (Less than 1% to 9%) 2861
▲ Anaprox/Naprosyn (3% to 9%) 2277
Navelbine Injection (Up to 3%) 1212
NegGram 2453
▲ Neupogen for Injection (9%) 495
Neurontin Capsules (Infrequent) 1978
▲ Nicotrol NS Nicotine Nasal Spray (5%) 1565
Nimotop Capsules (Up to 1.2%) 603
▲ Nipent for Injection (8% to 11%) 2733
Nolvadex Tablets 2957
Normodyne Injection (Rare) 2519
Normodyne Tablets (Rare; 2%) 2522
Noroxin Tablets 1758
Noroxin Tablets 2222
Norvasc Tablets (Less than 1% to 2%) 2020
Norvir (Less than 2%) 447
▲ Novantrone for Injection (6 to 18%) 1327
Nubain Injection (1% or less) 952
Nucofed 2225
Ocupress Ophthalmic Solution, 1% Sterile (Occasional) ⊙ 297
▲ Oncaspar (Greater than 5%) 2194
Oncovin Solution Vials & Hyporets 1521
OptiPranolol (Metipranolol 0.3%) Sterile Ophthalmic Solution (A small number of patients) ⊙ 256
▲ Orthoclone OKT3 Sterile Solution (21%) 1892
Orudis Capsules (Less than 1%) 2874
Oruvail Capsules (Less than 1%) 2874
OxyContin Tablets (Between 1% and 5%) 2163
Paxil Tablets (Infrequent) 2681
Penetrex Tablets (0.1% to 1%) 2196
Pentasa (One case) 1275
Pergonal (menotropins for injection, USP) 2618
▲ Permax Tablets (4.8%) 571
Plendil Extended-Release Tablets (0.5% to 1.5%) 514
Pondimin Tablets 2239
Ponstel (Rare) 1982
Pravachol Tablets (Rare) 770
Prevacid Delayed-Release Capsules (Less than 1%) 2746
Primaxin I.M. 1770
Primaxin I.V. (Less than 0.2%) 1772
Prinivil Tablets (Greater than 1%) 1776
Prinzide Tablets (0.3% to 1%) 1780
▲ Procardia Capsules (6%) 2024
▲ Procardia XL Extended Release Tablets (Less than 3% to 6%) 2026
Profasi (chorionic gonadotropin for injection, USP) 2620
▲ Prograf (3% to 29%) 1028
Prolastin Alpha$_1$-Proteinase Inhibitor (Human) (Occasional) 629
▲ Proleukin for Injection (52%) 812
ProSom Tablets (Infrequent) 457
Prostigmin Injectable 1305
Prostigmin Tablets 1306
Prostin E2 Suppository 2109
Protamine Sulfate Vials 1526
Proventil Inhalation Solution 0.083% (1.5%) 2527
Proventil Solution for Inhalation 0.5% (1.5%) 2525
Prozac Pulvules & Liquid, Oral Solution (1.4%) 935
Pulmozyme Inhalation 1054
Recombivax HB (Less than 1%) 1787
Redux Capsules (Infrequent) 2911
Reglan (Rare) 2243
Relafen Tablets (1%) 2688
Remeron Tablets (1%) 1878
RespiGam 1631
▲ Retrovir Capsules (5%) 1216
▲ Retrovir I.V. Infusion (5%) 1221
▲ Retrovir Syrup (5%) 1216
ReVia Tablets (Less than 1%) 957
Rhinocort Nasal Inhaler (Less than 1%) 552
Rilutek Tablets (More than 2%) 2198
Risperdal Tablets (Up to 1%) 1348
▲ Roferon-A Injection (8% to 12%) 2308
▲ Romazicon (3% to 9%) 2311
Rowasa 2727
▲ Rythmol Tablets–150mg, 225mg, 300mg (2.0 to 5.3%) 1399
Sandimmune 2416
Sansert Tablets 2424
▲ Sectral Capsules (4%) 2914
Ser-Ap-Es Tablets 867
Serophene (clomiphene citrate tablets, USP) 2621
Serzone Tablets (Frequent) 776
Sinemet Tablets 959
Sinemet CR Tablets (1.6%) 961
▲ Stadol (3% to 9%) 779
Streptase for Infusion (Rare) 557
Sular Tablets (Less than or equal to 1%) 2961
Suprane (desflurane, USP) (Less than 1%) 1865
Symmetrel Capsules (0.1% to 1%) 965
Symmetrel Syrup (0.1% to 1%) 963
Talwin Injection (Infrequent) 2465
▲ Tambocor Tablets (10.3%) 1555
Taxol Injection (2%) 723
▲ Taxotere for Injection Concentrate (6%) 2204
▲ Tegison Capsules (1 to 10%) 2314
Tegretol/Tegretol-XR 870
Tenex Tablets (3% or less) 2249
▲ Tenoretic Tablets (0.6% to 6%) 2963
▲ Tenormin Tablets and I.V. Injection (0.6% to 6%) 2965
Tetramune (Rare) 1449
Tiazac Capsules (Less than 1% to 2%) 1019
Tilade Inhaler (2.8%) 2207
Timolide Tablets (1.2%) 1791
Timoptic in Ocudose (Less frequent) 1796
Timoptic Sterile Ophthalmic Solution (Less frequent) 1794
Timoptic-XE 1798
Tonocard Tablets (Less than 1%) 519
Toprol-XL Tablets (About 1 of 100 patients) 560
Toradol (1% or less) 2319
Tornalate Solution for Inhalation, 0.2% (Less than 1%) 976
Tornalate Metered Dose Inhaler (Less than 1% to 1.0%) 978
Tracrium Injection 1155
Trandate (Rare) 1158
▲ Trasylol (3%) 607
Trental Tablets (Less than 1%) 1291
Tri-Immunol Adsorbed 1452
Tripedia 908
Ultram Tablets (50 mg) (Less than 1%) 1594
Univasc Tablets (Less than 1%) 2553
Uroqid-Acid No. 2 Tablets 633
Valium Injectable 2336
Vancocin HCl, Oral Solution & Pulvules 1536
Vancocin HCl, Vials & ADD-Vantage 1534
▲ Vascor Tablets (200 and 300 mg) (3.59 to 8.70%) 1597
Vaseretic Tablets (0.5% to 2.0%) 1810
Vasotec I.V. 1814
Vasotec Tablets (0.5% to 1.3%) 1816
Velban Vials 1537
Ventolin Inhalation Solution (1.5%) 1171
Ventolin Nebules Inhalation Solution (1.5%) 1172
VePesid Capsules and Injection (0.7% to 2%) 727
Verelan Capsules (1% or less) 1455
Versed Injection (Less than 1%) 2324
▲ Vesanoid Capsules (60%) 2327
▲ Videx Tablets, Powder for Oral Solution, & Pediatric Powder for Oral Solution (2% to 23%) 2980
Virazole 1310
▲ Visken Tablets (5%) 2428
▲ Vistide Injection (10% to 22%) 1057
Cataflam/Voltaren/Voltaren-XR (Less than 1%) 833
▲ Vumon for Injection (Approximately 5%) 729
Wellbutrin Tablets (Infrequent) 1177
Yutopar Intravenous Injection (Infrequent) 566
Zebeta Tablets (1.1% to 1.5%) 1457
▲ Zerit Capsules (Fewer than 1% to 13%) 731
Zestoretic Tablets (0.3 to 1%) 2968
Zestril Tablets (Greater than 1%) 2972
Ziac 1459
Zocor Tablets (Rare) 1821
Zoladex 3-month (1% to 5%) 2978
Zoloft Tablets (Infrequent) 2051
Zosyn (0.1% or less to 1.1%) 1463
Zyrtec Tablets (Less than 2%) 2053

Dyspnea, nocturnal

Prinivil Tablets (0.3% to 1.0%) 1776
Prinzide Tablets 1780
Zestoretic Tablets 2968
Zestril Tablets (0.3% to 1.0%) 2972

Dysrhythmia

Abbokinase (Occasional) 403
Anectine (Rare) 1062
Asendin Tablets 1419
▲ Brethaire Inhaler (About 4%) 830
Loxitane 1426
Mellaril 2398
Procardia Capsules (About 1 patient in 150) 2024
Procardia XL Extended Release Tablets (About 1 patient in 150) 2026
▲ Roferon-A Injection (7%) 2308
Taxotere for Injection Concentrate (Rare) 2204

Dystonia

Anafranil Capsules (Rare) 819
▲ Atamet Tablets (Among most common) 567
Betaseron for SC Injection 653
BuSpar Tablets (Rare) 738
Clozaril Tablets 2377
Cognex Capsules (Rare) 1961
Compazine 2644
Dilantin Infatabs (Rare) 1967
Dilantin Kapseals (Rare) 1965
Dilantin-125 Suspension (Rare) 1969
Diprivan Injectable Emulsion (Less than 1%) 2939
Doral Tablets 2773
Effexor (Rare) 2825
Eldepryl Capsules 2729
Eskalith (One report in a child) 2658
Etrafon 2495
Felbatol (Infrequent) 2774
Halcion Tablets 2093
Haldol Decanoate (Frequent) 1587
Haldol Injection, Tablets and Concentrate 1585
Imitrex Injection (Rare) 1095
Imitrex Tablets (Rare) 1099
Inapsine Injection 462
Lamictal Tablets (Rare) 1105
Larodopa Tablets (Frequent) 2296
Levoprome 1321
Lioresal Tablets 847
Lithium Carbonate Capsules & Tablets 2352
Lithonate/Lithotabs/Lithobid 2721
Loxitane 1426
LUVOX Tablets (Infrequent) 2723
Mellaril 2398
Moban Tablets and Concentrate (Infrequent) 1036
Navane Capsules and Concentrate 2018

(▣ Described in PDR For Nonprescription Drugs) Incidence data in parenthesis; ▲ 3% or more (⊙ Described in PDR For Ophthalmology)

Dystonia **Side Effects Index** 1320

Navane Intramuscular ... 2019
Neurontin Capsules (Infrequent) ... 1978
Orap Tablets (Less frequent) ... 1037
Paxil Tablets (Infrequent) ... 2681
▲ Permax Tablets (11.6%) ... 571
Prolixin ... 510
Prozac Pulvules & Liquid, Oral Solution (Rare) ... 935
Reglan (Approximately 0.2%) ... 2243
Remeron Tablets (Infrequent) ... 1878
▲ Risperdal Tablets (17% to 34%) .. 1348
Serentil ... 689
▲ Sinemet Tablets (Among most common) ... 959
Sinemet CR Tablets (1.8%) ... 961
Stelazine ... 2692
Thorazine ... 2701
Torecan ... 2367
Triavil Tablets ... 1800
Trilafon ... 2532
Wellbutrin Tablets (Frequent) ... 1177
Xanax Tablets ... 2115
Zoloft Tablets (Infrequent) ... 2051

Dystonia, tardive

Compazine ... 2644
Haldol Decanoate ... 1587
Haldol Injection, Tablets and Concentrate ... 1585
Thorazine ... 2701

Dystonic reactions (see under Dystonia)

Dysuria

Alferon N Injection (1%) ... 2142
Ambien Tablets (Rare) ... 2559
Anafranil Capsules (Up to 2%) ... 819
Androderm Testosterone Transdermal System (Less than 1%) ... 2634
Asacol Delayed-Release Tablets ... 2129
Atrohist Plus Tablets ... 1605
Atromid-S Capsules ... 2808
Avonex ... 662
Bontril Slow-Release Capsules ... 786
BuSpar Tablets (Infrequent) ... 738
Cardura Tablets (0.5%) ... 1993
Casodex Tablets (2% to 5%) ... 2934
Cedax (0.1% to 1%) ... 2480
Ceftin (0.1% to 1%) ... 1067
▲ CellCept Capsules (More than or equal to 3%) ... 2265
Cerebyx Injection (Infrequent) ... 1956
Claritin-D Tablets (Less frequent) .. 2487
Clinoril Tablets ... 1658
Cogentin ... 1661
Cognex Capsules (Infrequent) ... 1961
Combipres Tablets (Rare) ... 682
Crixivan Capsules (Less than 2%) .. 1670
Cytotec (Infrequent) ... 2576
D.A. II Tablets ... 972
D.A. Chewable Tablets ... 970
DaunoXome (Less than or equal to 5%) ... 1842
Daypro Caplets (1% to 3%) ... 2578
Deconsal II Tablets ... 1605
Demser Capsules (A few patients) .. 1690
Depakote Tablets (1% to 5%) ... 418
Desferal Vials ... 838
Dipentum Capsules (Rare) ... 2084
Diupres Tablets ... 1691
Dolobid Tablets (Less than 1 in 100) ... 1695
Doxil (Less than 1%) ... 2613
Dura-Tap/PD Capsules ... 970
Dura-Vent/DA Tablets ... 972
Dura-Vent Tablets ... 971
DynaCirc CR Tablets (0.5% to 1.0%) ... 2383
Effexor (Frequent) ... 2825
Engerix-B Unit-Dose Vials ... 2656
Estring Vaginal Ring (1% to 3%) ... 2086
Ethmozine Tablets (Less than 2%) 2217
Fedahist Gyrocaps ... 2545
Felbatol ... 2774
Feldene Capsules (Less than 1%) .. 2008
Flagyl 375 Capsules ... 2587
Floxin I.V. (Less than 1%) ... 1580
Floxin Tablets (200 mg, 300 mg, 400 mg) (Less than 1%) ... 1577
▲ Fludara for Injection (3% to 4%) ... 658
Foscavir Injection (Between 1% and 5%) ... 541
Gastrocrom Capsules (Infrequent) .. 1611
Gastrocrom Oral Concentrate (Less common) ... 1611
Glucotrol XL Extended Release Tablets (Less than 1%) ... 2012
Helidac Therapy ... 2135
Histussin D Liquid ... 670
Hivid Tablets (Less than 1%) ... 2287
Hydrea Capsules (Very rare) ... 705
Hydropres Tablets ... 1718
IFEX ... 706
Imitrex Injection (Rare) ... 1095
Imitrex Tablets (Up to 2%) ... 1099
Intal Inhaler (Infrequent) ... 2185
Intal Nebulizer Solution ... 2186
Ismo Tablets (Fewer than 1%) ... 2844
Kerlone Tablets (Less than 2%) ... 2588
Klonopin Tablets ... 2294
Lamictal Tablets (Rare) ... 1105
Lioresal Tablets (Rare) ... 847
Lodine Capsules and Tablets (1% to 3%) ... 2849
▲ Lupron Depot 3.75 mg (Among most frequent) ... 2739
Lupron Depot 7.5 mg (Less than 5%) ... 2741
Lupron Injection (Less than 5%) ... 2736
LUVOX Tablets (Infrequent) ... 2723
Maxaquin Tablets (Less than 1%) .. 2593
Merrem I.V. (0.1% to 1.0%) ... 2952
Methotrexate Sodium Tablets, Injection, for Injection and LPF Injection (Less common) ... 1322
MetroGel-Vaginal ... 917
Midamor Tablets (Less than or equal to 1%) ... 1746
Moduretic Tablets (Less than or equal to 1%) ... 1748
Nalfon 200 Pulvules & Nalfon Tablets (Less than 1%) ... 933
Naprelan Tablets (Less than 1%) .. 2861
Neurontin Capsules (Infrequent) ... 1978
Norpace (Less than 1%) ... 2596
Norvasc Tablets (Less than or equal to 0.1%) ... 2020
Norvir (Less than 2%) ... 447
Novahistine DMX ... 782
Novahistine Elixir ... 782
Oncovin Solution Vials & Hyporets 1521
Ornade Spansule Capsules ... 2678
OxyContin Tablets (Less than 1%) 2163
Paxil Tablets (Infrequent) ... 2681
Permax Tablets (Infrequent) ... 571
Plendil Extended-Release Tablets (0.5% to 1.5%) ... 514
Pondimin Tablets ... 2239
Ponstel ... 1982
Prinivil Tablets (0.3% to 1.0%) ... 1776
Prinzide Tablets ... 1780
Procardia XL Extended Release Tablets (1% or less) ... 2026
▲ Proleukin for Injection (3%) ... 812
Protostat Tablets ... 1939
Prozac Pulvules & Liquid, Oral Solution (Infrequent) ... 935
Pyrazinamide Tablets (Rare) ... 1442
Questran ... 774
Recombivax HB (Less than 1%) ... 1787
Relafen Tablets (Less than 1%) ... 2688
Remeron Tablets (Infrequent) ... 1878
Retrovir Capsules ... 1216
Retrovir I.V. Infusion ... 1221
Retrovir Syrup ... 1216
Rifater (Rare) ... 1280
Rilutek Tablets (Up to 1.2%) ... 2198
Risperdal Tablets (Infrequent) ... 1348
Rondec Oral Drops ... 974
Rondec Syrup ... 974
Rondec ... 974
Salagen Tablets (Less than 1%) ... 1546
Sanorex Tablets ... 2423
Sansert Tablets ... 2424
Sectral Capsules (Up to 2%) ... 2914
Seldane-D Extended-Release Tablets ... 1286
Ser-Ap-Es Tablets ... 867
Serzone Tablets ... 776
Sular Tablets (Less than or equal to 1%) ... 2961
Supprelin Injection (1% to 3%) ... 2230
Syn-Rx Tablets ... 1622
Syn-Rx DM Tablets ... 1623
Tegison Capsules (Less than 1%) .. 2314
▲ TheraCys BCG Live (Intravesical) (3.6% to 51.8%) ... 911
Thioplex (Thiotepa For Injection) ... 1329
▲ TICE BCG, USP (59.5%) ... 1881
Tolectin (200, 400 and 600 mg) (Less than 1%) ... 1591
Trinalin Repetabs Tablets ... 1373
Tussend ... 1830
Tussend Expectorant ... 1831
Ultram Tablets (50 mg) (Less than 1%) ... 1594
Unasyn (Less than 1%) ... 2035
Urispas Tablets ... 2710
Uroqid-Acid No. 2 Tablets (Occasional) ... 633
Vagistat-1 (Less than 1%) ... 783
▲ Vesanoid Capsules (9%) ... 2327
Wellbutrin Tablets (Rare) ... 1177
Zerit Capsules (Fewer than 1% to 3%) ... 731
Zestril Tablets (0.3% to 1.0%) ... 2972
Zofran Injection (2%) ... 1227
Zoloft Tablets (Infrequent) ... 2051
Zosyn (1.0% or less) ... 1463
Zyrtec Tablets (Less than 2%) ... 2053

E

Ear, discomfort

AeroBid Inhaler System (1% to 3%) ... 1004
Aerobid-M Inhaler System (1% to 3%) ... 1004
Bumex (0.1%) ... 2260
BuSpar Tablets (Rare) ... 738
Cytotec (Infrequent) ... 2576
Invirase Capsules (Less than 2%) .. 2291
Kerlone Tablets (Less than 2%) ... 2588
Ponstel ... 1982
ReVia Tablets (Less than 1%) ... 957
▲ Tegison Capsules (1-10%) ... 2314
Versed Injection (Less than 1%) ... 2324

Ear, drainage

Hivid Tablets (Less than 1%) ... 2287
Tegison Capsules (Less than 1%) .. 2314

Ear, external abnormalities, fetal

Accutane Capsules ... 2252
Depen Titratable Tablets ... 2770

Ear disease, unspecified

Cardene I.V. (Rare) ... 2815
Clozaril Tablets (Less than 1%) ... 2377
Depakote Tablets (1% to 5%) ... 418
Naprelan Tablets (Less than 1%) .. 2861
Salagen Tablets (Rare) ... 1546
▲ Vesanoid Capsules (6%) ... 2327
Videx Tablets, Powder for Oral Solution, & Pediatric Powder for Oral Solution (Less than 1%) ... 2980

Ears, blocked

Asacol Delayed-Release Tablets ... 2129
Chemet Capsules (1.0% to 3.7%) 666
Dalgan Injection ... 529
Hivid Tablets (Less than 1%) ... 2287
Neurontin Capsules (Infrequent) ... 1978
Orthoclone OKT3 Sterile Solution .. 1892
ReVia Tablets (Less than 1%) ... 957
Supprelin Injection (2% to 3%) ... 2230
Versed Injection (Less than 1%) ... 2324

Ears, ringing (see under Tinnitus)

Ears, roaring in

Amikacin Sulfate Injection, USP ... 523
Garamycin Injectable ... 2502
Nebcin Vials, Hyporets & ADD-Vantage ... 1518

Ebriety, feeling of

Intron A for Injection (Less than 5%) ... 2506

Ebstein's anomaly

Eskalith ... 2658
Lithium Carbonate Capsules & Tablets ... 2352

Ecchymoses

Activase (Less than 1% to 1%) ... 1045
▲ Anaprox/Naprosyn (3% to 9%) ... 2277
Avonex (2%) ... 662
BuSpar Tablets (Rare) ... 738
Calan SR Caplets (1% or less) ... 2571
Calan Tablets (1% or less) ... 2568
Caverject Injection (2%) ... 2064
Celestone Soluspan Suspension ... 2484
▲ CellCept Capsules (More than or equal to 3%) ... 2265
▲ Cerebyx Injection (7.3%) ... 1956
Clinoril Tablets (Less than 1%) ... 1658
Cordarone Tablets (Less than 1%) 2818
Cortifoam ... 2540
Cortone Acetate Sterile Suspension ... 1663
Cortone Acetate Tablets ... 1664
Covera-HS Tablets (Less than 2%) 2573
Cozaar Tablets (Less than 1%) ... 1668
Daypro Caplets (Less than 1%) ... 2578
Decadron Elixir ... 1676
Decadron Phosphate Injection ... 1680
Decadron Phosphate with Xylocaine Injection, Sterile ... 1683
Decadron-LA Sterile Suspension ... 1687
Depakote Tablets (1% to 5%) ... 418
▲ EC-Naprosyn Delayed-Release Tablets (3% to 9%) ... 2277
Effexor (Frequent) ... 2825
Engerix-B Unit-Dose Vials (Less than 1%) ... 2656
Feldene Capsules (Less than 1%) .. 2008
Floxin I.V. ... 1580
Floxin Tablets (200 mg, 300 mg, 400 mg) ... 1577
Hydeltrasol Injection, Sterile ... 1708
Hydeltra-T.B.A. Sterile Suspension 1710
Hydrocortone Acetate Sterile Suspension ... 1712
Hydrocortone Phosphate Injection, Sterile ... 1713
Hydrocortone Tablets ... 1715
Hyzaar Tablets ... 1720
Indocin Capsules (Less than 1%) ... 1723
Indocin I.V. (Less than 1%) ... 1727
Indocin (Less than 1%) ... 1723
Isoptin Oral Tablets (Less than 1%) ... 1393
Isoptin SR Tablets (1% or less) ... 1395
Lamictal Tablets (Infrequent) ... 1105
Lodine Capsules and Tablets (Less than 1%) ... 2849
Lumitene ... 799
▲ Lupron Depot 3.75 mg (Among most frequent) ... 2739
Lupron Injection (Less than 5%) ... 2736
LUVOX Tablets (Infrequent) ... 2723
Methotrexate Sodium Tablets, Injection, for Injection and LPF Injection ... 1322
Miltown Tablets ... 2780
▲ Naprelan Tablets (Less than 3% to 9%) ... 2861
▲ Anaprox/Naprosyn (3% to 9%) ... 2277
Norvir (Less than 2%) ... 447
▲ Novantrone for Injection (7 to 11%) ... 1327
Oncaspar ... 2194
Parafon Forte DSC Caplets (Rare) .. 1590
Paxil Tablets (Infrequent) ... 2681
Pentasa (Less than 1%) ... 1275
Pipracil (Less frequent) ... 1435
PMB 200 and PMB 400 ... 2890
▲ Prograf (Greater than 3%) ... 1028
Questran ... 774
Redux Capsules ... 2911
Rilutek Tablets (Infrequent) ... 2198
Roferon-A Injection (Rare) ... 2308
Serzone Tablets (Infrequent) ... 776
Sular Tablets (Less than or equal to 1%) ... 2961
Ticlid Tablets ... 2317
Trilisate (Rare) ... 2155
Vaqta (1.3%) ... 1805
Verelan Capsules (1% or less) ... 1455
▲ Videx Tablets, Powder for Oral Solution, & Pediatric Powder for Oral Solution (15%) ... 2980
Wellbutrin Tablets ... 1177
Zoladex (1% or greater) ... 2976
Zoladex 3-month ... 2978
Zosyn (1.0% or less) ... 1463
Zyloprim Tablets (Less than 1%) ... 1194

Ecchymosis, soft eyelid tissue

BOTOX (Botulinum Toxin Type A) Purified Neurotoxin Complex ... 473

Ectrodactylia

Cytoxan (2 cases) ... 700

Ectropion

BOTOX (Botulinum Toxin Type A) Purified Neurotoxin Complex (Less than 1%) ... 473
Demulen ... 2580

Eczema

▲ Accutane Capsules (Less than 1 patient in 10) ... 2252
▲ AeroBid Inhaler System (3% to 9%) ... 1004
▲ Aerobid-M Inhaler System (3% to 9%) ... 1004
Anafranil Capsules (Infrequent) ... 819
Benoquin Cream 20% ... 1298
Cardura Tablets (Less than 0.5% of 3960 patients) ... 1993
Cataflam Tablets (Less than 1%) ... 833
Cerumenex Drops (1% of 2,700 patients) ... 2148
Claritin-D Tablets (Less frequent) . 2487
Clozaril Tablets (Less than 1%) ... 2377
Cognex Capsules (Infrequent) ... 1961
Compazine ... 2644

(Described in PDR For Nonprescription Drugs) Incidence data in parenthesis; ▲ 3% or more (Described in PDR For Ophthalmology)

1321 Side Effects Index Edema

Dantrium Capsules (Less frequent) 2131
Effexor (Rare) 2825
Engerix-B Unit-Dose Vials 2656
Etrafon 2495
Glucotrol Tablets (About 1 in 70) 2011
Invirase Capsules (Less than 2%) 2291
Kwell Cream & Lotion (Relatively infrequent) 2172
Kwell Shampoo (Infrequent) 2173
Lac-Hydrin 12% Lotion (Less frequent) 2796
Lamictal Tablets (Infrequent) 1105
Lindane Lotion USP 1% (Relatively infrequent) 481
Lindane Shampoo USP 1% (Relatively infrequent) 483
Lopid Tablets (1.9%) 1974
LUVOX Tablets (Infrequent) 2723
Macrobid Capsules 2138
Macrodantin Capsules 2140
Maxaquin Tablets (Less than 1%) 2593
Miacalcin Nasal Spray (Less than 1%) 2403
Naprelan Tablets (Less than 1%) 2861
Neurontin Capsules (Infrequent) 1978
Nipent for Injection (Less than 3%) 2733
Norvir (Less than 2%) 447
Orudis Capsules (Less than 1%) 2874
Oruvail Capsules (Less than 1%) 2874
Oxistat Lotion (0.4%) 1139
Paxil Tablets (Infrequent) 2681
Pentasa (Less than 1%) 1275
Permax Tablets (Infrequent) 571
Prolixin 510
Prozac Pulvules & Liquid, Oral Solution (Rare) 935
Redux Capsules (Infrequent) 2911
RespiGam (Infrequent) 1631
Rilutek Tablets (0.8% to 1.6%) 2198
Serzone Tablets (Infrequent) 776
Stelazine 2692
Triavil Tablets 1800
Trilafon 2532
Varivax (Greater than or equal to 1%) 1807
▲ Videx Tablets, Powder for Oral Solution, & Pediatric Powder for Oral Solution (12%) 2980
Cataflam/Voltaren/Voltaren-XR (Less than 1%) 833
Zebeta Tablets 1457
Ziac 1459
▲ Zosyn (4.2%) 1463
Zyrtec Tablets (Less than 2%) 2053

Eczema, exacerbation of

▲ Zonalon Cream (Approximately 1% to 10%) 1042

Eczematous reactions (see under Eczema)

Edema

Accutane Capsules (Less than 1%) 2252
Adapin Capsules (Occasional) 1542
▲ AeroBid Inhaler System (3% to 9%) 1004
▲ Aerobid-M Inhaler System (3% to 9%) 1004
Aldoclor Tablets 1638
Aldomet Ester HCl Injection 1642
Aldomet Oral 1640
Aldoril Tablets 1644
Alferon N Injection (One patient) 2142
Alkeran for Injection 1196
Altace Capsules (Less than 1%) 1238
Alupent Tablets (0.2%) 672
Ambien Tablets (Infrequent) 2559
Amen Tablets (Occasional) 785
Americaine Anesthetic Lubricant 1603
Americaine Otic Topical Anesthetic Ear Drops 1603
Amicar Syrup, Tablets, and Injection 1312
Anafranil Capsules (Infrequent) 819
▲ Anaprox/Naprosyn (3% to 9%) 2277
Androderm Testosterone Transdermal System 2634
▲ Android Capsules, 10 mg (Among most common) 1297
Antivenin (Crotalidae) Polyvalent 2803
Apresazide Capsules (Less frequent) 824
Apresoline Hydrochloride Tablets (Less frequent) 826
Aredia for Injection (Up to 1%) 827
▲ Arimidex Tablets (7.3% to 11.4%) 2932
Asacol Delayed-Release Tablets 2129
Asendin Tablets (Less frequent) 1419
Atamet Tablets 567
Atretol Tablets 569
Aygestin Tablets 990
▲ Betapace Tablets (2% to 8%) 637
▲ Betaseron for SC Injection (8%) 653
Bicillin C-R Injection 2810
Bicillin C-R 900/300 Injection 2812
Bicillin L-A Injection 2813
Blocadren Tablets (0.6%) 1654
Brevibloc (esmolol HCl) Injection (Less than 1%) 1860
Brevicon 2563
BuSpar Tablets (Infrequent) 738
Calan SR Caplets (1.9%) 2571
Calan Tablets (1.9%) 2568
Capoten Tablets 740
Capozide Tablets 744
Cardene Capsules (0.6% to 1.0%) 2261
▲ Cardizem CD Capsules (2.6% to 4.6%) 1251
▲ Cardizem SR Capsules (5.4% to 9%) 1255
Cardizem Injectable (Less than 1%) 1253
Cardizem Tablets (2.4%) 1257
▲ Cardura Tablets (About 0.7% to 4%) 1993
Casodex Tablets (2% to 5%) 2934
Cataflam Tablets (1% to 3%) 833
Catapres-TTS (3 of 101 patients) 680
Ceclor Pulvules & Suspension 1470
Celestone Soluspan Suspension 2484
▲ CellCept Capsules (11.8% to 12.2%) 2265
Cerebyx Injection (Infrequent) 1956
Claritin-D Tablets (Less frequent) 2487
Climara Transdermal System 640
Clinoril Tablets (Greater than 1%) 1658
Clomid 1262
Clozaril Tablets (Less than 1%) 2377
Cognex Capsules (Infrequent) 1961
Condylox Topical Solution (Less than 5%) 1853
Cordarone Tablets (1 to 3%) 2818
CORTENEMA 2713
Cortifoam 2540
Cortone Acetate Sterile Suspension 1663
Cortone Acetate Tablets 1664
Covera-HS Tablets (1.9% to 3.0%) 2573
Cozaar Tablets (1% or greater) 1668
Cycrin Tablets (Occasional) 991
Cytotec (Infrequent) 2576
Cytovene (1% or less) 2270
Dalalone D.P. Injectable 1009
Dalgan Injection (Less than 1%) 529
Danocrine Capsules 2437
▲ DaunoXome (2% to 9%) 1842
Daypro Caplets (Less than 1%) 2578
Decadron Elixir 1676
Decadron Phosphate Injection 1680
Decadron Phosphate with Xylocaine Injection, Sterile 1683
Decadron Tablets 1678
Decadron-LA Sterile Suspension 1687
Demadex Tablets and Injection (1.1%) 691
Demulen 2580
Depakote Tablets (1% to 5%) 418
Depo-Provera Contraceptive Injection (1% to 5%) 2079
Depo-Provera Sterile Aqueous Suspension 2083
Dermatop Emollient Cream 0.1% (Less than 1%) 1264
Desogen Tablets 1867
Desquam-E Gel 2792
Desquam-X Gel 2792
Desquam-X 10 Bar 2792
Desquam-X Wash 2792
▲ Desyrel and Desyrel Dividose (2.8% to 7.0%) 504
Dexacort Phosphate in Respihaler 1606
Dexacort Phosphate in Turbinaire 1607
Diethylstilbestrol Tablets 1477
Dilacor XR Extended-release Capsules (Infrequent) 2183
Diphtheria & Tetanus Toxoids Adsorbed Purogenated (Mild) 1422
Diprivan Injectable Emulsion (Less than 1%) 2939
Dolobid Tablets (Less than 1 in 100) 1695
Doxil (Less than 1%) 2613
Duragesic Transdermal System (1% or greater) 1336
Duranest Injections 533
Dyclone 0.5% and 1% Topical Solutions, USP 535
Dynabac (0.1% to 1%) 668
▲ DynaCirc Capsules (3.5% to 8.7%) 2381
▲ DynaCirc CR Tablets (8.9% to 35.9%) 2383
▲ EC-Naprosyn Delayed-Release Tablets (3% to 9%) 2277
Effexor (Infrequent) 2825
Elavil 2945
▲ Emcyt Capsules (19%) 2085
▲ Epogen for Injection (9% to 17%) 489
Ergamisol Tablets (1%) 1340
Esimil Tablets 840
Estrace Cream and Tablets 751
Estraderm Transdermal System 842
ESTRATAB Tablets (0.3, 0.625, 1.25, 2.5 mg) 2715
Estratest 2718
▲ Eulexin Capsules (4%) 2498
Felbatol 2774
Feldene Capsules (Greater than 1%) 2008
Fioricet with Codeine Capsules 2387
Fiorinal with Codeine Capsules 2390
Flexeril Tablets (Rare) 1701
▲ Flolan for Injection (60%) 1085
Florinef Acetate Tablets 506
Floxin I.V. (Less than 1%) 1580
Floxin Tablets (200 mg, 300 mg, 400 mg) (Less than 1%) 1577
▲ Fludara for Injection (8% to 19%) 658
Foscavir Injection (Between 1% and 5%) 541
Gammar-P I.V., Immune Globulin Intravenous (Human) 798
Gantanol Tablets 2285
Gantrisin 2286
Gastrocrom Capsules (Infrequent) 1611
Gastrocrom Oral Concentrate (Less common) 1611
▲ Gemzar for Injection (Less than 1% to 13%) 1482
Glucotrol XL Extended Release Tablets (Less than 1%) 2012
▲ Habitrol Nicotine Transdermal System (4%) 884
Halotestin Tablets 2095
Hismanal Tablets (Less frequent) 1341
Hivid Tablets (Less than 1%) 2287
Humatrope Vials (2.5%) 1490
Hydeltrasol Injection, Sterile 1708
Hydeltra-T.B.A. Sterile Suspension 1710
Hydralazine Hydrochloride Injection USP (Less frequent) 2712
Hydrocortone Acetate Sterile Suspension 1712
Hydrocortone Phosphate Injection, Sterile 1713
Hydrocortone Tablets 1715
Hytrin Capsules (0.9%) 434
Hyzaar Tablets (1.3%) 1720
IBU Tablets (Greater than 1%) 1389
Imdur (Less than or equal to 5%) 1362
Imitrex Tablets (Rare to infrequent) 1099
Indocin Capsules (Less than 1%) 1723
Indocin I.V. (Less than 1%) 1727
Indocin (Less than 1%) 1723
Invirase Capsules (Less than 2%) 2291
Iopidine 0.5% (Less than 1%) ◉ 219
Ismelin Tablets 845
Ismo Tablets (Fewer than 1%) 2844
Isoptin Oral Tablets (1.9%) 1393
Isoptin SR Tablets (1.9%) 1395
Kadian Capsules (Less than 3%) 2948
Kerlone Tablets (1.3% to 1.8%) 2588
Klonopin Tablets 2294
Lamictal Tablets (Rare) 1105
Lamprene Capsules (Less than 1%) 846
Larodopa Tablets (Rare) 2296
▲ Leukine (13% to 34%) 1317
▲ Leustatin (6%) 1889
Levlen/Tri-Levlen 646
Librax Capsules (Rare) 2330
Librium Capsules (Isolated cases) 2331
Librium Injectable (Isolated cases) 2332
Lioresal Tablets 847
Lodine Capsules and Tablets (Less than 1%) 2849
Lo/Ovral Tablets 2852
Lo/Ovral-28 Tablets 2857
Lopressor HCT Tablets (1 in 100 patients) 850
Lotrel Capsules (0.6% to 3.2%) 858
Lotrimin 2514
Lotrisone Cream (1 of 270 patients) 2515
Lovenox Injection (2%) 2187
Ludiomil Tablets (Rare) 861
▲ Lupron Depot 3.75 mg (5.4%) 2739
▲ Lupron Depot 7.5 mg (12.5%) 2741
▲ Lupron Depot - 3 Month 22.5 mg (Less than 5%) 2743
LUVOX Tablets (Frequent) 2723
MS Contin Tablets (Less frequent) 2149
MSIR (Infrequent) 2152
Matulane Capsules 2300
Mavik Tablets (0.3% to 1.0%) 1407
Maxair Autohaler 1550
Maxair Inhaler (Less than 1%) 1552
Maxaquin Tablets (Less than 1%) 2593
Megace Oral Suspension (1% to 3%) 708
Megace Tablets 710
Mellaril 2398
Menest Tablets 2671
Mesantoin Tablets 2400
Methadone Hydrochloride Oral Concentrate 2356
Methadone Hydrochloride Oral Solution & Tablets 2357
Metubine Iodide Vials 932
▲ Mexitil Capsules (About 2 in 1,000 to 3.8%) 684
Minipress Capsules (1-4%) 2015
Minizide Capsules 2016
Modicon 1928
8-MOP Capsules 1294
Monoket Tablets (Fewer than 1%) 2550
Monopril Tablets (0.2% to 1.0% or more) 762
Motrin Ibuprofen Suspension, Oral Drops, Chewable Tablets, Caplets (1% to less than 3%) 1563
Mutamycin for Injection 712
Mykrox Tablets (Less than 2%) 1617
▲ Naprelan Tablets (Less than 3% to 9%) 2861
▲ Anaprox/Naprosyn (3% to 9%) 2277
Nardil (Common) 1977
Neoral (2% or less) 2405
Neurontin Capsules (Infrequent) 1978
Nimotop Capsules (Up to 1.2%) 603
▲ Nolvadex Tablets (3.8% to 32.4%) 2957
Nordette-21 Tablets 2863
Nordette-28 Tablets 2866
Norinyl 2563
▲ Normodyne Injection (Up to 2%) 2519
Normodyne Tablets (Up to 2%) 2522
Noroxin Tablets (Less frequent) 1758
Noroxin Tablets (Less frequent) 2222
Norpace (1 to 3%) 2596
Norpramin Tablets 1273
Nor-Q D Tablets 2598
▲ Norvasc Tablets (1.8% to 10.8%) 2020
Norvir (Less than 2%) 447
Novocain Hydrochloride for Spinal Anesthesia 2457
Nubain Injection (1% or less) 952
Ogen Tablets 2103
Ogen Vaginal Cream 2106
▲ Oncaspar (Greater than 5%) 2194
Oncovin Solution Vials & Hyporets (Rare) 1521
OptiPranolol (Metipranolol 0.3%) Sterile Ophthalmic Solution (A small number of patients) ◉ 256
Oramorph SR (Morphine Sulfate Sustained Release Tablets) (Less frequent) 2359
Orlaam Oral Solution (1% to 3%) 2361
Ortho-Cept 1907
Ortho-Cyclen/Ortho-Tri-Cyclen 1914
Ortho Dienestrol Cream 1922
Ortho-Est 1925
Ortho-Novum 1928
Ortho-Cyclen/Ortho Tri-Cyclen 1914
▲ Orudis Capsules (3% to 9%) 2874
▲ Oruvail Capsules (3% to 9%) 2874
Ovcon 765
Ovral Tablets 2877
Ovral-28 Tablets 2878
Ovrette Tablets 2878
Oxandrin 783
Oxsoralen-Ultra Capsules 1302
OxyContin Tablets (Less than 1%) 2163
Pamelor 2409
Parnate Tablets 2679
Paxil Tablets (Frequent) 2681
Pediapred Oral Solution 1618
Pediazole Suspension 2340
Penetrex Tablets (0.1% to 1%) 2196
Pentasa (Less than 1%) 1275
Pentaspan Injection 954
Permax Tablets (1.6%) 571
Pfizerpen for Injection 2022
PMB 200 and PMB 400 2890
Pontocaine Hydrochloride for Spinal Anesthesia 2460

(Described in PDR For Nonprescription Drugs) Incidence data in parenthesis; ▲ 3% or more (◉ Described in PDR For Ophthalmology)

Pregnyl for Injection ... 1878
Prelone Syrup ... 1834
Premarin Intravenous ... 2893
Premarin Tablets ... 2896
Premarin Vaginal Cream ... 2898
Premphase ... 2900
Prempro ... 2905
Prevacid Delayed-Release Capsules (Less than 1%) ... 2746
Prinivil Tablets (0.3% to 1.0%) ... 1776
Prinzide Tablets ... 1780
Priscoline Hydrochloride Ampuls ... 864
▲ Procardia XL Extended Release Tablets (10% to about 30%) ... 2026
▲ Procrit for Injection (17%) ... 1896
Profasi (chorionic gonadotropin for injection, USP) ... 2620
Proglycem (Frequent) ... 575
▲ Proleukin for Injection (47%) ... 812
Propulsid (1% or less) ... 1346
ProSom Tablets (Rare) ... 457
Provera Tablets ... 2110
Prozac Pulvules & Liquid, Oral Solution (Infrequent) ... 935
Quadrinal Tablets ... 1398
Questran ... 774
RMS Suppositories CII ... 2766
Recombivax HB (Less than 1%) ... 1787
Redux Capsules (Infrequent) ... 2911
Reglan ... 2243
▲ Relafen Tablets (3% to 9%) ... 2688
Remeron Tablets (1%) ... 1878
RespiGam (Infrequent) ... 1631
Retrovir Capsules (0.8%) ... 1216
Retrovir I.V. Infusion (1%) ... 1221
Retrovir Syrup (0.8%) ... 1216
ReVia Tablets (Less than 1%) ... 957
Rilutek Tablets (Rare to frequent) ... 2198
Risperdal Tablets (Infrequent) ... 1348
▲ Roferon-A Injection (11%) ... 2308
Rowasa (1.2%) ... 2727
Roxanol ... 2365
Rythmol Tablets–150mg, 225mg, 300mg (0.6 to 1.4%) ... 1399
▲ Salagen Tablets (5%) ... 1546
Sandimmune (2% or less) ... 2416
Sandostatin Injection (1% to 4%) ... 2421
Sanorex Tablets ... 2423
Sansert Tablets ... 2424
Sectral Capsules (2%) ... 2914
Ser-Ap-Es Tablets ... 867
Serax Capsules ... 2916
Serax Tablets ... 2916
Serentil ... 689
Serzone Tablets ... 776
Sinemet Tablets ... 959
Sinemet CR Tablets ... 961
Sinequan (Occasional) ... 2028
Soma Compound w/Codeine Tablets ... 2784
Soma Compound Tablets ... 2783
Sporanox Capsules (0.4% to 3.5%) ... 1352
Stadol (Less than 1%) ... 779
Stimate, (desmopressin acetate) Nasal Spray, 1.5 mg/mL ... 806
Supprelin Injection (2% to 3%) ... 2230
▲ Synarel Nasal Solution for Endometriosis (8% of patients) ... 2605
▲ Tambocor Tablets (3.5%) ... 1555
Tapazole Tablets ... 1361
▲ Taxol Injection (21%) ... 723
▲ Taxotere for Injection Concentrate (6%) ... 2204
▲ Tegison Capsules (1 to 10%) ... 2314
Tegretol/Tegretol-XR ... 870
Tenex Tablets (Less frequent) ... 2249
Testoderm Testosterone Transdermal System ... 486
Tetanus Toxoid Adsorbed Purogenated ... 1447
Thyro-Block Tablets (A few people) 2785
Tiazac Capsules (2%) ... 1019
Timolide Tablets ... 1791
Timoptic in Ocudose ... 1796
Timoptic Sterile Ophthalmic Solution ... 1794
Timoptic-XE ... 1798
Tofranil Ampuls ... 873
Tofranil Tablets ... 875
Tofranil-PM Capsules ... 876
▲ Tolectin (200, 400 and 600 mg) (3 to 9%) ... 1591
Tonocard Tablets (Less than 1%) ... 519
▲ Toradol (4%) ... 2319
Trancopal Caplets ... 2468
Trandate Tablets (Up to 2%) ... 1158
Trental Tablets (Less than 1%) ... 1291
Triavil Tablets ... 1800
Levlen/Tri-Levlen ... 646
Trilisate (Less than 1%) ... 2155
Tri-Norinyl ... 2607
▲ Tripedia (1% to 21%) ... 908
Triphasil-21 Tablets ... 2919
Triphasil-28 Tablets ... 2924
Tympagesic Ear Drops ... 2476
Unasyn (Less than 1%) ... 2035
Vaqta (Less than 1%) ... 1805
Vascor Tablets (200 and 300 mg) (0.5 to 2.0%) ... 1597
Verelan Capsules (1.9%) ... 1455
▲ Vesanoid Capsules (29% to 32%) 2327
Videx Tablets, Powder for Oral Solution, & Pediatric Powder for Oral Solution (Up to 2%) ... 2980
▲ Visken Tablets (6%) ... 2428
Vistide Injection ... 1057
Vivactil Tablets ... 1820
Vivelle Transdermal System ... 880
Cataflam/Voltaren/Voltaren-XR (1% to 3%) ... 833
Wellbutrin Tablets (Frequent) ... 1177
Winstrol Tablets ... 2468
▲ Xanax Tablets (4.9%) ... 2115
Xylocaine Injections (Extremely rare) ... 562
Zebeta Tablets ... 1457
Zestoretic Tablets ... 2968
Zestril Tablets (0.3% to 1.0%) ... 2972
Ziac ... 1459
▲ Zoladex (1% to 7%) ... 2976
Zoladex 3-month ... 2978
Zoloft Tablets (Infrequent) ... 2051
▲ Zonalon Cream (Approximately 1% to 10%) ... 1042
Zosyn (0.1% to 1.9%) ... 1463
Zovirax Capsules (0.3%) ... 1187
Zovirax Sterile Powder (Less than 1%) ... 1191
Zovirax (0.3%) ... 1187
Zyrtec Tablets (Less than 2%) ... 2053

Edema, allergic

Cytosar-U Sterile Powder (Less frequent) ... 2077
Periactin ... 1767

Edema, angioneurotic

Accupril Tablets ... 1950
Achromycin V Capsules ... 1417
Airet Albuterol Sulfate Inhalation Solution (Rare) ... 1602
Albuterol Sulfate, USP Solution for Inhalation, Arm-a-Med (Rare) ... 522
Altace Capsules (0.3%) ... 1238
Anaprox/Naprosyn (Less than 1%) ... 2277
Atrovent Nasal Spray 0.06% (Rare) ... 678
Augmentin ... 2637
Augmentin Tablets ... 2640
Azactam for Injection (Less than 1%) ... 736
Brontex (Infrequent) ... 2130
Carafate Suspension ... 1250
Carafate Tablets ... 1249
Carbocaine Injection ... 2432
Cardizem SR Capsules (Infrequent) ... 1255
Cardizem Tablets (Infrequent) ... 1257
Catapres Tablets (About 5 in 1,000 patients) ... 679
Catapres-TTS ... 680
Ceclor Pulvules & Suspension ... 1470
Ceftin Tablets ... 1067
Ceptaz (Very rare) ... 1070
Ceredase ... 1055
Chibroxin Sterile Ophthalmic Solution (With oral form) ... 1657
Chloroptic S.O.P. ... ⊙ 236
Chloroptic Sterile Ophthalmic Solution ... ⊙ 236
Cipro I.V. Pharmacy Bulk Package (Less than 1%) ... 590
Claritin Tablets (2% or fewer patients) ... 2485
Claritin-D Tablets ... 2487
Clinoril Tablets (Less than 1 in 100) ... 1658
Combipres Tablets (About 5 in 1,000) ... 682
Compazine ... 2644
Cortone Acetate Sterile Suspension ... 1663
Cortone Acetate Tablets ... 1664
Cozaar Tablets (Rare) ... 1668
CytoGam (A possibility) ... 1630
Dalalone D.P. Injectable ... 1009
Decadron Elixir ... 1676
Decadron Phosphate Injection ... 1680
Decadron Phosphate with Xylocaine Injection, Sterile ... 1683
Decadron Tablets ... 1678
Decadron-LA Sterile Suspension ... 1687
Declomycin Tablets ... 1421
Demadex Tablets and Injection (One patient) ... 691
Dexacort Phosphate in Respihaler ... 1606
Dexacort Phosphate in Turbinaire ... 1607
DiaBeta Tablets ... 1265
Diflucan Tablets, Injection, and Oral Suspension (Rare) ... 2003
Diprivan Injectable Emulsion (Rare) ... 2939
Disalcid ... 1549
Dolobid Tablets (Less than 1 in 100) ... 1695
Doryx Capsules ... 1970
Duricef Capsules, Tablets, and Oral Suspension ... 750
DYNACIN Capsules ... 1627
EC-Naprosyn Delayed-Release Tablets (Less than 1%) ... 2277
Eminase ... 2215
EMLA Cream ... 536
Engerix-B Unit-Dose Vials ... 2656
Etrafon ... 2495
Flexeril Tablets ... 1701
Flovent (Rare) ... 1089
Floxin I.V. (Less than 1%) ... 1580
Floxin Tablets (200 mg, 300 mg, 400 mg) (Less than 1%) ... 1577
Fluvirin (Influenza Virus Vaccine) (Rare) ... 1608
Fulvicin P/G Tablets (Rare) ... 2499
Fulvicin P/G 165 & 330 Tablets (Rare) ... 2500
Fungizone Oral Suspension (Rare) ... 704
Gastrocrom Capsules (Infrequent) ... 1611
Gastrocrom Oral Concentrate (Less common) ... 1611
Glynase PresTab Tablets ... 2091
Grifulvin V (griseofulvin tablets) Microsize (griseofulvin oral suspension) Microsize (Rare) ... 1944
Gris-PEG Tablets, 125 mg & 250 mg (Rare) ... 476
Havrix (Rare) ... 2663
Helidac Therapy ... 2135
Hespan Injection ... 945
Hismanal Tablets (Less frequent) ... 1341
Hydeltrasol Injection, Sterile ... 1708
Hydeltra-T.B.A. Sterile Suspension 1710
Hydrocortone Acetate Sterile Suspension ... 1712
Hydrocortone Phosphate Injection, Sterile ... 1713
Hydrocortone Tablets ... 1715
Hyperab Rabies Immune Globulin (Human) (Rare) ... 618
HyperHep Hepatitis B Immune Globulin (Human) ... 619
Hyper-Tet Tetanus Immune Globulin (Human) (Few isolated cases) ... 621
IBU Tablets (Less than 1%) ... 1389
Imitrex Tablets ... 1099
Imogam Rabies Immune Globulin (Human) ... 897
▲ Imovax Rabies Vaccine (Up to 6%) 899
Influenza Virus Vaccine, Trivalent, Types A and B (chromatograph- and filter-purified subviron antigen) FluShield, 1996-1997 Formula (Rare) ... 2842
Intal Nebulizer Solution ... 2186
Intron A for Injection (Rare) ... 2506
JE-VAX ... 904
Lamictal Tablets (Rare) ... 1105
Lescol Capsules (Rare) ... 2395
Levoprome ... 1321
Lithonate/Lithotabs/Lithobid ... 2721
Lodine Capsules and Tablets (Less than 1%) ... 2849
Lomotil ... 2591
Lopid Tablets ... 1974
Lotensin Tablets ... 852
Lotensin HCT Tablets ... 855
Lutrepulse for Injection ... 998
Marcaine (Rare) ... 2446
Marcaine Spinal (Rare) ... 2449
Mavik Tablets (0.13%) ... 1407
Mefoxin ... 1734
Mefoxin Premixed Intravenous Solution ... 1737
Mellaril ... 2398
Mevacor Tablets (Rare) ... 1742
Micronase Tablets ... 2099
Miltown Tablets (Rare) ... 2780
Minocin Intravenous ... 1428
Minocin Oral Suspension ... 1431
Minocin Pellet-Filled Capsules ... 1429
Monodox Capsules ... 1858
Monopril Tablets (0.2% to 1.0%) ... 762
Motofen Tablets ... 789
Motrin Ibuprofen Suspension, Oral Drops, Chewable Tablets, Caplets (Less than 1%) ... 1563
Mykrox Tablets ... 1617
Myochrysine Injection ... 1754
Nalfon 200 Pulvules & Nalfon Tablets (Less than 1%) ... 933
▲ Naprelan Tablets (3% to 9%) ... 2861
Anaprox/Naprosyn (Less than 1%) ... 2277
Navelbine Injection ... 1212
Nescaine/Nescaine MPF ... 549
Normodyne Injection (Rare) ... 2519
Normodyne Tablets (Rare) ... 2522
Noroxin Tablets ... 1758
Noroxin Tablets ... 2222
Orthoclone OKT3 Sterile Solution ... 1892
Parafon Forte DSC Caplets (Extremely rare) ... 1590
Paxil Tablets (Rare) ... 2681
Pediazole Suspension ... 2340
Pepcid Injection (Infrequent) ... 1765
Pepcid (Infrequent) ... 1763
Pergonal (menotropins for injection, USP) ... 2618
Phenergan with Codeine (Infrequent) ... 2883
Phenergan Injection ... 2880
Phenergan Tablets ... 2882
Phenergan VC with Codeine ... 2888
PMB 200 and PMB 400 (Rare) ... 2890
Pravachol Tablets (Rare) ... 770
Prilosec Delayed-Release Capsules (Less than 1%) ... 516
Primaxin I.M. ... 1770
Primaxin I.V. (Less than 0.2%) ... 1772
Prinzide Tablets (Rare) ... 1780
Procanbid Extended-Release Tablets (Occasional) ... 1983
Procardia Capsules (Less than 0.5%) ... 2024
Profasi (chorionic gonadotropin for injection, USP) ... 2620
Prolixin ... 510
Proventil Inhalation Solution 0.083% (Rare) ... 2527
Proventil Solution for Inhalation 0.5% (Rare) ... 2525
Proventil Syrup (Rare) ... 2528
Quadrinal Tablets ... 1398
▲ Rabies Vaccine, Imovax Rabies I.D. (Less frequent; up to 6%) ... 901
Redux Capsules ... 2911
Relafen Tablets (1%) ... 2688
Rilutek Tablets (Rare) ... 2198
Risperdal Tablets ... 1348
Robaxisal Tablets ... 2246
Salflex Tablets ... 791
Seldane Tablets ... 1284
Seldane-D Extended-Release Tablets ... 1286
Semprex-D Capsules (Rare) ... 1620
Sensorcaine (Rare) ... 554
Serentil ... 689
Serevent Inhalation Aerosol (Rare) 1149
Solganal Suspension ... 2530
Soma Compound w/Codeine Tablets ... 2784
Soma Compound Tablets ... 2783
Soma Tablets ... 2782
Sporanox Capsules ... 1352
Stelazine ... 2692
Streptase for Infusion (Rare) ... 557
Supprelin Injection ... 2230
Talwin Compound ... 2466
Taxol Injection (2%) ... 723
Tazicef for Injection (Very rare) ... 2697
Tazidime Vials, Faspak & ADD-Vantage (Very rare) ... 1531
Terramycin Intramuscular Solution 2034
Thorazine ... 2701
Torecan ... 2367
Trandate (Rare) ... 1158
Triavil Tablets ... 1800
Trilafon ... 2532
Trusopt Sterile Ophthalmic Solution ... 1803
Ultram Tablets (50 mg) ... 1594
Univasc Tablets (Less than 0.5%) ... 2553
Velosulin BR Human Insulin 10 ml Vials ... 1847
Ventolin Inhalation Solution (Rare) ... 1171
Ventolin Nebules Inhalation Solution (Rare) ... 1172
Ventolin Rotacaps for Inhalation (Rare) ... 1173
Ventolin Syrup (Rare) ... 1175
Ventolin Tablets (Rare) ... 1176
Vermox Chewable Tablets (Rare) ... 1357

(▭ Described in PDR For Nonprescription Drugs) Incidence data in parenthesis; ▲ 3% or more (⊙ Described in PDR For Ophthalmology)

Side Effects Index — Edema, oropharyngeal

Vibramycin ... 2038
Vibramycin Hyclate Intravenous ... 2040
Vibramycin ... 2038
Videx Tablets, Powder for Oral Solution, & Pediatric Powder for Oral Solution (Less than 1%) ... 2980
Volmax Extended-Release Tablets (Rare) ... 1835
Wellbutrin Tablets ... 1177
Zantac (Rare) ... 1182
Zantac Injection (Rare) ... 1180
Zantac Syrup (Rare) ... 1182
Zaroxolyn Tablets ... 1625
Zebeta Tablets ... 1457
Zestoretic Tablets ... 2968
Ziac ... 1459
Zocor Tablets (Rare) ... 1821
Zofran Injection (Rare) ... 1227
Zyloprim Tablets (Less than 1%) ... 1194
Zyrtec Tablets (Less than 2%) ... 2053

Edema, ankle
Verelan Capsules (1.4%) ... 1455

Edema, aphakic cystoid macular
Timoptic in Ocudose (Less frequent) ... 1796
Timoptic Sterile Ophthalmic Solution (Less frequent) ... 1794
Timoptic-XE ... 1798

Edema, arm
Torecan ... 2367

Edema, cerebral
Betaseron for SC Injection ... 653
Cerebyx Injection (2.2%) ... 1956
Compazine ... 2644
Etrafon (Extremely rare) ... 2495
Felbatol ... 2774
Foscavir Injection (Less than 1%) ... 541
Levoprome ... 1321
Navane Capsules and Concentrate ... 2018
Navane Intramuscular ... 2019
Orthoclone OKT3 Sterile Solution ... 1892
Permax Tablets (Rare) ... 571
Proleukin for Injection (Less than 1%) ... 812
Prolixin ... 510
Stelazine ... 2692
Thorazine ... 2701
Triavil Tablets ... 1800
Trilafon (Extremely rare) ... 2532
▲ Vesanoid Capsules (3%) ... 2327

Edema, conjunctival
Cipro Tablets ... 584
Cortisporin Ophthalmic Ointment Sterile ... 1074
Effexor (Rare) ... 2825
Paxil Tablets (Rare) ... 2681
Vexol 1% Ophthalmic Suspension (Less than 1%) ... ⊚ 227

Edema, corneal
AMVISC Plus ... ⊚ 327
Healon (Rare) ... ⊚ 302
Healon GV ... ⊚ 303
Miochol-E with Iocare Steri-Tags and Miochol-E System Pak (Infrequent) ... ⊚ 263
OcuCoat ... ⊚ 321
Plaquenil Sulfate Tablets ... 2459
▲ Rev-Eyes Ophthalmic Eyedrops 0.5% (10% to 40%) ... ⊚ 324
Symmetrel Capsules (0.1% to 1%) ... 965
Symmetrel Syrup (0.1% to 1%) ... 963
Vexol 1% Ophthalmic Suspension (Less than 1%) ... ⊚ 227
Viroptic Ophthalmic Solution, 1% Sterile ... 1177

Edema, cystoid macular
AdatoSil 5000 (Less than 2%) ... ⊚ 265

Edema, dependent
Anafranil Capsules (Rare) ... 819
Zoloft Tablets (Infrequent) ... 2051

Edema, digitus
Alupent Tablets (0.2%) ... 672

Edema, extremities
Ceclor Pulvules & Suspension ... 1470
Cipro I.V. (1% or less) ... 587
Cipro Tablets (Less than 1%) ... 584
Depakene ... 416
Depakote Tablets ... 418
Mavik Tablets (0.13%) ... 1407
Rifadin ... 1276

Rifater ... 1280
Taxotere for Injection Concentrate ... 2204
Teslac Tablets ... 727

Edema, facial
Adalat CC (Less than 1.0%) ... 582
Ambien Tablets (Rare) ... 2559
Antivenin (Crotalidae) Polyvalent ... 2803
Asacol Delayed-Release Tablets ... 2129
Avonex ... 662
Azmacort Oral Inhaler (Infrequent) ... 2175
BuSpar Tablets (Infrequent) ... 738
Cardizem SR Capsules (Infrequent) ... 1255
Cardizem Tablets (Infrequent) ... 1257
Cardura Tablets (1%) ... 1993
Ceclor Pulvules & Suspension ... 1470
▲ CellCept Capsules (More than or equal to 3%) ... 2265
Cerebyx Injection (Frequent) ... 1956
Cipro I.V. (1% or less) ... 587
Cipro I.V. Pharmacy Bulk Package (Less than 1%) ... 590
Cipro Tablets (Less than 1%) ... 584
Cognex Capsules (Infrequent) ... 1961
Cozaar Tablets (Rare) ... 1668
Cytovene (1% or less) ... 2270
Depakene ... 416
Depakote Tablets (1% to 5%) ... 418
Doxil (Less than 1%) ... 2613
Effexor (Infrequent) ... 2825
Elavil ... 2945
Etopophos for Injection (Sometimes) ... 701
Etoposide Injection (Sometimes) ... 539
Etrafon ... 2495
▲ Felbatol (3.4%) ... 2774
Flexeril Tablets (Less than 1%) ... 1701
Flonase Nasal Spray ... 1088
Floxin I.V. ... 1580
Floxin Tablets (200 mg, 300 mg, 400 mg) ... 1577
Foscavir Injection (Between 1 and 5%) ... 541
Hespan Injection ... 945
Hytrin Capsules (At least 1%) ... 434
Imitrex Tablets ... 1099
▲ Intron A for Injection (Up to 10%) ... 2506
Iopidine 0.5% (Less than 1%) ... ⊚ 219
Klonopin Tablets ... 2294
Lamictal Tablets (Infrequent) ... 1105
Limbitrol ... 2333
Lioresal Intrathecal ... 1634
Loxitane ... 1426
Mavik Tablets (0.13%) ... 1407
Maxaquin Tablets (Less than 1%) ... 2593
NegGram ... 2453
Neupogen for Injection ... 495
Neurontin Capsules (Frequent) ... 1978
▲ Nipent for Injection (3% to 10%) ... 2733
Noroxin Tablets ... 1758
Noroxin Tablets ... 2222
Norpramin Tablets ... 1273
Norvir (Less than 2%) ... 447
Ocuflox Ophthalmic Solution ... 478
Oncaspar (Less than 1%) ... 2194
Orudis Capsules (Less than 1%) ... 2874
Oruvail Capsules (Less than 1%) ... 2874
OxyContin Tablets (Less than 1%) ... 2163
Pamelor ... 2409
Paxil Tablets (Infrequent) ... 2681
Pepcid Injection (Infrequent) ... 1765
Pepcid (Infrequent) ... 1763
Pergonal (menotropins for injection, USP) ... 2618
Permax Tablets (1.1%) ... 571
Platinol for Injection (Occasional) ... 717
Platinol-AQ Injection (Occasional) ... 719
Plendil Extended-Release Tablets (0.5% to 1.5%) ... 514
Ponstel ... 1982
Primaxin I.V. (Less than 0.2%) ... 1772
Prinivil Tablets (0.3% to 1.0%) ... 1776
Prinzide Tablets ... 1780
Procardia XL Extended Release Tablets (1% or less) ... 2026
Prozac Pulvules & Liquid, Oral Solution (Infrequent) ... 935
Redux Capsules ... 2911
Remeron Tablets (Infrequent) ... 1878
Rhinocort Nasal Inhaler (Less than 1%) ... 552
Rifadin ... 1276
Rifater ... 1280
Rilutek Tablets (Infrequent) ... 2198
Serzone Tablets (Infrequent) ... 776
Sular Tablets (Less than or equal to 1%) ... 2961
Sulfamylon Cream ... 940
Surmontil Capsules ... 2917
Talacen Caplets (Rare) ... 2464

Talwin Injection (Rare) ... 2465
Talwin Compound (Rare) ... 2466
Talwin Injection (Rare) ... 2465
Talwin Nx Tablets ... 2467
Thyro-Block Tablets (A few people) ... 2785
Tofranil Ampuls ... 873
Tofranil Tablets ... 875
Tofranil-PM Capsules ... 876
Torecan ... 2367
Triavil Tablets ... 1800
VePesid Capsules and Injection (Sometimes) ... 727
▲ Vesanoid Capsules (6%) ... 2327
Videx Tablets, Powder for Oral Solution, & Pediatric Powder for Oral Solution (Less than 1%) ... 2980
Vistide Injection ... 1057
Zestoretic Tablets ... 2968
Zestril Tablets (0.3% to 1.0%) ... 2972
Zoloft Tablets (Infrequent) ... 2051
Zyloprim Tablets (Less than 1%) ... 1194
Zyrtec Tablets (Less than 2%) ... 2053

Edema, fibrinous
Blenoxane ... 697

Edema, genital
Cerebyx Injection (Infrequent) ... 1956
Doxil (Less than 1%) ... 2613
Estring Vaginal Ring (At least 1 report) ... 2086

Edema, heart failure
(see under Congestive heart failure)

Edema, laryngeal
Activase (Very rare) ... 1045
Antivenin (Crotalidae) Polyvalent ... 2803
Axid Pulvules (Rare) ... 1468
Bicillin C-R Injection ... 2810
Bicillin C-R 900/300 Injection ... 2812
Bicillin L-A Injection ... 2813
Brontex (Infrequent) ... 2130
Capozide Tablets ... 744
Carbocaine Injection ... 2432
Cataflam Tablets (Less than 1%) ... 833
Cipro I.V. (1% or less) ... 587
Cipro Tablets (Less than 1%) ... 584
Compazine ... 2644
Etrafon ... 2495
Floxin I.V. ... 1580
Garamycin Injectable ... 2502
Hespan Injection ... 945
Intal Inhaler (Rare) ... 2185
Intal Nebulizer Solution (Rare) ... 2186
Levoprome ... 1321
Lopid Tablets ... 1974
Lotrel Capsules (About 0.5%) ... 858
Marcaine (Rare) ... 2446
Marcaine Spinal (Rare) ... 2449
Mavik Tablets (0.13%) ... 1407
Maxaquin Tablets ... 2593
Mellaril ... 2398
Nardil ... 1977
Nescaine/Nescaine MPF ... 549
Nipent for Injection (Less than 3%) ... 2733
Nubain Injection (1% or less) ... 952
Orthoclone OKT3 Sterile Solution ... 1892
Orudis Capsules (Less than 1%) ... 2874
Oruvail Capsules (Less than 1%) ... 2874
Pen•Vee K ... 2879
Penetrex Tablets ... 2196
Pergonal (menotropins for injection, USP) ... 2618
Permax Tablets (Rare) ... 571
Phenergan with Codeine (Infrequent) ... 2883
Phenergan VC with Codeine ... 2888
Prinivil Tablets (0.3% to 1.0%) ... 1776
Prinzide Tablets (Rare) ... 1780
Prolixin ... 510
Prozac Pulvules & Liquid, Oral Solution (Rare) ... 935
Redux Capsules ... 2911
Reglan (Rare) ... 2243
Sensorcaine ... 554
Serentil ... 689
Stelazine ... 2692
Thioplex (Thiotepa For Injection) ... 1329
Thorazine ... 2701
Toradol ... 2319
Torecan ... 2367
Triavil Tablets ... 1800
Trilafon ... 2532
Vaseretic Tablets ... 1810
Vasotec I.V. ... 1814
Vasotec Tablets ... 1816
▲ Vesanoid Capsules (3%) ... 2327

Cataflam/Voltaren/Voltaren-XR (Less than 1%) ... 833
Zestoretic Tablets ... 2968
Zestril Tablets (0.3% to 1.0%) ... 2972

Edema, lesional
Oncaspar (Less than 1%) ... 2194

Edema, lips
Cipro I.V. (1% or less) ... 587
Cipro I.V. Pharmacy Bulk Package (Less than 1%) ... 590
Cipro Tablets (Less than 1%) ... 584
Cozaar Tablets (Rare) ... 1668
Ethmozine Tablets (Less than 2%) ... 2217
Imitrex Tablets ... 1099
Mavik Tablets (0.13%) ... 1407
▲ Oncaspar (Greater than 1% but less than 5%) ... 2194
Orthoclone OKT3 Sterile Solution ... 1892
Retrovir Capsules ... 1216
Retrovir I.V. Infusion ... 1221
Retrovir Syrup ... 1216

Edema, local
Anafranil Capsules (Up to 2%) ... 819
Cafergot ... 2376
Celestone Soluspan Suspension ... 2484
D.H.E. 45 Injection ... 2381
▲ EMLA Cream (6% to 56%) ... 536
Ergomar Tablets ... 1543
Furacin Soluble Dressing (Approximately 1%) ... 2220
Furacin Topical Cream (Approximately 1%) ... 2220
Havrix (Rare) ... 2663
Oncaspar ... 2194
▲ Prostep (nicotine transdermal system) (8%) ... 1439
Retin-A (tretinoin) Cream/Gel/Liquid ... 1947
Wigraine Tablets ... 1884
Zovirax Ointment 5% ... 1190

Edema, lower extremities
▲ Cardene Capsules (7.1% to 8.0%) ... 2261
▲ Cardene SR Capsules (4.4% to 5.9%) ... 2264
Cipro I.V. Pharmacy Bulk Package (Less than 1%) ... 590
Eldepryl Capsules ... 2729
Eminase ... 2215
Estring Vaginal Ring (1% to 3%) ... 2086
Foscavir Injection (Less than 1%) ... 541
Ganite ... 2711
Miacalcin Injection ... 2402
Monopril Tablets (0.4% to 1.0%) ... 762
Parlodel ... 2411
Pondimin Tablets ... 2239
▲ Procardia Capsules (About 1 in 10 patients) ... 2024
Redux Capsules ... 2911
Sansert Tablets ... 2424
Taxotere for Injection Concentrate ... 2204
Zyrtec Tablets (Less than 2%) ... 2053

Edema, macular
Clomid ... 1262
Retrovir Capsules (A single case) ... 1216
Retrovir I.V. Infusion (A single case) ... 1221
Retrovir Syrup (A single case) ... 1216

Edema, nasal
▲ Atrovent Nasal Spray 0.03% (3.1%) ... 676

Edema, non-specific
(see under Edema)

Edema, oropharyngeal
Airet Albuterol Sulfate Inhalation Solution (Rare) ... 1602
Albuterol Sulfate, USP Solution for Inhalation, Arm-a-Med (Rare) ... 522
Anafranil Capsules (Rare) ... 819
Atrovent Nasal Spray 0.06% (Rare) ... 678
Cataflam Tablets (Less than 1%) ... 833
Cipro I.V. (1% or less) ... 587
Cipro Tablets (Less than 1%) ... 584
Procardia Capsules (Less than 0.5%) ... 2024
Proventil Inhalation Aerosol (Rare) ... 2524
Proventil Inhalation Solution 0.083% (Rare) ... 2527
Proventil Solution for Inhalation 0.5% (Rare) ... 2525
Proventil Syrup (Rare) ... 2528
Ventolin Inhalation Aerosol and Refill (Rare) ... 1170

(▄ Described in PDR For Nonprescription Drugs)   Incidence data in parenthesis; ▲ 3% or more   (⊚ Described in PDR For Ophthalmology)

Edema, oropharyngeal — Side Effects Index — 1324

Ventolin Inhalation Solution (Rare) 1171
Ventolin Nebules Inhalation Solution (Rare) 1172
Ventolin Rotacaps for Inhalation (Rare) 1173
Ventolin Syrup (Rare) 1175
Ventolin Tablets (Rare) 1176
Volmax Extended-Release Tablets (Rare) 1835
Cataflam/Voltaren/Voltaren-XR (Less than 1%) 833

Edema, palpebral

▲ AKTOB (Among most frequent; less than 3 of 100 patients) ⊙ 207
Alomide Ophthalmic Solution (Less than 1%) 465
Aralen Phosphate Tablets 2431
Aredia for Injection (One patient) 827
Betoptic Ophthalmic Solution (Rare) 465
Betoptic S Ophthalmic Suspension 467
Cipro I.V. (1% or less) 587
Cipro I.V. Pharmacy Bulk Package (Less than 1%) 590
Cortisporin Ophthalmic Ointment Sterile 1074
Crixivan Capsules (Less than 2%) 1670
Crolom (Infrequent) ⊙ 254
DDAVP (Up to 2%) 2180
Desmopressin Acetate Rhinal Tube (Up to 2%) 997
Feldene Capsules (Less than 1%) 2008
Imitrex Tablets 1099
Iopidine 0.5% (Less than 3%) ⊙ 219
Livostin (Approximately 1% to 3%) ⊙ 262
Mavik Tablets 1407
Monopril Tablets 762
▲ Ocupress Ophthalmic Solution, 1% Sterile (About 1 of 4 patients) ⊙ 297
Orthoclone OKT3 Sterile Solution 1892
▲ Polysporin Ophthalmic Ointment Sterile (Among those occurring most often) 1140
Prinzide Tablets 1780
ProSom Tablets (Infrequent) 457
Quadrinal Tablets 1398
ReVia Tablets (Less than 1%) 957
Vaseretic Tablets 1810
Vasotec Tablets 1816
Viroptic Ophthalmic Solution, 1% Sterile (2.8%) 1177

Edema, penile

Caverject Injection (1%) 2064

Edema, periorbital (see under Edema, peripheral)

Edema, peripheral

▲ Adalat Capsules (10 mg and 20 mg) (7% to about 10%) 580
▲ Adalat CC (18% to 29%) 582
AeroBid Inhaler System (1% to 3%) 1004
Aerobid-M Inhaler System (1% to 3%) 1004
Ambien Tablets (Rare) 2559
Anaprox/Naprosyn (Some patients) 2277
▲ Arimidex Tablets (5.3% to 8.5%) 2932
▲ Asacol Delayed-Release Tablets (3%) 2129
Azulfidine (Rare) 2059
Betimol 0.25%, 0.5% (1% to 5%) ⊙ 259
Cardene I.V. (Rare) 2815
Cardizem SR Capsules (Infrequent) 1255
Cardizem Tablets (Infrequent) 1257
Cartrol Tablets (1.7%) 413
▲ Casodex Tablets (8%) 2934
▲ CellCept Capsules (27.0% to 28.6%) 2265
Celontin Kapseals 1955
Ceredase 1055
Claritin Tablets (Rare) 2485
Claritin-D Tablets (Less frequent) 2487
Clozaril Tablets 2377
Cognex Capsules (Frequent) 1961
Compazine 2644
Crixivan Capsules (Less than 2%) 1670
Demser Capsules (Rare) 1690
Depakote Tablets (1% to 5%) 418
Dilacor XR Extended-release Capsules (2.2% to 2.3%) 2183
Dipentum Capsules (Rare) 2084
Dynabac (0.1% to 1%) 668
▲ DynaCirc CR Tablets (9% to 36%) 2383
EC-Naprosyn Delayed-Release Tablets (Some patients) 2277
Effexor (Frequent) 2825
Eldepryl Capsules 2729
Emcyt Capsules 2085
Ergamisol Tablets (Less frequent) 1340
Ethmozine Tablets (Less than 2%) 2217
Etrafon 2495
Fansidar Tablets 2281
Feldene Capsules (Approximately 2%) 2008
Foscavir Injection (Less than 1%) 541
Gantanol Tablets 2285
▲ Gemzar for Injection (20%) 1482
Hespan Injection 945
Humatrope Vials (Infrequent) 1490
▲ Hylorel Tablets (28.6%) 1613
Hyskon Hysteroscopy Fluid (Rare) 1633
▲ Hytrin Capsules (0.6% to 5.5%) 434
Imitrex Tablets 1099
Infumorph 200 and Infumorph 500 Sterile Solutions (Several reports) 985
Intron A for Injection (Less than or equal to 5%) 2506
Iopidine 0.5% (Less than 1%) ⊙ 219
Kadian Capsules (Less than 3%) 2948
Lamictal Tablets (Infrequent) 1105
▲ Leukine (11% to 15%) 1317
Levoprome 1321
Lioresal Intrathecal (Up to 3.3%) 1634
Lopressor (1%) 848
Lotensin Tablets 852
▲ Lovenox Injection (3%) 2187
Lupron Depot-PED 7.5 mg, 11.25 mg and 15 mg (Less than 2%) 2744
▲ Lupron Injection (5% or more) 2736
Lupron Injection Pediatric (Less than 2%) 2737
Megace Oral Suspension (1% to 3%) 708
Mellaril 2398
Merrem I.V. (0.1% to 1.0%) 2952
Miacalcin Nasal Spray (Less than 1%) 2403
Miltown Tablets 2780
▲ Nalfon 200 Pulvules & Nalfon Tablets (5%) 933
Naprelan Tablets (Less than 3%) 2861
Anaprox/Naprosyn (Some patients) 2277
Navane Capsules and Concentrate 2018
Navane Intramuscular 2019
Neurontin Capsules (1.7%) 1978
Nicotrol NS Nicotine Nasal Spray (Less than 1%) 1565
▲ Nipent for Injection (3% to 10%) 2733
Nolvadex Tablets (Infrequent) 2957
Norvir (Less than 2%) 447
Nutropin (Infrequent) 1049
Nutropin AQ Injection (Infrequent) 1051
▲ Oncaspar (Greater than 1% but less than 5%) 2194
Orap Tablets 1037
Orudis Capsules (Approximately 2%) 2874
Oruvail Capsules (Approximately 2%) 2874
OxyContin Tablets (Less than 1%) 2163
Paxil Tablets (Infrequent) 2681
Pediazole Suspension 2340
Pepcid Injection (Infrequent) 1765
Pepcid (Infrequent) 1763
▲ Permax Tablets (7.4%) 571
▲ Plendil Extended-Release Tablets (2.0% to 17.4%) 514
PMB 200 and PMB 400 2890
Prilosec Delayed-Release Capsules (Less than 1%) 516
Prinivil Tablets (0.3% to 1.0%) 1776
Prinzide Tablets 1780
▲ Procardia Capsules (7% to approximately 10%; about 1 in 8 to about 1 in 25 patients) 2024
▲ Procardia XL Extended Release Tablets (1% or less to about 30%) 2026
▲ Prograf (10% to 26%) 1028
Prolixin 510
Protropin (Infrequent) 1053
Prozac Pulvules & Liquid, Oral Solution (Infrequent) 935
Remeron Tablets (2%) 1878
ReoPro Vials (1.6%) 1526
▲ Rilutek Tablets (3.3% to 4.2%) 2198
Rowasa (0.61%) 2727
Sansert Tablets 2424
▲ Serzone Tablets (3%) 776
Stelazine 2692
▲ Sular Tablets (22%) 2961
Symmetrel Capsules (1% to 5%) 965
▲ Symmetrel Syrup (1% to 5%) 963
▲ Taxotere for Injection Concentrate (6%) 2204
Thorazine 2701
▲ Tiazac Capsules (8%) 1019
Tolectin (200, 400 and 600 mg) (Some patients) 1591
Toprol-XL Tablets (About 1 of 100 patients) 560
Torecan 2367
▲ Trasylol (3%) 607
Triavil Tablets 1800
Trilafon 2532
Univasc Tablets (More than 1%) 2553
▲ Vesanoid Capsules (52%) 2327
Videx Tablets, Powder for Oral Solution, & Pediatric Powder for Oral Solution (Less than 1%) 2980
▲ Zebeta Tablets (3.0% to 3.7%) 1457
Zestoretic Tablets 2968
Zestril Tablets (0.3% to 1.0%) 2972
Ziac (0.9% to 1.1%) 1459
▲ Zoladex (21%) 2976
Zoladex 3-month (1% to 5%) 2978
Zoloft Tablets (Infrequent) 2051
Zovirax 1187
Zyrtec Tablets (Less than 2%) 2053

Edema, pharyngeal

Avonex 662
Cipro Tablets 584
Maxaquin Tablets 2593
NegGram 2453
Noroxin Tablets 1758
Noroxin Tablets 2222

Edema, pulmonary

Abelcet Injection 1540
Activase 1045
Adalat Capsules (10 mg and 20 mg) (About 2%) 580
Aldoclor Tablets 1638
Aldoril Tablets 1644
Ambien Tablets (Rare) 2559
Apresazide Capsules 824
Betapace Tablets (Rare) 637
Betaseron for SC Injection 653
Blocadren Tablets 1654
Brevibloc (esmolol HCl) Injection (Less than 1%) 1860
Calan SR Caplets (1.8%) 2571
Calan Tablets (1.8%) 2568
▲ CellCept Capsules (More than or equal to 3%) 2265
Cipro I.V. (1% or less) 587
Cipro I.V. Pharmacy Bulk Package (Less than 1%) 590
Cipro Tablets (Less than 1%) 584
Clomid 1262
Cognex Capsules (Rare) 1961
Cordarone Intravenous (Less than 2%) 2821
Covera-HS Tablets (1.8% to 2%) 2573
Cytosar-U Sterile Powder 2077
Dantrium Intravenous (Rare) 2132
Diprivan Injectable Emulsion (Rare) 2939
Diupres Tablets 1691
Diuril Oral Suspension 1694
Diuril Sodium Intravenous 1693
Diuril Tablets 1694
Dyazide Capsules 2653
▲ Eminase (Less than 10%) 2215
Enduron Tablets 424
Esidrix Tablets 839
Esimil Tablets 840
Floxin I.V. 1580
Floxin Tablets (200 mg, 300 mg, 400 mg) 1577
Fungizone Intravenous 507
HydroDIURIL Tablets 1716
Hydropres Tablets 1718
Hyskon Hysteroscopy Fluid (Rare; 0.11% to 1.4%) 1633
Hyzaar Tablets 1720
Indocin Capsules (Less than 1%) 1723
Indocin I.V. (Less than 1%) 1727
Indocin (Less than 1%) 1723
Inversine Tablets 1729
Isoptin Oral Tablets (1.8%) 1393
Isoptin SR Tablets (1.8%) 1395
Isuprel Injection 2441
Lopressor HCT Tablets 850
Lotensin HCT Tablets 855
Maxaquin Tablets 2593
Moduretic Tablets 1748
Mutamycin for Injection 712
Nalfon 200 Pulvules & Nalfon Tablets (Less than 1%) 933
Naprelan Tablets (Less than 1%) 2861
Narcan Injection (Several instances) 950
Neurontin Capsules (Rare) 1978
Nubain Injection (1% or less) 952
Oretic Tablets 450
Orthoclone OKT3 Sterile Solution (Less than 2%) 1892
Paxil Tablets (Rare) 2681
Penetrex Tablets 2196
Permax Tablets (Infrequent) 571
Placidyl Capsules 456
Prinivil Tablets (Greater than 1%) 1776
Prinzide Tablets 1780
Procardia Capsules (About 2%) 2024
Procardia XL Extended Release Tablets (About 2%) 2026
▲ Prograf (Greater than 3%) 1028
▲ Proleukin for Injection (Less than 1% to 10%) 812
Protamine Sulfate Vials 1526
Prozac Pulvules & Liquid, Oral Solution (Rare) 935
Redux Capsules 2911
ReoPro Vials (1.5%) 1526
Rilutek Tablets (Infrequent) 2198
▲ Roferon-A Injection (9%) 2308
Ser-Ap-Es Tablets 867
Taxotere for Injection Concentrate (Rare) 2204
Timolide Tablets 1791
Timoptic in Ocudose (Less frequent) 1796
Timoptic Sterile Ophthalmic Solution (Less frequent) 1794
Timoptic-XE 1798
Tonocard Tablets (Less than 1%) 519
Toradol (1% or less) 2319
Trasylol (1.2%) 607
Vaseretic Tablets 1810
Vasotec I.V. 1814
Vasotec Tablets (0.5% to 1.0%) 1816
Verelan Capsules (1.8%) 1455
▲ Vesanoid Capsules (3%) 2327
Virazole (Infrequent) 1310
Yutopar Intravenous Injection 566
Zestoretic Tablets 2968
Zestril Tablets (Greater than 1%) 2972
Ziac 1459
Zosyn (1.0% or less) 1463
Zovirax Sterile Powder (Less than 1%) 1191

Edema, pulmonary, non-cardiogenic

Hespan Injection 945
Kadian Capsules (Less than 3%) 2948
Streptase for Infusion (Rare) 557

Edema, retinal

Aralen Phosphate Tablets 2431
Lopid Tablets 1974
Plaquenil Sulfate Tablets 2459

Edema, scrotal

Caverject Injection (Less than 1%) 2064
Intron A for Injection (Less than or equal to 5%) 2506

Edema, skin (see under Edema, angioneurotic)

Edema, tongue

Antivenin (Crotalidae) Polyvalent 2803
Cataflam Tablets (Less than 1%) 833
Cerebyx Injection (Infrequent) 1956
Cozaar Tablets (Rare) 1668
Effexor (Infrequent) 2825
Elavil 2945
Ethmozine Tablets (Less than 2%) 2217
Etopophos for Injection (Sometimes) 701
Etoposide Injection (Sometimes) 539
Etrafon 2495
Flexeril Tablets (Less than 1%) 1701
Flonase Nasal Spray 1088
Lamictal Tablets (Rare) 1105
Limbitrol 2333
Mavik Tablets (0.13%) 1407
Norpramin Tablets 1273
Pamelor 2409
Paxil Tablets (Rare) 2681
Prozac Pulvules & Liquid, Oral Solution (Rare) 935
Reglan 2243
Remeron Tablets (Rare) 1878
Retrovir Capsules 1216
Retrovir I.V. Infusion 1221
Retrovir Syrup 1216
Risperdal Tablets (Rare) 1348
Surmontil Capsules 2917
Tofranil Ampuls 873

(Described in PDR For Nonprescription Drugs)   Incidence data in parenthesis; ▲ 3% or more   (⊙ Described in PDR For Ophthalmology)

Side Effects Index

Tofranil Tablets	875
Tofranil-PM Capsules	876
Toradol	2319
Triavil Tablets	1800
VePesid Capsules and Injection (Sometimes)	727
Cataflam/Voltaren/Voltaren-XR (Less than 1%)	833
Zoloft Tablets (Rare)	2051
Zyloprim Tablets (Less than 1%)	1194
Zyrtec Tablets (Less than 2%)	2053

Efficacy, lack of
Neoral (1.4%)	2405

Ejaculation, inhibition
Demser Capsules (Infrequent)	1690
Dibenzyline Capsules	2650
Esimil Tablets	840
Etrafon	2495
Ismelin Tablets	845
Lioresal Tablets (Rare)	847
▲ LUVOX Tablets (8%)	2723
Mellaril	2398
Normodyne Injection (Up to 5%)	2519
▲ Normodyne Tablets (Up to 5%)	2522
Parnate Tablets	2679
▲ Paxil Tablets (3.7% to 10.0%)	2681
Serentil	689
▲ Trandate Tablets (Up to 5%)	1158
Triavil Tablets	1800
Trilafon	2532
Wellbutrin Tablets (Infrequent)	1177

Ejaculation, premature
Anafranil Capsules (Rare)	819
Bumex (0.1%)	2260

Ejaculation disturbances
Amicar Syrup, Tablets, and Injection	1312
▲ Anafranil Capsules (6% to 42%)	819
Asendin Tablets (Less than 1%)	1419
BuSpar Tablets (Rare)	738
Caverject Injection (Less than 1%)	2064
Clozaril Tablets (1%)	2377
Compazine	2644
Desyrel and Desyrel Dividose	504
▲ Effexor (3% to 12.5%)	2825
▲ Hylorel Tablets (7.0%)	1613
Lamictal Tablets (Rare)	1105
Lioresal Intrathecal (1% or more)	1634
▲ LUVOX Tablets (8%)	2723
Nardil	1977
Neurontin Capsules (Infrequent)	1978
Norpramin Tablets	1273
▲ Orlaam Oral Solution (3% to 9%)	2361
▲ Paxil Tablets (1.6% to 23%)	2681
Proscar Tablets (2.8%)	1784
Prozac Pulvules & Liquid, Oral Solution (Infrequent)	935
Redux Capsules	2911
Remeron Tablets (Rare)	1878
▲ ReVia Tablets (Less than 10%)	957
Risperdal Tablets (Infrequent)	1348
Serzone Tablets (Infrequent)	776
Stelazine	2692
Surmontil Capsules	2917
Thorazine	2701
▲ Trandate Injection (Up to 5%)	1158
Wellbutrin Tablets (Rare)	1177

Ejection fraction reduction
Adriamycin PFS	2056
Adriamycin RDF	2056
Novantrone for Injection	1327

Elastosis perforans, serpiginosa
Cuprimine Capsules (Rare)	1673
Depen Titratable Tablets (Rare)	2770

Elation
▲ Marinol (Dronabinol) Capsules (8% to 24%)	2353

Electrocardiographic changes
(see under EKG changes)

Electroencephalographic changes
(see under EEG changes)

Electrolyte disturbances
(see under Electrolyte imbalance)

Electrolyte imbalance
Aldactone Tablets	2558
Aldoclor Tablets	1638
Aldoril Tablets	1644
Apresazide Capsules	824

Atromid-S Capsules	2808
Capastat Sulfate Injection (1 patient)	968
Capozide Tablets	744
Celestone Soluspan Suspension	2484
CORTENEMA	2713
Cytosar-U Sterile Powder (Less than 7 patients)	2077
Dalalone D.P. Injectable	1009
Daranide Tablets	1676
Decadron Elixir	1676
Decadron Phosphate Injection	1680
Decadron Phosphate with Xylocaine Injection, Sterile	1683
Demadex Tablets and Injection	691
Diamox Intravenous	⊙ 317
Diamox Sequels (Sustained Release)	⊙ 318
Diamox Tablets	⊙ 317
Diupres Tablets	1691
Diuril Oral Suspension	1694
Diuril Sodium Intravenous	1693
Diuril Tablets	1694
Dyazide Capsules	2653
Enduron Tablets	424
Esidrix Tablets	839
▲ Foscavir Injection (5% or greater)	541
GlaucTabs	⊙ 209
Humegon for Injection	1873
HydroDIURIL Tablets	1716
Hydropres Tablets	1718
Lutrepulse for Injection	998
Macrobid Capsules	2138
Macrodantin Capsules	2140
Maxaquin Tablets (Less than or equal to 0.1%)	2593
Metrodin (urofollitropin for injection)	2616
Moduretic Tablets	1748
Neptazane Tablets	⊙ 320
Oretic Tablets	450
Permax Tablets (Rare)	571
Platinol for Injection	717
Platinol-AQ Injection	719
Pravachol Tablets	770
Prevacid Delayed-Release Capsules (Less than 1%)	2746
Prinzide Tablets	1780
Risperdal Tablets	1348
Serophene (clomiphene citrate tablets, USP)	2621
Sodium Polystyrene Sulfonate Suspension	2367
Tenoretic Tablets	2963
Thalitone (Common)	1293
Timolide Tablets	1791
Vaseretic Tablets	1810
Winstrol Tablets	2468
Zaroxolyn Tablets	1625
Zestoretic Tablets	2968
Zosyn	1463

Elevated bilirubin levels
(see under Hyperbilirubinemia)

Embolism
Activase	1045
Amen Tablets	785
Cycrin Tablets	991
Demadex Tablets and Injection	691
Desogen Tablets	1867
▲ Eminase (Less than 10%)	2215
Sterile FUDR	2284
Lasix Injection, Oral Solution and Tablets	1267
LUVOX Tablets (Rare)	2723
Metrodin (urofollitropin for injection)	2616
Ortho-Cept	1907
Ortho-Cyclen/Ortho-Tri-Cyclen	1914
Ortho-Cyclen/Ortho Tri-Cyclen	1914
Paraplatin for Injection	713
Premphase	2900
Prempro	2905
Provera Tablets	2110
Zosyn (1.0% or less)	1463

Embolism, arterial
Metrodin (urofollitropin for injection)	2616

Embolism, cholesterol
Activase (Rare)	1045

Embolism, limb
Felbatol	2774
ReoPro Vials (0.3%)	1526

Embolism, lower extremities
Rilutek Tablets (Infrequent)	2198

Embolism, pulmonary
Abelcet Injection	1540
Actimmune (Rare)	1043
Ambien Tablets (Rare)	2559
Amen Tablets	785
Amicar Syrup, Tablets, and Injection	1312
Avonex	662
Brevicon	2563
Cerebyx Injection (Infrequent)	1956
Cipro I.V. (1% or less)	587
Cipro I.V. Pharmacy Bulk Package (Less than 1%)	590
Cipro Tablets (Less than 1%)	584
Climara Transdermal System	640
Clomid	1262
Clozaril Tablets	2377
Cognex Capsules (Infrequent)	1961
Cycrin Tablets	991
Cytovene-IV (One report)	2270
Demulen	2580
Depo-Provera Contraceptive Injection (Fewer than 1%)	2079
Depo-Provera Sterile Aqueous Suspension	2083
Desogen Tablets	1867
Effexor (Rare)	2825
Emcyt Capsules (2%)	2085
Epogen for Injection (Rare)	489
Estrace Cream and Tablets	751
Estraderm Transdermal System	842
ESTRATAB Tablets (0.3, 0.625, 1.25, 2.5 mg)	2715
Estratest	2718
Ethmozine Tablets (Less than 2%)	2217
Foscavir Injection (Less than 1%)	541
Heparin Lock Flush Solution	2831
Heparin Sodium Injection	2832
Heparin Sodium Vials	1486
Humegon for Injection	1873
Imitrex Tablets	1099
Levlen/Tri-Levlen	646
Lioresal Intrathecal (1% or more)	1634
Lo/Ovral Tablets	2852
Lo/Ovral-28 Tablets	2857
Lupron Injection (Less than 5%)	2736
Maxaquin Tablets (Less than 1%)	2593
Megace Tablets (Rare)	710
Menest Tablets	2671
Merrem I.V. (0.1% to 1%)	2952
Metrodin (urofollitropin for injection)	2616
Modicon	1928
Mononine, Coagulation Factor IX (Human), Monoclonal Antibody Purified	804
Neurontin Capsules (Rare)	1978
Nipent for Injection (Less than 3%)	2733
Nolvadex Tablets (0.4%)	2957
Nordette-21 Tablets	2863
Nordette-28 Tablets	2866
Norinyl	2563
Norplant System	2868
Nor-Q D Tablets	2598
Ogen Tablets	2103
Ogen Vaginal Cream	2106
Ortho-Cept	1907
Ortho-Cyclen/Ortho-Tri-Cyclen	1914
Ortho Dienestrol Cream	1922
Ortho-Est	1925
Ortho-Novum	1928
Ortho-Cyclen/Ortho Tri-Cyclen	1914
Ovcon	765
Ovral Tablets	2877
Ovral-28 Tablets	2878
Ovrette Tablets	2878
Paxil Tablets (Rare)	2681
Permax Tablets (Infrequent)	571
PMB 200 and PMB 400	2890
Premarin Intravenous	2893
Premarin Tablets	2896
Premarin Vaginal Cream	2898
Premphase	2900
Prempro	2905
Prinivil Tablets (0.3% to 1.0%)	1776
Prinzide Tablets	1780
▲ Procrit for Injection (3.2%)	1896
Proleukin for Injection (Less than 1%)	812
Provera Tablets (Occasional)	2110
Prozac Pulvules & Liquid, Oral Solution	935
Redux Capsules (Rare)	2911
Remeron Tablets (Rare)	1878
ReoPro Vials (0.3%)	1526
Risperdal Tablets	1348
Scleromate Injection	1234
Serophene (clomiphene citrate tablets, USP) (Rare)	2621

Sotradecol (Sodium Tetradecyl Sulfate Injection) (One patient)	987
Taxol Injection (Rare)	723
Taxotere for Injection Concentrate	2204
Tenormin Tablets and I.V. Injection (1.2%)	2965
Tonocard Tablets (Less than 1%)	519
Levlen/Tri-Levlen	646
Tri-Norinyl	2607
Triphasil-21 Tablets	2919
Triphasil-28 Tablets	2924
Vaseretic Tablets	1810
Vasotec I.V.	1814
Vasotec Tablets (0.5% to 1.0%)	1816
Vivelle Transdermal System	880
Wellbutrin Tablets (Rare)	1177
Zestoretic Tablets	2968
Zestril Tablets (0.3% to 1.0%)	2972
Zoladex 3-month (1% to 5%)	2978
Zosyn (1.0% or less)	1463

Embolism, retinal artery
Xalatan (Extremely rare)	⊙ 304

Embryotoxicity
Methotrexate Sodium Tablets, Injection, for Injection and LPF Injection	1322
Mycelex Troches	601
Terramycin Intramuscular Solution	2034

Emergence delirium
Versed Injection (Less than 1%)	2324

Emesis
(see under Vomiting)

Emotional disturbances
Accutane Capsules	2252
CORTENEMA	2713
Depakene	416
Depakote Tablets	418
Efudex (Infrequent)	2280
Florinef Acetate Tablets	506
Lariam Tablets (Less than 1%)	2295
Mysoline (Occasional)	2860
Paxil Tablets (Infrequent)	2681
Phenobarbital Elixir and Tablets	1523
Plaquenil Sulfate Tablets	2459
Prelone Syrup	1834
Tofranil Tablets	875
▲ Yutopar Intravenous Injection (5% to 6%)	566
▲ Zonalon Cream (Approximately 1% to 10%)	1042

Emotional lability
Adenoscan (Less than 1%)	1022
Ambien Tablets (Infrequent)	2559
Anafranil Capsules (Up to 2%)	819
Asacol Delayed-Release Tablets	2129
Betapace Tablets (Rare)	637
Blocadren Tablets	1654
BuSpar Tablets (Rare)	738
Cardura Tablets (Less than 0.5% of 3960 patients)	1993
Cartrol Tablets	413
Cerebyx Injection (Infrequent)	1956
Claritin-D Tablets (Less frequent)	2487
Danocrine Capsules	2437
DaunoXome (Less than or equal to 5%)	1842
Depakote Tablets (1% to 5%)	418
Diprivan Injectable Emulsion (Less than 1%)	2939
Doxil (1% to 5%)	2613
Effexor (Frequent)	2825
Emcyt Capsules (2%)	2085
▲ Felbatol (6.5%)	2774
Floxin I.V.	1580
Floxin Tablets (200 mg, 300 mg, 400 mg)	1577
Foscavir Injection (Less than 1%)	541
Hivid Tablets (Less than 1%)	2287
IBU Tablets (Less than 1%)	1389
Inderal	2834
Inderal LA Long Acting Capsules	2836
Inderide Tablets	2838
Inderide LA Long Acting Capsules	2840
Intron A for Injection (Less than 5%)	2506
Kerlone Tablets (Less than 2%)	2588
Lamictal Tablets (1.3%)	1105
Levatol Tablets	2547
Lioresal Intrathecal (1% or more)	1634
Lopressor HCT Tablets	850
▲ Lupron Depot 3.75 mg (10.8%)	2739
Lupron Depot-PED 7.5 mg, 11.25 mg and 15 mg (Less than 2%)	2744
Lupron Injection Pediatric (Less than 2%)	2737

(⊞ Described in PDR For Nonprescription Drugs)   Incidence data in parenthesis; ▲ 3% or more   (⊙ Described in PDR For Ophthalmology)

Emotional lability Side Effects Index 1326

LUVOX Tablets (Infrequent) 2723
Monoket Tablets (Up to 2%) 2550
Motrin Ibuprofen Suspension, Oral Drops, Chewable Tablets, Caplets (Less than 1%) 1563
Naprelan Tablets (Less than 1%) .. 2861
Neurontin Capsules (More than 1%) 1978
▲ Nicotrol NS Nicotine Nasal Spray (Over 5%) 1565
Nipent for Injection (Less than 3%) 2733
Normodyne Tablets 2522
Norplant System (Less than 1%).... 2868
Norvir (Less than 2%) 447
Oncaspar (Less than 1%) 2194
OxyContin Tablets (Less than 1%) 2163
Paxil Tablets (Frequent) 2681
Pediapred Oral Solution 1618
Penetrex Tablets (Less than 0.1%) 2196
Permax Tablets (Infrequent)............ 571
▲ Prograf (Greater than 3%) 1028
ProSom Tablets (Infrequent) 457
Proventil Syrup (1%)............ 2528
Prozac Pulvules & Liquid, Oral Solution (Infrequent) 935
▲ Redux Capsules (3.1%) 2911
Remeron Tablets (Infrequent) 1878
Retrovir Capsules 1216
Retrovir I.V. Infusion............ 1221
Retrovir Syrup............ 1216
Rilutek Tablets (Infrequent) 2198
Risperdal Tablets (Rare)............ 1348
Roferon-A Injection (Less than 3%) 2308
Romazicon (1% to 3%) 2311
Sectral Capsules 2914
Serzone Tablets 776
▲ Synarel Nasal Solution for Central Precocious Puberty (6%) 2603
▲ Synarel Nasal Solution for Endometriosis (15% of patients) 2605
Tegison Capsules (Less than 1%) .. 2314
Tenoretic Tablets............ 2963
Tenormin Tablets and I.V. Injection 2965
Timolide Tablets............ 1791
Timoptic in Ocudose 1796
Timoptic Sterile Ophthalmic Solution 1794
Timoptic-XE 1798
Toprol-XL Tablets 560
Trandate Tablets 1158
▲ Ultram Tablets (50 mg) (7% to 14%) 1594
Ventolin Syrup (1% of children)...... 1175
Videx Tablets, Powder for Oral Solution, & Pediatric Powder for Oral Solution (Up to 1%)............ 2980
Visken Tablets............ 2428
Zebeta Tablets 1457
Ziac 1459
▲ Zoladex (60%) 2976
Zoladex 3-month 2978
Zoloft Tablets (Infrequent) 2051
Zyrtec Tablets (Less than 2%) 2053

Emphysema

Avonex 662
▲ Exosurf Neonatal for Intratracheal Suspension (7% to 44%) 1081
Paxil Tablets (Rare)............ 2681
Permax Tablets (Infrequent)............ 571

Encephalitis

Attenuvax 1650
Biavax II 1653
Cerebyx Injection (Infrequent) 1956
Cognex Capsules (Rare)............ 1961
JE-VAX (1 to 2.3 per million vaccines) 904
M-M-R II (Very rare)............ 1730
M-R-VAX II (Rare)............ 1732
Mumpsvax (Very rare)............ 1751
Nipent for Injection (Less than 3%) 2733
Orthoclone OKT3 Sterile Solution .. 1892
Solganal Suspension............ 2530
Varivax 1807
Videx Tablets, Powder for Oral Solution, & Pediatric Powder for Oral Solution (Less than 1%)............ 2980

Encephalomyelitis

JE-VAX (Two cases.)............ 904

Encephalopathy

Abelcet Injection............ 1540
Acel-Imune Diphtheria and Tetanus Toxoids and Acellular Pertussis Vaccine Adsorbed 1415
Anafranil Capsules (Infrequent) 819
Betaseron for SC Injection............ 653
Bumex (0.6%) 2260
Ceptaz 1070
Cerebyx Injection (Infrequent)............ 1956
Cytovene-IV (Two or more reports) 2270
Depakene (Rare) 416
Depakote Tablets (Rare instances) 418
Diphtheria and Tetanus Toxoids and Pertussis Vaccine Adsorbed.. 2650
Ergamisol Tablets 1340
Felbatol 2774
Fortaz 1092
Foscavir Injection (Less than 1%) .. 541
Fungizone Intravenous 507
Garamycin Injectable 2502
Havrix (Rare)............ 2663
Influenza Virus Vaccine, Trivalent, Types A and B (chromatograph- and filter-purified subviron antigen) FluShield, 1996-1997 Formula 2842
JE-VAX (1 to 2.3 per million vaccines) 904
Lariam Tablets 2295
Lithonate/Lithotabs/Lithobid............ 2721
M-M-R II (Very rare) 1730
M-R-VAX II (Once for every million doses) 1732
Maxipime for Injection............ 758
Methotrexate Sodium Tablets, Injection, for Injection and LPF Injection 1322
Midamor Tablets (Between 1% and 3%) 1746
Moduretic Tablets 1748
MSTA Mumps Skin Test Antigen 2988
Netromycin Injection 100 mg/ml... 2516
Neurontin Capsules (Rare) 1978
Orthoclone OKT3 Sterile Solution .. 1892
PASER Granules............ 1333
Primaxin I.M. 1770
Primaxin I.V. (Less than 0.2%) 1772
Redux Capsules 2911
Roferon-A Injection (Infrequent) 2308
Streptomycin Sulfate Injection............ 2031
Tapazole Tablets (Rare) 1361
Tazidime Vials, Faspak & ADD-Vantage 1531
Tetramune (Rare) 1449
Tri-Immunol Adsorbed (Rare) 1452
Tripedia 908
▲ Vesanoid Capsules (3%) 2327
Videx Tablets, Powder for Oral Solution, & Pediatric Powder for Oral Solution (Less than 1%)............ 2980
Zovirax Sterile Powder (Approximately 1%)............ 1191

Encephalopathy, hepatic

Eulexin Capsules 2498
Intron A for Injection (Very rare)...... 2506
Prilosec Delayed-Release Capsules (Rare) 516
Taxol Injection (Rare)............ 723

Encephalopathy, hypertensive

Catapres-TTS (Rare) 680
Combipres Tablets 682
Epogen for Injection (On occasion) 489
Procrit for Injection (Occasional) 1896

Encephalopathy, toxic

Nydrazid Injection (Uncommon)...... 509
Rifamate Capsules (Uncommon) 1278
Rifater (Uncommon)............ 1280

Endocardial fibrosis

Myleran Tablets (One case) 1209

Endocarditis

Betaseron for SC Injection............ 653
Cytovene-IV (One report)............ 2270
Oncaspar (Less than 1%) 2194
Proleukin for Injection (1%)............ 812

Endocrine disturbances

▲ Cleocin Vaginal Cream (4%) 2070
Compazine 2644
Levoprome 1321
Norplant System 2868
Permax Tablets (Rare) 571
Pravachol Tablets 770
Stelazine 2692

Endometrial carcinoma (see under Carcinoma, endometrial)

Endometrial hyperplasia

Anafranil Capsules (Rare) 819
Nolvadex Tablets 2957
Ogen Vaginal Cream............ 2106

Endometriosis

Anafranil Capsules (Infrequent) 819
Clomid 1262
Nolvadex Tablets (A few reports).... 2957

Endometritis

▲ Cleocin Vaginal Cream (5%) 2070
ParaGard T 380A Intrauterine Copper Contraceptive 1936
Prostin E2 Suppository............ 2109

Endophthalmitis

AdatoSil 5000 (Less than 2%).... ◉ 265
Healon GV............ ◉ 303
ISPAN Perfluoropropane .... ◉ 267
ISPAN Sulfur Hexafluoride............ ◉ 266

Endotracheal tube occlusion

Survanta Beractant Intratracheal Suspension (Less than 1%) 2346

Endotracheal tube, reflux into

Exosurf Neonatal for Intratracheal Suspension............ 1081
Survanta Beractant Intratracheal Suspension (Less than 1%) 2346

Energy, high

Axocet Capsules (Infrequent)............ 2469
Eldepryl Capsules 2729
Esgic-plus Capsules (Infrequent) 1012
Esgic-plus Tablets (Infrequent) 1012
Fioricet Tablets (Infrequent)............ 2386
Fioricet with Codeine Capsules (Infrequent) 2387
Fiorinal with Codeine Capsules (Infrequent) 2390
Phrenilin (Infrequent)............ 790
▲ ReVia Tablets (Less than 10%) 957
Sedapap Tablets 50 mg/650 mg (Infrequent) 1826

Energy, loss of

Demulen 2580
Levlen/Tri-Levlen 646
▲ Minipress Capsules (6.9%) 2015
▲ Minizide Capsules (6.9%)............ 2016
Modicon............ 1928
Ortho-Cyclen/Ortho-Tri-Cyclen 1914
Ortho-Novum............ 1928
Ortho-Cyclen/Ortho Tri-Cyclen 1914
▲ ReVia Tablets (More than 10%)...... 957
Levlen/Tri-Levlen............ 646

Enteritis

Ambien Tablets (Rare) 2559
Anafranil Capsules (Rare) 819
Betaseron for SC Injection............ 653
Felbatol 2774
Foscavir Injection (Less than 1%) .. 541
▲ Sterile FUDR (Among more common)............ 2284
Lamprene Capsules (Less than 1%)............ 846
Methotrexate Sodium Tablets, Injection, for Injection and LPF Injection 1322
Paxil Tablets (Rare) 2681
Prozac Pulvules & Liquid, Oral Solution (Rare) 935
Redux Capsules (Infrequent) 2911

Enteritis, staphylococci

Furoxone 2221

Enterocolitis

Achromycin V Capsules (Rare) 1417
Augmentin 2637
Augmentin Tablets 2640
Chloromycetin Sodium Succinate.... 1960
Declomycin Tablets............ 1421
Doryx Capsules............ 1970
DYNACIN Capsules............ 1627
Foscavir Injection (Less than 1%) .. 541
Helidac Therapy............ 2135
Indocin I.V. (Less than 3%)............ 1727
Leucovorin Calcium Tablets, Wellcovorin Brand 1204
Minocin Intravenous............ 1428
Minocin Oral Suspension 1431
Minocin Pellet-Filled Capsules 1429
Monodox Capsules 1858
Myochrysine Injection (Rare) 1754
Omnipen Capsules 2872
Omnipen for Oral Suspension 2873
ProSom Tablets (Rare) 457
Spectrobid Tablets 2030
Terramycin Intramuscular Solution 2034
Unasyn 2035
Vibramycin 2038
Vibramycin Hyclate Intravenous 2040
Vibramycin 2038

Enterocolitis with perforation

Idamycin Injection (Rare)............ 2096

Enterocolitis, hemorrhagic

Velban Vials 1537

Enterocolitis, necrotizing

▲ Exosurf Neonatal for Intratracheal Suspension (2% to 13%) 1081
▲ Survanta Beractant Intratracheal Suspension (6.1%)............ 2346

Enterocolitis, neutropenic

Azulfidine (Rare) 2059

Enterocolitis, ulcerative

Ridaura Capsules (Less than 1%) .. 2691
Solganal Suspension (Rare) 2530

Entropion

BOTOX (Botulinum Toxin Type A) Purified Neurotoxin Complex (Less than 1%)............ 473

Enuresis

BuSpar Tablets (Rare)............ 738
Depakene 416
Depakote Tablets............ 418
Klonopin Tablets 2294
Lioresal Tablets (Rare) 847
Mintezol............ 1747
Serentil............ 689
Wellbutrin Tablets (Rare)............ 1177

Eosinophilia

Abelcet Injection............ 1540
Achromycin V Capsules 1417
Adapin Capsules (A few patients).... 1542
Altace Capsules (Scattered incidents; less than 1%)............ 1238
Amikacin Sulfate Injection, USP (Rare) 523
Amikacin Sulfate Injection, USP (Rare) 981
Amikin Injectable (Rare)............ 502
Amoxil............ 2631
Anaprox/Naprosyn (Less than 1%)............ 2277
Ancef Injection 2632
Ancobon Capsules............ 2254
Apresazide Capsules (Less frequent)............ 824
Apresoline Hydrochloride Tablets (Less frequent)............ 826
Asacol Delayed-Release Tablets 2129
Asendin Tablets (Very rare) 1419
Atretol Tablets 569
Atromid-S Capsules 2808
Augmentin 2637
Augmentin Tablets 2640
▲ Avonex (5%)............ 662
Axid Pulvules (Rare)............ 1468
Azactam for Injection............ 736
Azulfidine (Rare) 2059
Bactrim DS Tablets............ 2257
Bactrim I.V. Infusion............ 2255
Bactrim 2257
Beclovent Inhalation Aerosol and Refill 1063
Betapace Tablets (Rare)............ 637
Bicillin C-R Injection 2810
Bicillin C-R 900/300 Injection 2812
Bicillin L-A Injection 2813
BuSpar Tablets (Rare)............ 738
▲ Capastat Sulfate Injection (Majority of patients)............ 968
▲ Capoten Tablets (About 4 to 7 of 100 patients) 740
Capozide Tablets (Sometimes) 744
Cataflam Tablets (Rare) 833
Ceclor Pulvules & Suspension (1 in 50)............ 1470
▲ Cedax (3%) 2480
Cefizox for Intramuscular or Intravenous Use (1% to 5%)............ 1025
▲ Cefobid Intravenous/Intramuscular (1 in 10) 1996
▲ Cefobid Pharmacy Bulk Package - Not for Direct Infusion (1 in 10).. 1999
Cefotan (1 in 200)............ 2936
Ceftin (0.1% to 1%)............ 1067
Cefzil Tablets and Oral Suspension (2.3%)............ 747
Celontin Kapseals 1955
Ceptaz (One in 13)............ 1070
Chemet Capsules (0.5% to 1.5%) 666
▲ Cipro I.V. (Among most frequent) .. 587

(Described in PDR For Nonprescription Drugs) Incidence data in parenthesis; ▲ 3% or more (◉ Described in PDR For Ophthalmology)

▲ Cipro I.V. Pharmacy Bulk Package (Among most frequent) 590
Cipro Tablets (0.6%; rare) 584
Claforan Sterile and Injection (Less than 1% to 2.4%) 1259
Cleocin Phosphate Injection 2068
Cleocin Vaginal Cream 2070
Clinoril Tablets (Less than 1 in 100) 1658
Clozaril Tablets (1%) 2377
Compazine 2644
Cuprimine Capsules 1673
Cytosar-U Sterile Powder (Less than 7 patients) 2077
Cytovene (1% or less) 2270
Danocrine Capsules 2437
Daypro Caplets (Rare) 2578
Declomycin Tablets 1421
Demser Capsules (Rare) 1690
Depakene 416
Depakote Tablets 418
Depen Titratable Tablets 2770
Diabinese Tablets 2002
Dilantin Infatabs 1967
Dilantin Kapseals 1965
Dilantin-125 Suspension 1969
Dipentum Capsules (Rare) 2084
Dobutrex Solution Vials (Occasional) 1480
Dolobid Tablets (Less than 1 in 100) 1695
Doryx Capsules 1970
Doxil (Less than 1%) 2613
Duricef Capsules, Tablets, and Oral Suspension 750
Dynabac (1.2%) 668
DYNACIN Capsules 1627
EC-Naprosyn Delayed-Release Tablets (Less than 1%) 2277
Effexor (Rare) 2825
Efudex 2280
Elavil 2945
Eminase (Occasional) 2215
Etrafon 2495
Fansidar Tablets 2281
Felbatol 2774
Feldene Capsules (Greater than 1%) 2008
Flexeril Tablets (Rare) 1701
Floxin I.V. (More than or equal to 1%) 1580
Floxin Tablets (200 mg, 300 mg, 400 mg) (More than or equal to 1%) 1577
▲ Fortaz (1 in 13) 1092
Fungizone Intravenous 507
Gantanol Tablets 2285
Gantrisin 2286
Garamycin Injectable 2502
Geocillin Tablets 2009
Helidac Therapy 2135
Hivid Tablets (2.5%) 2287
Hydralazine Hydrochloride Injection USP (Less frequent) 2712
IBU Tablets (Less than 1%) 1389
Intal Inhaler (Infrequent) 2185
Intal Nebulizer Solution (Rare) 2186
Keflex Pulvules & Oral Suspension 930
Keftab Tablets 931
▲ Kefurox Vials, Faspak & ADD-Vantage (1 in 14) 1509
Kefzol Vials, Faspak & ADD-Vantage 1511
Klonopin Tablets 2294
Lamictal Tablets (Infrequent) 1105
Lamprene Capsules (Less than 1%) 846
Lescol Capsules (Rare) 2395
Leukine 1317
Levoprome 1321
Limbitrol 2333
Lopid Tablets 1974
Lorabid Suspension and Pulvules 1513
Lotensin Tablets (Scattered incidents) 852
Lotensin HCT Tablets (Scattered accounts) 855
Ludiomil Tablets (Isolated reports) 861
Macrobid Capsules (1% to 5%) 2138
Macrodantin Capsules (Less often) 2140
Mandol Vials, Faspak & ADD-Vantage 1516
Matulane Capsules 2300
Maxaquin Tablets (Less than or equal to 0.1%) 2593
Maxipime for Injection (1.7%) 758
Mefoxin 1734
Mefoxin Premixed Intravenous Solution 1737
Mellaril 2398
Merrem I.V. (Greater than 0.2%) 2952
Mesantoin Tablets 2400
Mevacor Tablets 1742
Mezlin 594
Mezlin Pharmacy Bulk Package 597
Miltown Tablets 2780
Minocin Intravenous 1428
Minocin Oral Suspension 1431
Minocin Pellet-Filled Capsules 1429
Monocid Injection (2.9%) 2674
Monodox Capsules 1858
Monopril Tablets (2 patients) 762
Motrin Ibuprofen Suspension, Oral Drops, Chewable Tablets, Caplets (Less than 1%) 1563
Mycobutin Capsules (1%) 2101
Myochrysine Injection 1754
Naprelan Tablets (Less than 1%) 2861
Anaprox/Naprosyn (Less than 1%) 2277
Navane Capsules and Concentrate 2018
Navane Intramuscular 2019
Nebcin Vials, Hyporets & ADD-Vantage 1518
NegGram 2453
Netromycin Injection 100 mg/ml (4 of 1000 patients) 2516
Noroxin Tablets (0.6% to 1.5%) 1758
Noroxin Tablets (0.6% to 1.5%) 2222
Norpramin Tablets 1273
Nydrazid Injection 509
Omnipen Capsules 2872
Omnipen for Oral Suspension 2873
Orthoclone OKT3 Sterile Solution 1892
Pamelor 2409
▲ PASER Granules (55% of 38 patients with drug-induced hepatitis) 1333
Paxil Tablets (Rare) 2681
Pediazole Suspension 2340
Pen•Vee K (Frequent) 2879
Penetrex Tablets (Less than 1%) 2196
Permax Tablets (Rare) 571
Pipracil 1435
PMB 200 and PMB 400 2890
Ponstel (Occasional) 1982
Pravachol Tablets (Rare) 770
Prevacid Delayed-Release Capsules (Less than 1%) 2746
Primaxin I.M. 1770
Primaxin I.V. 1772
Prinivil Tablets (0.3% to 1.0%) 1776
Prinzide Tablets 1780
Proglycem 575
▲ Proleukin for Injection (6%) 812
Prolixin 510
Quadrinal Tablets 1398
Rifadin (Occasional) 1276
Rifamate Capsules 1278
Rifater (Occasional) 1280
Rimactane Capsules 865
▲ Rocephin Injectable Vials, ADD-Vantage, Galaxy Container (6%) 2305
Sansert Tablets 2424
Septra 1146
Septra I.V. Infusion 1142
Septra I.V. Infusion ADD-Vantage Vials 1144
Septra 1146
Ser-Ap-Es Tablets 867
Serentil 689
Sinequan (A few patients) 2028
Solganal Suspension (Rare) 2530
Soma Compound w/Codeine Tablets 2784
Soma Compound Tablets 2783
Soma Tablets 2782
Spectrobid Tablets 2030
Stelazine 2692
Sulfamylon Cream 940
Suprax (Less than 2%) 1443
Surmontil Capsules 2917
▲ Synarel Nasal Solution for Endometriosis (10% to 15%) 2605
Talacen Caplets (Rare) 2464
Talwin Injection (Rare) 2465
Talwin Compound 2466
Talwin Injection (Rare) 2465
Talwin Nx Tablets (Rare) 2467
Tao Capsules 2033
▲ Tazicef for Injection (1 in 13 patients) 2697
▲ Tazidime Vials, Faspak & ADD-Vantage (1 in 13) 1531
Tegretol/Tegretol-XR 870
Terramycin Intramuscular Solution 2034
Thorazine 2701
Ticar for Injection 2704
Ticlid Tablets 2317
Timentin for Injection 2706
Tofranil Ampuls 873
Tofranil Tablets 875
Tofranil-PM Capsules 876
Tonocard Tablets (Less than 1%) 519
Toradol (1% or less) 2319
Torecan 2367
Triavil Tablets 1800
Trilafon 2532
Unasyn 2035
Urispas Tablets 2710
Vancocin HCl, Oral Solution & Pulvules (Infrequent) 1536
Vancocin HCl, Vials & ADD-Vantage (Infrequent) 1534
Vantin for Oral Suspension and Vantin Tablets 2112
Vaqta (Isolated reports) 1805
Vascor Tablets (200 and 300 mg) 1597
Vaseretic Tablets 1810
Vasotec I.V. 1814
Vasotec Tablets (0.5% to 1.0%) 1816
Vibramycin 2038
Vibramycin Hyclate Intravenous 2040
Vibramycin 2038
Vivactil Tablets 1820
Cataflam/Voltaren/Voltaren-XR (Rare) 833
▲ Xanax Tablets (3.2% to 9.5%) 2115
Zantac (Rare) 1182
Zantac Injection 1180
Zantac Syrup (Rare) 1182
Zarontin Capsules 1986
Zarontin Syrup 1986
Zestoretic Tablets 2968
Zestril Tablets (0.3% to 1.0%) 2972
▲ Zinacef (1 in 14 patients) 1184
Zocor Tablets 1821
Zosyn 1463
Zyloprim Tablets (Less than 1%) 1194

Eosinophilia, myoclonus

Atretol Tablets (One case) 569
▲ Avonex (5%) 662
Tegretol/Tegretol-XR (One case) 870

Eosinophilia, peripheral

Atretol Tablets (One case) 569
Tegretol/Tegretol-XR (One case) 870

Eosinophilia, pulmonary

Dapsone Tablets USP 1331
Daraprim Tablets (Rare) 1199
DYNACIN Capsules (Rare) 1627

Eosinophilic pneumonitis

Anaprox/Naprosyn (Less than 1%) 2277
Capoten Tablets 740
Capozide Tablets 744
Anaprox/Naprosyn (Less than 1%) 2277

Epidermal necrolysis (see also under Necrolysis, epidermal)

Aldoclor Tablets 1638
Aldomet Ester HCl Injection 1642
Aldomet Oral 1640
Aldoril Tablets 1644
Anaprox/Naprosyn (Less than 1%) 2277
Bactrim DS Tablets (Rare) 2257
Bactrim I.V. Infusion (Rare) 2255
Bactrim (Rare) 2257
Clinoril Tablets (Less than 1%) 1658
Cuprimine Capsules 1673
Diamox ⊙ 317
EC-Naprosyn Delayed-Release Tablets (Less than 1%) 2277
Fansidar Tablets 2281
Fioricet with Codeine Capsules (Several cases) 2387
Gantanol Tablets 2285
Gantrisin 2286
Keflex Pulvules & Oral Suspension (Rare) 930
Keftab Tablets 931
Anaprox/Naprosyn (Less than 1%) 2277
Neptazane Tablets ⊙ 320
Prinzide Tablets 1780
Tagamet (Very rare) 2694
Talacen Caplets (Rare) 2464
Talwin Injection (Rare) 2465
Talwin Compound 2466
Talwin Injection 2465
Tenoretic Tablets 2963
Trancopal Caplets (Rare) 2468
Vasotec I.V. 1814

Epidermolysis bullosa

Anaprox/Naprosyn (Less than 1%) 2277
▲ Naprelan Tablets (3% to 9%) 2861
Anaprox/Naprosyn (Less than 1%) 2277

Epididymitis

Anafranil Capsules (Infrequent) 819
Asacol Delayed-Release Tablets 2129
Avonex 662
Betaseron for SC Injection 653
Cognex Capsules (Rare) 1961
Cordarone Tablets (Rare) 2818
Lamictal Tablets (Rare) 1105
Maxaquin Tablets (Less than 1%) 2593
Neurontin Capsules (Rare) 1978
Oxandrin 783
Paxil Tablets (Rare) 2681
Permax Tablets (Rare) 571
Prozac Pulvules & Liquid, Oral Solution (Rare) 935
TICE BCG, USP (0.3%) 1881
Winstrol Tablets 2468

Epigastric pain (see under Distress, epigastric)

Epilation

Velban Vials 1537

Epilepsy, aggravation

Estrace Cream and Tablets 751
Indocin Capsules (Less than 1%) 1723
Indocin I.V. (Less than 1%) 1727
Indocin (Less than 1%) 1723

Epileptiform movements, unspecified

Clozaril Tablets (1%) 2377

Epinephrine effect, reversal

Compazine 2644
Etrafon 2495
Stelazine 2692
Triavil Tablets 1800

Epiphora

Betimol 0.25%, 0.5% (1% to 5%) ⊙ 259

Epiphyseal closure

Accutane Capsules (Two children) 2252
Aquasol A Vitamin A Capsules, USP 525
Aquasol A Parenteral 526
Estratest 2718
Oxandrin 783
Winstrol Tablets 2468

Epistaxis

▲ Accutane Capsules (Up to 80%) 2252
Activase (Less than 1%) 1045
Adalat CC (3% or less) 582
AeroBid Inhaler System (1% to 3%) 1004
Aerobid-M Inhaler System (1% to 3%) 1004
Alferon N Injection (1%) 2142
Altace Capsules (Less than 1%) 1238
Ambien Tablets (Rare) 2559
Anafranil Capsules (Up to 2%) 819
▲ Atrovent Nasal Spray 0.03% (7.0% to 9.0%) 676
▲ Atrovent Nasal Spray 0.06% (8.2%) 678
Bactroban Nasal (Less than 1%) 2643
Beconase (Fewer than 3 per 100 patients) 1065
Bioclate, Antihemophilic Factor (Recombinant) (One patient out of 13,394) 797
BuSpar Tablets (Rare) 738
Cardizem CD Capsules (Less than 1%) 1251
Cardizem SR Capsules (Less than 1%) 1255
Cardizem Injectable 1253
Cardizem Tablets (Less than 1%) 1257
Cardura Tablets (1%) 1993
Cataflam Tablets (Less than 1%) 833
Cerebyx Injection (Infrequent) 1956
Cipro I.V. (1% or less) 587
Cipro I.V. Pharmacy Bulk Package (Less than 1%) 590
Cipro Tablets (Less than 1%) 584
Claritin Tablets (2% or fewer patients) 2485
Claritin-D Tablets (Less frequent) 2487
Clinoril Tablets (Less than 1%) 1658
Clozaril Tablets (Less than 1%) 2377

(Described in PDR For Nonprescription Drugs) Incidence data in parenthesis; ▲ 3% or more (⊙ Described in PDR For Ophthalmology)

Cognex Capsules (Infrequent) 1961
Coumadin 941
Cozaar Tablets (Less than 1%) 1668
Cytotec (Infrequent) 2576
DDAVP (Up to 3%) 2180
Desmopressin Acetate Rhinal Tube (Up to 3%) 997
Dexacort Phosphate in Turbinaire .. 1607
Dilacor XR Extended-release Capsules (Infrequent) 2183
Diupres Tablets 1691
Dynabac (0.1% to 1%) 668
DynaCirc CR Tablets (0.5% to 1.0%) 2383
Effexor (Infrequent) 2825
Eminase (Less than 1%) 2215
Ergamisol Tablets (Up to 1%) 1340
Felbatol 2774
Feldene Capsules (Less than 1%) .. 2008
Fioricet with Codeine Capsules 2387
Fiorinal with Codeine Capsules 2390
▲ Flolan for Injection (4%) 1085
▲ Flonase Nasal Spray (3% to 6%) 1088
Floxin I.V. (Less than 1%) 1580
Floxin Tablets (200 mg, 300 mg, 400 mg) (Less than 1%) 1577
Fludara for Injection (Up to 1%) 658
Fluorouracil Injection 2282
Foscavir Injection (Less than 1%) .. 541
Sterile FUDR (Remote possibility) .. 2284
Hismanal Tablets (Less frequent) 1341
Hivid Tablets (Less than 1%) 2287
Hydropres Tablets 1718
Hytrin Capsules (At least 1%) 434
Hyzaar Tablets 1720
IBU Tablets (Less than 1%) 1389
Indocin Capsules (Less than 1%) 1723
Indocin I.V. (Less than 1%) 1727
Indocin (Less than 1%) 1723
Intal Inhaler (Rare) 2185
Intal Nebulizer Solution 2186
Intron A for Injection (Less than or equal to 5%) 2506
Invirase Capsules (Less than 2%) .. 2291
Kerlone Tablets (Less than 2%) 2588
Lamictal Tablets (Infrequent) 1105
▲ Leukine (17%) 1317
▲ Leustatin (5%) 1889
Lotensin HCT Tablets (0.3% to 1.0%) 855
Lupron Depot - 3 Month 22.5 mg (Less than 5%) 2743
Lupron Depot-PED 7.5 mg, 11.25 mg and 15 mg (Less than 2%) 2744
Lupron Injection Pediatric (Less than 2%) 2737
LUVOX Tablets (Infrequent) 2723
Matulane Capsules 2300
Mavik Tablets (0.3% to 1.0%) 1407
Maxaquin Tablets (Less than 1%) .. 2593
Merrem I.V. (0.7%) 2952
Methotrexate Sodium Tablets, Injection, for Injection and LPF Injection (Less common) 1322
▲ Miacalcin Nasal Spray (3.5%) 2403
Minipress Capsules (1-4%) 2015
Minizide Capsules 2016
Mithracin 599
Monopril Tablets (0.2% to 1.0%) .. 762
Motrin Ibuprofen Suspension, Oral Drops, Chewable Tablets, Caplets (Less than 1%) 1563
Mykrox Tablets (Less than 2%) 1617
Naprelan Tablets (Less than 1%) .. 2861
Nasacort AQ Nasal Spray (2.7%) .. 2191
Nasacort Nasal Inhaler (Fewer than 5%) 2189
Nasalcrom Nasal Solution (Less than 1%) 2192
Nasalide Nasal Solution 0.025% (5% or less) 2301
▲ Nasarel Nasal Solution (3% to 9%) 2302
▲ Neupogen for Injection (15%) 495
Neurontin Capsules (Infrequent) 1978
Nicotrol NS Nicotine Nasal Spray (More common) 1565
Norvasc Tablets (More than 0.1% to 1%) 2020
Norvir (Less than 2%) 447
Oncaspar (Less than 1%) 2194
OptiPranolol (Metipranolol 0.3%) Sterile Ophthalmic Solution (A small number of patients) ⊙ 256
Orudis Capsules (Less than 1%) 2874
Oruvail Capsules (Less than 1%) 2874
Paxil Tablets (Infrequent) 2681
Penetrex Tablets (0.1% to 1%) 2196
Permax Tablets (1.6%) 571
Plendil Extended-Release Tablets (0.5% to 1.5%) 514
Prevacid Delayed-Release Capsules (Less than 1%) 2746
Prilosec Delayed-Release Capsules (Less than 1%) 516
Prinivil Tablets (0.3% to 1.0%) 1776
Prinzide Tablets 1780
Procardia XL Extended Release Tablets (1% or less) 2026
ProSom Tablets (Rare) 457
Proventil Syrup (1 of 100 patients) 2528
Prozac Pulvules & Liquid, Oral Solution (Infrequent) 935
Redux Capsules (Infrequent) 2911
Remeron Tablets (Infrequent) 1878
ReoPro Vials (9 to 11 events) 1526
Retrovir Capsules 1216
Retrovir I.V. Infusion 1221
Retrovir Syrup 1216
ReVia Tablets (Less than 1%) 957
▲ Rhinocort Nasal Inhaler (3 to 9%) .. 552
Rilutek Tablets (Infrequent) 2198
Risperdal Tablets (Infrequent) 1348
Rocephin Injectable Vials, ADD-Vantage, Galaxy Container (Rare) 2305
Roferon-A Injection (Rare) 2308
Salagen Tablets (2%) 1546
Sandostatin Injection (Less than 1%) 2421
Seldane Tablets (Up to 0.7%) 1284
Seldane-D Extended-Release Tablets 1286
Ser-Ap-Es Tablets 867
Serzone Tablets (Infrequent) 776
▲ Stadol (3% to 9%) 779
Stimate, (desmopressin acetate) Nasal Spray, 1.5 mg/mL 806
Sular Tablets (Less than or equal to 1%) 2961
Supprelin Injection (1% to 3%) 2230
▲ Tegison Capsules (25-50%) 2314
Tiazac Capsules (Less than 1%) 1019
Ticlid Tablets (0.5% to 1.0%) 2317
Tolectin (200, 400 and 600 mg) (Less than 1%) 1591
Toradol (1% or less) 2319
Trental Tablets (Less than 1%) 1291
Trilisate (Less than 1%) 2155
Unasyn (Less than 1%) 2035
Vancenase AQ Nasal Spray 0.042% (Fewer than 3 per 100 patients) 2535
▲ Vancenase AQ Double Strength Nasal Spray 0.084% (2% to 5%) 2536
Vancenase PocketHaler Nasal Inhaler (2 per 100 patients) 2534
Vantin for Oral Suspension and Vantin Tablets (Less than 1%) 2112
▲ Ventolin Inhalation Aerosol and Refill (3%) 1170
Ventolin Rotacaps for Inhalation (2%) 1173
Ventolin Syrup (1 of 100 patients) 1175
▲ Videx Tablets, Powder for Oral Solution, & Pediatric Powder for Oral Solution (Less than 1% to 14%) 2980
Cataflam/Voltaren/Voltaren-XR (Less than 1%) 833
Wellbutrin Tablets (Rare) 1177
Zestoretic Tablets 2968
Zestril Tablets (0.3% to 1.0%) 2972
Zoladex (1% or greater) 2976
Zoladex 3-month 2978
Zoloft Tablets (Infrequent) 2051
Zosyn (1.0% or less) 1463
Zyloprim Tablets (Less than 1%) 1194
Zyrtec Tablets (Less than 2%) 2053

Epithelial cells, atypical

Blenoxane 697
Cytoxan 700

Epitheliopathy

Alomide Ophthalmic Solution 465

Equilibrium, dysfunction

Calan SR Caplets (1% or less) 2571
Calan Tablets (1% or less) 2568
Covera-HS Tablets (Less than 2%) 2573
Floxin I.V. 1580
Floxin Tablets (200 mg, 300 mg, 400 mg) 1577
Hivid Tablets (Less than 1%) 2287
Isoptin Oral Tablets (Less than 1%) 1393
Isoptin SR Tablets (1% or less) 1395
Lariam Tablets 2295
Oncovin Solution Vials & Hyporets (Rare) 1521
Procardia Capsules (2% or less) 2024
Restoril Capsules (Less than 1%) .. 2413
Rifater 1280
Streptomycin Sulfate Injection 2031
Tegison Capsules (Less than 1%) .. 2314
Transderm Scōp Transdermal Therapeutic System (Few patients) 890
Velban Vials (Rare) 1537
Verelan Capsules (1% or less) 1455

Erection disturbances

Aldactazide Tablets 2556
Aldactone Tablets 2558
Bumex (0.1%) 2260
Dantrium Capsules (Less frequent) 2131
Desyrel and Desyrel Dividose 504
Effexor (Rare) 2825
Lescol Capsules 2395
Mevacor Tablets (0.5% to 1.0%) .. 1742
▲ Paxil Tablets (3.7% to 10.0%) 2681
Pravachol Tablets 770
Risperdal Tablets (Frequent) 1348
Wellbutrin Tablets (Infrequent) 1177
Winstrol Tablets 2468
Zocor Tablets 1821
▲ Zoladex (18%) 2976
Zoladex 3-month 2978

Ergotism

Cafergot (Rare) 2376
Parlodel (Rare) 2411

Erosion, genital

▲ Condylox Topical Solution (67%) .. 1853

Eructation

Ambien Tablets (Rare) 2559
Anafranil Capsules (Up to 2%) 819
▲ Asacol Delayed-Release Tablets (16%) 2129
Cedax (0.1% to 1%) 2480
Claritin-D Tablets (Less frequent) .. 2487
Clozaril Tablets (Less than 1%) 2377
Crixivan Capsules (Less than 2%) .. 1670
Cytovene (1% or less) 2270
Dilacor XR Extended-release Capsules (Infrequent) 2183
Dolobid Tablets (Less than 1 in 100) 1695
Effexor (Frequent) 2825
Hivid Tablets (Less than 1%) 2287
Imitrex Injection (Rare) 1095
Intron A for Injection (Less than 5%) 2506
Invirase Capsules (Less than 2%) .. 2291
Lamictal Tablets (Rare) 1105
Lodine Capsules and Tablets (Less than 1%) 2849
LUVOX Tablets (Infrequent) 2723
▲ Mycobutin Capsules (3%) 2101
Naprelan Tablets (Less than 1%) .. 2861
Neurontin Capsules (Rare) 1978
Norvir (Less than 2%) 447
Orap Tablets 1037
Orudis Capsules (Less than 1%) 2874
Oruvail Capsules (Less than 1%) 2874
OxyContin Tablets (Less than 1%) 2163
Paxil Tablets (Infrequent) 2681
Pentasa (Less than 1%) 1275
Permax Tablets (Infrequent) 571
Prevacid Delayed-Release Capsules (Less than 1%) 2746
Procardia XL Extended Release Tablets (1% or less) 2026
Prozac Pulvules & Liquid, Oral Solution (Infrequent) 935
Questran (Less frequent) 774
Redux Capsules (Infrequent) 2911
Relafen Tablets (Less than 1%) 2688
Remeron Tablets (Infrequent) 1878
Retrovir Capsules 1216
Retrovir I.V. Infusion 1221
Retrovir Syrup 1216
Risperdal Tablets (Rare) 1348
Serzone Tablets (Infrequent) 776
Toradol (1% or less) 2319
Trental Tablets (0.6%) 1291
Videx Tablets, Powder for Oral Solution, & Pediatric Powder for Oral Solution (Less than 1%) 2980
Zoloft Tablets (Infrequent) 2051

Eruptions

Cuprimine Capsules 1673
Diabinese Tablets (Approximately 1% or less) 2002
Norpace (1 to 3%) 2596

Eruptions, acneiform (see under Acneiform eruptions)

Eruptions, bullous

Ambien Tablets (Rare) 2559
Cataflam Tablets (Rare) 833
Coumadin (Infrequent) 941
Dynabac 668
Eulexin Capsules 2498
Felbatol (Infrequent) 2774
Fragmin Injection (Rare) 2088
Hivid Tablets (Less than 1%) 2287
LUVOX Tablets 2723
Redux Capsules 2911
Relafen Tablets (1%) 2688
Risperdal Tablets (Rare) 1348
▲ Tegison Capsules (1-10%) 2314
Cataflam/Voltaren/Voltaren-XR (Rare) 833
Yodoxin Tablets 1235
Zoloft Tablets (Rare) 2051
Zyrtec Tablets (Less than 2%) 2053

Eruptions, cutaneous

Aldactazide Tablets 2556
Aldactone Tablets 2558
Cardizem SR Capsules (Infrequent) 1255
Rifater (Rare) 1280
Seldane-D Extended-Release Tablets 1286
Taxotere for Injection Concentrate 2204

Eruptions, eczematoid (see under Eczema)

Eruptions, erythema annulare centrifugum

Plaquenil Sulfate Tablets 2459

Eruptions, erythematous

Aldactazide Tablets 2556
Aldactone Tablets 2558
Benoquin Cream 20% 1298
Macrobid Capsules 2138
Macrodantin Capsules 2140

Eruptions, exfoliative

Nydrazid Injection 509
Quinidex Extentabs 2240
Rifater 1280

Eruptions, fixed drug

Achromycin V Capsules (Rare) 1417
Cytovene (1% or less) 2270
Declomycin Tablets 1421
Depen Titratable Tablets 2770
Deponit NTG Transdermal Delivery System 2541
DYNACIN Capsules (Rare) 1627
Ergamisol Tablets (Less frequent) .. 1340
Miltown Tablets 2780
Minocin Intravenous (Rare) 1428
Minocin Oral Suspension (Rare) 1431
Minocin Pellet-Filled Capsules (Rare) 1429
Nitro-Bid IV 1270
Nitro-Bid Ointment (Uncommon) 1272
Nitro-Dur (nitroglycerin) Transdermal Infusion System (Uncommon) 1365
PMB 200 and PMB 400 2890
Soma Compound w/Codeine Tablets 2784
Soma Compound Tablets 2783
Soma Tablets 2782

Eruptions, hemorrhagic

Amen Tablets 785
Brevicon 2563
Climara Transdermal System 640
Cycrin Tablets 991
Demulen 2580
Depo-Provera Sterile Aqueous Suspension 2083
Desogen Tablets 1867
Diethylstilbestrol Tablets 1477
Estrace Cream and Tablets 751
Estraderm Transdermal System 842
ESTRATAB Tablets (0.3, 0.625, 1.25, 2.5 mg) 2715
Estratest 2718
Levlen/Tri-Levlen 646
Lo/Ovral Tablets 2852
Lo/Ovral-28 Tablets 2857
Menest Tablets 2671
Modicon 1928
Nolvadex Tablets (Rare) 2957
Nordette-21 Tablets 2863
Nordette-28 Tablets 2866
Norinyl 2563

(Described in PDR For Nonprescription Drugs) Incidence data in parenthesis; ▲ 3% or more (⊙ Described in PDR For Ophthalmology)

Side Effects Index — Erythema, facial

Nor-Q D Tablets ... 2598
Ogen Tablets ... 2103
Ogen Vaginal Cream ... 2106
Ortho-Cept ... 1907
Ortho-Cyclen/Ortho-Tri-Cyclen ... 1914
Ortho Dienestrol Cream ... 1922
Ortho-Est ... 1925
Ortho-Novum ... 1928
Ortho-Cyclen/Ortho Tri-Cyclen ... 1914
Ovcon ... 765
Ovral Tablets ... 2877
Ovral-28 Tablets ... 2878
Ovrette Tablets ... 2878
PMB 200 and PMB 400 ... 2890
Premarin Intravenous ... 2893
Premarin Tablets ... 2896
Premarin Vaginal Cream ... 2898
Premphase ... 2900
Prempro ... 2905
Provera Tablets ... 2110
Levlen/Tri-Levlen ... 646
Tri-Norinyl ... 2607
Triphasil-21 Tablets ... 2919
Triphasil-28 Tablets ... 2924
Vivelle Transdermal System ... 880

Eruptions, herpetic
▲ Chemet Capsules (2.6% to 11.2%) ... 666

Eruptions, lichenoid
Plaquenil Sulfate Tablets ... 2459

Eruptions, maculopapular
Aldactazide Tablets ... 2556
Aldactone Tablets ... 2558
Amaryl Tablets (Less than 1%) ... 1241
Bicillin C-R Injection ... 2810
Bicillin C-R 900/300 Injection ... 2812
Bicillin L-A Injection ... 2813
DiaBeta Tablets (1.5%) ... 1265
Glucotrol Tablets (About 1 in 70) ... 2011
Glynase PresTab Tablets (1.5%) ... 2091
Macrobid Tablets ... 2138
Macrodantin Capsules ... 2140
Micronase Tablets (1.5%) ... 2099
Mustargen (Occasional) ... 1752
Nydrazid Injection ... 509
Pen•Vee K ... 2879
Pfizerpen for Injection ... 2022
Plaquenil Sulfate Tablets ... 2459
Rifater ... 1280

Eruptions, morbilliform
Amaryl Tablets (Less than 1%) ... 1241
Ceclor Pulvules & Suspension (1 in 100) ... 1470
DiaBeta Tablets (1.5%) ... 1265
Glucotrol Tablets (About 1 in 70) ... 2011
Glynase PresTab Tablets (1.5%) ... 2091
Micronase Tablets (1.5%) ... 2099
Mysoline ... 2860
Nydrazid Injection ... 509
Plaquenil Sulfate Tablets ... 2459
Rifater ... 1280

Eruptions, mucocutaneous
▲ Chemet Capsules (2.6% to 11.2%) ... 666

Eruptions, purpuric
Nydrazid Injection ... 509
Plaquenil Sulfate Tablets ... 2459
Rifater ... 1280

Eruptions, vascular
Pipracil (Less frequent) ... 1435

Erythema
▲ Accutane Capsules (Less than 1 patient in 10) ... 2252
▲ Acel-Imune Diphtheria and Tetanus Toxoids and Acellular Pertussis Vaccine Adsorbed (4% to 10%) ... 1415
Aclovate (Approximately 2%) ... 1061
Amaryl Tablets (Less than 1%) ... 1241
Americaine Anesthetic Lubricant ... 1603
Americaine Otic Topical Anesthetic Ear Drops ... 1603
Ativan Injection ... 2805
A/T/S 2% Acne Topical Gel (Occasional) ... 1244
A/T/S 2% Acne Topical Solution (Occasional) ... 1244
Avonex ... 662
Azelex (Less than 1%) ... 471
Bactroban Ointment (Less than 1%) ... 2642
Benzamycin Topical Gel (Occasional) ... 919

Betoptic Ophthalmic Solution (Rare) ... 465
Betoptic S Ophthalmic Suspension (Small number of patients) ... 467
Biavax II ... 1653
▲ Blenoxane (Approximately 50%) ... 697
Brevibloc (esmolol HCl) Injection (Less than 1%) ... 1860
Brevoxyl ... 2732
▲ Brevoxyl Cleansing Lotion (5 of 100 patients) ... 2732
Carbocaine Injection ... 2432
▲ Catapres-TTS (26 of 101 patients) ... 680
Caverject Injection (Less than 1%) ... 2064
Ceftin (0.1% to 1%) ... 1067
Cerumenex Drops (1% of 2,700 patients) ... 2148
Cholera Vaccine ... 2818
Cipro I.V. (1% or less) ... 587
Cipro I.V. Pharmacy Bulk Package (Less than 1%) ... 590
Claritin-D Tablets (Less frequent) ... 2487
▲ Cleocin T Topical (7%) ... 2072
▲ Climara Transdermal System (9%) ... 640
Clomid ... 1262
Clozaril Tablets (Less than 1%) ... 2377
Collagenase Santyl Ointment ... 1381
Compazine ... 2644
Cormax Ointment (Approximately 0.3%) ... 1856
Cortone Acetate Sterile Suspension ... 1663
Cortone Acetate Tablets ... 1664
Cosmegen Injection ... 1666
Cozaar Tablets (Less than 1%) ... 1668
Cutivate Ointment (Less than 1%) ... 1078
Dalalone D.P. Injectable ... 1009
Dalgan Injection (Less than 1%) ... 529
Dantrium Intravenous (Rare) ... 2132
Decadron Elixir ... 1676
Decadron Phosphate Injection ... 1680
Decadron Phosphate with Xylocaine Injection, Sterile ... 1683
Decadron Tablets ... 1678
Decadron-LA Sterile Suspension ... 1687
Desferal Vials ... 838
DesOwen Cream, Ointment and Lotion (Less than 2%) ... 1032
Desquam-E Gel ... 2792
Desquam-X Gel ... 2792
Desquam-X 10 Bar ... 2792
Desquam-X Wash ... 2792
Dexacort Phosphate in Respihaler ... 1606
Dexacort Phosphate in Turbinaire ... 1607
DiaBeta Tablets (1.5%) ... 1265
Digibind (One patient) ... 1079
Dipentum Capsules (Rare) ... 2084
Diphtheria & Tetanus Toxoids Adsorbed Purogenated (Mild) ... 1422
Diprivan Injectable Emulsion (Rare) ... 2939
Diprolene Gel 0.05% (Less frequent) ... 2490
Diprolene Ointment 0.05% (3 per 767 patients) ... 2491
▲ Dovonex Ointment 0.005% (1% to 10%) ... 2793
▲ Doxil (3.4%) ... 2613
Duragesic Transdermal System (1% or greater) ... 1336
▲ Efudex (Among most frequent) ... 2280
Elimite (permethrin) 5% Cream (1 to 2% or less) ... 475
▲ EMLA Cream (30% to 56%) ... 536
Engerix-B Unit-Dose Vials (Less than 1%) ... 2656
Erycette (erythromycin 2%) Topical Solution ... 1943
Etrafon ... 2495
Eulexin Capsules ... 2498
Exelderm Cream 1.0% (1%) ... 2794
Feldene Capsules (Less than 1%) ... 2008
Fioricet with Codeine Capsules ... 2387
Fiorinal with Codeine Capsules ... 2390
Fluorouracil Injection ... 2282
Fosamax Tablets (Rare) ... 1703
▲ Sterile FUDR (Among more common) ... 2284
Gammar-P I.V., Immune Globulin Intravenous (Human) ... 798
Garamycin 0.1% ... 2501
Glucotrol Tablets (About 1 in 70) ... 2011
Glynase PresTab Tablets (1.5%) ... 2091
▲ Habitrol Nicotine Transdermal System (Once in 35% of patients; 22 of 220 patients) ... 884
Heparin Lock Flush Solution ... 2831
Heparin Sodium Injection ... 2832
Heparin Sodium Vials ... 1486
Hycamtin for Injection ... 2665

Hydeltrasol Injection, Sterile ... 1708
Hydeltra-T.B.A. Sterile Suspension ... 1710
Hydrea Capsules ... 705
Hydrocortone Acetate Sterile Suspension ... 1712
Hydrocortone Phosphate Injection, Sterile ... 1713
Hydrocortone Tablets ... 1715
Hyzaar Tablets ... 1720
Imitrex Injection (Infrequent) ... 1095
Imitrex Tablets (Infrequent) ... 1099
Intron A for Injection (Less than 5%) ... 2506
Invirase Capsules (Less than 2%) ... 2291
▲ IPOL Poliovirus Vaccine Inactivated (3.2%) ... 903
▲ Lac-Hydrin 12% Lotion (1 in 10 to 50 patients) ... 2796
Lamictal Tablets (Infrequent) ... 1105
Lamprene Capsules (Less than 1%) ... 846
▲ Leustatin (6%) ... 1889
Levoprome ... 1321
Livostin (Approximately 1% to 3%) ... ⊙ 262
Lotrimin ... 2514
Lotrisone Cream ... 2515
Lovenox Injection ... 2187
Lupron Injection ... 2736
M-M-R II ... 1730
M-R-VAX II ... 1732
Marcaine (Rare) ... 2446
Marcaine Spinal (Rare) ... 2449
Melanex Topical Solution ... 1842
Mellaril ... 2398
Menomune-A/C/Y/W-135 ... 906
Meruvax II ... 1740
MetroGel ... 1034
Metubine Iodide Vials ... 932
▲ Miacalcin Nasal Spray (10.6%) ... 2403
Micronase Tablets (1.5%) ... 2099
8-MOP Capsules ... 1294
Monocid Injection (Less than 1%) ... 2674
Mutamycin for Injection ... 712
Naftin Cream 1% (2%) ... 477
Naftin Gel 1% (0.5%) ... 477
NegGram ... 2453
Nescaine/Nescaine MPF ... 549
Nolvadex Tablets ... 2957
Noroxin Tablets (Less frequent) ... 1758
Noroxin Tablets (Less frequent) ... 2222
▲ Oncaspar (Greater than 5%) ... 2194
Orthoclone OKT3 Sterile Solution ... 1892
Oxistat Cream (0.2%) ... 1139
Oxsoralen-Ultra Capsules ... 1302
Paraplatin for Injection ... 713
PedvaxHIB ... 1761
Pipracil ... 1435
Plendil Extended-Release Tablets (0.5% to 1.5%) ... 514
Prinivil Tablets (0.3% to 1.0%) ... 1776
Prinzide Tablets ... 1780
Profasi (chorionic gonadotropin for injection, USP) ... 2620
▲ Proleukin for Injection (41%) ... 812
Prolixin ... 510
Prostep (nicotine transdermal system) (At least once in 22% of patients) ... 1439
Recombivax HB (Equal to or greater than 1%) ... 1787
Renova (tretinoin emollient cream) 0.05% (Almost all subjects) ... 1945
Retin-A (tretinoin) Cream/Gel/Liquid ... 1947
Rifater ... 1280
Sensorcaine (Rare) ... 554
Serentil ... 689
Solganal Suspension ... 2530
▲ Spectazole (econazole nitrate 1%) Cream (3%) ... 1947
Stelazine ... 2692
Sufenta Injection (0.3% to 1%) ... 1355
Sulfamylon Cream ... 940
Supprelin Injection (1%) ... 2230
T-Stat 2.0% Topical Solution and Pads ... 2797
Taxotere for Injection Concentrate (0.9%) ... 2204
Temovate E Emollient (Less than 2%) ... 1154
▲ Temovate Gel (Among most frequent) ... 1153
Temovate Ointment (Less frequent) ... 1152
Tetanus Toxoid Adsorbed Purogenated ... 1447
THERAMYCIN Z 2% Solution ... 1629
Topicort LP Emollient Cream 0.05% (0.8%) ... 1289
Torecan ... 2367

Tracrium Injection (0.6%) ... 1155
Transderm Scōp Transdermal Therapeutic System (Infrequent) ... 890
Triavil Tablets ... 1800
Trilafon ... 2532
▲ Tripedia (3% to 25%) ... 908
Tympagesic Ear Drops ... 2476
Ultravate Cream 0.05% (Less frequent) ... 2797
Ultravate Ointment 0.05% (Less frequent) ... 2798
Unasyn (Less than 1%) ... 2035
Vaqta (Less than 1%) ... 1805
▲ Videx Tablets, Powder for Oral Solution, & Pediatric Powder for Oral Solution (4%) ... 2980
▲ Vivelle Transdermal System (One of the two most common) ... 880
Westcort Ointment 0.2% (2%) ... 2800
▲ Yutopar Intravenous Injection (10 to 15%) ... 566
Zestoretic Tablets ... 2968
Zestril Tablets (0.3% to 1.0%) ... 2972
▲ Zinecard Injection (4% to 5%) ... 2120

Erythema at injection site
▲ ActHIB (Up to 24.0%) ... 893
▲ Actimmune (14%) ... 1043
Attenuvax ... 1650
DDAVP Injection (Occasional) ... 2178
DDAVP Injection 15 mcg/mL (Occasional) ... 2179
Desmopressin Acetate Injection (Occasional) ... 996
Diphtheria and Tetanus Toxoids and Pertussis Vaccine Adsorbed ... 2650
Engerix-B Unit-Dose Vials (1% to 10%) ... 2656
Floxin I.V. (Approximately 2%) ... 1580
Gamimune N, 5% Immune Globulin Intravenous (Human), 5% (Some cases) ... 612
Gamimune N, 10% Immune Globulin Intravenous (Human), 10% (Some cases) ... 615
Helixate, Antihemophilic Factor (Recombinant) (Two reports out of 3,254 patients) ... 799
HibTITER (Less than 1% to 2.0%) ... 1423
▲ Imovax Rabies Vaccine (About 25%) ... 899
KOGENATE Antihemophilic Factor (Recombinant) ... 626
▲ Leustatin (9%) ... 1889
Mivacron (Less than 1%) ... 1125
▲ Navelbine Injection (Approximately one-third of patients) ... 1212
▲ OmniHIB (0.3% to 24.0%) ... 2676
Pneumovax 23 (Common) ... 1768
Primaxin I.V. (0.4%) ... 1772
Rabies Vaccine Adsorbed (A few patients) ... 2686
▲ Rabies Vaccine, Imovax Rabies I.D. (About 25%) ... 901
Taxol Injection ... 723
Taxotere for Injection Concentrate ... 2204
▲ Tetramune (19% to 40%) ... 1449
Tubersol (Tuberculin Purified Protein Derivative (Mantoux)) (Infrequent) ... 2988
▲ Typhim Vi (Up to 11%) ... 914
▲ Vaqta (0.8% to 12.9%) ... 1805
▲ Varivax (19.3% to 32.5%) ... 1807
Velosulin BR Human Insulin 10 ml Vials ... 1847

Erythema, conjunctival
▲ AK-Spore (Among most frequent) ... ⊙ 205
▲ AKTOB (Among most frequent; less than 3 of 100 patients) ... ⊙ 207
Neosporin Ophthalmic Ointment Sterile ... 1130
Neosporin Ophthalmic Solution Sterile ... 1131
▲ Polysporin Ophthalmic Ointment Sterile (Among those occurring most often) ... 1140
▲ Rev-Eyes Ophthalmic Eyedrops 0.5% (10% to 40%) ... ⊙ 324
TobraDex Ophthalmic Suspension and Ointment (Less than 4%) ... 469
Tobrex Ophthalmic Ointment and Solution (Less than 3 of 100 patients) ... ⊙ 226

Erythema, facial
Celestone Soluspan Suspension ... 2484
CORTENEMA ... 2713
Florinef Acetate Tablets ... 506
Hydrea Capsules (Less frequent) ... 705

(▣ Described in PDR For Nonprescription Drugs)   Incidence data in parenthesis; ▲ 3% or more   (⊙ Described in PDR For Ophthalmology)

Erythema, facial

- Normodyne Tablets (Less common) ... 2522
- Pediapred Oral Solution ... 1618
- Prelone Syrup ... 1834
- Trandate Tablets (Less common) ... 1158

Erythema, hemorrhagic exudative
(see under Henoch-Schonlein purpura)

Erythema, maculopapular

- Teslac Tablets ... 727

Erythema multiforme

- Abelcet Injection ... 1540
- Acel-Imune Diphtheria and Tetanus Toxoids and Acellular Pertussis Vaccine Adsorbed ... 1415
- Aldactazide Tablets ... 2556
- Aldoclor Tablets ... 1638
- Aldoril Tablets ... 1644
- Altace Capsules (Less than 1%) ... 1238
- Amen Tablets ... 785
- Amoxil ... 2631
- Anaprox/Naprosyn (Less than 1%) ... 2277
- Atretol Tablets ... 569
- Atromid-S Capsules ... 2808
- Attenuvax (Rare) ... 1650
- Augmentin ... 2637
- Augmentin Suspension ... 2640
- Axocet Capsules (Infrequent) ... 2469
- Azactam for Injection (Less than 1%) ... 736
- Azulfidine (Rare) ... 2059
- Bactrim DS Tablets ... 2257
- Bactrim I.V. Infusion ... 2255
- Bactrim ... 2257
- Biavax II (Rare) ... 1653
- Brevicon ... 2563
- Calan SR Caplets (1% or less) ... 2571
- Calan Tablets (1% or less) ... 2568
- Capoten Tablets ... 740
- Capozide Tablets ... 744
- Cardizem CD Capsules (Infrequent) ... 1251
- Cardizem SR Capsules (Infrequent) ... 1255
- Cardizem Injectable ... 1253
- Cardizem Tablets (Infrequent) ... 1257
- Cataflam Tablets (Rare) ... 833
- Ceclor Pulvules & Suspension ... 1470
- Cefizox for Intramuscular or Intravenous Use ... 1025
- Cefotan ... 2936
- Ceftin ... 1067
- Cefzil Tablets and Oral Suspension (Rare) ... 747
- Ceptaz ... 1070
- Chibroxin Sterile Ophthalmic Solution (With oral form) ... 1657
- Cipro I.V. (1% or less) ... 587
- Cipro I.V. Pharmacy Bulk Package (Less than 1%) ... 590
- Cipro Tablets ... 584
- Claritin Tablets (Rare) ... 2485
- Claritin-D Tablets ... 2487
- Cleocin Phosphate Injection (Rare) ... 2068
- Climara Transdermal System ... 640
- Cleocin Vaginal Cream (Rare) ... 2070
- Clinoril Tablets (Less than 1%) ... 1658
- Clomid ... 1262
- Clozaril Tablets ... 2377
- Covera-HS Tablets (Less than 2%) ... 2573
- Cycrin Tablets ... 991
- Daypro Caplets (Less than 1%) ... 2578
- Decadron Phosphate with Xylocaine Injection, Sterile ... 1683
- Demulen ... 2580
- Depakene ... 416
- Depakote Tablets ... 418
- Depo-Provera Sterile Aqueous Suspension ... 2083
- Desogen Tablets ... 1867
- Diabinese Tablets ... 2002
- Diamox ... ⊚ 317
- Diethylstilbestrol Tablets ... 1477
- Diphtheria and Tetanus Toxoids and Pertussis Vaccine Adsorbed ... 2650
- Diupres Tablets ... 1691
- Diuril Oral Suspension ... 1694
- Diuril Sodium Intravenous ... 1693
- Diuril Tablets ... 1694
- Dolobid Tablets (Less than 1 in 100) ... 1695
- Doxil (Less than 1%) ... 2613
- Duricef Capsules, Tablets, and Oral Suspension ... 750
- DYNACIN Capsules ... 1627
- EC-Naprosyn Delayed-Release Tablets (Less than 1%) ... 2277
- Engerix-B Unit-Dose Vials ... 2656
- Esgic-plus Capsules (Several cases) ... 1012
- Esgic-plus Tablets (Several cases) ... 1012
- Estrace Cream and Tablets ... 751
- Estraderm Transdermal System ... 842
- ESTRATAB Tablets (0.3, 0.625, 1.25, 2.5 mg) ... 2715
- Estratest ... 2718
- Fansidar Tablets ... 2281
- Feldene Capsules (Less than 1%) ... 2008
- Fioricet Tablets (Several cases) ... 2386
- Fioricet with Codeine Capsules (Several cases) ... 2387
- Fiorinal Capsules (Several cases) ... 2388
- Fiorinal with Codeine Capsules ... 2390
- Fiorinal Tablets (Several cases) ... 2388
- Floxin I.V. ... 1580
- Floxin Tablets (200 mg, 300 mg, 400 mg) ... 1577
- Fortaz ... 1092
- Foscavir Injection (Rare) ... 541
- Gantanol Tablets ... 2285
- Gantrisin ... 2286
- GlaucTabs ... ⊚ 209
- Gris-PEG Tablets, 125 mg & 250 mg (Rare) ... 476
- Havrix (Rare) ... 2663
- Hespan Injection ... 945
- HibTITER ... 1423
- HydroDIURIL Tablets ... 1716
- Hydropres Tablets ... 1718
- Hyzaar Tablets ... 1720
- IBU Tablets (Less than 1%) ... 1389
- Indocin Capsules (Less than 1%) ... 1723
- Indocin I.V. (Less than 1%) ... 1727
- Indocin (Less than 1%) ... 1723
- Isoptin Oral Tablets (Less than 1%) ... 1393
- Isoptin SR Tablets (1% or less) ... 1395
- Keflex Pulvules & Oral Suspension (Rare) ... 930
- Keftab Tablets (Rare) ... 931
- Kefurox Vials, Faspak & ADD-Vantage ... 1509
- Lamictal Tablets ... 1105
- Lariam Tablets ... 2295
- Lasix Injection, Oral Solution and Tablets ... 1267
- Lescol Capsules (Rare) ... 2395
- Leukeran Tablets (Rare) ... 1205
- Levlen/Tri-Levlen ... 646
- Lodine Capsules and Tablets (Less than 1%) ... 2849
- Lo/Ovral Tablets ... 2852
- Lo/Ovral-28 Tablets ... 2857
- Lorabid Suspension and Pulvules ... 1513
- Lupron Depot-PED 7.5 mg, 11.25 mg and 15 mg (2%) ... 2744
- Lupron Injection Pediatric ... 2737
- M-M-R II (Rare) ... 1730
- M-R-VAX II (Rare) ... 1732
- Macrobid Capsules (Rare) ... 2138
- Macrodantin Capsules (Rare) ... 2140
- Maxipime for Injection ... 758
- Menest Tablets ... 2671
- Meruvax II (Rare) ... 1740
- Mesantoin Tablets (Rare) ... 2400
- Methotrexate Sodium Tablets, Injection, for Injection and LPF Injection ... 1322
- Mevacor Tablets (Rare) ... 1742
- Miltown Tablets (Rare) ... 2780
- Minocin Intravenous ... 1428
- Minocin Oral Suspension ... 1431
- Minocin Pellet-Filled Capsules ... 1429
- Mintezol ... 1747
- Modicon ... 1928
- Moduretic Tablets ... 1748
- Motrin Ibuprofen Suspension, Oral Drops, Chewable Tablets, Caplets (Less than 1%) ... 1563
- Mumpsvax (Rare) ... 1751
- Mustargen ... 1752
- Myleran Tablets (Rare) ... 1209
- Anaprox/Naprosyn (Less than 1%) ... 2277
- NegGram ... 2453
- Neptazane Tablets ... ⊚ 320
- Nordette-21 Tablets ... 2863
- Nordette-28 Tablets ... 2866
- Norinyl ... 2563
- Noroxin Tablets ... 1758
- Noroxin Tablets ... 2222
- Nor-Q D Tablets ... 2598
- Ogen Tablets ... 2103
- Ogen Vaginal Cream ... 2106
- Omnipen Capsules ... 2872
- Omnipen for Oral Suspension ... 2873
- Ortho-Cept ... 1907
- Ortho-Cyclen/Ortho Tri-Cyclen ... 1914
- Ortho Dienestrol Cream ... 1922
- Ortho-Est ... 1925
- Ortho-Novum ... 1928
- Ortho-Cyclen/Ortho Tri-Cyclen ... 1914
- Ovcon ... 765
- Ovral Tablets ... 2877
- Ovral-28 Tablets ... 2878
- Ovrette Tablets ... 2878
- PCE Dispertab Tablets (Rare) ... 453
- Paxil Tablets (Rare) ... 2681
- Pediazole Suspension ... 2340
- Penetrex Tablets (0.1% to 1%) ... 2196
- Phrenilin (Several cases) ... 790
- Pipracil (Rare) ... 1435
- PMB 200 and PMB 400 ... 2890
- Pravachol Tablets (Rare) ... 770
- Premarin Intravenous ... 2893
- Premarin Tablets ... 2896
- Premarin Vaginal Cream ... 2898
- Premphase ... 2900
- Prempro ... 2905
- Prilosec Delayed-Release Capsules (Very rare) ... 516
- Primaxin I.M. ... 1770
- Primaxin I.V. (Less than 0.2%) ... 1772
- Prinzide Tablets ... 1780
- Proloprim Tablets (Rare) ... 1141
- Proventil Syrup (Rare) ... 2528
- Provera Tablets ... 2110
- Prozac Pulvules & Liquid, Oral Solution (Rare) ... 935
- Redux Capsules ... 2911
- Relafen Tablets (Rare) ... 2688
- Rilutek Tablets (Rare) ... 2198
- Ritalin ... 866
- Rocaltrol Capsules (One case) ... 2303
- SSD (Infrequent) ... 1402
- Sedapap Tablets 50 mg/650 mg (Several cases) ... 1826
- Semprex-D Capsules (Rare) ... 1620
- Septra ... 1146
- Septra I.V. Infusion ... 1142
- Septra I.V. Infusion ADD-Vantage Vials ... 1144
- Septra ... 1146
- Silvadene Cream 1% (Infrequent) ... 1288
- Soma Compound w/Codeine Tablets ... 2784
- Soma Compound Tablets ... 2783
- Soma Tablets ... 2782
- Spectrobid Tablets ... 2030
- Suprax (Less than 2%) ... 1443
- Tagamet (Very rare) ... 2694
- Tazicef for Injection ... 2697
- Tazidime Vials, Faspak & ADD-Vantage ... 1531
- Tegretol/Tegretol-XR ... 870
- Tetramune ... 1449
- Tiazac Capsules (Infrequent) ... 1019
- Ticlid Tablets (Rare) ... 2317
- Timolide Tablets ... 1791
- Tolectin (200, 400 and 600 mg) (Less than 1%) ... 1591
- Tonocard Tablets (Less than 1%) ... 519
- Trancopal Caplets (Rare) ... 2468
- Tri-Immunol Adsorbed ... 1452
- Levlen/Tri-Levlen ... 646
- Trilisate (Rare) ... 2155
- Trimpex Tablets (Rare) ... 2323
- Tri-Norinyl ... 2607
- Triphasil-21 Tablets ... 2919
- Triphasil-28 Tablets ... 2924
- Unasyn ... 2035
- Vantin for Oral Suspension and Vantin Tablets ... 2112
- Varivax ... 1807
- Vaseretic Tablets ... 1810
- Vasotec I.V. ... 1814
- Vasotec Tablets (0.5% to 1.0%) ... 1816
- Ventolin Syrup (Rare) ... 1175
- Verelan Capsules (1% or less) ... 1455
- Vivelle Transdermal System ... 880
- Cataflam/Voltaren/Voltaren-XR (Rare) ... 833
- Zantac (Rare) ... 1182
- Zantac Injection (Rare) ... 1180
- Zantac Syrup (Rare) ... 1182
- Zestoretic Tablets ... 2968
- Zinacef (Rare) ... 1184
- Zocor Tablets (Rare) ... 1821
- Zoloft Tablets (Rare) ... 2051
- Zosyn (Rare) ... 1463
- Zyloprim Tablets (Less than 1%) ... 1194

Erythema nodosum

- Accutane Capsules (Less than 1%) ... 2252
- Amen Tablets ... 785
- Asacol Delayed-Release Tablets ... 2129
- Atretol Tablets ... 569
- Betaseron for SC Injection ... 653
- Brevicon ... 2563
- Cipro I.V. (1% or less) ... 587
- Cipro I.V. Pharmacy Bulk Package (Less than 1%) ... 590
- Cipro Tablets (Less than 1%) ... 584
- Climara Transdermal System ... 640
- Clomid ... 1262
- Cycrin Tablets ... 991
- Demulen ... 2580
- Depo-Provera Sterile Aqueous Suspension ... 2083
- Desogen Tablets ... 1867
- Diethylstilbestrol Tablets ... 1477
- Dipentum Capsules (Rare) ... 2084
- Doxil (Less than 1%) ... 2613
- Engerix-B Unit-Dose Vials ... 2656
- Estrace Cream and Tablets ... 751
- Estraderm Transdermal System ... 842
- ESTRATAB Tablets (0.3, 0.625, 1.25, 2.5 mg) ... 2715
- Estratest ... 2718
- Floxin I.V. ... 1580
- Floxin Tablets (200 mg, 300 mg, 400 mg) ... 1577
- Indocin Capsules (Less than 1%) ... 1723
- Indocin I.V. (Less than 1%) ... 1727
- Indocin (Less than 1%) ... 1723
- Levlen/Tri-Levlen ... 646
- Lo/Ovral Tablets ... 2852
- Lo/Ovral-28 Tablets ... 2857
- Maxaquin Tablets ... 2593
- Menest Tablets ... 2671
- Modicon ... 1928
- Myleran Tablets (Rare) ... 1209
- Neupogen for Injection (One event) ... 495
- Nordette-21 Tablets ... 2863
- Nordette-28 Tablets ... 2866
- Norinyl ... 2563
- Nor-Q D Tablets ... 2598
- Ogen Tablets ... 2103
- Ogen Vaginal Cream ... 2106
- Ortho-Cept ... 1907
- Ortho-Cyclen/Ortho-Tri-Cyclen ... 1914
- Ortho Dienestrol Cream ... 1922
- Ortho-Est ... 1925
- Ortho-Novum ... 1928
- Ortho-Cyclen/Ortho Tri-Cyclen ... 1914
- Ovcon ... 765
- Ovral Tablets ... 2877
- Ovral-28 Tablets ... 2878
- Ovrette Tablets ... 2878
- Paxil Tablets (Rare) ... 2681
- Penetrex Tablets ... 2196
- Pentasa (Less than 1%) ... 1275
- PMB 200 and PMB 400 ... 2890
- Premarin Intravenous ... 2893
- Premarin Tablets ... 2896
- Premarin Vaginal Cream ... 2898
- Premphase ... 2900
- Prempro ... 2905
- Provera Tablets ... 2110
- Recombivax HB (Less than 1%) ... 1787
- Tegretol/Tegretol-XR ... 870
- Levlen/Tri-Levlen ... 646
- Tri-Norinyl ... 2607
- Triphasil-21 Tablets ... 2919
- Triphasil-28 Tablets ... 2924
- Vesanoid Capsules (Isolated cases) ... 2327
- Vivelle Transdermal System ... 880

Erythema simplex

- Oncaspar (Less than 1%) ... 2194

Erythematous streaking

- Adriamycin PFS ... 2056
- Adriamycin RDF ... 2056
- Doxorubicin Astra ... 531
- Rubex for Injection ... 721
- ▲ Zinecard Injection (4% to 5%) ... 2120

Erythrocyte survival time, shortened

- Easprin ... 1971

Erythrocytes, abnormal

- Effexor (Rare) ... 2825
- Hydrea Capsules ... 705
- Paxil Tablets (Rare) ... 2681

Erythrocytes, vacuolation of

- Pyrazinamide Tablets (Rare) ... 1442
- Rifater (Rare) ... 1280

Erythrocytosis

- Danocrine Capsules ... 2437
- Moban Tablets and Concentrate ... 1036
- Pergonal (menotropins for injection, USP) (One patient) ... 2618
- Ponstel ... 1982

(⊛ Described in PDR For Nonprescription Drugs)   Incidence data in parenthesis; ▲ 3% or more   (⊚ Described in PDR For Ophthalmology)

1331 Side Effects Index Exanthema

Erythrocyturia
Amikacin Sulfate Injection, USP 523
Amikacin Sulfate Injection, USP 981
Amikin Injectable 502
Netromycin Injection 100 mg/ml...... 2516
Quadrinal Tablets 1398

Erythroderma, exfoliative
Tagamet...... 2694

Erythroid hyperplasia
Pyrazinamide Tablets (Rare) 1442
Rifater (Rare)...... 1280

Erythromelalgia
Adalat Capsules (10 mg and 20 mg) (Less than 0.5%)...... 580
Adalat CC (Rare) 582
Parlodel 2411
Procardia Capsules (Approximately 0.5%) 2024

Erythropenia
▲ Accutane Capsules (1 in 5 to 1 in 10 patients)...... 2252
Apresazide Capsules (Less frequent) 824
Dopram Injectable...... 2235
Haldol Decanoate...... 1587
Moban Tablets and Concentrate...... 1036
Mustargen...... 1752
Ponstel 1982
Primaxin I.M. 1770
Ser-Ap-Es Tablets 867
Unasyn 2035

Escharotic effect
Cetacaine Topical Anesthetic 812

Esophageal disease, unspecified
Myleran Tablets 1209

Esophageal necrosis
Ethamolin Injection (0.1 to 0.4%).. 2544

Esophageal stenosis
Rilutek Tablets (Infrequent) 2198

Esophageal stricture
▲ Ethamolin Injection (Among most common; 1.3%)...... 2544
Lodine Capsules and Tablets (Less than 1%)...... 2849
Prevacid Delayed-Release Capsules (Less than 1%)...... 2746

Esophageal ulceration
Cytosar-U Sterile Powder (Less frequent) 2077
Doryx Capsules (Rare)...... 1970
Mexitil Capsules (About 1 in 10,000) 684
Micro-K...... 2237
Micro-K LS Packets...... 2238
Minocin Pellet-Filled Capsules (Rare) 1429
Pediapred Oral Solution 1618
Prevacid Delayed-Release Capsules (Less than 1%)...... 2746
Slow-K Extended-Release Tablets...... 869

Esophagitis
Achromycin V Capsules (Rare) 1417
Adalat CC (Less than 1.0%)...... 582
Adriamycin PFS 2056
Adriamycin RDF 2056
Anafranil Capsules (Up to 1%) 819
Betaseron for SC Injection...... 653
▲ Cardioquin Tablets (Among most frequent) 2146
▲ CellCept Capsules (More than or equal to 3%)...... 2265
Cleocin Vaginal Cream...... 2070
Cognex Capsules (Infrequent) 1961
Cosmegen Injection 1666
Cytosar-U Sterile Powder (Less frequent) 2077
Didronel Tablets...... 2133
Doryx Capsules (Rare)...... 1970
Doxil (Less than 1%)...... 2613
Doxorubicin Astra 531
DYNACIN Capsules (Rare)...... 1627
Effexor (Infrequent) 2825
Ethamolin Injection (0.1 to 0.4%).. 2544
Felbatol (Infrequent)...... 2774
Fioricet with Codeine Capsules 2387
Fiorinal with Codeine Capsules 2390
Fludara for Injection (Up to 3%) 658
Fosamax Tablets 1703
Helidac Therapy (Rare)...... 2135
Hivid Tablets (Less than 1%) 2287
Intron A for Injection (Less than 5%)...... 2506
Lamictal Tablets...... 1105
Lodine Capsules and Tablets (Less than 1%)...... 2849
Lotrel Capsules...... 858
LUVOX Tablets (Infrequent) 2723
Minocin Pellet-Filled Capsules (Rare) 1429
Monodox Capsules (Rare) 1858
Motrin Ibuprofen Suspension, Oral Drops, Chewable Tablets, Caplets (Less than 1%) 1563
Naprelan Tablets (Less than 1%) .. 2861
Neurontin Capsules (Rare) 1978
Norvir (Less than 2%) 447
Paxil Tablets (Rare) 2681
Permax Tablets (Infrequent)...... 571
Prevacid Delayed-Release Capsules (Less than 1%)...... 2746
Prozac Pulvules & Liquid, Oral Solution (Infrequent) 935
▲ Quinaglute Dura-Tabs Tablets (Among most frequent) 644
▲ Quinidex Extentabs (Among most frequent) 2240
Risperdal Tablets (Rare)...... 1348
Rubex for Injection 721
Rythmol Tablets–150mg, 225mg, 300mg (1.9%) 1399
Salagen Tablets (Less than 1%)...... 1546
Serzone Tablets (Infrequent) 776
Taxotere for Injection Concentrate 2204
Trilisate (Rare) 2155
Urobiotic-250 Capsules (Rare) 2038
Vibramycin (Rare) 2038
Videx Tablets, Powder for Oral Solution, & Pediatric Powder for Oral Solution (Less than 1%)...... 2980
Wellbutrin Tablets 1177
▲ Zinecard Injection (3% to 6%) 2120

Esophagitis, ulcerative
Achromycin V Capsules (Rare) 1417
Celestone Soluspan Suspension 2484
CORTENEMA...... 2713
Cortone Acetate Sterile Suspension 1663
Cortone Acetate Tablets 1664
Dalalone D.P. Injectable 1009
Decadron Elixir 1676
Decadron Phosphate Injection 1680
Decadron Phosphate with Xylocaine Injection, Sterile...... 1683
Decadron Tablets...... 1678
Decadron-LA Sterile Suspension...... 1687
DYNACIN Capsules (Rare)...... 1627
Florinef Acetate Tablets 506
Foscavir Injection (Less than 1%) .. 541
Hydeltrasol Injection, Sterile...... 1708
Hydeltra-T.B.A. Sterile Suspension 1710
Hydrocortone Phosphate Injection, Sterile 1713
Hydrocortone Tablets 1715
Indocin I.V. (Less than 1%)...... 1727
Monodox Capsules (Rare) 1858
Prelone Syrup 1834
Vibramycin (Rare) 2038

Esophagopharyngitis
Ergamisol Tablets 1340
Fluorouracil Injection (Common)...... 2282
Sterile FUDR 2284

Esophagospasm
Ambien Tablets (Rare) 2559
Gastrocrom Capsules (Infrequent).. 1611
Gastrocrom Oral Concentrate 1611
Neurontin Capsules (Rare) 1978

Esophagus, perforation
Ethamolin Injection (0.1 to 0.4%).. 2544

Estrogen, decrease
Cytoxan 700

Euphoria
Adderall Tablets...... 2209
Adipex-P Tablets and Capsules 1035
Akineton 1380
Alfenta Injection (0.3% to 1%) 1334
Ambien Tablets (Frequent) 2559
Anafranil Capsules (Infrequent) 819
Artane...... 1418
Atamet Tablets 567
Axocet Capsules (Infrequent)...... 2469
Benadryl Injection 1955
Betaseron for SC Injection...... 653
▲ Bromfed-DM Cough Syrup (Among most frequent) 1832
Brontex 2130
BuSpar Tablets (Infrequent)...... 738
Celestone Soluspan Suspension 2484
Claritin-D Tablets (Less frequent) .. 2487
CORTENEMA...... 2713
Cortone Acetate Sterile Suspension 1663
Cortone Acetate Tablets 1664
Cytovene (1% or less)...... 2270
Dalmane Capsules (Rare)...... 2329
Darvon-N/Darvocet-N 1473
Darvon 1475
Darvon-N Suspension & Tablets 1473
Decadron Elixir 1676
Decadron Phosphate Injection 1680
Decadron Phosphate with Xylocaine Injection, Sterile...... 1683
Decadron Tablets...... 1678
Decadron-LA Sterile Suspension...... 1687
Demerol 2438
Desoxyn Gradumet Tablets 422
Dexacort Phosphate in Respihaler .. 1606
Dexacort Phosphate in Turbinaire .. 1607
Dexedrine 2648
DextroStat-Dextroamphetamine Sulfate Tablets 2211
Dilaudid-HP Injection (Less frequent) 1384
Dilaudid-HP Lyophilized Powder 250 mg (Less frequent)...... 1384
Dilaudid Tablets and Liquid...... 1386
Dimetane-DC Cough Syrup 2232
Dimetane-DX Cough Syrup 2233
Diprivan Injectable Emulsion (Less than 1%)...... 2939
Doral Tablets 2773
▲ Duragesic Transdermal System (3% to 10%) 1336
Duramorph Injection 983
Duranest Injections...... 533
Dyclone 0.5% and 1% Topical Solutions, USP 535
Effexor (Infrequent) 2825
Eldepryl Capsules 2729
EMLA Cream (Unlikely with cream) 536
Ergamisol Tablets 1340
Esgic-plus Capsules (Infrequent) 1012
Esgic-plus Tablets (Infrequent) 1012
Ethmozine Tablets (Less than 2%) 2217
Fastin Capsules 2662
Felbatol (Infrequent)...... 2774
Fioricet Tablets (Infrequent)...... 2386
Fioricet with Codeine Capsules (Infrequent) 2387
Florinef Acetate Tablets 506
Floxin I.V. (Less than 1%) 1580
Floxin Tablets (200 mg, 300 mg, 400 mg) (Less than 1%)...... 1577
Flumadine Tablets & Syrup (Less than 0.3%)...... 1013
Fluorouracil Injection 2282
Sterile FUDR (Remote possibility) .. 2284
Halcion Tablets (0.9% to 0.5%) ... 2093
Haldol Decanoate...... 1587
Haldol Injection, Tablets and Concentrate 1585
Hivid Tablets (Less than 1%) 2287
Hydeltrasol Injection, Sterile...... 1708
Hydeltra-T.B.A. Sterile Suspension 1710
Hydrocortone Acetate Sterile Suspension 1712
Hydrocortone Phosphate Injection, Sterile 1713
Hydrocortone Tablets 1715
Hyperstat I.V. Injection 2504
Imitrex Injection (Infrequent) 1095
Imitrex Tablets (Infrequent) 1099
Infumorph 200 and Infumorph 500 Sterile Solutions...... 985
Invirase Capsules (Less than 2%) .. 2291
Ionamin Capsules 1615
Kadian Capsules (Less than 3%) 2948
Lamictal Tablets (Infrequent)...... 1105
Larodopa Tablets (Relatively frequent) 2296
Levsin/Levsinex/Levbid 2549
Limbitrol 2333
Lioresal Intrathecal (1% or more) .. 1634
Lioresal Tablets 847
Lomotil 2591
LUVOX Tablets (Infrequent) 2723
▲ MS Contin Tablets (Among most frequent) 2149
▲ MSIR (Among most frequent) 2152
▲ Marinol (Dronabinol) Capsules (3% to 10%) 2353
Mepergan Injection 2859
Methadone Hydrochloride Oral Concentrate 2356
Methadone Hydrochloride Oral Solution & Tablets...... 2357
Miltown Tablets 2780
Moban Tablets and Concentrate (Less frequent) 1036
Motofen Tablets 789
Nardil (Less common) 1977
Neurontin Capsules (Infrequent)...... 1978
Norvir (Less than 2%) 447
Nubain Injection (1% or less) 952
▲ Oramorph SR (Morphine Sulfate Sustained Release Tablets) (Among most frequent) 2359
Orlaam Oral Solution (1% to 3%).. 2361
Ornade Spansule Capsules 2678
OxyContin Tablets (Between 1% and 5%) 2163
OxyIR Capsules...... 2167
PBZ Tablets 863
PBZ-SR Tablets...... 862
Paxil Tablets (Rare) 2681
Percocet Tablets 955
Percodan Tablets...... 955
Percodan-Demi Tablets...... 956
Periactin 1767
Permax Tablets (Infrequent)...... 571
Phenergan with Codeine...... 2883
Phenergan Injection 2880
Phenergan Tablets 2882
Phenergan VC with Codeine 2888
Phrenilin (Infrequent)...... 790
PMB 200 and PMB 400 2890
Prelone Syrup 1834
Prelu-2 Timed Release Capsules...... 687
ProSom Tablets (Infrequent) 457
Prozac Pulvules & Liquid, Oral Solution (Infrequent) 935
RMS Suppositories CII...... 2766
Redux Capsules (Infrequent) 2911
Remeron Tablets (Infrequent) 1878
Restoril Capsules (2-3%) 2413
Rilutek Tablets (Rare) 2198
Risperdal Tablets (Infrequent)...... 1348
Romazicon (1% to 3%) 2311
Roxanol 2365
Roxicodone Tablets, Oral Solution & Intensol (Oxycodone) 2366
Sansert Tablets...... 2424
Sedapap Tablets 50 mg/650 mg (Infrequent) 1826
Serax Capsules 2916
Serax Tablets...... 2916
Serzone Tablets (Infrequent) 776
Sinemet Tablets 959
Sinemet CR Tablets 961
Soma Compound w/Codeine Tablets 2784
Soma Compound Tablets (Very rare) 2783
Soma Tablets...... 2782
Stadol (1% or greater) 779
Sublimaze Injection...... 463
Symmetrel Capsules (0.1% to 1%) 965
Symmetrel Syrup (0.1% to 1%) 963
Talacen Caplets 2464
▲ Talwin Injection (Most common)...... 2465
Talwin Compound 2466
▲ Talwin Injection (Most common)...... 2465
Talwin Nx Tablets 2467
Tambocor Tablets (Less than 1%) 1555
Tavist Syrup...... 2426
Tavist Tablets 2427
Toradol (1% or less) 2319
Tornalate Solution for Inhalation, 0.2% (Less than 1%) 976
Trinalin Repetabs Tablets 1373
Tussend 1830
Tussionex Pennkinetic Extended-Release Suspension 1624
Tylenol with Codeine 1592
Tylox Capsules 1593
▲ Ultram Tablets (50 mg) (1% to 14%) 1594
Versed Injection (Less than 1%) 2324
Wellbutrin Tablets (1.2%)...... 1177
Wygesic Tablets 2930
▲ Xylocaine Injections (Among most common)...... 562
Zarontin Capsules 1986
Zarontin Syrup 1986
Zoloft Tablets (Infrequent) 2051
Zyrtec Tablets (Less than 2%) 2053

Eventration
Redux Capsules 2911

Exanthema
Calan SR Caplets (1% or less) 2571
Calan Tablets (1% or less) 2568
Covera-HS Tablets (Less than 2%) 2573
Isoptin Oral Tablets (Less than 1%)...... 1393
Isoptin SR Tablets (1% or less) 1395

Side Effects Index

Exanthema
- Verelan Capsules (1% or less) 1455

Excitability
- Actifed Cold & Allergy Tablets ...... ⓝ 807
- Actifed Cold & Sinus Caplets and Tablets ...... ⓝ 808
- Alka-Seltzer Plus Cold Medicine .. ⓝ 611
- Alka-Seltzer Plus Cold Medicine Liqui-Gels ...... ⓝ 612
- Alka-Seltzer Plus Cold & Cough Medicine ...... ⓝ 611
- Alka-Seltzer Plus Cold & Cough Medicine Liqui-Gels ...... ⓝ 612
- Alka-Seltzer Plus Night-Time Cold Medicine ...... ⓝ 611
- Alka-Seltzer Plus Night-Time Cold Medicine Liqui-Gels ...... ⓝ 612
- Alka-Seltzer Plus Sinus Medicine ... ⓝ 611
- Allerest Maximum Strength .... ⓝ 649
- Allerest No Drowsiness ...... ⓝ 649
- Allerest Sinus Pain Formula ...... ⓝ 649
- Asendin Tablets (Less frequent) 1419
- Astramorph/PF Injection, USP (Preservative-Free) 526
- Atrohist Pediatric Capsules 1603
- Atrohist Pediatric Suspension 1604
- Atrohist Pediatric Suspension Dye-Free 1604
- Axocet Capsules (Infrequent) 2469
- Benadryl Allergy Chewables ...... ⓝ 811
- Benadryl Allergy Decongestant Liquid Medication ...... ⓝ 812
- Benadryl Allergy Decongestant Tablets ...... ⓝ 812
- Benadryl Allergy Liquid Medication ...... ⓝ 813
- Benadryl Allergy ...... ⓝ 811
- Benadryl Dye-Free Allergy Liqui-gel Softgels ...... ⓝ 813
- Benadryl Dye-Free Allergy Liquid Medication ...... ⓝ 814
- Benadryl Injection 1955
- Bentyl 1246
- Bromfed Capsules (Extended-Release) 1832
- Bromfed Syrup ...... ⓝ 712
- Bromfed Tablets 1832
- Bromfed-DM Cough Syrup 1832
- Bromfed-PD Capsules (Extended-Release) 1832
- Bronkometer Aerosol 2432
- Bronkosol Solution 2432
- BuSpar Tablets (2%) 738
- Cerose DM ...... ⓝ 853
- Cheracol Plus Head Cold/Cough Formula ...... ⓝ 741
- Children's TYLENOL Cold Multi-Symptom Chewable Tablets and Liquid 1559
- Children's TYLENOL Cold Plus Cough Multi Symptom Chewable Tablets and Liquid 1560
- Children's Vicks DayQuil Allergy Relief ...... ⓝ 730
- Children's Vicks NyQuil Cold/Cough Relief ...... ⓝ 731
- Chlor-Trimeton Allergy Decongestant Tablets ...... ⓝ 759
- Chlor-Trimeton Allergy Tablets .... ⓝ 758
- Claritin-D Tablets 2487
- Cocaine Hydrochloride Topical Solutions 529
- Cogentin 1661
- Allergy-Sinus Comtrex Multi-Symptom Allergy-Sinus Formula Tablets and Caplets ... ⓝ 639
- Contac Continuous Action Nasal Decongestant/Antihistamine 12 Hour Capsules ...... ⓝ 773
- Contac Maximum Strength Continuous Action Decongestant/Antihistamine 12 Hour Caplets ...... ⓝ 772
- Contac Night Allergy/Sinus Caplets ...... ⓝ 771
- Contac Severe Cold and Flu Formula Caplets ...... ⓝ 773
- Coricidin Cold + Flu Tablets ...... ⓝ 760
- Coricidin 'D' Decongestant Tablets ...... ⓝ 760
- Crixivan Capsules (Less than 2%)... 1670
- D.A. Chewable Tablets 970
- Dalmane Capsules (Rare) 2329
- ▲ Desyrel and Desyrel Dividose (1.4% to 5.1%) 504
- Dimetapp Allergy Dye-Free Elixir.. ⓝ 838
- Dimetapp Allergy Sinus Caplets .. ⓝ 838
- Dimetapp Cold & Allergy Chewable Tablets ...... ⓝ 838
- Dimetapp Cold & Cough Liqui-Gels ...... ⓝ 839
- Dimetapp Cold & Fever Suspension ...... ⓝ 839
- Dimetapp Elixir ...... ⓝ 840
- Dimetapp Extentabs ...... ⓝ 841
- Dimetapp Tablets/Liqui-Gels ...... ⓝ 841
- Donnatal (In elderly patients) 2234
- Donnatal Extentabs (In elderly patients) 2234
- Donnatal Tablets (In elderly patients) 2234
- Drixoral Cold and Allergy Sustained-Action Tablets ...... ⓝ 763
- Drixoral Cold and Flu Extended-Release Tablets ...... ⓝ 764
- Drixoral Allergy/Sinus Extended Release Tablets ...... ⓝ 765
- Duramorph Injection 983
- Dura-Tap/PD Capsules 970
- Elavil 2945
- Emete-con Intramuscular/Intravenous 2007
- Entex PSE Tablets 973
- Esgic-plus Capsules (Infrequent) 1012
- Esgic-plus Tablets (Infrequent) 1012
- Etrafon 2495
- Fioricet Tablets (Infrequent) 2386
- Fioricet with Codeine Capsules (Infrequent) 2387
- Flexeril Tablets (Less than 1%) 1701
- Guaifed 1833
- Guaimax-D Tablets 809
- Infumorph 200 and Infumorph 500 Sterile Solutions 985
- Isoetharine Inhalation Solution, USP, Arm-a-Med 545
- Levsin/Levsinex/Levbid 2549
- Lioresal Tablets 847
- Marax Tablets & DF Syrup 2015
- Marcaine 2446
- Marcaine Spinal 2449
- Mebaral Tablets 2452
- Mellaril 2398
- Mobigesic Tablets ...... ⓝ 607
- Narcan Injection 950
- Neo-Synephrine Hydrochloride 1% Carpuject 2455
- Neo-Synephrine Hydrochloride 1% Injection 2455
- Nescaine/Nescaine MPF 549
- Nolahist Tablets 790
- Orap Tablets 1037
- Ornade Spansule Capsules 2678
- Orudis Capsules (Greater than 1%) 2874
- Oruvail Capsules (Greater than 1%) 2874
- Oxandrin 783
- PBZ Tablets 863
- PBZ-SR Tablets 862
- PediaCare 1569
- Pediatric Vicks 44m Cough & Cold Relief ...... ⓝ 737
- Percogesic Analgesic Tablets ...... ⓝ 727
- Periactin 1767
- Phenergan Injection 2880
- Phenergan Tablets 2882
- Phenobarbital Elixir and Tablets 1523
- Phrenilin (Infrequent) 790
- Pontocaine Hydrochloride for Spinal Anesthesia 2460
- Prolixin 510
- Protopam Chloride for Injection (Several cases) 2909
- ▲ Proventil Syrup (2 of 100 patients; children 2 to 6 years, approximately 20%) 2528
- Pyrroxate Caplets ...... ⓝ 742
- Quadrinal Tablets 1398
- Robinul Injectable 2247
- Robitussin Night-Time Cold Formula ...... ⓝ 847
- Rondec Oral Drops (Rare) 974
- Rondec Syrup (Rare) 974
- Rondec Tablet (Rare) 974
- Rondec Chewable Tablets 974
- Rondec-TR Tablet (Rare) 974
- Ryna ...... ⓝ 804
- Rynatan 2781
- Rynatuss 2782
- Sedapap Tablets 50 mg/650 mg (Infrequent) 1826
- Sensorcaine 554
- Serentil 689
- Serevent Inhalation Aerosol 1149
- Sinarest ...... ⓝ 663
- Sine-Off Sinus Medicine ...... ⓝ 784
- Singlet Tablets ...... ⓝ 785
- Sinulin Tablets 792
- Sudafed Cold & Allergy Tablets .... ⓝ 826
- Talacen Caplets (Rare) 2464
- Talwin Injection (Rare) 2465
- Talwin Compound (Rare) 2466
- Talwin Injection (Rare) 2465
- Talwin Nx Tablets 2467
- Tavist Syrup 2426
- Tavist Tablets 2427
- Teldrin 12 Hour Antihistamine/Nasal Decongestant Allergy Relief Capsules ...... ⓝ 786
- TheraFlu ...... ⓝ 750
- TheraFlu Maximum Strength Nighttime Flu, Cold & Cough Medicine ...... ⓝ 751
- Torecan 2367
- Trancopal Caplets 2468
- Triaminic Night Time ...... ⓝ 754
- Triaminic Syrup ...... ⓝ 755
- Triaminic Triaminicol Cold & Cough ...... ⓝ 756
- Triaminicin Tablets ...... ⓝ 756
- Triavil Tablets 1800
- Trinalin Repetabs Tablets 1373
- Tussend 1830
- TYLENOL Allergy Sinus, Maximum Strength Caplets and Gelcaps 1571
- TYLENOL Cold Medication, Multi-Symptom Formula Tablets and Caplets 1572
- TYLENOL Cold Medication, Multi-Symptom Hot Liquid Packets 1572
- TYLENOL Flu NightTime, Maximum Strength Gelcaps 1575
- TYLENOL Flu NightTime, Maximum Strength Hot Medication Packets 1575
- Ventolin Syrup (2 of 100 patients) 1175
- Vicks 44 LiquiCaps Cough, Cold & Flu Relief ...... ⓝ 728
- Vicks 44M Cough, Cold & Flu Relief ...... ⓝ 729
- Vicks DayQuil Allergy Relief 12-Hour Extended Release Tablets ...... ⓝ 733
- Vicks DayQuil Allergy Relief 4-Hour Tablets ...... ⓝ 733
- Vicks Nyquil Hot Therapy ...... ⓝ 735
- Vicks NyQuil LiquiCaps/Liquid Multi-Symptom Cold/Flu Relief, Original and Cherry Flavors ...... ⓝ 736
- Winstrol Tablets 2468
- Yohimex Tablets 1414

Excitement, paradoxical
- Dizac (diazepam injectable emulsion) CIV (Less frequent) 1862
- Etrafon 2495
- Halcion Tablets 2093
- Librium Capsules 2331
- Miltown Tablets 2780
- Placidyl Capsules (Occasional) 456
- PMB 200 and PMB 400 2890
- ProSom Tablets 457
- Restoril Capsules (Less than 0.5%) 2413
- Serax Capsules 2916
- Serax Tablets 2916
- Triavil Tablets 1800
- Valium Injectable 2336
- Valium Tablets 2335

Excoriation
- Catapres-TTS (3 of 101 patients).. 680
- Flonase Nasal Spray (Less than 1%) 1088
- Sulfamylon Cream (Rare) 940
- ▲ Videx Tablets, Powder for Oral Solution, & Pediatric Powder for Oral Solution (4%) 2980

Exercise tolerance, decreased
- Blocadren Tablets 1654
- Lopressor HCT Tablets (1 in 100 patients) 850
- Timoptic in Ocudose (Less frequent) 1796
- Timoptic Sterile Ophthalmic Solution (Less frequent) 1794
- Timoptic-XE 1798

Exophthalmos
- Anafranil Capsules (Rare) 819
- Aquasol A Vitamin A Capsules, USP 525
- Aquasol A Parenteral 526
- Celestone Soluspan Suspension 2484
- CORTENEMA 2713
- Cortone Acetate Sterile Suspension 1663
- Cortone Acetate Tablets 1664
- Dalalone D.P. Injectable 1009
- Decadron Elixir 1676
- Decadron Phosphate Injection 1680
- Decadron Phosphate with Xylocaine Injection, Sterile 1683
- Decadron Tablets 1678
- Decadron-LA Sterile Suspension 1687
- Dexacort Phosphate in Respihaler .. 1606
- Dexacort Phosphate in Turbinaire .. 1607
- Effexor (Infrequent) 2825
- Eskalith 2658
- Florinef Acetate Tablets 506
- Hydeltrasol Injection, Sterile 1708
- Hydeltra-T.B.A. Sterile Suspension 1710
- Hydrocortone Acetate Sterile Suspension 1712
- Hydrocortone Phosphate Injection, Sterile 1713
- Hydrocortone Tablets 1715
- Lithonate/Lithotabs/Lithobid 2721
- Paxil Tablets (Rare) 2681
- Pediapred Oral Solution 1618
- Prelone Syrup 1834
- Zoloft Tablets (Rare) 2051

Extrapyramidal symptoms
- Abelcet Injection 1540
- Adapin Capsules (Infrequent) 1542
- Anafranil Capsules (Infrequent) 819
- Asendin Tablets (Less than 1%) 1419
- BuSpar Tablets (Rare) 738
- Cardizem CD Capsules (Infrequent) 1251
- Cardizem SR Capsules (Infrequent) 1255
- Cardizem Injectable 1253
- Cardizem Tablets (Infrequent) 1257
- ▲ Cerebyx Injection (4.4%) 1956
- Clozaril Tablets 2377
- Cognex Capsules (Infrequent) 1961
- Compazine 2644
- ▲ Demser Capsules (10%) 1690
- Desyrel and Desyrel Dividose 504
- Elavil 2945
- Eskalith 2658
- Etrafon (More common) 2495
- Felbatol 2774
- Flexeril Tablets (Rare) 1701
- Floxin Tablets (200 mg, 300 mg, 400 mg) 1577
- Foscavir Injection (Less than 1%) .. 541
- Haldol Decanoate (Frequent) 1587
- Haldol Injection, Tablets and Concentrate (Frequent) 1585
- Inapsine Injection 462
- Intron A for Injection (Less than 5%) 2506
- Kytril Injection (Rare) 2667
- Kytril Tablets (One case) 2669
- Levoprome 1321
- Librax Capsules (Rare) 2330
- Librium Capsules (Isolated cases) ... 2331
- Librium Injectable (Isolated cases) .. 2332
- Limbitrol 2333
- Lithonate/Lithotabs/Lithobid 2721
- ▲ Loxitane (Frequent) 1426
- Ludiomil Tablets (Rare) 861
- LUVOX Tablets (Infrequent) 2723
- Mellaril (Infrequent) 2398
- Mepergan Injection (Rare) 2859
- Moban Tablets and Concentrate ... 1036
- Navane Capsules and Concentrate 2018
- Navane Intramuscular 2019
- Norpramin Tablets 1273
- Orap Tablets (Frequent) 1037
- Pamelor 2409
- Paxil Tablets (Rare) 2681
- Permax Tablets (1.6%) 571
- Phenergan with Codeine 2883
- Phenergan Injection 2880
- Phenergan Suppositories 2882
- Phenergan Syrup 2881
- Phenergan Tablets 2882
- Proglycem 575
- Prolixin 510
- Propulsid (Rare) 1346
- Prozac Pulvules & Liquid, Oral Solution (Rare) 935
- Reglan (Approximately 0.2%) 2243
- Remeron Tablets (Infrequent) 1878
- Rilutek Tablets (Infrequent) 2198
- ▲ Risperdal Tablets (17% to 34%) .. 1348
- Ser-Ap-Es Tablets (Rare) 867
- Serentil 689
- Sinemet CR Tablets 961
- Sinequan (Infrequent) 2028
- Stelazine 2692
- Surmontil Capsules 2917
- Thorazine 2701
- Tiazac Capsules (Infrequent) 1019
- Tigan 2231

(ⓝ Described in PDR For Nonprescription Drugs)   Incidence data in parenthesis; ▲ 3% or more   (ⓞ Described in PDR For Ophthalmology)

Side Effects Index

Eyes, redness

Tofranil Ampuls	873
Tofranil Tablets	875
Tofranil-PM Capsules	876
Toradol (1% or less)	2319
Torecan	2367
Triavil Tablets	1800
Trilafon	2532
Vivactil Tablets	1820
Zofran Injection (Rare)	1227
Zofran Tablets (Rare)	1231

Extrasystoles

Adalat CC (Less than 1.0%)	582
Ambien Tablets (Rare)	2559
Anafranil Capsules (Infrequent)	819
Benadryl Injection	1955
Cardene Capsules (Rare)	2261
Cardene I.V. (0.7%)	2815
Cardioquin Tablets (Frequent)	2146
Dilacor XR Extended-release Capsules	2183
Diprivan Injectable Emulsion (Less than 1%)	2939
Effexor (Infrequent)	2825
Foscavir Injection (Less than 1%)	541
Imdur (Less than or equal to 5%)	1362
Intron A for Injection (Less than 5%)	2506
Lariam Tablets (Less than 1%)	2295
Levo-Dromoran	2297
Lopid Tablets	1974
Lufyllin & Lufyllin-400 Tablets	2778
Lufyllin-GG Elixir & Tablets	2779
Maxaquin Tablets (Less than 1%)	2593
Norvasc Tablets (Less than or equal to 0.1%)	2020
Ornade Spansule Capsules	2678
PBZ Tablets	863
PBZ-SR Tablets	862
Periactin	1767
Quadrinal Tablets	1398
Quibron	2227
Quinidex Extentabs	2240
Redux Capsules (Infrequent)	2911
Respbid Tablets	687
Slo-bid Gyrocaps	2201
Tavist Syrup	2426
Tavist Tablets	2427
Theo-Dur Extended-Release Tablets	1367
Theo-X Extended-Release Tablets	793
Trinalin Repetabs Tablets	1373
Tussend	1830
Uni-Dur Extended-Release Tablets	1374

Extrasystoles, supraventricular

Caverject Injection (Less than 1%)	2064
Corvert Injection (0.9% to 5.1%)	2075
LUVOX Tablets (Rare)	2723

Extravasation

Adriamycin PFS	2056
Adriamycin RDF	2056
Brevibloc (esmolol HCl) Injection (Less than 1%)	1860
Cerubidine for Injection	634
Claforan Sterile and Injection (Rare)	1259
Cosmegen Injection	1666
DaunoXome	1842
Doxil	2613
Doxorubicin Astra	531
▲ Etopophos for Injection (5%)	701
Fluorescite	⊞ 217
Gemzar for Injection (Infrequent)	1482
Hyperstat I.V. Injection	2504
Idamycin Injection	2096
Levophed Bitartrate Injection	2445
Mutamycin for Injection	712
Platinol for Injection	717
Platinol-AQ Injection	719
Romazicon	2311
Rubex for Injection	721
Taxol Injection	723
Taxotere for Injection Concentrate	2204
Velban Vials	1537
Zinecard Injection (1% to 3%)	2120

Extroversion

| Ambien Tablets | 2559 |
| Halcion Tablets | 2093 |

Exudate, increased

Bactroban Ointment (Less than 1%)	2642
▲ THROMBATE III Antithrombin III (Human) (1 of 17)	631
Xalatan (Less than 1%)	⊙ 304

Eye abnormalities, fetal

| Accutane Capsules | 2252 |

| Clomid | 1262 |

Eye globe, perforation
(see under Bulbus oculi, perforation)

Eye movements, abnormal

Klonopin Tablets	2294
Mevacor Tablets (0.5% to 1.0%)	1742
Zocor Tablets	1821

Eyeball, perforation
(see under Bulbus oculi, perforation)

Eyelashes, matting of

Alomide Ophthalmic Solution (Less than 1%)	465
Betoptic Ophthalmic Solution	465
Betoptic S Ophthalmic Suspension (Small number of patients)	467
Iopidine 0.5% (Less than 1%)	⊙ 219
Lacrisert Sterile Ophthalmic Insert	1730

Eyelids, cyclic, movement of

| Versed Injection | 2324 |

Eyelids, deposits in

Alomide Ophthalmic Solution (Less than 1%)	465
Iopidine 0.5% (Less than 3%)	⊙ 219
Xalatan (1% to 4%)	⊙ 304

Eyelids, edema of

BOTOX (Botulinum Toxin Type A) Purified Neurotoxin Complex (2 cases)	473
Ciloxan Ophthalmic Solution (Less than 1%)	468
Hyzaar Tablets	1720
Lacrisert Sterile Ophthalmic Insert	1730
Phenobarbital Elixir and Tablets	1523
Polytrim Ophthalmic Solution Sterile (Multiple reports)	479
▲ Rev-Eyes Ophthalmic Eyedrops 0.5% (10% to 40%)	⊙ 324
Tobrex Ophthalmic Ointment and Solution (Less than 3 of 100 patients)	⊙ 226
Xalatan (1% to 4%)	⊙ 304

Eyelids, erythema

| ▲ Betimol 0.25%, 0.5% (More than 5%) | ⊙ 259 |
| Xalatan (1% to 4%) | ⊙ 304 |

Eyelids, heavy

Axocet Capsules (Infrequent)	2469
Esgic-plus Capsules (Infrequent)	1012
Esgic-plus Tablets (Infrequent)	1012
Fioricet Tablets (Infrequent)	2386
Fioricet with Codeine Capsules (Infrequent)	2387
Fiorinal with Codeine Capsules (Infrequent)	2390
Phrenilin (Infrequent)	790
Sedapap Tablets 50 mg/650 mg (Infrequent)	1826

Eyes, burning

▲ AKPRO (6%)	⊙ 206
▲ Betagan (About 1 in 3 patients)	⊙ 230
Bleph-10	472
Catapres Tablets	679
Catapres-TTS	680
▲ Ciloxan Ophthalmic Solution (Among most frequent)	468
Cleocin T Topical	2072
Combipres Tablets	682
Cozaar Tablets (Less than 1%)	1668
Dalmane Capsules (Rare)	2329
FML Forte Liquifilm	⊙ 237
FML Liquifilm	⊙ 238
FLUORACAINE (Occasional)	⊙ 208
FLURESS (Occasional)	⊙ 208
▲ Genoptic Sterile Ophthalmic Solution (Among most frequent)	⊙ 241
▲ Genoptic Sterile Ophthalmic Ointment (Among most frequent)	⊙ 241
HMS Liquifilm	⊙ 241
Hivid Tablets (Less than 1%)	2287
Hyzaar Tablets	1720
IOPIDINE Sterile Ophthalmic Solution	⊙ 218
Isopto Carpine Ophthalmic Solution	⊙ 221
Lamprene Capsules (Greater than 1%)	846
▲ Livostin (29%)	⊙ 262

Motofen Tablets (Less frequent)	789
Muro 128 Ophthalmic Ointment	⊙ 256
Muro 128 Solution 2% and 5%	⊙ 255
Nicotrol NS Nicotine Nasal Spray (More common)	1565
Ocufen	⊙ 242
▲ Ocuflox Ophthalmic Solution (One of the two most frequent)	478
▲ Ocupress Ophthalmic Solution, 1% Sterile (About 1 of 4 patients)	⊙ 297
Ophthetic	⊙ 244
Phospholine Iodide	⊙ 323
Pilopine HS Ophthalmic Gel	⊙ 224
▲ Polytrim Ophthalmic Solution Sterile (Among most frequent)	479
Pred Forte	⊙ 247
Pred Mild	⊙ 250
▲ PROPINE with C CAP Compliance Cap (6%)	⊙ 251
ReVia Tablets (Less than 1%)	957
Soma Compound w/Codeine Tablets	2784
Soma Compound Tablets	2783
Tessalon Perles	1018
▲ Timoptic in Ocudose (Approximately 1 in 8 patients)	1796
▲ Timoptic Sterile Ophthalmic Solution (Approximately 1 in 8 patients)	1794
▲ Trusopt Sterile Ophthalmic Solution (Among most frequent)	1803
Vira-A Ophthalmic Ointment, 3%	⊙ 299
Visken Tablets (2% or fewer patients)	2428
▲ Voltaren Ophthalmic Sterile Ophthalmic Solution (15%)	⊙ 264
Xalatan (5% to 15%)	⊙ 304

Eyes, dilatation of pupil
(see under Mydriasis)

Eyes, disorders

AeroBid Inhaler System (1% to 3%)	1004
Aerobid-M Inhaler System (1% to 3%)	1004
Ativan Tablets (Less frequent)	2807
Atretol Tablets	569
Cartrol Tablets (Less common)	413
Clinoril Tablets (Less than 1%)	1658
Cordarone Tablets	2818
Desferal Vials	838
Desyrel and Desyrel Dividose (Up to 2.8%)	504
Dynabac (0.1% to 1%)	668
Flonase Nasal Spray (Less than 1%)	1088
Foscavir Injection (Between 1% and 5%)	541
Hivid Tablets (Less than 1%)	2287
Loxitane	1426
Lupron Depot 3.75 mg	2739
Lupron Injection (Less than 5%)	2736
Mintezol	1747
Nasalide Nasal Solution 0.025% (5% or less)	2301
Neurontin Capsules (Rare)	1978
▲ Novantrone for Injection (2 to 7%)	1327
Permax Tablets (1.1%)	571
Redux Capsules (Infrequent)	2911
ReVia Tablets (Less than 1%)	957
Tambocor Tablets	1555
▲ Tegison Capsules (50-75%)	2314
Tegretol/Tegretol-XR	870
▲ THROMBATE III Antithrombin III (Human) (1 of 17)	631
Urispas Tablets	2710
Varivax (Greater than or equal to 1%)	1807
Versed Injection (Less than 1%)	2324
▲ Vesanoid Capsules (17%)	2327
Videx Tablets, Powder for Oral Solution, & Pediatric Powder for Oral Solution (Less than 1%)	2980
Vistide Injection	1057

Eyes, dry
(see also under Xerophthalmia)

Accutane Capsules	2252
Blocadren Tablets	1654
Cordarone Tablets	2818
Inderal (Rare)	2834
Inderal LA Long Acting Capsules (Rare)	2836
Inderide LA Long Acting Capsules (Rare)	2840
Kerlone Tablets (Less than 1%)	2588
Lamprene Capsules (Greater than 1%)	846
Lopressor (Rare)	848

Normodyne Tablets	2522
▲ Norpace (3 to 9%)	2596
Sectral Capsules (Up to 2%)	2914
Tenoretic Tablets	2963
Tenormin Tablets and I.V. Injection	2965
Trandate Tablets (Less common)	1158
Transderm Scōp Transdermal Therapeutic System (Infrequent)	890
Vexol 1% Ophthalmic Suspension (Less than 1%)	⊙ 227

Eyes, irritation

AK-Spore	⊙ 205
Bleph-10	472
Blocadren Tablets (1.1%)	1654
▲ BOTOX (Botulinum Toxin Type A) Purified Neurotoxin Complex (10.0%)	473
Cardizem CD Capsules (Less than 1%)	1251
Cardizem SR Capsules (Less than 1%)	1255
Cardizem Injectable	1253
Cardizem Tablets (Less than 1%)	1257
Clear Eyes ACR Astringent/Lubricant Eye Redness Reliever Eye Drops	⊙ 314
Cleocin T Topical	2072
Crolom (Infrequent)	⊙ 254
Emgel 2% Topical Gel	1081
Eye-Stream Eye Irrigating Solution	469
Feldene Capsules (Less than 1%)	2008
▲ Genoptic Sterile Ophthalmic Solution (Among most frequent)	⊙ 241
▲ Genoptic Sterile Ophthalmic Ointment (Among most frequent)	⊙ 241
▲ Ilotycin Ophthalmic Ointment (Among most frequent)	928
Imitrex Injection (Infrequent)	1095
Imitrex Tablets (Up to 2%)	1099
Invirase Capsules (Less than 2%)	2291
Iopidine 0.5% (Less than 3%)	⊙ 219
Isopto Carbachol Ophthalmic Solution	⊙ 221
Lamprene Capsules (Greater than 1%)	846
Methotrexate Sodium Tablets, Injection, for Injection and LPF Injection (Less common)	1322
Mevacor Tablets (0.5% to 1.0%)	1742
Muro 128 Ophthalmic Ointment	⊙ 256
Muro 128 Solution 2% and 5%	⊙ 255
Nicotrol NS Nicotine Nasal Spray (More common)	1565
Ocufen	⊙ 242
▲ Ocupress Ophthalmic Solution, 1% Sterile (About 1 of 4 patients)	⊙ 297
Ocusert Pilo-20 and Pilo-40 Ocular Therapeutic Systems (Infrequent)	⊙ 252
Ophthalgan	⊙ 323
▲ Polytrim Ophthalmic Solution Sterile (Among most frequent)	479
Pondimin Tablets	2239
Ponstel	1982
Quadrinal Tablets	1398
Roferon-A Injection (Less than 1%)	2308
T-Stat 2.0% Topical Solution and Pads	2797
Tambocor Tablets (Less than 1%)	1555
▲ Tegison Capsules (50-75%)	2314
THERAMYCIN Z 2% Solution	1629
Tiazac Capsules (Less than 1%)	1019
Timolide Tablets	1791
Tornalate Solution for Inhalation, 0.2% (Less than 1%)	976
Vaqta (Less than 1%)	1805
Vira-A Ophthalmic Ointment, 3%	⊙ 299
Visine L.R. Eye Drops	⊙ 301
Visken Tablets (2% or fewer patients)	2428
Viva-Drops	⊙ 326

Eyes, nonreactive

| Nipent for Injection (Less than 3%) | 2733 |

Eyes, redness

AK-Spore	⊙ 205
Albalon Solution with Liquifilm	⊙ 229
All-Flex Arcing Spring Diaphragm (See also Ortho Diaphragm Kits)	1921
BuSpar Tablets (Infrequent)	738
Clozaril Tablets (Less than 1%)	2377
Eye-Stream Eye Irrigating Solution	469
FLUORACAINE (Occasional)	⊙ 208
Hivid Tablets (Less than 1%)	2287

(⊞ Described in PDR For Nonprescription Drugs)   Incidence data in parenthesis; ▲ 3% or more   (⊙ Described in PDR For Ophthalmology)

Eyes, redness

- Humorsol Sterile Ophthalmic Solution ... 1707
- Livostin (Approximately 1% to 3%) ... ⊚ 262
- Ocuflox Ophthalmic Solution ... 478
- Ortho Diaphragm Kits—All-Flex Arcing Spring; Ortho Coil Spring; Ortho-White Flat Spring ... 1921
- Ortho Diaphragm Kit ... 1921
- ▲ Polytrim Ophthalmic Solution Sterile (Among most frequent) ... 479
- Transderm Scōp Transdermal Therapeutic System (Infrequent) ... 890
- Visine L.R. Eye Drops ... ⊛ 301
- Viva-Drops ... ⊛ 326

Eyes, "spots" before the

- Clomid (Occasional) ... 1262
- Depakene ... 416
- Depakote Tablets ... 418
- Tambocor Tablets ... 1555

Eyes, swollen

(see under Edema, palpebral)

Eyes, tearing

- ▲ Alomide Ophthalmic Solution (1% to 5%) ... 465
- Amicar Syrup, Tablets, and Injection ... 1312
- Beconase AQ Nasal Spray (Fewer than 3 per 100 patients) ... 1065
- Betoptic Ophthalmic Solution (Occasional) ... 465
- Betoptic S Ophthalmic Suspension (Small number of patients) ... 467
- Chemet Capsules (1.0% to 3.7%) ... 666
- Ciloxan Ophthalmic Solution (Less than 1%) ... 468
- Dantrium Capsules (Less frequent) ... 2131
- Dipentum Capsules (Rare) ... 2084
- Emcyt Capsules (1%) ... 2085
- ▲ Iopidine 0.5% (4%) ... ⊚ 219
- Nasalide Nasal Solution 0.025% ... 2301
- Nipent for Injection (Less than 3%) ... 2733
- Ocuflox Ophthalmic Solution ... 478
- ▲ Ocupress Ophthalmic Solution, 1% Sterile (About 1 of 4 patients) ... ⊚ 297
- Polytrim Ophthalmic Solution Sterile (Multiple reports) ... 479
- Rev-Eyes Ophthalmic Eyedrops 0.5% (Less frequently) ... ⊚ 324
- Timoptic in Ocudose (Less frequent) ... 1796
- Timoptic Sterile Ophthalmic Solution (Less frequent) ... 1794
- Timoptic-XE (1% to 5% of patients) ... 1798
- Vancenase AQ Nasal Spray 0.042% (Fewer than 3 per 100 patients) ... 2535
- Xalatan (1% to 4%) ... ⊚ 304

ECG changes

(see under EKG changes)

EEG changes

- Anafranil Capsules (Infrequent) ... 819
- Asendin Tablets (Less frequent) ... 1419
- Clozaril Tablets ... 2377
- Compazine ... 2644
- Dizac (diazepam injectable emulsion) CIV ... 1862
- Elavil ... 2945
- Eskalith ... 2658
- Etrafon ... 2495
- Flexeril Tablets (Rare) ... 1701
- Foscavir Injection (Between 1% and 5%) ... 541
- Halcion Tablets ... 2093
- Librax Capsules ... 2330
- Librium Capsules (Isolated cases) ... 2331
- Librium Injectable ... 2332
- Limbitrol ... 2333
- Lithium Carbonate Capsules & Tablets ... 2352
- Lithonate/Lithotabs/Lithobid ... 2721
- Ludiomil Tablets (Rare) ... 861
- Miltown Tablets ... 2780
- Norpramin Tablets ... 1273
- Pamelor ... 2409
- Paxil Tablets (Rare) ... 2681
- Penetrex Tablets ... 2196
- PMB 200 and PMB 400 ... 2890
- Prolixin ... 510
- ProSom Tablets ... 457
- Prozac Pulvules & Liquid, Oral Solution (Rare) ... 935

- Serax Capsules ... 2916
- Serax Tablets ... 2916
- Solganal Suspension ... 2530
- Surmontil Capsules ... 2917
- Tofranil Ampuls ... 873
- Tofranil Tablets ... 875
- Tofranil-PM Capsules ... 876
- Triavil Tablets ... 1800
- Tripedia ... 908
- Valium Injectable ... 2336
- Valium Tablets (Infrequent) ... 2335
- Vivactil Tablets ... 1820
- Wellbutrin Tablets (Rare) ... 1177

EKG changes

- Anafranil Capsules (Infrequent) ... 819
- Apresazide Capsules ... 824
- Aralen Hydrochloride Injection (Rare) ... 2430
- Aralen Phosphate Tablets (Rare) ... 2431
- Azactam for Injection (Less than 1%) ... 736
- ▲ Betapace Tablets (4% to 7%) ... 637
- Bumex (0.4%) ... 2260
- Cafergot ... 2376
- Cardene Capsules (0.6%) ... 2261
- Cardene I.V. (1.4%) ... 2815
- Cardizem CD Capsules (Less than 1% to 1.6%) ... 1251
- ▲ Cardizem SR Capsules (4.1%) ... 1255
- Cardizem Injectable ... 1253
- Cardizem Tablets (Less than 1%) ... 1257
- Catapres Tablets (Rare) ... 679
- Catapres-TTS ... 680
- Clozaril Tablets (1%) ... 2377
- Combipres Tablets (Rare) ... 682
- Compazine ... 2644
- Demadex Tablets and Injection (2.0%) ... 691
- Dilacor XR Extended-release Capsules (Infrequent) ... 2183
- Diprivan Injectable Emulsion (Less than 1%) ... 2939
- Elavil ... 2945
- Eskalith ... 2658
- Ethmozine Tablets (1.6%) ... 2217
- Etrafon (Occasional) ... 2495
- Foscavir Injection (Between 1% and 5%) ... 541
- Haldol Decanoate ... 1587
- Haldol Injection, Tablets and Concentrate ... 1585
- Hydralazine Hydrochloride Injection USP ... 2712
- Hyperstat I.V. Injection ... 2504
- Imitrex Tablets (Infreqent) ... 1099
- Kytril Injection (Rare) ... 2667
- Lanoxicaps ... 1110
- Lanoxin Elixir Pediatric ... 1113
- Lanoxin Injection ... 1116
- Lanoxin Injection Pediatric ... 1119
- Lanoxin Tablets ... 1121
- Lithium Carbonate Capsules & Tablets ... 2352
- Lithonate/Lithotabs/Lithobid ... 2721
- Lotensin Tablets (Scattered incidents) ... 852
- Lotensin HCT Tablets (Scattered accounts) ... 855
- Loxitane (A few cases) ... 1426
- ▲ Lupron Injection (5% or more) ... 2736
- Macrobid Capsules ... 2138
- Macrodantin Capsules ... 2140
- Mellaril ... 2398
- Midamor Tablets ... 1746
- Miltown Tablets ... 2780
- Nalfon 200 Pulvules & Nalfon Tablets (Less than 1%) ... 933
- Naprelan Tablets (Less than 1%) ... 2861
- Navane Capsules and Concentrate ... 2018
- Navane Intramuscular ... 2019
- Nimotop Capsules (Up to 1.4%) ... 603
- Novantrone for Injection ... 1327
- Orap Tablets (2.7%) ... 1037
- Paxil Tablets (Infrequent) ... 2681
- Permax Tablets (Infrequent) ... 571
- PMB 200 and PMB 400 ... 2890
- Polycitra-K Crystals ... 574
- Polycitra-K Oral Solution ... 575
- ▲ Prograf (Greater than 3%) ... 1028
- Prolixin ... 510
- Prostigmin Injectable ... 1305
- Prostigmin Tablets ... 1306
- ▲ Quinaglute Dura-Tabs Tablets (3%) ... 644
- Quinidex Extentabs ... 2240
- Redux Capsules ... 2911
- Retrovir Capsules (2.4%) ... 1216
- ▲ Retrovir I.V. Infusion (3%) ... 1221
- Retrovir Syrup (2.4%) ... 1216

- ReVia Tablets (Less than 1%) ... 957
- Salagen Tablets (Less than 1%) ... 1546
- Stelazine ... 2692
- Suprane (desflurane, USP) (Less than 1%) ... 1865
- ▲ Taxol Injection (Common; 14% to 23%) ... 723
- Taxotere for Injection Concentrate ... 2204
- Thorazine ... 2701
- Tiazac Capsules (Less than 1%) ... 1019
- Tofranil Ampuls ... 873
- Tofranil Tablets ... 875
- Tofranil-PM Capsules ... 876
- Torecan ... 2367
- Tornalate Solution for Inhalation, 0.2% (Less than 1%) ... 976
- Triavil Tablets ... 1800
- Trilafon (Occasional) ... 2532
- Ultram Tablets (50 mg) (Infrequent) ... 1594
- Wellbutrin Tablets (Infrequent) ... 1177
- Zemuron Injection (Less than 1%) ... 1885
- Zofran Injection (Rare) ... 1227
- Zofran Tablets (Rare) ... 1231

EKG changes, PR prolongation

- Imitrex Injection (Infrequent) ... 1095
- Lanoxin Injection Pediatric ... 1119
- Respbid Tablets ... 687

EKG changes, Q wave disturbances

- Compazine ... 2644
- ▲ Imdur (Less than or equal to 5%) ... 1362
- Stelazine ... 2692
- Thorazine ... 2701

EKG changes, QRS interval prolonged

- Aralen Hydrochloride Injection (Rare) ... 2430
- Aralen Phosphate Tablets (Rare) ... 2431
- Doxorubicin Astra ... 531
- Haldol Injection, Tablets and Concentrate ... 1585
- Norpace (1 to 3%) ... 2596
- Quinaglute Dura-Tabs Tablets ... 644
- Rum-K Syrup ... 1004
- Rythmol Tablets–150mg, 225mg, 300mg (0.5 to 1.9%) ... 1399
- Tonocard Tablets (Less than 1%) ... 519

EKG changes, QT interval prolonged

- Cardioquin Tablets ... 2146
- Cerebyx Injection (Infrequent) ... 1956
- Cordarone Intravenous (Less than 2%) ... 2821
- Corvert Injection (1.2%) ... 2075
- Foscavir Injection (Rare) ... 541
- Haldol Decanoate ... 1587
- Imitrex Injection (Infrequent) ... 1095
- Inapsine Injection ... 462
- Mellaril ... 2398
- Norpace (1 to 3%) ... 2596
- Orap Tablets ... 1037
- Orlaam Oral Solution (Low frequency) ... 2361
- Propulsid (Rare) ... 1346
- Prozac Pulvules & Liquid, Oral Solution ... 935
- Quinidex Extentabs ... 2240
- Risperdal Tablets ... 1348
- Seldane Tablets (Rare) ... 1284
- Seldane-D Extended-Release Tablets (Rare) ... 1286
- Serentil ... 689
- Tonocard Tablets (Less than 1%) ... 519
- Vascor Tablets (200 and 300 mg) (0.5 to 2.0%) ... 1597

EKG changes, reversible flattening

- Eskalith ... 2658
- Lithium Carbonate Capsules & Tablets ... 2352
- Lithonate/Lithotabs/Lithobid ... 2721

EKG changes, sinus pause

- Brethaire Inhaler ... 830
- Ethmozine Tablets (1.6%) ... 2217
- Tambocor Tablets (1% to less than 3%) ... 1555

EKG changes, ST section

- ▲ Adenoscan (3%) ... 1022
- Brethaire Inhaler ... 830
- Cardene I.V. (Rare) ... 2815
- Clozaril Tablets ... 2377
- Dilacor XR Extended-release Capsules (Infrequent) ... 2183

- Diprivan Injectable Emulsion (Less than 1%) ... 2939
- Doxorubicin Astra ... 531
- Foscavir Injection (Between 1% and 5%) ... 541
- Imitrex Injection (Infrequent) ... 1095
- Lanoxicaps ... 1110
- Lanoxin Elixir Pediatric ... 1113
- Lanoxin Injection ... 1116
- Lanoxin Injection Pediatric ... 1119
- Lanoxin Tablets ... 1121
- LUVOX Tablets (Infrequent) ... 2723
- Macrobid Capsules ... 2138
- Macrodantin Capsules ... 2140
- Orlaam Oral Solution (Low frequency) ... 2361
- OxyContin Tablets (Less than 1%) ... 2163
- Risperdal Tablets (Rare) ... 1348
- Rum-K Syrup ... 1004

EKG changes, T-wave

- Adenoscan (Less than 1%) ... 1022
- Aralen Hydrochloride Injection (Rare) ... 2430
- Aralen Phosphate Tablets (Rare) ... 2431
- Brethaire Inhaler ... 830
- Cardene I.V. (Rare) ... 2815
- Clozaril Tablets ... 2377
- Compazine ... 2644
- Dopram Injectable ... 2235
- Doxorubicin Astra ... 531
- Eskalith ... 2658
- Flagyl 375 Capsules ... 2587
- Flagyl I.V. ... 2373
- Helidac Therapy ... 2135
- Imitrex Injection (Infrequent) ... 1095
- Lithium Carbonate Capsules & Tablets ... 2352
- Lithonate/Lithotabs/Lithobid ... 2721
- Macrobid Capsules ... 2138
- Macrodantin Capsules ... 2140
- Mellaril ... 2398
- MetroGel-Vaginal ... 917
- Moban Tablets and Concentrate (Rare) ... 1036
- Mycobutin Capsules (More than one patient) ... 2101
- Orap Tablets ... 1037
- Orlaam Oral Solution (Low frequency) ... 2361
- Pentasa (Infrequent) ... 1275
- Protostat Tablets ... 1939
- Risperdal Tablets (Rare) ... 1348
- Rum-K Syrup ... 1004
- Serentil ... 689
- Stelazine ... 2692
- Sular Tablets (Less than or equal to 1%) ... 2961
- Thorazine ... 2701
- Tornalate Solution for Inhalation, 0.2% (Less than 1%) ... 976

ESR, elevation

- ▲ Accutane Capsules (Approximately 40%) ... 2252
- Altace Capsules (Less than 1%) ... 1238
- Ambien Tablets (Rare) ... 2559
- Capoten Tablets ... 740
- Capozide Tablets ... 744
- Cipro I.V. (Rare) ... 587
- Cipro I.V. Pharmacy Bulk Package (Rare) ... 590
- Clozaril Tablets ... 2377
- Cytotec (Infrequent) ... 2576
- Floxin I.V. (More than or equal to 1%) ... 1580
- Floxin Tablets (200 mg, 300 mg, 400 mg) (More than or equal to 1%) ... 1577
- Inocor Lactate Injection (1 case) ... 2439
- Lamprene Capsules (Greater than 1%) ... 846
- Lescol Capsules (Rare) ... 2395
- Maxaquin Tablets ... 2593
- Mevacor Tablets (Rare) ... 1742
- Monopril Tablets ... 762
- Pravachol Tablets (Rare) ... 770
- Prinivil Tablets (0.3% to 1.0%) ... 1776
- Prinzide Tablets ... 1780
- Prozac Pulvules & Liquid, Oral Solution (Rare) ... 935
- Recombivax HB ... 1787
- Sansert Tablets ... 2424
- ▲ Tegison Capsules (25-50%) ... 2314
- Vaseretic Tablets ... 1810
- Vasotec I.V. ... 1814
- Vasotec Tablets (0.5% to 1.0%) ... 1816
- Zestoretic Tablets ... 2968
- Zestril Tablets (0.3% to 1.0%) ... 2972
- Zocor Tablets (Rare) ... 1821

(⊛ Described in PDR For Nonprescription Drugs) Incidence data in parenthesis; ▲ 3% or more (⊚ Described in PDR For Ophthalmology)

1335 **Side Effects Index** **Fatigue**

F

Face, red scaly
▲ Tegison Capsules (50-75%) ... 2314

Face, rhythmical involuntary movements
Compazine ... 2644
Etrafon ... 2495
Haldol Decanoate ... 1587
Lithonate/Lithotabs/Lithobid ... 2721
Mellaril ... 2398
Moban Tablets and Concentrate ... 1036
Orap Tablets ... 1037
Reglan ... 2243
Stelazine ... 2692
Thorazine ... 2701

Facial dysmorphia, fetal
Accutane Capsules ... 2252

Facial features, coarsening
Dilantin Infatabs ... 1967
Dilantin Kapseals ... 1965
Dilantin-125 Suspension ... 1969

Facial swelling
Altace Capsules ... 1238
Alupent Tablets (0.2%) ... 672
Carafate Suspension ... 1250
Carafate Tablets ... 1249
Cortifoam ... 2540
▲ Doxil (Approximately 6.8%) ... 2613
Hivid Tablets (Less than 1%) ... 2287
JE-VAX (0.1%) ... 904
Stelazine ... 2692
Unasyn (Less than 1%) ... 2035

Facies, mask-like
Compazine ... 2644
Loxitane ... 1426
Reglan ... 2243
Stelazine ... 2692
Thorazine ... 2701

Factors II, V, VII, X, decrease
Androderm Testosterone Transdermal System ... 2634
▲ Android Capsules, 10 mg (Among most common) ... 1297
Estratest ... 2718
Halotestin Tablets ... 2095
Oxandrin ... 783
Testoderm Testosterone Transdermal System ... 486
Testred Capsules, 10 mg ... 1308

Factors VII, VIII, IX, X, increase
Amen Tablets ... 785
Aygestin Tablets ... 990
Brevicon ... 2563
Depo-Provera Sterile Aqueous Suspension ... 2083
Estratest ... 2718
Norinyl ... 2563
Nor-Q D Tablets ... 2598
Ortho-Cyclen/Ortho-Tri-Cyclen ... 1914
Ortho-Cyclen/Ortho Tri-Cyclen ... 1914
Tri-Norinyl ... 2607

Fainting (see under Syncope)

Falling
Ambien Tablets (Infrequent) ... 2559
Dalmane Capsules ... 2329
Eldepryl Capsules ... 2729
Halcion Tablets ... 2093
Matulane Capsules ... 2300
Monopril Tablets (0.4% to 1.0%) .. 762
Restoril Capsules ... 2413
Sinemet CR Tablets ... 961
Tofranil Ampuls ... 873
Tofranil Tablets ... 875
Tofranil-PM Capsules ... 876

Fanconi syndrome
Depakene (Rare) ... 416
Depakote Tablets (Rare) ... 418
Garamycin Injectable ... 2502
IFEX ... 706
Vistide Injection (2%) ... 1057

Fasciculations
Anectine ... 1062
Crixivan Capsules (Less than 2%) .. 1670
Eskalith ... 2658
Lithium Carbonate Capsules & Tablets ... 2352
Lithonate/Lithotabs/Lithobid ... 2721
Mestinon Injectable ... 1300
Mestinon ... 1300
Myochrysine Injection (Rare) ... 1754
Paxil Tablets (Rare) ... 2681
▲ Prostigmin Injectable (Among most common) ... 1305
▲ Prostigmin Tablets (Among most common) ... 1306
Tensilon Injectable ... 1307

Fasciitis, necrotizing fulminant
Clinoril Tablets (Rare) ... 1658
Dolobid Tablets ... 1695
Indocin (Rare) ... 1723

Fatality, hepatic related
Cylert Tablets (Rare) ... 415
Macrobid Capsules ... 2138
Macrodantin Capsules ... 2140

Fatality, non-cardiovascular related
Atromid-S Capsules ... 2808

Fatigue
Accupril Tablets (2.6%) ... 1950
▲ Accutane Capsules (Approximately 1 patient in 20) ... 2252
▲ Actigall Capsules (4.5%) ... 818
▲ Actimmune (14%) ... 1043
▲ Adalat CC (4%) ... 582
Adapin Capsules (Occasional) ... 1542
AeroBid Inhaler System (1% to 3%) ... 1004
Aerobid-M Inhaler System (1% to 3%) ... 1004
▲ Alferon N Injection (6% to 14%) ... 2142
Altace Capsules (2.0%) ... 1238
Alupent Tablets (1.4%) ... 672
Ambien Tablets (1%) ... 2559
Amen Tablets ... 785
Amicar Syrup, Tablets, and Injection ... 1312
▲ Anafranil Capsules (35% to 39%) ... 819
Ancobon Capsules ... 2254
Androderm Testosterone Transdermal System (Less than 1%) ... 2634
Antabuse Tablets (Small number of patients) ... 2802
Aquasol A Vitamin A Capsules, USP ... 525
Aquasol A Parenteral ... 526
▲ Aredia for Injection (Up to 22.7%) ... 827
Asendin Tablets (Less frequent) ... 1419
Atamet Tablets ... 567
Atretol Tablets ... 569
Atromid-S Capsules (Less often) ... 2808
Atrovent Inhalation Aerosol (Less than 1%) ... 674
Axocet Capsules (Infrequent) ... 2469
Bactrim DS Tablets ... 2257
Bactrim I.V. Infusion ... 2255
Bactrim ... 2257
Benadryl Injection ... 1955
▲ Betapace Tablets (5% to 20%) ... 637
Bioclate, Antihemophilic Factor (Recombinant) (One patient out of 13,394) ... 797
▲ Blocadren Tablets (3.4% to 5%) ... 1654
Brevibloc (esmolol HCl) Injection (About 1%) ... 1860
Bumex (0.1%) ... 2260
▲ BuSpar Tablets (4%) ... 738
Calan SR Caplets (1.7%) ... 2571
Calan Tablets (1.7%) ... 2568
Capoten Tablets (About 0.5 to 2%) ... 740
Capozide Tablets (0.5 to 2%) ... 744
▲ Cardioquin Tablets (7%) ... 2146
▲ Cardura Tablets (0.7% to 12%) ... 1993
▲ Cartrol Tablets (7.1%) ... 413
Cataflam Tablets ... 833
▲ Catapres Tablets (About 4 in 100 patients) ... 679
▲ Catapres-TTS (6 of 101 patients) .. 680
Cedax (0.1% to 1%) ... 2480
Ceredase ... 1055
▲ Chemet Capsules (5.2% to 15.7%) ... 666
▲ Claritin Tablets (4%) ... 2485
▲ Claritin-D Tablets (4%) ... 2487
Clinoril Tablets (Less than 1 in 100) ... 1658
Clomid (Fewer than 1%) ... 1262
Clozaril Tablets (2%) ... 2377
▲ Cognex Capsules (4%) ... 1961
Colestid (Infrequent) ... 2073
▲ Combipres Tablets (About 4%) ... 682
▲ Cordarone Tablets (4 to 9%) ... 2818
Cortifoam ... 2540
Cosmegen Injection ... 1666
▲ Covera-HS Tablets (1.7% to 4.5%) ... 2573
Cozaar Tablets (1% or greater) ... 1668
▲ Crixivan Capsules (3.6%) ... 1670
Cycrin Tablets ... 991
Cytotec (Infrequent) ... 2576
Danocrine Capsules ... 2437
▲ Dantrium Capsules (Among most frequent) ... 2131
▲ DaunoXome (6% to 43%) ... 1842
Daypro Caplets ... 2578
▲ Depo-Provera Contraceptive Injection (More than 5%) ... 2079
Depo-Provera Sterile Aqueous Suspension ... 2083
▲ Desyrel and Desyrel Dividose (5.7% to 11.3%) ... 504
Dibenzyline Capsules ... 2650
Dipentum Capsules (1.8%) ... 2084
Diprivan Injectable Emulsion (Less than 1%) ... 2939
▲ Dizac (diazepam injectable emulsion) CIV (Among most common) ... 1862
Dolobid Tablets (Greater than 1 in 100) ... 1695
Doral Tablets (1.9%) ... 2773
Doxil ... 2613
Dyazide Capsules ... 2653
▲ DynaCirc Capsules (2.0% to 8.5%) ... 2381
DynaCirc CR Tablets (2.5% to 4.3%) ... 2383
Dyrenium Capsules (Rare) ... 2655
Edecrin ... 1698
Elavil ... 2945
Eldepryl Capsules ... 2729
Elspar ... 1700
Emete-con Intramuscular/Intravenous ... 2007
▲ Engerix-B Unit-Dose Vials (14%) ... 2656
▲ Epivir (27%) ... 1200
▲ Epogen for Injection (9% to 25%) ... 489
▲ Ergamisol Tablets (6% to 11%) ... 1340
Esgic-plus Capsules (Infrequent) ... 1012
Esgic-plus Tablets (Infrequent) ... 1012
Esimil Tablets ... 840
Eskalith ... 2658
▲ Ethmozine Tablets (3.1% to 5.9%) ... 2217
Etrafon ... 2495
▲ Famvir Tablets (Among most frequent; 4.4% to 6.3%) ... 2660
Fansidar Tablets ... 2281
▲ Felbatol (6.9% to 16.8%) ... 2774
Feldene Capsules (Occasional) ... 2008
Fioricet Tablets (Infrequent) ... 2386
Fioricet with Codeine Capsules (Infrequent) ... 2387
Fiorinal with Codeine Capsules (Infrequent) ... 2390
Flexeril Tablets (1% to 3%) ... 1701
Flolan for Injection ... 1085
▲ Flovent (22% to 28%) ... 1089
Floxin I.V. (1% to 3%) ... 1580
Floxin Tablets (200 mg, 300 mg, 400 mg) (1% to 3%) ... 1577
▲ Fludara for Injection (10% to 38%) ... 658
Flumadine Tablets & Syrup (1.0%) 1013
▲ Foscavir Injection (5% or greater) .. 541
Fulvicin P/G Tablets (Occasional) .. 2499
Fulvicin P/G 165 & 330 Tablets (Occasional) ... 2500
Gammagard S/D, Immune Globulin, Intravenous (Human) (Occasional) ... 577
Gammar-P I.V., Immune Globulin Intravenous (Human) ... 798
Gantanol Tablets ... 2285
Gantrisin ... 2286
Gastrocrom Capsules (Infrequent) .. 1611
Gastrocrom Oral Concentrate (Less common) ... 1611
GlaucTabs ... ⊙ 209
Grifulvin V (griseofulvin tablets) Microsize (griseofulvin oral suspension) Microsize (Occasional) ... 1944
Gris-PEG Tablets, 125 mg & 250 mg (Occasional) ... 476
Halcion Tablets (0.9% to 0.5%) ... 2093
▲ Havrix (1% to 10%) ... 2663
Hexalen Capsules (1%) ... 2760
▲ Hismanal Tablets (4.2%) ... 1341
▲ Hivid Tablets (Less than 1% to 3.8%) ... 2287
▲ Hycamtin for Injection (Up to 37%) ... 2665
▲ Hylorel Tablets (25.7% to 63.6%) 1613
▲ Hytrin Capsules (7.4% to 11.3%) 434
Hyzaar Tablets (1% or greater) ... 1720
IFEX (Less than 1%) ... 706
Imdur (Less than or equal to 5%) .. 1362
Imitrex Injection (1.1%) ... 1095
Imitrex Tablets ... 1099
Imodium Capsules ... 1343
Inderal ... 2834
Inderal LA Long Acting Capsules ... 2836
Inderide Tablets ... 2838
Inderide LA Long Acting Capsules .. 2840
Indocin (Greater than 1%) ... 1723
▲ Intron A for Injection (4% to 96%) ... 2506
Inversine Tablets ... 1729
IOPIDINE Sterile Ophthalmic Solution ... ⊙ 218
Ismelin Tablets ... 845
Isoptin Oral Tablets (1.7%) ... 1393
Isoptin SR Tablets (1.7%) ... 1395
K-Phos Neutral Tablets ... 633
K-Phos Original Formula 'Sodium Free' Tablets (Less frequent) ... 633
Keflex Pulvules & Oral Suspension ... 930
Keftab Tablets ... 931
▲ Kerlone Tablets (2.9% to 9.7%) ... 2588
Lamprene Capsules (Less than 1%) ... 846
▲ Lariam Tablets (Among most frequent) ... 2295
Larodopa Tablets (Relatively frequent) ... 2296
Lescol Capsules (2.7%) ... 2395
▲ Leucovorin Calcium for Injection (2% to 13%) ... 1313
▲ Leustatin (11% to 45%) ... 1889
▲ Levatol Tablets (4.4%) ... 2547
Levbid Extended-Release Tablets ... 2549
Levlen/Tri-Levlen ... 646
Levsin/Levsinex/Levbid ... 2549
Limbitrol ... 2333
Lioresal Tablets (2% to 4%) ... 847
Lithium Carbonate Capsules & Tablets ... 2352
Lithonate/Lithotabs/Lithobid ... 2721
Livostin (Approximately 1% to 3%) ... ⊙ 262
▲ Lopid Tablets (3.8%) ... 1974
▲ Lopressor (10%) ... 848
▲ Lopressor HCT Tablets (10 in 100 patients) ... 850
Lotensin Tablets (2.4%) ... 852
▲ Lotensin HCT Tablets (5.2%) ... 855
Lotrel Capsules ... 858
▲ Ludiomil Tablets (4%) ... 861
Lupron Injection (Less than 5%) ... 2736
Matulane Capsules ... 2300
Mavik Tablets (More than 1%) ... 1407
Maxair Autohaler ... 1550
Maxair Inhaler (Less than 1%) ... 1552
Maxaquin Tablets (Less than 1%) .. 2593
Mesantoin Tablets ... 2400
▲ Mesnex Injection (33%) ... 711
Methotrexate Sodium Tablets, Injection, for Injection and LPF Injection (Frequent) ... 1322
Metrodin (urofollitropin for injection) ... 2616
▲ Mexitil Capsules (1.9% to 3.8%) .. 684
Miacalcin Nasal Spray (1% to 3%) 2403
Midamor Tablets (Between 1% and 3%) ... 1746
Mintezol ... 1747
Modicon ... 1928
Moduretic Tablets (Greater than 1%, less than 3%) ... 1748
Monoket Tablets (Up to 4%) ... 2550
Monopril Tablets (Less than 1.0% to 1.0% or more) ... 762
Motofen Tablets (1 in 200 to 1 in 600) ... 789
Motrin Ibuprofen Suspension, Oral Drops, Chewable Tablets, Caplets ... 1563
Mutamycin for Injection ... 712
▲ Mykrox Tablets (4.4%) ... 1617
Myleran Tablets ... 1209
Mysoline (Occasional) ... 2860
Nalfon 200 Pulvules & Nalfon Tablets (1.7%) ... 933
Nardil (Common) ... 1977
Navane Capsules and Concentrate 2018
Navane Intramuscular ... 2019
▲ Navelbine Injection (27%) ... 1212
Neptazane Tablets ... ⊙ 320
▲ Neupogen for Injection (11%) ... 495
▲ Neurontin Capsules (Among most common; 11%) ... 1978
Neutrexin for Injection (1.8%) ... 2761
▲ Nicotrol NS Nicotine Nasal Spray (Over 5%) ... 1565

(▭ Described in PDR For Nonprescription Drugs) Incidence data in parenthesis; ▲ 3% or more (⊙ Described in PDR For Ophthalmology)

Fatigue

- ▲ Nipent for Injection (29% to 42%) ... 2733
- Nizoral Tablets ... 1345
- ▲ Nolvadex Tablets (3.8%) ... 2957
- ▲ Normodyne Injection (1% to 10%) ... 2519
- ▲ Normodyne Tablets (1% to 10%) ... 2522
- ▲ Norpace (3 to 9%) ... 2596
- Norpramin Tablets ... 1273
- ▲ Norvasc Tablets (4.5%) ... 2020
- Nydrazid Injection ... 509
- Oncaspar ... 2194
- Ornade Spansule Capsules ... 2678
- Ortho-Cyclen/Ortho-Tri-Cyclen ... 1914
- Ortho-Novum ... 1928
- Ortho-Cyclen/Ortho Tri-Cyclen ... 1914
- Orthoclone OKT3 Sterile Solution ... 1892
- PBZ Tablets ... 863
- PBZ-SR Tablets ... 862
- Pamelor ... 2409
- ▲ Parlodel (1.0% to 7%) ... 2411
- Pediazole Suspension ... 2340
- Peganone Tablets ... 455
- Penetrex Tablets (0.1% to 1%) ... 2196
- Pentaspan Injection ... 954
- Pepcid Injection (Infrequent) ... 1765
- Pepcid (Infrequent) ... 1763
- Peptavlon ... 2997
- Periactin ... 1767
- Phenergan Injection ... 2880
- Phenurone Tablets (Less than 1%) ... 455
- Phrenilin (Infrequent) ... 790
- Pipracil ... 1435
- Pondimin Tablets ... 2239
- ▲ Pravachol Tablets (1.9% to 3.8%) ... 770
- Pregnyl for Injection ... 1878
- Premphase ... 2900
- Prempro ... 2905
- Prilosec Delayed-Release Capsules (Less than 1%) ... 516
- Prinivil Tablets (2.5%) ... 1776
- ▲ Prinzide Tablets (3.7%) ... 1780
- ▲ Procardia XL Extended Release Tablets (5.9%) ... 2026
- ▲ Procrit for Injection (9% to 25%) ... 1896
- Profasi (chorionic gonadotropin for injection, USP) ... 2620
- ▲ Proleukin for Injection (53%) ... 812
- Propulsid (More than 1%) ... 1346
- Proventil Syrup (Children 2 to 6 years, 1%) ... 2528
- Provera Tablets ... 2110
- ▲ Prozac Pulvules & Liquid, Oral Solution (4.2%) ... 935
- Quadrinal Tablets ... 1398
- Questran ... 774
- ▲ Quinidex Extentabs (7%) ... 2240
- ▲ Rabies Vaccine Adsorbed (8% to 10%) ... 2686
- Recombivax HB (Equal to or greater than 1%) ... 1787
- ▲ Reglan (Approximately 10%) ... 2243
- Relafen Tablets (1% to 3%) ... 2688
- ReVia Tablets (Less than 1% to 4%) ... 957
- RhoGAM Rh₀(D) Immune Globulin (Human) ... 1902
- Rifadin ... 1276
- Rifamate Capsules ... 1278
- Rifater ... 1280
- Rimactane Capsules ... 865
- Risperdal Tablets (Frequent) ... 1348
- Roferon-A Injection (86% to 95%) ... 2308
- Romazicon (1% to 3%) ... 2311
- Rowasa (3.44%) ... 2727
- ▲ Rythmol Tablets–150mg, 225mg, 300mg (1.8 to 6.0%) ... 1399
- SSKI Solution (Less frequent) ... 2767
- Sandostatin Injection (1% to 4%) ... 2421
- Sansert Tablets ... 2424
- ▲ Sectral Capsules (11%) ... 2914
- Sedapap Tablets 50 mg/650 mg (Infrequent) ... 1826
- ▲ Seldane Tablets (2.9% to 4.5%) ... 1284
- Seldane-D Extended-Release Tablets (2.1%) ... 1286
- Septra ... 1146
- Septra I.V. Infusion ... 1142
- Septra I.V. Infusion ADD-Vantage Vials ... 1144
- Septra ... 1146
- Serevent Inhalation Aerosol (1% to 3%) ... 1149
- Serophene (clomiphene citrate tablets, USP) (Less than 1 in 100 patients) ... 2621
- Sinemet Tablets ... 959
- Sinemet CR Tablets ... 961
- Sinequan (Occasional) ... 2028
- Sporanox Capsules (0.5% to 2.8%) ... 1352
- Stelazine ... 2692
- ▲ Supprelin Injection (1% to 10%) ... 2230
- Surmontil Capsules ... 2917
- Symmetrel Capsules (0.1% to 5%) ... 965
- Symmetrel Syrup (0.1% to 5%) ... 963
- ▲ Tambocor Tablets (7.7%) ... 1555
- Tavist Syrup ... 2426
- Tavist Tablets ... 2427
- ▲ Tegison Capsules (50-75%) ... 2314
- Tegretol/Tegretol-XR ... 870
- ▲ Tenex Tablets (2% to 12%) ... 2249
- ▲ Tenoretic Tablets (0.6% to 26%) ... 2963
- ▲ Tenormin Tablets and I.V. Injection (0.6% to 26%) ... 2965
- TheraCys BCG Live (Intravesical) (Up to 0.9%) ... 911
- Thioplex (Thiotepa For Injection) ... 1329
- ▲ TICE BCG, USP (7.4%) ... 1881
- Tilade Inhaler (1.1%) ... 2207
- Timolide Tablets (1.9%) ... 1791
- Timoptic in Ocudose (Less frequent) ... 1796
- Timoptic Sterile Ophthalmic Solution (Less frequent) ... 1794
- Timoptic-XE ... 1798
- Tofranil Ampuls ... 873
- Tofranil Tablets ... 875
- Tofranil-PM Capsules ... 876
- Tonocard Tablets (0.8% to 1.6%) ... 519
- ▲ Toprol-XL Tablets (About 10 of 100 patients) ... 560
- Tornalate Solution for Inhalation, 0.2% (1.5%) ... 976
- ▲ Trandate Tablets (1% to 11%) ... 1158
- Tranxene ... 459
- Triavil Tablets ... 1800
- Levlen/Tri-Levlen ... 646
- ▲ Trinalin Repetabs Tablets ... 1373
- Trusopt Sterile Ophthalmic Solution (Infrequent) ... 1803
- Tussend ... 1830
- Unasyn (Less than 1%) ... 2035
- Univasc Tablets (2.4%) ... 2553
- Uroqid-Acid No. 2 Tablets ... 633
- ▲ Valium Injectable (Among most common) ... 2336
- ▲ Valium Tablets (Among most common) ... 2335
- Vantin for Oral Suspension and Vantin Tablets (Less than 1%) ... 2112
- ▲ Vaqta (3.9%) ... 1805
- Varivax (Greater than or equal to 1%) ... 1807
- ▲ Vaseretic Tablets (3.9%) ... 1810
- Vasotec I.V. (0.5 to 1%) ... 1814
- Vasotec Tablets (1.8% to 3.0%) ... 1816
- Ventolin Syrup (1% of children) ... 1175
- Verelan Capsules (1.7%) ... 1455
- Vesanoid Capsules ... 2327
- ▲ Visken Tablets (8%) ... 2428
- Vivactil Tablets ... 1820
- Cataflam/Voltaren/Voltaren-XR ... 833
- ▲ Wellbutrin Tablets (5.0%) ... 1177
- ▲ Xanax Tablets (48.6%) ... 2115
- Zarontin Capsules ... 1986
- Zarontin Syrup ... 1986
- Zaroxolyn Tablets ... 1625
- ▲ Zebeta Tablets (6.6% to 8.2%) ... 1457
- ▲ Zestoretic Tablets (3.7%) ... 2968
- Zestril Tablets (2.5%) ... 2972
- ▲ Ziac (3.0% to 4.6%) ... 1459
- ▲ Zinecard Injection (48% to 61%) ... 2120
- Zithromax (1% or less) ... 2043
- Zithromax (1% or less) ... 2046
- ▲ Zofran Injection (5%) ... 1227
- ▲ Zofran Tablets (9% to 13%) ... 1231
- ▲ Zoladex (5%) ... 2976
- ▲ Zoloft Tablets (10.6%) ... 2051
- ▲ Zonalon Cream (Approximately 1% to 10%) ... 1042
- Zovirax (0.4%) ... 1187
- ▲ Zyrtec Tablets (5.9%) ... 2053

Fatigue, muscular

- Apresazide Capsules ... 824
- Axocet Capsules (Infrequent) ... 2469
- Capozide Tablets ... 744
- Demadex Tablets and Injection ... 691
- Dyazide Capsules ... 2653
- Esgic-plus Capsules (Infrequent) ... 1012
- Esgic-plus Tablets (Infrequent) ... 1012
- Esidrix Tablets ... 839
- Fioricet Tablets (Infrequent) ... 2386
- Fioricet with Codeine Capsules (Infrequent) ... 2387
- Fiorinal with Codeine Capsules (Infrequent) ... 2390
- Imitrex Injection (Rare) ... 1095
- Isoptin Injectable ... 1391
- Lasix Injection, Oral Solution and Tablets ... 1267
- Oretic Tablets ... 450
- Phrenilin (Infrequent) ... 790
- Prinzide Tablets ... 1780
- Sedapap Tablets 50 mg/650 mg (Infrequent) ... 1826
- ▲ Tenoretic Tablets (3% to 6%) ... 2963
- ▲ Tenormin Tablets and I.V. Injection (3% to 6%) ... 2965
- Thalitone (Common) ... 1293
- Vaseretic Tablets ... 1810
- Zaroxolyn Tablets ... 1625
- Zestoretic Tablets ... 2968

Fat intolerance

- Anafranil Capsules (Rare) ... 819

Fear

- BuSpar Tablets (Infrequent) ... 738
- Claritin-D Tablets ... 2487
- D.A. II Tablets ... 972
- D.A. Chewable Tablets ... 970
- Deconsal II Tablets ... 1605
- Dilaudid Ampules ... 1382
- Dilaudid Cough Syrup ... 1383
- Dilaudid ... 1382
- Dura-Tap/PD Capsules ... 970
- Dura-Vent/DA Tablets ... 972
- Dura-Vent Tablets ... 971
- Entex PSE Tablets ... 973
- EpiPen–Epinephrine Auto-Injector ... 808
- Fedahist Gyrocaps ... 2545
- Guaimax-D Tablets ... 809
- Histussin D Liquid ... 670
- Hycodan Tablets and Syrup ... 946
- Hycomine Compound Tablets ... 948
- Hycomine ... 947
- Hycotuss Expectorant Syrup ... 950
- Hydrocet Capsules ... 787
- Lorcet 10/650 Tablets ... 1016
- Lortab ... 2751
- Novahistine DMX ... 782
- Novahistine Elixir ... 782
- Phenobarbital Elixir and Tablets ... 1523
- Seldane-D Extended-Release Tablets ... 1286
- Syn-Rx Tablets ... 1622
- Syn-Rx DM Tablets ... 1623
- Trinalin Repetabs Tablets ... 1373
- Tussend ... 1830
- Tussend Expectorant ... 1831
- Tussionex Pennkinetic Extended-Release Suspension ... 1624
- Vicodin Tablets ... 1404
- Vicodin ES Tablets ... 1405
- Vicodin HP Tablets ... 1403
- Vicodin Tuss Expectorant ... 1406
- Xanax Tablets (1.4%) ... 2115
- Zydone Capsules ... 967

Febrile reactions

- Albuminar-5, Albumin (Human) U.S.P. 5% (Occasional) ... 795
- Albuminar-25, Albumin (Human) U.S.P. 25% ... 796
- Capastat Sulfate Injection ... 968
- Digibind ... 1079
- Humegon for Injection ... 1873
- INFeD (Iron Dextran Injection, USP) ... 2478
- ▲ JE-VAX (5.5%) ... 904
- ▲ Leustatin (11%) ... 1889
- Metrodin (urofollitropin for injection) ... 2616
- Mumpsvax (Very rare) ... 1751
- NephrAmine Injection ... 2169
- PedvaxHIB ... 1761
- Pergonal (menotropins for injection, USP) ... 2618
- Thioplex (Thiotepa For Injection) ... 1329
- Tri-Immunol Adsorbed ... 1452
- Varivax (Less than 0.1%) ... 1807

Fecal fat, increase
(see under Steatorrhea)

Fecal impaction

- Betaseron for SC Injection ... 653
- Clozaril Tablets ... 2377
- Cognex Capsules (Infrequent) ... 1961
- Doxil (Less than 1%) ... 2613
- Etrafon ... 2495
- Kayexalate (At large doses in elderly individuals) ... 2444
- Paxil Tablets (Rare) ... 2681
- Prolixin ... 510
- Questran ... 774
- Rilutek Tablets (Infrequent) ... 2198
- Sodium Polystyrene Sulfonate Suspension ... 2367
- Trilafon (Occasional) ... 2532

Feces, color change

- Prilosec Delayed-Release Capsules (Less than 1%) ... 516
- Rifadin ... 1276

Feces, discoloration

- Derifil Tablets ... 2371
- Lamprene Capsules (Greater than 1%) ... 846
- Mycobutin Capsules ... 2101
- Prevacid Delayed-Release Capsules (Less than 1%) ... 2746
- Risperdal Tablets (Rare) ... 1348
- Urised Tablets ... 2123

Feeling, intoxicated

- Ambien Tablets (Rare) ... 2559
- ▲ Axocet Capsules (Among most frequent) ... 2469
- ▲ Esgic-plus Capsules (Among most frequent) ... 1012
- ▲ Esgic-plus Tablets (Among most frequent) ... 1012
- ▲ Fioricet Tablets (Among most frequent) ... 2386
- Fioricet with Codeine Capsules (Frequent) ... 2387
- Fiorinal with Codeine Capsules (1.0%) ... 2390
- Imitrex Injection (Rare) ... 1095
- ▲ Phrenilin (Among most frequent) ... 790
- ▲ Sedapap Tablets 50 mg/650 mg (Among the most frequent) ... 1826

Feelings, drugged

- ▲ Ambien Tablets (3%) ... 2559
- Paxil Tablets (Infrequent; 2%) ... 2681

Feeling, shaky

- Esgic-plus Capsules (Infrequent) ... 1012
- Esgic-plus Tablets (Infrequent) ... 1012
- Fioricet Tablets (Infrequent) ... 2386
- Fioricet with Codeine Capsules (Infrequent) ... 2387
- Fiorinal with Codeine Capsules (Infrequent) ... 2390
- Phrenilin (Infrequent) ... 790

Feeling, strange

- Ambien Tablets (Rare) ... 2559
- Imitrex Injection (2.2%) ... 1095
- Imitrex Tablets ... 1099
- Neurontin Capsules (Rare) ... 1978
- ▲ ReVia Tablets (Less than 10%) ... 957

Feet, cold

- Hivid Tablets (Less than 1%) ... 2287
- KOGENATE Antihemophilic Factor (Recombinant) ... 626
- Parlodel ... 2411

Female genitalia, tenderness

- Supprelin Injection (2% to 3%) ... 2230

Fertility, impairment of

- Amen Tablets ... 785
- Depo-Provera Contraceptive Injection (Fewer than 1%) ... 2079
- Depo-Provera Sterile Aqueous Suspension ... 2083
- Halotestin Tablets ... 2095
- Intron A for Injection ... 2506

Fertility, male, decrease

- Lopid Tablets ... 1974

Festination

- Eldepryl Capsules ... 2729

Fetal acidosis

- Prepidil Gel ... 2108

Fetal circulation, persistent

- Exosurf Neonatal for Intratracheal Suspension (Less than 1% to 2%) ... 1081

Fetal death
(see under Death, fetal)

Fetal defects

- Accupril Tablets ... 1950
- ▲ Accutane Capsules (Potentially all exposed fetuses) ... 2252
- Butisol Sodium Elixir & Tablets ... 2768
- Capozide Tablets ... 744
- Climara Transdermal System ... 640
- Clomid (Less than 1%) ... 1262
- Cytoxan ... 700

(▫ Described in PDR For Nonprescription Drugs)   Incidence data in parenthesis; ▲ 3% or more   (◉ Described in PDR For Ophthalmology)

Side Effects Index

Fetal depression
- Prepidil Gel ... 2108

Fetal harm
- Accupril Tablets ... 1950
- ▲ Accutane Capsules (Potentially all exposed fetuses) ... 2252
- Advil Cold and Sinus Caplets and Tablets ... ⊗ 837
- Albenza Tablets ... 2629
- Alkeran for Injection ... 1196
- Alkeran Tablets ... 1198
- Amen Tablets ... 785
- Amikacin Sulfate Injection, USP ... 523
- Amikacin Sulfate Injection, USP ... 981
- Amikin Injectable ... 502
- Aquasol A Vitamin A Capsules, USP ... 525
- Aquasol A Parenteral ... 526
- Arimidex Tablets ... 2932
- Ativan Injection ... 2805
- Aygestin Tablets ... 990
- Azathioprine Tablets ... 2349
- BiCNU ... 696
- Cafergot ... 2376
- Capoten Tablets ... 740
- CeeNU Capsules ... 699
- Cerubidine for Injection ... 634
- Clomid ... 1262
- Cozaar Tablets ... 1668
- Cycrin Tablets ... 991
- Cystospaz ... 2123
- Cytadren Tablets ... 837
- Cytosar-U Sterile Powder ... 2077
- Cytotec ... 2576
- Cytoxan ... 700
- Danocrine Capsules ... 2437
- DaunoXome ... 1842
- Depen Titratable Tablets ... 2770
- Depo-Provera Sterile Aqueous Suspension ... 2083
- Diethylstilbestrol Tablets ... 1477
- Diucardin Tablets ... 2824
- Doral Tablets ... 2773
- DYNACIN Capsules ... 1627
- Efudex ... 2280
- Enduron Tablets ... 424
- Ergomar Tablets ... 1543
- Eskalith ... 2658
- Estrace Cream and Tablets ... 751
- Estraderm Transdermal System ... 842
- Estratest ... 2718
- Etopophos for Injection ... 701
- Etoposide Injection ... 539
- Eulexin Capsules ... 2498
- Fiorinal ... 2388
- Fludara for Injection ... 658
- Fluoroplex Topical Solution & Cream 1% ... 475
- Fluorouracil Injection ... 2282
- Sterile FUDR ... 2284
- Garamycin Injectable ... 2502
- Gemzar for Injection ... 1482
- Habitrol Nicotine Transdermal System ... 884
- Humegon for Injection ... 1873
- Hycamtin for Injection ... 2665
- Hyzaar Tablets ... 1720
- IFEX ... 706
- Imuran ... 1103
- Lescol Capsules ... 2395
- Leukeran Tablets ... 1205
- Lithium Carbonate Capsules & Tablets ... 2352
- Lithonate/Lithotabs/Lithobid ... 2721
- Lotensin Tablets ... 852
- Lotensin HCT Tablets ... 855
- Lotrel Capsules ... 858
- Lupron Depot 3.75 mg ... 2739
- Lysodren Tablets ... 707
- Matulane Capsules ... 2300
- Mavik Tablets ... 1407
- Mebaral Tablets ... 2452
- Megace Oral Suspension ... 708
- Megace Tablets ... 710
- Menest Tablets ... 2671
- Metrodin (urofollitropin for injection) ... 2616
- Mevacor Tablets ... 1742
- Minocin Oral Suspension ... 1431
- Minocin Pellet-Filled Capsules ... 1429
- Mithracin ... 599
- Monopril Tablets ... 762
- Mustargen ... 1752
- Myleran Tablets ... 1209
- Navelbine Injection ... 1212
- Nebcin Vials, Hyporets & ADD-Vantage ... 1518
- Nembutal Sodium Capsules ... 440
- Nembutal Sodium Solution ... 442
- Nembutal Sodium Suppositories ... 444
- Neosporin G.U. Irrigant Sterile ... 1130
- Netromycin Injection 100 mg/ml ... 2516
- Neutrexin for Injection ... 2761
- Nicotrol NS Nicotine Nasal Spray ... 1565
- Nolvadex Tablets ... 2957
- Norisodrine with Calcium Iodide Syrup ... 446
- Novantrone for Injection ... 1327
- Oncovin Solution Vials & Hyporets ... 1521
- Oretic Tablets ... 450
- Ortho Dienestrol Cream ... 1922
- ParaGard T 380A Intrauterine Copper Contraceptive ... 1936
- Paraplatin for Injection ... 713
- Peganone Tablets ... 455
- Pergonal (menotropins for injection, USP) ... 2618
- Phenobarbital Elixir and Tablets ... 1523
- Phenurone Tablets ... 455
- Platinol for Injection ... 717
- Platinol-AQ Injection ... 719
- PMB 200 and PMB 400 ... 2890
- Pravachol Tablets ... 770
- Premarin Intravenous ... 2893
- Premarin Tablets ... 2896
- Prinivil Tablets ... 1776
- Prinzide Tablets ... 1780
- Profasi (chorionic gonadotropin for injection, USP) ... 2620
- ProSom Tablets ... 457
- Prostep (nicotine transdermal system) ... 1439
- Purinethol Tablets ... 1214
- Quadrinal Tablets ... 1398
- ReoPro Vials ... 1526
- Restoril Capsules ... 2413
- SSKI Solution ... 2767
- Seconal Sodium Pulvules ... 1529
- Serax Capsules ... 2916
- Serax Tablets ... 2916
- Soma Compound w/Codeine Tablets ... 2784
- Soma Compound Tablets ... 2783
- Streptomycin Sulfate Injection ... 2031
- Synarel Nasal Solution for Endometriosis ... 2605
- Tapazole Tablets ... 1361
- Taxol Injection ... 723
- Taxotere for Injection Concentrate ... 2204
- Tenoretic Tablets ... 2963
- Tenormin Tablets and I.V. Injection ... 2965
- Testoderm Testosterone Transdermal System ... 486
- Testred Capsules, 10 mg ... 1308
- Thioguanine Tablets, Tabloid Brand ... 1225
- Thioplex (Thiotepa For Injection) ... 1329
- Univasc Tablets ... 2553
- Vaseretic Tablets ... 1810
- Vasotec I.V. ... 1814
- Vasotec Tablets ... 1816
- Velban Vials ... 1537
- VePesid Capsules and Injection ... 727
- Vesanoid Capsules ... 2327
- Virazole ... 1310
- Vivelle Transdermal System ... 880
- Vumon for Injection ... 729
- Wigraine Tablets ... 1884
- Winstrol Tablets ... 2468
- Xanax Tablets ... 2115
- Zestoretic Tablets ... 2968
- Zestril Tablets ... 2972
- Zocor Tablets ... 1821
- Zoladex ... 2976

Fetal heart rate, deceleration
- Prepidil Gel (2.1% to 4.3%) ... 2108

Fetal hemorrhage
- Coumadin ... 941
- Soma Compound w/Codeine Tablets ... 2784
- Soma Compound Tablets ... 2783

Fetal hydantoin syndrome
- Dilantin Infatabs ... 1967
- Dilantin Kapseals ... 1965
- Dilantin-125 Suspension ... 1969

Fetal problems, unspecified
- Actron Caplets and Tablets ... ⊗ 608
- Aleve ... 2124
- Alka-Seltzer Plus ... ⊗ 611
- Alka-Seltzer Plus Sinus Medicine ... ⊗ 611
- Ascriptin ... ⊗ 650
- BC Powder ... ⊗ 631
- Genuine Bayer Aspirin Tablets & Caplets ... ⊗ 618
- Extra Strength Bayer Arthritis Pain Regimen Formula ... ⊗ 615
- Extra Strength Bayer Aspirin Caplets & Tablets ... ⊗ 617
- Extended-Release Bayer 8-Hour Aspirin ... ⊗ 616
- Extra Strength Bayer Plus Aspirin Caplets ... ⊗ 617
- Extra Strength Bayer PM Aspirin Plus Sleep Aid ... ⊗ 617
- Aspirin Regimen Bayer Children's Chewable Aspirin ... ⊗ 616
- Aspirin Regimen Bayer Regular Strength 325 mg Caplets ... ⊗ 613
- Cipro I.V. ... 587
- Dalmane Capsules ... 2329
- Empirin Aspirin Tablets ... ⊗ 818
- Humorsol Sterile Ophthalmic Solution ... 1707
- Motrin IB Caplets, Tablets, and Gelcaps ... ⊗ 802
- Nuprin Ibuprofen/Analgesic Tablets & Caplets ... ⊗ 645
- Orudis KT ... ⊗ 842
- Polytrim Ophthalmic Solution Sterile ... 479
- Vaseretic Tablets ... 1810
- Vasotec I.V. ... 1814
- Vasotec Tablets ... 1816

Fetal sepsis, intrauterine
- Prepidil Gel ... 2108

Fever
- Abbokinase ... 403
- Abbokinase Open-Cath ... 405
- ▲ Abelcet Injection (12% to 15%) ... 1540
- ▲ Acel-Imune Diphtheria and Tetanus Toxoids and Acellular Pertussis Vaccine Adsorbed (7% to 19%) ... 1415
- ▲ ActHIB (0.5% to 24.6%) ... 893
- ▲ Actimmune (52%) ... 1043
- ▲ Actimmune ... 1045
- Adalat Capsules (10 mg and 20 mg) (2% or less) ... 580
- Adalat CC (Rare) ... 582
- Adriamycin PFS (Occasional) ... 2056
- Adriamycin RDF (Occasional) ... 2056
- ▲ AeroBid Inhaler System (3% to 9%) ... 1004
- ▲ Aerobid-M Inhaler System (3% to 9%) ... 1004
- Albenza Tablets (Up to 1.0%) ... 2629
- Aldomet Ester HCI Injection ... 1642
- Aldomet Oral ... 1640
- Aldoril Tablets ... 1644
- ▲ Alferon N Injection (18% to 81%) ... 2142
- Alkeran for Injection ... 1196
- Alkeran Tablets ... 1198
- All-Flex Arcing Spring Diaphragm (See also Ortho Diaphragm Kits) ... 1921
- Altace Capsules (Less than 1%) ... 1238
- Alupent Tablets (0.4%) ... 672
- Ambien Tablets (Infrequent) ... 2559
- Amen Tablets (Rare) ... 785
- Amicar Syrup, Tablets, and Injection ... 1312
- Anafranil Capsules (2% to 4%) ... 819
- Anaprox/Naprosyn (Less than 1%) ... 2277
- Ancobon Capsules ... 2254
- Antivenin (Crotalidae) Polyvalent ... 2803
- Apresazide Capsules (Less frequent) ... 824
- Apresoline Hydrochloride Tablets (Less frequent) ... 826
- ▲ Aredia for Injection (At least 5% to 31.5%) ... 827
- Arimidex Tablets (2% to 5%) ... 2932
- ▲ Asacol Delayed-Release Tablets (6%) ... 2129
- Asendin Tablets ... 1419
- Atretol Tablets ... 569
- Attenuvax (Occasional) ... 1650
- Augmentin (Frequent) ... 2637
- Augmentin Tablets (Frequent) ... 2640
- ▲ Avonex (23%) ... 662
- Axid Pulvules (1.6%) ... 1468
- Axocet Capsules (Infrequent) ... 2469
- Azactam for Injection (Less than 1%) ... 736
- Azathioprine Tablets (Less than 1%) ... 2349
- Azulfidine (One in every 30 patients or less) ... 2059
- Benemid Tablets ... 1651
- Betapace Tablets (Rare; 1% to 4%) ... 637
- ▲ Betaseron for SC Injection (59%) ... 653
- Biavax II (Occasional) ... 1653
- Bicillin C-R Injection ... 2810
- Bicillin C-R 900/300 Injection ... 2812
- Bicillin L-A Injection ... 2813
- Bioclate, Antihemophilic Factor (Recombinant) (Extremely rare) ... 797
- Blenoxane (Frequent) ... 697
- Bleph-10 Ophthalmic Solution 10% ... 472
- Blocadren Tablets ... 1654
- Brevibloc (esmolol HCI) Injection (Less than 1%) ... 1860
- BuSpar Tablets (Infrequent) ... 738
- Butisol Sodium Elixir & Tablets (1 to 3 patients per 100) ... 2768
- Calan SR Caplets ... 2571
- Calan Tablets ... 2568
- ▲ Capoten Tablets (About 4 to 7 of 100) ... 740
- Capozide Tablets (Sometimes) ... 744
- Carbocaine Injection ... 2432
- Cardene I.V. (Rare) ... 2815
- Cardioquin Tablets ... 2146
- Cardura Tablets (Less than 0.5% of 3960 patients) ... 1993
- Cartrol Tablets (Less common) ... 413
- Casodex Tablets (2% to 5%) ... 2934
- Cataflam Tablets (Rare) ... 833
- Catapres Tablets ... 679
- Catapres-TTS ... 680
- Ceclor Pulvules & Suspension (Frequently) ... 1470
- Cedax (0.1% to 1%) ... 2480
- Cefizox for Intramuscular or Intravenous Use (1% to 5%) ... 1025
- Cefotan ... 2936
- Ceftin for Oral Suspension (0.1% to 1%) ... 1067
- Cefzil Tablets and Oral Suspension (Rare) ... 747
- Celestone Soluspan Suspension ... 2484
- ▲ CellCept Capsules (More than or equal to 3%; 21.4% to 23.3%) ... 2265
- Ceptaz (2% of patients) ... 1070
- Cerebyx Injection (Frequent) ... 1956
- Ceredase ... 1055
- Cerubidine for Injection (Rare) ... 634
- Cervidil (Less than 1%) ... 1008
- ▲ Chemet Capsules (5.2% to 15.7%) ... 666
- Cipro I.V. (1% or less) ... 587
- Cipro I.V. Pharmacy Bulk Package (Less than 1%) ... 590
- Cipro Tablets (Less than 1%; rare) ... 584
- Claforan Sterile and Injection (2.4%) ... 1259
- Claritin Tablets (2% or fewer patients) ... 2485
- Claritin-D Tablets (Less frequent) ... 2487
- Clinoril Tablets (Less than 1%) ... 1658
- Clomid ... 1262
- ▲ Clozaril Tablets (5% or more) ... 2377
- Cogentin ... 1661
- Cognex Capsules (Frequent) ... 1961
- ColBENEMID Tablets ... 1662
- Combipres Tablets ... 682
- Compazine ... 2644
- Cordarone Intravenous (2.0%) ... 2821
- Cosmegen Injection ... 1666
- Coumadin (Infrequent) ... 941
- Cozaar Tablets (Less than 1%) ... 1668
- Crixivan Capsules (Less than 2%) ... 1670
- Cuprimine Capsules (Rare) ... 1673
- Cycrin Tablets ... 991
- Cystospaz ... 2123
- Cytadren Tablets (Several) ... 837
- CytoGam (Less than 5.0%) ... 1630
- ▲ Cytosar-U Sterile Powder (Among most frequent) ... 2077
- Cytotec (Infrequent) ... 2576
- ▲ Cytovene (38%) ... 2270
- Cytoxan ... 700
- DTIC-Dome (Infrequent) ... 593
- Danocrine Capsules (Rare) ... 2437
- Dantrium Capsules (Less frequent) ... 2131
- Dapsone Tablets USP ... 1331
- Daranide Tablets ... 1676
- Daraprim Tablets (Rare) ... 1199
- ▲ DaunoXome (5% to 42%) ... 1842
- Daypro Caplets (Rare) ... 2578
- Depakene ... 416
- Depakote Tablets (1% to 5%) ... 418
- Depen Titratable Tablets (Rare) ... 2770

(⊗ Described in PDR For Nonprescription Drugs)   Incidence data in parenthesis; ▲ 3% or more   (◉ Described in PDR For Ophthalmology)

Fever
Side Effects Index
1338

Depo-Provera Contraceptive Injection (Fewer than 1%) 2079
Depo-Provera Sterile Aqueous Suspension 2083
Desferal Vials 838
Diamox .... ◉ 317
Dilacor XR Extended-release Capsules (Infrequent) 2183
Dilantin Infatabs 1967
Dilantin Kapseals 1965
Dilantin-125 Suspension 1969
Dipentum Capsules (Rare) 2084
Diphtheria & Tetanus Toxoids Adsorbed Purogenated (Mild) 1422
▲ Diphtheria and Tetanus Toxoids and Pertussis Vaccine Adsorbed (0.3% to approximately 50%) 2650
Diprivan Injectable Emulsion (Less than 1%) 2939
Diucardin Tablets 2824
Diupres Tablets 1691
Diuril Oral Suspension 1694
Diuril Sodium Intravenous 1693
Diuril Tablets 1694
Dobutrex Solution Vials (Occasional) 1480
Dolobid Tablets (Less than 1 in 100) 1695
Dopram Injectable 2235
▲ Doxil (7.8% to 9.1%) 2613
Doxorubicin Astra (Occasional) 531
Duricef Capsules, Tablets, and Oral Suspension 750
Dynabac (0.1% to 1%) 668
Easprin 1971
EC-Naprosyn Delayed-Release Tablets (Less than 1%) 2277
Edecrin 1698
Effexor 2825
Elavil 2945
Elspar 1700
Emete-con Intramuscular/Intravenous (Rare) 2007
▲ Eminase (Less than 10%) 2215
Enduron Tablets 424
▲ Engerix-B Unit-Dose Vials (1% to 10%) 2656
▲ Epivir (10%) 1200
▲ Epogen for Injection (29% to 38%) 489
▲ Ergamisol Tablets (3% to 5%) 1340
Esgic-plus Capsules (Infrequent) 1012
Esgic-plus Tablets (Infrequent) 1012
Eskalith 2658
▲ Ethamolin Injection (Among most common; 1.8%) 2544
Ethmozine Tablets (Rare) 2217
▲ Etopophos for Injection (3% to 24%) 701
Etoposide Injection (0.7% to 2%) 539
Etrafon 2495
Famvir Tablets (0.8% to 3.3%) 2660
▲ Felbatol (2.6% to 22.6%) 2774
Feldene Capsules (Less than 1%) 2008
Fioricet Tablets (Infrequent) 2386
Fioricet with Codeine Capsules (Infrequent) 2387
Fiorinal with Codeine Capsules (Infrequent) 2390
Flagyl 375 Capsules 2587
Flagyl I.V. 2373
▲ Flolan for Injection (25%) 1085
Flovent (1% to 3%) 1089
Floxin I.V. (1% to 3%) 1580
Floxin Tablets (200 mg, 300 mg, 400 mg) (1% to 3%) 1577
▲ Fludara for Injection (60% to 69%) 658
Flumadine Tablets & Syrup 1013
Fluothane 2830
Fluvirin (Influenza Virus Vaccine) (Infrequent) 1608
Fortaz (2%) 1092
▲ Foscavir Injection (Less than 1% to 65%) 541
Fragmin Injection (Rare) 2088
Sterile FUDR 2284
▲ Fungizone Intravenous (Among most common) 507
Furoxone 2221
▲ Gamimune N, 5% Immune Globulin Intravenous (Human), 5% (Among most common; 24.4%) 612
▲ Gamimune N, 10% Immune Globulin Intravenous (Human), 10% (Among most common; 24.4%) 615
Gammagard S/D, Immune Globulin, Intravenous (Human) (Occasional) 577
Gammar-P I.V., Immune Globulin Intravenous (Human) 798
Ganite 2711
Gantanol Tablets 2285
Gantrisin 2286
Garamycin Injectable 2502
▲ Gemzar for Injection (16% to 41%) 1482
GlaucTabs .... ◉ 209
Haldol Decanoate 1587
Haldol Injection, Tablets and Concentrate 1585
▲ Havrix (1% to 10%) 2663
Helidac Therapy 2135
Heparin Lock Flush Solution 2831
Heparin Sodium Injection 2832
▲ Heparin Sodium Vials (Among most common) 1486
Hespan Injection 945
Helixate, Antihemophilic Factor (Recombinant) (Two reports out of 3,254 patients) 799
HibTITER (0.6% to 1.4%) 1423
Hivid Tablets (Less than 1% to 1.7%) 2287
Humegon for Injection 1873
▲ Hycamtin for Injection (Less than 1% to 34%) 2665
Hydralazine Hydrochloride Injection USP (Less frequent) 2712
Hydrea Capsules (Rare) 705
HydroDIURIL Tablets 1716
Hydropres Tablets 1718
Hyperstat I.V. Injection 2504
Hyskon Hysteroscopy Fluid (Rare) 1633
Hytrin Capsules (0.5% to at least 1%) 434
Hyzaar Tablets 1720
IBU Tablets (Rare; less than 1%) 1389
▲ Idamycin Injection (26%) 2096
IFEX (1%) 706
Imdur (Less than or equal to 5%) 1362
Imitrex Injection (Rare) 1095
Imitrex Tablets (Infrequent) 1099
▲ Imovax Rabies Vaccine (Up to 6%) 899
Imuran (Less than 1%) 1103
Inderal 2834
Inderal LA Long Acting Capsules 2836
Inderide Tablets 2838
Inderide LA Long Acting Capsules 2840
INFeD (Iron Dextran Injection, USP) 2478
Influenza Virus Vaccine, Trivalent, Types A and B (chromatograph- and filter-purified subviron antigen) FluShield, 1996-1997 Formula (Infrequent) 2842
Inocor Lactate Injection (0.9%) 2439
▲ Intron A for Injection (3% to 86%) 2506
Invirase Capsules (Less than 2%) 2291
▲ IPOL Poliovirus Vaccine Inactivated (Up to 38%) 903
Isoptin SR Tablets 1395
▲ JE-VAX (Less than 3% to approximately 10%) 904
Kadian Capsules (Less than 3%) 2948
Keftab Tablets 931
Kefurox Vials, Faspak & ADD-Vantage 1509
Kerlone Tablets 2588
Klonopin Tablets 2294
KOGENATE Antihemophilic Factor (Recombinant) (Two reports) 626
Konyne 80 Factor IX Complex 627
▲ Kytril Injection (3%; 8.6%) 2667
▲ Kytril Tablets (5%) 2669
▲ Lamictal Tablets (5.5%) 1105
Lamprene Capsules (Less than 1%) 846
▲ Lariam Tablets (Among most frequent) 2295
Lasix Injection, Oral Solution and Tablets 1267
Lescol Capsules (Rare) 2395
Leucovorin Calcium Tablets, Wellcovorin Brand 1204
Leukeran Tablets 1205
▲ Leukine (77% to 95%) 1317
▲ Leustatin (Frequent; 11% to 69%) 1889
Levatol Tablets 2547
Levbid Extended-Release Tablets 2549
Levlen/Tri-Levlen 646
Levoprome 1321
Levsin/Levsinex/Levbid 2549
Lioresal Intrathecal (0.2% to 0.7%) 1634
Lithonate/Lithotabs/Lithobid 2721
Lodine Capsules and Tablets (Greater than or equal to 1%) 2849
Lopressor HCT Tablets 850
Lotensin HCT Tablets (0.3% or more) 855
▲ Lovenox Injection (5%) 2187
Loxitane 1426
Lupron Depot 7.5 mg (Less than 5%) 2741
Lupron Depot - 3 Month 22.5 mg (Less than 5%) 2743
Lupron Depot-PED 7.5 mg, 11.25 mg and 15 mg (Less than 2%) 2744
Lupron Injection (Less than 5%) 2736
Lupron Injection Pediatric (Less than 2%) 2737
LUVOX Tablets 2723
M-M-R II 1730
M-R-VAX II 1732
Macrobid Capsules (Rare to less than 1%) 2138
Macrodantin Capsules (Rare) 2140
Massengill Disposable Douche 2627
Massengill Medicated Disposable Douche 2628
Matulane Capsules 2300
Maxipime for Injection (0.1% to 1%) 758
Mebaral Tablets (Less than 1 in 100) 2452
Mefoxin 1734
Mefoxin Premixed Intravenous Solution 1737
▲ Megace Oral Suspension (1% to 6%) 708
Mellaril 2398
Menomune-A/C/Y/W-135 (Up to 2%) 906
▲ Mepron Suspension (14% to 40%) 1206
Merrem I.V. (0.1% to 1.0%) 2952
Meruvax II 1740
Methadone Hydrochloride Oral Concentrate 2356
Methotrexate Sodium Tablets, Injection, for Injection and LPF Injection (Less common to frequent) 1322
MetroGel-Vaginal 917
Mevacor Tablets (Rare) 1742
Mexitil Capsules (1.2%) 684
Miacalcin Nasal Spray (Less than 1%) 2403
Miltown Tablets (Rare) 2780
Minipress Capsules 2015
Minizide Capsules 2016
Mintezol 1747
Mithracin 599
Moban Tablets and Concentrate 1036
Modicon 1928
Moduretic Tablets 1748
Monocid Injection (Less than 1%) 2674
Mononine, Coagulation Factor IX (Human), Monoclonal Antibody Purified 804
Monopril Tablets (0.4% to 1.0%) 762
Motrin Ibuprofen Suspension, Oral Drops, Chewable Tablets, Caplets (Rare; less than 1%) 1563
Mumpsvax (Uncommon) 1751
▲ Mutamycin for Injection (14%) 712
Myambutol Tablets 1432
Mycobutin Capsules (2%) 2101
Myochrysine Injection 1754
Nalfon 200 Pulvules & Nalfon Tablets (Less than 1%) 933
Naprelan Tablets (Less than 3%) 2861
Anaprox/Naprosyn (Less than 1%) 2277
Nardil (Less frequent) 1977
Navane Capsules and Concentrate 2018
Navane Intramuscular 2019
Navelbine Injection 1212
Nebcin Vials, Hyporets & ADD-Vantage 1518
Nembutal Sodium Capsules 440
Nembutal Sodium Solution 442
Nembutal Sodium Suppositories (Less than 1%) 444
Neoral (2% or less) 2405
Neptazane Tablets .... ◉ 320
Netromycin Injection 100 mg/ml (1 of 1000 patients) 2516
▲ Neupogen for Injection (12%) 495
Neurontin Capsules (More than 1%) 1978
▲ Neutrexin for Injection (8.3%) 2761
▲ Nipent for Injection (42% to 46%) 2733
Nizoral Tablets (Less than 1%) 1345
Normodyne Tablets 2522
Noroxin Tablets (0.3% to 1.0%) 1758
Noroxin Tablets (0.3% to 1.0%) 2222
Norpace (Infrequent) 2596
Norpramin Tablets 1273
▲ Norvir (0.9% to 4.4%) 447
▲ Novantrone for Injection (24 to 78%) 1327
Nuromax Injection (Less than or equal to 0.1%) 1136
Nydrazid Injection 509
▲ OmniHIB (0.6% to 20.1%) 2676
Omnipen for Oral Suspension 2873
▲ Oncaspar (Greater than 5%) 2194
Oncovin Solution Vials & Hyporets 1521
Orap Tablets 1037
Orlaam Oral Solution 2361
Ortho-Cyclen/Ortho-Tri-Cyclen 1914
Ortho Diaphragm Kits—All-Flex Arcing Spring; Ortho Coil Spring; Ortho-White Flat Spring 1921
Ortho Diaphragm Kit-Coil Spring 1921
Ortho-Novum 1928
Ortho-Cyclen/Ortho Tri-Cyclen 1914
Ortho-White Diaphragm Kit-Flat Spring (See also Ortho Diaphragm Kits) 1921
▲ Orthoclone OKT3 Sterile Solution (89% to 90%) 1892
OxyContin Tablets (Between 1% and 5%) 2163
Panhematin 452
ParaGard T 380A Intrauterine Copper Contraceptive 1936
Paraplatin for Injection 713
PASER Granules 1333
Paxil Tablets (2%) 2681
Pediazole Suspension 2340
PedvaxHIB 1761
Peganone Tablets 455
Pen•Vee K (Frequent) 2879
Penetrex Tablets (0.1% to 1%) 2196
Pentasa (0.9%) 1275
Pentaspan Injection 954
Pepcid Injection (Infrequent) 1765
Pepcid (Infrequent) 1763
Pergonal (menotropins for injection, USP) 2618
Permax Tablets (Frequent) 571
Pfizerpen for Injection 2022
Phenobarbital Elixir and Tablets (Less than 1 in 100 patients) 1523
Phenurone Tablets (Less than 1%) 455
Phrenilin (Infrequent) 790
Platinol for Injection 717
Platinol-AQ Injection 719
PMB 200 and PMB 400 (Rare) 2890
Pneumovax 23 (Rare) 1768
Pnu-Imune 23 (Occasional) 1437
Podocon-25 1949
Pondimin Tablets 2239
Potaba Capsules, Envules, Powder, and Tablets (Infrequent) 1234
Pravachol Tablets (Rare) 770
Premphase 2900
Prempro 2905
Prepidil Gel (1.4%) 2108
Prevacid Delayed-Release Capsules (Less than 1%) 2746
Prilosec Delayed-Release Capsules (Less than 1%) 516
Primaxin I.M. 1770
Primaxin I.V. (0.5%) 1772
Prinivil Tablets (0.3% to 1.1%) 1776
Prinzide Tablets (0.3 to 1%) 1780
Procanbid Extended-Release Tablets (Fairly common) 1983
Procardia Capsules (2% or less) 2024
Procardia XL Extended Release Tablets (1% or less) 2026
▲ Procrit for Injection (29% to 38%) 1896
Proglycem 575
▲ Prograf (15% to 48%) 1028
Prolastin Alpha$_1$-Proteinase Inhibitor (Human) (0.77%) 629
▲ Proleukin for Injection (89%) 812
Prolixin 510
Proloprim Tablets 1141
Propulsid (2.2%) 1346
ProSom Tablets (Infrequent) 457
▲ Prostin E2 Suppository (Approximately one-half) 2109
Protostat Tablets 1939
Provera Tablets 2110
Prozac Pulvules & Liquid, Oral Solution (1.4% to 2%) 935
Pulmozyme Inhalation 1054
Pyrazinamide Tablets (Rare) 1442
Quadrinal Tablets 1398

(▣ Described in PDR For Nonprescription Drugs)   Incidence data in parenthesis; ▲ 3% or more   (◉ Described in PDR For Ophthalmology)

Side Effects Index — Fissuring, fingertips

▲ Quinaglute Dura-Tabs Tablets (6%) ... 644
Quinidex Extentabs ... 2240
▲ Rabies Vaccine Adsorbed (8% to 10%) ... 2686
▲ Rabies Vaccine, Imovax Rabies I.D. (Less frequent; up to 6%) ... 901
Recombivax HB (Greater than 1%) ... 1787
Redux Capsules (Frequent) ... 2911
Relafen Tablets (Less than 1%) ... 2688
Remeron Tablets (Infrequent) ... 1878
▲ RespiGam (6%) ... 1631
▲ Retrovir Capsules (3.2% to 16%) ... 1216
▲ Retrovir I.V. Infusion (4% to 16%) ... 1221
▲ Retrovir Syrup (3.2% to 16%) ... 1216
ReVia Tablets (Less than 1%) ... 957
▲ Revex (nalmefene hydrochloride injection) (3%) ... 1863
▲ RhoGAM Rh₀(D) Immune Globulin (Human) (25% in one study) ... 1902
Ridaura Capsules (Rare) ... 2691
Rifadin ... 1276
Rifamate Capsules ... 1278
Rifater ... 1280
Rimactane Capsules ... 865
Risperdal Tablets (2% to 3%) ... 1348
Ritalin ... 866
Robaxin Injectable ... 2245
Robaxin Tablets ... 2246
Robaxisal Tablets ... 2246
Rocephin Injectable Vials, ADD-Vantage, Galaxy Container (Less than 1%) ... 2305
▲ Roferon-A Injection (74% to 92%) 2308
▲ Rowasa (1.2% to 3.19%) ... 2727
Rubex for Injection (Occasional) ... 721
Rythmol Tablets–150mg, 225mg, 300mg (1.9%) ... 1399
SSKI Solution (Less frequent) ... 2767
Sandimmune (2% or less) ... 2416
Sandoglobulin I.V. (Less than 1%) .. 2419
Sansert Tablets ... 2424
Seconal Sodium Pulvules (Less than 1 in 100) ... 1529
Sectral Capsules ... 2914
Sedapap Tablets 50 mg/650 mg (Infrequent) ... 1826
Septra I.V. Infusion ... 1142
Septra I.V. Infusion ADD-Vantage Vials ... 1144
Ser-Ap-Es Tablets ... 867
Serax Capsules ... 2916
Serax Tablets ... 2916
Serentil ... 689
Serzone Tablets (2%) ... 776
Sinequan (Occasional) ... 2028
Solganal Suspension ... 2530
Soma Compound w/Codeine Tablets ... 2784
Soma Compound Tablets ... 2783
Soma Tablets ... 2782
Sporanox Capsules (0.3% to 2.5%) ... 1352
Stelazine ... 2692
▲ Streptase for Infusion (Among most common; 1% to 4%) ... 557
Sular Tablets (Less than or equal to 1%) ... 2961
▲ Supprelin Injection (6% to 12%) 2230
Suprane (desflurane, USP) (Less than 1%) ... 1865
Symmetrel Capsules (Uncommon).. 965
Symmetrel Syrup (Uncommon) ... 963
Tagamet (Rare) ... 2694
Tambocor Tablets (1% to less than 3%) ... 1555
Tao Capsules ... 2033
Tapazole Tablets ... 1361
▲ Taxol Injection (12%) ... 723
Taxotere for Injection Concentrate 2204
Tazicef for Injection (2%) ... 2697
Tazidime Vials, Faspak & ADD-Vantage (2%) ... 1531
▲ Tegison Capsules (10-25%) ... 2314
Tegretol/Tegretol-XR ... 870
Tenoretic Tablets ... 2963
Tenormin Tablets and I.V. Injection 2965
Terazol 3 Vaginal Cream (1%) ... 1941
Terazol 3 Vaginal Suppositories (2.8% of 284 patients) ... 1942
Terazol 7 Vaginal Cream (1.7% of 521 patients) ... 1943
Tetanus & Diphtheria Toxoids Adsorbed Purogenated (Rare) ... 1446
Tetanus Toxoid Adsorbed Purogenated ... 1447
▲ Tetramune (24% to 40%) ... 1449
▲ TheraCys BCG Live (Intravesical) (2.6% to 38.4%) ... 911
Thioplex (Thiotepa For Injection) ... 1329
Thorazine (Occasional) ... 2701

▲ THROMBATE III Antithrombin III (Human) (1 of 17) ... 631
Thyro-Block Tablets (A few people) 2785
▲ TICE BCG, USP (19.9%) ... 1881
Ticlid Tablets ... 2317
Timolide Tablets ... 1791
Timoptic in Ocudose ... 1796
Timoptic Sterile Ophthalmic Solution ... 1794
Timoptic-XE ... 1798
Tofranil Tablets ... 875
Tofranil-PM Capsules ... 876
Tolectin (200, 400 and 600 mg) (Less than 1%) ... 1591
Tonocard Tablets (Less than 1%) .. 519
Toprol-XL Tablets ... 560
Toradol (1% or less) ... 2319
Torecan (Occasional) ... 2367
Trandate Tablets (Less common) .. 1158
Trasylol (12%) ... 607
Triavil Tablets ... 1800
▲ Tri-Immunol Adsorbed (50%) ... 1452
Trilafon ... 2532
Levlen/Tri-Levlen ... 646
Trimpex Tablets ... 2323
Triostat Injection (Approximately 1%) ... 2708
Tripedia (1% to 4%) ... 908
Typhim Vi (Up to 2%) ... 914
Univasc Tablets ... 2553
Urispas Tablets ... 2710
Vancocin HCl, Vials & ADD-Vantage ... 1534
Vantin for Oral Suspension and Vantin Tablets (Less than 1%) ... 2112
Vaqta (2.6% to 3.1%) ... 1805
Vascor Tablets (200 and 300 mg) (0.5 to 2.0%) ... 1597
Vaseretic Tablets ... 1810
Vasotec I.V. (0.5 to 1%) ... 1814
Vasotec Tablets (0.5% to 1.0%) ... 1816
VePesid Capsules and Injection (0.7% to 2%; infrequent) ... 727
Verelan Capsules ... 1455
▲ Vesanoid Capsules (83%) ... 2327
▲ Videx Tablets, Powder for Oral Solution, & Pediatric Powder for Oral Solution (9% tp 82%) ... 2980
▲ Viramune Tablets (Among most frequent; 3%) ... 2368
Visken Tablets ... 2428
▲ Vistide Injection (15% to 57%) ... 1057
Vivactil Tablets ... 1820
Vivotif Berna ... 660
Cataflam/Voltaren/Voltaren-XR (Rare) ... 833
▲ Vumon for Injection (3%) ... 729
Wellbutrin Tablets (1.2%) ... 1177
WinRho SD (A small number of cases) ... 1839
WinRho SD (1%) ... 1840
Yodoxin Tablets ... 1235
Zantac (Rare) ... 1182
Zantac Injection ... 1180
Zantac Syrup (Rare) ... 1182
Zebeta Tablets ... 1457
▲ Zerit Capsules (5% to 38%) ... 731
Zestoretic Tablets (0.3 to 1%) ... 2968
Zestril Tablets (0.3% to 1.0%) ... 2972
Ziac ... 1459
▲ Zinecard Injection (22% to 34%) .. 2120
Zithromax (1% or less) ... 2043
Zocor Tablets (Rare) ... 1821
▲ Zofran Injection (2% to 8%) ... 1227
▲ Zofran Tablets (8%) ... 1231
Zoladex (1% or greater but less than 5%) ... 2976
Zoladex 3-month ... 2978
Zoloft (1.6%) ... 2051
Zonalon Cream (Less than 1%) ... 1042
Zosyn (2.4% to 3.2%) ... 1463
Zovirax Capsules ... 1187
Zovirax Sterile Powder (Less than 1%) ... 1191
Zovirax ... 1187
Zyloprim Tablets (Less than 1%) 1194
Zyrtec Tablets (Less than 2%) ... 2053

Fever, neutropenic
▲ Neupogen for Injection (13%) ... 495

Fibrillations
LUVOX Tablets (Rare) ... 2723
Tambocor Tablets ... 1555
Tenex Tablets (Rare) ... 2249

Fibrillations, atrial
Adalat CC (Less than 1.0%) ... 582
▲ Aredia for Injection (Up to 6%) ... 827
Betaseron for SC Injection ... 653

Cardene Capsules (Less than 0.4%) ... 2261
▲ CellCept Capsules (More than or equal to 3%) ... 2265
Clozaril Tablets ... 2377
Cognex Capsules (Infrequent) ... 1961
Cordarone Intravenous (Less than 2%) ... 2821
Cozaar Tablets (Less than 1%) ... 1668
Demadex Tablets and Injection ... 691
Desyrel and Desyrel Dividose ... 504
Dilacor XR Extended-release Capsules (1.4%) ... 2183
Diprivan Injectable Emulsion (Less than 1%) ... 2939
DynaCirc Capsules (0.5% to 1%) .. 2381
DynaCirc CR Tablets (0.5% to 1.0%) ... 2383
Emete-con Intramuscular/Intravenous ... 2007
Ethmozine Tablets (Less than 2%) 2217
Felbatol ... 2774
Foscavir Injection (Less than 1%) .. 541
Hivid Tablets (Less than 1%) ... 2287
Hyzaar Tablets ... 1720
Idamycin Injection ... 2096
Imdur (Less than or equal to 5%) ... 1362
Imitrex Injection (Extremely rare) ... 1095
Imitrex Tablets (Rare) ... 1099
Intron A for Injection (Less than 5%) ... 2506
Ismo Tablets (Fewer than 1%) ... 2844
Kadian Capsules (Less than 3%) ... 2948
Kytril Injection (Rare) ... 2667
Kytril Tablets (Rare) ... 2669
Lamictal Tablets ... 1105
Lopid Tablets (0.7%) ... 1974
Nalfon 200 Pulvules & Nalfon Tablets (Less than 1%) ... 933
Neurontin Capsules (Rare) ... 1978
Norvasc Tablets (More than 0.1% to 1%) ... 2020
OptiPranolol (Metipranolol 0.3%) Sterile Ophthalmic Solution (A small number of patients) ... ⊚ 256
Paxil Tablets (Rare) ... 2681
Permax Tablets (Infrequent) ... 571
Prinivil Tablets (0.3% to 1.0%) ... 1776
Prinzide Tablets ... 1780
Prozac Pulvules & Liquid, Oral Solution ... 935
Redux Capsules ... 2911
▲ ReoPro Vials (3.5%) ... 1526
Rilutek Tablets (Infrequent) ... 2198
Risperdal Tablets ... 1348
Rythmol Tablets–150mg, 225mg, 300mg (0.7 to 1.2%) ... 1399
Sular Tablets (Less than or equal to 1%) ... 2961
Taxol Injection (Rare) ... 723
Taxotere for Injection Concentrate 2204
Tegison Capsules (Less than 1%) .. 2314
▲ Tenormin Tablets and I.V. Injection (5%) ... 2965
▲ Trasylol (24%) ... 607
Vaseretic Tablets ... 1810
Vasotec I.V. ... 1814
Vasotec Tablets (0.5% to 1.0%) ... 1816
Zestril Tablets (0.3% to 1.0%) ... 2972
Zosyn (1.0% or less) ... 1463

Fibrillations, ventricular
Abelcet Injection ... 1540
Adenocard Injection (Rare) ... 1021
Ana-Kit Anaphylaxis Emergency Treatment Kit ... 611
Betapace Tablets ... 637
Betaseron for SC Injection ... 653
Calan SR Caplets ... 2571
Calan Tablets ... 2568
Cardioquin Tablets ... 2146
Cardizem Injectable (Less than 1%) ... 1253
Clozaril Tablets ... 2377
Cordarone Intravenous (Less than 2%) ... 2821
Covera-HS Tablets ... 2573
Diprivan Injectable Emulsion (Less than 1%) ... 2939
DynaCirc Capsules (0.5% to 1%) .. 2381
DynaCirc CR Tablets (0.5% to 1.0%) ... 2383
Eminase ... 2215
Fungizone Intravenous ... 507
Hespan Injection ... 945
Hyzaar Tablets ... 1720
Imitrex Injection (Rare) ... 1095
Imitrex Tablets (Rare) ... 1099
Isoptin SR Tablets ... 1395
Lanoxicaps ... 1110

Marcaine ... 2446
Narcan Injection (Several instances) ... 950
Norpace ... 2596
Norpramin Tablets ... 1273
Nuromax Injection (Less than or equal to 0.1%) ... 1136
Primacor Injection (0.2%) ... 2461
Procanbid Extended-Release Tablets ... 1983
Propulsid (Rare) ... 1346
Quinaglute Dura-Tabs Tablets ... 644
Quinidex Extentabs ... 2240
Redux Capsules ... 2911
Rilutek Tablets (Rare) ... 2198
Seldane Tablets (Rare) ... 1284
Seldane-D Extended-Release Tablets (Rare) ... 1286
Sensorcaine ... 554
Tonocard Tablets (Less than 1%) .. 519
Trasylol (2%) ... 607
Zosyn (1.0% or less) ... 1463

Fibromyalgia
Cozaar Tablets (Less than 1%) ... 1668
Hyzaar Tablets ... 1720

Fibrosing colonopathy
Creon ... 2714
Ultrase Capsules ... 2476
Ultrase MT Capsules ... 2477

Fibrosis
Cafergot (Rare) ... 2376
Genotropin Injection (Infrequent) ... 2090
Inversine Tablets ... 1729
Methotrexate Sodium Tablets, Injection, for Injection and LPF Injection ... 1322
Myochrysine Injection ... 1754
Ocufen ... ⊚ 242
Platinol for Injection ... 717
Platinol-AQ Injection ... 719
Ridaura Capsules (Rare) ... 2691
Solganal Suspension ... 2530
Taxol Injection (Rare) ... 723

Fibrosis, bladder
Cytoxan ... 700

Fibrosis, interstitial pulmonary (see under Pulmonary fibrosis)

Fibrosis, ovary
Cytoxan ... 700

Fibrosis, pelvic
Lupron Injection ... 2736

Fibrosis, periportal
Tagamet (A single case) ... 2694

Fibrosis, pleural
D.H.E. 45 Injection (Occasional) ... 2381
Intron A for Injection (Less than or equal to 5%) ... 2506
Taxol Injection (Rare) ... 723

Fibrosis, pleuropulmonary
Cafergot ... 2376

Fibrosis, retroperitoneal
Cafergot ... 2376

Fibrotendinitis
Naprelan Tablets (Less than 1%) .. 2861

Fingernails, brittle
Neoral (2% or less) ... 2405
Sandimmune (2% or less) ... 2416
Trental Tablets (Less than 1%) ... 1291

Fingernails, darkening
Drithocreme 0.1%, 0.25%, 0.5%, 1.0% (HP) ... 920
Dritho-Scalp 0.25%, 0.5% ... 921

Fingers, discoloration
Eskalith ... 2658
Lithium Carbonate Capsules & Tablets (A single report) ... 2352
Lithonate/Lithotabs/Lithobid ... 2721

Fissures, lips
Aquasol A Vitamin A Capsules, USP ... 525
Aquasol A Parenteral ... 526

Fissuring, fingertips
FLUORACAINE ... ⊚ 208
FLURESS ... ⊚ 208

(⊡ Described in PDR For Nonprescription Drugs) Incidence data in parenthesis; ▲ 3% or more (⊚ Described in PDR For Ophthalmology)

Fissuring, fingertips | **Side Effects Index** | **1340**

- Ophthetic ◉ 244

Fissuring, unspecified
- Ergamisol Tablets 1340
- Fluorouracil Injection 2282
- Sterile FUDR (Remote possibility) 2284
- Melanex Topical Solution 1842
- Oxistat Cream (0.1%) 1139
- Temovate Cream (1 of 421 patients) 1152
- Temovate E Emollient (Less than 2%) 1154
- ▲ Temovate Gel (Among most frequent) 1153

Fistula, regional lymph node
- TICE BCG, USP (Rare) 1881

Fistula, tracheo-esophageal
- Proleukin for Injection (Less than 1%) 812

Flaccidity
- Streptomycin Sulfate Injection 2031

Flare
- Dipentum Capsules (Rare) 2084
- Nolvadex Tablets 2957

Flare, postinjection
- Attenuvax (Rare) 1650
- Biavax II 1653
- Celestone Soluspan Suspension 2484
- Dalalone D.P. Injectable 1009
- Decadron Phosphate Injection 1680
- Decadron-LA Sterile Suspension 1687
- Demerol 2438
- Dilaudid-HP Injection (Less frequent) 1384
- Dilaudid-HP Lyophilized Powder 250 mg (Less frequent) 1384
- Hydeltrasol Injection, Sterile 1708
- Hydeltra-T.B.A. Sterile Suspension 1710
- Hydrocortone Acetate Sterile Suspension 1712
- M-M-R II 1730
- M-R-VAX II 1732
- Mepergan Injection 2859
- Meruvax II 1740
- Mumpsvax (Rare) 1751

Flatulence
- ▲ Actigall Capsules (7.7%) 818
- Adalat Capsules (10 mg and 20 mg) (2% or less) 580
- Adalat CC (Less than 1.0%) 582
- AeroBid Inhaler System (1% to 3%) 1004
- Aerobid-M Inhaler System (1% to 3%) 1004
- Aldoclor Tablets 1638
- Aldomet Ester HCl Injection 1642
- Aldomet Oral 1640
- Aldoril Tablets 1644
- Ambien Tablets (Infrequent) 2559
- Anafranil Capsules (Up to 6%) 819
- ▲ Asacol Delayed-Release Tablets (3%) 2129
- Asendin Tablets (Less than 1%) 1419
- Atamet Tablets 567
- Atromid-S Capsules (Less frequent) 2808
- Augmentin (Less frequent) 2637
- Augmentin Tablets (Less frequent) 2640
- ▲ Axid Pulvules (4.9%) 1468
- Axocet Capsules (Infrequent) 2469
- Betapace Tablets (1% to 2%) 637
- Betaseron for SC Injection 653
- Buprenex Injectable (Infrequent) 2170
- BuSpar Tablets (Infrequent) 738
- Carafate Suspension (Less than 0.5%) 1250
- Carafate Tablets (Less than 0.5%) 1249
- Cardura Tablets (1%) 1993
- Cartrol Tablets (Less common) 413
- ▲ Casodex Tablets (5%) 2934
- Cataflam Tablets (1% to 3%) 833
- Cedax (0.1% to 1%) 2480
- Ceftin (0.1% to 1%) 1067
- ▲ CellCept Capsules (More than or equal to 3%) 2265
- Cerebyx Injection (Infrequent) 1956
- Cipro I.V. (1% or less) 587
- Cipro I.V. Pharmacy Bulk Package (Less than 1%) 590
- Cipro Tablets 584
- Claritin Tablets (2% or fewer patients) 2485
- Claritin-D Tablets (Less frequent) 2487
- Clinoril Tablets (1% to 3%) 1658
- ▲ Cognex Capsules (4%) 1961
- Colestid (Less frequent) 2073
- Cozaar Tablets (Less than 1%) 1668
- Crixivan Capsules (Less than 2%) 1670
- Cytotec (2.9%) 2576
- ▲ Cytovene (6%) 2270
- Daypro Caplets (1% to 3%) 2578
- Depakote Tablets (1% to 5%) 418
- Desyrel and Desyrel Dividose 504
- Dilacor XR Extended-release Capsules 2183
- Dipentum Capsules (Rare) 2084
- Dolobid Tablets (Greater than 1 in 100) 1695
- DUPHALAC Solution 2714
- Duragesic Transdermal System (1% or greater) 1336
- Dynabac (1.5%) 668
- ▲ Effexor (3%) 2825
- Emcyt Capsules (2%) 2085
- Ergamisol Tablets (Less than 1% to 2%) 1340
- Esgic-plus Capsules (Infrequent) 1012
- Esgic-plus Tablets (Infrequent) 1012
- Eskalith 2658
- Estring Vaginal Ring (1% to 3%) 2086
- Ethmozine Tablets (Less than 2%) 2217
- Famvir Tablets (1.5% to 1.9%) 2660
- Felbatol 2774
- Feldene Capsules (Greater than 1%) 2008
- Fioricet Tablets (Infrequent) 2386
- Fioricet with Codeine Capsules (Infrequent) 2387
- Fiorinal (Less frequent) 2388
- Flexeril Tablets (Less than 1%) 1701
- Floxin I.V. (1% to 3%) 1580
- Floxin Tablets (200 mg, 300 mg, 400 mg) (1% to 3%) 1577
- Fosamax Tablets (2.6%) 1703
- Foscavir Injection (Between 1% and 5%) 541
- Gastrocrom Capsules (Infrequent) 1611
- Gastrocrom Oral Concentrate (Infrequent) 1611
- Geocillin Tablets 2009
- ▲ Glucophage Tablets (Among most common) 754
- ▲ Glucotrol XL Extended Release Tablets (3.2%) 2012
- Helidac Therapy (Less than 1%) 2135
- Hivid Tablets (Less than 1%) 2287
- ▲ Hylorel Tablets (32.0%) 1613
- Hytrin Capsules (At least 1%) 434
- Hyzaar Tablets 1720
- IBU Tablets (Greater than 1%) 1389
- Imdur (Less than or equal to 5%) 1362
- Imitrex Injection (Rare) 1095
- Indocin Capsules (Less than 1%) 1723
- Indocin I.V. (Less than 1%) 1727
- Indocin (Less than 1%) 1723
- Intron A for Injection (Less than 5%) 2506
- K-Dur Microburst Release System (potassium chloride, USP) E.R. Tablets 1364
- ▲ K-Lor Powder Packets (Among most common) 438
- ▲ K-Norm Capsules (Among most common) 1615
- ▲ K-Tab Filmtab (Most common) 439
- Lamictal Tablets (More than 1%) 1105
- Lamisil Tablets (2.2%) 2394
- Larodopa Tablets (Infrequent) 2296
- Lescol Capsules (2.6%) 2395
- Lioresal Intrathecal (1% or more) 1634
- Lithonate/Lithotabs/Lithobid 2721
- ▲ Lodine Capsules and Tablets (3% to 9%) 2849
- Lopressor (1%) 848
- Lopressor HCT Tablets (1 in 100) 850
- Lotensin HCT Tablets (0.3% or more) 855
- ▲ LUVOX Tablets (4%) 2723
- Macrobid Capsules (1.5%) 2138
- Maxaquin Tablets (Less than 1%) 2593
- ▲ Megace Oral Suspension (Up to 10%) 708
- Merrem I.V. (0.1% to 1.0%) 2952
- ▲ Mevacor Tablets (3.7% to 6.4%) 1742
- Miacalcin Nasal Spray (Less than 1%) 2403
- ▲ Micro-K LS Packets (Among most common) 2238
- Midamor Tablets (Less than or equal to 1%) 1746
- Moduretic Tablets (Less than or equal to 1%) 1748
- Monopril Tablets (0.2% to 1.0%) 762
- Motrin Ibuprofen Suspension, Oral Drops, Chewable Tablets, Caplets (1% to less than 3%) 1563
- Mycobutin Capsules (2%) 2101
- Nalfon 200 Pulvules & Nalfon Tablets (Less than 1%) 933
- Naprelan Tablets (Less than 3%) 2861
- Nephro-Fer Rx Tablets 2168
- Neurontin Capsules (Frequent) 1978
- ▲ Nipent for Injection (3% to 10%) 2733
- Noroxin Tablets (0.3% to 1.0%) 1758
- Noroxin Tablets (0.3% to 1.0%) 2222
- ▲ Norpace (3 to 9%) 2596
- Norvasc Tablets (More than 0.1% to 1%) 2020
- Norvir (0.9%) 447
- Oncaspar (Less than 1%) 2194
- ▲ Orudis Capsules (3% to 9%) 2874
- ▲ Oruvail Capsules (3% to 9%) 2874
- OxyContin Tablets (Less than 1%) 2163
- ▲ Paxil Tablets (4.0%) 2681
- Pediazole Suspension 2340
- Penetrex Tablets (0.1% to 1%) 2196
- Permax Tablets (Infrequent) 571
- Phrenilin (Less frequent) 790
- Plendil Extended-Release Tablets (0.5% to 1.5%) 514
- Ponstel (Less frequent) 1982
- ▲ Pravachol Tablets (2.7% to 3.3%) 770
- ▲ Precose (77%) 604
- Prevacid Delayed-Release Capsules (Less than 1%) 2746
- Prilosec Delayed-Release Capsules (Less than 1 to 2.7%) 516
- Prinivil Tablets (0.3% to 1.0%) 1776
- Prinzide Tablets 1780
- Procardia Capsules (2% or less) 2024
- Procardia XL Extended Release Tablets (Less than 3%) 2026
- ▲ Prograf (Greater than 3%) 1028
- ▲ Propulsid (3.5%) 1346
- ProSom Tablets (Infrequent) 457
- Prostigmin Injectable 1305
- Prostigmin Tablets 1306
- Prozac Pulvules & Liquid, Oral Solution (1.6%) 935
- Questran (Less frequent) 774
- Redux Capsules (Frequent) 2911
- ▲ Relafen Tablets (3% to 9%) 2688
- Retrovir Capsules 1216
- Retrovir I.V. Infusion 1221
- Retrovir Syrup 1216
- ReVia Tablets (Less than 1%) 957
- ▲ Ridaura Capsules (3 to 9%) 2691
- Rifadin (Some patients) 1276
- Rifamate Capsules (Some patients) 1278
- Rifater 1280
- Rilutek Tablets (2.0% to 2.5%) 2198
- Rimactane Capsules 865
- Risperdal Tablets (Infrequent) 1348
- Rocephin Injectable Vials, ADD-Vantage, Galaxy Container (Rare) 2305
- Roferon-A Injection (Less than 3%) 2308
- ▲ Rowasa (3.6 to 6.13%) 2727
- Rythmol Tablets–150mg, 225mg, 300mg (0.3 to 1.9%) 1399
- ▲ Sandostatin Injection (Less than 10%) 2421
- ▲ Sectral Capsules (3%) 2914
- Sedapap Tablets 50 mg/650 mg (Infrequent) 1826
- Serzone Tablets 776
- Sinemet Tablets 959
- Sinemet CR Tablets 961
- Sporanox Capsules (Less than 1%) 1352
- Sular Tablets (Less than or equal to 1%) 2961
- ▲ Supprelin Injection (3%) 2230
- ▲ Suprax (4%) 1443
- Tambocor Tablets (Less than 1%) 1555
- Tegison Capsules (Less than 1%) 2314
- Ticlid Tablets (1.5%) 2317
- Timentin for Injection 2706
- ▲ Tolectin (200, 400 and 600 mg) (3 to 9%) 1591
- Toprol-XL Tablets (About 1 of 100 patients) 560
- Toradol (Greater than 1%) 2319
- Ultram Tablets (50 mg) (1% to less than 5%) 1594
- Ultrase MT Capsules (1.5%) 2477
- Unasyn (Less than 1%) 2035
- Urecholine 1804
- Vantin for Oral Suspension and Vantin Tablets (Less than 1%) 2112
- Vascor Tablets (200 and 300 mg) (0.5 to 2.0%) 1597
- Vaseretic Tablets (0.5% to 2.0%) 1810
- Videx Tablets, Powder for Oral Solution, & Pediatric Powder for Oral Solution (Up to 2%) 2980
- Vistide Injection 1057
- Cataflam/Voltaren/Voltaren-XR (1% to 3%) 833
- Zestoretic Tablets 2968
- Zestril Tablets (0.3% to 1.0%) 2972
- Zithromax (1% or less) 2043
- Zithromax Tablets (1% or less) 2046
- Zocor Tablets (1.9%) 1821
- Zoladex (1% or greater) 2976
- Zoladex 3-month 2978
- ▲ Zoloft Tablets (3.3%) 2051
- Zosyn (1.0% or less to 1.3%) 1463
- Zovirax (0.4%) 1187
- Zyrtec Tablets (Less than 2%) 2053

Flatus
- Trental Tablets (0.6%) 1291

Floating feeling
- Dilaudid-HP Injection (Less frequent) 1384
- Dilaudid-HP Lyophilized Powder 250 mg (Less frequent) 1384
- Dilaudid Tablets and Liquid (Less frequent) 1386
- MS Contin Tablets (Less frequent) 2149
- MSIR (Infrequent) 2152
- Nubain Injection (1% or less) 952
- Oramorph SR (Morphine Sulfate Sustained Release Tablets) (Less frequent) 2359
- Stadol (1% or greater) 779

Fluid depletion
- Capoten Tablets 740
- Capozide Tablets 744
- DUPHALAC Solution 2714

Fluid imbalance
- Apresazide Capsules 824
- Capozide Tablets 744
- Dalalone D.P. Injectable 1009
- Demadex Tablets and Injection 691
- Esidrix Tablets 839
- Lutrepulse for Injection 998
- Prinzide Tablets 1780
- Tenoretic Tablets 2963
- Vaseretic Tablets 1810
- ▲ Vesanoid Capsules (6%) 2327
- Zestoretic Tablets 2968

Fluid overload
- ▲ Aredia for Injection (Up to at least 15%) 827
- Orthoclone OKT3 Sterile Solution 1892
- Prinivil Tablets (0.3% to 1.0%) 1776
- RespiGam (1%) 1631
- Zestoretic Tablets 2968
- Zestril Tablets (0.3% to 1.0%) 2972
- Zosyn (1.9%) 1463

Fluid retention (see under Edema)

Flu-like symptoms
- ▲ Actimmune (Most common) 1043
- ▲ AeroBid Inhaler System (10%) 1004
- ▲ Aerobid-M Inhaler System (10%) 1004
- ▲ Alferon N Injection (30%) 2142
- Altace Capsules 1238
- Alupent Tablets (0.2%) 672
- Arimidex Tablets (2% to 5%) 2932
- ▲ Asacol Delayed-Release Tablets (3%) 2129
- Atromid-S Capsules 2808
- ▲ Avonex (61%) 662
- ▲ Betaseron for SC Injection (53% to 76%) 653
- Cartrol Tablets (Less common) 413
- ▲ Casodex Tablets (4%) 2934
- Cataflam Tablets 833
- Caverject Injection (2%) 2064
- ▲ CellCept Capsules (More than or equal to 3%) 2265
- Cerebyx Injection (Infrequent) 1956
- ▲ Chemet Capsules (5.2% to 15.7%) 666
- Claritin-D Tablets (Less frequent) 2487
- Clozaril Tablets 2377
- Crixivan Capsules (Less than 2%) 1670
- DTIC-Dome 593
- DaunoXome (Up to 5%) 1842
- ▲ Depakote Tablets (At least 5%) 418
- Dilacor XR Extended-release Capsules (2.3%) 2183
- Doxil (Less than 1%) 2613
- Dynabac (0.1% to 1%) 668
- Effexor 2825

(▣ Described in PDR For Nonprescription Drugs) Incidence data in parenthesis; ▲ 3% or more (◉ Described in PDR For Ophthalmology)

1341 **Side Effects Index** **Flushing**

Engerix-B Unit-Dose Vials (Less than 1%) ... 2656
Epogen for Injection (Rare) ... 489
Ergamisol Tablets (5 out of 463 patients) ... 1340
▲ Estring Vaginal Ring (3%) ... 2086
Eulexin Capsules ... 2498
Felbatol (Frequent) ... 2774
Feldene Capsules (Less than 1%) .. 2008
▲ Flolan for Injection (25%) ... 1085
▲ Gemzar for Injection (19%) ... 1482
Hivid Tablets (Less than 1%) ... 2287
Humegon for Injection ... 1873
Hytrin Capsules (At least 1% to 2.4%) ... 434
Imdur (Less than or equal to 5%) .. 1362
▲ Intron A for Injection (Up to 79%) 2506
JE-VAX (Less than 3%) ... 904
Kadian Capsules (Less than 3%) ... 2948
Kerlone Tablets (Less than 2%) ... 2588
▲ Lamictal Tablets (7.0%) ... 1105
▲ Lescol Capsules (5.1%) ... 2395
Lioresal Intrathecal (1% or more) .. 1634
▲ Lopressor HCT Tablets (10 in 100 patients) ... 850
Lotensin HCT Tablets (More than 1.0%) ... 855
Lupron Depot 3.75 mg (Less than 5%) ... 2739
▲ LUVOX Tablets (3%) ... 2723
Miacalcin Nasal Spray (1% to 3%) 2403
Mycobutin Capsules (Less than 1%) ... 2101
▲ Naprelan Tablets (10%) ... 2861
Nipent for Injection (Less than 3%) ... 2733
Normodyne Injection ... 2519
Normodyne Tablets ... 2522
Norvir (Less than 2%) ... 447
Orlaam Oral Solution (1% to 3%).. 2361
Orthoclone OKT3 Sterile Solution .. 1892
ParaGard T 380A Intrauterine Copper Contraceptive ... 1936
Paxil Tablets (Infrequent) ... 2681
Pergonal (menotropins for injection, USP) ... 2618
▲ Permax Tablets (3.2%) ... 571
Prevacid Delayed-Release Capsules (Less than 1%) ... 2746
Prilosec Delayed-Release Capsules (1%) ... 516
Procrit for Injection (Rare) ... 1896
Prolastin Alpha$_1$-Proteinase Inhibitor (Human) (Occasional) ... 629
▲ Prozac Pulvules & Liquid, Oral Solution (2.8% to 10%) ... 935
Pulmozyme Inhalation ... 1054
Redux Capsules (Frequent) ... 2911
▲ Remeron Tablets (5%) ... 1878
Retrovir Capsules ... 1216
Retrovir I.V. Infusion ... 1221
Retrovir Syrup ... 1216
Rifadin ... 1276
Rifater ... 1280
Rilutek Tablets (More than 2%) ... 2198
Risperdal Tablets (Infrequent) ... 1348
▲ Roferon-A Injection (16%) ... 2308
▲ Rowasa (5.28%) ... 2727
Sandostatin Injection (1% to 4%).. 2421
▲ Serzone Tablets (3%) ... 776
Slo-Niacin Tablets ... 2767
Sular Tablets (Less than or equal to 1%) ... 2961
Tegison Capsules (Less than 1%) .. 2314
Tiazac Capsules (1%) ... 1019
▲ TICE BCG, USP (33.2%) ... 1881
Trandate ... 1158
Trental Tablets (Less than 1%) ... 1291
Typhim Vi ... 914
▲ Univasc Tablets (3.1%) ... 2553
Vascor Tablets (200 and 300 mg) (0.5 to 2.08%) ... 1597
▲ Videx Tablets, Powder for Oral Solution, & Pediatric Powder for Oral Solution (Less than 1% to 7%) ... 2980
Cataflam/Voltaren/Voltaren-XR ... 833
Wellbutrin Tablets (Frequent) ... 1177
▲ Xalatan (Approximately 4%) ... ◉ 304
▲ Zerit Capsules (Fewer than 1% to 9%) ... 731

Flushing

Accutane Capsules (Less than 1%) ... 2252
▲ Acthrel for Injection (16%) ... 2990
▲ Adalat Capsules (10 mg and 20 mg) (About 10% to 25%) ... 580
▲ Adalat CC (4%) ... 582
Adapin Capsules (Occasional) ... 1542
▲ Adenoscan (44%) ... 1022
Ambien Tablets (Rare) ... 2559
Americaine Hemorrhoidal Ointment ... ▣ 649
Aminohippurate Sodium Injection .. 1646
▲ Anafranil Capsules (7% to 8%) ... 819
Antivenin (Crotalidae) Polyvalent ... 2803
Apresazide Capsules (Less frequent) ... 824
Apresoline Hydrochloride Tablets (Less frequent) ... 826
AquaMEPHYTON Injection ... 1648
Atamet Tablets ... 567
Atrohist Pediatric Capsules ... 1603
Atrovent Inhalation Aerosol (Less frequent) ... 674
Azactam for Injection (One patient) ... 736
Bellergal-S Tablets (Rare) ... 2375
Benemid Tablets ... 1651
BiCNU ... 696
Bioclate, Antihemophilic Factor (Recombinant) (One patient out of 13,394) ... 797
Bontril Slow-Release Capsules ... 786
Brethine Ampuls (0.0 to 2.4%) ... 832
Brevibloc (esmolol HCl) Injection (Less than 1%) ... 1860
Bromfed ... 1832
Buprenex Injectable (Less than 1%) ... 2170
BuSpar Tablets (Infrequent) ... 738
Calan SR Caplets (0.6%) ... 2571
Calan Tablets (0.6%) ... 2568
Capoten Tablets (2 to 5 of 1000 patients) ... 740
Capozide Tablets (2 to 5 of 1000 patients) ... 744
Carbastat Intraocular Solution ... ◉ 260
▲ Cardene Capsules (5.6% to 9.7%) 2261
Cardioquin Tablets ... 2146
Cardizem CD Capsules (1.4%) ... 1251
Cardizem SR Capsules (1.7% to 3%) ... 1255
Cardizem Injectable (1.7%) ... 1253
Cardizem Tablets (Less than 1%) .. 1257
Cardura Tablets (Less than 0.5% of 3960 patients to 1%) ... 1993
Cataflam Tablets (Rare) ... 833
Ceredase ... 1055
Chromagen Capsules ... 2470
Cipro I.V. (1% or less) ... 587
Cipro I.V. Pharmacy Bulk Package (Less than 1%) ... 590
Cipro Tablets (Less than 1%) ... 584
Claritin Tablets (2% or fewer patients) ... 2485
Claritin-D Tablets (Less frequent) .. 2487
Clinoril Tablets (Less than 1 in 100) ... 1658
▲ Cognex Capsules (3%) ... 1961
ColBENEMID Tablets ... 1662
Cordarone Tablets (1 to 3%) ... 2818
Covera-HS Tablets (0.6% to 0.8%) ... 2573
Cozaar Tablets (Less than 1%) ... 1668
Crixivan Capsules (Less than 2%).. 1670
CytoGam (Less than 5.0%) ... 1630
DDAVP (Occasional) ... 2180
DDAVP Tablets ... 2182
D.H.E. 45 Injection (Occasional) ... 2381
Dalgan Injection (Less than 1%) ... 529
Dalmane Capsules (Rare) ... 2329
Danocrine Capsules ... 2437
▲ DaunoXome (13.8% to 16%) ... 1842
Desmopressin Acetate Rhinal Tube (Occasional) ... 997
Dilaudid Tablets and Liquid ... 1386
Diprivan Injectable Emulsion (Less than 1%) ... 2939
Dolobid Tablets ... 1695
Donnagel Liquid and Donnagel Chewable Tablets (Rare) ... ▣ 854
Dopram Injectable ... 2235
▲ Doxil (Approximately 6.8%) ... 2613
▲ DynaCirc Capsules (2.0% to 5.1%) ... 2381
DynaCirc CR Tablets (1.3% to 2.5%) ... 2383
Effexor ... 2825
Emcyt Capsules (1%) ... 2085
Emete-con Intramuscular/Intravenous ... 2007
Eminase (Occasional) ... 2215
Engerix-B Unit-Dose Vials (Less than 1%) ... 2656
Ethyol (amifostine) for Injection ... 485
Etopophos for Injection ... 701
Etoposide Injection ... 539
Factrel (Rare) ... 2996
Felbatol ... 2774
Fioricet with Codeine Capsules ... 2387
Fiorinal with Codeine Capsules ... 2390
Flagyl 375 Capsules ... 2587
Flagyl I.V. ... 2373
▲ Flolan for Injection (42% to 58%) 1085
Foscavir Injection (Between 1% and 5%) ... 541
Fungizone Intravenous ... 507
Furoxone (Rare) ... 2221
Gamimune N, 5% Immune Globulin Intravenous (Human), 5% ... 612
Gamimune N, 10% Immune Globulin Intravenous (Human), 10% ... 615
Gammagard S/D, Immune Globulin, Intravenous (Human) (Occasional) ... 577
Gammar-P I.V., Immune Globulin Intravenous (Human) ... 798
Gastrocrom Capsules (Infrequent).. 1611
Gastrocrom Oral Concentrate (Less common) ... 1611
Glucotrol XL Extended Release Tablets (Less than 1%) ... 2012
Helidac Therapy ... 2135
Hespan Injection ... 945
Hivid Tablets (Less than 1%) ... 2287
Hydralazine Hydrochloride Injection USP ... 2712
Hyperstat I.V. Injection ... 2504
Hyskon Hysteroscopy Fluid (Rare).. 1633
Hyzaar Tablets ... 1720
Imdur (Less than or equal to 5%) .. 1362
▲ Imitrex Injection (6.6%) ... 1095
Imitrex Tablets (Up to 4%) ... 1099
Indocin Capsules (Less than 1%) ... 1723
Indocin I.V. (Less than 1%) ... 1727
Indocin (Less than 1%) ... 1723
INFeD (Iron Dextran Injection, USP) ... 2478
Intron A for Injection (Less than 5%) ... 2506
Isoptin Oral Tablets (0.6%) ... 1393
Isoptin SR Tablets (0.6%) ... 1395
Kerlone Tablets (Less than 2%) ... 2588
Konÿne 80 Factor IX Complex ... 627
Lamictal Tablets (Infrequent) ... 1105
Larodopa Tablets (Infrequent) ... 2296
Lescol Capsules (Rare) ... 2395
Leukine ... 1317
Lodine Capsules and Tablets (Less than 1%) ... 2849
Lomotil ... 2591
Lotensin Tablets ... 852
Lotensin HCT Tablets (0.3% to 1.0%) ... 855
Lotrel Capsules (Up to 0.3%) ... 858
Ludiomil Tablets (Rare) ... 861
Lufyllin & Lufyllin-400 Tablets ... 2778
Lufyllin-GG Elixir & Tablets ... 2779
Lutrepulse for Injection ... 998
▲ LUVOX Tablets (3%) ... 2723
Lysodren Tablets ... 707
Marinol (Dronabinol) Capsules (0.3% to 1%) ... 2353
Matulane Capsules ... 2300
Mavik Tablets (0.3% to 1.0%) ... 1407
Maxair Autohaler ... 1550
Maxair Inhaler (Less than 1%) ... 1552
Maxaquin Tablets (Less than 1%) .. 2593
Mephyton Tablets ... 1739
MetroGel-Vaginal ... 917
Metubine Iodide Vials ... 932
Mevacor Tablets (Rare) ... 1742
Miacalcin Nasal Spray (Less than 1%) ... 2403
Miochol-E with Iocare Steri-Tags and Miochol-E System Pak (Rare) ... ◉ 263
MIOSTAT Intraocular Solution ... ◉ 222
▲ Mivacron (15%) ... 1125
Moduretic Tablets (Less than or equal to 1%) ... 1748
Monoket Tablets (Up to 2%) ... 2550
Mononine, Coagulation Factor IX (Human), Monoclonal Antibody Purified ... 804
Monopril Tablets (0.2% to 1.0%).. 762
Motofen Tablets ... 789
Myochrysine Injection ... 1754
Neoral (Up to 4%) ... 2405
Nimbex Injection (0.2%) ... 1131
Nimotop Capsules (Less than 1% to 2.1%) ... 603
Nitrolingual Spray ... 2193
Nitrostat Tablets ... 1981
▲ Nolvadex Tablets (32.7%) ... 2957
Norisodrine with Calcium Iodide Syrup ... 446
Normodyne Injection (1%) ... 2519
Norpramin Tablets ... 1273
▲ Norvasc Tablets (0.7% to 4.5%) .. 2020
Nubain Injection (1% or less) ... 952
Nuromax Injection (0.3%) ... 1136
Orlaam Oral Solution ... 2361
Orthoclone OKT3 Sterile Solution .. 1892
Pamelor ... 2409
Pediazole Suspension ... 2340
Pepcid Injection (Infrequent) ... 1765
Pepcid (Infrequent) ... 1763
Peptavlon ... 2997
Persantine Tablets ... 686
▲ Plendil Extended-Release Tablets (3.9% to 6.9%) ... 514
Pravachol Tablets (Rare) ... 770
Primaxin I.M. ... 1770
Primaxin I.V. (Less than 0.2%) ... 1772
Prinivil Tablets (0.3% to 1.0%) ... 1776
Prinzide Tablets (0.3 to 1%) ... 1780
Priscoline Hydrochloride Ampuls ... 864
Procanbid Extended-Release Tablets (Occasional) ... 1983
▲ Procardia Capsules (Approximately 10% to 25%; 1 in 8 patients) ... 2024
▲ Procardia XL Extended Release Tablets (Less than 3% to 25%).. 2026
ProSom Tablets (Infrequent) ... 457
Prostigmin Injectable ... 1305
Prostigmin Tablets ... 1306
Prostin E2 Suppository ... 2109
Protamine Sulfate Vials ... 1526
Protostat Tablets ... 1939
Proventil (Less than 1%) ... 2529
Quadrinal Tablets ... 1398
Quibron ... 2227
Quinaglute Dura-Tabs Tablets ... 644
Recombivax HB (Less than 1%) ... 1787
Regitine Vials ... 864
Reglan ... 2243
Respbid Tablets ... 687
RespiGam ... 1631
Rifadin ... 1276
Rifater ... 1280
Risperdal Tablets (Rare) ... 1348
Robaxin Injectable ... 2245
Rocephin Injectable Vials, ADD-Vantage, Galaxy Container (Occasional) ... 2305
Roferon-A Injection (Less than 0.5%) ... 2308
Romazicon (1% to 3%) ... 2311
Rondec Chewable Tablets ... 974
Rythmol Tablets–150mg, 225mg, 300mg (Less than 1%) ... 1399
▲ Salagen Tablets (8% to 13%) ... 1546
▲ Sandimmune (Less than 1 to 4%).. 2416
Sandostatin Injection (1% to 4%).. 2421
Ser-Ap-Es Tablets ... 867
Sinemet Tablets ... 959
Sinemet CR Tablets ... 961
Sinequan (Occasional) ... 2028
Slo-bid Gyrocaps ... 2201
Slo-Niacin Tablets ... 2767
Solganal Suspension ... 2530
Sorbitrate ... 2959
Stimate, (desmopressin acetate) Nasal Spray, 1.5 mg/mL (Occasional) ... 806
Streptase for Infusion ... 557
Supprelin Injection (2%) ... 2230
Surmontil Capsules ... 2917
Talacen Caplets (Infrequent) ... 2464
Talwin Compound (Infrequent) ... 2466
Talwin Nx Tablets (Infrequent) ... 2467
Tambocor Tablets (1% to less than 3%) ... 1555
▲ Taxol Injection (28%) ... 723
Taxotere for Injection Concentrate 2204
Theo-Dur Extended-Release Tablets ... 1367
Theo-X Extended-Release Tablets .. 793
THYREL TRH ... 2992
Tofranil Ampuls ... 873
Tofranil Tablets ... 875
Tofranil-PM Capsules ... 876
Toradol ... 2319
Tornalate Solution for Inhalation, 0.2% (Less than 1%) ... 976
Tornalate Metered Dose Inhaler (Rare) ... 978
Trancopal Caplets ... 2468
Trandate Injection (1 of 100 patients) ... 1158
Trental Tablets ... 1291
Uni-Dur Extended-Release Tablets.. 1374
Univasc Tablets (1.6%) ... 2553
Urised Tablets ... 2123
Vancocin HCl, Vials & ADD-Vantage ... 1534
Vantin for Oral Suspension and Vantin Tablets (Less than 1%) 2112

(▣ Described in PDR For Nonprescription Drugs) Incidence data in parenthesis; ▲ 3% or more (◉ Described in PDR For Ophthalmology)

Vaseretic Tablets 1810
Vasotec I.V. 1814
Vasotec Tablets (0.5% to 1.0%) 1816
Ventolin Tablets (Fewer than 1 of 100 patients) 1176
VePesid Capsules and Injection 727
Verelan Capsules (0.6%) 1455
▲ Vesanoid Capsules (23%) 2327
Vivactil Tablets 1820
Volmax Extended-Release Tablets (Less frequent) 1835
Cataflam/Voltaren/Voltaren-XR (Rare) 833
▲ Vumon for Injection (Approximately 5%) 729
Wellbutrin Tablets (Rare) 1177
Yocon Tablets 1235
Yohimex Tablets 1414
Zebeta Tablets 1457
Zestoretic Tablets (0.3 to 1%) 2968
Zestril Tablets (0.3% to 1.0%) 2972
Ziac 1459
Zocor Tablets (Rare) 1821
Zoloft Tablets (Infrequent) 2051
Zosyn (1.0% or less) 1463
Zyrtec Tablets (Less than 2%) 2053

Flushing, cutaneous

Diupres Tablets 1691
Hydropres Tablets 1718
Isuprel Hydrochloride Solution 2443
Isuprel Injection 2441
Isuprel Mistometer 2442
Kadian Capsules (Less than 3%) 2948
▲ Mivacron (About 25%) 1125
Nicotinex Elixir ◙ 671
Nitrolingual Spray 2193
Quinidex Extentabs 2240
Roferon-A Injection (Less than 0.5%) 2308
Talwin Nx Tablets 2467
▲ Tracrium Injection (5%) 1155
Urecholine 1804

Flushing, facial

▲ Acthrel for Injection (16%) 2990
▲ Adenocard Injection (18%) 1021
Adriamycin PFS 2056
Adriamycin RDF 2056
Alferon N Injection (One patient) 2142
Brontex 2130
▲ Calcimar Injection, Synthetic (2% to 5%) 2176
Chromagen Capsules 2470
Chromagen FA 2471
Chromagen Forte 2471
▲ Cognex Capsules (3%) 1961
DDAVP Injection (Occasional) 2178
DDAVP Injection 15 mcg/mL (Occasional) 2179
DTIC-Dome 593
Demerol 2438
Desmopressin Acetate Injection (Occasional) 996
Dilaudid-HP Injection (Less frequent) 1384
Dilaudid-HP Lyophilized Powder 250 mg (Less frequent) 1384
Doxil 2613
Doxorubicin Astra 531
Geref (sermorelin acetate for injection) 2995
Helixate, Antihemophilic Factor (Recombinant) (One report out of 3,254 patients) 799
Imitrex Tablets 1099
Kadian Capsules (Less than 3%) 2948
KOGENATE Antihemophilic Factor (Recombinant) (One report) 626
Loxitane 1426
MS Contin Tablets (Less frequent) 2149
MSIR (Infrequent) 2152
Marinol (Dronabinol) Capsules (Greater than 1%) 2353
Mepergan Injection 2859
Methadone Hydrochloride Oral Concentrate 2356
Methadone Hydrochloride Oral Solution & Tablets 2357
Miacalcin Injection (About 2-5%) .. 2402
Mintezol 1747
Mithracin 599
Nicotrol NS Nicotine Nasal Spray (More common) 1565
Oramorph SR (Morphine Sulfate Sustained Release Tablets) (Less frequent) 2359
Papaverine Hydrochloride Vials and Ampoules 1523
Phenergan with Codeine 2883
Phenergan VC with Codeine 2888
RMS Suppositories CII 2766
Roxanol 2365
Rubex for Injection 721
Sandimmune 2416
Sandoglobulin I.V. (Less than 1%) .. 2419
Sansert Tablets (Rare) 2424
Soma Compound w/Codeine Tablets 2784
Soma Compound Tablets 2783
Stimate, (desmopressin acetate) Nasal Spray, 1.5 mg/mL (Occasional) 806
Tonocard Tablets (Less than 1%) .. 519
Urecholine 1804

Flushing, hands

▲ Calcimar Injection, Synthetic (2% to 5%) 2176
Miacalcin Injection (About 2-5%) .. 2402

Flushing, upper thorax

▲ Acthrel for Injection (16%) 2990
Sandimmune 2416

Folic acid absorption, impaired

Azulfidine (Rare) 2059

Follicle development, multiple

Lutrepulse for Injection (Some incidents) 998
Micronor Tablets 1903

Follicular atresia, delayed

Micronor Tablets 1903
Norplant System 2868

Folliculitis

Aclovate (Infrequent) 1061
Anafranil Capsules (Rare) 819
Analpram-HC Rectal Cream 1% and 2.5% 993
Anusol-HC Cream 2.5% (Infrequent to frequent) 1953
Anusol-HC Suppositories 1954
Cleocin T Topical 2072
Cleocin Vaginal Cream 2070
Cordran Lotion (Infrequent) 1854
Cordran Tape (Infrequent) 1855
Cormax Ointment (Approximately 0.3%) 1856
Cormax Scalp Application (Approximately 0.6%) 1857
Cortisporin Cream 1073
Cortisporin Ointment 1074
Cortisporin Otic Solution Sterile 1076
Cortisporin Otic Suspension Sterile 1077
Crixivan Capsules (Less than 2%) .. 1670
Cutivate Cream 1078
Cutivate Ointment (Infrequent to more frequent) 1078
DaunoXome (Less than or equal to 5%) 1842
Decadron Phosphate Topical Cream 1686
Decaspray Topical Aerosol 1689
Dermatop Emollient Cream 0.1% (Infrequent to frequent) 1264
DesOwen Cream, Ointment and Lotion (Infrequent) 1032
Didronel Tablets 2133
Diprolene AF Cream 0.05% (Infrequent) 2489
Diprolene Gel 0.05% (Less frequent) 2490
Diprolene Lotion 0.05% (2%) 2491
Diprolene Ointment 0.05% (2 per 767 patients) 2491
Dovonex Ointment 0.005% (Less than 1%) 2793
Elocon Cream 0.1% (Infrequent) 2492
Elocon Lotion 0.1% (4 in 156 subjects) 2493
Elocon Ointment 0.1% (Infrequent) 2494
Epifoam (Infrequent) 2543
Eskalith 2658
Florone/Florone E 921
Halog (Infrequent) 2795
Hytone 922
Hytone Ointment 2 ½% 923
Intron A for Injection (Less than 5%) 2506
Invirase Capsules (Less than 2%) .. 2291
Lidex (Infrequent) 2299
Lithium Carbonate Capsules & Tablets 2352
Lithonate/Lithotabs/Lithobid 2721
Locoid Cream, Ointment and Topical Solution (Infrequent) 994
Lotrisone Cream (Infrequent) 2515
Mantadil Cream 1124
8-MOP Capsules 1294
NeoDecadron Topical Cream 1757
Norvir (Less than 2%) 447
Oxistat Cream (0.3%) 1139
Oxsoralen-Ultra Capsules 1302
Pandel Cream, 0.1% 2475
Pediotic Suspension Sterile 1140
Pramosone Cream, Lotion & Ointment 995
ProctoCream-HC 2.5% (Infrequent to frequent) 2552
ProctoFoam-HC 2552
Psorcon Cream 0.05% (Infrequent) 924
Psorcon Ointment 0.05% 923
Synalar (Infrequent) 2299
Temovate E Emollient (Less than 2%) 1154
▲ Temovate Gel (Among most frequent) 1153
Temovate Ointment (Less frequent) 1152
Temovate Scalp Application (2 of 294 patients; infrequent) 1153
Topicort Emollient Cream 0.25% (0.8%) 1289
Topicort Gel 0.05% (Infrequent) 1290
Topicort LP Emollient Cream 0.05% (Infrequent) 1289
Topicort Ointment 0.25% (Infrequent) 1291
Tridesilon Cream 0.05% (infrequent) 609
Tridesilon Ointment 0.05% (infrequent) 610
Ultravate Cream 0.05% (Infrequent) 2797
Ultravate Ointment 0.05% (Infrequent) 2798
Westcort Cream 0.2% (Infrequent) 2799
Westcort Ointment 0.2% 2800

Fontanels, bulging

Achromycin V Capsules 1417
Aquasol A Vitamin A Capsules, USP 525
Aquasol A Parenteral 526
Declomycin Tablets 1421
Diphtheria and Tetanus Toxoids and Pertussis Vaccine Adsorbed .. 2650
Doryx Capsules 1970
DYNACIN Capsules 1627
Helidac Therapy 2135
Macrobid Capsules (Rare) 2138
Macrodantin Capsules 2140
Minocin Intravenous 1428
Minocin Oral Suspension 1431
Minocin Pellet-Filled Capsules 1429
Monodox Capsules 1858
NegGram (Occasional) 2453
Nizoral Tablets (Less than 1%) 1345
Terramycin Intramuscular Solution 2034
Tetramune 1449
Tri-Immunol Adsorbed 1452
Urobiotic-250 Capsules 2038
Vibramycin 2038
Vibramycin Hyclate Intravenous 2040
Vibramycin 2038

Foot drop

Betaseron for SC Injection 653
Kadian Capsules (Less than 3%) 2948
Matulane Capsules 2300
Oncovin Solution Vials & Hyporets 1521
Videx Tablets, Powder for Oral Solution, & Pediatric Powder for Oral Solution (Less than 1%) 2980
Zyloprim Tablets (Less than 1%) 1194

Forceps delivery, increased incidence

Carbocaine Injection 2432
Marcaine 2446
Sensorcaine 554

Foreign body reaction

Anafranil Capsules (Infrequent) 819
▲ Ciloxan Ophthalmic Solution (Less than 10%) 468
Ethiodol Injection (Infrequent) 2472
Vexol 1% Ophthalmic Suspension (1% to 5%) .... ⊙ 227
▲ Xalatan (5% to 15%) .... ⊙ 304

Foreskin irretraction (see under Preputium, irretraction of)

Foveal reflex, loss of

Aralen Phosphate Tablets 2431
Plaquenil Sulfate Tablets 2459

Fracture, pathological

Arimidex Tablets (2% to 5%) 2932
Casodex Tablets (2% to 5%) 2934
Lamictal Tablets (Rare) 1105
LUVOX Tablets (Rare) 2723
Prozac Pulvules & Liquid, Oral Solution (Rare) 935
Remeron Tablets (Rare) 1878

Fractures, long bones

Celestone Soluspan Suspension 2484
CORTENEMA 2713
Cortifoam 2540
Cortone Acetate Sterile Suspension 1663
Cortone Acetate Tablets 1664
Dalalone D.P. Injectable 1009
Decadron Phosphate Injection 1680
Decadron Tablets 1678
Decadron-LA Sterile Suspension 1687
Dexacort Phosphate in Respihaler .. 1606
Dexacort Phosphate in Turbinaire .. 1607
Hydeltrasol Injection, Sterile 1708
Hydeltra-T.B.A. Sterile Suspension 1710
Hydrocortone Acetate Sterile Suspension 1712
Hydrocortone Phosphate Injection, Sterile 1713
Hydrocortone Tablets 1715
Pediapred Oral Solution 1618
Prelone Syrup 1834

Fractures, unspecified

Cognex Capsules (Frequent) 1961
Neurontin Capsules (1.1%) 1978

Fractures, vertebral compression

Celestone Soluspan Suspension 2484
CORTENEMA 2713
Dalalone D.P. Injectable 1009
Decadron Tablets 1678
Decadron-LA Sterile Suspension 1687
Hydeltrasol Injection, Sterile 1708
Hydeltra-T.B.A. Sterile Suspension 1710
Hydrocortone Acetate Sterile Suspension 1712
Hydrocortone Phosphate Injection, Sterile 1713
Hydrocortone Tablets 1715
Prelone Syrup 1834

Freckling

Cytosar-U Sterile Powder (Less frequent) 2077

Free fatty acids, elevation

▲ Yutopar Intravenous Injection (80% to 100%) 566

Free T3 resin uptake, decrease (see under T3, decrease)

Fretfulness (see under Anxiety)

Frigidity, unspecified

DynaCirc CR Tablets (0.5% to 1.0%) 2383
Wellbutrin Tablets (Infrequent) 1177

Fullness, abdominal (see under Abdominal bloating)

Fungal invasion

Blephamide Liquifilm Sterile Ophthalmic Suspension 472
Blephamide Ointment .... ⊙ 234
Cortisporin Ophthalmic Ointment Sterile (Possible) 1074
Cortisporin Ophthalmic Suspension Sterile (Possible) 1075
Econopred & Econopred Plus Ophthalmic Suspensions (Possibility) .... ⊙ 216
FML Forte Liquifilm (Possibility) .. ⊙ 237
FML Liquifilm (Possibility) .... ⊙ 238
FML S.O.P. (Possibility) .... ⊙ 239
FML-S Liquifilm .... ⊙ 240
Pred Mild .... ⊙ 250
Pred-G Liquifilm Sterile Ophthalmic Suspension .... ⊙ 248
Pred-G S.O.P. Sterile Ophthalmic Ointment .... ⊙ 249
TobraDex Ophthalmic Suspension and Ointment 469

Furunculosis

Ambien Tablets (Rare) 2559
Avonex 662

(◙ Described in PDR For Nonprescription Drugs) Incidence data in parenthesis; ▲ 3% or more (⊙ Described in PDR For Ophthalmology)

Side Effects Index

(continued)

Betaseron for SC Injection ... 653
Cognex Capsules (Infrequent) ... 1961
Depakote Tablets (1% to 5%) ... 418
Doxil (Less than 1%) ... 2613
Effexor (Rare) ... 2825
▲ Elocon Cream 0.1%
 (Approximately 7%) ... 2492
▲ Elocon Ointment 0.1% (4.8% to approximately 7%) ... 2494
Hivid Tablets (Less than 1%) ... 2287
Intron A for Injection (Less than 5%) ... 2506
Invirase Capsules (Less than 2%) .. 2291
LUVOX Tablets (Infrequent) ... 2723
Methotrexate Sodium Tablets, Injection, for Injection and LPF Injection ... 1322
▲ Nipent for Injection (4%) ... 2733
Paxil Tablets (Infrequent) ... 2681
Rilutek Tablets (Rare) ... 2198
Risperdal Tablets (Rare) ... 1348
Zyloprim Tablets (Less than 1%) ... 1194
Zyrtec Tablets (Less than 2%) ... 2053

G

Gait, abnormal

Actimmune (Rare) ... 1043
Ambien Tablets (Rare) ... 2559
Anafranil Capsules (Infrequent) ... 819
Ativan Injection ... 2805
Avonex ... 662
Betaseron for SC Injection ... 653
Cardizem CD Capsules (Less than 1%) ... 1251
Cardizem SR Capsules (Less than 1%) ... 1255
Cardizem Injectable ... 1253
Cardizem Tablets (Less than 1%) .. 1257
Compazine ... 2644
▲ Cordarone Tablets (4 to 9%) ... 2818
Cytovene (1% or less) ... 2270
DaunoXome (Less than or equal to 5%) ... 1842
Depakote Tablets (1% to 5%) ... 418
Duragesic Transdermal System (1% or greater) ... 1336
Ethmozine Tablets (Less than 2%) 2217
▲ Felbatol (5.3% to 9.7%) ... 2774
Flexeril Tablets (Rare) ... 1701
Flumadine Tablets & Syrup (Less than 0.3%) ... 1013
Foscavir Injection (Less than 1%) .. 541
Glucotrol XL Extended Release Tablets (Less than 1%) ... 2012
Intron A for Injection (Less than 5%) ... 2506
Lamictal Tablets (Infrequent) ... 1105
Lioresal Intrathecal (1% or more) .. 1634
Loxitane ... 1426
LUVOX Tablets (Infrequent) ... 2723
Norvir (Less than 2%) ... 447
Oncovin Solution Vials & Hyporets 1521
OxyContin Tablets (Less than 1%) 2163
Paxil Tablets (Rare) ... 2681
Permax Tablets (1.6%) ... 571
Prozac Pulvules & Liquid, Oral Solution (Infrequent) ... 935
Redux Capsules (Less than 2%) ... 2911
Rilutek Tablets (Infrequent) ... 2198
▲ Risperdal Tablets (17% to 34%) .. 1348
Roferon-A Injection (Infrequent) ... 2308
Serzone Tablets (Infrequent) ... 776
Sinemet CR Tablets ... 961
Stelazine ... 2692
Thorazine ... 2701
Tiazac Capsules (Less than 1%) ... 1019
Torecan ... 2367
Ultram Tablets (50 mg) (Less than 1%) ... 1594
▲ Vesanoid Capsules (3%) ... 2327
Videx Tablets, Powder for Oral Solution, & Pediatric Powder for Oral Solution (Less than 1%) ... 2980
Vistide Injection ... 1057
Zantac 150 Tablets ... 1182
Zantac Injection ... 1180
Zoloft Tablets (Infrequent) ... 2051

Galactorrhea

Adapin Capsules ... 1542
Amen Tablets (Rare) ... 785
Asendin Tablets (Less than 1%) ... 1419
BuSpar Tablets (Rare) ... 738
Calan SR Caplets (1% or less) ... 2571
Calan Tablets (1% or less) ... 2568
Compazine ... 2644
Covera-HS Tablets (Less than 2%) 2573
Cycrin Tablets (Rare) ... 991
Demser Capsules (Infrequent) ... 1690
Depakene ... 416

Depakote Tablets ... 418
Depo-Provera Contraceptive Injection (Fewer than 1%) ... 2079
Depo-Provera Sterile Aqueous Suspension ... 2083
Elavil ... 2945
Etrafon ... 2495
Flexeril Tablets (Rare) ... 1701
Haldol Decanoate ... 1587
Haldol Injection, Tablets and Concentrate ... 1585
Imitrex Tablets (Rare) ... 1099
Isoptin SR Tablets (1% or less) ... 1395
Limbitrol ... 2333
Loxitane (Rare) ... 1426
Ludiomil Tablets (Isolated reports) .. 861
Mellaril ... 2398
Moban Tablets and Concentrate (Infrequent) ... 1036
Norpramin Tablets ... 1273
Pamelor ... 2409
Paxil Tablets ... 2681
Premphase ... 2900
Prempro ... 2905
Proglycem ... 575
Prolixin Oral Concentrate ... 510
Provera Tablets (Rare) ... 2110
Reglan ... 2243
Sandostatin Injection (Less than 1%) ... 2421
Seldane Tablets ... 1284
Seldane-D Extended-Release Tablets ... 1286
Serentil ... 689
Sinequan ... 2028
Stelazine ... 2692
Surmontil Capsules ... 2917
Tofranil Ampuls ... 873
Tofranil Tablets ... 875
Tofranil-PM Capsules ... 876
Triavil Tablets ... 1800
Trilafon ... 2532
Vivactil Tablets ... 1820
Xanax Tablets ... 2115
Zoloft Tablets ... 2051

Gallbladder, calcification

Questran (Occasional) ... 774

Gallbladder, sonographic abnormalities

Rocephin Injectable Vials, ADD-Vantage, Galaxy Container .. 2305

Gallbladder disease

Avonex ... 662
Brevicon ... 2563
Climara Transdermal System ... 640
Demulen ... 2580
Desogen Tablets ... 1867
Diethylstilbestrol Tablets ... 1477
Estrace Cream and Tablets ... 751
Estraderm Transdermal System ... 842
ESTRATAB Tablets (0.3, 0.625, 1.25, 2.5 mg) ... 2715
Estratest ... 2718
Levlen/Tri-Levlen ... 646
Lo/Ovral Tablets ... 2852
Lo/Ovral-28 Tablets ... 2857
Lopid Tablets (0.9%) ... 1974
Menest Tablets ... 2671
Modicon ... 1928
Nordette-21 Tablets ... 2863
Nordette-28 Tablets ... 2866
Norinyl ... 2563
Nor-Q D Tablets ... 2598
Ogen Tablets ... 2103
Ogen Vaginal Cream ... 2106
Ortho-Cept ... 1907
Ortho-Cyclen/Ortho-Tri-Cyclen ... 1914
Ortho Dienestrol Cream ... 1922
Ortho-Est ... 1925
Ortho-Novum ... 1928
Ortho-Cyclen/Ortho Tri-Cyclen ... 1914
Ovcon ... 765
Ovral Tablets ... 2877
Ovral-28 Tablets ... 2878
Ovrette Tablets ... 2878
PMB 200 and PMB 400 ... 2890
Premarin Intravenous ... 2893
Premarin Tablets ... 2896
Premarin Vaginal Cream ... 2898
Premphase (A 2- to 4-fold increase) ... 2900
Prempro (A 2- to 4-fold increase) .. 2905
Pulmozyme Inhalation ... 1054
Rocephin Injectable Vials, ADD-Vantage, Galaxy Container .. 2305
Sandostatin Injection ... 2421
Levlen/Tri-Levlen ... 646
Tri-Norinyl ... 2607

Triphasil-21 Tablets ... 2919
Triphasil-28 Tablets ... 2924
Vivelle Transdermal System ... 880

Gallstones

Atromid-S Capsules ... 2808
Imitrex Injection (Rare) ... 1095
Intron A for Injection (Less than 5%) ... 2506
Relafen Tablets (Less than 1%) ... 2688
▲ Sandostatin Injection (27% to 52%) ... 2421

Gamma-glutamyl transpeptidase, elevation

▲ Accutane Capsules (1 in 5 to 1 in 10 patients) ... 2252
Arimidex Tablets (2% to 5%) ... 2932
Biaxin (Less than 1%) ... 406
▲ CellCept Capsules (More than or equal to 3%) ... 2265
Ceftaz (One in 19) ... 1070
Cipro I.V. (Infrequent) ... 587
▲ Cipro I.V. Pharmacy Bulk Package (Among most frequent) ... 590
Cipro Tablets (Less than 0.1%) ... 584
Cordarone Intravenous (Two cases) ... 2821
Dynabac (0.1% to 1%) ... 668
Felbatol (Rare) ... 2774
Floxin I.V. ... 1580
Floxin Tablets (200 mg, 300 mg, 400 mg) ... 1577
▲ Fortaz (1 in 19) ... 1092
Fungizone Intravenous ... 507
Hivid Tablets (Less than 1%) ... 2287
Lescol Capsules ... 2395
Maxaquin Tablets (Less than or equal to 0.1%) ... 2593
Mevacor Tablets ... 1742
Monocid Injection (1.6%) ... 2674
Oncaspar ... 2194
Parlodel ... 2411
Pentasa (Less than 1%) ... 1275
Prevacid Delayed-Release Capsules (Less than 1%) ... 2746
Prilosec Delayed-Release Capsules (Rare) ... 516
▲ Prograf (Greater than 3%) ... 1028
Rilutek Tablets (Infrequent) ... 2198
▲ Tazicef for Injection (1 in 19 patients) ... 2697
▲ Tazidime Vials, Faspak & ADD-Vantage (1 in 19) ... 1531
▲ Tegison Capsules (10-25%) ... 2314
Vantin for Oral Suspension and Vantin Tablets ... 2112
Viramune Tablets (2.4%) ... 2368
Zithromax (1% to 2%) ... 2043
Zithromax Tablets (1% to 2%) ... 2046
Zocor Tablets ... 1821

Gangrene

Cafergot ... 2376
Cytovene-IV (One report) ... 2270
Felbatol ... 2774
Heparin Lock Flush Solution ... 2831
Heparin Sodium Injection ... 2832
Heparin Sodium Vials ... 1486
Levophed Bitartrate Injection (Rare) ... 2445
Mepergan Injection ... 2859
Phenergan Injection ... 2880
Proleukin for Injection (1%) ... 812

Gastric acid, regurgitation

Prilosec Delayed-Release Capsules (1.9%) ... 516

Gastric dilation

Anafranil Capsules (Rare) ... 819
Felbatol ... 2774

Gastric discomfort (see under Distress, gastrointestinal)

Gastric disorder (see under Distress, gastrointestinal)

Gastric erosion

Robaxisal Tablets ... 2246
Soma Compound w/Codeine Tablets (Rare) ... 2784
Soma Compound Tablets (Less common) ... 2783

Gastric secretions, increase

Sansert Tablets ... 2424
Tensilon Injectable ... 1307

Gastritis

Aldactazide Tablets ... 2556
Aldactone Tablets ... 2558
Ambien Tablets (Rare) ... 2559
Anafranil Capsules (Infrequent) ... 819
Asacol Delayed-Release Tablets ... 2129
Atromid-S Capsules ... 2808
Augmentin ... 2637
Augmentin Tablets ... 2640
Avonex ... 662
Betaseron for SC Injection ... 653
Carnitor Injection (Less frequent) .. 2623
▲ CellCept Capsules (More than or equal to 3%) ... 2265
Cerebyx Injection (Infrequent) ... 1956
Claritin Tablets (2% or fewer patients) ... 2485
Claritin-D Tablets (Less frequent) .. 2487
Clinoril Tablets (Less than 1%) ... 1658
Cognex Capsules (Infrequent) ... 1961
Cozaar Tablets (Less than 1%) ... 1668
Crixivan Capsules (Less than 2%) .. 1670
DaunoXome (Less than or equal to 5%) ... 1842
Dolobid Tablets (Less than 1 in 100) ... 1695
Doxil (Less than 1%) ... 2613
Dynabac (0.1% to 1%) ... 668
Effexor (Infrequent) ... 2825
Eskalith ... 2658
Estring Vaginal Ring (1% to 3%) ... 2086
Etrafon ... 2495
Felbatol ... 2774
Flexeril Tablets (Less than 1%) ... 1701
Fosamax Tablets (0.5%) ... 1703
Sterile FUDR ... 2284
Hivid Tablets (Less than 1%) ... 2287
Hyzaar Tablets ... 1720
IBU Tablets (Less than 1%) ... 1389
Imdur (Less than or equal to 5%) .. 1362
Invirase Capsules (Less than 2%) .. 2291
Keflex Pulvules & Oral Suspension ... 930
Keftab Tablets ... 931
Klonopin Tablets ... 2294
Lamictal Tablets (Rare) ... 1105
Lithonate/Lithotabs/Lithobid ... 2721
Lodine Capsules and Tablets (1% to 3%) ... 2849
Lotensin Tablets ... 852
LUVOX Tablets (Infrequent) ... 2723
Miacalcin Nasal Spray (Less than 1%) ... 2403
Motrin Ibuprofen Suspension, Oral Drops, Chewable Tablets, Caplets (Less than 1%) ... 1563
Nalfon 200 Pulvules & Nalfon Tablets (Less than 1%) ... 933
Naprelan Tablets (Less than 3%) .. 2861
Neoral (2% or less) ... 2405
Norvasc Tablets (Less than or equal to 0.1%) ... 2020
Norvir (Less than 2%) ... 447
Orudis Capsules (Less than 1%) ... 2874
Oruvail Capsules (Less than 1%) ... 2874
OxyContin Tablets (Between 1% and 5%) ... 2163
Permax Tablets (Infrequent) ... 571
Prinivil Tablets (0.3% to 1.0%) ... 1776
Prinzide Tablets ... 1780
Prolixin ... 510
ProSom Tablets (Infrequent) ... 457
Prozac Pulvules & Liquid, Oral Solution (Infrequent) ... 935
Redux Capsules (Frequent) ... 2911
Relafen Tablets (1% to 3%) ... 2688
Remeron Tablets (Rare) ... 1878
Rilutek Tablets (Infrequent) ... 2198
Risperdal Tablets (Infrequent) ... 1348
Robaxisal Tablets ... 2246
Sandimmune (2% or less) ... 2416
Serzone Tablets (Infrequent) ... 776
Solganal Suspension ... 2530
Soma Compound w/Codeine Tablets ... 2784
▲ Soma Compound Tablets (Among most common) ... 2783
Spectrobid Tablets ... 2030
Sporanox Capsules (Infrequent) ... 1352
Sular Tablets (Less than or equal to 1%) ... 2961
Supprelin Injection (2% to 3%) ... 2230
Tolectin (200, 400 and 600 mg) (1 to 3%) ... 1591
Toradol (1% or less) ... 2319
Unasyn ... 2035
Vascor Tablets (200 and 300 mg) (0.5 to 2.0%) ... 1597
Videx Tablets, Powder for Oral Solution, & Pediatric Powder for Oral Solution (Less than 1%) ... 2980
Vistide Injection ... 1057

(⊡ Described in PDR For Nonprescription Drugs)   Incidence data in parenthesis; ▲ 3% or more   (⊚ Described in PDR For Ophthalmology)

Gastritis Side Effects Index 1344

Zebeta Tablets ... 1457
Zestoretic Tablets ... 2968
Zestril Tablets (0.3% to 1.0%) ... 2972
Ziac ... 1459
Zithromax (1% or less) ... 2043
Zoloft Tablets (Rare) ... 2051
Zosyn (1.0% or less) ... 1463
Zyloprim Tablets (Less than 1%) ... 1194
Zyrtec Tablets (Less than 2%) ... 2053

Gastroenteritis

Altace Capsules (Less than 1%) ... 1238
Ambien Tablets (Infrequent) ... 2559
Asacol Delayed-Release Tablets ... 2129
Cardura Tablets (Less than 0.5% of 3960 patients) ... 1993
▲ CellCept Capsules (More than or equal to 3%) ... 2265
Clinoril Tablets (Less than 1%) ... 1658
Clozaril Tablets (Less than 1%) ... 2377
Cognex Capsules (Infrequent) ... 1961
Cytosar-U Sterile Powder (One case) ... 2077
Danocrine Capsules ... 2437
Depakote Tablets (1% to 5%) ... 418
Dynabac (0.1% to 1%) ... 668
Effexor (Infrequent) ... 2825
Fioricet with Codeine Capsules ... 2387
Fiorinal with Codeine Capsules ... 2390
Foscavir Injection (Less than 1%) ... 541
Sterile FUDR ... 2284
Indocin Capsules (Less than 1%) ... 1723
Indocin I.V. (Less than 1%) ... 1727
Indocin (Less than 1%) ... 1723
Intron A for Injection (Less than 5%) ... 2506
Invirase Capsules (Less than 2%) ... 2291
Lioresal Intrathecal (1% or more) ... 1634
Lotensin HCT Tablets (0.3% or more) ... 855
LUVOX Tablets (Infrequent) ... 2723
Maxaquin Tablets ... 2593
Naprelan Tablets (Less than 1%) ... 2861
Neurontin Capsules (Infrequent) ... 1978
Norvir (Less than 2%) ... 447
Paxil Tablets (Rare) ... 2681
Permax Tablets (Infrequent) ... 571
Prevacid Delayed-Release Capsules (Less than 1%) ... 2746
Primaxin I.M. ... 1770
Primaxin I.V. (Less than 0.2%) ... 1772
Prozac Pulvules & Liquid, Oral Solution (1.0%) ... 935
Redux Capsules (Frequent) ... 2911
Relafen Tablets (1%) ... 2688
Remeron Tablets (Rare) ... 1878
RespiGam (1%) ... 1631
Risperdal Tablets (Rare) ... 1348
Rythmol Tablets—150mg, 225mg, 300mg (0.03 to 1.9%) ... 1399
Serzone Tablets (Frequent) ... 776
Videx Tablets, Powder for Oral Solution, & Pediatric Powder for Oral Solution (Less than 1%) ... 2980
Zoloft Tablets (Rare) ... 2051

Gastroenteritis, hemorrhagic

Fungizone Intravenous ... 507

Gastroesophageal reflux

Anafranil Capsules (Infrequent) ... 819
Felbatol ... 2774
Imitrex Injection (Infrequent) ... 1095
Imitrex Tablets (Infrequent) ... 1099
Kadian Capsules (Less than 3%) ... 2948
Procardia XL Extended Release Tablets (1% or less) ... 2026
Risperdal Tablets (Rare) ... 1348

Gastrointestinal bleeding

(see under Bleeding, gastrointestinal)

Gastrointestinal disorders

▲ Accutane Capsules (Approximately 1 patient in 20) ... 2252
▲ Actigall Capsules (3.9%) ... 818
Adderall Tablets ... 2209
▲ Adenoscan (13%) ... 1022
Adipex-P Tablets and Capsules ... 1035
▲ AeroBid Inhaler System (1% to 10%) ... 1004
▲ Aerobid-M Inhaler System (1% to 10%) ... 1004
Aldactone Tablets ... 2558
Aldoclor Tablets ... 1638
▲ Alka-Seltzer Cherry Effervescent Antacid and Pain Reliever (4.9% at doses of 1000 mg/day) ... 609
▲ Alka-Seltzer Lemon Lime Effervescent Antacid and Pain Reliever (4.9% at doses of 1000 mg/day) ... 609
▲ Alka-Seltzer Original Effervescent Antacid and Pain Reliever (4.9% at doses of 1000 mg/day) ... 609
Alkeran for Injection (Infrequent) ... 1196
Alkeran Tablets (Infrequent) ... 1198
Anafranil Capsules (Up to 2%) ... 819
Ana-Kit Anaphylaxis Emergency Treatment Kit ... 611
Anaprox/Naprosyn ... 2277
▲ Anturane (Most frequent) ... 823
Apresazide Capsules ... 824
Aralen Hydrochloride Injection ... 2430
Aralen Phosphate Tablets ... 2431
Regular Strength Ascriptin Tablets ... 650
Ativan Tablets ... 2807
▲ Atrohist Pediatric Suspension (Among most common) ... 1604
▲ Atrohist Pediatric Suspension Dye-Free (Among most common) ... 1604
Atromid-S Capsules (Less frequent) ... 2808
Axid Pulvules (1.1%) ... 1468
▲ Genuine Bayer Aspirin Tablets & Caplets (4.9% at doses of 1000 mg/day) ... 618
▲ Aspirin Regimen Bayer Regular Strength 325 mg Caplets (4.9% of 4500 people tested) ... 613
Benemid Tablets ... 1651
Berocca Plus Tablets ... 2259
▲ Betaseron for SC Injection (6%) ... 653
Bio-Ginkgo (Less than 1%) ... 2984
Bleph-10 Ophthalmic Solution 10% ... 472
Brethaire Inhaler ... 830
Brevicon ... 2563
▲ Bufferin Analgesic Tablets (4.8%) ... 636
BuSpar Tablets ... 738
Capoten Tablets ... 740
Capozide Tablets ... 744
▲ Cardioquin Tablets (22%) ... 2146
Carnitor Tablets and Solution ... 2624
Cartrol Tablets (Less common) ... 413
▲ Cataflam Tablets (About 20%) ... 833
Ceclor Pulvules & Suspension (About 2.5%) ... 1470
Cefotan (1.5%) ... 2936
▲ Ceptaz (Among most common) ... 1070
▲ Chemet Capsules (About 10%) ... 666
Cleocin T Topical ... 2072
Cleocin Vaginal Cream ... 2070
▲ Clinoril Tablets (3% to 9%) ... 1658
Colestid (Most common) ... 2073
▲ CREON 5 Capsules (Among most frequent) ... 2714
▲ Cuprimine Capsules (17%) ... 1673
DDAVP (Up to 2%) ... 2180
Dalmane Capsules ... 2329
▲ Daranide Tablets (Among the most common effects) ... 1676
Decadron Elixir ... 1676
Decadron Phosphate Injection ... 1680
Decadron Phosphate with Xylocaine Injection, Sterile ... 1683
Demulen ... 2580
Depakote Tablets (1% to 5%) ... 418
Depo-Provera Contraceptive Injection (Fewer than 1%) ... 2079
Desmopressin Acetate Rhinal Tube (Up to 2%) ... 997
Desyrel and Desyrel Dividose ... 504
Dexedrine ... 2648
DextroStat-Dextroamphetamine Sulfate Tablets ... 2211
Diamox Intravenous ... 317
Diamox Sequels (Sustained Release) ... 318
Diamox Tablets ... 317
Didronel Tablets ... 2133
Duricef Capsules, Tablets, and Oral Suspension ... 750
Dyazide Capsules ... 2653
Dynabac (1.6%) ... 668
EC-Naprosyn Delayed-Release Tablets ... 2277
▲ Ecotrin (4.9% at 1000 mg/day) ... 2625
Eminase ... 2215
Esgic-plus Capsules (Infrequent) ... 1012
Esgic-plus Tablets (Infrequent) ... 1012
Esidrix Tablets ... 839
Ethmozine Tablets (0.3% to 0.4%) ... 2217
▲ Eulexin Capsules (6%) ... 2498
▲ Feldene Capsules (Approximately 20%) ... 2008
Fioricet Tablets (Infrequent) ... 2386
Fiorinal (Less frequent) ... 2388
▲ Flagyl 375 Capsules (Most frequent) ... 2587
Flovent (1% to 3%) ... 1089
▲ Fortaz (Among most common) ... 1092
Fosamax Tablets ... 1703
Fungizone Oral Suspension ... 704
GlaucTabs ... 209
▲ Glucophage Tablets (Among most common) ... 754
Halfprin Tablets ... 1413
▲ Histussin D Liquid (Among most frequent) ... 670
Humegon for Injection ... 1873
Hydrea Capsules (Less frequent) ... 705
▲ IBU Tablets (4% to 16%) ... 1389
Ionamin Capsules ... 1615
Isoptin Oral Tablets (Less than 1%) ... 1393
K-Dur Microburst Release System (potassium chloride, USP) E.R. Tablets ... 1364
K-Phos Neutral Tablets ... 633
Kefurox Vials, Faspak & ADD-Vantage (1 in 150) ... 1509
Kemadrin Tablets ... 1105
▲ Lamprene Capsules (40-50%) ... 846
Lanoxicaps ... 1110
Lanoxin Elixir Pediatric ... 1113
Lanoxin Injection ... 1116
Lanoxin Injection Pediatric ... 1119
Lanoxin Tablets ... 1121
Lasix Injection, Oral Solution and Tablets ... 1267
Leukeran Tablets (Infrequent) ... 1205
▲ Leukine (37%) ... 1317
▲ Lopid Tablets (34.2%) ... 1974
▲ Lorabid Suspension and Pulvules (Most common) ... 1513
Lupron Depot 3.75 mg (Less than 5%) ... 2739
▲ Lupron Depot - 3 Month 22.5 mg (16.0%) ... 2743
Lupron Injection (Less than 5%) ... 2736
Metrodin (urofollitropin for injection) ... 2616
Midamor Tablets (Less than or equal to 1%) ... 1746
Modicon ... 1928
Moduretic Tablets (Less than or equal to 1%) ... 1748
8-MOP Capsules ... 1294
▲ Motrin Ibuprofen Suspension, Oral Drops, Chewable Tablets, Caplets (Most frequent; 4% to 16%) ... 1563
Myambutol Tablets ... 1432
Mycostatin Pastilles (Occasional) ... 713
Nalfon 200 Pulvules & Nalfon Tablets ... 933
Naprelan Tablets (Less than 1%) ... 2861
Anaprox/Naprosyn ... 2277
Neptazane Tablets ... 320
Nimotop Capsules (Up to 2.4%) ... 603
Nipent for Injection ... 2733
Norinyl ... 2563
Nor-Q D Tablets ... 2598
Norvir (Less than 2%) ... 447
▲ Novahistine DMX (Infrequent) ... 782
▲ Novantrone for Injection (58 to 88%) ... 1327
Orap Tablets ... 1037
Oretic Tablets ... 450
Ortho-Cyclen/Ortho-Tri-Cyclen ... 1914
Ortho-Novum ... 1928
Ortho-Cyclen/Ortho Tri-Cyclen ... 1914
Ovcon ... 765
Oxsoralen-Ultra Capsules ... 1302
OxyContin Tablets (Less than 1%) ... 2163
▲ Pancrease Capsules (Most frequent) ... 1589
▲ Pancrease MT Capsules (Most frequent) ... 1589
▲ Paraplatin for Injection (21% to 50%) ... 713
Phenergan with Dextromethorphan ... 2885
Pilopine HS Ophthalmic Gel (Occasional) ... 224
Pima Syrup ... 1004
Plaquenil Sulfate Tablets ... 2459
▲ Precose (Most common) ... 604
▲ Prepidil Gel (5.7%) ... 2108
Prinzide Tablets (0.3 to 1%) ... 1780
Prodium ... 695
Proglycem (Frequent) ... 575
Proleukin for Injection ... 812
Proventil Syrup (Children 2 to 6 years, 2%) ... 2528
▲ Prozac Pulvules & Liquid, Oral Solution (6%) ... 935
Pyrazinamide Tablets ... 1442
Quadrinal Tablets ... 1398
Redux Capsules ... 2911
▲ Retrovir Capsules (20%) ... 1216
▲ Retrovir I.V. Infusion (20%) ... 1221
▲ Retrovir Syrup (20%) ... 1216
Rifadin ... 1276
Rifater ... 1280
Rimactane Capsules ... 865
Robaxin Injectable ... 2245
▲ Rynatan (Among most common) ... 2781
▲ Rynatuss (Among most common) ... 2782
SSD ... 1402
▲ SSKI Solution (Among most frequent) ... 2767
Salagen Tablets (Less than 1%) ... 1546
Serophene (clomiphene citrate tablets, USP) ... 2621
Silvadene Cream 1% ... 1288
Skelaxin Tablets ... 793
Slo-Niacin Tablets (Less common) ... 2767
Soma Compound Tablets ... 2783
▲ Sporanox Capsules (4%) ... 1352
St. Joseph Adult Chewable Aspirin (81 mg.) ... 768
▲ Supprelin Injection (3% to 10%) ... 2230
▲ Suprax (30%) ... 1443
Taxotere for Injection Concentrate ... 2204
▲ Tazicef for Injection (Among most common) ... 2697
Tenoretic Tablets ... 2963
Tessalon Perles ... 1018
Thalitone (Common) ... 1293
TICE BCG, USP (1.0%) ... 1881
▲ Ticlid Tablets (30% to 40%) ... 2317
Timoptic-XE ... 1798
Tofranil Ampuls ... 873
Tofranil Tablets ... 875
▲ Tolectin (200, 400 and 600 mg) (10%) ... 1591
Tonocard Tablets (Less than 1%) ... 519
Toprol-XL Tablets ... 560
Tranxene (Less common) ... 459
▲ Trecator-SC Tablets (Among most common) ... 2919
▲ Trilisate (Less than 20%) ... 2155
Tri-Norinyl ... 2607
Trinsicon Capsules (Rare) ... 2759
Trisoralen Tablets ... 1309
Tussend Expectorant ... 1831
Tussi-Organidin DM NR Liquid and DM-S NR Liquid (Rare) ... 2786
▲ Ultrase Capsules (Most frequent) ... 2476
▲ Ultrase MT Capsules (Among most frequent) ... 2477
Uroqid-Acid No. 2 Tablets ... 633
Vantin for Oral Suspension and Vantin Tablets ... 2112
▲ Vascor Tablets (200 and 300 mg) (4.35 to 6.98%) ... 1597
Vaseretic Tablets ... 1810
Ventolin Syrup (2% of children) ... 1175
▲ Vesanoid Capsules (26%) ... 2327
Viokase ... 2251
▲ Cataflam/Voltaren/Voltaren-XR (About 20%) ... 833
Zestoretic Tablets (0.3 to 1.0%) ... 2968
Zinacef (1 in 150 patients) ... 1184
▲ Zoloft Tablets (Most common) ... 2051
Zosyn ... 1463

Gastrointestinal motility, decreased

Ditropan ... 1267

Gastrointestinal obstruction

K-Dur Microburst Release System (potassium chloride, USP) E.R. Tablets ... 1364
K-Norm Capsules ... 1615
K-Tab Filmtab ... 439
Micro-K ... 2237
Micro-K LS Packets ... 2238
Pancrease MT Capsules ... 1589
Slow-K Extended-Release Tablets ... 869

Gastrointestinal perforation

Anaprox/Naprosyn (Approximately 1% to 4%) ... 2277
Cataflam Tablets (Approximately 1% to about 4%) ... 833
Clinoril Tablets (Rare) ... 1658
Cortone Acetate Sterile Suspension ... 1663
Cortone Acetate Tablets ... 1664
Daypro Caplets ... 2578
Dolobid Tablets (Less than 1 in 100) ... 1695
EC-Naprosyn Delayed-Release Tablets (Approximately 1% to 4%) ... 2277
Feldene Capsules (Less than 1%) ... 2008

(▣ Described in PDR For Nonprescription Drugs)   Incidence data in parenthesis; ▲ 3% or more   (⊙ Described in PDR For Ophthalmology)

1345 **Side Effects Index** **Glossitis**

Indocin (Approximately 1%) 1723
K-Dur Microburst Release System (potassium chloride, USP) E.R. Tablets 1364
K-Norm Capsules 1615
K-Tab Filmtab 439
Lodine Capsules and Tablets 2849
Micro-K 2237
Micro-K LS Packets 2238
Motrin Ibuprofen Suspension, Oral Drops, Chewable Tablets, Caplets (Less than 1% to 4%) 1563
Naprelan Tablets (Approximately 1% to 4%) 2861
Anaprox/Naprosyn (Approximately 1% to 4%) 2277
Oncovin Solution Vials & Hyporets 1521
Orudis Capsules (Less than 1%) 2874
Oruvail Capsules (Less than 1%) 2874
Ponstel 1982
▲ Prograf (Greater than 3%) 1028
Relafen Tablets 2688
Slow-K Extended-Release Tablets 869
Tolectin (200, 400 and 600 mg) (Less than 1%) 1591
Toradol 2319
Cataflam/Voltaren/Voltaren-XR (Approximately 1% to about 4%) 833

Gastrointestinal reactions (see under Gastrointestinal disorders)

Gastrointestinal reflux

Cytotec (Infrequent) 2576

Gastrointestinal symptoms (see under Gastrointestinal disorders)

Gastrointestinal toxicity

Alkeran for Injection 1196
Alkeran Tablets 1198
Anaprox/Naprosyn 2277
BiCNU 696
CeeNU Capsules 699
Cytosar-U Sterile Powder (With experimental doses) 2077
EC-Naprosyn Delayed-Release Tablets 2277
Naprelan Tablets 2861
Anaprox/Naprosyn 2277
Neutrexin for Injection 2761
Toradol 2319

Gastrointestinal upset (see under Gastrointestinal disorders)

Genital abnormalities

Clomid 1262
Danocrine Capsules 2437
Felbatol 2774
Hivid Tablets (Less than 1%) 2287
Megace Oral Suspension (Several reports) 708
Megace Tablets 710

Genital eruptions

Estring Vaginal Ring (1% to 3%) 2086

Genital moniliasis

Duricef Capsules, Tablets, and Oral Suspension 750

Genitalia, external, labial fusion of

Danocrine Capsules 2437

Genitalia, male, external, abnormalities of

Proscar Tablets 1784

Genitourinary disturbances

Betapace Tablets (1% to 3%) 637
Dalmane Capsules 2329
Eulexin Capsules (2%) 2498
▲ Leukine (50%) 1317
▲ Nipent for Injection (Up to 15%) 2733
▲ Paraplatin for Injection (10% to 11%) 713
▲ Paxil Tablets (3%) 2681
Tranxene 459

Germinal aplasia

Mustargen 1752

Giddiness (see under Dizziness)

Gingival hyperplasia

Adalat Capsules (10 mg and 20 mg) (Less than 0.5%) 580
Adalat CC (Rare) 582
Calan SR Caplets (1% or less) 2571
Calan Tablets (1% or less) 2568
Cardizem CD Capsules (Infrequent) 1251
Cardizem SR Capsules (Infrequent) 1255
Cardizem Injectable 1253
Cardizem Tablets (Infrequent) 1257
▲ CellCept Capsules (More than or equal to 3%) 2265
Covera-HS Tablets (Less than 2%) 2573
Dilantin Infatabs 1967
Dilantin Kapseals 1965
Dilantin-125 Suspension 1969
Intron A for Injection (Less than 5%) 2506
Isoptin Oral Tablets (Less than 1%) 1393
Isoptin SR Tablets (1% or less) 1395
Lamictal Tablets (Infrequent) 1105
Mesantoin Tablets 2400
▲ Neoral (5% to 16%) 2405
Norvasc Tablets (More than 0.1% to 1%) 2020
Orap Tablets (One patient) 1037
Plendil Extended-Release Tablets (Less than 0.5%) 514
Procardia Capsules (Less than 0.5%) 2024
Procardia XL Extended Release Tablets (1% or less) 2026
▲ Sandimmune (4 to 16%) 2416
Sular Tablets (Less than or equal to 1%) 2961
Tiazac Capsules (Infrequent) 1019
Verelan Capsules (1% or less) 1455
Zoloft Tablets (Rare) 2051

Gingival swelling

Lomotil 2591
Motofen Tablets 789

Gingival ulcer

Motrin Ibuprofen Suspension, Oral Drops, Chewable Tablets, Caplets (Less than 1%) 1563

Gingivitis

Accutane Capsules (Less than 1%) 2252
Anafranil Capsules (Infrequent) 819
Avonex 662
Benemid Tablets 1651
Betaseron for SC Injection 653
▲ CellCept Capsules (More than or equal to 3%) 2265
Cognex Capsules (Infrequent) 1961
ColBENEMID Tablets 1662
Crixivan Capsules (Less than 2%) 1670
Cytotec (Infrequent) 2576
Doxil (Less than 1%) 2613
Effexor (Infrequent) 2825
Hivid Tablets (Less than 1%) 2287
▲ Intron A for Injection (Up to 14%) 2506
Invirase Capsules (Less than 2%) 2291
Klonopin Tablets 2294
Lamictal Tablets (Infrequent) 1105
Lupron Depot-PED 7.5 mg, 11.25 mg and 15 mg (Less than 2%) 2744
Lupron Injection Pediatric (Less than 2%) 2737
LUVOX Tablets (Infrequent) 2723
Methotrexate Sodium Tablets, Injection, for Injection and LPF Injection 1322
Myochrysine Injection 1754
Neurontin Capsules (Frequent) 1978
▲ Nipent for Injection (3% to 10%) 2733
Norvir (Less than 2%) 447
Paxil Tablets (Rare) 2681
Permax Tablets (Infrequent) 571
Prozac Pulvules & Liquid, Oral Solution (Infrequent) 935
Relafen Tablets (Less than 1%) 2688
Ridaura Capsules (0.1 to 1%) 2691
Risperdal Tablets (Rare) 1348
Serzone Tablets (Infrequent) 776
Solganal Suspension 2530
▲ Tegison Capsules (1-10%) 2314
Videx Tablets, Powder for Oral Solution, & Pediatric Powder for Oral Solution (Less than 1%) 2980

Gingivostomatitis

Cuprimine Capsules (Rare) 1673
Depen Titratable Tablets (Rare) 2770

Glandular enlargement

Hespan Injection 945
Questran 774
ReVia Tablets (Less than 1%) 957

Glassy-eyed appearance

Klonopin Tablets 2294

Glaucoma (see also under IOP, elevation)

▲ AdatoSil 5000 (0.6% to approximately 30%) .... ⊙ 265
AK-PRED .... ⊙ 204
AK-Trol Ointment & Suspension .... ⊙ 205
Ambien Tablets (Rare) 2559
Amicar Syrup, Tablets, and Injection 1312
Anafranil Capsules (Rare) 819
Anectine 1062
Artane 1418
Beclovent Inhalation Aerosol and Refill (Rare) 1063
Beconase (Rare) 1065
Blephamide Liquifilm Sterile Ophthalmic Suspension 472
Blephamide Ointment (A possibility) .... ⊙ 234
Celestone Soluspan Suspension 2484
CORTENEMA 2713
Cortifoam 2540
Cortisporin Ophthalmic Ointment Sterile 1074
Cortisporin Ophthalmic Suspension Sterile 1075
Cortone Acetate Sterile Suspension 1663
Cortone Acetate Tablets 1664
Dalalone D.P. Injectable 1009
Decadron Elixir 1676
Decadron Phosphate Injection 1680
Decadron Phosphate Sterile Ophthalmic Ointment 1684
Decadron Phosphate Sterile Ophthalmic Solution 1685
Decadron Phosphate with Xylocaine Injection, Sterile 1683
Decadron Tablets 1678
Decadron-LA Sterile Suspension 1687
Dexacort Phosphate in Respihaler 1606
Dexacort Phosphate in Turbinaire 1607
Diupres Tablets 1691
Econopred & Econopred Plus Ophthalmic Suspensions .... ⊙ 216
Eflone Sterile Ophthalmic Suspension .... ⊙ 261
Elavil 2945
Etrafon 2495
FML Forte Liquifilm .... ⊙ 237
FML S.O.P. .... ⊙ 239
▲ FML-S Liquifilm (Among most often) .... ⊙ 240
Flarex Ophthalmic Suspension .... ⊙ 217
Florinef Acetate Tablets 506
HMS Liquifilm (Rare) .... ⊙ 241
Healon .... ⊙ 302
Humorsol Sterile Ophthalmic Solution 1707
Hydeltrasol Injection, Sterile 1708
Hydeltra-T.B.A. Sterile Suspension 1710
Hydrocortone Acetate Sterile Suspension 1712
Hydrocortone Phosphate Injection, Sterile 1713
Hydrocortone Tablets 1715
Hydropres Tablets 1718
ISPAN Perfluoropropane .... ⊙ 267
ISPAN Sulfur Hexafluoride .... ⊙ 266
▲ Maxitrol Ophthalmic Ointment and Suspension (Most often) .... ⊙ 222
Midamor Tablets (Less than or equal to 1%) 1746
Moduretic Tablets 1748
Nardil (Less common) 1977
NeoDecadron Sterile Ophthalmic Ointment 1755
NeoDecadron Sterile Ophthalmic Solution 1756
Norpramin Tablets 1273
Ornade Spansule Capsules 2678
Pediapred Oral Solution 1618
Poly-Pred Liquifilm .... ⊙ 246
Pred Mild .... ⊙ 250
Pred-G Liquifilm Sterile Ophthalmic Suspension .... ⊙ 248
Pred-G S.O.P. Sterile Ophthalmic Ointment .... ⊙ 249
Prelone Syrup 1834
Prolixin 510
Prozac Pulvules & Liquid, Oral Solution (Rare) 935
Redux Capsules (Infrequent) 2911
Remeron Tablets (Infrequent) 1878
Rhinocort Nasal Inhaler (Rare) 552
Rilutek Tablets (Rare) 2198
Ser-Ap-Es Tablets 867
Sular Tablets (Less than or equal to 1%) 2961
Terra-Cortril Ophthalmic Suspension 2033
TobraDex Ophthalmic Suspension and Ointment 469
Triavil Tablets 1800
Trilafon (Occasional) 2532
Vancenase AQ Nasal Spray 0.042% (Extremely rare) 2535
Vancenase PocketHaler Nasal Inhaler (Extremely rare) 2534
Vexol 1% Ophthalmic Suspension (1% to 5%) .... ⊙ 227
Viroptic Ophthalmic Solution, 1% Sterile 1177
Vivactil Tablets 1820
Zyrtec Tablets (Less than 2%) 2053

Glaucoma, angle closure precipitation

Atrovent Nasal Spray 0.03% 676
Atrovent Nasal Spray 0.06% 678
Ocusert Pilo-20 and Pilo-40 Ocular Therapeutic Systems .... ⊙ 252
Transderm Scōp Transdermal Therapeutic System (Infrequent) 890

Glaucoma, corticosteroid-induced

AK-Trol Ointment & Suspension .... ⊙ 205
Blephamide Liquifilm Sterile Ophthalmic Suspension 472
Econopred & Econopred Plus Ophthalmic Suspensions .... ⊙ 216
FML Forte Liquifilm .... ⊙ 237
FML Liquifilm .... ⊙ 238
FML-S Liquifilm .... ⊙ 240
HMS Liquifilm .... ⊙ 241
Maxitrol Ophthalmic Ointment and Suspension .... ⊙ 222
Poly-Pred Liquifilm .... ⊙ 246
Pred Forte .... ⊙ 247
Pred-G Liquifilm Sterile Ophthalmic Suspension .... ⊙ 248
TobraDex Ophthalmic Suspension and Ointment 469

Glaucoma, secondary

AMO Vitrax Viscoelastic Solution ⊙ 229

Glaucoma, worsening of narrow angle

Atrovent Inhalation Aerosol 674
Atrovent Inhalation Solution 675
Atrovent Nasal Spray 0.03% 676
Atrovent Nasal Spray 0.06% 678

Globus hystericus

Daranide Tablets 1676
Imitrex Injection (Rare) 1095

Glomerular filtration rate, decrease

Capoten Tablets 740
Capozide Tablets 744
Monopril Tablets 762

Glomerulitis

Feldene Capsules (Less than 1%) 2008
Motrin Ibuprofen Suspension, Oral Drops, Chewable Tablets, Caplets (Less than 1%) 1563
Ridaura Capsules 2691
Solganal Suspension 2530

Glomerulonephritis

Anaprox/Naprosyn (Less than 1%) 2277
Apresazide Capsules 824
Cuprimine Capsules 1673
Depen Titratable Tablets (Rare) 2770
EC-Naprosyn Delayed-Release Tablets (Less than 1%) 2277
Foscavir Injection (Less than 1%) 541
Myochrysine Injection 1754
▲ Naprelan Tablets (3% to 9%) 2861
Anaprox/Naprosyn (Less than 1%) 2277
Orthoclone OKT3 Sterile Solution 1892
Ser-Ap-Es Tablets 867
Zyrtec Tablets (Rare) 2053

Glossitis

Achromycin V Capsules (Rare) 1417

(▭ Described in PDR For Nonprescription Drugs) Incidence data in parenthesis; ▲ 3% or more (⊙ Described in PDR For Ophthalmology)

AeroBid Inhaler System (1% to 3%) ... 1004
Aerobid-M Inhaler System (1% to 3%) ... 1004
Anafranil Capsules (Infrequent) ... 819
Atretol Tablets ... 569
Augmentin ... 2637
Augmentin Tablets ... 2640
Bactrim DS Tablets ... 2257
Bactrim I.V. Infusion ... 2255
Bactrim ... 2257
Betaseron for SC Injection ... 653
Betoptic Ophthalmic Solution (Rare) ... 465
Betoptic S Ophthalmic Suspension (Rare) ... 467
Biaxin ... 406
Capoten Tablets ... 740
Capozide Tablets ... 744
Chloromycetin Sodium Succinate ... 1960
Clinoril Tablets (Less than 1%) ... 1658
Cognex Capsules (Infrequent) ... 1961
Cuprimine Capsules ... 1673
Daraprim Tablets ... 1199
Declomycin Tablets ... 1421
Depakote Tablets (1% to 5%) ... 418
Depen Titratable Tablets (Rare) ... 2770
Didronel Tablets ... 2133
Doryx Capsules ... 1970
Doxil (1% to 5%) ... 2613
DYNACIN Capsules ... 1627
Effexor (Infrequent) ... 2825
Fansidar Tablets ... 2281
Felbatol ... 2774
Flagyl 375 Capsules ... 2587
Flagyl I.V. ... 2373
Foscavir Injection (Less than 1%) ... 541
Sterile FUDR ... 2284
Gantanol Tablets ... 2285
Gantrisin ... 2286
Gastrocrom Oral Concentrate ... 1611
Geocillin Tablets ... 2009
Halcion Tablets ... 2093
Helidac Therapy (Less than 1%) ... 2135
Hivid Tablets (Less than 1%) ... 2287
▲ Hylorel Tablets (8.4%) ... 1613
Imdur (Less than or equal to 5%) ... 1362
Inversine Tablets ... 1729
Invirase Capsules (Less than 2%) ... 2291
Lamictal Tablets (Infrequent) ... 1105
Lupron Depot 3.75 mg ... 2739
LUVOX Tablets (Infrequent) ... 2723
Maxair Autohaler ... 1550
Maxair Inhaler (Less than 1%) ... 1552
Merrem I.V. (1.0%) ... 2952
MetroGel-Vaginal ... 917
Minocin Intravenous ... 1428
Minocin Oral Suspension ... 1431
Minocin Pellet-Filled Capsules ... 1429
Monodox Capsules ... 1858
Myochrysine Injection ... 1754
Neurontin Capsules (Infrequent) ... 1978
Nipent for Injection (Less than 3%) ... 2733
Omnipen Capsules ... 2872
Omnipen for Oral Suspension ... 2873
Paxil Tablets (Infrequent) ... 2681
Pediazole Suspension ... 2340
Permax Tablets (Rare) ... 571
Primaxin I.M. ... 1770
Primaxin I.V. (Less than 0.2%) ... 1772
Proloprim Tablets ... 1141
Protostat Tablets ... 1939
Prozac Pulvules & Liquid, Oral Solution (Infrequent) ... 935
Relafen Tablets (Less than 1%) ... 2688
Remeron Tablets (Infrequent) ... 1878
Ridaura Capsules (1 to 3%) ... 2691
Rilutek Tablets (Infrequent) ... 2198
Septra ... 1146
Septra I.V. Infusion ... 1142
Septra I.V. Infusion ADD-Vantage Vials ... 1144
Septra ... 1146
Serzone Tablets (Rare) ... 776
Solganal Suspension ... 2530
Spectrobid Tablets ... 2030
Sular Tablets (Less than or equal to 1%) ... 2961
Tegretol/Tegretol-XR ... 870
Terramycin Intramuscular Solution ... 2034
Teslac Tablets ... 727
Tolectin (200, 400 and 600 mg) (Less than 1%) ... 1591
Trimpex Tablets ... 2323
Unasyn (Less than 1%) ... 2035
Urobiotic-250 Capsules (Rare) ... 2038
Vaseretic Tablets ... 1810
Vasotec I.V. ... 1814
Vasotec Tablets (0.5% to 1.0%) ... 1816
Vibramycin ... 2038
Vibramycin Hyclate Intravenous ... 2040
Vibramycin ... 2038
Wellbutrin Tablets (Rare) ... 1177
Zoloft Tablets (Rare) ... 2051

Glossodynia

Adenoscan (Less than 1%) ... 1022
Aldoclor Tablets ... 1638
Aldomet Ester HCl Injection ... 1642
Aldomet Oral ... 1640
Aldoril Tablets ... 1644
Clozaril Tablets (1%) ... 2377
Crixivan Capsules (Less than 2%) ... 1670
Etrafon ... 2495
Hivid Tablets (Less than 1%) ... 2287
▲ Imitrex Injection (4.9%) ... 1095
Imitrex Tablets ... 1099
Omnipen for Oral Suspension (Occasional) ... 2873
Questran (Less frequent) ... 774
Rifadin (Occasional) ... 1276
Rifamate Capsules (Occasional) ... 1278
Rifater (Occasional) ... 1280
Rimactane Capsules ... 865
▲ Tegison Capsules (10-25%) ... 2314
Trilafon ... 2532

Glossoncus

Altace Capsules ... 1238
Calcimar Injection, Synthetic (A few cases) ... 2176
Cataflam Tablets (Less than 1%) ... 833
Ceftin (0.1% to 1%) ... 1067
Fluvirin (Influenza Virus Vaccine) ... 1608
Miacalcin Injection (A few cases) ... 2402
Myochrysine Injection ... 1754
Romazicon (Less than 1%) ... 2311
Solganal Suspension ... 2530
Tambocor Tablets (Less than 1%) ... 1555
Cataflam/Voltaren/Voltaren-XR (Less than 1%) ... 833
Zarontin Capsules ... 1986
Zarontin Syrup ... 1986

Glossoplegia

Risperdal Tablets (Rare) ... 1348

Glossotrichia

Aldomet Ester HCl Injection ... 1642
Asendin Tablets ... 1419
Augmentin ... 2637
Augmentin Tablets ... 2640
Elavil ... 2945
Etrafon ... 2495
Helidac Therapy ... 2135
Klonopin Tablets ... 2294
Limbitrol ... 2333
Ludiomil Tablets (Isolated reports) ... 861
Norpramin Tablets ... 1273
Pamelor ... 2409
▲ Pen•Vee K (Among most common) ... 2879
Spectrobid Tablets ... 2030
Surmontil Capsules ... 2917
Tofranil Ampuls ... 873
Tofranil Tablets ... 875
Tofranil-PM Capsules ... 876
Unasyn ... 2035
Vivactil Tablets ... 1820

Glucose tolerance, changes

Brevicon ... 2563
Cortifoam ... 2540
Danocrine Capsules ... 2437
Demulen (Significant percentage of patients) ... 2580
Estrace Cream and Tablets ... 751
Estratest ... 2718
Foscavir Injection (Less than 1%) ... 541
Glynase PresTab Tablets ... 2091
Lasix Injection, Oral Solution and Tablets ... 1267
Levlen/Tri-Levlen ... 646
Micronor Tablets ... 1903
Modicon ... 1928
Norinyl ... 2563
Nor-Q D Tablets ... 2598
Ortho Dienestrol Cream ... 1922
Ortho-Novum ... 1928
Ovcon ... 765
Phenergan Injection ... 2880
PMB 200 and PMB 400 ... 2890
Premarin Intravenous ... 2893
Levlen/Tri-Levlen ... 646
Tri-Norinyl ... 2607
Winstrol Tablets ... 2468
Zanosar Sterile Powder (Some patients) ... 2119

Glucose tolerance, decreased

Amen Tablets ... 785
Cycrin Tablets ... 991
Depo-Provera Contraceptive Injection (Some patients) ... 2079
Emcyt Capsules ... 2085
Estraderm Transdermal System ... 842
ESTRATAB Tablets (0.3, 0.625, 1.25, 2.5 mg) ... 2715
Lo/Ovral Tablets ... 2852
Lo/Ovral-28 Tablets ... 2857
Lotensin HCT Tablets ... 855
Menest Tablets ... 2671
Naprelan Tablets (Less than 1%) ... 2861
Nordette-21 Tablets ... 2863
Nordette-28 Tablets ... 2866
Nutropin ... 1049
Nutropin AQ Injection ... 1051
Ogen Tablets ... 2103
Ogen Vaginal Cream ... 2106
Ortho-Cyclen/Ortho-Tri-Cyclen ... 1914
Ortho-Cyclen/Ortho Tri-Cyclen ... 1914
Ovral Tablets ... 2877
Ovral-28 Tablets ... 2878
Ovrette Tablets ... 2878
Oxandrin ... 783
PMB 200 and PMB 400 ... 2890
Premarin Intravenous ... 2893
Premarin Vaginal Cream ... 2898
Premphase ... 2900
Prempro ... 2905
Provera Tablets (A small percentage of patients) ... 2110
Triphasil-21 Tablets ... 2919
Triphasil-28 Tablets ... 2924
Vivelle Transdermal System ... 880

Glucosuria

Aclovate ... 1061
Bumex ... 2260
▲ Cipro I.V. Pharmacy Bulk Package (Among most frequent) ... 590
Combipres Tablets (Rare) ... 682
Cormax Ointment ... 1856
Cormax Scalp Application ... 1857
Dermatop Emollient Cream 0.1% ... 1264
Diprolene AF Cream 0.05% (Some patients) ... 2489
Diprolene Lotion 0.05% (Some patients) ... 2491
Diprolene Ointment 0.05% (Some patients) ... 2491
Elspar (Low) ... 1700
Floxin I.V. (More than or equal to 1%) ... 1580
Floxin Tablets (200 mg, 300 mg, 400 mg) (More than or equal to 1%) ... 1577
Hivid Tablets (Less than 1%) ... 2287
Humatrope Vials (Infrequent) ... 1490
Naprelan Tablets (Less than 1%) ... 2861
ProctoCream-HC 2.5% ... 2552
Rythmol Tablets–150mg, 225mg, 300mg (Less than 1%) ... 1399
Sinemet CR Tablets ... 961
Temovate Cream ... 1152
Temovate Gel ... 1153
Temovate Ointment ... 1152
Temovate Scalp Application ... 1153
Ultravate Cream 0.05% ... 2797
Ultravate Ointment 0.05% ... 2798

Glycosuria

Aldoclor Tablets ... 1638
Aldoril Tablets ... 1644
Anafranil Capsules (Rare) ... 819
Apresazide Capsules ... 824
Atretol Tablets ... 569
Betaseron for SC Injection ... 653
Capozide Tablets ... 744
Cognex Capsules (Infrequent) ... 1961
Combipres Tablets ... 682
Compazine ... 2644
Cytotec (Infrequent) ... 2576
Diamox Intravenous (Occasional) ... ◎ 317
Diamox Sequels (Sustained Release) ... ◎ 318
Diamox Tablets (Occasional) ... ◎ 317
Diucardin Tablets ... 2824
Diupres Tablets ... 1691
Diuril Oral Suspension ... 1694
Diuril Sodium Intravenous ... 1693
Diuril Tablets ... 1694
Doxil (Less than 1%) ... 2613
Dyazide Capsules ... 2653
Effexor (Infrequent) ... 2825
Enduron Tablets ... 424
Esidrix Tablets ... 839
Esimil Tablets ... 840
Eskalith ... 2658
Etrafon ... 2495
Florinef Acetate Tablets ... 506
Foscavir Injection (Less than 1%) ... 541
GlaucTabs (Occasional) ... ◎ 209
Hivid Tablets (Less than 1%) ... 2287
HydroDIURIL Tablets ... 1716
Hydropres Tablets ... 1718
Hyzaar Tablets ... 1720
Inderide Tablets ... 2838
Inderide LA Long Acting Capsules ... 2840
Indocin Capsules (Less than 1%) ... 1723
Indocin I.V. (Less than 1%) ... 1727
Indocin (Less than 1%) ... 1723
Lasix Injection, Oral Solution and Tablets ... 1267
Lithium Carbonate Capsules & Tablets ... 2352
Lithonate/Lithotabs/Lithobid ... 2721
Lopressor HCT Tablets ... 850
Lotensin HCT Tablets ... 855
Minizide Capsules ... 2016
Moduretic Tablets ... 1748
Mykrox Tablets ... 1617
Navane Capsules and Concentrate ... 2018
Navane Intramuscular ... 2019
Neptazane Tablets ... ◎ 320
Neurontin Capsules (Rare) ... 1978
Noroxin Tablets (Less frequent) ... 1758
Noroxin Tablets (Less frequent) ... 2222
Norvir (Less than 2%) ... 447
Oretic Tablets ... 450
Prevacid Delayed-Release Capsules (Less than 1%) ... 2746
Prilosec Delayed-Release Capsules (Less than 1%) ... 516
Proglycem (Frequent) ... 575
Rocephin Injectable Vials, ADD-Vantage, Galaxy Container (Rare) ... 2305
Ser-Ap-Es Tablets ... 867
Stelazine ... 2692
Supprelin Injection (1%) ... 2230
▲ Tegison Capsules (1-10%) ... 2314
Tegretol/Tegretol-XR ... 870
Tenoretic Tablets ... 2963
Thalitone ... 1293
Thorazine ... 2701
Timolide Tablets ... 1791
Trilafon ... 2532
Vistide Injection ... 1057
Wellbutrin Tablets (Rare) ... 1177
Yutopar Intravenous Injection (Infrequent) ... 566
Zanosar Sterile Powder ... 2119
Zaroxolyn Tablets ... 1625

Goiter

Anafranil Capsules (Rare) ... 819
Azulfidine (Rare) ... 2059
Betaseron for SC Injection (2%) ... 653
Effexor (Rare) ... 2825
Lamictal Tablets (Rare) ... 1105
LUVOX Tablets (Rare) ... 2723
Neurontin Capsules (Rare) ... 1978
Pediazole Suspension ... 2340
Pima Syrup (Rare) ... 1004
Prevacid Delayed-Release Capsules (Less than 1%) ... 2746
Prozac Pulvules & Liquid, Oral Solution (Rare) ... 935
Quadrinal Tablets ... 1398
Redux Capsules (Infrequent) ... 2911
Remeron Tablets (Rare) ... 1878
SSKI Solution ... 2767
▲ Sandostatin Injection (6% to 8%) ... 2421
Supprelin Injection (1%) ... 2230
Thyro-Block Tablets (Rare) ... 2785

Goiter, diffuse

Lithium Carbonate Capsules & Tablets ... 2352

Goiter, euthyroid

Eskalith ... 2658
Lithium Carbonate Capsules & Tablets ... 2352
Lithonate/Lithotabs/Lithobid ... 2721

Goiter, fetal

Quadrinal Tablets ... 1398
Tapazole Tablets ... 1361

Goiter production (see under Goiter)

Gold deposits, ocular

Ridaura Capsules ... 2691

Gold toxicity

Myochrysine Injection (Common) ... 1754
Ridaura Capsules ... 2691

Gonadotropin secretion, increase

Cytoxan ... 700

(▭ Described in PDR For Nonprescription Drugs) Incidence data in parenthesis; ▲ 3% or more (◎ Described in PDR For Ophthalmology)

Gonadotropin secretion, inhibition
- ▲ Android Capsules, 10 mg (Among most common) ... 1297
- ▲ Estratest (Among most common) ... 2718
- Foscavir Injection (Less than 1%) ... 541
- Halotestin Tablets ... 2095
- Oxandrin ... 783
- Testred Capsules, 10 mg ... 1308

Goodpasture's syndrome
- Cuprimine Capsules ... 1673
- Depen Titratable Tablets (Rare) ... 2770

Gout
- Adalat CC (Less than 1.0%) ... 582
- Ambien Tablets (Rare) ... 2559
- Anafranil Capsules (Infrequent) ... 819
- Apresazide Capsules ... 824
- Asacol Delayed-Release Tablets ... 2129
- Capozide Tablets ... 744
- Cardura Tablets (Less than 0.5% of 3960 patients) ... 1993
- Cartrol Tablets (Less common) ... 413
- Casodex Tablets (2% to 5%) ... 2934
- Cipro I.V. (1% or less) ... 587
- Cipro I.V. Pharmacy Bulk Package (Less than 1%) ... 590
- Cipro Tablets (Less than 1%) ... 584
- Cognex Capsules (Infrequent) ... 1961
- Combipres Tablets ... 682
- Cozaar Tablets (Less than 1%) ... 1668
- Cytotec (Infrequent) ... 2576
- Demadex Tablets and Injection ... 691
- Dilacor XR Extended-release Capsules (Infrequent) ... 2183
- Edecrin ... 1698
- Effexor (Rare) ... 2825
- Esidrix Tablets ... 839
- Hivid Tablets (Less than 1%) ... 2287
- Hytrin Capsules (At least 1%) ... 434
- Hyzaar Tablets ... 1720
- Lasix Injection, Oral Solution and Tablets (Rare) ... 1267
- Lopressor HCT Tablets (1 in 100 patients) ... 850
- Lotensin HCT Tablets (0.3% to 1.0%) ... 855
- Lotrel Capsules (Infrequent) ... 858
- Mavik Tablets (0.3% to 1.0%) ... 1407
- Maxaquin Tablets (Less than 1%) ... 2593
- Moduretic Tablets (Less than or equal to 1%) ... 1748
- Monopril Tablets (0.2% to 1.0%) ... 762
- Myambutol Tablets ... 1432
- Mykrox Tablets ... 1617
- Nipent for Injection (Less than 3%) ... 2733
- Norvir (Less than 2%) ... 447
- Oretic Tablets ... 450
- Paxil Tablets (Rare) ... 2681
- Permax Tablets (Infrequent) ... 571
- Prevacid Delayed-Release Capsules (Less than 1%) ... 2746
- Prinivil Tablets (0.3% to 1.0%) ... 1776
- Prinzide Tablets ... 1780
- Procardia XL Extended Release Tablets (1% or less) ... 2026
- Proglycem ... 575
- Prozac Pulvules & Liquid, Oral Solution (Rare) ... 935
- Pyrazinamide Tablets ... 1442
- Redux Capsules (Infrequent) ... 2911
- Remeron Tablets (Rare) ... 1878
- Rifater ... 1280
- Rilutek Tablets (Infrequent) ... 2198
- Serzone Tablets (Infrequent) ... 776
- Sular Tablets (Less than or equal to 1%) ... 2961
- Tegison Capsules (Less than 1%) ... 2314
- Tenoretic Tablets ... 2963
- Timolide Tablets ... 1791
- Vaseretic Tablets (0.5% to 2.0%) ... 1810
- Zaroxolyn Tablets ... 1625
- Zebeta Tablets ... 1457
- Zestoretic Tablets ... 2968
- Zestril Tablets (0.3% to 1.0%) ... 2972
- Ziac ... 1459
- Zoladex (Greater than 1% but less than 5%) ... 2976
- Zoladex 3-month ... 2978
- Zosyn (1.0% or less) ... 1463
- Zyloprim Tablets (Less than 1%) ... 1194

Granulocytopenia
- Albenza Tablets (Rare) ... 2629
- Aldoclor Tablets ... 1638
- Aldomet Ester HCI Injection (Rare) ... 1642
- Aldomet Oral ... 1640
- Aldoril Tablets ... 1644
- Anaprox/Naprosyn (Less than 1%) ... 2277

- Chloromycetin Sodium Succinate ... 1960
- Claforan Sterile and Injection (Rare) ... 1259
- Cytosar-U Sterile Powder ... 2077
- Cytovene-IV ... 2270
- Dalmane Capsules (Rare) ... 2329
- Dilantin Infatabs (Occasional) ... 1967
- Dilantin Kapseals (Occasional) ... 1965
- Dilantin-125 Suspension (Occasional) ... 1969
- EC-Naprosyn Delayed-Release Tablets (Less than 1%) ... 2277
- Ergamisol Tablets (Less than 1% to 2%) ... 1340
- Felbatol (Infrequent) ... 2774
- ▲ Foscavir Injection (5% or greater up to 17%) ... 541
- Fulvicin P/G Tablets ... 2499
- Fulvicin P/G 165 & 330 Tablets ... 2500
- Garamycin Injectable ... 2502
- Grifulvin V (griseofulvin tablets) Microsize (griseofulvin oral suspension) Microsize ... 1944
- Gris-PEG Tablets, 125 mg & 250 mg ... 476
- Intron A for Injection (Less than 5%) ... 2506
- Leucovorin Calcium Tablets, Wellcovorin Brand ... 1204
- Limbitrol (Rare) ... 2333
- Macrobid Capsules ... 2138
- Macrodantin Capsules ... 2140
- Mefoxin ... 1734
- Mefoxin Premixed Intravenous Solution ... 1737
- Methotrexate Sodium Tablets, Injection, for Injection and LPF Injection ... 1322
- Mustargen ... 1752
- Myochrysine Injection ... 1754
- Mysoline (Rare) ... 2860
- ▲ Naprelan Tablets (3% to 9%) ... 2861
- Anaprox/Naprosyn (Less than 1%) ... 2277
- ▲ Navelbine Injection (29% to 80%) ... 1212
- Nebcin Vials, Hyporets & ADD-Vantage ... 1518
- Propulsid (Rare) ... 1346
- Relafen Tablets (Less than 1%) ... 2688
- ▲ Retrovir Capsules (1.8% to 47%) ... 1216
- ▲ Retrovir I.V. Infusion (1.8% to 47%) ... 1221
- ▲ Retrovir Syrup (1.8% to 47%) ... 1216
- Ridaura Capsules ... 2691
- Rythmol Tablets–150mg, 225mg, 300mg (Less than 1%) ... 1399
- Serentil (A single case) ... 689
- Solganal Suspension (Rare) ... 2530
- Talacen Caplets ... 2464
- Talwin Injection ... 2465
- Talwin Compound (Rare) ... 2466
- Talwin Injection ... 2465
- Talwin Nx Tablets ... 2467
- Tapazole Tablets ... 1361
- Tolectin (200, 400 and 600 mg) (Less than 1%) ... 1591
- Velban Vials ... 1537
- ▲ Videx Tablets, Powder for Oral Solution, & Pediatric Powder for Oral Solution (6% to 8%) ... 2980
- Vistide Injection ... 1057
- Zantac (A few patients) ... 1182
- Zantac Injection (Few patients) ... 1180
- Zantac Syrup (A few patients) ... 1182
- Zinecard Injection ... 2120

Granulocytosis
- Hivid Tablets (Less than 1%) ... 2287
- Vantin for Oral Suspension and Vantin Tablets ... 2112

Granuloma, unspecified
- Fluorescite ... ⊙ 217

Granulomatosis, Wegener's
- Accutane Capsules ... 2252

Gray syndrome
- Chloromycetin Sodium Succinate (2 cases) ... 1960

Grogginess
- Versed Injection (Less than 1%) ... 2324

Groin, itch
- Miltown Tablets ... 2780
- PMB 200 and PMB 400 ... 2890

Groin, rash
- Miltown Tablets ... 2780
- PMB 200 and PMB 400 ... 2890

Growth, retardation
- Aquasol A Vitamin A Capsules, USP ... 525
- Clomid ... 1262
- Depen Titratable Tablets (One infant) ... 2770

Growth, suppression in children
- Azmacort Oral Inhaler ... 2175
- Beclovent Inhalation Aerosol and Refill ... 1063
- Celestone Soluspan Suspension ... 2484
- CORTENEMA ... 2713
- Cortifoam ... 2540
- Cortone Acetate Sterile Suspension ... 1663
- Cortone Acetate Tablets ... 1664
- Cylert Tablets ... 415
- Dalalone D.P. Injectable ... 1009
- Decadron Elixir ... 1676
- Decadron Phosphate Injection ... 1680
- Decadron Phosphate with Xylocaine Injection, Sterile ... 1683
- Decadron Tablets ... 1678
- Decadron-LA Sterile Suspension ... 1687
- Desoxyn Gradumet Tablets ... 422
- Dexacort Phosphate in Respihaler ... 1606
- Dexacort Phosphate in Turbinaire ... 1607
- Florinef Acetate Tablets ... 506
- Hydeltrasol Injection, Sterile ... 1708
- Hydeltra-T.B.A. Sterile Suspension ... 1710
- Hydrocortone Acetate Sterile Suspension ... 1712
- Hydrocortone Phosphate Injection, Sterile ... 1713
- Hydrocortone Tablets ... 1715
- Nasacort Nasal Inhaler ... 2189
- Pediapred Oral Solution ... 1618
- Prelone Syrup ... 1834
- ProctoCream-HC 2.5% (With chronic therapy) ... 2552

Growth retardation, intrauterine
- Accupril Tablets ... 1950
- Altace Capsules ... 1238
- Capoten Tablets ... 740
- Capozide Tablets ... 744
- Cozaar Tablets ... 1668
- Dilantin Kapseals ... 1965
- Dilantin-125 Suspension ... 1969
- Elavil ... 2945
- Hyzaar Tablets ... 1720
- Lotensin Tablets ... 852
- Lotensin HCT Tablets ... 855
- Metubine Iodide Vials ... 932
- Monopril Tablets ... 762
- Prinivil Tablets ... 1776
- Prinzide Tablets ... 1780
- Tenoretic Tablets ... 2963
- Tenormin Tablets and I.V. Injection ... 2965
- Univasc Tablets ... 2553
- Vaseretic Tablets ... 1810
- Vasotec I.V. ... 1814
- Vasotec Tablets ... 1816
- Yutopar Intravenous Injection ... 566
- Zestoretic Tablets ... 2968
- Zestril Tablets ... 2972

Guillain-Barre syndrome
- Acel-Imune Diphtheria and Tetanus Toxoids and Acellular Pertussis Vaccine Adsorbed ... 1415
- ActHIB ... 893
- Asacol Delayed-Release Tablets (Rare) ... 2129
- Attenuvax (Rare) ... 1650
- Azulfidine (Rare) ... 2059
- Biavax II (Isolated reports) ... 1653
- Cuprimine Capsules ... 1673
- Cytovene-IV (One report) ... 2270
- Danocrine Capsules (Rare) ... 2437
- Depen Titratable Tablets ... 2770
- Diphtheria and Tetanus Toxoids and Pertussis Vaccine Adsorbed ... 2650
- Eminase (Less than 1 in 1,000) ... 2215
- Engerix-B Unit-Dose Vials (Less than 1%) ... 2656
- Fluvirin (Influenza Virus Vaccine) (Less than one case per 100,000) ... 1608
- Havrix (Rare) ... 2663
- HibTITER ... 1423
- Imovax Rabies Vaccine (Two cases) ... 899
- Influenza Virus Vaccine, Trivalent, Types A and B (chromatograph- and filter-purified subviron antigen) FluShield, 1996-1997 Formula (Rare) ... 2842
- IPOL Poliovirus Vaccine Inactivated ... 903

- M-M-R II (Rare) ... 1730
- M-R-VAX II (Rare) ... 1732
- Meruvax II (Isolated reports) ... 1740
- Myochrysine Injection (Rare) ... 1754
- Noroxin Tablets ... 1758
- Noroxin Tablets ... 2222
- OmniHIB ... 2676
- Orimune ... 1433
- Paxil Tablets ... 2681
- PedvaxHIB ... 1761
- Pneumovax 23 (Rare) ... 1768
- Pnu-Imune 23 ... 1437
- Recombivax HB ... 1787
- Redux Capsules ... 2911
- Tetramune ... 1449
- Tri-Immunol Adsorbed ... 1452

Gums, sore
- Hivid Tablets (Less than 1%) ... 2287
- Prolixin ... 510
- Thyro-Block Tablets ... 2785
- Wellbutrin Tablets (Infrequent) ... 1177

Gustatory sensation
- Torecan (Occasional) ... 2367
- ▲ Wellbutrin Tablets (3.1%) ... 1177

Gynecological disorders, unspecified
- ▲ Zofran Tablets (7%) ... 1231

Gynecomastia
- Adalat Capsules (10 mg and 20 mg) (Less than 0.5%) ... 580
- Adalat CC (Rare) ... 582
- Adapin Capsules ... 1542
- Aldactazide Tablets (Not infrequent) ... 2556
- Aldactone Tablets (Not infrequent) ... 2558
- Aldoclor Tablets ... 1638
- Aldomet Ester HCI Injection ... 1642
- Aldomet Oral ... 1640
- Aldoril Tablets ... 1644
- Anafranil Capsules (Rare) ... 819
- Androderm Testosterone Transdermal System ... 2634
- ▲ Android Capsules, 10 mg (Among most common) ... 1297
- Asendin Tablets ... 1419
- Atromid-S Capsules ... 2808
- Avonex ... 662
- Axid Pulvules (Rare) ... 1468
- Betaseron for SC Injection ... 653
- Calan SR Caplets (1% or less) ... 2571
- Calan Tablets (1% or less) ... 2568
- Capoten Tablets ... 740
- Capozide Tablets ... 744
- ▲ Casodex Tablets (5%) ... 2934
- Catapres Tablets (About 1 in 1,000 patients) ... 679
- Catapres-TTS ... 680
- Cipro I.V. (1% or less) ... 587
- Cipro I.V. Pharmacy Bulk Package (Less than 1%) ... 590
- Clinoril Tablets (Rare) ... 1658
- Combipres Tablets (About 1 in 1,000) ... 682
- Compazine ... 2644
- Covera-HS Tablets (Less than 2%) ... 2573
- Elavil ... 2945
- Etrafon ... 2495
- ▲ Eulexin Capsules (9%) ... 2498
- Flexeril Tablets (Rare) ... 1701
- Foscavir Injection (Less than 1%) ... 541
- Haldol Decanoate ... 1587
- Haldol Injection, Tablets and Concentrate ... 1585
- Halotestin Tablets ... 2095
- Humatrope Vials (Rare) ... 1490
- Humegon for Injection (Occasional) ... 1873
- IBU Tablets (Less than 1%) ... 1389
- Indocin Capsules (Less than 1%) ... 1723
- Indocin I.V. (Less than 1%) ... 1727
- Indocin (Less than 1%) ... 1723
- Intron A for Injection (Less than 5%) ... 2506
- Isoptin Oral Tablets (Less than 1%) ... 1393
- Isoptin SR Tablets (1% or less) ... 1395
- Kadian Capsules (Less than 3%) ... 2948
- Lanoxicaps (Occasional) ... 1110
- Lanoxin Elixir Pediatric (Occasional) ... 1113
- Lanoxin Injection (Occasional) ... 1116
- Lanoxin Injection Pediatric (Occasional) ... 1119
- Lanoxin Tablets (Occasional) ... 1121
- Lescol Capsules ... 2395
- Limbitrol ... 2333
- Loxitane (Rare) ... 1426

Side Effects Index

Gynecomastia

- Ludiomil Tablets (Isolated reports) ... 861
- Lupron Depot 7.5 mg (Less than 5%) ... 2741
- Lupron Depot - 3 Month 22.5 mg (Less than 5%) ... 2743
- Lupron Depot-PED 7.5 mg, 11.25 mg and 15 mg (Less than 2%) ... 2744
- ▲ Lupron Injection (5% or more) ... 2736
- Lupron Injection Pediatric (Less than 2%) ... 2737
- Matulane Capsules (In prepubertal and early pubertal boys) ... 2300
- Megace Oral Suspension (1% to 3%) ... 708
- Mellaril ... 2398
- Mevacor Tablets (0.5% to 1.0%) ... 1742
- Midamor Tablets ... 1746
- Moban Tablets and Concentrate (Infrequent) ... 1036
- Moduretic Tablets ... 1748
- Motrin Ibuprofen Suspension, Oral Drops, Chewable Tablets, Caplets (Less than 1%) ... 1563
- Myleran Tablets (Rare) ... 1209
- Navane Capsules and Concentrate ... 2018
- Navane Intramuscular ... 2019
- Neoral (Less than 1% to 4%) ... 2405
- Nizoral Tablets (Less than 1%) ... 1345
- Norpace (Rare) ... 2596
- Norpramin Tablets ... 1273
- Nutropin (Rare) ... 1049
- Nutropin AQ Injection (Rare) ... 1051
- Nydrazid Injection ... 509
- Orudis Capsules (Rare) ... 2874
- Oruvail Capsules (Rare) ... 2874
- Oxandrin ... 783
- Pamelor ... 2409
- Pepcid Injection (Rare) ... 1765
- Pepcid (Rare) ... 1763
- Pergonal (menotropins for injection, USP) (Occasional) ... 2618
- Pravachol Tablets ... 770
- Pregnyl for Injection ... 1878
- Prevacid Delayed-Release Capsules (Less than 1%) ... 2746
- Prilosec Delayed-Release Capsules (Less than 1%) ... 516
- Procardia Capsules (Less than 0.5%) ... 2024
- Profasi (chorionic gonadotropin for injection, USP) ... 2620
- Prolixin ... 510
- Protropin (Rare) ... 1053
- Prozac Pulvules & Liquid, Oral Solution ... 935
- Redux Capsules ... 2911
- Reglan ... 2243
- Rifamate Capsules ... 1278
- Rifater ... 1280
- Risperdal Tablets (Rare) ... 1348
- ▲ Sandimmune (Less than 1 to 4%) ... 2416
- Sandostatin Injection (Less than 1%) ... 2421
- Ser-Ap-Es Tablets ... 867
- Serentil ... 689
- Sinequan ... 2028
- Sporanox Capsules (Less than 1%) ... 1352
- Stelazine ... 2692
- Surmontil Capsules ... 2917
- ▲ Tagamet (4%; 0.3% to 1%) ... 2694
- Testoderm Testosterone Transdermal System (Five in 104 patients; frequent) ... 486
- Testred Capsules, 10 mg ... 1308
- Thorazine ... 2701
- Tofranil Ampuls ... 873
- Tofranil Tablets ... 875
- Tofranil-PM Capsules ... 876
- Torecan ... 2367
- Trecator-SC Tablets ... 2919
- Triavil Tablets ... 1800
- Trilafon ... 2532
- Vaseretic Tablets ... 1810
- Vasotec I.V. ... 1814
- Vasotec Tablets (0.5% to 1.0%) ... 1816
- Verelan Capsules (1% or less) ... 1455
- Vivactil Tablets ... 1820
- Wellbutrin Tablets (Infrequent) ... 1177
- Winstrol Tablets ... 2468
- Xanax Tablets ... 2115
- Zantac (Occasional) ... 1182
- Zantac Injection ... 1180
- Zantac Syrup (Occasional) ... 1182
- Zocor Tablets ... 1821
- ▲ Zoladex 3-month (8%) ... 2978
- Zoloft Tablets (Rare) ... 2051
- Zyloprim Tablets (Less than 1%) ... 1194

GGTP, elevation
(see under Gamma-glutamyl transpeptidase, elevation)

H

Haemophilus B disease
- PedvaxHIB ... 1761

Hair, abnormal growth
(see under Hirsutism)

Hair, dry brittle
- Atromid-S Capsules (Less often) ... 2808
- Claritin Tablets (2% or fewer patients) ... 2485
- Claritin-D Tablets ... 2487
- Clomid (Fewer than 1%) ... 1262
- Eskalith ... 2658
- Lithium Carbonate Capsules & Tablets ... 2352
- Lithonate/Lithotabs/Lithobid ... 2721
- Neoral (Rare) ... 2405
- Nizoral 2% Shampoo ... 1344
- Sandimmune (Rare) ... 2416
- Selsun Rx 2.5% Selenium Sulfide Lotion, USP ... 2345

Hair, oily
- Nizoral 2% Shampoo ... 1344
- Selsun Rx 2.5% Selenium Sulfide Lotion, USP ... 2345

Hair discoloration
- Drithocreme 0.1%, 0.25%, 0.5%, 1.0% (HP) ... 920
- Dritho-Scalp 0.25%, 0.5% ... 921
- Effexor (Rare) ... 2825
- Fototar Cream ... 1300
- MG 217 Medicated Tar Shampoo ... 800
- Plaquenil Sulfate Tablets ... 2459
- Selsun Rx 2.5% Selenium Sulfide Lotion, USP ... 2345
- Wellbutrin Tablets (Rare) ... 1177

Hair loss
(see under Alopecia)

Hair problems, unspecified
- Accutane Capsules ... 2252
- Emcyt Capsules (1%) ... 2085
- Invirase Capsules (Less than 2%) ... 2291
- Lescol Capsules ... 2395
- ▲ Lupron Depot 3.75 mg (Among most frequent) ... 2739
- Mevacor Tablets ... 1742
- Pravachol Tablets ... 770
- ▲ Roferon-A Injection (18%) ... 2308
- Zocor Tablets ... 1821
- ▲ Zoladex (4%) ... 2976
- Zoladex 3-month ... 2978

Hair texture, abnormal
- Imdur (Less than or equal to 5%) ... 1362
- Intron A for Injection (Less than 5%) ... 2506
- Nizoral 2% Shampoo (One occurrence in 41 patients) ... 1344
- Zoloft Tablets (Rare) ... 2051

Hair thinning
- ▲ Accutane Capsules (Less than 1 patient in 10) ... 2252
- Actigall Capsules ... 818
- Arimidex Tablets (2% to 5%) ... 2932
- Combipres Tablets ... 682
- Cortifoam ... 2540
- Eskalith ... 2658
- Intron A for Injection ... 2506
- Lithium Carbonate Capsules & Tablets ... 2352
- Lithonate/Lithotabs/Lithobid ... 2721
- Nolvadex Tablets (Infrequent) ... 2957
- Seldane Tablets ... 1284
- Seldane-D Extended-Release Tablets ... 1286
- Trilafon Tablets ... 2532

Halitosis
- Anafranil Capsules (Up to 2%) ... 819
- Azactam for Injection (Less than 1%) ... 736
- Claritin-D Tablets (Less frequent) ... 2487
- Crixivan Capsules (Less than 2%) ... 1670
- Effexor (Rare) ... 2825
- ▲ Intron A for Injection (Less than 5%) ... 2506
- Lamictal Tablets (Infrequent) ... 1105

Hallucinations
- Actimmune (Rare) ... 1043
- Adapin Capsules (Infrequent) ... 1542
- Ambien Tablets (Infrequent) ... 2559
- Amicar Syrup, Tablets, and Injection ... 1312
- Anafranil Capsules (Infrequent) ... 819
- Ancobon Capsules ... 2254
- Artane (Rare) ... 1418
- Asendin Tablets (Very rare) ... 1419
- Atamet Tablets ... 567
- Ativan Injection (1%) ... 2805
- Azulfidine (Rare) ... 2059
- Bactrim DS Tablets ... 2257
- Bactrim I.V. Infusion ... 2255
- Bactrim ... 2257
- Betaseron for SC Injection ... 653
- Biaxin ... 406
- Blocadren Tablets (Less than 1%) ... 1654
- Brontex ... 2130
- Buprenex Injectable (Infrequent) ... 2170
- BuSpar Tablets (Infrequent) ... 738
- Butisol Sodium Elixir & Tablets (Less than 1 in 100) ... 2768
- Cardizem CD Capsules (Less than 1%) ... 1251
- Cardizem SR Capsules (Less than 1%) ... 1255
- Cardizem Injectable ... 1253
- Cardizem Tablets (Less than 1%) ... 1257
- Ceclor Pulvules & Suspension (Rare) ... 1470
- Celontin Kapseals (Rare) ... 1955
- Chibroxin Sterile Ophthalmic Solution (With oral form) ... 1657
- Cipro I.V. (1% or less) ... 587
- Cipro I.V. Pharmacy Bulk Package (Less than 1%) ... 590
- Cipro Tablets (Less than 1%) ... 584
- Claritin-D Tablets ... 2487
- Clozaril Tablets (Less than 1%) ... 2377
- Cogentin ... 1661
- Cognex Capsules (2%) ... 1961
- Cylert Tablets ... 415
- D.A. II Tablets ... 972
- D.A. Chewable Tablets ... 970
- Dalmane Capsules (Rare) ... 2329
- Darvon-N/Darvocet-N ... 1473
- Darvon ... 1475
- Darvon-N Suspension & Tablets ... 1473
- DaunoXome (Less than or equal to 5%) ... 1842
- Deconsal II Tablets ... 1605
- Demerol ... 2438
- Demser Capsules ... 1690
- Depakene ... 416
- Depakote Tablets (1% to 5%) ... 418
- Desyrel and Desyrel Dividose ... 504
- Didronel Tablets ... 2133
- Dilaudid-HP Injection (Less frequent) ... 1384
- Dilaudid-HP Lyophilized Powder 250 mg (Less frequent) ... 1384
- Dilaudid Tablets and Liquid (Less frequent) ... 1386
- Dimetane-DC Cough Syrup ... 2232
- Dimetane-DX Cough Syrup ... 2233
- Diprivan Injectable Emulsion (Less than 1%) ... 2939
- Ditropan ... 1267
- Dizac (diazepam injectable emulsion) CIV (Less frequent) ... 1862
- Dolobid Tablets (Less than 1 in 100) ... 1695
- Doral Tablets (Rare) ... 2773
- ▲ Duragesic Transdermal System (3% to 10%) ... 1336
- Dura-Tap/PD Capsules ... 970
- Dura-Vent/DA Tablets ... 972
- Dura-Vent Tablets ... 971
- E.E.S. (Isolated reports) ... 427
- Effexor (Infrequent) ... 2825
- Elavil ... 2945
- ▲ Eldepryl Capsules (3 of 49 patients) ... 2729
- Elspar ... 1700
- Entex PSE Tablets ... 973
- Ergamisol Tablets (Less frequent) ... 1340
- EryPed (Isolated reports) ... 425
- Ery-Tab Tablets (Isolated reports) ... 426
- Erythrocin Stearate Filmtab (Isolated reports) ... 429
- Erythromycin Base Filmtab (Isolated reports) ... 430
- Erythromycin Delayed-Release Capsules, USP (Isolated reports) ... 431
- Eskalith ... 2658
- Ethmozine Tablets (Less than 2%) ... 2217
- Etrafon ... 2495
- Fansidar Tablets ... 2281
- Fedahist Gyrocaps ... 2545
- Felbatol (Infrequent) ... 2774
- Feldene Capsules (Less than 1%) ... 2008
- Fioricet with Codeine Capsules ... 2387
- Fiorinal with Codeine Capsules ... 2390
- Flexeril Tablets (Less than 1%) ... 1701
- Floxin I.V. (Less than 1%) ... 1580
- Floxin Tablets (200 mg, 300 mg, 400 mg) (Less than 1%) ... 1577
- Flumadine Tablets & Syrup (Less than 0.3%) ... 1013
- Foscavir Injection (Between 1% and 5%) ... 541
- Ganite ... 2711
- Gantanol Tablets ... 2285
- Gantrisin ... 2286
- Garamycin Ophthalmic ... 2501
- Gastrocrom Capsules (Infrequent) ... 1611
- Gastrocrom Oral Concentrate (Less common) ... 1611
- Genoptic Sterile Ophthalmic Solution (Rare) ... 241
- Genoptic Sterile Ophthalmic Ointment (Rare) ... 241
- Gentak (Rare) ... 209
- Guaimax-D Tablets ... 809
- Halcion Tablets ... 2093
- Haldol Decanoate ... 1587
- Haldol Injection, Tablets and Concentrate ... 1585
- Histussin D Liquid ... 670
- Hivid Tablets (Less than 1%) ... 2287
- Hydrea Capsules (Extremely rare) ... 705
- IBU Tablets (Less than 1%) ... 1389
- ▲ IFEX (Among most common) ... 706
- Imitrex Tablets (Rare) ... 1099
- Inapsine Injection ... 462
- Inderal ... 2834
- Inderal LA Long Acting Capsules ... 2836
- Inderide Tablets ... 2838
- Inderide LA Long Acting Capsules ... 2840
- Invirase Capsules (Less than 2%) ... 2291
- Kadian Capsules (Less than 3%) ... 2948
- Keflex Pulvules & Oral Suspension ... 930
- Keftab Tablets ... 931
- Kerlone Tablets (Less than 2%) ... 2588
- Klonopin Tablets ... 2294
- Lamictal Tablets (Infrequent) ... 1105
- Lariam Tablets ... 2295
- Larodopa Tablets (Relatively frequent) ... 2296
- Leukeran Tablets (Rare) ... 1205
- Levsin/Levsinex/Levbid ... 2549
- Limbitrol ... 2333
- Lioresal Intrathecal (0.3% to 0.5%) ... 1634
- Lioresal Tablets ... 847
- Lithonate/Lithotabs/Lithobid ... 2721
- Lopressor ... 848
- Lopressor HCT Tablets ... 850
- Ludiomil Tablets (Rare) ... 861
- LUVOX Tablets (Infrequent) ... 2723
- MS Contin Tablets (Less frequent) ... 2149
- MSIR (Infrequent) ... 2152
- Marinol (Dronabinol) Capsules (Greater than 1%) ... 2353
- Matulane Capsules ... 2300
- Maxaquin Tablets ... 2593
- Mebaral Tablets (Less than 1 in 100) ... 2452
- Mepergan Injection ... 2859
- Merrem I.V. (0.1% to 1.0%) ... 2952
- Methergine (Rare) ... 2401
- Mexitil Capsules (About 3 in 1,000) ... 684
- Minipress Capsules (Less than 1%) ... 2015
- Minizide Capsules (Rare) ... 2016
- Motrin Ibuprofen Suspension, Oral Drops, Chewable Tablets, Caplets (Less than 1%) ... 1563
- Myambutol Tablets ... 1432
- Myochrysine Injection (Rare) ... 1754
- NegGram ... 2453
- Nembutal Sodium Capsules (Less than 1%) ... 440
- Nembutal Sodium Solution (Less than 1%) ... 442
- Nembutal Sodium Suppositories (Less than 1%) ... 444
- Neurontin Capsules (Infrequent) ... 1978
- Nipent for Injection (Less than 3%) ... 2733
- Norflex ... 1554
- Norgesic (Occasional) ... 1554
- Noroxin Tablets ... 1758
- Noroxin Tablets ... 2222

(Described in PDR For Nonprescription Drugs) Incidence data in parenthesis; ▲ 3% or more (Described in PDR For Ophthalmology)

Side Effects Index

Norpramin Tablets ... 1273
Norvir (Less than 2%) ... 447
Novahistine DMX ... ⊠ 782
Novahistine Elixir ... ⊠ 782
Nubain Injection (1% or less) ... 952
Oramorph SR (Morphine Sulfate Sustained Release Tablets) (Less frequent) ... 2359
Orudis Capsules (Rare) ... 2874
Oruvail Capsules (Rare) ... 2874
OxyContin Tablets (Less than 1%) ... 2163
Pamelor ... 2409
Parlodel ... 2411
Paxil Tablets (Infrequent) ... 2681
Pediazole Suspension ... 2340
Penetrex Tablets (Less than 0.1%) ... 2196
Pepcid Injection (Infrequent) ... 1765
Pepcid (Infrequent) ... 1763
Periactin ... 1767
▲ Permax Tablets (13.8%) ... 571
Phenergan with Codeine ... 2883
Phenergan VC with Codeine ... 2888
Phenobarbital Elixir and Tablets (Less than 1 in 100 patients) ... 1523
Placidyl Capsules ... 456
Prevacid Delayed-Release Capsules (Less than 1%) ... 2746
Prilosec Delayed-Release Capsules (Less than 1%) ... 516
Primaxin I.M. ... 1770
Primaxin I.V. ... 1772
Procanbid Extended-Release Tablets (Occasional) ... 1983
▲ Prograf (Greater than 3%) ... 1028
ProSom Tablets (Rare) ... 457
Prozac Pulvules & Liquid, Oral Solution (Infrequent) ... 935
Redux Capsules (Rare) ... 2911
Reglan (Rare) ... 2243
Remeron Tablets (Infrequent) ... 1878
Restoril Capsules (Less than 0.5%) ... 2413
ReVia Tablets (Less than 1%) ... 957
Rilutek Tablets (Infrequent) ... 2198
Roferon-A Injection (Infrequent) ... 2308
Rondec Oral Drops ... 974
Rondec Syrup ... 974
Rondec ... 974
Sansert Tablets ... 2424
Seconal Sodium Pulvules (Less than 1 in 100) ... 1529
Seldane-D Extended-Release Tablets ... 1286
Septra ... 1146
Septra I.V. Infusion ... 1142
Septra I.V. Infusion ADD-Vantage Vials ... 1144
Septra ... 1146
Serax Capsules ... 2916
Serax Tablets ... 2916
Serzone Tablets (Infrequent) ... 776
Sinemet Tablets ... 959
▲ Sinemet CR Tablets (3.9%) ... 961
Sinequan (Infrequent) ... 2028
Stadol (Less than 1%) ... 779
Surmontil Capsules ... 2917
Symmetrel Capsules (1% to 5%) .. 965
Symmetrel Syrup (1% to 5%) ... 963
Syn-Rx Tablets ... 1622
Syn-Rx DM Tablets ... 1623
Tagamet ... 2694
Talacen Caplets ... 2464
Talwin Injection ... 2465
Talwin Compound ... 2466
Talwin Injection ... 2465
Talwin Nx Tablets ... 2467
Tenoretic Tablets ... 2963
Tenormin Tablets and I.V. Injection 2965
Tiazac Capsules (Less than 1%) ... 1019
Timolide Tablets ... 1791
Timoptic in Ocudose (Less frequent) ... 1796
Timoptic Sterile Ophthalmic Solution (Less frequent) ... 1794
Timoptic-XE ... 1798
Tofranil Ampuls ... 873
Tofranil Tablets ... 875
Tofranil-PM Capsules ... 876
▲ Tonocard Tablets (2.1% to 11.2%) ... 519
Toradol (1% or less) ... 2319
Transderm Scōp Transdermal Therapeutic System (Infrequent) ... 890
Triavil Tablets ... 1800
Trilisate (Rare) ... 2155
Trinalin Repetabs Tablets ... 1373
Tussend ... 1830
Tussend Expectorant ... 1831
▲ Ultram Tablets (50 mg) (Less than 1% to 14%) ... 1594
Valium Injectable ... 2336
Valium Tablets ... 2335
Versed Injection ... 2324
▲ Vesanoid Capsules (6%) ... 2327
Visken Tablets (Less than 1%) ... 2428
Vistide Injection ... 1057
Vivactil Tablets ... 1820
Wellbutrin Tablets (Frequent) ... 1177
Xanax Tablets (Rare) ... 2115
Zantac (Rare) ... 1182
Zantac Injection ... 1180
Zantac Syrup (Rare) ... 1182
Zebeta Tablets ... 1457
Ziac ... 1459
Zoloft Tablets (Infrequent) ... 2051
Zosyn (1.0% or less) ... 1463
Zovirax Capsules ... 1187
Zovirax Sterile Powder (Approximately 1%) ... 1191
Zovirax ... 1187

Hallucinations, auditory

Catapres Tablets (Rare) ... 679
Catapres-TTS ... 680
Combipres Tablets ... 682
Orthoclone OKT3 Sterile Solution .. 1892

Hallucinations, hypnagogic

Anafranil Capsules (Infrequent) ... 819

Hallucinations, visual

Atretol Tablets ... 569
Catapres Tablets (Rare) ... 679
Catapres-TTS ... 680
Combipres Tablets ... 682
Orthoclone OKT3 Sterile Solution .. 1892
Parlodel (Less than 1%) ... 2411
Salagen Tablets (Rare) ... 1546
Talwin Compound ... 2466
Talwin Nx Tablets ... 2467
Tegretol/Tegretol-XR ... 870
Tessalon Perles ... 1018

Halos

Cordarone Tablets ... 2818
Plaquenil Sulfate Tablets (Fairly common) ... 2459

Hand-foot syndrome

(see under Palmar-plantar erythrodysesthesia syndrome)

Hangover

Effexor (Infrequent) ... 2825
Neurontin Capsules (Rare) ... 1978
Nipent for Injection (Less than 3%) ... 2733
Phenobarbital Elixir and Tablets ... 1523
Placidyl Capsules ... 456
▲ ProSom Tablets (3%) ... 457
Prozac Pulvules & Liquid, Oral Solution (Infrequent) ... 935
Serzone Tablets (Infrequent) ... 776

Head, roaring sensation

BuSpar Tablets (Infrequent) ... 738

Head, tight feeling

Adenocard Injection (Less than 1%) ... 1021
Imitrex Injection (2.2%) ... 1095
Imitrex Tablets (Infrequent) ... 1099

Headache

▲ Abelcet Injection (4% to 7%) ... 1540
▲ Accupril Tablets (1.7% to 5.6%) .. 1950
▲ Accutane Capsules (Approximately 1 patient in 20) ... 2252
Achromycin V Capsules ... 1417
▲ Actigall Capsules (18.1%) ... 818
▲ Actimmune (33%) ... 1043
Acutrim ... ⊠ 648
Adagen (pegademase bovine) Injection (One patient) ... 988
▲ Adalat Capsules (10 mg and 20 mg) (About 10% to 23%) ... 580
▲ Adalat CC (19%) ... 582
Adapin Capsules (Occasional) ... 1542
Adderall Tablets ... 2209
Adenocard Injection (2%) ... 1021
▲ Adenoscan (18%) ... 1022
Adipex-P Tablets and Capsules ... 1035
▲ AeroBid Inhaler System (25%) ... 1004
▲ Aerobid-M Inhaler System (25%) .. 1004
Aerolate ... 1003
▲ Airet Albuterol Sulfate Inhalation Solution (3% to 3.1%) ... 1602
AK-FLUOR Injection 10% and 25% ... ⊚ 204
Albalon Solution with Liquifilm... ⊚ 229
▲ Albenza Tablets (1.3% to 11.0%) 2629
▲ Albuterol Sulfate, USP Solution for Inhalation, Arm-a-Med (3% to 3.1%) ... 522
Aldactazide Tablets ... 2556
Aldactone Tablets ... 2558
Aldoclor Tablets ... 1638
Aldomet Ester HCl Injection ... 1642
Aldomet Oral ... 1640
Aldoril Tablets ... 1644
Alfenta Injection (0.3% to 1%) ... 1334
▲ Alferon N Injection (3% to 31%)... 2142
Alomide Ophthalmic Solution (1.5%) ... 465
▲ Altace Capsules (1.2% to 5.4%)... 1238
Alupent (1% to 4%) ... 672
Amaryl Tablets (1.5%) ... 1241
Ambien Tablets (7% to 19%) ... 2559
Amen Tablets (Rare) ... 785
Amicar Syrup, Tablets, and Injection ... 1312
Amikacin Sulfate Injection, USP (Rare) ... 523
Amikacin Sulfate Injection, USP (Rare) ... 981
Amikin Injectable (Rare) ... 502
▲ Anafranil Capsules (28% to 52%) 819
Ana-Kit Anaphylaxis Emergency Treatment Kit (Common) ... 611
▲ Anaprox/Naprosyn (3% to 9%)... 2277
Ancobon Capsules ... 2254
▲ Androderm Testosterone Transdermal System (4%) ... 2634
▲ Android Capsules, 10 mg (Among most common) ... 1297
Antabuse Tablets (Small number of patients) ... 2802
Apresazide Capsules (Common) ... 824
Apresoline Hydrochloride Tablets (Common) ... 826
Aquasol A Vitamin A Capsules, USP ... 525
Aquasol A Parenteral ... 526
Aralen Hydrochloride Injection ... 2430
Aralen Phosphate Tablets ... 2431
▲ Aredia for Injection (At least 10% to 17.7%) ... 827
▲ Arimidex Tablets (13.0% to 17.9%) ... 2932
Artane ... 1418
▲ Asacol Delayed-Release Tablets (35%) ... 2129
Asendin Tablets (Less frequent) ... 1419
Astramorph/PF Injection, USP (Preservative-Free) ... 526
Atamet Tablets ... 567
Ativan Tablets (Less frequent) ... 2807
Atretol Tablets ... 569
Atrohist Plus Tablets ... 1605
Atromid-S Capsules (Less often) ... 2808
Atrovent Inhalation Aerosol (2,4%; about 2 in 100) ... 674
▲ Atrovent Inhalation Solution (6.4%) ... 675
▲ Atrovent Nasal Spray 0.03% (9.8%) ... 676
Augmentin (Less frequent) ... 2637
Augmentin Tablets (Less frequent) 2640
▲ Avonex (67%) ... 662
▲ Axid Pulvules (16.6%) ... 1468
Axocet Capsules (Infrequent) ... 2469
Azactam for Injection (Less than 1%) ... 736
▲ Azulfidine (Approximately one-third of patients) ... 2059
Bactrim DS Tablets ... 2257
Bactrim I.V. Infusion ... 2255
Bactrim ... 2257
▲ Bactroban Nasal (9%) ... 2643
Beclovent Inhalation Aerosol and Refill ... 1063
Beconase (Fewer than 5 per 100 patients) ... 1065
Benadryl Injection ... 1955
Benemid Tablets ... 1651
Bentyl ... 1246
Betagan (Rare) ... ⊚ 230
▲ Betapace Tablets (3% to 8%) ... 637
▲ Betaseron for SC Injection (84%) .. 653
▲ Betimol 0.25%, 0.5% (More than 5%) ... ⊚ 259
Betoptic Ophthalmic Solution (Rare) ... 465
Betoptic S Ophthalmic Suspension (Rare) ... 467
Biavax II ... 1653
Biaxin (2%) ... 406
Biltricide Tablets ... 584
Blocadren Tablets (Greater than 1%) ... 1654
Bontril Slow-Release Capsules ... 786
Brethaire Inhaler ... 830
Brethine Ampuls ... 832
Brethine Tablets ... 831
Brevibloc (esmolol HCl) Injection (About 2%) ... 1860
Brevicon ... 2563
Bricanyl Subcutaneous Injection ... 1247
Bricanyl Tablets ... 1248
▲ Bromfed-DM Cough Syrup (Among most frequent) ... 1832
Bronkometer Aerosol ... 2432
Bronkosol Solution ... 2432
Brontex ... 2130
Bumex (0.6%) ... 2260
▲ Buprenex Injectable (1-5%) ... 2170
▲ BuSpar Tablets (6%) ... 738
Butisol Sodium Elixir & Tablets (Less than 1 in 100) ... 2768
Calan SR Caplets (2.2%) ... 2571
Calan Tablets (2.2%) ... 2568
Calcijex Injection ... 412
Capoten Tablets (About 0.5 to 2%) ... 740
Capozide Tablets (0.5 to 2%) ... 744
Carafate Suspension (Less than 0.5%) ... 1250
Carafate Tablets (Less than 0.5%) 1249
Carbastat Intraocular Solution ... ⊚ 260
Carbocaine Injection ... 2432
▲ Cardene Capsules (6.4% to 8.2%) 2261
▲ Cardene I.V. (14.6) ... 2815
▲ Cardene SR Capsules (6.2%) ... 2264
Cardioquin Tablets ... 2146
▲ Cardizem CD Capsules (4.6% to 5.4%) ... 1251
▲ Cardizem SR Capsules (4.5% to 12%) ... 1255
Cardizem Injectable (Less than 1%) ... 1253
Cardizem Tablets (2.1%) ... 1257
▲ Cardura Tablets (9.9% to 14%) ... 1993
Cartrol Tablets (0.7%) ... 413
▲ Casodex Tablets (4%) ... 2934
▲ Cataflam Tablets (3% to 9%) ... 833
Catapres Tablets (About 1 in 100 patients) ... 679
▲ Catapres-TTS (5 of 101 patients) .. 680
Caverject Injection (2%) ... 2064
Cedax (0.1% to 3%) ... 2480
Ceftin (0.1% to 1%) ... 1067
Cefzil Tablets and Oral Suspension (Less than 1%) ... 747
Celestone Soluspan Suspension ... 2484
▲ CellCept Capsules (16.1% to 21.1%) ... 2265
Celontin Kapseals ... 1955
Ceptaz (Fewer than 1%) ... 1070
▲ Cerebyx Injection (2.2% to 8.9%) 1956
Ceredase ... 1055
Cerezyme (Three patients) ... 1056
▲ Chemet Capsules (5.2% to 15.7%) ... 666
Chloromycetin Sodium Succinate... 1960
Cholera Vaccine ... 2818
▲ Cipro I.V. (Among most frequent) .. 587
Cipro I.V. Pharmacy Bulk Package (Greater than 1%) ... 590
Cipro Tablets (1% to 1.2%) ... 584
Claforan Sterile and Injection (Less than 1%) ... 1259
▲ Claritin Tablets (12%) ... 2485
▲ Claritin-D Tablets (19%) ... 2487
Climara Transdermal System ... 640
Cleocin Vaginal Cream (Less than 1% to 2%) ... 2070
▲ Clinoril Tablets (3% to 9%) ... 1658
Clomid (1.3%) ... 1262
▲ Clozaril Tablets (More than 5 to 7%) ... 2377
▲ Cognex Capsules (11%) ... 1961
ColBENEMID Tablets ... 1662
Colestid ... 2073
Combipres Tablets (About 1 in 100) ... 682
Compazine ... 2644
Cordarone Tablets (1 to 3%) ... 2818
Cormax Scalp Application (Approximately 0.3%) ... 1857
CORTENEMA ... 2713
Cortifoam ... 2540
Cortone Acetate Sterile Suspension ... 1663
Cortone Acetate Tablets ... 1664
▲ Corvert Injection (3.6%) ... 2075
Coumadin (Infrequent) ... 941
▲ Covera-HS Tablets (2.2% to 6.6%) ... 2573
Cozaar Tablets (1% or greater) ... 1668
▲ Crixivan Capsules (5.6%) ... 1670
Cycrin Tablets ... 991
Cylert Tablets ... 415
▲ Cytadren Tablets (1 in 20) ... 837
CytoGam (Infrequent) ... 1630

(⊠ Described in PDR For Nonprescription Drugs)   Incidence data in parenthesis; ▲ 3% or more   (⊚ Described in PDR For Ophthalmology)

Headache — **Side Effects Index** — **1350**

Cytosar-U Sterile Powder (Less frequent) 2077
Cytotec (2.4%) 2576
▲ Cytovene (4%) 2270
D.A. II Tablets 972
D.A. Chewable Tablets 970
DDAVP Injection (Infrequent) 2178
DDAVP Injection 15 mcg/mL (Infrequent) 2179
▲ DDAVP (2 to 5%) 2180
DDAVP Tablets 2182
D.H.E. 45 Injection (Occasional) 2381
Dalalone D.P. Injectable 1009
Dalgan Injection (Less than 1%) 529
Dalmane Capsules 2329
Danocrine Capsules 2437
Dantrium Capsules (Less frequent) 2131
Dapsone Tablets USP 1331
Daranide Tablets 1676
Daraprim Tablets (Rare) 1199
Darvon-N/Darvocet-N 1473
Darvon 1475
Darvon-N Suspension & Tablets 1473
▲ DaunoXome (3% to 22%) 1842
Decadron Elixir 1676
Decadron Phosphate Injection 1680
Decadron Phosphate with Xylocaine Injection, Sterile 1683
Decadron Tablets 1678
Decadron-LA Sterile Suspension 1687
Declomycin Tablets 1421
Deconsal II Tablets 1605
▲ Demadex Tablets and Injection (7.3%) 691
Demerol 2438
Demser Capsules (Infrequent) 1690
Demulen 2580
Depakene 416
Depakote Tablets 418
▲ Depo-Provera Contraceptive Injection (More than 5%) 2079
Depo-Provera Sterile Aqueous Suspension 2083
▲ Deponit NTG Transdermal Delivery System (Most common; 63%) 2541
Desmopressin Acetate Injection (Infrequent) 996
▲ Desmopressin Acetate Rhinal Tube (2% to 5%) 997
Desogen Tablets 1867
Desoxyn Gradumet Tablets 422
▲ Desyrel and Desyrel Dividose (9.9% to 19.8%) 504
Dexacort Phosphate in Respihaler 1606
Dexacort Phosphate in Turbinaire 1607
Dexatrim ▣ 795
Dexatrim Plus Vitamins Caplets ▣ 796
Dexedrine 2648
DextroStat-Dextroamphetamine Sulfate Tablets 2211
Diethylstilbestrol Tablets 1477
▲ Diflucan Tablets, Injection, and Oral Suspension (1.9% to 13% of patients) 2003
▲ Dilacor XR Extended-release Capsules (2.9% to 8.9%) 2183
Dilantin Infatabs 1967
Dilantin Kapseals 1965
Dilantin-125 Suspension 1969
▲ Dilatrate-SR Capsules (Most common) 2542
Dilaudid-HP Injection (Less frequent) 1384
Dilaudid-HP Lyophilized Powder 250 mg (Less frequent) 1384
Dilaudid Tablets and Liquid (Less frequent) 1386
Dimetane-DC Cough Syrup 2232
Dimetane-DX Cough Syrup 2233
▲ Dipentum Capsules (5.0%) 2084
Diprivan Injectable Emulsion (Less than 1%) 2939
Diucardin Tablets 2824
Diupres Tablets 1691
Diuril Oral Suspension 1694
Diuril Sodium Intravenous 1693
Diuril Tablets 1694
Dizac (diazepam injectable emulsion) CIV (Less frequent) 1862
Dobutrex Solution Vials (1% to 3%) 1480
▲ Dolobid Tablets (3% to 9%) 1695
Donnatal 2234
Donnatal Extentabs 2234
Donnatal Tablets 2234
Dopram Injectable 2235
▲ Doral Tablets (4.5%) 2773
▲ Doxil (Approximately 6.8%) 2613
▲ Duragesic Transdermal System (3% to 10%) 1336
Duramorph Injection (A significant minority of cases) 983
Duranest Injections 533
Dura-Tap/PD Capsules 970
Duratuss Tablets 2750
Dura-Vent/DA Tablets 972
Dura-Vent Tablets 971
Dyazide Capsules 2653
▲ Dynabac (8.6%) 668
DYNACIN Capsules 1627
▲ DynaCirc Capsules (10.7% to 22.0%) 2381
▲ DynaCirc CR Tablets (10.3% to 13.9%) 2383
Dyrenium Capsules (Rare) 2655
Easprin 1971
▲ EC-Naprosyn Delayed-Release Tablets (3% to 9%) 2277
Edecrin 1698
▲ Effexor (3% to 25%) 2825
Elavil 2945
▲ Eldepryl Capsules (2 of 49 patients) 2729
Elspar 1700
Emcyt Capsules (1%) 2085
Emete-con Intramuscular/Intravenous 2007
▲ Eminase (Less than 10%) 2215
Enduron Tablets 424
▲ Engerix-B Unit-Dose Vials (1% to 10%) 2656
Entex LA Tablets 972
Entex PSE Tablets 973
EPIFRIN ⊙ 237
EpiPen 808
▲ Epivir (35%) 1200
▲ Epogen for Injection (0.4% to 19%) 489
▲ Ergamisol Tablets (3% to 4%) 1340
Esgic-plus Capsules (Infrequent) 1012
Esgic-plus Tablets (Infrequent) 1012
Esidrix Tablets 839
Esimil Tablets 840
Eskalith 2658
Estrace Cream and Tablets 751
Estraderm Transdermal System 842
ESTRATAB Tablets (0.3, 0.625, 1.25, 2.5 mg) 2715
Estratest 2718
▲ Estring Vaginal Ring (13%) 2086
▲ Ethmozine Tablets (5.8% to 8.0%) 2217
Etrafon 2495
Exgest LA Tablets 787
Factrel (Rare) 2996
▲ Famvir Tablets (Among most frequent; 22.7% to 23.6%) 2660
Fansidar Tablets 2281
Fastin Capsules 2662
Fedahist Gyrocaps 2545
▲ Felbatol (Among most common; 6.5% to 36.8%) 2774
Feldene Capsules (Greater than 1%) 2008
Fioricet Tablets (Infrequent) 2386
Fioricet with Codeine Capsules (Infrequent) 2387
Fiorinal with Codeine Capsules (Infrequent) 2390
Flagyl 375 Capsules (Sometimes) 2587
Flagyl I.V. 2373
Flexeril Tablets (1% to 3%) 1701
▲ Flolan for Injection (49% to 83%) 1085
Flonase Nasal Spray (1% to 3%) 1088
Florinef Acetate Tablets 506
▲ Flovent (17% to 34%) 1089
▲ Floxin I.V. (1% to 9%) 1580
▲ Floxin Tablets (200 mg, 300 mg, 400 mg) (1% to 9%) 1577
Fludara for Injection (Up to 3%) 658
Flumadine Tablets & Syrup (1.4%) 1013
Fluorescite ⊙ 217
Fluorouracil Injection 2282
Fortaz (Less than 1%) 1092
▲ Fosamax Tablets (2.6%) 1703
▲ Foscavir Injection (5% or greater up to 26%) 541
Sterile FUDR (Remote possibility) 2284
Fulvicin P/G Tablets (Occasional) 2499
Fulvicin P/G 165 & 330 Tablets (Occasional) 2500
▲ Fungizone Intravenous (Among most common) 507
Furoxone (Occasional) 2221
Gamimune N, 5% Immune Globulin Intravenous (Human), 5% 612
Gamimune N, 10% Immune Globulin Intravenous (Human), 10% 615
Gammagard S/D, Immune Globulin, Intravenous (Human) (Occasional; 12 of 16 patients) 577
▲ Gammar-P I.V., Immune Globulin Intravenous (Human) (5.4%) 798
Gantanol Tablets 2285
Gantrisin 2286
Garamycin Injectable 2502
▲ Gastrocrom Capsules (4 of 87 patients) 1611
▲ Gastrocrom Oral Concentrate (4 of 87 patients) 1611
Gemzar for Injection (Common) 1482
Genotropin Injection (Infrequent) 2090
Geocillin Tablets 2009
Geref (sermorelin acetate for injection) 2995
Glucotrol Tablets (About 1 in 50) 2011
▲ Glucotrol XL Extended Release Tablets (8.6%) 2012
Grifulvin V (griseofulvin tablets) Microsize (griseofulvin oral suspension) Microsize (Occasional) 1944
Gris-PEG Tablets, 125 mg & 250 mg (Occasional) 476
Guaifed 1833
Guaimax-D Tablets 809
▲ Habitrol Nicotine Transdermal System (17%) 884
▲ Halcion Tablets (9.7%) 2093
Haldol Decanoate 1587
Haldol Injection, Tablets and Concentrate 1585
Halotestin Tablets 2095
▲ Havrix (14% of adults; less than 9% of children) 2663
Helidac Therapy (Sometimes) 2135
Heparin Lock Flush Solution 2831
Heparin Sodium Injection 2832
Heparin Sodium Vials (Rare) 1486
Hespan Injection 945
▲ Hismanal Tablets (6.7%) 1341
Histussin D Liquid 670
Hivid Tablets (Less than 1% to 2.1%) 2287
Humatrope Vials (Infrequent) 1490
Humegon for Injection 1873
Humorsol Sterile Ophthalmic Solution 1707
▲ Hycamtin for Injection (0.2% to 21%) 2665
Hydeltrasol Injection, Sterile 1708
Hydeltra-T.B.A. Sterile Suspension 1710
Hydralazine Hydrochloride Injection USP (Common) 2712
Hydrea Capsules (Extremely rare) 705
Hydrocortone Acetate Sterile Suspension 1712
Hydrocortone Phosphate Injection, Sterile 1713
Hydrocortone Tablets 1715
HydroDIURIL Tablets 1716
Hydropres Tablets 1718
▲ Hylorel Tablets (58.1%) 1613
Hyperstat I.V. Injection 2504
▲ Hytrin Capsules (1.1% to 16.2%) 434
Hyzaar Tablets (1% or greater) 1720
IBU Tablets (Greater than 1%) 1389
▲ Idamycin Injection (20%) 2096
▲ Imdur (38% to 57%) 1362
Imitrex Injection (2.2%) 1095
Imitrex Tablets 1099
▲ Imovax Rabies Vaccine (About 20%) 899
Inderide Tablets 2838
Inderide LA Long Acting Capsules 2840
▲ Indocin (11.7%) 1723
INFeD (Iron Dextran Injection, USP) 2478
Infumorph 200 and Infumorph 500 Sterile Solutions (A significant minority of cases) 985
Intal Inhaler (Infrequent) 2185
Intal Nebulizer Solution 2186
▲ Intron A for Injection (4% to 62%) 2506
Invirase Capsules (Rare; 0.6%) 2291
Ionamin Capsules 1615
IOPIDINE Sterile Ophthalmic Solution ⊙ 218
Iopidine 0.5% (Less than 3%) ⊙ 219
▲ Ismo Tablets (19% to 38%) 2844
ISMOTIC 45% w/v Solution ⊙ 221
Isoetharine Inhalation Solution, USP, Arm-a-Med 545
Isoptin Injectable (1.2%) 1391
Isoptin Oral Tablets (2.2%) 1393
Isoptin SR Tablets (2.2%) 1395
Isopto Carbachol Ophthalmic Solution ⊙ 221
▲ Isordil Sublingual Tablets (Most common) 2845
▲ Isordil Tembids (Most common) 2847
▲ Isordil Titradose Tablets (Most common) 2848
Isuprel Hydrochloride Solution 2443
Isuprel Injection 2441
Isuprel Mistometer 2442
▲ JE-VAX (Less than 3% to approximately 15.2%) 904
K-Phos Neutral Tablets 633
Kadian Capsules (Less than 3%) 2948
Keflex Pulvules & Oral Suspension 930
Keftab Tablets 931
▲ Kerlone Tablets (6.5% to 14.8%) 2588
Klonopin Tablets 2294
Konȳne 80 Factor IX Complex 627
Kutrase Capsules 2546
▲ Kytril Injection (14%) 2667
▲ Kytril Tablets (14% to 21%) 2669
▲ Lamictal Tablets (Among most common; 29.1%) 1105
▲ Lamisil Tablets (12.9%) 2394
Lamprene Capsules (Less than 1%) 846
Lanoxicaps 1110
Lanoxin Elixir Pediatric 1113
Lanoxin Injection 1116
Lanoxin Injection Pediatric 1119
Lanoxin Tablets 1121
▲ Lariam Tablets (Among most frequent) 2295
Larodopa Tablets (Relatively frequent) 2296
Lasix Injection, Oral Solution and Tablets 1267
▲ Lescol Capsules (8.9%) 2395
▲ Leukine (26%) 1317
▲ Leustatin (7% to 22%) 1889
▲ Levatol Tablets (7.8%) 2547
Levbid Extended-Release Tablets 2549
Levlen/Tri-Levlen 646
Levophed Bitartrate Injection 2445
Levsin/Levsinex/Levbid 2549
Limbitrol 2333
▲ Lioresal Intrathecal (1.6% to 10.7%) 1634
▲ Lioresal Tablets (4% to 8%) 847
Lithium Carbonate Capsules & Tablets 2352
Lithonate/Lithotabs/Lithobid 2721
▲ Livostin (5%) ⊙ 262
Lodine Capsules and Tablets (Less Than 1%) 2849
Lomotil 2591
Lo/Ovral Tablets 2852
Lo/Ovral-28 Tablets 2857
Lopid Tablets (1.2%) 1974
Lopressor 848
▲ Lopressor HCT Tablets (10 in 100 patients) 850
Lorabid Suspension and Pulvules (0.9% to 3.2%) 1513
▲ Lotensin Tablets (6.2%) 852
▲ Lotensin HCT Tablets (3.1%) 855
Lotrel Capsules (2.2%) 858
Loxitane 1426
▲ Ludiomil Tablets (4%) 861
Lufyllin & Lufyllin-400 Tablets 2778
Lufyllin-GG Elixir & Tablets 2779
▲ Lupron Depot 3.75 mg (25.9%) 2739
▲ Lupron Depot - 3 Month 22.5 mg (6.4%) 2743
Lupron Depot-PED 7.5 mg, 11.25 mg and 15 mg (Less than 2%) 2744
▲ Lupron Injection (5% or more) 2736
Lupron Injection Pediatric (Less than 2%) 2737
▲ LUVOX Tablets (22%) 2723
M-M-R II 1730
M-R-VAX II 1732
MS Contin Tablets (Less frequent) 2149
MSIR (Infrequent) 2152
▲ Macrobid Capsules (6%) 2138
Marax Tablets & DF Syrup 2015
Marcaine 2446
Marcaine Spinal 2449
Marinol (Dronabinol) Capsules (Less than 1%) 2353
Matulane Capsules 2300
Mavik Tablets (More than 1%) 1407
Maxair Autohaler (1.3% to 2.0%) 1550
Maxair Inhaler (2.0%) 1552
▲ Maxaquin Tablets (3.2%) 2593
Maxipime for Injection (0.1% to 1%) 758
Mebaral Tablets (Less than 1 in 100) 2452
▲ Megace Oral Suspension (Up to 10%) 708
Mellaril (Extremely rare) 2398

(▣ Described in PDR For Nonprescription Drugs) Incidence data in parenthesis; ▲ 3% or more (⊙ Described in PDR For Ophthalmology)

Menest Tablets 2671
Mepergan Injection 2859
▲ Mepron Suspension (16% to 18%) 1206
Merrem I.V. (2.8%) 2952
Meruvax II 1740
▲ Mesnex Injection (50%) 711
Methadone Hydrochloride Oral Concentrate 2356
Methadone Hydrochloride Oral Solution & Tablets 2357
Methergine 2401
Methotrexate Sodium Tablets, Injection, for Injection and LPF Injection (Less common) 1322
Metrodin (urofollitropin for injection) 2616
MetroGel-Vaginal (Equal to or less than 2%) 917
▲ Mevacor Tablets (2.1% to 9.3%) 1742
▲ Mexitil Capsules (5.7% to 7.5%) 684
▲ Miacalcin Nasal Spray (3.2%) 2403
Micronor Tablets (Less common) 1903
▲ Midamor Tablets (3% to 8%) 1746
Miltown Tablets 2780
▲ Minipress Capsules (7.8%) 2015
▲ Minizide Capsules (7.8%) 2016
Minocin Intravenous 1428
Minocin Oral Suspension 1431
Minocin Pellet-Filled Capsules 1429
Mintezol 1747
MIOSTAT Intraocular Solution ⊙ 222
Mithracin 599
Modicon 1928
▲ Moduretic Tablets (3% to 8%) 1748
8-MOP Capsules 1294
Monistat Dual-Pak (1.3%) 1906
Monistat 3 Vaginal Suppositories (1.3%) 1905
Mono-Gesic Tablets 810
▲ Monoket Tablets (13% to 35%) 2550
Mononine, Coagulation Factor IX (Human), Monoclonal Antibody Purified 804
Monopril Tablets (Less than 1.0% to 1.0% or more) 762
Motofen Tablets (1 in 40) 789
Motrin Ibuprofen Suspension, Oral Drops, Chewable Tablets, Caplets (1% to less than 3%) 1563
MSTA Mumps Skin Test Antigen 2988
Mutamycin for Injection 712
Myambutol Tablets 1432
▲ Mycobutin Capsules (3%) 2101
▲ Mykrox Tablets (9.3%) 1617
Myochrysine Injection 1754
▲ Nalfon 200 Pulvules & Nalfon Tablets (8.7%) 933
▲ Naprelan Tablets (15%) 2861
▲ Anaprox/Naprosyn (3% to 9%) 2277
Nardil (Common) 1977
Nasacort AQ Nasal Spray (2% or greater) 2191
▲ Nasacort Nasal Inhaler (Approximately 18%) 2189
Nasalcrom Nasal Solution (1 in 50) 2192
Nasalide Nasal Solution 0.025% (5% or less) 2301
Nebcin Vials, Hyporets & ADD-Vantage 1518
NegGram (Occasional) 2453
Nembutal Sodium Capsules 440
Nembutal Sodium Solution 442
Nembutal Sodium Suppositories (Less than 1%) 444
▲ Neoral (2% to 15%) 2405
Neo-Synephrine Hydrochloride 1% Carpuject 2455
Neo-Synephrine Hydrochloride 1% Injection 2455
Nescaine/Nescaine MPF 549
Netromycin Injection 100 mg/ml (Fewer than 1 of 1000 patients) 2516
▲ Neupogen for Injection (7%) 495
Neurontin Capsules (More than 1%) 1978
▲ Nicotrol NS Nicotine Nasal Spray (18%) 1565
▲ Nimotop Capsules (Up to 4.1%) 603
▲ Nipent for Injection (13% to 17%) 2733
▲ Nitro-Bid IV (Most common) 1270
▲ Nitro-Bid Ointment (Most common) 1272
▲ Nitro-Dur (nitroglycerin) Transdermal Infusion System (Most common) 1365
▲ Nitrolingual Spray (50%) 2193
Nitrostat Tablets 1981
Nizoral Tablets (Less than 1%) 1345
Nolvadex Tablets (Infrequent) 2957
Nordette-21 Tablets 2863
Nordette-28 Tablets 2866
Norflex 1554
Norgesic 1554
Norinyl 2563
Norisodrine with Calcium Iodide Syrup 446
Normodyne Tablets (2%) 2522
Noroxin Tablets (2.0% to 2.8%) 1758
Noroxin Tablets (2.0% to 2.8%) 2222
▲ Norpace (3 to 9%) 2596
Norplant System 2868
Norpramin Tablets 1273
Nor-Q D Tablets 2598
▲ Norvasc Tablets (7.3%) 2020
▲ Norvir (5.1% to 6.3%) 447
Novahistine DMX ◘ 782
Novahistine Elixir ◘ 782
▲ Novantrone for Injection (10 to 13%) 1327
Novocain Hydrochloride for Spinal Anesthesia 2457
▲ Nubain Injection (3%) 952
Nucofed 2225
Numorphan Injection 953
Numorphan Suppositories 953
Nutropin (A small number of patients) 1049
Nutropin AQ Injection (A small number of patients) 1051
Ocupress Ophthalmic Solution, 1% Sterile (Occasional) ⊙ 297
Ogen Tablets 2103
Ogen Vaginal Cream 2106
▲ Oncaspar (Greater than 1% but less than 5%) 2194
Oncovin Solution Vials & Hyporets 1521
OptiPranolol (Metipranolol 0.3%) Sterile Ophthalmic Solution (A small number of patients) ⊙ 256
Oramorph SR (Morphine Sulfate Sustained Release Tablets) (Less frequent) 2359
▲ Orap Tablets (1 of 20 patients; 22.2%) 1037
Oretic Tablets 450
Organidin NR Tablets and Liquid (Rare) 2781
▲ Orlaam Oral Solution (1% to 3%) 2361
Ornade Spansule Capsules 2678
Ortho-Cept 1907
Ortho-Cyclen/Ortho-Tri-Cyclen 1914
Ortho Dienestrol Cream 1922
Ortho-Est 1925
Ortho-Novum 1928
Ortho-Cyclen/Ortho Tri-Cyclen 1914
▲ Orthoclone OKT3 Sterile Solution (11% to 44%) 1892
▲ Orudis Capsules (3% to 9%) 2874
▲ Oruvail Capsules (3% to 9%) 2874
OSMOGLYN Oral Osmotic Agent ⊙ 225
Ovcon 765
Ovral Tablets 2877
Ovral-28 Tablets 2878
Ovrette Tablets 2878
Oxsoralen-Ultra Capsules 1302
▲ OxyContin Tablets (7%) 2163
PBZ Tablets 863
PBZ-SR Tablets 862
Pamelor 2409
Papaverine Hydrochloride Vials and Ampoules 1523
Paremyd ⊙ 244
▲ Parlodel (Less than 2% to 19%) 2411
Parnate Tablets 2679
▲ Paxil Tablets (18%) 2681
Pediapred Oral Solution 1618
Pediazole Suspension 2340
Peganone Tablets 455
Penetrex Tablets (Up to 2%) 2196
Pentasa (2.0% to 2.2%) 1275
Pentaspan Injection 954
▲ Pepcid Injection (4.7%) 1765
▲ Pepcid (4.7%) 1763
Peptavlon 2997
Pergonal (menotropins for injection, USP) 2618
Periactin 1767
▲ Permax Tablets (5.3%) 571
Persantine Tablets (2.3%) 686
Phenergan with Codeine 2883
Phenergan VC with Codeine 2888
Phenobarbital Elixir and Tablets (Less than 1 in 100 patients) 1523
Phenurone Tablets (2%) 455
Phrenilin (Infrequent) 790
Pipracil 1435
Plaquenil Sulfate Tablets 2459
▲ Plendil Extended-Release Tablets (10.6% to 14.7%) 514
PMB 200 and PMB 400 2890
Pneumovax 23 1768
Pondimin Tablets 2239
Ponstel 1982
Pontocaine Hydrochloride for Spinal Anesthesia 2460
▲ Pravachol Tablets (1.7% to 6.2%) 770
Pregnyl for Injection 1878
Prelone Syrup 1834
Prelu-2 Timed Release Capsules 687
Premarin Intravenous 2893
Premarin Tablets 2896
Premarin Vaginal Cream 2898
Premphase 2900
Prempro 2905
Prevacid Delayed-Release Capsules (Greater than 1%) 2746
▲ Prilosec Delayed-Release Capsules (2.9% to 6.9%) 516
Primacor Injection (2.9%) 2461
Primaxin I.M. 1770
Primaxin I.V. (Less than 0.2%) 1772
▲ Prinivil Tablets (4.4% to 5.7%) 1776
▲ Prinzide Tablets (5.2%) 1780
Pro-Banthine Tablets 2226
▲ Procardia Capsules (Approximately 10% to 23%; 1 in 8 patients) 2024
▲ Procardia XL Extended Release Tablets (15.8% to 23%) 2026
▲ Procrit for Injection (0.40% to 19%) 1896
Profasi (chorionic gonadotropin for injection, USP) 2620
Proglycem 575
▲ Prograf (31% to 64%) 1028
▲ Proleukin for Injection (12%) 812
Prolixin 510
PROPINE with C CAP Compliance Cap ⊙ 251
▲ Propulsid (19.3%) 1346
▲ ProSom Tablets (16%) 457
▲ Prostep (nicotine transdermal system) (11%) 1439
Prostigmin Injectable 1305
Prostigmin Tablets 1306
▲ Prostin E2 Suppository (Approximately one-tenth) 2109
Protopam Chloride for Injection 2909
Protostat Tablets 1939
Proventil Inhalation Aerosol 2524
▲ Proventil Inhalation Solution 0.083% (3% to 3.1%) 2527
▲ Proventil Repetabs Tablets (7%) 2529
▲ Proventil Solution for Inhalation 0.5% (3% to 3.1%) 2525
▲ Proventil Syrup (4 of 100 patients) 2528
▲ Proventil Tablets (7%) 2529
Provera Tablets 2110
▲ Prozac Pulvules & Liquid, Oral Solution (20.3% to 33%) 935
Pyridium 1985
Quadrinal Tablets 1398
Questran 774
Quibron 2227
▲ Quinaglute Dura-Tabs Tablets (3%) 644
▲ Quinidex Extentabs (7%) 2240
RMS Suppositories CII 2766
▲ Rabies Vaccine Adsorbed (8% to 10%) 2686
▲ Rabies Vaccine, Imovax Rabies I.D. (About 20%) 901
Recombivax HB (Equal to or greater than 1%) 1787
▲ Redux Capsules (16.1%) 2911
Reglan (Less frequent) 2243
▲ Relafen Tablets (3% to 9%) 2688
Respbid Tablets 687
▲ Retrovir Capsules (1.6% to 62.5%) 1216
▲ Retrovir I.V. Infusion (2% to 62.5%) 1221
▲ Retrovir Syrup (1.6% to 62.5%) 1216
▲ Rev-Eyes Ophthalmic Eyedrops 0.5% (10% to 40%) ⊙ 324
▲ ReVia Tablets (7% to more than 10%) 957
Revex (nalmefene hydrochloride injection) (1%) 1863
Rifadin 1276
Rifamate Capsules 1278
Rifater 1280
▲ Rilutek Tablets (7.0% to 8.0%) 2198
Rimactane Capsules 865
▲ Risperdal Tablets (12% to 14%) 1348
Ritalin 866
Robaxin Injectable 2245
Robaxin Tablets 2246
Robaxisal Tablets 2246
Robinul Forte Tablets 2247
Robinul Injectable 2247
Robinul Tablets 2247
Rocaltrol Capsules 2303
Rocephin Injectable Vials, ADD-Vantage, Galaxy Container (Occasional) 2305
▲ Roferon-A Injection (44% to 66%) 2308
▲ Romazicon (1% to 9%) 2311
Rondec Oral Drops 974
Rondec Syrup 974
Rondec 974
▲ Rowasa (6.50%) 2727
Roxanol 2365
▲ Rythmol Tablets–150mg, 225mg, 300mg (1.5 to 4.5%) 1399
▲ Salagen Tablets (11%) 1546
▲ Sandimmune (2 to 15%) 2416
▲ Sandoglobulin I.V. (Most common; 2%) 2419
▲ Sandostatin Injection (6%) 2421
Sanorex Tablets 2423
Scleromate Injection (Rare) 1234
Seconal Sodium Pulvules (Less than 1 in 100) 1529
▲ Sectral Capsules (6%) 2914
Sedapap Tablets 50 mg/650 mg (Infrequent) 1826
▲ Seldane Tablets (6.3% to 15.8%) 1284
▲ Seldane-D Extended-Release Tablets (17.4%) 1286
▲ Semprex-D Capsules (19%) 1620
Sensorcaine 554
Septra 1146
Septra I.V. Infusion 1142
Septra I.V. Infusion ADD-Vantage Vials 1144
Septra 1146
Ser-Ap-Es Tablets 867
Serax Capsules (In few instances) 2916
Serax Tablets (In few instances) 2916
▲ Serevent Inhalation Aerosol (28%) 1149
Seromycin Capsules 975
Serophene (clomiphene citrate tablets, USP) (Less than 1 in 100 patients) 2621
▲ Serzone Tablets (36%) 776
Sinemet Tablets 959
Sinemet CR Tablets (2.0%) 961
Sinequan (Occasional) 2028
Skelaxin Tablets 793
Slo-bid Gyrocaps 2201
Slo-Niacin Tablets 2767
Solganal Suspension (Rare) 2530
Soma Compound w/Codeine Tablets (Infrequent or rare) 2784
Soma Compound Tablets (Infrequent or rare) 2783
Soma Tablets 2782
▲ Sorbitrate (Most common) 2959
Sotradecol (Sodium Tetradecyl Sulfate Injection) 987
▲ Sporanox Capsules (1.5% to 3.8%) 1352
▲ Stadol (3% to 9%) 779
Stelazine 2692
Streptase for Infusion 557
Streptomycin Sulfate Injection 2031
▲ Sular Tablets (22%) 2961
▲ Supprelin Injection (22%) 2230
Suprane (desflurane, USP) (Greater than 1%) 1865
Suprax (Less than 2%) 1443
Surmontil Capsules 2917
Sus-Phrine Injection 1017
Symmetrel Capsules (1% to 5%) 965
Symmetrel Syrup (1% to 5%) 963
▲ Synarel Nasal Solution for Endometriosis (19% of patients) 2605
Syn-Rx Tablets 1622
Syn-Rx DM Tablets 1623
Tagamet (2.1% to 3.5%) 2694
Talacen Caplets 2464
Talwin Injection 2465
Talwin Compound 2466
Talwin Injection 2465
Talwin Nx Tablets 2467
▲ Tambocor Tablets (9.6%) 1555
Tapazole Tablets 1361
Tavist Syrup 2426
Tavist Tablets 2427
Tazicef for Injection (Less than 1%) 2697
Tazidime Vials, Faspak & ADD-Vantage (Less than 1%) 1531
▲ Tegison Capsules (25-50%) 2314
Tegretol/Tegretol-XR 870
Temovate Scalp Application (1 of 294 patients) 1153

(◘ Described in PDR For Nonprescription Drugs) Incidence data in parenthesis; ▲ 3% or more (⊙ Described in PDR For Ophthalmology)

Headache Side Effects Index 1352

▲ Tenex Tablets (1% to 13%) 2249
Tenoretic Tablets 2963
Tenormin Tablets and I.V. Injection 2965
▲ Terazol 3 Vaginal Cream (21%)...... 1941
▲ Terazol 3 Vaginal Suppositories (30.3% of 284 patients)........... 1942
▲ Terazol 7 Vaginal Cream (26% of 521 patients) 1943
Tessalon Perles........... 1018
Testoderm Testosterone Transdermal System 486
Testred Capsules, 10 mg........... 1308
Thalitone 1293
Theo-24 Extended Release Capsules 2753
Theo-Dur Extended-Release Tablets 1367
Theo-X Extended-Release Tablets .. 793
TheraCys BCG Live (Intravesical) (Up to 1.8%)........... 911
Thioplex (Thiotepa For Injection) 1329
THYREL TRH........... 2992
▲ Tiazac Capsules (18%) 1019
TICE BCG, USP (2.4%) 1881
Ticlid Tablets (0.5% to 1.0%) 2317
Tigan........... 2231
▲ Tilade Inhaler (6.0%) 2207
Timentin for Injection........... 2706
Timolide Tablets (Less than 1%).... 1791
Timoptic in Ocudose (Less frequent) 1796
Timoptic Sterile Ophthalmic Solution (Less frequent) 1794
Timoptic-XE (1% to 5% of patients) 1798
Tofranil Ampuls 873
Tofranil Tablets 875
Tofranil-PM Capsules........... 876
▲ Tolectin (200, 400 and 600 mg) (3 to 9%) 1591
Tonocard Tablets (2.1% to 4.6%) 519
Toprol-XL Tablets 560
▲ Toradol (17%) 2319
Torecan (Occasional)........... 2367
▲ Tornalate Solution for Inhalation, 0.2% (8.4%) 976
▲ Tornalate Metered Dose Inhaler (3.5% to 4%)........... 978
Trancopal Caplets........... 2468
Trandate 1158
Transderm Scōp Transdermal Therapeutic System (Few patients) 890
▲ Transderm-Nitro Transdermal Therapeutic System (63%) 878
Tranxene (Less common)........... 459
Trental Tablets (1.2%)........... 1291
Triavil Tablets 1800
Trilafon........... 2532
Levlen/Tri-Levlen........... 646
Trilisate (Less than 2%)........... 2155
Trinalin Repetabs Tablets 1373
Tri-Norinyl........... 2607
Triphasil-21 Tablets........... 2919
Triphasil-28 Tablets........... 2924
Trusopt Sterile Ophthalmic Solution (Infrequent) 1803
Tussend 1830
Tussend Expectorant........... 1831
Tussi-Organidin DM NR Liquid and DM-S NR Liquid (Rare) 2786
Tympagesic Ear Drops 2476
▲ Typhim Vi (Up to 27%) 914
Typhoid Vaccine........... 2929
▲ Ultram Tablets (50 mg) (18% to 32%) 1594
Unasyn (Less than 1%) 2035
Uni-Dur Extended-Release Tablets.. 1374
Uniphyl 400 mg and 600 mg Tablets 2157
Univasc Tablets (More than 1%) 2553
Urecholine........... 1804
Urispas Tablets........... 2710
Uroqid-Acid No. 2 Tablets 633
Valium Injectable 2336
Valium Tablets (Infrequent) 2335
▲ Valtrex Caplets (13% to 17%)........... 1167
Vancenase AQ Nasal Spray 0.042% (Fewer than 5 per 100 patients) 2535
▲ Vancenase AQ Double Strength Nasal Spray 0.084% (33% to 34%) 2536
Vantin for Oral Suspension and Vantin Tablets (Less than 1% to 1.1%)........... 2112
▲ Vaqta (0.4% to 16.8%)........... 1805
Varivax (Greater than or equal to 1%)........... 1807
▲ Vascor Tablets (200 and 300 mg) (6.98 to 13.64%) 1597
▲ Vaseretic Tablets (5.5%)........... 1810
Vasotec I.V. (2.9%) 1814
▲ Vasotec Tablets (1.8% to 5.2%).... 1816
Vasoxyl Injection 1169
Velban Vials 1537
▲ Ventolin Inhalation Aerosol and Refill (3%) 1170
▲ Ventolin Inhalation Solution (3.1%) 1171
▲ Ventolin Nebules Inhalation Solution (3% to 3.1%)........... 1172
▲ Ventolin Rotacaps for Inhalation (2% to 5%)........... 1173
▲ Ventolin Syrup (4 of 100 patients) 1175
▲ Ventolin Tablets (7 of 100 patients) 1176
▲ Verelan Capsules (2.2% to 5.3%) 1455
Versed Injection (1.3% to 1.5%).... 2324
▲ Vesanoid Capsules (86%)........... 2327
Vexol 1% Ophthalmic Suspension (Less than 2%) ...... ⊙ 227
▲ Videx Tablets, Powder for Oral Solution, & Pediatric Powder for Oral Solution (6% to 55%) 2980
▲ Viramune Tablets (Among most frequent; 3%) 2368
▲ Vistide Injection (27%)........... 1057
Vivactil Tablets 1820
▲ Vivelle Transdermal System (Approximately 36%) 880
Vivotif Berna 660
▲ Volmax Extended-Release Tablets (18.8%) 1835
▲ Cataflam/Voltaren/Voltaren-XR (3% to 9%)........... 833
WinRho SD (2%)........... 1840
Wygesic Tablets 2930
▲ Xanax Tablets (12.9% to 29.2%).. 2115
▲ Xylocaine Injections (3%) 562
Yocon Tablets 1235
Yodoxin Tablets 1235
Yohimex Tablets........... 1414
▲ Yutopar Intravenous Injection (10 to 15%)........... 566
Zantac........... 1182
Zantac Injection 1180
Zantac Syrup 1182
Zarontin Capsules 1986
Zarontin Syrup 1986
Zaroxolyn Tablets 1625
▲ Zebeta Tablets (8.8% to 10.9%) .. 1457
▲ Zerit Capsules (3% to 54%) 731
▲ Zestoretic Tablets (5.2%)........... 2968
▲ Zestril Tablets (4.4% to 5.7%) 2972
Ziac (0.4% to 4.5%)........... 1459
Zithromax (1% or less)........... 2043
Zithromax Tablets (1% or less) 2046
▲ Zocor Tablets (3.5%) 1821
▲ Zofran Injection (17% to 25%) 1227
▲ Zofran Tablets (9% to 27%) 1231
▲ Zoladex (Greater than 1% to 75%) 2976
Zoladex 3-month (1% to 5%)........... 2978
▲ Zoloft Tablets (20.3%)........... 2051
▲ Zonalon Cream (Approximately 1% to 10%) 1042
▲ Zosyn (4.5% to 7.7%)........... 1463
▲ Zovirax Capsules (0.6% to 5.9%).. 1187
Zovirax Sterile Powder (Less than 1%) 1191
▲ Zovirax (0.6% to 5.9%)........... 1187
Zyloprim Tablets (Less than 1%).... 1194
Zyrtec Tablets (Greater than 2%) .. 2053

Headache, migraine

Norvasc Tablets (Less than or equal to 0.1%)........... 2020
Paxil Tablets (Rare)........... 2681
Prozac Pulvules & Liquid, Oral Solution (Rare) 935
Sansert Tablets........... 2424
▲ Wellbutrin Tablets (25.7%) 1177

Headache, periorbital

Pilopine HS Ophthalmic Gel .... ⊙ 224

Headache, positional

▲ Xylocaine Injections (3%) 562

Headache, sinus

Avonex 662
Colestid 2073
Prozac Pulvules & Liquid, Oral Solution (2.3%) 935
▲ Serevent Inhalation Aerosol (4%) .. 1149

Headache, supraorbital

Isopto Carpine Ophthalmic Solution .... ⊙ 221

Headache, temporal

Isopto Carpine Ophthalmic Solution .... ⊙ 221
Pilopine HS Ophthalmic Gel .... ⊙ 224

Headache, throbbing

Hyperstat I.V. Injection 2504
ReVia Tablets (Less than 1%)........... 957

Headache, transient

Aralen Hydrochloride Injection 2430
Aralen Phosphate Tablets 2431
Bio-Ginkgo (Sometimes)........... 2984
DDAVP Injection (Infrequent)........... 2178
DDAVP (Infrequent) 2180
Desmopressin Acetate Injection (Infrequent) 996
Levophed Bitartrate Injection........... 2445
Plaquenil Sulfate Tablets 2459
Stimate, (desmopressin acetate) Nasal Spray, 1.5 mg/mL (Infrequent) 806
▲ Transderm-Nitro Transdermal Therapeutic System (Most common)........... 878

Headedness, heavy

Desyrel and Desyrel Dividose (Up to 2.8%) 504
Parlodel (Less than 1%)........... 2411

Hearing, decrease

Aralen Hydrochloride Injection 2430
Aralen Phosphate Tablets 2431
Ativan Injection (Infrequent)........... 2805
▲ Avonex (3%)........... 662
Clinoril Tablets (Less than 1%)........ 1658
Daypro Caplets (Less than 1%) 2578
DYNACIN Capsules (Rare)........... 1627
Felbatol 2774
Floxin I.V. (Less than 1%) 1580
Invirase Capsules (Less than 2%) .. 2291
Minocin Intravenous (Rare)........... 1428
Minocin Oral Suspension (Rare) 1431
Minocin Pellet-Filled Capsules (Rare) 1429
Nalfon 200 Pulvules & Nalfon Tablets (1.6%)........... 933
Platinol for Injection (Occasional).... 717
Platinol-AQ Injection (Occasional) .. 719
ProSom Tablets (Rare) 457
Risperdal Tablets (Rare)........... 1348
Ziac 1459

Hearing, disturbances

Anaprox/Naprosyn (Less than 3%)........... 2277
Diamox........... ⊙ 317
EC-Naprosyn Delayed-Release Tablets (Less than 3%) 2277
Floxin I.V. 1580
Floxin Tablets (200 mg, 300 mg, 400 mg) 1577
GlaucTabs........... ⊙ 209
Imitrex Tablets (Infrequent) 1099
Indocin Capsules (Less than 1%)..... 1723
Indocin I.V. (Less than 1%)........... 1727
Indocin (Less than 1%) 1723
Intron A for Injection (Less than 5%)........... 2506
Lupron Injection 2736
Naprelan Tablets (Less than 3%) .. 2861
Anaprox/Naprosyn (Less than 3%)........... 2277
Roferon-A Injection (Less than 4%)........... 2308

Hearing, impaired

Anaprox/Naprosyn (Less than 1%)........... 2277
Arthritis Strength Bufferin Analgesic Caplets .... ▣ 637
Bumex (0.5%) 2260
Desferal Vials........... 838
Diamox Sequels (Sustained Release)........... ⊙ 318
▲ Disalcid (Among most common)...... 1549
EC-Naprosyn Delayed-Release Tablets (Less than 1%) 2277
Kefurox Vials, Faspak & ADD-Vantage 1509
Mustargen........... 1752
Anaprox/Naprosyn (Less than 1%) 2277
Norvir (Less than 2%) 447
Orudis Capsules (Less than 1%) 2874
Oruvail Capsules (Less than 1%).... 2874
Prostin E2 Suppository........... 2109
Salflex Tablets........... 791
Streptomycin Sulfate Injection.......... 2031
Trilisate (Less than 2%)........... 2155
Vesanoid Capsules (Less than 1%) 2327

Hearing, loss of

Abelcet Injection........... 1540
Alka-Seltzer Cherry Effervescent Antacid and Pain Reliever .... ▣ 609
Alka-Seltzer Extra Strength Effervescent Antacid and Pain Reliever .... ▣ 609
Alka-Seltzer Lemon Lime Effervescent Antacid and Pain Reliever .... ▣ 609
Alka-Seltzer Original Effervescent Antacid and Pain Reliever .... ▣ 609
Altace Capsules (Less than 1%)...... 1238
Amikacin Sulfate Injection, USP 523
Amikacin Sulfate Injection, USP 981
Amikin Injectable 502
Ancobon Capsules........... 2254
Aralen Hydrochloride Injection (1 patient)........... 2430
Ascriptin .... ▣ 650
Azulfidine (Rare) 2059
Genuine Bayer Aspirin Tablets & Caplets .... ▣ 618
Extra Strength Bayer Arthritis Pain Regimen Formula .... ▣ 615
Extra Strength Bayer Aspirin Caplets & Tablets .... ▣ 617
Extended-Release Bayer 8-Hour Aspirin .... ▣ 616
Extra Strength Bayer PM Aspirin Plus Sleep Aid .... ▣ 617
Aspirin Regimen Bayer Children's Chewable Aspirin ...... ▣ 616
Aspirin Regimen Bayer Regular Strength 325 mg Caplets .... ▣ 613
Cama Arthritis Pain Reliever........... ▣ 748
▲ Capastat Sulfate Injection (3%) 968
Cataflam Tablets (Less than 1%).... 833
Cipro I.V. (1% or less)........... 587
Cipro I.V. Pharmacy Bulk Package (Less than 1%)........... 590
Cipro Tablets (Less than 1%) 584
Demadex Tablets and Injection 691
Depakene 416
Depakote Tablets........... 418
Desferal Vials........... 838
Doan's Regular Strength Analgesic........... ▣ 654
Ecotrin 2625
Floxin Tablets (200 mg, 300 mg, 400 mg) (Less than 1%)........... 1577
▲ Fludara for Injection (2% to 6%).... 658
Fungizone Intravenous 507
Garamycin Injectable 2502
Hivid Tablets (Less than 1%) 2287
IBU Tablets (Less than 1%) 1389
Lasix Injection, Oral Solution and Tablets 1267
Matulane Capsules 2300
Miacalcin Nasal Spray (Less than 1%)........... 2403
Mobigesic Tablets .... ▣ 607
Mono-Gesic Tablets 810
Motrin Ibuprofen Suspension, Oral Drops, Chewable Tablets, Caplets (Less than 1%) 1563
Nebcin Vials, Hyporets & ADD-Vantage........... 1518
Neoral (2% or less) 2405
Netromycin Injection 100 mg/ml (1 of 250 patients)........... 2516
Neurontin Capsules (Infrequent)........... 1978
Orthoclone OKT3 Sterile Solution .. 1892
Pediazole Suspension 2340
Platinol for Injection 717
Platinol-AQ Injection........... 719
Primaxin I.M. 1770
Primaxin I.V. (Less than 0.2%)....... 1772
Quinidex Extentabs........... 2240
Retrovir Capsules 1216
Retrovir I.V. Infusion........... 1221
Retrovir Syrup........... 1216
Salflex Tablets........... 791
Sandimmune (2% or less)........... 2416
Sandostatin Injection (Less than 1%)........... 2421
Supprelin Injection (1% to 3%) 2230
Tegison Capsules (Less than 1%) .. 2314
Tonocard Tablets (0.4% to 1.5%) 519
Toradol (1% or less) 2319
Trilisate (Rare) 2155
Vancocin HCl, Oral Solution & Pulvules (A few dozen cases) 1536
Vancocin HCl, Vials & ADD-Vantage (Few dozen cases) 1534
▲ Vesanoid Capsules (6%) 2327
Cataflam/Voltaren/Voltaren-XR (Less than 1%)........... 833

(▣ Described in PDR For Nonprescription Drugs) Incidence data in parenthesis; ▲ 3% or more (⊙ Described in PDR For Ophthalmology)

1353 **Side Effects Index** **Heat stroke**

Zinacef (A few pediatric patients) .. 1184

Hearing loss, reversible
Biaxin (Isolated reports) 406
Cardioquin Tablets 2146
Cataflam Tablets (Less than 1%) 833
Chibroxin Sterile Ophthalmic Solution (With oral form) 1657
Depakene 416
Depakote Tablets 418
E.E.S. 427
E-Mycin Tablets (Isolated reports) .. 1388
Easprin 1971
ERYC (Isolated reports) 1972
EryPed (Isolated reports) 425
Ery-Tab Tablets (Isolated reports) .. 426
Erythrocin Stearate Filmtab (Isolated reports) 429
Erythromycin Base Filmtab (Isolated reports) 430
Erythromycin Delayed-Release Capsules, USP (Isolated reports) 431
Feldene Capsules (Less than 1%) .. 2008
Hyperstat I.V. Injection 2504
Ilosone (Isolated reports) 927
Ilotycin Gluceptate, IV, Vials (Rare) 929
Lasix Injection, Oral Solution and Tablets 1267
Noroxin Tablets (Rare) 1758
Noroxin Tablets (Rare) 2222
PCE Dispertab Tablets (Isolated reports) 453
Pediazole Suspension (Isolated reports) 2340
Quinaglute Dura-Tabs Tablets 644
Romazicon (Less than 1%) 2311
Salflex Tablets 791
Cataflam/Voltaren/Voltaren-XR (Less than 1%) 833

Heartbeat, irregular
Adenocard Injection 1021
Brethaire Inhaler 830
IOPIDINE Sterile Ophthalmic Solution (0.7%) ⊙ 218
K-Phos Neutral Tablets 633
K-Phos Original Formula 'Sodium Free' Tablets (Less frequent) 633
Maxair Inhaler (Less than 1%) 1552
Quadrinal Tablets 1398
SSKI Solution (Less frequent) 2767
Slo-Niacin Tablets 2767
Uroqid-Acid No. 2 Tablets 633

Heartbeats, ectopic
Imitrex Injection (Infrequent) 1095

Heartbeats, premature
Plendil Extended-Release Tablets (0.5% to 1.5%) 514
▲ Taxol Injection (23%) 723

Heart block (see also under Sinoatrial block)
Actimmune (Rare) 1043
Adenocard Injection 1021
Anafranil Capsules (Rare) 819
Asendin Tablets (Very rare) 1419
Betagan ⊙ 230
Betimol 0.25%, 0.5% ⊙ 259
Betoptic Ophthalmic Solution (Rare) 465
Betoptic S Ophthalmic Suspension (Rare) 467
Brevibloc (esmolol HCl) Injection (Less than 1%) 1860
Carbocaine Injection 2432
Cardene Capsules (Less than 0.4%) 2261
Cordarone Tablets (2 to 5%) 2818
Diprivan Injectable Emulsion (Less than 1%) 2939
Elavil 2945
Etrafon 2495
Flexeril Tablets (Rare) 1701
Imitrex Tablets (Rare) 1099
Limbitrol 2333
Ludiomil Tablets (Rare) 861
Marcaine 2446
Marcaine Spinal 2449
Normodyne Injection (Rare) 2519
Normodyne Tablets (Less common) 2522
Norpace 2596
Norpramin Tablets 1273
Ocupress Ophthalmic Solution, 1% Sterile ⊙ 297
Pamelor 2409
Paxil Tablets (Rare) 2681
Permax Tablets (Rare) 571
Redux Capsules (Rare) 2911
Rum-K Syrup 1004
Sensorcaine 554
Surmontil Capsules 2917
Tenex Tablets (Rare) 2249
▲ Tenormin Tablets and I.V. Injection (4.5%) 2965
Timoptic in Ocudose (Less frequent) 1796
Timoptic Sterile Ophthalmic Solution (Less frequent) 1794
Tofranil Ampuls 873
Tofranil Tablets 875
Tofranil-PM Capsules 876
Trandate (Rare) 1158
Triavil Tablets 1800
Vascor Tablets (200 and 300 mg) 1597
Visken Tablets (2% or fewer patients) 2428
Vivactil Tablets 1820

Heart block, second degree
Cartrol Tablets (Rare) 413
Dipentum Capsules (Rare) 2084
Procanbid Extended-Release Tablets (Two of almost 500 patients) 1983
Zofran Injection (Rare) 1227

Heart block, third degree
Wellbutrin Tablets 1177

Heartburn
▲ Adalat Capsules (10 mg and 20 mg) (11%) 580
▲ AeroBid Inhaler System (3% to 9%) 1004
▲ Aerobid-M Inhaler System (3% to 9%) 1004
Aleve 2124
▲ Alferon N Injection (3%) 2142
▲ Alka-Seltzer Cherry Effervescent Antacid and Pain Reliever (11.9% at doses of 1000 mg/day) ◘ 609
▲ Alka-Seltzer Lemon Lime Effervescent Antacid and Pain Reliever (11.9% at doses of 1000 mg/day) ◘ 609
▲ Alka-Seltzer Original Effervescent Antacid and Pain Reliever (11.9% at doses of 1000 mg/day) ◘ 609
▲ Anaprox/Naprosyn (3% to 9%) 2277
▲ Regular Strength Ascriptin Tablets (11.9%) ◘ 650
Axocet Capsules (Infrequent) 2469
▲ Genuine Bayer Aspirin Tablets & Caplets (11.9% at doses of 1000 mg/day) ◘ 618
▲ Aspirin Regimen Bayer Regular Strength 325 mg Caplets (11.9% of 4500 people tested) ◘ 613
▲ Bufferin Analgesic Tablets (11.9%) ◘ 636
▲ Cardioquin Tablets (Among most frequent) 2146
Cleocin Vaginal Cream (Less than 1%) 2070
▲ Clozaril Tablets (4%) 2377
Colestid (Less frequent) 2073
Dalmane Capsules 2329
DiaBeta Tablets (1.8%) 1265
Dipentum Capsules 2084
▲ EC-Naprosyn Delayed-Release Tablets (3% to 9%) 2277
▲ Ecotrin (11.9% at 1000 mg/day) 2625
Eldepryl Capsules 2729
Esgic-plus Capsules (Infrequent) 1012
Esgic-plus Tablets (Infrequent) 1012
Etrafon 2495
Fedahist Gyrocaps 2545
Fioricet Tablets (Infrequent) 2386
Fioricet with Codeine Capsules (Infrequent) 2387
Fiorinal with Codeine Capsules (Infrequent) 2390
Floxin I.V. 1580
Floxin Tablets (200 mg, 300 mg, 400 mg) 1577
Glynase PresTab Tablets (1.8%) 2091
▲ Halfprin Tablets (11.9%) 1413
Hivid Tablets (Less than 1%) 2287
▲ IBU Tablets (3% to 9%) 1389
▲ Indocin (3% to 9%) 1723
Lopressor (1%) 848
Lopressor HCT Tablets (1 in 100) 850
Mevacor Tablets (1.6%) 1742
▲ Mexitil Capsules (39.3% to 39.6%) 684
Micronase Tablets (1.8%) 2099
Midamor Tablets (Less than or equal to 1%) 1746
Moduretic Tablets 1748
Monopril Tablets (0.2% to 1.0%) .. 762
▲ Motrin Ibuprofen Suspension, Oral Drops, Chewable Tablets, Caplets (3% to 9%) 1563
▲ Naprelan Tablets (3% to 9%) 2861
▲ Anaprox/Naprosyn (3% to 9%) 2277
Noroxin Tablets (0.3% to 1.0%) 1758
Noroxin Tablets (0.3% to 1.0%) 2222
Novahistine Elixir ◘ 782
Phrenilin (Infrequent) 790
Ponstel (Less frequent) 1982
Pravachol Tablets (2.0% to 2.9%) 770
Primaxin I.M. 1770
Primaxin I.V. (Less than 0.2%) 1772
Prinivil Tablets (0.3% to 1.0%) 1776
Prinzide Tablets (0.3% to 1%) 1780
▲ Procardia Capsules (11%) 2024
▲ Procardia XL Extended Release Tablets (11%) 2026
Proventil Inhalation Aerosol (Less than 5%) 2524
▲ Quinaglute Dura-Tabs Tablets (Among most frequent) 644
▲ Quinidex Extentabs (Among most frequent) 2240
Rifadin (Some patients) 1276
Rifamate Capsules (Some patients) 1278
Rifater 1280
Rimactane Capsules 865
Rondec Oral Drops 974
Rondec Syrup 974
Rondec 974
Sansert Tablets 2424
Sedapap Tablets 50 mg/650 mg (Infrequent) 1826
Sinemet CR Tablets 961
▲ St. Joseph Adult Chewable Aspirin (81 mg.) (11.9% of 4500 patients) ◘ 768
Syprine Capsules 1790
Toprol-XL Tablets (About 1 of 100 patients) 560
▲ Trilisate (Less than 20%) 2155
▲ Ventolin Inhalation Aerosol and Refill (Fewer than 5 in 100 patients) 1170
Zestoretic Tablets (0.3 to 1%) 2968
Zestril Tablets (0.3% to 1.0%) 2972

Heart defects, congenital
Clomid 1262
ESTRATAB Tablets (0.3, 0.625, 1.25, 2.5 mg) 2715

Heart failure
Accupril Tablets (Rare) 1950
Actimmune (Rare) 1043
Activase 1045
Altace Capsules (2.0%) 1238
Betapace Tablets (2% to 5%) 637
Betaseron for SC Injection 653
Calan SR Caplets 2571
Calan Tablets 2568
Cartrol Tablets (Rare) 413
Cognex Capsules (Infrequent) 1961
Dantrium Capsules (Less frequent) 2131
Dantrium Intravenous 2132
Dexatrim Plus Vitamins Caplets .. ◘ 796
DynaCirc Capsules (0.5% to 1%) .. 2381
DynaCirc CR Tablets (0.5% to 1.0%) 2383
Isoptin Oral Tablets (1.8%) 1393
Isoptin SR Tablets 1395
Kerlone Tablets (Less than 2%) 2588
Merrem I.V. (0.1% to 1.0%) 2952
Neurontin Capsules (Rare) 1978
Nipent for Injection (Less than 3%) 2733
Orthoclone OKT3 Sterile Solution .. 1892
Procardia XL Extended Release Tablets (Rare) 2026
Pulmozyme Inhalation 1054
Redux Capsules 2911
Remeron Tablets (Rare) 1878
Rilutek Tablets (Infrequent) 2198
Sectral Capsules (Up to 2%) 2914
Taxotere for Injection Concentrate (Rare) 2204
▲ Tenormin Tablets and I.V. Injection (19%) 2965
▲ Trasylol (10%) 607
Verelan Capsules 1455
Videx Tablets, Powder for Oral Solution, & Pediatric Powder for Oral Solution (Less than 1%) 2980
Visken Tablets (Less than 1%) 2428

Heart failure, congestive (see under Congestive heart failure)

Heart failure, worsening of
Prinivil Tablets (Greater than 1%).. 1776
Prinzide Tablets 1780
Vascor Tablets (200 and 300 mg) (1.9%) 1597
Zestoretic Tablets 2968
Zestril Tablets (Greater than 1%) .. 2972

Heart murmur
Cipro I.V. (1% or less) 587
Imdur (Less than or equal to 5%) .. 1362
Invirase Capsules (Less than 2%) .. 2291
RespiGam (Infrequent) 1631
Roferon-A Injection (Rare) 2308
Sansert Tablets 2424
▲ Vesanoid Capsules (3%) 2327
Yutopar Intravenous Injection (Infrequent) 566

Heart rate, changes
▲ Blocadren Tablets (5%) 1654
Cafergot 2376
Cardura Tablets (About 0.7%) 1993
D.H.E. 45 Injection 2381
Dopram Injectable 2235
Ergomar Tablets 1543
Invirase Capsules (Less than 2%) .. 2291
Nucofed 2225
▲ Yutopar Intravenous Injection (80 to 100%) 566
Zemuron Injection 1885

Heart rate, changes fetal
Brethine Ampuls 832
Brethine Tablets 831
▲ Prepidil Gel (17.0%) 2108
Sectral Capsules 2914
▲ Yutopar Intravenous Injection (80 to 100%) 566

Heart rate, decrease
Betagan ⊙ 230
Cocaine Hydrochloride Topical Solutions 529
Guaifed 1833
Levatol Tablets (1 in 25%) 2547
Tornalate Solution for Inhalation, 0.2% (Less than 1%) 976
Tracrium Injection (0.6%) 1155

Heart rate, increase
Brethine Tablets 831
Bricanyl Subcutaneous Injection (Common) 1247
Bricanyl Tablets (Common) 1248
Cocaine Hydrochloride Topical Solutions 529
DDAVP Injection (Infrequent) 2178
Desmopressin Acetate Injection (Infrequent) 996
▲ Dobutrex Solution Vials (7.5% to approximately 10%) 1480
Effexor (Four beats per minute) 2825
Hivid Tablets (Less than 1%) 2287
Papaverine Hydrochloride Vials and Ampoules 1523
Pentaspan Injection 954
Pro-Banthine Tablets 2226
Rondec Oral Drops 974
Rondec Syrup 974
Rondec 974
Serevent Inhalation Aerosol 1149
Stimate, (desmopressin acetate) Nasal Spray, 1.5 mg/mL (Infrequent) 806
Tracrium Injection (2.1%) 1155
Yohimex Tablets 1414

Heart spasms (see under Cardiospasm)

Heat intolerance
Alferon N Injection (1%) 2142
Imitrex Tablets 1099
Maxaquin Tablets (Less than 1%).. 2593

Heat stroke
Asendin Tablets 1419
Clozaril Tablets 2377
Cogentin 1661
Compazine 2644
Cystospaz 2123
Haldol Decanoate 1587
Haldol Injection, Tablets and Concentrate 1585
Levsin/Levsinex/Levbid 2549
Loxitane 1426

(◘ Described in PDR For Nonprescription Drugs) Incidence data in parenthesis; ▲ 3% or more (⊙ Described in PDR For Ophthalmology)

Heat stroke

Orap Tablets ... 1037
Prolixin ... 510
Serentil ... 689
Stelazine ... 2692

Heavy sensation, arms

Adenocard Injection (Less than 1%) ... 1021
Peptavlon ... 2997

Heavy sensation, legs

Eldepryl Capsules ... 2729
K-Phos Neutral Tablets ... 633
K-Phos Original Formula 'Sodium Free' Tablets (Less frequent) ... 633
Peptavlon ... 2997

Hematemesis

Anaprox/Naprosyn (Less than 1%) ... 2277
Betaseron for SC Injection ... 653
Clozaril Tablets (Less than 1%) ... 2377
EC-Naprosyn Delayed-Release Tablets (Less than 1%) ... 2277
Effexor (Rare) ... 2825
Felbatol ... 2774
Feldene Capsules (Less than 1%) ... 2008
Foscavir Injection (Less than 1%) ... 541
Imitrex Tablets (Rare) ... 1099
Lamictal Tablets ... 1105
▲ Leukine (13%) ... 1317
Lufyllin & Lufyllin-400 Tablets ... 2778
Lufyllin-GG Elixir & Tablets ... 2779
LUVOX Tablets (Rare) ... 2723
Matulane Capsules ... 2300
Methotrexate Sodium Tablets, Injection, for Injection and LPF Injection ... 1322
Mithracin ... 599
Motrin Ibuprofen Suspension, Oral Drops, Chewable Tablets, Caplets (Less than 1%) ... 1563
Mutamycin for Injection ... 712
▲ Naprelan Tablets (3% to 9%) ... 2861
Anaprox/Naprosyn (Less than 1%) ... 2277
Neurontin Capsules (Rare) ... 1978
Orudis Capsules (Less than 1%) ... 2874
Oruvail Capsules (Less than 1%) ... 2874
Paxil Tablets (Rare) ... 2681
Permax Tablets (Infrequent) ... 571
Prevacid Delayed-Release Capsules (Less than 1%) ... 2746
Prozac Pulvules & Liquid, Oral Solution (Rare) ... 935
Quadrinal Tablets ... 1398
Quibron ... 2227
ReoPro Vials (5 to 11 events) ... 1526
Respbid Tablets ... 687
Rilutek Tablets (Rare) ... 2198
Risperdal Tablets (Rare) ... 1348
Slo-bid Gyrocaps ... 2201
Theo-Dur Extended-Release Tablets ... 1367
Theo-X Extended-Release Tablets ... 793
Uni-Dur Extended-Release Tablets ... 1374
Zoladex 3-month (1% to 5%) ... 2978

Hematochezia

Adriamycin PFS ... 2056
Adriamycin RDF ... 2056
Anafranil Capsules (Infrequent) ... 819
Avonex ... 662
Cataflam Tablets (Less than 1%) ... 833
Cognex Capsules (Infrequent) ... 1961
Colestid (Infrequent) ... 2073
Coumadin ... 941
Dipentum Capsules (Rare) ... 2084
Doxorubicin Astra ... 531
Glucotrol XL Extended Release Tablets (Less than 1%) ... 2012
Hivid Tablets (Less than 1%) ... 2287
Invirase Capsules (Less than 2%) ... 2291
Nalfon 200 Pulvules & Nalfon Tablets (Less than 1%) ... 933
Neurontin Capsules (Infrequent) ... 1978
Orudis Capsules (Less than 1%) ... 2874
Oruvail Capsules (Less than 1%) ... 2874
Penetrex Tablets (0.1% to 1%) ... 2196
Ridaura Capsules (0.1 to 1%) ... 2691
Rowasa ... 2727
Rubex for Injection ... 721
Cataflam/Voltaren/Voltaren-XR (Less than 1%) ... 833

Hematocrit, decrease

Altace Capsules (Rare; 0.4% to 1.5%) ... 1238
Blocadren Tablets ... 1654
Cefobid Pharmacy Bulk Package - Not for Direct Infusion (1 in 20) ... 1999

▲ Cipro I.V. (Among most frequent) ... 587
▲ Cipro I.V. Pharmacy Bulk Package (Among most frequent) ... 590
Dopram Injectable ... 2235
Dynabac (0.1% to 1%) ... 668
▲ Feldene Capsules (3% to 9%) ... 2008
Hespan Injection ... 945
Hivid Tablets (Less than 1%) ... 2287
Hyzaar Tablets (Frequent but rare clinical importance) ... 1720
IBU Tablets (Less than 1%) ... 1389
▲ Kefurox Vials, Faspak & ADD-Vantage (1 in 10) ... 1509
▲ Lariam Tablets (Among most frequent) ... 2295
Larodopa Tablets ... 2296
Lopid Tablets (Occasional) ... 1974
Merrem I.V. (Greater than 0.2%) ... 2952
Methotrexate Sodium Tablets, Injection, for Injection and LPF Injection (Less common) ... 1322
Mezlin ... 594
Mezlin Pharmacy Bulk Package ... 597
Monopril Tablets ... 762
Motrin Ibuprofen Suspension, Oral Drops, Chewable Tablets, Caplets (Less than 1%) ... 1563
Noroxin Tablets (Less frequent) ... 1758
Noroxin Tablets (Less frequent) ... 2222
Norpace (Less than 1%) ... 2596
Penetrex Tablets (Less than 1%) ... 2196
▲ Ponstel (2-5%) ... 1982
Precose ... 604
Primaxin I.M. ... 1770
Primaxin I.V. ... 1772
Prinivil Tablets (Frequent) ... 1776
Prinzide Tablets (Frequent) ... 1780
Proglycem ... 575
ReoPro Vials (7 to 11 events) ... 1526
Serzone Tablets (2.8%) ... 776
Sinemet CR Tablets (1% or greater) ... 961
Timentin for Injection ... 2706
Tolectin (200, 400 and 600 mg) (1 to 3%) ... 1591
Tornalate Solution for Inhalation, 0.2% (Infrequent) ... 976
Tranxene ... 459
Unasyn ... 2035
Vantin for Oral Suspension and Vantin Tablets ... 2112
Vaseretic Tablets (0.5% to 2.0%) ... 1810
Vasotec I.V. (Frequent) ... 1814
Vasotec Tablets (Frequent) ... 1816
Xanax Tablets (Less than 1%) ... 2115
Zanosar Sterile Powder ... 2119
Zestoretic Tablets (Frequent) ... 2968
Zestril Tablets (Frequent) ... 2972
▲ Zinacef (1 in 10 patients) ... 1184
Zosyn ... 1463

Hematocrit, increase

Clozaril Tablets ... 2377
Epogen for Injection ... 489
Maxipime for Injection (0.1% to 1%) ... 758
Procrit for Injection ... 1896
Synarel Nasal Solution for Endometriosis ... 2605

Hematocrit, transient decrease

Cytosar-U Sterile Powder (Less than 7 patients) ... 2077

Hematocrit content, deviation

▲ Avonex (3%) ... 662
Bumex (0.6%) ... 2260
Doral Tablets (1.5%) ... 2773

Hematologic reactions

Ana-Kit Anaphylaxis Emergency Treatment Kit (Rare) ... 611
Cefotan (1.4%) ... 2936
Dapsone Tablets USP ... 1331
Daraprim Tablets ... 1199
Feldene Capsules ... 2008
Floxin I.V. ... 1580
Floxin Tablets (200 mg, 300 mg, 400 mg) ... 1577
Lopid Tablets ... 1974
Procanbid Extended-Release Tablets (Fairly common) ... 1983
Thalitone ... 1293

Hematologic toxicity

Adriamycin PFS ... 2056
Adriamycin RDF ... 2056
Ana-Kit Anaphylaxis Emergency Treatment Kit (Rare) ... 611
Depen Titratable Tablets ... 2770
Doxil ... 2613

Doxorubicin Astra ... 531
Sterile FUDR ... 2284
Hivid Tablets (Less than 1%) ... 2287
Imuran ... 1103
Neutrexin for Injection ... 2761
Retrovir I.V. Infusion ... 1221
Solganal Suspension ... 2530
Zanosar Sterile Powder (Rare) ... 2119

Hematoma

▲ Caverject Injection (3%) ... 2064
Claritin-D Tablets (Less frequent) ... 2487
Depakene ... 416
Depakote Tablets ... 418
Eldepryl Capsules ... 2729
Eminase (2.8%) ... 2215
▲ Fragmin Injection (Most common) ... 2088
Havrix (Less than 1%) ... 2663
Heparin Lock Flush Solution ... 2831
Heparin Sodium Injection ... 2832
Heparin Sodium Vials ... 1486
Imitrex Tablets (Rare) ... 1099
Lovenox Injection ... 2187
Lutrepulse for Injection ... 998
Netromycin Injection 100 mg/ml (4 of 1000 patients) ... 2516
Nimotop Capsules (Less than 1%) ... 603
Paxil Tablets (Infrequent) ... 2681
Pipracil ... 1435
ReoPro Vials ... 1526
Sandostatin Injection (1% to 4%) ... 2421
▲ THROMBATE III Antithrombin III (Human) (1 of 17) ... 631
Toradol ... 2319
▲ Varivax (24.4% to 32.5%) ... 1807
Versed Injection (Less than 1%) ... 2324

Hematoma, pelvic

Syntocinon Injection ... 2425

Hematoma, subdermal

Redux Capsules ... 2911

Hematoma, subdural

Cerebyx Injection (Infrequent) ... 1956
Naprelan Tablets (Less than 1%) ... 2861
Rilutek Tablets (Infrequent) ... 2198

Hematopoietic depression

Cosmegen Injection ... 1666
▲ DTIC-Dome (Among most common) ... 593
Methotrexate Sodium Tablets, Injection, for Injection and LPF Injection ... 1322
Mustargen (Occasional) ... 1752

Hematospermia

LUVOX Tablets (Rare) ... 2723

Hematuria

▲ Accutane Capsules (Less than 1 in 10) ... 2252
Anafranil Capsules (Infrequent) ... 819
Anaprox/Naprosyn (Less than 1%) ... 2277
Androderm Testosterone Transdermal System (Less than 1%) ... 2634
Asacol Delayed-Release Tablets ... 2129
Atromid-S Capsules ... 2808
Augmentin (Rare) ... 2637
Augmentin Tablets (Rare) ... 2640
Avonex ... 662
Azulfidine (Rare) ... 2059
Benemid Tablets ... 1651
Betaseron for SC Injection ... 653
Cardene I.V. (0.7%) ... 2815
▲ Casodex Tablets (7%) ... 2934
Cataflam Tablets (Less than 1%) ... 833
Caverject Injection (Less than 1%) ... 2064
Cedax (0.1% to 1%) ... 2480
▲ CellCept Capsules (12.1% to 14.0%) ... 2265
Cipro I.V. (1% or less) ... 587
Cipro I.V. Pharmacy Bulk Package (Less than 1%) ... 590
Cipro Tablets ... 584
Clinoril Tablets (Less than 1%) ... 1658
Cognex Capsules (Infrequent) ... 1961
ColBENEMID Tablets ... 1662
Condylox Topical Solution (Less than 5%) ... 1853
Coumadin ... 941
Crixivan Capsules (Less than 2% to approximately 4%) ... 1670
Cuprimine Capsules ... 1673
Cytotec (Infrequent) ... 2576
Cytovene (1% or less) ... 2270
Cytoxan ... 700
Danocrine Capsules ... 2437

Dantrium Capsules (Less frequent) ... 2131
Daraprim Tablets ... 1199
Daypro Caplets (Less than 1%) ... 2578
Demser Capsules (A few patients) ... 1690
Depen Titratable Tablets ... 2770
Desyrel and Desyrel Dividose ... 504
Diamox Intravenous (Occasional) ⊙ 317
Diamox Sequels (Sustained Release) ⊙ 318
Diamox Tablets (Occasional) ⊙ 317
Dipentum Capsules (Rare) ... 2084
Diuril Sodium Intravenous (1 case) ... 1693
Dolobid Tablets (Less than 1 in 100) ... 1695
Doxil (Less than 1%) ... 2613
EC-Naprosyn Delayed-Release Tablets (Less than 1%) ... 2277
Edecrin ... 1698
Effexor (Frequent) ... 2825
Eminase ... 2215
▲ Eulexin Capsules (7%) ... 2498
Felbatol ... 2774
Feldene Capsules (Less than 1%) ... 2008
Floxin I.V. (More than or equal to 1%) ... 1580
Floxin Tablets (200 mg, 300 mg, 400 mg) (More than or equal to 1%) ... 1577
Fludara for Injection (2% to 3%) ... 658
Foscavir Injection (Less than 1%) ... 541
▲ Gemzar for Injection (Up to 35%) ... 1482
Genotropin Injection (Infrequent) ... 2090
GlaucTabs (Occasional) ⊙ 209
Hylorel Tablets (2.3%) ... 1613
IBU Tablets (Less than 1%) ... 1389
▲ IFEX (6% to 92%) ... 706
Imitrex Tablets (Rare) ... 1099
Indocin Capsules (Less than 1%) ... 1723
Indocin I.V. (Less than 1%) ... 1727
Indocin (Less than 1%) ... 1723
INFeD (Iron Dextran Injection, USP) ... 2478
Intron A for Injection (Less than 5%) ... 2506
Lamictal Tablets (Infrequent) ... 1105
▲ Leukine (9%) ... 1317
Lioresal Intrathecal (1% or more) ... 1634
Lioresal Tablets (Rare) ... 847
Lodine Capsules and Tablets (Less than 1%) ... 2849
Lufyllin & Lufyllin-400 Tablets ... 2778
Lufyllin-GG Elixir & Tablets ... 2779
Lupron Depot 7.5 mg (Less than 5%) ... 2741
▲ Lupron Injection (5% or more) ... 2736
LUVOX Tablets (Infrequent) ... 2723
Lysodren Tablets (Infrequent) ... 707
Matulane Capsules ... 2300
Maxaquin Tablets (Less than 1%) ... 2593
Methergine (Rare) ... 2401
Methotrexate Sodium Tablets, Injection, for Injection and LPF Injection ... 1322
Miacalcin Nasal Spray (Less than 1%) ... 2403
Mintezol ... 1747
Motrin Ibuprofen Suspension, Oral Drops, Chewable Tablets, Caplets (Less than 1%) ... 1563
Myochrysine Injection ... 1754
Nalfon 200 Pulvules & Nalfon Tablets (Less than 1%) ... 933
Naprelan Tablets (Less than 1%) ... 2861
Anaprox/Naprosyn (Less than 1%) ... 2277
Neoral (Rare) ... 2405
Neptazane Tablets ⊙ 320
Neupogen for Injection (Infrequent) ... 495
Neurontin Capsules (Infrequent) ... 1978
Noroxin Tablets ... 1758
Noroxin Tablets ... 2222
Norvir (Less than 2%) ... 447
Oncaspar (Less than 1%) ... 2194
Ortho Diaphragm Kit ... 1921
Orudis Capsules (Less than 1%) ... 2874
Oruvail Capsules (Less than 1%) ... 2874
OxyContin Tablets (Less than 1%) ... 2163
Paxil Tablets (Infrequent) ... 2681
Pediazole Suspension ... 2340
Pentasa (Less than 1%) ... 1275
Permax Tablets (1.1%) ... 571
Ponstel ... 1982
Prevacid Delayed-Release Capsules (Less than 1%) ... 2746
Prilosec Delayed-Release Capsules (Less than 1%) ... 516
Primaxin I.M. ... 1770
Primaxin I.V. ... 1772
Priscoline Hydrochloride Ampuls ... 864

(⌘ Described in PDR For Nonprescription Drugs)   Incidence data in parenthesis; ▲ 3% or more   (⊙ Described in PDR For Ophthalmology)

1355 Side Effects Index Hemolytic anemia

Procardia XL Extended Release Tablets (1% or less) 2026
Proglycem 575
▲ Prograf (Greater than 3%) 1028
▲ Proleukin for Injection (9%) 812
ProSom Tablets (Rare) 457
Prozac Pulvules & Liquid, Oral Solution (Rare) 935
Questran 774
Redux Capsules (Rare) 2911
Relafen Tablets (Less than 1%) 2688
Remeron Tablets (Infrequent) 1878
ReoPro Vials (4 events) 1526
Retrovir Capsules (0.8%) 1216
Retrovir I.V. Infusion (1%) 1221
Retrovir Syrup (0.8%) 1216
Ridaura Capsules (1 to 3%) 2691
Rifadin (Rare) 1276
Rifamate Capsules (Rare) 1278
Rifater (Rare) 1280
Rilutek Tablets (Infrequent) 2198
Rimactane Capsules 865
Risperdal Tablets (Infrequent) 1348
Rocephin Injectable Vials, ADD-Vantage, Galaxy Container (Rare) 2305
Sandimmune (Rare) 2416
Sandostatin Injection (Less than 1%) 2421
Serzone Tablets (Infrequent) 776
Sinemet CR Tablets (1% or greater) 961
Solganal Suspension 2530
Sular Tablets (Less than or equal to 1%) 2961
Supprelin Injection (1% to 3%) 2230
Tazicef for Injection (Occasional) 2697
▲ Tegison Capsules (1-10%) 2314
Testoderm Testosterone Transdermal System (One in 104 patients) 486
▲ TheraCys BCG Live (Intravesical) (17.0% to 39.3%) 911
▲ TICE BCG, USP (26.0%) 1881
Ticlid Tablets 2317
Tolectin (200, 400 and 600 mg) (Less than 1%) 1591
Toradol (1% or less) 2319
Unasyn 2035
Urobiotic-250 Capsules 2038
Uroqid-Acid No. 2 Tablets (Rare) 633
Videx Tablets, Powder for Oral Solution, & Pediatric Powder for Oral Solution (Less than 1%) 2980
Vistide Injection 1057
Cataflam/Voltaren/Voltaren-XR (Less than 1%) 833
Zarontin Capsules 1986
Zarontin Syrup 1986
Zerit Capsules (Fewer than 1%) 731
Zoladex 3-month (1% to 5%) 2978
Zosyn (1.0% or less) 1463
Zovirax Sterile Powder (Less than 1%) 1191
Zyloprim Tablets (Less than 1%) 1194
Zyrtec Tablets (Less than 2%) 2053

Hematuria, genitourinary

Eminase (2.4%) 2215

Hematuria, microscopic

Calcium Disodium Versenate Injection 1548
Celontin Kapseals 1955
▲ Crixivan Capsules (Approximately 4%) 1670

Hemianopsia

Felbatol 2774

Hemiparesis

Anafranil Capsules (Rare) 819
Foscavir Injection (Less than 1%) 541
Klonopin Tablets 2294
Methotrexate Sodium Tablets, Injection, for Injection and LPF Injection 1322
Orthoclone OKT3 Sterile Solution 1892
Videx Tablets, Powder for Oral Solution, & Pediatric Powder for Oral Solution (Less than 1%) 2980

Hemiplegia

Betaseron for SC Injection 653
Cerebyx Injection (Infrequent) 1956
Cognex Capsules (Infrequent) 1961
Doxil (Less than 1%) 2613
Imitrex Injection (Rare) 1095
Lamictal Tablets (Rare) 1105
LUVOX Tablets (Infrequent) 2723
Neurontin Capsules (Infrequent) 1978
Orthoclone OKT3 Sterile Solution 1892
Permax Tablets (Rare) 571
Prevacid Delayed-Release Capsules (Less than 1%) 2746
Redux Capsules 2911
Rilutek Tablets (Infrequent) 2198
▲ Vesanoid Capsules (3%) 2327

Hemochromatosis

Effexor (Rare) 2825

Hemoconcentration

Haldol Decanoate 1587
Humegon for Injection 1873
Lutrepulse for Injection 998
Metrodin (urofollitropin for injection) 2616
Mykrox Tablets 1617
Serophene (clomiphene citrate tablets, USP) 2621
Zaroxolyn Tablets 1625

Hemodilution

Hespan Injection 945

Hemoglobin, decrease

Altace Capsules (Rare; 0.4% to 1.5%) 1238
Apresazide Capsules (Less frequent) 824
Apresoline Hydrochloride Tablets (Less frequent) 826
Betaseron for SC Injection 653
Blocadren Tablets 1654
Casodex Tablets (2% to 5%) 2934
Cataflam Tablets (Less than 1%) 833
Cedax (1% to 2%) 2480
▲ Cefobid Intravenous/Intramuscular (1 in 20) 1996
▲ Cefobid Pharmacy Bulk Package - Not for Direct Infusion (1 in 20) 1999
▲ Cipro I.V. (Among most frequent) 587
▲ Cipro I.V. Pharmacy Bulk Package (Among most frequent) 590
Cipro Tablets (Less than 0.1%) 584
Crixivan Capsules (0.5%) 1670
Cytadren Tablets (1 patient) 837
▲ Dapsone Tablets USP (Almost all patients) 1331
Dopram Injectable 2235
Dynabac (0.1% to 1%) 668
Easprin 1971
▲ Feldene Capsules (3% to 9%) 2008
Hydralazine Hydrochloride Injection USP (Less frequent) 2712
Hyzaar Tablets (Frequent but rare clinical importance) 1720
IBU Tablets (Less than 1%) 1389
Invirase Capsules (Less than 1%) 2291
▲ Kefurox Vials, Faspak & ADD-Vantage (1 in 10) 1509
Larodopa Tablets (Occasional) 2296
Lopid Tablets (Occasional) 1974
Lotensin Tablets (Rare; 1 of 2014 patients) 852
Macrobid Capsules (1% to 5%) 2138
Macrodantin Capsules 2140
Maxaquin Tablets (Less than or equal to 0.1%) 2593
Merrem I.V. (Greater than 0.2%) 2952
Mezlin 594
Mezlin Pharmacy Bulk Package 597
Mithracin 599
Monopril Tablets 762
▲ Motrin Ibuprofen Suspension, Oral Drops, Chewable Tablets, Caplets (Less than 1% to 22.8%) 1563
Mustargen 1752
Noroxin Tablets (0.6%) 1758
Noroxin Tablets (0.6%) 2222
Norpace (1 to 3%) 2596
Penetrex Tablets (Less than 1%) 2196
Pentaspan Injection 954
Primaxin I.M. 1770
Primaxin I.V. 1772
Prinivil Tablets (Frequent) 1776
Prinzide Tablets (Frequent) 1780
Proglycem 575
ReoPro Vials (7 to 11 events) 1526
Ridaura Capsules 2691
Rifadin 1276
Rifamate Capsules 1278
Rifater 1280
Rimactane Capsules (Rare) 865
▲ Roferon-A Injection (4% to 31%) 2308
Ser-Ap-Es Tablets 867
Sinemet CR Tablets (1% or greater) 961
▲ Tegison Capsules (10-25%) 2314
Timentin for Injection 2706
Tolectin (200, 400 and 600 mg) (1 to 3%) 1591
Tornalate Solution for Inhalation, 0.2% (Infrequent) 976
Ultram Tablets (50 mg) (Infrequent) 1594
Unasyn 2035
Vantin for Oral Suspension and Vantin Tablets 2112
Vaseretic Tablets (0.5% to 2.0%) 1810
Vasotec I.V. (Frequent) 1814
Vasotec Tablets (Frequent) 1816
▲ Videx Tablets, Powder for Oral Solution, & Pediatric Powder for Oral Solution (2% to 9%) 2980
Viramune Tablets (1.2%) 2368
Cataflam/Voltaren/Voltaren-XR (Less than 1%) 833
WinRho SD 1840
Zestoretic Tablets (Frequent) 2968
Zestril Tablets (Frequent) 2972
▲ Zinacef (1 in 10 patients) 1184
Zosyn 1463

Hemoglobin content, deviation

Bumex (0.8%) 2260
Doral Tablets (1.4%) 2773
▲ Intron A for Injection (Up to 32%) 2506
Xanax Tablets (Less than 1%) 2115

Hemoglobinemia

Clozaril Tablets 2377
Hivid Tablets (Less than 1%) 2287
Zovirax Sterile Powder (Less than 1%) 1191

Hemoglobinuria

Rifadin (Rare) 1276
Rifamate Capsules 1278
Rifater (Rare) 1280
Rimactane Capsules (Rare) 865
▲ Tegison Capsules (1-10%) 2314

Hemolysis

Cognex Capsules (Rare) 1961
Cozaar Tablets (One subject) 1668
▲ Dapsone Tablets USP (Most common) 1331
Doxil (1% to 5%) 2613
Foscavir Injection (Less than 1%) 541
Furoxone 2221
Hespan Injection (Rare) 945
Hyzaar Tablets (One subject) 1720
Kefurox Vials, Faspak & ADD-Vantage 1509
Macrobid Capsules 2138
Macrodantin Capsules 2140
Mycobutin Capsules (Less than 1%) 2101
Orudis Capsules (Less than 1%) 2874
Oruvail Capsules (Less than 1%) 2874
Plaquenil Sulfate Tablets 2459
Platinol for Injection 717
Platinol-AQ Injection 719
Prevacid Delayed-Release Capsules (Less than 1%) 2746
Rifadin (Rare) 1276
Rifamate Capsules (Rare) 1278
Rifater (Rare) 1280
Rimactane Capsules 865
Trasylol (0.3%) 607
Vaseretic Tablets (A few cases) 1810
Vasotec I.V. (A few cases) 1814
Vasotec Tablets (A few cases) 1816

Hemolysis, neonatal

AquaMEPHYTON Injection 1648
Dapsone Tablets USP 1331
Mephyton Tablets 1739

Hemolytic anemia

Accupril Tablets 1950
Achromycin V Capsules 1417
Aldoclor Tablets 1638
Aldomet Ester HCl Injection 1642
Aldomet Oral 1640
Aldoril Tablets 1644
Alkeran for Injection 1196
Alkeran Tablets 1198
Altace Capsules (Less than 1%) 1238
Amaryl Tablets 1241
Anaprox/Naprosyn (Less than 1%) 2277
Atamet Tablets (Rare) 567
▲ Azulfidine (One in every 30 patients or less) 2059
Bactrim DS Tablets 2257
Bactrim I.V. Infusion 2255
Bactrim 2257
Benadryl Injection 1955
Benemid Tablets 1651
Bicillin C-R Injection 2810
Bicillin C-R 900/300 Injection 2812
Bicillin L-A Injection (Infrequent) 2813
▲ Bromfed-DM Cough Syrup (Among most frequent) 1832
Capoten Tablets 740
Capozide Tablets 744
Cardioquin Tablets 2146
Cardizem CD Capsules (Infrequent) 1251
Cardizem SR Capsules (Infrequent) 1255
Cardizem Injectable 1253
Cardizem Tablets (Infrequent) 1257
Cataflam Tablets (Rare) 833
Ceclor Pulvules & Suspension (Rare) 1470
Cedax 2480
Cefizox for Intramuscular or Intravenous Use (Rare) 1025
Cefotan 2936
Ceftin 1067
Cefzil Tablets and Oral Suspension 747
Ceptaz (Exceedingly rare cases) 1070
Cipro I.V. (Rare) 587
Cipro I.V. Pharmacy Bulk Package (Rare) 590
Cipro Tablets 584
Claforan Sterile and Injection (Rare) 1259
Clinoril Tablets (Less than 1 in 100) 1658
ColBENEMID Tablets 1662
Compazine 2644
Cuprimine Capsules 1673
Declomycin Tablets 1421
Depen Titratable Tablets 2770
Desyrel and Desyrel Dividose 504
DiaBeta Tablets (Occasional) 1265
Diabinese Tablets 2002
Diamox ◉ 317
Dimetane-DC Cough Syrup 2232
Dimetane-DX Cough Syrup 2233
Dipentum Capsules (Rare) 2084
Diucardin Tablets 2824
Diupres Tablets 1691
Diuril Oral Suspension 1694
Diuril Sodium Intravenous 1693
Diuril Tablets 1694
Dolobid Tablets (Less than 1 in 100) 1695
Doryx Capsules 1970
Duricef Capsules, Tablets, and Oral Suspension 750
Dyazide Capsules 2653
DYNACIN Capsules 1627
EC-Naprosyn Delayed-Release Tablets (Less than 1%) 2277
Enduron Tablets 424
Etrafon 2495
Eulexin Capsules 2498
Fansidar Tablets 2281
Felbatol 2774
Feldene Capsules (Less than 1%) 2008
Fiorinal with Codeine Capsules 2390
Floxin I.V. 1580
Floxin Tablets (200 mg, 300 mg, 400 mg) 1577
Fludara for Injection (Rare) 658
Fortaz (Rare) 1092
Furoxone 2221
Gantanol Tablets 2285
Gantrisin 2286
GlaucTabs ◉ 209
Glucotrol Tablets 2011
Glucotrol XL Extended Release Tablets 2012
Glynase PresTab Tablets 2091
Helidac Therapy 2135
HydroDIURIL Tablets 1716
Hydropres Tablets 1718
Hyzaar Tablets 1720
IBU Tablets (Less than 1%) 1389
Indocin Capsules (Less than 1%) 1723
Indocin I.V. (Less than 1%) 1727
Indocin (Less than 1%) 1723
Intron A for Injection (Less than 5%) 2506
Invirase Capsules (Rare) 2291
Lamictal Tablets 1105
Larodopa Tablets (Rare) 2296
Lasix Injection, Oral Solution and Tablets 1267
Lescol Capsules (Rare) 2395
Leustatin (Some reports) 1889
Lodine Capsules and Tablets (Less than 1%) 2849
Lorabid Suspension and Pulvules 1513
Lotensin Tablets (Rare) 852
Lotensin HCT Tablets (Rare) 855

(■ Described in PDR For Nonprescription Drugs) Incidence data in parenthesis; ▲ 3% or more (◉ Described in PDR For Ophthalmology)

Hemolytic anemia — Side Effects Index — 1356

Lotrel Capsules (Rare) 858
Macrobid Capsules 2138
Macrodantin Capsules 2140
Matulane Capsules 2300
Maxaquin Tablets 2593
Maxipime for Injection 758
Mefoxin 1734
Mefoxin Premixed Intravenous Solution 1737
Mesantoin Tablets (Uncommon) 2400
Mevacor Tablets (Rare) 1742
Micronase Tablets 2099
Minocin Intravenous 1428
Minocin Oral Suspension 1431
Minocin Pellet-Filled Capsules 1429
Moduretic Tablets 1748
Monodox Capsules 1858
Monopril Tablets 762
Motrin Ibuprofen Suspension, Oral Drops, Chewable Tablets, Caplets (Less than 1%) 1563
Mustargen (Rare) 1752
Mutamycin for Injection 712
Nalfon 200 Pulvules & Nalfon Tablets (Less than 1%) 933
Anaprox/Naprosyn (Less than 1%) 2277
Navane Capsules and Concentrate 2018
Navane Intramuscular 2019
NegGram (Rare) 2453
NephrAmine Injection 2169
Neptazane Tablets ⊙ 320
Nipent for Injection (Less than 3%) 2733
Nizoral Tablets (Less than 1%) 1345
Noroxin Tablets (Rare) 1758
Noroxin Tablets (Rare) 2222
Nydrazid Injection 509
▲ Oncaspar (Greater than 1% but less than 5%) 2194
Orap Tablets 1037
Ornade Spansule Capsules 2678
Orthoclone OKT3 Sterile Solution 1892
PBZ Tablets 863
PBZ-SR Tablets 862
PASER Granules 1333
Pediazole Suspension 2340
Pen•Vee K (Infrequent) 2879
Periactin 1767
Pfizerpen for Injection (Rare) 2022
Platinol for Injection 717
Platinol-AQ Injection 719
Ponstel 1982
Pravachol Tablets (Rare) 770
Prilosec Delayed-Release Capsules (Rare) 516
Primaxin I.M. 1770
Primaxin I.V. 1772
Prinivil Tablets 1776
Prinzide Tablets 1780
Procanbid Extended-Release Tablets (Rare) 1983
Procardia Capsules 2024
Procardia XL Extended Release Tablets 2026
Prozac Pulvules & Liquid, Oral Solution 935
Pyridium 1985
Quinaglute Dura-Tabs Tablets 644
Quinidex Extentabs 2240
Redux Capsules 2911
ReoPro Vials (0.3%) 1526
Rifadin 1276
Rifamate Capsules 1278
Rifater 1280
Rimactane Capsules (Rare) 865
Rocephin Injectable Vials, ADD-Vantage, Galaxy Container (Less than 1%) 2305
Roferon-A Injection (Rare) 2308
SSD 1402
Septra 1146
Septra I.V. Infusion 1142
Septra I.V. Infusion ADD-Vantage Vials 1144
Septra 1146
Silvadene Cream 1% 1288
Sinemet Tablets (Rare) 959
Sinemet CR Tablets 961
Skelaxin Tablets 793
Stelazine 2692
Sulfamylon Cream 940
Suprax 1443
Talacen Caplets (Rare) 2464
Tavist Syrup 2426
Tavist Tablets 2427
Tazicef for Injection 2697
Tazidime Vials, Faspak & ADD-Vantage (Rare) 1531
Terramycin Intramuscular Solution 2034
Thorazine 2701
Tiazac Capsules (Infrequent) 1019
Ticlid Tablets (Rare) 2317
Timolide Tablets 1791
Tolectin (200, 400 and 600 mg) (Less than 1%) 1591
Tonocard Tablets (Less than 1%) 519
Trilafon 2532
Trinalin Repetabs Tablets 1373
Tussend 1830
Univasc Tablets (Less than 1%) 2553
Vantin for Oral Suspension and Vantin Tablets 2112
Vaseretic Tablets 1810
Vasotec I.V. 1814
Vasotec Tablets 1816
Vibramycin 2038
Vibramycin Hyclate Intravenous 2040
Vibramycin 2038
Virazole 1310
Cataflam/Voltaren/Voltaren-XR (Rare) 833
Zestoretic Tablets 2968
Zestril Tablets (Rare) 2972
Zinacef 1184
Zocor Tablets (Rare) 1821
Zyloprim Tablets (Less than 1%) 1194
Zyrtec Tablets (Rare) 2053

Hemolytic icterus (see under Jaundice)

Hemolytic sideroblastic anemia (see under Anemia, hemolytic, sideroblastic)

Hemolytic-uremic syndrome

Azulfidine (Rare) 2059
Brevicon 2563
Cytovene-IV (One report) 2270
Demulen 2580
Desogen Tablets 1867
Felbatol 2774
Gemzar for Injection (0.25%) 1482
Levlen/Tri-Levlen 646
Lo/Ovral Tablets 2852
Lo/Ovral-28 Tablets 2857
Modicon 1928
Mutamycin for Injection 712
Nordette-21 Tablets 2863
Nordette-28 Tablets 2866
Norinyl 2563
Nor-Q D Tablets 2598
Ortho-Cept 1907
Ortho-Cyclen/Ortho-Tri-Cyclen 1914
Ortho-Novum 1928
Ortho-Cyclen/Ortho Tri-Cyclen 1914
Ovcon 765
Ovral Tablets 2877
Ovral-28 Tablets 2878
Ovrette Tablets 2878
Paraplatin for Injection (Rare) 713
Toradol 2319
Levlen/Tri-Levlen 646
Tri-Norinyl 2607
Valtrex Caplets 1167

Hemopericardium

Cardene I.V. (0.7%) 2815
Cytoxan 700

Hemoperitoneum

Humegon for Injection 1873
Merrem I.V. (0.7%) 2952
Metrodin (urofollitropin for injection) 2616
Pergonal (menotropins for injection, USP) 2618
Serophene (clomiphene citrate tablets, USP) 2621

Hemophilus

Intron A for Injection (Less than 5%) 2506

Hemoptysis

Abelcet Injection 1540
Anafranil Capsules (Rare) 819
Avonex 662
Betaseron for SC Injection 653
Cerebyx Injection (Infrequent) 1956
Cipro I.V. (1% or less) 587
Cipro I.V. Pharmacy Bulk Package (Less than 1%) 590
Cipro Tablets (Less than 1%) 584
Claritin Tablets (2% or fewer patients) 2485
Claritin-D Tablets 2487
Cognex Capsules (Rare) 1961
DaunoXome (Less than or equal to 5%) 1842
Duragesic Transdermal System (1% or greater) 1336
Dynabac (0.1% to 1%) 668
Effexor (Rare) 2825
Eminase (2.2%) 2215
▲ Fludara for Injection (1% to 6%) 658
Foscavir Injection (Between 1% and 5%) 541
Hivid Tablets (Less than 1%) 2287
Intal Inhaler (Rare) 2185
Intal Nebulizer Solution (Rare) 2186
Intron A for Injection (Less than or equal to 5%) 2506
Invirase Capsules (Less than 2%) 2291
Lupron Depot 7.5 mg (Less than 5%) 2741
Lupron Injection 2736
LUVOX Tablets (Rare) 2723
Matulane Capsules 2300
Orudis Capsules (Less than 1%) 2874
Oruvail Capsules (Less than 1%) 2874
Paxil Tablets (Rare) 2681
Permax Tablets (Infrequent) 571
Prevacid Delayed-Release Capsules (Less than 1%) 2746
Prinivil Tablets (0.3% to 1.0%) 1776
Prinzide Tablets 1780
Proleukin for Injection (1%) 812
Prozac Pulvules & Liquid, Oral Solution (Rare) 935
Pulmozyme Inhalation 1054
ReoPro Vials (9 to 11 events) 1526
Rifater 1280
Rilutek Tablets (Infrequent) 2198
Videx Tablets, Powder for Oral Solution, & Pediatric Powder for Oral Solution (Less than 1%) 2980
Zestoretic Tablets 2968
Zestril Tablets (0.3% to 1.0%) 2972
Zosyn (1.0% or less) 1463

Hemorrhage (see under Bleeding)

Hemorrhage, adrenal

Heparin Lock Flush Solution 2831
Heparin Sodium Injection 2832

Hemorrhage, cerebral (see under Cerebral hemorrhage)

Hemorrhage, eye, anterior chamber

Zoloft Tablets (Rare) 2051

Hemorrhage, eyes

AdatoSil 5000 (Greater than 2%) ⊙ 265
Dilacor XR Extended-release Capsules 2183
Eminase (Less than 1%) 2215
Hivid Tablets (Less than 1%) 2287
Kerlone Tablets (Less than 2%) 2588
Neurontin Capsules (Infrequent) 1978
Ocufen ⊙ 242
Paxil Tablets (Rare) 2681
Permax Tablets (Infrequent) 571
Proglycem 575
Prozac Pulvules & Liquid, Oral Solution (Rare) 935
ReoPro Vials (9 to 11 events) 1526
Ticlid Tablets 2317
Zyrtec Tablets (Less than 2%) 2053

Hemorrhage, gastrointestinal (see under Bleeding, gastrointestinal)

Hemorrhage, intra-alveolar

Depen Titratable Tablets 2770

Hemorrhage, intramuscular

Abbokinase 403
Abbokinase Open-Cath 405

Hemorrhage, intraventricular

▲ Exosurf Neonatal for Intratracheal Suspension (4% to 57%) 1081

Hemorrhage, muscle

Prozac Pulvules & Liquid, Oral Solution (Rare) 935

Hemorrhage, neonatal

Fiorinal 2388
Mebaral Tablets 2452
Mysoline 2860
Quadrinal Tablets 1398
Rifadin 1276
Rifater 1280
Soma Compound Tablets 2783

Hemorrhage, ovarian

Clomid 1262
Heparin Lock Flush Solution 2831
Heparin Sodium Injection 2832
Heparin Sodium Vials 1486

Hemorrhage, postpartum

Fiorinal 2388
Rifadin 1276
Rifater 1280
Syntocinon Injection 2425

Hemorrhage, pulmonary

▲ Exosurf Neonatal for Intratracheal Suspension (1% to 10%) 1081
Felbatol 2774
Foscavir Injection (Less than 1%) 541
ReoPro Vials (9 to 11 events) 1526
▲ Survanta Beractant Intratracheal Suspension (7.2%) 2346

Hemorrhage, purpuric

Atretol Tablets 569
Tegretol/Tegretol-XR 870

Hemorrhage, retinal

Clomid 1262
Glucotrol XL Extended Release Tablets (Less than 1%) 2012
Intron A for Injection (Rare) 2506
Matulane Capsules 2300
Orudis Capsules (Less than 1%) 2874
Oruvail Capsules (Less than 1%) 2874
Paxil Tablets (Rare) 2681

Hemorrhage, retroperitoneal

Abbokinase 403
Abbokinase Open-Cath 405
Activase (Less than 1%) 1045
Eminase 2215
Heparin Lock Flush Solution 2831
Heparin Sodium Injection 2832
Heparin Sodium Vials 1486

Hemorrhage, subarachnoid

Betaseron for SC Injection 653
Brevicon 2563
Demulen 2580
Hivid Tablets (Less than 1%) 2287
Imitrex Injection 1095
Imitrex Tablets 1099
Norinyl 2563
Nor-Q D Tablets 2598
Orthoclone OKT3 Sterile Solution 1892
Rilutek Tablets (Rare) 2198
Tri-Norinyl 2607

Hemorrhage, subconjunctival

Effexor (Infrequent) 2825

Hemorrhage, subcutaneous

Mustargen 1752
Ticlid Tablets 2317

Hemorrhage, vitreous

Xalatan (Extremely rare) ⊙ 304

Hemorrhagic colitis

Cytoxan (Isolated reports) 700
Lamictal Tablets (Rare) 1105
Primaxin I.M. 1770
Primaxin I.V. (Less than 0.2%) 1772

Hemorrhagic complications

Coumadin 941
Fragmin Injection (Low incidence) 2088
Heparin Sodium Vials 1486
Lovenox Injection (Low incidence) 2187
▲ Paraplatin for Injection (5%) 713

Hemorrhagic diathesis

▲ Mithracin (5.4 to 11.9%) 599
Solganal Suspension (Rare) 2530

Hemorrhagic disturbances

Cytovene-IV (One report) 2270

Hemorrhagic eruptions (see under Eruptions, hemorrhagic)

Hemorrhagic syndrome (see under Bleeding syndrome)

Hemorrhagic tendency

Mithracin 599
Mustargen 1752

Hemorrhoids

Ambien Tablets (Rare) 2559
Anafranil Capsules (Infrequent) 819

(▣ Described in PDR For Nonprescription Drugs) Incidence data in parenthesis; ▲ 3% or more (⊙ Described in PDR For Ophthalmology)

▲ Chemet Capsules (12.0% to 20.9%) 666
Claritin-D Tablets (Less frequent) .. 2487
Cognex Capsules (Infrequent) 1961
DaunoXome (Less than or equal to 5%) 1842
Effexor (Infrequent) 2825
Estring Vaginal Ring (1% to 3%) 2086
Hivid Tablets (Less than 1%) 2287
Imdur (Less than or equal to 5%) .. 1362
Invirase Capsules (Less than 2%) .. 2291
LUVOX Tablets (Infrequent) 2723
Neurontin Capsules (Infrequent) 1978
ReVia Tablets (Less than 1%) 957
Risperdal Tablets (Infrequent) 1348
Rowasa (1.35%) 2727
Sandostatin Injection (Less than 1%) 2421
Zoloft Tablets (Rare) 2051
Zyrtec Tablets (Less than 2%) 2053

Hemorrhoids, aggravation

Colestid 2073
Questran 774

Hemostasis, interference

Depakote Tablets 418

Hemothorax

Permax Tablets (Rare) 571

Henoch-Schonlein purpura

Bactrim DS Tablets 2257
Bactrim I.V. Infusion 2255
Bactrim 2257
LUVOX Tablets 2723
Septra 1146
Septra I.V. Infusion 1142
Septra I.V. Infusion ADD-Vantage Vials 1144
Septra 1146

Henoch-Schonlein vasculitis

IBU Tablets (Less than 1%) 1389
Motrin Ibuprofen Suspension, Oral Drops, Chewable Tablets, Caplets (Less than 1%) 1563

Hepatic adenoma

Brevicon 2563
Danocrine Capsules 2437
Desogen Tablets 1867
Estraderm Transdermal System (Rare) 842
ESTRATAB Tablets (0.3, 0.625, 1.25, 2.5 mg) (Rare) 2715
Estratest (Rare) 2718
Halotestin Tablets 2095
Lo/Ovral Tablets 2852
Lo/Ovral-28 Tablets 2857
Menest Tablets 2671
Nordette-21 Tablets 2863
Nordette-28 Tablets 2866
Norinyl 2563
Nor-Q D Tablets 2598
Ortho-Cept 1907
Ortho-Cyclen/Ortho-Tri-Cyclen 1914
Ortho-Cyclen/Ortho Tri-Cyclen 1914
Ovcon (Rare) 765
Ovral Tablets 2877
Ovral-28 Tablets 2878
Ovrette Tablets 2878
PMB 200 and PMB 400 2890
Premarin Intravenous 2893
Premarin Vaginal Cream 2898
Tri-Norinyl 2607
Triphasil-21 Tablets 2919
Triphasil-28 Tablets 2924

Hepatic coma

Capozide Tablets 744
Esidrix Tablets 839
Prinzide Tablets 1780
Ritalin (Some instances) 866
Tenoretic Tablets 2963
Vaseretic Tablets 1810
Zestoretic Tablets 2968

Hepatic dysfunction

Ambien Tablets (Infrequent) 2559
Anafranil Capsules (Infrequent) 819
Anaprox/Naprosyn (Less than 1%) 2277
Ancobon Capsules 2254
Atretol Tablets 569
Augmentin (Infrequent) 2637
Augmentin Tablets (Infrequent) 2640
Biaxin (Infrequent) 406
BiCNU 696
Cefotan 2936
Ceftin Tablets 1067
Ceptaz 1070
▲ Cipro I.V. (Among most frequent) .. 587
Claritin Tablets (Rare) 2485
Clomid 1262
Cuprimine Capsules 1673
Cylert Tablets 415
▲ Cytosar-U Sterile Powder (Among most frequent) 2077
Cytotec (Infrequent) 2576
Cytovene (2%) 2270
Danocrine Capsules 2437
Dantrium Capsules 2131
Daranide Tablets 1676
Darvon-N/Darvocet-N 1473
Darvon 1475
Darvon-N Suspension & Tablets 1473
Depakene 416
Depakote Tablets 418
Depen Titratable Tablets (Isolated cases) 2770
Diamox Intravenous (Occasional) .... ◉ 317
Diamox Sequels (Sustained Release) .... ◉ 318
Diamox Tablets (Occasional) .... ◉ 317
Dilantin Infatabs 1967
Dilantin Kapseals 1965
Dilantin-125 Suspension 1969
Disalcid 1549
Dolobid Tablets (Less than 1 in 100) 1695
Duricef Capsules, Tablets, and Oral Suspension 750
Dyazide Capsules 2653
E.E.S. 427
E-Mycin Tablets 1388
EC-Naprosyn Delayed-Release Tablets (Less than 1%) 2277
ERYC 1972
EryPed 425
Ery-Tab Tablets 426
Erythrocin Stearate Filmtab 429
Erythromycin Base Filmtab 430
Erythromycin Delayed-Release Capsules, USP 431
Ethmozine Tablets (Rare) 2217
Feldene Capsules (Less than 1%) .. 2008
Floxin I.V. 1580
Floxin Tablets (200 mg, 300 mg, 400 mg) 1577
Fludara for Injection (1% to 3%) 658
Fluothane 2830
Fortaz 1092
Foscavir Injection (Between 1% and 5%) 541
GlaucTabs (Occasional) .... ◉ 209
Halcion Tablets (Rare) 2093
▲ IFEX (3%) 706
Intron A for Injection (Less than 5%) 2506
Keftab Tablets 931
Librax Capsules (Occasional) 2330
Librium Capsules (Occasional) 2331
Librium Injectable (Occasional) 2332
Limbitrol (Rare) 2333
Lorabid Suspension and Pulvules (Rare) 1513
Lupron Injection 2736
Matulane Capsules 2300
Maxipime for Injection 758
Metrodin (urofollitropin for injection) 2616
Anaprox/Naprosyn (Less than 1%) 2277
Neutrexin for Injection 2761
▲ Nipent for Injection (2% to 19%) .. 2733
Nizoral Tablets (Rare) 1345
Normodyne Injection 2519
Normodyne Tablets 2522
▲ Novantrone for Injection (10 to 14%) 1327
Nydrazid Injection 509
Orudis Capsules (Less than 1%) 2874
Oruvail Capsules (Less than 1%) 2874
PCE Dispertab Tablets 453
Paxil Tablets 2681
Pediazole Suspension 2340
Pergonal (menotropins for injection, USP) 2618
Persantine Tablets (Rare) 686
▲ Prograf (5% to 36%) 1028
Proleukin for Injection 812
ReVia Tablets 957
Rifater (Rare) 1280
Salflex Tablets 791
Serax Capsules 2916
Serax Tablets 2916
Serophene (clomiphene citrate tablets, USP) 2621
Sporanox Capsules (0.3% to 2.7%) 1352
Suprax 1443
Tambocor Tablets (Rare) 1555
Tapazole Tablets 1361
Tazicef for Injection 2697
Tazidime Vials, Faspak & ADD-Vantage 1531
Tegretol/Tegretol-XR 870
Tenex Tablets (Less frequent) 2249
TheraCys BCG Live (Intravesical) (Up to 2.7%) 911
Tolectin (200, 400 and 600 mg) (Less than 1%) 1591
Toradol 2319
Trandate 1158
Vantin for Oral Suspension and Vantin Tablets 2112
Vumon for Injection (Less than 1%) 729
Wygesic Tablets 2930
Zanosar Sterile Powder 2119
Zinacef 1184
Zyrtec Tablets (Less than 2%) 2053

Hepatic enzymes, elevation (see also under SGOT elevation; SGPT elevation; Serum transaminase, elevation)

▲ Accutane Capsules (1 in 5 to 5 in 10 patients; approximately 15%) 2252
Achromycin V Capsules (Rare) 1417
Altace Capsules (Rare) 1238
▲ Anaprox/Naprosyn (Up to 15%) 2277
Atamet Tablets 567
Azathioprine Tablets 2349
Biaxin (Infrequent) 406
Biltricide Tablets 584
Brethine Ampuls 832
Brethine Tablets 831
Bricanyl Subcutaneous Injection (Rare) 1247
Bricanyl Tablets (Rare) 1248
Calan SR Caplets 2571
Calan Tablets 2568
Capoten Tablets 740
Capozide Tablets (Rare) 744
▲ Casodex Tablets (6%) 2934
Cataflam Tablets (Rare) 833
Cefobid Pharmacy Bulk Package - Not for Direct Infusion (1 patient in 1285) 1999
Cefotan (1.2%) 2936
Ceptaz 1070
▲ Cipro I.V. Pharmacy Bulk Package (Among most frequent) 590
Cordarone Intravenous (Common) .. 2821
Coumadin (Infrequent) 941
Covera-HS Tablets (1.4%) 2573
Cylert Tablets 415
Danocrine Capsules 2437
Dantrium Capsules 2131
Depakote Tablets 418
Dyazide Capsules 2653
DYNACIN Capsules 1627
Dyrenium Capsules (Rare) 2655
▲ EC-Naprosyn Delayed-Release Tablets (Up to 15%) 2277
Ergamisol Tablets (Rare) 1340
Helidac Therapy (Rare) 2135
Hismanal Tablets (Less frequent) 1341
Hydrea Capsules 705
Hyzaar Tablets (Occasional) 1720
▲ IFEX (3%) 706
Inocor Lactate Injection (Rare) 2439
Isoptin Oral Tablets 1393
Isoptin SR Tablets 1395
Lescol Capsules 2395
Lithonate/Lithotabs/Lithobid 2721
Lodine Capsules and Tablets (Less than 1%) 2849
Lotensin Tablets 852
Lotrel Capsules (Scattered incidents) 858
Ludiomil Tablets 861
Methotrexate Sodium Tablets, Injection, for Injection and LPF Injection (Frequent) 1322
Minocin Intravenous 1428
Minocin Oral Suspension 1431
Minocin Pellet-Filled Capsules 1429
Monopril Tablets 762
▲ Anaprox/Naprosyn (Up to 15%) 2277
Navelbine Injection 1212
Neoral 2405
Nolvadex Tablets 2957
Norpace (Less than 1%) 2596
Norvasc Tablets 2020
Pediazole Suspension 2340
Pipracil (Less frequent) 1435
Platinol for Injection 717
Platinol-AQ Injection 719
Prinivil Tablets (Rare) 1776
Prinzide Tablets (Rare) 1780
Propulsid (Rare) 1346
Recombivax HB 1787
Ridaura Capsules (Less than 1%) .. 2691
Roferon-A Injection (Frequent) 2308
Rowasa 2727
Rythmol Tablets–150mg, 225mg, 300mg (Less than 1%) 1399
Sandostatin Injection (Less than 1%) 2421
Sinemet Tablets 959
Sporanox Capsules 1352
Tenoretic Tablets 2963
Tenormin Tablets and I.V. Injection 2965
Testoderm Testosterone Transdermal System (One in 104 patients) 486
Thioguanine Tablets, Tabloid Brand (Occasional) 1225
Toradol 2319
Tornalate Solution for Inhalation, 0.2% (Infrequent) 976
Trental Tablets (Rare) 1291
Ultram Tablets (50 mg) (Infrequent) 1594
Univasc Tablets 2553
Vascor Tablets (200 and 300 mg) (Approximately 1%) 1597
Vaseretic Tablets (Rare) 1810
Vasotec I.V. 1814
Vasotec Tablets 1816
Verelan Capsules 1455
Vermox Chewable Tablets (Rare) 1357
Cataflam/Voltaren/Voltaren-XR (Rare) 833
Xanax Tablets 2115
▲ Zanosar Sterile Powder (A number of patients) 2119
Zestoretic Tablets (Rare) 2968
Zestril Tablets (Rare) 2972
Zoloft Tablets (One or more patients) 2051

Hepatic failure

Abelcet Injection 1540
Biaxin (Very rare) 406
Capoten Tablets (Rare) 740
Clinoril Tablets (Less than 1 in 100) 1658
Depakene 416
Depakote Tablets 418
Diflucan Tablets, Injection, and Oral Suspension (Rare) 2003
Doxil (Less than 1%) 2613
DYNACIN Capsules (Rare) 1627
Elavil 2945
Felbatol (A marked increase) 2774
Floxin I.V. 1580
Floxin Tablets (200 mg, 300 mg, 400 mg) 1577
Fludara for Injection (Up to 1%) 658
Fungizone Intravenous 507
Helidac Therapy 2135
Hivid Tablets (Rare) 2287
Intron A for Injection (Very rare) 2506
Lodine Capsules and Tablets (Rare; less than 1%) 2849
Lotensin Tablets (Rare) 852
Mavik Tablets (Rare) 1407
Merrem I.V. (0.1% to 1.0%) 2952
Minocin Intravenous (Rare) 1428
Minocin Oral Suspension (Rare) 1431
Minocin Pellet-Filled Capsules (Rare) 1429
Monopril Tablets 762
Motrin Ibuprofen Suspension, Oral Drops, Chewable Tablets, Caplets (Less than 1%) 1563
Oncaspar 2194
Prilosec Delayed-Release Capsules (Rare) 516
Prinivil Tablets (Rare) 1776
Prinzide Tablets (Rare) 1780
Proleukin for Injection (Less than 1%) 812
Prozac Pulvules & Liquid, Oral Solution 935
Redux Capsules 2911
Risperdal Tablets (Rare) 1348
Tambocor Tablets (Rare) 1555
Toradol 2319
Univasc Tablets (Rare) 2553
Vaseretic Tablets (Rare) 1810
Vasotec I.V. (Rare) 1814
Vasotec Tablets (Rare; 0.5% to 1.0%) 1816
Videx Tablets, Powder for Oral Solution, & Pediatric Powder for Oral Solution (Less than 1%) 2980
Vistide Injection (Less than 1%) 1057
Zestoretic Tablets (Rare) 2968

Side Effects Index

Hepatic failure

- Zestril Tablets (Rare) ... 2972
- Zofran Injection ... 1227
- Zofran Tablets ... 1231
- Zoloft Tablets (One or more patients) ... 2051

Hepatic function tests, impaired
(see under Liver function, impaired)

Hepatic veno-occlusive disease, life threatening

- Abelcet Injection ... 1540
- Alkeran for Injection ... 1196
- Azathioprine Tablets (1 patient) ... 2349
- Imuran (Rare) ... 1103
- Myleran Tablets ... 1209
- Thioguanine Tablets, Tabloid Brand ... 1225

Hepatitis

- Abelcet Injection ... 1540
- Accupril Tablets (0.5% to 1.0%) .. 1950
- Accutane Capsules (Several cases) 2252
- Aldoclor Tablets ... 1638
- Aldomet Ester HCl Injection ... 1642
- Aldomet Oral ... 1640
- Aldoril Tablets ... 1644
- Altace Capsules (Less than 1%) ... 1238
- Anafranil Capsules (Infrequent) ... 819
- Anaprox/Naprosyn (Rare) ... 2277
- Antabuse Tablets (Multiple cases) .. 2802
- Apresazide Capsules (Rare) ... 824
- Apresoline Hydrochloride Tablets (Rare) ... 826
- Asacol Delayed-Release Tablets (Rare) ... 2129
- Asendin Tablets (Very rate) ... 1419
- Atretol Tablets ... 569
- Augmentin (Rare) ... 2637
- Augmentin Tablets (Rare) ... 2640
- Axid Pulvules ... 1468
- Azactam for Injection (Less than 1%) ... 736
- Azulfidine (Rare) ... 2059
- Bactrim DS Tablets ... 2257
- Bactrim I.V. Infusion ... 2255
- Bactrim ... 2257
- Betaseron for SC Injection ... 653
- Capoten Tablets ... 740
- Capozide Tablets ... 744
- Cartrol Tablets (Rare) ... 413
- Cataflam Tablets (Less than 1%) ... 833
- Catapres Tablets (Rare) ... 679
- Ceclor Pulvules & Suspension (Rare) ... 1470
- ▲ CellCept Capsules (More than or equal to 3%) ... 2265
- Chibroxin Sterile Ophthalmic Solution (With oral form) ... 1657
- Claritin Tablets (Rare) ... 2485
- Claritin-D Tablets ... 2487
- Clinoril Tablets (Less than 1%) ... 1658
- Clomid ... 1262
- Clozaril Tablets ... 2377
- Combipres Tablets (Rare) ... 682
- Cosmegen Injection ... 1666
- Coumadin (Infrequent) ... 941
- Cylert Tablets ... 415
- Cytovene (1% or less) ... 2270
- Dantrium Capsules (Less frequent) 2131
- Daypro Caplets (Less than 1%) ... 2578
- DiaBeta Tablets (Rare) ... 1265
- Diflucan Tablets, Injection, and Oral Suspension (Rare) ... 2003
- Dipentum Capsules (Rare) ... 2084
- Disalcid ... 1549
- Dolobid Tablets (Less than 1 in 100) ... 1695
- Doxil (Less than 1%) ... 2613
- DYNACIN Capsules (Rare) ... 1627
- EC-Naprosyn Delayed-Release Tablets (Rare) ... 2277
- Effexor (Rare) ... 2825
- Elavil (Rare) ... 2945
- Ethmozine Tablets (Rare) ... 2217
- Etrafon (Rare) ... 2495
- Eulexin Capsules (Less than 1%) ... 2498
- Fansidar Tablets ... 2281
- Felbatol ... 2774
- Feldene Capsules (Less than 1%) ... 2008
- Fiorinal with Codeine Capsules ... 2390
- Flexeril Tablets (Rare) ... 1701
- Floxin I.V. ... 1580
- Floxin Tablets (200 mg, 300 mg, 400 mg) ... 1577
- Foscavir Injection (Less than 1%) ... 541
- Fungizone Intravenous ... 507
- Gantanol Tablets ... 2285
- Gantrisin ... 2286

- Halotestin Tablets ... 2095
- Havrix (Rare) ... 2663
- Hivid Tablets (Less than 1%) ... 2287
- Hydralazine Hydrochloride Injection USP (Rare) ... 2712
- IBU Tablets (Less than 1%) ... 1389
- Invirase Capsules (Less than 2%) .. 2291
- Keflex Pulvules & Oral Suspension (Rare) ... 930
- Keftab Tablets (Rare) ... 931
- Kefzol Vials, Faspak & ADD-Vantage (Rare) ... 1511
- Konyne 80 Factor IX Complex ... 627
- Lamictal Tablets (Rare) ... 1105
- Lamprene Capsules (Less than 1%) ... 846
- Lescol Capsules ... 2395
- Lodine Capsules and Tablets (Less than 1%) ... 2849
- Loxitane (Rare) ... 1426
- LUVOX Tablets ... 2723
- Macrobid Capsules (Rare) ... 2138
- Macrodantin Capsules (Rare) ... 2140
- Mandol Vials, Faspak & ADD-Vantage (Rare) ... 1516
- Maxaquin Tablets ... 2593
- Mesantoin Tablets ... 2400
- Mevacor Tablets ... 1742
- Mexitil Capsules (Rare) ... 684
- Miacalcin Nasal Spray (Less than 1%) ... 2403
- Micronase Tablets (Rare) ... 2099
- Minocin Intravenous (Rare) ... 1428
- Minocin Oral Suspension (Rare) ... 1431
- Minocin Pellet-Filled Capsules (Rare) ... 1429
- Monopril Tablets (0.2% to 1.0%) .. 762
- Motrin Ibuprofen Suspension, Oral Drops, Chewable Tablets, Caplets (Rare; less than 1%) ... 1563
- Mycobutin Capsules (Less than 1%) ... 2101
- Myochrysine Injection ... 1754
- Anaprox/Naprosyn (Rare) ... 2277
- Nimotop Capsules (Less than 1%) ... 603
- Nizoral Tablets (Several cases) ... 1345
- Nolvadex Tablets (Rare) ... 2957
- Normodyne Injection (Less common) ... 2519
- Normodyne Tablets (Less common) ... 2522
- Noroxin Tablets ... 1758
- Noroxin Tablets ... 2222
- Norpramin Tablets ... 1273
- Norvir (Less than 2%) ... 447
- Orlaam Oral Solution (Low frequency) ... 2361
- Orthoclone OKT3 Sterile Solution .. 1892
- Papaverine Hydrochloride Vials and Ampoules (Infrequent) ... 1523
- Parnate Tablets (Rare) ... 2679
- PASER Granules ... 1333
- Paxil Tablets (Rare) ... 2681
- Pediazole Suspension ... 2340
- Pentasa (Infrequent) ... 1275
- Permax Tablets (Infrequent) ... 571
- Phenurone Tablets (2%) ... 455
- Pravachol Tablets ... 770
- Prilosec Delayed-Release Capsules (Rare) ... 516
- Primaxin I.M. ... 1770
- Primaxin I.V. (Less than 0.2%) ... 1772
- Prinivil Tablets (0.3% to 1.0%) ... 1776
- Prinzide Tablets ... 1780
- Priscoline Hydrochloride Ampuls ... 864
- ▲ Prograf (Greater than 3%) ... 1028
- Propulsid (Rare) ... 1346
- Prozac Pulvules & Liquid, Oral Solution (Rare) ... 935
- Redux Capsules (Infrequent) ... 2911
- Retrovir Capsules (Rare) ... 1216
- Retrovir I.V. Infusion (Rare) ... 1221
- Retrovir Syrup ... 1216
- Rifadin (Rare) ... 1276
- Rifamate Capsules (Rare) ... 1278
- Rifater (Rare; occasional) ... 1280
- Rilutek Tablets (Infrequent) ... 2198
- Rimactane Capsules (Rare) ... 865
- Risperdal Tablets (Rare) ... 1348
- Roferon-A Injection (Infrequent) ... 2308
- Rythmol Tablets—150mg, 225mg, 300mg (0.03%) ... 1399
- SSD ... 1402
- Salflex Tablets ... 791
- Sandostatin Injection (Less than 1%) ... 2421
- Seldane Tablets (Isolated reports) .. 1284
- Seldane-D Extended-Release Tablets (Isolated reports) ... 1286
- Septra ... 1146
- Septra I.V. Infusion ... 1142

- Septra I.V. Infusion ADD-Vantage Vials ... 1144
- Septra ... 1146
- Ser-Ap-Es Tablets ... 867
- Serzone Tablets (Rare) ... 776
- Silvadene Cream 1% ... 1288
- Solganal Suspension ... 2530
- Sporanox Capsules (Rare) ... 1352
- Stelazine ... 2692
- Tapazole Tablets ... 1361
- ▲ Tegison Capsules (1-10%) ... 2314
- Tegretol/Tegretol-XR ... 870
- TICE BCG, USP (0.2%) ... 1881
- Ticlid Tablets (Rare) ... 2317
- Timentin for Injection (Rare) ... 2706
- Tolectin (200, 400 and 600 mg) (Less than 1%) ... 1591
- Tonocard Tablets (Less than 1%) ... 519
- Toradol ... 2319
- Trandate (Less common) ... 1158
- Trecator-SC Tablets ... 2919
- Trental Tablets (Rare) ... 1291
- Triavil Tablets (Rare) ... 1800
- Trilisate (Rare) ... 2155
- Ultram Tablets (50 mg) (Infrequent) ... 1594
- Univasc Tablets (Less than 1%) ... 2553
- Urobiotic-250 Capsules ... 2038
- Vaseretic Tablets ... 1810
- Vasotec I.V. ... 1814
- Vasotec Tablets (0.5% to 1.0%) ... 1816
- Vermox Chewable Tablets (Rare) ... 1357
- ▲ Vesanoid Capsules (3%) ... 2327
- Viramune Tablets (1%) ... 2368
- Cataflam/Voltaren/Voltaren-XR (Less than 1%) ... 833
- Wellbutrin Tablets ... 1177
- Yutopar Intravenous Injection (Less than 1%) ... 566
- Zantac (Occasional) ... 1182
- Zantac Injection ... 1180
- Zantac Syrup (Occasional) ... 1182
- Zaroxolyn Tablets ... 1625
- Zestoretic Tablets ... 2968
- Zestril Tablets (0.3% to 1.0%) ... 2972
- Zocor Tablets ... 1821
- Zoloft Tablets (One or more patients) ... 2051
- Zyrtec Tablets (Rare) ... 2053

Hepatitis, allergic

- Adalat Capsules (10 mg and 20 mg) (Less than 0.5%) ... 580
- Adalat CC (Rare) ... 582
- Procardia Capsules (Rare; less than 0.5%) ... 2024
- Procardia XL Extended Release Tablets (Rare instances) ... 2026

Hepatitis, cholestatic

- Android Capsules, 10 mg ... 1297
- Antabuse Tablets (Multiple cases) .. 2802
- Biaxin (Infrequent) ... 406
- Ceptaz ... 1070
- Cordarone Tablets (Rare) ... 2818
- Dipentum Capsules (One case) ... 2084
- Dynabac (Rare) ... 668
- Estratest ... 2718
- Foscavir Injection (Less than 1%) .. 541
- Glynase PresTab Tablets (Rare) ... 2091
- Lamisil Tablets (Rare) ... 2394
- Lodine Capsules and Tablets (Less than 1%) ... 2849
- Nalfon 200 Pulvules & Nalfon Tablets (Less than 1%) ... 933
- Oxandrin ... 783
- Pipracil (Less frequent) ... 1435
- Prilosec Delayed-Release Capsules (Rare) ... 516
- Risperdal Tablets (Rare) ... 1348
- Seldane Tablets (Isolated reports) .. 1284
- Seldane-D Extended-Release Tablets (Isolated reports) ... 1286
- Tao Capsules ... 2033
- Testoderm Testosterone Transdermal System ... 486
- Zosyn ... 1463

Hepatitis, fulminant

- Antabuse Tablets (Multiple cases) .. 2802
- Cataflam Tablets (Rare) ... 833
- Sporanox Capsules (One patient) ... 1352
- Tapazole Tablets (Rare) ... 1361
- Cataflam/Voltaren/Voltaren-XR (Rare) ... 833

Hepatitis, granulomatous

- Cardioquin Tablets (A few cases) ... 2146
- Dipentum Capsules (Rare) ... 2084
- Quinaglute Dura-Tabs Tablets ... 644
- Quinidex Extentabs ... 2240

- Zyloprim Tablets (Less than 1%) ... 1194

Hepatitis, idiosyncratic, reversible

- Sporanox Capsules (Three cases) .. 1352

Hepatitis, overt

- Prilosec Delayed-Release Capsules (Rare) ... 516

Hepatitis, reactive

- Dipentum Capsules (Rare) ... 2084
- Macrobid Capsules (Rare) ... 2138
- Macrodantin Capsules (Rare) ... 2140

Hepatitis, toxic

- Alkeran for Injection ... 1196
- Cuprimine Capsules (Rare) ... 1673
- Dapsone Tablets USP ... 1331
- Depen Titratable Tablets (Rare) ... 2770
- Dilantin Infatabs ... 1967
- Dilantin Kapseals ... 1965
- Dilantin-125 Suspension ... 1969
- Indocin Capsules (Less than 1%) ... 1723
- Indocin I.V. (Less than 1%) ... 1727
- Indocin (Less than 1%) ... 1723
- Rifamate Capsules ... 1278
- Solganal Suspension ... 2530

Hepatitis, viral

- Koāte-HP Antihemophilic Factor (Human) ... 624
- Prolastin Alpha₁-Proteinase Inhibitor (Human) ... 629

Hepatobiliary dysfunction

- Azactam for Injection (Less than 1%) ... 736
- Lamisil Tablets (Rare) ... 2394

Hepatomas

- Avonex ... 662
- Brevicon ... 2563
- Demulen (Rare) ... 2580
- Lescol Capsules (Rare) ... 2395
- Lopid Tablets ... 1974
- Mevacor Tablets (Rare) ... 1742
- Norinyl ... 2563
- Nor-Q D Tablets (Extremely rare) .. 2598
- Ovcon ... 765
- PMB 200 and PMB 400 ... 2890
- Pravachol Tablets (Rare) ... 770
- Premarin Intravenous ... 2893
- Premarin Vaginal Cream ... 2898
- Tri-Norinyl ... 2607
- Zocor Tablets (Rare) ... 1821

Hepatomas, benign

- Desogen Tablets ... 1867
- Levlen/Tri-Levlen (Rare) ... 646
- Lo/Ovral Tablets ... 2852
- Lo/Ovral-28 Tablets ... 2857
- Micronor Tablets (Rare) ... 1903
- Modicon ... 1928
- Nordette-21 Tablets ... 2863
- Nordette-28 Tablets ... 2866
- Ortho-Cept ... 1907
- Ortho-Cyclen/Ortho-Tri-Cyclen (Rare) ... 1914
- Ortho-Novum ... 1928
- Ortho-Cyclen/Ortho Tri-Cyclen (Rare) ... 1914
- Ovral Tablets ... 2877
- Ovral-28 Tablets ... 2878
- Ovrette Tablets ... 2878
- Levlen/Tri-Levlen (Rare) ... 646
- Triphasil-21 Tablets ... 2919
- Triphasil-28 Tablets ... 2924

Hepatomas, malignant

- Danocrine Capsules (Rare) ... 2437
- Demulen ... 2580

Hepatomegaly

- Atromid-S Capsules ... 2808
- Avonex ... 662
- Betaseron for SC Injection ... 653
- Blocadren Tablets ... 1654
- Cosmegen Injection ... 1666
- DaunoXome (Less than or equal to 5%) ... 1842
- Garamycin Injectable ... 2502
- Hivid Tablets (Rare; less than 3%) 2287
- Invirase Capsules (Less than 2%) .. 2291
- Klonopin Tablets ... 2294
- Megace Oral Suspension (1% to 3%) ... 708
- Monopril Tablets (0.4% to 1.0%) .. 762
- Neupogen for Injection (Infrequent) ... 495
- Neurontin Capsules (Infrequent) ... 1978
- Norvir (Less than 2%) ... 447

(⊞ Described in PDR For Nonprescription Drugs)   Incidence data in parentheses; ▲ 3% or more   (⊛ Described in PDR For Ophthalmology)

Oncaspar (Less than 1%) 2194
Orthoclone OKT3 Sterile Solution 1892
PASER Granules 1333
Permax Tablets (Infrequent) 571
Procanbid Extended-Release Tablets 1983
Proleukin for Injection (1%) 812
Prozac Pulvules & Liquid, Oral Solution (Rare) 935
Redux Capsules (Infrequent) 2911
Retrovir Capsules (Rare) 1216
Retrovir I.V. Infusion (Rare) 1221
Retrovir Syrup 1216
Sular Tablets (Less than or equal to 1%) 2961
Thioguanine Tablets, Tabloid Brand 1225
Timolide Tablets 1791
Timoptic in Ocudose 1796
Timoptic Sterile Ophthalmic Solution 1794
Timoptic-XE 1798
Tornalate Solution for Inhalation, 0.2% (One patient) 976
Videx Tablets, Powder for Oral Solution, & Pediatric Powder for Oral Solution (Less than 1%) 2980
Vistide Injection 1057
Zoloft Tablets (One or more patients) 2051
Zyloprim Tablets (Less than 1%) 1194

Hepatorenal syndrome, unspecified

Cataflam Tablets (Less than 1%) 833
Felbatol 2774
Motrin Ibuprofen Suspension, Oral Drops, Chewable Tablets, Caplets (Less than 1%) 1563
Cataflam/Voltaren/Voltaren-XR (Less than 1%) 833

Hepatosplenomegaly

Aquasol A Vitamin A Capsules, USP 525
Aquasol A Parenteral 526
Doxil (Less than 1%) 2613
Foscavir Injection (Less than 1%) 541
Invirase Capsules (Less than 2%) 2291
Naprelan Tablets (Less than 1%) 2861
▲ Vesanoid Capsules (9%) 2327

Hepatotoxicity

▲ Accutane Capsules (1 in 5 to 1 in 10 patients) 2252
Adriamycin PFS 2056
Adriamycin RDF 2056
Alkeran Tablets (Rare) 1198
Android Capsules, 10 mg 1297
Azathioprine Tablets (Less than 1%) 2349
BiCNU 696
Cardioquin Tablets (A few cases) 2146
Cataflam Tablets 833
CeeNU Capsules 699
Cognex Capsules 1961
Cosmegen Injection 1666
Cytadren Tablets (Less than 1 in 1000) 837
Dantrium Capsules 2131
Demulen 2580
Depakene 416
Depakote Tablets 418
Diflucan Tablets, Injection, and Oral Suspension (Rare) 2003
Easprin 1971
Estratest 2718
Fulvicin P/G Tablets (Rare) 2499
Fulvicin P/G 165 & 330 Tablets (Rare) 2500
Furoxone 2221
Helidac Therapy (Rare) 2135
Hivid Tablets 2287
Imuran (Less than 1%) 1103
Inocor Lactate Injection (0.2%) 2439
Intron A for Injection (Rare) 2506
Leukeran Tablets 1205
Levoprome 1321
Loxitane 1426
Methotrexate Sodium Tablets, Injection, for Injection and LPF Injection 1322
Minocin Intravenous 1428
Minocin Oral Suspension 1431
Motrin Ibuprofen Suspension, Oral Drops, Chewable Tablets, Caplets 1563
▲ Neoral (4% to 7%) 2405
Neutrexin for Injection 2761
Nizoral Tablets 1345
Platinol for Injection 717
Platinol-AQ Injection 719
Purinethol Tablets (Frequent) 1214
Pyrazinamide Tablets 1442
Quinaglute Dura-Tabs Tablets 644
Quinidex Extentabs (A few cases) 2240
Reglan (Rare) 2243
ReVia Tablets 957
Rifater 1280
Roferon-A Injection (Unusual) 2308
▲ Sandimmune (Less than 1 to 7%) 2416
Tapazole Tablets 1361
Tigan 2231
Torecan 2367
Vibramycin (Rare) 2038
Vibramycin Hyclate Intravenous (Rare) 2040
Vibramycin (Rare) 2038
Cataflam/Voltaren/Voltaren-XR 833
▲ Zanosar Sterile Powder (A number of patients) 2119
Zyloprim Tablets (A few cases) 1194

Hernia, hiatal

Cognex Capsules (Infrequent) 1961
Neurontin Capsules (Rare) 1978

Hernia, unspecified

Avonex 662
Betaseron for SC Injection 653
▲ CellCept Capsules (More than or equal to 3%) 2265
Effexor (Infrequent) 2825
Permax Tablets (Infrequent) 571
▲ Prograf (Greater than 3%) 1028
Rilutek Tablets (Infrequent) 2198
Serzone Tablets (Infrequent) 776
Videx Tablets, Powder for Oral Solution, & Pediatric Powder for Oral Solution (Less than 1%) 2980
Zoloft Tablets (Rare) 2051

Herpes labialis

Alferon N Injection (1%) 2142

Herpes labialis, recurrent, exacerbation of

Azelex (Rare) 471

Herpes, precipitation

Matulane Capsules 2300
Oxsoralen-Ultra Capsules 1302

Herpes simplex

Ambien Tablets (Rare) 2559
Avonex (2%) 662
Blephamide Ointment ⊙ 234
▲ CellCept Capsules (16.7% to 20.0%; 12.5% to 15.2%) 2265
Cognex Capsules (Infrequent) 1961
Cortisporin Ophthalmic Ointment Sterile 1074
Crixivan Capsules (Less than 2%) 1670
Cytovene (1% or less) 2270
Doxil (1% to 5%) 2613
Effexor (Infrequent) 2825
Efudex (Infrequent) 2280
FML S.O.P. ⊙ 239
Foscavir Injection (Less than 1%) 541
Intron A for Injection (Up to 5%) 2506
Invirase Capsules (Less than 2%) 2291
8-MOP Capsules 1294
Naprelan Tablets (Less than 1%) 2861
Neurontin Capsules (Infrequent) 1978
▲ Nipent for Injection (4%) 2733
Oncaspar 2194
Paxil Tablets (Rare) 2681
Permax Tablets (Infrequent) 571
Proglycem 575
▲ Prograf (Greater than 3%) 1028
Prozac Pulvules & Liquid, Oral Solution (Infrequent) 935
Remeron Tablets (Infrequent) 1878
Rhinocort Nasal Inhaler (Less than 1%) 552
Sular Tablets (Less than or equal to 1%) 2961
Tegison Capsules (Less than 1%) 2314
Vexol 1% Ophthalmic Suspension ⊙ 227
Videx Tablets, Powder for Oral Solution, & Pediatric Powder for Oral Solution (Up to 2%) 2980
Vistide Injection 1057
Zoladex 3-month (1% to 5%) 2978

Herpes simplex, disseminated

Accutane Capsules (Less than 1%) 2252

Herpes zoster

Ambien Tablets (Rare) 2559
▲ Avonex (3%) 662
▲ CellCept Capsules (6.0% to 7.6%; 6.7% to 6.9%) 2265
Cognex Capsules (Infrequent) 1961
Crixivan Capsules (Less than 2%) 1670
Doxil (Less than 1%) 2613
Effexor (Infrequent) 2825
Engerix-B Unit-Dose Vials 2656
Intron A for Injection (Less than 5%) 2506
Invirase Capsules (Less than 2%) 2291
Lamictal Tablets (Rare) 1105
Leustatin (8 episodes) 1889
Mustargen 1752
Naprelan Tablets (Less than 1%) 2861
Neurontin Capsules (Rare) 1978
▲ Nipent for Injection (8%) 2733
Paxil Tablets (Rare) 2681
Permax Tablets (Infrequent) 571
Prinivil Tablets (0.3% to 1.0%) 1776
Prinzide Tablets 1780
Prozac Pulvules & Liquid, Oral Solution (Rare) 935
Recombivax HB 1787
Remeron Tablets (Rare) 1878
Sular Tablets (Less than or equal to 1%) 2961
Varivax 1807
Vaseretic Tablets 1810
Vasotec I.V. 1814
Vasotec Tablets (0.5% to 1.0%) 1816
Videx Tablets, Powder for Oral Solution, & Pediatric Powder for Oral Solution (Up to 2%) 2980
Zestoretic Tablets 2968
Zestril Tablets (0.3% to 1.0%) 2972

Herpes, unspecified

Megace Oral Suspension (1% to 3%) 708

Herxheimer's reaction

Bicillin L-A Injection 2813
Chloromycetin Sodium Succinate 1960
Pfizerpen for Injection 2022

Hiccups

Ambien Tablets (Frequent) 2559
Anafranil Capsules (Rare) 819
Atamet Tablets 567
Avonex 662
Betaseron for SC Injection 653
BuSpar Tablets (Rare) 738
Celontin Kapseals 1955
Cipro I.V. (1% or less) 587
Cipro I.V. Pharmacy Bulk Package (Less than 1%) 590
Cipro Tablets (Less than 1%) 584
Dalalone D.P. Injectable 1009
Dalgan Injection (Less than 1%) 529
DaunoXome (Less than or equal to 5%) 1842
Decadron Elixir 1676
Decadron Phosphate Injection 1680
Decadron Phosphate with Xylocaine Injection, Sterile 1683
Decadron Tablets 1678
Decadron-LA Sterile Suspension (Low) 1687
Dexacort Phosphate in Respihaler 1606
Dexacort Phosphate in Turbinaire 1607
Diprivan Injectable Emulsion (Less than 1%) 2939
Dizac (diazepam injectable emulsion) CIV (Less frequent) 1862
Dopram Injectable 2235
Duragesic Transdermal System (1% or greater) 1336
Emete-con Intramuscular/Intravenous 2007
Ethyol (amifostine) for Injection 485
▲ Felbatol (9.7%) 2774
Fioricet with Codeine Capsules 2387
Fiorinal with Codeine Capsules 2390
Floxin I.V. 1580
Floxin Tablets (200 mg, 300 mg, 400 mg) 1577
Imitrex Injection (Rare) 1095
Imitrex Tablets (Rare) 1099
ISMOTIC 45% w/v Solution (Very rare) ⊙ 221
Kadian Capsules (Less than 3%) 2948
Lamictal Tablets (Rare) 1105
Larodopa Tablets (Rare) 2296
LUVOX Tablets (Rare) 2723
Maxaquin Tablets 2593
Mexitil Capsules (About 1 in 1,000) 684
Moduretic Tablets (Less than or equal to 1%) 1748
Neoral (2% or less) 2405
Neurontin Capsules (Rare) 1978
Nicotrol NS Nicotine Nasal Spray (Less than 1%) 1565
Norvir (Less than 2%) 447
▲ OxyContin Tablets (Between 1% and 5%) 2163
Paxil Tablets (Rare) 2681
Permax Tablets (1.1%) 571
Platinol for Injection 717
Platinol-AQ Injection (Infrequent) 719
Prevacid Delayed-Release Capsules (Less than 1%) 2746
Prozac Pulvules & Liquid, Oral Solution (Infrequent) 935
Questran 774
Redux Capsules 2911
Remeron Tablets (Rare) 1878
Rilutek Tablets (Infrequent) 2198
Romazicon (Less than 1%) 2311
Sandimmune (2% or less) 2416
Serzone Tablets (Infrequent) 776
Sinemet Tablets 959
Sinemet CR Tablets 961
Soma Compound w/Codeine Tablets 2784
Soma Compound Tablets 2783
Soma Tablets 2782
Tonocard Tablets (Less than 1%) 519
Valium Injectable 2336
▲ Versed Injection (3.9%) 2324
Vistide Injection 1057
Zarontin Capsules 1986
Zarontin Syrup 1986
Zemuron Injection (Less than 1%) 1885
Zoloft Tablets (Rare) 2051
Zosyn (1.0% or less to 2.6%) 1463

Hirsutism

Accutane Capsules (Less than 1%) 2252
Aldactazide Tablets 2556
Aldactone Tablets 2558
Amen Tablets (Few cases) 785
Androderm Testosterone Transdermal System 2634
▲ Android Capsules, 10 mg (Among most common) 1297
Betaseron for SC Injection 653
Brevicon 2563
▲ CellCept Capsules (More than or equal to 3%) 2265
Climara Transdermal System 640
Cortone Acetate Sterile Suspension 1663
Cortone Acetate Tablets 1664
Cycrin Tablets (A few cases) 991
Cytadren Tablets (Rare) 837
Dalalone D.P. Injectable 1009
Danocrine Capsules 2437
Dantrium Capsules (Less frequent) 2131
Decadron Elixir 1676
Decadron Phosphate Injection 1680
Decadron Phosphate with Xylocaine Injection, Sterile 1683
Decadron Tablets 1678
Decadron-LA Sterile Suspension 1687
Demulen 2580
Depo-Provera Contraceptive Injection (Fewer than 1%) 2079
Depo-Provera Sterile Aqueous Suspension 2083
Desogen Tablets 1867
Desyrel and Desyrel Dividose 504
Dexacort Phosphate in Respihaler 1606
Dexacort Phosphate in Turbinaire 1607
Diethylstilbestrol Tablets 1477
Effexor (Rare) 2825
Eldepryl Capsules 2729
Estrace Cream and Tablets 751
Estraderm Transdermal System 842
ESTRATAB Tablets (0.3, 0.625, 1.25, 2.5 mg) 2715
Estratest 2718
Florinef Acetate Tablets 506
Halotestin Tablets 2095
Hydeltrasol Injection, Sterile 1708
Hydeltra-T.B.A. Sterile Suspension 1710
Hydrocortone Acetate Sterile Suspension 1712
Hydrocortone Phosphate Injection, Sterile 1713
Hydrocortone Tablets 1715
Hyperstat I.V. Injection 2504
Intron A for Injection (Less than 5%) 2506
Klonopin Tablets 2294
Lamictal Tablets (Infrequent) 1105
Levlen/Tri-Levlen 646
Lo/Ovral Tablets 2852
Lo/Ovral-28 Tablets 2857
Lupron Depot 7.5 mg (Less than 5%) 2741

(▭ Described in PDR For Nonprescription Drugs) Incidence data in parenthesis; ▲ 3% or more (⊙ Described in PDR For Ophthalmology)

Hirsutism

- Lupron Injection ... 2736
- Menest Tablets ... 2671
- Micronor Tablets (Rare) ... 1903
- Modicon ... 1928
- ▲ Neoral (21% to 45%) ... 2405
- Neurontin Capsules (Infrequent) ... 1978
- Nordette-21 Tablets ... 2863
- Nordette-28 Tablets ... 2866
- Norinyl ... 2563
- Norplant System ... 2868
- Nor-Q D Tablets ... 2598
- Ogen Tablets ... 2103
- Ogen Vaginal Cream ... 2106
- Ortho-Cept ... 1907
- Ortho-Cyclen/Ortho-Tri-Cyclen ... 1914
- Ortho Dienestrol Cream ... 1922
- Ortho-Est ... 1925
- Ortho-Novum ... 1928
- Ortho-Cyclen/Ortho Tri-Cyclen ... 1914
- Ovcon ... 765
- Ovral Tablets ... 2877
- Ovral-28 Tablets ... 2878
- Ovrette Tablets ... 2878
- Oxandrin ... 783
- Paxil Tablets (Rare) ... 2681
- Permax Tablets (Infrequent) ... 571
- PMB 200 and PMB 400 ... 2890
- Premarin Intravenous ... 2893
- Premarin Tablets ... 2896
- Premarin Vaginal Cream ... 2898
- Premphase ... 2900
- Prempro ... 2905
- Proglycem (Frequent) ... 575
- ▲ Prograf (Greater than 3%) ... 1028
- Provera Tablets (A few cases) ... 2110
- Prozac Pulvules & Liquid, Oral Solution (Rare) ... 935
- Redux Capsules (Infrequent) ... 2911
- ▲ Sandimmune (21 to 45%) ... 2416
- Synarel Nasal Solution for Endometriosis (2.5% of patients) ... 2605
- ▲ Tegison Capsules (1-10%) ... 2314
- Tegretol/Tegretol-XR (Isolated cases) ... 870
- Testoderm Testosterone Transdermal System ... 486
- Testred Capsules, 10 mg ... 1308
- Levlen/Tri-Levlen ... 646
- Tri-Norinyl ... 2607
- Triphasil-21 Tablets ... 2919
- Triphasil-28 Tablets ... 2924
- Vivelle Transdermal System ... 880
- Wellbutrin Tablets (Rare) ... 1177
- Winstrol Tablets ... 2468
- Zarontin Capsules ... 1986
- Zarontin Syrup ... 1986
- ▲ Zoladex (7%) ... 2976

Hives

(see also under Urticaria)

- AeroBid Inhaler System (1% to 3%) ... 1004
- Aerobid-M Inhaler System (1% to 3%) ... 1004
- Alferon N Injection ... 2142
- Alupent Tablets (0.2%) ... 672
- Atrovent Inhalation Aerosol (Less frequent) ... 674
- Betoptic Ophthalmic Solution (Rare) ... 465
- Betoptic S Ophthalmic Suspension (Rare) ... 467
- Bumex (0.2%) ... 2260
- Carafate Tablets ... 1249
- Catapres Tablets (About 5 in 1,000 patients) ... 679
- Catapres-TTS ... 680
- Combipres Tablets (About 5 in 1,000) ... 682
- Cutivate Ointment (Less than 1%) ... 1078
- Emete-con Intramuscular/Intravenous ... 2007
- Fioricet with Codeine Capsules ... 2387
- Fiorinal with Codeine Capsules ... 2390
- Fluorescite (Very rare) ... ⊚ 217
- Fluvirin (Influenza Virus Vaccine) (Rare) ... 1608
- Habitrol Nicotine Transdermal System (Once in 35% of patients) ... 884
- HibTITER ... 1423
- Imitrex Tablets (Rare) ... 1099
- Influenza Virus Vaccine, Trivalent, Types A and B (chromatograph- and filter-purified subviron antigen) FluShield, 1996-1997 Formula (Rare) ... 2842
- JE-VAX (0.2%) ... 904
- Metrodin (urofollitropin for injection) ... 2616
- Monistat Dual-Pak (Less than 0.5%) ... 1906
- Monistat 3 Vaginal Suppositories (Less than 0.5%) ... 1905
- Quadrinal Tablets ... 1398
- Soma Compound w/Codeine Tablets ... 2784
- Soma Compound Tablets ... 2783
- Sotradecol (Sodium Tetradecyl Sulfate Injection) ... 987
- Stadol (Less than 1%) ... 779
- Thioplex (Thiotepa For Injection) (Rare) ... 1329
- ▲ THROMBATE III Antithrombin III (Human) (1 of 17) ... 631
- Tracrium Injection (0.1%) ... 1155
- Varivax (Greater than or equal to 1%) ... 1807
- Versed Injection (Less than 1%) ... 2324
- Zovirax Sterile Powder (Approximately 2%) ... 1191

Hives at injection site

- Diprivan Injectable Emulsion (Less than 1%) ... 2939
- Idamycin Injection ... 2096

Hoarseness

- ▲ AeroBid Inhaler System (3% to 9%) ... 1004
- ▲ Aerobid-M Inhaler System (3% to 9%) ... 1004
- Android Capsules, 10 mg ... 1297
- Atamet Tablets ... 567
- Atrovent Inhalation Aerosol (Less than 1%) ... 674
- Atrovent Nasal Spray 0.03% (Less than 2%) ... 676
- Atrovent Nasal Spray 0.06% (Less than 1%) ... 678
- Azmacort Oral Inhaler (Infrequent) ... 2175
- Beclovent Inhalation Aerosol and Refill (A few patients) ... 1063
- Capoten Tablets ... 740
- Capozide Tablets ... 744
- Danocrine Capsules ... 2437
- Depo-Provera Contraceptive Injection (Fewer than 1%) ... 2079
- Dexacort Phosphate in Respihaler ... 1606
- Emcyt Capsules (1%) ... 2085
- Halotestin Tablets ... 2095
- Intal Inhaler (Rare) ... 2185
- Intal Nebulizer Solution (Rare) ... 2186
- Larodopa Tablets (Rare) ... 2296
- LUVOX Tablets (Infrequent) ... 2723
- Matulane Capsules ... 2300
- Monopril Tablets (0.2% to 1.0%) ... 762
- Nasarel Nasal Solution (1% or less) ... 2302
- Nicotrol NS Nicotine Nasal Spray (More common) ... 1565
- Oxandrin ... 783
- Retrovir Capsules ... 1216
- Retrovir I.V. Infusion ... 1221
- Retrovir Syrup ... 1216
- ReVia Tablets (Less than 1%) ... 957
- Rhinocort Nasal Inhaler (Less than 1%) ... 552
- Sinemet Tablets ... 959
- Sinemet CR Tablets ... 961
- Vanceril Inhaler (Few patients) ... 2538
- Vaseretic Tablets ... 1810
- Vasotec I.V. ... 1814
- Vasotec Tablets (0.5% to 1.0%) ... 1816
- Ventolin Inhalation Aerosol and Refill (Rare) ... 1170
- Ventolin Rotacaps for Inhalation (Rare to 2%) ... 1173

Hodgkin's disease

- Clomid ... 1262
- Dilantin Infatabs ... 1967
- Dilantin Kapseals ... 1965
- Dilantin-125 Suspension ... 1969

Hormonal imbalance

- Norvir (Less than 2%) ... 447
- ParaGard T 380A Intrauterine Copper Contraceptive ... 1936
- Wellbutrin Tablets (Rare) ... 1177

Horner's syndrome

- Atamet Tablets ... 567
- Larodopa Tablets (Rare) ... 2296
- Sinemet Tablets ... 959
- Sinemet CR Tablets ... 961

Hostility

- Anafranil Capsules (Infrequent) ... 819
- BuSpar Tablets (2%) ... 738
- Cerebyx Injection (Infrequent) ... 1956
- Cognex Capsules (2%) ... 1961
- Desyrel and Desyrel Dividose (1.3% to 3.5%) ... 504
- Duragesic Transdermal System (Less than 1%) ... 1336
- Effexor (Infrequent) ... 2825
- Floxin I.V. ... 1580
- Floxin Tablets (200 mg, 300 mg, 400 mg) ... 1577
- Lamictal Tablets (Frequent) ... 1105
- LUVOX Tablets (Infrequent) ... 2723
- Neurontin Capsules (Frequent) ... 1978
- Nipent for Injection (Less than 3%) ... 2733
- Nubain Injection (1% or less) ... 952
- Paxil Tablets (Infrequent) ... 2681
- Permax Tablets (Infrequent) ... 571
- Prevacid Delayed-Release Capsules (Less than 1%) ... 2746
- ProSom Tablets (Infrequent) ... 457
- Prozac Pulvules & Liquid, Oral Solution (Infrequent) ... 935
- Redux Capsules (Infrequent) ... 2911
- Remeron Tablets (Infrequent) ... 1878
- Rilutek Tablets (Frequent) ... 2198
- Serzone Tablets (Infrequent) ... 776
- Stadol (Less than 1%) ... 779
- ▲ Wellbutrin Tablets (5.6%) ... 1177
- Xanax Tablets (Rare) ... 2115

Hot flashes

- Alferon N Injection (1%) ... 2142
- Ambien Tablets (Rare) ... 2559
- Anafranil Capsules (2% to 5%) ... 819
- ▲ Arimidex Tablets (11.8% to 12.6%) ... 2932
- Atamet Tablets ... 567
- Axocet Capsules (Infrequent) ... 2469
- Cardene Capsules (Rare) ... 2261
- Cardene SR Capsules (Rare) ... 2264
- ▲ Casodex Tablets (49%) ... 2934
- Ceredase ... 1055
- Clozaril Tablets (Less than 1%) ... 2377
- DaunoXome (Less than or equal to 5%) ... 1842
- Depo-Provera Contraceptive Injection (1% to 5%) ... 2079
- Dipentum Capsules (Rare) ... 2084
- Esgic-plus Capsules (Infrequent) ... 1012
- Esgic-plus Tablets (Infrequent) ... 1012
- Estring Vaginal Ring (2%) ... 2086
- ▲ Eulexin Capsules (46% to 61% with LHRH-agonist) ... 2498
- Fioricet Tablets (Infrequent) ... 2386
- Fioricet with Codeine Capsules (Infrequent) ... 2387
- Fiorinal with Codeine Capsules (Infrequent) ... 2390
- Hivid Tablets (Less than 1%) ... 2287
- Imdur (Less than or equal to 5%) ... 1362
- Intron A for Injection (Less than 5%) ... 2506
- Invirase Capsules (Less than 2%) ... 2291
- Lamictal Tablets (1.3%) ... 1105
- Larodopa Tablets (Infrequent) ... 2296
- Lotrel Capsules ... 858
- ▲ Lupron Depot 3.75 mg (72.9%) ... 2739
- ▲ Lupron Depot 7.5 mg (58.9%) ... 2741
- ▲ Lupron Depot - 3 Month 22.5 mg (58.5%) ... 2743
- ▲ Lupron Injection (5% or more) ... 2736
- Mexitil Capsules (Less than 1% or about 2 in 1,000) ... 684
- ▲ Nolvadex Tablets (2.8% to 63.9%) ... 2957
- Norvasc Tablets (More than 0.1% to 1%) ... 2020
- Orlaam Oral Solution (Males 2:1) ... 2361
- Phrenilin (Infrequent) ... 790
- Procardia XL Extended Release Tablets (1% or less) ... 2026
- Prostin E2 Suppository ... 2109
- Prozac Pulvules & Liquid, Oral Solution (1.8%) ... 935
- ReVia Tablets (Less than 1%) ... 957
- Roferon-A Injection (Infrequent) ... 2308
- ▲ Romazicon (1% to 3%) ... 2311
- Rythmol Tablets–150mg, 225mg, 300mg (Less than 1%) ... 1399
- Sanorex Tablets ... 2423
- Sedapap Tablets 50 mg/650 mg (Infrequent) ... 1826
- Sinemet Tablets ... 959
- Sinemet CR Tablets ... 961
- Supprelin Injection (2%) ... 2230
- Synarel Nasal Solution for Central Precocious Puberty (3%) ... 2603
- ▲ Synarel Nasal Solution for Endometriosis (90% of patients) ... 2605
- ▲ Zoladex (62% to 96%) ... 2976
- ▲ Zoladex 3-month (64%) ... 2978

- Zoloft Tablets (2.2%) ... 2051
- Zyrtec Tablets (Less than 2%) ... 2053

Hunger

- Diabinese Tablets (Less than 2%) ... 2002
- Imitrex Injection (Rare) ... 1095
- Imitrex Tablets (Rare) ... 1099
- Respbid Tablets ... 687

Hydrocephalus

- Betaseron for SC Injection ... 653
- Pergonal (menotropins for injection, USP) (One report) ... 2618
- Prozac Pulvules & Liquid, Oral Solution (Rare) ... 935

Hydrocephalus, fetal

- Accutane Capsules ... 2252

Hydronephrosis

- ▲ CellCept Capsules (More than or equal to 3%) ... 2265
- Crixivan Capsules (Less than 2%) ... 1670

Hydrothorax

- Clomid ... 1262
- Humegon for Injection ... 1873
- Metrodin (urofollitropin for injection) ... 2616
- Serophene (clomiphene citrate tablets, USP) ... 2621

Hyperactive deep tendon reflexes

- Eskalith ... 2658
- Lithium Carbonate Capsules & Tablets ... 2352
- Lithonate/Lithotabs/Lithobid ... 2721

Hyperactivity

- AeroBid Inhaler System (1% to 3%) ... 1004
- Aerobid-M Inhaler System (1% to 3%) ... 1004
- Amoxil (Rare) ... 2631
- Augmentin (Rare) ... 2637
- Augmentin Tablets (Rare) ... 2640
- Ceclor Pulvules & Suspension (Rare) ... 1470
- Ceftin for Oral Suspension (0.1% to 1%) ... 1067
- Cefzil Tablets and Oral Suspension (Less than 1%) ... 747
- Dalmane Capsules (Rare) ... 2329
- Depakene ... 416
- Depakote Tablets ... 418
- Dopram Injectable ... 2235
- Etrafon ... 2495
- Fioricet with Codeine Capsules ... 2387
- Fiorinal with Codeine Capsules ... 2390
- ▲ Inapsine Injection (Among most common) ... 462
- Infumorph 200 and Infumorph 500 Sterile Solutions ... 985
- Ludiomil Tablets (Rare) ... 861
- Mellaril (Extremely rare) ... 2398
- Moban Tablets and Concentrate (Less frequent) ... 1036
- Phenobarbital Elixir and Tablets ... 1523
- Proventil Syrup (2 of 100 patients) ... 2528
- Roferon-A Injection (Infrequent) ... 2308
- Seldane-D Extended-Release Tablets (1.1%) ... 1286
- Trilafon ... 2532
- Ventolin Inhalation Aerosol and Refill (1%) ... 1170
- Ventolin Rotacaps for Inhalation (Less than 1%) ... 1173
- Ventolin Syrup (2 of 100 patients) ... 1175
- Versed Injection ... 2324
- Yocon Tablets ... 1235
- Zarontin Capsules ... 1986
- Zarontin Syrup ... 1986

Hyperactivity, paradoxical

- Restoril Capsules (Less than 0.5%) ... 2413

Hyperacusis

- Anafranil Capsules (Infrequent) ... 819
- Atretol Tablets ... 569
- Cerebyx Injection (Infrequent) ... 1956
- Effexor (Rare) ... 2825
- Paxil Tablets (Rare) ... 2681
- Remeron Tablets (Rare) ... 1878
- Rilutek Tablets (Rare) ... 2198
- Risperdal Tablets (Rare) ... 1348
- Romazicon (Less than 1%) ... 2311
- Serzone Tablets (Infrequent) ... 776
- Tegretol/Tegretol-XR ... 870

(⊞ Described in PDR For Nonprescription Drugs)   Incidence data in parentheses; ▲ 3% or more   (⊚ Described in PDR For Ophthalmology)

Hyperalgesia

- Betaseron for SC Injection ... 653
- Lamictal Tablets (Rare) ... 1105
- Paxil Tablets (Rare) ... 2681
- Retrovir Capsules ... 1216
- Retrovir I.V. Infusion ... 1221
- Retrovir Syrup ... 1216

Hyperammonemia

- Depakene ... 416
- Depakote Tablets ... 418
- Felbatol ... 2774
- Haldol Decanoate ... 1587
- NephrAmine Injection (Infrequent) ... 2169
- Oncaspar (Less than 1%) ... 2194

Hyperbilirubinemia

- Abelcet Injection ... 1540
- Altace Capsules ... 1238
- Ancobon Capsules ... 2254
- AquaMEPHYTON Injection ... 1648
- Atamet Tablets ... 567
- Augmentin (Infrequent) ... 2637
- Augmentin Tablets (Infrequent) ... 2640
- Azathioprine Tablets (Less than 1%) ... 2349
- Bactrim DS Tablets ... 2257
- Bactrim I.V. Infusion ... 2255
- Bactrim ... 2257
- ▲ Betaseron for SC Injection (6%) ... 653
- Biaxin (Less than 1%) ... 406
- BiCNU ... 696
- Calan SR Caplets ... 2571
- Calan Tablets ... 2568
- Capoten Tablets ... 740
- Capozide Tablets ... 744
- Casodex Tablets (2% to 5%) ... 2934
- Cedax (0.1% to 1%) ... 2480
- CeeNU Capsules (Small percentage) ... 699
- Cefizox for Intramuscular or Intravenous Use (Rare) ... 1025
- Cefotan ... 2936
- Ceftin ... 1067
- Ceptaz ... 1070
- ▲ Cipro I.V. (Among most frequent) ... 587
- ▲ Cipro I.V. Pharmacy Bulk Package (Among most frequent) ... 590
- Cipro Tablets (0.3%) ... 584
- Covera-HS Tablets ... 2573
- ▲ Crixivan Capsules (7.8% to approximately 10%) ... 1670
- Cytosar-U Sterile Powder (With experimental doses) ... 2077
- Dalmane Capsules (Rare) ... 2329
- Dapsone Tablets USP ... 1331
- Depakene (Occasional) ... 416
- Depakote Tablets (Occasional) ... 418
- Desyrel and Desyrel Dividose ... 504
- Dilacor XR Extended-release Capsules ... 2183
- Doxil (1% to 5%) ... 2613
- Duricef Capsules, Tablets, and Oral Suspension ... 750
- Dynabac (0.1% to 1%) ... 668
- Elspar ... 1700
- Epivir (0.8%) ... 1200
- Ergamisol Tablets (Less than 1% to 1%) ... 1340
- Ethmozine Tablets (Rare) ... 2217
- Eulexin Capsules ... 2498
- ▲ Exosurf Neonatal for Intratracheal Suspension (10% to 61%) ... 1081
- Floxin I.V. ... 1580
- Floxin Tablets (200 mg, 300 mg, 400 mg) ... 1577
- Fortaz ... 1092
- ▲ Sterile FUDR (Among more common) ... 2284
- Fungizone Intravenous ... 507
- Garamycin Injectable ... 2502
- ▲ Gemzar for Injection (13% to 26%) ... 1482
- Hycamtin for Injection (Less than 3%) ... 2665
- Hyperstat I.V. Injection ... 2504
- HypRho-D Full Dose Rho (D) Immune Globulin (Human) ... 623
- Hyzaar Tablets (Occasional) ... 1720
- ▲ IFEX (3%) ... 706
- Inocor Lactate Injection (Rare) ... 2439
- Invirase Capsules (Less than 1%) ... 2291
- Isoptin Oral Tablets ... 1393
- Isoptin SR Tablets ... 1395
- Lamprene Capsules (Less than 1%) ... 846
- Larodopa Tablets (Rare) ... 2296
- Lescol Capsules ... 2395
- ▲ Leukine (30%) ... 1317
- Leustatin ... 1889
- Lopid Tablets (Occasional) ... 1974

- Lotensin Tablets ... 852
- Lotrel Capsules (Rare) ... 858
- Mavik Tablets (0.2% of patients) ... 1407
- Maxaquin Tablets ... 2593
- Mephyton Tablets (Rare) ... 1739
- Merrem I.V. (Greater than 0.2%) ... 2952
- Mevacor Tablets ... 1742
- Mezlin ... 594
- Mezlin Pharmacy Bulk Package ... 597
- Mithracin ... 599
- Monopril Tablets ... 762
- ▲ Navelbine Injection (2% to 9%) ... 1212
- Nebcin Vials, Hyporets & ADD-Vantage ... 1518
- Neoral ... 2405
- Netromycin Injection 100 mg/ml (15 of 1000 patients) ... 2516
- Neutrexin for Injection (1.8%) ... 2761
- Nolvadex Tablets (1.8%) ... 2957
- Nydrazid Injection ... 509
- Oncaspar ... 2194
- Oxandrin ... 783
- ▲ Paraplatin for Injection (5%) ... 713
- Penetrex Tablets (Less than 1%) ... 2196
- Pipracil (Less frequent) ... 1435
- Platinol for Injection ... 717
- Platinol-AQ Injection ... 719
- Pravachol Tablets ... 770
- Prilosec Delayed-Release Capsules (Rare) ... 516
- Primaxin I.M. ... 1770
- Primaxin I.V. ... 1772
- Prinivil Tablets (Rare) ... 1776
- Prinzide Tablets (Rare) ... 1780
- Proglycem Suspension ... 575
- ▲ Proleukin for Injection (64%) ... 812
- Proloprim Tablets ... 1141
- Retrovir Capsules (Rare) ... 1216
- Retrovir I.V. Infusion (Rare) ... 1221
- Retrovir Syrup (Rare) ... 1216
- RhoGAM Rh₀(D) Immune Globulin (Human) ... 1902
- Rifadin (Some cases) ... 1276
- Rifamate Capsules ... 1278
- Rifater (Some cases) ... 1280
- Rimactane Capsules (Rare) ... 865
- Rocephin Injectable Vials, ADD-Vantage, Galaxy Container (Less than 1%) ... 2305
- Sectral Capsules ... 2914
- Septra ... 1146
- Septra I.V. Infusion ... 1142
- Septra I.V. Infusion ADD-Vantage Vials ... 1144
- Septra ... 1146
- Sinemet Tablets ... 959
- Suprax ... 1443
- ▲ Taxol Injection (7%) ... 723
- Tazicef for Injection ... 2697
- Tazidime Vials, Faspak & ADD-Vantage ... 1531
- Tenoretic Tablets ... 2963
- Tenormin Tablets and I.V. Injection ... 2965
- Timentin for Injection ... 2706
- Trimpex Tablets ... 2323
- Vantin for Oral Suspension and Vantin Tablets ... 2112
- Vaseretic Tablets (Rare) ... 1810
- Vasotec I.V. ... 1814
- Vasotec Tablets ... 1816
- Verelan Capsules ... 1455
- Videx Tablets, Powder for Oral Solution, & Pediatric Powder for Oral Solution (1% to 2%) ... 2980
- Viramune Tablets (0.4%) ... 2368
- Winstrol Tablets ... 2468
- Xanax Tablets ... 2115
- Zerit Capsules (Up to 2%) ... 731
- Zestoretic Tablets (Rare) ... 2968
- Zestril Tablets (Rare) ... 2972
- Zinacef (1 in 500 patients) ... 1184
- Zithromax (1 in 1%) ... 2043
- Zithromax Tablets (Less than 1%) ... 2046
- Zocor Tablets ... 1821
- Zoloft Tablets (One or more patients) ... 2051
- Zosyn ... 1463
- Zyloprim Tablets (Less than 1%) ... 1194
- Zyrtec Tablets (A single case) ... 2053

Hypercalcemia

- Androderm Testosterone Transdermal System ... 2634
- ▲ Android Capsules, 10 mg (Among most common) ... 1297
- Apresazide Capsules ... 824
- Betaseron for SC Injection ... 653
- Calcijex Injection ... 412
- Capozide Tablets (A few patients) ... 744
- ▲ CellCept Capsules (More than or equal to 3%) ... 2265

- Cipro I.V. (Infrequent) ... 587
- ▲ Cipro I.V. Pharmacy Bulk Package (Among most frequent) ... 590
- Climara Transdermal System ... 640
- Dovonex Ointment 0.005% (Less than 1%) ... 2793
- Doxil (Less than 1%) ... 2613
- Enduron Tablets ... 424
- Esidrix Tablets ... 839
- Eskalith ... 2658
- Estrace Cream and Tablets ... 751
- Estraderm Transdermal System ... 842
- ESTRATAB Tablets (0.3, 0.625, 1.25, 2.5 mg) ... 2715
- Estratest ... 2718
- Foscavir Injection (Between 1% and 5%) ... 541
- Halotestin Tablets ... 2095
- Hivid Tablets (Less than 1%) ... 2287
- Hyzaar Tablets ... 1720
- Intron A for Injection (Less than or equal to 5%) ... 2506
- Lithonate/Lithotabs/Lithobid ... 2721
- Lupron Depot 7.5 mg (Less than 5%) ... 2741
- Maxipime for Injection (0.1% to 1%) ... 758
- Megace Tablets ... 710
- Menest Tablets ... 2671
- Mykrox Tablets (A few patients) ... 1617
- Nipent for Injection (Less than 3%) ... 2733
- Nolvadex Tablets (Infrequent) ... 2957
- Ogen Tablets ... 2103
- Ogen Vaginal Cream ... 2106
- Oretic Tablets (Rare occasions) ... 450
- Ortho Dienestrol Cream ... 1922
- Ortho-Est ... 1925
- Oxandrin ... 783
- Paxil Tablets (Rare) ... 2681
- PhosLo Tablets ... 695
- PMB 200 and PMB 400 ... 2890
- Premarin Intravenous ... 2893
- Premarin Tablets ... 2896
- Premarin Vaginal Cream ... 2898
- Premphase ... 2900
- Prempro ... 2905
- Prinzide Tablets ... 1780
- Proleukin for Injection (1%) ... 812
- Rilutek Tablets (Rare) ... 2198
- ▲ Rocaltrol Capsules (1 in 3) ... 2303
- Tenoretic Tablets ... 2963
- Teslac Tablets ... 727
- Testoderm Testosterone Transdermal System ... 486
- Vaseretic Tablets ... 1810
- Vesanoid Capsules (Isolated cases) ... 2327
- Vivelle Transdermal System ... 880
- Winstrol Tablets ... 2468
- Zaroxolyn Tablets (Infrequent) ... 1625
- Zestoretic Tablets ... 2968
- Zoladex ... 2976
- Zoladex 3-month (Rare) ... 2978
- Zosyn ... 1463
- Zyloprim Tablets (Less than 1%) ... 1194

Hypercalciuria

- Calcijex Injection (Some instances) ... 412
- Prelone Syrup ... 1834
- ▲ Rocaltrol Capsules (1 in 7) ... 2303

Hypercarbia

- Alfenta Injection (0.3% to 1%) ... 1334
- Survanta Beractant Intratracheal Suspension (Less than 1%) ... 2346

Hyperchloremia

- Androderm Testosterone Transdermal System ... 2634
- ▲ Android Capsules, 10 mg (Among most common) ... 1297
- Daranide Tablets ... 1676
- Demadex Tablets and Injection ... 691
- Primaxin I.M. ... 1770
- Primaxin I.V. ... 1772
- Sulfamylon Cream ... 940
- Testoderm Testosterone Transdermal System ... 486
- Winstrol Tablets ... 2468

Hyperchloremic acidosis

- Questran (Less frequent) ... 774

Hyperchlorhydria

- Prozac Pulvules & Liquid, Oral Solution (Rare) ... 935

Hypercholesterolemia

- ▲ Accutane Capsules (About 7%) ... 2252
- Ambien Tablets (Rare) ... 2559
- Anafranil Capsules (Infrequent) ... 819

- Androderm Testosterone Transdermal System ... 2634
- ▲ Android Capsules, 10 mg (Among most common) ... 1297
- Arimidex Tablets (2% to 5%) ... 2932
- Atretol Tablets (Occasional reports) ... 569
- Bumex (0.4%) ... 2260
- Calcijex Injection ... 412
- ▲ CellCept Capsules (8.5% to 12.8%) ... 2265
- ▲ Chemet Capsules (4.2% to 10.4%) ... 666
- Cipro I.V. (Infrequent) ... 587
- Cipro I.V. Pharmacy Bulk Package (Less than 1%) ... 590
- Cipro Tablets ... 584
- Cognex Capsules (Infrequent) ... 1961
- Diflucan Tablets, Injection, and Oral Suspension ... 2003
- Effexor (Infrequent) ... 2825
- Ergamisol Tablets ... 1340
- Estratest ... 2718
- Floxin I.V. ... 1580
- Floxin Tablets (200 mg, 300 mg, 400 mg) ... 1577
- Halotestin Tablets ... 2095
- Hyzaar Tablets ... 1720
- Kerlone Tablets (Less than 2%) ... 2588
- ▲ Leukine (17%) ... 1317
- Lotensin HCT Tablets ... 855
- LUVOX Tablets (Infrequent) ... 2723
- Maxaquin Tablets ... 2593
- Naprelan Tablets (Less than 1%) ... 2861
- Neurontin Capsules (Rare) ... 1978
- Noroxin Tablets ... 1758
- Noroxin Tablets ... 2222
- Norpace (1 to 3%) ... 2596
- Norvir (Less than 2%) ... 447
- Oxandrin ... 783
- Paxil Tablets (Rare) ... 2681
- Penetrex Tablets ... 2196
- Permax Tablets (Infrequent) ... 571
- Prevacid Delayed-Release Capsules (Less than 1%) ... 2746
- Prinzide Tablets ... 1780
- Prozac Pulvules & Liquid, Oral Solution (Rare) ... 935
- Rilutek Tablets (Rare) ... 2198
- Rocaltrol Capsules ... 2303
- Serzone Tablets (Rare) ... 776
- Synarel Nasal Solution for Endometriosis ... 2605
- ▲ Tegison Capsules (19%) ... 2314
- Tegretol/Tegretol-XR (Occasional) ... 870
- Testoderm Testosterone Transdermal System ... 486
- Testred Capsules, 10 mg ... 1308
- Ticlid Tablets ... 2317
- Timolide Tablets ... 1791
- Vaseretic Tablets ... 1810
- ▲ Vesanoid Capsules (Up to 60%) ... 2327
- Zestoretic Tablets ... 2968
- Zoladex ... 2976
- Zoladex 3-month ... 2978
- Zoloft Tablets (Rare) ... 2051

Hypercorticism

- Beconase ... 1065
- Blephamide Liquifilm Sterile Ophthalmic Suspension (Rare) ... 472
- Blephamide Ointment (Rare) ... ⊚ 234
- Econopred & Econopred Plus Ophthalmic Suspensions (Rare) ... ⊚ 216
- FML Forte Liquifilm (Rare) ... ⊚ 237
- FML Liquifilm (Rare) ... ⊚ 238
- FML S.O.P. (Rare) ... ⊚ 239
- Nasacort Nasal Inhaler ... 2189
- Nasalide Nasal Solution 0.025% ... 2301
- Pred Forte (Rare) ... ⊚ 247
- Pred Mild (Rare) ... ⊚ 250

Hyperdipsia

(see under Dipsesis)

Hyperemia

- ▲ Alomide Ophthalmic Solution (1% to 5%) ... 465
- Celontin Kapseals ... 1955
- ▲ Iopidine 0.5% (13%) ... ⊚ 219
- Lacrisert Sterile Ophthalmic Insert ... 1730
- Vexol 1% Ophthalmic Suspension (1% to 5%) ... ⊚ 227
- Vироptic Ophthalmic Solution, 1% Sterile ... 1177

Hyperemia, conjunctival

- Chibroxin Sterile Ophthalmic Solution ... 1657

Hyperemia, conjunctival Side Effects Index 1362

Diprivan Injectable Emulsion (Less than 1%) 2939
Econopred & Econopred Plus Ophthalmic Suspensions (Occasional) ◉ 216
FML Forte Liquifilm (Occasional) ◉ 237
FML Liquifilm (Occasional) ◉ 238
FML S.O.P. (Occasional) ◉ 239
▲ Genoptic Sterile Ophthalmic Solution (Among most frequent) ◉ 241
▲ Genoptic Sterile Ophthalmic Ointment (Among most frequent) ◉ 241
▲ Ocupress Ophthalmic Solution, 1% Sterile (About 1 of 4 patients) ◉ 297
Tensilon Injectable 1307
▲ Xalatan (5% to 15%) ◉ 304

Hyperesthesia

Anafranil Capsules (Rare) 819
Asacol Delayed-Release Tablets 2129
Avonex 662
Betaseron for SC Injection 653
Cerebyx Injection (Infrequent) 1956
Effexor (Infrequent) 2825
▲ Flolan for Injection (12%) 1085
Foscavir Injection (Less than 1%) 541
Imitrex Injection (Rare) 1095
Imitrex Tablets (Rare) 1099
Intron A for Injection (Less than 5%) 2506
Invirase Capsules (Less than 2%) 2291
Lamictal Tablets (Rare) 1105
Neurontin Capsules (Rare) 1978
Norvir (Less than 2%) 447
Redux Capsules (Infrequent) 2911
Sansert Tablets 2424
Sectral Capsules (Up to 2%) 2914
Serzone Tablets (Rare) 776
Videx Tablets, Powder for Oral Solution, & Pediatric Powder for Oral Solution (Less than 1%) 2980
Ziac 1459
Zoloft Tablets (Infrequent) 2051
Zyrtec Tablets (Less than 2%) 2053

Hyperesthesia, tongue

Alferon N Injection (1%) 2142

Hyperexcitability

Lufyllin & Lufyllin-400 Tablets 2778
Lufyllin-GG Elixir & Tablets 2779

Hyperexcitability, reflex

Quadrinal Tablets 1398
Quibron 2227
Respbid Tablets 687
Slo-bid Gyrocaps 2201
Theo-Dur Extended-Release Tablets 1367
Theo-X Extended-Release Tablets 793
Uni-Dur Extended-Release Tablets 1374

Hyperferremia

Pyrazinamide Tablets (Rare) 1442

Hypergammaglobulinemia

Prevacid Delayed-Release Capsules (Less than 1%) 2746

Hyperglycemia

Abelcet Injection 1540
▲ Accutane Capsules (Less than 1 in 10) 2252
Aclovate 1061
Actimmune (Rare) 1043
Adapin Capsules 1542
Albalon Solution with Liquifilm ◉ 229
Aldoclor Tablets 1638
Aldoril Tablets 1644
Altace Capsules 1238
Ambien Tablets (Infrequent) 2559
Anafranil Capsules (Infrequent) 819
Anaprox/Naprosyn (Less than 1%) 2277
Apresazide Capsules 824
▲ Betaseron for SC Injection (15%) 653
Blocadren Tablets 1654
▲ Bumex (6.6%) 2260
Capozide Tablets 744
Cardizem CD Capsules (Less than 1%) 1251
Cardizem SR Capsules (Less than 1%) 1255
Cardizem Injectable 1253
Cardizem Tablets (Less than 1%) 1257
▲ Casodex Tablets (5%) 2934
Catapres Tablets (Rare) 679
▲ CellCept Capsules (8.6% to 12.4%) 2265
Cerebyx Injection (Infrequent) 1956
▲ Cipro I.V. (Among most frequent) 587
Cipro Tablets 584
Clinoril Tablets (Rare) 1658
Clozaril Tablets 2377
Combipres Tablets 682
Compazine 2644
Cormax Ointment 1856
Cormax Scalp Application 1857
Demadex Tablets and Injection (Uncommon) 691
Dermatop Emollient Cream 0.1% 1264
Dilantin Kapseals 1965
Dilantin-125 Suspension 1969
Diprivan Injectable Emulsion (Less than 1%) 2939
Diprolene AF Cream 0.05% (Some patients) 2489
Diprolene Lotion 0.05% (Some patients) 2491
Diprolene Ointment 0.05% (Some patients) 2491
Diucardin Tablets 2824
Diupres Tablets 1691
Diuril Oral Suspension 1694
Diuril Sodium Intravenous 1693
Diuril Tablets 1694
Doxil (1% to 5%) 2613
Dyazide Capsules 2653
EC-Naprosyn Delayed-Release Tablets (Less than 1%) 2277
Edecrin 1698
Effexor (Infrequent) 2825
Elavil 2945
Elspar (Low) 1700
Enduron Tablets 424
Esgic-plus Capsules 1012
Esgic-plus Tablets 1012
Esidrix Tablets 839
Esimil Tablets 840
Etrafon 2495
Felbatol 2774
Feldene Capsules (Less than 1%) 2008
Fioricet Tablets 2386
Fioricet with Codeine Capsules 2387
Fiorinal with Codeine Capsules 2390
Flexeril Tablets (Rare) 1701
Florinef Acetate Tablets 506
Floxin I.V. (More than or equal to 1%) 1580
Floxin Tablets (200 mg, 300 mg, 400 mg) (More than or equal to 1%) 1577
▲ Fludara for Injection (1% to 6%) 658
Genotropin Injection (Infrequent) 2090
Haldol Decanoate 1587
Haldol Injection, Tablets and Concentrate 1585
Hivid Tablets (Less than 1%) 2287
Humatrope Vials (Infrequent) 1490
HydroDIURIL Tablets 1716
Hydropres Tablets 1718
Hyperstat I.V. Injection 2504
Hyzaar Tablets 1720
Imitrex Tablets (Rare) 1099
Inderide LA Long Acting Capsules 2840
Indocin Capsules (Less than 1%) 1723
Indocin I.V. (1% to 3%) 1727
Indocin (Less than 1%) 1723
Invirase Capsules (Less than 1% to less than 2%) 2291
Kerlone Tablets (Less than 2%) 2588
Lamictal Tablets (Rare) 1105
Lamprene Capsules (Greater than 1%) 846
Lasix Injection, Oral Solution and Tablets 1267
▲ Leukine (25% to 41%) 1317
Limbitrol 2333
Lioresal Intrathecal (1% or more) 1634
Lioresal Tablets 847
Lodine Capsules and Tablets (Less than 1%) 2849
Lo/Ovral Tablets 2852
Lo/Ovral-28 Tablets 2857
Lopressor HCT Tablets 850
Lotensin Tablets 852
Lotensin HCT Tablets 855
Ludiomil Tablets (Rare) 861
Lufyllin & Lufyllin-400 Tablets 2778
Lufyllin-GG Elixir & Tablets 2779
▲ Lupron Depot - 3 Month 22.5 mg (More than or equal to 5%) 2743
LUVOX Tablets (Rare) 2723
▲ Megace Oral Suspension (Up to 6%) 708
Megace Tablets 710
▲ Mepron Suspension (9%) 1206
Minizide Capsules 2016
Mintezol 1747
Moduretic Tablets 1748
Mykrox Tablets 1617
Naprelan Tablets (Less than 3%) 2861
Anaprox/Naprosyn (Less than 1%) 2277
Navane Capsules and Concentrate 2018
Navane Intramuscular 2019
Neoral (2% or less) 2405
Nimotop Capsules (0.8%; rare) 603
Noroxin Tablets 1758
Noroxin Tablets 2222
Norpramin Tablets 1273
Nydrazid Injection 509
▲ Oncaspar (Greater than 1% but less than 5%) 2194
Oretic Tablets 450
Ovral Tablets 2877
Ovral-28 Tablets 2878
Ovrette Tablets 2878
Pamelor 2409
Paxil Tablets (Infrequent) 2681
Permax Tablets (Infrequent) 571
Prevacid Delayed-Release Capsules (Less than 1%) 2746
Prinzide Tablets 1780
ProctoCream-HC 2.5% 2552
Proglycem (Frequent) 575
▲ Prograf (Many patients; 29% to 47%) 1028
Proleukin for Injection (2%) 812
Prozac Pulvules & Liquid, Oral Solution (Rare) 935
Quadrinal Tablets 1398
Quibron 2227
Redux Capsules (Rare) 2911
Relafen Tablets (Less than 1%) 2688
Respbid Tablets 687
Rifamate Capsules 1278
Rifater 1280
Sandimmune (2% or less) 2416
▲ Sandostatin Injection (1.5%; 16%) 2421
Ser-Ap-Es Tablets 867
Sinemet CR Tablets (1% or greater) 961
Sinequan 2028
Slo-bid Gyrocaps 2201
Slo-Niacin Tablets 2767
Stelazine 2692
Suprane (desflurane, USP) 1865
Surmontil Capsules 2917
Temovate Cream 1152
Temovate Gel 1153
Temovate Ointment 1152
Temovate Scalp Application 1153
Tenoretic Tablets 2963
Thalitone 1293
Theo-Dur Extended-Release Tablets 1367
Theo-X Extended-Release Tablets 793
Thorazine 2701
Tiazac Capsules (Less than 1%) 1019
Timolide Tablets 1791
Timoptic in Ocudose 1796
Timoptic Sterile Ophthalmic Solution 1794
Timoptic-XE 1798
Tofranil Ampuls 873
Tofranil Tablets 875
Tofranil-PM Capsules 876
Tornalate Solution for Inhalation, 0.2% (Infrequent) 976
▲ Trasylol (3%) 607
Triavil Tablets 1800
Trilafon 2532
Triphasil-21 Tablets 2919
Triphasil-28 Tablets 2924
Ultravate Cream 0.05% 2797
Ultravate Ointment 0.05% 2798
Uni-Dur Extended-Release Tablets 1374
Vantin for Oral Suspension and Vantin Tablets 2112
Vaseretic Tablets 1810
Videx Tablets, Powder for Oral Solution, & Pediatric Powder for Oral Solution (1% to 5%) 2980
Vistide Injection 1057
Vivactil Tablets 1820
Yutopar Intravenous Injection 566
Zaroxolyn Tablets 1625
Zebeta Tablets 1457
Zestoretic Tablets 2968
Zithromax (Less than 1%) 2043
Zithromax Tablets (Less than 1%) 2046
Zoladex (Greater than 1% but less than 5%) 2976
Zoladex 3-month 2978
Zosyn 1463

Hyperglycemia, transient

Eskalith 2658
Lithium Carbonate Capsules & Tablets 2352
Lithonate/Lithotabs/Lithobid 2721

Hyperglycinemia

Asendin Tablets (Very rare) 1419
Depakene 416
Depakote Tablets 418
Moban Tablets and Concentrate 1036

Hyperhemoglobinemia

Ambien Tablets (Rare) 2559

Hyperheparinemia

Mustargen (Rare) 1752
Protamine Sulfate Vials (Some patients) 1526

Hyperhidrosis

Accutane Capsules (Less than 1%) 2252
Axocet Capsules (Infrequent) 2469
Decadron Phosphate with Xylocaine Injection, Sterile 1683
DynaCirc Capsules (0.5% to 1%) 2381
DynaCirc CR Tablets (0.5% to 1.0%) 2383
Esgic-plus Capsules (Infrequent) 1012
Esgic-plus Tablets (Infrequent) 1012
Fioricet Tablets (Infrequent) 2386
Fioricet with Codeine Capsules (Infrequent) 2387
Fiorinal with Codeine Capsules (Infrequent) 2390
Havrix (Rare) 2663
Miacalcin Nasal Spray (Less than 1%) 2403
Monopril Tablets (0.4% to 1.0%) 762
Noroxin Tablets (0.3% to 1.0%) 1758
Noroxin Tablets (0.3% to 1.0%) 2222
Penetrex Tablets (0.1% to 1%) 2196
Phrenilin (Infrequent) 790
Prilosec Delayed-Release Capsules (Less than 1%) 516
Primaxin I.M. 1770
Primaxin I.V. (Less than 0.2%) 1772
Prinivil Tablets 1776
Prinzide Tablets (0.3 to 1%) 1780
Quadrinal Tablets 1398
Sedapap Tablets 50 mg/650 mg (Infrequent) 1826
Tussend 1830
Vaseretic Tablets 1810
Vasotec Tablets 1816
Visken Tablets (2% or fewer patients) 2428
Zestoretic Tablets 2968

Hyperhistaminemia

▲ Vesanoid Capsules (3%) 2327

Hyperirritability

Atrohist Plus Tablets 1605
Mintezol 1747
Mysoline (Occasional) 2860
Seromycin Capsules 975

Hyperirritability, muscle

Eskalith 2658
Lithium Carbonate Capsules & Tablets 2352
Lithonate/Lithotabs/Lithobid 2721

Hyperirritability, neuromuscular

Mezlin 594
Mezlin Pharmacy Bulk Package 597
Timentin for Injection 2706

Hyperkalemia

Abelcet Injection 1540
Accupril Tablets (Rare) 1950
Altace Capsules (Approximately 1%) 1238
Anaprox/Naprosyn (Less than 1%) 2277
Androderm Testosterone Transdermal System 2634
▲ Android Capsules, 10 mg (Among most common) 1297
Anectine (Rare) 1062
Atromid-S Capsules 2808
Blocadren Tablets 1654
Capoten Tablets 740
Capozide Tablets 744
▲ CellCept Capsules (8.9% to 10.3%) 2265
Ceptaz 1070
Cerebyx Injection (Infrequent) 1956
Cipro I.V. (Infrequent) 587

(▭ Described in PDR For Nonprescription Drugs) Incidence data in parenthesis; ▲ 3% or more (◉ Described in PDR For Ophthalmology)

Cipro I.V. Pharmacy Bulk Package (Less than 1%) 590
Cipro Tablets 584
Clinoril Tablets (Less than 1 in 100) 1658
Demadex Tablets and Injection 691
Diprivan Injectable Emulsion (Less than 1%) 2939
Doxil (Less than 1%) 2613
Dyazide Capsules 2653
Dynabac (2.6%) 668
Dyrenium Capsules (Rare) 2655
EC-Naprosyn Delayed-Release Tablets (Less than 1%) 2277
Effexor (Rare) 2825
Epogen for Injection (Approximately 0.11%) 489
Estratest 2718
Feldene Capsules (Less than 1%) 2008
Floxin I.V. 1580
Floxin Tablets (200 mg, 300 mg, 400 mg) 1577
Fludara for Injection 658
Fungizone Intravenous 507
Halotestin Tablets 2095
Hivid Tablets (Less than 1%) 2287
Hyzaar Tablets (0.4%) 1720
Indocin Capsules (Less than 1%) 1723
Indocin I.V. (Less than 1%) 1727
Indocin (Less than 1%) 1723
Invirase Capsules (Less than 1%) 2291
K-Dur Microburst Release System (potassium chloride, USP) E.R. Tablets 1364
▲ K-Lor Powder Packets (Among most severe) 438
K-Norm Capsules 1615
▲ K-Tab Filmtab (Most common) 439
Kerlone Tablets (Less than 2%) 2588
Lotensin Tablets (Approximately 1%) 852
Lotensin HCT Tablets (Approximately 1%) 855
Lotrel Capsules (Approximately 1.5%) 858
Mavik Tablets (Rare) 1407
Maxaquin Tablets 2593
Maxipime for Injection (0.1% to 1%) 758
Micro-K 2237
▲ Micro-K LS Packets (Most severe) 2238
Midamor Tablets (Between 1% and 3%) 1746
Moduretic Tablets (Greater than 1%, less than 3%) 1748
Monopril Tablets (Approximately 2.6%) 762
▲ Naprelan Tablets (3% to 9%) 2861
Anaprox/Naprosyn (Less than 1%) 2277
Neoral (Occasional) 2405
Netromycin Injection 100 mg/ml (Fewer than 1 of 1000 patients) 2516
Noroxin Tablets 1758
Noroxin Tablets 2222
Oxandrin 783
Paxil Tablets (Rare) 2681
Penetrex Tablets (Less than 1%) 2196
Polycitra Syrup 574
Polycitra-K Crystals 574
Polycitra-K Oral Solution 575
Polycitra-LC 574
Primaxin I.M. 1770
Primaxin I.V. 1772
▲ Prinivil Tablets (Approximately 2.2% to 4.8%) 1776
Prinzide Tablets (Approximately 1.4%) 1780
Procrit for Injection (0.11%) 1896
▲ Prograf (10% to 45%) 1028
▲ Proleukin for Injection (4%) 812
Proloprim Tablets 1141
Redux Capsules (Rare) 2911
Rum-K Syrup 1004
Sandimmune (Occasional) 2416
Septra 1146
Septra I.V. Infusion 1142
Septra I.V. Infusion ADD-Vantage Vials 1144
Septra 1146
Slow-K Extended-Release Tablets 869
▲ Tegison Capsules (25-50%) 2314
Testoderm Testosterone Transdermal System 486
Testred Capsules, 10 mg 1308
Toradol 2319
Univasc Tablets (Approximately 1.3%) 2553
Vaseretic Tablets 1810
Vasotec I.V. (Approximately 1%) 1814
Vasotec Tablets (Approximately 1%) 1816
Winstrol Tablets 2468
Zebeta Tablets 1457
Zestoretic Tablets (Approximately 1.4%) 2968
▲ Zestril Tablets (Approximately 2.2% to 4.8%) 2972
Zithromax (1% to 2%) 2043
Zithromax Tablets (1% to 2%) 2046
Zosyn 1463

Hyperkalemia, neonatal

Altace Capsules 1238
Capozide Tablets 744
Lotensin Tablets 852
Monopril Tablets 762
Prograf 1028
Zestril Tablets 2972

Hyperkeratosis

Blenoxane 697
Calan SR Caplets (1% or less) 2571
Calan Tablets (1% or less) 2568
Cognex Capsules (Infrequent) 1961
Covera-HS Tablets (Less than 2%) 2573
Isoptin Oral Tablets (Less than 1%) 1393
Isoptin SR Tablets (1% or less) 1395
Risperdal Tablets (Infrequent) 1348
Verelan Capsules (1% or less) 1455
Zyrtec Tablets (Less than 2%) 2053

Hyperkinesia

Anafranil Capsules (Infrequent) 819
Betaseron for SC Injection (2%) 653
Butisol Sodium Elixir & Tablets (Less than 1 in 100) 2768
Cardene Capsules (Rare) 2261
Cardene SR Capsules (Rare) 2264
Cedax (0.1% to 1%) 2480
Cerebyx Injection (Infrequent) 1956
Claritin Tablets (2% or fewer patients) 2485
Claritin-D Tablets (Less frequent) 2487
Clozaril Tablets (1%) 2377
Cognex Capsules (Frequent) 1961
DaunoXome (Less than or equal to 5%) 1842
Doral Tablets 2773
Effexor (Infrequent) 2825
Flumadine Tablets & Syrup (Less than 0.3%) 1013
Foscavir Injection (Less than 1%) 541
Hivid Tablets (Less than 1%) 2287
Intron A for Injection (Less than 5%) 2506
Lamictal Tablets (Infrequent) 1105
Levo-Dromoran 2297
LUVOX Tablets (Frequent) 2723
Maxair Autohaler 1550
Maxair Inhaler (Less than 1%) 1552
Maxaquin Tablets (Less than 1%) 2593
Mebaral Tablets (Less than 1 in 100) 2452
Nembutal Sodium Capsules (Less than 1%) 440
Nembutal Sodium Solution (Less than 1%) 442
Nembutal Sodium Suppositories (Less than 1%) 444
Neurontin Capsules (Frequent) 1978
Nipent for Injection (Less than 3%) 2733
▲ Orap Tablets (5.5%) 1037
OxyContin Tablets (Less than 1%) 2163
Paxil Tablets (Infrequent) 2681
Penetrex Tablets (Less than 0.1%) 2196
Permax Tablets (Infrequent) 571
Phenobarbital Elixir and Tablets (Less than 1 in 100 patients) 1523
▲ Proventil Syrup (Children 2 to 6 years, 4%) 2528
Prozac Pulvules & Liquid, Oral Solution (Infrequent) 935
Redux Capsules (Infrequent) 2911
Remeron Tablets (Frequent) 1878
▲ Risperdal Tablets (17% to 34%) 1348
Salagen Tablets (Less than 1%) 1546
Seconal Sodium Pulvules (Less than 1 in 100) 1529
Seldane-D Extended-Release Tablets (1.1%) 1286
Serzone Tablets (Rare) 776
Supprelin Injection (1% to 3%) 2230
Symmetrel Capsules (0.1% to 1%) 965
Symmetrel Syrup (0.1% to 1%) 963
Tegison Capsules (Less than 1%) 2314
Toradol (1% or less) 2319
Tornalate Solution for Inhalation, 0.2% (Less than 1%) 976
Tornalate Metered Dose Inhaler (Less than 1%) 978
▲ Ventolin Syrup (4% in children) 1175
Zithromax (1% or less) 2043
Zoloft Tablets (Infrequent) 2051
Zyrtec Tablets (Less than 2%) 2053

Hyperlipidemia

Ambien Tablets (Rare) 2559
Betapace Tablets (Rare) 637
▲ CellCept Capsules (More than or equal to 3%) 2265
▲ Diprivan Injectable Emulsion (Less than 1% to 10%) 2939
Doxil (Less than 1%) 2613
Effexor (Infrequent) 2825
Ergamisol Tablets 1340
Estrace Cream and Tablets 751
Heparin Lock Flush Solution 2831
Heparin Sodium Injection 2832
Heparin Sodium Vials 1486
Hivid Tablets (Less than 1%) 2287
Kerlone Tablets (Less than 2%) 2588
▲ Lupron Depot - 3 Month 22.5 mg (More than or equal to 5%) 2743
LUVOX Tablets (Rare) 2723
Neurontin Capsules (Rare) 1978
Nolvadex Tablets (Infrequent) 2957
Norvir (1.7% to 4.1%) 447
Ogen Tablets 2103
Prevacid Delayed-Release Capsules (Less than 1%) 2746
▲ Prograf (Greater than 3%) 1028
Prozac Pulvules & Liquid, Oral Solution (Rare) 935
Redux Capsules (Rare) 2911
Sandimmune 2416
Supprelin Injection (1%) 2230
▲ Videx Tablets, Powder for Oral Solution, & Pediatric Powder for Oral Solution (2% to 7%) 2980
Vistide Injection 1057
Zyloprim Tablets (Less than 1%) 1194

Hypermenorrhea

Cytotec (0.5%) 2576

Hypermetabolic syndrome

Nardil (Less frequent) 1977

Hypermotility, gastrointestinal

Roferon-A Injection (Infrequent) 2308

Hypernatremia

Androderm Testosterone Transdermal System 2634
▲ Android Capsules, 10 mg (Among most common) 1297
Cytovene-IV (One report) 2270
Demadex Tablets and Injection 691
Doxil (Less than 1%) 2613
DUPHALAC Solution 2714
Felbatol 2774
Fleet Enema 1001
Hivid Tablets (Less than 1%) 2287
ISMOTIC 45% w/v Solution (Very rare) ◉ 221
Nardil (Less common) 1977
Proleukin for Injection (1%) 812
Testoderm Testosterone Transdermal System 486
Timentin for Injection 2706
Toradol 2319
Zosyn 1463

Hyperosmolarity

Diprivan Injectable Emulsion (Less than 1%) 2939
ISMOTIC 45% w/v Solution (Very rare) ◉ 221

Hyperostosis, skeletal

Accutane Capsules 2252
Anafranil Capsules (Rare) 819
▲ Tegison Capsules (Greater than 75%) 2314

Hyperoxia

Exosurf Neonatal for Intratracheal Suspension 1081

Hyperparathyroidism

Apresazide Capsules 824
Eskalith 2658
Lithonate/Lithotabs/Lithobid 2721
Prinzide Tablets 1780
Vaseretic Tablets 1810

Hyperphenylalaninemia

Daraprim Tablets (Rare) 1199

Hyperphosphatemia

Achromycin V Capsules 1417
Androderm Testosterone Transdermal System 2634
▲ Android Capsules, 10 mg (Among most common) 1297
Didronel Tablets 2133
Effexor (Rare) 2825
Estratest 2718
Fleet Enema 1001
Fludara for Injection 658
▲ Foscavir Injection (5% or greater) 541
Halotestin Tablets 2095
▲ Lupron Depot - 3 Month 22.5 mg (More than or equal to 5%) 2743
Minocin Intravenous 1428
Minocin Oral Suspension 1431
Minocin Pellet-Filled Capsules 1429
Oxandrin 783
Paxil Tablets (Rare) 2681
▲ Prograf (Greater than 3%) 1028
Proleukin for Injection (1%) 812
Risperdal Tablets (Rare) 1348
▲ Roferon-A Injection (9%) 2308
▲ Synarel Nasal Solution for Endometriosis (10% to 15%) 2605
Testoderm Testosterone Transdermal System 486
Testred Capsules, 10 mg 1308
Winstrol Tablets 2468
Zithromax (Less than 1%) 2043
Zithromax Tablets (Less than 1%) 2046

Hyperpigmentation

Accutane Capsules (Less than 1%) 2252
BiCNU 696
▲ Blenoxane (Approximately 50%) 697
Blocadren Tablets 1654
▲ Catapres-TTS (5 of 101 patients) 680
Celestone Soluspan Suspension 2484
Cipro I.V. (1% or less) 587
Cipro I.V. Pharmacy Bulk Package (Less than 1%) 590
Cipro Tablets (Less than 1%) 584
Cortone Acetate Sterile Suspension 1663
Dalalone D.P. Injectable 1009
Decadron Phosphate Injection 1680
Decadron Phosphate with Xylocaine Injection, Sterile 1683
Decadron-LA Sterile Suspension 1687
Dovonex Ointment 0.005% (Less than 1%) 2793
▲ Efudex (Among most frequent) 2280
EMLA Cream (Rare) 536
Florinef Acetate Tablets 506
Floxin I.V. 1580
Floxin Tablets (200 mg, 300 mg, 400 mg) 1577
Fluoroplex Topical Solution & Cream 1% (Occasional) 475
Hydeltrasol Injection, Sterile 1708
Hydeltra-T.B.A. Sterile Suspension 1710
Hydrocortone Acetate Sterile Suspension 1712
Hydrocortone Phosphate Injection, Sterile 1713
Lac-Hydrin 12% Lotion (Less frequent) 2796
▲ Lamprene Capsules (75-100%) 846
Lodine Capsules and Tablets (Less than 1%) 2849
Matulane Capsules 2300
Maxaquin Tablets 2593
▲ Myleran Tablets (5-10%) 1209
Norplant System 2868
Penetrex Tablets 2196
Purinethol Tablets 1214
Retin-A (tretinoin) Cream/Gel/Liquid 1947
Taxotere for Injection Concentrate 2204
T.R.U.E. Test (Occasional; 2 to 9 reports) 1162

Hyperpigmentation, dermal creases

Adriamycin PFS (A few cases primarily in children) 2056
Adriamycin RDF (A few cases primarily in children) 2056
Rubex for Injection (A few cases) 721

Hyperpigmentation, nail beds

Adriamycin PFS (A few cases primarily in children) 2056
Adriamycin RDF (A few cases primarily in children) 2056
Doxorubicin Astra (a few cases) 531

(▣ Described in PDR For Nonprescription Drugs) Incidence data in parenthesis; ▲ 3% or more (◉ Described in PDR For Ophthalmology)

Hyperpigmentation, nail beds — Side Effects Index

Florinef Acetate Tablets ... 506
Rubex for Injection (A few cases) ... 721

Hyperplasia, endocervical
Demulen ... 2580
Depo-Provera Contraceptive Injection (Fewer than 1%) ... 2079

Hyperplasia, endometrial
Estraderm Transdermal System ... 842

Hyperplasia, gingival
(see under Gingival hyperplasia)

Hyperplasia, mammary
Cuprimine Capsules (Rare) ... 1673
Depen Titratable Tablets (Rare) ... 2770

Hyperprolactinemia
Aldoclor Tablets ... 1638
Aldomet Ester HCl Injection ... 1642
Aldomet Oral ... 1640
Aldoril Tablets ... 1644
Asendin Tablets (Less frequent) ... 1419
Calan SR Caplets (1% or less) ... 2571
Calan Tablets (1% or less) ... 2568
Compazine ... 2644
Covera-HS Tablets (Less than 2%) ... 2573
Haldol Decanoate ... 1587
Haldol Injection, Tablets and Concentrate ... 1585
Isoptin SR Tablets (1% or less) ... 1395
Mellaril ... 2398
Moban Tablets and Concentrate ... 1036
Paxil Tablets ... 2681
Prolixin Oral Concentrate ... 510
Prozac Pulvules & Liquid, Oral Solution ... 935
Redux Capsules ... 2911
Reglan ... 2243
Risperdal Tablets ... 1348
Stelazine ... 2692
Thorazine ... 2701
Torecan ... 2367
Trilafon ... 2532
Zoloft Tablets ... 2051

Hyperprothrombinemia
Brevicon ... 2563
Doxil (1% to 5%) ... 2613
Eminase ... 2215
Estratest ... 2718
Maxipime for Injection (1.4%) ... 758
Norinyl ... 2563
Nor-Q D Tablets ... 2598
Tri-Norinyl ... 2607
Zyloprim Tablets (Less than 1%) ... 1194

Hyperpyrexia
(see under Fever)

Hyperreflexia
Anafranil Capsules (Rare) ... 819
Cerebyx Injection (Frequent) ... 1956
Compazine ... 2644
Depakote Tablets (1% to 5%) ... 418
Effexor (Rare) ... 2825
Foscavir Injection (Less than 1%) ... 541
Haldol Injection, Tablets and Concentrate ... 1585
Invirase Capsules (Less than 2%) ... 2291
Levoprome ... 1321
Lithonate/Lithotabs/Lithobid (One report) ... 2721
Nardil (Common) ... 1977
Navane Capsules and Concentrate ... 2018
Navane Intramuscular ... 2019
Neurontin Capsules (Frequent) ... 1978
Orap Tablets (Less frequent) ... 1037
Orthoclone OKT3 Sterile Solution ... 1892
Paxil Tablets (Rare) ... 2681
Pfizerpen for Injection ... 2022
Placidyl Capsules ... 456
Prolixin ... 510
Redux Capsules ... 2911
Remeron Tablets (Infrequent) ... 1878
Risperdal Tablets (Rare) ... 1348
Seromycin Capsules ... 975
Stelazine ... 2692
Triavil Tablets ... 1800
Trilafon ... 2532
Videx Tablets, Powder for Oral Solution, & Pediatric Powder for Oral Solution (Less than 1%) ... 2980

Hyperreflexia, neonatal
Compazine ... 2644
Etrafon ... 2495
Stelazine ... 2692
Thorazine ... 2701

Hypersecretion
Diupres Tablets ... 1691
Hydropres Tablets ... 1718
Ser-Ap-Es Tablets ... 867

Hypersensitivity
AK-FLUOR Injection 10% and 25% (Rare) ... 204
AK-PRED ... 204
AK-Spore ... 205
▲ AKTOB (Among most frequent; less than 3 of 100 patients) ... 207
Alkeran for Injection ... 1196
Americaine Otic Topical Anesthetic Ear Drops ... 1603
Amoxil ... 2631
Anectine (Rare) ... 1062
Atrohist Plus Tablets ... 1605
Azulfidine ... 2059
Beclovent Inhalation Aerosol and Refill ... 1063
Beconase Inhalation Aerosol (Rare) ... 1065
Betagan ... 230
Bicillin C-R Injection ... 2810
Bicillin C-R 900/300 Injection ... 2812
Bicillin L-A Injection ... 2813
Bleph-10 ... 472
Butisol Sodium Elixir & Tablets (Less than 1 in 100) ... 2768
Cefizox for Intramuscular or Intravenous Use (Less than 1%) ... 1025
Cefobid Intravenous/Intramuscular ... 1996
Cefobid Pharmacy Bulk Package - Not for Direct Infusion ... 1999
Cefotan (1.2%) ... 2936
Chloromycetin Ophthalmic Ointment, 1% ... 298
Clinoril Tablets (Less than 1%) ... 1658
Cocaine Hydrochloride Topical Solutions ... 529
Collagenase Santyl Ointment (One case) ... 1381
Cortisporin Ophthalmic Ointment Sterile ... 1074
Cortisporin Ophthalmic Suspension Sterile ... 1075
Cortone Acetate Sterile Suspension ... 1663
Cortone Acetate Tablets ... 1664
Daranide Tablets ... 1676
Daraprim Tablets ... 1199
Decadron Elixir ... 1676
Decadron Phosphate Injection ... 1680
Decadron Phosphate with Xylocaine Injection, Sterile ... 1683
Decadron Tablets ... 1678
Decadron-LA Sterile Suspension ... 1687
Demser Capsules (Rare) ... 1690
Dexacort Phosphate in Respihaler ... 1606
Dexacort Phosphate in Turbinaire ... 1607
Dolobid Tablets (Less than 1 in 100) ... 1695
Elspar ... 1700
Estratest (Rare) ... 2718
FML-S Liquifilm ... 240
Flexeril Tablets ... 1701
Floxin I.V. ... 1580
Floxin Tablets (200 mg, 300 mg, 400 mg) (Less than 1%) ... 1577
Fluorescite ... 217
Fortaz (Immediate in 1 in 285 patients) ... 1092
Geocillin Tablets ... 2009
Gris-PEG Tablets, 125 mg & 250 mg ... 476
Halotestin Tablets ... 2095
Heparin Sodium Vials ... 1486
Hep-B-Gammagee (Rare) ... 1706
Hibistat Germicidal Hand Rinse (Very rare) ... 2948
Hydeltrasol Injection, Sterile ... 1708
Hydeltra-T.B.A. Sterile Suspension ... 1710
Hydrocortone Acetate Sterile Suspension ... 1712
Hydrocortone Phosphate Injection, Sterile ... 1713
Hydrocortone Tablets ... 1715
Hyperstat I.V. Injection ... 2504
Imitrex Injection (Infrequent) ... 1095
Imitrex Tablets (Frequent) ... 1099
Imodium Capsules ... 1343
Inderide Tablets ... 2838
Indocin (Less than 1%) ... 1723
Inocor Lactate Injection (Several reports) ... 2439
ISMOTIC 45% w/v Solution ... 221
Kefurox Vials, Faspak & ADD-Vantage (Less than 1%) ... 1509
Kefzol Vials, Faspak & ADD-Vantage ... 1511
Lacrisert Sterile Ophthalmic Insert ... 1730

Leukeran Tablets ... 1205
Lopressor HCT Tablets ... 850
Lupron Injection ... 2736
Maxitrol Ophthalmic Ointment and Suspension ... 222
Mesnex Injection ... 711
Metubine Iodide Vials ... 932
Miacalcin Injection ... 2402
Miltown Tablets ... 2780
Mustargen ... 1752
Nembutal Sodium Capsules ... 440
Nembutal Sodium Solution ... 442
Nembutal Sodium Suppositories (Less than 1%) ... 444
NeoDecadron Topical Cream ... 1757
Nizoral Tablets (Several cases) ... 1345
Norflex ... 1554
Normodyne Injection (Rare) ... 2519
Normodyne Tablets (Rare) ... 2522
Noroxin Tablets (A few patients) ... 1758
Noroxin Tablets (A few patients) ... 2222
Novocain Hydrochloride for Spinal Anesthesia (Rare) ... 2457
Ocupress Ophthalmic Solution, 1% Sterile ... 297
PBZ Tablets ... 863
PBZ-SR Tablets ... 862
Paraplatin for Injection (2%) ... 713
Peptavlon ... 2997
Peridex (Rare) ... 2127
Periogard Oral Rinse (Rare) ... 892
Phenobarbital Elixir and Tablets ... 1523
Pontocaine Hydrochloride for Spinal Anesthesia ... 2460
Prinzide Tablets ... 1780
Prolopim Tablets ... 1141
Recombivax HB ... 1787
Rifadin ... 1276
Rimactane Capsules ... 865
Ritalin ... 866
Sandoglobulin I.V. ... 2419
Seromycin Capsules ... 975
Synarel Nasal Solution for Endometriosis (0.2%) ... 2605
Talacen Caplets (A few cases) ... 2464
Tenoretic Tablets ... 2963
TERAK Ointment (Rare) ... 210
Tetanus Toxoid Adsorbed Purogenated ... 1447
TheraCys BCG Live (Intravesical) (Up to 1.8%) ... 911
Tigan ... 2231
Timoptic in Ocudose (Less frequent) ... 1796
Timoptic Sterile Ophthalmic Solution (Less frequent) ... 1794
TobraDex Ophthalmic Suspension and Ointment (Less than 4%) ... 469
Tobrex Ophthalmic Ointment and Solution (Less than 3 of 100 patients) ... 226
Tonocard Tablets (Less than 1%) ... 519
Toradol (1% or less) ... 2319
Trandate (Rare) ... 1158
Trimpex Tablets (Rare) ... 2323
Urobiotic-250 Capsules ... 2038
Vancenase AQ Nasal Spray 0.042% (Rare) ... 2535
Vanceril Inhaler (Rare) ... 2538
Viroptic Ophthalmic Solution, 1% Sterile ... 1177
Xylocaine Injections ... 562
Zantac (Rare) ... 1182
Zantac Injection (Rare) ... 1180
Zantac Syrup (Rare) ... 1182
Zinacef (Fewer than 1%) ... 1184
Zyloprim Tablets (Less than 1%) ... 1194

Hypersensitivity pancreatitis
Azathioprine Tablets (Rare) ... 2349
Imuran ... 1103

Hypersensitivity pneumonitis
Fungizone Intravenous ... 507
Pentasa (Infrequent) ... 1275
Relafen Tablets (Rarer) ... 2688

Hypersensitivity reactions, Arthus-type
Diphtheria and Tetanus Toxoids and Pertussis Vaccine Adsorbed (Rare) ... 2650
Tripedia ... 908

Hypersensitivity reactions, general
Alferon N Injection ... 2142
Alkeran Tablets ... 1198
Altace Capsules (Less than 1%) ... 1238
Ancef Injection ... 2632
Asacol Delayed-Release Tablets (Some patients) ... 2129

Augmentin ... 2637
Augmentin Tablets ... 2640
▲ Avonex (3%) ... 662
Axid Pulvules (Rare) ... 1468
Beconase AQ Nasal Spray (Rare) ... 1065
Betaseron for SC Injection ... 653
Betimol 0.25%, 0.5% ... 259
Bioclate, Antihemophilic Factor (Recombinant) ... 797
Brethine Ampuls ... 832
Brethine Tablets ... 831
Carafate Suspension ... 1250
Carafate Tablets ... 1249
Ceclor Pulvules & Suspension (About 1.5%) ... 1470
Ceftin ... 1067
Ceptaz (2% of patients) ... 1070
Ceredase (A limited number of patients) ... 1055
Chibroxin Sterile Ophthalmic Solution (With oral form) ... 1657
Cipro Tablets ... 584
Cleocin Phosphate Injection ... 2068
Cleocin Vaginal Cream ... 2070
Clozaril Tablets ... 2377
Coumadin (Infrequent) ... 941
Dalalone D.P. Injectable ... 1009
Didronel Tablets ... 2133
Digibind ... 1079
Dilantin-125 Suspension ... 1969
Dobutrex Solution Vials (Occasional) ... 1480
Doryx Capsules ... 1970
Duranest Injections ... 533
Ethiodol Injection (Infrequent) ... 2472
Etrafon (Extremely rare) ... 2495
Factrel (Rare) ... 2996
Flonase Nasal Spray ... 1088
Flovent (Rare) ... 1089
▲ Fulvicin P/G Tablets (Among most common) ... 2499
Fulvicin P/G 165 & 330 Tablets ... 2500
Gamimune N, 5% Immune Globulin Intravenous (Human), 5% (One patient) ... 612
Gamimune N, 10% Immune Globulin Intravenous (Human), 10% (One patient) ... 615
Gammagard S/D, Immune Globulin, Intravenous (Human) (A remote possibility) ... 577
Gammar-P I.V., Immune Globulin Intravenous (Human) ... 798
Gantrisin ... 2286
GlaucTabs ... 209
Grifulvin V (griseofulvin tablets) Microsize (griseofulvin oral suspension) Microsize ... 1944
Heparin Lock Flush Solution ... 2831
Heparin Sodium Injection ... 2832
Hespan Injection ... 945
Hyzaar Tablets ... 1720
▲ Ilotycin Ophthalmic Ointment (Among most frequent) ... 928
INFeD (Iron Dextran Injection, USP) ... 2478
Keflex Pulvules & Oral Suspension ... 930
Kytril Injection (Rare) ... 2667
Kytril Tablets (Rare) ... 2669
Lasix Injection, Oral Solution and Tablets ... 1267
Lescol Capsules (Rare) ... 2395
Levoprome ... 1321
Lorabid Suspension and Pulvules ... 1513
Lotensin Tablets ... 852
Lutrepulse for Injection ... 998
Mebaral Tablets (Less than 1 in 100) ... 2452
Menomune-A/C/Y/W-135 ... 906
Metaproterenol Sulfate Inhalation Solution, USP, Arm-a-Med (Rare) ... 547
Mevacor Tablets ... 1742
Minocin Pellet-Filled Capsules ... 1429
Monocid Injection (Less than 1%) ... 2674
Neosporin Ophthalmic Solution Sterile (Rare) ... 1131
Norcuron for Injection ... 1875
Nubain Injection (1% or less) ... 952
Ogen Vaginal Cream ... 2106
Omnipen Capsules ... 2872
Oncaspar (Greater than 1% but less than 5%) ... 2194
Orthoclone OKT3 Sterile Solution ... 1892
Pen•Vee K (Occasional) ... 2879
Pentaspan Injection ... 954
Pergonal (menotropins for injection, USP) (Some patients) ... 2618
Phenobarbital Elixir and Tablets (Less than 1 in 100 patients) ... 1523
Polytrim Ophthalmic Solution Sterile (Multiple reports) ... 479

(⊞ Described in PDR For Nonprescription Drugs)   Incidence data in parenthesis; ▲ 3% or more   (⊙ Described in PDR For Ophthalmology)

Side Effects Index

(continued)

Profasi (chorionic gonadotropin for injection, USP) ... 2620
Proscar Tablets ... 1784
▲ Prostep (nicotine transdermal system) (3% of patients) ... 1439
Rabies Vaccine Adsorbed (Less than 1%) ... 2686
ReoPro Vials ... 1526
RespiGam ... 1631
Rifater ... 1280
Seconal Sodium Pulvules (Less than 1 in 100) ... 1529
Semprex-D Capsules (Rare) ... 1620
Serevent Inhalation Aerosol (Rare) ... 1149
Skelaxin Tablets ... 793
Spectrobid Tablets ... 2030
Streptase for Infusion ... 557
Supprelin Injection ... 2230
▲ Taxol Injection (2% to 41%) ... 723
Taxotere for Injection Concentrate (0.9%) ... 2204
Tessalon Perles ... 1018
Timoptic-XE ... 1798
Tornalate Solution for Inhalation, 0.2% ... 976
Tornalate Metered Dose Inhaler ... 978
Trasylol ... 607
Tympagesic Ear Drops ... 2476
Unasyn ... 2035
Univasc Tablets (Less than 1%) ... 2553
Vancenase AQ Double Strength Nasal Spray 0.084% (Rare) ... 2536
Vancenase PocketHaler Nasal Inhaler ... 2534
Vermox Chewable Tablets (Rare) ... 1357
Vistide Injection ... 1057
▲ Vumon for Injection (5%) ... 729
Zocor Tablets (Rare) ... 1821
Zofran Injection (Rare) ... 1227

Hypersensitivity vasculitis

Aldoclor Tablets ... 1638
Aldomet Ester HCl Injection ... 1642
Aldomet Oral Suspension ... 1640
Aldoril Tablets ... 1644
Brethine Ampuls (Rare) ... 832
Brethine Tablets (Rare) ... 831
Bricanyl Subcutaneous Injection (Rare) ... 1247
Bricanyl Tablets (Rare) ... 1248
Clinoril Tablets (Less than 1 in 100) ... 1658
Dolobid Tablets (Less than 1 in 100) ... 1695
Streptase for Infusion ... 557
Tagamet (Rare) ... 2694

Hypersomnia

LUVOX Tablets (Infrequent) ... 2723
Nardil (Common) ... 1977
Prinivil Tablets (0.3% to 1.0%) ... 1776
Prinzide Tablets ... 1780
Zestoretic Tablets ... 2968
Zestril Tablets (0.3% to 1.0%) ... 2972

Hypertension

Abbokinase ... 403
Abbokinase Open-Cath ... 405
Abelcet Injection ... 1540
Activase ... 1045
Adderall Tablets ... 2209
Adenocard Injection ... 1021
Adenoscan (Less than 1%) ... 1022
Adipex-P Tablets and Capsules ... 1035
AeroBid Inhaler System (1% to 3%) ... 1004
Aerobid-M Inhaler System (1% to 3%) ... 1004
Airet Albuterol Sulfate Inhalation Solution (1% to 3.1%) ... 1602
AKPRO ... ⊙ 206
Albalon Solution with Liquifilm ... ⊙ 229
Albuterol Sulfate, USP Solution for Inhalation, Arm-a-Med (1% to 3.1%) ... 522
▲ Alfenta Injection (18%) ... 1334
Alupent ... 672
Ambien Tablets (Infrequent) ... 2559
Amen Tablets ... 785
Ana-Kit Anaphylaxis Emergency Treatment Kit ... 611
Androderm Testosterone Transdermal System (Less than 1%) ... 2634
Anectine ... 1062
▲ Aredia for Injection (Up to at least 15%) ... 827
Arimidex Tablets (2% to 5%) ... 2932
Regular Strength Ascriptin Tablets ... ⊞ 650
Asendin Tablets (Less than 1%) ... 1419

Atamet Tablets (Rare) ... 567
Ativan Injection (0.1%) ... 2805
Atretol Tablets ... 569
Atrohist Plus Tablets ... 1605
Atrovent Inhalation Solution (0.9%) ... 675
Genuine Bayer Aspirin Tablets & Caplets (Small increases at doses of 1000 mg/day) ... ⊞ 618
Betapace Tablets (Less than 1% to 2%) ... 637
▲ Betaseron for SC Injection (7%) ... 653
Betimol 0.25%, 0.5% (1% to 5%) ... ⊙ 259
Bontril Slow-Release Capsules ... 786
Brethaire Inhaler (Fewer than 1 per 100) ... 830
Brevicon ... 2563
▲ Bromfed-DM Cough Syrup (Among most frequent) ... 1832
Buprenex Injectable (Less than 1%) ... 2170
BuSpar Tablets (Infrequent) ... 738
Cafergot ... 2376
Calcijex Injection ... 412
Carbocaine Injection ... 2432
Cardene I.V. (0.7%) ... 2815
▲ Casodex Tablets (5%) ... 2934
Cataflam Tablets (Less than 1%) ... 833
Catapres-TTS ... 680
Caverject Injection (2%) ... 2064
Celestone Soluspan Suspension ... 2484
▲ CellCept Capsules (28.2% to 32.4%; 16.9% to 17.6%) ... 2265
Cerebyx Injection (Frequent) ... 1956
Cipro I.V. (1% or less) ... 587
Cipro I.V. Pharmacy Bulk Package (Less than 1%) ... 590
Cipro Tablets (Less than 1%) ... 584
Claritin Tablets (2% or fewer patients) ... 2485
Claritin-D Tablets (Less frequent) ... 2487
Climara Transdermal System (Occasional) ... 640
Clinoril Tablets (Less than 1%) ... 1658
Clomid ... 1262
▲ Clozaril Tablets (4%) ... 2377
Cognex Capsules (Frequent) ... 1961
CORTENEMA ... 2713
Cortifoam ... 2540
Cortone Acetate Sterile Suspension ... 1663
Cortone Acetate Tablets ... 1664
Corvert Injection (1.2%) ... 2075
Cycrin Tablets ... 991
Cytotec (Infrequent) ... 2576
Cytovene (1% or less) ... 2270
DDAVP Injection (Infrequent) ... 2178
DDAVP Rhinal Tube (Infrequent) ... 2180
D.H.E. 45 Injection (Occasional) ... 2381
Dalalone D.P. Injectable ... 1009
Dalgan Injection (Less than 1%) ... 529
Danocrine Capsules ... 2437
DaunoXome (Less than or equal to 5%) ... 1842
Decadron Elixir ... 1676
Decadron Phosphate Injection ... 1680
Decadron Phosphate with Xylocaine Injection, Sterile ... 1683
Decadron Tablets ... 1678
Decadron-LA Sterile Suspension ... 1687
Demulen ... 2580
Depakote Tablets (1% to 5%) ... 418
Depo-Provera Sterile Aqueous Suspension ... 2083
Desmopressin Acetate Injection (Infrequent) ... 996
Desmopressin Acetate Rhinal Tube (Infrequent) ... 997
Desogen Tablets ... 1867
Desoxyn Gradumet Tablets ... 422
Desyrel and Desyrel Dividose (1.3% to 2.1%) ... 504
Dexacort Phosphate in Respihaler ... 1606
Dexacort Phosphate in Turbinaire ... 1607
Dexedrine ... 2648
DextroStat-Dextroamphetamine Sulfate Tablets ... 2211
Dilacor XR Extended-release Capsules ... 2183
Dilaudid-HP Injection (Less frequent) ... 1384
Dilaudid-HP Lyophilized Powder 250 mg (Less frequent) ... 1384
Diladuid Tablets and Liquid ... 1386
Dimetane-DC Cough Syrup ... 2232
Dimetane-DX Cough Syrup ... 2233
Dipentum Capsules (Rare) ... 2084
▲ Diprivan Injectable Emulsion (Less than 1% to 8%) ... 2939

▲ Dobutrex Solution Vials (Most patients) ... 1480
Dopram Injectable ... 2235
Duragesic Transdermal System (1% to 3%) ... 1336
Ecotrin ... 2625
▲ Effexor (1.1% to 4.5%) ... 2825
Elavil ... 2945
Eldepryl Capsules ... 2729
Emcyt Capsules ... 2085
Emete-con Intramuscular/Intravenous ... 2007
▲ Epogen for Injection (0.75% to 24%) ... 489
Estrace Cream and Tablets (Occasional) ... 751
Estraderm Transdermal System ... 842
ESTRATAB Tablets (0.3, 0.625, 1.25, 2.5 mg) (Not uncommon) ... 2715
Estratest (Common) ... 2718
Ethmozine Tablets (Less than 2%) ... 2217
▲ Etopophos for Injection (3%) ... 701
Etoposide Injection ... 539
Etrafon ... 2495
Eulexin Capsules (1%) ... 2498
Fastin Capsules ... 2662
Felbatol ... 2774
Feldene Capsules (Less than 1%) ... 2008
Flexeril Tablets (Rare) ... 1701
Florinef Acetate Tablets ... 506
Floxin I.V. (Less than 1%) ... 1580
Floxin Tablets (200 mg, 300 mg, 400 mg) (Less than 1%) ... 1577
Flumadine Tablets & Syrup (Less than 0.3%) ... 1013
Foscavir Injection (Between 1% and 5%) ... 541
Fungizone Intravenous ... 507
Gammagard S/D, Immune Globulin, Intravenous (Human) (Occasional) ... 577
Garamycin Injectable ... 2502
Gemzar for Injection (2%) ... 1482
Glucotrol XL Extended Release Tablets (Less than 1%) ... 2012
▲ Habitrol Nicotine Transdermal System (3% to 9% of patients) ... 884
Haldol Decanoate ... 1587
Haldol Injection, Tablets and Concentrate ... 1585
Halfprin Tablets ... 1413
Helidac Therapy (Less than 1%) ... 2135
Hivid Tablets (Less than 1%) ... 2287
Hycomine Compound Tablets ... 948
Hycomine ... 947
Hycotuss Expectorant Syrup ... 950
Hydeltrasol Injection, Sterile ... 1708
Hydeltra-T.B.A. Sterile Suspension ... 1710
Hydrocortone Acetate Sterile Suspension ... 1712
Hydrocortone Phosphate Injection, Sterile ... 1713
Hydrocortone Tablets ... 1715
IBU Tablets (Less than 1%) ... 1389
IFEX (Less than 1%) ... 706
Imdur (Less than or equal to 5%) ... 1362
Imitrex Injection (Infrequent) ... 1095
Imitrex Tablets (Infrequent) ... 1099
Inapsine Injection ... 462
Indocin Capsules (Less than 1%) ... 1723
Indocin I.V. (Less than 1%) ... 1727
Indocin (Less than 1%) ... 1723
INFeD (Iron Dextran Injection, USP) ... 2478
Intron A for Injection (Less than 5%) ... 2506
Invirase Capsules (Less than 2%) ... 2291
Ionamin Capsules ... 1615
Isuprel Injection ... 2441
Kadian Capsules (Less than 3%) ... 2948
Kerlone Tablets (Less than 2%) ... 2588
Kytril Injection (2%) ... 2667
Kytril Tablets (1%) ... 2669
Lamictal Tablets (Rare) ... 1105
Larodopa Tablets (Rare) ... 2296
▲ Leukine (25% to 34%) ... 1317
Levlen/Tri-Levlen ... 646
Levophed Bitartrate Injection ... 2445
Limbitrol ... 2333
Lioresal Intrathecal (0.2% to 0.6%) ... 1634
Lodine Capsules and Tablets (Less than 1%) ... 2849
Lo/Ovral Tablets ... 2852
Lo/Ovral-28 Tablets ... 2857
Loxitane ... 1426
Ludiomil Tablets (Rare) ... 861
Lupron Depot - 3 Month 22.5 mg (Less than 5%) ... 2743
▲ Lupron Injection (5% or more) ... 2736
LUVOX Tablets (Frequent) ... 2723

Lysodren Tablets (Infrequent) ... 707
MS Contin Tablets (Less frequent) ... 2149
MSIR (Infrequent) ... 2152
Maxaquin Tablets (Less than 1%) ... 2593
▲ Megace Oral Suspension (Up to 8%) ... 708
Megace Tablets ... 710
Menest Tablets ... 2671
Mepergan Injection (Rare) ... 2859
Merrem I.V. (0.1% to 1.0%) ... 2952
Metaproterenol Sulfate Inhalation Solution, USP, Arm-a-Med (1 in 300 patients) ... 547
▲ Methergine (Most common) ... 2401
Mexitil Capsules (Less than 1% or about 1 in 1,000) ... 684
Miacalcin Nasal Spray (1% to 3%) ... 2403
Modicon ... 1928
Monoket Tablets (Fewer than 1%) ... 2550
Monopril Tablets (0.4% to 1.0%) ... 762
Motrin Ibuprofen Suspension, Oral Drops, Chewable Tablets, Caplets (Less than 1%) ... 1563
Mutamycin for Injection ... 712
Naprelan Tablets (Less than 3%) ... 2861
Narcan Injection (Several instances) ... 950
▲ Neoral (Approximately 50% to most patients) ... 2405
Neo-Synephrine Hydrochloride (Ophthalmic) (Rare) ... 2456
▲ Neupogen for Injection (4%) ... 495
Neurontin Capsules (Frequent) ... 1978
Nimotop Capsules (Less than 1%) ... 603
Nipent for Injection (Less than 3%) ... 2733
Nordette-21 Tablets ... 2863
Nordette-28 Tablets ... 2866
Norinyl ... 2563
Norpramin Tablets ... 1273
Nor-Q D Tablets ... 2598
Novocain Hydrochloride for Spinal Anesthesia ... 2457
Nubain Injection (1% or less) ... 952
Ogen Tablets (Occasional) ... 2103
Ogen Vaginal Cream (Occasional) ... 2106
Oncaspar (Less than 1%) ... 2194
Oncovin Solution Vials & Hyporets ... 1521
OptiPranolol (Metipranolol 0.3%) Sterile Ophthalmic Solution (A small number of patients) ... ⊙ 256
Oramorph SR (Morphine Sulfate Sustained Release Tablets) (Less frequent) ... 2359
Orap Tablets ... 1037
Orlaam Oral Solution (Low frequency) ... 2361
Ornade Spansule Capsules ... 2678
Ortho-Cept ... 1907
Ortho-Cyclen/Ortho-Tri-Cyclen ... 1914
Ortho Dienestrol Cream ... 1922
Ortho-Est (Occasional) ... 1925
Ortho-Novum ... 1928
Ortho-Cyclen/Ortho Tri-Cyclen ... 1914
▲ Orthoclone OKT3 Sterile Solution (8%) ... 1892
Orudis Capsules (Less than 1%) ... 2874
Oruvail Capsules (Less than 1%) ... 2874
Ovcon ... 765
Ovral Tablets ... 2877
Ovral-28 Tablets ... 2878
Ovrette Tablets ... 2878
Pamelor ... 2409
Papaverine Hydrochloride Vials and Ampoules ... 1523
Parlodel ... 2411
Paxil Tablets (Frequent) ... 2681
Pediapred Oral Solution ... 1618
Permax Tablets (1.6%) ... 571
Phenergan with Codeine ... 2883
Phenergan with Dextromethorphan ... 2885
Phenergan Injection ... 2880
Phenergan Suppositories ... 2882
Phenergan Syrup ... 2881
Phenergan Tablets ... 2882
Phenergan VC ... 2886
Phenergan VC with Codeine ... 2888
PMB 200 and PMB 400 ... 2890
Pondimin Tablets ... 2239
Prelone Syrup ... 1834
Prelu-2 Timed Release Capsules ... 687
Premarin Intravenous ... 2893
Premarin Tablets ... 2896
Premarin Vaginal-Cream ... 2898
Prevacid Delayed-Release Capsules (Less than 1%) ... 2746
Prilosec Delayed-Release Capsules (Less than 1%) ... 516
Priscoline Hydrochloride Ampuls ... 864

(⊞ Described in PDR For Nonprescription Drugs)   Incidence data in parenthesis; ▲ 3% or more   (⊙ Described in PDR For Ophthalmology)

Hypertension Side Effects Index 1366

▲ Procrit for Injection (0.75% to 24%) 1896
Proglycem (A few cases) 575
▲ Prograf (Common; 31% to 47%) .. 1028
Prolixin 510
Propagest Tablets 791
PROPINE with C CAP Compliance Cap .... ⊙ 251
Protopam Chloride for Injection 2909
Proventil Inhalation Aerosol (Less than 5%) 2524
Proventil Inhalation Solution 0.083% (1% to 3.1%) 2527
Proventil Repetabs Tablets 2529
Proventil Solution for Inhalation 0.5% (1% to 3.1%) 2525
Proventil Syrup 2528
Proventil Tablets 2529
Provera Tablets 2110
Prozac Pulvules & Liquid, Oral Solution (Infrequent) 935
Redux Capsules (Frequent) 2911
Reglan 2243
Relafen Tablets (Less than 1%) 2688
Remeron Tablets (Frequent) 1878
RespiGam (1%) 1631
ReVia Tablets (Less than 1%) 957
▲ Revex (nalmefene hydrochloride injection) (5%) 1863
▲ Rilutek Tablets (3.3% to 6.8%) 2198
Risperdal Tablets (Infrequent) 1348
Rocaltrol Capsules 2303
▲ Roferon-A Injection (11%) 2308
Romazicon (Less than 1%) 2311
Rondec Oral Drops 974
Rondec Syrup 974
Rondec 974
▲ Salagen Tablets (3%) 1546
▲ Sandimmune (13 to 53%) 2416
Sandostatin Injection (Less than 1%) 2421
Serevent Inhalation Aerosol 1149
Serzone Tablets (Infrequent) 776
Sinemet Tablets (Rare) 959
Sinemet CR Tablets 961
Sinequan (Occasional) 2028
Sinulin Tablets 792
Sporanox Capsules (2% to 3.2%) .. 1352
Stadol (Less than 1%) 779
Stimate, (desmopressin acetate) Nasal Spray, 1.5 mg/mL (Infrequent) 806
Sublimaze Injection 463
▲ Sufenta Injection (3% to 9%) 1355
Sular Tablets (Less than or equal to 1%) 2961
Supprelin Injection (1% to 3%) 2230
Suprane (desflurane, USP) (Greater than 1%) 1865
Surmontil Capsules 2917
Survanta Beractant Intratracheal Suspension (Less than 1%) 2346
Symmetrel Capsules (0.1% to 1%) 965
Symmetrel Syrup (0.1% to 1%) 963
Talwin Injection (Infrequent) 2465
Tambocor Tablets (Less than 1%) 1555
Taxol Injection (1%) 723
Taxotere for Injection Concentrate (Rare) 2204
Tegretol/Tegretol-XR 870
Teslac Tablets 727
THYREL TRH (A small number of patients) 2992
Timoptic in Ocudose (Less frequent) 1796
Timoptic Sterile Ophthalmic Solution (Less frequent) 1794
Timoptic-XE 1798
Tofranil Ampuls 873
Tofranil Tablets 875
Tofranil-PM Capsules 876
▲ Tolectin (200, 400 and 600 mg) (3 to 9%) 1591
Tonocard Tablets (Less than 1%) .. 519
Toradol (Greater than 1%) 2319
Tornalate Solution for Inhalation, 0.2% (Less than 1%) 976
Trasylol (2%) 607
Triavil Tablets 1800
Trilafon (Occasional) 2532
Levlen/Tri-Levlen 646
Trinalin Repetabs Tablets 1373
Tri-Norinyl 2607
Triostat Injection (Approximately 1%) 2708
Triphasil-21 Tablets 2919
Triphasil-28 Tablets 2924
Ultram Tablets (50 mg) (Infrequent) 1594
Vascor Tablets (200 and 300 mg) (0.5 to 2.0%) 1597
Vasotec I.V. 1814
Vasoxyl Injection 1169
▲ Velban Vials (Among most common) 1537
▲ Ventolin Inhalation Aerosol and Refill (Fewer than 5 per 100 patients) 1170
Ventolin Inhalation Solution (1% to 3.1%) 1171
Ventolin Nebules Inhalation Solution (1% to 3.1%) 1172
Ventolin Rotacaps for Inhalation 1173
Ventolin Syrup 1175
Ventolin Tablets 1176
VePesid Capsules and Injection 727
Versed Injection 2324
▲ Vesanoid Capsules (11%) 2327
Vicodin Tuss Expectorant 1406
Videx Tablets, Powder for Oral Solution, & Pediatric Powder for Oral Solution (1%) 2980
Vivactil Tablets 1820
Vivelle Transdermal System 880
Volmax Extended-Release Tablets .. 1835
Cataflam/Voltaren/Voltaren-XR (Less than 1%) 833
Vumon for Injection 729
▲ Wellbutrin Tablets (4.3%) 1177
Yocon Tablets 1235
Yohimex Tablets 1414
Zemuron Injection (0.1%; 2%) 1885
Zerit Capsules (Fewer than 1% to 2%) 731
▲ Zestril Tablets (5.7%) 2972
Zoladex (1% or greater but less than 5%) 2976
Zoladex 3-month 2978
Zoloft Tablets (Infrequent) 2051
Zosyn (1.3% to 1.6%) 1463
Zyrtec Tablets (Less than 2%) 2053

Hypertension, aggravation

Ambien Tablets (Rare) 2559
Atretol Tablets 569
Atrovent Inhalation Solution (0.9%) 675
Tegretol/Tegretol-XR 870
Zoloft Tablets (Rare) 2051

Hypertension, intracranial

Aclovate 1061
Amicar Syrup, Tablets, and Injection 1312
Betaseron for SC Injection 653
Cerebyx Injection (Frequent) 1956
Cutivate Cream 1078
Cutivate Ointment 1078
Cytovene-IV (Two or more reports) 2270
Danocrine Capsules (Rare) 2437
Dermatop Emollient Cream 0.1% .. 1264
Diprivan Injectable Emulsion (Less than 1%) 2939
Doryx Capsules 1970
DYNACIN Capsules 1627
Genotropin Injection (A small number of patients) 2090
Humatrope Vials (A small number of patients) 1490
Macrobid Capsules (Rare) 2138
Macrodantin Capsules (Rare) 2140
Minocin Intravenous 1428
Minocin Oral Suspension 1431
Minocin Pellet-Filled Capsules 1429
Monodox Capsules 1858
Norplant System (Less than 1%) 2868
Pediazole Suspension 2340
Permax Tablets (Rare) 571
ProctoCream-HC 2.5% 2552
Terramycin Intramuscular Solution 2034
Urobiotic-250 Capsules 2038
▲ Vesanoid Capsules (9%) 2327
Vibramycin 2038
Vibramycin Hyclate Intravenous 2040
Vibramycin 2038

Hypertension, rebound

Deponit NTG Transdermal Delivery System (Uncommon) 2541
Dilatrate-SR Capsules (Uncommon) 2542
Isordil Sublingual Tablets (Uncommon) 2845
Isordil Tembids (Uncommon) 2847
Isordil Titradose Tablets (Uncommon) 2848
Nitro-Bid IV (Uncommon) 1270
Nitro-Bid Ointment (Uncommon) 1272
Nitro-Dur (nitroglycerin) Transdermal Infusion System (Uncommon) 1365
Sorbitrate (Uncommon) 2959
Tenex Tablets (Less common) 2249
Transderm-Nitro Transdermal Therapeutic System (Uncommon) 878

Hypertensive crises

Accupril Tablets (Rare) 1950
Emete-con Intramuscular/Intravenous 2007
Imitrex Injection (Rare) 1095
Monopril Tablets (0.2% to 1.0%) .. 762
Sandostatin Injection (Less than 1%) 2421

Hyperthermia

Anafranil Capsules (More than 30 cases) 819
Asendin Tablets (Less than 1%) 1419
Biltricide Tablets 584
Calcijex Injection 412
Cholera Vaccine 2818
Cogentin 1661
Effexor 2825
Elspar 1700
Emete-con Intramuscular/Intravenous 2007
Furoxone (Rare) 2221
Geocillin Tablets 2009
Humate-P, Antihemophilic Factor (Human), Dried Pasteurized (Rare) 801
Hyperab Rabies Immune Globulin (Human) 618
Hyper-Tet Tetanus Immune Globulin (Human) 621
HypRho-D Full Dose Rho (D) Immune Globulin (Human) 623
HypRho-D Mini-Dose Rho (D) Immune Globulin (Human) 622
Lomotil 2591
MICRhoGAM Rh_o(D) Immune Globulin (Human) (Reported in a small number of women) 1902
Marcaine (Rare) 2446
Marcaine Spinal (Rare) 2449
Motofen Tablets 789
Nescaine/Nescaine MPF 549
Prolixin 510
Reglan 2243
Rocaltrol Capsules 2303
Sensorcaine (Rare) 554
Stelazine 2692
Typhoid Vaccine 2929

Hyperthyroidism

Anafranil Capsules (Rare) 819
Cartrol Tablets 413
Cognex Capsules (Rare) 1961
Cordarone Tablets (1 to 3%) 2818
Cytomel Tablets 2647
Effexor (Rare) 2825
Eltroxin Tablets (Rare) 2214
Eskalith (Rare) 2658
Intron A for Injection (Less than 5%) 2506
Levothroid Tablets (Rare) 1015
Levothyroxine Sodium, USP for Injection 546
Levoxyl Tablets 918
Lithium Carbonate Capsules & Tablets (Rare cases) 2352
Lithonate/Lithotabs/Lithobid (Rare) 2721
Miacalcin Nasal Spray (Less than 1%) 2403
Neurontin Capsules (Rare) 1978
Paxil Tablets (Rare) 2681
Prozac Pulvules & Liquid, Oral Solution (Rare) 935
Roferon-A Injection (Infrequent) 2308
Synthroid (Rare) 1410
Tenoretic Tablets 2963
Tenormin Tablets and I.V. Injection 2965
Thyro-Block Tablets (Rare) 2785

Hypertonia

Adalat CC (Less than 1.0%) 582
Anafranil Capsules (2% to 4%) 819
▲ Asacol Delayed-Release Tablets (5%) 2129
▲ Betaseron for SC Injection (26%) .. 653
Cardene I.V. (Rare) 2815
Cardura Tablets (1%) 1993
Casodex Tablets (2% to 5%) 2934
Ceclor Pulvules & Suspension (Rare) 1470
▲ CellCept Capsules (More than or equal to 3%) 2265
Claritin-D Tablets (Less frequent) .. 2487
Cognex Capsules (Frequent) 1961
Cytovene (1% or less) 2270
DaunoXome (Less than or equal to 5%) 1842
Depakote Tablets (1% to 5%) 418
Dilacor XR Extended-release Capsules (Infrequent) 2183
Diprivan Injectable Emulsion (Less than 1%) 2939
Doxil (Less than 1%) 2613
Duragesic Transdermal System (Less than 1%) 1336
▲ Effexor (3%; infrequent) 2825
Eskalith 2658
Flexeril Tablets (Less than 1%) 1701
Foscavir Injection (Less than 1%) .. 541
Glucotrol XL Extended Release Tablets (Less than 1%) 2012
Havrix (Less than 1%) 2663
Hivid Tablets (Less than 1%) 2287
Intron A for Injection (Less than 5%) 2506
Lamictal Tablets (Rare) 1105
Lioresal Intrathecal (Up to 6.0%) .. 1634
Lithonate/Lithotabs/Lithobid 2721
Lotensin Tablets 852
Lotensin HCT Tablets (1.5%) 855
LUVOX Tablets (2%) 2723
Naprelan Tablets (Less than 1%) .. 2861
Norvasc Tablets (Less than or equal to 0.1%) 2020
Paxil Tablets (Infrequent) 2681
Penetrex Tablets (0.1% to 1%) 2196
Permax Tablets (1.1%) 571
Procardia XL Extended Release Tablets (1% or less) 2026
▲ Prograf (Greater than 3%) 1028
Prozac Pulvules & Liquid, Oral Solution (Rare) 935
Redux Capsules (Frequent) 2911
▲ Rilutek Tablets (5.3% to 5.9%) 2198
▲ Risperdal Tablets (17% to 34%) .. 1348
Serzone Tablets (1%) 776
Sular Tablets (Less than or equal to 1%) 2961
Tegison Capsules (Less than 1%) .. 2314
▲ Ultram Tablets (50 mg) (1% to less than 5%) 1594
Videx Tablets, Powder for Oral Solution, & Pediatric Powder for Oral Solution (Less than 1%) 2980
Zoladex (1%) 2976
Zoladex 3-month 2978
Zoloft Tablets (1.3%) 2051
Zyrtec Tablets (Less than 2%) 2053

Hypertrichosis

Anafranil Capsules (Rare) 819
Analpram-HC Rectal Cream 1% and 2.5% 993
Anusol-HC Cream 2.5% (Infrequent to frequent) 1953
Azelex (Rare) 471
Clomid 1262
Cordran Lotion (Infrequent) 1854
Cordran Tape (Infrequent) 1855
Cormax Ointment (Infrequent) 1856
Cormax Scalp Application (Infrequent) 1857
Cortifoam 2540
Cortisporin Cream 1073
Cortisporin Ointment 1074
Cortisporin Otic Solution Sterile 1076
Cortisporin Otic Suspension Sterile 1077
Cutivate Ointment (Less than 1%) 1078
Decadron Phosphate Topical Cream 1686
Decaspray Topical Aerosol 1689
Dilantin Infatabs 1967
Dilantin Kapseals 1965
Dilantin-125 Suspension 1969
Diprolene AF Cream 0.05% (Infrequent) 2489
Diprolene Lotion 0.05% (Infrequent) 2491
Diprolene Ointment 0.05% (Infrequent) 2491
Elocon Cream 0.1% (Infrequent) 2492
Elocon Lotion 0.1% (Infrequent) 2493
Elocon Ointment 0.1% (Infrequent) 2494
Epifoam (Infrequent) 2543
Florone/Florone E 921
Halog (Infrequent) 2795
Hytone 922
Hytone Ointment 2 ½% 923
Kerlone Tablets (Less than 2%) 2588
Lidex (Infrequent) 2299

(▣ Described in PDR For Nonprescription Drugs) Incidence data in parenthesis; ▲ 3% or more (⊙ Described in PDR For Ophthalmology)

Side Effects Index

(continued from Hypertriglyceridemia and related)

Locoid Cream, Ointment and Topical Solution (Infrequent) ... 994
Lotrisone Cream (Infrequent) ... 2515
Mantadil Cream ... 1124
NeoDecadron Topical Cream ... 1757
Norplant System ... 2868
Pandel Cream, 0.1% ... 2475
Pediotic Suspension Sterile ... 1140
Pramosone Cream, Lotion & Ointment ... 995
ProctoCream-HC 2.5% (Infrequent to frequent) ... 2552
ProctoFoam-HC ... 2552
Proglycem ... 575
Psorcon Ointment 0.05% ... 923
Risperdal Tablets (Rare) ... 1348
Synalar (Infrequent) ... 2299
Temovate E Emollient (Infrequent) ... 1154
Temovate Gel (Infrequent) ... 1153
Temovate Scalp Application (Infrequent) ... 1153
Topicort Emollient Cream 0.25% (Infrequent) ... 1289
Topicort Gel 0.05% (Infrequent) ... 1290
Topicort LP Emollient Cream 0.05% (Infrequent) ... 1289
Topicort Ointment 0.25% (Infrequent) ... 1291
Tridesilon Cream 0.05% (Infrequent) ... 609
Tridesilon Ointment 0.05% (Infrequent) ... 610
Ultravate Cream 0.05% (Infrequent) ... 2797
Ultravate Ointment 0.05% (Infrequent) ... 2798
Westcort Cream 0.2% (Infrequent) ... 2799
Zoloft Tablets (Rare) ... 2051
Zyrtec Tablets (Less than 2%) ... 2053

Hypertriglyceridemia

▲ Accutane Capsules (Approximately 25%) ... 2252
Atretol Tablets (Occasional reports) ... 569
Blocadren Tablets ... 1654
Brevicon ... 2563
▲ Cipro I.V. (Among most frequent) ... 587
▲ Cipro I.V. Pharmacy Bulk Package (Among most frequent) ... 590
Cipro Tablets ... 584
Cytovene-IV (One report) ... 2270
Demulen ... 2580
Diflucan Tablets, Injection, and Oral Suspension ... 2003
Ergamisol Tablets ... 1340
Estratest ... 2718
Floxin I.V. ... 1580
Floxin Tablets (200 mg, 300 mg, 400 mg) ... 1577
Hivid Tablets (Less than 1%) ... 2287
Hyzaar Tablets ... 1720
Intron A for Injection (Less than 5%) ... 2506
Levlen/Tri-Levlen (A small portion of women) ... 646
Lo/Ovral Tablets ... 2852
Lo/Ovral-28 Tablets ... 2857
Lotensin HCT Tablets ... 855
Maxaquin Tablets ... 2593
Modicon ... 1928
Nizoral Tablets ... 1345
Nordette-21 Tablets ... 2863
Nordette-28 Tablets ... 2866
Norinyl ... 2563
Noroxin Tablets ... 1758
Noroxin Tablets ... 2222
Norpace (1 to 3%) ... 2596
Nor-Q D Tablets ... 2598
Ortho-Cyclen/Ortho-Tri-Cyclen ... 1914
Ortho-Novum ... 1928
Ortho-Cyclen/Ortho Tri-Cyclen ... 1914
Ovcon ... 765
Ovral Tablets ... 2877
Ovral-28 Tablets ... 2878
Ovrette Tablets ... 2878
Penetrex Tablets ... 2196
Premarin Tablets ... 2896
Premarin Vaginal Cream ... 2898
Prinzide Tablets ... 1780
Risperdal Tablets (Rare) ... 1348
Roferon-A Injection (Rare) ... 2308
Sporanox Capsules (Rare) ... 1352
▲ Synarel Nasal Solution for Endometriosis (12%) ... 2605
▲ Tegison Capsules (46%) ... 2314
Tegretol/Tegretol-XR (Occasional) ... 870
Ticlid Tablets ... 2317
Timolide Tablets ... 1791
Levlen/Tri-Levlen (A small portion of women) ... 646
Tri-Norinyl ... 2607
Triphasil-21 Tablets ... 2919
Triphasil-28 Tablets ... 2924
Vaseretic Tablets ... 1810
▲ Vesanoid Capsules (Up to 60%) ... 2327
▲ Zebeta Tablets (Most frequent laboratory change) ... 1457
Zestoretic Tablets ... 2968
Zoladex ... 2976
Zoladex 3-month ... 2978
Zoloft Tablets ... 2051

Hypertrophic papillae of the tongue

Primaxin I.M. ... 1770
Primaxin I.V. (Less than 0.2%) ... 1772
Serentil ... 689

Hypertrophy, genital

Supprelin Injection (2% to 3%) ... 2230

Hypertrophy, gum

Cytovene-IV (One report) ... 2270
Peganone Tablets ... 455
Zarontin Capsules ... 1986
Zarontin Syrup ... 1986

Hyperuricemia

▲ Accutane Capsules (1 in 10 patients) ... 2252
Adriamycin PFS ... 2056
Adriamycin RDF ... 2056
Aldoclor Tablets ... 1638
Aldoril Tablets ... 1644
Alka-Seltzer Cherry Effervescent Antacid and Pain Reliever (Less than 1%) ... 609
Alka-Seltzer Lemon Lime Effervescent Antacid and Pain Reliever (Less than 1%) ... 609
Alka-Seltzer Original Effervescent Antacid and Pain Reliever (Less than 1%) ... 609
Altace Capsules ... 1238
Anafranil Capsules (Infrequent) ... 819
Apresazide Capsules ... 824
Regular Strength Ascriptin Tablets ... 650
Axid Pulvules ... 1468
Genuine Bayer Aspirin Tablets & Caplets (Less than 1.0% at doses of 1000 mg/day) ... 618
Benemid Tablets ... 1651
Blocadren Tablets ... 1654
Bufferin Analgesic Tablets ... 636
▲ Bumex (18.4%) ... 2260
Capozide Tablets ... 744
Cardizem CD Capsules (Less than 1%) ... 1251
Cardizem SR Capsules (Less than 1%) ... 1255
Cardizem Injectable (Less than 1%) ... 1253
Cardizem Tablets (Less than 1%) ... 1257
▲ CellCept Capsules (More than or equal to 3%) ... 2265
Cerubidine for Injection ... 634
▲ Cipro I.V. (Among most frequent) ... 587
▲ Cipro I.V. Pharmacy Bulk Package (Among most frequent) ... 590
Cipro Tablets (Less than 0.1%) ... 584
Clozaril Tablets ... 2377
Combipres Tablets ... 682
Cotazym Capsules ... 1866
Creon ... 2714
Cytosar-U Sterile Powder ... 2077
Daranide Tablets ... 1676
Demadex Tablets and Injection ... 691
Diucardin Tablets ... 2824
Diupres Tablets ... 1691
Diuril Oral Suspension ... 1694
Diuril Sodium Intravenous ... 1693
Diuril Tablets ... 1694
Doxil (1% to 5%) ... 2613
Doxorubicin Astra ... 531
Dyazide Capsules ... 2653
Dynabac (0.1% to 1%) ... 668
Ecotrin ... 2625
Edecrin ... 1698
Effexor (Infrequent) ... 2825
Enduron Tablets ... 424
Esidrix Tablets ... 839
Esimil Tablets ... 840
Fludara for Injection ... 658
Halfprin Tablets (Less than 1%) ... 1413
Hivid Tablets (Less than 1%) ... 2287
Hydrea Capsules (Occasional) ... 705
HydroDIURIL Tablets ... 1716
Hydropres Tablets ... 1718
Hyzaar Tablets ... 1720
Imdur (Less than or equal to 5%) ... 1362
Inderide Tablets ... 2838
Inderide LA Long Acting Capsules ... 2840
Kerlone Tablets (Less than 2%) ... 2588
Larodopa Tablets ... 2296
Lasix Injection, Oral Solution and Tablets ... 1267
Lopressor HCT Tablets ... 850
Lotensin Tablets ... 852
Lotensin HCT Tablets ... 855
Lotrel Capsules (Rare) ... 858
Lupron Depot 7.5 mg (Less than 5%) ... 2741
Lupron Injection ... 2736
Minizide Capsules ... 2016
Moduretic Tablets ... 1748
Myambutol Tablets ... 1432
Mykrox Tablets ... 1617
Myleran Tablets ... 1209
Naprelan Tablets (Less than 1%) ... 2861
Neoral (Occasional) ... 2405
▲ Neupogen for Injection (27% to 58%) ... 495
Novantrone for Injection ... 1327
▲ Oncaspar (Greater than 1% but less than 5%) ... 2194
Oretic Tablets ... 450
Pancrease MT Capsules (With extremely high dose) ... 1589
Parlodel ... 2411
Permax Tablets (Rare) ... 571
Platinol for Injection ... 717
Platinol-AQ Injection ... 719
Prinzide Tablets ... 1780
Proglycem (Common) ... 575
▲ Prograf (Greater than 3%) ... 1028
Proleukin for Injection (9%) ... 812
Purinethol Tablets ... 1214
Pyrazinamide Tablets ... 1442
Redux Capsules (Rare) ... 2911
Relafen Tablets (Less than 1%) ... 2688
Rifadin ... 1276
Rifamate Capsules ... 1278
Rifater ... 1280
Rimactane Capsules ... 865
Risperdal Tablets (Rare) ... 1348
▲ Roferon-A Injection (10%) ... 2308
Rubex for Injection ... 721
Sandimmune (Occasional) ... 2416
Ser-Ap-Es Tablets ... 867
Slo-Niacin Tablets ... 2767
Tenoretic Tablets ... 2963
Thalitone ... 1293
Thioguanine Tablets, Tabloid Brand (Frequent) ... 1225
Tiazac Capsules (Less than 1%) ... 1019
Timolide Tablets ... 1791
Ultrase Capsules ... 2476
Ultrase MT Capsules ... 2477
Univasc Tablets ... 2553
Vaseretic Tablets ... 1810
Videx Tablets, Powder for Oral Solution, & Pediatric Powder for Oral Solution (1% to 3%) ... 2980
Viokase ... 2251
Zaroxolyn Tablets ... 1625
Zebeta Tablets ... 1457
Zestoretic Tablets ... 2968
Ziac ... 1459
Zymase Capsules (With extremely high doses) ... 1889

Hyperuricosuria

Creon ... 2714
Myleran Tablets ... 1209
Pancrease Capsules ... 1589
Pancrease MT Capsules (With extremely high dose) ... 1589
Ultrase Capsules ... 2476
Ultrase MT Capsules ... 2477

Hyperuricuria

Cotazym Capsules ... 1866
Pancrease Capsules ... 1589
Viokase ... 2251
Zymase Capsules (With extremely high doses) ... 1889

Hyperventilation

Adenocard Injection (Less than 1%) ... 1021
Anafranil Capsules (Infrequent) ... 819
Avonex ... 662
Betaseron for SC Injection ... 653
Bumex (0.1%) ... 2260
BuSpar Tablets (Infrequent) ... 738
Cataflam Tablets (Less than 1%) ... 833
Cerebyx Injection (Infrequent) ... 1956
Clozaril Tablets (Less than 1%) ... 2377
Cognex Capsules (Infrequent) ... 1961

Hypoactivity

Diprivan Injectable Emulsion (Less than 1%) ... 2939
Dizac (diazepam injectable emulsion) CIV (Less frequent) ... 1862
Doxil (Less than 1%) ... 2613
Dynabac (0.1% to 1%) ... 668
Effexor (Infrequent) ... 2825
Ethmozine Tablets (Less than 2%) ... 2217
Glucophage Tablets ... 754
Lamictal Tablets (Infrequent) ... 1105
Lioresal Intrathecal (1% or more) ... 1634
LUVOX Tablets (Infrequent) ... 2723
Mono-Gesic Tablets ... 810
Neurontin Capsules (Rare) ... 1978
Orthoclone OKT3 Sterile Solution ... 1892
Paxil Tablets (Infrequent) ... 2681
Permax Tablets (Infrequent) ... 571
Primaxin I.M. ... 1770
Primaxin I.V. (Less than 0.2%) ... 1772
ProSom Tablets (Rare) ... 457
Protopam Chloride for Injection ... 2909
Prozac Pulvules & Liquid, Oral Solution (Infrequent) ... 935
Redux Capsules (Rare) ... 2911
Rilutek Tablets (Infrequent) ... 2198
Risperdal Tablets (Infrequent) ... 1348
▲ Romazicon (3% to 9%) ... 2311
Serzone Tablets (Rare) ... 776
Sulfamylon Cream ... 940
Supprelin Injection (1% to 3%) ... 2230
Valium Injectable ... 2336
Versed Injection (Less than 1%) ... 2324
Cataflam/Voltaren/Voltaren-XR (Less than 1%) ... 833
▲ Xanax Tablets (9.7%) ... 2115
Yutopar Intravenous Injection (Infrequent) ... 566
Zoloft Tablets (Rare) ... 2051
Zyrtec Tablets (Less than 2%) ... 2053

Hypervitaminosis A syndrome

Aquasol A Vitamin A Capsules, USP ... 525
Aquasol A Parenteral ... 526

Hypervolemia

▲ CellCept Capsules (More than or equal to 3%) ... 2265
Foscavir Injection (Less than 1%) ... 541
NephrAmine Injection ... 2169

Hypesthesia

Cardene I.V. (0.7%) ... 2815
Caverject Injection (Less than 1%) ... 2064
Cerebyx Injection (2.2% frequent) ... 1956
Cognex Capsules (Infrequent) ... 1961
Cozaar Tablets (Less than 1%) ... 1668
Crixivan Capsules (Less than 2%) ... 1670
Cytovene (1% or less) ... 2270
Effexor ... 2825
▲ Ethmozine Tablets (2% to 5%) ... 2217
▲ Flolan for Injection (1% to 12%) ... 1085
Flumadine Tablets & Syrup ... 1013
Glucotrol XL Extended Release Tablets (Less than 3%) ... 2012
Hyzaar Tablets ... 1720
Kadian Capsules (Less than 3%) ... 2948
Lamictal Tablets (Infrequent) ... 1105
▲ Lopid Tablets (More common) ... 1974
Lotensin HCT Tablets (0.3% or more) ... 855
Lupron Depot 3.75 mg ... 2739
Lupron Depot - 3 Month 22.5 mg (Less than 5%) ... 2743
Megace Oral Suspension (1% to 3%) ... 708
▲ Navelbine Injection (Among most frequent) ... 1212
Neurontin Capsules (Infrequent) ... 1978
Orlaam Oral Solution (1% to 3%) ... 2361
OxyContin Tablets (Less than 1%) ... 2163
Paxil Tablets (Infrequent) ... 2681
Prozac Pulvules & Liquid, Oral Solution (Infrequent) ... 935
Recombivax HB ... 1787
Remeron Tablets (Frequent) ... 1878
ReoPro Vials (0.3%) ... 1526
Rilutek Tablets (Infrequent) ... 2198
Salagen Tablets (Less than 1%) ... 1546
Serzone Tablets ... 776
Sular Tablets (Less than or equal to 1%) ... 2961

Hypnotic effects

Placidyl Capsules (Occasional) ... 456
Trilafon ... 2532

Hypoactivity

AeroBid Inhaler System (1% to 3%) ... 1004

(⊞ Described in PDR For Nonprescription Drugs)   Incidence data in parenthesis; ▲ 3% or more   (⊚ Described in PDR For Ophthalmology)

Hypoactivity

- Aerobid-M Inhaler System (1% to 3%) ... 1004
- Dizac (diazepam injectable emulsion) CIV (Less frequent) ... 1862
- Valium Injectable ... 2336

Hypoadrenalism

- Sandostatin Injection (Less than 1%) ... 2421

Hypoadrenalism, neonatal

- Azmacort Oral Inhaler ... 2175
- Beconase ... 1065
- Celestone Soluspan Suspension ... 2484
- Cortone Acetate Tablets ... 1664
- Dalalone D.P. Injectable ... 1009
- Decadron Elixir ... 1676
- Decadron Phosphate Injection ... 1680
- Decadron Phosphate with Xylocaine Injection, Sterile ... 1683
- Decadron Tablets ... 1678
- Decadron-LA Sterile Suspension ... 1687
- Dexacort Phosphate in Respihaler ... 1606
- Dexacort Phosphate in Turbinaire ... 1607
- Florinef Acetate Tablets ... 506
- Hydeltrasol Injection, Sterile ... 1708
- Hydeltra-T.B.A. Sterile Suspension ... 1710
- Hydrocortone Acetate Sterile Suspension ... 1712
- Hydrocortone Phosphate Injection, Sterile ... 1713
- Hydrocortone Tablets ... 1715
- Nasacort Nasal Inhaler ... 2189
- Prelone Syrup ... 1834
- Rhinocort Nasal Inhaler ... 552
- Vancenase AQ Nasal Spray 0.042% ... 2535
- Vancenase PocketHaler Nasal Inhaler ... 2534
- Vanceril Inhaler ... 2538

Hypoalbuminemia

- Cipro I.V. Pharmacy Bulk Package (Less than 1%) ... 590
- Dapsone Tablets USP ... 1331
- Dynabac (0.1% to 1%) ... 668
- ▲ Leukine (27%) ... 1317
- Maxaquin Tablets (Less than or equal to 0.1%) ... 2593
- Oncaspar ... 2194
- ▲ Proleukin for Injection (8%) ... 812
- Vantin for Oral Suspension and Vantin Tablets ... 2112
- Zanosar Sterile Powder (A number of patients) ... 2119
- Zosyn ... 1463

Hypoalbuminuria

- Elspar ... 1700
- Unasyn ... 2035

Hypocalcemia

- Abelcet Injection ... 1540
- ▲ Aredia for Injection (Up to 12%) ... 827
- ▲ CellCept Capsules (More than or equal to 3%) ... 2265
- Cortifoam ... 2540
- Cosmegen Injection ... 1666
- Doxil (1% to 5%) ... 2613
- Ethyol (amifostine) for Injection (Rare; less than 1%) ... 485
- Felbatol ... 2774
- Fleet Enema ... 1001
- Fludara for Injection ... 658
- ▲ Fosamax Tablets (Approximately 18%) ... 1703
- ▲ Foscavir Injection (5% or greater up to 15%) ... 541
- Fungizone Intravenous ... 507
- Ganite ... 2711
- Garamycin Injectable ... 2502
- Hivid Tablets (Less than 1%) ... 2287
- Kayexalate ... 2444
- Lasix Injection, Oral Solution and Tablets ... 1267
- Leukine (2%) ... 1317
- Maxipime for Injection (0.1% to 1%) ... 758
- Mithracin ... 599
- Nebcin Vials, Hyporets & ADD-Vantage ... 1518
- Neutrexin for Injection (1.8%) ... 2761
- ▲ Paraplatin for Injection (16% to 31%) ... 713
- Paxil Tablets (Rare) ... 2681
- Platinol for Injection ... 717
- Platinol-AQ Injection ... 719
- Precose ... 604
- ▲ Prograf (Greater than 3%) ... 1028
- ▲ Proleukin for Injection (15%) ... 812
- ▲ Roferon-A Injection (28%) ... 2308

- Sodium Polystyrene Sulfonate Suspension ... 2367
- Synarel Nasal Solution for Endometriosis ... 2605
- Tegretol-XR Tablets ... 870
- Vistide Injection ... 1057
- Zosyn ... 1463

Hypocalcemia, neonatal

- Yutopar Intravenous Injection (Infrequent) ... 566

Hypocarbia

- Exosurf Neonatal for Intratracheal Suspension ... 1081
- Survanta Beractant Intratracheal Suspension (Less than 1%) ... 2346

Hypochloremia

- ▲ Bumex (14.9%) ... 2260
- Demadex Tablets and Injection ... 691
- Dyazide Capsules ... 2653
- Dynabac (0.1% to 1%) ... 668
- Enduron Tablets ... 424
- Esidrix Tablets ... 839
- Foscavir Injection (Less than 1%) ... 541
- Mykrox Tablets ... 1617
- Oretic Tablets ... 450
- Zaroxolyn Tablets ... 1625

Hypochloremic alkalosis

- Apresazide Capsules ... 824
- Capozide Tablets ... 744
- Diuril Sodium Intravenous ... 1693
- Esidrix Tablets ... 839
- Lasix Injection, Oral Solution and Tablets ... 1267
- Lotensin HCT Tablets ... 855
- Mykrox Tablets ... 1617
- Prinzide Tablets ... 1780
- Tenoretic Tablets ... 2963
- Thalitone (Common) ... 1293
- Vaseretic Tablets ... 1810
- Zaroxolyn Tablets ... 1625
- Zestoretic Tablets ... 2968

Hypocholesterolemia

- Bumex (0.4%) ... 2260
- Prevacid Delayed-Release Capsules (Less than 1%) ... 2746
- Proleukin for Injection (1%) ... 812

Hypochondriasis

- LUVOX Tablets (Infrequent) ... 2723

Hypocoagulability

- Orudis Capsules (Less than 1%) ... 2874
- Oruvail Capsules (Less than 1%) ... 2874

Hypoesthesia

- Ambien Tablets (Infrequent) ... 2559
- Anafranil Capsules (Rare) ... 819
- Cardura Tablets (0.5% to 1%) ... 1993
- Claritin Tablets (2% or fewer patients) ... 2485
- Claritin-D Tablets (Less frequent) ... 2487
- Engerix-B Unit-Dose Vials ... 2656
- ▲ Foscavir Injection (5% or greater) ... 541
- Gastrocrom Oral Concentrate (Less common) ... 1611
- Imdur (Less than or equal to 5%) ... 1362
- ▲ Intron A for Injection (Up to 10%) ... 2506
- Ismo Tablets (Fewer than 1%) ... 2844
- Normodyne Injection (1%) ... 2519
- Norvasc Tablets (More than 0.1% to 1%) ... 2020
- Procardia XL Extended Release Tablets (1% or less) ... 2026
- Redux Capsules ... 2911
- Risperdal Tablets (Rare) ... 1348
- Romazicon (1% to 3%) ... 2311
- Sectral Capsules (Up to 2%) ... 2914
- Tambocor Tablets (1% to less than 3%) ... 1555
- Tornalate Solution for Inhalation, 0.2% (Less than 1%) ... 976
- Trandate Injection (1 of 100 patients) ... 1158
- Zebeta Tablets (1.1% to 1.5%) ... 1457
- Zoloft Tablets (1.7%) ... 2051
- Zyrtec Tablets (Less than 2%) ... 2053

Hypoestrogeneism

- ▲ Lupron Depot 3.75 mg (Among most frequent) ... 2739
- Neurontin Capsules (Rare) ... 1978
- ▲ Synarel Nasal Solution for Endometriosis (Most frequent) ... 2605

Hypofibrinogenemia

- Depakene ... 416

- Depakote Tablets ... 418
- Elspar ... 1700
- Lamictal Tablets ... 1105
- Oncaspar ... 2194
- Panhematin ... 452
- Pediazole Suspension ... 2340

Hypogammaglobulinemia

- Methotrexate Sodium Tablets, Injection, for Injection and LPF Injection (Rare) ... 1322

Hypogeusia

- Cuprimine Capsules (Some patients) ... 1673
- Depen Titratable Tablets (Some patients) ... 2770

Hypoglycemia

- Abelcet Injection ... 1540
- Adapin Capsules ... 1542
- Amaryl Tablets (0.9% to 1.7%) ... 1241
- Anaprox/Naprosyn (Less than 1%) ... 2277
- Ancobon Capsules ... 2254
- Asendin Tablets (Very rare) ... 1419
- Avonex ... 662
- Azulfidine (Rare) ... 2059
- Bactrim DS Tablets (Rare) ... 2257
- Bactrim I.V. Infusion (Rare) ... 2255
- Bactrim (Rare) ... 2257
- Betaseron for SC Injection ... 653
- Blocadren Tablets ... 1654
- Cartrol Tablets ... 413
- Cataflam Tablets (Less than 1%) ... 833
- ▲ CellCept Capsules (More than or equal to 3%) ... 2265
- Cipro I.V. (Rare) ... 587
- Cipro I.V. Pharmacy Bulk Package (Rare) ... 590
- Cipro Tablets (Less than 0.1%) ... 584
- Compazine ... 2644
- Cuprimine Capsules ... 1673
- Cytovene (1% or less) ... 2270
- Depen Titratable Tablets (Extremely rare) ... 2770
- DiaBeta Tablets ... 1265
- Diabinese Tablets ... 2002
- Doxil (Less than 1%) ... 2613
- EC-Naprosyn Delayed-Release Tablets (Less than 1%) ... 2277
- Edecrin (In 2 uremic patients) ... 1698
- Effexor (Infrequent) ... 2825
- Elavil ... 2945
- Etrafon ... 2495
- Fansidar Tablets (Rare) ... 2281
- Felbatol ... 2774
- Feldene Capsules (Less than 1%) ... 2008
- Flexeril Tablets (Rare) ... 1701
- Floxin I.V. (More than or equal to 1%) ... 1580
- Floxin Tablets (200 mg, 300 mg, 400 mg) (More than or equal to 1%) ... 1577
- Furoxone ... 2221
- Gantanol Tablets (Rare) ... 2285
- Gantrisin (Rare) ... 2286
- Glucophage Tablets ... 754
- Glucotrol Tablets ... 2011
- Glucotrol XL Extended Release Tablets (Rare; less than 1%; less than 3%) ... 2012
- Glynase PresTab Tablets ... 2091
- Haldol Decanoate ... 1587
- Haldol Injection, Tablets and Concentrate ... 1585
- Hivid Tablets (Less than 1%) ... 2287
- ▲ Humalog Injection (Most common) ... 1488
- Humulin 50/50, 100 Units ... 1491
- Humulin 70/30, 100 Units ... 1492
- Humulin L, 100 Units ... 1494
- IBU Tablets (Less than 1%) ... 1389
- Regular, 100 Units ... 1503
- Pork Regular, 100 Units ... 1507
- Imitrex Tablets (Rare) ... 1099
- Indocin I.V. (1% to 3%) ... 1727
- ▲ Invirase Capsules (5%) ... 2291
- Limbitrol ... 2333
- Ludiomil Tablets (Rare) ... 861
- Lupron Injection (Less than 5%) ... 2736
- LUVOX Tablets (Rare) ... 2723
- Maxaquin Tablets (Less than or equal to 0.1%) ... 2593
- Mepron Suspension (1%) ... 1206
- Micronase Tablets ... 2099
- Mithracin ... 599
- Moban Tablets and Concentrate ... 1036
- Motrin Ibuprofen Suspension, Oral Drops, Chewable Tablets, Caplets (Less than 1%) ... 1563
- ▲ Naprelan Tablets (3% to 9%) ... 2861

- Anaprox/Naprosyn (Less than 1%) ... 2277
- Navane Capsules and Concentrate ... 2018
- Navane Intramuscular ... 2019
- Normodyne Injection ... 2519
- Normodyne Tablets ... 2522
- Noroxin Tablets ... 1758
- Noroxin Tablets ... 2222
- Norpace ... 2596
- Norpramin Tablets ... 1273
- ▲ Oncaspar (Greater than 1% but less than 5%) ... 2194
- Pamelor ... 2409
- PASER Granules ... 1333
- Paxil Tablets (Rare) ... 2681
- Pediazole Suspension (Rare) ... 2340
- Permax Tablets (Infrequent) ... 571
- Precose ... 604
- Prevacid Delayed-Release Capsules (Less than 1%) ... 2746
- Prilosec Delayed-Release Capsules (Less than 1%) ... 516
- Proleukin for Injection (2%) ... 812
- Prozac Pulvules & Liquid, Oral Solution (Infrequent) ... 935
- Redux Capsules (Infrequent) ... 2911
- Risperdal Tablets (Rare) ... 1348
- Sandostatin Injection (Approximately 2% to 3%) ... 2421
- Septra (Rare) ... 1146
- Septra I.V. Infusion (Rare) ... 1142
- Septra I.V. Infusion ADD-Vantage Vials (Rare) ... 1144
- Septra (Rare) ... 1146
- Serzone Tablets (Rare) ... 776
- Sinequan ... 2028
- Stelazine ... 2692
- Surmontil Capsules ... 2917
- Tenoretic Tablets ... 2963
- Tenormin Tablets and I.V. Injection ... 2965
- Thorazine ... 2701
- Timolide Tablets ... 1791
- Timoptic-XE ... 1798
- Tofranil Ampuls ... 873
- Tofranil Tablets ... 875
- Tofranil-PM Capsules ... 876
- Triavil Tablets ... 1800
- Trilafon ... 2532
- Vantin for Oral Suspension and Vantin Tablets ... 2112
- Videx Tablets, Powder for Oral Solution, & Pediatric Powder for Oral Solution (Up to 1%) ... 2980
- Vivactil Tablets ... 1820
- Cataflam/Voltaren/Voltaren-XR (Less than 1%) ... 833
- Zanosar Sterile Powder ... 2119
- Zoloft Tablets (Rare) ... 2051
- Zosyn (1.0% or less) ... 1463

Hypoglycemia, masked symptoms of

- Betagan ... ⊙ 230
- Betimol 0.25%, 0.5% ... ⊙ 259
- Timoptic in Ocudose (Less frequent) ... 1796
- Timoptic-XE ... 1798

Hypoglycemia, neonatal

- Brethine Ampuls ... 832
- Brethine Tablets ... 831
- Bricanyl Subcutaneous Injection ... 1247
- DiaBeta Tablets ... 1265
- Normodyne Injection ... 2519
- Normodyne Tablets (Rare) ... 2522
- Trandate ... 1158
- Yutopar Intravenous Injection (Infrequent) ... 566

Hypogonadism

- Permax Tablets (Rare) ... 571
- Virazole ... 1310

Hypohidrosis

- Bellergal-S Tablets (Rare) ... 2375
- Bentyl ... 1246
- Ditropan ... 1267
- Donnatal ... 2234
- Donnatal Extentabs ... 2234
- Donnatal Tablets ... 2234
- Kutrase Capsules ... 2546
- Levsin/Levsinex/Levbid ... 2549
- Pro-Banthine Tablets ... 2226
- Risperdal Tablets (Infrequent) ... 1348
- Robinul Forte Tablets ... 2247
- Robinul Injectable ... 2247
- Robinul Tablets ... 2247

Hypokalemia

- ▲ Abelcet Injection (4% to 6%) ... 1540
- Aldactazide Tablets ... 2556

1369 Side Effects Index Hypophosphatemia

Aldoclor Tablets 1638
Aldoril Tablets 1644
Anafranil Capsules (Infrequent) 819
Ancobon Capsules 2254
Apresazide Capsules 824
▲ Aredia for Injection (4% to 18%) 827
Avonex 662
▲ Bumex (14.7%) 2260
Capozide Tablets 744
Cardene I.V. (0.7%) 2815
Cardura Tablets (Less than 0.5% of 3960 patients) 1993
Celestone Soluspan Suspension 2484
▲ CellCept Capsules (10.0% to 10.1%) 2265
Cerebyx Injection (Frequent) 1956
Cipro I.V. (Infrequent) 587
Combipres Tablets 682
CORTENEMA 2713
Cortifoam 2540
Cortone Acetate Sterile Suspension 1663
Cortone Acetate Tablets 1664
Cytovene (1% or less) 2270
Dalalone D.P. Injectable 1009
Daranide Tablets 1676
Decadron Elixir 1676
Decadron Phosphate Injection 1680
Decadron Phosphate with Xylocaine Injection, Sterile 1683
Decadron Tablets 1678
Decadron-LA Sterile Suspension 1687
Demadex Tablets and Injection 691
Dexacort Phosphate in Respihaler 1606
Dexacort Phosphate in Turbinaire 1607
Diflucan Tablets, Injection, and Oral Suspension 2003
Digibind 1079
Diuril Sodium Intravenous 1693
Dobutrex Solution Vials (Rare) 1480
Doxil (Less than 1%) 2613
DUPHALAC Solution 2714
Dyazide Capsules (Uncommon) 2653
Dyrenium Capsules (Rare) 2655
Effexor (Infrequent) 2825
Enduron Tablets 424
Esidrix Tablets 839
Felbatol (Infrequent) 2774
▲ Flolan for Injection (6%) 1085
Florinef Acetate Tablets 506
▲ Foscavir Injection (5% or greater up to 16%) 541
▲ Fungizone Intravenous (Among most common) 507
Garamycin Injectable 2502
Hivid Tablets (Less than 1%) 2287
Hydeltrasol Injection, Sterile 1708
Hydeltra-T.B.A. Sterile Suspension 1710
Hydrocortone Acetate Sterile Suspension 1712
Hydrocortone Phosphate Injection, Sterile 1713
Hydrocortone Tablets 1715
HydroDIURIL Tablets 1716
▲ Hyzaar Tablets (6.7%) 1720
Imdur (Less than or equal to 5%) 1362
Invirase Capsules (Less than 1%) 2291
Kayexalate 2444
Kerlone Tablets (Less than 2%) 2588
Lamprene Capsules (Less than 1%) 846
Lanoxicaps 1110
Lasix Injection, Oral Solution and Tablets 1267
Lopressor HCT Tablets (Less than 10 in 100 patients) 850
Lotensin HCT Tablets 855
Lotrel Capsules 858
▲ Lupron Depot - 3 Month 22.5 mg (More than or equal to 5%) 2743
LUVOX Tablets (Rare) 2723
Maxaquin Tablets 2593
Mezlin (Rare) 594
Mezlin Pharmacy Bulk Package 597
Mithracin 599
Mykrox Tablets 1617
Naprelan Tablets (Less than 1%) 2861
Nebcin Vials, Hyporets & ADD-Vantage 1518
Norpace (1 to 3%) 2596
Oretic Tablets 450
▲ Paraplatin for Injection (16% to 28%) 713
Paxil Tablets (Rare) 2681
Pediapred Oral Solution 1618
Permax Tablets (Infrequent) 571
Pipracil (Rare with high doses) 1435
Platinol for Injection 717
Platinol-AQ Injection 719
Prelone Syrup 1834
Primacor Injection (0.6%) 2461
Prinzide Tablets 1780
▲ Prograf (11% to 29%) 1028
▲ Proleukin for Injection (9%) 812
Prozac Pulvules & Liquid, Oral Solution (Rare) 935
Redux Capsules (Infrequent) 2911
Relafen Tablets (Less than 1%) 2688
Rilutek Tablets (Infrequent) 2198
Risperdal Tablets (Rare) 1348
Septra 1146
Sinemet CR Tablets 961
Sodium Polystyrene Sulfonate Suspension 2367
Sporanox Capsules (0.2% to 2.0%) 1352
Sular Tablets (Less than or equal to 1%) 2961
▲ Tegison Capsules (25-50%) 2314
Tenoretic Tablets 2963
Thalitone (Common) 1293
Timentin for Injection 2706
Timolide Tablets 1791
Tornalate Solution for Inhalation, 0.2% (Infrequent) 976
Vaseretic Tablets 1810
Ventolin Inhalation Aerosol and Refill 1170
Ventolin Inhalation Solution 1171
Ventolin Nebules Inhalation Solution 1172
Ventolin Rotacaps for Inhalation 1173
Ventolin Tablets 1176
Vistide Injection 1057
Yutopar Intravenous Injection 566
Zaroxolyn Tablets 1625
Zestoretic Tablets 2968
Ziac 1459
Zofran Injection (Rare) 1227
Zofran Tablets (Rare) 1231
Zosyn 1463
Zovirax Sterile Powder (Less than 1%) 1191

Hypokalemic alkalosis

Celestone Soluspan Suspension 2484
CORTENEMA 2713
Cortone Acetate Sterile Suspension 1663
Cortone Acetate Tablets 1664
Dalalone D.P. Injectable 1009
Decadron Elixir 1676
Decadron Phosphate Injection 1680
Decadron Phosphate with Xylocaine Injection, Sterile 1683
Decadron Tablets 1678
Decadron-LA Sterile Suspension 1687
Dexacort Phosphate in Respihaler 1606
Dexacort Phosphate in Turbinaire 1607
Florinef Acetate Tablets 506
Hydeltrasol Injection, Sterile 1708
Hydeltra-T.B.A. Sterile Suspension 1710
Hydrocortone Acetate Sterile Suspension 1712
Hydrocortone Phosphate Injection, Sterile 1713
Hydrocortone Tablets 1715
Pediapred Oral Solution 1618
Prelone Syrup 1834

Hypokinesia

Ambien Tablets (Rare) 2559
Anafranil Capsules (Infrequent) 819
Cerebyx Injection (Infrequent) 1956
▲ Clozaril Tablets (4%) 2377
Depakote Tablets (1% to 5%) 418
Doral Tablets 2773
Doxil (Less than 1%) 2613
Effexor (Rare) 2825
Hivid Tablets (Less than 1%) 2287
Intron A for Injection (Less than 5%) 2506
Ismo Tablets (Fewer than 1%) 2844
Lamictal Tablets (Rare) 1105
Levo-Dromoran 2297
LUVOX Tablets (Frequent) 2723
Neurontin Capsules (Rare) 1978
Paxil Tablets (Rare) 2681
Permax Tablets (Infrequent) 571
▲ ProSom Tablets (8%) 457
Redux Capsules (Infrequent) 2911
Remeron Tablets (Frequent) 1878
Rilutek Tablets (Infrequent) 2198
▲ Risperdal Tablets (17% to 34%) 1348
Tenex Tablets (3% or less) 2249
Zoloft Tablets (Infrequent) 2051

Hypomagnesemia

Abelcet Injection 1540
Apresazide Capsules 824
▲ Aredia for Injection (3.4% to at least 15%) 827
Avonex 662
Bumex 2260
Capozide Tablets 744
Cytovene-IV (One report) 2270
Demadex Tablets and Injection (One case) 691
Diucardin Tablets 2824
Diuril Sodium Intravenous 1693
Doxil (Less than 1%) 2613
Esidrix Tablets 839
Esimil Tablets 840
Felbatol 2774
▲ Foscavir Injection (5% or greater up to 15%) 541
Fungizone Intravenous 507
Garamycin Injectable 2502
Hivid Tablets (Less than 1%) 2287
HydroDIURIL Tablets 1716
Hyzaar Tablets 1720
Lanoxicaps 1110
Lasix Injection, Oral Solution and Tablets 1267
▲ Leukine (15%) 1317
Lopressor HCT Tablets 850
Lotensin HCT Tablets 855
Mykrox Tablets 1617
Nebcin Vials, Hyporets & ADD-Vantage 1518
Neoral 2405
▲ Paraplatin for Injection (29% to 63%) 713
Platinol for Injection 717
Platinol-AQ Injection 719
Prinzide Tablets 1780
▲ Prograf (15% to 48%) 1028
▲ Proleukin for Injection (16%) 812
Sandimmune (In some patients) 2416
Ser-Ap-Es Tablets 867
Vaseretic Tablets 1810
Zaroxolyn Tablets 1625
Zestoretic Tablets 2968

Hypomania

Anafranil Capsules (Several patients) 819
Asendin Tablets (Less than 1%) 1419
Desyrel and Desyrel Dividose 504
Effexor (0.5%) 2825
Elavil (Rare) 2945
Lamictal Tablets (Rare) 1105
Limbitrol 2333
Ludiomil Tablets (Rare) 861
▲ Nardil (Most common) 1977
Norpramin Tablets 1273
Pamelor 2409
Paxil Tablets (Approximately 1.0%) 2681
Remeron Tablets (Approximately 0.2%) 1878
Serzone Tablets (0.3% to 1.6%) 776
Surmontil Capsules 2917
Tofranil Ampuls 873
Tofranil Tablets 875
Tofranil-PM Capsules 876
Triavil Tablets (Rare) 1800
Vivactil Tablets 1820
Wellbutrin Tablets (Frequent) 1177
Xanax Tablets 2115
Zoloft Tablets (0.4%) 2051

Hypomenorrhea

Aquasol A Vitamin A Capsules, USP 525
Aquasol A Parenteral 526
Effexor (Rare) 2825
Pentasa (Less than 1%) 1275
Prozac Pulvules & Liquid, Oral Solution (Rare) 935
Redux Capsules 2911

Hyponatremia

Actimmune (Rare) 1043
Aldactone Tablets 2558
Altace Capsules 1238
Amaryl Tablets 1241
Apresazide Capsules 824
Atretol Tablets 569
▲ Bumex (9.2%) 2260
Capoten Tablets 740
Capozide Tablets 744
Clozaril Tablets 2377
Cytovene-IV (Two or more reports) 2270
DDAVP Injection 2178
DDAVP 2180
DDAVP Tablets 2182
Demadex Tablets and Injection 691
Depakene 416
Depakote Tablets 418
Desmopressin Acetate Injection 996
DiaBeta Tablets 1265
Diuril Sodium Intravenous 1693
Doxil (Less than 1%) 2613
Dyazide Capsules 2653
Effexor (Rare) 2825
Enduron Tablets 424
Esidrix Tablets 839
Felbatol (Infrequent) 2774
Foscavir Injection (Between 1% and 5%) 541
Garamycin Injectable 2502
Glucotrol Tablets 2011
Glucotrol XL Extended Release Tablets 2012
Glynase PresTab Tablets 2091
Haldol Decanoate 1587
Haldol Injection, Tablets and Concentrate 1585
Hivid Tablets (Less than 1%) 2287
▲ Indocin I.V. (3% to 9%) 1727
Kadian Capsules (Less than 3%) 2948
Lasix Injection, Oral Solution and Tablets 1267
Lotensin Tablets (Scattered incidents) 852
Lotensin HCT Tablets (Scattered accounts) 855
LUVOX Tablets 2723
Mavik Tablets (0.3% to 1.0%) 1407
▲ Mepron Suspension (7% to 10%) 1206
Micronase Tablets 2099
Moduretic Tablets 1748
Monopril Tablets 762
Mykrox Tablets 1617
Nebcin Vials, Hyporets & ADD-Vantage 1518
▲ Neutrexin for Injection (4.6%) 2761
Nimotop Capsules (Less than 1%) 603
Nipent for Injection (Less than 3%) 2733
Oncaspar (Less than 1%) 2194
Oncovin Solution Vials & Hyporets 1521
Orap Tablets 1037
Oretic Tablets 450
Orudis Capsules (Less than 1%) 2874
Oruvail Capsules (Less than 1%) 2874
OxyContin Tablets (Less than 1%) 2163
▲ Paraplatin for Injection (10% to 47%) 713
Paxil Tablets (Rare) 2681
Platinol for Injection 717
Platinol-AQ Injection 719
Primaxin I.M. 1770
Primaxin I.V. 1772
Prinivil Tablets 1776
Prinzide Tablets 1780
▲ Prograf (Greater than 3%) 1028
▲ Proleukin for Injection (4%) 812
Proloprim Tablets 1141
Prozac Pulvules & Liquid, Oral Solution (Rare) 935
Rilutek Tablets (Infrequent) 2198
Risperdal Tablets (Infrequent; 2 patients) 1348
Rythmol Tablets–150mg, 225mg, 300mg (Less than 1%) 1399
Septra 1146
Septra I.V. Infusion 1142
Septra I.V. Infusion ADD-Vantage Vials 1144
Septra 1146
Stimate, (desmopressin acetate) Nasal Spray, 1.5 mg/mL 806
Tegretol/Tegretol-XR 870
Tenoretic Tablets 2963
Thalitone (Common) 1293
Ticlid Tablets (Rare) 2317
Toradol 2319
Vaseretic Tablets 1810
Vasotec I.V. 1814
Vasotec Tablets 1816
Zaroxolyn Tablets 1625
Zestoretic Tablets 2968
Zestril Tablets 2972
Zoloft Tablets (Several cases) 2051
Zosyn 1463

Hyponatremia, dilutional

Apresazide Capsules 824
Capozide Tablets 744
Diuril Sodium Intravenous 1693
Esidrix Tablets 839
Hyzaar Tablets 1720
Oretic Tablets 450
Prinzide Tablets 1780
Tenoretic Tablets 2963
Vaseretic Tablets 1810
Zestoretic Tablets 2968

Hypophosphatemia

ALternaGEL Liquid 1358
Apresazide Capsules 824
▲ Aredia for Injection (Up to 18%) 827

(▣ Described in PDR For Nonprescription Drugs) Incidence data in parenthesis; ▲ 3% or more (◉ Described in PDR For Ophthalmology)

Hypophosphatemia

- Basaljel ... 2810
- Capozide Tablets (A few patients) ... 744
- Cardene I.V. (Rare) ... 2815
- ▲ CellCept Capsules (12.5% to 15.8%) ... 2265
- Cerebyx Injection (Frequent) ... 1956
- Doxil (Less than 1%) ... 2613
- Effexor (Rare) ... 2825
- Esidrix Tablets ... 839
- ▲ Felbatol (3.4%; infrequent) ... 2774
- ▲ Fosamax Tablets (Approximately 10%) ... 1703
- ▲ Foscavir Injection (5% or greater up to 8%) ... 541
- ▲ Ganite (Up to 79%) ... 2711
- Gelusil Antacid-Anti-gas Liquid ... 819
- Gelusil Antacid-Anti-gas Tablets ... 819
- Hivid Tablets (Less than 1%) ... 2287
- Maalox Antacid/Anti-Gas Tablets ... 889
- Maalox Heartburn Relief Suspension ... 658
- Maalox Antacid Liquid ... 888
- Extra Strength Maalox Antacid/Anti-Gas Liquid and Tablets ... 888
- Mithracin ... 599
- Mykrox Tablets ... 1617
- Mylanta ... 1359
- Platinol for Injection ... 717
- Platinol-AQ Injection ... 719
- ▲ Prograf (Greater than 3%) ... 1028
- ▲ Proleukin for Injection (11%) ... 812
- ▲ Roferon-A Injection (22%) ... 2308
- Rolaids Antacid Tablets ... 807
- Tenoretic Tablets ... 2963
- Zanosar Sterile Powder ... 2119
- Zaroxolyn Tablets ... 1625

Hypopigmentation

- Accutane Capsules (Less than 1%) ... 2252
- Aclovate (Infrequent) ... 1061
- Analpram-HC Rectal Cream 1% and 2.5% ... 993
- Anusol-HC Cream 2.5% (Infrequent to frequent) ... 1953
- Anusol-HC Suppositories ... 1954
- Catapres-TTS ... 680
- Celestone Soluspan Suspension ... 2484
- Cordran Lotion (Infrequent) ... 1854
- Cordran Tape (Infrequent) ... 1855
- Cormax Ointment (Infrequent) ... 1856
- Cormax Scalp Application (Infrequent) ... 1857
- Cortisporin Cream ... 1073
- Cortisporin Ointment ... 1074
- Cortisporin Otic Solution Sterile ... 1076
- Cortisporin Otic Suspension Sterile ... 1077
- Cortone Acetate Sterile Suspension ... 1663
- Cutivate Cream ... 1078
- Cutivate Ointment (Infrequent to more frequent) ... 1078
- Dalalone D.P. Injectable ... 1009
- Decadron Phosphate Injection ... 1680
- Decadron Phosphate Topical Cream ... 1686
- Decadron Phosphate with Xylocaine Injection, Sterile ... 1683
- Decadron-LA Sterile Suspension ... 1687
- Decaspray Topical Aerosol ... 1689
- Dermatop Emollient Cream 0.1% (Infrequent to frequent) ... 1264
- DesOwen Cream, Ointment and Lotion (Infrequent) ... 1032
- Diprolene AF Cream 0.05% (Infrequent) ... 2489
- Diprolene Gel 0.05% (Infrequent) ... 2490
- Diprolene Lotion 0.05% (Infrequent) ... 2491
- Diprolene Ointment 0.05% (Infrequent) ... 2491
- Elocon Cream 0.1% (Infrequent) ... 2492
- Elocon Lotion 0.1% (Infrequent) ... 2493
- Elocon Ointment 0.1% (Infrequent) ... 2494
- Epifoam (Infrequent) ... 2543
- Florone/Florone E ... 921
- Halog (Infrequent) ... 2795
- Hydeltrasol Injection, Sterile ... 1708
- Hydeltra-T.B.A. Sterile Suspension ... 1710
- Hydrocortone Acetate Sterile Suspension ... 1712
- Hydrocortone Phosphate Injection, Sterile ... 1713
- Hytone ... 922
- Hytone Ointment 2 ½% ... 923
- Lidex (Infrequent) ... 2299
- Locoid Cream, Ointment and Topical Solution (Infrequent) ... 994
- Lotrisone Cream (Infrequent) ... 2515
- Mantadil Cream ... 1124
- 8-MOP Capsules ... 1294
- NeoDecadron Topical Cream ... 1757
- Oxsoralen-Ultra Capsules ... 1302
- Pandel Cream, 0.1% ... 2475
- Pediotic Suspension Sterile ... 1140
- Pramosone Cream, Lotion & Ointment ... 995
- ProctoCream-HC 2.5% (Infrequent to frequent) ... 2552
- ProctoFoam-HC ... 2552
- Psorcon Cream 0.05% (Infrequent) ... 924
- Psorcon Ointment 0.05% (Infrequent) ... 923
- Retin-A (tretinoin) Cream/Gel/Liquid ... 1947
- Synalar (Infrequent) ... 2299
- Taxotere for Injection Concentrate ... 2204
- Temovate Cream ... 1152
- Temovate E Emollient (Infrequent) ... 1154
- Temovate Gel (Infrequent) ... 1153
- Temovate Ointment ... 1152
- Temovate Scalp Application (Infrequent) ... 1153
- Topicort Emollient Cream 0.25% (Infrequent) ... 1289
- Topicort Gel 0.05% (Infrequent) ... 1290
- Topicort LP Emollient Cream 0.05% (Infrequent) ... 1289
- Topicort Ointment 0.25% (Infrequent) ... 1291
- Tridesilon Cream 0.05% (Infrequent) ... 609
- Tridesilon Ointment 0.05% (Infrequent) ... 610
- Ultravate Cream 0.05% (Infrequent) ... 2797
- Ultravate Ointment 0.05% (Infrequent) ... 2798
- Westcort Cream 0.2% (Infrequent) ... 2799
- Westcort Ointment 0.2% (Infrequent) ... 2800

Hypoplasia, enamel

- Achromycin V Capsules ... 1417
- Declomycin Tablets ... 1421
- Doryx Capsules ... 1970
- DYNACIN Capsules ... 1627
- Helidac Therapy ... 2135
- Minocin Intravenous ... 1428
- Minocin Oral Suspension ... 1431
- Minocin Pellet-Filled Capsules ... 1429
- Monodox Capsules ... 1858
- Terramycin Intramuscular Solution ... 2034
- Vibramycin ... 2038
- Vibramycin Hyclate Intravenous ... 2040
- Vibramycin ... 2038

Hypoplasia, erythroid

- Capoten Tablets ... 740
- Capozide Tablets ... 744

Hypoplasia, myeloid
(see under Bone marrow hypoplasia)

Hypoplastic anemia

- Eminase (Less than 1%) ... 2215
- Mykrox Tablets ... 1617
- Myochrysine Injection ... 1754
- Procanbid Extended-Release Tablets (Approximately 0.5%) ... 1983
- Solganal Suspension (Rare) ... 2530
- Tonocard Tablets (Less than 1%) ... 519
- Trinalin Repetabs Tablets ... 1373
- Zaroxolyn Tablets ... 1625

Hypopnea

- Stadol (Less than 1%) ... 779

Hypoproteinemia

- ▲ CellCept Capsules (More than or equal to 3%) ... 2265
- Cipro I.V. ... 587
- Cipro I.V. Pharmacy Bulk Package (Less than 1%) ... 590
- Cortifoam ... 2540
- Doxil (Less than 1%) ... 2613
- Effexor (Rare) ... 2825
- Foscavir Injection (Less than 1%) ... 541
- Lupron Injection ... 2736
- Maxaquin Tablets (Less than or equal to 0.1%) ... 2593
- ▲ Oncaspar (Greater than 1% but less than 5%) ... 2194
- ▲ Prograf (Greater than 3%) ... 1028
- ▲ Proleukin for Injection (7%) ... 812
- Risperdal Tablets (Rare) ... 1348
- Unasyn ... 2035
- Vantin for Oral Suspension and Vantin Tablets ... 2112
- Zosyn ... 1463

Hypoprothrombinemia

- Azulfidine (Rare) ... 2059
- Bactrim DS Tablets ... 2257
- Bactrim I.V. Infusion ... 2255
- Bactrim ... 2257
- Cipro I.V. (Rare) ... 587
- Fansidar Tablets ... 2281
- Felbatol ... 2774
- Foscavir Injection (Less than 1%) ... 541
- Gantanol Tablets ... 2285
- Gantrisin ... 2286
- Limbitrol (Rare) ... 2333
- Merrem I.V. (Greater than 0.2%) ... 2952
- Mithracin ... 599
- PASER Granules ... 1333
- Pediazole Suspension ... 2340
- ▲ Prograf (Greater than 3%) ... 1028
- Questran ... 774
- Rocephin Injectable Vials, ADD-Vantage, Galaxy Container (Rare) ... 2305
- Septra ... 1146
- Septra I.V. Infusion ... 1142
- Septra I.V. Infusion ADD-Vantage Vials ... 1144
- Septra ... 1146
- Tapazole Tablets ... 1361

Hypoptyalism

- Demser Capsules ... 1690
- Risperdal Tablets (Frequent) ... 1348
- Vantin for Oral Suspension and Vantin Tablets (Less than 1%) ... 2112
- ▲ Xanax Tablets (32.8%) ... 2115

Hypopyon

- Healon (Rare) ... ⊙ 302
- Healon GV (Rare) ... ⊙ 303
- OcuCoat (Rare) ... ⊙ 321

Hyporeflexia

- Betaseron for SC Injection ... 653
- Cerebyx Injection (2.8%) ... 1956
- Cognex Capsules (Infrequent) ... 1961
- Compazine ... 2644
- Foscavir Injection (Less than 1%) ... 541
- Invirase Capsules (Less than 2%) ... 2291
- Lioresal Intrathecal (1% or more) ... 1634
- LUVOX Tablets (Rare) ... 2723
- Matulane Capsules ... 2300
- Navelbine Injection (Less than 5%) ... 1212
- Neurontin Capsules (Frequent) ... 1978
- Paxil Tablets (Rare) ... 2681
- ProSom Tablets (Rare) ... 457
- Prozac Pulvules & Liquid, Oral Solution (Rare) ... 935
- Redux Capsules ... 2911
- ▲ Retrovir Capsules (5.6%) ... 1216
- ▲ Retrovir I.V. Infusion (7%) ... 1221
- ▲ Retrovir Syrup (5.6%) ... 1216
- ▲ Risperdal Tablets (17% to 34%) ... 1348
- Stelazine ... 2692
- Thorazine ... 2701
- ▲ Vesanoid Capsules (3%) ... 2327
- Videx Tablets, Powder for Oral Solution, & Pediatric Powder for Oral Solution (Less than 1%) ... 2980
- Xanax Tablets (2.7%) ... 2115
- Zoloft Tablets (Rare) ... 2051

Hyporeflexia, neonatal

- Compazine ... 2644
- Stelazine Concentrate ... 2692
- Thorazine ... 2701

Hyporesponsive episode, unspecified

- Diphtheria and Tetanus Toxoids and Pertussis Vaccine Adsorbed ... 2650
- HibTITER (One case) ... 1423
- Tetramune ... 1449

Hypospadias

- Amen Tablets (Approximately 10 to 16 per 1,000 male births) ... 785
- Cycrin Tablets (Approximately 10 to 16 per 1,000 male births) ... 991
- Depo-Provera Contraceptive Injection (5 to 8 per 1,000 male births) ... 2079
- Depo-Provera Sterile Aqueous Suspension (About 5 to 8 per 1,000) ... 2083
- Megace Oral Suspension (Approximately 10 to 16 male births per 1,000) ... 708
- Megace Tablets ... 710
- Provera Tablets ... 2110

Hyposthenuria

- Floxin I.V. (More than or equal to 1%) ... 1580
- Floxin Tablets (200 mg, 300 mg, 400 mg) (More than or equal to 1%) ... 1577
- ▲ Fungizone Intravenous (Among most common) ... 507

Hypotaxia

- ▲ Vesanoid Capsules (3%) ... 2327

Hypotension

- Abbokinase ... 403
- Abbokinase Open-Cath ... 405
- ▲ Abelcet Injection (6% to 7%) ... 1540
- Accupril Tablets (2.9%) ... 1950
- Acel-Imune Diphtheria and Tetanus Toxoids and Acellular Pertussis Vaccine Adsorbed (Rare) ... 1415
- Acthrel for Injection ... 2990
- Actimmune (Rare) ... 1043
- Activase ... 1045
- ▲ Adalat Capsules (10 mg and 20 mg) (Approximately 5%) ... 580
- Adalat CC (Less than 1.0%) ... 582
- Adapin Capsules (Occasional) ... 1542
- Adenocard Injection (Less than 1%) ... 1021
- Adenoscan (2%) ... 1022
- AK-FLUOR Injection 10% and 25% ... ⊙ 204
- Aldoclor Tablets ... 1638
- Aldomet Oral ... 1640
- Aldoril Tablets ... 1644
- ▲ Alfenta Injection (10%) ... 1334
- ▲ Alferon N Injection (6%) ... 2142
- Alkeran for Injection (In some patients) ... 1196
- ▲ Altace Capsules (10.7%) ... 1238
- Ambien Tablets (Rare) ... 2559
- Amicar Syrup, Tablets, and Injection ... 1312
- Amikacin Sulfate Injection, USP (Rare) ... 523
- Amikacin Sulfate Injection, USP (Rare) ... 981
- Amikin Injectable (Rare) ... 502
- Anectine ... 1062
- Apresazide Capsules (Less frequent) ... 824
- Apresoline Hydrochloride Tablets (Less frequent) ... 826
- AquaMEPHYTON Injection ... 1648
- Aralen Hydrochloride Injection (Rare) ... 2430
- Aralen Phosphate Tablets (Rare) ... 2431
- Asendin Tablets (Less than 1%) ... 1419
- Ativan Injection (0.1%) ... 2805
- Ativan Tablets (Rare) ... 2807
- Atretol Tablets ... 569
- Atrohist Plus Tablets ... 1605
- Atrovent Inhalation Aerosol ... 674
- Avonex ... 662
- Azactam for Injection (Less than 1%) ... 736
- Azathioprine Tablets (Occasional) ... 2349
- Benadryl Injection ... 1955
- Betagan ... ⊙ 230
- ▲ Betapace Tablets (3% to 6%) ... 637
- Betaseron for SC Injection ... 653
- Betimol 0.25%, 0.5% ... ⊙ 259
- Bioclate, Antihemophilic Factor (Recombinant) ... 797
- Blenoxane (Approximately 1%) ... 697
- ▲ Blocadren Tablets (3%) ... 1654
- ▲ Brevibloc (esmolol HCl) Injection (20% to 50%) ... 1860
- ▲ Bromfed-DM Cough Syrup (Among most frequent) ... 1832
- Brontex ... 2130
- Bumex (0.8%) ... 2260
- ▲ Buprenex Injectable (1-5%) ... 2170
- BuSpar Tablets (Infrequent) ... 738
- Butisol Sodium Elixir & Tablets (Less than 1 in 100) ... 2768
- Calan SR Caplets (2.5%) ... 2571
- Calan Tablets (2.5%) ... 2568
- Capoten Tablets (Rare) ... 740
- Capozide Tablets (Rare) ... 744
- Carbocaine Injection ... 2432
- Cardene Capsules (Rare) ... 2261
- ▲ Cardene I.V. (5.6%) ... 2815
- Cardene SR Capsules (Rare) ... 2264
- Cardizem CD Capsules (Less than 1%) ... 1251
- Cardizem SR Capsules (1%) ... 1255
- Cardizem Tablets (Less than 1%) ... 1257
- Cardura Tablets (1% to 1.7%) ... 1993
- Cataflam Tablets (Rare) ... 833
- Caverject Injection (Less than 1%) ... 2064

(⊞ Described in PDR For Nonprescription Drugs)   Incidence data in parenthesis; ▲ 3% or more   (⊙ Described in PDR For Ophthalmology)

1371 Side Effects Index Hypotension

▲ CellCept Capsules (More than or equal to 3%) 2265
Ceptaz (Very rare) 1070
▲ Cerebyx Injection (7.7%) 1956
Ceredase (A few events) 1055
Cerezyme (One patient) 1056
Cipro I.V. (1% or less) 587
Cipro I.V. Pharmacy Bulk Package (Less than 1%) 590
Claritin Tablets (2% or fewer patients) 2485
Claritin-D Tablets (Less frequent) .. 2487
Cleocin Phosphate Injection (Rare) 2068
Clinoril Tablets (Less than 1 in 100) 1658
Clomid 1262
▲ Clozaril Tablets (More than 5 to 9%) 2377
Cognex Capsules (Frequent) 1961
Compazine 2644
▲ Cordarone Intravenous (Most common; 15.6% to 16%) 2821
Cordarone Tablets (Less than 1%) 2818
Corvert Injection (2.0%) 2075
Coumadin 941
Covera-HS Tablets (0.7% to 2.5%) 2573
Cozaar Tablets (Less than 1%) 1668
▲ Cytadren Tablets (1 in 30) 837
CytoGam 1630
Cytotec (Infrequent) 2576
Cytovene (1% or less) 2270
D.A. II Tablets 972
D.A. Chewable Tablets 970
DDAVP Injection (Infrequent) 2178
DDAVP Nasal Spray (Infrequent) 2180
Dalgan Injection (Less than 1%) 529
Dalmane Capsules (Rare) 2329
Decadron Phosphate with Xylocaine Injection, Sterile 1683
Deconsal II Tablets 1605
Demadex Tablets and Injection 691
Demerol 2438
Depakote Tablets (1% to 5%) 418
Deponit NTG Transdermal Delivery System (Infrequent; 4%) 2541
Desferal Vials 838
Desmopressin Acetate Injection (Infrequent) 996
▲ Desyrel and Desyrel Dividose (3.8% to 7.0%) 504
Dilacor XR Extended-release Capsules 2183
Dilatrate-SR Capsules (Infrequent) 2542
Dilaudid Ampules 1382
Dilaudid-HP Injection (Less frequent) 1384
Dilaudid-HP Lyophilized Powder 250 mg (Less frequent) 1384
Dilaudid 1382
Dilaudid Oral Liquid 1386
Dilaudid 1382
Dilaudid Tablets - 8 mg 1386
Dimetane-DC Cough Syrup 2232
Dimetane-DX Cough Syrup 2233
Diphtheria and Tetanus Toxoids and Pertussis Vaccine Adsorbed (Rare) 2650
▲ Diprivan Injectable Emulsion (Rare; 1% to 26%) 2939
Disalcid 1549
Diupres Tablets 1691
Diuril Oral Suspension 1694
Diuril Sodium Intravenous 1693
Diuril Tablets 1694
Dizac (diazepam injectable emulsion) CIV (Less frequent) 1862
Dobutrex Solution Vials (Occasional) 1480
▲ Doxil (Approximately 6.8%) 2613
Duragesic Transdermal System (1% to 3%) 1336
Duranest Injections 533
Dura-Tap/PD Capsules 970
Dura-Vent/DA Tablets 972
Dura-Vent Tablets 971
Dyazide Capsules 2653
Dyclone 0.5% and 1% Topical Solutions, USP 535
DynaCirc Capsules (0.5% to 1%) .. 2381
DynaCirc CR Tablets (0.5% to 1.0%) 2383
Effexor (Infrequent) 2825
Elavil 2945
Eldepryl Capsules 2729
Emete-con Intramuscular/Intravenous 2007
▲ Eminase (10.4%) 2215
EMLA Cream (Unlikely with cream) 536
Engerix-B Unit-Dose Vials (Less than 1%) 2656
Esidrix Tablets 839
Eskalith 2658
Ethmozine Tablets (Less than 2%) 2217
▲ Ethyol (amifostine) for Injection (62%) 485
Etopophos for Injection (One episode; 3%) 701
Etoposide Injection (0.7% to 2%) .. 539
Etrafon 2495
▲ Exosurf Neonatal for Intratracheal Suspension (39% to 77%) 1081
Fedahist Gyrocaps 2545
Felbatol 2774
Fioricet with Codeine Capsules 2387
Flexeril Tablets (Less than 1%) .. 1701
▲ Flolan for Injection (16% to 27%) 1085
Floxin I.V. (Less than 1%) 1580
Floxin Tablets (200 mg, 300 mg, 400 mg) (Less than 1%) 1577
Fluorescite .... ⊙ 217
Fluothane 2830
Fortaz (Very rare) 1092
Foscavir Injection (Between 1% and 5%) 541
▲ Fungizone Intravenous (Among most common) 507
Furoxone 2221
Gamimune N, 5% Immune Globulin Intravenous (Human), 5% (Rare) 612
Garamycin Injectable 2502
Glucophage Tablets 754
Haldol Decanoate 1587
Haldol Injection, Tablets and Concentrate 1585
Hespan Injection 945
Helixate, Antihemophilic Factor (Recombinant) 799
Hismanal Tablets (Rare) 1341
Histussin D Liquid 670
Humalog Injection (Less common) .. 1488
Humulin 50/50, 100 Units 1491
Humulin 70/30, 100 Units (Less common) 1492
Humulin L, 100 Units (Less common) 1494
Hydralazine Hydrochloride Injection USP (Less frequent) 2712
HydroDIURIL Tablets 1716
Hydropres Tablets 1718
▲ Hyperstat I.V. Injection (7%) 2504
Hyskon Hysteroscopy Fluid (Rare) .. 1633
▲ Hytrin Capsules (0.6%; 21%) 434
Hyzaar Tablets 1720
IFEX (Less than 1%) 706
Regular, 100 Units (Less common) 1503
Pork Regular, 100 Units (Less common) 1507
Imdur (Less than or equal to 5%) .. 1362
Imitrex Injection (Infrequent) 1095
Imitrex Tablets (Infrequent) 1099
Imuran (Occasional) 1103
▲ Inapsine Injection (Among most common) 462
Inderal 2834
Inderal LA Long Acting Capsules 2836
Inderide Tablets 2838
Inderide LA Long Acting Capsules .. 2840
Indocin Capsules (Less than 1%) 1723
Indocin I.V. (Less than 1%) 1727
Indocin (Less than 1%) 1723
INFeD (Iron Dextran Injection, USP) 2478
Inocor Lactate Injection (1.3%) 2439
Intron A for Injection (Less than 5%) 2506
Invirase Capsules (Less than 2%) .. 2291
Ismelin Tablets 845
Ismo Tablets (Fewer than 1%) 2844
Isoptin Oral Tablets (2.5%) 1393
Isoptin SR Tablets (2.5%) 1395
Isopto Carbachol Ophthalmic Solution .... ⊙ 221
Isordil Sublingual Tablets (Infrequent) 2845
Isordil Tembids (Infrequent) 2847
Isordil Titradose Tablets (Infrequent) 2848
Isuprel Injection 2441
Kadian Capsules (Less than 3%) 2948
Kerlone Tablets (Less than 2%) 2588
KOGENATE Antihemophilic Factor (Recombinant) 626
Kytril Injection (Rare) 2667
Kytril Tablets (Rare) 2669
Lasix Injection, Oral Solution and Tablets 1267
▲ Leukine (13%) 1317
Levo-Dromoran 2297
Librium Injectable (Isolated cases) 2332
Limbitrol 2333
Lioresal Intrathecal (0.7% to 2.0%) 1634
▲ Lioresal Tablets (Up to 9%) 847
Lithium Carbonate Capsules & Tablets 2352
Lithonate/Lithotabs/Lithobid 2721
Lopressor (1%) 848
Lopressor HCT Tablets 850
Lotensin HCT Tablets (0.6%; rare) 855
Lotrel Capsules (Rare) 858
Loxitane 1426
Ludiomil Tablets (Rare) 861
Lufyllin & Lufyllin-400 Tablets 2778
Lufyllin-GG Elixir & Tablets 2779
Lupron Depot 3.75 mg 2739
Lupron Depot 7.5 mg 2741
Lupron Depot - 3 Month 22.5 mg (Less than 5%) 2743
Lupron Depot-PED 7.5 mg, 11.25 mg and 15 mg 2744
Lupron Injection 2736
Lutrepulse for Injection 998
LUVOX Tablets (Frequent) 2723
MS Contin Tablets (Less frequent) 2149
MSIR (Infrequent) 2152
Marcaine 2446
Marcaine Spinal 2449
Marinol (Dronabinol) Capsules (0.3 to 1%) 2353
Matulane Capsules 2300
Mavik Tablets (0.3% to 1.0%) 1407
Maxair Autohaler 1550
Maxair Inhaler (Less than 1%) 1552
Maxaquin Tablets (Less than 1%) .. 2593
Mebaral Tablets (Less than 1 in 100) 2452
Mefoxin 1734
Mefoxin Premixed Intravenous Solution 1737
Mellaril 2398
Mepergan Injection (Rare) 2859
Mephyton Tablets (Rare) 1739
Mepron Suspension (1%) 1206
Merrem I.V. (0.1% to 1.0%) 2952
▲ Mesnex Injection (17%) 711
Methadone Hydrochloride Oral Concentrate 2356
Methergine 2401
Metubine Iodide Vials 932
Mexitil Capsules (Less than 1% or about 6 in 1,000) 684
Mintezol 1747
Miochol-E with Iocare Steri-Tags and Miochol-E System Pak (Rare) .... ⊙ 263
Mivacron (Two patients; less than 1%) 1125
Moban Tablets and Concentrate (Rare) 1036
8-MOP Capsules 1294
Monoclate-P, Factor VIII:C Pasteurized, Monoclonal Antibody Purified Antihemophilic Factor (Human) 802
Monoket Tablets (Fewer than 1%) 2550
Mononine, Coagulation Factor IX (Human), Monoclonal Antibody Purified 804
▲ Monopril Tablets (0.2% to 4.4%) .. 762
Motrin Ibuprofen Suspension, Oral Drops, Chewable Tablets, Caplets (Less than 1%) 1563
Narcan Injection (Several instances) 950
Navane Capsules and Concentrate 2018
Navane Intramuscular 2019
Nembutal Sodium Capsules (Less than 1%) 440
Nembutal Sodium Solution (Less than 1%) 442
Nembutal Sodium Suppositories (Less than 1%) 444
Nescaine/Nescaine MPF 549
Netromycin Injection 100 mg/ml (Fewer than 1 of 1000 patients) 2516
Neurontin Capsules (Infrequent) 1978
Nimbex Injection (0.2%) 1131
▲ Nimotop Capsules (1.2%-50.0%) 603
▲ Nipent for Injection (3% to 10%) .. 2733
Nitro-Bid IV (Infrequent) 1270
Nitro-Bid Ointment (Infrequent) 1272
Nitro-Dur (nitroglycerin) Transdermal Infusion System (Infrequent) 1365
Nitrolingual Spray 2193
Norcuron for Injection (Rare) 1875
Normodyne Injection (1%) 2519
Normodyne Tablets 2522
Norpace (1 to 3%) 2596
Norpramin Tablets 1273
Norvasc Tablets (0.1% to 1%; rare) 2020
Norvir (Less than 2%) 447
Novahistine DMX .... ◙ 782
Novahistine Elixir .... ◙ 782
Novantrone for Injection (Occasional) 1327
Novocain Hydrochloride for Spinal Anesthesia 2457
Novolin 70/30 Prefilled Disposable Insulin Delivery System (Rare) 1850
Nubain Injection (1% or less) 952
Nuromax Injection (0.3%) 1136
Ocupress Ophthalmic Solution, 1% Sterile .... ⊙ 297
Ogen Tablets 2103
Ogen Vaginal Cream 2106
▲ Oncaspar (Greater than 1% but less than 5%) 2194
Oncovin Solution Vials & Hyporets 1521
Oramorph SR (Morphine Sulfate Sustained Release Tablets) (Less frequent) 2359
Orap Tablets 1037
Oretic Tablets 450
Ornade Spansule Capsules 2678
Orthoclone OKT3 Sterile Solution .. 1892
Oxsoralen-Ultra Capsules 1302
OxyContin Tablets 2163
PBZ Tablets 863
PBZ-SR Tablets 862
Pamelor 2409
Paraplatin for Injection (Rare) 713
▲ Parlodel (28%) 2411
Paxil Tablets (Infrequent) 2681
Pentaspan Injection 954
Periactin 1767
Permax Tablets (2.1%) 571
Phenergan with Codeine 2883
Phenergan with Dextromethorphan 2885
Phenergan Injection 2880
Phenergan Suppositories 2882
Phenergan Syrup 2881
Phenergan Tablets 2882
Phenergan VC 2886
Phenergan VC with Codeine 2888
Phenobarbital Elixir and Tablets (Less than 1 in 100 patients) 1523
Placidyl Capsules 456
Plasma-Plex, Plasma Protein Fraction (Human) U.S.P. 5% Solution Heat-Treated 806
Platinol for Injection (Occasional) 717
Platinol-AQ Injection (Occasional) .. 719
Plendil Extended-Release Tablets (0.5% to 1.5%) 514
Pondimin Tablets 2239
Pontocaine Hydrochloride for Spinal Anesthesia 2460
Pravachol Tablets 770
Prevacid Delayed-Release Capsules (Less than 1%) 2746
Primacor Injection (2.9%) 2461
Primaxin I.M. 1770
Primaxin I.V. (0.4%) 1772
Prinivil Tablets (0.3% to 4.4%; rare) 1776
Prinzide Tablets (1.4%) 1780
Priscoline Hydrochloride Ampuls 864
Procanbid Extended-Release Tablets (Rare) 1983
▲ Procardia Capsules (Approximately 5%; about 1 in 20 to 1 in 50 patients) 2024
Procardia XL Extended Release Tablets (Occasional) 2026
Proglycem (Occasional) 575
▲ Prograf (Greater than 3%) 1028
Prolastin Alpha$_1$-Proteinase Inhibitor (Human) (Rare) 629
▲ Proleukin for Injection (85%) 812
Prolixin (Rare) 510
Prostigmin Injectable 1305
Prostigmin Tablets 1306
Prostin E2 Suppository 2109
Protamine Sulfate Vials 1526
Prozac Pulvules & Liquid, Oral Solution (Infrequent) 935
Quadrinal Tablets 1398
Quibron 2227
RMS Suppositories CII 2766
Recombivax HB (Less than 1%) 1787
Redux Capsules (Infrequent) 2911
Regitine Vials 864
Reglan 2243
Remeron Tablets (Infrequent) 1878
▲ ReoPro Vials (21.1%) 1526
Respbid Tablets 687
RespiGam (Infrequent) 1631

(◙ Described in PDR For Nonprescription Drugs) Incidence data in parenthesis; ▲ 3% or more (⊙ Described in PDR For Ophthalmology)

Revex (nalmefene hydrochloride injection) (1%) 1863
Rifadin 1276
Rifater 1280
Rilutek Tablets (Infrequent) 2198
Risperdal Tablets (Infrequent) 1348
Robaxin Injectable 2245
Roferon-A Injection (Less than 4%) 2308
Roxanol 2365
Rum-K Syrup 1004
Rythmol Tablets–150mg, 225mg, 300mg (0.1 to 1.1%) 1399
Salflex Tablets 791
Sandoglobulin I.V. (Less than 1%) 2419
Seconal Sodium Pulvules (Less than 1 in 100) 1529
Sectral Capsules (Up to 2%) 2914
Seldane Tablets (Rare) 1284
Seldane-D Extended-Release Tablets (Rare) 1286
Sensorcaine 554
Ser-Ap-Es Tablets 867
▲ Serentil (One of the two most prevalent) 689
Serzone Tablets (2%) 776
Sinemet CR Tablets 961
Sinequan (Occasional) 2028
Slo-bid Gyrocaps 2201
Soma Compound w/Codeine Tablets 2784
Soma Compound Tablets 2783
Soma Tablets 2782
Sorbitrate (Infrequent) 2959
Stadol (Less than 1%) 779
Stelazine 2692
Stimate, (desmopressin acetate) Nasal Spray, 1.5 mg/mL (Infrequent) 806
▲ Streptase for Infusion (1% to 10%) 557
Sublimaze Injection 463
▲ Sufenta Injection (3% to 9%) 1355
Sular Tablets (Less than or equal to 1%) 2961
Surmontil Capsules 2917
Survanta Beractant Intratracheal Suspension (Less than 1%) 2346
Symmetrel Capsules (Uncommon) 965
Symmetrel Syrup (Uncommon) 963
Syn-Rx Tablets 1622
Syn-Rx DM Tablets 1623
Tagamet Injection (Rare) 2694
Talacen Caplets (Infrequent) 2464
Talwin Compound (Infrequent) 2466
Talwin Nx Tablets 2467
Tambocor Tablets (Less than 1%) 1555
Tavist Syrup 2426
Tavist Tablets 2427
▲ Taxol Injection (2% to 12%) 723
Taxotere for Injection Concentrate (0.9% to 3.6%) 2204
Tazicef for Injection (Very rare) 2697
Tazidime Vials, Faspak & ADD-Vantage (Very rare) 1531
Tegretol/Tegretol-XR 870
Tenoretic Tablets 2963
▲ Tenormin Tablets and I.V. Injection (25%) 2965
Tensilon Injectable 1307
Tetramune (Rare) 1449
Thalitone (Common) 1293
Theo-Dur Extended-Release Tablets 1367
Theo-X Extended-Release Tablets 793
THYREL TRH (A small number of patients) 2992
Tiazac Capsules (Less than 1%) 1019
Timolide Tablets (1.6%) 1791
Timoptic in Ocudose (Less frequent) 1796
Timoptic Sterile Ophthalmic Solution (Less frequent) 1794
Timoptic-XE 1798
Tonocard Tablets (1.8% to 3.4%) 519
Toprol-XL Tablets (About 1 of 100 patients) 560
Toradol 2319
Torecan 2367
Tornalate Solution for Inhalation, 0.2% 976
Tracrium Injection (5 out of 875 patients) 1155
Trandate (Less common; 1 of 100 patients) 1158
▲ Transderm-Nitro Transdermal Therapeutic System (4%) 878
Tranxene 459
▲ Trasylol (6%) 607
Trental Tablets (Less than 1%) 1291
Triavil Tablets 1800
Tri-Immunol Adsorbed (Rare) 1452
Trilafon (Rare) 2532
Trinalin Repetabs Tablets 1373
Triostat Injection (Approximately 2%) 2708
Tripedia 908
Tussend 1830
Tussend Expectorant 1831
Typhim Vi 914
Uni-Dur Extended-Release Tablets 1374
Urecholine 1804
Valium Injectable 2336
Valium Tablets (Infrequent) 2335
Vancocin HCl, Oral Solution & Pulvules 1536
Vancocin HCl, Vials & ADD-Vantage (Infrequent) 1534
Vantin for Oral Suspension and Vantin Tablets (Less than 1%) 2112
Vaseretic Tablets (Rare; 0.9%) 1810
Vasotec I.V. (Rare) 1814
▲ Vasotec Tablets (0.5% to 6.7%) 1816
Velosulin BR Human Insulin 10 ml Vials 1847
VePesid Capsules and Injection (0.7% to 2%) 727
Verelan Capsules (2.5%) 1455
Versed Injection 2324
▲ Vesanoid Capsules (14%; occasional) 2327
Vexol 1% Ophthalmic Suspension (Less than 2%) ◉ 227
Videx Tablets, Powder for Oral Solution, & Pediatric Powder for Oral Solution (1% to 4%) 2980
Virazole 1310
Visken Tablets (2% or fewer patients) 2428
Vistide Injection 1057
Vivactil Tablets 1820
Cataflam/Voltaren/Voltaren-XR (Rare) 833
Vumon for Injection (2%) 729
Wellbutrin Tablets (2.5%) 1177
▲ Xanax Tablets (4.7%) 2115
▲ Xylocaine Injections (3%) 562
▲ Yutopar Intravenous Injection (80 to 100%) 566
Zantac Injection 1180
Zaroxolyn Tablets 1625
Zebeta Tablets 1457
Zemuron Injection (0.1%; 2%) 1885
Zestoretic Tablets (1.4%; rare) 2968
Zestril Tablets (Rare; 0.3% to 9.7%) 2972
Ziac 1459
Zofran Injection (Rare; 2%) 1227
▲ Zofran Tablets (5%) 1231
Zoloft Tablets (Infrequent) 2051
Zosyn (1.0% or less) 1463
Zovirax Sterile Powder (Less than 1%) 1191
Zyrtec Tablets (Rare) 2053

Hypotension, asymptomatic

▲ Brevibloc (esmolol HCl) Injection (About 25%) 1860
▲ Cardizem Injectable (4.3%) 1253
▲ Isoptin SR Tablets (5%) 1395
▲ Neupogen for Injection (7 of 176 patients) 495
▲ Verelan Capsules (5%) 1455

Hypotension, exertional

Cardene Capsules (Less than 0.4%) 2261
Esimil Tablets 840

Hypotension, neonatal

Accupril Tablets 1950
Altace Capsules 1238
Capoten Tablets 740
Capozide Tablets 744
Cozaar Tablets 1668
Hyzaar Tablets 1720
Lotensin Tablets 852
Lotensin HCT Tablets (0.6%; rare) 855
Lotrel Capsules 858
Monopril Tablets 762
Normodyne Injection 2519
Normodyne Tablets (Rare) 2522
Prinivil Tablets 1776
Prinzide Tablets 1780
Sectral Capsules 2914
Trandate 1158
Univasc Tablets 2553
Vaseretic Tablets 1810
Vasotec I.V. 1814
Vasotec Tablets 1816
Yutopar Intravenous Injection (Infrequent) 566
Zestoretic Tablets 2968
Zestril Tablets 2972

Hypotension, orthostatic

Accupril Tablets (Rare) 1950
▲ Adalat Capsules (10 mg and 20 mg) (Approximately 5%) 580
Aldactazide Tablets 2556
Aldoclor Tablets 1638
Aldomet Ester HCl Injection 1642
Aldomet Oral 1640
Aldoril Tablets 1644
▲ Anafranil Capsules (Approximately 20%) 819
Apresazide Capsules 824
Atamet Tablets (Less frequent) 567
Brontex 2130
Capoten Tablets 740
Capozide Tablets 744
▲ Cardura Tablets (Up to 23%) 1993
Catapres-TTS 680
Clozaril Tablets 2377
Combipres Tablets (About 3 in 100) 682
Desyrel and Desyrel Dividose 504
Dipentum Capsules (Rare) 2084
Diucardin Tablets 2824
Diupres Tablets 1691
Diuril Oral Suspension 1694
Diuril Sodium Intravenous 1693
Diuril Tablets 1694
Elavil 2945
Eldepryl Capsules 2729
Enduron Tablets 424
Esidrix Tablets 839
Esimil Tablets 840
Furoxone 2221
HydroDIURIL Tablets 1716
Hydropres Tablets 1718
▲ Hylorel Tablets (6.6% to 7.5%) 1613
Hyperstat I.V. Injection 2504
Hytrin Capsules 434
Inderide Tablets 2838
Inderide LA Long Acting Capsules 2840
IOPIDINE Sterile Ophthalmic Solution ◉ 218
Kadian Capsules 2948
Larodopa Tablets 2296
Lasix Injection, Oral Solution and Tablets 1267
Levoprome (Among the most important) 1321
Lopressor HCT Tablets 850
Lotensin HCT Tablets 855
Loxitane 1426
Lysodren Tablets (Infrequent) 707
MS Contin Tablets 2149
Mellaril 2398
Methadone Hydrochloride Oral Concentrate 2356
Midamor Tablets (Less than or equal to 1%) 1746
Minipress Capsules (1-4%) 2015
Minizide Capsules 2016
Moduretic Tablets (Less than or equal to 1%) 1748
Monopril Tablets (1.4% to 1.9%) 762
Mykrox Tablets (Less than 2%) 1617
Oretic Tablets 450
▲ Parlodel (6%) 2411
Phenergan with Codeine 2883
Phenergan VC with Codeine 2888
Prinivil Tablets (0.3% to 1.2%) 1776
Prinzide Tablets (0.5% to 1.0%) 1780
Regitine Vials 864
Risperdal Tablets 1348
Roxanol 2365
Sandostatin Injection (Less than 1%) 2421
Ser-Ap-Es Tablets 867
Sinemet Tablets (Less frequent) 959
Sinemet CR Tablets (1.0%) 961
Slo-Niacin Tablets (Less common) 2767
Sporanox Capsules (1%) 1352
Symmetrel Capsules (1% to 5%) 965
Symmetrel Syrup (1% to 5%) 963
Tenoretic Tablets 2963
Thalitone 1293
Timolide Tablets 1791
Tofranil Ampuls 873
Tofranil Tablets 875
Tofranil-PM Capsules 876
Tonocard Tablets (Less than 1%) 519
Trandate 1158
Triavil Tablets 1800
Ultram Tablets (50 mg) (Less than 1%) 1594
Vaseretic Tablets (0.5% to 2.0%) 1810
Vasotec I.V. 1814
Vasotec Tablets (0.5% to 1.6%) 1816
Vivactil Tablets 1820
Wellbutrin Tablets 1177
Zaroxolyn Tablets 1625
Zebeta Tablets 1457
Zestoretic Tablets (0.3 to 1%) 2968
Zestril Tablets (0.3% to 1.2%) 2972
Ziac 1459

Hypotension, postural

Adalat CC (Less than 1.0%) 582
Akineton 1380
Altace Capsules (2.2%) 1238
Ambien Tablets (Infrequent) 2559
▲ Anafranil Capsules (4% to 6%) 819
Avonex 662
Betaseron for SC Injection 653
Cardene Capsules (Rare) 2261
Cardene I.V. (1.4%) 2815
Cardene SR Capsules (0.9%) 2264
▲ Cardura Tablets (0.3% to 29%) 1993
▲ CellCept Capsules (More than or equal to 3%) 2265
Cerebyx Injection (Infrequent) 1956
Cipro Tablets 584
Corvert Injection (2.0%) 2075
Covera-HS Tablets (0.4%) 2573
Depakote Tablets (1% to 5%) 418
Dibenzyline Capsules 2650
Dilacor XR Extended-release Capsules (Infrequent) 2183
Dyazide Capsules 2653
Effexor (1%) 2825
Esimil Tablets 840
Etrafon 2495
Hycomine Compound Tablets 948
Hycomine 947
Hycotuss Expectorant Syrup 950
▲ Hytrin Capsules (0.5% to 21%) 434
Intron A for Injection (Less than 5%) 2506
Inversine Tablets 1729
Ismelin Tablets 845
Ismo Tablets (Fewer than 1%) 2844
Isordil Tembids 2847
Isordil Titradose Tablets 2848
Kadian Capsules (Less than 3%) 2948
Lamictal Tablets (Infrequent) 1105
Lioresal Intrathecal (1% or more) 1634
Lotensin Tablets (0.4%) 852
Lotensin HCT Tablets (0.3%) 855
LUVOX Tablets 2723
Nardil (Common) 1977
Nitrolingual Spray (Occasional) 2193
Nitrostat Tablets (Occasional) 1981
▲ Normodyne Injection (58%) 2519
Normodyne Tablets (1%) 2522
Noroxin Tablets 1758
Noroxin Tablets 2222
Norvasc Tablets (More than 0.1% to 1%) 2020
Norvir (Less than 2%) 447
Orap Tablets 1037
Orlaam Oral Solution (Less than 1%) 2361
OxyContin Tablets (Between 1% and 5%) 2163
▲ Parlodel (6%) 2411
Paxil Tablets (1.2%) 2681
▲ Permax Tablets (9.0%) 571
Prozac Pulvules & Liquid, Oral Solution (Infrequent) 935
Redux Capsules (Infrequent) 2911
Rilutek Tablets (0.8% to 1.6%) 2198
Sansert Tablets 2424
▲ Serzone Tablets (2.8% to 4%) 776
Soma Compound w/Codeine Tablets 2784
Soma Compound Tablets 2783
Soma Tablets 2782
Sorbitrate 2959
Sular Tablets (Less than or equal to 1%) 2961
Tegison Capsules (Less than 1%) 2314
▲ Tenoretic Tablets (2% to 4%) 2963
▲ Tenormin Tablets and I.V. Injection (2% to 4%) 2965
Thorazine 2701
Torecan 2367
▲ Trandate (58%) 1158
Trecator-SC Tablets 2919
Trilafon 2532
Univasc Tablets (Less than 1%; 0.51%) 2553
Vasotec I.V. (2.3%) 1814
Vicodin Tuss Expectorant 1406
Vistide Injection 1057
Zoloft Tablets (Infrequent) 2051

Hypotension, secondary to spinal block

Duranest Injections 533
Marcaine 2446

(▣ Described in PDR For Nonprescription Drugs) Incidence data in parenthesis; ▲ 3% or more (◉ Described in PDR For Ophthalmology)

Side Effects Index

Hypotension, symptomatic
- Accupril Tablets ... 1950
- Altace Capsules (0.5%) ... 1238
- ▲ Brevibloc (esmolol HCl) Injection (12%) ... 1860
- Calan SR Caplets ... 2571
- Calan Tablets ... 2568
- Cardizem CD Capsules (Occasional) ... 1251
- Cardizem SR Capsules (Occasional) ... 1255
- ▲ Cardizem Injectable (3.2%) ... 1253
- Cardizem Tablets (Occasional) ... 1257
- Covera-HS Tablets ... 2573
- Cozaar Tablets ... 1668
- Hyzaar Tablets ... 1720
- Isoptin Injectable (1.5%) ... 1391
- Lotensin Tablets (Rare to 0.3%) ... 852
- Lotensin HCT Tablets ... 855
- Lotrel Capsules ... 858
- Mavik Tablets (Rare) ... 1407
- Monopril Tablets ... 762
- Prinivil Tablets ... 1776
- Univasc Tablets (Less than 1%; 0.5%) ... 2553

Hypotensive crisis
- Acthrel for Injection (One patient) ... 2990
- Fiorinal with Codeine Capsules ... 2390
- Miltown Tablets ... 2780
- PMB 200 and PMB 400 (One instance) ... 2890
- Prolixin ... 510

Hypothermia
- Betaseron for SC Injection ... 653
- Clozaril Tablets (Less than 1%) ... 2377
- Doxil (Less than 1%) ... 2613
- Ethmozine Tablets (Less than 2%) ... 2217
- Felbatol ... 2774
- Foscavir Injection (Less than 1%) ... 541
- Ganite ... 2711
- Glucophage Tablets ... 754
- Lioresal Intrathecal (1% or more) ... 1634
- Norvir (Less than 2%) ... 447
- Permax Tablets (Infrequent) ... 571
- Prozac Pulvules & Liquid, Oral Solution (Rare) ... 935
- Redux Capsules ... 2911
- Rilutek Tablets (Rare) ... 2198
- Salagen Tablets (Less than 1%) ... 1546
- Urecholine ... 1804
- ▲ Vesanoid Capsules (3%) ... 2327

Hypothyroidism
- Anafranil Capsules (Infrequent) ... 819
- Aredia for Injection (Up to 6%) ... 827
- Avonex ... 662
- Betaseron for SC Injection ... 653
- Cognex Capsules (Rare) ... 1961
- Cordarone Tablets (1 to 3%) ... 2818
- Effexor (Rare) ... 2825
- Eskalith ... 2658
- Genotropin Injection (Infrequent) ... 2090
- Humatrope Vials ... 1490
- Imitrex Tablets (Rare) ... 1099
- Intron A for Injection (Less than 5%) ... 2506
- Lamictal Tablets (Rare) ... 1105
- Lithium Carbonate Capsules & Tablets ... 2352
- Lithonate/Lithotabs/Lithobid ... 2721
- LUVOX Tablets (Infrequent) ... 2723
- Neurontin Capsules (Rare) ... 1978
- Paxil Tablets (Rare) ... 2681
- Permax Tablets (Infrequent) ... 571
- Proleukin for Injection (Less than 1%) ... 812
- Protropin ... 1053
- Prozac Pulvules & Liquid, Oral Solution (Infrequent) ... 935
- Redux Capsules (Rare) ... 2911
- Remeron Tablets (Rare) ... 1878
- Roferon-A Injection (Rare to infrequent) ... 2308
- ▲ Sandostatin Injection (Several isolated patients up to 12%) ... 2421
- Thyro-Block Tablets (Rare) ... 2785

Hypotonia
- Ambien Tablets (Rare) ... 2559
- Cerebyx Injection (Infrequent) ... 1956
- Diphtheria and Tetanus Toxoids and Pertussis Vaccine Adsorbed ... 2650
- Diprivan Injectable Emulsion (Less than 1%) ... 2939
- Doxil (Less than 1%) ... 2613
- Duragesic Transdermal System (Less than 1%) ... 1336
- Effexor (Infrequent) ... 2825
- Klonopin Tablets ... 2294
- Lamictal Tablets (Rare) ... 1105
- ▲ Lioresal Intrathecal (2.4% to 34.7%) ... 1634
- LUVOX Tablets (Infrequent) ... 2723
- Neurontin Capsules (Infrequent) ... 1978
- Orthoclone OKT3 Sterile Solution ... 1892
- OxyContin Tablets (Less than 1%) ... 2163
- Penetrex Tablets (Less than 0.1%) ... 2196
- Permax Tablets (Infrequent) ... 571
- Redux Capsules (Rare) ... 2911
- Remeron Tablets (Rare) ... 1878
- Rilutek Tablets (Rare) ... 2198
- Risperdal Tablets (Rare) ... 1348
- Serzone Tablets (Rare) ... 776
- Supprelin Injection (1%) ... 2230
- Tetramune ... 1449
- Vistide Injection (1 Patient) ... 1057
- Zoloft Tablets (Rare) ... 2051

Hypouresis
- Amikacin Sulfate Injection, USP ... 523
- Atromid-S Capsules ... 2808
- Chemet Capsules (Up to 3.7%) ... 666
- Dilaudid-HP Injection ... 1384
- Dilaudid-HP Lyophilized Powder 250 mg ... 1384
- ▲ Indocin I.V. (41% of infants) ... 1727
- K-Phos Neutral Tablets ... 633
- Proglycem ... 575
- Prograf ... 1028
- Slo-Niacin Tablets ... 2767
- Uroqid-Acid No. 2 Tablets ... 633
- Yocon Tablets ... 1235

Hypouricemia
- Cipro I.V. (Infrequent) ... 587
- Cipro I.V. Pharmacy Bulk Package (Less than 1%) ... 590
- Timentin for Injection ... 2706
- Vistide Injection ... 1057
- Zoloft Tablets ... 2051

Hypoventilation
- Anafranil Capsules (Rare) ... 819
- Betaseron for SC Injection ... 653
- ▲ Buprenex Injectable (1-5%) ... 2170
- Butisol Sodium Elixir & Tablets (Less than 1 in 100) ... 2768
- Carbocaine Injection ... 2432
- Diprivan Injectable Emulsion (Less than 1%) ... 2939
- Dopram Injectable ... 2235
- ▲ Duragesic Transdermal System (2% to 10%) ... 1336
- Levo-Dromoran ... 2297
- Lioresal Intrathecal (0.2% to 4.0%) ... 1634
- Marcaine ... 2446
- Marcaine Spinal ... 2449
- Mebaral Tablets (Less than 1 in 100) ... 2452
- Nembutal Sodium Capsules (Less than 1%) ... 440
- Nembutal Sodium Solution (Less than 1%) ... 442
- Nembutal Sodium Suppositories (Less than 1%) ... 444
- Nescaine/Nescaine MPF ... 549
- Neurontin Capsules (Rare) ... 1978
- Norvir (Less than 2%) ... 447
- Permax Tablets (Rare) ... 571
- Phenobarbital Elixir and Tablets (Less than 1 in 100 patients) ... 1523
- Rilutek Tablets (Infrequent) ... 2198
- Seconal Sodium Pulvules (Less than 1 in 100) ... 1529
- Sensorcaine ... 554
- Versed Injection ... 2324
- ▲ Videx Tablets, Powder for Oral Solution, & Pediatric Powder for Oral Solution (Less than 1% to 8%) ... 2980
- Virazole (Infrequent) ... 1310

Hypovolemia
- Demadex Tablets and Injection ... 691
- Estratest ... 2718
- Humegon for Injection ... 1873
- Inapsine Injection ... 462
- Metrodin (urofollitropin for injection) ... 2616
- Mykrox Tablets ... 1617
- Serophene (clomiphene citrate tablets, USP) ... 2621
- Zaroxolyn Tablets ... 1625

Hypoxemia
- Abbokinase ... 403
- Abbokinase Open-Cath ... 405
- Glucophage Tablets ... 754
- Inocor Lactate Injection (1 case) ... 2439
- Isuprel Hydrochloride Solution ... 2443
- Methotrexate Sodium Tablets, Injection, for Injection and LPF Injection ... 1322
- Mivacron (Less than 1%) ... 1125
- Orthoclone OKT3 Sterile Solution ... 1892
- RespiGam (1%) ... 1631

Hypoxia
- Alfenta Injection ... 1334
- Ambien Tablets (Rare) ... 2559
- Atretol Tablets ... 569
- Betaseron for SC Injection ... 653
- Cerebyx Injection (Infrequent) ... 1956
- Depakene ... 416
- Dilantin-125 Suspension ... 1969
- Diprivan Injectable Emulsion (Less than 1%) ... 2939
- Effexor (Rare) ... 2825
- Felbatol ... 2774
- Fludara for Injection (Up to 1%) ... 658
- Kadian Capsules (Less than 3%) ... 2948
- Leukine ... 1317
- Levophed Bitartrate Injection ... 2445
- Merrem I.V. (0.1% to 1.0%) ... 2952
- Nardil (Less frequent) ... 1977
- Orthoclone OKT3 Sterile Solution ... 1892
- Permax Tablets (Rare) ... 571
- Prozac Pulvules & Liquid, Oral Solution (Rare) ... 935
- Pulmozyme Inhalation ... 1054
- RespiGam (1%) ... 1631
- Rilutek Tablets (Infrequent) ... 2198
- Suprane (desflurane, USP) (Less than 1%) ... 1865
- Tegretol/Tegretol-XR ... 870
- Videx Tablets, Powder for Oral Solution, & Pediatric Powder for Oral Solution (Less than 1%) ... 2980
- ▲ Zofran Tablets (9%) ... 1231
- Zosyn (1.0% or less) ... 1463

Hysteria
- Ambien Tablets (Rare) ... 2559
- Cognex Capsules (Rare) ... 1961
- Diprivan Injectable Emulsion (Less than 1%) ... 2939
- Imitrex Injection (Rare) ... 1095
- Imitrex Tablets (Rare) ... 1099
- Klonopin Tablets ... 2294
- Lioresal Intrathecal (1% or more) ... 1634
- LUVOX Tablets (Infrequent) ... 2723
- Neurontin Capsules (Rare) ... 1978
- Ornade Spansule Capsules ... 2678
- PBZ Tablets ... 863
- PBZ-SR Tablets ... 862
- Paxil Tablets (Rare) ... 2681
- Periactin ... 1767
- Phenergan Injection ... 2880
- Phenergan Tablets ... 2882
- Placidyl Capsules (Occasional) ... 456
- Prozac Pulvules & Liquid, Oral Solution (Rare) ... 935
- Tavist Syrup ... 2426
- Tavist Tablets ... 2427
- Trinalin Repetabs Tablets ... 1373
- Tussend ... 1830
- Zoloft Tablets (Rare) ... 2051

HPA axis suppression
- Aclovate ... 1061
- Cormax Ointment ... 1856
- Cormax Scalp Application ... 1857
- Cutivate Cream ... 1078
- Cutivate Ointment ... 1078
- Dermatop Emollient Cream 0.1% ... 1264
- Diprolene AF Cream 0.05% (Some patients) ... 2489
- Diprolene Lotion 0.05% (Some patients) ... 2491
- Diprolene Ointment 0.05% (Some patients) ... 2491
- Elocon Cream 0.1% ... 2492
- ProctoCream-HC 2.5% ... 2552
- Temovate Cream ... 1152
- Temovate E Emollient ... 1154
- Temovate Gel ... 1153
- Temovate Ointment ... 1152
- Temovate Scalp Application ... 1153
- Ultravate Cream 0.05% ... 2797
- Ultravate Ointment 0.05% ... 2798

HPA function suppression
- Azmacort Oral Inhaler ... 2175
- Beclovent Inhalation Aerosol and Refill ... 1063
- Vanceril Inhaler ... 2538

I

Ichthyosis
- Efudex (Infrequent) ... 2280
- ▲ Lamprene Capsules (8-28%) ... 846

Idiosyncrasy
- Berocca Plus Tablets (Possible) ... 2259
- Berocca Tablets ... 2259
- Blenoxane (Approximately 1%) ... 697
- Cocaine Hydrochloride Topical Solutions ... 529
- Cystospaz ... 2123
- Donnatal ... 2234
- Donnatal Extentabs ... 2234
- Donnatal Tablets ... 2234
- Duranest Injections ... 533
- Etrafon (Extremely rare) ... 2495
- Lasix Injection, Oral Solution and Tablets ... 1267
- Luride Lozi-Tabs Tablets (Rare) ... 892
- Miltown Tablets ... 2780
- Novocain Hydrochloride for Spinal Anesthesia (Rare) ... 2457
- PMB 200 and PMB 400 ... 2890
- Pontocaine Hydrochloride for Spinal Anesthesia ... 2460
- Robinul Forte Tablets ... 2247
- Robinul Injectable ... 2247
- Robinul Tablets ... 2247
- Soma Compound w/Codeine Tablets (Very rare) ... 2784
- Soma Compound Tablets (Very rare) ... 2783
- Soma Tablets (Occasional) ... 2782
- Tympagesic Ear Drops (Infrequently) ... 2476
- Xylocaine Injections ... 562

Idiosyncratic reactions
(see under Idiosyncrasy)

Idioventricular rhythms
- Activase ... 1045
- Corvert Injection (0.2%) ... 2075
- Eminase ... 2215

Ileitis, regional
- Accutane Capsules ... 2252
- Indocin (Less than 1%) ... 1723
- Norvir (Less than 2%) ... 447

Ileus
- Betaseron for SC Injection ... 653
- ▲ CellCept Capsules (More than or equal to 3%) ... 2265
- Cerebyx Injection (Infrequent) ... 1956
- Cipro I.V. (Less than 1%) ... 587
- Cipro I.V. Pharmacy Bulk Package (Less than 1%) ... 590
- Cogentin ... 1661
- Dilaudid Tablets and Liquid ... 1386
- Diprivan Injectable Emulsion (Less than 1%) ... 2939
- Effexor (Rare) ... 2825
- Ethmozine Tablets (Less than 2%) ... 2217
- Felbatol ... 2774
- Hyperstat I.V. Injection ... 2504
- Indocin I.V. (1% to 3%) ... 1727
- Inversine Tablets ... 1729
- Lioresal Intrathecal ... 1634
- Merrem I.V. (0.1% to 1.0%) ... 2952
- Nimotop Capsules (Rare) ... 603
- Nipent for Injection (Less than 3%) ... 2733
- Paxil Tablets (Rare) ... 2681
- Proglycem (Frequent) ... 575
- ▲ Prograf (Greater than 3%) ... 1028
- Proleukin for Injection (2%) ... 812
- ReoPro Vials (0.3%) ... 1526
- Rilutek Tablets (Rare) ... 2198
- Taxotere for Injection Concentrate ... 2204
- Vaseretic Tablets ... 1810
- Vasotec I.V. ... 1814
- Vasotec Tablets (0.5% to 1.0%) ... 1816
- Velban Vials ... 1537
- Videx Tablets, Powder for Oral Solution, & Pediatric Powder for Oral Solution (Less than 1%) ... 2980
- Yutopar Intravenous Injection (Infrequent) ... 566
- Zosyn (1.0% or less) ... 1463

Ileus, adynamic
- Compazine ... 2644
- Etrafon ... 2495
- Navane Capsules and Concentrate ... 2018
- Navane Intramuscular ... 2019
- Stelazine ... 2692

(℞ Described in PDR For Nonprescription Drugs) Incidence data in parenthesis; ▲ 3% or more (⊚ Described in PDR For Ophthalmology)

Thorazine 2701
Trilafon (Occasional) 2532

Ileus, neonatal
Yutopar Intravenous Injection (Infrequent) 566

Ileus, paralytic
Anafranil Capsules (Rare) 819
Apresazide Capsules (Less frequent) 824
Apresoline Hydrochloride Tablets (Less frequent) 826
Artane (Rare) 1418
Asendin Tablets (Very rare) 1419
Calan SR Caplets (Infrequent) 2571
Calan Tablets (Infrequent) 2568
Clozaril Tablets 2377
Cogentin 1661
Covera-HS Tablets (Infrequent) 2573
Elavil 2945
Etrafon 2495
Flexeril Tablets (Rare) 1701
Foscavir Injection (Less than 1%) 541
Hydralazine Hydrochloride Injection USP (Less frequent) 2712
Imodium Capsules (Rare) 1343
Isoptin SR Tablets (Infrequent) 1395
Limbitrol 2333
Lomotil 2591
Loxitane 1426
Ludiomil Tablets (Isolated reports) 861
Mellaril 2398
Motofen Tablets 789
Navelbine Injection (1%) 1212
Norpramin Tablets 1273
Oncovin Solution Vials & Hyporets 1521
Pamelor 2409
Podocon-25 1949
Prolixin 510
Ser-Ap-Es Tablets 867
Serentil 689
Surmontil Capsules 2917
Taxol Injection (Rare) 723
Tofranil Ampuls 873
Tofranil Tablets (Rare) 875
Tofranil-PM Capsules 876
Torecan 2367
Triavil Tablets 1800
Verelan Capsules (Infrequent) 1455
Vivactil Tablets 1820

Illusion, unspecified
Ambien Tablets (Infrequent) 2559
Anafranil Capsules (Rare) 819

Immobility
Moban Tablets and Concentrate 1036

Immunoglobulin, abnormalities
Dilantin Infatabs 1967
Dilantin Kapseals 1965
Dilantin-125 Suspension 1969
Proglycem 575
Rilutek Tablets (Infrequent) 2198

Immunosuppression
Cytoxan 700
Purinethol Tablets 1214
Rifamate Capsules 1278
Rimactane Capsules 865

Immunosuppression, progressive
Lamictal Tablets 1105

Impetigo
Hivid Tablets (Less than 1%) 2287
▲ Videx Tablets, Powder for Oral Solution, & Pediatric Powder for Oral Solution (6%) 2980

Impotence
Abelcet Injection 1540
Accupril Tablets (0.5% to 1.0%) 1950
Adalat CC (3% or less) 582
Adderall Tablets 2209
Adipex-P Tablets and Capsules 1035
Aldoclor Tablets 1638
Aldomet Ester HCl Injection 1642
Aldomet Oral 1640
Aldoril Tablets 1644
Altace Capsules (Less than 1%) 1238
Ambien Tablets (Rare) 2559
▲ Anafranil Capsules (Up to 20%) 819
Androderm Testosterone Transdermal System (Less than 1%) 2634
Antabuse Tablets (Small number of patients) 2802
Asendin Tablets (Less than 1%) 1419
Atretol Tablets 569
Atromid-S Capsules 2808
Axid Pulvules 1468
Bentyl 1246
Betagan ◉ 230
Betaseron for SC Injection 653
Betimol 0.25%, 0.5% ◉ 259
Blocadren Tablets (Less than 1%) 1654
BuSpar Tablets (Rare) 738
Calan SR Caplets (1% or less) 2571
Calan Tablets (1% or less) 2568
Capoten Tablets 740
Capozide Tablets 744
Cardene Capsules (Rare) 2261
Cardene SR Capsules (Rare) 2264
Cardizem CD Capsules (Less than 1%) 1251
Cardizem SR Capsules (Less than 1%) 1255
Cardizem Injectable 1253
Cardizem Tablets (Less than 1%) 1257
Cardura Tablets (1.1%) 1993
Cartrol Tablets (Less common) 413
▲ Casodex Tablets (5%) 2934
Cataflam Tablets (Less than 1%) 833
Catapres Tablets (About 3 in 100 patients) 679
Catapres-TTS (2 of 101 patients) 680
▲ CellCept Capsules (More than or equal to 3%) 2265
Claritin Tablets (2% or fewer patients) 2485
Claritin-D Tablets (Less frequent) 2487
Clozaril Tablets (Less than 1%) 2377
Cognex Capsules (Infrequent) 1961
Combipres Tablets (About 3%) 682
Compazine 2644
Covera-HS Tablets (Less than 2%) 2573
Cozaar Tablets (Less than 1%) 1668
Cytotec (Infrequent) 2576
Cytovene-IV (Two or more reports) 2270
Demadex Tablets and Injection 691
Demser Capsules (Infrequent) 1690
Desoxyn Gradumet Tablets 422
Desyrel and Desyrel Dividose 504
Dexedrine 2648
DextroStat-Dextroamphetamine Sulfate Tablets 2211
Dilacor XR Extended-release Capsules (Infrequent) 2183
Dipentum Capsules (Rare) 2084
Ditropan 1267
Diupres Tablets 1691
Diuril Oral Suspension 1694
Diuril Sodium Intravenous 1693
Diuril Tablets 1694
Donnatal 2234
Donnatal Extentabs 2234
Donnatal Tablets 2234
Doral Tablets 2773
Dyazide Capsules 2653
DynaCirc Capsules (0.5% to 1%) 2381
DynaCirc CR Tablets (0.5% to 1.0%) 2383
▲ Effexor (2.1% to 6%) 2825
Elavil 2945
Esimil Tablets (A few instances) 840
Eskalith 2658
Ethmozine Tablets (Less than 2%) 2217
Etrafon 2495
▲ Eulexin Capsules (33%) 2498
Fastin Capsules 2662
Flexeril Tablets (Rare) 1701
Haldol Decanoate 1587
Haldol Injection, Tablets and Concentrate 1585
HydroDIURIL Tablets 1716
Hydropres Tablets 1718
Hytrin Capsules (1.2% to 1.6%) 434
Hyzaar Tablets 1720
Imdur (Less than or equal to 5%) 1362
Inderal (Rare) 2834
Inderal LA Long Acting Capsules (Rare) 2836
Inderide Tablets (Rare) 2838
Inderide LA Long Acting Capsules (Rare) 2840
Intron A for Injection (Less than 5%) 2506
Inversine Tablets 1729
Ionamin Capsules 1615
Ismelin Tablets 845
Ismo Tablets (Fewer than 1%) 2844
Isoptin Oral Tablets (Less than 1%) 1393
Isoptin SR Tablets (1% or less) 1395
Kerlone Tablets (1.2%) 2588
Lamictal Tablets (Infrequent) 1105
Levatol Tablets (0.5%) 2547
Levsin/Levsinex/Levbid 2549
Limbitrol (Less common) 2333
Lioresal Intrathecal (0.2% to 1.6%) 1634
Lioresal Tablets (Rare) 847
Lithonate/Lithotabs/Lithobid 2721
Lopid Tablets 1974
Lopressor HCT Tablets (1 in 100 patients) 850
Lotensin Tablets 852
Lotensin HCT Tablets (1.2%) 855
Lotrel Capsules 858
Ludiomil Tablets (Rare) 861
▲ Lupron Depot 7.5 mg (5.4%) 2741
Lupron Depot - 3 Month 22.5 mg (Less than 5%) 2743
▲ Lupron Injection (5% or more) 2736
LUVOX Tablets (2%) 2723
MS Contin Tablets (Less frequent) 2149
MSIR (Infrequent) 2152
Mavik Tablets (0.3% to 1.0%) 1407
▲ Megace Oral Suspension (4% to 14%) 708
Methotrexate Sodium Tablets, Injection, for Injection and LPF Injection (Rare) 1322
Mexitil Capsules (Less than 1% or about 4 in 1,000) 684
Midamor Tablets (Between 1% and 3%) 1746
Minipress Capsules (Less than 1%) 2015
Minizide Capsules (Rare) 2016
Moduretic Tablets (Less than or equal to 1%) 1748
Mykrox Tablets (Less than 2%) 1617
Mysoline (Occasional) 2860
Navane Capsules and Concentrate 2018
Navane Intramuscular 2019
Neurontin Capsules (1.5%) 1978
Nipent for Injection (Less than 3%) 2733
Nizoral Tablets (Less than 1%) 1345
Nolvadex Tablets 2957
▲ Normodyne Injection (1% to 4%) 2519
▲ Normodyne Tablets (1% to 4%) 2522
Norpace (1 to 3%) 2596
Norpramin Tablets 1273
Norvir (Less than 2%) 447
Oramorph SR (Morphine Sulfate Sustained Release Tablets) (Less frequent) 2359
▲ Orap Tablets (3 of 20 patients) 1037
▲ Orlaam Oral Solution (3% to 9%) 2361
Orudis Capsules (Less than 1%) 2874
Oruvail Capsules (Less than 1%) 2874
Oxandrin 783
OxyContin Tablets (Less than 1%) 2163
Pamelor 2409
Parnate Tablets 2679
▲ Paxil Tablets (5% to 10.0%) 2681
Pepcid Injection (Rare) 1765
Pepcid (Rare) 1763
Permax Tablets (Infrequent) 571
Plendil Extended-Release Tablets (0.5% to 1.5%) 514
Prelu-2 Timed Release Capsules 687
Prevacid Delayed-Release Capsules (Less than 1%) 2746
Prinivil Tablets (1.0%) 1776
Prinzide Tablets (1.2%) 1780
Pro-Banthine Tablets 2226
Procardia XL Extended Release Tablets (Less than 3%) 2026
Prolixin 510
▲ Proscar Tablets (3.7%) 1784
Prozac Pulvules & Liquid, Oral Solution (1.7%) 935
Redux Capsules (Rare) 2911
Reglan 2243
Relafen Tablets (Less than 1%) 2688
Remeron Tablets (Infrequent) 1878
Rilutek Tablets (Infrequent) 2198
Robinul Forte Tablets 2247
Robinul Injectable 2247
Robinul Tablets 2247
Roferon-A Injection (Less than 4%) 2308
Rythmol Tablets–150mg, 225mg, 300mg (Less than 1%) 1399
Sanorex Tablets (Rare) 2423
Sectral Capsules (Up to 2%) 2914
Sensorcaine 554
Ser-Ap-Es Tablets 867
Serentil 689
Serzone Tablets (Frequent) 776
Sporanox Capsules (0.2% to 1.2%) 1352
Stelazine 2692
Sular Tablets (Less than or equal to 1%) 2961
Surmontil Capsules 2917
Tagamet 2694
Tambocor Tablets (Less than 1%) 1555
Tegretol/Tegretol-XR 870
▲ Tenex Tablets (Up to 7%) 2249
Tenoretic Tablets 2963
Tenormin Tablets and I.V. Injection 2965
Thalitone 1293
Thorazine 2701
Tiazac Capsules (Less than 1%) 1019
Timolide Tablets 1791
Timoptic in Ocudose (Less frequent) 1796
Timoptic Sterile Ophthalmic Solution (Less frequent) 1794
Timoptic-XE 1798
Tofranil Ampuls 873
Tofranil Tablets 875
Tofranil-PM Capsules 876
Trandate Tablets (1% to 4%) 1158
Trecator-SC Tablets 2919
Trilafon 2532
Vascor Tablets (200 and 300 mg) (0.5 to 2.0%) 1597
Vaseretic Tablets (2.2%) 1810
Vasotec I.V. 1814
Vasotec Tablets (0.5% to 1.0%) 1816
Verelan Capsules (1% or less) 1455
Videx Tablets, Powder for Oral Solution, & Pediatric Powder for Oral Solution (Less than 1%) 2980
Visken Tablets (2% or fewer patients) 2428
Vivactil Tablets 1820
Cataflam/Voltaren/Voltaren-XR (Less than 1%) 833
▲ Wellbutrin Tablets (3.4%) 1177
Winstrol Tablets 2468
Zantac (Occasional) 1182
Zantac Injection 1180
Zantac Syrup (Occasional) 1182
Zaroxolyn Tablets 1625
Zebeta Tablets 1457
Zerit Capsules (Fewer than 1% to 1%) 731
Zestoretic Tablets (1.2%) 2968
Zestril Tablets (1.0%) 2972
Ziac (1.1%) 1459
Zoladex 3-month (1% to 5%) 2978
Zyloprim Tablets (Less than 1%) 1194

Impulse control, impaired
Anafranil Capsules (Rare) 819

Incontinence
Doral Tablets 2773
Halcion Tablets 2093
MetroGel-Vaginal 917
Minipress Capsules (Less than 1%) 2015
Minizide Capsules (Rare) 2016
Moduretic Tablets (Less than or equal to 1%) 1748
Protostat Tablets 1939
Serax Capsules 2916
Serax Tablets 2916
Serentil 689
Supprelin Injection (1% to 3%) 2230
Tensilon Injectable 1307
Valium Injectable 2336
Valium Tablets (Infrequent) 2335
Xanax Tablets (1.5%) 2115

Incontinence, fecal
Betaseron for SC Injection 653
Carbocaine Injection 2432
Cardura Tablets (Less than 0.5% of 3960 patients) 1993
Cognex Capsules (Infrequent) 1961
Cytovene (1% or less) 2270
Depakote Tablets (1% to 5%) 418
Eskalith 2658
Klonopin Tablets 2294
Lioresal Intrathecal (1% or more) 1634
Lithium Carbonate Capsules & Tablets 2352
Lithonate/Lithotabs/Lithobid 2721
LUVOX Tablets (Rare) 2723
Marcaine 2446
Marcaine Spinal 2449
Marinol (Dronabinol) Capsules (Less than 1%) 2353
Neurontin Capsules (Infrequent) 1978
Paxil Tablets (Rare) 2681
Pentasa (Less than 1%) 1275
Permax Tablets (Rare) 571
Prozac Pulvules & Liquid, Oral Solution (Rare) 935
Redux Capsules (Rare) 2911
Rilutek Tablets (Infrequent) 2198
Risperdal Tablets (Rare) 1348
Sensorcaine 554
Zoloft Tablets (Rare) 2051

(▣ Described in PDR For Nonprescription Drugs) Incidence data in parenthesis; ▲ 3% or more (◉ Described in PDR For Ophthalmology)

1375 Side Effects Index Infection, fungal

Zosyn (1.0% or less) 1463

Incontinence, urinary
Ambien Tablets (Infrequent) 2559
Anafranil Capsules (Infrequent) 819
Androderm Testosterone Transdermal System (Less than 1%) 2634
Atamet Tablets 567
Avonex 662
Betaseron for SC Injection 653
Carbocaine Injection 2432
Cardura Tablets (1%) 1993
Casodex Tablets (2%) 2934
Cerebyx Injection (Infrequent) 1956
Clozaril Tablets (1%) 2377
▲Cognex Capsules (3%) 1961
Dantrium Capsules (Less frequent) 2131
Depakote Tablets (1% to 5%) 418
Desyrel and Desyrel Dividose 504
Dizac (diazepam injectable emulsion) CIV (Less frequent) 1862
Doral Tablets 2773
Effexor (Infrequent) 2825
Esimil Tablets 840
Eskalith 2658
Estring Vaginal Ring (1% to 3%) 2086
Ethmozine Tablets (Less than 2%) 2217
Etrafon 2495
▲Felbatol (6.5%) 2774
Flagyl 375 Capsules 2587
Flagyl I.V. 2373
Foscavir Injection (Less than 1%) 541
Helidac Therapy 2135
Humorsol Sterile Ophthalmic Solution (Rare) 1707
Hytrin Capsules (At least 1%) 434
Intron A for Injection (Less than 5%) 2506
Ismelin Tablets 845
Lamictal Tablets (Infrequent) 1105
Larodopa Tablets (Infrequent) 2296
Lioresal Intrathecal (Up to 2.0%) 1634
Lithium Carbonate Capsules & Tablets 2352
Lithonate/Lithotabs/Lithobid 2721
Lupron Depot-PED 7.5 mg, 11.25 mg and 15 mg (Less than 2%) 2744
Lupron Injection (Less than 5%) 2736
Lupron Injection Pediatric (Less than 2%) 2737
LUVOX Tablets (Infrequent) 2723
Marcaine 2446
Marcaine Spinal 2449
Megace Oral Suspension (1% to 3%) 708
Mellaril 2398
Naprelan Tablets (Less than 1%) 2861
Neurontin Capsules (Infrequent) 1978
Parlodel 2411
Parnate Tablets 2679
Paxil Tablets (Infrequent) 2681
Penetrex Tablets (0.1% to 1%) 2196
Permax Tablets (Frequent) 571
ProSom Tablets (Rare) 457
Prozac Pulvules & Liquid, Oral Solution (Infrequent) 935
Redux Capsules (Rare) 2911
Reglan 2243
Remeron Tablets (Infrequent) 1878
Rilutek Tablets (Infrequent) 2198
Risperdal Tablets (Infrequent) 1348
Sensorcaine 554
Serentil 689
Serzone Tablets (Infrequent) 776
Sinemet Tablets 959
Sinemet CR Tablets 961
Tenex Tablets (3% or less) 2249
Tensilon Injectable 1307
▲TheraCys BCG Live (Intravesical) (Up to 6.3%) 911
TICE BCG, USP (2.4%) 1881
Torecan 2367
Vistide Injection 1057
Wellbutrin Tablets (Rare) 1177
Zoladex 3-month (1% to 5%) 2978
Zoloft Tablets (Infrequent) 2051
Zosyn (1.0% or less) 1463

Incoordination (see under Ataxia)

Indecisiveness
Anafranil Capsules (Rare) 819

Indigestion
Adapin Capsules 1542
Asacol Delayed-Release Tablets 2129
Augmentin 2637
Augmentin Tablets 2640
Carafate Suspension (Less than 0.5%) 1250
Carafate Tablets (Less than 0.5%) 1249
▲Cataflam Tablets (3% to 9%) 833
Ceftin (0.1% to 1%) 1067
Colestid (Less frequent) 2073
▲Depakene (Among most common) 416
▲Depakote Tablets (One of the most common) 418
Eskalith 2658
Feldene Capsules (Greater than 1%) 2008
▲Hylorel Tablets (23.7%) 1613
IBU Tablets (Greater than 1%) 1389
▲Indocin (3% to 9%) 1723
Lithonate/Lithotabs/Lithobid 2721
Lopressor HCT Tablets (1 in 100 patients) 850
Motrin Ibuprofen Suspension, Oral Drops, Chewable Tablets, Caplets (1% to less than 3%) 1563
Oncaspar 2194
▲Parlodel (4%) 2411
Sinequan 2028
▲Trilisate (Less than 20%) 2155
▲Cataflam/Voltaren/Voltaren-XR (3% to 9%) 833

Induration at injection site
▲Acel-Imune Diphtheria and Tetanus Toxoids and Acellular Pertussis Vaccine Adsorbed (1.5% to 7%) 1415
▲ActHIB (0.8% to 38.2%) 893
Ancef Injection 2632
▲Aredia for Injection (Up to 41%) 827
Biavax II 1653
▲Brevibloc (esmolol HCl) Injection (About 8%) 1860
Capastat Sulfate Injection 968
Cefizox for Intramuscular or Intravenous Use (1% to 5%) 1025
Cholera Vaccine 2818
▲Claforan Sterile and Injection (4.3%) 1259
Cleocin Phosphate Injection 2068
Dalalone D.P. Injectable 1009
Decadron-LA Sterile Suspension 1687
Demerol 2438
Desferal Vials 838
Diphtheria and Tetanus Toxoids and Pertussis Vaccine Adsorbed 2650
▲Engerix-B Unit-Dose Vials (1% to 10%) 2656
Factrel (Rare) 2996
Fluvirin (Influenza Virus Vaccine) (Less than one-third) 1608
▲Havrix (1% to 10%) 2663
IPOL Poliovirus Vaccine Inactivated (1%) 903
Kefzol Vials, Faspak & ADD-Vantage (Infrequent) 1511
Lupron Depot 3.75 mg 2739
Lupron Depot 7.5 mg 2741
Lupron Depot - 3 Month 22.5 mg 2743
Lupron Depot-PED 7.5 mg, 11.25 mg and 15 mg 2744
Lupron Injection 2736
Lutrepulse for Injection 998
M-M-R II 1730
M-R-VAX II 1732
Mefoxin 1734
Mepergan Injection 2859
Meruvax II 1740
Netromycin Injection 100 mg/ml (4 of 1000 patients) 2516
▲OmniHIB (0.8% to 22.5%) 2676
Oncaspar 2194
PedvaxHIB 1761
Pipracil (2%) 1435
Pneumovax 23 1768
Primaxin I.V. (0.2%) 1772
Rabies Vaccine Adsorbed (A few patients) 2686
Rocephin Injectable Vials, ADD-Vantage, Galaxy Container (1%) 2305
Talwin Injection 2465
Taxol Injection (Rare) 723
Tetanus & Diphtheria Toxoids Adsorbed Purogenated 1446
Ticar for Injection 2704
Timentin for Injection 2706
Tri-Immunol Adsorbed (Common) 1452
Tripedia 908
▲Typhim Vi (Up to 18%) 914
Typhoid Vaccine 2929
▲Varivax (19.35 to 32.5%) 1807
Versed Injection (0.5%-1.7%) 2324

Infantile spasms
Diphtheria and Tetanus Toxoids and Pertussis Vaccine Adsorbed 2650
Tetramune 1449

Infection at injection site
▲Cytovene-IV (9%) 2270
NephrAmine Injection 2169

Infection, bacterial
▲CellCept Capsules (More than or equal to 3%) 2265
Claritin-D Tablets (Less frequent) 2487
Cytosar-U Sterile Powder 2077
Econopred & Econopred Plus Ophthalmic Suspensions ⊙ 216
Foscavir Injection (Between 1% and 5%) 541
Imdur (Less than or equal to 5%) 1362
Invirase Capsules (Less than 2%) 2291
▲Leustatin (42%) 1889
▲Lopid Tablets (More common) 1974
▲Nipent for Injection (5%) 2733
Orthoclone OKT3 Sterile Solution 1892
▲Paraplatin for Injection (14% to 18%) 713

Infection, body as a whole
▲Abelcet Injection (4% to 6%) 1540
Alkeran for Injection 1196
Ambien Tablets (1%) 2559
▲Avonex (11%) 662
Axid Pulvules (1.7%) 1468
Betapace Tablets (1% to 4%) 637
Betaseron for SC Injection 653
Cardene Capsules (Rare) 2261
Cardene SR Capsules (Rare) 2264
Cardura Tablets (Less than 0.5% of 3960 patients) 1993
Cartrol Tablets (Less common) 413
▲Casodex Tablets (10%) 2934
▲CellCept Capsules (18.2% to 20.9%; 12.7% to 15.6%) 2265
Cerebyx Injection (Frequent) 1956
Clozaril Tablets 2377
Compazine 2644
Coumadin 941
▲Cytovene (9%) 2270
Depakote Tablets (1% to 5%) 418
Dilacor XR Extended-release Capsules 2183
Doxil (1% to 5%) 2613
▲Effexor (2.2% to 6%) 2825
▲Fludara for Injection (33% to 44%) 658
▲Foscavir Injection (5% or greater) 541
▲Idamycin Injection (95%) 2096
▲IFEX (8%) 706
▲Lamictal Tablets (4.4%) 1105
▲Leukine (65%) 1317
▲Leustatin (28%) 1889
Lodine Capsules and Tablets (Less than 1%) 2849
Lotensin Tablets 852
Lotensin HCT Tablets (0.3% or more) 855
Lupron Depot-PED 7.5 mg, 11.25 mg and 15 mg (Less than 2%) 2744
Lupron Injection (Less than 5%) 2736
Lupron Injection Pediatric (Less than 2%) 2737
Megace Oral Suspension (1% to 3%) 708
▲Naprelan Tablets (3% to 9%) 2861
Orudis Capsules (Less than 1%) 2874
Oruvail Capsules (Less than 1%) 2874
Permax Tablets (1.1%) 571
Prelone Syrup 1834
Prevacid Delayed-Release Capsules (Less than 1%) 2746
Redux Capsules (Frequent) 2911
Serentil 689
▲Serzone Tablets (8%) 776
Stelazine 2692
TheraCys BCG Live (Intravesical) (2.0% to 2.7%) 911
Toradol (1% or less) 2319
▲Trasylol (6%) 607
▲Videx Tablets, Powder for Oral Solution, & Pediatric Powder for Oral Solution (4% to 7%) 2980
▲Vumon for Injection (12%) 729
Xanax Tablets (1.3%) 2115

Infection, candida albicans
AeroBid Inhaler System 1004
Aerobid-M Inhaler System 1004
▲Cleocin Vaginal Cream (11% to 26%) 2070
Flonase Nasal Spray (Rare) 1088
Rhinocort Nasal Inhaler (Rare) 552

Infection, cecum
Rubex for Injection 721

Infection, colon
Rubex for Injection 721

Infection, conjunctiva
Urobiotic-250 Capsules 2038

Infection, cryptococcus
Orthoclone OKT3 Sterile Solution (1.6%) 1892

Infection, cytomegalovirus
▲CellCept Capsules (8.3% to 13.4%; 3.6% to 15.2%) 2265
▲Doxil (20.1%) 2613
▲Neoral (4.8%) 2405
▲Orthoclone OKT3 Sterile Solution (3% to 19%) 1892
▲Sandimmune (4.8 to 12.3%) 2416

Infection, decreased resistance
Anafranil Capsules (Infrequent) 819
CORTENEMA 2713
Cortifoam 2540
Cytoxan 700
Dalalone D.P. Injectable 1009
Dexacort Phosphate in Respihaler 1606
Dexacort Phosphate in Turbinaire 1607
Methotrexate Sodium Tablets, Injection, for Injection and LPF Injection (Frequent) 1322
Orthoclone OKT3 Sterile Solution 1892
Prelone Syrup 1834
Prograf 1028
Sandimmune 2416

Infection, ears
▲AeroBid Inhaler System (3% to 9%) 1004
▲Aerobid-M Inhaler System (3% to 9%) 1004
Claritin-D Tablets (Less frequent) 2487
Cognex Capsules (Infrequent) 1961
Cytovene-IV (One report) 2270
Neurontin Capsules (Infrequent) 1978
▲PedvaxHIB (Among most frequent) 1761
Tegison Capsules (Less than 1%) 2314

Infection, eyes
Acular Sterile Ophthalmic Solution (0.5%) 470
AeroBid Inhaler System (1% to 3%) 1004
Aerobid-M Inhaler System (1% to 3%) 1004
Decadron Phosphate Sterile Ophthalmic Ointment 1684
Decadron Phosphate Sterile Ophthalmic Solution 1685
Humorsol Sterile Ophthalmic Solution 1707

Infection, eyes, fungal
Blephamide Liquifilm Sterile Ophthalmic Suspension 472
CORTENEMA 2713
Cortisporin Ophthalmic Ointment Sterile 1074
Cortisporin Ophthalmic Suspension Sterile 1075
Pred-G S.O.P. Sterile Ophthalmic Ointment ⊙ 249

Infection, fungal
AK-Trol Ointment & Suspension ⊙ 205
Blephamide Liquifilm Sterile Ophthalmic Suspension 472
Crixivan Capsules (Less than 2%) 1670
Cytosar-U Sterile Powder 2077
Econopred & Econopred Plus Ophthalmic Suspensions ⊙ 216
FML Forte Liquifilm ⊙ 237
FML Liquifilm ⊙ 238
FML S.O.P. ⊙ 239
FML-S Liquifilm ⊙ 240
Foscavir Injection (Between 1% and 5%) 541
Intron A for Injection (Less than 5%) 2506
Invirase Capsules (Less than 2%) 2291
▲Leustatin (20%) 1889
Maxitrol Ophthalmic Ointment and Suspension ⊙ 222
▲Novantrone for Injection (9 to 15%) 1327
▲Orthoclone OKT3 Sterile Solution (4% to 34%) 1892
Penetrex Tablets (0.1% to 1%) 2196
Poly-Pred Liquifilm ⊙ 246

Side Effects Index

Infection, fungal, local
- Doxil (Less than 1%) 2613
- ▲ Neoral (7.5%) 2405
- ▲ Sandimmune (7.5 to 9.6%) 2416
- Vancenase AQ Double Strength Nasal Spray 0.084% (Single cases) 2536
- Vantin for Oral Suspension and Vantin Tablets (Less than 1%) 2112

Infection, fungal, systemic
- Neoral (2.2%) 2405
- Sandimmune (2.2 to 3.9%) 2416

Infection, gastrointestinal
- Adriamycin PFS 2056
- Adriamycin RDF 2056
- Ceftin for Oral Suspension (0.1% to 1%) 1067
- Cytotec (Infrequent) 2576
- Doxorubicin Astra 531

Infection, gram-negative bacteria
- ▲ Orthoclone OKT3 Sterile Solution (1.6% to 7.5%) 1892

Infection, gram-positive bacteria
- ▲ Orthoclone OKT3 Sterile Solution (9.0%) 1892

Infection, herpes simplex
- ▲ Orthoclone OKT3 Sterile Solution (5% to 31%) 1892

Infection, Legionella
- Orthoclone OKT3 Sterile Solution (0.7% to 1.6%) 1892

Infection, localized
- Dermatop Emollient Cream 0.1% 1264
- ▲ Flolan for Injection (21%) 1085
- Norplant System (0.7%) 2868
- ProctoCream-HC 2.5% 2552
- ▲ Proleukin for Injection (23%) 812
- TheraCys BCG Live (Intravesical) (Up to 0.9%) 911

Infection, masking signs of
- AK-PRED .... ⊙ 204
- AK-Trol Ointment & Suspension .. ⊙ 205
- Blephamide Liquifilm Sterile Ophthalmic Suspension 472
- Blephamide Ointment .... ⊙ 234
- CORTENEMA 2713
- Dalalone D.P. Injectable 1009
- Dexacort Phosphate in Respihaler .. 1606
- Dexacort Phosphate in Turbinaire .. 1607
- FML Forte Liquifilm .... ⊙ 237
- FML Liquifilm .... ⊙ 238
- FML S.O.P. .... ⊙ 239
- FML-S Liquifilm .... ⊙ 240
- Florinef Acetate Tablets 506
- Maxitrol Ophthalmic Ointment and Suspension .... ⊙ 222
- NeoDecadron Topical Cream 1757
- Pred Forte .... ⊙ 247
- Pred Mild .... ⊙ 250
- Prelone Syrup 1834
- TobraDex Ophthalmic Suspension and Ointment 469

Infection, mononucleosis-like syndrome
- PASER Granules 1333

Infection, nasal
- Beconase Inhalation Aerosol (Rare) 1065
- Flonase Nasal Spray (Rare) 1088
- Miacalcin Nasal Spray (1% to 3%) 2403

Infection, non-pulmonary
- ▲ Exosurf Neonatal for Intratracheal Suspension (13% to 35%) 1081

Infection, opportunistic
- ▲ Doxil (50.4%) 2613
- Leustatin 1889
- Methotrexate Sodium Tablets, Injection, for Injection and LPF Injection (Rare) 1322

Infection, parasitic
- Cytosar-U Sterile Powder 2077

Infection, pelvis
- ParaGard T 380A Intrauterine Copper Contraceptive 1936
- Wellbutrin Tablets (Rare) 1177

Infection, pharyngeal
- Beconase Inhalation Aerosol (Rare) 1065
- Flonase Nasal Spray (Rare) 1088

Infection, Pneumocystis carinii
(see under Pneumocystis carinii, susceptibility)

Infection, post-treatment, unspecified
- ▲ Survanta Beractant Intratracheal Suspension (10.2 to 20.7%) 2346

Infection, protozoan
- Orthoclone OKT3 Sterile Solution .. 1892

Infection, respiratory
- Accutane Capsules 2252
- Betimol 0.25%, 0.5% (1% to 5%) .... ⊙ 259
- ▲ CellCept Capsules (22.0% to 23.9%; 13.1% to 15.8%) 2265
- Cognex Capsules (Infrequent) 1961
- DDAVP 2180
- Daypro Caplets (Less than 1%) 2578
- Desmopressin Acetate Rhinal Tube 997
- Maxaquin Tablets 2593
- Nalfon 200 Pulvules & Nalfon Tablets (1.5%) 933
- Plendil Extended-Release Tablets (0.5% to 1.5%) 514
- ▲ Serevent Inhalation Aerosol (4%) .. 1149
- TheraCys BCG Live (Intravesical) (Up to 2.7%) 911
- Vascor Tablets (200 and 300 mg) (2.84%) 1597

Infection, sapraphytic
- Cytosar-U Sterile Powder 2077

Infection, secondary
- Aclovate (Infrequent) 1061
- AK-PRED .... ⊙ 204
- AK-Trol Ointment & Suspension .. ⊙ 205
- Analpram-HC Rectal Cream 1% and 2.5% 993
- Anusol-HC Cream 2.5% (Infrequent to frequent) 1953
- Anusol-HC Suppositories 1954
- Bleph-10 Ophthalmic Solution 10% 472
- Blephamide Liquifilm Sterile Ophthalmic Suspension 472
- Blephamide Ointment .... ⊙ 234
- ▲ Cordran Lotion (More frequent) 1854
- ▲ Cordran Tape (More frequent) 1855
- Cormax Ointment (Infrequent) 1856
- Cormax Scalp Application (Infrequent) 1857
- Cortisporin Cream 1073
- Cortisporin Ointment 1074
- Cortisporin Ophthalmic Ointment Sterile 1074
- Cortisporin Ophthalmic Suspension Sterile 1075
- Cortisporin Otic Solution Sterile 1076
- Cortisporin Otic Suspension Sterile 1077
- Cutivate Cream 1078
- Cutivate Ointment (Infrequent to more frequent) 1078
- Decadron Phosphate Sterile Ophthalmic Ointment 1684
- Decadron Phosphate Sterile Ophthalmic Solution 1685
- Decadron Phosphate Topical Cream 1686
- Decaspray Topical Aerosol 1689
- Dermatop Emollient Cream 0.1% (Infrequent to frequent) 1264
- DesOwen Cream, Ointment and Lotion (Infrequent) 1032
- Diprolene AF Cream 0.05% (Infrequent) 2489
- Diprolene Gel 0.05% (Infrequent) .. 2490
- Diprolene Lotion 0.05% (Infrequent) 2491
- Diprolene Ointment 0.05% (Infrequent) 2491
- E.E.S. 427
- Eflone Sterile Ophthalmic Suspension .... ⊙ 261
- Elocon Cream 0.1% (Infrequent) 2492
- Elocon Lotion 0.1% (Infrequent) 2493
- Elocon Ointment 0.1% (Infrequent) 2494
- Epifoam (Infrequent) 2543
- EryPed 200 & EryPed 400 Granules 425
- Ery-Tab Tablets 428
- Erythrocin Stearate Filmtab 429
- FML Forte Liquifilm .... ⊙ 237
- FML Liquifilm .... ⊙ 238
- FML S.O.P. .... ⊙ 239
- FML-S Liquifilm .... ⊙ 240
- Flarex Ophthalmic Suspension .... ⊙ 217
- Florone/Florone E 921
- Halog (Infrequent) 2795
- Hytone 922
- Hytone Ointment 2 ½ % 923
- Ilosone 927
- Ilotycin Gluceptate, IV, Vials 929
- Imuran 1103
- Lidex (Infrequent) 2299
- Locoid Cream, Ointment and Topical Solution (Infrequent) 994
- Lotrisone Cream (1 of 270 patients) 2515
- Mantadil Cream 1124
- Maxitrol Ophthalmic Ointment and Suspension .... ⊙ 222
- NeoDecadron Sterile Ophthalmic Ointment 1755
- NeoDecadron Topical Cream 1757
- Pandel Cream, 0.1% 2475
- Pediotic Suspension Sterile 1140
- Pipracil 1435
- Poly-Pred Liquifilm .... ⊙ 246
- Pramosone Cream, Lotion & Ointment 995
- Pred Forte .... ⊙ 247
- Pred Mild .... ⊙ 250
- Pred-G Liquifilm Sterile Ophthalmic Suspension .... ⊙ 248
- Pred-G S.O.P. Sterile Ophthalmic Ointment .... ⊙ 249
- Prelone Syrup 1834
- ProctoCream-HC 2.5% (Infrequent to frequent) 2552
- ProctoFoam-HC 2552
- Psorcon Cream 0.05% (Infrequent) 924
- Psorcon Ointment 0.05% 923
- Synalar (Infrequent) 2299
- Temovate Cream 1152
- Temovate E Emollient (Infrequent) 1154
- Temovate Gel (Infrequent) 1153
- Temovate Ointment 1152
- Temovate Scalp Application (Infrequent) 1153
- TobraDex Ophthalmic Suspension and Ointment 469
- Topicort Emollient Cream 0.25% (Infrequent) 1289
- Topicort Gel 0.05% (Infrequent) 1290
- Topicort LP Emollient Cream 0.05% (Infrequent) 1289
- Topicort Ointment 0.25% (Infrequent) 1291
- Tridesilon Cream 0.05% (Infrequent) 609
- Tridesilon Ointment 0.05% (Infrequent) 610
- Ultravate Cream 0.05% (Infrequent) 2797
- Ultravate Ointment 0.05% (Less frequent) 2798
- Vexol 1% Ophthalmic Suspension .... ⊙ 227
- Westcort Cream 0.2% (Infrequent) 2799
- Westcort Ointment 0.2% 2800

Infection, Serratia
- Alkeran Tablets 1198
- Orthoclone OKT3 Sterile Solution (1.6%) 1892

Infection, Staphylococcus epidermidis
- ▲ Orthoclone OKT3 Sterile Solution (4.8%) 1892

Infection, trichomonas vaginalis
- Cleocin Vaginal Cream (1%) 2070
- Zosyn (1.0% or less) 1463

Infection, unspecified
- Arimidex Tablets (2% to 5%) 2932
- ▲ Azathioprine Tablets (Less than 1% to 20%) 2349
- Betadine Ointment 2145
- BiCNU 696
- CORTENEMA 2713
- ▲ Ergamisol Tablets (5% to 12%) 1340
- Etopophos for Injection 701
- Etoposide Injection 539
- Etrafon 2495
- Felbatol 2774
- ▲ Gemzar for Injection (3% to 16%) 1482
- Hivid Tablets (Less than 1%) 2287
- ▲ Hycamtin for Injection (26%) 2665
- ▲ Imuran (Less than 1% to 20%) 1103
- ▲ Leucovorin Calcium for Injection (1% to 8%) 1313
- LUVOX Tablets 2723
- Methotrexate Sodium Tablets, Injection, for Injection and LPF Injection (Less common) 1322
- Neoral (0.9%) 2405
- ▲ Nipent for Injection (7% to 36%) .. 2733
- ▲ Paraplatin for Injection (5%) 713
- Paxil Tablets 2681
- Platinol for Injection 717
- ▲ Proleukin for Injection (23%) 812
- ▲ Taxol Injection (30%) 723
- Taxotere for Injection Concentrate 2204
- Tiazac Capsules (2%) 1019
- VePesid Capsules and Injection 727
- ▲ Vesanoid Capsules (58%) 2327
- ▲ Videx Tablets, Powder for Oral Solution, & Pediatric Powder for Oral Solution (4% to 7%) 2980
- ▲ Vistide Injection (12% to 25%) 1057
- Wellbutrin Tablets (Rare) 1177
- ▲ Zinecard Injection (19% to 23%) .. 2120
- ▲ Zoladex (13%) 2976
- Zoladex 3-month 2978

Infection, upper respiratory
- ▲ Acel-Imune Diphtheria and Tetanus Toxoids and Acellular Pertussis Vaccine Adsorbed (6%) 1415
- ▲ Actigall Capsules (15.5%) 818
- ▲ AeroBid Inhaler System (25%) 1004
- ▲ Aerobid-M Inhaler System (25%) .. 1004
- Altace Capsules 1238
- ▲ Ambien Tablets (5%) 2559
- ▲ Aredia for Injection (Up to 23.2%) 827
- ▲ Atrovent Inhalation Solution (13.2%) 675
- ▲ Atrovent Nasal Spray 0.03% (9.8%) 676
- ▲ Avonex (31%) 662
- ▲ Caverject Injection (4%) 2064
- Ceftin for Oral Suspension (0.1% to 1%) 1067
- Claritin Tablets (2% or fewer patients) 2485
- Claritin-D Tablets (Less frequent) .. 2487
- ▲ Cleocin Vaginal Cream (3%) 2070
- Cognex Capsules (3%) 1961
- ▲ Covera-HS Tablets (5.4%) 2573
- ▲ Cozaar Tablets (7.9%) 1668
- Crixivan Capsules (Less than 2%) .. 1670
- Cytotec (Infrequent) 2576
- DDAVP 2180
- Daypro Caplets (Less than 1%) 2578
- Dipentum Capsules (1.5%) 2084
- ▲ Epogen for Injection (11%) 489
- ▲ Estring Vaginal Ring (5%) 2086
- Famvir Tablets (.07% to 3.3%) 2660
- ▲ Felbatol (5.3% to 45.2%) 2774
- ▲ Flovent (15% to 31%) 1089
- ▲ Fludara for Injection (2% to 16%) 658
- Havrix (Less than 1%) 2663
- Helidac Therapy (1.0%) 2135
- ▲ Hyzaar Tablets (6.1%) 1720
- Invirase Capsules (Less than 2%) .. 2291
- Ismo Tablets (Fewer than 1%) 2844
- Kerlone Tablets (2.6%) 2588
- ▲ Lescol Capsules (16.2%) 2395
- Levatol Tablets (2.5%) 2547
- Lotensin HCT Tablets (More than 1%) 855
- ▲ LUVOX Tablets (9%) 2723
- Mavik Tablets (0.3% to 1.0%) 1407
- Methotrexate Sodium Tablets, Injection, for Injection and LPF Injection (Less common) 1322
- Miacalcin Nasal Spray (1% to 3%) 2403
- Monoket Tablets (Up to 4%) 2550
- Monopril Tablets (2.2%) 762
- ▲ Nipent for Injection (13% to 16%) 2733
- Oncaspar (Less than 1%) 2194
- ▲ PedvaxHIB (Among most frequent) 1761
- ▲ Plendil Extended-Release Tablets (0.7% to 3.9%) 514
- Prevacid Delayed-Release Capsules (Less than 1%) 2746
- Prilosec Delayed-Release Capsules (1.9%) 516
- Prinivil Tablets (1.2% to 1.5%) 1776
- Prinzide Tablets (2.2%) 1780
- Procardia XL Extended Release Tablets (1% or less) 2026
- ▲ Procrit for Injection (11%) 1896
- Prolixin 510
- ▲ Propulsid (3.1%) 1346
- ▲ Prozac Pulvules & Liquid, Oral Solution (7.6%) 935
- Recombivax HB (Equal to or greater than 1%) 1787
- ▲ Risperdal Tablets (3%) 1348
- Rowasa (1.8%) 2727

(⊙ Described in PDR For Nonprescription Drugs)   Incidence data in parenthesis; ▲ 3% or more   (⊙ Described in PDR For Ophthalmology)

Seldane-D Extended-Release Tablets (1.3%) 1286
▲ Serevent Inhalation Aerosol (14%) 1149
Sinemet CR Tablets (1.8%) 961
▲ Stadol (3% to 9%) 779
Stimate, (desmopressin acetate) Nasal Spray, 1.5 mg/mL 806
▲ Supprelin Injection (1% to 10%) 2230
▲ Taxol Injection (One of the two most frequently reported infectious complications) 723
▲ Tetramune (Among most common) 1449
▲ Tilade Inhaler (3.9%) 2207
Timoptic in Ocudose (Less frequent) 1796
Timoptic Sterile Ophthalmic Solution (Less frequent) 1794
Timoptic-XE (1% to 5% of patients) 1798
Univasc Tablets (More than 1%) 2553
Vaqta (1.1% to 2.8%) 1805
Vaseretic Tablets 1810
Vasotec I.V. 1814
Vasotec Tablets (0.5% to 1.0%) 1816
▲ Xalatan (Approximately 4%) ⊙ 304
▲ Xanax Tablets (4.3%) 2115
▲ Zebeta Tablets (4.8% to 5.0%) 1457
Zestoretic Tablets (2.2%) 2968
Zestril Tablets (1.5% to 2.0%) 2972
Ziac (Up to 2.1%) 1459
Zocor Tablets (2.1%) 1821
▲ Zoladex (7%) 2976
Zoladex 3-month 2978
Zyrtec Tablets (Less than 2%) 2053

Infection, urinary tract

▲ Actigall Capsules (6.5%) 818
All-Flex Arcing Spring Diaphragm (See also Ortho Diaphragm Kits) 1921
Ambien Tablets (2%) 2559
Androderm Testosterone Transdermal System (Less than 1%) 2634
▲ Aredia for Injection (At least 15%) 827
Arimidex Tablets (2% to 5%) 2932
Atrovent Inhalation Solution (Less than 3%) 675
Cardura Tablets (1.4%) 1993
▲ Casodex Tablets (6%) 2934
Ceftin for Oral Suspension (0.1% to 1%) 1067
▲ CellCept Capsules (37.0% to 37.2%; 44.4% to 45.5%) 2265
▲ Cleocin Vaginal Cream (8%) 2070
▲ Cognex Capsules (3%) 1961
Cozaar Tablets (Less than 1%) 1668
Crixivan Capsules (Less than 2%) 1670
Cytovene (1% or less) 2270
Depo-Provera Contraceptive Injection (Fewer than 1%) 2079
Dilacor XR Extended-release Capsules 2183
Effexor 2825
Ergamisol Tablets (1 out of 463 patients) 1340
Estring Vaginal Ring (2%) 2086
▲ Felbatol (3.4%) 2774
▲ Fludara for Injection (2% to 15%) 658
Foscavir Injection (Between 1% and 5%) 541
Hytrin Capsules (0.5% to 1.3%) 434
Hyzaar Tablets 1720
Imdur (Less than or equal to 5%) 1362
Intron A for Injection (Less than 5%) 2506
Invirase Capsules (Less than 2%) 2291
Lamictal Tablets (More than 1%; infrequent) 1105
▲ Lopid Tablets (More common) 1974
Lotensin Tablets 852
Lotensin HCT Tablets (0.3% or more) 855
▲ Lupron Injection (5% or more) 2736
LUVOX Tablets (Infrequent) 2723
Megace Oral Suspension (1% to 3%) 708
▲ Naprelan Tablets (3% to 9%) 2861
▲ Neoral (21.1%) 2405
▲ Nipent for Injection (3%) 2733
▲ Novantrone for Injection (7%) 1327
Ortho Diaphragm Kits—All-Flex Arcing Spring; Ortho Coil Spring; Ortho-White Flat Spring 1921
Paxil Tablets (2%) 2681
Prilosec Delayed-Release Capsules (Less than 1%) 516
Prinivil Tablets (0.3% to 1.0%) 1776
Prinzide Tablets (0.3 to 1%) 1780
▲ Prograf (16% to 19%) 1028
▲ Proleukin for Injection (23%) 812
Propulsid (2.4%) 1346
Prozac Pulvules & Liquid, Oral Solution (1.2%) 935
Redux Capsules (Frequent) 2911
Remeron Tablets (Frequent) 1878
ReoPro Vials (1.9%) 1526
▲ Rilutek Tablets (2.5% to 4.5%) 2198
▲ Sandimmune (20.2 to 21.1%) 2416
Sandostatin Injection (1% to 4%) 2421
Serzone Tablets (2%) 776
Sinemet CR Tablets (2.2%) 961
▲ Taxol Injection (One of the two most frequently reported infectious complications) 723
Testoderm Testosterone Transdermal System (Four in 104 patients) 486
TICE BCG, USP (1.5%) 1881
Tolectin (200, 400 and 600 mg) (1 to 3%) 1591
▲ Trasylol (3%) 607
Vaseretic Tablets (0.5% to 2.0%) 1810
Vasotec I.V. 1814
Vasotec Tablets (1.3%) 1816
Vistide Injection 1057
Wellbutrin Tablets (Infrequent) 1177
Zestoretic Tablets (0.3 to 1%) 2968
Zestril Tablets (0.3% to 1.0%) 2972
Zoladex (1% or greater but less than 5%) 2976
Zoladex 3-month (1% to 5%) 2978
Zyrtec Tablets (Less than 2%) 2053

Infection, vagina

Micronor Tablets 1903
Modicon 1928
Norplant System (Uncommon) 2868
Ortho-Cyclen/Ortho-Tri-Cyclen 1914
Ortho-Novum 1928
Ortho-Cyclen/Ortho Tri-Cyclen 1914
Supprelin Injection (1% to 3%) 2230

Infection, viral

Accupril Tablets (0.5 to 1.0%) 1950
▲ Actigall Capsules (19.4%) 818
Blephamide Liquifilm Sterile Ophthalmic Suspension 472
Blephamide Ointment ⊙ 234
Claritin-D Tablets (Less frequent) 2487
Cortisporin Ophthalmic Ointment Sterile 1074
Cortisporin Ophthalmic Suspension Sterile 1075
Cytosar-U Sterile Powder 2077
Econopred & Econopred Plus Ophthalmic Suspensions ⊙ 216
FML Forte Liquifilm ⊙ 237
FML Liquifilm ⊙ 238
FML S.O.P. ⊙ 239
Foscavir Injection (Less than 1%) 541
Imdur (Less than or equal to 5%) 1362
Intron A for Injection (Less than 5%) 2506
Koāte-HP Antihemophilic Factor (Human) 624
Konȳne 80 Factor IX Complex 627
▲ Leustatin (20%) 1889
▲ Lopid Tablets (More common) 1974
▲ Neoral (15.9%) 2405
Neurontin Capsules (More than 1%) 1978
▲ Nipent for Injection (Up to 8%) 2733
Orthoclone OKT3 Sterile Solution (1.5%) 1892
Prinivil Tablets (0.3% to 1.0%) 1776
Prinzide Tablets (0.3% to 1%) 1780
Prolastin Alpha$_1$-Proteinase Inhibitor (Human) 629
▲ Propulsid (3.6%) 1346
▲ Prozac Pulvules & Liquid, Oral Solution (3.4%) 935
▲ Sandimmune (15.9 to 18.4%) 2416
▲ Supprelin Injection (1% to 10%) 2230
Tilade Inhaler (2.4%) 2207
Voltaren Ophthalmic Sterile Ophthalmic Solution (Less than or equal to 1%) ⊙ 264
Zestoretic Tablets (0.3 to 1%) 2968
Zestril Tablets (0.3% to 1.0%) 2972

Infectious-mononucleosis-like syndrome

Dapsone Tablets USP 1331

Infertility

Cytovene-IV (Two or more reports) 2270
Leukeran Tablets 1205
Lo/Ovral Tablets 2852
Lo/Ovral-28 Tablets 2857
Methotrexate Sodium Tablets, Injection, for Injection and LPF Injection 1322
Nordette-21 Tablets (discontinued) 2863
Nordette-28 Tablets 2866
Ovral Tablets 2877
Ovral-28 Tablets 2878
Ovrette Tablets 2878
ParaGard T 380A Intrauterine Copper Contraceptive 1936
Zyloprim Tablets (Less than 1%) 1194

Infertility, male

Azulfidine 2059
Dapsone Tablets USP 1331

Infertility, temporary

Brevicon 2563
Demulen 2580
Desogen Tablets 1867
Levlen/Tri-Levlen 646
Modicon 1928
Norinyl 2563
Nor-Q D Tablets 2598
Ortho-Cept 1907
Ortho-Cyclen/Ortho-Tri-Cyclen 1914
Ortho-Novum 1928
Ortho-Cyclen/Ortho Tri-Cyclen 1914
Ovcon 765
Levlen/Tri-Levlen 646
Tri-Norinyl 2607
Triphasil-21 Tablets 2919
Triphasil-28 Tablets 2924

Inflammation

AMVISC Plus (Rare) ⊙ 327
Adalat Capsules (10 mg and 20 mg) (2% or less) 580
▲ Calcimar Injection, Synthetic (10%) 2176
Ceptaz (1 in 69 patients) 1070
Chloromycetin Ophthalmic Ointment, 1% ⊙ 298
Decadron-LA Sterile Suspension 1687
Exact ■ 722
Fluoroplex Topical Solution & Cream 1% 475
Lupron Injection (Less than 5%) 2736
ParaGard T 380A Intrauterine Copper Contraceptive 1936
Prilosec Delayed-Release Capsules (Less than 1%) 516
Procardia Capsules (2% or less) 2024
Terramycin with Polymyxin B Sulfate Ophthalmic Ointment (Rare) 2035
Zestoretic Tablets (0.3 to 1%) 2968

Inflammation, genital

▲ Condylox Topical Solution (71% to 63%) 1853
TICE BCG, USP (1.8%) 1881

Inflammation, ocular

AMO Vitrax Viscoelastic Solution ⊙ 229
Benzamycin Topical Gel (Occasional) 919
Betoptic Ophthalmic Solution 465
Betoptic S Ophthalmic Suspension (Small number of patients) 467
Dilacor XR Extended-release Capsules 2183
▲ Ilotycin Ophthalmic Ointment (Among most frequent) 928
IOPIDINE Sterile Ophthalmic Solution (0.45%) ⊙ 218
Rilutek Tablets (Infrequent) 2198
TERAK Ointment (Rare) ⊙ 210

Inflammation, oral (see under Stomatitis)

Inflammation, perianal

▲ Cytosar-U Sterile Powder (Among most frequent) 2077
Doryx Capsules 1970
Rubex for Injection 721

Inflammation, upper respiratory tract

Prevacid Delayed-Release Capsules (Less than 1%) 2746
Solganal Suspension 2530

Inflammation, uterine

Anafranil Capsules (Rare) 819

Inflammation at application site

▲ Androderm Testosterone Transdermal System (7%) 2634
Benzamycin Topical Gel (Occasional) 919
▲ Estraderm Transdermal System (About 17%) 842
Vivelle Transdermal System 880

Inflammation at injection site

Abelcet Injection 1540
Ambien Tablets (Rare) 2559
▲ Aredia for Injection (Up to 41%) 827
▲ Avonex (3%) 662
▲ Betaseron for SC Injection (85%) 653
▲ Brevibloc (esmolol HCl) Injection (About 8%) 1860
▲ Calcimar Injection, Synthetic (About 10%) 2176
Caverject Injection 2064
Ceptaz (One in 69 patients) 1070
Cerebyx Injection (Infrequent) 1956
▲ Claforan Sterile and Injection (4.3%) 1259
Cytovene-IV (2%) 2270
Dalalone D.P. Injectable 1009
▲ Dalgan Injection (3 to 9%) 529
DaunoXome (Two patients) 1842
Diprivan Injectable Emulsion (Less than 1%) 2939
Dobutrex Solution Vials 1480
Estratest 2718
Fluvirin (Influenza Virus Vaccine) (Less than one-third) 1608
Fortaz (1 in 69 patients) 1092
Foscavir Injection (Between 1% and 5%) 541
Genotropin Injection (Infrequent) 2090
Geref (sermorelin acetate for injection) 2995
▲ Havrix (1% to 10%) 2663
Humalog Injection 1488
Humulin 50/50, 100 Units 1491
Humulin 70/30, 100 Units 1492
Humulin L, 100 Units 1494
Regular, 100 Units 1503
Pork Regular, 100 Units 1507
INFeD (Iron Dextran Injection, USP) 2478
▲ Intron A for Injection (Up to 7%) 2506
▲ JE-VAX (2.9% to approximately 20%) 904
Levoprome 1321
Lutrepulse for Injection 998
Maxipime for Injection (0.6%) 758
▲ Merrem I.V. (3.0%) 2952
▲ Miacalcin Injection (About 10%) 2402
RespiGam (1%) 1631
Rifadin I.V. 1276
Roferon-A Injection (Rare) 2308
Romazicon 2311
Septra I.V. Infusion 1142
▲ Supprelin Injection (45%) 2230
Taxotere for Injection Concentrate 2204
Tazicef for Injection (Less than 2%) 2697
Tazidime Vials, Faspak & ADD-Vantage (1 in 69) 1531
Testred Capsules, 10 mg 1308
Tetanus & Diphtheria Toxoids Adsorbed Purogenated (Mild to moderate) 1446
Vancocin HCl, Vials & ADD-Vantage 1534
Varivax (Less than 0.05%) 1807
Versed Injection (0.5%-2.6%) 2324
▲ Zofran Injection (4%) 1227
Zosyn (0.2% to 1.3%) 1463
▲ Zovirax Sterile Powder (Approximately 9%) 1191

Influenza-like symptoms

Ambien Tablets (2%) 2559
▲ Atrovent Inhalation Solution (3.7%) 675
Cardura Tablets (Less than 0.5% of 3960 patients to 1.1%) 1993
Engerix-B Unit-Dose Vials (Less than 1%) 2656
▲ Flovent (Up to 13%) 1089
Foscavir Injection (Between 1% and 5%) 541
Hespan Injection 945
Imitrex Injection (Rare) 1095
Invirase Capsules (Less than 2%) 2291
Maxaquin Tablets (Less than 1%) 2593
Monopril Tablets (0.4% to 1.0%) 762
Plendil Extended-Release Tablets (0.5% to 1.5%) 514
Pravachol Tablets (Up to 2.4%) 770
Prinivil Tablets (0.3%) 1776
Prinzide Tablets (0.3% to 1%) 1780
Prozac Pulvules & Liquid, Oral Solution (1.2%) 935

(■ Described in PDR For Nonprescription Drugs) Incidence data in parenthesis; ▲ 3% or more (⊙ Described in PDR For Ophthalmology)

Influenza-like symptoms Side Effects Index 1378

Recombivax HB (Less than 1%) 1787
Zestoretic Tablets (0.3 to 1%) 2968
Zestril Tablets (0.3%) 2972
▲ Zoladex (5%) 2976
Zoladex 3-month (1% to 5%) 2978

Insomnia

Accupril Tablets (0.5% to 1.0%) .. 1950
Accutane Capsules 2252
Actifed Cold & Allergy Tablets .... ▣ 807
Actifed Cold & Sinus Caplets and Tablets .... ▣ 808
▲ Actigall Capsules (1.9%) 818
Acutrim .... ▣ 648
Adalat CC (Less than 1.0%) 582
Adderall Tablets 2209
Adipex-P Tablets and Capsules 1035
Advil Cold and Sinus Caplets and Tablets .... ▣ 837
AeroBid Inhaler System (1% to 3%) 1004
Aerobid-M Inhaler System (1% to 3%) 1004
Airet Albuterol Sulfate Inhalation Solution (1% to 3.1%) 1602
Albuterol Sulfate, USP Solution for Inhalation, Arm-a-Med (1% to 3.1%) 522
Alferon N Injection (2%) 2142
Alka-Seltzer Plus .... ▣ 611
Alka-Seltzer Plus Sinus Medicine ▣ 611
Allerest Maximum Strength .... ▣ 649
Allerest No Drowsiness .... ▣ 649
Allerest Sinus Pain Formula .... ▣ 649
Altace Capsules (Less than 1%) 1238
Alupent Tablets (1.8%) 672
Ambien Tablets (Frequent) 2559
Amen Tablets 785
Amoxil (Rare) 2631
▲ Anafranil Capsules (11% to 25%) 819
Anaprox/Naprosyn (Less than 1%) 2277
Aredia for Injection (Up to 1%) 827
Arimidex Tablets (2% to 5%) 2932
Asacol Delayed-Release Tablets 2129
Asendin Tablets (Less frequent) 1419
Atamet Tablets 567
Atrohist Plus Tablets 1605
Atrovent Inhalation Aerosol (Less than 1%) 674
Atrovent Inhalation Solution (0.9%) 675
Augmentin (Rare) 2637
Augmentin Tablets (Rare) 2640
Axid Pulvules (2.7%) 1468
Azactam for Injection (Less than 1%) 736
Azulfidine (Rare) 2059
Bactrim DS Tablets 2257
Bactrim I.V. Infusion 2255
Bactrim 2257
Benadryl Allergy Decongestant Liquid Medication .... ▣ 812
Benadryl Allergy Decongestant Tablets .... ▣ 812
Benadryl Allergy Sinus Headache Caplets .... ▣ 813
Benadryl Injection 1955
Bentyl 1246
Benylin Multisymptom .... ▣ 816
Betoptic Ophthalmic Solution (Rare) 465
Betoptic S Ophthalmic Suspension (Rare) 467
Biaxin 406
Blocadren Tablets (Less than 1%) 1654
Bontril Slow-Release Capsules 786
Brethaire Inhaler 830
Bromfed 1832
▲ Bromfed-DM Cough Syrup (Among most frequent) 1832
Bromfed-PD Capsules (Extended-Release) 1832
Bronkometer Aerosol 2432
Bronkosol Solution 2432
▲ BuSpar Tablets (3%) 738
Butisol Sodium Elixir & Tablets (Less than 1 in 100) 2768
Calan SR Caplets (1% or less) 2571
Calan Tablets (1% or less) 2568
Capoten Tablets (About 0.5 to 2%) 740
Capozide Tablets (0.5 to 2%) 744
Carafate Suspension (Less than 0.5%) 1250
Carafate Tablets (Less than 0.5%) 1249
Cardene Capsules (0.6%) 2261
Cardizem CD Capsules (Less than 1%) 1251
Cardizem SR Capsules (1%) 1255
Cardizem Injectable 1253
Cardizem Tablets (Less than 1%) .. 1257
Cardura Tablets (1% to 1.2%) 1993
Cartrol Tablets (1.7%) 413
▲ Casodex Tablets (5%) 2934
Cataflam Tablets (Less than 1%) 833
Catapres Tablets (About 5 in 1,000 patients) 679
Catapres-TTS (2 of 101 patients) .. 680
Ceclor Pulvules & Suspension (Rare) 1470
Cedax (0.1% to 1%) 2480
Cefzil Tablets and Oral Suspension (Less than 1%) 747
Celestone Soluspan Suspension 2484
▲ CellCept Capsules (8.9% to 11.8%) 2265
Celontin Kapseals 1955
Cerebyx Injection (Infrequent) 1956
Cerose DM .... ▣ 853
Children's TYLENOL Cold Multi-Symptom Chewable Tablets and Liquid 1559
Children's Vicks DayQuil Allergy Relief .... ▣ 730
Children's Vicks NyQuil Cold/Cough Relief .... ▣ 731
Chlor-Trimeton Allergy Decongestant Tablets .... ▣ 759
Cipro I.V. (1% or less) 587
Cipro I.V. Pharmacy Bulk Package (Less than 1%) 590
Cipro Tablets (Less than 1%) 584
Claritin Tablets (2% or fewer patients) 2485
▲ Claritin-D Tablets (16%) 2487
Clinoril Tablets (Less than 1%) 1658
Clomid (Fewer than 1%) 1262
Clozaril Tablets (2%) 2377
▲ Cognex Capsules (6%) 1961
Colestid (Infrequent) 2073
Combipres Tablets (About 5 in 1,000) 682
Compazine (Sometimes) 2644
Allergy-Sinus Comtrex Multi-Symptom Allergy-Sinus Formula Tablets and Caplets .... ▣ 639
Condylox Topical Solution (Less than 5%) 1853
Contac Continuous Action Nasal Decongestant/Antihistamine 12 Hour Capsules .... ▣ 773
Contac Maximum Strength Continuous Action Decongestant/Antihistamine 12 Hour Caplets .... ▣ 772
Contac Severe Cold and Flu Formula Caplets .... ▣ 773
Cordarone Tablets (1 to 3%) 2818
Coricidin 'D' Decongestant Tablets .... ▣ 760
CORTENEMA 2713
Cortifoam 2540
Cortone Acetate Sterile Suspension 1663
Cortone Acetate Tablets 1664
Covera-HS Tablets (Less than 2%) 2573
Cozaar Tablets (1.4%) 1668
▲ Crixivan Capsules (3.1%) 1670
Cycrin Tablets 991
▲ Cylert Tablets (Most frequent) 415
Cytovene (1% or less) 2270
D.A. II Tablets 972
D.A. Chewable Tablets 970
Dantrium Capsules (Less frequent) 2131
Dapsone Tablets USP 1331
Daraprim Tablets (Rare) 1199
DaunoXome (Up to 6%) 1842
Decadron Elixir 1676
Decadron Phosphate Injection 1680
Decadron Phosphate with Xylocaine Injection, Sterile 1683
Decadron Tablets 1678
Decadron-LA Sterile Suspension 1687
Deconsal II Tablets 1605
Demadex Tablets and Injection (1.2%) 691
Demser Capsules 1690
Demulen 2580
Depakote Tablets (1% to 5%) 418
Depo-Provera Contraceptive Injection (1% to 5%) 2079
Depo-Provera Sterile Aqueous Suspension 2083
Desoxyn Gradumet Tablets 422
▲ Desyrel and Desyrel Dividose (6.4% to 9.9%) 504
Dexacort Phosphate in Respihaler .. 1606
Dexacort Phosphate in Turbinaire .. 1607
Dexatrim .... ▣ 795
Dexatrim Plus Vitamins Caplets .. ▣ 796
Dexedrine 2648
DextroStat-Dextroamphetamine Sulfate Tablets 2211
Dilacor XR Extended-release Capsules (1.0%) 2183
Dilantin Infatabs 1967
Dilantin Kapseals 1965
Dilantin-125 Suspension 1969
Dilaudid-HP Injection (Less frequent) 1384
Dilaudid-HP Lyophilized Powder 250 mg (Less frequent) 1384
Dilaudid Tablets and Liquid (Less frequent) 1386
Dimetane-DC Cough Syrup 2232
Dimetane-DX Cough Syrup 2233
Dimetapp Cold & Allergy Chewable Tablets .... ▣ 838
Dimetapp Extentabs .... ▣ 841
Dimetapp Tablets/Liqui-Gels .... ▣ 841
Dipentum Capsules (Rare) 2084
Diprivan Injectable Emulsion (Less than 1%) 2939
Ditropan 1267
Dizac (diazepam injectable emulsion) CIV (Less frequent) 1862
Dolobid Tablets (Greater than 1 in 100) 1695
Donnatal 2234
Donnatal Extentabs 2234
Donnatal Tablets 2234
Dorcol Children's Cough Syrup .... ▣ 748
Doxil (Less than 1%) 2613
Drixoral Cold and Allergy Sustained-Action Tablets .... ▣ 763
Drixoral Cold and Flu Extended-Release Tablets .... ▣ 764
Dura-Tap/PD Capsules 970
Duratuss Tablets 2750
Dura-Vent/DA Tablets 972
Dura-Vent Tablets 971
Dynabac (1.0%) 668
DynaCirc Capsules (0.5% to 1%) .. 2381
DynaCirc CR Tablets (0.5% to 1.0%) 2383
EC-Naprosyn Delayed-Release Tablets (Less than 1%) 2277
▲ Effexor (3% to 22.5%) 2825
Efidac/24 .... ▣ 655
Efudex 2280
Elavil 2945
Eldepryl Capsules (1 of 49 patients) 2729
▲ Emcyt Capsules (3%) 2085
Emete-con Intramuscular/Intravenous 2007
Engerix-B Unit-Dose Vials (Less than 1%) 2656
Entex LA Tablets 972
Entex PSE Tablets 973
▲ Epivir (11%) 1200
Ergamisol Tablets (1%) 1340
▲ Estring Vaginal Ring (4%) 2086
Etrafon 2495
Exgest LA Tablets 787
Famvir Tablets (1.5% to 2.5%) 2660
Fansidar Tablets 2281
Fastin Capsules 2662
Fedahist Gyrocaps 2545
▲ Felbatol (Among most common; 8.6% to 17.5%) 2774
Feldene Capsules (Less than 1%) .. 2008
Fioricet with Codeine Capsules 2387
Fiorinal with Codeine Capsules 2390
Flagyl 375 Capsules 2587
Flagyl I.V. 2373
Flexeril Tablets (Less than 1%) 1701
▲ Flolan for Injection (4%) 1085
Florinef Acetate Tablets 506
▲ Flovent (3% to 13%) 1089
▲ Floxin I.V. (3% to 7%) 1580
▲ Floxin Tablets (200 mg, 300 mg, 400 mg) (3% to 7%) 1577
Flumadine Tablets & Syrup (2.1% to 3.4%) 1013
Foscavir Injection (Between 1% and 5%) 541
Fulvicin P/G Tablets (Occasional) .. 2499
Fulvicin P/G 165 & 330 Tablets (Occasional) 2500
Gantanol Tablets 2285
Gantrisin 2286
Gastrocrom Capsules (Infrequent) .. 1611
Gastrocrom Oral Concentrate (Less common) 1611
Gemzar for Injection (Infrequent) 1482
Glucotrol XL Extended Release Tablets (Less than 3%) 2012
Grifulvin V (griseofulvin tablets) Microsize (griseofulvin oral suspension) Microsize (Occasional) 1944
Gris-PEG Tablets, 125 mg & 250 mg (Occasional) 476
Guaimax-D Tablets 809
▲ Habitrol Nicotine Transdermal System (3% to 9% of patients) .. 884
Halcion Tablets (Rare) 2093
Haldol Decanoate 1587
Haldol Injection, Tablets and Concentrate 1585
Havrix (Less than 1%) 2663
Helidac Therapy (1.0%) 2135
Histussin D Liquid 670
Hivid Tablets (Less than 1%) 2287
Hydeltrasol Injection, Sterile 1708
Hydeltra-T.B.A. Sterile Suspension 1710
Hydrocortone Acetate Sterile Suspension 1712
Hydrocortone Phosphate Injection, Sterile 1713
Hydrocortone Tablets 1715
Hytrin Capsules (At least 1%) 434
Hyzaar Tablets 1720
IBU Tablets (Less than 1%) 1389
Imdur (Less than or equal to 5%) .. 1362
Inderal 2834
Inderal LA Long Acting Capsules 2836
Inderide Tablets 2838
Inderide LA Long Acting Capsules .. 2840
Indocin (Less than 1%) 1723
▲ Intron A for Injection (Up to 11%) 2506
Invirase Capsules (Less than 2%) .. 2291
Ionamin Capsules 1615
IOPIDINE Sterile Ophthalmic Solution .... ⊙ 218
Iopidine 0.5% (Less than 1%) .... ⊙ 219
Ismo Tablets (Fewer than 1%) 2844
Isoetharine Inhalation Solution, USP, Arm-a-Med 545
Isoptin Oral Tablets (Less than 1%) 1393
Isoptin SR Tablets (1% or less) 1395
Kadian Capsules (Less than 3%) 2948
▲ Kerlone Tablets (1.2% to 5%) 2588
Klonopin Tablets 2294
Kytril Injection (Less than 2%) 2667
▲ Kytril Tablets (3%) 2669
▲ Lamictal Tablets (5.6%) 1105
Larodopa Tablets (Relatively frequent) 2296
Lescol Capsules (2.7%) 2395
▲ Leukine (11%) 1317
▲ Leustatin (7%) 1889
Levatol Tablets (1.9%) 2547
Levbid Extended-Release Tablets 2549
Levlen/Tri-Levlen 646
Levo-Dromoran 2297
Levsin/Levsinex/Levbid 2549
Lioresal Intrathecal (Up to 1.6%) .. 1634
▲ Lioresal Tablets (2% to 7%) 847
Lodine Capsules and Tablets (Less than 1%) 2849
Lopressor 848
Lopressor HCT Tablets 850
Lorabid Suspension and Pulvules 1513
Lotensin Tablets 852
Lotensin HCT Tablets (0.3% to 1.0%) 855
Lotrel Capsules 858
Loxitane 1426
Ludiomil Tablets (2%) 861
Lufyllin & Lufyllin-400 Tablets 2778
Lufyllin-GG Elixir & Tablets 2779
Lupron Depot 3.75 mg (Less than 5%) 2739
Lupron Depot 7.5 mg (Less than 5%) 2741
▲ Lupron Depot - 3 Month 22.5 mg (8.5%) 2743
▲ Lupron Injection (5% or more) 2736
▲ LUVOX Tablets (21%) 2723
MS Contin Tablets (Less frequent) 2149
MSIR (Infrequent) 2152
Marax Tablets & DF Syrup 2015
Matulane Capsules 2300
Mavik Tablets (0.3% to 1.0%) 1407
Maxair Autohaler 1550
Maxair Inhaler (Less than 1%) 1552
Maxaquin Tablets (Less than 1%) .. 2593
Mebaral Tablets (Less than 1 in 100) 2452
▲ Megace Oral Suspension (Up to 6%) 708
▲ Mepron Suspension (10% to 19%) 1206
Merrem I.V. (0.1% to 1.0%) 2952
Mesantoin Tablets 2400
Methadone Hydrochloride Oral Concentrate 2356
Methadone Hydrochloride Oral Solution & Tablets 2357
MetroGel-Vaginal 917

(▣ Described in PDR For Nonprescription Drugs) Incidence data in parenthesis; ▲ 3% or more (⊙ Described in PDR For Ophthalmology)

Mevacor Tablets (0.5% to 1.0%) .. 1742
Miacalcin Nasal Spray (Less than 1%) 2403
Midamor Tablets (Less than or equal to 1%) 1746
Modicon 1928
Moduretic Tablets (Less than or equal to 1%) 1748
8-MOP Capsules 1294
Monoket Tablets (Fewer than 1%) 2550
Monopril Tablets (1.0% or more) .. 762
Motofen Tablets (1 in 200 to 1 in 600) 789
Motrin Ibuprofen Suspension, Oral Drops, Chewable Tablets, Caplets (Less than 1%) 1563
Mycobutin Capsules (1%) 2101
Mykrox Tablets 1617
Nalfon 200 Pulvules & Nalfon Tablets (Less than 1%) 933
Naprelan Tablets (Less than 3%) .. 2861
Anaprox/Naprosyn (Less than 1%) 2277
Nardil (Common) 1977
Navane Capsules and Concentrate 2018
Navane Intramuscular 2019
Nembutal Sodium Capsules (Less than 1%) 440
Nembutal Sodium Solution (Less than 1%) 442
Nembutal Sodium Suppositories (Less than 1%) 444
Neurontin Capsules (More than 1%) 1978
Nicotrol NS Nicotine Nasal Spray 1565
▲Nipent for Injection (3% to 10%) .. 2733
Nolahist Tablets 790
Nolamine Timed-Release Tablets (Occasional) 790
Noroxin Tablets (Less frequent) 1758
Noroxin Tablets (Less frequent) 2222
Norpace (Less than 1%) 2596
Norpramin Tablets 1273
Norvasc Tablets (More than 0.1% to 1%) 2020
Norvir (1.3% to 2.6%) 447
Novahistine DMX ▣ 782
Novahistine Elixir ▣ 782
Nucofed 2225
Ocupress Ophthalmic Solution, 1% Sterile (Occasional) ⊙ 297
Oramorph SR (Morphine Sulfate Sustained Release Tablets) (Less frequent) 2359
▲Orap Tablets (2 of 20 patients) 1037
▲Orlaam Oral Solution (9.1%) 2361
Ornade Spansule Capsules 2678
Ortho-Cyclen/Ortho-Tri-Cyclen 1914
Ortho-Novum 1928
Ortho-Cyclen/Ortho Tri-Cyclen 1914
▲Orudis Capsules (3% to 9%) 2874
▲Oruvail Capsules (3% to 9%) 2874
Oxandrin 783
Oxsoralen-Ultra Capsules 1302
OxyContin Tablets (Between 1% and 5%) 2163
PBZ Tablets 863
PBZ-SR Tablets 862
Pamelor 2409
Parlodel (Less than 1%) 2411
Parnate Tablets 2679
▲Paxil Tablets (1.3% to 24%) 2681
Pediatric Vicks 44d Cough & Head Congestion Relief ▣ 736
Pediatric Vicks 44m Cough & Cold Relief ▣ 737
Pediazole Suspension 2340
Peganone Tablets 455
Penetrex Tablets (1%) 2196
Pentasa (Less than 1%) 1275
Pentaspan Injection 954
Pepcid Injection (Infrequent) 1765
Pepcid (Infrequent) 1763
Periactin 1767
▲Permax Tablets (7.9%) 571
Phenergan with Dextromethorphan 2885
Phenergan Injection 2880
Phenergan VC 2886
Phenobarbital Elixir and Tablets (Less than 1 in 100 patients) 1523
Phenurone Tablets (1%) 455
Placidyl Capsules 456
Plendil Extended-Release Tablets (0.5% to 1.5%) 514
Pondimin Tablets 2239
Ponstel 1982
Pravachol Tablets 770
Prelone Syrup 1834
Prelu-2 Timed Release Capsules 687
Premphase 2900
Prempro 2905
Prilosec Delayed-Release Capsules (Less than 1%) 516
Primatene Tablets ▣ 844
Prinivil Tablets (0.3% to 1.0%) 1776
Prinzide Tablets 1780
Pro-Banthine Tablets 2226
Procardia XL Extended Release Tablets (Less than 3%) 2026
Proglycem 575
▲Prograf (29% to 64%) 1028
Propagest Tablets 791
Propulsid (1.9%) 1346
▲Prostep (nicotine transdermal system) (3% to 9% of patients) .. 1439
Protostat Tablets 1939
Proventil Inhalation Aerosol 2524
Proventil Inhalation Solution 0.083% (1% to 3.1%) 2527
Proventil Repetabs Tablets (2%) 2529
Proventil Solution for Inhalation 0.5% (1% to 3.1%) 2525
Proventil Syrup (1 of 100 patients; children 2 to 6 years, 2%) 2528
Proventil Tablets (2%) 2529
Provera Tablets 2110
▲Prozac Pulvules & Liquid, Oral Solution (13.8% to 30%) 935
Pyrroxate Caplets ▣ 742
Quadrinal Tablets 1398
Quibron 2227
RMS Suppositories CII 2766
Recombivax HB (Less to greater than 1%) 1787
▲Redux Capsules (19.9%) 2911
Reglan (Less frequent) 2243
Relafen Tablets (1% to 3%) 2688
ReoPro Vials (0.3%) 1526
Respbid Tablets 687
▲Retrovir Capsules (2.4% to 5%) 1216
▲Retrovir I.V. Infusion (3% to 5%) .. 1221
▲Retrovir Syrup (2.4% to 5%) 1216
▲ReVia Tablets (3%) 957
Rifater 1280
Rilutek Tablets (2.1% to 2.9%) 2198
▲Risperdal Tablets (23% to 26%) .. 1348
▲Ritalin (One of the two most common) 866
Robinul Forte Tablets 2247
Robinul Injectable 2247
Robinul Tablets 2247
Robitussin Maximum Strength Cough & Cold ▣ 847
Robitussin Pediatric Cough & Cold Formula ▣ 848
Robitussin-CF ▣ 846
Robitussin-DAC Syrup 2249
Robitussin-PE ▣ 846
▲Romazicon (3% to 9%) 2311
Rondec Oral Drops 974
Rondec Syrup 974
Rondec 974
Rowasa (0.12%) 2727
Roxanol 2365
Ryna ▣ 804
Rythmol Tablets–150mg, 225mg, 300mg (0.3 to 1.5%) 1399
▲Sanorex Tablets (Among most common) 2423
Sansert Tablets 2424
Seconal Sodium Pulvules (Less than 1 in 100) 1529
▲Sectral Capsules (3%) 2914
Seldane Tablets 1284
▲Seldane-D Extended-Release Tablets (25.9%) 1286
▲Semprex-D Capsules (4%) 1620
Septra 1146
Septra I.V. Infusion 1142
Septra I.V. Infusion ADD-Vantage Vials 1144
Septra 1146
Serophene (clomiphene citrate tablets, USP) (Approximately 1 in 50 patients) 2621
▲Serzone Tablets (11%) 776
Sinarest ▣ 663
Sine-Aid Maximum Strength Sinus Headache Gelcaps, Caplets and Tablets 1570
Sine-Off No Drowsiness Formula Caplets ▣ 784
Sinemet Tablets 959
Sinemet CR Tablets (1.2%) 961
Sinulin Tablets 792
Sinutab Non-Drying Liquid Caps .. ▣ 823
Slo-bid Gyrocaps 2201
Soma Compound w/Codeine Tablets (Infrequent or rare) 2784
Soma Compound Tablets (Infrequent or rare) 2783
Soma Tablets 2782
Sporanox Capsules (Infrequent) 1352
▲Stadol (11%) 779
Stelazine (Sometimes) 2692
Stimate, (desmopressin acetate) Nasal Spray, 1.5 mg/mL 806
Sudafed Cold & Allergy Tablets ▣ 826
Sudafed Nasal Decongestant Tablets, 30 mg ▣ 825
Sudafed Nasal Decongestant Tablets, 60 mg ▣ 825
Sudafed Sinus Caplets ▣ 829
Sudafed Sinus Tablets ▣ 829
Sudafed 12 Hour Caplets ▣ 824
Sular Tablets (Less than or equal to 1%) 2961
▲Supprelin Injection (3% to 10%) 2230
Surmontil Capsules 2917
▲Symmetrel Capsules (5% to 10%) 965
▲Symmetrel Syrup (5% to 10%) 963
▲Synarel Nasal Solution for Endometriosis (8% of patients) .. 2605
Syn-Rx Tablets 1622
Syn-Rx DM Tablets 1623
Talacen Caplets (Infrequent) 2464
Talwin Injection 2465
Talwin Compound (Infrequent) 2466
Talwin Injection 2465
Talwin Nx Tablets 2467
Tambocor Tablets (1% to less than 3%) 1555
Tavist Syrup 2426
Tavist Tablets 2427
Teldrin 12 Hour Antihistamine/Nasal Decongestant Allergy Relief Capsules ▣ 786
▲Tenex Tablets (Less than 3% to 4%) 2249
Theo-24 Extended Release Capsules 2753
Theo-Dur Extended-Release Tablets 1367
Theo-X Extended-Release Tablets .. 793
TheraFlu ▣ 750
TheraFlu Maximum Strength Nighttime Flu, Cold & Cough Medicine ▣ 751
Thorazine 2701
Tiazac Capsules (Less than 1%) 1019
Timolide Tablets (Less than 1%) 1791
Timoptic in Ocudose (Less frequent) 1796
Timoptic Sterile Ophthalmic Solution 1794
Timoptic-XE 1798
Tofranil Ampuls 873
Tofranil Tablets 875
Tofranil-PM Capsules 876
Tonocard Tablets (Less than 1%) .. 519
Toprol-XL Tablets 560
Toradol (1% or less) 2319
Tornalate Solution for Inhalation, 0.2% (Less than 1%) 976
Tornalate Metered Dose Inhaler (0.5%; less than 1%) 978
Tranxene 459
Trental Tablets 1291
Triaminic Syrup ▣ 755
Triaminic DM Syrup ▣ 756
Triaminicin Tablets ▣ 756
Triavil Tablets 1800
Trilafon 2532
Levlen/Tri-Levlen 646
Trinalin Repetabs Tablets 1373
Tussend 1830
Tussend Expectorant 1831
TYLENOL Cold Medication, Multi-Symptom Formula Tablets and Caplets 1572
TYLENOL Cold Medication, Multi-Symptom Hot Liquid Packets 1572
TYLENOL Cold Medication, No Drowsiness Formula Caplets and Gelcaps 1572
TYLENOL Cough Medication with Decongestant, Multi Symptom 1574
TYLENOL Flu NightTime, Maximum Strength Hot Medication Packets 1575
TYLENOL Sinus, Maximum Strength Geltabs, Gelcaps, Caplets and Tablets 1576
Uni-Dur Extended-Release Tablets .. 1374
Uniphyl 400 mg and 600 mg Tablets 2157
Valium Injectable 2336
Valium Tablets 2335
Vantin for Oral Suspension and Vantin Tablets (Less than 1%) 2112
Vascor Tablets (200 and 300 mg) (0.5 to 2.65%) 1597
Vaseretic Tablets (0.5% to 2.0%) 1810
Vasotec I.V. 1814
Vasotec Tablets (0.5% to 1.0%) 1816
Ventolin Inhalation Aerosol and Refill 1170
Ventolin Inhalation Solution (1% to 3.1%) 1171
Ventolin Nebules Inhalation Solution (1% to 3.1%) 1172
Ventolin Rotacaps for Inhalation (Less than 1%) 1173
Ventolin Syrup (1 of 100 patients; 2% in children) 1175
Ventolin Tablets (2 of 100 patients) 1176
Verelan Capsules (1% or less) 1455
Versed Injection (Less than 1%) 2324
▲Vesanoid Capsules (14%) 2327
Vicks 44 LiquiCaps Cough, Cold & Flu Relief ▣ 728
Vicks 44 LiquiCaps Non-Drowsy Cough & Cold Relief ▣ 729
Vicks 44D Cough & Head Congestion Relief ▣ 728
Vicks 44M Cough, Cold & Flu Relief ▣ 729
Vicks DayQuil Allergy Relief 4-Hour Tablets ▣ 733
Vicks DayQuil LiquiCaps/Liquid Multi-Symptom Cold/Flu Relief ▣ 734
Vicks DayQuil SINUS Pressure & CONGESTION Relief ▣ 734
Vicks Nyquil Hot Therapy ▣ 735
Vicks NyQuil LiquiCaps/Liquid Multi-Symptom Cold/Flu Relief, Original and Cherry Flavors ▣ 736
▲Videx Tablets, Powder for Oral Solution, & Pediatric Powder for Oral Solution (Less than 1% to 8%) 2980
▲Visken Tablets (10%) 2428
Vistide Injection 1057
Vivactil Tablets 1820
Volmax Extended-Release Tablets (2.4%) 1835
Cataflam/Voltaren/Voltaren-XR (Less than 1%) 833
▲Wellbutrin Tablets (18.6%) 1177
Winstrol Tablets 2468
▲Xanax Tablets (8.9% to 29.4%) 2115
Zantac (Rare) 1182
Zantac Injection 1180
Zantac Syrup (Rare) 1182
Zaroxolyn Tablets 1625
Zebeta Tablets (1.5% to 2.5%) 1457
▲Zerit Capsules (2% to 31%) 731
Zestoretic Tablets 2968
Zestril Tablets (0.3% to 1.0%) 2972
Ziac (1.1% to 1.2%) 1459
Zithromax (1% or less) 2043
Zithromax Tablets (1% or less) 2046
Zocor Tablets 1821
▲Zoladex (5% to 11%) 2976
Zoladex 3-month 2978
▲Zoloft Tablets (16.4%) 2051
▲Zosyn (4.5% to 6.6%) 1463
Zyloprim Tablets (Less than 1%) 1194
Zyrtec Tablets (Less than 2%) 2053

Insomnia, early morning

Hydropres Tablets 1718

Insulin allergy

Velosulin BR Human Insulin 10 ml Vials (Very rare) 1847

Insulin autoimmune syndrome

Tapazole Tablets 1361

Insulin reaction

Modicon 1928
Ortho-Cyclen/Ortho-Tri-Cyclen 1914
Ortho-Novum 1928
Ortho-Cyclen/Ortho Tri-Cyclen 1914
Velosulin BR Human Insulin 10 ml Vials 1847

Insulin requirement, changes

Ana-Kit Anaphylaxis Emergency Treatment Kit 611
Celestone Soluspan Suspension 2484
CORTENEMA 2713
Cortone Acetate Sterile Suspension 1663
Cortone Acetate Tablets 1664
Dalalone D.P. Injectable 1009
Danocrine Capsules 2437
Decadron Elixir 1676

(▣ Described in PDR For Nonprescription Drugs) Incidence data in parenthesis; ▲ 3% or more (⊙ Described in PDR For Ophthalmology)

Insulin requirement, changes — Side Effects Index — 1380

Decadron Phosphate Injection 1680
Decadron Phosphate with Xylocaine Injection, Sterile 1683
Decadron Tablets 1678
Decadron-LA Sterile Suspension 1687
Dexacort Phosphate in Respihaler 1606
Dexacort Phosphate in Turbinaire 1607
Florinef Acetate Tablets 506
Hydrocortone Phosphate Injection, Sterile 1713
Hydrocortone Tablets 1715
Oretic Tablets 450
Pediapred Oral Solution 1618
Prelone Syrup 1834
Prinzide Tablets 1780
Tenoretic Tablets 2963
Vaseretic Tablets 1810

Insulin shock

Zanosar Sterile Powder 2119

Intercourse, sexual, painful (see under Pain with coitus)

Intestinal motility, decrease

Bellergal-S Tablets (Rare) 2375

Intestinal obstruction

Ambien Tablets (Rare) 2559
Anafranil Capsules (Rare) 819
Avonex 662
Betaseron for SC Injection 653
Clozaril Tablets 2377
Effexor (Rare) 2825
Felbatol 2774
Hycamtin for Injection (1.1% to 4.5%) 2665
Kayexalate 2444
Lamprene Capsules (Less than 1%) 846
Levsin/Levsinex/Levbid 2549
LUVOX Tablets (Rare) 2723
ParaGard T 380A Intrauterine Copper Contraceptive 1936
Paxil Tablets (Rare) 2681
Permax Tablets (Infrequent) 571
Pulmozyme Inhalation 1054
Remeron Tablets (Rare) 1878
Rilutek Tablets (Infrequent) 2198
Risperdal Tablets 1348
Sodium Polystyrene Sulfonate Suspension (Rare) 2367
Taxol Injection (Rare) 723
Taxotere for Injection Concentrate 2204

Intestinal obstruction, pseudo

Catapres Tablets (Rare) 679
Nimotop Capsules (Rare) 603

Intestinal penetration

ParaGard T 380A Intrauterine Copper Contraceptive 1936

Intestinal perforation

Avonex 662
Cataflam Tablets (Rare) 833
Cipro I.V. (Less than 1%) 587
Cipro I.V. Pharmacy Bulk Package (Less than 1%) 590
Cipro Tablets (Less than 1%) 584
Cytovene-IV (One report) 2270
Floxin I.V. 1580
Floxin Tablets (200 mg, 300 mg, 400 mg) 1577
Hydrocortone Tablets 1715
Maxaquin Tablets 2593
Penetrex Tablets 2196
Proleukin for Injection (Less than 1% to 2%) 812
Taxol Injection (Rare) 723
Thioguanine Tablets, Tabloid Brand 1225
Cataflam/Voltaren/Voltaren-XR (Rare) 833
Wellbutrin Tablets (Rare) 1177

Intestinal strictures

Clinoril Tablets (Rare) 1658
Indocin Capsules (Less than 1%) 1723
Indocin I.V. (Less than 1%) 1727
Indocin SR Capsules (Less than 1%) 1723

Intoxication, chronic

Miltown Tablets 2780
Placidyl Capsules 456

Intracranial pressure, increase

Albenza Tablets (Up to 1.5%) 2629
Anectine 1062
Brontex 2130
Calcium Disodium Versenate Injection 1548
Celestone Soluspan Suspension 2484
Chibroxin Sterile Ophthalmic Solution (With oral form) 1657
Cipro I.V. 587
Cipro Tablets 584
Cortifoam 2540
Cortone Acetate Sterile Suspension 1663
Cortone Acetate Tablets 1664
Decadron Elixir 1676
Decadron Phosphate Injection 1680
Decadron Phosphate with Xylocaine Injection, Sterile 1683
Decadron Tablets 1678
Decadron-LA Sterile Suspension 1687
Dilaudid Ampules 1382
Dilaudid Cough Syrup 1383
Dilaudid-HP Injection (Less frequent) 1384
Dilaudid-HP Lyophilized Powder 250 mg (Less frequent) 1384
Dilaudid 1382
Dilaudid Oral Liquid (Less frequent) 1386
Dilaudid 1382
Dilaudid Tablets - 8 mg (Less frequent) 1386
Eskalith 2658
Floxin Tablets (200 mg, 300 mg, 400 mg) 1577
Hydeltrasol Injection, Sterile 1708
Hydeltra-T.B.A. Sterile Suspension 1710
Hydrocortone Acetate Sterile Suspension 1712
Hydrocortone Phosphate Injection, Sterile 1713
Hydrocortone Tablets 1715
Lithium Carbonate Capsules & Tablets 2352
MS Contin Tablets (Less frequent) 2149
MSIR (Infrequent) 2152
NegGram (Occasional) 2453
Nizoral Tablets (Rare) 1345
Noroxin Tablets 1758
Noroxin Tablets 2222
Oramorph SR (Morphine Sulfate Sustained Release Tablets) (Less frequent) 2359
Penetrex Tablets 2196

Intracranial pressure with papilledema

CORTENEMA 2713
Dalalone D.P. Injectable 1009
Dexacort Phosphate in Respihaler 1606
Dexacort Phosphate in Turbinaire 1607
Florinef Acetate Tablets 506
Lithonate/Lithotabs/Lithobid 2721
Nutropin (A small number of patients) 1049
Nutropin AQ Injection (A small number of patients) 1051
Prelone Syrup 1834

Intraocular pressure, increase (see under Glaucoma)

Intraocular pressure, paradoxical increase

Humorsol Sterile Ophthalmic Solution 1707
Phospholine Iodide ◉ 323

Intravascular coagulation, disseminated

Clinoril Tablets (Less than 1 in 100) 1658
Dolobid Tablets (Less than 1 in 100) 1695
Felbatol 2774
Hespan Injection (Rare) 945
Indocin Capsules (Less than 1%) 1723
Indocin I.V. 1727
Indocin (Less than 1%) 1723
Oncaspar (Greater than 1% but less than 5%) 2194
Parlodel 2411
Sulfamylon Cream 940
TheraCys BCG Live (Intravesical) (Up to 2.7%) 911
▲ Vesanoid Capsules (26%) 2327

Involuntary movements, abnormal

Atamet Tablets 567
Atretol Tablets 569
Clozaril Tablets (Less than 1%) 2377
Cordarone Tablets 2818
Dopram Injectable 2235
Elavil 2945
Eldepryl Capsules 2729
Haldol Decanoate 1587
Methadone Hydrochloride Oral Concentrate 2356
Moban Tablets and Concentrate 1036
Orap Tablets 1037
Parlodel 2411
Prolixin Oral Concentrate 510
▲ Roferon-A Injection (Less than 0.5% to 7%) 2308
Sinemet Tablets 959
Symmetrel Capsules (Uncommon) 965
Symmetrel Syrup (Uncommon) 963
Tegretol/Tegretol-XR 870
▲ Xanax Tablets (14.8%) 2115

Involuntary movements, extremities

Compazine 2644
Etrafon 2495
Haldol Decanoate 1587
Haldol Injection, Tablets and Concentrate 1585
Moban Tablets and Concentrate 1036
Navane Capsules and Concentrate 2018
Navane Intramuscular 2019
Orap Tablets 1037
Prolixin 510
Reglan 2243
Serentil 689
Stelazine 2692
Thorazine 2701

Involuntary movements, trunk

Haldol Decanoate 1587
Mellaril 2398
Orap Tablets 1037
Prolixin 510
Reglan 2243
Serentil 689

Iodine uptake, elevated

Lithonate/Lithotabs/Lithobid 2721

Iodism

Norisodrine with Calcium Iodide Syrup 446
Quadrinal Tablets 1398
Thyro-Block Tablets 2785

Iridocyclitis (see also under Iritis)

Betagan (Rare) ◉ 230
Trusopt Sterile Ophthalmic Solution (Rare) 1803

Iris cysts

Humorsol Sterile Ophthalmic Solution 1707
Phospholine Iodide (Rare) ◉ 323
Salagen Tablets (Rare) 1546

Iritis (see also under Uveitis)

Aredia for Injection (Rare) 827
Carbastat Intraocular Solution (Occasional) ◉ 260
FLUORACAINE ◉ 208
FLURESS (Sometimes) ◉ 208
Healon (Rare) ◉ 302
Kerlone Tablets (Less than 2%) 2588
MIOSTAT Intraocular Solution ◉ 222
Myochrysine Injection (Rare) 1754
Norvir (Less than 2%) 447
OcuCoat (Rare) ◉ 321
Ophthetic (Sometimes) ◉ 244
Prozac Pulvules & Liquid, Oral Solution (Rare) 935
Solganal Suspension (Rare) 2530
Tenex Tablets (3% or less) 2249
Videx Tablets, Powder for Oral Solution, & Pediatric Powder for Oral Solution (Less than 1%) 2980
Vistide Injection 1057
Zyloprim Tablets (Less than 1%) 1194

Iritis, activation of latent

Humorsol Sterile Ophthalmic Solution 1707
Phospholine Iodide ◉ 323

Iron deficiency

Cuprimine Capsules 1673
Depen Titratable Tablets 2770
Epogen for Injection 489
Risperdal Tablets (Rare) 1348
Sandostatin Injection (Less than 1%) 2421
Syprine Capsules 1790

Iron deficiency anemia

Permax Tablets (Infrequent) 571

Irritability

▲ ActHIB (10.1% to 77.9%) 893
▲ AeroBid Inhaler System (3% to 9%) 1004
▲ Aerobid-M Inhaler System (3% to 9%) 1004
Anafranil Capsules (2%) 819
Aquasol A Vitamin A Capsules, USP 525
Aquasol A Parenteral 526
Atrohist Pediatric Capsules 1603
Benadryl Injection 1955
Bromfed 1832
▲ Bromfed-DM Cough Syrup (Among most frequent) 1832
Bromfed-PD Capsules (Extended-Release) 1832
Cataflam Tablets (Less than 1%) 833
Catapres-TTS 680
Cedax (0.1% to 1%) 2480
Ceftin for Oral Suspension (0.1% to 1%) 1067
Celontin Kapseals 1955
Cipro I.V. (1% or less) 587
Cipro I.V. Pharmacy Bulk Package (Less than 1%) 590
Cipro Tablets (Less than 1%) 584
Claritin-D Tablets (Less frequent) 2487
Clomid 1262
Clozaril Tablets (Less than 1%) 2377
Cylert Tablets 415
Cytovene-IV (One report) 2270
D.A. II Tablets 972
D.A. Chewable Tablets 970
Dalmane Capsules 2329
Dimetane-DC Cough Syrup 2232
Dimetane-DX Cough Syrup 2233
Dipentum Capsules (Rare) 2084
Doral Tablets 2773
Dura-Tap/PD Capsules 970
Dura-Vent/DA Tablets 972
Dura-Vent Tablets 971
Efudex 2280
Elavil 2945
Eldepryl Capsules 2729
Elspar 1700
Engerix-B Unit-Dose Vials (Less than 1%) 2656
Entex PSE Tablets 973
Esgic-plus Capsules 1012
Esgic-plus Tablets 1012
Fioricet Tablets 2386
Fioricet with Codeine Capsules 2387
Fiorinal with Codeine Capsules 2390
Flagyl 375 Capsules 2587
Flagyl I.V. 2373
▲ Gamimune N, 5% Immune Globulin Intravenous (Human), 5% (Among most common; 11.5%) 612
▲ Gamimune N, 10% Immune Globulin Intravenous (Human), 10% (Among most common; 11.5%) 615
Gastrocrom Capsules (2 of 87 patients) 1611
Gastrocrom Oral Concentrate (2 of 87 patients) 1611
Guaifed 1833
Guaimax-D Tablets 809
Halcion Tablets 2093
Helidac Therapy 2135
HibTITER (133 of 1,118 vaccinations) 1423
▲ Intron A for Injection (Up to 16%) 2506
Invirase Capsules (Less than 2%) 2291
IOPIDINE Sterile Ophthalmic Solution ◉ 218
IPOL Poliovirus Vaccine Inactivated 903
ISMOTIC 45% w/v Solution (Very rare) ◉ 221
▲ Lamictal Tablets (3.0%) 1105
Lufyllin & Lufyllin-400 Tablets 2778
Lufyllin-GG Elixir & Tablets 2779
Mebaral Tablets 2452
Mesantoin Tablets 2400
Methadone Hydrochloride Oral Concentrate 2356
Methotrexate Sodium Tablets, Injection, for Injection and LPF Injection 1322
▲ Nicotrol NS Nicotine Nasal Spray (Over 5%) 1565
▲ OmniHIB (10.1% to 72.6%) 2676
Orlaam Oral Solution 2361
Ornade Spansule Capsules 2678
PBZ Tablets 863
PBZ-SR Tablets 862
Periactin 1767
Phenobarbital Elixir and Tablets 1523

(Described in PDR For Nonprescription Drugs)   Incidence data in parenthesis; ▲ 3% or more   (◉ Described in PDR For Ophthalmology)

Side Effects Index

Irritation, nasal

Drug	Page
Placidyl Capsules	456
Plaquenil Sulfate Tablets	2459
Plendil Extended-Release Tablets (0.5% to 1.5%)	514
Pregnyl for Injection	1878
Prinivil Tablets (0.3% to 1.0%)	1776
Prinzide Tablets	1780
Profasi (chorionic gonadotropin for injection, USP)	2620
Proleukin for Injection	812
Protostat Tablets	1939
Proventil Repetabs Tablets (Less than 1%)	2529
Proventil Syrup (Less than 100 to 1 of 100 patients)	2528
Proventil Tablets (Less than 1%)	2529
Quadrinal Tablets	1398
Quibron	2227
Recombivax HB	1787
Respbid Tablets	687
Retrovir Capsules (1.6%)	1216
Retrovir I.V. Infusion (2%)	1221
Retrovir Syrup (1.6%)	1216
▲ReVia Tablets (Less than 10%)	957
Roferon-A Injection (Infrequent)	2308
Rondec Chewable Tablets	974
Seldane-D Extended-Release Tablets (1.1%)	1286
Skelaxin Tablets	793
Slo-bid Gyrocaps	2201
Soma Compound w/Codeine Tablets (Infrequent or rare)	2784
Soma Compound Tablets (Infrequent or rare)	2783
Soma Tablets	2782
Symmetrel Capsules (1% to 5%)	965
Symmetrel Syrup (1% to 5%)	963
Talacen Caplets (Rare)	2464
Talwin Injection	2465
Talwin Compound (Rare)	2466
Talwin Injection	2465
Talwin Nx Tablets	2467
Tavist Syrup	2426
Tavist Tablets	2427
▲Tetramune (42% to 54%)	1449
Theo-24 Extended Release Capsules	2753
Theo-Dur Extended-Release Tablets	1367
Theo-X Extended-Release Tablets	793
Tranxene	459
Triavil Tablets	1800
Trinalin Repetabs Tablets	1373
▲Tripedia (5% to 15%)	908
Tussend	1830
Uni-Dur Extended-Release Tablets	1374
Uniphyl 400 mg and 600 mg Tablets	2157
Vantin for Oral Suspension and Vantin Tablets (Less than 1%)	2112
Varivax (Greater than or equal to 1%)	1807
Ventolin Syrup (Less than 1 of 100 patients)	1175
Ventolin Tablets (Fewer than 1 of 100 patients)	1176
Volmax Extended-Release Tablets (Less frequent)	1835
Cataflam/Voltaren/Voltaren-XR (Less than 1%)	833
▲Xanax Tablets (33.1%)	2115
Yocon Tablets	1235
Yohimex Tablets	1414
Zarontin Capsules	1986
Zarontin Syrup	1986
Zestoretic Tablets	2968
Zestril Tablets (0.3% to 1.0%)	2972

Irritation

Drug	Page
Aclovate Cream (Approximately 2%)	1061
Americaine Hemorrhoidal Ointment	▣649
Analpram-HC Rectal Cream 1% and 2.5%	993
Anusol Hemorrhoidal Ointment	▣810
Anusol-HC Cream 2.5% (Infrequent to frequent)	1953
Anusol-HC Suppositories	1954
Atrovent Inhalation Aerosol (1.6%)	674
Azelex (Less than 1%)	471
Benoquin Cream 20%	1298
BiCozene Creme	▣747
Bleph-10 Ophthalmic Ointment 10%	472
Caverject Injection (Less than 1%)	2064
Chloresium (A few instances)	2371
Cordran Lotion (Infrequent)	1854
Cordran Tape (Infrequent)	1855
Cormax Ointment (0.5%)	1856
Cormax Scalp Application (Infrequent)	1857
Cortisporin Otic Solution Sterile	1076
Cortisporin Otic Suspension Sterile	1077
Cutivate Cream	1078
Cutivate Ointment (Less than 1%)	1078
Decadron Phosphate Topical Cream	1686
Decaspray Topical Aerosol	1689
Desenex	▣652
Desenex Foot & Sneaker Deodorant Spray	▣653
DesOwen Cream, Ointment and Lotion (Less than 2%)	1032
Diprolene Gel 0.05% (Less frequent)	2490
Dyclone 0.5% and 1% Topical Solutions, USP	535
▲Efudex (Among most frequent)	2280
Elocon Lotion 0.1% (Infrequent)	2493
Eurax Cream & Lotion	2794
Exact	▣722
Florone/Florone E	921
Fluoroplex Topical Solution & Cream 1%	475
Furacin Soluble Dressing	2220
Hibiclens Antimicrobial Skin Cleanser	2947
Hibistat Towelette	2948
Hytone	922
Hytone Ointment 2 ½%	923
Kwell Shampoo	2173
Lac-Hydrin 12% Lotion (Less frequent)	2796
Lamisil Cream 1% (1%)	2393
Lidex (Infrequent)	2299
Lindane Lotion USP 1% (Relatively infrequent)	481
Lindane Shampoo USP 1% (Relatively infrequent)	483
Locoid Cream, Ointment and Topical Solution (Infrequent)	994
Lotrimin AF Antifungal Cream Liquid, Spray Powder, Spray Deodorant Powder, Powder and Jock Itch Spray Powder	▣766
Lotrisone Cream (Infrequent)	2515
Melanex Topical Solution	1842
Monistat 3 Vaginal Suppositories	1905
Monistat-Derm (miconazole nitrate 2%) Cream (Isolated reports)	1944
Mycelex OTC Cream Antifungal	▣622
NeoDecadron Topical Cream	1757
▲Nizoral 2% Cream (5%)	1344
Nizoral 2% Shampoo (Less than 1%)	1344
Nystop (Nystatin Topical Powder, USP)	1948
Oil of Olay Daily UV Protectant SPF 15 Beauty Fluid-Original and Fragrance Free (Olay Co. Inc.)	▣725
Oncovin Solution Vials & Hyporets	1521
Oxistat Cream (0.4%)	1139
Pandel Cream, 0.1%	2475
Pediotic Suspension Sterile	1140
Pramosone Cream, Lotion & Ointment	995
Pred-G Liquifilm Sterile Ophthalmic Suspension	⊚248
Psorcon Cream 0.05% (Infrequent)	924
Psorcon Ointment 0.05%	923
Serevent Inhalation Aerosol (Rare)	1149
Solbar PF Ultra Liquid SPF 30	1989
Synalar (Infrequent)	2299
Temovate Cream	1152
Temovate E Emollient (Less than 2%)	1154
▲Temovate Gel (Among most frequent)	1153
Temovate Ointment (0.5%)	1152
Temovate Scalp Application (Infrequent)	1153
Testoderm Testosterone Transdermal System (2%)	486
Tridesilon Cream 0.05% (Infrequent)	609
Tridesilon Ointment 0.05% (Infrequent)	610
Tympagesic Ear Drops	2476
Vagistat-1 (Less than 1%)	783
Westcort Cream 0.2% (Infrequent)	2799
Westcort Ointment 0.2% (1%)	2800

Irritation, anal

Drug	Page
Anusol Hemorrhoidal Ointment	▣810
Colyte and Colyte-flavored	2540
GoLYTELY (Infrequent)	694
NuLYTELY (Less frequent)	694
Cherry Flavor NuLYTELY (Less frequent)	694
Questran (Less frequent)	774
Zosyn (1.0% or less)	1463

Irritation, gastric

Drug	Page
Akineton	1380
Aldoclor Tablets	1638
Aldoril Tablets	1644
Apresazide Capsules	824
Capoten Tablets (About 0.5 to 2%)	740
Capozide Tablets (0.5 to 2%)	744
Combipres Tablets	682
D.A. II Tablets	972
D.A. Chewable Tablets	970
Dantrium Capsules (Less frequent)	2131
Diucardin Tablets	2824
Diupres Tablets	1691
Diuril Oral Suspension	1694
Diuril Sodium Intravenous	1693
Diuril Tablets	1694
Dura-Tap/PD Capsules	970
Dura-Vent/DA Tablets	972
Dura-Vent Tablets	971
Enduron Tablets	424
Entex LA Tablets	972
Esidrix Tablets	839
Esimil Tablets	840
Exgest LA Tablets	787
Hydrea Capsules	705
HydroDIURIL Tablets	1716
Hydropres Tablets	1718
Hyzaar Tablets	1720
Inderide Tablets	2838
Inderide LA Long Acting Capsules	2840
Kayexalate	2444
Lasix Injection, Oral Solution and Tablets	1267
Lopressor HCT Tablets	850
Lotensin HCT Tablets	855
Marax Tablets & DF Syrup	2015
Minizide Capsules	2016
Moduretic Tablets	1748
Nalfon 200 Pulvules & Nalfon Tablets (Less than 1%)	933
Norflex	1554
Oretic Tablets	450
Prinzide Tablets	1780
Quadrinal Tablets	1398
Ser-Ap-Es Tablets	867
Sodium Polystyrene Sulfonate Suspension	2367
Thalitone	1293
Timolide Tablets	1791
Vaseretic Tablets	1810
Zestoretic Tablets	2968
Ziac	1459

Irritation, gastrointestinal

Drug	Page
Dibenzyline Capsules	2650
Glucotrol XL Extended Release Tablets (Rare)	2012
▲K-Lor Powder Packets (Among most common)	438
▲K-Norm Capsules (Among most common)	1615
▲Micro-K Extencaps (Among most common)	2237
Procardia XL Extended Release Tablets (Less than 1%)	2026
Tenoretic Tablets	2963
Urocit-K Tablets (Some patients)	1828

Irritation, glossal

(see under Irritation, oral)

Irritation, local

Drug	Page
AK-Spore	⊚205
Androderm Testosterone Transdermal System (Less than 1%)	2634
Aspercreme Creme, Lotion Analgesic Rub	▣794
Astramorph/PF Injection, USP (Preservative-Free)	526
Auralgan Otic Solution	2810
Bentyl Injection	1246
BENZASHAVE Medicated Shave Cream 5% and 10%	1627
Betasept Surgical Scrub	2145
Bleph-10	472
Blephamide Liquifilm Sterile Ophthalmic Suspension	472
Blephamide Ointment	⊚234
▲Cipro I.V. Pharmacy Bulk Package (Among most frequent)	590
Claforan Sterile and Injection	1259
▲Climara Transdermal System (31%)	640
▲Cleocin Vaginal Cream (7%)	2070
Cortisporin Ophthalmic Ointment Sterile	1074
Cortisporin Ophthalmic Suspension Sterile	1075
Demerol	2438
Deponit NTG Transdermal Delivery System	2541
Dermatop Emollient Cream 0.1%	1264
Desenex Prescription	▣653
Desferal Vials	838
Drithocreme 0.1%, 0.25%, 0.5%, 1.0% (HP)	920
Dritho-Scalp 0.25%, 0.5% (More frequent)	921
Duramorph Injection	983
Edecrin (Occasionally)	1698
▲Estraderm Transdermal System (About 17%)	842
Eurax Cream & Lotion	2794
Garamycin Cream 0.1%	2501
Garamycin Injectable (Rare)	2502
Garamycin Ointment 0.1%	2501
Heparin Lock Flush Solution	2831
Heparin Sodium Injection	2832
Heparin Sodium Vials	1486
HibTITER	1423
Infumorph 200 and Infumorph 500 Sterile Solutions	985
Lovenox Injection	2187
Mepergan Injection	2859
Monistat Dual-Pak	1906
Naftin Cream 1% (2%)	477
Neosporin Ophthalmic Ointment Sterile	1130
Neosporin Ophthalmic Solution Sterile	1131
Nitro-Dur (nitroglycerin) Transdermal Infusion System	1365
▲Nizoral 2% Cream (5%)	1344
Novacet Lotion (Rare)	1041
Novolin 70/30 Prefilled Disposable Insulin Delivery System	1850
Nydrazid Injection	509
Occlusal-HP	1041
Ogen Vaginal Cream	2106
Otic Domeboro Solution	604
Polysporin Ophthalmic Ointment Sterile	1140
▲Polytrim Ophthalmic Solution Sterile (Most frequent)	479
ProctoCream-HC 2.5% (Infrequent to frequent)	2552
Retin-A (tretinoin) Cream/Gel/Liquid	1947
Rifadin I.V.	1276
Selsun Rx 2.5% Selenium Sulfide Lotion, USP	2345
Shade Gel SPF 30 Sunblock	▣767
Shade UVAGUARD SPF 15 Suncreen Lotion	▣768
Sulfacet-R Lotion (Rare)	925
Sulfacet-R Tint Free Lotion (Rare)	925
Sultrin (Frequent)	1941
Terramycin Intramuscular Solution	2034
Topicort Emollient Cream 0.25% (Infrequent)	1289
Topicort Gel 0.05% (Infrequent)	1290
Topicort LP Emollient Cream 0.05% (Infrequent)	1289
Topicort Ointment 0.25% (Infrequent)	1291
Transderm-Nitro Transdermal Therapeutic System	878
Viroptic Ophthalmic Solution, 1% Sterile	1177
Vivelle Transdermal System	880
VōSol (Very rare)	2786
Zebeta Tablets	1457
Zonalon Cream (Less than 1%)	1042

Irritation, nasal

Drug	Page
AeroBid Inhaler System (1% to 3%)	1004
Aerobid-M Inhaler System (1% to 3%)	1004
Atrovent Nasal Spray 0.03% (2.0%)	676
Beconase	1065
Claritin-D Tablets (Less frequent)	2487
▲Dexacort Phosphate in Turbinaire (One of the two most common)	1607
Efudex (Infrequent)	2280
Flonase Nasal Spray (1% to 3%)	1088
Miacalcin Nasal Spray (10.6%)	2403
Nasacort Nasal Inhaler (2.8%)	2189
Nasalcrom Nasal Solution (1 in 40)	2192
Nasalide Nasal Solution 0.025% (5% or less)	2301
Nicotrol NS Nicotine Nasal Spray	1565

(▣ Described in PDR For Nonprescription Drugs)   Incidence data in parenthesis; ▲ 3% or more   (⊚ Described in PDR For Ophthalmology)

Side Effects Index

Irritation, nasal
- Stadol (3% to 9%) ... 779
- ▲ Synarel Nasal Solution for Endometriosis (10% of patients) 2605
- Vancenase AQ Nasal Spray 0.042% ... 2535
- Vancenase AQ Double Strength Nasal Spray 0.084% ... 2536
- ▲ Vancenase PocketHaler Nasal Inhaler (11 per 100 patients) 2534

Irritation, nasopharyngeal
- Beclovent Inhalation Aerosol and Refill ... 1063
- ▲ Beconase AQ Nasal Spray (24% of patients) ... 1065
- ▲ Intal Inhaler (Among most frequent) ... 2185
- Intal Nebulizer Solution ... 2186
- ▲ Rhinocort Nasal Inhaler (3 to 9%).. 552
- ▲ Vancenase AQ Nasal Spray 0.042% (Up to 24%) ... 2535

Irritation, ocular
- ▲ Acular Sterile Ophthalmic Solution (3%) ... 470
- Albalon Solution with Liquifilm ... ⊙ 229
- Ambien Tablets (Infrequent) ... 2559
- Atrovent Nasal Spray 0.03% (Less than 2%) ... 676
- A/T/S 2% Acne Topical Gel ... 1244
- ▲ A/T/S 2% Acne Topical Solution (17 out of 90 patients) ... 1244
- Benzamycin Topical Gel (Occasional) ... 919
- Cormax Scalp Application (Approximately 0.3%) ... 1857
- Erycette (erythromycin 2%) Topical Solution ... 1943
- FML Forte Liquifilm ... ⊙ 237
- FML Liquifilm ... ⊙ 238
- Flovent (1% to 3%) ... 1089
- ▲ Garamycin Ophthalmic (Among most frequent) ... 2501
- ▲ Gentak (Among most frequent) ... ⊙ 209
- Hivid Tablets (Less than 1%) ... 2287
- Lacrisert Sterile Ophthalmic Insert 1730
- Monopril Tablets (0.2% to 1.0%).. 762
- Oncovin Solution Vials & Hyporets 1521
- Pred Forte ... ⊙ 247
- Pred Mild ... ⊙ 250
- ProSom Tablets (Infrequent) ... 457
- Rythmol Tablets–150mg, 225mg, 300mg (Less than 1%) ... 1399
- Temovate Scalp Application (1 of 294 patients) ... 1153
- Timoptic in Ocudose (Less frequent) ... 1796
- Timoptic Sterile Ophthalmic Solution (Less frequent) ... 1794
- Timoptic-XE ... 1798
- Vexol 1% Ophthalmic Suspension (Less than 1%) ... ⊙ 227

Irritation, oral
- AeroBid Inhaler System (1% to 3%) ... 1004
- Aerobid-M Inhaler System (1% to 3%) ... 1004
- Kutrase Capsules ... 2546
- Lasix Injection, Oral Solution and Tablets ... 1267
- Mycostatin Pastilles ... 713
- Peridex ... 2127
- Periogard Oral Rinse ... 892
- Sandimmune (Rare) ... 2416

Irritation, oropharynx
- Brethaire Inhaler ... 830
- Proventil Inhalation Aerosol ... 2524
- Proventil Repetabs Tablets ... 2529
- Proventil Syrup ... 2528
- Proventil Tablets ... 2529
- Ventolin Syrup ... 1175
- Ventolin Tablets ... 1176
- Volmax Extended-Release Tablets .. 1835

Irritation, perianal
(see under Irritation, anal)

Irritation, skin
(see under Irritation, local)

Irritation, vaginal
- Ceftin for Oral Suspension (0.1% to 1%) ... 1067
- Danocrine Capsules ... 2437
- Encare Vaginal Contraceptive Suppositories ... ⊡ 797
- Floxin I.V. (Less than 1%) ... 1580
- Floxin Tablets (200 mg, 300 mg, 400 mg) (Less than 1%) ... 1577
- Massengill ... 2627
- Massengill Medicated Disposable Douche ... 2628
- Massengill Powder ... 2627
- Monistat Dual-Pak (2%) ... 1906
- Monistat 3 Vaginal Suppositories (2%) ... 1905
- Mycelex-G 500 mg Vaginal Tablets (1 in 149 patients) ... 602
- Sultrin (Frequent) ... 1941
- Supprelin Injection (1% to 3%) ... 2230
- ▲ Terazol 3 Vaginal Cream (5%) ... 1941
- ▲ Terazol 7 Vaginal Cream (3.1% of 521 patients) ... 1943

Irritation, vulvovaginal
(see under Irritation, vaginal)

Irritation at injection site
- Bactrim I.V. Infusion (Infrequent) ... 2255
- Bentyl Injection ... 1246
- ▲ Eulexin Capsules (3%) ... 2498
- ▲ Gammagard S/D, Immune Globulin, Intravenous (Human) (16%) ... 577
- Humegon for Injection ... 1873
- Metrodin (urofollitropin for injection) ... 2616
- Nembutal Sodium Capsules ... 440
- Nembutal Sodium Solution ... 442
- Nembutal Sodium Suppositories (Less than 1%) ... 444
- Pepcid Injection Premixed (Infrequent) ... 1765
- Pergonal (menotropins for injection, USP) ... 2618
- Retrovir I.V. Infusion (Infrequent) 1221
- Romazicon ... 2311
- Septra I.V. Infusion (Infrequent) ... 1142
- Septra I.V. Infusion ADD-Vantage Vials (Infrequent) ... 1144

Ischemia
- Amicar Syrup, Tablets, and Injection ... 1312
- Cafergot ... 2376
- Heparin Sodium Vials ... 1486
- ▲ Lupron Injection (5% or more) ... 2736
- Sandostatin Injection (Less than 1%) ... 2421
- Sensorcaine ... 554
- Trandate ... 1158
- ▲ Vesanoid Capsules (3%) ... 2327

Ischemia, arteria basilaris
- AK-FLUOR Injection 10% and 25% ... ⊙ 204
- Fluorescite ... ⊙ 217

Ischemia, cerebral
- Betagan ... ⊙ 230
- Betaseron for SC Injection ... 653
- Betimol 0.25%, 0.5% ... ⊙ 259
- Cardene Capsules (Less than 0.4%) ... 2261
- Hyperstat I.V. Injection ... 2504
- Imitrex Tablets (Rare) ... 1099
- Lioresal Intrathecal (1% or more) 1634
- Nitrolingual Spray (Occasional) ... 2193
- Ocupress Ophthalmic Solution, 1% Sterile ... ⊙ 297
- Paxil Tablets (Rare) ... 2681
- Permax Tablets (Infrequent) ... 571
- Prozac Pulvules & Liquid, Oral Solution (Rare) ... 935
- Quinaglute Dura-Tabs Tablets (2%) ... 644
- Redux Capsules ... 2911
- Remeron Tablets (Rare) ... 1878
- ReoPro Vials (0.3%) ... 1526
- Rilutek Tablets (Rare) ... 2198
- Sorbitrate ... 2959
- Sular Tablets (Less than or equal to 1%) ... 2961
- Timolide Tablets ... 1791
- Timoptic in Ocudose ... 1796
- Timoptic Sterile Ophthalmic Solution (Less frequent) ... 1794
- Timoptic-XE ... 1798
- Zoladex 3-month (1% to 5%) ... 2978

Ischemia, myocardial
- Anafranil Capsules (Rare) ... 819
- Dilacor XR Extended-release Capsules ... 2183
- Diprivan Injectable Emulsion (Less than 1%) ... 2939
- Ergamisol Tablets ... 1340
- Flolan for Injection (2%) ... 1085
- Fluorouracil Injection ... 2282
- Sterile FUDR (Remote possibility) .. 2284
- Hyperstat I.V. Injection ... 2504
- Imitrex Injection (Extremely rare) ... 1095
- Imitrex Tablets (Rare) ... 1099
- Levlen/Tri-Levlen ... 646
- Modicon (An increased incidence) .. 1928
- Ortho-Cyclen/Ortho-Tri-Cyclen ... 1914
- Ortho-Novum (An increased incidence) ... 1928
- Ortho-Cyclen/Ortho Tri-Cyclen ... 1914
- Ovcon ... 765
- Paxil Tablets (Rare) ... 2681
- ▲ Proleukin for Injection (3%) ... 812
- Rilutek Tablets (Infrequent) ... 2198
- Suprane (desflurane, USP) (Less than 1%) ... 1865
- Levlen/Tri-Levlen ... 646
- Ultram Tablets (50 mg) (Infrequent) ... 1594

Ischemia, peripheral
- Anafranil Capsules (Rare) ... 819
- Avonex ... 662
- Brevibloc (esmolol HCl) Injection (Approximately 1%) ... 1860
- Cardura Tablets (0.3%) ... 1993
- Cytovene-IV (One report) ... 2270
- Felbatol ... 2774
- Intron A for Injection (Less than 5%) ... 2506
- Kerlone Tablets (Less than 2%) ... 2588
- Norvasc Tablets (More than 0.1% to 1%) ... 2020
- Ziac (0.4% to 0.7%) ... 1459
- Zoloft Tablets (Infrequent) ... 2051

Ischemia of digits
- Zovirax Sterile Powder (Less than 1%) ... 1191

Ischemic attacks, transient
- Actimmune (Rare) ... 1043
- Clozaril Tablets (Several patients) .. 2377
- Cognex Capsules (Infrequent) ... 1961
- Demulen ... 2580
- DynaCirc Capsules (0.5% to 1%) .. 2381
- DynaCirc CR Tablets (0.5% to 1.0%) ... 2383
- Epogen for Injection (0.4%) ... 489
- Fludara for Injection (Up to 1%) ... 658
- Imitrex Injection ... 1095
- Lupron Injection ... 2736
- Monopril Tablets (0.4% to 1.0%) ... 762
- Orthoclone OKT3 Sterile Solution .. 1892
- Prinivil Tablets (0.3% to 1.0%) ... 1776
- Prinzide Tablets ... 1780
- Procrit for Injection (0.4%) ... 1896
- Proleukin for Injection (Less than 1%) ... 812
- Roferon-A Injection ... 2308
- Tonocard Tablets ... 519
- Zestoretic Tablets ... 2968
- Zestril Tablets (0.3% to 1.0%) ... 2972

Ischemic colitis
- Inderal ... 2834
- Inderal LA Long Acting Capsules ... 2836
- Inderide Tablets ... 2838
- Inderide LA Long Acting Capsules . 2840
- Kerlone Tablets ... 2588
- Levatol Tablets ... 2547
- Normodyne Tablets ... 2522
- Sectral Capsules ... 2914
- Timolide Tablets ... 1791
- Timoptic in Ocudose ... 1796
- Timoptic Sterile Ophthalmic Solution ... 1794

Ischemic injury
- Levophed Bitartrate Injection ... 2445

Itching
(see under Pruritus)

Itching, eyes
- ▲ AK-Spore (Among most frequent) ... ⊙ 205
- ▲ Alomide Ophthalmic Solution (1% to 5%) ... 465
- ▲ Betimol 0.25%, 0.5% (More than 5%) ... ⊙ 259
- Betoptic Ophthalmic Solution (Rare) ... 465
- Betoptic S Ophthalmic Suspension (Small number of patients) ... 467
- BuSpar Tablets (Infrequent) ... 738
- Chloroptic Sterile Ophthalmic Solution ... ⊙ 236
- Ciloxan Ophthalmic Solution (Less than 10%) ... 468
- Combipres Tablets ... 682
- Crolom (Infrequent) ... 254
- Geocillin Tablets ... 2009
- Lamprene Capsules (Greater than 1%) ... 846
- Mykrox Tablets (Less than 2%) ... 1617
- Neurontin Capsules (Rare) ... 1978
- Sular Tablets (Less than or equal to 1%) ... 2961
- Timoptic in Ocudose (Less frequent) ... 1796
- Timoptic Sterile Ophthalmic Solution (Less frequent) ... 1794
- Timoptic-XE (1% to 5% of patients) ... 1798
- TobraDex Ophthalmic Suspension and Ointment (Less than 4%) ... 469
- Transderm Scōp Transdermal Therapeutic System (Infrequent) 890
- Vantin for Oral Suspension and Vantin Tablets (Less than 1%) 2112
- Vaqta (Less than 1%) ... 1805
- ▲ Xalatan (5% to 15%) ... ⊙ 304

Itching, vulvovaginal
- Clozaril Tablets (Less than 1%) ... 2377
- Hivid Tablets (Less than 1%) ... 2287
- Kefzol Vials, Faspak & ADD-Vantage ... 1511
- MetroGel-Vaginal (Equal to or less than 2%) ... 917
- Monistat Dual-Pak (2%) ... 1906
- Monistat 3 Vaginal Suppositories (2%) ... 1905
- Terazol 3 Vaginal Cream ... 1941
- Terazol 7 Vaginal Cream (2.3% of 521 patients) ... 1943

IOP, elevation
- AMO Vitrax Viscoelastic Solution ... ⊙ 229
- AMVISC Plus ... ⊙ 327
- AdatoSil 5000 (Greater than 2%) ... ⊙ 265
- AK-CIDE ... ⊙ 203
- AK-CIDE Ointment ... ⊙ 203
- AK-Trol Ointment & Suspension .. ⊙ 205
- Albalon Solution with Liquifilm ... ⊙ 229
- Beclovent Inhalation Aerosol and Refill (Rare) ... 1063
- Beconase (Rare) ... 1065
- Blephamide Liquifilm Sterile Ophthalmic Suspension ... 472
- Blephamide Ointment ... ⊙ 234
- Celestone Soluspan Suspension ... 2484
- Cognex Capsules (Infrequent) ... 1961
- Cystospaz ... 2123
- Cytovene (1% or less) ... 2270
- Dalalone D.P. Injectable ... 1009
- Effexor (Rare) ... 2825
- FML Forte Liquifilm ... ⊙ 237
- FML Liquifilm ... ⊙ 238
- FML S.O.P. ... ⊙ 239
- FML-S Liquifilm ... ⊙ 240
- Florinef Acetate Tablets ... 506
- HMS Liquifilm ... ⊙ 241
- Healon (Some cases) ... ⊙ 302
- Healon GV ... ⊙ 303
- ▲ Maxitrol Ophthalmic Ointment and Suspension (Most often) ... ⊙ 222
- Neurontin Capsules (Rare) ... 1978
- OcuCoat (Some cases) ... ⊙ 321
- Paremyd ... ⊙ 244
- Paxil Tablets (Rare) ... 2681
- Permax Tablets (Infrequent) ... 571
- Poly-Pred Liquifilm ... ⊙ 246
- Pred Forte ... ⊙ 247
- Pred Mild ... ⊙ 250
- Pred-G Liquifilm Sterile Ophthalmic Suspension ... ⊙ 248
- Prelone Syrup ... 1834
- Salagen Tablets (Less than 1%) ... 1546
- Sandostatin Injection (Less than 1%) ... 2421
- Serzone Tablets (Rare) ... 776
- TobraDex Ophthalmic Suspension and Ointment ... 469
- Vancenase AQ Double Strength Nasal Spray 0.084% (Rare) ... 2536
- Videx Tablets, Powder for Oral Solution, & Pediatric Powder for Oral Solution (Less than 1%) ... 2980
- Viroptic Ophthalmic Solution, 1% Sterile ... 1177
- ▲ Voltaren Ophthalmic Sterile Ophthalmic Solution (15%) ... ⊙ 264

IUD, difficult removal
- ParaGard T 380A Intrauterine Copper Contraceptive ... 1936

IUD, embedment
- ParaGard T 380A Intrauterine Copper Contraceptive ... 1936

(⊡ Described in PDR For Nonprescription Drugs)   Incidence data in parenthesis; ▲ 3% or more   (⊙ Described in PDR For Ophthalmology)

Side Effects Index

IUD, expulsion (complete)
ParaGard T 380A Intrauterine Copper Contraceptive ... 1936

IUD, expulsion (partial)
ParaGard T 380A Intrauterine Copper Contraceptive ... 1936

IUD, fragmentation
ParaGard T 380A Intrauterine Copper Contraceptive ... 1936

J

Jaundice
Abelcet Injection ... 1540
Adapin Capsules (Occasional) ... 1542
Aldactazide Tablets ... 2556
Aldoclor Tablets ... 1638
Aldomet Ester HCl Injection ... 1642
Aldomet Oral ... 1640
Aldoril Tablets ... 1644
Altace Capsules ... 1238
Amen Tablets (A few instances) ... 785
Anaprox/Naprosyn (Rare; less than 1%) ... 2277
Ancobon Capsules ... 2254
Androderm Testosterone Transdermal System ... 2634
Android Capsules, 10 mg ... 1297
Apresazide Capsules ... 824
AquaMEPHYTON Injection ... 1648
Aquasol A Vitamin A Capsules, USP ... 525
Aquasol A Parenteral ... 526
Asendin Tablets (Very rare) ... 1419
Axid Pulvules ... 1468
Azactam for Injection (Less than 1%) ... 736
Azulfidine ... 2059
Biaxin (Infrequent) ... 406
Brevicon ... 2563
Capoten Tablets ... 740
Capozide Tablets ... 744
Cartrol Tablets (Rare) ... 413
Cataflam Tablets (Less than 1%) ... 833
Cedax ... 2480
Ceftin Tablets (Very rare) ... 1067
Chibroxin Sterile Ophthalmic Solution (With oral form) ... 1657
Cipro I.V. (1% or less) ... 587
Cipro I.V. Pharmacy Bulk Package (Less than 1%) ... 590
Cipro Tablets (Rare) ... 584
Claritin Tablets (2% or fewer patients) ... 2485
Claritin-D Tablets ... 2487
Cleocin Phosphate Injection ... 2068
Cleocin Vaginal Cream ... 2070
Clinoril Tablets (Less than 1%) ... 1658
Clozaril Tablets ... 2377
Combipres Tablets ... 682
Coumadin (Infrequent) ... 941
Crixivan Capsules (Less than 2%) ... 1670
Cylert Tablets ... 415
Cytosar-U Sterile Powder (Less frequent) ... 2077
Cytovene-IV (One report) ... 2270
Cytoxan (Isolated reports) ... 700
Danocrine Capsules ... 2437
Dantrium Capsules ... 2131
Dapsone Tablets USP ... 1331
Darvon-N/Darvocet-N (Rare) ... 1473
Darvon ... 1475
Darvon-N Suspension & Tablets ... 1473
Daypro Caplets ... 2578
Demulen ... 2580
Depo-Provera Contraceptive Injection (Fewer than 1%) ... 2079
Desyrel and Desyrel Dividose ... 504
Diflucan Tablets, Injection, and Oral Suspension ... 2003
Diucardin Tablets ... 2824
Dizac (diazepam injectable emulsion) CIV (Less frequent) ... 1862
Dolobid Tablets (Less than 1 in 100) ... 1695
Doral Tablets ... 2773
Doxil (Less than 1%) ... 2613
Dyazide Capsules ... 2653
Dyrenium Capsules (Rare) ... 2655
E.E.S. ... 427
E-Mycin Tablets ... 1388
EC-Naprosyn Delayed-Release Tablets (Rare; less than 1%) ... 2277
Edecrin (Rare) ... 1698
Effexor (Rare) ... 2825
Elavil (Rare) ... 2945
Enduron Tablets ... 424
ERYC ... 1972
EryPed 200 & EryPed 400 Granules ... 425
Ery-Tab Tablets ... 426
Erythrocin Stearate Filmtab ... 429
Esidrix Tablets ... 839
Esimil Tablets ... 840
Estraderm Transdermal System ... 842
ESTRATAB Tablets (0.3, 0.625, 1.25, 2.5 mg) ... 2715
Ethmozine Tablets (Rare) ... 2217
Etrafon (Less frequent; rare) ... 2495
Eulexin Capsules (Less than 1%) ... 2498
Felbatol ... 2774
Feldene Capsules (Less than 1%) ... 2008
Flexeril Tablets (Rare) ... 1701
Floxin I.V. ... 1580
Floxin Tablets (200 mg, 300 mg, 400 mg) ... 1577
Foscavir Injection (Less than 1%) ... 541
Fungizone Intravenous ... 507
Gantrisin ... 2286
Glucotrol Tablets (One case) ... 2011
Glucotrol XL Extended Release Tablets (One case) ... 2012
Halcion Tablets ... 2093
Haldol Decanoate ... 1587
Haldol Injection, Tablets and Concentrate ... 1585
Halotestin Tablets ... 2095
Havrix (Rare) ... 2663
HydroDIURIL Tablets ... 1716
Hydropres Tablets ... 1718
Hyzaar Tablets ... 1720
IBU Tablets (Less than 1%) ... 1389
Inderide Tablets ... 2838
Inderide LA Long Acting Capsules ... 2840
Indocin Capsules (Less than 1%) ... 1723
Indocin I.V. (Less than 1%) ... 1727
Indocin (Less than 1%) ... 1723
Inocor Lactate Injection (Rare) ... 2439
Intron A for Injection (Less than 5%) ... 2506
Invirase Capsules (Rare) ... 2291
Lamprene Capsules (Less than 1%) ... 846
Lasix Injection, Oral Solution and Tablets ... 1267
Leukeran Tablets ... 1205
Levlen/Tri-Levlen ... 646
Levoprome ... 1321
Librax Capsules (Occasional) ... 2330
Librium Capsules (Occasional) ... 2331
Librium Injectable (Occasional) ... 2332
Limbitrol (Rare) ... 2333
Lodine Capsules and Tablets (Less than 1%) ... 2849
Lopressor HCT Tablets ... 850
Loxitane (Rare) ... 1426
Ludiomil Tablets (Rare) ... 861
LUVOX Tablets (Rare) ... 2723
Matulane Capsules ... 2300
Mavik Tablets (Rare) ... 1407
Mefoxin ... 1734
Mefoxin Premixed Intravenous Solution ... 1737
Mellaril ... 2398
Merrem I.V. (0.1% to 1.0%) ... 2952
Mesantoin Tablets ... 2400
Midamor Tablets (Less than or equal to 1%) ... 1746
Mintezol ... 1747
Modicon ... 1928
Moduretic Tablets ... 1748
Monopril Tablets ... 762
Motrin Ibuprofen Suspension, Oral Drops, Chewable Tablets, Caplets (Rare; less than 1%) ... 1563
Mustargen (Infrequent) ... 1752
Myochrysine Injection ... 1754
Nalfon 200 Pulvules & Nalfon Tablets (Less than 1%) ... 933
▲ Naprelan Tablets (3% to 9%) ... 2861
Anaprox/Naprosyn (Rare; less than 1%) ... 2277
Nardil (Less frequent) ... 1977
Nimotop Capsules (Less than 1%) ... 603
Nizoral Tablets ... 1345
Norinyl ... 2563
Normodyne Injection ... 2519
Normodyne Tablets ... 2522
Noroxin Tablets ... 1758
Noroxin Tablets ... 2222
Norpramin Tablets ... 1273
Nor-Q D Tablets ... 2598
Norvasc Tablets ... 2020
▲ Novantrone for Injection (3 to 7%) ... 1327
Nydrazid Injection ... 509
▲ Oncaspar (Greater than 1% but less than 5%) ... 2194
Ortho-Cyclen/Ortho Tri-Cyclen ... 1914
Ortho-Novum ... 1928
Ortho-Cyclen/Ortho Tri-Cyclen ... 1914
Orudis Capsules (Rare) ... 2874
Oruvail Capsules (Rare) ... 2874
Ovcon ... 765
Oxandrin ... 783
PCE Dispertab Tablets ... 453
Pamelor ... 2409
PASER Granules ... 1333
Paxil Tablets (Rare) ... 2681
Pediazole Suspension ... 2340
Periactin ... 1767
Permax Tablets (Rare) ... 571
Phenergan Injection ... 2880
Phenergan Tablets ... 2882
Prilosec Delayed-Release Capsules (Rare) ... 516
Primaxin I.M. ... 1770
Primaxin I.V. (Less than 0.2%) ... 1772
Prinivil Tablets ... 1776
Prinzide Tablets ... 1780
▲ Prograf (Greater than 3%) ... 1028
▲ Proleukin for Injection (11%) ... 812
Prozac Pulvules & Liquid, Oral Solution (Rare) ... 935
Redux Capsules ... 2911
Reglan (Rare) ... 2243
Ridaura Capsules (Less than 1%) ... 2691
Rifadin (Some patients) ... 1276
Rifamate Capsules ... 1278
Rifater ... 1280
Rilutek Tablets (Infrequent) ... 2198
Risperdal Tablets ... 1348
Rocephin Injectable Vials, ADD-Vantage, Galaxy Container (Rare) ... 2305
Sandostatin Injection (Less than 1%) ... 2421
Seldane Tablets (Isolated reports) ... 1284
Seldane-D Extended-Release Tablets (Isolated reports) ... 1286
Septra I.V. Infusion ... 1142
Septra I.V. Infusion ADD-Vantage Vials ... 1144
Ser-Ap-Es Tablets ... 867
Serax Capsules ... 2916
Serax Tablets ... 2916
Serentil ... 689
Sinequan (Occasional) ... 2028
Skelaxin Tablets ... 793
Solganal Suspension ... 2530
Sporanox Capsules ... 1352
Stelazine ... 2692
Surmontil Capsules ... 2917
Tambocor Tablets ... 1555
Tao Capsules ... 2033
Tapazole Tablets ... 1361
Tenoretic Tablets ... 2963
Testoderm Testosterone Transdermal System ... 486
Thalitone ... 1293
Thioguanine Tablets, Tabloid Brand ... 1225
Thorazine ... 2701
Tigan ... 2231
Tofranil Ampuls ... 873
Tofranil Tablets ... 875
Tofranil-PM Capsules ... 876
Tonocard Tablets (Less than 1%) ... 519
Torecan ... 2367
Trancopal Caplets (Rare) ... 2468
Trandate ... 1158
Trecator-SC Tablets ... 2919
Trental Tablets (Rare) ... 1291
Triavil Tablets ... 1800
Trilafon (Low incidence) ... 2532
Levlen/Tri-Levlen ... 646
Tri-Norinyl ... 2607
Univasc Tablets ... 2553
Valium Injectable (Isolated reports) ... 2336
Valium Tablets (Isolated reports) ... 2335
Vaseretic Tablets ... 1810
Vasotec I.V. ... 1814
Vasotec Tablets ... 1816
Vivactil Tablets ... 1820
Cataflam/Voltaren/Voltaren-XR (Less than 1%) ... 833
Wellbutrin Tablets (Infrequent) ... 1177
Wygesic Tablets (Rare) ... 2930
Xanax Tablets ... 2115
Yutopar Intravenous Injection (Infrequent) ... 566
Zantac (Occasional) ... 1182
Zantac Injection ... 1180
Zantac Syrup (Occasional) ... 1182
Zestoretic Tablets ... 2968
Ziac ... 1459
Zoloft Tablets (One or more patients) ... 2051

Jaundice, cholestatic
Accupril Tablets (Rare) ... 1950
Altace Capsules (Rare) ... 1238
Amaryl Tablets (Rare) ... 1241
Amen Tablets ... 785
Androderm Testosterone Transdermal System ... 2634
▲ Android Capsules, 10 mg (Among most common) ... 1297
Atretol Tablets ... 569
Augmentin ... 2637
Augmentin Tablets ... 2640
Axid Pulvules (Rare) ... 1468
Aygestin Tablets ... 990
Bactrim DS Tablets ... 2257
Bactrim I.V. Infusion ... 2255
Bactrim ... 2257
Brevicon ... 2563
Capoten Tablets (Rare) ... 740
Capozide Tablets (Rare) ... 744
Ceclor Pulvules & Suspension (Rare) ... 1470
Cefzil Tablets and Oral Suspension (Rare) ... 747
Chibroxin Sterile Ophthalmic Solution (With oral form) ... 1657
Cipro Tablets ... 584
Climara Transdermal System ... 640
Compazine ... 2644
Cycrin Tablets ... 991
Danocrine Capsules ... 2437
Dapsone Tablets USP ... 1331
Darvon-N/Darvocet-N (Rare) ... 1473
Darvon ... 1475
Darvon-N Suspension & Tablets (Rare) ... 1473
Demulen ... 2580
Depo-Provera Sterile Aqueous Suspension ... 2083
Desogen Tablets ... 1867
DiaBeta Tablets (Rare) ... 1265
Diabinese Tablets (Rare) ... 2002
Diethylstilbestrol Tablets ... 1477
Doxil (Less than 1%) ... 2613
Estrace Cream and Tablets ... 751
Estraderm Transdermal System ... 842
ESTRATAB Tablets (0.3, 0.625, 1.25, 2.5 mg) ... 2715
Estratest ... 2718
Eulexin Capsules (Less than 1%) ... 2498
Floxin I.V. ... 1580
Floxin Tablets (200 mg, 300 mg, 400 mg) ... 1577
Glucotrol Tablets (Rare) ... 2011
Glynase PresTab Tablets (Rare) ... 2091
Halotestin Tablets ... 2095
Keflex Pulvules & Oral Suspension (Rare) ... 930
Keftab Tablets (Rare) ... 931
Kefzol Vials, Faspak & ADD-Vantage (Rare) ... 1511
Lescol Capsules ... 2395
Levlen/Tri-Levlen ... 646
Lodine Capsules and Tablets (Less than 1%) ... 2849
Lo/Ovral Tablets ... 2852
Lo/Ovral-28 Tablets ... 2857
Lopid Tablets ... 1974
Lotensin Tablets (Rare) ... 852
Lotensin HCT Tablets (Rare) ... 855
Lotrel Capsules (Rare) ... 858
Macrobid Capsules (Rare) ... 2138
Macrodantin Capsules (Rare) ... 2140
Mandol Vials, Faspak & ADD-Vantage (Rare) ... 1516
Mavik Tablets (Rare) ... 1407
Menest Tablets ... 2671
Merrem I.V. (0.1% to 1.0%) ... 2952
Mevacor Tablets ... 1742
Micronase Tablets (Rare) ... 2099
Modicon ... 1928
Monopril Tablets ... 762
Myleran Tablets (Rare) ... 1209
Myochrysine Injection ... 1754
Nordette-21 Tablets ... 2863
Nordette-28 Tablets ... 2866
Norinyl ... 2563
Normodyne Injection (Less common) ... 2519
Normodyne Tablets (Less common) ... 2522
Noroxin Tablets ... 1758
Noroxin Tablets ... 2222
Norpace (Infrequent) ... 2596
Nor-Q D Tablets ... 2598
Ogen Tablets ... 2103
Ogen Vaginal Cream ... 2106
Ortho-Cept ... 1907
Ortho-Cyclen/Ortho-Tri-Cyclen ... 1914
Ortho Dienestrol Cream ... 1922
Ortho-Est ... 1925
Ortho-Novum ... 1928
Ortho-Cyclen/Ortho Tri-Cyclen ... 1914

Side Effects Index

Jaundice, cholestatic

Drug	Page
Ovcon	765
Ovral Tablets	2877
Ovral-28 Tablets	2878
Ovrette Tablets	2878
Oxandrin	783
Pepcid Injection (Infrequent)	1765
Pepcid (Infrequent)	1763
Placidyl Capsules	456
PMB 200 and PMB 400	2890
Pravachol Tablets	770
Premarin Intravenous	2893
Premarin Tablets	2896
Premarin Vaginal Cream	2898
Premphase	2900
Prempro	2905
Prilosec Delayed-Release Capsules (Rare)	516
Prinivil Tablets (0.3% to 1.0%)	1776
Prinzide Tablets (Rare)	1780
Procardia Capsules	2024
Procardia XL Extended Release Tablets	2026
▲ Prograf (Greater than 3%)	1028
Prolixin	510
Proloprim Tablets (Rare)	1141
Provera Tablets	2110
Prozac Pulvules & Liquid, Oral Solution	935
Relafen Tablets (1%)	2688
Ridaura Capsules (Rare)	2691
Septra	1146
Septra I.V. Infusion	1142
Septra I.V. Infusion ADD-Vantage Vials	1144
Septra	1146
Stelazine	2692
Tegretol/Tegretol-XR	870
Testoderm Testosterone Transdermal System	486
Testred Capsules, 10 mg	1308
Ticlid Tablets (Rare)	2317
Timentin for Injection (Rare)	2706
Toradol	2319
Torecan (Occasional case)	2367
Trancopal Caplets	2468
Trandate (Less common)	1158
Levlen/Tri-Levlen	646
Tri-Norinyl	2607
Triphasil-21 Tablets	2919
Triphasil-28 Tablets	2924
Univasc Tablets (Rare)	2553
Vaseretic Tablets (Rare)	1810
Vasotec I.V. (Rare)	1814
Vasotec Tablets (0.5% to 1.0%; rare)	1816
Vivelle Transdermal System	880
Winstrol Tablets (Rare)	2468
Zestoretic Tablets (Rare)	2968
Zestril Tablets (0.3% to 1.0%)	2972
Zithromax (1% or less; rare)	2043
Zithromax Tablets (1% or less; rare)	2046
Zocor Tablets	1821
Zyloprim Tablets (Less than 1%)	1194

Jaundice, fetal

Drug	Page
Diupres Tablets	1691
Diuril Oral Suspension	1694
Diuril Sodium Intravenous	1693
Diuril Tablets	1694
HydroDIURIL Tablets	1716
Hydropres Tablets	1718

Jaundice, hepatocellular

Drug	Page
Atretol Tablets	569
Augmentin	2637
Augmentin Tablets	2640
Axid Pulvules (Rare)	1468
Biaxin (Infrequent)	406
Floxin I.V.	1580
Floxin Tablets (200 mg, 300 mg, 400 mg)	1577
Monopril Tablets	762
Prilosec Delayed-Release Capsules (Rare)	516
Prinivil Tablets (0.3% to 1.0%)	1776
Prinzide Tablets	1780
Tegretol/Tegretol-XR	870
Ticlid Tablets (Rare)	2317
Vaseretic Tablets	1810
Vasotec I.V.	1814
Vasotec Tablets (0.5% to 1.0%)	1816
Zantac (Occasional)	1182
Zestoretic Tablets	2968
Zestril Tablets (0.3% to 1.0%)	2972

Jaundice, intrahepatic

Drug	Page
Minizide Capsules	2016
Solganal Suspension	2530

Jaundice, intrahepatic cholestatic

Drug	Page
Aldoclor Tablets	1638
Apresazide Capsules	824
Augmentin	2637
Augmentin Tablets	2640
Capozide Tablets	744
Combipres Tablets	682
Diucardin Tablets	2824
Diupres Tablets	1691
Diuril Oral Suspension	1694
Diuril Sodium Intravenous	1693
Diuril Tablets	1694
Enduron Tablets	424
Esidrix Tablets	839
Esimil Tablets	840
HydroDIURIL Tablets	1716
Hydropres Tablets	1718
Hyzaar Tablets	1720
Inderide Tablets	2838
Inderide LA Long Acting Capsules	2840
Lasix Injection, Oral Solution and Tablets	1267
Lopressor HCT Tablets	850
Lotensin HCT Tablets	855
Moduretic Tablets	1748
Mykrox Tablets	1617
Oretic Tablets	450
Prinzide Tablets	1780
Ser-Ap-Es Tablets	867
Solganal Suspension	2530
Tenoretic Tablets	2963
Thalitone	1293
Timolide Tablets	1791
Vaseretic Tablets	1810
Zaroxolyn Tablets	1625
Zestoretic Tablets	2968
Ziac	1459

Jaundice, neonatal

Drug	Page
Aldactazide Tablets	2556
Aldoclor Tablets	1638
Aldoril Tablets	1644
Apresazide Capsules	824
AquaMEPHYTON Injection	1648
Capozide Tablets	744
Compazine	2644
Depo-Provera Sterile Aqueous Suspension	2083
Diucardin Tablets	2824
Diupres Tablets	1691
Diuril Oral Suspension	1694
Diuril Sodium Intravenous	1693
Diuril Tablets	1694
Dyazide Capsules	2653
Enduron Tablets	424
Esidrix Tablets	839
Esimil Tablets	840
HydroDIURIL Tablets	1716
Hydropres Tablets	1718
Inderide Tablets	2838
Inderide LA Long Acting Capsules	2840
Levlen/Tri-Levlen	646
Lopressor HCT Tablets	850
Lotensin HCT Tablets	855
Mephyton Tablets	1739
Modicon	1928
Moduretic Tablets	1748
Mykrox Tablets	1617
Oretic Tablets	450
Ortho-Novum	1928
Prinzide Tablets	1780
Ser-Ap-Es Tablets	867
Stelazine	2692
Syntocinon Injection	2425
Tenoretic Tablets	2963
Thorazine	2701
Timolide Tablets	1791
Levlen/Tri-Levlen	646
Vaseretic Tablets	1810
Zestoretic Tablets	2968

Jaundice, obstructive

Drug	Page
Thorazine	2701
Tofranil Ampuls	873
Tofranil Tablets	875
Tofranil-PM Capsules	876

Jaw tightness

Drug	Page
Anectine	1062
Imitrex Injection (Relatively common)	1095
Respbid Tablets	687

Jerks
(see under Twitching)

Jitteriness

Drug	Page
Adalat Capsules (10 mg and 20 mg) (2% or less)	580
Compazine	2644
Etrafon	2495

Drug	Page
Nardil (Less common)	1977
Procardia Capsules (2% or less)	2024
Reglan	2243
Stelazine	2692
Thorazine	2701
▲ Yutopar Intravenous Injection (5% to 6%)	566

Joint disorder

Drug	Page
▲ CellCept Capsules (More than or equal to 3%)	2265
Naprelan Tablets (Less than 3%)	2861
Oncaspar (Less than 1%)	2194
Redux Capsules (Infrequent)	2911

Joint disorder, unspecified

Drug	Page
Cartrol Tablets (Less common)	413
Effexor (Infrequent)	2825
Hytrin Capsules (At least 1%)	434
Keflex Pulvules & Oral Suspension	930
Keftab Tablets	931
Lamictal Tablets (1.3%)	1105
▲ Lupron Depot 3.75 mg (7.8%)	2739
▲ Lupron Depot - 3 Month 22.5 mg (11.7%)	2743
Norvir (Less than 2%)	447
Videx Tablets, Powder for Oral Solution, & Pediatric Powder for Oral Solution (Less than 1%)	2980
Zoladex (1% or greater)	2976
Zoladex 3-month	2978

Joint effusion

Drug	Page
Sandostatin Injection (Less than 1%)	2421

Joint pain
(see under Arthralgia)

Joint stiffness

Drug	Page
Adalat Capsules (10 mg and 20 mg) (2% or less)	580
Cipro I.V. (1% or less)	587
Cipro I.V. Pharmacy Bulk Package (Less than 1%)	590
Cipro Tablets (Less than 1%)	584
Danocrine Capsules	2437
Imitrex Injection (Infrequent)	1095
NegGram	2453
Neurontin Capsules (Infrequent)	1978
Oncaspar	2194
Procardia Capsules (2% or less)	2024
Supprelin Injection (2% to 3%)	2230

K

Kawasaki-like syndrome

Drug	Page
Pentasa (Less than 1%)	1275

Keratitis

Drug	Page
Acular Sterile Ophthalmic Solution (1%)	470
Alomide Ophthalmic Solution (Less than 1%)	465
Anafranil Capsules (Rare)	819
Betagan	⊚ 230
Betimol 0.25%, 0.5% (1% to 5%)	⊚ 259
Betoptic Ophthalmic Solution (Rare)	465
Betoptic S Ophthalmic Suspension (Rare)	467
BOTOX (Botulinum Toxin Type A) Purified Neurotoxin Complex (Less than 1%)	473
Ciloxan Ophthalmic Solution (Less than 1%)	468
Econopred & Econopred Plus Ophthalmic Suspensions (Occasional)	⊚ 216
Effexor (Rare)	2825
Engerix-B Unit-Dose Vials	2656
FML Forte Liquifilm (Occasional)	⊚ 237
FML Liquifilm (Occasional)	⊚ 238
FML S.O.P. (Occasional)	⊚ 239
Iopidine 0.5% (Less than 3%)	⊚ 219
Ocuflox Ophthalmic Solution	478
Ocupress Ophthalmic Solution, 1% Sterile	⊚ 297
Pilopine HS Ophthalmic Gel	⊚ 224
Pred Forte (Occasional)	⊚ 247
Pred Mild (Occasional)	⊚ 250
Timoptic Sterile Ophthalmic Solution (Less frequent)	1794
Timoptic-XE	1798
Vexol 1% Ophthalmic Suspension (Less than 1%)	⊚ 227
▲ Voltaren Ophthalmic Sterile Ophthalmic Solution (28%)	⊚ 264

Keratitis, bacterial

Drug	Page
Cortisporin Ophthalmic Ointment Sterile	1074
Decadron Phosphate Sterile Ophthalmic Ointment	1684
Decadron Phosphate Sterile Ophthalmic Solution	1685
Humorsol Sterile Ophthalmic Solution	1707
NeoDecadron Sterile Ophthalmic Ointment	1755
Neosporin Ophthalmic Ointment Sterile	1130
Trusopt Sterile Ophthalmic Solution	1803
Xalatan	⊚ 304

Keratitis, epithelial

Drug	Page
FLUORACAINE (Rare)	⊚ 208
FLURESS (Rare)	⊚ 208
Ophthetic	⊚ 244

Keratitis, punctate

Drug	Page
Albalon Solution with Liquifilm	⊚ 229
Pred-G Liquifilm Sterile Ophthalmic Suspension (Occasional)	⊚ 248
Pred-G S.O.P. Sterile Ophthalmic Ointment	⊚ 249
▲ Rev-Eyes Ophthalmic Eyedrops 0.5% (10% to 40%)	⊚ 324

Keratitis, superficial punctate

Drug	Page
▲ Trusopt Sterile Ophthalmic Solution (10% to 15%)	1803
Vira-A Ophthalmic Ointment, 3%	⊚ 299
Viroptic Ophthalmic Solution, 1% Sterile	1177

Keratitis nigricans

Drug	Page
Timoptic in Ocudose (Less frequent)	1796

Keratoconjunctivitis

Drug	Page
Betaseron for SC Injection	653
Naprelan Tablets (Less than 1%)	2861
Paxil Tablets (Rare)	2681
Remeron Tablets (Infrequent)	1878
Serzone Tablets (Infrequent)	776
Sular Tablets (Less than or equal to 1%)	2961
Viroptic Ophthalmic Solution, 1% Sterile	1177

Keratopathy

Drug	Page
▲ AdatoSil 5000 (0.6% to 30%)	⊚ 265
Alomide Ophthalmic Solution (Less than 1%)	465
Ciloxan Ophthalmic Solution (Less than 1%)	468
Iopidine 0.5% (Less than 3%)	⊚ 219
Trilafon	2532

Keratopathy, bullous

Drug	Page
AMO Endosol (Balanced Salt Solution)	⊚ 229
Carbastat Intraocular Solution (Occasional)	⊚ 260
MIOSTAT Intraocular Solution	⊚ 222

Keratopathy, epithelial

Drug	Page
Compazine	2644
Etrafon	2495
Stelazine	2692
Thorazine	2701
Viroptic Ophthalmic Solution, 1% Sterile	1177
▲ Xalatan (5% to 15%)	⊚ 304

Keratosis pilaris

Drug	Page
Azelex (Rare)	471

Kernicterus, neonatal

Drug	Page
AVC	1245
Azulfidine	2059
Bactrim DS Tablets	2257
Bactrim I.V. Infusion	2255
Bactrim	2257
Blephamide Ointment	⊚ 234
Fansidar Tablets	2281
Gantanol Tablets	2285
Gantrisin	2286
Pediazole Suspension	2340
Septra	1146
Silvadene Cream 1%	1288

Ketosis

Drug	Page
Betaseron for SC Injection	653
Cerebyx Injection (Infrequent)	1956
Doxil	2613
Paxil Tablets (Rare)	2681

(⊞ Described in PDR For Nonprescription Drugs)   Incidence data in parenthesis; ▲ 3% or more   (⊚ Described in PDR For Ophthalmology)

Kidney, decrease in size
BiCNU 696
CeeNU Capsules 699

Kidney damage
Azulfidine 2059
BiCNU (Occasional) 696
CeeNU Capsules (Occasional) 699
Lasix Injection, Oral Solution and Tablets 1267

Kidney stones (see under Renal stones)

L

Labia, fusion
Depo-Provera Sterile Aqueous Suspension (Rare) 2083
Provera Tablets (Rare) 2110

Labor, preterm, delayed
Airet Albuterol Sulfate Inhalation Solution 1602
Ventolin Inhalation Solution 1171
Ventolin Nebules Inhalation Solution 1172
Ventolin Rotacaps for Inhalation 1173
Ventolin Syrup 1175
Ventolin Tablets 1176

Labor, slowing
Astramorph/PF Injection, USP (Preservative-Free) 526
Brontex 2130
Carbocaine Injection 2432
Kadian Capsules (Occasional; less than 3%) 2948
Marcaine 2446
Marcaine Spinal 2449
Proventil Inhalation Solution 0.083% (Some reports) 2527
Proventil Repetabs Tablets (Some reports) 2529
Proventil Solution for Inhalation 0.5% (Some reports) 2525
Proventil Syrup (Some reports) 2528
Proventil Tablets (Some patients) 2529
Sensorcaine 554

Laboratory abnormalities, unspecified
Betapace Tablets (1% to 4%) 637
Cartrol Tablets (1.2%) 413

Labyrinth disorder
Anafranil Capsules (Rare) 819

Labyrinthitis
Avonex 662
Benadryl Injection 1955
Cognex Capsules (Rare) 1961
Effexor (Rare) 2825
Kerlone Tablets (Less than 2%) 2588
Neurontin Capsules (Rare) 1978
Nipent for Injection (Less than 3%) 2733
Ornade Spansule Capsules 2678
Periactin 1767
Tavist Syrup 2426
Tavist Tablets 2427
Trinalin Repetabs Tablets 1373

Lacrimal duct, stenosis
Ergamisol Tablets 1340
Fluorouracil Injection 2282
Sterile FUDR (Remote possibility) 2284

Lacrimal gland, disorders
DDAVP (Up to 2%) 2180
Intron A for Injection (Less than 5%) 2506
Neurontin Capsules (Rare) 1978

Lacrimation
Adriamycin PFS (Rare) 2056
Adriamycin RDF (Rare) 2056
Albalon Solution with Liquifilm ⊙ 229
Apresazide Capsules (Less frequent) 824
Apresoline Hydrochloride Tablets (Less frequent) 826
Asendin Tablets (Less than 1%) 1419
▲BOTOX (Botulinum Toxin Type A) Purified Neurotoxin Complex (10.0%) 473
Claritin Tablets (Rare) 2485
Crolom (Infrequent) ⊙ 254
Doxorubicin Astra (Rare) 531
Efudex 2280
Fluorouracil Injection 2282
Sterile FUDR (Remote possibility) 2284
Heparin Lock Flush Solution 2831
Heparin Sodium Injection 2832
Heparin Sodium Vials (Rare) 1486
Hivid Tablets (Less than 1%) 2287
Humorsol Sterile Ophthalmic Solution 1707
Hydralazine Hydrochloride Injection USP 2712
Hyperstat I.V. Injection 2504
Imitrex Injection (Infrequent) 1095
Imitrex Tablets (Infrequent) 1099
Intal Inhaler (Infrequent) 2185
Intal Nebulizer Solution 2186
Livostin (Approximately 1% to 3%) ⊙ 262
Methadone Hydrochloride Oral Concentrate 2356
Neurontin Capsules (Rare) 1978
Nipent for Injection (Less than 3%) 2733
OptiPranolol (Metipranolol 0.3%) Sterile Ophthalmic Solution (A small number of patients) ⊙ 256
Orlaam Oral Solution (Less than 1%) 2361
Phospholine Iodide ⊙ 323
Pilopine HS Ophthalmic Gel ⊙ 224
Procardia XL Extended Release Tablets (1% or less) 2026
Proglycem 575
ReVia Tablets (A small fraction of patients) 957
Rubex for Injection (Rare) 721
▲Salagen Tablets (6%) 1546
Ser-Ap-Es Tablets 867
▲Tegison Capsules (1-10%) 2314
Tensilon Injectable 1307
Trusopt Sterile Ophthalmic Solution (Approximately 1% to 5%) 1803
Urecholine 1804
Vaseretic Tablets 1810
Vasotec I.V. 1814
Vasotec Tablets (0.5% to 1.0%) 1816
Vexol 1% Ophthalmic Suspension (Less than 1%) ⊙ 227
Vira-A Ophthalmic Ointment, 3% ⊙ 299

Lacrimation, abnormal
Ambien Tablets (Rare) 2559
Anafranil Capsules (Up to 3%) 819
Cardura Tablets (Less than 0.5% of 3960 patients) 1993
Claritin-D Tablets (Less frequent) 2487
Desmopressin Acetate Rhinal Tube (Up to 2%) 997
Ergamisol Tablets (Up to 4%) 1340
Flumadine Tablets & Syrup 1013
Kerlone Tablets (Less than 2%) 2588
Lamictal Tablets (Rare) 1105
Miacalcin Nasal Spray (1% to 3%) 2403
Naprelan Tablets (Less than 1%) 2861
Nicotrol NS Nicotine Nasal Spray (Common) 1565
Redux Capsules (Rare) 2911
Remeron Tablets (Infrequent) 1878
Risperdal Tablets (Rare) 1348
Romazicon (1% to 3%) 2311
Zebeta Tablets 1457
Ziac 1459
Zoloft Tablets (Rare) 2051

Lacrimation, decrease
Ditropan 1267

Lactation
Aldoclor Tablets 1638
Aldomet Ester HCl Injection 1642
Aldomet Oral 1640
Aldoril Tablets 1644
Compazine 2644
Desyrel and Desyrel Dividose 504
Effexor (Rare) 2825
Etrafon 2495
Haldol Decanoate 1587
Haldol Injection, Tablets and Concentrate 1585
Lamictal Tablets (Infrequent) 1105
▲Lupron Depot 3.75 mg (Among most frequent) 2739
LUVOX Tablets (Infrequent) 2723
Mellaril 2398
Navane Capsules and Concentrate 2018
Navane Intramuscular 2019
Paxil Tablets (Rare) 2681
Permax Tablets (Infrequent) 571
Prozac Pulvules & Liquid, Oral Solution (Rare) 935
Serentil 689
Stelazine 2692
Synarel Nasal Solution for Endometriosis (Less than 1%) 2605
Thorazine 2701
Triavil Tablets 1800
Trilafon 2532

Lactation, non-puerperal
Anafranil Capsules (Up to 4%) 819
Diupres Tablets 1691
Flumadine Tablets & Syrup (Less than 0.3%) 1013
Hydropres Tablets 1718
Risperdal Tablets (Infrequent) 1348

Lactation, possible diminution
Brevicon 2563
Demulen 2580
Desogen Tablets 1867
Levlen/Tri-Levlen 646
Lo/Ovral Tablets 2852
Lo/Ovral-28 Tablets 2857
Modicon 1928
Nordette-21 Tablets 2863
Nordette-28 Tablets 2866
Norinyl 2563
Nor-Q D Tablets 2598
Ortho-Cept 1907
Ortho-Cyclen/Ortho-Tri-Cyclen 1914
Ortho-Novum 1928
Ortho-Cyclen/Ortho Tri-Cyclen 1914
Ovral Tablets 2877
Ovral-28 Tablets 2878
Ovrette Tablets 2878
Levlen/Tri-Levlen 646
Tri-Norinyl 2607
Triphasil-21 Tablets 2919
Triphasil-28 Tablets 2924

Lactation, suppression
Bentyl 1246
Cystospaz 2123
Depo-Provera Contraceptive Injection (Fewer than 1%) 2079
Ditropan 1267
Donnatal 2234
Donnatal Extentabs 2234
Donnatal Tablets 2234
Kutrase Capsules 2546
Levsin/Levsinex/Levbid 2549
Ovcon 765
Pro-Banthine Tablets 2226
Robinul Forte Tablets 2247
Robinul Injectable 2247
Robinul Tablets 2247

Lactation abnormalities
Demulen 2580
Levoprome 1321
Prolixin 510
THYREL TRH (Less frequent) 2992

Lactic acidosis
Glucophage Tablets (Rare) 754
Hivid Tablets (Rare) 2287
Retrovir Capsules (Rare) 1216
Retrovir I.V. Infusion (Rare) 1221
Retrovir Syrup (Rare) 1216
Yutopar Intravenous Injection (Infrequent) 566

Lagophthalmos
BOTOX (Botulinum Toxin Type A) Purified Neurotoxin Complex 473

Laryngeal changes
Alupent Tablets (0.2%) 672
Mexitil Capsules (About 1 in 1,000) 684

Laryngeal stridor
Lotrel Capsules (About 0.5%) 858
Monopril Tablets 762
Omnipen for Oral Suspension 2873

Laryngismus
Anafranil Capsules (Rare) 819
Effexor (Infrequent) 2825
LUVOX Tablets (Rare) 2723

Laryngitis
AeroBid Inhaler System (1% to 3%) 1004
Aerobid-M Inhaler System (1% to 3%) 1004
Ambien Tablets (Rare) 2559
Anafranil Capsules (Up to 2%) 819
Avonex 662
▲Betaseron for SC Injection (6%) 653
Claritin Tablets (2% or fewer patients) 2485
Claritin-D Tablets 2487
Clozaril Tablets (Less than 1%) 2377
Effexor (Infrequent) 2825
Foscavir Injection (Less than 1%) 541
Invirase Capsules (Less than 2%) 2291
Monopril Tablets (0.2% to 1.0%) 762
Naprelan Tablets (Less than 1%) 2861
Neurontin Capsules (Rare) 1978
Permax Tablets (Infrequent) 571
Prinivil Tablets (0.3% to 1.0%) 1776
Prinzide Tablets 1780
ProSom Tablets (Rare) 457
Prostin E2 Suppository 2109
▲Pulmozyme Inhalation (3% to 4%) 1054
Redux Capsules (Infrequent) 2911
Remeron Tablets (Rare) 1878
Rilutek Tablets (Infrequent) 2198
Serevent Inhalation Aerosol (1% to 3%) 1149
Serzone Tablets (Infrequent) 776
Sular Tablets (Less than or equal to 1%) 2961
Trental Tablets (Less than 1%) 1291
Videx Tablets, Powder for Oral Solution, & Pediatric Powder for Oral Solution (Less than 1%) 2980
Zestoretic Tablets 2968
Zestril Tablets (0.3% to 1.0%) 2972

Laryngospasm
Alfenta Injection (0.3% to 1%) 1334
Atrovent Inhalation Aerosol 674
Atrovent Nasal Spray 0.06% 678
Blocadren Tablets 1654
Carafate Suspension 1250
Carafate Tablets 1249
Cartrol Tablets 413
Dilaudid-HP Injection (Less frequent) 1384
Dilaudid-HP Lyophilized Powder 250 mg (Less frequent) 1384
Dilaudid Tablets and Liquid 1386
Diprivan Injectable Emulsion (Less than 1%) 2939
Dizac (diazepam injectable emulsion) CIV 1862
Dopram Injectable 2235
Etopophos for Injection (Sometimes) 701
Etoposide Injection (Sometimes) 539
Haldol Decanoate 1587
Haldol Injection, Tablets and Concentrate 1585
Inapsine Injection (Less common) 462
Inderal 2834
Inderal LA Long Acting Capsules 2836
Inderide Tablets 2838
Inderide LA Long Acting Capsules 2840
Isoptin Injectable (Rare) 1391
Kerlone Tablets 2588
Levatol Tablets 2547
Lopressor HCT Tablets 850
MS Contin Tablets (Less frequent) 2149
MSIR (Infrequent) 2152
Normodyne Tablets 2522
Oramorph SR (Morphine Sulfate Sustained Release Tablets) (Less frequent) 2359
Orthoclone OKT3 Sterile Solution 1892
Reglan 2243
Sectral Capsules 2914
Serevent Inhalation Aerosol (Rare) 1149
Sublimaze Injection 463
▲Suprane (desflurane, USP) (3% to 50%) 1865
Tenoretic Tablets 2963
Tenormin Tablets and I.V. Injection 2965
Tensilon Injectable 1307
Tessalon Perles 1018
Timolide Tablets 1791
Timoptic in Ocudose 1796
Timoptic Sterile Ophthalmic Solution 1794
Timoptic-XE 1798
Toprol-XL Tablets 560
Tracrium Injection 1155
Trandate Tablets 1158
Valium Injectable 2336
VePesid Capsules and Injection (Sometimes) 727
Versed Injection (Less than 1.0%) 2324
Visken Tablets 2428
Zebeta Tablets 1457
Ziac 1459

Lassitude
Atrohist Pediatric Capsules 1603
Atrohist Plus Tablets 1605
Azmacort Oral Inhaler 2175

(▭ Described in PDR For Nonprescription Drugs) Incidence data in parenthesis; ▲ 3% or more (⊙ Described in PDR For Ophthalmology)

Lassitude

- Beconase ... 1065
- Bromfed ... 1832
- ▲ Cartrol Tablets (7.1%) ... 413
- Codiclear DH Syrup ... 808
- Daranide Tablets ... 1676
- Dexedrine ... 2648
- Esimil Tablets ... 840
- Felbatol ... 2774
- ▲ Hytrin Capsules (7.4% to 11.3%) ... 434
- Inderal ... 2834
- Inderal LA Long Acting Capsules ... 2836
- Inderide Tablets ... 2838
- Inderide LA Long Acting Capsules ... 2840
- Ismelin Tablets ... 845
- ▲ Mykrox Tablets (4.4%) ... 1617
- Nasacort Nasal Inhaler ... 2189
- Neurontin Capsules (Rare) ... 1978
- Parlodel (Less than 1%) ... 2411
- Pediazole Suspension ... 2340
- Phenergan Injection ... 2880
- Phenergan Tablets ... 2882
- Plaquenil Sulfate Tablets ... 2459
- Protamine Sulfate Vials ... 1526
- ▲ Reglan (Approximately 10%) ... 2243
- Risperdal Tablets ... 1348
- Rondec Chewable Tablets ... 974
- Tonocard Tablets (0.8% to 1.6%) ... 519
- Triavil Tablets ... 1800

Laughing, easy

- ▲ Marinol (Dronabinol) Capsules (8% to 24%) ... 2353

Laxative effect

- Beelith Tablets ... 632
- Derifil Tablets ... 2371
- Mag-Ox 400 ... 666
- Phillips' Milk of Magnesia Liquid ... ▣ 627
- Uro-Mag ... 666

Left ventricular dysfunction

- Orthoclone OKT3 Sterile Solution ... 1892
- Rubex for Injection ... 721

Left ventricular ejection fraction, asymptomatic declines in

- Idamycin Injection ... 2096

Left ventricular ejection fraction, change

- Novantrone for Injection ... 1327

Leg cramps, nocturnal

- Prostin E2 Suppository ... 2109

Legs, heaviness

- Rum-K Syrup ... 1004
- SSKI Solution (Less frequent) ... 2767
- Uroqid-Acid No. 2 Tablets ... 633

Legs, restless

- Ambien Tablets (Rare) ... 2559

Legs, stiffness

- Gastrocrom Capsules (Infrequent) ... 1611
- Gastrocrom Oral Concentrate (Less common) ... 1611

Legs, weakness

- Gastrocrom Capsules (Infrequent) ... 1611
- Gastrocrom Oral Concentrate (Less common) ... 1611

Lens, pigmentation

- Triavil Tablets ... 1800

Lens opacities, changes

- Etrafon ... 2495
- Floxin I.V. ... 1580
- Humorsol Sterile Ophthalmic Solution ... 1707
- Isopto Carpine Ophthalmic Solution ... ⊙ 221
- Lamisil Tablets ... 2394
- Lescol Capsules ... 2395
- Mevacor Tablets ... 1742
- Pilopine HS Ophthalmic Gel ... ⊙ 224
- Pravachol Tablets ... 770
- Zocor Tablets ... 1821

Lens opacities, irregular

- Floxin Tablets (200 mg, 300 mg, 400 mg) ... 1577
- Lysodren Tablets (Infrequent) ... 707
- Mellaril ... 2398
- Serentil ... 689
- Thorazine ... 2701
- Torecan ... 2367

Lenticular deposits

- Compazine ... 2644

- Etrafon ... 2495
- Levoprome ... 1321
- Prolixin ... 510
- Ridaura Capsules (Less than 1%) ... 2691
- Stelazine ... 2692
- Thorazine ... 2701
- Trilafon ... 2532

Leriche's syndrome

- Sansert Tablets ... 2424

Lesions, anogenital

- Achromycin V Capsules (Rare) ... 1417
- Declomycin Tablets ... 1421
- DYNACIN Capsules ... 1627
- Helidac Therapy ... 2135
- Minocin Intravenous ... 1428
- Minocin Oral Suspension ... 1431
- Minocin Pellet-Filled Capsules ... 1429
- Monodox Capsules ... 1858
- Vibramycin ... 2038

Lesions, cardiac

- Amicar Syrup, Tablets, and Injection (One case) ... 1312

Lesions, corneal

- Effexor (Infrequent) ... 2825

Lesions, cutaneous

- Duranest Injections ... 533
- Dyclone 0.5% and 1% Topical Solutions, USP ... 535
- Lupron Depot - 3 Month 22.5 mg ... 2743
- Novocain Hydrochloride for Spinal Anesthesia ... 2457
- Pontocaine Hydrochloride for Spinal Anesthesia ... 2460
- Quadrinal Tablets ... 1398
- ▲ Tonocard Tablets (0.4% to 12.2%) ... 519
- Xylocaine Injections (Extremely rare) ... 562
- Zestril Tablets (0.3% to 1.0%) ... 2972

Lesions, erythema perstans-like

- AquaMEPHYTON Injection ... 1648

Lesions, esophageal

- Cataflam/Voltaren/Voltaren-XR (Rare) ... 833

Lesions, follicular-pustular

- Topicort Emollient Cream 0.25% (0.8%) ... 1289

Lesions, gastrointestinal

- K-Dur Microburst Release System (potassium chloride, USP) E.R. Tablets ... 1364
- K-Norm Capsules ... 1615
- K-Tab Filmtab ... 439
- Micro-K ... 2237
- Micro-K LS Packets ... 2238
- Slow-K Extended-Release Tablets ... 869

Lesions, hepatic

- Amicar Syrup, Tablets, and Injection (One case) ... 1312

Lesions, neuro-ocular

- Cycrin Tablets ... 991
- Modicon ... 1928
- Ortho-Novum ... 1928
- Premphase ... 2900
- Prempro ... 2905
- Provera Tablets ... 2110

Lesions, rectal mucosal

- Testoderm Testosterone Transdermal System (One in 104 patients) ... 486

Lesions, retinal vascular

- Amen Tablets ... 785
- Brevicon ... 2563
- Cycrin Tablets ... 991
- Demulen ... 2580
- Depo-Provera Contraceptive Injection ... 2079
- Depo-Provera Sterile Aqueous Suspension ... 2083
- Levlen/Tri-Levlen ... 646
- Modicon ... 1928
- Norinyl ... 2563
- Nor-Q D Tablets ... 2598
- Ortho-Cyclen/Ortho-Tri-Cyclen ... 1914
- Ortho-Novum ... 1928
- Ortho-Cyclen/Ortho Tri-Cyclen ... 1914
- Premphase ... 2900
- Prempro ... 2905

- Provera Tablets ... 2110
- Levlen/Tri-Levlen ... 646
- Tri-Norinyl ... 2607

Lesions, sceloderma-like

- AquaMEPHYTON Injection ... 1648

Lesions, spinal column, posterior

- Azulfidine (Rare) ... 2059

Lesions, stenotic

- K-Norm Capsules ... 1615

Lethargy

- Accutane Capsules ... 2252
- ▲ ActHIB (17.0% to 18.6%) ... 893
- Aldactazide Tablets ... 2556
- Aldactone Tablets ... 2558
- ▲ Ambien Tablets (3%) ... 2559
- Apresazide Capsules ... 824
- Aquasol A Vitamin A Capsules, USP ... 525
- Aquasol A Parenteral ... 526
- Asacol Delayed-Release Tablets ... 2129
- Bentyl ... 1246
- Betagan (Rare) ... ⊙ 230
- Betoptic Ophthalmic Solution (Rare) ... 465
- Betoptic S Ophthalmic Suspension (Rare) ... 467
- Capozide Tablets ... 744
- Cataflam Tablets ... 833
- Catapres-TTS (3 of 101 patients) ... 680
- CeeNU Capsules ... 699
- Cipro I.V. (1% or less) ... 587
- Cipro I.V. Pharmacy Bulk Package (Less than 1%) ... 590
- Cipro Tablets (Less than 1%) ... 584
- Clozaril Tablets (1%) ... 2377
- Cosmegen Injection ... 1666
- Dalmane Capsules ... 2329
- Demadex Tablets and Injection ... 691
- Depakene ... 416
- Depakote Tablets ... 418
- Dilaudid Ampules ... 1382
- Dilaudid Cough Syrup ... 1383
- Dilaudid ... 1382
- Dipentum Capsules (1.8%) ... 2084
- Diupres Tablets ... 1691
- Diuril Sodium Intravenous ... 1693
- Dyazide Capsules ... 2653
- DynaCirc Capsules (0.5% to 1%) ... 2381
- DynaCirc CR Tablets (0.5% to 1.0%) ... 2383
- Eldepryl Capsules (1 of 49 patients) ... 2729
- ▲ Emcyt Capsules (4%) ... 2085
- Ergamisol Tablets ... 1340
- Esidrix Tablets ... 839
- Eskalith ... 2658
- Etrafon ... 2495
- Sterile FUDR ... 2284
- Ganite ... 2711
- Garamycin Injectable ... 2502
- Gastrocrom Capsules (Infrequent) ... 1611
- Gastrocrom Oral Concentrate (Less common) ... 1611
- Haldol Decanoate ... 1587
- Haldol Injection, Tablets and Concentrate ... 1585
- Hycodan Tablets and Syrup ... 946
- Hycomine Compound Tablets ... 948
- Hycomine ... 947
- Hycotuss Expectorant Syrup ... 950
- Hydrocet Capsules ... 787
- Hydropres Tablets ... 1718
- Hyperstat I.V. Injection ... 2504
- Inderal ... 2834
- Inderal LA Long Acting Capsules ... 2836
- Inderide Tablets ... 2838
- Invirase Capsules (Less than 2%) ... 2291
- ISMOTIC 45% w/v Solution (Very rare) ... ⊙ 221
- Kadian Capsules (Less than 3%) ... 2948
- Kerlone Tablets (2.8%) ... 2588
- Lasix Injection, Oral Solution and Tablets ... 1267
- ▲ Leucovorin Calcium for Injection (2% to 13%) ... 1313
- Levo-Dromoran ... 2297
- Limbitrol ... 2333
- Lioresal Intrathecal ... 1634
- Lithium Carbonate Capsules & Tablets ... 2352
- Lithonate/Lithotabs/Lithobid ... 2721
- Lomotil ... 2591
- Lopressor HCT Tablets (10 in 100 patients) ... 850
- Lorcet 10/650 Tablets ... 1016
- Lortab ... 2751
- Lupron Injection (Less than 5%) ... 2736

- Lysodren Tablets (25%) ... 707
- Matulane Capsules ... 2300
- Mellaril (Extremely rare) ... 2398
- Mithracin ... 599
- Mononine, Coagulation Factor IX (Human), Monoclonal Antibody Purified ... 804
- ▲ Mykrox Tablets (4.4%) ... 1617
- Nebcin Vials, Hyporets & ADD-Vantage ... 1518
- Neoral (Rare) ... 2405
- ▲ OmniHIB (17.0% to 18.6%) ... 2676
- Oretic Tablets ... 450
- Orthoclone OKT3 Sterile Solution ... 1892
- Parlodel ... 2411
- Phenobarbital Elixir and Tablets ... 1523
- Prinzide Tablets ... 1780
- Proleukin for Injection ... 812
- Prolixin ... 510
- ▲ Restoril Capsules (5%) ... 2413
- ▲ RhoGAM Rho(D) Immune Globulin (Human) (25% in one study) ... 1902
- Roferon-A Injection (Less than 0.5% to 6%) ... 2308
- Sandimmune (Rare) ... 2416
- Serax Capsules ... 2916
- Serax Tablets ... 2916
- Solganal Suspension (Rare) ... 2530
- ▲ Stadol (3% to 9%) ... 779
- Supprelin Injection (1% to 3%) ... 2230
- ▲ Tegison Capsules (1-10%) ... 2314
- Tenoretic Tablets (1% to 3%) ... 2963
- Tenormin Tablets and I.V. Injection (1% to 3%) ... 2965
- Thalitone (Common) ... 1293
- Tonocard Tablets (0.8% to 1.6%) ... 519
- Trilafon ... 2532
- Trilisate (Less than 2%) ... 2155
- Tussend ... 1830
- Tussionex Pennkinetic Extended-Release Suspension ... 1624
- Vaseretic Tablets ... 1810
- ▲ Verelan Capsules (3.2%) ... 1455
- Versed Injection (Less than 1.0%) ... 2324
- Vicodin Tablets ... 1404
- Vicodin ES Tablets ... 1405
- Vicodin HP Tablets ... 1403
- Vicodin Tuss Expectorant ... 1406
- ▲ Videx Tablets, Powder for Oral Solution, & Pediatric Powder for Oral Solution (4%) ... 2980
- Visken Tablets (2% or fewer patients) ... 2428
- Cataflam/Voltaren/Voltaren-XR ... 833
- WinRho SD (One report) ... 1839
- Zarontin Capsules ... 1986
- Zarontin Syrup ... 1986
- Zaroxolyn Tablets ... 1625
- Zestoretic Tablets ... 2968
- ▲ Zoladex (5% to 8%) ... 2976
- Zoladex 3-month ... 2978
- Zovirax Sterile Powder (Approximately 1%) ... 1191
- Zydone Capsules ... 967

Leucoencephalopathy

- Fungizone Intravenous ... 507
- Methotrexate Sodium Tablets, Injection, for Injection and LPF Injection ... 1322

Leukemia, acute

- BiCNU ... 696
- CeeNU Capsules ... 699
- Etopophos for Injection (Rare) ... 701
- Etoposide Injection (Rare) ... 539
- Leukeran Tablets ... 1205
- Nipent for Injection (Less than 3%) ... 2733
- Platinol for Injection (Rare) ... 717
- Platinol-AQ Injection (Rare) ... 719
- VePesid Capsules and Injection (Rare) ... 727

Leukemia, lymphoblastic

- Permax Tablets (Rare) ... 571

Leukemia, lymphocytic

- Betaseron for SC Injection ... 653
- Clomid ... 1262
- Mustargen ... 1752

Leukemia, myeloblastic, acute

- Invirase Capsules (Rare) ... 2291

Leukemia, unspecified

- Cytovene-IV (Two or more reports) ... 2270
- Depen Titratable Tablets ... 2770
- Felbatol ... 2774
- Genotropin Injection (A small number of children) ... 2090

(▣ Described in PDR For Nonprescription Drugs)   Incidence data in parenthesis; ▲ 3% or more   (⊙ Described in PDR For Ophthalmology)

Humatrope Vials (A small number of children) 1490
Indocin (Rare) 1723
Nutropin (A small number of patients) 1049
Nutropin AQ Injection (A small number of patients) 1051
Protropin (A small number) 1053
Trental Tablets (Rare) 1291

Leukemoid reaction

Anafranil Capsules (Rare) 819
Netromycin Injection 100 mg/ml (Fewer than 1 in 1000 patients) 2516

Leukocytosis

Abelcet Injection 1540
▲Adriamycin PFS (High incidence) 2056
▲Adriamycin RDF (High incidence) 2056
Atretol Tablets 569
Azactam for Injection (Less than 1%) 736
Capastat Sulfate Injection 968
▲CellCept Capsules (7.1% to 10.9%) 2265
Cerebyx Injection (Infrequent) 1956
Cipro I.V. (Rare) 587
Cipro I.V. Pharmacy Bulk Package (Rare) 590
Cipro Tablets (Less than 0.1%) 584
Clinoril Tablets (Less than 1 in 100) 1658
Clomid 1262
Clozaril Tablets (Less than 1%) 2377
Cuprimine Capsules 1673
Danocrine Capsules 2437
Depen Titratable Tablets 2770
Desyrel and Desyrel Dividose 504
Diprivan Injectable Emulsion (Less than 1%) 2939
Dynabac (0.1% to 1%) 668
Effexor (Infrequent) 2825
▲Efudex (Among most frequent) 2280
Eskalith 2658
Felbatol (Infrequent) 2774
Floxin I.V. (More than or equal to 1%) 1580
Floxin Tablets (200 mg, 300 mg, 400 mg) (More than or equal to 1%) 1577
Foscavir Injection (Less than 1%) 541
Fungizone Intravenous 507
Haldol Decanoate 1587
Haldol Injection, Tablets and Concentrate 1585
INFeD (Iron Dextran Injection, USP) 2478
Kerlone Tablets (Less than 2%) 2588
Lamictal Tablets (Infrequent) 1105
Lariam Tablets (Occasional) 2295
Lioresal Intrathecal (1% or more) 1634
Lithium Carbonate Capsules & Tablets 2352
Lithonate/Lithotabs/Lithobid 2721
LUVOX Tablets (Infrequent) 2723
Mesantoin Tablets 2400
Moban Tablets and Concentrate 1036
Monopril Tablets 762
Navane Capsules and Concentrate (Occasional) 2018
Navane Intramuscular 2019
Nebcin Vials, Hyporets & ADD-Vantage 1518
Neupogen for Injection (Approximately 2%) 495
Orthoclone OKT3 Sterile Solution 1892
Panhematin 452
▲PASER Granules (79% of 38 patients with drug-induced hepatitis) 1333
Paxil Tablets (Rare) 2681
Penetrex Tablets (Less than 1%) 2196
Permax Tablets (Infrequent) 571
Prilosec Delayed-Release Capsules (Rare) 516
Primaxin I.V. 1772
Prinivil Tablets (0.3% to 1.0%) 1776
Prinzide Tablets 1780
▲Prograf (8% to 32%) 1028
Prolastin Alpha$_1$-Proteinase Inhibitor (Human) 629
▲Proleukin for Injection (9%) 812
Prolixin 510
ReoPro Vials (1.0%) 1526
Rilutek Tablets (Infrequent) 2198
Risperdal Tablets (Rare) 1348
Rocephin Injectable Vials, ADD-Vantage, Galaxy Container (Rare) 2305
Suprane (desflurane, USP) 1865
Symmetrel Capsules (Uncommon) 965
Symmetrel Syrup (Uncommon) 963
Tao Capsules 2033
▲Tegison Capsules (10-25%) 2314
Tegretol/Tegretol-XR 870
Torecan 2367
▲Trasylol (3%) 607
Vantin for Oral Suspension and Vantin Tablets 2112
Vaseretic Tablets 1810
Vasotec I.V. 1814
Vasotec Tablets (0.5% to 1.0%) 1816
▲Vesanoid Capsules (About 40%) 2327
Wellbutrin Tablets 1177
Zestoretic Tablets 2968
Zestril Tablets (0.3% to 1.0%) 2972
Zovirax Sterile Powder (Less than 1%) 1191
Zyloprim Tablets (Less than 1%) 1194

Leukocyturia

Amikacin Sulfate Injection, USP 523
Amikacin Sulfate Injection, USP 981
Amikin Injectable 502
Primaxin I.M. 1770
Primaxin I.V. 1772
Sinemet CR Tablets (1% or greater) 961

Leukoderma

Betaseron for SC Injection 653
Effexor (Rare) 2825
Lamictal Tablets (Rare) 1105
Ultravate Cream 0.05% (Less frequent) 2797
Ultravate Ointment 0.05% (Less frequent) 2798

Leukoencephalopathy, multifocal progressive

Ergamisol Tablets 1340
Invirase Capsules (Less than 2%) 2291

Leukonychia

Desyrel and Desyrel Dividose 504

Leukopenia

▲Abelcet Injection (4%) 1540
▲Accutane Capsules (1 in 5 to 1 in 10 patients) 2252
Adalat Capsules (10 mg and 20 mg) (Less than 0.5%) 580
Adalat CC (Rare) 582
Adapin Capsules (Occasional) 1542
Adriamycin PFS 2056
Adriamycin RDF 2056
Aldactazide Tablets 2556
Aldoclor Tablets 1638
Aldomet Ester HCl Injection 1642
Aldomet Oral 1640
Aldoril Tablets 1644
▲Alferon N Injection (11%) 2142
Alkeran Tablets 1198
Altace Capsules (Scattered incidents) 1238
Amaryl Tablets 1241
Ambien Tablets (Rare) 2559
Amicar Syrup, Tablets, and Injection 1312
Amoxil 2631
Anafranil Capsules 819
Anaprox/Naprosyn (Less than 1%) 2277
Ancef Injection 2632
Ancobon Capsules 2254
Anturane (Rare) 823
Apresazide Capsules (Less frequent) 824
Apresoline Hydrochloride Tablets (Less frequent) 826
Aquasol A Vitamin A Capsules, USP 525
Aquasol A Parenteral 526
Aredia for Injection (Up to 4%) 827
Arimidex Tablets (2% to 5%) 2932
Asacol Delayed-Release Tablets 2129
Asendin Tablets (Less than 1%) 1419
Atamet Tablets (Rare) 567
Atretol Tablets 569
Atrohist Plus Tablets 1605
Atromid-S Capsules 2808
Augmentin 2637
Augmentin Tablets 2640
▲Azathioprine Tablets (5.3% to more than 50%) 2349
Azulfidine (Rare) 2059
Bactrim DS Tablets 2257
Bactrim I.V. Infusion 2255
Bactrim 2257
Benemid Tablets 1651
Betapace Tablets (Rare) 637
Bicillin C-R Injection 2810
Bicillin C-R 900/300 Injection 2812
Bicillin L-A Injection (Infrequent) 2813
BiCNU 696
BuSpar Tablets (Rare) 738
Capastat Sulfate Injection 968
Capozide Tablets 744
Cardizem CD Capsules (Infrequent) 1251
Cardizem SR Capsules (Infrequent) 1255
Cardizem Injectable 1253
Cardizem Tablets (Infrequent) 1257
Cardura Tablets 1993
Casodex Tablets (2% to 5%) 2934
Cataflam Tablets (Less than 1%) 833
Ceclor Pulvules & Suspension 1470
Cedax (0.1% to 1%) 2480
CeeNU Capsules 699
Cefizox for Intramuscular or Intravenous Use (Rare) 1025
Cefotan 2936
Ceftin 1067
Cefzil Tablets and Oral Suspension (0.2%) 747
▲CellCept Capsules (23.2% to 34.5%; 11.5% to 16.3%) 2265
Celontin Kapseals 1955
Ceptaz (Very rare) 1070
Cerebyx Injection (Infrequent) 1956
Chibroxin Sterile Ophthalmic Solution (With oral form) 1657
Chloromycetin Sodium Succinate 1960
Cipro I.V. (Infrequent) 587
▲Cipro I.V. Pharmacy Bulk Package (Among most frequent) 590
Cipro Tablets (0.4%) 584
Claforan Sterile and Injection (Less than 1%) 1259
Cleocin Phosphate Injection 2068
Cleocin Vaginal Cream 2070
Clinoril Tablets (Less than 1%) 1658
▲Clozaril Tablets (3%) 2377
Cognex Capsules (Rare) 1961
ColBENEMID Tablets 1662
Combipres Tablets 682
Compazine 2644
Cosmegen Injection 1666
Cuprimine Capsules (2%) 1673
Cytadren Tablets (Rare) 837
▲Cytosar-U Sterile Powder (Among most frequent) 2077
▲Cytovene (29%) 2270
Cytoxan (Less frequent to common) 700
Dalmane Capsules (Rare) 2329
Danocrine Capsules 2437
Dantrium Capsules (Less frequent) 2131
Dantrium Intravenous 2132
Daranide Tablets 1676
Daraprim Tablets 1199
Daypro Caplets (Less than 1%) 2578
Depakene 416
Depakote Tablets 418
▲Depen Titratable Tablets (2%; up to 5%) 2770
DiaBeta Tablets 1265
Diabinese Tablets 2002
Diamox ⊙ 317
Didronel Tablets (One report) 2133
Diflucan Tablets, Injection, and Oral Suspension 2003
Dilantin Infatabs (Occasional) 1967
Dilantin Kapseals (Occasional) 1965
Dilantin-125 Suspension (Occasional) 1969
Dipentum Capsules (Rare) 2084
Diucardin Tablets 2824
Diupres Tablets 1691
Diuril Oral Suspension 1694
Diuril Sodium Intravenous 1693
Diuril Tablets 1694
Dolobid Tablets (Less than 1 in 100) 1695
▲Doxil (About 60%) 2613
Doxorubicin Astra 531
Dyazide Capsules 2653
DynaCirc Capsules (0.5% to 1%) 2381
DynaCirc CR Tablets (0.5% to 1.0%) 2383
Easprin 1971
EC-Naprosyn Delayed-Release Tablets (Less than 1%) 2277
Effexor (Infrequent) 2825
Elavil 2945
Elspar 1700
▲Emcyt Capsules (4%) 2085
Enduron Tablets 424
▲Ergamisol Tablets (Less than 1% to 33%) 1340
Esidrix Tablets 839
Esimil Tablets (A few instances) 840
▲Etopophos for Injection (3% to 91%) 701
▲Etoposide Injection (3% to 91%) 539
Etrafon 2495
▲Eulexin Capsules (3%) 2498
Fansidar Tablets 2281
▲Felbatol (6.5%; infrequent) 2774
Feldene Capsules (Greater than 1%) 2008
Flagyl I.V. 2373
Flexeril Tablets (Rare) 1701
Floxin I.V. (More than or equal to 1%) 1580
Floxin Tablets (200 mg, 300 mg, 400 mg) (More than or equal to 1%) 1577
Fluorouracil Injection 2282
Fortaz (Very rare) 1092
▲Foscavir Injection (5% or greater) 541
▲Sterile FUDR (Among more common) 2284
Fulvicin P/G Tablets (Rare) 2499
Fulvicin P/G 165 & 330 Tablets (Rare) 2500
Fungizone Intravenous 507
Ganite 2711
Gantanol Tablets 2285
Gantrisin 2286
Garamycin Injectable 2502
▲Gemzar for Injection (15% to 71%) 1482
Geocillin Tablets 2009
GlaucTabs ⊙ 209
Glucotrol Tablets 2011
Glucotrol XL Extended Release Tablets 2012
Glynase PresTab Tablets 2091
Grifulvin V (griseofulvin tablets) Microsize (griseofulvin oral suspension) Microsize (Rare) 1944
Gris-PEG Tablets, 125 mg & 250 mg (Rare) 476
Haldol Decanoate 1587
Haldol Injection, Tablets and Concentrate 1585
Helidac Therapy 2135
▲Hexalen Capsules (1% to 15%) 2760
▲Hivid Tablets (Less than 1% to 13.1%) 2287
▲Hycamtin for Injection (32% to 98%) 2665
Hydralazine Hydrochloride Injection USP (Less frequent) 2712
▲Hydrea Capsules (Most common) 705
HydroDIURIL Tablets 1716
Hydropres Tablets 1718
Hyperstat I.V. Injection 2504
Hyzaar Tablets 1720
▲IFEX (Almost universal) 706
▲Imuran (28% to more than 50%) 1103
Inderide Tablets 2838
Inderide LA Long Acting Capsules 2840
Indocin Capsules (Less than 1%) 1723
Indocin I.V. (Less than 1%) 1727
Indocin (Less than 1%) 1723
▲Intron A for Injection (Less than 5% to 68%) 2506
Ismelin Tablets 845
Kadian Capsules (Less than 3%) 2948
Keftab Tablets 931
Kefurox Vials, Faspak & ADD-Vantage (1 in 750) 1509
Kefzol Vials, Faspak & ADD-Vantage 1511
Klonopin Tablets 2294
▲Kytril Tablets (11%) 2669
Lamictal Tablets (Infrequent) 1105
▲Lariam Tablets (Among most frequent) 2295
Larodopa Tablets 2296
Lasix Injection, Oral Solution and Tablets 1267
Lescol Capsules (Rare) 2395
▲Leucovorin Calcium for Injection (14% to 93%) 1313
▲Leukine (17%) 1317
Levoprome 1321
Lodine Capsules and Tablets (Less than 1%) 2849
Lopid Tablets (Rare to occasional) 1974
Lopressor HCT Tablets 850
Lorabid Suspension and Pulvules 1513
Lotensin Tablets (Scattered incidents) 852
Lotensin HCT Tablets (Scattered accounts) 855
Loxitane (Rare) 1426
LUVOX Tablets (Rare) 2723
Macrobid Capsules 2138
Macrodantin Capsules 2140
Matulane Capsules (Frequent) 2300

(▣ Described in PDR For Nonprescription Drugs) Incidence data in parenthesis; ▲ 3% or more (⊙ Described in PDR For Ophthalmology)

Mavik Tablets (Rare) ... 1407
Maxaquin Tablets (Less than or equal to 0.1%) ... 2593
Mefoxin ... 1734
Mefoxin Premixed Intravenous Solution ... 1737
Mellaril (Infrequent) ... 2398
Mepergan Injection (Very rare) ... 2859
▲ Mepron Suspension (4%) ... 1206
Mesantoin Tablets ... 2400
▲ Methotrexate Sodium Tablets, Injection, for Injection and LPF Injection (Among most frequent; 1% to 3%) ... 1322
Mevacor Tablets (Rare) ... 1742
Mexitil Capsules (About 1 in 1,000) ... 684
Mezlin ... 594
Mezlin Pharmacy Bulk Package ... 597
Micronase Tablets ... 2099
Miltown Tablets ... 2780
Minizide Capsules ... 2016
Mintezol ... 1747
▲ Mithracin (6%) ... 599
Moban Tablets and Concentrate ... 1036
Moduretic Tablets ... 1748
Monocid Injection (Less than 1%) ... 2674
Monopril Tablets ... 762
Mutamycin for Injection ... 712
▲ Mycobutin Capsules (17%) ... 2101
Mykrox Tablets ... 1617
Myleran Tablets ... 1209
Naprelan Tablets (Less than 1%) ... 2861
Anaprox/Naprosyn (Less than 1%) ... 2277
Nardil (Less frequent) ... 1977
Navane Capsules and Concentrate (Occasional) ... 2018
Navane Intramuscular (Occasional) ... 2019
▲ Navelbine Injection (12% to 81%) ... 1212
Nebcin Vials, Hyporets & ADD-Vantage ... 1518
NegGram (Rare) ... 2453
▲ Neoral (Up to 6%) ... 2405
Neptazane Tablets ... ◉ 320
Netromycin Injection 100 mg/ml (Fewer than 1 in 1000 patients) ... 2516
Neurontin Capsules (1.1%) ... 1978
▲ Nipent for Injection (22% to 60%) ... 2733
Nizoral Tablets (Less than 1%) ... 1345
Nolvadex Tablets (0.4%) ... 2957
Noroxin Tablets ... 1758
Noroxin Tablets ... 2222
Norvir (Less than 2%) ... 447
Omnipen Capsules ... 2872
Omnipen for Oral Suspension ... 2873
▲ Oncaspar (Greater than 1% but less than 5%) ... 2194
Oncovin Solution Vials & Hyporets ... 1521
Oretic Tablets ... 450
Ornade Spansule Capsules ... 2678
Orthoclone OKT3 Sterile Solution ... 1892
PBZ Tablets ... 863
PBZ-SR Tablets ... 862
▲ Paraplatin for Injection (26% to 98%) ... 713
Parnate Tablets ... 2679
PASER Granules ... 1333
Paxil Tablets (Infrequent) ... 2681
Pediazole Suspension ... 2340
Pen•Vee K (Infrequent) ... 2879
Penetrex Tablets (Less than 1%) ... 2196
Pentasa ... 1275
Pepcid Injection (Rare) ... 1765
Pepcid (Rare) ... 1763
Periactin ... 1767
Permax Tablets (Infrequent) ... 571
Pfizerpen for Injection (Rare) ... 2022
Phenergan with Codeine (Rare) ... 2883
Phenergan with Dextromethorphan (Rare) ... 2885
Phenergan Injection ... 2880
Phenergan Suppositories (Rare) ... 2882
Phenergan Syrup (Rare) ... 2881
Phenergan Tablets (Rare) ... 2882
Phenergan VC (Rare) ... 2886
Phenergan VC with Codeine (Rare) ... 2888
Phenurone Tablets (2%) ... 455
Pipracil ... 1435
Plaquenil Sulfate Tablets ... 2459
Platinol for Injection ... 717
Platinol-AQ Injection ... 719
PMB 200 and PMB 400 ... 2890
Podocon-25 ... 1949
Ponstel (Occasional) ... 1982
Pravachol Tablets (Rare) ... 770
Primaxin I.M. ... 1770
Primaxin I.V. (Less than 0.2%) ... 1772
Prinzide Tablets ... 1780
Priscoline Hydrochloride Ampuls ... 864
Procardia Capsules (Less than 0.5%) ... 2024
▲ Prograf (Greater than 3%) ... 1028
▲ Proleukin for Injection (34%) ... 812
Prolixin ... 510
Proloprim Tablets ... 1141
Propulsid (Rare) ... 1346
ProSom Tablets (Rare) ... 457
Protostat Tablets ... 1939
Prozac Pulvules & Liquid, Oral Solution (Rare) ... 935
Purinethol Tablets (Frequent) ... 1214
Reglan (A few cases) ... 2243
Relafen Tablets (Less than 1%) ... 2688
Remeron Tablets (Rare) ... 1878
Ridaura Capsules ... 2691
Rifadin ... 1276
Rifamate Capsules ... 1278
Rifater (Rare) ... 1280
Rilutek Tablets (Infrequent) ... 2198
Rimactane Capsules (Rare) ... 865
Risperdal Tablets (Rare) ... 1348
Ritalin ... 866
Rocephin Injectable Vials, ADD-Vantage, Galaxy Container (2.1%) ... 2305
▲ Roferon-A Injection (3% to 20%) ... 2308
Rythmol Tablets–150mg, 225mg, 300mg (Less than 1%) ... 1399
▲ SSD (About 20%) ... 1402
Salagen Tablets (Less than 1%) ... 1546
▲ Sandimmune (Up to 6%) ... 2416
Septra ... 1146
Septra I.V. Infusion ... 1142
Septra I.V. Infusion ADD-Vantage Vials ... 1144
Septra ... 1146
Ser-Ap-Es Tablets ... 867
Serax Capsules (Rare) ... 2916
Serax Tablets (Rare) ... 2916
Serentil ... 689
Serzone Tablets (Infrequent) ... 776
Silvadene Cream 1% (Several cases) ... 1288
Sinemet Tablets (Rare) ... 959
Sinemet CR Tablets ... 961
Sinequan (Occasional) ... 2028
Skelaxin Tablets ... 793
Solganal Suspension (Rare) ... 2530
Soma Compound w/Codeine Tablets (Very rare) ... 2784
Soma Compound Tablets (Very rare) ... 2783
Soma Tablets ... 2782
Spectrobid Tablets ... 2030
Stelazine ... 2692
Sular Tablets (Less than or equal to 1%) ... 2961
Suprax (Less than 2%) ... 1443
Symmetrel Capsules (Less than 0.1%) ... 965
Symmetrel Syrup (Less than 0.1%) ... 963
Tagamet (Approximately 1 per 100,000) ... 2694
Tambocor Tablets (Less than 1%) ... 1555
Tapazole Tablets ... 1361
▲ Taxol Injection (17% to 90%) ... 723
Taxotere for Injection Concentrate ... 2204
Tazicef for Injection (Very rare) ... 2697
Tazidime Vials, Faspak & ADD-Vantage (Very rare) ... 1531
▲ Tegison Capsules (10-25%) ... 2314
Tegretol/Tegretol-XR ... 870
Tenoretic Tablets ... 2963
Thalitone ... 1293
▲ TheraCys BCG Live (Intravesical) (Up to 5.4%) ... 911
Thioguanine Tablets, Tabloid Brand ... 1225
Thioplex (Thiotepa For Injection) ... 1329
Thorazine ... 2701
Tiazac Capsules (Infrequent) ... 1019
Ticar for Injection ... 2704
TICE BCG, USP (0.3%) ... 1881
Timentin for Injection ... 2706
Timolide Tablets ... 1791
Tonocard Tablets (Less than 1%) ... 519
Toradol ... 2319
Torecan ... 2367
Trental Tablets (Less than 1%) ... 1291
Triavil Tablets ... 1800
Trilafon ... 2532
Trimpex Tablets ... 2323
Unasyn ... 2035
Urispas Tablets (1 case) ... 2710
Vantin for Oral Suspension and Vantin Tablets ... 2112
Vascor Tablets (200 and 300 mg) (2 cases) ... 1597
Vaseretic Tablets ... 1810
▲ Velban Vials (Among most common) ... 1537
▲ VePesid Capsules and Injection (3% to 91%) ... 727
▲ Videx Tablets, Powder for Oral Solution, & Pediatric Powder for Oral Solution (13% to 16%) ... 2980
Vivactil Tablets ... 1820
Cataflam/Voltaren/Voltaren-XR (Less than 1%) ... 833
▲ Vumon for Injection (89%) ... 729
Wellbutrin Tablets ... 1177
Yutopar Intravenous Injection ... 566
Zanosar Sterile Powder ... 2119
Zantac (A few patients) ... 1182
Zantac Injection (Few patients) ... 1180
Zantac Syrup (A few patients) ... 1182
Zarontin Capsules ... 1986
Zarontin Syrup ... 1986
Zaroxolyn Tablets ... 1625
Zerit Capsules (Up to 1%) ... 731
Zestoretic Tablets (Rare) ... 2968
Zestril Tablets (Rare) ... 2972
Zinacef (1 in 750 patients) ... 1184
Zinecard Injection ... 2120
Zithromax (Less than 1%) ... 2043
Zithromax Tablets (Less than 1%) ... 2046
Zocor Tablets (Rare) ... 1821
Zosyn ... 1463
Zovirax Capsules ... 1187
Zovirax Sterile Powder ... 1191
Zovirax ... 1187
Zyloprim Tablets (Less than 1%) ... 1194

Leukopenia, transient

Rifater ... 1280

Leukoplakia, oral

Betaseron for SC Injection ... 653
Doxil (Less than 1%) ... 2613
Foscavir Injection (Less than 1%) ... 541
Intron A for Injection (Less than 5%) ... 2506
Videx Tablets, Powder for Oral Solution, & Pediatric Powder for Oral Solution (Less than 1%) ... 2980

Leukorrhea

Anafranil Capsules (Up to 2%) ... 819
Avonex ... 662
Betaseron for SC Injection ... 653
Depo-Provera Contraceptive Injection (1% to 5%) ... 2079
Effexor (Infrequent) ... 2825
▲ Estring Vaginal Ring (7%) ... 2086
Intron A for Injection (Less than 5%) ... 2506
Lodine Capsules and Tablets (Less than 1%) ... 2849
Maxaquin Tablets (Less than 1%) ... 2593
Neurontin Capsules (Rare) ... 1978
▲ Norplant System (5% or greater) ... 2868
ParaGard T 380A Intrauterine Copper Contraceptive ... 1936
Paxil Tablets (Rare) ... 2681
Permax Tablets (Rare) ... 571
Prozac Pulvules & Liquid, Oral Solution (Infrequent) ... 935
Remeron Tablets (Infrequent) ... 1878
Risperdal Tablets (Infrequent) ... 1348
▲ Supprelin Injection (6% to 12%) ... 2230
Zoloft Tablets (Rare) ... 2051
Zosyn (1.0% or less) ... 1463
Zyrtec Tablets (Less than 2%) ... 2053

Lhermitte's sign

Platinol for Injection ... 717
Platinol-AQ Injection ... 719

Libido, changes

Adapin Capsules ... 1542
Adderall Tablets ... 2209
Adipex-P Tablets and Capsules ... 1035
Amen Tablets ... 785
▲ Anafranil Capsules (Up to 21%) ... 819
▲ Android Capsules, 10 mg (Among most common) ... 1297
Asendin Tablets (Less than 1%) ... 1419
Brevicon ... 2563
Climara Transdermal System ... 640
Cycrin Tablets ... 991
Danocrine Capsules ... 2437
Demulen ... 2580
Depo-Provera Sterile Aqueous Suspension ... 2083
Desogen Tablets ... 1867
Desoxyn Gradumet Tablets ... 422
Dexedrine ... 2648
DextroStat-Dextroamphetamine Sulfate Tablets ... 2211
Diethylstilbestrol Tablets ... 1477
Dizac (diazepam injectable emulsion) CIV (Less frequent) ... 1862
Doral Tablets ... 2773
Elavil ... 2945
Estrace Cream and Tablets ... 751
Estraderm Transdermal System ... 842
ESTRATAB Tablets (0.3, 0.625, 1.25, 2.5 mg) ... 2715
Estratest ... 2718
Etrafon ... 2495
Fastin Capsules ... 2662
Flexeril Tablets (Rare) ... 1701
Halcion Tablets ... 2093
Halotestin Tablets ... 2095
Invirase Capsules (Less than 2%) ... 2291
Ionamin Capsules ... 1615
Levlen/Tri-Levlen ... 646
Librax Capsules (Rare) ... 2330
Librium Capsules (Isolated cases) ... 2331
Librium Injectable (Isolated cases) ... 2332
Limbitrol ... 2333
Lo/Ovral Tablets ... 2852
Lo/Ovral-28 Tablets ... 2857
Mellaril ... 2398
Menest Tablets ... 2671
Modicon ... 1928
Neurontin Capsules (Infrequent) ... 1978
Nipent for Injection (Less than 3%) ... 2733
Nordette-21 Tablets ... 2863
Nordette-28 Tablets ... 2866
Norinyl ... 2563
Nor-Q D Tablets ... 2598
Ogen Tablets ... 2103
Ogen Vaginal Cream ... 2106
Ortho-Cept ... 1907
Ortho-Cyclen/Ortho-Tri-Cyclen ... 1914
Ortho Dienestrol Cream ... 1922
Ortho-Est ... 1925
Ortho-Novum ... 1928
Ortho-Cyclen/Ortho Tri-Cyclen ... 1914
Orudis Capsules (Rare) ... 2874
Oruvail Capsules (Rare) ... 2874
Ovcon ... 765
Ovral Tablets ... 2877
Ovral-28 Tablets ... 2878
Ovrette Tablets ... 2878
Oxandrin ... 783
PMB 200 and PMB 400 ... 2890
Prelu-2 Timed Release Capsules ... 687
Premarin Intravenous ... 2893
Premarin Tablets ... 2896
Premarin Vaginal Cream ... 2898
Premphase ... 2900
Prempro ... 2905
Provera Tablets ... 2110
Roferon-A Injection (Less than 4%) ... 2308
Sanorex Tablets (Rare) ... 2423
Serax Capsules ... 2916
Serax Tablets ... 2916
Serentil ... 689
Sinequan ... 2028
▲ Supprelin Injection (3% to 10%) ... 2230
Torecan ... 2367
Triavil Tablets ... 1800
Trilafon ... 2532
Levlen/Tri-Levlen ... 646
Tri-Norinyl ... 2607
Triphasil-21 Tablets ... 2919
Triphasil-28 Tablets ... 2924
Valium Injectable ... 2336
Valium Tablets (Infrequent) ... 2335
Vivactil Tablets ... 1820
Vivelle Transdermal System ... 880
▲ Xanax Tablets (7.1%) ... 2115

Libido, decrease

Adalat CC (Less than 1.0%) ... 582
Aldoclor Tablets ... 1638
Aldomet Ester HCl Injection ... 1642
Aldomet Oral ... 1640
Aldoril Tablets ... 1644
Ambien Tablets (Rare) ... 2559
Androderm Testosterone Transdermal System (Less than 1%) ... 2634
Atromid-S Capsules ... 2808
Axid Pulvules ... 1468
Betaseron for SC Injection ... 653
Blocadren Tablets (0.6%) ... 1654
Bontril Slow-Release Capsules ... 786
BuSpar Tablets (Infrequent) ... 738
Calcijex Injection ... 412
Cardura Tablets (0.8%) ... 1993
▲ Casodex Tablets (2% to 5%) ... 2934
Claritin Tablets (2% or fewer patients) ... 2485
Claritin-D Tablets (Less frequent) ... 2487
Clozaril Tablets (Less than 1%) ... 2377
▲ Cordarone Tablets (1 to 3%) ... 2818

(■ Described in PDR For Nonprescription Drugs) Incidence data in parenthesis; ▲ 3% or more (◉ Described in PDR For Ophthalmology)

1389 **Side Effects Index** **Light-headedness**

Cozaar Tablets (Less than 1%) 1668
Cytotec (Infrequent) 2576
Cytovene (1% or less) 2270
Depo-Provera Contraceptive Injection (1% to 5%) 2079
Desyrel and Desyrel Dividose (Less than 1% to 1.3%) 504
Diupres Tablets 1691
DynaCirc Capsules (0.5% to 1%) 2381
DynaCirc CR Tablets (0.5% to 1.0%) 2383
▲ Effexor (2% to 5.7%) 2825
Estring Vaginal Ring (At least 1 report) 2086
Ethmozine Tablets (Less than 2%) 2217
Fioricet with Codeine Capsules 2387
Fiorinal with Codeine Capsules 2390
Flagyl 375 Capsules 2587
Glucotrol XL Extended Release Tablets (Less than 1%) 2012
Helidac Therapy 2135
Hydropres Tablets 1718
Hyperstat I.V. Injection 2504
Hytrin Capsules (0.6%) 434
Hyzaar Tablets 1720
Imdur (Less than or equal to 5%) 1362
Intron A for Injection (Up to 5%) 2506
Inversine Tablets 1729
IOPIDINE Sterile Ophthalmic Solution ⊙ 218
Kadian Capsules (Less than 3%) 2948
Kerlone Tablets (Less than 2%) 2588
Lamictal Tablets (Rare) 1105
Lopid Tablets 1974
Lopressor 848
Lotensin Tablets 852
Lotensin HCT Tablets (0.3% to 1.0%) 855
Lotrel Capsules 858
Ludiomil Tablets (Rare) 861
Lupron Depot 3.75 mg (Less than 5%) 2739
Lupron Depot 7.5 mg (Less than 5%) 2741
Lupron Depot - 3 Month 22.5 mg (Less than 5%) 2743
Lupron Injection (Less than 5%) 2736
LUVOX Tablets (2%) 2723
MS Contin Tablets (Less frequent) 2149
MSIR 2152
Mavik Tablets (0.3% to 1.0%) 1407
▲ Megace Oral Suspension (Up to 5%) 708
Methadone Hydrochloride Oral Concentrate 2356
Methadone Hydrochloride Oral Solution & Tablets 2357
MetroGel-Vaginal 917
Mexitil Capsules (Less than 1% or about 4 in 1,000) 684
Midamor Tablets (Less than or equal to 1%) 1746
Moduretic Tablets 1748
Monopril Tablets (0.2% to 1.0%) 762
Norpramin Tablets 1273
Norvir (Less than 2%) 447
Oramorph SR (Morphine Sulfate Sustained Release Tablets) (Less frequent) 2359
Pamelor 2409
▲ Paxil Tablets (3% to 9%) 2681
Pepcid Injection (Infrequent) 1765
Pepcid (Infrequent) 1763
Permax Tablets (Infrequent) 571
Plendil Extended-Release Tablets (0.5% to 1.5%) 514
Pondimin Tablets 2239
Prevacid Delayed-Release Capsules (Less than 1%) 2746
Prinivil Tablets (0.4%) 1776
Prinzide Tablets (0.3% to 1%) 1780
Procardia XL Extended Release Tablets (1% or less) 2026
▲ Proscar Tablets (3.3%) 1784
ProSom Tablets (Rare) 457
Protostat Tablets 1939
▲ Prozac Pulvules & Liquid, Oral Solution (1.6% to 11%) 935
RMS Suppositories CII 2766
Redux Capsules (Infrequent) 2911
Rilutek Tablets (Infrequent) 2198
Rocaltrol Capsules 2303
Roxanol 2365
Sandostatin Injection (Less than 1%) 2421
Ser-Ap-Es Tablets 867
Serzone Tablets (1%) 776
Sporanox Capsules (0.2% to 1.2%) 1352
Sular Tablets (Less than or equal to 1%) 2961
Surmontil Capsules 2917
Symmetrel Capsules (0.1% to 1%) 965
Symmetrel Syrup (0.1% to 1%) 963
▲ Synarel Nasal Solution for Endometriosis (22% of patients) 2605
Tambocor Tablets (Less than 1%) 1555
Tenex Tablets (3% or less) 2249
Testoderm Testosterone Transdermal System 486
Testred Capsules, 10 mg 1308
Timolide Tablets (Less than 1%) 1791
Timoptic in Ocudose 1796
Timoptic Sterile Ophthalmic Solution 1794
Timoptic-XE 1798
Tofranil Ampuls 873
Tofranil Tablets 875
Tofranil-PM Capsules 876
Toprol-XL Tablets 560
Vaseretic Tablets (0.5% to 2.0%) 1810
Videx Tablets, Powder for Oral Solution, & Pediatric Powder for Oral Solution (Less than 1%) 2980
▲ Wellbutrin Tablets (3.1%) 1177
Winstrol Tablets 2468
▲ Xanax Tablets (14.4%) 2115
Zantac Injection 1180
Zebeta Tablets 1457
Zestoretic Tablets (0.3 to 1%) 2968
Zestril Tablets (0.4%) 2972
▲ Zoladex (61%) 2976
Zyloprim Tablets (Less than 1%) 1194
Zyrtec Tablets (Less than 2%) 2053

Libido, increase

Androderm Testosterone Transdermal System 2634
Avonex 662
Bontril Slow-Release Capsules 786
BuSpar Tablets (Infrequent) 738
Clozaril Tablets (Less than 1%) 2377
Cognex Capsules (Infrequent) 1961
Depo-Provera Contraceptive Injection (Fewer than 1%) 2079
Desyrel and Desyrel Dividose 504
Effexor (Infrequent) 2825
Haldol Decanoate 1587
Haldol Injection, Tablets and Concentrate 1585
Klonopin Tablets 2294
Lamictal Tablets (Rare) 1105
Ludiomil Tablets (Rare) 861
Lupron Injection 2736
LUVOX Tablets (Infrequent) 2723
Moban Tablets and Concentrate 1036
Norpramin Tablets 1273
Pamelor 2409
Paxil Tablets (Rare) 2681
Permax Tablets (Infrequent) 571
Pondimin Tablets 2239
Prolixin 510
Prozac Pulvules & Liquid, Oral Solution (Infrequent) 935
Questran 774
Redux Capsules (Frequent) 2911
Remeron Tablets (Infrequent) 1878
Rilutek Tablets (Infrequent) 2198
Risperdal Tablets (Infrequent) 1348
Serzone Tablets (Infrequent) 776
Surmontil Capsules 2917
Synarel Nasal Solution for Endometriosis (1% of patients) 2605
Testoderm Testosterone Transdermal System 486
Testred Capsules, 10 mg 1308
Tofranil Ampuls 873
Tofranil Tablets 875
Tofranil-PM Capsules 876
Wellbutrin Tablets (Frequent) 1177
Winstrol Tablets 2468
▲ Xanax Tablets (7.7%) 2115
Zarontin Capsules (Rare) 1986
Zarontin Syrup (Rare) 1986
▲ Zoladex (12%) 2976

Libido, loss

Catapres Tablets (About 3 in 100 patients) 679
Catapres-TTS 680
Combipres Tablets (About 3%) 682
▲ Eulexin Capsules (36%) 2498
Lescol Capsules 2395
Methotrexate Sodium Tablets, Injection, for Injection and LPF Injection (Rare) 1322
Mevacor Tablets (0.5% to 1.0%) 1742
Nolvadex Tablets 2957
Orap Tablets 1037
Pravachol Tablets 770
Roferon-A Injection (Infrequent) 2308
Vascor Tablets (200 and 300 mg) (0.5 to 2.0%) 1597
Zantac (Occasional) 1182
Ziac (0.4%) 1459
Zocor Tablets 1821

Lichen planus

Aralen Hydrochloride Injection 2430
Aralen Phosphate Tablets 2431
Cuprimine Capsules 1673
Depen Titratable Tablets (Rare) 2770
Felbatol 2774
Minipress Capsules (Less than 1%) 2015
Minizide Capsules (Rare) 2016
Pentasa (Less than 1%) 1275
Trandate Tablets 1158
Zyloprim Tablets (Less than 1%) 1194

Lichen planus, bullous

Normodyne Tablets 2522
Trandate Tablets 1158

Light-headedness

Accupril Tablets 1950
▲ Adalat Capsules (10 mg and 20 mg) (About 10% to 27%) 580
Adenocard Injection (2%) 1021
▲ Adenoscan (12%) 1022
Aldoclor Tablets 1638
Aldomet Ester HCl Injection 1642
Aldomet Oral 1640
Alferon N Injection (One patient to 3%) 2142
Altace Capsules 1238
Ambien Tablets (2%) 2559
Anaprox/Naprosyn (Less than 3%) 2277
▲ Axocet Capsules (Among most frequent) 2469
Beclovent Inhalation Aerosol and Refill 1063
Beconase (Fewer than 5 per 100 patients) 1065
▲ Bentyl (11%) 1246
▲ Betapace Tablets (4% to 12%) 637
Brevibloc (esmolol HCl) Injection (Less than 1%) 1860
Brontex 2130
▲ BuSpar Tablets (3%) 738
Capoten Tablets 740
▲ Cardioquin Tablets (15%) 2146
▲ Cardura Tablets (Up to 23%) 1993
Ceredase 1055
Chibroxin Sterile Ophthalmic Solution (With oral form) 1657
Cipro I.V. (1% or less) 587
Cipro I.V. Pharmacy Bulk Package (Less than 1%) 590
Cipro Tablets (Less than 1%) 584
Clomid (Fewer than 1%) 1262
Colestid (Infrequent) 2073
Cutivate Ointment (Less than 1%) 1078
▲ DHCplus Capsules (Among most frequent) 2148
Dalmane Capsules 2329
Dantrium Capsules (Less frequent) 2131
Dantrium Intravenous 2132
Daraprim Tablets (Rare) 1199
Darvon-N/Darvocet-N 1473
Darvon 1475
Darvon-N Suspension & Tablets 1473
▲ Demerol (Among most frequent) 2438
Deponit NTG Transdermal Delivery System (Occasional; 4%) 2541
▲ Desyrel and Desyrel Dividose (19.7% to 28.0%) 504
Dexacort Phosphate in Turbinaire 1607
Dilatrate-SR Capsules (Occasional) 2542
▲ Dilaudid-HP Injection (Among most frequent) 1384
▲ Dilaudid-HP Lyophilized Powder 250 mg (Among most frequent) 1384
Dilaudid Tablets and Liquid 1386
Dipentum Capsules 2084
Dolobid Tablets (Less than 1 in 100) 1695
Duranest Injections 533
Dyclone 0.5% and 1% Topical Solutions, USP 535
DYNACIN Capsules 1627
EC-Naprosyn Delayed-Release Tablets (Less than 3%) 2277
▲ Eldepryl Capsules (7 of 49 patients) 2729
EMLA Cream (Unlikely with cream) 536
Entex PSE Tablets 973
▲ Esgic-plus Capsules (Among most frequent) 1012
▲ Esgic-plus Tablets (Among most frequent) 1012
Factrel (Rare) 2996
▲ Fioricet Tablets (Among most frequent) 2386
Fioricet with Codeine Capsules (Frequent) 2387
Fiorinal Capsules (Less frequent) 2388
Fiorinal with Codeine Capsules (2.6%) 2390
Fiorinal Tablets (Less frequent) 2388
Floxin I.V. 1580
Floxin Tablets (200 mg, 300 mg, 400 mg) 1577
Gammagard S/D, Immune Globulin, Intravenous (Human) (Occasional) 577
Gastrocrom Capsules (Infrequent) 1611
Gastrocrom Oral Concentrate (Less common) 1611
Guaimax-D Tablets 809
▲ Halcion Tablets (4.9%) 2093
Hydrocet Capsules 787
Hyperstat I.V. Injection 2504
▲ Hytrin Capsules (28%) 434
Hyzaar Tablets 1720
Inderal 2834
Inderal LA Long Acting Capsules 2836
Inderide Tablets 2838
Inderide LA Long Acting Capsules 2840
Indocin (Less than 1%) 1723
Inversine Tablets 1729
Ismo Tablets 2844
ISMOTIC 45% w/v Solution (Very rare) ⊙ 221
Isordil Sublingual Tablets 2845
Isordil Tembids 2847
Isordil Titradose Tablets 2848
Kemadrin Tablets 1105
Lioresal Intrathecal 1634
▲ Lorcet 10/650 Tablets (Among most frequent) 1016
▲ Lortab (Among most frequent) 2751
Lotensin HCT Tablets 855
Loxitane 1426
▲ Lupron Injection (5% or more) 2736
▲ MS Contin Tablets (Among most frequent) 2149
▲ MSIR (Among most frequent) 2152
Marcaine Spinal 2449
Mavik Tablets (1.3%) 1407
Maxaquin Tablets 2593
▲ Mepergan Injection (Among most frequent) 2859
▲ Methadone Hydrochloride Oral Concentrate (Among most frequent) 2356
Methadone Hydrochloride Oral Solution & Tablets 2357
▲ Mexitil Capsules (10.5 to 26.4%) 684
Minocin Intravenous 1428
Minocin Oral Suspension 1431
Minocin Pellet-Filled Capsules 1429
Monoket Tablets 2550
Monopril Tablets 762
Motofen Tablets (1 in 20) 789
▲ Mykrox Tablets (10.2%) 1617
Naprelan Tablets (Less than 3%) 2861
Anaprox/Naprosyn (Less than 3%) 2277
Navane Capsules and Concentrate 2018
Navane Intramuscular 2019
NegGram 2453
Nimotop Capsules (Less than 1%) 603
Nitro-Bid IV 1270
Nitro-Bid Ointment 1272
Nitro-Dur (nitroglycerin) Transdermal Infusion System (Occasional) 1365
Nolvadex Tablets (Infrequent) 2957
Norflex 1554
Norgesic 1554
Noroxin Tablets 1758
Noroxin Tablets 2222
Nucofed 2225
Numorphan Injection 953
Numorphan Suppositories 953
▲ Oramorph SR (Morphine Sulfate Sustained Release Tablets) (Among most frequent) 2359
▲ OxyIR Capsules (Among most frequent) 2167
Parafon Forte DSC Caplets (Occasional) 1590
▲ Parlodel (Less than 1% to 5%) 2411
Penetrex Tablets 2196
Peptavlon 2997
▲ Percocet Tablets (Among most frequent) 955
▲ Percodan Tablets (Among most frequent) 955
▲ Percodan-Demi Tablets (Among most frequent) 956

(▣ Described in PDR For Nonprescription Drugs) Incidence data in parenthesis; ▲ 3% or more (⊙ Described in PDR For Ophthalmology)

Light-headedness — Side Effects Index

Drug	Page
Phenergan with Codeine	2883
Phenergan VC with Codeine	2888
▲ Phrenilin (Among most frequent)	790
Prinivil Tablets	1776
Prinzide Tablets	1780
▲ Procardia Capsules (Approximately 10% to 27%; 1 in 8 patients)	2024
▲ Procardia XL Extended Release Tablets (27%; 1 in 8 patients)	2026
Prolastin Alpha₁-Proteinase Inhibitor (Human) (0.19%)	629
Prozac Pulvules & Liquid, Oral Solution (1.6%)	935
Quadrinal Tablets	1398
▲ Quinidex Extentabs (15%)	2240
▲ RMS Suppositories CII (Among most frequent)	2766
Recombivax HB (Less than 1%)	1787
Robaxin Injectable	2245
Robaxin Tablets	2246
▲ Robaxisal Tablets (One in 20-25)	2246
▲ Roxanol (Among most frequent)	2365
▲ Roxicodone Tablets, Oral Solution & Intensol (Oxycodone) (Among most frequent)	2366
Sansert Tablets	2424
▲ Sedapap Tablets 50 mg/650 mg (Among the most frequent)	1826
Sensorcaine	554
Serophene (clomiphene citrate tablets, USP) (Less than 1 in 100 patients)	2621
▲ Serzone Tablets (10%)	776
Sorbitrate	2959
▲ Symmetrel Capsules (5% to 10%)	965
▲ Symmetrel Syrup (5% to 10%)	963
Talacen Caplets	2464
▲ Talwin Injection (Most common)	2465
Talwin Compound	2466
▲ Talwin Injection (Most common)	2465
Talwin Nx Tablets	2467
Tambocor Tablets	1555
Tenoretic Tablets (1% to 3%)	2963
Tenormin Tablets and I.V. Injection (1% to 3%)	2965
▲ THROMBATE III Antithrombin III (Human) (1 of 17)	631
THYREL TRH	2992
▲ Tornalate Solution for Inhalation, 0.2% (6.8%)	976
▲ Tornalate Metered Dose Inhaler (3%)	978
Trandate	1158
▲ Transderm-Nitro Transdermal Therapeutic System (6%)	878
Trilisate (Less than 2%)	2155
Tussend	1830
▲ Tylenol with Codeine (Among most frequent)	1592
▲ Tylox Capsules (Among most frequent)	1593
Urecholine	1804
Vancenase AQ Nasal Spray 0.042% (Fewer than 5 per 100 patients)	2535
Vaseretic Tablets	1810
Vasotec Tablets	1816
Ventolin Inhalation Aerosol and Refill (1%)	1170
Ventolin Rotacaps for Inhalation (Less than 1%)	1173
Versed Injection (Less than 1%)	2324
▲ Vicodin Tablets (Among most frequent)	1404
▲ Vicodin ES Tablets (Among most frequent)	1405
▲ Vicodin HP Tablets (Among most frequent)	1403
Wygesic Tablets	2930
▲ Xanax Tablets (20.8% to 29.8%)	2115
▲ Xylocaine Injections (Among most common)	562
Zaroxolyn Tablets	1625
Zestoretic Tablets	2968
Zestril Tablets	2972
Zovirax Sterile Powder (Less than 1%)	1191
▲ Zydone Capsules (Among most frequent)	967

Limb reduction defects

Drug	Page
Accupril Tablets	1950
Altace Capsules	1238
Capoten Tablets	740
Capozide Tablets	744
Cozaar Tablets	1668
Diethylstilbestrol Tablets	1477
Elavil	2945
ESTRATAB Tablets (0.3, 0.625, 1.25, 2.5 mg) (Less than 1 per 1,000)	2715
Hyzaar Tablets	1720
Lo/Ovral Tablets	2852
Lo/Ovral-28 Tablets	2857
Lotensin Tablets	852
Lotensin HCT Tablets	855
Lotrel Capsules	858
Metubine Iodide Vials	932
Monopril Tablets	762
Nordette-21 Tablets	2863
Nordette-28 Tablets	2866
Ovral Tablets	2877
Ovral-28 Tablets	2878
Ovrette Tablets	2878
Prinivil Tablets	1776
Prinzide Tablets	1780
Proventil Inhalation Aerosol	2524
Proventil Inhalation Solution 0.083%	2527
Proventil Repetabs Tablets	2529
Proventil Syrup	2528
Univasc Tablets	2553
Vaseretic Tablets	1810
Vasotec I.V.	1814
Vasotec Tablets	1816
Ventolin Inhalation Aerosol and Refill	1170
Ventolin Inhalation Solution (Rare)	1171
Ventolin Nebules Inhalation Solution (Rare)	1172
Ventolin Rotacaps for Inhalation	1173
Ventolin Syrup	1175
Ventolin Tablets	1176
Zestoretic Tablets	2968
Zestril Tablets	2972

Lipoatrophy

Drug	Page
Imitrex Injection (Rare)	1095

Lipodystrophy

Drug	Page
Genotropin Injection (Infrequent)	2090
Humalog Injection	1488
Humulin 50/50, 100 Units (Rare)	1491
Humulin 70/30, 100 Units (Rare)	1492
Humulin L, 100 Units (Rare)	1494
Regular, 100 Units (Rare)	1503
Pork Regular, 100 Units (Rare)	1507

Lipohypertrophy

Drug	Page
Imitrex Injection (Rare)	1095

Lipoma

Drug	Page
Avonex	662
Cognex Capsules (Infrequent)	1961
Intron A for Injection (Less than 5%)	2506

Lipoprotein levels, changes

Drug	Page
▲ Accutane Capsules (About 16%)	2252
Atretol Tablets	569
Danocrine Capsules	2437
Demulen	2580
Humegon for Injection (Occasional)	1873
Levlen/Tri-Levlen	646
Nor-Q D Tablets	2598
Synarel Nasal Solution for Endometriosis	2605
Tegretol/Tegretol-XR (Occasional)	870
Timolide Tablets	1791
Levlen/Tri-Levlen	646
Triphasil-21 Tablets	2919
Vivelle Transdermal System	880
Winstrol Tablets	2468
Zoladex	2976
Zoladex 3-month	2978

Lipoproteins, electrophoretic abnormalities

Drug	Page
Sandimmune	2416

Lipotrophy

Drug	Page
Humulin 50/50, 100 Units (Rare)	1491
Humulin 70/30, 100 Units (Rare)	1492
Humulin L, 100 Units (Rare)	1494
Regular, 100 Units (Rare)	1503
Pork Regular, 100 Units (Rare)	1507

Lips, dry
(see under Xerochilia)

Lips, enlargement

Drug	Page
Dilantin Infatabs	1967
Dilantin Kapseals	1965
Dilantin-125 Suspension	1969
Eskalith	2658

Lips, swelling

Drug	Page
Altace Capsules	1238
Cataflam Tablets (Less than 1%)	833
Fluvirin (Influenza Virus Vaccine)	1608
Lithonate/Lithotabs/Lithobid	2721
Phenobarbital Elixir and Tablets	1523
Proscar Tablets	1784
Quadrinal Tablets	1398
Tambocor Tablets (Less than 1%)	1555
Cataflam/Voltaren/Voltaren-XR (less than 1%)	833

Listlessness

Drug	Page
Indocin (Greater than 1%)	1723
Polycitra Syrup	574
Polycitra-K Crystals	574
Polycitra-K Oral Solution	575
Polycitra-LC	574
Rum-K Syrup	1004

Livedo reticularis

Drug	Page
Activase	1045
Felbatol	2774
Symmetrel Capsules (1% to 5%)	965
Symmetrel Syrup (1% to 5%)	963

Liver abnormalities

Drug	Page
Cardene Capsules (Rare)	2261
Cardene SR Capsules (Rare)	2264
Catapres Tablets (About 1 in 100 patients)	679
Clozaril Tablets (1%)	2377
Combipres Tablets	682
Compazine (A few observations)	2644
Cytadren Tablets (Rare)	837
Lamprene Capsules (Less than 1%)	846
Methotrexate Sodium Tablets, Injection, for Injection and LPF Injection	1322
Nolvadex Tablets (Rare)	2957
Oncaspar (Less than 1%)	2194
Pepcid Injection (Infrequent)	1765
Pepcid (Infrequent)	1763
Pravachol Tablets	770
Relafen Tablets (1%)	2688
ReVia Tablets	957
Ridaura Capsules (1 to 3%)	2691
Sectral Capsules	2914
▲ Videx Tablets, Powder for Oral Solution, & Pediatric Powder for Oral Solution (38%)	2980
Zocor Tablets	1821

Liver abscess

Drug	Page
Cytosar-U Sterile Powder (With experimental doses)	2077

Liver damage

Drug	Page
Atretol Tablets	569
Azulfidine	2059
Butisol Sodium Elixir & Tablets (Less than 1 in 100)	2768
Compazine	2644
Cytosar-U Sterile Powder	2077
Dilantin Infatabs	1967
Dilantin Kapseals	1965
Dilantin-125 Suspension	1969
Etrafon	2495
Hivid Tablets (Less than 1%)	2287
Lasix Injection, Oral Solution and Tablets	1267
▲ Leukine (13%)	1317
Mebaral Tablets (Less than 1 in 100)	2452
Mintezol	1747
Nardil (Very few patients)	1977
Nembutal Sodium Capsules	440
Nembutal Sodium Solution	442
Nembutal Sodium Suppositories (Less than 1%)	444
Norvir (Less than 2%)	447
Nydrazid Injection (Occasional)	509
Phenobarbital Elixir and Tablets (Less than 1 in 100 patients)	1523
▲ Prograf (Greater than 3%)	1028
Prolixin	510
Redux Capsules	2911
Rifater (Occasional instances)	1280
Risperdal Tablets (Rare)	1348
Seconal Sodium Pulvules (Less than 1 in 100)	1529
Stelazine	2692
Tegretol/Tegretol-XR	870
Trasylol (0.5%)	607
Triavil Tablets	1800
Trilafon	2532
Unisom With Pain Relief-Nighttime Sleep Aid and Pain Reliever	1991
Wellbutrin Tablets (Infrequent)	1177

Liver disorders

Drug	Page
Aldoclor Tablets	1638
Aldomet Oral	1640
Aldoril Tablets	1644
Cosmegen Injection	1666
Intal Inhaler (Rare)	2185
Invirase Capsules (Rare)	2291
▲ Leukine (77%)	1317
Lo/Ovral Tablets	2852
Lo/Ovral-28 Tablets	2857
Ludiomil Tablets (Rare)	861
Ovral Tablets	2877
Ovral-28 Tablets	2878
Ovrette Tablets	2878
Prozac Pulvules & Liquid, Oral Solution (Rare)	935
Pulmozyme Inhalation	1054
Triphasil-21 Tablets	2919
Triphasil-28 Tablets	2924
▲ Vesanoid Capsules (3%)	2327

Liver dysfunction
(see under Hepatic dysfunction)

Liver function, changes

Drug	Page
Aldoclor Tablets	1638
Aldomet Ester HCl Injection	1642
Aldomet Oral	1640
Aldoril Tablets	1644
▲ Android Capsules, 10 mg (Among most common)	1297
Asendin Tablets (Less than 1%)	1419
Atretol Tablets	569
Aygestin Tablets	990
Blocadren Tablets	1654
Capoten Tablets	740
▲ Cataflam Tablets (3% to 9%)	833
Cefobid Intravenous/Intramuscular (1 patient in 1285)	1996
Clinoril Tablets (Less than 1 in 100)	1658
Cosmegen Injection	1666
Dantrium Capsules	2131
Depakene (Occasional)	416
Depakote Tablets (Occasional)	418
DiaBeta Tablets (Isolated cases)	1265
Dolobid Tablets (Less than 1 in 100)	1695
Emcyt Capsules	2085
EryPed Drops and Chewable Tablets	425
Erythromycin Base Filmtab	430
Erythromycin Delayed-Release Capsules, USP	431
ESTRATAB Tablets (0.3, 0.625, 1.25, 2.5 mg)	2715
Estratest	2718
Feldene Capsules (Less than 1%)	2008
Ilotycin Gluceptate, IV, Vials	929
▲ Methotrexate Sodium Tablets, Injection, for Injection and LPF Injection (15%)	1322
Mevacor Tablets	1742
Minipress Capsules (Less than 1%)	2015
Minizide Capsules (Rare)	2016
Mithracin	599
Moban Tablets and Concentrate (Rare)	1036
Modicon	1928
Normodyne Injection (Less common)	2519
Ortho-Novum	1928
Oxandrin	783
Pipracil (Less than 2%)	1435
▲ Prograf (5% to 36%)	1028
Prolixin	510
Reglan (Rare)	2243
Surmontil Capsules	2917
Tegretol/Tegretol-XR	870
Timolide Tablets	1791
Tonocard Tablets (Less than 1%)	519
Toradol	2319
Tornalate Solution for Inhalation, 0.2% (One patient)	976
Vaqta (Isolated reports)	1805
▲ Cataflam/Voltaren/Voltaren-XR (3% to 9%)	833
Winstrol Tablets	2468
Zestril Tablets (Rare)	2972
Zovirax Capsules	1187
Zovirax Sterile Powder	1191
Zovirax	1187

Liver function, impaired

Drug	Page
Accupril Tablets (Rare)	1950
Actimmune (Rare)	1043
▲ Albenza Tablets (Less than 1.0% to 15.6%)	2629
Aldoclor Tablets	1638
Aldomet Ester HCl Injection	1642
Aldomet Oral	1640
Aldoril Tablets	1644

(▣ Described in PDR For Nonprescription Drugs) Incidence data in parenthesis; ▲ 3% or more (◉ Described in PDR For Ophthalmology)

Side Effects Index

(continued from previous column)

Amen Tablets ... 785
Androderm Testosterone Transdermal System ... 2634
Atretol Tablets ... 569
Atromid-S Capsules ... 2808
Capastat Sulfate Injection ... 968
Catapres Tablets (About 1 in 100 patients) ... 679
▲ CellCept Capsules (More than or equal to 3%) ... 2265
Cerebyx Injection (Infrequent) ... 1956
Claritin-D Tablets (Less frequent) ... 2487
Cleocin Phosphate Injection ... 2068
Cleocin Vaginal Cream ... 2070
▲ Cordarone Intravenous (3.4%) ... 2821
▲ Cordarone Tablets (4 to 9%) ... 2818
Cycrin Tablets ... 991
DTIC-Dome (Few reports) ... 593
▲ Daypro Caplets (Up to 15%) ... 2578
Demulen ... 2580
Depo-Provera Sterile Aqueous Suspension ... 2083
Desyrel and Desyrel Dividose ... 504
Diflucan Tablets, Injection, and Oral Suspension ... 2003
Diprivan Injectable Emulsion (Less than 1%) ... 2939
DynaCirc Capsules (0.5% to 1%) ... 2381
DynaCirc CR Tablets (0.5% to 1.0%) ... 2383
E.E.S. ... 427
Edecrin (Rare) ... 1698
Elavil (Rare) ... 2945
Engerix-B Unit-Dose Vials ... 2656
ERYC ... 1972
EryPed 200 & EryPed 400 Granules ... 425
Ery-Tab Tablets ... 426
Erythrocin Stearate Filmtab ... 429
Ethmozine Tablets (Rare) ... 2217
Etrafon (Rare) ... 2495
Eulexin Capsules ... 2498
▲ Feldene Capsules (Up to 15%) ... 2008
Flexeril Tablets (Less than 1%) ... 1701
Floxin Tablets (200 mg, 300 mg, 400 mg) ... 1577
Gastrocrom Capsules (Infrequent) ... 1611
Gastrocrom Oral Concentrate (Less common) ... 1611
Glynase PresTab Tablets ... 2091
Haldol Decanoate ... 1587
Haldol Injection, Tablets and Concentrate ... 1585
Halotestin Tablets ... 2095
▲ Hivid Tablets (Less than 1% to 8.9%) ... 2287
▲ IBU Tablets (Less than 1% up to 15%) ... 1389
Idamycin Injection (Less than 5%) ... 2096
Imitrex Injection (Infrequent) ... 1095
Imitrex Tablets ... 1099
Intron A for Injection (Less than 5%) ... 2506
Lamictal Tablets (Infrequent) ... 1105
▲ Lamisil Tablets (3.3%) ... 2394
Leukine ... 1317
Lopid Tablets (Occasional) ... 1974
▲ Lupron Depot - 3 Month 22.5 mg (More than or equal to 5%) ... 2743
Mevacor Tablets ... 1742
Mexitil Capsules (About 5 in 1,000) ... 684
Micronase Tablets ... 2099
Midamor Tablets (Rare) ... 1746
Moduretic Tablets ... 1748
Motrin Ibuprofen Suspension, Oral Drops, Chewable Tablets, Caplets (Less than 1%) ... 1563
Myambutol Tablets ... 1432
Mycelex Troches ... 601
Naprelan Tablets (Less than 1%) ... 2861
Nimotop Capsules (Up to 1.2%) ... 603
▲ Nipent for Injection (2% to 19%) ... 2733
Normodyne Tablets (Less common) ... 2522
Norpramin Tablets ... 1273
Norvir (Less than 2%) ... 447
▲ Oncaspar (Greater than 1% but less than 5%) ... 2194
Orlaam Oral Solution (Low frequency) ... 2361
▲ Orudis Capsules (Greater than 3%) ... 2874
▲ Oruvail Capsules (Greater than 3%) ... 2874
PCE Dispertab Tablets ... 453
Pamelor ... 2409
Paxil Tablets (Infrequent) ... 2681
Pediazole Suspension ... 2340
Permax Tablets (Infrequent) ... 571
Premarin Vaginal Cream ... 2898

Prevacid Delayed-Release Capsules (Less than 1%) ... 2746
Provera Tablets ... 2110
Prozac Pulvules & Liquid, Oral Solution (Infrequent) ... 935
Questran ... 774
▲ Relafen Tablets (Up to 15%) ... 2688
Remeron Tablets (Infrequent) ... 1878
Rifadin (Rare) ... 1276
Rifamate Capsules ... 1278
Rifater (Rare) ... 1280
Rilutek Tablets (Infrequent) ... 2198
Rimactane Capsules (Rare) ... 865
Ritalin (Some instances) ... 866
Serzone Tablets (Infrequent) ... 776
Slo-Niacin Tablets ... 2767
Sular Tablets (Less than or equal to 1%) ... 2961
Tegretol/Tegretol-XR ... 870
Testoderm Testosterone Transdermal System ... 486
Thioguanine Tablets, Tabloid Brand (Occasional) ... 1225
Ticlid Tablets (1.0%) ... 2317
Tofranil Ampuls ... 873
Tofranil Tablets ... 875
Tofranil-PM Capsules ... 876
Trandate (Less common) ... 1158
Tranxene ... 459
▲ Trasylol (5%) ... 607
Triavil Tablets (Rare) ... 1800
Vascor Tablets (200 and 300 mg) (0.5 to 2.0%) ... 1597
▲ Vesanoid Capsules (50% to 60%) ... 2327
▲ Viramune Tablets (Among most frequent) ... 2368
Vistide Injection ... 1057
Vivactil Tablets ... 1820
Wygesic Tablets ... 2930
Yutopar Intravenous Injection (Less than 1%) ... 566

Liver injury

Anafranil Capsules (Rare) ... 819
Cordarone Tablets (Common) ... 2818
Eulexin Capsules ... 2498
Mexitil Capsules (Rare) ... 684
ReVia Tablets ... 957
Trandate Tablets (Rare) ... 1158
Vantin for Oral Suspension and Vantin Tablets ... 2112

Liver tumors
(see under Hepatomas)

Liver, degenerative changes in

Lescol Capsules ... 2395
Phenobarbital Elixir and Tablets ... 1523

Loffler's syndrome

PASER Granules ... 1333

Loss of balance
(see under Balance, loss of)

Lower spinal segments deficit

Duranest Injections (Rare) ... 533

Lumbago

Prinivil Tablets (0.3% to 1.0%) ... 1776
Prinzide Tablets ... 1780
Zestoretic Tablets ... 2968
Zestril Tablets (0.3% to 1.0%) ... 2972

Lung, carcinoma

Betaseron for SC Injection ... 653
Cognex Capsules (Rare) ... 1961
Permax Tablets (Rare) ... 571
Prinivil Tablets (0.3% to 1.0%) ... 1776
Rilutek Tablets (Infrequent) ... 2198

Lung consolidation

Survanta Beractant Intratracheal Suspension ... 2346

Lung development, hypoplastic

Accupril Tablets ... 1950
Altace Capsules ... 1238
Capoten Tablets ... 740
Capozide Tablets ... 744
Cozaar Tablets ... 1668
Hyzaar Tablets ... 1720
Lotensin Tablets ... 852
Lotensin HCT Tablets ... 855
Lotrel ... 858
Monopril Tablets ... 762
Prinivil Tablets ... 1776
Prinzide Tablets ... 1780
Univasc Tablets ... 2553
Vaseretic Tablets ... 1810
Vasotec I.V. ... 1814

Vasotec Tablets ... 1816
Zestoretic Tablets ... 2968
Zestril Tablets ... 2972

Lung disorders, unspecified

Cartrol Tablets ... 413
Casodex Tablets (2% to 5%) ... 2934
▲ CellCept Capsules (More than or equal to 3%) ... 2265
▲ Leukine (20%) ... 1317
Megace Oral Suspension (1% to 3%) ... 708
Naprelan Tablets (Less than 1%) ... 2861
▲ Nipent for Injection (Up to 12%) ... 2733
Norvir (Less than 2%) ... 447
▲ Prograf (Greater than 3%) ... 1028
Pulmozyme Inhalation ... 1054
▲ Trasylol (7%) ... 607
Videx Tablets, Powder for Oral Solution, & Pediatric Powder for Oral Solution (Less than 1%) ... 2980
Vistide Injection ... 1057

Lung neoplasms, malignant

Prinzide Tablets ... 1780
Zestoretic Tablets ... 2968
Zestril Tablets (0.3% to 1.0%) ... 2972

Lupus erythematosus

Aldoclor Tablets ... 1638
Aldomet Ester HCl Injection ... 1642
Aldomet Oral ... 1640
Aldoril Tablets ... 1644
Anafranil Capsules (Rare) ... 819
Dapsone Tablets USP ... 1331
Depakene ... 416
Depakote Tablets (1% to 5%) ... 418
Dilantin Infatabs ... 1967
Dilantin Kapseals ... 1965
Dilantin-125 Suspension ... 1969
Fansidar Tablets ... 2281
Gris-PEG Tablets, 125 mg & 250 mg ... 476
Inderal (Rare) ... 2834
Inderal LA Long Acting Capsules (Rare) ... 2836
Inderide LA Long Acting Capsules (Rare) ... 2840
Peganone Tablets ... 455
Rythmol Tablets—150mg, 225mg, 300mg (Less than 1%) ... 1399
Tonocard Tablets (1.6%) ... 519

Lupus erythematosus, systemic

Achromycin V Capsules ... 1417
AK-CIDE (Some instances) ... ⊙ 203
AK-CIDE Ointment (Some instances) ... ⊙ 203
Atromid-S Capsules ... 2808
Bactrim DS Tablets ... 2257
Bactrim I.V. Infusion ... 2255
Bactrim ... 2257
Cardioquin Tablets ... 2146
Celontin Kapseals ... 1955
Compazine ... 2644
Declomycin Tablets ... 1421
Dilantin Infatabs ... 1967
Dilantin Kapseals ... 1965
Dilantin-125 Suspension ... 1969
Etrafon ... 2495
Gantanol Tablets ... 2285
Gantrisin ... 2286
Inderal (Extremely rare) ... 2834
Inderal LA Long Acting Capsules (Extremely rare) ... 2836
Inderide Tablets (Extremely rare) ... 2838
Inderide LA Long Acting Capsules (Extremely rare) ... 2840
Mellaril ... 2398
Mexitil Capsules (About 4 in 10,000) ... 684
Monodox Capsules ... 1858
Normodyne Tablets (Less common) ... 2522
Norplant System (Rare) ... 2868
Pediazole Suspension ... 2340
Procanbid Extended-Release Tablets (Fairly common) ... 1983
Prolixin ... 510
Quinaglute Dura-Tabs Tablets ... 644
Quinidex Extentabs ... 2240
Sectral Capsules ... 2914
Septra ... 1146
Septra I.V. Infusion ... 1142
Septra I.V. Infusion ADD-Vantage Vials ... 1144
Septra ... 1146
Serentil ... 689
Stelazine ... 2692
Syprine Capsules ... 1790
Terramycin Intramuscular Solution ... 2034

Thorazine ... 2701
Timoptic in Ocudose (Less frequent) ... 1796
Timoptic Sterile Ophthalmic Solution (Less frequent) ... 1794
Timoptic-XE ... 1798
Trandate (Less common) ... 1158
Trilafon ... 2532
Vibramycin Hyclate Intravenous ... 2040
Zarontin Capsules ... 1986
Zarontin Syrup ... 1986

Lupus erythematosus, systemic, exacerbation or activation of

Apresazide Capsules ... 824
Atretol Tablets ... 569
Capozide Tablets ... 744
Doryx Capsules ... 1970
Dyazide Capsules ... 2653
DYNACIN Capsules ... 1627
Esidrix Tablets ... 839
Fulvicin P/G Tablets ... 2499
Fulvicin P/G 165 & 330 Tablets ... 2500
Helidac Therapy ... 2135
Lasix Injection, Oral Solution and Tablets ... 1267
Lotensin HCT Tablets ... 855
Minocin Intravenous ... 1428
Minocin Oral Suspension ... 1431
Minocin Pellet-Filled Capsules ... 1429
Prinzide Tablets ... 1780
Ser-Ap-Es Tablets ... 867
Tegretol/Tegretol-XR ... 870
Tenoretic Tablets ... 2963
Thalitone ... 1293
Vaseretic Tablets ... 1810
Vibramycin ... 2038
Zaroxolyn Tablets ... 1625
Zestoretic Tablets ... 2968

Lupus erythematosus syndrome

Atretol Tablets (Isolated cases) ... 569
Azulfidine (Rare) ... 2059
Cuprimine Capsules ... 1673
Depen Titratable Tablets ... 2770
Felbatol ... 2774
Fulvicin P/G Tablets ... 2499
Fulvicin P/G 165 & 330 Tablets ... 2500
IBU Tablets (Less than 1%) ... 1389
Mesantoin Tablets ... 2400
Mexitil Capsules (About 4 in 10,000) ... 684
Motrin Ibuprofen Suspension, Oral Drops, Chewable Tablets, Caplets (Less than 1%) ... 1563
Naprelan Tablets (Less than 1%) ... 2861
Navane Capsules and Concentrate ... 2018
Navane Intramuscular ... 2019
Norpace (Some cases) ... 2596
Permax Tablets (Rare) ... 571
Prozac Pulvules & Liquid, Oral Solution (Rare) ... 935
Rifamate Capsules ... 1278
Roferon-A Injection (Rare; less than 3%) ... 2308
Tegretol/Tegretol-XR (Isolated cases) ... 870
Thorazine ... 2701

Lupus-like syndrome

Aldoclor Tablets ... 1638
Aldomet Ester HCl Injection ... 1642
Aldomet Oral ... 1640
Aldoril Tablets ... 1644
Cuprimine Capsules ... 1673
Depen Titratable Tablets ... 2770
DYNACIN Capsules ... 1627
Elavil ... 2945
Fulvicin P/G Tablets ... 2499
Fulvicin P/G 165 & 330 Tablets ... 2500
Gastrocrom Oral Concentrate (Less common) ... 1611
Gris-PEG Tablets, 125 mg & 250 mg ... 476
Lescol Capsules (Rare) ... 2395
Levlen/Tri-Levlen ... 646
Lopid Tablets ... 1974
Macrobid Capsules ... 2138
Macrodantin Capsules ... 2140
Mevacor Tablets (Rare) ... 1742
Minocin Intravenous ... 1428
Minocin Oral Suspension ... 1431
Minocin Pellet-Filled Capsules ... 1429
Nardil (Less frequent) ... 1977
Nydrazid Injection ... 509
Pravachol Tablets (Rare) ... 770
Recombivax HB ... 1787
Rifater ... 1280
Tapazole Tablets ... 1361
Tegretol-XR Tablets (Isolated cases) ... 870

(▥ Described in PDR For Nonprescription Drugs)   Incidence data in parenthesis; ▲ 3% or more   (⊙ Described in PDR For Ophthalmology)

Side Effects Index

Lupus-like syndrome

- Tenoretic Tablets ... 2963
- Tenormin Tablets and I.V. Injection ... 2965
- TICE BCG, USP (Rare) ... 1881
- Tonocard Tablets (1.6%) ... 519
- Levlen/Tri-Levlen ... 646
- Zocor Tablets (Rare) ... 1821

Lyell's syndrome

- Atretol Tablets ... 569
- Azulfidine (Rare) ... 2059
- Combipres Tablets ... 682
- Daypro Caplets (Less than 1 %) ... 2578
- Fulvicin P/G Tablets (Rare) ... 2499
- Fulvicin P/G 165 & 330 Tablets (Rare) ... 2500
- Motrin Ibuprofen Suspension, Oral Drops, Chewable Tablets, Caplets (Less than 1%) ... 1563
- Pediazole Suspension ... 2340
- Proloprim Tablets (Rare) ... 1141
- Rifater ... 1280
- Tegretol/Tegretol-XR (Extremely rare) ... 870
- Tenoretic Tablets ... 2963
- Thalitone ... 1293
- Toradol ... 2319
- Trimpex Tablets (Rare) ... 2323
- Zyloprim Tablets (Less than 1%) ... 1194

Lymph nodes, tender

- ProSom Tablets (Rare) ... 457

Lymphadenitis

- Intron A for Injection (Less than or equal to 5%) ... 2506

Lymphadenopathy

- Accutane Capsules (Less than 1%) ... 2252
- Adalat CC (Less than 1.0%) ... 582
- AeroBid Inhaler System (1% to 3%) ... 1004
- Aerobid-M Inhaler System (1% to 3%) ... 1004
- Alferon N Injection (1%) ... 2142
- Ambien Tablets (Rare) ... 2559
- Anafranil Capsules (Infrequent) ... 819
- Antivenin (Crotalidae) Polyvalent ... 2803
- Apresazide Capsules (Less frequent) ... 824
- Apresoline Hydrochloride Tablets (Less frequent) ... 826
- Asacol Delayed-Release Tablets ... 2129
- Atretol Tablets ... 569
- Attenuvax (Less common) ... 1650
- Avonex ... 662
- ▲ Betaseron for SC Injection (14%) ... 653
- Biavax II ... 1653
- Cardioquin Tablets ... 2146
- Cardura Tablets (Less than 0.5% of 3960 patients) ... 1993
- Ceclor Pulvules & Suspension (Infrequent) ... 1470
- Cerebyx Injection (Infrequent) ... 1956
- Cipro Tablets (0.3% to 1%) ... 584
- Claritin-D Tablets (Less frequent) ... 2487
- Cognex Capsules (Infrequent) ... 1961
- Crixivan Capsules (Less than 2%) ... 1670
- Cuprimine Capsules ... 1673
- DaunoXome (Less than or equal to 5%) ... 1842
- Depen Titratable Tablets ... 2770
- Dilacor XR Extended-release Capsules (Infrequent) ... 2183
- Dilantin Infatabs ... 1967
- Dilantin Kapseals ... 1965
- Dilantin-125 Suspension ... 1969
- Doxil (Less than 1%) ... 2613
- Effexor (Infrequent) ... 2825
- Engerix-B Unit-Dose Vials (Less than 1%) ... 2656
- Felbatol (Infrequent) ... 2774
- Foscavir Injection (Between 1% and 5%) ... 541
- Havrix (Less than 1%; rare) ... 2663
- Hivid Tablets (Less than 1%) ... 2287
- Hydralazine Hydrochloride Injection USP (Less frequent) ... 2712
- Imitrex Tablets (Rare) ... 1099
- INFeD (Iron Dextran Injection, USP) ... 2478
- Intron A for Injection (Less than or equal to 5%) ... 2506
- Invirase Capsules (Less than 2%) ... 2291
- Kerlone Tablets (Less than 2%) ... 2588
- Klonopin Tablets ... 2294
- Lamictal Tablets (Infrequent) ... 1105
- Lamprene Capsules (Less than 1%) ... 846
- ▲ Lupron Depot 3.75 mg (Among most frequent) ... 2739
- LUVOX Tablets (Infrequent) ... 2723
- M-M-R II ... 1730
- M-R-VAX II ... 1732
- Maxaquin Tablets (Less than 1%) ... 2593
- Meruvax II ... 1740
- Mesantoin Tablets ... 2400
- Miacalcin Nasal Spray (1% to 3%) ... 2403
- Mintezol ... 1747
- Monopril Tablets (0.2% to 1.0%) ... 762
- MSTA Mumps Skin Test Antigen ... 2988
- Mumpsvax ... 1751
- Nalfon 200 Pulvules & Nalfon Tablets (Less than 1%) ... 933
- Neurontin Capsules (Infrequent) ... 1978
- Norvir (Less than 2%) ... 447
- Nydrazid Injection ... 509
- Orthoclone OKT3 Sterile Solution ... 1892
- OxyContin Tablets (Less than 1%) ... 2163
- ▲ PASER Granules (46% of 38 patients with drug-induced hepatitis) ... 1333
- Paxil Tablets (Infrequent) ... 2681
- PedvaxHIB ... 1761
- Peganone Tablets ... 455
- Permax Tablets (Infrequent) ... 571
- Proglycem ... 575
- Prozac Pulvules & Liquid, Oral Solution (2%) ... 935
- Quadrinal Tablets ... 1398
- Quinaglute Dura-Tabs Tablets ... 644
- Quinidex Extentabs ... 2240
- Recombivax HB (Less than 1%) ... 1787
- Redux Capsules (Rare) ... 2911
- Remeron Tablets (Rare) ... 1878
- Retrovir Capsules ... 1216
- Retrovir I.V. Infusion ... 1221
- Retrovir Syrup ... 1216
- Rifamate Capsules ... 1278
- Rifater ... 1280
- Rilutek Tablets (Rare) ... 2198
- Risperdal Tablets (Rare) ... 1348
- Salagen Tablets (Less than 1%) ... 1546
- Ser-Ap-Es Tablets ... 867
- Serzone Tablets (Infrequent) ... 776
- Tapazole Tablets ... 1361
- Tegretol/Tegretol-XR ... 870
- TICE BCG, USP (Occasional) ... 1881
- Tolectin (200, 400 and 600 mg) (Less than 1%) ... 1591
- Typhim Vi ... 914
- Varivax (Greater than or equal to 1%) ... 1807
- Wellbutrin Tablets (Rare) ... 1177
- ▲ Zerit Capsules (Fewer than 1% to 5%) ... 731
- Zoloft Tablets (Infrequent) ... 2051
- Zovirax ... 1187
- Zyloprim Tablets (Less than 1%) ... 1194
- Zyrtec Tablets (Less than 2%) ... 2053

Lymphadenopathy, post-cervical

- Diphtheria and Tetanus Toxoids and Pertussis Vaccine Adsorbed ... 2650
- Foscavir Injection (Less than 1%) ... 541

Lymphangitis, regional

- Doxil (Less than 1%) ... 2613

Lymphedema

- Doxil (Less than 1%) ... 2613
- Lupron Depot - 3 Month 22.5 mg (Less than 5%) ... 2743
- Paxil Tablets (Rare) ... 2681
- Redux Capsules (Infrequent) ... 2911

Lymphocytes, decrease

(see under Lymphocytopenia)

Lymphocytes, increase

(see under Lymphocytosis)

Lymphocytopenia

- ▲ Betaseron for SC Injection (82%) ... 653
- Dipentum Capsules (Rare) ... 2084
- Floxin I.V. (More than or equal to 1%) ... 1580
- Floxin Tablets (200 mg, 300 mg, 400 mg) (More than or equal to 1%) ... 1577
- Foscavir Injection (Less than 1%) ... 541
- Leukeran Tablets ... 1205
- Mavik Tablets (0.3% to 1.0%) ... 1407
- Mustargen ... 1752
- Orthoclone OKT3 Sterile Solution ... 1892
- Paxil Tablets (Rare) ... 2681
- Rocephin Injectable Vials, ADD-Vantage, Galaxy Container (Less than 1%) ... 2305
- Stelazine Tablets ... 2692
- Talwin Injection (Rare) ... 2465
- Unasyn ... 2035
- Vantin for Oral Suspension and Vantin Tablets ... 2112
- ▲ Xanax Tablets (5.5% to 7.4%) ... 2115

Lymphocytosis

- Ceclor Pulvules & Suspension ... 1470
- Ceptaz (Very rare) ... 1070
- Cipro I.V. (Infrequent) ... 587
- ▲ Cipro I.V. Pharmacy Bulk Package (Among most frequent) ... 590
- Depakene ... 416
- Depakote Tablets ... 418
- Dynabac (0.1% to 1%) ... 668
- Effexor (Infrequent) ... 2825
- Floxin I.V. (More than or equal to 1%) ... 1580
- Floxin Tablets (200 mg, 300 mg, 400 mg) (More than or equal to 1%) ... 1577
- Fortaz (Very rare) ... 1092
- Neurontin Capsules (Rare) ... 1978
- Norvir (Less than 2%) ... 447
- Paxil Tablets (Rare) ... 2681
- Permax Tablets (Rare) ... 571
- Primaxin I.M. ... 1770
- Primaxin I.V. ... 1772
- Prozac Pulvules & Liquid, Oral Solution (Rare) ... 935
- Remeron Tablets (Rare) ... 1878
- Rocephin Injectable Vials, ADD-Vantage, Galaxy Container (Rare) ... 2305
- Tazicef for Injection (Very rare) ... 2697
- Tazidime Vials, Faspak & ADD-Vantage (Very rare) ... 1531
- Unasyn ... 2035
- Vantin for Oral Suspension and Vantin Tablets ... 2112
- Zyloprim Tablets (Less than 1%) ... 1194

Lymphoma

- Azathioprine Tablets (0.5%) ... 2349
- Cytovene-IV (Two or more reports) ... 2270
- Dilantin Infatabs ... 1967
- Dilantin Kapseals ... 1965
- Dilantin-125 Suspension ... 1969
- Imuran (0.5%) ... 1103
- Methotrexate Sodium Tablets, Injection, for Injection and LPF Injection (Rare) ... 1322
- ▲ Neoral (1% to 6%) ... 2405
- Orthoclone OKT3 Sterile Solution ... 1892
- Prograf ... 1028
- ▲ Sandimmune (Less than 1 to 6%) ... 2416

Lymphoma, lymphocytic

- CellCept Capsules (0.6% to 1.0%) ... 2265
- Dantrium Capsules (Less frequent) ... 2131
- Dantrium Intravenous ... 2132

Lymphoma-like disorder

- Anafranil Capsules (Rare) ... 819
- Foscavir Injection (Between 1% and 5%) ... 541
- PASER Granules ... 1333
- Videx Tablets, Powder for Oral Solution, & Pediatric Powder for Oral Solution (Up to 2%) ... 2980

Lymphomonocytosis

- Haldol Decanoate ... 1587
- Haldol Injection, Tablets and Concentrate ... 1585

LDH abnormalities

- Bumex (1.0%) ... 2260
- Ceftin Tablets (1.0%) ... 1067
- ▲ Emcyt Capsules (2% to 31%) ... 2085
- Hivid Tablets (Less than 1%) ... 2287
- Nimotop Capsules (0.4%; rare) ... 603
- Sinemet CR Tablets ... 961
- Zithromax (Less than 1%) ... 2043
- Zithromax Tablets (Less than 1%) ... 2046

LDH increase

- Accutane Capsules ... 2252
- Adalat CC (Rare) ... 582
- Atamet Tablets ... 567
- Biaxin (Less than 1%) ... 406
- Cardizem CD Capsules (Less than 1%) ... 1251
- Cardizem SR Capsules (Less than 1%) ... 1255
- Cardizem Injectable ... 1253
- Cardizem Tablets (Less than 1%) ... 1257
- Cefizox for Intramuscular or Intravenous Use ... 1025
- Cefotan (1 in 700) ... 2936
- Ceftin for Oral Suspension (1.0%) ... 1067
- Cefzil Tablets and Oral Suspension ... 747
- ▲ CellCept Capsules (More than or equal to 3%) ... 2265
- Ceptaz (One in 18) ... 1070
- Chibroxin Sterile Ophthalmic Solution (With oral form) ... 1657
- ▲ Cipro I.V. (Among most frequent) ... 587
- ▲ Cipro I.V. Pharmacy Bulk Package (Among most frequent) ... 590
- Cipro Tablets (0.4%) ... 584
- Claforan Sterile and Injection (Less than 1%) ... 1259
- Cuprimine Capsules (Few cases) ... 1673
- Cytovene (1% or less) ... 2270
- Demulen ... 2580
- Depakene (Frequent) ... 416
- Depakote Tablets (Frequent) ... 418
- Depen Titratable Tablets (Few reports) ... 2770
- Dilacor XR Extended-release Capsules (Rare) ... 2183
- Doxil (Less than 1%) ... 2613
- Duricef Capsules, Tablets, and Oral Suspension ... 750
- Felbatol (Infrequent) ... 2774
- Floxin I.V. ... 1580
- Floxin Tablets (200 mg, 300 mg, 400 mg) ... 1577
- ▲ Fortaz (1 in 18) ... 1092
- Foscavir Injection (Between 1% and 5%) ... 541
- ▲ Sterile FUDR (Among more common) ... 2284
- Garamycin Injectable ... 2502
- Glucotrol Tablets (Occasional) ... 2011
- Glucotrol XL Extended Release Tablets (Occasional) ... 2012
- Inderide Tablets ... 2838
- Kefurox Vials, Faspak & ADD-Vantage (1 in 75) ... 1509
- Kerlone Tablets (Less than 2%) ... 2588
- Larodopa Tablets ... 2296
- Lopid Capsules (Occasional) ... 1974
- Lorabid Suspension and Pulvules ... 1513
- LUVOX Tablets (Rare) ... 2723
- Mefoxin ... 1734
- Mefoxin Premixed Intravenous Solution ... 1737
- Megace Oral Suspension (1% to 3%) ... 708
- Merrem I.V. (Greater than 0.2%) ... 2952
- Monocid Injection (1.6%) ... 2674
- Monopril Tablets ... 762
- Nalfon 200 Pulvules & Nalfon Tablets (Less than 1%) ... 933
- Nebcin Vials, Hyporets & ADD-Vantage ... 1518
- ▲ Neupogen for Injection (27% to 58%) ... 495
- Noroxin Tablets (Less frequent) ... 1758
- Noroxin Tablets (Less frequent) ... 2222
- Paxil Tablets (Rare) ... 2681
- Pentasa (Less than 1%) ... 1275
- Pipracil (Less frequent) ... 1435
- Prevacid Delayed-Release Capsules (Less than 1%) ... 2746
- Primaxin I.M. ... 1770
- Primaxin I.V. ... 1772
- Procardia Capsules (Rare) ... 2024
- Procardia XL Extended Release Tablets (Rare) ... 2026
- Rilutek Tablets (Rare) ... 2198
- Roferon-A Injection (Less than 1%) ... 2308
- Sectral Capsules ... 2914
- Serzone Tablets (Infrequent) ... 776
- Sinemet Tablets ... 959
- Sinemet CR Tablets ... 961
- Suprax ... 1443
- ▲ Tazicef for Injection (1 in 18 patients) ... 2697
- ▲ Tazidime Vials, Faspak & ADD-Vantage (1 in 18) ... 1531
- ▲ Tegison Capsules (15%) ... 2314
- Tiazac Capsules (Less than 1%) ... 1019
- Timentin for Injection ... 2706
- Toprol-XL Tablets ... 560
- Tornalate Solution for Inhalation, 0.2% (Rare) ... 976
- Unasyn ... 2035
- Vantin for Oral Suspension and Vantin Tablets ... 2112
- Zanosar Sterile Powder (A number of patients) ... 2119
- Zinacef (1 in 75 patients) ... 1184

(⊠ Described in PDR For Nonprescription Drugs)   Incidence data in parenthesis; ▲ 3% or more   (⊙ Described in PDR For Ophthalmology)

1393 **Side Effects Index** **Malaise**

LE cells test positive
(see under Lupus erythematosus)

LE-like reactions
(see under Lupus erythematosus)

M

Maceration
Monistat-Derm (miconazole nitrate 2%) Cream (Isolated reports) 1944
Oxistat Cream (0.1%) 1139

Maceration, skin
Cortisporin Otic Solution Sterile 1076
Cortisporin Otic Suspension Sterile 1077
DesOwen Cream, Ointment and Lotion (Infrequent) 1032
Locoid Cream, Ointment and Topical Solution (Infrequent) 994
Neurontin Capsules (Rare) 1978
Pediotic Suspension Sterile 1140

Macrocytic anemia
Ambien Tablets (Rare) 2559
Azathioprine Tablets (2 patients) 2349
Depakene 416
Depakote Tablets 418
Dilantin Infatabs 1967
Dilantin-125 Suspension 1969
Eulexin Capsules 2498
Imuran (2 cases) 1103
Lamictal Tablets (Rare) 1105

Macrocytosis
Depakene 416
Depakote Tablets (1% to 5%) 418
Dilantin Kapseals 1965
Retrovir Capsules (The majority of children) 1216
Retrovir I.V. Infusion (The majority of children) 1221
Retrovir Syrup (The majority of children) 1216

Macrophages, reactive
Blenoxane 697

Maculae
Calan SR Caplets (1% or less) 2571
Calan Tablets (1% or less) 2568
Covera-HS Tablets (Less than 2%) 2573
Isoptin Oral Tablets (Less than 1%) 1393
Isoptin SR Tablets (1% or less) 1395
Verelan Capsules (1% or less) 1455

Maculopathy
Tolectin (200, 400 and 600 mg) (Less than 1%) 1591

Malabsorption syndrome
Elspar 1700
Purinethol Tablets (Occasional) 1214
Sandostatin Injection (1% to 4%) .. 2421

Malaise
Abelcet Injection 1540
Accupril Tablets (0.5%-1.0%) 1950
Accutane Capsules 2252
AeroBid Inhaler System (1% to 3%) 1004
Aerobid-M Inhaler System (1% to 3%) 1004
Airet Albuterol Sulfate Inhalation Solution (1.5%) 1602
Albuterol Sulfate, USP Solution for Inhalation, Arm-a-Med (1.5%) 522
▲ Alferon N Injection (9% to 65%) 2142
Altace Capsules (Less than 1%) 1238
Ambien Tablets (Infrequent) 2559
Amicar Syrup, Tablets, and Injection 1312
Anafranil Capsules (Infrequent) 819
Anaprox/Naprosyn (Less than 1%) 2277
Antivenin (Crotalidae) Polyvalent 2803
Apresazide Capsules 824
Aquasol A Vitamin A Capsules, USP 525
Aquasol A Parenteral 526
▲ Arimidex Tablets (2% to 5%) 2932
Asacol Delayed-Release Tablets (1% to 2%) 2129
Atamet Tablets 567
▲ Avonex (4%) 662
Azactam for Injection (Less than 1%) 736
Azathioprine Tablets 2349
▲ Betaseron for SC Injection (15%) .. 653
Biavax II 1653
Biltricide Tablets 584
Buprenex Injectable (Infrequent) 2170
BuSpar Tablets (Infrequent) 738
Calan SR Caplets 2571
Calan Tablets 2568
Capoten Tablets (0.5 to 2%) 740
Capozide Tablets (0.5 to 2%) 744
Cardene Capsules (0.6%) 2261
▲ Cardura Tablets (About 0.7% to 12%) 1993
Cartrol Tablets (Less common) 413
Cataflam Tablets (Less than 1%) 833
Catapres Tablets (About 1 in 100 patients) 679
Catapres-TTS 680
Celestone Soluspan Suspension 2484
▲ CellCept Capsules (More than or equal to 3%) 2265
Cerebyx Injection (Infrequent) 1956
Cholera Vaccine 2818
Cipro I.V. (1% or less) 587
Cipro I.V. Pharmacy Bulk Package (Less than 1%) 590
Cipro Tablets (Less than 1%) 584
Claritin Tablets (2% or fewer patients) 2485
Claritin-D Tablets (Less frequent) .. 2487
Clinoril Tablets (Less than 1 in 100) 1658
Clozaril Tablets (Less than 1%) 2377
Cognex Capsules (Frequent) 1961
Combipres Tablets (About 1%) 682
▲ Cordarone Tablets (4 to 9%) 2818
Cortone Acetate Sterile Suspension 1663
Cortone Acetate Tablets 1664
Cosmegen Injection 1666
Crixivan Capsules (0.5% to less than 2%) 1670
Cytosar-U Sterile Powder (Occasional) 2077
Cytovene-IV (1% or less) 2270
DTIC-Dome (Infrequent) 593
Dalalone D.P. Injectable 1009
▲ Dantrium Capsules (Among most frequent) 2131
Daraprim Tablets (Rare) 1199
▲ DaunoXome (1% to 9%) 1842
Daypro Caplets (Less than 1%) 2578
Decadron Elixir 1676
Decadron Phosphate Injection 1680
Decadron Phosphate with Xylocaine Injection, Sterile 1683
Decadron Tablets 1678
Decadron-LA Sterile Suspension 1687
Depakene 416
Depakote Tablets (1% to 5%) 418
Desyrel and Desyrel Dividose (Up to 2.8%) 504
Dexacort Phosphate in Respihaler .. 1606
Dexacort Phosphate in Turbinaire .. 1607
Dilacor XR Extended-release Capsules (Infrequent) 2183
Diphtheria & Tetanus Toxoids Adsorbed Purogenated (Mild) 1422
Dolobid Tablets (Less than 1 in 100) 1695
Doral Tablets 2773
Dynabac (0.1% to 1%) 668
EC-Naprosyn Delayed-Release Tablets (Less than 1%) 2277
Edecrin 1698
Effexor (Frequent) 2825
Elavil 2945
Eldepryl Capsules 2729
Engerix-B Unit-Dose Vials (Less than 1%) 2656
▲ Epivir (27%) 1200
Ergamisol Tablets 1340
▲ Etopophos for Injection (39%) 701
Etrafon 2495
Felbatol (Frequent) 2774
Feldene Capsules (Greater than 1%) 2008
Flexeril Tablets (Less than 1%) 1701
▲ Flovent (22% to 28%) 1089
Floxin I.V. (Less than 1%) 1580
Floxin Tablets (200 mg, 300 mg, 400 mg) (Less than 1%) 1577
▲ Fludara for Injection (6% to 8%) 658
Fluvirin (Influenza Virus Vaccine) (Infrequent) 1608
▲ Foscavir Injection (5% or greater) .. 541
Sterile FUDR 2284
▲ Fungizone Intravenous (Among most common) 507
Furoxone (Occasional) 2221
Gamimune N, 5% Immune Globulin Intravenous (Human), 5% 612
Gamimune N, 10% Immune Globulin Intravenous (Human), 10% 615
Gammar-P I.V., Immune Globulin Intravenous (Human) 798
Gastrocrom Capsules (1 report) 1611
Gastrocrom Oral Concentrate (1 report) 1611
Gemzar for Injection (Infrequent) 1482
GlaucTabs ...... ⊙ 209
Glucophage Tablets 754
▲ Havrix (1% to 10%) 2663
Helidac Therapy (Less than 1%) 2135
Hivid Tablets (Less than 1%) 2287
Humegon for Injection 1873
Hycamtin for Injection (0.5% to 1.8%) 2665
Hydeltrasol Injection, Sterile 1708
Hydeltra-T.B.A. Sterile Suspension 1710
Hydrea Capsules 705
Hydrocortone Acetate Sterile Suspension 1712
Hydrocortone Phosphate Injection, Sterile 1713
Hydrocortone Tablets 1715
Hyperstat I.V. Injection 2504
IFEX (Less than 1%) 706
Imdur (Less than or equal to 5%) .. 1362
Imitrex Injection (1.1%) 1095
Imitrex Tablets 1099
▲ Imovax Rabies Vaccine (Up to 6%) 899
Imuran 1103
Indocin (Greater than 1%) 1723
INFeD (Iron Dextran Injection, USP) 2478
Influenza Virus Vaccine, Trivalent, Types A and B (chromatograph- and filter-purified subviron antigen) FluShield, 1996-1997 Formula (Infrequent) 2842
▲ Intron A for Injection (Up to 14%) 2506
Iopidine 0.5% (Less than 1%) .... ⊙ 219
Ismo Tablets (Fewer than 1%) 2844
Isoptin SR Tablets 1395
▲ JE-VAX (Approximately 10%) 904
Kadian Capsules (Less than 3%) 2948
Kerlone Tablets (Less than 2%) 2588
Lamictal Tablets (2.3%) 1105
Larodopa Tablets (Relatively frequent) 2296
Lescol Capsules (Rare) 2395
▲ Leucovorin Calcium for Injection (2% to 13%) 1313
▲ Leukine (57%) 1317
▲ Leustatin (5% to 7%) 1889
Lioresal Intrathecal (1% or more) .. 1634
▲ Lodine Capsules and Tablets (3% to 9%) 2849
Lomotil 2591
LUVOX Tablets (Frequent) 2723
M-M-R II 1730
M-R-VAX II 1732
Macrobid Capsules (Less than 1% to common) 2138
Macrodantin Capsules (Common) .. 2140
Marinol (Dronabinol) Capsules (Less than 1%) 2353
Maxaquin Tablets (Less than 1%) .. 2593
Meruvax II 1740
Methotrexate Sodium Tablets, Injection, for Injection and LPF Injection (Frequent) 1322
Metrodin (urofollitropin for injection) 2616
Mevacor Tablets (Rare) 1742
Mexitil Capsules (Less than 1% or about 3 in 1,000) 684
Mithracin 599
Moduretic Tablets (Less than or equal to 1%) 1748
8-MOP Capsules 1294
Motrin Ibuprofen Suspension, Oral Drops, Chewable Tablets, Caplets 1563
Myambutol Tablets 1432
▲ Mykrox Tablets (4.4%) 1617
Myochrysine Injection 1754
Nalfon 200 Pulvules & Nalfon Tablets (Less than 1%) 933
Naprelan Tablets (Less than 1%) .. 2861
Anaprox/Naprosyn (Less than 1%) 2277
Nardil 1977
Neptazane Tablets ...... ⊙ 320
Neurontin Capsules (Frequent) 1978
▲ Norpace (3 to 9%) 2596
Norpramin Tablets 1273
Norvasc Tablets (More than 0.1% to 1%) 2020
Norvir (0.7% to 1.7%) 447
Nydrazid Injection 509
▲ Oncaspar (Greater than 5%) 2194
▲ Orlaam Oral Solution (11%) 2361
Orthoclone OKT3 Sterile Solution .. 1892
Orudis Capsules (Greater than 1%) 2874
Oruvail Capsules (Greater than 1%) 2874
Oxsoralen-Ultra Capsules 1302
OxyContin Tablets (Less than 1%) 2163
Pamelor 2409
Papaverine Hydrochloride Vials and Ampoules 1523
Parafon Forte DSC Caplets (Occasional) 1590
Paxil Tablets (Frequent) 2681
Penetrex Tablets (0.1% to 1%) 2196
Pentasa (Less than 1%) 1275
Pentaspan Injection 954
Pergonal (menotropins for injection, USP) 2618
Permax Tablets (Infrequent) 571
Pneumovax 23 1768
Pravachol Tablets (Rare) 770
Prevacid Delayed-Release Capsules (Less than 1%) 2746
Prilosec Delayed-Release Capsules (Less than 1%) 516
Prinivil Tablets (0.3% to 1.0%) 1776
Prinzide Tablets 1780
Procardia XL Extended Release Tablets (1% or less) 2026
Proglycem 575
▲ Proleukin for Injection (53%) 812
▲ ProSom Tablets (5%) 457
Proventil Inhalation Solution 0.083% (1.5%) 2527
Proventil Solution for Inhalation 0.5% (1.5%) 2525
Prozac Pulvules & Liquid, Oral Solution (Infrequent) 935
Pulmozyme Inhalation 1054
Pyrazinamide Tablets 1442
▲ Rabies Vaccine, Imovax Rabies I.D. (Less frequent; up to 6%) 901
Recombivax HB (Equal to or greater than 1%) 1787
Redux Capsules (Infrequent) 2911
Relafen Tablets (1%) 2688
Remeron Tablets (Frequent) 1878
RespiGam (One child) 1631
▲ Retrovir Capsules (8% to 53.2%) 1216
▲ Retrovir I.V. Infusion (8% to 53.2%) 1221
▲ Retrovir Syrup (8% to 53.2%) 1216
Rifadin 1276
Rifamate Capsules 1278
Rifater 1280
Rilutek Tablets (0.4% to 1.2%) 2198
Risperdal Tablets (Infrequent) 1348
Romazicon (1% to 3%) 2311
▲ Rowasa (3.44%) 2727
Sansert Tablets 2424
Sectral Capsules 2914
Serevent Inhalation Aerosol (1% to 3%) 1149
Serzone Tablets (Infrequent) 776
Sinemet Tablets 959
Sinemet CR Tablets 961
Solganal Suspension 2530
Sporanox Capsules (1% to 1.2%) .. 1352
Sular Tablets (Less than or equal to 1%) 2961
Supprelin Injection (1% to 3%) 2230
Surmontil Capsules 2917
Tambocor Tablets (1% to less than 3%) 1555
Tenex Tablets (3% or less) 2249
Tetanus & Diphtheria Toxoids Adsorbed Purogenated (Rare) 1446
Tetanus Toxoid Adsorbed Purogenated 1447
▲ TheraCys BCG Live (Intravesical) (2.0% to 40.2%) 911
▲ TICE BCG, USP (7.4%) 1881
Tofranil Ampuls 873
Tofranil Tablets 875
Tofranil-PM Capsules 876
Tonocard Tablets (Less than 1%) .. 519
Trandate 1158
Trental Tablets (Less than 1%) 1291
Triavil Tablets 1800
▲ Typhim Vi (4.1% to 37%) 914
Typhoid Vaccine 2929
Ultram Tablets (50 mg) (1% to less than 5%) 1594
Unasyn (Less than 1%) 2035
Univasc Tablets (Less than 1%) 2553
Urecholine 1804
Vantin for Oral Suspension and Vantin Tablets (Less than 1%) 2112

(▣ Described in PDR For Nonprescription Drugs) Incidence data in parenthesis; ▲ 3% or more (⊙ Described in PDR For Ophthalmology)

Varivax (Greater than or equal to 1%) 1807
▲ Velban Vials (Among most common) 1537
Ventolin Inhalation Solution (1.5%) 1171
Ventolin Nebules Inhalation Solution (1.5%) 1172
Verelan Capsules 1455
▲ Vesanoid Capsules (66%) 2327
▲ Videx Tablets, Powder for Oral Solution, & Pediatric Powder for Oral Solution (Up to 29%) 2980
Viramune Tablets 2368
Vistide Injection 1057
Cataflam/Voltaren/Voltaren-XR (Less than 1%) 833
▲ Yutopar Intravenous Injection (5% to 6%) 566
Zantac (Rare) 1182
Zantac Injection (Rare) 1180
Zantac Syrup (Rare) 1182
Zebeta Tablets 1457
▲ Zerit Capsules (1% to 17%) 731
Zestoretic Tablets 2968
Zestril Tablets (0.3% to 1.0%) 2972
Ziac 1459
▲ Zinecard Injection (48% to 61%) 2120
Zithromax (1% or less) 2043
Zocor Tablets (Rare) 1821
▲ Zofran Injection (5%) 1227
▲ Zofran Tablets (9% to 13%) 1231
Zoladex (1% to 5%) 2976
Zoladex 3-month 2978
Zoloft Tablets (Infrequent) 2051
Zosyn (1.0% or less) 1463
▲ Zovirax (11.5%) 1187
Zyloprim Tablets (Less than 1%) 1194
Zyrtec Tablets (Less than 2%) 2053

Malaria relapse
Aramine Injection 1649

Male pattern baldness (see under Alopecia, hereditaria)

Malignancies, secondary
Cytoxan (Isolated reports) 700
Leukeran Tablets 1205

Malignant hyperthermia
Anectine 1062
Foscavir Injection (Less than 1%) 541
Proleukin for Injection (Less than 1%) 812

Malignant hyperthermia, familial
Sensorcaine 554

Malignant melanoma
Atamet Tablets 567
Sinemet Tablets 959
Sinemet CR Tablets 961

Malignant neoplasms
CellCept Capsules (0.8% to 1.4%) 2265
Orthoclone OKT3 Sterile Solution 1892
▲ Tegison Capsules (1 to 10%) 2314

Malodor, unspecified
Condylox Topical Solution (Less than 5%) 1853

Manic behavior
Ambien Tablets (Rare) 2559
Anafranil Capsules (Infrequent) 819
Betaseron for SC Injection 653
Cipro I.V. (1% or less) 587
Cipro I.V. Pharmacy Bulk Package (Less than 1%) 590
Cipro Tablets (Less than 1%) 584
Cytovene (1% or less) 2270
Effexor (0.5%) 2825
Elavil (Rare) 2945
Felbatol 2774
Floxin I.V. 1580
Floxin Tablets (200 mg, 300 mg, 400 mg) 1577
Halcion Tablets 2093
Hivid Tablets (Less than 1%) 2287
Lamictal Tablets (Rare) 1105
Levsin/Levsinex/Levbid 2549
Ludiomil Tablets (Rare) 861
LUVOX Tablets (Frequent) 2723
Maxaquin Tablets 2593
Nardil (Less frequent) 1977
Neurontin Capsules (Rare) 1978
Orthoclone OKT3 Sterile Solution 1892
Pamelor 2409
Parnate Tablets 2679
Paxil Tablets (Approximately 1.0%; infrequent) 2681
Permax Tablets (Infrequent) 571
Protopam Chloride for Injection (Several cases) 2909
Prozac Pulvules & Liquid, Oral Solution (Infrequent) 935
Redux Capsules 2911
Remeron Tablets (Infrequent) 1878
Rilutek Tablets (Infrequent) 2198
Risperdal Tablets 1348
Roferon-A Injection 2308
Rythmol Tablets–150mg, 225mg, 300mg (Less than 1%) 1399
Serzone Tablets (0.3% to 1.6%) 776
Tofranil Ampuls 873
Tofranil Tablets 875
Tofranil-PM Capsules 876
Triavil Tablets (Rare) 1800
Videx Tablets, Powder for Oral Solution, & Pediatric Powder for Oral Solution (Less than 1%) 2980
Wellbutrin Tablets (Frequent) 1177
Xanax Tablets 2115
Zoloft Tablets (0.4%) 2051

Masculinization, female fetus
Oxandrin 783

Mass, abdominal (see under Abdominal mass)

Mastalgia (see under Mastodynia)

Mastitis
Humegon for Injection (Occasional) 1873
Intron A for Injection (Less than or equal to 5%) 2506
Paxil Tablets (Rare) 2681
Redux Capsules (Rare) 2911
Risperdal Tablets (Infrequent) 1348

Mastodynia
Climara Transdermal System 640
Estrace Cream and Tablets 751
Estraderm Transdermal System 842
ESTRATAB Tablets (0.3, 0.625, 1.25, 2.5 mg) 2715
Estratest 2718
Estring Vaginal Ring (Uncommon) 2086
Haldol Decanoate 1587
Menest Tablets 2671
Nalfon 200 Pulvules & Nalfon Tablets (Less than 1%) 933
Norplant System 2868
Ogen Tablets 2103
Ogen Vaginal Cream 2106
Ortho-Est 1925
Premarin Intravenous 2893
Premarin Tablets 2896
Premarin Vaginal Cream 2898
Premphase 2900
Prempro 2905

Medullary hypoplasia
Novantrone for Injection 1327

Megacolon, acquired
Felbatol 2774

Megacolon, toxic
Lomotil 2591
Motofen Tablets 789

Megaloblastic anemia
Azulfidine (Rare) 2059
Bactrim DS Tablets 2257
Bactrim I.V. Infusion 2255
Bactrim 2257
Daraprim Tablets 1199
Dilantin Infatabs 1967
Dilantin Kapseals 1965
Dilantin-125 Suspension 1969
Dyazide Capsules 2653
Dyrenium Capsules (Rare) 2655
Eminase (Less than 1%) 2215
Fansidar Tablets 2281
Glucophage Tablets (Five cases) 754
Macrobid Capsules 2138
Macrodantin Capsules 2140
Mebaral Tablets (Less than 1 in 100) 2452
Mesantoin Tablets (Uncommon) 2400
Mysoline (Rare idiosyncrasy) 2860
Nembutal Sodium Capsules 440
Nembutal Sodium Solution 442
Nembutal Sodium Suppositories (Less than 1%) 444
Permax Tablets (Infrequent) 571
Phenobarbital Elixir and Tablets (A few cases) 1523
Proloprim Tablets 1141
Seconal Sodium Pulvules 1529
Septra 1146
Septra I.V. Infusion 1142
Septra I.V. Infusion ADD-Vantage Vials 1144
Septra 1146
Trimpex Tablets 2323
Zovirax Sterile Powder (Less than 1%) 1191

Megaloblastosis
Cytosar-U Sterile Powder 2077

Melanoma, malignant, activation of
Larodopa Tablets 2296

Melanoma, skin
Clomid 1262
Cognex Capsules (Rare) 1961
8-MOP Capsules 1294

Melanosis
Intron A for Injection (Less than 5%) 2506
Neurontin Capsules (Rare) 1978

Melasma
Amen Tablets 785
Aygestin Tablets 990
Depo-Provera Contraceptive Injection (Fewer than 1%) 2079
Diethylstilbestrol Tablets 1477
Estratest 2718
Modicon 1928
Ortho Dienestrol Cream 1922
Ortho-Novum 1928

Melasma, possibly persistent
Brevicon 2563
Climara Transdermal System 640
Demulen 2580
Desogen Tablets 1867
Estrace Cream and Tablets 751
Estraderm Transdermal System 842
ESTRATAB Tablets (0.3, 0.625, 1.25, 2.5 mg) 2715
Levlen/Tri-Levlen 646
Menest Tablets 2671
Micronor Tablets 1903
Modicon 1928
Norinyl 2563
Nor-Q D Tablets 2598
Ogen Tablets 2103
Ogen Vaginal Cream 2106
Ortho-Cept 1907
Ortho-Cyclen/Ortho-Tri-Cyclen 1914
Ortho-Est 1925
Ortho-Novum 1928
Ortho-Cyclen/Ortho Tri-Cyclen 1914
Ovcon 765
PMB 200 and PMB 400 2890
Premarin Intravenous 2893
Premarin Tablets 2896
Premarin Vaginal Cream 2898
Premphase 2900
Prempro 2905
Levlen/Tri-Levlen 646
Tri-Norinyl 2607
Vivelle Transdermal System 880

Melena
Abelcet Injection 1540
Anaprox/Naprosyn (Less than 1%) 2277
Betaseron for SC Injection 653
Casodex Tablets (2% to 5%) 2934
Cataflam Tablets (Less than 1%) 833
Cedax 2480
Cytovene (1% or less) 2270
DaunoXome (Less than or equal to 5%) 1842
Diamox Intravenous (Occasional) ◉ 317
Diamox Sequels (Sustained Release) ◉ 318
Diamox Tablets (Occasional) ◉ 317
EC-Naprosyn Delayed-Release Tablets (Less than 1%) 2277
Effexor (Infrequent) 2825
Feldene Capsules (Less than 1%) 2008
Foscavir Injection (Between 1% and 5%) 541
Fungizone Intravenous 507
GlaucTabs (Occasional) ◉ 209
Helidac Therapy (2.5%) 2135
Hivid Tablets (Less than 1%) 2287
IBU Tablets (Less than 1%) 1389
Imdur (Less than or equal to 5%) 1362
Imitrex Tablets (Rare) 1099
Intron A for Injection (Less than 5%) 2506
Invirase Capsules (Less than 2%) 2291
Lamictal Tablets (Rare) 1105
Lodine Capsules and Tablets (1% to 3%) 2849
Lotensin Tablets 852
Lotensin HCT Tablets (Scattered accounts) 855
LUVOX Tablets (Infrequent) 2723
Merrem I.V. (0.7%) 2952
Methotrexate Sodium Tablets, Injection, for Injection and LPF Injection 1322
Motrin Ibuprofen Suspension, Oral Drops, Chewable Tablets, Caplets (Less than 1%) 1563
Naprelan Tablets (Less than 1%) 2861
Anaprox/Naprosyn (Less than 1%) 2277
Neptazane Tablets ◉ 320
Orudis Capsules (Less than 1%) 2874
Oruvail Capsules (Less than 1%) 2874
Paxil Tablets (Rare) 2681
Pediazole Suspension 2340
Permax Tablets (Infrequent) 571
Prevacid Delayed-Release Capsules (Less than 1%) 2746
Procardia XL Extended Release Tablets (1% or less) 2026
ProSom Tablets (Rare) 457
Prozac Pulvules & Liquid, Oral Solution (2%) 935
Redux Capsules (Rare) 2911
Relafen Tablets (1%) 2688
Ridaura Capsules (0.1 to 1%) 2691
Rilutek Tablets (Rare) 2198
Risperdal Tablets (Infrequent) 1348
Sular Tablets (Less than or equal to 1%) 2961
Tegison Capsules (Less than 1%) 2314
Toradol 2319
Vaseretic Tablets 1810
Vasotec I.V. 1814
Vasotec Tablets (0.5% to 1.0%) 1816
▲ Videx Tablets, Powder for Oral Solution, & Pediatric Powder for Oral Solution (Up to 7%) 2980
Vistide Injection 1057
Cataflam/Voltaren/Voltaren-XR (Less than 1%) 833
Zithromax (1% or less) 2043
Zithromax Tablets (1% or less) 2046
Zoloft Tablets (Rare) 2051
Zosyn (1.0% or less) 1463
Zyrtec Tablets (Less than 2%) 2053

Memory impairment
▲ Anafranil Capsules (7% to 9%) 819
Cataflam Tablets (Less than 1%) 833
Cogentin 1661
Cozaar Tablets (Less than 1%) 1668
Desyrel and Desyrel Dividose (Less than 1% to 1.4%) 504
Eldepryl Capsules 2729
Eskalith 2658
Halcion Tablets (0.9% to 0.5%) 2093
Hyzaar Tablets 1720
Imitrex Tablets (Rare) 1099
Klonopin Tablets 2294
Lamictal Tablets (2.4%) 1105
Lithonate/Lithotabs/Lithobid 2721
Lopressor 848
Ludiomil Tablets (Rare) 861
▲ Lupron Depot 3.75 mg (Among most frequent) 2739
Lupron Injection (Less than 5%) 2736
Monopril Tablets (0.2% to 1.0%) 762
Nydrazid Injection (Uncommon) 509
Prinivil Tablets (0.3% to 1.0%) 1776
Prinzide Tablets 1780
Rifamate Capsules (Uncommon) 1278
Rifater (Uncommon) 1280
Roferon-A Injection (Less than 4%) 2308
Serax Capsules 2916
Serax Tablets 2916
Seromycin Capsules 975
▲ Serzone Tablets (4%) 776
Sinemet CR Tablets 961
Timolide Tablets 1791
Tonocard Tablets (Less than 1%) 519
Transderm Scōp Transdermal Therapeutic System (Infrequent) 890
▲ Vesanoid Capsules (3%) 2327
Cataflam/Voltaren/Voltaren-XR (Less than 1%) 833
Wellbutrin Tablets (Infrequent) 1177
▲ Xanax Tablets (33.1%) 2115
Zestoretic Tablets 2968
Ziac 1459

1395 Side Effects Index Mental clouding

Memory loss, short-term
Blocadren Tablets 1654
Cartrol Tablets 413
Clozaril Tablets (Less than 1%) 2377
Cytovene-IV (One report) 2270
Ergamisol Tablets (10 out of 463 patients) 1340
Ethmozine Tablets (Less than 2%) 2217
Hivid Tablets (Less than 1%) 2287
Inderal 2834
Inderal LA Long Acting Capsules 2836
Inderide Tablets 2838
Inderide LA Long Acting Capsules 2840
Kerlone Tablets 2588
Lescol Capsules 2395
Levatol Tablets 2547
Levsin/Levsinex/Levbid 2549
Lopressor HCT Tablets 850
Mevacor Tablets (0.5% to 1.0%) 1742
Mexitil Capsules (About 9 in 1,000) 684
Normodyne Tablets 2522
Parnate Tablets 2679
Placidyl Capsules 456
Pravachol Tablets 770
Redux Capsules 2911
Rythmol Tablets–150mg, 225mg, 300mg (Less than 1%) 1399
Sectral Capsules 2914
Tenoretic Tablets 2963
Tenormin Tablets and I.V. Injection 2965
Testoderm Testosterone Transdermal System (One in 104 patients) 486
Timoptic in Ocudose 1796
Timoptic Sterile Ophthalmic Solution 1794
Timoptic-XE 1798
Toprol-XL Tablets 560
Trandate Tablets 1158
Visken Tablets 2428
Zocor Tablets 1821

Meniere's syndrome
Netromycin Injection 100 mg/ml 2516

Meningism
Albenza Tablets (Up to 1.0%) 2629
Antivenin (Crotalidae) Polyvalent (Occasional) 2803
Marcaine 2446
Marcaine Spinal 2449
Neurontin Capsules (Rare) 1978
Nipent for Injection (Less than 3%) 2733
Novocain Hydrochloride for Spinal Anesthesia 2457
Pontocaine Hydrochloride for Spinal Anesthesia 2460
Redux Capsules 2911
Sensorcaine 554

Meningitis
Azulfidine (Rare) 2059
Betaseron for SC Injection 653
Carbocaine Injection 2432
Cerebyx Injection (Infrequent) 1956
DaunoXome (Less than or equal to 5%) 1842
▲ Exosurf Neonatal for Intratracheal Suspension (Less than 1% to 6%) 1081
Foscavir Injection (Between 1% and 5%) 541
Lioresal Intrathecal (2 cases of 244 patients) 1634
Marcaine with Epinephrine 2446
Marcaine Spinal 2449
Orthoclone OKT3 Sterile Solution 1892
Paxil Tablets (Rare) 2681
Permax Tablets (Infrequent) 571
Proleukin for Injection (Less than 1%) 812
Redux Capsules 2911

Meningitis, aseptic
Anaprox/Naprosyn (Less than 1%) 2277
Atretol Tablets (One case) 569
Bactrim 2257
Cataflam Tablets (Rare) 833
EC-Naprosyn Delayed-Release Tablets (Less than 1%) 2277
IBU Tablets (Rare; less than 1%) 1389
Motrin Ibuprofen Suspension, Oral Drops, Chewable Tablets, Caplets (Rare; less than 1%) 1563
Anaprox/Naprosyn (Less than 1%) 2277
Orudis Capsules (Less than 1%) 2874
Oruvail Capsules (Less than 1%) 2874
Proloprim Tablets (Rare) 1141
Sandoglobulin I.V. (Infrequent) 2419
Septra 1146
Septra I.V. Infusion 1142
Septra I.V. Infusion ADD-Vantage Vials 1144
Septra 1146
Tegretol/Tegretol-XR (One case) 870
Toradol 2319
Cataflam/Voltaren/Voltaren-XR (Rare) 833

Meningitis, septic
Carbocaine Injection 2432
Marcaine 2446
Sensorcaine 554

Menometrorrhagia
Orudis Capsules (Less than 1%) 2874
Oruvail Capsules (Less than 1%) 2874

Menopause
Avonex 662
Effexor (Rare) 2825
LUVOX Tablets (Infrequent) 2723
Permax Tablets (Infrequent) 571
Prozac Pulvules & Liquid, Oral Solution (Infrequent) 935
Ultram Tablets (50 mg) (1% to less than 5%) 1594
Wellbutrin Tablets (Rare) 1177

Menorrhagia
Asacol Delayed-Release Tablets 2129
▲ Betaseron for SC Injection (6%) 653
Claritin Tablets (2% or fewer patients) 2485
Claritin-D Tablets 2487
Clomid (1.3%) 1262
Dipentum Capsules (Rare) 2084
Effexor (Infrequent) 2825
Floxin I.V. (Less than 1%) 1580
Floxin Tablets (200 mg, 300 mg, 400 mg) (Less than 1%) 1577
IBU Tablets (Less than 1%) 1389
Intron A for Injection (Less than 5%) 2506
Lamictal Tablets (Rare) 1105
LUVOX Tablets (Infrequent) 2723
Motrin Ibuprofen Suspension, Oral Drops, Chewable Tablets, Caplets (Less than 1%) 1563
Naprelan Tablets (Less than 1%) 2861
Neurontin Capsules (Infrequent) 1978
Paxil Tablets (Infrequent) 2681
Pentasa (Less than 1%) 1275
Permax Tablets (Infrequent) 571
Prozac Pulvules & Liquid, Oral Solution (Infrequent) 935
Remeron Tablets (Rare) 1878
Risperdal Tablets (Frequent) 1348
Serzone Tablets (Infrequent) 776
Zoloft Tablets (Rare) 2051
Zyrtec Tablets (Less than 2%) 2053

Menstrual disorders
AeroBid Inhaler System 1004
▲ Aerobid-M Inhaler System (3% to 9%) 1004
Ambien Tablets (Infrequent) 2559
Anafranil Capsules (Up to 4%) 819
Anaprox/Naprosyn (Less than 1%) 2277
▲ Betaseron for SC Injection (17%) 653
Ceredase 1055
Cortifoam 2540
Cytotec (0.3%) 2576
Danocrine Capsules 2437
EC-Naprosyn Delayed-Release Tablets (Less than 1%) 2277
Effexor (1%) 2825
Etrafon 2495
Felbatol 2774
Halcion Tablets 2093
Halotestin Tablets 2095
Kerlone Tablets (Less than 2%) 2588
Lamictal Tablets (More than 1%) 1105
Lupron Depot 3.75 mg (Less than 5%) 2739
Mustargen 1752
▲ Naprelan Tablets (3% to 9%) 2861
Anaprox/Naprosyn (Less than 1%) 2277
▲ Nicotrol NS Nicotine Nasal Spray (4%) 1565
▲ Nolvadex Tablets (5.7%) 2957
ParaGard T 380A Intrauterine Copper Contraceptive 1936
Redux Capsules (Frequent) 2911
Rifadin 1276
Rifater 1280
Rimactane Capsules 865
Seldane-D Extended-Release Tablets 1286
Sporanox Capsules (Infrequent) 1352
Tegison Capsules (Less than 1%) 2314
Trilafon 2532
Ultram Tablets (50 mg) (Less than 1%) 1594
Vaqta (1.1%) 1805
▲ Wellbutrin Tablets (4.7%) 1177
▲ Xanax Tablets (10.4%) 2115
Zoladex 2976
Zoloft Tablets (1.0%) 2051

Menstrual dysfunction
LUVOX Tablets (Infrequent) 2723
Methotrexate Sodium Tablets, Injection, for Injection and LPF Injection 1322

Menstrual flow, changes
Amen Tablets 785
Aygestin Tablets 990
Coumadin 941
Cycrin Tablets 991
Danocrine Capsules 2437
Daypro Caplets (Less than 1%) 2578
Demulen 2580
Depo-Provera Sterile Aqueous Suspension 2083
Desogen Tablets 1867
Estraderm Transdermal System 842
ESTRATAB Tablets (0.3, 0.625, 1.25, 2.5 mg) 2715
Estratest 2718
Levlen/Tri-Levlen 646
Lo/Ovral Tablets 2852
Lo/Ovral-28 Tablets 2857
Menest Tablets 2671
Micronor Tablets (Common) 1903
Moban Tablets and Concentrate 1036
Modicon 1928
Nordette-21 Tablets 2863
Nordette-28 Tablets 2866
Ortho-Cept 1907
Ortho-Cyclen/Ortho-Tri-Cyclen 1914
Ortho Dienestrol Cream 1922
Ortho-Est 1925
Ortho-Novum 1928
Ortho-Cyclen/Ortho Tri-Cyclen 1914
Ovcon 765
Ovral Tablets 2877
Ovral-28 Tablets 2878
Ovrette Tablets 2878
ParaGard T 380A Intrauterine Copper Contraceptive 1936
PMB 200 and PMB 400 2890
Premarin Intravenous 2893
Premarin Vaginal Cream 2898
Provera Tablets 2110
Levlen/Tri-Levlen 646
Triphasil-21 Tablets 2919
Triphasil-28 Tablets 2924
Vivelle Transdermal System 880

Menstrual irregularities
Accutane Capsules (Less than 1%) 2252
Aldactazide Tablets 2556
Aldactone Tablets 2558
▲ Android Capsules, 10 mg (Among most common) 1297
Asendin Tablets (Less than 1%) 1419
Brevicon 2563
BuSpar Tablets (Infrequent) 738
Calan SR Caplets (1% or less) 2571
Calan Tablets (1% or less) 2568
Celestone Soluspan Suspension 2484
Claritin-D Tablets (Less frequent) 2487
Compazine 2644
CORTENEMA 2713
Cortone Acetate Sterile Suspension 1663
Cortone Acetate Tablets 1664
Covera-HS Tablets (Less than 2%) 2573
Dalalone D.P. Injectable 1009
Decadron Elixir 1676
Decadron Phosphate Injection 1680
Decadron Phosphate with Xylocaine Injection, Sterile 1683
Decadron Tablets 1678
Decadron-LA Sterile Suspension 1687
Demulen 2580
Depakene 416
Depakote Tablets 418
▲ Depo-Provera Contraceptive Injection (More than 5%) 2079
Desyrel and Desyrel Dividose 504
Dexacort Phosphate in Respihaler 1606
Dexacort Phosphate in Turbinaire 1607
Doral Tablets 2773
▲ Estratest (Among most common) 2718
Florinef Acetate Tablets 506
Fulvicin P/G Tablets (Rare) 2499
Fulvicin P/G 165 & 330 Tablets (Rare) 2500
Haldol Decanoate 1587
Haldol Injection, Tablets and Concentrate 1585
Hydeltrasol Injection, Sterile 1708
Hydeltra-T.B.A. Sterile Suspension 1710
Hydrocortone Acetate Sterile Suspension 1712
Hydrocortone Phosphate Injection, Sterile 1713
Hydrocortone Tablets 1715
Intron A for Injection (Less than 5%) 2506
Isoptin Oral Tablets (Less than 1%) 1393
Isoptin SR Tablets (1% or less) 1395
Levoprome 1321
Librax Capsules (Rare) 2330
Librium Capsules (Isolated cases) 2331
Librium Injectable (Isolated cases) 2332
Limbitrol (Rare) 2333
Loxitane (Rare) 1426
Mellaril 2398
▲ Micronor Tablets (Most frequent) 1903
▲ Nolvadex Tablets (12.5% to 24.6%) 2957
Norinyl 2563
Nor-Q D Tablets 2598
Oxandrin 783
ParaGard T 380A Intrauterine Copper Contraceptive 1936
Pediapred Oral Solution 1618
Prelone Syrup 1834
Prevacid Delayed-Release Capsules (Less than 1%) 2746
Prolixin 510
Rifamate Capsules 1278
Rimactane Capsules 865
Seldane Tablets 1284
Serax Capsules 2916
Serax Tablets 2916
Serentil 689
Stelazine 2692
Testred Capsules, 10 mg 1308
Torecan 2367
Triavil Tablets 1800
Tri-Norinyl 2607
Vantin for Oral Suspension and Vantin Tablets (Less than 1%) 2112
Winstrol Tablets 2468
Xanax Tablets 2115

Menstruation, early
Benadryl Injection 1955
Desyrel and Desyrel Dividose 504
Ornade Spansule Capsules 2678
Periactin 1767
Tavist Syrup 2426
Tavist Tablets 2427
Trinalin Repetabs Tablets 1373
Tussend 1830

Menstruation, painful
ProSom Tablets (Infrequent) 457
Prozac Pulvules & Liquid, Oral Solution (2.6%) 935

Mental acuity, loss of
Crixivan Capsules (Less than 2%) 1670
Retrovir Capsules 1216
Retrovir I.V. Infusion 1221
Retrovir Syrup 1216
Sinemet CR Tablets 961

Mental clouding
Compazine 2644
Halcion Tablets 2093
Hycodan Tablets and Syrup 946
Hycomine Compound Tablets 948
Hycomine 947
Hycotuss Expectorant Syrup 950
Hydrocet Capsules 787
Lorcet 10/650 Tablets 1016
Lortab 2751
Tussend 1830
Tussionex Pennkinetic Extended-Release Suspension 1624
Vicodin Tablets 1404
Vicodin ES Tablets 1405
Vicodin HP Tablets 1403
Vicodin Tuss Expectorant 1406
Zydone Capsules 967

(Described in PDR For Nonprescription Drugs) Incidence data in parenthesis; ▲ 3% or more (◉ Described in PDR For Ophthalmology)

Side Effects Index

Mental confusion
(see under Confusion)

Mental depression
(see under Depression, mental)

Mental perception, altered
Mykrox Tablets ... 1617

Mental performance, impairment
Aldoclor Tablets ... 1638
Aldomet Ester HCl Injection ... 1642
Aldomet Oral ... 1640
Aldoril Tablets ... 1644
Alferon N Injection (1%) ... 2142
Ambien Tablets (Infrequent) ... 2559
Anafranil Capsules (Up to 5%) ... 819
Anaprox/Naprosyn (Less than 1%) ... 2277
Asendin Tablets (Less than 1%) ... 1419
Atamet Tablets ... 567
Ativan Injection ... 2805
Beclovent Inhalation Aerosol and Refill ... 1063
Bentyl ... 1246
Bromfed-DM Cough Syrup ... 1832
Brontex ... 2130
BuSpar Tablets (2%) ... 738
Butisol Sodium Elixir & Tablets ... 2768
Cardura Tablets (Less than 0.5% of 3960 patients) ... 1993
Claritin Tablets (2% or fewer patients) ... 2485
Claritin-D Tablets (Less frequent) ... 2487
Clozaril Tablets ... 2377
Compazine ... 2644
DHCplus Capsules ... 2148
Demerol ... 2438
Desyrel and Desyrel Dividose ... 504
Dilaudid Ampules ... 1382
Dilaudid Cough Syrup ... 1383
Dilaudid ... 1382
EC-Naprosyn Delayed-Release Tablets (Less than 1%) ... 2277
Elavil ... 2945
Ergamisol Tablets (Less frequent) ... 1340
Esgic-plus Capsules ... 1012
Esgic-plus Tablets ... 1012
Eskalith ... 2658
Etrafon ... 2495
Felbatol ... 2774
Fioricet Tablets ... 2386
Fioricet with Codeine Capsules ... 2387
Fiorinal with Codeine Capsules ... 2390
Fludara for Injection (Up to 1%) ... 658
Flumadine Tablets & Syrup (0.3% to 2.1%) ... 1013
Foscavir Injection (Less than 1%) ... 541
Grifulvin V (griseofulvin tablets) Microsize (griseofulvin oral suspension) Microsize ... 1944
Hivid Tablets (Less than 1%) ... 2287
Hycodan Tablets and Syrup ... 946
Hycomine Compound Tablets ... 948
Hycomine ... 947
Hycotuss Expectorant Syrup ... 950
Hydrocet Capsules ... 787
Imdur (Less than or equal to 5%) ... 1362
Imitrex Injection (Rare) ... 1095
Imitrex Tablets (Infrequent) ... 1099
▲ Intron A for Injection (Up to 14%) ... 2506
Inversine Tablets ... 1729
Invirase Capsules (Less than 2%) ... 2291
Kadian Capsules (Less than 3%) ... 2948
Lamictal Tablets (1.7%) ... 1105
Levsin/Levsinex/Levbid ... 2549
Limbitrol ... 2333
Lioresal Intrathecal ... 1634
Lithonate/Lithotabs/Lithobid ... 2721
Lorcet 10/650 Tablets ... 1016
Lortab ... 2751
Loxitane ... 1426
MS Contin Tablets ... 2149
Mebaral Tablets ... 2452
Methadone Hydrochloride Oral Concentrate ... 2356
Miltown Tablets ... 2780
Monoket Tablets (Fewer than 1%) ... 2550
▲ Naprelan Tablets (3% to 9%) ... 2861
Anaprox/Naprosyn (Less than 1%) ... 2277
▲ Nicotrol NS Nicotine Nasal Spray (Over 5%) ... 1565
Norpramin Tablets ... 1273
Orap Tablets ... 1037
PBZ-SR Tablets ... 862
Paxil Tablets (Frequent) ... 2681
Percocet Tablets ... 955
Percodan Tablets ... 955
Phenergan with Codeine ... 2883
Phenergan with Dextromethorphan ... 2885
Phenergan Injection ... 2880
Phenergan Suppositories ... 2882
Phenergan Syrup ... 2881
Phenergan Tablets ... 2882
Phenergan VC ... 2886
Phenergan VC with Codeine ... 2888
PMB 200 and PMB 400 ... 2890
ProSom Tablets ... 457
Prozac Pulvules & Liquid, Oral Solution (1.6%) ... 935
RMS Suppositories CII ... 2766
Remeron Tablets ... 1878
Restoril Capsules (Less than 1%) ... 2413
Rifadin ... 1276
Rifamate Capsules ... 1278
Rifater ... 1280
Rimactane Capsules ... 865
Risperdal Tablets (Infrequent) ... 1348
Ryna ... 804
▲ Serzone Tablets (3%) ... 776
Sinemet Tablets ... 959
Surmontil Capsules ... 2917
Timolide Tablets ... 1791
Timoptic in Ocudose ... 1796
Timoptic Sterile Ophthalmic Solution ... 1794
Timoptic-XE ... 1798
Tofranil Tablets ... 875
Tofranil-PM Capsules ... 876
Toradol (1% or less) ... 2319
Tussend ... 1830
Tussionex Pennkinetic Extended-Release Suspension ... 1624
Tylenol with Codeine ... 1592
Tylox Capsules ... 1593
Ultram Tablets (50 mg) (Less than 1%) ... 1594
Vicodin Tablets ... 1404
Vicodin ES Tablets ... 1405
Vicodin HP Tablets ... 1403
Vicodin Tuss Expectorant ... 1406
Vistaril Intramuscular Solution (Seldom) ... 2042
Vivactil Tablets ... 1820
Wygesic Tablets ... 2930
Xanax Tablets ... 2115
Zarontin Capsules ... 1986
Zarontin Syrup ... 1986
Zebeta Tablets ... 1457
Zestril Tablets (0.3% to 1.0%) ... 2972
Ziac ... 1459
Zoloft Tablets (1.3%) ... 2051
Zydone Capsules ... 967
Zyrtec Tablets (Less than 2%) ... 2053

Mental slowness
BuSpar Tablets (Infrequent) ... 738
Celontin Kapseals ... 1955
Tonocard Tablets (Less than 1%) ... 519

Mental status, altered
Clozaril Tablets ... 2377
Eldepryl Capsules ... 2729
Etrafon ... 2495
Florinef Acetate Tablets ... 506
Haldol Decanoate ... 1587
▲ Idamycin Injection (41%) ... 2096
Ludiomil Tablets ... 861
Mellaril ... 2398
Moban Tablets and Concentrate ... 1036
Navane Capsules and Concentrate ... 2018
Navane Intramuscular ... 2019
Oncaspar ... 2194
Orap Tablets ... 1037
Orthoclone OKT3 Sterile Solution ... 1892
▲ Prograf (Approximately 55%) ... 1028
▲ Proleukin for Injection (73%) ... 812
Risperdal Tablets ... 1348
▲ Roferon-A Injection (10% to 17%) ... 2308
Serentil ... 689
Sinemet CR Tablets ... 961
Stelazine ... 2692
Torecan ... 2367
Triavil Tablets ... 1800

Mesenteric arterial thrombosis
Blocadren Tablets ... 1654
Inderal ... 2834
Inderal LA Long Acting Capsules ... 2836
Inderide Tablets ... 2838
Inderide LA Long Acting Capsules ... 2840
Kerlone Tablets ... 2588
Levatol Tablets ... 2547
Lo/Ovral Tablets ... 2852
Lo/Ovral-28 Tablets ... 2857
Nordette-21 Tablets ... 2863
Nordette-28 Tablets ... 2866
Normodyne Tablets ... 2522
Ovral Tablets ... 2877
Ovral-28 Tablets ... 2878
Ovrette Tablets ... 2878
Rilutek Tablets (Rare) ... 2198
Sectral Capsules ... 2914
Tenoretic Tablets ... 2963
Tenormin Tablets and I.V. Injection ... 2965
Timolide Tablets ... 1791
Timoptic in Ocudose ... 1796
Timoptic Sterile Ophthalmic Solution ... 1794
Triphasil-21 Tablets ... 2919
Triphasil-28 Tablets ... 2924
Ziac ... 1459

Metabolic acidosis
(see under Acidosis, metabolic)

Metabolic changes
Clinoril Tablets (Rare) ... 1658
▲ Leukine (58%) ... 1317
Pravachol Tablets ... 770
Vumon for Injection (Less than 1%) ... 729

Metaplasia, bronchiolar squamous
Blenoxane ... 697

Methemoglobinemia
Americaine Anesthetic Lubricant (Rare) ... 1603
Americaine Otic Topical Anesthetic Ear Drops (Rare) ... 1603
Azulfidine (Rare) ... 2059
Bactrim DS Tablets ... 2257
Bactrim I.V. Infusion ... 2255
Bactrim ... 2257
Cipro Tablets ... 584
Deponit NTG Transdermal Delivery System (Extremely rare) ... 2541
Desyrel and Desyrel Dividose ... 504
Dilatrate-SR Capsules (Infrequent) ... 2542
Eulexin Capsules ... 2498
Fansidar Tablets ... 2281
Gantanol Tablets ... 2285
Gantrisin ... 2286
Ismo Tablets (Extremely rare) ... 2844
Isordil Sublingual Tablets (Extremely rare) ... 2845
Isordil Tembids (Extremely rare) ... 2847
Isordil Titradose Tablets (Extremely rare) ... 2848
Macrobid Capsules ... 2138
Macrodantin Capsules (Rare) ... 2140
Monoket Tablets (Extremely rare) ... 2550
Nitro-Bid IV (Extremely rare) ... 1270
Nitro-Bid Ointment (Extremely rare) ... 1272
Nitro-Dur (nitroglycerin) Transdermal Infusion System (Very rare) ... 1365
Pediazole Suspension ... 2340
Proloprim Tablets ... 1141
Pyridium ... 1985
Reglan ... 2243
Septra ... 1146
Septra I.V. Infusion ... 1142
Septra I.V. Infusion ADD-Vantage Vials ... 1144
Septra ... 1146
Sorbitrate (Extremely rare) ... 2959
Transderm-Nitro Transdermal Therapeutic System (Extremely rare) ... 878
Trimpex Tablets ... 2323

Metrorrhagia
▲ Betaseron for SC Injection (15%) ... 653
Depakote Tablets (1% to 5%) ... 418
Floxin I.V. (Less than 1%) ... 1580
Floxin Tablets (200 mg, 300 mg, 400 mg) (Less than 1%) ... 1577
LUVOX Tablets (Infrequent) ... 2723
Naprelan Tablets (Less than 1%) ... 2861
Paxil Tablets (Rare) ... 2681
Pentasa (Less than 1%) ... 1275
Permax Tablets (Infrequent) ... 571
Prozac Pulvules & Liquid, Oral Solution (Rare) ... 935
Remeron Tablets (Rare) ... 1878
Rilutek Tablets (Infrequent) ... 2198
Salagen Tablets (Less than 1%) ... 1546
Serzone Tablets (Infrequent) ... 776

Metyrapone test, altered results
Amen Tablets ... 785
Aygestin Tablets ... 990
Cycrin Tablets ... 991
Depo-Provera Sterile Aqueous Suspension ... 2083
Estrace Cream and Tablets ... 751
Estratest ... 2718
Provera Tablets ... 2110

Microcephaly
Felbatol ... 2774

Microcephaly, fetal
Accutane Capsules ... 2252
Dilantin Infatabs ... 1967
Dilantin Kapseals ... 1965
Dilantin-125 Suspension ... 1969

Microphthalmia, fetal
Accutane Capsules ... 2252

Micropinna, fetal
Accutane Capsules ... 2252

Micturition, difficulty
Apresazide Capsules (Less frequent) ... 824
Apresoline Hydrochloride Tablets (Less frequent) ... 826
Atrovent Inhalation Aerosol (Less than 1%) ... 674
Benadryl Injection ... 1955
Blocadren Tablets ... 1654
▲ Bromfed-DM Cough Syrup (Among most frequent) ... 1832
Casodex Tablets (2% to 5%) ... 2934
Catapres Tablets (About 2 in 1,000 patients) ... 679
Catapres-TTS ... 680
Chemet Capsules (Up to 3.7%) ... 666
Combipres Tablets (About 2 in 1,000) ... 682
Dantrium Capsules (Less frequent) ... 2131
Dimetane-DC Cough Syrup ... 2232
Dimetane-DX Cough Syrup ... 2233
Donnagel Liquid and Donnagel Chewable Tablets (Rare) ... 854
Effexor (2%) ... 2825
Fioricet with Codeine Capsules ... 2387
Fiorinal with Codeine Capsules ... 2390
Flexeril Tablets (Rare) ... 1701
Hydralazine Hydrochloride Injection USP (Less frequent) ... 2712
▲ Hylorel Tablets (33.6%) ... 1613
Kutrase Capsules ... 2546
Levo-Dromoran ... 2297
Levoprome (Sometimes) ... 1321
Lioresal Intrathecal (Up to 2.0%) ... 1634
Maxaquin Tablets (Less than 1%) ... 2593
Normodyne Tablets (Less common) ... 2522
Norpramin Tablets ... 1273
Nucofed ... 2225
OxyContin Tablets (Less than 1%) ... 2163
PBZ Tablets ... 863
PBZ-SR Tablets ... 862
▲ Paxil Tablets (3%) ... 2681
Periactin ... 1767
Proventil (Less than 1%) ... 2529
Quadrinal Tablets ... 1398
Ser-Ap-Es Tablets ... 867
Stadol (Less than 1%) ... 779
Tavist Syrup ... 2426
Tavist Tablets ... 2427
Timolide Tablets ... 1791
Timoptic in Ocudose ... 1796
Timoptic Sterile Ophthalmic Solution ... 1794
Timoptic-XE ... 1798
Tofranil Ampuls ... 873
Tofranil Tablets (Rare) ... 875
Tofranil-PM Capsules ... 876
Trancopal Caplets ... 2468
Trandate Tablets (Less common) ... 1158
Transderm Scōp Transdermal Therapeutic System (Infrequent) ... 890
Tussend ... 1830
Urised Tablets ... 2123
Uroqid-Acid No. 2 Tablets (Occasional) ... 633
Ventolin Tablets (Fewer than 1 of 100 patients) ... 1176
Vivactil Tablets ... 1820
Volmax Extended-Release Tablets (Less frequent) ... 1835
▲ Xanax Tablets (12.2%) ... 2115
Zovirax Sterile Powder (Less than 1%) ... 1191

Micturition, painful
Nucofed ... 2225
Ortho Diaphragm Kit ... 1921
▲ TheraCys BCG Live (Intravesical) (More common) ... 911
Uroqid-Acid No. 2 Tablets (Occasional) ... 633
Zovirax Sterile Powder (Less than 1%) ... 1191

(▣ Described in PDR For Nonprescription Drugs)   Incidence data in parenthesis; ▲ 3% or more   (◉ Described in PDR For Ophthalmology)

Micturition disturbances

- Adalat CC (3% or less) 582
- Ambien Tablets (Rare) 2559
- ▲ Anafranil Capsules (4% to 14%) 819
- Asendin Tablets (Very rare) 1419
- Atretol Tablets 569
- Atrohist Plus Tablets 1605
- Benadryl Injection 1955
- Benemid Tablets 1651
- Bontril Slow-Release Capsules 786
- ▲ Bromfed-DM Cough Syrup (Among most frequent) 1832
- BuSpar Tablets (Infrequent) 738
- Calan SR Caplets (1% or less) 2571
- Calan Tablets (1% or less) 2568
- Capoten Tablets (Approximately 1 to 2 of 1000 patients) 740
- Capozide Tablets (Approximately 1 to 2 of 1000 patients) 744
- Cardene Capsules (Rare) 2261
- Cardene I.V. (Rare) 2815
- Cardene SR Capsules (0.6%) 2264
- Cardura Tablets 1993
- Cartrol Tablets (Less common) 413
- Casodex Tablets (2% to 5%) 2934
- Cataflam Tablets (Less than 1%) 833
- Caverject Injection (Less than 1%) 2064
- ▲ CellCept Capsules (More than or equal to 3%) 2265
- Cerezyme (One patient) 1056
- Cipro I.V. (1% or less) 587
- Cipro I.V. Pharmacy Bulk Package (Less than 1%) 590
- Claritin Tablets (2% or fewer patients) 2485
- Claritin-D Tablets (Less frequent) 2487
- Clomid (Fewer than 1%) 1262
- Clozaril Tablets (1%) 2377
- ▲ Cognex Capsules (3%) 1961
- ColBENEMID Tablets 1662
- Covera-HS Tablets (Less than 2%) 2573
- Cozaar Tablets (Less than 1%) 1668
- Crixivan Capsules (Less than 2%) 1670
- Cytovene (1% or less) 2270
- Dalgan Injection (Less than 1%) 529
- Dantrium Capsules (Less frequent) 2131
- Daranide Tablets 1676
- Daypro Caplets (1% to 3%) 2578
- ▲ Demadex Tablets and Injection (6.7%) 691
- Desyrel and Desyrel Dividose 504
- Dimetane-DC Cough Syrup 2232
- Dimetane-DX Cough Syrup 2233
- Dipentum Capsules (Rare) 2084
- Dopram Injectable 2235
- Duragesic Transdermal System (Less than 1%) 1336
- Duramorph Injection 983
- Dynabac (0.1% to 1%) 668
- ▲ Effexor (3%) 2825
- Elavil 2945
- Eldepryl Capsules 2729
- Eskalith 2658
- Estring Vaginal Ring (At least 1 report) 2086
- Ethmozine Tablets (Less than 2%) 2217
- Etrafon 2495
- Flexeril Tablets (Less than 1%) 1701
- Floxin I.V. (Less than 1%) 1580
- Floxin Tablets (200 mg, 300 mg, 400 mg) (Less than 1%) 1577
- Flumadine Tablets & Syrup 1013
- Foscavir Injection (Less than 1%) 541
- Gastrocrom Oral Concentrate (Less common) 1611
- Hivid Tablets (Less than 1%) 2287
- Hydrocet Capsules 787
- Hytrin Capsules (At least 1%) 434
- Hyzaar Tablets 1720
- IFEX 706
- Imitrex Injection (Rare) 1095
- Imitrex Tablets (Infrequent) 1099
- Indocin (Rare) 1723
- Intal Inhaler (Infrequent) 2185
- Intal Nebulizer Solution 2186
- Intron A for Injection (Less than 5%) 2506
- Invirase Capsules (Less than 2%) 2291
- Ismo Tablets (Fewer than 1%) 2844
- Isoptin Oral Tablets (Less than 1%) 1393
- Isoptin SR Tablets (1% or less) 1395
- Kerlone Tablets (Less than 2%) 2588
- Lamictal Tablets (Infrequent) 1105
- Limbitrol 2333
- Lioresal Intrathecal (Up to 0.9%) 1634
- ▲ Lioresal Tablets (2% to 6%) 847
- Lodine Capsules and Tablets (1% to 3%) 2849
- Lotensin HCT Tablets (0.3% to more than 1%) 855
- Ludiomil Tablets (Rare) 861
- Lupron Depot 7.5 mg (Less than 5%) 2741
- ▲ Lupron Injection (5% or more) 2736
- ▲ LUVOX Tablets (3%) 2723
- Matulane Capsules 2300
- Maxaquin Tablets (Less than 1%) 2593
- Megace Oral Suspension (Up to 2%) 708
- Midamor Tablets (Less than or equal to 1%) 1746
- Minipress Capsules (1-4%) 2015
- Minizide Capsules (Rare) 2016
- Moduretic Tablets 1748
- Monopril Tablets (0.2% to 1.0%) 762
- Mycelex-G 500 mg Vaginal Tablets (Rare) 602
- Naprelan Tablets (Less than 1%) 2861
- Neurontin Capsules (Infrequent) 1978
- ▲ Norpace (3 to 9%) 2596
- Norpramin Tablets 1273
- Norvasc Tablets (More than 0.1% to 1%) 2020
- Norvir (Less than 2%) 447
- Oncaspar (Less than 1%) 2194
- Orap Tablets 1037
- Ornade Spansule Capsules 2678
- Ortho Diaphragm Kit 1921
- PBZ Tablets 863
- PBZ-SR Tablets 862
- Pamelor 2409
- Parlodel 2411
- Parnate Tablets 2679
- ▲ Paxil Tablets (3%) 2681
- Pentasa (Less than 1%) 1275
- Permax Tablets (2.7%) 571
- Plendil Extended-Release Tablets (0.5% to 1.5%) 514
- Pondimin Tablets 2239
- Prilosec Delayed-Release Capsules (Less than 1%) 516
- Proleukin for Injection (1%) 812
- Propulsid (1.2%) 1346
- ProSom Tablets (Infrequent) 457
- Prostigmin Injectable 1305
- Prostigmin Tablets 1306
- Prozac Pulvules & Liquid, Oral Solution (1.6% to 4%) 935
- Redux Capsules (2.8%) 2911
- Reglan 2243
- Remeron Tablets (2%) 1878
- Retrovir Capsules 1216
- Retrovir I.V. Infusion 1221
- Retrovir Syrup 1216
- ReVia Tablets (Less than 1%) 957
- Risperdal Tablets 1348
- ▲ Salagen Tablets (9% to 12%) 1546
- ▲ Sectral Capsules (3%) 2914
- Seldane Tablets 1284
- Seldane-D Extended-Release Tablets 1286
- Serophene (clomiphene citrate tablets, USP) (Less than 1 in 100 patients) 2621
- Serzone Tablets (2%) 776
- Sinemet CR Tablets (0.8%) 961
- Supprelin Injection (1% to 3%) 2230
- Surmontil Capsules 2917
- Tavist Syrup 2426
- Tavist Tablets 2427
- Tegretol/Tegretol-XR 870
- Tenex Tablets (Less frequent) 2249
- Tensilon Injectable 1307
- ▲ TheraCys BCG Live (Intravesical) (1.8% to 40.2%) 911
- ▲ TICE BCG, USP (40.4%) 1881
- Tofranil Ampuls 873
- Tofranil Tablets 875
- Tofranil-PM Capsules 876
- Toradol (1% or less) 2319
- Triavil Tablets 1800
- Trinalin Repetabs Tablets 1373
- Tussend 1830
- Ultram Tablets (50 mg) (1% to less than 5%) 1594
- Univasc Tablets (More than 1%) 2553
- Urecholine 1804
- Verelan Capsules (1% or less) 1455
- ▲ Vesanoid Capsules (3%) 2327
- Videx Tablets, Powder for Oral Solution, & Pediatric Powder for Oral Solution (Less than 1% to 4%) 2980
- Vivactil Tablets 1820
- Cataflam/Voltaren/Voltaren-XR (Less than 1%) 833
- Wellbutrin Tablets (2.5%) 1177
- Zerit Capsules (Fewer than 1% to 1%) 731
- Zoladex (1% or greater) 2976
- Zoladex 3-month (1% to 5%) 2978
- Zoloft Tablets (1.4%; 2.0%) 2051

Migraine

- Ambien Tablets (Infrequent) 2559
- Amen Tablets 785
- ▲ Anafranil Capsules (Up to 3%) 819
- Asacol Delayed-Release Tablets 2129
- ▲ Betaseron for SC Injection (12%) 653
- Brevicon 2563
- Cardura Tablets (Less than 0.5% of 3960 patients) 1993
- Cerebyx Injection (Infrequent) 1956
- Claritin Tablets (2% or fewer patients) 2485
- Claritin-D Tablets (Less frequent) 2487
- Climara Transdermal System 640
- Clomid 1262
- Cognex Capsules (Infrequent) 1961
- Colestid 2073
- Cozaar Tablets (Less than 1%) 1668
- Cycrin Tablets 991
- Cytovene (1% or less) 2270
- Demulen 2580
- Depo-Provera Contraceptive Injection 2079
- Depo-Provera Sterile Aqueous Suspension 2083
- Desogen Tablets 1867
- Diethylstilbestrol Tablets 1477
- Doxil (Less than 1%) 2613
- Effexor (Frequent) 2825
- Eldepryl Capsules 2729
- Engerix-B Unit-Dose Vials 2656
- Estrace Cream and Tablets 751
- Estraderm Transdermal System 842
- ESTRATAB Tablets (0.3, 0.625, 1.25, 2.5 mg) 2715
- Estratest 2718
- Estring Vaginal Ring (1% to 3%) 2086
- Felbatol (Infrequent) 2774
- Gastrocrom Capsules (Infrequent) 1611
- Gastrocrom Oral Concentrate (Less common) 1611
- Glucotrol XL Extended Release Tablets (Less than 1%) 2012
- Hivid Tablets (Less than 1%) 2287
- Hyzaar Tablets 1720
- Imdur (Less than or equal to 5%) 1362
- Imitrex Tablets 1099
- Intron A for Injection (Less than 5%) 2506
- Lamictal Tablets (Infrequent) 1105
- Levlen/Tri-Levlen 646
- Lo/Ovral Tablets 2852
- Lo/Ovral-28 Tablets 2857
- LUVOX Tablets 2723
- Maxair Autohaler 1550
- Maxair Inhaler (Less than 1%) 1552
- Menest Tablets 2671
- Miacalcin Nasal Spray (Less than 1%) 2403
- Micronor Tablets 1903
- Modicon 1928
- Naprelan Tablets (Less than 1%) 2861
- Neurontin Capsules (Infrequent) 1978
- Nicotrol NS Nicotine Nasal Spray (Less than 1%) 1565
- Nordette-21 Tablets 2863
- Nordette-28 Tablets 2866
- Norinyl 2563
- Norplant System 2868
- Nor-Q D Tablets 2598
- Norvir (Less than 2%) 447
- Ogen Tablets 2103
- Ogen Vaginal Cream 2106
- Ortho-Cept 1907
- Ortho-Cyclen/Ortho-Tri-Cyclen 1914
- Ortho Dienestrol Cream 1922
- Ortho-Est 1925
- Ortho-Novum 1928
- Ortho-Cyclen/Ortho Tri-Cyclen 1914
- Orudis Capsules (Less than 1%) 2874
- Oruvail Capsules (Less than 1%) 2874
- Ovcon 765
- Ovral Tablets 2877
- Ovral-28 Tablets 2878
- Ovrette Tablets 2878
- OxyContin Tablets (Less than 1%) 2163
- Paxil Tablets (Infrequent) 2681
- Permax Tablets (Rare) 571
- PMB 200 and PMB 400 2890
- Premarin Intravenous 2893
- Premarin Tablets 2896
- Premarin Vaginal Cream 2898
- Premphase 2900
- Prempro 2905
- Procardia XL Extended Release Tablets (1% or less) 2026
- Propulsid (1% or less) 1346
- Provera Tablets 2110
- Prozac Pulvules & Liquid, Oral Solution (Infrequent) 935
- Recombivax HB 1787
- Redux Capsules (Frequent) 2911
- Remeron Tablets (Infrequent) 1878
- Rilutek Tablets (Infrequent) 2198
- Risperdal Tablets (Rare) 1348
- Serzone Tablets 776
- Sular Tablets (Less than or equal to 1%) 2961
- Supprelin Injection (1% to 3%) 2230
- Levlen/Tri-Levlen 646
- Tri-Norinyl 2607
- Triphasil-21 Tablets 2919
- Triphasil-28 Tablets 2924
- Ultram Tablets (50 mg) (Infrequent) 1594
- Videx Tablets, Powder for Oral Solution, & Pediatric Powder for Oral Solution (Less than 1%) 2980
- Vivelle Transdermal System 880
- Zerit Capsules (Fewer than 1% to 3%) 731
- Zoladex (1% or greater) 2976
- Zoladex 3-month 2978
- Zoloft Tablets (Infrequent) 2051
- Zyrtec Tablets (Less than 2%) 2053

Miliaria

- Aclovate (Infrequent) 1061
- Analpram-HC Rectal Cream 1% and 2.5% 993
- Anusol-HC Cream 2.5% (Infrequent to frequent) 1953
- ▲ Cordran Lotion (More frequent) 1854
- ▲ Cordran Tape (More frequent) 1855
- Cormax Ointment (Infrequent) 1856
- Cormax Scalp Application (Infrequent) 1857
- Cortisporin Cream 1073
- Cortisporin Ointment 1074
- Cortisporin Otic Solution Sterile 1076
- Cortisporin Otic Suspension Sterile 1077
- Cutivate Cream 1078
- Cutivate Ointment (Infrequent to more frequent) 1078
- Decadron Phosphate Topical Cream 1686
- Decaspray Topical Aerosol 1689
- Dermatop Emollient Cream 0.1% (Infrequent to frequent) 1264
- DesOwen Cream, Ointment and Lotion (Infrequent) 1032
- Diprolene AF Cream 0.05% (Infrequent) 2489
- Diprolene Gel 0.05% (Infrequent) 2490
- Diprolene Lotion 0.05% (Infrequent) 2491
- Diprolene Ointment 0.05% (Infrequent) 2491
- Elocon Cream 0.1% (Infrequent) 2492
- Elocon Lotion 0.1% (Infrequent) 2493
- Elocon Ointment 0.1% (Infrequent) 2494
- Epifoam (Infrequent) 2543
- Florone/Florone E 921
- Halog (Infrequent) 2795
- Hytone 922
- Hytone Ointment 2 ½% 923
- Lidex (Infrequent) 2299
- Locoid Cream, Ointment and Topical Solution (Infrequent) 994
- Lotrisone Cream (Infrequent) 2515
- Mantadil Cream 1124
- 8-MOP Capsules 1294
- NeoDecadron Topical Cream 1757
- Oxsoralen-Ultra Capsules 1302
- Pandel Cream, 0.1% 2475
- Pediotic Suspension Sterile 1140
- Pramosone Cream, Lotion & Ointment 995
- ProctoCream-HC 2.5% (Infrequent to frequent) 2552
- ProctoFoam-HC 2552
- Psorcon Cream 0.05% (Infrequent) 924
- Psorcon Ointment 0.05% 923
- Synalar (Infrequent) 2299
- Temovate Cream 1152
- Temovate E Emollient (Infrequent) 1154
- Temovate Gel (Infrequent) 1153
- Temovate Ointment 1152
- Temovate Scalp Application (Infrequent) 1153
- Topicort Emollient Cream 0.25% (Infrequent) 1289
- Topicort Gel 0.05% (Infrequent) 1290
- Topicort LP Emollient Cream 0.05% (Infrequent) 1289
- Topicort Ointment 0.25% (Infrequent) 1291

(▣ Described in PDR For Nonprescription Drugs) Incidence data in parenthesis; ▲ 3% or more (◉ Described in PDR For Ophthalmology)

Miliaria

Side Effects Index

Tridesilon Cream 0.05% (Infrequent) ... 609
Tridesilon Ointment 0.05% (Infrequent) ... 610
Ultravate Cream 0.05% (Infrequent) ... 2797
Ultravate Ointment 0.05% (Less frequent) ... 2798
Westcort Cream 0.2% (Infrequent) ... 2799
Westcort Ointment 0.2% ... 2800

Miosis

▲ Buprenex Injectable (1-5%) ... 2170
Carbocaine Injection ... 2432
Compazine ... 2644
Dibenzyline Capsules ... 2650
Dilaudid-HP Injection (Less frequent) ... 1384
Dilaudid-HP Lyophilized Powder 250 mg (Less frequent) ... 1384
Dilaudid Tablets and Liquid (Less frequent) ... 1386
Duramorph Injection ... 983
Effexor (Rare) ... 2825
▲ Felbatol (6.5%) ... 2774
Fioricet with Codeine Capsules ... 2387
Fiorinal with Codeine Capsules ... 2390
Kadian Capsules (Less than 3%) ... 2948
Lioresal Tablets ... 847
MS Contin Tablets (Less frequent) ... 2149
MSIR (Infrequent) ... 2152
Marcaine ... 2446
Mellaril ... 2398
Mestinon Injectable ... 1300
Mestinon ... 1300
Navane Capsules and Concentrate ... 2018
Navane Intramuscular ... 2019
Neurontin Capsules (Rare) ... 1978
Numorphan Injection ... 953
Numorphan Suppositories ... 953
Ocufen ... ⊚ 242
Oramorph SR (Morphine Sulfate Sustained Release Tablets) (Less frequent) ... 2359
Pilagan ... ⊚ 245
Pontocaine Hydrochloride for Spinal Anesthesia ... 2460
Prostigmin Injectable ... 1305
Prostigmin Tablets ... 1306
Redux Capsules (Rare) ... 2911
Sensorcaine ... 554
Serentil ... 689
Soma Compound w/Codeine Tablets ... 2784
Stelazine ... 2692
Sublimaze Injection ... 463
Talwin Injection (Rare) ... 2465
Tensilon Injectable ... 1307
Thorazine ... 2701
Torecan ... 2367
Urecholine ... 1804
Versed Injection (Less than 1%) ... 2324

Miscarriage

Cytotec ... 2576
Vantin for Oral Suspension and Vantin Tablets ... 2112

Mitral valve prolapse

Effexor (Rare) ... 2825
Levlen/Tri-Levlen ... 646

Moaning

Diprivan Injectable Emulsion (Less than 1%) ... 2939

Molluscum contagiosum

Norvir (Less than 2%) ... 447

Moniliasis

▲ Aredia for Injection (Up to 6%) ... 827
Betaseron for SC Injection ... 653
Biaxin ... 406
Cedax (0.1% to 1%) ... 2480
▲ CellCept Capsules (10.1% to 12.1%) ... 2265
▲ Chemet Capsules (5.2% to 15.7%) ... 666
▲ Doxil (Less than 1% to 5.5%) ... 2613
Effexor (Infrequent) ... 2825
Foscavir Injection (Between 1% and 5%) ... 541
Hivid Tablets (Less than 1%) ... 2287
Imdur (Less than or equal to 5%) ... 1362
▲ Intron A for Injection (Up to 17%) ... 2506
Maxipime for Injection (0.1% to 1%) ... 758
▲ Megace Oral Suspension (1% to 3%) ... 708

▲ Mepron Suspension (5% to 10%) ... 1206
Merrem I.V. (0.1% to 2.0%) ... 2952
Monodox Capsules ... 1858
Nipent for Injection (2%) ... 2733
Norvir (Less than 2%) ... 447
Paxil Tablets (Infrequent) ... 2681
Pentasa (Less than 1%) ... 1275
Permax Tablets (Infrequent) ... 571
Prozac Pulvules & Liquid, Oral Solution (Rare) ... 935
Remeron Tablets (Rare) ... 1878
Rhinocort Nasal Inhaler (Less than 1%) ... 552
Rilutek Tablets (0.4% to 1.2%) ... 2198
Serzone Tablets (Rare) ... 776
Vibramycin ... 2038
Vistide Injection ... 1057
Zithromax (1% or less) ... 2043
Zithromax Tablets (1% or less) ... 2046
Zosyn (1.6%) ... 1463

Moniliasis, genital

Achromycin V Capsules ... 1417
Ancef Injection ... 2632
Cerebyx Injection (Infrequent) ... 1956
Claforan Sterile and Injection (Less than 1%) ... 1259
Dynabac (0.1% to 1%) ... 668
DYNACIN Capsules ... 1627
Effexor (Infrequent) ... 2825
▲ Estring Vaginal Ring (6%) ... 2086
Keflex Pulvules & Oral Suspension ... 930
Keftab Tablets ... 931
Kefzol Vials, Faspak & ADD-Vantage ... 1511
Lamictal Tablets (Infrequent) ... 1105
Lorabid Suspension and Pulvules (1.1%) ... 1513
Maxaquin Tablets (Less than 1%) ... 2593
Minocin Intravenous ... 1428
Minocin Oral Suspension ... 1431
Minocin Pellet-Filled Capsules ... 1429
Paxil Tablets (Rare) ... 2681
Penetrex Tablets (0.1% to 1%) ... 2196
Rilutek Tablets (Rare) ... 2198
Rocephin Injectable Vials, ADD-Vantage, Galaxy Container (Occasional) ... 2305

Monoclonal B-lymphoproliferative disorder

Orthoclone OKT3 Sterile Solution ... 1892

Monocytosis

Celontin Kapseals ... 1955
Cipro Tablets (Less than 0.1%) ... 584
Cuprimine Capsules ... 1673
Depen Titratable Tablets ... 2770
Dynabac (0.1% to 1%) ... 668
Maxaquin Tablets ... 2593
Mesantoin Tablets ... 2400
Paxil Tablets (Rare) ... 2681
Primaxin I.M. ... 1770
Primaxin I.V. ... 1772
Rocephin Injectable Vials, ADD-Vantage, Galaxy Container (Rare) ... 2305
Unasyn ... 2035
Vantin for Oral Suspension and Vantin Tablets ... 2112

Mononeuropathy

Acel-Imune Diphtheria and Tetanus Toxoids and Acellular Pertussis Vaccine Adsorbed ... 1415
Diphtheria and Tetanus Toxoids and Pertussis Vaccine Adsorbed ... 2650
Felbatol ... 2774
Tetramune ... 1449
Tri-Immunol Adsorbed ... 1452

Monoplegia

Imitrex Injection (Rare) ... 1095
Imitrex Tablets (Infrequent) ... 1099

Mood changes

▲ Adalat Capsules (10 mg and 20 mg) (7%) ... 580
Adalat CC (Rare) ... 582
AeroBid Inhaler System (1% to 3%) ... 1004
Aerobid-M Inhaler System (1% to 3%) ... 1004
Betapace Tablets (Less than 1% to 3%) ... 637
Celestone Soluspan Suspension ... 2484
Clomid ... 1262
CORTENEMA ... 2713
Cortone Acetate Sterile Suspension ... 1663

Cortone Acetate Tablets ... 1664
Decadron Elixir ... 1676
Decadron Phosphate Injection ... 1680
Decadron Phosphate with Xylocaine Injection, Sterile ... 1683
Decadron Tablets ... 1678
Decadron-LA Sterile Suspension ... 1687
Demulen ... 2580
Dexacort Phosphate in Respihaler ... 1606
Dexacort Phosphate in Turbinaire ... 1607
Dilaudid Ampules ... 1382
Dilaudid Cough Syrup ... 1383
Dilaudid-HP Injection (Less frequent) ... 1384
Dilaudid-HP Lyophilized Powder 250 mg (Less frequent) ... 1384
Dilaudid ... 1382
Dilaudid Oral Liquid (Less frequent) ... 1386
Dilaudid ... 1382
Dilaudid Tablets - 8 mg (Less frequent) ... 1386
Dipentum Capsules (Rare) ... 2084
Eldepryl Capsules ... 2729
Feldene Capsules (Less than 1%) ... 2008
Florinef Acetate Tablets ... 506
Hexalen Capsules ... 2760
Hivid Tablets (Less than 1%) ... 2287
Hycodan Tablets and Syrup ... 946
Hycomine Compound Tablets ... 948
Hycomine ... 947
Hycotuss Expectorant Syrup ... 950
Hydeltrasol Injection, Sterile ... 1708
Hydelta-T.B.A. Sterile Suspension ... 1710
Hydrocet Capsules ... 787
Hydrocortone Acetate Sterile Suspension ... 1712
Hydrocortone Phosphate Injection, Sterile ... 1713
Hydrocortone Tablets ... 1715
Levlen/Tri-Levlen ... 646
Lorcet 10/650 Tablets ... 1016
Lortab ... 2751
Lupron Depot 3.75 mg ... 2739
Lupron Injection (Less than 5%) ... 2736
MS Contin Tablets (Less frequent) ... 2149
MSIR (Infrequent) ... 2152
Marinol (Dronabinol) Capsules ... 2353
Methotrexate Sodium Tablets, Injection, for Injection and LPF Injection (Occasional) ... 1322
Modicon ... 1928
Monopril Tablets (0.2% to 1.0%) ... 762
Oncaspar ... 2194
Oramorph SR (Morphine Sulfate Sustained Release Tablets) (Less frequent) ... 2359
Ortho-Cyclen/Ortho Tri-Cyclen ... 1914
Ortho-Novum ... 1928
Ortho-Cyclen/Ortho Tri-Cyclen ... 1914
Orthoclone OKT3 Sterile Solution ... 1892
Pondimin Tablets ... 2239
Prelone Syrup ... 1834
▲ Procardia Capsules (7%) ... 2024
▲ Procardia XL Extended Release Tablets (7%) ... 2026
▲ Supprelin Injection (2% to 10%) ... 2230
▲ Tonocard Tablets (1.5% to 11.0%) ... 519
Levlen/Tri-Levlen ... 646
Tussend ... 1830
Tussionex Pennkinetic Extended-Release Suspension ... 1624
Univasc Tablets (Less than 1%) ... 2553
Vicodin Tablets ... 1404
Vicodin ES Tablets ... 1405
Vicodin HP Tablets ... 1403
Vicodin Tuss Expectorant ... 1406
Wellbutrin Tablets (Infrequent) ... 1177
Zydone Capsules ... 967

Moro reflex, depressed

Diupres Tablets ... 1691
Hydropres Tablets ... 1718

Motor and phonic tics, exacerbations

Adderall Tablets ... 2209
Dexedrine ... 2648
DextroStat-Dextroamphetamine Sulfate Tablets ... 2211

Motor disturbances, reversible involuntary

Zantac (Rare) ... 1182
Zantac Injection (Rare) ... 1180
Zantac Syrup (Rare) ... 1182

Motor restlessness

Compazine ... 2644

Etrafon ... 2495
Haldol Injection, Tablets and Concentrate ... 1585
Mellaril ... 2398
Moban Tablets and Concentrate ... 1036
Navane Capsules and Concentrate ... 2018
Navane Intramuscular ... 2019
Orap Tablets (Less frequent) ... 1037
Prolixin ... 510
Reglan ... 2243
Serentil ... 689
Stelazine ... 2692
Thorazine ... 2701
Torecan ... 2367

Motor skills, impairment

Ambien Tablets ... 2559
Cogentin ... 1661
Compazine ... 2644
Dapsone Tablets USP ... 1331
Desyrel and Desyrel Dividose ... 504
Dexacort Phosphate in Respihaler ... 1606
Dexacort Phosphate in Turbinaire ... 1607
Dilaudid Cough Syrup ... 1383
Doral Tablets ... 2773
Duranest Injections ... 533
Effexor ... 2825
Fulvicin P/G Tablets ... 2499
Fulvicin P/G 165 & 330 Tablets (Occasional) ... 2500
Halcion Tablets ... 2093
Levsin/Levsinex/Levbid ... 2549
Moban Tablets and Concentrate ... 1036
Neurontin Capsules (Rare) ... 1978
Oncovin Solution Vials & Hyporets ... 1521
Orap Tablets ... 1037
Platinol for Injection ... 717
Platinol-AQ Injection ... 719
▲ Prograf (Approximately 55%) ... 1028
Proleukin for Injection (2%) ... 812
Remeron Tablets ... 1878
Risperdal Tablets ... 1348
Robaxin Injectable ... 2245
Serzone Tablets ... 776
Soma Compound w/Codeine Tablets ... 2784
Soma Compound Tablets ... 2783
Tonocard Tablets (Up to 1.2%) ... 519

Mouth, burning

Eldepryl Capsules ... 2729
Fioricet with Codeine Capsules ... 2387
Fiorinal with Codeine Capsules ... 2390
Gastrocrom Capsules (Infrequent) ... 1611
Thyro-Block Tablets ... 2785

Mouth, dry
(see under Xerostomia)

Mouth, fissuring in corner of

Parnate Tablets ... 2679

Mouth, puckering

Compazine ... 2644
Etrafon ... 2495
Haldol Decanoate ... 1587
Haldol Injection, Tablets and Concentrate ... 1585
Mellaril ... 2398
Moban Tablets and Concentrate ... 1036
Navane Capsules and Concentrate ... 2018
Navane Intramuscular ... 2019
Orap Tablets ... 1037
Prolixin ... 510
Serentil ... 689
Stelazine ... 2692
Thorazine ... 2701
Triavil Tablets ... 1800
Trilafon ... 2532

Mouth sensations, unpleasant

Mycelex Troches ... 601

Mouth, sore

Alferon N Injection (One patient) ... 2142
▲ Imitrex Injection (4.9%) ... 1095
Neoral (Rare) ... 2405
Omnipen for Oral Suspension (Occasional) ... 2873
Oncaspar ... 2194
Prolixin ... 510
Rifadin (Occasional) ... 1276
Rifamate Capsules ... 1278
Rifater (Occasional) ... 1280
Rimactane Capsules ... 865
Tegison Capsules ... 2314
Tornalate Solution for Inhalation, (0.2%, 1.9%) ... 976
▲ Videx Tablets, Powder for Oral Solution, & Pediatric Powder for Oral Solution (16%) ... 2980

(🅟 Described in PDR For Nonprescription Drugs)   Incidence data in parenthesis; ▲ 3% or more   (⊚ Described in PDR For Ophthalmology)

Side Effects Index / Myalgia

Movement, abnormal
- BuSpar Tablets (Infrequent) ... 738
- Cognex Capsules (Infrequent) ... 1961
- ▲ Diprivan Injectable Emulsion (3% to 17%) ... 2939
- Hivid Tablets (Less than 1%) ... 2287
- Lamictal Tablets (Rare) ... 1105
- Oramorph SR (Morphine Sulfate Sustained Release Tablets) (Less frequent) ... 2359
- Orthoclone OKT3 Sterile Solution ... 1892

Mucha-Habermann syndrome
- Azulfidine (Rare) ... 2059

Mucocutaneous lymph node syndrome
(see under Kawasaki-like syndrome)

Mucosal pigmentation, changes
- Aralen Hydrochloride Injection ... 2430
- Aralen Phosphate Tablets ... 2431
- Intron A for Injection (Less than 5%) ... 2506
- Minocin Oral Suspension ... 1431
- Minocin Pellet-Filled Capsules ... 1429
- Plaquenil Sulfate Tablets ... 2459

Mucositis
- Adriamycin PFS ... 2056
- Adriamycin RDF ... 2056
- Alferon N Injection (One patient) ... 2142
- Cerubidine for Injection ... 634
- Doxorubicin Astra ... 531
- ▲ Etopophos for Injection (11%) ... 701
- Fludara for Injection (Up to 2%) ... 658
- Hydrea Capsules ... 705
- ▲ Idamycin Injection (50%) ... 2096
- ▲ Neupogen for Injection (12%) ... 495
- Neurontin Capsules (Rare) ... 1978
- Oncaspar ... 2194
- ▲ Paraplatin for Injection (1% to 10%) ... 713
- Rubex for Injection ... 721
- ▲ Taxol Injection (31%) ... 723
- ▲ Vesanoid Capsules (26%) ... 2327
- ▲ Vumon for Injection (76%) ... 729

Mucous membrane, abnormalities
- Atrohist Plus Tablets ... 1605
- Capoten Tablets (Approximately 1 in 1000 patients) ... 740
- Clinoril Tablets ... 1658
- DYNACIN Capsules ... 1627
- Lescol Capsules ... 2395
- ▲ Leukine (75%) ... 1317
- Mevacor Tablets ... 1742
- Mexitil Capsules (About 1 in 1,000) ... 684
- Minocin Intravenous ... 1428
- Minocin Oral Suspension ... 1431
- Minocin Pellet-Filled Capsules ... 1429
- Monopril Tablets ... 762
- Naprelan Tablets (Less than 1%) ... 2861
- Norisodrine with Calcium Iodide Syrup ... 446
- ▲ Novantrone for Injection (18 to 29%) ... 1327
- Remeron Tablets ... 1878
- Salagen Tablets (Less than 1%) ... 1546
- ▲ Tegison Capsules (1-10%) ... 2314
- Zocor Tablets ... 1821

Mucous plugs
- Exosurf Neonatal for Intratracheal Suspension ... 1081

Mucus, blood-tinted
- Atrovent Nasal Spray 0.03% (2.0%) ... 676
- Flonase Nasal Spray (1% to 3%) ... 1088
- Peptavlon ... 2997

Mucus, excess
- ReVia Tablets (Less than 1%) ... 957

Mucus secretion, decreased
- Tegison Capsules (Less than 1%) ... 2314

Murmur
- Cipro I.V. Pharmacy Bulk Package (Less than 1%) ... 590
- ▲ Lupron Injection (5% or more) ... 2736
- Neurontin Capsules (Infrequent) ... 1978

Muscle atrophy
- Betaseron for SC Injection ... 653
- Norcuron for Injection ... 1875
- Permax Tablets (Rare) ... 571

- ▲ Videx Tablets, Powder for Oral Solution, & Pediatric Powder for Oral Solution (8%) ... 2980
- Virazole ... 1310

Muscle cramp
(see under Cramping, muscular)

Muscle hypotonia
- Pipracil (Rare) ... 1435
- ▲ Xanax Tablets (6.3%) ... 2115

Muscle mass, loss
- Celestone Soluspan Suspension ... 2484
- CORTENEMA ... 2713
- Cortone Acetate Sterile Suspension ... 1663
- Cortone Acetate Tablets ... 1664
- Dalalone D.P. Injectable ... 1009
- Decadron Elixir ... 1676
- Decadron Phosphate Injection ... 1680
- Decadron Phosphate with Xylocaine Injection, Sterile ... 1683
- Decadron Tablets ... 1678
- Decadron-LA Sterile Suspension ... 1687
- Dexacort Phosphate in Respihaler ... 1606
- Dexacort Phosphate in Turbinaire ... 1607
- Florinef Acetate Tablets ... 506
- Hydeltrasol Injection, Sterile ... 1708
- Hydeltra-T.B.A. Sterile Suspension ... 1710
- Hydrocortone Phosphate Injection, Sterile ... 1713
- Hydrocortone Tablets ... 1715
- Oncovin Solution Vials & Hyporets ... 1521
- Pediapred Oral Solution ... 1618
- Prelone Syrup ... 1834

Muscle movement, intraoperative
- Dilaudid Tablets and Liquid (Less frequent) ... 1386
- Sufenta Injection (0.3% to 1%) ... 1355

Muscle rigidity
- ▲ Alfenta Injection (One of the two most common) ... 1334
- Asendin Tablets ... 1419
- BuSpar Tablets (Infrequent) ... 738
- Ceftin (0.1% to 1%) ... 1067
- Clozaril Tablets ... 2377
- Compazine ... 2644
- Cozaar Tablets (Less than 1%) ... 1668
- Cytotec (Infrequent) ... 2576
- Dilaudid-HP Injection (Less frequent) ... 1384
- Dilaudid-HP Lyophilized Powder 250 mg (Less frequent) ... 1384
- Dilaudid Tablets and Liquid (Less frequent) ... 1386
- Etrafon ... 2495
- Haldol Decanoate ... 1587
- Hivid Tablets (Less than 1%) ... 2287
- Imitrex Injection (Rare) ... 1095
- Imogam Rabies Immune Globulin (Human) (Uncommon) ... 897
- Inapsine Injection (Very rare) ... 462
- Invirase Capsules (Less than 2%) ... 2291
- Loxitane ... 1426
- MS Contin Tablets (Less frequent) ... 2149
- MSIR (Infrequent) ... 2152
- Mellaril ... 2398
- Miacalcin Nasal Spray (Less than 1%) ... 2403
- Nardil (Less frequent) ... 1977
- Navane Capsules and Concentrate ... 2018
- Navane Intramuscular ... 2019
- Oramorph SR (Morphine Sulfate Sustained Release Tablets) (Less frequent) ... 2359
- ▲ Orap Tablets (3 of 20 patients) ... 1037
- Orthoclone OKT3 Sterile Solution ... 1892
- Paremyd ... ⊚ 244
- Permax Tablets ... 571
- Prolixin ... 510
- ProSom Tablets (1%) ... 457
- Reglan ... 2243
- Risperdal Tablets ... 1348
- Serentil ... 689
- Serzone Tablets (Infrequent) ... 776
- Stelazine ... 2692
- Sublimaze Injection (Infrequent) ... 463
- ▲ Sufenta Injection (One of the two most common) ... 1355
- Supprelin Injection (2% to 3%) ... 2230
- Symmetrel Capsules (Uncommon) ... 965
- Symmetrel Syrup (Uncommon) ... 963
- Thorazine ... 2701
- Torecan ... 2367
- Trilafon ... 2532
- Versed Injection (0.3%) ... 2324
- Wellbutrin Tablets ... 1177
- Xanax Tablets (2.2%) ... 2115

Muscle spasms
- Aldactazide Tablets ... 2556
- Aldoclor Tablets ... 1638
- Aldoril Tablets ... 1644
- Alupent Tablets (0.2%) ... 672
- Apresazide Capsules ... 824
- ▲ Avonex (7%) ... 662
- BuSpar Tablets (Infrequent) ... 738
- Capozide Tablets ... 744
- Clozaril Tablets (1%) ... 2377
- Combipres Tablets ... 682
- Danocrine Capsules ... 2437
- Diucardin Tablets ... 2824
- Diupres Tablets ... 1691
- Diuril Oral Suspension ... 1694
- Diuril Sodium Intravenous ... 1693
- Diuril Tablets ... 1694
- Dizac (diazepam injectable emulsion) CIV (Less frequent) ... 1862
- Dopram Injectable ... 2235
- Doral Tablets (Rare) ... 2773
- Enduron Tablets ... 424
- Esidrix Tablets ... 839
- Esimil Tablets ... 840
- Etrafon ... 2495
- Halcion Tablets ... 2093
- HydroDIURIL Tablets ... 1716
- Hydropres Tablets ... 1718
- Hyzaar Tablets ... 1720
- Inderide Tablets ... 2838
- Inderide LA Long Acting Capsules ... 2840
- Indocin I.V. (Less than 1%) ... 1727
- Lamictal Tablets (1.0%) ... 1105
- Lasix Injection, Oral Solution and Tablets ... 1267
- Lopressor HCT Tablets ... 850
- Lotensin HCT Tablets ... 855
- Loxitane ... 1426
- Mestinon Injectable ... 1300
- Minizide Capsules ... 2016
- Mivacron (Less than 1%) ... 1125
- Moduretic Tablets (Less than or equal to 1%) ... 1748
- Oretic Tablets ... 450
- Parnate Tablets ... 2679
- Prinzide Tablets ... 1780
- Proleukin for Injection (1%) ... 812
- ProSom Tablets (Infrequent) ... 457
- Prostigmin Injectable ... 1305
- Prostigmin Tablets ... 1306
- Proventil Syrup (Less than 1 of 100 patients) ... 2528
- Retrovir Capsules ... 1216
- Retrovir I.V. Infusion ... 1221
- Retrovir Syrup ... 1216
- Ser-Ap-Es Tablets ... 867
- Tenoretic Tablets ... 2963
- Thalitone ... 1293
- Timolide Tablets ... 1791
- Tonocard Tablets (Less than 1%) ... 519
- Valium Injectable ... 2336
- Valium Tablets ... 2335
- Vancocin HCl, Oral Solution & Pulvules ... 1536
- Vancocin HCl, Vials & ADD-Vantage ... 1534
- Vaseretic Tablets ... 1810
- Ventolin Syrup (Less than 1 of 100 patients) ... 1175
- Wellbutrin Tablets (1.9%) ... 1177
- Xanax Tablets (Rare) ... 2115
- Zaroxolyn Tablets ... 1625
- Zestoretic Tablets ... 2968
- Ziac ... 1459

Muscle twitching
- Atamet Tablets ... 567
- Clozaril Tablets (Less than 1%) ... 2377
- Dalalone D.P. Injectable ... 1009
- Decadron-LA Sterile Suspension (Low) ... 1687
- Desyrel and Desyrel Dividose ... 504
- Dilaudid-HP Injection ... 1384
- Dilaudid-HP Lyophilized Powder 250 mg ... 1384
- Dilaudid Tablets and Liquid (Less frequent) ... 1386
- Dopram Injectable ... 2235
- Flexeril Tablets (Less than 1%) ... 1701
- Garamycin Injectable ... 2502
- Humorsol Sterile Ophthalmic Solution ... 1707
- Larodopa Tablets (Infrequent) ... 2296
- Loxitane ... 1426
- Lufyllin & Lufyllin-400 Tablets ... 2778
- Lufyllin-GG Elixir & Tablets ... 2779
- MS Contin Tablets (Less frequent) ... 2149
- Netromycin Injection 100 mg/ml ... 2516
- Placidyl Capsules ... 456
- Quadrinal Tablets ... 1398
- Quibron ... 2227

- Respbid Tablets ... 687
- Retrovir Syrup ... 1216
- Sinemet Tablets ... 959
- Sinemet CR Tablets ... 961
- Theo-Dur Extended-Release Tablets ... 1367
- Theo-X Extended-Release Tablets ... 793
- Tonocard Tablets (Less than 1%) ... 519
- Uni-Dur Extended-Release Tablets ... 1374
- Uniphyl 400 mg and 600 mg Tablets ... 2157
- ▲ Xanax Tablets (7.9%) ... 2115

Muscle weakness
(see also under Asthenia; Weakness, muscle)
- Anaprox/Naprosyn (Less than 1%) ... 2277
- Antivenin (Crotalidae) Polyvalent (Frequent) ... 2803
- BuSpar Tablets (Rare) ... 738
- Celestone Soluspan Suspension ... 2484
- Clozaril Tablets (1%) ... 2377
- CORTENEMA ... 2713
- Dalalone D.P. Injectable ... 1009
- Decadron Tablets ... 1678
- Decadron-LA Sterile Suspension ... 1687
- Depakene ... 416
- Depakote Tablets ... 418
- EC-Naprosyn Delayed-Release Tablets (Less than 1%) ... 2277
- Enduron Tablets ... 424
- Etrafon ... 2495
- Fansidar Tablets ... 2281
- Garamycin Injectable ... 2502
- Hydrocortone Acetate Sterile Suspension ... 1712
- Hyzaar Tablets ... 1720
- Intron A for Injection (Less than 5%) ... 2506
- Klonopin Tablets ... 2294
- Mestinon Injectable ... 1300
- Mestinon ... 1300
- Anaprox/Naprosyn (Less than 1%) ... 2277
- ▲ Norpace (3 to 9%) ... 2596
- Norvasc Tablets (Less than or equal to 0.1%) ... 2020
- Norvir (Less than 2%) ... 447
- Pediapred Oral Solution ... 1618
- Placidyl Capsules (Occasional) ... 456
- Plaquenil Sulfate Tablets ... 2459
- Prelone Syrup ... 1834
- Prostigmin Injectable ... 1305
- Prostigmin Tablets ... 1306
- Proventil (2%) ... 2529
- Recombivax HB ... 1787
- Rifadin ... 1276
- Rifamate Capsules ... 1278
- Rythmol Tablets–150mg, 225mg, 300mg (Less than 1%) ... 1399
- Tensilon Injectable ... 1307
- Triavil Tablets ... 1800
- Trilafon ... 2532
- Xanax Tablets ... 2115

Muscular disturbances
- Felbatol ... 2774
- ▲ Foscavir Injection (5% or greater) ... 541
- Hivid Tablets (Less than 1%) ... 2287
- Lescol Capsules ... 2395
- ▲ Risperdal Tablets (17% to 34%) ... 1348
- Roferon-A Injection (Less than 0.5%) ... 2308
- Serevent Inhalation Aerosol (1% to 3%) ... 1149
- Slo-Niacin Tablets ... 2767
- Zosyn (1.0% or less) ... 1463

Musculoskeletal symptoms, unspecified
- ▲ Accutane Capsules (Approximately 16%) ... 2252
- Demadex Tablets and Injection ... 691
- ▲ Epivir (12%) ... 1200
- ▲ Flovent (1% to 22%) ... 1089
- Imdur (Less than or equal to 5%) ... 1362
- Invirase Capsules (0.6% to less than 2%) ... 2291
- Seldane Tablets ... 1284
- Seldane-D Extended-Release Tablets ... 1286

Mutism
- Anafranil Capsules (Rare) ... 819
- Lopid Tablets ... 1974
- LUVOX Tablets (Rare) ... 2723

Myalgia
- Abelcet Injection ... 1540
- Accupril Tablets (1.5%) ... 1950

(▣ Described in PDR For Nonprescription Drugs)   Incidence data in parenthesis; ▲ 3% or more   (⊚ Described in PDR For Ophthalmology)

Myalgia Side Effects Index 1400

▲ Actigall Capsules (5.8%) ... 818
▲ Actimmune (6%) ... 1043
Adalat Capsules (10 mg and 20 mg) (Less than 0.5%) ... 580
Adalat CC (Less than 1.0%) ... 582
Aldoclor Tablets ... 1638
Aldomet Ester HCl Injection ... 1642
Aldomet Oral ... 1640
Aldoril Tablets ... 1644
▲ Alferon N Injection (One patient to 45%) ... 2142
All-Flex Arcing Spring Diaphragm (See also Ortho Diaphragm Kits) 1921
Altace Capsules (Less than 1%) ... 1238
Alupent Tablets (0.2%) ... 672
▲ Ambien Tablets (1% to 7%) ... 2559
Amicar Syrup, Tablets, and Injection ... 1312
▲ Anafranil Capsules (Up to 13%) ... 819
Anaprox/Naprosyn (Less than 1%) ... 2277
Anectine ... 1062
Apresazide Capsules ... 824
▲ Aredia for Injection (Up to 14.8%) 827
Arimidex Tablets (2% to 5%) ... 2932
▲ Asacol Delayed-Release Tablets (3%) ... 2129
Atretol Tablets ... 569
Atromid-S Capsules (Less often) ... 2808
Augmentin ... 2637
Augmentin Tablets ... 2640
▲ Avonex (34%) ... 662
Axid Pulvules (1.7%) ... 1468
Azactam for Injection (Less than 1%) ... 736
Azathioprine Tablets ... 2349
Azmacort Oral Inhaler ... 2175
Bactrim DS Tablets ... 2257
Bactrim I.V. Infusion ... 2255
Bactrim ... 2257
Beconase ... 1065
Betapace Tablets (Rare) ... 637
▲ Betaseron for SC Injection (44%) .. 653
Biavax II ... 1653
Bumex (0.2%) ... 2260
BuSpar Tablets (1%) ... 738
Cafergot ... 2376
Calcijex Injection ... 412
Capoten Tablets ... 740
Capozide Tablets ... 744
Cardene Capsules (1.0%) ... 2261
Cardioquin Tablets ... 2146
Cardura Tablets (1%) ... 1993
Casodex Tablets (2% to 5%) ... 2934
Catapres Tablets (About 6 in 1,000 patients) ... 679
Catapres-TTS ... 680
▲ CellCept Capsules (More than or equal to 3%) ... 2265
Cerebyx Injection (Infrequent) ... 1956
Chibroxin Sterile Ophthalmic Solution (With oral form) ... 1657
Cipro Tablets ... 584
Claritin Tablets (2% or fewer patients) ... 2485
Claritin-D Tablets (Less frequent) .. 2487
Clinoril Tablets (Less than 1 in 100) ... 1658
Clomid ... 1262
Clozaril Tablets (1%) ... 2377
▲ Cognex Capsules (9%) ... 1961
Colestid ... 2073
Combipres Tablets (About 6 in 1,000) ... 682
Cosmegen Injection ... 1666
Coumadin ... 941
Cozaar Tablets (1.0%) ... 1668
Crixivan Capsules (Less than 2%) .. 1670
Cytosar-U Sterile Powder ... 2077
Cytotec (Infrequent) ... 2576
Cytovene (1% or less) ... 2270
D.H.E. 45 Injection ... 2381
DTIC-Dome (Infrequent) ... 593
Dalgan Injection (Less than 1%) ... 529
Dantrium Capsules (Less frequent) 2131
▲ DaunoXome (Up to 7%) ... 1842
Demadex Tablets and Injection (1.6%) ... 691
Depakote Tablets (1% to 5%) ... 418
▲ Desyrel and Desyrel Dividose (5.1% to 5.6%) ... 504
DiaBeta Tablets ... 1265
Dilacor XR Extended-release Capsules (2.3%) ... 2183
Diprivan Injectable Emulsion (Less than 1%) ... 2939
Diupres Tablets ... 1691
Dolobid Tablets (Less than 1 in 100) ... 1695
Donnatal ... 2234
Donnatal Extentabs ... 2234
Donnatal Tablets ... 2234
Doxil (Less than 1%) ... 2613
Dyazide Capsules ... 2653
Dynabac (0.1% to 1%) ... 668
EC-Naprosyn Delayed-Release Tablets (Less than 1%) ... 2277
Effexor ... 2825
Engerix-B Unit-Dose Vials (Less than 1%) ... 2656
▲ Epivir (8%) ... 1200
Epogen for Injection (Rare) ... 489
Ergamisol Tablets (2% to 3%) ... 1340
Esidrix Tablets ... 839
Esimil Tablets ... 840
▲ Ethmozine Tablets (2% to 5%) ... 2217
Felbatol (2.6%) ... 2774
Flexeril Tablets (Rare) ... 1701
▲ Flolan for Injection (3% to 44%) ... 1085
Floxin I.V. (Less than 1%) ... 1580
Floxin Tablets (200 mg, 300 mg, 400 mg) (Less than 1%) ... 1577
▲ Fludara for Injection (4% to 16%) 658
Fluvirin (Influenza Virus Vaccine) (Infrequent) ... 1608
▲ Fosamax Tablets (4.1% to 6%) ... 1703
Foscavir Injection (Between 1% and 5%) ... 541
▲ Fungizone Intravenous (Among most common) ... 507
Gamimune N, 5% Immune Globulin Intravenous (Human), 5% ... 612
Gamimune N, 10% Immune Globulin Intravenous (Human), 10% ... 615
Gammar-P I.V., Immune Globulin Intravenous (Human) ... 798
Gantanol Tablets ... 2285
Gantrisin ... 2286
▲ Gastrocrom Capsules (3 of 87 patients) ... 1611
▲ Gastrocrom Oral Concentrate (3 of 87 patients) ... 1611
Gemzar for Injection (Common) ... 1482
Glucophage Tablets ... 754
Glucotrol XL Extended Release Tablets (Less than 3%) ... 2012
Glynase PresTab Tablets ... 2091
▲ Habitrol Nicotine Transdermal System (3% to 9% of patients) .. 884
Havrix (Less than 1%) ... 2663
Hespan Injection ... 945
Hismanal Tablets (Less frequent) ... 1341
Hivid Tablets (Less than 1%; 0.4%) ... 2287
Humatrope Vials (Infrequent) ... 1490
Hytrin Capsules (At least 1%) ... 434
Hyzaar Tablets ... 1720
Imdur (Less than or equal to 5%) .. 1362
Imitrex Injection (1.8%) ... 1095
Imitrex Tablets (Frequent) ... 1099
▲ Imovax Rabies Vaccine (About 20%) ... 899
Imuran ... 1103
INFeD (Iron Dextran Injection, USP) ... 2478
Influenza Virus Vaccine, Trivalent, Types A and B (chromatograph- and filter-purified subviron antigen) FluShield, 1996-1997 Formula (Infrequent) ... 2842
Intal Inhaler (Rare) ... 2185
Intal Nebulizer Solution (Rare) ... 2186
▲ Intron A for Injection (3% to 75%) ... 2506
Iopidine 0.5% (0.2%) ... ◉ 219
Ismelin Tablets ... 845
▲ JE-VAX (Approximately 10%) ... 904
▲ Kerlone Tablets (3.2%) ... 2588
Lamictal Tablets (More than 1%) .. 1105
▲ Lariam Tablets (Among most frequent) ... 2295
Lasix Injection, Oral Solution and Tablets ... 1267
▲ Lescol Capsules (5.0%) ... 2395
▲ Leukine (18%) ... 1317
▲ Leustatin (5%) ... 1889
Lioresal Tablets ... 847
Lopid Tablets ... 1974
Lopressor ... 848
Lopressor HCT Tablets (1 in 100 patients) ... 850
Lotensin Tablets ... 852
Lotensin HCT Tablets (0.3% or more) ... 855
Lotrel Capsules ... 858
Lupron Depot 3.75 mg (Less than 5%) ... 2739
Lupron Depot 7.5 mg (Less than 5%) ... 2741
▲ Lupron Injection (5% or more) ... 2736
LUVOX Tablets ... 2723
M-M-R II ... 1730
M-R-VAX II ... 1732
Macrobid Capsules ... 2138
Macrodantin Capsules ... 2140
Marinol (Dronabinol) Capsules (Less than 1%) ... 2353
Matulane Capsules ... 2300
Maxaquin Tablets (Less than 1%) .. 2593
Meruvax II ... 1740
Methotrexate Sodium Tablets, Injection, for Injection and LPF Injection (Rare) ... 1322
Metrodin (urofollitropin for injection) ... 2616
Mevacor Tablets (1.8% to 2.4%) .. 1742
Miacalcin Nasal Spray (1% to 3%) 2403
Micronase Tablets ... 2099
Monocid Injection (Less than 1%) .. 2674
▲ Monopril Tablets (0.2% to 3.3%) .. 762
Mycobutin Capsules (2%) ... 2101
Naprelan Tablets (Less than 3%) .. 2861
Anaprox/Naprosyn (Less than 1%) ... 2277
Nasacort Nasal Inhaler ... 2189
Navelbine Injection (Less than 5%) 1212
Neoral (2% or less) ... 2405
Neupogen for Injection ... 495
Neurontin Capsules (2.0%) ... 1978
▲ Nicotrol NS Nicotine Nasal Spray (3%) ... 1565
Nimotop Capsules (Up to 1.4%) ... 603
▲ Nipent for Injection (11% to 19%) ... 2733
Nolvadex Tablets (2.8%) ... 2957
Noroxin Tablets ... 1758
Noroxin Tablets ... 2222
▲ Norplant System (5% or greater) .. 2868
Norvasc Tablets (More than 0.1% to 1%) ... 2020
Norvir (1.7% to 2.2%) ... 447
▲ Oncaspar (Greater than 1% but less than 5%) ... 2194
Oncovin Solution Vials & Hyporets 1521
OptiPranolol (Metipranolol 0.3%) Sterile Ophthalmic Solution (A small number of patients) ... ◉ 256
Orap Tablets (2.7%) ... 1037
Oretic Tablets ... 450
Orlaam Oral Solution (Less than 1%) ... 2361
Ortho Diaphragm Kits—All-Flex Arcing Spring; Ortho Coil Spring; Ortho-White Flat Spring ... 1921
Ortho Diaphragm Kit ... 1921
Orthoclone OKT3 Sterile Solution .. 1892
Orudis Capsules (Less than 1%) ... 2874
Oruvail Capsules (Less than 1%) ... 2874
Paxil Tablets (2%) ... 2681
Penetrex Tablets (0.1% to 1%) ... 2196
Pentasa (Less than 1%) ... 1275
Pepcid Injection (Infrequent) ... 1765
Pepcid (Infrequent) ... 1763
Permax Tablets (1.1%) ... 571
Phenobarbital Elixir and Tablets (Rare) ... 1523
Phenurone Tablets (Less than 1%) 455
Plendil Extended-Release Tablets (0.5% to 1.5%) ... 514
Pneumovax 23 ... 1768
Pnu-Imune 23 (Occasional) ... 1437
Pondimin Tablets ... 2239
Pravachol Tablets (0.6% to 2.7%) 770
Prevacid Delayed-Release Capsules (Less than 1%) ... 2746
Prilosec Delayed-Release Capsules (Less than 1%) ... 516
Prinivil Tablets (0.3% to greater than 1%) ... 1776
Prinzide Tablets (0.3% to 1%) ... 1780
Procanbid Extended-Release Tablets (Fairly common) ... 1983
Procardia Capsules (Less than 0.5%) ... 2024
Procardia XL Extended Release Tablets (1% or less) ... 2026
Procrit for Injection (Rare) ... 1896
▲ Prograf (Greater than 3%) ... 1028
▲ Proleukin for Injection (6%) ... 812
Propulsid (More than 1%) ... 1346
ProSom Tablets (Infrequent) ... 457
Prostep (nicotine transdermal system) (1% to 3% of patients) .. 1439
Prostin E2 Suppository ... 2109
Prozac Pulvules & Liquid, Oral Solution (1.2% to 5%) ... 935
Pyrazinamide Tablets (Frequent) ... 1442
Questran ... 774
Quinaglute Dura-Tabs Tablets ... 644
Quinidex Extentabs ... 2240
▲ Rabies Vaccine, Imovax Rabies I.D. (About 20%) ... 901
Recombivax HB (Less than 1%) ... 1787
Redux Capsules (Frequent) ... 2911
Remeron Tablets (2%) ... 1878
ReoPro Vials (0.3%) ... 1526
RespiGam ... 1631
▲ Retrovir Capsules (8%) ... 1216
▲ Retrovir I.V. Infusion (8%) ... 1221
▲ Retrovir Syrup (8%) ... 1216
▲ ReVia Tablets (More than 10%) ... 957
Revex (nalmefene hydrochloride injection) ... 1863
Rhinocort Nasal Inhaler (Less than 1%) ... 552
▲ RhoGAM $Rh_o(D)$ Immune Globulin (Human) (25% in one study) ... 1902
Rifater (Frequent) ... 1280
Risperdal Tablets (Infrequent) ... 1348
Rocaltrol Capsules ... 2303
▲ Roferon-A Injection (68% to 69%) 2308
Salagen Tablets (1%) ... 1546
Sandimmune (2% or less) ... 2416
Sandostatin Injection (Less than 1%) ... 2421
Sansert Tablets ... 2424
Sectral Capsules (2%) ... 2914
Septra ... 1146
Septra I.V. Infusion ... 1142
Septra I.V. Infusion ADD-Vantage Vials ... 1144
Septra ... 1146
Ser-Ap-Es Tablets ... 867
Serevent Inhalation Aerosol (1% to 3%) ... 1149
Serzone Tablets ... 776
Sporanox Capsules (1%) ... 1352
Streptase for Infusion ... 557
Sular Tablets (Less than or equal to 1%) ... 2961
Supprelin Injection (2% to 3%) ... 2230
Suprane (desflurane, USP) (Less than 1%) ... 1865
▲ Synarel Nasal Solution for Endometriosis (10% of patients) 2605
Tagamet (Rare) ... 2694
Tambocor Tablets (Less than 1%) 1555
Tapazole Tablets ... 1361
▲ Taxol Injection (8% to 60%) ... 723
Taxotere for Injection Concentrate 2204
▲ Tegison Capsules (1-10%) ... 2314
Tegretol/Tegretol-XR ... 870
Tenex Tablets (Less frequent) ... 2249
Tenoretic Tablets ... 2963
Thalitone (Common) ... 1293
▲ TheraCys BCG Live (Intravesical) (1.0% to 7.1%) ... 911
Timentin for Injection ... 2706
Timolide Tablets (Less than 1%) ... 1791
Tonocard Tablets (1.7%) ... 519
Toprol-XL Tablets ... 560
Toradol ... 2319
▲ Typhim Vi (2% to 7.4%) ... 914
Typhoid Vaccine ... 2929
Univasc Tablets (1.3%) ... 2553
Vancenase AQ Double Strength Nasal Spray 0.084% (1% to 2%) ... 2536
Vaqta (2.0%) ... 1805
Varivax (Greater than or equal to 1%) ... 1807
Vaseretic Tablets ... 1810
Vasotec I.V. ... 1814
Vasotec Tablets (0.5% to 1.0%) ... 1816
Verelan Capsules (1.1%) ... 1455
▲ Vesanoid Capsules (14%) ... 2327
▲ Videx Tablets, Powder for Oral Solution, & Pediatric Powder for Oral Solution (9%) ... 2980
Viramune Tablets ... 2368
▲ Visken Tablets (10%) ... 2428
Vistide Injection ... 1057
Wellbutrin Tablets ... 1177
Wigraine Tablets ... 1884
WinRho SD (One report) ... 1839
Xalatan (1% to 2%) ... ◉ 304
Zantac (Rare) ... 1182
Zantac Injection (Rare) ... 1180
Zantac Syrup (Rare) ... 1182
Zebeta Tablets ... 1457
▲ Zerit Capsules (2% to 35%) ... 731
Zestoretic Tablets (0.3 to 1%) ... 2968
Zestril Tablets (0.3% to 1.0%) ... 2972
Ziac (Up to 2.4%) ... 1459
Zocor Tablets ... 1821
▲ Zofran Injection (10%) ... 1227
▲ Zoladex (3%) ... 2976
Zoladex 3-month ... 2978
Zoloft Tablets (1.7%) ... 2051
Zosyn (1.0% or less) ... 1463
Zovirax ... 1187

(▣ Described in PDR For Nonprescription Drugs) Incidence data in parenthesis; ▲ 3% or more (◉ Described in PDR For Ophthalmology)

1401 Side Effects Index Myocardial infarction

Zyloprim Tablets (Less than 1%) 1194
Zyrtec Tablets (Less than 2%) 2053

Myasthenia gravis
Abelcet Injection 1540
Avonex 662
▲ Betaseron for SC Injection (13%) 653
Blocadren Tablets (Less than 1%) 1654
Capoten Tablets 740
Capozide Tablets 744
Casodex Tablets (2% to 5%) 2934
▲ CellCept Capsules (More than or equal to 3%) 2265
Cerebyx Injection (Frequent) 1956
Cuprimine Capsules 1673
Cytovene (1% or less) 2270
Depen Titratable Tablets 2770
Effexor (Infrequent) 2825
Eskalith (Rare) 2658
Lamictal Tablets (1.3%) 1105
Lopid Tablets 1974
LUVOX Tablets (Infrequent) 2723
Myleran Tablets (Rare) 1209
Naprelan Tablets (Less than 1%) 2861
Netromycin Injection 100 mg/ml 2516
Paxil Tablets (1%) 2681
▲ Prograf (Greater than 3%) 1028
Redux Capsules (Infrequent) 2911
Remeron Tablets (Frequent) 1878
Rilutek Tablets (Infrequent) 2198
Sular Tablets (Less than or equal to 1%) 2961
Timolide Tablets 1791
Tonocard Tablets (Less than 1%) 519
Vistide Injection 1057

Myasthenia gravis, exacerbation of
Betoptic Ophthalmic Solution (Rare) 465
Betoptic S Ophthalmic Suspension 467
Chibroxin Sterile Ophthalmic Solution (With oral form) 1657
Cipro I.V. 587
Cipro I.V. Pharmacy Bulk Package (Less than 1%) 590
Cipro Tablets 584
Floxin I.V. (Possible) 1580
Floxin Tablets (200 mg, 300 mg, 400 mg) 1577
Maxaquin Tablets 2593
Mefoxin (A possibility) 1734
Mefoxin Premixed Intravenous Solution 1737
Mykrox Tablets (exacerbation of) 1617
Noroxin Tablets 1758
Noroxin Tablets 2222
Norpace 2596
Penetrex Tablets 2196
Timoptic Sterile Ophthalmic Solution (Less frequent) 1794
Timoptic-XE 1798

Myasthenia gravis, increase
Betagan ⊙ 230
Betimol 0.25%, 0.5% ⊙ 259
Timoptic in Ocudose (Less frequent) 1796

Myasthenia gravis-like syndrome
Achromycin V Capsules (Rare) 1417
Clozaril Tablets 2377
Garamycin Injectable 2502
Helidac Therapy (Rare) 2135

Mydriasis
AK-CIDE (Occasional) ⊙ 203
AK-CIDE Ointment (Occasional) ⊙ 203
AKPRO (Infrequent) ⊙ 206
Albalon Solution with Liquifilm ⊙ 229
Anafranil Capsules (Up to 2%) 819
Artane 1418
Asendin Tablets (Less than 1%) 1419
Atamet Tablets 567
Atrohist Plus Tablets 1605
Bentyl 1246
Betaseron for SC Injection 653
Blephamide Liquifilm Sterile Ophthalmic Suspension 472
Blephamide Ointment (Occasional) ⊙ 234
Cardioquin Tablets (Occasional) 2146
Caverject Injection (Less than 1%) 2064
Cerebyx Injection (Infrequent) 1956
Claritin-D Tablets (Less frequent) 2487
Clozaril Tablets (Less than 1%) 2377
Cocaine Hydrochloride Topical Solutions 529
Cogentin 1661
Compazine 2644
Cystospaz 2123
Ditropan 1267
Donnatal 2234
Donnatal Extentabs 2234
Donnatal Tablets 2234
Dopram Injectable 2235
Econopred & Econopred Plus Ophthalmic Suspensions (Occasional) ⊙ 216
Effexor (2%) 2825
Elavil 2945
Etrafon 2495
FML Forte Liquifilm (Occasional) ⊙ 237
FML Liquifilm (Occasional) ⊙ 238
FML S.O.P. (Occasional) ⊙ 239
Foscavir Injection (Less than 1%) 541
Healon GV ⊙ 303
Imitrex Tablets (Rare) 1099
Inversine Tablets 1729
IOPIDINE Sterile Ophthalmic Solution (0.4%) ⊙ 218
Kemadrin Tablets 1105
Kutrase Capsules 2546
Larodopa Tablets (Infrequent) 2296
Levsin/Levsinex/Levbid 2549
Limbitrol 2333
Lioresal Tablets 847
Ludiomil Tablets (Rare) 861
LUVOX Tablets (Infrequent) 2723
Methadone Hydrochloride Oral Concentrate 2356
Navane Capsules and Concentrate 2018
Navane Intramuscular 2019
Norflex 1554
Norgesic 1554
Norpramin Tablets 1273
Ocufen ⊙ 242
Orlaam Oral Solution 2361
Pamelor 2409
Paxil Tablets (Infrequent) 2681
Pred Forte (Occasional) ⊙ 247
Pred Mild (Occasional) ⊙ 250
Pro-Banthine Tablets 2226
PROPINE with C CAP Compliance Cap ⊙ 251
Proventil Syrup (Less than 1 of 100 patients) 2528
Prozac Pulvules & Liquid, Oral Solution (Infrequent) 935
Quinaglute Dura-Tabs Tablets (Occasional) 644
Quinidex Extentabs (Occasional) 2240
Redux Capsules (Infrequent) 2911
Robinul Forte Tablets 2247
Robinul Injectable 2247
Robinul Tablets 2247
Sansert Tablets 2424
Serzone Tablets (Infrequent) 776
Sinemet Tablets 959
Soma Compound w/Codeine Tablets (Very rare) 2784
Soma Compound Tablets (Very rare) 2783
Soma Tablets 2782
Stelazine 2692
Surmontil Capsules 2917
Testoderm Testosterone Transdermal System (One in 104 patients) 486
Thorazine 2701
Tofranil Ampuls 873
Tofranil Tablets 875
Tofranil-PM Capsules 876
Transderm Scōp Transdermal Therapeutic System 890
Triavil Tablets 1800
Trilafon (Occasional) 2532
Trinalin Repetabs Tablets 1373
Ventolin Syrup (Less than 1 of 100 patients) 1175
Vivactil Tablets 1820
Wellbutrin Tablets (Infrequent) 1177
Zoloft Tablets (Infrequent) 2051

Myelitis
Havrix (Rare) 2663
Paxil Tablets (Rare) 2681
Permax Tablets (Rare) 571
Recombivax HB 1787
Zyrtec Tablets (Less than 2%) 2053

Myelitis, transverse
Asacol Delayed-Release Tablets (Rare) 2129
Azulfidine (Rare) 2059
Cytovene-IV (Two or more reports) 2270
Engerix-B Unit-Dose Vials 2656
JE-VAX (One case) 904
Recombivax HB 1787

Myelodysplastic syndrome
Azulfidine (Rare) 2059
▲ Neupogen for Injection (Approximately 3%) 495

Myelofibrosis
Mexitil Capsules (About 2 in 10,000) 684

Myelopathy, dorsal column
Platinol for Injection 717
Platinol-AQ Injection 719

Myelosuppression
Adriamycin PFS 2056
Adriamycin RDF 2056
Alkeran for Injection 1196
▲ BiCNU (Most frequent) 696
CeeNU Capsules 699
▲ Cerubidine for Injection (All patients) 634
DaunoXome 1842
Doxil 2613
Doxorubicin Astra 531
Etopophos for Injection 701
Etoposide Injection 539
▲ Fludara for Injection (Among most common) 658
Gemzar for Injection 1482
Hexalen Capsules 2760
Idamycin Injection 2096
IFEX 706
Leukeran Tablets 1205
Leustatin (Frequent) 1889
Mutamycin for Injection 712
▲ Myleran Tablets (Most frequent) 1209
▲ Navelbine Injection (53%) 1212
Novantrone for Injection 1327
▲ Platinol for Injection (25% to 30%) 717
▲ Platinol-AQ Injection (25% to 30% of patients) 719
Purinethol Tablets 1214
Roferon-A Injection 2308
Rubex for Injection 721
▲ Thioguanine Tablets, Tabloid Brand (Most frequent) 1225
Velban Vials 1537
VePesid Capsules and Injection 727
▲ Vumon for Injection (75%) 729
Zinecard Injection 2120

Myelosuppression, persistent severe
Adriamycin PFS 2056
Adriamycin RDF 2056
Novantrone for Injection 1327

Myocardial failure
Protamine Sulfate Vials 1526

Myocardial infarction
Abbokinase (Rare) 403
Abbokinase Open-Cath (Rare) 405
Abelcet Injection 1540
Accupril Tablets (Rare) 1950
Actimmune (Rare) 1043
Activase 1045
▲ Adalat Capsules (10 mg and 20 mg) (About 4%) 580
Adenoscan (Less than 1%) 1022
Altace Capsules (Less than 1% to 1.7%) 1238
Ambien Tablets (Rare) 2559
Anafranil Capsules (Rare) 819
Asendin Tablets (Very rare) 1419
Atretol Tablets 569
Betaseron for SC Injection 653
Blenoxane (Rare) 697
Brevicon 2563
BuSpar Tablets (Rare) 738
Calan SR Caplets (1% or less) 2571
Calan Tablets (1% or less) 2568
Capoten Tablets (2 to 3 of 1000 patients) 740
Capozide Tablets (2 to 3 of 1000 patients) 744
Cardene Capsules (Less than 0.4%) 2261
Cardene I.V. 2815
Cardizem CD Capsules (Infrequent) 1251
Cardizem SR Capsules (Infrequent) 1255
Cardizem Tablets (Infrequent) 1257
Cardura Tablets (Less than 0.5% of 3960 patients) 1993
Cartrol Tablets 413
Cataflam Tablets (Less than 1%) 833
Cipro I.V. (1% or less) 587
Cipro I.V. Pharmacy Bulk Package (Less than 1%) 590
Cipro Tablets (Less than 1%) 584
Climara Transdermal System 640
Clozaril Tablets 2377
Cognex Capsules (Infrequent) 1961
Covera-HS Tablets (Less than 2%) 2573
Cozaar Tablets (Less than 1%) 1668
Cytovene-IV (Two or more reports) 2270
DDAVP Injection (Rare) 2178
DDAVP Injection 15 mcg/mL (Rare) 2179
D.H.E. 45 Injection (Extremely rare) 2381
Demulen 2580
Desmopressin Acetate Injection (Rare) 996
Desogen Tablets 1867
Desyrel and Desyrel Dividose 504
Dilacor XR Extended-release Capsules 2183
Diprivan Injectable Emulsion (Less than 1%) 2939
DynaCirc Capsules (0.5% to 1%) 2381
DynaCirc CR Tablets (0.5% to 1.0%) 2383
Elavil 2945
▲ Emcyt Capsules (3%) 2085
Epogen for Injection (0.4%) 489
Estrace Cream and Tablets 751
Estraderm Transdermal System 842
ESTRATAB Tablets (0.3, 0.625, 1.25, 2.5 mg) 2715
Estratest 2718
Ethmozine Tablets (Less than 2%) 2217
Etrafon 2495
Flexeril Tablets (Rare) 1701
Fludara for Injection (Up to 3%) 658
Gemzar for Injection (2%) 1482
Glucophage Tablets 754
Helidac Therapy (Less than 1%) 2135
Heparin Lock Flush Solution 2831
Heparin Sodium Injection 2832
Heparin Sodium Vials 1486
Hydralazine Hydrochloride Injection USP 2712
Hyperstat I.V. Injection 2504
Hyzaar Tablets 1720
Idamycin Injection 2096
Imdur (Less than or equal to 5%) 1362
Imitrex Injection (Extremely rare) 1095
Imitrex Tablets (Rare) 1099
Isoptin Oral Tablets (Less than 1%) 1393
Isoptin SR Tablets (1% or less) 1395
Kerlone Tablets (Less than 2%) 2588
Lamictal Tablets (Rare) 1105
Levlen/Tri-Levlen 646
Limbitrol 2333
Lodine Capsules and Tablets (Less than 1%) 2849
Lo/Ovral Tablets 2852
Lo/Ovral-28 Tablets 2857
Lotrel Capsules (Rare) 858
Ludiomil Tablets (Isolated reports) 861
Lupron Injection (Less than 5%) 2736
LUVOX Tablets (Infrequent) 2723
Maxaquin Tablets (Less than 1%) 2593
Menest Tablets 2671
Merrem I.V. (0.1% to 1.0%) 2952
Methergine (Rare) 2401
Miacalcin Nasal Spray (Less than 1%) 2403
Modicon 1928
Monoket Tablets (Fewer than 1%) 2550
Mononine, Coagulation Factor IX (Human), Monoclonal Antibody Purified 804
Monopril Tablets (0.2% to 1.0%) 762
Naprelan Tablets (Less than 1%) 2861
Navelbine Injection (Rare) 1212
Neoral (Rare) 2405
Neupogen for Injection (11 of 375 cancer patients) 495
Neurontin Capsules (Rare) 1978
Nordette-21 Tablets 2863
Nordette-28 Tablets 2866
Norinyl 2563
Normodyne Injection 2519
Normodyne Tablets 2522
Noroxin Tablets (Less frequent) 1758
Noroxin Tablets (Less frequent) 2222
Norplant System 2868
Norpramin Tablets 1273
Nor-Q D Tablets 2598
Norvasc Tablets (Rare) 2020
Nuromax Injection (Less than or equal to 0.1%) 1136
Ogen Tablets 2103
Ogen Vaginal Cream 2106
Oncovin Solution Vials & Hyporets 1521
OptiPranolol (Metipranolol 0.3%) Sterile Ophthalmic

(▣ Described in PDR For Nonprescription Drugs) Incidence data in parenthesis; ▲ 3% or more (⊙ Described in PDR For Ophthalmology)

Myocardial infarction Side Effects Index 1402

Solution (A small number of patients) ⊙ 256
Ortho-Cept 1907
Ortho-Cyclen/Ortho-Tri-Cyclen 1914
Ortho Dienestrol Cream 1922
Ortho-Est 1925
Ortho-Novum 1928
Ortho-Cyclen/Ortho Tri-Cyclen 1914
Orthoclone OKT3 Sterile Solution 1892
Orudis Capsules (Rare) 2874
Oruvail Capsules (Rare) 2874
Ovcon 765
Ovral Tablets 2877
Ovral-28 Tablets 2878
Ovrette Tablets 2878
Pamelor 2409
Parlodel (9 cases) 2411
Paxil Tablets (Rare) 2681
Permax Tablets (1.1%) 571
Platinol for Injection (Rare) 717
Platinol-AQ Injection (Rare) 719
Plendil Extended-Release Tablets (0.5% to 1.5%) 514
PMB 200 and PMB 400 2890
Premarin Intravenous 2893
Premarin Tablets 2896
Premarin Vaginal Cream 2898
Premphase 2900
Prempro 2905
Prevacid Delayed-Release Capsules (Less than 1%) 2746
Prinivil Tablets (0.3% to 1.0%) 1776
Prinzide Tablets 1780
▲ Procardia Capsules (About 4%; rare; about 1 patient in 15) 2024
Procardia XL Extended Release Tablets (Rare) 2026
Procrit for Injection (0.4%) 1896
Proleukin for Injection (2%) 812
Prostin E2 Suppository (Two cases) 2109
Prozac Pulvules & Liquid, Oral Solution (Rare) 935
Redux Capsules 2911
Relafen Tablets (Less than 1%) 2688
Remeron Tablets (Infrequent) 1878
Rilutek Tablets (Infrequent) 2198
Risperdal Tablets (Infrequent) 1348
Roferon-A Injection (Rare to infrequent) 2308
Salagen Tablets (One patient) 1546
Sandimmune (Rare) 2416
Sinemet CR Tablets 961
Stimate, (desmopressin acetate) Nasal Spray, 1.5 mg/mL (Rare) 806
Sular Tablets (Less than or equal to 1%) 2961
Suprane (desflurane, USP) (Less than 1%) 1865
Surmontil Capsules 2917
Taxol Injection (Rare) 723
Tegretol/Tegretol-XR 870
Tenex Tablets (Rare) 2249
Tiazac Capsules 1019
Tofranil Ampuls 873
Tofranil Tablets 875
Tofranil-PM Capsules 876
Tonocard Tablets (Less than 1%) 519
Toprol-XL Tablets (Some cases) 560
▲ Trasylol (11%) 607
Triavil Tablets 1800
Levlen/Tri-Levlen 646
Tri-Norinyl 2607
Triostat Injection (Approximately 2%) 2708
Triphasil-21 Tablets 2919
Triphasil-28 Tablets 2924
Univasc Tablets (Less than 1%) 2553
Vascor Tablets (200 and 300 mg) (About 3% of patients) 1597
Vaseretic Tablets 1810
Vasotec I.V. (0.5 to 1%) 1814
Vasotec Tablets (0.5% to 1.2%) 1816
Velban Vials 1537
Verelan Capsules (1% or less) 1455
▲ Vesanoid Capsules (3%) 2327
Videx Tablets, Powder for Oral Solution, & Pediatric Powder for Oral Solution (Less than 1%) 2980
Vivactil Tablets 1820
Cataflam/Voltaren/Voltaren-XR (Less than 1%) 833
Wellbutrin Tablets (Rare) 1177
Zestoretic Tablets 2968
Zestril Tablets (0.3% to 1.0%) 2972
Zoladex (Greater than 1% but less than 5%) 2976
Zoladex 3-month 2978
Zoloft Tablets (Rare) 2051
Zosyn (1.0% or less) 1463

Myocardial infarction, post-abrupt discontinuation
Inderal (Some cases) 2834
Inderal LA Long Acting Capsules (Some cases) 2836
Tenoretic Tablets 2963
Tenormin Tablets and I.V. Injection 2965
Trandate 1158
Visken Tablets 2428

Myocardial insufficiency
Idamycin Injection 2096
Orthoclone OKT3 Sterile Solution 1892

Myocardial necrosis
Cytoxan 700

Myocardial rupture, following recent MI
Activase 1045
Cortone Acetate Sterile Suspension 1663
Cortone Acetate Tablets 1664
Dalalone D.P. Injectable 1009
Decadron Elixir 1676
Decadron Phosphate Injection 1680
Decadron Phosphate with Xylocaine Injection, Sterile 1683
Decadron Tablets 1678
Decadron-LA Sterile Suspension 1687
Dexacort Phosphate in Respihaler 1606
Dexacort Phosphate in Turbinaire 1607
Hydeltrasol Injection, Sterile 1708
Hydeltra-T.B.A. Sterile Suspension 1710
Hydrocortone Acetate Sterile Suspension 1712
Hydrocortone Phosphate Injection, Sterile 1713
Hydrocortone Tablets 1715

Myocarditis
Aldoclor Tablets 1638
Aldomet Ester HCl Injection 1642
Aldomet Oral 1640
Aldoril Tablets 1644
Asacol Delayed-Release Tablets (Rare) 2129
Cerubidine for Injection (Rare) 634
Clozaril Tablets 2377
Cytovene-IV (One report) 2270
Dipentum Capsules (One patient) 2084
Gantrisin 2286
Pentasa (Infrequent) 1275
Proleukin for Injection (Less than 1% to 1%) 812
Redux Capsules 2911
Risperdal Tablets (Rare) 1348
▲ Vesanoid Capsules (3%) 2327

Myocarditis, allergic
Azulfidine (Rare) 2059
Bactrim DS Tablets 2257
Bactrim I.V. Infusion 2255
Bactrim 2257
Fansidar Tablets 2281
Gantanol Tablets 2285
Pediazole Suspension 2340
Septra 1146
Septra I.V. Infusion 1142
Septra I.V. Infusion ADD-Vantage Vials 1144
Septra 1146

Myocarditis, hemorrhagic
Cytoxan 700

Myocardium, depression
Carbocaine Injection 2432
Decadron Phosphate with Xylocaine Injection, Sterile 1683
Marcaine 2446
Marcaine Spinal 2449
Nescaine/Nescaine MPF 549
Normodyne Tablets 2522
Novocain Hydrochloride for Spinal Anesthesia 2457
Pontocaine Hydrochloride for Spinal Anesthesia 2460
Sensorcaine 554

Myoclonia
Alfenta Injection 1334
▲ Anafranil Capsules (2% to 13%) 819
Cerebyx Injection (Infrequent) 1956
Chibroxin Sterile Ophthalmic Solution (With oral form) 1657
Cipro Tablets 584
Clozaril Tablets (1%) 2377
Diprivan Injectable Emulsion (Less than 1%) 2939
Duramorph Injection 983
Effexor (Infrequent) 2825
Eldepryl Capsules 2729
Imitrex Injection (Rare) 1095
Infumorph 200 and Infumorph 500 Sterile Solutions 985
Kadian Capsules (Less than 3%) 2948
Lamictal Tablets (Infrequent) 1105
LUVOX Tablets (Frequent) 2723
Nardil (Common) 1977
Neurontin Capsules (Rare) 1978
Noroxin Tablets 1758
Noroxin Tablets 2222
Orthoclone OKT3 Sterile Solution 1892
▲ Paxil Tablets (3%) 2681
Penetrex Tablets (0.1% to 1%) 2196
Permax Tablets (Infrequent) 571
Primaxin I.M. 1770
Primaxin I.V. (Less than 0.2%) 1772
▲ Prograf (Greater than 3%) 1028
Prozac Pulvules & Liquid, Oral Solution (2%) 935
Remeron Tablets (Rare) 1878
Revex (nalmefene hydrochloride injection) (Less than 1%) 1863
Rilutek Tablets (Infrequent) 2198
Serzone Tablets (Infrequent) 776
Wellbutrin Tablets (Frequent) 1177

Myoglobinemia
Anectine 1062
Symmetrel Capsules (Uncommon) 965
Symmetrel Syrup (Uncommon) 963

Myoglobinuria
Amicar Syrup, Tablets, and Injection 1312
Anectine 1062
Haldol Decanoate 1587
Lescol Capsules 2395
Orap Tablets 1037
Risperdal Tablets 1348
Zocor Tablets (Rare) 1821

Myopathy
Amicar Syrup, Tablets, and Injection 1312
Anafranil Capsules (Rare) 819
Atromid-S Capsules 2808
Betaseron for SC Injection 653
Cerebyx Injection (Infrequent) 1956
Cognex Capsules (Rare) 1961
Cortone Acetate Tablets 1664
Darvon-N/Darvocet-N 1473
Darvon 1475
Darvon-N Suspension & Tablets 1473
Foscavir Injection (Rare) 541
Hivid Tablets (Less than 1%) 2287
Hydeltrasol Injection, Sterile 1708
Intal Inhaler (Infrequent) 2185
Lescol Capsules (Occasional) 2395
Lopid Tablets (Occasional) 1974
LUVOX Tablets (Rare) 2723
Mevacor Tablets 1742
Normodyne Tablets (Less common) 2522
Paxil Tablets (2%) 2681
Pediapred Oral Solution 1618
Pravachol Tablets (Rare) 770
Redux Capsules 2911
ReoPro Vials (0.4%) 1526
Retrovir Capsules 1216
Retrovir I.V. Infusion 1221
Retrovir Syrup 1216
Rifadin (Rare) 1276
Rifater (Rare) 1280
Trandate Tablets (Less common) 1158
Videx Tablets, Powder for Oral Solution, & Pediatric Powder for Oral Solution (2% to 4%) 2980
Zocor Tablets 1821
Zyloprim Tablets (Less than 1%) 1194

Myopathy, steroid
Celestone Soluspan Suspension 2484
CORTENEMA 2713
Cortone Acetate Sterile Suspension 1663
Dalalone D.P. Injectable 1009
Decadron Elixir 1676
Decadron Phosphate Injection 1680
Decadron Phosphate with Xylocaine Injection, Sterile 1683
Decadron Tablets 1678
Decadron-LA Sterile Suspension 1687
Dexacort Phosphate in Respihaler 1606
Dexacort Phosphate in Turbinaire 1607
Florinef Acetate Tablets 506
Hydeltra-T.B.A. Sterile Suspension 1710
Hydrocortone Acetate Sterile Suspension 1712
Hydrocortone Phosphate Injection, Sterile 1713
Hydrocortone Tablets 1715
Prelone Syrup 1834

Myopia
Humorsol Sterile Ophthalmic Solution 1707
Isopto Carpine Ophthalmic Solution ⊙ 221
Neptazane Tablets ⊙ 320
Phospholine Iodide ⊙ 323
Pilopine HS Ophthalmic Gel ⊙ 224
Zarontin Capsules 1986
Zarontin Syrup 1986

Myopia, transient
Combipres Tablets (Occasional) 682
Diamox Intravenous ⊙ 317
Diamox Sequels (Sustained Release) ⊙ 318
Diamox Tablets ⊙ 317
GlaucTabs ⊙ 209
Trusopt Sterile Ophthalmic Solution 1803

Myosis
Etrafon 2495
Trilafon 2532

Myositis
Amicar Syrup, Tablets, and Injection 1312
Anafranil Capsules (Rare) 819
Atromid-S Capsules 2808
Betaseron for SC Injection 653
Doxil (Less than 1%) 2613
Foscavir Injection (Rare) 541
Hivid Tablets (Less than 1%) 2287
Imdur (Less than or equal to 5%) 1362
Inocor Lactate Injection (1 case) 2439
Lopid Tablets 1974
Mycobutin Capsules (Less than 1%; rare) 2101
Norvir (Less than 2%) 447
Paxil Tablets (Rare) 2681
Permax Tablets (Infrequent) 571
Prozac Pulvules & Liquid, Oral Solution (Rare) 935
Remeron Tablets (Rare) 1878
Retrovir Capsules 1216
Retrovir I.V. Infusion 1221
Retrovir Syrup 1216
Serevent Inhalation Aerosol (1% to 3%) 1149
Sular Tablets (Less than or equal to 1%) 2961
Ticlid Tablets (Rare) 2317
Vaseretic Tablets 1810
Vasotec I.V. 1814
Vasotec Tablets (0.5% to 1.0%) 1816
Vesanoid Capsules (Isolated cases) 2327
Videx Tablets, Powder for Oral Solution, & Pediatric Powder for Oral Solution (Less than 1%) 2980

Myxedema
Eskalith 2658
Lithium Carbonate Capsules & Tablets 2352
Lithonate/Lithotabs/Lithobid 2721
Quadrinal Tablets 1398
SSKI Solution 2767

N

Nails, changes
Accutane Capsules (Less than 1%) 2252
Blenoxane 697
BuSpar Tablets (Rare) 738
Cytoxan 700
Effexor (Infrequent) 2825
Ergamisol Tablets 1340
Fluorouracil Injection 2282
Sterile FUDR (Remote possibility) 2284
Hivid Tablets (Less than 1%) 2287
Intron A for Injection (Less than 5%) 2506
Lescol Capsules 2395
Lupron Depot 3.75 mg (Less than 5%) 2739
Mevacor Tablets 1742
Naprelan Tablets (Less than 1%) 2861
Oncaspar 2194
Pentasa (Less than 1%) 1275
Pravachol Tablets 770
Taxol Injection (Uncommon; 2%) 723
Taxotere for Injection Concentrate (2.6%) 2204
▲ Tegison Capsules (10-25%) 2314

(▣ Described in PDR For Nonprescription Drugs) Incidence data in parenthesis; ▲ 3% or more (⊙ Described in PDR For Ophthalmology)

Side Effects Index — Nausea

Nails, discoloration
- Teslac Tablets (Rare) ... 727
- Zocor Tablets ... 1821

Nails, discoloration
- Helidac Therapy (Rare) ... 2135
- Retrovir Capsules ... 1216
- Retrovir I.V. Infusion ... 1221
- Retrovir Syrup ... 1216

Nails, loss of
- Fluorouracil Injection ... 2282
- Sterile FUDR (Remote possibility) ... 2284

Nasal burning
- Atrovent Nasal Spray 0.03% (2.0%) ... 676
- Atrovent Nasal Spray 0.06% (Less than 1%) ... 678
- ▲ Beconase Inhalation Aerosol (11 in 100 patients) ... 1065
- Duration 12 Hour Nasal Spray ... ▣ 766
- ▲ Flonase Nasal Spray (3% to 6%) ... 1088
- Intal Inhaler (Rare) ... 2185
- Intal Nebulizer Solution ... 2186
- IOPIDINE Sterile Ophthalmic Solution ... ⊙ 218
- Nasacort Nasal Inhaler (Rare) ... 2189
- ▲ Nasalcrom Nasal Solution (1 in 25) ... 2192
- ▲ Nasalide Nasal Solution 0.025% (Approximately 45%) ... 2301
- ▲ Nasarel Nasal Solution (13% to 44%) ... 2302
- Neo-Synephrine Maximum Strength 12 Hour Nasal Spray ... ▣ 624
- Neo-Synephrine 12 Hour ... ▣ 624
- Neo-Synephrine ... ▣ 624
- Nicotrol NS Nicotine Nasal Spray (More common) ... 1565
- Rhinocort Nasal Inhaler (Rare) ... 552
- Vancenase AQ Double Strength Nasal Spray 0.084% (4% to 5%) ... 2536
- Vancenase PocketHaler Nasal Inhaler (11 per 100 patients) ... 2534
- Vicks Sinex Nasal Spray and Ultra Fine Mist ... ▣ 738

Nasal congestion
- ▲ Adalat Capsules (10 mg and 20 mg) (2% or less to 6%) ... 580
- Adenoscan (Less than 1%) ... 1022
- ▲ AeroBid Inhaler System (15%) ... 1004
- ▲ Aerobid-M Inhaler System (15%) ... 1004
- Airet Albuterol Sulfate Inhalation Solution (1%) ... 1602
- Albuterol Sulfate, USP Solution for Inhalation, Arm-a-Med (1%) ... 522
- Aldoclor Tablets ... 1638
- Aldomet Ester HCl Injection ... 1642
- Aldomet Oral ... 1640
- Aldoril Tablets ... 1644
- Amicar Syrup, Tablets, and Injection ... 1312
- Apresazide Capsules (Less frequent) ... 824
- Apresoline Hydrochloride Tablets (Less frequent) ... 826
- Asacol Delayed-Release Tablets ... 2129
- ▲ Atrovent Nasal Spray 0.03% (3.1%) ... 676
- Atrovent Nasal Spray 0.06% (1.1%) ... 678
- Axocet Capsules (Infrequent) ... 2469
- Azactam for Injection (Less than 1%) ... 736
- Bentyl ... 1246
- Betagan ... ⊙ 230
- Betimol 0.25%, 0.5% ... ⊙ 259
- Brevibloc (esmolol HCl) Injection (Less than 1%) ... 1860
- BuSpar Tablets (Frequent) ... 738
- Cardizem CD Capsules (Less than 1%) ... 1251
- Cardizem SR Capsules (Less than 1%) ... 1255
- Cardizem Injectable ... 1253
- Cardizem Tablets (Less than 1%) ... 1257
- Cartrol Tablets (1.1%) ... 413
- Caverject Injection (1%) ... 2064
- Cedax (0.1% to 1%) ... 2480
- Chemet Capsules (0.7% to 3.7%) ... 666
- Claritin Tablets (2% or fewer patients) ... 2485
- Claritin-D Tablets (Less frequent) ... 2487
- Clozaril Tablets (1%) ... 2377
- Compazine ... 2644
- Cozaar Tablets (2.0%) ... 1668
- DDAVP (Occasional) ... 2180
- Danocrine Capsules (Rare) ... 2437
- Demser Capsules (Infrequent) ... 1690
- Desmopressin Acetate Rhinal Tube (Occasional) ... 997
- Desyrel and Desyrel Dividose (2.8% to 5.7%) ... 504
- Dibenzyline Capsules ... 2650
- Diupres Tablets ... 1691
- DynaCirc CR Tablets (0.5% to 1.0%) ... 2383
- Esgic-plus Capsules (Infrequent) ... 1012
- Esgic-plus Tablets (Infrequent) ... 1012
- Esimil Tablets ... 840
- Etrafon ... 2495
- Fioricet Tablets (Infrequent) ... 2386
- Fioricet with Codeine Capsules (Infrequent) ... 2387
- Fiorinal with Codeine Capsules (Infrequent) ... 2390
- Flagyl 375 Capsules ... 2587
- Flagyl I.V. ... 2373
- Flonase Nasal Spray (Less than 1%) ... 1088
- ▲ Flovent (8% to 22%) ... 1089
- Helidac Therapy ... 2135
- Hydralazine Hydrochloride Injection USP ... 2712
- Hydropres Tablets ... 1718
- Hyskon Hysteroscopy Fluid (Rare) ... 1633
- ▲ Hytrin Capsules (0.6% to 5.9%) ... 434
- Hyzaar Tablets ... 1720
- Imdur (Less than or equal to 5%) ... 1362
- ▲ Intal Inhaler (Among most frequent) ... 2185
- Intal Nebulizer Solution (Rare) ... 2186
- ▲ Intron A for Injection (Up to 10%) ... 2506
- Ismelin Tablets ... 845
- Levoprome (Sometimes) ... 1321
- Limbitrol (Less common) ... 2333
- Lioresal Tablets ... 847
- Loxitane ... 1426
- Ludiomil Tablets (Rare) ... 861
- Methergine (Rare) ... 2401
- MetroGel-Vaginal ... 917
- ▲ Miacalcin Nasal Spray (10.6%) ... 2403
- Midamor Tablets (Less than or equal to 1%) ... 1746
- Minipress Capsules (1-4%) ... 2015
- Minizide Capsules ... 2016
- Moduretic Tablets (Less than or equal to 1%) ... 1748
- Nasalcrom Nasal Solution (Less than 1%) ... 2192
- Nasalide Nasal Solution 0.025% (5% or less) ... 2301
- Navane Capsules and Concentrate ... 2018
- Navane Intramuscular ... 2019
- Orlaam Oral Solution ... 2361
- Ornade Spansule Capsules ... 2678
- Orthoclone OKT3 Sterile Solution ... 1892
- Pentaspan Injection ... 954
- Periactin ... 1767
- Phrenilin (Infrequent) ... 790
- Prinivil Tablets (0.4%) ... 1776
- Prinzide Tablets (0.3% to 1%) ... 1780
- ▲ Procardia Capsules (2% or less to 6%) ... 2024
- ▲ Procardia XL Extended Release Tablets (6%) ... 2026
- Prolixin ... 510
- Protostat Tablets ... 1939
- Proventil Inhalation Solution 0.083% (1%) ... 2527
- Proventil Solution for Inhalation 0.5% (1%) ... 2525
- Prozac Pulvules & Liquid, Oral Solution (2.6%) ... 935
- Regitine Vials ... 864
- ReVia Tablets (Less than 1%) ... 957
- Robaxin Injectable ... 2245
- Robaxin Tablets ... 2246
- Sedapap Tablets 50 mg/650 mg (Infrequent) ... 1826
- Ser-Ap-Es Tablets ... 867
- ▲ Stadol (13%) ... 779
- Stelazine ... 2692
- Stimate, (desmopressin acetate) Nasal Spray, 1.5 mg/mL (Occasional) ... 806
- Tavist Syrup ... 2426
- Tavist Tablets ... 2427
- Tessalon Perles ... 1018
- Thorazine ... 2701
- Tiazac Capsules (Less than 1%) ... 1019
- Timoptic in Ocudose (Less frequent) ... 1796
- Timoptic Sterile Ophthalmic Solution (Less frequent) ... 1794
- Timoptic-XE ... 1798
- Trental Tablets (Less than 1%) ... 1291
- Trilafon (Occasional) ... 2532
- Vaqta (1.1%) ... 1805
- Ventolin Inhalation Solution (1%) ... 1171
- Ventolin Nebules Inhalation Solution (1%) ... 1172
- Ventolin Rotacaps for Inhalation (2%) ... 1173
- ▲ Xanax Tablets (7.3% to 17.4%) ... 2115
- Zestoretic Tablets (0.3 to 1%) ... 2968
- Zestril Tablets (0.4%) ... 2972

Nasal discharge, increase
- Aredia for Injection (One patient) ... 827
- ▲ Flovent (4% to 16%) ... 1089
- Hivid Tablets (Less than 1%) ... 2287
- IOPIDINE Sterile Ophthalmic Solution (0.45%) ... ⊙ 218
- ▲ Miacalcin Nasal Spray (10.6%) ... 2403
- Neo-Synephrine Maximum Strength 12 Hour Nasal Spray ... ▣ 624
- Neo-Synephrine 12 Hour ... ▣ 624
- Neo-Synephrine ... ▣ 624
- Vicks Sinex Nasal Spray and Ultra Fine Mist ... ▣ 738

Nasal drainage
- Alferon N Injection (2%) ... 2142

Nasal drip, posterior
- ▲ Atrovent Nasal Spray 0.03% (3.1%) ... 676

Nasal itching
(see under Pruritus, rhinal)

Nasal mucosa, dryness
(see under Xeromycteria)

Nasal septum, perforation
- Beconase (Rare) ... 1065
- Dexacort Phosphate in Turbinaire ... 1607
- Nasacort AQ Nasal Spray (One patient) ... 2191
- Nasacort Nasal Inhaler (Rare) ... 2189
- Nasalide Nasal Solution 0.025% (Rare) ... 2301
- Nasarel Nasal Solution (Rare) ... 2302
- Rhinocort Nasal Inhaler (Less than 1%) ... 552
- Vancenase AQ Nasal Spray 0.042% (Extremely rare) ... 2535
- Vancenase AQ Double Strength Nasal Spray 0.084% (Rare) ... 2536
- Vancenase PocketHaler Nasal Inhaler (Extremely rare) ... 2534

Nasal stinging
- Duration 12 Hour Nasal Spray ... ▣ 766
- Nasacort Nasal Inhaler (Rare) ... 2189
- ▲ Nasalcrom Nasal Solution (1 in 20) ... 2192
- ▲ Nasarel Nasal Solution (13% to 44%) ... 2302
- Neo-Synephrine Maximum Strength 12 Hour Nasal Spray ... ▣ 624
- Neo-Synephrine 12 Hour ... ▣ 624
- Neo-Synephrine ... ▣ 624
- 12 Hour Nostrilla ... ▣ 660
- Otrivin ... ▣ 662
- Vicks Sinex Nasal Spray and Ultra Fine Mist ... ▣ 738

Nasal stuffiness
- Asendin Tablets (Less than 1%) ... 1419
- Beconase AQ Nasal Spray (Fewer than 3 per 100 patients) ... 1065
- Benadryl Injection ... 1955
- Bentyl ... 1246
- Loxitane ... 1426
- Mellaril ... 2398
- ▲ Normodyne Injection (1% to 6%) ... 2519
- ▲ Normodyne Tablets (1% to 6%) ... 2522
- PBZ Tablets ... 863
- PBZ-SR Tablets ... 862
- ▲ Parlodel (3% to 4%) ... 2411
- Phenergan Injection ... 2880
- Phenergan Tablets ... 2882
- Serentil ... 689
- ▲ Trandate Tablets (1% to 6%) ... 1158
- Trinalin Repetabs Tablets ... 1373
- Tussend ... 1830
- Vancenase AQ Nasal Spray 0.042% (Fewer than 3 per 100 patients) ... 2535

Nasal ulceration
- Beconase (Rare) ... 1065
- Flonase Nasal Spray (Less than 1%) ... 1088
- Nasarel Nasal Solution (1% or less) ... 2302
- Nicotrol NS Nicotine Nasal Spray (More common) ... 1565

Nasal Spray 0.084% (Rare) (Vancenase AQ Double Strength) ... 2536
Vancenase PocketHaler Nasal Inhaler (Rare) ... 2534

Nasolacrimal canals, obstruction
- Humorsol Sterile Ophthalmic Solution ... 1707
- Phospholine Iodide ... ⊙ 323

Nasopharyngitis
- Hivid Tablets (Less than 1%) ... 2287
- Nalfon 200 Pulvules & Nalfon Tablets (1.2%) ... 933
- ▲ Serevent Inhalation Aerosol (14%) ... 1149

Nausea
- Abbokinase ... 403
- Abbokinase Open-Cath ... 405
- ▲ Abelcet Injection (6% to 8%) ... 1540
- Accupril Tablets (1.4% to 2.4%) ... 1950
- Accutane Capsules ... 2252
- Achromycin V Capsules (Rare) ... 1417
- ▲ Actigall Capsules (14.2%) ... 818
- ▲ Actimmune (10%) ... 1043
- Activase ... 1045
- ▲ Adalat Capsules (10 mg and 20 mg) (About 10% to 11%) ... 580
- Adalat CC (2%) ... 582
- Adapin Capsules ... 1542
- ▲ Adenocard Injection (3%) ... 1021
- ▲ Adriamycin PFS (Frequent) ... 2056
- ▲ Adriamycin RDF (Frequent) ... 2056
- ▲ AeroBid Inhaler System (25%) ... 1004
- ▲ Aerobid-M Inhaler System (25%) ... 1004
- Aerolate ... 1003
- ▲ Airet Albuterol Sulfate Inhalation Solution (3.1% to 4%) ... 1602
- AK-FLUOR Injection 10% and 25% ... ⊙ 204
- Albalon Solution with Liquifilm ... ⊙ 229
- ▲ Albenza Tablets (3.7% to 6.2%) ... 2629
- Albuminar-5, Albumin (Human) U.S.P. 5% (Occasional) ... 795
- Albuminar-25, Albumin (Human) U.S.P. 25% ... 796
- ▲ Albuterol Sulfate, USP Solution for Inhalation, Arm-a-Med (3.1% to 4%) ... 522
- Aldactazide Tablets ... 2556
- Aldoclor Tablets ... 1638
- Aldomet Ester HCl Injection ... 1642
- Aldomet Oral ... 1640
- Aldoril Tablets ... 1644
- ▲ Alfenta Injection (28%) ... 1334
- ▲ Alferon N Injection (4% to 48%) ... 2142
- Alka-Seltzer Cherry Effervescent Antacid and Pain Reliever (7.6% at doses of 1000 mg/day) ... ▣ 609
- Alka-Seltzer Lemon Lime Effervescent Antacid and Pain Reliever (7.6% at doses of 1000 mg/day) ... ▣ 609
- Alka-Seltzer Original Effervescent Antacid and Pain Reliever (7.6% at doses of 1000 mg/day) ... ▣ 609
- Alkeran for Injection ... 1196
- Alkeran Tablets (Infrequent) ... 1198
- Alomide Ophthalmic Solution (Less than 1%) ... 465
- Altace Capsules (Less than 1% to 2.2%) ... 1238
- Alupent (1% to 4%) ... 672
- Amaryl Tablets (1.1%) ... 1241
- ▲ Ambien Tablets (2% to 6%) ... 2559
- Amen Tablets (Rare) ... 785
- Amicar Syrup, Tablets, and Injection ... 1312
- Amikacin Sulfate Injection, USP (Rare) ... 523
- Amikacin Sulfate Injection, USP (Rare) ... 981
- Amikin Injectable (Rare) ... 502
- Aminohippurate Sodium Injection ... 1646
- Amoxil ... 2631
- ▲ Anafranil Capsules (9% to 33%) ... 819
- Ana-Kit Anaphylaxis Emergency Treatment Kit (Common) ... 611
- ▲ Anaprox/Naprosyn (3% to 9%) ... 2277
- Ancef Injection (Rare) ... 2632
- Ancobon Capsules ... 2254
- Androderm Testosterone Transdermal System ... 2634
- ▲ Android Capsules, 10 mg (Among most common) ... 1297
- Antabuse Tablets ... 2802
- Antilirium Injectable ... 1007
- Antivenin (Crotalidae) Polyvalent ... 2803
- Apresazide Capsules (Common) ... 824

(▣ Described in PDR For Nonprescription Drugs) Incidence data in parentheses; ▲ 3% or more (⊙ Described in PDR For Ophthalmology)

Nausea Side Effects Index 1404

Apresoline Hydrochloride Tablets (Common) 826
Aralen Hydrochloride Injection 2430
Aralen Phosphate Tablets 2431
▲ Aredia for Injection (Up to 26.6%) 827
▲ Arimidex Tablets (15.6% to 19.5%) 2932
▲ Artane (30% to 50%) 1418
▲ Asacol Delayed-Release Tablets (13%) 2129
▲ Regular Strength Ascriptin Tablets (7.6%) ▣ 650
Asendin Tablets (Less frequent) 1419
Astramorph/PF Injection, USP (Preservative-Free) (Frequent) 526
Atamet Tablets (Common) 567
Ativan Injection (Occasional) 2805
Ativan Tablets (Less frequent) 2807
▲ Atretol Tablets (Among most frequent) 569
Atrohist Pediatric Capsules 1603
Atrohist Plus Tablets 1605
▲ Atromid-S Capsules (Most common) 2808
Atrovent Inhalation Aerosol (2.8%) 674
▲ Atrovent Inhalation Solution (4.1%) 675
Atrovent Nasal Spray 0.03% (2.2%) 676
▲ Augmentin (3%) 2637
▲ Augmentin Tablets (3%) 2640
▲ Avonex (33%) 662
▲ Axid Pulvules (1.2% to 5.4%) 1468
▲ Axocet Capsules (Among most frequent) 2469
Azactam for Injection (1 to 1.3%) 736
▲ Azathioprine Tablets (Approximately 12%) 2349
▲ Azulfidine (Approximately one-third of patients) 2059
▲ Bactrim DS Tablets (Among most common) 2257
▲ Bactrim I.V. Infusion (Among most common) 2255
▲ Bactrim (Among most common) 2257
Bactroban Nasal (Less than 1%) 2643
Bactroban Ointment (Less than 1%) 2642
▲ Genuine Bayer Aspirin Tablets & Caplets (7.6% at doses of 1000 mg/day) ▣ 618
▲ Aspirin Regimen Bayer Regular Strength 325 mg Caplets (7.6% of 4500 people tested) ▣ 613
Beconase AQ Nasal Spray (Fewer than 5 in 100 patients) 1065
Benadryl Injection 1955
Benemid Tablets 1651
▲ Bentyl (14%) 1246
Betagan ⊚ 230
▲ Betapace Tablets (5% to 10%) 637
Betaseron for SC Injection 653
Betimol 0.25%, 0.5% (1% to 5%) ⊚ 259
Biavax II 1653
▲ Biaxin (3%) 406
BiCNU (Frequent) 696
Biltricide Tablets 584
Bioclate, Antihemophilic Factor (Recombinant) (Extremely rare; one patient out of 13,394) 797
Blocadren Tablets (0.6%) 1654
Bontril Slow-Release Capsules 786
Brethaire Inhaler 830
Brethine Ampuls (1.3 to 3.9%) 832
Brethine Tablets 831
▲ Brevibloc (esmolol HCl) Injection (7%) 1860
Brevicon 2563
Bricanyl Subcutaneous Injection 1247
Bricanyl Tablets 1248
Bromfed 1832
▲ Bromfed-DM Cough Syrup (Among most frequent) 1832
Bromfed-PD Capsules (Extended-Release) 1832
Bronkometer Aerosol 2432
Bronkosol Solution 2432
Brontex 2130
▲ Bufferin Analgesic Tablets (7.6%) ▣ 636
Bumex (0.6%) 2260
▲ Buprenex Injectable (5-10%) 2170
▲ BuSpar Tablets (8%) 738
Butisol Sodium Elixir & Tablets (Less than 1 in 100) 2768
Cafergot 2376
Calan SR Caplets (2.7%) 2571
Calan Tablets (2.7%) 2568
Calcijex Injection 412
▲ Calcimar Injection, Synthetic (About 10%) 2176
Capoten Tablets (About 0.5 to 2%) 740
Capozide Tablets (0.5 to 2%) 744
Carafate Suspension (Less than 0.5%) 1250
Carafate Tablets (Less than 0.5%) 1249
Carbocaine Injection 2432
Cardene Capsules (1.9% to 2.2%) 2261
▲ Cardene I.V. (4.9%) 2815
Cardene SR Capsules (1.9%) 2264
▲ Cardioquin Tablets (Among most frequent) 2146
Cardizem CD Capsules (1.4%) 1251
Cardizem SR Capsules (1.3% to 1.6%) 1255
Cardizem Injectable (Less than 1%) 1253
Cardizem Tablets (1.9%) 1257
Cardura Tablets (1.5% to 3%) 1993
Carnitor Injection (Less frequent) 2623
Carnitor Tablets and Solution 2624
Cartrol Tablets (2.1%) 413
▲ Casodex Tablets (11%) 2934
▲ Cataflam Tablets (3% to 9%) 833
▲ Catapres Tablets (About 5 in 100 patients) 679
Catapres-TTS (1 of 101 patients) 680
Caverject Injection (Less than 1%) 2064
Ceclor Pulvules & Suspension (Rare) 1470
▲ Cedax (4%) 2480
CeeNU Capsules 699
Cefizox for Intramuscular or Intravenous Use (Occasional) 1025
Cefobid Intravenous/Intramuscular (Rare) 1996
Cefobid Pharmacy Bulk Package - Not for Direct Infusion (Rare) 1999
Cefotan (1 in 700) 2936
▲ Ceftin (2.6% to 6.7%) 1067
▲ Cefzil Tablets and Oral Suspension (3.5%) 747
▲ CellCept Capsules (19.9% to 23.6%) 2265
Celontin Kapseals (Frequent) 1955
Ceptaz (One in 156 patients) 1070
▲ Cerebyx Injection (4.5% to 8.9%) 1956
Ceredase 1055
Cerezyme (One patient) 1056
Cerubidine for Injection 634
Cervidil (Less than 1%) 1008
▲ Chemet Capsules (12.0% to 20.9%) 666
Chloromycetin Sodium Succinate 1960
Chromagen Capsules 2470
Chromagen FA 2471
Chromagen Forte 2471
Ciloxan Ophthalmic Solution (Less than 1%) 468
▲ Cipro I.V. (Among most frequent) 587
▲ Cipro I.V. Pharmacy Bulk Package (Among most frequent) 590
▲ Cipro Tablets (5.2%) 584
Claforan Sterile and Injection (1.4%; rare) 1259
Claritin Tablets (2% or fewer patients) 2485
▲ Claritin-D Tablets (3%) 2487
Cleocin Phosphate Injection 2068
Climara Transdermal System 640
Cleocin Vaginal Cream (Less than 1%) 2070
▲ Clinoril Tablets (3% to 9%) 1658
Clomid (2.2%) 1262
▲ Clozaril Tablets (5% or more) 2377
Codiclear DH Syrup 808
Cogentin 1661
▲ Cognex Capsules (28%) 1961
Colace Capsules, Syrup, Liquid 2212
ColBENEMID Tablets 1662
Colestid (Less frequent) 2073
▲ Colyte and Colyte-flavored (Among most frequent) 2540
▲ Combipres Tablets (About 5%) 682
Compazine 2644
▲ Cordarone Intravenous (3.9%) 2821
▲ Cordarone Tablets (10 to 33%) 2818
Cortone Acetate Sterile Suspension 1663
Cortone Acetate Tablets 1664
Corvert Injection (1.9%) 2075
Cosmegen Injection (Common) 1666
Coumadin (Infrequent) 941
Covera-HS Tablets (2.1% to 2.7%) 2573
Cozaar Tablets (1% or greater) 1668
▲ Creon (Among most frequent) 2714
▲ Crixivan Capsules (11.7%) 1670
Crystodigin Tablets 1472
Cuprimine Capsules (Greater than 1%) 1673
Cycrin Tablets 991
Cylert Tablets 415
▲ Cytadren Tablets (1 in 8) 837
CytoGam (Less than 5.0%) 1630
▲ Cytosar-U Sterile Powder (Among most frequent) 2077
▲ Cytotec (3.2%) 2576
▲ Cytovene (26%) 2270
Cytoxan (Common) 700
DDAVP Injection (Infrequent) 2178
DDAVP Injection 15 mcg/mL (Infrequent) 2179
DDAVP (Up to 2%) 2180
DDAVP Tablets 2182
▲ DHCplus Capsules (Among most frequent) 2148
D.H.E. 45 Injection 2381
▲ DTIC-Dome (90% with the initial few doses) 593
Dalalone D.P. Injectable 1009
▲ Dalgan Injection (3 to 9%) 529
Dalmane Capsules 2329
Danocrine Capsules 2437
Dantrium Capsules (Less frequent) 2131
Dapsone Tablets USP 1331
▲ Daranide Tablets (Among the most common effects) 1676
▲ Darvon-N/Darvocet-N (Among most frequent) 1473
▲ Darvon (Among most frequent) 1475
▲ Darvon-N Suspension & Tablets (Among most frequent) 1473
▲ DaunoXome (3% to 51%) 1842
▲ Daypro Caplets (3% to 9%) 2578
Decadron Elixir 1676
Decadron Phosphate Injection 1680
Decadron Phosphate with Xylocaine Injection, Sterile 1683
Decadron Tablets 1678
Decadron-LA Sterile Suspension 1687
Declomycin Tablets 1421
Deconsal II Tablets 1605
Demadex Tablets and Injection (1.8%) 691
▲ Demerol (Among most frequent) 2438
Demser Capsules (Infrequent) 1690
▲ Demulen (Among most common) 2580
▲ Depakene (Among most common) 416
▲ Depakote Tablets (22% to 31%) 418
▲ Depen Titratable Tablets (17%) 2770
Depo-Provera Contraceptive Injection (1% to 5%) 2079
Depo-Provera Sterile Aqueous Suspension 2083
Desmopressin Acetate Injection (Infrequent) 996
Desmopressin Acetate Rhinal Tube (Up to 2%) 997
Desogen Tablets 1867
▲ Desyrel and Desyrel Dividose (9.9% to 12.7%) 504
Dexacort Phosphate in Respihaler 1606
Dexacort Phosphate in Turbinaire 1607
DiaBeta Tablets (1.8%) 1265
▲ Diabinese Tablets (Less than 5%) 2002
Diamox Intravenous ⊚ 317
Diamox Sequels (Sustained Release) ⊚ 318
Diamox Tablets ⊚ 317
▲ Didronel Tablets (About 1 patient in 15; possibly 2 or 3 in 10) 2133
Diethylstilbestrol Tablets 1477
▲ Diflucan Tablets, Injection, and Oral Suspension (2% to 7%) 2003
Dilacor XR Extended-release Capsules (1.7% to 2.2%) 2183
Dilantin Infatabs 1967
Dilantin Kapseals 1965
Dilantin-125 Suspension 1969
Dilaudid Ampules 1382
Dilaudid Cough Syrup 1383
▲ Dilaudid-HP Injection (Among most frequent) 1384
▲ Dilaudid-HP Lyophilized Powder 250 mg (Among most frequent) 1384
Dilaudid 1382
Dilaudid Oral Liquid 1386
Dilaudid 1382
Dilaudid Tablets - 8 mg 1386
Dimetane-DC Cough Syrup 2232
Dimetane-DX Cough Syrup 2233
▲ Dipentum Capsules (5.0%) 2084
Diprivan Injectable Emulsion (Less than 1%) 2939
▲ Disalcid (Among most common) 1549
Ditropan 1267
Diucardin Tablets 2824
Diupres Tablets 1691
Diuril Oral Suspension 1694
Diuril Sodium Intravenous 1693
Diuril Tablets 1694
Dizac (diazepam injectable emulsion) CIV (Less frequent) 1862
Dobutrex Solution Vials (1% to 3%) 1480
▲ Dolobid Tablets (3% to 9%) 1695
Donnatal 2234
Donnatal Extentabs 2234
Donnatal Tablets 2234
Dopram Injectable 2235
Doral Tablets 2773
Doryx Capsules 1970
▲ Doxil (16.9% to 18.2%) 2613
Doxorubicin Astra (Frequent) 531
DUPHALAC Solution 2714
▲ Duragesic Transdermal System (10% or more) 1336
Duramorph Injection (Frequent) 983
Duratuss HD Elixir 2750
Dura-Vent Tablets 971
Duricef Capsules, Tablets, and Oral Suspension (Rare) 750
Dyazide Capsules 2653
▲ Dynabac (8.3%) 668
DYNACIN Capsules 1627
▲ DynaCirc Capsules (1.0% to 5.1%) 2381
DynaCirc CR Tablets (1.2%) 2383
Dyrenium Capsules (Rare) 2655
E.E.S. 427
E-Mycin Tablets (Infrequent) 1388
Easprin 1971
▲ EC-Naprosyn Delayed-Release Tablets (3% to 9%) 2277
▲ Ecotrin (7.6% at 1000 mg/day) 2625
Edecrin 1698
▲ Effexor (6% to 58.0%) 2825
Elavil 2945
▲ Eldepryl Capsules (10 of 49 patients) 2729
Elspar 1700
▲ Emcyt Capsules (15%) 2085
Emete-con Intramuscular/Intravenous 2007
▲ Eminase (Less than 10%) 2215
Enduron Tablets 424
Engerix-B Unit-Dose Vials (Less than 1%) 2656
Ensure Plus High Calorie Complete Nutrition 2338
Entex LA Tablets 972
Entex PSE Tablets 973
EpiPen Jr.- Epinephrine Auto-Injector 808
▲ Epivir (13% to 33%) 1200
▲ Epogen for Injection (0.26% to 17%) 489
▲ Ergamisol Tablets (22% to 65%) 1340
▲ Ergomar Tablets (Up to 10%) 1543
▲ ERYC (Among most frequent) 1972
▲ EryPed (Among most frequent) 425
▲ Ery-Tab Tablets (Among most frequent) 426
▲ Erythrocin Stearate Filmtab (Among most frequent) 429
▲ Erythromycin Base Filmtab (Among most frequent) 430
▲ Erythromycin Delayed-Release Capsules, USP (Among most frequent) 431
▲ Esgic-plus Capsules (Among most frequent) 1012
▲ Esgic-plus Tablets (Among most frequent) 1012
Esidrix Tablets 839
Esimil Tablets 840
Eskalith 2658
Estrace Cream and Tablets 751
Estraderm Transdermal System 842
ESTRATAB Tablets (0.3, 0.625, 1.25, 2.5 mg) 2715
Estratest 2718
▲ Estring Vaginal Ring (3%) 2086
▲ Ethmozine Tablets (6.9% to 9.6%) 2217
Ethyol (amifostine) for Injection (Frequent) 485
▲ Etopophos for Injection (3% to 43%) 701
▲ Etoposide Injection (31% to 43%) 539
Etrafon 2495
▲ Eulexin Capsules (9% to 11%) 2498
Exgest LA Tablets 787
Factrel (Rare) 2996
▲ Famvir Tablets (Among most frequent; 10.0% to 12.5%) 2660
Fansidar Tablets 2281
Fedahist Gyrocaps 2545
▲ Felbatol (Among most common; 6.5% to 34.2%) 2774

(▣ Described in PDR For Nonprescription Drugs) Incidence data in parenthesis; ▲ 3% or more (⊚ Described in PDR For Ophthalmology)

▲ Feldene Capsules (3% to 9%) 2008
Feosol Caplets 2626
Feosol Elixir (Occasional) 2627
Feosol Tablets (Occasional) 2627
▲ Fioricet Tablets (Among most frequent) 2386
Fioricet with Codeine Capsules (Frequent) 2387
Fiorinal Capsules (Less frequent) 2388
▲ Fiorinal with Codeine Capsules (3.7%) 2390
Fiorinal Tablets (Less frequent) 2388
▲ Flagyl 375 Capsules (About 12%) 2587
Flagyl I.V. 2373
Flexeril Tablets (1% to 3%) 1701
▲ Flolan for Injection (32% to 67%) 1085
Flonase Nasal Spray (Less than 1%) 1088
▲ Flovent (1% to 22%) 1089
▲ Floxin I.V. (3% to 10%) 1580
▲ Floxin Tablets (200 mg, 300 mg, 400 mg) (3% to 10%) 1577
▲ Fludara for Injection (31% to 36%) 658
Flumadine Tablets & Syrup (2.8%) 1013
Fluorescite .... ⊙ 217
Fluorouracil Injection (Common) 2282
Fluothane 2830
Fortaz (1 in 156 patients) 1092
▲ Fosamax Tablets (3.6%) 1703
▲ Foscavir Injection (5% or greater up to 47%) 541
▲ Sterile FUDR (Among more common) 2284
Fulvicin P/G Tablets (Occasional) .. 2499
Fulvicin P/G 165 & 330 Tablets (Occasional) 2500
▲ Fungizone Intravenous (Among most common) 507
Fungizone Oral Suspension 704
Furoxone (Occasional) 2221
Gamimune N, 5% Immune Globulin Intravenous (Human), 5% 612
Gamimune N, 10% Immune Globulin Intravenous (Human), 10% 615
Gammagard S/D, Immune Globulin, Intravenous (Human) (Occasional) 577
Gammar-P I.V., Immune Globulin Intravenous (Human) 798
Ganite 2711
Gantanol Tablets 2285
Gantrisin 2286
Garamycin Injectable 2502
▲ Gastrocrom Capsules (3 of 87 patients) 1611
▲ Gastrocrom Oral Concentrate (3 of 87 patients) 1611
▲ Gemzar for Injection (58% to 71%) 1482
Genotropin Injection (A small number of patients) 2090
Geocillin Tablets 2009
Geref (sermorelin acetate for injection) 2995
GlaucTabs .... ⊙ 209
Glucagon for Injection Vials and Emergency Kit (Occasional) 1485
▲ Glucophage Tablets (Among most common) 754
Glucotrol Tablets (1 in 70) 2011
Glucotrol XL Extended Release Tablets (Less than 3%) 2012
Glynase PresTab Tablets (1.8%) 2091
▲ GoLYTELY (Up to 50%) 694
Grifulvin V (griseofulvin tablets) Microsize (griseofulvin oral suspension) Microsize (Occasional) 1944
Gris-PEG Tablets, 125 mg & 250 mg (Occasional) 476
Guaifed 1833
Guaimax-D Tablets 809
▲ Habitrol Nicotine Transdermal System (3% to 9% of patients) .. 884
▲ Halcion Tablets (4.6%) 2093
Haldol Decanoate 1587
Haldol Injection, Tablets and Concentrate 1585
▲ Halfprin Tablets (7.6%) 1413
Halotestin Tablets 2095
▲ Havrix (1% to 10%) 2663
▲ Helidac Therapy (10.2% to approximately 12%) 2135
Heparin Lock Flush Solution 2831
Heparin Sodium Injection 2832
Heparin Sodium Vials (Rare) 1486
▲ Hexalen Capsules (1% to 33%) 2760
Helixate, Antihemophilic Factor (Recombinant) 799
Hismanal Tablets (2.5%) 1341
▲ Histussin D Liquid (Among most frequent) 670
Hivid Tablets (Less than 1% to 3.4%) 2287
Humatrope Vials (A small number of patients) 1490
Humegon for Injection 1873
Humorsol Sterile Ophthalmic Solution (Rare) 1707
▲ Hycamtin for Injection (Less than 1% to 77%) 2665
Hycodan Tablets and Syrup 946
Hycomine Compound Tablets 948
Hycomine 947
Hycotuss Expectorant Syrup 950
Hydeltrasol Injection, Sterile 1708
Hydeltra-T.B.A. Sterile Suspension 1710
Hydergine 2392
Hydralazine Hydrochloride Injection USP (Common) 2712
Hydrea Capsules (Less frequent) 705
Hydrocet Capsules 787
Hydrocortone Acetate Sterile Suspension 1712
Hydrocortone Phosphate Injection, Sterile 1713
Hydrocortone Tablets 1715
HydroDIURIL Tablets 1716
Hydropres Tablets 1718
▲ Hylorel Tablets (3.9%) 1613
▲ Hyperstat I.V. Injection (4%) 2504
Hyskon Hysteroscopy Fluid (Rare) .. 1633
▲ Hytrin Capsules (0.5% to 4.4%) 434
Hyzaar Tablets (1% or greater) 1720
▲ IBU Tablets (3% to 9%) 1389
▲ Idamycin Injection (82%) 2096
▲ IFEX (58%) 706
Ilosone (Infrequent) 927
Imdur (Less than or equal to 5%) .. 1362
▲ Imitrex Injection (4%) 1095
Imitrex Tablets 1099
Imodium Capsules 1343
▲ Imovax Rabies Vaccine (Up to 6%) 899
▲ Imuran (Approximately 12%) 1103
Inderal 2834
Inderal LA Long Acting Capsules 2836
Inderide Tablets 2838
Inderide LA Long Acting Capsules .. 2840
▲ Indocin (3% to 9%) 1723
INFeD (Iron Dextran Injection, USP) 2478
Infumorph 200 and Infumorph 500 Sterile Solutions 985
Inocor Lactate Injection (1.7%) 2439
Intal Inhaler (Infrequent) 2185
Intal Nebulizer Solution (Rare) 2186
▲ Intron A for Injection (1% to 66%) 2506
Inversine Tablets 1729
Invirase Capsules (1.9%) 2291
Iopidine 0.5% (Less than 1%) .... ⊙ 219
Ismelin Tablets 845
Ismo Tablets (2% to 4%) 2844
ISMOTIC 45% w/v Solution .... ⊙ 221
Isoetharine Inhalation Solution, USP, Arm-a-Med 545
Isoptin Injectable (0.9%) 1391
Isoptin Oral Tablets (2.7%) 1393
Isoptin SR Tablets (2.7%) 1395
Isuprel Hydrochloride Solution 2443
Isuprel Mistometer 2442
▲ JE-VAX (Approximately 10%) 904
K-Dur Microburst Release System (potassium chloride, USP) E.R. Tablets 1364
▲ K-Lor Powder Packets (Among most common) 438
▲ K-Norm Capsules (Among most common) 1615
K-Phos Neutral Tablets 633
K-Phos Original Formula 'Sodium Free' Tablets 633
▲ K-Tab Filmtab (Most common) 439
▲ Kadian Capsules (Among most frequent) 2948
Kayexalate 2444
Keflex Pulvules & Oral Suspension (Rare) 930
Keftab Tablets (Rare) 931
Kefurox Vials, Faspak & ADD-Vantage (1 in 440) 1509
Kefzol Vials, Faspak & ADD-Vantage (Rare) 1511
Kemadrin Tablets 1105
▲ Kerlone Tablets (1.6% to 5.8%) 2588
Klonopin Tablets 2294
KOGENATE Antihemophilic Factor (Recombinant) 626
Ku-Zyme HP Capsules 2547
▲ Kytril Tablets (15%) 2669
▲ Lamictal Tablets (Among most common; 18% to 25%) 1105
Lamisil Tablets (2.6%) 2394
▲ Lamprene Capsules (40-50%) 846
Lanoxicaps (Common) 1110
Lanoxin Elixir Pediatric 1113
Lanoxin Injection (Common) 1116
Lanoxin Injection Pediatric 1119
Lanoxin Tablets (Common) 1121
▲ Lariam Tablets (Among most frequent) 2295
Larodopa Tablets (Relatively frequent) 2296
Lasix Injection, Oral Solution and Tablets 1267
▲ Lescol Capsules (3.2%) 2395
▲ Leucovorin Calcium for Injection (6% to 74%) 1313
Leukeran Tablets (Infrequent) 1205
▲ Leukine (58% to 90%) 1317
▲ Leustatin (28%) 1889
▲ Levatol Tablets (4.3%) 2547
Levbid Extended-Release Tablets 2549
Levlen/Tri-Levlen 646
Levo-Dromoran 2297
Levoprome (Sometimes) 1321
Levsin/Levsinex/Levbid 2549
Librax Capsules (Infrequent) 2330
Librium Capsules (Isolated cases) .. 2331
Librium Injectable (Isolated cases) 2332
Limbitrol 2333
▲ Lioresal Intrathecal (1.4% to 10.5%) 1634
▲ Lioresal Tablets (4% to 12%) 847
Lithium Carbonate Capsules & Tablets 2352
Lithonate/Lithotabs/Lithobid 2721
Livostin (Approximately 1% to 3%) .... ⊙ 262
▲ Lodine Capsules and Tablets (3% to 9%) 2849
Lomotil 2591
▲ Lo/Ovral Tablets (10% or less) 2852
▲ Lo/Ovral-28 Tablets (10% or less) 2857
Lopid Tablets (2.5%) 1974
Lopressor (1%) 848
Lopressor HCT Tablets (1 in 100 patients) 850
Lorabid Suspension and Pulvules (Up to 2.5%) 1513
▲ Lorcet 10/650 Tablets (Among most frequent) 1016
▲ Lortab (Among most frequent) 2751
Lotensin Tablets (1.3%) 852
Lotensin HCT Tablets (1.4%) 855
Lotrel Capsules 858
▲ Lovenox Injection (3%) 2187
Loxitane 1426
Ludiomil Tablets (2%) 861
Lufyllin & Lufyllin-400 Tablets 2778
Lufyllin-GG Elixir & Tablets 2779
Lupron Depot 3.75 mg (Less than 5%) 2739
▲ Lupron Depot 7.5 mg (5.4%) 2741
Lupron Depot-PED 7.5 mg, 11.25 mg and 15 mg (Less than 2%) 2744
▲ Lupron Injection (5% or more) 2736
Lupron Injection Pediatric (Less than 2%) 2737
▲ LUVOX Tablets (40%) 2723
Lysodren Tablets 707
M-M-R II 1730
M-R-VAX II 1732
▲ MS Contin Tablets (Among most frequent) 2149
▲ MSIR (Among most frequent) 2152
▲ Macrobid Capsules (8%) 2138
▲ Macrodantin Capsules (Among most often) 2140
Mandol Vials, Faspak & ADD-Vantage (Rare) 1516
Marax Tablets & DF Syrup (Frequent, on empty stomach) 2015
Marcaine 2446
Marcaine Spinal (Rare) 2449
▲ Marinol (Dronabinol) Capsules (3% to 10%) 2353
Massengill Disposable Douche 2627
Massengill Medicated Disposable Douche 2628
Matulane Capsules (Frequent) 2300
Maxair Autohaler (1.3% to 1.7%) .. 1550
Maxair Inhaler (1.7%) 1552
▲ Maxaquin Tablets (3.7%) 2593
Maxipime for Injection (0.1% to 1%) 758
Mebaral Tablets (Less than 1 in 100) 2452
Mefoxin (Rare) 1734
Mefoxin Premixed Intravenous Solution (Rare) 1737
▲ Megace Oral Suspension (Up to 5%) 708
Megace Tablets 710
Mellaril 2398
Menest Tablets 2671
▲ Mepergan Injection (Among most frequent) 2859
▲ Mepron Suspension (21% to 22%) 1206
▲ Merrem I.V. (3.9%) 2952
Meruvax II 1740
Mesantoin Tablets 2400
▲ Mesnex Injection (33%) 711
Mestinon Injectable 1300
Mestinon 1300
Metaproterenol Sulfate Inhalation Solution, USP, Arm-a-Med (About 1 in 50 patients) 547
▲ Methadone Hydrochloride Oral Concentrate (Among most frequent) 2356
Methadone Hydrochloride Oral Solution & Tablets 2357
Methergine (Occasional) 2401
▲ Methotrexate Sodium Tablets, Injection, for Injection and LPF Injection (Among most frequent; 10%) 1322
MetroCream 1034
Metrodin (urofollitropin for injection) 2616
MetroGel 1034
MetroGel-Vaginal (Equal to or less than 2%) 917
▲ Mevacor Tablets (1.9% to 4.7%) .. 1742
▲ Mexitil Capsules (39.3% to 39.6%) 684
Mezlin 594
Mezlin Pharmacy Bulk Package 597
▲ Miacalcin Injection (About 10%) 2402
Miacalcin Nasal Spray (Less than 1%; 1.8%) 2403
▲ Micro-K (Among most common) 2237
▲ Micro-K LS Packets (Among most common) 2238
Micronase Tablets (1.8%) 2099
Micronor Tablets (Less common) 1903
▲ Midamor Tablets (3% to 8%) 1746
Miltown Tablets 2780
▲ Minipress Capsules (4.9%) 2015
▲ Minizide Capsules (4.9%) 2016
Minocin Intravenous 1428
Minocin Oral Suspension 1431
Minocin Pellet-Filled Capsules 1429
Mintezol 1747
Mithracin 599
Moban Tablets and Concentrate (Occasional) 1036
Modicon 1928
▲ Moduretic Tablets (3% to 8%) 1748
▲ 8-MOP Capsules (Most common; approximately 10%) 1294
Monoclate-P, Factor VIII:C Pasteurized, Monoclonal Antibody Purified Antihemophilic Factor (Human) 802
Monodox Capsules 1858
Monoket Tablets (Up to 3%) 2550
Mononine, Coagulation Factor IX (Human), Monoclonal Antibody Purified 804
Monopril Tablets (1.2% to 2.2%) .. 762
Motofen Tablets (1 in 15) 789
▲ Motrin Ibuprofen Suspension, Oral Drops, Chewable Tablets, Caplets (3% to 9%) 1563
MSTA Mumps Skin Test Antigen 2988
Mustargen 1752
▲ Mutamycin for Injection (14%) 712
Myambutol Tablets 1432
Mycelex Troches 601
▲ Mycobutin Capsules (6%) 2101
Mycostatin Pastilles (Occasional) 713
Mykrox Tablets (Less than 2%) 1617
Myleran Tablets 1209
Myochrysine Injection 1754
Mysoline (Occasional) 2860
▲ Nalfon 200 Pulvules & Nalfon Tablets (7.7%) 933
▲ Naprelan Tablets (3% to 9%) 2861
▲ Anaprox/Naprosyn (3% to 9%) 2277
Narcan Injection 950
Nardil 1977
Nasalide Nasal Solution 0.025% (5% or less) 2301
Nasarel Nasal Solution (Greater than 1%) 2302
Navane Capsules and Concentrate .. 2018
Navane Intramuscular 2019

(▣ Described in PDR For Nonprescription Drugs) Incidence data in parenthesis; ▲ 3% or more (⊙ Described in PDR For Ophthalmology)

Nausea
Side Effects Index
1406

▲ Navelbine Injection (Up to 34%) ... 1212
Nebcin Vials, Hyporets & ADD-Vantage ... 1518
NegGram ... 2453
Nembutal Sodium Capsules (Less than 1%) ... 440
Nembutal Sodium Solution (Less than 1%) ... 442
Nembutal Sodium Suppositories (Less than 1%) ... 444
▲ Neoral (4% to 10%) ... 2405
Nephro-Fer Rx Tablets ... 2168
Neptazane Tablets ... ⊙ 320
Nescaine/Nescaine MPF ... 549
Netromycin Injection 100 mg/ml ... 2516
▲ Neupogen for Injection (10%; 57%) ... 495
Neurontin Capsules (More than 1%) ... 1978
▲ Neutrexin for Injection (4.6%) ... 2761
▲ Nicotrol NS Nicotine Nasal Spray (5%) ... 1565
Nimotop Capsules (Up to 1.4%) ... 603
▲ Nipent for Injection (53% to 63%) ... 2733
Nitrolingual Spray (Uncommon) ... 2193
Nitrostat Tablets ... 1981
Nizoral Tablets (Approximately 3%) ... 1345
▲ Nolvadex Tablets (2.1% to 25.7%) ... 2957
▲ Nordette-21 Tablets (10% or less) 2863
▲ Nordette-28 Tablets (10% or less) 2866
Norflex ... 1554
Norgesic ... 1554
Norinyl ... 2563
Norisodrine with Calcium Iodide Syrup ... 446
▲ Normodyne Injection (Less than 1% to 19%) ... 2519
▲ Normodyne Tablets (Less than 1% to 19%) ... 2522
▲ Noroxin Tablets (2.6% to 4.2%) ... 1758
▲ Noroxin Tablets (2.6% to 4.2%) ... 2222
▲ Norpace (3 to 9%) ... 2596
Norplant System ... 2868
Norpramin Tablets ... 1273
Nor-Q D Tablets ... 2598
Norvasc Tablets (2.9%) ... 2020
▲ Norvir (23.1% to 26.2%) ... 447
Novahistine DMX (Infrequent) ... ▣ 782
Novahistine Elixir ... ▣ 782
▲ Novantrone for Injection (31 to 72%) ... 1327
Novocain Hydrochloride for Spinal Anesthesia ... 2457
▲ Nubain Injection (6%) ... 952
Nucofed ... 2225
▲ NuLYTELY (Up to 50% of patients) ... 694
▲ Cherry Flavor NuLYTELY (Among most common) ... 694
Numorphan Injection ... 953
Numorphan Suppositories ... 953
Nutropin (A small number of patients) ... 1049
Nutropin AQ Injection (A small number of patients) ... 1051
Nydrazid Injection (Common) ... 509
Ocupress Ophthalmic Solution, 1% Sterile ... ⊙ 297
Ogen Tablets ... 2103
Ogen Vaginal Cream ... 2106
Omnipen Capsules ... 2872
Omnipen for Oral Suspension ... 2873
▲ Oncaspar (Greater than 5%) ... 2194
Oncovin Solution Vials & Hyporets 1521
OptiPranolol (Metipranolol 0.3%) Sterile Ophthalmic Solution (A small number of patients) ... ⊙ 256
▲ Oramorph SR (Morphine Sulfate Sustained Release Tablets) (Among most frequent) ... 2359
Orap Tablets ... 1037
Oretic Tablets ... 450
▲ Organidin NR Tablets and Liquid (One of the two most common) ... 2781
Orlaam Oral Solution (1% to 3%) ... 2361
Ornade Spansule Capsules ... 2678
Ortho-Cept ... 1907
Ortho-Cyclen/Ortho-Tri-Cyclen ... 1914
Ortho Dienestrol Cream ... 1922
Ortho-Est ... 1925
Ortho-Novum ... 1928
Ortho-Cyclen/Ortho Tri-Cyclen ... 1914
▲ Orthoclone OKT3 Sterile Solution (19%) ... 1892
▲ Orudis Capsules (3% to 9%) ... 2874
▲ Oruvail Capsules (3% to 9%) ... 2874
OSMOGLYN Oral Osmotic Agent ⊙ 225
Osmolite HN High Nitrogen Isotonic Liquid Nutrition ... 2339
Ovcon ... 765
▲ Ovral Tablets (10% or less) ... 2877
▲ Ovral-28 Tablets (10% or less) ... 2878
▲ Ovrette Tablets (10% or less) ... 2878
Oxandrin ... 783
▲ Oxsoralen-Ultra Capsules (10%) ... 1302
▲ OxyContin Tablets (Less than 1% to 23%) ... 2163
▲ OxyIR Capsules (Among most frequent) ... 2167
PBZ Tablets ... 863
PBZ-SR Tablets ... 862
▲ PCE Dispertab Tablets (Among most frequent) ... 453
Pamelor ... 2409
Papaverine Hydrochloride Vials and Ampoules ... 1523
▲ Paraplatin for Injection (75% to 94%) ... 713
Paremyd ... ⊙ 244
▲ Parlodel (7% to 49%) ... 2411
Parnate Tablets ... 2679
▲ PASER Granules (Among most common) ... 1333
▲ Paxil Tablets (1.9% to 36.3%) ... 2681
▲ Pediazole Suspension (Among most frequent) ... 2340
Peganone Tablets ... 455
▲ Pen•Vee K (Among most common) 2879
▲ Penetrex Tablets (2% to 8%) ... 2196
Pentasa (1.8% to 3.1%) ... 1275
Pentaspan Injection ... 954
Pepcid Injection (Infrequent) ... 1765
Pepcid (Infrequent) ... 1763
Peptavlon ... 2997
▲ Percocet Tablets (Among most frequent) ... 955
▲ Percodan Tablets (Among most frequent) ... 955
▲ Percodan-Demi Tablets (Among most frequent) ... 956
Pergonal (menotropins for injection, USP) ... 2618
Periactin ... 1767
Peri-Colace Capsules and Syrup ... 2226
▲ Permax Tablets (24.3%) ... 571
Phenergan with Codeine ... 2883
Phenergan with Dextromethorphan 2885
Phenergan Injection ... 2880
Phenergan Suppositories ... 2882
Phenergan Syrup ... 2881
Phenergan Tablets ... 2882
Phenergan VC ... 2886
Phenergan VC with Codeine ... 2888
Phenobarbital Elixir and Tablets (Less than 1 in 100 patients) ... 1523
PhosChol ... 488
PhosLo Tablets (Occasional) ... 695
▲ Phrenilin (Among most frequent) ... 790
Pima Syrup ... 1004
Pipracil (Less frequent) ... 1435
Placidyl Capsules ... 456
Plaquenil Sulfate Tablets ... 2459
Plasma-Plex, Plasma Protein Fraction (Human) U.S.P. 5% Solution Heat-Treated ... 806
▲ Platinol for Injection (Almost all patients) ... 717
▲ Platinol-AQ Injection (Almost all patients) ... 719
Plendil Extended-Release Tablets (1.0% to 1.7%) ... 514
PMB 200 and PMB 400 ... 2890
Pneumovax 23 ... 1768
Pondimin Tablets ... 2239
Ponstel ... 1982
Pontocaine Hydrochloride for Spinal Anesthesia ... 2460
Potaba Capsules, Envules, Powder, and Tablets (Infrequent) ... 1234
▲ Pravachol Tablets (2.9% to 7.3%) 770
Premarin Intravenous ... 2893
Premarin Tablets ... 2896
Premarin Vaginal Cream ... 2898
Premphase ... 2900
Prempro ... 2905
Prevacid Delayed-Release Capsules (1.4%) ... 2746
▲ Prilosec Delayed-Release Capsules (2.2% to 4.0%) ... 516
Primaxin I.M. (0.6%) ... 1770
Primaxin I.V. (2.0%) ... 1772
Prinivil Tablets (Greater than 1% to 2.0%) ... 1776
Prinzide Tablets (2.2%) ... 1780
Priscoline Hydrochloride Ampuls ... 864
Pro-Banthine Tablets ... 2226
▲ Procanbid Extended-Release Tablets (3% to 4%) ... 1983
▲ Procardia Capsules (Approximately 10% to 11%) ... 2024
▲ Procardia XL Extended Release Tablets (3.3% to 11%) ... 2026
▲ Procrit for Injection (0.26% to 17%) ... 1896
Proglycem (Frequent) ... 575
▲ Prograf (30% to 46%) ... 1028
▲ Proleukin for Injection (87%) ... 812
Prolixin ... 510
Proloprim Tablets ... 1141
▲ Propulsid (7.6%) ... 1346
▲ ProSom Tablets (4%) ... 457
Prostep (nicotine transdermal system) (1% to 3% of patients) ... 1439
Prostigmin Injectable ... 1305
Prostigmin Tablets ... 1306
▲ Prostin E2 Suppository (Approximately one-third) ... 2109
Protamine Sulfate Vials ... 1526
Protopam Chloride for Injection ... 2909
▲ Protostat Tablets (About 12% of patients) ... 1939
▲ Proventil Inhalation Aerosol (Less than 15%) ... 2524
▲ Proventil Inhalation Solution 0.083% (3.1% to 4%) ... 2527
Proventil Repetabs Tablets (2% to 4%) ... 2529
▲ Proventil Solution for Inhalation 0.5% (3.1% to 4%) ... 2525
Proventil Tablets (2%) ... 2529
Provera Tablets ... 2110
▲ Prozac Pulvules & Liquid, Oral Solution (5% to 27%) ... 935
Purinethol Tablets (Uncommon) ... 1214
Pyrazinamide Tablets ... 1442
Quadrinal Tablets ... 1398
Questran (Less frequent) ... 774
Quibron ... 2227
▲ Quinaglute Dura-Tabs Tablets (3%) ... 644
▲ Quinidex Extentabs (Among most frequent) ... 2240
▲ RMS Suppositories CII (Among most frequent) ... 2766
▲ Rabies Vaccine Adsorbed (8% to 10%) ... 2686
Rabies Vaccine, Imovax Rabies I.D. (Less frequent; up to 2%) ... 901
Recombivax HB (Equal to or greater than 1%) ... 1787
Redux Capsules (Frequent) ... 2911
Regitine Vials ... 864
Reglan ... 2243
▲ Relafen Tablets (3% to 9%) ... 2688
Remeron Tablets (1.5%) ... 1878
▲ ReoPro Vials (18.4%) ... 1526
Respbid Tablets ... 687
▲ Retrovir Capsules (0.8% to 61%) 1216
▲ Retrovir I.V. Infusion (1% to 61%) 1221
▲ Retrovir Syrup (0.8% to 61%) ... 1216
▲ ReVia Tablets (10% to more than 10%) ... 957
▲ Revex (nalmefene hydrochloride injection) (18%) ... 1863
Rhinocort Nasal Inhaler (Less than 1%) ... 552
▲ Ridaura Capsules (10%) ... 2691
Rifadin (Some patients) ... 1276
Rifamate Capsules (Some patients) ... 1278
Rifater ... 1280
▲ Rilutek Tablets (12.2% to 20.5%) 2198
Rimactane Capsules ... 865
▲ Risperdal Tablets (4% to 6%) ... 1348
Ritalin ... 866
Robaxin Tablets ... 2246
▲ Robaxisal Tablets (One in 20-25) .. 2246
Robinul Forte Tablets ... 2247
Robinul Injectable ... 2247
Robinul Tablets ... 2247
Rocaltrol Capsules ... 2303
Rocephin Injectable Vials, ADD-Vantage, Galaxy Container (Less than 1%) ... 2305
▲ Roferon-A Injection (37% to 51%) 2308
▲ Romazicon (11%) ... 2311
Rondec Oral Drops ... 974
Rondec Syrup ... 974
Rondec Tablet ... 974
Rondec Chewable Tablets ... 974
Rondec-TR Tablet ... 974
▲ Rowasa (1.2% to 5.77%) ... 2727
▲ Roxanol (Among most frequent) ... 2365
▲ Roxicodone Tablets, Oral Solution & Intensol (Oxycodone) (Among most frequent) ... 2366
Rum-K Syrup ... 1004
▲ Rythmol Tablets–150mg, 225mg, 300mg (2.4 to 10.7%) ... 1399
▲ SSKI Solution (Among most frequent) ... 2767
▲ Salagen Tablets (6% to 15%) ... 1546
Salflex Tablets ... 791
▲ Sandimmune (2 to 10%) ... 2416
Sandoglobulin I.V. (Less than 1%) .. 2419
▲ Sandostatin Injection (4% to 61%) ... 2421
Sanorex Tablets ... 2423
Sansert Tablets ... 2424
Seconal Sodium Pulvules (Less than 1 in 100) ... 1529
▲ Sectral Capsules (4%) ... 2914
▲ Sedapap Tablets 50 mg/650 mg (Among the most frequent) ... 1826
▲ Seldane Tablets (4.6% to 7.6%) ... 1284
▲ Seldane-D Extended-Release Tablets (4.5%) ... 1286
Semprex-D Capsules (2%) ... 1620
Senna X-Prep Bowel Evacuant Liquid ... 1236
Sensorcaine (Rare) ... 554
▲ Septra (Among most common) ... 1146
▲ Septra I.V. Infusion (Among the most common) ... 1142
▲ Septra I.V. Infusion ADD-Vantage Vials (Among most common) ... 1144
▲ Septra (Among most common) ... 1146
Ser-Ap-Es Tablets ... 867
Serax Capsules ... 2916
Serax Tablets ... 2916
Serentil ... 689
Serevent Inhalation Aerosol (1% to 3%) ... 1149
Serophene (clomiphene citrate tablets, USP) (Approximately 1 in 50 patients) ... 2621
▲ Serzone Tablets (14% to 23%) ... 776
Sinemet Tablets (Common) ... 959
▲ Sinemet CR Tablets (5.5%) ... 961
Sinequan ... 2028
Skelaxin Tablets ... 793
Slo-bid Gyrocaps ... 2201
Slo-Niacin Tablets ... 2767
▲ Slow-K Extended-Release Tablets (Among most common) ... 869
Sodium Polystyrene Sulfonate Suspension ... 2367
Solganal Suspension (Rare) ... 2530
Soma Compound w/Codeine Tablets ... 2784
▲ Soma Compound Tablets (Among most common) ... 2783
Soma Tablets ... 2782
Sotradecol (Sodium Tetradecyl Sulfate Injection) ... 987
Spectrobid Tablets (2%) ... 2030
▲ Sporanox Capsules (2.4% to 10.6%) ... 1352
▲ St. Joseph Adult Chewable Aspirin (81 mg.) (7.3% of 4500 patients) ... ▣ 768
▲ Stadol (13%) ... 779
Stelazine ... 2692
Stimate, (desmopressin acetate) Nasal Spray, 1.5 mg/mL (Infrequent) ... 806
Streptase for Infusion ... 557
Streptomycin Sulfate Injection ... 2031
Sublimaze Injection ... 463
▲ Sufenta Injection (3% to 9%) ... 1355
Sular Tablets (2%) ... 2961
▲ Supprelin Injection (3% to 10%) ... 2230
▲ Suprane (desflurane, USP) (27%) .. 1865
▲ Suprax (7%) ... 1443
Surmontil Capsules ... 2917
Sus-Phrine Injection ... 1017
▲ Symmetrel Capsules (5% to 10%) 965
▲ Symmetrel Syrup (5% to 10%) ... 963
Syn-Rx Tablets ... 1622
Syn-Rx DM Tablets ... 1623
Syntocinon Injection ... 2425
Talacen Caplets (Rare) ... 2464
▲ Talwin Injection (Most common) ... 2465
Talwin Compound ... 2466
▲ Talwin Injection (Most common) ... 2465
Talwin Nx Tablets ... 2467
▲ Tambocor Tablets (8.9%) ... 1555
Tao Capsules (Infrequent) ... 2033
Tapazole Tablets ... 1361
Tavist Syrup ... 2426
Tavist Tablets ... 2427
▲ Taxol Injection (52%) ... 723
Taxotere for Injection Concentrate 2204
Tazicef for Injection (Less than 2%; 1 in 156 patients) ... 2697
Tazidime Vials, Faspak & ADD-Vantage (1 in 156) ... 1531
▲ Tegison Capsules (10-25%) ... 2314
▲ Tegretol/Tegretol-XR (Among most frequent) ... 870

(▣ Described in PDR For Nonprescription Drugs) Incidence data in parenthesis; ▲ 3% or more (⊙ Described in PDR For Ophthalmology)

1407 Side Effects Index Necrolysis, epidermal

Tenex Tablets (3% or less) 2249
▲ Tenoretic Tablets (3% to 4%) 2963
▲ Tenormin Tablets and I.V. Injection (3% to 4%) 2965
Tensilon Injectable 1307
Terramycin Intramuscular Solution 2034
Teslac Tablets 727
Tessalon Perles 1018
Testoderm Testosterone Transdermal System 486
Testred Capsules, 10 mg 1308
Thalitone 1293
Theo-24 Extended Release Capsules 2753
Theo-Dur Extended-Release Tablets 1367
Theo-X Extended-Release Tablets 793
▲ TheraCys BCG Live (Intravesical) (Up to 16.1%) 911
Thioguanine Tablets, Tabloid Brand (Less frequent) 1225
Thioplex (Thiotepa For Injection) 1329
Thorazine 2701
▲ THROMBATE III Antithrombin III (Human) (3 of 17) 631
THYREL TRH 2992
Tiazac Capsules (2%) 1019
Ticar for Injection 2704
▲ TICE BCG, USP (3.0%) 1881
▲ Ticlid Tablets (7.0%) 2317
▲ Tilade Inhaler (4.0%) 2207
Timentin for Injection 2706
Timolide Tablets (Less than 1%) 1791
Timoptic in Ocudose (Less frequent) 1796
Timoptic Sterile Ophthalmic Solution (Less frequent) 1794
Timoptic-XE 1798
Tofranil Ampuls 873
Tofranil Tablets 875
Tofranil-PM Capsules 876
▲ Tolectin (200, 400 and 600 mg) (11%) 1591
▲ Tonocard Tablets (14.5% to 24.6%) 519
Toprol-XL Tablets (About 1 of 100 patients) 560
▲ Toradol (12%) 2319
Tornalate Solution for Inhalation, 0.2% (1.9%) 976
Tornalate Metered Dose Inhaler (0.5% to 3%) 978
Trancopal Caplets 2468
▲ Trandate (13 of 100 patients) 1158
Transderm Scōp Transdermal Therapeutic System (Few patients) 890
▲ Trasylol (3%) 607
Trental Tablets (2.2%) 1291
Triavil Tablets 1800
Trilafon (Occasional) 2532
Levlen/Tri-Levlen 646
▲ Trilisate (Less than 20%) 2155
Trimpex Tablets 2323
Trinalin Repetabs Tablets 1373
Tri-Norinyl 2607
▲ Triphasil-21 Tablets (10% or less) 2919
▲ Triphasil-28 Tablets (10% or less) 2924
Trusopt Sterile Ophthalmic Solution (Infrequent) 1803
Tussend 1830
Tussend Expectorant 1831
Tussionex Pennkinetic Extended-Release Suspension 1624
▲ Tussi-Organidin DM NR Liquid and DM-S NR Liquid (One of the two most common) 2786
▲ Tylenol with Codeine (Among most frequent) 1592
▲ Tylox Capsules (Among most frequent) 1593
Tympagesic Ear Drops 2476
▲ Typhim Vi (2% to 8.2%) 914
▲ Ultram Tablets (50 mg) (24% to 40%) 1594
Unasyn (Less than 1%) 2035
Uni-Dur Extended-Release Tablets 1374
Uniphyl 400 mg and 600 mg Tablets 2157
Univasc Tablets (More than 1%) 2553
Urecholine 1804
Urispas Tablets 2710
Urobiotic-250 Capsules (Rare) 2038
Urocit-K Tablets (Some patients) 1828
Uroqid-Acid No. 2 Tablets 633
Valium Injectable 2336
Valium Tablets (Infrequent) 2335
▲ Valtrex Caplets (6% to 16%) 1167
Vancenase AQ Nasal Spray 0.042% (Fewer than 5 per 100 patients) 2535
Vancocin HCl, Oral Solution & Pulvules (Infrequent) 1536
Vancocin HCl, Vials & ADD-Vantage (Infrequent) 1534
Vantin for Oral Suspension and Vantin Tablets (Less than 1%) 2112
Vaqta (2.3%) 1805
Varivax (Greater than or equal to 1%) 1807
▲ Vascor Tablets (200 and 300 mg) (12.29 to 26.09%) 1597
Vaseretic Tablets (2.5%) 1810
Vasotec I.V. (1.1%) 1814
Vasotec Tablets (1.3% to 1.4%) 1816
Vasoxyl Injection 1169
Velban Vials 1537
▲ Ventolin Inhalation Aerosol and Refill (Fewer than 15 per 100 patients; 6%) 1170
▲ Ventolin Inhalation Solution (3.1% to 4%) 1171
▲ Ventolin Nebules Inhalation Solution (3.1% to 4%) 1172
▲ Ventolin Rotacaps for Inhalation (4%) 1173
Ventolin Tablets (2 of 100 patients) 1176
▲ VePesid Capsules and Injection (31% to 43%) 727
Verelan Capsules (2.7%) 1455
Versed Injection (2.8%) 2324
▲ Vesanoid Capsules (57%) 2327
Vibramycin 2038
Vibramycin Hyclate Intravenous 2040
Vibramycin 2038
▲ Vicodin Tablets (Among most frequent) 1404
▲ Vicodin ES Tablets (Among most frequent) 1405
▲ Vicodin HP Tablets (Among most frequent) 1403
Vicodin Tuss Expectorant (More frequently in ambulatory than in recumbent patients) 1406
▲ Videx Tablets, Powder for Oral Solution, & Pediatric Powder for Oral Solution (6% to 58%) 2980
▲ Viramune Tablets (Among most frequent; 5%) 2368
▲ Visken Tablets (5%) 2428
▲ Vistide Injection (8% to 65%) 1057
Vivactil Tablets 1820
Vivelle Transdermal System 880
Vivotif Berna (Infrequent) 660
▲ Volmax Extended-Release Tablets (4.2%) 1835
Voltaren Ophthalmic Sterile Ophthalmic Solution (1%) ⊙ 264
▲ Cataflam/Voltaren/Voltaren-XR (3% to 9%) 833
▲ Vumon for Injection (29%) 729
▲ Wellbutrin Tablets (22.9%) 1177
Wigraine Tablets 1884
WinRho SD (One report) 1839
Winstrol Tablets 2468
▲ Wygesic Tablets (Most frequent) 2930
▲ Xanax Tablets (9.6% to 22.0%) 2115
Xylocaine Injections (Less than 1%) 562
Yocon Tablets (Common) 1235
Yodoxin Tablets 1235
▲ Yutopar Intravenous Injection (10% to 15%) 566
▲ Zanosar Sterile Powder (Most patients) 2119
Zantac 1182
Zantac Injection 1180
Zantac Syrup 1182
Zarontin Capsules (Frequent) 1986
Zarontin Syrup (Frequent) 1986
Zaroxolyn Tablets 1625
Zebeta Tablets (1.5% to 2.2%) 1457
Zemuron Injection (Less than 1%) 1885
▲ Zerit Capsules (6% to 44%) 731
Zestoretic Tablets (2.2%) 2968
Zestril Tablets (Greater than 1% to 2.0%) 2972
Ziac (0.9% to 1.1%) 1459
Zinacef (1 in 440 patients) 1184
▲ Zinecard Injection (51% to 77%) 2120
Zithromax (1% to 5%) 2043
▲ Zithromax Tablets (3% to 5%) 2046
Zocor Tablets (1.3%) 1821
▲ Zoladex (5% to 11%) 2976
Zoladex 3-month 2978
▲ Zoloft Tablets (26.1%) 2051
Zonalon Cream (Less than 1%) 1042
▲ Zosyn (5.8% to 6.9%) 1463
▲ Zovirax Capsules (2.4% to 8%) 1187
▲ Zovirax Sterile Powder (Approximately 7%) 1191
▲ Zovirax (2.4% to 8.0%) 1187
▲ Zydone Capsules (Among most frequent) 967
Zyloprim Tablets (Less than 1%) 1194
Zyrtec Tablets (Greater than 2%) 2053

Nausea, acute/severe

Doxorubicin Astra (Frequent) 531
Rubex for Injection (Frequent) 721

Neck tightness

Imitrex Injection (Relatively common) 1095
Respbid Tablets 687

Neck, rigidity of

Cytovene (1% or less) 2270
Depakote Tablets (1% to 5%) 418
Dilacor XR Extended-release Capsules (Infrequent) 2183
Diprivan Injectable Emulsion (Less than 1%) 2939
DynaCirc CR Tablets (0.5% to 1.0%) 2383
Effexor (Infrequent) 2825
Hivid Tablets (Less than 1%) 2287
▲ Imitrex Injection (4.8%) 1095
Imitrex Tablets 1099
Ismo Tablets (Fewer than 1%) 2844
Lioresal Intrathecal (1% or more) 1634
LUVOX Tablets (Infrequent) 2723
Naprelan Tablets (Less than 1%) 2861
Norvir (Less than 2%) 447
Paxil Tablets (Rare) 2681
Prostin E2 Suppository 2109
Prozac Pulvules & Liquid, Oral Solution (Infrequent) 935
Redux Capsules (Rare) 2911
Remeron Tablets (Infrequent) 1878
Serzone Tablets (1%) 776
Varivax (Greater than or equal to 1%) 1807
Videx Tablets, Powder for Oral Solution, & Pediatric Powder for Oral Solution (Less than 1%) 2980

Necrolysis, digitus

▲ Tegison Capsules (Greater than 75%) 2314

Necrolysis, epidermal

▲ Accutane Capsules (Approximately 1 in 20) 2252
Amoxil 2631
Atretol Tablets (Extremely rare) 569
Atromid-S Capsules 2808
A/T/S 2% Acne Topical Gel (Occasional) 1244
Augmentin (Occasional) 2637
Augmentin Tablets (Occasional) 2640
Axocet Capsules (Infrequent) 2469
Azactam for Injection (Less than 1%) 736
Azelex (Less than 1%) 471
Azulfidine (Rare) 2059
Benzamycin Topical Gel (Occasional) 919
Betoptic Ophthalmic Solution (Rare) 465
Betoptic S Ophthalmic Suspension (Rare) 467
Blephamide Liquifilm Sterile Ophthalmic Suspension 472
▲ Blephamide Ointment (Among most often) ⊙ 234
Brevoxyl 2732
▲ Brevoxyl Cleansing Lotion (5 of 100 patients) 2732
Cardizem SR Capsules (Infrequent) 1255
Cardizem Tablets (Infrequent) 1257
Ceclor Pulvules & Suspension (Rare) 1470
Cedax 2480
Cefizox for Intramuscular or Intravenous Use 1025
Cefotan 2936
Ceftin 1067
Cefzil Tablets and Oral Suspension 747
Ceptaz 1070
Chibroxin Sterile Ophthalmic Solution (With oral form) 1657
Cipro I.V. (1% or less) 587
Cipro I.V. Pharmacy Bulk Package (Less than 1%) 590
Cipro Tablets 584
Claritin-D Tablets (Less frequent) 2487
Cleocin T Topical 2072
Cleocin Vaginal Cream 2070
Combipres Tablets 682
Condylox Topical Solution (Less than 5%) 1853
Cozaar Tablets (One subject) 1668
Daypro Caplets (Less than 1%) 2578
Depakene (One case) 416
Depakote Tablets (One case) 418
Depen Titratable Tablets (Rare) 2770
DesOwen Cream, Ointment and Lotion (Less than 2%) 1032
Desquam-E Gel 2792
Desquam-X Gel 2792
Desquam-X 10 Bar 2792
Desquam-X Wash 2792
Diamox Sequels (Sustained Release) ⊙ 318
Diflucan Tablets, Injection, and Oral Suspension 2003
Dilacor XR Extended-release Capsules 2183
Dilantin Infatabs 1967
Dilantin Kapseals 1965
Dilantin-125 Suspension 1969
Diupres Tablets 1691
Diuril Oral Suspension 1694
Diuril Sodium Intravenous 1693
Diuril Tablets 1694
Dolobid Tablets (Less than 1 in 100) 1695
▲ Dovonex Ointment 0.005% (1% to 10%) 2793
Duricef Capsules, Tablets, and Oral Suspension 750
Emcyt Capsules (1%) 2085
Emgel 2% Topical Gel (Occasional) 1081
Esgic-plus Capsules (Several cases) 1012
Esgic-plus Tablets (Several cases) 1012
Eulexin Capsules 2498
Exact ◘ 722
FML-S Liquifilm ⊙ 240
Felbatol 2774
Feldene Capsules (Less than 1%) 2008
Fioricet Tablets (Several cases) 2386
Fiorinal Capsules (Several cases) 2388
Fiorinal with Codeine Capsules 2390
Fiorinal Tablets (Several cases) 2388
Floxin I.V. 1580
Floxin Tablets (200 mg, 300 mg, 400 mg) 1577
Fortaz 1092
Foscavir Injection (Rare) 541
Fulvicin P/G Tablets (Rare) 2499
Fungizone Oral Suspension (Rare) 704
Gantrisin (Rare) 2286
GlaucTabs ⊙ 209
HydroDIURIL Tablets 1716
Hydropres Tablets 1718
Hyzaar Tablets (One subject) 1720
IBU Tablets (Less than 1%) 1389
Indocin Capsules (Less than 1%) 1723
Indocin I.V. (Less than 1%) 1727
Indocin (Less than 1%) 1723
Intron A for Injection (Less than 5%) 2506
Lac-Hydrin 12% Lotion (1 in 60 patients) 2796
Lamisil Tablets (Isolated reports) 2394
Lescol Capsules (Rare) 2395
Leukeran Tablets (Rare) 1205
Lodine Capsules and Tablets (Less than 1%) 2849
Lorabid Suspension and Pulvules 1513
Lotrimin 2514
Lotrisone Cream 2515
LUVOX Tablets 2723
Maxaquin Tablets 2593
Maxipime for Injection 758
Mefoxin 1734
Mefoxin Premixed Intravenous Solution 1737
Mesantoin Tablets (Rare) 2400
Methotrexate Sodium Tablets, Injection, for Injection and LPF Injection 1322
Mevacor Tablets (Rare) 1742
Moduretic Tablets 1748
Motrin Ibuprofen Suspension, Oral Drops, Chewable Tablets, Caplets (Less than 1%) 1563
Nalfon 200 Pulvules & Nalfon Tablets (Less than 1%) 933
Noroxin Tablets 1758
Noroxin Tablets 2222
PCE Dispertab Tablets (Rare) 453
Paxil Tablets 2681
Pediazole Suspension 2340
Penetrex Tablets (0.1% to 1%) 2196
Pepcid Injection (Very rare) 1765
Pepcid (very rare) 1763

(◘ Described in PDR For Nonprescription Drugs) Incidence data in parenthesis; ▲ 3% or more (⊙ Described in PDR For Ophthalmology)

Necrolysis, epidermal — Side Effects Index — 1408

Phenobarbital Elixir and Tablets (Rare) 1523
Phenurone Tablets (One case) 455
Phrenilin (Several cases) 790
Pravachol Tablets (Rare) 770
Prilosec Delayed-Release Capsules (Very rare) 516
Primaxin I.M. 1770
Primaxin I.V. (Less than 0.2%) 1772
Prinivil Tablets (Rare) 1776
Prinzide Tablets (Rare) 1780
Proloprim Tablets (Rare) 1141
Prozac Pulvules & Liquid, Oral Solution 935
Relafen Tablets (Rarer) 2688
Renova (tretinoin emollient cream) 0.05% (Almost all subjects) 1945
Retin-A (tretinoin) Cream/Gel/Liquid 1947
Sedapap Tablets 50 mg/650 mg (Several cases) 1826
Septra 1146
Septra I.V. Infusion 1142
Septra I.V. Infusion ADD-Vantage Vials (Rare) 1144
Septra 1146
Suprax 1443
Tazicef for Injection 2697
Tazidime Vials, Faspak & ADD-Vantage 1531
▲ Tegison Capsules (Greater than 75%) 2314
Tegretol/Tegretol-XR (Extremely rare) 870
Thalitone 1293
Tiazac Capsules (Less than 1%) 1019
Timolide Tablets 1791
Tolectin (200, 400 and 600 mg) (Less than 1%) 1591
Trusopt Sterile Ophthalmic Solution (Rare) 1803
Ultram Tablets (50 mg) (Less than 1%) 1594
Vancocin HCl, Oral Solution & Pulvules (Infrequent) 1536
Vancocin HCl, Vials & ADD-Vantage (Infrequent) 1534
Vantin for Oral Suspension and Vantin Tablets (Less than 1%) 2112
Vaseretic Tablets 1810
Vasotec I.V. 1814
Vasotec Tablets (0.5% to 1.0%) 1816
Zestoretic Tablets 2968
Zestril Tablets (Rare) 2972
Zinacef (Rare) 1184
Zocor Tablets (Rare) 1821
Zonalon Cream (Less than 1%) 1042
Zyloprim Tablets (Less than 1%) 1194

Necrosis

Amicar Syrup, Tablets, and Injection 1312
Benadryl Parenteral 1955
Betaseron for SC Injection (2%) 653
Capoten Tablets (Rare) 740
Capozide Tablets (Rare) 744
Ceptaz 1070
Fortaz 1092
Levophed Bitartrate Injection 2445
MSTA Mumps Skin Test Antigen 2988
▲ Naprelan Tablets (3% to 9%) 2861
Platinol for Injection 717
Platinol-AQ Injection 719
PPD Tine Test 2993
Scleromate Injection 1234
Sensorcaine 554
Taxol Injection (Rare) 723
▲ Tegison Capsules (Greater than 75%) 2314
Tuberculin, Old, Tine Test 2994
Tubersol (Tuberculin Purified Protein Derivative (Mantoux)) 2988

Necrosis, aseptic

Cortifoam 2540
Cortone Acetate Tablets 1664

Necrosis, bone

Avonex 662
Prozac Pulvules & Liquid, Oral Solution (Rare) 935
Rilutek Tablets (Rare) 2198

Necrosis, bowel

Cytosar-U Sterile Powder (Less frequent) 2077
Proleukin for Injection (Less than 1%) 812

Necrosis, buccal

Orudis Capsules (Less than 1%) 2874
Oruvail Capsules (Less than 1%) 2874

Necrosis, cecal

Adriamycin PFS 2056
Adriamycin RDF 2056
Doxorubicin Astra 531
Rubex for Injection 721

Necrosis, colon

Adriamycin PFS 2056
Adriamycin RDF 2056
Doxorubicin Astra 531
Kayexalate 2444
Rubex for Injection 721
Sodium Polystyrene Sulfonate Suspension (Rare) 2367

Necrosis, cutaneous

▲ Androderm Testosterone Transdermal System (12%) 2634
Aramine Injection 1649
Betaseron for SC Injection 653
Brevibloc (esmolol HCl) Injection (Less than 1%) 1860
Cognex Capsules (Rare) 1961
Coumadin (Less frequent) 941
Dobutrex Solution Vials (Isolated cases) 1480
Doxil (Less than 1%) 2613
Heparin Lock Flush Solution 2831
Heparin Sodium Injection 2832
Heparin Sodium Vials 1486
Lovenox Injection 2187
Mutamycin for Injection 712
Naprelan Tablets (Less than 1%) 2861
Neurontin Capsules (Rare) 1978
SSD (Infrequent) 1402
Vancocin HCl, Vials & ADD-Vantage 1534

Necrosis, fat

Garamycin Injectable (Rare) 2502

Necrosis, hepatic

Accupril Tablets (Rare) 1950
Altace Capsules (Rare) 1238
Azulfidine (Rare) 2059
Bactrim DS Tablets (Rare) 2257
Bactrim I.V. Infusion (Rare) 2255
Bactrim (Rare) 2257
Benemid Tablets 1651
Blephamide Liquifilm Sterile Ophthalmic Suspension 472
▲ Blephamide Ointment (Among most often) ⊙ 234
Capoten Tablets (Rare) 740
Capozide Tablets (Rare) 744
Cataflam Tablets (Rare) 833
Cipro I.V. (1% or less) 587
Cipro I.V. Pharmacy Bulk Package (Less than 1%) 590
Cipro Tablets (Rare) 584
Claritin Tablets (Rare) 2485
Claritin-D Tablets 2487
ColBENEMID Tablets 1662
Cordarone Intravenous 2821
DTIC-Dome 593
Darvon-N/Darvocet-N 1473
Darvon Compound-65 Pulvules 1475
Darvon-N Suspension & Tablets 1473
Diamox Intravenous (Occasional) ⊙ 317
Diamox Sequels (Sustained Release) ⊙ 318
Diamox Tablets (Occasional) ⊙ 317
Eulexin Capsules 2498
FML-S Liquifilm ⊙ 240
Fansidar Tablets 2281
Floxin I.V. 1580
Floxin Tablets (200 mg, 300 mg, 400 mg) 1577
Fluothane 2830
Sterile FUDR 2284
Gantanol Tablets 2285
Gantrisin (Rare) 2286
GlaucTabs ⊙ 209
Inocor Lactate Injection 2439
Lescol Capsules (Rare) 2395
Lodine Capsules and Tablets (Rare; less than 1%) 2849
Lotensin Tablets (Rare) 852
Lotensin HCT Tablets 855
Lotrel Capsules (Rare) 858
Macrobid Capsules (Rare) 2138
Macrodantin Capsules (Rare) 2140
Mavik Tablets (Rare) 1407
Maxaquin Tablets 2593
Mevacor Tablets (Rare) 1742
Mexitil Capsules (Rare) 684
Monopril Tablets 762
Motrin Ibuprofen Suspension, Oral Drops, Chewable Tablets, Caplets (Less than 1%) 1563
Nardil (Less frequent) 1977
Neptazane Tablets ⊙ 320
Nolvadex Tablets (Rare) 2957
Normodyne Injection 2519
Normodyne Tablets (Less common) 2522
Noroxin Tablets 1758
Noroxin Tablets 2222
Oxandrin (Rare) 783
Paxil Tablets 2681
Pediazole Suspension 2340
Penetrex Tablets 2196
Pravachol Tablets (Rare) 770
Prilosec Delayed-Release Capsules (Rare) 516
Prinivil Tablets (Rare) 1776
Prinzide Tablets (Rare) 1780
Prozac Pulvules & Liquid, Oral Solution 935
SSD 1402
Septra 1146
Septra I.V. Infusion 1142
Septra I.V. Infusion ADD-Vantage Vials (Rare) 1144
Septra 1146
Silvadene Cream 1% 1288
Tapazole Tablets (Rare) 1361
Taxol Injection (Rare) 723
Ticlid Tablets (Rare) 2317
Trandate (Less common) 1158
Trusopt Sterile Ophthalmic Solution (Rare) 1803
Univasc Tablets (Rare) 2553
Vaseretic Tablets (Rare) 1810
Vasotec I.V. (Rare) 1814
Vasotec Tablets (Rare) 1816
Cataflam/Voltaren/Voltaren-XR (Rare) 833
Winstrol Tablets (Rare) 2468
Wygesic Tablets 2930
Zestoretic Tablets (Rare) 2968
Zestril Tablets (Rare) 2972
Zocor Tablets (Rare) 1821
Zyloprim Tablets (Less than 1%) 1194

Necrosis, intestinal

Lanoxicaps (Very rare) 1110
Lanoxin Elixir Pediatric (Very rare) 1113
Lanoxin Injection (Very rare) 1116
Lanoxin Injection Pediatric (Very rare) 1119
Lanoxin Tablets (Very rare) 1121
Oncovin Solution Vials & Hyporets 1521
Thioguanine Tablets, Tabloid Brand 1225

Necrosis, ischemic

Felbatol 2774

Necrosis, macular

Nebcin Vials, Hyporets & ADD-Vantage 1518

Necrosis, pancreatic

Proglycem 575

Necrosis, papillary

Cataflam Tablets (Rare) 833
Feldene Capsules (Less than 1%) 2008
Nalfon 200 Pulvules & Nalfon Tablets (Less than 1%) 933
Ponstel 1982
Cataflam/Voltaren/Voltaren-XR (Rare) 833

Necrosis, renal papillary

Anaprox/Naprosyn (Less than 1%) 2277
Dapsone Tablets USP 1331
Darvon-N/Darvocet-N 1473
Darvon 1475
Darvon-N Suspension & Tablets 1473
EC-Naprosyn Delayed-Release Tablets (Less than 1%) 2277
Feldene Capsules 2008
IBU Tablets (Less than 1%) 1389
Lodine Capsules and Tablets (Less than 1%) 2849
Motrin Ibuprofen Suspension, Oral Drops, Chewable Tablets, Caplets (Less than 1%) 1563
▲ Naprelan Tablets (3% to 9%) 2861
Anaprox/Naprosyn (Less than 1%) 2277
Relafen Tablets 2688

Necrosis, renal tubular

Calcium Disodium Versenate Injection 1548
Capastat Sulfate Injection 968
▲ CellCept Capsules (6.3% to 10.0%) 2265
Cytoxan 700
Motrin Ibuprofen Suspension, Oral Drops, Chewable Tablets, Caplets (Less than 1%) 1563
Neoral (1.0%) 2405
Trasylol (0.9%) 607
▲ Vesanoid Capsules (3%) 2327

Necrosis, tissue

Adriamycin PFS 2056
Adriamycin RDF 2056
Cerubidine for Injection 634
Coumadin (Less frequent) 941
DaunoXome 1842
Doxorubicin Astra (Occasional) 531
Fragmin Injection (Rare) 2088
Idamycin Injection 2096
Mepergan Injection 2859
Novantrone for Injection (Rare reports) 1327
Phenergan Injection 2880
Phenergan Tablets 2882
Rubex for Injection 721
Silvadene Cream 1% (Infrequent) 1288
Sotradecol (Sodium Tetradecyl Sulfate Injection) 987

Necrotizing angiitis

Aldactazide Tablets 2556
Aldoclor Tablets 1638
Aldoril Tablets 1644
Apresazide Capsules 824
Capozide Tablets 744
Combipres Tablets 682
Cortifoam 2540
Diucardin Tablets 2824
Diupres Tablets 1691
Diuril Sodium Intravenous 1693
Dyazide Capsules 2653
Enduron Tablets 424
Esidrix Tablets 839
Esimil Tablets 840
Florinef Acetate Tablets 506
HydroDIURIL Tablets 1716
Hydropres Tablets 1718
Hyzaar Tablets 1720
Inderide Tablets 2838
Inderide LA Long Acting Capsules 2840
Lasix Injection, Oral Solution and Tablets 1267
Lodine Capsules and Tablets (Less than 1%) 2849
Lopressor HCT Tablets 850
Lotensin HCT Tablets 855
Minizide Capsules 2016
Moduretic Tablets 1748
Mykrox Tablets 1617
Oretic Tablets 450
Prinzide Tablets 1780
Ser-Ap-Es Tablets 867
Tenoretic Tablets 2963
Thalitone 1293
Vaseretic Tablets 1810
Zaroxolyn Tablets 1625
Zestoretic Tablets 2968
Ziac 1459
Zyloprim Tablets (Less than 1%) 1194

Neonatal morbidity

Altace Capsules (Several dozen cases) 1238
Capoten Tablets 740
Capozide Tablets 744
Cozaar Tablets 1668
Hyzaar Tablets 1720
Lotensin Tablets 852
Lotensin HCT Tablets (Several dozen cases) 855
Lotrel Capsules 858
Mavik Tablets 1407
Monopril Tablets 762
Prinivil Tablets 1776
Prinzide Tablets 1780
Univasc Tablets 2553
Vaseretic Tablets 1810
Vasotec I.V. 1814
Vasotec Tablets 1816
Zestoretic Tablets 2968
Zestril Tablets 2972

Neonatal prematurity

Accupril Tablets 1950
Adderall Tablets 2209
Altace Capsules 1238
Capoten Tablets 740

(▣ Described in PDR For Nonprescription Drugs) Incidence data in parenthesis; ▲ 3% or more (⊙ Described in PDR For Ophthalmology)

Side Effects Index

Capozide Tablets ... 744
Cozaar Tablets ... 1668
Hyzaar Tablets ... 1720
Lotensin Tablets ... 852
Lotensin HCT Tablets ... 855
Monopril Tablets ... 762
Prinivil Tablets ... 1776
Prinzide Tablets ... 1780
Univasc Tablets ... 2553
Vaseretic Tablets ... 1810
Vasotec I.V. ... 1814
Vasotec Tablets ... 1816
Zestoretic Tablets ... 2968
Zestril Tablets ... 2972

Neoplasm
(see under Carcinoma)

Neoplasm, malignant
Estratest ... 2718
Ortho Dienestrol Cream ... 1922
Orthoclone OKT3 Sterile Solution .. 1892
Pergonal (menotropins for injection, USP) ... 2618

Neoplasms, hepatic
Androderm Testosterone Transdermal System (Rare) ... 2634
Android Capsules, 10 mg (Rare) ... 1297
Betaseron for SC Injection ... 653
Brevicon ... 2563
Estratest (Rare) ... 2718
Norinyl ... 2563
Nor-Q D Tablets ... 2598
Ortho-Cyclen/Ortho-Tri-Cyclen ... 1914
Ortho-Cyclen/Ortho-Tri-Cyclen ... 1914
Oxandrin ... 783
Testoderm Testosterone Transdermal System (Rare) ... 486
Testred Capsules, 10 mg (Rare) ... 1308
Tri-Norinyl ... 2607
Winstrol Tablets ... 2468

Nephritis
Azulfidine (Rare) ... 2059
Betaseron for SC Injection ... 653
Capastat Sulfate Injection (1 patient) ... 968
Cipro Tablets (Less than 1%) ... 584
Disalcid ... 1549
Paxil Tablets (Rare) ... 2681
Pediazole Suspension ... 2340
Phenurone Tablets (1%) ... 455
Redux Capsules (Rare) ... 2911
Rilutek Tablets (Rare) ... 2198
Salflex Tablets ... 791
Solganal Suspension ... 2530
Tapazole Tablets (Very rare) ... 1361
Timolide Tablets ... 1791
Toradol ... 2319
Zithromax (1% or less) ... 2043
Zithromax (1% or less) ... 2046
Zyloprim Tablets (Less than 1%) ... 1194

Nephritis, interstitial
Aldoclor Tablets ... 1638
Aldoril Tablets ... 1644
Anaprox/Naprosyn (Less than 1%) ... 2277
Asacol Delayed-Release Tablets ... 2129
Augmentin (Rare) ... 2637
Augmentin Tablets (Rare) ... 2640
Bactrim DS Tablets ... 2257
Bactrim I.V. Infusion ... 2255
Bactrim ... 2257
Capoten Tablets ... 740
Capozide Tablets ... 744
Cataflam Tablets (Rare) ... 833
Ceclor Pulvules & Suspension (Rare) ... 1470
Chibroxin Sterile Ophthalmic Solution (With oral form) ... 1657
Cipro I.V. (1% or less) ... 587
Cipro I.V. Pharmacy Bulk Package (Less than 1%) ... 590
Cipro Tablets (Less than 1%) ... 584
Claforan Sterile and Injection (Occasional) ... 1259
Clinoril Tablets (Less than 1 in 100) ... 1658
Clozaril Tablets ... 2377
Daypro Caplets (Less than 1%) ... 2578
Dipentum Capsules (Rare) ... 2084
Diupres Tablets ... 1691
Diuril Oral Suspension ... 1694
Diuril Sodium Intravenous ... 1693
Diuril Tablets ... 1694
Dolobid Tablets (Less than 1 in 100) ... 1695
Dyazide Capsules ... 2653
Dyrenium Capsules (Rare) ... 2655

EC-Naprosyn Delayed-Release Tablets (Less than 1%) ... 2277
Feldene Capsules (Less than 1%) .. 2008
Floxin I.V. ... 1580
Floxin Tablets (200 mg, 300 mg, 400 mg) ... 1577
HydroDIURIL Tablets ... 1716
Hydropres Tablets ... 1718
Hyzaar Tablets ... 1720
Indocin (Less than 1%) ... 1723
Keflex Pulvules & Oral Suspension (Rare) ... 930
Keftab Tablets (Rare) ... 931
Kefzol Vials, Faspak & ADD-Vantage ... 1511
Lasix Injection, Oral Solution and Tablets ... 1267
Lodine Capsules and Tablets (Less than 1%) ... 2849
Maxaquin Tablets ... 2593
Mefoxin ... 1734
Mefoxin Premixed Intravenous Solution ... 1737
Mezlin (Rare) ... 594
Mezlin Pharmacy Bulk Package (Rare) ... 597
Moduretic Tablets ... 1748
Monocid Injection (Rare) ... 2674
Motrin Ibuprofen Suspension, Oral Drops, Chewable Tablets, Caplets ... 1563
Nalfon 200 Pulvules & Nalfon Tablets (Less than 1%) ... 933
▲ Naprelan Tablets (3% to 9%) ... 2861
Anaprox/Naprosyn (Less than 1%) ... 2277
Noroxin Tablets ... 1758
Noroxin Tablets ... 2222
Orthoclone OKT3 Sterile Solution .. 1892
Orudis Capsules (Less than 1%) ... 2874
Oruvail Capsules (Less than 1%) ... 2874
Penetrex Tablets ... 2196
Pentasa (Infrequent) ... 1275
Pipracil (Rare) ... 1435
Prilosec Delayed-Release Capsules (Less than 1%) ... 516
Prinzide Tablets ... 1780
Proleukin for Injection (Less than 1%) ... 812
Pyrazinamide Tablets (Rare) ... 1442
Relafen Tablets (Less than 1%) ... 2688
Rifadin ... 1276
Rifamate Capsules (Rare) ... 1278
Rifater (Rare) ... 1280
SSD (Infrequent) ... 1402
Septra ... 1146
Septra I.V. Infusion ... 1142
Septra I.V. Infusion ADD-Vantage Vials ... 1144
Septra ... 1146
Silvadene Cream 1% (Infrequent) ... 1288
Streptase for Infusion ... 557
Tagamet (Rare) ... 2694
Vancocin HCl, Oral Solution & Pulvules (Rare) ... 1536
Vancocin HCl, Vials & ADD-Vantage (Rare) ... 1534
Vaseretic Tablets ... 1810
Cataflam/Voltaren/Voltaren-XR (Rare) ... 833
Zestoretic Tablets ... 2968
Ziac ... 1459
Zinacef (Rare) ... 1184
Zosyn (Rare) ... 1463

Nephritis, purpuric
Vantin for Oral Suspension and Vantin Tablets ... 2112

Nephrocalcinosis
▲ Fungizone Intravenous (Among most common) ... 507
Rocaltrol Capsules ... 2303

Nephrolithiasis
Axid Pulvules ... 1468
▲ Crixivan Capsules (Approximately 4%) ... 1670
Invirase Capsules (Rare) ... 2291
Sandostatin Injection (Less than 1%) ... 2421

Nephropathy
Asacol Delayed-Release Tablets ... 2129
Bicillin C-R Injection ... 2810
Bicillin C-R 900/300 Injection ... 2812
Bicillin L-A Injection (Infrequent) ... 2813
Cedax ... 2480
Cefizox for Intramuscular or Intravenous Use ... 1025
Cefotan ... 2936

Ceftin ... 1067
Cefzil Tablets and Oral Suspension ... 747
Ceptaz ... 1070
Duricef Capsules, Tablets, and Oral Suspension ... 750
Fortaz ... 1092
Foscavir Injection (Less than 1%) ... 541
Hivid Tablets (Less than 1%) ... 2287
Keftab Tablets ... 931
Lorabid Suspension and Pulvules ... 1513
Maxipime for Injection ... 758
Nipent for Injection (Less than 3%) ... 2733
Pen•Vee K (Infrequent) ... 2879
Pfizerpen for Injection (Rare) ... 2022
Suprax ... 1443
Tazicef for Injection ... 2697
Tazidime Vials, Faspak & ADD-Vantage ... 1531
Vantin for Oral Suspension and Vantin Tablets ... 2112
Zinacef ... 1184

Nephropathy, acute uric acid
Oncaspar ... 2194
Oncovin Solution Vials & Hyporets ... 1521

Nephropathy, severe
Methotrexate Sodium Tablets, Injection, for Injection and LPF Injection ... 1322

Nephrosclerosis, malignant
Naprelan Tablets (Less than 1%) .. 2861

Nephrosis, toxic
Azulfidine (Rare) ... 2059
Bactrim DS Tablets ... 2257
Bactrim I.V. Infusion ... 2255
Bactrim ... 2257
Fansidar Tablets ... 2281
Felbatol ... 2774
Foscavir Injection (Less than 1%) ... 541
Fulvicin P/G Tablets (Rare) ... 2499
Fulvicin P/G 165 & 330 Tablets (Rare) ... 2500
Gantanol Tablets ... 2285
Gantrisin ... 2286
Intal Inhaler (Rare) ... 2185
Intal Nebulizer Solution (Rare) ... 2186
Mesantoin Tablets ... 2400
Nalfon 200 Pulvules & Nalfon Tablets (Less than 1%) ... 933
Neurontin Capsules (Rare) ... 1978
Pediazole Suspension ... 2340
Permax Tablets (Rare) ... 571
SSD ... 1402
Septra ... 1146
Septra I.V. Infusion ... 1142
Septra I.V. Infusion ADD-Vantage Vials ... 1144
Septra ... 1146
Silvadene Cream 1% ... 1288

Nephrotic syndrome
Anaprox/Naprosyn (Occasional; less than 1%) ... 2277
Azulfidine (Rare) ... 2059
Benemid Tablets ... 1651
Capoten Tablets (Approximately 1 to 2 of 1000 patients) ... 740
Capozide Tablets (Approximately 1 to 2 of 1000 patients) ... 744
Cataflam Tablets (Rare) ... 833
Clinoril Tablets (Less than 1 in 100) ... 1658
ColBENEMID Tablets ... 1662
Cuprimine Capsules ... 1673
Dapsone Tablets USP ... 1331
Depen Titratable Tablets ... 2770
Dipentum Capsules (Rare) ... 2084
Dolobid Tablets (Rare) ... 1695
EC-Naprosyn Delayed-Release Tablets (Occasional; less than 1%) ... 2277
Feldene Capsules (Less than 1%) .. 2008
Hyperab Rabies Immune Globulin (Human) (Rare) ... 618
Hyper-Tet Tetanus Immune Globulin (Human) (Few isolated cases) ... 621
Indocin (Less than 1%) ... 1723
Motrin Ibuprofen Suspension, Oral Drops, Chewable Tablets, Caplets (Occasional) ... 1563
Myochrysine Injection ... 1754
▲ Naprelan Tablets (3% to 9%) ... 2861
Anaprox/Naprosyn (Occasional; less than 1%) ... 2277
Orudis Capsules (Less than 1%) ... 2874
Oruvail Capsules (Less than 1%) ... 2874

Pentasa (Infrequent) ... 1275
Proglycem ... 575
Relafen Tablets (Less than 1%) ... 2688
Ridaura Capsules ... 2691
Rythmol Tablets–150mg, 225mg, 300mg (Less than 1%) ... 1399
Solganal Suspension ... 2530
Ticlid Tablets (Rare) ... 2317
Toradol ... 2319
Cataflam/Voltaren/Voltaren-XR (Rare) ... 833

Nephrotoxicity
Amikacin Sulfate Injection, USP ... 523
Amikacin Sulfate Injection, USP ... 981
Amikin Injectable ... 502
BiCNU ... 696
Capastat Sulfate Injection ... 968
CeeNU Capsules ... 699
Cefotan (Rare) ... 2936
Cortisporin Cream ... 1073
Cortisporin Ointment ... 1074
Cortisporin Otic Solution Sterile ... 1076
Cortisporin Otic Suspension Sterile ... 1077
Esgic-plus Capsules ... 1012
Esgic-plus Tablets ... 1012
Fioricet Tablets ... 2386
Fioricet with Codeine Capsules ... 2387
Fiorinal with Codeine Capsules ... 2390
Furoxone ... 2221
Garamycin Injectable ... 2502
IBU Tablets ... 1389
Leustatin ... 1889
Methotrexate Sodium Tablets, Injection, for Injection and LPF Injection ... 1322
Nebcin Vials, Hyporets & ADD-Vantage ... 1518
NeoDecadron Topical Cream ... 1757
▲ Neoral (25% to 38%) ... 2405
Neosporin G.U. Irrigant Sterile ... 1130
Netromycin Injection 100 mg/ml ... 2516
Neutrexin for Injection ... 2761
Paraplatin for Injection (Uncommon) ... 713
Pediotic Suspension Sterile ... 1140
Platinol for Injection ... 717
Platinol-AQ Injection ... 719
▲ Prograf (33% to 40%) ... 1028
Rowasa ... 2727
▲ Sandimmune (25 to 38%) ... 2416
Streptomycin Sulfate Injection (Rare) ... 2031
Vancocin HCl, Oral Solution & Pulvules ... 1536
Vancocin HCl, Vials & ADD-Vantage ... 1534
▲ Vistide Injection (53%) ... 1057
Zanosar Sterile Powder ... 2119
Zinacef ... 1184

Nerve deafness
Biavax II ... 1653
M-M-R II ... 1730
Mumpsvax ... 1751
Plaquenil Sulfate Tablets ... 2459

Nervousness
Accupril Tablets (0.5% to 1.0%) .. 1950
Accutane Capsules ... 2252
Actifed Cold & Allergy Tablets ... ⊞ 807
Actifed Cold & Sinus Caplets and Tablets ... ⊞ 808
Acutrim ... ⊞ 648
▲ Adalat Capsules (10 mg and 20 mg) (2% or less to 7%) ... 580
Adalat CC (Rare) ... 582
Adenoscan (2%) ... 1022
Advil Cold and Sinus Caplets and Tablets ... ⊞ 837
▲ AeroBid Inhaler System (3% to 9%) ... 1004
▲ Aerobid-M Inhaler System (3% to 9%) ... 1004
▲ Airet Albuterol Sulfate Inhalation Solution (4%) ... 1602
Albalon Solution with Liquifilm ... ⊚ 229
▲ Albuterol Sulfate, USP Solution for Inhalation, Arm-a-Med (4%) ... 522
Alferon N Injection (1%) ... 2142
Alka-Seltzer Plus ... ⊞ 611
Alka-Seltzer Plus Sinus Medicine ... ⊞ 611
Allerest Maximum Strength ... ⊞ 649
Allerest No Drowsiness ... ⊞ 649
Allerest Sinus Pain Formula ... ⊞ 649
Altace Capsules (Less than 1%) ... 1238
▲ Alupent (6.8%) ... 672
Ambien Tablets (1%) ... 2559
Amen Tablets ... 785
▲ Anafranil Capsules (4% to 18%) ... 819
Arimidex Tablets (2% to 5%) ... 2932

(⊞ Described in PDR For Nonprescription Drugs)   Incidence data in parenthesis; ▲ 3% or more   (⊚ Described in PDR For Ophthalmology)

Nervousness Side Effects Index 1410

▲ Artane (30% to 50%) 1418
Asacol Delayed-Release Tablets 2129
Asendin Tablets (Less frequent) 1419
Atrohist Plus Tablets 1605
▲ Atrovent Inhalation Aerosol (3.1%) 674
Atrovent Inhalation Solution (0.5%) 675
Axid Pulvules (1.1%) 1468
Bactrim DS Tablets 2257
Bactrim I.V. Infusion 2255
Bactrim 2257
Benadryl Allergy Decongestant Liquid Medication ...... ◘ 812
Benadryl Allergy Decongestant Tablets ...... ◘ 812
Benadryl Allergy Sinus Headache Caplets ...... ◘ 813
Benadryl Injection 1955
▲ Bentyl (6%) 1246
Benylin Multisymptom ...... ◘ 816
▲ Betaseron for SC Injection (8%) 653
Blocadren Tablets (Less than 1%) 1654
Brethaire Inhaler 830
▲ Brethine Ampuls (16.9 to 38.0%) 832
Brethine Tablets (Common) 831
Brevicon 2563
▲ Bricanyl Subcutaneous Injection (Among most common) 1247
▲ Bricanyl Tablets (One of the two most common) 1248
Bromfed 1832
▲ Bromfed-DM Cough Syrup (Among most frequent) 1832
Bromfed-PD Capsules (Extended-Release) 1832
▲ BuSpar Tablets (5%) 738
Butisol Sodium Elixir & Tablets (Less than 1 in 100) 2768
Capoten Tablets 740
Capozide Tablets 744
Cardene Capsules (0.6%) 2261
Cardioquin Tablets (2%) 2146
Cardizem CD Capsules (Less than 1%) 1251
Cardizem SR Capsules (Less than 1%) 1255
Cardizem Injectable 1253
Cardizem Tablets (Less than 1%) 1257
Cardura Tablets (2%) 1993
Cartrol Tablets (Less common) 413
Casodex Tablets (2% to 5%) 2934
Catapres Tablets (About 3 in 100 patients) 679
Catapres-TTS (1 of 101 patients) 680
Ceclor Pulvules & Suspension (Rare) 1470
Cefzil Tablets and Oral Suspension (Less than 1%) 747
Celontin Kapseals 1955
Cerebyx Injection (Frequent) 1956
Cerose DM ...... ◘ 853
Children's TYLENOL Cold Multi-Symptom Chewable Tablets and Liquid 1559
Children's Vicks DayQuil Allergy Relief ...... ◘ 730
Children's Vicks NyQuil Cold/Cough Relief ...... ◘ 731
Chlor-Trimeton Allergy Decongestant Tablets ...... ◘ 759
Claritin Tablets (2% or fewer patients) 2485
▲ Claritin-D Tablets (5%) 2487
Clinoril Tablets (Greater than 1%) 1658
Cocaine Hydrochloride Topical Solutions 529
Cogentin 1661
Cognex Capsules (Frequent) 1961
Combipres Tablets (About 3%) 682
Compazine 2644
Allergy-Sinus Comtrex Multi-Symptom Allergy-Sinus Formula Tablets and Caplets ...... ◘ 639
Contac Continuous Action Nasal Decongestant/Antihistamine 12 Hour Capsules ...... ◘ 773
Contac Maximum Strength Continuous Action Decongestant/Antihistamine 12 Hour Caplets ...... ◘ 772
Contac Severe Cold and Flu Formula Caplets ...... ◘ 773
Coricidin 'D' Decongestant Tablets ...... ◘ 760
Cozaar Tablets (Less than 1%) 1668
Crixivan Capsules (Less than 2%) 1670
Cycrin Tablets 991
Cystospaz 2123
Cytovene (1% or less) 2270
D.A. II Tablets 972
D.A. Chewable Tablets 970
Dalmane Capsules 2329
Danocrine Capsules 2437
Dantrium Capsules (Less frequent) 2131
Daranide Tablets 1676
Decadron Phosphate with Xylocaine Injection, Sterile 1683
Deconsal II Tablets 1605
Demadex Tablets and Injection (1.1%) 691
Demulen 2580
Depakote Tablets (1% to 5%) 418
▲ Depo-Provera Contraceptive Injection (More than 5%) 2079
Depo-Provera Sterile Aqueous Suspension 2083
Desogen Tablets 1867
▲ Desyrel and Desyrel Dividose (6.4% to 14.8%) 504
Dexatrim ...... ◘ 795
Dexatrim Plus Vitamins Caplets ...... ◘ 796
Dilantin Infatabs 1967
Dilantin Kapseals 1965
Dilantin-125 Suspension 1969
Dilaudid-HP Injection 1384
Dilaudid-HP Lyophilized Powder 250 mg 1384
Dilaudid Tablets and Liquid (Less frequent) 1386
Dimetane-DC Cough Syrup 2232
Dimetane-DX Cough Syrup 2233
Dimetapp Cold & Allergy Chewable Tablets ...... ◘ 838
Dimetapp Extentabs ...... ◘ 841
Dimetapp Tablets/Liqui-Gels ...... ◘ 841
Diupres Tablets 1691
Dolobid Tablets (Less than 1 in 100) 1695
Donnatal 2234
Donnatal Extentabs 2234
Donnatal Tablets 2234
Doral Tablets 2773
Dorcol Children's Cough Syrup ...... ◘ 748
Drixoral Cold and Allergy Sustained-Action Tablets ...... ◘ 763
Drixoral Cold and Flu Extended-Release Tablets ...... ◘ 764
Drixoral Allergy/Sinus Extended Release Tablets ...... ◘ 765
▲ Duragesic Transdermal System (3% to 10%) 1336
Duranest Injections 533
Dura-Tap/PD Capsules 970
Duratuss Tablets 2750
Dura-Vent/DA Tablets 972
Dura-Vent Tablets 971
Dyclone 0.5% and 1% Topical Solutions, USP 535
Dynabac (0.1% to 1%) 668
DynaCirc Capsules (0.5% to 1%) 2381
DynaCirc CR Tablets (0.5% to 1.0%) 2383
▲ Effexor (2% to 21.3%) 2825
Efidac/24 ...... ◘ 655
Eldepryl Capsules 2729
Emete-con Intramuscular/Intravenous 2007
EMLA Cream (Unlikely with cream) 536
Entex LA Tablets 972
Entex PSE Tablets 973
EpiPen Jr.- Epinephrine Auto-Injector 808
Ergamisol Tablets (1% to 2%) 1340
Estring Vaginal Ring (At least 1 report) 2086
▲ Ethmozine Tablets (2% to 5%) 2217
Eulexin Capsules (1%) 2498
Exgest LA Tablets 787
Fansidar Tablets 2281
Fedahist Gyrocaps 2545
▲ Felbatol (7.0% to 16.1%) 2774
Feldene Capsules (Less than 1%) 2008
Fioricet with Codeine Capsules 2387
Fiorinal with Codeine Capsules 2390
▲ Flexeril Tablets (1% to 3%) 1701
▲ Flolan for Injection (11% to 21%) 1085
▲ Floxin I.V. (1% to 3%) 1580
▲ Floxin Tablets (200 mg, 300 mg, 400 mg) (1% to 3%) 1577
Flumadine Tablets & Syrup (1.3% to 2.1%) 1013
▲ Foscavir Injection (Between 1% and 5%) 541
Gastrocrom Oral Concentrate (Less common) 1611
▲ Glucotrol XL Extended Release Tablets (3.6%) 2012
Guaimax-D Tablets 809
▲ Halcion Tablets (5.2%) 2093
Helidac Therapy (Less than 1%) 2135
Hismanal Tablets (2.1%) 1341
Hivid Tablets (Less than 1%) 2287
Hydropres Tablets 1718
Hytrin Capsules (2.3%) 434
Hyzaar Tablets 1720
IBU Tablets (Greater than 1%) 1389
Imdur (Less than or equal to 5%) 1362
Indocin (Less than 1%) 1723
Intron A for Injection (Up to 3%) 2506
Iopidine 0.5% (Less than 1%) ...... ⊙ 219
Ismo Tablets (Fewer than 1%) 2844
Isuprel Hydrochloride Solution 2443
Isuprel Injection 2441
Isuprel Mistometer 2442
Kerlone Tablets (0.8%) 2588
Kutrase Capsules 2546
Lamictal Tablets (Frequent) 1105
Levbid Extended-Release Tablets 2549
Levlen/Tri-Levlen 646
Levo-Dromoran 2297
Levsin/Levsinex/Levbid 2549
Lodine Capsules and Tablets (1% to 3%) 2849
Lo/Ovral Tablets 2852
Lo/Ovral-28 Tablets 2857
Lorabid Suspension and Pulvules 1513
Lotensin Tablets 852
Lotensin HCT Tablets (0.3% to 1.0%) 855
Lotrel Capsules 858
▲ Ludiomil Tablets (6%) 861
Lupron Depot 3.75 mg (Less than 5%) 2739
Lupron Depot - 3 Month 22.5 mg (Less than 5%) 2743
Lupron Depot-PED 7.5 mg, 11.25 mg and 15 mg (Less than 2%) 2744
Lupron Injection (Less than 5%) 2736
Lupron Injection Pediatric (Less than 2%) 2737
▲ LUVOX Tablets (12%) 2723
MS Contin Tablets (Less frequent) 2149
MSIR (Infrequent) 2152
Marax Tablets & DF Syrup 2015
Marinol (Dronabinol) Capsules (Greater than 1%) 2353
Matulane Capsules 2300
▲ Maxair Autohaler (4.5% to 6.9%) 1550
▲ Maxair Inhaler (6.9%) 1552
Maxaquin Tablets (Less than 1%) 2593
Mebaral Tablets (Less than 1 in 100) 2452
Merrem I.V. (0.1% to 1.0%) 2952
Mesantoin Tablets 2400
▲ Metaproterenol Sulfate Inhalation Solution, USP, Arm-a-Med (About 1 in 7 patients) 547
▲ Mexitil Capsules (5% to 11.3%) 684
Midamor Tablets (Less than or equal to 1%) 1746
Minipress Capsules (1-4%) 2015
Minizide Capsules 2016
Modicon 1928
Moduretic Tablets (Less than or equal to 1%) 1748
8-MOP Capsules 1294
Monoket Tablets (Fewer than 1%) 2550
Motofen Tablets (1 in 200 to 1 in 600) 789
Motrin Ibuprofen Suspension, Oral Drops, Chewable Tablets, Caplets (1% to less than 3%) 1563
Mykrox Tablets (Less than 2%) 1617
▲ Nalfon 200 Pulvules & Nalfon Tablets (5.7%) 933
Naprelan Tablets (Less than 1%) 2861
Nembutal Sodium Capsules (Less than 1%) 440
Nembutal Sodium Solution (Less than 1%) 442
Nembutal Sodium Suppositories (Less than 1%) 444
Neurontin Capsules (2.4%) 1978
▲ Nipent for Injection (3% to 10%) 2733
Nolahist Tablets 790
Nolamine Timed-Release Tablets (Occasional) 790
Nordette-21 Tablets 2863
Nordette-28 Tablets 2866
Norinyl 2563
Norisodrine with Calcium Iodide Syrup 446
▲ Norpace (1 to 3%) 2596
Norplant System 2868
Nor-Q D Tablets 2598
Norvasc Tablets (More than 0.1% to 1%) 2020
Norvir (Less than 2%) 447
Novahistine DMX ...... ◘ 782
Novahistine Elixir ...... ◘ 782
Novocain Hydrochloride for Spinal Anesthesia 2457
Nubain Injection (1% or less) 952
Nucofed 2225
OptiPranolol (Metipranolol 0.3%) Sterile Ophthalmic Solution (A small number of patients) ...... ⊙ 256
Oramorph SR (Morphine Sulfate Sustained Release Tablets) (Less frequent) 2359
▲ Orap Tablets (8.3%) 1037
▲ Orlaam Oral Solution (3% to 9%) 2361
Ornade Spansule Capsules 2678
Ortho-Cept 1907
Ortho-Cyclen/Ortho-Tri-Cyclen 1914
Ortho-Novum 1928
Ortho-Cyclen/Ortho Tri-Cyclen 1914
▲ Orudis Capsules (3% to 9%) 2874
▲ Oruvail Capsules (3% to 9%) 2874
Ovcon 765
Ovral Tablets 2877
Ovral-28 Tablets 2878
Ovrette Tablets 2878
Oxsoralen-Ultra Capsules 1302
OxyContin Tablets (Between 1% and 5%) 2163
PBZ Tablets 863
PBZ-SR Tablets 862
Parlodel 2411
▲ Paxil Tablets (4% to 9%) 2681
Pediatric Vicks 44d Cough & Head Congestion Relief ...... ◘ 736
Pediatric Vicks 44m Cough & Cold Relief ...... ◘ 737
Penetrex Tablets (1%) 2196
Periactin 1767
Permax Tablets (Frequent) 571
Phenergan Injection 2880
Phenergan Tablets 2882
Phenergan VC 2886
Phenergan VC with Codeine 2888
Phenobarbital Elixir and Tablets (Less than 1 in 100 patients) 1523
Plaquenil Sulfate Tablets 2459
Plendil Extended-Release Tablets (0.5% to 1.5%) 514
Pondimin Tablets 2239
Ponstel 1982
Pontocaine Hydrochloride for Spinal Anesthesia 2460
Premphase 2900
Prempro 2905
Prevacid Delayed-Release Capsules (Less than 1%) 2746
Prilosec Delayed-Release Capsules (Less than 1%) 516
Primatene Tablets ...... ◘ 844
Prinivil Tablets (0.3% to 1.0%) 1776
Prinzide Tablets 1780
Pro-Banthine Tablets 2226
▲ Procardia Capsules (2% or less to 7%) 2024
▲ Procardia XL Extended Release Tablets (Less than 3% to 7%) 2026
▲ Prograf (Greater than 3%) 1028
Propagest Tablets 791
Propulsid (1.4%) 1346
▲ ProSom Tablets (8%) 457
▲ Proventil Inhalation Aerosol (Less than 10%) 2524
▲ Proventil Inhalation Solution 0.083% (4%) 2527
▲ Proventil Repetabs Tablets (2% to 20%) 2529
▲ Proventil Solution for Inhalation 0.5% (4%) 2525
▲ Proventil Syrup (9 of 100 patients; children 2 to 6 years, 15%) 2528
▲ Proventil Tablets (20%) 2529
Provera Tablets 2110
▲ Prozac Pulvules & Liquid, Oral Solution (14.9%) 935
Pyrroxate Caplets ...... ◘ 742
Quadrinal Tablets 1398
Quinidex Extentabs (2%) 2240
Redux Capsules (Frequent) 2911
▲ Relafen Tablets (1% to 3%) 2688
Retrovir Capsules (1.6%) 1216
Retrovir I.V. Infusion (2%) 1221
Retrovir Syrup (1.6%) 1216
▲ ReVia Tablets (4% to more than 10%) 957
Revex (nalmefene hydrochloride injection) (Less than 1%) 1863
Rhinocort Nasal Inhaler (Less than 1%) 552
Risperdal Tablets (Frequent) 1348
▲ Ritalin (One of the two most common) 866
Robinul Forte Tablets 2247
Robinul Injectable 2247

(◘ Described in PDR For Nonprescription Drugs) Incidence data in parenthesis; ▲ 3% or more (⊙ Described in PDR For Ophthalmology)

Robinul Tablets 2247
Robitussin Maximum Strength Cough & Cold ■ 847
Robitussin Pediatric Cough & Cold Formula ■ 848
Robitussin-CF ■ 846
Robitussin-DAC Syrup 2249
Robitussin-PE ■ 846
Roferon-A Injection (Less than 3% to less than 5%) 2308
▲ Romazicon (3% to 9%) 2311
Rondec Oral Drops 974
Rondec Syrup 974
Rondec 974
Ryna ■ 804
Salagen Tablets (Less than 1%) 1546
▲ Sanorex Tablets (Among most common) 2423
Seconal Sodium Pulvules (Less than 1 in 100) 1529
Seldane Tablets (1.4% to 1.5%) 1284
▲ Seldane-D Extended-Release Tablets (6.7%) 1286
▲ Semprex-D Capsules (3%) 1620
Septra 1146
Septra I.V. Infusion 1142
Septra I.V. Infusion ADD-Vantage Vials 1144
Septra 1146
Ser-Ap-Es Tablets 867
Serevent Inhalation Aerosol (1% to 3%) 1149
Serophene (clomiphene citrate tablets, USP) (Approximately 1 in 50 patients) 2621
Sinarest ■ 663
Sine-Aid Maximum Strength Sinus Headache Gelcaps, Caplets and Tablets 1570
Sine-Off No Drowsiness Formula Caplets ■ 784
Sinemet CR Tablets 961
Sinulin Tablets 792
Sinutab Non-Drying Liquid Caps ■ 823
Skelaxin Tablets 793
Stadol (1% or greater) 779
Sudafed Cold & Allergy Tablets ■ 826
Sudafed Nasal Decongestant Tablets, 30 mg ■ 825
Sudafed Nasal Decongestant Tablets, 60 mg ■ 825
Sudafed Sinus Caplets ■ 829
Sudafed Sinus Tablets ■ 829
Sudafed 12 Hour Caplets ■ 824
Sular Tablets (Less than or equal to 1%) 2961
Supprelin Injection (1% to 3%) 2230
Symmetrel Capsules (1% to 5%) 965
Symmetrel Syrup (1% to 5%) 963
Syn-Rx Tablets 1622
Syn-Rx DM Tablets 1623
Tavist Syrup 2426
Tavist Tablets 2427
Teldrin 12 Hour Antihistamine/Nasal Decongestant Allergy Relief Capsules ■ 786
Tenex Tablets (Less frequent) 2249
TheraFlu ■ 750
TheraFlu Maximum Strength Nighttime Flu, Cold & Cough Medicine ■ 751
Tiazac Capsules (Less than 1% to 2%) 1019
Timolide Tablets (Less than 1%) 1791
Timoptic in Ocudose (Less frequent) 1796
Timoptic Sterile Ophthalmic Solution (Less frequent) 1794
Timoptic-XE 1798
Tofranil Tablets 875
▲ Tonocard Tablets (0.4% to 11.5%) 519
Toradol (1% or less) 2319
▲ Tornalate Solution for Inhalation, 0.2% (11.1%) 976
Tornalate Metered Dose Inhaler (1.5% to 5%) 978
Tranxene (Less common) 459
Trental Tablets 1291
Triaminic Syrup ■ 755
Triaminic Triaminicol Cold & Cough ■ 756
Triaminic DM Syrup ■ 756
Triaminicin Tablets ■ 756
Levlen/Tri-Levlen 646
Trinalin Repetabs Tablets 1373
Tri-Norinyl 2607
Triphasil-21 Tablets 2919
Triphasil-28 Tablets 2924
Tussend 1830
TYLENOL Cold Medication, Multi-Symptom Formula Tablets and Caplets 1572
TYLENOL Cold Medication, Multi-Symptom Hot Liquid Packets 1572
TYLENOL Cold Medication, No Drowsiness Formula Caplets and Gelcaps 1572
TYLENOL Cough Medication with Decongestant, Multi Symptom 1574
TYLENOL Flu NightTime, Maximum Strength Hot Medication Packets 1575
TYLENOL Sinus, Maximum Strength Geltabs, Gelcaps, Caplets and Tablets 1576
Tympagesic Ear Drops 2476
▲ Ultram Tablets (50 mg) (1% to 14%) 1594
Univasc Tablets (Less than 1%) 2553
Urispas Tablets 2710
Varivax (Greater than or equal to 1%) 1807
▲ Vascor Tablets (200 and 300 mg) (7.37 to 11.63%) 1597
Vaseretic Tablets (0.5% to 2.0%) 1810
Vasotec I.V. 1814
Vasotec Tablets (0.5% to 1.0%) 1816
▲ Ventolin Inhalation Aerosol and Refill (1%; fewer than 10 per 100 patients) 1170
▲ Ventolin Inhalation Solution (4%) 1171
▲ Ventolin Nebules Inhalation Solution (4%) 1172
Ventolin Rotacaps for Inhalation (1%) 1173
▲ Ventolin Syrup (9 of 100 patients; 15% in children) 1175
▲ Ventolin Tablets (Approximately 20 of 100 patients) 1176
Versed Injection (Less than 1%) 2324
Vicks 44 LiquiCaps Cough, Cold & Flu Relief ■ 728
Vicks 44 LiquiCaps Non-Drowsy Cough & Cold Relief ■ 729
Vicks 44D Cough & Head Congestion Relief ■ 728
Vicks 44M Cough, Cold & Flu Relief ■ 729
Vicks DayQuil Allergy Relief 4-Hour Tablets ■ 733
Vicks DayQuil LiquiCaps/Liquid Multi-Symptom Cold/Flu Relief ■ 734
Vicks DayQuil SINUS Pressure & CONGESTION Relief ■ 734
Vicks Nyquil Hot Therapy ■ 735
Vicks NyQuil LiquiCaps/Liquid Multi-Symptom Cold/Flu Relief, Original and Cherry Flavors ■ 736
▲ Videx Tablets, Powder for Oral Solution, & Pediatric Powder for Oral Solution (Up to 27%) 2980
▲ Visken Tablets (7%) 2428
▲ Volmax Extended-Release Tablets (8.5%) 1835
▲ Xanax Tablets (4.1%) 2115
▲ Xylocaine Injections (Among most common) 562
▲ Yutopar Intravenous Injection (5% to 6%) 566
Zaroxolyn Tablets (Less than 2%) 1625
▲ Zerit Capsules (Fewer than 1% to 10%) 731
Zestoretic Tablets 2968
Zestril Tablets (0.3% to 1.0%) 2972
Zithromax (1% or less) 2043
▲ Zoladex (3%) 2976
Zoladex 3-month 2978
▲ Zoloft Tablets (3.4%) 2051
Zyrtec Tablets (Less than 2%) 2053

Neuralgia

Altace Capsules (Less than 1%) 1238
Ambien Tablets (Rare) 2559
Anafranil Capsules (Infrequent) 819
Betaseron for SC Injection 653
Crixivan Capsules (Less than 2%) 1670
Effexor (Infrequent) 2825
Foscavir Injection (Less than 1%) 541
Hivid Tablets (Less than 1%) 2287
Imitrex Tablets (Rare) 1099
Kerlone Tablets (Less than 2%) 2588
Lamictal Tablets (Rare) 1105
Lamprene Capsules (Less than 1%) 846
LUVOX Tablets (Infrequent) 2723
Miacalcin Nasal Spray (Less than 1%) 2403
Naprelan Tablets (Less than 1%) 2861
Nipent for Injection (Less than 3%) 2733
Norvir (Less than 2%) 447
Paxil Tablets (Rare) 2681
Permax Tablets (1.1%) 571
Phenobarbital Elixir and Tablets (Rare) 1523
Prozac Pulvules & Liquid, Oral Solution (Infrequent) 935
Redux Capsules (Infrequent) 2911
Serzone Tablets (Infrequent) 776
Videx Tablets, Powder for Oral Solution, & Pediatric Powder for Oral Solution (Less than 1%) 2980
Zerit Capsules (Fewer than 1% to 1%) 731

Neural tube defects, unspecified

Clomid 1262
Serophene (clomiphene citrate tablets, USP) 2621

Neuritis

Ambien Tablets (Rare) 2559
Benadryl Injection 1955
Clinoril Tablets (Rare) 1658
Cognex Capsules (Infrequent) 1961
Cytosar-U Sterile Powder (Less frequent) 2077
Effexor (Rare) 2825
Fluorescite ⊙ 217
Foscavir Injection (Less than 1%) 541
Hivid Tablets (Less than 1%) 2287
Imdur (Less than or equal to 5%) 1362
Lotrel Capsules (Infrequent) 858
Naprelan Tablets (Less than 1%) 2861
Nipent for Injection (Less than 3%) 2733
Ornade Spansule Capsules 2678
Periactin 1767
Permax Tablets (Rare) 571
ProSom Tablets (Rare) 457
Redux Capsules (Rare) 2911
Sandostatin Injection (Less than 1%) 2421
Tapazole Tablets 1361
Tavist Syrup 2426
Tavist Tablets 2427
Trinalin Repetabs Tablets 1373
Tussend 1830
Zyloprim Tablets (Less than 1%) 1194

Neuritis, optic

Accutane Capsules (Less than 1%) 2252
Amen Tablets 785
Antabuse Tablets 2802
Attenuvax 1650
Biavax II 1653
Cardioquin Tablets (Occasional) 2146
Chloromycetin Sodium Succinate 1960
Clomid 1262
Cordarone Tablets (Rare) 2818
Cuprimine Capsules 1673
Cycrin Tablets 991
Decadron Phosphate Sterile Ophthalmic Ointment 1684
Decadron Phosphate Sterile Ophthalmic Solution 1685
Demulen 2580
Depen Titratable Tablets 2770
Depo-Provera Sterile Aqueous Suspension 2083
Doxil (1% to 5%) 2613
Engerix-B Unit-Dose Vials 2656
ESTRATAB Tablets (0.3, 0.625, 1.25, 2.5 mg) 2715
Estratest 2718
Etopophos for Injection (Infrequent) 701
Etoposide Injection 539
Ganite (Less than 1%) 2711
IBU Tablets (Less than 1%) 1389
Levlen/Tri-Levlen 646
Lo/Ovral Tablets 2852
Lo/Ovral-28 Tablets 2857
M-M-R II (Infrequent) 1730
M-R-VAX II 1732
Macrobid Capsules (Rare) 2138
Macrodantin Capsules (Rare) 2140
Menest Tablets 2671
Motrin Ibuprofen Suspension, Oral Drops, Chewable Tablets, Caplets (Less than 1%) 1563
Mumpsvax 1751
Myambutol Tablets 1432
Nalfon 200 Pulvules & Nalfon Tablets (Less than 1%) 933
Nordette-21 Tablets 2863
Nordette-28 Tablets 2866
Nydrazid Injection (Uncommon) 509
Ortho Dienestrol Cream 1922
Ovral Tablets 2877
Ovral-28 Tablets 2878
Ovrette Tablets 2878
PASER Granules 1333
Platinol for Injection (Infrequent) 717
Platinol-AQ Injection (Infrequent) 719
PMB 200 and PMB 400 2890
Premarin Intravenous 2893
Premarin Vaginal Cream 2898
Premphase 2900
Prempro 2905
Proleukin for Injection (Less than 1%) 812
Provera Tablets 2110
Quinaglute Dura-Tabs Tablets (Occasional) 644
Quinidex Extentabs (Occasional) 2240
Recombivax HB 1787
Rifamate Capsules (Uncommon) 1278
Rifater (Uncommon) 1280
Trecator-SC Tablets 2919
Levlen/Tri-Levlen 646
VePesid Capsules and Injection 727
Videx Tablets, Powder for Oral Solution, & Pediatric Powder for Oral Solution (Several patients) 2980
Yodoxin Tablets 1235
Zyloprim Tablets (Less than 1%) 1194

Neuritis, peripheral

Antabuse Tablets 2802
Antivenin (Crotalidae) Polyvalent (Occasional) 2803
Apresazide Capsules (Less frequent) 824
Apresoline Hydrochloride Tablets (Less frequent) 826
Atretol Tablets 569
Bactrim DS Tablets 2257
Bactrim I.V. Infusion 2255
Bactrim 2257
Chloromycetin Sodium Succinate 1960
ColBENEMID Tablets 1662
Doxil (Less than 1%) 2613
Fansidar Tablets 2281
Gantanol Tablets 2285
Gantrisin 2286
Hydralazine Hydrochloride Injection USP (Less frequent) 2712
Intal Inhaler (Rare) 2185
Intal Nebulizer Solution (Rare) 2186
Lopid Tablets 1974
Myambutol Tablets 1432
Nasalcrom Nasal Solution (Rare) 2192
Paxil Tablets (Rare) 2681
Pediazole Suspension 2340
Redux Capsules (Infrequent) 2911
Rilutek Tablets (Rare) 2198
Septra 1146
Septra I.V. Infusion 1142
Septra I.V. Infusion ADD-Vantage Vials 1144
Septra 1146
Ser-Ap-Es Tablets 867
Solganal Suspension 2530
Streptomycin Sulfate Injection 2031
Tegretol/Tegretol-XR 870
Trecator-SC Tablets 2919
Velban Vials 1537

Neuritis, retrobulbar

Attenuvax 1650
Biavax II 1653
M-M-R II 1730
M-R-VAX II 1732
Meruvax II 1740
Mumpsvax (Infrequent) 1751
Redux Capsules 2911

Neuroencephalopathy

Taxol Injection (Rare; less than 1%) 723

Neuroleptic malignant syndrome

Asendin Tablets (Less than 1%) 1419
Atamet Tablets 567
Clozaril Tablets (Several cases) 2377
Compazine 2644
Etrafon 2495
Haldol Decanoate 1587
Haldol Injection, Tablets and Concentrate 1585
Inapsine Injection (Very rare) 462
Loxitane 1426
Mellaril 2398
Moban Tablets and Concentrate 1036
Navane Capsules and Concentrate (Rare) 2018
Navane Intramuscular (Rare) 2019
Norpramin Tablets 1273

(■ Described in PDR For Nonprescription Drugs) Incidence data in parenthesis; ▲ 3% or more (⊙ Described in PDR For Ophthalmology)

Neuroleptic malignant syndrome — Side Effects Index

Orap Tablets	1037
Paxil Tablets	2681
Permax Tablets	571
Prolixin	510
Prozac Pulvules & Liquid, Oral Solution	935
Reglan (Rare)	2243
Risperdal Tablets	1348
Serentil	689
Serzone Tablets (Rare)	776
Sinemet Tablets	959
Sinemet CR Tablets	961
Stelazine	2692
Symmetrel Capsules (Sporadic cases)	965
Symmetrel Syrup (Sporadic cases)	963
Tegretol-XR Tablets (Isolated cases)	870
Thorazine	2701
Torecan	2367
Triavil Tablets	1800
Trilafon	2532
Zoloft Tablets	2051

Neurological disability, unspecified

Abelcet Injection	1540
Acel-Imune Diphtheria and Tetanus Toxoids and Acellular Pertussis Vaccine Adsorbed (Rare)	1415
Fungizone Intravenous	507
Hivid Tablets (Less than 1%)	2287
JE-VAX (Two cases)	904
▲ Nipent for Injection (1% to 11%)	2733
Rabies Vaccine, Imovax Rabies I.D. (Two cases)	901
Tetramune (Rare)	1449
TICE BCG, USP (0.9%)	1881

Neuromuscular block reversal, difficult

Nuromax Injection (Less than or equal to 0.1%)	1136

Neuromuscular blockade

Amikacin Sulfate Injection, USP	523
Amikacin Sulfate Injection, USP	981
Amikin Injectable	502
Mivacron (3 of 2,074 patients)	1125
Nebcin Vials, Hyporets & ADD-Vantage	1518
Netromycin Injection 100 mg/ml	2516
Zemuron Injection	1885

Neuromuscular excitability

Ceptaz	1070
Fortaz	1092
Tazidime Vials, Faspak & ADD-Vantage	1531
Ticar for Injection (With very high doses)	2704
Zosyn	1463

Neuromuscular symptoms

Azulfidine	2059
Eulexin Capsules (2%)	2498
Lupron Depot 3.75 mg (Less than 5%)	2739
▲ Lupron Depot - 3 Month 22.5 mg (9.6%)	2743

Neuromyopathy

Aralen Hydrochloride Injection	2430
Aralen Phosphate Tablets	2431

Neuro-ocular lesions

Amen Tablets	785
Demulen	2580
Triphasil-21 Tablets	2919
Triphasil-28 Tablets	2924

Neuropathy

Altace Capsules (Less than 1%)	1238
Ambien Tablets (Rare)	2559
Anafranil Capsules (Rare)	819
Betaseron for SC Injection	653
Bicillin C-R Injection	2810
Bicillin C-R 900/300 Injection	2812
Bicillin L-A Injection (Infrequent)	2813
Casodex Tablets (2% to 5%)	2934
▲ Chemet Capsules (1.0% to 12.7%)	666
Cognex Capsules (Infrequent)	1961
Cortifoam	2540
Cuprimine Capsules	1673
Cytosar-U Sterile Powder (Two patients)	2077
Cytotec (Infrequent)	2576
▲ Cytovene (8%)	2270
▲ DaunoXome (1% to 13%)	1842
Depen Titratable Tablets	2770

Dilacor XR Extended-release Capsules	2183
Diprivan Injectable Emulsion (Less than 1%)	2939
Doxil (Less than 1%)	2613
Effexor (Infrequent)	2825
Engerix-B Unit-Dose Vials	2656
▲ Epivir (12%)	1200
Fioricet with Codeine Capsules	2387
Fiorinal with Codeine Capsules	2390
▲ Foscavir Injection (5% or greater)	541
Havrix (Rare)	2663
Intron A for Injection (Less than 5%)	2506
Kerlone Tablets (Less than 2%)	2588
LUVOX Tablets	2723
Matulane Capsules	2300
Megace Oral Suspension (1% to 3%)	708
Mutamycin for Injection	712
Mykrox Tablets (Less than 2%)	1617
Nimotop Capsules (Less than 1%)	603
Nipent for Injection (Less than 3%)	2733
Norvir (Less than 2%)	447
Paxil Tablets (Rare)	2681
Pen•Vee K (Infrequent)	2879
Permax Tablets (Infrequent)	571
Pfizerpen for Injection (Rare)	2022
Platinol for Injection	717
Platinol-AQ Injection	719
▲ Prograf (Greater than 3%)	1028
Prozac Pulvules & Liquid, Oral Solution (Infrequent)	935
Redux Capsules	2911
Roferon-A Injection (Less than 0.5%)	2308
Sporanox Capsules (Isolated cases)	1352
Tambocor Tablets (Less than 1%)	1555
Urobiotic-250 Capsules	2038
▲ Videx Tablets, Powder for Oral Solution, & Pediatric Powder for Oral Solution (Rare in children; 17% to 21%)	2980
Vistide Injection	1057
Zaroxolyn Tablets	1625
▲ Zerit Capsules (15% to 21%)	731

Neuropathy, autonomic

Platinol for Injection	717
Platinol-AQ Injection	719
Taxol Injection (Rare)	723

Neuropathy, optic

Decadron Phosphate Injection	1680
Decadron Phosphate Sterile Ophthalmic Ointment	1684
Decadron Phosphate Sterile Ophthalmic Solution	1685
Healon GV	⊚ 303
Tolectin (200, 400 and 600 mg) (Less than 1%)	1591

Neuropathy, peripheral

Abelcet Injection	1540
Ancobon Capsules	2254
Antabuse Tablets	2802
Asacol Delayed-Release Tablets (Rare)	2129
Azulfidine (Rare)	2059
Betapace Tablets (One case)	637
Cordarone Tablets (Common)	2818
Cozaar Tablets (Less than 1%)	1668
Crixivan Capsules (Less than 2%)	1670
Cuprimine Capsules	1673
Dapsone Tablets USP	1331
Depen Titratable Tablets	2770
Diphtheria and Tetanus Toxoids and Pertussis Vaccine Adsorbed (A few cases)	2650
Elavil	2945
▲ Epivir (13%)	1200
Ergamisol Tablets	1340
Etrafon	2495
Flagyl 375 Capsules	2587
Flagyl I.V.	2373
Flexeril Tablets (Rare)	1701
Floxin I.V.	1580
Floxin Tablets (200 mg, 300 mg, 400 mg)	1577
Fludara for Injection	658
Foscavir Injection (Less than 1%)	541
Fungizone Intravenous	507
Garamycin Injectable	2502
Helidac Therapy	2135
▲ Hexalen Capsules (9% to 31%)	2760
▲ Hivid Tablets (28.3% up to 1/3 of patients)	2287
Hyzaar Tablets	1720
▲ Idamycin Injection (7%)	2096

Indocin Capsules (Less than 1%)	1723
Indocin I.V. (Less than 1%)	1727
Indocin (Less than 1%)	1723
JE-VAX (1 to 2.3 per million vaccines)	904
Lescol Capsules	2395
Leukeran Tablets	1205
Ludiomil Tablets (Isolated reports)	861
Lupron Depot 3.75 mg	2739
Lupron Depot 7.5 mg	2741
Lupron Depot - 3 Month 22.5 mg	2743
Lupron Depot-PED 7.5 mg, 11.25 mg and 15 mg	2744
Lupron Injection (Less than 5%)	2736
Macrobid Capsules	2138
Macrodantin Capsules	2140
Mevacor Tablets (0.5% to 1.0%)	1742
Myochrysine Injection (Rare)	1754
▲ Navelbine Injection (Up to 20%)	1212
Netromycin Injection 100 mg/ml	2516
Noroxin Tablets	1758
Noroxin Tablets	2222
Norpramin Tablets	1273
Norvir (Less than 2%)	447
▲ Nydrazid Injection (Among most common)	509
Pamelor	2409
▲ Paraplatin for Injection (4% to 16%)	713
Placidyl Capsules	456
Platinol for Injection	717
Platinol-AQ Injection	719
Pravachol Tablets	770
Prinivil Tablets (0.3% to 1.0%)	1776
Prinzide Tablets	1780
Protostat Tablets	1939
Recombivax HB	1787
Ridaura Capsules (Less than 1%)	2691
Rifamate Capsules	1278
Rifater	1280
Surmontil Capsules	2917
▲ Taxol Injection (Frequent; 3% to 60%)	723
Ticlid Tablets (Rare)	2317
Tofranil Ampuls	873
Tofranil Tablets	875
Tofranil-PM Capsules	876
Triavil Tablets	1800
Tripedia (A few cases)	908
Vaseretic Tablets	1810
Vasotec I.V.	1814
Vasotec Tablets (0.5% to 1.0%)	1816
▲ Videx Tablets, Powder for Oral Solution, & Pediatric Powder for Oral Solution (12% to 51%)	2980
Vivactil Tablets	1820
Yodoxin Tablets	1235
▲ Zerit Capsules (14% to 24%)	731
Zestoretic Tablets	2968
Zestril Tablets (0.3% to 1.0%)	2972
Zocor Tablets	1821
Zyloprim Tablets (Less than 1%)	1194

Neuropathy, peripheral sensory

Norvir (Less than 2%)	447

Neuropsychometrics performance, decrease

Blocadren Tablets	1654
Cartrol Tablets	413
Inderal	2834
Inderal LA Long Acting Capsules	2836
Inderide Tablets	2838
Inderide LA Long Acting Capsules	2840
Kerlone Tablets	2588
Levatol Tablets	2547
Lopressor HCT Tablets	850
Normodyne Tablets	2522
Sectral Capsules	2914
Tenoretic Tablets	2963
Tenormin Tablets and I.V. Injection	2965
Timoptic in Ocudose	1796
Timoptic Sterile Ophthalmic Solution	1794
Timoptic-XE	1798
Toprol-XL Tablets	560
Trandate Tablets	1158
Visken Tablets	2428

Neuroretinitis

BiCNU	696

Neurosis, unspecified

Ambien Tablets (Rare)	2559
Avonex	662
Betaseron for SC Injection	653
Cerebyx Injection (Infrequent)	1956
Cognex Capsules (Infrequent)	1961
Intron A for Injection (Less than 5%)	2506

Lamictal Tablets (Rare)	1105
Neurontin Capsules (Rare)	1978
Nipent for Injection (Less than 3%)	2733
Paxil Tablets (Infrequent)	2681
Permax Tablets (Infrequent)	571
Redux Capsules (Rare)	2911
Remeron Tablets (Infrequent)	1878
Zoloft Tablets (Infrequent)	2051

Neurotoxicity

Amikacin Sulfate Injection, USP	523
Amikacin Sulfate Injection, USP	981
Amikin Injectable	502
Cytosar-U Sterile Powder (Less frequent)	2077
Fluorouracil Injection (Rare)	2282
Foscavir Injection	541
Garamycin Injectable	2502
Helidac Therapy (Rare)	2135
Hexalen Capsules	2760
Leustatin (Rare)	1889
Nebcin Vials, Hyporets & ADD-Vantage	1518
Netromycin Injection 100 mg/ml	2516
Oncovin Solution Vials & Hyporets	1521
▲ Paraplatin for Injection (5% to 28%)	713
Platinol for Injection	717
Platinol-AQ Injection	719
▲ Prograf (Approximately 55%)	1028
Streptomycin Sulfate Injection	2031
Velban Vials (Not common)	1537
Vumon for Injection (Less than 1%)	729
▲ Zinecard Injection (10% to 17%)	2120

Neurotoxicity, peripheral

Etopophos for Injection (1% to 2%)	701
Etoposide Injection (1% to 2%)	539
VePesid Capsules and Injection (1% to 2%)	727

Neurovascular episodes

ParaGard T 380A Intrauterine Copper Contraceptive	1936

Neutropenia

Accupril Tablets (Rare)	1950
Achromycin V Capsules	1417
Altace Capsules	1238
Ancef Injection	2632
Aredia for Injection (Up to 1%)	827
Azactam for Injection (Less than 1%)	736
Bactrim DS Tablets	2257
Bactrim I.V. Infusion	2255
Bactrim	2257
▲ Betaseron for SC Injection (18%)	653
Capoten Tablets	740
Capozide Tablets	744
Cardura Tablets	1993
Ceclor Pulvules & Suspension (Rare)	1470
Cedax	2480
Cefizox for Intramuscular or Intravenous Use (Rare)	1025
Cefobid Intravenous/Intramuscular (1 in 50)	1996
Cefobid Pharmacy Bulk Package - Not for Direct Infusion (1 in 50)	1999
Cefotan	2936
Ceftin	1067
Cefzil Tablets and Oral Suspension	747
CellCept Capsules (Up to 2.0%)	2265
Ceptaz (Very rare)	1070
Chemet Capsules (0.5% to 1.5%)	666
Chibroxin Sterile Ophthalmic Solution (With oral form)	1657
Claforan Sterile and Injection (Less than 1%)	1259
Cleocin Phosphate Injection	2068
Cleocin Vaginal Cream	2070
Clinoril Tablets (Less than 1 in 100)	1658
▲ Clozaril Tablets (3%)	2377
Crixivan Capsules (1.1%)	1670
▲ Cytovene-IV (7% to 41%)	2270
Cytoxan	700
▲ DaunoXome (15% to 36%)	1842
Declomycin Tablets	1421
Desyrel and Desyrel Dividose (Occasional)	504
Diflucan Tablets, Injection, and Oral Suspension	2003
Dipentum Capsules (Rare)	2084
Dizac (diazepam injectable emulsion) CIV (Less frequent)	1862
Doryx Capsules	1970
▲ Doxil (44.2% to 49.9%)	2613

(⊡ Described in PDR For Nonprescription Drugs)   Incidence data in parenthesis; ▲ 3% or more   (⊚ Described in PDR For Ophthalmology)

Side Effects Index

Duricef Capsules, Tablets, and Oral Suspension ... 750
DYNACIN Capsules ... 1627
Edecrin ... 1698
▲ Epivir (7.2% to 22%) ... 1200
Ergamisol Tablets (2 out of 463 patients) ... 1340
▲ Etopophos for Injection (37% to 88%) ... 701
Flagyl 375 Capsules ... 2587
Floxin I.V. (More than or equal to 1%) ... 1580
Floxin Tablets (200 mg, 300 mg, 400 mg) (More than or equal to 1%) ... 1577
▲ Fludara for Injection (Among most common) ... 658
Fluorouracil Injection (Rare) ... 2282
Fortaz (Very rare) ... 1092
Gantanol Tablets ... 2285
Gastrocrom Capsules (Infrequent) ... 1611
Gastrocrom Oral Concentrate (Less common) ... 1611
▲ Gemzar for Injection (18% to 63%) ... 1482
Geocillin Tablets ... 2009
Halcion Tablets (1.5%) ... 2093
Helidac Therapy ... 2135
Hivid Tablets (16.9%) ... 2287
▲ Hycamtin for Injection (Most common; 26% to 98%) ... 2665
IBU Tablets (Less than 1%) ... 1389
▲ Intron A for Injection (26% to 92%) ... 2506
Keflex Pulvules & Oral Suspension ... 930
Keftab Tablets ... 931
Kefurox Vials, Faspak & ADD-Vantage (Less than 1 in 100) ... 1509
Kefzol Vials, Faspak & ADD-Vantage ... 1511
Lamictal Tablets ... 1105
Lamisil Tablets (Isolated case) ... 2394
Leukeran Tablets ... 1205
▲ Leustatin (Common; 70%) ... 1889
Lodine Capsules and Tablets (Less than 1%) ... 2849
Lorabid Suspension and Pulvules ... 1513
Lotensin Tablets (Rare) ... 852
Lotensin HCT Tablets ... 855
Lotrel Capsules ... 858
Mandol Vials, Faspak & ADD-Vantage ... 1516
Mavik Tablets (Rare) ... 1407
Mefoxin ... 1734
Mefoxin Premixed Intravenous Solution ... 1737
▲ Mepron Suspension (5%) ... 1206
Mesantoin Tablets ... 2400
MetroGel-Vaginal ... 917
Mexitil Capsules (About 1 in 1,000) ... 684
Mezlin ... 594
Mezlin Pharmacy Bulk Package ... 597
Midamor Tablets (Rare) ... 1746
Minocin Intravenous ... 1428
Minocin Oral Suspension ... 1431
Minocin Pellet-Filled Capsules ... 1429
Moduretic Tablets ... 1748
Monocid Injection (Less than 1%) .. 2674
Monodox Capsules ... 1858
Monopril Tablets ... 762
Motrin Ibuprofen Suspension, Oral Drops, Chewable Tablets, Caplets (Less than 1%) ... 1563
▲ Mycobutin Capsules (25%) ... 2101
▲ Neutrexin for Injection (30.3%) ... 2761
Nolvadex Tablets (Rare) ... 2957
Noroxin Tablets (1.4%) ... 1758
Noroxin Tablets (1.4%) ... 2222
Orthoclone OKT3 Sterile Solution .. 1892
▲ Paraplatin for Injection (16% to 97%) ... 713
Pipracil ... 1435
Platinol for Injection ... 717
Platinol-AQ Injection ... 719
Prilosec Delayed-Release Capsules (Rare) ... 516
Primaxin I.M. ... 1770
Primaxin I.V. (Less than 0.2%) ... 1772
Prinivil Tablets (Rare) ... 1776
Prinzide Tablets (Rare) ... 1780
Procanbid Extended-Release Tablets (Approximately 0.5%) ... 1983
Proglycem ... 575
Proleukin for Injection ... 812
Proloprim Tablets ... 1141
Protostat Tablets ... 1939
Reglan (A few cases) ... 2243
Retrovir ... 1216
Ridaura Capsules (0.1 to 1%) ... 2691

Rilutek Tablets (3 cases) ... 2198
Rocephin Injectable Vials, ADD-Vantage, Galaxy Container (Less than 1%) ... 2305
▲ Roferon-A Injection (Up to 68%) ... 2308
Sansert Tablets ... 2424
Septra ... 1146
Septra I.V. Infusion ... 1142
Septra I.V. Infusion ADD-Vantage Vials ... 1144
Septra ... 1146
Suprax ... 1443
Symmetrel Capsules (Less than 0.1%) ... 965
Symmetrel Syrup (Less than 0.1%) ... 963
▲ Taxol Injection (52% to 90%) ... 723
▲ Taxotere for Injection Concentrate (76%) ... 2204
Tazicef for Injection (Very rare) ... 2697
Tazidime Vials, Faspak & ADD-Vantage (Very rare) ... 1531
Terramycin Intramuscular Solution ... 2034
Ticar for Injection ... 2704
Ticlid Tablets (0.8% to 2.4%) ... 2317
Timentin for Injection ... 2706
Tonocard Tablets (Less than 1%) .. 519
Trimpex Tablets ... 2323
Unasyn ... 2035
Univasc Tablets (More than 1%) ... 2553
Valium Injectable (Isolated reports) ... 2336
Valium Tablets (Isolated reports) ... 2335
Vancocin HCl, Oral Solution & Pulvules (Several dozen cases) ... 1536
Vancocin HCl, Vials & ADD-Vantage (Several dozen cases) ... 1534
Vantin for Oral Suspension and Vantin Tablets ... 2112
Vascor Tablets (200 and 300 mg) (2 cases) ... 1597
Vaseretic Tablets (Rare; several cases) ... 1810
Vasotec I.V. (Several cases) ... 1814
Vasotec Tablets (Rare; several cases) ... 1816
Vermox Chewable Tablets (Rare) ... 1357
Vibramycin ... 2038
Vibramycin Hyclate Intravenous ... 2040
Vibramycin ... 2038
▲ Viramune Tablets (11.1%) ... 2368
▲ Vistide Injection (20% to 31%) ... 1057
▲ Vumon for Injection (95%) ... 729
Xanax Tablets (2.3% to 3.0%) ... 2115
▲ Zerit Capsules (5% to 13%) ... 731
Zestoretic Tablets (Rare) ... 2968
Zestril Tablets (Rare) ... 2972
Zinacef (Fewer than 1 in 100) ... 1184
Zithromax (Less than 1%) ... 2043
Zithromax Tablets (Less than 1%) ... 2046
Zosyn ... 1463
Zovirax Sterile Powder (Less than 1%) ... 1191

Neutropenia, congenital
Azulfidine (Rare) ... 2059

Neutrophilia
Dynabac (1.2%) ... 668
Floxin I.V. (More than or equal to 1%) ... 1580
Floxin Tablets (200 mg, 300 mg, 400 mg) (More than or equal to 1%) ... 1577
Hivid Tablets (Less than 1%) ... 2287
Maxipime for Injection (0.1% to 1%) ... 758
Zovirax Sterile Powder (Less than 1%) ... 1191

Neutrophils, decrease
(see under Neutropenia)

Nevi, pre-existing, increased growth of
Nutropin AQ Injection (Rare) ... 1051

Night blindness
(see under Nyctalopia)

Nightmares
Aldoclor Tablets ... 1638
Aldomet Ester HCl Injection ... 1642
Aldomet Oral ... 1640
Aldoril Tablets ... 1644
Asendin Tablets (Less frequent) ... 1419
Atamet Tablets ... 567
Biaxin ... 406
Blocadren Tablets ... 1654
Butisol Sodium Elixir & Tablets (Less than 1 in 100) ... 2768

Cataflam Tablets (Less than 1%) ... 833
Catapres Tablets ... 679
Catapres-TTS ... 680
Cipro I.V. (1% or less) ... 587
Cipro I.V. Pharmacy Bulk Package (Less than 1%) ... 590
Cipro Tablets (Less than 1%) ... 584
▲ Clozaril Tablets (4%) ... 2377
Combipres Tablets ... 682
Desyrel and Desyrel Dividose (Less than 1% to 5.1%) ... 504
Diupres Tablets ... 1691
Doral Tablets ... 2773
Elavil ... 2945
Eldepryl Capsules ... 2729
Etrafon ... 2495
Floxin I.V. ... 1580
Floxin Tablets (200 mg, 300 mg, 400 mg) ... 1577
Halcion Tablets (Rare) ... 2093
Hydropres Tablets ... 1718
Ismo Tablets (Fewer than 1%) ... 2844
Larodopa Tablets (Relatively frequent) ... 2296
Lopressor ... 848
Lopressor HCT Tablets (1 in 100 patients) ... 850
Ludiomil Tablets (Rare) ... 861
Marinol (Dronabinol) Capsules (Less than 1%) ... 2353
Matulane Capsules ... 2300
Mebaral Tablets (Less than 1 in 100) ... 2452
Monoket Tablets (Fewer than 1%) ... 2550
Nardil (Infrequent) ... 1977
Nembutal Sodium Capsules (Less than 1%) ... 440
Nembutal Sodium Solution (Less than 1%) ... 442
Nembutal Sodium Suppositories (Less than 1%) ... 444
Norpramin Tablets ... 1273
Orudis Capsules (Rare) ... 2874
Oruvail Capsules (Rare) ... 2874
Pamelor ... 2409
Parlodel ... 2411
Penetrex Tablets ... 2196
Phenobarbital Elixir and Tablets (Less than 1 in 100 patients) ... 1523
Plaquenil Sulfate Tablets ... 2459
Relafen Tablets (Less than 1%) ... 2688
ReVia Tablets (Less than 1%) ... 957
Risperdal Tablets (Rare) ... 1348
Seconal Sodium Pulvules (Less than 1 in 100) ... 1529
Seldane Tablets ... 1284
Seldane-D Extended-Release Tablets ... 1286
Ser-Ap-Es Tablets ... 867
Sinemet Tablets ... 959
Surmontil Capsules ... 2917
Timolide Tablets ... 1791
Timoptic in Ocudose ... 1796
Timoptic Sterile Ophthalmic Solution ... 1794
Timoptic-XE ... 1798
Tofranil Ampuls ... 873
Tofranil Tablets ... 875
Tofranil-PM Capsules ... 876
Toprol-XL Tablets ... 560
Triavil Tablets ... 1800
Vantin for Oral Suspension and Vantin Tablets (Less than 1%) ... 2112
Ventolin Inhalation Aerosol and Refill (1%) ... 1170
Versed Injection (Less than 1%) ... 2324
Vivactil Tablets ... 1820
Cataflam/Voltaren/Voltaren-XR (Less than 1%) ... 833

Night sweat
Crixivan Capsules (Less than 2%) .. 1670
Hivid Tablets (Less than 1%) ... 2287
Neoral (Rare) ... 2405
▲ Oncaspar (Greater than 1% but less than 5%) ... 2194
▲ Roferon-A Injection (8%) ... 2308
Sandimmune (Rare) ... 2416

Night terrors
(see under Pavor nocturnus)

Nitritoid reactions
Myochrysine Injection ... 1754

Nitrogen balance, changes
(see under BUN levels, changes)

Nocturia
Adalat Capsules (10 mg and 20 mg) (Less than 0.5%) ... 580

Adalat CC (Less than 1.0%) ... 582
Ambien Tablets (Rare) ... 2559
Anafranil Capsules (Infrequent) ... 819
Avonex ... 662
Betaseron for SC Injection ... 653
BuSpar Tablets (Rare) ... 738
Calcijex Injection ... 412
Cardene Capsules (0.4%) ... 2261
Cardizem CD Capsules (Less than 1%) ... 1251
Cardizem SR Capsules (Less than 1%) ... 1255
Cardizem Injectable ... 1253
Cardizem Tablets (Less than 1%) .. 1257
▲ Casodex Tablets (9%) ... 2934
Cataflam Tablets (Less than 1%) ... 833
Catapres Tablets (About 1 in 100 patients) ... 679
Claritin-D Tablets (Less frequent) ... 2487
Cognex Capsules (Infrequent) ... 1961
Combipres Tablets (About 1%) ... 682
Cozaar Tablets (Less than 1%) ... 1668
Crixivan Capsules (Less than 2%) .. 1670
Dantrium Capsules (Less frequent) ... 2131
DaunoXome (Less than or equal to 5%) ... 1842
DynaCirc Capsules (0.5% to 1%) .. 2381
DynaCirc CR Tablets (0.5% to 1.0%) ... 2383
Effexor (Infrequent) ... 2825
Eldepryl Capsules ... 2729
Esimil Tablets ... 840
Foscavir Injection (Between 1% and 5%) ... 541
Hivid Tablets (Less than 1%) ... 2287
▲ Hylorel Tablets (48.4%) ... 1613
Hyperstat I.V. Injection ... 2504
Hyzaar Tablets ... 1720
Intron A for Injection (Less than 5%) ... 2506
Ismelin Tablets ... 845
Klonopin Tablets ... 2294
Lioresal Tablets (Rare) ... 847
LUVOX Tablets (Infrequent) ... 2723
Matulane Capsules ... 2300
Miacalcin Injection ... 2402
Moduretic Tablets (Less than or equal to 1%) ... 1748
Mykrox Tablets (Less than 2%) ... 1617
Naprelan Tablets (Less than 1%) .. 2861
Neurontin Capsules (Rare) ... 1978
Norpramin Tablets ... 1273
Norvasc Tablets (More than 0.1% to 1%) ... 2020
Norvir (Less than 2%) ... 447
Orap Tablets ... 1037
Pamelor ... 2409
Paxil Tablets (Infrequent) ... 2681
Procardia Capsules (Less than 0.5%) ... 2024
Procardia XL Extended Release Tablets (1% or less) ... 2026
ProSom Tablets (Rare) ... 457
Redux Capsules (Frequent) ... 2911
Rilutek Tablets (Rare) ... 2198
Rocaltrol Capsules ... 2303
Sectral Capsules (Up to 2%) ... 2914
Serzone Tablets (Infrequent) ... 776
Sular Tablets (Less than or equal to 1%) ... 2961
Supprelin Injection (1% to 3%) ... 2230
Tenex Tablets (Less frequent) ... 2249
Tiazac Capsules (Less than 1%) ... 1019
▲ TICE BCG, USP (4.5%) ... 1881
Trilafon ... 2532
Vagistat-1 (Less than 1%) ... 783
Videx Tablets, Powder for Oral Solution, & Pediatric Powder for Oral Solution (Less than 1%) ... 2980
Vivactil Tablets ... 1820
Cataflam/Voltaren/Voltaren-XR (Less than 1%) ... 833
Wellbutrin Tablets (Frequent) ... 1177
Zoloft Tablets (Infrequent) ... 2051

Nodal rhythm
Covera-HS Tablets ... 2573
Isoptin SR Tablets ... 1395
Lanoxicaps (Common) ... 1110
Lanoxin Elixir Pediatric (Common) .. 1113
Lanoxin Injection (Common) ... 1116
▲ Lanoxin Injection Pediatric (Among most common) ... 1119
Lanoxin Tablets (Common) ... 1121
Prostigmin Injectable ... 1305
Prostigmin Tablets ... 1306
Romazicon (Less than 1%) ... 2311
Sodium Polystyrene Sulfonate Suspension ... 2367
Suprane (desflurane, USP) (Greater than 1%) ... 1865

(▣ Described in PDR For Nonprescription Drugs)   Incidence data in parenthesis; ▲ 3% or more   (⊙ Described in PDR For Ophthalmology)

Nodal rhythm Side Effects Index 1414

Versed Injection (Less than 1%) 2324

Nodule at injection site

Depo-Provera Sterile Aqueous Suspension 2083
Diphtheria and Tetanus Toxoids and Pertussis Vaccine Adsorbed (Occasional) 2650
Genotropin Injection (Infrequent) 2090
Lovenox Injection 2187
Tetramune (Occasional) 1449

Nodule, subcutaneous

Naprelan Tablets (Less than 1%) 2861
Neurontin Capsules (Rare) 1978
Permax Tablets (Rare) 571
Prozac Pulvules & Liquid, Oral Solution (Rare) 935

Noise intolerance

BuSpar Tablets (Infrequent) 738
Neurontin Capsules (Rare) 1978

Nuchal rigidity

CytoGam (Infrequent) 1630
Gamimune N, 5% Immune Globulin Intravenous (Human), 5% (Infrequent) 612
Gamimune N, 10% Immune Globulin Intravenous (Human), 10% (Infrequent) 615
Gammar-P I.V., Immune Globulin Intravenous (Human) (Infrequent) 798
Methotrexate Sodium Tablets, Injection, for Injection and LPF Injection 1322
Sandoglobulin I.V. (Infrequent) 2419

Numbness

Adapin Capsules (Infrequent) 1542
Adenocard Injection (1%) 1021
AeroBid Inhaler System (1% to 3%) 1004
Aerobid-M Inhaler System (1% to 3%) 1004
Alferon N Injection (One patient to 3%) 2142
Amikacin Sulfate Injection, USP 523
Apresazide Capsules (Less frequent) 824
Apresoline Hydrochloride Tablets (Less frequent) 826
Asendin Tablets (Less than 1%) 1419
Atamet Tablets 567
Axocet Capsules (Infrequent) 2469
Bentyl 1246
BuSpar Tablets (2%) 738
Cafergot 2376
Catapres-TTS 680
Caverject Injection (Less than 1%) 2064
Cefizox for Intramuscular or Intravenous Use (Rare) 1025
Clozaril Tablets (Less than 1%) 2377
Demulen 2580
Desyrel and Desyrel Dividose 504
DynaCirc Capsules (0.5% to 1%) .. 2381
Elavil 2945
Elimite (permethrin) 5% Cream (1 to 2% or less) 475
EMLA Cream (Unlikely with cream) 536
Esgic-plus Capsules (Infrequent) 1012
Esgic-plus Tablets (Infrequent) 1012
Fioricet Tablets (Infrequent) 2386
Fioricet with Codeine Capsules (Infrequent) 2387
Fiorinal with Codeine Capsules (Infrequent) 2390
Garamycin Injectable 2502
Hydralazine Hydrochloride Injection USP (Less frequent) 2712
▲ Imitrex Injection (4.6%) 1095
Imitrex Tablets (Frequent) 1099
INFeD (Iron Dextran Injection, USP) 2478
K-Phos Neutral Tablets 633
K-Phos Original Formula 'Sodium Free' Tablets (Less frequent) 633
Kerlone Tablets (Less than 2%) 2588
Larodopa Tablets (Relatively frequent) 2296
Limbitrol 2333
Loxitane 1426
Ludiomil Tablets (Rare) 861
Lupron Injection (Less than 5%) 2736
▲ Mexitil Capsules (2.4% to 3.8%) .. 684
Mintezol 1747
Moduretic Tablets (Less than or equal to 1%) 1748
Monopril Tablets (0.4% to 1.0%) .. 762
Nebcin Vials, Hyporets & ADD-Vantage 1518
Netromycin Injection 100 mg/ml 2516
Nicotrol NS Nicotine Nasal Spray (Less than 1%) 1565
Normodyne Injection (1%) 2519
Norpace (Less than 1%) 2596
Norplant System 2868
Norpramin Tablets 1273
Nubain Injection (1% or less) 952
Pamelor 2409
Parlodel 2411
Parnate Tablets 2679
Peganone Tablets 455
Phrenilin (Infrequent) 790
Rifadin 1276
Rifamate Capsules 1278
Rifater 1280
Rimactane Capsules 865
▲ Roferon-A Injection (3% to 12%) .. 2308
Rythmol Tablets–150mg, 225mg, 300mg (Less than 1%) 1399
SSKI Solution (Less frequent) 2767
Sedapap Tablets 50 mg/650 mg (Infrequent) 1826
Ser-Ap-Es Tablets 867
Sinemet Tablets 959
Sinemet CR Tablets 961
Sinequan (Infrequent) 2028
Surmontil Capsules 2917
Tofranil Ampuls 873
Tofranil Tablets 875
Tofranil-PM Capsules 876
Tonocard Tablets (Less than 1%) .. 519
Trandate Injection (1 of 100 patients) 1158
Triavil Tablets 1800
Vivactil Tablets 1820

Numbness, buccal mucosa

Azactam for Injection (Less than 1%) 736
Clozaril Tablets (1%) 2377
Marcaine Spinal 2449
Nicotrol NS Nicotine Nasal Spray (More common) 1565

Numbness, extremities

Cogentin 1661
Estrace Cream and Tablets 751
Etrafon 2495
Flagyl 375 Capsules 2587
Flagyl I.V. 2373
Foscavir Injection 541
Helidac Therapy 2135
IOPIDINE Sterile Ophthalmic Solution ..... ◉ 218
Levlen/Tri-Levlen 646
Lomotil 2591
Maxair Autohaler 1550
Maxair Inhaler (Less than 1%) 1552
MetroCream 1034
Modicon 1928
Myambutol Tablets 1432
Norpramin Tablets 1273
Ortho-Cyclen/Ortho-Tri-Cyclen 1914
Ortho-Est 1925
Ortho-Novum 1928
Ortho-Cyclen/Ortho Tri-Cyclen 1914
Protostat Tablets 1939
Sansert Tablets 2424
Trilafon 2532
Levlen/Tri-Levlen 646
Videx Tablets, Powder for Oral Solution, & Pediatric Powder for Oral Solution (Less than 1%) 2980
Zerit Capsules 731

Numbness, face

Invirase Capsules (Less than 2%) .. 2291
Nicotrol NS Nicotine Nasal Spray (More common) 1565
Placidyl Capsules 456

Numbness, feet

Uroqid-Acid No. 2 Tablets 633

Numbness, fingers

Alferon N Injection (One patient) 2142
Cormax Ointment (Approximately 0.3%) 1856
Cutivate Cream (1.0%) 1078
Hivid Tablets 2287
Temovate E Emollient (Less than 2%) 1154
▲ Temovate Gel (Among most frequent) 1153
Temovate Ointment (Less frequent) 1152
Wigraine Tablets 1884

Numbness, hands

Alferon N Injection (One patient) 2142
Hyperstat I.V. Injection 2504
Uroqid-Acid No. 2 Tablets 633

Numbness, lips

K-Phos Neutral Tablets 633
K-Phos Original Formula 'Sodium Free' Tablets (Less frequent) 633
Marcaine Spinal 2449
Oncaspar 2194
Sensorcaine 554
Uroqid-Acid No. 2 Tablets 633

Numbness, mouth (see under Numbness, buccal mucosa)

Numbness, nose

Nicotrol NS Nicotine Nasal Spray (More common) 1565

Numbness, skin

Eskalith 2658
Lithium Carbonate Capsules & Tablets 2352
Lithonate/Lithotabs/Lithobid 2721

Numbness, toes

Hivid Tablets 2287
Wigraine Tablets 1884

Numbness, tongue (see under Numbness, buccal mucosa)

Numbness/tingling, fingers and toes

Cafergot 2376
D.H.E. 45 Injection 2381
Eldepryl Capsules 2729
Ergomar Tablets 1543
MetroGel 1034

Nyctalopia

Accutane Capsules 2252
Anafranil Capsules (Rare) 819
Aralen Hydrochloride Injection 2430
Aralen Phosphate Tablets 2431
Cardioquin Tablets (Occasional) 2146
Cataflam Tablets (Less than 1%) 833
Mellaril 2398
Paxil Tablets (Rare) 2681
Questran (One case) 774
Quinaglute Dura-Tabs Tablets (Occasional) 644
Quinidex Extentabs (Occasional) 2240
Serzone Tablets (Rare) 776
Tegison Capsules (Less than 1%) .. 2314
Cataflam/Voltaren/Voltaren-XR (Less than 1%) 833

Nystagmus

Anafranil Capsules (Rare) 819
Atretol Tablets 569
Betaseron for SC Injection 653
▲ Cerebyx Injection (15.1% to 44.4%) 1956
Cipro I.V. (1% or less) 587
Cipro I.V. Pharmacy Bulk Package (Less than 1%) 590
Cipro Tablets 584
Clozaril Tablets (Less than 1%) 2377
Cylert Tablets 415
Dalalone D.P. Injectable 1009
Decadron-LA Sterile Suspension (Low) 1687
Depakene 416
Depakote Tablets 418
▲ Dilantin Infatabs (Among most common) 1967
▲ Dilantin Kapseals (Among most common) 1965
▲ Dilantin-125 Suspension (Among most common) 1969
Dilaudid-HP Injection (Less frequent) 1384
Dilaudid-HP Lyophilized Powder 250 mg (Less frequent) 1384
Dilaudid Tablets and Liquid (Less frequent) 1386
Diprivan Injectable Emulsion (Less than 1%) 2939
Dizac (diazepam injectable emulsion) CIV (Less frequent) 1862
Effexor (Rare) 2825
Ergamisol Tablets 1340
Eskalith 2658
Ethmozine Tablets (Less than 2%) 2217
Felbatol 2774
Floxin I.V. 1580
Floxin Tablets (200 mg, 300 mg, 400 mg) 1577
Fluorouracil Injection 2282
Foscavir Injection (Less than 1%) .. 541
Sterile FUDR (Remote possibility) .. 2284
Isoptin Injectable 1391
Kadian Capsules (Less than 3%) 2948
Klonopin Tablets 2294
Lamictal Tablets (1.0%) 1105
Lioresal Intrathecal (1% or more) .. 1634
Lioresal Tablets 847
Lithium Carbonate Capsules & Tablets 2352
Lithonate/Lithotabs/Lithobid 2721
MS Contin Tablets (Less frequent) 2149
MSIR (Infrequent) 2152
Macrobid Capsules 2138
Macrodantin Capsules 2140
Matulane Capsules 2300
Maxaquin Tablets 2593
Mebaral Tablets 2452
Mesantoin Tablets 2400
Mysoline (Occasional) 2860
Nardil (Less common) 1977
Netromycin Injection 100 mg/ml 2516
▲ Neurontin Capsules (Among most common; 8.3%) 1978
Noroxin Tablets 1758
Noroxin Tablets 2222
Oncovin Solution Vials & Hyporets (Rare) 1521
Oramorph SR (Morphine Sulfate Sustained Release Tablets) (Less frequent) 2359
Paxil Tablets (Rare) 2681
Peganone Tablets 455
Penetrex Tablets 2196
Placidyl Capsules 456
Plaquenil Sulfate Tablets 2459
ProSom Tablets (Rare) 457
Prozac Pulvules & Liquid, Oral Solution (Rare) 935
Remeron Tablets (Rare) 1878
Robaxin Injectable 2245
Talwin Injection (Rare) 2465
Tambocor Tablets (Less than 1%) 1555
Tegretol/Tegretol-XR 870
Tonocard Tablets (Up to 1.1%) 519
Valium Injectable 2336
Velban Vials (Rare) 1537
Versed Injection (Less than 1%) 2324
Zoloft Tablets (Infrequent) 2051

Nystagmus, horizontal (see also under Nystagmus)

Restoril Capsules (Less than 0.5%) 2413

NMS (see under Neuroleptic malignant syndrome)

NPN elevation

Garamycin Injectable 2502
Nebcin Vials, Hyporets & ADD-Vantage 1518

O

Obstipation

Compazine 2644
Etrafon 2495
Mellaril 2398
Serentil 689
Stelazine 2692
Thorazine 2701
Torecan 2367
Triavil Tablets 1800
Trilafon (Occasional) 2532

Obtundation

Orthoclone OKT3 Sterile Solution .. 1892
Roferon-A Injection (Rare) 2308
Zovirax Sterile Powder (Approximately 1%) 1191

Occult bleeding

Fiorinal with Codeine Capsules 2390
Soma Compound w/Codeine Tablets 2784
▲ Soma Compound Tablets (Among most common) 2783

Occult blood in stool, positive test

Lioresal Tablets 847

Ocular allergy

Alomide Ophthalmic Solution (Less than 1%) 465
Anafranil Capsules (Up to 2%) 819

1415 Side Effects Index Opisthotonos

▲ Trusopt Sterile Ophthalmic Solution (Approximately 10%) 1803
Voltaren Ophthalmic Sterile Ophthalmic Solution .... ⊙ 264

Ocular discomfort
▲ Alomide Ophthalmic Solution (Among most frequent) 465
Betoptic Ophthalmic Solution 465
▲ Betoptic S Ophthalmic Suspension (Most frequent) 467
BuSpar Tablets (Rare) 738
▲ Iopidine 0.5% (6%) .... ⊙ 219
▲ Ocuflox Ophthalmic Solution (One of the two most frequent) 478
▲ Trusopt Sterile Ophthalmic Solution (Among most frequent) .. 1803
Vexol 1% Ophthalmic Suspension (1% to 5%) .... ⊙ 227

Ocular, foreign body sensation
▲ Alomide Ophthalmic Solution (1% to 5%) 465
▲ Betimol 0.25%, 0.5% (More than 5%) .... ⊙ 259
Betoptic Ophthalmic Solution 465
Betoptic S Ophthalmic Suspension (Small number of patients) 467
IOPIDINE Sterile Ophthalmic Solution .... ⊙ 218
Iopidine 0.5% (Less than 3%) .... ⊙ 219
Ocuflox Ophthalmic Solution 478
Timoptic in Ocudose (Less frequent) 1796
Timoptic Sterile Ophthalmic Solution (Less frequent) 1794
Timoptic-XE (1% to 5% of patients) 1798

Ocular exudate
▲ Alomide Ophthalmic Solution (1% to 5%) 465
Betoptic Ophthalmic Solution 465
Betoptic S Ophthalmic Suspension (Small number of patients) 467
Iopidine 0.5% (Less than 3%) .... ⊙ 219
Livostin (Approximately 1% to 3%) .... ⊙ 262
Timoptic in Ocudose (Less frequent) 1796
Timoptic Sterile Ophthalmic Solution (Less frequent) 1794
Timoptic-XE (1% to 5% of patients) 1798
Vexol 1% Ophthalmic Suspension (1% to 5%) .... ⊙ 227

Ocular hypotony
IOPIDINE Sterile Ophthalmic Solution .... ⊙ 218

Ocular infection
CORTENEMA 2713
NeoDecadron Sterile Ophthalmic Ointment 1755
NeoDecadron Sterile Ophthalmic Solution 1756
Prelone Syrup 1834
Terra-Cortril Ophthalmic Suspension 2033
Trilafon 2532

Ocular lesions
Brevicon 2563
Decadron Phosphate Sterile Ophthalmic Ointment 1684
Decadron Phosphate Sterile Ophthalmic Solution 1685
Norinyl 2563
Nor-Q D Tablets 2598
Ovcon 765
Tri-Norinyl 2607

Ocular palsies
Attenuvax (Rare) 1650
M-M-R II (Rare) 1730
M-R-VAX II (Rare) 1732
Plaquenil Sulfate Tablets 2459

Ocular perforation
Decadron Phosphate Sterile Ophthalmic Ointment 1684
Decadron Phosphate Sterile Ophthalmic Solution 1685
Eflone Sterile Ophthalmic Suspension .... ⊙ 261
Flarex Ophthalmic Suspension .... ⊙ 217

Ocular pressure
Zebeta Tablets 1457

Ocular tension, increase
Bentyl 1246
Cortisporin Ophthalmic Ointment Sterile 1074
Cortisporin Ophthalmic Suspension Sterile 1075
Decadron Phosphate Sterile Ophthalmic Ointment 1684
Decadron Phosphate Sterile Ophthalmic Solution 1685
Donnatal 2234
Donnatal Extentabs 2234
Donnatal Tablets 2234
Kutrase Capsules 2546
Levsin/Levsinex/Levbid 2549
Norflex 1554
Norgesic 1554
Pro-Banthine Tablets 2226
Robinul Forte Tablets 2247
Robinul Injectable 2247
Robinul Tablets 2247
Urispas Tablets 2710
Ziac 1459

Ocular toxicity
AKTOB (Less than 3 of 100 patients) .... ⊙ 207
Plaquenil Sulfate Tablets 2459
Platinol for Injection 717
Platinol-AQ Injection 719
Ridaura Capsules 2691
TobraDex Ophthalmic Suspension and Ointment (Less than 4%) 469
Tobrex Ophthalmic Ointment and Solution (Less than 3 of 100 patients) .... ⊙ 226

Oculogyric crises
Anafranil Capsules (Rare) 819
Atamet Tablets 567
Betaseron for SC Injection 653
Cognex Capsules (Rare) 1961
Compazine 2644
Cylert Tablets 415
Etrafon 2495
Haldol Decanoate (Frequent) 1587
Haldol Injection, Tablets and Concentrate 1585
Inapsine Injection 462
Larodopa Tablets (Rare) 2296
Mellaril 2398
Orap Tablets (Less frequent) 1037
Paxil Tablets 2681
Phenergan with Codeine 2883
Phenergan with Dextromethorphan 2885
Phenergan Injection 2880
Phenergan Suppositories 2882
Phenergan Syrup 2881
Phenergan Tablets 2882
Phenergan VC 2886
Phenergan VC with Codeine 2888
Prolixin 510
Reglan 2243
▲ Risperdal Tablets (17% to 34%) .. 1348
Serentil 689
Sinemet Tablets 959
Stelazine 2692
Symmetrel Capsules (Less than 0.1%) 965
Symmetrel Syrup (Less than 0.1%) 963
Thorazine 2701
Timolide Tablets 1791
Torecan 2367
Triavil Tablets 1800
Trilafon 2532

Oculomotor disturbances
Atretol Tablets 569
Levoprome 1321
Pravachol Tablets 770
Tegretol/Tegretol-XR 870

Oiliness
A/T/S 2% Acne Topical Gel (Occasional) 1244
Erycette (erythromycin 2%) Topical Solution 1943
T-Stat 2.0% Topical Solution and Pads 2797
THERAMYCIN Z 2% Solution 1629

Oligohydramnios
Accupril Tablets 1950
Altace Capsules 1238
Capoten Tablets 740
Capozide Tablets 744
Cleocin Vaginal Cream (2%) 2070
Clinoril Tablets 1658
Cozaar Tablets 1668
Dolobid Tablets 1695
Hyzaar Tablets 1720
Lotensin Tablets 852
Lotensin HCT Tablets 855
Lotrel Capsules 858
Monopril Tablets 762
Prinivil Tablets 1776
Prinzide Tablets 1780
Univasc Tablets 2553
Vaseretic Tablets 1810
Vasotec I.V. 1814
Vasotec Tablets 1816
Zestoretic Tablets 2968
Zestril Tablets 2972

Oligomenorrhea
Brevicon 2563
Levlen/Tri-Levlen 646
Modicon 1928
Mustargen 1752
▲ Nolvadex Tablets (8.7%) 2957
Norinyl 2563
Nor-Q D Tablets 2598
Ortho-Cyclen/Ortho-Tri-Cyclen 1914
Ortho-Novum 1928
Ortho-Cyclen/Ortho Tri-Cyclen 1914
Sandostatin Injection (Less than 1%) 2421
Levlen/Tri-Levlen 646
Tri-Norinyl 2607

Oligospermia
Androderm Testosterone Transdermal System 2634
Android Capsules, 10 mg (At high dosages) 1297
▲ Azulfidine (Approximately one-third of patients) 2059
Cytoxan 700
Halotestin Tablets 2095
Methotrexate Sodium Tablets, Injection, for Injection and LPF Injection 1322
Nizoral Tablets 1345
Oxandrin 783
Testoderm Testosterone Transdermal System 486
Testred Capsules, 10 mg 1308
Winstrol Tablets 2468

Oliguria
Abelcet Injection 1540
Altace Capsules 1238
Amikacin Sulfate Injection, USP 523
Amikacin Sulfate Injection, USP 981
Amikin Injectable 502
Anafranil Capsules (Infrequent) 819
Apresazide Capsules 824
Astramorph/PF Injection, USP (Preservative-Free) 526
Atretol Tablets 569
Azulfidine (Rare) 2059
Bactrim DS Tablets 2257
Bactrim I.V. Infusion 2255
Bactrim 2257
Betaseron for SC Injection 653
Brontex 2130
Calcium Disodium Versenate Injection 1548
Capastat Sulfate Injection (1 patient) 968
Capoten Tablets (Approximately 1 to 2 of 1000 patients) 740
Capozide Tablets (Approximately 1 to 2 of 1000 patients) 744
Cataflam Tablets (Rare) 833
Cerebyx Injection (Infrequent) 1956
Cleocin Phosphate Injection (Rare) 2068
Cleocin Vaginal Cream (Rare) 2070
Clomid 1262
ColBENEMID Tablets 1662
Demadex Tablets and Injection 691
Diprivan Injectable Emulsion (Less than 1%) 2939
Duragesic Transdermal System (Less than 1%) 1336
Duramorph Injection 983
Dyazide Capsules 2653
Esidrix Tablets 839
Eskalith 2658
Fansidar Tablets 2281
Fungizone Intravenous 507
Gantanol Tablets 2285
Gantrisin 2286
Garamycin Injectable 2502
Humegon for Injection 1873
Hyskon Hysteroscopy Fluid (Rare) .. 1633
Hyzaar Tablets 1720
Infumorph 200 and Infumorph 500 Sterile Solutions 985
Kerlone Tablets (Less than 2%) 2588
Lasix Injection, Oral Solution and Tablets 1267
Lioresal Intrathecal (1% or more) .. 1634
Lithium Carbonate Capsules & Tablets 2352
Lithonate/Lithotabs/Lithobid 2721
Lotrel Capsules 858
LUVOX Tablets (Rare) 2723
Metrodin (urofollitropin for injection) 2616
Miltown Tablets (Rare) 2780
Monopril Tablets 762
Mykrox Tablets 1617
Nalfon 200 Pulvules & Nalfon Tablets (Less than 1%) 933
Nebcin Vials, Hyporets & ADD-Vantage 1518
Netromycin Injection 100 mg/ml 2516
Oretic Tablets 450
Orthoclone OKT3 Sterile Solution .. 1892
Paxil Tablets (Rare) 2681
Pediazole Suspension 2340
Phenergan with Codeine 2883
Phenergan VC with Codeine 2888
PMB 200 and PMB 400 (Rare) 2890
Primaxin I.M. 1770
Primaxin I.V. (Less than 0.2%) 1772
Prinivil Tablets (0.3% to 1.0%) 1776
Prinzide Tablets 1780
Priscoline Hydrochloride Ampuls 864
▲ Prograf (16% to 18%) 1028
▲ Proleukin for Injection (76%) 812
ProSom Tablets (Rare) 457
Redux Capsules (Infrequent) 2911
Sansert Tablets 2424
Septra 1146
Septra I.V. Infusion 1142
Septra I.V. Infusion ADD-Vantage Vials 1144
Septra 1146
Serophene (clomiphene citrate tablets, USP) 2621
Serzone Tablets (Rare) 776
Tegretol/Tegretol-XR 870
Tenoretic Tablets 2963
Thalitone (Common) 1293
Toradol (1% or less) 2319
Univasc Tablets (Less than 1%) 2553
Vaseretic Tablets 1810
Vasotec I.V. 1814
Vasotec Tablets (0.5% to 1.0%) 1816
Cataflam/Voltaren/Voltaren-XR (Rare) 833
Zaroxolyn Tablets 1625
Zestoretic Tablets 2968
Zestril Tablets (0.3% to 1.0%) 2972
Zoloft Tablets (Rare) 2051
Zosyn (1.0% or less) 1463

Oliguria, neonatal
Altace Capsules 1238
Capoten Tablets 740
Capozide Tablets 744
Lotensin Tablets 852
Monopril Tablets 762
Zestril Tablets 2972

"On-off" phenomenon
Atamet Tablets 567
Larodopa Tablets 2296
Parlodel 2411
Sinemet Tablets 959
Sinemet CR Tablets (1.6%) 961

Onycholysis
Adriamycin PFS (A few cases) 2056
Adriamycin RDF (A few cases) 2056
Doxorubicin Astra (A few cases) 531
Feldene Capsules (Less than 1%) .. 2008
Helidac Therapy (Rare) 2135
Orudis Capsules (Less than 1%) 2874
Oruvail Capsules (Less than 1%) 2874
Rubex for Injection (A few cases) 721
Taxotere for Injection Concentrate (0.8%) 2204
▲ Tegison Capsules (1-10%) 2314
Zyloprim Tablets (Less than 1%) 1194

Oogenesis, defective
Cytoxan 700
Methotrexate Sodium Tablets, Injection, for Injection and LPF Injection 1322

Ophthalmoplegia
Betaseron for SC Injection 653
Cytovene-IV (One report) 2270
Lescol Capsules 2395
Mevacor Tablets 1742
Pravachol Tablets 770

(▣ Described in PDR For Nonprescription Drugs) Incidence data in parenthesis; ▲ 3% or more (⊙ Described in PDR For Ophthalmology)

Side Effects Index

Opisthotonos
- Redux Capsules ... 2911
- Zocor Tablets ... 1821

Opisthotonos
- Compazine ... 2644
- Diprivan Injectable Emulsion (Rare; less than 1%) ... 2939
- Etrafon ... 2495
- Haldol Decanoate (Frequent) ... 1587
- Haldol Injection, Tablets and Concentrate ... 1585
- Levoprome ... 1321
- Lioresal Intrathecal (1% or more) ... 1634
- Mellaril ... 2398
- Orap Tablets (Less frequent) ... 1037
- Prolixin ... 510
- Reglan ... 2243
- Serentil ... 689
- Stelazine ... 2692
- Thorazine ... 2701
- Tigan ... 2231
- Torecan ... 2367
- Triavil Tablets ... 1800
- Trilafon ... 2532

Optic atrophy
- Aralen Phosphate Tablets ... 2431
- Diupres Tablets ... 1691
- Eskalith ... 2658
- Hydropres Tablets ... 1718
- Lithium Carbonate Capsules & Tablets ... 2352
- Oncovin Solution Vials & Hyporets ... 1521
- Plaquenil Sulfate Tablets ... 2459
- Rifater (Uncommon) ... 1280
- Ser-Ap-Es Tablets ... 867
- Yodoxin Tablets ... 1235

Optic disorders
- Effexor (Rare) ... 2825

Optic nerve, damage
- AK-CIDE (Infrequent) ... ⊚ 203
- AK-CIDE Ointment (Infrequent) ... ⊚ 203
- AK-PRED ... ⊚ 204
- AK-Trol Ointment & Suspension (Infrequent) ... ⊚ 205
- Blephamide Liquifilm Sterile Ophthalmic Suspension (Infrequent) ... 472
- Blephamide Ointment (Infrequent) ... ⊚ 234
- Celestone Soluspan Suspension (Possible) ... 2484
- CORTENEMA ... 2713
- Cortisporin Ophthalmic Ointment Sterile (Infrequent) ... 1074
- Cortisporin Ophthalmic Suspension Sterile (Infrequent) ... 1075
- Dapsone Tablets USP ... 1331
- Dexacort Phosphate in Respihaler ... 1606
- Dexacort Phosphate in Turbinaire ... 1607
- Econopred & Econopred Plus Ophthalmic Suspensions ... ⊚ 216
- Eflone Sterile Ophthalmic Suspension ... ⊚ 261
- FML Forte Liquifilm (Infrequent) ... ⊚ 237
- FML Liquifilm (Infrequent) ... ⊚ 238
- FML S.O.P. (Infrequent) ... ⊚ 239
- FML-S Liquifilm (Infrequent) ... ⊚ 240
- Flarex Ophthalmic Suspension ... ⊚ 217
- Florinef Acetate Tablets ... 506
- HMS Liquifilm (Rare) ... ⊚ 241
- Maxitrol Ophthalmic Ointment and Suspension (Infrequent) ... ⊚ 222
- NeoDecadron Sterile Ophthalmic Ointment ... 1755
- NeoDecadron Sterile Ophthalmic Solution (Infrequent) ... 1756
- Poly-Pred Liquifilm (Infrequent) ... ⊚ 246
- Pred Forte (Infrequent) ... ⊚ 247
- Pred Mild (Infrequent) ... ⊚ 250
- Pred-G Liquifilm Sterile Ophthalmic Suspension (Infrequent) ... ⊚ 248
- Pred-G S.O.P. Sterile Ophthalmic Ointment ... ⊚ 249
- Prelone Syrup ... 1834
- Streptomycin Sulfate Injection ... 2031
- Taxol Injection (Rare) ... 723
- Terra-Cortril Ophthalmic Suspension (Infrequent) ... 2033
- TobraDex Ophthalmic Suspension and Ointment (Infrequent) ... 469
- Vexol 1% Ophthalmic Suspension ... ⊚ 227

Optic nerve, infarction
- Hyperstat I.V. Injection ... 2504
- Trandate ... 1158

Orchitis
- Biavax II ... 1653
- M-M-R II ... 1730
- Maxaquin Tablets (Less than 1%) ... 2593
- Mumpsvax (Rare) ... 1751
- Prozac Pulvules & Liquid, Oral Solution (Rare) ... 935
- TICE BCG, USP (0.2%) ... 1881

Organic brain syndrome
- Eskalith ... 2658
- Lithium Carbonate Capsules & Tablets ... 2352

Organomegaly
- ▲ Vesanoid Capsules (3%) ... 2327

Oropharyngitis
- ▲ Roferon-A Injection (14%) ... 2308

Oropharynx, dry
- ▲ Atrovent Inhalation Aerosol (About 5 in 100) ... 674
- Brethaire Inhaler ... 830
- Proventil Inhalation Aerosol ... 2524
- Proventil Repetabs Tablets ... 2529
- Proventil Syrup ... 2528
- Proventil Tablets ... 2529
- ▲ Roferon-A Injection (14%) ... 2308
- Tussionex Pennkinetic Extended-Release Suspension ... 1624
- Ventolin Syrup ... 1175
- Ventolin Tablets ... 1176
- Volmax Extended-Release Tablets ... 1835

Orthopnea
- Prinivil Tablets (0.3% to 1.0%) ... 1776
- Prinzide Tablets ... 1780
- Zestoretic Tablets ... 2968
- Zestril Tablets (0.3% to 1.0%) ... 2972

Oscillopsia
- Lamictal Tablets (Infrequent) ... 1105

Osteoarticular pain
- Cardizem CD Capsules (Less than 1%) ... 1251
- Cardizem SR Capsules (Less than 1%) ... 1255
- Cardizem Injectable ... 1253
- Cardizem Tablets (Less than 1%) ... 1257
- Tiazac Capsules (Less than 1%) ... 1019

Osteomalacia
- Didronel Tablets ... 2133
- Dilantin Kapseals ... 1965
- Dilantin-125 Suspension ... 1969
- Phenobarbital Elixir and Tablets ... 1523

Osteomalacia, phosphate-induced
- K-Phos Neutral Tablets ... 633
- K-Phos Original Formula 'Sodium Free' Tablets ... 633
- Uroqid-Acid No. 2 Tablets ... 633

Osteomalacia syndromes
- Amphojel ... 2802
- Basaljel ... 2810
- Gelusil Antacid-Anti-gas Liquid ... ⊞ 819
- Gelusil Antacid-Anti-gas Tablets ... ⊞ 819
- Maalox Antacid/Anti-Gas Tablets ... 889
- Maalox Heartburn Relief Suspension ... ⊞ 658
- Maalox Antacid Liquid ... 888
- Extra Strength Maalox Antacid/Anti-Gas Liquid and Tablets ... 888
- Mylanta ... 1359
- Rolaids Antacid Tablets ... ⊞ 807

Osteomyelitis
- Nipent for Injection (1%) ... 2733
- Permax Tablets (Rare) ... 571
- TICE BCG, USP (Rare; about 1 per 1,000,000 vaccinees) ... 1881

Osteoporosis
- Celestone Soluspan Suspension ... 2484
- Cognex Capsules (Infrequent) ... 1961
- CORTENEMA ... 2713
- Cortifoam ... 2540
- Cortone Acetate Sterile Suspension ... 1663
- Cortone Acetate Tablets ... 1664
- Dalalone D.P. Injectable ... 1009
- Decadron Elixir ... 1676
- Decadron Phosphate Injection ... 1680
- Decadron Phosphate with Xylocaine Injection, Sterile ... 1683
- Decadron Tablets ... 1678

- Decadron-LA Sterile Suspension ... 1687
- Depo-Provera Contraceptive Injection (Fewer than 1%) ... 2079
- Dexacort Phosphate in Respihaler ... 1606
- Dexacort Phosphate in Turbinaire ... 1607
- Effexor (Rare) ... 2825
- Florinef Acetate Tablets ... 506
- Fludara for Injection (Up to 2%) ... 658
- Heparin Lock Flush Solution ... 2831
- Heparin Sodium Injection ... 2832
- Heparin Sodium Vials ... 1486
- Hydeltrasol Injection, Sterile ... 1708
- Hydeltra-T.B.A. Sterile Suspension ... 1710
- Hydrocortone Acetate Sterile Suspension ... 1712
- Hydrocortone Phosphate Injection, Sterile ... 1713
- Hydrocortone Tablets ... 1715
- Methotrexate Sodium Tablets, Injection, for Injection and LPF Injection (Rare) ... 1322
- Neupogen for Injection (Infrequent) ... 495
- Neurontin Capsules (Rare) ... 1978
- Paxil Tablets (Rare) ... 2681
- Pediapred Oral Solution ... 1618
- Permax Tablets (Rare) ... 571
- Prelone Syrup ... 1834
- ▲ Prograf (Greater than 3%) ... 1028
- Prozac Pulvules & Liquid, Oral Solution (Rare) ... 935
- Questran (Less frequent) ... 774
- Rilutek Tablets (Rare) ... 2198
- Zoladex 3-month (1% to 5%) ... 2978

Otitis externa
- Ambien Tablets (Rare) ... 2559
- Betaseron for SC Injection ... 653
- Neurontin Capsules (Rare) ... 1978
- Paxil Tablets (Rare) ... 2681
- ▲ Tegison Capsules (1-10%) ... 2314
- Videx Tablets, Powder for Oral Solution, & Pediatric Powder for Oral Solution (Less than 1%) ... 2980

Otitis media
- Ambien Tablets (Rare) ... 2559
- Anafranil Capsules (Up to 4%) ... 819
- ▲ Avonex (6%) ... 662
- Betaseron for SC Injection ... 653
- Chemet Capsules (1.0% to 3.7%) ... 666
- Cognex Capsules (Infrequent) ... 1961
- Dilacor XR Extended-release Capsules ... 2183
- Doxil (Less than 1%) ... 2613
- Effexor (Infrequent) ... 2825
- Estring Vaginal Ring (1% to 3%) ... 2086
- ▲ Felbatol (3.4% to 9.7%) ... 2774
- Foscavir Injection (Less than 1%) ... 541
- Invirase Capsules (Less than 2%) ... 2291
- LUVOX Tablets (Infrequent) ... 2723
- M-M-R II ... 1730
- Naprelan Tablets (Less than 1%) ... 2861
- Neurontin Capsules (Infrequent) ... 1978
- Orthoclone OKT3 Sterile Solution ... 1892
- Paxil Tablets (Infrequent) ... 2681
- ▲ PedvaxHIB (Among most frequent) ... 1761
- Permax Tablets (Infrequent) ... 571
- Prevacid Delayed-Release Capsules (Less than 1%) ... 2746
- Remeron Tablets (Rare) ... 1878
- Sandostatin Injection (Less than 1%) ... 2421
- Sular Tablets (Less than or equal to 1%) ... 2961
- ▲ Tetramune (Among most common) ... 1449
- Varivax (Greater than or equal to 1%) ... 1807
- ▲ Videx Tablets, Powder for Oral Solution, & Pediatric Powder for Oral Solution (Up to 11%) ... 2980
- Zoloft Tablets (Rare) ... 2051

Ototoxicity
- Amikacin Sulfate Injection, USP ... 523
- Amikacin Sulfate Injection, USP ... 981
- Amikin Injectable ... 502
- Cortisporin Cream ... 1073
- Cortisporin Ointment ... 1074
- Cortisporin Otic Solution Sterile ... 1076
- Cortisporin Otic Suspension Sterile ... 1077
- Demadex Tablets and Injection ... 691
- Garamycin Injectable ... 2502
- Lasix Injection, Oral Solution and Tablets ... 1267
- Nebcin Vials, Hyporets & ADD-Vantage ... 1518
- NeoDecadron Topical Cream ... 1757
- Neosporin G.U. Irrigant Sterile ... 1130
- Netromycin Injection 100 mg/ml ... 2516

- ▲ Paraplatin for Injection (1% to 13%) ... 713
- Pediotic Suspension Sterile ... 1140
- ▲ Platinol for Injection (Up to 31%) ... 717
- ▲ Platinol-AQ Injection (Up to 31% of patients) ... 719
- Streptomycin Sulfate Injection ... 2031
- Vancocin HCl, Oral Solution & Pulvules ... 1536
- Vancocin HCl, Vials & ADD-Vantage ... 1534
- Zyrtec Tablets (Less than 2%) ... 2053

Ovarian cyst formation
- Anafranil Capsules (Infrequent) ... 819
- ▲ Avonex (3%) ... 662
- Clomid ... 1262
- Humegon for Injection ... 1873
- Metrodin (urofollitropin for injection) ... 2616
- Micronor Tablets ... 1903
- Nolvadex Tablets (2.8%; a small number of premenopausal patients) ... 2957
- Pergonal (menotropins for injection, USP) ... 2618
- Profasi (chorionic gonadotropin for injection, USP) ... 2620
- Serophene (clomiphene citrate tablets, USP) (Less than 1 in 100 patients) ... 2621

Ovarian cysts, enlargement of existing
- Profasi (chorionic gonadotropin for injection, USP) ... 2620
- Synarel Nasal Solution for Central Precocious Puberty ... 2603
- Synarel Nasal Solution for Endometriosis ... 2605

Ovarian disorder
- Neurontin Capsules (Rare) ... 1978
- Prozac Pulvules & Liquid, Oral Solution (Infrequent) ... 935
- Wellbutrin Tablets (Rare) ... 1177

Ovarian enlargement
- ▲ Clomid (13.6%) ... 1262
- ▲ Humegon for Injection (Approximately 20%) ... 1873
- Lutrepulse for Injection (Rare) ... 998
- ▲ Metrodin (urofollitropin for injection) (Approximately 20%) ... 2616
- ▲ Pergonal (menotropins for injection, USP) (Approximately 20%) ... 2618
- Profasi (chorionic gonadotropin for injection, USP) ... 2620
- ▲ Serophene (clomiphene citrate tablets, USP) (Approximately 1 in 7 patients) ... 2621

Ovarian hyperstimulation syndrome
- Clomid ... 1262
- Humegon for Injection (Approximately 0.4%) ... 1873
- Lutrepulse for Injection (One case) ... 998
- ▲ Metrodin (urofollitropin for injection) (Approximately 6%) ... 2616
- Pergonal (menotropins for injection, USP) ... 2618
- Profasi (chorionic gonadotropin for injection, USP) ... 2620
- Serophene (clomiphene citrate tablets, USP) ... 2621

Oversedation
- RespiGam (1%) ... 1631
- Versed Injection (1.6%) ... 2324

Overstimulation
- Adderall Tablets ... 2209
- Adipex-P Tablets and Capsules ... 1035
- Ana-Kit Anaphylaxis Emergency Treatment Kit (Common) ... 611
- Bontril Slow-Release Capsules ... 786
- Desoxyn Gradumet Tablets ... 422
- Dexedrine ... 2648
- DextroStat-Dextroamphetamine Sulfate Tablets ... 2211
- Eldepryl Capsules ... 2729
- Fastin Capsules ... 2662
- Halcion Tablets ... 2093
- Ionamin Capsules ... 1615
- Miltown Tablets ... 2780
- Parafon Forte DSC Caplets (Occasional) ... 1590
- Parnate Tablets ... 2679
- PMB 200 and PMB 400 ... 2890
- Prelu-2 Timed Release Capsules ... 687

(⊞ Described in PDR For Nonprescription Drugs)   Incidence data in parenthesis; ▲ 3% or more   (⊚ Described in PDR For Ophthalmology)

Side Effects Index

Sanorex Tablets ... 2423

Oxyhemoglobin desaturation
▲ Suprane (desflurane, USP) (3% to 26%) ... 1865

P

Pain
▲ Abelcet Injection (4%) ... 1540
Adalat CC (Less than 1.0%) ... 582
Ambien Tablets (Rare) ... 2559
Americaine Hemorrhoidal Ointment ... 649
▲ Anafranil Capsules (3% to 4%) ... 819
Androderm Testosterone Transdermal System (Less than 1%) ... 2634
Antivenin (Crotalidae) Polyvalent (Frequent) ... 2803
▲ Aredia for Injection (At least 15%) ... 827
▲ Arimidex Tablets (10.7% to 15.4%) ... 2932
▲ Asacol Delayed-Release Tablets (14%) ... 2129
▲ Atrovent Inhalation Solution (4.1%) ... 675
▲ Avonex (24%) ... 662
▲ Axid Pulvules (4.2%) ... 1468
Bactroban Ointment (1.5%) ... 2642
Betapace Tablets (1% to 3%) ... 637
▲ Betaseron for SC Injection (52%) ... 653
Cardene SR Capsules (0.6%) ... 2264
Cardura Tablets (2%) ... 1993
Cartrol Tablets (Less common) ... 413
▲ Casodex Tablets (27%) ... 2934
▲ CellCept Capsules (More than or equal to 3%; 31.2% to 33.0%) ... 2265
Cipro I.V. Pharmacy Bulk Package (Less than 1%) ... 590
▲ Condylox Topical Solution (50% to 72%) ... 1853
Coumadin ... 941
Crixivan Capsules (Less than 2%) ... 1670
Cytotec (Infrequent) ... 2576
Cytovene (2%) ... 2270
Dalalone D.P. Injectable ... 1009
Dalmane Capsules ... 2329
Danocrine Capsules ... 2437
Decadron-LA Sterile Suspension ... 1687
▲ Depakote Tablets (At least 5%) ... 418
Desferal Vials ... 838
Dilacor XR Extended-release Capsules (Infrequent) ... 2183
▲ Doxil (3.4%) ... 2613
Dynabac (2.2%) ... 668
Effexor ... 2825
▲ Efudex (Among most frequent) ... 2280
▲ Ethmozine Tablets (3.5%) ... 2217
Famvir Tablets (2.0% to 2.6%) ... 2660
▲ Felbatol (6.5%) ... 2774
Feldene Capsules (Less than 1%) ... 2008
Floxin I.V. (Less than 1%) ... 1580
Floxin Tablets (200 mg, 300 mg, 400 mg) (Less than 1%) ... 1577
▲ Fludara for Injection (20% to 22%) ... 658
Fluorescite ... ⊙ 217
Fluoroplex Topical Solution & Cream 1% ... 475
Fluorouracil Injection ... 2282
▲ Foscavir Injection (5% or greater) ... 541
▲ Fungizone Intravenous (Among most common) ... 507
▲ Gemzar for Injection (7% to 48%) ... 1482
Glucotrol XL Extended Release Tablets (Less than 3%) ... 2012
Helidac Therapy (1.0%) ... 2135
Heparin Sodium Vials ... 1486
Hivid Tablets (Less than 1%) ... 2287
Humegon for Injection ... 1873
Hycamtin for Injection (1.1% to 5.4%) ... 2665
▲ Intron A for Injection (Up to 18%) ... 2506
K-Phos Neutral Tablets ... 633
K-Phos Original Formula 'Sodium Free' Tablets (Less frequent) ... 633
Kadian Capsules (Less than 3%) ... 2948
Kerlone Tablets (Less than 2%) ... 2588
Klonopin Tablets ... 2294
Lamprene Capsules (Less than 1%) ... 846
▲ Leukine (17%) ... 1317
▲ Leustatin (6%) ... 1889
Librium Injectable ... 2332
Lioresal Intrathecal (Up to 4.0%) ... 1634
Lotensin HCT Tablets (0.3% or more) ... 855
Lovenox Injection ... 2187
▲ Lupron Depot 3.75 mg (8.4%) ... 2739
▲ Lupron Depot 7.5 mg (7.1%) ... 2741
▲ Lupron Depot - 3 Month 22.5 mg (26.6%) ... 2743
Lupron Depot-PED 7.5 mg, 11.25 mg and 15 mg (2%) ... 2744
▲ Lupron Injection (5% or more) ... 2736
Lupron Injection Pediatric ... 2737
LUVOX Tablets ... 2723
Marax Tablets & DF Syrup ... 2015
Matulane Capsules ... 2300
▲ Megace Oral Suspension (Up to 6%) ... 708
▲ Mepron Suspension (10%) ... 1206
Merrem I.V. (0.1% to 1.0%) ... 2952
Monoket Tablets (Less than 1% to 4%) ... 2550
Monopril Tablets (0.4% to 1.0%) ... 762
Mutamycin for Injection ... 712
Mycobutin Capsules (1%) ... 2101
▲ Naprelan Tablets (3% to 9%) ... 2861
Neupogen for Injection (2%) ... 495
Nicotrol NS Nicotine Nasal Spray (Less than 1%) ... 1565
▲ Nipent for Injection (8% to 20%) ... 2733
Nolvadex Tablets (2.8%) ... 2957
▲ Norpace (3 to 9%) ... 2596
▲ Norplant System (3.7%) ... 2868
Norvasc Tablets (More than 0.1% to 1%) ... 2020
Norvir (Less than 2%) ... 447
▲ Oncaspar (Greater than 5%) ... 2194
Orthoclone OKT3 Sterile Solution ... 1892
Orudis Capsules (Less than 1%) ... 2874
Oruvail Capsules (Less than 1%) ... 2874
Oxistat Lotion (0.4%) ... 1139
OxyContin Tablets (Less than 1%) ... 2163
ParaGard T 380A Intrauterine Copper Contraceptive ... 1936
▲ Paraplatin for Injection (17% to 54%) ... 713
Pergonal (menotropins for injection, USP) ... 2618
▲ Permax Tablets (7.0%) ... 571
PPD Tine Test ... 2993
▲ Pravachol Tablets (1.4% to 10.0%) ... 770
Prilosec Delayed-Release Capsules (Less than 1%) ... 516
Prinivil Tablets (0.3% to 1.0%) ... 1776
Prinzide Tablets ... 1780
Procardia XL Extended Release Tablets (Less than 3%) ... 2026
▲ Prograf (19% to 63%) ... 1028
▲ Proleukin for Injection (54%) ... 812
▲ Propulsid (3.4%) ... 1346
ProSom Tablets (2%) ... 457
▲ Prostep (nicotine transdermal system) (3% to 9% of patients) ... 1439
▲ Prozac Pulvules & Liquid, Oral Solution (6%) ... 935
Redux Capsules (Frequent) ... 2911
▲ ReoPro Vials (3.4%) ... 1526
▲ Roferon-A Injection (24%) ... 2308
Rythmol Tablets—150mg, 225mg, 300mg (Less than 1%) ... 1399
Serzone Tablets ... 776
Stimate, (desmopressin acetate) Nasal Spray, 1.5 mg/mL ... 806
▲ Supprelin Injection (1% to 10%) ... 2230
▲ Taxotere for Injection Concentrate (7% of 134 patients) ... 2204
▲ Tegison Capsules (1-10%) ... 2314
▲ Terazol 3 Vaginal Suppositories (3.9% of 284 patients) ... 1942
Terazol 7 Vaginal Cream (2.1% of 521 patients) ... 1943
Tetanus Toxoid Adsorbed Purogenated ... 1447
▲ Tiazac Capsules (7%) ... 1019
Ticlid Tablets (0.5% to 1.0%) ... 2317
Tripedia ... 908
Tuberculin, Old, Tine Test ... 2994
Univasc Tablets (More than 1%) ... 2553
Vancenase AQ Double Strength Nasal Spray 0.084% (2% to 4%) ... 2536
Vascor Tablets (200 and 300 mg) (0.5 to 2.0%) ... 1597
▲ Versed Injection (3.7-5.0%) ... 2324
▲ Vesanoid Capsules (37%) ... 2327
▲ Videx Tablets, Powder for Oral Solution, & Pediatric Powder for Oral Solution (6% to 31%) ... 2980
Wellbutrin Tablets (Infrequent) ... 1177
▲ Zerit Capsules (3% to 18%) ... 731
Zestoretic Tablets ... 2968
Zestril Tablets (0.3% to 1.0%) ... 2972
▲ Zoladex (8% to 17%) ... 2976
▲ Zoladex 3-month (14%) ... 2978
Zosyn (1.7% to 3.2%) ... 1463
Zovirax Capsules ... 1187
Zovirax Ointment 5% ... 1190
Zovirax Sterile Powder ... 1191
Zovirax ... 1187

Pain, abdominal
(see under Abdominal pain/cramps)

Pain, arm
Cozaar Tablets (Less than 1%) ... 1668
Hyzaar Tablets ... 1720
Norplant System ... 2868
Plendil Extended-Release Tablets (0.5% to 1.5%) ... 514
Prinzide Tablets ... 1780
Vaqta (1.3%) ... 1805
Zestoretic Tablets ... 2968
Zestril Tablets (0.3% to 1.0%) ... 2972

Pain, back
(see under Backache)

Pain, biliary
Actigall Capsules ... 818
LUVOX Tablets (Rare) ... 2723
Rilutek Tablets (Rare) ... 2198

Pain, bone
Abelcet Injection ... 1540
▲ Aredia for Injection (At least 5% to at least 15%) ... 827
▲ Arimidex Tablets (6.5% to 11.8%) ... 2932
Avonex ... 662
Calcijex Injection ... 412
▲ Casodex Tablets (4%) ... 2934
Cytosar-U Sterile Powder (Occasional) ... 2077
▲ Didronel Tablets (About 1 patient in 10 to about 2 in 10) ... 2133
Dilacor XR Extended-release Capsules (Infrequent) ... 2183
Doxil (Less than 1%) ... 2613
Effexor (Infrequent) ... 2825
Estring Vaginal Ring (2%) ... 2086
Hivid Tablets (Less than 1%) ... 2287
▲ Hylorel Tablets (42.9%) ... 1613
▲ Intron A for Injection (Less than 5%) ... 2506
K-Phos Neutral Tablets ... 633
K-Phos Original Formula 'Sodium Free' Tablets (Less frequent) ... 633
Kadian Capsules (Less than 3%) ... 2948
Lamprene Capsules (Less than 1%) ... 846
▲ Leukine (21%) ... 1317
Levatol Tablets (2.4%) ... 2547
▲ Lupron Depot 7.5 mg (Less than 5%) ... 2741
▲ Lupron Injection (5% or more) ... 2736
Naprelan Tablets (Less than 1%) ... 2861
▲ Neupogen for Injection (22% to 33%) ... 495
▲ Nolvadex Tablets (5.7%) ... 2957
Oncaspar (Less than 1%) ... 2194
Oncovin Solution Vials & Hyporets ... 1521
Permax Tablets (Infrequent) ... 571
Prozac Pulvules & Liquid, Oral Solution (Infrequent) ... 935
Remeron Tablets (Rare) ... 1878
ReVia Tablets (A small fraction of patients) ... 957
Rifadin ... 1276
Rifater ... 1280
Risperdal Tablets (Rare) ... 1348
Rocaltrol Capsules ... 2303
▲ Roferon-A Injection (25% to 47%) ... 2308
▲ Tegison Capsules (50-75%) ... 2314
Uroqid-Acid No. 2 Tablets ... 633
▲ Velban Vials (Among most common) ... 1537
▲ Vesanoid Capsules (77%) ... 2327
Zoladex (Small number of patients) ... 2976
▲ Zoladex 3-month (6%) ... 2978

Pain, breast
Ambien Tablets (Rare) ... 2559
Casodex Tablets (2% to 5%) ... 2934
Claritin Tablets (2% or fewer patients) ... 2485
Cytotec (Infrequent) ... 2576
Depo-Provera Contraceptive Injection (1% to 5%) ... 2079
Kerlone Tablets (Less than 2%) ... 2588
▲ Lupron Injection (5% or more) ... 2736
Neurontin Capsules (Rare) ... 1978
Permax Tablets (Infrequent) ... 571
Prinivil Tablets (0.3% to 1.0%) ... 1776
Risperdal Tablets (Rare to infrequent) ... 1348
Serzone Tablets (1%) ... 776

▲ Supprelin Injection (1% to 12%) ... 2230
Zestril Tablets (0.3% to 1.0%) ... 2972
Zyrtec Tablets (Less than 2%) ... 2053

Pain, burning
DDAVP Injection 15 mcg/mL (Occasional) ... 2179

Pain, cancer related
TICE BCG, USP ... 1881
Zoladex (Occasional) ... 2976
Zoladex 3-month ... 2978

Pain, cervical
Typhim Vi ... 914

Pain, dental
Claritin-D Tablets (Less frequent) ... 2487
Cozaar Tablets (Less than 1%) ... 1668
Estring Vaginal Ring (1% to 3%) ... 2086
Flovent (1% to 3%) ... 1089
Hivid Tablets (Less than 1%) ... 2287
Hyzaar Tablets ... 1720
▲ LUVOX Tablets (3%) ... 2723
Risperdal Tablets (Up to 2%) ... 1348
Serevent Inhalation Aerosol (1% to 3%) ... 1149
Wellbutrin Tablets (Infrequent) ... 1177

Pain, ear
Adenoscan (Less than 1%) ... 1022
Anafranil Capsules (Infrequent) ... 819
Asacol Delayed-Release Tablets ... 2129
Avonex ... 662
Axocet Capsules (Infrequent) ... 2469
Bactroban Nasal (Less than 1%) ... 2643
Betaseron for SC Injection ... 653
Cardura Tablets (Less than 0.5% of 3960 patients) ... 1993
Cerebyx Injection (Infrequent) ... 1956
Claritin Tablets (2% or fewer patients) ... 2485
Claritin-D Tablets (Less frequent) ... 2487
Cognex Capsules (Infrequent) ... 1961
DaunoXome (Less than or equal to 5%) ... 1842
Depakote Tablets (1% to 5%) ... 418
Dilacor XR Extended-release Capsules (Infrequent) ... 2183
Diprivan Injectable Emulsion (Less than 1%) ... 2939
Effexor (Frequent) ... 2825
Engerix-B Unit-Dose Vials ... 2656
Esgic-plus Capsules (Infrequent) ... 1012
Esgic-plus Tablets (Infrequent) ... 1012
Fioricet Tablets (Infrequent) ... 2386
Fioricet with Codeine Capsules (Infrequent) ... 2387
Fiorinal with Codeine Capsules (Infrequent) ... 2390
Foscavir Injection (Less than 1%) ... 541
Hivid Tablets (Less than 1%) ... 2287
Imdur (Less than or equal to 5%) ... 1362
Imitrex Tablets (Infrequent) ... 1099
Intron A for Injection (Less than or equal to 5%) ... 2506
Invirase Capsules (Less than 2%) ... 2291
Lamictal Tablets (1.8%) ... 1105
Lopressor HCT Tablets (1 in 100 patients) ... 850
LUVOX Tablets (Infrequent) ... 2723
Maxaquin Tablets (Less than 1%) ... 2593
Miacalcin Nasal Spray (Less than 1%) ... 2403
Neurontin Capsules (Infrequent) ... 1978
Nicotrol NS Nicotine Nasal Spray (More common) ... 1565
Nipent for Injection (Less than 3%) ... 2733
Norvir (Less than 2%) ... 447
Paxil Tablets (Infrequent) ... 2681
Permax Tablets (Infrequent) ... 571
Phrenilin (Infrequent) ... 790
Prinzide Tablets (0.3 to 1%) ... 1780
ProSom Tablets (Infrequent) ... 457
Prozac Pulvules & Liquid, Oral Solution (Infrequent) ... 935
Recombivax HB (Less than 1%) ... 1787
Remeron Tablets (Infrequent) ... 1878
Rilutek Tablets (Rare) ... 2198
Roferon-A Injection (Less than 1%) ... 2308
Sedapap Tablets 50 mg/650 mg (Infrequent) ... 1826
Serzone Tablets (Infrequent) ... 776
Stadol (1% or greater) ... 779
Sular Tablets (Less than or equal to 1%) ... 2961
Supprelin Injection (1% to 3%) ... 2230
Timolide Tablets ... 1791
Tonocard Tablets (Less than 1%) ... 519

(⊡ Described in PDR For Nonprescription Drugs)   Incidence data in parenthesis; ▲ 3% or more   (⊙ Described in PDR For Ophthalmology)

Pain, ear

Trental Tablets (Less than 1%) 1291
▲ Vesanoid Capsules (23%) 2327
▲ Videx Tablets, Powder for Oral Solution, & Pediatric Powder for Oral Solution (Less than 1% to 11%) 2980
Zebeta Tablets 1457
Zestoretic Tablets (0.3 to 1%) 2968
Ziac 1459
Zoloft Tablets (Infrequent) 2051
Zosyn (1.0% or less) 1463
Zyrtec Tablets (Less than 2%) 2053

Pain, epigastric
(see under Distress, epigastric)

Pain, esophageal

Hivid Tablets (Less than 1%) 2287

Pain, extremities

▲ Betapace Tablets (2% to 7%) 637
Betimol 0.25%, 0.5% (1% to 5%) .... ⊚ 259
Blocadren Tablets 1654
Cartrol Tablets (Less common) 413
Cipro I.V. Pharmacy Bulk Package (Less than 1%) 590
Colestid 2073
Danocrine Capsules 2437
Diprivan Injectable Emulsion (Less than 1%) 2939
Ergomar Tablets (Frequent) 1543
Flovent (1% to 3%) 1089
Floxin I.V. (Less than 1%) 1580
Floxin Tablets (200 mg, 300 mg, 400 mg) (Less than 1%) 1577
Fluorouracil Injection 2282
Heparin Sodium Vials 1486
▲ Hytrin Capsules (3.5%) 434
IOPIDINE Sterile Ophthalmic Solution .... ⊚ 218
Levlen/Tri-Levlen 646
Mavik Tablets (0.3% to 1.0%) 1407
▲ Mesnex Injection (50%) 711
▲ Oncaspar (Greater than 1% but less than 5%) 2194
Oncovin Solution Vials & Hyporets 1521
Rifadin 1276
Rifater 1280
SSKI Solution (Less frequent) 2767
Sansert Tablets 2424
▲ Supprelin Injection (6% to 10%) 2230
Teslac Tablets 727
Timoptic-XE 1798
Levlen/Tri-Levlen 646
Uroqid-Acid No. 2 Tablets 633
Videx Tablets, Powder for Oral Solution, & Pediatric Powder for Oral Solution 2980
Zerit Capsules 731

Pain, eye

AK-Spore .... ⊚ 205
Alomide Ophthalmic Solution (Less than 1%) 465
Ambien Tablets (Infrequent) 2559
Anafranil Capsules (Infrequent) 819
Asacol Delayed-Release Tablets 2129
Atrovent Inhalation Aerosol 674
Atrovent Inhalation Solution (Less than 3%) 675
Atrovent Nasal Spray 0.06% 678
Avonex 662
Betimol 0.25%, 0.5% (1% to 5%) .... ⊚ 259
Betoptic Ophthalmic Solution 465
Betoptic S Ophthalmic Suspension (Small number of patients) 467
BuSpar Tablets (Rare) 738
Cardura Tablets (1%) 1993
Cerebyx Injection (Infrequent) 1956
Cipro I.V. (1% or less) 587
Cipro I.V. Pharmacy Bulk Package (Less than 1%) 590
Cipro Tablets (Less than 1%) 584
Claritin Tablets (2% or fewer patients) 2485
Claritin-D Tablets (Less frequent) .. 2487
Clear Eyes ACR Astringent/Lubricant Eye Redness Reliever Eye Drops ...... ⊚ 314
Clomid 1262
Cognex Capsules (Infrequent) 1961
Crixivan Capsules (Less than 2%).. 1670
Cytovene (1% or less) 2270
DaunoXome (Less than or equal to 5%) 1842
Depakote Tablets (1% to 5%) 418
Diprivan Injectable Emulsion (Less than 1%) 2939
Doxil (Less than 1%) 2613

Effexor (Infrequent) 2825
Eldepryl Capsules 2729
EPIFRIN .... ⊚ 237
Ethmozine Tablets (Less than 2%) . 2217
Eye-Stream Eye Irrigating Solution.. 469
Flumadine Tablets & Syrup 1013
Foscavir Injection (Between 1% and 5%) 541
Glucotrol XL Extended Release Tablets (Less than 1%) 2012
Hivid Tablets (Less than 1%) 2287
Intron A for Injection (Less than 5%) 2506
Iopidine 0.5% (Less than 1%) .... ⊚ 219
Livostin (Approximately 1% to 3%) .... ⊚ 262
LUVOX Tablets (Infrequent) 2723
Maxaquin Tablets (Less than 1%) .. 2593
Miacalcin Injection 2402
Naprelan Tablets (Less than 1%) .. 2861
Neurontin Capsules (Infrequent) ... 1978
Norvasc Tablets (More than 0.1% to 1%) 2020
Norvir (Less than 2%) 447
Ocuflox Ophthalmic Solution 478
Ophthalgan .... ⊚ 323
Orudis Capsules (Less than 1%) 2874
Oruvail Capsules (Less than 1%) ... 2874
Paxil Tablets (Infrequent) 2681
Permax Tablets (Infrequent) 571
Prevacid Delayed-Release Capsules (Less than 1%) 2746
ProSom Tablets (Infrequent) 457
Prostin E2 Suppository 2109
Prozac Pulvules & Liquid, Oral Solution (Infrequent) 935
Remeron Tablets (Infrequent) 1878
ReVia Tablets (Less than 1%) 957
Risperdal Tablets (Rare) 1348
Salagen Tablets (Less than 1%) 1546
Sectral Capsules (Up to 2%) 2914
Serzone Tablets (Frequent) 776
Soma Tablets 2782
Synarel Nasal Solution for Endometriosis (Less than 1%) 2605
Tambocor Tablets (Less than 1%) .. 1555
Tegison Capsules (Frequent) 2314
Timoptic in Ocudose (Less frequent) 1796
Timoptic Sterile Ophthalmic Solution (Less frequent) 1794
Timoptic-XE (1% to 5% of patients) 1798
Vexol 1% Ophthalmic Suspension (1% to 5%) .... ⊚ 227
Videx Tablets, Powder for Oral Solution, & Pediatric Powder for Oral Solution (Less than 1%) 2980
Visine L.R. Eye Drops .... ⊚ 301
Viva-Drops .... ⊚ 326
Xalatan (1% to 4%) .... ⊚ 304
Zebeta Tablets 1457
Ziac 1459
Zoloft Tablets (Infrequent) 2051
Zyrtec Tablets (Less than 2%) 2053

Pain, facial

Hivid Tablets (Less than 1%) 2287
Imitrex Injection (Infrequent) 1095
Imitrex Tablets (Infrequent) 1099
Invirase Capsules (Less than 2%) .. 2291
Norvir (Less than 2%) 447
Supprelin Injection (2% to 3%) 2230

Pain, female genitalia

Floxin Tablets (200 mg, 300 mg, 400 mg) (Less than 1%) 1577
▲ Supprelin Injection (3% to 10%)... 2230

Pain, femoral nerve

Questran 774

Pain, flank

▲ Chemet Capsules (5.2% to 15.7%) 666
Crixivan Capsules (Less than 2% to approximately 4%) 1670
Fludara for Injection 658
Hivid Tablets (Less than 1%) 2287
Neupogen for Injection (Infrequent) 495
Prinivil Tablets (0.3% to 1.0%) 1776
Prinzide Tablets 1780
ReVia Tablets (Less than 1%) 957
Sansert Tablets 2424
TheraCys BCG Live (Intravesical) (Up to 4.9%) 911
Toradol 2319
Vaseretic Tablets 1810
Vasotec I.V. 1814
Vasotec Tablets (0.5% to 1.0%) 1816

▲ Vesanoid Capsules (9%) 2327
Zestoretic Tablets 2968
Zestril Tablets (0.3% to 1.0%) 2972

Pain, genital

▲ Condylox Topical Solution (50% to 72%) 1853
▲ TheraCys BCG Live (Intravesical) (Up to 9.8%) 911
Zerit Capsules (Up to 2%) 731

Pain, hip

Cozaar Tablets (Less than 1%) 1668
Gamimune N, 5% Immune Globulin Intravenous (Human), 5% 612
Gamimune N, 10% Immune Globulin Intravenous (Human), 10% 615
Hyzaar Tablets 1720
Plendil Extended-Release Tablets (0.5% to 1.5%) 514
Prinivil Tablets (0.3% to 1.0%) 1776
Prinzide Tablets 1780
Zestoretic Tablets 2968
Zestril Tablets (0.3% to 1.0%) 2972

Pain, inguinal

Hivid Tablets (Less than 1%) 2287
ReVia Tablets (Less than 1%) 957

Pain, jaw

Cipro I.V. (1% or less) 587
Cipro I.V. Pharmacy Bulk Package (Less than 1%) 590
▲ Flolan for Injection (54%) 1085
Navelbine Injection (Less than 5%) 1212
Oncovin Solution Vials & Hyporets 1521
Permax Tablets (Infrequent) 571
ProSom Tablets (Rare) 457
Prozac Pulvules & Liquid, Oral Solution (Infrequent) 935
▲ Velban Vials (Among most common) 1537

Pain, kidney

Avonex 662
Ceftin (0.1% to 1%) 1067
Effexor (Infrequent) 2825
Lamictal Tablets (Rare) 1105
Monopril Tablets (0.4% to 1.0%).. 762
Naprelan Tablets (Less than 1%) .. 2861
Norvir (Less than 2%) 447
Paxil Tablets (Rare) 2681
Redux Capsules (Infrequent) 2911
Rilutek Tablets (Infrequent) 2198
Videx Tablets, Powder for Oral Solution, & Pediatric Powder for Oral Solution (Less than 1%) 2980

Pain, knee

Cozaar Tablets (Less than 1%) 1668
Hyzaar Tablets 1720
Plendil Extended-Release Tablets (0.5% to 1.5%) 514
Prinivil Tablets (0.3% to 1.0%) 1776
Zestril Tablets (0.3% to 1.0%) 2972

Pain, lower extremities

Adalat CC (3% or less) 582
Axocet Capsules (Infrequent) 2469
Cartrol Tablets (1.2%) 413
Chemet Capsules (Up to 3.0%) 666
Cipro Tablets (0.3% to 1%) 584
Clozaril Tablets (1%) 2377
Cozaar Tablets (1.0%) 1668
Crixivan Capsules (Less than 2%).. 1670
DynaCirc CR Tablets (0.5% to 1.0%) 2383
Eldepryl Capsules (1 of 49 patients) 2729
Esgic-plus Capsules (Infrequent) 1012
Esgic-plus Tablets (Infrequent) 1012
Estrace Cream and Tablets 751
Fioricet Tablets (Infrequent) 2386
Fioricet with Codeine Capsules (Infrequent) 2387
Fiorinal with Codeine Capsules (Infrequent) 2390
Hivid Tablets (Less than 1%) 2287
Hyzaar Tablets 1720
Lopid Tablets 1974
Mevacor Tablets (0.5% to 1.0%) 1742
Midamor Tablets (Less than or equal to 1%) 1746
Moduretic Tablets 1748
Ortho-Est 1925
Phrenilin (Infrequent) 790
Plendil Extended-Release Tablets (0.5% to 1.5%) 514

Prilosec Delayed-Release Capsules (Less than 1%) 516
Prinivil Tablets (0.3% to 1.0%) 1776
Prinzide Tablets (0.3% to 1%) 1780
▲ ProSom Tablets (3%) 457
Prozac Pulvules & Liquid, Oral Solution (1.6%) 935
ReVia Tablets (Less than 1%) 957
Rifamate Capsules 1278
Rimactane Capsules 865
Rowasa (2.09%) 2727
Sedapap Tablets 50 mg/650 mg (Infrequent) 1826
Sinemet CR Tablets 961
Tenex Tablets (Less frequent) 2249
Tenoretic Tablets (Up to 3%) 2963
Tenormin Tablets and I.V. Injection (Up to 3%) 2965
Timolide Tablets 1791
Timoptic in Ocudose 1796
Timoptic Sterile Ophthalmic Solution 1794
Vivelle Transdermal System 880
Zestoretic Tablets (0.3 to 1%) 2968
Zestril Tablets (0.3% to 1.0%) 2972
Zovirax (0.3%) 1187

Pain, medullary bone

▲ Neupogen for Injection (33%) 495

Pain, Mittelschmerz

Serophene (clomiphene citrate tablets, USP) 2621

Pain, muscle
(see under Myalgia)

Pain, nasal sinus(es)

▲ Flovent (Up to 13%) 1089

Pain, neck
(see under Torticollis)

Pain, neuritic

Oncovin Solution Vials & Hyporets 1521

Pain, nostril

DDAVP (Up to 2%) 2180
Desmopressin Acetate Rhinal Tube (Up to 2%) 997

Pain, oral mucosa

Cipro Tablets (Less than 1%) 584
Floxin I.V. 1580
Floxin Tablets (200 mg, 300 mg, 400 mg) 1577
Maxaquin Tablets 2593

Pain, parotid gland

Oncovin Solution Vials & Hyporets 1521

Pain, pelvic

Adalat CC (Less than 1.0%) 582
Androderm Testosterone Transdermal System (Less than 1%) 2634
▲ Arimidex Tablets (5.3% to 6.9%).. 2932
▲ Betaseron for SC Injection (6%)..... 653
▲ Casodex Tablets (13%) 2934
Caverject Injection (Less than 1%) 2064
▲ CellCept Capsules (More than or equal to 3%) 2265
▲ Cerebyx Injection (4.4%) 1956
Clomid 1262
Danocrine Capsules 2437
Depo-Provera Contraceptive Injection (1% to 5%) 2079
Effexor (Infrequent) 2825
Hivid Tablets (Less than 1%) 2287
Humegon for Injection 1873
Intron A for Injection (Less than 5%) 2506
Invirase Capsules (Less than 2%) .. 2291
LUVOX Tablets (Rare) 2723
Massengill Disposable Douche 2627
Massengill Medicated Disposable Douche 2628
Naprelan Tablets (Less than 1%) .. 2861
Nolvadex Tablets 2957
Paxil Tablets (Rare) 2681
Permax Tablets (Infrequent) 571
Prinivil Tablets (0.3% to 1.0%) 1776
Prinzide Tablets 1780
Prozac Pulvules & Liquid, Oral Solution (Infrequent) 935
Redux Capsules (Infrequent) 2911
Serophene (clomiphene citrate tablets, USP) 2621
Serzone Tablets (Infrequent) 776
Zerit Capsules (Up to 2%) 731
Zestoretic Tablets 2968

(⊞ Described in PDR For Nonprescription Drugs)   Incidence data in parenthesis; ▲ 3% or more   (⊚ Described in PDR For Ophthalmology)

Zestril Tablets (0.3% to 1.0%) 2972
▲ Zoladex 3-month (6%) 2978

Pain, penile
▲ Caverject Injection (2% to 37%) 2064
Hivid Tablets (Less than 1%) 2287

Pain, perineal
Anafranil Capsules (Infrequent) 819
Foscavir Injection (Less than 1%) 541
Maxaquin Tablets (Less than 1%) 2593
Risperdal Tablets (Infrequent) 1348
Zosyn (1.0% or less) 1463

Pain, pharynx
Oncovin Solution Vials & Hyporets 1521
Prilosec Delayed-Release Capsules (Less than 1%) 516
Primaxin I.M. 1770
Primaxin I.V. (Less than 0.2%) 1772
Prinivil Tablets (0.3% to 1.0%) 1776
Prinzide Tablets (0.3% to 1%) 1780
Sinemet CR Tablets 961
Zestoretic Tablets (0.3 to 1%) 2968
Zestril Tablets (0.3% to 1.0%) 2972

Pain, postoperative
▲ Revex (nalmefene hydrochloride injection) (4%) 1863

Pain, precordium
Cafergot 2376
Chromagen Capsules 2470
Chromagen FA 2471
Chromagen Forte 2471
D.H.E. 45 Injection 2381
Ergomar Tablets 1543
Imitrex Tablets 1099
Mykrox Tablets (2.7%) 1617
Phenergan VC with Codeine 2888
Wigraine Tablets 1884
Zoloft Tablets (Rare) 2051

Pain, prostate
Lupron Depot 3.75 mg 2739
Lupron Depot 7.5 mg 2741
Lupron Depot - 3 Month 22.5 mg 2743
Lupron Depot-PED 7.5 mg, 11.25 mg and 15 mg 2744
Lupron Injection 2736

Pain, rectum
CORTENEMA (Rare) 2713
Hivid Tablets (Less than 1%) 2287
Noroxin Tablets (0.3% to 1.0%) 1758
Noroxin Tablets (0.3% to 1.0%) 2222
Questran 774
Rowasa (0.61% to 1.23%) 2727

Pain, renal
Ambien Tablets (Rare) 2559
Anafranil Capsules (Infrequent) 819
Neurontin Capsules (Rare) 1978
Zoloft Tablets (Rare) 2051

Pain, retrosternal
▲ Ethamolin Injection (Among most common) 2544
Invirase Capsules (Less than 2%) 2291
Zofran Injection (2%) 1227

Pain, right upper quadrant
Calan SR Caplets 2571
Calan Tablets 2568
Intron A for Injection (Less than 5%) 2506
Invirase Capsules (Rare) 2291
Isoptin SR Tablets 1395
Tapazole Tablets 1361

Pain, shoulder
Brevibloc (esmolol HCl) Injection (Less than 1%) 1860
Cartrol Tablets (Less common) 413
Cozaar Tablets (Less than 1%) 1668
Crixivan Capsules (Less than 2%) 1670
Engerix-B Unit-Dose Vials (Less than 1%) 2656
Hytrin Capsules (At least 1%) 434
Hyzaar Tablets 1720
Mevacor Tablets (0.5% to 1.0%) 1742
Moduretic Tablets 1748
Prinivil Tablets (0.3% to 1.0%) 1776
Prinzide Tablets (0.3% to 1%) 1780
Recombivax HB (Less than 1%) 1787
ReVia Tablets (Less than 1%) 957
Sinemet CR Tablets (1.0%) 961
Tonocard Tablets (Less than 1%) 519
Zestoretic Tablets (0.3 to 1%) 2968
Zestril Tablets (0.3% to 1.0%) 2972
Zofran Injection (2%) 1227

Pain, stomach (see under Stomachache)

Pain, substernal
Aerolate 1003
Tenex Tablets (3% or less) 2249
Unasyn (Less than 1%) 2035

Pain, testicular
Caverject Injection (Less than 1%) 2064
Lupron Depot 7.5 mg (Less than 5%) 2741
Lupron Injection (Less than 5%) 2736
Neurontin Capsules (Rare) 1978
Prilosec Delayed-Release Capsules (Less than 1%) 516

Pain, thoracic spine
▲ Chemet Capsules (5.2% to 15.7%) 666
Primaxin I.M. 1770
Primaxin I.V. (Less than 0.2%) 1772

Pain, throat
DDAVP 2180
Desmopressin Acetate Rhinal Tube 997
Dizac (diazepam injectable emulsion) CIV 1862

Pain, trunk
Diprivan Injectable Emulsion (Less than 1%) 2939
▲ Epogen for Injection (3%) 489
Floxin I.V. (1% to 3%) 1580
Floxin Tablets (200 mg, 300 mg, 400 mg) (1% to 3%) 1577
▲ Leustatin (6%) 1889
▲ Procrit for Injection (3%) 1896
▲ Supprelin Injection (1% to 10%) 2230

Pain, tumor site
Blenoxane (Infrequent) 697
Navelbine Injection 1212
Nolvadex Tablets 2957
Velban Vials 1537

Pain, upper extremities
Cipro I.V. (1% or less) 587
Engerix-B Unit-Dose Vials (Less than 1%) 2656
Hivid Tablets (Less than 1%) 2287
Lopid Tablets 1974
Midamor Tablets (Less than or equal to 1%) 1746
Moduretic Tablets 1748
Prinivil Tablets (0.3% to 1.0%) 1776
ProSom Tablets (Infrequent) 457
Prozac Pulvules & Liquid, Oral Solution (1.6%) 935
Rifamate Capsules 1278
Rimactane Capsules 865
Timolide Tablets 1791
Timoptic in Ocudose 1796
Timoptic Sterile Ophthalmic Solution 1794

Pain, urethral
Avonex 662
Ceftin (0.1% to 1%) 1067
Cerebyx Injection (Infrequent) 1956
Permax Tablets (Rare) 571
Prozac Pulvules & Liquid, Oral Solution (Rare) 935

Pain, urinary bladder
Duragesic Transdermal System (Less than 1%) 1336
Effexor (Infrequent) 2825
Hivid Tablets (Less than 1%) 2287
TICE BCG, USP 1881

Pain, vaginal
▲ Estring Vaginal Ring (5%) 2086
Floxin I.V. (Less than 1%) 1580
Hivid Tablets (Less than 1%) 2287
Neurontin Capsules (Rare) 1978
Prostin E2 Suppository 2109
Vagistat-1 (Less than 1%) 783

Pain, vascular
Lamprene Capsules (Less than 1%) 846

Pain, vulva
DDAVP Injection (Infrequent) 2178
DDAVP Injection 15 mcg/mL (Infrequent) 2179
Desmopressin Acetate Injection (Infrequent) 996
Stimate, (desmopressin acetate) Nasal Spray, 1.5 mg/mL (Infrequent) 806
▲ Terazol 3 Vaginal Suppositories (4.2% of 284 patients) 1942

Pain at application site
Rowasa (1.35%) 2727
▲ Sulfamylon Cream (One of two most frequent) 940
Zovirax Ointment 5% 1190

Pain at injection site
▲ ActHIB (6.4% to 9.0%) 893
Actimmune 1043
Adagen (pegademase bovine) Injection (Two patients) 988
Alfenta Injection (0.3% to 1%) 1334
▲ Alferon N Injection (12%) 2142
Amicar Syrup, Tablets, and Injection 1312
Ancef Injection (Infrequent) 2632
AquaMEPHYTON Injection 1648
▲ Aredia for Injection (Up to 41%) 827
▲ Ativan Injection (17%) 2805
Attenuvax 1650
Bactrim I.V. Infusion (Infrequent) 2255
Biavax II 1653
Brethine Ampuls (0.5 to 2.6%) 832
Calcijex Injection (Occasional) 412
Capastat Sulfate Injection 968
Cardene I.V. (0.7%) 2815
Cefizox for Intramuscular or Intravenous Use (1% to 5%) 1025
Cefobid Intravenous/Intramuscular (Occasional) 1996
Cefobid Pharmacy Bulk Package - Not for Direct Infusion (Occasional) 1999
Cerebyx Injection (Frequent) 1956
Cholera Vaccine 2818
Cipro I.V. (1% or less) 587
▲ Claforan Sterile and Injection (4.3%) 1259
Cleocin Phosphate Injection 2068
Cytovene-IV (1% or less) 2270
Demerol 2438
Depo-Provera Contraceptive Injection (Fewer than 1%) 2079
Desferal Vials 838
Dilaudid-HP Injection (Rare) 1384
Dilaudid-HP Lyophilized Powder 250 mg (Rare) 1384
Diphtheria and Tetanus Toxoids and Pertussis Vaccine Adsorbed 2650
▲ Diprivan Injectable Emulsion (10% to 17.6%) 2939
Doxil (Less than 1%) 2613
Edecrin (Occasional) 1698
Engerix-B Unit-Dose Vials (Less than 1%) 2656
Factrel (Occasional) 2996
▲ Flolan for Injection (13%) 1085
Fluorescite ...... ◉ 217
Foscavir Injection (Between 1% and 5%) 541
Fragmin Injection (up to 4.5%) 2088
▲ Fungizone Intravenous (Among most common) 507
▲ Gammagard S/D, Immune Globulin, Intravenous (Human) (16%) 577
Garamycin Injectable (Occasional) 2502
Genotropin Injection (Infrequent) 2090
Hep-B-Gammagee 1706
Humatrope Vials (Infrequent) 1490
Humegon for Injection 1873
HyperHep Hepatitis B Immune Globulin (Human) 619
Hyperstat I.V. Injection 2504
▲ Imovax Rabies Vaccine (About 25%) 899
INFeD (Iron Dextran Injection, USP) 2478
Intron A for Injection (Less than 5%) 2506
▲ IPOL Poliovirus Vaccine Inactivated (13%) 903
Kefzol Vials, Faspak & ADD-Vantage (Infrequent) 1511
▲ Leustatin (9% to 19%) 1889
Levoprome (Frequent) 1321
Mandol Vials, Faspak & ADD-Vantage (Infrequent) 1516
Maxipime for Injection (0.6%) 758
Mefoxin 1734
Mepergan Injection 2859
Merrem I.V. (0.4%) 2952
Meruvax II 1740
Metrodin (urofollitropin for injection) 2616
Mezlin 594
Mezlin Pharmacy Bulk Package 597
▲ Monocid Injection (5.7%) 2674
Mononine, Coagulation Factor IX (Human), Monoclonal Antibody Purified 804
▲ Navelbine Injection (Up to 13%) 1212
Nebcin Vials, Hyporets & ADD-Vantage 1518
Netromycin Injection 100 mg/ml (4 of 1000 patients) 2516
Nutropin (Infrequent) 1049
Nutropin AQ Injection (Infrequent) 1051
▲ OmniHIB (6.4% to 9.0%) 2676
▲ Oncaspar (Greater than 1% but less than 5%) 2194
PedvaxHIB 1761
Peptavlon 2997
Pergonal (menotropins for injection, USP) 2618
Pipracil (2%) 1435
Pneumovax 23 (Common) 1768
▲ Pnu-Imune 23 (72%) 1437
Pregnyl for Injection 1878
Primaxin I.M. (1.2%) 1770
Primaxin I.V. (0.7%) 1772
Profasi (chorionic gonadotropin for injection, USP) 2620
Protropin (Infrequent) 1053
Rabies Vaccine Adsorbed (A few patients) 2686
▲ Rabies Vaccine, Imovax Rabies I.D. (About 25%) 901
Recombivax HB (Equal to or greater than 1%) 1787
Retrovir I.V. Infusion (Infrequent) 1221
Robaxin Injectable 2245
Rocephin Injectable Vials, ADD-Vantage, Galaxy Container (1%) 2305
Roferon-A Injection (Less than 1%) 2308
▲ Romazicon (3% to 9%) 2311
▲ Sandostatin Injection (7.7%) 2421
Septra I.V. Infusion (Infrequent) 1142
Septra I.V. Infusion ADD-Vantage Vials (Infrequent) 1144
Sotradecol (Sodium Tetradecyl Sulfate Injection) 987
Testred Capsules, 10 mg 1308
▲ Tetramune (21% to 65%) 1449
Thioplex (Thiotepa For Injection) 1329
Ticar for Injection 2704
Timentin for Injection 2706
Toradol (2%) 2319
Tubersol (Tuberculin Purified Protein Derivative (Mantoux)) 2988
▲ Typhim Vi (Up to 56%) 914
▲ Unasyn (3% to 16%) 2035
Vancocin HCl, Vials & ADD-Vantage 1534
▲ Vaqta (1.2% to 51.1%) 1805
▲ Varivax (19.3% to 32.5%; less than 0.05%) 1807
▲ Versed Injection (3.7% to 5.0%) 2324
Zantac Injection 1180
▲ Zinecard Injection (12% to 13%) 2120
▲ Zofran Injection (4%) 1227
Zosyn (0.2%) 1463

Pain with coitus
Condylox Topical Solution (Less than 5%) 1853

Paleness, unusual
Geref (sermorelin acetate for injection) 2995
Nucofed 2225

Palilalia
Nardil (Less common) 1977

Pallor
Ambien Tablets (Infrequent) 2559
Anafranil Capsules (Infrequent) 819
Ana-Kit Anaphylaxis Emergency Treatment Kit (Common) 611
Azulfidine 2059
Brevibloc (esmolol HCl) Injection (Less than 1%) 1860
Buprenex Injectable (Infrequent) 2170
Capoten Tablets (2 to 5 of 1000 patients) 740
Capozide Tablets (2 to 5 of 1000 patients) 744
Cardura Tablets (Less than 0.5% of 3960 patients) 1993
Catapres Tablets 679
Catapres-TTS 680
Claritin-D Tablets 2487
Clozaril Tablets (Less than 1%) 2377

(▣ Described in PDR For Nonprescription Drugs) Incidence data in parenthesis; ▲ 3% or more (◉ Described in PDR For Ophthalmology)

Pallor **Side Effects Index** 1420

Combipres Tablets ... 682
Cytotec (Infrequent) ... 2576
D.A. II Tablets ... 972
D.A. Chewable Tablets ... 970
Dalgan Injection (Less than 1%) ... 529
Dapsone Tablets USP ... 1331
Deconsal II Tablets ... 1605
Dilacor XR Extended-release Capsules (Infrequent) ... 2183
Dura-Tap/PD Capsules ... 970
Dura-Vent/DA Tablets ... 972
Dura-Vent Tablets ... 971
▲ EMLA Cream (37%) ... 536
EpiPen ... 808
Etrafon ... 2495
Fedahist Gyrocaps ... 2545
▲ Flolan for Injection (21%) ... 1085
Flumadine Tablets & Syrup (Less than 0.3%) ... 1013
Gantrisin ... 2286
Histussin D Liquid ... 670
Imitrex Injection (Rare) ... 1095
Imitrex Tablets (Infrequent) ... 1099
Kadian Capsules (Less than 3%) ... 2948
Levophed Bitartrate Injection ... 2445
Lioresal Intrathecal (1% or more) ... 1634
LUVOX Tablets (Infrequent) ... 2723
Mellaril ... 2398
▲ Miacalcin Nasal Spray (10.6%) ... 2403
Monoket Tablets (Fewer than 1%) ... 2550
Nitrolingual Spray ... 2193
Nitrostat Tablets ... 1981
Novahistine DMX ... ▣ 782
Novahistine Elixir ... ▣ 782
Paremyd ... ⊙ 244
Paxil Tablets (Rare) ... 2681
Proloprim Tablets ... 1141
Proventil Syrup (Children 2 to 6 years, 1%) ... 2528
RespiGam (Infrequent) ... 1631
Risperdal Tablets (Rare) ... 1348
Rondec Oral Drops ... 974
Rondec Syrup ... 974
Rondec ... 974
Seldane-D Extended-Release Tablets ... 1286
Septra I.V. Infusion ... 1142
Septra I.V. Infusion ADD-Vantage Vials ... 1144
Serzone Tablets (Rare) ... 776
Supprelin Injection (1% to 3%) ... 2230
Survanta Beractant Intratracheal Suspension (Less than 1%) ... 2346
Sus-Phrine Injection ... 1017
Syn-Rx Tablets ... 1622
Syn-Rx DM Tablets ... 1623
Tonocard Tablets (Less than 1%) ... 519
Toradol (1% or less) ... 2319
Trilafon (Occasional) ... 2532
Trinalin Repetabs Tablets ... 1373
Tussend ... 1830
Tussend Expectorant ... 1831
Tympagesic Ear Drops ... 2476
Ventolin Syrup (1% of children) ... 1175
▲ Vesanoid Capsules (6%) ... 2327
Vistide Injection ... 1057
Wellbutrin Tablets (Rare) ... 1177
Zoloft Tablets (Rare) ... 2051

Pallor, facial

Parlodel (Less than 1%) ... 2411

Pallor, optic disc

Aralen Phosphate Tablets ... 2431
Plaquenil Sulfate Tablets ... 2459

Palmar-plantar erythrodysesthesia syndrome

▲ Doxil (3.4%) ... 2613
Fluorouracil Injection ... 2282

Palpebra superior, elevation

IOPIDINE Sterile Ophthalmic Solution (1.3%) ... ⊙ 218

Palpitations

Accupril Tablets (0.5% to 1.0%) ... 1950
Accutane Capsules (Less than 1%) ... 2252
Acutrim ... ▣ 648
▲ Adalat Capsules (10 mg and 20 mg) (2% or less to 7%) ... 580
Adalat CC (Less than 1.0%) ... 582
Adderall Tablets ... 2209
Adenocard Injection (Less than 1%) ... 1021
Adenoscan (Less than 1%) ... 1022
Adipex-P Tablets and Capsules ... 1035
▲ AeroBid Inhaler System (3% to 9%) ... 1004
▲ Aerobid-M Inhaler System (3% to 9%) ... 1004
Aerolate ... 1003
Altace Capsules (Less than 1%) ... 1238
Alupent (1% to 4%) ... 672
Ambien Tablets (2%) ... 2559
▲ Anafranil Capsules (4%) ... 819
Ana-Kit Anaphylaxis Emergency Treatment Kit (Common) ... 611
Anaprox/Naprosyn (Less than 3%) ... 2277
Apresazide Capsules (Common) ... 824
Apresoline Hydrochloride Tablets (Common) ... 826
Asendin Tablets (Less frequent) ... 1419
Atamet Tablets (Less frequent) ... 567
Atrohist Pediatric Capsules ... 1603
Atrohist Plus Tablets ... 1605
Atrovent Inhalation Aerosol (1.8%) ... 674
Atrovent Inhalation Solution (Less than 3%) ... 675
Atrovent Nasal Spray 0.06% (Less than 1%) ... 678
Avonex ... 662
Bellergal-S Tablets (Rare) ... 2375
Benadryl Injection ... 1955
Bentyl ... 1246
Betagan ... ⊙ 230
▲ Betapace Tablets (3% to 14%) ... 637
▲ Betaseron for SC Injection (8%) ... 653
Betimol 0.25%, 0.5% ... ⊙ 259
Blocadren Tablets ... 1654
Bontril Slow-Release Capsules ... 786
▲ Brethine Ampuls (7.8 to 22.9%) ... 832
Brethine Tablets ... 831
Bricanyl Subcutaneous Injection (Common) ... 1247
Bricanyl Tablets (Common) ... 1248
Bromfed ... 1832
▲ Bromfed-DM Cough Syrup (Among most frequent) ... 1832
Bromfed-PD Capsules (Extended-Release) ... 1832
Bronkometer Aerosol ... 2432
Bronkosol Solution ... 2432
Brontex ... 2130
BuSpar Tablets (1%) ... 738
Calan SR Caplets (1% or less) ... 2571
Calan Tablets (1% or less) ... 2568
Capoten Tablets (Approximately 1 of 100 patients) ... 740
Capozide Tablets (Approximately 1 of 100 patients) ... 744
▲ Cardene Capsules (3.3% to 3.4%) 2261
Cardene SR Capsules (2.8%) ... 2264
▲ Cardioquin Tablets (7%) ... 2146
Cardizem CD Capsules (Less than 1%) ... 1251
Cardizem SR Capsules (1.3%) ... 1255
Cardizem Injectable ... 1253
Cardizem Tablets (Less than 1%) ... 1257
Cardura Tablets (1.2% to 2%) ... 1993
Cartrol Tablets (Less common) ... 413
Cataflam Tablets (Less than 1%) ... 833
Catapres Tablets (About 5 in 1,000 patients) ... 679
Catapres-TTS ... 680
▲ CellCept Capsules (More than or equal to 3%) ... 2265
Cerebyx Injection (Infrequent) ... 1956
Cipro I.V. (1% or less) ... 587
Cipro I.V. Pharmacy Bulk Package (Less than 1%) ... 590
Cipro Tablets (Less than 1%) ... 584
Claritin Tablets (2% or fewer patients) ... 2485
Claritin-D Tablets (Less frequent) ... 2487
Clinoril Tablets (Less than 1 in 100) ... 1658
Clomid ... 1262
Clozaril Tablets (Less than 1%) ... 2377
Cognex Capsules (Infrequent) ... 1961
Combipres Tablets (About 5 in 1,000) ... 682
Corvert Injection (1.0%) ... 2075
Covera-HS Tablets (Less than 2%) 2573
Cozaar Tablets (Less than 1%) ... 1668
Crixivan Capsules (Less than 2%) ... 1670
Cystospaz ... 2123
D.A. II Tablets ... 972
D.A. Chewable Tablets ... 970
Dalmane Capsules ... 2329
DaunoXome (Less than or equal to 5%) ... 1842
Daypro Caplets (Less than 1%) ... 2578
Deconsal II Tablets ... 1605
Demerol ... 2438
Depakote Tablets (1% to 5%) ... 418
Desoxyn Gradumet Tablets ... 422
Desyrel and Desyrel Dividose (Up to 7%) ... 504
Dexatrim ... ▣ 795
Dexatrim Plus Vitamins Caplets ... ▣ 796
Dexedrine ... 2648
DextroStat-Dextroamphetamine Sulfate Tablets ... 2211
Dilacor XR Extended-release Capsules (Infrequent) ... 2183
Dilaudid-HP Injection (Less frequent) ... 1384
Dilaudid-HP Lyophilized Powder 250 mg (Less frequent) ... 1384
Dilaudid Tablets and Liquid ... 1386
Dimetane-DX Cough Syrup ... 2233
Dipentum Capsules (Rare) ... 2084
Ditropan ... 1267
Dobutrex Solution Vials (1% to 3%) ... 1480
Dolobid Tablets (Rare) ... 1695
Donnatal ... 2234
Donnatal Extentabs ... 2234
Donnatal Tablets ... 2234
Doral Tablets ... 2773
Doxil (Less than 1%) ... 2613
Dura-Tap/PD Capsules ... 970
Dura-Vent/DA Tablets ... 972
Dura-Vent Tablets ... 971
Dynabac (0.1% to 1%) ... 668
▲ DynaCirc Capsules (1.0% to 5.1%) ... 2381
DynaCirc CR Tablets (1.2%) ... 2383
E.E.S. (Isolated reports) ... 427
EC-Naprosyn Delayed-Release Tablets (Less than 3%) ... 2277
Effexor ... 2825
Elavil ... 2945
Eldepryl Capsules (1 of 49 patients) ... 2729
Engerix-B Unit-Dose Vials ... 2656
Entex PSE Tablets ... 973
EpiPen ... 808
EryPed (Isolated reports) ... 425
Ery-Tab Tablets (Isolated reports) ... 426
Erythrocin Stearate Filmtab (Isolated reports) ... 429
Erythromycin Base Filmtab (Isolated reports) ... 430
Erythromycin Delayed-Release Capsules, USP (Isolated reports) 431
▲ Ethmozine Tablets (5.8%) ... 2217
Etrafon ... 2495
Fastin Capsules ... 2662
Fedahist Gyrocaps ... 2545
Felbatol (Frequent) ... 2774
Feldene Capsules (Less than 1%) ... 2008
Fioricet with Codeine Capsules ... 2387
Fiorinal with Codeine Capsules ... 2390
Flexeril Tablets (Less than 1%) ... 1701
▲ Flolan for Injection (63%) ... 1085
Floxin I.V. (Less than 1%) ... 1580
Floxin Tablets (200 mg, 300 mg, 400 mg) (Less than 1%) ... 1577
Flumadine Tablets & Syrup (Less than 0.3%) ... 1013
Foscavir Injection (Between 1% and 5%) ... 541
Gammar-P I.V., Immune Globulin Intravenous (Human) ... 798
Gastrocrom Oral Concentrate (Less common) ... 1611
Guaifed ... 1833
Guaimax-D Tablets ... 809
Hismanal Tablets (Rare to less frequent) ... 1341
Histussin D Liquid ... 670
Hivid Tablets (Less than 1%) ... 2287
Hycomine Compound Tablets ... 948
Hycomine ... 947
Hycotuss Expectorant Syrup ... 950
Hydralazine Hydrochloride Injection USP (Common) ... 2712
▲ Hylorel Tablets (29.5%) ... 1613
Hyperstat I.V. Injection ... 2504
▲ Hytrin Capsules (0.9% to 28%) ... 434
Hyzaar Tablets (1.4%) ... 1720
IBU Tablets (Less than 1%) ... 1389
Imdur (Less than or equal to 5%) ... 1362
Imitrex Injection (Infrequent) ... 1095
Imitrex Tablets (Up to 2%) ... 1099
Indocin (Less than 1%) ... 1723
Intron A for Injection (Less than 5%) ... 2506
Ionamin Capsules ... 1615
IOPIDINE Sterile Ophthalmic Solution ... ⊙ 218
Ismo Tablets (Fewer than 1%) ... 2844
Isoetharine Inhalation Solution, USP, Arm-a-Med ... 545
Isoptin Oral Tablets (Less than 1%) ... 1393
Isoptin SR Tablets (1% or less) ... 1395
Isuprel Hydrochloride Solution ... 2443
Isuprel Injection ... 2441
Isuprel Mistometer ... 2442
Kadian Capsules (Less than 3%) ... 2948
Kerlone Tablets (1.9%) ... 2588
Klonopin Tablets ... 2294
Kutrase Capsules ... 2546
Lamictal Tablets (1.0%) ... 1105
Larodopa Tablets (Infrequent) ... 2296
Levbid Extended-Release Tablets ... 2549
Levo-Dromoran ... 2297
Levsin/Levsinex/Levbid ... 2549
Limbitrol ... 2333
Lioresal Intrathecal (1% or more) ... 1634
Lioresal Tablets (Rare) ... 847
Lodine Capsules and Tablets (Less than 1%) ... 2849
Lopressor (1%) ... 848
Lopressor HCT Tablets ... 850
Lotensin Tablets ... 852
Lotensin HCT Tablets (0.3% to 1.0%) ... 855
Lotrel Capsules (0.5% to 0.3%) ... 858
Ludiomil Tablets (Rare) ... 861
Lufyllin & Lufyllin-400 Tablets ... 2778
Lufyllin-GG Elixir & Tablets ... 2779
▲ Lupron Depot 3.75 mg (Among most frequent) ... 2739
▲ LUVOX Tablets (3%) ... 2723
MS Contin Tablets (Less frequent) 2149
MSIR (Infrequent) ... 2152
Marax Tablets & DF Syrup ... 2015
Marinol (Dronabinol) Capsules (Greater than 1%) ... 2353
Mavik Tablets (0.3% to 1.0%) ... 1407
Maxair Autohaler (1.3% to 1.7%) ... 1550
Maxair Inhaler (1.7%) ... 1552
Megace Oral Suspension (1% to 3%) ... 708
Mepergan Injection ... 2859
Metaproterenol Sulfate Inhalation Solution, USP, Arm-a-Med (Approximately 1 in 300 patients) ... 547
Methadone Hydrochloride Oral Concentrate ... 2356
Methadone Hydrochloride Oral Solution & Tablets ... 2357
Methergine (Rare) ... 2401
▲ Mexitil Capsules (4.3% to 7.5%) ... 684
Miacalcin Nasal Spray (Less than 1%) ... 2403
Midamor Tablets (Less than or equal to 1%) ... 1746
Miltown Tablets ... 2780
▲ Minipress Capsules (5.3%) ... 2015
▲ Minizide Capsules (5.3%) ... 2016
Moduretic Tablets ... 1748
Monoket Tablets (Fewer than 1%) 2550
Monopril Tablets (0.2% to 1.0%) ... 762
Motrin Ibuprofen Suspension, Oral Drops, Chewable Tablets, Caplets (Less than 1%) ... 1563
Mykrox Tablets (Less than 2%) ... 1617
Nalfon 200 Pulvules & Nalfon Tablets (2.5%) ... 933
Naprelan Tablets (Less than 3%) ... 2861
Anaprox/Naprosyn (Less than 3%) ... 2277
Netromycin Injection 100 mg/ml (Fewer than 1 of 1000 patients) 2516
Neurontin Capsules (Infrequent) ... 1978
▲ Nicotrol NS Nicotine Nasal Spray (4%) ... 1565
Nimotop Capsules (Less than 1%) 603
Nitrostat Tablets (Occasional) ... 1981
Norflex ... 1554
Norgesic ... 1554
Norisodrine with Calcium Iodide Syrup ... 446
Noroxin Tablets (Less frequent) ... 1758
Noroxin Tablets (Less frequent) ... 2222
Norpramin Tablets ... 1273
Norvasc Tablets (0.7% to 4.5%) ... 2020
Norvir (Less than 2%) ... 447
Novahistine DMX ... ▣ 782
Novahistine Elixir ... ▣ 782
Ocupress Ophthalmic Solution, 1% Sterile (Occasional) ... ⊙ 297
OptiPranolol (Metipranolol 0.3%) Sterile Ophthalmic Solution (A small number of patients) ... ⊙ 256
Oramorph SR (Morphine Sulfate Sustained Release Tablets) (Less frequent) ... 2359
Orap Tablets ... 1037
Ornade Spansule Capsules ... 2678
Orudis Capsules (Less than 1%) ... 2874
Oruvail Capsules (Less than 1%) ... 2874

(▣ Described in PDR For Nonprescription Drugs) Incidence data in parenthesis; ▲ 3% or more (⊙ Described in PDR For Ophthalmology)

PBZ Tablets 863
PBZ-SR Tablets 862
Pamelor 2409
Parnate Tablets 2679
Paxil Tablets (2% to 3%) 2681
Pediazole Suspension 2340
Penetrex Tablets (0.1% to 1%) 2196
Pentasa (Less than 1%) 1275
Pepcid Injection (Infrequent) 1765
Pepcid (Infrequent) 1763
Periactin 1767
Permax Tablets (2.1%) 571
Phenergan with Codeine 2883
Phenergan VC with Codeine 2888
Phenurone Tablets (Less than 1%) 455
Plendil Extended-Release Tablets (0.4% to 2.5%) 514
PMB 200 and PMB 400 2890
Pondimin Tablets 2239
Ponstel (Rare) 1982
Prelu-2 Timed Release Capsules 687
Prevacid Delayed-Release Capsules (Less than 1%) 2746
Prilosec Delayed-Release Capsules (Less than 1%) 516
Primaxin I.M. 1770
Primaxin I.V. (Less than 0.2%) 1772
Prinivil Tablets (0.3% to 1.0%) 1776
Prinzide Tablets (0.3 to 1%) 1780
Pro-Banthine Tablets 2226
▲ Procardia Capsules (2% or less to 7%) 2024
▲ Procardia XL Extended Release Tablets (Less than 3% to 7%) 2026
Proglycem (Common) 575
Propulsid (1% or less) 1346
ProSom Tablets (Infrequent) 457
▲ Proventil Inhalation Aerosol (Less than 10%) 2524
▲ Proventil Repetabs Tablets (5%) 2529
Proventil Syrup (Less than 1 of 100 patients) 2528
▲ Proventil Tablets (5%) 2529
Prozac Pulvules & Liquid, Oral Solution (1.3% to 2%) 935
Quadrinal Tablets 1398
▲ Quinidex Extentabs (7%) 2240
RMS Suppositories CII 2766
Recombivax HB (Less than 1%) 1787
Redux Capsules (Frequent) 2911
Relafen Tablets (Less than 1%) 2688
ReoPro Vials (0.7%) 1526
Respbid Tablets 687
RespiGam 1631
Restoril Capsules (Less than 1%) 2413
ReVia Tablets (Less than 1%) 957
Rifater 1280
Rilutek Tablets (0.4% to 1.2%) 2198
Risperdal Tablets (Infrequent) 1348
Ritalin 866
Robinul Forte Tablets 2247
Robinul Injectable 2247
Robinul Tablets 2247
Rocephin Injectable Vials, ADD-Vantage, Galaxy Container (Rare) 2305
Roferon-A Injection (Less than 3%) 2308
▲ Romazicon (3% to 9%) 2311
Rondec Oral Drops 974
Rondec Syrup 974
Rondec Tablet 974
Rondec Chewable Tablets 974
Rondec-TR Tablet 974
Roxanol 2365
▲ Rythmol Tablets–150mg, 225mg, 300mg (0.6 to 3.4%) 1399
Salagen Tablets (Less than 1%) 1546
Sandostatin Injection (Less than 1%) 2421
Sanorex Tablets 2423
Seldane Tablets (Rare) 1284
▲ Seldane-D Extended-Release Tablets (2.4%) 1286
Semprex-D Capsules 1620
Ser-Ap-Es Tablets 867
Serevent Inhalation Aerosol (1% to 3%) 1149
Serzone Tablets 776
Sinemet Tablets (Less frequent) 959
Sinemet CR Tablets 961
Slo-bid Gyrocaps 2201
Stadol (1% or greater) 779
Stimate, (desmopressin acetate) Nasal Spray, 1.5 mg/mL 806
▲ Sular Tablets (3%) 2961
Supprelin Injection (1% to 3%) 2230
Surmontil Capsules 2917
Sus-Phrine Injection 1017
Synarel Nasal Solution for Endometriosis (Less than 1%) 2605
Syn-Rx Tablets 1622
Syn-Rx DM Tablets 1623
▲ Tambocor Tablets (6.1%) 1555
Tavist Syrup 2426
Tavist Tablets 2427
Tenex Tablets (3% or less) 2249
Thalitone (Common) 1293
Theo-Dur Extended-Release Tablets 1367
Theo-X Extended-Release Tablets 793
Tiazac Capsules (Less than 1% to 2%) 1019
Timolide Tablets 1791
Timoptic in Ocudose (Less frequent) 1796
Timoptic Sterile Ophthalmic Solution (Less frequent) 1794
Timoptic-XE 1798
Tofranil Ampuls 873
Tofranil Tablets 875
Tofranil-PM Capsules 876
Tonocard Tablets (0.4% to 1.8%) 519
Toprol-XL Tablets (About 1 of 100 patients) 560
Toradol (1% or less) 2319
▲ Tornalate Solution for Inhalation, 0.2% (3.1%) 976
Tornalate Metered Dose Inhaler (1.5% to approximately 3%) 978
Trandate 1158
Trental Tablets 1291
Triavil Tablets 1800
Trinalin Repetabs Tablets 1373
Tussend Expectorant 1831
Ultram Tablets (50 mg) (Infrequent) 1594
Uni-Dur Extended-Release Tablets 1374
Univasc Tablets (Less than 1%) 2553
Urispas Tablets 2710
▲ Vascor Tablets (200 and 300 mg) (2.27 to 6.52%) 1597
Vaseretic Tablets (0.5% to 2.0%) 1810
Vasotec I.V. 1814
Vasotec Tablets (0.5% to 1.0%) 1816
▲ Ventolin Inhalation Aerosol and Refill (Fewer than 10 in 100 patients) 1170
Ventolin Inhalation Solution 1171
Ventolin Nebules Inhalation Solution 1172
Ventolin Syrup (Less than 1 of 100 patients) 1175
▲ Ventolin Tablets (5 of 100 patients) 1176
Verelan Capsules (1% or less) 1455
Vicodin Tuss Expectorant 1406
Videx Tablets, Powder for Oral Solution, & Pediatric Powder for Oral Solution (Less than 1%) 2980
Visken Tablets (Less than 1%) 2428
Vivactil Tablets 1820
Volmax Extended-Release Tablets (2.4%) 1835
Cataflam/Voltaren/Voltaren-XR (Less than 1%) 833
▲ Wellbutrin Tablets (3.7%) 1177
▲ Xanax Tablets (7.7%) 2115
▲ Yutopar Intravenous Injection (About one-third) 566
Zaroxolyn Tablets 1625
Zebeta Tablets 1457
Zestoretic Tablets (0.3 to 1%) 2968
Zestril Tablets (0.3% to 1.0%) 2972
Ziac 1459
Zithromax (1% or less) 2043
Zithromax Tablets (1% or less) 2046
Zoladex (1% or greater) 2976
Zoladex 3-month 2978
▲ Zoloft Tablets (3.5%) 2051
Zyrtec Tablets (Less than 2%) 2053

Palsy, cranial nerve

Carbocaine Injection 2432
Marcaine Spinal 2449
NegGram (A few cases) 2453
Orthoclone OKT3 Sterile Solution 1892
Pontocaine Hydrochloride for Spinal Anesthesia 2460
Sensorcaine 554

Palsy, optic nerve

Symmetrel Capsules (0.1% to 1%) 965
Symmetrel Syrup (0.1% to 1%) 963

Palsy, peripheral nerve

Lescol Capsules 2395
Mevacor Tablets 1742
Pravachol Tablets 770
Zocor Tablets 1821

Pancolitis

Rowasa 2727

Pancreatic disease, unspecified

Pulmozyme Inhalation 1054

Pancreatic enzymes, increased

Norpramin Tablets 1273

Pancreatitis

Accupril Tablets (Rare) 1950
Achromycin V Capsules (Rare) 1417
Actimmune (Rare) 1043
Activase 1045
Aldactazide Tablets 2556
Aldoclor Tablets 1638
Aldomet Ester HCl Injection 1642
Aldomet Oral 1640
Aldoril Tablets 1644
Altace Capsules (Less than 1%) 1238
Anaprox/Naprosyn (Less than 1%) 2277
Apresazide Capsules 824
Asacol Delayed-Release Tablets 2129
Asendin Tablets (Very rare) 1419
Atromid-S Capsules 2808
Azulfidine (Rare) 2059
Bactrim DS Tablets 2257
Bactrim I.V. Infusion 2255
Bactrim 2257
Betaseron for SC Injection 653
Calcijex Injection 412
Capoten Tablets 740
Capozide Tablets 744
Cataflam Tablets (Less than 1%) 833
Celestone Soluspan Suspension 2484
Chibroxin Sterile Ophthalmic Solution (With oral form) 1657
Cipro I.V. (1% or less) 587
Cipro I.V. Pharmacy Bulk Package (Less than 1%) 590
Cipro Tablets 584
Clinoril Tablets (Less than 1 in 100) 1658
Clozaril Tablets 2377
Cognex Capsules 1961
Combipres Tablets 682
CORTENEMA 2713
Cortifoam 2540
Cortone Acetate Sterile Suspension 1663
Cortone Acetate Tablets 1664
Cuprimine Capsules 1673
Cytosar-U Sterile Powder (Two cases) 2077
Cytovene (1% or less) 2270
Dalalone D.P. Injectable 1009
Danocrine Capsules (Rare) 2437
Dapsone Tablets USP 1331
Daypro Caplets (Less than 1%) 2578
Decadron Elixir 1676
Decadron Phosphate Injection 1680
Decadron Phosphate with Xylocaine Injection, Sterile 1683
Decadron Tablets 1678
Decadron-LA Sterile Suspension 1687
Declomycin Tablets 1421
Depakene 416
Depakote Tablets 418
Depen Titratable Tablets (Isolated cases) 2770
Dexacort Phosphate in Respihaler 1606
Dexacort Phosphate in Turbinaire 1607
Dipentum Capsules (Rare) 2084
Diucardin Tablets 2824
Diupres Tablets 1691
Diuril Oral Suspension 1694
Diuril Sodium Intravenous 1693
Diuril Tablets 1694
Doxil (Less than 1%) 2613
Dyazide Capsules 2653
DYNACIN Capsules 1627
EC-Naprosyn Delayed-Release Tablets (Less than 1%) 2277
Edecrin (Rare) 1698
Elspar 1700
Enduron Tablets 424
Epivir (Less than 0.5%) 1200
Ergamisol Tablets (Less frequent) 1340
Esidrix Tablets 839
Esimil Tablets 840
Estrace Cream and Tablets 751
Fansidar Tablets 2281
Felbatol 2774
Feldene Capsules (Less than 1%) 2008
Flagyl 375 Capsules (Rare) 2587
Flagyl I.V. (Rare) 2373
Florinef Acetate Tablets 506
Floxin I.V. 1580
Floxin Tablets (200 mg, 300 mg, 400 mg) 1577
Foscavir Injection (Between 1% and 5%) 541
Gantanol Tablets 2285
Gantrisin 2286
Helidac Therapy (Rare) 2135
Hivid Tablets (Less than 1% rare) 2287
Humatrope Vials (Rare) 1490
Hydeltrasol Injection, Sterile 1708
Hydeltra-T.B.A. Sterile Suspension 1710
Hydrocortone Acetate Sterile Suspension 1712
Hydrocortone Phosphate Injection, Sterile 1713
Hydrocortone Tablets 1715
HydroDIURIL Tablets 1716
Hydropres Tablets 1718
Hyperstat I.V. Injection 2504
Hyzaar Tablets 1720
IBU Tablets (Less than 1%) 1389
Inderide Tablets 2838
Inderide LA Long Acting Capsules 2840
Invirase Capsules (Rare) 2291
Lamictal Tablets 1105
Lasix Injection, Oral Solution and Tablets 1267
Lescol Capsules 2395
Lodine Capsules and Tablets (Less than 1%) 2849
Lomotil 2591
Lopid Tablets 1974
Lopressor HCT Tablets 850
Lotensin Tablets 852
Lotensin HCT Tablets (Rare) 855
Lotrel Capsules (Rare) 858
Macrobid Capsules 2138
Macrodantin Capsules 2140
Mavik Tablets (Rare) 1407
Methotrexate Sodium Tablets, Injection, for Injection and LPF Injection 1322
MetroGel-Vaginal 917
Mevacor Tablets 1742
Mexitil Capsules (Rare) 684
Minipress Capsules (Less than 1%) 2015
Minizide Capsules (Rare) 2016
Minocin Intravenous 1428
Minocin Oral Suspension 1431
Minocin Pellet-Filled Capsules 1429
Moduretic Tablets 1748
Monopril Tablets (0.2% to 1.0%) 762
Motofen Tablets 789
Motrin Ibuprofen Suspension, Oral Drops, Chewable Tablets, Caplets (Less than 1%) 1563
Mykrox Tablets 1617
Nalfon 200 Pulvules & Nalfon Tablets (Less than 1%) 933
▲ Naprelan Tablets (3% to 9%) 2861
Anaprox/Naprosyn (Less than 1%) 2277
Neoral (Rare) 2405
Neurontin Capsules (Rare) 1978
Noroxin Tablets (Rare) 1758
Noroxin Tablets (Rare) 2222
Norvir (Less than 2%) 447
Nutropin AQ Injection (Rare) 1051
Ogen Tablets 2103
Oncaspar (1%) 2194
Oretic Tablets 450
Orudis Capsules (Rare) 2874
Oruvail Capsules (Rare) 2874
Paxil Tablets 2681
Pediapred Oral Solution 1618
Pediazole Suspension 2340
Pentasa (Infrequent to less than 1%) 1275
Permax Tablets (Rare) 571
Pravachol Tablets 770
Prelone Syrup 1834
Premarin Tablets 2896
Premarin Vaginal Cream 2898
Premphase 2900
Prempro 2905
Prilosec Delayed-Release Capsules (Less than 1%) 516
Prinivil Tablets (0.3% to 1.0%) 1776
Prinzide Tablets 1780
Proglycem 575
Proleukin for Injection (Less than 1%) 812
Prozac Pulvules & Liquid, Oral Solution 935
Purinethol Tablets 1214
Questran 774
Redux Capsules (Rare) 2911
Relafen Tablets (Less than 1%) 2688
Remeron Tablets (Rare) 1878
Retrovir Capsules (Rare) 1216
Retrovir I.V. Infusion (Rare) 1221
Retrovir Syrup (Rare) 1216

(Described in PDR For Nonprescription Drugs) Incidence data in parenthesis; ▲ 3% or more (◉ Described in PDR For Ophthalmology)

Pancreatitis

Rilutek Tablets (Infrequent)	2198
Risperdal Tablets	1348
Rocaltrol Capsules	2303
Roferon-A Injection (Infrequent)	2308
Rowasa	2727
Sandimmune (Rare)	2416
Septra	1146
Septra I.V. Infusion	1142
Septra I.V. Infusion ADD-Vantage Vials	1144
Septra	1146
Ser-Ap-Es Tablets	867
Tagamet (Rare)	2694
Tenoretic Tablets	2963
Thalitone	1293
Timolide Tablets	1791
Tonocard Tablets (Less than 1%)	519
Toradol	2319
Univasc Tablets (Less than 1%)	2553
Urobiotic-250 Capsules	2038
Vaseretic Tablets	1810
Vasotec I.V.	1814
Vasotec Tablets (0.5% to 1.0%)	1816
Vesanoid Capsules (Isolated cases)	2327
▲ Videx Tablets, Powder for Oral Solution, & Pediatric Powder for Oral Solution (2% to 10%)	2980
Vistide Injection (Less than 1%)	1057
Cataflam/Voltaren/Voltaren-XR (Less than 1%)	833
Zantac (Rare)	1182
Zantac Injection (Rare)	1180
Zantac Syrup (Rare)	1182
Zaroxolyn Tablets	1625
Zerit Capsules (Up to 2%)	731
Zestoretic Tablets	2968
Zestril Tablets (0.3% to 1.0%)	2972
Ziac	1459
Zocor Tablets	1821
Zoloft Tablets (Rare)	2051
Zosyn (1.0% or less)	1463

Pancreatitis, hemorrhagic

Hivid Tablets (Less than 1%)	2287
Videx Tablets, Powder for Oral Solution, & Pediatric Powder for Oral Solution (Less than 1%)	2980
Zyloprim Tablets (Less than 1%)	1194

Pancytopenia

Albenza Tablets (Rare)	2629
Altace Capsules (Less than 1%)	1238
Amaryl Tablets	1241
Anafranil Capsules	819
Ancobon Capsules	2254
Atretol Tablets	569
Azactam for Injection (Less than 1%)	736
Capoten Tablets	740
Capozide Tablets	744
Cedax	2480
Cefizox for Intramuscular or Intravenous Use	1025
Cefotan	2936
Ceftin	1067
Cefzil Tablets and Oral Suspension	747
Celontin Kapseals	1955
Ceptaz	1070
Chloromycetin Sodium Succinate	1960
Cipro I.V. (Rare)	587
Cipro I.V. Pharmacy Bulk Package (Rare)	590
Cipro Tablets (0.1%)	584
Cognex Capsules (Rare)	1961
Compazine	2644
Cosmegen Injection	1666
Cytosar-U Sterile Powder (Less than 7 patients)	2077
Cytovene (1% or less)	2270
Daraprim Tablets	1199
DiaBeta Tablets (Occasional)	1265
Diabinese Tablets	2002
Diamox	⊚ 317
Didronel Tablets (Rare)	2133
Dilantin Infatabs (Occasional)	1967
Dilantin Kapseals (Occasional)	1965
Dilantin-125 Suspension (Occasional)	1969
Duricef Capsules, Tablets, and Oral Suspension	750
Ergamisol Tablets	1340
Etrafon	2495
Felbatol (May be more than 100 fold)	2774
Floxin I.V.	1580
Floxin Tablets (200 mg, 300 mg, 400 mg)	1577
Fluorouracil Injection	2282
Fortaz	1092
Foscavir Injection (Less than 1%)	541
Sterile FUDR (Remote possibility)	2284

Gastrocrom Oral Concentrate (Less common)	1611
GlaucTabs	⊚ 209
Glucotrol Tablets	2011
Glucotrol XL Extended Release Tablets	2012
Glynase PresTab Tablets	2091
Imitrex Tablets	1099
Invirase Capsules (Less than 2%)	2291
Kefurox Vials, Faspak & ADD-Vantage	1509
Lamictal Tablets	1105
Leustatin	1889
Levoprome	1321
Lodine Capsules and Tablets (Less than 1%)	2849
Lorabid Suspension and Pulvules	1513
Matulane Capsules	2300
Maxipime for Injection	758
Mellaril	2398
Mesantoin Tablets	2400
Methotrexate Sodium Tablets, Injection, for Injection and LPF Injection (1% to 3%)	1322
Micronase Tablets	2099
Monopril Tablets	762
Motrin Ibuprofen Suspension, Oral Drops, Chewable Tablets, Caplets (Less than 1%)	1563
Mustargen	1752
Nalfon 200 Pulvules & Nalfon Tablets (Less than 1%)	933
Navane Capsules and Concentrate	2018
Navane Intramuscular	2019
Neptazane Tablets	⊚ 320
Nolvadex Tablets (Rare)	2957
▲ Oncaspar (Greater than 1% but less than 5%)	2194
Orthoclone OKT3 Sterile Solution	1892
Pentasa	1275
Pepcid Injection (Rare)	1765
Pepcid (Rare)	1763
Ponstel (Occasional)	1982
Prilosec Delayed-Release Capsules (Rare)	516
Primaxin I.M.	1770
Primaxin I.V.	1772
Prolixin	510
Propulsid (Rare)	1346
Prozac Pulvules & Liquid, Oral Solution	935
Redux Capsules	2911
Remeron Tablets (Rare)	1878
Retrovir I.V. Infusion	1221
Ridaura Capsules (Less than 0.1%)	2691
Serentil	689
Soma Compound w/Codeine Tablets (Very rare)	2784
Soma Compound Tablets (Very rare)	2783
Soma Tablets	2782
Stelazine	2692
Suprax	1443
Tagamet (Very rare)	2694
Tapazole Tablets	1361
Tazicef for Injection	2697
Tazidime Vials, Faspak & ADD-Vantage	1531
Tegretol/Tegretol-XR	870
▲ Thioguanine Tablets, Tabloid Brand (Nearly all patients)	1225
Thorazine	2701
Ticlid Tablets (Rare)	2317
Torecan	2367
Trental Tablets (Rare)	1291
Triavil Tablets	1800
Trilafon	2532
Vantin for Oral Suspension and Vantin Tablets	2112
Wellbutrin Tablets (Rare)	1177
Zantac (Rare)	1182
Zantac Injection (Rare)	1180
Zantac Syrup (Rare)	1182
Zarontin Capsules	1986
Zarontin Syrup	1986
Zinacef	1184
Zyloprim Tablets (Less than 1%)	1194

Panencephalitis, sclerosing, subacute

M-M-R II	1730

Panic

Ambien Tablets (Rare)	2559
Anafranil Capsules (1% to 2%)	819
Cozaar Tablets (Less than 1%)	1668
Hyzaar Tablets	1720
Imitrex Tablets	1099
Lamictal Tablets (Infrequent)	1105
Pamelor	2409

Panmyelopathy

Solganal Suspension (Rare)	2530

Papilledema

Accutane Capsules	2252
Amen Tablets	785
Aquasol A Vitamin A Capsules, USP	525
Aquasol A Parenteral	526
Betaseron for SC Injection	653
Brevicon	2563
Celestone Soluspan Suspension	2484
Cortone Acetate Sterile Suspension	1663
Cortone Acetate Tablets	1664
Cycrin Tablets	991
Danocrine Capsules	2437
Decadron Elixir	1676
Decadron Phosphate Injection	1680
Decadron Phosphate with Xylocaine Injection, Sterile	1683
Decadron Tablets	1678
Decadron-LA Sterile Suspension	1687
Demulen	2580
Depo-Provera Contraceptive Injection	2079
Depo-Provera Sterile Aqueous Suspension	2083
Effexor (Rare)	2825
Eskalith	2658
Genotropin Injection (A small number of patients)	2090
Humatrope Vials (A small number of patients)	1490
Hydeltrasol Injection, Sterile	1708
Hydeltra-T.B.A. Sterile Suspension	1710
Hydrocortone Acetate Sterile Suspension	1712
Hydrocortone Phosphate Injection, Sterile	1713
Hydrocortone Tablets	1715
Hyperstat I.V. Injection (1 patient)	2504
Levlen/Tri-Levlen	646
Lithium Carbonate Capsules & Tablets	2352
Matulane Capsules	2300
Modicon	1928
NegGram (Occasional)	2453
Nizoral Tablets (Rare)	1345
Norinyl	2563
Norplant System	2868
Nor-Q D Tablets	2598
Ortho-Cyclen/Ortho-Tri-Cyclen	1914
Ortho-Novum	1928
Ortho-Cyclen/Ortho Tri-Cyclen	1914
Ovcon	765
Platinol for Injection (Infrequent)	717
Platinol-AQ Injection (Infrequent)	719
Premphase	2900
Prempro	2905
Provera Tablets	2110
Redux Capsules	2911
Levlen/Tri-Levlen	646
Tri-Norinyl	2607

Papillitis

Attenuvax	1650
Biavax II	1653
M-M-R II (Infrequent)	1730
M-R-VAX II	1732
Mumpsvax (Infrequent)	1751

Papilloma, scrotum

Testoderm Testosterone Transdermal System (One in 104 patients)	486

Papules

Catapres-TTS (1 of 101 patients)	680
Depen Titratable Tablets	2770
Duragesic Transdermal System (1% or greater)	1336
Oxistat Cream (0.1%)	1139
Yodoxin Tablets	1235

Papules, erythematous

(see under Erythema multiforme)

Paralysis

Atretol Tablets	569
Betapace Tablets (Rare)	637
Betaseron for SC Injection	653
Carbocaine Injection	2432
Cerebyx Injection (Infrequent)	1956
Cognex Capsules (Infrequent)	1961
Coumadin	941
Depo-Provera Contraceptive Injection (Fewer than 1%)	2079
Felbatol	2774
Foscavir Injection (Less than 1%)	541
Hivid Tablets (Less than 1%)	2287

Hyperstat I.V. Injection	2504
Imitrex Tablets (Rare)	1099
Lamictal Tablets	1105
Lovenox Injection (1.9%)	2187
Lupron Depot 3.75 mg	2739
Lupron Depot 7.5 mg	2741
Lupron Depot - 3 Month 22.5 mg	2743
Lupron Depot-PED 7.5 mg, 11.25 mg and 15 mg	2744
Lupron Injection	2736
LUVOX Tablets (Infrequent)	2723
Naprelan Tablets (Less than 1%)	2861
Nipent for Injection (Less than 3%)	2733
Norvir (Less than 2%)	447
Novocain Hydrochloride for Spinal Anesthesia	2457
Oncovin Solution Vials & Hyporets	1521
Orimune (Rare)	1433
Paxil Tablets (Infrequent)	2681
Permax Tablets (Infrequent)	571
Pontocaine Hydrochloride for Spinal Anesthesia	2460
Prozac Pulvules & Liquid, Oral Solution (Rare)	935
Redux Capsules (Rare)	2911
Remeron Tablets (Rare)	1878
Sodium Polystyrene Sulfonate Suspension	2367
Tegretol/Tegretol-XR	870
Videx Tablets, Powder for Oral Solution, & Pediatric Powder for Oral Solution (Less than 1%)	2980
Zyrtec Tablets (Less than 2%)	2053

Paralysis, bladder

Etrafon	2495
Prolixin	510

Paralysis, extraocular muscles

Lescol Capsules	2395
Plaquenil Sulfate Tablets	2459
Pravachol Tablets	770

Paralysis, facial

Avonex	662
Betaseron for SC Injection	653
Depo-Provera Contraceptive Injection (Fewer than 1%)	2079
Imitrex Tablets (Rare)	1099
Neurontin Capsules (Infrequent)	1978
Rilutek Tablets (Infrequent)	2198
▲ Vesanoid Capsules (3%)	2327

Paralysis, flaccid

Diamox Intravenous (Occasional)	⊚ 317
Diamox Sequels (Sustained Release)	⊚ 318
Diamox Tablets (Occasional)	⊚ 317
GlaucTabs (Occasional)	⊚ 209
Neptazane Tablets	⊚ 320
Rum-K Syrup	1004

Paralysis, legs
(see under Paralysis, lower extremities)

Paralysis, lower extremities

Carbocaine Injection	2432
Marcaine	2446
Marcaine Spinal	2449
Sensorcaine	554

Paralysis, oculomotor nerve

Anafranil Capsules (Rare)	819

Paralysis, radial nerve

Tripedia	908

Paralysis, respiratory

Amikacin Sulfate Injection, USP	523
Amikacin Sulfate Injection, USP	981
Amikin Injectable	502
Carbocaine Injection	2432
Marcaine	2446
Marcaine Spinal	2449
Novocain Hydrochloride for Spinal Anesthesia	2457
Pontocaine Hydrochloride for Spinal Anesthesia	2460
Sensorcaine	554
Tensilon Injectable	1307

Paralysis, sensory motor

Demerol	2438

Paralysis, skeletal muscle

Amikacin Sulfate Injection, USP	523
Amikacin Sulfate Injection, USP	981
Amikin Injectable	502
Anectine	1062

(⊞ Described in PDR For Nonprescription Drugs)   Incidence data in parenthesis; ▲ 3% or more   (⊚ Described in PDR For Ophthalmology)

1423 **Side Effects Index** **Paresthesia**

Netromycin Injection 100 mg/ml.... 2516
Norcuron for Injection 1875
Nuromax Injection 1136

Paralysis, spinal cord

Ethamolin Injection (One child) 2544

Paralysis, spinal nerve

Novocain Hydrochloride for Spinal Anesthesia 2457
Pontocaine Hydrochloride for Spinal Anesthesia 2460

Paralysis, vocal cord

Foscavir Injection (Less than 1%) .. 541

Paralysis agitans (see under Parkinsonism)

Paranoia

Adalat Capsules (10 mg and 20 mg) (Less than 0.5%) 580
Adalat CC (Rare) 582
Anafranil Capsules (Infrequent) 819
Artane (One case) 1418
Atamet Tablets 567
Betaseron for SC Injection 653
Cipro I.V. (1% or less) 587
Cipro I.V. Pharmacy Bulk Package (Less than 1%) 590
Clozaril Tablets (Less than 1%) 2377
Cognex Capsules (Infrequent) 1961
Desyrel and Desyrel Dividose 504
Doral Tablets 2773
Duragesic Transdermal System (1% or greater) 1336
Effexor (Infrequent) 2825
Etrafon 2495
Felbatol 2774
Floxin I.V. 1580
Floxin Tablets (200 mg, 300 mg, 400 mg) 1577
Hivid Tablets (Less than 1%) 2287
Lamictal Tablets (Infrequent) 1105
Larodopa Tablets (Infrequent) 2296
Lioresal Intrathecal (1% or more) .. 1634
LUVOX Tablets (Infrequent) 2723
▲ Marinol (Dronabinol) Capsules (3% to 10%) 2353
Neurontin Capsules (Infrequent) 1978
Orthoclone OKT3 Sterile Solution .. 1892
Parlodel (Less than 1%) 2411
Paxil Tablets (Infrequent) 2681
Permax Tablets (Frequent) 571
Procardia Capsules (Less than 0.5%) 2024
Prozac Pulvules & Liquid, Oral Solution (Infrequent) 935
Remeron Tablets (Infrequent) 1878
ReVia Tablets (Less than 1%) 957
Rilutek Tablets (Infrequent) 2198
Romazicon (1% to 3%) 2311
Sandostatin Injection (Less than 1%) 2421
Serzone Tablets (Infrequent) 776
Sinemet Tablets 959
Sinemet CR Tablets 961
Trilafon 2532
Videx Tablets, Powder for Oral Solution, & Pediatric Powder for Oral Solution (Less than 1%) 2980
Wellbutrin Tablets (Infrequent) 1177
Zoloft Tablets (Infrequent) 2051

Paraparesis

Leustatin 1889
Orthoclone OKT3 Sterile Solution .. 1892

Paraplegia

Foscavir Injection (Less than 1%) .. 541
Methotrexate Sodium Tablets, Injection, for Injection and LPF Injection 1322
Orthoclone OKT3 Sterile Solution .. 1892
Redux Capsules 2911

Parapsoriasis varioliformis acuta

Azulfidine (Rare) 2059

Parathyroid hormone deficiency, fetal

Accutane Capsules 2252

Parenchymatous organs, toxic damage

Phenobarbital Elixir and Tablets 1523
Tagamet (Highly unlikely) 2694

Paresis

Ambien Tablets (Rare) 2559
Anafranil Capsules (Up to 2%) 819
Cardura Tablets (Less than 0.5% of 3960 patients) 1993
Cognex Capsules (Infrequent) 1961
Engerix-B Unit-Dose Vials 2656
Imdur (Less than or equal to 5%) .. 1362
Intron A for Injection (Less than 5%) 2506
Invirase Capsules (Less than 2%) .. 2291
Leukeran Tablets (Rare) 1205
Methotrexate Sodium Tablets, Injection, for Injection and LPF Injection 1322
Neurontin Capsules (Infrequent) 1978
Oncovin Solution Vials & Hyporets 1521
Seromycin Capsules 975
Tambocor Tablets (1% to less than 3%) 1555
Tenex Tablets (3% or less) 2249

Paresthesia

Accupril Tablets (0.5% to 1.0%) .. 1950
Accutane Capsules 2252
Adalat CC (3% or less) 582
Adapin Capsules (Infrequent) 1542
Adenoscan (2%) 1022
Aldactazide Tablets 2556
Aldoclor Tablets 1638
Aldomet Ester HCl Injection 1642
Aldomet Oral 1640
Aldoril Tablets 1644
Altace Capsules (Less than 1%) 1238
Ambien Tablets (Infrequent) 2559
Amikacin Sulfate Injection, USP (Rare) 523
Amikacin Sulfate Injection, USP (Rare) 981
Amikin Injectable (Rare) 502
▲ Anafranil Capsules (2% to 9%) 819
Ancobon Capsules 2254
Androderm Testosterone Transdermal System (Less than 1%) 2634
▲ Android Capsules, 10 mg (Among most common) 1297
Apresazide Capsules (Less frequent) 824
Apresoline Hydrochloride Tablets (Less frequent) 826
Aredia for Injection 827
▲ Arimidex Tablets (4.6% to 6.1%) .. 2932
Asacol Delayed-Release Tablets 2129
Atretol Tablets 569
Atrovent Inhalation Aerosol (Less frequent) 674
Azactam for Injection (Less than 1%) 736
Benadryl Injection 1955
Betagan .... ⊙ 230
Betapace Tablets (1% to 4%) 637
Betimol 0.25%, 0.5% .... ⊙ 259
Biavax II 1653
Blocadren Tablets (0.6%) 1654
Brevibloc (esmolol HCl) Injection (Less than 1%) 1860
BuSpar Tablets (1%) 738
Cafergot 2376
Calan SR Caplets (1% or less) 2571
Calan Tablets (1% or less) 2568
Capoten Tablets (About 0.5 to 2%) 740
Capozide Tablets (0.5 to 2%) 744
Carbocaine Injection 2432
Cardene Capsules (1.0%) 2261
Cardene I.V. (0.7%) 2815
Cardizem CD Capsules (Less than 1%) 1251
Cardizem SR Capsules (Less than 1%) 1255
Cardizem Injectable (Less than 1%) 1253
Cardizem Tablets (Less than 1%) .. 1257
Cardura Tablets (1%) 1993
Cartrol Tablets (2.0%) 413
▲ Casodex Tablets (6%) 2934
Cataflam Tablets (Less than 1%) 833
Ceclor Pulvules & Suspension 1470
Cedax (0.1% to 1%) 2480
Cefizox for Intramuscular or Intravenous Use (1% to 5%) 1025
▲ CellCept Capsules (More than or equal to 3%) 2265
Ceptaz (Fewer than 1%) 1070
▲ Cerebyx Injection (7 of 16 volunteers; 3.9% to 4.4%) 1956
▲ Chemet Capsules (1.0% to 12.7%) 666
Cipro I.V. (1% or less) 587
Cipro I.V. Pharmacy Bulk Package (Less than 1%) 590
Cipro Tablets (Less than 1%) 584
Claritin Tablets (2% or fewer patients) 2485
Claritin-D Tablets (Less frequent) .. 2487
Clinoril Tablets (Less than 1%) 1658
Clomid 1262
Clozaril Tablets 2377
Cognex Capsules (Frequent) 1961
Combipres Tablets 682
▲ Cordarone Tablets (4 to 9%) 2818
Coumadin 941
Covera-HS Tablets (1.0%) 2573
Cozaar Tablets (Less than 1%) 1668
Crixivan Capsules (Less than 2%) .. 1670
▲ Cytovene (6%) 2270
D.H.E. 45 Injection (Occasional) 2381
Dalalone D.P. Injectable 1009
Danocrine Capsules 2437
▲ Daranide Tablets (Among the most common effects) 1676
Decadron-LA Sterile Suspension 1687
Depakote Tablets (1% to 5%) 418
Depo-Provera Contraceptive Injection (Fewer than 1%) 2079
Dermatop Emollient Cream 0.1% (Less than 1%) 1264
Desyrel and Desyrel Dividose (Up to 1.4%) 504
Diamox Sequels (Sustained Release) .... ⊙ 318
Didronel Tablets 2133
Dilacor XR Extended-release Capsules (Infrequent) 2183
Dilaudid-HP Injection (Less frequent) 1384
Dilaudid-HP Lyophilized Powder 250 mg (Less frequent) 1384
Dilaudid Tablets and Liquid (Less frequent) 1386
Dipentum Capsules (Rare) 2084
Diprivan Injectable Emulsion (Less than 1%) 2939
Diucardin Tablets 2824
Diupres Tablets 1691
Diuril Oral Suspension 1694
Diuril Sodium Intravenous 1693
Diuril Tablets 1694
Dolobid Tablets (Less than 1 in 100) 1695
Doxil (Less than 1%) 2613
Duragesic Transdermal System (1% or greater) 1336
Dyazide Capsules 2653
Dynabac (0.1% to 1%) 668
DynaCirc Capsules (0.5% to 1%) .. 2381
DynaCirc CR Tablets (0.5% to 1.0%) 2383
▲ Effexor (3%) 2825
▲ Eminase (Less than 10%) 2215
EMLA Cream 536
Enduron Tablets 424
Engerix-B Unit-Dose Vials 2656
▲ Epivir (13%) 1200
▲ Epogen for Injection (11%) 489
Ergamisol Tablets (2% to 3%) 1340
Esidrix Tablets 839
Esimil Tablets 840
Estratest 2718
▲ Ethmozine Tablets (2% to 5%) 2217
Famvir Tablets (1.3% to 2.65%) 2660
▲ Felbatol (3.5%) 2774
Feldene Capsules (Less than 1%) .. 2008
Flagyl I.V. 2373
Flexeril Tablets (Less than 1%) 1701
▲ Flolan for Injection (1% to 12%) 1085
Floxin I.V. (Less than 1%) 1580
Floxin Tablets (200 mg, 300 mg, 400 mg) (Less than 1%) 1577
▲ Fludara for Injection (4% to 12%) 658
Fortaz (Less than 1%) 1092
▲ Foscavir Injection (5% or greater) .. 541
Ganite 2711
Gastrocrom Capsules (Infrequent) .. 1611
Gastrocrom Oral Concentrate (Less common) 1611
Gemzar for Injection (Less than 1%) 1482
GlaucTabs .... ⊙ 209
Glucotrol XL Extended Release Tablets (Less than 3%) 2012
Halcion Tablets (Rare) 2093
Halotestin Tablets 2095
Havrix (Rare) 2663
Helidac Therapy (1.5%) 2135
Hismanal Tablets (Less frequent) 1341
▲ Hycamtin for Injection (9%) 2665
Hydralazine Hydrochloride Injection USP (Less frequent) 2712
HydroDIURIL Tablets 1716
Hydropres Tablets 1718
▲ Hylorel Tablets (25.1%) 1613
Hytrin Capsules (0.8% to 2.9%) 434
Hyzaar Tablets 1720
IBU Tablets (Less than 1%) 1389
Imdur (Less than or equal to 5%) .. 1362
▲ Imitrex Injection (5%) 1095
Imitrex Tablets (Frequent) 1099
Inderide Tablets 2838
Inderide LA Long Acting Capsules .. 2840
Indocin (Less than 1%) 1723
INFeD (Iron Dextran Injection, USP) 2478
▲ Intron A for Injection (1% to 21%) 2506
Inversine Tablets 1729
Invirase Capsules (1.0%) 2291
IOPIDINE Sterile Ophthalmic Solution .... ⊙ 218
Iopidine 0.5% (Less than 1%) .... ⊙ 219
Ismelin Tablets 845
Isoptin Oral Tablets (Less than 1%) 1393
Isoptin SR Tablets (1% or less) 1395
Kadian Capsules (Less than 3%) 2948
Kerlone Tablets (1.9%) 2588
Lamictal Tablets (More than 1%) .. 1105
Lasix Injection, Oral Solution and Tablets 1267
Lescol Capsules 2395
▲ Leukine (11%) 1317
▲ Lioresal Intrathecal (0.7% to 6.7%) 1634
Lioresal Tablets 847
Lodine Capsules and Tablets (Less than 1%) 2849
▲ Lopid Tablets (More common) 1974
Lopressor HCT Tablets 850
Lotensin Tablets 852
Lotensin HCT Tablets (0.3% to 1.0%) 855
Lotrisone Cream (5 of 270 patients) 2515
Loxitane 1426
Lupron Depot 3.75 mg (Less than 5%) 2739
Lupron Depot 7.5 mg (Less than 5%) 2741
Lupron Depot - 3 Month 22.5 mg (Less than 5%) 2743
Lupron Injection (Less than 5%) 2736
LUVOX Tablets 2723
M-M-R II 1730
M-R-VAX II 1732
MS Contin Tablets (Less frequent) 2149
MSIR (Infrequent) 2152
Marcaine Spinal 2449
Matulane Capsules 2300
Mavik Tablets (0.3% to 1.0%) 1407
Maxaquin Tablets (Less than 1%) .. 2593
Megace Oral Suspension (1% to 3%) 708
Merrem I.V. (0.1% to 1.0%) 2952
Meruvax II 1740
Mevacor Tablets (0.5% to 1.0%) .. 1742
▲ Mexitil Capsules (2.4% to 3.8%) .. 684
Miacalcin Nasal Spray (1% to 3%) 2403
Midamor Tablets (Less than or equal to 1%) 1746
Miltown Tablets 2780
Minipress Capsules (Less than 1%) 2015
Minizide Capsules (Rare) 2016
Moduretic Tablets (Less than or equal to 1%) 1748
Monoket Tablets (Fewer than 1%) 2550
Monopril Tablets (0.2% to 1.0%) .. 762
Motrin Ibuprofen Suspension, Oral Drops, Chewable Tablets, Caplets (Less than 1%) 1563
Mycobutin Capsules (More than one patient) 2101
Mykrox Tablets 1617
Naprelan Tablets (Less than 3%) .. 2861
Nardil (Less common) 1977
▲ Navelbine Injection (Among most frequent) 1212
NegGram (Rare) 2453
Neoral (1% to 2%) 2405
Neptazane Tablets .... ⊙ 320
Netromycin Injection 100 mg/ml (Fewer than 1 of 1000 patients) 2516
Neurontin Capsules (Frequent) 1978
Nicotrol NS Nicotine Nasal Spray (Common) 1565
▲ Nipent for Injection (3% to 10%) .. 2733
Nizoral Tablets (Rare) 1345
▲ Normodyne Injection (Up to 5%) 2519
Normodyne Tablets (Up to 5%) 2522
Noroxin Tablets 1758
Noroxin Tablets 2222
Norvasc Tablets (More than 0.1% to 1%) 2020
Norvir (2.0% to 2.6%) 447

Paresthesia | Side Effects Index | 1424

Paresthesia

- ▲ Oncaspar (Greater than 1% but less than 5%) ... 2194
- Oncovin Solution Vials & Hyporets ... 1521
- Oramorph SR (Morphine Sulfate Sustained Release Tablets) (Less frequent) ... 2359
- Oretic Tablets ... 450
- Ornade Spansule Capsules ... 2678
- Orudis Capsules (Less than 1%) ... 2874
- Oruvail Capsules (Less than 1%) ... 2874
- OxyContin Tablets (Less than 1%) ... 2163
- Pandel Cream, 0.1% (1 of 226 patients) ... 2475
- Paraplatin for Injection (1%) ... 713
- Parlodel (Less than 1%) ... 2411
- Parnate Tablets ... 2679
- ▲ Paxil Tablets (1.0% to 5.9%) ... 2681
- Pediazole Suspension ... 2340
- Penetrex Tablets (0.1% to 1%) ... 2196
- Pentasa (Less than 1%) ... 1275
- Pentaspan Injection ... 954
- Pepcid Injection (Infrequent) ... 1765
- Pepcid (Infrequent) ... 1763
- Periactin ... 1767
- Permax Tablets (1.6%) ... 571
- Phenurone Tablets (Less than 1%) ... 455
- Platinol for Injection ... 717
- Platinol-AQ Injection ... 719
- Plendil Extended-Release Tablets (1.2% to 1.6%) ... 514
- PMB 200 and PMB 400 ... 2890
- Pneumovax 23 (Rare) ... 1768
- Pnu-Imune 23 ... 1437
- Podocon-25 ... 1949
- Pravachol Tablets ... 770
- Prevacid Delayed-Release Capsules (Less than 1%) ... 2746
- Prilosec Delayed-Release Capsules (Less than 1%) ... 516
- Primaxin I.M. ... 1770
- Primaxin I.V. (Less than 0.2%) ... 1772
- Prinivil Tablets (0.3% to 1.0%) ... 1776
- Prinzide Tablets (1.5%) ... 1780
- Procardia XL Extended Release Tablets (Less than 3%) ... 2026
- ▲ Procrit for Injection (11%) ... 1896
- Proglycem ... 575
- ▲ Prograf (15% to 40%) ... 1028
- ProSom Tablets (Infrequent) ... 457
- Prostin E2 Suppository ... 2109
- Prozac Pulvules & Liquid, Oral Solution (1.7%) ... 935
- Questran ... 774
- Redux Capsules (Frequent) ... 2911
- Relafen Tablets (1%) ... 2688
- Remeron Tablets (Frequent) ... 1878
- ▲ Retrovir Capsules (6%) ... 1216
- ▲ Retrovir I.V. Infusion (6%) ... 1221
- ▲ Retrovir Syrup (6%) ... 1216
- Risperdal Tablets (Infrequent) ... 1348
- ▲ Roferon-A Injection (8% to 12%) .. 2308
- Romazicon (1% to 3%) ... 2311
- Rythmol Tablets—150mg, 225mg, 300mg (Less than 1%) ... 1399
- Salagen Tablets (Less than 1%) ... 1546
- Sandimmune (1 to 3%) ... 2416
- Sanorex Tablets ... 2423
- Sansert Tablets ... 2424
- Seldane Tablets ... 1284
- Seldane-D Extended-Release Tablets ... 1286
- Sensorcaine ... 554
- Ser-Ap-Es Tablets ... 867
- Seromycin Capsules ... 975
- ▲ Serzone Tablets (4%) ... 776
- Sinemet CR Tablets (0.8%) ... 961
- Sinequan (Infrequent) ... 2028
- Stadol (1% or greater) ... 779
- Sular Tablets (Less than or equal to 1%) ... 2961
- Supprelin Injection (2% to 3%) ... 2230
- Synarel Nasal Solution for Endometriosis (Less than 1%) ... 2605
- Talacen Caplets (Rare) ... 2464
- Talwin Injection (Infrequent) ... 2465
- Talwin Compound ... 2466
- Talwin Injection ... 2465
- Talwin Nx Tablets ... 2467
- Tambocor Tablets (1% to less than 3%) ... 1555
- Tapazole Tablets ... 1361
- Tavist Syrup ... 2426
- Tavist Tablets ... 2427
- ▲ Taxotere for Injection Concentrate (7% of 134 patients) ... 2204
- Tazicef for Injection (Less than 1%) ... 2697
- Tazidime Vials, Faspak & ADD-Vantage (Less than 1%) ... 1531
- ▲ Tegison Capsules (1-10%) ... 2314
- Tegretol/Tegretol-XR ... 870
- Tenex Tablets (3% or less) ... 2249
- Tenoretic Tablets ... 2963
- Teslac Tablets ... 727
- Testoderm Testosterone Transdermal System ... 486
- Testred Capsules, 10 mg. ... 1308
- Thalitone ... 1293
- Tiazac Capsules (Less than 1% to 2%) ... 1019
- Timolide Tablets ... 1791
- Timoptic in Ocudose (Less frequent) ... 1796
- Timoptic Sterile Ophthalmic Solution (Less frequent) ... 1794
- Timoptic-XE ... 1798
- ▲ Tonocard Tablets (3.5% to 9.2%) ... 519
- Toradol (1% or less) ... 2319
- Tornalate Solution for Inhalation, 0.2% (1.5%) ... 976
- ▲ Trandate Tablets (Up to 5%) ... 1158
- Trinalin Repetabs Tablets ... 1373
- Trusopt Sterile Ophthalmic Solution ... 1803
- Tussend ... 1830
- Ultram Tablets (50 mg) (Less than 1%) ... 1594
- Ultravate Ointment 0.05% (Less frequent) ... 2798
- Vascor Tablets (200 and 300 mg) (2.46%) ... 1597
- Vaseretic Tablets (0.5% to 2.0%) ... 1810
- Vasotec I.V. ... 1814
- Vasotec Tablets (0.5% to 1.0%) ... 1816
- Velban Vials ... 1537
- Verelan Capsules (1% or less) ... 1455
- Versed Injection (Less than 1%) ... 2324
- ▲ Vesanoid Capsules (17%) ... 2327
- ▲ Visken Tablets (3%) ... 2428
- Vistide Injection ... 1057
- Cataflam/Voltaren/Voltaren-XR (Less than 1%) ... 833
- Wellbutrin Tablets ... 1177
- Xanax Tablets (2.4%) ... 2115
- Zaroxolyn Tablets ... 1625
- Zebeta Tablets ... 1457
- Zestoretic Tablets (1.5%) ... 2968
- Zestril Tablets (0.3% to 1.0%) ... 2972
- Ziac ... 1459
- Zocor Tablets ... 1821
- Zofran Injection (2%) ... 1227
- Zoladex (1% or greater) ... 2976
- Zoladex 3-month (1% to 5%) ... 2978
- Zoloft Tablets (2.0%) ... 2051
- ▲ Zonalon Cream (Approximately 1% to 10%) ... 1042
- Zovirax (0.8% to 1.2%) ... 1187
- Zyloprim Tablets (Less than 1%) ... 1194
- Zyrtec Tablets (Less than 2%) ... 2053

Paresthesia, chest

- Esimil Tablets ... 840
- Ismelin Tablets ... 845

Paresthesia, circumoral

- Cerebyx Injection (Infrequent) ... 1956
- Effexor (Infrequent) ... 2825
- ▲ Norvir (2.6% to 5.9%) ... 447
- Paxil Tablets (Rare) ... 2681
- ProSom Tablets (Rare) ... 457
- Prozac Pulvules & Liquid, Oral Solution (Rare) ... 935
- Rilutek Tablets (1.3% to 3.3%) ... 2198

Paresthesia, extremities

- Asendin Tablets (Less than 1%) ... 1419
- Bellergal-S Tablets (Rare) ... 2375
- Diamox ... ⊚ 317
- Elavil ... 2945
- Etrafon ... 2495
- Flagyl 375 Capsules ... 2587
- Flagyl I.V. ... 2373
- Fulvicin P/G Tablets (Rare) ... 2499
- Fulvicin P/G 165 & 330 Tablets (Rare) ... 2500
- Helidac Therapy ... 2135
- Limbitrol ... 2333
- Motofen Tablets ... 789
- Norpramin Tablets ... 1273
- Pamelor ... 2409
- Protostat Tablets ... 1939
- Rifater ... 1280
- Rum-K Syrup ... 1004
- Surmontil Capsules ... 2917
- Tofranil Ampuls ... 873
- Tofranil Tablets ... 875
- Tofranil-PM Capsules ... 876
- Triavil Tablets ... 1800
- Velban Vials ... 1537
- Vivactil Tablets ... 1820

Paresthesia, facial

- DTIC-Dome ... 593
- ▲ Nicotrol NS Nicotine Nasal Spray (More common) ... 1565

Paresthesia, feet

- Grifulvin V (griseofulvin tablets) Microsize (griseofulvin oral suspension) Microsize (Rare) ... 1944
- Gris-PEG Tablets, 125 mg & 250 mg (Rare) ... 476
- Lupron Depot 7.5 mg ... 2741
- Nydrazid Injection ... 509
- Rifamate Capsules ... 1278

Paresthesia, hands

- Grifulvin V (griseofulvin tablets) Microsize (griseofulvin oral suspension) Microsize (Rare) ... 1944
- Gris-PEG Tablets, 125 mg & 250 mg (Rare) ... 476
- Inderal ... 2834
- Inderal LA Long Acting Capsules ... 2836
- Inderide Tablets ... 2838
- Inderide LA Long Acting Capsules ... 2840
- Nydrazid Injection ... 509
- Oncaspar ... 2194
- Rifamate Capsules ... 1278

Paresthesia, peripheral

- Norvir (5% to 6%) ... 447

Parkinsonism

- Aldoclor Tablets ... 1638
- Aldomet Ester HCl Injection ... 1642
- Aldomet Oral ... 1640
- Aldoril Tablets ... 1644
- Ancobon Capsules ... 2254
- Clozaril Tablets (Less than 1%) ... 2377
- Cognex Capsules (Infrequent) ... 1961
- Compazine ... 2644
- Demser Capsules ... 1690
- Diupres Tablets ... 1691
- Etrafon ... 2495
- Hydropres Tablets ... 1718
- Indocin (Less than 1%) ... 1723
- Levoprome ... 1321
- Orap Tablets ... 1037
- Risperdal Tablets (0.6% to 4.1%) ... 1348
- Serentil ... 689
- Stelazine ... 2692
- Tigan ... 2231
- Trilafon ... 2532

Parkinsonism, aggravation of

- Ana-Kit Anaphylaxis Emergency Treatment Kit ... 611
- Cognex Capsules (Rare) ... 1961
- Reglan ... 2243
- Risperdal Tablets ... 1348

Parkinson-like symptoms

- Actimmune (Rare) ... 1043
- Compazine ... 2644
- Cytovene-IV (One report) ... 2270
- Elspar (Rare) ... 1700
- Haldol Decanoate ... 1587
- Haldol Injection, Tablets and Concentrate ... 1585
- Moban Tablets and Concentrate ... 1036
- Navane Capsules and Concentrate ... 2018
- Navane Intramuscular ... 2019
- Oncaspar ... 2194
- Orap Tablets (Frequent) ... 1037
- Prolixin ... 510
- Reglan ... 2243
- Ser-Ap-Es Tablets (Rare) ... 867
- Triavil Tablets ... 1800

Paroniria

- Cardura Tablets (Less than 0.5% of 3960 patients) ... 1993
- Claritin Tablets (2% or fewer patients) ... 2485
- Claritin-D Tablets (Less frequent) ... 2487
- Imdur (Less than or equal to 5%) .. 1362
- Intron A for Injection (Less than 5%) ... 2506
- Maxaquin Tablets (Less than 1%) .. 2593
- Procardia XL Extended Release Tablets (1% or less) ... 2026
- Zyrtec Tablets (Less than 2%) ... 2053

Paronychia

- Accutane Capsules (Less than 1%) ... 2252
- ▲ Tegison Capsules (1-10%) ... 2314

Parosmia

- Ambien Tablets (Rare) ... 2559
- Anafranil Capsules (Infrequent) ... 819

Parotid gland, enlargement

- Betaseron for SC Injection ... 653
- Cardura Tablets (Less than 0.5% of 3960 patients) ... 1993
- Cerebyx Injection (Infrequent) ... 1956
- Effexor (Infrequent) ... 2825
- Flumadine Tablets & Syrup (Less than 0.3%) ... 1013
- Hivid Tablets (Less than 1%) ... 2287
- Intron A for Injection (Less than 5%) ... 2506
- Iopidine 0.5% (0.2%) ... ⊚ 219
- Lamictal Tablets (Rare) ... 1105
- LUVOX Tablets (Infrequent) ... 2723
- Miacalcin Nasal Spray (Less than 1%) ... 2403
- Norvasc Tablets (Less than or equal to 0.1%) ... 2020
- Norvir (Less than 2%) ... 447
- Paxil Tablets (Rare) ... 2681
- Redux Capsules (Rare) ... 2911
- Remeron Tablets (Rare) ... 1878
- Zyrtec Tablets (Less than 2%) ... 2053

Parotid gland, enlargement

- Asendin Tablets (Very rare) ... 1419
- Depakene ... 416
- Depakote Tablets ... 418
- Diprivan Injectable Emulsion (Less than 1%) ... 2939
- Elavil ... 2945
- Etrafon (Rare) ... 2495
- Hyperstat I.V. Injection ... 2504
- Intal Inhaler (Infrequent) ... 2185
- Intal Nebulizer Solution ... 2186
- Limbitrol ... 2333
- Mellaril (Rare) ... 2398
- Norisodrine with Calcium Iodide Syrup ... 446
- Norpramin Tablets ... 1273
- Pamelor ... 2409
- Surmontil Capsules ... 2917
- Tofranil Ampuls ... 873
- Tofranil Tablets ... 875
- Tofranil-PM Capsules ... 876
- Trental Tablets (Less than 1%) ... 1291
- Videx Tablets, Powder for Oral Solution, & Pediatric Powder for Oral Solution (Less than 1%) ... 2980

Parotid tenderness

- Esimil Tablets ... 840
- Ismelin Tablets ... 845
- Trilafon (Rare) ... 2532

Parotitis

- Artane (Rare) ... 1418
- Biavax II ... 1653
- Catapres Tablets (Rare) ... 679
- Combipres Tablets (Rare) ... 682
- Kemadrin Tablets ... 1105
- M-M-R II ... 1730
- Mumpsvax (Very low) ... 1751
- Peridex ... 2127
- Periogard Oral Rinse ... 892
- Vivactil Tablets ... 1820

"Pasty mass," presence of, in the transverse colon

- Questran ... 774

Patent ductus arteriosus

- Accupril Tablets ... 1950
- Altace Capsules ... 1238
- Capoten Tablets ... 740
- Capozide Tablets ... 744
- Cozaar Tablets ... 1668
- ▲ Exosurf Neonatal for Intratracheal Suspension (45% to 59%) ... 1081
- Hyzaar Tablets ... 1720
- Lotensin Tablets ... 852
- Lotensin HCT Tablets ... 855
- Lotrel Capsules ... 858
- Monopril Tablets ... 762
- Prinivil Tablets ... 1776
- Prinzide Tablets ... 1780
- ▲ Survanta Beractant Intratracheal Suspension (46.9%) ... 2346
- Univasc Tablets ... 2553
- Vaseretic Tablets ... 1810
- Vasotec I.V. ... 1814
- Vasotec Tablets ... 1816
- Zestoretic Tablets ... 2968
- Zestril Tablets ... 2972

Pavor nocturnus

- Zarontin Capsules ... 1986
- Zarontin Syrup ... 1986

Peeling

(see under Necrolysis, epidermal)

Pelger-Huet anomaly

- Risperdal Tablets (Rare) ... 1348

(℞ Described in PDR For Nonprescription Drugs)   Incidence data in parenthesis; ▲ 3% or more   (⊚ Described in PDR For Ophthalmology)

Peliosis hepatis
Androderm Testosterone Transdermal System (Rare) 2634
Android Capsules, 10 mg (Rare) 1297
Danocrine Capsules 2437
Estratest 2718
Halotestin Tablets 2095
Oxandrin 783
Testoderm Testosterone Transdermal System (Rare) 486
Testred Capsules, 10 mg (Rare)...... 1308
Winstrol Tablets 2468

Pellagra
Nydrazid Injection 509
Rifamate Capsules 1278
Rifater.......... 1280
Trecator-SC Tablets 2919

Pelvic inflammatory disease
Avonex 662
BuSpar Tablets (Rare).......... 738
Massengill.......... 2627
Massengill Medicated Disposable Douche.......... 2628
Massengill Powder.......... 2627
ParaGard T 380A Intrauterine Copper Contraceptive 1936

Pelvic pressure
Flagyl 375 Capsules.......... 2587
Helidac Therapy 2135
MetroGel-Vaginal (Equal to or less than 2%).......... 917
Nolvadex Tablets 2957
Protostat Tablets 1939
▲ Zoladex (18%).......... 2976

Pemphigoid-like lesion
Capoten Tablets.......... 740
Capozide Tablets 744
Timoptic in Ocudose 1796
Timoptic Sterile Ophthalmic Solution 1794
Timoptic-XE 1798

Pemphigus
Accupril Tablets (0.5% to 1.0%) .. 1950
Cuprimine Capsules 1673
Depen Titratable Tablets 2770
Lotensin Tablets (Rare).......... 852
Lotensin HCT Tablets (Rare) 855
Lotrel Capsules (Rare).......... 858
Mavik Tablets (0.3% to 1.0%)....... 1407
Prinivil Tablets (0.3% to 1.0%)...... 1776
Prinzide Tablets 1780
Rifadin (Occasional).......... 1276
Rifamate Capsules (Occasional) 1278
Rifater (Occasional).......... 1280
Rimactane Capsules.......... 865
Univasc Tablets (Less than 1%)...... 2553
Vaseretic Tablets 1810
Vasotec I.V.......... 1814
Vasotec Tablets (0.5% to 1.0%).... 1816
Zestril Tablets (0.3% to 1.0%) 2972

Pemphigus, bullous
Capoten Tablets 740
Capozide Tablets 744
Efudex (Infrequent).......... 2280
Monopril Tablets 762

Penile angulation
Caverject Injection.......... 2064

Penile discharge, unspecified
Alferon N Injection (1%) 2142
▲ Caverject Injection (3%) 2064
ProSom Tablets (Rare) 457

Penile disorder, unspecified
Avonex 662
Lupron Depot - 3 Month 22.5 mg (Less than 5%).......... 2743
Norvir (Less than 2%) 447
Videx Tablets, Powder for Oral Solution, & Pediatric Powder for Oral Solution (Less than 1%)........ 2980

Penile erection, decrease
▲ Zoladex (18%) 2976
▲ Zoladex 3-month (One of the two most common) 2978

Penile erection, prolonged or inappropriate
Androderm Testosterone Transdermal System 2634
▲ Android Capsules, 10 mg (Among most common) 1297
▲ Caverject Injection (4%) 2064
Desyrel and Desyrel Dividose 504
Oxandrin 783
Testoderm Testosterone Transdermal System 486

Penile erections, increase (see under Priapism)

Penile fibrosis
▲ Caverject Injection (3% to 7.8%) .. 2064

Penile inflammation
Foscavir Injection (Less than 1%) .. 541

Penis, decreased sensation
Eldepryl Capsules 2729

Penis, enlargement
Caverject Injection (2%) 2064
Intron A for Injection (Less than or equal to 5%).......... 2506
Lupron Injection.......... 2736
Oxandrin 783
Winstrol Tablets.......... 2468

Penis, fibrotic plaques (see under Peyronie's disease)

Perforation, cervix (partial)
ParaGard T 380A Intrauterine Copper Contraceptive 1936

Perforation, cervix (total)
ParaGard T 380A Intrauterine Copper Contraceptive 1936

Perforation, uterine wall
ParaGard T 380A Intrauterine Copper Contraceptive 1936

Perforation, uterine wall (partial)
ParaGard T 380A Intrauterine Copper Contraceptive 1936

Perforation, uterine wall (total)
ParaGard T 380A Intrauterine Copper Contraceptive 1936

Perianal sensation, loss of
Carbocaine Injection.......... 2432
Marcaine 2446
Marcaine Spinal 2449
Nescaine/Nescaine MPF.......... 549
Sensorcaine 554
Xylocaine Injections 562

Periarteritis
Nasalcrom Nasal Solution (Rare) 2192
Tapazole Tablets 1361

Periarteritis nodosum
Bactrim DS Tablets.......... 2257
Bactrim I.V. Infusion.......... 2255
Bactrim 2257
Dilantin Infatabs.......... 1967
Dilantin Kapseals 1965
Dilantin-125 Suspension 1969
Fansidar Tablets.......... 2281
Gantanol Tablets 2285
Gantrisin 2286
Pediazole Suspension 2340
Septra 1146
Septra I.V. Infusion 1142
Septra I.V. Infusion ADD-Vantage Vials.......... 1144
Septra 1146

Pericardial effusion
Activase 1045
Betaseron for SC Injection.......... 653
Clomid 1262
Clozaril Tablets.......... 2377
Doxil (1% to 5%) 2613
Fludara for Injection (One patient).. 658
▲ Leukine (25%).......... 1317
Neurontin Capsules (Rare) 1978
Nipent for Injection (Less than 3%).......... 2733
Proleukin for Injection (1%) 812
ReoPro Vials (0.4%) 1526
Taxotere for Injection Concentrate (Less frequent).......... 2204
Vesanoid Capsules 2327

Pericardial tamponade
Azulfidine (Rare).......... 2059

Pericarditis
Achromycin V Capsules 1417
Activase.......... 1045
Aldoclor Tablets 1638
Aldomet Ester HCl Injection 1642
Aldomet Oral 1640
Aldoril Tablets.......... 1644
Asacol Delayed-Release Tablets (Rare) 2129
Avonex 662
Azulfidine (Rare) 2059
Cardene Capsules (Less than 0.4%).......... 2261
Cerubidine for Injection (Rare) 634
Clozaril Tablets.......... 2377
Cytosar-U Sterile Powder (Less frequent) 2077
Cytovene-IV (Two or more reports) 2270
Cytoxan 700
Declomycin Tablets.......... 1421
Dipentum Capsules (Rare).......... 2084
Doryx Capsules.......... 1970
DYNACIN Capsules.......... 1627
Helidac Therapy 2135
Inocor Lactate Injection (1 case) 2439
Intal Inhaler (Rare) 2185
Intal Nebulizer Solution (Rare)......... 2186
LUVOX Tablets (Rare).......... 2723
Minocin Intravenous.......... 1428
Minocin Oral Suspension 1431
Minocin Pellet-Filled Capsules 1429
Monodox Capsules 1858
Nasalcrom Nasal Solution (Rare) 2192
Neurontin Capsules (Rare) 1978
PASER Granules.......... 1333
Pentasa (Infrequent to less than 1%).......... 1275
Permax Tablets (Rare) 571
Procanbid Extended-Release Tablets (Fairly common).......... 1983
Proleukin for Injection (Less than 1%).......... 812
Rilutek Tablets (Infrequent) 2198
Rowasa (Rare).......... 2727
Terramycin Intramuscular Solution 2034
Tonocard Tablets (Less than 1%).. 519
▲ Trasylol (5%) 607
▲ Vesanoid Capsules (3%) 2327
Vibramycin 2038
Vibramycin Hyclate Intravenous 2040
Vibramycin 2038
Zyloprim Tablets (Less than 1%).... 1194

Perinatal disorder, unspecified
Diprivan Injectable Emulsion (Less than 1%).......... 2939

Periodontitis
Avonex 662

Peripheral nerve symptoms
MSTA Mumps Skin Test Antigen 2988
Xylocaine Injections (Less than 1%).......... 562

Peripheral vascular disorder, unspecified
Androderm Testosterone Transdermal System (Less than 1%).......... 2634
Avonex 662
Betapace Tablets (1% to 3%).......... 637
▲ Betaseron for SC Injection (5%)...... 653
Cardene Capsules (Rare).......... 2261
Cardene SR Capsules (Rare) 2264
Caverject Injection (Less than 1%) 2064
▲ CellCept Capsules (More than or equal to 3%).......... 2265
Effexor (Infrequent) 2825
▲ Lopid Tablets (More common).......... 1974
Lotensin HCT Tablets (0.3% or more) 855
Neurontin Capsules (Infrequent)...... 1978
Norvir (Less than 2%) 447
Orudis Capsules (Less than 1%) 2874
Oruvail Capsules (Less than 1%)..... 2874
Paxil Tablets (Infrequent).......... 2681
Redux Capsules (Infrequent) 2911
Rilutek Tablets (Infrequent) 2198
Videx Tablets, Powder for Oral Solution, & Pediatric Powder for Oral Solution (Less than 1%)........ 2980
Zerit Capsules (Fewer than 1%)...... 731
Zoladex (Greater than 1% but less than 5%).......... 2976
Zoladex 3-month 2978

Peristalsis, increase
Mestinon Injectable.......... 1300
Mestinon 1300
Prostigmin Injectable 1305
Prostigmin Tablets 1306
Tensilon Injectable 1307

Peritonitis
Betaseron for SC Injection.......... 653
Cytosar-U Sterile Powder.......... 2077
Neupogen for Injection (2%) 495
ParaGard T 380A Intrauterine Copper Contraceptive 1936
Paxil Tablets (Rare) 2681
▲ Prograf (Greater than 3%) 1028
Redux Capsules 2911
Rilutek Tablets (Infrequent) 2198
▲ Taxol Injection (30%) 723

Peritonitis, chemical
Vancocin HCl, Vials & ADD-Vantage 1534

Perivasculitis
Etopophos for Injection.......... 701
Etoposide Injection 539
VePesid Capsules and Injection........ 727

Perleche
Neurontin Capsules (Rare) 1978

Personality changes
Ambien Tablets (Rare) 2559
Cardizem CD Capsules (Less than 1%).......... 1251
Cardizem SR Capsules (Less than 1%).......... 1255
Cardizem Injectable 1253
Cardizem Tablets (Less than 1%).. 1257
Celestone Soluspan Suspension 2484
Cerebyx Injection (Infrequent) 1956
CORTENEMA.......... 2713
Cortone Acetate Sterile Suspension 1663
Cortone Acetate Tablets.......... 1664
Cytosar-U Sterile Powder (With experimental doses).......... 2077
Decadron Elixir 1676
Decadron Phosphate with Xylocaine Injection, Sterile.......... 1683
Decadron Tablets.......... 1678
Decadron-LA Sterile Suspension...... 1687
Dexacort Phosphate in Respihaler .. 1606
Dexacort Phosphate in Turbinaire .. 1607
Eldepryl Capsules 2729
Florinef Acetate Tablets 506
Foscavir Injection (Less than 1%) .. 541
Hydeltrasol Injection, Sterile.......... 1708
Hydeltra-T.B.A. Sterile Suspension 1710
Hydrocortone Acetate Sterile Suspension.......... 1712
Hydrocortone Phosphate Injection, Sterile 1713
Hydrocortone Tablets 1715
Imitrex Tablets (Rare) 1099
Intron A for Injection (Less than 5%).......... 2506
Lamictal Tablets (Infrequent).......... 1105
Levo-Dromoran.......... 2297
Lioresal Intrathecal (1% or more) .. 1634
▲ Lupron Depot 3.75 mg (Among most frequent) 2739
Lupron Depot-PED 7.5 mg, 11.25 mg and 15 mg (Less than 2%)..... 2744
Lupron Injection Pediatric (Less than 2%).......... 2737
Nalfon 200 Pulvules & Nalfon Tablets (Less than 1%) 933
Neurontin Capsules (Rare) 1978
Norvir (Less than 2%) 447
Orudis Capsules (Rare).......... 2874
Oruvail Capsules (Rare) 2874
Permax Tablets (2.1%) 571
Prelone Syrup 1834
Redux Capsules 2911
Rilutek Tablets (Infrequent) 2198
Tiazac Capsules (Less than 1%) 1019

Perspiration (see under Diaphoresis)

Petechiae
Asendin Tablets (Very rare) 1419
Avonex 662
Azactam for Injection (Less than 1%).......... 736
Betaseron for SC Injection.......... 653
Cardizem CD Capsules (Less than 1%).......... 1251
Cardizem SR Capsules (Less than 1%).......... 1255
Cardizem Injectable 1253
Cardizem Tablets (Less than 1%).. 1257
Celestone Soluspan Suspension (No incidence in labeling).......... 2484
Cerebyx Injection (Infrequent) 1956
Clozaril Tablets (Less than 1%) 2377
▲ Cognex Capsules (7%).......... 1961

(▭ Described in PDR For Nonprescription Drugs) Incidence data in parenthesis; ▲ 3% or more (◉ Described in PDR For Ophthalmology)

Petechiae Side Effects Index 1426

Cortone Acetate Sterile Suspension 1663
Cortone Acetate Tablets 1664
Danocrine Capsules 2437
Decadron Elixir 1676
Decadron Phosphate Injection 1680
Decadron Phosphate with Xylocaine Injection, Sterile 1683
Decadron-LA Sterile Suspension 1687
Depakene 416
Depakote Tablets 418
Doxil (Less than 1%) 2613
Engerix-B Unit-Dose Vials (Less than 1%) 2656
Feldene Capsules (Less than 1%) 2008
Floxin I.V. 1580
Floxin Tablets (200 mg, 300 mg, 400 mg) 1577
▲ Gemzar for Injection (16%) 1482
Hydeltrasol Injection, Sterile 1708
Hydeltra-T.B.A. Sterile Suspension 1710
Hydrocortone Acetate Sterile Suspension 1712
Hydrocortone Phosphate Injection, Sterile 1713
Hydrocortone Tablets 1715
Indocin Capsules (Less than 1%) 1723
Indocin I.V. (Less than 1%) 1727
Indocin (Less than 1%) 1723
Lac-Hydrin 12% Lotion (Less frequent) 2796
Lamictal Tablets (Rare to infrequent) 1105
▲ Leukine (6%) 1317
▲ Leustatin (8%) 1889
Lioresal Intrathecal (1% or more) 1634
Ludiomil Tablets (Rare) 861
Matulane Capsules 2300
Miltown Tablets 2780
Mustargen 1752
Nipent for Injection (Less than 3%) 2733
Norpramin Tablets 1273
▲ Novantrone for Injection (7 to 11%) 1327
Oncaspar (Less than 1%) 2194
Pamelor (No incidence in labeling) 2409
Parafon Forte DSC Caplets (Rare) 1590
Permax Tablets (Infrequent) 571
PMB 200 and PMB 400 2890
▲ Proleukin for Injection (4%) 812
Prozac Pulvules & Liquid, Oral Solution (Rare) 935
Recombivax HB 1787
Remeron Tablets (Rare) 1878
ReoPro Vials (0.3%) 1526
Rilutek Tablets (Rare) 2198
Roferon-A Injection (Rare) 2308
Sandostatin Injection (Less than 1%) 2421
Solganal Suspension 2530
Sular Tablets (Less than or equal to 1%) 2961
Surmontil Capsules 2917
Tiazac Capsules (Less than 1%) 1019
Tofranil Ampuls 873
Tofranil Tablets 875
Tofranil-PM Capsules 876
Urobiotic-250 Capsules 2038
▲ Videx Tablets, Powder for Oral Solution, & Pediatric Powder for Oral Solution (7%) 2980
Vivactil Tablets 1820

Petechiae and ecchymosis

CORTENEMA 2713
Dalalone D.P. Injectable 1009
Decadron Tablets 1678
Dexacort Phosphate in Respihaler 1606
Dexacort Phosphate in Turbinaire 1607
Florinef Acetate Tablets 506
Pediapred Oral Solution 1618
Prelone Syrup 1834

Petechial hemorrhage

Atretol Tablets 569
Tegretol/Tegretol-XR 870

Peyronie's disease

Avonex 662
Blocadren Tablets 1654
Cartrol Tablets 413
▲ Caverject Injection (3%) 2064
Dilantin Infatabs 1967
Dilantin Kapseals 1965
Dilantin-125 Suspension 1969
Inderal (Rare) 2834
Inderal LA Long Acting Capsules (Rare) 2836
Inderide Tablets (Rare) 2838
Inderide LA Long Acting Capsules (Rare) 2840
Kerlone Tablets (Less than 2%) 2588
Levatol Tablets 2547
Lopressor (1 of 100,000 patients) 848
Lopressor HCT Tablets (1 in 100,000) 850
Normodyne Tablets (Less common) 2522
Sansert Tablets 2424
Sectral Capsules 2914
Tenoretic Tablets 2963
Tenormin Tablets and I.V. Injection 2965
Timolide Tablets 1791
Timoptic in Ocudose 1796
Timoptic Sterile Ophthalmic Solution 1794
Timoptic-XE 1798
Toprol-XL Tablets (Fewer than 1 of 100,000 patients) 560
Trandate Tablets (Less common) 1158
Visken Tablets 2428
Zebeta Tablets 1457
Ziac (Very rare) 1459

Pharyngeal changes

Mexitil Capsules (About 1 in 1,000) 684

Pharyngeal discomfort

Cozaar Tablets (Less than 1%) 1668
Hyzaar Tablets 1720
Prinzide Tablets (0.3% to 1.0%) 1780
Zestoretic Tablets (0.3% to 1.0%) 2968

Pharyngeal secretion, increase

IOPIDINE Sterile Ophthalmic Solution ◉ 218
Prostigmin Injectable 1305
Prostigmin Tablets 1306

Pharyngitis

Accupril Tablets (0.5% to 1.0%) 1950
▲ Actigall Capsules (8.4%) 818
Adalat CC (Less than 1.0%) 582
AeroBid Inhaler System (1% to 3%) 1004
Aerobid-M Inhaler System (1% to 3%) 1004
Airet Albuterol Sulfate Inhalation Solution (Less than 1%) 1602
Albuterol Sulfate, USP Solution for Inhalation, Arm-a-Med (Less than 1%) 522
Alferon N Injection (1%) 2142
▲ Ambien Tablets (3%) 2559
▲ Anafranil Capsules (Up to 14%) 819
▲ Arimidex Tablets (6.1% to 9.3%) 2932
▲ Asacol Delayed-Release Tablets (11%) 2129
▲ Atrovent Inhalation Solution (3.7%) 675
▲ Atrovent Nasal Spray 0.03% (8.1%) 676
Atrovent Nasal Spray 0.06% (Less than 1%) 678
▲ Axid Pulvules (3.3%) 1468
Bactroban Nasal (0.5% to 4%) 2643
Cardura Tablets (Less than 0.5% of 3960 patients) 1993
Cartrol Tablets (1.1%) 413
Casodex Tablets (2% to 5%) 2934
▲ CellCept Capsules (9.5% to 11.2%) 2265
Cerebyx Injection (Infrequent) 1956
Claritin Tablets (2% or fewer patients) 2485
▲ Claritin-D Tablets (3%) 2487
Cognex Capsules (Frequent) 1961
Cosmegen Injection 1666
Cozaar Tablets (1% or greater) 1668
Crixivan Capsules (Less than 2%) 1670
▲ Depakote Tablets (At least 5%) 418
▲ Dilacor XR Extended-release Capsules (1.4% to 5.6%) 2183
Diprivan Injectable Emulsion (Less than 1%) 2939
Doxil (Less than 1%) 2613
Duragesic Transdermal System (1% or greater) 1336
Effexor 2825
Estring Vaginal Ring (1%) 2086
Ethmozine Tablets (Less than 2%) 2217
Famvir Tablets (2.6% to 2.7%) 2660
▲ Felbatol (2.6% to 9.7%) 2774
Flonase Nasal Spray (1% to 3%) 1088
▲ Flovent (9% to 25%) 1089
Floxin I.V. (1% to 3%) 1580
Floxin Tablets (200 mg, 300 mg, 400 mg) (1% to 3%) 1577
▲ Fludara for Injection (Up to 9%) 658
Foscavir Injection (Between 1% and 5%) 541
Sterile FUDR 2284
Gastrocrom Oral Concentrate (Less common) 1611
Glucotrol XL Extended Release Tablets (Less than 1%) 2012
▲ Habitrol Nicotine Transdermal System (3% to 9% of patients) 884
Havrix (Less than 1%) 2663
Hismanal Tablets (1.7%) 1341
Hivid Tablets (Less than 1%) 2287
Hytrin Capsules (At least 1%) 434
Hyzaar Tablets (1% or greater) 1720
Imdur (Less than or equal to 5%) 1362
Inderal 2834
Inderal LA Long Acting Capsules 2836
Inderide Tablets 2838
Inderide LA Long Acting Capsules 2840
▲ Intron A for Injection (1% to 31%) 2506
Invirase Capsules (Less than 2%) 2291
Iopidine 0.5% (Less than 1%) ◉ 219
Kerlone Tablets (2.0%) 2588
▲ Lamictal Tablets (9.8%) 1105
▲ Lescol Capsules (3.8%) 2395
▲ Leukine (23%) 1317
Livostin (Approximately 1% to 3%) ◉ 262
Lodine Capsules and Tablets (Less than 1%) 2849
Lotrel Capsules 858
Lupron Depot - 3 Month 22.5 mg (Less than 5%) 2743
LUVOX Tablets 2723
Megace Oral Suspension (1% to 3%) 708
Methotrexate Sodium Tablets, Injection, for Injection and LPF Injection 1322
Mexitil Capsules (Less than 1%) 684
Miacalcin Nasal Spray (Less than 1%) 2403
Monopril Tablets (0.2% to 1.0%) 762
▲ Naprelan Tablets (3% to 9%) 2861
▲ Nasacort AQ Nasal Spray (5.1%) 2191
▲ Nasarel Nasal Solution (3% to 9%) 2302
Neurontin Capsules (2.8%) 1978
Nicotrol NS Nicotine Nasal Spray (More common) 1565
▲ Nipent for Injection (8% to 10%) 2733
Norvir (0.4% to 2.6%) 447
Orudis Capsules (Less than 1%) 2874
Oruvail Capsules (Less than 1%) 2874
OxyContin Tablets (Less than 1%) 2163
Paxil Tablets (2.1%) 2681
Permax Tablets (Frequent) 571
Plendil Extended-Release Tablets (0.5% to 1.5%) 514
Prilosec Delayed-Release Capsules (1%) 516
Prinivil Tablets (0.3% to 1.0%) 1776
Prinzide Tablets 1780
▲ Prograf (Greater than 3%) 1028
Propulsid (More than 1%) 1346
ProSom Tablets (1%) 457
▲ Prostep (nicotine transdermal system) (3% to 9% of patients) 1439
Prostin E2 Suppository 2109
Proventil Inhalation Solution 0.083% (Less than 1%) 2527
Proventil Solution for Inhalation 0.5% (Less than 1%) 2525
▲ Prozac Pulvules & Liquid, Oral Solution (2.7% to 11%) 935
▲ Pulmozyme Inhalation (36% to 40%) 1054
Recombivax HB (Equal to or greater than 1%) 1787
▲ Redux Capsules (6.1%) 2911
Retrovir Capsules 1216
Retrovir I.V. Infusion 1221
Retrovir Syrup 1216
Revex (nalmefene hydrochloride injection) (Less than 1%) 1863
▲ Rhinocort Nasal Inhaler (3 to 9%) 552
Risperdal Tablets (2% to 3%) 1348
▲ Salagen Tablets (3%) 1546
Sectral Capsules (Up to 2%) 2914
▲ Semprex-D Capsules (3%) 1620
▲ Serzone Tablets (6%) 776
Solganal Suspension 2530
▲ Stadol (3% to 9%) 779
Sular Tablets (Less than 1% to 5%) 2961
▲ Supprelin Injection (3% to 10%) 2230
▲ Suprane (desflurane, USP) (3% to 10%) 1865
Tegison Capsules (Less than 1%) 2314
▲ Tiazac Capsules (3%) 1019
▲ Tilade Inhaler (5.7%) 2207
Univasc Tablets (1.8%) 2553
▲ Vancenase AQ Double Strength Nasal Spray 0.084% (11% to 12%) 2536
Vaqta (Up to 2.7%) 1805
Varivax 1807
Vascor Tablets (200 and 300 mg) (0.5 to 2.0%) 1597
Velban Vials 1537
Ventolin Inhalation Solution (Less than 1%) 1171
Ventolin Nebules Inhalation Solution (Less than 1%) 1172
Vexol 1% Ophthalmic Suspension (Less than 2%) ◉ 227
▲ Videx Tablets, Powder for Oral Solution, & Pediatric Powder for Oral Solution (Less than 1% to 14%) 2980
Vistide Injection 1057
Zebeta Tablets (2.2%) 1457
Zestoretic Tablets 2968
Zestril Tablets (0.3% to 1.0%) 2972
Ziac 1459
▲ Zoladex (5%) 2976
Zoloft Tablets (1.2%) 2051
Zosyn (1.0% or less) 1463
Zyloprim Tablets (Less than 1%) 1194
Zyrtec Tablets (2%) 2053

Pharyngoxerosis

Atretol Tablets 569
Tegretol/Tegretol-XR 870

Phimosis

Caverject Injection (Less than 1%) 2064

Phlebitis

Adalat CC (Less than 1.0%) 582
Ambien Tablets (Rare) 2559
Ancef Injection (Rare) 2632
Atamet Tablets (Rare) 567
Atromid-S Capsules 2808
Azactam for Injection (1.9%) 736
Blenoxane (Infrequent) 697
Cefizox for Intramuscular or Intravenous Use (1% to 5%) 1025
Cefobid Intravenous/Intramuscular (1 in 120) 1996
Cefobid Pharmacy Bulk Package - Not for Direct Infusion (1 in 120) 1999
Cefotan (1 in 300) 2936
Ceptaz (Fewer than 2%) 1070
Clomid 1262
Clozaril Tablets (Less than 1%) 2377
Cognex Capsules (Infrequent) 1961
Cytotec (Infrequent) 2576
Cytovene (2%) 2270
Dantrium Capsules (Less frequent) 2131
Demerol 2438
Dilacor XR Extended-release Capsules (Infrequent) 2183
Diprivan Injectable Emulsion (Rare; less than 1%) 2939
Dizac (diazepam injectable emulsion) CIV (Less frequent) 1862
Dobutrex Solution Vials (Occasional) 1480
Dopram Injectable 2235
▲ Etopophos for Injection (5%) 701
Floxin I.V. (Approximately 2%) 1580
Fludara for Injection (1% to 3%) 658
Fluorescite ◉ 217
Fortaz (1 in 69 patients) 1092
Foscavir Injection (Less than 1%) 541
▲ Fungizone Intravenous (Among most common) 507
IFEX (2%) 706
INFeD (Iron Dextran Injection, USP) 2478
Kefzol Vials, Faspak & ADD-Vantage 1511
Larodopa Tablets (Rare) 2296
Leustatin (2%) 1889
▲ Lupron Injection (5% or more) 2736
Lutrepulse for Injection 998
LUVOX Tablets (Rare) 2723
Maxaquin Tablets (Less than 1%) 2593
Maxipime for Injection (1.3%) 758
Merrem I.V. (1.2%) 2952
Mithracin 599
Mivacron (Less than 1%) 1125
Monocid Injection (Less often) 2674
▲ Navelbine Injection (Up to 10%) 1212
Nipent for Injection (Less than 3%) 2733
Nolvadex Tablets (0.3%) 2957
Novantrone for Injection (Infrequent) 1327

(▣ Described in PDR For Nonprescription Drugs) Incidence data in parenthesis; ▲ 3% or more (◉ Described in PDR For Ophthalmology)

1427 Side Effects Index Photosensitivity

Panhematin 452
Paxil Tablets (Rare) 2681
▲ Primaxin I.V. (3.1%) 1772
▲ Proleukin for Injection (23%) 812
Remeron Tablets (Rare) 1878
Retrovir Capsules (1.6%) 1216
Retrovir I.V. Infusion (2%) 1221
Retrovir Syrup (1.6%) 1216
ReVia Tablets (Less than 1%) 957
Rifater 1280
Rilutek Tablets (0.4% to 0.8%) 2198
Risperdal Tablets (Rare) 1348
Rocephin Injectable Vials, ADD-Vantage, Galaxy Container (Less than 1%) 2305
Serophene (clomiphene citrate tablets, USP) (Rare) 2621
Sinemet Tablets (Rare) 959
Sinemet CR Tablets 961
Taxol Injection (Rare) 723
Taxotere for Injection Concentrate 2204
Tazicef for Injection (Less than 2%) 2697
Tazidime Vials, Faspak & ADD-Vantage (Less than 2%) 1531
Tegison Capsules (Less than 1%) 2314
Testoderm Testosterone Transdermal System (One in 104 patients) 486
Ticar for Injection 2704
Trasylol (1.0%) 607
Triostat Injection (Approximately 1%) 2708
▲ Valium Injectable (Among most common) 2336
Vancocin HCl, Vials & ADD-Vantage 1534
Velban Vials 1537
Versed Injection (0.4%) 2324
▲ Vesanoid Capsules (11%) 2327
Wellbutrin Tablets (Rare) 1177
▲ Zinecard Injection (3% to 6%) 2120
Zosyn (1.3%) 1463
▲ Zovirax Sterile Powder (Approximately 9%) 1191

Phlebosclerosis

Adriamycin PFS 2056
Adriamycin RDF 2056
Doxorubicin Astra 531
Rubex for Injection 721

Phobic disorder

Anafranil Capsules (Infrequent) 819
Cipro I.V. (1% or less) 587
Cipro I.V. Pharmacy Bulk Package (Less than 1%) 590
Cipro Tablets (Less than 1%) 584
Floxin I.V. 1580
Floxin Tablets (200 mg, 300 mg, 400 mg) 1577
Imitrex Tablets (Rare) 1099
LUVOX Tablets (Infrequent) 2723
Maxaquin Tablets 2593

Phonophobia

Imitrex Tablets (Frequent) 1099

Phosphaturia

Daranide Tablets 1676

Phosphenes

Clomid (1.5%) 1262
Serophene (clomiphene citrate tablets, USP) 2621

Phospholipid concentration, increase

Demulen 2580
Estratest 2718
Triphasil-21 Tablets 2919
Triphasil-28 Tablets 2924

Photodynamic reaction

Urobiotic-250 Capsules 2038

Photophobia

Accutane Capsules (Less than 1%) 2252
Anafranil Capsules (Infrequent) 819
Betaseron for SC Injection 653
Betimol 0.25%, 0.5% (1% to 5%) ⊛ 259
Betoptic Ophthalmic Solution (Rare) 465
Betoptic S Ophthalmic Suspension (Small number of patients) 467
BOTOX (Botulinum Toxin Type A) Purified Neurotoxin Complex 473
BuSpar Tablets (Rare) 738
Calcijex Injection 412
Cardioquin Tablets 2146
Cardura Tablets (Less than 0.5% of 3960 patients) 1993
Celontin Kapseals 1955
Cerebyx Injection (Infrequent) 1956
Chibroxin Sterile Ophthalmic Solution 1657
Ciloxan Ophthalmic Solution (Less than 1%) 468
Claritin-D Tablets (Less frequent) 2487
Clomid (1.5%) 1262
▲ Cordarone Tablets (4 to 9%) 2818
CytoGam (Infrequent) 1630
Cytovene (1% or less) 2270
Effexor (Infrequent) 2825
Ergamisol Tablets 1340
Etrafon 2495
Floxin I.V. (Less than 1%) 1580
Floxin Tablets (200 mg, 300 mg, 400 mg) (Less than 1%) 1577
Fluorouracil Injection 2282
Foscavir Injection (Less than 1%) 541
Sterile FUDR (Remote possibility) 2284
Gamimune N, 5% Immune Globulin Intravenous (Human), 5% (Infrequent) 612
Gamimune N, 10% Immune Globulin Intravenous (Human), 10% (Infrequent) 615
Gammar-P I.V., Immune Globulin Intravenous (Human) (Infrequent) 798
Havrix (Less than 1%) 2663
Hivid Tablets (Less than 1%) 2287
Imdur (Less than or equal to 5%) 1362
Imitrex Injection (Infrequent) 1095
Imitrex Tablets (Frequent) 1099
Intron A for Injection (Less than 5%) 2506
Iopidine 0.5% (Less than 3%) ⊛ 219
Lacrisert Sterile Ophthalmic Insert 1730
Lamictal Tablets (Infrequent) 1105
Levophed Bitartrate Injection 2445
Lioresal Intrathecal (1% or more) 1634
Lodine Capsules and Tablets (Less than 1%) 2849
LUVOX Tablets (Infrequent) 2723
Matulane Capsules 2300
Maxaquin Tablets 2593
Mesantoin Tablets 2400
Neurontin Capsules (Infrequent) 1978
Nipent for Injection (Less than 3%) 2733
Nizoral Tablets (Less than 1%) 1345
Norvir (Less than 2%) 447
Ocuflox Ophthalmic Solution 478
Ocupress Ophthalmic Solution, 1% Sterile (Occasional) ⊛ 297
OptiPranolol (Metipranolol 0.3%) Sterile Ophthalmic Solution (A small number of patients) ⊛ 256
▲ Orthoclone OKT3 Sterile Solution (10%) 1892
Paremyd ⊛ 244
Paxil Tablets (Rare) 2681
Permax Tablets (Infrequent) 571
Plaquenil Sulfate Tablets (Fairly common) 2459
Prinivil Tablets (0.3% to 1.0%) 1776
Prinzide Tablets 1780
ProSom Tablets (Infrequent) 457
Prozac Pulvules & Liquid, Oral Solution (Infrequent) 935
Quinaglute Dura-Tabs Tablets 644
Quinidex Extentabs 2240
Redux Capsules 2911
Retrovir Capsules 1216
Retrovir I.V. Infusion 1221
Retrovir Syrup 1216
▲ Rev-Eyes Ophthalmic Eyedrops 0.5% (10% to 40%) ⊛ 324
Rilutek Tablets (Rare) 2198
Risperdal Tablets (Rare) 1348
Rocaltrol Capsules 2303
Sandoglobulin I.V. (Infrequent) 2419
Serentil 689
Serophene (clomiphene citrate tablets, USP) 2621
Serzone Tablets (Infrequent) 776
Supprelin Injection (1% to 3%) 2230
Tambocor Tablets (Less than 1%) 1555
Tegison Capsules (Less than 1%) 2314
Triavil Tablets 1800
Trilafon 2532
Trusopt Sterile Ophthalmic Solution (Approximately 1% to 5%) 1803
Vexol 1% Ophthalmic Suspension (Less than 1%) ⊛ 227
Videx Tablets, Powder for Oral Solution, & Pediatric Powder for Oral Solution (Less than 1% to 5%) 2980
Vira-A Ophthalmic Ointment, 3% ⊛ 299
Xalatan (1% to 4%) ⊛ 304
Zestoretic Tablets 2968
Zestril Tablets (0.3% to 1.0%) 2972
Zoloft Tablets (Rare) 2051
Zosyn (1.0% or less) 1463

Photopsia

Ambien Tablets (Rare) 2559
Clomid 1262
Risperdal Tablets (Rare) 1348

Photosensitivity

Accupril Tablets (Rare) 1950
Achromycin V Capsules 1417
Adapin Capsules (Occasional) 1542
Aldactazide Tablets 2556
Aldoclor Tablets 1638
Aldoril Tablets 1644
Alferon N Injection (1%) 2142
Altace Capsules (Less than 1%) 1238
Amaryl Tablets (Less than 1%) 1241
Ambien Tablets (Rare) 2559
Anafranil Capsules (Infrequent) 819
Anaprox/Naprosyn (Less than 1%) 2277
Ancobon Capsules 2254
Apresazide Capsules 824
Asendin Tablets (Less than 1%) 1419
Atretol Tablets 569
Avonex 662
Azulfidine (Rare) 2059
Bactrim DS Tablets 2257
Bactrim I.V. Infusion 2255
Bactrim 2257
Benadryl Injection 1955
Betapace Tablets (Rare) 637
Betaseron for SC Injection 653
▲ Bromfed-DM Cough Syrup (Among most frequent) 1832
Capoten Tablets 740
Capozide Tablets 744
Cardioquin Tablets (Occasional) 2146
Cardizem CD Capsules (Less than 1%) 1251
Cardizem SR Capsules (Less than 1%) 1255
Cardizem Injectable 1253
Cardizem Tablets (Less than 1%) 1257
Cataflam Tablets (Less than 1%) 833
Cerebyx Injection (Infrequent) 1956
Chibroxin Sterile Ophthalmic Solution (With oral form) 1657
Cipro I.V. (1% or less) 587
Cipro I.V. Pharmacy Bulk Package (Less than 1%) 590
Cipro Tablets (Less than 1%) 584
Claritin Tablets (2% or fewer patients) 2485
Claritin-D Tablets 2487
Clinoril Tablets (Less than 1 in 100) 1658
Clozaril Tablets 2377
Combipres Tablets 682
Compazine 2644
▲ Cordarone Tablets (4 to 9%) 2818
Cozaar Tablets (Less than 1%) 1668
Cytovene (1% or less) 2270
Dantrium Capsules 2131
Daypro Caplets (Less than 1%) 2578
Declomycin Tablets 1421
Depakene 416
Depakote Tablets 418
DiaBeta Tablets 1265
Diabinese Tablets 2002
Diamox Intravenous (Occasional) ⊛ 317
Diamox Sequels (Sustained Release) ⊛ 318
Diamox Tablets (Occasional) ⊛ 317
Dimetane-DC Cough Syrup 2232
Dimetane-DX Cough Syrup 2233
Dipentum Capsules (Rare) 2084
Diucardin Tablets 2824
Diupres Tablets 1691
Diuril Oral Suspension 1694
Diuril Sodium Intravenous 1693
Diuril Tablets 1694
Dolobid Tablets (Less than 1 in 100) 1695
Doryx Capsules 1970
Dyazide Capsules 2653
DYNACIN Capsules (Rare) 1627
Dyrenium Capsules (Rare) 2655
EC-Naprosyn Delayed-Release Tablets (Less than 1%) 2277
Effexor (Infrequent) 2825
▲ Efudex (Among most frequent) 2280
Elavil 2945
Eldepryl Capsules 2729
Enduron Tablets 424
Ergamisol Tablets 1340
Esidrix Tablets 839
Esimil Tablets 840
Etrafon 2495
Eulexin Capsules 2498
Fansidar Tablets 2281
Felbatol (Rare) 2774
Flexeril Tablets (Rare) 1701
Floxin I.V. 1580
Floxin Tablets (200 mg, 300 mg, 400 mg) 1577
Fluorouracil Injection 2282
Sterile FUDR (Remote possibility) 2284
Fulvicin P/G Tablets (Occasional) 2499
Fulvicin P/G 165 & 330 Tablets (Occasional) 2500
Gantanol Tablets 2285
Gantrisin 2286
Garamycin 0.1% 2501
Gastrocrom Oral Concentrate (Less common) 1611
GlaucTabs (Occasional) ⊛ 209
Glucotrol Tablets 2011
Glynase PresTab Tablets 2091
Grifulvin V (griseofulvin tablets) Microsize (griseofulvin oral suspension) Microsize 1944
Gris-PEG Tablets, 125 mg & 250 mg (Occasional) 476
Haldol Decanoate (Isolated cases) 1587
Haldol Injection, Tablets and Concentrate (Isolated cases) 1585
Helidac Therapy (Rare) 2135
Hibistat Germicidal Hand Rinse (Rare) 2948
Hismanal Tablets (Less frequent) 1341
Hivid Tablets (Less than 1%) 2287
HydroDIURIL Tablets 1716
Hydropres Tablets 1718
Hyzaar Tablets 1720
Imitrex Injection 1095
Imitrex Tablets 1099
Inderide Tablets 2838
Inderide LA Long Acting Capsules 2840
Intron A for Injection (Less than 5%) 2506
Invirase Capsules (Less than 2%) 2291
Lamictal Tablets (Rare) 1105
Lasix Injection, Oral Solution and Tablets 1267
Lescol Capsules (Rare) 2395
Levoprome 1321
Limbitrol 2333
Lodine Capsules and Tablets (Less than 1%) 2849
Lopressor HCT Tablets 850
Lotensin Tablets 852
Lotensin HCT Tablets (0.3% or more) 855
Ludiomil Tablets (Rare) 861
Lupron Depot 3.75 mg 2739
Lupron Depot 7.5 mg 2741
Lupron Depot - 3 Month 22.5 mg 2743
Lupron Depot-PED 7.5 mg, 11.25 mg and 15 mg 2744
LUVOX Tablets (Infrequent) 2723
Maxaquin Tablets (2.4%) 2593
Mellaril (Extremely rare) 2398
Mepergan Injection (Extremely rare) 2859
▲ Methotrexate Sodium Tablets, Injection, for Injection and LPF Injection (3% to 10%) 1322
Mevacor Tablets (Rare) 1742
Micronase Tablets 2099
Minizide Capsules 2016
Minocin Intravenous (Rare) 1428
Minocin Oral Suspension (Rare) 1431
Minocin Pellet-Filled Capsules (Rare) 1429
Moduretic Tablets 1748
Monodox Capsules 1858
Monopril Tablets (0.2% to 1.0%) 762
Motrin Ibuprofen Suspension, Oral Drops, Chewable Tablets, Caplets (Less than 1%) 1563
Mykrox Tablets 1617
▲ Naprelan Tablets (3% to 9%) 2861
Anaprox/Naprosyn (Less than 1%) 2277
Navane Capsules and Concentrate 2018
Navane Intramuscular 2019
NegGram (Infrequent) 2453
Neptazane Tablets ⊛ 320
Neurontin Capsules (Rare) 1978
Nipent for Injection (Less than 3%) 2733
Noroxin Tablets 1758

(▣ Described in PDR For Nonprescription Drugs) Incidence data in parenthesis; ▲ 3% or more (⊛ Described in PDR For Ophthalmology)

Photosensitivity — Side Effects Index — 1428

Noroxin Tablets ... 2222
Norpramin Tablets ... 1273
Norvir (Less than 2%) ... 447
Oretic Tablets ... 450
Ornade Spansule Capsules ... 2678
Orudis Capsules (Less than 1%) ... 2874
Oruvail Capsules (Less than 1%) ... 2874
PBZ Tablets ... 863
PBZ-SR Tablets ... 862
pHisoHex ... 2458
Pamelor (No incidence in labeling) ... 2409
Paxil Tablets (Rare) ... 2681
Pediazole Suspension ... 2340
Penetrex Tablets (0.1% to 1%) ... 2196
Pentasa (Less than 1%) ... 1275
Periactin ... 1767
Phenergan with Codeine (Rare) ... 2883
Phenergan with Dextromethorphan (Rare) ... 2885
Phenergan Injection ... 2880
Phenergan Suppositories (Rare) ... 2882
Phenergan Syrup (Rare) ... 2881
Phenergan Tablets (Rare) ... 2882
Phenergan VC (Rare) ... 2886
Phenergan VC with Codeine (Rare) 2888
Polytrim Ophthalmic Solution Sterile ... 479
Pravachol Tablets (Rare) ... 770
Prinivil Tablets (0.3% to 1.0%) ... 1776
Prinzide Tablets ... 1780
▲Prograf (Greater than 3%) ... 1028
Prolixin ... 510
ProSom Tablets (Rare) ... 457
Pyrazinamide Tablets (Rare) ... 1442
Quinaglute Dura-Tabs Tablets (Occasional) ... 644
Quinidex Extentabs (Occasional) ... 2240
Relafen Tablets (1%) ... 2688
Remeron Tablets (Infrequent) ... 1878
Rifater (Rare) ... 1280
Rilutek Tablets (Infrequent) ... 2198
Risperdal Tablets (Frequent) ... 1348
Seldane Tablets ... 1284
Seldane-D Extended-Release Tablets ... 1286
Septra ... 1146
Septra I.V. Infusion ... 1142
Septra I.V. Infusion ADD-Vantage Vials ... 1144
Septra ... 1146
Ser-Ap-Es Tablets ... 867
Serzone Tablets (Infrequent) ... 776
Sinequan (Occasional) ... 2028
Solganal Suspension ... 2530
Stelazine (Occasional) ... 2692
Surmontil Capsules ... 2917
Symmetrel Syrup (0.1% to 1%) ... 963
Tavist Syrup ... 2426
Tavist Tablets ... 2427
Tegretol/Tegretol-XR ... 870
Tenoretic Tablets ... 2963
Terramycin Intramuscular Solution 2034
Thalitone ... 1293
Thorazine (Occasional) ... 2701
Tiazac Capsules (Less than 1%) ... 1019
Timolide Tablets ... 1791
Tofranil Ampuls ... 873
Tofranil Tablets ... 875
Tofranil-PM Capsules ... 876
Triavil Tablets ... 1800
Trilafon ... 2532
Trinalin Repetabs Tablets ... 1373
Tussend ... 1830
Univasc Tablets (Less than 1%) ... 2553
Vaseretic Tablets ... 1810
Vasotec I.V. ... 1814
Vasotec Tablets (0.5% to 1.0%) ... 1816
Velban Vials (1 case) ... 1537
Vibramycin ... 2038
Vibramycin Hyclate Intravenous ... 2040
Vibramycin ... 2038
Vivactil Tablets ... 1820
Cataflam/Voltaren/Voltaren-XR (Less than 1%) ... 833
Zaroxolyn Tablets ... 1625
Zestoretic Tablets ... 2968
Zestril Tablets (0.3% to 1.0%) ... 2972
Ziac ... 1459
Zithromax (1% or less) ... 2043
Zithromax Tablets (1% or less) ... 2046
Zocor Tablets (Rare) ... 1821
Zoloft Tablets (Rare) ... 2051
Zyrtec Tablets (Less than 2%) ... 2053

Phototoxicity

Cipro Tablets ... 584
Dapsone Tablets USP ... 1331
Floxin Tablets (200 mg, 300 mg, 400 mg) ... 1577
Lamprene Capsules (Less than 1%) ... 846
Maxaquin Tablets ... 2593
Noroxin Tablets ... 1758
Noroxin Tablets ... 2222
Zyrtec Tablets (Less than 2%) ... 2053

Physical performance, impairment

Adipex-P Tablets and Capsules ... 1035
Brontex ... 2130
Butisol Sodium Elixir & Tablets ... 2768
Clozaril Tablets ... 2377
Compazine ... 2644
DHCplus Capsules ... 2148
Demerol ... 2438
Desyrel and Desyrel Dividose ... 504
Esgic-plus Capsules ... 1012
Esgic-plus Tablets ... 1012
Etrafon ... 2495
Fioricet Tablets ... 2386
Fioricet with Codeine Capsules ... 2387
Fiorinal with Codeine Capsules ... 2390
Gris-PEG Tablets, 125 mg & 250 mg (Occasional) ... 476
Hycodan Tablets and Syrup ... 946
Hycomine Compound Tablets ... 948
Hycomine ... 947
Hycotuss Expectorant Syrup ... 950
Hydrocet Capsules ... 787
Kadian Capsules ... 2948
Lithonate/Lithotabs/Lithobid ... 2721
Lorcet 10/650 Tablets ... 1016
Lortab ... 2751
Loxitane ... 1426
MS Contin Tablets ... 2149
Mebaral Tablets ... 2452
Methadone Hydrochloride Oral Concentrate ... 2356
Miltown Tablets ... 2780
Norpramin Tablets ... 1273
Percocet Tablets ... 955
Percodan Tablets ... 955
Phenergan with Codeine ... 2883
Phenergan with Dextromethorphan 2885
Phenergan Injection ... 2880
Phenergan Suppositories ... 2882
Phenergan Syrup ... 2881
Phenergan Tablets ... 2882
Phenergan VC ... 2886
Phenergan VC with Codeine ... 2888
PMB 200 and PMB 400 ... 2890
RMS Suppositories CII ... 2766
Soma Compound Tablets ... 2783
Surmontil Capsules ... 2917
Tofranil Tablets ... 875
Tofranil-PM Capsules ... 876
Tussend ... 1830
Tussionex Pennkinetic Extended-Release Suspension ... 1624
Tylenol with Codeine ... 1592
Tylox Capsules ... 1593
Ultram Tablets (50 mg) ... 1594
Vicodin Tablets ... 1404
Vicodin ES Tablets ... 1405
Vicodin HP Tablets ... 1403
Vicodin Tuss Expectorant ... 1406
Vivactil Tablets ... 1820
Wygesic Tablets ... 2930
Zydone Capsules ... 967

Pigmentary deposits, conjuctiva

Mellaril ... 2398

Pigmentary deposits, cornea

Lamprene Capsules (Greater than 1%) ... 846
Triavil Tablets ... 1800

Pigmentation

Aquasol A Vitamin A Capsules, USP ... 525
Aquasol A Parenteral ... 526
Cortifoam ... 2540
Cosmegen Injection ... 1666
Etopophos for Injection (Infrequent) ... 701
Etoposide Injection (Infrequent) ... 539
Etrafon ... 2495
Genotropin Injection (Infrequent) ... 2090
Levoprome ... 1321
Lupron Injection (Less than 5%) ... 2736
Mesantoin Tablets ... 2400
Minipress Capsules (Single report) 2015
Minizide Capsules (Single report) ... 2016
Plaquenil Sulfate Tablets ... 2459
Prolixin ... 510
Risperdal Tablets (Frequent) ... 1348
Timolide Tablets (Less than 1%) ... 1791
Timoptic in Ocudose ... 1796
Timoptic Sterile Ophthalmic Solution ... 1794
Timoptic-XE ... 1798
Triavil Tablets ... 1800
Trilafon ... 2532
VePesid Capsules and Injection (Infrequent) ... 727

Pigmentation disorders

Accutane Capsules (Less than 1%) ... 2252
Aralen Hydrochloride Injection ... 2430
Aralen Phosphate Tablets ... 2431
Atretol Tablets ... 569
Cardioquin Tablets (Occasional) ... 2146
Cordarone Tablets (Occasional) ... 2818
Cytoxan ... 700
Daraprim Tablets (Rare) ... 1199
DYNACIN Capsules ... 1627
Ethyl Chloride, U.S.P. ... 1040
Fluori-Methane ... 1040
Fluorouracil Injection ... 2282
Sterile FUDR (Remote possibility) .. 2284
Mellaril ... 2398
Methotrexate Sodium Tablets, Injection, for Injection and LPF Injection ... 1322
Minocin Intravenous ... 1428
Minocin Oral Suspension ... 1431
Minocin Pellet-Filled Capsules ... 1429
Orudis Capsules (Less than 1%) ... 2874
Oruvail Capsules (Less than 1%) ... 2874
Quinaglute Dura-Tabs Tablets ... 644
Quinidex Extentabs (Occasional) ... 2240
Retrovir Capsules ... 1216
Retrovir I.V. Infusion ... 1221
Retrovir Syrup ... 1216
Supprelin Injection (1% to 3%) ... 2230
Tapazole Tablets ... 1361
Tegretol/Tegretol-XR ... 870
Thorazine ... 2701
▲Xalatan (5% to 15%) ... ⊙ 304

Pill rolling motion

Compazine ... 2644
Stelazine ... 2692
Thorazine ... 2701

Piloerection

Anafranil Capsules (Rare) ... 819
Vasoxyl Injection ... 1169
Yohimex Tablets ... 1414

Pituitary apoplexy

Factrel ... 2996
Sandostatin Injection (Less than 1%) ... 2421
THYREL TRH (Infrequent) ... 2992

Pituitary tumors

Clomid ... 1262

Pituitary unresponsiveness, secondary

Celestone Soluspan Suspension ... 2484
CORTENEMA ... 2713
Cortone Acetate Sterile Suspension ... 1663
Cortone Acetate Tablets ... 1664
Dalalone D.P. Injectable ... 1009
Decadron Elixir ... 1676
Decadron Phosphate Injection ... 1680
Decadron Phosphate with Xylocaine Injection, Sterile ... 1683
Decadron Tablets ... 1678
Decadron-LA Sterile Suspension ... 1687
Dexacort Phosphate in Respihaler .. 1606
Dexacort Phosphate in Turbinaire .. 1607
Florinef Acetate Tablets ... 506
Hydeltrasol Injection, Sterile ... 1708
Hydeltra-T.B.A. Sterile Suspension 1710
Hydrocortone Acetate Sterile Suspension ... 1712
Hydrocortone Phosphate Injection, Sterile ... 1713
Hydrocortone Tablets ... 1715
Pediapred Oral Solution ... 1618
Prelone Syrup ... 1834

Placenta previa

Redux Capsules ... 2911

Placental disorder, unspecified

Felbatol ... 2774

Plaques, erythematous

AquaMEPHYTON Injection ... 1648

Plaques, indurated

AquaMEPHYTON Injection ... 1648

Plaques, pruritic

AquaMEPHYTON Injection ... 1648

Platelet, decrease (see under Thrombocytopenia)

Platelet, increase (see under Thrombocytosis)

Platelet disorder, unspecified

Felbatol (Rare) ... 2774
▲Foscavir Injection (1% to 5% or greater) ... 541
Hivid Tablets (Less than 1%) ... 2287
Zoloft Tablets (Rare) ... 2051

Plethora

Talwin Injection ... 2465
Talwin Nx Tablets ... 2467

Pleural effusion

Betaseron for SC Injection ... 653
▲CellCept Capsules (More than or equal to 3%) ... 2265
Cipro I.V. (1% or less) ... 587
Cipro I.V. Pharmacy Bulk Package (Less than 1%) ... 590
Clinoril Tablets (Less than 1 in 100) ... 1658
Clomid ... 1262
Clozaril Tablets ... 2377
Doxil (Less than 1%) ... 2613
▲Ethamolin Injection (Among most common; 2.1%) ... 2544
Felbatol ... 2774
▲Flolan for Injection (4%) ... 1085
Foscavir Injection (Less than 1%) .. 541
Ganite ... 2711
Humegon for Injection ... 1873
Hyskon Hysteroscopy Fluid (Rare) .. 1633
Leukine (1%) ... 1317
Lupron Depot - 3 Month 22.5 mg (Less than 5%) ... 2743
Lutrepulse for Injection ... 998
Macrobid Capsules ... 2138
Macrodantin Capsules ... 2140
Matulane Capsules ... 2300
Metrodin (urofollitropin for injection) ... 2616
Permax Tablets (Infrequent) ... 571
Prinivil Tablets (0.3% to 1.0%) ... 1776
Prinzide Tablets ... 1780
Procanbid Extended-Release Tablets (Fairly common) ... 1983
Profasi (chorionic gonadotropin for injection, USP) ... 2620
▲Prograf (30% to 32%) ... 1028
▲Proleukin for Injection (7%) ... 812
Prozac Pulvules & Liquid, Oral Solution (Rare) ... 935
ReoPro Vials (1.3%) ... 1526
Rilutek Tablets (Infrequent) ... 2198
Sansert Tablets ... 2424
Serophene (clomiphene citrate tablets, USP) ... 2621
Sular Tablets (Less than or equal to 1%) ... 2961
▲Taxotere for Injection Concentrate (6%) ... 2204
▲Trasylol (5%) ... 607
▲Vesanoid Capsules (20%) ... 2327
Zestoretic Tablets ... 2968
Zestril Tablets (0.3% to 1.0%) ... 2972
Zosyn (1.3%) ... 1463

Pleural effusion with pericarditis

Dantrium Capsules (Less frequent) 2131

Pleural friction rubs

Lupron Injection (Less than 5%) ... 2736
Sansert Tablets ... 2424

Pleural infiltration

▲Ethamolin Injection (Among most common; 2.1%) ... 2544

Pleuralgia

Intron A for Injection (Less than 5%) ... 2506
Monopril Tablets (0.4% to 1.0%) .. 762
Procanbid Extended-Release Tablets (Fairly common) ... 1983

Pleurisy

AeroBid Inhaler System (1% to 3%) ... 1004
Aerobid-M Inhaler System (1% to 3%) ... 1004
Effexor (Rare) ... 2825
ReoPro Vials (1.3%) ... 1526
Tonocard Tablets (Less than 1%) .. 519

Pleuritis

Azulfidine (Rare) ... 2059

(Described in PDR For Nonprescription Drugs) Incidence data in parenthesis; ▲ 3% or more (⊙ Described in PDR For Ophthalmology)

1429 Side Effects Index Polyps, rectal

Inocor Lactate Injection (1 case) 2439

Pneumatosis cystoides intestinalis

Cytosar-U Sterile Powder 2077

Pneumocystis carinii

CellCept Capsules (Up to 0.3%) 2265

Pneumocystis carinii, susceptibility

▲Doxil (9.2%) 2613
▲Orthoclone OKT3 Sterile Solution (3.1%) 1892

Pneumomediastinum

Exosurf Neonatal for Intratracheal Suspension (1% to 4%) 1081

Pneumonia

▲Abelcet Injection (3% to 5%) 1540
AeroBid Inhaler System (1% to 3%) 1004
Aerobid-M Inhaler System (1% to 3%) 1004
Ambien Tablets (Rare) 2559
Anafranil Capsules (Infrequent) 819
Atretol Tablets 569
Avonex 662
Betaseron for SC Injection 653
Casodex Tablets (2% to 5%) 2934
▲CellCept Capsules (3.6% to 10.6%) 2265
Cerebyx Injection (Frequent) 1956
Clozaril Tablets (Less than 1%) 2377
Cognex Capsules (Frequent) 1961
Compazine 2644
Crixivan Capsules (Less than 2%) 1670
Cytosar-U Sterile Powder (Less frequent) 2077
Cytotec (Infrequent) 2576
▲Cytovene (6%) 2270
Doxil (1% to 5%) 2613
Effexor (Infrequent) 2825
▲Ethamolin Injection (Among most common; 1.2%) 2544
Felbatol 2774
▲Fludara for Injection (16% to 22%) 658
Foscavir Injection (Between 1% and 5%) 541
Imdur (Less than or equal to 5%) 1362
Intron A for Injection (Rare; less than or equal to 5%) 2506
Invirase Capsules (Less than 2%) 2291
Ismo Tablets (Fewer than 1%) 2844
Kerlone Tablets (Less than 2%) 2588
Lamictal Tablets (Rare) 1105
▲Leustatin (6%) 1889
Lioresal Intrathecal (Up to 2.0%) 1634
Lupron Depot - 3 Month 22.5 mg (Less than 5%) 2743
Lupron Injection (Less than 5%) 2736
LUVOX Tablets (Rare) 2723
Megace Oral Suspension (Up to 2%) 708
Miacalcin Nasal Spray (Less than 1%) 2403
Naprelan Tablets (Less than 1%) 2861
▲Neoral (6.2%) 2405
Neurontin Capsules (Frequent) 1978
▲Nipent for Injection (5%) 2733
▲Novantrone for Injection (9%) 1327
Orthoclone OKT3 Sterile Solution 1892
Paxil Tablets (Infrequent) 2681
Permax Tablets (Frequent) 571
Prevacid Delayed-Release Capsules (Less than 1%) 2746
Prinivil Tablets (0.3% to 1.0%) 1776
Prinzide Tablets 1780
▲Prograf (Greater than 3%) 1028
Prolixin 510
Prozac Pulvules & Liquid, Oral Solution (Infrequent) 935
Pulmozyme Inhalation 1054
Remeron Tablets (Infrequent) 1878
ReoPro Vials (1.0%) 1526
Rilutek Tablets (More than 2%) 2198
Risperdal Tablets (Infrequent) 1348
▲Roferon-A Injection (Less than 3% to 11%) 2308
▲Sandimmune (6.2 to 9.2%) 2416
Sandostatin Injection (Less than 1%) 2421
Serentil 689
Serzone Tablets (Infrequent) 776
Stelazine 2692
▲Taxol Injection (30%) 723
Tegretol/Tegretol-XR 870
▲Tetramune (Among most common) 1449
Tonocard Tablets (Less than 1%) 519
▲Trasylol (4%) 607
Vaseretic Tablets 1810
Vasotec I.V. 1814
Vasotec Tablets (1.0%) 1816
▲Vesanoid Capsules (14%) 2327
▲Videx Tablets, Powder for Oral Solution, & Pediatric Powder for Oral Solution (5% to 8%) 2980
Virazole 1310
▲Vistide Injection (9%) 1057
Wellbutrin Tablets (Rare) 1177
▲Zerit Capsules (3% to 4%) 731
Zestoretic Tablets 2968
Zestril Tablets (0.3% to 1.0%) 2972
Zoladex 3-month (1% to 5%) 2978
Zyrtec Tablets (Less than 2%) 2053

Pneumonia, aspiration

Cerebyx Injection (Infrequent) 1956
Ethamolin Injection 2544
Lioresal Intrathecal (1% or more) 1634
Neurontin Capsules (Rare) 1978

Pneumonia, congenital

Exosurf Neonatal for Intratracheal Suspension (1% to 4%) 1081

Pneumonia, eosinophilic

Prozac Pulvules & Liquid, Oral Solution 935
Relafen Tablets (Rarer) 2688

Pneumonia, interstitial

Betaseron for SC Injection 653
Leukeran Tablets 1205
Norvir (Less than 2%) 447
Taxol Injection (Rare) 723
Videx Tablets, Powder for Oral Solution, & Pediatric Powder for Oral Solution (Less than 1%) 2980

Pneumonia, nosocomial

▲Exosurf Neonatal for Intratracheal Suspension (2% to 15%) 1081

Pneumonitis

Aldoclor Tablets 1638
Aldoril Tablets 1644
Apresazide Capsules 824
Atretol Tablets 569
Azulfidine (Rare) 2059
▲Blenoxane (Approximately 10%) 697
Capozide Tablets 744
Cardioquin Tablets 2146
Clinoril Tablets (Less than 1 in 100) 1658
Diucardin Tablets 2824
Diupres Tablets 1691
Diuril Oral Suspension 1694
Diuril Sodium Intravenous 1693
Diuril Tablets 1694
Enduron Tablets 424
Esidrix Tablets 839
Esimil Tablets 840
Felbatol 2774
Foscavir Injection (Less than 1%) 541
HydroDIURIL Tablets 1716
Hydropres Tablets 1718
Hyzaar Tablets 1720
Inderide Tablets 2838
Inderide LA Long Acting Capsules 2840
Intron A for Injection (Rare) 2506
Lopressor HCT Tablets 850
Lotensin HCT Tablets 855
Matulane Capsules 2300
Methotrexate Sodium Tablets, Injection, for Injection and LPF Injection 1322
Moduretic Tablets 1748
Mykrox Tablets (Rare) 1617
Myochrysine Injection 1754
Oretic Tablets 450
Orthoclone OKT3 Sterile Solution 1892
Pediazole Suspension 2340
Prinzide Tablets 1780
Prolixin 510
Quinaglute Dura-Tabs Tablets 644
Quinidex Extentabs 2240
Roferon-A Injection (Infrequent) 2308
Ser-Ap-Es Tablets 867
Solganal Suspension 2530
Tegretol/Tegretol-XR 870
TICE BCG, USP (1.2%) 1881
Timolide Tablets 1791
Varivax (Less than 1%) 1807
Vaseretic Tablets 1810
Zaroxolyn Tablets 1625
Zestoretic Tablets 2968
Ziac 1459

Pneumonitis, allergic

Dyazide Capsules 2653
Floxin I.V. 1580
Floxin Tablets (200 mg, 300 mg, 400 mg) 1577
▲Fludara for Injection (Up to 6%) 658
Ticlid Tablets (Rare) 2317

Pneumonitis, eosinophilic

Monopril Tablets 762
▲Naprelan Tablets (3% to 9%) 2861
Tilade Inhaler (Isolated cases) 2207

Pneumonitis, interstitial

Actimmune (Rare) 1043
Alkeran for Injection 1196
Alkeran Tablets 1198
Asacol Delayed-Release Tablets 2129
Cordarone Tablets 2818
Cuprimine Capsules (Rare) 1673
Cytosar-U Sterile Powder (Ten patients) 2077
Depen Titratable Tablets 2770
Imuran (Less than 1%) 1103
Ludiomil Tablets (Several voluntary reports) 861
Macrobid Capsules (Rare to common) 2138
Macrodantin Capsules (Rare) 2140
Methotrexate Sodium Tablets, Injection, for Injection and LPF Injection 1322
Redux Capsules 2911
Ridaura Capsules (Less than 0.1%) 2691
Tonocard Tablets (Less than 1%) 519

Pneumopericardium

Exosurf Neonatal for Intratracheal Suspension (1% to 4%) 1081

Pneumothorax

Betaseron for SC Injection 653
Cerebyx Injection (Infrequent) 1956
Cytovene-IV (One report) 2270
Doxil (Less than 1%) 2613
▲Exosurf Neonatal for Intratracheal Suspension (6% to 20%) 1081
Foscavir Injection (Between 1% and 5%) 541
Intron A for Injection (Less than or equal to 5%) 2506
Permax Tablets (Rare) 571
Proleukin for Injection (1%) 812
Pulmozyme Inhalation 1054
Remeron Tablets (Rare) 1878
Rifater 1280
Rilutek Tablets (Infrequent) 2198
▲Trasylol (3%) 607
Videx Tablets, Powder for Oral Solution, & Pediatric Powder for Oral Solution (Less than 1%) 2980
Virazole 1310
Zosyn (1.3%) 1463

Poliomyelitis

Invirase Capsules (Less than 2%) 2291

Pollakiuria

DynaCirc Capsules (1.3% to 3.4%) 2381
DynaCirc CR Tablets (0.5% to 1.0%) 2383
Sandostatin Injection (1% to 4%) 2421
Sanorex Tablets 2423
Visken Tablets (2% or fewer patients) 2428

Polyarteritis nodosa

Anafranil Capsules (Rare) 819
Azulfidine (Rare) 2059

Polyarthralgia

Eskalith 2658
Lithonate/Lithotabs/Lithobid 2721
Minocin Intravenous 1428
Minocin Oral Suspension 1431
Minocin Pellet-Filled Capsules 1429
Primaxin I.M. 1770
Primaxin I.V. (Less than 0.2%) 1772

Polyarthralgia, migratory

Cuprimine Capsules (Some patients) 1673
Depen Titratable Tablets 2770

Polyarthritis

Cleocin Phosphate Injection (Rare) 2068
Cleocin Vaginal Cream (Rare) 2070
▲Roferon-A Injection (5%) 2308

Polyarthropathy

Mesantoin Tablets 2400

Polycythemia

Androderm Testosterone Transdermal System 2634
▲Android Capsules, 10 mg (Among most common) 1297
▲CellCept Capsules (More than or equal to 3%) 2265
Danocrine Capsules 2437
Estratest 2718
Gastrocrom Capsules (Infrequent) 1611
Gastrocrom Oral Concentrate (Less common) 1611
Halotestin Tablets 2095
Oxandrin 783
Permax Tablets (Rare) 571
Redux Capsules (Rare) 2911
Testoderm Testosterone Transdermal System 486
Testred Capsules, 10 mg 1308

Polydipsia

Calcijex Injection 412
Clozaril Tablets (Less than 1%) 2377
Eskalith 2658
Imitrex Injection (Rare) 1095
Imitrex Tablets (Rare) 1099
Lithium Carbonate Capsules & Tablets 2352
Lithonate/Lithotabs/Lithobid (Occasional) 2721
Loxitane 1426
Navane Capsules and Concentrate 2018
Navane Intramuscular 2019
Risperdal Tablets (Frequent) 1348
Rocaltrol Capsules 2303

Polymenorrhea

Sandostatin Injection (Less than 1%) 2421

Polymyalgia rheumatica

Lescol Capsules (Rare) 2395
Mevacor Tablets (Rare) 1742
Miacalcin Nasal Spray (Less than 1%) 2403
Pravachol Tablets (Rare) 770
Zocor Tablets (Rare) 1821

Polymyositis

Cuprimine Capsules (Rare) 1673
Depen Titratable Tablets (Rare) 2770
Intal Inhaler (Rare) 2185
Intal Nebulizer Solution (Rare) 2186
Nasalcrom Nasal Solution (Rare) 2192
Tagamet (Rare) 2694

Polyneuritis

Antabuse Tablets 2802
Biavax II 1653
M-M-R II 1730
M-R-VAX II 1732
Meruvax II 1740
Podocon-25 1949
Proglycem 575

Polyneuropathy

Acel-Imune Diphtheria and Tetanus Toxoids and Acellular Pertussis Vaccine Adsorbed 1415
Biavax II (Isolated reports) 1653
Dilantin Infatabs 1967
Dilantin Kapseals 1965
Dilantin-125 Suspension 1969
Diphtheria and Tetanus Toxoids and Pertussis Vaccine Adsorbed 2650
IFEX (Less than 1%) 706
Intron A for Injection (Less than 5%) 2506
M-M-R II 1730
M-R-VAX II 1732
Meruvax II (Isolated reports) 1740
Tetramune 1449
Tri-Immunol Adsorbed 1452

Polyphagia

Atromid-S Capsules 2808
Etrafon 2495
Triavil Tablets 1800
Trilafon 2532

Polyps, endometrial

Nolvadex Tablets 2957

Polyps, nasal

▲Atrovent Nasal Spray 0.03% (3.1%) 676
Pulmozyme Inhalation 1054
Zyrtec Tablets (Less than 2%) 2053

Polyps, rectal

Lupron Injection (Less than 5%) 2736

(▣ Described in PDR For Nonprescription Drugs) Incidence data in parenthesis; ▲ 3% or more (⊙ Described in PDR For Ophthalmology)

Polyradiculoneuropathy Side Effects Index 1430

Polyradiculoneuropathy
Depen Titratable Tablets 2770

Polyuria
Adalat Capsules (10 mg and 20 mg) (Less than 0.5%) 580
Ambien Tablets (Rare) 2559
Anafranil Capsules (Infrequent) 819
Avonex 662
Betaseron for SC Injection 653
Calcijex Injection 412
Capoten Tablets (Approximately 1 to 2 of 1000 patients) 740
Capozide Tablets (Approximately 1 to 2 of 1000 patients) 744
Cardizem CD Capsules (Less than 1%) 1251
Cardizem SR Capsules (1.3%) 1255
Cardizem Injectable 1253
Cardizem Tablets (Less than 1%) 1257
Cardura Tablets (2%) 1993
Cerebyx Injection (Infrequent) 1956
Cipro I.V. (1% or less) 587
Cipro I.V. Pharmacy Bulk Package (Less than 1%) 590
Cipro Tablets (Less than 1%) 584
Claritin-D Tablets (Less frequent) 2487
Clomid (Fewer than 1%) 1262
Cognex Capsules (Infrequent) 1961
Cytotec (Infrequent) 2576
DaunoXome (Less than or equal to 5%) 1842
Diamox Intravenous ⊙ 317
Diamox Sequels (Sustained Release) ⊙ 318
Diamox Tablets ⊙ 317
Effexor (Infrequent) 2825
Elspar (Low) 1700
Eskalith 2658
Etrafon 2495
Flagyl 375 Capsules 2587
Flagyl I.V. 2373
Floxin I.V. 1580
Floxin Tablets (200 mg, 300 mg, 400 mg) 1577
Foscavir Injection (Between 1% and 5%) 541
GlaucTabs ⊙ 209
Glucotrol XL Extended Release Tablets (Less than 3%) 2012
Helidac Therapy 2135
Hivid Tablets (Less than 1%) 2287
IBU Tablets (Less than 1%) 1389
Imdur (Less than or equal to 5%) 1362
Intron A for Injection (Less than 5%) 2506
Lamictal Tablets (Infrequent) 1105
Lithium Carbonate Capsules & Tablets 2352
Lithonate/Lithotabs/Lithobid (Occasional) 2721
Lotrel Capsules 858
LUVOX Tablets (Infrequent) 2723
Maxaquin Tablets 2593
MetroGel-Vaginal 917
Midamor Tablets (Less than or equal to 1%) 1746
Moduretic Tablets 1748
Motrin Ibuprofen Suspension, Oral Drops, Chewable Tablets, Caplets (Less than 1%) 1563
Neptazane Tablets ⊙ 320
Norvasc Tablets (Less than or equal to 0.1%) 2020
Norvir (Less than 2%) 447
Novahistine Elixir ▣ 782
Oncovin Solution Vials & Hyporets 1521
OxyContin Tablets (Less than 1%) 2163
Paxil Tablets (Infrequent) 2681
Penetrex Tablets 2196
Plendil Extended-Release Tablets (0.5% to 1.5%) 514
Primaxin I.M. 1770
Primaxin I.V. (Less than 0.2%) 1772
Procardia XL Extended Release Tablets (Less than 3%) 2026
Prolixin 510
Protostat Tablets 1939
Prozac Pulvules & Liquid, Oral Solution (Rare) 935
Redux Capsules (2.1%) 2911
Remeron Tablets (Rare) 1878
Retrovir Capsules 1216
Retrovir I.V. Infusion 1221
Retrovir Syrup 1216
Risperdal Tablets (Frequent) 1348
Rocaltrol Capsules 2303
Rondec Oral Drops 974
Rondec Syrup 974
Rondec 974
Sansert Tablets 2424
Serzone Tablets (Infrequent) 776
Supprelin Injection (1% to 3%) 2230
Tambocor Tablets (Less than 1%) 1555
Tegison Capsules (Less than 1%) 2314
Tiazac Capsules (Less than 1% to 1%) 1019
Tonocard Tablets (Less than 1%) 519
Toradol (1% or less) 2319
Trilafon (Occasional) 2532
Videx Tablets, Powder for Oral Solution, & Pediatric Powder for Oral Solution (Less than 1%) 2980
Ziac 1459
Zoloft Tablets (Infrequent) 2051
Zyrtec Tablets (Less than 2%) 2053

Porphyria
Brevicon 2563
Demulen 2580
Desogen Tablets 1867
Levlen/Tri-Levlen 646
Lo/Ovral Tablets 2852
Lo/Ovral-28 Tablets 2857
Modicon 1928
Nordette-21 Tablets 2863
Nordette-28 Tablets 2866
Norinyl 2563
Nor-Q D Tablets 2598
Ortho-Cept 1907
Ortho-Cyclen/Ortho-Tri-Cyclen 1914
Ortho-Novum 1928
Ortho-Cyclen/Ortho Tri-Cyclen 1914
Ovcon 765
Ovral Tablets 2877
Ovral-28 Tablets 2878
Ovrette Tablets 2878
Plaquenil Sulfate Tablets 2459
Pyrazinamide Tablets (Rare) 1442
Reglan 2243
Rifater (Rare) 1280
Sulfamylon Cream (A single case) 940
Levlen/Tri-Levlen 646
Tri-Norinyl 2607
Triphasil-21 Tablets 2919
Triphasil-28 Tablets 2924

Porphyria, aggravation
Cataflam Tablets (One patient) 833
Cerebyx Injection (Infrequent) 1956
Climara Transdermal System 640
Danocrine Capsules 2437
Dilantin Infatabs 1967
Dilantin Kapseals (Isolated reports) 1965
Dilantin-125 Suspension (Isolated reports) 1969
Epogen for Injection (Rare) 489
Estrace Cream and Tablets 751
Estraderm Transdermal System 842
ESTRATAB Tablets (0.3, 0.625, 1.25, 2.5 mg) 2715
Estratest 2718
Menest Tablets 2671
Miltown Tablets 2780
Ogen Tablets 2103
Ogen Vaginal Cream 2106
Ortho Dienestrol Cream 1922
Ortho-Est 1925
Plaquenil Sulfate Tablets 2459
PMB 200 and PMB 400 2890
Premarin Intravenous 2893
Premarin Tablets 2896
Premarin Vaginal Cream 2898
Premphase 2900
Prempro 2905
Procrit for Injection (Rare) 1896
Rifadin (Isolated reports) 1276
Rifater (Isolated reports) 1280
Vivelle Transdermal System 880
Cataflam/Voltaren/Voltaren-XR (One patient) 833
Zantac (Rare) 1182
Zantac Injection (Rare) 1180
Zantac Syrup (Rare) 1182

Porphyria, hepatic cutaneous
Diabinese Tablets 2002
Glucotrol Tablets 2011
Glucotrol XL Extended Release Tablets 2012

Porphyria, intermittent, acute
Atretol Tablets 569
Depakene 416
Depakote Tablets 418
Tegretol/Tegretol-XR 870

Porphyria, pseudo
Daypro Caplets (Less than 1%) 2578

Porphyria cutanea tarda
Amaryl Tablets (Less than 1%) 1241
Anaprox/Naprosyn (Less than 1%) 2277
DiaBeta Tablets 1265
Diabinese Tablets 2002
EC-Naprosyn Delayed-Release Tablets (Less than 1%) 2277
Glucotrol Tablets 2011
Glynase PresTab Tablets 2091
Micronase Tablets 2099
Myleran Tablets (Rare) 1209
▲Naprelan Tablets (3% to 9%) 2861
Anaprox/Naprosyn (Less than 1%) 2277

Porphyria cutanea tarda, pseudo
Relafen Tablets (1%) 2688

Potassium loss (see under Hypokalemia)

Potassium retention (see under Hyperkalemia)

Potentia, decrease
Kadian Capsules (Less than 3%) 2948
Methadone Hydrochloride Oral Concentrate 2356
RMS Suppositories CII 2766
▲ReVia Tablets (Less than 10%) 957
Roxanol 2365

Precocious puberty
Pregnyl for Injection 1878
Profasi (chorionic gonadotropin for injection, USP) 2620

Pregnancy, accidental
Depo-Provera Contraceptive Injection (Fewer than 1%) 2079

Pregnancy, ectopic
Clomid 1262
Depo-Provera Contraceptive Injection 2079
Humegon for Injection 1873
Metrodin (urofollitropin for injection) 2616
Micronor Tablets 1903
Modicon 1928
Norplant System 2868
Ortho-Novum 1928
ParaGard T 380A Intrauterine Copper Contraceptive 1936
Pergonal (menotropins for injection, USP) 2618
Serophene (clomiphene citrate tablets, USP) 2621

Pregnancy, multiple
Clomid (An increased chance) 1262
Lutrepulse for Injection (Some incidents) 998

Pregnancy, sensation of
Depo-Provera Contraceptive Injection (Fewer than 1%) 2079

Pregnancy, spontaneous termination of
Lutrepulse for Injection (Some incidents) 998

Pregnancy tests, false positive
Ceredase 1055
Compazine 2644
Etrafon 2495
Mellaril 2398
Navane Capsules and Concentrate 2018
Navane Intramuscular 2019
Phenergan Injection 2880
Serentil 689
Stelazine 2692
Thorazine 2701
Triavil Tablets 1800

Pregnancy tests, false results
Phenergan Injection 2880
Prolixin 510
Torecan 2367
Trilafon 2532

Premature ventricular contractions
Diprivan Injectable Emulsion (Less than 1%) 2939
Imitrex Injection (Infrequent) 1095
Mexitil Capsules (1.0% to 1.9%) 684
Prinivil Tablets (0.3% to 1.0%) 1776
Prinzide Tablets 1780
Rythmol Tablets–150mg, 225mg, 300mg (0.6 to 1.5%) 1399
Versed Injection (Less than 1%) 2324
Zestril Tablets (0.3% to 1.0%) 2972

Premenstrual-like syndrome
Amen Tablets 785
Brevicon 2563
Crixivan Capsules (Less than 2%) 1670
Cycrin Tablets 991
Demulen 2580
Depo-Provera Sterile Aqueous Suspension 2083
Desogen Tablets 1867
Diethylstilbestrol Tablets 1477
ESTRATAB Tablets (0.3, 0.625, 1.25, 2.5 mg) 2715
Estratest 2718
Levlen/Tri-Levlen 646
Lo/Ovral Tablets 2852
Lo/Ovral-28 Tablets 2857
LUVOX Tablets (Infrequent) 2723
Menest Tablets 2671
Modicon 1928
Nordette-21 Tablets 2863
Nordette-28 Tablets 2866
Norinyl 2563
Nor-Q D Tablets 2598
Ortho-Cept 1907
Ortho-Cyclen/Ortho-Tri-Cyclen 1914
Ortho Dienestrol Cream 1922
Ortho-Novum 1928
Ortho-Cyclen/Ortho Tri-Cyclen 1914
Ovcon 765
Ovral Tablets 2877
Ovral-28 Tablets 2878
Ovrette Tablets 2878
PMB 200 and PMB 400 2890
Premarin Intravenous 2893
Premarin Vaginal Cream 2898
Premphase 2900
Prempro 2905
Provera Tablets 2110
Levlen/Tri-Levlen 646
Tri-Norinyl 2607
Triphasil-21 Tablets 2919
Triphasil-28 Tablets 2924

Preputium, irretraction of
Condylox Topical Solution (Less than 5%) 1853

Pressor response, paradoxical
Aldomet Ester HCl Injection 1642
Apresazide Capsules (Less frequent) 824
Apresoline Hydrochloride Tablets (Less frequent) 826
Hydralazine Hydrochloride Injection USP (Less frequent) 2712
Ser-Ap-Es Tablets 867

Pre syncope
Betapace Tablets (1% to 4%) 637

Priapism
Androderm Testosterone Transdermal System 2634
Atamet Tablets 567
▲Caverject Injection (4%) 2064
Clozaril Tablets 2377
Compazine 2644
Coumadin 941
Desyrel and Desyrel Dividose 504
Esimil Tablets (A few instances) 840
Haldol Decanoate 1587
Haldol Injection, Tablets and Concentrate 1585
Halotestin Tablets 2095
Heparin Lock Flush Solution 2831
Heparin Sodium Injection 2832
Heparin Sodium Vials 1486
Hytrin Capsules 434
Ismelin Tablets 845
Larodopa Tablets (Rare) 2296
LUVOX Tablets 2723
Mellaril 2398
Minipress Capsules (Less than 1%) 2015
Minizide Capsules (Rare) 2016
Moban Tablets and Concentrate 1036
Oxandrin 783
Papaverine Hydrochloride Vials and Ampoules 1523
Paxil Tablets 2681
Permax Tablets (Infrequent) 571
Prozac Pulvules & Liquid, Oral Solution 935
Rilutek Tablets (Infrequent) 2198
Risperdal Tablets (Rare) 1348
Serzone Tablets 776
Sinemet Tablets 959
Sinemet CR Tablets 961
Stelazine 2692

(▣ Described in PDR For Nonprescription Drugs) Incidence data in parenthesis; ▲ 3% or more (⊙ Described in PDR For Ophthalmology)

Side Effects Index — Pruritus

Proarrhythmia
- Betapace Tablets (Less than 1% to 5%) ... 637
- ▲ Ethmozine Tablets (3.7% of 1072 patients) ... 2217
- Procanbid Extended-Release Tablets ... 1983
- ▲ Rythmol Tablets–150mg, 225mg, 300mg (1.2 to 4.7%) ... 1399

Proctitis
- Avonex ... 662
- Betaseron for SC Injection ... 653
- Cosmegen Injection ... 1666
- Effexor (Rare) ... 2825
- ▲ Eulexin Capsules (8%) ... 2498
- Flagyl 375 Capsules ... 2587
- Foscavir Injection (Less than 1%) ... 541
- Furoxone ... 2221
- Helidac Therapy ... 2135
- Indocin Capsules (Less than 1%) ... 1723
- Indocin I.V. (Less than 1%) ... 1727
- Indocin (Less than 1%) ... 1723
- MetroGel-Vaginal ... 917
- Miltown Tablets (Rare) ... 2780
- Neurontin Capsules (Rare) ... 1978
- PMB 200 and PMB 400 (Rare) ... 2890
- Protostat Tablets ... 1939
- Rilutek Tablets (Rare) ... 2198
- Urobiotic-250 Capsules (Rare) ... 2038
- Zoloft Tablets (Rare) ... 2051

Proctitis, ulceration
- Doxil (Less than 1%) ... 2613
- Foscavir Injection (Less than 1%) ... 541

Proctocolitis
- Diabinese Tablets (Less than 1%) ... 2002

Prolactin levels, elevated
(see under Hyperprolactinemia)

Prolactin secretion, inhibition of
- Bellergal-S Tablets ... 2375

Proprioception, loss of
- Platinol for Injection ... 717
- Platinol-AQ Injection ... 719

Proptosis
- Amen Tablets ... 785
- Brevicon ... 2563
- Cycrin Tablets ... 991
- Demulen ... 2580
- Depo-Provera Contraceptive Injection ... 2079
- Depo-Provera Sterile Aqueous Suspension ... 2083
- Levlen/Tri-Levlen ... 646
- Modicon ... 1928
- Norinyl ... 2563
- Nor-Q D Tablets ... 2598
- Ortho-Cyclen/Ortho-Tri-Cyclen ... 1914
- Ortho-Novum ... 1928
- Ortho-Cyclen/Ortho Tri-Cyclen ... 1914
- Ovcon ... 765
- Premphase ... 2900
- Prempro ... 2905
- Provera Tablets ... 2110
- Levlen/Tri-Levlen ... 646
- Tri-Norinyl ... 2607

Prostate disease, unspecified
- ▲ Androderm Testosterone Transdermal System (5%) ... 2634
- Dilacor XR Extended-release Capsules (Infrequent) ... 2183

Prostatic cancer, transient worsening symptoms
- Zoladex (A small percentage) ... 2976
- Zoladex 3-month (A small percentage) ... 2978

Prostatic disorder
- Anafranil Capsules (Infrequent) ... 819
- Atrovent Nasal Spray 0.03% ... 676
- Atrovent Nasal Spray 0.06% ... 678
- Avonex ... 662
- Caverject Injection (2%) ... 2064
- Monoket Tablets (Fewer than 1%) ... 2550
- Naprelan Tablets (Less than 1%) ... 2861
- Redux Capsules (Rare) ... 2911
- Testoderm Testosterone Transdermal System ... 486
- Testred Capsules, 10 mg ... 1308
- Thorazine ... 2701
- Winstrol Tablets ... 2468

Prostatic hypertrophy
- Android Capsules, 10 mg ... 1297
- Caverject Injection (2%) ... 2064
- Eldepryl Capsules ... 2729
- Halotestin Tablets ... 2095
- Invirase Capsules (Less than 2%) ... 2291
- Testoderm Testosterone Transdermal System (One in 104 patients) ... 486
- ▲ Vesanoid Capsules (3%) ... 2327
- Winstrol Tablets ... 2468

Prostatitis
- Caverject Injection (2%) ... 2064
- Effexor (Infrequent) ... 2825
- Kerlone Tablets (Less than 2%) ... 2588
- Testoderm Testosterone Transdermal System (Four in 104 patients) ... 486
- TICE BCG, USP (0.3%) ... 1881

Prostration
- Bicillin C-R Injection ... 2810
- Bicillin C-R 900/300 Injection ... 2812
- Bicillin L-A Injection ... 2813
- Pfizerpen for Injection ... 2022

Protein bound iodine, lowered
(see under PBI decrease)

Protein catabolism
- Celestone Soluspan Suspension ... 2484
- CORTENEMA ... 2713
- Dexacort Phosphate in Respihaler ... 1606
- Dexacort Phosphate in Turbinaire ... 1607
- Florinef Acetate Tablets ... 506
- Hydeltrasol Injection, Sterile ... 1708
- Hydeltra-T.B.A. Sterile Suspension ... 1710
- Hydrocortone Acetate Sterile Suspension ... 1712
- Hydrocortone Phosphate Injection, Sterile ... 1713
- Hydrocortone Tablets ... 1715

Proteinuria
- ▲ Accutane Capsules (Less than 1 patient in 10) ... 2252
- Altace Capsules (Scattered incidents) ... 1238
- Anaprox/Naprosyn ... 2277
- Atromid-S Capsules ... 2808
- Azulfidine (Rare) ... 2059
- ▲ Betaseron for SC Injection (5%) ... 653
- Calcium Disodium Versenate Injection ... 1548
- Capoten Tablets (Approximately 1 of 100 patients) ... 740
- Capozide Tablets (About 1 of 100 patients) ... 744
- Cataflam Tablets (Less than 1%) ... 833
- Ceclor Pulvules & Suspension (Infrequent) ... 1470
- Celontin Kapseals ... 1955
- Cleocin Phosphate Injection (Rare) ... 2068
- Cleocin Vaginal Cream (Rare) ... 2070
- Clinoril Tablets (Less than 1 in 100) ... 1658
- Crixivan Capsules (Less than 2%) ... 1670
- ▲ Cuprimine Capsules (6%) ... 1673
- Cytovene-IV (One report) ... 2270
- Daypro Caplets ... 2578
- ▲ Depen Titratable Tablets (6%) ... 2770
- Dipentum Capsules (Rare) ... 2084
- Dolobid Tablets (Less than 1 in 100) ... 1695
- EC-Naprosyn Delayed-Release Tablets ... 2277
- Elspar (Infrequent) ... 1700
- Eminase ... 2215
- Feldene Capsules (Less than 1%) ... 2008
- Floxin I.V. (More than or equal to 1%) ... 1580
- Floxin Tablets (200 mg, 300 mg, 400 mg) (More than or equal to 1%) ... 1577
- Fludara for Injection (Up to 1%) ... 658
- Fulvicin P/G Tablets (Rare) ... 2499
- Fulvicin P/G 165 & 330 Tablets (Rare) ... 2500
- Garamycin Injectable ... 2502
- ▲ Gemzar for Injection (2% to 45%) ... 1482
- Grifulvin V (griseofulvin tablets) Microsize (griseofulvin oral suspension) Microsize (Rare) ... 1944
- Gris-PEG Tablets, 125 mg & 250 mg (Rare) ... 476
- IFEX (Rare) ... 706
- Indocin (Less than 1%) ... 1723
- Intron A for Injection (Less than 5%) ... 2506
- Kerlone Tablets (Less than 2%) ... 2588
- Lotensin Tablets (Scattered incidents) ... 852
- Lotensin HCT Tablets (Scattered accounts) ... 855
- Mithracin ... 599
- Motrin Ibuprofen Suspension, Oral Drops, Chewable Tablets, Caplets ... 1563
- Myochrysine Injection ... 1754
- Naprelan Tablets ... 2861
- Anaprox/Naprosyn ... 2277
- Nebcin Vials, Hyporets & ADD-Vantage ... 1518
- Netromycin Injection 100 mg/ml ... 2516
- Neupogen for Injection (Infrequent) ... 495
- Prilosec Delayed-Release Capsules (Less than 1%) ... 516
- Primaxin I.M. ... 1770
- Primaxin I.V. ... 1772
- ▲ Proleukin for Injection (12%) ... 812
- Ridaura Capsules (0.9%) ... 2691
- Roferon-A Injection (Infrequent) ... 2308
- Sinemet CR Tablets ... 961
- Solganal Suspension ... 2530
- ▲ Tegison Capsules (1-10%) ... 2314
- Tolectin (200, 400 and 600 mg) (Less than 1%) ... 1591
- Toradol (1% or less) ... 2319
- Tornalate Metered Dose Inhaler (Rare) ... 978
- Ultram Tablets (50 mg) (Infrequent) ... 1594
- Vaqta (Isolated reports) ... 1805
- ▲ Vistide Injection (48% to 80%) ... 1057
- Cataflam/Voltaren/Voltaren-XR (Less than 1%) ... 833
- Zosyn ... 1463

Proteinuria, increased
- Bumex ... 2260
- Chemet Capsules (Up to 3.7%) ... 666
- Noroxin Tablets (1.0%) ... 1758
- Noroxin Tablets (1.0%) ... 2222
- Penetrex Tablets (Less than 1%) ... 2196

Prothrombin, decrease
(see under Hypoprothrombinemia)

Prothrombin, increase
(see under Hyperprothrombinemia)

Prothrombin time, deviation
- Bumex (0.8%) ... 2260
- Lupron Depot - 3 Month 22.5 mg ... 2743
- Rythmol Tablets–150mg, 225mg, 300mg (Less than 1%) ... 1399

Prothrombin time, increase
(see under Prothrombin time prolongation)

Prothrombin time prolongation
- Azactam for Injection ... 736
- Biaxin (1%) ... 406
- Cefizox for Intramuscular or Intravenous Use ... 1025
- Cefotan ... 2936
- Ceftin ... 1067
- Cefzil Tablets and Oral Suspension ... 747
- Ceptaz ... 1070
- Cipro I.V. ... 587
- Cipro I.V. Pharmacy Bulk Package (Less than 1%) ... 590
- Cipro Tablets ... 584
- Clinoril Tablets ... 1658
- Duricef Capsules, Tablets, and Oral Suspension ... 750
- Felbatol ... 2774
- Floxin I.V. ... 1580
- Floxin Tablets (200 mg, 300 mg, 400 mg) ... 1577
- Fortaz ... 1092
- Sterile FUDR ... 2284
- Hespan Injection ... 945
- Keftab Tablets ... 931
- Kefurox Vials, Faspak & ADD-Vantage ... 1509
- Lorabid Suspension and Pulvules (Rare) ... 1513
- Maxaquin Tablets (Less than or equal to 0.1%) ... 2593
- Maxipime for Injection (1.6%) ... 758
- Merrem I.V. (Greater than 0.2%) ... 2952
- Netromycin Injection 100 mg/ml (1 of 1000 patients) ... 2516
- Noroxin Tablets ... 1758
- Noroxin Tablets ... 2222
- Oncaspar ... 2194
- Ortho-Cyclen/Ortho-Tri-Cyclen ... 1914
- Ortho-Cyclen/Ortho Tri-Cyclen ... 1914
- Oxandrin ... 783
- Panhematin ... 452
- Penetrex Tablets ... 2196
- Pentaspan Injection ... 954
- Primaxin I.M. ... 1770
- Primaxin I.V. ... 1772
- Provera Tablets ... 2110
- Questran ... 774
- Rocephin Injectable Vials, ADD-Vantage, Galaxy Container (Less than 1%) ... 2305
- Suprax (Rare) ... 1443
- Tazicef for Injection ... 2697
- Tazidime Vials, Faspak & ADD-Vantage ... 1531
- ▲ Tegison Capsules (10-25%) ... 2314
- Timentin for Injection ... 2706
- Vantin for Oral Suspension and Vantin Tablets ... 2112
- Zinacef ... 1184
- Zosyn ... 1463

Pruritus
- Abelcet Injection ... 1540
- Accupril Tablets (0.5% to 1.0%) ... 1950
- ▲ Accutane Capsules (Up to 80%) ... 2252
- Aclovate (Approximately 2%) ... 1061
- Actigall Capsules ... 818
- Adalat Capsules (10 mg and 20 mg) (2% or less) ... 580
- Adalat CC (Less than 1.0%) ... 582
- Adapin Capsules (Occasional) ... 1542
- ▲ AeroBid Inhaler System (3% to 9%) ... 1004
- ▲ Aerobid-M Inhaler System (3% to 9%) ... 1004
- AK-Spore ... ⊙ 205
- Aldactazide Tablets ... 2556
- Alfenta Injection (0.3% to 1%) ... 1334
- Alferon N Injection (2%) ... 2142
- Alkeran for Injection ... 1196
- Altace Capsules (Less than 1%) ... 1238
- Alupent Tablets (0.4%) ... 672
- Amaryl Tablets (Less than 1%) ... 1241
- Ambien Tablets (Infrequent) ... 2559
- Amen Tablets (Occasional) ... 785
- Americaine Anesthetic Lubricant ... 1603
- Americaine Otic Topical Anesthetic Ear Drops ... 1603
- Amicar Syrup, Tablets, and Injection ... 1312
- ▲ Anafranil Capsules (2% to 6%) ... 819
- Analpram-HC Rectal Cream 1% and 2.5% ... 993
- ▲ Anaprox/Naprosyn (3% to 9%) ... 2277
- Ancef Injection ... 2632
- Ancobon Capsules ... 2254
- Antivenin (Crotalidae) Polyvalent ... 2803
- Anusol-HC Cream 2.5% (Infrequent to frequent) ... 1953
- Anusol-HC Suppositories ... 1954
- Apresazide Capsules (Less frequent) ... 824
- Apresoline Hydrochloride Tablets (Less frequent) ... 826
- Aralen Hydrochloride Injection ... 2430
- Aralen Phosphate Tablets ... 2431
- Arimidex Tablets (2% to 5%) ... 2932
- ▲ Asacol Delayed-Release Tablets (3%) ... 2129
- Asendin Tablets (Less than 1%) ... 1419
- ▲ Astramorph/PF Injection, USP (Preservative-Free) (High incidence) ... 526
- Atromid-S Capsules (Less often) ... 2808
- Atrovent Inhalation Aerosol (Less frequent) ... 674
- A/T/S 2% Acne Topical Gel (Occasional) ... 1244
- A/T/S 2% Acne Topical Solution (Occasional) ... 1244
- Augmentin ... 2637
- Augmentin Tablets ... 2640
- Axid Pulvules (1.7%) ... 1468
- Axocet Capsules (Infrequent) ... 2469
- Aygestin Tablets ... 990
- Azactam for Injection (Less than 1%) ... 736
- Azelex (Approximately 1% to 5%) ... 471
- Azulfidine (One in every 30 patients or less) ... 2059
- Bactrim DS Tablets ... 2257
- Bactrim I.V. Infusion ... 2255
- Bactrim ... 2257

(▭ Described in PDR For Nonprescription Drugs)   Incidence data in parenthesis; ▲ 3% or more   (⊙ Described in PDR For Ophthalmology)

Pruritus
Side Effects Index
1432

Bactroban Nasal (1%) 2643
Bactroban Ointment (1%) 2642
Benemid Tablets 1651
Bentyl 1246
Benzamycin Topical Gel (Occasional) 919
Betagan (Rare) ◉ 230
Betapace Tablets (Rare) 637
Blenoxane 697
Blocadren Tablets (1.1%) 1654
▲Bromfed-DM Cough Syrup (Among most frequent) 1832
Brontex (Infrequent) 2130
Bumex (0.1% to 0.4%) 2260
Buprenex Injectable (Less than 1%) 2170
BuSpar Tablets (Infrequent) 738
Cafergot 2376
Calcijex Injection 412
Capoten Tablets (About 2 of 100 patients) 740
Capozide Tablets (About 2 of 100 patients) 744
Carafate Suspension (Less than 0.5%) 1250
Carafate Tablets (Less than 0.5%) 1249
Carbocaine Injection 2432
Cardioquin Tablets 2146
Cardizem CD Capsules (Less than 1%) 1251
Cardizem SR Capsules (Less than 1%) 1255
Cardizem Injectable (Less than 1%) 1253
Cardizem Tablets (Less than 1%) 1257
Cardura Tablets (1%) 1993
Casodex Tablets (2% to 5%) 2934
Cataflam Tablets (1% to 3%) 833
Catapres Tablets (About 7 in 1,000 patients) 679
▲Catapres-TTS (51 of 101 patients) 680
Caverject Injection (Less than 1%) 2064
Ceclor Pulvules & Suspension (Less than 1 in 200) 1470
Cedax (0.1% to 1%) 2480
Cefizox for Intramuscular or Intravenous Use (1% to 5%) 1025
Cefotan (1 in 700) 2936
Ceftin (0.1% to 1%) 1067
▲CellCept Capsules (More than or equal to 3%) 2265
Ceptaz (2% of patients) 1070
▲Cerebyx Injection (7 of 16 volunteers; 2.8% to 48.9%) 1956
Ceredase 1055
Cerezyme (One patient) 1056
Cerumenex Drops (1% of 2,700 patients) 2148
▲Chemet Capsules (2.6% to 11.2%) 666
Chloromium (A few instances) 2371
Chloroptic S.O.P. ◉ 236
Cipro I.V. (1% or less) 587
Cipro I.V. Pharmacy Bulk Package (Less than 1%) 590
Cipro Tablets (Less than 1%) 584
Claforan Sterile and Injection (2.4%) 1259
Claritin Tablets (2% or fewer patients) 2485
Claritin-D Tablets (Less frequent) 2487
▲Cleocin T Topical (10%) 2072
Cleocin Vaginal Cream (2%) 2070
Clinoril Tablets (Greater than 1%) 1658
Clomid 1262
Clozaril Tablets (Less than 1%) 2377
▲Cognex Capsules (7%) 1961
ColBENEMID Tablets 1662
Compazine 2644
Cordran Lotion (Infrequent) 1854
Cordran Tape (Infrequent) 1855
Cormax Ointment (0.5%) 1856
Cormax Scalp Application (Infrequent) 1857
Cortisporin Cream 1073
Cortisporin Ointment 1074
Cortisporin Ophthalmic Ointment Sterile 1074
Cortisporin Ophthalmic Suspension Sterile 1075
Cortisporin Otic Solution Sterile 1076
Cortisporin Otic Suspension Sterile 1077
Coumadin (Infrequent) 941
Cozaar Tablets (Less than 1%) 1668
Crixivan Capsules (Less than 2%) 1670
▲Cuprimine Capsules (5%) 1673
Cutivate Cream (2.9%) 1078
Cutivate Ointment (Less than 1%) 1078
Cycrin Tablets (Occasional) 991
▲Cytadren Tablets (1 in 20) 837
Cytosar-U Sterile Powder (Less frequent) 2077
▲Cytovene (6%) 2270
▲DHCplus Capsules (Among most frequent) 2148
D.H.E. 45 Injection 2381
Dalgan Injection (Less than 1%) 529
Dalmane Capsules (Rare) 2329
Danocrine Capsules 2437
Dantrium Capsules (Less frequent) 2131
Daranide Tablets 1676
▲DaunoXome (Up to 7%) 1842
Daypro Caplets (Less than 1%) 2578
Decadron Phosphate Topical Cream 1686
Decaspray Topical Aerosol 1689
Demerol 2438
Depakene 416
Depakote Tablets (1% to 5%) 418
▲Depen Titratable Tablets (5%) 2770
Depo-Provera Sterile Aqueous Suspension 2083
Dermatop Emollient Cream 0.1% (Less than 1%) 1264
Desferal Vials 838
DesOwen Cream, Ointment and Lotion (Less than 2%) 1032
Desyrel and Desyrel Dividose 504
DiaBeta Tablets (1.5%) 1265
Diabinese Tablets (Less than 3%) 2002
Didronel Tablets 2133
▲Differin Gel (10% to 40%) 1033
Dilacor XR Extended-release Capsules 2183
Dilaudid-HP Injection (Less frequent) 1384
Dilaudid-HP Lyophilized Powder 250 mg (Less frequent) 1384
Dilaudid Tablets and Liquid 1386
Dimetane-DC Cough Syrup 2232
Dimetane-DX Cough Syrup 2233
Dipentum Capsules (1.3%) 2084
Diprivan Injectable Emulsion (Less than 1%) 2939
Diprolene AF Cream 0.05% (Infrequent) 2489
Diprolene Gel 0.05% (2%) 2490
Diprolene Lotion 0.05% (Infrequent) 2491
Diprolene Ointment 0.05% (2 per 767 patients) 2491
Diupres Tablets 1691
Dolobid Tablets (Less than 1 in 100) 1695
Dopram Injectable 2235
Doral Tablets 2773
▲Dovonex Cream 0.005% (1% to 10%) 2792
▲Dovonex Ointment 0.005% (Approximately 10% to 15%) 2793
Doxil (1% to 5%) 2613
▲Duragesic Transdermal System (1% to 10%) 1336
▲Duramorph Injection (High incidence; occasional) 983
Dynabac (1.2%) 668
DynaCirc Capsules (0.5% to 1%) 2381
DynaCirc CR Tablets (0.5% to 1.0%) 2383
Easprin 1971
▲EC-Naprosyn Delayed-Release Tablets (3% to 9%) 2277
Effexor (1%) 2825
▲Efudex (Among most frequent) 2280
▲Elimite (permethrin) 5% Cream (7%) 475
▲Elocon Cream 0.1% (1.6% to approximately 7%) 2492
Elocon Lotion 0.1% (1 in 209 patients) 2493
▲Elocon Ointment 0.1% (4.8% to approximately 7%) 2494
Emcyt Capsules (2%) 2085
Emgel 2% Topical Gel (Occasional) 1081
Eminase (Occasional) 2215
EMLA Cream (2%) 536
Engerix-B Unit-Dose Vials (Less than 1%) 2656
Ergamisol Tablets (1% to 2%) 1340
Ergomar Tablets 1543
Erycette (erythromycin 2%) Topical Solution 1943
Esgic-plus Capsules (Infrequent) 1012
Esgic-plus Tablets (Infrequent) 1012
Estring Vaginal Ring (At least 1 report) 2086
Ethmozine Tablets (Less than 2%) 2217
Etopophos for Injection (Infrequent) 701
Etoposide Injection (Infrequent) 539
Etrafon 2495
Eulexin Capsules 2498
Exact ▣ 722
▲Exelderm Cream 1.0% (3%) 2794
Exelderm Solution 1.0% (Approximately 1%) 2795
Famvir Tablets (0.9% to 3.7%) 2660
Fansidar Tablets 2281
Felbatol (Frequent) 2774
Feldene Capsules (Occasional) 2008
Fioricet Tablets (Infrequent) 2386
Fioricet with Codeine Capsules (Infrequent) 2387
Fiorinal with Codeine Capsules (Infrequent) 2390
Flagyl I.V. 2373
Flexeril Tablets (Rare) 1701
▲Flolan for Injection (4%) 1085
Florone/Florone E 921
Floxin I.V. (1% to 3%) 1580
Floxin Tablets (200 mg, 300 mg, 400 mg) (1% to 3%) 1577
Fludara for Injection (1% to 3%) 658
Fluorescite ◉ 217
Fluoroplex Topical Solution & Cream 1% 475
Fortaz (2%) 1092
Foscavir Injection (Between 1% and 5%) 541
Fragmin Injection (Rare) 2088
Fungizone Intravenous 507
Furacin Soluble Dressing (Approximately 1%) 2220
Furacin Topical Cream (Approximately 1%) 2220
Gamimune N, 5% Immune Globulin Intravenous (Human), 5% 612
Gamimune N, 10% Immune Globulin Intravenous (Human), 10% (A single incidence) 615
Gammar-P I.V., Immune Globulin Intravenous (Human) 798
Gantanol Tablets 2285
Gantrisin 2286
Garamycin Cream 0.1% 2501
Garamycin Injectable 2502
Garamycin Ointment 0.1% 2501
▲Gastrocrom Capsules (3 of 87 patients) 1611
▲Gastrocrom Oral Concentrate (3 of 87 patients) 1611
▲Gemzar for Injection (13%) 1482
Geocillin Tablets (Infrequent) 2009
Glucotrol Tablets (About 1 in 70) 2011
Glucotrol XL Extended Release Tablets (Less than 3%) 2012
Glynase PresTab Tablets (1.5%) 2091
Habitrol Nicotine Transdermal System (Once in 35% of patients) 884
Halcion Tablets 2093
Halog (Infrequent) 2795
Havrix (Less than 1%) 2663
Heparin Lock Flush Solution 2831
Heparin Sodium Injection 2832
Heparin Sodium Vials 1486
Hespan Injection 945
Hexalen Capsules (Less than 1%) 2760
Hismanal Tablets (Less frequent) 1341
Hivid Tablets (Less than 1%) 2287
Humalog Injection (Less common) 1488
Hycodan Tablets and Syrup 946
Hycomine 947
Hydralazine Hydrochloride Injection USP (Less frequent) 2712
Hydrocet Capsules 787
Hydropres Tablets 1718
Hyskon Hysteroscopy Fluid (Rare) 1633
Hytone 922
Hytone Ointment 2 ½% 923
Hytrin Capsules (At least 1%) 434
Hyzaar Tablets 1720
IBU Tablets (Greater than 1%) 1389
Imdur (Less than or equal to 5%) 1362
Imitrex Injection (Infrequent) 1095
Imitrex Tablets (Infrequent) 1099
Indocin (Less than 1%) 1723
INFeD (Iron Dextran Injection, USP) 2478
Infumorph 200 and Infumorph 500 Sterile Solutions (Occasional) 985
▲Intron A for Injection (Up to 11%) 2506
IOPIDINE Sterile Ophthalmic Solution ◉ 218
Ismo Tablets (Fewer than 1%) 2844
Isoptin Injectable (Rare) 1391
JE-VAX 904
Kadian Capsules (Less than 3%) 2948
Kefurox Vials, Faspak & ADD-Vantage (Less than 1 in 250) 1509
Kerlone Tablets (Less than 2%) 2588
▲Lamictal Tablets (3.1%) 1105
Lamisil Cream 1% (0.2%) 2393
Lamisil Tablets (2.8%) 2394
▲Lamprene Capsules (1-5%) 846
Lariam Tablets (Less than 1%) 2295
Lasix Injection, Oral Solution and Tablets 1267
Lescol Capsules 2395
▲Leukine (23%) 1317
▲Leustatin (6%) 1889
Levo-Dromoran 2297
Levoprome 1321
Lidex (Infrequent) 2299
Limbitrol 2333
Lioresal Intrathecal (Up to 4.0%) 1634
Lioresal Tablets 847
Lithium Carbonate Capsules & Tablets 2352
Lithonate/Lithotabs/Lithobid 2721
Locoid Cream, Ointment and Topical Solution (Infrequent) 994
Lodine Capsules and Tablets (1% to 3%) 2849
Lomotil 2591
Lopid Tablets 1974
▲Lopressor (5%) 848
Lopressor HCT Tablets (Fewer than 1 in 100) 850
Lorabid Suspension and Pulvules 1513
Lortab 2751
Lotensin Tablets 852
Lotensin HCT Tablets (0.3% or more) 855
Lotrimin 2514
Lotrisone Cream 2515
Loxitane 1426
Ludiomil Tablets (Rare) 861
Lupron Injection (Less than 5%) 2736
Lutrepulse for Injection 998
LUVOX Tablets 2723
MS Contin Tablets (Less frequent) 2149
MSIR (Infrequent) 2152
Macrobid Capsules (Less than 1%) 2138
Macrodantin Capsules 2140
Marcaine (Rare) 2446
Marcaine Spinal (Rare) 2449
Matulane Capsules 2300
Mavik Tablets (0.3% to 1.0%) 1407
Maxair Autohaler 1550
Maxair Inhaler (Less than 1%) 1552
Maxaquin Tablets (Less than 1%) 2593
Maxipime for Injection (0.1% to 1%) 758
Mefoxin 1734
Mefoxin Premixed Intravenous Solution 1737
Megace Oral Suspension (1% to 3%) 708
▲Mepron Suspension (5%) 1206
Merrem I.V. (1.6%) 2952
Methadone Hydrochloride Oral Concentrate 2356
Methadone Hydrochloride Oral Solution & Tablets 2357
Methotrexate Sodium Tablets, Injection, for Injection and LPF Injection (1% to 3%) 1322
MetroCream (Less than 3%) 1034
MetroGel-Vaginal (Equal to or less than 2%) 917
▲Mevacor Tablets (0.5% to 5.2%) 1742
Mezlin 594
Mezlin Pharmacy Bulk Package 597
Miacalcin Nasal Spray (Less than 1%) 2403
Micronase Tablets (1.5%) 2099
Midamor Tablets (Less than or equal to 1%) 1746
Minipress Capsules (Less than 1%) 2015
Minizide Capsules (Rare) 2016
Mintezol 1747
Moduretic Tablets (Greater than 1%, less than 3%) 1748
▲8-MOP Capsules (Approximately 10%) 1294
Monocid Injection (Less than 1%) 2674
Monoket Tablets (Up to 2%) 2550
Monopril Tablets (0.2% to 1.0%) 762
Motofen Tablets 789
Motrin Ibuprofen Suspension, Oral Drops, Chewable Tablets, Caplets (1% to less than 3%) 1563
Myambutol Tablets 1432
Mycelex Troches 601
Mykrox Tablets (Less than 2%) 1617

(▣ Described in PDR For Nonprescription Drugs) Incidence data in parenthesis; ▲ 3% or more (◉ Described in PDR For Ophthalmology)

Myochrysine Injection 1754
Naftin Cream 1% (2%) 477
Naftin Gel 1% (1.0%) 477
▲ Nalfon 200 Pulvules & Nalfon Tablets (4.2%) 933
Naprelan Tablets (Less than 1%) 2861
▲ Anaprox/Naprosyn (3% to 9%) 2277
Navane Capsules and Concentrate 2018
Navane Intramuscular 2019
Navelbine Injection 1212
Nebcin Vials, Hyporets & ADD-Vantage 1518
NegGram 2453
NeoDecadron Topical Cream 1757
Neoral (Rare) 2405
Neosporin Ophthalmic Ointment Sterile 1130
Neosporin Ophthalmic Solution Sterile 1131
Nescaine/Nescaine MPF 549
Netromycin Injection 100 mg/ml (4 or 5 of 1000 patients) 2516
Neurontin Capsules (1.3%) 1978
▲ Neutrexin for Injection (5.5%) 2761
Nicotrol NS Nicotine Nasal Spray (2%) 1565
Nimotop Capsules (Less than 1%) 603
▲ Nipent for Injection (10% to 21%) 2733
▲ Nizoral 2% Cream (5%) 1344
Nizoral 2% Shampoo (One occurrence in 41 patients) 1344
Nizoral Tablets (1.5%) 1345
Norflex 1554
Normodyne Injection (Rare; 1%) 2519
Normodyne Tablets (Rare) 2522
Noroxin Tablets (0.3 to 1.0%) 1758
Noroxin Tablets (0.3% to 1.0%) 2222
Norpace (1 to 3%) 2596
Norplant System 2868
Norpramin Tablets 1273
Norvasc Tablets (More than 0.1% to 1%) 2020
Norvir (Less than 2%) 447
Nubain Injection (1% or less) 952
Numorphan Injection 953
Numorphan Suppositories 953
Omnipen for Oral Suspension 2873
Oncaspar (Less than 1%) 2194
Oramorph SR (Morphine Sulfate Sustained Release Tablets) (Less frequent) 2359
Orthoclone OKT3 Sterile Solution 1892
Orudis Capsules (Less than 1%) 2874
Oruvail Capsules (Less than 1%) 2874
Oxistat (1.6%) 1139
▲ Oxsoralen-Ultra Capsules (10%) 1302
▲ OxyContin Tablets (13%) 2163
OxyIR Capsules 2167
Pamelor 2409
Pandel Cream, 0.1% 2475
Paraplatin for Injection 713
Paxil Tablets (Frequent) 2681
Pediazole Suspension 2340
Pediotic Suspension Sterile 1140
Penetrex Tablets (1%) 2196
Pentasa (Less than 1%) 1275
Pepcid Injection (Infrequent) 1765
Pepcid (Infrequent) 1763
Percocet Tablets 955
Percodan Tablets 955
Percodan-Demi Tablets 956
Permax Tablets (Infrequent) 571
Persantine Tablets 686
Phenergan with Codeine (Infrequent) 2883
Phenergan VC with Codeine 2888
PhosLo Tablets (Isolated cases) 695
Phrenilin (Infrequent) 790
Pipracil (Less frequent) 1435
Plaquenil Sulfate Tablets 2459
PMB 200 and PMB 400 2890
PPD Tine Test 2993
Pramosone Cream, Lotion & Ointment 995
Pravachol Tablets 770
Premphase 2900
Prempro 2905
Prevacid Delayed-Release Capsules (Less than 1%) 2746
Prilosec Delayed-Release Capsules (Less than 1%) 516
Primaxin I.M. 1770
Primaxin I.V. (0.3%) 1772
Prinivil Tablets (Greater than 1%) 1776
Prinzide Tablets (0.3 to 1%) 1780
Procanbid Extended-Release Tablets (Occasional) 1983
Procardia Capsules (2% or less) 2024
Procardia XL Extended Release Tablets (Less than 3%) 2026
ProctoCream-HC 2.5% (Infrequent to frequent) 2552
Proglycem 575
▲ Prograf (11% to 36%) 1028
▲ Proleukin for Injection (48%) 812
Prolixin 510
▲ Proloprim Tablets (Most often) 1141
Propulsid (1.2%) 1346
ProSom Tablets (1%) 457
Prostep (nicotine transdermal system) 1439
Provera Tablets 2110
Prozac Pulvules & Liquid, Oral Solution (2.4% to 3%) 935
Psorcon Cream 0.05% (Infrequent) 924
Psorcon Ointment 0.05% 923
Pyrazinamide Tablets 1442
Pyridium 1985
Quinaglute Dura-Tabs Tablets 644
Quinidex Extentabs 2240
RMS Suppositories CII 2766
Recombivax HB (Less than 1%) 1787
Redux Capsules (Frequent) 2911
▲ Relafen Tablets (3% to 9%) 2688
Remeron Tablets (Frequent) 1878
Renova (tretinoin emollient cream) 0.05% (Almost all subjects) 1945
ReoPro Vials (0.3%) 1526
RespiGam 1631
Retrovir Capsules 1216
Retrovir I.V. Infusion 1221
Retrovir Syrup 1216
▲ Rev-Eyes Ophthalmic Eyedrops 0.5% (10% to 40%) ⊙ 324
ReVia Tablets (Less than 1%) 957
Revex (nalmefene hydrochloride injection) (Less than 1%) 1863
Rhinocort Nasal Inhaler (Less than 1%) 552
▲ Ridaura Capsules (17%) 2691
Rifadin (Occasional) 1276
Rifamate Capsules (Occasional) 1278
Rifater (Occasional) 1280
▲ Rilutek Tablets (2.5% to 3.8%) 2198
Rimactane Capsules (Occasional) 865
Risperdal Tablets (Infrequent) 1348
Robaxin Injectable 2245
Robaxin Tablets 2246
Robaxisal Tablets 2246
Rocaltrol Capsules 2303
Rocephin Injectable Vials, ADD-Vantage, Galaxy Container (Less than 1%) 2305
▲ Roferon-A Injection (5% to 13%) 2308
Rowasa (1.23%) 2727
Roxanol 2365
Roxicodone Tablets, Oral Solution & Intensol (Oxycodone) 2366
Rythmol Tablets–150mg, 225mg, 300mg (Less than 1%) 1399
Salagen Tablets (1%) 1546
Sandimmune (Rare) 2416
Sandostatin Injection (1% to 4%) 2421
Sectral Capsules (Up to 2%) 2914
Sedapap Tablets 50 mg/650 mg (Infrequent) 1826
Seldane Tablets (1.0% to 1.6%) 1284
Seldane-D Extended-Release Tablets 1286
Sensorcaine (Rare) 554
Septra 1146
Septra I.V. Infusion 1142
Septra I.V. Infusion ADD-Vantage Vials 1144
Septra 1146
Ser-Ap-Es Tablets 867
Serentil 689
Serzone Tablets (2%) 776
Sinequan (Occasional) 2028
Skelaxin Tablets 793
Slo-Niacin Tablets 2767
Solganal Suspension 2530
Soma Compound w/Codeine Tablets (Rare) 2784
Soma Compound Tablets (Less common) 2783
Soma Tablets 2782
▲ Spectazole (econazole nitrate 1%) Cream (3%) 1947
Sporanox Capsules (0.7% to 2.5%) 1352
Stadol (1% or greater) 779
Stelazine 2692
Streptase for Infusion 557
Sublimaze Injection 463
▲ Sufenta Injection (25%) 1355
Sular Tablets (Less than or equal to 1%) 2961
Sulfamylon Cream 940
Supprelin Injection (1% to 3%) 2230
Suprane (desflurane, USP) (Less than 1%) 1865
Suprax (Less than 2%) 1443
Surmontil Capsules 2917
Synalar (Infrequent) 2299
Synarel Nasal Solution for Central Precocious Puberty (2.6%) 2603
T-Stat 2.0% Topical Solution and Pads 2797
Talwin Injection 2465
Talwin Nx Tablets 2467
Tambocor Tablets (Less than 1%) 1555
Tapazole Tablets 1361
Taxotere for Injection Concentrate 2204
Tazicef for Injection (2%) 2697
Tazidime Vials, Faspak & ADD-Vantage (2%) 1531
▲ Tegison Capsules (50-75%) 2314
Temovate Cream (Less frequent) 1152
Temovate E Emollient (Less than 2%) 1154
▲ Temovate Gel (Among most frequent) 1153
Temovate Ointment (0.5%) 1152
Temovate Scalp Application (1 of 294 patients; infrequent) 1153
Tenex Tablets (3% or less) 2249
Terazol 3 Vaginal Suppositories (1.8% of 284 patients) 1942
Tessalon Perles 1018
▲ Testoderm Testosterone Transdermal System (7%) 486
THERAMYCIN Z 2% Solution 1629
Tiazac Capsules (Less than 1%) 1019
Ticar for Injection 2704
Ticlid Tablets (1.3%) 2317
Timentin for Injection 2706
Timolide Tablets 1791
Timoptic in Ocudose 1796
Timoptic Sterile Ophthalmic Solution 1794
Timoptic-XE 1798
Tofranil Ampuls 873
Tofranil Tablets 875
Tofranil-PM Capsules 876
Tonocard Tablets (Less than 1%) 519
Topicort Emollient Cream 0.25% (Infrequent) 1289
Topicort Gel 0.05% (Infrequent) 1290
Topicort LP Emollient Cream 0.05% (0.8%) 1289
Topicort Ointment 0.25% (Infrequent) 1291
▲ Toprol-XL Tablets (About 5 of 100 patients) 560
Toradol (Greater than 1%) 2319
Tornalate Solution for Inhalation, 0.2% 976
Tracrium Injection (0.2%) 1155
Trandate (Rare; 1 of 100 patients) 1158
Trasylol 607
Trental Tablets (Less than 1%) 1291
Triavil Tablets 1800
Tridesilon Cream 0.05% (Infrequent) 609
Tridesilon Ointment 0.05% (Infrequent) 610
Trilafon 2532
Trilisate (Less than 1%) 2155
Trimpex Tablets 2323
Trusopt Sterile Ophthalmic Solution 1803
T.R.U.E. Test (Common; up to 48 reports) 1162
Tuberculin, Old, Tine Test 2994
Tussionex Pennkinetic Extended-Release Suspension 1624
Tylenol with Codeine 1592
Tylox Capsules 1593
Tympagesic Ear Drops 2476
▲ Ultram Tablets (50 mg) (8% to 11%) 1594
▲ Ultravate Cream 0.05% (4.4%) 2797
Ultravate Ointment 0.05% (Less frequent) 2798
Unasyn (Less than 1%) 2035
Univasc Tablets (Less than 1%) 2553
▲ Vagistat-1 (Approximately 5%) 783
Vancocin HCl, Oral Solution & Pulvules 1536
Vancocin HCl, Vials & ADD-Vantage 1534
Vaqta (Less than 1%) 1805
Varivax (Greater than or equal to 1%) 1807
Vaseretic Tablets (0.5% to 2.0%) 1810
Vasotec I.V. 1814
Vasotec Tablets (0.5% to 1.0%) 1816
VePesid Capsules and Injection (Infrequent) 727
Versed Injection (Less than 1%) 2324
▲ Vesanoid Capsules (20%) 2327
Vexol 1% Ophthalmic Suspension (1% to 5%) ⊙ 227
Vicodin HP Tablets 1403
▲ Videx Tablets, Powder for Oral Solution, & Pediatric Powder for Oral Solution (7% to 70%) 2980
Viramune Tablets 2368
Visken Tablets (1%) 2428
Vistide Injection 1057
Vivactil Tablets 1820
Vivelle Transdermal System (One of the two most common) 880
Cataflam/Voltaren/Voltaren-XR (1% to 3%) 833
Wellbutrin Tablets (2.2%) 1177
Westcort Cream 0.2% (Infrequent) 2799
Westcort Ointment 0.2% (2%) 2800
Wigraine Tablets 1884
Xanax Tablets 2115
Xerac AC Solution 1990
Yodoxin Tablets 1235
Zantac Injection 1180
Zebeta Tablets 1457
Zemuron Injection (Less than 1%) 1885
▲ Zerit Capsules (Fewer than 1% to 12%) 731
Zestoretic Tablets (0.3 to 1%) 2968
Zestril Tablets (Greater than 1%) 2972
Ziac 1459
Zinacef (Fewer than 1 in 250 patients) 1184
Zocor Tablets 1821
Zofran Injection (2%) 1227
▲ Zofran Tablets (5%) 1231
Zoladex (2%) 2976
▲ Zoladex 3-month (1% to 5%) 2978
Zoloft Tablets (Infrequent) 2051
▲ Zosyn (3.1% to 3.2%) 1463
Zovirax Capsules 1187
Zovirax Ointment 5% 1190
Zovirax Sterile Powder (Approximately 2%) 1191
Zovirax 1187
Zyloprim Tablets (Less than 1%) 1194
Zyrtec Tablets (Less than 2%) 2053

Pruritus, ear lobes

Miacalcin Injection 2402

Pruritus, exacerbation of

Actigall Capsules (One patient) 818
▲ Zonalon Cream (Approximately 1% to 10%) 1042

Pruritus, genital

Anafranil Capsules (Infrequent) 819
Ancef Injection 2632
Avonex 662
Ceclor Pulvules & Suspension (Less than 1 in 100) 1470
Ceftin (0.1% to 1%) 1067
Cefzil Tablets and Oral Suspension (1.6%) 747
Cipro Tablets (1%) 584
Cognex Capsules (Infrequent) 1961
▲ Condylox Topical Solution (50% to 65%) 1853
Duricef Capsules, Tablets, and Oral Suspension 750
Estring Vaginal Ring (1% to 3%) 2086
▲ Floxin I.V. (1% to 6%) 1580
▲ Floxin Tablets (200 mg, 300 mg, 400 mg) (1% to 6%) 1577
Foscavir Injection (Less than 1%) 541
Keflex Pulvules & Oral Suspension 930
Keftab Tablets 931
Kefzol Vials, Faspak & ADD-Vantage 1511
Neurontin Capsules (Rare) 1978
Nolvadex Tablets (Infrequent) 2957
Primaxin I.M. 1770
Primaxin I.V. (Less than 0.2%) 1772
ProSom Tablets (Infrequent) 457
Risperdal Tablets (Rare) 1348
Supprelin Injection (1% to 3%) 2230
Suprax (Less than 2%) 1443
▲ Terazol 3 Vaginal Cream (5%) 1941
Terazol 3 Vaginal Suppositories (1.8% of 284 patients) 1942
Terazol 7 Vaginal Cream (2.3% of 521 patients) 1943
▲ Vagistat-1 (Approximately 5%) 783
Vantin for Oral Suspension and Vantin Tablets (Less than 1% to greater than 1%) 2112
Zosyn (1.0% or less) 1463

Pruritus, injection site

▲ Alferon N Injection (12%) 2142

(Described in PDR For Nonprescription Drugs) Incidence data in parenthesis; ▲ 3% or more (⊙ Described in PDR For Ophthalmology)

Pruritus, injection site
Side Effects Index
1434

▲ Cardizem Injectable (3.9%) 1253
Ceredase 1055
Cipro I.V. (1% or less) 587
Diprivan Injectable Emulsion (Less than 1%) 2939
Engerix-B Unit-Dose Vials (Less than 1%) 2656
Factrel (Occasional) 2996
Helixate, Antihemophilic Factor (Recombinant) 799
Humalog Injection 1488
Humulin 50/50, 100 Units 1491
Humulin 70/30, 100 Units 1492
Humulin L, 100 Units 1494
Regular, 100 Units 1503
Pork Regular, 100 Units 1507
▲ Imovax Rabies Vaccine (About 25%) 899
Intron A for Injection (Less than 5%) 2506
KOGENATE Antihemophilic Factor (Recombinant) 626
MSTA Mumps Skin Test Antigen 2988
▲ Rabies Vaccine, Imovax Rabies I.D. (About 25%) 901
▲ Supprelin Injection (45%) 2230
Tubersol (Tuberculin Purified Protein Derivative (Mantoux)) 2988
Vaqta (Less than 1%) 1805
▲ Varivax (19.3% to 32.5%) 1807
Velosulin BR Human Insulin 10 ml Vials 1847

Pruritus, localized

▲ Androderm Testosterone Transdermal System (37%) 2634
Epifoam (Infrequent) 2543
Eskalith 2658
Loprox 1% Cream and Lotion (1 out of 514 patients) 1269
▲ Norplant System (3.7%) 2868
▲ Polytrim Ophthalmic Solution Sterile (Among most frequent) 479
ProctoFoam-HC 2552

Pruritus, not associated with rash

Combipres Tablets (About 7 in 1,000) 682

Pruritus, ocular

▲ AKTOB (Among most frequent) ⊙ 207
▲ Alomide Ophthalmic Solution (1% to 5%) 465
Aredia for Injection (One patient) 827
▲ Iopidine 0.5% (10%) ⊙ 219
Ocuflox Ophthalmic Solution 478
▲ Polysporin Ophthalmic Ointment Sterile (Among those occurring most often) 1140
Stimate, (desmopressin acetate) Nasal Spray, 1.5 mg/mL 806
Tobrex Ophthalmic Ointment and Solution (Less than 3% of 100 patients) ⊙ 226

Pruritus, rhinal

Atrovent Nasal Spray 0.03% (2.0%) 676
Intal Inhaler (Rare) 2185
Intal Nebulizer Solution 2186
▲ Miacalcin Nasal Spray (10.6%) 2403

Pruritus ani

Ancef Injection 2632
Estring Vaginal Ring (At least 1 report) 2086
Foscavir Injection (Less than 1%) 541
Furoxone 2221
Keflex Pulvules & Oral Suspension 930
Keftab Tablets 931
Kefzol Vials, Faspak & ADD-Vantage 1511
Noroxin Tablets (Less frequent) 1758
Noroxin Tablets (Less frequent) 2222
Yodoxin Tablets 1235

Pseudolactation

Ser-Ap-Es Tablets 867

Pseudolymphoma

Dilantin Infatabs 1967
Dilantin Kapseals 1965
Dilantin-125 Suspension 1969

Pseudomembranous colitis

Amoxil 2631
Ancef Injection 2632
Augmentin 2637
Augmentin Tablets 2640
Azactam for Injection (Less than 1%) 736
Benzamycin Topical Gel 919
Biaxin 406
Ceclor Pulvules & Suspension 1470
Cedax 2480
Cefizox for Intravenous or Intravenous Use 1025
Cefobid Intravenous/Intramuscular 1996
Cefobid Pharmacy Bulk Package - Not for Direct Infusion 1999
▲ Cefotan (Most frequent) 2936
Ceftin 1067
Cefzil Tablets and Oral Suspension (Rare) 747
Ceptaz 1070
Chibroxin Sterile Ophthalmic Solution (With oral form) 1657
Cipro I.V. (1% or less) 587
Cipro I.V. Pharmacy Bulk Package (Less than 1%) 590
Cipro Tablets 584
Claforan Sterile and Injection 1259
Cleocin Phosphate Injection 2068
Cleocin T Topical (Rare) 2072
Cleocin Vaginal Cream 2070
Duricef Capsules, Tablets, and Oral Suspension 750
E.E.S. (Rare) 427
E-Mycin Tablets 1388
ERYC (Rare) 1972
EryPed (Rare) 425
Ery-Tab Tablets (Rare) 426
Erythrocin Stearate Filmtab (Rare) 429
Erythromycin Base Filmtab (Rare) 430
Erythromycin Delayed-Release Capsules, USP (Rare) 431
Floxin I.V. 1580
Floxin Tablets (200 mg, 300 mg, 400 mg) 1577
Fortaz (Less frequent) 1092
Foscavir Injection (Less than 1%) 541
Gantrisin 2286
Keflex Pulvules & Oral Suspension 930
Keftab Tablets 931
Kefurox Vials, Faspak & ADD-Vantage (1 in 440) 1509
Kefzol Vials, Faspak & ADD-Vantage 1511
Lorabid Suspension and Pulvules 1513
Macrobid Capsules (Sporadic reports) 2138
Macrodantin Capsules (Sporadic reports) 2140
Mandol Vials, Faspak & ADD-Vantage 1516
Maxaquin Tablets 2593
Maxipime for Injection (0.1% to 1%) 758
Mefoxin 1734
Mefoxin Premixed Intravenous Solution 1737
Merrem I.V. 2952
Mezlin 594
Mezlin Pharmacy Bulk Package 597
Monocid Injection (Less than 1%) 2674
NegGram 2453
Noroxin Tablets 1758
Noroxin Tablets 2222
Omnipen Capsules 2872
Omnipen for Oral Suspension 2873
PCE Dispertab Tablets (Rare) 453
Pediazole Suspension (Rare) 2340
Penetrex Tablets (Less than 0.1%) 2196
Pipracil (Rare) 1435
Primaxin I.M. 1770
Primaxin I.V. (Less than 0.2%) 1772
Rifadin 1276
Rifater 1280
Rocephin Injectable Vials, ADD-Vantage, Galaxy Container 2305
Spectrobid Tablets 2030
Suprax (Several patients) 1443
Tazicef for Injection 2697
Tazidime Vials, Faspak & ADD-Vantage 1531
Ticar for Injection 2704
Timentin for Injection 2706
Unasyn 2035
Vancocin HCl, Vials & ADD-Vantage 1534
Vantin for Oral Suspension and Vantin Tablets (Less than 1%) 2112
Zinacef 1184
Zithromax 2043
Zithromax Tablets 2046
Zosyn (One patient) 1463

Pseudomembranous enterocolitis

Bactrim DS Tablets 2257
Bactrim I.V. Infusion 2255
Bactrim 2257
Gantanol Tablets 2285
Rilutek Tablets (Rare) 2198
Rimactane Capsules (Rare) 865
Septra 1146
Septra I.V. Infusion 1142
Septra I.V. Infusion ADD-Vantage Vials 1144
Septra 1146
Videx Tablets, Powder for Oral Solution, & Pediatric Powder for Oral Solution (Less than 1%) 2980

Pseudoparkinsonism

BuSpar Tablets 738
Compazine 2644
Mellaril (Infrequent) 2398
Navane Capsules and Concentrate 2018
Navane Intramuscular 2019
Stelazine 2692
Thorazine 2701
Triavil Tablets 1800
Wellbutrin Tablets (1.5%) 1177

Pseudotumor cerebri

Accutane Capsules (A number of cases) 2252
Achromycin V Capsules 1417
Celestone Soluspan Suspension 2484
Cordarone Tablets (Rare) 2818
CORTENEMA 2713
Cortone Acetate Sterile Suspension 1663
Cortone Acetate Tablets 1664
Cytovene-IV (One report) 2270
Danocrine Capsules 2437
Decadron Elixir 1676
Decadron Phosphate Injection 1680
Decadron Phosphate with Xylocaine Injection, Sterile 1683
Decadron Tablets 1678
Declomycin Tablets 1421
Dexacort Phosphate in Respihaler 1606
Dexacort Phosphate in Turbinaire 1607
DYNACIN Capsules 1627
Eskalith 2658
Florinef Acetate Tablets 506
Garamycin Injectable 2502
Helidac Therapy 2135
Hydeltrasol Injection, Sterile 1708
Hydrocortone Tablets 1715
IBU Tablets (Less than 1%) 1389
Lithium Carbonate Capsules & Tablets 2352
Lithonate/Lithotabs/Lithobid 2721
Minocin Intravenous 1428
Minocin Oral Suspension 1431
Minocin Pellet-Filled Capsules 1429
Motrin Ibuprofen Suspension, Oral Drops, Chewable Tablets, Caplets (Less than 1%) 1563
Norplant System 2868
Pediapred Oral Solution 1618
Synthroid 1410
Tegison Capsules 2314
Vesanoid Capsules 2327

Psoriasis

Anafranil Capsules (Infrequent) 819
Asacol Delayed-Release Tablets (Rare) 2129
Betaseron for SC Injection 653
Cognex Capsules (Infrequent) 1961
Desyrel and Desyrel Dividose 504
Doxil (Less than 1%) 2613
Effexor (Rare) 2825
Eskalith 2658
Intron A for Injection (Less than 5%) 2506
Lithonate/Lithotabs/Lithobid 2721
Neurontin Capsules (Rare) 1978
Norvir (Less than 2%) 447
Prozac Pulvules & Liquid, Oral Solution (Rare) 935
Quinidex Extentabs 2240
Redux Capsules (Infrequent) 2911
Rilutek Tablets (Infrequent) 2198
Ziac 1459

Psoriasis, exacerbation

Cormax Ointment (Rare) 1856
Cormax Scalp Application (Rare) 1857
Cytovene-IV (One report) 2270
▲ Dovonex Cream 0.005% (1% to 10%) 2792
▲ Dovonex Ointment 0.005% (1% to 10%) 2793
Eskalith 2658
Foscavir Injection (Less than 1%) 541
Intron A for Injection 2506
Lithium Carbonate Capsules & Tablets 2352
Lithonate/Lithotabs/Lithobid 2721
Methotrexate Sodium Tablets, Injection, for Injection and LPF Injection 1322
Neupogen for Injection (Infrequent) 495
Oxsoralen-Ultra Capsules 1302
Plaquenil Sulfate Tablets 2459
Risperdal Tablets (Rare) 1348
Temovate Scalp Application (Rare) 1153
Tenoretic Tablets 2963
Tenormin Tablets and I.V. Injection 2965
Toprol-XL Tablets 560

Psoriasis, pustular

Cutivate Cream 1078
Cutivate Ointment 1078

Psoriasis, rapid flare of

Seldane Tablets 1284
Seldane-D Extended-Release Tablets 1286

Psychiatric disturbances

Aldoclor Tablets 1638
Aldomet Ester HCl Injection 1642
Aldomet Oral 1640
Aldoril Tablets 1644
Anafranil Capsules (Up to 3%) 819
Aralen Hydrochloride Injection 2430
Aralen Phosphate Tablets 2431
Artane (Rare) 1418
Clinoril Tablets (Less than 1 in 100) 1658
Cogentin 1661
Cortone Acetate Sterile Suspension 1663
Cortone Acetate Tablets 1664
Cuprimine Capsules 1673
Dalalone D.P. Injectable 1009
Decadron Elixir 1676
Decadron Phosphate Injection 1680
Decadron Phosphate with Xylocaine Injection, Sterile 1683
Decadron Tablets 1678
Decadron-LA Sterile Suspension 1687
Dexacort Phosphate in Respihaler 1606
Dexacort Phosphate in Turbinaire 1607
Didronel Tablets 2133
Hydeltrasol Injection, Sterile 1708
Hydeltra-T.B.A. Sterile Suspension 1710
Hydrocortone Acetate Sterile Suspension 1712
Hydrocortone Phosphate Injection, Sterile 1713
Hydrocortone Tablets 1715
▲ Hylorel Tablets (3.8%) 1613
Indocin (Less than 1%) 1723
Invirase Capsules (Less than 2%) 2291
Lescol Capsules 2395
▲ Leukine (15%) 1317
Mebaral Tablets (Less than 1 in 100) 2452
Mintezol 1747
Nembutal Sodium Capsules (Less than 1%) 440
Nembutal Sodium Solution (Less than 1%) 442
Nembutal Sodium Suppositories (Less than 1%) 444
Nizoral Tablets (Rare) 1345
Noroxin Tablets 1758
Noroxin Tablets 2222
Pepcid Injection (Infrequent) 1765
Pepcid (Infrequent) 1763
Phenobarbital Elixir and Tablets (Less than 1 in 100 patients) 1523
▲ Phenurone Tablets (17%) 455
Prilosec Delayed-Release Capsules (Less than 1%) 516
Primaxin I.M. 1770
Primaxin I.V. (Less than 0.2%) 1772
Seconal Sodium Pulvules (Less than 1 in 100) 1529
Ser-Ap-Es Tablets 867
Timoptic in Ocudose (Less frequent) 1796
Timoptic Sterile Ophthalmic Solution (Less frequent) 1794
Timoptic-XE 1798
Tonocard Tablets (Less than 1%) 519
Trecator-SC Tablets 2919
Zarontin Capsules 1986
Zarontin Syrup 1986

Psychic dependence (see under Dependence, psychological)

Psychomotor retardation

Lithonate/Lithotabs/Lithobid 2721
Serzone Tablets (2%) 776

(Described in PDR For Nonprescription Drugs)
Incidence data in parenthesis; ▲ 3% or more
(⊙ Described in PDR For Ophthalmology)

1435 Side Effects Index Pulmonary function, decreased

Psychoses

Adderall Tablets (Rare) 2209
Adipex-P Tablets and Capsules 1035
Aldoclor Tablets 1638
Aldomet Ester HCl Injection 1642
Aldomet Oral 1640
Aldoril Tablets 1644
Anafranil Capsules (Infrequent) 819
Ancobon Capsules 2254
Antabuse Tablets 2802
Apresazide Capsules (Less frequent) 824
Aralen Phosphate Tablets (Rare) 2431
Aredia for Injection (Up to 4%) 827
Atamet Tablets 567
Avonex 662
Bentyl 1246
Betaseron for SC Injection 653
Bontril Slow-Release Capsules (Rare) 786
Buprenex Injectable (Less than 1%) 2170
BuSpar Tablets (Rare) 738
Butisol Sodium Elixir & Tablets (Less than 1 in 100) 2768
Calan SR Caplets (1% or less) 2571
Calan Tablets (1% or less) 2568
Cataflam Tablets (Rare) 833
Cedax 2480
Celestone Soluspan Suspension 2484
Celontin Kapseals (Rare) 1955
Cerebyx Injection (Infrequent) 1956
Chibroxin Sterile Ophthalmic Solution (With oral form) 1657
Cipro I.V. Pharmacy Bulk Package (Less than 1%) 590
Clinoril Tablets (Less than 1 in 100) 1658
Clomid 1262
Cognex Capsules (Rare) 1961
CORTENEMA 2713
Cortone Acetate Sterile Suspension 1663
Cortone Acetate Tablets 1664
Covera-HS Tablets (Less than 2%) 2573
Cytovene (1% or less) 2270
Dapsone Tablets USP 1331
Decadron Elixir 1676
Decadron Phosphate Injection 1680
Decadron Phosphate with Xylocaine Injection, Sterile 1683
Decadron Tablets 1678
Decadron-LA Sterile Suspension 1687
Depakene 416
Depakote Tablets 418
Desoxyn Gradumet Tablets (Rare) 422
Desyrel and Desyrel Dividose 504
Dexatrim ▣ 795
Dexatrim Plus Vitamins Caplets ▣ 796
Dexedrine (Rare at recommended doses) 2648
DextroStat-Dextroamphetamine Sulfate Tablets (Rare) 2211
Effexor (Infrequent) 2825
Fastin Capsules (Rare) 2662
Felbatol 2774
Fioricet with Codeine Capsules 2387
Fiorinal with Codeine Capsules 2390
Florinef Acetate Tablets 506
Floxin I.V. 1580
Foscavir Injection (Less than 1%) 541
Gastrocrom Capsules (Infrequent) 1611
Gastrocrom Oral Concentrate (Less common) 1611
Hivid Tablets (Less than 1%) 2287
Hydeltrasol Injection, Sterile 1708
Hydeltra-T.B.A. Sterile Suspension 1710
Hydralazine Hydrochloride Injection USP (Less frequent) 2712
Hydrocortone Acetate Sterile Suspension 1712
Hydrocortone Phosphate Injection, Sterile 1713
Hydrocortone Tablets 1715
Hydropres Tablets 1718
Indocin (Less than 1%) 1723
Ionamin Capsules (Rare) 1615
Isoptin Oral Tablets (Less than 1%) 1393
Isoptin SR Tablets (1% or less) 1395
Klonopin Tablets 2294
Lamictal Tablets (Infrequent) 1105
Lanoxicaps 1110
Lanoxin Elixir Pediatric 1113
Lanoxin Injection 1116
Lanoxin Injection Pediatric 1119
Lanoxin Tablets 1121
Lariam Tablets 2295
Larodopa Tablets (Infrequent) 2296
Levsin/Levsinex/Levbid 2549
Ludiomil Tablets (Rare) 861
LUVOX Tablets (Infrequent to frequent) 2723
Macrobid Capsules (Rare) 2138
Macrodantin Capsules (Rare) 2140
Mellaril (Extremely rare) 2398
Mexitil Capsules (Less than 1% or about 2 in 1,000) 684
Nardil (Infrequent) 1977
Neurontin Capsules (Infrequent) 1978
Noroxin Tablets 1758
Noroxin Tablets 2222
Norpace (Rare) 2596
Orthoclone OKT3 Sterile Solution 1892
Paremyd ⊙ 244
Parlodel (Less than 1%) 2411
Paxil Tablets (Rare) 2681
Pediapred Oral Solution 1618
Pediazole Suspension 2340
Penetrex Tablets (Less than 0.1%) 2196
Permax Tablets (2.1%; frequent) 571
Plaquenil Sulfate Tablets 2459
Prelone Syrup 1834
Prelu-2 Timed Release Capsules (Rare) 687
Procanbid Extended-Release Tablets (Occasional) 1983
▲ Prograf (Greater than 3%) 1028
Prozac Pulvules & Liquid, Oral Solution (Infrequent) 935
Quinaglute Dura-Tabs Tablets 644
Quinidex Extentabs 2240
Rilutek Tablets (Rare) 2198
Ritalin 866
Rocaltrol Capsules (Rare) 2303
Roferon-A Injection 2308
Rythmol Tablets–150mg, 225mg, 300mg (Less than 1%) 1399
Seromycin Capsules 975
Sinemet Tablets 959
Sinemet CR Tablets 961
Symmetrel Capsules (0.1% to 1%) 965
Symmetrel Syrup (0.1% to 1%) 963
Tagamet 2694
Tenoretic Tablets 2963
Tenormin Tablets and I.V. Injection 2965
Tonocard Tablets (Less than 1%) 519
Toradol 2319
Trilafon 2532
Verelan Capsules (1% or less) 1455
Videx Tablets, Powder for Oral Solution, & Pediatric Powder for Oral Solution (Less than 1%) 2980
Cataflam/Voltaren/Voltaren-XR (Rare) 833
Wellbutrin Tablets (Infrequent) 1177
Zarontin Capsules 1986
Zarontin Syrup 1986
Zoloft Tablets 2051
Zovirax Sterile Powder 1191

Psychoses, aggravation

Clozaril Tablets 2377
CORTENEMA 2713
Cortone Acetate Sterile Suspension 1663
Cortone Acetate Tablets 1664
Decadron Elixir 1676
Decadron Phosphate Injection 1680
Decadron Phosphate with Xylocaine Injection, Sterile 1683
Decadron Tablets 1678
Decadron-LA Sterile Suspension 1687
Etrafon 2495
Florinef Acetate Tablets 506
Hydeltrasol Injection, Sterile 1708
Hydeltra-T.B.A. Sterile Suspension 1710
Hydrocortone Acetate Sterile Suspension 1712
Hydrocortone Phosphate Injection, Sterile 1713
Hydrocortone Tablets 1715
Mellaril 2398
Norpramin Tablets 1273
Pamelor 2409
Pediapred Oral Solution 1618
Prelone Syrup 1834
Prolixin 510
Serentil 689
Surmontil Capsules 2917
Tofranil Ampuls (Occasional) 873
Tofranil Tablets (Occasional) 875
Tofranil-PM Capsules (Occasional) 876
Torecan 2367
Vivactil Tablets 1820

Psychoses, toxic

Astramorph/PF Injection, USP (Preservative-Free) 526
Chibroxin Sterile Ophthalmic Solution (With oral form) 1657
Cipro I.V. (1% or less) 587
Cipro Tablets 584
Duramorph Injection 983
Floxin Tablets (200 mg, 300 mg, 400 mg) 1577
Infumorph 200 and Infumorph 500 Sterile Solutions 985
NegGram (Rare) 2453
Nydrazid Injection (Uncommon) 509
Penetrex Tablets 2196
Rifamate Capsules (Uncommon) 1278
Rifater (Uncommon) 1280
Ritalin 866

Psychosis, activation

Atretol Tablets 569
Compazine 2644
Levoprome 1321
Prolixin 510
Stelazine 2692
Tegretol/Tegretol-XR 870
Triavil Tablets 1800

Psychosis, overt

Calcijex Injection (Rare) 412
Pediapred Oral Solution 1618

Psychosis, paranoid

Zarontin Capsules (Rare) 1986
Zarontin Syrup (Rare) 1986

Psychotic episodes (see under Psychoses)

Psychotic symptoms, paradoxical exacerbation

Haldol Decanoate 1587
Haldol Injection, Tablets and Concentrate 1585
Navane Capsules and Concentrate (Infrequent) 2018
Navane Intramuscular (Infrequent) 2019

Ptosis, eyelids

AK-CIDE ⊙ 203
AK-CIDE Ointment ⊙ 203
Betagan ⊙ 230
Betaseron for SC Injection 653
Betimol 0.25%, 0.5% ⊙ 259
Blephamide Liquifilm Sterile Ophthalmic Suspension 472
Blephamide Ointment (Occasional) ⊙ 234
Blocadren Tablets 1654
▲ BOTOX (Botulinum Toxin Type A) Purified Neurotoxin Complex (0.3% to 15.7%) 473
Clozaril Tablets (Less than 1%) 2377
Cognex Capsules (Rare) 1961
Depen Titratable Tablets 2770
Econopred & Econopred Plus Ophthalmic Suspensions (Occasional) ⊙ 216
Esimil Tablets 840
FML Forte Liquifilm (Occasional) ⊙ 237
FML Liquifilm (Occasional) ⊙ 238
FML S.O.P. (Occasional) ⊙ 239
Imdur (Less than or equal to 5%) 1362
Ismelin Tablets 845
Lamictal Tablets (Rare) 1105
Lioresal Intrathecal (1% or more) 1634
Loxitane 1426
Naprelan Tablets (Less than 1%) 2861
Neurontin Capsules (Infrequent) 1978
Ocupress Ophthalmic Solution, 1% Sterile (Occasional) ⊙ 297
Paxil Tablets (Rare) 2681
Pred Forte (Occasional) ⊙ 247
Pred Mild ⊙ 250
Prozac Pulvules & Liquid, Oral Solution (Rare) 935
▲ Rev-Eyes Ophthalmic Eyedrops 0.5% (10% to 40%) ⊙ 324
Serzone Tablets (Rare) 776
Timolide Tablets 1791
Timoptic in Ocudose (Less frequent) 1796
Timoptic Sterile Ophthalmic Solution (Less frequent) 1794
Timoptic-XE 1798
Zoloft Tablets (Rare) 2051
Zyrtec Tablets (Less than 2%) 2053

Pubic hair, growth

▲ Synarel Nasal Solution for Central Precocious Puberty (5%) 2603

Pulmonary air leak

▲ Exosurf Neonatal for Intratracheal Suspension (Up to 48%) 1081
▲ Survanta Beractant Intratracheal Suspension (10.9%) 2346

Pulmonary allergy, unspecified

Idamycin Injection (2%) 2096

Pulmonary congestion

Prinzide Tablets 1780
▲ Proleukin for Injection (54%) 812
Zestoretic Tablets (0.3 to 1%) 2968

Pulmonary disease, chronic interstitial obstructive

Dipentum Capsules (Rare) 2084
Methotrexate Sodium Tablets, Injection, for Injection and LPF Injection (Occasional) 1322

Pulmonary disease, chronic obstructive

LUVOX Tablets (Rare) 2723
▲ Zoladex (5%) 2976
Zoladex 3-month 2978

Pulmonary distress

Betoptic Ophthalmic Solution (Rare) 465
Betoptic S Ophthalmic Suspension (Rare) 467
Humegon for Injection 1873
Metrodin (urofollitropin for injection) 2616
Serophene (clomiphene citrate tablets, USP) 2621

Pulmonary edema (see under Edema, pulmonary)

Pulmonary embolism (see under Embolism, pulmonary)

Pulmonary emphysema, interstitial

▲ Survanta Beractant Intratracheal Suspension (20.2%) 2346

Pulmonary fibrosis

Alkeran for Injection 1196
Alkeran Tablets 1198
BiCNU 696
▲ Blenoxane (10%) 697
Cafergot 2376
CeeNU Capsules 699
Cordarone Intravenous (One of more than 1,000 patients) 2821
▲ Cordarone Tablets (4 to 9%) 2818
Cuprimine Capsules (Rare) 1673
Cytovene-IV (One report) 2270
Cytoxan 700
Depen Titratable Tablets 2770
Garamycin Injectable 2502
Leukeran Tablets 1205
Lupron Injection (Less than 5%) 2736
Macrobid Capsules (Rare to common) 2138
Macrodantin Capsules (Rare; common) 2140
Mesantoin Tablets 2400
Mexitil Capsules (Isolated reports) 684
Myleran Tablets (Rare) 1209
Paxil Tablets (Rare) 2681
Pentasa (One case) 1275
Permax Tablets (Rare) 571
Prozac Pulvules & Liquid, Oral Solution (Rare) 935
Sansert Tablets 2424
Tonocard Tablets (Less than 1%) 519

Pulmonary function, changes

▲ Betapace Tablets (3% to 8%) 637
Diprivan Injectable Emulsion (Less than 1%) 2939
Eulexin Capsules (Less than 1%) 2498
Humegon for Injection 1873
IFEX (Less than 1%) 706
Intron A for Injection 2506
▲ Leukine (48%) 1317
Macrobid Capsules (Common) 2138
Macrodantin Capsules (Common) 2140
Mexitil Capsules (Isolated reports) 684
Navelbine Injection (A few patients) 1212
▲ Novantrone for Injection (24 to 43%) 1327
Pergonal (menotropins for injection, USP) 2618
Virazole 1310

Pulmonary function, decreased

▲ Rilutek Tablets (13.1% to 16%) 2198

(▣ Described in PDR For Nonprescription Drugs) Incidence data in parenthesis; ▲ 3% or more (⊙ Described in PDR For Ophthalmology)

Pulmonary hemorrhage

Pulmonary hemorrhage
(see under Hemorrhage, pulmonary)

Pulmonary hypersensitivity
Atretol Tablets	569
Cytadren Tablets (Rare)	837
Fludara for Injection	658
Septra I.V. Infusion	1142
Septra I.V. Infusion ADD-Vantage Vials	1144
Tegretol/Tegretol-XR	870

Pulmonary hypersensitivity, acute
Macrobid Capsules (Less than 1%)	2138
Macrodantin Capsules	2140

Pulmonary hypersensitivity, chronic
Macrodantin Capsules	2140
Timolide Tablets	1791

Pulmonary hypersensitivity, subacute
Macrodantin Capsules	2140

Pulmonary hypertension
Indocin I.V. (1% to 3%)	1727
Permax Tablets (Rare)	571
Pondimin Tablets	2239
Protamine Sulfate Vials	1526
Redux Capsules	2911
▲ Vesanoid Capsules (3%)	2327

Pulmonary infarction
Humegon for Injection	1873
LUVOX Tablets (Rare)	2723
Metrodin (urofollitropin for injection)	2616
Prinivil Tablets (0.3% to 1.0%)	1776
Prinzide Tablets	1780
Vaseretic Tablets	1810
Vasotec I.V.	1814
Vasotec Tablets (0.5% to 1.0%)	1816
Zestoretic Tablets	2968
Zestril Tablets (0.3% to 1.0%)	2972

Pulmonary infiltrates
Bactrim DS Tablets	2257
Bactrim I.V. Infusion	2255
Bactrim	2257
Beclovent Inhalation Aerosol and Refill	1063
BiCNU	696
CeeNU Capsules	699
DaunoXome (Less than or equal to 5%)	1842
DYNACIN Capsules (Rare)	1627
Fansidar Tablets	2281
Fludara for Injection	658
Foscavir Injection (Between 1% and 5%)	541
Ganite	2711
Gantanol Tablets	2285
Gantrisin	2286
Hydrea Capsules (Rare)	705
Imdur (Less than or equal to 5%)	1362
Intal Inhaler (Infrequent)	2185
Intal Nebulizer Solution (Rare)	2186
Intron A for Injection (Rare)	2506
Leustatin	1889
Lupron Injection	2736
Macrobid Capsules	2138
Macrodantin Capsules	2140
Minocin Intravenous (Rare)	1428
Minocin Oral Suspension (Rare)	1431
Minocin Pellet-Filled Capsules (Rare)	1429
Mutamycin for Injection	712
Pediazole Suspension	2340
Pentasa (Less than 1%)	1275
Prinivil Tablets (0.3% to 1.0%)	1776
Prinzide Tablets	1780
Septra (Rare)	1146
Septra I.V. Infusion	1142
Septra I.V. Infusion ADD-Vantage Vials	1144
Septra (Rare)	1146
Vantin for Oral Suspension and Vantin Tablets	2112
Vascor Tablets (200 and 300 mg)	1597
Vaseretic Tablets	1810
Vasotec I.V.	1814
Vasotec Tablets (0.5% to 1.0%)	1816
▲ Vesanoid Capsules (6%)	2327
Zestoretic Tablets	2968
Zestril Tablets (0.3% to 1.0%)	2972

Pulmonary inflammation
Cordarone Tablets	2818

Pulmonary toxicity, unspecified
Alkeran for Injection	1196
Alkeran Tablets	1198
BiCNU	696
CeeNU Capsules	699
▲ Cordarone Tablets (10% to 17%)	2818
Cytosar-U Sterile Powder	2077
Fungizone Intravenous	507
▲ Idamycin Injection (39%)	2096
Methotrexate Sodium Tablets, Injection, for Injection and LPF Injection (Less than 2.5%)	1322
Mutamycin for Injection	712

Pulse, fast
Arco-Lase Plus Tablets	513
Dextratrim Maximum Strength Plus Vitamin C/Caffeine-Free Caplets	795
Humalog Injection (Less common)	1488
Humulin 50/50, 100 Units	1491
Humulin 70/30, 100 Units (Less common)	1492
Humulin L, 100 Units (Less common)	1494
Regular, 100 Units (Less common)	1503
Pork Regular, 100 Units	1507
Novolin 70/30 Prefilled Disposable Insulin Delivery System (Rare)	1850
Propagest Tablets	791
RespiGam (1%)	1631
Sinulin Tablets	792
Urised Tablets	2123
Velosulin BR Human Insulin 10 ml Vials	1847

Pulse changes
AquaMEPHYTON Injection	1648
Asendin Tablets	1419
Clozaril Tablets	2377
Compazine	2644
Dalgan Injection (Less than 1%)	529
Effexor	2825
Etrafon	2495
Haldol Decanoate	1587
Imitrex Injection (Rare)	1095
Loxitane	1426
LUVOX Tablets (Infrequent)	2723
Mellaril	2398
Mephyton Tablets (Rare)	1739
Moban Tablets and Concentrate	1036
Navane Capsules and Concentrate	2018
Navane Intramuscular	2019
Norvasc Tablets (Less than or equal to 0.1%)	2020
Orap Tablets	1037
Prolixin	510
Risperdal Tablets	1348
Ritalin	866
Serentil	689
Stelazine	2692
Tornalate Solution for Inhalation, 0.2% (1.2%)	976
Triavil Tablets	1800
Trilafon (Occasional)	2532
▲ Versed Injection (Among most frequent)	2324
Yutopar Intravenous Injection (Common)	566

Pulse rate, depression
Acthrel for Injection (One patient)	2990
Cafergot	2376
Lanoxicaps	1110
Lanoxin Injection	1116
ReoPro Vials (1.0%)	1526
Sansert Tablets	2424

Pupillary atonia
Healon GV	303

Pupils, unequal-sized
Hivid Tablets (Less than 1%)	2287

Purple toes syndrome
Activase	1045
Coumadin (Infrequent)	941

Purpura
Adalat Capsules (10 mg and 20 mg) (Less than 0.5%)	580
Adalat CC (Rare)	582
Adapin Capsules (Occasional)	1542
Aldactazide Tablets	2556
Aldoclor Tablets	1638
Aldoril Tablets	1644
Altace Capsules (Less than 1%)	1238
Ambien Tablets (Rare)	2559
Anafranil Capsules (Up to 3%)	819
Anaprox/Naprosyn (Less than 3%)	2277
Apresazide Capsules (Less frequent)	824
Apresoline Hydrochloride Tablets (Less frequent)	826
Asendin Tablets (Very rare)	1419
Atretol Tablets	569
Attenuvax (Rare)	1650
Azactam for Injection (Less than 1%)	736
Azulfidine (Rare)	2059
Bactrim DS Tablets	2257
Bactrim I.V. Infusion	2255
Bactrim	2257
Biavax II	1653
Calan SR Caplets (1% or less)	2571
Calan Tablets (1% or less)	2568
Capozide Tablets	744
Cardizem CD Capsules (Infrequent)	1251
Cardizem SR Capsules (Infrequent)	1255
Cardizem Injectable	1253
Cardizem Tablets (Infrequent)	1257
Cardura Tablets (Less than 0.5% of 3960 patients)	1993
Cataflam Tablets (Less than 1%)	833
Cipro I.V. (1% or less)	587
Cipro I.V. Pharmacy Bulk Package (Less than 1%)	590
Claritin Tablets (2% or fewer patients)	2485
Claritin-D Tablets	2487
Clinoril Tablets (Less than 1 in 100)	1658
Cognex Capsules (2%)	1961
ColBENEMID Tablets	1662
Combipres Tablets (Few)	682
Covera-HS Tablets (Less than 2%)	2573
Cytotec (Infrequent)	2576
Dapsone Tablets USP	1331
DiaBeta Tablets (Occasional)	1265
Diucardin Tablets	2824
Diupres Tablets	1691
Diuril Oral Suspension	1694
Diuril Sodium Intravenous	1693
Diuril Tablets	1694
Dyazide Capsules	2653
Easprin	1971
EC-Naprosyn Delayed-Release Tablets (Less than 3%)	2277
Elavil	2945
▲ Eminase (Less than 10%)	2215
Enduron Tablets	424
Engerix-B Unit-Dose Vials	2656
Esidrix Tablets	839
Esimil Tablets	840
Etrafon	2495
Fansidar Tablets	2281
▲ Felbatol (12.9%)	2774
Flexeril Tablets (Rare)	1701
Florinef Acetate Tablets	506
Floxin I.V.	1580
Floxin Tablets (200 mg, 300 mg, 400 mg)	1577
Gantanol Tablets	2285
Gantrisin	2286
Garamycin Injectable	2502
Gastrocrom Oral Concentrate (Less common)	1611
Hivid Tablets (Less than 1%)	2287
Hydralazine Hydrochloride Injection USP (Less frequent)	2712
HydroDIURIL Tablets	1716
Hydropres Tablets	1718
Hyzaar Tablets	1720
Imdur (Less than or equal to 5%)	1362
Inderide Tablets	2838
Inderide LA Long Acting Capsules	2840
Indocin Capsules (Less than 1%)	1723
Indocin I.V. (Less than 1%)	1727
Indocin (Less than 1%)	1723
INFeD (Iron Dextran Injection, USP)	2478
Intron A for Injection (Less than 5%)	2506
Isoptin Oral Tablets (Less than 1%)	1393
Isoptin SR Tablets (1% or less)	1395
Kerlone Tablets (Less than 2%)	2588
Lasix Injection, Oral Solution and Tablets	1267
Lescol Capsules (Rare)	2395
▲ Leustatin (10%)	1889
Limbitrol	2333
Lodine Capsules and Tablets (Less than 1%)	2849
Lopressor HCT Tablets (1 in 100 patients)	850
Lotensin HCT Tablets	855
Lovenox Injection	2187
Ludiomil Tablets (Isolated reports)	861
LUVOX Tablets (Rare)	2723
M-M-R II	1730
M-R-VAX II	1732
Matulane Capsules	2300
Maxaquin Tablets (Less than 1%)	2593
Mevacor Tablets (Rare)	1742
Minizide Capsules	2016
Moduretic Tablets	1748
Motrin Ibuprofen Suspension, Oral Drops, Chewable Tablets, Caplets (Less than 1%)	1563
Mumpsvax (Extremely rare)	1751
Mykrox Tablets	1617
Myochrysine Injection	1754
Nalfon 200 Pulvules & Nalfon Tablets (Less than 1%)	933
Naprelan Tablets (Less than 3%)	2861
Anaprox/Naprosyn (Less than 3%)	2277
Neurontin Capsules (Frequent)	1978
Nicotrol NS Nicotine Nasal Spray (Less than 1%)	1565
Norpramin Tablets	1273
Norvasc Tablets (More than 0.1% to 1%)	2020
Oncaspar (Less than 1%)	2194
Oretic Tablets	450
Orudis Capsules (Less than 1%)	2874
Oruvail Capsules (Less than 1%)	2874
Pamelor	2409
Paxil Tablets (Infrequent)	2681
Pediazole Suspension	2340
Penetrex Tablets (0.1% to 1%)	2196
Permax Tablets (Rare)	571
Pravachol Tablets (Rare)	770
Prinzide Tablets	1780
Procardia Capsules (Less than 0.5%)	2024
Procardia XL Extended Release Tablets (1% or less)	2026
▲ Proleukin for Injection (4%)	812
Proloprim Tablets	1141
ProSom Tablets (Rare)	457
Prozac Pulvules & Liquid, Oral Solution (Rare)	935
Rifadin	1276
Rifater	1280
Rilutek Tablets (Rare)	2198
Risperdal Tablets (Infrequent)	1348
Rythmol Tablets–150mg, 225mg, 300mg (Less than 1%)	1399
Septra I.V. Infusion	1142
Ser-Ap-Es Tablets	867
Sinequan (Occasional)	2028
Solganal Suspension (Rare)	2530
▲ Supprelin Injection (2% to 12%)	2230
Surmontil Capsules	2917
Tegretol/Tegretol-XR	870
Tenex Tablets (3% or less)	2249
Tenoretic Tablets	2963
Tenormin Tablets and I.V. Injection	2965
Thalitone	1293
Tiazac Capsules (Infrequent)	1019
Ticlid Tablets (2.2%)	2317
Timolide Tablets	1791
Tofranil Ampuls	873
Tofranil Tablets	875
Tofranil-PM Capsules	876
Tolectin (200, 400 and 600 mg) (Less than 1%)	1591
Toradol (Greater than 1%)	2319
Trandate Tablets	1158
Trental Tablets (Rare)	1291
Triavil Tablets	1800
Urobiotic-250 Capsules	2038
Vaseretic Tablets	1810
Verelan Capsules (1% or less)	1455
Vivactil Tablets	1820
Cataflam/Voltaren/Voltaren-XR (Less than 1%)	833
Zaroxolyn Tablets	1625
Zebeta Tablets	1457
Zestoretic Tablets	2968
Ziac	1459
Zocor Tablets (Rare)	1821
Zoloft Tablets (Infrequent)	2051
Zosyn (1.0% or less)	1463
Zyloprim Tablets (Less than 1%)	1194
Zyrtec Tablets (Less than 2%)	2053

Purpura annularis
Redux Capsules	2911

Purpura, allergic
Cataflam/Voltaren/Voltaren-XR (Rare)	833

Purpura, anaphylactoid
Achromycin V Capsules	1417

1437 Side Effects Index Rash

- Declomycin Tablets 1421
- Doryx Capsules 1970
- DYNACIN Capsules 1627
- Helidac Therapy 2135
- Minocin Intravenous 1428
- Minocin Oral Suspension 1431
- Minocin Pellet-Filled Capsules 1429
- Monodox Capsules 1858
- Terramycin Intramuscular Solution 2034
- Vibramycin 2038
- Vibramycin Hyclate Intravenous 2040
- Vibramycin 2038

Purpura, fulminous
- Zovirax Sterile Powder (Less than 1%) 1191

Purpura, nonthrombocytopenic
- Blocadren Tablets 1654
- Cartrol Tablets 413
- Edecrin (Rare) 1698
- Inderal 2834
- Inderal LA Long Acting Capsules 2836
- Inderide Tablets 2838
- Inderide LA Long Acting Capsules 2840
- Kerlone Tablets 2588
- Levatol Tablets 2547
- Lopressor HCT Tablets 850
- Miltown Tablets 2780
- Normodyne Tablets 2522
- PMB 200 and PMB 400 2890
- Prolixin 510
- Sectral Capsules 2914
- Septra I.V. Infusion ADD-Vantage Vials 1144
- Timolide Tablets 1791
- Timoptic in Ocudose 1796
- Timoptic Sterile Ophthalmic Solution 1794
- Timoptic-XE 1798
- Toprol-XL Tablets 560
- Trandate Tablets 1158
- Visken Tablets 2428

Purpura, thrombocytopenic
- Amoxil 2631
- Atromid-S Capsules 2808
- Augmentin 2637
- Augmentin Tablets 2640
- Axid Pulvules (Rare) 1468
- Blocadren Tablets 1654
- Cardioquin Tablets 2146
- Cartrol Tablets 413
- Compazine 2644
- Cuprimine Capsules 1673
- Diamox ◉ 317
- Diupres Tablets 1691
- Etrafon 2495
- Garamycin Ophthalmic 2501
- Genoptic Sterile Ophthalmic Solution (Rare) ◉ 241
- Genoptic Sterile Ophthalmic Ointment (Rare) ◉ 241
- Gentak (Rare) ◉ 209
- GlaucTabs ◉ 209
- Helidac Therapy 2135
- Hydropres Tablets 1718
- IBU Tablets (Less than 1%) 1389
- Inderal 2834
- Inderal LA Long Acting Capsules 2836
- Inderide Tablets 2838
- Inderide LA Long Acting Capsules 2840
- Indocin Capsules (Less than 1%) 1723
- Indocin I.V. (Less than 1%) 1727
- Indocin (Less than 1%) 1723
- Kerlone Tablets 2588
- Levatol Tablets 2547
- Lopressor HCT Tablets 850
- Meruvax II 1740
- Miltown Tablets (Rare) 2780
- Neptazane Tablets ◉ 320
- Normodyne Tablets 2522
- Omnipen Capsules 2872
- Omnipen for Oral Suspension 2873
- Phenergan Injection 2880
- Phenergan Tablets 2882
- PMB 200 and PMB 400 (Rare) 2890
- Ponstel (Occasional) 1982
- Proglycem 575
- Prolixin 510
- Prozac Pulvules & Liquid, Oral Solution 935
- Quinaglute Dura-Tabs Tablets 644
- Quinidex Extentabs 2240
- ReVia Tablets (One patient) 957
- Ritalin 866
- Sectral Capsules 2914
- ▲ Septra I.V. Infusion (Among most frequent) 1142
- Septra I.V. Infusion ADD-Vantage Vials 1144
- Spectrobid Tablets 2030
- Stelazine 2692
- Talacen Caplets (A few cases) 2464
- Thorazine 2701
- Timolide Tablets 1791
- Timoptic in Ocudose 1796
- Timoptic Sterile Ophthalmic Solution 1794
- Timoptic-XE 1798
- Toprol-XL Tablets 560
- Trandate Tablets 1158
- Triavil Tablets 1800
- Trilafon 2532
- Visken Tablets 2428
- Zebeta Tablets 1457

Purpura, thrombocytopenic thrombotic
- Cuprimine Capsules 1673
- Depen Titratable Tablets 2770
- Floxin I.V. 1580
- Floxin Tablets (200 mg, 300 mg, 400 mg) 1577
- Mycobutin Capsules (One patient) 2101
- Norplant System 2868
- Risperdal Tablets (A single case) 1348
- Ticlid Tablets (Rare) 2317
- Valtrex Caplets 1167

Pustules, scalp
- Cormax Scalp Application (Approximately 1%) 1857
- Nizoral 2% Shampoo (One occurrence in 41 patients) 1344
- Temovate Scalp Application (3 of 294 patients) 1153

Pustules, unspecified
- Duragesic Transdermal System (Less than 1%) 1336
- Ultravate Ointment 0.05% (Less frequent) 2798

Pustulosis, provocation
- Cormax Ointment (Rare) 1856
- Cormax Scalp Application (Rare) 1857
- Temovate Scalp Application (Rare) 1153

Pyelonephritis
- Ambien Tablets (Rare) 2559
- Anafranil Capsules (Rare) 819
- Avonex 662
- ▲ CellCept Capsules (More than or equal to 3%) 2265
- Cleocin Vaginal Cream (2%) 2070
- Dilacor XR Extended-release Capsules 2183
- Effexor (Infrequent) 2825
- Foscavir Injection (Less than 1%) 541
- Lupron Depot 3.75 mg 2739
- Miacalcin Nasal Spray (Less than 1%) 2403
- Naprelan Tablets (Less than 1%) 2861
- Norvir (Less than 2%) 447
- Permax Tablets (Rare) 571
- Prinivil Tablets (0.3% to 1.0%) 1776
- Prinzide Tablets 1780
- Prozac Pulvules & Liquid, Oral Solution (Rare) 935
- Rilutek Tablets (Rare) 2198
- Zestril Tablets (0.3% to 1.0%) 2972

Pyoderma gangrenosum
- Asacol Delayed-Release Tablets (Rare) 2129

Pyrexia (see under Fever)

Pyridoxine deficiency
- Macrodantin Capsules 2140
- Nydrazid Injection 509
- Rifamate Capsules 1278
- Rifater 1280

Pyrogenic granuloma
- Accutane Capsules (A number of cases) 2252
- ▲ Tegison Capsules (1-10%) 2314

Pyrosis (see under Heartburn)

Pyuria
- Anafranil Capsules (Rare) 819
- Cognex Capsules (Infrequent) 1961
- Effexor (Infrequent) 2825
- Floxin I.V. (More than or equal to 1%) 1580
- Floxin Tablets (200 mg, 300 mg, 400 mg) (More than or equal to 1%) 1577
- Naprelan Tablets (Less than 1%) 2861
- Neurontin Capsules (Rare) 1978
- Orlaam Oral Solution (Low frequency) 2361
- Paxil Tablets (Rare) 2681
- Permax Tablets (Infrequent) 571
- Prilosec Delayed-Release Capsules (Less than 1%) 516
- Prozac Pulvules & Liquid, Oral Solution (Rare) 935
- TICE BCG, USP (0.7%) 1881
- Zosyn 1463

PBI decrease
- Atamet Tablets 567
- Capozide Tablets 744
- Dyazide Capsules 2653
- Estratest 2718
- Lysodren Tablets (Infrequent) 707
- Sinemet Tablets 959
- Sinemet CR Tablets 961

PBI increase
- Amen Tablets 785
- Aygestin Tablets 990
- Cycrin Tablets 991
- Depo-Provera Sterile Aqueous Suspension 2083
- Etrafon 2495
- Larodopa Tablets (Rare) 2296
- Provera Tablets 2110
- Trilafon 2532

PSP excretion, depression
- Capastat Sulfate Injection (Many instances) 968

Q

Quadriplegia
- Orthoclone OKT3 Sterile Solution 1892
- Soma Compound w/Codeine Tablets (Very rare) 2784
- Soma Compound Tablets (Very rare) 2783
- Soma Tablets 2782

R

Radiculoneuropathy
- Imitrex Tablets (Rare) 1099
- Pneumovax 23 (Rare) 1768
- Pnu-Imune 23 1437
- Recombivax HB 1787

Rage
- Dizac (diazepam injectable emulsion) CIV (Less frequent) 1862
- Librium Capsules 2331
- Serax Capsules 2916
- Serax Tablets 2916
- Valium Tablets 2335
- Xanax Tablets (Rare) 2115

Rales
- Adalat CC (Less than 1.0%) 582
- Aredia for Injection (Up to 6%) 827
- Blenoxane 697
- Blocadren Tablets (0.6%) 1654
- Brevibloc (esmolol HCl) Injection (Less than 1%) 1860
- Crixivan Capsules (Less than 2%) 1670
- Ganite 2711
- Hivid Tablets (Less than 1%) 2287
- Imdur (Less than or equal to 5%) 1362
- RespiGam (1%) 1631
- Sular Tablets (Less than or equal to 1%) 2961
- Survanta Beractant Intratracheal Suspension 2346
- Timolide Tablets (Less than 1%) 1791
- Timoptic in Ocudose 1796
- Timoptic Sterile Ophthalmic Solution 1794
- Timoptic-XE 1798
- ▲ Vesanoid Capsules (14%) 2327
- ▲ Videx Tablets, Powder for Oral Solution, & Pediatric Powder for Oral Solution (6%) 2980

Rash
- Abbokinase 403
- Abbokinase Open-Cath 405
- ▲ Abelcet Injection (3% to 5%) 1540
- Accupril Tablets (1.4%) 1950
- ▲ Accutane Capsules (Less than 1 patient in 10) 2252
- Acel-Imune Diphtheria and Tetanus Toxoids and Acellular Pertussis Vaccine Adsorbed (1.2%) 1415
- Actigall Capsules 818
- ▲ Actimmune (17%) 1043
- Activase (Very rare) 1045
- Adalat CC (3% or less) 582
- ▲ AeroBid Inhaler System (3% to 9%) 1004
- ▲ Aerobid-M Inhaler System (3% to 9%) 1004
- Airet Albuterol Sulfate Inhalation Solution (Rare) 1602
- AK-Spore ◉ 205
- AK-Trol Ointment & Suspension ◉ 205
- Albenza Tablets (Rare) 2629
- Albuterol Sulfate, USP Solution for Inhalation, Arm-a-Med (Rare) 522
- Aldoclor Tablets 1638
- Aldomet Ester HCl Injection 1642
- Aldomet Oral 1640
- Aldoril Tablets 1644
- Alkeran for Injection 1196
- Alkeran Tablets 1198
- All-Flex Arcing Spring Diaphragm (See also Ortho Diaphragm Kits) 1921
- Alomide Ophthalmic Solution (Less than 1%) 465
- Altace Capsules (Less than 1%) 1238
- Ambien Tablets (2%) 2559
- Amen Tablets (Occasional) 785
- Americaine Anesthetic Lubricant 1603
- Americaine Hemorrhoidal Ointment ▣ 649
- Americaine Otic Topical Anesthetic Ear Drops 1603
- Amoxil 2631
- ▲ Anafranil Capsules (4% to 8%) 819
- Anaprox/Naprosyn (Less than 1%) 2277
- Ancobon Capsules 2254
- Androderm Testosterone Transdermal System (Less than 1% to 2%) 2634
- Anectine 1062
- Apresazide Capsules (Less frequent) 824
- Apresoline Hydrochloride Tablets (Less frequent) 826
- ▲ Arimidex Tablets (5.7% to 6.1%) 2932
- ▲ Asacol Delayed-Release Tablets (6%) 2129
- Atrohist Plus Tablets 1605
- Atrovent Inhalation Aerosol (1.2%) 674
- Atrovent Nasal Spray 0.06% (Rare) 678
- Attenuvax (Occasional) 1650
- Axid Pulvules (1.9%) 1468
- Axocet Capsules 2469
- Azactam for Injection (1 to 1.3%) 736
- Azelex (Less than 1%) 471
- ▲ Bactrim DS Tablets (Among most common) 2257
- ▲ Bactrim I.V. Infusion (Among most common) 2255
- ▲ Bactrim (Among most common) 2257
- Bactroban Nasal (Less than 1%) 2643
- Bactroban Ointment (Less than 1%) 2642
- Bentyl 1246
- Betagan ◉ 230
- Betapace Tablets (2% to 5%) 637
- Betimol 0.25%, 0.5% ◉ 259
- Biavax II (Infrequent) 1653
- ▲ Biaxin (3%) 406
- BiCozene Creme ▣ 747
- ▲ Blenoxane (Approximately 50%) 697
- Bleph-10 Ophthalmic Solution 10% 472
- Blocadren Tablets (Less than 1%) 1654
- BOTOX (Botulinum Toxin Type A) Purified Neurotoxin Complex (7 cases) 473
- Brevicon 2563
- Bumex (0.2%) 2260
- Buprenex Injectable (Infrequent) 2170
- Butisol Sodium Elixir & Tablets (Less than 1 in 100) 2768
- Caladryl Cream For Kids ▣ 817
- Calan SR Caplets (1.2%) 2571
- Calan Tablets (1.2%) 2568
- ▲ Capoten Tablets (About 4 to 7 of 100 patients) 740
- ▲ Capozide Tablets (About 4 to 7 of 100 patients) 744
- Carafate Suspension (Less than 0.5%) 1250

(▣ Described in PDR For Nonprescription Drugs) Incidence data in parenthesis; ▲ 3% or more (◉ Described in PDR For Ophthalmology)

Carafate Tablets (Less than 0.5%) 1249	▲ Disalcid (Among most common) 1549	Gammar-P I.V., Immune Globulin Intravenous (Human) 798	Lodine Capsules and Tablets (1% to 3%) 2849
Cardene Capsules (0.4% to 1.2%) 2261	Ditropan 1267	Gantanol Tablets 2285	Lo/Ovral Tablets 2852
Cardene SR Capsules (0.6%) 2264	Diucardin Tablets 2824	Gantrisin 2286	Lo/Ovral-28 Tablets 2857
▲ Cardioquin Tablets (5%) 2146	Diupres Tablets 1691	Garamycin Injectable 2502	Lopid Tablets (1.7%) 1974
Cardizem CD Capsules (1.2%) 1251	Diuril Oral Suspension 1694	Gastrocrom Capsules (2 of 87 patients) 1611	Lopressor HCT Tablets 850
Cardizem SR Capsules (1% to 1.5%) 1255	Diuril Sodium Intravenous 1693	Gastrocrom Oral Concentrate (2 of 87 patients) 1611	Lorabid Suspension and Pulvules (0.7% to 2.9%) 1513
Cardizem Injectable 1253	Diuril Tablets 1694		Lortab 2751
Cardizem Tablets (1.3%) 1257	▲ Dolobid Tablets (3% to 9%) 1695	▲ Gemzar for Injection (28% to 30%) 1482	Lotensin Tablets 852
Cardura Tablets (1%) 1993	▲ Donnazyme Tablets (Most frequent) 2235	Genotropin Injection (Infrequent) 2090	Lotensin HCT Tablets (0.3% to 1.0%) 855
Cartrol Tablets (1.3%) 413	Doral Tablets 2773	GlaucTabs ⊙ 209	Lotrel Capsules 858
▲ Casodex Tablets (6%) 2934	▲ Dovonex Cream 0.005% (1% to 10%) 2792	Glucophage Tablets 754	Lupron Depot 3.75 mg 2739
Cataflam Tablets (1% to 3%) 833	▲ Dovonex Ointment 0.005% (1% to 10%) 2793	Glucotrol XL Extended Release Tablets (1% or greater) 2012	Lupron Depot 7.5 mg 2741
Catapres Tablets (About 1 in 100 patients) 679	Doxidan Liqui-Gels 801	Habitrol Nicotine Transdermal System (Once in 35% of patients) 884	Lupron Depot - 3 Month 22.5 mg 2743
Catapres-TTS 680	Doxil (1% to 5%) 2613		Lupron Depot-PED 7.5 mg, 11.25 mg and 15 mg (2%) 2744
Caverject Injection (Less than 1%) 2064	Duragesic Transdermal System (1% or greater) 1336	Havrix (Less than 1%) 2663	Lutrepulse for Injection 998
Ceclor Pulvules & Suspension 1470	Duricef Capsules, Tablets, and Oral Suspension 750	Helidac Therapy (Less than 1%) 2135	LUVOX Tablets 2723
Cedax (0.1% to 1%) 2480	Dyazide Capsules 2653	Hespan Injection 945	M-M-R II (Infrequent) 1730
Cefizox for Intramuscular or Intravenous Use 1025	Dynabac (1.4%) 668	Hexalen Capsules (Less than 1%) 2760	M-R-VAX II (Infrequent) 1732
Cefotan (1 in 150) 2936	DynaCirc Capsules (1.5% to 2.0%) 2381	Helixate, Antihemophilic Factor (Recombinant) (Two reports out of 3,254 patients) 799	Matulane Capsules 2300
Ceftin (0.1% to 1%) 1067	DynaCirc CR Tablets (1.3% to 2.6%) 2383		Mavik Tablets (0.3% to 1.0%) 1407
Cefzil Tablets and Oral Suspension (0.9%) 747	Dyrenium Capsules (Rare) 2655	HibTITER (1 of 1,118 vaccinations) 1423	Maxair Autohaler 1550
▲ CellCept Capsules (6.4% to 7.7%) 2265	E-Mycin Tablets 1388	Hismanal Tablets (Less frequent) 1341	Maxair Inhaler (Less than 1%) 1552
Ceptaz (2% of patients) 1070	▲ Effexor (3%) 2825	▲ Hivid Tablets (3.4%) 2287	Maxaquin Tablets (Less than 1%) 2593
Cerebyx Injection (Frequent) 1956	▲ Efudex (Among most frequent) 2280	Humalog Injection (Less common) 1488	Maxipime for Injection (1.1%) 758
Cerezyme (One patient) 1056	Eldepryl Capsules 2729	Humegon for Injection 1873	Mefoxin 1734
Cerumenex Drops 2148	Elimite (permethrin) 5% Cream (1 to 2% or less) 475	Humulin 50/50, 100 Units 1491	Mefoxin Premixed Intravenous Solution 1737
▲ Chemet Capsules (2.6% to 11.2%) 666	Emete-con Intramuscular/Intravenous 2007	Humulin 70/30, 100 Units (Less common) 1492	▲ Megace Oral Suspension (2% to 12%) 708
Chibroxin Sterile Ophthalmic Solution (With oral form) 1657	Eminase (Occasional) 2215	Humulin L, 100 Units (Less common) 1494	Megace Tablets 710
Cipro I.V. (Greater than 1%) 587	EMLA Cream (Less than 1%) 536	Hycodan Tablets and Syrup 946	▲ Mepron Suspension (22% to 23%) 1206
Cipro I.V. Pharmacy Bulk Package (Greater than 1%) 590	Enduron Tablets 424	Hycomine 947	Merrem I.V. (1.4% to 3.5%) 2952
Cipro Tablets (1.1%; rare) 584	Engerix-B Unit-Dose Vials (Less than 1%) 2656	Hydralazine Hydrochloride Injection USP (Less frequent) 2712	Meruvax II 1740
Claritin Tablets (2% or fewer patients) 2485	▲ Epivir (9%) 1200	Hydrocet Capsules 787	Mesantoin Tablets 2400
Claritin-D Tablets (Less frequent) 2487	▲ Epogen for Injection (Rare; Up to 16%) 489	HydroDIURIL Tablets 1716	Methadone Hydrochloride Oral Concentrate 2356
Cleocin Vaginal Cream (Less than 1%) 2070	Ergamisol Tablets (10 patients) 1340	Hydropres Tablets 1718	Methotrexate Sodium Tablets, Injection, for Injection and LPF Injection (1% to 3%) 1322
▲ Clinoril Tablets (3% to 9%) 1658	Esgic-plus Capsules 1012	Hyperab Rabies Immune Globulin (Human) (Rare) 618	
Clomid (Fewer than 1%) 1262	Esgic-plus Tablets 1012	Hyperstat I.V. Injection 2504	Metrodin (urofollitropin for injection) 2616
Clozaril Tablets (2%) 2377	Esidrix Tablets 839	Hytrin Capsules (At least 1%) 434	MetroGel-Vaginal (Equal to or less than 2%) 917
Cogentin 1661	Esimil Tablets 840	Hyzaar Tablets (1.4%) 1720	▲ Mevacor Tablets (0.8% to 5.2%) 1742
▲ Cognex Capsules (7%) 1961	Eskalith 2658	▲ IBU Tablets (3% to 9%) 1389	▲ Mexitil Capsules (3.8% to 4.2%) 684
Colace Capsules, Syrup, Liquid 2212	Estraderm Transdermal System (Rare) 842	Idamycin Injection 2096	Miacalcin Injection 2402
Colestid (Infrequent) 2073	Ethmozine Tablets (Less than 2%) 2217	Regular, 100 Units (Less common) 1503	Micro-K LS Packets (Rare) 2238
Combipres Tablets 682	Ethyol (amifostine) for Injection (Rare; less than 1%) 485	Pork Regular, 100 Units 1507	Mivacron (Less than 1%) 1125
Compazine 2644	Etopophos for Injection (Infrequent) 701	Imdur (Less than or equal to 5%) 1362	Moban Tablets and Concentrate 1036
Cordarone Tablets (Less than 1%) 2818	Etoposide Injection (Infrequent) 539	Imitrex Injection (Infrequent) 1095	Modicon 1928
Cortisporin Ophthalmic Ointment Sterile 1074	Etrafon 2495	Imitrex Tablets (Rare to infrequent) 1099	▲ Moduretic Tablets (3% to 8%) 1748
Covera-HS Tablets (1.2% to 2%) 2573	▲ Eulexin Capsules (3% to 8%) 2498	Inderide Tablets 2838	8-MOP Capsules 1294
Cozaar Tablets (Less than 1%) 1668	Ex-Lax Chocolated Laxative Tablets 748	Inderide LA Long Acting Capsules 2840	Monocid Injection (Less than 1%) 2674
Crixivan Capsules 1670	Extra Gentle Ex-Lax Laxative Pills 749	Indocin Capsules (Less than 1%) 1723	Monoket Tablets (Less than 1% to 4%) 2550
▲ Cuprimine Capsules (5%) 1673	Regular Strength Ex-Lax Laxative Pills 749	Indocin I.V. (Less than 1%) 1727	Monopril Tablets (0.2% to 1.0% or more) 762
Cycrin Tablets (Occasional) 991	Ex-Lax Gentle Nature Laxative Pills 749	Indocin (Less than 1%) 1723	▲ Motrin Ibuprofen Suspension, Oral Drops, Chewable Tablets, Caplets (3% to 9%) 1563
▲ Cytadren Tablets (1 in 6) 837	▲ Felbatol (3.4% to 9.7%) 2774	INFeD (Iron Dextran Injection, USP) 2478	
▲ ytosar-U Sterile Powder (Among most frequent) 2077	Feldene Capsules (Occasional) 2008	Intal Inhaler (Infrequent) 2185	MSTA Mumps Skin Test Antigen 2988
Cytotec (Infrequent) 2576	Fioricet Tablets 2386	Intal Nebulizer Solution 2186	Mutamycin for Injection (Rare) 712
▲ Cytovene (15%) 2270	Fioricet with Codeine Capsules 2387	Invirase Capsules (1.3%) 2291	▲ Mycobutin Capsules (11%) 2101
DDAVP 2180	Fiorinal with Codeine Capsules 2390	Ismo Tablets (Fewer than 1%) 2844	Mycostatin Pastilles (Rare) 713
D.H.E. 45 Injection (Occasional) 2381	▲ Flolan for Injection (10%) 1085	ISMOTIC 45% w/v Solution (Very rare) ⊙ 221	Mykrox Tablets (Less than 2%) 1617
Dalgan Injection (Less than 1%) 529	Flonase Nasal Spray 1088	Isoptin Oral Tablets (1.2%) 1393	Naftin Gel 1% (0.5%) 477
Danocrine Capsules 2437	Flovent (Rare) 1089	Isoptin SR Tablets (1.2% or less) 1395	Nalfon 200 Pulvules & Nalfon Tablets (3.7%) 933
Daypro Caplets (Rare to 9%) 2578	Floxin I.V. (1% to 3%) 1580	▲ JE-VAX (5% to approximately 10%) 904	
Demadex Tablets and Injection 691	Floxin Tablets (200 mg, 300 mg, 400 mg) (1% to 3%) 1577	K-Lor Powder Packets (Rare) 438	▲ Naprelan Tablets (3% to 9%) 2861
Depakene 416	Flumadine Tablets & Syrup (0.3% to 1%) 1013	K-Tab Filmtab (Rare) 439	Naprosyn Tablets (Less than 1%) 2277
▲ Depakote Tablets (1% to 6%) 418	Fosamax Tablets (Rare) 1703	Kadian Capsules (Less than 3%) 2948	Nasalcrom Nasal Solution (Less than 1%) 2192
▲ Depen Titratable Tablets (5%) 2770	▲ Foscavir Injection (5% or greater) 541	Keflex Pulvules & Oral Suspension 930	Navane Capsules and Concentrate 2018
Depo-Provera Contraceptive Injection (1% to 5%) 2079	Fragmin Injection (Rare) 2088	Keftab Tablets 931	Navane Intramuscular 2019
Depo-Provera Sterile Aqueous Suspension 2083	Sterile FUDR 2284	Kefurox Vials, Faspak & ADD-Vantage (1 in 125) 1509	Navelbine Injection (Less than 5%) 1212
Dermatop Emollient Cream 0.1% (Less than 1%) 1264	▲ Fulvicin P/G Tablets (Among most common) 2499	Kerlone Tablets (1.2%) 2588	▲ NegGram (Most frequent) 2453
Desferal Vials 838	▲ Fulvicin P/G 165 & 330 Tablets (Among most common) 2500	KOGENATE Antihemophilic Factor (Recombinant) (Two reports) 626	Neptazane Tablets ⊙ 320
Desmopressin Acetate Rhinal Tube 997	Fungizone Intravenous 507	Kytril Injection (Rare; 1%) 2667	Netromycin Injection 100 mg/ml (4 or 5 of 1000 patients) 2516
Desyrel and Desyrel Dividose 504	Fungizone Oral Suspension 704	▲ Lamictal Tablets (10%) 1105	▲ Neupogen for Injection (6%; 12%) 495
Diflucan Tablets, Injection, and Oral Suspension (1.8%) 2003	Furacin Soluble Dressing (Approximately 1%) 2220	▲ Lamisil Tablets (5.6%) 2394	Neurontin Capsules (More than 1%) 1978
Dilacor XR Extended-release Capsules (1.0%) 2183	Furacin Topical Cream (Approximately 1%) 2220	▲ Lariam Tablets (Among most frequent) 2295	▲ Neutrexin for Injection (5.5%) 2761
Dilantin Infatabs 1967	Gamimune N, 5% Immune Globulin Intravenous (Human), 5% (Rare) 612	Lescol Capsules (2.3%) 2395	Nicotrol NS Nicotine Nasal Spray (Less than 1%) 1565
Dilantin Kapseals 1965		Leukeran Tablets (Rare) 1205	Nimbex Injection (0.1%) 1131
Dilantin-125 Suspension 1969	Gamimune N, 10% Immune Globulin Intravenous (Human), 10% (Rare; a single incidence) 615	Leukine (44% to 70%) 1317	Nimotop Capsules (Up to 2.4%) 603
Dilaudid-HP Injection (Less frequent) 1384		Leustatin (10% to 27%) 1889	▲ Nipent for Injection (26% to 43%) 2733
Dilaudid-HP Lyophilized Powder 250 mg (Less frequent) 1384		Levoprome 1321	Nordette-21 Tablets 2863
Diaudid Tablets and Liquid 1386		Lioresal Intrathecal (1% or more) 1634	Nordette-28 Tablets 2866
Dipentum Capsules (2%) 2084		Lithium Carbonate Capsules & Tablets 2352	Norinyl 2563
Diphtheria and Tetanus Toxoids and Pertussis Vaccine Adsorbed 2650		Livostin (Approximately 1% to 3%) ⊙ 262	Normodyne Injection (Rare) 2519
Diprivan Injectable Emulsion (Less than 1% to 5%) 2939			Normodyne Tablets (1%) 2522
			Noroxin Tablets (0.3% to 1.0%) 1758

(📖 Described in PDR For Nonprescription Drugs)   Incidence data in parenthesis; ▲ 3% or more   (⊙ Described in PDR For Ophthalmology)

1439 Side Effects Index Rash, allergic

Noroxin Tablets (0.3% to 1.0%).... 2222
Norpace (1 to 3%) 2596
Norplant System 2868
Nor-Q D Tablets 2598
Norvasc Tablets (Less than 1% to 2%) 2020
Norvir (2.6%) 447
Novantrone for Injection (Occasional) 1327
Novolin 70/30 Prefilled Disposable Insulin Delivery System (Rare) 1850
Ocupress Ophthalmic Solution, 1% Sterile .... ⊙ 297
Oil of Olay Daily UV Protectant SPF 15 Beauty Fluid-Original and Fragrance Free (Olay Co. Inc.) .... ▣ 725
Omnipen for Oral Suspension 2873
▲ Oncaspar (Greater than 5%) 2194
Oncovin Solution Vials & Hyporets (Rare) 1521
OptiPranolol (Metipranolol 0.3%) Sterile Ophthalmic Solution (A small number of patients) .... ⊙ 256
▲ Orap Tablets (8.3%) 1037
Oretic Tablets 450
Organidin NR Tablets and Liquid (Rare) 2781
Orlaam Oral Solution (1% to 3%).. 2361
Ortho-Cyclen/Ortho-Tri-Cyclen 1914
Ortho Diaphragm Kits—All-Flex Arcing Spring; Ortho Coil Spring; Ortho-White Flat Spring 1921
Ortho Diaphragm Kit-Coil Spring 1921
Ortho-Novum 1928
Ortho-Cyclen/Ortho Tri-Cyclen 1914
Ortho-White Diaphragm Kit-Flat Spring (See also Ortho Diaphragm Kits) 1921
Orthoclone OKT3 Sterile Solution .. 1892
Orudis Capsules (Greater than 1%) 2874
Oruvail Capsules (Greater than 1%) 2874
Ovral Tablets 2877
Ovrette Tablets 2878
Oxistat Cream (0.1%) 1139
Oxsoralen-Ultra Capsules 1302
OxyContin Tablets (Between 1% and 5%) 2163
Pamelor 2409
Paraplatin for Injection 713
▲ PASER Granules (Among most common) 1333
Paxil Tablets (2% to 3%) 2681
Pediazole Suspension 2340
Penetrex Tablets (Less than 1% to 1%) 2196
Pentasa (1.0% to 1.3%) 1275
Pepcid Injection (Infrequent) 1765
Pepcid (Infrequent) 1763
Percocet Tablets 955
Pergonal (menotropins for injection, USP) 2618
Peri-Colace Capsules and Syrup 2226
▲ Permax Tablets (3.2%) 571
Persantine Tablets (2.3%) 686
Phenergan with Codeine 2883
Phenergan with Dextromethorphan 2885
Phenergan Suppositories 2882
Phenergan Syrup 2881
Phenergan VC 2886
Phenergan VC with Codeine 2888
Phillips' Gelcaps .... ▣ 627
Phrenilin (Infrequent) 790
Placidyl Capsules 456
Platinol for Injection (Infrequent) 717
Platinol-AQ Injection (Infrequent) 719
Plendil Extended-Release Tablets (0.2% to 2.0%) 514
Pneumovax 23 (Rare) 1768
Pnu-Imune 23 (Rare to infrequent) 1437
Polysporin Ophthalmic Ointment Sterile 1140
Pondimin Tablets 2239
Ponstel 1982
▲ Pravachol Tablets (1.3% to 4.0%) 770
Premarin Tablets 2896
Premphase 2900
Prempro 2905
Prevacid Delayed-Release Capsules (Less than 1%) 2746
Prilosec Delayed-Release Capsules (Less than 1% to 1.5%) 516
Primaxin I.M. (0.4%) 1770
Primaxin I.V. (0.9%) 1772
Prinivil Tablets (0.3% to 1.7%) 1776
Prinzide Tablets (1.2%) 1780
Priscoline Hydrochloride Ampuls 864
Procardia XL Extended Release Tablets (Less than 3%) 2026
▲ Procrit for Injection (Rare to 16%) 1896
Profasi (chorionic gonadotropin for injection, USP) 2620
▲ Prograf (8% to 24%) 1028
Prolastin Alpha$_1$-Proteinase Inhibitor (Human) (Occasional) 629
▲ Proleukin for Injection (26%) 812
▲ Proloprim Tablets (2.9% to 6.7%) 1141
Propulsid (1.6%) 1346
Proscar Tablets 1784
ProSom Tablets (Infrequent) 457
Prostep (nicotine transdermal system) (1% to 3% of patients).. 1439
Prostigmin Injectable 1305
Prostigmin Tablets 1306
Prostin E2 Suppository 2109
Proventil Inhalation Aerosol (Rare) 2524
Proventil Inhalation Solution 0.083% (Rare) 2527
Proventil Repetabs Tablets (2%) 2529
Proventil Solution for Inhalation 0.5% (Rare) 2525
Proventil Syrup (Rare) 2528
Proventil Tablets (2%) 2529
Provera Tablets 2110
▲ Prozac Pulvules & Liquid, Oral Solution (Approximately 4% of 5,600 patients) 935
▲ Pulmozyme Inhalation (10% to 12%) 1054
Pyrazinamide Tablets 1442
Pyridium 1985
Questran (Less frequent) 774
Quibron 2227
▲ Quinaglute Dura-Tabs Tablets (6%) 644
▲ Quinidex Extentabs (5%) 2240
RMS Suppositories CII 2766
Recombivax HB (Less than 1%) 1787
Redux Capsules (2.3%) 2911
▲ Relafen Tablets (3% to 9%) 2688
Remeron Tablets (Frequent) 1878
Respbid Tablets 687
RespiGam (1%) 1631
▲ Retrovir Capsules (17%) 1216
▲ Retrovir I.V. Infusion (17%) 1221
▲ Retrovir Syrup (17%) 1216
▲ ReVia Tablets (Less than 10%) 957
Rhinocort Nasal Inhaler (Less than 1%) 552
▲ Ridaura Capsules (24%) 2691
Rifadin (Occasional) 1276
Rifamate Capsules (Occasional) 1278
Rifater (Occasional) 1280
Rimactane Capsules 865
Risperdal Tablets (2% to 5%) 1348
Robaxin Injectable 2245
Robaxin Tablets 2246
Robaxisal Tablets 2246
Rocephin Injectable Vials, ADD-Vantage, Galaxy Container (1.7%) 2305
▲ Roferon-A Injection (11% to 44%) 2308
Romazicon (1% to 3%) 2311
Rowasa (1.2% to 2.82%) 2727
Rythmol Tablets–150mg, 225mg, 300mg (0.6 to 2.6%) 1399
▲ SSKI Solution (Among most frequent) 2767
Salagen Tablets (1%) 1546
Salflex Tablets 791
Sandostatin Injection (Less than 1%) 2421
Sanorex Tablets 2423
Sansert Tablets (Rare) 2424
Sectral Capsules (2%) 2914
Sedapap Tablets 50 mg/650 mg .. 1826
Seldane Tablets (1.0% to 1.6%) 1284
Seldane-D Extended-Release Tablets (1.1%) 1286
▲ Septra (Among most common) 1146
▲ Septra I.V. Infusion (Among most common) 1142
▲ Septra I.V. Infusion ADD-Vantage Vials (Among most common) 1144
▲ Septra (Among most common) 1146
Ser-Ap-Es Tablets 867
Serentil 689
Serevent Inhalation Aerosol (Rare; 1% to 3%) 1149
Serzone Tablets (2%) 776
Shade Gel SPF 30 Sunblock .... ▣ 767
Shade UVAGUARD SPF 15 Suncreen Lotion .... ▣ 768
Silvadene Cream 1% (Infrequent) .. 1288
Sinemet CR Tablets 961
Skelaxin Tablets 793
Slo-bid Gyrocaps 2201
Slo-Niacin Tablets (Less common).. 2767
Slow-K Extended-Release Tablets (Rare) 869
Solganal Suspension 2530
Soma Compound w/Codeine Tablets 2784
Soma Compound Tablets (Less common) 2783
▲ Sporanox Capsules (3% to 8.6%).. 1352
Stadol (Less than 1%) 779
Stelazine 2692
Sular Tablets (2%) 2961
Sulfamylon Cream 940
▲ Supprelin Injection (3% to 10%).... 2230
Suprax (Less than 2%) 1443
Synarel Nasal Solution for Central Precocious Puberty (2.6%) 2603
Synthroid 1410
Tagamet 2694
Talacen Caplets (Infrequent) 2464
Talwin Carpuject (Infrequent) 2465
Talwin Compound (Infrequent) 2466
Talwin Injection (Infrequent) 2465
Talwin Nx Tablets (Infrequent) 2467
▲ Taxol Injection (12%) 723
Taxotere for Injection Concentrate (0.9%) 2204
Tazicef for Injection (2%) 2697
▲ Tegison Capsules (50-75%) 2314
Tenex Tablets (Less frequent) 2249
Tetramune (Up to 3%) 1449
Thalitone 1293
Theo-Dur Extended-Release Tablets 1367
Theo-X Extended-Release Tablets .. 793
Tiazac Capsules (2%) 1019
TICE BCG, USP (0.6%) 1881
▲ Ticlid Tablets (5.1%) 2317
Tilade Inhaler (Less than 1%) 2207
Timolide Tablets (Less than 1%) 1791
Timoptic in Ocudose (Less frequent) 1796
Timoptic Sterile Ophthalmic Solution (Less frequent) 1794
Timoptic-XE 1798
Tolectin (200, 400 and 600 mg) .. 1591
▲ Tonocard Tablets (0.4% to 12.2%) 519
▲ Toprol-XL Tablets (About 5 of 100 patients) 560
Toradol (Greater than 1%) 2319
Tracrium Injection 1155
Trandate (Rare) 1158
Transderm Scōp Transdermal Therapeutic System (Infrequent) 890
Trental Tablets (Less than 1%) 1291
Tri-Immunol Adsorbed 1452
Trilisate (Less than 1%) 2155
▲ Trimpex Tablets (2.6% to 6.7%) .. 2323
Tri-Norinyl 2607
Triphasil-21 Tablets 2919
Triphasil-28 Tablets 2924
Trusopt Sterile Ophthalmic Solution (Rare) 1803
Tussionex Pennkinetic Extended-Release Suspension 1624
Tussi-Organidin DM NR Liquid and DM-S NR Liquid (Rare) 2786
Tylox Capsules 1593
Tympagesic Ear Drops 2476
Ultram Tablets (50 mg) (1% to less than 5%) 1594
Ultravate Cream 0.05% (Less frequent) 2797
Ultravate Ointment 0.05% (Less frequent) 2798
Unasyn (Less than 2%) 2035
Uni-Dur Extended-Release Tablets.. 1374
Univasc Tablets (Less than 1% to 1.6%) 2553
Urised Tablets 2123
Vancenase PocketHaler Nasal Inhaler (Rare) 2534
Vanceril Inhaler (Rare) 2538
Vancocin HCl, Oral Solution & Pulvules (Infrequent) 1536
Vancocin HCl, Vials & ADD-Vantage (Infrequent) 1534
Vantin for Oral Suspension and Vantin Tablets (Less than 1% to 3.5%) 2112
Vaqta (Less than 1%) 1805
Varivax (Greater than or equal to 1%) 1807
Vascor Tablets (200 and 300 mg) (0.5 to 2.0%) 1597
Vaseretic Tablets (0.5% to 2.0%) 1810
Vasotec I.V. (0.5% to 1.0%) 1814
Vasotec Tablets (0.5%; 1.3% to 1.4%) 1816
Velosulin BR Human Insulin 10 ml Vials 1847
Ventolin Inhalation Solution (Rare).. 1171
Ventolin Nebules Inhalation Solution (Rare) 1172
Ventolin Rotacaps for Inhalation (Rare) 1173
Ventolin Syrup (Rare) 1175
Ventolin Tablets (Rare) 1176
VePesid Capsules and Injection (Infrequent) 727
Verelan Capsules (1% or less to 1.4%) 1455
Vermox Chewable Tablets (Rare) 1357
Versed Injection (Less than 1%) 2324
▲ Vesanoid Capsules (54%) 2327
Vicodin HP Tablets 1403
▲ Videx Tablets, Powder for Oral Solution, & Pediatric Powder for Oral Solution (7% to 70%) 2980
▲ Viramune Tablets (Among most frequent; 8% to 37%) 2368
Virazole 1310
Visken Tablets (Less than 1%) 2428
Vistide Injection 1057
Vivelle Transdermal System (Rare) 880
Vivotif Berna 660
Volmax Extended-Release Tablets (Rare) 1835
Cataflam/Voltaren/Voltaren-XR (1% to 3%) 833
▲ Vumon for Injection (3%) 729
▲ Wellbutrin Tablets (8.0%) 1177
Xalatan (1% to 2%) .... ⊙ 304
▲ Xanax Tablets (10.8%) 2115
Yutopar Intravenous Injection (Infrequent) 566
Zaroxolyn Tablets 1625
Zebeta Tablets 1457
Zemuron Injection (Less than 1%) 1885
▲ Zerit Capsules (4% to 40%) 731
Zestoretic Tablets (1.2%) 2968
Zestril Tablets (0.01% to 1.7%) 2972
Ziac 1459
Zithromax (1% or less) 2043
Zithromax Tablets (1% or less) 2046
Zofran Injection (Approximately 1%) 1227
Zofran Tablets (Approximately 1%) 1231
▲ Zoladex (1% to 6%) 2976
Zoladex 3-month 2978
Zoloft Tablets (2.1%) 2051
Zosyn (1.3% to 4.2%) 1463
Zovirax Capsules (0.6% to 1.7%).. 1187
Zovirax Ointment 5% 1190
Zovirax Sterile Powder (Approximately 2%) 1191
Zovirax (0.6% to 1.7%) 1187
Zyrtec Tablets (Less than 2%) 2053

Rash, actinic

Solganal Suspension 2530

Rash, allergic

Amen Tablets 785
Aygestin Tablets 990
Brevicon 2563
Cycrin Tablets 991
Demulen 2580
Depo-Provera Sterile Aqueous Suspension 2083
Desogen Tablets 1867
Florinef Acetate Tablets 506
Levlen/Tri-Levlen 646
Luride Drops 50 ml (Rare) 891
Luride Lozi-Tabs Tablets (Rare) 892
Modicon 1928
Norinyl 2563
Nor-Q D Tablets 2598
Ortho-Cept 1907
Ortho-Cyclen/Ortho-Tri-Cyclen 1914
Ortho-Novum 1928
Ortho-Cyclen/Ortho Tri-Cyclen 1914
Ovcon 765
Parafon Forte DSC Caplets (Rare) .. 1590
Periactin 1767
Poly-Vi-Flor Drops (Rare) 1600
Poly-Vi-Flor Tablets (Rare) 1600
Premphase 2900
Prempro 2905
Levlen/Tri-Levlen 646
Tri-Norinyl 2607
Tri-Vi-Flor Drops (Rare) 1601
Varivax (Greater than or equal to 1%) 1807

(▣ Described in PDR For Nonprescription Drugs) Incidence data in parenthesis; ▲ 3% or more (⊙ Described in PDR For Ophthalmology)

Rash, bullous

Rash, bullous
- Orudis Capsules (Less than 1%) 2874
- Oruvail Capsules (Less than 1%) 2874
- Trandate Tablets (Less common) 1158
- ▲ Zosyn (4.2%) 1463

Rash, bullous erythrodermatous of the palms and soles
- Idamycin Injection 2096

Rash, circumocular
- Polytrim Ophthalmic Solution Sterile (Multiple reports) 479

Rash, diaper
- Cefzil Tablets and Oral Suspension (1.5%) 747

Rash, drug
- Benadryl Injection 1955
- Dimetane-DC Cough Syrup 2232
- Dimetane-DX Cough Syrup 2233
- Nitrolingual Spray 2193
- Nitrostat Tablets 1981
- Ornade Spansule Capsules 2678
- PBZ Tablets 863
- PBZ-SR Tablets 862
- Tavist Syrup 2426
- Tavist Tablets 2427
- Trancopal Caplets 2468
- Trinalin Repetabs Tablets 1373
- Tussend 1830

Rash, erythematous
- Achromycin V Capsules 1417
- Anafranil Capsules (Infrequent) 819
- Atretol Tablets 569
- Blocadren Tablets 1654
- Cartrol Tablets 413
- Celontin Kapseals 1955
- ▲ Cognex Capsules (7%) 1961
- DTIC-Dome (Infrequent) 593
- Declomycin Tablets 1421
- Doryx Capsules 1970
- DYNACIN Capsules 1627
- Flagyl 375 Capsules 2587
- Flagyl I.V. 2373
- Foscavir Injection (Between 1% and 5%) 541
- Helidac Therapy 2135
- Hivid Tablets (Less than 1%) 2287
- Inderal 2834
- Inderal LA Long Acting Capsules 2836
- Inderide Tablets 2838
- Inderide LA Long Acting Capsules 2840
- Kerlone Tablets (Less than 2%) 2588
- Levatol Tablets 2547
- Methotrexate Sodium Tablets, Injection, for Injection and LPF Injection 1322
- Miacalcin Nasal Spray (1% to 3%) 2403
- Minocin Intravenous 1428
- Minocin Oral Suspension 1431
- Minocin Pellet-Filled Capsules 1429
- Monodox Capsules 1858
- Norvasc Tablets (More than 0.1% to 1%) 2020
- Protostat Tablets 1939
- Sectral Capsules 2914
- Tegretol/Tegretol-XR 870
- Tenoretic Tablets 2963
- Tenormin Tablets and I.V. Injection 2965
- Terramycin Intramuscular Solution 2034
- Timolide Tablets 1791
- Timoptic in Ocudose 1796
- Timoptic Sterile Ophthalmic Solution 1794
- Timoptic-XE 1798
- Vibramycin 2038
- Vibramycin Hyclate Intravenous 2040
- Vibramycin 2038
- Visken Tablets 2428
- Zarontin Capsules 1986
- Zarontin Syrup 1986
- Zoloft Tablets (Infrequent) 2051
- ▲ Zosyn (3.9%) 1463
- Zyrtec Tablets (Less than 2%) 2053

Rash, erythematous maculopapular
- Aldactazide Tablets 2556
- Amoxil 2631
- Etopophos for Injection (Infrequent) 701
- Miltown Tablets 2780
- Omnipen Capsules (Frequent) 2872
- Omnipen for Oral Suspension (Frequent) 2873
- PMB 200 and PMB 400 2890
- Viramune Tablets 2368

Rash, exfoliative
- Cardioquin Tablets 2146
- Quinaglute Dura-Tabs Tablets 644

Rash, female genitalia
- Floxin I.V. (Less than 1%) 1580
- Floxin Tablets (200 mg, 300 mg, 400 mg) (Less than 1%) 1577

Rash, follicular
- Hivid Tablets (Less than 1%) 2287
- Zoloft Tablets (Rare) 2051

Rash, herpetic
(see under Eruptions, herpetic)

Rash, leg
- DDAVP 2180
- Desmopressin Acetate Rhinal Tube 997

Rash, lichenoid
- Normodyne Tablets (Less common) 2522
- Permax Tablets (Rare) 571
- Trandate Tablets (Less common) 1158

Rash, maculopapular
- Abelcet Injection 1540
- Achromycin V Capsules 1417
- Anafranil Capsules (Infrequent) 819
- Betaseron for SC Injection 653
- Capastat Sulfate Injection 968
- Capoten Tablets 740
- Capozide Tablets 744
- Catapres-TTS (1 of 101; 10 cases of 3,539 patients) 680
- Cerebyx Injection (Infrequent) 1956
- Chloromycetin Sodium Succinate 1960
- Cleocin Phosphate Injection 2068
- Cleocin Vaginal Cream 2070
- ▲ Cognex Capsules (7%) 1961
- Cytosar-U Sterile Powder (Occasional) 2077
- Cytovene (1% or less) 2270
- Danocrine Capsules 2437
- Declomycin Tablets 1421
- Depakote Tablets (1% to 5%) 418
- Didronel Tablets 2133
- Doryx Capsules 1970
- Doxil (Less than 1%) 2613
- DYNACIN Capsules 1627
- Effexor (Infrequent) 2825
- Fluorouracil Injection 2282
- Foscavir Injection (Between 1% and 5%) 541
- Sterile FUDR (Remote possibility) .. 2284
- Fungizone Intravenous 507
- Haldol Decanoate 1587
- Haldol Injection, Tablets and Concentrate 1585
- Helidac Therapy 2135
- Hivid Tablets (Less than 1%) 2287
- Hydrea Capsules (Less frequent) 705
- Hyskon Hysteroscopy Fluid (Rare) .. 1633
- ▲ IBU Tablets (3% to 9%) 1389
- Invirase Capsules (Less than 2%) .. 2291
- Lamictal Tablets (Infrequent) 1105
- Lanoxicaps (Rare) 1110
- Lanoxin Elixir Pediatric (Rare) 1113
- Lanoxin Injection (Rare) 1116
- Lanoxin Injection Pediatric (Rare) .. 1119
- Lanoxin Tablets (Rare) 1121
- Lodine Capsules and Tablets (Less than 1%) 2849
- Lotrisone Cream (1 of 270 patients) 2515
- Mandol Vials, Faspak & ADD-Vantage 1516
- Mesantoin Tablets 2400
- Minocin Intravenous 1428
- Minocin Oral Suspension 1431
- Minocin Pellet-Filled Capsules 1429
- Monodox Capsules 1858
- ▲ Motrin Ibuprofen Suspension, Oral Drops, Chewable Tablets, Caplets (3% to 9%) 1563
- Normodyne Tablets (Less common) 2522
- Norvasc Tablets (More than 0.1% to 1%) 2020
- Norvir (Less than 2%) 447
- Paxil Tablets (Rare) 2681
- Procanbid Extended-Release Tablets (Occasional) 1983
- Proloprim Tablets (Mild to moderate) 1141
- Prozac Pulvules & Liquid, Oral Solution (Infrequent) 935
- Rifamate Capsules 1278
- Serax Capsules 2916
- Serax Tablets 2916
- Serzone Tablets (Infrequent) 776
- Sular Tablets (Less than or equal to 1%) 2961
- Synarel Nasal Solution for Endometriosis (Less than 1%) 2605
- Terramycin Intramuscular Solution 2034
- Ticlid Tablets 2317
- Toradol 2319
- Trandate Tablets (Less common) 1158
- Vibramycin 2038
- Vibramycin Hyclate Intravenous 2040
- Vibramycin 2038
- ▲ Zerit Capsules (Fewer than 1% or 6%) 731
- Zoloft Tablets (Infrequent) 2051
- ▲ Zosyn (4.2%) 1463
- Zyloprim Tablets (Less than 1%) 1194
- Zyrtec Tablets (Less than 2%) 2053

Rash, morbilliform
- ▲ Cleocin Phosphate Injection (Most frequent) 2068
- ▲ Cleocin Vaginal Cream (Most frequent) 2070
- ▲ Dilantin Infatabs (Among most common) 1967
- ▲ Dilantin Kapseals (Among most common) 1965
- ▲ Dilantin-125 Suspension (Among most common) 1969
- Furoxone 2221
- Mesantoin Tablets 2400
- Proloprim Tablets (Mild to moderate) 1141
- Rifamate Capsules 1278
- Serax Capsules 2916
- Serax Tablets 2916

Rash, papular
- Alcovate Cream (Approximately 2%) 1061
- ▲ Chemet Capsules (2.6% to 11.2%) 666
- Danocrine Capsules 2437

Rash, papular, neck
- Alferon N Injection (1%) 2142

Rash, penile
- Caverject Injection (1%) 2064

Rash, perianal
- Mintezol 1747

Rash, pruritic
- Atretol Tablets 569
- ▲ Capoten Tablets (About 4 to 7 of 100 patients) 740
- ▲ Capozide Tablets (About 4 to 7 of 100 patients) 744
- Cycrin Tablets 991
- Etopophos for Injection (Infrequent) 701
- Fluorouracil Injection 2282
- Sterile FUDR (Remote possibility) .. 2284
- Hivid Tablets (Less than 1%) 2287
- Lithonate/Lithotabs/Lithobid 2721
- Miltown Tablets 2780
- PMB 200 and PMB 400 2890
- Premphase 2900
- Prempro 2905
- Proloprim Tablets (Mild to moderate) 1141
- Skelaxin Tablets 793
- Spectazole (econazole nitrate 1%) Cream (One case) 1947
- Tegretol/Tegretol-XR 870

Rash, psoriaform
- Cardioquin Tablets 2146
- Foscavir Injection (Less than 1%) .. 541
- Inderal (Rare) 2834
- Inderal LA Long Acting Capsules (Rare) 2836
- Inderide Tablets (Rare) 2838
- Inderide LA Long Acting Capsules (Rare) 2840
- Normodyne Tablets (Less common) 2522
- Quinaglute Dura-Tabs Tablets 644
- Tenoretic Tablets 2963
- Tenormin Tablets and I.V. Injection 2965
- Trandate Tablets (Less common) 1158

Rash, purpuric
- Danocrine Capsules 2437
- Dilantin Infatabs 1967
- Dilantin Kapseals 1965
- Dilantin-125 Suspension 1969
- Eminase (0.3%) 2215
- Mesantoin Tablets 2400

Rash, pustular
- Anafranil Capsules (Infrequent) 819
- Cerebyx Injection (Infrequent) 1956
- Doxil (Less than 1%) 2613
- Effexor (Rare) 2825
- Lamictal Tablets (Rare) 1105
- Prozac Pulvules & Liquid, Oral Solution (Rare) 935
- Sular Tablets (Less than or equal to 1%) 2961

Rash, scarlatiniform
- Dilantin Infatabs 1967
- Dilantin Kapseals 1965
- Dilantin-125 Suspension 1969
- Mesantoin Tablets 2400

Rash, skin
(see also under Rash)
- Adapin Capsules (Occasional) 1542
- Amicar Syrup, Tablets, and Injection 1312
- Amikacin Sulfate Injection, USP (Rare) 523
- Amikacin Sulfate Injection, USP (Rare) 981
- Amikin Injectable (Rare) 502
- Ancef Injection 2632
- Anturane 823
- Artane (Rare) 1418
- Asendin Tablets (Less frequent) 1419
- Atamet Tablets 567
- Ativan Injection (Occasional) 2805
- Atretol Tablets 569
- Atromid-S Capsules (Less often) 2808
- Atrovent Nasal Spray 0.03% (Infrequent) 676
- ▲ Augmentin (3%) 2637
- ▲ Augmentin Tablets (3%) 2640
- Azathioprine Tablets (Approximately 2%) 2349
- Azulfidine (One in every 30 patients or less) 2059
- Beclovent Inhalation Aerosol and Refill (Rare) 1063
- Beconase (Rare) 1065
- Bicillin C-R Injection 2810
- Bicillin C-R 900/300 Injection 2812
- Bicillin L-A Injection 2813
- BuSpar Tablets (1%) 738
- Calcimar Injection, Synthetic (Occasional) 2176
- Ceptaz (2% of patients) 1070
- Cerubidine for Injection (Rare) 634
- Chromagen Capsules 2470
- Chromagen FA 2471
- Chromagen Forte 2471
- Claforan Sterile and Injection (2.4%) 1259
- Combipres Tablets (About 1%) 682
- Cylert Tablets 415
- Cytosar-U Sterile Powder (Rare) 2077
- Cytoxan (Occurs occasionally) 700
- Dalmane Capsules (Rare) 2329
- Danocrine Capsules 2437
- Darvon-N/Darvocet-N 1473
- Darvon 1475
- Darvon-N Suspension & Tablets (Less than 1%) 1473
- Demerol 2438
- Dizac (diazepam injectable emulsion) CIV (Less frequent) 1862
- Dobutrex Solution Vials (Occasionally) 1480
- EC-Naprosyn Delayed-Release Tablets (Less than 1%) 2277
- Edecrin 1698
- Elavil 2945
- Elspar 1700
- Emcyt Capsules (1%) 2085
- Ery-Tab Tablets 426
- Factrel 2996
- Feldene Capsules (Occasional) 2008
- Flexeril Tablets (Less than 1%) 1701
- ▲ Fludara for Injection (15%) 658
- Fortaz (2%) 1092
- Ganite 2711
- Geocillin Tablets (Infrequent) 2009
- Grifulvin V (griseofulvin tablets) Microsize (griseofulvin oral suspension) Microsize 1944
- Gris-PEG Tablets, 125 mg & 250 mg 476
- Ilosone 927
- Imodium Capsules 1343

(⊞ Described in PDR For Nonprescription Drugs)   Incidence data in parentheses; ▲ 3% or more   (⊙ Described in PDR For Ophthalmology)

1441 Side Effects Index Renal failure

Imuran (Approximately 2%) 1103
▲ Intron A for Injection (Up to 25%) 2506
K-Norm Capsules (Rare) 1615
Kefzol Vials, Faspak & ADD-Vantage 1511
Kemadrin Tablets (Occasional) 1105
Klonopin Tablets 2294
Lamprene Capsules (1-5%) 846
Larodopa Tablets (Infrequent) 2296
Lasix Injection, Oral Solution and Tablets 1267
Levo-Dromoran 2297
Limbitrol 2333
Lioresal Tablets 847
▲ Lopressor (5%) 848
Lopressor HCT Tablets 850
Loxitane 1426
Ludiomil Tablets (Rare) 861
Lysodren Tablets 707
MS Contin Tablets (Less frequent) 2149
MSIR (Infrequent) 2152
Mebaral Tablets (Less than 1 in 100) 2452
Mepergan Injection 2859
Mestinon Injectable (Occasional) 1300
Mestinon (Occasional) 1300
Methadone Hydrochloride Oral Solution & Tablets 2357
Mezlin 594
Mezlin Pharmacy Bulk Package 597
Midamor Tablets (Less than or equal to 1%) 1746
Midrin Capsules 788
Minipress Capsules (1-4%) 2015
Minizide Capsules 2016
Mintezol 1747
Monistat Dual-Pak (Less than 0.5%) 1906
Monistat 3 Vaginal Suppositories (Less than 0.5%) 1905
Mycelex-G 500 mg Vaginal Tablets (Rare) 602
Naprosyn Suspension (Less than 1%) 2277
Nardil (Less common) 1977
Nebcin Vials, Hyporets & ADD-Vantage 1518
Nembutal Sodium Capsules 440
Nembutal Sodium Solution 442
Nembutal Sodium Suppositories (Less than 1%) 444
Neosporin Ophthalmic Ointment Sterile 1130
▲ Nolvadex Tablets (13%) 2957
Norpramin Tablets 1273
Oramorph SR (Morphine Sulfate Sustained Release Tablets) (Less frequent) 2359
OxyIR Capsules 2167
Papaverine Hydrochloride Vials and Ampoules 1523
Parlodel 2411
Parnate Tablets (Rare) 2679
Peganone Tablets 455
Pfizerpen for Injection 2022
Phenobarbital Elixir and Tablets (Less than 1 in 100 patients) 1523
▲ Phenurone Tablets (5%) 455
Pipracil (1%) 1435
Pnu-Imune 23 (Rare to infrequent) 1437
Pondimin Tablets 2239
Potaba Capsules, Envules, Powder, and Tablets (Infrequent) 1234
Proglycem 575
Proloprim Tablets 1141
Purinethol Tablets 1214
Quadrinal Tablets 1398
▲ Quinidex Extentabs (5%) 2240
Reglan (A few cases) 2243
Ritalin 866
Roxanol 2365
Roxicodone Tablets, Oral Solution & Intensol (Oxycodone) 2366
SSD (Infrequent) 1402
Seconal Sodium Pulvules (Less than 1 in 100) 1529
Serax Capsules (Rare) 2916
Serax Tablets (Rare) 2916
Seromycin Capsules 975
Sinemet Tablets 959
Sinequan (Occasional) 2028
Soma Compound w/Codeine Tablets 2784
Soma Compound Tablets 2783
Soma Tablets 2782
Spectrobid Tablets 2030
Surmontil Capsules 2917
Symmetrel Capsules (0.1% to 1%) 965
Symmetrel Syrup (0.1% to 1%) 963
Talacen Caplets (A few cases) 2464
Tambocor Tablets (1% to less than 3%) 1555
Tao Capsules 2033
Tapazole Tablets 1361
Tazidime Vials, Faspak & ADD-Vantage (2%) 1531
Tegretol/Tegretol-XR 870
Tenex Tablets (Less frequent) 2249
Tenoretic Tablets 2963
Tenormin Tablets and I.V. Injection 2965
TheraCys BCG Live (Intravesical) (Up to 1.8%; rare) 911
Thioplex (Thiotepa For Injection) (Occasional) 1329
Thyro-Block Tablets 2785
Ticar for Injection 2704
Timentin for Injection 2706
Tofranil Ampuls 873
Tofranil Tablets 875
Tofranil-PM Capsules 876
Trandate Tablets (Less common) 1158
Tranxene 459
Trecator-SC Tablets 2919
Trental Tablets (Less than 1%) 1291
Triavil Tablets 1800
Trinsicon Capsules (Extremely rare) 2759
Unasyn 2035
Urised Tablets 2123
Urobiotic-250 Capsules 2038
Uroqid-Acid No. 2 Tablets (Occasional) 633
Valium Injectable 2336
Valium Tablets (Infrequent) 2335
Vancocin HCl, Oral Solution & Pulvules (Infrequent) 1536
Vancocin HCl, Vials & ADD-Vantage (Infrequent) 1534
Ventolin Inhalation Aerosol and Refill (Rare) 1170
Ventolin Inhalation Solution (Rare) 1171
Ventolin Syrup (Rare) 1175
Ventolin Tablets (Rare) 1176
Vicodin HP Tablets 1403
Vivactil Tablets 1820
Wygesic Tablets 2930
Zantac (Rare) 1182
Zantac Injection 1180
Zantac Syrup (Rare) 1182
Zaroxolyn Tablets 1625
Zinacef (1 in 125 patients) 1184
Zovirax Capsules (0.3%) 1187
Zovirax Ointment 5% (0.3%) 1190
Zovirax (0.3%) 1187
Zyloprim Tablets (Less than 1%) 1194

Rash, urticarial
Capoten Tablets (Rare) 740
Capozide Tablets (Rare) 744
DTIC-Dome (Infrequent) 593
Mesantoin Tablets 2400
Miltown Tablets 2780
Normodyne Tablets (Less common) 2522
PMB 200 and PMB 400 2890
Serax Capsules 2916
Serax Tablets 2916
Ticlid Tablets 2317
Trandate Tablets (Less common) 1158
▲ Zosyn (4.2%) 1463

Rash, varicella-like
Varivax (0.9% to 5.5%) 1807

Rash, vesiculobullous
Betaseron for SC Injection 653
▲ Cognex Capsules (7%) 1961
Cytovene (1% or less) 2270
Doxil (Less than 1%) 2613
Effexor (Rare) 2825
Foscavir Injection (Rare) 541
IBU Tablets (Less than 1%) 1389
Lamictal Tablets (Infrequent) 1105
Lodine Capsules and Tablets (Less than 1%) 2849
Megace Oral Suspension (1% to 3%) 708
Norvir (Less than 2%) 447
Paxil Tablets (Rare) 2681
Permax Tablets (Rare) 571
Prozac Pulvules & Liquid, Oral Solution (Rare) 935
Serzone Tablets (Infrequent) 776
Videx Tablets, Powder for Oral Solution, & Pediatric Powder for Oral Solution (Less than 1%) 2980

Raynaud's phenomenon
Blenoxane 697
Blocadren Tablets 1654
Capoten Tablets (2 to 3 of 1000 patients) 740
Capozide Tablets (2 to 3 of 1000 patients) 744
Catapres Tablets (Rare) 679
Catapres-TTS 680
Combipres Tablets (Rare) 682
Imitrex Injection (Rare) 1095
Inderal 2834
Inderal LA Long Acting Capsules 2836
Inderide Tablets 2838
Inderide LA Long Acting Capsules 2840
Kerlone Tablets 2588
Lopressor HCT Tablets 850
Parlodel (Less than 2%) 2411
Platinol for Injection 717
Platinol-AQ Injection 719
Roferon-A Injection (Infrequent) 2308
Sandostatin Injection (Less than 1%) 2421
Tenoretic Tablets 2963
Tenormin Tablets and I.V. Injection 2965
Timolide Tablets 1791
Timoptic in Ocudose 1796
Timoptic Sterile Ophthalmic Solution 1794
Timoptic-XE 1798
Toprol-XL Tablets (About 1 of 100 patients) 560
Velban Vials 1537

Rectal bleeding
Accutane Capsules 2252
Ambien Tablets (Rare) 2559
Anafranil Capsules (Infrequent) 819
Betaseron for SC Injection 653
BuSpar Tablets (Infrequent) 738
Casodex Tablets (2% to 5%) 2934
Clozaril Tablets (Less than 1%) 2377
Cognex Capsules (Infrequent) 1961
CORTENEMA (Rare) 2713
Daypro Caplets (Less than 1%) 2578
Demadex Tablets and Injection 691
Depo-Provera Contraceptive Injection (Fewer than 1%) 2079
Dipentum Capsules (Rare) 2084
Effexor (Infrequent) 2825
Eldepryl Capsules 2729
▲ Eulexin Capsules (14%) 2498
Felbatol 2774
Foscavir Injection (Between 1% and 5%) 541
Geocillin Tablets 2009
Hivid Tablets (Less than 1%) 2287
Indocin Capsules (Less than 1%) 1723
Indocin I.V. (Less than 1%) 1727
Indocin (Less than 1%) 1723
Intron A for Injection (Less than 5%) 2506
Invirase Capsules (Less than 2%) 2291
LUVOX Tablets (Infrequent) 2723
Naprelan Tablets (Less than 1%) 2861
Neurontin Capsules (Rare) 1978
Orudis Capsules (Less than 1%) 2874
Oruvail Capsules (Less than 1%) 2874
Paxil Tablets (Infrequent) 2681
Pentasa (Less than 1%) 1275
Prevacid Delayed-Release Capsules (Less than 1%) 2746
Questran 774
Redux Capsules (Rare) 2911
Relafen Tablets (Less than 1%) 2688
Retrovir Capsules 1216
Retrovir I.V. Infusion 1221
Retrovir Syrup 1216
Serzone Tablets (Infrequent) 776
Toradol (1% or less) 2319
Vantin for Oral Suspension and Vantin Tablets 2112
Velban Vials 1537
Videx Tablets, Powder for Oral Solution, & Pediatric Powder for Oral Solution (Less than 1%) 2980
Zyrtec Tablets (Less than 2%) 2053

Rectal discomfort
Fleet Babylax 1000
Helidac Therapy (1.5%) 2135

Rectal disorders, unspecified
▲ CellCept Capsules (More than or equal to 3%) 2265
Cytotec (Infrequent) 2576
Dipentum Capsules (Rare) 2084
Foscavir Injection (Less than 1%) 541
Kerlone Tablets (Less than 2%) 2588
Naprelan Tablets (Less than 1%) 2861
Norvir (Less than 2%) 447
Redux Capsules (Frequent) 2911
Vistide Injection 1057
Wellbutrin Tablets (Rare) 1177

Rectal urgency (see under Defecate, desire to)

Red blood cell, aplasia
Mysoline (Rare) 2860

Red blood cell, hypoplasia of
Mysoline (Rare) 2860

"Red neck" syndrome
Vancocin HCl, Oral Solution & Pulvules 1536
Vancocin HCl, Vials & ADD-Vantage 1534

Reflexes, increased (see under Hyperreflexia)

Regurgitation
Crixivan Capsules (Less than 2% to 2%) 1670
Fosamax Tablets (2.0%) 1703
IPOL Poliovirus Vaccine Inactivated 903
Mevacor Tablets (0.5% to 1.0%) 1742
Mylanta (Occasional) 1359
Plendil Extended-Release Tablets (0.5% to 1.5%) 514

Renal agenesis, unilateral, neonatal
Leukeran Tablets 1205

Renal calculi (see also under Renal stones)
Anafranil Capsules (Infrequent) 819
Avonex 662
Cardura Tablets (Less than 0.5% of 3960 patients) 1993
Cipro I.V. (1% or less) 587
Cipro I.V. Pharmacy Bulk Package (Less than 1%) 590
Cipro Tablets 584
Clinoril Tablets (Rare) 1658
Cognex Capsules (Infrequent) 1961
Daranide Tablets 1676
Diamox ⊙ 317
Dilacor XR Extended-release Capsules (Infrequent) 2183
Effexor (Infrequent) 2825
Floxin I.V. 1580
Floxin Tablets (200 mg, 300 mg, 400 mg) 1577
Imitrex Injection (Rare) 1095
Lioresal Intrathecal (1% or more) 1634
Lodine Capsules and Tablets (Less than 1%) 2849
Maxaquin Tablets 2593
Miacalcin Nasal Spray (Less than 1%) 2403
Naprelan Tablets (Less than 1%) 2861
Neptazane Tablets ⊙ 320
Neurontin Capsules (Rare) 1978
Paxil Tablets (Rare) 2681
Penetrex Tablets 2196
Permax Tablets (Infrequent) 571
Prevacid Delayed-Release Capsules (Less than 1%) 2746
Prozac Pulvules & Liquid, Oral Solution (Rare) 935
Rilutek Tablets (Infrequent) 2198

Renal colic
Benemid Tablets 1651
ColBENEMID Tablets 1662
Crixivan Capsules (Less than 2%) 1670
Daranide Tablets 1676
Ethmozine Tablets (Less than 2%) 2217
Kerlone Tablets (Less than 2%) 2588
Noroxin Tablets (Less frequent) 1758
Noroxin Tablets (Less frequent) 2222
Timolide Tablets (Less than 1%) 1791
Zebeta Tablets 1457
Ziac 1459

Renal disease
Anaprox/Naprosyn (Less than 1%) 2277
▲ Naprelan Tablets (3% to 9%) 2861
Anaprox/Naprosyn (Less than 1%) 2277

Renal failure
▲ Abelcet Injection (4% to 5%) 1540
ActHIB 893
Aldoclor Tablets 1638
Aldoril Tablets 1644
Amicar Syrup, Tablets, and Injection 1312
Anaprox/Naprosyn (Less than 1%) 2277
Ancobon Capsules 2254

(▭ Described in PDR For Nonprescription Drugs) Incidence data in parenthesis; ▲ 3% or more (⊙ Described in PDR For Ophthalmology)

Atretol Tablets 569
Bactrim DS Tablets 2257
Bactrim I.V. Infusion 2255
Bactrim 2257
Betaseron for SC Injection 653
BiCNU 696
Bumex (0.1%) 2260
Capoten Tablets (Approximately 1 to 2 of 1000 patients) 740
Capozide Tablets (Approximately 1 to 2 of 1000 patients) 744
Cataflam Tablets 833
CeeNU Capsules 699
Cerebyx Injection (Infrequent) 1956
Chibroxin Sterile Ophthalmic Solution (With oral form) 1657
Cipro I.V. (1% or less) 587
Cipro I.V. Pharmacy Bulk Package (Less than 1%) 590
Cipro Tablets (Less than 1%) 584
Clinoril Tablets (Less than 1 in 100) 1658
Clomid 1262
Cognex Capsules (Rare) 1961
Corvert Injection (0.3%) 2075
Cytovene (1% or less) 2270
Dilacor XR Extended-release Capsules 2183
Diprivan Injectable Emulsion (Less than 1%) 2939
Diupres Tablets 1691
Diuril Oral Suspension 1694
Diuril Sodium Intravenous 1693
Diuril Tablets 1694
Dolobid Tablets (Less than 1 in 100) 1695
Dyrenium Capsules (One case) 2655
EC-Naprosyn Delayed-Release Tablets (Less than 1%) 2277
Ergamisol Tablets (Less frequent) 1340
Feldene Capsules (Less than 1%) 2008
Floxin I.V. 1580
Fludara for Injection (Up to 1%) 658
HydroDIURIL Tablets 1716
Hydropres Tablets 1718
Hyzaar Tablets 1720
IFEX (1 episode) 706
Indocin (Less than 1%) 1723
Lamictal Tablets (Rare) 1105
Levo-Dromoran 2297
Lioresal Intrathecal (1% or more) 1634
Lodine Capsules and Tablets (Less than 1%) 2849
Maxaquin Tablets 2593
Merrem I.V. (0.1% to 1.0%) 2952
Methotrexate Sodium Tablets, Injection, for Injection and LPF Injection 1322
Moduretic Tablets (Less than or equal to 1%) 1748
Mutamycin for Injection 712
Nalfon 200 Pulvules & Nalfon Tablets (Less than 1%) 933
▲ Naprelan Tablets (Less than 1% to 9%) 2861
Anaprox/Naprosyn (Less than 1%) 2277
Nipent for Injection (Less than 3%) 2733
Noroxin Tablets 1758
Noroxin Tablets 2222
Norvir (Less than 2%) 447
▲ Novantrone for Injection (Up to 8%) 1327
OmniHIB 2676
Oncaspar 2194
Orthoclone OKT3 Sterile Solution 1892
Orudis Capsules (Less than 1%) 2874
Oruvail Capsules (Less than 1%) 2874
Penetrex Tablets (0.1% to 1%) 2196
Permax Tablets (Infrequent) 571
Ponstel 1982
Prinzide Tablets 1780
▲ Prograf (Greater than 3%) 1028
Proleukin for Injection (Less than 1%) 812
Prozac Pulvules & Liquid, Oral Solution 935
Redux Capsules 2911
Rifadin 1276
Rythmol Tablets–150mg, 225mg, 300mg (Less than 1%) 1399
Septra 1146
Septra I.V. Infusion 1142
Septra I.V. Infusion ADD-Vantage Vials 1144
Septra 1146
Tegretol/Tegretol-XR 870
Tenormin Tablets and I.V. Injection (0.4%) 2965
Ticlid Tablets (Rare) 2317
Timolide Tablets 1791
Tolectin (200, 400 and 600 mg) (Less than 1%) 1591
Tonocard Tablets 519
Trasylol (2%) 607
Vancocin HCl, Oral Solution & Pulvules (Rare) 1536
Vancocin HCl, Vials & ADD-Vantage (Rare) 1534
Vaseretic Tablets 1810
Vasotec I.V. 1814
Vasotec Tablets (0.5% to 1.0%) 1816
Videx Tablets, Powder for Oral Solution, & Pediatric Powder for Oral Solution (Less than 1%) 2980
Cataflam/Voltaren/Voltaren-XR 833
Zestoretic Tablets 2968
Ziac 1459
Zovirax Sterile Powder 1191
Zyloprim Tablets (Less than 1%) 1194

Renal failure, acute

Abelcet Injection 1540
Accupril Tablets (Rare) 1950
Activase 1045
Albenza Tablets 2629
Altace Capsules (Rare) 1238
Ambien Tablets (Rare) 2559
Anectine 1062
Cataflam Tablets (Rare) 833
Daypro Caplets (Less than 1%) 2578
Didronel I.V. Infusion (Rare) 1545
Dyazide Capsules 2653
Dyrenium Capsules 2655
Elspar 1700
Ethamolin Injection (Two women) 2544
Felbatol 2774
Floxin I.V. 1580
Floxin Tablets (200 mg, 300 mg, 400 mg) 1577
Foscavir Injection (Between 1% and 5%) 541
Fungizone Intravenous 507
Gammar-P I.V., Immune Globulin Intravenous (Human) (Several reports) 798
Ganite (Two patients) 2711
Haldol Decanoate 1587
Hivid Tablets (Less than 1%) 2287
IBU Tablets (Less than 1%) 1389
Imitrex Injection 1095
Imitrex Tablets 1099
Indocin I.V. (Less than 1%) 1727
Lotrel Capsules (Rare) 858
LUVOX Tablets 2723
Mefoxin (Rare) 1734
Mefoxin Premixed Intravenous Solution (Rare) 1737
Methotrexate Sodium Tablets, Injection, for Injection and LPF Injection 1322
Mevacor Tablets 1742
Minocin Intravenous (Rare) 1428
Minocin Oral Suspension (Rare) 1431
Minocin Pellet-Filled Capsules (Rare) 1429
Monocid Injection (Rare) 2674
Monopril Tablets (Rare) 762
Motrin Ibuprofen Suspension, Oral Drops, Chewable Tablets, Caplets (Less than 1%) 1563
Neurontin Capsules (Rare) 1978
Orap Tablets 1037
Pediazole Suspension 2340
Pravachol Tablets (Rare) 770
Primaxin I.M. 1770
Primaxin I.V. (Less than 0.2%) 1772
Prinivil Tablets (Rare; 0.3% to 1.3%) 1776
Prinzide Tablets 1780
Prolixin 510
Rifadin (Rare) 1276
Rifamate Capsules (Rare) 1278
Rifater (Rare) 1280
Rimactane Capsules (Rare) 865
Risperdal Tablets 1348
Tenex Tablets (Rare) 2249
Toradol 2319
Trasylol (0.5%) 607
Vaseretic Tablets (Rare) 1810
Vasotec I.V. (Rare) 1814
Vasotec Tablets (Rare) 1816
▲ Vesanoid Capsules (3%) 2327
Videx Tablets, Powder for Oral Solution, & Pediatric Powder for Oral Solution (Less than 1%) 2980
Cataflam/Voltaren/Voltaren-XR (Rare) 833
Zestoretic Tablets (Rare) 2968
Zestril Tablets (0.3% to 1.0%) 2972
Zocor Tablets (Rare) 1821

Renal failure, neonatal

Accupril Tablets 1950
Altace Capsules 1238
Capoten Tablets 740
Capozide Tablets 744
Cozaar Tablets 1668
Etopophos for Injection 701
Etoposide Injection 539
Hyzaar Tablets 1720
Lotensin Tablets 852
Lotensin HCT Tablets 855
Lotrel Capsules 858
Monopril Tablets 762
Prinivil Tablets 1776
Prinzide Tablets 1780
Univasc Tablets 2553
Vaseretic Tablets 1810
Vasotec I.V. 1814
Vasotec Tablets 1816
VePesid Capsules and Injection 727
Zestoretic Tablets 2968
Zestril Tablets 2972

Renal failure, worsening of

Accupril Tablets (Rare) 1950

Renal function impairment

Abelcet Injection 1540
Aldoclor Tablets 1638
Aldoril Tablets 1644
Altace Capsules (Rare; 1.2%) 1238
Amikacin Sulfate Injection, USP 523
Amikin Injectable 502
Brevicon 2563
Cedax 2480
Cefotan 2936
Ceftin 1067
Cefzil Tablets and Oral Suspension 747
Ceptaz 1070
Cleocin Phosphate Injection (Rare) 2068
Cleocin Vaginal Cream 2070
Cordarone Intravenous (Less than 2%) 2821
Cytosar-U Sterile Powder (Less frequent) 2077
Cytovene (1% or less) 2270
DTIC-Dome (Few reports) 593
Demulen 2580
Desogen Tablets 1867
▲ Didronel I.V. Infusion (Approximately 10%) 1545
Diupres Tablets 1691
Diuril Oral Suspension 1694
Diuril Sodium Intravenous 1693
Diuril Tablets 1694
Duricef Capsules, Tablets, and Oral Suspension 750
Estrace Cream and Tablets 751
Felbatol 2774
Fludara for Injection (Up to 1%) 658
Fortaz 1092
▲ Foscavir Injection (5% or greater up to approximately 33%) 541
▲ Fungizone Intravenous (Among most common) 507
Garamycin Injectable 2502
Hivid Tablets (Less than 1%) 2287
HydroDIURIL Tablets 1716
Hydropres Tablets 1718
Hyzaar Tablets 1720
Idamycin Injection (More than 1%) 2096
Keftab Tablets 931
Kerlone Tablets (Less than 2%) 2588
Lescol Capsules 2395
▲ Leukine (8%) 1317
Levlen/Tri-Levlen 646
Lithonate/Lithotabs/Lithobid 2721
Lopid Tablets 1974
Lorabid Suspension and Pulvules 1513
Maxipime for Injection 758
Modicon 1928
Moduretic Tablets (Less than or equal to 1%) 1748
Mutamycin for Injection 712
Naprelan Tablets (Less than 1%) 2861
Nebcin Vials, Hyporets & ADD-Vantage 1518
▲ Neoral (25% to 38%) 2405
Neutrexin for Injection 2761
Nipent for Injection (Less than 3%) 2733
Nolvadex Tablets 2957
Norinyl 2563
Nor-Q D Tablets 2598
Oncaspar 2194
Ortho-Cept 1907
Ortho-Cyclen/Ortho-Tri-Cyclen 1914
Ortho-Novum 1928
Ortho-Cyclen/Ortho Tri-Cyclen 1914
Orudis Capsules (Greater than 1%) 2874
Oruvail Capsules (Greater than 1%) 2874
Ovcon 765
Paxil Tablets (Rare) 2681
Platinol for Injection 717
Platinol-AQ Injection 719
Prinivil Tablets (0.3% to 1.0%) 1776
Prinzide Tablets 1780
▲ Prograf (33% to 40%) 1028
ReoPro Vials (0.3%) 1526
▲ Sandimmune (25 to 38%) 2416
Suprax 1443
Tazicef for Injection 2697
Tazidime Vials, Faspak & ADD-Vantage 1531
Timolide Tablets 1791
Tonocard Tablets 519
Tranxene 459
▲ Trasylol (5% to 30%) 607
Levlen/Tri-Levlen 646
Tri-Norinyl 2607
Vantin for Oral Suspension and Vantin Tablets 2112
Vaseretic Tablets 1810
Vasotec I.V. 1814
Vasotec Tablets (0.5% to 1.0%) 1816
Videx Tablets, Powder for Oral Solution, & Pediatric Powder for Oral Solution (Less than 1%) 2980
Vumon for Injection (Less than 1%) 729
Zestoretic Tablets 2968
Zestril Tablets (0.3% to 1.0%) 2972
Ziac 1459

Renal impairment

Asacol Delayed-Release Tablets 2129
Capozide Tablets 744
Clinoril Tablets (Less than 1 in 100) 1658
ColBENEMID Tablets 1662
Dolobid Tablets (Less than 1 in 100) 1695
Fioricet with Codeine Capsules 2387
Fiorinal with Codeine Capsules 2390
▲ IFEX (6%) 706
▲ Indocin I.V. (41% of infants) 1727
Kefzol Vials, Faspak & ADD-Vantage 1511
Macrobid Capsules 2138
Macrodantin Capsules 2140
▲ Netromycin Injection 100 mg/ml (7%) 2516
PCE Dispertab Tablets 453
Panhematin 452
Proleukin for Injection (2%) 812
Vistide Injection 1057

Renal insufficiency

Capastat Sulfate Injection (1 patient) 968
Capoten Tablets (Approximately 1 to 2 of 1000 patients) 740
Capozide Tablets (Approximately 1 to 2 of 1000 patients) 744
Daypro Caplets (Less than 1%) 2578
E.E.S. (Isolated reports) 427
Elspar 1700
Erythrocin Stearate Filmtab (Isolated reports) 429
Floxin I.V. 1580
Floxin Tablets (200 mg, 300 mg, 400 mg) 1577
Indocin Capsules (Less than 1%) 1723
Indocin I.V. (Less than 1%) 1727
Indocin (Less than 1%) 1723
Lodine Capsules and Tablets (Less than 1%) 2849
Lopid Tablets 1974
Monopril Tablets (0.2% to 1.0%) 762
Neupogen for Injection (Two events) 495
Nipent for Injection (Less than 3%) 2733
Orthoclone OKT3 Sterile Solution 1892
▲ Platinol for Injection (28% to 36%) 717
Proleukin for Injection 812
Rifadin (Rare) 1276
Rifamate Capsules (Rare) 1278
Rifater (Rare) 1280
Rimactane Capsules (Rare) 865
Risperdal Tablets (Rare) 1348
Taxotere for Injection Concentrate 2204
Univasc Tablets (Less than 1%) 2553
▲ Vesanoid Capsules (11%) 2327
Zoladex (Greater than 1% but less than 5%) 2976
Zoladex 3-month 2978

(▭ Described in PDR For Nonprescription Drugs) — Incidence data in parenthesis; ▲ 3% or more — (◉ Described in PDR For Ophthalmology)

1443 Side Effects Index Retinal detachment

Renal insufficiency, reversible
Actimmune (Rare) 1043

Renal rickets
IFEX 706

Renal stones (see also under Renal calculi)
Betaseron for SC Injection 653
Clinoril Tablets 1658
Dyazide Capsules 2653
Dyrenium Capsules (Rare) 2655
Effexor (Infrequent) 2825
GlaucTabs ⊙ 209
Hivid Tablets (Less than 1%) 2287
Imdur (Less than or equal to 5%) 1362
LUVOX Tablets (Rare) 2723
Nipent for Injection (Less than 3%) 2733
Norvir (Less than 2%) 447
Redux Capsules (Infrequent) 2911
Relafen Tablets (Less than 1%) 2688
Remeron Tablets (Infrequent) 1878
Serzone Tablets (Infrequent) 776
Tegison Capsules 2314
Videx Tablets, Powder for Oral Solution, & Pediatric Powder for Oral Solution (Less than 1%) 2980

Renal tubular cells excretion, increase
Quadrinal Tablets 1398

Renal tubular damage
Betaseron for SC Injection 653
Foscavir Injection (Less than 1%) 541
Hydrea Capsules (Occasional) 705
Platinol for Injection 717
Platinol-AQ Injection 719
Vistide Injection 1057

Respiration, painful
Prinivil Tablets (0.3% to 1.0%) 1776
Prinzide Tablets 1780
Zestoretic Tablets 2968
Zestril Tablets (0.3% to 1.0%) 2972

Respiratory alkalosis
▲ Ganite (40% to 50%) 2711

Respiratory arrest
Alfenta Injection 1334
Ancobon Capsules 2254
AquaMEPHYTON Injection 1648
Carbocaine Injection 2432
Cipro I.V. (1% or less) 587
Cipro I.V. Pharmacy Bulk Package (Less than 1%) 590
Clozaril Tablets (Rare) 2377
Decadron Phosphate with Xylocaine Injection, Sterile 1683
Demerol 2438
Dilaudid-HP Injection 1384
Dilaudid-HP Lyophilized Powder 250 mg 1384
Dilaudid Tablets and Liquid 1386
Duranest Injections 533
Dyclone 0.5% and 1% Topical Solutions, USP 535
EMLA Cream (Unlikely with cream) 536
Floxin I.V. (Less than 1%) 1580
Floxin Tablets (200 mg, 300 mg, 400 mg) (Less than 1%) 1577
Fluothane 2830
INFeD (Iron Dextran Injection, USP) 2478
Kadian Capsules 2948
MS Contin Tablets 2149
MSIR 2152
Marcaine 2446
Marcaine Spinal 2449
Mepergan Injection 2859
Methadone Hydrochloride Oral Solution & Tablets 2357
Nescaine/Nescaine MPF 549
Novocain Hydrochloride for Spinal Anesthesia 2457
Nubain Injection (1% or less) 952
Orthoclone OKT3 Sterile Solution 1892
OxyContin Tablets 2163
Pontocaine Hydrochloride for Spinal Anesthesia 2460
Proleukin for Injection (Less than 1%) 812
Prostigmin Injectable 1305
Prostigmin Tablets 1306
RMS Suppositories CII 2766
Roxanol 2365
Sensorcaine 554
Sublimaze Injection 463
Tonocard Tablets (Less than 1%) 519
▲ Xylocaine Injections (Among most common) 562

Respiratory congestion, unspecified
Cozaar Tablets (Less than 1%) 1668
▲ Epogen for Injection (15%) 489
Hyzaar Tablets 1720
▲ Procrit for Injection (15%) 1896
▲ Supprelin Injection (3% to 10%) 2230
Videx Tablets, Powder for Oral Solution, & Pediatric Powder for Oral Solution (Up to 3%) 2980

Respiratory depression (see under Depression, respiratory)

Respiratory depression, postoperative
Alfenta Injection (1% to 3%) 1334
Sublimaze Injection (Occasional) 463
Sufenta Injection (0.3% to 1%) 1355

Respiratory difficulty
▲ Abelcet Injection (3% to 4%) 1540
▲ Acthrel for Injection (6%) 2990
Ambien Tablets 2559
Ana-Kit Anaphylaxis Emergency Treatment Kit 611
Carafate Suspension 1250
Carafate Tablets 1249
Cardene I.V. (Rare) 2815
Claritin-D Tablets 2487
D.A. II Tablets 972
D.A. Chewable Tablets 970
Deconsal II Tablets 1605
Diphtheria and Tetanus Toxoids and Pertussis Vaccine Adsorbed 2650
Dura-Tap/PD Capsules 970
Dura-Vent/DA Tablets 972
Dura-Vent Tablets 971
Entex PSE Tablets 973
EpiPen 808
Fedahist Gyrocaps 2545
Felbatol 2774
Guaimax-D Tablets 809
Haldol Decanoate 1587
Haldol Injection, Tablets and Concentrate 1585
Histussin D Liquid 670
Humorsol Sterile Ophthalmic Solution (Infrequent) 1707
INFeD (Iron Dextran Injection, USP) 2478
Invirase Capsules (Less than 2%) 2291
Kadian Capsules (Less than 3%) 2948
Levophed Bitartrate Injection 2445
Lioresal Intrathecal (1% or more) 1634
Norpace (Infrequent) 2596
Novahistine DMX ▣ 782
Novahistine Elixir ▣ 782
Novocain Hydrochloride for Spinal Anesthesia 2457
Papaverine Hydrochloride Vials and Ampoules 1523
Pontocaine Hydrochloride for Spinal Anesthesia 2460
Rilutek Tablets (More than 2%) 2198
Rondec Oral Drops 974
Rondec Syrup 974
Rondec 974
Seldane-D Extended-Release Tablets 1286
Solganal Suspension 2530
Sus-Phrine Injection 1017
Syn-Rx Tablets 1622
Syn-Rx DM Tablets 1623
Tetramune (Rare) 1449
▲ Trasylol (3%) 607
Triavil Tablets 1800
Tri-Immunol Adsorbed 1452
Trinalin Repetabs Tablets 1373
Tussend 1830
Tussend Expectorant 1831
Versed Injection (Less than 1%) 2324
▲ Vesanoid Capsules (26%) 2327

Respiratory discharge, upper, unspecified
Emcyt Capsules (1%) 2085

Respiratory distress
Aldoclor Tablets 1638
Aldoril Tablets 1644
Americaine Otic Topical Anesthetic Ear Drops 1603
Apresazide Capsules 824
Atrovent Inhalation Solution (1.4%) 675
Blocadren Tablets 1654
Capozide Tablets 744
Cardura Tablets (1.1%) 1993
Cartrol Tablets 413
Ceredase 1055
Cipro I.V. (1% or less) 587
Cipro I.V. Pharmacy Bulk Package (Less than 1%) 590
Clomid 1262
Cordarone Intravenous (2%) 2821
Cytosar-U Sterile Powder 2077
Cytovene-IV (One report) 2270
Dalgan Injection (Less than 1%) 529
Dantrium Capsules (Less frequent) 2131
Dilacor XR Extended-release Capsules (Infrequent) 2183
Diucardin Tablets 2824
Diupres Tablets 1691
Diuril Oral Suspension 1694
Diuril Sodium Intravenous 1693
Diuril Tablets 1694
Duragesic Transdermal System (Less than 1%) 1336
Dyazide Capsules 2653
Elspar 1700
Eminase (Less than 1 in 1,000) 2215
Enduron Tablets 424
Esidrix Tablets 839
Esimil Tablets 840
Floxin I.V. 1580
Floxin Tablets (200 mg, 300 mg, 400 mg) 1577
Fluvirin (Influenza Virus Vaccine) 1608
Foscavir Injection (Between 1% and 5%) 541
Glucophage Tablets 754
Hivid Tablets (Less than 1%) 2287
Humegon for Injection 1873
HydroDIURIL Tablets 1716
Hydropres Tablets 1718
Hyzaar Tablets 1720
Inderal 2834
Inderal LA Long Acting Capsules 2836
Inderide Tablets 2838
Inderide LA Long Acting Capsules 2840
Indocin Capsules (Less than 1%) 1723
Indocin I.V. (Less than 1%) 1727
Indocin (Less than 1%) 1723
Kerlone Tablets 2588
Lamictal Tablets (More than 1%) 1105
Leukine 1317
Levatol Tablets 2547
Lopressor HCT Tablets 850
Lotensin HCT Tablets 855
▲ Lupron Depot - 3 Month 22.5 mg (6.4%) 2743
Maxaquin Tablets (Less than 1%) 2593
Metrodin (urofollitropin for injection) 2616
▲ Mexitil Capsules (3.3% to 5.7%) 684
Moduretic Tablets 1748
Mutamycin for Injection (Few cases) 712
Mykrox Tablets (Rare) 1617
Naprelan Tablets (Less than 1%) 2861
Normodyne Tablets 2522
Nubain Injection (1% or less) 952
Nuromax Injection 1136
Oretic Tablets 450
▲ Paraplatin for Injection (6% to 12%) 713
Paxil Tablets 2681
Pergonal (menotropins for injection, USP) 2618
Phenergan VC 2886
Phenergan VC with Codeine 2888
Prinzide Tablets 1780
Procardia XL Extended Release Tablets (1% or less) 2026
▲ Prograf (Greater than 3%) 1028
Protamine Sulfate Vials 1526
RespiGam (2%) 1631
Sandimmune 2416
Sectral Capsules 2914
Serevent Inhalation Aerosol 1149
Taxotere for Injection Concentrate 2204
Tenoretic Tablets 2963
Tenormin Tablets and I.V. Injection 2965
TICE BCG, USP (1.6%) 1881
Timolide Tablets 1791
Timoptic in Ocudose 1796
Timoptic Sterile Ophthalmic Solution (Less frequent) 1794
Timoptic-XE 1798
Toprol-XL Tablets 560
Trandate Tablets 1158
Vaseretic Tablets 1810
Videx Tablets, Powder for Oral Solution, & Pediatric Powder for Oral Solution (Up to 2%) 2980
Virazole 1310
Visken Tablets 2428
Zaroxolyn Tablets 1625
Zebeta Tablets 1457
Zestoretic Tablets 2968
Ziac 1459

Respiratory distress, neonatal
Hycodan Tablets and Syrup 946
Hycomine Compound Tablets 948
Hycomine 947
Hycotuss Expectorant Syrup 950
Stadol (Rare) 779

Respiratory failure
▲ Abelcet Injection (9% to 10%) 1540
Betagan ⊙ 230
Betimol 0.25%, 0.5% ⊙ 259
Betoptic Ophthalmic Solution (Rare) 465
Betoptic S Ophthalmic Suspension (Rare) 467
Cocaine Hydrochloride Topical Solutions 529
Crixivan Capsules (Less than 2%) 1670
Isoptin Injectable 1391
Ocupress Ophthalmic Solution, 1% Sterile ⊙ 297
Orthoclone OKT3 Sterile Solution 1892
▲ Proleukin for Injection (Less than 1% to 9%) 812
Pulmozyme Inhalation 1054
Survanta Beractant Intratracheal Suspension 2346
Timoptic in Ocudose (Less frequent) 1796
Timoptic Sterile Ophthalmic Solution (Less frequent) 1794
Timoptic-XE 1798

Respiratory moniliasis
Rilutek Tablets (Infrequent) 2198

Respiratory tract, hypersensitivity
Septra 1146
Septra I.V. Infusion 1142
Septra I.V. Infusion ADD-Vantage Vials (Rare) 1144
Septra 1146

Restlessness (see under Dysphoria)

Retardation, psychomotor
Eskalith 2658
Lithium Carbonate Capsules & Tablets 2352
Roferon-A Injection (Infrequent) 2308

Retching
Imitrex Injection (Rare) 1095
Versed Injection (Less than 1%) 2324

Reticulocytopenia
Chloromycetin Sodium Succinate 1960
Cosmegen Injection 1666
Cytosar-U Sterile Powder 2077
Garamycin Injectable 2502

Reticulocytosis
▲ Dapsone Tablets USP (Almost all patients) 1331
Dipentum Capsules (Rare) 2084
Garamycin Injectable 2502
▲ Tegison Capsules (25-50%) 2314
Ticlid Tablets (Rare) 2317
Virazole 1310
Zyloprim Tablets (Less than 1%) 1194

Retinal artery occlusion
Activase 1045

Retinal atrophy
Aralen Phosphate Tablets 2431
Clinoril Tablets 1658
Plaquenil Sulfate Tablets 2459

Retinal damage
Aralen Hydrochloride Injection 2430
Aralen Phosphate Tablets 2431
Dapsone Tablets USP 1331
Neurontin Capsules (Rare) 1978
Plaquenil Sulfate Tablets 2459

Retinal detachment
Carbastat Intraocular Solution ⊙ 260
▲ Cytovene (8%) 2270
Foscavir Injection (Less than 1%) 541
Humorsol Sterile Ophthalmic Solution (Occasional) 1707
Isopto Carpine Ophthalmic Solution (Rare) ⊙ 221
LUVOX Tablets (Rare) 2723

(▣ Described in PDR For Nonprescription Drugs) Incidence data in parenthesis; ▲ 3% or more (⊙ Described in PDR For Ophthalmology)

Retinal detachment — Side Effects Index — 1444

MIOSTAT Intraocular Solution ◉ 222
Ocusert Pilo-20 and Pilo-40 Ocular Therapeutic Systems ◉ 252
Permax Tablets (Rare) 571
Phospholine Iodide (A few cases) ◉ 323
Pilopine HS Ophthalmic Gel ◉ 224
Sular Tablets (Less than or equal to 1%) 2961
Videx Tablets, Powder for Oral Solution, & Pediatric Powder for Oral Solution (Less than 1%) 2980
Vistide Injection 1057
Xalatan (Extremely rare) ◉ 304

Retinal disorder, unspecified
Anafranil Capsules (Rare) 819
Lamisil Tablets 2394
Lotensin HCT Tablets (0.3% or more) 855
Redux Capsules (Rare) 2911

Retinal hemorrhage, neonatal
Syntocinon Injection 2425

Retinal pigmentation disorders
Aralen Phosphate Tablets 2431
Desferal Vials 838
ISPAN Perfluoropropane ◉ 267
ISPAN Sulfur Hexafluoride ◉ 266
Plaquenil Sulfate Tablets 2459
Platinol for Injection 717
Platinol-AQ Injection 719
Videx Tablets, Powder for Oral Solution, & Pediatric Powder for Oral Solution (Several patients) 2980

Retinal vascular disorder
Betimol 0.25%, 0.5% ◉ 259
Clomid 1262
Intron A for Injection (Rare) 2506
Permax Tablets 571
Virazole 1310

Retinitis
Attenuvax (Infrequent) 1650
Betaseron for SC Injection 653
Cytovene (1% or less) 2270
Doxil (1% to 5%) 2613
Indocin (Less than 1%) 1723
M-M-R II (Infrequent) 1730
M-R-VAX II 1732
Videx Tablets, Powder for Oral Solution, & Pediatric Powder for Oral Solution (Up to 1%) 2980

Retinitis, bilateral
Typhim Vi 914

Retinitis, macular
Zyloprim Tablets (Less than 1%) 1194

Retinoic-acid-APL syndrome
▲ Vesanoid Capsules (Up to 25%) 2327

Retinopathy
Aralen Hydrochloride Injection 2430
Aralen Phosphate Tablets 2431
Cardizem CD Capsules (Infrequent) 1251
Cardizem SR Capsules (Infrequent) 1255
Cardizem Injectable 1253
Cardizem Tablets (Infrequent) 1257
Clinoril Tablets 1658
Haldol Decanoate 1587
Haldol Injection, Tablets and Concentrate 1585
Lysodren Tablets (Infrequent) 707
Minipress Capsules (Single report) 2015
Minizide Capsules (Single report) 2016
Neurontin Capsules (Rare) 1978
Nipent for Injection (Less than 3%) 2733
Nolvadex Tablets 2957
Plaquenil Sulfate Tablets (Rare) 2459
Roferon-A Injection (Rare) 2308
▲ Tegison Capsules (10-25%) 2314
Tiazac Capsules (Infrequent) 1019
Tolectin (200, 400 and 600 mg) (Less than 1%) 1591

Retinopathy, pigmentary
Aralen Phosphate Tablets 2431
Compazine 2644
Etrafon 2495
Levoprome 1321
Mellaril 2398
Prolixin 510
Stelazine 2692
Thorazine 2701
Triavil Tablets 1800
Trilafon 2532

Retrocollis
Etrafon 2495
Trilafon 2532

Retrolental fibroplasia
▲ Indocin I.V. (3% to 9%) 1727

Retroperitoneal fibrosis
Blocadren Tablets 1654
D.H.E. 45 Injection (Occasional) 2381
Parlodel (A few patients) 2411
Redux Capsules 2911
Sansert Tablets (Very rare) 2424
Timolide Tablets 1791
Timoptic in Ocudose (Less frequent) 1796
Timoptic Sterile Ophthalmic Solution (Less frequent) 1794
Timoptic-XE 1798

Retrosternal discomfort
IOPIDINE Sterile Ophthalmic Solution ◉ 218
Levophed Bitartrate Injection 2445

Reye's Syndrome, potential for development of
Alka-Seltzer Cherry Effervescent Antacid and Pain Reliever ▣ 609
Alka-Seltzer Extra Strength Effervescent Antacid and Pain Reliever ▣ 609
Alka-Seltzer Lemon Lime Effervescent Antacid and Pain Reliever ▣ 609
Alka-Seltzer Original Effervescent Antacid and Pain Reliever ▣ 609
Alka-Seltzer Plus ▣ 611
Alka-Seltzer Plus Sinus Medicine ▣ 611
Ascriptin ▣ 650
Arthritis Strength BC Powder ▣ 631
BC Cold Powder Multi-Symptom Formula (Cold-Sinus-Allergy) ▣ 631
BC Cold Powder Non-Drowsy Formula (Cold-Sinus) ▣ 631
BC Powder ▣ 631
Backache Caplets ▣ 635
Genuine Bayer Aspirin Tablets & Caplets ▣ 618
Extra Strength Bayer Arthritis Pain Regimen Formula ▣ 615
Extra Strength Bayer Aspirin Caplets & Tablets ▣ 617
Extended-Release Bayer 8-Hour Aspirin ▣ 616
Extra Strength Bayer Plus Aspirin Caplets ▣ 617
Extra Strength Bayer PM Aspirin Plus Sleep Aid ▣ 617
Aspirin Regimen Bayer 81 mg Tablets with Calcium ▣ 615
Aspirin Regimen Bayer Adult Low Strength 81 mg Tablets ▣ 613
Aspirin Regimen Bayer Children's Chewable Aspirin ▣ 616
Arthritis Strength Bufferin Analgesic Caplets ▣ 637
Extra Strength Bufferin Analgesic Tablets ▣ 637
Cama Arthritis Pain Reliever ▣ 748
Darvon 1475
Disalcid 1549
Doan's Extra-Strength Analgesic ▣ 653
Extra Strength Doan's P.M. ▣ 653
Doan's Regular Strength Analgesic ▣ 654
Easprin 1971
Ecotrin 2625
Empirin Aspirin Tablets ▣ 818
Excedrin Extra-Strength Analgesic Tablets, Caplets, and Geltabs 734
Fiorinal with Codeine Capsules 2390
Goody's Extra Strength Headache Powders ▣ 632
Goody's Extra Strength Pain Relief Tablets ▣ 632
Helidac Therapy (Rare) 2135
Norgesic Tablets 1554
Pepto-Bismol Original Liquid, Original and Cherry Tablets and Easy-To-Swallow Caplets (Rare) 2126
Pepto-Bismol Maximum Strength Liquid (Rare) 2126
Percodan Tablets 955
St. Joseph Adult Chewable Aspirin (81 mg.) ▣ 768
Vanquish Analgesic Caplets ▣ 627

Rhabdomyolysis
Activase 1045
Amicar Syrup, Tablets, and Injection 1312
Anectine (Rare) 1062
Atromid-S Capsules 2808
Azulfidine (Rare) 2059
Clozaril Tablets 2377
Cytovene-IV (One report) 2270
Felbatol 2774
Floxin I.V. 1580
Floxin Tablets (200 mg, 300 mg, 400 mg) 1577
Foscavir Injection (Rare) 541
Lescol Capsules 2395
Lopid Tablets 1974
Mevacor Tablets 1742
Orap Tablets 1037
PCE Dispertab Tablets 453
Pravachol Tablets (Rare) 770
Risperdal Tablets 1348
Videx Tablets, Powder for Oral Solution, & Pediatric Powder for Oral Solution (Rare) 2980
Wellbutrin Tablets 1177
Zocor Tablets (Rare) 1821

Rheumatic syndrome
Nydrazid Injection 509
Rifamate Capsules 1278
Rifater 1280

Rheumatoid arthritis
Atromid-S Capsules 2808
Helidac Therapy (Less than 1%) 2135
Norplant System (Rare) 2868
Prozac Pulvules & Liquid, Oral Solution (Rare) 935
Redux Capsules (Infrequent) 2911
Rilutek Tablets (Rare) 2198

Rheumatoid factor, positive
Aldoclor Tablets 1638
Aldomet Ester HCl Injection 1642
Aldomet Oral 1640
Aldoril Tablets 1644
Elavil 2945

Rhinitis
▲ Acel-Imune Diphtheria and Tetanus Toxoids and Acellular Pertussis Vaccine Adsorbed (6%) 1415
▲ Actigall Capsules (5.2%) 818
Adalat CC (3% or less) 582
▲ AeroBid Inhaler System (3% to 9%) 1004
▲ Aerobid-M Inhaler System (3% to 9%) 1004
Ambien Tablets (1%) 2559
▲ Anafranil Capsules (7% to 12%) 819
Aredia for Injection (Up to 6%) 827
Arimidex Tablets (2% to 5%) 2932
▲ Asacol Delayed-Release Tablets (5%) 2129
Atrovent Inhalation Solution (2.3%) 675
▲ Atrovent Nasal Spray 0.03% (2.0% to 5.1%) 676
▲ Axid Pulvules (9.8%) 1468
▲ Bactroban Nasal (1.0% to 6%) 2643
Capoten Tablets 740
Capozide Tablets 744
Carafate Suspension 1250
Carafate Tablets 1249
Cardene Capsules (Rare) 2261
Cardene SR Capsules (Rare) 2264
▲ Cardura Tablets (3%) 1993
Cartrol Tablets (Less common) 413
Casodex Tablets (2% to 5%) 2934
▲ CellCept Capsules (More than or equal to 3%) 2265
Cerebyx Injection (Infrequent) 1956
Claritin Tablets (2% or fewer patients) 2485
▲ Cognex Capsules (8%) 1961
Cozaar Tablets (Less than 1%) 1668
▲ DDAVP (3 to 8%) 2180
▲ DaunoXome (Up to 12%) 1842
Demadex Tablets and Injection (2.8%) 691
Depakote Tablets (1% to 5%) 418
▲ Desmopressin Acetate Rhinal Tube (3% to 8%) 997
▲ Dilacor XR Extended-release Capsules (2.9% to 9.6%) 2183
Doxil (Less than 1%) 2613
Effexor 2825
▲ Felbatol (6.9%) 2774
Flovent (1% to 3%) 1089
Foscavir Injection (Between 1% and 5%) 541
Gemzar for Injection (Infrequent) 1482
Glucotrol XL Extended Release Tablets (Less than 3%) 2012
Heparin Lock Flush Solution 2831
Heparin Sodium Injection 2832
Heparin Sodium Vials (Rare) 1486
Hytrin Capsules (At least 1% to 1.9%) 434
Hyzaar Tablets 1720
IBU Tablets (Less than 1%) 1389
Imdur (Less than or equal to 5%) 1362
Intron A for Injection (Less than 5%) 2506
Invirase Capsules (Less than 2%) 2291
Iopidine 0.5% (Less than 1%) ◉ 219
Kadian Capsules (Less than 3%) 2948
Kerlone Tablets (1.4%) 2588
▲ Lamictal Tablets (13.6%) 1105
▲ Lescol Capsules (4.7%) 2395
▲ Leukine (11%) 1317
Lioresal Intrathecal (1% or more) 1634
Lodine Capsules and Tablets (Less than 1%) 2849
▲ Lorabid Suspension and Pulvules (1.6% to 6.3%) 1513
Lotensin HCT Tablets (More than 1%) 855
Lupron Depot 3.75 mg (Less than 5%) 2739
LUVOX Tablets 2723
Marinol (Dronabinol) Capsules (Less than 1%) 2353
▲ Mepron Suspension (5%) 1206
▲ Miacalcin Nasal Spray (12%) 2403
Monopril Tablets (0.2% to 1.0%) 762
Motrin Ibuprofen Suspension, Oral Drops, Chewable Tablets, Caplets (Less than 1%) 1563
Mumpsvax 1751
▲ Naprelan Tablets (3% to 9%) 2861
Nasacort AQ Nasal Spray (2% or greater) 2191
▲ Neurontin Capsules (4.1%) 1978
▲ Nipent for Injection (10% to 11%) 2733
Norvasc Tablets (Less than or equal to 0.1%) 2020
Norvir (Less than 2%) 447
OptiPranolol (Metipranolol 0.3%) Sterile Ophthalmic Solution (A small number of patients) ◉ 256
Orlaam Oral Solution (1% to 3%) 2361
Orudis Capsules (Less than 1%) 2874
Oruvail Capsules (Less than 1%) 2874
Pandel Cream, 0.1% (7 of 226 patients) 2475
Paxil Tablets (Frequent) 2681
▲ Permax Tablets (12.2%) 571
Pravachol Tablets (0.1% to 4.0%) 770
Prilosec Delayed-Release Capsules (2%) 516
Prinivil Tablets (0.3% to 1.0%) 1776
Prinzide Tablets (0.3 to 1%) 1780
▲ Prograf (Greater than 3%) 1028
▲ Propulsid (7.3%) 1346
ProSom Tablets (Infrequent) 457
Prozac Pulvules & Liquid, Oral Solution (Frequent) 935
Pulmozyme Inhalation 1054
Recombivax HB (Less than 1%) 1787
Redux Capsules (Frequent) 2911
Retrovir Capsules 1216
Retrovir I.V. Infusion 1221
Retrovir Syrup 1216
▲ Rilutek Tablets (7.8% to 8.9%) 2198
▲ Risperdal Tablets (8% to 10%) 1348
Roferon-A Injection (Less than 1%) 2308
▲ Salagen Tablets (5% to 14%) 1546
Sectral Capsules 2914
Serevent Inhalation Aerosol (1% to 3%) 1149
Serzone Tablets 776
▲ Stadol (3% to 9%) 779
Stimate, (desmopressin acetate) Nasal Spray, 1.5 mg/mL (Occasional) 806
Sular Tablets (Less than or equal to 1%) 2961
▲ Synarel Nasal Solution for Central Precocious Puberty (5%) 2603
Tenex Tablets (3% or less) 2249
Tiazac Capsules (2%) 1019
▲ Tilade Inhaler (4.6%) 2207
Toradol (1% or less) 2319
Tornalate Solution for Inhalation, 0.2% (1.5%) 976
Univasc Tablets (More than 1%) 2553
Vascor Tablets (200 and 300 mg) (0.5 to 2.0%) 1597

(▣ Described in PDR For Nonprescription Drugs) Incidence data in parenthesis; ▲ 3% or more (◉ Described in PDR For Ophthalmology)

1445 Side Effects Index Sclerosis, subcutaneous tissues

Vexol 1% Ophthalmic Suspension (Less than 2%) ...... ⊙ 227
▲ Videx Tablets, Powder for Oral Solution, & Pediatric Powder for Oral Solution (48%) 2980
Vistide Injection 1057
▲ Zebeta Tablets (2.9% to 4.0%) 1457
Zestoretic Tablets (0.3 to 1%) 2968
Zestril Tablets (0.3% to 1.0%) 2972
Ziac (0.7% to 0.9%) 1459
Zoladex (1% or greater) 2976
Zoladex 3-month 2978
Zoloft Tablets (2.0%) 2051
Zosyn (1.2%) 1463
Zyloprim Tablets (Less than 1%) 1194
Zyrtec Tablets (Less than 2%) 2053

Rhinitis, ulcerative

Atrovent Nasal Spray 0.03% (2.0%) 676

Rhinorrhea

▲ ActHIB (21.3% to 24.5%) 893
▲ AeroBid Inhaler System (3% to 9%) 1004
▲ Aerobid-M Inhaler System (3% to 9%) 1004
▲ Atrovent Nasal Spray 0.03% (3.1%) 676
Beconase (Fewer than 3 per 100 patients) 1065
Calcijex Injection 412
Chemet Capsules (0.7% to 3.7%) 666
Clozaril Tablets (Less than 1%) 2377
Colyte and Colyte-flavored (Isolated cases) 2540
4-Way Fast Acting Nasal Spray (regular & mentholated) ...... ▣ 644
4-Way 12 Hour Nasal Spray ...... ▣ 644
Flonase Nasal Spray (Less than 1%) 1088
Floxin I.V. (Less than 1%) 1580
Floxin Tablets (200 mg, 300 mg, 400 mg) (Less than 1%) 1577
GoLYTELY (Isolated cases) 694
Intron A for Injection (Less than 5%) 2506
Klonopin Tablets 2294
Methadone Hydrochloride Oral Concentrate 2356
Nicotrol NS Nicotine Nasal Spray (Common) 1565
NuLYTELY (Isolated cases) 694
Cherry Flavor NuLYTELY (Isolated cases) 694
▲ OmniHIB (21.3 to 24.5%) 2676
Orlaam Oral Solution 2361
Plendil Extended-Release Tablets (0.2% to 1.6%) 514
Prinivil Tablets (0.3% to 1.0%) 1776
Prinzide Tablets 1780
RespiGam (Infrequent) 1631
ReVia Tablets (Less than 1%) 957
Rocaltrol Capsules 2303
▲ Roferon-A Injection (4% to 12%) .. 2308
Soma Compound w/Codeine Tablets 2784
Soma Compound Tablets 2783
Supprelin Injection (2% to 3%) 2230
Tegison Capsules (Less than 1%) .. 2314
Vancenase AQ Nasal Spray 0.042% (Fewer than 3 per 100 patients) 2535
Vancenase PocketHaler Nasal Inhaler (1 per 100 patients) 2534
Vaseretic Tablets 1810
Vasotec I.V. 1814
Vasotec Tablets (0.5% to 1.0%) 1816
▲ Videx Tablets, Powder for Oral Solution, & Pediatric Powder for Oral Solution (21%) 2980
Yohimex Tablets 1414
Zestoretic Tablets 2968
Zestril Tablets (0.3% to 1.0%) 2972

Rhonchi

Brevibloc (esmolol HCl) Injection (Less than 1%) 1860
Crixivan Capsules (Less than 2%) .. 1670
Ganite 2711
Hivid Tablets (Less than 1%) 2287
Survanta Beractant Intratracheal Suspension 2346
▲ Videx Tablets, Powder for Oral Solution, & Pediatric Powder for Oral Solution (6%) 2980
Zemuron Injection (Less than 1%) 1885

Rigidity

Abbokinase 403
Abbokinase Open-Cath 405
Alfenta Injection 1334
Ambien Tablets (Rare) 2559
Brevibloc (esmolol HCl) Injection (Less than 1%) 1860
Cardura Tablets (Less than 0.5% of 3960 patients) 1993
Cedax (0.1% to 1%) 2480
Claritin Tablets (2% or fewer patients) 2485
Claritin-D Tablets (Less frequent) .. 2487
▲ Clozaril Tablets (3%) 2377
Cytotec (Infrequent) 2576
▲ DaunoXome (Up to 19%) 1842
Dipentum Capsules (Rare) 2084
Diprivan Injectable Emulsion (Less than 1%) 2939
▲ Ergamisol Tablets (3% to 5%) 1340
Ethmozine Tablets (Rare) 2217
Ethyol (amifostine) for Injection (Rare; less than 1%) 485
▲ Etopophos for Injection (3%) 701
Famvir Tablets (0.5% to 1.5%) 2660
Felbatol 2774
Flumadine Tablets & Syrup 1013
▲ Foscavir Injection (5% or greater) .. 541
Hivid Tablets (Less than 1%) 2287
Hyzaar Tablets 1720
Imdur (Less than or equal to 5%) .. 1362
Imitrex Tablets (Rare) 1099
▲ Intron A for Injection (Up to 42%) 2506
Ismo Tablets (Fewer than 1%) 2844
Kerlone Tablets (Less than 2%) 2588
Lioresal Tablets 847
Moban Tablets and Concentrate 1036
Norvasc Tablets (More than 0.1% to 1%) 2020
▲ Orap Tablets (2 of 20 patients) 1037
▲ Orthoclone OKT3 Sterile Solution (8%) 1892
Pediazole Suspension 2340
Procardia XL Extended Release Tablets (1% or less) 2026
Proleukin for Injection 812
Risperdal Tablets (Infrequent) 1348
Romazicon (Less than 1%) 2311
▲ Sublimaze Injection (Among most common) 463
▲ Tegison Capsules (1-10%) 2314
▲ Xanax Tablets (4.2%) 2115
Zoloft Tablets (Infrequent) 2051
Zosyn (1.0% or less) 1463
Zovirax Sterile Powder (Less than 1%) 1191
Zyrtec Tablets (Less than 2%) 2053

Rosacea

Elocon Cream 0.1% (1.6%) 2492

Rosacea, worsening of

MetroCream (Less than 3%) 1034

S

Salicylism

Easprin 1971

Saliva, discoloration

Mycobutin Capsules 2101
Rifadin 1276

Salivary gland enlargement

Anafranil Capsules (Rare) 819
Betaseron for SC Injection 653
Clozaril Tablets 2377
Hivid Tablets (Less than 1%) 2287
Lithonate/Lithotabs/Lithobid 2721
Neurontin Capsules (Rare) 1978
Pediazole Suspension 2340
Permax Tablets (Infrequent) 571
Prozac Pulvules & Liquid, Oral Solution (Rare) 935
Remeron Tablets (Rare) 1878
Rilutek Tablets (Rare) 2198
▲ SSKI Solution (Among most frequent) 2767
Thyro-Block Tablets 2785

Salivation

Alferon N Injection (1%) 2142
Altace Capsules (Less than 1%) 1238
Ambien Tablets (Rare) 2559
Anafranil Capsules (Infrequent) 819
Anectine 1062
Antilirium Injectable 1007
Betaseron for SC Injection 653
BuSpar Tablets (Infrequent) 738
Ceftin for Oral Suspension (0.1% to 1%) 1067
Cerebyx Injection (Infrequent) 1956
Claritin Tablets (2% or fewer patients) 2485
▲ Clozaril Tablets (More than 5 to 31%) 2377
Cognex Capsules (Infrequent) 1961
Cordarone Tablets (1 to 3%) 2818
Dalmane Capsules (Rare) 2329
Desyrel and Desyrel Dividose 504
Diupres Tablets 1691
Dizac (diazepam injectable emulsion) CIV (Less frequent) 1862
Effexor (Rare) 2825
Emete-con Intramuscular/Intravenous 2007
Eskalith 2658
Etrafon 2495
Fioricet with Codeine Capsules 2387
Fiorinal with Codeine Capsules 2390
Garamycin Injectable 2502
Haldol Injection, Tablets and Concentrate 1585
Hivid Tablets (Less than 1%) 2287
Humorsol Sterile Ophthalmic Solution (Rare) 1707
Hydropres Tablets 1718
Hyperstat I.V. Injection 2504
IFEX (Less than 1%) 706
Intron A for Injection (Less than 5%) 2506
Isopto Carbachol Ophthalmic Solution ...... ⊙ 221
Kerlone Tablets (Less than 2%) 2588
Lamictal Tablets (Infrequent) 1105
Lioresal Intrathecal (Up to 2.7%) .. 1634
Lithonate/Lithotabs/Lithobid 2721
Loxitane 1426
Ludiomil Tablets (Rare) 861
LUVOX Tablets (Infrequent) 2723
Megace Oral Suspension (1% to 3%) 708
Mestinon Injectable 1300
Mestinon 1300
Mexitil Capsules (About 4 in 1,000) 684
Moban Tablets and Concentrate (Occasional) 1036
Navane Capsules and Concentrate 2018
Navane Intramuscular 2019
Neurontin Capsules (Infrequent) 1978
▲ Orap Tablets (13.8%) 1037
Orudis Capsules (Less than 1%) 2874
Oruvail Capsules (Less than 1%) 2874
Paxil Tablets (Infrequent) 2681
PhosChol 488
Prevacid Delayed-Release Capsules (Less than 1%) 2746
Primaxin I.M. 1770
Primaxin I.V. (Less than 0.2%) 1772
Prinivil Tablets (Greater than 1%) .. 1776
Prinzide Tablets 1780
Prolixin 510
▲ Prostigmin Injectable (Among most common) 1305
▲ Prostigmin Tablets (Among most common) 1306
Prozac Pulvules & Liquid, Oral Solution (Rare) 935
Quadrinal Tablets 1398
Remeron Tablets (Rare) 1878
Risperdal Tablets (Up to 2%) 1348
Roferon-A Injection (Infrequent) 2308
Serzone Tablets (Rare) 776
Suprane (desflurane, USP) (Greater than 1%) 1865
Tensilon Injectable 1307
Trental Tablets (Less than 1%) 1291
Triavil Tablets 1800
Trilafon 2532
Urecholine 1804
Valium Injectable (Rare) 2336
Valium Tablets (Infrequent) 2335
▲ Wellbutrin Tablets (3.4%) 1177
▲ Xanax Tablets (4.2% to 5.6%) 2115
Zestril Tablets (Greater than 1%) .. 2972
Zoloft Tablets (Infrequent) 2051
Zyrtec Tablets (Less than 2%) 2053

Salivation, increase (see under Salivation)

Salpingitis

Betaseron for SC Injection 653
Permax Tablets (Infrequent) 571
Prozac Pulvules & Liquid, Oral Solution (Rare) 935

Sarcoidosis

Risperdal Tablets (Rare) 1348

Sarcoma, bone

Permax Tablets (Infrequent) 571

Sarcoma, unspecified

Foscavir Injection (Between 1% and 5%) 541
Megace Oral Suspension (1% to 3%) 708
▲ Videx Tablets, Powder for Oral Solution, & Pediatric Powder for Oral Solution (3% to 5%) 2980
Vistide Injection 1057

Scalp, dry

Nizoral 2% Shampoo 1344
Selsun Rx 2.5% Selenium Sulfide Lotion, USP 2345

Scalp, oily

Nizoral 2% Shampoo 1344
Selsun Rx 2.5% Selenium Sulfide Lotion, USP 2345

Scalp, tightness

Cormax Scalp Application (Approximately 0.3%) 1857
Temovate Scalp Application (1 of 294 patients) 1153

Scalp defects, fetal

Tapazole Tablets (Rare) 1361

Scarring

Condylox Topical Solution (Less than 5%) 1853
Dalalone D.P. Injectable 1009
Decadron-LA Sterile Suspension 1687
▲ Efudex (Among most frequent) 2280
Fluoroplex Topical Solution & Cream 1% (Occasional) 475
Stimate, (desmopressin acetate) Nasal Spray, 1.5 mg/mL 806
T.R.U.E. Test (Two reports) 1162
Tubersol (Tuberculin Purified Protein Derivative (Mantoux)) 2988

Schizophrenia, precipitation

Anafranil Capsules (Rare) 819
Nardil (Less frequent) 1977
Redux Capsules 2911

Sciatica

Ambien Tablets (Rare) 2559
Wellbutrin Tablets (Rare) 1177

Sclera, discoloration

Hivid Tablets (Less than 1%) 2287
Mellaril 2398
Minipress Capsules (1-4%) 2015
Minizide Capsules 2016
Novantrone for Injection 1327
Serentil 689
Ticlid Tablets 2317
Torecan 2367

Sclera, infection

Urobiotic-250 Capsules 2038

Scleral injection

Azulfidine (Rare) 2059
Bactrim DS Tablets 2257
Bactrim I.V. Infusion 2255
Bactrim 2257
Fansidar Tablets 2281
Gantanol Tablets 2285
Pediazole Suspension 2340
Prelone Syrup 1834
Septra 1146
Septra I.V. Infusion 1142
Septra I.V. Infusion ADD-Vantage Vials 1144
Septra 1146

Scleritis

Ambien Tablets (Infrequent) 2559
Anafranil Capsules (Infrequent) 819
Aredia for Injection (Rare) 827
Effexor (Rare) 2825

Scleroderma

Depo-Provera Contraceptive Injection (Fewer than 1%) 2079
Redux Capsules 2911

Sclerosis, multiple

Engerix-B Unit-Dose Vials (Less than 1%) 2656
Havrix (Rare) 2663
Recombivax HB 1787

Sclerosis, skin

Norplant System (Rare) 2868
Parnate Tablets 2679
Talwin Injection 2465

Sclerosis, subcutaneous tissues

Talwin Injection 2465

(▣ Described in PDR For Nonprescription Drugs) Incidence data in parenthesis; ▲ 3% or more (⊙ Described in PDR For Ophthalmology)

Scotomata
Side Effects Index
1446

Scotomata

Adenoscan (Less than 1%) 1022
Aralen Hydrochloride Injection 2430
Aralen Phosphate Tablets 2431
Cardioquin Tablets (Occasional) 2146
Cataflam Tablets (Less than 1%) 833
Eskalith 2658
IBU Tablets (Less than 1%) 1389
Kerlone Tablets (Less than 2%) 2588
Lithium Carbonate Capsules & Tablets 2352
Lithonate/Lithotabs/Lithobid 2721
Motrin Ibuprofen Suspension, Oral Drops, Chewable Tablets, Caplets (Less than 1%) 1563
Placidyl Capsules 456
Plaquenil Sulfate Tablets 2459
Proglycem 575
ProSom Tablets (Rare) 457
Quinaglute Dura-Tabs Tablets (Occasional) 644
Quinidex Extentabs (Occasional) 2240
Tegison Capsules (Less than 1%) 2314
Trental Tablets (Less than 1%) 1291
Cataflam/Voltaren/Voltaren-XR (Less than 1%) 833

Scotomata, scintillating

Clomid (1.5%) 1262
Serophene (clomiphene citrate tablets, USP) 2621
Taxol Injection (Rare) 723

Screaming, excessive

Tri-Immunol Adsorbed (Rare) 1452

Seborrhea

▲ Accutane Capsules (Less than 1 patient in 10) 2252
Anafranil Capsules (Rare) 819
Androderm Testosterone Transdermal System 2634
Avonex 662
Betaseron for SC Injection 653
Cognex Capsules (Rare) 1961
Crixivan Capsules (Less than 2%) 1670
Danocrine Capsules 2437
DaunoXome (Less than or equal to 5%) 1842
Depakote Tablets (1% to 5%) 418
Fludara for Injection (Up to 1%) 658
Foscavir Injection (Between 1% and 5%) 541
Halotestin Tablets 2095
Invirase Capsules (Less than 2%) 2291
Lamictal Tablets (Rare) 1105
Loxitane 1426
Lupron Depot-PED 7.5 mg, 11.25 mg and 15 mg (2%) 2744
Lupron Injection Pediatric 2737
LUVOX Tablets (Infrequent) 2723
Neurontin Capsules (Infrequent) 1978
Norvir (Less than 2%) 447
Paxil Tablets (Rare) 2681
Permax Tablets (Infrequent) 571
Prolixin 510
Prozac Pulvules & Liquid, Oral Solution (Rare) 935
Remeron Tablets (Rare) 1878
Rilutek Tablets (Infrequent) 2198
Risperdal Tablets (Up to 1%) 1348
Salagen Tablets (Less than 1%) 1546
▲ Synarel Nasal Solution for Central Precocious Puberty (3%) 2603
▲ Synarel Nasal Solution for Endometriosis (8% of patients) 2605
Testoderm Testosterone Transdermal System 486
▲ Zoladex (26%) 2976
Zoladex 3-month 2978
Zyrtec Tablets (Less than 2%) 2053

Sedation

Aldoclor Tablets 1638
Aldomet Ester HCl Injection 1642
Aldomet Oral 1640
Aldoril Tablets 1644
Ancobon Capsules 2254
Ativan Injection 2805
▲ Ativan Tablets (15.9%) 2807
▲ Atrohist Pediatric Suspension (Among most common) 1604
▲ Atrohist Pediatric Suspension Dye-Free (Among most common) 1604
▲ Axocet Capsules (Among most frequent) 2469
▲ Benadryl Injection (Among most frequent) 1955
▲ Bromfed-DM Cough Syrup (Among most frequent) 1832
Brontex 2130
▲ Buprenex Injectable (Most frequent) 2170
▲ Catapres Tablets (About 10 in 100 patients) 679
Catapres-TTS (3 of 101 patients) 680
▲ Clozaril Tablets (More than 5 to 39%) 2377
▲ Combipres Tablets (About 10%) 682
▲ DHCplus Capsules (Among most frequent) 2148
▲ Dalgan Injection (3 to 9%) 529
Dalmane Capsules 2329
▲ Darvon-N/Darvocet-N (Among most frequent) 1473
▲ Darvon (Among most frequent) 1475
▲ Darvon-N Suspension & Tablets (Among most frequent) 1473
Daypro Caplets (1% to 3%) 2578
▲ Demerol (Among most frequent) 2438
▲ Demser Capsules (Almost all patients) 1690
Depakene 416
Depakote Tablets 418
Dilaudid Ampules 1382
Dilaudid Cough Syrup 1383
▲ Dilaudid-HP Injection (Among most frequent) 1384
▲ Dilaudid-HP Lyophilized Powder 250 mg (Among most frequent) 1384
Dilaudid 1382
Dilaudid Oral Liquid 1386
Dilaudid 1382
Dilaudid Tablets - 8 mg 1386
▲ Dimetane-DC Cough Syrup (Most frequent) 2232
▲ Dimetane-DX Cough Syrup (Among most frequent) 2233
Diupres Tablets 1691
▲ Esgic-plus Capsules (Among most frequent) 1012
▲ Esgic-plus Tablets (Among most frequent) 1012
Etrafon (Less frequent) 2495
Fedahist Gyrocaps 2545
▲ Fioricet Tablets (Among most frequent) 2386
Fioricet with Codeine Capsules (Frequent) 2387
Fiorinal with Codeine Capsules 2390
Halcion Tablets 2093
Hycodan Tablets and Syrup 946
Hycomine Compound Tablets 948
Hycomine 947
Hycotuss Expectorant Syrup 950
Hydrocet Capsules 787
Hydropres Tablets 1718
Imitrex Injection (2.7%) 1095
Imitrex Tablets 1099
Kadian Capsules (Less than 3%) 2948
Lioresal Tablets 847
Lomotil 2591
▲ Lorcet 10/650 Tablets (Among most frequent) 1016
▲ Lortab (Among most frequent) 2751
▲ MS Contin Tablets (Among most frequent) 2149
▲ MSIR (Among most frequent) 2152
▲ Mepergan Injection (Among most frequent) 2859
▲ Methadone Hydrochloride Oral Concentrate (Among most frequent) 2356
Methadone Hydrochloride Oral Solution & Tablets 2357
Motofen Tablets 789
Navane Capsules and Concentrate 2018
Navane Intramuscular 2019
▲ Nubain Injection (36%) 952
▲ Oramorph SR (Morphine Sulfate Sustained Release Tablets) (Among most frequent) 2359
▲ Orap Tablets (14 of 20 patients) 1037
Ornade Spansule Capsules 2678
▲ OxyIR Capsules (Among most frequent) 2167
Papaverine Hydrochloride Vials and Ampoules 1523
▲ Percocet Tablets (Among most frequent) 955
▲ Percodan Tablets (Among most frequent) 955
▲ Percodan-Demi Tablets (Among most frequent) 956
Periactin 1767
Phenergan with Codeine 2883
Phenergan with Dextromethorphan 2885
Phenergan Suppositories 2882
Phenergan Syrup 2881
Phenergan VC 2886
Phenergan VC with Codeine 2888
Phenobarbital Elixir and Tablets 1523
▲ Phrenilin (Among most frequent) 790
Prozac Pulvules & Liquid, Oral Solution (1.9%) 935
▲ RMS Suppositories CII (Among most frequent) 2766
Roferon-A Injection (Infrequent) 2308
Rondec Oral Drops 974
Rondec Syrup 974
Rondec 974
▲ Roxanol (Among most frequent) 2365
▲ Roxicodone Tablets, Oral Solution & Intensol (Oxycodone) (Among most frequent) 2366
▲ Rynatan (Among most common) 2781
▲ Rynatuss (Among most common) 2782
▲ Sedapap Tablets 50 mg/650 mg (Among the most frequent) 1826
▲ Seldane-D Extended-Release Tablets (7.2%) 1286
▲ Semprex-D Capsules (6% more common than with placebo) 1620
Soma Compound w/Codeine Tablets 2784
Talacen Caplets 2464
Talwin Injection 2465
Talwin Compound 2466
Talwin Injection 2465
Talwin Nx Tablets 2467
▲ Tavist Syrup (Among most frequent) 2426
▲ Tavist Tablets (Among most frequent) 2427
▲ Tenex Tablets (5% to 39%) 2249
Tessalon Perles 1018
Triavil Tablets 1800
▲ Trinalin Repetabs Tablets (Among most frequent) 1373
Tussend 1830
Tussionex Pennkinetic Extended-Release Suspension 1624
▲ Tylenol with Codeine (Among most frequent) 1592
▲ Tylox Capsules (Among most frequent) 1593
Versed Injection (1.6%) 2324
▲ Vicodin Tablets (Among most frequent) 1404
▲ Vicodin ES Tablets (Among most frequent) 1405
▲ Vicodin HP Tablets (Among most frequent) 1403
Vicodin Tuss Expectorant 1406
▲ Wellbutrin Tablets (19.8%) 1177
▲ Wygesic Tablets (Most frequent) 2930
Xanax Tablets 2115
▲ Zofran Injection (8%) 1227
▲ Zofran Tablets (20%) 1231
▲ Zydone Capsules (Among most frequent) 967

Seizure control, loss of

Depakene 416

Seizures (see also under Convulsions)

Accutane Capsules 2252
Acel-Imune Diphtheria and Tetanus Toxoids and Acellular Pertussis Vaccine Adsorbed (One child) 1415
Actimmune (Rare) 1043
Adapin Capsules (Infrequent) 1542
▲ Aredia for Injection (3% to 4%) 827
Asendin Tablets (Less than 1%) 1419
Atretol Tablets 569
Attenuvax (Rare) 1650
▲ Avonex (3%) 662
Axocet Capsules (Infrequent) 2469
Azactam for Injection (Less than 1%) 736
Brethine Ampuls (Rare) 832
Brethine Tablets (Rare) 831
BuSpar Tablets (Infrequent) 738
Ceftin Tablets 1067
Cefzil Tablets and Oral Suspension 747
Ceptaz (Fewer than 1%) 1070
Cipro I.V. Pharmacy Bulk Package (Less than 1%) 590
Claritin Tablets (Rare) 2485
Clomid 1262
▲ Clozaril Tablets (3.5 to approximately 5%) 2377
DDAVP Injection (Rare) 2178
DDAVP (Rare) 2180
Dantrium Capsules (Less frequent) 2131
Daraprim Tablets (Rare) 1199
Desmopressin Acetate Injection (Rare) 996
Diflucan Tablets, Injection, and Oral Suspension 2003
Diprivan Injectable Emulsion (Less than 1%) 2939
Duricef Capsules, Tablets, and Oral Suspension 750
E.E.S. (Isolated reports) 427
Elavil 2945
Eldepryl Capsules 2729
Epogen for Injection (1.1% to approximately 2.5%) 489
EryPed (Isolated reports) 425
Ery-Tab Tablets (Isolated reports) 426
Erythrocin Stearate Filmtab (Isolated reports) 429
Erythromycin Base Filmtab (Isolated reports) 430
Erythromycin Delayed-Release Capsules, USP (Isolated reports) 431
Ethmozine Tablets (Less than 2%) 2217
Etrafon 2495
▲ Exosurf Neonatal for Intratracheal Suspension (2% to 10%) 1081
Fioricet with Codeine Capsules (Infrequent) 2387
Floxin I.V. (Less than 1%) 1580
Fortaz 1092
▲ Foscavir Injection (5% or greater up to 10%) 541
Guaifed 1833
Hexalen Capsules (1%) 2760
HibTITER (One case) 1423
Hivid Tablets (Less than 1% to 1.3%) 2287
▲ Idamycin Injection (4%) 2096
IFEX (Occasional) 706
Imitrex Tablets (Rare) 1099
INFeD (Iron Dextran Injection, USP) 2478
Isoptin Injectable (Occasional) 1391
JE-VAX (1 to 2.3 per million vaccines) 904
K-Phos Neutral Tablets 633
Keftab Tablets 931
Kwell Cream & Lotion (Exceedingly rare) 2172
Lariam Tablets 2295
Leukeran Tablets (Rare) 1205
Lindane Lotion USP 1% (Exceedingly rare) 481
Lindane Shampoo USP 1% (Exceedingly rare) 483
Lioresal Intrathecal (1% or more) 1634
Lorabid Suspension and Pulvules 1513
Loxitane 1426
Ludiomil Tablets (Rare) 861
M-M-R II (Rare) 1730
M-R-VAX II (Rare) 1732
MS Contin Tablets (Less frequent) 2149
MSIR (Infrequent) 2152
Merrem I.V. (0.1% to 1.0%) 2952
Methergine 2401
Mexitil Capsules (About 2 in 1,000) 684
Myleran Tablets 1209
Nalfon 200 Pulvules & Nalfon Tablets (Less than 1%) 933
Narcan Injection 950
Navane Capsules and Concentrate (Infrequent) 2018
Navane Intramuscular (Infrequent) 2019
Noroxin Tablets 1758
Noroxin Tablets 2222
Norpramin Tablets 1273
Novantrone for Injection (2 to 4%) 1327
Oramorph SR (Morphine Sulfate Sustained Release Tablets) (Less frequent) 2359
Orap Tablets 1037
Orthoclone OKT3 Sterile Solution 1892
OxyContin Tablets (Less than 1%) 2163
Pamelor 2409
Parlodel (72 cases) 2411
PedvaxHIB (Infrequent) 1761
Penetrex Tablets 2196
Platinol for Injection 717
Platinol-AQ Injection 719
Primaxin I.M. 1770
Primaxin I.V. (0.4%) 1772
Prinzide Tablets 1780
▲ Procrit for Injection (1.1% to 10%) 1896
ProSom Tablets (Infrequent) 457
Prozac Pulvules & Liquid, Oral Solution (12 among 6,000 patients) 935
Remeron Tablets (One patient) 1878
Retrovir Capsules (Rare; 0.8%) 1216
Retrovir I.V. Infusion (Rare; 1%) 1221
Retrovir Syrup (Rare; 0.8%) 1216
Risperdal Tablets (0.3%) 1348
Roferon-A Injection (Less than 1% to less than 4%) 2308
Romazicon 2311

(▣ Described in PDR For Nonprescription Drugs) Incidence data in parenthesis; ▲ 3% or more (◉ Described in PDR For Ophthalmology)

Side Effects Index

Rythmol Tablets—150mg, 225mg, 300mg (0.3%) ... 1399
Seldane Tablets ... 1284
Seldane-D Extended-Release Tablets ... 1286
Seromycin Capsules ... 975
Serzone Tablets (One patient) ... 776
Sinequan (Infrequent) ... 2028
Suprax ... 1443
Surmontil Capsules ... 2917
Talwin Injection ... 2465
Talwin Compound ... 2466
Talwin Injection ... 2465
Tazidime Vials, Faspak & ADD-Vantage ... 1531
Tegretol/Tegretol-XR ... 870
Tofranil Ampuls ... 873
Tofranil Tablets ... 875
Tofranil-PM Capsules ... 876
Tonocard Tablets (Less than 1%) .. 519
Triavil Tablets ... 1800
Ultram Tablets (50 mg) (Less than 1%) ... 1594
Uroqid-Acid No. 2 Tablets ... 633
Vaseretic Tablets ... 1810
Versed Injection ... 2324
Videx Tablets, Powder for Oral Solution, & Pediatric Powder for Oral Solution (1%) ... 2980
Vivactil Tablets ... 1820
Wellbutrin Tablets (Frequent) ... 1177
Xanax Tablets ... 2115
Zinacef ... 1184
Zovirax Capsules ... 1187
Zovirax Sterile Powder (Approximately 1%) ... 1191
Zovirax ... 1187

Seizures, convulsive

Aralen Hydrochloride Injection ... 2430
Aralen Phosphate Tablets ... 2431
Cipro I.V. (1% or less) ... 587
Cipro Tablets (Less than 1%) ... 584
Cylert Tablets ... 415
Etrafon ... 2495
Flagyl 375 Capsules ... 2587
Flagyl I.V. ... 2373
Helidac Therapy ... 2135
Mellaril (Infrequent) ... 2398
Mezlin ... 594
Mezlin Pharmacy Bulk Package ... 597
Phenergan Injection ... 2880
Phenergan Tablets ... 2882
Protostat Tablets ... 1939
Reglan (Isolated reports) ... 2243
Robaxin Injectable ... 2245
Serentil ... 689
Thorazine ... 2701
Timentin for Injection ... 2706
Trilafon ... 2532

Seizures, epileptiform

Eskalith ... 2658
Etrafon (A few instances) ... 2495
Lioresal Tablets ... 847
Lithium Carbonate Capsules & Tablets ... 2352
Lithonate/Lithotabs/Lithobid ... 2721
Pamelor ... 2409
Parlodel (4 cases) ... 2411

Seizures, exacerbation of

Lamictal Tablets (2.3%) ... 1105
Serzone Tablets (One patient) ... 776

Seizures, grand mal

Desyrel and Desyrel Dividose ... 504
▲ Foscavir Injection (5% or greater) .. 541
Haldol Decanoate ... 1587
Haldol Injection, Tablets and Concentrate ... 1585
Hivid Tablets (Less than 1%) ... 2287
Orap Tablets ... 1037
Pepcid Injection (Infrequent) ... 1765
Pepcid (Infrequent) ... 1763
Proleukin for Injection (1%) ... 812
Prolixin ... 510
Sodium Polystyrene Sulfonate Suspension (One case) ... 2367
Taxol Injection (Rare; less than 1%) ... 723
Thorazine ... 2701
Zofran Injection (Rare) ... 1227
Zofran Tablets (Rare) ... 1231

Seizures, neonatal

Capoten Tablets ... 740
Capozide Tablets ... 744
Esgic-plus Capsules (One 2-day-old male infant) ... 1012

Esgic-plus Tablets (One 2-day-old male infant) ... 1012

Self-deprecation

Hydropres Tablets ... 1718

Sensation, abnormal
(see under Paresthesia)

Sensation, disturbance of temperature

Dopram Injectable ... 2235
Duranest Injections ... 533
Dyclone 0.5% and 1% Topical Solutions, USP ... 535
Ethmozine Tablets (Less than 2%) ... 2217
▲ Imitrex Injection (10.8%) ... 1095
Imitrex Tablets (2% to 3%; rare) .. 1099
IOPIDINE Sterile Ophthalmic Solution ... ⊚ 218
Tonocard Tablets (0.5% to 1.5%) ... 519
Xylocaine Injections ... 562

Sensation, heavy

▲ Imitrex Injection (7.3%) ... 1095
Imitrex Tablets (Less than 1% to 2%) ... 1099

Sensation of pressure/tightness

▲ Imitrex Injection (5.1 to 7.1%) ... 1095
Imitrex Tablets (Less than 1% to 2%) ... 1099

Sensations, numbness

Duranest Injections ... 533
Dyclone 0.5% and 1% Topical Solutions, USP ... 535
Xylocaine Injections ... 562

Sensations, pulsating

Imitrex Injection (Infrequent) ... 1095
Imitrex Tablets (Infrequent) ... 1099

Sensitivity, light

Cipro Tablets ... 584
▲ Orap Tablets (1 of 20 patients) ... 1037
ReVia Tablets (Less than 1%) ... 957
Stimate, (desmopressin acetate) Nasal Spray, 1.5 mg/mL ... 806
Symmetrel Capsules (0.1% to 1%) ... 965
Symmetrel Syrup (Sensitivity, light 0.17% to 1%) ... 963

Sensitivity, sun

Cipro Tablets ... 584
Danocrine Capsules (Rare) ... 2437
Minocin Oral Suspension ... 1431
Renova (tretinoin emollient cream) 0.05% ... 1945
Retin-A (tretinoin) Cream/Gel/Liquid ... 1947
Tegrin Dandruff Shampoo ... ⊞ 634
Tegrin Skin Cream & Tegrin Medicated Soap ... ⊞ 634
Thorazine ... 2701

Sensitivity reactions

AVC (Occasional) ... 1245
Anusol Hemorrhoidal Ointment (Rare) ... ⊞ 810
Auralgan Otic Solution ... 2810
Bactroban Ointment ... 2642
Benoquin Cream 20% ... 1298
Betadine Skin Cleanser (Rare) ... 2145
Betadine 5% Sterile Ophthalmic Prep Solution (Occasional instances) ... ⊚ 266
Betasept Surgical Scrub ... 2145
Bleph-10 (Rare) ... 472
Brevoxyl ... 2732
Capozide Tablets ... 744
Caverject Injection (Less than 1%) ... 2064
Children's TYLENOL acetaminophen Chewable Tablets, Elixir, Suspension Liquid, and Suspension Drops (Rare) ... 1559
Coly-Mycin S Otic w/Neomycin & Hydrocortisone ... 1965
Congess ... 1003
CORTENEMA (Rare) ... 2713
Cortisporin Otic Solution Sterile (Occasional) ... 1076
Creon ... 2714
Cycrin Tablets (Occasional) ... 991
Drithocreme 0.1%, 0.25%, 0.5%, 1.0% (HP) ... 920
Dritho-Scalp 0.25%, 0.5% ... 921
Dyclone 0.5% and 1% Topical Solutions, USP ... 535

Esidrix Tablets ... 839
Ethyl Chloride, U.S.P. (Extremely rare) ... 1040
FML-S Liquifilm ... ⊚ 240
Fero-Folic-500 Filmtab ... 433
Fluori-Methane (Extremely rare) ... 1040
Hibiclens Antimicrobial Skin Cleanser ... 2947
Hibistat Towelette ... 2948
Humatrope Vials ... 1490
Humegon for Injection ... 1873
Hyperab Rabies Immune Globulin (Human) (Occasional) ... 618
Hyper-Tet Tetanus Immune Globulin (Human) (Extremely rare) ... 621
HypRho-D Full Dose Rho (D) Immune Globulin (Human) (Extremely rare) ... 623
HypRho-D Mini-Dose Rho (D) Immune Globulin (Human) (Extremely rare) ... 622
Iberet-Folic-500 Filmtab ... 433
Infants' TYLENOL acetaminophen Suspension Drops (Rare) ... 1559
Junior Strength TYLENOL acetaminophen Coated Caplets and Chewable Tablets (Rare) ... 1562
Melanex Topical Solution ... 1842
Metrodin (urofollitropin for injection) ... 2616
Monistat Dual-Pak ... 1906
Monistat 3 Vaginal Suppositories ... 1905
Mycostatin Pastilles (Rare) ... 713
Mykrox Tablets ... 1617
Nescaine/Nescaine MPF ... 549
pHisoHex ... 2458
Pediotic Suspension Sterile (Occasional) ... 1140
Pergonal (menotropins for injection, USP) ... 2618
Polysporin Ophthalmic Ointment Sterile ... 1140
Polytrim Ophthalmic Solution Sterile (Rare) ... 479
Prinzide Tablets ... 1780
Provera Tablets (An occasional patient) ... 2110
Retrovir Capsules (Rare) ... 1216
Retrovir I.V. Infusion (Rare) ... 1221
Retrovir Syrup ... 1216
Sensorcaine ... 554
Sine-Aid Maximum Strength Sinus Headache Gelcaps, Caplets and Tablets (Rare) ... 1570
Sinulin Tablets (Rare) ... 792
Solbar PF Ultra Liquid SPF 30 ... 1989
Trusopt Sterile Ophthalmic Solution ... 1803
T.R.U.E. Test (One report) ... 1162
Tylenol (Rare) ... 1570
TYLENOL Allergy Sinus, Maximum Strength Caplets and Gelcaps (Rare) ... 1571
TYLENOL Cold Medication, No Drowsiness Formula Caplets and Gelcaps (Rare) ... 1572
TYLENOL Flu NightTime, Maximum Strength Hot Medication Packets (Rare) ... 1575
TYLENOL Severe Allergy Medication Caplets (Rare) ... 1571
TYLENOL Sinus, Maximum Strength Geltabs, Gelcaps, Caplets and Tablets (Rare) ... 1576
Tympagesic Ear Drops ... 2476
Vaseretic Tablets ... 1810
Zaroxolyn Tablets ... 1625
Zestoretic Tablets ... 2968

Sensorium, clouded

Betapace Tablets (Rare) ... 637
Blocadren Tablets ... 1654
Cartrol Tablets ... 413
Inderal ... 2834
Inderal LA Long Acting Capsules ... 2836
Inderide Tablets ... 2838
Inderide LA Long Acting Capsules ... 2840
Kerlone Tablets ... 2588
Levatol Tablets (Slight) ... 2547
Lopressor HCT Tablets ... 850
Mexitil Capsules (1.9% to 2.6%) ... 684
Normodyne Tablets ... 2522
Sectral Capsules ... 2914
Tenoretic Tablets ... 2963
Tenormin Tablets and I.V. Injection ... 2965
Timolide Tablets ... 1791
Timoptic in Ocudose ... 1796
Timoptic Sterile Ophthalmic Solution ... 1794
Timoptic-XE ... 1798

Toprol-XL Tablets ... 560
Trandate Tablets ... 1158
Visken Tablets ... 2428
Xanax Tablets ... 2115
Zebeta Tablets ... 1457
Ziac ... 1459

Sensorium, dull

Diupres Tablets ... 1691
Hydropres Tablets ... 1718
Ser-Ap-Es Tablets ... 867

Sensory deficit

Oncovin Solution Vials & Hyporets ... 1521

Sensory deficit, persistent

Duranest Injections ... 533
Nescaine/Nescaine MPF ... 549
Videx Tablets, Powder for Oral Solution, & Pediatric Powder for Oral Solution (1% to 4%) ... 2980

Sensory disturbances

Alupent Tablets (0.2%) ... 672
Anafranil Capsules (Infrequent) ... 819
Foscavir Injection (Between 1% and 5%) ... 541
▲ Leukine (6%) ... 1317
Paxil Tablets ... 2681
▲ Prograf (Approximately 55%) ... 1028
▲ Proleukin for Injection (10%) ... 812
▲ Wellbutrin Tablets (4.0%) ... 1177
Xanax Tablets ... 2115

Sepsis

▲ Abelcet Injection (7% to 9%) ... 1540
Avonex ... 662
Betaseron for SC Injection ... 653
Casodex Tablets (2% to 5%) ... 2934
▲ CellCept Capsules (17.6% to 19.7%; 17.5% to 21.8%) ... 2265
Cerebyx Injection (Infrequent) ... 1956
Clozaril Tablets ... 2377
Cognex Capsules (Rare) ... 1961
Cytosar-U Sterile Powder (One case; less frequent) ... 2077
▲ Cytovene (4%) ... 2270
Diprivan Injectable Emulsion (Less than 1%) ... 2939
Doxil (Less than 1% to 5%) ... 2613
Ergamisol Tablets (2 out of 463 patients) ... 1340
Exosurf Neonatal for Intratracheal Suspension (24% to 34%) ... 1081
Felbatol ... 2774
▲ Flolan for Injection (25%) ... 1085
▲ Foscavir Injection (5% or greater) .. 541
Gemzar for Injection (Less than 1%) ... 1482
▲ Hycamtin for Injection (26%) ... 2665
Intron A for Injection (Less than 5%) ... 2506
▲ Leukine (11%) ... 1317
Lutrepulse for Injection ... 998
Merrem I.V. (0.1% to 1.0%) ... 2952
▲ Navelbine Injection (8%) ... 1212
▲ Nipent for Injection (3%) ... 2733
▲ Novantrone for Injection (31 to 34%) ... 1327
Oncaspar (Less than 1%) ... 2194
Orthoclone OKT3 Sterile Solution ... 1892
Permax Tablets (Infrequent) ... 571
Pravachol Tablets ... 770
▲ Proleukin for Injection (23%) ... 812
Pulmozyme Inhalation ... 1054
Rilutek Tablets (Infrequent) ... 2198
Rythmol Tablets—150mg, 225mg, 300mg (One case) ... 1399
Survanta Beractant Intratracheal Suspension ... 2346
▲ Taxol Injection (30%) ... 723
Ticlid Tablets (Rare) ... 2317
Trasylol (3%) ... 607
Vistide Injection ... 1057
▲ Zinecard Injection (12% to 17%) .. 2120
Zoladex 3-month (1% to 5%) ... 2978

Sepsis, intestinal

Questran (One case) ... 774

Septicemia

▲ Leustatin (6%) ... 1889
▲ Neoral (5.3%) ... 2405
Orudis Capsules (Rare) ... 2874
Oruvail Capsules (Rare) ... 2874
ParaGard T 380A Intrauterine Copper Contraceptive ... 1936
▲ Sandimmune (4.8 to 5.3%) ... 2416
Thioplex (Thiotepa For Injection) ... 1329
Tonocard Tablets (Less than 1%) .. 519
Vesanoid Capsules ... 2327

(⊞ Described in PDR For Nonprescription Drugs)   Incidence data in parenthesis; ▲ 3% or more   (⊚ Described in PDR For Ophthalmology)

Side Effects Index

Septic shock
- Oncaspar (Less than 1%) ... 2194
- Tonocard Tablets (Less than 1%) .. 519

Serositis
- Monopril Tablets ... 762
- Vaseretic Tablets ... 1810
- Vasotec I.V. ... 1814
- Vasotec Tablets (0.5% to 1.0%) ... 1816

Serum alkaline phosphatase, elevation
- Abelcet Injection ... 1540
- ▲ Accutane Capsules (1 in 5 to 1 in 10 patients) ... 2252
- Adalat CC (Rare) ... 582
- Ambien Tablets (Rare) ... 2559
- Arimidex Tablets (2% to 5%) ... 2932
- Asacol Delayed-Release Tablets ... 2129
- Atamet Tablets ... 567
- Augmentin (Infrequent) ... 2637
- Augmentin Tablets (Infrequent) ... 2640
- Axid Pulvules (Less common) ... 1468
- Azactam for Injection (Less than 1%) ... 736
- Azathioprine Tablets (Less than 1%) ... 2349
- Betaseron for SC Injection ... 653
- Biaxin (Less than 1%) ... 406
- BiCNU ... 696
- Bumex (0.4%) ... 2260
- Calan SR Caplets ... 2571
- Calan Tablets ... 2568
- Capoten Tablets ... 740
- Capozide Tablets ... 744
- Cardizem CD Capsules (Less than 1%) ... 1251
- Cardizem SR Capsules (1%) ... 1255
- Cardizem Injectable (Less than 1%) ... 1253
- Cardizem Tablets (Less than 1%) ... 1257
- Casodex Tablets (2% to 5%) ... 2934
- Ceclor Pulvules & Suspension (1 in 40) ... 1470
- Cedax (0.1% to 1%) ... 2480
- Cefizox for Intramuscular or Intravenous Use (1% to 5%) ... 1025
- Cefotan (1 in 700) ... 2936
- Ceftin ... 1067
- Cefzil Tablets and Oral Suspension (0.2%) ... 747
- ▲ CellCept Capsules (More than or equal to 3%) ... 2265
- Ceptaz (One in 23) ... 1070
- ▲ Chemet Capsules (4.2% to 10.4%) ... 666
- Chibroxin Sterile Ophthalmic Solution (With oral form) ... 1657
- ▲ Cipro I.V. (Among most frequent) .. 587
- ▲ Cipro I.V. Pharmacy Bulk Package (Among most frequent) ... 590
- Cipro Tablets (0.8%) ... 584
- Claforan Sterile and Injection (Less than 1%) ... 1259
- Colestid (One or more occasions) .. 2073
- Covera-HS Tablets ... 2573
- Cytotec (Infrequent) ... 2576
- Cytovene (1% or less) ... 2270
- Dalgan Injection ... 529
- Dalmane Capsules (Rare) ... 2329
- Depen Titratable Tablets (Few reports) ... 2770
- Dilacor XR Extended-release Capsules (Rare) ... 2183
- ▲ Doxil (1.3% to 7.8%) ... 2613
- Duricef Capsules, Tablets, and Oral Suspension ... 750
- Dynabac (0.1% to 1%) ... 668
- Effexor (Infrequent) ... 2825
- Elspar ... 1700
- Ergamisol Tablets (Less frequent) .. 1340
- Felbatol (Infrequent) ... 2774
- Floxin I.V. (More than or equal to 1%) ... 1580
- Floxin Tablets (200 mg, 300 mg, 400 mg) (More than or equal to 1%) ... 1577
- ▲ Fortaz (1 in 23) ... 1092
- Foscavir Injection (Between 1% and 5%) ... 541
- ▲ Sterile FUDR (Among more common) ... 2284
- Fungizone Intravenous ... 507
- ▲ Gemzar for Injection (55% to 77%) ... 1482
- Glucotrol Tablets (Occasional) ... 2011
- Glucotrol XL Extended Release Tablets (Occasional) ... 2012
- ▲ Hexalen Capsules (9%) ... 2760
- Hivid Tablets (Less than 1%) ... 2287

- Imuran ... 1103
- Inderide Tablets ... 2838
- ▲ Intron A for Injection (Up to 13%) ... 2506
- Isoptin Oral Tablets ... 1393
- Isoptin SR Tablets ... 1395
- Keftab Tablets ... 931
- Kefzol Vials, Faspak & ADD-Vantage (Rare) ... 1511
- Klonopin Tablets ... 2294
- Lamictal Tablets (Infrequent) ... 1105
- Larodopa Tablets ... 2296
- Lescol Capsules ... 2395
- ▲ Leukine (8%) ... 1317
- Lopid Tablets (Occasional) ... 1974
- Lorabid Suspension and Pulvules ... 1513
- Mandol Vials, Faspak & ADD-Vantage ... 1516
- Maxaquin Tablets ... 2593
- Maxipime for Injection (0.1% to 1%) ... 758
- Mefoxin ... 1734
- Mefoxin Premixed Intravenous Solution ... 1737
- ▲ Mepron Suspension (5% to 8%) ... 1206
- Merrem I.V. (Greater than 0.2%) ... 2952
- Mevacor Tablets ... 1742
- Mezlin ... 594
- Mezlin Pharmacy Bulk Package ... 597
- Mithracin ... 599
- Monocid Injection (1.6%) ... 2674
- Monopril Tablets ... 762
- Mycobutin Capsules (Less than 1%) ... 2101
- Nalfon 200 Pulvules & Nalfon Tablets (Less than 1%) ... 933
- Navane Capsules and Concentrate ... 2018
- Navane Intramuscular ... 2019
- ▲ Neupogen for Injection (21% to 58%) ... 495
- ▲ Neutrexin for Injection (4.6%) ... 2761
- Nimotop Capsules (0.2%; rare) ... 603
- ▲ Nolvadex Tablets (3.0%) ... 2957
- Noroxin Tablets (1.1%) ... 1758
- Noroxin Tablets (1.1%) ... 2222
- Norpramin Tablets ... 1273
- Nutropin ... 1049
- Nutropin AQ Injection ... 1051
- Oxandrin ... 783
- ▲ Paraplatin for Injection (24% to 37%) ... 713
- Parlodel ... 2411
- Paxil Tablets (Rare) ... 2681
- Penetrex Tablets (Less than 1%) ... 2196
- Pentasa (Less than 1%) ... 1275
- Pravachol Tablets ... 770
- Prevacid Delayed-Release Capsules (Less than 1%) ... 2746
- Prilosec Delayed-Release Capsules (Rare) ... 516
- Primaxin I.M. ... 1770
- Primaxin I.V. ... 1772
- Procardia Capsules (Rare) ... 2024
- Procardia XL Extended Release Tablets (Rare) ... 2026
- Proglycem ... 575
- ▲ Prograf (Greater than 3%) ... 1028
- ▲ Proleukin for Injection (56%) ... 812
- Rifadin ... 1276
- Rifamate Capsules ... 1278
- Rilutek Tablets (Infrequent) ... 2198
- Rimactane Capsules (Rare) ... 865
- Rocephin Injectable Vials, ADD-Vantage, Galaxy Container (Less than 1%) ... 2305
- ▲ Roferon-A Injection (1% to 11%; up to 50%) ... 2308
- Rythmol Tablets–150mg, 225mg, 300mg (0.2%) ... 1399
- Sectral Capsules ... 2914
- Sinemet Tablets ... 959
- Sinemet CR Tablets ... 961
- Suprax (Less than 2%) ... 1443
- Tambocor Tablets (Rare) ... 1555
- ▲ Taxol Injection (22%) ... 723
- ▲ Tazicef for Injection (1 in 23 patients) ... 2697
- ▲ Tazidime Vials, Faspak & ADD-Vantage (1 in 23) ... 1531
- ▲ Tegison Capsules (10-25%) ... 2314
- Tiazac Capsules (Less than 1%) ... 1019
- Timentin for Injection ... 2706
- Toprol-XL Tablets ... 560
- Unasyn ... 2035
- Vantin for Oral Suspension and Vantin Tablets ... 2112
- Verelan Capsules ... 1455
- Videx Tablets, Powder for Oral Solution, & Pediatric Powder for Oral Solution (1% to 4%) ... 2980
- Vistide Injection ... 1057
- Winstrol Tablets ... 2468

- Xanax Tablets (Less than 1% to 1.7%) ... 2115
- Zerit Capsules (1% to 4%) ... 731
- Zinacef (1 in 50 patients) ... 1184
- Zithromax (Less than 1%) ... 2043
- Zithromax Tablets (Less than 1%) ... 2046
- Zocor Tablets ... 1821
- Zosyn ... 1463

Serum aminotransferase, elevation
- Procanbid Extended-Release Tablets ... 1983

Serum amylase, elevation
- Cipro I.V. (Rare) ... 587
- Cipro I.V. Pharmacy Bulk Package (Rare) ... 590
- Cipro Tablets (Less than 0.1%) ... 584
- Crixivan Capsules (1.0%) ... 1670
- Cuprimine Capsules (Few cases) ... 1673
- Cytotec (Infrequent) ... 2576
- Desyrel and Desyrel Dividose ... 504
- ▲ Epivir (3% to 4.2%) ... 1200
- Foscavir Injection (Less than 1%) ... 541
- Hespan Injection ... 945
- ▲ Hivid Tablets (5.1%) ... 2287
- Invirase Capsules (Less than 1%) ... 2291
- Kadian Capsules ... 2948
- ▲ Mepron Suspension (1% to 8%) ... 1206
- Oncaspar (Less than 1%) ... 2194
- Pentasa (Less than 1%) ... 1275
- Pentaspan Injection ... 954
- Platinol for Injection (Infrequent) ... 717
- Platinol-AQ Injection (Infrequent) ... 719
- ▲ Videx Tablets, Powder for Oral Solution, & Pediatric Powder for Oral Solution (22%) ... 2980
- Zerit Capsules (Up to 14%) ... 731

Serum bicarbonate content, variations
- ▲ Bumex (3.1%) ... 2260
- Dynabac (1.4%) ... 668
- Hivid Tablets (Less than 1%) ... 2287
- ▲ Vistide Injection (9%) ... 1057

Serum bilirubin, elevation
(see under Hyperbilirubinemia)

Serum bilirubin levels, abnormalities
- Atamet Tablets ... 567
- Bumex (0.8%) ... 2260
- Cefzil Tablets and Oral Suspension (Less than 0.1%) ... 747
- Doral Tablets (Less than 1%) ... 2773
- Emcyt Capsules (1% to 2%) ... 2085
- Imuran ... 1103
- Kefurox Vials, Faspak & ADD-Vantage (1 in 500) ... 1509
- Roferon-A Injection (Up to less than 1%) ... 2308
- Sinemet Tablets ... 959
- Sinemet CR Tablets ... 961
- Xanax Tablets (Less than 1% to 1.6%) ... 2115

Serum calcium, depression
(see under Hypocalcemia)

Serum calcium content, variations
- Bumex (2.4%) ... 2260

Serum calcium decrease
(see under Hypocalcemia)

Serum cholesterol, increase
(see under Hypercholesterolemia)

Serum creatine phosphokinase, elevation
- Catapres Tablets (Rare) ... 679
- ▲ Cipro I.V. (Among most frequent) ... 587
- ▲ Cipro I.V. Pharmacy Bulk Package (Among most frequent) ... 590
- Combipres Tablets (Rare) ... 682
- Cytovene (1% or less) ... 2270
- Foscavir Injection (Less than 1%) ... 541
- Haldol Decanoate ... 1587
- Havrix (Less than 1%) ... 2663
- Hivid Tablets (Less than 1%) ... 2287
- ▲ Invirase Capsules (4%) ... 2291
- Norvir (0.9% to 3.4%) ... 447
- Quinidex Extentabs ... 2240
- Risperdal Tablets (Infrequent) ... 1348
- Sular Tablets (Less than or equal to 1%) ... 2961
- Suprane (desflurane, USP) (Less than 1%) ... 1865

- Symmetrel Capsules (Uncommon) ... 965
- Symmetrel Syrup (Uncommon) ... 963
- ▲ Trasylol (5%) ... 607
- Zithromax (1% to 2%) ... 2043
- Zithromax Tablets (1% to 2%) ... 2046
- ▲ Zocor Tablets (About 5% of patients) ... 1821

Serum creatinine, elevation
- ▲ Abelcet Injection (11% to 12%) ... 1540
- Accupril Tablets (2%) ... 1950
- Altace Capsules (1.2% to 1.5%) ... 1238
- Amikacin Sulfate Injection, USP ... 523
- Amikacin Sulfate Injection, USP ... 981
- Amikin Injectable ... 502
- Ancobon Capsules ... 2254
- Asacol Delayed-Release Tablets ... 2129
- Azactam for Injection ... 736
- Bactrim DS Tablets ... 2257
- Bactrim I.V. Infusion ... 2255
- Bactrim ... 2257
- Biaxin (Less than 1%) ... 406
- ▲ Bumex (7.4%) ... 2260
- Capastat Sulfate Injection (A significant number of patients) ... 968
- Capoten Tablets ... 740
- Capozide Tablets ... 744
- Casodex Tablets (2% to 5%) ... 2934
- Caverject Injection (Less than 1%) ... 2064
- Ceclor Pulvules & Suspension (Less than 1 in 500) ... 1470
- Cedax (0.1% to 1%) ... 2480
- Cefizox for Intramuscular or Intravenous Use (Occasional) ... 1025
- Cefobid Intravenous/Intramuscular (1 in 48) ... 1996
- Cefobid Pharmacy Bulk Package - Not for Direct Infusion (1 in 48) .. 1999
- Cefotan ... 2936
- Ceftin ... 1067
- Cefzil Tablets and Oral Suspension (0.1%) ... 747
- ▲ CellCept Capsules (More than or equal to 3%) ... 2265
- Ceptaz (Occasional) ... 1070
- Chibroxin Sterile Ophthalmic Solution (With oral form) ... 1657
- ▲ Cipro I.V. (Among most frequent) .. 587
- ▲ Cipro I.V. Pharmacy Bulk Package (Among most frequent) ... 590
- Cipro Tablets (1.1%) ... 584
- Claforan Sterile and Injection (Occasional) ... 1259
- Cozaar Tablets (Less than 0.1%) ... 1668
- Cytovene (1% or less) ... 2270
- Daypro Caplets (Occasional) ... 2578
- Didronel I.V. Infusion (Occasional) .. 1545
- Didronel Tablets ... 2133
- Diprivan Injectable Emulsion (Less than 1%) ... 2939
- Doxil (Less than 1%) ... 2613
- Duricef Capsules, Tablets, and Oral Suspension ... 750
- Dyazide Capsules ... 2653
- Dynabac (0.1% to 1%) ... 668
- Dyrenium Capsules (Rare) ... 2655
- Effexor (Infrequent) ... 2825
- Ergamisol Tablets (Less frequent) .. 1340
- Eulexin Capsules ... 2498
- Feldene Capsules (Greater than 1%) ... 2008
- Floxin I.V. (More than or equal to 1%) ... 1580
- Floxin Tablets (200 mg, 300 mg, 400 mg) (More than or equal to 1%) ... 1577
- Fortaz (Occasional) ... 1092
- ▲ Foscavir Injection (5% or greater up to 27%) ... 541
- Fungizone Intravenous ... 507
- ▲ Ganite (About 12.5%) ... 2711
- Gantanol Tablets ... 2285
- Gantrisin ... 2286
- Garamycin Injectable ... 2502
- ▲ Gemzar for Injection (Up to 8%) ... 1482
- Glucotrol Tablets (Occasional) ... 2011
- Glucotrol XL Extended Release Tablets ... 2012
- ▲ Hexalen Capsules (7%) ... 2760
- Hivid Tablets (Less than 1%) ... 2287
- Hydrea Capsules (Occasional) ... 705
- Hyzaar Tablets (0.8%) ... 1720
- IFEX ... 706
- Indocin I.V. ... 1727
- Intron A for Injection (Up to 3%) ... 2506
- Keftab Tablets ... 931
- Kefurox Vials, Faspak & ADD-Vantage ... 1509
- Lamictal Tablets (Rare) ... 1105
- ▲ Leukine (15%) ... 1317

(ⓝ Described in PDR For Nonprescription Drugs)   Incidence data in parenthesis; ▲ 3% or more   (ⓞ Described in PDR For Ophthalmology)

1449 Side Effects Index Sexual dysfunction

Lodine Capsules and Tablets (Less than 1%) 2849
Lorabid Suspension and Pulvules 1513
Lotensin Tablets (About 2%) 852
Lotensin HCT Tablets 855
Lotrel Capsules 858
Lupron Injection (Less than 5%) 2736
Macrobid Capsules 2138
Macrodantin Capsules 2140
Mandol Vials, Faspak & ADD-Vantage 1516
Mavik Tablets (Rare) 1407
Maxipime for Injection (0.1% to 1%) 758
Mefoxin 1734
Mefoxin Premixed Intravenous Solution 1737
Mepron Suspension (1%) 1206
Merrem I.V. (Greater than 0.2%) 2952
Mezlin 594
Mezlin Pharmacy Bulk Package 597
Mithracin 599
Monocid Injection (Occasional) 2674
Monopril Tablets 762
Motrin Ibuprofen Suspension, Oral Drops, Chewable Tablets, Caplets 1563
Mutamycin for Injection (2%) 712
Mykrox Tablets 1617
Naprelan Tablets (Less than 1%) 2861
Nebcin Vials, Hyporets & ADD-Vantage 1518
Neoral 2405
Neutrexin for Injection (0.9%) 2761
▲ Nipent for Injection (3% to 10%) 2733
Nolvadex Tablets (1.7%) 2957
▲ Normodyne Injection (8%) 2519
Noroxin Tablets (Less frequent) 1758
Noroxin Tablets (Less frequent) 2222
Norpace (Less than 1%) 2596
Oncaspar 2194
Oxandrin 783
▲ Paraplatin for Injection (5% to 10%) 713
Pediazole Suspension 2340
Phenurone Tablets (1% or less) 455
Pipracil 1435
Platinol for Injection 717
Platinol-AQ Injection 719
Prevacid Delayed-Release Capsules (Less than 1%) 2746
Prilosec Delayed-Release Capsules (Less than 1%) 516
Primaxin I.M. 1770
Primaxin I.V. 1772
▲ Prinivil Tablets (About 2.0% to approximately 11.6%) 1776
Prinzide Tablets 1780
Procardia Capsules (Rare) 2024
Procardia XL Extended Release Tablets (Rare) 2026
▲ Prograf (19% to 39%) 1028
▲ Proleukin for Injection (61%) 812
Proloprim Tablets 1141
▲ Rocaltrol Capsules (1 in 6) 2303
Rocephin Injectable Vials, ADD-Vantage, Galaxy Container (Less than 1%) 2305
Roferon-A Injection (Up to less than 1%) 2308
Sandimmune 2416
Septra 1146
Septra I.V. Infusion 1142
Septra I.V. Infusion ADD-Vantage Vials 1144
Septra 1146
Sinemet CR Tablets 961
Sular Tablets (Less than or equal to 1%) 2961
Suprax (Less than 2%) 1443
Tagamet 2694
Tazicef for Injection (Occasional) 2697
Tazidime Vials, Faspak & ADD-Vantage (Occasional) 1531
▲ Tegison Capsules (1-10%) 2314
Timentin for Injection 2706
Toradol 2319
▲ Trandate Injection (8 of 100 patients) 1158
▲ Trasylol (18% to 21%) 607
Trilisate (Less than 1%) 2155
Trimpex Tablets 2323
Ultram Tablets (50 mg) (Infrequent) 1594
Unasyn 2035
Univasc Tablets (1% to 2%) 2553
Vancocin HCl, Oral Solution & Pulvules (Rare) 1536
Vancocin HCl, Vials & ADD-Vantage (Rare) 1534
Vantin for Oral Suspension and Vantin Tablets 2112
▲ Vaseretic Tablets (About 0.6% to 20%) 1810
▲ Vasotec I.V. (0.2% to 20%) 1814
▲ Vasotec Tablets (About 0.2% to 20%) 1816
▲ Vistide Injection (18% to 53%) 1057
Xanax Tablets (1.9% to 2.2%) 2115
Zantac (Rare) 1182
Zantac Injection 1180
Zantac Syrup (Rare) 1182
Zaroxolyn Tablets 1625
Zebeta Tablets 1457
Zestoretic Tablets 2968
Zestril Tablets (About 2.0%) 2972
Zinacef 1184
Zithromax (Less than 1%) 2043
Zithromax Tablets (Less than 1%) 2046
Zosyn 1463
Zovirax Capsules 1187
▲ Zovirax Sterile Powder (5% to 10%) 1191
Zovirax 1187

Serum electrolyte changes (see under Electrolyte imbalance)

Serum fibrogen, decrease

Trental Tablets (Rare) 1291

Serum lipase, elevation

Hivid Tablets (Less than 1%) 2287
Oncaspar 2194
Pentasa (Less than 1%) 1275
Redux Capsules 2911

Serum PBI levels, decrease (see under PBI decrease)

Serum phosphorus, elevation

Macrodantin Capsules 2140
Nutropin 1049
Nutropin AQ Injection 1051
Zebeta Tablets 1457

Serum phosphorus content, variations

▲ Bumex (4.5%) 2260
Dynabac (0.1% to 1%) 668
Macrobid Capsules (1% to 5%) 2138
Maxipime for Injection (Up to 2.8%) 758

Serum potassium, reduction (see under Hypokalemia)

Serum proteins, changes

Brevicon 2563
Bumex (0.7%) 2260
Doral Tablets (Less than 1%) 2773
Dynabac (0.1% to 1%) 668
Norinyl 2563
Tri-Norinyl 2607

Serum sickness

Amoxil 2631
Antivenin (Black Widow Spider) 1647
Antivenin (Crotalidae) Polyvalent 2803
Augmentin 2637
Augmentin Tablets 2640
Axid Pulvules (Rare) 1468
Azulfidine (Rare) 2059
Bactrim DS Tablets 2257
Bactrim I.V. Infusion 2255
Bactrim 2257
Bicillin C-R Injection 2810
Bicillin C-R 900/300 Injection 2812
Bicillin L-A Injection 2813
Ceclor Pulvules & Suspension (0.05% to 0.024%) 1470
Cefizox for Intramuscular or Intravenous Use 1025
Ceftin 1067
Cefzil Tablets and Oral Suspension (Rare) 747
Daypro Caplets (Less than 1%) 2578
Duricef Capsules, Tablets, and Oral Suspension (Rare) 750
Fansidar Tablets 2281
Feldene Capsules (Less than 1%) 2008
Flagyl 375 Capsules 2587
Flagyl I.V. 2373
Floxin I.V. 1580
Floxin Tablets (200 mg, 300 mg, 400 mg) 1577
Gantanol Tablets 2285
Gantrisin 2286
Helidac Therapy 2135
IBU Tablets (Less than 1%) 1389
Intal Inhaler (Rare) 2185
Intal Nebulizer Solution 2186
Lorabid Suspension and Pulvules (Rare) 1513
Motrin Ibuprofen Suspension, Oral Drops, Chewable Tablets, Caplets (Less than 1%) 1563
Nasalcrom Nasal Solution (Rare) 2192
Omnipen Capsules 2872
Omnipen for Oral Suspension 2873
Orthoclone OKT3 Sterile Solution 1892
Pediazole Suspension 2340
Pen•Vee K 2879
Pfizerpen for Injection 2022
Pneumovax 23 (Rare) 1768
Protostat Tablets 1939
Prozac Pulvules & Liquid, Oral Solution (Rare) 935
Quadrinal Tablets 1398
Rabies Vaccine Adsorbed (Less than 1%) 2686
Recombivax HB (Less than 1%) 1787
Rocephin Injectable Vials, ADD-Vantage, Galaxy Container (Rare) 2305
Septra 1146
Septra I.V. Infusion 1142
Septra I.V. Infusion ADD-Vantage Vials 1144
Septra 1146
Suprax (Less than 2%) 1443
Ticlid Tablets (Rare) 2317
Tolectin (200, 400 and 600 mg) (Less than 1%) 1591
Vantin for Oral Suspension and Vantin Tablets 2112
Vibramycin 2038

Serum transaminase, elevation

Amaryl Tablets (Isolated cases) 1241
Atromid-S Capsules 2808
Augmentin (Infrequent) 2637
Augmentin Tablets (Infrequent) 2640
Azathioprine Tablets (Less than 1%) 2349
Bactrim DS Tablets 2257
Bactrim I.V. Infusion 2255
Bactrim 2257
BiCNU 696
Calan SR Caplets 2571
Calan Tablets 2568
Capoten Tablets 740
Capozide Tablets 744
CeeNU Capsules (Small percentage) 699
▲ Chemet Capsules (6% to 10% of patients) 666
Clomid 1262
▲ Cognex Capsules (29%) 1961
Cordarone Tablets 2818
Covera-HS Tablets 2573
Danocrine Capsules 2437
Depakene (Frequent) 416
Depakote Tablets (Frequent) 418
DiaBeta Tablets (Isolated cases) 1265
Diflucan Tablets, Injection, and Oral Suspension (Rare) 2003
Dilacor XR Extended-release Capsules 2183
Duratuss HD Elixir (A single elevation) 2750
Duricef Capsules, Tablets, and Oral Suspension 750
▲ Eminase (Less than 10%) 2215
Ethmozine Tablets (Rare) 2217
Eulexin Capsules 2498
▲ Sterile FUDR (Among more common) 2284
Garamycin Injectable 2502
▲ Gemzar for Injection (Approximately two-thirds) 1482
Glynase PresTab Tablets (Isolated reports) 2091
Imuran 1103
Inderide Tablets 2838
Inderide LA Long Acting Capsules 2840
Intron A for Injection (Less than 5%) 2506
Invirase Capsules (Isolated cases) 2291
Isoptin Oral Tablets (Less than 1%) 1393
Isoptin SR Tablets 1395
Klonopin Tablets 2294
▲ Lariam Tablets (Among most frequent) 2295
Lescol Capsules 2395
Leustatin 1889
Lopid Tablets 1974
Lotensin Tablets 852
LUVOX Tablets (Frequent) 2723
Marinol (Dronabinol) Capsules (Less than 1%) 2353
Mavik Tablets (0.8% of patients) 1407
Methotrexate Sodium Tablets, Injection, for Injection and LPF Injection 1322
Mevacor Tablets (1.9%) 1742
Micronase Tablets 2099
Mithracin 599
Monopril Tablets 762
Nardil (Common) 1977
Navane Capsules and Concentrate (Infrequent) 2018
Navane Intramuscular (Infrequent) 2019
Nebcin Vials, Hyporets & ADD-Vantage 1518
Netromycin Injection 100 mg/ml (15 of 1000 patients) 2516
▲ Normodyne Injection (4%) 2519
▲ Normodyne Tablets (4%) 2522
▲ Nydrazid Injection (10% to 20%) 509
Paxil Tablets 2681
Plendil Extended-Release Tablets (Two episodes) 514
Pravachol Tablets 770
▲ Proleukin for Injection (56%) 812
Proloprim Tablets 1141
Rifadin 1276
▲ Rifamate Capsules (10% to 20%) 1278
▲ Rifater (10% to 20% of patients) 1280
Rimactane Capsules (Rare) 865
Ritalin (Some instances) 866
▲ Roferon-A Injection (Up to 50%) 2308
Rythmol Tablets–150mg, 225mg, 300mg (0.2%) 1399
Seldane Tablets (One case) 1284
Seldane-D Extended-Release Tablets (One case) 1286
Septra 1146
Septra I.V. Infusion 1142
Septra I.V. Infusion ADD-Vantage Vials 1144
Septra 1146
Seromycin Capsules 975
Streptase for Infusion 557
Tagamet 2694
Tambocor Tablets (Rare) 1555
Tapazole Tablets 1361
Toprol-XL Tablets 560
▲ Trandate (4% of patients) 1158
▲ Trasylol (5%) 607
Trilisate (Rare) 2155
Trimpex Tablets 2323
Tussend Expectorant 1831
Vascor Tablets (200 and 300 mg) (Approximately 1%) 1597
Verelan Capsules 1455
Yutopar Intravenous Injection (Less than 1%) 566
Zocor Tablets (1%) 1821
Zofran Tablets 1231
Zovirax Sterile Powder (1% to 2%) 1191
Zyrtec Tablets (Occasional) 2053

Serum triglyceride, elevation (see under Hypertriglyceridemia)

Serum vitamin B_{12} levels, subnormal

Glucophage Tablets 754

Sexual activity, decrease

Catapres Tablets (About 3 in 100 patients) 679
Catapres-TTS 680
Combipres Tablets (About 3%) 682
Orlaam Oral Solution (1% to 3%) 2361
Propulsid (Less than 1%) 1346
ReVia Tablets (Less than 1%) 957
Risperdal Tablets (Frequent) 1348

Sexual activity, increase

Fioricet with Codeine Capsules 2387
Fiorinal with Codeine Capsules 2390
Halotestin Tablets 2095
ReVia Tablets (Less than 1%) 957

Sexual dysfunction

Adalat Capsules (10 mg and 20 mg) (2% or less) 580
▲ Anafranil Capsules (20% to 42%) 819
Betapace Tablets (Less than 1% to 2%) 637
Carbocaine Injection 2432
Cardizem CD Capsules (Less than 1%) 1251
Cardizem SR Capsules (Less than 1%) 1255
Cardizem Injectable 1253
Cardizem Tablets (Less than 1%) 1257

Sexual dysfunction

Cardura Tablets (2%) ... 1993
Catapres-TTS (2 of 101 patients) .. 680
Duranest Injections ... 533
Effexor (2%) ... 2825
Eldepryl Capsules ... 2729
Eskalith ... 2658
Hivid Tablets (Less than 1%) ... 2287
Levatol Tablets (0.5%) ... 2547
Lithonate/Lithotabs/Lithobid ... 2721
Marcaine ... 2446
Marcaine Spinal ... 2449
Monopril Tablets (Less than 1.0% to 1.0%) ... 762
Nardil (Common) ... 1977
Nescaine/Nescaine MPF ... 549
Norvasc Tablets (Less than 1% to 2%) ... 2020
▲ Paxil Tablets (3.7% to 10.0%) ... 2681
Procardia Capsules (2% or less) ... 2024
Prozac Pulvules & Liquid, Oral Solution (1.9%) ... 935
Risperdal Tablets (Frequent) ... 1348
Sensorcaine ... 554
Tiazac Capsules (Less than 1%) ... 1019
Wellbutrin Tablets (Frequent) ... 1177
▲ Xanax Tablets (7.4%) ... 2115
Xylocaine Injections ... 562
Ziac ... 1459
▲ Zoladex (21%) ... 2976
▲ Zoladex 3-month (One of the two most common) ... 2978
▲ Zoloft Tablets (1.7%; 15.5%) ... 2051

Sexual maturity, accelerated

Lupron Depot-PED 7.5 mg, 11.25 mg and 15 mg (Less than 2%) ... 2744
Lupron Injection Pediatric (Less than 2%) ... 2737

Shivering
(see under Trembling)

Shock

Abelcet Injection ... 1540
Acel-Imune Diphtheria and Tetanus Toxoids and Acellular Pertussis Vaccine Adsorbed (Rare) ... 1415
AK-FLUOR Injection 10% and 25% ... ⊚ 204
Antivenin (Crotalidae) Polyvalent ... 2803
AquaMEPHYTON Injection ... 1648
Aralen Hydrochloride Injection ... 2430
Betaseron for SC Injection ... 653
Cerebyx Injection (Infrequent) ... 1956
Cordarone Intravenous (Less than 2%) ... 2821
Coumadin ... 941
Demerol ... 2438
Demulen ... 2580
Desferal Vials ... 838
Dilaudid-HP Injection ... 1384
Dilaudid-HP Lyophilized Powder 250 mg ... 1384
Dilaudid Tablets and Liquid ... 1386
Diphtheria and Tetanus Toxoids and Pertussis Vaccine Adsorbed (Rare) ... 2650
▲ Eminase (Less than 10%) ... 2215
EMLA Cream ... 536
Etrafon (Occasional) ... 2495
Floxin I.V. ... 1580
Floxin Tablets (200 mg, 300 mg, 400 mg) ... 1577
Fluorescite ... ⊚ 217
Fungizone Intravenous ... 507
Heparin Lock Flush Solution (Rare) ... 2831
Heparin Sodium Injection (Rare) ... 2832
Heparin Sodium Vials (Rare) ... 1486
Humorsol Sterile Ophthalmic Solution (Infrequent) ... 1707
Hyperstat I.V. Injection ... 2504
Imitrex Tablets ... 1099
Indocin Capsules (Less than 1%) ... 1723
Indocin I.V. (Less than 1%) ... 1727
Indocin (Less than 1%) ... 1723
INFeD (Iron Dextran Injection, USP) ... 2478
Kadian Capsules ... 2948
Levo-Dromoran ... 2297
MS Contin Tablets ... 2149
MSIR ... 2152
Mepergan Injection ... 2859
Merrem I.V. (0.1% to 1.0%) ... 2952
Methadone Hydrochloride Oral Solution & Tablets ... 2357
Midamor Tablets ... 1746
Monopril Tablets (0.2%) ... 762
Nitro-Bid IV ... 1270
Nubain Injection (1% or less) ... 952

Oramorph SR (Morphine Sulfate Sustained Release Tablets) (Less frequent) ... 2359
Orthoclone OKT3 Sterile Solution ... 1892
Orudis Capsules (Rare) ... 2874
Oruvail Capsules (Rare) ... 2874
OxyContin Tablets ... 2163
Permax Tablets (Infrequent) ... 571
RMS Suppositories CII ... 2766
Redux Capsules ... 2911
Rifadin (Rare) ... 1276
Rifamate Capsules (Rare) ... 1278
Rifater ... 1280
Rilutek Tablets (Infrequent) ... 2198
Roxanol ... 2365
Salagen Tablets (Rare) ... 1546
Sandoglobulin I.V. (Rare) ... 2419
Sus-Phrine Injection ... 1017
Talwin Injection (Infrequent) ... 2465
Thorazine ... 2701
Trasylol (1.7%) ... 607
Tri-Immunol Adsorbed (1 per 1,750) ... 1452
Trilafon ... 2532
Videx Tablets, Powder for Oral Solution, & Pediatric Powder for Oral Solution (Less than 1%) ... 2980
Zofran Injection (Rare) ... 1227

Shock, anaphylactic
(see under Anaphylactic shock)

Shock, hypovolemic

Diethylstilbestrol Tablets ... 1477
PMB 200 and PMB 400 ... 2890
Prevacid Delayed-Release Capsules (Less than 1%) ... 2746

Sialadenitis

Aldoclor Tablets ... 1638
Aldomet Ester HCl Injection ... 1642
Aldomet Oral ... 1640
Aldoril Tablets ... 1644
Apresazide Capsules ... 824
Capozide Tablets ... 744
Diucardin Tablets ... 2824
Diupres Tablets ... 1691
Diuril Oral Suspension ... 1694
Diuril Sodium Intravenous ... 1693
Diuril Tablets ... 1694
Dyazide Capsules ... 2653
Enduron Tablets ... 424
Esidrix Tablets ... 839
Esimil Tablets ... 840
HydroDIURIL Tablets ... 1716
Hydropres Tablets ... 1718
Hyzaar Tablets ... 1720
Inderide Tablets ... 2838
Inderide LA Long Acting Capsules ... 2840
Lopressor HCT Tablets ... 850
Lotensin HCT Tablets ... 855
Macrobid Capsules ... 2138
Macrodantin Capsules ... 2140
Moduretic Tablets ... 1748
Mykrox Tablets (Rare) ... 1617
Permax Tablets (Rare) ... 571
Prinzide Tablets ... 1780
Redux Capsules (Rare) ... 2911
Ser-Ap-Es Tablets ... 867
Timolide Tablets ... 1791
Vaseretic Tablets ... 1810
Videx Tablets, Powder for Oral Solution, & Pediatric Powder for Oral Solution (Up to 2%) ... 2980
Zaroxolyn Tablets ... 1625
Zestoretic Tablets ... 2968
Ziac ... 1459

Sialadenopathy

Tapazole Tablets ... 1361

Sialism
(see under Salivation)

Sialorrhea

Albuminar-5, Albumin (Human) U.S.P. 5% (Occasional) ... 795
Albuminar-25, Albumin (Human) U.S.P. 25% ... 796
Atamet Tablets ... 567
Diprivan Injectable Emulsion (Less than 1%) ... 2939
Haldol Decanoate ... 1587
Larodopa Tablets (Relatively frequent) ... 2296
Mestinon Injectable ... 1300
Prostigmin Injectable ... 1305
Prostigmin Tablets ... 1306
Sinemet Tablets ... 959
Sinemet CR Tablets ... 961
Tensilon Injectable ... 1307

Torecan (Occasional) ... 2367
Versed Injection ... 2324

Sialosis
(see under Salivation)

Sickle cell disease

Levlen/Tri-Levlen ... 646

Sinoatrial block

Blocadren Tablets (Less than 1%) ... 1654
Flumadine Tablets & Syrup (Less than 0.3%) ... 1013
Neurontin Capsules (Rare) ... 1978
Timoptic in Ocudose (Less frequent) ... 1796
Timoptic-XE ... 1798

Sinoatrial node dysfunction

Cardene I.V. ... 2815
Cordarone Tablets ... 2818
Eskalith ... 2658
Lithonate/Lithotabs/Lithobid ... 2721

Sinus arrest

Catapres Tablets (Rare) ... 679
Cordarone Tablets ... 2818
Nipent for Injection (Less than 3%) ... 2733
Rythmol Tablets—150mg, 225mg, 300mg (Less than 1%) ... 1399
Tambocor Tablets (1% to less than 3%) ... 1555
Tonocard Tablets (Less than 1%) ... 519

Sinus bradycardia

Activase ... 1045
Adenocard Injection ... 1021
Adenoscan ... 1022
Brethaire Inhaler ... 830
▲ Cardizem SR Capsules (3%) ... 1255
Catapres Tablets (Rare) ... 679
Catapres-TTS ... 680
Cerebyx Injection (Infrequent) ... 1956
Combipres Tablets (Rare) ... 682
Cordarone Intravenous (Less than 2%) ... 2821
Cordarone Tablets (2 to 5%) ... 2818
Corvert Injection (1.2%) ... 2075
Cozaar Tablets (Less than 1%) ... 1668
Desyrel and Desyrel Dividose (Occasional) ... 504
Dilacor XR Extended-release Capsules ... 2183
Effexor (Rare) ... 2825
Eldepryl Capsules ... 2729
Eminase ... 2215
Hyzaar Tablets ... 1720
IBU Tablets (Less than 1%) ... 1389
Kytril Injection (Rare) ... 2667
Lanoxicaps ... 1110
Lanoxin Elixir Pediatric ... 1113
Lanoxin Injection ... 1116
Lanoxin Injection Pediatric ... 1119
Lanoxin Tablets ... 1121
Motrin Ibuprofen Suspension, Oral Drops, Chewable Tablets, Caplets (Less than 1%) ... 1563
▲ Sandostatin Injection (25%) ... 2421
Serzone Tablets (1.5%) ... 776
▲ Taxol Injection (23%) ... 723
Vascor Tablets (200 and 300 mg) (0.5 to 2.0%) ... 1597

Sinus congestion

▲ AeroBid Inhaler System (3% to 9%) ... 1004
▲ Aerobid-M Inhaler System (3% to 9%) ... 1004
▲ Desyrel and Desyrel Dividose (2.8% to 5.7%) ... 504
Hivid Tablets (Less than 1%) ... 2287
▲ Lupron Injection (5% or more) ... 2736
Mykrox Tablets (Less than 2%) ... 1617
Nasacort Nasal Inhaler (Fewer than 5%) ... 2189
▲ Stadol (3% to 9%) ... 779

Sinus discomfort

AeroBid Inhaler System (1% to 3%) ... 1004
Aerobid-M Inhaler System (1% to 3%) ... 1004
Cozaar Tablets (1.5%) ... 1668
Hivid Tablets (Less than 1%) ... 2287
Imitrex Injection (2.2%) ... 1095
Nicotrol NS Nicotine Nasal Spray (More common) ... 1565
ReVia Tablets (Less than 1%) ... 957

Sinus drainage

▲ AeroBid Inhaler System (3% to 9%) ... 1004
▲ Aerobid-M Inhaler System (3% to 9%) ... 1004
Alferon N Injection (2%) ... 2142

Sinusitis

▲ Actigall Capsules (11.0%) ... 818
▲ AeroBid Inhaler System (3% to 9%) ... 1004
▲ Aerobid-M Inhaler System (3% to 9%) ... 1004
▲ Ambien Tablets (4%) ... 2559
▲ Anafranil Capsules (2% to 6%) ... 819
▲ Arimidex Tablets (2% to 5%) ... 2932
Asacol Delayed-Release Tablets (2.3%) ... 2129
Atrovent Inhalation Solution (2.3%) ... 675
▲ Avonex (18%) ... 662
Axid Pulvules (2.4%) ... 1468
▲ Betaseron for SC Injection (36%) ... 653
Betimol 0.25%, 0.5% (1% to 5%) ... ⊚ 259
Cardene Capsules (Rare) ... 2261
Cardene SR Capsules (Rare) ... 2264
Cardura Tablets (Less than 0.5% of 3960 patients) ... 1993
Cartrol Tablets (Less common) ... 413
Caverject Injection (2%) ... 2064
Ceftin for Oral Suspension (0.1% to 1%) ... 1067
▲ CellCept Capsules (More than or equal to 3%) ... 2265
Cerebyx Injection (Infrequent) ... 1956
Claritin Tablets (2% or fewer patients) ... 2485
Claritin-D Tablets (Less frequent) ... 2487
Cognex Capsules (Frequent) ... 1961
Cozaar Tablets (1.0%) ... 1668
Crixivan Capsules (Less than 2%) ... 1670
▲ DaunoXome (Up to 8%) ... 1842
Daypro Caplets (Less than 1%) ... 2578
Depakote Tablets (1% to 5%) ... 418
Dilacor XR Extended-release Capsules (2.0%) ... 2183
Doxil (Less than 1%) ... 2613
▲ Estring Vaginal Ring (4%) ... 2086
Ethmozine Tablets (Less than 2%) ... 2217
Famvir Tablets (1.3% to 2.6%) ... 2660
▲ Felbatol (3.5%) ... 2774
Flonase Nasal Spray (Less than 1%) ... 1088
▲ Flovent (3% to 22%) ... 1089
Fludara for Injection (Up to 5%) ... 658
Foscavir Injection (Between 1% and 5%) ... 541
▲ Habitrol Nicotine Transdermal System (3% to 9% of patients) ... 884
Hivid Tablets (Less than 1%) ... 2287
Hytrin Capsules (2.6%) ... 434
Hyzaar Tablets (1.2%) ... 1720
Imdur (Less than or equal to 5%) ... 1362
▲ Intron A for Injection (Up to 21%) ... 2506
Invirase Capsules (Less than 2%) ... 2291
Kerlone Tablets (Less than 2%) ... 2588
Lescol Capsules (2.6%) ... 2395
Lodine Capsules and Tablets (Less than 1%) ... 2849
Lotensin Tablets ... 852
Lotensin HCT Tablets (More than 1%) ... 855
LUVOX Tablets (Frequent) ... 2723
Marinol (Dronabinol) Capsules (Less than 1%) ... 2353
▲ Mepron Suspension (7%) ... 1206
Miacalcin Nasal Spray (1% to 3%) ... 2403
Monoket Tablets (Fewer than 1%) ... 2550
Monopril Tablets (0.2% to 1.0%) ... 762
▲ Naprelan Tablets (3% to 9%) ... 2861
Nasarel Nasal Solution (1% or less) ... 2302
▲ Neoral (3% to 7%) ... 2405
▲ Nipent for Injection (6%) ... 2733
Ocupress Ophthalmic Solution, 1% Sterile (Occasional) ... ⊚ 297
Paxil Tablets (Infrequent) ... 2681
Permax Tablets (Infrequent) ... 571
Plendil Extended-Release Tablets (0.5% to 1.5%) ... 514
Prinivil Tablets (0.3% to 1.0%) ... 1776
Prinzide Tablets (0.3 to 1%) ... 1780
Procardia XL Extended Release Tablets (1% or less) ... 2026
▲ Prograf (Greater than 3%) ... 1028
▲ Propulsid (3.6%) ... 1346
ProSom Tablets (Infrequent) ... 457
▲ Prostep (nicotine transdermal system) (3% to 9% of patients) ... 1439
Prozac Pulvules & Liquid, Oral Solution (2.1% to 5%) ... 935

(☒ Described in PDR For Nonprescription Drugs)   Incidence data in parenthesis; ▲ 3% or more   (⊚ Described in PDR For Ophthalmology)

Side Effects Index — Skin, eruptions

Pulmozyme Inhalation ... 1054
Redux Capsules (Frequent) ... 2911
Remeron Tablets (Frequent) ... 1878
Retrovir Capsules ... 1216
Retrovir I.V. Infusion ... 1221
Retrovir Syrup ... 1216
Rilutek Tablets (0.4% to 1.6%) ... 2198
Risperdal Tablets (1% to 2%) ... 1348
▲ Roferon-A Injection (Less than 3% to 11%) ... 2308
Salagen Tablets (1%) ... 1546
▲ Sandimmune (Less than 1 to 7%) .. 2416
Serzone Tablets ... 776
Stadol (1% or greater) ... 779
▲ Sular Tablets (3%) ... 2961
Supprelin Injection (2% to 3%) ... 2230
Univasc Tablets (More than 1%) ... 2553
▲ Videx Tablets, Powder for Oral Solution, & Pediatric Powder for Oral Solution (7%) ... 2980
Vistide Injection ... 1057
Zebeta Tablets (2.2%) ... 1457
Zestoretic Tablets (0.3 to 1%) ... 2968
Zestril Tablets (0.3% to 1.0%) ... 2972
Ziac ... 1459
Zoladex (1% or greater) ... 2976
Zoladex 3-month ... 2978
Zoloft Tablets (Rare) ... 2051
Zyrtec Tablets (Less than 2%) ... 2053

Sinus syndrome, sick

Cardizem Injectable (Less than 1%) ... 1253
Rythmol Tablets—150mg, 225mg, 300mg (Less than 1%) ... 1399

Sinus tachycardia

Adenocard Injection ... 1021
Aramine Injection ... 1649
Corvert Injection (2.7%) ... 2075
Etrafon ... 2495
Foscavir Injection (Between 1% and 5%) ... 541
IBU Tablets (Less than 1%) ... 1389
Motrin Ibuprofen Suspension, Oral Drops, Chewable Tablets, Caplets (Less than 1%) ... 1563
▲ Proleukin for Injection (70%) ... 812
Propulsid (Rare cases) ... 1346
Seldane Tablets ... 1284
Seldane-D Extended-Release Tablets ... 1286
▲ Taxol Injection (23%) ... 723
Taxotere for Injection Concentrate (Rare) ... 2204
Vascor Tablets (200 and 300 mg) (0.5 to 2.0%) ... 1597

Skin, anesthesia
(see under Numbness, skin)

Skin, bleeding

Sulfamylon Cream (Rare) ... 940

Skin, burning

▲ Cleocin T Topical (10%) ... 2072
Cleocin Vaginal Cream ... 2070
▲ Differin Gel (10% to 40%) ... 1033
Diprolene AF Cream 0.05% (Infrequent) ... 2489
Diprolene Lotion 0.05% (1%) ... 2491
Diprolene Ointment 0.05% (Infrequent) ... 2491
▲ Dovonex Ointment 0.005% (Approximately 10% to 15%) ... 2793
Drysol Solution ... 1989
▲ Emgel 2% Topical Gel (Most common) ... 1081
Epifoam (Infrequent) ... 2543
▲ Exelderm Cream 1.0% (3%) ... 2794
Exelderm Solution 1.0% (Approximately 1%) ... 2795
Gastrocrom Capsules (Infrequent) .. 1611
Gastrocrom Oral Concentrate (Less common) ... 1611
Halog (Infrequent) ... 2795
Maxaquin Tablets ... 2593
MetroCream (Less than 3%) ... 1034
MetroGel ... 1034
8-MOP Capsules ... 1294
Monistat Dual-Pak ... 1906
Nubain Injection (1% or less) ... 952
Oxsoralen Lotion 1% ... 1301
Oxsoralen-Ultra Capsules ... 1302
ProctoFoam-HC ... 2552
Trisoralen Tablets ... 1309
▲ Ultravate Cream 0.05% (4.4%) ... 2797
Ultravate Ointment 0.05% (1.6%) 2798

Skin, cracking

Aquasol A Vitamin A Capsules, USP ... 525
Aquasol A Parenteral ... 526
Cormax Ointment (Approximately 0.3%) ... 1856
Diprolene Gel 0.05% (Less frequent) ... 2490
Hivid Tablets (Less than 1%) ... 2287
Temovate Cream (Less frequent) ... 1152
Temovate E Emollient (Less than 2%) ... 1154
▲ Temovate Gel (Among most frequent) ... 1153
Temovate Ointment (Less frequent) ... 1152
Zonalon Cream (Less than 1%) ... 1042

Skin, discoloration

AK-FLUOR Injection 10% and 25% ... ⊚ 204
Anafranil Capsules (Infrequent) ... 819
Android Capsules, 10 mg ... 1297
Atretol Tablets ... 569
Avonex ... 662
Azulfidine (Rare) ... 2059
Benzamycin Topical Gel ... 919
Brevibloc (esmolol HCl) Injection (Less than 1%) ... 1860
Cerebyx Injection (Infrequent) ... 1956
Compazine ... 2644
Cordarone Tablets (Less than 1%) ... 2818
Cytovene (1% or less) ... 2270
Doxil (Less than 1%) ... 2613
Ergamisol Tablets (Up to 2%) ... 1340
Estrace Cream and Tablets ... 751
Estratest ... 2718
Fluorescite ... ⊚ 217
Foscavir Injection (Between 1% and 5%) ... 541
Halotestin Tablets ... 2095
INFeD (Iron Dextran Injection, USP) ... 2478
Intron A for Injection (Less than 5%) ... 2506
Invirase Capsules (Less than 2%) .. 2291
Lamictal Tablets (Rare) ... 1105
Lamprene Capsules (More than 1%) ... 846
Lescol Capsules ... 2395
Lumitene ... ▣ 799
LUVOX Tablets (Infrequent) ... 2723
Mevacor Tablets ... 1742
Minocin Oral Suspension ... 1431
Mycobutin Capsules (Less than 1%) ... 2101
Neurontin Capsules (Rare) ... 1978
Norvasc Tablets (Less than or equal to 0.1%) ... 2020
Ortho-Est ... 1925
Orudis Capsules (Less than 1%) ... 2874
Oruvail Capsules (Less than 1%) ... 2874
Oxandrin ... 783
Parlodel ... 2411
Paxil Tablets (Rare) ... 2681
Permax Tablets (Infrequent) ... 571
Pravachol Tablets ... 770
Prostin E2 Suppository ... 2109
Prozac Pulvules & Liquid, Oral Solution (Rare) ... 935
Quadrinal Tablets ... 1398
Retin-A (tretinoin) Cream/Gel/Liquid ... 1947
Retrovir I.V. Infusion ... 1221
Rifater ... 1280
SSD (Infrequent) ... 1402
Silvadene Cream 1% (Infrequent) .. 1288
Sotradecol (Sodium Tetradecyl Sulfate Injection) ... 987
Stelazine ... 2692
Sular Tablets (Less than or equal to 1%) ... 2961
Taxol Injection ... 723
Tegretol/Tegretol-XR ... 870
Testoderm Testosterone Transdermal System ... 486
Ticlid Tablets ... 2317
Torecan ... 2367
Videx Tablets, Powder for Oral Solution, & Pediatric Powder for Oral Solution (Less than 1%) ... 2980
Vistide Injection ... 1057
Zocor Tablets ... 1821
Zoladex (1% or greater) ... 2976
Zoladex 3-month ... 2978
Zoloft Tablets (Rare) ... 2051

Skin, dryness

▲ Accutane Capsules (Up to 80%) ... 2252
Actigall Capsules ... 818
Anafranil Capsules (Up to 2%) ... 819
Aquasol A Vitamin A Capsules, USP ... 525
Aquasol A Parenteral ... 526
Asacol Delayed-Release Tablets ... 2129
Atromid-S Capsules ... 2808
▲ A/T/S 2% Acne Topical Solution (17 out of 90 patients) ... 1244
Bactroban Ointment (Less than 1%) ... 2642
Benzac ... 1031
Benzamycin Topical Gel (Approximately 3%) ... 919
BuSpar Tablets (Infrequent) ... 738
Cardura Tablets (Less than 0.5% of 3960 patients) ... 1993
Casodex Tablets (2% to 5%) ... 2934
Claritin Tablets (2% or fewer patients) ... 2485
Claritin-D Tablets (Less frequent) ... 2487
▲ Cleocin T Topical (23%) ... 2072
Cognex Capsules (Infrequent) ... 1961
Cortifoam ... 2540
Cozaar Tablets (Less than 1%) ... 1668
Crixivan Capsules (Less than 2%).. 1670
Cytovene (1% or less) ... 2270
DaunoXome (Less than or equal to 5%) ... 1842
Depakote Tablets (1% to 5%) ... 418
Depo-Provera Contraceptive Injection (Fewer than 1%) ... 2079
Dermatop Emollient Cream 0.1% (Infrequent to frequent) ... 1264
DesOwen Cream, Ointment and Lotion (Less than 2%) ... 1032
▲ Desquam-E Gel (2 in 50 patients) .. 2792
▲ Desquam-X Gel (2 in 50 patients) .. 2792
▲ Desquam-X 10 Bar (2 in 50 patients) ... 2792
▲ Desquam-X Wash (2 in 50 patients) ... 2792
▲ Differin Gel (10% to 40%) ... 1033
Diprolene AF Cream 0.05% (Infrequent) ... 2489
▲ Diprolene Gel 0.05% (4%) ... 2490
Diprolene Lotion 0.05% (Infrequent) ... 2491
Diprolene Ointment 0.05% (Infrequent) ... 2491
Donnagel Liquid and Donnagel Chewable Tablets (Rare) ... ▣⊚ 854
▲ Dovonex Ointment 0.005% (1% to 10%) ... 2793
Effexor (Infrequent) ... 2825
Elocon Cream 0.1% (Infrequent) 2492
Elocon Ointment 0.1% (Infrequent) ... 2494
Emcyt Capsules (2%) ... 2085
Emgel 2% Topical Gel (Occasional) ... 1081
Epifoam (Infrequent) ... 2543
Ergamisol Tablets ... 1340
Ethmozine Tablets (Less than 2%) 2217
Florone/Florone E ... 921
Fluorouracil Injection ... 2282
Foscavir Injection (Less than 1%) .. 541
Sterile FUDR (Remote possibility) .. 2284
Halog (Infrequent) ... 2795
Hivid Tablets (Less than 1%) ... 2287
Hytone ... 922
Hytone Ointment 2 ½% ... 923
Hyzaar Tablets ... 1720
Imitrex Tablets (Rare) ... 1099
▲ Intron A for Injection (Up to 10%) .. 2506
Invirase Capsules (Less than 2%) .. 2291
Lac-Hydrin 12% Lotion (Less frequent) ... 2796
Lamictal Tablets (Rare) ... 1105
▲ Lamprene Capsules (8-28%) ... 846
Lescol Capsules ... 2395
Lomotil ... 2591
Lotrisone Cream (Infrequent) ... 2515
Lupron Injection (Less than 5%) 2736
LUVOX Tablets (Infrequent) ... 2723
MetroCream ... 1034
Metrodin (urofollitropin for injection) ... 2616
MetroGel ... 1034
Mevacor Tablets ... 1742
Mexitil Capsules (About 1 in 1,000) ... 684
Motofen Tablets ... 789
Mykrox Tablets (Less than 2%) ... 1617
Mylerran Tablets (Rare) ... 1209
Naprelan Tablets (Less than 1%) ... 2861
Neurontin Capsules (Infrequent) ... 1978
▲ Nipent for Injection (3% to 10%) ... 2733
Nizoral 2% Shampoo (One occurrence in 41 patients) ... 1344
Norvasc Tablets (Less than or equal to 0.1%) ... 2020
Norvir (Less than 2%) ... 447
OxyContin Tablets (Less than 1%) 2163
pHisoHex ... 2458
Pandel Cream, 0.1% ... 2475
Paxil Tablets (Infrequent) ... 2681
Pentasa (Less than 1%) ... 1275
Pepcid Injection (Infrequent) ... 1765
Pepcid (Infrequent) ... 1763
Permax Tablets (Infrequent) ... 571
Pravachol Tablets ... 770
Prilosec Delayed-Release Capsules (Less than 1%) ... 516
ProctoCream-HC 2.5% (Infrequent to frequent) ... 2552
ProctoFoam-HC ... 2552
▲ Proleukin for Injection (15%) ... 812
ProSom Tablets (Rare) ... 457
Prozac Pulvules & Liquid, Oral Solution (Infrequent) ... 935
Psorcon Ointment 0.05% ... 923
Remeron Tablets (Infrequent) ... 1878
Renova (tretinoin emollient cream) 0.05% (Almost all subjects) ... 1945
Risperdal Tablets (2% to 4%) ... 1348
▲ Roferon-A Injection (5% to 17%) ... 2308
Serzone Tablets (Infrequent) ... 776
Sular Tablets (Less than or equal to 1%) ... 2961
Taxotere for Injection Concentrate ... 2204
▲ Tegison Capsules (50-75%) ... 2314
Ultravate Cream 0.05% (Less frequent) ... 2797
Ultravate Ointment 0.05% (Less frequent) ... 2798
Varivax (Greater than or equal to 1%) ... 1807
▲ Vesanoid Capsules (77%) ... 2327
Vistide Injection ... 1057
Wellbutrin Tablets (Infrequent) ... 1177
Zocor Tablets ... 1821
Zoladex (1% or greater) ... 2976
Zoladex 3-month ... 2978
Zoloft Tablets (Infrequent) ... 2051
▲ Zonalon Cream (Approximately 1% to 10%) ... 1042
Zyrtec Tablets (Less than 2%) ... 2053

Skin, eruptions

▲ Anaprox/Naprosyn (3% to 9%) ... 2277
Antabuse Tablets (Occasional) ... 2802
Aralen Hydrochloride Injection ... 2430
Bactrim DS Tablets ... 2257
Bactrim I.V. Infusion ... 2255
Bactrim ... 2257
Biaxin ... 406
Cardizem CD Capsules (Infrequent) ... 1251
Cosmegen Injection ... 1666
Daranide Tablets ... 1676
Depen Titratable Tablets (Rare) 2770
E.E.S. ... 427
Easprin ... 1971
▲ EC-Naprosyn Delayed-Release Tablets (3% to 9%) ... 2277
EryPed 200 & EryPed 400 Granules ... 425
Ery-Tab Tablets ... 426
Erythrocin Stearate Filmtab ... 429
Fansidar Tablets ... 2281
Flovent (1% to 3%) ... 1089
Floxin Tablets (200 mg, 300 mg, 400 mg) ... 1577
Gantanol Tablets ... 2285
Gantrisin ... 2286
Halotestin Tablets ... 2095
Ilotycin Gluceptate, IV, Vials ... 929
Imitrex Injection (Infrequent) ... 1095
Librax Capsules (Rare) ... 2330
Librium Capsules (Isolated cases) .. 2331
Librium Injectable (Isolated instances) ... 2332
Mellaril (Infrequent) ... 2398
Micronase Tablets (1.5%) ... 2099
Mysoline (Occasional) ... 2860
▲ Naprelan Tablets (3% to 9%) ... 2861
▲ Anaprox/Naprosyn (3% to 9%) ... 2277
Nydrazid Injection ... 509
PCE Dispertab Tablets ... 453
PASER Granules ... 1333
Pediazole Suspension ... 2340
Pen•Vee K ... 2879
Phenobarbital Elixir and Tablets (Rare) ... 1523
Pima Syrup ... 1004
Plaquenil Sulfate Tablets ... 2459
Rifamate Capsules ... 1278
Seldane Tablets (1.0% to 1.6%) ... 1284
Septra ... 1146
Septra I.V. Infusion ... 1142
Septra I.V. Infusion ADD-Vantage Vials ... 1144
Septra ... 1146

(▣ Described in PDR For Nonprescription Drugs)   Incidence data in parenthesis; ▲ 3% or more   (⊚ Described in PDR For Ophthalmology)

Skin, eruptions — Side Effects Index — 1452

Serevent Inhalation Aerosol (1% to 3%) 1149
Tapazole Tablets 1361
Tessalon Perles 1018
Trasylol 607
Yodoxin Tablets 1235
Zyloprim Tablets (Less than 1%) 1194

Skin, erythema

Cleocin Vaginal Cream 2070
▲ Differin Gel (10% to 40%) 1033
DYNACIN Capsules (Rare) 1627
Emgel 2% Topical Gel (Occasional) 1081
Gastrocrom Capsules (Infrequent) 1611
Gastrocrom Oral Concentrate (Less common) 1611
Maxaquin Tablets 2593
MetroCream (Less than 3%) 1034
Minocin Intravenous 1428
Minocin Oral Suspension 1431
Minocin Pellet-Filled Capsules 1429
Monodox Capsules 1858
pHisoHex 2458
Plaquenil Sulfate Tablets 2459
Terramycin Intramuscular Solution 2034
T.R.U.E. Test (Two to 27 reports) 1162
Vibramycin Hyclate Intravenous 2040

Skin, fluorescence

AK-FLUOR Injection 10% and 25% ⊙ 204

Skin, fragile

▲ Accutane Capsules (Up to 80%) 2252
Dalalone D.P. Injectable 1009
Dexacort Phosphate in Respihaler 1606
Dexacort Phosphate in Turbinaire 1607
Florinef Acetate Tablets 506

Skin, fragility

Celestone Soluspan Suspension 2484
CORTENEMA 2713
Cortone Acetate Sterile Suspension 1663
Cortone Acetate Tablets 1664
Cuprimine Capsules 1673
Decadron Elixir 1676
Decadron Phosphate Injection 1680
Decadron Phosphate with Xylocaine Injection, Sterile 1683
Decadron Tablets 1678
Decadron-LA Sterile Suspension 1687
Depen Titratable Tablets 2770
Hydeltrasol Injection, Sterile 1708
Hydeltra-T.B.A. Sterile Suspension 1710
Hydrocortone Acetate Sterile Suspension 1712
Hydrocortone Phosphate Injection, Sterile 1713
Hydrocortone Tablets 1715
Pediapred Oral Solution 1618
Prelone Syrup 1834
▲ Tegison Capsules (50-75%) 2314

Skin, hypertrophy

Anafranil Capsules (Rare) 819
Betaseron for SC Injection 653
▲ CellCept Capsules (More than or equal to 3%) 2265
Dilacor XR Extended-release Capsules (Infrequent) 2183
Effexor (Rare) 2825
Estring Vaginal Ring (1% to 3%) 2086
Foscavir Injection (Less than 1%) 541
Paxil Tablets (Rare) 2681
Prozac Pulvules & Liquid, Oral Solution (Rare) 935
Redux Capsules (Rare) 2911
Remeron Tablets (Rare) 1878
Supprelin Injection (1% to 3%) 2230
Videx Tablets, Powder for Oral Solution, & Pediatric Powder for Oral Solution (Less than 1%) 2980

Skin, infection

▲ Accutane Capsules (Approximately 1 patient in 20 patients) 2252
Crixivan Capsules (Less than 2%) 1670
▲ Neoral (7.0%) 2405
Prinivil Tablets (0.3% to 1.0%) 1776
Prinzide Tablets 1780
Pronto Lice Killing Shampoo & Conditioner in One Kit ▣ 669
▲ Sandimmune (7.0 to 10.1%) 2416
Zestoretic Tablets 2968
Zestril Tablets (0.3% to 1.0%) 2972

Skin, irritation

Accuzyme Ointment (Occasional) 1236
▲ Androderm Testosterone Transdermal System (5%) 2634
Benzamycin Topical Gel (Occasional) 919
Betadine Solution 2145
Betadine Surgical Scrub (Rare) 2145
Blocadren Tablets 1654
Compazine 2644
Cortisporin Cream 1073
Cortisporin Ointment 1074
Differin Gel (Approximately 1% or less) 1033
Diprolene AF Cream 0.05% (Infrequent) 2489
Diprolene Lotion 0.05% (Less than 1%) 2491
Diprolene Ointment 0.05% (Infrequent) 2491
▲ Dovonex Cream 0.005% (Approximately 10% to 15%) 2792
▲ Dovonex Ointment 0.005% (Approximately 10% to 15%) 2793
Drithocreme 0.1%, 0.25%, 0.5%, 1.0% (HP) 920
Dritho-Scalp 0.25%, 0.5% (More frequent) 921
Elocon Cream 0.1% (Infrequent) 2492
Elocon Ointment 0.1% (Infrequent) 2494
Epifoam (Infrequent) 2543
Halog (Infrequent) 2795
Lotrimin 2514
Lotrisone Cream 2515
Mantadil Cream 1124
MetroCream (Less than 3%) 1034
MetroGel 1034
MG 217 ▣ 800
Occlusal-HP 1041
Orap Tablets 1037
Panafil Ointment (Occasional) 2372
Panafil-White Ointment (Occasional) 2372
ProctoFoam-HC 2552
Pronto Lice Killing Shampoo & Conditioner in One Kit ▣ 669
Questran (Less frequent) 774
SalAc 1042
Selsun Rx 2.5% Selenium Sulfide Lotion, USP 2345
Sportscreme External Analgesic Rub Cream & Lotion ▣ 798
Stelazine 2692
▲ Tegison Capsules (50-75%) 2314
Timolide Tablets 1791
Timoptic in Ocudose 1796
Timoptic Sterile Ophthalmic Solution 1794
Timoptic-XE 1798
Tolectin (200, 400 and 600 mg) (1 to 3%) 1591
Vascor Tablets (200 and 300 mg) (0.5 to 2.0%) 1597
Xerac AC Solution 1990
Ziac 1459

Skin, lesions

Hivid Tablets (Less than 1%) 2287
Lupron Injection (Less than 5%) 2736
Prinivil Tablets (0.3% to 1.0%) 1776
Prinzide Tablets 1780
Procanbid Extended-Release Tablets (Fairly common) 1983
Zestoretic Tablets 2968

Skin, maceration

Analpram-HC Rectal Cream 1% and 2.5% 993
Anusol-HC Cream 2.5% (Infrequent to frequent) 1953
▲ Cordran Lotion (More frequent) 1854
▲ Cordran Tape (More frequent) 1855
Cormax Ointment (Infrequent) 1856
Cormax Scalp Application (Infrequent) 1857
Cortisporin Cream 1073
Cortisporin Ointment 1074
Decadron Phosphate Topical Cream 1686
Decaspray Topical Aerosol 1689
Diprolene AF Cream 0.05% (Infrequent) 2489
Diprolene Lotion 0.05% (Infrequent) 2491
Diprolene Ointment 0.05% (Infrequent) 2491
Elocon Lotion 0.1% (Infrequent) 2493
Epifoam (Infrequent) 2543
Florone/Florone E 921
Halog (Infrequent) 2795
Hytone 922
Hytone Ointment 2 ½% 923
Lidex (Infrequent) 2299
Lotrisone Cream (Infrequent) 2515
Monistat Dual-Pak 1906
NeoDecadron Topical Cream 1757
Pramosone Cream, Lotion & Ointment 995
ProctoCream-HC 2.5% (Infrequent to frequent) 2552
ProctoFoam-HC 2552
Psorcon Ointment 0.05% 923
Synalar (Infrequent) 2299
Temovate Scalp Application (Infrequent) 1153
Topicort Emollient Cream 0.25% (Infrequent) 1289
Topicort Gel 0.05% (Infrequent) 1290
Topicort LP Emollient Cream 0.05% (Infrequent) 1289
Topicort Ointment 0.25% (Infrequent) 1291
Tridesilon Cream 0.05% (Infrequent) 609
Tridesilon Ointment 0.05% (Infrequent) 610
Westcort Cream 0.2% (Infrequent) 2799

Skin, nodule

Cerebyx Injection (Infrequent) 1956
Imdur (Less than or equal to 5%) 1362
Imitrex Tablets (Rare) 1099
Invirase Capsules (Less than 2%) 2291
Lescol Capsules 2395
Lotrel Capsules 858
Mevacor Tablets 1742
Neurontin Capsules (Rare) 1978
Permax Tablets (Rare) 571
Pravachol Tablets 770
Rilutek Tablets (Rare) 2198
Zocor Tablets 1821

Skin, oiliness

A/T/S 2% Acne Topical Solution 1244
Benzamycin Topical Gel 919
▲ Cleocin T Topical (18%) 2072
Cleocin Vaginal Cream 2070
Emgel 2% Topical Gel (Occasional) 1081
Propulsid (Less than 1%) 1346
ReVia Tablets (Less than 1%) 957

Skin, photoallergic reactions

Feldene Capsules (Less than 1%) 2008
IBU Tablets (Less than 1%) 1389

Skin, phototoxic eruptions

Proloprim Tablets 1141
Trimpex Tablets 2323

Skin, tenderness

A/T/S 2% Acne Topical Gel 1244
A/T/S 2% Acne Topical Solution 1244
Benzamycin Topical Gel 919
▲ Blenoxane (Approximately 50%) 697
Efudex 2280
Emgel 2% Topical Gel 1081
Imitrex Injection (Rare) 1095
Imitrex Tablets (Infrequent) 1099
Naftin Gel 1% (0.5%) 477

Skin, wrinkling

Depen Titratable Tablets 2770
Imitrex Tablets (Rare) 1099

Skin atrophy

Aclovate (Infrequent) 1061
Analpram-HC Rectal Cream 1% and 2.5% 993
Cormax Ointment (Approximately 0.3%) 1856
Cormax Scalp Application (Infrequent) 1857
Cortisporin Cream 1073
Cortisporin Ointment 1074
Cortisporin Otic Solution Sterile 1076
Cortisporin Otic Suspension Sterile 1077
Cutivate Cream 1078
Cutivate Ointment (Infrequent to more frequent) 1078
Decadron Phosphate Topical Cream 1686
Decaspray Topical Aerosol 1689
Dermatop Emollient Cream 0.1% (1%) 1264
DesOwen Cream, Ointment and Lotion (Infrequent) 1032
Diprolene AF Cream 0.05% (Infrequent) 2489
Diprolene Gel 0.05% (Less frequent) 2490
Diprolene Lotion 0.05% (Infrequent) 2491
Diprolene Ointment 0.05% (Infrequent) 2491
Dovonex Ointment 0.005% (Less than 1%) 2793
Effexor (Rare) 2825
Elocon Cream 0.1% (1.6%) 2492
Elocon Lotion 0.1% (Infrequent) 2493
▲ Elocon Ointment 0.1% (4.8%) 2494
Epifoam (Infrequent) 2543
Etrafon 2-10 Tablets 2495
Florone/Florone E 921
Halog (Infrequent) 2795
Hytone 922
Hytone Ointment 2 ½% 923
Lidex (Infrequent) 2299
Locoid Cream, Ointment and Topical Solution (Infrequent) 994
Lotrisone Cream (Infrequent) 2515
Mantadil Cream 1124
NeoDecadron Topical Cream 1757
Pandel Cream, 0.1% 2475
Pediotic Suspension Sterile 1140
Pramosone Cream, Lotion & Ointment 995
ProctoCream-HC 2.5% (Infrequent to frequent) 2552
ProctoFoam-HC 2552
Psorcon Ointment 0.05% 923
Synalar (Infrequent) 2299
Tegison Capsules (Less than 1%) 2314
Temovate Cream (Less frequent) 1152
Temovate E Emollient (Less than 2%) 1154
▲ Temovate Gel (Among most frequent) 1153
Temovate Ointment (Less frequent) 1152
Temovate Scalp Application (Infrequent) 1153
Topicort Emollient Cream 0.25% (Infrequent) 1289
Topicort Gel 0.05% (Infrequent) 1290
Topicort LP Emollient Cream 0.05% (Infrequent) 1289
Topicort Ointment 0.25% (Infrequent) 1291
Tridesilon Cream 0.05% (Infrequent) 609
Tridesilon Ointment 0.05% (Infrequent) 610
Ultravate Cream 0.05% (Less frequent) 2797
Ultravate Ointment 0.05% (Less frequent) 2798
Westcort Cream 0.2% (Infrequent) 2799
Westcort Ointment 0.2% 2800

Skin eruptions, pleomorphic

Aralen Phosphate Tablets 2431

Skin odor, abnormal

Anafranil Capsules (Up to 2%) 819
Zoloft Tablets (Rare) 2051

Skin reactions

▲ Catapres-TTS (51 of 101 patients) 680
Cefobid Intravenous/Intramuscular (1 in 45) 1996
Cefobid Pharmacy Bulk Package - Not for Direct Infusion (1 in 45) 1999
Compazine 2644
Cortisporin Ophthalmic Ointment Sterile 1074
Cortisporin Otic Suspension Sterile (Occasional) 1077
Crixivan Capsules (Less than 2%) 1670
▲ DHCplus Capsules (Among most frequent) 2148
Doxorubicin Astra 531
▲ Epogen for Injection (7% to 10%) 489
Exelderm Cream 1.0% (Infrequent) 2794
Exelderm Solution 1.0% (Infrequent) 2795
Floxin Tablets (200 mg, 300 mg, 400 mg) 1577
Foscavir Injection (Less than 1%) 541
Hivid Tablets (Less than 1%) 2287
Lamisil Tablets (Isolated reports) 2394
Lanoxicaps (Rare) 1110
Lanoxin Elixir Pediatric (Rare) 1113
Lanoxin Injection (Rare) 1116
Lanoxin Injection Pediatric (Rare) 1119
Lanoxin Tablets (Rare) 1121
▲ Leukine (77%) 1317
Lupron Depot 3.75 mg (Less than 5%) 2739

1453 **Side Effects Index** **Soreness, injection site**

Lupron Depot 7.5 mg (Less than 5%) 2741
▲ Lupron Depot - 3 Month 22.5 mg (8.5%) 2743
Lupron Injection (Less than 5%) 2736
Maxaquin Tablets (Less than 1%) 2593
Megace Oral Suspension (1% to 3%) 708
▲ Nipent for Injection (4% to 17%) 2733
▲ Nolvadex Tablets (18.7%) 2957
ParaGard T 380A Intrauterine Copper Contraceptive 1936
Prilosec Delayed-Release Capsules (Very rare) 516
Primaxin I.M. 1770
Primaxin I.V. (Less than 0.2%) 1772
Prinivil Tablets (Rare) 1776
Prinzide Tablets (Rare) 1780
▲ Procrit for Injection (7% to 10%) 1896
▲ Prograf (Greater than 3%) 1028
Redux Capsules (Infrequent) 2911
Rifadin 1276
Rifater 1280
Rilutek Tablets (Infrequent) 2198
Romazicon (1% to 3%) 2311
Septra I.V. Infusion 1142
Streptomycin Sulfate Injection 2031
▲ Supprelin Injection (45%) 2230
Taxol Injection 723
Taxotere for Injection Concentrate 2204
Tegison Capsules (Less than 1%) 2314
▲ Ultrase MT Capsules (Among most frequent) 2477
▲ Vesanoid Capsules (14%) 2327
Videx Tablets, Powder for Oral Solution, & Pediatric Powder for Oral Solution (Less than 1% to 13%) 2980
Xalatan (1% to 2%) ⊙ 304
Zestoretic Tablets (Rare) 2968
Zestril Tablets (Rare) 2972
Zinecard Injection (1%) 2120

Skin test reactions, suppression

Celestone Soluspan Suspension 2484
CORTENEMA 2713
Cortone Acetate Sterile Suspension 1663
Cortone Acetate Tablets 1664
Dalalone D.P. Injectable 1009
Decadron Elixir 1676
Decadron Phosphate Injection 1680
Decadron Phosphate with Xylocaine Injection, Sterile 1683
Decadron Tablets 1678
Decadron-LA Sterile Suspension 1687
Dexacort Phosphate in Respihaler 1606
Dexacort Phosphate in Turbinaire 1607
Florinef Acetate Tablets 506
Hydeltrasol Injection, Sterile 1708
Hydeltra-T.B.A. Sterile Suspension 1710
Hydrocortone Acetate Sterile Suspension 1712
Hydrocortone Phosphate Injection, Sterile 1713
Hydrocortone Tablets 1715
Pediapred Oral Solution 1618
Prelone Syrup 1834
T.R.U.E. Test (Up to 2 reports) 1162

Skull abnormalities, fetal

Accupril Tablets 1950
Accutane Capsules 2252
Altace Capsules 1238
Capoten Tablets 740
Capozide Tablets 744
Cozaar Tablets 1668
Hyzaar Tablets 1720
Lotensin Tablets 852
Lotensin HCT Tablets 855
Lotrel Capsules 858
Monopril Tablets 762
Prinivil Tablets 1776
Prinzide Tablets 1780
Univasc Tablets 2553
Vaseretic Tablets 1810
Vasotec I.V. 1814
Vasotec Tablets 1816
Zestoretic Tablets 2968
Zestril Tablets 2972

Sleep, disturbances

Actigall Capsules 818
Adalat Capsules (10 mg and 20 mg) (2% or less) 580
Adalat CC (Rare) 582
Ambien Tablets (Infrequent; 1%) 2559
▲ Anafranil Capsules (4% to 9%) 819
Ativan Tablets (Less frequent) 2807
▲ Avonex (19%) 662
▲ Betapace Tablets (1% to 8%) 637
▲ Cardioquin Tablets (3%) 2146
▲ Clozaril Tablets (4%) 2377
Cordarone Tablets (1 to 3%) 2818
Cozaar Tablets (Less than 1%) 1668
Crixivan Capsules (Less than 2%) 1670
Dalgan Injection (Less than 1%) 529
Danocrine Capsules 2437
Daypro Caplets (1% to 3%) 2578
Dizac (diazepam injectable emulsion) CIV (Less frequent) 1862
Doral Tablets (Rare) 2773
Effexor (Infrequent) 2825
Elavil 2945
Eldepryl Capsules 2729
▲ Epivir (11%) 1200
▲ Ethmozine Tablets (2% to 5%) 2217
Floxin I.V. (1% to 3%) 1580
Floxin Tablets (200 mg, 300 mg, 400 mg) (1% to 3%) 1577
Fludara for Injection (1% to 3%) 658
Foscavir Injection (Less than 1%) 541
Halcion Tablets 2093
HibTITER 1423
Hylorel Tablets (2.1%) 1613
Hyzaar Tablets 1720
Imitrex Injection (Rare) 1095
Imitrex Tablets (Rare to infrequent) 1099
Lamictal Tablets (1.4%) 1105
Lithium Carbonate Capsules & Tablets 2352
Lopressor 848
Lupron Depot 3.75 mg (Less than 5%) 2739
▲ Lupron Depot - 3 Month 22.5 mg (8.5%) 2743
▲ Lupron Injection (5% or more) 2736
LUVOX Tablets (Infrequent) 2723
▲ Mexitil Capsules (7.1% to 7.5%) 684
Monopril Tablets (0.2% to 1.0%) 762
Nardil (Common) 1977
Noroxin Tablets (Less frequent) 1758
Noroxin Tablets (Less frequent) 2222
Parlodel (Less than 1%) 2411
Procardia Capsules (2% or less) 2024
ProSom Tablets (Infrequent) 457
Proventil Syrup (Less than 1 of 100 patients) 2528
▲ Prozac Pulvules & Liquid, Oral Solution (3%) 935
▲ Quinidex Extentabs (3%) 2240
Recombivax HB (Less than 1%) 1787
Redux Capsules (Infrequent) 2911
▲ ReVia Tablets (More than 10%) 957
Risperdal Tablets (Frequent) 1348
▲ Roferon-A Injection (5% to 11%) 2308
Sinemet CR Tablets 961
▲ Tetramune (Up to 28%) 1449
Tofranil Tablets 875
Tonocard Tablets (Less than 1%) 519
Triavil Tablets 1800
Trinalin Repetabs Tablets 1373
Ultram Tablets (50 mg) (1% to less than 5%) 1594
Univasc Tablets (Less than 1%) 2553
Valium Tablets 2335
Varivax (Greater than or equal to 1%) 1807
Ventolin Syrup (Less than 1 of 100 patients) 1175
Verelan Capsules (1.4%) 1455
Versed Injection (Less than 1%) 2324
Videx Tablets, Powder for Oral Solution, & Pediatric Powder for Oral Solution (Less than 1%) 2980
▲ Wellbutrin Tablets (4.0%) 1177
Xanax Tablets (Rare) 2115
Zarontin Capsules 1986
Zarontin Syrup 1986
Ziac 1459

Sleepiness (see under Drowsiness)

Sleeplessness (see under Insomnia)

Sloughing

Aramine Injection 1649
Efudex 2280
FLUORACAINE (Rare) ⊙ 208
Fluorescite ⊙ 217
Fluorouracil Injection (Common) 2282
FLURESS (Rare) ⊙ 208
Gamimune N, 5% Immune Globulin Intravenous (Human), 5% (One patient) 612
Gamimune N, 10% Immune Globulin Intravenous (Human), 10% (One patient) 615
MSTA Mumps Skin Test Antigen 2988
Norplant System 2868
Ophthetic ⊙ 244
Robaxin Injectable 2245
Scleromate Injection 1234
Sotradecol (Sodium Tetradecyl Sulfate Injection) 987
Talwin Injection 2465
Velban Vials 1537

Sluggishness

Axocet Capsules (Infrequent) 2469
Esgic-plus Capsules (Infrequent) 1012
Esgic-plus Tablets (Infrequent) 1012
Fioricet Tablets (Infrequent) 2386
Fioricet with Codeine Capsules (Infrequent) 2387
Fiorinal with Codeine Capsules (Infrequent) 2390
Parlodel Capsules (Less than 1%) 2411
Phrenilin (Infrequent) 790
Sedapap Tablets 50 mg/650 mg (Infrequent) 1826

Smell, disturbances

Beclovent Inhalation Aerosol and Refill 1063
Beconase 1065
Biaxin 406
BuSpar Tablets (Infrequent) 738
Ceredase 1055
Cordarone Tablets (1 to 3%) 2818
Ergamisol Tablets (1%) 1340
Floxin I.V. 1580
Floxin Tablets (200 mg, 300 mg, 400 mg) 1577
Hivid Tablets (Less than 1%) 2287
Imitrex Injection (Rare) 1095
Imitrex Tablets (Infrequent) 1099
Maxair Autohaler (0.6%) 1550
Maxair Inhaler (Less than 1%) 1552
Nasalide Nasal Solution 0.025% (5% or less) 2301
Nicotrol NS Nicotine Nasal Spray (More common) 1565
Rhinocort Nasal Inhaler (Less than 1%) 552
Rythmol Tablets–150mg, 225mg, 300mg (Less than 1%) 1399
Timentin for Injection 2706
Tonocard Tablets (Less than 1%) 519
Tornalate Solution for Inhalation, 0.2% 976
Tornalate Metered Dose Inhaler 978
Xanax Tablets 2115

Smell, loss of the sense (see under Anosmia)

Smoker's tongue (see under Leukoplakia, oral)

Sneezing

▲ AeroBid Inhaler System (3% to 9%) 1004
▲ Aerobid-M Inhaler System (3% to 9%) 1004
Afrin ▣ 757
Alomide Ophthalmic Solution (Less than 1%) 465
▲ Atrovent Nasal Spray 0.03% (3.1%) 676
Azactam for Injection (Less than 1%) 736
▲ Beconase (4%) 1065
Bentyl 1246
Carbocaine Injection 2432
Claritin Tablets (2% or fewer patients) 2485
Claritin-D Tablets (Less frequent) 2487
Clozaril Tablets (Less than 1%) 2377
Diprivan Injectable Emulsion (Less than 1%) 2939
Duration 12 Hour Nasal Spray ▣ 766
Ethyol (amifostine) for Injection 485
4-Way Fast Acting Nasal Spray (regular & mentholated) ▣ 644
4-Way 12 Hour Nasal Spray ▣ 644
Flonase Nasal Spray (Less than 1%) 1088
Hespan Injection 945
Intal Inhaler (Rare) 2185
Intal Nebulizer Solution (Rare) 2186
Intron A for Injection (Less than or equal to 5%) 2506
Marcaine (Rare) 2446
Marcaine Spinal (Rare) 2449
Methadone Hydrochloride Oral Concentrate 2356
Nasacort Nasal Inhaler (Fewer than 5%) 2189
▲ Nasalcrom Nasal Solution (1 in 10) 2192
Nasalide Nasal Solution 0.025% (5% or less) 2301
Neo-Synephrine Maximum Strength 12 Hour Nasal Spray ▣ 624
Neo-Synephrine 12 Hour ▣ 624
Neo-Synephrine ▣ 624
Nescaine/Nescaine MPF 549
Nicotrol NS Nicotine Nasal Spray (Common) 1565
12 Hour Nōstrilla ▣ 660
Orlaam Oral Solution 2361
Otrivin ▣ 662
Plendil Extended-Release Tablets (Up to 1.6%) 514
Quadrinal Tablets 1398
ReVia Tablets (Less than 1%) 957
Rhinocort Nasal Inhaler (Less than 1%) 552
Sensorcaine (Rare) 554
Vancenase AQ Nasal Spray 0.042% 2535
▲ Vancenase PocketHaler Nasal Inhaler (10 per 100 patients) 2534
Vicks Sinex Nasal Spray and Ultra Fine Mist ▣ 738

Social reaction, anti (see under Sociopathy)

Sociopathy

BuSpar Tablets (Infrequent) 738
DextroStat-Dextroamphetamine Sulfate Tablets 2211
Neurontin Capsules (Rare) 1978
Paxil Tablets (Rare) 2681
Prozac Pulvules & Liquid, Oral Solution (Rare) 935
Redux Capsules 2911

Sodium depletion (see under Hyponatremia)

Sodium loss (see under Hyponatremia)

Sodium retention

Celestone Soluspan Suspension 2484
CORTENEMA 2713
Cortone Acetate Sterile Suspension 1663
Cortone Acetate Tablets 1664
Dalalone D.P. Injectable 1009
Decadron Elixir 1676
Decadron Phosphate Injection 1680
Decadron Phosphate with Xylocaine Injection, Sterile 1683
Decadron Tablets 1678
Decadron-LA Sterile Suspension 1687
Dexacort Phosphate in Respihaler 1606
Dexacort Phosphate in Turbinaire 1607
▲ Estratest (Among most common) 2718
Florinef Acetate Tablets 506
Halotestin Tablets 2095
Hydeltrasol Injection, Sterile 1708
Hydeltra-T.B.A. Sterile Suspension 1710
Hydrocortone Acetate Sterile Suspension 1712
Hydrocortone Phosphate Injection, Sterile 1713
Hydrocortone Tablets 1715
Hyperstat I.V. Injection 2504
Kayexalate 2444
Oxandrin 783
Pediapred Oral Solution 1618
Prelone Syrup 1834
Proglycem (Frequent) 575
Sodium Polystyrene Sulfonate Suspension 2367
Testred Capsules, 10 mg 1308
Winstrol Tablets 2468

Somnambulism

Ambien Tablets (Rare) 2559
Anafranil Capsules (Infrequent) 819
Halcion Tablets 2093
Zoloft Tablets (Rare) 2051

Somnolence (see under Drowsiness)

Soreness, injection site

▲ Alferon N Injection (10%) 2142
▲ Engerix-B Unit-Dose Vials (22%) 2656
▲ Havrix (56% of adults; 21% of children) 2663
Hyperab Rabies Immune Globulin (Human) 618
Hyper-Tet Tetanus Immune Globulin (Human) 621

(▣ Described in PDR For Nonprescription Drugs) Incidence data in parenthesis; ▲ 3% or more (⊙ Described in PDR For Ophthalmology)

Soreness, injection site

- HypRho-D Full Dose Rho (D) Immune Globulin (Human) ... 623
- HypRho-D Mini-Dose Rho (D) Immune Globulin (Human) ... 622
- Imogam Rabies Immune Globulin (Human) (Uncommon) ... 897
- INFeD (Iron Dextran Injection, USP) ... 2478
- ▲ Influenza Virus Vaccine, Trivalent, Types A and B (chromatograph- and filter-purified subviron antigen) FluShield, 1996-1997 Formula (Most frequent) ... 2842
- ▲ JE-VAX (5.9% to 24.5%) ... 904
- Pneumovax 23 (Common) ... 1768
- ▲ Typhim Vi (13%) ... 914
- ▲ Varivax (19.3% to 32.5%) ... 1807

Soreness, vaginal

- Mycelex-G 500 mg Vaginal Tablets (1 in 149 patients) ... 602

Sore throat
(see under Throat, soreness)

Spasm, biliary tract

- Brontex ... 2130
- Demerol ... 2438
- Dilaudid-HP Injection (Less frequent) ... 1384
- Dilaudid-HP Lyophilized Powder 250 mg (Less frequent) ... 1384
- Dilaudid Tablets and Liquid ... 1386
- MS Contin Tablets (Less frequent) ... 2149
- MSIR (Infrequent) ... 2152
- Methadone Hydrochloride Oral Solution & Tablets ... 2357
- Oramorph SR (Morphine Sulfate Sustained Release Tablets) (Less frequent) ... 2359
- Phenergan with Codeine ... 2883
- Phenergan VC with Codeine ... 2888
- RMS Suppositories CII ... 2766
- Roxanol ... 2365
- Trilafon ... 2532

Spasm, gastrointestinal

- Fioricet with Codeine Capsules ... 2387
- Fiorinal with Codeine Capsules ... 2390
- Methadone Hydrochloride Oral Concentrate ... 2356

Spasm, generalized

- Anafranil Capsules (Rare) ... 819
- Foscavir Injection (Between 1% and 5%) ... 541
- Invirase Capsules (Less than 2%) ... 2291
- LUVOX Tablets (Infrequent) ... 2723
- Naprelan Tablets (Less than 1%) ... 2861
- Paxil Tablets (Rare) ... 2681
- Prinivil Tablets (0.3% to 1.0%) ... 1776
- Prinzide Tablets ... 1780
- ▲ Prograf (Greater than 3%) ... 1028
- Zestoretic Tablets ... 2968
- Zestril Tablets (0.3% to 1.0%) ... 2972

Spasm, vesical sphincters

- Lorcet 10/650 Tablets ... 1016
- Lortab ... 2751
- Tussend ... 1830
- Tussionex Pennkinetic Extended-Release Suspension ... 1624
- Vicodin ES Tablets ... 1405
- Vicodin HP Tablets ... 1403
- Vicodin Tuss Expectorant ... 1406
- Zydone Capsules ... 967

Spatial disorientation

- Serophene (clomiphene citrate tablets, USP) ... 2621

Speech, bulbar type

- Reglan ... 2243

Speech, incoherent

- Clozaril Tablets (Less than 1%) ... 2377
- Marcaine Spinal ... 2449
- Sensorcaine ... 554

Speech, slurring

- BuSpar Tablets (Rare) ... 738
- Clozaril Tablets (1%) ... 2377
- Dalgan Injection (Less than 1%) ... 529
- Dalmane Capsules (Rare) ... 2329
- ▲ Dilantin Infatabs (Among most common) ... 1967
- ▲ Dilantin Kapseals (Among most common) ... 1965
- ▲ Dilantin-125 Suspension (Among most common) ... 1969

- Dizac (diazepam injectable emulsion) CIV (Less frequent) ... 1862
- Doral Tablets ... 2773
- Eskalith ... 2658
- Etrafon ... 2495
- Fioricet with Codeine Capsules ... 2387
- Fiorinal with Codeine Capsules ... 2390
- Halcion Tablets ... 2093
- Kadian Capsules (Less than 3%) ... 2948
- Klonopin Tablets ... 2294
- Levoprome (Sometimes) ... 1321
- Lioresal Tablets ... 847
- Lithium Carbonate Capsules & Tablets ... 2352
- Lithonate/Lithotabs/Lithobid ... 2721
- Loxitane ... 1426
- LUVOX Tablets (Rare) ... 2723
- Matulane Capsules ... 2300
- Mebaral Tablets ... 2452
- Miltown Tablets ... 2780
- Placidyl Capsules ... 456
- PMB 200 and PMB 400 ... 2890
- Serax Capsules ... 2916
- Serax Tablets ... 2916
- Serentil ... 689
- Symmetrel Capsules (0.1% to 1%) ... 965
- Symmetrel Syrup (0.1% to 1%) ... 963
- Tonocard Tablets (Less than 1%) ... 519
- Tranxene ... 459
- Trilafon ... 2532
- Valium Injectable ... 2336
- Valium Tablets (Infrequent) ... 2335
- Versed Injection (Less than 1%) ... 2324
- Xanax Tablets ... 2115

Speech difficulties

- Clozaril Tablets (Less than 1%) ... 2377
- ▲ Demser Capsules (10%) ... 1690
- Ethmozine Tablets (Less than 2%) ... 2217
- Marinol (Dronabinol) Capsules (Less than 1%) ... 2353
- Mexitil Capsules (2.6%) ... 684
- Nubain Injection (1% or less) ... 952
- Stadol (Less than 1%) ... 779

Speech disturbances

- Ambien Tablets (Infrequent) ... 2559
- Anafranil Capsules (Up to 3%) ... 819
- Atretol Tablets ... 569
- ▲ Avonex (3%) ... 662
- Bentyl ... 1246
- ▲ Betaseron for SC Injection (3%) ... 653
- Brevibloc (esmolol HCl) Injection (Less than 1%) ... 1860
- Cerebyx Injection (Frequent) ... 1956
- Dantrium Capsules (Less frequent) ... 2131
- Demulen ... 2580
- Depakote Tablets (1% to 5%) ... 418
- Desyrel and Desyrel Dividose ... 504
- Doral Tablets ... 2773
- Duragesic Transdermal System (1% or greater) ... 1336
- Effexor (Infrequent) ... 2825
- Eldepryl Capsules ... 2729
- Ergamisol Tablets ... 1340
- Estrace Cream and Tablets ... 751
- Foscavir Injection (Less than 1%) ... 541
- Hivid Tablets (Less than 1%) ... 2287
- Intron A for Injection (Less than 5%) ... 2506
- Invirase Capsules (Less than 2%) ... 2291
- Kerlone Tablets (Less than 2%) ... 2588
- Lamictal Tablets (2.5%) ... 1105
- Levbid Extended-Release Tablets ... 2549
- Levlen/Tri-Levlen ... 646
- Levsin/Levsinex/Levbid ... 2549
- Lioresal Intrathecal (Up to 3.5%) ... 1634
- Modicon ... 1928
- ▲ Orap Tablets (2 of 20 patients) ... 1037
- Ortho-Cyclen/Ortho Tri-Cyclen ... 1914
- Ortho-Est ... 1925
- Ortho-Novum ... 1928
- Ortho-Cyclen/Ortho Tri-Cyclen ... 1914
- OxyContin Tablets (Less than 1%) ... 2163
- Permax Tablets (1.1%) ... 571
- ▲ Proleukin for Injection (7%) ... 812
- Redux Capsules (Infrequent) ... 2911
- Romazicon (Less than 1%) ... 2311
- Rythmol Tablets—150mg, 225mg, 300mg (Less than 1%) ... 1399
- Salagen Tablets (Less than 1%) ... 1546
- Tambocor Tablets (Less than 1%) ... 1555
- Tegretol/Tegretol-XR ... 870
- Tonocard Tablets (Less than 1%) ... 519
- Levlen/Tri-Levlen ... 646
- ▲ Vesanoid Capsules (3%) ... 2327
- Videx Tablets, Powder for Oral Solution, & Pediatric Powder for Oral Solution (Less than 1%) ... 2980

Spermatogenesis, changes

- Cytovene-IV (One report) ... 2270
- Danocrine Capsules ... 2437
- Thioplex (Thiotepa For Injection) ... 1329

Spermatogenesis, defective

- Methotrexate Sodium Tablets, Injection, for Injection and LPF Injection ... 1322
- Mustargen ... 1752

Spermatogenesis, inhibition

- Cytovene-IV ... 2270
- Cytoxan ... 700

Spermatozoa, changes

- Dexacort Phosphate in Respihaler ... 1606
- Dexacort Phosphate in Turbinaire ... 1607

Spinal block

- Carbocaine Injection ... 2432
- Duranest Injections ... 533
- Marcaine ... 2446
- Marcaine Spinal ... 2449
- Nescaine/Nescaine MPF ... 549
- Novocain Hydrochloride for Spinal Anesthesia ... 2457
- Sensorcaine ... 554
- Xylocaine Injections ... 562

Spinal cord infarction

- Activase ... 1045

Spinal cord, compression

- Zoladex ... 2976
- Zoladex 3-month (Isolated cases) ... 2978

Spinal fracture

- Lupron Depot 3.75 mg ... 2739
- Lupron Depot 7.5 mg ... 2741
- Lupron Depot - 3 Month 22.5 mg ... 2743
- Lupron Depot-PED 7.5 mg, 11.25 mg and 15 mg ... 2744
- Lupron Injection ... 2736

Splenic infarction

- Lamprene Capsules (Less than 1%) ... 846

Splenomegaly

- Apresazide Capsules (Less frequent) ... 824
- Apresoline Hydrochloride Tablets (Less frequent) ... 826
- Betaseron for SC Injection ... 653
- DaunoXome (Less than or equal to 5%) ... 1842
- Garamycin Injectable ... 2502
- Hydralazine Hydrochloride Injection USP (Less frequent) ... 2712
- Invirase Capsules (Less than 2%) ... 2291
- ▲ Neupogen for Injection (Approximately 30%) ... 495
- Orthoclone OKT3 Sterile Solution ... 1892
- Permax Tablets (Rare) ... 571
- RhoGAM Rho(D) Immune Globulin (Human) (One patient) ... 1902
- Ser-Ap-Es Tablets ... 867

Spotting

- Amen Tablets ... 785
- Aygestin Tablets ... 990
- Brevicon ... 2563
- BuSpar Tablets (Infrequent) ... 738
- Climara Transdermal System ... 640
- Clomid (1.3%) ... 1262
- Cycrin Tablets ... 991
- Cytotec (0.7%) ... 2576
- Danocrine Capsules ... 2437
- Demulen ... 2580
- Depo-Provera Contraceptive Injection ... 2079
- Depo-Provera Sterile Aqueous Suspension ... 2083
- Desogen Tablets ... 1867
- Estrace Cream and Tablets ... 751
- Estraderm Transdermal System ... 842
- ESTRATAB Tablets (0.3, 0.625, 1.25, 2.5 mg) ... 2715
- Estratest ... 2718
- Levlen/Tri-Levlen (Sometimes) ... 646
- Lo/Ovral Tablets ... 2852
- Lo/Ovral-28 Tablets ... 2857
- Menest Tablets ... 2671
- Micronor Tablets ... 1903
- Modicon (Sometimes) ... 1928
- Nordette-21 Tablets ... 2863
- Nordette-28 Tablets ... 2866
- Norinyl ... 2563
- ▲ Norplant System (17.1%) ... 2868

- Nor-Q D Tablets ... 2598
- Ogen Tablets ... 2103
- Ogen Vaginal Cream ... 2106
- Ortho-Cept ... 1907
- Ortho-Cyclen/Ortho-Tri-Cyclen ... 1914
- Ortho-Est ... 1925
- Ortho-Novum (Sometimes) ... 1928
- Ortho-Cyclen/Ortho Tri-Cyclen ... 1914
- Ovcon (Sometimes) ... 765
- Ovral Tablets ... 2877
- Ovral-28 Tablets ... 2878
- Ovrette Tablets ... 2878
- ParaGard T 380A Intrauterine Copper Contraceptive ... 1936
- PMB 200 and PMB 400 ... 2890
- Premarin Intravenous ... 2893
- Premarin Tablets ... 2896
- Premarin Vaginal Cream ... 2898
- Premphase ... 2900
- Prempro ... 2905
- Provera Tablets ... 2110
- Levlen/Tri-Levlen (Sometimes) ... 646
- Tri-Norinyl (Sometimes) ... 2607
- Triphasil-21 Tablets ... 2919
- Triphasil-28 Tablets ... 2924
- Verelan Capsules (1% or less) ... 1455
- Vivelle Transdermal System ... 880

Sputum, discoloration

- Lamprene Capsules (Greater than 1%) ... 846
- Mycobutin Capsules ... 2101
- Rifadin ... 1276
- Rifater ... 1280

Sputum, increase

- ▲ AeroBid Inhaler System (3% to 9%) ... 1004
- ▲ Aerobid-M Inhaler System (3% to 9%) ... 1004
- Airet Albuterol Sulfate Inhalation Solution (1.5%) ... 1602
- Albuterol Sulfate, USP Solution for Inhalation, Arm-a-Med (1.5%) ... 522
- Anafranil Capsules (Infrequent) ... 819
- Atrovent Inhalation Solution (1.4%) ... 675
- Cerebyx Injection (Infrequent) ... 1956
- Claritin-D Tablets (Less frequent) ... 2487
- DaunoXome (Less than or equal to 5%) ... 1842
- Effexor (Rare) ... 2825
- Imdur (Less than or equal to 5%) ... 1362
- Maxaquin Tablets (Less than 1%) ... 2593
- Nicotrol NS Nicotine Nasal Spray (Less than 1%) ... 1565
- Paxil Tablets (Rare) ... 2681
- Proventil Inhalation Solution 0.083% (1.5%) ... 2527
- Proventil Solution for Inhalation 0.5% (1.5%) ... 2525
- Pulmozyme Inhalation ... 1054
- Rilutek Tablets (More than 2%) ... 2198
- Risperdal Tablets (Rare) ... 1348
- Salagen Tablets (Less than 1%) ... 1546
- Tegison Capsules (Less than 1%) ... 2314
- Tilade Inhaler (1.7%) ... 2207
- Tornalate Solution for Inhalation, 0.2% (Less than 1%) ... 976
- Ventolin Inhalation Solution (1.5%) ... 1171
- Ventolin Nebules Inhalation Solution (1.5%) ... 1172
- Vistide Injection ... 1057
- Zyrtec Tablets (Less than 2%) ... 2053

Status epilepticus

- Atretol Tablets ... 569
- Clozaril Tablets ... 2377
- Depakene ... 416
- Dilantin-125 Suspension ... 1969
- Felbatol ... 2774
- Hivid Tablets (Less than 1%) ... 2287
- Oncaspar ... 2194
- Tegretol/Tegretol-XR ... 870
- Xanax Tablets ... 2115

Steatorrhea

- Azathioprine Tablets (Less than 1%) ... 2349
- Fungizone Oral Suspension ... 704
- Imuran (Less than 1%) ... 1103
- Questran (Less frequent) ... 774

Steatosis, hepatic

- Ergamisol Tablets (Rare) ... 1340
- Hivid Tablets (Rare) ... 2287
- Retrovir Capsules ... 1216
- Retrovir I.V. Infusion (Rare) ... 1221
- Retrovir Syrup ... 1216

(℞ Described in PDR For Nonprescription Drugs)   Incidence data in parentheses; ▲ 3% or more   (⊙ Described in PDR For Ophthalmology)

1455 **Side Effects Index** **Stinging**

Steatosis, microvesicular
Orudis Capsules (Rare) 2874
Oruvail Capsules (Rare) 2874

Stenosis, aortic
Naprelan Tablets (Less than 1%) 2861
Videx Tablets, Powder for Oral Solution, & Pediatric Powder for Oral Solution (Less than 1%) 2980

Stenosis, subglottic
Survanta Beractant Intratracheal Suspension 2346

Stevens-Johnson syndrome
AK-CIDE (Some instances) ⊚ 203
AK-CIDE Ointment (Some instances) ⊚ 203
Aldoclor Tablets 1638
Aldoril Tablets 1644
Amoxil 2631
Anaprox/Naprosyn (Less than 1%) 2277
Ancef Injection 2632
Apresazide Capsules 824
Atretol Tablets (Extremely rare) 569
Atromid-S Capsules 2808
Augmentin (Rare) 2637
Augmentin Tablets (Rare) 2640
Azulfidine (Rare) 2059
Bactrim DS Tablets (Rare) 2257
Bactrim I.V. Infusion 2255
Bactrim (Rare) 2257
Betagan ⊚ 230
Biaxin (Rare) 406
Bleph-10 (Isolated incident) 472
Blephamide Liquifilm Sterile Ophthalmic Suspension 472
▲ Blephamide Ointment (Among most often) ⊚ 234
Calan SR Caplets (1% or less) 2571
Calan Tablets (1% or less) 2568
Capoten Tablets 740
Capozide Tablets 744
Cardizem SR Capsules (Infrequent) 1255
Cardizem Tablets (Infrequent) 1257
Cataflam Tablets (Rare) 833
Ceclor Pulvules & Suspension (Rare) 1470
Cedax 2480
Cefizox for Intramuscular or Intravenous Use 1025
Cefotan 2936
Ceftin 1067
Cefzil Tablets and Oral Suspension (Rare) 747
Celontin Kapseals 1955
Ceptaz 1070
Chibroxin Sterile Ophthalmic Solution (With oral form) 1657
Cipro I.V. (1% or less) 587
Cipro I.V. Pharmacy Bulk Package (Less than 1%) 590
Cipro Tablets 584
Cleocin Phosphate Injection 2068
Cleocin Vaginal Cream (Some cases) 2070
Clinoril Tablets (Less than 1 in 100) 1658
Clozaril Tablets 2377
Cordarone Intravenous (Less than 2%) 2821
Covera-HS Tablets (Less than 2%) 2573
Cytovene-IV (Two or more reports) 2270
Danocrine Capsules (Rare) 2437
Daypro Caplets (Less than 1%) 2578
Depakene 416
Depakote Tablets 418
Diamox Intravenous ⊚ 317
Diamox Sequels (Sustained Release) ⊚ 318
Diamox Tablets ⊚ 317
Didronel Tablets (A single case) 2133
Diflucan Tablets, Injection, and Oral Suspension 2003
Dilacor XR Extended-release Capsules 2183
Dilantin Infatabs 1967
Dilantin Kapseals 1965
Dilantin-125 Suspension 1969
Diupres Tablets 1691
Diuril Oral Suspension 1694
Diuril Sodium Intravenous 1693
Diuril Tablets 1694
Dolobid Tablets (Less than 1 in 100) 1695
Duricef Capsules, Tablets, and Oral Suspension (Rare) 750
DYNACIN Capsules (Rare) 1627
EC-Naprosyn Delayed-Release Tablets (Less than 1%) 2277
Enduron Tablets 424
Engerix-B Unit-Dose Vials 2656
Esidrix Tablets 839
Esimil Tablets 840
FML-S Liquifilm (Rare) ⊚ 240
Fansidar Tablets 2281
Felbatol (Rare) 2774
Feldene Capsules (Less than 1%) 2008
Floxin I.V. 1580
Floxin Tablets (200 mg, 300 mg, 400 mg) 1577
Fortaz 1092
Foscavir Injection (Rare) 541
Fungizone Oral Suspension (Rare) 704
Gantanol Tablets 2285
Gantrisin (Rare) 2286
GlaucTabs ⊚ 209
HydroDIURIL Tablets 1716
Hydropres Tablets 1718
Hyzaar Tablets 1720
IBU Tablets (Less than 1%) 1389
Indocin Capsules (Less than 1%) 1723
Indocin I.V. (Less than 1%) 1727
Indocin (Less than 1%) 1723
Invirase Capsules (Rare) 2291
Isoptin Oral Tablets (Less than 1%) 1393
Isoptin SR Tablets (1% or less) 1395
Keflex Pulvules & Oral Suspension (Rare) 930
Keftab Tablets 931
Kefurox Vials, Faspak & ADD-Vantage 1509
Lamictal Tablets (Rare) 1105
Lamisil Tablets (Isolated reports) 2394
Lariam Tablets 2295
Lescol Capsules (Rare) 2395
Leukeran Tablets (Rare) 1205
Lodine Capsules and Tablets (Less than 1%) 2849
Lopressor HCT Tablets 850
Lorabid Suspension and Pulvules 1513
Lotensin Tablets 852
Lotensin HCT Tablets (Rare) 855
Lotrel Capsules (Rare) 858
LUVOX Tablets 2723
Macrobid Capsules (Rare) 2138
Macrodantin Capsules (Rare) 2140
Maxaquin Tablets 2593
Maxipime for Injection 758
Mesantoin Tablets 2400
Methotrexate Sodium Tablets, Injection, for Injection and LPF Injection 1322
Mevacor Tablets (Rare) 1742
Mexitil Capsules (Rare) 684
Miltown Tablets (Rare) 2780
Minocin Intravenous (Rare) 1428
Minocin Oral Suspension (Rare) 1431
Minocin Pellet-Filled Capsules (Rare) 1429
Mintezol 1747
Moduretic Tablets 1748
Motrin Ibuprofen Suspension, Oral Drops, Chewable Tablets, Caplets (Less than 1%) 1563
Mycostatin Pastilles (Very rare) 713
Nalfon 200 Pulvules & Nalfon Tablets (Less than 1%) 933
Anaprox/Naprosyn (Less than 1%) 2277
NegGram 2453
Neptazane Tablets ⊚ 320
Noroxin Tablets 1758
Noroxin Tablets 2222
Orthoclone OKT3 Sterile Solution 1892
PCE Dispertab Tablets (Rare) 453
Pediazole Suspension 2340
Penetrex Tablets (0.1% to 1%) 2196
Phenobarbital Elixir and Tablets (Rare) 1523
Phenurone Tablets (One case) 455
Pipracil (Rare) 1435
PMB 200 and PMB 400 (Rare) 2890
Pravachol Tablets (Rare) 770
Prilosec Delayed-Release Capsules (Very rare) 516
Primaxin I.M. 1770
Primaxin I.V. 1772
Prinivil Tablets (Rare) 1776
Prinzide Tablets (Rare) 1780
Proloprim Tablets (Rare) 1141
Proventil Syrup (Rare) 2528
Recombivax HB 1787
Redux Capsules 2911
Relafen Tablets (Rare) 2688
SSD 1402
Septra 1146
Septra I.V. Infusion 1142
Septra I.V. Infusion ADD-Vantage Vials (Rare) 1144
Septra 1146
Ser-Ap-Es Tablets 867
Silvadene Cream 1% 1288
Sporanox Capsules (Rare) 1352
Sultrin (Frequent) 1941
Suprax (Less than 2%) 1443
Tagamet (Very rare) 2694
Tazicef for Injection 2697
Tazidime Vials, Faspak & ADD-Vantage 1531
Tegretol/Tegretol-XR (Extremely rare) 870
Tiazac Capsules (Less than 1%) 1019
Ticlid Tablets (Rare) 2317
Timolide Tablets 1791
Tonocard Tablets (Less than 1%) 519
Toradol 2319
Trancopal Caplets (Rare) 2468
Trimpex Tablets (Rare) 2323
Trusopt Sterile Ophthalmic Solution (Rare) 1803
Ultram Tablets (50 mg) (Less than 1%) 1594
Vancocin HCl, Oral Solution & Pulvules (Infrequent) 1536
Vancocin HCl, Vials & ADD-Vantage (Infrequent) 1534
Vantin for Oral Suspension and Vantin Tablets 2112
Vaseretic Tablets 1810
Vasotec I.V. 1814
Vasotec Tablets (0.5% to 1.0%) 1816
Ventolin Syrup (Rare) 1175
Verelan Capsules (1% or less) 1455
Viramune Tablets 2368
Cataflam/Voltaren/Voltaren-XR (Rare) 833
Wellbutrin Tablets 1177
Zarontin Capsules 1986
Zarontin Syrup 1986
Zestoretic Tablets 2968
Zinacef (Rare) 1184
Zocor Tablets (Rare) 1821
Zosyn (Rare) 1463
Zyloprim Tablets (Less than 1%) 1194

Stimulation
Anafranil Capsules (Infrequent) 819
Atamet Tablets 567
Dalmane Capsules (Rare) 2329
Dizac (diazepam injectable emulsion) CIV (Less frequent) 1862
Placidyl Capsules (Occasional) 456
Proventil Tablets 2529
Serax Capsules 2916
Serax Tablets 2916
Sinemet Tablets 959
Sinemet CR Tablets 961
Valium Injectable 2336
Valium Tablets 2335
Xanax Tablets (Rare) 2115

Stinging
Aci-Jel Therapeutic Vaginal Jelly (Occasional cases) 1903
▲ Acular Sterile Ophthalmic Solution (Approximately 40%) 470
Afrin ▣ 757
▲ AKPRO (6%) ⊚ 206
▲ Alomide Ophthalmic Solution (Among most frequent) 465
Americaine Anesthetic Lubricant 1603
Americaine Otic Topical Anesthetic Ear Drops 1603
Attenuvax 1650
Azelex (Approximately 1% to 5%) 471
Bactroban Nasal (2%) 2643
Bactroban Ointment (1.5%) 2642
▲ Betagan (About 1 in 3 patients) ⊚ 230
▲ Betimol 0.25%, 0.5% (One of the two most frequent) ⊚ 259
Biavax II 1653
Bleph-10 472
Chloromycetin Ophthalmic Ointment, 1% (Occasional) ⊚ 298
Chloromycetin Ophthalmic Solution ⊚ 299
Chloroptic S.O.P. ⊚ 236
Chloroptic Sterile Ophthalmic Solution ⊚ 236
Cormax Ointment (Approximately 0.3%) 1856
▲ Cormax Scalp Application (Approximately 10%) 1857
Cortisporin Otic Solution Sterile 1076
Cortisporin Otic Suspension Sterile (Rare) 1077
Cozaar Tablets (Less than 1%) 1668
DesOwen Cream, Ointment and Lotion (Approximately 3%) 1032
Differin Gel (Approximately 1% or less) 1033
▲ Diprivan Injectable Emulsion (10% to 17.6%) 2939
Diprolene AF Cream 0.05% (0.4%) 2489
▲ Diprolene Gel 0.05% (6%) 2490
Doxil 2613
Doxorubicin Astra 531
Dyclone 0.5% and 1% Topical Solutions, USP 535
▲ Elimite (permethrin) 5% Cream (10%) 475
▲ Elocon Cream 0.1% (Approximately 7%) 2492
▲ Elocon Ointment 0.1% (4.8% to approximately 7%) 2494
▲ Exelderm Cream 1.0% (3%) 2794
Exelderm Solution 1.0% (Approximately 1%) 2795
4-Way Fast Acting Nasal Spray (regular & mentholated) ▣ 644
4-Way 12 Hour Nasal Spray ▣ 644
FML Forte Liquifilm ⊚ 237
FML Liquifilm ⊚ 238
FLUORACAINE (Occasional) ⊚ 208
FLURESS (Occasional) ⊚ 208
HMS Liquifilm (Occasional) ⊚ 241
Humorsol Sterile Ophthalmic Solution 1707
Hyzaar Tablets 1720
Idamycin Injection 2096
Imitrex Injection (Infrequent) 1095
Isopto Carpine Ophthalmic Solution ⊚ 221
▲ Lac-Hydrin 12% Lotion (1 in 10 to 30 patients) 2796
▲ Livostin (29%) ⊚ 262
Lotrimin 2514
Lotrisone Cream 2515
M-M-R II 1730
M-R-VAX II 1732
Melanex Topical Solution 1842
Meruvax II 1740
MetroCream (Less than 3%) 1034
Monoclate-P, Factor VIII:C Pasteurized, Monoclonal Antibody Purified Antihemophilic Factor (Human) 802
Mumpsvax 1751
Mutamycin for Injection 712
▲ Naftin Cream 1% (6%) 477
▲ Naftin Gel 1% (5.0%) 477
▲ Nasalide Nasal Solution 0.025% (Approximately 45%) 2301
▲ Nizoral 2% Cream (5%) 1344
Ocufen ⊚ 242
Ocuflox Ophthalmic Solution 478
Ophthetic (Occasional) ⊚ 244
Oxistat (0.1%) 1139
Pandel Cream, 0.1% (2 of 226 patients) 2475
Paremyd ⊚ 244
Pediotic Suspension Sterile (Rare) 1140
Phospholine Iodide ⊚ 323
Polytrim Ophthalmic Solution Sterile 479
Pred Forte ⊚ 247
Pred Mild ⊚ 250
Pred-G Liquifilm Sterile Ophthalmic Suspension ⊚ 248
▲ PROPINE with C CAP Compliance Cap (6%) ⊚ 251
Renova (tretinoin emollient cream) 0.05% (Almost all subjects) 1945
Rubex for Injection 721
▲ Spectazole (econazole nitrate 1%) Cream (3%) 1947
Talwin Injection 2465
Temovate Cream (1%) 1152
▲ Temovate E Emollient (5%) 1154
▲ Temovate Gel (Among most frequent) 1153
Temovate Ointment (Less frequent) 1152
▲ Temovate Scalp Application (29 of 294 patients) 1153
▲ Timoptic in Ocudose (Approximately 1 in 8 patients) 1796
▲ Timoptic Sterile Ophthalmic Solution (Approximately 1 in 8 patients) 1794
▲ Timoptic-XE (1 in 8 patients) 1798
▲ Trusopt Sterile Ophthalmic Solution (Among most frequent) 1803
▲ Ultravate Cream 0.05% (4.4%) 2797
Ultravate Ointment 0.05% (1.6%) 2798
▲ Viroptic Ophthalmic Solution, 1% Sterile (4.6%) 1177

(▣ Described in PDR For Nonprescription Drugs) Incidence data in parenthesis; ▲ 3% or more (⊚ Described in PDR For Ophthalmology)

Stinging · Side Effects Index · 1456

- ▲ Voltaren Ophthalmic Sterile Ophthalmic Solution (15%) ... ⊙ 264
- VōSol (Occasional) ... 2786
- ▲ Xalatan (5% to 15%) ... ⊙ 304
- Xerac AC Solution ... 1990
- ▲ Zonalon Cream (Approximately 21%) ... 1042
- ▲ Zovirax Ointment 5% (28.3%) ... 1190

Stomach, nervous

- Clozaril Tablets (Less than 1%) ... 2377

Stomachache

- ▲ AeroBid Inhaler System (10%) ... 1004
- ▲ Aerobid-M Inhaler System (10%) ... 1004
- Aleve ... 2124
- ▲ Alka-Seltzer Cherry Effervescent Antacid and Pain Reliever (14.5% at doses of 1000 mg/day) ... ▣ 609
- ▲ Alka-Seltzer Lemon Lime Effervescent Antacid and Pain Reliever (14.5% at doses of 1000 mg/day) ... ▣ 609
- ▲ Alka-Seltzer Original Effervescent Antacid and Pain Reliever (14.5% at doses of 1000 mg/day) ... ▣ 609
- Alomide Ophthalmic Solution (Less than 1%) ... 465
- ▲ Regular Strength Ascriptin Tablets (14.5%) ... ▣ 650
- ▲ Genuine Bayer Aspirin Tablets & Caplets (14.5% at doses of 1000 mg/day) ... ▣ 618
- ▲ Aspirin Regimen Bayer Regular Strength 325 mg Caplets (14.5% of 4500 people tested) ... ▣ 613
- Bontril Slow-Release Capsules ... 786
- Brontex ... 2130
- ▲ Bufferin Analgesic Tablets (14.5%) ... ▣ 636
- ▲ Chemet Capsules (5.2% to 15.7%) ... 666
- Cylert Tablets ... 415
- ▲ Ecotrin (14.5% at 1000 mg/day) ... 2625
- Guaifed ... 1833
- ▲ Halfprin Tablets (14.5%) ... 1413
- Intal Inhaler (Rare) ... 2185
- Intal Nebulizer Solution ... 2186
- Invirase Capsules (Less than 2%) ... 2291
- K-Phos Neutral Tablets ... 633
- K-Phos Original Formula 'Sodium Free' Tablets ... 633
- Ortho-Cyclen/Ortho-Tri-Cyclen ... 1914
- Ortho-Cyclen/Ortho Tri-Cyclen ... 1914
- PhosChol ... 488
- Proventil Syrup (Less than 1 of 100 patients) ... 2528
- ▲ SSKI Solution (Among most frequent) ... 2767
- ▲ Serevent Inhalation Aerosol (4%) ... 1149
- ▲ St. Joseph Adult Chewable Aspirin (81 mg.) (14.3% of 4500 patients) ... ▣ 768
- Stadol (1% or greater) ... 779
- Thyro-Block Tablets (Sometimes) ... 2785
- Uroqid-Acid No. 2 Tablets ... 633
- ▲ Ventolin Inhalation Aerosol and Refill (3%) ... 1170
- Ventolin Inhalation Solution (2% to 3%) ... 1171
- Ventolin Rotacaps for Inhalation (2%) ... 1173
- Ventolin Syrup (Less than 1 of 100 patients) ... 1175
- Zofran Injection (2%) ... 1227

Stomatitis

- Actigall Capsules ... 818
- Adapin Capsules ... 1542
- Adriamycin PFS ... 2056
- Adriamycin RDF ... 2056
- ▲ Alferon N Injection (6%) ... 2142
- Anaprox/Naprosyn (Less than 3%) ... 2277
- Aredia for Injection (Up to 1%) ... 827
- Asendin Tablets ... 1419
- Atretol Tablets ... 569
- Atromid-S Capsules ... 2808
- Augmentin ... 2637
- Augmentin Tablets ... 2640
- Azulfidine (Rare) ... 2059
- Bactrim DS Tablets ... 2257
- Bactrim I.V. Infusion ... 2255
- Bactrim ... 2257
- Biaxin ... 406
- Blenoxane ... 697
- CeeNU Capsules (Infrequent) ... 699
- Chloromycetin Sodium Succinate ... 1960
- Claritin Tablets (2% or fewer patients) ... 2485
- Claritin-D Tablets (Less frequent) ... 2487
- Clinoril Tablets (Less than 1 in 100) ... 1658
- Cognex Capsules (Infrequent) ... 1961
- ▲ Cytosar-U Sterile Powder (Among most frequent) ... 2077
- ▲ DaunoXome (1% to 9%) ... 1842
- Daypro Caplets (Less than 1%) ... 2578
- Depakote Tablets (1% to 5%) ... 418
- Dipentum Capsules (1.0%) ... 2084
- Dolobid Tablets (Less than 1 in 100) ... 1695
- ▲ Doxil (5.2% to 6.8%) ... 2613
- Doxorubicin Astra ... 531
- EC-Naprosyn Delayed-Release Tablets (Less than 3%) ... 2277
- Effexor (Infrequent) ... 2825
- Efudex ... 2280
- Elavil ... 2945
- ▲ Ergamisol Tablets (3% to 39%) ... 1340
- Estratest ... 2718
- ▲ Etopophos for Injection (1% to 6%) ... 701
- ▲ Etoposide Injection (1% to 6%) ... 539
- Etrafon ... 2495
- Fansidar Tablets ... 2281
- Feldene Capsules (Greater than 1%) ... 2008
- Flagyl 375 Capsules ... 2587
- Flagyl I.V. ... 2373
- Flexeril Tablets (Rare) ... 1701
- ▲ Fludara for Injection (Up to 9%) ... 658
- Flumadine Tablets & Syrup ... 1013
- Fluorouracil Injection (Rare to common) ... 2282
- Foscavir Injection (Less than 1%) ... 541
- ▲ Sterile FUDR (Among more common) ... 2284
- Gantanol Tablets ... 2285
- Gantrisin ... 2286
- Garamycin Injectable ... 2502
- Gastrocrom Oral Concentrate ... 1611
- ▲ Gemzar for Injection (10% to 15%) ... 1482
- Halcion Tablets ... 2093
- Helidac Therapy (Less than 1%) ... 2135
- ▲ Hivid Tablets (Less than 1% to 3.0%) ... 2287
- ▲ Hycamtin for Injection (Less than 1% to 24%) ... 2665
- Hydrea Capsules (Less frequent) ... 705
- IFEX (Less than 1%) ... 706
- ▲ Intron A for Injection (Less than 5%) ... 2506
- Invirase Capsules (Less than 2%) ... 2291
- Lamictal Tablets (Infrequent) ... 1105
- ▲ Leucovorin Calcium for Injection (16% to 84%) ... 1313
- ▲ Leukine (24% to 62%) ... 1317
- Limbitrol ... 2333
- Ludiomil Tablets (Isolated reports) ... 861
- LUVOX Tablets (Infrequent) ... 2723
- Matulane Capsules ... 2300
- Maxair Autohaler ... 1550
- Maxair Inhaler (Less than 1%) ... 1552
- ▲ Methotrexate Sodium Tablets, Injection, for Injection and LPF Injection (3% to 10%) ... 1322
- MetroGel-Vaginal ... 917
- Miltown Tablets (Rare) ... 2780
- Mithracin ... 599
- Mutamycin for Injection (Frequent) ... 712
- Myochrysine Injection ... 1754
- Naprelan Tablets (Less than 3%) ... 2861
- Anaprox/Naprosyn (Less than 3%) ... 2277
- ▲ Navelbine Injection (Less than 20%) ... 1212
- ▲ Neupogen for Injection (5%) ... 495
- Neurontin Capsules (Infrequent) ... 1978
- Nicotrol NS Nicotine Nasal Spray (Common) ... 1565
- ▲ Nipent for Injection (5% to 12%) ... 2733
- Noroxin Tablets ... 1758
- Noroxin Tablets ... 2222
- Norpramin Tablets ... 1273
- ▲ Novantrone for Injection (18 to 29%) ... 1327
- Omnipen Capsules ... 2872
- Omnipen for Oral Suspension ... 2873
- Orudis Capsules (Greater than 1%) ... 2874
- Oruvail Capsules (Greater than 1%) ... 2874
- OxyContin Tablets (Less than 1%) ... 2163
- Pamelor ... 2409
- Paxil Tablets (Rare) ... 2681
- Pediazole Suspension ... 2340
- Penetrex Tablets (0.1% to 1%) ... 2196
- PMB 200 and PMB 400 (Rare) ... 2890
- Prevacid Delayed-Release Capsules (Less than 1%) ... 2746
- ▲ Proleukin for Injection (32%) ... 812
- Protostat Tablets ... 1939
- Prozac Pulvules & Liquid, Oral Solution (Infrequent) ... 935
- Quadrinal Tablets ... 1398
- Relafen Tablets (1% to 3%) ... 2688
- Remeron Tablets (Infrequent) ... 1878
- ▲ Ridaura Capsules (13%) ... 2691
- Rilutek Tablets (0.8% to 1.2%) ... 2198
- Risperdal Tablets (Infrequent) ... 1348
- Roferon-A Injection (Infrequent) ... 2308
- Rubex for Injection ... 721
- Septra ... 1146
- Septra I.V. Infusion ... 1142
- Septra I.V. Infusion ADD-Vantage Vials ... 1144
- Septra ... 1146
- Serzone Tablets (Infrequent) ... 776
- Sinequan ... 2028
- Solganal Suspension ... 2530
- Spectrobid Tablets ... 2030
- Surmontil Capsules ... 2917
- ▲ Taxotere for Injection Concentrate (42.3%) ... 2204
- Tegretol/Tegretol-XR ... 870
- Testred Capsules, 10 mg ... 1308
- Thioguanine Tablets, Tabloid Brand (Less frequent) ... 1225
- Timentin for Injection ... 2706
- Tofranil Ampuls ... 873
- Tofranil Tablets ... 875
- Tofranil-PM Capsules ... 876
- Tolectin (200, 400 and 600 mg) (Less than 1%) ... 1591
- Tonocard Tablets (Less than 1%) ... 519
- Toradol (Greater than 1%) ... 2319
- Trecator-SC Tablets ... 2919
- Triavil Tablets ... 1800
- Ultram Tablets (50 mg) (Infrequent) ... 1594
- Unasyn ... 2035
- Urobiotic-250 Capsules (Rare) ... 2038
- Vaseretic Tablets ... 1810
- Vasotec I.V. ... 1814
- Vasotec Tablets (0.5% to 1.0%) ... 1816
- Velban Vials (Not common) ... 1537
- ▲ VePesid Capsules and Injection (1% to 6%) ... 727
- ▲ Videx Tablets, Powder for Oral Solution, & Pediatric Powder for Oral Solution (16%) ... 2980
- Vistide Injection ... 1057
- Vivactil Tablets ... 1820
- Wellbutrin Tablets (Frequent) ... 1177
- ▲ Zinecard Injection (26% to 34%) ... 2120
- Zoloft Tablets (Rare) ... 2051
- Zyloprim Tablets (Less than 1%) ... 1194
- Zyrtec Tablets (Less than 2%) ... 2053

Stomatitis, ulcerative

- Anafranil Capsules (Up to 2%) ... 819
- Anaprox/Naprosyn (Less than 1%) ... 2277
- Betaseron for SC Injection ... 653
- Cataflam Tablets (Less than 1%) ... 833
- Cosmegen Injection ... 1666
- Crixivan Capsules (Less than 2%) ... 1670
- Depen Titratable Tablets ... 2770
- Doxil (1% to 5%) ... 2613
- EC-Naprosyn Delayed-Release Tablets (Less than 1%) ... 2277
- Felbatol ... 2774
- Foscavir Injection (Between 1% and 5%) ... 541
- Indocin Capsules (Less than 1%) ... 1723
- Indocin I.V. (Less than 1%) ... 1727
- Indocin (Less than 1%) ... 1723
- Intron A for Injection (Less than 5%) ... 2506
- Lodine Capsules and Tablets (Less than 1%) ... 2849
- ▲ Methotrexate Sodium Tablets, Injection, for Injection and LPF Injection (Among most frequent) ... 1322
- ▲ Naprelan Tablets (Less than 1% to 9%) ... 2861
- Anaprox/Naprosyn (Less than 1%) ... 2277
- Neurontin Capsules (Rare) ... 1978
- Paxil Tablets (Rare to infrequent) ... 2681
- Permax Tablets (Rare) ... 571
- Prozac Pulvules & Liquid, Oral Solution (Infrequent) ... 935
- Remeron Tablets (Rare) ... 1878
- Videx Tablets, Powder for Oral Solution, & Pediatric Powder for Oral Solution (Less than 1%) ... 2980
- Vistide Injection ... 1057
- Cataflam/Voltaren/Voltaren-XR (Less than 1%) ... 833
- Zerit Capsules (Fewer than 1% to 3%) ... 731
- Zoloft Tablets (Rare) ... 2051
- Zosyn (1.0% or less) ... 1463
- Zyrtec Tablets (Less than 2%) ... 2053

Stool, bloody (see under Hematochezia)

Stool, color changes

- Anafranil Capsules (Rare) ... 819
- Coumadin ... 941
- Helidac Therapy ... 2135
- Invirase Capsules (Less than 2%) ... 2291
- Levlen/Tri-Levlen ... 646
- Modicon ... 1928
- Nizoral Tablets ... 1345
- Ortho-Cyclen/Ortho-Tri-Cyclen ... 1914
- Ortho-Novum ... 1928
- Ortho-Cyclen/Ortho Tri-Cyclen ... 1914
- Pepto-Bismol Original Liquid, Original and Cherry Tablets and Easy-To-Swallow Caplets ... 2126
- Pepto-Bismol Maximum Strength Liquid ... 2126
- Questran ... 774
- ReVia Tablets ... 957
- Sporanox Capsules ... 1352
- Ticlid Tablets ... 2317
- Levlen/Tri-Levlen ... 646

Stools, abnormal

- Clozaril Tablets (Less than 1%) ... 2377
- Dynabac (0.1% to 1%) ... 668
- Effexor (Rare) ... 2825
- Hivid Tablets (Less than 1%) ... 2287
- Norvir (Less than 2%) ... 447
- Pentasa (Less than 1%) ... 1275
- ▲ Relafen Tablets (3% to 9%) ... 2688
- ▲ Sandostatin Injection (Less than 10%) ... 2421
- Ultrase MT Capsules (1.5%) ... 2477
- Videx Tablets, Powder for Oral Solution, & Pediatric Powder for Oral Solution (Less than 1%) ... 2980
- Zosyn (1.9% to 2.4%) ... 1463

Stools, loose

- ▲ Acel-Imune Diphtheria and Tetanus Toxoids and Acellular Pertussis Vaccine Adsorbed (3.5%) ... 1415
- Atromid-S Capsules (Less frequent) ... 2808
- ▲ Augmentin (9%) ... 2637
- ▲ Augmentin Tablets (9%) ... 2640
- Cedax (0.1% to 2%) ... 2480
- Cefobid Pharmacy Bulk Package - Not for Direct Infusion (1 in 30) ... 1999
- ▲ Ceftin (3.7% to 8.6%) ... 1067
- ▲ Chemet Capsules (12.0% to 20.9%) ... 666
- Cognex Capsules ... 1961
- Colestid (Less frequent) ... 2073
- Dipentum Capsules ... 2084
- Fluorouracil Injection ... 2282
- Geocillin Tablets ... 2009
- Hivid Tablets (Less than 1%) ... 2287
- Imdur (Less than or equal to 5%) ... 1362
- ▲ Intron A for Injection (Up to 10%) ... 2506
- Kutrase Capsules (Occasional) ... 2546
- Ku-Zyme Capsules ... 2546
- Lumitene ... ▣ 799
- MagTab SR Caplets ... 1844
- ▲ Mesnex Injection (70%) ... 711
- Micro-K LS Packets (Frequent) ... 2238
- Noroxin Tablets (0.3% to 1.0%) ... 1758
- Noroxin Tablets (0.3% to 1.0%) ... 2222
- Norvasc Tablets (Less than or equal to 0.1%) ... 2020
- Pipracil (2%) ... 1435
- ▲ Ridaura Capsules (approx. 50%) ... 2691
- ▲ Sandostatin Injection (4% to 61%) ... 2421
- ▲ Suprax (6%) ... 1443
- Tonocard Tablets (Up to 6.8%) ... 519
- Urocit-K Tablets (Some patients) ... 1828
- ▲ Vantin for Oral Suspension and Vantin Tablets (5.9% to 10.6%) ... 2112
- ▲ Zithromax (2% to 7%) ... 2043
- ▲ Zithromax Tablets (5% to 7%) ... 2046
- ▲ Zoloft Tablets (17.7%) ... 2051

Strabismus

- Anafranil Capsules (Rare) ... 819
- Lamictal Tablets (Rare) ... 1105
- Lioresal Tablets ... 847
- Neurontin Capsules (Rare) ... 1978
- Prozac Pulvules & Liquid, Oral Solution (Rare) ... 935

(▣ Described in PDR For Nonprescription Drugs) Incidence data in parenthesis; ▲ 3% or more (⊙ Described in PDR For Ophthalmology)

1457 **Side Effects Index** **Sulfite, sensitivity to**

▲Videx Tablets, Powder for Oral Solution, & Pediatric Powder for Oral Solution (5%) ... 2980

Striae

Aclovate (Infrequent) ... 1061
Analpram-HC Rectal Cream 1% and 2.5% ... 993
Anusol-HC Cream 2.5% (Infrequent to frequent) ... 1953
▲Blenoxane (Approximately 50%) ... 697
▲Cordran Lotion (More frequent) ... 1854
▲Cordran Tape (More frequent) ... 1855
Cormax Ointment (Infrequent) ... 1856
Cormax Scalp Application (Infrequent) ... 1857
Cortisporin Cream ... 1073
Cortisporin Ointment ... 1074
Cortisporin Otic Solution Sterile ... 1076
Cortisporin Otic Suspension Sterile 1077
Cutivate Cream ... 1078
Cutivate Ointment (Infrequent to more frequent) ... 1078
Decadron Phosphate Topical Cream ... 1686
Decaspray Topical Aerosol ... 1689
Dermatop Emollient Cream 0.1% (Infrequent to frequent) ... 1264
DesOwen Cream, Ointment and Lotion (Infrequent) ... 1032
Diprolene AF Cream 0.05% (Infrequent) ... 2489
Diprolene Gel 0.05% (Infrequent) .. 2490
Diprolene Lotion 0.05% (Infrequent) ... 2491
Diprolene Ointment 0.05% (Infrequent) ... 2491
Elocon Cream 0.1% (Infrequent) ... 2492
Elocon Lotion 0.1% (Infrequent) ... 2493
Elocon Ointment 0.1% (Infrequent) ... 2494
Epifoam (Infrequent) ... 2543
Florinef Acetate Tablets ... 506
Florone/Florone E ... 921
Halog (Infrequent) ... 2795
Hytone ... 922
Hytone Ointment 2 ½% ... 923
Lidex (Infrequent) ... 2299
Locoid Cream, Ointment and Topical Solution (Infrequent) ... 994
Lotrisone Cream (Infrequent) ... 2515
Lupron Depot-PED 7.5 mg, 11.25 mg and 15 mg (Less than 2%) ... 2744
Lupron Injection Pediatric (Less than 2%) ... 2737
Mantadil Cream ... 1124
NeoDecadron Topical Cream ... 1757
Pandel Cream, 0.1% ... 2475
Pediotic Suspension Sterile ... 1140
Pramosone Cream, Lotion & Ointment ... 995
ProctoCream-HC 2.5% (Infrequent to frequent) ... 2552
ProctoFoam-HC ... 2552
Psorcon Cream 0.05% (Infrequent) ... 924
Psorcon Ointment 0.05% ... 923
Synalar (Infrequent) ... 2299
Temovate Cream ... 1152
Temovate E Emollient (Infrequent) 1154
Temovate Gel (Infrequent) ... 1153
Temovate Ointment ... 1152
Temovate Scalp Application (Infrequent) ... 1153
Topicort Emollient Cream 0.25% (Infrequent) ... 1289
Topicort Gel 0.05% (Infrequent) ... 1290
Topicort LP Emollient Cream 0.05% (Infrequent) ... 1289
Topicort Ointment 0.25% (Infrequent) ... 1291
Tridesilon Cream 0.05% (Infrequent) ... 609
Tridesilon Ointment 0.05% (Infrequent) ... 610
Ultravate Cream 0.05% (Infrequently) ... 2797
Ultravate Ointment 0.05% (Infrequent) ... 2798
Westcort Cream 0.2% (Infrequent) ... 2799
Westcort Ointment 0.2% ... 2800

Stridor

Cedax ... 2480
Floxin I.V. ... 1580
Foscavir Injection (Between 1% and 5%) ... 541
Hespan Injection ... 945
Maxaquin Tablets (Less than 1%) .. 2593
Nubain Injection (1% or less) ... 952
Reglan (Rare) ... 2243
Rilutek Tablets (Infrequent) ... 2198
Risperdal Tablets (Infrequent) ... 1348
Salagen Tablets (Less than 1%) ... 1546
Serevent Inhalation Aerosol (Rare) 1149
Zoloft Tablets (Rare) ... 2051

Stroke

Activase (0.9%) ... 1045
Amicar Syrup, Tablets, and Injection ... 1312
Asendin Tablets (Very rare) ... 1419
Betapace Tablets (Less than 1% to 1%) ... 637
Brevicon ... 2563
Clomid ... 1262
Cytovene-IV (Two or more reports) 2270
Danocrine Capsules ... 2437
Demulen ... 2580
Dexatrim ... ◘ 795
Dexatrim Plus Vitamins Caplets .. ◘ 796
DynaCirc Capsules (0.5% to 1%) .. 2381
DynaCirc CR Tablets (0.5% to 1.0%) ... 2383
Elavil ... 2945
Estraderm Transdermal System ... 842
ESTRATAB Tablets (0.3, 0.625, 1.25, 2.5 mg) ... 2715
Estratest ... 2718
Etrafon ... 2495
Flexeril Tablets (Rare) ... 1701
Heparin Lock Flush Solution ... 2831
Heparin Sodium Injection ... 2832
Heparin Sodium Vials ... 1486
Humegon for Injection ... 1873
Imitrex Injection ... 1095
Imitrex Tablets ... 1099
Intron A for Injection (Less than 5%) ... 2506
Limbitrol ... 2333
Ludiomil Tablets (Isolated reports) 861
Lupron Injection ... 2736
Menest Tablets ... 2671
Metrodin (urofollitropin for injection) ... 2616
Modicon ... 1928
Monoket Tablets (Fewer than 1%) 2550
Norinyl ... 2563
Norplant System ... 2868
Norpramin Tablets ... 1273
Nor-Q D Tablets ... 2598
Ortho-Cyclen/Ortho-Tri-Cyclen ... 1914
Ortho Dienestrol Cream ... 1922
Ortho-Novum ... 1928
Ortho-Cyclen/Ortho Tri-Cyclen ... 1914
Ovcon ... 765
Pamelor ... 2409
Parlodel (30 cases) ... 2411
Premarin Intravenous ... 2893
Premarin Vaginal Cream ... 2898
Prinivil Tablets (0.3% to 1.0%) ... 1776
Prinzide Tablets ... 1780
Proleukin for Injection (Less than 1% to 1%) ... 812
Roferon-A Injection (Infrequent) ... 2308
Surmontil Capsules ... 2917
Testoderm Testosterone Transdermal System (Two in 104 patients) ... 486
Tofranil Ampuls ... 873
Tofranil Tablets ... 875
Tofranil-PM Capsules ... 876
Triavil Tablets ... 1800
Tri-Norinyl ... 2607
▲Vesanoid Capsules (3%) ... 2327
Vivactil Tablets ... 1820
Vivelle Transdermal System ... 880
Zestoretic Tablets ... 2968
Zestril Tablets (0.3% to 1.0%) ... 2972

Stroke, hemorrhagic

Activase (0.7%) ... 1045
Demulen ... 2580
Levlen/Tri-Levlen ... 646
Modicon ... 1928
Nor-Q D Tablets ... 2598
Ortho-Cyclen/Ortho-Tri-Cyclen ... 1914
Ortho-Novum ... 1928
Ortho-Cyclen/Ortho Tri-Cyclen ... 1914
Levlen/Tri-Levlen ... 646
Triphasil-21 Tablets ... 2919
Triphasil-28 Tablets ... 2924

Stroke, thrombotic

Levlen/Tri-Levlen ... 646
Ortho-Cyclen/Ortho-Tri-Cyclen ... 1914
Ortho-Cyclen/Ortho Tri-Cyclen ... 1914
Levlen/Tri-Levlen ... 646
Triphasil-21 Tablets ... 2919
Triphasil-28 Tablets ... 2924

Strongyloidiasis hyperinfection

Tagamet (Extremely rare) ... 2694

Stuffiness, nasal (see under Nasal congestion)

Stupor

Ambien Tablets (Infrequent) ... 2559
Anafranil Capsules (Rare) ... 819
Betaseron for SC Injection ... 653
BuSpar Tablets (Rare) ... 738
▲Cerebyx Injection (7.7%) ... 1956
Desyrel and Desyrel Dividose ... 504
Duragesic Transdermal System (Less than 1%) ... 1336
Effexor (Infrequent) ... 2825
Eskalith ... 2658
Felbatol (2.6%) ... 2774
Foscavir Injection (Between 1% and 5%) ... 541
Hivid Tablets (Less than 1%) ... 2287
Kerlone Tablets (Less than 2%) ... 2588
Lamictal Tablets (Infrequent) ... 1105
Lithium Carbonate Capsules & Tablets ... 2352
Lithonate/Lithotabs/Lithobid ... 2721
LUVOX Tablets (Infrequent) ... 2723
Moduretic Tablets (Less than or equal to 1%) ... 1748
Neurontin Capsules (Infrequent) ... 1978
Orthoclone OKT3 Sterile Solution .. 1892
OxyContin Tablets (Less than 1%) 2163
Paxil Tablets (Rare) ... 2681
Permax Tablets (Rare) ... 571
PhosLo Tablets ... 695
ProSom Tablets (Infrequent) ... 457
Prozac Pulvules & Liquid, Oral Solution (Rare) ... 935
Redux Capsules ... 2911
Remeron Tablets (Rare) ... 1878
Rilutek Tablets (Infrequent) ... 2198
Risperdal Tablets (Infrequent) ... 1348
Romazicon (Less than 1%) ... 2311
Serax Capsules ... 2916
Serax Tablets ... 2916
Streptomycin Sulfate Injection ... 2031
Tambocor Tablets (Less than 1%) 1555
Toradol (1% or less) ... 2319

Stye

Cognex Capsules (Infrequent) ... 1961
Crolom (Infrequent) ... ⊙ 254
Intron A for Injection (Less than 5%) ... 2506
Neurontin Capsules (Infrequent) ... 1978

Sudden Infant Death Syndrome

Diphtheria and Tetanus Toxoids and Pertussis Vaccine Adsorbed .. 2650
Felbatol ... 2774

Suicide, attempt of

Ambien Tablets (Rare) ... 2559
Anafranil Capsules (Infrequent) ... 819
Avonex (One patient) ... 662
Betaseron for SC Injection (2%; 1 suicide, 4 attempts) ... 653
Effexor (Infrequent) ... 2825
Felbatol (Infrequent) ... 2774
Floxin I.V. ... 1580
Foscavir Injection (Less than 1%) .. 541
Hivid Tablets (Less than 1%) ... 2287
Imitrex Tablets (Rare) ... 1099
Intron A for Injection (Rare; less than 5%) ... 2506
Invirase Capsules (Rare) ... 2291
Lamictal Tablets (Rare) ... 1105
Levo-Dromoran ... 2297
Lioresal Intrathecal ... 1634
Lupron Depot 3.75 mg (Rare) ... 2739
LUVOX Tablets (Infrequent) ... 2723
Neurontin Capsules (Rare) ... 1978
Paxil Tablets ... 2681
Penetrex Tablets (Rare) ... 2196
Proleukin for Injection ... 812
Redux Capsules (Rare) ... 2911
ReVia Tablets (Less than 1%) ... 957
Rilutek Tablets (Infrequent) ... 2198
Risperdal Tablets (1.2%) ... 1348
Roferon-A Injection ... 2308
Serzone Tablets (Infrequent) ... 776
Symmetrel Capsules (Less than 0.1%) ... 965
Symmetrel Syrup (Less than 0.1%) ... 963
Videx Tablets, Powder for Oral Solution, & Pediatric Powder for Oral Solution (Less than 1%) ... 2980
Vivactil Tablets ... 1820
Xanax Tablets ... 2115
Zoloft Tablets (Infrequent) ... 2051

Suicidal ideation

Ambien Tablets ... 2559
Anafranil Capsules (Infrequent) ... 819
Atamet Tablets ... 567
▲Avonex (4%) ... 662
Betaseron for SC Injection ... 653
BuSpar Tablets (Infrequent) ... 738
Celontin Kapseals (Rare) ... 1955
Cognex Capsules (Rare) ... 1961
Depakote Tablets ... 418
Desyrel and Desyrel Dividose ... 504
Floxin I.V. ... 1580
Floxin Tablets (200 mg, 300 mg, 400 mg) (Rare) ... 1577
Halcion Tablets ... 2093
Hydropres Tablets ... 1718
Intron A for Injection (Rare) ... 2506
Klonopin Tablets ... 2294
Lamictal Tablets (Rare) ... 1105
Lamprene Capsules (Less than 1%) ... 846
Larodopa Tablets (Infrequent) ... 2296
Lioresal Intrathecal ... 1634
Lupron Depot 3.75 mg (Rare) ... 2739
Miltown Tablets ... 2780
Neurontin Capsules (Infrequent) ... 1978
Nizoral Tablets (Rare) ... 1345
Penetrex Tablets (Rare) ... 2196
Prozac Pulvules & Liquid, Oral Solution ... 935
Reglan (Less frequent) ... 2243
Remeron Tablets ... 1878
ReVia Tablets (2%) ... 957
Roferon-A Injection ... 2308
Seromycin Capsules ... 975
Serzone Tablets (Infrequent) ... 776
Sinemet Tablets ... 959
Sinemet CR Tablets ... 961
Symmetrel Capsules (Less than 0.1%) ... 965
Symmetrel Syrup (Less than 0.1%) ... 963
Trilafon ... 2532
Ultram Tablets (50 mg) (Infrequent) ... 1594
Wellbutrin Tablets (Rare) ... 1177
Xanax Tablets ... 2115
Zarontin Capsules (Rare) ... 1986
Zarontin Syrup (Rare) ... 1986
Zoloft Tablets (Infrequent) ... 2051

Sulfhemoglobinemia

Pediazole Suspension ... 2340

Sulfite, sensitivity to

Aldomet Ester HCl Injection ... 1642
Aldomet Oral Suspension ... 1640
Amikacin Sulfate Injection, USP ... 523
Amikacin Sulfate Injection, USP ... 981
Amikin Injectable ... 502
Ana-Kit Anaphylaxis Emergency Treatment Kit ... 611
Antilirium Injectable ... 1007
Aramine Injection ... 1649
Compazine ... 2644
Cortisporin Otic Solution Sterile ... 1076
Dalalone D.P. Injectable ... 1009
Dalgan Injection ... 529
Decadron Phosphate Injection ... 1680
Decadron Phosphate with Xylocaine Injection, Sterile ... 1683
Decadron-LA Sterile Suspension ... 1687
Dilaudid Tablets and Liquid ... 1386
Dobutrex Solution Vials ... 1480
Duranest Injections ... 533
Eldopaque Forte 4% Cream ... 1299
EpiPen ... 808
Garamycin Injectable ... 2502
Hydrocortone Phosphate Injection, Sterile ... 1713
Isuprel Hydrochloride Solution ... 2443
Isuprel Injection ... 2441
Levoprome ... 1321
Mepergan Injection ... 2859
Minocin Oral Suspension ... 1431
Moban Tablets and Concentrate ... 1036
Nebcin Vials, Hyporets & ADD-Vantage ... 1518
NeoDecadron Sterile Ophthalmic Solution ... 1756
Neo-Synephrine Hydrochloride 1% Carpuject ... 2455
Neo-Synephrine Hydrochloride 1% Injection ... 2455
NephrAmine Injection ... 2169
Norflex Injection ... 1554
Novocain Hydrochloride for Spinal Anesthesia ... 2457
Nubain Injection ... 952
Numorphan Injection ... 953
Phenergan Injection ... 2880

(◘ Described in PDR For Nonprescription Drugs) Incidence data in parenthesis; ▲ 3% or more (⊙ Described in PDR For Ophthalmology)

Sulfite, sensitivity to / Side Effects Index

Sulfite, sensitivity to

Pontocaine Hydrochloride for Spinal Anesthesia	2460
Pred Forte	⊙ 247
Pred Mild	⊙ 250
Rowasa	2727
Sensorcaine	554
Septra I.V. Infusion	1142
Septra I.V. Infusion ADD-Vantage Vials	1144
Eldopaque/Eldoquin/Solaquin/Viquin	1299
Stelazine	2692
Streptomycin Sulfate Injection	2031
Sulfacet-R Lotion	925
Sulfacet-R Tint Free Lotion	925
Sulfamylon Cream	940
Talwin Injection	2465
Tensilon Injectable	1307
Tofranil Ampuls	873
Torecan	2367
Tylenol with Codeine (Probably low)	1592
Tylox Capsules	1593
Tympagesic Ear Drops	2476
Vibramycin	2038
Viquin Forte 4% Cream	1299
Xylocaine with Epinephrine Injections	562
Yutopar Intravenous Injection	566

Sunburn

▲ Accutane Capsules (Approximately 1 patient in 20)	2252
Differin Gel (Approximately 1% or less)	1033
Methotrexate Sodium Tablets, Injection, for Injection and LPF Injection	1322
▲ Tegison Capsules (25-50%)	2314

Sunburn, exacerbation of

Imitrex Injection (Rare)	1095

Superinfection

Achromycin V Capsules	1417
Adriamycin PFS	2056
Adriamycin RDF	2056
Ancef Injection	2632
Augmentin	2637
Augmentin Tablets	2640
Ceclor Pulvules & Suspension	1470
Cefotan	2936
Ceftin	1067
Cefzil Tablets and Oral Suspension (1.5%)	747
Ceptaz	1070
Doxorubicin Astra	531
Duricef Capsules, Tablets, and Oral Suspension	750
E-Mycin Tablets	1388
ERYC	1972
Fortaz	1092
Helidac Therapy	2135
Keflex Pulvules & Oral Suspension	930
Kefzol Vials, Faspak & ADD-Vantage	1511
Lorabid Suspension and Pulvules	1513
Macrobid Capsules	2138
Macrodantin Capsules	2140
Minocin Intravenous	1428
Minocin Oral Suspension	1431
Minocin Pellet-Filled Capsules	1429
Monodox Capsules	1858
Pipracil	1435
Primaxin I.M.	1770
Rubex for Injection	721
Streptomycin Sulfate Injection	2031
Suprax	1443
TERAK Ointment	⊙ 210
Vancocin HCl, Vials & ADD-Vantage	1534
Vascor Tablets (200 and 300 mg) (0.5 to 2.0%)	1597
Zinacef	1184

Suppuration

Efudex	2280

Supraventricular contractions, premature

Paxil Tablets (Rare)	2681

Susurrus aurium

Monoket Tablets (Fewer than 1%)	2550

Swallowing

Diprivan Injectable Emulsion (Less than 1%)	2939

Swallowing, impairment

Axocet Capsules (Infrequent)	2469

Capoten Tablets	740
Capozide Tablets	744
Compazine	2644
Coumadin	941
Dantrium Capsules (Less frequent)	2131
Dantrium Intravenous	2132
Esgic-plus Capsules (Infrequent)	1012
Esgic-plus Tablets (Infrequent)	1012
Fioricet Tablets (Infrequent)	2386
Fioricet with Codeine Capsules (Infrequent)	2387
Fiorinal with Codeine Capsules (Infrequent)	2390
Lutrepulse for Injection	998
Mavik Tablets	1407
Monopril Tablets	762
Myochrysine Injection	1754
Neoral (Rare)	2405
Orthoclone OKT3 Sterile Solution	1892
Phrenilin (Infrequent)	790
Prinivil Tablets	1776
Prinzide Tablets	1780
Sandimmune (Rare)	2416
Sedapap Tablets 50 mg/650 mg (Infrequent)	1826
Solganal Suspension	2530
Stelazine	2692
Thorazine	2701
Vaseretic Tablets	1810
Vasotec Tablets	1816
Zestoretic Tablets	2968
Zestril Tablets	2972

Sweat discoloration

Atamet Tablets	567
Lamprene Capsules (Greater than 1%)	846
Mycobutin Capsules	2101
Rifadin	1276
Rifater	1280
Sinemet Tablets	959
Sinemet CR Tablets	961

Sweating
(see under Diaphoresis)

Sweet's syndrome

▲ Vesanoid Capsules (3%)	2327

Swelling

▲ AK-Spore (Among most frequent)	⊙ 205
Americaine Hemorrhoidal Ointment	▥ 649
Atromid-S Capsules	2808
Bactroban Ointment (Less than 1%)	2642
Cafergot	2376
Cipro I.V. Pharmacy Bulk Package (Less than 1%)	590
Cortisporin Ophthalmic Ointment Sterile	1074
Cortisporin Ophthalmic Suspension Sterile	1075
Coumadin	941
D.H.E. 45 Injection	2381
Demulen	2580
Desferal Vials	838
▲ Doxil (3.4%)	2613
Efudex	2280
Exact	▥ 722
Fluorouracil Injection	2282
Hyzaar Tablets (1.3%)	1720
Maxaquin Tablets	2593
Nasalcrom Nasal Solution	2192
Neosporin Ophthalmic Ointment Sterile	1130
Neosporin Ophthalmic Solution Sterile	1131
Oncaspar	2194
Oxandrin	783
PedvaxHIB	1761
Phenobarbital Elixir and Tablets	1523
Quadrinal Tablets	1398
Recombivax HB (Equal to or greater than 1%)	1787
Serevent Inhalation Aerosol (Rare)	1149
Sulfamylon Cream	940
TobraDex Ophthalmic Suspension and Ointment (Less than 4%)	469
Vaqta (Less than 1%)	1805
Versed Injection (Less than 1%)	2324
Viramune Tablets	2368

Swelling, axillary

Depo-Provera Contraceptive Injection (Fewer than 1%)	2079

Swelling, edematous, ankles

Androderm Testosterone Transdermal System	2634

Android Capsules, 10 mg	1297
Eskalith	2658
Estratest	2718
Halotestin Tablets	2095
Lithium Carbonate Capsules & Tablets	2352
Lithonate/Lithotabs/Lithobid	2721
Lo/Ovral Tablets	2852
Lo/Ovral-28 Tablets	2857
Modicon	1928
Ortho-Cyclen/Ortho-Tri-Cyclen	1914
Ortho-Novum	1928
Ortho-Cyclen/Ortho Tri-Cyclen	1914
Ovral Tablets	2877
Ovral-28 Tablets	2878
Ovrette Tablets	2878
Testoderm Testosterone Transdermal System	486
Triphasil-21 Tablets	2919
Triphasil-28 Tablets	2924

Swelling, edematous, wrists

Eskalith	2658
Lithium Carbonate Capsules & Tablets	2352
Lithonate/Lithotabs/Lithobid	2721

Swelling, extremities

Colestid (Infrequent)	2073
Imitrex Injection (Rare)	1095
Noroxin Tablets (Less frequent)	1758
Noroxin Tablets (Less frequent)	2222

Swelling, feet

K-Phos Neutral Tablets	633
Uroqid-Acid No. 2 Tablets	633

Swelling, joint

Ceftin for Oral Suspension (0.1% to 1%)	1067
Cozaar Tablets (Less than 1%)	1668
Danocrine Capsules	2437
Hivid Tablets (1% to 3%)	2287
Hyzaar Tablets	1720
Imitrex Injection (Infrequent)	1095
Intal Inhaler (Infrequent)	2185
Intal Nebulizer Solution	2186
Lithonate/Lithotabs/Lithobid	2721
▲ Mykrox Tablets (3.1%)	1617
NegGram	2453
Neurontin Capsules (Infrequent)	1978
Rifater	1280

Swelling, legs

K-Phos Neutral Tablets	633
Uroqid-Acid No. 2 Tablets	633

Swelling, lower legs
(see under Swelling, legs)

Swelling, mouth

Acel-Imune Diphtheria and Tetanus Toxoids and Acellular Pertussis Vaccine Adsorbed (Rare)	1415
Diphtheria and Tetanus Toxoids and Pertussis Vaccine Adsorbed (Rare)	2650
Felbatol (Rare)	2774
Tambocor Tablets (Less than 1%)	1555
Tetramune (Rare)	1449
Tripedia	908

Swelling, periorbital

Ocuflox Ophthalmic Solution	478
Streptase for Infusion (Rare)	557

Swelling, salivary gland

Eskalith	2658
Flexeril Tablets (Rare)	1701
Norisodrine with Calcium Iodide Syrup	446
Zyloprim Tablets (Less than 1%)	1194

Swelling at injection site

▲ Aredia for Injection (Up to 41%)	827
Attenuvax	1650
Avonex	662
Azactam for Injection (2.4%)	736
Caverject Injection (Less than 1%)	2064
Cerebyx Injection (Infrequent)	1956
Ceredase	1055
Cipro I.V. (1% or less)	587
Cytovene-IV (1% or less)	2270
DDAVP Injection (Occasional)	2178
DDAVP Injection 15 mcg/mL (Occasional)	2179
Desmopressin Acetate Injection (Occasional)	996
Diphtheria and Tetanus Toxoids and Pertussis Vaccine Adsorbed	2650

▲ Engerix-B Unit-Dose Vials (1% to 10%)	2656
Factrel	2996
Floxin I.V. (Approximately 2%)	1580
Geref (sermorelin acetate for injection)	2995
Havrix (1% to 10%)	2663
HibTITER (Less than 1% to 1.7%)	1423
Humalog Injection	1488
Humegon for Injection	1873
Humulin 50/50, 100 Units	1491
Humulin 70/30, 100 Units (Occasional)	1492
Humulin L, 100 Units (Occasional)	1494
Regular, 100 Units (Occasional)	1503
Pork Regular, 100 Units	1507
▲ Imovax Rabies Vaccine (About 25%)	899
INFeD (Iron Dextran Injection, USP)	2478
▲ JE-VAX (2.9% to approximately 20%)	904
▲ Leustatin (9% to 19%)	1889
Levoprome	1321
M-M-R II	1730
M-R-VAX II	1732
Merrem I.V. (0.2%)	2952
Metrodin (urofollitropin for injection)	2616
Pergonal (menotropins for injection, USP)	2618
Pneumovax 23 (Common)	1768
Pnu-Imune 23 (Rare)	1437
Rabies Vaccine Adsorbed (A few patients)	2686
▲ Rabies Vaccine, Imovax Rabies I.D. (About 25%)	901
▲ Supprelin Injection (45%)	2230
Taxol Injection	723
▲ Tetramune (20% to 43%)	1449
Timentin for Injection	2706
▲ Vaqta (1.5% to 13.6%)	1805
▲ Varivax (19.3% to 32.5%)	1807
Velosulin BR Human Insulin 10 ml Vials	1847
WinRho SD (A small number of cases)	1839
Zemuron Injection (Less than 1%)	1885

Syncope

Accupril Tablets (0.5% to 1.0%)	1950
Actimmune (Rare)	1043
Adalat Capsules (10 mg and 20 mg) (Approximately 0.5%)	580
Adalat CC (Rare)	582
AeroBid Inhaler System (1% to 3%)	1004
Aerobid-M Inhaler System (1% to 3%)	1004
AK-FLUOR Injection 10% and 25%	⊙ 204
All-Flex Arcing Spring Diaphragm (See also Ortho Diaphragm Kits)	1921
Altace Capsules (Less than 1% to 2.1%)	1238
Alupent Tablets (0.4%)	672
Ambien Tablets (Infrequent)	2559
Amicar Syrup, Tablets, and Injection	1312
Anafranil Capsules (Up to 2%)	819
Antabuse Tablets	2802
Aredia for Injection (Up to 6%)	827
Asendin Tablets (Less than 1%)	1419
Atamet Tablets	567
Atretol Tablets	569
Atrohist Plus Tablets	1605
▲ Avonex (4%)	662
Axocet Capsules (Infrequent)	2469
Bentyl	1246
Betagan	⊙ 230
Betapace Tablets (1% to 5%)	637
Betaseron for SC Injection	653
Betimol 0.25%, 0.5%	⊙ 259
Blocadren Tablets (0.6%)	1654
Brevibloc (esmolol HCl) Injection (Less than 1%)	1860
Brontex	2130
BuSpar Tablets (Infrequent)	738
Butisol Sodium Elixir & Tablets (Less than 1 in 100)	2768
Calan SR Caplets (1% or less)	2571
Calan Tablets (1% or less)	2568
Capoten Tablets	740
Capozide Tablets	744
Carbocaine Injection	2432
Cardene Capsules (0.8%)	2261
Cardene I.V. (0.7%)	2815
Cardizem CD Capsules (Less than 1%)	1251
Cardizem SR Capsules (Less than 1%)	1255

(▥ Described in PDR For Nonprescription Drugs)   Incidence data in parenthesis; ▲ 3% or more   (⊙ Described in PDR For Ophthalmology)

1459 Side Effects Index Synovitis

Cardizem Injectable (Less than 1%) 1253
Cardizem Tablets (Less than 1%) 1257
▲ Cardura Tablets (0.5% to 23%) 1993
Catapres Tablets (Rare) 679
Catapres-TTS 680
Ceclor Pulvules & Suspension 1470
Cerebyx Injection (Infrequent) 1956
Cipro I.V. (1% or less) 587
Cipro I.V. Pharmacy Bulk Package (Less than 1%) 590
Cipro Tablets (Less than 1%) 584
Claritin Tablets (2% or fewer patients) 2485
Claritin-D Tablets (Less frequent) 2487
Clinoril Tablets (Less than 1%) 1658
Clomid 1262
▲ Clozaril Tablets (More than 5 to 6%) 2377
Cognex Capsules (Frequent) 1961
Corvert Injection (0.3%) 2075
Covera-HS Tablets (Less than 2%) 2573
Cozaar Tablets (Less than 1%) 1668
Crixivan Capsules (Less than 2%) 1670
Cytotec (Infrequent) 2576
Dalmane Capsules (Rare) 2329
Danocrine Capsules 2437
DaunoXome (Less than or equal to 5%) 1842
Demadex Tablets and Injection 691
Demerol 2438
Demulen 2580
Depo-Provera Contraceptive Injection (Fewer than 1%) 2079
Deponit NTG Transdermal Delivery System (Uncommon) 2541
▲ Desyrel and Desyrel Dividose (2.8% to 4.5%) 504
Dilacor XR Extended-release Capsules 2183
Dilatrate-SR Capsules (Uncommon) 2542
Dilaudid-HP Injection (Less frequent) 1384
Dilaudid-HP Lyophilized Powder 250 mg (Less frequent) 1384
Dilaudid Tablets and Liquid 1386
Diprivan Injectable Emulsion (Less than 1%) 2939
Diupres Tablets 1691
Dizac (diazepam injectable emulsion) CIV (Less frequent) 1862
Dolobid Tablets (Rare) 1695
Doxil (Less than 1%) 2613
Duragesic Transdermal System (1% or greater) 1336
Dynabac (0.1% to 1%) 668
DynaCirc Capsules (0.5% to 1%) 2381
DynaCirc CR Tablets (0.5% to 1.0%) 2383
Effexor (Infrequent) 2825
Elavil 2945
▲ Eldepryl Capsules (7 of 49 patients) 2729
Engerix-B Unit-Dose Vials 2656
Esgic-plus Capsules (Infrequent) 1012
Esgic-plus Tablets (Infrequent) 1012
Esimil Tablets 840
Eskalith 2658
Estrace Cream and Tablets 751
Estring Vaginal Ring (1% to 3%) 2086
Ethmozine Tablets (Less than 2%) 2217
Etrafon 2495
Fioricet Tablets (Infrequent) 2386
Fioricet with Codeine Capsules (Infrequent) 2387
Fiorinal with Codeine Capsules (Infrequent) 2390
Flagyl I.V. 2373
Fleet Bisacodyl Enema 1000
Flexeril Tablets (Less than 1%) 1701
Flolan for Injection 1085
Florinef Acetate Tablets 506
Floxin I.V. (Less than 1%) 1580
Floxin Tablets (200 mg, 300 mg, 400 mg) (Less than 1%) 1577
Flumadine Tablets & Syrup (Less than 0.3%) 1013
Fluorescite ◉ 217
Foscavir Injection (Less than 1%) 541
Gamimune N, 5% Immune Globulin Intravenous (Human), 5% 612
Gamimune N, 10% Immune Globulin Intravenous (Human), 10% 615
Glucotrol XL Extended Release Tablets (Less than 3%) 2012
Halcion Tablets 2093
Havrix (Rare) 2663
Helidac Therapy (Less than 1%) 2135
Hismanal Tablets 1341
Hivid Tablets (Less than 1%) 2287
Hydropres Tablets 1718
▲ Hylorel Tablets (7.8%) 1613
▲ Hytrin Capsules (0.5% to 21%) 434
Hyzaar Tablets 1720
Imdur 1362
Imitrex Injection (Infrequent) 1095
Imitrex Tablets (Rare to infrequent) 1099
Indocin (Less than 1%) 1723
INFeD (Iron Dextran Injection, USP) 2478
Intron A for Injection (Less than 5%) 2506
Inversine Tablets 1729
Invirase Capsules (Less than 2%) 2291
Ismelin Tablets 845
Ismo Tablets (Fewer than 1%) 2844
ISMOTIC 45% w/v Solution (Very rare) ◉ 221
Isoptin Oral Tablets (Less than 1%) 1393
Isoptin SR Tablets (1% or less) 1395
Isopto Carbachol Ophthalmic Solution ◉ 221
Isordil Sublingual Tablets (Uncommon) 2845
Isordil Tembids (Uncommon) 2847
Isordil Titradose Tablets (Uncommon) 2848
Kadian Capsules (Less than 3%) 2948
Kerlone Tablets (Less than 2%) 2588
Kytril Tablets (Rare) 2669
Lamictal Tablets (Infrequent) 1105
Lariam Tablets (Less than 1%) 2295
Larodopa Tablets (Relatively frequent) 2296
▲ Leukine (13%) 1317
Levlen/Tri-Levlen 646
▲ Levoprome (Among the most important) 1321
Librax Capsules (Few) 2330
Librium Capsules (Few instances) 2331
Librium Injectable (Isolated instances) 2332
Limbitrol 2333
Lioresal Intrathecal (1% or more) 1634
Lioresal Tablets (Rare) 847
Lodine Capsules and Tablets (Less than 1%) 2849
Lopid Tablets 1974
Lotensin Tablets (0.1%) 852
Lotensin HCT Tablets (0.3% or more) 855
Loxitane 1426
Ludiomil Tablets (Rare) 861
▲ Lupron Depot 3.75 mg (Among most frequent) 2739
Lupron Depot-PED 7.5 mg, 11.25 mg and 15 mg (Less than 2%) 2744
Lupron Injection (Less than 5%) 2736
Lupron Injection Pediatric (Less than 2%) 2737
LUVOX Tablets (Frequent) 2723
MS Contin Tablets (Less frequent) 2149
MSIR (Infrequent) 2152
Marcaine (Rare) 2446
Marcaine Spinal (Rare) 2449
Matulane Capsules 2300
Mavik Tablets (0.2%) 1407
Maxair Autohaler 1550
Maxair Inhaler (Less than 1%) 1552
Maxaquin Tablets (Less than 1%) 2593
Mebaral Tablets (Less than 1 in 100) 2452
Mepergan Injection 2859
Merrem I.V. (0.1% to 1.0%) 2952
Methadone Hydrochloride Oral Concentrate 2356
Methadone Hydrochloride Oral Solution & Tablets 2357
Mexitil Capsules (Less than 1% or about 6 in 1,000) 684
Miltown Tablets 2780
Minipress Capsules (1-4%) 2015
Minizide Capsules (Rare) 2016
Modicon 1928
Moduretic Tablets (Less than or equal to 1%) 1748
Monopril Tablets (0.2% to 1.0%) 762
Mumpsvax 1751
Mutamycin for Injection 712
Mykrox Tablets 1617
Myochrysine Injection 1754
Naprelan Tablets (Less than 1%) 2861
Navane Capsules and Concentrate 2018
Navane Intramuscular 2019
Nembutal Sodium Capsules (Less than 1%) 440
Nembutal Sodium Solution (Less than 1%) 442
Nembutal Sodium Suppositories (Less than 1%) 444
Nescaine/Nescaine MPF 549
Neurontin Capsules (Infrequent) 1978
Nipent for Injection (Less than 3%) 2733
Nitro-Bid IV (Uncommon) 1270
Nitro-Bid Ointment (Uncommon) 1272
Nitro-Dur (nitroglycerin) Transdermal Infusion System (Uncommon) 1365
Nitrostat Tablets 1981
Norflex 1554
Norgesic 1554
Normodyne Injection (Rare) 2519
Normodyne Tablets (Rare) 2522
Norpace (1 to 3%) 2596
Norvasc Tablets (More than 0.1% to 1%) 2020
Norvir (Less than 2%) 447
Nubain Injection (1% or less) 952
Ocupress Ophthalmic Solution, 1% Sterile ◉ 297
Oramorph SR (Morphine Sulfate Sustained Release Tablets) (Less frequent) 2359
Orap Tablets 1037
Ortho-Cyclen/Ortho-Tri-Cyclen 1914
Ortho Diaphragm Kits—All-Flex Arcing Spring; Ortho Coil Spring; Ortho-White Flat Spring 1921
Ortho Diaphragm Kit-Coil Spring 1921
Ortho-Est 1925
Ortho-Novum 1928
Ortho-Cyclen/Ortho Tri-Cyclen 1914
Ortho-White Diaphragm Kit-Flat Spring (See also Ortho Diaphragm Kits) 1921
OxyContin Tablets (Less than 1%) 2163
ParaGard T 380A Intrauterine Copper Contraceptive 1936
▲ Parlodel (0.7% to 8%) 2411
Paxil Tablets (Frequent) 2681
Pediazole Suspension 2340
Penetrex Tablets (0.1% to 1%) 2196
Peptavlon 2997
Periactin 1767
Permax Tablets (2.1%) 571
Phenergan with Codeine 2883
Phenergan Injection 2880
Phenergan Tablets 2882
Phenergan VC with Codeine 2888
Phenobarbital Elixir and Tablets (Less than 1 in 100 patients) 1523
Phrenilin (Infrequent) 790
Placidyl Capsules (Occasional) 456
Plendil Extended-Release Tablets (0.5% to 1.5%) 514
PMB 200 and PMB 400 2890
Pondimin Tablets 2239
Prevacid Delayed-Release Capsules (Less than 1%) 2746
Prinivil Tablets (0.3% to 1.0%) 1776
Prinzide Tablets (0.8% to 0.1%) 1780
Procardia Capsules (Approximately 0.5%; approximately 1 patient in 250) 2024
Procardia XL Extended Release Tablets (1% or less) 2026
▲ Proleukin for Injection (3%) 812
ProSom Tablets (Rare) 457
Prostigmin Injectable 1305
Prostigmin Tablets 1306
Prostin E2 Suppository 2109
Prozac Pulvules & Liquid, Oral Solution (Infrequent) 935
Questran 774
Quinaglute Dura-Tabs Tablets 644
Quinidex Extentabs (Many reports) 2240
RMS Suppositories CII 2766
Recombivax HB 1787
Redux Capsules (Infrequent) 2911
Relafen Tablets (Less than 1%) 2688
Remeron Tablets (Infrequent) 1878
Retrovir Capsules 1216
Retrovir I.V. Infusion 1221
Retrovir Syrup 1216
Rilutek Tablets (Infrequent) 2198
Risperdal Tablets (0.2%) 1348
Robaxin Injectable 2245
Roferon-A Injection (Less than 0.5% to less than 5%) 2308
Roxanol 2365
Rythmol Tablets–150mg, 225mg, 300mg (0.8 to 2.2%) 1399
Salagen Tablets (Less than 1%) 1546
Sandostatin Injection (Less than 1%) 2421
Sanorex Tablets 2423
Sedapap Tablets 50 mg/650 mg (Infrequent) 1826
Seldane Tablets (Rare) 1284
Seldane-D Extended-Release Tablets (Rare) 1286
Sensorcaine 554
Ser-Ap-Es Tablets 867
Serax Capsules (Rare) 2916
Serax Tablets (Rare) 2916
Serentil 689
Serzone Tablets (Infrequent) 776
Sinemet Tablets 959
Sinemet CR Tablets 961
Solganal Suspension 2530
Soma Compound w/Codeine Tablets (Infrequent or rare) 2784
Soma Compound Tablets (Infrequent or rare) 2783
Soma Tablets 2782
Sorbitrate (Uncommon) 2959
Stadol 779
Sular Tablets (Less than or equal to 1%) 2961
Supprelin Injection (1% to 3%) 2230
Talacen Caplets (Infrequent) 2464
Talwin Injection (Rare) 2465
Talwin Compound (Infrequent) 2466
Talwin Injection 2465
Talwin Nx Tablets 2467
Tambocor Tablets (1% to less than 3%) 1555
Taxol Injection (Approximately 1%; rare) 723
Taxotere for Injection Concentrate 2204
Tegison Capsules (Less than 1%) 2314
Tegretol/Tegretol-XR 870
Tenex Tablets (Less frequent) 2249
Tenoretic Tablets 2963
Tenormin Tablets and I.V. Injection 2965
Thorazine 2701
THYREL TRH (A small number of patients) 2992
Tiazac Capsules (Less than 1%) 1019
Timolide Tablets (Less than 1%) 1791
Timoptic in Ocudose (Less frequent) 1796
Timoptic Sterile Ophthalmic Solution (Less frequent) 1794
Timoptic-XE 1798
Tofranil Tablets 875
Tonocard Tablets (Less than 1%) 519
Toprol-XL Tablets (About 1 of 100 patients) 560
Toradol (1% or less) 2319
Trandate (Rare) 1158
▲ Transderm-Nitro Transdermal Therapeutic System (4%) 878
Levlen/Tri-Levlen 646
Ultram Tablets (50 mg) (Less than 1%) 1594
Univasc Tablets (Less than 1%; 0.51%) 2553
Urecholine 1804
Valium Injectable 2336
Vantin for Oral Suspension and Vantin Tablets (Less than 1%) 2112
Vascor Tablets (200 and 300 mg) (0.5 to 2.0%) 1597
Vaseretic Tablets (0.5% to 2.0%) 1810
Vasotec I.V. (0.5%) 1814
Vasotec Tablets (0.5% to 2.2%) 1816
Verelan Capsules (1% or less) 1455
Versed Injection (Less than 1%) 2324
Videx Tablets, Powder for Oral Solution, & Pediatric Powder for Oral Solution (Up to 3%) 2980
Visken Tablets (2% or fewer patients) 2428
Vistide Injection 1057
Vivelle Transdermal System 880
Wellbutrin Tablets (1.2%) 1177
▲ Xanax Tablets (3.1% to 3.8%) 2115
Zaroxolyn Tablets 1625
Zerit Capsules (Fewer than 1% to 1%) 731
Zestoretic Tablets (0.1 to 0.8%) 2968
Zestril Tablets (0.1% to 1.8%) 2972
Ziac 1459
Zofran Injection (Rare) 1227
Zoloft Tablets (Infrequent) 2051
Zosyn (1.0% or less) 1463

Synovia, immunological destruction

Solganal Suspension 2530

Synovitis

Avonex 662
Cuprimine Capsules (Some patients) 1673
Depen Titratable Tablets 2770
Foscavir Injection (Less than 1%) 541

(▣ Described in PDR For Nonprescription Drugs) Incidence data in parenthesis; ▲ 3% or more (◉ Described in PDR For Ophthalmology)

Synovitis Side Effects Index 1460

Lopid Tablets 1974

Systemic lupus erythematosus (see under Lupus erythematosus, systemic)

SGOT changes

Atamet Tablets 567
▲ Avonex (3%) 662
Bumex (0.6%) 2260
Doral Tablets (1.3%) 2773
▲ Emcyt Capsules (2% to 34%) 2085
Epivir (Up to 1.7%) 1200
Humegon for Injection (Occasional) 1873
▲ Roferon-A Injection (1% to 46%) 2308
Sinemet Tablets 959
Sinemet CR Tablets 961

SGOT elevation

Abelcet Injection 1540
Accutane Capsules 2252
Adalat CC (Rare) 582
Ambien Tablets (Rare) 2559
Amoxil 2631
Anafranil Capsules (Approximately 1%) 819
Anaprox/Naprosyn (Less than 1%) 2277
Ancef Injection 2632
Arimidex Tablets (2% to 5%) 2932
Asacol Delayed-Release Tablets 2129
Atamet Tablets 567
Atromid-S Capsules 2808
Augmentin 2637
Augmentin Tablets 2640
Axid Pulvules (Less common) 1468
Azactam for Injection (Less than 1%) 736
▲ Betaseron for SC Injection (4%) 653
Biaxin (Less than 1%) 406
BuSpar Tablets (Infrequent) 738
Calan SR Caplets 2571
Calan Tablets 2568
Calcijex Injection 412
Cardizem CD Capsules (Less than 1%) 1251
Cardizem SR Capsules (Less than 1%) 1255
Cardizem Injectable (Less than 1%) 1253
Cardizem Tablets (Less than 1%) 1257
Casodex Tablets (2% to 5%) 2934
Cataflam Tablets (About 1% to about 4%) 833
Ceclor Pulvules & Suspension (1 in 40) 1470
Cedax (0.1% to 1%) 2480
Cefizox for Intramuscular or Intravenous Use (1% to 5%) 1025
Cefotan (1 in 300) 2936
Ceftin (2.0%) 1067
Cefzil Tablets and Oral Suspension (2%) 747
▲ CellCept Capsules (More than or equal to 3%) 2265
Ceptaz (One in 16) 1070
▲ Chemet Capsules (4.2% to 10.4%) 666
Chibroxin Sterile Ophthalmic Solution (With oral form) 1657
▲ Cipro I.V. (Among most frequent) 587
▲ Cipro I.V. Pharmacy Bulk Package (Among most frequent) 590
Cipro Tablets (1.7%) 584
Claforan Sterile and Injection (Less than 1%) 1259
Colestid (One or more occasions) 2073
Cordarone Intravenous (Common) 2821
Cordarone Tablets 2818
Covera-HS Tablets (1.4%) 2573
Crixivan Capsules (Less than 1% to 3.1%) 1670
Cytovene (1% or less) 2270
DDAVP Tablets 2182
Dalgan Injection (Less than 1%) 529
Dalmane Capsules (Rare) 2329
Daypro Caplets (Under 1% of patients) 2578
Demser Capsules (Rare) 1690
Depakene (Frequent) 416
Depakote Tablets (Frequent) 418
Diflucan Tablets, Injection, and Oral Suspension 2003
Dilacor XR Extended-release Capsules (Rare) 2183
Dipentum Capsules (Rare) 2084
Duricef Capsules, Tablets, and Oral Suspension 750
Dynabac (0.1% to 1%) 668
EC-Naprosyn Delayed-Release Tablets (Less than 1%) 2277
Effexor (Infrequent) 2825
Elspar 1700
Eulexin Capsules 2498
Felbatol (Frequent) 2774
Feldene Capsules (Less than 1%) 2008
Floxin I.V. (More than or equal to 1%) 1580
Floxin Tablets (200 mg, 300 mg, 400 mg) (More than or equal to 1%) 1577
▲ Fortaz (1 in 16) 1092
Foscavir Injection (Between 1% and 5%) 541
Fungizone Intravenous 507
Garamycin Injectable 2502
▲ Gemzar for Injection (52% to 78%) 1482
Geocillin Tablets 2009
Glucotrol Tablets (Occasional) 2011
Glucotrol XL Extended Release Tablets (Occasional) 2012
Heparin Lock Flush Solution 2831
Heparin Sodium Injection 2832
Heparin Sodium Vials (A high percentage of patients) 1486
▲ Hivid Tablets (Less than 1% to 7.6%) 2287
Hycamtin for Injection (Less than 1% to 5%) 2665
▲ Imdur (Less than or equal to 5%) 1362
Imuran 1103
▲ Intron A for Injection (Up to 63% of patients) 2506
Invirase Capsules (Less than 1%) 2291
Isoptin Oral Tablets 1393
Isoptin SR Tablets 1395
Keflex Pulvules & Oral Suspension 930
Keftab Tablets 931
▲ Kefurox Vials, Faspak & ADD-Vantage (1 in 25) 1509
Kefzol Vials, Faspak & ADD-Vantage (Rare) 1511
Kerlone Tablets (Less than 2%) 2588
Kytril Injection (2.8%) 2667
▲ Kytril Tablets (5%) 2669
Lamprene Capsules (Less than 1%) 846
Larodopa Tablets (Rare) 2296
Lioresal Tablets 847
Lopid Tablets (Occasional) 1974
Lorabid Suspension and Pulvules 1513
Lotensin HCT Tablets 855
Lovenox Injection (Up to 4% of patients) 2187
Loxitane 1426
Macrobid Capsules (1% to 5%) 2138
Macrodantin Capsules 2140
Mandol Vials, Faspak & ADD-Vantage 1516
Marinol (Dronabinol) Capsules (Less than 1%) 2353
Maxaquin Tablets 2593
Maxipime for Injection (2.4%) 758
Mefoxin 1734
Mefoxin Premixed Intravenous Solution 1737
▲ Mepron Suspension (4%) 1206
Merrem I.V. (Greater than 0.2%) 2952
Mexitil Capsules (About 1%) 684
Mezlin 594
Mezlin Pharmacy Bulk Package 597
Mithracin 599
Monocid Injection (1.6%) 2674
Motrin Ibuprofen Suspension, Oral Drops, Chewable Tablets, Caplets (Less than 1%) 1563
▲ Mycelex Troches (About 15%) 601
▲ Mycobutin Capsules (7%) 2101
Nalfon 200 Pulvules & Nalfon Tablets (Less than 1%) 933
Naprelan Tablets (Less than 1%) 2861
Anaprox/Naprosyn (Less than 1%) 2277
▲ Navelbine Injection (1% to 54%) 1212
Nebcin Vials, Hyporets & ADD-Vantage 1518
▲ Neutrexin for Injection (13.8%) 2761
▲ Nolvadex Tablets (4.8%) 2957
Noroxin Tablets (1.4% to 1.6%) 1758
Noroxin Tablets (1.4% to 1.6%) 2222
Nydrazid Injection 509
Omnipen Capsules 2872
Omnipen for Oral Suspension 2873
Oncaspar (Greater than 1% but less than 5%) 2194
Orthoclone OKT3 Sterile Solution 1892
Orudis Capsules 2874
Oruvail Capsules 2874
Oxandrin 783
▲ Paraplatin for Injection (15% to 23%) 713
Parlodel 2411
Paxil Tablets (Infrequent) 2681
Penetrex Tablets (Less than 1% but more than or equal to 0.1%) 2196
Pentasa (Less than 1%) 1275
Pipracil (Less frequent) 1435
Platinol for Injection 717
Platinol-AQ Injection 719
Pravachol Tablets 770
Prevacid Delayed-Release Capsules (Less than 1%) 2746
Prilosec Delayed-Release Capsules (Rare) 516
Primaxin I.M. 1770
Primaxin I.V. 1772
Procardia Capsules (Rare) 2024
Procardia XL Extended Release Tablets (Rare) 2026
Proglycem Suspension 575
▲ Prograf (Greater than 3%) 1028
ProSom Tablets (Rare) 457
Remeron Tablets (Rare) 1878
Revex (nalmefene hydrochloride injection) (0.3%) 1863
Rifamate Capsules 1278
Rifater 1280
Risperdal Tablets (Infrequent) 1348
Rocaltrol Capsules 2303
▲ Rocephin Injectable Vials, ADD-Vantage, Galaxy Container (3.1%) 2305
Sectral Capsules 2914
Serzone Tablets (Infrequent) 776
Sinemet Tablets 959
Spectrobid Tablets 2030
Suprax (Less than 2%) 1443
Synarel Nasal Solution for Endometriosis (One patient) 2605
▲ Taxol Injection (19%) 723
▲ Tazicef for Injection (1 in 16 patients) 2697
▲ Tazidime Vials, Faspak & ADD-Vantage (1 in 16) 1531
▲ Tegison Capsules (18%) 2314
Tiazac Capsules (Less than 1%) 1019
Ticar for Injection 2704
Timentin for Injection 2706
Tornalate Solution for Inhalation, 0.2% (Less than 1%) 976
Tornalate Metered Dose Inhaler (Rare) 978
Unasyn 2035
Vantin for Oral Suspension and Vantin Tablets 2112
Verelan Capsules 1455
▲ Videx Tablets, Powder for Oral Solution, & Pediatric Powder for Oral Solution (6% to 9%) 2980
Viramune Tablets (2.0%) 2368
Vistide Injection 1057
Cataflam/Voltaren/Voltaren-XR (About 1% to about 4%) 833
Winstrol Tablets 2468
Xanax Tablets (Less than 1% to 3.2%) 2115
▲ Zanosar Sterile Powder (A number of patients) 2119
Zebeta Tablets (One to two times normal) 1457
▲ Zerit Capsules (6% to 63%) 731
▲ Zinacef (1 in 25 patients) 1184
Zithromax (1% to 2%) 2043
Zithromax Tablets (1% to 2%) 2046
Zocor Tablets 1821
▲ Zofran Injection (Approximately 5% of patients) 1227
Zofran Tablets (Approximately 1% to 2%) 1231
Zoladex (Less than 1% of all patients) 2976
Zoladex 3-month 2978
Zoloft Tablets (Infrequent) 2051
Zosyn 1463
Zyloprim Tablets (Less than 1%) 1194

SGPT changes

Atamet Tablets 567
Bumex (0.5%) 2260
Cataflam Tablets (About 1% to about 4%) 833
Humegon for Injection (Occasional) 1873
Sinemet Tablets 959
Sinemet CR Tablets 961
Cataflam/Voltaren/Voltaren-XR (About 1% to about 4%) 833

SGPT elevation

Abelcet Injection 1540
Accutane Capsules 2252
Adalat CC (Rare) 582
Ambien Tablets (Infrequent) 2559
Anafranil Capsules (Approximately 3%) 819
Anaprox/Naprosyn (Less than 1%) 2277
Ancef Injection 2632
Arimidex Tablets (2% to 5%) 2932
Asacol Delayed-Release Tablets 2129
Atamet Tablets 567
Atromid-S Capsules 2808
Augmentin 2637
Augmentin Tablets 2640
Axid Pulvules (Less common) 1468
Azactam for Injection (Less than 1%) 736
▲ Betaseron for SC Injection (19%) 653
Biaxin (Less than 1%) 406
BuSpar Tablets (Infrequent) 738
Calan SR Caplets 2571
Calan Tablets 2568
Calcijex Injection 412
Cardizem CD Capsules (Less than 1%) 1251
Cardizem SR Capsules (Less than 1%) 1255
Cardizem Injectable 1253
Cardizem Tablets (Less than 1%) 1257
Casodex Tablets (2% to 5%) 2934
Ceclor Pulvules & Suspension (1 in 40) 1470
Cedax (0.1% to 1%) 2480
Cefizox for Intramuscular or Intravenous Use (1% to 5%) 1025
Cefotan (1 in 150) 2936
Ceftin (1.6%) 1067
Cefzil Tablets and Oral Suspension (2%) 747
▲ CellCept Capsules (More than or equal to 3%) 2265
Ceptaz (One in 15) 1070
▲ Chemet Capsules (4.2% to 10.4%) 666
Chibroxin Sterile Ophthalmic Solution (With oral form) 1657
▲ Cipro I.V. (Among most frequent) 587
▲ Cipro I.V. Pharmacy Bulk Package (Among most frequent) 590
Cipro Tablets (1.9%) 584
Claforan Sterile and Injection (Less than 1%) 1259
Colestid (One or more occasions) 2073
Cordarone Intravenous (Common) 2821
Cordarone Tablets 2818
Covera-HS Tablets (1.4%) 2573
Crixivan Capsules (Less than 1% to 2.1%) 1670
Cytovene (1% or less) 2270
Dalmane Capsules (Rare) 2329
Depakene (Frequent) 416
Depakote Tablets (Frequent) 418
Dilacor XR Extended-release Capsules (Rare) 2183
Dipentum Capsules (Rare) 2084
Doral Tablets (Less than 1%) 2773
Doxil (1% to 5%) 2613
Duricef Capsules, Tablets, and Oral Suspension 750
Dynabac (0.1% to 1%) 668
EC-Naprosyn Delayed-Release Tablets (Less than 1%) 2277
Effexor (Rare) 2825
Elspar 1700
▲ Epivir (3.7% to 4%) 1200
Eulexin Capsules 2498
▲ Felbatol (3.5% to 5.2%) 2774
Feldene Capsules (Less than 1%) 2008
Floxin I.V. (More than or equal to 1%) 1580
Floxin Tablets (200 mg, 300 mg, 400 mg) (More than or equal to 1%) 1577
▲ Fortaz (1 in 15) 1092
Foscavir Injection (Between 1% and 5%) 541
Fungizone Intravenous 507
Garamycin Injectable 2502
▲ Gemzar for Injection (38% to 72%) 1482
Heparin Lock Flush Solution 2831
Heparin Sodium Injection 2832
▲ Heparin Sodium Vials (A high percentage of patients) 1486
Hivid Tablets (Less than 1%) 2287
Hycamtin for Injection (Less than 1% to 5%) 2665
Imdur (Less than or equal to 5%) 1362
Imuran 1103
▲ Intron A for Injection (Up to 15% of patients) 2506

1461 **Side Effects Index** **Tachycardia**

Invirase Capsules (Less than 1%) .. 2291
Isoptin Oral Tablets ... 1393
Isoptin SR Tablets ... 1395
Keflex Pulvules & Oral Suspension 930
Keftab Tablets ... 931
▲Kefurox Vials, Faspak & ADD-Vantage (1 in 25) ... 1509
Kefzol Vials, Faspak & ADD-Vantage (Rare) ... 1511
Kerlone Tablets (Less than 2%) ... 2588
▲Kytril Injection (3.3%) ... 2667
▲Kytril Tablets (6%) ... 2669
Larodopa Tablets (Rare) ... 2296
▲Leukine (13%) ... 1317
Lopid Tablets (Occasional) ... 1974
Lorabid Suspension and Pulvules ... 1513
Lotensin HCT Tablets ... 855
Lovenox Injection (Up to 4% of patients) ... 2187
Loxitane ... 1426
Macrobid Capsules (1% to 5%) ... 2138
Macrodantin Capsules ... 2140
Mandol Vials, Faspak & ADD-Vantage ... 1516
Marinol (Dronabinol) Capsules (Less than 1%) ... 2353
Mavik Tablets (0.3% to 1.0%) ... 1407
Maxaquin Tablets ... 2593
Maxipime for Injection (2.8%) ... 758
Mefoxin ... 1734
Mefoxin Premixed Intravenous Solution ... 1737
▲Mepron Suspension (6%) ... 1206
Merrem I.V. (Greater than 0.2%) ... 2952
Mezlin ... 594
Mezlin Pharmacy Bulk Package ... 597
Mithracin ... 599
Monocid Injection (1.6%) ... 2674
Motrin Ibuprofen Suspension, Oral Drops, Chewable Tablets, Caplets (Less than 1%) ... 1563
▲Mycobutin Capsules (9%) ... 2101
Naprelan Tablets (Less than 1%) .. 2861
Anaprox/Naprosyn (Less than 1%) ... 2277
Nebcin Vials, Hyporets & ADD-Vantage ... 1518
▲Neutrexin for Injection (11.0%) ... 2761
Nimotop Capsules (0.2%; rare) ... 603
Noroxin Tablets (1.4%) ... 1758
Noroxin Tablets (1.4%) ... 2222
Nydrazid Injection ... 509
▲Oncaspar (Greater than 5%) ... 2194
Orthoclone OKT3 Sterile Solution .. 1892
Orudis Capsules ... 2874
Oruvail Capsules ... 2874
Parlodel ... 2411
Paxil Tablets (Infrequent) ... 2681
Penetrex Tablets (Less than 1% but more than or equal to 0.1%) 2196
Pentasa (Less than 1%) ... 1275
Pipracil (Less frequent) ... 1435
Plendil Extended-Release Tablets (0.5% to 1.5%) ... 514
Pravachol Tablets ... 770
Prevacid Delayed-Release Capsules (Less than 1%) ... 2746
Prilosec Delayed-Release Capsules (Rare) ... 516
Primaxin I.M. ... 1770
Primaxin I.V. ... 1772
Procardia Capsules (Rare) ... 2024
Procardia XL Extended Release Tablets (Rare) ... 2026
Proglycem Capsules ... 575
▲Prograf (Greater than 3%) ... 1028
Remeron Tablets (Rare; 2.0%) ... 1878
Rifamate Capsules ... 1278
Rifater ... 1280
Risperdal Tablets (Infrequent) ... 1348
Rocaltrol Capsules ... 2303
▲Rocephin Injectable Vials, ADD-Vantage, Galaxy Container (3.3%) ... 2305
Sectral Capsules ... 2914
Serzone Tablets (Infrequent) ... 776
Sinemet Tablets ... 959
Suprax (Less than 2%) ... 1443
Synarel Nasal Solution for Endometriosis (One patient) ... 2605
▲Tazicef for Injection (1 in 15 patients) ... 2697
▲Tazidime Vials, Faspak & ADD-Vantage (1 in 15) ... 1531
▲Tegison Capsules (23%) ... 2314
Tiazac Capsules (Less than 1%) ... 1019
Ticar for Injection ... 2704
▲Tilade Inhaler (3.3%) ... 2207
Timentin for Injection ... 2706
Tornalate Solution for Inhalation, 0.2% (Less than 1%) ... 976
Trasylol ... 607
Unasyn ... 2035
Vantin for Oral Suspension and Vantin Tablets ... 2112
Vascor Tablets (200 and 300 mg) (0.5 to 2.0%) ... 1597
Verelan Capsules ... 1455
▲Videx Tablets, Powder for Oral Solution, & Pediatric Powder for Oral Solution (6% to 9%) ... 2980
▲Viramune Tablets (3.4%) ... 2368
Vistide Injection ... 1057
Zantac ... 1182
Zantac Injection ... 1180
Zantac Syrup ... 1182
Zebeta Tablets (One to two times normal) ... 1457
▲Zerit Capsules (10% to 65%) ... 731
▲Zinacef (1 in 25 patients) ... 1184
Zithromax (1% to 2%) ... 2043
Zithromax Tablets (1% to 2%) ... 2046
Zocor Tablets ... 1821
▲Zofran Injection (Approximately 5% of patients) ... 1227
Zofran Tablets (Approximately 1% to 2%) ... 1231
Zoladex (Less than 1% of all patients) ... 2976
Zoladex 3-month ... 2978
Zoloft Tablets (Infrequent) ... 2051
Zosyn ... 1463
Zyloprim Tablets (Less than 1%) ... 1194

SIADH secretion syndrome
(see under ADH syndrome, inappropriate)

SLE-like syndrome
(see under Lupus erythematosus, systemic)

ST section changes
(see under EKG changes, ST section)

S_3 gallop
(see under Ventricular gallop)

T

T-wave flattening
(see under EKG changes, T-wave)

Tachyarrhythmia

Actimmune (Rare) ... 1043
Isuprel Injection ... 2441

Tachyarrhythmia, ventricular

Seldane Tablets (Rare) ... 1284
Seldane-D Extended-Release Tablets (Rare) ... 1286

Tachyarrhythmias, supraventricular

Claritin Tablets (Rare) ... 2485
Lanoxicaps ... 1110
Lanoxin Elixir Pediatric ... 1113
Lanoxin Injection ... 1116
Lanoxin Injection Pediatric ... 1119
Lanoxin Tablets ... 1121

Tachycardia

Abbokinase ... 403
Abbokinase Open-Cath ... 405
Accupril Tablets (0.5% to 1.0%) .. 1950
Accutane Capsules (Less than 1%) ... 2252
Acthrel for Injection ... 2990
Adalat CC (Less than 1.0%) ... 582
Adapin Capsules (Occasional) ... 1542
Adderall Tablets ... 2209
Adipex-P Tablets and Capsules ... 1035
AeroBid Inhaler System (1% to 3%) ... 1004
Aerobid-M Inhaler System (1% to 3%) ... 1004
Airet Albuterol Sulfate Inhalation Solution (1%) ... 1602
AKPRO ... ⊙ 206
Albuterol Sulfate, USP Solution for Inhalation, Arm-a-Med (1%) ... 522
▲Alfenta Injection (12%) ... 1334
Alkeran for Injection (In some patients) ... 1196
Alupent (Less than 1%) ... 672
Ambien Tablets (Infrequent) ... 2559
▲Anafranil Capsules (2% to approximately 20%) ... 819
Anectine ... 1062
Apresazide Capsules (Common) ... 824
Apresoline Hydrochloride Tablets (Common) ... 826
Aredia for Injection (Up to 6%) ... 827
Artane ... 1418
Asendin Tablets (Less than 1%) ... 1419
Atrohist Plus Tablets ... 1605
Atrovent Inhalation Aerosol (Less frequent) ... 674
Atrovent Inhalation Solution (Less than 3%) ... 675
Atrovent Nasal Spray 0.03% ... 676
Atrovent Nasal Spray 0.06% (Less than 1%) ... 678
Axocet Capsules (Infrequent) ... 2469
Bellergal-S Tablets (Rare) ... 2375
Benadryl Injection ... 1955
Bentyl ... 1246
▲Betaseron for SC Injection (6%) ... 653
Bontril Slow-Release Capsules ... 786
▲Brethaire Inhaler (About 5 per 100) ... 830
Brethine Ampuls (1.3 to 1.5%) ... 832
Bronkometer Aerosol ... 2432
Bronkosol Solution ... 2432
Brontex ... 2130
Buprenex Injectable (Less than 1%) ... 2170
BuSpar Tablets (1%) ... 738
Cafergot ... 2376
Capoten Tablets (Approximately 1 of 100 patients) ... 740
Capozide Tablets (Approximately 1 of 1000 patients) ... 744
Carbocaine Injection ... 2432
Cardene Capsules (0.8% to 3.4%) 2261
▲Cardene I.V. (3.5%) ... 2815
Cardizem CD Capsules (Less than 1%) ... 1251
Cardizem SR Capsules (Less than 1%) ... 1255
Cardizem Injectable ... 1253
Cardizem Tablets (Less than 1%) .. 1257
Cardura Tablets (0.3% to 0.9%) .. 1993
Cartrol Tablets ... 413
Cataflam Tablets (Less than 1%) ... 833
Catapres Tablets (About 5 in 1,000 patients) ... 679
Catapres-TTS ... 680
Ceftin (0.1% to 1%) ... 1067
▲CellCept Capsules (More than or equal to 3%) ... 2265
Cerebyx Injection (2.2%) ... 1956
Cipro I.V. (1% or less) ... 587
Cipro I.V. Pharmacy Bulk Package (Less than 1%) ... 590
Claritin Tablets (2% or fewer patients) ... 2485
Claritin-D Tablets (Less frequent) .. 2487
Clinoril Tablets (Less than 1 in 100) ... 1658
Clomid ... 1262
▲Clozaril Tablets (More than 5 to 25%) ... 2377
Cogentin ... 1661
Cognex Capsules (Infrequent) ... 1961
Colestid (Infrequent) ... 2073
Combipres Tablets (About 5 in 1,000) ... 682
Compazine ... 2644
Corvert Injection (2.7%) ... 2075
Cozaar Tablets (Less than 1%) ... 1668
Cystospaz ... 2123
Cytadren Tablets (1 in 40) ... 837
D.A. II Tablets ... 972
D.A. Chewable Tablets ... 970
D.H.E. 45 Injection ... 2381
Dantrium Capsules (Less frequent) 2131
Dapsone Tablets USP ... 1331
DaunoXome (Less than or equal to 5%) ... 1842
Deconsal II Tablets ... 1605
Demadex Tablets and Injection ... 691
Demerol ... 2438
Depakote Tablets (1% to 5%) ... 418
Depo-Provera Contraceptive Injection (Fewer than 1%) ... 2079
Desferal Vials ... 838
Desoxyn Gradumet Tablets ... 422
Desyrel and Desyrel Dividose (Up to 7%) ... 504
Dexedrine ... 2648
DextroStat-Dextroamphetamine Sulfate Tablets ... 2211
Dibenzyline Capsules ... 2650
Dilacor XR Extended-release Capsules (Infrequent) ... 2183
Dilaudid-HP Injection (Less frequent) ... 1384
Dilaudid-HP Lyophilized Powder 250 mg (Less frequent) ... 1384
Dilaudid Tablets and Liquid ... 1386
Dipentum Capsules (Rare) ... 2084
Diprivan Injectable Emulsion (Less than 1%) ... 2939
Ditropan ... 1267
Donnagel Liquid and Donnagel Chewable Tablets (Rare) ... ▣ 854
Donnatal ... 2234
Donnatal Extentabs ... 2234
Donnatal Tablets ... 2234
Doxil (1% to 5%) ... 2613
Dura-Tap/PD Capsules ... 970
Dura-Vent/DA Tablets ... 972
Dura-Vent Tablets ... 971
Dyazide Capsules ... 2653
DynaCirc Capsules (1.0% to 3.4%) ... 2381
DynaCirc CR Tablets (0.5% to 1.0%) ... 2383
Effexor (2%) ... 2825
Elavil ... 2945
Eldepryl Capsules ... 2729
Engerix-B Unit-Dose Vials ... 2656
Entex PSE Tablets ... 973
EpiPen Jr.- Epinephrine Auto-Injector ... 808
Epogen for Injection (0.31%) ... 489
Esgic-plus Capsules (Infrequent) ... 1012
Esgic-plus Tablets (Infrequent) ... 1012
Esidrix Tablets ... 839
▲Etopophos for Injection (3%) ... 701
Etoposide Injection (0.7% to 2%) .. 539
Etrafon ... 2495
Factrel (Rare) ... 2996
Fastin Capsules ... 2662
Fedahist Gyrocaps ... 2545
Felbatol (Frequent) ... 2774
Fioricet Tablets (Infrequent) ... 2386
Fioricet with Codeine Capsules (Infrequent) ... 2387
Fiorinal with Codeine Capsules (Infrequent) ... 2390
Flexeril Tablets (Less than 1%) ... 1701
▲Flolan for Injection (1% to 35%) ... 1085
Floxin I.V. ... 1580
Floxin Tablets (200 mg, 300 mg, 400 mg) ... 1577
Flumadine Tablets & Syrup (Less than 0.3%) ... 1013
Gamimune N, 5% Immune Globulin Intravenous (Human), 5% (One patient) ... 612
Gamimune N, 10% Immune Globulin Intravenous (Human), 10% (One patient) ... 615
Gammar-P I.V., Immune Globulin Intravenous (Human) ... 798
Ganite ... 2711
Gastrocrom Oral Concentrate (Less common) ... 1611
Guaifed ... 1833
Guaimax-D Tablets ... 809
Habitrol Nicotine Transdermal System (Occasionally) ... 884
Halcion Tablets (0.9% to 0.5%) ... 2093
Haldol Decanoate ... 1587
Haldol Injection, Tablets and Concentrate ... 1585
Hespan Injection ... 945
Histussin D Liquid ... 670
Hivid Tablets (Less than 1%) ... 2287
Humegon for Injection ... 1873
Hycomine Compound Tablets ... 948
Hycomine ... 947
Hydralazine Hydrochloride Injection USP (Common) ... 2712
Hytrin Capsules (0.6% to 1.9%) ... 434
Hyzaar Tablets ... 1720
Imdur (Less than or equal to 5%) .. 1362
Imitrex Injection (Infrequent) ... 1095
Imitrex Tablets (Infrequent) ... 1099
▲Inapsine Injection (Among most common) ... 462
Indocin Capsules (Less than 1%) ... 1723
Indocin I.V. (Less than 1%) ... 1727
Indocin (Less than 1%) ... 1723
INFeD (Iron Dextran Injection, USP) ... 2478
Intron A for Injection (Less than 5%) ... 2506
Ionamin Capsules ... 1615
Isoetharine Inhalation Solution, USP, Arm-a-Med ... 545
Isoptin Injectable (1.0%) ... 1391
Isuprel Hydrochloride Solution ... 2443
Isuprel Injection ... 2441
Isuprel Mistometer ... 2442
K-Phos Neutral Tablets ... 633
Kadian Capsules (Less than 3%) ... 2948
Kutrase Capsules ... 2546
Kytril Injection (Rare) ... 2667
Lamictal Tablets (Infrequent) ... 1105

(▣ Described in PDR For Nonprescription Drugs) Incidence data in parenthesis; ▲ 3% or more (⊙ Described in PDR For Ophthalmology)

Tachycardia Side Effects Index 1462

Lasix Injection, Oral Solution and Tablets 1267
▲ Leukine (11%) 1317
▲ Leustatin (6%) 1889
Levbid Extended-Release Tablets (No incidence data in labeling) 2549
Levo-Dromoran 2297
Levoprome 1321
Levsin/Levsinex/Levbid 2549
Librium Injectable 2332
Limbitrol 2333
Lioresal Intrathecal (1% or more) 1634
Lomotil 2591
Lotensin HCT Tablets (0.3% or more) 855
Loxitane 1426
Ludiomil Tablets (Rare) 861
Lufyllin & Lufyllin-400 Tablets 2778
Lufyllin-GG Elixir & Tablets 2779
▲ Lupron Depot 3.75 mg (Among most frequent; less than 5%) 2739
Lutrepulse for Injection 998
LUVOX Tablets (Frequent) 2723
MS Contin Tablets (Less frequent) 2149
MSIR (Infrequent) 2152
Marax Tablets & DF Syrup 2015
Marcaine (Rare) 2446
Marcaine Spinal (Rare) 2449
Marinol (Dronabinol) Capsules (1%) 2353
Matulane Capsules 2300
Maxair Autohaler (1.2% to 1.3%) 1550
Maxair Inhaler (1.2%) 1552
Maxaquin Tablets (Less than 1%) 2593
Mellaril 2398
Mepergan Injection 2859
Merrem I.V. (0.1% to 1.0%) 2952
▲ Metaproterenol Sulfate Inhalation Solution, USP, Arm-a-Med (About 1 in 7 patients) 547
Methadone Hydrochloride Oral Concentrate 2356
Metubine Iodide Vials 932
Miacalcin Nasal Spray (Less than 1%) 2403
Miltown Tablets 2780
Minipress Capsules (Less than 1%) 2015
Minizide Capsules (Rare) 2016
Mivacron (Less than 1%) 1125
Moban Tablets and Concentrate 1036
Moduretic Tablets (Less than or equal to 1%) 1748
Monoket Tablets (Fewer than 1%) 2550
Monopril Tablets (0.4% to 1.0%) 762
Motofen Tablets 789
Nalfon 200 Pulvules & Nalfon Tablets (Less than 1%) 933
Naprelan Tablets (Less than 1%) 2861
Narcan Injection 950
Nardil (Less frequent) 1977
Navane Capsules and Concentrate 2018
Navane Intramuscular 2019
Nescaine/Nescaine MPF 549
Neupogen for Injection 495
Neurontin Capsules (Infrequent) 1978
Nicotrol NS Nicotine Nasal Spray 1565
Nimotop Capsules (Up to 1.4%) 603
Nipent for Injection (Less than 3%) 2733
Norcuron for Injection (Rare) 1875
Norflex 1554
Norgesic 1554
Norisodrine with Calcium Iodide Syrup 446
Normodyne Injection 2519
Normodyne Tablets 2522
Norpramin Tablets 1273
Norvasc Tablets (More than 0.1% to 1%) 2020
Norvir (Less than 2%) 447
Novahistine DMX ▣ 782
Novahistine Elixir ▣ 782
Novantrone for Injection 1327
Nubain Injection (1% or less) 952
Oncaspar (Greater than 1% but less than 5%) 2194
Oramorph SR (Morphine Sulfate Sustained Release Tablets) (Less frequent) 2359
Orap Tablets 1037
Oretic Tablets 450
Orlaam Oral Solution 2361
Ornade Spansule Capsules 2678
▲ Orthoclone OKT3 Sterile Solution (10%) 1892
Orudis Capsules (Less than 1%) 2874
Oruvail Capsules (Less than 1%) 2874
PBZ Tablets 863
PBZ-SR Tablets 862
Pamelor 2409
Paremyd ⊙ 244
Parnate Tablets 2679
Paxil Tablets (Frequent) 2681
Pediazole Suspension 2340
Penetrex Tablets (0.1% to 1%) 2196
Peptavlon 2997
Pergonal (menotropins for injection, USP) 2618
Periactin 1767
Permax Tablets (Infrequent) 571
Phenergan with Codeine 2883
Phenergan Injection 2880
Phenergan Tablets 2882
Phenergan VC with Codeine 2888
Phrenilin (Infrequent) 790
Platinol for Injection (Occasional) 717
Platinol-AQ Injection (Occasional) 719
Plendil Extended-Release Tablets (0.5% to 1.5%) 514
PMB 200 and PMB 400 2890
Prelu-2 Timed Release Capsules 687
Prilosec Delayed-Release Capsules (Less than 1%) 516
Primaxin I.M. 1770
Primaxin I.V. (Less than 0.2%) 1772
Prinzide Tablets 1780
Priscoline Hydrochloride Ampuls 864
Pro-Banthine Tablets 2226
Procardia XL Extended Release Tablets (1% or less) 2026
Procrit for Injection (0.31%) 1896
Proglycem (Common) 575
▲ Prograf (Greater than 3%) 1028
Prolastin Alpha$_1$-Proteinase Inhibitor (Human) (Occasional) 629
Prolixin 510
PROPINE with C CAP Compliance Cap ⊙ 251
Propulsid (Rare) 1346
Prostep (nicotine transdermal system) (Occasional) 1439
Prostigmin Injectable 1305
Prostigmin Tablets 1306
Protopam Chloride for Injection 2909
▲ Proventil Inhalation Aerosol (10%) 2524
Proventil Inhalation Solution 0.083% (1%) 2527
▲ Proventil Repetabs Tablets (5%) 2529
Proventil Solution for Inhalation 0.5% (1%) 2525
Proventil Syrup (1 of 100 patients; children 2 to 6 years, 2%) 2528
▲ Proventil Tablets (5%) 2529
Prozac Pulvules & Liquid, Oral Solution (Infrequent) 935
Quadrinal Tablets 1398
Quibron 2227
Recombivax HB 1787
Redux Capsules (Infrequent) 2911
Regitine Vials 864
Respbid Tablets 687
RespiGam (1%) 1631
ReVia Tablets (Less than 1%) 957
▲ Revex (nalmefene hydrochloride injection) (5%) 1863
Rilutek Tablets (1.3% to 2.0%) 2198
▲ Risperdal Tablets (3% to 5%) 1348
Ritalin 866
Robinul Forte Tablets 2247
Robinul Injectable 2247
Robinul Tablets 2247
Romazicon (Less than 1%) 2311
Salagen Tablets (2%) 1546
Sandimmune 2416
Sandostatin Injection (Less than 1%) 2421
▲ Sanorex Tablets (Among most common) 2423
Sansert Tablets 2424
Sedapap Tablets 50 mg/650 mg (Infrequent) 1826
Seldane-D Extended-Release Tablets 1286
Semprex-D Capsules 1620
Sensorcaine (Rare) 554
Ser-Ap-Es Tablets 867
Serentil 689
Serevent Inhalation Aerosol (1% to 3%) 1149
Serzone Tablets (Infrequent) 776
Sinequan (Occasional) 2028
Slo-bid Gyrocaps 2201
Soma Compound w/Codeine Tablets 2784
Soma Compound Tablets 2783
Soma Tablets 2782
Stadol (Infrequent) 779
Stelazine 2692
Stimate, (desmopressin acetate) Nasal Spray, 1.5 mg/mL 806
Sufenta Injection (0.3% to 1%) 1355
Supprelin Injection (1% to 3%) 2230
Suprane (desflurane, USP) (Greater than 1%) 1865
Surmontil Capsules 2917
Survanta Beractant Intratracheal Suspension 2346
Symmetrel Capsules (Uncommon) 965
Symmetrel Syrup (Uncommon) 963
Syn-Rx Tablets 1622
Syn-Rx DM Tablets 1623
Tagamet (Rare) 2694
Talacen Caplets (Infrequent) 2464
Talwin Injection (Rare) 2465
Talwin Compound (Infrequent) 2466
Talwin Injection 2465
Talwin Nx Tablets 2467
Tambocor Tablets (1% to less than 3%) 1555
Tavist Syrup 2426
Tavist Tablets 2427
Taxol Injection (2%) 723
Taxotere for Injection Concentrate 2204
Tenex Tablets (Less frequent) 2249
Tenoretic Tablets 2963
Tenormin Tablets and I.V. Injection 2965
Thalitone (Common) 1293
Theo-24 Extended Release Capsules 2753
Theo-X Extended-Release Tablets 793
Thorazine 2701
Tiazac Capsules (Less than 1% to 1%) 1019
Tofranil Ampuls 873
Tofranil Tablets 875
Tofranil-PM Capsules 876
▲ Tonocard Tablets (3.2%) 519
▲ Tornalate Solution for Inhalation, 0.2% (3.7%) 976
Tornalate Metered Dose Inhaler (Less than 1%) 978
Tracrium Injection 1155
Trasylol (2%) 607
Trental Tablets (Rare) 1291
Triavil Tablets 1800
Trilafon 2532
Trinalin Repetabs Tablets 1373
▲ Triostat Injection (3%) 2708
Tussend 1830
Tussend Expectorant 1831
Ultram Tablets (50 mg) (Less than 1%) 1594
Urispas Tablets 2710
Uroqid-Acid No. 2 Tablets 633
Vaseretic Tablets (0.5% to 2.0%) 1810
▲ Ventolin Inhalation Aerosol and Refill (10 in 100 patients) 1170
Ventolin Inhalation Solution (1%) 1171
Ventolin Nebules Inhalation Solution (1%) 1172
Ventolin Syrup (1 of 100 patients; 2% in children) 1175
▲ Ventolin Tablets (5 of 100 patients) 1176
VePesid Capsules and Injection (0.7% to 2%) 727
Versed Injection (Less than 1%) 2324
Videx Tablets, Powder for Oral Solution, & Pediatric Powder for Oral Solution (Less than 1%) 2980
Virazole (Infrequent) 1310
Visken Tablets (2% or fewer patients) 2428
Vistide Injection 1057
Vivactil Tablets 1820
Volmax Extended-Release Tablets (2.7%) 1835
Cataflam/Voltaren/Voltaren-XR (Less than 1%) 833
▲ Vumon for Injection (Approximately 5%) 729
▲ Wellbutrin Tablets (10.8%) 1177
Wigraine Tablets 1884
▲ Xanax Tablets (7.7% to 15.4%) 2115
Yocon Tablets 1235
Zantac (Rare) 1182
Zantac Injection (Rare) 1180
Zantac Syrup (Rare) 1182
Zaroxolyn Tablets 1625
Zemuron Injection (Less than 1%) 1885
Zestoretic Tablets 2968
Zofran Injection (Rare) 1227
Zofran Tablets (Rare) 1231
Zoladex (1% or greater) 2976
Zoladex 3-month 2978
Zoloft Tablets (Infrequent) 2051
Zosyn (1.0% or less) 1463
Zyrtec Tablets (Less than 2%) 2053

Tachycardia, junctional

▲ Lanoxicaps (Among most common) 1110
▲ Lanoxin Injection Pediatric (Among most common) 1119
Romazicon (1 of 446 patients) 2311

Tachycardia, persistent (maternal)

▲ Yutopar Intravenous Injection (80% to 100%) 566

Tachycardia, reflux

Urecholine 1804

Tachycardia, supraventricular

Cardene I.V. (0.7%) 2815
Corvert Injection (2.7%) 2075
Diprivan Injectable Emulsion (Less than 1%) 2939
Felbatol (Rare) 2774
▲ Flolan for Injection (8%) 1085
Fludara for Injection (Up to 3%) 658
Hytrin Capsules (Occasional) 434
Ismo Tablets (Fewer than 1%) 2844
Proleukin for Injection (Less than 1%) 812
Reglan 2243
ReoPro Vials (1.0%) 1526
Rilutek Tablets (Rare) 2198
Rythmol Tablets–150mg, 225mg, 300mg (Less than 1%) 1399
Sodium Polystyrene Sulfonate Suspension 2367
Sular Tablets (Less than or equal to 1%) 2961
Taxol Injection (Rare) 723
▲ Tenormin Tablets and I.V. Injection (11.5%) 2965
▲ Trasylol (4%) 607
Zosyn (1.0% or less) 1463

Tachycardia, ventricular

Activase 1045
Adenocard Injection 1021
Adenoscan 1022
Ambien Tablets (Rare) 2559
Anafranil Capsules (Rare) 819
Aramine Injection 1649
Axid Pulvules (2 individuals) 1468
Betapace Tablets 637
Biaxin (Rare) 406
Cardene Capsules (Less than 0.4%) 2261
Cardene I.V. (0.7%) 2815
Cardene SR Capsules (Rare) 2264
Cardioquin Tablets 2146
Cardizem Injectable (Less than 1%) 1253
Cordarone Intravenous (2.4%) 2821
Corvert Injection (0.2% to 4.9%) 2075
Cozaar Tablets (Less than 1%) 1668
Demadex Tablets and Injection 691
Desyrel and Desyrel Dividose (Two patients) 504
Diprivan Injectable Emulsion (Less than 1%) 2939
Dobutrex Solution Vials (Rare) 1480
Dynabac (Rare) 668
E.E.S. (Occasional reports) 427
Eminase 2215
EryPed (Occasional reports) 425
Ery-Tab Tablets (Occasional reports) 426
Erythrocin Stearate Filmtab (Occasional reports) 429
Erythromycin Base Filmtab (Occasional reports) 430
Erythromycin Delayed-Release Capsules, USP (Occasional reports) 431
▲ Ethmozine Tablets (2% to 5%) 2217
Hyperstat I.V. Injection 2504
Hyzaar Tablets 1720
Ilosone (Rare) 927
Ilotycin Gluceptate, IV, Vials (Rare) 929
Imdur (Less than or equal to 5%) 1362
Imitrex Injection (Extremely rare) 1095
Imitrex Tablets (Rare) 1099
Lanoxicaps 1110
Lanoxin Elixir Pediatric 1113
Lanoxin Injection 1116
Lanoxin Injection Pediatric 1119
Lanoxin Tablets 1121
Marcaine 2446
Nalfon 200 Pulvules & Nalfon Tablets (Less than 1%) 933
Narcan Injection (Several instances) 950
Norpace 2596
Norpramin Tablets 1273

(▣ Described in PDR For Nonprescription Drugs) Incidence data in parenthesis; ▲ 3% or more (⊙ Described in PDR For Ophthalmology)

Side Effects Index — Taste, bad

Norvasc Tablets (More than 0.1% to 1%) ... 2020
PCE Dispertab Tablets (Rare) ... 453
Parlodel (Less than 1%) ... 2411
Pediazole Suspension ... 2340
Permax Tablets (Infrequent) ... 571
Primacor Injection (1% to 2.8%) ... 2461
Prinivil Tablets (0.3% to 1.0%) ... 1776
Prinzide Tablets ... 1780
Propulsid (Rare) ... 1346
Quinaglute Dura-Tabs Tablets ... 644
Quinidex Extentabs ... 2240
Redux Capsules ... 2911
Rilutek Tablets (Rare) ... 2198
Risperdal Tablets (Rare) ... 1348
Romazicon (1 of 446 patients) ... 2311
Rythmol Tablets–150mg, 225mg, 300mg (1.4 to 3.4%) ... 1399
Seldane Tablets (Rare) ... 1284
Seldane-D Extended-Release Tablets (Rare) ... 1286
Sensorcaine ... 554
Sodium Polystyrene Sulfonate Suspension ... 2367
Survanta Beractant Intratracheal Suspension ... 2346
Tambocor Tablets (0.4%) ... 1555
Taxol Injection (Approximately 1%) ... 723
▲ Tenormin Tablets and I.V. Injection (16%) ... 2965
▲ Trasylol (6%) ... 607
Vascor Tablets (200 and 300 mg) (0.5 to 2.0%) ... 1597
Yutopar Intravenous Injection ... 566
Zestril Tablets (0.3% to 1.0%) ... 2972
Zosyn (1.0% or less) ... 1463

Tachypnea

Abelcet Injection ... 1540
Actimmune (Rare) ... 1043
Diprivan Injectable Emulsion (Less than 1%) ... 2939
Dopram Injectable ... 2235
▲ Fungizone Intravenous (Among most common) ... 507
Hespan Injection ... 945
Humegon for Injection ... 1873
Lufyllin & Lufyllin-400 Tablets ... 2778
Lufyllin-GG Elixir & Tablets ... 2779
Nardil (Less frequent) ... 1977
Orthoclone OKT3 Sterile Solution ... 1892
Pergonal (menotropins for injection, USP) ... 2618
▲ Proleukin for Injection (8%) ... 812
Quadrinal Tablets ... 1398
Quibron ... 2227
Respbid Tablets ... 687
RespiGam (1%) ... 1631
Retrovir Capsules ... 1216
Retrovir I.V. Infusion ... 1221
Retrovir Syrup ... 1216
Roferon-A Injection (Infrequent) ... 2308
Sensorcaine ... 554
Slo-bid Gyrocaps ... 2201
Sulfamylon Cream ... 940
Survanta Beractant Intratracheal Suspension ... 2346
Symmetrel Capsules (Uncommon) ... 965
Symmetrel Syrup (Uncommon) ... 963
Theo-Dur Extended-Release Tablets ... 1367
Theo-X Extended-Release Tablets ... 793
Uni-Dur Extended-Release Tablets ... 1374
Versed Injection (Less than 1%) ... 2324

Talkativeness

Alupent Tablets (0.2%) ... 672
Atretol Tablets ... 569
Dalmane Capsules ... 2329
Tegretol/Tegretol-XR ... 870
Xanax Tablets (2.2%) ... 2115

Tardive dyskinesia

Asendin Tablets (Rare) ... 1419
BuSpar Tablets (Rare) ... 738
Clozaril Tablets ... 2377
Cognex Capsules (Rare) ... 1961
Compazine ... 2644
Depakote Tablets (1% to 5%) ... 418
Desyrel and Desyrel Dividose ... 504
Elavil ... 2945
Eldepryl Capsules ... 2729
Etrafon ... 2495
Haldol Decanoate ... 1587
Haldol Injection, Tablets and Concentrate ... 1585
Loxitane ... 1426
LUVOX Tablets (Rare) ... 2723
Mellaril ... 2398
Moban Tablets and Concentrate ... 1036

Navane Capsules and Concentrate ... 2018
Navane Intramuscular ... 2019
Orap Tablets ... 1037
Prolixin ... 510
Reglan ... 2243
Risperdal Tablets ... 1348
Serentil ... 689
Sinequan (Infrequent) ... 2028
Stelazine ... 2692
Thorazine ... 2701
Triavil Tablets ... 1800
Trilafon ... 2532
Wellbutrin Tablets ... 1177

Tardive dystonia
(see under Dystonia, tardive)

Taste, altered

Adalat CC (Rare) ... 582
Adapin Capsules ... 1542
Alferon N Injection (1%) ... 2142
Altace Capsules (Less than 1%) ... 1238
Ambien Tablets (Infrequent) ... 2559
▲ Anafranil Capsules (4% to 8%) ... 819
AquaMEPHYTON Injection ... 1648
Asacol Delayed-Release Tablets ... 2129
Atrovent Nasal Spray 0.03% (Less than 2%) ... 676
Atrovent Nasal Spray 0.06% (Less than 1%) ... 678
Azactam for Injection (Less than 1%) ... 736
Bactroban Nasal (0.8% to 3%) ... 2643
Betaseron for SC Injection ... 653
▲ Biaxin (3%) ... 406
Brevibloc (esmolol HCl) Injection ... 1860
BuSpar Tablets (Infrequent) ... 738
Capoten Tablets (Approximately 2 to 4 of 100 patients) ... 740
Capozide Tablets (Approximately 2 to 4 of 100 patients) ... 744
Cardura Tablets (Less than 0.5% of 3960 patients) ... 1993
Cataflam Tablets (Less than 1%) ... 833
Catapres-TTS (1 of 101 patients) ... 680
Cedax (0.1% to 1%) ... 2480
▲ Cerebyx Injection (3.3%; frequent) ... 1956
Claritin Tablets (2% or fewer patients) ... 2485
Claritin-D Tablets (Less frequent) ... 2487
Cognex Capsules (Infrequent) ... 1961
Cordarone Tablets (1 to 3%) ... 2818
Cozaar Tablets (Less than 1%) ... 1668
Crixivan Capsules (Less than 2% to 2.6%) ... 1670
▲ Cuprimine Capsules (12%) ... 1673
Cytotec (Infrequent) ... 2576
Cytovene (1% or less) ... 2270
Dantrium Capsules (Less frequent) ... 2131
DaunoXome (Less than or equal to 5%) ... 1842
Daypro Caplets (Less than 1%) ... 2578
Depakote Tablets (1% to 5%) ... 418
Diamox Intravenous ... ⊚ 317
Diamox Sequels (Sustained Release) ... ⊚ 318
Diamox Tablets ... ⊚ 317
▲ Didronel I.V. Infusion (5%) ... 1545
Diflucan Tablets, Injection, and Oral Suspension (1%) ... 2003
Dilacor XR Extended-release Capsules ... 2183
Dilaudid-HP Injection (Less frequent) ... 1384
Dilaudid-HP Lyophilized Powder 250 mg (Less frequent) ... 1384
Dilaudid Tablets and Liquid ... 1386
Diprivan Injectable Emulsion (Less than 1%) ... 2939
Doral Tablets ... 2773
Doxil (Less than 1%) ... 2613
Dynabac (0.1% to 1%) ... 668
Effexor (2%) ... 2825
Eldepryl Capsules ... 2729
▲ Ergamisol Tablets (8%) ... 1340
Eskalith ... 2658
▲ Etopophos for Injection (6%) ... 701
FML Forte Liquifilm ... ⊚ 237
FML Liquifilm ... ⊚ 238
▲ Felbatol (6.1%) ... 2774
Floxin I.V. ... 1580
Floxin Tablets (200 mg, 300 mg, 400 mg) ... 1577
Flumadine Tablets & Syrup (Less than 0.3%) ... 1013
Fosamax Tablets (0.5%) ... 1703
Foscavir Injection (Between 1% and 5%) ... 541
Gastrocrom Capsules (Infrequent) ... 1611
Gastrocrom Oral Concentrate (Less common) ... 1611

Geref (sermorelin acetate for injection) ... 2995
GlaucTabs ... ⊚ 209
Halcion Tablets (Rare) ... 2093
Helixate, Antihemophilic Factor (Recombinant) ... 799
Hivid Tablets (Less than 1%) ... 2287
Hyperstat I.V. Injection ... 2504
Hyzaar Tablets ... 1720
Imitrex Injection (Infrequent) ... 1095
Imitrex Tablets ... 1099
INFeD (Iron Dextran Injection, USP) ... 2478
▲ Intron A for Injection (Up to 24%) ... 2506
Invirase Capsules (Less than 2%) ... 2291
IOPIDINE Sterile Ophthalmic Solution ... ⊚ 218
▲ Iopidine 0.5% (3%) ... ⊚ 219
Kerlone Tablets (Less than 2%) ... 2588
KOGENATE Antihemophilic Factor (Recombinant) ... 626
Kytril Injection (2%) ... 2667
Lamictal Tablets (Infrequent) ... 1105
Lamisil Tablets (2.8%) ... 2394
Lamprene Capsules (Less than 1%) ... 846
Lescol Capsules ... 2395
Limbitrol ... 2333
Lioresal Tablets (Rare) ... 847
Lithonate/Lithotabs/Lithobid ... 2721
Lodine Capsules and Tablets (Less than 1%) ... 2849
▲ Lopid Tablets (More common) ... 1974
Lotensin HCT Tablets (0.3% to 1.0%) ... 855
Lupron Depot 3.75 mg (Less than 5%) ... 2739
Lupron Injection (Less than 5%) ... 2736
▲ LUVOX Tablets (3%) ... 2723
MS Contin Tablets (Less frequent) ... 2149
MSIR (Infrequent) ... 2152
Maxair Autohaler (0.6%) ... 1550
Maxair Inhaler (Less than 1%) ... 1552
Maxaquin Tablets (Less than 1%) ... 2593
▲ Mepron Suspension (3%) ... 1206
MetroGel-Vaginal ... 917
Mevacor Tablets ... 1742
Mexitil Capsules (About 5 in 1,000) ... 684
Mezlin ... 594
Mezlin Pharmacy Bulk Package ... 597
Miacalcin Nasal Spray (Less than 1%) ... 2403
Monopril Tablets (0.2% to 1.0%) ... 762
▲ Mycobutin Capsules (3%) ... 2101
Neptazane Tablets ... ⊚ 320
Neurontin Capsules (Infrequent) ... 1978
Nicotrol NS Nicotine Nasal Spray (More common) ... 1565
Nipent for Injection (Less than 3%) ... 2733
Normodyne Injection (1%) ... 2519
Normodyne Tablets (1%) ... 2522
Norvasc Tablets (Less than or equal to 0.1%) ... 2020
▲ Norvir (5.4% to 10.3%) ... 447
Ocupress Ophthalmic Solution, 1% Sterile (Occasional) ... ⊚ 297
Oramorph SR (Morphine Sulfate Sustained Release Tablets) (Less frequent) ... 2359
▲ Orap Tablets (1 of 20 patients) ... 1037
Orudis Capsules (Less than 1%) ... 2874
Oruvail Capsules (Less than 1%) ... 2874
OxyContin Tablets (Less than 1%) ... 2163
Paraplatin for Injection (1%) ... 713
Paxil Tablets (2%) ... 2681
Penetrex Tablets (1%) ... 2196
Pepcid Injection (Infrequent) ... 1765
Pepcid (Infrequent) ... 1763
Peridex ... 2127
Periogard Oral Rinse ... 892
Permax Tablets (1.6%) ... 571
Pravachol Tablets ... 770
Prevacid Delayed-Release Capsules (Less than 1%) ... 2746
▲ Prilosec Delayed-Release Capsules (Less than 1% to 15%) ... 516
Primaxin I.M. ... 1770
Primaxin I.V. (Less than 0.2%) ... 1772
Procardia XL Extended Release Tablets (1% or less) ... 2026
▲ Proleukin for Injection (7%) ... 812
ProSom Tablets (Infrequent) ... 457
Proventil Inhalation Aerosol ... 2524
Proventil Repetabs Tablets ... 2529
Proventil Syrup ... 2528
Proventil Tablets ... 2529
Prozac Pulvules & Liquid, Oral Solution (1.8% to 2%) ... 935
Quadrinal Tablets ... 1398

Redux Capsules (Frequent) ... 2911
Relafen Tablets (Less than 1%) ... 2688
▲ Retrovir Capsules (5%) ... 1216
▲ Retrovir I.V. Infusion (5%) ... 1221
▲ Retrovir Syrup (5%) ... 1216
▲ Roferon-A Injection (Less than 4% to 25%) ... 2308
▲ Rythmol Tablets–150mg, 225mg, 300mg (2.5 to 22.6%) ... 1399
Salagen Tablets (1%) ... 1546
Seldane-D Extended-Release Tablets (1.1%) ... 1286
Serzone Tablets (2%) ... 776
Sinequan ... 2028
Sular Tablets (Less than or equal to 1%) ... 2961
Surmontil Capsules ... 2917
Talwin Injection (Rare) ... 2465
Tambocor Tablets (Less than 1%) ... 1555
Tegison Capsules (Less than 1%) ... 2314
Tenex Tablets (3% or less) ... 2249
Timentin for Injection ... 2706
Tofranil Ampuls ... 873
Tofranil Tablets ... 875
Tofranil-PM Capsules ... 876
Tonocard Tablets (Less than 1%) ... 519
Toradol (1% or less) ... 2319
Tornalate Solution for Inhalation, 0.2% ... 976
Tornalate Metered Dose Inhaler ... 978
Trandate (1 of 100 patients) ... 1158
Triavil Tablets ... 1800
Univasc Tablets (Less than 1%) ... 2553
Vantin for Oral Suspension and Vantin Tablets (Less than 1%) ... 2112
Vascor Tablets (200 and 300 mg) (0.5 to 2.0%) ... 1597
Vaseretic Tablets ... 1810
Vasotec I.V. ... 1814
Vasotec Tablets (0.5% to 1.0%) ... 1816
Ventolin Inhalation Aerosol and Refill ... 1170
Ventolin Rotacaps for Inhalation (2%) ... 1173
Ventolin Syrup ... 1175
Vexol 1% Ophthalmic Suspension (Less than 2%) ... ⊚ 227
Videx Tablets, Powder for Oral Solution, & Pediatric Powder for Oral Solution (Less than 1%) ... 2980
Vistide Injection ... 1057
Volmax Extended-Release Tablets ... 1835
Cataflam/Voltaren/Voltaren-XR (Less than 1%) ... 833
Xanax Tablets ... 2115
Zebeta Tablets ... 1457
Zestoretic Tablets ... 2968
Zestril Tablets (0.3% to 1.0%) ... 2972
Ziac ... 1459
Zocor Tablets ... 1821
Zoloft Tablets (1.2%) ... 2051
▲ Zonalon Cream (Approximately 1% to 10%) ... 1042
Zosyn (1.0% or less) ... 1463
Zyloprim Tablets (Less than 1%) ... 1194
Zyrtec Tablets (Less than 2%) ... 2053

Taste, bad

Alupent (Less frequent; approximately 1 in 300 patients) ... 672
▲ Ciloxan Ophthalmic Solution (Less than 10%) ... 468
Cipro I.V. (1% or less) ... 587
Cipro I.V. Pharmacy Bulk Package (Less than 1%) ... 590
Cipro Tablets (Less than 1%) ... 584
Cleocin Phosphate Injection (Occasional) ... 2068
Desyrel and Desyrel Dividose (Up to 1.4%) ... 504
Fluorescite ... ⊚ 217
Imitrex Tablets ... 1099
▲ Intal Inhaler (Among most frequent) ... 2185
▲ Mesnex Injection (100%) ... 711
Metaproterenol Sulfate Inhalation Solution, USP, Arm-a-Med (Approximately 1 in 300 patients) ... 547
Methergine (Rare) ... 2401
Moduretic Tablets (Less than or equal to 1%) ... 1748
Nasalcrom Nasal Solution (1 in 50) ... 2192
Pondimin Tablets ... 2239
Rhinocort Nasal Inhaler (Less than 1%) ... 552
▲ THROMBATE III Antithrombin III (Human) (3 of 17) ... 631
THYREL TRH ... 2992

(▣ Described in PDR For Nonprescription Drugs)   Incidence data in parenthesis; ▲ 3% or more   (⊚ Described in PDR For Ophthalmology)

Side Effects Index

Taste, bad
- Trental Tablets (Less than 1%) 1291
- Zovirax (0.3%) 1187

Taste, bitter
- Atamet Tablets 567
- Ceftin Tablets 1067
- Chibroxin Sterile Ophthalmic Solution 1657
- Clinoril Tablets (Less than 1 in 100) 1658
- Clozaril Tablets (Less than 1%) 2377
- Colace Capsules, Syrup, Liquid 2212
- Dalmane Capsules (Rare) 2329
- Ethmozine Tablets (Less than 2%) 2217
- Larodopa Tablets (Infrequent) 2296
- Ludiomil Tablets (Rare) 861
- Monoket Tablets (Fewer than 1%) 2550
- Mykrox Tablets (Less than 2%) 1617
- Noroxin Tablets (Less frequent) 1758
- Noroxin Tablets (Less frequent) 2222
- Nubain Injection (1% or less) 952
- Procanbid Extended-Release Tablets (Occasional) 1983
- Risperdal Tablets (Rare) 1348
- Sinemet Tablets 959
- Sinemet CR Tablets 961
- ▲Trusopt Sterile Ophthalmic Solution (Approximately one-quarter of patients) 1803
- Versed Injection (Less than 1%) 2324
- Zaroxolyn Tablets 1625

Taste, changes
(see under Taste, altered)

Taste, loss
(see under Ageusia)

Taste, metallic
- Actigall Capsules 818
- Adenocard Injection (Less than 1%) 1021
- Adenoscan (Less than 1%) 1022
- Antabuse Tablets (Small number of patients) 2802
- Calcijex Injection 412
- ▲Chemet Capsules (12.0% to 20.9%) 666
- Cleocin Phosphate Injection (Occasional) 2068
- Clinoril Tablets (Less than 1 in 100) 1658
- ▲Didronel I.V. Infusion (5%) 1545
- Eskalith 2658
- Flagyl 375 Capsules (Not unusual) 2587
- Flagyl I.V. 2373
- Glucophage Tablets (Approximately 3%) 754
- Helidac Therapy (Not unusual) 2135
- Lithium Carbonate Capsules & Tablets 2352
- Lithonate/Lithotabs/Lithobid 2721
- Marcaine Spinal 2449
- MetroCream 1034
- MetroGel 1034
- MetroGel-Vaginal (Equal to or less than 2%) 917
- Myochrysine Injection 1754
- Nalfon 200 Pulvules & Nalfon Tablets (Less than 1%) 933
- Norisodrine with Calcium Iodide Syrup 446
- Pima Syrup 1004
- Protostat Tablets 1939
- Ridaura Capsules 2691
- Robaxin Injectable 2245
- Rocaltrol Capsules 2303
- Sensorcaine 554
- Solganal Suspension 2530
- Thyro-Block Tablets 2785

Taste, salty
- Lithonate/Lithotabs/Lithobid 2721
- Miacalcin Injection 2402

Taste, unpleasant
- Adderall Tablets 2209
- Adipex-P Tablets and Capsules 1035
- ▲AeroBid Inhaler System (10%) 1004
- ▲Aerobid-M Inhaler System (10%) 1004
- Asendin Tablets (Less than 1%) 1419
- Beclovent Inhalation Aerosol and Refill 1063
- Beconase 1065
- Brethaire Inhaler 830
- ▲Ceftin for Oral Suspension (5.0%) 1067
- Desoxyn Gradumet Tablets 422
- Dexedrine 2648
- DextroStat-Dextroamphetamine Sulfate Tablets 2211
- Efudex 2280
- Elavil 2945
- Etrafon 2495
- Fastin Capsules 2662
- Flagyl I.V. 2373
- Flexeril Tablets (1% to 3%) 1701
- Flonase Nasal Spray (Less than 1%) 1088
- Ionamin Capsules 1615
- Mephyton Tablets 1739
- Norpramin Tablets 1273
- Pamelor 2409
- Prelu-2 Timed Release Capsules 687
- Quadrinal Tablets 1398
- Questran 774
- Sanorex Tablets 2423
- ▲Stadol (3% to 9%) 779
- ▲Tilade Inhaler (12.6%) 2207
- Vivactil Tablets 1820

Tears, discoloration
- Mycobutin Capsules 2101
- Rifadin 1276
- Rifater 1280

Teeth, discoloration
- Achromycin V Capsules 1417
- Declomycin Tablets 1421
- Doryx Capsules 1970
- DYNACIN Capsules (In children less than 8 years of age; rare in adults) 1627
- Feosol Elixir 2627
- Helidac Therapy 2135
- Minocin Intravenous (Rare) 1428
- Minocin Oral Suspension (Rare) 1431
- Minocin Pellet-Filled Capsules (Rare) 1429
- Monodox Capsules 1858
- Neurontin Capsules (Rare) 1978
- Peridex 2127
- Periogard Oral Rinse 892
- Primaxin I.M. 1770
- Primaxin I.V. (Less than 0.2%) 1772
- Terramycin Intramuscular Solution 2034
- Urobiotic-250 Capsules 2038
- Ventolin Inhalation Aerosol and Refill (1%) 1170
- Vibramycin 2038
- Vibramycin Hyclate Intravenous 2040
- Vibramycin 2038

Teeth, mottling of enamel
(see under Teeth, discoloration)

Teeth grinding
- Anafranil Capsules (Infrequent) 819
- Zoloft Tablets (Infrequent) 2051

Telangiectasia
- Avonex 662
- Cormax Ointment (Approximately 0.3%) 1856
- Diprolene Gel 0.05% (Less frequent) 2490
- Efudex 2280
- Fluoroplex Topical Solution & Cream 1% 475
- Methotrexate Sodium Tablets, Injection, for Injection and LPF Injection 1322
- Redux Capsules 2911
- Sansert Tablets (Rare) 2424
- Temovate E Emollient (Less than 2%) 1154
- ▲Temovate Gel (Among most frequent) 1153
- Temovate Ointment (Less frequent) 1152
- Ultravate Ointment 0.05% (Less frequent) 2798

Telogen effluvium
- Lariam Tablets 2295

Temperature disturbances, cutaneous
- ▲EMLA Cream (7%) 536
- Wellbutrin Tablets (1.9%) 1177

Temperature elevation
(see under Hyperthermia)

Temporal bone, swelling
- Lupron Injection (Less than 5%) 2736

Tenderness
- Americaine Anesthetic Lubricant 1603
- Americaine Otic Topical Anesthetic Ear Drops 1603
- Bactroban Ointment (Less than 1%) 2642
- Biavax II 1653
- Condylox Topical Solution (Less than 5%) 1853
- Cormax Scalp Application (Approximately 0.3%) 1857
- Efudex (Infrequent) 2280
- Hep-B-Gammagee 1706
- HibTITER (0.3% to 3.7%) 1423
- M-M-R 1730
- M-R-VAX II 1732
- Mevacor Tablets 1742
- ▲Miacalcin Nasal Spray (10.6%) 2403
- Oncaspar 2194
- Recombivax HB (Equal to or greater than 1%) 1787
- T-Stat 2.0% Topical Solution and Pads 2797
- Temovate Scalp Application (1 of 294 patients) 1153
- Tetanus Toxoid Adsorbed Purogenated 1447
- Thioguanine Tablets, Tabloid Brand 1225
- ▲Versed Injection (5.6%) 2324
- Vivelle Transdermal System 880
- Zocor Tablets 1821

Tenderness, elbow
- Temovate E Emollient (Less than 2%) 1154

Tenderness, right upper quadrant
- Cataflam Tablets 833
- Eulexin Capsules 2498
- Normodyne Injection 2519
- Trandate 1158
- Cataflam/Voltaren/Voltaren-XR 833

Tendinitis
- Ambien Tablets (Rare) 2559
- Cipro Tablets 584
- Cognex Capsules (Infrequent) 1961
- Floxin I.V. 1580
- Floxin Tablets (200 mg, 300 mg, 400 mg) 1577
- Kerlone Tablets 2588
- Maxaquin Tablets 2593
- Neurontin Capsules 1978
- Noroxin Tablets 1758
- Noroxin Tablets 2222

Tenderness at injection site
- ▲Acel-Imune Diphtheria and Tetanus Toxoids and Acellular Pertussis Vaccine Adsorbed (26%) 1415
- ▲ActHIB (1.1% to 66.9%) 893
- ▲Actimmune (14%) 1043
- Cefizox for Intramuscular or Intravenous Use (1% to 5%) 1025
- Cholera Vaccine 2818
- ▲Claforan Sterile and Injection (4.3%) 1259
- Diphtheria and Tetanus Toxoids and Pertussis Vaccine Adsorbed .. 2650
- Fluvirin (Influenza Virus Vaccine) (Less than one-third) 1608
- HyperHep Hepatitis B Immune Globulin (Human) 619
- Imogam Rabies Immune Globulin (Human) (Uncommon) 897
- ▲JE-VAX (Approximately 20%) 904
- Mefoxin 1734
- MSTA Mumps Skin Test Antigen 2988
- ▲OmniHIB (1.1% to 46.3%) 2676
- Rocephin Injectable Vials, ADD-Vantage, Galaxy Container (1%) 2305
- Taxol Injection 723
- ▲Tetramune (21% to 65%) 1449
- ▲Tripedia (2% to 35%) 908
- ▲Typhim Vi (Up to 98%) 914
- Typhoid Vaccine 2929
- Vancocin HCl, Vials & ADD-Vantage 1534
- ▲Vaqta (1.7% to 16.8%) 1805

Tendinous contracture
- Lamictal Tablets (Rare) 1105
- LUVOX Tablets (Infrequent) 2723
- Serzone Tablets (Rare) 776

Tendon disorder, unspecified
- Imdur (Less than or equal to 5%) 1362
- Naprelan Tablets (Less than 3%) 2861

Tendon rupture
- Cipro Tablets 584
- Cortone Acetate Sterile Suspension 1663
- Cortone Acetate Tablets 1664
- Dalalone D.P. Injectable 1009
- Decadron Elixir 1676
- Decadron Phosphate Injection 1680
- Decadron Phosphate with Xylocaine Injection, Sterile 1683
- Decadron Tablets 1678
- Decadron-LA Sterile Suspension 1687
- Dexacort Phosphate in Respihaler 1606
- Dexacort Phosphate in Turbinaire 1607
- Hydeltrasol Injection, Sterile 1708
- Hydeltra-T.B.A. Sterile Suspension 1710
- Hydrocortone Acetate Sterile Suspension 1712
- Hydrocortone Phosphate Injection, Sterile 1713
- Hydrocortone Tablets 1715
- Noroxin Tablets 1758
- Penetrex Tablets 2196
- Remeron Tablets (Rare) 1878

Tenesmus
- Ambien Tablets (Rare) 2559
- Asacol Delayed-Release Tablets 2129
- Betaseron for SC Injection 653
- Cerebyx Injection (Infrequent) 1956
- DaunoXome (1% to 4%) 1842
- Doxil (Less than 1%) 2613
- Foscavir Injection (Less than 1%) 541
- Ismo Tablets (Fewer than 1%) 2844
- Norvir (Less than 2%) 447
- Prevacid Delayed-Release Capsules (Less than 1%) 2746
- Rilutek Tablets (Infrequent) 2198
- Zoloft Tablets (Rare) 2051

Tenosynovitis
- Betaseron for SC Injection 653
- Effexor 2825
- Lupron Depot 3.75 mg 2739
- Lupron Depot 7.5 mg 2741
- Lupron Depot - 3 Month 22.5 mg 2743
- Lupron Depot-PED 7.5 mg, 11.25 mg and 15 mg 2744
- LUVOX Tablets (Infrequent) 2723
- Paxil Tablets (Rare) 2681
- Permax Tablets (Infrequent) 571
- Prozac Pulvules & Liquid, Oral Solution (Infrequent) 935
- Redux Capsules (Infrequent) 2911
- Remeron Tablets (Infrequent) 1878
- Serzone Tablets (Infrequent) 776
- Sular Tablets (Less than or equal to 1%) 2961
- Videx Tablets, Powder for Oral Solution, & Pediatric Powder for Oral Solution (Less than 1%) 2980

Tenseness
- Bronkometer Aerosol 2432
- Bronkosol Solution 2432
- Claritin-D Tablets 2487
- Clomid (Fewer than 1%) 1262
- D.A. II Tablets 972
- D.A. Chewable Tablets 970
- Dura-Tap/PD Capsules 970
- Dura-Vent/DA Tablets 972
- Dura-Vent Tablets 971
- EpiPen–Epinephrine Auto-Injector 808
- Fedahist Gyrocaps 2545
- Histussin D Liquid 670
- Loxitane 1426
- Novahistine DMX 782
- Novahistine Elixir 782
- Prostin E2 Suppository 2109
- Seldane-D Extended-Release Tablets 1286
- Trinalin Repetabs Tablets 1373
- Tussend 1830
- Tussend Expectorant 1831

Testes, size decrease
- ▲Lupron Depot 7.5 mg (5.4%) 2741
- ▲Lupron Injection (5% or more) 2736

Testicular atrophy
- Cytoxan 700
- ▲Lupron Depot - 3 Month 22.5 mg (20.2%) 2743
- Oxandrin 783
- Winstrol Tablets 2468

Testicular disorder, unspecified
- Androderm Testosterone Transdermal System (Less than 1%) 2634
- Avonex 662
- Caverject Injection (Less than 1%) 2064
- Lupron Depot - 3 Month 22.5 mg (Less than 5%) 2743
- Redux Capsules (Rare) 2911
- Tenex Tablets (3% or less) 2249
- Vivelle Transdermal System 880

(⊞ Described in PDR For Nonprescription Drugs)   Incidence data in parenthesis; ▲ 3% or more   (⊙ Described in PDR For Ophthalmology)

1465 Side Effects Index Throbbing, head

Testicular function, inhibited
Alkeran for Injection 1196
Oxandrin 783
Winstrol Tablets 2468

Testicular hypertrophy
Cytovene-IV (One report) 2270

Testicular swelling
Adapin Capsules 1542
Asendin Tablets (Very rare) 1419
Elavil 2945
Etrafon 2495
Flexeril Tablets (Rare) 1701
Hivid Tablets (Less than 1%) 2287
Limbitrol 2333
Ludiomil Tablets (Isolated reports) 861
Neurontin Capsules (Rare) 1978
Norpramin Tablets 1273
Pamelor 2409
Sinequan 2028
Surmontil Capsules 2917
Tofranil Ampuls 873
Tofranil Tablets 875
Tofranil-PM Capsules 876
Triavil Tablets 1800
Vivactil Tablets 1820
Wellbutrin Tablets (Infrequent) 1177

Testosterone, decreased physiologic effects
Lupron Injection 2736
Zoladex 2976

Testosterone serum levels, transient increase
Zoladex 2976
Zoladex 3-month 2978

Tetany
Ambien Tablets (Rare) 2559
Aredia for Injection (Rare) 827
Foscavir Injection (Less than 1%) 541
Garamycin Injectable 2502
Imitrex Tablets (Rare) 1099
Lasix Injection, Oral Solution and Tablets (Rare) 1267
Paxil Tablets (Rare) 2681
Platinol for Injection (Occasional) 717
Platinol-AQ Injection (Occasional) 719
Redux Capsules (Rare) 2911
Rilutek Tablets (Rare) 2198
Syntocinon Injection 2425

Thermoregulatory mechanisms, interference
Astramorph/PF Injection, USP (Preservative-Free) 526
Compazine 2644
Duramorph Injection 983
Infumorph 200 and Infumorph 500 Sterile Solutions 985

Thinking, abnormality
Ambien Tablets (Rare) 2559
Anafranil Capsules (Frequent) 819
Androderm Testosterone Transdermal System (Less than 1%) 2634
Brevibloc (esmolol HCl) Injection (Less than 1%) 1860
Butisol Sodium Elixir & Tablets (Less than 1 in 100) 2768
Cardura Tablets (Less than 0.5% of 3960 patients) 1993
Cerebyx Injection (Frequent) 1956
▲ Cognex Capsules (3%) 1961
Cytovene (1% or less) 2270
DaunoXome (Less than or equal to 5%) 1842
Depakote Tablets (1% to 5%) 418
Dilacor XR Extended-release Capsules 2183
Diprivan Injectable Emulsion (Less than 1%) 2939
Doral Tablets 2773
Duragesic Transdermal System (1% or greater) 1336
Effexor (2%) 2825
▲ Felbatol (6.5%) 2774
Flexeril Tablets (Less than 1%) 1701
Halcion Tablets 2093
Hivid Tablets (Less than 1%) 2287
Intron A for Injection (Less than 5%) 2506
Kadian Capsules (Less than 3%) 2948
Kerlone Tablets (Less than 2%) 2588
Lamictal Tablets (Frequent) 1105
Levo-Dromoran 2297
Lioresal Intrathecal (0.5% to 1.3%) 1634
Lithonate/Lithotabs/Lithobid 2721
▲ Marinol (Dronabinol) Capsules (3% to 10%) 2353
Mebaral Tablets (Less than 1 in 100) 2452
Megace Oral Suspension (1% to 3%) 708
Nembutal Sodium Capsules (Less than 1%) 440
Nembutal Sodium Solution (Less than 1%) 442
Nembutal Sodium Suppositories (Less than 1%) 444
Neurontin Capsules (1.7%) 1978
Nipent for Injection (Less than 3%) 2733
Norvir (0.7%) 447
OxyContin Tablets (Between 1% and 5%) 2163
Paxil Tablets (Infrequent) 2681
Permax Tablets (Frequent) 571
Phenobarbital Elixir and Tablets (Less than 1 in 100 patients) 1523
Prevacid Delayed-Release Capsules (Less than 1%) 2746
▲ Prograf (Greater than 3%) 1028
ProSom Tablets (2%) 457
▲ Prozac Pulvules & Liquid, Oral Solution (4%) 935
Redux Capsules (2.0%) 2911
▲ Remeron Tablets (3%) 1878
ReoPro Vials (2.1%) 1526
Rilutek Tablets (Infrequent) 2198
Seconal Sodium Pulvules (Less than 1 in 100) 1529
Serzone Tablets (Infrequent) 776
Sular Tablets (Less than or equal to 1%) 2961
Symmetrel Capsules (0.1% to 1%) 965
Symmetrel Syrup (0.1% to 1%) 963
Tegison Capsules (Less than 1%) 2314
Toradol (1% or less) 2319
Videx Tablets, Powder for Oral Solution, & Pediatric Powder for Oral Solution (1% to 2%) 2980
Wellbutrin Tablets (Infrequent) 1177
Zoladex (1% or greater) 2976
Zoladex 3-month 2978
Zoloft Tablets (Infrequent) 2051
Zyrtec Tablets (Less than 2%) 2053

Thirst (see under Dipsesis)

Thrashing
Diprivan Injectable Emulsion (Less than 1%) 2939

Throat, aching
Zebeta Tablets 1457

Throat, burning
Diprivan Injectable Emulsion (Less than 1%) 2939
Eldepryl Capsules 2729
Emcyt Capsules (1%) 2085
Gastrocrom Capsules (Infrequent) 1611
Thyro-Block Tablets 2785

Throat, congestion
Bentyl 1246

Throat, dryness
Accupril Tablets (0.5% to 1.0%) 1950
AeroBid Inhaler System (1% to 3%) 1004
Aerobid-M Inhaler System (1% to 3%) 1004
Alupent Tablets (0.4%) 672
Atrovent Nasal Spray 0.03% (Less than 2%) 676
Atrovent Nasal Spray 0.06% (1.4%) 678
Azmacort Oral Inhaler 2175
Beclovent Inhalation Aerosol and Refill 1063
Beconase 1065
Benadryl Injection 1955
▲ Bromfed-DM Cough Syrup (Among most frequent) 1832
Catapres-TTS (2 of 101 patients) 680
Claritin-D Tablets (Less frequent) 2487
Clozaril Tablets (Less than 1%) 2377
Cognex Capsules (Infrequent) 1961
D.A. II Tablets 972
D.A. Chewable Tablets 970
Daraprim Tablets (Rare) 1199
▲ Dimetane-DC Cough Syrup (Most frequent) 2232
▲ Dimetane-DX Cough Syrup (Among most frequent) 2233
Dura-Tap/PD Capsules 970
Dura-Vent/DA Tablets 972
Hylorel Tablets (1.7%) 1613
▲ Intal Inhaler (Among most frequent) 2185
Marax Tablets & DF Syrup 2015
Neurontin Capsules (1.7%) 1978
▲ Norpace (3 to 9%) 2596
Ornade Spansule Capsules 2678
PBZ Tablets 863
PBZ-SR Tablets 862
Penetrex Tablets (0.1% to 1%) 2196
Periactin 1767
Robinul Injectable 2247
▲ Seldane Tablets (2.3% to 4.8%) 1284
▲ Seldane-D Extended-Release Tablets (21.7%) 1286
Tavist Syrup 2426
Tavist Tablets 2427
Trinalin Repetabs Tablets 1373
Tussend 1830

Throat, irritation
AeroBid Inhaler System (1% to 3%) 1004
Aerobid-M Inhaler System (1% to 3%) 1004
Alupent (1% to 4%) 672
Aredia for Injection (One patient) 827
Azmacort Oral Inhaler 2175
Beconase Inhalation Aerosol 1065
Clozaril Tablets (1%) 2377
Colace Capsules, Syrup, Liquid 2212
Dexacort Phosphate in Respihaler 1606
▲ Intal Inhaler (Among most frequent) 2185
Isuprel Mistometer (Occasional) 2442
Nasacort Nasal Inhaler (Fewer than 5%) 2189
Nicotrol NS Nicotine Nasal Spray (Common) 1565
Norvir (1.7% to 2.6%) 447
Paxil Tablets (2%) 2681
▲ Roferon-A Injection (21%) 2308
Tornalate Solution for Inhalation, 0.2% (2.5%) 976
▲ Tornalate Metered Dose Inhaler (3.0% to 5%) 978
▲ Ventolin Inhalation Aerosol and Refill (6%) 1170
Ventolin Rotacaps for Inhalation (2%) 1173

Throat, presence of hard nodule
Lupron Depot 7.5 mg (Less than 5%) 2741
Lupron Injection 2736

Throat, soreness
▲ Adalat Capsules (10 mg and 20 mg) (6%) 580
▲ Adenoscan (15%) 1022
▲ AeroBid Inhaler System (20%) 1004
▲ Aerobid-M Inhaler System (20%) 1004
All-Flex Arcing Spring Diaphragm (See also Ortho Diaphragm Kits) 1921
Altace Capsules 1238
Atretol Tablets 569
Azulfidine 2059
Biavax II 1653
Blocadren Tablets 1654
BuSpar Tablets (Frequent) 738
Capoten Tablets 740
Capozide Tablets 744
Cardene Capsules (Rare) 2261
Cardene SR Capsules (Rare) 2264
Cartrol Tablets 413
Chemet Capsules (0.7% to 3.7%) 666
Clozaril Tablets 2377
Compazine 2644
Cytosar-U Sterile Powder (Less frequent) 2077
Danocrine Capsules 2437
Dapsone Tablets USP 1331
Demadex Tablets and Injection (1.6%) 691
Depen Titratable Tablets 2770
DynaCirc Capsules (0.5% to 1%) 2381
Etrafon 2495
Gantrisin 2286
Helixate, Antihemophilic Factor (Recombinant) 799
Hivid Tablets (Less than 1%) 2287
▲ Imitrex Injection (3.3%) 1095
Inderal 2834
Inderal LA Long Acting Capsules 2836
Inderide Tablets 2838
Inderide LA Long Acting Capsules 2840
Kerlone Tablets 2588
KOGENATE Antihemophilic Factor (Recombinant) 626
Levatol Tablets 2547
Lopressor HCT Tablets 850
M-M-R II 1730
M-R-VAX II 1732
Mavik Tablets (0.3% to 1.0%) 1407
Maxair Autohaler 1550
Maxair Inhaler (Less than 1%) 1552
Meruvax II 1740
Monopril Tablets 762
Mykrox Tablets (Less than 2%) 1617
Nasalide Nasal Solution 0.025% (5% or less) 2301
▲ Neupogen for Injection (4%) 495
Normodyne Tablets 2522
Ortho Diaphragm Kits—All-Flex Arcing Spring; Ortho Coil Spring; Ortho-White Flat Spring 1921
Ortho Diaphragm Kit 1921
Prinivil Tablets 1776
Prinzide Tablets 1780
▲ Procardia Capsules (6%) 2024
▲ Procardia XL Extended Release Tablets (6%) 2026
Prolixin 510
Proloprim Tablets 1141
Quadrinal Tablets 1398
Remeron Tablets 1878
ReVia Tablets (Less than 1%) 957
Rowasa (2.33%) 2727
Rythmol Tablets–150mg, 225mg, 300mg 1399
Sectral Capsules 2914
Seldane Tablets (0.5% to 3.2%) 1284
Seldane-D Extended-Release Tablets (1.9%) 1286
Septra I.V. Infusion 1142
Septra I.V. Infusion ADD-Vantage Vials 1144
Stelazine 2692
Stimate, (desmopressin acetate) Nasal Spray, 1.5 mg/mL 806
Tapazole Tablets 1361
Tegretol/Tegretol-XR 870
Tenoretic Tablets 2963
Tenormin Tablets and I.V. Injection 2965
Ticlid Tablets 2317
Timoptic in Ocudose 1796
Timoptic Sterile Ophthalmic Solution 1794
Timoptic-XE 1798
Tofranil Ampuls 873
Tofranil Tablets 875
Tofranil-PM Capsules 876
Tonocard Tablets 519
Toprol-XL Tablets 560
Trandate Tablets 1158
Trental Tablets (Less than 1%) 1291
Univasc Tablets 2553
Valium Injectable 2336
Vaseretic Tablets 1810
Vasotec I.V. 1814
Vasotec Tablets (0.5% to 1.0%) 1816
Visken Tablets 2428
Zebeta Tablets 1457
Zestoretic Tablets 2968
Zestril Tablets 2972
Ziac 1459
Zovirax (0.3%) 1187

Throat, swelling of
Calcimar Injection, Synthetic (A few cases) 2176
Floxin I.V. 1580
Floxin Tablets (200 mg, 300 mg, 400 mg) 1577
Miacalcin Injection (A few cases) 2402
SSKI Solution (Less frequent) 2767

Throat, tightness
Adenocard Injection (Less than 1%) 1021
Alferon N Injection (1%) 2142
▲ Doxil (Approximately 6.8%) 2613
Etopophos for Injection (Sometimes) 701
Etoposide Injection (Sometimes) 539
Etrafon 2495
Paxil Tablets (2%) 2681
THYREL TRH (Less frequent) 2992
Trilafon 2532
Unasyn (Less than 1%) 2035
VePesid Capsules and Injection (Sometimes) 727

Throbbing, head
EpiPen–Epinephrine Auto-Injector 808

Throbbing, localized

Catapres-TTS (1 of 101 patients) ... 680

Thrombocythemia (see under Thrombocytosis)

Thrombocytopenia

▲ Abelcet Injection (4% to 5%) ... 1540
Accupril Tablets (Rare) ... 1950
Accutane Capsules (Less than 1 in 10 patients) ... 2252
Achromycin V Capsules ... 1417
Adalat Capsules (10 mg and 20 mg) (Less than 0.5%) ... 580
Adalat CC (Rare) ... 582
Adapin Capsules (Occasional) ... 1542
Albenza Tablets (Rare) ... 2629
Aldactazide Tablets ... 2556
Aldoclor Tablets ... 1638
Aldomet Ester HCl Injection ... 1642
Aldomet Oral ... 1640
Aldoril Tablets ... 1644
Alkeran Tablets ... 1198
Altace Capsules (Less than 1%) ... 1238
Amaryl Tablets ... 1241
Amicar Syrup, Tablets, and Injection ... 1312
Amoxil ... 2631
Anafranil Capsules ... 819
Anaprox/Naprosyn (Less than 1%) ... 2277
Ancef Injection ... 2632
Ancobon Capsules ... 2254
Anturane (Rare) ... 823
Apresazide Capsules ... 824
Aredia for Injection (Up to 1%) ... 827
Asacol Delayed-Release Tablets ... 2129
Asendin Tablets (Very rare) ... 1419
Atamet Tablets (Rare) ... 567
Atretol Tablets ... 569
Atrohist Plus Tablets ... 1605
Attenuvax (Rare) ... 1650
Augmentin ... 2637
Augmentin Tablets ... 2640
Axid Pulvules (One patient) ... 1468
Axocet Capsules ... 2469
Azactam for Injection (Less than 1%) ... 736
Azathioprine Tablets ... 2349
Azulfidine (Rare) ... 2059
Bactrim DS Tablets ... 2257
Bactrim I.V. Infusion ... 2255
Bactrim ... 2257
Benadryl Injection ... 1955
Betapace Tablets (Rare) ... 637
Betaseron for SC Injection ... 653
Biavax II ... 1653
Bicillin C-R Injection ... 2810
Bicillin C-R 900/300 Injection ... 2812
Bicillin L-A Injection (Infrequent) ... 2813
BiCNU ... 696
▲ Bromfed-DM Cough Syrup (Among most frequent) ... 1832
Bumex (0.2%) ... 2260
BuSpar Tablets (Rare) ... 738
Capastat Sulfate Injection (Rare) ... 968
Capoten Tablets ... 740
Capozide Tablets ... 744
Cardene I.V. (Rare) ... 2815
Cardizem CD Capsules (Infrequent) ... 1251
Cardizem SR Capsules (Infrequent) ... 1255
Cardizem Injectable ... 1253
Cardizem Tablets (Infrequent) ... 1257
Cataflam Tablets (Less than 1%) ... 833
Catapres Tablets (Rare) ... 679
Ceclor Pulvules & Suspension (Rare) ... 1470
Cedax (0.1% to 1%) ... 2480
CeeNU Capsules ... 699
Cefizox for Intramuscular or Intravenous Use (Rare) ... 1025
Cefotan ... 2936
Ceftin ... 1067
Cefzil Tablets and Oral Suspension (Rare) ... 747
▲ CellCept Capsules (8.2% to 10.1%) ... 2265
Ceptaz (Very rare) ... 1070
Cerebyx Injection (Infrequent) ... 1956
Chibroxin Sterile Ophthalmic Solution (With oral form) ... 1657
Chloromycetin Sodium Succinate ... 1960
▲ Cipro I.V. (Among most frequent) ... 587
▲ Cipro I.V. Pharmacy Bulk Package (Among most frequent) ... 590
Cipro Tablets (0.1%) ... 584
Claforan Sterile and Injection (Less than 1%) ... 1259
Cleocin Phosphate Injection ... 2068
Cleocin Vaginal Cream ... 2070
Clinoril Tablets (Less than 1 in 100) ... 1658
Clozaril Tablets ... 2377
Cognex Capsules (Rare) ... 1961
Combipres Tablets ... 682
Cordarone Intravenous (Less than 2%) ... 2821
Cordarone Tablets (Rare) ... 2818
Cosmegen Injection ... 1666
Crixivan Capsules (0.5%) ... 1670
▲ Cuprimine Capsules (4%) ... 1673
Cytosar-U Sterile Powder (Less than 7 patients) ... 2077
Cytotec (Infrequent) ... 2576
▲ Cytovene (6%) ... 2270
Cytoxan (Occasional) ... 700
Danocrine Capsules ... 2437
Daranide Tablets ... 1676
Daraprim Tablets ... 1199
Daypro Caplets (Less than 1%) ... 2578
Declomycin Tablets ... 1421
Demser Capsules (Rare) ... 1690
Depakene ... 416
Depakote Tablets ... 418
▲ Depen Titratable Tablets (4%; up to 5%) ... 2770
DiaBeta Tablets ... 1265
Diabinese Tablets ... 2002
Diflucan Tablets, Injection, and Oral Suspension ... 2003
Dilantin Infatabs (Occasional) ... 1967
Dilantin Kapseals (Occasional) ... 1965
Dilantin-125 Suspension (Occasional) ... 1969
Dimetane-DC Cough Syrup ... 2232
Dimetane-DX Cough Syrup ... 2233
Dipentum Capsules (Rare) ... 2084
Diucardin Tablets ... 2824
Diupres Tablets ... 1691
Diuril Oral Suspension ... 1694
Diuril Sodium Intravenous ... 1693
Diuril Tablets ... 1694
Dobutrex Solution Vials (Isolated cases) ... 1480
Dolobid Tablets (Less than 1 in 100) ... 1695
Doryx Capsules ... 1970
▲ Doxil (6.5% to 9.2%) ... 2613
Duricef Capsules, Tablets, and Oral Suspension ... 750
Dyazide Capsules ... 2653
Dynabac (0.1% to 1%) ... 668
DYNACIN Capsules ... 1627
Dyrenium Capsules (Rare) ... 2655
Easprin ... 1971
EC-Naprosyn Delayed-Release Tablets (Less than 1%) ... 2277
Edecrin (Rare) ... 1698
Effexor (Infrequent) ... 2825
Efudex ... 2280
Elavil ... 2945
Emcyt Capsules (1%) ... 2085
▲ Eminase (Less than 10%) ... 2215
Enduron Tablets ... 424
Engerix-B Unit-Dose Vials ... 2656
Epivir (Up to 0.4%) ... 1200
▲ Ergamisol Tablets (Up to 10%) ... 1340
Esgic-plus Capsules ... 1012
Esgic-plus Tablets ... 1012
Esidrix Tablets ... 839
Esimil Tablets (A few instances) ... 840
Ethmozine Tablets (2 patients) ... 2217
▲ Etopophos for Injection (1% to 41%) ... 701
▲ Etoposide Injection (1% to 41%) ... 539
Etrafon ... 2495
Eulexin Capsules (1%) ... 2498
▲ Exosurf Neonatal for Intratracheal Suspension (Less than 1% to 25%) ... 1081
Fansidar Tablets ... 2281
Felbatol (Infrequent) ... 2774
Feldene Capsules (Less than 1%) ... 2008
Fioricet Tablets ... 2386
Fioricet with Codeine Capsules ... 2387
Flagyl 375 Capsules (Rare) ... 2587
Flagyl I.V. (Rare) ... 2373
Flexeril Tablets (Rare) ... 1701
Flolan for Injection ... 1085
Floxin I.V. (More than or equal to 1%) ... 1580
Floxin Tablets (200 mg, 300 mg, 400 mg) (More than or equal to 1%) ... 1577
▲ Fludara for Injection (Among most common) ... 658
Fluorouracil Injection ... 2282
Fortaz (Very rare) ... 1092
Foscavir Injection (Between 1% and 5%) ... 541
Fragmin Injection (Less than 1%) ... 2088
▲ Sterile FUDR (Among more common) ... 2284
Fungizone Intravenous ... 507
Gantanol Tablets ... 2285
Gantrisin ... 2286
Garamycin Injectable ... 2502
▲ Gemzar for Injection (15% to 47%) ... 1482
Geocillin Tablets ... 2009
Glucotrol Tablets ... 2011
Glucotrol XL Extended Release Tablets ... 2012
Glynase PresTab Tablets ... 2091
Helidac Therapy (Rare) ... 2135
▲ Heparin Lock Flush Solution (0 to 30%) ... 2831
▲ Heparin Sodium Injection (0 to 30%) ... 2832
▲ Heparin Sodium Vials (0 to 30%) ... 1486
▲ Hexalen Capsules (3% to 10%) ... 2760
Hivid Tablets (Less than 1% to 1.3%) ... 2287
▲ Hycamtin for Injection (26% to 63%) ... 2665
Hydralazine Hydrochloride Injection USP (Less frequent) ... 2712
Hydrea Capsules (Occasional; less often; rare) ... 705
Hydrocet Capsules ... 787
HydroDIURIL Tablets ... 1716
Hydropres Tablets ... 1718
Hyperstat I.V. Injection ... 2504
Hyzaar Tablets ... 1720
IBU Tablets (Less than 1%) ... 1389
▲ IFEX (About 20%) ... 706
Imdur (Less than or equal to 5%) ... 1362
Imitrex Tablets ... 1099
Imuran ... 1103
Inderide Tablets ... 2838
Inderide LA Long Acting Capsules ... 2840
Indocin I.V. (1% to 3%) ... 1727
Inocor Lactate Injection (2.4%) ... 2439
▲ Intron A for Injection (Less than 5% to 15%) ... 2506
Invirase Capsules (Rare) ... 2291
Ismelin Tablets ... 845
Kadian Capsules (Less than 3%) ... 2948
Keflex Pulvules & Oral Suspension ... 930
Keftab Tablets ... 931
Kefurox Vials, Faspak & ADD-Vantage ... 1509
Kerlone Tablets (Less than 2%) ... 2588
Klonopin Tablets ... 2294
▲ Kytril Tablets (3%) ... 2669
Lamictal Tablets (Rare) ... 1105
▲ Lariam Tablets (Among most frequent; occasional) ... 2295
Lasix Injection, Oral Solution and Tablets ... 1267
Lescol Capsules (Rare) ... 2395
▲ Leucovorin Calcium for Injection (1% to 18%) ... 1313
▲ Leukine (19%) ... 1317
▲ Leustatin (Common; 12%) ... 1889
Levoprome ... 1321
Limbitrol ... 2333
Lodine Capsules and Tablets (Less than 1%) ... 2849
Lopid Tablets (Rare) ... 1974
Lopressor HCT Tablets ... 850
Lorabid Suspension and Pulvules ... 1513
Lortab ... 2751
Lotensin Tablets ... 852
Lotensin HCT Tablets (Rare) ... 855
Lotrel Capsules (Rare) ... 858
Lovenox Injection (1.9%) ... 2187
Loxitane (Rare) ... 1426
Ludiomil Tablets (Isolated reports) ... 861
▲ Lupron Depot - 3 Month 22.5 mg (More than or equal to 5%) ... 2743
LUVOX Tablets (Infrequent) ... 2723
M-M-R II ... 1730
M-R-VAX II ... 1732
Macrobid Capsules ... 2138
Macrodantin Capsules ... 2140
Mandol Vials, Faspak & ADD-Vantage (Rare) ... 1516
Matulane Capsules (Frequent) ... 2300
Mavik Tablets (0.3% to 1.0%) ... 1407
Maxaquin Tablets (Less than or equal to 0.1%) ... 2593
Mefoxin ... 1734
Mefoxin Premixed Intravenous Solution ... 1737
Mellaril ... 2398
Merrem I.V. (Greater than 0.2%) ... 2952
Mesantoin Tablets ... 2400
▲ Methotrexate Sodium Tablets, Injection, for Injection and LPF Injection (3% to 10%) ... 1322
MetroGel-Vaginal ... 917
Mevacor Tablets (Rare) ... 1742
Mexitil Capsules (About 2 in 1,000) ... 684
Mezlin ... 594
Mezlin Pharmacy Bulk Package ... 597
Micronase Tablets ... 2099
Minizide Capsules ... 2016
Minocin Intravenous ... 1428
Minocin Oral Suspension ... 1431
Minocin Pellet-Filled Capsules ... 1429
Mithracin ... 599
Moduretic Tablets ... 1748
Monocid Injection (Less than 1%) ... 2674
Monodox Capsules ... 1858
Monopril Tablets ... 762
Motrin Ibuprofen Suspension, Oral Drops, Chewable Tablets, Caplets (Less than 1%) ... 1563
Mustargen ... 1752
Mutamycin for Injection ... 712
▲ Mycobutin Capsules (5%; rare) ... 2101
Mykrox Tablets (Rare) ... 1617
Myleran Tablets ... 1209
Myochrysine Injection ... 1754
Nalfon 200 Pulvules & Nalfon Tablets (Less than 1%) ... 933
Naprelan Tablets (Less than 1%) ... 2861
Anaprox/Naprosyn (Less than 1%) ... 2277
Navane Capsules and Concentrate ... 2018
Navane Intramuscular ... 2019
Navelbine Injection (1% to 4%) ... 1212
Nebcin Vials, Hyporets & ADD-Vantage ... 1518
NegGram (Rare) ... 2453
Neoral (2% or less) ... 2405
Netromycin Injection 100 mg/ml (1 per 1000 patients) ... 2516
▲ Neupogen for Injection (Fewer than 6% to 12%) ... 495
Neurontin Capsules (Infrequent) ... 1978
▲ Neutrexin for Injection (10.1%) ... 2761
Nimotop Capsules (0.3%; rare) ... 603
▲ Nipent for Injection (6% to 32%) ... 2733
Nizoral Tablets (Less than 1%) ... 1345
Nolvadex Tablets (Occasional; 1.5%) ... 2957
Noroxin Tablets (1.0%) ... 1758
Noroxin Tablets (1.0%) ... 2222
Norpace (Rare) ... 2596
Norpramin Tablets ... 1273
Norvir (Less than 2%) ... 447
Nydrazid Injection ... 509
Omnipen Capsules ... 2872
Omnipen for Oral Suspension ... 2873
▲ Oncaspar (Greater than 1% but less than 5%) ... 2194
Oncovin Solution Vials & Hyporets ... 1521
Oretic Tablets ... 450
Ornade Spansule Capsules ... 2678
Orthoclone OKT3 Sterile Solution ... 1892
Orudis Capsules (Less than 1%) ... 2874
Oruvail Capsules (Less than 1%) ... 2874
PBZ Tablets ... 863
PBZ-SR Tablets ... 862
Pamelor ... 2409
Panhematin ... 452
▲ Paraplatin for Injection (22% to 70%) ... 713
Parnate Tablets ... 2679
PASER Granules ... 1333
Paxil Tablets ... 2681
Pediazole Suspension ... 2340
PedvaxHIB (One child) ... 1761
Pen•Vee K (Infrequent) ... 2879
Pentasa (Less than 1%) ... 1275
Pentaspan Injection ... 954
Pepcid Injection (Rare) ... 1765
Pepcid (Rare) ... 1763
Periactin ... 1767
Permax Tablets (Infrequent) ... 571
Pfizerpen for Injection (Rare) ... 2022
Phenergan with Codeine (Rare) ... 2883
Phenergan with Dextromethorphan (Rare) ... 2885
Phenergan Suppositories (Rare) ... 2882
Phenergan Syrup ... 2881
Phenergan VC ... 2886
Phenergan VC with Codeine ... 2888
Phrenilin (Infrequent) ... 790
Pipracil ... 1435
Placidyl Capsules (One case) ... 456
Plaquenil Sulfate Tablets ... 2459
Platinol for Injection ... 717
Platinol-AQ Injection ... 719
Pneumovax 23 ... 1768
Pnu-Imune 23 (Rare) ... 1437
Podocon-25 ... 1949
Pravachol Tablets (Rare) ... 770

Side Effects Index

(continued)

Entry	Page
Prevacid Delayed-Release Capsules (Less than 1%)	2746
Prilosec Delayed-Release Capsules (Rare)	516
Primacor Injection (0.4%)	2461
Primaxin I.M.	1770
Primaxin I.V. (Less than 0.2%)	1772
Prinivil Tablets (Rare)	1776
Prinzide Tablets (Rare)	1780
Priscoline Hydrochloride Ampuls	864
Procanbid Extended-Release Tablets (Approximately 0.5%)	1983
Procardia Capsules (Less than 0.5%)	2024
Procardia XL Extended Release Tablets (Some patients)	2026
Proglycem	575
▲ Prograf (10% to 24%)	1028
▲ Proleukin for Injection (64%)	812
Proloprim Tablets	1141
Propulsid (Rare)	1346
Protostat Tablets (Rare)	1939
Prozac Pulvules & Liquid, Oral Solution (Rare)	935
Purinethol Tablets (Frequent)	1214
Pyrazinamide Tablets (Rare)	1442
Recombivax HB	1787
Relafen Tablets (Less than 1%)	2688
Remeron Tablets (Rare)	1878
ReoPro Vials (0.7% to 5.2%)	1526
▲ Retrovir Capsules (12%)	1216
▲ Retrovir I.V. Infusion (12%)	1221
▲ Retrovir Syrup (12%)	1216
Ridaura Capsules (1 to 3%)	2691
Rifadin (Rare)	1276
Rifamate Capsules	1278
Rifater (Rare)	1280
Rimactane Capsules (Rare)	865
Risperdal Tablets (Rare)	1348
Rocephin Injectable Vials, ADD-Vantage, Galaxy Container (Less than 1%)	2305
▲ Roferon-A Injection (5% to 62%)	2308
Rythmol Tablets—150mg, 225mg, 300mg (Less than 1%)	1399
SSD	1402
Sandimmune (2% or less; occasional)	2416
Sansert Tablets	2424
Sedapap Tablets 50 mg/650 mg	1826
Seldane Tablets	1284
Seldane-D Extended-Release Tablets	1286
Septra	1146
▲ Septra I.V. Infusion (Among most frequent)	1142
Septra I.V. Infusion ADD-Vantage Vials	1144
Septra	1146
Ser-Ap-Es Tablets	867
Serentil	689
Silvadene Cream 1%	1288
Sinemet Tablets (Rare)	959
Sinemet CR Tablets	961
Sinequan (Occasional)	2028
Solganal Suspension (Rare)	2530
Spectrobid Tablets	2030
Stelazine	2692
Suprax (Less than 2%)	1443
Surmontil Capsules	2917
Tagamet (Approximately 3 per 1,000,000)	2694
Tambocor Tablets (Less than 1%)	1555
Tapazole Tablets	1361
Tavist Syrup	2426
Tavist Tablets	2427
▲ Taxol Injection (7% to 20%; uncommon)	723
▲ Taxotere for Injection Concentrate (7.5%)	2204
Tazicef for Injection (Very rare)	2697
Tazidime Vials, Faspak & ADD-Vantage (Very rare)	1531
▲ Tegison Capsules (1-10%)	2314
Tegretol/Tegretol-XR	870
Tenoretic Tablets	2963
Tenormin Tablets and I.V. Injection	2965
Terramycin Intramuscular Solution	2034
Thalitone	1293
TheraCys BCG Live (Intravesical) (Up to 0.9%)	911
Thioguanine Tablets, Tabloid Brand	1225
Thioplex (Thiotepa For Injection)	1329
Tiazac Capsules (Infrequent)	1019
Ticar for Injection	2704
TICE BCG, USP (0.3%)	1881
Ticlid Tablets (Rare)	2317
Timentin for Injection	2706
Timolide Tablets	1791
Tofranil Ampuls	873
Tofranil Tablets	875
Tofranil-PM Capsules	876
Tolectin (200, 400 and 600 mg) (Less than 1%)	1591
Tonocard Tablets (Less than 1%)	519
Toradol	2319
Torecan	2367
Tornalate Metered Dose Inhaler (Rare)	978
Trasylol (2%)	607
Trecator-SC Tablets	2919
Trental Tablets (Rare)	1291
Triavil Tablets	1800
Trimpex Tablets	2323
Trinalin Repetabs Tablets	1373
Tussend	1830
Unasyn	2035
Vancocin HCl, Oral Solution & Pulvules (Rare)	1536
Vancocin HCl, Vials & ADD-Vantage (Rare)	1534
Vantin for Oral Suspension and Vantin Tablets	2112
Vaseretic Tablets (Rare)	1810
Vasotec I.V. (Rare)	1814
Vasotec Tablets (Rare)	1816
Velban Vials	1537
▲ VePesid Capsules and Injection (1% to 41%)	727
Vibramycin	2038
Vibramycin Hyclate Intravenous	2040
Vibramycin	2038
Vicodin HP Tablets	1403
Videx Tablets, Powder for Oral Solution, & Pediatric Powder for Oral Solution (1% to 2%)	2980
Viramune Tablets (0.8%)	2368
Vistide Injection	1057
Vivactil Tablets	1820
Cataflam/Voltaren/Voltaren-XR (Less than 1%)	833
▲ Vumon for Injection (85%)	729
Zanosar Sterile Powder	2119
Zantac (A few patients)	1182
Zantac Injection (Few patients)	1180
Zantac Syrup (A few patients)	1182
Zaroxolyn Tablets	1625
Zebeta Tablets	1457
▲ Zerit Capsules (3% to 5%)	731
Zestoretic Tablets (Rare)	2968
Zestril Tablets (Rare)	2972
Ziac	1459
Zinacef (Rare)	1184
Zinecard Injection	2120
Zithromax (Less than 1%)	2043
Zithromax Tablets (Less than 1%)	2046
Zocor Tablets (Rare)	1821
Zosyn	1463
Zovirax Sterile Powder (Less than 1%)	1191
Zyloprim Tablets (Less than 1%)	1194
Zyrtec Tablets (Rare)	2053

Thrombocytopenia, immune

Entry	Page
Ticlid Tablets (Rare)	2317

Thrombocytopenia, neonatal

Entry	Page
Capozide Tablets	744
Diupres Tablets	1691
Dyazide Capsules (Rare)	2653
Etopophos for Injection	701
Etoposide Injection	539
HydroDIURIL Tablets	1716
Hydropres Tablets	1718
Lopressor HCT Tablets	850
Lotensin HCT Tablets	855
Prinzide Tablets	1780
VePesid Capsules and Injection	727
Zestoretic Tablets	2968

Thrombocytopenic purpura
(see under Purpura, thrombocytopenic)

Thrombocytosis

Entry	Page
▲ Accutane Capsules (1 in 5 to 1 in 10 patients)	2252
Ancef Injection	2632
Augmentin (Less than 1%)	2637
Augmentin Tablets (Less than 1%)	2640
Azactam for Injection (Less than 1%)	736
Cedax (0.1% to 1%)	2480
Cefizox for Intramuscular or Intravenous Use (1% to 5%)	1025
Cefotan (1 in 300)	2936
Ceptaz (One in 45)	1070
Chemet Capsules (0.5% to 1.5%)	666
▲ Cipro I.V. (Among most frequent)	587
▲ Cipro I.V. Pharmacy Bulk Package (Among most frequent)	590
Cipro Tablets (0.1%)	584
Clozaril Tablets	2377
Cuprimine Capsules	1673
Danocrine Capsules	2437
Demser Capsules (Rare)	1690
Depakote Tablets (1% to 5%)	418
Depen Titratable Tablets	2770
▲ Dynabac (3.8%)	668
Effexor (Infrequent)	2825
Estratest	2718
Floxin I.V. (More than or equal to 1%)	1580
Floxin Tablets (200 mg, 300 mg, 400 mg) (More than or equal to 1%)	1577
Fortaz (1 in 45)	1092
Kefzol Vials, Faspak & ADD-Vantage	1511
Lovenox Injection	2187
Maxaquin Tablets (Less than 1%)	2593
Maxipime for Injection (0.1% to 1%)	758
Merrem I.V. (Greater than 0.2%)	2952
Monocid Injection (1.7%)	2674
Motrin Ibuprofen Suspension, Oral Drops, Chewable Tablets, Caplets	1563
Netromycin Injection 100 mg/ml (2 of 1000 patients)	2516
Paxil Tablets (Rare)	2681
Penetrex Tablets (Less than 1%)	2196
Pentasa (Less than 1%)	1275
Permax Tablets (Rare)	571
Prevacid Delayed-Release Capsules (Less than 1%)	2746
Primaxin I.M.	1770
Primaxin I.V.	1772
Redux Capsules (Rare)	2911
▲ Rocephin Injectable Vials, ADD-Vantage, Galaxy Container (5.1%)	2305
Tazicef for Injection (1 in 45 patients)	2697
Tazidime Vials, Faspak & ADD-Vantage (1 in 45)	1531
Ticlid Tablets	2317
Unasyn	2035
Vantin for Oral Suspension and Vantin Tablets	2112
Zosyn	1463
Zovirax Sterile Powder (Less than 1%)	1191

Thromboembolic complications

Entry	Page
Arimidex Tablets (1.6% to 3.4%)	2932
Atromid-S Capsules	2808
Brevicon	2563
Cycrin Tablets	991
Demulen	2580
Depo-Provera Sterile Aqueous Suspension	2083
Estraderm Transdermal System	842
Estratest	2718
Heparin Lock Flush Solution	2831
Heparin Sodium Injection	2832
Heparin Sodium Vials	1486
Humegon for Injection	1873
Levlen/Tri-Levlen	646
Menest Tablets	2671
Metrodin (urofollitropin for injection)	2616
Modicon	1928
Mononine, Coagulation Factor IX (Human), Monoclonal Antibody Purified	804
Nordette-21 Tablets	2863
Nordette-28 Tablets	2866
Norinyl	2563
Norplant System	2868
Nor-Q D Tablets	2598
Ogen Vaginal Cream	2106
Ortho-Cyclen/Ortho-Tri-Cyclen	1914
Ortho Dienestrol Cream	1922
Ortho-Est	1925
Ortho-Novum	1928
Ortho-Cyclen/Ortho Tri-Cyclen	1914
Ovcon	765
PMB 200 and PMB 400	2890
Premarin Intravenous	2893
Premarin Vaginal Cream	2898
Premphase	2900
Prempro	2905
Provera Tablets (Occasional)	2110
Serophene (clomiphene citrate tablets, USP) (Rare)	2621
Ticlid Tablets	2317
Levlen/Tri-Levlen	646
Tri-Norinyl	2607
Triphasil-21 Tablets	2919
Triphasil-28 Tablets	2924

Thromboembolic disease
(see under Thromboembolic complications)

Thromboembolism

Entry	Page
Amen Tablets	785
Brevicon	2563
Cortone Acetate Sterile Suspension	1663
Cortone Acetate Tablets	1664
Cycrin Tablets	991
Dalalone D.P. Injectable	1009
Danocrine Capsules	2437
Decadron Elixir	1676
Decadron Phosphate Injection	1680
Decadron Phosphate with Xylocaine Injection, Sterile	1683
Decadron Tablets	1678
Decadron-LA Sterile Suspension	1687
Demulen	2580
Dexacort Phosphate in Respihaler	1606
Dexacort Phosphate in Turbinaire	1607
Diethylstilbestrol Tablets	1477
Estrace Cream and Tablets	751
Estraderm Transdermal System	842
Estratest	2718
Hydeltrasol Injection, Sterile	1708
Hydeltra-T.B.A. Sterile Suspension	1710
Hydrocortone Acetate Sterile Suspension	1712
Hydrocortone Phosphate Injection, Sterile	1713
Hydrocortone Tablets	1715
Lamprene Capsules (Less than 1%)	846
Lo/Ovral Tablets	2852
Lo/Ovral-28 Tablets	2857
Modicon	1928
Nordette-21 Tablets	2863
Nordette-28 Tablets	2866
Norinyl	2563
Ortho-Cyclen/Ortho-Tri-Cyclen	1914
Ortho Dienestrol Cream	1922
Ortho-Est	1925
Ortho-Novum	1928
Ortho-Cyclen/Ortho Tri-Cyclen	1914
Ovcon	765
Ovral Tablets	2877
Ovral-28 Tablets	2878
Ovrette Tablets	2878
Premarin Tablets	2896
Premarin Vaginal Cream	2898
Tegretol-XR Tablets	870
Tri-Norinyl	2607
Triphasil-21 Tablets	2919
Triphasil-28 Tablets	2924

Thromboembolism, arterial

Entry	Page
Brevicon	2563
Demulen	2580
Desogen Tablets	1867
Levlen/Tri-Levlen	646
Metrodin (urofollitropin for injection)	2616
Modicon	1928
Norinyl	2563
Nor-Q D Tablets	2598
Ortho-Cept	1907
Ortho-Cyclen/Ortho-Tri-Cyclen	1914
Ortho-Novum	1928
Ortho-Cyclen/Ortho Tri-Cyclen	1914
Ovcon	765
Pergonal (menotropins for injection, USP)	2618
Profasi (chorionic gonadotropin for injection, USP)	2620
Levlen/Tri-Levlen	646
Tri-Norinyl	2607

Thrombopenia
(see under Thrombocytopenia)

Thrombophlebitis

Entry	Page
Abelcet Injection	1540
AK-FLUOR Injection 10% and 25%	⊙ 204
Amen Tablets	785
Amicar Syrup, Tablets, and Injection	1312
Anafranil Capsules (Rare)	819
Arimidex Tablets (2% to 5%)	2932
Atretol Tablets	569
Azactam for Injection (1.9%)	736
Bactrim I.V. Infusion (Rare)	2255
Betaseron for SC Injection	653
Brevibloc (esmolol HCl) Injection (Less than 1%)	1860
Brevicon	2563
Cerebyx Injection (Infrequent)	1956
Cipro I.V. (1% or less)	587

(▣ Described in PDR For Nonprescription Drugs) Incidence data in parenthesis; ▲ 3% or more (⊙ Described in PDR For Ophthalmology)

Thrombophlebitis

Cipro I.V. Pharmacy Bulk Package
(Less than 1%) ... 590
Cleocin Phosphate Injection ... 2068
Climara Transdermal System ... 640
Clomid ... 1262
Clozaril Tablets (Less than 1%) ... 2377
Cortifoam ... 2540
Cuprimine Capsules (Rare) ... 1673
Cycrin Tablets ... 991
▲ Cytosar-U Sterile Powder (Among most frequent) ... 2077
Dalgan Injection (Less than 1%) ... 529
Dantrium Intravenous ... 2132
Demulen ... 2580
Depen Titratable Tablets (Rare) ... 2770
Depo-Provera Contraceptive Injection (Fewer than 1%) ... 2079
Depo-Provera Sterile Aqueous Suspension ... 2083
Desogen Tablets ... 1867
Doxil (Less than 1%) ... 2613
Effexor (Infrequent) ... 2825
▲ Emcyt Capsules (3%) ... 2085
Epogen for Injection (Rare) ... 489
Ergamisol Tablets ... 1340
Estrace Cream and Tablets ... 751
Estraderm Transdermal System ... 842
ESTRATAB Tablets (0.3, 0.625, 1.25, 2.5 mg) ... 2715
Estratest ... 2718
Estring Vaginal Ring (At least 1 report) ... 2086
Ethmozine Tablets (Less than 2%) ... 2217
Felbatol ... 2774
Flagyl I.V. ... 2373
Florinef Acetate Tablets ... 506
Fluorescite ... ⊚ 217
Fluorouracil Injection ... 2282
Foscavir Injection (Less than 1%) ... 541
Sterile FUDR ... 2284
▲ Fungizone Intravenous (Among most common) ... 507
Indocin Capsules (Rare) ... 1723
Indocin I.V. ... 1727
Indocin (Rare) ... 1723
Invirase Capsules (Rare) ... 2291
Kefurox Vials, Faspak & ADD-Vantage (1 in 60) ... 1509
Kerlone Tablets (Less than 2%) ... 2588
Lasix Injection, Oral Solution and Tablets ... 1267
Levlen/Tri-Levlen ... 646
Lo/Ovral Tablets ... 2852
Lo/Ovral-28 Tablets ... 2857
Mandol Vials, Faspak & ADD-Vantage (Rare) ... 1516
Mefoxin ... 1734
Mefoxin Premixed Intravenous Solution ... 1737
Megace Tablets (Rare) ... 710
Menest Tablets ... 2671
Merrem I.V. (1.2%) ... 2952
Mestinon Injectable ... 1300
Methergine (Rare) ... 2401
Mezlin ... 594
Mezlin Pharmacy Bulk Package ... 597
Miacalcin Nasal Spray (Less than 1%) ... 2403
Modicon ... 1928
Mustargen ... 1752
Mutamycin for Injection ... 712
Neurontin Capsules (Rare) ... 1978
Nordette-21 Tablets ... 2863
Nordette-28 Tablets ... 2866
Norinyl ... 2563
Norplant System ... 2868
Nor-Q D Tablets ... 2598
Ogen Tablets ... 2103
Ogen Vaginal Cream ... 2106
Ortho-Cept ... 1907
Ortho-Cyclen/Ortho-Tri-Cyclen ... 1914
Ortho Dienestrol Cream ... 1922
Ortho-Est ... 1925
Ortho-Novum ... 1928
Ortho-Cyclen/Ortho Tri-Cyclen ... 1914
Ovcon ... 765
Ovral Tablets ... 2877
Ovral-28 Tablets ... 2878
Ovrette Tablets ... 2878
Paxil Tablets (Rare) ... 2681
Permax Tablets (Infrequent) ... 571
▲ Pipracil (4%) ... 1435
PMB 200 and PMB 400 ... 2890
Premarin Intravenous ... 2893
Premarin Tablets ... 2896
Premarin Vaginal Cream ... 2898
Premphase ... 2900
Prempro ... 2905
▲ Primaxin I.V. (3.1%) ... 1772
Procrit for Injection (Rare) ... 1896
Provera Tablets (Occasional) ... 2110

Prozac Pulvules & Liquid, Oral Solution (Rare) ... 935
Redux Capsules (Infrequent) ... 2911
Relafen Tablets (Less than 1%) ... 2688
Risperdal Tablets (Rare) ... 1348
Robaxin Injectable ... 2245
Roferon-A Injection (Rare) ... 2308
Romazicon (1% to 3%) ... 2311
Sandostatin Injection (Less than 1%) ... 2421
Sansert Tablets ... 2424
Septra I.V. Infusion (Rare) ... 1142
Septra I.V. Infusion ADD-Vantage Vials (Rare) ... 1144
Taxotere for Injection Concentrate ... 2204
Tegretol/Tegretol-XR ... 870
Timentin for Injection ... 2706
Levlen/Tri-Levlen ... 646
Tri-Norinyl ... 2607
Triphasil-21 Tablets ... 2919
Triphasil-28 Tablets ... 2924
▲ Unasyn (3%) ... 2035
Vancocin HCl, Vials & ADD-Vantage ... 1534
Zinacef (1 in 60 patients) ... 1184
Zosyn (0.2% to 1.3%) ... 1463
Zyloprim Tablets (Less than 1%) ... 1194

Thrombophlebitis, deep-vein

Cardene I.V. (Rare) ... 2815
Cytovene (1% or less) ... 2270
Humegon for Injection ... 1873
Lamictal Tablets (Rare) ... 1105
Lioresal Intrathecal (1% or more) ... 1634
Naprelan Tablets (Less than 1%) ... 2861
Nipent for Injection (Less than 3%) ... 2733

Thromboplastin time, increase

Azactam for Injection ... 736
Eminase ... 2215
Hespan Injection ... 945
Merrem I.V. (Greater than 0.2%) ... 2952
▲ Oncaspar (Greater than 1% but less than 5%) ... 2194
Pentaspan Injection ... 954
Zosyn ... 1463

Thrombosis

Ambien Tablets (Rare) ... 2559
Amicar Syrup, Tablets, and Injection ... 1312
Betaseron for SC Injection ... 653
BiCNU (Rare) ... 696
▲ CellCept Capsules (More than or equal to 3%) ... 2265
Demadex Tablets and Injection ... 691
Demulen ... 2580
Diprivan Injectable Emulsion (Rare; less than 1%) ... 2939
Doxil (Less than 1%) ... 2613
Emcyt Capsules ... 2085
Estratest ... 2718
Foscavir Injection (Between 1% and 5%) ... 541
Hivid Tablets (Less than 1%) ... 2287
Humegon for Injection ... 1873
Imitrex Tablets (Rare) ... 1099
Kerlone Tablets (Less than 2%) ... 2588
Konÿne 80 Factor IX Complex ... 627
Leukine ... 1317
Leustatin (2%) ... 1889
Lovenox Injection (Rare) ... 2187
Lupron Injection (5% or more) ... 2736
Metrodin (urofollitropin for injection) ... 2616
Mustargen ... 1752
▲ Oncaspar (Greater than 1% but less than 5%) ... 2194
Ovcon ... 765
Paxil Tablets (Rare) ... 2681
Pipracil ... 1435
PMB 200 and PMB 400 ... 2890
Premarin Intravenous ... 2893
Premarin Vaginal Cream ... 2898
Proleukin for Injection (1%) ... 812
Redux Capsules (Rare) ... 2911
Rilutek Tablets (Rare) ... 2198
Stimate, (desmopressin acetate) Nasal Spray, 1.5 mg/mL (Rare) ... 806
▲ Valium Injectable (Among most common) ... 2336

Thrombosis, arterial

Orthoclone OKT3 Sterile Solution ... 1892

Thrombosis, cerebral
(see under Cerebral thrombosis)

Thrombosis, coronary
(see under Coronary thrombosis)

Thrombosis, glomerular capillary

Amicar Syrup, Tablets, and Injection ... 1312
Neoral ... 2405
Sandimmune ... 2416

Thrombosis, mesenteric

Brevicon ... 2563
Cartrol Tablets ... 413
Demulen ... 2580
ESTRATAB Tablets (0.3, 0.625, 1.25, 2.5 mg) ... 2715
Estratest ... 2718
Levatol Tablets ... 2547
Levlen/Tri-Levlen ... 646
Menest Tablets ... 2671
Norinyl ... 2563
Nor-Q D Tablets ... 2598
Ortho Dienestrol Cream ... 1922
Ovcon ... 765
PMB 200 and PMB 400 ... 2890
Premarin Intravenous ... 2893
Premarin Vaginal Cream ... 2898
Trandate Tablets ... 1158
Levlen/Tri-Levlen ... 646
Tri-Norinyl ... 2607

Thrombosis, mesenteric arterial

Timoptic-XE ... 1798
Visken Tablets ... 2428
Zebeta Tablets ... 1457

Thrombosis, renal artery

Epogen for Injection (Rare) ... 489
Procrit for Injection ... 1896

Thrombosis, retinal

Amen Tablets ... 785
Brevicon ... 2563
Clomid ... 1262
Cycrin Tablets ... 991
Demulen ... 2580
Depo-Provera Contraceptive Injection ... 2079
Depo-Provera Sterile Aqueous Suspension ... 2083
Epogen for Injection (Rare) ... 489
ESTRATAB Tablets (0.3, 0.625, 1.25, 2.5 mg) ... 2715
Estratest ... 2718
Levlen/Tri-Levlen ... 646
Lo/Ovral Tablets ... 2852
Lo/Ovral-28 Tablets ... 2857
Menest Tablets ... 2671
Modicon ... 1928
Nordette-21 Tablets ... 2863
Nordette-28 Tablets ... 2866
Norinyl ... 2563
Nor-Q D Tablets ... 2598
Ortho-Cyclen/Ortho-Tri-Cyclen ... 1914
Ortho Dienestrol Cream ... 1922
Ortho-Novum ... 1928
Ortho-Cyclen/Ortho Tri-Cyclen ... 1914
Ovcon ... 765
Ovral Tablets ... 2877
Ovral-28 Tablets ... 2878
Ovrette Tablets ... 2878
PMB 200 and PMB 400 ... 2890
Premarin Intravenous ... 2893
Premarin Vaginal Cream ... 2898
Premphase ... 2900
Prempro ... 2905
Procrit for Injection (Rare) ... 1896
Provera Tablets (Occasional) ... 2110
Levlen/Tri-Levlen ... 646
Tri-Norinyl ... 2607
Triphasil-21 Tablets ... 2919
Triphasil-28 Tablets ... 2924

Thrombosis, sagittal sinus

Danocrine Capsules ... 2437
Oncaspar ... 2194

Thrombosis, venous

Actimmune (Rare) ... 1043
Activase ... 1045
Clomid ... 1262
Clozaril Tablets ... 2377
Demulen ... 2580
Depo-Provera Contraceptive Injection (Fewer than 1%) ... 2079
Desogen Tablets ... 1867
Dizac (diazepam injectable emulsion) CIV (Less frequent) ... 1862
Epogen for Injection (Rare) ... 489
Fludara for Injection (1% to 3%) ... 658
Mepergan Injection ... 2859
Modicon ... 1928

Mononine, Coagulation Factor IX (Human), Monoclonal Antibody Purified ... 804
Mykrox Tablets ... 1617
Nimotop Capsules (Less than 1%) ... 603
Nolvadex Tablets (0.8%) ... 2957
Norplant System ... 2868
Oncaspar ... 2194
Ortho-Cept ... 1907
Ortho-Cyclen/Ortho-Tri-Cyclen ... 1914
Ortho-Novum ... 1928
Ortho-Cyclen/Ortho Tri-Cyclen ... 1914
Orthoclone OKT3 Sterile Solution ... 1892
Phenergan Injection ... 2880
Pipracil (Less frequent) ... 1435
Taxol Injection (Approximately 1%) ... 723
Taxotere for Injection Concentrate ... 2204
Zaroxolyn Tablets ... 1625

Thrombosis of vascular access

▲ Epogen for Injection (0.25% to 7%) ... 489
Lasix Injection, Oral Solution and Tablets ... 1267
Procrit for Injection ... 1896

Thrombotic events, unspecified

DDAVP Injection (Rare) ... 2178
DDAVP Injection 15 mcg/mL (Rare) ... 2179
Danocrine Capsules ... 2437
Desmopressin Acetate Injection (Rare) ... 996
Procrit for Injection ... 1896

Thrombotic microangiopathy

Blenoxane (Rare) ... 697
Platinol for Injection (Rare) ... 717
Platinol-AQ Injection (Rare) ... 719

Thrombotic vascular disease

Ortho-Cyclen/Ortho-Tri-Cyclen ... 1914
Ortho Dienestrol Cream ... 1922
Ortho-Cyclen/Ortho Tri-Cyclen ... 1914
▲ Tegison Capsules (1 to 10%) ... 2314

Thrush, oral
(see under Candidiasis, oral)

Thymol turbidity test, positive

Atromid-S Capsules ... 2808
Cuprimine Capsules ... 1673
Depen Titratable Tablets (Few reports) ... 2770

Thymus gland abnormalities, fetal

Accutane Capsules ... 2252

Thyroid adenoma

Permax Tablets (Rare) ... 571
Quadrinal Tablets ... 1398
SSKI Solution ... 2767

Thyroid binding globulin, increase
(see under T4, increase)

Thyroid disease, exacerbation

Proleukin for Injection ... 812

Thyroid
(see under T4, decrease; T4, increase; T3, decrease)

Thyroid function test, abnormal

BuSpar Tablets (Rare) ... 738
Depakene ... 416
Depakote Tablets ... 418
Depo-Provera Sterile Aqueous Suspension ... 2083
DYNACIN Capsules (Very rare) ... 1627
Lescol Capsules ... 2395
Mevacor Tablets ... 1742
Minocin Intravenous (Very rare) ... 1428
Minocin Oral Suspension (Very rare) ... 1431
Minocin Pellet-Filled Capsules (Very rare) ... 1429
Pravachol Tablets ... 770
Proleukin for Injection ... 812
Provera Tablets ... 2110
Roferon-A Injection (Infrequent) ... 2308
SSKI Solution ... 2767
Zocor Tablets ... 1821

Thyroid gland discoloration

Achromycin V Capsules ... 1417
Declomycin Tablets ... 1421
Doryx Capsules ... 1970
DYNACIN Capsules ... 1627
Helidac Therapy ... 2135
Minocin Intravenous ... 1428

(⊠ Described in PDR For Nonprescription Drugs) Incidence data in parenthesis; ▲ 3% or more (⊚ Described in PDR For Ophthalmology)

1469 **Side Effects Index** **Tinnitus**

Minocin Oral Suspension ... 1431
Minocin Pellet-Filled Capsules ... 1429
Monodox Capsules ... 1858
Terramycin Intramuscular Solution 2034
Vibramycin ... 2038
Vibramycin Hyclate Intravenous ... 2040
Vibramycin ... 2038

Thyroid gland enlargement

Lupron Injection (Less than 5%) ... 2736

Thyroid hormone, changes (see under T4, decrease; T4, increase; T3, decrease)

Thyroid nodule

ProSom Tablets (Rare) ... 457

Thyroiditis

Cuprimine Capsules ... 1673
Depen Titratable Tablets (Extremely rare) ... 2770
Paxil Tablets (Rare) ... 2681
Sular Tablets (Less than or equal to 1%) ... 2961

Tingling

Apresazide Capsules (Less frequent) ... 824
Apresoline Hydrochloride Tablets (Less frequent) ... 826
Asendin Tablets (Less than 1%) ... 1419
Axocet Capsules (Infrequent) ... 2469
Azelex (Approximately 1% to 5%) ... 471
Bentyl ... 1246
Cipro I.V. ... 587
Cipro Tablets ... 584
Condylox Topical Solution (Less than 5%) ... 1853
Decadron Phosphate Injection ... 1680
DynaCirc Capsules (0.5% to 1%) .. 2381
Elimite (permethrin) 5% Cream (1 to 2% or less) ... 475
▲ Elocon Ointment 0.1% (4.8%) ... 2494
Engerix-B Unit-Dose Vials (Less than 1%) ... 2656
Esgic-plus Capsules (Infrequent) ... 1012
Esgic-plus Tablets (Infrequent) ... 1012
Fioricet Tablets (Infrequent) ... 2386
Fioricet with Codeine Capsules (Infrequent) ... 2387
Fiorinal with Codeine Capsules (Infrequent) ... 2390
Floxin I.V. ... 1580
Floxin Tablets (200 mg, 300 mg, 400 mg) ... 1577
Hydralazine Hydrochloride Injection USP (Less frequent) ... 2712
▲ Imitrex Injection (13.5%) ... 1095
▲ Imitrex Tablets (4% to 8%) ... 1099
K-Phos Neutral Tablets ... 633
K-Phos Original Formula 'Sodium Free' Tablets (Less frequent) ... 633
Konÿne 80 Factor IX Complex ... 627
Ludiomil Tablets (Rare) ... 861
Maxaquin Tablets ... 2593
Mononine, Coagulation Factor IX (Human), Monoclonal Antibody Purified ... 804
NegGram ... 2453
Neoral (Rare) ... 2405
Noroxin Tablets ... 1758
Norpace (Less than 1%) ... 2596
Norplant System ... 2868
Norpramin Tablets ... 1273
Nubain Injection (1% or less) ... 952
Oxistat Lotion (0.4%) ... 1139
Pamelor ... 2409
Phrenilin (Infrequent) ... 790
Priscoline Hydrochloride Ampuls ... 864
SSKI Solution (Less frequent) ... 2767
Sandimmune (Rare) ... 2416
Sedapap Tablets 50 mg/650 mg (Infrequent) ... 1826
Ser-Ap-Es Tablets ... 867
Slo-Niacin Tablets ... 2767
THYREL TRH (Less frequent) ... 2992
Tofranil Ampuls ... 873
Tofranil Tablets ... 875
Tofranil-PM Capsules ... 876
Zonalon Cream (Less than 1%) ... 1042

Tingling, ears

Parlodel (Less than 1%) ... 2411

Tingling, extremities

Bellergal-S Tablets (Rare) ... 2375
Diamox Sequels (Sustained Release) ... ◉ 318
Elavil ... 2945
Etrafon ... 2495
GlaucTabs ... ◉ 209
Hivid Tablets ... 2287
Hydrocortone Phosphate Injection, Sterile ... 1713
Limbitrol ... 2333
MetroCream ... 1034
Myambutol Tablets ... 1432
Neptazane Tablets ... ◉ 320
Nicotrol NS Nicotine Nasal Spray (Common) ... 1565
Norpramin Tablets ... 1273
Polycitra Syrup ... 574
Polycitra-K Crystals ... 574
Polycitra-K Oral Solution ... 575
Polycitra-LC ... 574
Surmontil Capsules ... 2917
Triavil Tablets ... 1800
Videx Tablets, Powder for Oral Solution, & Pediatric Powder for Oral Solution ... 2980
Vivactil Tablets ... 1820
Zerit Capsules ... 731

Tingling, feet

Alferon N Injection (1%) ... 2142
Fluorouracil Injection ... 2282
Uroqid-Acid No. 2 Tablets ... 633

Tingling, fingers

Noroxin Tablets (0.3% to 1.0%) ... 1758
Noroxin Tablets (0.3% to 1.0%) ... 2222
Parlodel (Rare) ... 2411
Peptavlon ... 2997
Wigraine Tablets ... 1884

Tingling, hands

Adenocard Injection (1%) ... 1021
Fluorouracil Injection ... 2282
Uroqid-Acid No. 2 Tablets ... 633

Tingling, legs

Alferon N Injection (1%) ... 2142

Tingling, lips

K-Phos Neutral Tablets ... 633
K-Phos Original Formula 'Sodium Free' Tablets (Less frequent) ... 633
Marcaine Spinal ... 2449
Sensorcaine ... 554
Uroqid-Acid No. 2 Tablets ... 633

Tingling, mouth

Foscavir Injection ... 541
Marcaine Spinal ... 2449
Sensorcaine ... 554

Tingling, perineal area

Hydeltrasol Injection, Sterile ... 1708

Tingling, scalp

Cormax Scalp Application (Approximately 0.6%) ... 1857
▲ Normodyne Injection (7%) ... 2519
Normodyne Tablets (Less common) ... 2522
Temovate Scalp Application (2 of 294 patients) ... 1153
▲ Trandate (7 of 100 patients) ... 1158

Tingling, skin

Amikacin Sulfate Injection, USP ... 523
Garamycin Injectable ... 2502
Nebcin Vials, Hyporets & ADD-Vantage ... 1518
Netromycin Injection 100 mg/ml ... 2516
▲ Normodyne Injection (7%) ... 2519
▲ Trandate Injection (7 of 100 patients) ... 1158

Tingling, toes

Wigraine Tablets ... 1884

Tinnitus

Abelcet Injection ... 1540
Accutane Capsules (Less than 1%) ... 2252
Achromycin V Capsules ... 1417
Adalat CC (Less than 1.0%) ... 582
Adapin Capsules (Occasional) ... 1542
Alferon N Injection (One patient) ... 2142
Alka-Seltzer Cherry Effervescent Antacid and Pain Reliever ... ▣ 609
Alka-Seltzer Extra Strength Effervescent Antacid and Pain Reliever ... ▣ 609
Alka-Seltzer Lemon Lime Effervescent Antacid and Pain Reliever ... ▣ 609
Alka-Seltzer Original Effervescent Antacid and Pain Reliever ... ▣ 609
Altace Capsules (Less than 1%) ... 1238
Ambien Tablets (Infrequent) ... 2559
Amicar Syrup, Tablets, and Injection ... 1312
Amikacin Sulfate Injection, USP ... 523
▲ Anafranil Capsules (4% to 6%) ... 819
▲ Anaprox/Naprosyn (3% to 9%) ... 2277
Aralen Hydrochloride Injection (1 patient) ... 2430
Aralen Phosphate Tablets (1 patient) ... 2431
Asacol Delayed-Release Tablets ... 2129
Ascriptin ... ▣ 650
Asendin Tablets (Less than 1%) ... 1419
Atretol Tablets ... 569
Atrohist Plus Tablets ... 1605
Atrovent Nasal Spray 0.06% (Less than 1%) ... 678
Axocet Capsules (Infrequent) ... 2469
Azactam for Injection (Less than 1%) ... 736
Azulfidine (Rare) ... 2059
Arthritis Strength BC Powder ... ▣ 631
BC Powder ... ▣ 631
Backache Caplets ... ▣ 635
Bactrim DS Tablets ... 2257
Bactrim I.V. Infusion ... 2255
Bactrim ... 2257
Genuine Bayer Aspirin Tablets & Caplets ... ▣ 618
Extra Strength Bayer Arthritis Pain Regimen Formula ... ▣ 615
Extra Strength Bayer Aspirin Caplets & Tablets ... ▣ 617
Extended-Release Bayer 8-Hour Aspirin ... ▣ 616
Extra Strength Bayer PM Aspirin Plus Sleep Aid ... ▣ 617
Aspirin Regimen Bayer 81 mg Tablets with Calcium ... ▣ 615
Aspirin Regimen Bayer Children's Chewable Aspirin ... ▣ 616
Aspirin Regimen Bayer Regular Strength 325 mg Caplets ... ▣ 613
Benadryl Injection ... 1955
Biaxin ... 406
Blocadren Tablets (Less than 1%) 1654
Arthritis Strength Bufferin Analgesic Caplets ... ▣ 637
Buprenex Injectable (Less than 1%) ... 2170
BuSpar Tablets (Frequent) ... 738
Cama Arthritis Pain Reliever ... ▣ 748
Capastat Sulfate Injection ... 968
Carbocaine Injection ... 2432
Cardene Capsules (Rare) ... 2261
Cardene I.V. (Rare) ... 2815
Cardene SR Capsules (Rare) ... 2264
Cardioquin Tablets ... 2146
Cardizem CD Capsules (Less than 1%) ... 1251
Cardizem SR Capsules (Less than 1%) ... 1255
Cardizem Injectable ... 1253
Cardizem Tablets (Less than 1%) .. 1257
Cardura Tablets (1%) ... 1993
Cartrol Tablets (Less common) ... 413
Cataflam Tablets (1% to 3%) ... 833
▲ Cerebyx Injection (8.9%) ... 1956
Cipro I.V. (1% or less) ... 587
Cipro I.V. Pharmacy Bulk Package (Less than 1%) ... 590
Cipro Tablets (Less than 1%) ... 584
Claritin Tablets (2% or fewer patients) ... 2485
Claritin-D Tablets (Less frequent) .. 2487
Clinoril Tablets (Greater than 1%) 1658
Clomid ... 1262
Cognex Capsules (Infrequent) ... 1961
Cozaar Tablets (Less than 1%) ... 1668
Cuprimine Capsules (Greater than 1%) ... 1673
Cytotec (Infrequent) ... 2576
Cytovene (1% or less) ... 2270
Dalgan Injection (Less than 1%) ... 529
Dapsone Tablets USP ... 1331
Daranide Tablets ... 1676
DaunoXome (Less than or equal to 5%) ... 1842
Daypro Caplets (1% to 3%) ... 2578
Demadex Tablets and Injection ... 691
Depakote Tablets (1% to 5%) ... 418
Depen Titratable Tablets ... 2770
Desferal Vials ... 838
Desyrel and Desyrel Dividose (1.4%) ... 504
Diamox Intravenous ... ◉ 317
Diamox Sequels (Sustained Release) ... ◉ 318
Diamox Tablets ... ◉ 317
Dilacor XR Extended-release Capsules (1.0%) ... 2183
Dipentum Capsules (Rare) ... 2084
Diprivan Injectable Emulsion (Less than 1%) ... 2939
▲ Disalcid (Among most common) ... 1549
Doan's Extra-Strength Analgesic .. ▣ 653
Extra Strength Doan's P.M. ... ▣ 653
Doan's Regular Strength Analgesic ... ▣ 654
Dolobid Tablets (Greater than 1 in 100) ... 1695
Doxil (Less than 1%) ... 2613
Duranest Injections ... 533
Dyclone 0.5% and 1% Topical Solutions, USP ... 535
Dynabac (0.1% to 1%) ... 668
Easprin ... 1971
▲ EC-Naprosyn Delayed-Release Tablets (3% to 9%) ... 2277
Ecotrin ... 2625
Edecrin ... 1698
Effexor (2%) ... 2825
Elavil ... 2945
Eldepryl Capsules ... 2729
EMLA Cream (Unlikely with cream) 536
Engerix-B Unit-Dose Vials ... 2656
Esgic-plus Capsules (Infrequent) ... 1012
Esgic-plus Tablets (Infrequent) ... 1012
Eskalith ... 2658
Ethmozine Tablets (Less than 2%) 2217
Etrafon ... 2495
Excedrin Extra-Strength Analgesic Tablets, Caplets, and Geltabs ... 734
Fansidar Tablets ... 2281
Feldene Capsules (Greater than 1%) ... 2008
Fioricet Tablets (Infrequent) ... 2386
Fioricet with Codeine Capsules (Infrequent) ... 2387
Fiorinal with Codeine Capsules (Infrequent) ... 2390
Flexeril Tablets (Less than 1%) ... 1701
Floxin I.V. (Less than 1%) ... 1580
Floxin Tablets (200 mg, 300 mg, 400 mg) (Less than 1%) ... 1577
Flumadine Tablets & Syrup (0.3% to 1%) ... 1013
Foscavir Injection (Less than 1%) .. 541
Fungizone Intravenous ... 507
Gantanol Tablets ... 2285
Gantrisin ... 2286
Garamycin Injectable ... 2502
Gastrocrom Oral Concentrate (Less common) ... 1611
GlaucTabs ... ◉ 209
Halcion Tablets (Rare) ... 2093
Helidac Therapy ... 2135
Hivid Tablets (Less than 1%) ... 2287
Hyperstat I.V. Injection ... 2504
Hytrin Capsules (At least 1%) ... 434
Hyzaar Tablets ... 1720
IBU Tablets (Greater than 1%) ... 1389
Ilosone (Isolated reports) ... 927
Imdur (Less than or equal to 5%) .. 1362
Indocin (Greater than 1%) ... 1723
Intron A for Injection (Less than 5%) ... 2506
Invirase Capsules (Less than 2%) .. 2291
Kerlone Tablets (Less than 2%) ... 2588
Lamictal Tablets (1.1%) ... 1105
▲ Lariam Tablets (Among most frequent) ... 2295
Lasix Injection, Oral Solution and Tablets ... 1267
Lioresal Intrathecal (1% or more) .. 1634
Lioresal Tablets ... 847
Lithium Carbonate Capsules & Tablets ... 2352
Lithonate/Lithotabs/Lithobid ... 2721
Lodine Capsules and Tablets (1% to 3%) ... 2849
Lopressor ... 848
Lopressor HCT Tablets (1 in 100 patients) ... 850
Lotensin HCT Tablets (0.3% to 1.0%) ... 855
Lotrel Capsules (Infrequent) ... 858
Ludiomil Tablets (Rare) ... 861
Lupron Depot - 3 Month 22.5 mg (Less than 5%) ... 2743
LUVOX Tablets ... 2723
Marcaine ... 2446
Marcaine Spinal ... 2449
Marinol (Dronabinol) Capsules (Less than 1%) ... 2353
Maxaquin Tablets (Less than 1%) .. 2593
Methergine (Rare) ... 2401
Methotrexate Sodium Tablets, Injection, for Injection and LPF Injection (Less common) ... 1322

(▣ Described in PDR For Nonprescription Drugs) Incidence data in parenthesis; ▲ 3% or more (◉ Described in PDR For Ophthalmology)

Tinnitus

Mexitil Capsules (1.9% to 2.4%) .. 684
Miacalcin Nasal Spray (Less than
    1%) 2403
Midamor Tablets (Less than or
    equal to 1%) 1746
Minipress Capsules (Less than
    1%) 2015
Minizide Capsules (Rare) 2016
Mintezol 1747
Mobigesic Tablets .... 🕮 607
Moduretic Tablets 1748
Mono-Gesic Tablets 810
Monopril Tablets (0.2% to 1.0%)... 762
Motrin Ibuprofen Suspension, Oral
    Drops, Chewable Tablets,
    Caplets (1% to less than 3%) 1563
Mustargen (Infrequent) 1752
Mykrox Tablets (Less than 2%) 1617
▲ Nalfon 200 Pulvules & Nalfon
    Tablets (4.5%) 933
▲ Naprelan Tablets (3% to 9%)....... 2861
▲ Anaprox/Naprosyn (3% to 9%)..... 2277
Nebcin Vials, Hyporets &
    ADD-Vantage 1518
Neoral (2% or less) 2405
Neptazane Tablets .... ⊙ 320
Nescaine/Nescaine MPF 549
Netromycin Injection 100 mg/ml... 2516
Neurontin Capsules (Infrequent) ... 1978
Nipent for Injection (Less than
    3%) 2733
Noroxin Tablets 1758
Noroxin Tablets 2222
Norpramin Tablets 1273
Norvasc Tablets (More than 0.1%
    to 1%) 2020
Norvir (Less than 2%) 447
Ornade Spansule Capsules 2678
Orthoclone OKT3 Sterile Solution .. 1892
Orudis Capsules (Greater than
    1%) 2874
Oruvail Capsules (Greater than
    1%) 2874
OxyContin Tablets (Less than 1%) 2163
PBZ Tablets 863
PBZ-SR Tablets 862
Pamelor 2409
Parnate Tablets 2679
Paxil Tablets (Frequent) 2681
Pediazole Suspension 2340
Penetrex Tablets (0.1% to 1%) 2196
Pepcid Injection (Infrequent) 1765
Pepcid (Infrequent) 1763
Pepto-Bismol Original Liquid,
    Original and Cherry Tablets and
    Easy-To-Swallow Caplets 2126
Pepto-Bismol Maximum Strength
    Liquid 2126
Periactin 1767
Permax Tablets (Infrequent) 571
Phenergan Injection 2880
Phenergan Tablets 2882
Phrenilin (Infrequent) 790
Plaquenil Sulfate Tablets 2459
Platinol for Injection 717
Platinol-AQ Injection 719
Pontocaine Hydrochloride for
    Spinal Anesthesia 2460
Prevacid Delayed-Release
    Capsules (Less than 1%) 2746
Prilosec Delayed-Release Capsules
    (Less than 1%) 516
Primaxin I.M. 1770
Primaxin I.V. (Less than 0.2%) 1772
Prinivil Tablets (0.3% to 1.0%)...... 1776
Prinzide Tablets (0.3 to 1%) 1780
Procardia Capsules (Less than
    0.5%) 2024
Procardia XL Extended Release
    Tablets (1% or less) 2026
▲ Prograf (Greater than 3%) 1028
ProSom Tablets (Infrequent) 457
Proventil (2%) 2529
Prozac Pulvules & Liquid, Oral
    Solution (2%) 935
Questran 774
Quinaglute Dura-Tabs Tablets 644
Quinidex Extentabs 2240
Recombivax HB (Less than 1%)... 1787
Redux Capsules (Infrequent) 2911
▲ Relafen Tablets (3% to 9%) 2688
ReVia Tablets (Less than 1%) 957
Rifater 1280
Risperdal Tablets (Rare) 1348
Romazicon (Less than 1%) 2311
Rythmol Tablets—150mg, 225mg,
    300mg (Less than 1 to 1.9%) 1399
Salflex Tablets (Common) 791
Sandimmune (2% or less) 2416
Sedapap Tablets 50 mg/650 mg
    (Infrequent) 1826

Sensorcaine 554
Septra 1146
Septra I.V. Infusion 1142
Septra I.V. Infusion ADD-Vantage
    Vials 1144
Septra 1146
Serzone Tablets (Up to 3%) 776
Sinequan (Occasional) 2028
Soma Compound w/Codeine
    Tablets 2784
Soma Compound Tablets 2783
Sporanox Capsules (Infrequent) ... 1352
▲ Stadol (3% to 9%) 779
Streptomycin Sulfate Injection..... 2031
Sular Tablets (Less than or equal
    to 1%) 2961
Surmontil Capsules 2917
Talacen Caplets (Rare) 2464
Talwin Injection (Rare) 2465
Talwin Compound 2466
Talwin Injection 2465
Talwin Nx Tablets 2467
Tambocor Tablets (1% to less
    than 3%) 1555
Tavist Syrup 2426
Tavist Tablets 2427
Tegretol/Tegretol-XR 870
Tenex Tablets (3% or less) 2249
Tiazac Capsules (Less than 1%) ... 1019
Ticlid Tablets (0.5% to 1.0%) 2317
Timolide Tablets 1791
Timoptic in Ocudose 1796
Timoptic Sterile Ophthalmic
    Solution 1794
Timoptic-XE 1798
Tofranil Ampuls 873
Tofranil Tablets 875
Tofranil-PM Capsules 876
Tolectin (200, 400 and 600 mg)
    (1 to 3%) 1591
Tonocard Tablets (0.4% to 1.5%)   519
Toprol-XL Tablets 560
Toradol (1% or less) 2319
Torecan 2367
Triavil Tablets 1800
▲ Trilisate (Less than 20%) 2155
Trinalin Repetabs Tablets 1373
Tussend 1830
Tympagesic Ear Drops 2476
Ultram Tablets (50 mg)
    (Infrequent) 1594
Univasc Tablets (Less than 1%)... 2553
Vancenase AQ Double Strength
    Nasal Spray 0.084% (2% to
    3%) 2536
Vancocin HCl, Oral Solution &
    Pulvules (Rare) 1536
Vancocin HCl, Vials &
    ADD-Vantage (Rare) 1534
Vantin for Oral Suspension and
    Vantin Tablets (Less than 1%) ... 2112
▲ Vascor Tablets (200 and 300 mg)
    (Up to 6.52%) 1597
Vaseretic Tablets (0.5% to 2.0%) 1810
Vasotec I.V. 1814
Vasotec Tablets (0.5% to 1.0%)... 1816
Videx Tablets, Powder for Oral
    Solution, & Pediatric Powder for
    Oral Solution (Less than 1%)..... 2980
Vivactil Tablets 1820
Cataflam/Voltaren/Voltaren-XR
    (1% to 3%) 833
Wellbutrin Tablets 1177
▲ Xanax Tablets (6.6%) 2115
▲ Xylocaine Injections (Among most
    common) 562
Zebeta Tablets 1457
Zestoretic Tablets (0.3 to 1%) 2968
Zestril Tablets (0.3% to 1.0%) 2972
Ziac 1459
Zoloft Tablets (1.4%) 2051
Zosyn (1.0% or less) 1463
Zyloprim Tablets (Less than 1%)... 1194
Zyrtec Tablets (Less than 2%) 2053

Tiredness
(see under Fatigue)

Tissue damage, ischemic

Sansert Tablets (Rare) 2424

Toes, discoloration

Eskalith (A few reports) 2658
Lithium Carbonate Capsules &
    Tablets (A single report) 2352
Lithonate/Lithotabs/Lithobid 2721

Tolerance

Adipex-P Tablets and Capsules 1035
Astramorph/PF Injection, USP
    (Preservative-Free) 526

Axocet Capsules 2469
Bellergal-S Tablets 2375
Brontex 2130
Butisol Sodium Elixir & Tablets..... 2768
Carnitor Tablets and Solution........ 2624
DHCplus Capsules 2148
DextroStat-Dextroamphetamine
    Sulfate Tablets 2211
Dilatrate-SR Capsules 2542
Dilaudid Tablets and Liquid........... 1386
Duragesic Transdermal System..... 1336
Duramorph Injection 983
Dyclone 0.5% and 1% Topical
    Solutions, USP 535
Esgic-plus Capsules 1012
Esgic-plus Tablets 1012
Fioricet Tablets 2386
Fiorinal Capsules 2388
Fiorinal with Codeine Capsules 2390
Fiorinal Tablets 2388
Hycodan Tablets and Syrup 946
Hycomine Compound Tablets 948
Hycomine 947
Hycotuss Expectorant Syrup 950
Hydrocet Capsules 787
Infumorph 200 and Infumorph
    500 Sterile Solutions 985
Isordil Sublingual Tablets 2845
Isordil Tembids 2847
Isordil Titradose Tablets 2848
Kadian Capsules (Less than 3%) ... 2948
Lorcet 10/650 Tablets 1016
Lortab 2751
MS Contin Tablets 2149
Mebaral Tablets 2452
Methadone Hydrochloride Oral
    Solution & Tablets 2357
Nembutal Sodium Solution 442
Nembutal Sodium Suppositories... 444
Nitrostat Tablets 1981
Oramorph SR (Morphine Sulfate
    Sustained Release Tablets) 2359
Percocet Tablets 955
Percodan Tablets 955
Phrenilin 790
Placidyl Capsules 456
Ritalin 866
Roxanol 2365
Seconal Sodium Pulvules 1529
Sedapap Tablets 50 mg/650 mg
    (Infrequent) 1826
Sorbitrate 2959
Tylenol with Codeine 1592
Vicodin Tablets 1404
Vicodin HP Tablets 1403
Vicodin Tuss Expectorant 1406
Zemuron Injection (Rare) 1885

Tolerance, diminished

Cocaine Hydrochloride Topical
    Solutions 529
Duranest Injections 533
▲ Fungizone Intravenous (Most
    patients) 507
Sensorcaine 554
Timolide Tablets 1791
Xylocaine Injections 562

Tongue, black "hairy"
(see under Glossotrichia)

Tongue, burning

Atamet Tablets 567
BuSpar Tablets (Rare) 738
Halcion Tablets 2093
Larodopa Tablets (Infrequent) 2296
Nalfon 200 Pulvules & Nalfon
    Tablets (Less than 1%) 933
Sinemet Tablets 959
Sinemet CR Tablets 961

Tongue, discoloration

Aldomet Ester HCl Injection 1642
Aldomet Oral 1640
Claritin-D Tablets (Less frequent)... 2487
Effexor (Rare) 2825
Etrafon 2495
Helidac Therapy 2135
Maxaquin Tablets (Less than 1%)... 2593
Paxil Tablets (Rare) 2681
Pepto-Bismol Original Liquid,
    Original and Cherry Tablets and
    Easy-To-Swallow Caplets 2126
Pepto-Bismol Maximum Strength
    Liquid 2126
Peridex 2127
Periogard Oral Rinse 892
Prilosec Delayed-Release Capsules
    (2%) 516
Prozac Pulvules & Liquid, Oral
    Solution (Rare) 935

Remeron Tablets (Rare) 1878
Rilutek Tablets (Rare) 2198
Risperdal Tablets (Rare) 1348
Trilafon 2532
Vistide Injection 1057
Zyrtec Tablets (Less than 2%) 2053

Tongue, fine vermicular movements

Compazine 2644
Eskalith 2658
Etrafon 2495
Haldol Decanoate 1587
Haldol Injection, Tablets and
    Concentrate 1585
Lithonate/Lithotabs/Lithobid 2721
Mellaril 2398
Moban Tablets and Concentrate ... 1036
Navane Capsules and Concentrate 2018
Navane Intramuscular 2019
Orap Tablets 1037
Reglan 2243
Stelazine 2692
Thorazine 2701

Tongue, furry

Flagyl 375 Capsules 2587
Geocillin Tablets 2009
MetroGel-Vaginal 917
Protostat Tablets 1939

Tongue, mucosal atrophy

Prilosec Delayed-Release Capsules
    (Less than 1%) 516

Tongue, protrusion

Compazine 2644
Etrafon 2495
Haldol Decanoate 1587
Haldol Injection, Tablets and
    Concentrate 1585
Loxitane 1426
Mellaril 2398
Moban Tablets and Concentrate ... 1036
Navane Capsules and Concentrate 2018
Navane Intramuscular 2019
Orap Tablets 1037
Phenergan with Codeine 2883
Phenergan with Dextromethorphan 2885
Phenergan Suppositories 2882
Phenergan Syrup 2881
Phenergan VC 2886
Phenergan VC with Codeine 2888
Prolixin 510
Prozac Pulvules & Liquid, Oral
    Solution (One case) 935
Reglan 2243
Serentil 689
Stelazine 2692
Thorazine 2701
Triavil Tablets 1800
Trilafon 2532

Tongue, rounding

Etrafon 2495
Trilafon 2532

Tongue, sore
(see under Glossodynia)

Tongue, swelling
(see under Glossoncus)

Tongue disorder, unspecified

Avonex 662
▲ Cerebyx Injection (4.4%) 1956
Cytovene (1% or less) 2270
Hivid Tablets (Less than 1%) 2287
Lioresal Intrathecal (1% or more) .. 1634
Redux Capsules 2911
Salagen Tablets (Less than 1%)... 1546
Videx Tablets, Powder for Oral
    Solution, & Pediatric Powder for
    Oral Solution (Less than 1%) 2980

Tooth development, impaired

Terramycin Intramuscular Solution 2034
Urobiotic-250 Capsules 2038
Vibramycin Hyclate Intravenous ... 2040

Tooth discoloration

Questran Powder for Oral
    Suspension 774
Urobiotic-250 Capsules
    (Contraindicated in pregnancy)... 2038

Tooth disorder

Anafranil Capsules (Up to 5%) 819
Avonex 662
Axid Pulvules (1.0%) 1468
Dilacor XR Extended-release
    Capsules (Infrequent) 2183

(🕮 Described in PDR For Nonprescription Drugs)   Incidence data in parenthesis; ▲ 3% or more   (⊙ Described in PDR For Ophthalmology)

Estring Vaginal Ring (1% to 3%).... 2086
Invirase Capsules (Less than 2%) .. 2291
Ismo Tablets (Fewer than 1%) 2844
▲ Lamictal Tablets (3.2%) 1105
Lescol Capsules (2.1%) 2395
Lotensin HCT Tablets (0.3% or
more) 855
▲ LUVOX Tablets (3%) 2723
Naprelan Tablets (Less than 1%) .. 2861
▲ Nicotrol NS Nicotine Nasal Spray
(4%) 1565
▲ Nipent for Injection (3% to 10%) .. 2733
Paxil Tablets (Rare) 2681
Questran Powder for Oral
Suspension 774
Rilutek Tablets (Up to 1.2%) 2198
Serzone Tablets 776
Versed Injection 2324
Zyrtec Tablets (Less than 2%) 2053

Torsade de pointes
Betapace Tablets (Up to 5.8%) 637
Biaxin (Rare) 406
Cardioquin Tablets 2146
Cordarone Intravenous 2821
Corvert Injection 2075
Dynabac (Rare) 668
Felbatol 2774
Haldol Decanoate 1587
Haldol Injection, Tablets and
Concentrate 1585
Ilosone (Rare) 927
Ilotycin Gluceptate, IV, Vials (Rare) 929
Inapsine Injection (At least one
case) 462
Norpace 2596
PCE Dispertab Tablets (Rare) 453
Pediazole Suspension 2340
Propulsid (Rare) 1346
Quinidex Extentabs 2240
Seldane Tablets (Rare) 1284
Seldane-D Extended-Release
Tablets (Rare) 1286
Tambocor Tablets (Rare) 1555
Vascor Tablets (200 and 300 mg) 1597

Torticollis
Adalat CC (Less than 1.0%) 582
Adenocard Injection (Less than
1%) 1021
▲ Adenoscan (15%) 1022
Anafranil Capsules (Rare) 819
Arimidex Tablets (2% to 5%) 2932
Asacol Delayed-Release Tablets ... 2129
Betaseron for SC Injection 653
Cardene I.V. (Rare) 2815
Cartrol Tablets (Less common) 413
Casodex Tablets (2% to 5%) 2934
Cipro I.V. (1% or less) 587
Cipro I.V. Pharmacy Bulk Package
(Less than 1%) 590
Cipro Tablets (Less than 1%) 584
Claritin-D Tablets (Less frequent) 2487
Clozaril Tablets (1%) 2377
Compazine 2644
Cytovene (1% or less) 2270
Danocrine Capsules 2437
Depakote Tablets (1% to 5%) 418
Dilacor XR Extended-release
Capsules (Infrequent) 2183
Diprivan Injectable Emulsion (Less
than 1%) 2939
Dynabac (0.1% to 1%) 668
DynaCirc CR Tablets (0.5% to
1.0%) 2383
Effexor (Frequent; infrequent) 2825
Eldepryl Capsules 2729
Engerix-B Unit-Dose Vials (Less
than 1%) 2656
Etrafon 2495
Foscavir Injection (Less than 1%) .. 541
▲ Gammar-P I.V., Immune Globulin
Intravenous (Human) (3.6%) 798
Hivid Tablets (Less than 1%) 2287
Hylorel Tablets (1.5%) 1613
Hytrin Capsules (At least 1%) 434
Imdur (Less than or equal to 5%) .. 1362
▲ Imitrex Injection (4.8%) 1095
Kerlone Tablets (Less than 2%) 2588
Lamictal Tablets (2.4%) 1105
Lotensin HCT Tablets (0.3% or
more) 855
LUVOX Tablets (Rare to
infrequent) 2723
Mellaril 2398
Moduretic Tablets 1748
Monoket Tablets (Fewer than 1%) 2550
Naprelan Tablets (Less than 1%) .. 2861
Norvir (Less than 2%) 447
Orap Tablets (2.7%) 1037

▲ Orthoclone OKT3 Sterile Solution
(14%) 1892
OxyContin Tablets (Less than 1%) 2163
Paxil Tablets (Infrequent) 2681
Permax Tablets (2.7%) 571
Phenergan with Codeine 2883
Phenergan with Dextromethorphan 2885
Phenergan Suppositories 2882
Phenergan Syrup 2881
Phenergan VC 2886
Phenergan VC with Codeine 2888
Prinivil Tablets (0.3% to 1.0%) 1776
Prinzide Tablets 1780
ProSom Tablets (Infrequent) 457
Prozac Pulvules & Liquid, Oral
Solution (Rare to infrequent) 935
Recombivax HB (Less than 1%) 1787
Redux Capsules (Infrequent) 2911
Reglan 2243
Remeron Tablets (Infrequent) 1878
Risperdal Tablets (Rare) 1348
Serentil 689
Serzone Tablets 776
Stelazine 2692
▲ Supprelin Injection (1% to 10%) ... 2230
Thorazine 2701
Tiazac Capsules (1%) 1019
Tonocard Tablets (Less than 1%) .. 519
Torecan 2367
Triavil Tablets 1800
Trilafon 2532
Vistide Injection 1057
Zebeta Tablets 1457
Zestoretic Tablets 2968
Zestril Tablets (0.3% to 1.0%) 2972
Ziac 1459

Total proteins, decrease
(see under Hypoproteinemia)

Tourette's syndrome
Adderall Tablets 2209
Cylert Tablets 415
Desoxyn Gradumet Tablets 422
Dexedrine 2648
DextroStat-Dextroamphetamine
Sulfate Tablets 2211
Ritalin (Rare) 866

Toxic granulation
Efudex 2280

Toxicity, bone marrow
▲ Mutamycin for Injection (64.4%) ... 712

Toxicity, cutaneous
▲ Lysodren Tablets (15%) 707
Platinol for Injection (Rare) 717
Platinol-AQ Injection (Rare) 719

Toxicity, hepatic
Achromycin V Capsules (Rare) 1417
BiCNU 696
Blenoxane (Infrequent) 697
CeeNU Capsules 699
Cordarone Tablets 2818
Danocrine Capsules 2437
Declomycin Tablets (Rare) 1421
Etopophos for Injection (Rare)...... 701
Etoposide Injection (Up to 3%) 539
Hexalen Capsules (Less than 1%) 2760
Methotrexate Sodium Tablets,
Injection, for Injection and LPF
Injection 1322
Parafon Forte DSC Caplets (Rare) .. 1590
Ponstel 1982
Pyridium 1985
Terramycin Intramuscular Solution 2034
Urobiotic-250 Capsules 2038
VePesid Capsules and Injection
(Up to 3%) 727

Toxicity, renal
Achromycin V Capsules 1417
Amikacin Sulfate Injection, USP ... 523
Anaprox/Naprosyn 2277
Blenoxane (Infrequent) 697
Declomycin Tablets (No incidence,
dose related) 1421
Depen Titratable Tablets 2770
Doryx Capsules 1970
EC-Naprosyn Delayed-Release
Tablets 2277
Feldene Capsules 2008
Fiorinal with Codeine Capsules ... 2390
▲ IFEX (6%) 706
Minocin Intravenous 1428
Minocin Oral Suspension 1431
Minocin Pellet-Filled Capsules 1429
Mutamycin for Injection (2%) 712
Anaprox/Naprosyn 2277

Orudis Capsules 2874
Oruvail Capsules 2874
▲ Platinol for Injection (28% to
36%) 717
▲ Platinol-AQ Injection (28% to
36% of patients) 719
Pyridium 1985
Relafen Tablets 2688
Roferon-A Injection (Unusual) 2308
▲ TheraCys BCG Live (Intravesical)
(2.0% to 9.8%) 911

Toxicity, vascular
Blenoxane (Rare) 697
Platinol for Injection (Rare) 717
Platinol-AQ Injection (Rare) 719

Toxic shock syndrome
All-Flex Arcing Spring Diaphragm
(See also Ortho Diaphragm Kits) 1921
Ortho Diaphragm Kits—All-Flex
Arcing Spring; Ortho Coil Spring;
Ortho-White Flat Spring 1921
Ortho Diaphragm Kit 1921

Toxoplasmosis
Doxil 2613
Foscavir Injection (Less than 1%) .. 541

Tracheitis
PedvaxHIB (One case) 1761
Serevent Inhalation Aerosol (1% to
3%) 1149
Solganal Suspension 2530

Tracheobronchitis
Monopril Tablets (0.4% to 1.0%) .. 762

Transaminase, elevation
(see under Serum transaminase,
elevation)

Trauma, unspecified
Ambien Tablets (Infrequent) 2559
Caverject Injection (2%) 2064
Decadron Phosphate Sterile
Ophthalmic Ointment 1684
Decadron Phosphate Sterile
Ophthalmic Solution 1685
Effexor (2%) 2825
Humorsol Sterile Ophthalmic
Solution 1707
Invirase Capsules (Less than 2%) .. 2291
▲ Lescol Capsules (5.1%) 2395
Neurontin Capsules (Frequent) ... 1978
Paxil Tablets (1.4%) 2681
Pravachol Tablets 770
Prinzide Tablets (0.3 to 1%) 1780
▲ Tetramune (Among most
common) 1449
Zestoretic Tablets (0.3 to 1%) 2968

Trembling
Adalat Capsules (10 mg and 20
mg) (2% or less) 580
▲ AeroBid Inhaler System (3% to
9%) 1004
▲ Aerobid-M Inhaler System (3% to
9%) 1004
Alfenta Injection (0.3% to 1%) 1334
Alferon N Injection (One patient) .. 2142
Axocet Capsules (Infrequent) 2469
Calan SR Caplets 2571
Calan Tablets 2568
Clozaril Tablets (Less than 1%) 2377
Covera-HS Tablets (Less than 2%) 2573
Diprivan Injectable Emulsion (Less
than 1%) 2939
Emete-con
Intramuscular/Intravenous 2007
Fluothane 2830
Gammar-P I.V., Immune Globulin
Intravenous (Human) 798
Imitrex Injection (Infrequent) 1095
Imitrex Tablets (Rare to
infrequent) 1099
Inapsine Injection (Less common) .. 462
INFeD (Iron Dextran Injection,
USP) 2478
Invirase Capsules (Less than 2%) .. 2291
Marax Tablets & DF Syrup 2015
Marcaine Spinal 2449
Nucofed 2225
Paxil Tablets 2681
Procardia Capsules (2% or less) .. 2024
▲ Prostin E2 Suppository
(Approximately one-tenth) 2109
▲ Proventil Syrup (9 of 100
patients) 2528
Quadrinal Tablets 1398
Romazicon (Less than 1%) 2311

▲ Streptase for Infusion (Among
most common; 1% to 4%) 557
▲ Ventolin Syrup (9 of 100 patients) 1175
▲ Vesanoid Capsules (63%) 2327
WinRho SD (One report) 1839
Xylocaine Injections (2%) 562
▲ Zofran Injection (7%) 1227
▲ Zofran Tablets (5%) 1231

Tremor, fine hand
Atamet Tablets 567
Eskalith 2658
Lithium Carbonate Capsules &
Tablets 2352
Lithonate/Lithotabs/Lithobid 2721
Sinemet Tablets 959
Sinemet CR Tablets 961
▲ Vascor Tablets (200 and 300 mg)
(3.02 to 9.30%) 1597

Tremors
▲ Adalat Capsules (10 mg and 20
mg) (8%) 580
Adalat CC (Rare) 582
Adderall Tablets 2209
Adenoscan (Less than 1%) 1022
Adipex-P Tablets and Capsules ... 1035
▲ Airet Albuterol Sulfate Inhalation
Solution (10.7% to 20%) 1602
▲ Albuterol Sulfate, USP Solution for
Inhalation, Arm-a-Med (10.7%
to 20%) 522
Altace Capsules (Less than 1%) ... 1238
Alupent (1% to 4%) 672
Ambien Tablets (Infrequent) 2559
Amikacin Sulfate Injection, USP
(Rare) 523
Amikacin Sulfate Injection, USP
(Rare) 981
Amikin Injectable (Rare) 502
▲ Anafranil Capsules (33% to 54%) 819
Ana-Kit Anaphylaxis Emergency
Treatment Kit (Occasional to
common) 611
Apresazide Capsules (Less
frequent) 824
Apresoline Hydrochloride Tablets
(Less frequent) 826
Asacol Delayed-Release Tablets ... 2129
Asendin Tablets (Less frequent) ... 1419
Atarax Tablets & Syrup (Rare) 1992
Atromid-S Capsules 2808
Atrovent Inhalation Aerosol (Less
frequent) 674
Atrovent Inhalation Solution
(0.9%) 675
Benadryl Injection 1955
Betaseron for SC Injection 653
Bontril Slow-Release Capsules 786
Brethaire Inhaler 830
▲ Brethine Ampuls (7.8 to 38.0%) ... 832
Brethine Tablets (Common) 831
▲ Bricanyl Subcutaneous Injection
(Among most common) 1247
▲ Bricanyl Tablets (One of the two
most common) 1248
▲ Bromfed-DM Cough Syrup (Among
most frequent) 1832
Bronkometer Aerosol 2432
Bronkosol Solution 2432
Buprenex Injectable (Infrequent) .. 2170
BuSpar Tablets (1%) 738
Carbocaine Injection 2432
Cardene Capsules (0.6%) 2261
Cardioquin Tablets (2%) 2146
Cardizem CD Capsules (Less than
1%) 1251
Cardizem SR Capsules (Less than
1%) 1255
Cardizem Injectable 1253
Cardizem Tablets (Less than 1%) . 1257
Cardura Tablets (Less than 0.5%
of 3960 patients) 1993
Cataflam Tablets (Less than 1%) .. 833
▲ CellCept Capsules (11.0% to
11.8%) 2265
▲ Cerebyx Injection (3.3% to 9.5%) 1956
Chibroxin Sterile Ophthalmic
Solution (With oral form) 1657
Cipro I.V. (1% or less) 587
Cipro I.V. Pharmacy Bulk Package
(Less than 1%) 590
Cipro Tablets (Less than 1%) 584
Claritin Tablets (2% or fewer
patients) 2485
Claritin-D Tablets (Less frequent) 2487
▲ Clozaril Tablets (More than 5 to
6%) 2377
Cocaine Hydrochloride Topical
Solutions 529
Cognex Capsules (2%) 1961

(▫ Described in PDR For Nonprescription Drugs)   Incidence data in parenthesis; ▲ 3% or more   (⊚ Described in PDR For Ophthalmology)

Compazine ... 2644
▲ Cordarone Tablets (4 to 9%) ... 2818
Cozaar Tablets (Less than 1%) ... 1668
Crixivan Capsules (Less than 2%) .. 1670
Cytovene (1% or less) ... 2270
D.A. II Tablets ... 972
D.A. Chewable Tablets ... 970
Danocrine Capsules ... 2437
Daranide Tablets ... 1676
DaunoXome (Less than or equal to 5%) ... 1842
Decadron Phosphate with Xylocaine Injection, Sterile ... 1683
Deconsal II Tablets ... 1605
Demerol ... 2438
▲ Demser Capsules (10%) ... 1690
Depakene ... 416
▲ Depakote Tablets (9%) ... 418
Desoxyn Gradumet Tablets ... 422
▲ Desyrel and Desyrel Dividose (2.8% to 5.1%) ... 504
Dexedrine ... 2648
DextroStat-Dextroamphetamine Sulfate Tablets ... 2211
Dilantin Infatabs (Rare) ... 1967
Dilantin Kapseals (Rare) ... 1965
Dilantin-125 Suspension (Rare) ... 1969
Dilaudid-HP Injection (Less frequent) ... 1384
Dilaudid-HP Lyophilized Powder 250 mg (Less frequent) ... 1384
Dilaudid Tablets and Liquid (Less frequent) ... 1386
Dimetane-DC Cough Syrup ... 2232
Dimetane-DX Cough Syrup ... 2233
Dipentum Capsules (Rare) ... 2084
Diprivan Injectable Emulsion (Less than 1%) ... 2939
Dizac (diazepam injectable emulsion) CIV (Less frequent) ... 1862
Doral Tablets ... 2773
Duragesic Transdermal System (1% or greater) ... 1336
Duranest Injections ... 533
Dura-Tap/PD Capsules ... 970
Dura-Vent/DA Tablets ... 972
Dura-Vent Tablets ... 971
Dyazide Capsules ... 2653
Dyclone 0.5% and 1% Topical Solutions, USP ... 535
Dynabac (0.1% to 1%) ... 668
▲ Effexor (5% to 10.2%) ... 2825
Elavil ... 2945
Eldepryl Capsules ... 2729
Elspar ... 1700
Emete-con Intramuscular/Intravenous ... 2007
▲ Eminase (Less than 10%) ... 2215
EMLA Cream (Unlikely with cream) ... 536
Entex PSE Tablets ... 973
EpiPen ... 808
Esgic-plus Capsules ... 1012
Esgic-plus Tablets ... 1012
Esimil Tablets ... 840
Eskalith ... 2658
Ethmozine Tablets (Less than 2%) ... 2217
Etrafon ... 2495
Fastin Capsules ... 2662
Fedahist Gyrocaps ... 2545
▲ Felbatol (6.1%) ... 2774
Fioricet Tablets ... 2386
Fioricet with Codeine Capsules ... 2387
Fiorinal with Codeine Capsules ... 2390
Flexeril Tablets (Less than 1%) ... 1701
▲ Flolan for Injection (21%) ... 1085
Floxin I.V. (Less than 1%) ... 1580
Floxin Tablets (200 mg, 300 mg, 400 mg) (Less than 1%) ... 1577
Flumadine Tablets & Syrup (Less than 0.3%) ... 1013
Foscavir Injection (Between 1% and 5%) ... 541
▲ Glucotrol XL Extended Release Tablets (3.6%) ... 2012
Guaimax-D Tablets ... 809
Histussin D Liquid ... 670
Hivid Tablets (Less than 1%) ... 2287
Hydralazine Hydrochloride Injection USP (Less frequent) ... 2712
Hyzaar Tablets ... 1720
Imdur (Less than or equal to 5%) .. 1362
Imitrex Injection (Infrequent) ... 1095
Imitrex Tablets (Rare to infrequent) ... 1099
Intron A for Injection (Less than 5%) ... 2506
Inversine Tablets ... 1729
Invirase Capsules (Less than 2%) .. 2291
Ionamin Capsules ... 1615
Ismelin Tablets ... 845
Isoetharine Inhalation Solution, USP, Arm-a-Med ... 545
Isoptin Oral Tablets (Less than 1%) ... 1393
Isoptin SR Tablets (1% or less) ... 1395
Isuprel Hydrochloride Solution ... 2443
Isuprel Injection ... 2441
Isuprel Mistometer ... 2442
Kadian Capsules (Less than 3%) ... 2948
Kerlone Tablets (Less than 2%) ... 2588
Klonopin Tablets ... 2294
▲ Lamictal Tablets (4.4%) ... 1105
Larodopa Tablets (Relatively frequent) ... 2296
Lescol Capsules ... 2395
Leukeran Tablets (Rare) ... 1205
Limbitrol (Less common) ... 2333
Lioresal Intrathecal (Up to 1.3%) .. 1634
Lioresal Tablets ... 847
Lithium Carbonate Capsules & Tablets ... 2352
Lithonate/Lithotabs/Lithobid ... 2721
Lotrel Capsules ... 858
Loxitane ... 1426
▲ Ludiomil Tablets (3%) ... 861
▲ LUVOX Tablets (5%) ... 2723
MS Contin Tablets (Less frequent) 2149
MSIR (Infrequent) ... 2152
Marcaine ... 2446
Marcaine Spinal ... 2449
Marinol (Dronabinol) Capsules (Less than 1%) ... 2353
Matulane Capsules ... 2300
▲ Maxair Autohaler (1.3% to 6.0%) .. 1550
▲ Maxair Inhaler (6.0%) ... 1552
Maxaquin Tablets (Less than 1%) .. 2593
Mellaril ... 2398
Mepergan Injection ... 2859
Mesantoin Tablets ... 2400
▲ Metaproterenol Sulfate Inhalation Solution, USP, Arm-a-Med (About 1 in 20 patients) ... 547
Methadone Hydrochloride Oral Concentrate ... 2356
Mevacor Tablets (0.5% to 1.0%) .. 1742
▲ Mexitil Capsules (12.6%) ... 684
Midamor Tablets (Less than or equal to 1%) ... 1746
Moban Tablets and Concentrate ... 1036
Moduretic Tablets ... 1748
Monoket Tablets (Fewer than 1%) 2550
Monopril Tablets (0.2% to 1.0%) .. 762
Nalfon 200 Pulvules & Nalfon Tablets (2.2%) ... 933
Nardil (Common) ... 1977
NegGram ... 2453
▲ Neoral (21% to 55%) ... 2405
Nescaine/Nescaine MPF ... 549
▲ Neurontin Capsules (6.8%) ... 1978
Nicotrol NS Nicotine Nasal Spray (Under 5%) ... 1565
Nolamine Timed-Release Tablets (Occasional) ... 790
Norflex ... 1554
Norisodrine with Calcium Iodide Syrup ... 446
Noroxin Tablets ... 1758
Noroxin Tablets ... 2222
Norpramin Tablets ... 1273
Norvasc Tablets (More than 0.1% to 1%) ... 2020
Norvir (Less than 2%) ... 447
Novahistine DMX ... (▣) 782
Novahistine Elixir ... (▣) 782
Novocain Hydrochloride for Spinal Anesthesia ... 2457
Oramorph SR (Morphine Sulfate Sustained Release Tablets) (Less frequent) ... 2359
Orap Tablets (2.7%) ... 1037
Orlaam Oral Solution ... 2361
Ornade Spansule Capsules ... 2678
▲ Orthoclone OKT3 Sterile Solution (13%) ... 1892
OxyContin Tablets (Less than 1%) 2163
Pamelor ... 2409
Parnate Tablets ... 2679
▲ Paxil Tablets (Up to 14.7%) ... 2681
Penetrex Tablets (0.1% to 1%) ... 2196
Pentaspan Injection ... 954
Periactin ... 1767
▲ Permax Tablets (4.2%) ... 571
Phenergan Injection ... 2880
Phenergan Tablets ... 2882
Phenergan VC ... 2886
Phenergan VC with Codeine ... 2888
Placidyl Capsules ... 456
Pontocaine Hydrochloride for Spinal Anesthesia ... 2460
Pravachol Tablets ... 770
Prelu-2 Timed Release Capsules ... 687
Prilosec Delayed-Release Capsules (Less than 1%) ... 516
Primacor Injection (0.4%) ... 2461
Primaxin I.M. ... 1770
Primaxin I.V. (Less than 0.2%) ... 1772
Prinivil Tablets (0.3% to 1.0%) ... 1776
Prinzide Tablets ... 1780
▲ Procardia Capsules (2% or less to 8%) ... 2024
▲ Procardia XL Extended Release Tablets (1% or less to 8%) ... 2026
▲ Prograf (44% to 56%) ... 1028
Propulsid (1% or less) ... 1346
ProSom Tablets (Rare) ... 457
Prostin E2 Suppository ... 2109
▲ Proventil Inhalation Aerosol (Less than 15%) ... 2524
▲ Proventil Inhalation Solution 0.083% (10.7% to 20%) ... 2527
▲ Proventil Repetabs Tablets (6% to 20%) ... 2529
▲ Proventil Solution for Inhalation 0.5% (10.7% to 20%) ... 2525
▲ Proventil Syrup (10 of 100 patients) ... 2528
▲ Proventil Tablets (20%) ... 2529
▲ Prozac Pulvules & Liquid, Oral Solution (5% to 9%) ... 935
Quinidex Extentabs (2%) ... 2240
Redux Capsules (Infrequent) ... 2911
Reglan ... 2243
Relafen Tablets (1%) ... 2688
Remeron Tablets (2%) ... 1878
Restoril Capsules (Less than 1%) .. 2413
Retrovir Capsules ... 1216
Retrovir I.V. Infusion ... 1221
Retrovir Syrup ... 1216
ReVia Tablets (Less than 1%) ... 957
Revex (nalmefene hydrochloride injection) (Less than 1%) ... 1863
Rilutek Tablets (Frequent) ... 2198
▲ Risperdal Tablets (17% to 34%) .. 1348
Roferon-A Injection (Less than 0.5%) ... 2308
▲ Romazicon (3% to 9%) ... 2311
Rondec Oral Drops ... 974
Rondec Syrup ... 974
Rondec ... 974
Rythmol Tablets–150mg, 225mg, 300mg (0.3 to 1.4%) ... 1399
Salagen Tablets (2%) ... 1546
▲ Sandimmune (12 to 55%) ... 2416
Sandostatin Injection (Less than 1%) ... 2421
Sanorex Tablets ... 2423
Seldane Tablets ... 1284
Seldane-D Extended-Release Tablets ... 1286
Sensorcaine ... 554
Ser-Ap-Es Tablets ... 867
Serax Capsules ... 2916
Serax Tablets ... 2916
Serentil ... 689
▲ Serevent Inhalation Aerosol (4%) .. 1149
Seromycin Capsules ... 975
Serzone Tablets (2%) ... 776
Sinequan (Infrequent) ... 2028
Soma Compound w/Codeine Tablets (Infrequent or rare) ... 2784
Soma Compound Tablets (Infrequent or rare) ... 2783
Soma Tablets ... 2782
Stadol (1% or greater) ... 779
Stelazine ... 2692
Sular Tablets (Less than or equal to 1%) ... 2961
Supprelin Injection (1% to 3%) ... 2230
Surmontil Capsules ... 2917
Sus-Phrine Injection ... 1017
Syn-Rx Tablets ... 1622
Syn-Rx DM Tablets ... 1623
Talacen Caplets (Rare) ... 2464
Talwin Injection (Rarely) ... 2465
Talwin Compound (Rare) ... 2466
Talwin Injection (Rare) ... 2465
Talwin Nx Tablets (Rare) ... 2467
▲ Tambocor Tablets (4.7%) ... 1555
Tavist Syrup ... 2426
Tavist Tablets ... 2427
Tenex Tablets (Less frequent) ... 2249
Theo-Dur Extended-Release Tablets ... 1367
Thorazine ... 2701
Tiazac Capsules (Less than 1%) 1019
Tilade Inhaler (Less than 1%) ... 2207
Tofranil Ampuls ... 873
Tofranil Tablets ... 875
Tofranil-PM Capsules ... 876
▲ Tonocard Tablets (2.9% to 21.6%) ... 519
Toradol (1% or less) ... 2319
Torecan ... 2367
▲ Tornalate Solution for Inhalation, 0.2% (26.6% decreasing to 9%) ... 976
▲ Tornalate Metered Dose Inhaler (9.1% to 14%) ... 978
Trancopal Caplets ... 2468
Tranxene ... 459
Trental Tablets (0.3%) ... 1291
Triavil Tablets ... 1800
Trinalin Repetabs Tablets ... 1373
Tussend ... 1830
Tussend Expectorant ... 1831
Typhim Vi ... 914
▲ Ultram Tablets (50 mg) (Less than 1% to 14%) ... 1594
Valium Injectable ... 2336
Valium Tablets (Infrequent) ... 2335
▲ Vascor Tablets (200 and 300 mg) (0.5 to 6.98%) ... 1597
▲ Ventolin Inhalation Aerosol and Refill (Fewer than 15 per 100 patients; 1%) ... 1170
▲ Ventolin Inhalation Solution (10.7% to 20%) ... 1171
▲ Ventolin Nebules Inhalation Solution (10.7% to 20%) ... 1172
Ventolin Rotacaps for Inhalation (1%) ... 1173
▲ Ventolin Syrup (10 of 100 patients) ... 1175
▲ Ventolin Tablets (Aproximately 20 of 100 patients) ... 1176
▲ Vesanoid Capsules (3%) ... 2327
Videx Tablets, Powder for Oral Solution, & Pediatric Powder for Oral Solution (Less than 1%) ... 2980
Vistaril Capsules (Rare) ... 2042
Vistaril Intramuscular Solution (Rare) ... 2042
Vistaril Oral Suspension (Rare) ... 2042
Vivactil Tablets ... 1820
▲ Volmax Extended-Release Tablets (24.2%) ... 1835
Cataflam/Voltaren/Voltaren-XR (Less than 1%) ... 833
▲ Wellbutrin Tablets (21.1%) ... 1177
▲ Xanax Tablets (4.0%) ... 2115
▲ Xylocaine Injections (Among most common) ... 562
Yocon Tablets ... 1235
Yohimex Tablets ... 1414
▲ Yutopar Intravenous Injection (10% to 15%) ... 566
Zebeta Tablets ... 1457
Zerit Capsules (Fewer than 1% to 2%) ... 731
Zestoretic Tablets ... 2968
Zestril Tablets (0.3% to 1.0%) ... 2972
Ziac ... 1459
Zocor Tablets ... 1821
▲ Zoloft Tablets (10.7%) ... 2051
Zosyn (1.0% or less) ... 1463
Zovirax Sterile Powder (Approximately 1%) ... 1191
Zyrtec Tablets (Less than 2%) ... 2053

Tremulousness

Adalat CC (Rare) ... 582
Etrafon ... 2495
Lithonate/Lithotabs/Lithobid ... 2721
Narcan Injection ... 950
Nubain Injection (1% or less) ... 952
Prolixin ... 510
Sedapap Tablets 50 mg/650 mg (Infrequent) ... 1826
Trandate ... 1158
Verelan Capsules (1% or less) ... 1455

Trigeminal neuralgia

Nalfon 200 Pulvules & Nalfon Tablets (Less than 1%) ... 933
Torecan (Occasional case) ... 2367

Triglycerides, increase (see under Hypertriglyceridemia)

Trismus

Atamet Tablets ... 567
Ceftin (0.1% to 1%) ... 1067
Compazine ... 2644
Cytovene (1% or less) ... 2270
Demser Capsules ... 1690
Duranest Injections (Rare) ... 533
Effexor (Frequent) ... 2825
Etrafon ... 2495
Larodopa Tablets (Infrequent) ... 2296
LUVOX Tablets (Rare) ... 2723
Mellaril ... 2398
Paxil Tablets (Rare) ... 2681
Reglan ... 2243

(▣ Described in PDR For Nonprescription Drugs) Incidence data in parenthesis; ▲ 3% or more (◉ Described in PDR For Ophthalmology)

1473 Side Effects Index Ulcers, gastrointestinal

Rilutek Tablets (Rare) 2198
Serentil 689
Sinemet Tablets 959
Sinemet CR Tablets 961
Stelazine 2692
Thorazine 2701
Torecan 2367
Triavil Tablets 1800
Trilafon 2532

Tubal damage

ParaGard T 380A Intrauterine Copper Contraceptive 1936

Tubulopathy

Orudis Capsules (Rare) 2874
Oruvail Capsules (Rare) 2874

Tumor flare

Invirase Capsules (Less than 2%) 2291
Megace Tablets 710
▲ Zoladex (23%) 2976

Tumor lysis syndrome

Adriamycin PFS 2056
Adriamycin RDF 2056
Fludara for Injection (Up to 1%) 658
Leustatin (Rare) 1889

Twins, conjoined

Fulvicin P/G Tablets (Rare) 2499
Fulvicin P/G 165 & 330 Tablets (Rare) 2500
Gris-PEG Tablets, 125 mg & 250 mg (Two cases) 476

Twitching

▲ Anafranil Capsules (4% to 7%) 819
Cardura Tablets (Less than 0.5% of 3960 patients) 1993
Cataflam Tablets (Less than 1%) 833
Cerebyx Injection (Infrequent) 1956
Cognex Capsules (Infrequent) 1961
Compazine 2644
Depakote Tablets (1% to 5%) 418
Desoxyn Gradumet Tablets 422
Dilantin Infatabs 1967
Dilantin Kapseals 1965
Dilantin-125 Suspension 1969
Diprivan Injectable Emulsion (Less than 1%) 2939
Duranest Injections 533
Dyclone 0.5% and 1% Topical Solutions, USP 535
Effexor (1%) 2825
EMLA Cream (Unlikely with cream) 536
Eskalith 2658
Fioricet with Codeine Capsules 2387
Fiorinal with Codeine Capsules 2390
Hivid Tablets (Less than 1%) 2287
Imitrex Tablets (Rare) 1099
Kerlone Tablets (Less than 2%) 2588
Lamictal Tablets (Infrequent) 1105
Lioresal Intrathecal (1% or more) 1634
Lithium Carbonate Capsules & Tablets 2352
Lithonate/Lithotabs/Lithobid 2721
LUVOX Tablets (Infrequent) 2723
Methadone Hydrochloride Oral Concentrate 2356
Nardil (Common) 1977
Neurontin Capsules (1.3%) 1978
Nipent for Injection (Less than 3%) 2733
Norvasc Tablets (Less than or equal to 0.1%) 2020
Norvir (Less than 2%) 447
OxyContin Tablets (Between 1% and 5%) 2163
Permax Tablets (1.1%) 571
ProSom Tablets (Infrequent) 457
Prozac Pulvules & Liquid, Oral Solution (Infrequent) 935
Redux Capsules 2911
Remeron Tablets (Frequent) 1878
Retrovir Capsules 1216
Retrovir I.V. Infusion 1221
Retrovir Syrup 1216
Salagen Tablets (Less than 1%) 1546
Sensorcaine 554
Serzone Tablets (Infrequent) 776
Stelazine 2692
Tambocor Tablets (Less than 1%) 1555
Trilafon 2532
Triostat Injection (Approximately 1%) 2708
Videx Tablets, Powder for Oral Solution, & Pediatric Powder for Oral Solution (Up to 2%) 2980
Cataflam/Voltaren/Voltaren-XR (Less than 1%) 833
▲ Xylocaine Injections (Among most common) 562
Zebeta Tablets 1457
Ziac 1459
Zoloft Tablets (1.4%) 2051
Zyrtec Tablets (Less than 2%) 2053

Twitching, lid muscle

Humorsol Sterile Ophthalmic Solution 1707
Neurontin Capsules (Infrequent) 1978
Phospholine Iodide ⊙ 323
Salagen Tablets (Rare) 1546

Twitching, muscle

Amikacin Sulfate Injection, USP 523
Eldepryl Capsules 2729
Leukeran Tablets (Rare) 1205
Nebcin Vials, Hyporets & ADD-Vantage 1518
Parnate Tablets 2679
ReVia Tablets (Less than 1%) 957
Slo-bid Gyrocaps 2201
Theo-24 Extended Release Capsules 2753

Tympanic membrane perforation

Imdur (Less than or equal to 5%) 1362

Typhlitis

Adriamycin PFS 2056
Adriamycin RDF 2056
Doxorubicin Astra 531
Rubex for Injection 721

T4, decrease

Eskalith 2658
Intron A for Injection (Less than 5%) 2506
Lithium Carbonate Capsules & Tablets 2352
Lithonate/Lithotabs/Lithobid 2721
Redux Capsules (Infrequent) 2911

T4, increase

Brevicon 2563
Danocrine Capsules 2437
Estratest 2718
Nolvadex Tablets (A few postmenopausal women) 2957
Norinyl 2563
Nor-Q D Tablets 2598
Ortho-Cyclen/Ortho-Tri-Cyclen 1914
Ortho-Cyclen/Ortho Tri-Cyclen 1914
Redux Capsules (Infrequent) 2911
Tri-Norinyl 2607

T3, decrease

Amen Tablets 785
Aygestin Tablets 990
Brevicon 2563
Cycrin Tablets 991
Depo-Provera Sterile Aqueous Suspension 2083
Eskalith 2658
Estratest 2718
Intron A for Injection (Less than 5%) 2506
Lithium Carbonate Capsules & Tablets 2352
Lithonate/Lithotabs/Lithobid 2721
Norinyl 2563
Nor-Q D Tablets 2598
Provera Tablets 2110
Tri-Norinyl 2607

U

Ulceration

Aldactazide Tablets 2556
Aldactone Tablets 2558
Cerumenex Drops 2148
Condylox Topical Solution (Less than 5%) 1853
Cytosar-U Sterile Powder (Less frequent) 2077
Daypro Caplets (Less than 1%) 2578
Doxorubicin Astra 531
▲ Efudex (Among most frequent) 2280
Eulexin Capsules 2498
Fluorouracil Injection (Common) 2282
Heparin Lock Flush Solution 2831
Heparin Sodium Injection 2832
Heparin Sodium Vials 1486
K-Tab Filmtab 439
Micro-K 2237
Mutamycin for Injection 712
Norplant System 2868
PPD Tine Test 2993
Rubex for Injection 721
Sotradecol (Sodium Tetradecyl Sulfate Injection) 987
Talwin Injection 2465
Tuberculin, Old, Tine Test 2994
Tubersol (Tuberculin Purified Protein Derivative (Mantoux)) 2988

Ulceration, tongue

Foscavir Injection (Less than 1%) 541
Hivid Tablets (Less than 1%) 2287
Invirase Capsules (2.5%) 2291

Ulcerative esophagitis

Dexacort Phosphate in Respihaler 1606
Dexacort Phosphate in Turbinaire 1607
Hydrocortone Acetate Sterile Suspension 1712
Vibramycin (Rare) 2038

Ulcer attack

Questran 774

Ulcers

Effexor (Rare) 2825
Paxil Tablets (Rare) 2681
Remeron Tablets (Infrequent) 1878
ReVia Tablets (Less than 1%) 957
▲ Vesanoid Capsules (3%) 2327
Zoladex (Greater than 1% but less than 5%) 2976
Zoladex 3-month 2978

Ulcers, anal

Cafergot (Rare) 2376
▲ Cytosar-U Sterile Powder (Among most frequent) 2077
Hivid Tablets (Less than 1%) 2287

Ulcers, aphthous

Capoten Tablets (About 0.5 to 2%) 740
Capozide Tablets (0.5 to 2%) 744

Ulcers, corneal

AK-PRED ⊙ 204
FML Forte Liquifilm (Occasional) ⊙ 237
FML Liquifilm (Occasional) ⊙ 238
FML S.O.P. (Occasional) ⊙ 239
▲ Garamycin Ophthalmic (Among most frequent) 2501
Genoptic Sterile Ophthalmic Solution ⊙ 241
Genoptic Sterile Ophthalmic Ointment ⊙ 241
LUVOX Tablets (Rare) 2723
Myochrysine Injection (Rare) 1754
Oncovin Solution Vials & Hyporets 1521
Poly-Pred Liquifilm ⊙ 246
Solganal Suspension (Rare) 2530

Ulcers, cutaneous

Anafranil Capsules (Rare) 819
Avonex 662
Betaseron for SC Injection 653
▲ CellCept Capsules (More than or equal to 3%) 2265
Cognex Capsules (Rare) 1961
Cytosar-U Sterile Powder (Less frequent) 2077
Doxil (Less than 1%) 2613
Eskalith 2658
Foscavir Injection (Between 1% and 5%) 541
Hivid Tablets (Less than 1%) 2287
Hydrea Capsules 705
Invirase Capsules (Less than 2%) 2291
Lioresal Intrathecal (1% or more) 1634
Lithium Carbonate Capsules & Tablets 2352
Lithonate/Lithotabs/Lithobid 2721
Miacalcin Nasal Spray (Less than 1%) 2403
Naprelan Tablets (Less than 1%) 2861
Paxil Tablets (Rare) 2681
Permax Tablets (Infrequent) 571
Remeron Tablets (Rare) 1878
Rilutek Tablets (Infrequent) 2198
Risperdal Tablets (Rare) 1348
Sular Tablets (Less than or equal to 1%) 2961
T.R.U.E. Test 1162
Videx Tablets, Powder for Oral Solution, & Pediatric Powder for Oral Solution (Less than 1%) 2980

Ulcers, duodenal

Ancobon Capsules 2254
Atamet Tablets (Rare) 567
Betaseron for SC Injection 653
Cognex Capsules (Rare) 1961
Fioricet with Codeine Capsules 2387
Foscavir Injection (Less than 1%) 541
Sterile FUDR 2284
IBU Tablets (Less than 1%) 1389
Indocin Capsules (Less than 1%) 1723
Indocin I.V. (Less than 1%) 1727
Indocin (Less than 1%) 1723
Larodopa Tablets (Rare) 2296
Lupron Depot - 3 Month 22.5 mg (Less than 5%) 2743
Motrin Ibuprofen Suspension, Oral Drops, Chewable Tablets, Caplets (Less than 1%) 1563
Pentasa (Less than 1%) 1275
Proleukin for Injection (Less than 1%) 812
Prozac Pulvules & Liquid, Oral Solution (Rare) 935
Relafen Tablets (1%) 2688
Sinemet Tablets (Rare) 959
Sinemet CR Tablets 961
Taxotere for Injection Concentrate 2204
Trilisate (Rare) 2155
Zosyn (1.3%) 1463

Ulcers, esophageal

Doxil (Less than 1%) 2613
Effexor (Rare) 2825
▲ Ethamolin Injection (Among most common; 2.1%) 2544
Fosamax Tablets (1.5%) 1703
Helidac Therapy (Rare) 2135
Hivid Tablets (Less than 1%) 2287
Naprelan Tablets (Less than 1%) 2861
Pentasa (Less than 1%) 1275
Permax Tablets (Rare) 571
Urobiotic-250 Capsules (Rare) 2038

Ulcers, gastrointestinal

Adriamycin PFS 2056
Adriamycin RDF 2056
Anafranil Capsules (Infrequent) 819
Anaprox/Naprosyn (Less than 1% to 4%) 2277
Cataflam Tablets 833
Clinoril Tablets 1658
Clozaril Tablets (Less than 1%) 2377
Cosmegen Injection 1666
Cytosar-U Sterile Powder 2077
Dolobid Tablets 1695
Easprin 1971
EC-Naprosyn Delayed-Release Tablets (Less than 1% to 4%) 2277
Ergamisol Tablets 1340
Felbatol 2774
Feldene Capsules 2008
Fiorinal with Codeine Capsules 2390
Fluorouracil Injection 2282
Sterile FUDR 2284
IBU Tablets (Less than 1%) 1389
Indocin Capsules (Less than 1%) 1723
Indocin I.V. (Less than 1%) 1727
Indocin (Less than 1%) 1723
Intron A for Injection (Less than 5%) 2506
K-Dur Microburst Release System (potassium chloride, USP) E.R. Tablets 1364
K-Norm Capsules 1615
K-Tab Filmtab 439
Larodopa Tablets (Rare) 2296
Lodine Capsules and Tablets 2849
LUVOX Tablets (Infrequent) 2723
Methotrexate Sodium Tablets, Injection, for Injection and LPF Injection 1322
Micro-K 2237
Micro-K LS Packets 2238
Motrin Ibuprofen Suspension, Oral Drops, Chewable Tablets, Caplets (Less than 1% to 4%) 1563
Nalfon 200 Pulvules & Nalfon Tablets 933
▲ Naprelan Tablets (3% to 9%) 2861
Anaprox/Naprosyn (Less than 1% to 4%) 2277
Neutrexin for Injection 2761
Orudis Capsules (Less than 1%) 2874
Oruvail Capsules (Less than 1%) 2874
Paxil Tablets (Rare) 2681
Ponstel 1982
Purinethol Tablets 1214
Relafen Tablets (1%) 2688
Rilutek Tablets (Infrequent) 2198
Sandostatin Injection (Less than 1%) 2421
Slow-K Extended-Release Tablets (1 per 100,000 patient-years) 869
Tolectin (200, 400 and 600 mg) (Less than 1%) 1591
Toradol 2319
Trilisate (Less than 1%) 2155

(▣ Described in PDR For Nonprescription Drugs) Incidence data in parenthesis; ▲ 3% or more (⊙ Described in PDR For Ophthalmology)

Ulcers, gastrointestinal

Side Effects Index

Ulcers, gastrointestinal
- Cataflam/Voltaren/Voltaren-XR ... 833
- Wellbutrin Tablets (Rare) ... 1177

Ulcers, intestinal
- Lodine Capsules and Tablets (Less than 1%) ... 2849

Ulcers, leg
- Imdur (Less than or equal to 5%) .. 1362
- Neurontin Capsules (Rare) ... 1978

Ulcers, oral mucosal
- Alkeran for Injection (Infrequent) ... 1196
- Alkeran Tablets (Infrequent) ... 1198
- Anafranil Capsules (Infrequent) ... 819
- Asacol Delayed-Release Tablets ... 2129
- Atretol Tablets ... 569
- Atrovent Inhalation Aerosol (Less frequent) ... 674
- Azactam for Injection (Less than 1%) ... 736
- Ceftin (0.1% to 1%) ... 1067
- ▲ CellCept Capsules (More than or equal to 3%) ... 2265
- Ceredase ... 1055
- Cipro I.V. (1% or less) ... 587
- Cipro I.V. Pharmacy Bulk Package (Less than 1%) ... 590
- Clozaril Tablets ... 2377
- Cuprimine Capsules (Some patients) ... 1673
- ▲ Cytosar-U Sterile Powder (Among most frequent) ... 2077
- Cytovene (1% or less) ... 2270
- Cytoxan (Isolated reports) ... 700
- Depen Titratable Tablets (Some patients) ... 2770
- Doxil (1% to 5%) ... 2613
- Dynabac (0.1% to 1%) ... 668
- Effexor (Infrequent) ... 2825
- Hivid Tablets (Less than 1% up to 3.0%) ... 2287
- IBU Tablets (Less than 1%) ... 1389
- Kerlone Tablets (Less than 2%) ... 2588
- Lamictal Tablets (Infrequent) ... 1105
- Leukeran Tablets (Infrequent) ... 1205
- Myochrysine Injection ... 1754
- Nalfon 200 Pulvules & Nalfon Tablets (Less than 1%) ... 933
- Naprelan Tablets (Less than 1%) .. 2861
- Neutrexin for Injection ... 2761
- Noroxin Tablets (Less frequent) ... 1758
- Noroxin Tablets (Less frequent) ... 2222
- Norvir (Less than 2%) ... 447
- Oncovin Solution Vials & Hyporets 1521
- Paxil Tablets (Infrequent) ... 2681
- Pentasa (Less than 1%) ... 1275
- ProSom Tablets (Rare) ... 457
- Prozac Pulvules & Liquid, Oral Solution (Rare) ... 935
- Redux Capsules (Rare) ... 2911
- Retrovir Capsules ... 1216
- Retrovir I.V. Infusion ... 1221
- Retrovir Syrup ... 1216
- Serzone Tablets (Infrequent) ... 776
- Solganal Suspension ... 2530
- Sular Tablets (Less than or equal to 1%) ... 2961
- Tegison Capsules (Less than 1%) .. 2314
- Tegretol/Tegretol-XR ... 870
- Vistide Injection ... 1057
- Zoloft Tablets (Rare) ... 2051

Ulcers, peptic
- Anafranil Capsules (Infrequent) ... 819
- Atromid-S Capsules ... 2808
- Betaseron for SC Injection ... 653
- Capoten Tablets (About 0.5 to 2%) ... 740
- Capozide Tablets (0.5 to 2%) ... 744
- Cataflam Tablets (0.6% to 4%) ... 833
- Clinoril Tablets (Less than 1 in 100) ... 1658
- Cognex Capsules (Infrequent) ... 1961
- Colestid (Rare) ... 2073
- Cortifoam ... 2540
- Cuprimine Capsules (Less than 1%) ... 1673
- Daypro Caplets (Less than 1%) ... 2578
- Dilacor XR Extended-release Capsules ... 2183
- Dolobid Tablets (Less than 1 in 100) ... 1695
- Effexor (Infrequent) ... 2825
- Feldene Capsules (About 1%) ... 2008
- Fiorinal with Codeine Capsules ... 2390
- Hydeltra-T.B.A. Sterile Suspension 1710
- Hydrocortone Acetate Sterile Suspension ... 1712
- Hydrocortone Phosphate Injection, Sterile ... 1713
- Hydrocortone Tablets ... 1715
- Imdur (Less than or equal to 5%) .. 1362
- Imitrex Injection (Rare) ... 1095
- Imitrex Tablets (Rare) ... 1099
- Indocin Capsules (Less than 1%) 1723
- Indocin I.V. (Less than 1%) ... 1727
- Indocin (Less than 1%) ... 1723
- Lamictal Tablets (Rare) ... 1105
- Lupron Injection (Less than 5%) ... 2736
- Mexitil Capsules (About 8 in 10,000) ... 684
- Midamor Tablets (Rare) ... 1746
- Moduretic Tablets ... 1748
- Naprelan Tablets (Less than 1%) .. 2861
- Neoral (2% or less) ... 2405
- Neurontin Capsules (Rare) ... 1978
- Orudis Capsules (Less than 1%) ... 2874
- Oruvail Capsules (Less than 1%) ... 2874
- Paxil Tablets (Rare) ... 2681
- Permax Tablets (Rare to infrequent) ... 571
- Prozac Pulvules & Liquid, Oral Solution (Rare) ... 935
- Redux Capsules (Infrequent) ... 2911
- Relafen Tablets (0.3%) ... 2688
- Sandimmune (2% or less) ... 2416
- Sandostatin Injection (Less than 1%) ... 2421
- Serzone Tablets (Infrequent) ... 776
- Ticlid Tablets (Rare) ... 2317
- Tolectin (200, 400 and 600 mg) (1 to 3%) ... 1591
- Toradol ... 2319
- Cataflam/Voltaren/Voltaren-XR (0.6% to 4%) ... 833
- Ziac ... 1459
- Zosyn (1.0% or less) ... 1463

Ulcers, peptic, aggravation of
- Anturane ... 823
- Eldepryl Capsules ... 2729

Ulcers, peptic, hemorrhagic
- Imdur (Less than or equal to 5%) .. 1362
- Videx Tablets, Powder for Oral Solution, & Pediatric Powder for Oral Solution (Less than 1%) ... 2980
- Zoloft Tablets (Rare) ... 2051

Ulcers, peptic, reactivation of
- Anturane ... 823
- Depen Titratable Tablets (Isolated cases) ... 2770
- Didronel Tablets (A few patients) 2133
- Velban Vials ... 1537

Ulcers, peptic with or without perforation
- Asacol Delayed-Release Tablets (Rare) ... 2129
- Cataflam Tablets (Approximately 1% to 4%) ... 833
- Didronel Tablets (One report) ... 2133
- Lodine Capsules and Tablets (Less than 1%) ... 2849
- Nalfon 200 Pulvules & Nalfon Tablets (Less than 1%) ... 933
- Cataflam/Voltaren/Voltaren-XR (Approximately 1% to 4%) ... 833

Ulcers, peptic with perforation and hemorrhage
- Anaprox/Naprosyn (Approximately 1% to 4%) ... 2277
- Cataflam Tablets (Approximately 1% to 4%) ... 833
- Celestone Soluspan Suspension ... 2484
- CORTENEMA ... 2713
- Cortone Acetate Sterile Suspension ... 1663
- Cortone Acetate Tablets ... 1664
- Dalalone D.P. Injectable ... 1009
- Decadron Elixir ... 1676
- Decadron Phosphate Injection ... 1680
- Decadron Phosphate with Xylocaine Injection, Sterile ... 1683
- Decadron Tablets ... 1678
- Decadron-LA Sterile Suspension ... 1687
- Dexacort Phosphate in Respihaler .. 1606
- Dexacort Phosphate in Turbinaire .. 1607
- EC-Naprosyn Delayed-Release Tablets (Approximately 1% to 4%) ... 2277
- Florinef Acetate Tablets ... 506
- Hydeltrasol Injection, Sterile ... 1708
- Hydrocortone Tablets ... 1715
- IBU Tablets (Less than 1%) ... 1389
- Lodine Capsules and Tablets (Less than 1%) ... 2849
- Motrin Ibuprofen Suspension, Oral Drops, Chewable Tablets, Caplets (Less than 1%) ... 1563
- Anaprox/Naprosyn (Approximately 1% to 4%) ... 2277
- Pediapred Oral Solution ... 1618
- Prelone Syrup ... 1834
- Cataflam/Voltaren/Voltaren-XR (Approximately 1% to 4%) ... 833

Ulcers, pharyngeal
- Myochrysine Injection ... 1754

Ulcers, vulvovaginal
- Foscavir Injection (One case) ... 541
- Hivid Tablets (Less than 1%) ... 2287

Unconsciousness
(see under Consciousness, loss of)

Underventilation
(see under Hypoventilation)

Unsteadiness
- Ativan Injection ... 2805
- ▲ Ativan Tablets (3.4%) ... 2807
- ▲ Atretol Tablets (Among most frequent) ... 569
- Kadian Capsules ... 2948
- MSTA Mumps Skin Test Antigen ... 2988
- Restoril Capsules (Less than 1%) .. 2413
- Tambocor Tablets ... 1555
- ▲ Tegretol/Tegretol-XR (Among most frequent) ... 870
- Tonocard Tablets (Up to 1.2%) ... 519

Upper respiratory symptoms
- ▲ Bactroban Nasal (5%) ... 2643
- Betapace Tablets (1% to 5%) ... 637
- Engerix-B Unit-Dose Vials (Less than 1%) ... 2656
- Varivax (Greater than or equal to 1%) ... 1807
- ▲ Vesanoid Capsules (63%) ... 2327
- ▲ Wellbutrin Tablets (5.0%) ... 1177

Urate excretion, impaired
- Fiorinal with Codeine Capsules ... 2390

Uremia
(see under Azotemia)

Ureteral obstruction
- Halotestin Tablets ... 2095
- Zoladex ... 2976
- Zoladex 3-month (Isolated cases) .. 2978

Ureteral spasm
- Dilaudid Ampules ... 1382
- Dilaudid Cough Syrup ... 1383
- Dilaudid ... 1382
- Hycodan Tablets and Syrup ... 946
- Hycomine Compound Tablets ... 948
- Hycomine ... 947
- Hycotuss Expectorant Syrup ... 950
- Hydrocet Capsules ... 787
- Lorcet 10/650 Tablets ... 1016
- Lortab ... 2751
- Tussend ... 1830
- Tussionex Pennkinetic Extended-Release Suspension ... 1624
- Vicodin Tablets ... 1404
- Vicodin ES Tablets ... 1405
- Vicodin HP Tablets ... 1403
- Vicodin Tuss Expectorant ... 1406
- Zydone Capsules ... 967

Ureteritis, hemorrhagic
- Cytoxan ... 700

Urethral disorder
- Anafranil Capsules (Infrequent) ... 819
- Estring Vaginal Ring (At least 1 report) ... 2086
- Foscavir Injection (Between 1% and 5%) ... 541

Urethritis
- Betaseron for SC Injection ... 653
- Dyclone 0.5% and 1% Topical Solutions, USP ... 535
- Norvir (Less than 2%) ... 447
- Paxil Tablets (Rare to infrequent)... 2681
- Prozac Pulvules & Liquid, Oral Solution (Rare) ... 935
- Remeron Tablets (Rare) ... 1878
- TICE BCG, USP (1.2%) ... 1881

Uric acid level, increase
(see under Hyperuricemia)

Uric acid stones
- Benemid Tablets ... 1651
- ColBENEMID Tablets ... 1662

Uricaciduria
- Permax Tablets (Rare) ... 571

Urinary bladder, irritability
- MIOSTAT Intraocular Solution ... Ⓞ 222
- Neosporin G.U. Irrigant Sterile ... 1130
- Winstrol Tablets ... 2468

Urinary bladder malignancies
- Permax Tablets (Rare) ... 571

Urinary calculi
- Adalat CC (Less than 1.0%) ... 582

Urinary cytology, abnormal
- Orthoclone OKT3 Sterile Solution .. 1892

Urinary difficulty
(see under Micturition, difficulty)

Urinary disturbances
- Esimil Tablets ... 840
- Ismelin Tablets ... 845
- ▲ Lupron Depot - 3 Month 22.5 mg (14.9%) ... 2743
- Prozac Pulvules & Liquid, Oral Solution (Infrequent) ... 935
- ReVia Tablets (Less than 1%) ... 957
- Sansert Tablets ... 2424
- ▲ TheraCys BCG Live (Intravesical) (Up to 17.9%) ... 911
- Trilafon (Occasional) ... 2532

Urinary findings, abnormal
- Capastat Sulfate Injection (A high percentage of cases) ... 968
- Ceclor Pulvules & Suspension (Less than 1 in 200) ... 1470
- Clozaril Tablets (2%) ... 2377
- Phenurone Tablets (1 in 100 patients or less) ... 455

Urinary frequency
(see under Micturition disturbances)

Urinary glucose, false-positive
- Augmentin ... 2637
- Augmentin Tablets ... 2640
- Ceclor Pulvules & Suspension ... 1470
- Cedax ... 2480
- Ceftin ... 1067
- Ceptaz ... 1070
- Fortaz ... 1092
- Keflex Pulvules & Oral Suspension ... 930
- Omnipen for Oral Suspension ... 2873
- Tazicef for Injection ... 2697
- Tazidime Vials, Faspak & ADD-Vantage ... 1531

Urinary hesitancy
- Artane ... 1418
- Bentyl ... 1246
- BuSpar Tablets (Infrequent) ... 738
- Cystospaz ... 2123
- Dalgan Injection (Less than 1%) ... 529
- Dilaudid-HP Injection (Less frequent) ... 1384
- Dilaudid-HP Lyophilized Powder 250 mg (Less frequent) ... 1384
- Dilaudid Tablets and Liquid ... 1386
- Ditropan ... 1267
- Donnatal ... 2234
- Donnatal Extentabs ... 2234
- Donnatal Tablets ... 2234
- Eldepryl Capsules ... 2729
- Fludara for Injection (Up to 3%) ... 658
- Kadian Capsules (Less than 3%) ... 2948
- Kutrase Capsules ... 2546
- Levsin/Levsinex/Levbid ... 2549
- Librax Capsules ... 2330
- Ludiomil Tablets ... 861
- MS Contin Tablets (Less frequent) 2149
- MSIR (Infrequent) ... 2152
- Marax Tablets & DF Syrup ... 2015
- Methadone Hydrochloride Oral Concentrate ... 2356
- Methadone Hydrochloride Oral Solution & Tablets ... 2357
- Mexitil Capsules (Less than 1% or about 2 in 1,000) ... 684
- Norflex ... 1554
- Norgesic ... 1554
- ▲ Norpace (14%) ... 2596

(🆁 Described in PDR For Nonprescription Drugs)   Incidence data in parenthesis; ▲ 3% or more   (Ⓞ Described in PDR For Ophthalmology)

Side Effects Index — Urine, color change

Oramorph SR (Morphine Sulfate Sustained Release Tablets) (Less frequent)	2359
Pamelor	2409
▲ Paxil Tablets (3%)	2681
Pro-Banthine Tablets	2226
ProSom Tablets (Infrequent)	457
RMS Suppositories CII	2766
Retrovir Capsules	1216
Retrovir I.V. Infusion	1221
Retrovir Syrup	1216
Robinul Forte Tablets	2247
Robinul Injectable	2247
Robinul Tablets	2247
Roxanol	2365
Valium Injectable	2336
Valium Tablets (Infrequent)	2335

Urinary obstruction

Caverject Injection (Less than 1%)	2064
LUVOX Tablets (Infrequent)	2723
Ortho Diaphragm Kit	1921
Salagen Tablets (Less than 1%)	1546
TICE BCG, USP (0.3%)	1881

Urinary retention

Adapin Capsules	1542
Akineton	1380
Ambien Tablets (Rare)	2559
▲ Anafranil Capsules (2% to 7%)	819
Artane	1418
Asendin Tablets (Less than 1%)	1419
▲ Astramorph/PF Injection, USP (Preservative-Free) (Approximately 90% of males; somewhat less in females)	526
Atamet Tablets	567
Atretol Tablets	569
Atrovent Inhalation Solution (Less than 3%)	675
Atrovent Nasal Spray 0.03%	676
Atrovent Nasal Spray 0.06%	678
Avonex	662
Bellergal-S Tablets (Rare)	2375
Benadryl Injection	1955
Bentyl	1246
Betaseron for SC Injection	653
Brevibloc (esmolol HCl) Injection (Less than 1%)	1860
Brontex	2130
Buprenex Injectable (Less than 1%)	2170
BuSpar Tablets (Rare)	738
Carbocaine Injection	2432
Casodex Tablets (2% to 5%)	2934
Catapres Tablets (About 1 in 1,000 patients)	679
Cerebyx Injection (Infrequent)	1956
Cipro I.V. (1% or less)	587
Cipro I.V. Pharmacy Bulk Package (Less than 1%)	590
Cipro Tablets (Less than 1%)	584
Claritin-D Tablets (Less frequent)	2487
Clozaril (1%)	2377
Cogentin	1661
Cognex Capsules (Infrequent)	1961
Combipres Tablets (About 1 in 1,000)	682
Compazine	2644
Cystospaz	2123
Cytosar-U Sterile Powder (Less frequent)	2077
D.A. II Tablets	972
D.A. Chewable Tablets	970
Dalgan Injection (Less than 1%)	529
Dantrium Capsules (Less frequent)	2131
Demerol	2438
Desyrel and Desyrel Dividose	504
Dilaudid Ampules	1382
Dilaudid Cough Syrup	1383
Dilaudid-HP Injection (Less frequent)	1384
Dilaudid-HP Lyophilized Powder 250 mg (Less frequent)	1384
Dilaudid	1382
Dilaudid Oral Liquid	1386
Dilaudid	1382
Dilaudid Tablets - 8 mg	1386
Diprivan Injectable Emulsion (Less than 1%)	2939
Ditropan	1267
Dizac (diazepam injectable emulsion) CIV (Less frequent)	1862
Donnatal	2234
Donnatal Extentabs	2234
Donnatal Tablets	2234
Dopram Injectable	2235
Doral Tablets	2773
▲ Duragesic Transdermal System (3% to 10%)	1336
Duramorph Injection (Frequent in males; less frequent in females)	983
Dura-Tap/PD Capsules	970
Duratuss Tablets	2750
Dura-Vent/DA Tablets	972
Dura-Vent Tablets	971
Effexor (1%)	2825
Elavil	2945
Eldepryl Capsules (1 of 49 patients)	2729
Entex LA Tablets	972
Ethmozine Tablets (Less than 2%)	2217
Etrafon	2495
Exgest LA Tablets	787
Felbatol	2774
Flexeril Tablets (Less than 1%)	1701
Floxin I.V. (Less than 1%)	1580
Floxin Tablets (200 mg, 300 mg, 400 mg) (Less than 1%)	1577
Foscavir Injection (Between 1% and 5%)	541
Halcion Tablets	2093
Haldol Decanoate	1587
Haldol Injection, Tablets and Concentrate	1585
Hivid Tablets (Less than 1%)	2287
Hycodan Tablets and Syrup	946
Hycomine Compound Tablets	948
Hycomine	947
Hycotuss Expectorant Syrup	950
Hydrocet Capsules	787
Infumorph 200 and Infumorph 500 Sterile Solutions (Frequent)	985
Inversine Tablets	1729
Kadian Capsules (Less than 3%)	2948
Klonopin Tablets	2294
Kutrase Capsules	2546
Lamictal Tablets (Infrequent)	1105
Larodopa Tablets (Infrequent)	2296
Levbid Extended-Release Tablets	2549
Levo-Dromoran	2297
Levsin/Levsinex/Levbid	2549
Limbitrol	2333
▲ Lioresal Intrathecal (0.7% to 8.0%)	1634
Lioresal Tablets (Rare)	847
Lomotil	2591
Lorcet 10/650 Tablets	1016
Lortab	2751
Loxitane	1426
Ludiomil Tablets (Rare)	861
▲ LUVOX Tablets (3%)	2723
MS Contin Tablets (Less frequent)	2149
MSIR (Infrequent)	2152
Marax Tablets & DF Syrup (Occasional)	2015
Marcaine	2446
Marcaine Spinal	2449
Maxaquin Tablets	2593
Mellaril	2398
Mepergan Injection	2859
Methadone Hydrochloride Oral Concentrate	2356
Methadone Hydrochloride Oral Solution & Tablets	2357
Mexitil Capsules (Less than 1% or about 2 in 1,000)	684
Moban Tablets and Concentrate	1036
Motofen Tablets	789
Naprelan Tablets (Less than 1%)	2861
Nardil (Less common)	1977
Neurontin Capsules (Infrequent)	1978
Norflex	1554
Norgesic	1554
Normodyne Tablets (Less common)	2522
▲ Norpace (3 to 9%)	2596
Norpramin Tablets	1273
Norvir (Less than 2%)	447
Oncovin Solution Vials & Hyporets	1521
Oramorph SR (Morphine Sulfate Sustained Release Tablets) (Less frequent)	2359
Ornade Spansule Capsules	2678
OxyContin Tablets (Less than 1%)	2163
PBZ Tablets	863
PBZ-SR Tablets	862
Pamelor	2409
Parlodel	2411
Parnate Tablets	2679
Paxil Tablets (Infrequent)	2681
Pediazole Suspension	2340
Penetrex Tablets	2196
Periactin	1767
Permax Tablets (Infrequent)	571
Phenergan with Codeine	2883
Phenergan VC with Codeine	2888
Pro-Banthine Tablets	2226
Proleukin for Injection (1%)	812
Prostin E2 Suppository	2109
Prozac Pulvules & Liquid, Oral Solution (Infrequent)	935
RMS Suppositories CII	2766
Redux Capsules (Rare)	2911
Remeron Tablets (Infrequent)	1878
ReoPro Vials (0.4%)	1526
Revex (nalmefene hydrochloride injection) (Less than 1%)	1863
Rilutek Tablets (Infrequent)	2198
Risperdal Tablets (Rare)	1348
Robinul Forte Tablets	2247
Robinul Injectable	2247
Robinul Tablets	2247
Roxanol	2365
Sensorcaine	554
Serentil	689
Serzone Tablets (2%)	776
Sinemet Tablets	959
Sinemet CR Tablets	961
Sinequan	2028
Stelazine	2692
Sufenta Injection	1355
Surmontil Capsules	2917
Symmetrel Capsules (0.1% to 1%)	965
Symmetrel Syrup (0.1% to 1%)	963
Tagamet (Rare)	2694
Talacen Caplets (Rare)	2464
Talwin Injection (Infrequent)	2465
Talwin Compound	2466
Talwin Injection	2465
Talwin Nx Tablets	2467
Tambocor Tablets (Less than 1%)	1555
Tavist Syrup	2426
Tavist Tablets	2427
Tegison Capsules (Less than 1%)	2314
Tegretol/Tegretol-XR	870
Thioplex (Thiotepa For Injection)	1329
Thorazine	2701
Tofranil Ampuls	873
Tofranil Tablets (Rare)	875
Tofranil-PM Capsules	876
Tonocard Tablets (Less than 1%)	519
Toradol (1% or less)	2319
Torecan	2367
Trandate Tablets (Less common)	1158
Triavil Tablets	1800
Trinalin Repetabs Tablets	1373
Tussend	1830
Tussionex Pennkinetic Extended-Release Suspension	1624
Ultram Tablets (50 mg) (1% to less than 5%)	1594
Unasyn (Less than 1%)	2035
Urised Tablets	2123
Vicodin Tablets	1404
Vicodin ES Tablets	1405
Vicodin HP Tablets	1403
Vicodin Tuss Expectorant	1406
Vivactil Tablets	1820
Wellbutrin Tablets (1.9%)	1177
Xanax Tablets	2115
▲ Zofran Injection (3%)	1227
▲ Zofran Tablets (5%)	1231
Zoladex 3-month (1% to 5%)	2978
Zoloft Tablets (Rare)	2051
Zosyn (1.0% or less)	1463
Zydone Capsules	967
Zyrtec Tablets (Less than 2%)	2053

Urinary sediment, abnormalities

Crixivan Capsules (Less than 2%)	1670
Dyazide Capsules	2653
Roferon-A Injection (Infrequent)	2308

Urinary tract, burning

| Rowasa (0.61%) | 2727 |

Urinary tract, infection

Anafranil Capsules (Up to 6%)	819
Cartrol Tablets (Less common)	413
Cytotec (Infrequent)	2576
Ortho Diaphragm Kit	1921
Permax Tablets (2.7%)	571
Rowasa (0.61%)	2727
▲ TheraCys BCG Live (Intravesical) (1.0% to 17.9%)	911
Zoladex (Greater than 1% but less than 5%)	2976
Zoladex 3-month (1% to 5%)	2978

Urinary tract, obstruction

Cognex Capsules (Rare)	1961
Lupron Injection (Less than 5%)	2736
Zoladex (Greater than 1% but less than 5%)	2976
Zoladex 3-month (1% to 5%)	2978

Urinary tract dilatation

| Asendin Tablets | 1419 |
| Elavil | 2945 |

Etrafon	2495
Limbitrol	2333
Norpramin Tablets	1273
Pamelor	2409
Surmontil Capsules	2917
Tofranil Ampuls	873
Tofranil Tablets (Rare)	875
Tofranil-PM Capsules	876
Triavil Tablets	1800

Urinary tract disorder, unspecified

▲ CellCept Capsules (More than or equal to 3%; 6.7% to 10.6%)	2265
▲ Cleocin Vaginal Cream (11%)	2070
▲ Leukine (14%)	1317
Lupron Depot 3.75 mg	2739
Pravachol Tablets (0.7% to 2.4%)	770
Prozac Pulvules & Liquid, Oral Solution (Rare)	935
Redux Capsules	2911
▲ Zoladex (13%)	2976
Zoladex 3-month (1% to 5%)	2978

Urinary tract irritation

| Orudis Capsules (Greater than 1%) | 2874 |
| Oruvail Capsules (Greater than 1%) | 2874 |

Urinary urgency

Adenoscan (Less than 1%)	1022
Asacol Delayed-Release Tablets	2129
Avonex	662
▲ Betaseron for SC Injection (4%)	653
Casodex Tablets (2% to 5%)	2934
Caverject Injection (Less than 1%)	2064
Clozaril (1%)	2377
Cognex Capsules (Infrequent)	1961
Effexor (Infrequent)	2825
▲ Hylorel Tablets (33.6%)	1613
Isopto Carbachol Ophthalmic Solution (Frequent)	⊙ 221
Lupron Depot 7.5 mg (Less than 5%)	2741
▲ Lupron Injection (5% or more)	2736
LUVOX Tablets (Infrequent)	2723
Neurontin Capsules (Rare)	1978
Nubain Injection (1% or less)	952
Paxil Tablets (Infrequent)	2681
Plendil Extended-Release Tablets (0.5% to 1.5%)	514
ProSom Tablets (Infrequent)	457
Prozac Pulvules & Liquid, Oral Solution (Infrequent)	935
Remeron Tablets (Rare)	1878
Rilutek Tablets (Infrequent)	2198
Serzone Tablets (Infrequent)	776
▲ TheraCys BCG Live (Intravesical) (Up to 17.9%)	911
THYREL TRH	2992
▲ TICE BCG, USP (5.8%)	1881
Vasoxyl Injection	1169

Urination, difficult
(see under Micturition, difficulty)

Urination, painful
(see under Micturition, painful)

Urine, abnormal

Crixivan Capsules (Less than 2%)	1670
Diprivan Injectable Emulsion (Less than 1%)	2939
Lamictal Tablets (Rare)	1105
Lithonate/Lithotabs/Lithobid	2721
Maxaquin Tablets (Less than or equal to 0.1%)	2593
Naprelan Tablets (Less than 1%)	2861
Rilutek Tablets (Infrequent)	2198
Tornalate Solution for Inhalation, 0.2% (Infrequent)	976

Urine, burnt odor

| Questran | 774 |

Urine, cells in

▲ Accutane Capsules (1 in 5 to 1 in 10 patients)	2252
Merrem I.V. (Greater than 0.2%)	2952
TheraCys BCG Live (Intravesical) (Up to 0.9%)	911
Zovirax Sterile Powder (Less than 1%)	1191

Urine, color change

Adriamycin PFS	2056
Adriamycin RDF	2056
AK-FLUOR Injection 10% and 25%	⊙ 204
Atamet Tablets	567
Azulfidine (Rare)	2059

(▥ Described in PDR For Nonprescription Drugs)   Incidence data in parenthesis; ▲ 3% or more   (⊙ Described in PDR For Ophthalmology)

Side Effects Index

Urine, color change

- Cerubidine for Injection ... 634
- Claritin Tablets (2% or fewer patients) ... 2485
- Claritin-D Tablets ... 2487
- Clinoril Tablets (Less than 1%) ... 1658
- Coumadin ... 941
- Demulen ... 2580
- Desferal Vials ... 838
- Diprivan Injectable Emulsion (Less than 1%) ... 2939
- Doxorubicin Astra ... 531
- Eulexin Capsules ... 2498
- Flagyl 375 Capsules (Approximately 1 patient in 100,000) ... 2587
- Flagyl I.V. ... 2373
- Fluorescite ... ⊙ 217
- Helidac Therapy ... 2135
- Lamprene Capsules (Greater than 1%) ... 846
- Larodopa Tablets (Infrequent) ... 2296
- Levlen/Tri-Levlen ... 646
- MetroGel-Vaginal ... 917
- Modicon ... 1928
- ▲ Mycobutin Capsules (30%) ... 2101
- Nizoral Tablets ... 1345
- Normodyne Injection ... 2519
- Novantrone for Injection ... 1327
- Ortho-Cyclen/Ortho-Tri-Cyclen ... 1914
- Ortho-Novum ... 1928
- Ortho-Cyclen/Ortho Tri-Cyclen ... 1914
- Parafon Forte DSC Caplets (Rare) ... 1590
- Primaxin I.M. ... 1770
- Primaxin I.V. (Less than 0.2%) ... 1772
- Prodium ... 695
- Protostat Tablets (Approximately one patient in 100,000) ... 1939
- Pyrazinamide Tablets ... 1442
- Pyridium ... 1985
- ReVia Tablets ... 957
- Rifadin ... 1276
- Rifater ... 1280
- Rubex for Injection ... 721
- Sectral Capsules ... 2914
- Sinemet Tablets ... 959
- Sinemet CR Tablets ... 961
- Slo-Niacin Tablets ... 2767
- Sporanox Capsules ... 1352
- Ticlid Tablets ... 2317
- Trandate ... 1158
- Levlen/Tri-Levlen ... 646
- Urised Tablets ... 2123

Urine, fluorescence

- AK-FLUOR Injection 10% and 25% ... ⊙ 204

Urine, microscopic deposits

- Atretol Tablets ... 569
- Tegretol/Tegretol-XR ... 870

Urine, output low
(see under Hypouresis)

Urine, presence of granular casts

- Amikacin Sulfate Injection, USP ... 523
- Amikacin Sulfate Injection, USP ... 981
- Amikin Injectable ... 502
- Primaxin I.M. ... 1770
- Primaxin I.V. ... 1772
- Rocephin Injectable Vials, ADD-Vantage, Galaxy Container (Less than 1%) ... 2305
- Unasyn ... 2035

Urine, presence of RBCs
(see under Hematuria)

Urine, presence of urobilinogen

- Primaxin I.M. ... 1770
- Primaxin I.V. ... 1772

Urolithiasis

- Crixivan Capsules (Less than 2%) ... 1670
- Kytril Injection (Rare) ... 2667
- Paxil Tablets (Rare) ... 2681
- Permax Tablets (Infrequent) ... 571
- Prozac Pulvules & Liquid, Oral Solution (Rare) ... 935
- Trusopt Sterile Ophthalmic Solution (Rare) ... 1803

Urticaria

- Accutane Capsules (Less than 1%) ... 2252
- Acel-Imune Diphtheria and Tetanus Toxoids and Acellular Pertussis Vaccine Adsorbed ... 1415
- Achromycin V Capsules ... 1417
- ActHIB ... 893
- Actigall Capsules ... 818
- Activase (Very rare) ... 1045
- Adalat Capsules (10 mg and 20 mg) (2% or less) ... 580
- Adalat CC (Rare) ... 582
- Adderall Tablets ... 2209
- Adipex-P Tablets and Capsules ... 1035
- Adriamycin PFS (Occasional) ... 2056
- Adriamycin RDF (Occasional) ... 2056
- AeroBid Inhaler System (1% to 3%) ... 1004
- Aerobid-M Inhaler System (1% to 3%) ... 1004
- Airet Albuterol Sulfate Inhalation Solution (Rare) ... 1602
- Albenza Tablets (Rare) ... 2629
- Albuminar-5, Albumin (Human) U.S.P. 5% ... 795
- Albuminar-25, Albumin (Human) U.S.P. 25% ... 796
- Albuterol Sulfate, USP Solution for Inhalation, Arm-a-Med (Rare) ... 522
- Aldactazide Tablets ... 2556
- Aldactone Tablets ... 2558
- Aldoclor Tablets ... 1638
- Aldoril Tablets ... 1644
- Alfenta Injection (0.3% to 1%) ... 1334
- Alkeran for Injection ... 1196
- Altace Capsules (Less than 1%) ... 1238
- Amaryl Tablets (Less than 1%) ... 1241
- Ambien Tablets (Rare) ... 2559
- Amen Tablets (Occasional) ... 785
- Americaine Anesthetic Lubricant ... 1603
- Americaine Otic Topical Anesthetic Ear Drops ... 1603
- Amoxil ... 2631
- Anafranil Capsules (Up to 1%) ... 819
- Anaprox/Naprosyn (Less than 1%) ... 2277
- Ancobon Capsules ... 2254
- Antivenin (Crotalidae) Polyvalent ... 2803
- Apresazide Capsules (Less frequent) ... 824
- Apresoline Hydrochloride Tablets (Less frequent) ... 826
- Asacol Delayed-Release Tablets ... 2129
- Asendin Tablets (Less than 1%) ... 1419
- Astramorph/PF Injection, USP (Preservative-Free) ... 526
- Atretol Tablets ... 569
- Atrohist Plus Tablets ... 1605
- Atromid-S Capsules (Less often) ... 2808
- Atrovent Inhalation Aerosol ... 674
- Atrovent Inhalation Solution (Less than 3%) ... 675
- Atrovent Nasal Spray 0.06% (Rare) ... 678
- A/T/S 2% Acne Topical Gel ... 1244
- A/T/S 2% Acne Topical Solution (One case) ... 1244
- Attenuvax (Rare) ... 1650
- ▲ Augmentin (3%) ... 2637
- ▲ Augmentin Tablets (3%) ... 2640
- ▲ Avonex (5%) ... 662
- ▲ Axid Pulvules (More frequent) ... 1468
- Azactam for Injection (Less than 1%) ... 736
- Azulfidine (One in every 30 patients or less) ... 2059
- ▲ Bactrim DS Tablets (Among most common) ... 2257
- ▲ Bactrim I.V. Infusion (Among most common) ... 2255
- ▲ Bactrim (Among most common) ... 2257
- Beclovent Inhalation Aerosol and Refill (Rare) ... 1063
- Beconase (Rare) ... 1065
- Benadryl Injection ... 1955
- Benemid Tablets ... 1651
- Bentyl ... 1246
- Benzamycin Topical Gel (Approximately 3%) ... 919
- Betagan ... ⊙ 230
- Betaseron for SC Injection ... 653
- Betimol 0.25%, 0.5% ... ⊙ 259
- Biavax II ... 1653
- Biaxin ... 406
- Bicillin C-R Injection ... 2810
- Bicillin C-R 900/300 Injection ... 2812
- Bicillin L-A Injection ... 2813
- Biltricide Tablets (Rare) ... 584
- Bioclate, Antihemophilic Factor (Recombinant) (Extremely rare) ... 797
- ▲ Bromfed-DM Cough Syrup (Among most frequent) ... 1832
- Brontex (Infrequent) ... 2130
- Buprenex Injectable (Rare) ... 2170
- BuSpar Tablets (Rare) ... 738
- Calan SR Caplets (1% or less) ... 2571
- Calan Tablets (1% or less) ... 2568
- Capastat Sulfate Injection ... 968
- Capozide Tablets ... 744
- Carafate Suspension ... 1250
- Carafate Tablets ... 1249
- Carbocaine Injection ... 2432
- Cardioquin Tablets ... 2146
- Cardizem CD Capsules (Less than 1%) ... 1251
- Cardizem SR Capsules (Less than 1%) ... 1255
- Cardizem Injectable ... 1253
- Cardizem Tablets (Less than 1%) ... 1257
- Cataflam Tablets (Less than 1%) ... 833
- Catapres Tablets (About 5 in 1,000 patients) ... 679
- Catapres-TTS (2 cases of 3,539 patients) ... 680
- Ceclor Pulvules & Suspension (Less than 1 in 200) ... 1470
- Cedax (0.1% to 1%) ... 2480
- Cefotan ... 2936
- Ceftin (0.1% to 1%) ... 1067
- Cefzil Tablets and Oral Suspension (0.1%) ... 747
- Ceptaz ... 1070
- Cerebyx Injection (Infrequent) ... 1956
- Ceredase ... 1055
- Chibroxin Sterile Ophthalmic Solution (With oral form) ... 1657
- Chloroptic S.O.P. ... ⊙ 236
- Chloroptic Sterile Ophthalmic Solution ... ⊙ 236
- Cipro I.V. (1% or less) ... 587
- Cipro I.V. Pharmacy Bulk Package (Less than 1%) ... 590
- Cipro Tablets (Less than 1%) ... 584
- Claforan Sterile and Injection (Less frequent) ... 1259
- Claritin Tablets (2% or fewer patients) ... 2485
- Claritin-D Tablets (Less frequent) ... 2487
- Cleocin Phosphate Injection ... 2068
- Cleocin Vaginal Cream (Less than 1%) ... 2070
- Clozaril Tablets (Less than 1%) ... 2377
- ▲ Cognex Capsules (7%) ... 1961
- ColBENEMID Tablets ... 1662
- Colestid (Rare) ... 2073
- Colyte and Colyte-flavored (Isolated cases) ... 2540
- Combipres Tablets (About 5 in 1,000) ... 682
- Compazine ... 2644
- Cortone Acetate Sterile Suspension ... 1663
- Cortone Acetate Tablets ... 1664
- Coumadin (Infrequent) ... 941
- Covera-HS Tablets (Less than 2%) ... 2573
- Cozaar Tablets (Less than 1%) ... 1668
- Crixivan Capsules (Less than 2%) ... 1670
- Cuprimine Capsules ... 1673
- Cycrin Tablets (Occasional) ... 991
- Cystospaz ... 2123
- Cytadren Tablets (Rare) ... 837
- Cytosar-U Sterile Powder (Less frequent) ... 2077
- Cytovene (1% or less) ... 2270
- Dalalone D.P. Injectable ... 1009
- Danocrine Capsules ... 2437
- Dantrium Capsules (Less frequent) ... 2131
- Dantrium Intravenous (Rare) ... 2132
- Daypro Caplets (Less than 1%) ... 2578
- Decadron Elixir ... 1676
- Decadron Phosphate Injection ... 1680
- Decadron Phosphate with Xylocaine Injection, Sterile ... 1683
- Decadron Tablets ... 1678
- Decadron-LA Sterile Suspension ... 1687
- Declomycin Tablets ... 1421
- Demerol ... 2438
- Demser Capsules (Rare) ... 1690
- Depen Titratable Tablets ... 2770
- Depo-Provera Sterile Aqueous Suspension ... 2083
- Dermatop Emollient Cream 0.1% (Less than 1%) ... 1264
- Desferal Vials ... 838
- Desoxyn Gradumet Tablets ... 422
- Desyrel and Desyrel Dividose ... 504
- Dexacort Phosphate in Respihaler ... 1606
- Dexacort Phosphate in Turbinaire ... 1607
- Dexedrine ... 2648
- DextroStat-Dextroamphetamine Sulfate Tablets ... 2211
- DiaBeta Tablets (1.5%) ... 1265
- Diabinese Tablets (Approximately 1% or less) ... 2002
- Diamox Intravenous (Occasional) ... ⊙ 317
- Diamox Sequels (Sustained Release) ... ⊙ 318
- Diamox (Occasional) ... ⊙ 317
- Didronel Tablets ... 2133
- Dilacor XR Extended-release Capsules (Infrequent) ... 2183
- Dilaudid-HP Injection (Less frequent) ... 1384
- Dilaudid-HP Lyophilized Powder 250 mg (Less frequent) ... 1384
- Dilaudid Tablets and Liquid ... 1386
- Dimetane-DC Cough Syrup ... 2232
- Dimetane-DX Cough Syrup ... 2233
- Diphtheria and Tetanus Toxoids and Pertussis Vaccine Adsorbed (Rare) ... 2650
- Diprivan Injectable Emulsion (Less than 1%) ... 2939
- Disalcid ... 1549
- Diucardin Tablets ... 2824
- Diupres Tablets ... 1691
- Diuril Oral Suspension ... 1694
- Diuril Sodium Intravenous ... 1693
- Diuril Tablets ... 1694
- Dizac (diazepam injectable emulsion) CIV (Less frequent) ... 1862
- Dolobid Tablets (Less than 1 in 100) ... 1695
- Donnatal ... 2234
- Donnatal Extentabs ... 2234
- Donnatal Tablets ... 2234
- Doryx Capsules ... 1970
- Doxil (1% to 5%) ... 2613
- Doxorubicin Astra (Occasional) ... 531
- Duramorph Injection ... 983
- Duranest Injections ... 533
- Duricef Capsules, Tablets, and Oral Suspension ... 750
- Dyazide Capsules ... 2653
- Dyclone 0.5% and 1% Topical Solutions, USP ... 535
- Dynabac (1.2%) ... 668
- DYNACIN Capsules ... 1627
- DynaCirc Capsules (0.5% to 1%) ... 2381
- DynaCirc CR Tablets (0.5% to 1.0%) ... 2383
- E.E.S. ... 427
- E-Mycin Tablets ... 1388
- Easprin ... 1971
- EC-Naprosyn Delayed-Release Tablets (Less than 1%) ... 2277
- Effexor (Infrequent) ... 2825
- Efudex ... 2280
- Elavil ... 2945
- Elspar ... 1700
- Emete-con Intramuscular/Intravenous (Rare) ... 2007
- Eminase (Occasional) ... 2215
- EMLA Cream ... 536
- Enduron Tablets ... 424
- Engerix-B Unit-Dose Vials (Less than 1%) ... 2656
- Epogen for Injection (Rare) ... 489
- Ergamisol Tablets (Less than 1%) ... 1340
- ERYC ... 1972
- Erycette (erythromycin 2%) Topical Solution ... 1943
- EryPed ... 425
- Ery-Tab Tablets ... 426
- Erythrocin Stearate Filmtab ... 429
- Erythromycin Base Filmtab ... 430
- Erythromycin Delayed-Release Capsules, USP ... 431
- Esidrix Tablets ... 839
- Esimil Tablets ... 840
- Ethmozine Tablets (Less than 2%) ... 2217
- Etopophos for Injection (Infrequent) ... 701
- Etoposide Injection (Infrequent) ... 539
- Etrafon ... 2495
- Factrel (Rare) ... 2996
- Fansidar Tablets ... 2281
- Fastin Capsules ... 2662
- Felbatol (Infrequent) ... 2774
- Feldene Capsules (Less than 1%) ... 2008
- Flagyl 375 Capsules ... 2587
- Flagyl I.V. ... 2373
- Flexeril Tablets (Less than 1%) ... 1701
- Flonase Nasal Spray (Less than 1%) ... 1088
- Florinef Acetate Tablets ... 506
- Flovent (Rare) ... 1089
- Floxin I.V. (Less than 1%) ... 1580
- Floxin Tablets (200 mg, 300 mg, 400 mg) (Less than 1%) ... 1577
- Fortaz ... 1092
- Foscavir Injection (Less than 1%) ... 541
- ▲ Fulvicin P/G Tablets (Among most common) ... 2499
- ▲ Fulvicin P/G 165 & 330 Tablets (Among most common) ... 2500
- Fungizone Oral Suspension (Rare) ... 704
- Furoxone ... 2221

(⊡ Described in PDR For Nonprescription Drugs)   Incidence data in parenthesis; ▲ 3% or more   (⊙ Described in PDR For Ophthalmology)

1477 **Side Effects Index** **Urticaria**

Gamimune N, 10% Immune Globulin Intravenous (Human), 10% (A single incidence) 615
Gammagard S/D, Immune Globulin, Intravenous (Human) (Occasional) 577
Gantanol Tablets 2285
Gantrisin 2286
Garamycin Injectable 2502
Gastrocrom Capsules (Infrequent) 1611
Gastrocrom Oral Concentrate (Less common) 1611
Geocillin Tablets (Infrequent) 2009
Geref (sermorelin acetate for injection) (One patient) 2995
GlaucTabs (Occasional) ⊙ 209
Glucotrol Tablets (About 1 in 70) 2011
Glucotrol XL Extended Release Tablets (Less than 1%) 2012
Glynase PresTab Tablets (1.5%) 2091
GoLYTELY (Isolated cases) 694
Grifulvin V (griseofulvin tablets) Microsize (griseofulvin oral suspension) Microsize (Occasional) 1944
Gris-PEG Tablets, 125 mg & 250 mg 476
Habitrol Nicotine Transdermal System (Once in 35% of patients) 884
Havrix (Less than 1%) 2663
Helidac Therapy 2135
Heparin Lock Flush Solution 2831
Heparin Sodium Injection 2832
▲ Heparin Sodium Vials (Among most common) 1486
Hep-B-Gammagee 1706
Hespan Injection 945
Hivid Tablets (Less than 1% to 3.4%) 2287
Hydeltrasol Injection, Sterile 1708
Hydeltra-T.B.A. Sterile Suspension 1710
Hydralazine Hydrochloride Injection USP (Less frequent) 2712
Hydrocortone Acetate Sterile Suspension 1712
Hydrocortone Phosphate Injection, Sterile 1713
Hydrocortone Tablets 1715
HydroDIURIL Tablets 1716
Hydropres Tablets 1718
HyperHep Hepatitis B Immune Globulin (Human) 619
Hyskon Hysteroscopy Fluid (Rare) 1633
Hyzaar Tablets 1720
IBU Tablets (Less than 1%) 1389
Idamycin Injection 2096
Ilosone 927
Ilotycin Gluceptate, IV, Vials 929
Imitrex Injection 1095
Imitrex Tablets 1099
Imogam Rabies Immune Globulin (Human) 897
▲ Imovax Rabies Vaccine (Up to 6%) 899
Inderide Tablets 2838
Inderide LA Long Acting Capsules 2840
Indocin Capsules (Less than 1%) 1723
Indocin I.V. (Less than 1%) 1727
Indocin (Less than 1%) 1723
INFeD (Iron Dextran Injection, USP) 2478
Infumorph 200 and Infumorph 500 Sterile Solutions 985
Intal Inhaler (Infrequent) 2185
Intal Nebulizer Solution 2186
Intron A for Injection (Less than 5%) 2506
Invirase Capsules (Less than 2%) 2291
Ionamin Capsules 1615
Isoptin Injectable (Rare) 1391
Isoptin Oral Tablets (Less than 1%) 1393
Isoptin SR Tablets (1% or less) 1395
JE-VAX 904
Keflex Pulvules & Oral Suspension 930
Keftab Tablets 931
Kefurox Vials, Faspak & ADD-Vantage (Less than 1 in 250) 1509
Kutrase Capsules 2546
Kytril Tablets (Rare) 2669
Lamictal Tablets (Infrequent) 1105
Lamisil Tablets (1.1%) 2394
Lasix Injection, Oral Solution and Tablets 1267
Lescol Capsules (Rare) 2395
Leucovorin Calcium for Injection 1313
Leucovorin Calcium Tablets 1315
Levbid Extended-Release Tablets 2549
Levo-Dromoran 2297
Levoprome 1321
Levsin/Levsinex/Levbid 2549
Limbitrol 2333
Lioresal Intrathecal (0.2% to 1.2%) 1634
Lodine Capsules and Tablets (Less than 1%) 2849
Lomotil 2591
Lopid Tablets 1974
Lopressor HCT Tablets 850
Lorabid Suspension and Pulvules 1513
Lotensin HCT Tablets 855
Lotrimin 2514
Lotrisone Cream 2515
Lupron Depot 3.75 mg 2739
Lupron Depot 7.5 mg 2741
Lupron Depot - 3 Month 22.5 mg 2743
Lupron Depot-PED 7.5 mg, 11.25 mg and 15 mg 2744
Lutrepulse for Injection 998
LUVOX Tablets (Infrequent) 2723
M-M-R II 1730
M-R-VAX II 1732
MS Contin Tablets (Less frequent) 2149
MSIR (Infrequent) 2152
Macrobid Capsules (Less than 1%) 2138
Macrodantin Capsules 2140
Mandol Vials, Faspak & ADD-Vantage 1516
Marcaine (Rare) 2446
Marcaine Spinal (Rare) 2449
Matulane Capsules 2300
Maxaquin Tablets (Less than 1%) 2593
Maxipime for Injection (0.1% to 1%) 758
Mellaril (Infrequent) 2398
Mepergan Injection 2859
Merrem I.V. (0.1% to 1.0%) 2952
Meruvax II 1740
Methadone Hydrochloride Oral Concentrate 2356
Methadone Hydrochloride Oral Solution & Tablets 2357
Methotrexate Sodium Tablets, Injection, for Injection and LPF Injection 1322
Mevacor Tablets (Rare) 1742
Mezlin 594
Mezlin Pharmacy Bulk Package 597
Micronase Tablets (1.5%) 2099
Minizide Capsules 2016
Minocin Intravenous 1428
Minocin Oral Suspension 1431
Minocin Pellet-Filled Capsules 1429
Mivacron (Less than 1%) 1125
Moduretic Tablets 1748
8-MOP Capsules 1294
Monoclate-P, Factor VIII:C Pasteurized, Monoclonal Antibody Purified Antihemophilic Factor (Human) 802
Monodox Capsules 1858
Mononine, Coagulation Factor IX (Human), Monoclonal Antibody Purified 804
Monopril Tablets (0.2% to 1.0%) 762
Motofen Tablets 789
Motrin Ibuprofen Suspension, Oral Drops, Chewable Tablets, Caplets (Less than 1%) 1563
Mumpsvax (Extremely rare) 1751
Mycostatin Pastilles (Rare) 713
Mykrox Tablets 1617
Myleran Tablets 1209
Nalfon 200 Pulvules & Nalfon Tablets (Less than 1%) 933
Naprelan Tablets (Less than 1%) 2861
Anaprox/Naprosyn (Less than 1%) 2277
Nasalcrom Nasal Solution 2192
Navane Capsules and Concentrate 2018
Navane Intramuscular 2019
Navelbine Injection 1212
Nebcin Vials, Hyporets & ADD-Vantage 1518
NegGram 2453
Neptazane Tablets ⊙ 320
Nescaine/Nescaine MPF 549
Neupogen for Injection 495
Neurontin Capsules (Infrequent) 1978
▲ Nipent for Injection (3% to 10%) 2733
Nizoral Tablets (Several cases) 1345
Norflex (Rare) 1554
Norgesic (Rare) 1554
Normodyne Injection (Rare) 2519
Normodyne Tablets (Rare) 2522
Noroxin Tablets (Less frequent) 1758
Noroxin Tablets (Less frequent) 2222
Norplant System 2868
Norpramin Tablets 1273
Norvasc Tablets (Less than or equal to 0.1%) 2020
Norvir (Less than 2%) 447
Novantrone for Injection (Occasional) 1327
Novocain Hydrochloride for Spinal Anesthesia 2457
Nubain Injection (1% or less) 952
NuLYTELY (Isolated cases) 694
Cherry Flavor NuLYTELY (Isolated cases) 694
Nuromax Injection (Less than or equal to 0.1%) 1136
OmniHIB 2676
Omnipen Capsules 2872
Omnipen for Oral Suspension 2873
▲ Oncaspar (Greater than 5%) 2194
Oramorph SR (Morphine Sulfate Sustained Release Tablets) (Less frequent) 2359
Oretic Tablets 450
Organidin NR Tablets and Liquid (Rare) 2781
Ornade Spansule Capsules 2678
Orthoclone OKT3 Sterile Solution 1892
Orudis Capsules (Less than 1%) 2874
Oruvail Capsules (Less than 1%) 2874
Oxsoralen-Ultra Capsules 1302
PBZ Tablets 863
PBZ-SR Tablets 862
PCE Dispertab Tablets 453
Pamelor 2409
ParaGard T 380A Intrauterine Copper Contraceptive 1936
Paraplatin for Injection 713
Parnate Tablets 2679
Paxil Tablets (Infrequent) 2681
Pediazole Suspension 2340
PedvaxHIB (Two children) 1761
Pen•Vee K 2879
Penetrex Tablets (0.1% to 1%) 2196
Pentasa (Less than 1%) 1275
Pentaspan Injection 954
Pepcid Injection (Infrequent) 1765
Pepcid (Infrequent) 1763
Pergonal (menotropins for injection, USP) 2618
Periactin 1767
Pfizerpen for Injection 2022
Phenergan with Codeine 2883
Phenergan Injection 2880
Phenergan Tablets 2882
Phenergan VC with Codeine 2888
Placidyl Capsules 456
Plaquenil Sulfate Tablets 2459
Plendil Extended-Release Tablets (0.5% to 1.5%) 514
Pneumovax 23 (Rare) 1768
Pnu-Imune 23 (Rare) 1437
Pondimin Tablets 2239
Ponstel 1982
Pontocaine Hydrochloride for Spinal Anesthesia 2460
Pravachol Tablets (Rare) 770
Prelu-2 Timed Release Capsules 687
Premphase 2900
Prempro 2905
Prevacid Delayed-Release Capsules (Less than 1%) 2746
Prilosec Delayed-Release Capsules (Less than 1%) 516
Primaxin I.M. 1770
Primaxin I.V. (0.2%) 1772
Prinivil Tablets (0.3% to 1.0%) 1776
Prinzide Tablets 1780
Pro-Banthine Tablets 2226
Procanbid Extended-Release Tablets (Occasional) 1983
Procardia Capsules (2% or less) 2024
Procardia XL Extended Release Tablets (1% or less) 2026
Procrit for Injection (Rare) 1896
Profasi (chorionic gonadotropin for injection, USP) 2620
Proleukin for Injection (2%) 812
Prolixin 510
ProSom Tablets (Infrequent) 457
Prostigmin Injectable 1305
Prostigmin Tablets 1306
Protostat Tablets 1939
Proventil Inhalation Aerosol (Rare) 2524
Proventil Inhalation Solution 0.083% (Rare) 2527
Proventil Solution for Inhalation 0.5% (Rare) 2525
Proventil Syrup (Rare) 2528
Provera Tablets 2110
▲ Prozac Pulvules & Liquid, Oral Solution (Infrequent; approximately 4% of 5,600 patients) 935
Pyrazinamide Tablets 1442
Questran 774
Quinaglute Dura-Tabs Tablets 644
Quinidex Extentabs 2240
RMS Suppositories CII 2766
▲ Rabies Vaccine, Imovax Rabies I.D. (Less frequent; up to 6%) 901
Recombivax HB (Less than 1%) 1787
Redux Capsules (Frequent) 2911
Reglan (A few cases) 2243
Relafen Tablets (1%) 2688
Remeron Tablets (Rare) 1878
Retrovir Capsules 1216
Retrovir I.V. Infusion 1221
Retrovir Syrup 1216
Ridaura Capsules (1 to 3%) 2691
Rifadin (Occasional) 1276
Rifamate Capsules (Occasional) 1278
Rifater (Occasional) 1280
Rilutek Tablets (Infrequent) 2198
Rimactane Capsules 865
Risperdal Tablets (Rare) 1348
Ritalin 866
Robaxin Injectable 2245
Robaxin Tablets 2246
Robaxisal Tablets 2246
Robinul Forte Tablets 2247
Robinul Injectable 2247
Robinul Tablets 2247
Roferon-A Injection (Less than 3%; rare) 2308
Roxanol 2365
Rubex for Injection (Occasional) 721
Salflex Tablets 791
Sandostatin Injection (Less than 1%) 2421
Seldane Tablets (1.0% to 1.6%) 1284
Seldane-D Extended-Release Tablets 1286
Sensorcaine (Rare) 554
▲ Septra (Among most common) 1146
▲ Septra I.V. Infusion (Among most common) 1142
▲ Septra I.V. Infusion ADD-Vantage Vials (Among most common) 1144
▲ Septra (Among most common) 1146
Ser-Ap-Es Tablets 867
Serax Capsules 2916
Serax Tablets 2916
Serevent Inhalation Aerosol (Rare; 1% to 3%) 1149
Serophene (clomiphene citrate tablets, USP) (Less than 1 in 100 patients) 2621
Serzone Tablets (Infrequent) 776
Soma Compound w/Codeine Tablets 2784
Soma Compound Tablets (Less common) 2783
Sotradecol (Sodium Tetradecyl Sulfate Injection) 987
Spectrobid Tablets 2030
Sporanox Capsules 1352
Stelazine 2692
Streptase for Infusion 557
Sublimaze Injection 463
Sular Tablets (Less than or equal to 1%) 2961
Sulfamylon Cream 940
Supprelin Injection (Less than 2% to 4%) 2230
Suprax (Less than 2%) 1443
Surmontil Capsules 2917
Sus-Phrine Injection 1017
Synarel Nasal Solution for Central Precocious Puberty (2.6%) 2603
Synarel Nasal Solution for Endometriosis (Less than 1%) 2605
Synthroid 1410
T-Stat 2.0% Topical Solution and Pads 2797
Talacen Caplets (Rare) 2464
Talwin Carpuject 2465
Talwin Compound (Rare) 2466
Talwin Injection 2465
Talwin Nx Tablets (Rare) 2467
Tambocor Tablets (Less than 1%) 1555
Tao Capsules (Infrequent) 2033
Tapazole Tablets 1361
Tavist Syrup 2426
Tavist Tablets 2427
Taxol Injection (2%) 723
Tazicef for Injection 2697
Tazidime Vials, Faspak & ADD-Vantage 1531
Tegison Capsules (Less than 1%) 2314
Tegretol/Tegretol-XR 870
Tenoretic Tablets 2963
Terramycin Intramuscular Solution 2034
Tetramune 1449
Thalitone 1293

(■ Described in PDR For Nonprescription Drugs) Incidence data in parenthesis; ▲ 3% or more (⊙ Described in PDR For Ophthalmology)

Thioplex (Thiotepa For Injection) 1329
Thorazine (Occasional) 2701
Ticar for Injection 2704
Ticlid Tablets (0.5% to 1.0%) 2317
Timentin for Injection 2706
Timolide Tablets 1791
Timoptic in Ocudose (Less frequent) 1796
Timoptic Sterile Ophthalmic Solution (Less frequent) 1794
Timoptic-XE 1798
Tofranil Ampuls 873
Tofranil Tablets 875
Tofranil-PM Capsules 876
Tolectin (200, 400 and 600 mg) (Less than 1%) 1591
Tonocard Tablets (Less than 1%) .. 519
Toradol (1% or less) 2319
Tornalate Solution for Inhalation, 0.2% (Less than 1%) 976
Tracrium Injection 1155
Trandate (Rare) 1158
Trental Tablets (Less than 1%) 1291
Triavil Tablets 1800
Tri-Immunol Adsorbed 1452
Trilafon 2532
Trilisate (Rare) 2155
Trinalin Repetabs Tablets 1373
Tripedia 908
Trusopt Sterile Ophthalmic Solution 1803
T.R.U.E. Test (One report) 1162
Tussend 1830
Tussi-Organidin DM NR Liquid and DM-S NR Liquid (Rare) 2786
Tympagesic Ear Drops 2476
Typhim Vi 914
Ultram Tablets (50 mg) (Less than 1%) 1594
Ultravate Ointment 0.05% (Less frequent) 2798
Unasyn 2035
Univasc Tablets (Less than 1%) 2553
Urispas Tablets 2710
Valium Injectable 2336
Vancenase PocketHaler Nasal Inhaler (Rare) 2534
Vanceril Inhaler (Rare) 2538
Vancocin HCl, Oral Solution & Pulvules 1536
Vancocin HCl, Vials & ADD-Vantage 1534
Vaqta (Less than 1%) 1805
Vaseretic Tablets 1810
Vasotec I.V. 1814
Vasotec Tablets (0.5% to 1.0%) 1816
Velosulin BR Human Insulin 10 ml Vials 1847
Ventolin Inhalation Aerosol and Refill (Rare) 1170
Ventolin Inhalation Solution (Rare) .. 1171
Ventolin Nebules Inhalation Solution (Rare) 1172
Ventolin Rotacaps for Inhalation (Rare) 1173
Ventolin Syrup (Rare) 1175
Ventolin Tablets (Rare) 1176
VePesid Capsules and Injection (Infrequent) 727
Verelan Capsules (1% or less) 1455
Vermox Chewable Tablets (Rare) 1357
Vibramycin 2038
Vibramycin Hyclate Intravenous 2040
Vibramycin 2038
Videx Tablets, Powder for Oral Solution, & Pediatric Powder for Oral Solution (Less than 1%) 2980
Vistide Injection 1057
Vivactil Tablets 1820
Vivotif Berna (Infrequent) 660
Volmax Extended-Release Tablets (Rare) 1835
Cataflam/Voltaren/Voltaren-XR (Less than 1%) 833
Vumon for Injection 729
Wellbutrin Tablets 1177
Xylocaine Injections (Extremely rare) 562
Yodoxin Tablets 1235
Zarontin Capsules 1986
Zarontin Syrup 1986
Zaroxolyn Tablets 1625
Zerit Capsules (Fewer than 1% to 3%) 731
Zestoretic Tablets 2968
Zestril Tablets (0.3% to 1.0%) 2972
Ziac 1459
Zinacef (Fewer than 1 in 250 patients) 1184
Zinecard Injection (2%) 2120
Zocor Tablets (Rare) 1821
Zofran Injection (Rare) 1227
Zoloft Tablets (Rare) 2051
Zovirax 1187
Zyloprim Tablets (Less than 1%) 1194
Zyrtec Tablets (Less than 2%) 2053

Urticaria, hemorrhagic

Methadone Hydrochloride Oral Concentrate 2356
Methadone Hydrochloride Oral Solution & Tablets (Rare) 2357
RMS Suppositories CII (Rare) 2766
Roxanol (Rare) 2365

Urticarial reaction, generalized

Celontin Kapseals 1955
Chloromycetin Sodium Succinate 1960
Emgel 2% Topical Gel 1081
Scleromate Injection 1234
T-Stat 2.0% Topical Solution and Pads (One case) 2797
THERAMYCIN Z 2% Solution (One case) 1629

Uterine contractions, abnormal

Cervidil (2.0% to 4.7%) 1008
▲ Prepidil Gel (6.6%) 2108

Uterine contractions, altered

Astramorph/PF Injection, USP (Preservative-Free) 526
Proventil Inhalation Solution 0.083% 2527
Proventil Repetabs Tablets 2529
Proventil Solution for Inhalation 0.5% 2525
Proventil Syrup 2528
Proventil Tablets 2529
Talwin Injection 2465

Uterine contractions, cessation of

Proglycem 575

Uterine contractions, production of

Cytotec 2576

Uterine contractions, prolonged

Wigraine Tablets 1884

Uterine fibromyomata, increase in size

Betaseron for SC Injection 653
Climara Transdermal System 640
Diethylstilbestrol Tablets 1477
Effexor (Infrequent) 2825
Estrace Cream and Tablets 751
Estraderm Transdermal System 842
ESTRATAB Tablets (0.3, 0.625, 1.25, 2.5 mg) 2715
Estratest 2718
Menest Tablets 2671
Nolvadex Tablets (A few reports) 2957
Ogen Tablets 2103
Ogen Vaginal Cream 2106
Ortho Dienestrol Cream 1922
Ortho-Est 1925
PMB 200 and PMB 400 2890
Premarin Intravenous 2893
Premarin Tablets 2896
Premarin Vaginal Cream 2898
Premphase 2900
Prempro 2905
Serzone Tablets (Rare) 776
Vivelle Transdermal System 880

Uterine hypertonus

Syntocinon Injection 2425
Vasoxyl Injection 1169

Uterine inertia

Levoprome (Sometimes) 1321

Uterine rupture

Prepidil Gel 2108
Prostin E2 Suppository 2109
Syntocinon Injection 2425

Uterine spasm

Effexor (Rare) 2825
Paxil Tablets (Rare) 2681
Prozac Pulvules & Liquid, Oral Solution (Rare) 935
Syntocinon Injection 2425

Uterotonic effect

Bellergal-S Tablets 2375
D.H.E. 45 Injection 2381

Uveitis

AK-CIDE .... ⊚ 203
AK-CIDE Ointment .... ⊚ 203
Aredia for Injection (Rare) 827
Betaseron for SC Injection 653
Blephamide Liquifilm Sterile Ophthalmic Suspension 472
Blephamide Ointment .... ⊚ 234
Cardioquin Tablets 2146
Diupres Tablets 1691
Econopred & Econopred Plus Ophthalmic Suspensions .... ⊚ 216
FML Forte Liquifilm .... ⊚ 237
FML Liquifilm .... ⊚ 238
FML S.O.P. .... ⊚ 239
Healon GV (Rare) .... ⊚ 303
Humorsol Sterile Ophthalmic Solution 1707
Hydropres Tablets 1718
ISPAN Perfluoropropane .... ⊚ 267
ISPAN Sulfur Hexafluoride .... ⊚ 266
Lamictal Tablets (Rare) 1105
Mycobutin Capsules (Rare) 2101
Neurontin Capsules (Rare) 1978
Nipent for Injection (Less than 3%) 2733
Norvir (Less than 2%) 447
OptiPranolol (Metipranolol 0.3%) Sterile Ophthalmic Solution .... ⊚ 256
Phospholine Iodide .... ⊚ 323
Pred Forte .... ⊚ 247
Pred Mild .... ⊚ 250
Questran 774
Quinaglute Dura-Tabs Tablets 644
Quinidex Extentabs 2240
Ser-Ap-Es Tablets 867
Vira-A Ophthalmic Ointment, 3% .... ⊚ 299
Vistide Injection 1057

V

Vagina, dryness

Arimidex Tablets (1.2% to 1.9%) .. 2932
Clomid (Fewer than 1%) 1262
Danocrine Capsules 2437
Flagyl 375 Capsules 2587
Flagyl I.V. 2373
Helidac Therapy 2135
Massengill 2627
Massengill Medicated Disposable Douche 2628
Massengill Powder 2627
MetroGel-Vaginal 917
Nolvadex Tablets (Infrequent) 2957
Protostat Tablets 1939
Risperdal Tablets (Frequent) 1348
▲ Supprelin Injection (12%) 2230
▲ Synarel Nasal Solution for Endometriosis (19% of patients) 2605
Vagistat-1 (Less than 1%) 783

Vagina, warm feeling in

Prepidil Gel (1.5%) 2108

Vaginal adenosis

Estrace Cream and Tablets 751
Ortho-Est 1925
Premarin Tablets 2896
Vivelle Transdermal System 880

Vaginal burning

Floxin I.V. (Less than 1%) 1580
Floxin Tablets (200 mg, 300 mg, 400 mg) 1577
MetroGel-Vaginal (Equal to or less than 2%) 917
Monistat Dual-Pak (2%) 1906
Monistat 3 Vaginal Suppositories (2%) 1905
Mycelex-G 500 mg Vaginal Tablets (1 in 149 patients) 602
▲ Terazol 3 Vaginal Cream (5%) 1941
▲ Terazol 3 Vaginal Suppositories (15.2% of 284 patients) 1942
▲ Terazol 7 Vaginal Cream (5.2% of 521 patients) 1943
▲ Vagistat-1 (Approximately 6%) 783

Vaginal candidiasis

Azactam for Injection (Less than 1%) 736
Brevicon 2563
Cefotan 2936
Ceftin (0.1% to 1%) 1067
Cipro Tablets 584
Climara Transdermal System 640
Clozaril Tablets (Less than 1%) 2377
Demulen 2580
Desogen Tablets 1867
Diethylstilbestrol Tablets 1477
Estrace Cream and Tablets 751
Estraderm Transdermal System 842
ESTRATAB Tablets (0.3, 0.625, 1.25, 2.5 mg) 2715
Estratest 2718
Flagyl 375 Capsules 2587
Floxin I.V. 1580
Floxin Tablets (200 mg, 300 mg, 400 mg) 1577
Helidac Therapy 2135
Levlen/Tri-Levlen 646
Lo/Ovral Tablets 2852
Lo/Ovral-28 Tablets 2857
Menest Tablets 2671
▲ MetroGel-Vaginal (6.1%) 917
Modicon 1928
Nordette-21 Tablets 2863
Nordette-28 Tablets 2866
Norinyl 2563
Noroxin Tablets 1758
Noroxin Tablets 2222
Nor-Q D Tablets 2598
Ogen Tablets 2103
Ogen Vaginal Cream 2106
Ortho-Cept 1907
Ortho-Cyclen/Ortho-Tri-Cyclen 1914
Ortho Dienestrol Cream 1922
Ortho-Est 1925
Ortho-Novum 1928
Ortho-Cyclen/Ortho Tri-Cyclen 1914
Ovcon 765
Ovral Tablets 2877
Ovral-28 Tablets 2878
Ovrette Tablets 2878
PMB 200 and PMB 400 2890
Premarin Tablets 2896
Premarin Vaginal Cream 2898
Premphase 2900
Prempro 2905
Protostat Tablets 1939
Levlen/Tri-Levlen 646
Tri-Norinyl 2607
Triphasil-21 Tablets 2919
Triphasil-28 Tablets 2924
▲ Vantin for Oral Suspension and Vantin Tablets (3.1%) 2112
Vivelle Transdermal System 880
Zinacef 1184

Vaginal discharge

Ceftin (0.1% to 1%) 1067
Floxin I.V. (1% to 3%) 1580
Floxin Tablets (200 mg, 300 mg, 400 mg) (1% to 3%) 1577
Hivid Tablets (Less than 1%) 2287
Invirase Capsules (Less than 2%) .. 2291
Keflex Pulvules & Oral Suspension 930
Keftab Tablets 931
Lupron Depot-PED 7.5 mg, 11.25 mg and 15 mg (2%) 2744
Lupron Injection Pediatric 2737
Massengill Disposable Douche 2627
Methotrexate Sodium Tablets, Injection, for Injection and LPF Injection (Less common) 1322
MetroGel-Vaginal (Equal to or less than 2%) 917
▲ Nolvadex Tablets (29.6%) 2957
ParaGard T 380A Intrauterine Copper Contraceptive 1936
ProSom Tablets (Infrequent) 457
▲ Synarel Nasal Solution for Central Precocious Puberty (3%) 2603
Vagistat-1 (Less than 1%) 783

Vaginismus

Prostin E2 Suppository 2109

Vaginitis

Ambien Tablets (Infrequent) 2559
Anafranil Capsules (Up to 2%) 819
Ancef Injection 2632
Augmentin (1%) 2637
Augmentin Tablets (1%) 2640
▲ Avonex (4%) 662
Azactam for Injection (Less than 1%) 736
Brevicon 2563
Ceclor Pulvules & Suspension (Less than 1 in 100) 1470
Cedax (0.1% to 1%) 2480
Cefizox for Intramuscular or Intravenous Use (Rare) 1025
Cefotan 2936
Ceftin (0.1% to 1%) 1067
Cefzil Tablets and Oral Suspension (1.6%) 747
Ceptaz (Fewer than 1%) 1070
Cerebyx Injection (Infrequent) 1956
Cipro I.V. (1% or less) 587
Cipro I.V. Pharmacy Bulk Package (Less than 1%) 590

1479 **Side Effects Index** **Vasodilation**

Cipro Tablets (Less than 1% to 2%) 584
Claforan Sterile and Injection (Less than 1%) 1259
Claritin Tablets (2% or fewer patients) 2485
Claritin-D Tablets (Less frequent) 2487
▲Cleocin Vaginal Cream (16% to 33%) 2070
Demulen 2580
Depo-Provera Contraceptive Injection (1% to 5%) 2079
Desogen Tablets 1867
Dilacor XR Extended-release Capsules (Infrequent) 2183
Duricef Capsules, Tablets, and Oral Suspension 750
Dynabac (0.1% to 1%) 668
Effexor (Frequent) 2825
▲Estring Vaginal Ring (5%) 2086
▲Floxin I.V. (1% to 5%) 1580
▲Floxin Tablets (200 mg, 300 mg, 400 mg) (1% to 5%) 1577
Fortaz (Less than 1%) 1092
Geocillin Tablets 2009
Keflex Pulvules & Oral Suspension 930
Keftab Tablets 931
Kefzol Vials, Faspak & ADD-Vantage 1511
▲Lamictal Tablets (4.1%) 1105
Levlen/Tri-Levlen 646
Lioresal Intrathecal (1% or more) 1634
Lo/Ovral Tablets 2852
Lo/Ovral-28 Tablets 2857
Lorabid Suspension and Pulvules (1.3%) 1513
▲Lupron Depot 3.75 mg (11.4%) 2739
Lupron Depot-PED 7.5 mg, 11.25 mg and 15 mg (2%) 2744
Lupron Injection Pediatric 2737
LUVOX Tablets (Infrequent) 2723
Maxaquin Tablets (Less than 1%) 2593
Modicon 1928
Naprelan Tablets (Less than 1%) 2861
Nordette-21 Tablets 2863
Nordette-28 Tablets 2866
Norinyl 2563
▲Norplant System (5% or greater) 2868
Nor-Q D Tablets 2598
Ortho-Cept 1907
Ortho-Cyclen/Ortho-Tri-Cyclen 1914
Ortho-Novum 1928
Ortho-Cyclen/Ortho Tri-Cyclen 1914
Ovcon 765
Ovral Tablets 2877
Ovral-28 Tablets 2878
Ovrette Tablets 2878
ParaGard T 380A Intrauterine Copper Contraceptive 1936
Paxil Tablets (Infrequent) 2681
Penetrex Tablets (0.1% to 1%) 2196
Permax Tablets (Infrequent) 571
Propulsid (1.2%) 1346
Prostin E2 Suppository 2109
Prozac Pulvules & Liquid, Oral Solution (Infrequent) 935
Remeron Tablets (Infrequent) 1878
Rocephin Injectable Vials, ADD-Vantage, Galaxy Container (Occasional) 2305
Sandostatin Injection (Less than 1%) 2421
Serzone Tablets (2%) 776
Solganal Suspension 2530
Sular Tablets (Less than or equal to 1%) 2961
▲Supprelin Injection (3% to 10%) 2230
Suprax (Less than 2%) 1443
Tazicef for Injection (Less than 1%) 2697
Tazidime Vials, Faspak & ADD-Vantage (Less than 1%) 1531
Tegison Capsules (Less than 1%) 2314
Levlen/Tri-Levlen 646
Tri-Norinyl 2607
Triphasil-21 Tablets 2919
Triphasil-28 Tablets 2924
Urobiotic-250 Capsules (Rare) 2038
Vantin for Oral Suspension and Vantin Tablets (Less than 1% greater than 1%) 2112
Wellbutrin Tablets (Infrequent) 1177
Zerit Capsules (Up to 2%) 731
Zinacef 1184
Zithromax (1% or less to 1%) 2043
Zithromax Tablets (1% or less to 1%) 2046
▲Zoladex (75%) 2976
Zosyn (1.0% or less) 1463
Zyrtec Tablets (Less than 2%) 2053

Vaginitis, atrophic

Imdur (Less than or equal to 5%) 1362
Zoloft Tablets (Rare) 2051

Varices, esophageal

Myleran Tablets 1209
Thioguanine Tablets, Tabloid Brand 1225

Vascular access, clotting

▲Epogen for Injection (0.25 to 7%) 489
▲Procrit for Injection (0.25 to 7%) 1896

Vascular insufficiency, lower extremities

Sansert Tablets 2424

Vascular complications, unspecified

Avonex 662
Depakote Tablets (1% to 5%) 418
Metrodin (urofollitropin for injection) 2616
Ortho-Cyclen/Ortho-Tri-Cyclen 1914
Ortho-Cyclen/Ortho Tri-Cyclen 1914
Pergonal (menotropins for injection, USP) 2618
ReoPro Vials (1.8%) 1526
Zofran Tablets 1231

Vascular stenosis

Zyloprim Tablets (Less than 1%) 1194

Vasculitis

Accutane Capsules 2252
Aldoclor Tablets 1638
Aldomet Ester HCl Injection 1642
Aldomet Oral 1640
Aldoril Tablets 1644
Alkeran for Injection 1196
Alkeran Tablets 1198
Altace Capsules (Less than 1%) 1238
Anaprox/Naprosyn (Less than 1%) 2277
Asendin Tablets (Rare) 1419
Axid Pulvules (Rare) 1468
Azulfidine (Rare) 2059
Calan SR Caplets (1% or less) 2571
Calan Tablets (1% or less) 2568
Capoten Tablets 740
Capozide Tablets 744
Cardioquin Tablets 2146
Chibroxin Sterile Ophthalmic Solution (With oral form) 1657
Cipro I.V. (1% or less) 587
Cipro I.V. Pharmacy Bulk Package (Less than 1%) 590
Cipro Tablets 584
Clozaril Tablets 2377
ColBENEMID Tablets 1662
Combipres Tablets 682
Cordarone Tablets (Rare) 2818
Coumadin (Infrequent) 941
Covera-HS Tablets (Less than 2%) 2573
Depen Titratable Tablets (Rare) 2770
DiaBeta Tablets 1265
Diucardin Tablets 2824
Diupres Tablets 1691
Diuril Oral Suspension 1694
Diuril Sodium Intravenous 1693
Diuril Tablets 1694
Dyazide Capsules 2653
EC-Naprosyn Delayed-Release Tablets (Less than 1%) 2277
Eminase 2215
Enduron Tablets 424
Felbatol 2774
Feldene Capsules (Less than 1%) 2008
Floxin I.V. (Less than 1%) 1580
Floxin Tablets (200 mg, 300 mg, 400 mg) (Less than 1%) 1577
Glynase PresTab Tablets 2091
HydroDIURIL Tablets 1716
Hydropres Tablets 1718
Hyzaar Tablets 1720
Inderide Tablets 2838
Inderide LA Long Acting Capsules 2840
Inocor Lactate Injection (1 case) 2439
Isoptin Oral Tablets (Less than 1%) 1393
Isoptin SR Tablets (1% or less) 1395
Lasix Injection, Oral Solution and Tablets 1267
Lescol Capsules (Rare) 2395
Lodine Capsules and Tablets (Less than 1%) 2849
Lopid Tablets 1974
Maxaquin Tablets 2593
Methotrexate Sodium Tablets, Injection, for Injection and LPF Injection (Rare) 1322
Mevacor Tablets (Rare) 1742
Micronase Tablets 2099
Minizide Capsules 2016
Moduretic Tablets 1748
Monopril Tablets 762
Mumpsvax (Rare) 1751
Anaprox/Naprosyn (Less than 1%) 2277
Nipent for Injection (Less than 3%) 2733
Noroxin Tablets 1758
Noroxin Tablets 2222
Nydrazid Injection 509
Oretic Tablets 450
Orthoclone OKT3 Sterile Solution 1892
PASER Granules 1333
Pediazole Suspension 2340
Permax Tablets (Rare) 571
Pravachol Tablets (Rare) 770
Prinivil Tablets (0.3% to 1.0%) 1776
Prinzide Tablets 1780
Quinaglute Dura-Tabs Tablets 644
Quinidex Extentabs 2240
Relafen Tablets (1%) 2688
Retrovir Capsules (Rare) 1216
Retrovir I.V. Infusion (Rare) 1221
Retrovir Syrup (Rare) 1216
Rifamate Capsules 1278
Rifater 1280
Ritalin 866
Roferon-A Injection (Rare; less than 3%) 2308
Sporanox Capsules (1%) 1352
Tenoretic Tablets 2963
Thalitone 1293
Ticlid Tablets (Rare) 2317
Timolide Tablets 1791
Tonocard Tablets (Less than 1%) 519
Vancocin HCl, Oral Solution & Pulvules (Rare) 1536
Vancocin HCl, Vials & ADD-Vantage (Rare) 1534
Vaseretic Tablets 1810
Vasotec I.V. 1814
Vasotec Tablets (0.5% to 1.0%) 1816
Verelan Capsules (1% or less) 1455
Zestoretic Tablets 2968
Zestril Tablets (0.3% to 1.0%) 2972
Ziac 1459
Zocor Tablets (Rare) 1821
Zyloprim Tablets (Less than 1%) 1194

Vasculitis, allergic

Lodine Capsules and Tablets (Less than 1%) 2849

Vasculitis, cutaneous

Capozide Tablets 744
Combipres Tablets 682
Diucardin Tablets 2824
Diupres Tablets 1691
Diuril Oral Suspension 1694
Diuril Sodium Intravenous 1693
Diuril Tablets 1694
Enduron Tablets 424
HydroDIURIL Tablets 1716
Hydropres Tablets 1718
Hyzaar Tablets 1720
Inderide Tablets 2838
Inderide LA Long Acting Capsules 2840
Lodine Capsules and Tablets (Rare) 2849
Minizide Capsules 2016
Moduretic Tablets 1748
Mykrox Tablets 1617
Neupogen for Injection (Infrequent) 495
Oretic Tablets 450
Prinzide Tablets 1780
Tenoretic Tablets 2963
Thalitone 1293
Timolide Tablets 1791
Vaseretic Tablets 1810
Zaroxolyn Tablets 1625
Zebeta Tablets 1457
Zestoretic Tablets 2968
Ziac 1459

Vasculitis, leukocytoclastic

Cardizem CD Capsules (A number of cases) 1251
Cardizem SR Capsules 1255
Cardizem Injectable 1253
Cardizem Tablets 1257
Tiazac Capsules (A number of cases) 1019

Vasculitis, periarteritic

Intal Inhaler (Rare) 2185
Intal Nebulizer Solution (Rare) 2186
Nasalcrom Nasal Solution 2192

Vasculitis, renal

Cuprimine Capsules (Rare) 1673
Depen Titratable Tablets 2770

Vasoconstriction

Cocaine Hydrochloride Topical Solutions 529
Survanta Beractant Intratracheal Suspension (Less than 1%) 2346

Vasodilation

Accupril Tablets (0.5% to 1.0%) 1950
Asacol Delayed-Release Tablets 2129
▲Avonex (4%) 662
Betapace Tablets (1% to 3%) 637
Cardene I.V. (0.7%) 2815
▲Cardene SR Capsules (4.7% to 5.5%) 2264
Cardizem Injectable (1.7%) 1253
Cartrol Tablets (Less common) 413
Caverject Injection (Less than 1%) 2064
Ceclor Pulvules & Suspension 1470
▲CellCept Capsules (More than or equal to 3%) 2265
▲Cerebyx Injection (5.6%) 1956
Cytovene (1% or less) 2270
DDAVP 2180
Depakote Tablets (1% to 5%) 418
Desmopressin Acetate Rhinal Tube 997
Desyrel and Desyrel Dividose 504
Dilacor XR Extended-release Capsules 2183
Ditropan 1267
Dynabac (0.1% to 1%) 668
▲Effexor (2.3% to 5.6%) 2825
Ethmozine Tablets (Less than 2%) 2217
Flexeril Tablets (Less than 1%) 1701
▲Flolan for Injection (Most common) 1085
Floxin I.V. (Less than 1%) 1580
Floxin Tablets (200 mg, 300 mg, 400 mg) (Less than 1%) 1577
Hyperstat I.V. Injection 2504
Hytrin Capsules (At least 1%) 434
Imitrex Injection (Rare) 1095
Imitrex Tablets (Rare) 1099
Kadian Capsules (Less than 3%) 2948
Lamictal Tablets (Infrequent) 1105
Lioresal Intrathecal (1% or more) 1634
Lorabid Suspension and Pulvules 1513
Lotrel Capsules 858
Lupron Depot-PED 7.5 mg, 11.25 mg and 15 mg (Less than 2%) 2744
Lupron Injection Pediatric (Less than 2%) 2737
▲LUVOX Tablets (3%) 2723
Marcaine Spinal 2449
Marinol (Dronabinol) Capsules (Greater than 1%) 2353
Naprelan Tablets (Less than 1%) 2861
Neurontin Capsules (1.1%) 1978
Norvir (1.3% to 1.7%) 447
Novocain Hydrochloride for Spinal Anesthesia 2457
Orudis Capsules (Less than 1%) 2874
Oruvail Capsules (Less than 1%) 2874
OxyContin Tablets (Less than 1%) 2163
▲Paxil Tablets (3% to 4%) 2681
Penetrex Tablets (0.1% to 1%) 2196
Pentasa (Less than 1%) 1275
▲Permax Tablets (3.2%) 571
Prevacid Delayed-Release Capsules (Less than 1%) 2746
▲Prozac Pulvules & Liquid, Oral Solution (At least 5%) 935
Redux Capsules (Frequent) 2911
Remeron Tablets (Frequent) 1878
Retrovir Capsules 1216
Retrovir I.V. Infusion 1221
Retrovir Syrup 1216
Revex (nalmefene hydrochloride injection) (1%) 1863
▲Serzone Tablets (4%) 776
Sorbitrate 2959
▲Stadol (3% to 9%) 779
▲Sular Tablets (4%) 2961
▲Supprelin Injection (35%) 2230
Suprane (desflurane, USP) (Less than 1%) 1865
▲Tiazac Capsules (4%) 1019
Timolide Tablets 1791
Timoptic in Ocudose 1796
Timoptic Sterile Ophthalmic Solution 1794
Timoptic-XE 1798
Tracrium Injection 1155
Ultram Tablets (50 mg) (1% to less than 5%) 1594
Vascor Tablets (200 and 300 mg) (0.5 to 2.0%) 1597
▲Videx Tablets, Powder for Oral

(Described in PDR For Nonprescription Drugs) Incidence data in parenthesis; ▲ 3% or more (◉ Described in PDR For Ophthalmology)

Vasodilation Side Effects Index 1480

Solution, & Pediatric Powder for Oral Solution (22%) 2980
Vistide Injection 1057
Zerit Capsules (Fewer than 1% to 3%) 731
Zyloprim Tablets (Less than 1%) 1194

Vasodilation, peripheral
Persantine Tablets 686

Vasomotor disturbances
Aminohippurate Sodium Injection .. 1646
Ceredase 1055
Paremyd ⊙ 244
Xanax Tablets (2.0%) 2115

Vasomotor flushes
▲ Clomid (10.4%) 1262
▲ Serophene (clomiphene citrate tablets, USP) (Approximately 1 in 10 patients) 2621

Vasospasm, digital
▲ Parlodel (3%) 2411

Vasospasm, rebound
Nimotop Capsules (Less than 1%) 603

Vasospasm, unspecified
Anafranil Capsules (Rare) 819
Betaseron for SC Injection 653
D.H.E. 45 Injection (Occasional) 2381

Vasovagal episode
Alferon N Injection (2%) 2142
Caverject Injection (Less than 1%) 2064
IOPIDINE Sterile Ophthalmic Solution ⊙ 218
Parlodel (Less than 1%) 2411
Tonocard Tablets (Less than 1%) .. 519
Versed Injection (Less than 1%) 2324

Vein, pigmentation of
Fluorouracil Injection 2282

Veins, varicoses
Ambien Tablets (Rare) 2559
Betaseron for SC Injection 653
Depo-Provera Contraceptive Injection (Fewer than 1%) 2079
Effexor (Rare) 2825
Imdur (Less than or equal to 5%) .. 1362
Lupron Depot - 3 Month 22.5 mg (Less than 5%) 2743
Paxil Tablets (Rare) 2681
Permax Tablets (Infrequent) 571
Redux Capsules (Infrequent) 2911
Serzone Tablets (Rare) 776
Zoladex 3-month (1% to 5%) 2978
Zoloft Tablets (Rare) 2051

Venous infection at injection site
Primaxin I.V. (0.1%) 1772

Venous thrombophlebitis
Metrodin (urofollitropin for injection) 2616

Ventilator dependence
Virazole 1310

Ventricular arrhythmias
Adalat Capsules (10 mg and 20 mg) (Fewer than 0.5%) 580
Adenoscan (Less than 1%) 1022
Anectine (Rare) 1062
▲ Betapace Tablets (4.3% of 3,257 patients) 637
Biaxin (Rare) 406
Carbocaine Injection 2432
Cardioquin Tablets 2146
Cardizem Injectable (Less than 1%) 1253
Corvert Injection 2075
Diethylstilbestrol Tablets 1477
Doxil (Less than 1%) 2613
Dynabac (Rare) 668
EpiPen–Epinephrine Auto-Injector .. 808
Foscavir Injection (Rare) 541
Hismanal Tablets 1341
Hyperstat I.V. Injection 2504
Ilosone (Rare) 927
Ilotycin Gluceptate, IV, Vials (Rare) 929
Isuprel Injection 2441
Lanoxicaps (Less common) 1110
Lanoxin Elixir Pediatric (Less common) 1113
Lanoxin Injection 1116
Lanoxin Injection Pediatric (Less common) 1119
Lanoxin Tablets (Less common) 1121
Lioresal Intrathecal (1% or more) .. 1634
Lufyllin & Lufyllin-400 Tablets 2778
Lufyllin-GG Elixir & Tablets 2779
Marcaine 2446
Marcaine Spinal 2449
Mexitil Capsules (1.0% to 1.9%) .. 684
Nescaine/Nescaine MPF 549
Normodyne Injection (1%) 2519
Pediazole Suspension (Rare) 2340
▲ Primacor Injection (12.1%) 2461
Procardia Capsules (Fewer than 0.5%) 2024
Procardia XL Extended Release Tablets (Fewer than 0.5%) 2026
▲ Proleukin for Injection (3%) 812
Propulsid (Rare) 1346
Prozac Pulvules & Liquid, Oral Solution (Rare) 935
Quadrinal Tablets 1398
Quibron 2227
ReoPro Vials (0.3%) 1526
Respbid Tablets 687
Seldane Tablets (Rare) 1284
Seldane-D Extended-Release Tablets (Rare) 1286
Sensorcaine 554
Slo-bid Gyrocaps 2201
▲ Tambocor Tablets (7% to 13%) 1555
Theo-Dur Extended-Release Tablets 1367
Theo-X Extended-Release Tablets .. 793
▲ Tonocard Tablets (10.9%) 519
Trandate Injection (1 of 100 patients) 1158
Uni-Dur Extended-Release Tablets .. 1374

Ventricular arrhythmias, post-abrupt discontinuation
Tenormin Tablets and I.V. Injection 2965

Ventricular bigeminy
Azactam for Injection (Less than 1%) 736

Ventricular contractions
Sodium Polystyrene Sulfonate Suspension 2367
Versed Injection (Less than 1%) 2324
Yutopar Intravenous Injection 566

Ventricular contractions, premature
Adenocard Injection 1021
Azactam for Injection (Less than 1%) 736
Brethaire Inhaler 830
Cataflam Tablets (Less than 1%) 833
Clozaril Tablets (Less than 1%) 2377
Diupres Tablets 1691
▲ Dobutrex Solution Vials (Approximately 5%) 1480
Emete-con Intramuscular/Intravenous 2007
Gastrocrom Oral Concentrate (Less common) 1611
Hydropres Tablets 1718
Ismo Tablets (Fewer than 1%) 2844
▲ Lanoxin Injection (Most common) 1116
Lanoxin Injection Pediatric (Less common) 1119
Norpramin Tablets 1273
▲ Proleukin for Injection (5%) 812
Syntocinon Injection 2425
▲ Tonocard Tablets (10.9%) 519
Tornalate Solution for Inhalation, 0.2% (Less than 1%) 976
Tornalate Metered Dose Inhaler (Rare; 0.5%) 978
Vascor Tablets (200 and 300 mg) (0.5 to 2.0%) 1597
Cataflam/Voltaren/Voltaren-XR (Less than 1%) 833
Zantac (Rare) 1182
Zantac Injection (Rare) 1180
Zantac Syrup (Rare) 1182

Ventricular contractions, premature, multifocal
Lanoxicaps (Common) 1110
Lanoxin Elixir Pediatric (Less common) 1113
Lanoxin Injection 1116
Lanoxin Injection Pediatric (Less common) 1119
▲ Lanoxin Tablets (Among most common) 1121

Ventricular contractions, premature, unifocal
Lanoxicaps (Common) 1110
Lanoxin Elixir Pediatric (Less common) 1113
Lanoxin Injection 1116
Lanoxin Injection Pediatric (Less common) 1119
▲ Lanoxin Tablets (Among most common) 1121

Ventricular dilation, left-side
Retrovir Capsules (0.8%) 1216
Retrovir I.V. Infusion (1%) 1221
Retrovir Syrup (0.8%) 1216

Ventricular ectopic beats
Cipro Tablets (Less than 1%) 584
Desyrel and Desyrel Dividose 504
Digibind 1079
Dobutrex Solution Vials 1480
Hivid Tablets (Less than 1%) 2287
Kytril Injection (Rare) 2667
▲ Primacor Injection (8.5%) 2461
Quinaglute Dura-Tabs Tablets 644
Vasoxyl Injection 1169

Ventricular extrasystoles
Betaseron for SC Injection 653
Cardene Capsules (Rare) 2261
Cardene I.V. (1.4%) 2815
Cardene SR Capsules (Rare) 2264
Cardizem CD Capsules (Less than 1%) 1251
Cardizem SR Capsules (Less than 1%) 1255
Cardizem Injectable 1253
Cardizem Tablets (Less than 1%) .. 1257
Cerebyx Injection (Infrequent) 1956
Claritin-D Tablets (Less frequent) .. 2487
▲ Corvert Injection (5.1%) 2075
Dilacor XR Extended-release Capsules 2183
Lotrel Capsules (Infrequent) 858
Neurontin Capsules (Rare) 1978
Nipent for Injection (Less than 3%) 2733
Paxil Tablets (Rare) 2681
Permax Tablets (Infrequent) 571
Remeron Tablets (Infrequent) 1878
Rilutek Tablets (Infrequent) 2198
Risperdal Tablets (Rare) 1348
Romazicon (Less than 1%) 2311
Serzone Tablets (Infrequent) 776
Sular Tablets (Less than or equal to 1%) 2961
Tiazac Capsules (Less than 1%) 1019
▲ Trasylol (5%) 607

Ventricular failure
Doxorubicin Astra (Uncommon) 531
Flolan for Injection 1085
Tonocard Tablets (Up to 1.4%) 519

Ventricular fibrillation (see under Fibrillations, ventricular)

Ventricular flutter
Cardioquin Tablets (Frequent) 2146
Quinidex Extentabs 2240

Ventricular gallop
Retrovir Capsules (0.8%) 1216
Retrovir I.V. Infusion (1%) 1221
Retrovir Syrup (0.8%) 1216

Ventricular irregularities
▲ Calan SR Caplets (15%) 2571
▲ Calan Tablets (15%) 2568
Cerubidine for Injection 634
Eminase 2215
Isoptin Injectable 1391
Isoptin Oral Tablets (Greater than 1%) 1393
Verelan Capsules (1% or less) 1455

Ventricular irritation
Tenoretic Tablets 2963
Timolide Tablets 1791
Vaseretic Tablets 1810
Zestoretic Tablets 2968

Ventricular response, rapid
Calan SR Caplets 2571
Calan Tablets 2568
Verelan Capsules 1455

Venus sequelae
Diprivan Injectable Emulsion (Rare; less than 1%) 2939

Verruca
Foscavir Injection (Less than 1%) .. 541
Invirase Capsules (Less than 2%) .. 2291
Risperdal Tablets (Rare) 1348

Vertebral compression fractures
Cortone Acetate Sterile Suspension 1663
Cortone Acetate Tablets 1664
Decadron Elixir 1676
Decadron Phosphate Injection 1680
Decadron Phosphate with Xylocaine Injection, Sterile 1683
Dexacort Phosphate in Respihaler .. 1606
Dexacort Phosphate in Turbinaire .. 1607
Florinef Acetate Tablets 506
Pediapred Oral Solution 1618

Vertical deviation
▲ BOTOX (Botulinum Toxin Type A) Purified Neurotoxin Complex (2.1% to 16.9%) 473

Vertigo
Abelcet Injection 1540
Accupril Tablets (0.5% to 1.0%) .. 1950
Adalat CC (3% or less) 582
AeroBid Inhaler System (1% to 3%) 1004
Aerobid-M Inhaler System (1% to 3%) 1004
Albenza Tablets (Less than 1.0% to 1.2%) 2629
Aldactazide Tablets 2556
Aldoclor Tablets 1638
Aldoril Tablets 1644
Altace Capsules (Less than 1% to 1.5%) 1238
Ambien Tablets (Frequent) 2559
Amikacin Sulfate Injection, USP 523
Anafranil Capsules (Frequent) 819
Anaprox/Naprosyn (Less than 3%) 2277
Ancobon Capsules 2254
Androderm Testosterone Transdermal System (Less than 1%) 2634
Apresazide Capsules 824
Asacol Delayed-Release Tablets 2129
Azactam for Injection (Less than 1%) 736
Azulfidine (Rare) 2059
Bactrim DS Tablets 2257
Bactrim I.V. Infusion 2255
Bactrim 2257
Benadryl Injection 1955
Betapace Tablets (Rare) 637
Betoptic Ophthalmic Solution (Rare) 465
Betoptic S Ophthalmic Suspension (Rare) 467
Biaxin 406
Blocadren Tablets (0.6%) 1654
Brethaire Inhaler 830
Bumex (0.1%) 2260
▲ Buprenex Injectable (5-10%) 2170
Cafergot 2376
Capastat Sulfate Injection 968
Capozide Tablets 744
Carafate Suspension (Less than 0.5%) 1250
Carafate Tablets (Less than 0.5%) 1249
Cardene Capsules (Rare) 2261
Cardene SR Capsules (Rare) 2264
Cardioquin Tablets 2146
▲ Cardura Tablets (2% to 23%) 1993
Celestone Soluspan Suspension 2484
Cerebyx Injection (2.2%) 1956
Claritin Tablets (2% or fewer patients) 2485
Claritin-D Tablets (Less frequent) .. 2487
Cleocin Vaginal Cream (Less than 1%) 2070
Clinoril Tablets (Less than 1 in 100) 1658
Clomid (Fewer than 1%) 1262
▲ Clozaril Tablets (More than 5 to 19%) 2377
Cognex Capsules (Frequent) 1961
Combipres Tablets 682
CORTENEMA 2713
Cortone Acetate Sterile Suspension 1663
Cortone Acetate Tablets 1664
Cozaar Tablets (Less than 1%) 1668
Crixivan Capsules (Less than 2%) .. 1670
Dalalone D.P. Injectable 1009
Dalgan Injection (1 to less than 3%) 529
Dapsone Tablets USP 1331
Decadron Elixir 1676
Decadron Phosphate Injection 1680
Decadron Phosphate with Xylocaine Injection, Sterile 1683
Decadron Tablets 1678
Decadron-LA Sterile Suspension 1687

(Described in PDR For Nonprescription Drugs) Incidence data in parenthesis; ▲ 3% or more (⊙ Described in PDR For Ophthalmology)

Depakote Tablets (1% to 5%) 418
Desyrel and Desyrel Dividose 504
Dexacort Phosphate in Respihaler 1606
Dexacort Phosphate in Turbinaire 1607
Dilacor XR Extended-release Capsules (Infrequent) 2183
Dipentum Capsules (1.0%) 2084
▲ Disalcid (Among most common) 1549
Diucardin Tablets 2824
Diupres Tablets 1691
Diuril Oral Suspension 1694
Diuril Sodium Intravenous 1693
Diuril Tablets 1694
Dizac (diazepam injectable emulsion) CIV (Less frequent) 1862
Dolobid Tablets (Less than 1 in 100) 1695
Doxil (Less than 1%) 2613
Duragesic Transdermal System (Less than 1%) 1336
Dyazide Capsules 2653
Dynabac (2.3%) 668
DYNACIN Capsules 1627
E.E.S. (Isolated reports) 427
Easprin 1971
EC-Naprosyn Delayed-Release Tablets (Less than 3%) 2277
Edecrin 1698
Effexor (Frequent) 2825
Eldepryl Capsules 2729
▲ Eminase (Less than 10%) 2215
Enduron Tablets 424
Engerix-B Unit-Dose Vials 2656
EryPed (Isolated reports) 425
Ery-Tab Tablets (Isolated reports) 426
Erythrocin Stearate Filmtab (Isolated reports) 429
Erythromycin Base Filmtab (Isolated reports) 430
Erythromycin Delayed-Release Capsules, USP (Isolated reports) 431
Esidrix Tablets 839
Esimil Tablets 840
Eskalith 2658
Ethmozine Tablets (Less than 2%) 2217
Fansidar Tablets 2281
Feldene Capsules (Greater than 1%) 2008
Fioricet with Codeine Capsules 2387
Fiorinal with Codeine Capsules 2390
Flagyl 375 Capsules 2587
Flagyl I.V. 2373
Flexeril Tablets (Less than 1%) 1701
Florinef Acetate Tablets 506
Floxin I.V. (Less than 1%) 1580
Floxin Tablets (200 mg, 300 mg, 400 mg) (Less than 1%) 1577
Foscavir Injection (Less than 1%) 541
Fungizone Intravenous 507
Gantanol Tablets 2285
Gantrisin 2286
Garamycin Injectable 2502
Glucotrol XL Extended Release Tablets (Less than 1%) 2012
Haldol Decanoate 1587
Haldol Injection, Tablets and Concentrate 1585
Havrix (Less than 1%) 2663
Helidac Therapy 2135
Hexalen Capsules 2760
Hivid Tablets (Less than 1%) 2287
Hydeltrasol Injection, Sterile 1708
Hydeltra-T.B.A. Sterile Suspension 1710
Hydrocortone Acetate Sterile Suspension 1712
Hydrocortone Phosphate Injection, Sterile 1713
Hydrocortone Tablets 1715
HydroDIURIL Tablets 1716
Hydropres Tablets 1718
▲ Hytrin Capsules (0.5% to 21%) 434
Hyzaar Tablets 1720
Imdur (Less than or equal to 5%) 1362
▲ Imitrex Injection (11.9%) 1095
Imitrex Tablets 1099
Inderide Tablets 2838
Inderide LA Long Acting Capsules 2840
Indocin (Greater than 1%) 1723
Intal Inhaler (Rare) 2185
Intal Nebulizer Solution (Rare) 2186
▲ Intron A for Injection (Less than 5% to 23%) 2506
ISMOTIC 45% w/v Solution (Very rare) ⊙ 221
Isoptin Injectable 1391
Kadian Capsules (Less than 3%) 2948
Klonopin Tablets 2294
Lamictal Tablets (1.1%) 1105
Lariam Tablets 2295
Lasix Injection, Oral Solution and Tablets 1267
Lescol Capsules 2395
Lithium Carbonate Capsules & Tablets 2352
Lithonate/Lithotabs/Lithobid 2721
Lopid Tablets (1.5%) 1974
Lopressor 848
▲ Lopressor HCT Tablets (10 in 100 patients) 850
Lotensin HCT Tablets (1.5%) 855
▲ Lupron Depot - 3 Month 22.5 mg (6.4%) 2743
LUVOX Tablets (Infrequent) 2723
▲ Lysodren Tablets (15%) 707
Macrobid Capsules 2138
Macrodantin Capsules 2140
Marax Tablets & DF Syrup 2015
Mavik Tablets (0.3% to 1.0%) 1407
Maxaquin Tablets (Less than 1%) 2593
MetroGel-Vaginal 917
Mevacor Tablets (0.5% to 1.0%) 1742
Miacalcin Nasal Spray (Less than 1%) 2403
Midamor Tablets (Less than or equal to 1%) 1746
Miltown Tablets 2780
Minipress Capsules (1-4%) 2015
Minizide Capsules 2016
Minocin Intravenous 1428
Minocin Oral Suspension 1431
Minocin Pellet-Filled Capsules 1429
Moduretic Tablets (Less than or equal to 1%) 1748
Mono-Gesic Tablets 810
Monoket Tablets (Fewer than 1%) 2550
Monopril Tablets (0.2% to 1.0%) 762
Mustargen (Infrequent) 1752
▲ Mysoline (Among most frequent) 2860
Naprelan Tablets (Less than 1%) 2861
Anaprox/Naprosyn (Less than 3%) 2277
Nebcin Vials, Hyporets & ADD-Vantage 1518
NegGram 2453
Netromycin Injection 100 mg/ml 2516
Neurontin Capsules (Frequent) 1978
Nipent for Injection (Less than 3%) 2733
Nitrostat Tablets (Occasional) 1981
Normodyne Injection (1%) 2519
Normodyne Tablets (2%) 2522
Norvasc Tablets (More than 0.1% to 1%) 2020
Norvir (Less than 2%) 447
▲ Nubain Injection (5%) 952
Oncovin Solution Vials & Hyporets (Rare) 1521
Oretic Tablets 450
Ornade Spansule Capsules 2678
Orthoclone OKT3 Sterile Solution 1892
Orudis Capsules (Less than 1%) 2874
Oruvail Capsules (Less than 1%) 2874
OxyContin Tablets (Less than 1%) 2163
PBZ Tablets 863
PBZ-SR Tablets 862
Papaverine Hydrochloride Vials and Ampoules 1523
Parlodel (Less than 1%) 2411
Paxil Tablets (Frequent) 2681
Pediapred Oral Solution 1618
Pediazole Suspension 2340
▲ Penetrex Tablets (3%) 2196
Periactin 1767
Permax Tablets (Infrequent) 571
Phenobarbital Elixir and Tablets 1523
Plaquenil Sulfate Tablets 2459
PMB 200 and PMB 400 2890
Pravachol Tablets 770
Prelone Syrup 1834
Prilosec Delayed-Release Capsules (Less than 1%) 516
Primaxin I.M. 1770
Primaxin I.V. (Less than 0.2%) 1772
Prinivil Tablets (0.2%) 1776
Prinzide Tablets (0.3% to 1%) 1780
Procardia XL Extended Release Tablets (1% or less) 2026
Protostat Tablets 1939
Proventil Inhalation Aerosol 2524
Proventil Repetabs Tablets 2529
Proventil Syrup 2528
Proventil Tablets 2529
Prozac Pulvules & Liquid, Oral Solution (Infrequent) 935
Questran 774
Quinaglute Dura-Tabs Tablets 644
Quinidex Extentabs 2240
▲ Redux Capsules (3.1%) 2911
Relafen Tablets (1%) 2688
Remeron Tablets (Frequent) 1878
Retrovir Capsules 1216
Retrovir I.V. Infusion 1221
Retrovir Syrup 1216
Rifater 1280
▲ Rilutek Tablets (2.5% to 4.5%) 2198
Risperdal Tablets (Infrequent) 1348
Robaxin Injectable 2245
Roferon-A Injection (Less than 3%) 2308
▲ Romazicon (10%) 2311
Rythmol Tablets–150mg, 225mg, 300mg (Less than 1%) 1399
Salflex Tablets 791
Sandostatin Injection (Less than 1%) 2421
Septra 1146
Septra I.V. Infusion 1142
Septra I.V. Infusion ADD-Vantage Vials 1144
Septra 1146
Ser-Ap-Es Tablets 867
Serax Capsules (In few instances) 2916
Serax Tablets (In few instances) 2916
Seromycin Capsules 975
Serzone Tablets (Infrequent) 776
Soma Compound w/Codeine Tablets 2784
Soma Compound Tablets (Less frequent) 2783
Soma Tablets 2782
Sporanox Capsules (1%) 1352
Sular Tablets (Less than or equal to 1%) 2961
Tambocor Tablets (1% to less than 3%) 1555
Tapazole Tablets 1361
Tavist Syrup 2426
Tavist Tablets 2427
Tenex Tablets (Less frequent) 2249
Tenoretic Tablets (2%) 2963
Tenormin Tablets and I.V. Injection (2%) 2965
Thalitone 1293
Timolide Tablets 1791
Timoptic in Ocudose 1796
Timoptic Sterile Ophthalmic Solution 1794
Timoptic-XE 1798
▲ Tonocard Tablets (8.0% to 25.3%) 519
Toradol (1% or less) 2319
Tornalate Solution for Inhalation, 0.2% (Less than 1%) 976
Trandate (1 of 100 patients) 1158
Trinalin Repetabs Tablets 1373
Tussend 1830
▲ Ultram Tablets (50 mg) (26% to 33%) 1594
Urispas Tablets 2710
Valium Injectable 2336
Valium Tablets (Infrequent) 2335
Vancocin HCl, Oral Solution & Pulvules (Rare) 1536
Vancocin HCl, Vials & ADD-Vantage (Rare) 1534
Vascor Tablets (200 and 300 mg) (0.5 to 2.0%) 1597
Vaseretic Tablets (0.5% to 2.0%) 1810
Vasotec I.V. 1814
Vasotec Tablets (1.6%) 1816
Velban Vials (Rare) 1537
Ventolin Rotacaps for Inhalation 1173
Ventolin Syrup 1175
Ventolin Tablets 1176
Volmax Extended-Release Tablets 1835
Wellbutrin Tablets (Infrequent) 1177
Yodoxin Tablets 1235
Zantac (Rare) 1182
Zantac Injection 1180
Zantac Syrup (Rare) 1182
Zaroxolyn Tablets 1625
Zebeta Tablets 1457
Zestoretic Tablets (0.3 to 1%) 2968
Zestril Tablets (0.2%) 2972
Ziac 1459
Zithromax (1% or less) 2043
Zithromax Tablets (1% or less) 2046
Zocor Tablets 1821
Zoloft Tablets (Infrequent) 2051
Zosyn (1.0% or less) 1463
Zyloprim Tablets (Less than 1%) 1194
Zyrtec Tablets (Less than 2%) 2053

Vesical spasm

Dilaudid Ampules 1382
Dilaudid Cough Syrup 1383
Dilaudid 1382
Hycodan Tablets and Syrup 946
Hycomine Compound Tablets 948
Hycomine 947
Hycotuss Expectorant Syrup 950
Hydrocet Capsules 787
Vicodin Tablets 1404

Vesiculation

Adriamycin PFS 2056
Adriamycin RDF 2056
Attenuvax 1650
▲ Blenoxane (Approximately 50%) 697
▲ Catapres-TTS (7 of 101 patients) 680
Cipro I.V. (1% or less) 587
Condylox Topical Solution (Less than 5%) 1853
Diprolene Ointment 0.05% (1 per 767 patients) 2491
M-M-R II 1730
M-R-VAX II 1732
8-MOP Capsules 1294
MSTA Mumps Skin Test Antigen 2988
Oxsoralen-Ultra Capsules 1302
PPD Tine Test 2993
Rubex for Injection 721
Topicort LP Emollient Cream 0.05% (0.8%) 1289
T.R.U.E. Test (Two to 27 reports) 1162
Tuberculin, Old, Tine Test 2994
Tubersol (Tuberculin Purified Protein Derivative (Mantoux)) 2988
Tympagesic Ear Drops 2476
Ultram Tablets (50 mg) (Less than 1%) 1594
Ultravate Cream 0.05% (Less frequent) 2797
Velban Vials 1537

Vesiculobullous reaction

Feldene Capsules (Less than 1%; occasional) 2008
Floxin I.V. 1580
Floxin Tablets (200 mg, 300 mg, 400 mg) 1577
Motrin Ibuprofen Suspension, Oral Drops, Chewable Tablets, Caplets (Less than 1%) 1563

Vestibular dysfunction

Amikacin Sulfate Injection, USP 523
Anafranil Capsules (Up to 2%) 819
Cipro I.V. Pharmacy Bulk Package (Less than 1%) 590
Oncovin Solution Vials & Hyporets (Rare) 1521
Platinol for Injection 717
Platinol-AQ Injection 719
Redux Capsules (Infrequent) 2911
Rilutek Tablets (Rare) 2198
Streptomycin Sulfate Injection 2031
Velban Vials (Rare) 1537

Vibratory sensation, loss of

Platinol for Injection 717
Platinol-AQ Injection 719

Virilization

Androderm Testosterone Transdermal System 2634
▲ Android Capsules, 10 mg (Among most common) 1297
▲ Estratest (Among most common) 2718
Halotestin Tablets 2095
Intron A for Injection (Less than 5%) 2506
Oxandrin 783
Testoderm Testosterone Transdermal System 486
Testred Capsules, 10 mg 1308
Winstrol Tablets 2468

Virilization, female fetus

Amen Tablets 785
▲ Android Capsules, 10 mg (Among most common) 1297
Cycrin Tablets 991
Depo-Provera Sterile Aqueous Suspension 2083
Megace Tablets 710
Testred Capsules, 10 mg 1308

Vision, blurred

(see under Blurred vision)

Vision, changes

(see under Visual disturbances)

Vision, complete loss

Amen Tablets 785
Brevicon 2563
Cycrin Tablets 991
Demulen 2580
Depo-Provera Contraceptive Injection 2079
Depo-Provera Sterile Aqueous Suspension 2083
Levlen/Tri-Levlen 646
Modicon 1928

(Described in PDR For Nonprescription Drugs) Incidence data in parenthesis; ▲ 3% or more (⊙ Described in PDR For Ophthalmology)

Vision, complete loss Side Effects Index 1482

Norinyl 2563
Nor-Q D Tablets 2598
Ortho-Cyclen/Ortho-Tri-Cyclen 1914
Ortho-Novum 1928
Ortho-Cyclen/Ortho Tri-Cyclen 1914
Ovcon 765
Plaquenil Sulfate Tablets (One case) 2459
Premphase 2900
Prempro 2905
Provera Tablets 2110
Levlen/Tri-Levlen 646
Tri-Norinyl 2607

Vision, double (see under Diplopia)

Vision, loss of

Cognex Capsules (Rare) 1961
Nipent for Injection (Less than 3%) 2733
Paraplatin for Injection 713
Prinivil Tablets (0.3% to 1.0%) 1776
Prinzide Tablets 1780
Procardia Capsules 2024
Zestoretic Tablets 2968
Zestril Tablets (0.3% to 1.0%) 2972

Vision, loss of color

Cipro I.V. (1% or less) 587
Cipro Tablets (Less than 1%) 584
Mellaril 2398
Motrin Ibuprofen Suspension, Oral Drops, Chewable Tablets, Caplets 1563
Ponstel (Rare) 1982

Vision, obscured by enlarged iris cysts

Humorsol Sterile Ophthalmic Solution 1707

Vision, partial loss

Amen Tablets 785
Brevicon 2563
Cycrin Tablets 991
Demulen 2580
Depo-Provera Contraceptive Injection 2079
Depo-Provera Sterile Aqueous Suspension 2083
IBU Tablets (Less than 1%) 1389
Levlen/Tri-Levlen 646
Modicon 1928
Motrin Ibuprofen Suspension, Oral Drops, Chewable Tablets, Caplets (Less than 1%) 1563
Norinyl 2563
Nor-Q D Tablets 2598
Ortho-Cyclen/Ortho-Tri-Cyclen 1914
Ortho-Novum 1928
Ortho-Cyclen/Ortho Tri-Cyclen 1914
Ovcon 765
Premphase 2900
Prempro 2905
Provera Tablets 2110
Levlen/Tri-Levlen 646
Tri-Norinyl 2607

Vision, temporary loss

Clomid 1262
Soma Compound w/Codeine Tablets 2784
Soma Compound Tablets (Very rare) 2783
Soma Tablets 2782
Sular Tablets (Less than or equal to 1%) 2961

Vision, tunnel

BuSpar Tablets (Rare) 738
Serophene (clomiphene citrate tablets, USP) 2621

Vision abnormalities (see under Visual disturbances)

Visual acuity, defects

AK-CIDE ◉ 203
AK-CIDE Ointment ◉ 203
AK-PRED ◉ 204
AK-Trol Ointment & Suspension ◉ 205
Betoptic Ophthalmic Solution 465
Betoptic S Ophthalmic Suspension (Small number of patients) 467
Blephamide Liquifilm Sterile Ophthalmic Suspension 472
Blephamide Ointment ◉ 234
Cipro I.V. (1% or less) 587
Cipro I.V. Pharmacy Bulk Package (Less than 1%) 590
Cipro Tablets (Less than 1%) 584
Cortisporin Ophthalmic Ointment Sterile 1074
Cortisporin Ophthalmic Suspension Sterile 1075
Cozaar Tablets (Less than 1%) 1668
Eflone Sterile Ophthalmic Suspension ◉ 261
FML Forte Liquifilm ◉ 237
FML Liquifilm ◉ 238
FML S.O.P. ◉ 239
FML-S Liquifilm ◉ 240
Flarex Ophthalmic Suspension ◉ 217
HMS Liquifilm ◉ 241
Hyzaar Tablets 1720
Intron A for Injection 2506
Isopto Carbachol Ophthalmic Solution ◉ 221
Isopto Carpine Ophthalmic Solution (Frequent) ◉ 221
Maxitrol Ophthalmic Ointment and Suspension ◉ 222
Mellaril 2398
Myambutol Tablets 1432
NegGram 2453
Pilopine HS Ophthalmic Gel ◉ 224
Plaquenil Sulfate Tablets 2459
Pred Forte ◉ 247
Pred Mild ◉ 250
Pred-G Liquifilm Sterile Ophthalmic Suspension ◉ 248
Pred-G S.O.P. Sterile Ophthalmic Ointment ◉ 249
Serophene (clomiphene citrate tablets, USP) 2621
Symmetrel Capsules (0.1% to 1%) 965
Symmetrel Syrup (0.1% to 1%) 963
TobraDex Ophthalmic Suspension and Ointment 469
▲ Vesanoid Capsules (6%) 2327
Vexol 1% Ophthalmic Suspension ◉ 227

Visual disturbances

Accutane Capsules 2252
Achromycin V Capsules 1417
Adalat CC (Less than 1.0%) 582
AK-PRED ◉ 204
AK-Trol Ointment & Suspension ◉ 205
Alferon N Injection (1%) 2142
Altace Capsules (Less than 1%) 1238
Ambien Tablets (Frequent) 2559
Amicar Syrup, Tablets, and Injection 1312
▲ Anafranil Capsules (7% to 18%) 819
Anaprox/Naprosyn (Less than 3%) 2277
Aralen Hydrochloride Injection 2430
Aralen Phosphate Tablets 2431
Atrohist Plus Tablets 1605
Avonex 662
Betagan ◉ 230
Betapace Tablets (1% to 5%) 637
▲ Betaseron for SC Injection (7%) 653
Betimol 0.25%, 0.5% (1% to 5%) ◉ 259
Blephamide Liquifilm Sterile Ophthalmic Suspension 472
Blocadren Tablets 1654
Brevibloc (esmolol HCl) Injection (Less than 1%) 1860
Brevicon (Rare) 2563
▲ Bromfed-DM Cough Syrup (Among most frequent) 1832
Brontex 2130
Buprenex Injectable (Less than 1%) 2170
Cardene Capsules (Rare) 2261
Cardene SR Capsules (Rare) 2264
▲ Cardioquin Tablets (3%) 2146
Cardura Tablets (1.4% to 2%) 1993
Cipro I.V. (1% or less) 587
Cipro I.V. Pharmacy Bulk Package (Less than 1%) 590
Cipro Tablets (Less than 1%) 584
Clear Eyes ACR Astringent/Lubricant Eye Redness Reliever Eye Drops ◉ 314
Clinoril Tablets (Less than 1 in 100) 1658
Clomid (1.5%) 1262
▲ Clozaril Tablets (5% or more) 2377
▲ Cordarone Tablets (4 to 9%) 2818
Cuprimine Capsules 1673
Cytotec (Infrequent) 2576
Cytovene (1% or less) 2270
Danocrine Capsules 2437
Dantrium Capsules (Less frequent) 2131
Darvon-N/Darvocet-N 1473
Darvon 1475
Darvon-N Suspension & Tablets 1473
▲ DaunoXome (3%) 1842
Demerol 2438
Demulen (Rare) 2580
Depakote Tablets (1% to 5%) 418
Desferal Vials 838
Dilaudid-HP Injection (Less frequent) 1384
Dilaudid-HP Lyophilized Powder 250 mg (Less frequent) 1384
Dilaudid Tablets and Liquid (Less frequent) 1386
Dimetane-DC Cough Syrup 2232
Dimetane-DX Cough Syrup 2233
Dolobid Tablets (Less than 1 in 100) 1695
Doral Tablets 2773
Doxil (Less than 1%) 2613
DynaCirc Capsules (0.5% to 1%) 2381
DynaCirc CR Tablets (0.5% to 1.0%) 2383
Easprin 1971
EC-Naprosyn Delayed-Release Tablets (Less than 3%) 2277
Effexor (Frequent) 2825
Engerix-B Unit-Dose Vials 2656
Estrace Cream and Tablets 751
Estring Vaginal Ring (At least 1 report) 2086
Eye-Stream Eye Irrigating Solution 469
FML Forte Liquifilm ◉ 237
FML Liquifilm ◉ 238
FML-S Liquifilm ◉ 240
▲ Felbatol (5.3%) 2774
Feldene Capsules 2008
▲ Flolan for Injection (4%) 1085
Floxin I.V. (1% to 3%) 1580
Floxin Tablets (200 mg, 300 mg, 400 mg) (1% to 3%) 1577
▲ Fludara for Injection (3% to 15%) 658
Fluorouracil Injection 2282
▲ Foscavir Injection (5% or greater) 541
Sterile FUDR (Remote possibility) 2284
Garamycin Injectable 2502
Genotropin Injection (A small number of patients) 2090
Halcion Tablets (0.9% to 0.5%) 2093
Haldol Decanoate 1587
Haldol Injection, Tablets and Concentrate 1585
Helidac Therapy 2135
Hivid Tablets (Less than 1%) 2287
Humatrope Vials (A small number of patients) 1490
▲ Hylorel Tablets (29.2%) 1613
Hytrin Capsules (At least 1%) 434
Imdur (Less than or equal to 5%) 1362
Imitrex Injection (1.1%) 1095
Imitrex Tablets (Up to 3%) 1099
Inderal 2834
Inderal LA Long Acting Capsules 2836
Inderide Tablets 2838
Inderide LA Long Acting Capsules 2840
Intron A for Injection (Less than 5%) 2506
Invirase Capsules (Less than 2%) 2291
IOPIDINE Sterile Ophthalmic Solution ◉ 218
Iopidine 0.5% (Less than 1%) ◉ 219
Kerlone Tablets (Less than 2%) 2588
▲ Lamictal Tablets (3.4%) 1105
Lamisil Tablets (1.1%) 2394
Lamprene Capsules (Less than 1%) 846
Lanoxicaps 1110
Lanoxin Elixir Pediatric 1113
Lanoxin Injection 1116
Lanoxin Injection Pediatric 1119
Lanoxin Tablets 1121
Lariam Tablets 2295
Levlen/Tri-Levlen 646
Levo-Dromoran 2297
Lioresal Intrathecal (1% or more) 1634
Livostin (Approximately 1% to 3%) ◉ 262
Lodine Capsules and Tablets (Less than 1%) 2849
Lopressor 848
Lopressor HCT Tablets 850
Lotensin HCT Tablets (0.3% or more) 855
Lupron Depot - 3 Month 22.5 mg (Less than 5%) 2743
MS Contin Tablets (Less frequent) 2149
MSIR (Infrequent) 2152
Marinol (Dronabinol) Capsules (Less than 1%) 2353
Matulane Capsules 2300
Maxaquin Tablets (Less than 1%) 2593
Mepergan Injection 2859
Methadone Hydrochloride Oral Concentrate 2356
Methadone Hydrochloride Oral Solution & Tablets 2357
Methotrexate Sodium Tablets, Injection, for Injection and LPF Injection 1322
▲ Mexitil Capsules (5.7% to 7.5%) 684
Midamor Tablets (Less than or equal to 1%) 1746
Miltown Tablets 2780
Modicon (Rare) 1928
Moduretic Tablets (Less than or equal to 1%) 1748
Monopril Tablets (0.2% to 1.0%) 762
Myambutol Tablets 1432
Naprelan Tablets (Less than 3%) 2861
Anaprox/Naprosyn (Less than 3%) 2277
NegGram (Infrequent) 2453
Neoral (Rare) 2405
Neurontin Capsules (Frequent) 1978
Nicotrol NS Nicotine Nasal Spray (Less than 1%) 1565
Nipent for Injection (Less than 3%) 2733
Nolvadex Tablets 2957
Norinyl 2563
Normodyne Tablets (1%) 2522
Noroxin Tablets 1758
Noroxin Tablets 2222
Norplant System 2868
Nor-Q D Tablets 2598
Norvasc Tablets (More than 0.1% to 1%) 2020
Norvir (Less than 2%) 447
Nutropin (A small number of patients) 1049
Nutropin AQ Injection (A small number of patients) 1051
Ocupress Ophthalmic Solution, 1% Sterile (Occasional) ◉ 297
OptiPranolol (Metipranolol 0.3%) Sterile Ophthalmic Solution (A small number of patients) ◉ 256
Oramorph SR (Morphine Sulfate Sustained Release Tablets) (Less frequent) 2359
▲ Orap Tablets (4 of 20 patients; 5.5%) 1037
Ortho-Cyclen/Ortho-Tri-Cyclen 1914
Ortho-Est 1925
Ortho-Novum (Rare) 1928
Ortho-Cyclen/Ortho Tri-Cyclen 1914
Orudis Capsules (Greater than 1%) 2874
Oruvail Capsules (Greater than 1%) 2874
OxyContin Tablets (Less than 1%) 2163
Paraplatin for Injection (1%) 713
Parlodel 2411
▲ Paxil Tablets (4%) 2681
Penetrex Tablets (0.1% to 1%) 2196
▲ Permax Tablets (5.8%) 571
Phenergan with Codeine 2883
Phenergan VC with Codeine 2888
Phospholine Iodide (More frequent in children) ◉ 323
Plaquenil Sulfate Tablets 2459
Plendil Extended-Release Tablets (0.5% to 1.5%) 514
PMB 200 and PMB 400 2890
Pred Forte ◉ 247
Premphase 2900
Prempro 2905
Procardia XL Extended Release Tablets (1% or less) 2026
▲ Prograf (Greater than 3%) 1028
▲ Proleukin for Injection (7%) 812
Propulsid (1.4%) 1346
ProSom Tablets (Infrequent) 457
Prostigmin Injectable 1305
Prostigmin Tablets 1306
▲ Prozac Pulvules & Liquid, Oral Solution (2% to 5%) 935
▲ Quinidex Extentabs (3%) 2240
RMS Suppositories CII 2766
Recombivax HB (Less than 1%) 1787
Redux Capsules 2911
Reglan 2243
Relafen Tablets (1%) 2688
ReoPro Vials (0.7%) 1526
Ridaura Capsules 2691
Rifadin 1276
Rifamate Capsules 1278
Rifater 1280
Rimactane Capsules 865
Risperdal Tablets (1% to 2%) 1348
Ritalin (Rare) 866
▲ Roferon-A Injection (5% to 6%) 2308

(Described in PDR For Nonprescription Drugs) Incidence data in parenthesis; ▲ 3% or more (◉ Described in PDR For Ophthalmology)

▲ Romazicon (1% to 9%) 2311
Roxanol 2365
Rythmol Tablets–150mg, 225mg, 300mg (Less than 1% to 1.9%) 1399
Salagen Tablets (1%) 1546
Sandimmune (Rare) 2416
Sandostatin Injection (1% to 4%) 2421
Sectral Capsules (2%) 2914
Seldane Tablets 1284
Seldane-D Extended-Release Tablets 1286
Serophene (clomiphene citrate tablets, USP) (Approximately 1 in 50 patients) 2621
▲ Serzone Tablets (Up to 10%) 776
Slo-Niacin Tablets 2767
Sular Tablets (Less than or equal to 1%) 2961
▲ Supprelin Injection (2% to 6%) 2230
Symmetrel Capsules (0.1% to 1%) 965
Symmetrel Syrup (0.1% to 1%) 963
Talacen Caplets (Infrequent) 2464
Talwin Injection 2465
Talwin Compound (Infrequent) 2466
Talwin Injection 2465
Talwin Nx Tablets 2467
▲ Tambocor Tablets (15.9%) 1555
Taxol Injection (Rare) 723
▲ Tegison Capsules (10-25%) 2314
Tenex Tablets (3% or less) 2249
Tenoretic Tablets 2963
Tenormin Tablets and I.V. Injection 2965
Terra-Cortril Ophthalmic Suspension 2033
Thorazine 2701
Timolide Tablets 1791
Timoptic in Ocudose (Less frequent) 1796
Timoptic Sterile Ophthalmic Solution (Less frequent) 1794
Timoptic-XE 1798
Tolectin (200, 400 and 600 mg) (1 to 3%) 1591
▲ Tonocard Tablets (1.3% to 10.0%) 519
Toradol (1% or less) 2319
Trandate Tablets (1%) 1158
Levlen/Tri-Levlen 646
Tri-Norinyl 2607
Ultram Tablets (50 mg) (1% to less than 5%) 1594
Urispas Tablets 2710
Versed Injection (Less than 1%) 2324
▲ Vesanoid Capsules (17%) 2327
Videx Tablets, Powder for Oral Solution, & Pediatric Powder for Oral Solution (Less than 1% to 5%) 2980
Vira-A Ophthalmic Ointment, 3% ⊙ 299
Visine L.R. Eye Drops ⊙ 301
Visken Tablets (2% or fewer patients) 2428
Vistide Injection 1057
Viva-Drops ⊙ 326
Vivelle Transdermal System 880
Wellbutrin Tablets (Infrequent) 1177
Wygesic Tablets 2930
Zebeta Tablets 1457
Zerit Capsules (Fewer than 1% to 3%) 731
Ziac 1459
▲ Zoloft Tablets (4.2%) 2051
Zovirax 1187

Visual disturbances, flashing lights

Clomid (1.5%) 1262

Visual field, defects

AK-CIDE ⊙ 203
AK-CIDE Ointment ⊙ 203
AK-PRED ⊙ 204
AK-Trol Ointment & Suspension ⊙ 205
Anafranil Capsules (Rare) 819
Betaseron for SC Injection 653
Blephamide Liquifilm Sterile Ophthalmic Suspension 472
Blephamide Ointment ⊙ 234
Cardioquin Tablets (Occasional) 2146
Cerebyx Injection (Infrequent) 1956
Cognex Capsules (Infrequent) 1961
Cortisporin Ophthalmic Ointment Sterile 1074
Cortisporin Ophthalmic Suspension Sterile 1075
Doxil (Less than 1%) 2613
Effexor (Infrequent) 2825
Eflone Sterile Ophthalmic Suspension ⊙ 261
Eskalith 2658
FML Forte Liquifilm ⊙ 237
FML Liquifilm ⊙ 238
FML S.O.P. ⊙ 239
FML-S Liquifilm ⊙ 240
Flarex Ophthalmic Suspension ⊙ 217
Foscavir Injection (Less than 1%) 541
HMS Liquifilm ⊙ 241
Intron A for Injection 2506
LUVOX Tablets (Infrequent) 2723
Maxitrol Ophthalmic Ointment and Suspension ⊙ 222
Neurontin Capsules (Infrequent) 1978
Norvir (Less than 2%) 447
Paxil Tablets (Infrequent) 2681
Permax Tablets (Infrequent) 571
Pred Forte ⊙ 247
Pred Mild ⊙ 250
Pred-G Liquifilm Sterile Ophthalmic Suspension ⊙ 248
Prevacid Delayed-Release Capsules (Less than 1%) 2746
Quinaglute Dura-Tabs Tablets 644
Quinidex Extentabs 2240
Redux Capsules 2911
Romazicon (1% to 3%) 2311
Serzone Tablets (2%) 776
TobraDex Ophthalmic Suspension and Ointment 469
▲ Vesanoid Capsules (3%) 2327
Vexol 1% Ophthalmic Suspension ⊙ 227
Videx Tablets, Powder for Oral Solution, & Pediatric Powder for Oral Solution (Less than 1%) 2980
Zoloft Tablets (Rare) 2051
Zyrtec Tablets (Less than 2%) 2053

Visual impairment

Abelcet Injection 1540
Ciloxan Ophthalmic Solution (Less than 1%) 468
Fungizone Intravenous 507
Levlen/Tri-Levlen (Rare) 646
Ocusert Pilo-20 and Pilo-40 Ocular Therapeutic Systems ⊙ 252
Ortho-Cyclen/Ortho-Tri-Cyclen (Rare) 1914
Ortho-Cyclen/Ortho Tri-Cyclen (Rare) 1914
Ridaura Capsules 2691
Levlen/Tri-Levlen (Rare) 646

Vitamin D, increased requirement

Mebaral Tablets 2452

Vitamins, fat-soluble, absorption impaired

Questran 774

Vitiligo

Azelex (Rare) 471
Intron A for Injection (Less than 5%) 2506
Proleukin for Injection 812

Vitreous disorder, unspecified

Clomid 1262
▲ Cytovene (6%) 2270

Vitreous floaters

Avonex 662
Cataflam Tablets (Less than 1%) 833
ISPAN Perfluoropropane ⊙ 267
ISPAN Sulfur Hexafluoride ⊙ 266
Miacalcin Nasal Spray (Less than 1%) 2403
Sular Tablets (Less than or equal to 1%) 2961
Cataflam/Voltaren/Voltaren-XR (Less than 1%) 833

Voice, alteration

Accutane Capsules (Less than 1%) 2252
Danocrine Capsules 2437
Effexor (Infrequent) 2825
Imitrex Tablets (Rare) 1099
Kadian Capsules (Less than 3%) 2948
Lotensin HCT Tablets (0.3% or more) 855
Monopril Tablets (0.4% to 1.0%) 762
OxyContin Tablets (Less than 1%) 2163
Paxil Tablets (Infrequent) 2681
Permax Tablets (Infrequent) 571
▲ Prograf (Greater than 3%) 1028
▲ Pulmozyme Inhalation (12% to 16%) 1054
Salagen Tablets (2%) 1546
Serzone Tablets (Infrequent) 776
Ventolin Rotacaps for Inhalation (Less than 1%) 1173
▲ Zoladex (3%) 2976
Zoladex 3-month 2978

Voice, deepening

Aldactazide Tablets 2556
Aldactone Tablets 2558
▲ Android Capsules, 10 mg (Among most common) 1297
Danocrine Capsules 2437
Estratest 2718
Halotestin Tablets 2095
Oxandrin 783
Testred Capsules, 10 mg 1308
Winstrol Tablets 2468

Voice, hoarseness

Danocrine Capsules 2437
Estratest 2718

Voice, loss of (see under Aphonia)

Vomiting

Abbokinase 403
Abbokinase Open-Cath 405
▲ Abelcet Injection (6%) 1540
Accupril Tablets (1.4% to 2.4%) 1950
Accutane Capsules 2252
Acel-Imune Diphtheria and Tetanus Toxoids and Acellular Pertussis Vaccine Adsorbed (2% to 3%) 1415
Achromycin V Capsules (Rare) 1417
▲ ActHIB (1.5% to 5.4%) 893
▲ Actigall Capsules (9.7%) 818
▲ Actimmune (13%) 1043
Activase 1045
Adalat CC (Less than 1.0%) 582
Adapin Capsules 1542
Adriamycin PFS (Frequent) 2056
Adriamycin RDF (Frequent) 2056
▲ AeroBid Inhaler System (25%) 1004
▲ Aerobid-M Inhaler System (25%) 1004
Aerolate 1003
AK-FLUOR Injection 10% and 25% ⊙ 204
▲ Albenza Tablets (3.7% to 6.2%) 2629
Albuminar-5, Albumin (Human) U.S.P. 5% (Occasional) 795
Albuminar-25, Albumin (Human) U.S.P. 25% 796
Aldactazide Tablets 2556
Aldactone Tablets 2558
Aldoclor Tablets 1638
Aldomet Ester HCl Injection 1642
Aldomet Oral 1640
Aldoril Tablets 1644
▲ Alfenta Injection (18%) 1334
▲ Alferon N Injection (3% to 29%) 2142
▲ Alka-Seltzer Cherry Effervescent Antacid and Pain Reliever (7.6% at doses of 1000 mg/day) ▣ 609
▲ Alka-Seltzer Lemon Lime Effervescent Antacid and Pain Reliever (7.6% at doses of 1000 mg/day) ▣ 609
▲ Alka-Seltzer Original Effervescent Antacid and Pain Reliever (7.6% at doses of 1000 mg/day) ▣ 609
Alkeran for Injection 1196
Alkeran Tablets (Infrequent) 1198
All-Flex Arcing Spring Diaphragm (See also Ortho Diaphragm Kits) 1921
Altace Capsules (Less than 1% to 1.6%) 1238
Alupent (1% to 4%) 672
Amaryl Tablets (Less than 1%) 1241
Ambien Tablets (1%) 2559
Amicar Syrup, Tablets, and Injection 1312
Amikacin Sulfate Injection, USP (Rare) 523
Amikacin Sulfate Injection, USP (Rare) 981
Amikin Injectable (Rare) 502
Aminohippurate Sodium Injection 1646
Amoxil 2631
▲ Anafranil Capsules (7%) 819
Ana-Kit Anaphylaxis Emergency Treatment Kit 611
Anaprox/Naprosyn (Less than 1%) 2277
Ancef Injection (Rare) 2632
Ancobon Capsules 2254
Androderm Testosterone Transdermal System 2634
Antilirium Injectable 1007
Antivenin (Crotalidae) Polyvalent 2803
Apresazide Capsules (Common) 824
Apresoline Hydrochloride Tablets (Common) 826
Aquasol A Vitamin A Capsules, USP 525
Aquasol A Parenteral 526
Aralen Hydrochloride Injection 2430
Aralen Phosphate Tablets 2431
▲ Aredia for Injection (Up to at least 15%) 827
▲ Arimidex Tablets (9.2% to 10.6%) 2932
Artane 1418
▲ Asacol Delayed-Release Tablets (5%) 2129
▲ Regular Strength Ascriptin Tablets (7.6%) ▣ 650
Asendin Tablets (Less than 1%) 1419
Astramorph/PF Injection, USP (Preservative-Free) (Frequent) 526
Atamet Tablets 567
Ativan Injection (Occasional) 2805
▲ Atretol Tablets (Among most frequent) 569
Atrohist Plus Tablets 1605
Atromid-S Capsules (Less frequent) 2808
Atrovent Inhalation Aerosol 674
Augmentin (1%) 2637
Augmentin Tablets (1%) 2640
Axid Pulvules (1.2% to 3.6%) 1468
▲ Axocet Capsules (Among most frequent) 2469
Azactam for Injection (1 to 1.3%) 736
▲ Azathioprine Tablets (Approximately 12%) 2349
▲ Azulfidine (Approximately one-third of patients) 2059
▲ Bactrim DS Tablets (Among most common) 2257
▲ Bactrim I.V. Infusion (Among most common) 2255
▲ Bactrim (Among most common) 2257
▲ Genuine Bayer Aspirin Tablets & Caplets (7.6% at doses of 1000 mg/day) ▣ 618
▲ Aspirin Regimen Bayer Regular Strength 325 mg Caplets (7.6% of 4500 people tested) ▣ 613
Benadryl Injection 1955
Benemid Tablets 1651
Bentyl 1246
▲ Betapace Tablets (5% to 10%) 637
▲ Betaseron for SC Injection (21%) 653
Biavax II 1653
▲ Biaxin (6%) 406
BiCNU (Frequent) 696
Blenoxane (Frequent) 697
Blocadren Tablets (Less than 1%) 1654
Brethaire Inhaler 830
Brethine Ampuls (1.3 to 3.9%) 832
Brethine Tablets 831
Brevibloc (esmolol HCl) Injection (About 1%) 1860
Brevicon 2563
Bricanyl Subcutaneous Injection 1247
Bricanyl Tablets 1248
▲ Bromfed-DM Cough Syrup (Among most frequent) 1832
Brontex 2130
▲ Bufferin Analgesic Tablets (7.6%) ▣ 636
Bumex (0.2%) 2260
Buprenex Injectable (1-5%) 2170
BuSpar Tablets (1%) 738
Butisol Sodium Elixir & Tablets (Less than 1 in 100) 2768
Cafergot 2376
Calcijex Injection 412
▲ Calcimar Injection, Synthetic (About 10%) 2176
Capoten Tablets (About 0.5 to 2%) 740
Capozide Tablets (0.5 to 2%) 744
Carafate Suspension (Less than 0.5%) 1250
Carafate Tablets (Less than 0.5%) 1249
Carbocaine Injection 2432
Cardene Capsules (0.4%) 2261
▲ Cardene I.V. (4.9%) 2815
Cardene SR Capsules (0.6%) 2264
▲ Cardioquin Tablets (Among most frequent) 2146
Cardizem CD Capsules (Less than 1%) 1251
Cardizem SR Capsules (Less than 1%) 1255
Cardizem Injectable (Less than 1%) 1253
Cardizem Tablets (Less than 1%) 1257
Cardura Tablets 1993
Carnitor Injection 2623
Carnitor Tablets and Solution 2624
▲ Casodex Tablets (5%) 2934

(▣ Described in PDR For Nonprescription Drugs) Incidence data in parenthesis; ▲ 3% or more (⊙ Described in PDR For Ophthalmology)

Vomiting — Side Effects Index — 1484

Cataflam Tablets (Less than 1%) 833
▲ Catapres Tablets (About 5 in 100 patients) 679
Catapres-TTS 680
Ceclor Pulvules & Suspension (Rare) 1470
Cedax (1% to 2%) 2480
CeeNU Capsules 699
Cefizox for Intramuscular or Intravenous Use (Occasional) 1025
Cefobid Intravenous/Intramuscular (Rare) 1996
Cefobid Pharmacy Bulk Package - Not for Direct Infusion (Rare) 1999
Cefotan 2936
▲ Ceftin (2.6% to 6.7%) 1067
Cefzil Tablets and Oral Suspension (1%) 747
▲ CellCept Capsules (12.5% to 13.6%) 2265
Celontin Kapseals (Frequent) 1955
Ceptaz (One in 500 patients) 1070
Cerebyx Injection (2.2% to 2.8%) 1956
Ceredase 1055
Cerubidine for Injection 634
Cervidil (Less than 1%) 1008
▲ Chemet Capsules (12.0% to 20.9%) 666
Chloromycetin Sodium Succinate 1960
Chromagen Capsules 2470
Chromagen FA 2471
Chromagen Forte 2471
Cipro I.V. (1% or less) 587
Cipro I.V. Pharmacy Bulk Package (Less than 1%) 590
Cipro Tablets (2.0%) 584
Claforan Sterile and Injection (1.4%; rare) 1259
Claritin Tablets (2% or fewer patients) 2485
Claritin-D Tablets (Less frequent) 2487
Cleocin Phosphate Injection 2068
Climara Transdermal System 640
Cleocin Vaginal Cream (Less than 1%) 2070
Clinoril Tablets (Greater than 1%) 1658
Clomid (2.2%) 1262
▲ Clozaril Tablets (3%) 2377
Cocaine Hydrochloride Topical Solutions 529
Cogentin 1661
▲ Cognex Capsules (28%) 1961
ColBENEMID Tablets 1662
Colestid (Less frequent) 2073
Colyte and Colyte-flavored 2540
▲ Combipres Tablets (About 5%) 682
Compazine 2644
Condylox Topical Solution (Less than 5%) 1853
Cordarone Intravenous (Less than 2%) 2821
▲ Cordarone Tablets (10 to 33%) 2818
Cosmegen Injection (Common) 1666
Coumadin (Infrequent) 941
Cozaar Tablets (Less than 1%) 1668
▲ Creon (Among most frequent) 2714
▲ Crixivan Capsules (4.1%) 1670
Crystodigin Tablets 1472
Cuprimine Capsules (Greater than 1%) 1673
▲ Cytadren Tablets (1 in 30) 837
CytoGam (Less than 5.0%) 1630
▲ Cytosar-U Sterile Powder (Among most frequent) 2077
Cytotec (1.3%) 2576
▲ Cytovene (13%) 2270
Cytoxan (Common) 700
▲ DHCplus Capsules (Among most frequent) 2148
D.H.E. 45 Injection 2381
▲ DTIC-Dome (90% with the initial few doses) 593
▲ Dalgan Injection (3 to 9%) 529
Dalmane Capsules 2329
Danocrine Capsules 2437
Dantrium Capsules (Less frequent) 2131
Dapsone Tablets USP 1331
▲ Daranide Tablets (Among the most common effects) 1676
Daraprim Tablets 1199
▲ Darvon-N/Darvocet-N (Among most frequent) 1473
▲ Darvon (Among most frequent) 1475
▲ Darvon-N Suspension & Tablets (Among most frequent) 1473
▲ DaunoXome (3% to 20%) 1842
Daypro Caplets (1% to 3%) 2578
Declomycin Tablets 1421
Demadex Tablets and Injection 691
▲ Demerol (Among most frequent) 2438
Demser Capsules (Infrequent) 1690
▲ Demulen (Among most common) 2580
▲ Depakene (Among most common) 416
▲ Depakote Tablets (11% to 12%) 418
▲ Depen Titratable Tablets (17%) 2770
Desogen Tablets 1867
▲ Desyrel and Desyrel Dividose (9.9% to 12.7%) 504
Diabinese Tablets (Less than 2%) 2002
Diamox Intravenous ◉ 317
Diamox Sequels (Sustained Release) ◉ 318
Diamox Tablets ◉ 317
Diethylstilbestrol Tablets 1477
▲ Diflucan Tablets, Injection, and Oral Suspension (1.7% to 5.4%) 2003
Dilacor XR Extended-release Capsules (2.0%) 2183
Dilantin Infatabs 1967
Dilantin Kapseals 1965
Dilantin-125 Suspension 1969
Dilaudid Ampules 1382
Dilaudid Cough Syrup 1383
▲ Dilaudid-HP Injection (Among most frequent) 1384
▲ Dilaudid-HP Lyophilized Powder 250 mg (Among most frequent) 1384
Dilaudid 1382
Dilaudid Oral Liquid 1386
Dilaudid 1382
Dilaudid Tablets - 8 mg 1386
Dimetane-DC Cough Syrup 2232
Dimetane-DX Cough Syrup 2233
Dipentum Capsules (1.0%) 2084
Diphtheria and Tetanus Toxoids and Pertussis Vaccine Adsorbed 2650
Diprivan Injectable Emulsion (Less than 1%) 2939
Diucardin Tablets 2824
Diupres Tablets 1691
Diuril Oral Suspension 1694
Diuril Sodium Intravenous 1693
Diuril Tablets 1694
Dolobid Tablets (Greater than 1 in 100) 1695
Donnatal 2234
Donnatal Extentabs 2234
Donnatal Tablets 2234
Dopram Injectable 2235
Doryx Capsules 1970
▲ Doxil (7.8%) 2613
Doxorubicin Astra (Frequent) 531
DUPHALAC Solution 2714
▲ Duragesic Transdermal System (10% or more) 1336
Duramorph Injection (Frequent) 983
Duranest Injections 533
Dura-Vent Tablets 971
Duricef Capsules, Tablets, and Oral Suspension (Rare) 750
Dyazide Capsules 2653
Dyclone 0.5% and 1% Topical Solutions, USP 535
▲ Dynabac (3.0%) 668
DYNACIN Capsules 1627
DynaCirc Capsules (Up to 1.3%) 2381
DynaCirc CR Tablets (0.5% to 1.0%) 2383
Dyrenium Capsules (Rare) 2655
E.E.S. 427
E-Mycin Tablets (Infrequent) 1388
Easprin 1971
EC-Naprosyn Delayed-Release Tablets (Less than 1%) 2277
▲ Ecotrin (7.6% at 1000 mg/day) 2625
Edecrin 1698
▲ Effexor (6% to 7.9%) 2825
Elavil 2945
Eldepryl Capsules 2729
Elspar 1700
Emcyt Capsules (1%) 2085
▲ Eminase (Less than 10%) 2215
EMLA Cream (Unlikely with cream) 536
Enduron Tablets 424
Engerix-B Unit-Dose Vials (Less than 1%) 2656
Entex PSE Tablets 973
▲ Epivir (13%) 1200
▲ Epogen for Injection (0.26% to 17%) 489
▲ Ergamisol Tablets (6% to 20%) 1340
▲ Ergomar Tablets (Up to 10%) 1543
▲ ERYC (Among most frequent) 1972
▲ EryPed (Among most frequent) 425
▲ Ery-Tab Tablets (Among most frequent) 426
▲ Erythrocin Stearate Filmtab (Among most frequent) 429
▲ Erythromycin Base Filmtab (Among most frequent) 430
▲ Erythromycin Delayed-Release Capsules, USP (Among most frequent) 431
▲ Esgic-plus Capsules (Among most frequent) 1012
▲ Esgic-plus Tablets (Among most frequent) 1012
Esidrix Tablets 839
Esimil Tablets 840
Eskalith 2658
Estrace Cream and Tablets 751
Estraderm Transdermal System 842
ESTRATAB Tablets (0.3, 0.625, 1.25, 2.5 mg) 2715
Estratest 2718
Estring Vaginal Ring (At least 1 report) 2086
▲ Ethmozine Tablets (2% to 5%) 2217
Ethyol (amifostine) for Injection (Frequent) 485
▲ Etopophos for Injection (3% to 43%) 701
▲ Etoposide Injection (31% to 43%) 539
Etrafon 2495
▲ Eulexin Capsules (11%) 2498
Famvir Tablets (1.3% to 4.8%) 2660
Fansidar Tablets 2281
▲ Felbatol (Among most common; 8.6% to 38.7%) 2774
Feldene Capsules (Less than 1%) 2008
▲ Fioricet Tablets (Among most frequent) 2386
Fioricet with Codeine Capsules (Frequent) 2387
Fiorinal Capsules (Less frequent) 2388
Fiorinal with Codeine Capsules (Infrequent) 2390
Fiorinal Tablets (Less frequent) 2388
Flagyl 375 Capsules (Occasional) 2587
Flagyl I.V. 2373
Flexeril Tablets (Less than 1%) 1701
▲ Flolan for Injection (32% to 67%) 1085
Flonase Nasal Spray (Less than 1%) 1088
▲ Flovent (1% to 22%) 1089
Floxin I.V. (1% to 4%) 1580
Floxin Tablets (200 mg, 300 mg, 400 mg) (1% to 4%) 1577
▲ Fludara for Injection (31% to 36%) 658
Flumadine Tablets & Syrup (1.7%) 1013
Fluorescite ◉ 217
Fluorouracil Injection (Common) 2282
Fluothane 2830
Fortaz (1 in 500 patients) 1092
Fosamax Tablets (1.0%) 1703
▲ Foscavir Injection (5% or greater up to 26%) 541
▲ Sterile FUDR (Among more common) 2284
Fulvicin P/G Tablets (Occasional) 2499
Fulvicin P/G 165 & 330 Tablets (Occasional) 2500
▲ Fungizone Intravenous (Among most common) 507
Fungizone Oral Suspension 704
Furoxone (Occasional) 2221
Gamimune N, 5% Immune Globulin Intravenous (Human), 5% 612
Gamimune N, 10% Immune Globulin Intravenous (Human), 10% 615
Gammagard S/D, Immune Globulin, Intravenous (Human) (Occasional) 577
Gammar-P I.V., Immune Globulin Intravenous (Human) 798
Ganite 2711
Gantanol Tablets 2285
Gantrisin 2286
Garamycin Injectable 2502
Gastrocrom Oral Concentrate 1611
▲ Gemzar for Injection (58% to 71%) 1482
Genotropin Injection (A small number of patients) 2090
Geocillin Tablets 2009
Geref (sermorelin acetate for injection) 2995
GlaucTabs ◉ 209
Glucagon for Injection Vials and Emergency Kit (Occasional) 1485
▲ Glucophage Tablets (Among most common) 754
Glucotrol XL Extended Release Tablets (Less than 3%) 2012
GoLYTELY (Infrequent) 694
Grifulvin V (griseofulvin tablets) Microsize (griseofulvin oral suspension) Microsize (Occasional) 1944
Gris-PEG Tablets, 125 mg & 250 mg (Occasional) 476
Guaimax-D Tablets 809
▲ Habitrol Nicotine Transdermal System (3% to 9% of patients) 884
▲ Halcion Tablets (4.6%) 2093
Haldol Decanoate 1587
Haldol Injection, Tablets and Concentrate 1585
▲ Halfprin Tablets (7.6%) 1413
Halotestin Tablets 2095
Havrix (Less than 1%) 2663
Helidac Therapy (1.5%) 2135
Heparin Lock Flush Solution 2831
Heparin Sodium Injection 2832
Heparin Sodium Vials (Rare) 1486
Hespan Injection 945
▲ Hexalen Capsules (1% to 33%) 2760
Helixate, Antihemophilic Factor (Recombinant) (Three reports out of 3,254 patients) 799
HibTITER (9 of 1,118 vaccinations) 1423
Hivid Tablets (Less than 1%) 2287
Humatrope Vials (A small number of patients) 1490
Humegon for Injection 1873
Humorsol Sterile Ophthalmic Solution (Rare) 1707
▲ Hycamtin for Injection (Less than 1% to 58%) 2665
Hycodan Tablets and Syrup 946
Hycomine Compound Tablets 948
Hycomine 947
Hycotuss Expectorant Syrup 950
Hydralazine Hydrochloride Injection USP (Common) 2712
Hydrea Capsules (Less frequent) 705
Hydrocet Capsules 787
HydroDIURIL Tablets 1716
Hydropres Tablets 1718
▲ Hylorel Tablets (3.9%) 1613
▲ Hyperstat I.V. Injection (4%) 2504
Hyskon Hysteroscopy Fluid (Rare) 1633
Hytrin Capsules (At least 1%) 434
Hyzaar Tablets 1720
IBU Tablets (Less than 1%) 1389
▲ Idamycin Injection (82%) 2096
▲ IFEX (58%) 706
Ilosone (Infrequent) 927
Imdur (Less than or equal to 5%) 1362
▲ Imitrex Injection (4%) 1095
Imitrex Tablets 1099
Imodium Capsules 1343
▲ Imovax Rabies Vaccine (Up to 6%) 899
▲ Imuran (Approximately 12%) 1103
Inderal 2834
Inderal LA Long Acting Capsules 2836
Inderide Tablets 2838
Inderide LA Long Acting Capsules 2840
Indocin I.V. (1% to 3%) 1727
INFeD (Iron Dextran Injection, USP) 2478
Infumorph 200 and Infumorph 500 Sterile Solutions 985
Inocor Lactate Injection (0.9%) 2439
▲ Intron A for Injection (1% to 66%) 2506
Inversine Tablets 1729
Invirase Capsules (Less than 2%) 2291
IOPIDINE Sterile Ophthalmic Solution ◉ 218
Ismelin Tablets 845
Ismo Tablets (Fewer than 1% to 4%) 2844
ISMOTIC 45% w/v Solution ◉ 221
Isopto Carbachol Ophthalmic Solution ◉ 221
Isuprel Hydrochloride Solution 2443
Isuprel Mistometer 2442
▲ JE-VAX (Approximately 10%) 904
K-Dur Microburst Release System (potassium chloride, USP) E.R. Tablets 1364
▲ K-Lor Powder Packets (Among most common) 438
▲ K-Norm Capsules (Among most common) 1615
K-Phos Neutral Tablets 633
K-Phos Original Formula 'Sodium Free' Tablets 633
▲ K-Tab Filmtab (Most common) 439
Kadian Capsules (Less than 3%) 2948
Kayexalate 2444
Keflex Pulvules & Oral Suspension (Rare) 930
Keftab Tablets (Rare) 931
Kefurox Vials, Faspak & ADD-Vantage 1509
Kefzol Vials, Faspak & ADD-Vantage (Rare) 1511

(▭ Described in PDR For Nonprescription Drugs) Incidence data in parenthesis; ▲ 3% or more (◉ Described in PDR For Ophthalmology)

1485 **Side Effects Index** **Vomiting**

Kemadrin Tablets ... 1105
Kerlone Tablets (Less than 2%) ... 2588
KOGENATE Antihemophilic Factor (Recombinant) (Three reports) ... 626
▲ Kytril Tablets (9%) ... 2669
▲ Lamictal Tablets (Among most common; 11% to 18%) ... 1105
▲ Lamprene Capsules (40-50%) ... 846
Lanoxicaps (Common) ... 1110
Lanoxin Elixir Pediatric ... 1113
Lanoxin Injection (Common) ... 1116
Lanoxin Injection Pediatric ... 1119
Lanoxin Tablets (Common) ... 1121
▲ Lariam Tablets (Among most frequent) ... 2295
Larodopa Tablets (Relatively frequent) ... 2296
Lasix Injection, Oral Solution and Tablets ... 1267
Lescol Capsules ... 2395
▲ Leucovorin Calcium for Injection (7% to 46%) ... 1313
Leukeran Tablets (Infrequent) ... 1205
▲ Leukine (46% to 85%) ... 1317
▲ Leustatin (13%) ... 1889
Levbid Extended-Release Tablets ... 2549
Levlen/Tri-Levlen ... 646
Levo-Dromoran ... 2297
Levophed Bitartrate Injection ... 2445
Levoprome (Sometimes) ... 1321
Levsin/Levsinex/Levbid ... 2549
Limbitrol ... 2333
▲ Lioresal Intrathecal (1.6% to 10.5%) ... 1634
Lioresal Tablets (Rare) ... 847
Lithium Carbonate Capsules & Tablets ... 2352
Lithonate/Lithotabs/Lithobid ... 2721
Lodine Capsules and Tablets (1% to 3%) ... 2849
Lomotil ... 2591
▲ Lo/Ovral Tablets (10% or less) ... 2852
▲ Lo/Ovral-28 Tablets (10% or less) ... 2857
Lopid Tablets (2.5%) ... 1974
Lopressor HCT Tablets (1 in 100 patients) ... 850
Lorabid Suspension and Pulvules (0.5% to 3.3%) ... 1513
▲ Lorcet 10/650 Tablets (Among most frequent) ... 1016
▲ Lortab (Among most frequent) ... 2751
Lotensin Tablets ... 852
Lotensin HCT Tablets (0.3% to 1.0%) ... 855
Loxitane ... 1426
Ludiomil Tablets (Rare) ... 861
Lufyllin & Lufyllin-400 Tablets ... 2778
Lufyllin-GG Elixir & Tablets ... 2779
Lupron Depot 3.75 mg (Less than 5%) ... 2739
▲ Lupron Depot 7.5 mg (5.4%) ... 2741
Lupron Depot-PED 7.5 mg, 11.25 mg and 15 mg (Less than 2%) ... 2744
▲ Lupron Injection (5% or more) ... 2736
Lupron Injection Pediatric (Less than 2%) ... 2737
▲ LUVOX Tablets (5%) ... 2723
Lysodren Tablets ... 707
M-M-R II ... 1730
M-R-VAX II ... 1732
▲ MS Contin Tablets (Among most frequent) ... 2149
▲ MSIR (Among most frequent) ... 2152
Macrobid Capsules (Less than 1%) ... 2138
▲ Macrodantin Capsules (Among most often) ... 2140
Mandol Vials, Faspak & ADD-Vantage (Rare) ... 1516
Marax Tablets & DF Syrup (Frequent, on empty stomach) ... 2015
Marcaine (Rare) ... 2446
Marcaine Spinal (Rare) ... 2449
▲ Marinol (Dronabinol) Capsules (3% to 10%) ... 2353
▲ Matulane Capsules (Frequent) ... 2300
Mavik Tablets (0.3% to 1.0%) ... 1407
Maxair Autohaler ... 1550
Maxair Inhaler (Less than 1%) ... 1552
Maxaquin Tablets (Less than 1%) ... 2593
Maxipime for Injection (0.1% to 1%) ... 758
Mebaral Tablets (Less than 1 in 100) ... 2452
Mefoxin (Rare) ... 1734
Mefoxin Premixed Intravenous Solution (Rarely) ... 1737
▲ Megace Oral Suspension (Up to 6%) ... 708
Megace Tablets ... 710
Mellaril ... 2398
Menest Tablets ... 2671
▲ Mepergan Injection (Among most frequent) ... 2859
▲ Mepron Suspension (14%) ... 1206
Merrem I.V. (1.0% to 3.9%) ... 2952
Meruvax II ... 1740
Mesantoin Tablets ... 2400
Mesnex Injection ... 711
Mestinon Injectable ... 1300
Mestinon ... 1300
Metaproterenol Sulfate Inhalation Solution, USP, Arm-a-Med (Approximately 1 in 300 patients) ... 547
▲ Methadone Hydrochloride Oral Concentrate (Among most frequent) ... 2356
Methadone Hydrochloride Oral Solution & Tablets ... 2357
Methergine (Occasional) ... 2401
▲ Methotrexate Sodium Tablets, Injection, for Injection and LPF Injection (10%) ... 1322
Metrodin (urofollitropin for injection) ... 2616
MetroGel-Vaginal ... 917
Mevacor Tablets (0.5% to 1.0%; rare) ... 1742
▲ Mexitil Capsules (39.3% to 39.6%) ... 684
Mezlin ... 594
Mezlin Pharmacy Bulk Package ... 597
▲ Miacalcin Injection (About 10%) ... 2402
Miacalcin Nasal Spray (Less than 1%) ... 2403
▲ Micro-K (Among most common) ... 2237
▲ Micro-K LS Packets (Among most common) ... 2238
▲ Midamor Tablets (3% to 8%) ... 1746
Miltown Tablets ... 2780
Minipress Capsules (1-4%) ... 2015
Minizide Capsules (Rare) ... 2016
Minocin Intravenous ... 1428
Minocin Oral Suspension ... 1431
Minocin Pellet-Filled Capsules ... 1429
Mintezol ... 1747
Mithracin ... 599
Modicon ... 1928
Moduretic Tablets (Less than or equal to 1%) ... 1748
Monodox Capsules ... 1858
Mono-Gesic Tablets ... 810
Monoket Tablets (Fewer than 1%) ... 2550
Mononine, Coagulation Factor IX (Human), Monoclonal Antibody Purified ... 804
Monopril Tablets (1.2% to 2.2%) ... 762
▲ Motofen Tablets (1 in 30) ... 789
Motrin Ibuprofen Suspension, Oral Drops, Chewable Tablets, Caplets (1% to less than 3%) ... 1563
Mustargen ... 1752
▲ Mutamycin for Injection (14%) ... 712
Myambutol Tablets ... 1432
Mycelex Troches ... 601
Mycelex-G 500 mg Vaginal Tablets (1 in 149 patients) ... 602
Mycobutin Capsules (1%) ... 2101
Mycostatin Pastilles (Occasional) ... 713
Mykrox Tablets (Less than 2%) ... 1617
Myleran Tablets ... 1209
Myochrysine Injection ... 1754
Mysoline (Occasional) ... 2860
Nalfon 200 Pulvules & Nalfon Tablets (2.6%) ... 933
Naprelan Tablets (Less than 3%) ... 2861
Anaprox/Naprosyn (Less than 1%) ... 2277
Narcan Injection ... 950
Nardil ... 1977
Nasalide Nasal Solution 0.025% (5% or less) ... 2301
Navane Capsules and Concentrate ... 2018
Navane Intramuscular ... 2019
▲ Navelbine Injection (Up to 15% but less than 20%) ... 1212
Nebcin Vials, Hyporets & ADD-Vantage ... 1518
NegGram ... 2453
Nembutal Sodium Capsules (Less than 1%) ... 440
Nembutal Sodium Solution (Less than 1%) ... 442
Nembutal Sodium Suppositories (Less than 1%) ... 444
▲ Neoral (4% to 10%) ... 2405
Nephro-Fer Rx Tablets ... 2168
Neptazane Tablets ... ⊙ 320
Nesacaine Injections ... 549
Netromycin Injection 100 mg/ml (1 in 1000 patients) ... 2516
▲ Neupogen for Injection (7% to 57%) ... 495
Neurontin Capsules (More than 1%) ... 1978
▲ Neutrexin for Injection (4.6%) ... 2761
Nimotop Capsules (Less than 1%) ... 603
▲ Nipent for Injection (53% to 63%) ... 2733
Nitrolingual Spray (Uncommon) ... 2193
Nitrostat Tablets ... 1981
Nizoral Tablets (Approximately 3%) ... 1345
▲ Nolvadex Tablets (2.1% to 25%) ... 2957
▲ Nordette-21 Tablets (10% or less) ... 2863
▲ Nordette-28 Tablets (10% or less) ... 2866
Norflex ... 1554
Norgesic ... 1554
Norinyl ... 2563
Norisodrine with Calcium Iodide Syrup ... 446
▲ Normodyne Injection (Up to 4%) ... 2519
Normodyne Tablets (Up to 3%) ... 2522
Noroxin Tablets (0.3 to 1.0%) ... 1758
Noroxin Tablets (0.3% to 1.0%) ... 2222
Norpace (1 to 3%) ... 2596
Norplant System ... 2868
Norpramin Tablets ... 1273
Nor-Q D Tablets ... 2598
Norvasc Tablets (More than 0.1% to 1%) ... 2020
▲ Norvir (12.8% to 15.2%) ... 447
Novahistine Elixir ... ▣ 782
▲ Novantrone for Injection (31 to 72%) ... 1327
Novocain Hydrochloride for Spinal Anesthesia ... 2457
▲ Nubain Injection (6%) ... 952
Nucofed ... 2225
NuLYTELY (Less frequent) ... 694
Cherry Flavor NuLYTELY (Less frequent) ... 694
Numorphan Injection ... 953
Numorphan Suppositories ... 953
Nutropin (A small number of patients) ... 1049
Nutropin AQ Injection (A small number of patients) ... 1051
Nydrazid Injection (Common) ... 509
Ogen Tablets ... 2103
Ogen Vaginal Cream ... 2106
▲ OmniHIB (1.9% to 4.3%) ... 2676
Omnipen Capsules ... 2872
Omnipen for Oral Suspension ... 2873
▲ Oncaspar (Greater than 5%) ... 2194
Oncovin Solution Vials & Hyporets ... 1521
▲ Oramorph SR (Morphine Sulfate Sustained Release Tablets) (Among most frequent) ... 2359
Orap Tablets ... 1037
Oretic Tablets ... 450
▲ Organidin NR Tablets and Liquid (One of the two most common) ... 2781
Orlaam Oral Solution (1% to 3%) ... 2361
Ornade Spansule Capsules ... 2678
Ortho-Cept ... 1907
Ortho-Cyclen/Ortho-Tri-Cyclen ... 1914
Ortho Diaphragm Kits—All-Flex Arcing Spring; Ortho Coil Spring; Ortho-White Flat Spring ... 1921
Ortho Diaphragm Kit-Coil Spring ... 1921
Ortho Dienestrol Cream ... 1922
Ortho-Est ... 1925
Ortho-Novum ... 1928
Ortho-Cyclen/Ortho Tri-Cyclen ... 1914
Ortho-White Diaphragm Kit-Flat Spring (See also Ortho Diaphragm Kits) ... 1921
▲ Orthoclone OKT3 Sterile Solution (19%) ... 1892
Orudis Capsules (Greater than 1%) ... 2874
Oruvail Capsules (Greater than 1%) ... 2874
OSMOGLYN Oral Osmotic Agent ... ⊙ 225
Ovcon ... 765
▲ Ovral Tablets (10% or less) ... 2877
▲ Ovral-28 Tablets (10% or less) ... 2878
▲ Ovrette Tablets (10% or less) ... 2878
Oxandrin ... 783
▲ OxyContin Tablets (Less than 1% to 12%) ... 2163
▲ OxyIR Capsules (Among most frequent) ... 2167
PBZ Tablets ... 863
PBZ-SR Tablets ... 862
▲ PCE Dispertab Tablets (Among most frequent) ... 453
Pamelor ... 2409
▲ Paraplatin for Injection (65% to 84%) ... 713
Paremyd ... ⊙ 244
▲ Parlodel (2% to 5%) ... 2411
▲ PASER Granules (Among most common) ... 1333
Paxil Tablets (1.0%) ... 2681
▲ Pediazole Suspension (Among most frequent) ... 2340
Peganone Tablets ... 455
▲ Pen•Vee K (Among most common) ... 2879
▲ Penetrex Tablets (2% to 8%) ... 2196
Pentasa (1.5%) ... 1275
Pepcid Injection (Infrequent) ... 1765
Pepcid (Infrequent) ... 1763
Peptavlon ... 2997
▲ Percocet Tablets (Among most frequent) ... 955
▲ Percodan Tablets (Among most frequent) ... 955
▲ Percodan-Demi Tablets (Among most frequent) ... 956
Pergonal (menotropins for injection, USP) ... 2618
Periactin ... 1767
Permax Tablets (2.7%; frequent) ... 571
Persantine Tablets ... 686
Phenergan with Codeine ... 2883
Phenergan with Dextromethorphan ... 2885
Phenergan Injection ... 2880
Phenergan Suppositories ... 2882
Phenergan Syrup ... 2881
Phenergan Tablets ... 2882
Phenergan VC ... 2886
Phenergan VC with Codeine ... 2888
Phenobarbital Elixir and Tablets (Less than 1 in 100 patients) ... 1523
PhosLo Tablets ... 695
▲ Phrenilin (Among most frequent) ... 790
Pima Syrup ... 1004
Pipracil (Less than 2%) ... 1435
Placidyl Capsules ... 456
Plaquenil Sulfate Tablets (Rare) ... 2459
▲ Platinol for Injection (Almost all patients) ... 717
▲ Platinol-AQ Injection (Almost all patients) ... 719
Plendil Extended-Release Tablets (0.5% to 1.5%) ... 514
PMB 200 and PMB 400 (Rare) ... 2890
Pneumovax 23 ... 1768
Ponstel ... 1982
Pontocaine Hydrochloride for Spinal Anesthesia ... 2460
▲ Pravachol Tablets (2.9% to 7.3%) ... 770
Premarin Intravenous ... 2893
Premarin Tablets ... 2896
Premarin Vaginal Cream ... 2898
Premphase ... 2900
Prempro ... 2905
Prevacid Delayed-Release Capsules (Less than 1%) ... 2746
Prilosec Delayed-Release Capsules (1.5% to 3.2%) ... 516
Primaxin I.M. (0.3%) ... 1770
Primaxin I.V. (1.5%) ... 1772
Prinivil Tablets (0.3% to 1.0%) ... 1776
Prinzide Tablets (1.4%) ... 1780
Priscoline Hydrochloride Ampuls ... 864
Pro-Banthine Tablets ... 2226
▲ Procanbid Extended-Release Tablets (3% to 4%) ... 1983
Procardia XL Extended Release Tablets (1% or less) ... 2026
▲ Procrit for Injection (0.26% to 17%) ... 1896
Proglycem (Frequent) ... 575
▲ Prograf (12% to 27%) ... 1028
▲ Proleukin for Injection (87%) ... 812
Prolixin ... 510
Proloprim Tablets ... 1141
Propulsid (More than 1%) ... 1346
ProSom Tablets (Infrequent) ... 457
Prostigmin Injectable ... 1305
Prostigmin Tablets ... 1306
▲ Prostin E2 Suppository (Approximately two-thirds) ... 2109
Protamine Sulfate Vials ... 1526
Protostat Tablets (Occasional) ... 1939
Proventil Inhalation Aerosol ... 2524
Proventil Repetabs Tablets (1% to 4%) ... 2529
Proventil Syrup ... 2528
Proventil Tablets (2%) ... 2529
Prozac Pulvules & Liquid, Oral Solution (2.4%) ... 935
Purinethol Tablets (Uncommon) ... 1214
Pyrazinamide Tablets ... 1442
Quadrinal Tablets ... 1398
Questran (Less frequent) ... 774
Quibron ... 2227

(▣ Described in PDR For Nonprescription Drugs) Incidence data in parenthesis; ▲ 3% or more (⊙ Described in PDR For Ophthalmology)

▲ Quinaglute Dura-Tabs Tablets (3%) 644
▲ Quinidex Extentabs (Among most frequent) 2240
▲ RMS Suppositories CII (Among most frequent) 2766
▲ Rabies Vaccine, Imovax Rabies I.D. (Less frequent; up to 6%) 901
Recombivax HB (Less to greater than 1%) 1787
▲ Redux Capsules (3.2%) 2911
Regitine Vials 864
Relafen Tablets (1% to 3%) 2688
Remeron Tablets (Frequent) 1878
▲ ReoPro Vials (11.4%) 1526
Respbid Tablets 687
RespiGam (2%) 1631
▲ Retrovir Capsules (4.8% to 25%) 1216
▲ Retrovir I.V. Infusion (6% to 25%) 1221
▲ Retrovir Syrup (4.8% to 25%) 1216
▲ ReVia Tablets (3% to more than 10%) 957
▲ Revex (nalmefene hydrochloride injection) (9%) 1863
▲ Ridaura Capsules (10%) 2691
Rifadin (Some patients) 1276
Rifamate Capsules (Some patients) 1278
Rifater 1280
▲ Rilutek Tablets (4.2% to 4.5%) 2198
Rimactane Capsules 865
▲ Risperdal Tablets (5% to 7%) 1348
Robaxisal Tablets 2246
Robinul Forte Tablets 2247
Robinul Injectable 2247
Robinul Tablets 2247
Rocaltrol Capsules 2303
Rocephin Injectable Vials, ADD-Vantage, Galaxy Container (Less than 1%) 2305
▲ Roferon-A Injection (17% to 39%) 2308
▲ Romazicon (11%) 2311
Rondec Oral Drops 974
Rondec Syrup 974
Rondec 974
▲ Roxanol (Among most frequent) 2365
▲ Roxicodone Tablets, Oral Solution & Intensol (Oxycodone) (Among most frequent) 2366
Rubex for Injection (Frequent) 721
Rum-K Syrup 1004
▲ Rythmol Tablets–150mg, 225mg, 300mg (2.4 to 10.7%) 1399
▲ SSKI Solution (Among most frequent) 2767
▲ Salagen Tablets (4%) 1546
▲ Sandimmune (2 to 10%) 2416
Sandoglobulin I.V. 2419
▲ Sandostatin Injection (Less than 10%) 2421
Sanorex Tablets 2423
Sansert Tablets 2424
Seconal Sodium Pulvules (Less than 1 in 100) 1529
Sectral Capsules (Up to 2%) 2914
▲ Sedapap Tablets 50 mg/650 mg (Among the most frequent) 1826
▲ Seldane Tablets (4.6% to 7.6%) 1284
Seldane-D Extended-Release Tablets 1286
Senna X-Prep Bowel Evacuant Liquid (Rare) 1236
Sensorcaine (Rare) 554
▲ Septra (Among most common) 1146
▲ Septra I.V. Infusion (Among most common) 1142
▲ Septra I.V. Infusion ADD-Vantage Vials (Among most common) 1144
▲ Septra (Among most common) 1146
Ser-Ap-Es Tablets 867
Serentil 689
Serevent Inhalation Aerosol (1% to 3%) 1149
Serophene (clomiphene citrate tablets, USP) (Approximately 1 in 50 patients) 2621
Serzone Tablets (Up to 2%) 776
Sinemet Tablets (Less frequent) 959
Sinemet CR Tablets (1.8%) 961
Sinequan 2028
Skelaxin Tablets 793
Slo-bid Gyrocaps 2201
Slo-Niacin Tablets 2767
▲ Slow-K Extended-Release Tablets (Among most common) 869
Sodium Polystyrene Sulfonate Suspension 2367
Solganal Suspension (Rare) 2530
Soma Compound w/Codeine Tablets 2784
▲ Soma Compound Tablets (Among most common) 2783
Soma Tablets 2782
Sotradecol (Sodium Tetradecyl Sulfate Injection) 987
Spectrobid Tablets 2030
Sporanox Capsules (0.8% to 5.1%) 1352
▲ St. Joseph Adult Chewable Aspirin (81 mg.) (7.3% of 4500 patients) ▣ 768
▲ Stadol (13%) 779
Stelazine 2692
Stimate, (desmopressin acetate) Nasal Spray, 1.5 mg/mL 806
Streptomycin Sulfate Injection 2031
Sublimaze Injection 463
▲ Sufenta Injection (3% to 9%) 1355
▲ Supprelin Injection (3% to 10%) 2230
▲ Suprane (desflurane, USP) (16%) 1865
Suprax (Less than 2%) 1443
Surmontil Capsules 2917
Sus-Phrine Injection 1017
Symmetrel Capsules (0.1% to 1%) 965
Symmetrel Syrup (0.1% to 1%) 963
Syntocinon Injection 2425
Talacen Caplets (Occasional) 2464
▲ Talwin Injection (Most common) 2465
Talwin Compound 2466
▲ Talwin Injection (Most common) 2465
Talwin Nx Tablets 2467
Tambocor Tablets (1% to less than 3%) 1555
Tao Capsules (Infrequent) 2033
Tapazole Tablets 1361
Tavist Syrup 2426
Tavist Tablets 2427
▲ Taxol Injection (52%) 723
Taxotere for Injection Concentrate 2204
Tazicef for Injection (Less than 2%; 1 in 500 patients) 2697
Tazidime Vials, Faspak & ADD-Vantage (1 in 500) 1531
▲ Tegretol/Tegretol-XR (Among most frequent) 870
Tenoretic Tablets 2963
Tensilon Injectable 1307
Terramycin Intramuscular Solution 2034
Teslac Tablets 727
Testoderm Testosterone Transdermal System 486
Tetramune (1% to 5%) 1449
Thalitone 1293
Theo-24 Extended Release Capsules 2753
Theo-Dur Extended-Release Tablets 1367
Theo-X Extended-Release Tablets 793
▲ TheraCys BCG Live (Intravesical) (Up to 16.1%) 911
Thioguanine Tablets, Tabloid Brand (Less frequent) 1225
Thioplex (Thiotepa For Injection) 1329
Tiazac Capsules (Less than 1%) 1019
Ticar for Injection 2704
▲ TICE BCG, USP (3.0%) 1881
Ticlid Tablets (1.9%) 2317
Tilade Inhaler (1.7%) 2207
Timentin for Injection 2706
Timolide Tablets 1791
Timoptic in Ocudose 1796
Timoptic Sterile Ophthalmic Solution 1794
Timoptic-XE 1798
Tofranil Ampuls 873
Tofranil Tablets 875
Tofranil-PM Capsules 876
▲ Tolectin (200, 400 and 600 mg) (3 to 9%) 1591
▲ Tonocard Tablets (4.6% to 9.0%) 519
Toradol (Greater than 1%) 2319
▲ Trandate (4 of 100 patients; up to 3%) 1158
Transderm Scōp Transdermal Therapeutic System (Few patients) 890
Trasylol (2%) 607
Trental Tablets (1.2%) 1291
Triavil Tablets 1800
Tri-Immunol Adsorbed 1452
Trilafon (Occasional) 2532
Levlen/Tri-Levlen 646
▲ Trilisate (Less than 20%) 2155
Trimpex Tablets 2323
Trinalin Repetabs Tablets 1373
Tri-Norinyl 2607
Tripedia (Up to 2%) 908
▲ Triphasil-21 Tablets (10% or less) 2919
▲ Triphasil-28 Tablets (10% or less) 2924
Tussend 1830
Tussionex Pennkinetic Extended-Release Suspension 1624
▲ Tussi-Organidin DM NR Liquid and DM-S NR Liquid (One of the two most common) 2786
▲ Tylenol with Codeine (Among most frequent) 1592
▲ Tylox Capsules (Among most frequent) 1593
Tympagesic Ear Drops 2476
Typhim Vi (Up to 1.9%) 914
▲ Ultram Tablets (50 mg) (9% to 17%) 1594
Unasyn (Less than 1%) 2035
Uni-Dur Extended-Release Tablets 1374
Uniphyl 400 mg and 600 mg Tablets 2157
Univasc Tablets (less than 1%) 2553
Urecholine 1804
Urispas Tablets 2710
Urobiotic-250 Capsules 2038
Urocit-K Tablets (Some patients) 1828
Uroqid-Acid No. 2 Tablets 633
▲ Valtrex Caplets (Less than 1% to 7%) 1167
Vantin for Oral Suspension and Vantin Tablets (1.1% to 1.7%) 2112
Vaqta (1.0%) 1805
Varivax (Greater than or equal to 1%) 1807
Vaseretic Tablets (0.5% to 2.0%) 1810
Vasotec I.V. 1814
Vasotec Tablets (1.3%) 1816
Vasoxyl Injection 1169
Velban Vials 1537
▲ Ventolin Inhalation Aerosol and Refill (6%) 1170
▲ Ventolin Rotacaps for Inhalation (4%) 1173
Ventolin Syrup 1175
Ventolin Tablets 1176
▲ VePesid Capsules and Injection (31% to 43%) 727
Versed Injection (2.6%) 2324
▲ Vesanoid Capsules (57%) 2327
Vibramycin 2038
Vibramycin Hyclate Intravenous 2040
Vibramycin 2038
▲ Vicodin Tablets (Among most frequent) 1404
▲ Vicodin ES Tablets (Among most frequent) 1405
▲ Vicodin HP Tablets (Among most frequent) 1403
Vicodin Tuss Expectorant (More frequently in ambulatory than in recumbent patients) 1406
▲ Videx Tablets, Powder for Oral Solution, & Pediatric Powder for Oral Solution (6% to 58%) 2980
Visken Tablets (2% or fewer patients) 2428
▲ Vistide Injection (8% to 65%) 1057
Vivactil Tablets 1820
Vivelle Transdermal System 880
Vivotif Berna (Infrequent) 660
▲ Volmax Extended-Release Tablets (4.2%) 1835
Voltaren Ophthalmic Sterile Ophthalmic Solution (1%) ◉ 264
Cataflam/Voltaren/Voltaren-XR (Less than 1%) 833
▲ Vumon for Injection (29%) 729
▲ Wellbutrin Tablets (22.9%) 1177
Wigraine Tablets 1884
WinRho SD (One report) 1839
Winstrol Tablets 2468
▲ Wygesic Tablets (Most frequent) 2930
▲ Xanax Tablets (9.6% to 22.0%) 2115
▲ Xylocaine Injections (Among most common) 562
Yocon Tablets (Common) 1235
Yodoxin Tablets 1235
▲ Yutopar Intravenous Injection (10% to 15%) 566
▲ Zanosar Sterile Powder (Most patients) 2119
Zantac 1182
Zantac Injection 1180
Zantac Syrup 1182
Zarontin Capsules (Frequent) 1986
Zarontin Syrup (Frequent) 1986
Zaroxolyn Tablets 1625
Zebeta Tablets (1.1% to 1.5%) 1457
Zemuron Injection (Less than 1%) 1885
▲ Zerit Capsules (6% to 44%) 731
Zestoretic Tablets (1.4%) 2968
Zestril Tablets (0.3% to 1.0%) 2972
Ziac 1459
Zinacef 1184
▲ Zinecard Injection (42% to 59%) 2120
Zithromax (1% or less to 5%) 2043
Zithromax Tablets (1% or less to 2%) 2046
Zocor Tablets 1821
Zoladex (Greater than 1% but less than 5%) 2976
Zoladex 3-month 2978
▲ Zoloft Tablets (3.8%) 2051
Zosyn (2.6% to 3.3%) 1463
Zovirax Capsules (0.7% to 2.7%) 1187
▲ Zovirax Sterile Powder (Approximately 7%) 1191
Zovirax (0.7% to 2.7%) 1187
▲ Zydone Capsules (Among most frequent) 967
Zyloprim Tablets (Less than 1%) 1194
Zyrtec Tablets (Less than 2%) 2053

von Willebrand's-like syndrome, acquired

Hespan Injection 945

Vulva, dryness (see under Vagina, dryness)

Vulva, edema

Vagistat-1 (Less than 1%) 783

Vulva, swelling

MetroGel-Vaginal (Equal to or less than 2%) 917
Vagistat-1 (Less than 1%) 783

Vulvar disorder

Anafranil Capsules (Rare) 819
▲ Cleocin Vaginal Cream (6%) 2070
Estring Vaginal Ring (At least 1 report) 2086
Hivid Tablets (Less than 1% to 3.4%) 2287

Vulvitis

Prostin E2 Suppository 2109
Zovirax Ointment 5% (0.3%) 1190

W

Walking disorders

Oncovin Solution Vials & Hyporets 1521
Tonocard Tablets (Up to 1.2%) 519

Warmth

▲ Adalat Capsules (10 mg and 20 mg) (25%) 580
▲ Adalat CC (4%) 582
Alomide Ophthalmic Solution (Less than 1%) 465
Buprenex Injectable (Less than 1%) 2170
Caverject Injection (Less than 1%) 2064
Dopram Injectable 2235
EMLA Cream (Unlikely with cream) 536
Ethyol (amifostine) for Injection 485
Geref (sermorelin acetate for injection) 2995
Hyperstat I.V. Injection 2504
▲ Imitrex Injection (10.8%) 1095
▲ LUVOX Tablets (3%) 2723
Marax Tablets & DF Syrup 2015
Miacalcin Injection 2402
MSTA Mumps Skin Test Antigen 2988
Nubain Injection (1% or less) 952
Peptavlon 2997
Plendil Extended-Release Tablets (Up to 1.5%) 514
▲ Procardia Capsules (25%) 2024
▲ Procardia XL Extended Release Tablets (25%) 2026
Protamine Sulfate Vials 1526
Quadrinal Tablets 1398
Recombivax HB (Less than 1%) 1787
Sarapin 1237
Slo-Niacin Tablets 2767
Stadol (1% or greater) 779
Stimate, (desmopressin acetate) Nasal Spray, 1.5 mg/mL 806
Tilade Inhaler (Less than 1%) 2207
Tripedia 908
Versed Injection (Less than 1%) 2324
Xanax Tablets (1.3%) 2115

Warmth at injection site

Diphtheria and Tetanus Toxoids and Pertussis Vaccine Adsorbed 2650
HibTITER (Less than 1% to 1.8%) 1423
▲ Pneumovax 23 (Common) 1768
▲ Tetramune (16% to 35%) 1449
▲ Vaqta (0.6% to 17.3%) 1805

Wasting syndrome

Invirase Capsules (Less than 2%) 2291

(▣ Described in PDR For Nonprescription Drugs) Incidence data in parenthesis; ▲ 3% or more (◉ Described in PDR For Ophthalmology)

1487 Side Effects Index Weight gain

Water intoxication
Atretol Tablets 569
DDAVP Injection 2178
DDAVP 2180
DDAVP Tablets 2182
Desmopressin Acetate Injection 996
Methergine (Rare) 2401
Stimate, (desmopressin acetate) Nasal Spray, 1.5 mg/mL 806
Syntocinon Injection 2425
Tegretol/Tegretol-XR 870

Water retention (see also under Edema)
Hyperstat I.V. Injection 2504
Testred Capsules, 10 mg 1308

Weakness (see under Asthenia)

Weakness, feet
K-Phos Neutral Tablets 633
K-Phos Original Formula 'Sodium Free' Tablets (Less frequent) 633
Monopril Tablets (0.4% to 1.0%) 762
SSKI Solution (Less frequent) 2767
Uroqid-Acid No. 2 Tablets 633

Weakness, hands
K-Phos Neutral Tablets 633
K-Phos Original Formula 'Sodium Free' Tablets (Less frequent) 633
Monopril Tablets (0.4% to 1.0%) 762
SSKI Solution (Less frequent) 2767
Uroqid-Acid No. 2 Tablets 633

Weakness, legs
D.H.E. 45 Injection 2381
Dantrium Intravenous 2132
Ergomar Tablets (Frequent) 1543
K-Phos Neutral Tablets 633
K-Phos Original Formula 'Sodium Free' Tablets (Less frequent) 633
Lupron Injection (A few cases) 2736
SSKI Solution (Less frequent) 2767
Uroqid-Acid No. 2 Tablets 633
▲ Vesanoid Capsules (3%) 2327
Wigraine Tablets 1884

Weakness, local
Timoptic in Ocudose (Less frequent) 1796
Timoptic Sterile Ophthalmic Solution 1794
Timoptic-XE 1798

Weakness, muscle
Ambien Tablets (Rare) 2559
Amicar Syrup, Tablets, and Injection 1312
Anafranil Capsules (1% to 2%) 819
Anectine 1062
Atromid-S Capsules (Less often) 2808
Betagan ⊙ 230
Cardura Tablets (1%) 1993
Compazine 2644
Cozaar Tablets (Less than 1%) 1668
Crixivan Capsules (Less than 2%) 1670
Decadron Phosphate Injection 1680
Depen Titratable Tablets 2770
Dexacort Phosphate in Respihaler 1606
Dexacort Phosphate in Turbinaire 1607
Dizac (diazepam injectable emulsion) CIV (Some patients) 1862
Ergamisol Tablets 1340
Eskalith 2658
Felbatol 2774
Florinef Acetate Tablets 506
Foscavir Injection (Rare) 541
Hivid Tablets (Less than 1%) 2287
Humorsol Sterile Ophthalmic Solution (Infrequent) 1707
Hydeltra-T.B.A. Sterile Suspension 1710
Hydrocortone Phosphate Injection, Sterile 1713
Hydrocortone Tablets 1715
Imdur (Less than or equal to 5%) 1362
Kemadrin Tablets 1105
Lescol Capsules 2395
Lithium Carbonate Capsules & Tablets 2352
Lithonate/Lithotabs/Lithobid 2721
Metubine Iodide Vials 932
Mevacor Tablets 1742
▲ Naprelan Tablets (3% to 9%) 2861
Norcuron for Injection 1875
Nuromax Injection 1136
Ocupress Ophthalmic Solution, 1% Sterile ⊙ 297
Pravachol Tablets 770
Prilosec Delayed-Release Capsules (Less than 1%) 516
Protopam Chloride for Injection 2909
Retrovir Capsules 1216
Retrovir I.V. Infusion 1221
Retrovir Syrup 1216
Rifater 1280
Rimactane Capsules 865
Sodium Polystyrene Sulfonate Suspension 2367
Stelazine 2692
▲ Videx Tablets, Powder for Oral Solution, & Pediatric Powder for Oral Solution (6%) 2980
Zocor Tablets 1821
Zoloft Tablets (Infrequent) 2051
Zyrtec Tablets (Less than 2%) 2053

Weight change, increase or decrease
Amen Tablets 785
Asendin Tablets (Less than 1%) 1419
Climara Transdermal System 640
Cycrin Tablets 991
Demulen 2580
Depo-Provera Sterile Aqueous Suspension 2083
Desogen Tablets 1867
ESTRATAB Tablets (0.3, 0.625, 1.25, 2.5 mg) 2715
Estratest 2718
Estring Vaginal Ring (At least 1 report) 2086
Levlen/Tri-Levlen 646
Menest Tablets 2671
Moban Tablets and Concentrate 1036
Ogen Tablets 2103
Ogen Vaginal Cream 2106
Ortho-Cept 1907
Ortho-Cyclen/Ortho-Tri-Cyclen 1914
Ortho-Est 1925
Ortho-Cyclen/Ortho Tri-Cyclen 1914
Ovcon 765
Premphase 2900
Prempro 2905
Provera Tablets 2110
Levlen/Tri-Levlen 646

Weight changes, unspecified
Aygestin Tablets 990
Betapace Tablets (1% to 2%) 637
Cytotec (Infrequent) 2576
▲ Depo-Provera Contraceptive Injection (More than 5%) 2079
Diethylstilbestrol Tablets 1477
Estraderm Transdermal System 842
Flexeril Tablets (Rare) 1701
Klonopin Tablets 2294
Larodopa Tablets (Infrequent) 2296
Lodine Capsules and Tablets (Less than 1%) 2849
Lo/Ovral Tablets 2852
Lo/Ovral-28 Tablets 2857
Loxitane 1426
Marax Tablets & DF Syrup (Possible, with large doses) 2015
Monopril Tablets (0.2% to 1.0% or more) 762
Nordette-21 Tablets 2863
Nordette-28 Tablets 2866
Norpramin Tablets 1273
Ovral Tablets 2877
Ovral-28 Tablets 2878
Ovrette Tablets 2878
Prolixin 510
Trental Tablets (Less than 1%) 1291
Triavil Tablets 1800
Triphasil-21 Tablets 2919
Triphasil-28 Tablets 2924
Univasc Tablets (Less than 1%) 2553
Vivactil Tablets 1820

Weight decrease (see under Weight loss)

Weight gain
Adapin Capsules (Occasional) 1542
AeroBid Inhaler System (1% to 3%) 1004
Aerobid-M Inhaler System (1% to 3%) 1004
Aldoclor Tablets 1638
Aldomet Ester HCl Injection 1642
Aldomet Oral 1640
Aldoril Tablets 1644
Altace Capsules (Less than 1%) 1238
▲ Anafranil Capsules (2% to 18%) 819
Arimidex Tablets (1.5% to 4.1%) 2932
Atamet Tablets 567
Atromid-S Capsules 2808
Beclovent Inhalation Aerosol and Refill 1063
▲ Betaseron for SC Injection (4%) 653
Brevicon 2563
BuSpar Tablets (Infrequent) 738
Cardizem CD Capsules (Less than 1%) 1251
Cardizem SR Capsules (Less than 1%) 1255
Cardizem Injectable 1253
Cardizem Tablets (Less than 1%) 1257
Cardura Tablets (0.5% to 1%) 1993
Casodex Tablets (2% to 5%) 2934
Catapres Tablets (About 1 in 100 patients) 679
Catapres-TTS 680
▲ CellCept Capsules (More than or equal to 3%) 2265
Claritin Tablets (2% or fewer patients) 2485
Claritin-D Tablets (Less frequent) 2487
Clomid (Fewer than 1%) 1262
▲ Clozaril Tablets (4%) 2377
Cognex Capsules (Infrequent) 1961
Combipres Tablets (About 1%) 682
Compazine 2644
Cortifoam 2540
Cortone Acetate Sterile Suspension 1663
Cortone Acetate Tablets 1664
Dalalone D.P. Injectable 1009
Danocrine Capsules 2437
Daypro Caplets (Less than 1%) 2578
Decadron Elixir 1676
Decadron Phosphate Injection 1680
Decadron Phosphate with Xylocaine Injection, Sterile 1683
Decadron Tablets 1678
Decadron-LA Sterile Suspension 1687
▲ Demulen (Among most common) 2580
Depakene 416
▲ Depakote Tablets (8%) 418
Desyrel and Desyrel Dividose (1.4% to 4.5%) 504
Dexacort Phosphate in Respihaler 1606
Dexacort Phosphate in Turbinaire 1607
Dilacor XR Extended-release Capsules 2183
Diupres Tablets 1691
Doxil (Less than 1%) 2613
DynaCirc CR Tablets (0.5% to 1.0%) 2383
Effexor (Frequent) 2825
Elavil 2945
Esimil Tablets 840
Eskalith 2658
Estrace Cream and Tablets 751
Etrafon 2495
Felbatol (Frequent) 2774
Feldene Capsules (Less than 1%) 2008
▲ Flolan for Injection (6%) 1085
▲ Hismanal Tablets (3.6%) 1341
Humegon for Injection 1873
Hydeltrasol Injection, Sterile 1708
Hydeltra-T.B.A. Sterile Suspension 1710
Hydrocortone Acetate Sterile Suspension 1712
Hydrocortone Phosphate Injection, Sterile 1713
Hydrocortone Tablets 1715
Hydropres Tablets 1718
▲ Hylorel Tablets (44.3%) 1613
Hytrin Capsules (0.5%) 434
Imitrex Tablets (Rare) 1099
Indocin Capsules (Less than 1%) 1723
Indocin I.V. (Less than 1%) 1727
Indocin (Less than 1%) 1723
Invirase Capsules (Less than 2%) 2291
Ismelin Tablets 845
K-Phos Neutral Tablets 633
Kerlone Tablets (Less than 2%) 2588
Lamictal Tablets (Frequent) 1105
▲ Leukine (8%) 1317
Limbitrol 2333
Lioresal Tablets 847
Lithium Carbonate Capsules & Tablets 2352
Lithonate/Lithotabs/Lithobid 2721
Ludiomil Tablets (Rare) 861
Lupron Depot 3.75 mg (Less than 5%) 2739
Lupron Depot 7.5 mg (Less than 5%) 2741
Lupron Depot-PED 7.5 mg, 11.25 mg and 15 mg (Less than 2%) 2744
Lupron Injection 2736
Lupron Injection Pediatric (Less than 2%) 2737
LUVOX Tablets (Frequent) 2723
Maxair Autohaler 1550
Maxair Inhaler (Less than 1%) 1552
Megace Tablets (Frequent) 710
Mellaril 2398
Mesantoin Tablets 2400
Metrodin (urofollitropin for injection) 2616
Miacalcin Nasal Spray (Less than 1%) 2403
Micronor Tablets (Rare) 1903
Modicon 1928
Motrin Ibuprofen Suspension, Oral Drops, Chewable Tablets, Caplets 1563
Nardil (Common) 1977
Navane Capsules and Concentrate 2018
Navane Intramuscular 2019
Neurontin Capsules (2.9%) 1978
▲ Nicotrol NS Nicotine Nasal Spray (Over 5%) 1565
▲ Nolvadex Tablets (38.1%) 2957
Norinyl 2563
Norpace (1 to 3%) 2596
Norplant System 2868
Nor-Q D Tablets 2598
Norvasc Tablets (More than 0.1% to 1%) 2020
Orap Tablets 1037
Ortho Dienestrol Cream 1922
Ortho-Novum 1928
Orudis Capsules (Less than 1%) 2874
Oruvail Capsules (Less than 1%) 2874
Pamelor 2409
Paxil Tablets (Frequent) 2681
Pentaspan Injection 954
Periactin 1767
Permax Tablets (1.6%; frequent) 571
PMB 200 and PMB 400 2890
Premarin Intravenous 2893
Premarin Tablets 2896
Premarin Vaginal Cream 2898
Prevacid Delayed-Release Capsules (Less than 1%) 2746
Prilosec Delayed-Release Capsules (Less than 1%) 516
Prinivil Tablets (0.3% to 1.0%) 1776
Prinzide Tablets 1780
Procardia XL Extended Release Tablets (1% or less) 2026
▲ Proleukin for Injection (23%) 812
ProSom Tablets (Rare) 457
Prozac Pulvules & Liquid, Oral Solution (Infrequent) 935
Questran 774
Redux Capsules 2911
Relafen Tablets (1%) 2688
▲ Remeron Tablets (7.5% to 12%) 1878
ReVia Tablets (Less than 1%) 957
Rilutek Tablets (Infrequent) 2198
▲ Risperdal Tablets (18% or infrequent) 1348
Sansert Tablets 2424
Ser-Ap-Es Tablets 867
Serentil 689
Serophene (clomiphene citrate tablets, USP) (Less than 1 in 100 patients) 2621
Serzone Tablets 776
Sinemet Tablets 959
Sinemet CR Tablets 961
Sinequan (Occasional) 2028
Stelazine (Occasional) 2692
Sular Tablets (Less than or equal to 1%) 2961
▲ Supprelin Injection (3% to 10%) 2230
Surmontil Capsules 2917
▲ Synarel Nasal Solution for Endometriosis (8% of patients) 2605
Taxotere for Injection Concentrate 2204
Tiazac Capsules (Less than 1%) 1019
Tofranil Ampuls 873
Tofranil Tablets 875
Tofranil-PM Capsules 876
▲ Tolectin (200, 400 and 600 mg) (3 to 9%) 1591
Toradol (1% or less) 2319
Torecan 2367
Trilafon 2532
Trilisate (Less than 1%) 2155
Tri-Norinyl 2607
Uroqid-Acid No. 2 Tablets 633
▲ Vesanoid Capsules (23%) 2327
Visken Tablets (2% or fewer patients) 2428
Vivelle Transdermal System 880
▲ Wellbutrin Tablets (9.4% to 13.6%) 1177
▲ Xanax Tablets (2.7% to 27.2%) 2115
Zebeta Tablets 1457
Zestoretic Tablets 2968
Zestril Tablets (0.3% to 1.0%) 2972
Ziac 1459

(◘ Described in PDR For Nonprescription Drugs) Incidence data in parenthesis; ▲ 3% or more (⊙ Described in PDR For Ophthalmology)

Weight gain Side Effects Index 1488

Zoladex (Greater than 1% but less than 5%) 2976
Zoladex 3-month 2978
Zoloft Tablets (Infrequent) 2051
Zyrtec Tablets (Less than 2%) 2053

Weight loss

Abelcet Injection 1540
Accutane Capsules (Less than 1%) 2252
▲ Actimmune (6%) 1043
Adalat CC (Less than 1.0%) 582
Adderall Tablets 2209
Alferon N Injection (1%) 2142
Alkeran for Injection 1196
Alkeran Tablets 1198
Ambien Tablets (Rare) 2559
▲ Anafranil Capsules (Up to 7%) 819
Arimidex Tablets (2% to 5%) 2932
Atamet Tablets 567
▲ Betaseron for SC Injection (4%) 653
Blenoxane (Common) 697
Blocadren Tablets 1654
Brevicon 2563
BuSpar Tablets (Infrequent) 738
Calcijex Injection 412
Capoten Tablets 740
Capozide Tablets 744
Cardura Tablets (Less than 0.5% of 3960 patients) 1993
▲ Casodex Tablets (4%) 2934
Cataflam Tablets (Rare) 833
Celontin Kapseals 1955
Clomid (Fewer than 1%) 1262
Clozaril Tablets 2377
Cogentin 1661
▲ Cognex Capsules (3%) 1961
Cylert Tablets 415
Daranide Tablets 1676
Daypro Caplets (Less than 1%) 2578
Depakene 416
Depakote Tablets 418
Desyrel and Desyrel Dividose (Less than 1% to 5.7%) 504
Dexedrine 2648
DextroStat-Dextroamphetamine Sulfate Tablets 2211
Doxil (1% to 5%) 2613
Effexor (1%) 2825
Elavil 2945
Eldepryl Capsules (1 of 49 patients) 2729
Elspar 1700
Eskalith 2658
Estrace Cream and Tablets 751
Etrafon 2495
▲ Felbatol (3.4% to 6.5%) 2774
Feldene Capsules (Less than 1%) 2008
▲ Flolan for Injection (26%) 1085
Floxin I.V. (Less than 1%) 1580
Floxin Tablets (200 mg, 300 mg, 400 mg) (Less than 1%) 1577
Foscavir Injection (Between 1% and 5%) 541
▲ Fungizone Intravenous (Among most common) 507
Garamycin Injectable 2502
Hivid Tablets (Less than 1%) 2287
▲ Hylorel Tablets (42.2%) 1613
Imitrex Tablets (Rare) 1099
Intron A for Injection (Less than 1% to 5%) 2506
Invirase Capsules (Less than 2%) 2291
Kerlone Tablets (Less than 2%) 2588
Lamictal Tablets (Infrequent) 1105
Lamprene Capsules 846
▲ Leukine (37%) 1317
Limbitrol 2333
Lioresal Intrathecal (1% or more) 1634
Lithium Carbonate Capsules & Tablets 2352
Lithonate/Lithotabs/Lithobid 2721
Lopid Tablets 1974
Ludiomil Tablets (Rare) 861
Lupron Depot 3.75 mg (Less than 5%) 2739
LUVOX Tablets (Frequent) 2723
Methadone Hydrochloride Oral Concentrate 2356
Micronor Tablets 1903
Modicon 1928
Monoket Tablets (Fewer than 1%) 2550
Myleran Tablets 1209
Naprelan Tablets (Less than 1%) 2861
Neoral (Rare) 2405
Neurontin Capsules (Infrequent) 1978
▲ Nolvadex Tablets (22.6%) 2957
Norinyl 2563
Nor-Q D Tablets 2598
Norvir (Less than 2%) 447
Oncaspar (Less than 1%) 2194
Oncovin Solution Vials & Hyporets 1521
Orap Tablets 1037
Orlaam Oral Solution 2361
Ortho Dienestrol Cream 1922
Ortho-Novum 1928
Orudis Capsules (Less than 1%) 2874
Oruvail Capsules (Less than 1%) 2874
Pamelor 2409
Paxil Tablets (Frequent) 2681
Permax Tablets (Frequent) 571
Phenurone Tablets (Less than 1%) 455
Placidyl Capsules 456
Plaquenil Sulfate Tablets 2459
PMB 200 and PMB 400 2890
Premarin Intravenous 2893
Premarin Tablets 2896
Premarin Vaginal Cream 2898
Prevacid Delayed-Release Capsules (Less than 1%) 2746
Prinivil Tablets (0.3% to 1.0%) 1776
Prinzide Tablets 1780
▲ Proleukin for Injection (5%) 812
ProSom Tablets (Rare) 457
▲ Prozac Pulvules & Liquid, Oral Solution (5%) 935
Pulmozyme Inhalation 1054
Questran 774
Relafen Tablets (Less than 1%) 2688
Remeron Tablets (Infrequent) 1878
Retrovir Capsules (0.8%) 1216
Retrovir I.V. Infusion (1%) 1221
Retrovir Syrup (0.8%) 1216
ReVia Tablets (Less than 1%) 957
▲ Rilutek Tablets (3.7% to 4.6%) 2198
Risperdal Tablets (Infrequent) 1348
Ritalin 866
Rocaltrol Capsules 2303
▲ Roferon-A Injection (25% to 33%) 2308
Sandimmune (Rare) 2416
Sandostatin Injection (Less than 1%) 2421
Sansert Tablets 2424
Serzone Tablets (Infrequent) 776
Sinemet Tablets 959
Sinemet CR Tablets 961
Sular Tablets (Less than or equal to 1%) 2961
Surmontil Capsules 2917
Synarel Nasal Solution for Endometriosis (1% of patients) 2605
Tegison Capsules 2314
TICE BCG, USP (2.2%) 1881
Timolide Tablets 1791
Timoptic in Ocudose 1796
Timoptic Sterile Ophthalmic Solution 1794
Timoptic-XE 1798
Tofranil Ampuls 873
Tofranil Tablets 875
Tofranil-PM Capsules 876
▲ Tolectin (200, 400 and 600 mg) (3 to 9%) 1591
Tri-Norinyl 2607
Ultram Tablets (50 mg) (Less than 1%) 1594
▲ Vesanoid Capsules (17%) 2327
▲ Videx Tablets, Powder for Oral Solution, & Pediatric Powder for Oral Solution (Less than 1% to 8%) 2980
Vistide Injection 1057
Vivelle Transdermal System 880
Cataflam/Voltaren/Voltaren-XR (Rare) 833
▲ Wellbutrin Tablets (23.2% to 28%) 1177
▲ Xanax Tablets (2.3% to 22.6%) 2115
Zarontin Capsules (Frequent) 1986
Zarontin Syrup (Frequent) 1986
▲ Zerit Capsules (Fewer than 1% to 10%) 731
Zestoretic Tablets 2968
Zestril Tablets (0.3% to 1.0%) 2972
Zoloft Tablets (Infrequent) 2051

Wenckebach block

Buprenex Injectable (Less than 1%) 2170
Lanoxin Elixir Pediatric 1113
Lanoxin Injection 1116
▲ Lanoxin Injection Pediatric (Among most common) 1119
Lanoxin Tablets 1121

Wenckebach's period (see under A-V conduction, prolongation)

Wheals

Astramorph/PF Injection, USP (Preservative-Free) 526
Attenuvax (Rare) 1650
Biavax II 1653
Demerol 2438
Desferal Vials 838
Dilaudid-HP Injection (Less frequent) 1384
Dilaudid-HP Lyophilized Powder 250 mg (Less frequent) 1384
Duramorph Injection 983
Infumorph 200 and Infumorph 500 Sterile Solutions 985
M-M-R II 1730
M-R-VAX II 1732
Mepergan Injection 2859
Meruvax II 1740
Mumpsvax (Extremely rare) 1751

Wheezing

Abelcet Injection 1540
▲ Adalat Capsules (10 mg and 20 mg) (6%) 580
▲ AeroBid Inhaler System (3% to 9%) 1004
▲ Aerobid-M Inhaler System (3% to 9%) 1004
Airet Albuterol Sulfate Inhalation Solution (1% to 1.5%) 1602
Albuterol Sulfate, USP Solution for Inhalation, Arm-a-Med (1% to 1.5%) 522
Alferon N Injection 2142
Azmacort Oral Inhaler (Infrequent) 2175
Beclovent Inhalation Aerosol and Refill (Rare) 1063
Beconase (Rare) 1065
Bioclate, Antihemophilic Factor (Recombinant) 797
Blenoxane (Approximately 1%) 697
Brethaire Inhaler 830
Brevibloc (esmolol HCl) Injection (Less than 1%) 1860
▲ Bromfed-DM Cough Syrup (Among most frequent) 1832
Cartrol Tablets (Rare) 413
Claritin-D Tablets (Less frequent) 2487
Clozaril Tablets (Less than 1%) 2377
CytoGam (Less than 5.0%) 1630
Depen Titratable Tablets 2770
Dimetane-DC Cough Syrup 2232
Dimetane-DX Cough Syrup 2233
Diprivan Injectable Emulsion (Less than 1%) 2939
Fungizone Intravenous 507
Gamimune N, 5% Immune Globulin Intravenous (Human), 5% 612
Gamimune N, 10% Immune Globulin Intravenous (Human), 10% 615
Gammar-P I.V., Immune Globulin Intravenous (Human) 798
Hespan Injection 945
Hivid Tablets (Less than 1%) 2287
Humalog Injection (Less common) 1488
Humulin 50/50, 100 Units 1491
Humulin 70/30, 100 Units (Less common) 1492
Humulin L, 100 Units (Less common) 1494
Hyskon Hysteroscopy Fluid (Rare) 1633
Regular, 100 Units (Less Common) 1503
Pork Regular, 100 Units 1507
Imitrex Tablets 1099
▲ Intal Inhaler (Among most frequent) 2185
Intal Nebulizer Solution (Rare) 2186
Intron A for Injection (Less than or equal to 5%) 2506
JE-VAX 904
Lopressor (1%) 848
Lopressor HCT Tablets (Fewer than 1 in 100 patients) 850
Maxair Autohaler 1550
Maxair Inhaler (Less than 1%) 1552
Mivacron (One patient; less than 1%) 1125
Monoclate-P, Factor VIII:C Pasteurized, Monoclonal Antibody Purified Antihemophilic Factor (Human) 802
Mononine, Coagulation Factor IX (Human), Monoclonal Antibody Purified 804
Nasalcrom Nasal Solution 2192
Neupogen for Injection 495
Nimotop Capsules (Less than 1%) 603
Normodyne Injection (1%) 2519
Nubain Injection (1% or less) 952
Nuromax Injection (Less than or equal to 0.1%) 1136
Ornade Spansule Capsules 2678
▲ Orthoclone OKT3 Sterile Solution (13%) 1892
PBZ Tablets 863
PBZ-SR Tablets 862
Pentaspan Injection 954
Periactin 1767
Platinol for Injection (Occasional) 717
Platinol-AQ Injection (Occasional) 719
Prinivil Tablets (0.3% to 1.0%) 1776
Prinzide Tablets 1780
▲ Procardia Capsules (6%) 2024
▲ Procardia XL Extended Release Tablets (6%) 2026
▲ Proleukin for Injection (6%) 812
Prostin E2 Suppository 2109
Proventil Inhalation Solution 0.083% (1% to 1.5%) 2527
Proventil Solution for Inhalation 0.5% (1% to 1.5%) 2525
Pulmozyme Inhalation 1054
Quadrinal Tablets 1398
Questran 774
RespiGam (2%) 1631
Rhinocort Nasal Inhaler (Less than 1%) 552
Rifadin 1276
Rifater 1280
Sandimmune 2416
Sectral Capsules (Up to 2%) 2914
Sular Tablets (Less than or equal to 1%) 2961
Survanta Beractant Intratracheal Suspension 2346
Tavist Syrup 2426
Tavist Tablets 2427
Tenoretic Tablets (Up to 3%) 2963
Tenormin Tablets and I.V. Injection (Up to 3%) 2965
Thioplex (Thiotepa For Injection) 1329
Tonocard Tablets 519
Toprol-XL Tablets (About 1 of 100 patients) 560
Tracrium Injection (1 out of 875 patients; 0.2%) 1155
Trandate Injection (1 of 100 patients) 1158
Trinalin Repetabs Tablets 1373
Tussend 1830
Vancenase AQ Nasal Spray 0.042% (Extremely rare) 2535
Vancenase AQ Double Strength Nasal Spray 0.084% (Rare) 2536
Vancocin HCl, Oral Solution & Pulvules 1536
Vancocin HCl, Vials & ADD-Vantage 1534
Vaqta (Less than 1%) 1805
Ventolin Inhalation Solution (1% to 1.5%) 1171
Ventolin Nebules Inhalation Solution (1% to 1.5%) 1172
Versed Injection (Less than 1%) 2324
▲ Vesanoid Capsules (14%) 2327
Visken Tablets (2% or fewer patients) 2428
Zemuron Injection (Less than 1%) 1885
Zestoretic Tablets 2968
Zestril Tablets (0.3% to 1.0%) 2972

White-clot syndrome

Heparin Lock Flush Solution 2831
Heparin Sodium Injection 2832

Withdrawal reactions

Adapin Capsules (Possibility) 1542
Anafranil Capsules (Rare) 819
Astramorph/PF Injection, USP (Preservative-Free) 526
Betapace Tablets 637
Butisol Sodium Elixir & Tablets 2768
Catapres Tablets (About 1 in 100 patients) 679
Dalmane Capsules 2329
Darvon-N/Darvocet-N 1473
Darvon Compound-65 Pulvules 1475
Darvon-N Suspension & Tablets 1473
Dexacort Phosphate in Respihaler 1606
Dexacort Phosphate in Turbinaire 1607
Dexedrine 2648
Dilaudid Ampules 1382
Dilaudid Cough Syrup 1383
Dilaudid 1382
Dizac (diazepam injectable emulsion) CIV 1862
Doral Tablets 2773
Effexor (Rare) 2825
Fioricet Tablets (One report) 2386
Fioricet with Codeine Capsules (One report) 2387

(Described in PDR For Nonprescription Drugs) Incidence data in parenthesis; ▲ 3% or more (⊙ Described in PDR For Ophthalmology)

Fiorinal with Codeine Capsules (One report) 2390
Halcion Tablets 2093
Infumorph 200 and Infumorph 500 Sterile Solutions 985
Kadian Capsules (Less than 3%) 2948
Klonopin Tablets 2294
Levo-Dromoran 2297
Librium Capsules 2331
Librium Injectable 2332
Lortab 2751
LUVOX Tablets (Rare) 2723
MS Contin Tablets 2149
MSIR 2152
Mebaral Tablets 2452
Nembutal Sodium Capsules 440
Nembutal Sodium Solution 442
Nembutal Sodium Suppositories 444
Orlaam Oral Solution 2361
OxyContin Tablets (Less than 1%) 2163
Pamelor 2409
Paxil Tablets (Rare) 2681
Phenobarbital Elixir and Tablets 1523
Placidyl Capsules 456
Procardia XL Extended Release Tablets 2026
ProctoCream-HC 2.5% 2552
ProSom Tablets 457
Redux Capsules 2911
Remeron Tablets (Rare) 1878
ReVia Tablets (A small fraction of patients) 957
Revex (nalmefene hydrochloride injection) (Less than 1%) 1863
Risperdal Tablets (Rare) 1348
Stadol (2 patients) 779
Tranxene 459
Valium Injectable 2336
Valium Tablets 2335
Videx Tablets, Powder for Oral Solution, & Pediatric Powder for Oral Solution (Less than 1%) 2980
Xanax Tablets 2115
Zoloft Tablets (Rare) 2051

Wolff-Parkinson-White syndrome

Cytovene-IV (One report) 2270

Wound healing, impaired

AK-CIDE (Infrequent) ⊙ 203
AK-CIDE Ointment (Infrequent) ⊙ 203
AK-Trol Ointment & Suspension ⊙ 205
Blephamide Liquifilm Sterile Ophthalmic Suspension 472
Blephamide Ointment (Infrequent) ⊙ 234
Celestone Soluspan Suspension 2484
CORTENEMA 2713
Cortifoam 2540
Cortisporin Ophthalmic Ointment Sterile 1074
Cortisporin Ophthalmic Suspension Sterile 1075
Cortone Acetate Sterile Suspension 1663
Cortone Acetate Tablets 1664
Cytoxan 700
Dalalone D.P. Injectable 1009
Decadron Elixir 1676
Decadron Phosphate Injection 1680
Decadron Phosphate with Xylocaine Injection, Sterile 1683
Decadron Tablets 1678
Decadron-LA Sterile Suspension 1687
Dexacort Phosphate in Respihaler 1606
Dexacort Phosphate in Turbinaire 1607
Econopred & Econopred Plus Ophthalmic Suspensions ⊙ 216
FML Forte Liquifilm (Infrequent) ⊙ 237
FML Liquifilm ⊙ 238
FML S.O.P. (Infrequent) ⊙ 239
FML-S Liquifilm ⊙ 240
Florinef Acetate Tablets 506
FLUORACAINE ⊙ 208
Hydeltrasol Injection, Sterile 1708
Hydeltra-T.B.A. Sterile Suspension 1710
Hydrocortone Acetate Sterile Suspension 1712
Hydrocortone Phosphate Injection, Sterile 1713
Hydrocortone Tablets 1715
Maxitrol Ophthalmic Ointment and Suspension ⊙ 222
NeoDecadron Sterile Ophthalmic Ointment 1755
NeoDecadron Sterile Ophthalmic Solution 1756
Ocufen ⊙ 242
Pediapred Oral Solution 1618
Poly-Pred Liquifilm ⊙ 246
Pred Forte ⊙ 247
Pred Mild (Infrequent) ⊙ 250
Pred-G Liquifilm Sterile Ophthalmic Suspension ⊙ 248
Pred-G S.O.P. Sterile Ophthalmic Ointment ⊙ 249
Prelone Syrup 1834
Rhinocort Nasal Inhaler 552
Terra-Cortril Ophthalmic Suspension 2033
TobraDex Ophthalmic Suspension and Ointment 469
▲ Zofran Tablets (28%) 1231

Wound infection

▲ Neoral (7.0%) 2405
▲ Sandimmune (7.0 to 10.1%) 2416

Wrist-drop

Fludara for Injection (One case) 658
Rilutek Tablets (Rare) 2198

WBC, immature

▲ Betaseron for SC Injection (16%) 653
Biaxin (Less than 1%) 406
Cipro I.V. (Infrequent) 587
▲ Cipro I.V. Pharmacy Bulk Package (Among most frequent) 590
▲ Clozaril Tablets (3%) 2377
Cytosar-U Sterile Powder (Less than 7 patients) 2077
Lupron Depot 3.75 mg 2739
Lupron Depot 7.5 mg 2741
Lupron Depot-PED 7.5 mg, 11.25 mg and 15 mg 2744
Merrem I.V. (Greater than 0.2%) 2952
Naprelan Tablets (Less than 1%) 2861
Neurontin Capsules (1.1%) 1978
Zebeta Tablets 1457

WBC counts, fluctuation

Bumex (0.3%) 2260
Cytotec (Infrequent) 2576
Dopram Injectable 2235
Doral Tablets (2.6%) 2773
Effexor (Infrequent) 2825
Foscavir Injection (Between 1% and 5%) 541
Sterile FUDR 2284
Halcion Tablets (1.7 to 2.1%) 2093
Hivid Tablets (Less than 1%) 2287
Lopid Tablets 1974
▲ Lupron Depot - 3 Month 22.5 mg (More than or equal to 5%) 2743
MetroGel-Vaginal (Equal to or less than 2%) 917
Neurontin Capsules (Rare) 1978
Noroxin Tablets (1.3% to 1.4%) 1758
Noroxin Tablets (1.3% to 1.4%) 2222
Prevacid Delayed-Release Capsules (Less than 1%) 2746
Primaxin I.M. 1770
▲ Synarel Nasal Solution for Endometriosis (10% to 15%) 2605
Talwin Compound (Rare) 2466
▲ Tegison Capsules (10-25%) 2314
Tornalate Solution for Inhalation, 0.2% (Infrequent) 976
Tornalate Metered Dose Inhaler (Rare) 978
Xanax Tablets (1.4% to 2.3%) 2115

X

Xanthopsia

Aldactazide Tablets 2556
Aldoclor Tablets 1638
Aldoril Tablets 1644
Apresazide Capsules 824
Capozide Tablets 744
Combipres Tablets 682
Diucardin Tablets 2824
Diupres Tablets 1691
Diuril Oral Suspension 1694
Diuril Sodium Intravenous 1693
Diuril Tablets 1694
Dyazide Capsules 2653
Enduron Tablets 424
Esidrix Tablets 839
Esimil Tablets 840
HydroDIURIL Tablets 1716
Hydropres Tablets 1718
Hyzaar Tablets (One subject) 1720
Inderide Tablets 2838
Inderide LA Long Acting Capsules 2840
Lanoxicaps 1110
Lanoxin Elixir Pediatric 1113
Lanoxin Injection 1116
Lanoxin Injection Pediatric 1119
Lanoxin Tablets 1121
Lasix Injection, Oral Solution and Tablets 1267
Lopressor HCT Tablets 850
Lotensin HCT Tablets 855
Minizide Capsules 2016
Mintezol 1747
Moduretic Tablets 1748
Mykrox Tablets (Rare) 1617
Normodyne Tablets (Less common) 2522
Oretic Tablets 450
Prinzide Tablets 1780
Quadrinal Tablets 1398
Ser-Ap-Es Tablets 867
Tenoretic Tablets 2963
Thalitone 1293
Timolide Tablets 1791
Vaseretic Tablets 1810
Zaroxolyn Tablets 1625
Zestoretic Tablets 2968
Ziac 1459

Xerochilia

▲ Zonalon Cream (Approximately 1% to 10%) 1042

Xeromycteria

▲ Accutane Capsules (Up to 80%) 2252
Alomide Ophthalmic Solution (Less than 1%) 465
▲ Atrovent Nasal Spray 0.03% (5.1%) 676
▲ Atrovent Nasal Spray 0.06% (4.8%) 678
Beclovent Inhalation Aerosol and Refill 1063
Beconase 1065
Benadryl Injection 1955
▲ Bromfed-DM Cough Syrup (Among most frequent) 1832
Catapres Tablets 679
Claritin Tablets (2% or fewer patients) 2485
Claritin-D Tablets 2487
Combipres Tablets 682
D.A. II Tablets 972
D.A. Chewable Tablets 970
▲ Dexacort Phosphate in Turbinaire (One of the two most common) 1607
▲ Dimetane-DC Cough Syrup (Most frequent) 2232
Dimetane-DX Cough Syrup (Among most frequent) 2233
Dura-Tap/PD Capsules 970
Dura-Vent/DA Tablets 972
Flonase Nasal Spray (Less than 1%) 1088
Hivid Tablets (Less than 1%) 2287
IOPIDINE Sterile Ophthalmic Solution ⊙ 218
Iopidine 0.5% (2%) ⊙ 219
Marax Tablets & DF Syrup 2015
▲ Miacalcin Nasal Spray (10.6%) 2403
▲ Nasarel Nasal Solution (3% to 9%) 2302
▲ Norpace (3 to 9%) 2596
Ornade Spansule Capsules 2678
PBZ Tablets 863
PBZ-SR Tablets 862
Periactin 1767
▲ Seldane Tablets (2.3% to 4.8%) 1284
▲ Seldane-D Extended-Release Tablets (21.7%) 1286
Symmetrel Capsules (1% to 5%) 965
Symmetrel Syrup (1% to 5%) 963
Tavist Syrup 2426
Tavist Tablets 2427
▲ Tegison Capsules (Greater than 75%) 2314
Torecan 2367
Trinalin Repetabs Tablets 1373
Tussend 1830

Xerophthalmia

Accutane Capsules 2252
▲ Alomide Ophthalmic Solution (1% to 5%) 465
Betaseron for SC Injection 653
▲ Betimol 0.25%, 0.5% (More than 5%) ⊙ 259
Betoptic Ophthalmic Solution 465
Betoptic S Ophthalmic Suspension (Small number of patients) 467
Blocadren Tablets 1654
BOTOX (Botulinum Toxin Type A) Purified Neurotoxin Complex 473
Catapres Tablets 679
Catapres-TTS 680
Cognex Capsules (Infrequent) 1961
Combipres Tablets 682
Cytovene-IV (One report) 2270
Depakote Tablets (1% to 5%) 418
Dipentum Capsules (Rare) 2084
Effexor (Infrequent) 2825
Hivid Tablets (Less than 1%) 2287
IBU Tablets (Less than 1%) 1389
Inderal (Rare) 2834
Inderal LA Long Acting Capsules (Rare) 2836
Inderide Tablets (Rare) 2838
Inderide LA Long Acting Capsules 2840
Intron A for Injection (Less than 5%) 2506
Invirase Capsules (Less than 2%) 2291
IOPIDINE Sterile Ophthalmic Solution ⊙ 218
Iopidine 0.5% (Less than 3%) ⊙ 219
Kerlone Tablets (Less than 2%) 2588
Lamictal Tablets (Rare) 1105
Livostin (Approximately 1% to 3%) ⊙ 262
Lupron Depot - 3 Month 22.5 mg (Less than 5%) 2743
LUVOX Tablets (Infrequent) 2723
Mintezol 1747
Motrin Ibuprofen Suspension, Oral Drops, Chewable Tablets, Caplets (Less than 1%) 1563
Neurontin Capsules (Infrequent) 1978
Nipent for Injection (Less than 3%) 2733
Norvasc Tablets (Less than or equal to 0.1%) 2020
Ocuflox Ophthalmic Solution 478
Redux Capsules (Infrequent) 2911
Rev-Eyes Ophthalmic Eyedrops 0.5% (Less frequently) ⊙ 324
Risperdal Tablets (Infrequent) 1348
Sectral Capsules (Up to 2%) 2914
Serzone Tablets (Infrequent) 776
▲ Tegison Capsules (1-10%) 2314
Tenormin Tablets and I.V. Injection 2965
Timolide Tablets 1791
Timoptic in Ocudose 1796
Timoptic Sterile Ophthalmic Solution 1794
Timoptic-XE 1798
Toprol-XL Tablets (Rare) 560
Trusopt Sterile Ophthalmic Solution (Approximately 1% to 5%) 1803
Vaseretic Tablets 1810
Vasotec I.V. 1814
Vasotec Tablets (0.5% to 1.0%) 1816
Videx Tablets, Powder for Oral Solution, & Pediatric Powder for Oral Solution (Less than 1%) 2980
Xalatan (1% to 4%) ⊙ 304
Zoladex (1% or greater) 2976
Zoladex 3-month 2978
Zoloft Tablets (Infrequent) 2051
Zyrtec Tablets (Less than 2%) 2053

Xerosis cutis

Eskalith 2658
Lithium Carbonate Capsules & Tablets 2352
Lithonate/Lithotabs/Lithobid 2721
Zosyn (1.0% or less) 1463

Xerostomia

Accupril Tablets (0.5% to 1.0%) 1950
▲ Accutane Capsules (Up to 80%) 2252
Adalat CC (Less than 1.0%) 582
Adapin Capsules 1542
Adderall Tablets 2209
Adenoscan (Less than 1%) 1022
Adipex-P Tablets and Capsules 1035
Akineton 1380
Aldactone Tablets 2558
Aldoclor Tablets 1638
Aldomet Ester HCl Injection 1642
Aldomet Oral 1640
Aldoril Tablets 1644
Alferon N Injection (One patient) 2142
Altace Capsules (Less than 1%) 1238
Alupent Tablets (0.4%) 672
▲ Ambien Tablets (3%) 2559
▲ Anafranil Capsules (63% to 84%) 819
Ana-Kit Anaphylaxis Emergency Treatment Kit 611
Ancobon Capsules 2254
Antivert, Antivert/25 Tablets, & Antivert/50 Tablets 1992
Apresazide Capsules 824
Arco-Lase Plus Tablets 513
▲ Arimidex Tablets (4.5% to 5.7%) 2932
▲ Artane (30% to 50%) 1418
Asacol Delayed-Release Tablets 2129
▲ Asendin Tablets (14%) 1419
Atamet Tablets 567
Atarax Tablets & Syrup 1992
Atretol Tablets 569
Atrohist Pediatric Capsules 1603

(▣ Described in PDR For Nonprescription Drugs) Incidence data in parenthesis: ▲ 3% or more (⊙ Described in PDR For Ophthalmology)

Xerostomia **Side Effects Index** 1490

▲ Atrohist Pediatric Suspension (Among most common) 1604
Atrohist Plus Tablets 1605
Atrovent Inhalation Aerosol (2.4%) 674
▲ Atrovent Inhalation Solution (3.2%) 675
Atrovent Nasal Spray 0.03% (Less than 2%) 676
Atrovent Nasal Spray 0.06% (1.4%) 678
Avonex 662
Axid Pulvules (1.4%) 1468
Axocet Capsules (Infrequent) 2469
Azmacort Oral Inhaler 2175
Bactroban Nasal (Less than 1%) 2643
Beclovent Inhalation Aerosol and Refill (A few patients) 1063
Bellergal-S Tablets (Rare) 2375
Benadryl Injection 1955
▲ Bentyl (33%) 1246
Betaseron for SC Injection 653
Betimol 0.25%, 0.5% (1% to 5%) ⊙ 259
Bonine Tablets 1990
Bontril Slow-Release Capsules 786
Brethine Ampuls (Less than 0.5%) 832
Brevibloc (esmolol HCl) Injection (Less than 1%) 1860
Bromfed 1832
▲ Bromfed-DM Cough Syrup (Among most frequent) 1832
Bromfed-PD Capsules (Extended-Release) 1832
Bumex (0.1%) 2260
▲ BuSpar Tablets (3%) 738
Calan SR Caplets (1% or less) 2571
Calan Tablets (1% or less) 2568
Calcijex Injection 412
Capoten Tablets (About 0.5 to 2%) 740
Capozide Tablets (0.5 to 2%) 744
Carafate Suspension (Less than 0.5%) 1250
Carafate Tablets (Less than 0.5%) 1249
Cardene Capsules (0.4% to 1.4%) 2261
Cardizem CD Capsules (Less than 1%) 1251
Cardizem SR Capsules (Less than 1%) 1255
Cardizem Injectable (Less than 1%) 1253
Cardizem Tablets (Less than 1%) 1257
Cardura Tablets (1.4% to 2%) 1993
Casodex Tablets (2% to 5%) 2934
Cataflam Tablets (Less than 1%) 833
▲ Catapres Tablets (40 of 100 patients) 679
▲ Catapres-TTS (25 of 101 patients) 680
Caverject Injection (Less than 1%) 2064
Cedax (0.1% to 1%) 2480
▲ Cerebyx Injection (4.4%) 1956
Cipro I.V. (1% or less) 587
Cipro I.V. Pharmacy Bulk Package (Less than 1%) 590
▲ Claritin Tablets (3%) 2485
▲ Claritin-D Tablets (14%) 2487
Clinoril Tablets (Less than 1%) 1658
▲ Clozaril Tablets (More than 5 to 6%) 2377
Cogentin 1661
Cognex Capsules (Infrequent) 1961
▲ Combipres Tablets (40%) 682
Compazine 2644
Covera-HS Tablets (Less than 2%) 2573
Cozaar Tablets (Less than 1%) 1668
Crixivan Capsules (0.5% to less than 2%) 1670
Cystospaz 2123
Cytovene (1% or less) 2270
D.A. II Tablets 972
D.A. Chewable Tablets 970
Dalgan Injection (Less than 1%) 529
Dalmane Capsules (Rare) 2329
Daraprim Tablets (Rare) 1199
DaunoXome (Less than or equal to 5%) 1842
Demadex Tablets and Injection 691
Demerol 2438
Demser Capsules (Infrequent) 1690
Depakote Tablets (1% to 5%) 418
Desoxyn Gradumet Tablets 422
▲ Desyrel and Desyrel Dividose (14.8% to 33.8%) 504
Dexedrine 2648
DextroStat-Dextroamphetamine Sulfate Tablets 2211
Dilacor XR Extended-release Capsules (Infrequent) 2183
Dilaudid-HP Injection (Less frequent) 1384
Dilaudid-HP Lyophilized Powder 250 mg (Less frequent) 1384
Dilaudid Tablets and Liquid 1386
▲ Dimetane-DC Cough Syrup (Most frequent) 2232
▲ Dimetane-DX Cough Syrup (Among most frequent) 2233
Dipentum Capsules (Rare) 2084
Diprivan Injectable Emulsion (Less than 1%) 2939
Ditropan 1267
Diupres Tablets 1691
Diuril Sodium Intravenous 1693
Donnagel Liquid and Donnagel Chewable Tablets (Rare) ▣ 854
Donnatal 2234
Donnatal Extentabs 2234
Donnatal Tablets 2234
Doral Tablets (1.5%) 2773
▲ Duragesic Transdermal System (10% or more) 1336
Dura-Tap/PD Capsules 970
Dura-Vent/DA Tablets 972
Dyazide Capsules 2653
Dynabac (0.1% to 1%) 668
DynaCirc Capsules (0.5% to 1%) 2381
DynaCirc CR Tablets (0.5% to 1.0%) 2383
Dyrenium Capsules (Rare) 2655
▲ Effexor (2% to 22%) 2825
Elavil 2945
▲ Eldepryl Capsules (3 of 49 patients) 2729
Emete-con Intramuscular/Intravenous 2007
Esgic-plus Capsules (Infrequent) 1012
Esgic-plus Tablets (Infrequent) 1012
Esidrix Tablets 839
Esimil Tablets 840
Eskalith 2658
▲ Ethmozine Tablets (2% to 5%) 2217
Etrafon 2495
Fastin Capsules 2662
Fedahist Gyrocaps 2545
Felbatol (2.6%) 2774
Feldene Capsules (Less than 1%) 2008
Fioricet Tablets (Infrequent) 2386
Fioricet with Codeine Capsules (Infrequent) 2387
Fiorinal with Codeine Capsules (Infrequent) 2390
Flagyl 375 Capsules 2587
▲ Flexeril Tablets (7% to 27%) 1701
Flonase Nasal Spray (Less than 1%) 1088
Floxin I.V. (1% to 3%) 1580
Floxin Tablets (200 mg, 300 mg, 400 mg) (1% to 3%) 1577
Flumadine Tablets & Syrup (1.5%) 1013
Foscavir Injection (Between 1% and 5%) 541
Geocillin Tablets 2009
Habitrol Nicotine Transdermal System (Less than 1% of patients) 884
Halcion Tablets (Rare) 2093
Haldol Decanoate 1587
Haldol Injection, Tablets and Concentrate 1585
Helidac Therapy (Less than 1%) 2135
▲ Hismanal Tablets (5.2%) 1341
Hivid Tablets (Less than 1%) 2287
HydroDIURIL Tablets 1716
Hydropres Tablets 1718
Hylorel Tablets (1.7%) 1613
Hyperstat I.V. Injection 2504
Hytrin Capsules (At least 1%) 434
Hyzaar Tablets 1720
IBU Tablets (Less than 1%) 1389
Imdur (Less than or equal to 5%) 1362
Imitrex Tablets 1099
Imodium Capsules 1343
▲ Intron A for Injection (Up to 28%) 2506
Inversine Tablets 1729
Invirase Capsules (Less than 2%) 2291
Ionamin Capsules 1615
IOPIDINE Sterile Ophthalmic Solution ⊙ 218
▲ Iopidine 0.5% (10%) ⊙ 219
Ismelin Tablets 845
Isoptin Oral Tablets (Less than 1%) 1393
Isoptin SR Tablets (1% or less) 1395
Kadian Capsules (Less than 3%) 2948
Kemadrin Tablets 1105
Kerlone Tablets (Less than 2%) 2588
Klonopin Tablets 2294
Kutrase Capsules 2546
Lamictal Tablets (1.0%) 1105
Larodopa Tablets (Relatively frequent) 2296
Lasix Injection, Oral Solution and Tablets 1267
Levbid Extended-Release Tablets 2549
Levo-Dromoran 2297
Levoprome (Sometimes) 1321
Levsin/Levsinex/Levbid 2549
Librax Capsules 2330
▲ Limbitrol (Among most frequent) 2333
Lioresal Intrathecal (Up to 3.3%) 1634
Lioresal Tablets (Rare) 847
Lithium Carbonate Capsules & Tablets 2352
Lithonate/Lithotabs/Lithobid 2721
Livostin (Approximately 1% to 3%) ⊙ 262
Lodine Capsules and Tablets (Less than 1%) 2849
Lopressor (1%) 848
Lopressor HCT Tablets (1 in 100 patients) 850
Lotensin HCT Tablets (0.3% to 1.0%) 855
Lotrel Capsules 858
Loxitane 1426
▲ Ludiomil Tablets (22%) 861
▲ Lupron Depot 3.75 mg (Among most frequent; less than 5%) 2739
Lupron Depot - 3 Month 22.5 mg (Less than 5%) 2743
▲ LUVOX Tablets (14%) 2723
MS Contin Tablets (Less frequent) 2149
MSIR (Infrequent) 2152
Marax Tablets & DF Syrup (Occasional) 2015
Matulane Capsules 2300
Maxair Autohaler (1.3%) 1550
Maxair Inhaler (Less than 1%) 1552
Maxaquin Tablets (Less than 1%) 2593
Megace Oral Suspension (1% to 3%) 708
Mellaril 2398
Mepergan Injection 2859
Methadone Hydrochloride Oral Concentrate 2356
Methadone Hydrochloride Oral Solution & Tablets 2357
MetroGel-Vaginal 917
Mevacor Tablets (0.5% to 1.0%) 1742
Mexitil Capsules (2.8%) 684
Miacalcin Nasal Spray (Less than 1%) 2403
Midamor Tablets (Less than or equal to 1%) 1746
Minipress Capsules (1-4%) 2015
Minizide Capsules (Rare) 2016
Mintezol 1747
Moban Tablets and Concentrate (Occasional) 1036
Moduretic Tablets 1748
Monoket Tablets (Fewer than 1%) 2550
Monopril Tablets (0.2% to 1.0%) 762
Motofen Tablets (1 in 30) 789
Motrin Ibuprofen Suspension, Oral Drops, Chewable Tablets, Caplets (Less than 1%) 1563
Mykrox Tablets (Less than 2%) 1617
Nalfon 200 Pulvules & Nalfon Tablets (Less than 1%) 933
Nardil (Common) 1977
Navane Capsules and Concentrate 2018
Navane Intramuscular 2019
Neurontin Capsules (1.7%) 1978
Nicotrol NS Nicotine Nasal Spray (Less than 1%) 1565
Norflex 1554
Norgesic 1554
Noroxin Tablets (0.3 to 1.0%) 1758
Noroxin Tablets (0.3% to 1.0%) 2222
▲ Norpace (32%) 2596
Norpramin Tablets 1273
Norvasc Tablets (More than 0.1% to 1%) 2020
Norvir (Less than 2%) 447
Novahistine Elixir ▣ 782
▲ Nubain Injection (4%) 952
Oramorph SR (Morphine Sulfate Sustained Release Tablets) (Less frequent) 2359
▲ Orap Tablets (5 of 20 patients) 1037
Oretic Tablets 450
Orlaam Oral Solution (1% to 3%) 2361
Ornade Spansule Capsules 2678
Orudis Capsules (Less than 1%) 2874
Oruvail Capsules (Less than 1%) 2874
▲ OxyContin Tablets (6%) 2163
▲ PBZ Tablets (Among most frequent) 863
▲ PBZ-SR Tablets (Among most frequent) 862
Pamelor 2409
Paremyd ⊙ 244
▲ Parlodel (4%) 2411
Parnate Tablets 2679
▲ Paxil Tablets (1.0% to 20.6%) 2681
Penetrex Tablets (0.1% to 1%) 2196
Pepcid Injection (Infrequent) 1765
Pepcid (Infrequent) 1763
Periactin 1767
▲ Permax Tablets (3.7%; frequent) 571
Phenergan with Codeine 2883
Phenergan with Dextromethorphan 2885
Phenergan Injection 2880
Phenergan Suppositories 2882
Phenergan Syrup 2881
Phenergan Tablets 2882
Phenergan VC 2886
Phenergan VC with Codeine 2888
Phrenilin (Infrequent) 790
Plendil Extended-Release Tablets (0.5% to 1.5%) 514
▲ Pondimin Tablets (Among most common) 2239
Prelu-2 Timed Release Capsules 687
Prevacid Delayed-Release Capsules (Less than 1%) 2746
Prilosec Delayed-Release Capsules (Less than 1%) 516
Prinivil Tablets (0.3% to 1.0%) 1776
Prinzide Tablets (0.3% to 1%) 1780
Pro-Banthine Tablets 2226
Procardia XL Extended Release Tablets (Less than 3%) 2026
Prolixin 510
Propulsid (1% or less) 1346
ProSom Tablets (Frequent) 457
Protostat Tablets 1939
▲ Prozac Pulvules & Liquid, Oral Solution (5.0% to 12%) 935
RMS Suppositories CII 2766
▲ Redux Capsules (12.5%) 2911
Relafen Tablets (1% to 3%) 2688
▲ Remeron Tablets (25%) 1878
ReVia Tablets (Less than 1%) 957
Revex (nalmefene hydrochloride injection) (Less than 1%) 1863
Rhinocort Nasal Inhaler (1 to 3%) 552
Rilutek Tablets (2.0% to 3.0%) 2198
Robinul Forte Tablets 2247
Robinul Injectable 2247
Robinul Tablets 2247
Rocaltrol Capsules 2303
▲ Romazicon (3% to 9%) 2311
Rondec Oral Drops 974
Rondec Syrup 974
Rondec Tablet 974
Rondec Chewable Tablets 974
Rondec-TR Tablet 974
Roxanol 2365
▲ Rythmol Tablets–150mg, 225mg, 300mg (0.9 to 5.7%) 1399
▲ Sanorex Tablets (Among most common) 2423
Sedapap Tablets 50 mg/650 mg (Infrequent) 1826
▲ Seldane Tablets (2.3% to 4.8%) 1284
▲ Seldane-D Extended-Release Tablets (21.7%) 1286
▲ Semprex-D Capsules (7%) 1620
Ser-Ap-Es Tablets 867
Serentil 689
▲ Serzone Tablets (25%) 776
Sinemet Tablets 959
Sinemet CR Tablets (1.4%) 961
Sinequan 2028
▲ Stadol (3% to 9%) 779
Stelazine 2692
Sular Tablets (Less than or equal to 1%) 2961
Surmontil Capsules (Rare) 2917
Symmetrel Capsules (1% to 5%) 965
Symmetrel Syrup (1% to 5%) 963
Talwin Injection 2465
Tambocor Tablets (Less than 1%) 1555
Tavist Syrup 2426
Tavist Tablets 2427
▲ Tegison Capsules (1-10%) 2314
Tegretol/Tegretol-XR 870
▲ Tenex Tablets (5% to 54%) 2249
Tenoretic Tablets 2963
Thalitone (Common) 1293
Thorazine (Occasional) 2701
THYREL TRH 2992
Tiazac Capsules (Less than 1% to 1%) 1019
Tilade Inhaler (1.0%) 2207
Timoptic in Ocudose (Less frequent) 1796
Timoptic Sterile Ophthalmic Solution (Less frequent) 1794
Timoptic-XE 1798

(▣ Described in PDR For Nonprescription Drugs) Incidence data in parenthesis; ▲ 3% or more (⊙ Described in PDR For Ophthalmology)

Side Effects Index

Tofranil Ampuls 873
Tofranil Tablets 875
Tofranil-PM Capsules 876
Tonocard Tablets (Less than 1%) .. 519
Toprol-XL Tablets (About 1 of 100 patients) 560
Toradol (1% or less) 2319
Torecan 2367
▲ Transderm Scōp Transdermal Therapeutic System (About two-thirds) 890
Tranxene (Less common) 459
Trental Tablets (Less than 1%) 1291
Triavil Tablets 1800
Trilafon 2532
Trinalin Repetabs Tablets 1373
Tussend 1830
▲ Ultram Tablets (50 mg) (5% to 10%) 1594
Univasc Tablets (Less than 1%) 2553
Urised Tablets 2123
Urispas Tablets 2710
Vanceril Inhaler (Few patients) 2538
Vascor Tablets (200 and 300 mg) (0.5 to 3.40%) 1597
Vaseretic Tablets (0.5% to 2.0%) 1810
Vasotec I.V. 1814
Vasotec Tablets (0.5% to 1.0%) 1816
Ventolin Rotacaps for Inhalation (Less than 1%) 1173
Ventolin Tablets (Less than 1%) ... 1176
Verelan Capsules (1% or less) 1455
Videx Tablets, Powder for Oral Solution, & Pediatric Powder for Oral Solution (1% to 4%) 2980
Vistaril Capsules 2042
Vistaril Intramuscular Solution 2042
Vistaril Oral Suspension 2042
Vistide Injection 1057
Vivactil Tablets 1820
Cataflam/Voltaren/Voltaren-XR (Less than 1%) 833
▲ Wellbutrin Tablets (27.6%) 1177
▲ Xanax Tablets (14.7%) 2115
Zaroxolyn Tablets 1625
Zebeta Tablets (0.7% to 1.3%) 1457
Zestoretic Tablets (0.3 to 1%) 2968
Zestril Tablets (0.3% to 1.0%) 2972
Ziac 1459
Zofran Tablets (1% to 2%) 1231
Zoladex (1% or greater) 2976
Zoladex 3-month 2978
▲ Zoloft Tablets (16.3%) 2051
▲ Zonalon Cream (Approximately 1% to 10%) 1042
Zyrtec Tablets (5%) 2053

Y

Yawning

Ambien Tablets (Rare) 2559
Anafranil Capsules (Up to 3%) 819
▲ Effexor (3% to 8%) 2825
Imitrex Injection (Rare) 1095
LUVOX Tablets (2%) 2723
Methadone Hydrochloride Oral Concentrate 2356
▲ Normodyne Injection (3%) 2519
Orlaam Oral Solution (1% to 3%) .. 2361
▲ Paxil Tablets (4%) 2681
▲ Prozac Pulvules & Liquid, Oral Solution (At least 5% to 7%) 935
ReVia Tablets (Less than 1%) 957
Rilutek Tablets (Infrequent) 2198
Risperdal Tablets (Rare) 1348
Salagen Tablets (Less than 1%) 1546
Serzone Tablets (Rare) 776
Tonocard Tablets (Less than 1%) .. 519
▲ Trandate Injection (3 of 100 patients) 1158
Versed Injection (Less than 1%) ... 2324
Zoloft Tablets (1.9%) 2051

(℞ Described in PDR For Nonprescription Drugs)   Incidence data in parenthesis; ▲ 3% or more   (⊚ Described in PDR For Ophthalmology)

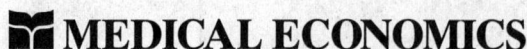

SECTION 4

INDICATIONS INDEX

This section lists in alphabetical order every indication cited in *PDR* and its companion volumes, with cross-references to each product entry in which the indication is found. For easy comparison, each listing includes the product's brand name, generic ingredients, and manufacturer. Page numbers refer to the 1997 editions of *PDR* and *PDR For Ophthalmology* and the 1996 edition of *PDR For Nonprescription Drugs*, which is published later each year. A key to the symbols denoting the companion volumes appears in the bottom margin.

Because *PDR* publishes only official product labeling, only approved indications are cited here. No unapproved uses are listed.

This index is intended to assist you in identifying the extent and nature of your prescribing alternatives as quickly and easily as possible. However, it is by its nature only an extract of the official labeling as it appears in *PDR*. For more definitive information, always consult the underlying *PDR* text.

A

Abdominal cramps
(see under Cramps, abdominal, symptomatic relief of)

Abdominal distention, unspecified
Gas-X Chewable Tablets (Simethicone) Sandoz Consumer .... 🆖 749
Ku-Zyme Capsules (Amylase, Lipase, Cellulase, Protease) Schwarz 2546

Abdominal distress, symptomatic relief of
Kutrase Capsules (Hyoscyamine Sulfate, Phenyltoloxamine Citrate, Amylase, Cellulase, Lipase, Protease) Schwarz 2546
Levsin/Levsinex/Levbid (Hyoscyamine Sulfate) Schwarz 2549

Abortion, inevitable or incomplete, adjunct to
Syntocinon Injection (Oxytocin) Sandoz Pharmaceuticals 2425

Abrasions, pain associated with
(see under Pain, topical relief of)

Abrasions, skin
(see under Infections, skin, bacterial, minor)

Abruptio placentae, to reduce fibrinolytic bleeding
Amicar Syrup, Tablets, and Injection (Aminocaproic Acid) Immunex 1312

Abscess, cutaneous
(see also under Infections, skin and skin structure)
Zosyn (Piperacillin Sodium, Tazobactam Sodium) Lederle 1463

Abscess, hepatic
(see also under Infections, intra-abdominal)
Flagyl 375 Capsules (Metronidazole) Searle 2587
Flagyl I.V. (Metronidazole Hydrochloride) SCS 2373
Mezlin (Mezlocillin Sodium) Bayer Pharmaceutical 594
Mezlin Pharmacy Bulk Package (Mezlocillin Sodium) Bayer Pharmaceutical 597

Abscess, intra-abdominal
(see also under Infections, intra-abdominal)
Cleocin Phosphate Injection (Clindamycin Phosphate) Pharmacia & Upjohn 2068
Flagyl 375 Capsules (Metronidazole) Searle 2587
Flagyl I.V. (Metronidazole Hydrochloride) SCS 2373
Mefoxin (Cefoxitin Sodium) Merck & Co., Inc. 1734
Mefoxin Premixed Intravenous Solution (Cefoxitin Sodium) Merck & Co., Inc. 1737
Mezlin (Mezlocillin Sodium) Bayer Pharmaceutical 594
Mezlin Pharmacy Bulk Package (Mezlocillin Sodium) Bayer Pharmaceutical 597
Netromycin Injection 100 mg/ml (Netilmicin Sulfate) Schering 2516

Abscess, lung
(see also under Infections, lower respiratory tract)
Cleocin Phosphate Injection (Clindamycin Phosphate) Pharmacia & Upjohn 2068
Flagyl 375 Capsules (Metronidazole) Searle 2587
Flagyl I.V. (Metronidazole Hydrochloride) SCS 2373
Mefoxin (Cefoxitin Sodium) Merck & Co., Inc. 1734
Mefoxin Premixed Intravenous Solution (Cefoxitin Sodium) Merck & Co., Inc. 1737
Mezlin (Mezlocillin Sodium) Bayer Pharmaceutical 594
Mezlin Pharmacy Bulk Package (Mezlocillin Sodium) Bayer Pharmaceutical 597
Ticar for Injection (Ticarcillin Disodium) SmithKline Beecham Pharmaceuticals 2704

Abscess, pelvic
Ticar for Injection (Ticarcillin Disodium) SmithKline Beecham Pharmaceuticals 2704

Abscess, tubo-ovarian
(see under Infections, gynecologic)

Accommodation, paralysis of
(see under Cycloplegia, production of)

Aches
(see under Pain, general)

Aches due to common cold
(see under Pain associated with upper respiratory infection)

Aches, muscular
(see under Pain, muscular, temporary relief of)

Acid indigestion
(see under Hyperacidity, gastric, symptomatic relief of)

Acidosis, metabolic
Bicitra (Sodium Citrate, Citric Acid) Baker Norton 573
Polycitra Syrup (Potassium Citrate, Sodium Citrate, Citric Acid) Baker Norton 574
Polycitra-K Crystals (Potassium Citrate, Citric Acid) Baker Norton 574
Polycitra-K Oral Solution (Potassium Citrate, Citric Acid) Baker Norton 575
Polycitra-LC (Potassium Citrate, Citric Acid, Sodium Citrate) Baker Norton 574

Acinetobacter calcoaceticus infections
Minocin Oral Suspension (Minocycline Hydrochloride) Lederle 1431
Primaxin I.M. (Cilastatin Sodium, Imipenem) Merck & Co., Inc. 1770
Rocephin Injectable Vials, ADD-Vantage, Galaxy Container (Ceftriaxone Sodium) Roche Pharmaceuticals 2305
Unasyn (Ampicillin Sodium, Sulbactam Sodium) Pfizer Inc 2035

Acinetobacter calcoaceticus infections, ocular
Chibroxin Sterile Ophthalmic Solution (Norfloxacin) Merck & Co., Inc. 1657

(🆖 Described in PDR For Nonprescription Drugs)   (⊚ Described in PDR For Ophthalmology)

Acinetobacter calcoaceticus infections — Indications Index — 1494

TobraDex Ophthalmic Suspension and Ointment (Dexamethasone, Tobramycin) Alcon Laboratories .. 469

Acinetobacter calcoaceticus skin and skin structure infections

Primaxin I.M. (Cilastatin Sodium, Imipenem) Merck & Co., Inc. 1770
Unasyn (Ampicillin Sodium, Sulbactam Sodium) Pfizer Inc 2035

Acinetobacter species infections

Achromycin V Capsules (Tetracycline Hydrochloride) Lederle 1417
Amikacin Sulfate Injection, USP (Amikacin Sulfate) Astra 523
Amikacin Sulfate Injection, USP (Amikacin Sulfate) Elkins-Sinn 981
Amikin Injectable (Amikacin Sulfate) Apothecon 502
Claforan Sterile and Injection (Cefotaxime Sodium) Hoechst Marion Roussel 1259
Declomycin Tablets (Demeclocycline Hydrochloride) Lederle 1421
Doryx Capsules (Doxycycline Hyclate) Parke-Davis........................ 1970
DYNACIN Capsules (Minocycline Hydrochloride) Medicis 1627
Minocin Intravenous (Minocycline Hydrochloride) Lederle 1428
Minocin Oral Suspension (Minocycline Hydrochloride) Lederle 1431
Minocin Pellet-Filled Capsules (Minocycline Hydrochloride) Lederle 1429
Monodox Capsules (Doxycycline Monohydrate) Oclassen.................. 1858
Primaxin I.M. (Cilastatin Sodium, Imipenem) Merck & Co., Inc. 1770
Primaxin I.V. (Cilastatin Sodium, Imipenem) Merck & Co., Inc. 1772
Terramycin Intramuscular Solution (Oxytetracycline) Pfizer Inc 2034
Vibramycin (Doxycycline Calcium) Pfizer Inc 2038
Vibramycin Hyclate Intravenous (Doxycycline Hyclate) Pfizer Inc.... 2040
Vibramycin (Doxycycline Monohydrate) Pfizer Inc 2038

Acinetobacter species lower respiratory tract infections

Primaxin I.V. (Cilastatin Sodium, Imipenem) Merck & Co., Inc. 1772

Acinetobacter species skin and skin structure infections

Claforan Sterile and Injection (Cefotaxime Sodium) Hoechst Marion Roussel 1259
Primaxin I.M. (Cilastatin Sodium, Imipenem) Merck & Co., Inc. 1770
Primaxin I.V. (Cilastatin Sodium, Imipenem) Merck & Co., Inc. 1772
Rocephin Injectable Vials, ADD-Vantage, Galaxy Container (Ceftriaxone Sodium) Roche Pharmaceuticals 2305

Acne rosacea

Novacet Lotion (Sulfur, Sulfacetamide Sodium) GenDerm 1041
Sulfacet-R Lotion (Sodium Sulfacetamide, Sulfur) Dermik 925
Sulfacet-R Tint Free Lotion (Sodium Sulfacetamide, Sulfur) Dermik 925

Acne rosacea, ocular

AK-PRED (Prednisolone Sodium Phosphate) Akorn .... ⊙ 204
Decadron Phosphate Sterile Ophthalmic Ointment (Dexamethasone Sodium Phosphate) Merck & Co., Inc. 1684
Decadron Phosphate Sterile Ophthalmic Solution (Dexamethasone Sodium Phosphate) Merck & Co., Inc. 1685
Econopred & Econopred Plus Ophthalmic Suspensions (Prednisolone Acetate) Alcon Laboratories .... ⊙ 216

Acne vulgaris

A/T/S 2% Acne Topical Gel (Erythromycin) Hoechst Marion Roussel 1244
A/T/S 2% Acne Topical Solution (Erythromycin) Hoechst Marion Roussel 1244
Azelex (Azelaic Acid) Allergan 471
Benzac (Benzoyl Peroxide) Galderma 1031
Benzamycin Topical Gel (Erythromycin, Benzoyl Peroxide) Dermik 919
BENZASHAVE Medicated Shave Cream 5% and 10% (Benzoyl Peroxide) Medicis................................ 1627
Brevoxyl (Benzoyl Peroxide) Stiefel 2732
Brevoxyl Cleansing Lotion (Benzoyl Peroxide) Stiefel 2732
Cleocin T Topical (Clindamycin Phosphate) Pharmacia & Upjohn 2072
Declomycin Tablets (Demeclocycline Hydrochloride) Lederle 1421
Desquam-E Gel (Benzoyl Peroxide) Westwood-Squibb.............................. 2792
Desquam-X Gel (Benzoyl Peroxide) Westwood-Squibb.............................. 2792
Desquam-X 10 Bar (Benzoyl Peroxide) Westwood-Squibb 2792
Desquam-X Wash (Benzoyl Peroxide) Westwood-Squibb 2792
Differin Gel (Adapalene) Galderma.. 1033
Doryx Capsules (Doxycycline Hyclate) Parke-Davis........................ 1970
Emgel 2% Topical Gel (Erythromycin) Glaxo Wellcome.... 1081
Erycette (erythromycin 2%) Topical Solution (Erythromycin) Ortho Dermatological 1943
Exact (Benzoyl Peroxide) Premier ▣ 722
Monodox Capsules (Doxycycline Monohydrate) Oclassen.................. 1858
Novacet Lotion (Sulfur, Sulfacetamide Sodium) GenDerm 1041
Retin-A (tretinoin) Cream/Gel/Liquid (Tretinoin) Ortho Dermatological 1947
SalAc (Salicylic Acid) GenDerm 1042
Sulfacet-R Lotion (Sodium Sulfacetamide, Sulfur) Dermik 925
Sulfacet-R Tint Free Lotion (Sodium Sulfacetamide, Sulfur) Dermik 925
T-Stat 2.0% Topical Solution and Pads (Erythromycin) Westwood-Squibb.............................. 2797
THERAMYCIN Z 2% Solution (Erythromycin) Medicis 1629
TRIAZ 6% and 10% Gels and 10% Cleanser (Benzoyl Peroxide) Medicis................................ 1629
Vibramycin (Doxycycline Calcium) Pfizer Inc 2038

Acne, cystic, severe recalcitrant

Accutane Capsules (Isotretinoin) Roche Pharmaceuticals 2252

Acne, nodulocystic, adjunctive treatment for

Desquam-X Gel (Benzoyl Peroxide) Westwood-Squibb.............................. 2792

Acne, pustular

Garamycin 0.1% (Gentamicin Sulfate) Schering 2501

Acne, unspecified

Hyland's ClearAc (Homeopathic Medications) Standard Homeopathic.. ▣ 789

Acneiform eruptions, severe, adjunct in

Achromycin V Capsules (Tetracycline Hydrochloride) Lederle 1417
DYNACIN Capsules (Minocycline Hydrochloride) Medicis 1627
Minocin Oral Suspension (Minocycline Hydrochloride) Lederle 1431
Minocin Pellet-Filled Capsules (Minocycline Hydrochloride) Lederle 1429

Acquired immunodeficiency syndrome (see under Infection, human immunodeficiency virus)

Acromegaly

Parlodel (Bromocriptine Mesylate) Sandoz Pharmaceuticals................ 2411
Sandostatin Injection (Octreotide Acetate) Sandoz Pharmaceuticals 2421

ACTH function, hypothalamic-pituitary, testing of (see under Addison's disease, diagnostic testing of)

Actinomyces species infection (see under Actinomycosis)

Actinomycosis

Achromycin V Capsules (Tetracycline Hydrochloride) Lederle 1417
Declomycin Tablets (Demeclocycline Hydrochloride) Lederle 1421
Doryx Capsules (Doxycycline Hyclate) Parke-Davis........................ 1970
DYNACIN Capsules (Minocycline Hydrochloride) Medicis 1627
Minocin Intravenous (Minocycline Hydrochloride) Lederle 1428
Minocin Oral Suspension (Minocycline Hydrochloride) Lederle 1431
Minocin Pellet-Filled Capsules (Minocycline Hydrochloride) Lederle 1429
Monodox Capsules (Doxycycline Monohydrate) Oclassen.................. 1858
Pfizerpen for Injection (Penicillin G Potassium) Pfizer Inc 2022
Terramycin Intramuscular Solution (Oxytetracycline) Pfizer Inc 2034
Vibramycin (Doxycycline Calcium) Pfizer Inc 2038
Vibramycin Hyclate Intravenous (Doxycycline Hyclate) Pfizer Inc.... 2040
Vibramycin (Doxycycline Monohydrate) Pfizer Inc 2038

Adam-Stokes attacks

Isuprel Injection (Isoproterenol Hydrochloride) Sanofi Winthrop .. 2441

Addison's disease (see under Adrenocortical insufficiency)

Adenocarcinoma, gastrointestinal, palliative management of (see under Carcinoma, gastrointestinal, palliative management of)

Adenomas, prolactin-secreting

Parlodel (Bromocriptine Mesylate) Sandoz Pharmaceuticals................ 2411

Adenosine deaminase, enzyme replacement therapy for

Adagen (pegademase bovine) Injection (Pegademase Bovine) Enzon.. 988

Adrenal cortical carcinoma (see under Carcinoma, adrenal cortex)

Adrenal hyperfunction, suppression of (see under Cushing's syndrome)

Adrenal hyperplasia, congenital

Celestone Soluspan Suspension (Betamethasone Sodium Phosphate, Betamethasone Acetate) Schering 2484
Cortone Acetate Sterile Suspension (Cortisone Acetate) Merck & Co., Inc. 1663
Cortone Acetate Tablets (Cortisone Acetate) Merck & Co., Inc. 1664
Dalalone D.P. Injectable (Dexamethasone Acetate) Forest 1009
Decadron Elixir (Dexamethasone) Merck & Co., Inc. 1676
Decadron Phosphate Injection (Dexamethasone Sodium Phosphate) Merck & Co., Inc. 1680
Decadron Tablets (Dexamethasone) Merck & Co., Inc. 1678
Decadron-LA Sterile Suspension (Dexamethasone Acetate) Merck & Co., Inc. 1687
Hydeltrasol Injection, Sterile (Prednisolone Sodium Phosphate) Merck & Co., Inc. 1708
Hydrocortone Phosphate Injection, Sterile (Hydrocortisone Sodium Phosphate) Merck & Co., Inc. 1713
Hydrocortone Tablets (Hydrocortisone) Merck & Co., Inc. 1715
Pediapred Oral Solution (Prednisolone Sodium Phosphate) Medeva 1618
Prelone Syrup (Prednisolone) Muro 1834

Adrenocortical hyperfunction, diagnostic testing of

Decadron Elixir (Dexamethasone) Merck & Co., Inc. 1676
Decadron Phosphate Injection (Dexamethasone Sodium Phosphate) Merck & Co., Inc. 1680
Decadron Tablets (Dexamethasone) Merck & Co., Inc. 1678

Adrenocortical insufficiency

Celestone Soluspan Suspension (Betamethasone Sodium Phosphate, Betamethasone Acetate) Schering 2484
Cortone Acetate Sterile Suspension (Cortisone Acetate) Merck & Co., Inc. 1663
Cortone Acetate Tablets (Cortisone Acetate) Merck & Co., Inc. 1664
Decadron Elixir (Dexamethasone) Merck & Co., Inc. 1676
Decadron Phosphate Injection (Dexamethasone Sodium Phosphate) Merck & Co., Inc. 1680
Decadron Tablets (Dexamethasone) Merck & Co., Inc. 1678
Florinef Acetate Tablets (Fludrocortisone Acetate) Apothecon 506
Hydeltrasol Injection, Sterile (Prednisolone Sodium Phosphate) Merck & Co., Inc. 1708
Hydrocortone Phosphate Injection, Sterile (Hydrocortisone Sodium Phosphate) Merck & Co., Inc. 1713
Hydrocortone Tablets (Hydrocortisone) Merck & Co., Inc. 1715
Pediapred Oral Solution (Prednisolone Sodium Phosphate) Medeva 1618
Prelone Syrup (Prednisolone) Muro 1834

Adrenogenital syndrome, salt-losing

Florinef Acetate Tablets (Fludrocortisone Acetate) Apothecon 506

Adynamic ileus (see under Ileus, paralytic)

Aerobacter aerogenes infections (see under Enterobacter aerogenes infections)

Aeromonas hydrophila infections, ocular

Chibroxin Sterile Ophthalmic Solution (Norfloxacin) Merck & Co., Inc. 1657

Agammaglobulinemias, congenital

Gamimune N, 5% Immune Globulin Intravenous (Human), 5% (Globulin, Immune (Human)) Bayer Biological.................................. 612
Gamimune N, 10% Immune Globulin Intravenous (Human), 10% (Globulin, Immune (Human)) Bayer Biological 615
Gammagard S/D, Immune Globulin, Intravenous (Human) (Globulin, Immune (Human)) Baxter Healthcare 577
Gammar-P I.V., Immune Globulin Intravenous (Human) (Globulin, Immune (Human)) Centeon 798

AIDS (see under Infection, human immunodeficiency virus)

AIDS related complex (see under Infection, acquired immunodeficiency syndrome-related complex)

Airway obstruction disorders (see under Bronchial asthma; Emphysema)

Albinism (see under Hypopigmentation, skin)

Alcohol withdrawal, acute, symptomatic relief of

Dizac (diazepam injectable emulsion) CIV (Diazepam) Ohmeda 1862

(▣ Described in PDR For Nonprescription Drugs) (⊙ Described in PDR For Ophthalmology)

Indications Index — Anemia

1495

Librium Capsules (Chlordiazepoxide Hydrochloride) Roche Products 2331
Librium Injectable (Chlordiazepoxide Hydrochloride) Roche Products 2332
Serax Capsules (Oxazepam) Wyeth-Ayerst 2916
Serax Tablets (Oxazepam) Wyeth-Ayerst 2916
Tranxene (Clorazepate Dipotassium) Abbott 459
Valium Injectable (Diazepam) Roche Products 2336
Valium Tablets (Diazepam) Roche Products 2335
Vistaril Intramuscular Solution (Hydroxyzine Hydrochloride) Pfizer Inc 2042

Alcoholism, acute, amelioration of manifestations of
Serentil (Mesoridazine Besylate) Boehringer Ingelheim 689
Vistaril Intramuscular Solution (Hydroxyzine Hydrochloride) Pfizer Inc 2042

Alcoholism, chronic, an aid in the management of
Antabuse Tablets (Disulfiram) Wyeth-Ayerst 2802
ReVia Tablets (Naltrexone Hydrochloride) DuPont 957
Serentil (Mesoridazine Besylate) Boehringer Ingelheim 689
Vistaril Intramuscular Solution (Hydroxyzine Hydrochloride) Pfizer Inc 2042

Allergic reactions associated with blood or plasma
Benadryl Injection (Diphenhydramine Hydrochloride) Parke-Davis 1955
PBZ Tablets (Tripelennamine Hydrochloride) CibaGeneva 863
PBZ-SR Tablets (Tripelennamine Hydrochloride) CibaGeneva 862
Periactin (Cyproheptadine Hydrochloride) Merck & Co., Inc. 1767
Phenergan Injection (Promethazine Hydrochloride) Wyeth-Ayerst 2880
Phenergan Suppositories (Promethazine Hydrochloride) Wyeth-Ayerst 2882
Phenergan Syrup (Promethazine Hydrochloride) Wyeth-Ayerst 2881
Phenergan Tablets (Promethazine Hydrochloride) Wyeth-Ayerst 2882

Allergic reactions, drug-induced
(see under Hypersensitivity reactions, drug-induced)

Allergic reactions, general
Ana-Kit Anaphylaxis Emergency Treatment Kit (Epinephrine Hydrochloride, Chlorpheniramine Maleate) Bayer Allergy 611
Celestone Soluspan Suspension (Betamethasone Sodium Phosphate, Betamethasone Acetate) Schering 2484
Cortone Acetate Sterile Suspension (Cortisone Acetate) Merck & Co., Inc. 1663
Cortone Acetate Tablets (Cortisone Acetate) Merck & Co., Inc. 1664
Dalalone D.P. Injectable (Dexamethasone Acetate) Forest 1009
Decadron Elixir (Dexamethasone) Merck & Co., Inc. 1676
Decadron Phosphate Injection (Dexamethasone Sodium Phosphate) Merck & Co., Inc. 1680
Decadron Tablets (Dexamethasone) Merck & Co., Inc. 1678
Decadron-LA Sterile Suspension (Dexamethasone Acetate) Merck & Co., Inc. 1687
EpiPen (Epinephrine) Center 808
Hydeltrasol Injection, Sterile (Prednisolone Sodium Phosphate) Merck & Co., Inc. 1708
Hydrocortone Phosphate Injection, Sterile (Hydrocortisone Sodium Phosphate) Merck & Co., Inc. 1713
Hydrocortone Tablets (Hydrocortisone) Merck & Co., Inc. 1715
Pediapred Oral Solution (Prednisolone Sodium Phosphate) Medeva 1618
Phenergan Injection (Promethazine Hydrochloride) Wyeth-Ayerst 2880
Prelone Syrup (Prednisolone) Muro 1834
Vistaril Intramuscular Solution (Hydroxyzine Hydrochloride) Pfizer Inc 2042

Allergic rhinitis
(see under Rhinitis, allergic)

Allescheriosis
(see under Pseudoallescheriosis)

Alopecia areata
Celestone Soluspan Suspension (Betamethasone Sodium Phosphate, Betamethasone Acetate) Schering 2484
Decadron Phosphate Injection (Dexamethasone Sodium Phosphate) Merck & Co., Inc. 1680
Decadron-LA Sterile Suspension (Dexamethasone Acetate) Merck & Co., Inc. 1687
Hydeltrasol Injection, Sterile (Prednisolone Sodium Phosphate) Merck & Co., Inc. 1708
Hydrocortone Acetate Sterile Suspension (Hydrocortisone Acetate) Merck & Co., Inc. 1712

Alzheimer's disease
(see under Dementia, Alzheimer's type)

Amebiasis, acute intestinal
E.E.S. (Erythromycin Ethylsuccinate) Abbott 427
E-Mycin Tablets (Erythromycin) Knoll Laboratories 1388
ERYC (Erythromycin) Parke-Davis 1972
EryPed (Erythromycin Ethylsuccinate) Abbott 425
Ery-Tab Tablets (Erythromycin) Abbott 426
Erythrocin Stearate Filmtab (Erythromycin Stearate) Abbott 429
Erythromycin Base Filmtab (Erythromycin) Abbott 430
Erythromycin Delayed-Release Capsules, USP (Erythromycin) Abbott 431
Flagyl 375 Capsules (Metronidazole) Searle 2587
Ilosone (Erythromycin Estolate) Dista 927
PCE Dispertab Tablets (Erythromycin) Abbott 453
Protostat Tablets (Metronidazole) Ortho Pharmaceutical 1939
Terramycin Intramuscular Solution (Oxytetracycline) Pfizer Inc 2034
Yodoxin Tablets (Iodoquinol) Glenwood-Palisades 1235

Amebiasis, acute intestinal, adjunct in
Achromycin V Capsules (Tetracycline Hydrochloride) Lederle 1417
Declomycin Tablets (Demeclocycline Hydrochloride) Lederle 1421
Doryx Capsules (Doxycycline Hyclate) Parke-Davis 1970
DYNACIN Capsules (Minocycline Hydrochloride) Medicis 1627
Minocin Intravenous (Minocycline Hydrochloride) Lederle 1428
Minocin Oral Suspension (Minocycline Hydrochloride) Lederle 1431
Minocin Pellet-Filled Capsules (Minocycline Hydrochloride) Lederle 1429
Monodox Capsules (Doxycycline Monohydrate) Oclassen 1858
Vibramycin (Doxycycline Calcium) Pfizer Inc 2038
Vibramycin Hyclate Intravenous (Doxycycline Hyclate) Pfizer Inc 2040
Vibramycin (Doxycycline Monohydrate) Pfizer Inc 2038

Amebiasis, extraintestinal
Aralen Hydrochloride Injection (Chloroquine Hydrochloride) Sanofi Winthrop 2430
Aralen Phosphate Tablets (Chloroquine Phosphate) Sanofi Winthrop 2431

Amebic liver abscess
Flagyl 375 Capsules (Metronidazole) Searle 2587
Protostat Tablets (Metronidazole) Ortho Pharmaceutical 1939

Amenorrhea-galactorrhea syndrome
Parlodel (Bromocriptine Mesylate) Sandoz Pharmaceuticals 2411

Amenorrhea, primary, hypothalamic
Lutrepulse for Injection (Gonadorelin Acetate) Ferring 998

Amenorrhea, secondary
Amen Tablets (Medroxyprogesterone Acetate) Carnrick 785
Aygestin Tablets (Norethindrone Acetate) ESI Lederle 990
Cycrin Tablets (Medroxyprogesterone Acetate) ESI Lederle 991
Provera Tablets (Medroxyprogesterone Acetate) Pharmacia & Upjohn 2110

Amyotrophic lateral sclerosis
(see under Sclerosis, amyotrophic lateral)

Analgesia
(see under Pain, general)

Anaphylactic reactions, adjunctive therapy in
Benadryl Injection (Diphenhydramine Hydrochloride) Parke-Davis 1955
PBZ Tablets (Tripelennamine Hydrochloride) CibaGeneva 863
PBZ-SR Tablets (Tripelennamine Hydrochloride) CibaGeneva 862
Periactin (Cyproheptadine Hydrochloride) Merck & Co., Inc. 1767
Phenergan Injection (Promethazine Hydrochloride) Wyeth-Ayerst 2880
Phenergan Suppositories (Promethazine Hydrochloride) Wyeth-Ayerst 2882
Phenergan Syrup (Promethazine Hydrochloride) Wyeth-Ayerst 2881
Phenergan Tablets (Promethazine Hydrochloride) Wyeth-Ayerst 2882

Anaphylactic shock, due to insect bite
Ana-Kit Anaphylaxis Emergency Treatment Kit (Epinephrine Hydrochloride, Chlorpheniramine Maleate) Bayer Allergy 611

Anaphylactoid reactions
Ana-Kit Anaphylaxis Emergency Treatment Kit (Epinephrine Hydrochloride, Chlorpheniramine Maleate) Bayer Allergy 611
EpiPen (Epinephrine) Center 808

Anaphylaxis, idiopathic
Ana-Kit Anaphylaxis Emergency Treatment Kit (Epinephrine Hydrochloride, Chlorpheniramine Maleate) Bayer Allergy 611
EpiPen (Epinephrine) Center 808

Anaphylaxis, treatment of
Ana-Kit Anaphylaxis Emergency Treatment Kit (Epinephrine Hydrochloride, Chlorpheniramine Maleate) Bayer Allergy 611
EpiPen (Epinephrine) Center 808

Ancylostoma duodenale infections
Mintezol (Thiabendazole) Merck & Co., Inc. 1747
Vermox Chewable Tablets (Mebendazole) Janssen 1357

Androgen, absence or deficiency of
Androderm Testosterone Transdermal System (Testosterone) SmithKline Beecham Pharmaceuticals 2634
Android Capsules, 10 mg (Methyltestosterone) ICN 1297
Halotestin Tablets (Fluoxymesterone) Pharmacia & Upjohn 2095

Anemia associated with chronic renal failure
Epogen for Injection (Epoetin Alfa) Amgen 489
Procrit for Injection (Epoetin Alfa) Ortho Biotech 1896

Anemia, chemotherapy-induced in cancer patients
Epogen for Injection (Epoetin Alfa) Amgen 489
Procrit for Injection (Epoetin Alfa) Ortho Biotech 1896

Anemia, hemolytic, acquired
Celestone Soluspan Suspension (Betamethasone Sodium Phosphate, Betamethasone Acetate) Schering 2484
Cortone Acetate Sterile Suspension (Cortisone Acetate) Merck & Co., Inc. 1663
Cortone Acetate Tablets (Cortisone Acetate) Merck & Co., Inc. 1664
Dalalone D.P. Injectable (Dexamethasone Acetate) Forest 1009
Decadron Elixir (Dexamethasone) Merck & Co., Inc. 1676
Decadron Phosphate Injection (Dexamethasone Sodium Phosphate) Merck & Co., Inc. 1680
Decadron Tablets (Dexamethasone) Merck & Co., Inc. 1678
Decadron-LA Sterile Suspension (Dexamethasone Acetate) Merck & Co., Inc. 1687
Hydeltrasol Injection, Sterile (Prednisolone Sodium Phosphate) Merck & Co., Inc. 1708
Hydrocortone Phosphate Injection, Sterile (Hydrocortisone Sodium Phosphate) Merck & Co., Inc. 1713
Hydrocortone Tablets (Hydrocortisone) Merck & Co., Inc. 1715
Pediapred Oral Solution (Prednisolone Sodium Phosphate) Medeva 1618
Prelone Syrup (Prednisolone) Muro 1834

Anemia, hypoplastic, congenital
Celestone Soluspan Suspension (Betamethasone Sodium Phosphate, Betamethasone Acetate) Schering 2484
Cortone Acetate Sterile Suspension (Cortisone Acetate) Merck & Co., Inc. 1663
Cortone Acetate Tablets (Cortisone Acetate) Merck & Co., Inc. 1664
Dalalone D.P. Injectable (Dexamethasone Acetate) Forest 1009
Decadron Elixir (Dexamethasone) Merck & Co., Inc. 1676
Decadron Phosphate Injection (Dexamethasone Sodium Phosphate) Merck & Co., Inc. 1680
Decadron Tablets (Dexamethasone) Merck & Co., Inc. 1678
Decadron-LA Sterile Suspension (Dexamethasone Acetate) Merck & Co., Inc. 1687
Hydeltrasol Injection, Sterile (Prednisolone Sodium Phosphate) Merck & Co., Inc. 1708
Hydrocortone Phosphate Injection, Sterile (Hydrocortisone Sodium Phosphate) Merck & Co., Inc. 1713
Hydrocortone Tablets (Hydrocortisone) Merck & Co., Inc. 1715
Pediapred Oral Solution (Prednisolone Sodium Phosphate) Medeva 1618
Prelone Syrup (Prednisolone) Muro 1834

Anemia, iron deficiency
Chromagen Capsules (Ferrous Fumarate, Vitamin C, Vitamin B_{12}) Savage 2470
Chromagen FA (Ascorbic Acid, Cyanocobalamin, Ferrous Fumarate, Folic Acid) Savage 2471
Chromagen Forte (Ascorbic Acid, Cyanocobalamin, Ferrous Fumarate, Folic Acid) Savage 2471
Feosol Caplets (Iron) SmithKline Beecham 2626
Feosol Capsules (Ferrous Sulfate) SmithKline Beecham Consumer 777
Feosol Elixir (Ferrous Sulfate) SmithKline Beecham 2627
Feosol Tablets (Ferrous Sulfate) SmithKline Beecham 2627
Fero-Grad-500 Filmtab (Ferrous Sulfate, Vitamin C) Abbott 434

(■ Described in PDR For Nonprescription Drugs)   (◉ Described in PDR For Ophthalmology)

Anemia

Anemia
- Fero-Gradumet Filmtab (Ferrous Sulfate) Abbott ... 434
- Iberet Tablets (Vitamin B Complex With Vitamin C, Ferrous Sulfate) Abbott ... 437
- Iberet (Vitamin B Complex With Vitamin C, Ferrous Sulfate) Abbott ... 438
- May-Vita Elixir (Vitamins with Minerals) Merz ... 1826
- Niferex-150 Capsules (Polysaccharide-Iron Complex) Central ... 811
- Niferex (Polysaccharide-Iron Complex) Central ... 811
- Nu-Iron 150 Capsules (Polysaccharide-Iron Complex) Merz ... 1826
- Nu-Iron Elixir (Polysaccharide-Iron Complex) Merz ... 1826
- Slow Fe Tablets (Ferrous Sulfate) Ciba Self-Medication ... 889
- Slow Fe with Folic Acid (Ferrous Sulfate, Folic Acid) Ciba Self-Medication ... 890
- Trinsicon Capsules (Vitamins with Iron) UCB ... 2759
- Vitron-C Tablets (Ferrous Fumarate, Vitamin C) Ciba Self-Medication ... [NP] 667

Anemia, megaloblastic, due to folic acid deficiency
- Leucovorin Calcium for Injection, Wellcovorin Brand (Leucovorin Calcium) Glaxo Wellcome Oncology/HIV ... 1203
- Leucovorin Calcium for Injection (Leucovorin Calcium) Immunex ... 1313

Anemia, pernicious
- Trinsicon Capsules (Vitamins with Iron) UCB ... 2759

Anemia, AZT-treated HIV-infected patients, treatment of
- Epogen for Injection (Epoetin Alfa) Amgen ... 489
- Procrit for Injection (Epoetin Alfa) Ortho Biotech ... 1896

Anemia, RBC (see under Erythroblastopenia)

Anemia, uterine leiomyomata-induced, preoperative adjunct
- Lupron Depot 3.75 mg (Leuprolide Acetate) TAP ... 2739

Anesthesia, general
- Alfenta Injection (Alfentanil Hydrochloride) Janssen ... 1334
- Diprivan Injectable Emulsion (Propofol) Zeneca ... 2939
- Fluothane (Halothane) Wyeth-Ayerst ... 2830
- Sublimaze Injection (Fentanyl Citrate) Akorn ... 463
- Sufenta Injection (Sufentanil Citrate) Janssen ... 1355
- Suprane (desflurane, USP) (Desflurane) Ohmeda ... 1865
- Versed Injection (Midazolam Hydrochloride) Roche Pharmaceuticals ... 2324

Anesthesia, general, adjunct in
- Alfenta Injection (Alfentanil Hydrochloride) Janssen ... 1334
- Anectine (Succinylcholine Chloride) Glaxo Wellcome ... 1062
- Atarax Tablets & Syrup (Hydroxyzine Hydrochloride) Pfizer Inc ... 1992
- Ativan Injection (Lorazepam) Wyeth-Ayerst ... 2805
- Demerol (Meperidine Hydrochloride) Sanofi Winthrop ... 2438
- Inapsine Injection (Droperidol) Akorn ... 462
- Levsin Injection (Hyoscyamine Sulfate) Schwarz ... 2549
- Mepergan Injection (Meperidine Hydrochloride, Promethazine Hydrochloride) Wyeth-Ayerst ... 2859
- Metubine Iodide Vials (Metocurine Iodide) Dista ... 932
- Mivacron (Mivacurium Chloride) Glaxo Wellcome ... 1125
- Nembutal Sodium Capsules (Pentobarbital Sodium) Abbott ... 440
- Nembutal Sodium Solution (Pentobarbital Sodium) Abbott ... 442
- Nimbex Injection (Cisatracurium Besylate) Glaxo Wellcome ... 1131
- Norcuron for Injection (Vecuronium Bromide) Organon ... 1875
- Nubain Injection (Nalbuphine Hydrochloride) DuPont ... 952
- Numorphan Injection (Oxymorphone Hydrochloride) DuPont ... 953
- Nuromax Injection (Doxacurium Chloride) Glaxo Wellcome ... 1136
- Phenergan Injection (Promethazine Hydrochloride) Wyeth-Ayerst ... 2880
- Phenergan Suppositories (Promethazine Hydrochloride) Wyeth-Ayerst ... 2882
- Phenergan Syrup (Promethazine Hydrochloride) Wyeth-Ayerst ... 2881
- Phenergan Tablets (Promethazine Hydrochloride) Wyeth-Ayerst ... 2882
- Robinul Injectable (Glycopyrrolate) Robins ... 2247
- Seconal Sodium Pulvules (Secobarbital Sodium) Lilly ... 1529
- Sublimaze Injection (Fentanyl Citrate) Akorn ... 463
- Talwin Injection (Pentazocine Lactate) Sanofi Winthrop ... 2465
- Thorazine (Chlorpromazine Hydrochloride) SmithKline Beecham Pharmaceuticals ... 2701
- Tracrium Injection (Atracurium Besylate) Glaxo Wellcome ... 1155
- Vasoxyl Injection (Methoxamine Hydrochloride) Glaxo Wellcome ... 1169
- Versed Injection (Midazolam Hydrochloride) Roche Pharmaceuticals ... 2324
- Zemuron Injection (Rocuronium Bromide) Organon ... 1885

Anesthesia, general, supplement to (see under Anesthesia, general, adjunct in)

Anesthesia, local
- Americaine Anesthetic Lubricant (Benzocaine) Medeva ... 1603
- Carbocaine Injection (Mepivacaine Hydrochloride Injection) Sanofi Winthrop ... 2432
- Cocaine Hydrochloride Topical Solutions (Cocaine Hydrochloride) Astra ... 529
- Duranest Injections (Etidocaine Hydrochloride) Astra ... 533
- Dyclone 0.5% and 1% Topical Solutions, USP (Dyclonine Hydrochloride) Astra ... 535
- Marcaine (Bupivacaine Hydrochloride, Epinephrine) Sanofi Winthrop ... 2446
- Nescaine/Nescaine MPF (Chloroprocaine Hydrochloride) Astra ... 549
- Sensorcaine (Bupivacaine Hydrochloride, Epinephrine Bitartrate) Astra ... 554
- Xylocaine Injections (Lidocaine Hydrochloride) Astra ... 562

Anesthesia, local, adjunct in
- Diprivan Injectable Emulsion (Propofol) Zeneca ... 2939
- Levsin Injection (Hyoscyamine Sulfate) Schwarz ... 2549
- Mepergan Injection (Meperidine Hydrochloride, Promethazine Hydrochloride) Wyeth-Ayerst ... 2859
- Neo-Synephrine Hydrochloride 1% Carpuject (Phenylephrine Hydrochloride) Sanofi Winthrop ... 2455
- Neo-Synephrine Hydrochloride 1% Injection (Phenylephrine Hydrochloride) Sanofi Winthrop ... 2455
- Phenergan Injection (Promethazine Hydrochloride) Wyeth-Ayerst ... 2880

Anesthesia, local, diagnostic procedures
- Marcaine (Bupivacaine Hydrochloride, Epinephrine) Sanofi Winthrop ... 2446
- Sensorcaine (Bupivacaine Hydrochloride, Epinephrine Bitartrate) Astra ... 554

Anesthesia, local, laryngeal
- Cocaine Hydrochloride Topical Solutions (Cocaine Hydrochloride) Astra ... 529

Anesthesia, local, nasal cavities
- Cocaine Hydrochloride Topical Solutions (Cocaine Hydrochloride) Astra ... 529

Anesthesia, local, obstetrical procedures
- Americaine Anesthetic Lubricant (Benzocaine) Medeva ... 1603
- Marcaine (Bupivacaine Hydrochloride, Epinephrine) Sanofi Winthrop ... 2446
- Sensorcaine (Bupivacaine Hydrochloride, Epinephrine Bitartrate) Astra ... 554

Anesthesia, local, ocular
- FLUORACAINE (Fluorescein Sodium, Proparacaine Hydrochloride) Akorn ... [O] 208
- Ophthetic (Proparacaine Hydrochloride) Allergan ... [O] 244

Anesthesia, local, oral cavity
- Cocaine Hydrochloride Topical Solutions (Cocaine Hydrochloride) Astra ... 529
- Dyclone 0.5% and 1% Topical Solutions, USP (Dyclonine Hydrochloride) Astra ... 535

Anesthesia, local, oral surgical procedures
- Marcaine (Bupivacaine Hydrochloride, Epinephrine) Sanofi Winthrop ... 2446
- Sensorcaine (Bupivacaine Hydrochloride, Epinephrine Bitartrate) Astra ... 554

Anesthesia, local, pharyngeal
- Americaine Anesthetic Lubricant (Benzocaine) Medeva ... 1603
- Dyclone 0.5% and 1% Topical Solutions, USP (Dyclonine Hydrochloride) Astra ... 535

Anesthesia, local, spinal
- Marcaine Spinal (Bupivacaine Hydrochloride) Sanofi Winthrop ... 2449
- Novocain Hydrochloride for Spinal Anesthesia (Procaine Hydrochloride) Sanofi Winthrop ... 2457
- Sensorcaine (Bupivacaine Hydrochloride, Epinephrine Bitartrate) Astra ... 554

Anesthesia, local, spinal, adjunct in
- Neo-Synephrine Hydrochloride 1% Carpuject (Phenylephrine Hydrochloride) Sanofi Winthrop ... 2455
- Neo-Synephrine Hydrochloride 1% Injection (Phenylephrine Hydrochloride) Sanofi Winthrop ... 2455

Anesthesia, local, surgical procedures
- Marcaine (Bupivacaine Hydrochloride, Epinephrine) Sanofi Winthrop ... 2446
- Sensorcaine (Bupivacaine Hydrochloride, Epinephrine Bitartrate) Astra ... 554

Anesthesia, local, therapeutic procedures
- Marcaine (Bupivacaine Hydrochloride, Epinephrine) Sanofi Winthrop ... 2446
- Sensorcaine (Bupivacaine Hydrochloride, Epinephrine Bitartrate) Astra ... 554

Anesthesia, regional
- Carbocaine Injection (Mepivacaine Hydrochloride Injection) Sanofi Winthrop ... 2432
- Marcaine (Bupivacaine Hydrochloride, Epinephrine) Sanofi Winthrop ... 2446
- Sensorcaine (Bupivacaine Hydrochloride, Epinephrine Bitartrate) Astra ... 554
- Xylocaine Injections (Lidocaine Hydrochloride) Astra ... 562

Anesthesia, regional, adjunct in
- Diprivan Injectable Emulsion (Propofol) Zeneca ... 2939
- Inapsine Injection (Droperidol) Akorn ... 462
- Neo-Synephrine Hydrochloride 1% Carpuject (Phenylephrine Hydrochloride) Sanofi Winthrop ... 2455
- Neo-Synephrine Hydrochloride 1% Injection (Phenylephrine Hydrochloride) Sanofi Winthrop ... 2455
- Sublimaze Injection (Fentanyl Citrate) Akorn ... 463

Anesthesia, spinal
- Pontocaine Hydrochloride for Spinal Anesthesia (Tetracaine Hydrochloride) Sanofi Winthrop ... 2460

Anesthesia care sedation, monitored
- Alfenta Injection (Alfentanil Hydrochloride) Janssen ... 1334
- Diprivan Injectable Emulsion (Propofol) Zeneca ... 2939

Angina (see under Angina pectoris)

Angina pectoris
- Adalat Capsules (10 mg and 20 mg) (Nifedipine) Bayer Pharmaceutical ... 580
- Calan Tablets (Verapamil Hydrochloride) Searle ... 2568
- Cardizem Tablets (Diltiazem Hydrochloride) Hoechst Marion Roussel ... 1257
- Covera-HS Tablets (Verapamil Hydrochloride) Searle ... 2573
- Dilatrate-SR Capsules (Isosorbide Dinitrate) Schwarz ... 2542
- Imdur (Isosorbide Mononitrate) Key ... 1362
- Inderal (Propranolol Hydrochloride) Wyeth-Ayerst ... 2834
- Inderal LA Long Acting Capsules (Propranolol Hydrochloride) Wyeth-Ayerst ... 2836
- Ismo Tablets (Isosorbide Mononitrate) Wyeth-Ayerst ... 2844
- Isoptin Oral Tablets (Verapamil Hydrochloride) Knoll Laboratories ... 1393
- Isordil Tembids (Isosorbide Dinitrate) Wyeth-Ayerst ... 2847
- Isordil Titradose Tablets (Isosorbide Dinitrate) Wyeth-Ayerst ... 2848
- Lopressor (Metoprolol Tartrate) CibaGeneva ... 848
- Monoket Tablets (Isosorbide Mononitrate) Schwarz ... 2550
- Nitro-Bid IV (Nitroglycerin) Hoechst Marion Roussel ... 1270
- Nitro-Bid Ointment (Nitroglycerin) Hoechst Marion Roussel ... 1272
- Nitro-Dur (nitroglycerin) Transdermal Infusion System (Nitroglycerin) Key ... 1365
- Nitrolingual Spray (Nitroglycerin) Rhone-Poulenc Rorer Pharmaceuticals ... 2193
- Procardia Capsules (Nifedipine) Pfizer Inc ... 2024
- Sorbitrate (Isosorbide Dinitrate) Zeneca ... 2959
- Tenormin Tablets and I.V. Injection (Atenolol) Zeneca ... 2965
- Toprol-XL Tablets (Metoprolol Succinate) Astra ... 560
- Transderm-Nitro Transdermal Therapeutic System (Nitroglycerin) CibaGeneva ... 878

Angina pectoris, acute, prophylaxis
- Isordil Sublingual Tablets (Isosorbide Dinitrate) Wyeth-Ayerst ... 2845
- Nitrolingual Spray (Nitroglycerin) Rhone-Poulenc Rorer Pharmaceuticals ... 2193
- Nitrostat Tablets (Nitroglycerin) Parke-Davis ... 1981

Angina pectoris, "conditionally" approved in
- Deponit NTG Transdermal Delivery System (Nitroglycerin) Schwarz ... 2541

Angina, chronic stable
- Adalat Capsules (10 mg and 20 mg) (Nifedipine) Bayer Pharmaceutical ... 580
- Calan Tablets (Verapamil Hydrochloride) Searle ... 2568
- Cardene Capsules (Nicardipine Hydrochloride) Roche Pharmaceuticals ... 2261

([NP] Described in PDR For Nonprescription Drugs)   ([O] Described in PDR For Ophthalmology)

Indications Index

Cardizem CD Capsules (Diltiazem Hydrochloride) Hoechst Marion Roussel ... 1251
Cardizem Tablets (Diltiazem Hydrochloride) Hoechst Marion Roussel ... 1257
Dilacor XR Extended-release Capsules (Diltiazem Hydrochloride) Rhone-Poulenc Rorer Pharmaceuticals ... 2183
Inderal Tablets (Propranolol Hydrochloride) Wyeth-Ayerst ... 2834
Isoptin Oral Tablets (Verapamil Hydrochloride) Knoll Laboratories ... 1393
Norvasc Tablets (Amlodipine Besylate) Pfizer Inc ... 2020
Procardia Capsules (Nifedipine) Pfizer Inc ... 2024
Procardia XL Extended Release Tablets (Nifedipine) Pfizer Inc ... 2026
Vascor Tablets (200 and 300 mg) (Bepridil Hydrochloride) McNeil Pharmaceutical ... 1597

Angina, classic effort-associated
(see under Angina, chronic stable)

Angina, crescendo
(see under Angina, unstable)

Angina, pre-infarction
(see under Angina, unstable)

Angina, Prinzmetal's
Adalat Capsules (10 mg and 20 mg) (Nifedipine) Bayer Pharmaceutical ... 580
Calan Tablets (Verapamil Hydrochloride) Searle ... 2568
Isoptin Oral Tablets (Verapamil Hydrochloride) Knoll Laboratories ... 1393
Norvasc Tablets (Amlodipine Besylate) Pfizer Inc ... 2020
Procardia Capsules (Nifedipine) Pfizer Inc ... 2024
Procardia XL Extended Release Tablets (Nifedipine) Pfizer Inc ... 2026

Angina, unstable
Calan Tablets (Verapamil Hydrochloride) Searle ... 2568
Isoptin Oral Tablets (Verapamil Hydrochloride) Knoll Laboratories ... 1393
Procardia Capsules (Nifedipine) Pfizer Inc ... 2024

Angina, variant
(see under Angina, Prinzmetal's)

Angina, vasospastic
(see under Angina, Prinzmetal's)

Angioedema, adjunctive therapy in
Extendryl (Chlorpheniramine Maleate, Methscopolamine Nitrate, Phenylephrine Hydrochloride) Fleming ... 1003
PBZ Tablets (Tripelennamine Hydrochloride) CibaGeneva ... 863
PBZ-SR Tablets (Tripelennamine Hydrochloride) CibaGeneva ... 862
Periactin (Cyproheptadine Hydrochloride) Merck & Co., Inc. 1767
Phenergan Suppositories (Promethazine Hydrochloride) Wyeth-Ayerst ... 2882
Phenergan Syrup (Promethazine Hydrochloride) Wyeth-Ayerst ... 2881
Phenergan Tablets (Promethazine Hydrochloride) Wyeth-Ayerst ... 2882
Tavist Syrup (Clemastine Fumarate) Sandoz Pharmaceuticals ... 2426
Tavist Tablets (Clemastine Fumarate) Sandoz Pharmaceuticals ... 2427

Angioedema, hereditary
Danocrine Capsules (Danazol) Sanofi Winthrop ... 2437
Winstrol Tablets (Stanozolol) Sanofi Winthrop ... 2468

Angiography, fluorescein, fundus
AK-FLUOR Injection 10% and 25% (Fluorescein Sodium) Akorn ... ⊚ 204

Fluorescite (Fluorescein Sodium) Alcon Laboratories ... ⊚ 217

Angiography, fluorescein, iris vasculature
AK-FLUOR Injection 10% and 25% (Fluorescein Sodium) Akorn ... ⊚ 204
Fluorescite (Fluorescein Sodium) Alcon Laboratories ... ⊚ 217

Ankylosing spondylitis
Anaprox/Naprosyn (Naproxen Sodium) Roche Pharmaceuticals.. 2277
Extra Strength Bayer Arthritis Pain Regimen Formula (Aspirin, Enteric Coated) Bayer Consumer ... ⊞ 615
Cataflam Tablets (Diclofenac Potassium) CibaGeneva ... 833
Celestone Soluspan Suspension (Betamethasone Sodium Phosphate, Betamethasone Acetate) Schering ... 2484
Clinoril Tablets (Sulindac) Merck & Co., Inc. ... 1658
Cortone Acetate Sterile Suspension (Cortisone Acetate) Merck & Co., Inc. ... 1663
Cortone Acetate Tablets (Cortisone Acetate) Merck & Co., Inc. ... 1664
Dalalone D.P. Injectable (Dexamethasone Acetate) Forest ... 1009
Decadron Elixir (Dexamethasone) Merck & Co., Inc. ... 1676
Decadron Phosphate Injection (Dexamethasone Sodium Phosphate) Merck & Co., Inc. ... 1680
Decadron Tablets (Dexamethasone) Merck & Co., Inc. ... 1678
Decadron-LA Sterile Suspension (Dexamethasone Acetate) Merck & Co., Inc. ... 1687
EC-Naprosyn Delayed-Release Tablets (Naproxen) Roche Pharmaceuticals ... 2277
Ecotrin (Aspirin) SmithKline Beecham ... 2625
Hydeltrasol Injection, Sterile (Prednisolone Sodium Phosphate) Merck & Co., Inc. ... 1708
Hydrocortone Phosphate Injection, Sterile (Hydrocortisone Sodium Phosphate) Merck & Co., Inc. ... 1713
Hydrocortone Tablets (Hydrocortisone) Merck & Co., Inc. ... 1715
Indocin (Indomethacin) Merck & Co., Inc. ... 1723
Naprelan Tablets (Naproxen Sodium) Wyeth-Ayerst ... 2861
Anaprox/Naprosyn (Naproxen) Roche Pharmaceuticals ... 2277
Pediapred Oral Solution (Prednisolone Sodium Phosphate) Medeva 1618
Prelone Syrup (Prednisolone) Muro 1834
Traumeel Injection Solution (Homeopathic Medications) Heel/BHI 1237
Voltaren Tablets (Diclofenac Sodium) CibaGeneva ... 833

Anorexia associated with weight loss, AIDS-induced
Marinol (Dronabinol) Capsules (Dronabinol) Roxane ... 2353
Megace Oral Suspension (Megestrol Acetate) Bristol-Myers Squibb Oncology/Immunology ... 708

Anterior segment inflammation
(see under Inflammation, anterior segment)

Anthrax
(see under B. anthracis infections)

Anticholinesterase drugs, overdosage, treatment of
Levsin/Levsinex/Levbid (Hyoscyamine Sulfate) Schwarz ... 2549
Protopam Chloride for Injection (Pralidoxime Chloride) Wyeth-Ayerst ... 2909

Antithrombin III deficiency, hereditary
THROMBATE III Antithrombin III (Human) (Antithrombin III) Bayer Biological ... 631

Anxiety and tension due to menopause
(see under Menopause, management of the manifestations of)

Anxiety disorders, management of
Ativan Tablets (Lorazepam) Wyeth-Ayerst ... 2807
BuSpar Tablets (Buspirone Hydrochloride) Bristol-Myers Squibb ... 738
Dizac (diazepam injectable emulsion) CIV (Diazepam) Ohmeda ... 1862
Etrafon (Perphenazine, Amitriptyline Hydrochloride) Schering ... 2495
Librium Capsules (Chlordiazepoxide Hydrochloride) Roche Products ... 2331
Librium Injectable (Chlordiazepoxide Hydrochloride) Roche Products ... 2332
Mebaral Tablets (Mephobarbital) Sanofi Winthrop ... 2452
Miltown Tablets (Meprobamate) Wallace ... 2780
Phenergan Injection (Promethazine Hydrochloride) Wyeth-Ayerst ... 2880
Phenergan Suppositories (Promethazine Hydrochloride) Wyeth-Ayerst ... 2882
Phenergan Syrup (Promethazine Hydrochloride) Wyeth-Ayerst ... 2881
Phenergan Tablets (Promethazine Hydrochloride) Wyeth-Ayerst ... 2882
Serax Capsules (Oxazepam) Wyeth-Ayerst ... 2916
Serax Tablets (Oxazepam) Wyeth-Ayerst ... 2916
Trancopal Caplets (Chlormezanone) Sanofi Winthrop ... 2468
Tranxene (Clorazepate Dipotassium) Abbott ... 459
Valium Injectable (Diazepam) Roche Products ... 2336
Valium Tablets (Diazepam) Roche Products ... 2335
Vistaril Intramuscular Solution (Hydroxyzine Hydrochloride) Pfizer Inc ... 2042
Xanax Tablets (Alprazolam) Pharmacia & Upjohn ... 2115

Anxiety, generalized non-psychotic, short-term treatment of
Compazine (Prochlorperazine) SmithKline Beecham Pharmaceuticals ... 2644
Stelazine (Trifluoperazine Hydrochloride) SmithKline Beecham Pharmaceuticals ... 2692

Anxiety, mental depression-induced
Adapin (Doxepin Hydrochloride) Lotus ... 1542
Ativan Tablets (Lorazepam) Wyeth-Ayerst ... 2807
Etrafon (Perphenazine, Amitriptyline Hydrochloride) Schering ... 2495
Limbitrol (Chlordiazepoxide, Amitriptyline Hydrochloride) Roche Products ... 2333
Ludiomil Tablets (Maprotiline Hydrochloride) CibaGeneva ... 861
Mellaril (Thioridazine Hydrochloride) Sandoz Pharmaceuticals ... 2398
Serax Capsules (Oxazepam) Wyeth-Ayerst ... 2916
Serax Tablets (Oxazepam) Wyeth-Ayerst ... 2916
Sinequan (Doxepin Hydrochloride) Pfizer Inc ... 2028
Triavil Tablets (Perphenazine, Amitriptyline Hydrochloride) Merck & Co., Inc. ... 1800
Vistaril Intramuscular Solution (Hydroxyzine Hydrochloride) Pfizer Inc ... 2042
Xanax Tablets (Alprazolam) Pharmacia & Upjohn ... 2115

Anxiety, preoperative
Ativan Injection (Lorazepam) Wyeth-Ayerst ... 2805
Dizac (diazepam injectable emulsion) CIV (Diazepam) Ohmeda ... 1862

Inapsine Injection (Droperidol) Akorn ... 462
Levoprome (Methotrimeprazine) Immunex ... 1321
Librium Capsules (Chlordiazepoxide Hydrochloride) Roche Products ... 2331
Librium Injectable (Chlordiazepoxide Hydrochloride) Roche Products ... 2332
Thorazine (Chlorpromazine Hydrochloride) SmithKline Beecham Pharmaceuticals ... 2701
Valium Injectable (Diazepam) Roche Products ... 2336
Vistaril Capsules (Hydroxyzine Pamoate) Pfizer Inc ... 2042
Vistaril Intramuscular Solution (Hydroxyzine Hydrochloride) Pfizer Inc ... 2042
Vistaril Oral Suspension (Hydroxyzine Pamoate) Pfizer Inc ... 2042

Anxiety, short-term symptomatic relief of
Atarax Tablets & Syrup (Hydroxyzine Hydrochloride) Pfizer Inc ... 1992
Ativan Tablets (Lorazepam) Wyeth-Ayerst ... 2807
BuSpar Tablets (Buspirone Hydrochloride) Bristol-Myers Squibb ... 738
Dizac (diazepam injectable emulsion) CIV (Diazepam) Ohmeda ... 1862
Librium Capsules (Chlordiazepoxide Hydrochloride) Roche Products ... 2331
Librium Injectable (Chlordiazepoxide Hydrochloride) Roche Products ... 2332
Miltown Tablets (Meprobamate) Wallace ... 2780
Serax Capsules (Oxazepam) Wyeth-Ayerst ... 2916
Serax Tablets (Oxazepam) Wyeth-Ayerst ... 2916
Tranxene (Clorazepate Dipotassium) Abbott ... 459
Valium Injectable (Diazepam) Roche Products ... 2336
Valium Tablets (Diazepam) Roche Products ... 2335
Vistaril Capsules (Hydroxyzine Pamoate) Pfizer Inc ... 2042
Vistaril Intramuscular Solution (Hydroxyzine Hydrochloride) Pfizer Inc ... 2042
Vistaril Oral Suspension (Hydroxyzine Pamoate) Pfizer Inc ... 2042
Xanax Tablets (Alprazolam) Pharmacia & Upjohn ... 2115

Aplastic anemia
(see under Anemia, aplastic)

Appendicitis, gangrenous
Primaxin I.M. (Cilastatin Sodium, Imipenem) Merck & Co., Inc. ... 1770

Appendicitis, perforated
Primaxin I.M. (Cilastatin Sodium, Imipenem) Merck & Co., Inc. ... 1770

Appendicitis with peritonitis
Merrem I.V. (Meropenem) Zeneca .. 2952
Primaxin I.M. (Cilastatin Sodium, Imipenem) Merck & Co., Inc. ... 1770
Zosyn (Piperacillin Sodium, Tazobactam Sodium) Lederle ... 1463

Appetite, suppression of
(see also under Obesity, exogenous)
Acutrim (Phenylpropanolamine Hydrochloride) Ciba Self-Medication ... ⊞ 648
Dexatrim (Phenylpropanolamine Hydrochloride) Thompson Medical ... ⊞ 795

Apprehension
(see under Anxiety disorders, management of)

ARC
(see under Infection, acquired immunodeficiency syndrome-related complex)

(⊞ Described in PDR For Nonprescription Drugs)   (⊚ Described in PDR For Ophthalmology)

Arrhythmias / Indications Index

Arrhythmias
- Calan Tablets (Verapamil Hydrochloride) Searle 2568
- Cardioquin Tablets (Quinidine Polygalacturonate) Purdue Frederick 2146
- Inderal (Propranolol Hydrochloride) Wyeth-Ayerst 2834
- Norpace (Disopyramide Phosphate) Searle 2596
- Quinidex Extentabs (Quinidine Sulfate) Robins 2240
- Tonocard Tablets (Tocainide Hydrochloride) Astra Merck 519

Arrhythmias associated with digitalis
- Calan Tablets (Verapamil Hydrochloride) Searle 2568
- Isoptin Oral Tablets (Verapamil Hydrochloride) Knoll Laboratories 1393

Arrhythmias due to thyrotoxicosis, adjunct to
- Inderal (Propranolol Hydrochloride) Wyeth-Ayerst 2834

Arrhythmias, supraventricular
- Inderal (Propranolol Hydrochloride) Wyeth-Ayerst 2834

Arrhythmias, ventricular
- Betapace Tablets (Sotalol Hydrochloride) Berlex 637
- Cardioquin Tablets (Quinidine Polygalacturonate) Purdue Frederick 2146
- Cordarone Intravenous (Amiodarone Hydrochloride) Wyeth-Ayerst 2821
- Ethmozine Tablets (Moricizine Hydrochloride) Roberts 2217
- Norpace (Disopyramide Phosphate) Searle 2596
- Procanbid Extended-Release Tablets (Procainamide Hydrochloride) Parke-Davis 1983
- Quinaglute Dura-Tabs Tablets (Quinidine Gluconate) Berlex 644
- Quinidex Extentabs (Quinidine Sulfate) Robins 2240
- Rythmol Tablets—150mg, 225mg, 300mg (Propafenone Hydrochloride) Knoll Laboratories 1399
- Sectral Capsules (Acebutolol Hydrochloride) Wyeth-Ayerst 2914
- Tambocor Tablets (Flecainide Acetate) 3M Pharmaceuticals 1555

Arrhythmias, ventricular, life-threatening
- Cordarone Tablets (Amiodarone Hydrochloride) Wyeth-Ayerst 2818
- Ethmozine Tablets (Moricizine Hydrochloride) Roberts 2217
- Mexitil Capsules (Mexiletine Hydrochloride) Boehringer Ingelheim 684
- Procanbid Extended-Release Tablets (Procainamide Hydrochloride) Parke-Davis 1983
- Tambocor Tablets (Flecainide Acetate) 3M Pharmaceuticals 1555
- Tonocard Tablets (Tocainide Hydrochloride) Astra Merck 519

Arteriovenous cannulae, occlusion of
- Streptase for Infusion (Streptokinase) Astra 557

Arthralgia, topical relief of
(see under Pain, topical relief of)

Arthritis
(see also under Osteoarthritis; Rheumatoid arthritis)
- Maximum Strength Ascriptin (Aspirin Buffered, Calcium Carbonate) Ciba Self-Medication 650
- Bufferin Analgesic Tablets (Aspirin) Bristol-Myers Products 636
- Arthritis Strength Bufferin Analgesic Caplets (Aspirin) Bristol-Myers Products 637
- Extra Strength Bufferin Analgesic Tablets (Aspirin) Bristol-Myers Products 637
- Cama Arthritis Pain Reliever (Aspirin, Aluminum Hydroxide, Magnesium Oxide) Sandoz Consumer 748
- Easprin (Aspirin) Parke-Davis 1971
- Trilisate (Choline Magnesium Trisalicylate) Purdue Frederick 2155

Arthritis, acute, gouty
- Celestone Soluspan Suspension (Betamethasone Sodium Phosphate, Betamethasone Acetate) Schering 2484
- Clinoril Tablets (Sulindac) Merck & Co., Inc. 1658
- Cortone Acetate Sterile Suspension (Cortisone Acetate) Merck & Co., Inc. 1663
- Cortone Acetate Tablets (Cortisone Acetate) Merck & Co., Inc. 1664
- Dalalone D.P. Injectable (Dexamethasone Acetate) Forest 1009
- Decadron Elixir (Dexamethasone) Merck & Co., Inc. 1676
- Decadron Phosphate Injection (Dexamethasone Sodium Phosphate) Merck & Co., Inc. 1680
- Decadron Tablets (Dexamethasone) Merck & Co., Inc. 1678
- Decadron-LA Sterile Suspension (Dexamethasone Acetate) Merck & Co., Inc. 1687
- Hydeltrasol Injection, Sterile (Prednisolone Sodium Phosphate) Merck & Co., Inc. 1708
- Hydeltra-T.B.A. Sterile Suspension (Prednisolone Tebutate) Merck & Co., Inc. 1710
- Hydrocortone Acetate Sterile Suspension (Hydrocortisone Acetate) Merck & Co., Inc. 1712
- Hydrocortone Phosphate Injection, Sterile (Hydrocortisone Sodium Phosphate) Merck & Co., Inc. 1713
- Hydrocortone Tablets (Hydrocortisone) Merck & Co., Inc. 1715
- Indocin (Indomethacin) Merck & Co., Inc. 1723
- Pediapred Oral Solution (Prednisolone Sodium Phosphate) Medeva 1618
- Prelone Syrup (Prednisolone) Muro 1834

Arthritis, chronic, gouty
- Anturane (Sulfinpyrazone) CibaGeneva 823
- ColBENEMID Tablets (Probenecid, Colchicine) Merck & Co., Inc. 1662

Arthritis, gonorrheal
- Pfizerpen for Injection (Penicillin G Potassium) Pfizer Inc 2022

Arthritis, intermittent, gouty
- Anturane (Sulfinpyrazone) CibaGeneva 823

Arthritis, juvenile
- Anaprox/Naprosyn (Naproxen Sodium) Roche Pharmaceuticals 2277
- Motrin Ibuprofen Suspension, Oral Drops, Chewable Tablets, Caplets (Ibuprofen) McNeil Consumer 1563
- Anaprox/Naprosyn (Naproxen) Roche Pharmaceuticals 2277
- Trilisate (Choline Magnesium Trisalicylate) Purdue Frederick 2155

Arthritis, osteo-
(see under Osteoarthritis)

Arthritis, psoriatic
- Extra Strength Bayer Arthritis Pain Regimen Formula (Aspirin, Enteric Coated) Bayer Consumer 615
- Celestone Soluspan Suspension (Betamethasone Sodium Phosphate, Betamethasone Acetate) Schering 2484
- Cortone Acetate Sterile Suspension (Cortisone Acetate) Merck & Co., Inc. 1663
- Cortone Acetate Tablets (Cortisone Acetate) Merck & Co., Inc. 1664
- Dalalone D.P. Injectable (Dexamethasone Acetate) Forest 1009
- Decadron Elixir (Dexamethasone) Merck & Co., Inc. 1676
- Decadron Phosphate Injection (Dexamethasone Sodium Phosphate) Merck & Co., Inc. 1680
- Decadron Tablets (Dexamethasone) Merck & Co., Inc. 1678
- Decadron-LA Sterile Suspension (Dexamethasone Acetate) Merck & Co., Inc. 1687
- Ecotrin (Aspirin) SmithKline Beecham 2625
- Hydeltrasol Injection, Sterile (Prednisolone Sodium Phosphate) Merck & Co., Inc. 1708
- Hydrocortone Phosphate Injection, Sterile (Hydrocortisone Sodium Phosphate) Merck & Co., Inc. 1713
- Hydrocortone Tablets (Hydrocortisone) Merck & Co., Inc. 1715
- Pediapred Oral Solution (Prednisolone Sodium Phosphate) Medeva 1618
- Prelone Syrup (Prednisolone) Muro 1834

Arthritis, rheumatoid
(see under Rheumatoid arthritis)

Arthritis, topical adjunct to
- BenGay External Analgesic Products (Menthol, Methyl Salicylate) Pfizer Consumer 714
- Mobisyl Analgesic Creme (Trolamine Salicylate) Ascher 607
- Thera-Gesic (Methyl Salicylate, Menthol) Mission 1830

Ascariasis, as secondary therapy in
- Mintezol (Thiabendazole) Merck & Co., Inc. 1747

Ascaris lumbricoides infections
- Vermox Chewable Tablets (Mebendazole) Janssen 1357

Aspergillosis
- Abelcet Injection (Amphotericin B) Liposome 1540
- Fungizone Intravenous (Amphotericin B) Apothecon 507
- Sporanox Capsules (Itraconazole) Janssen 1352

Aspergillus fumigatus infections
(see under Aspergillosis)

Asthma, bronchial
(see under Bronchial asthma)

Asthmatic attack, acute, in children age 6 years and older, treatment of
- Alupent (Metaproterenol Sulfate) Boehringer Ingelheim 672

Astrocytoma, palliative therapy in
- BiCNU (Carmustine (BCNU)) Bristol-Myers Squibb Oncology/Immunology 696

Athetosis, adjunctive therapy in
- Dizac (diazepam injectable emulsion) CIV (Diazepam) Ohmeda 1862
- Valium Injectable (Diazepam) Roche Products 2336
- Valium Tablets (Diazepam) Roche Products 2335

Athlete's foot
(see under Tinea pedis infections)

Atrial extrasystoles
- Inderal (Propranolol Hydrochloride) Wyeth-Ayerst 2834

Atrial fibrillation
- Brevibloc (esmolol HCl) Injection (Esmolol Hydrochloride) Ohmeda 1860
- Calan Tablets (Verapamil Hydrochloride) Searle 2568
- Cardioquin Tablets (Quinidine Polygalacturonate) Purdue Frederick 2146
- Cardizem Injectable (Diltiazem Hydrochloride) Hoechst Marion Roussel 1253
- Corvert Injection (Ibutilide Fumarate) Pharmacia & Upjohn 2075
- Crystodigin Tablets (Digitoxin) Lilly 1472
- Isoptin Injectable (Verapamil Hydrochloride) Knoll Laboratories 1391
- Isoptin Oral Tablets (Verapamil Hydrochloride) Knoll Laboratories 1393
- Lanoxicaps (Digoxin) Glaxo Wellcome 1110
- Lanoxin Elixir Pediatric (Digoxin) Glaxo Wellcome 1113
- Lanoxin Injection (Digoxin) Glaxo Wellcome 1116
- Lanoxin Injection Pediatric (Digoxin) Glaxo Wellcome 1119
- Lanoxin Tablets (Digoxin) Glaxo Wellcome 1121
- Quinaglute Dura-Tabs Tablets (Quinidine Gluconate) Berlex 644
- Quinidex Extentabs (Quinidine Sulfate) Robins 2240

Atrial fibrillation with embolism
- Coumadin (Warfarin Sodium) DuPont 941
- Heparin Sodium Vials (Heparin Sodium) Lilly 1486

Atrial fibrillation, paroxysmal
- Tambocor Tablets (Flecainide Acetate) 3M Pharmaceuticals 1555

Atrial flutter
- Brevibloc (esmolol HCl) Injection (Esmolol Hydrochloride) Ohmeda 1860
- Calan Tablets (Verapamil Hydrochloride) Searle 2568
- Cardioquin Tablets (Quinidine Polygalacturonate) Purdue Frederick 2146
- Cardizem Injectable (Diltiazem Hydrochloride) Hoechst Marion Roussel 1253
- Corvert Injection (Ibutilide Fumarate) Pharmacia & Upjohn 2075
- Crystodigin Tablets (Digitoxin) Lilly 1472
- Inderal (Propranolol Hydrochloride) Wyeth-Ayerst 2834
- Isoptin Injectable (Verapamil Hydrochloride) Knoll Laboratories 1391
- Isoptin Oral Tablets (Verapamil Hydrochloride) Knoll Laboratories 1393
- Lanoxicaps (Digoxin) Glaxo Wellcome 1110
- Lanoxin Elixir Pediatric (Digoxin) Glaxo Wellcome 1113
- Lanoxin Injection (Digoxin) Glaxo Wellcome 1116
- Lanoxin Injection Pediatric (Digoxin) Glaxo Wellcome 1119
- Lanoxin Tablets (Digoxin) Glaxo Wellcome 1121
- Quinaglute Dura-Tabs Tablets (Quinidine Gluconate) Berlex 644
- Quinidex Extentabs (Quinidine Sulfate) Robins 2240

Attention deficit disorders with hyperactivity
- Adderall Tablets (Amphetamine Aspartate, Amphetamine Sulfate, Dextroamphetamine Saccharate, Dextroamphetamine Sulfate) Richwood 2209
- Cylert Tablets (Pemoline) Abbott 415
- Desoxyn Gradumet Tablets (Methamphetamine Hydrochloride) Abbott 422
- Dexedrine (Dextroamphetamine Sulfate) SmithKline Beecham Pharmaceuticals 2648
- DextroStat-Dextroamphetamine Sulfate Tablets (Dextroamphetamine Sulfate) Richwood 2211
- Ritalin (Methylphenidate Hydrochloride) CibaGeneva 866

Autonomic response, exaggerated, management of disorders
- Bellergal-S Tablets (Phenobarbital, Ergotamine Tartrate, Belladonna Alkaloids) Sandoz Pharmaceuticals 2375

B

B. anthracis infections
- Achromycin V Capsules (Tetracycline Hydrochloride) Lederle 1417
- Declomycin Tablets (Demeclocycline Hydrochloride) Lederle 1421
- Doryx Capsules (Doxycycline Hyclate) Parke-Davis 1970

(▣ Described in PDR For Nonprescription Drugs) (◉ Described in PDR For Ophthalmology)

1499 Indications Index B. intermedius

DYNACIN Capsules (Minocycline Hydrochloride) Medicis ... 1627
Minocin Intravenous (Minocycline Hydrochloride) Lederle ... 1428
Minocin Oral Suspension (Minocycline Hydrochloride) Lederle ... 1431
Minocin Pellet-Filled Capsules (Minocycline Hydrochloride) Lederle ... 1429
Monodox Capsules (Doxycycline Monohydrate) Oclassen ... 1858
Pfizerpen for Injection (Penicillin G Potassium) Pfizer Inc ... 2022
Terramycin Intramuscular Solution (Oxytetracycline) Pfizer Inc ... 2034
Vibramycin (Doxycycline Calcium) Pfizer Inc ... 2038
Vibramycin Hyclate Intravenous (Doxycycline Hyclate) Pfizer Inc ... 2040
Vibramycin (Doxycycline Monohydrate) Pfizer Inc ... 2038

B. distasonis infections
Flagyl 375 Capsules (Metronidazole) Searle ... 2587
Flagyl I.V. (Metronidazole Hydrochloride) SCS ... 2373
Mefoxin (Cefoxitin Sodium) Merck & Co., Inc. ... 1734
Mefoxin Premixed Intravenous Solution (Cefoxitin Sodium) Merck & Co., Inc. ... 1737
Primaxin I.M. (Cilastatin Sodium, Imipenem) Merck & Co., Inc. ... 1770

B. distasonis intra-abdominal abscess
Flagyl 375 Capsules (Metronidazole) Searle ... 2587

B. distasonis intra-abdominal infections
Flagyl 375 Capsules (Metronidazole) Searle ... 2587
Flagyl I.V. (Metronidazole Hydrochloride) SCS ... 2373
Mefoxin (Cefoxitin Sodium) Merck & Co., Inc. ... 1734
Mefoxin Premixed Intravenous Solution (Cefoxitin Sodium) Merck & Co., Inc. ... 1737
Primaxin I.M. (Cilastatin Sodium, Imipenem) Merck & Co., Inc. ... 1770
Protostat Tablets (Metronidazole) Ortho Pharmaceutical ... 1939

B. distasonis liver abscess
Flagyl 375 Capsules (Metronidazole) Searle ... 2587
Flagyl I.V. (Metronidazole Hydrochloride) SCS ... 2373
Protostat Tablets (Metronidazole) Ortho Pharmaceutical ... 1939

B. distasonis peritonitis
Flagyl 375 Capsules (Metronidazole) Searle ... 2587
Flagyl I.V. (Metronidazole Hydrochloride) SCS ... 2373
Mefoxin (Cefoxitin Sodium) Merck & Co., Inc. ... 1734
Mefoxin Premixed Intravenous Solution (Cefoxitin Sodium) Merck & Co., Inc. ... 1737
Protostat Tablets (Metronidazole) Ortho Pharmaceutical ... 1939

B. fragilis bone and joint infections, adjunct to
Flagyl 375 Capsules (Metronidazole) Searle ... 2587
Flagyl I.V. (Metronidazole Hydrochloride) SCS ... 2373
Protostat Tablets (Metronidazole) Ortho Pharmaceutical ... 1939

B. fragilis brain abscess
Flagyl 375 Capsules (Metronidazole) Searle ... 2587
Flagyl I.V. (Metronidazole Hydrochloride) SCS ... 2373
Protostat Tablets (Metronidazole) Ortho Pharmaceutical ... 1939

B. fragilis central nervous system infections
Flagyl 375 Capsules (Metronidazole) Searle ... 2587
Flagyl I.V. (Metronidazole Hydrochloride) SCS ... 2373
Protostat Tablets (Metronidazole) Ortho Pharmaceutical ... 1939

B. fragilis empyema
Flagyl 375 Capsules (Metronidazole) Searle ... 2587
Flagyl I.V. (Metronidazole Hydrochloride) SCS ... 2373
Protostat Tablets (Metronidazole) Ortho Pharmaceutical ... 1939

B. fragilis endocarditis
Flagyl 375 Capsules (Metronidazole) Searle ... 2587
Flagyl I.V. (Metronidazole Hydrochloride) SCS ... 2373

B. fragilis endometritis
Flagyl 375 Capsules (Metronidazole) Searle ... 2587

B. fragilis endomyometritis
Flagyl 375 Capsules (Metronidazole) Searle ... 2587
Flagyl I.V. (Metronidazole Hydrochloride) SCS ... 2373
Protostat Tablets (Metronidazole) Ortho Pharmaceutical ... 1939

B. fragilis gynecologic infections
Cefobid Intravenous/Intramuscular (Cefoperazone Sodium) Pfizer Inc ... 1996
Cefobid Pharmacy Bulk Package - Not for Direct Infusion (Cefoperazone Sodium) Pfizer Inc ... 1999
Cefotan (Cefotetan) Zeneca ... 2936
Claforan Sterile and Injection (Cefotaxime Sodium) Hoechst Marion Roussel ... 1259
Flagyl I.V. (Metronidazole Hydrochloride) SCS ... 2373
Mefoxin (Cefoxitin Sodium) Merck & Co., Inc. ... 1734
Mefoxin Premixed Intravenous Solution (Cefoxitin Sodium) Merck & Co., Inc. ... 1737
Pipracil (Piperacillin Sodium) Lederle ... 1435
Primaxin I.V. (Cilastatin Sodium, Imipenem) Merck & Co., Inc. ... 1772
Protostat Tablets (Metronidazole) Ortho Pharmaceutical ... 1939
Unasyn (Ampicillin Sodium, Sulbactam Sodium) Pfizer Inc ... 2035

B. fragilis infections
Cefizox for Intramuscular or Intravenous Use (Ceftizoxime Sodium) Fujisawa ... 1025
Cefobid Intravenous/Intramuscular (Cefoperazone Sodium) Pfizer Inc ... 1996
Cefobid Pharmacy Bulk Package - Not for Direct Infusion (Cefoperazone Sodium) Pfizer Inc ... 1999
Cefotan (Cefotetan) Zeneca ... 2936
Claforan Sterile and Injection (Cefotaxime Sodium) Hoechst Marion Roussel ... 1259
Flagyl 375 Capsules (Metronidazole) Searle ... 2587
Flagyl I.V. (Metronidazole Hydrochloride) SCS ... 2373
Mefoxin (Cefoxitin Sodium) Merck & Co., Inc. ... 1734
Mefoxin Premixed Intravenous Solution (Cefoxitin Sodium) Merck & Co., Inc. ... 1737
Merrem I.V. (Meropenem) Zeneca ... 2952
Mezlin (Mezlocillin Sodium) Bayer Pharmaceutical ... 594
Mezlin Pharmacy Bulk Package (Mezlocillin Sodium) Bayer Pharmaceutical ... 597
Pipracil (Piperacillin Sodium) Lederle ... 1435
Primaxin I.M. (Cilastatin Sodium, Imipenem) Merck & Co., Inc. ... 1770
Primaxin I.V. (Cilastatin Sodium, Imipenem) Merck & Co., Inc. ... 1772
Rocephin Injectable Vials, ADD-Vantage, Galaxy Container (Ceftriaxone Sodium) Roche Pharmaceuticals ... 2305
Tazicef for Injection (Ceftazidime) SmithKline Beecham Pharmaceuticals ... 2697
Tazidime Vials, Faspak & ADD-Vantage (Ceftazidime) Lilly ... 1531
Timentin for Injection (Ticarcillin Disodium, Clavulanate Potassium) SmithKline Beecham Pharmaceuticals ... 2706
Unasyn (Ampicillin Sodium, Sulbactam Sodium) Pfizer Inc ... 2035
Zosyn (Piperacillin Sodium, Tazobactam Sodium) Lederle ... 1463

B. fragilis intra-abdominal abscess
Flagyl 375 Capsules (Metronidazole) Searle ... 2587

B. fragilis intra-abdominal infections
Cefizox for Intramuscular or Intravenous Use (Ceftizoxime Sodium) Fujisawa ... 1025
Cefobid Intravenous/Intramuscular (Cefoperazone Sodium) Pfizer Inc ... 1996
Cefobid Pharmacy Bulk Package - Not for Direct Infusion (Cefoperazone Sodium) Pfizer Inc ... 1999
Flagyl 375 Capsules (Metronidazole) Searle ... 2587
Flagyl I.V. (Metronidazole Hydrochloride) SCS ... 2373
Fortaz (Ceftazidime) Glaxo Wellcome ... 1092
Mefoxin (Cefoxitin Sodium) Merck & Co., Inc. ... 1734
Mefoxin Premixed Intravenous Solution (Cefoxitin Sodium) Merck & Co., Inc. ... 1737
Merrem I.V. (Meropenem) Zeneca ... 2952
Pipracil (Piperacillin Sodium) Lederle ... 1435
Primaxin I.M. (Cilastatin Sodium, Imipenem) Merck & Co., Inc. ... 1770
Primaxin I.V. (Cilastatin Sodium, Imipenem) Merck & Co., Inc. ... 1772
Protostat Tablets (Metronidazole) Ortho Pharmaceutical ... 1939
Rocephin Injectable Vials, ADD-Vantage, Galaxy Container (Ceftriaxone Sodium) Roche Pharmaceuticals ... 2305
Tazicef for Injection (Ceftazidime) SmithKline Beecham Pharmaceuticals ... 2697
Tazidime Vials, Faspak & ADD-Vantage (Ceftazidime) Lilly ... 1531
Timentin for Injection (Ticarcillin Disodium, Clavulanate Potassium) SmithKline Beecham Pharmaceuticals ... 2706
Unasyn (Ampicillin Sodium, Sulbactam Sodium) Pfizer Inc ... 2035

B. fragilis liver abscess
Flagyl I.V. (Metronidazole Hydrochloride) SCS ... 2373
Protostat Tablets (Metronidazole) Ortho Pharmaceutical ... 1939

B. fragilis lower respiratory tract infections
Flagyl 375 Capsules (Metronidazole) Searle ... 2587
Flagyl I.V. (Metronidazole Hydrochloride) SCS ... 2373
Mezlin (Mezlocillin Sodium) Bayer Pharmaceutical ... 594
Mezlin Pharmacy Bulk Package (Mezlocillin Sodium) Bayer Pharmaceutical ... 597
Protostat Tablets (Metronidazole) Ortho Pharmaceutical ... 1939

B. fragilis lung abscess
Flagyl 375 Capsules (Metronidazole) Searle ... 2587
Flagyl I.V. (Metronidazole Hydrochloride) SCS ... 2373
Mezlin (Mezlocillin Sodium) Bayer Pharmaceutical ... 594
Mezlin Pharmacy Bulk Package (Mezlocillin Sodium) Bayer Pharmaceutical ... 597
Protostat Tablets (Metronidazole) Ortho Pharmaceutical ... 1939

B. fragilis meningitis
Flagyl 375 Capsules (Metronidazole) Searle ... 2587
Flagyl I.V. (Metronidazole Hydrochloride) SCS ... 2373
Protostat Tablets (Metronidazole) Ortho Pharmaceutical ... 1939

B. fragilis peritonitis
Cefobid Intravenous/Intramuscular (Cefoperazone Sodium) Pfizer Inc ... 1996
Cefobid Pharmacy Bulk Package - Not for Direct Infusion (Cefoperazone Sodium) Pfizer Inc ... 1999
Flagyl 375 Capsules (Metronidazole) Searle ... 2587
Flagyl I.V. (Metronidazole Hydrochloride) SCS ... 2373
Mefoxin (Cefoxitin Sodium) Merck & Co., Inc. ... 1734
Mefoxin Premixed Intravenous Solution (Cefoxitin Sodium) Merck & Co., Inc. ... 1737
Merrem I.V. (Meropenem) Zeneca ... 2952
Protostat Tablets (Metronidazole) Ortho Pharmaceutical ... 1939
Timentin for Injection (Ticarcillin Disodium, Clavulanate Potassium) SmithKline Beecham Pharmaceuticals ... 2706
Zosyn (Piperacillin Sodium, Tazobactam Sodium) Lederle ... 1463

B. fragilis pneumonia
Flagyl 375 Capsules (Metronidazole) Searle ... 2587
Flagyl I.V. (Metronidazole Hydrochloride) SCS ... 2373
Mezlin (Mezlocillin Sodium) Bayer Pharmaceutical ... 594
Mezlin Pharmacy Bulk Package (Mezlocillin Sodium) Bayer Pharmaceutical ... 597
Protostat Tablets (Metronidazole) Ortho Pharmaceutical ... 1939

B. fragilis septicemia
Cefizox for Intramuscular or Intravenous Use (Ceftizoxime Sodium) Fujisawa ... 1025
Flagyl 375 Capsules (Metronidazole) Searle ... 2587
Flagyl I.V. (Metronidazole Hydrochloride) SCS ... 2373
Mefoxin (Cefoxitin Sodium) Merck & Co., Inc. ... 1734
Mefoxin Premixed Intravenous Solution (Cefoxitin Sodium) Merck & Co., Inc. ... 1737
Primaxin I.V. (Cilastatin Sodium, Imipenem) Merck & Co., Inc. ... 1772
Protostat Tablets (Metronidazole) Ortho Pharmaceutical ... 1939

B. fragilis skin and skin structure infections
Cefizox for Intramuscular or Intravenous Use (Ceftizoxime Sodium) Fujisawa ... 1025
Flagyl 375 Capsules (Metronidazole) Searle ... 2587
Flagyl I.V. (Metronidazole Hydrochloride) SCS ... 2373
Mefoxin (Cefoxitin Sodium) Merck & Co., Inc. ... 1734
Mefoxin Premixed Intravenous Solution (Cefoxitin Sodium) Merck & Co., Inc. ... 1737
Pipracil (Piperacillin Sodium) Lederle ... 1435
Primaxin I.M. (Cilastatin Sodium, Imipenem) Merck & Co., Inc. ... 1770
Primaxin I.V. (Cilastatin Sodium, Imipenem) Merck & Co., Inc. ... 1772
Protostat Tablets (Metronidazole) Ortho Pharmaceutical ... 1939
Rocephin Injectable Vials, ADD-Vantage, Galaxy Container (Ceftriaxone Sodium) Roche Pharmaceuticals ... 2305
Unasyn (Ampicillin Sodium, Sulbactam Sodium) Pfizer Inc ... 2035

B. fragilis tubo-ovarian abscess
Flagyl 375 Capsules (Metronidazole) Searle ... 2587
Flagyl I.V. (Metronidazole Hydrochloride) SCS ... 2373
Protostat Tablets (Metronidazole) Ortho Pharmaceutical ... 1939

B. fragilis vaginal cuff infection, post-surgical
Flagyl 375 Capsules (Metronidazole) Searle ... 2587
Flagyl I.V. (Metronidazole Hydrochloride) SCS ... 2373

B. intermedius infections
Primaxin I.M. (Cilastatin Sodium, Imipenem) Merck & Co., Inc. ... 1770

B. intermedius intra-abdominal infections
Primaxin I.M. (Cilastatin Sodium, Imipenem) Merck & Co., Inc. ... 1770

Indications Index

B. melaninogenicus endometritis
Timentin for Injection (Ticarcillin Disodium, Clavulanate Potassium) SmithKline Beecham Pharmaceuticals 2706

B. melaninogenicus infections
Timentin for Injection (Ticarcillin Disodium, Clavulanate Potassium) SmithKline Beecham Pharmaceuticals 2706

B. ovatus infections
Flagyl 375 Capsules (Metronidazole) Searle 2587
Flagyl I.V. (Metronidazole Hydrochloride) SCS 2373
Mefoxin (Cefoxitin Sodium) Merck & Co., Inc. 1734
Mefoxin Premixed Intravenous Solution (Cefoxitin Sodium) Merck & Co., Inc. 1737
Zosyn (Piperacillin Sodium, Tazobactam Sodium) Lederle 1463

B. ovatus intra-abdominal abscess
Flagyl 375 Capsules (Metronidazole) Searle 2587

B. ovatus intra-abdominal infections
Flagyl 375 Capsules (Metronidazole) Searle 2587
Flagyl I.V. (Metronidazole Hydrochloride) SCS 2373
Mefoxin (Cefoxitin Sodium) Merck & Co., Inc. 1734
Mefoxin Premixed Intravenous Solution (Cefoxitin Sodium) Merck & Co., Inc. 1737
Protostat Tablets (Metronidazole) Ortho Pharmaceutical 1939

B. ovatus liver abscess
Flagyl 375 Capsules (Metronidazole) Searle 2587
Flagyl I.V. (Metronidazole Hydrochloride) SCS 2373
Protostat Tablets (Metronidazole) Ortho Pharmaceutical 1939

B. ovatus peritonitis
Flagyl 375 Capsules (Metronidazole) Searle 2587
Flagyl I.V. (Metronidazole Hydrochloride) SCS 2373
Mefoxin (Cefoxitin Sodium) Merck & Co., Inc. 1734
Mefoxin Premixed Intravenous Solution (Cefoxitin Sodium) Merck & Co., Inc. 1737
Protostat Tablets (Metronidazole) Ortho Pharmaceutical 1939
Zosyn (Piperacillin Sodium, Tazobactam Sodium) Lederle 1463

B. pertussis infections
E.E.S. (Erythromycin Ethylsuccinate) Abbott 427
E-Mycin Tablets (Erythromycin) Knoll Laboratories 1388
ERYC (Erythromycin) Parke-Davis .. 1972
EryPed (Erythromycin Ethylsuccinate) Abbott 425
Ery-Tab Tablets (Erythromycin) Abbott 426
Erythrocin Stearate Filmtab (Erythromycin Stearate) Abbott 429
Erythromycin Base Filmtab (Erythromycin) Abbott 430
Erythromycin Delayed-Release Capsules, USP (Erythromycin) Abbott 431
Ilosone (Erythromycin Estolate) Dista 927
PCE Dispertab Tablets (Erythromycin) Abbott 453

B. pertussis respiratory tract infections
E.E.S. (Erythromycin Ethylsuccinate) Abbott 427
EryPed (Erythromycin Ethylsuccinate) Abbott 425
Ery-Tab Tablets (Erythromycin) Abbott 426
Erythrocin Stearate Filmtab (Erythromycin Stearate) Abbott 429
Erythromycin Base Filmtab (Erythromycin) Abbott 430
Erythromycin Delayed-Release Capsules, USP (Erythromycin) Abbott 431

PCE Dispertab Tablets (Erythromycin) Abbott 453

B. thetaiotaomicron infections
Flagyl 375 Capsules (Metronidazole) Searle 2587
Flagyl I.V. (Metronidazole Hydrochloride) SCS 2373
Mefoxin (Cefoxitin Sodium) Merck & Co., Inc. 1734
Mefoxin Premixed Intravenous Solution (Cefoxitin Sodium) Merck & Co., Inc. 1737
Merrem I.V. (Meropenem) Zeneca .. 2952
Primaxin I.M. (Cilastatin Sodium, Imipenem) Merck & Co., Inc. 1770
Zosyn (Piperacillin Sodium, Tazobactam Sodium) Lederle 1463

B. thetaiotaomicron intra-abdominal abscess
Flagyl 375 Capsules (Metronidazole) Searle 2587

B. thetaiotaomicron intra-abdominal infections
Flagyl 375 Capsules (Metronidazole) Searle 2587
Flagyl I.V. (Metronidazole Hydrochloride) SCS 2373
Mefoxin (Cefoxitin Sodium) Merck & Co., Inc. 1734
Mefoxin Premixed Intravenous Solution (Cefoxitin Sodium) Merck & Co., Inc. 1737
Merrem I.V. (Meropenem) Zeneca .. 2952
Primaxin I.M. (Cilastatin Sodium, Imipenem) Merck & Co., Inc. 1770
Protostat Tablets (Metronidazole) Ortho Pharmaceutical 1939

B. thetaiotaomicron liver abscess
Flagyl 375 Capsules (Metronidazole) Searle 2587
Flagyl I.V. (Metronidazole Hydrochloride) SCS 2373
Protostat Tablets (Metronidazole) Ortho Pharmaceutical 1939

B. thetaiotaomicron peritonitis
Flagyl 375 Capsules (Metronidazole) Searle 2587
Flagyl I.V. (Metronidazole Hydrochloride) SCS 2373
Mefoxin (Cefoxitin Sodium) Merck & Co., Inc. 1734
Mefoxin Premixed Intravenous Solution (Cefoxitin Sodium) Merck & Co., Inc. 1737
Merrem I.V. (Meropenem) Zeneca .. 2952
Protostat Tablets (Metronidazole) Ortho Pharmaceutical 1939
Zosyn (Piperacillin Sodium, Tazobactam Sodium) Lederle 1463

B. vulgatus infections
Cefotan (Cefotetan) Zeneca 2936
Flagyl 375 Capsules (Metronidazole) Searle 2587
Flagyl I.V. (Metronidazole Hydrochloride) SCS 2373
Mefoxin (Cefoxitin Sodium) Merck & Co., Inc. 1734
Mefoxin Premixed Intravenous Solution (Cefoxitin Sodium) Merck & Co., Inc. 1737
Zosyn (Piperacillin Sodium, Tazobactam Sodium) Lederle 1463

B. vulgatus intra-abdominal infections
Cefotan (Cefotetan) Zeneca 2936
Flagyl 375 Capsules (Metronidazole) Searle 2587
Flagyl I.V. (Metronidazole Hydrochloride) SCS 2373
Mefoxin (Cefoxitin Sodium) Merck & Co., Inc. 1734
Mefoxin Premixed Intravenous Solution (Cefoxitin Sodium) Merck & Co., Inc. 1737
Protostat Tablets (Metronidazole) Ortho Pharmaceutical 1939

B. vulgatus liver abscess
Flagyl 375 Capsules (Metronidazole) Searle 2587
Flagyl I.V. (Metronidazole Hydrochloride) SCS 2373
Protostat Tablets (Metronidazole) Ortho Pharmaceutical 1939

B. vulgatus peritonitis
Flagyl 375 Capsules (Metronidazole) Searle 2587
Flagyl I.V. (Metronidazole Hydrochloride) SCS 2373
Mefoxin (Cefoxitin Sodium) Merck & Co., Inc. 1734
Mefoxin Premixed Intravenous Solution (Cefoxitin Sodium) Merck & Co., Inc. 1737
Protostat Tablets (Metronidazole) Ortho Pharmaceutical 1939
Zosyn (Piperacillin Sodium, Tazobactam Sodium) Lederle 1463

Backache, systemic, symptomatic relief of
Actron Caplets and Tablets (Ketoprofen) Bayer Consumer .. 608
Aleve (Naproxen Sodium) Procter & Gamble 2124
Backache Caplets (Magnesium Salicylate) Bristol-Myers Products 635
Doan's Extra-Strength Analgesic (Magnesium Salicylate) Ciba Self-Medication 653
Extra Strength Doan's P.M. (Magnesium Salicylate, Diphenhydramine Hydrochloride) Ciba Self-Medication 653
Doan's Regular Strength Analgesic (Magnesium Salicylate) Ciba Self-Medication 654
Goody's Extra Strength Pain Relief Tablets (Aspirin, Acetaminophen, Caffeine) Block 632
Ibuprohm (Ibuprofen) Ohm 713
Nuprin Ibuprofen/Analgesic Tablets & Caplets (Ibuprofen) Bristol-Myers Products 645
Orudis KT (Ketoprofen) Whitehall-Robins 842
Panodol Tablets and Caplets (Acetaminophen) SmithKline Beecham Consumer 783
St. Joseph Adult Chewable Aspirin (81 mg.) (Aspirin) Schering-Plough HealthCare 768

Backache, temporary relief of
(see under Pain, topical relief of)

Bacteremia
(see under Septicemia, bacterial)

Bacterial shock, treatment adjunct
Isuprel Injection (Isoproterenol Hydrochloride) Sanofi Winthrop .. 2441
Narcan Injection (Naloxone Hydrochloride) DuPont 950

Bacteriuria associated with cystitis, elimination or suppression of
(see also under Infections, urinary tract)
Uroqid-Acid No. 2 Tablets (Methenamine Mandelate, Sodium Acid Phosphate) Beach 633

Bacteriuria, asymptomatic
Geocillin Tablets (Carbenicillin Indanyl Sodium) Pfizer Inc 2009

Bacteroides distasonis infections
(see under B. distasonis infections)

Bacteroides fragilis infections
(see under B. fragilis infections)

Bacteroides ovatus infections
(see under B. ovatus infections)

Bacteroides species bone and joint infections
Cefizox for Intramuscular or Intravenous Use (Ceftizoxime Sodium) Fujisawa 1025

Bacteroides species bone and joint infections, adjunct in
Flagyl 375 Capsules (Metronidazole) Searle 2587
Flagyl I.V. (Metronidazole Hydrochloride) SCS 2373
Protostat Tablets (Metronidazole) Ortho Pharmaceutical 1939

Bacteroides species CNS infection
Flagyl 375 Capsules (Metronidazole) Searle 2587
Flagyl I.V. (Metronidazole Hydrochloride) SCS 2373
Protostat Tablets (Metronidazole) Ortho Pharmaceutical 1939

Bacteroides species empyema
Flagyl 375 Capsules (Metronidazole) Searle 2587
Flagyl I.V. (Metronidazole Hydrochloride) SCS 2373
Protostat Tablets (Metronidazole) Ortho Pharmaceutical 1939

Bacteroides species endocarditis
Flagyl 375 Capsules (Metronidazole) Searle 2587
Flagyl I.V. (Metronidazole Hydrochloride) SCS 2373
Protostat Tablets (Metronidazole) Ortho Pharmaceutical 1939

Bacteroides species endomyometritis
Flagyl 375 Capsules (Metronidazole) Searle 2587
Flagyl I.V. (Metronidazole Hydrochloride) SCS 2373
Protostat Tablets (Metronidazole) Ortho Pharmaceutical 1939

Bacteroides species gynecologic infections
Cefobid Intravenous/Intramuscular (Cefoperazone Sodium) Pfizer Inc 1996
Cefobid Pharmacy Bulk Package - Not for Direct Infusion (Cefoperazone Sodium) Pfizer Inc 1999
Cefotan (Cefotetan) Zeneca 2936
Claforan Sterile and Injection (Cefotaxime Sodium) Hoechst Marion Roussel 1259
Flagyl 375 Capsules (Metronidazole) Searle 2587
Flagyl I.V. (Metronidazole Hydrochloride) SCS 2373
Mefoxin (Cefoxitin Sodium) Merck & Co., Inc. 1734
Mefoxin Premixed Intravenous Solution (Cefoxitin Sodium) Merck & Co., Inc. 1737
Mezlin (Mezlocillin Sodium) Bayer Pharmaceutical 594
Mezlin Pharmacy Bulk Package (Mezlocillin Sodium) Bayer Pharmaceutical 597
Primaxin I.M. (Cilastatin Sodium, Imipenem) Merck & Co., Inc. 1770
Primaxin I.V. (Cilastatin Sodium, Imipenem) Merck & Co., Inc. 1772
Protostat Tablets (Metronidazole) Ortho Pharmaceutical 1939
Unasyn (Ampicillin Sodium, Sulbactam Sodium) Pfizer Inc 2035

Bacteroides species infections
(see also under B. fragilis infections; B. distasonis infections; B. ovatus infections; B. thetaiotaomicron infections; B. vulgatus infections)
Achromycin V Capsules (Tetracycline Hydrochloride) Lederle 1417
Cefizox for Intramuscular or Intravenous Use (Ceftizoxime Sodium) Fujisawa 1025
Cefobid Intravenous/Intramuscular (Cefoperazone Sodium) Pfizer Inc 1996
Cefobid Pharmacy Bulk Package - Not for Direct Infusion (Cefoperazone Sodium) Pfizer Inc 1999
Cefotan (Cefotetan) Zeneca 2936
Ceptaz (Ceftazidime) Glaxo Wellcome 1070
Claforan Sterile and Injection (Cefotaxime Sodium) Hoechst Marion Roussel 1259
Declomycin Tablets (Demeclocycline Hydrochloride) Lederle 1421
Doryx Capsules (Doxycycline Hyclate) Parke-Davis 1970
Flagyl 375 Capsules (Metronidazole) Searle 2587
Flagyl I.V. (Metronidazole Hydrochloride) SCS 2373
Fortaz (Ceftazidime) Glaxo Wellcome 1092

(■ Described in PDR For Nonprescription Drugs)   (⊙ Described in PDR For Ophthalmology)

1501 **Indications Index** **Bites**

Mefoxin (Cefoxitin Sodium) Merck & Co., Inc. 1734
Mefoxin Premixed Intravenous Solution (Cefoxitin Sodium) Merck & Co., Inc. 1737
Mezlin (Mezlocillin Sodium) Bayer Pharmaceutical 594
Mezlin Pharmacy Bulk Package (Mezlocillin Sodium) Bayer Pharmaceutical 597
Minocin Intravenous (Minocycline Hydrochloride) Lederle 1428
Pipracil (Piperacillin Sodium) Lederle 1435
Primaxin I.M. (Cilastatin Sodium, Imipenem) Merck & Co., Inc. 1770
Primaxin I.V. (Cilastatin Sodium, Imipenem) Merck & Co., Inc. 1772
Protostat Tablets (Metronidazole) Ortho Pharmaceutical 1939
Tazicef for Injection (Ceftazidime) SmithKline Beecham Pharmaceuticals 2697
Tazidime Vials, Faspak & ADD-Vantage (Ceftazidime) Lilly .. 1531
Terramycin Intramuscular Solution (Oxytetracycline) Pfizer Inc 2034
Vibramycin Hyclate Intravenous (Doxycycline Hyclate) Pfizer Inc 2040

Bacteroides species intra-abdominal infections
Cefizox for Intramuscular or Intravenous Use (Ceftizoxime Sodium) Fujisawa 1025
Cefobid Intravenous/Intramuscular (Cefoperazone Sodium) Pfizer Inc 1996
Cefobid Pharmacy Bulk Package - Not for Direct Infusion (Cefoperazone Sodium) Pfizer Inc 1999
Cefotan (Cefotetan) Zeneca 2936
Ceptaz (Ceftazidime) Glaxo Wellcome 1070
Claforan Sterile and Injection (Cefotaxime Sodium) Hoechst Marion Roussel 1259
Flagyl 375 Capsules (Metronidazole) Searle 2587
Flagyl I.V. (Metronidazole Hydrochloride) SCS 2373
Fortaz (Ceftazidime) Glaxo Wellcome 1092
Mefoxin (Cefoxitin Sodium) Merck & Co., Inc. 1734
Mefoxin Premixed Intravenous Solution (Cefoxitin Sodium) Merck & Co., Inc. 1737
Mezlin (Mezlocillin Sodium) Bayer Pharmaceutical 594
Mezlin Pharmacy Bulk Package (Mezlocillin Sodium) Bayer Pharmaceutical 597
Pipracil (Piperacillin Sodium) Lederle 1435
Primaxin I.M. (Cilastatin Sodium, Imipenem) Merck & Co., Inc. 1770
Primaxin I.V. (Cilastatin Sodium, Imipenem) Merck & Co., Inc. 1772
Protostat Tablets (Metronidazole) Ortho Pharmaceutical 1939
Tazicef for Injection (Ceftazidime) SmithKline Beecham Pharmaceuticals 2697
Tazidime Vials, Faspak & ADD-Vantage (Ceftazidime) Lilly .. 1531
Unasyn (Ampicillin Sodium, Sulbactam Sodium) Pfizer Inc 2035

Bacteroides species liver abscess
Flagyl 375 Capsules (Metronidazole) Searle 2587
Flagyl I.V. (Metronidazole Hydrochloride) SCS 2373
Protostat Tablets (Metronidazole) Ortho Pharmaceutical 1939

Bacteroides species lower respiratory tract infections
Cefizox for Intramuscular or Intravenous Use (Ceftizoxime Sodium) Fujisawa 1025
Flagyl 375 Capsules (Metronidazole) Searle 2587
Flagyl I.V. (Metronidazole Hydrochloride) SCS 2373
Mefoxin (Cefoxitin Sodium) Merck & Co., Inc. 1734
Mefoxin Premixed Intravenous Solution (Cefoxitin Sodium) Merck & Co., Inc. 1737
Mezlin (Mezlocillin Sodium) Bayer Pharmaceutical 594
Mezlin Pharmacy Bulk Package (Mezlocillin Sodium) Bayer Pharmaceutical 597
Protostat Tablets (Metronidazole) Ortho Pharmaceutical 1939

Bacteroides species lung abscess
Flagyl 375 Capsules (Metronidazole) Searle 2587
Flagyl I.V. (Metronidazole Hydrochloride) SCS 2373
Mefoxin (Cefoxitin Sodium) Merck & Co., Inc. 1734
Mefoxin Premixed Intravenous Solution (Cefoxitin Sodium) Merck & Co., Inc. 1737
Mezlin (Mezlocillin Sodium) Bayer Pharmaceutical 594
Mezlin Pharmacy Bulk Package (Mezlocillin Sodium) Bayer Pharmaceutical 597
Protostat Tablets (Metronidazole) Ortho Pharmaceutical 1939

Bacteroides species meningitis
Flagyl 375 Capsules (Metronidazole) Searle 2587
Flagyl I.V. (Metronidazole Hydrochloride) SCS 2373
Protostat Tablets (Metronidazole) Ortho Pharmaceutical 1939

Bacteroides species peritonitis
Flagyl 375 Capsules (Metronidazole) Searle 2587
Flagyl I.V. (Metronidazole Hydrochloride) SCS 2373
Mefoxin (Cefoxitin Sodium) Merck & Co., Inc. 1734
Mefoxin Premixed Intravenous Solution (Cefoxitin Sodium) Merck & Co., Inc. 1737
Mezlin (Mezlocillin Sodium) Bayer Pharmaceutical 594
Mezlin Pharmacy Bulk Package (Mezlocillin Sodium) Bayer Pharmaceutical 597
Primaxin I.M. (Cilastatin Sodium, Imipenem) Merck & Co., Inc. 1770
Protostat Tablets (Metronidazole) Ortho Pharmaceutical 1939

Bacteroides species pneumonia
Flagyl 375 Capsules (Metronidazole) Searle 2587
Flagyl I.V. (Metronidazole Hydrochloride) SCS 2373
Mefoxin (Cefoxitin Sodium) Merck & Co., Inc. 1734
Mefoxin Premixed Intravenous Solution (Cefoxitin Sodium) Merck & Co., Inc. 1737
Mezlin (Mezlocillin Sodium) Bayer Pharmaceutical 594
Mezlin Pharmacy Bulk Package (Mezlocillin Sodium) Bayer Pharmaceutical 597
Protostat Tablets (Metronidazole) Ortho Pharmaceutical 1939

Bacteroides species septicemia
Cefizox for Intramuscular or Intravenous Use (Ceftizoxime Sodium) Fujisawa 1025
Flagyl 375 Capsules (Metronidazole) Searle 2587
Flagyl I.V. (Metronidazole Hydrochloride) SCS 2373
Mefoxin (Cefoxitin Sodium) Merck & Co., Inc. 1734
Mefoxin Premixed Intravenous Solution (Cefoxitin Sodium) Merck & Co., Inc. 1737
Mezlin (Mezlocillin Sodium) Bayer Pharmaceutical 594
Mezlin Pharmacy Bulk Package (Mezlocillin Sodium) Bayer Pharmaceutical 597
Pipracil (Piperacillin Sodium) Lederle 1435
Primaxin I.V. (Cilastatin Sodium, Imipenem) Merck & Co., Inc. 1772

Bacteroides species skin and skin structure infections
Cefizox for Intramuscular or Intravenous Use (Ceftizoxime Sodium) Fujisawa 1025
Claforan Sterile and Injection (Cefotaxime Sodium) Hoechst Marion Roussel 1259
Flagyl 375 Capsules (Metronidazole) Searle 2587
Flagyl I.V. (Metronidazole Hydrochloride) SCS 2373
Mefoxin (Cefoxitin Sodium) Merck & Co., Inc. 1734
Mefoxin Premixed Intravenous Solution (Cefoxitin Sodium) Merck & Co., Inc. 1737
Mezlin (Mezlocillin Sodium) Bayer Pharmaceutical 594
Mezlin Pharmacy Bulk Package (Mezlocillin Sodium) Bayer Pharmaceutical 597
Primaxin I.M. (Cilastatin Sodium, Imipenem) Merck & Co., Inc. 1770
Primaxin I.V. (Cilastatin Sodium, Imipenem) Merck & Co., Inc. 1772
Protostat Tablets (Metronidazole) Ortho Pharmaceutical 1939

Bacteroides species tubo-ovarian abscess
Flagyl 375 Capsules (Metronidazole) Searle 2587
Flagyl I.V. (Metronidazole Hydrochloride) SCS 2373
Protostat Tablets (Metronidazole) Ortho Pharmaceutical 1939

Bacteroides species vaginal cuff infection, post-surgical
Flagyl 375 Capsules (Metronidazole) Searle 2587
Flagyl I.V. (Metronidazole Hydrochloride) SCS 2373
Protostat Tablets (Metronidazole) Ortho Pharmaceutical 1939

Bacteroides thetaiotaomicron infections (see under B. thetaiotaomicron infections)

Bacteroides vulgatus infections (see under B. vulgatus infections)

Barber's itch (see under Folliculitis barbae)

Bartonella bacilliformis infections
Achromycin V Capsules (Tetracycline Hydrochloride) Lederle 1417
Declomycin Tablets (Demeclocycline Hydrochloride) Lederle 1421
Doryx Capsules (Doxycycline Hyclate) Parke-Davis 1970
DYNACIN Capsules (Minocycline Hydrochloride) Medicis 1627
Minocin Intravenous (Minocycline Hydrochloride) Lederle 1428
Minocin Oral Suspension (Minocycline Hydrochloride) Lederle 1431
Minocin Pellet-Filled Capsules (Minocycline Hydrochloride) Lederle 1429
Monodox Capsules (Doxycycline Monohydrate) Oclassen 1858
Terramycin Intramuscular Solution (Oxytetracycline) Pfizer Inc 2034
Vibramycin (Doxycycline Calcium) Pfizer Inc 2038
Vibramycin Hyclate Intravenous (Doxycycline Hyclate) Pfizer Inc 2040
Vibramycin (Doxycycline Monohydrate) Pfizer Inc 2038

Bartonellosis
DYNACIN Capsules (Minocycline Hydrochloride) Medicis 1627
Minocin Oral Suspension (Minocycline Hydrochloride) Lederle 1431
Minocin Pellet-Filled Capsules (Minocycline Hydrochloride) Lederle 1429
Monodox Capsules (Doxycycline Monohydrate) Oclassen 1858

Bedsores (see under Ulcers, decubitus, adjunctive therapy in)

Behavioral problems associated with chronic brain syndrome
Serentil (Mesoridazine Besylate) Boehringer Ingelheim 689

Behavioral problems associated with mental deficiency
Serentil (Mesoridazine Besylate) Boehringer Ingelheim 689

Behavioral problems, severe, in children
Haldol Injection, Tablets and Concentrate (Haloperidol) McNeil Pharmaceutical 1585
Mellaril (Thioridazine Hydrochloride) Sandoz Pharmaceuticals 2398
Thorazine (Chlorpromazine Hydrochloride) SmithKline Beecham Pharmaceuticals 2701

Bejel
Bicillin L-A Injection (Penicillin G Benzathine) Wyeth-Ayerst 2813

Belching (see under Eructation, relief of)

Benzodiazepine overdose, management of
Romazicon (Flumazenil) Roche Pharmaceuticals 2311

Berylliosis
Celestone Soluspan Suspension (Betamethasone Sodium Phosphate, Betamethasone Acetate) Schering 2484
Cortone Acetate Sterile Suspension (Cortisone Acetate) Merck & Co., Inc. 1663
Cortone Acetate Tablets (Cortisone Acetate) Merck & Co., Inc. 1664
Dalalone D.P. Injectable (Dexamethasone Acetate) Forest 1009
Decadron Elixir (Dexamethasone) Merck & Co., Inc. 1676
Decadron Phosphate Injection (Dexamethasone Sodium Phosphate) Merck & Co., Inc. 1680
Decadron Tablets (Dexamethasone) Merck & Co., Inc. 1678
Decadron-LA Sterile Suspension (Dexamethasone Acetate) Merck & Co., Inc. 1687
Hydeltrasol Injection, Sterile (Prednisolone Sodium Phosphate) Merck & Co., Inc. 1708
Hydrocortone Phosphate Injection, Sterile (Hydrocortisone Sodium Phosphate) Merck & Co., Inc. 1713
Hydrocortone Tablets (Hydrocortisone) Merck & Co., Inc. 1715
Pediapred Oral Solution (Prednisolone Sodium Phosphate) Medeva 1618
Prelone Syrup (Prednisolone) Muro 1834

Bifidobacterium species gynecologic infections
Primaxin I.V. (Cilastatin Sodium, Imipenem) Merck & Co., Inc. 1772

Bifidobacterium species infections
Primaxin I.V. (Cilastatin Sodium, Imipenem) Merck & Co., Inc. 1772

Bifidobacterium species intra-abdominal infections
Primaxin I.V. (Cilastatin Sodium, Imipenem) Merck & Co., Inc. 1772

Biliary calculi, chemical dissolution of
Actigall Capsules (Ursodiol) CibaGeneva 818

Biliary calculi, to prevent formation of
Actigall Capsules (Ursodiol) CibaGeneva 818

Bites, black widow spider
Antivenin (Black Widow Spider) (Black Widow Spider Antivenin (Equine)) Merck & Co., Inc. 1647

Bites, crotalidae (see under Envenomation, pit viper)

Bites, insect
Aquanil HC Lotion (Hydrocortisone) Persōn & Covey 1989
Benadryl Itch Stopping Cream Original Strength (Diphenhydramine Hydrochloride, Zinc Acetate) Warner Wellcome .... 📖 814

(📖 Described in PDR For Nonprescription Drugs) (◉ Described in PDR For Ophthalmology)

Bites

- Benadryl Gel (Diphenhydramine Hydrochloride, Zinc Acetate) Warner Wellcome ... 815
- Benadryl Spray (Diphenhydramine Hydrochloride, Zinc Acetate) Warner Wellcome ... 815
- Caldecort Anti-Itch Hydrocortisone Cream (Hydrocortisone Acetate) Ciba Self-Medication ... 651
- Cortaid (Hydrocortisone Acetate) Upjohn ... 800
- Cortizone-5 (Hydrocortisone) Thompson Medical ... 795
- Cortizone-10 Creme and Ointment (Hydrocortisone) Thompson Medical ... 795
- EpiPen (Epinephrine) Center ... 808
- Mantadil Cream (Chlorcyclizine Hydrochloride) Glaxo Wellcome ... 1124
- Unguentine Plus (Lidocaine Hydrochloride, Phenol) Mentholatum ... 712

Bites, pit vipers
(see under Envenomation, pit viper)

Blackheads, reduction of
(see under Histomoniasis, reduction of)

Bladder carcinoma, transitional cell
(see under Carcinoma, bladder, transitional cell)

Blastoma, medullary, palliative therapy in
- BiCNU (Carmustine (BCNU)) Bristol-Myers Squibb Oncology/Immunology ... 696

Blastomycosis
- Fungizone Intravenous (Amphotericin B) Apothecon ... 507
- Nizoral Tablets (Ketoconazole) Janssen ... 1345
- Sporanox Capsules (Itraconazole) Janssen ... 1352

Blastomycosis, North American
(see under Blastomycosis)

Bleeding associated with hemophilia A
- Konÿne 80 Factor IX Complex (Factor IX Complex) Bayer Biological ... 627

Bleeding, fibrinolytic
- Amicar Syrup, Tablets, and Injection (Aminocaproic Acid) Immunex ... 1312

Bleeding, upper gastrointestinal, in critically ill
- Tagamet (Cimetidine Hydrochloride) SmithKline Beecham Pharmaceuticals ... 2694

Blepharitis
- Garamycin Ophthalmic (Gentamicin Sulfate) Schering ... 2501
- Genoptic Sterile Ophthalmic Solution (Gentamicin Sulfate) Allergan ... 241
- Genoptic Sterile Ophthalmic Ointment (Gentamicin Sulfate) Allergan ... 241
- Gentak (Gentamicin Sulfate) Akorn ... 209
- Neosporin Ophthalmic Ointment Sterile (Polymyxin B Sulfate, Bacitracin Zinc, Neomycin Sulfate) Glaxo Wellcome ... 1130
- Neosporin Ophthalmic Solution Sterile (Polymyxin B Sulfate, Neomycin Sulfate, Gramicidin) Glaxo Wellcome ... 1131
- Polysporin Ophthalmic Ointment Sterile (Polymyxin B Sulfate, Bacitracin Zinc) Glaxo Wellcome ... 1140
- Pred Mild (Prednisolone Acetate) Allergan ... 250

Blepharitis, fungal
- Natacyn Antifungal Ophthalmic Suspension (Natamycin) Alcon Laboratories ... 223

Blepharoconjunctivitis
- Garamycin Ophthalmic (Gentamicin Sulfate) Schering ... 2501
- Genoptic Sterile Ophthalmic Solution (Gentamicin Sulfate) Allergan ... 241
- Genoptic Sterile Ophthalmic Ointment (Gentamicin Sulfate) Allergan ... 241
- Gentak (Gentamicin Sulfate) Akorn ... 209
- Neosporin Ophthalmic Ointment Sterile (Polymyxin B Sulfate, Bacitracin Zinc, Neomycin Sulfate) Glaxo Wellcome ... 1130
- Neosporin Ophthalmic Solution Sterile (Polymyxin B Sulfate, Neomycin Sulfate, Gramicidin) Glaxo Wellcome ... 1131
- Polysporin Ophthalmic Ointment Sterile (Polymyxin B Sulfate, Bacitracin Zinc) Glaxo Wellcome ... 1140
- Polytrim Ophthalmic Solution Sterile (Polymyxin B Sulfate, Trimethoprim Sulfate) Allergan ... 479

Blepharospasm
- BOTOX (Botulinum Toxin Type A) Purified Neurotoxin Complex (Botulinum Toxin Type A) Allergan ... 473

Blood clotting, prevention of in arterial surgery
- Heparin Sodium Injection (Heparin Sodium) Wyeth-Ayerst ... 2832
- Heparin Sodium Vials (Heparin Sodium) Lilly ... 1486

Blood clotting, prevention of in blood transfusion
- Heparin Lock Flush Solution (Heparin Sodium) Wyeth-Ayerst ... 2831
- Heparin Sodium Vials (Heparin Sodium) Lilly ... 1486

Blood clotting, prevention of in cardiac surgery
- Heparin Sodium Injection (Heparin Sodium) Wyeth-Ayerst ... 2832
- Heparin Sodium Vials (Heparin Sodium) Lilly ... 1486

Blood clotting, prevention of in dialysis procedures
- Heparin Lock Flush Solution (Heparin Sodium) Wyeth-Ayerst ... 2831
- Heparin Sodium Vials (Heparin Sodium) Lilly ... 1486

Blood clotting, prevention of in extracorporeal circulation
- Heparin Lock Flush Solution (Heparin Sodium) Wyeth-Ayerst ... 2831
- Heparin Sodium Vials (Heparin Sodium) Lilly ... 1486

Blood loss, perioperative, reduction of
- Trasylol (Aprotinin) Bayer Pharmaceutical ... 607

Blood pressure, maintaining during anesthesia
(see under Hypotension, acute)

Blood pressure, restoring during anesthesia
(see under Hypotension, acute)

Body aches
(see under Pain, general)

Boils, symptomatic relief of
(see under Furunculosis, symptomatic relief of)

Bone disease, metabolic, with chronic renal failure
(see under Osteodystrophy, renal)

Bone marrow transplantation, allogeneic or autologous, delayed or failed
- Leukine (Sargramostim) Immunex ... 1317

Bone marrow transplantation, to decrease the risk of septicemia
- Gamimune N, 5% Immune Globulin Intravenous (Human), 5% (Globulin, Immune (Human)) Bayer Biological ... 612
- Gamimune N, 10% Immune Globulin Intravenous (Human), 10% (Globulin, Immune (Human)) Bayer Biological ... 615

Bone mass, loss of
(see under Osteoporosis)

Bordetella pertussis
(see under B. pertussis infections)

Borrelia recurrentis infection
- Achromycin V Capsules (Tetracycline Hydrochloride) Lederle ... 1417
- Declomycin Tablets (Demeclocycline Hydrochloride) Lederle ... 1421
- Doryx Capsules (Doxycycline Hyclate) Parke-Davis ... 1970
- DYNACIN Capsules (Minocycline Hydrochloride) Medicis ... 1627
- Minocin Intravenous (Minocycline Hydrochloride) Lederle ... 1428
- Minocin Oral Suspension (Minocycline Hydrochloride) Lederle ... 1431
- Minocin Pellet-Filled Capsules (Minocycline Hydrochloride) Lederle ... 1429
- Monodox Capsules (Doxycycline Monohydrate) Oclassen ... 1858
- Terramycin Intramuscular Solution (Oxytetracycline) Pfizer Inc ... 2034
- Vibramycin (Doxycycline Calcium) Pfizer Inc ... 2038
- Vibramycin Hyclate Intravenous (Doxycycline Hyclate) Pfizer Inc ... 2040
- Vibramycin (Doxycycline Monohydrate) Pfizer Inc ... 2038

Bowel, evacuation of
- Colyte and Colyte-flavored (Polyethylene Glycol) Schwarz ... 2540
- Fleet Bisacodyl Enema (Bisacodyl) Fleet ... 1000
- Fleet Enema (Sodium Phosphate, Dibasic, Sodium Phosphate, Monobasic) Fleet ... 1001
- Fleet Mineral Oil Enema (Mineral Oil) Fleet ... 1001
- Fleet Phospho-Soda (Sodium Phosphate, Dibasic, Sodium Phosphate, Monobasic) Fleet ... 1002
- Fleet Prep Kits (Sodium Phosphate, Dibasic, Sodium Phosphate, Monobasic) Fleet ... 1002
- GoLYTELY (Polyethylene Glycol) Braintree ... 694
- NuLYTELY (Polyethylene Glycol, Sodium Bicarbonate, Sodium Chloride, Potassium Chloride) Braintree ... 694
- Cherry Flavor NuLYTELY (Polyethylene Glycol, Sodium Bicarbonate, Sodium Chloride, Potassium Chloride) Braintree ... 694
- Purge Concentrate (Castor Oil) Fleming ... 671
- Senna X-Prep Bowel Evacuant Liquid (Senna Concentrates) Gray ... 1236

Bowel, irritable, syndrome
- Bentyl (Dicyclomine Hydrochloride) Hoechst Marion Roussel ... 1246
- Konsyl Fiber Tablets (Calcium Polycarbophil) Konsyl ... 679
- Levsin/Levsinex/Levbid (Hyoscyamine Sulfate) Schwarz ... 2549
- Metamucil (Psyllium Preparations) Procter & Gamble ... 2125

Bowel, irritable, syndrome, "possibly" effective in, adjunctive therapy
- Cystospaz (Hyoscyamine) PolyMedica ... 2123
- Donnatal (Phenobarbital, Belladonna Alkaloids) Robins ... 2234
- Donnatal Extentabs (Phenobarbital, Belladonna Alkaloids) Robins ... 2234
- Donnatal Tablets (Phenobarbital, Belladonna Alkaloids) Robins ... 2234
- Librax Capsules (Chlordiazepoxide Hydrochloride, Clidinium Bromide) Roche Products ... 2330

Brain imaging
(see under Intracranial lesions imaging, magnetic resonance)

Brain tumors
(see under Tumors, brain, palliative therapy in)

Branhamella catarrhalis
(see under M. catarrhalis infections)

Breast cancer
(see under Carcinoma, breast)

Breast carcinoma
(see under Carcinoma, breast)

Breast disease, fibrocystic
- Danocrine Capsules (Danazol) Sanofi Winthrop ... 2437

Breathing, intermittent positive pressure-aid in
- Sodium Chloride Sterile Water for Inhalation, Arm-a-Vial (Sodium Chloride) Astra ... 557

Bromhidrosis, topical relief of
(see under Hyperhidrosis, topical relief of)

Bronchial asthma
- AeroBid Inhaler System (Flunisolide) Forest ... 1004
- Aerobid-M Inhaler System (Flunisolide) Forest ... 1004
- Aerolate (Theophylline Anhydrous) Fleming ... 1003
- Airet Albuterol Sulfate Inhalation Solution (Albuterol Sulfate) Medeva ... 1602
- Alupent (Metaproterenol Sulfate) Boehringer Ingelheim ... 672
- Ana-Kit Anaphylaxis Emergency Treatment Kit (Epinephrine Hydrochloride, Chlorpheniramine Maleate) Bayer Allergy ... 611
- Atrovent Inhalation Aerosol (Ipratropium Bromide) Boehringer Ingelheim ... 674
- Azmacort Oral Inhaler (Triamcinolone Acetonide) Rhone-Poulenc Rorer Pharmaceuticals ... 2175
- Beclovent Inhalation Aerosol and Refill (Beclomethasone Dipropionate) Glaxo Wellcome ... 1063
- Brethine Ampuls (Terbutaline Sulfate) CibaGeneva ... 832
- Brethine Tablets (Terbutaline Sulfate) CibaGeneva ... 831
- Bricanyl Subcutaneous Injection (Terbutaline Sulfate) Hoechst Marion Roussel ... 1247
- Bricanyl Tablets (Terbutaline Sulfate) Hoechst Marion Roussel ... 1248
- Bronkometer Aerosol (Isoetharine) Sanofi Winthrop ... 2432
- Bronkosol Solution (Isoetharine) Sanofi Winthrop ... 2432
- Celestone Soluspan Suspension (Betamethasone Sodium Phosphate, Betamethasone Acetate) Schering ... 2484
- Congess (Guaifenesin, Pseudoephedrine Hydrochloride) Fleming ... 1003
- Cortone Acetate Sterile Suspension (Cortisone Acetate) Merck & Co., Inc. ... 1663
- Cortone Acetate Tablets (Cortisone Acetate) Merck & Co., Inc. ... 1664
- Dalalone D.P. Injectable (Dexamethasone Acetate) Forest ... 1009
- Decadron Elixir (Dexamethasone) Merck & Co., Inc. ... 1676
- Decadron Phosphate Injection (Dexamethasone Sodium Phosphate) Merck & Co., Inc. ... 1680
- Decadron Tablets (Dexamethasone) Merck & Co., Inc. ... 1678
- Decadron-LA Sterile Suspension (Dexamethasone Acetate) Merck & Co., Inc. ... 1687
- Dexacort Phosphate in Respihaler (Dexamethasone Sodium Phosphate) Medeva ... 1606
- Flovent (Fluticasone Propionate) Glaxo Wellcome ... 1089

(■ Described in PDR For Nonprescription Drugs) (☉ Described in PDR For Ophthalmology)

Hydeltrasol Injection, Sterile (Prednisolone Sodium Phosphate) Merck & Co., Inc. 1708
Hydrocortone Phosphate Injection, Sterile (Hydrocortisone Sodium Phosphate) Merck & Co., Inc. 1713
Hydrocortone Tablets (Hydrocortisone) Merck & Co., Inc. 1715
Intal Inhaler (Cromolyn Sodium) Rhone-Poulenc Rorer Pharmaceuticals 2185
Intal Nebulizer Solution (Cromolyn Sodium) Rhone-Poulenc Rorer Pharmaceuticals 2186
Isoetharine Inhalation Solution, USP, Arm-a-Med (Isoetharine) Astra 545
Isuprel Hydrochloride Solution (Isoproterenol Hydrochloride) Sanofi Winthrop 2443
Isuprel Mistometer (Isoproterenol Hydrochloride) Sanofi Winthrop .. 2442
Lufyllin & Lufyllin-400 Tablets (Dyphylline) Wallace 2778
Lufyllin-GG Elixir & Tablets (Dyphylline, Guaifenesin) Wallace 2779
Maxair Autohaler (Pirbuterol Acetate) 3M Pharmaceuticals 1550
Maxair Inhaler (Pirbuterol Acetate) 3M Pharmaceuticals 1552
Metaproterenol Sulfate Inhalation Solution, USP, Arm-a-Med (Metaproterenol Sulfate) Astra 547
Norisodrine with Calcium Iodide Syrup (Calcium Iodide, Isoproterenol Sulfate) Abbott 446
Pediapred Oral Solution (Prednisolone Sodium Phosphate) Medeva 1618
Pima Syrup (Potassium Iodide) Fleming 1004
Prelone Syrup (Prednisolone) Muro 1834
Primatene Mist (Epinephrine) Whitehall-Robins .... ■ 843
Primatene Tablets (Theophylline Anhydrous, Ephedrine Hydrochloride) Whitehall-Robins .... ■ 844
Proventil Inhalation Aerosol (Albuterol) Schering 2524
Proventil Inhalation Solution 0.083% (Albuterol Sulfate) Schering 2527
Proventil Repetabs Tablets (Albuterol Sulfate) Schering 2529
Proventil Solution for Inhalation 0.5% (Albuterol Sulfate) Schering 2525
Proventil Syrup (Albuterol Sulfate) Schering 2528
Proventil Tablets (Albuterol Sulfate) Schering 2529
Quadrinal Tablets (Ephedrine Hydrochloride, Phenobarbital, Potassium Iodide, Theophylline Calcium Salicylate) Knoll Laboratories 1398
Quibron (Theophylline, Guaifenesin) Roberts 2227
Respbid Tablets (Theophylline Anhydrous) Boehringer Ingelheim 687
SSKI Solution (Potassium Iodide) Upsher-Smith 2767
Serevent Inhalation Aerosol (Salmeterol Xinafoate) Glaxo Wellcome 1149
Slo-bid Gyrocaps (Theophylline Anhydrous) Rhone-Poulenc Rorer Pharmaceuticals 2201
Sus-Phrine Injection (Epinephrine) Forest 1017
Theo-24 Extended Release Capsules (Theophylline Anhydrous) UCB 2753
Theo-Dur Extended-Release Tablets (Theophylline Anhydrous) Key 1367
Theo-X Extended-Release Tablets (Theophylline Anhydrous) Carnrick 793
Tilade Inhaler (Nedocromil Sodium) Rhone-Poulenc Rorer Pharmaceuticals 2207
Tornalate Solution for Inhalation, 0.2% (Bitolterol Mesylate) Dura .. 976
Tornalate Metered Dose Inhaler (Bitolterol Mesylate) Dura 978
Uni-Dur Extended-Release Tablets (Theophylline Anhydrous) Key 1374
Uniphyl 400 mg and 600 mg Tablets (Theophylline Anhydrous) Purdue Frederick 2157
Vanceril Inhaler (Beclomethasone Dipropionate) Schering 2538
Ventolin Inhalation Aerosol and Refill (Albuterol) Glaxo Wellcome 1170
Ventolin Inhalation Solution (Albuterol Sulfate) Glaxo Wellcome .. 1171
Ventolin Nebules Inhalation Solution (Albuterol Sulfate) Glaxo Wellcome 1172
Ventolin Rotacaps for Inhalation (Albuterol Sulfate) Glaxo Wellcome 1173
Ventolin Syrup (Albuterol Sulfate) Glaxo Wellcome 1175
Ventolin Tablets (Albuterol Sulfate) Glaxo Wellcome 1176
Volmax Extended-Release Tablets (Albuterol Sulfate) Muro 1835

Bronchial congestion

Dorcol Children's Cough Syrup (Pseudoephedrine Hydrochloride, Guaifenesin, Dextromethorphan Hydrobromide) Sandoz Consumer .... ■ 748
Entex LA Tablets (Phenylpropanolamine Hydrochloride, Guaifenesin) Dura 972
Guaifed (Guaifenesin, Pseudoephedrine Hydrochloride) Muro 1833
Guaifed Syrup (Guaifenesin, Pseudoephedrine Hydrochloride) Muro .... ■ 712
Humibid (Guaifenesin, Dextromethorphan Hydrobromide) Medeva 1612
Novahistine DMX (Dextromethorphan Hydrobromide, Guaifenesin, Pseudoephedrine Hydrochloride) SmithKline Beecham Consumer .... ■ 782
Organidin NR Tablets and Liquid (Guaifenesin) Wallace 2781
Pediatric Vicks 44e Cough & Chest Congestion Relief (Dextromethorphan Hydrobromide, Guaifenesin) Procter & Gamble ■ 737
Robitussin (Guaifenesin) Whitehall-Robins .... ■ 845
Robitussin A-C Syrup (Codeine Phosphate, Guaifenesin) Robins .. 2248
Robitussin Severe Congestion Liqui-Gels (Guaifenesin, Pseudoephedrine Hydrochloride) Whitehall-Robins .... ■ 845
Robitussin-DAC Syrup (Codeine Phosphate, Guaifenesin, Pseudoephedrine Hydrochloride) Robins 2249
Robitussin-DM (Dextromethorphan Hydrobromide, Guaifenesin) Whitehall-Robins .... ■ 846
Robitussin-PE (Guaifenesin, Pseudoephedrine Hydrochloride) Whitehall-Robins .... ■ 846
Sudafed Non-Drying Sinus Liquid Caps (Pseudoephedrine Hydrochloride, Guaifenesin) Warner Wellcome .... ■ 827
Syn-Rx Tablets (Pseudoephedrine Hydrochloride, Guaifenesin) Medeva 1622
Triaminic Expectorant (Phenylpropanolamine Hydrochloride, Guaifenesin) Sandoz Consumer ■ 753
Vicks 44E Cough & Chest Congestion Relief (Dextromethorphan Hydrobromide, Guaifenesin) Procter & Gamble ■ 729

Bronchitis, acute

Azactam for Injection (Aztreonam) Bristol-Myers Squibb 736
Ceftin Tablets (Cefuroxime Axetil) Glaxo Wellcome 1067
Cefzil Tablets and Oral Suspension (Cefprozil) Bristol-Myers Squibb .. 747
Dynabac (Dirithromycin) Bock 668
Lorabid Suspension and Pulvules (Loracarbef) Lilly 1513
Suprax (Cefixime) Lederle 1443

Bronchitis, chronic

Atrovent Inhalation Aerosol (Ipratropium Bromide) Boehringer Ingelheim 674
Brethine Ampuls (Terbutaline Sulfate) CibaGeneva 832
Brethine Tablets (Terbutaline Sulfate) CibaGeneva 831
Bricanyl Tablets (Terbutaline Sulfate) Hoechst Marion Roussel 1248
Norisodrine with Calcium Iodide Syrup (Calcium Iodide, Isoproterenol Sulfate) Abbott 446
Pima Syrup (Potassium Iodide) Fleming 1004
Quadrinal Tablets (Ephedrine Hydrochloride, Phenobarbital, Potassium Iodide, Theophylline Calcium Salicylate) Knoll Laboratories 1398
Respbid Tablets (Theophylline Anhydrous) Boehringer Ingelheim 687
SSKI Solution (Potassium Iodide) Upsher-Smith 2767
Slo-bid Gyrocaps (Theophylline Anhydrous) Rhone-Poulenc Rorer Pharmaceuticals 2201
Uniphyl 400 mg and 600 mg Tablets (Theophylline Anhydrous) Purdue Frederick 2157

Bronchitis, chronic, acute exacerbation of

Bactrim (Trimethoprim, Sulfamethoxazole) Roche Pharmaceuticals 2257
Biaxin (Clarithromycin) Abbott 406
Cedax (Ceftibuten Dihydrate) Schering 2480
Ceftin for Oral Suspension (Cefuroxime Axetil) Glaxo Wellcome 1067
Cefzil Tablets and Oral Suspension (Cefprozil) Bristol-Myers Squibb .. 747
Floxin I.V. (Ofloxacin) McNeil Pharmaceutical 1580
Floxin Tablets (200 mg, 300 mg, 400 mg) (Ofloxacin) McNeil Pharmaceutical 1577
Lorabid Suspension and Pulvules (Loracarbef) Lilly 1513
Maxaquin Tablets (Lomefloxacin Hydrochloride) Searle 2593
Primaxin I.M. (Cilastatin Sodium, Imipenem) Merck & Co., Inc. 1770
Septra (Trimethoprim, Sulfamethoxazole) Glaxo Wellcome 1146
Spectrobid Tablets (Bacampicillin Hydrochloride) Pfizer Inc 2030
Suprax (Cefixime) Lederle 1443
Vantin for Oral Suspension and Vantin Tablets (Cefpodoxime Proxetil) Pharmacia & Upjohn 2112

Bronchospasm during anesthesia

Isuprel Injection (Isoproterenol Hydrochloride) Sanofi Winthrop .. 2441

Bronchospasm, exercise-induced

Intal Nebulizer Solution (Cromolyn Sodium) Rhone-Poulenc Rorer Pharmaceuticals 2186
Proventil Inhalation Aerosol (Albuterol) Schering 2524
Serevent Inhalation Aerosol (Salmeterol Xinafoate) Glaxo Wellcome 1149
Ventolin Inhalation Aerosol and Refill (Albuterol) Glaxo Wellcome 1170

Bronchospasm, prevention and relief of

Albuterol Sulfate, USP Solution for Inhalation, Arm-a-Med (Albuterol Sulfate) Astra 522
Uni-Dur Extended-Release Tablets (Theophylline Anhydrous) Key 1374
Ventolin Inhalation Aerosol and Refill (Albuterol) Glaxo Wellcome 1170
Ventolin Rotacaps for Inhalation (Albuterol Sulfate) Glaxo Wellcome 1173

Bronchospasm, reversible (see also under Bronchial asthma)

Albuterol Sulfate, USP Solution for Inhalation, Arm-a-Med (Albuterol Sulfate) Astra 522
Alupent (Metaproterenol Sulfate) Boehringer Ingelheim 672
Atrovent Inhalation Aerosol (Ipratropium Bromide) Boehringer Ingelheim 674
Atrovent Inhalation Solution (Ipratropium Bromide) Boehringer Ingelheim 675
Brethaire Inhaler (Terbutaline Sulfate) CibaGeneva 830
Brethine Ampuls (Terbutaline Sulfate) CibaGeneva 832
Brethine Tablets (Terbutaline Sulfate) CibaGeneva 831
Bricanyl Subcutaneous Injection (Terbutaline Sulfate) Hoechst Marion Roussel 1247
Bricanyl Tablets (Terbutaline Sulfate) Hoechst Marion Roussel 1248
Bronkosol Solution (Isoetharine) Sanofi Winthrop 2432
Intal Inhaler (Cromolyn Sodium) Rhone-Poulenc Rorer Pharmaceuticals 2185
Isuprel Hydrochloride Solution (Isoproterenol Hydrochloride) Sanofi Winthrop 2443
Isuprel Mistometer (Isoproterenol Hydrochloride) Sanofi Winthrop .. 2442
Lufyllin & Lufyllin-400 Tablets (Dyphylline) Wallace 2778
Lufyllin-GG Elixir & Tablets (Dyphylline, Guaifenesin) Wallace 2779
Maxair Inhaler (Pirbuterol Acetate) 3M Pharmaceuticals 1552
Proventil Inhalation Aerosol (Albuterol) Schering 2524
Proventil Inhalation Solution 0.083% (Albuterol Sulfate) Schering 2527
Proventil Repetabs Tablets (Albuterol Sulfate) Schering 2529
Proventil Solution for Inhalation 0.5% (Albuterol Sulfate) Schering 2525
Proventil Syrup (Albuterol Sulfate) Schering 2528
Proventil Tablets (Albuterol Sulfate) Schering 2529
Quadrinal Tablets (Ephedrine Hydrochloride, Phenobarbital, Potassium Iodide, Theophylline Calcium Salicylate) Knoll Laboratories 1398
Respbid Tablets (Theophylline Anhydrous) Boehringer Ingelheim 687
Serevent Inhalation Aerosol (Salmeterol Xinafoate) Glaxo Wellcome 1149
Slo-bid Gyrocaps (Theophylline Anhydrous) Rhone-Poulenc Rorer Pharmaceuticals 2201
Sus-Phrine Injection (Epinephrine) Forest 1017
Theo-24 Extended Release Capsules (Theophylline Anhydrous) UCB 2753
Theo-Dur Extended-Release Tablets (Theophylline Anhydrous) Key 1367
Theo-X Extended-Release Tablets (Theophylline Anhydrous) Carnrick 793
Tornalate Solution for Inhalation, 0.2% (Bitolterol Mesylate) Dura .. 976
Tornalate Metered Dose Inhaler (Bitolterol Mesylate) Dura 978
Uniphyl 400 mg and 600 mg Tablets (Theophylline Anhydrous) Purdue Frederick 2157
Ventolin Inhalation Aerosol and Refill (Albuterol) Glaxo Wellcome 1170
Ventolin Inhalation Solution (Albuterol Sulfate) Glaxo Wellcome .. 1171
Ventolin Nebules Inhalation Solution (Albuterol Sulfate) Glaxo Wellcome 1172
Ventolin Rotacaps for Inhalation (Albuterol Sulfate) Glaxo Wellcome 1173
Ventolin Syrup (Albuterol Sulfate) Glaxo Wellcome 1175
Ventolin Tablets (Albuterol Sulfate) Glaxo Wellcome 1176
Volmax Extended-Release Tablets (Albuterol Sulfate) Muro 1835

Bronchospasm, reversible, associated with chronic bronchitis

Alupent (Metaproterenol Sulfate) Boehringer Ingelheim 672
Atrovent Inhalation Aerosol (Ipratropium Bromide) Boehringer Ingelheim 674
Atrovent Inhalation Solution (Ipratropium Bromide) Boehringer Ingelheim 675

(■ Described in PDR For Nonprescription Drugs) (◉ Described in PDR For Ophthalmology)

Bronchospasm

- Brethine Ampuls (Terbutaline Sulfate) CibaGeneva ... 832
- Brethine Tablets (Terbutaline Sulfate) CibaGeneva ... 831
- Bronkometer Aerosol (Isoetharine) Sanofi Winthrop ... 2432
- Bronkosol Solution (Isoetharine) Sanofi Winthrop ... 2432
- Isoetharine Inhalation Solution, USP, Arm-a-Med (Isoetharine) Astra ... 545
- Isuprel Hydrochloride Solution (Isoproterenol Hydrochloride) Sanofi Winthrop ... 2443
- Isuprel Mistometer (Isoproterenol Hydrochloride) Sanofi Winthrop ... 2442
- Lufyllin & Lufyllin-400 Tablets (Dyphylline) Wallace ... 2778
- Lufyllin-GG Elixir & Tablets (Dyphylline, Guaifenesin) Wallace ... 2779
- Metaproterenol Sulfate Inhalation Solution, USP, Arm-a-Med (Metaproterenol Sulfate) Astra ... 547
- Quibron (Theophylline, Guaifenesin) Roberts ... 2227
- Respbid Tablets (Theophylline Anhydrous) Boehringer Ingelheim ... 687
- Slo-bid Gyrocaps (Theophylline Anhydrous) Rhone-Poulenc Rorer Pharmaceuticals ... 2201
- Sus-Phrine Injection (Epinephrine) Forest ... 1017
- Theo-24 Extended Release Capsules (Theophylline Anhydrous) UCB ... 2753
- Theo-Dur Extended-Release Tablets (Theophylline Anhydrous) Key ... 1367
- Theo-X Extended-Release Tablets (Theophylline Anhydrous) Carnrick ... 793
- Uni-Dur Extended-Release Tablets (Theophylline Anhydrous) Key ... 1374
- Uniphyl 400 mg and 600 mg Tablets (Theophylline Anhydrous) Purdue Frederick ... 2157

Bronchospasm, reversible, associated with emphysema

- Alupent (Metaproterenol Sulfate) Boehringer Ingelheim ... 672
- Atrovent Inhalation Aerosol (Ipratropium Bromide) Boehringer Ingelheim ... 674
- Atrovent Inhalation Solution (Ipratropium Bromide) Boehringer Ingelheim ... 675
- Brethine Ampuls (Terbutaline Sulfate) CibaGeneva ... 832
- Brethine Tablets (Terbutaline Sulfate) CibaGeneva ... 831
- Bronkometer Aerosol (Isoetharine) Sanofi Winthrop ... 2432
- Bronkosol Solution (Isoetharine) Sanofi Winthrop ... 2432
- Isoetharine Inhalation Solution, USP, Arm-a-Med (Isoetharine) Astra ... 545
- Isuprel Hydrochloride Solution (Isoproterenol Hydrochloride) Sanofi Winthrop ... 2443
- Isuprel Mistometer (Isoproterenol Hydrochloride) Sanofi Winthrop ... 2442
- Lufyllin & Lufyllin-400 Tablets (Dyphylline) Wallace ... 2778
- Lufyllin-GG Elixir & Tablets (Dyphylline, Guaifenesin) Wallace ... 2779
- Maxair Autohaler (Pirbuterol Acetate) 3M Pharmaceuticals ... 1550
- Metaproterenol Sulfate Inhalation Solution, USP, Arm-a-Med (Metaproterenol Sulfate) Astra ... 547
- Quibron (Theophylline, Guaifenesin) Roberts ... 2227
- Respbid Tablets (Theophylline Anhydrous) Boehringer Ingelheim ... 687
- Slo-bid Gyrocaps (Theophylline Anhydrous) Rhone-Poulenc Rorer Pharmaceuticals ... 2201
- Sus-Phrine Injection (Epinephrine) Forest ... 1017
- Theo-24 Extended Release Capsules (Theophylline Anhydrous) UCB ... 2753
- Theo-Dur Extended-Release Tablets (Theophylline Anhydrous) Key ... 1367
- Theo-X Extended-Release Tablets (Theophylline Anhydrous) Carnrick ... 793
- Uni-Dur Extended-Release Tablets (Theophylline Anhydrous) Key ... 1374
- Uniphyl 400 mg and 600 mg Tablets (Theophylline Anhydrous) Purdue Frederick ... 2157

Bronchospastic disorders, "possibly" effective in

- Marax Tablets & DF Syrup (Ephedrine Sulfate, Theophylline, Hydroxyzine Hydrochloride) Pfizer Inc ... 2015

Brucella species infections

- Streptomycin Sulfate Injection (Streptomycin Sulfate) Pfizer Inc ... 2031

Brucella species infections, adjunct in

- Achromycin V Capsules (Tetracycline Hydrochloride) Lederle ... 1417
- Declomycin Tablets (Demeclocycline Hydrochloride) Lederle ... 1421
- Doryx Capsules (Doxycycline Hyclate) Parke-Davis ... 1970
- DYNACIN Capsules (Minocycline Hydrochloride) Medicis ... 1627
- Minocin Intravenous (Minocycline Hydrochloride) Lederle ... 1428
- Minocin Oral Suspension (Minocycline Hydrochloride) Lederle ... 1431
- Minocin Pellet-Filled Capsules (Minocycline Hydrochloride) Lederle ... 1429
- Monodox Capsules (Doxycycline Monohydrate) Oclassen ... 1858
- Terramycin Intramuscular Solution (Oxytetracycline) Pfizer Inc ... 2034
- Vibramycin (Doxycycline Calcium) Pfizer Inc ... 2038
- Vibramycin Hyclate Intravenous (Doxycycline Hyclate) Pfizer Inc ... 2040
- Vibramycin (Doxycycline Monohydrate) Pfizer Inc ... 2038

Brucellosis

- DYNACIN Capsules (Minocycline Hydrochloride) Medicis ... 1627
- Minocin Oral Suspension (Minocycline Hydrochloride) Lederle ... 1431
- Minocin Pellet-Filled Capsules (Minocycline Hydrochloride) Lederle ... 1429
- Monodox Capsules (Doxycycline Monohydrate) Oclassen ... 1858

Bruises, topical relief of
(see under Pain, topical relief of)

"Bubble boy" disease
(see under Adenosine deaminase, enzyme replacement therapy for)

Bulbar conjunctiva inflammation

- AK-PRED (Prednisolone Sodium Phosphate) Akorn ... ◉ 204
- AK-Trol Ointment & Suspension (Dexamethasone, Neomycin Sulfate, Polymyxin B Sulfate) Akorn ... ◉ 205
- Blephamide Liquifilm Sterile Ophthalmic Suspension (Prednisolone Acetate, Sulfacetamide Sodium) Allergan ... 472
- Cortisporin Ophthalmic Ointment Sterile (Polymyxin B Sulfate, Bacitracin Zinc, Neomycin Sulfate, Hydrocortisone) Glaxo Wellcome ... 1074
- Cortisporin Ophthalmic Suspension Sterile (Hydrocortisone, Polymyxin B Sulfate, Neomycin Sulfate) Glaxo Wellcome ... 1075
- Econopred & Econopred Plus Ophthalmic Suspensions (Prednisolone Acetate) Alcon Laboratories ... ◉ 216
- FML Forte Liquifilm (Fluorometholone) Allergan ... ◉ 237
- FML Liquifilm (Fluorometholone) Allergan ... ◉ 238
- FML S.O.P. (Fluorometholone) Allergan ... ◉ 239
- FML-S Liquifilm (Sulfacetamide Sodium, Fluorometholone) Allergan ... ◉ 240
- Maxitrol Ophthalmic Ointment and Suspension (Dexamethasone, Neomycin Sulfate, Polymyxin B Sulfate) Alcon Laboratories ... ◉ 222
- Poly-Pred Liquifilm (Neomycin Sulfate, Polymyxin B Sulfate, Prednisolone Acetate) Allergan ... ◉ 246
- Pred Forte (Prednisolone Acetate) Allergan ... ◉ 247
- Pred-G Liquifilm Sterile Ophthalmic Suspension (Gentamicin Sulfate, Prednisolone Acetate) Allergan ... ◉ 248
- Pred-G S.O.P. Sterile Ophthalmic Ointment (Gentamicin Sulfate, Prednisolone Acetate) Allergan ... ◉ 249
- TobraDex Ophthalmic Suspension and Ointment (Dexamethasone, Tobramycin) Alcon Laboratories ... 469

Burn wound infections
(see under Infections, burn wound)

Burns, maintenance of electrolyte balance

- Albuminar-25, Albumin (Human) U.S.P. 25% (Albumin (Human)) Centeon ... 796
- Plasma-Plex, Plasma Protein Fraction (Human) U.S.P. 5% Solution Heat-Treated (Plasma Protein Fraction (Human)) Centeon ... 806

Burns, minor

- A and D Medicated Diaper Rash Ointment (Petrolatum, White, Zinc Oxide) Schering-Plough HealthCare ... ▣ 757
- A and D Ointment (Petrolatum, Lanolin) Schering-Plough HealthCare ... ▣ 757
- Aquaphor Healing Ointment (Petrolatum, Mineral Oil) Beiersdorf ... 636
- Barri-Care Antimicrobial Barrier Ointment (Chloroxylenol) Care-Tech ... ▣ 646
- Betadine First Aid Cream (Povidone Iodine) Purdue Frederick ... 2144
- Betadine Ointment (Povidone Iodine) Purdue Frederick ... 2145
- Betadine Solution (Povidone Iodine) Purdue Frederick ... 2145
- Desitin Ointment (Cod Liver Oil, Zinc Oxide) Pfizer Consumer ... ▣ 715
- Medi-Quik (Benzalkonium Chloride, Lidocaine, Mentholatum ... ▣ 710
- Maximum Strength Mycitracin Triple Antibiotic First Aid Ointment (Bacitracin Zinc, Neomycin Sulfate, Polymyxin B Sulfate) Upjohn ... ▣ 803
- Polysporin Ointment (Bacitracin Zinc, Polymyxin B Sulfate) Warner Wellcome ... ▣ 822
- Polysporin Powder (Bacitracin Zinc, Polymyxin B Sulfate) Warner Wellcome ... ▣ 823

Burns, pain associated with
(see under Pain, topical relief of)

Burns, second- and third-degree, adjunctive therapy in

- Furacin Soluble Dressing (Nitrofurazone) Roberts ... 2220
- Furacin Topical Cream (Nitrofurazone) Roberts ... 2220
- Silvadene Cream 1% (Silver Sulfadiazine) Hoechst Marion Roussel ... 1288
- Sulfamylon Cream (Mafenide Acetate) Dow Hickam ... 940

Burns, to prevent marked hemoconcentration

- Albuminar-5, Albumin (Human) U.S.P. 5% (Albumin (Human)) Centeon ... 795
- Albuminar-25, Albumin (Human) U.S.P. 25% (Albumin (Human)) Centeon ... 796
- Plasma-Plex, Plasma Protein Fraction (Human) U.S.P. 5% Solution Heat-Treated (Plasma Protein Fraction (Human)) Centeon ... 806

Bursitis

- Anaprox/Naprosyn (Naproxen Sodium) Roche Pharmaceuticals ... 2277
- Celestone Soluspan Suspension (Betamethasone Sodium Phosphate, Betamethasone Acetate) Schering ... 2484
- Cortone Acetate Sterile Suspension (Cortisone Acetate) Merck & Co., Inc. ... 1663
- Cortone Acetate Tablets (Cortisone Acetate) Merck & Co., Inc. ... 1664
- Dalalone D.P. Injectable (Dexamethasone Acetate) Forest ... 1009
- Decadron Elixir (Dexamethasone) Merck & Co., Inc. ... 1676
- Decadron Phosphate Injection (Dexamethasone Sodium Phosphate) Merck & Co., Inc. ... 1680
- Decadron Phosphate with Xylocaine Injection, Sterile (Dexamethasone Sodium Phosphate, Lidocaine Hydrochloride) Merck & Co., Inc. ... 1683
- Decadron Tablets (Dexamethasone) Merck & Co., Inc. ... 1678
- Decadron-LA Sterile Suspension (Dexamethasone Acetate) Merck & Co., Inc. ... 1687
- Hydeltrasol Injection, Sterile (Prednisolone Sodium Phosphate) Merck & Co., Inc. ... 1708
- Hydeltra-T.B.A. Sterile Suspension (Prednisolone Tebutate) Merck & Co., Inc. ... 1710
- Hydrocortone Acetate Sterile Suspension (Hydrocortisone Acetate) Merck & Co., Inc. ... 1712
- Hydrocortone Phosphate Injection, Sterile (Hydrocortisone Sodium Phosphate) Merck & Co., Inc. ... 1713
- Hydrocortone Tablets (Hydrocortisone) Merck & Co., Inc. ... 1715
- Indocin (Indomethacin) Merck & Co., Inc. ... 1723
- Naprelan Tablets (Naproxen Sodium) Wyeth-Ayerst ... 2861
- Anaprox/Naprosyn (Naproxen) Roche Pharmaceuticals ... 2277
- Pediapred Oral Solution (Prednisolone Sodium Phosphate) Medeva ... 1618
- Prelone Syrup (Prednisolone) Muro ... 1834
- Traumeel Injection Solution (Homeopathic Medications) Heel/BHI ... 1237

Bursitis, subacromial, acute, symptomatic relief of

- Clinoril Tablets (Sulindac) Merck & Co., Inc. ... 1658
- Indocin (Indomethacin) Merck & Co., Inc. ... 1723
- Trilisate (Choline Magnesium Trisalicylate) Purdue Frederick ... 2155

C

C. difficile infection
(see under Colitis, pseudomembranous, antibiotic-associated)

C. diphtheriae infections

- E.E.S. (Erythromycin Ethylsuccinate) Abbott ... 427
- E-Mycin Tablets (Erythromycin) Knoll Laboratories ... 1388
- ERYC (Erythromycin) Parke-Davis ... 1972
- EryPed (Erythromycin Ethylsuccinate) Abbott ... 425
- Ery-Tab Tablets (Erythromycin) Abbott ... 426
- Erythrocin Stearate Filmtab (Erythromycin Stearate) Abbott ... 429
- Erythromycin Base Filmtab (Erythromycin) Abbott ... 430
- Erythromycin Delayed-Release Capsules, USP (Erythromycin) Abbott ... 431
- Ilosone (Erythromycin Estolate) Dista ... 927
- Ilotycin Gluceptate, IV, Vials (Erythromycin Gluceptate) Dista ... 929
- PCE Dispertab Tablets (Erythromycin) Abbott ... 453
- Pfizerpen for Injection (Penicillin G Potassium) Pfizer Inc ... 2022

C. minutissimum infections

- E.E.S. (Erythromycin Ethylsuccinate) Abbott ... 427
- E-Mycin Tablets (Erythromycin) Knoll Laboratories ... 1388
- ERYC (Erythromycin) Parke-Davis ... 1972
- EryPed (Erythromycin Ethylsuccinate) Abbott ... 425

(▣ Described in PDR For Nonprescription Drugs)   (◉ Described in PDR For Ophthalmology)

Ery-Tab Tablets (Erythromycin) Abbott 426
Erythrocin Stearate Filmtab (Erythromycin Stearate) Abbott 429
Erythromycin Base Filmtab (Erythromycin) Abbott 430
Erythromycin Delayed-Release Capsules, USP (Erythromycin) Abbott 431
Ilosone (Erythromycin Estolate) Dista 927
PCE Dispertab Tablets (Erythromycin) Abbott 453

Cachexia associated with weight loss, AIDS-induced
Megace Oral Suspension (Megestrol Acetate) Bristol-Myers Squibb Oncology/Immunology 708

Calcium deficiency
(see under Hypocalcemia)

Calluses
(see under Hyperkeratosis skin disorders)

Campylobacter fetus infections
Achromycin V Capsules (Tetracycline Hydrochloride) Lederle 1417
Declomycin Tablets (Demeclocycline Hydrochloride) Lederle 1421
Doryx Capsules (Doxycycline Hyclate) Parke-Davis 1970
DYNACIN Capsules (Minocycline Hydrochloride) Medicis 1627
Minocin Intravenous (Minocycline Hydrochloride) Lederle 1428
Minocin Oral Suspension (Minocycline Hydrochloride) Lederle 1431
Minocin Pellet-Filled Capsules (Minocycline Hydrochloride) Lederle 1429
Monodox Capsules (Doxycycline Monohydrate) Oclassen 1858
Terramycin Intramuscular Solution (Oxytetracycline) Pfizer Inc 2034
Vibramycin (Doxycycline Calcium) Pfizer Inc 2038
Vibramycin Hyclate Intravenous (Doxycycline Hyclate) Pfizer Inc .. 2040
Vibramycin (Doxycycline Monohydrate) Pfizer Inc 2038

Campylobacter jejuni infectious diarrhea
Cipro Tablets (Ciprofloxacin Hydrochloride) Bayer Pharmaceutical 584

Cancer, prostatic
(see under Carcinoma, prostatic, palliative treatment of)

Candida albicans infections
AVC (Sulfanilamide) Hoechst Marion Roussel 1245
Betadine Medicated Douche (Povidone Iodine) Purdue Frederick 2144
Betadine Medicated Gel (Povidone Iodine) Purdue Frederick 2144
Fungizone Oral Suspension (Amphotericin B) Bristol-Myers Squibb Oncology/Immunology 704
Loprox 1% Cream and Lotion (Ciclopirox Olamine) Hoechst Marion Roussel 1269
Lotrimin (Clotrimazole) Schering 2514
Mycelex-7 Vaginal Cream Antifungal (Clotrimazole) Bayer Consumer 622
Mycelex-7 Combination-Pack Vaginal Inserts & External Vulvar Cream (Clotrimazole) Bayer Consumer 623
Mycelex-G 500 mg Vaginal Tablets (Clotrimazole) Bayer Pharmaceutical 602
Mycostatin Cream & Topical Powder (Nystatin) Westwood-Squibb 2797
Nystop (Nystatin Topical Powder, USP) (Nystatin) Paddock 1948

Candida infections, serious
Ancobon Capsules (Flucytosine) Roche Pharmaceuticals 2254

Candida species urinary tract infections
Ancobon Capsules (Flucytosine) Roche Pharmaceuticals 2254

Candida strains pulmonary infections
Ancobon Capsules (Flucytosine) Roche Pharmaceuticals 2254

Candidemia
Diflucan Tablets, Injection, and Oral Suspension (Fluconazole) Pfizer Inc 2003

Candidiasis, bone marrow transplantation-induced, prophylactic therapy in
Diflucan Tablets, Injection, and Oral Suspension (Fluconazole) Pfizer Inc 2003

Candidiasis, cutaneous
Loprox 1% Cream and Lotion (Ciclopirox Olamine) Hoechst Marion Roussel 1269
Lotrimin (Clotrimazole) Schering 2514
Monistat Dual-Pak (Miconazole Nitrate) Ortho Pharmaceutical 1906
Monistat-Derm (miconazole nitrate 2%) Cream (Miconazole Nitrate) Ortho Dermatological 1944
Nizoral 2% Cream (Ketoconazole) Janssen 1344
Nystop (Nystatin Topical Powder, USP) (Nystatin) Paddock 1948
Spectazole (econazole nitrate 1%) Cream (Econazole Nitrate) Ortho Dermatological 1947

Candidiasis, disseminated
Diflucan Tablets, Injection, and Oral Suspension (Fluconazole) Pfizer Inc 2003

Candidiasis, esophageal
Diflucan Tablets, Injection, and Oral Suspension (Fluconazole) Pfizer Inc 2003

Candidiasis, mucocutaneous, chronic
Nizoral Tablets (Ketoconazole) Janssen 1345

Candidiasis, oral cavity
Fungizone Oral Suspension (Amphotericin B) Bristol-Myers Squibb Oncology/Immunology 704
Mycostatin Pastilles (Nystatin) Bristol-Myers Squibb Oncology/Immunology 713

Candidiasis, oropharyngeal
Diflucan Tablets, Injection, and Oral Suspension (Fluconazole) Pfizer Inc 2003
Mycelex Troches (Clotrimazole) Bayer Pharmaceutical 601
Nizoral Tablets (Ketoconazole) Janssen 1345

Candidiasis, oropharyngeal, prophylaxis of
Mycelex Troches (Clotrimazole) Bayer Pharmaceutical 601

Candidiasis, systemic
Fungizone Intravenous (Amphotericin B) Apothecon 507

Candidiasis, unspecified
Nizoral Tablets (Ketoconazole) Janssen 1345

Candidiasis, vaginal
Diflucan Tablets, Injection, and Oral Suspension (Fluconazole) Pfizer Inc 2003
Femstat 3 (Butoconazole Nitrate) Procter & Gamble 2124
Monistat Dual-Pak (Miconazole Nitrate) Ortho Pharmaceutical 1906
Monistat 3 Vaginal Suppositories (Miconazole Nitrate) Ortho Pharmaceutical 1905
Mycelex-7 Vaginal Antifungal Cream with 7 Disposable Applicators (Clotrimazole) Bayer Consumer 623
Mycelex-7 Vaginal Inserts Antifungal (Clotrimazole) Bayer Consumer 623
Mycelex-7 Combination-Pack Vaginal Inserts & External Vulvar Cream (Clotrimazole) Bayer Consumer 623
Mycelex-G 500 mg Vaginal Tablets (Clotrimazole) Bayer Pharmaceutical 602
Terazol 3 Vaginal Cream (Terconazole) Ortho Pharmaceutical 1941
Terazol 3 Vaginal Suppositories (Terconazole) Ortho Pharmaceutical 1942
Terazol 7 Vaginal Cream (Terconazole) Ortho Pharmaceutical 1943
Vagistat-1 (Tioconazole) Bristol-Myers Squibb 783

Candiduria
Nizoral Tablets (Ketoconazole) Janssen 1345

Canker sores
(see under Stomatitis, recurrent aphthous, symptomatic relief of)

Carbuncles
(see under Furunculosis, symptomatic relief of)

Carcinoma, adrenal cortex
Lysodren Tablets (Mitotane) Bristol-Myers Squibb Oncology/Immunology 707

Carcinoma, bladder, transitional cell
Adriamycin PFS (Doxorubicin Hydrochloride) Pharmacia & Upjohn 2056
Adriamycin RDF (Doxorubicin Hydrochloride) Pharmacia & Upjohn 2056
Doxorubicin Astra (Doxorubicin Hydrochloride) Astra 531
Platinol for Injection (Cisplatin) Bristol-Myers Squibb Oncology/Immunology 717
Platinol-AQ Injection (Cisplatin) Bristol-Myers Squibb Oncology/Immunology 719
Rubex for Injection (Doxorubicin Hydrochloride) Bristol-Myers Squibb Oncology/Immunology 721

Carcinoma, breast
Adriamycin PFS (Doxorubicin Hydrochloride) Pharmacia & Upjohn 2056
Adriamycin RDF (Doxorubicin Hydrochloride) Pharmacia & Upjohn 2056
Arimidex Tablets (Anastrozole) Zeneca 2932
Cytoxan (Cyclophosphamide) Bristol-Myers Squibb Oncology/Immunology 700
Doxorubicin Astra (Doxorubicin Hydrochloride) Astra 531
Methotrexate Sodium Tablets, Injection, for Injection and LPF Injection (Methotrexate Sodium) Immunex 1322
Nolvadex Tablets (Tamoxifen Citrate) Zeneca 2957
Rubex for Injection (Doxorubicin Hydrochloride) Bristol-Myers Squibb Oncology/Immunology 721
Thioplex (Thiotepa For Injection) (Thiotepa) Immunex 1329
Velban Vials (Vinblastine Sulfate) Lilly 1537

Carcinoma, breast, axillary node-negative, postsurgical and post-irradiation
Nolvadex Tablets (Tamoxifen Citrate) Zeneca 2957

Carcinoma, breast, metastatic, treatment of
Android Capsules, 10 mg (Methyltestosterone) ICN 1297
Nolvadex Tablets (Tamoxifen Citrate) Zeneca 2957
Taxol Injection (Paclitaxel) Bristol-Myers Squibb Oncology/Immunology 723
Taxotere for Injection Concentrate (Docetaxel) Rhone-Poulenc Rorer Pharmaceuticals 2204

Carcinoma, breast, palliative therapy in
Diethylstilbestrol Tablets (Diethylstilbestrol) Lilly 1477
Estrace Cream and Tablets (Estradiol) Bristol-Myers Squibb .. 751
ESTRATAB Tablets (0.3, 0.625, 1.25, 2.5 mg) (Estrogens, Esterified) Solvay 2715
Fluorouracil Injection (Fluorouracil) Roche Pharmaceuticals 2282
Halotestin Tablets (Fluoxymesterone) Pharmacia & Upjohn 2095
Megace Tablets (Megestrol Acetate) Bristol-Myers Squibb Oncology/Immunology 710
Menest Tablets (Estrogens, Esterified) SmithKline Beecham Pharmaceuticals 2671
Premarin Tablets (Estrogens, Conjugated) Wyeth-Ayerst 2896
Teslac Tablets (Testolactone) Bristol-Myers Squibb Oncology/Immunology 727
Testred Capsules, 10 mg (Methyltestosterone) ICN 1308
Zoladex (Goserelin Acetate) Zeneca 2976

Carcinoma, breast, postmenopausal women, postsurgical
Nolvadex Tablets (Tamoxifen Citrate) Zeneca 2957

Carcinoma, breast, postmenopausal women, post-tamoxifen therapy
Arimidex Tablets (Anastrozole) Zeneca 2932

Carcinoma, bronchogenic
Adriamycin PFS (Doxorubicin Hydrochloride) Pharmacia & Upjohn 2056
Adriamycin RDF (Doxorubicin Hydrochloride) Pharmacia & Upjohn 2056
Doxorubicin Astra (Doxorubicin Hydrochloride) Astra 531
Methotrexate Sodium Tablets, Injection, for Injection and LPF Injection (Methotrexate Sodium) Immunex 1322
Mustargen (Mechlorethamine Hydrochloride) Merck & Co., Inc. 1752
Rubex for Injection (Doxorubicin Hydrochloride) Bristol-Myers Squibb Oncology/Immunology 721

Carcinoma, cervix, palliative treatment in
Blenoxane (Bleomycin Sulfate) Bristol-Myers Squibb Oncology/Immunology 697

Carcinoma, colon, Dukes' stage C, adjunctive treatment in
Ergamisol Tablets (Levamisole Hydrochloride) Janssen 1340

Carcinoma, colon, palliative management of
Fluorouracil Injection (Fluorouracil) Roche Pharmaceuticals 2282

Carcinoma, colorectal, adjunctive therapy in
Leucovorin Calcium for Injection (Leucovorin Calcium) Immunex 1313

Carcinoma, endometrium, palliative treatment of
Depo-Provera Sterile Aqueous Suspension (Medroxyprogesterone Acetate) Pharmacia & Upjohn 2083
Megace Tablets (Megestrol Acetate) Bristol-Myers Squibb Oncology/Immunology 710

Carcinoma, epiglottis, palliative treatment in
Blenoxane (Bleomycin Sulfate) Bristol-Myers Squibb Oncology/Immunology 697

Carcinoma, gastric
Adriamycin PFS (Doxorubicin Hydrochloride) Pharmacia & Upjohn 2056

(▣ Described in PDR For Nonprescription Drugs)   (◉ Described in PDR For Ophthalmology)

Carcinoma

Carcinoma *(cont.)*
Adriamycin RDF (Doxorubicin Hydrochloride) Pharmacia & Upjohn.......... 2056
Doxorubicin Astra (Doxorubicin Hydrochloride) Astra 531
Rubex for Injection (Doxorubicin Hydrochloride) Bristol-Myers Squibb Oncology/Immunology 721

Carcinoma, gastrointestinal, palliative management of
Sterile FUDR (Floxuridine) Roche Pharmaceuticals 2284

Carcinoma, gingiva, palliative treatment in
Blenoxane (Bleomycin Sulfate) Bristol-Myers Squibb Oncology/Immunology 697

Carcinoma, head and neck
Blenoxane (Bleomycin Sulfate) Bristol-Myers Squibb Oncology/Immunology 697
Methotrexate Sodium Tablets, Injection, for Injection and LPF Injection (Methotrexate Sodium) Immunex 1322

Carcinoma, head and neck, adjunct in
Hydrea Capsules (Hydroxyurea) Bristol-Myers Squibb Oncology/Immunology 705

Carcinoma, larynx, palliative treatment in
Blenoxane (Bleomycin Sulfate) Bristol-Myers Squibb Oncology/Immunology 697

Carcinoma, lips, palliative treatment in
Blenoxane (Bleomycin Sulfate) Bristol-Myers Squibb Oncology/Immunology 697

Carcinoma, lung, non-small cell
Navelbine Injection (Vinorelbine Tartrate) Glaxo Wellcome Oncology/HIV 1212

Carcinoma, lung, small cell
Etopophos for Injection (Etoposide Phosphate) Bristol-Myers Squibb Oncology/Immunology 701
Etoposide Injection (Etoposide) Astra 539
Methotrexate Sodium Tablets, Injection, for Injection and LPF Injection (Methotrexate Sodium) Immunex 1322
VePesid Capsules and Injection (Etoposide) Bristol-Myers Squibb Oncology/Immunology 727

Carcinoma, metastatic, palliative treatment of
Estrace Cream and Tablets (Estradiol) Bristol-Myers Squibb .. 751
Mustargen (Mechlorethamine Hydrochloride) Merck & Co., Inc. 1752

Carcinoma, mouth, palliative treatment in
Blenoxane (Bleomycin Sulfate) Bristol-Myers Squibb Oncology/Immunology 697

Carcinoma, nasopharynx, palliative treatment in
Blenoxane (Bleomycin Sulfate) Bristol-Myers Squibb Oncology/Immunology 697

Carcinoma, oropharynx, palliative treatment in
Blenoxane (Bleomycin Sulfate) Bristol-Myers Squibb Oncology/Immunology 697

Carcinoma, ovary
Adriamycin PFS (Doxorubicin Hydrochloride) Pharmacia & Upjohn 2056
Adriamycin RDF (Doxorubicin Hydrochloride) Pharmacia & Upjohn 2056
Alkeran Tablets (Melphalan) Glaxo Wellcome Oncology/HIV 1198
Cytoxan (Cyclophosphamide) Bristol-Myers Squibb Oncology/Immunology 700
Doxorubicin Astra (Doxorubicin Hydrochloride) Astra 531
Hexalen Capsules (Altretamine) U.S. Bioscience 2760
Hycamtin for Injection (Topotecan Hydrochloride) SmithKline Beecham Pharmaceuticals 2665
Hydrea Capsules (Hydroxyurea) Bristol-Myers Squibb Oncology/Immunology 705
Paraplatin for Injection (Carboplatin) Bristol-Myers Squibb Oncology/Immunology 713
Platinol for Injection (Cisplatin) Bristol-Myers Squibb Oncology/Immunology 717
Platinol-AQ Injection (Cisplatin) Bristol-Myers Squibb Oncology/Immunology 719
Rubex for Injection (Doxorubicin Hydrochloride) Bristol-Myers Squibb Oncology/Immunology 721
Taxol Injection (Paclitaxel) Bristol-Myers Squibb Oncology/Immunology 723
Thioplex (Thiotepa For Injection) (Thiotepa) Immunex 1329

Carcinoma, palate, palliative treatment in
Blenoxane (Bleomycin Sulfate) Bristol-Myers Squibb Oncology/Immunology 697

Carcinoma, pancreas
Gemzar for Injection (Gemcitabine Hydrochloride) Lilly 1482
Mutamycin for Injection (Mitomycin (Mitomycin-C)) Bristol-Myers Squibb Oncology/Immunology 712

Carcinoma, pancreas, metastatic, islet cell
Zanosar Sterile Powder (Streptozocin) Pharmacia & Upjohn 2119

Carcinoma, pancreas, palliative management of
Fluorouracil Injection (Fluorouracil) Roche Pharmaceuticals 2282

Carcinoma, penis, palliative treatment in
Blenoxane (Bleomycin Sulfate) Bristol-Myers Squibb Oncology/Immunology 697

Carcinoma, prostate
Eulexin Capsules (Flutamide) Schering 2498

Carcinoma, prostate, adjunctive therapy in
Casodex Tablets (Bicalutamide) Zeneca 2934
Eulexin Capsules (Flutamide) Schering 2498

Carcinoma, prostatic, palliative treatment of
Diethylstilbestrol Tablets (Diethylstilbestrol) Lilly 1477
Emcyt Capsules (Estramustine Phosphate Sodium) Pharmacia & Upjohn 2085
Estrace Cream and Tablets (Estradiol) Bristol-Myers Squibb .. 751
ESTRATAB Tablets (0.3, 0.625, 1.25, 2.5 mg) (Estrogens, Esterified) Solvay 2715
Lupron Depot 7.5 mg (Leuprolide Acetate) TAP 2741
Lupron Depot - 3 Month 22.5 mg (Leuprolide Acetate) TAP 2743
Lupron Injection (Leuprolide Acetate) TAP 2736
Menest Tablets (Estrogens, Esterified) SmithKline Beecham Pharmaceuticals 2671
Premarin Tablets (Estrogens, Conjugated) Wyeth-Ayerst 2896
Zoladex (Goserelin Acetate) Zeneca 2976
Zoladex 3-month (Goserelin Acetate) Zeneca 2978

Carcinoma, rectum, palliative management of
Fluorouracil Injection (Fluorouracil) Roche Pharmaceuticals 2282

Carcinoma, renal, palliative treatment in
Depo-Provera Sterile Aqueous Suspension (Medroxyprogesterone Acetate) Pharmacia & Upjohn 2083

Carcinoma, renal cell, metastatic, in adults
Proleukin for Injection (Aldesleukin) Chiron 812

Carcinoma, sinus, palliative treatment in
Blenoxane (Bleomycin Sulfate) Bristol-Myers Squibb Oncology/Immunology 697

Carcinoma, skin, palliative treatment in
Blenoxane (Bleomycin Sulfate) Bristol-Myers Squibb Oncology/Immunology 697

Carcinoma, squamous cell, palliative treatment in
Blenoxane (Bleomycin Sulfate) Bristol-Myers Squibb Oncology/Immunology 697

Carcinoma, stomach
Mutamycin for Injection (Mitomycin (Mitomycin-C)) Bristol-Myers Squibb Oncology/Immunology 712

Carcinoma, stomach, palliative management of
Fluorouracil Injection (Fluorouracil) Roche Pharmaceuticals 2282

Carcinoma, superficial basal cell
Efudex (Fluorouracil) Roche Pharmaceuticals 2280

Carcinoma, testicular
Etopophos for Injection (Etoposide Phosphate) Bristol-Myers Squibb Oncology/Immunology 701
Etoposide Injection (Etoposide) Astra 539
Platinol for Injection (Cisplatin) Bristol-Myers Squibb Oncology/Immunology 717
Platinol-AQ Injection (Cisplatin) Bristol-Myers Squibb Oncology/Immunology 719
VePesid Capsules and Injection (Etoposide) Bristol-Myers Squibb Oncology/Immunology 727

Carcinoma, testicular, embryonic cell, palliative treatment in
Blenoxane (Bleomycin Sulfate) Bristol-Myers Squibb Oncology/Immunology 697

Carcinoma, testicular, germ cell
IFEX (Ifosfamide) Bristol-Myers Squibb Oncology/Immunology 706

Carcinoma, testicular, palliative treatment in
Blenoxane (Bleomycin Sulfate) Bristol-Myers Squibb Oncology/Immunology 697

Carcinoma, testis, advanced
Cosmegen Injection (Dactinomycin) Merck & Co., Inc. 1666
Mithracin (Plicamycin) Bayer Pharmaceutical 599
Velban Vials (Vinblastine Sulfate) Lilly 1537

Carcinoma, thyroid
Adriamycin PFS (Doxorubicin Hydrochloride) Pharmacia & Upjohn 2056
Adriamycin RDF (Doxorubicin Hydrochloride) Pharmacia & Upjohn 2056
Doxorubicin Astra (Doxorubicin Hydrochloride) Astra 531
Levothyroxine Sodium, USP for Injection (Levothyroxine Sodium) Astra 546
Rubex for Injection (Doxorubicin Hydrochloride) Bristol-Myers Squibb Oncology/Immunology 721
Synthroid (Levothyroxine Sodium) Knoll Pharmaceutical 1410

Carcinoma, tongue, palliative treatment in
Blenoxane (Bleomycin Sulfate) Bristol-Myers Squibb Oncology/Immunology 697

Carcinoma, tonsil, palliative treatment in
Blenoxane (Bleomycin Sulfate) Bristol-Myers Squibb Oncology/Immunology 697

Carcinoma, urinary bladder, in-situ
TheraCys BCG Live (Intravesical) (BCG, Live (Intravesical)) Connaught 911
TICE BCG, USP (BCG Vaccine) Organon 1881

Carcinoma, urinary bladder, superficial papillary
Thioplex (Thiotepa For Injection) (Thiotepa) Immunex 1329

Carcinoma, uterus
Cosmegen Injection (Dactinomycin) Merck & Co., Inc. 1666

Carcinoma, vulva, palliative treatment in
Blenoxane (Bleomycin Sulfate) Bristol-Myers Squibb Oncology/Immunology 697

Cardiac arrest
Isuprel Injection (Isoproterenol Hydrochloride) Sanofi Winthrop .. 2441

Cardiac arrest, an adjunct in
Levophed Bitartrate Injection (Norepinephrine Bitartrate) Sanofi Winthrop 2445

Cardiac arrhythmias
(see under Arrhythmias)

Cardiac decompensation
Dobutrex Solution Vials (Dobutamine Hydrochloride) Lilly 1480

Cardiac ischemic complications, acute, prevention of, adjunct to PTCA
ReoPro Vials (Abciximab) Lilly 1526

Cardiac output, low
Isuprel Injection (Isoproterenol Hydrochloride) Sanofi Winthrop .. 2441

Cardiogenic shock syndrome, correction of hemodynamic imbalance
Isuprel Injection (Isoproterenol Hydrochloride) Sanofi Winthrop .. 2441

Cardiomyopathy, doxorubicin-induced, to reduce the incidence and severity of
Zinecard Injection (Dexrazoxane) Pharmacia & Upjohn 2120

Carnitine, primary systemic deficiency of
L-Carnitine 250mg, 500mg Tablets and 500mg Chewable Wafers (Levocarnitine) Vitaline 2767
Carnitor Tablets and Solution (Levocarnitine) Sigma-Tau 2624

Carnitine deficiency, secondary
Carnitor Injection (Levocarnitine) Sigma-Tau 2623
Carnitor Tablets and Solution (Levocarnitine) Sigma-Tau 2624

Catabolic or tissue depleting processes, adjunctive therapy
Oxandrin (Oxandrolone) Bio-Technology General 783

Cataract extraction, surgical aid in
AMO Vitrax Viscoelastic Solution (Sodium Hyaluronate) Allergan.. ⊚ 229
AMVISC Plus (Sodium Hyaluronate) Chiron Vision .... ⊚ 327
Healon (Sodium Hyaluronate) Pharmacia & Upjohn .... ⊚ 302
Healon GV (Sodium Hyaluronate) Pharmacia & Upjohn .... ⊚ 303
OcuCoat (Hydroxypropyl Methylcellulose) Storz Ophthalmics .... ⊚ 321

(▣ Described in PDR For Nonprescription Drugs)   (⊚ Described in PDR For Ophthalmology)

1507 **Indications Index** **Cholecystitis**

Cellulitis, pelvic
(see under Pelvic cellulitis)

Central cranial diabetes insipidus
(see under Diabetes insipidus)

Central nervous system depression, drug-induced
Dopram Injectable (Doxapram Hydrochloride) Robins 2235

Cephalalgia, histaminic
Cafergot (Ergotamine Tartrate, Caffeine) Sandoz Pharmaceuticals 2376
D.H.E. 45 Injection (Dihydroergotamine Mesylate) Sandoz Pharmaceuticals 2381
Ergomar Tablets (Ergotamine Tartrate) Lotus 1543
Imitrex Injection (Sumatriptan Succinate) Glaxo Wellcome 1095
Wigraine Tablets (Ergotamine Tartrate, Caffeine) Organon 1884

Cerebral edema
(see under Edema, cerebral)

Cerumen, removal of
Auralgan Otic Solution (Antipyrine, Benzocaine, Glycerin) Wyeth-Ayerst 2810
Cerumenex Drops (Triethanolamine Polypeptide Oleate-Condensate) Purdue Frederick 2148
Debrox Drops (Carbamide Peroxide) SmithKline Beecham Consumer .... ▣ 775
Murine Ear Drops (Carbamide Peroxide) Ross .... ▣ 743

Cervicitis
Zithromax (Azithromycin) Pfizer Inc 2043
Zithromax Tablets (Azithromycin) Pfizer Inc 2046

Cervicitis, mild, adjunct
Amino-Cerv (Urea, Benzalkonium Chloride, L-Cystine, Sodium Propionate, Methionine, Inositol) Milex 1827

Cervicitis, postconization, adjunct
Amino-Cerv (Urea, Benzalkonium Chloride, L-Cystine, Sodium Propionate, Methionine, Inositol) Milex 1827

Cervicitis, postpartum, adjunct
Amino-Cerv (Urea, Benzalkonium Chloride, L-Cystine, Sodium Propionate, Methionine, Inositol) Milex 1827

Cervix, epithelialization, promotion of
Amino-Cerv (Urea, Benzalkonium Chloride, L-Cystine, Sodium Propionate, Methionine, Inositol) Milex 1827

Cervix, ripening of, in pregnant women at or near term
Cervidil (Dinoprostone) Forest 1008
Prepidil Gel (Dinoprostone) Pharmacia & Upjohn 2108

Chancroid
Achromycin V Capsules (Tetracycline Hydrochloride) Lederle 1417
Declomycin Tablets (Demeclocycline Hydrochloride) Lederle 1421
Doryx Capsules (Doxycycline Hyclate) Parke-Davis 1970
DYNACIN Capsules (Minocycline Hydrochloride) Medicis 1627
Gantanol Tablets (Sulfamethoxazole) Roche Pharmaceuticals 2285
Gantrisin (Acetyl Sulfisoxazole) Roche Pharmaceuticals 2286
Minocin Intravenous (Minocycline Hydrochloride) Lederle 1428
Minocin Oral Suspension (Minocycline Hydrochloride) Lederle 1431
Minocin Pellet-Filled Capsules (Minocycline Hydrochloride) Lederle 1429
Monodox Capsules (Doxycycline Monohydrate) Oclassen 1858
Terramycin Intramuscular Solution (Oxytetracycline) Pfizer Inc 2034
Vibramycin (Doxycycline Calcium) Pfizer Inc 2038
Vibramycin Hyclate Intravenous (Doxycycline Hyclate) Pfizer Inc 2040
Vibramycin (Doxycycline Monohydrate) Pfizer Inc 2038

Cheilitis, actinic
Aquaphor Healing Ointment, Original Formula (Mineral Oil, Petrolatum) Beiersdorf 636
Herpecin-L Cold Sore Lip Balm Stick (Allantoin) Chattem 812
Mentholatum Ointment (Camphor, Menthol) Mentholatum .... ▣ 711

Chickenpox
(see under Varicella, acute, treatment of)

Chlamydia psittaci infection
Achromycin V Capsules (Tetracycline Hydrochloride) Lederle 1417
Declomycin Tablets (Demeclocycline Hydrochloride) Lederle 1421
Doryx Capsules (Doxycycline Hyclate) Parke-Davis 1970
DYNACIN Capsules (Minocycline Hydrochloride) Medicis 1627
Minocin Intravenous (Minocycline Hydrochloride) Lederle 1428
Minocin Oral Suspension (Minocycline Hydrochloride) Lederle 1431
Minocin Pellet-Filled Capsules (Minocycline Hydrochloride) Lederle 1429
Monodox Capsules (Doxycycline Monohydrate) Oclassen 1858
Terramycin Intramuscular Solution (Oxytetracycline) Pfizer Inc 2034
Vibramycin (Doxycycline Calcium) Pfizer Inc 2038
Vibramycin Hyclate Intravenous (Doxycycline Hyclate) Pfizer Inc 2040
Vibramycin (Doxycycline Monohydrate) Pfizer Inc 2038

Chlamydia trachomatis conjunctivitis of the newborn
ERYC (Erythromycin) Parke-Davis .. 1972
Ery-Tab Tablets (Erythromycin) Abbott 426
Erythrocin Stearate Filmtab (Erythromycin Stearate) Abbott 429
Erythromycin Base Filmtab (Erythromycin) Abbott 430
Erythromycin Delayed-Release Capsules, USP (Erythromycin) Abbott 431
Ilosone (Erythromycin Estolate) Dista 927
Monodox Capsules (Doxycycline Monohydrate) Oclassen 1858
PCE Dispertab Tablets (Erythromycin) Abbott 453

Chlamydia trachomatis endocervical infections
Achromycin V Capsules (Tetracycline Hydrochloride) Lederle 1417
Doryx Capsules (Doxycycline Hyclate) Parke-Davis 1970
E-Mycin Tablets (Erythromycin) Knoll Laboratories 1388
ERYC (Erythromycin) Parke-Davis .. 1972
Ery-Tab Tablets (Erythromycin) Abbott 426
Erythrocin Stearate Filmtab (Erythromycin Stearate) Abbott 429
Erythromycin Base Filmtab (Erythromycin) Abbott 430
Erythromycin Delayed-Release Capsules, USP (Erythromycin) Abbott 431
Ilosone (Erythromycin Estolate) Dista 927
Minocin Oral Suspension (Minocycline Hydrochloride) Lederle 1431
Monodox Capsules (Doxycycline Monohydrate) Oclassen 1858
PCE Dispertab Tablets (Erythromycin) Abbott 453
Vibramycin (Doxycycline Calcium) Pfizer Inc 2038

Chlamydia trachomatis epididymo-orchitis, acute
Doryx Capsules (Doxycycline Hyclate) Parke-Davis 1970

Chlamydia trachomatis gynecologic infections
Floxin I.V. (Ofloxacin) McNeil Pharmaceutical 1580
Floxin Tablets (200 mg, 300 mg, 400 mg) (Ofloxacin) McNeil Pharmaceutical 1577

Chlamydia trachomatis infections
Achromycin V Capsules (Tetracycline Hydrochloride) Lederle 1417
Doryx Capsules (Doxycycline Hyclate) Parke-Davis 1970
DYNACIN Capsules (Minocycline Hydrochloride) Medicis 1627
E.E.S. (Erythromycin Ethylsuccinate) Abbott 427
E-Mycin Tablets (Erythromycin) Knoll Laboratories 1388
ERYC (Erythromycin) Parke-Davis .. 1972
EryPed (Erythromycin Ethylsuccinate) Abbott 425
Ery-Tab Tablets (Erythromycin) Abbott 426
Erythrocin Stearate Filmtab (Erythromycin Stearate) Abbott 429
Erythromycin Base Filmtab (Erythromycin) Abbott 430
Erythromycin Delayed-Release Capsules, USP (Erythromycin) Abbott 431
Floxin I.V. (Ofloxacin) McNeil Pharmaceutical 1580
Floxin Tablets (200 mg, 300 mg, 400 mg) (Ofloxacin) McNeil Pharmaceutical 1577
Minocin Oral Suspension (Minocycline Hydrochloride) Lederle 1431
Minocin Pellet-Filled Capsules (Minocycline Hydrochloride) Lederle 1429
Monodox Capsules (Doxycycline Monohydrate) Oclassen 1858
PCE Dispertab Tablets (Erythromycin) Abbott 453
Vibramycin (Doxycycline Calcium) Pfizer Inc 2038
Zithromax (Azithromycin) Pfizer Inc 2043
Zithromax Tablets (Azithromycin) Pfizer Inc 2046

Chlamydia trachomatis infections, ocular
(see under Trachoma)

Chlamydia trachomatis neonatal ophthalmia, prophylaxis of
Ilotycin Ophthalmic Ointment (Erythromycin) Dista 928

Chlamydia trachomatis nongonococcal cervicitis
Floxin I.V. (Ofloxacin) McNeil Pharmaceutical 1580
Floxin Tablets (200 mg, 300 mg, 400 mg) (Ofloxacin) McNeil Pharmaceutical 1577
Zithromax (Azithromycin) Pfizer Inc 2043
Zithromax Tablets (Azithromycin) Pfizer Inc 2046

Chlamydia trachomatis nongonococcal urethritis
DYNACIN Capsules (Minocycline Hydrochloride) Medicis 1627
Floxin I.V. (Ofloxacin) McNeil Pharmaceutical 1580
Floxin Tablets (200 mg, 300 mg, 400 mg) (Ofloxacin) McNeil Pharmaceutical 1577
Minocin Oral Suspension (Minocycline Hydrochloride) Lederle 1431
Minocin Pellet-Filled Capsules (Minocycline Hydrochloride) Lederle 1429
Zithromax (Azithromycin) Pfizer Inc 2043
Zithromax Tablets (Azithromycin) Pfizer Inc 2046

Chlamydia trachomatis pneumonia of infancy
ERYC (Erythromycin) Parke-Davis .. 1972
Ery-Tab Tablets (Erythromycin) Abbott 426
Erythrocin Stearate Filmtab (Erythromycin Stearate) Abbott 429
Erythromycin Base Filmtab (Erythromycin) Abbott 430
Erythromycin Delayed-Release Capsules, USP (Erythromycin) Abbott 431
Ilosone (Erythromycin Estolate) Dista 927
PCE Dispertab Tablets (Erythromycin) Abbott 453

Chlamydia trachomatis rectal infections
Achromycin V Capsules (Tetracycline Hydrochloride) Lederle 1417
Doryx Capsules (Doxycycline Hyclate) Parke-Davis 1970
E-Mycin Tablets (Erythromycin) Knoll Laboratories 1388
ERYC (Erythromycin) Parke-Davis .. 1972
Ery-Tab Tablets (Erythromycin) Abbott 426
Erythrocin Stearate Filmtab (Erythromycin Stearate) Abbott 429
Erythromycin Base Filmtab (Erythromycin) Abbott 430
Erythromycin Delayed-Release Capsules, USP (Erythromycin) Abbott 431
Ilosone (Erythromycin Estolate) Dista 927
Minocin Oral Suspension (Minocycline Hydrochloride) Lederle 1431
Monodox Capsules (Doxycycline Monohydrate) Oclassen 1858
PCE Dispertab Tablets (Erythromycin) Abbott 453
Vibramycin (Doxycycline Calcium) Pfizer Inc 2038

Chlamydia trachomatis urethral infections
Achromycin V Capsules (Tetracycline Hydrochloride) Lederle 1417
Doryx Capsules (Doxycycline Hyclate) Parke-Davis 1970
E.E.S. (Erythromycin Ethylsuccinate) Abbott 427
E-Mycin Tablets (Erythromycin) Knoll Laboratories 1388
ERYC (Erythromycin) Parke-Davis .. 1972
EryPed (Erythromycin Ethylsuccinate) Abbott 425
Ery-Tab Tablets (Erythromycin) Abbott 426
Erythrocin Stearate Filmtab (Erythromycin Stearate) Abbott 429
Erythromycin Base Filmtab (Erythromycin) Abbott 430
Erythromycin Delayed-Release Capsules, USP (Erythromycin) Abbott 431
Ilosone (Erythromycin Estolate) Dista 927
Monodox Capsules (Doxycycline Monohydrate) Oclassen 1858
PCE Dispertab Tablets (Erythromycin) Abbott 453
Vibramycin (Doxycycline Calcium) Pfizer Inc 2038

Chlamydia trachomatis urogenital infections during pregnancy
ERYC (Erythromycin) Parke-Davis .. 1972
Ery-Tab Tablets (Erythromycin) Abbott 426
Erythrocin Stearate Filmtab (Erythromycin Stearate) Abbott 429
Erythromycin Base Filmtab (Erythromycin) Abbott 430
Erythromycin Delayed-Release Capsules, USP (Erythromycin) Abbott 431
Ilosone (Erythromycin Estolate) Dista 927
PCE Dispertab Tablets (Erythromycin) Abbott 453

Chloasma
(see under Hyperpigmentation, skin, bleaching of)

Cholangitis
(see also under Infections, intra-abdominal)
Mezlin (Mezlocillin Sodium) Bayer Pharmaceutical 594
Mezlin Pharmacy Bulk Package (Mezlocillin Sodium) Bayer Pharmaceutical 597

Cholecystitis, acute
(see also under Infections, intra-abdominal)

(▣ Described in PDR For Nonprescription Drugs) (◉ Described in PDR For Ophthalmology)

Cholecystitis

Mezlin (Mezlocillin Sodium) Bayer Pharmaceutical ... 594
Mezlin Pharmacy Bulk Package (Mezlocillin Sodium) Bayer Pharmaceutical ... 597

Cholera
DYNACIN Capsules (Minocycline Hydrochloride) Medicis ... 1627
Minocin Oral Suspension (Minocycline Hydrochloride) Lederle ... 1431
Minocin Pellet-Filled Capsules (Minocycline Hydrochloride) Lederle ... 1429
Monodox Capsules (Doxycycline Monohydrate) Oclassen ... 1858
Vibramycin Hyclate Capsules (Doxycycline Hyclate) Pfizer Inc 2038

Cholesterol levels, elevated
(see under Hypercholesterolemia, primary, adjunct to diet)

Chorea, prophylaxis of
Bicillin L-A Injection (Penicillin G Benzathine) Wyeth-Ayerst ... 2813
Pen•Vee K (Penicillin V Potassium) Wyeth-Ayerst ... 2879

Choriocarcinoma
Blenoxane (Bleomycin Sulfate) Bristol-Myers Squibb Oncology/Immunology ... 697
Methotrexate Sodium Tablets, Injection, for Injection and LPF Injection (Methotrexate Sodium) Immunex ... 1322
Velban Vials (Vinblastine Sulfate) Lilly ... 1537

Chorioadenoma destruens
Methotrexate Sodium Tablets, Injection, for Injection and LPF Injection (Methotrexate Sodium) Immunex ... 1322

Chorioretinitis
Celestone Soluspan Suspension (Betamethasone Sodium Phosphate, Betamethasone Acetate) Schering ... 2484
Cortone Acetate Sterile Suspension (Cortisone Acetate) Merck & Co., Inc. ... 1663
Cortone Acetate Tablets (Cortisone Acetate) Merck & Co., Inc. ... 1664
Dalalone D.P. Injectable (Dexamethasone Acetate) Forest ... 1009
Decadron Elixir (Dexamethasone) Merck & Co., Inc. ... 1676
Decadron Phosphate Injection (Dexamethasone Sodium Phosphate) Merck & Co., Inc. ... 1680
Decadron Tablets (Dexamethasone) Merck & Co., Inc. ... 1678
Decadron-LA Sterile Suspension (Dexamethasone Acetate) Merck & Co., Inc. ... 1687
Hydeltrasol Injection, Sterile (Prednisolone Sodium Phosphate) Merck & Co., Inc. ... 1708
Hydrocortone Phosphate Injection, Sterile (Hydrocortisone Sodium Phosphate) Merck & Co., Inc. ... 1713
Hydrocortone Tablets (Hydrocortisone) Merck & Co., Inc. ... 1715
Pediapred Oral Solution (Prednisolone Sodium Phosphate) Medeva 1618
Prelone Syrup (Prednisolone) Muro 1834

Choroiditis
Celestone Soluspan Suspension (Betamethasone Sodium Phosphate, Betamethasone Acetate) Schering ... 2484
Cortone Acetate Sterile Suspension (Cortisone Acetate) Merck & Co., Inc. ... 1663
Cortone Acetate Tablets (Cortisone Acetate) Merck & Co., Inc. ... 1664
Dalalone D.P. Injectable (Dexamethasone Acetate) Forest ... 1009
Decadron Elixir (Dexamethasone) Merck & Co., Inc. ... 1676
Decadron Phosphate Injection (Dexamethasone Sodium Phosphate) Merck & Co., Inc. ... 1680
Decadron Tablets (Dexamethasone) Merck & Co., Inc. ... 1678
Decadron-LA Sterile Suspension (Dexamethasone Acetate) Merck & Co., Inc. ... 1687
Hydeltrasol Injection, Sterile (Prednisolone Sodium Phosphate) Merck & Co., Inc. ... 1708
Hydrocortone Phosphate Injection, Sterile (Hydrocortisone Sodium Phosphate) Merck & Co., Inc. ... 1713
Hydrocortone Tablets (Hydrocortisone) Merck & Co., Inc. ... 1715
Pediapred Oral Solution (Prednisolone Sodium Phosphate) Medeva 1618
Prelone Syrup (Prednisolone) Muro 1834

Christmas disease
(see under Hemophilia B)

Chromomycosis
Nizoral Tablets (Ketoconazole) Janssen ... 1345

Citrobacter diversus infections
Cipro I.V. (Ciprofloxacin) Bayer Pharmaceutical ... 587
Cipro I.V. Pharmacy Bulk Package (Ciprofloxacin) Bayer Pharmaceutical ... 590
Cipro Tablets (Ciprofloxacin Hydrochloride) Bayer Pharmaceutical ... 584
Floxin I.V. (Ofloxacin) McNeil Pharmaceutical ... 1580
Floxin Tablets (200 mg, 300 mg, 400 mg) (Ofloxacin) McNeil Pharmaceutical ... 1577
Maxaquin Tablets (Lomefloxacin Hydrochloride) Searle ... 2593

Citrobacter diversus urinary tract infections
Cipro I.V. (Ciprofloxacin) Bayer Pharmaceutical ... 587
Cipro I.V. Pharmacy Bulk Package (Ciprofloxacin) Bayer Pharmaceutical ... 590
Cipro Tablets (Ciprofloxacin Hydrochloride) Bayer Pharmaceutical ... 584
Floxin I.V. (Ofloxacin) McNeil Pharmaceutical ... 1580
Floxin Tablets (200 mg, 300 mg, 400 mg) (Ofloxacin) McNeil Pharmaceutical ... 1577
Maxaquin Tablets (Lomefloxacin Hydrochloride) Searle ... 2593

Citrobacter freundii infections
Azactam for Injection (Aztreonam) Bristol-Myers Squibb ... 736
Cipro I.V. (Ciprofloxacin) Bayer Pharmaceutical ... 587
Cipro I.V. Pharmacy Bulk Package (Ciprofloxacin) Bayer Pharmaceutical ... 590
Cipro Tablets (Ciprofloxacin Hydrochloride) Bayer Pharmaceutical ... 584
Claforan Sterile and Injection (Cefotaxime Sodium) Hoechst Marion Roussel ... 1259
Noroxin Tablets (Norfloxacin) Merck & Co., Inc. ... 1758
Noroxin Tablets (Norfloxacin) Roberts ... 2222

Citrobacter freundii intra-abdominal infections
Azactam for Injection (Aztreonam) Bristol-Myers Squibb ... 736

Citrobacter freundii skin and skin structure infections
Cipro I.V. (Ciprofloxacin) Bayer Pharmaceutical ... 587
Cipro I.V. Pharmacy Bulk Package (Ciprofloxacin) Bayer Pharmaceutical ... 590
Cipro Tablets (Ciprofloxacin Hydrochloride) Bayer Pharmaceutical ... 584
Claforan Sterile and Injection (Cefotaxime Sodium) Hoechst Marion Roussel ... 1259

Citrobacter freundii urinary tract infections
Cipro I.V. (Ciprofloxacin) Bayer Pharmaceutical ... 587
Cipro I.V. Pharmacy Bulk Package (Ciprofloxacin) Bayer Pharmaceutical ... 590
Cipro Tablets (Ciprofloxacin Hydrochloride) Bayer Pharmaceutical ... 584
Noroxin Tablets (Norfloxacin) Merck & Co., Inc. ... 1758
Noroxin Tablets (Norfloxacin) Roberts ... 2222

Citrobacter species infections
Azactam for Injection (Aztreonam) Bristol-Myers Squibb ... 736
Ceptaz (Ceftazidime) Glaxo Wellcome ... 1070
Claforan Sterile and Injection (Cefotaxime Sodium) Hoechst Marion Roussel ... 1259
Fortaz (Ceftazidime) Glaxo Wellcome ... 1092
Garamycin Injectable (Gentamicin Sulfate) Schering ... 2502
Nebcin Vials, Hyporets & ADD-Vantage (Tobramycin Sulfate) Lilly ... 1518
Netromycin Injection 100 mg/ml (Netilmicin Sulfate) Schering ... 2516
Primaxin I.M. (Cilastatin Sodium, Imipenem) Merck & Co., Inc. ... 1770
Primaxin I.V. (Cilastatin Sodium, Imipenem) Merck & Co., Inc. ... 1772
Tazicef for Injection (Ceftazidime) SmithKline Beecham Pharmaceuticals ... 2697
Tazidime Vials, Faspak & ADD-Vantage (Ceftazidime) Lilly .. 1531
Timentin for Injection (Ticarcillin Disodium, Clavulanate Potassium) SmithKline Beecham Pharmaceuticals ... 2706

Citrobacter species intra-abdominal infections
Azactam for Injection (Aztreonam) Bristol-Myers Squibb ... 736
Primaxin I.V. (Cilastatin Sodium, Imipenem) Merck & Co., Inc. ... 1772

Citrobacter species lower respiratory tract infections
Ceptaz (Ceftazidime) Glaxo Wellcome ... 1070
Fortaz (Ceftazidime) Glaxo Wellcome ... 1092
Tazicef for Injection (Ceftazidime) SmithKline Beecham Pharmaceuticals ... 2697
Tazidime Vials, Faspak & ADD-Vantage (Ceftazidime) Lilly .. 1531

Citrobacter species skin and skin structure infections
Azactam for Injection (Aztreonam) Bristol-Myers Squibb ... 736
Claforan Sterile and Injection (Cefotaxime Sodium) Hoechst Marion Roussel ... 1259
Primaxin I.M. (Cilastatin Sodium, Imipenem) Merck & Co., Inc. ... 1770
Primaxin I.V. (Cilastatin Sodium, Imipenem) Merck & Co., Inc. ... 1772

Citrobacter species urinary tract infections
Azactam for Injection (Aztreonam) Bristol-Myers Squibb ... 736
Claforan Sterile and Injection (Cefotaxime Sodium) Hoechst Marion Roussel ... 1259
Nebcin Vials, Hyporets & ADD-Vantage (Tobramycin Sulfate) Lilly ... 1518
Netromycin Injection 100 mg/ml (Netilmicin Sulfate) Schering ... 2516
Timentin for Injection (Ticarcillin Disodium, Clavulanate Potassium) SmithKline Beecham Pharmaceuticals ... 2706

Claudication, intermittent
Trental Tablets (Pentoxifylline) Hoechst Marion Roussel ... 1291

Clonorchiasis
Biltricide Tablets (Praziquantel) Bayer Pharmaceutical ... 584

Clonorchis sinensis/Opisthorchis viverrini infections
Biltricide Tablets (Praziquantel) Bayer Pharmaceutical ... 584

Clostridium species endomyometritis
Flagyl 375 Capsules (Metronidazole) Searle ... 2587
Flagyl I.V. (Metronidazole Hydrochloride) SCS ... 2373
Protostat Tablets (Metronidazole) Ortho Pharmaceutical ... 1939

Clostridium species gynecologic infections
Cefobid Intravenous/Intramuscular (Cefoperazone Sodium) Pfizer Inc ... 1996
Cefobid Pharmacy Bulk Package - Not for Direct Infusion (Cefoperazone Sodium) Pfizer Inc ... 1999
Claforan Sterile and Injection (Cefotaxime Sodium) Hoechst Marion Roussel ... 1259
Flagyl 375 Capsules (Metronidazole) Searle ... 2587
Flagyl I.V. (Metronidazole Hydrochloride) SCS ... 2373
Mefoxin (Cefoxitin Sodium) Merck & Co., Inc. ... 1734
Mefoxin Premixed Intravenous Solution (Cefoxitin Sodium) Merck & Co., Inc. ... 1737
Protostat Tablets (Metronidazole) Ortho Pharmaceutical ... 1939

Clostridium species infections
Achromycin V Capsules (Tetracycline Hydrochloride) Lederle ... 1417
Cefobid Intravenous/Intramuscular (Cefoperazone Sodium) Pfizer Inc ... 1996
Cefobid Pharmacy Bulk Package - Not for Direct Infusion (Cefoperazone Sodium) Pfizer Inc ... 1999
Cefotan (Cefotetan) Zeneca ... 2936
Claforan Sterile and Injection (Cefotaxime Sodium) Hoechst Marion Roussel ... 1259
Declomycin Tablets (Demeclocycline Hydrochloride) Lederle ... 1421
Doryx Capsules (Doxycycline Hyclate) Parke-Davis ... 1970
DYNACIN Capsules (Minocycline Hydrochloride) Medicis ... 1627
Flagyl 375 Capsules (Metronidazole) Searle ... 2587
Flagyl I.V. (Metronidazole Hydrochloride) SCS ... 2373
Mefoxin (Cefoxitin Sodium) Merck & Co., Inc. ... 1734
Mefoxin Premixed Intravenous Solution (Cefoxitin Sodium) Merck & Co., Inc. ... 1737
Minocin Intravenous (Minocycline Hydrochloride) Lederle ... 1428
Minocin Oral Suspension (Minocycline Hydrochloride) Lederle ... 1431
Minocin Pellet-Filled Capsules (Minocycline Hydrochloride) Lederle ... 1429
Monodox Capsules (Doxycycline Monohydrate) Oclassen ... 1858
Pfizerpen for Injection (Penicillin G Potassium) Pfizer Inc ... 2022
Pipracil (Piperacillin Sodium) Lederle ... 1435
Primaxin I.V. (Cilastatin Sodium, Imipenem) Merck & Co., Inc. ... 1772
Rocephin Injectable Vials, ADD-Vantage, Galaxy Container (Ceftriaxone Sodium) Roche Pharmaceuticals ... 2305
Terramycin Intramuscular Solution (Oxytetracycline) Pfizer Inc ... 2034
Vibramycin (Doxycycline Calcium) Pfizer Inc ... 2038
Vibramycin Hyclate Intravenous (Doxycycline Hyclate) Pfizer Inc.... 2040
Vibramycin (Doxycycline Monohydrate) Pfizer Inc ... 2038

Clostridium species intra-abdominal infections
Cefotan (Cefotetan) Zeneca ... 2936
Claforan Sterile and Injection (Cefotaxime Sodium) Hoechst Marion Roussel ... 1259
Flagyl 375 Capsules (Metronidazole) Searle ... 2587
Flagyl I.V. (Metronidazole Hydrochloride) SCS ... 2373
Mefoxin (Cefoxitin Sodium) Merck & Co., Inc. ... 1734

Mefoxin Premixed Intravenous Solution (Cefoxitin Sodium) Merck & Co., Inc. 1737
Primaxin I.V. (Cilastatin Sodium, Imipenem) Merck & Co., Inc. 1772
Protostat Tablets (Metronidazole) Ortho Pharmaceutical 1939
Rocephin Injectable Vials, ADD-Vantage, Galaxy Container (Ceftriaxone Sodium) Roche Pharmaceuticals 2305

Clostridium species liver abscess
Flagyl 375 Capsules (Metronidazole) Searle 2587
Flagyl I.V. (Metronidazole Hydrochloride) SCS 2373
Protostat Tablets (Metronidazole) Ortho Pharmaceutical 1939

Clostridium species peritonitis
Flagyl 375 Capsules (Metronidazole) Searle 2587
Flagyl I.V. (Metronidazole Hydrochloride) SCS 2373
Mefoxin (Cefoxitin Sodium) Merck & Co., Inc. 1734
Mefoxin Premixed Intravenous Solution (Cefoxitin Sodium) Merck & Co., Inc. 1737
Protostat Tablets (Metronidazole) Ortho Pharmaceutical 1939

Clostridium species septicemia
Cefobid Intravenous/Intramuscular (Cefoperazone Sodium) Pfizer Inc 1996
Cefobid Pharmacy Bulk Package - Not for Direct Infusion (Cefoperazone Sodium) Pfizer Inc 1999
Flagyl 375 Capsules (Metronidazole) Searle 2587
Flagyl I.V. (Metronidazole Hydrochloride) SCS 2373
Protostat Tablets (Metronidazole) Ortho Pharmaceutical 1939

Clostridium species skin and skin structure infections
Flagyl 375 Capsules (Metronidazole) Searle 2587
Flagyl I.V. (Metronidazole Hydrochloride) SCS 2373
Mefoxin (Cefoxitin Sodium) Merck & Co., Inc. 1734
Mefoxin Premixed Intravenous Solution (Cefoxitin Sodium) Merck & Co., Inc. 1737
Protostat Tablets (Metronidazole) Ortho Pharmaceutical 1939

Clostridium species tubo-ovarian abscess
Flagyl 375 Capsules (Metronidazole) Searle 2587
Flagyl I.V. (Metronidazole Hydrochloride) SCS 2373
Protostat Tablets (Metronidazole) Ortho Pharmaceutical 1939

Clostridium species vaginal cuff infection, post-surgical
Flagyl 375 Capsules (Metronidazole) Searle 2587
Flagyl I.V. (Metronidazole Hydrochloride) SCS 2373
Protostat Tablets (Metronidazole) Ortho Pharmaceutical 1939

CNS depression
(see under Central nervous system depression, drug-induced)

Coagulation, disseminated intravascular
(see under Coagulopathies, consumptive)

Coagulopathies, consumptive
Heparin Sodium Injection (Heparin Sodium) Wyeth-Ayerst 2832
Heparin Sodium Vials (Heparin Sodium) Lilly 1486

Coccidioidomycosis
Fungizone Intravenous (Amphotericin B) Apothecon 507
Nizoral Tablets (Ketoconazole) Janssen 1345

Coitus, adjunct in
Replens Vaginal Moisturizer (Glycerin, Lubricant) Warner Wellcome 823

Cold sores
(see under Herpetic manifestations, oral, symptomatic relief of)

Cold, common, symptomatic relief of
(see also under Influenza syndrome, symptomatic relief of)
Actifed Cold & Allergy Tablets (Pseudoephedrine Hydrochloride, Triprolidine Hydrochloride) Warner Wellcome 807
Actifed Cold & Sinus Caplets and Tablets (Acetaminophen, Pseudoephedrine Hydrochloride, Triprolidine Hydrochloride) Warner Wellcome 808
Afrin (Oxymetazoline Hydrochloride) Schering-Plough HealthCare 757
Alka-Seltzer Plus Cold Medicine (Chlorpheniramine Maleate, Aspirin, Phenylpropanolamine Bitartrate) Bayer Consumer 611
Atrohist Pediatric Suspension (Chlorpheniramine Tannate, Phenylephrine Tannate, Pyrilamine Tannate) Medeva 1604
Atrohist Pediatric Suspension Dye-Free (Chlorpheniramine Tannate, Phenylephrine Tannate, Pyrilamine Tannate) Medeva 1604
Atrohist Plus Tablets (Chlorpheniramine Maleate, Phenylpropanolamine Hydrochloride, Phenylephrine Hydrochloride, Hyoscyamine Sulfate, Atropine Sulfate, Scopolamine Hydrobromide) Medeva 1605
BC Cold Powder Multi-Symptom Formula (Cold-Sinus-Allergy) (Aspirin, Phenylpropanolamine Hydrochloride, Chlorpheniramine Maleate) Block 631
BC Cold Powder Non-Drowsy Formula (Cold-Sinus) (Aspirin, Phenylpropanolamine Hydrochloride) Block 631
Benadryl Allergy Chewables (Diphenhydramine Hydrochloride) Warner Wellcome 811
Benadryl Allergy/Cold Tablets (Acetaminophen, Diphenhydramine Hydrochloride, Pseudoephedrine Hydrochloride) Warner Wellcome 811
Benadryl Allergy Decongestant Liquid Medication (Diphenhydramine Hydrochloride, Pseudoephedrine Hydrochloride) Warner Wellcome 812
Benadryl Allergy Decongestant Tablets (Diphenhydramine Hydrochloride, Pseudoephedrine Hydrochloride) Warner Wellcome 812
Benadryl Allergy Liquid Medication (Diphenhydramine Hydrochloride) Warner Wellcome 813
Benadryl Allergy Sinus Headache Caplets (Diphenhydramine Hydrochloride, Pseudoephedrine Hydrochloride, Acetaminophen) Warner Wellcome 813
Benadryl Dye-Free Allergy Liqui-gel Softgels (Diphenhydramine Hydrochloride) Warner Wellcome 813
Bromfed Syrup (Brompheniramine Maleate, Pseudoephedrine Hydrochloride) Muro 712
Children's TYLENOL Cold Multi-Symptom Chewable Tablets and Liquid (Acetaminophen, Chlorpheniramine Maleate, Pseudoephedrine Hydrochloride) McNeil Consumer 1559
Chlor-Trimeton Allergy Decongestant Tablets (Chlorpheniramine Maleate, Pseudoephedrine Sulfate) Schering-Plough HealthCare 759
Congess (Guaifenesin, Pseudoephedrine Hydrochloride) Fleming 1003
Contac Continuous Action Nasal Decongestant/Antihistamine 12 Hour Capsules (Chlorpheniramine Maleate, Phenylpropanolamine Hydrochloride) SmithKline Beecham Consumer 773
Contac Maximum Strength Continuous Action Decongestant/Antihistamine 12 Hour Caplets (Chlorpheniramine Maleate, Phenylpropanolamine Hydrochloride) SmithKline Beecham Consumer 772
Coricidin Cold + Flu Tablets (Acetaminophen, Chlorpheniramine Maleate) Schering-Plough HealthCare 760
Coricidin 'D' Decongestant Tablets (Acetaminophen, Chlorpheniramine Maleate, Phenylpropanolamine Hydrochloride) Schering-Plough HealthCare 760
D.A. II Tablets (Chlorpheniramine Maleate, Methscopolamine Nitrate, Phenylephrine Hydrochloride) Dura 972
D.A. Chewable Tablets (Chlorpheniramine Maleate, Phenylephrine Hydrochloride, Methscopolamine Nitrate) Dura 970
Dimetapp Allergy Sinus Caplets (Acetaminophen, Brompheniramine Maleate, Phenylpropanolamine Hydrochloride) Whitehall-Robins 838
Dimetapp Cold & Cough Liqui-Gels (Brompheniramine Maleate, Dextromethorphan Hydrobromide, Phenylpropanolamine Hydrochloride) Whitehall-Robins 839
Dimetapp Cold & Fever Suspension (Acetaminophen, Brompheniramine Maleate, Pseudoephedrine Hydrochloride) Whitehall-Robins 839
Dimetapp Elixir (Brompheniramine Maleate, Phenylpropanolamine Hydrochloride) Whitehall-Robins 840
Dimetapp Extentabs (Brompheniramine Maleate, Phenylpropanolamine Hydrochloride) Whitehall-Robins 841
Dimetapp Tablets/Liqui-Gels (Brompheniramine Maleate, Phenylpropanolamine Hydrochloride) Whitehall-Robins 841
Drixoral Cold and Allergy Sustained-Action Tablets (Dexbrompheniramine Maleate, Pseudoephedrine Sulfate) Schering-Plough HealthCare 763
Drixoral Cold and Flu Extended-Release Tablets (Acetaminophen, Dexbrompheniramine Maleate, Pseudoephedrine Sulfate) Schering-Plough HealthCare 764
Drixoral Allergy/Sinus Extended Release Tablets (Acetaminophen, Pseudoephedrine Sulfate, Dexbrompheniramine Maleate) Schering-Plough HealthCare 765
Dura-Tap/PD Capsules (Chlorpheniramine Maleate, Pseudoephedrine Hydrochloride) Dura 970
Duration 12 Hour Nasal Spray (Oxymetazoline Hydrochloride) Schering-Plough HealthCare 766
Dura-Vent/DA Tablets (Chlorpheniramine Maleate, Phenylephrine Hydrochloride, Methscopolamine Nitrate) Dura 972
Dura-Vent Tablets (Phenylpropanolamine Hydrochloride, Guaifenesin) Dura 971
Efidac 24 Chlorpheniramine (Chlorpheniramine Maleate) Ciba Self-Medication 655
Entex LA Tablets (Phenylpropanolamine Hydrochloride, Guaifenesin) Dura 972
Exgest LA Tablets (Phenylpropanolamine Hydrochloride, Guaifenesin) Carnrick 787
4-Way Fast Acting Nasal Spray (regular & mentholated) (Naphazoline Hydrochloride, Phenylephrine Hydrochloride, Pyrilamine Maleate) Bristol-Myers Products 644
4-Way 12 Hour Nasal Spray (Oxymetazoline Hydrochloride) Bristol-Myers Products 644
Fedahist Gyrocaps (Pseudoephedrine Hydrochloride, Chlorpheniramine Maleate) Schwarz 2545
Guaifed Syrup (Guaifenesin, Pseudoephedrine Hydrochloride) Muro 712
Hyland's C-Plus Cold Tablets (Homeopathic Medications) Standard Homeopathic 789
Neo-Synephrine Maximum Strength 12 Hour Nasal Spray (Oxymetazoline Hydrochloride) Bayer Consumer 624
Neo-Synephrine Maximum Strength 12 Hour Nasal Spray Pump (Oxymetazoline Hydrochloride) Bayer Consumer 624
Neo-Synephrine (Phenylephrine Hydrochloride) Bayer Consumer 624
Nolamine Timed-Release Tablets (Phenindamine Tartrate, Phenylpropanolamine Hydrochloride, Chlorpheniramine Maleate) Carnrick 790
Novahistine Elixir (Chlorpheniramine Maleate, Phenylephrine Hydrochloride) SmithKline Beecham Consumer 782
PediaCare Cough-Cold Chewable Tablets and Liquid (Pseudoephedrine Hydrochloride, Chlorpheniramine Maleate, Dextromethorphan Hydrobromide) McNeil Consumer 1569
Propagest Tablets (Phenylpropanolamine Hydrochloride) Carnrick 791
Robitussin-PE (Guaifenesin, Pseudoephedrine Hydrochloride) Whitehall-Robins 846
Rynatan (Chlorpheniramine Tannate, Pyrilamine Tannate, Phenylephrine Tannate) Wallace 2781
Sinarest (Acetaminophen, Chlorpheniramine Maleate, Pseudoephedrine Hydrochloride) Ciba Self-Medication 663
Sine-Off No Drowsiness Formula Caplets (Acetaminophen, Pseudoephedrine Hydrochloride) SmithKline Beecham Consumer 784
Sine-Off Sinus Medicine (Acetaminophen, Chlorpheniramine Maleate, Pseudoephedrine Hydrochloride) SmithKline Beecham Consumer 784
Sinulin Tablets (Acetaminophen, Phenylpropanolamine Hydrochloride, Chlorpheniramine Maleate) Carnrick 792
Sinutab Sinus Allergy Medication, Maximum Strength Tablets and Caplets (Acetaminophen, Chlorpheniramine Maleate, Pseudoephedrine Hydrochloride) Warner Wellcome 823
Sudafed Children's Nasal Decongestant Liquid Medication (Pseudoephedrine Hydrochloride) Warner Wellcome 826
Sudafed Cold & Allergy Tablets (Chlorpheniramine Maleate, Pseudoephedrine Hydrochloride) Warner Wellcome 826
Sudafed Nasal Decongestant Tablets, 30 mg (Pseudoephedrine Hydrochloride) Warner Wellcome 825
Sudafed Nasal Decongestant Tablets, 60 mg (Pseudoephedrine Hydrochloride) Warner Wellcome 825

(▣ Described in PDR For Nonprescription Drugs) (◉ Described in PDR For Ophthalmology)

Cold — Indications Index — 1510

Sudafed Pediatric Nasal Decongestant Liquid Oral Drops (Pseudoephedrine Hydrochloride) Warner Wellcome 827
Triaminic Syrup (Phenylpropanolamine Hydrochloride, Chlorpheniramine Maleate) Sandoz Consumer 755
Triaminicin Tablets (Acetaminophen, Chlorpheniramine Maleate, Phenylpropanolamine Hydrochloride) Sandoz Consumer 756
Trinalin Repetabs Tablets (Azatadine Maleate, Pseudoephedrine Sulfate) Key 1373
Vicks Sinex 12-Hour Nasal Decongestant Spray and Ultra Fine Mist (Oxymetazoline Hydrochloride) Procter & Gamble 738
Vicks Sinex Nasal Spray and Ultra Fine Mist (Phenylephrine Hydrochloride) Procter & Gamble 738
Vicks Vapor Inhaler (Desoxyephedrine-Levo) Procter & Gamble 738

Colic, biliary, symptomatic relief of
Cystospaz (Hyoscyamine) PolyMedica 2123
Levsin/Levsinex/Levbid (Hyoscyamine Sulfate) Schwarz 2549

Colic, renal, symptomatic relief of
Cystospaz (Hyoscyamine) PolyMedica 2123
Levsin/Levsinex/Levbid (Hyoscyamine Sulfate) Schwarz 2549

Colic, symptomatic relief of
Hyland's Colic Tablets (Homeopathic Medications) Standard Homeopathic 789
Levsin/Levsinex/Levbid (Hyoscyamine Sulfate) Schwarz 2549

Colitis, mucous
(see under Bowel, irritable, syndrome)

Colitis, pseudomembranous, antibiotic-associated
Vancocin HCl, Oral Solution & Pulvules (Vancomycin Hydrochloride) Lilly 1536
Vancocin HCl, Vials & ADD-Vantage (Vancomycin Hydrochloride) Lilly 1534

Colitis, ulcerative, adjunctive therapy in
Anusol-HC Suppositories (Hydrocortisone Acetate) Parke-Davis 1954
Azulfidine (Sulfasalazine) Pharmacia & Upjohn 2059
CORTENEMA (Hydrocortisone) Solvay 2713

Colitis, ulcerative, left-sided adjunctive therapy in
CORTENEMA (Hydrocortisone) Solvay 2713

Colitis, ulcerative, systemic therapy for
Asacol Delayed-Release Tablets (Mesalamine) Procter & Gamble Pharmaceuticals 2129
Azulfidine (Sulfasalazine) Pharmacia & Upjohn 2059
Celestone Soluspan Suspension (Betamethasone Sodium Phosphate, Betamethasone Acetate) Schering 2484
Cortone Acetate Sterile Suspension (Cortisone Acetate) Merck & Co., Inc. 1663
Cortone Acetate Tablets (Cortisone Acetate) Merck & Co., Inc. 1664
Dalalone D.P. Injectable (Dexamethasone Acetate) Forest 1009
Decadron Elixir (Dexamethasone) Merck & Co., Inc. 1676
Decadron Phosphate Injection (Dexamethasone Sodium Phosphate) Merck & Co., Inc. 1680
Decadron Tablets (Dexamethasone) Merck & Co., Inc. 1678
Decadron-LA Sterile Suspension (Dexamethasone Acetate) Merck & Co., Inc. 1687
Dipentum Capsules (Olsalazine Sodium) Pharmacia & Upjohn 2084
Hydeltrasol Injection, Sterile (Prednisolone Sodium Phosphate) Merck & Co., Inc. 1708
Hydrocortone Phosphate Injection, Sterile (Hydrocortisone Sodium Phosphate) Merck & Co., Inc. 1713
Hydrocortone Tablets (Hydrocortisone) Merck & Co., Inc. 1715
Pediapred Oral Solution (Prednisolone Sodium Phosphate) Medeva 1618
Pentasa (Mesalamine) Hoechst Marion Roussel 1275
Prelone Syrup (Prednisolone) Muro 1834
ROWASA Rectal Suspension Enema 4.0 grams/unit (60 mL) (Mesalamine) Solvay 2727

Collagen disease
Celestone Soluspan Suspension (Betamethasone Sodium Phosphate, Betamethasone Acetate) Schering 2484
Cortone Acetate Sterile Suspension (Cortisone Acetate) Merck & Co., Inc. 1663
Cortone Acetate Tablets (Cortisone Acetate) Merck & Co., Inc. 1664
Dalalone D.P. Injectable (Dexamethasone Acetate) Forest 1009
Decadron Elixir (Dexamethasone) Merck & Co., Inc. 1676
Decadron Phosphate Injection (Dexamethasone Sodium Phosphate) Merck & Co., Inc. 1680
Decadron Tablets (Dexamethasone) Merck & Co., Inc. 1678
Decadron-LA Sterile Suspension (Dexamethasone Acetate) Merck & Co., Inc. 1687
Hydeltrasol Injection, Sterile (Prednisolone Sodium Phosphate) Merck & Co., Inc. 1708
Hydrocortone Phosphate Injection, Sterile (Hydrocortisone Sodium Phosphate) Merck & Co., Inc. 1713
Hydrocortone Tablets (Hydrocortisone) Merck & Co., Inc. 1715
Pediapred Oral Solution (Prednisolone Sodium Phosphate) Medeva 1618
Prelone Syrup (Prednisolone) Muro 1834

Colon, irritable
(see under Bowel, irritable, syndrome)

Colon, spastic
(see under Bowel, irritable, syndrome)

Colostomies, reduction in odor, adjunct to
Devrom Chewable Tablets (Bismuth Subgallate) Parthenon 714

Condylomata acuminata
Alferon N Injection (Interferon Alfa-N3 (Human Leukocyte Derived)) Purdue Frederick 2142
Intron A for Injection (Interferon alfa-2B, Recombinant) Schering .. 2506

Condylomata acuminata, topical treatment of
Condylox Topical Solution (Podofilox) Oclassen 1853
Podocon-25 (Podophyllin) Paddock 1949

Congestive heart failure
(see also under Edema, congestive heart failure-induced, adjunctive therapy in; Edema, congestive heart failure-induced, treatment of)
Aldactazide Tablets (Spironolactone, Hydrochlorothiazide) Searle 2556
Aldactone Tablets (Spironolactone) Searle 2558
Capoten Tablets (Captopril) Bristol-Myers Squibb 740
Crystodigin Tablets (Digitoxin) Lilly 1472
Inocor Lactate Injection (Amrinone Lactate) Sanofi Winthrop 2439
Lanoxicaps (Digoxin) Glaxo Wellcome 1110
Lanoxin Elixir Pediatric (Digoxin) Glaxo Wellcome 1113
Lanoxin Injection (Digoxin) Glaxo Wellcome 1116
Lanoxin Injection Pediatric (Digoxin) Glaxo Wellcome 1119
Lanoxin Tablets (Digoxin) Glaxo Wellcome 1121
Moduretic Tablets (Amiloride Hydrochloride, Hydrochlorothiazide) Merck & Co., Inc. 1748
Nitro-Bid IV (Nitroglycerin) Hoechst Marion Roussel 1270
Primacor Injection (Milrinone Lactate) Sanofi Winthrop 2461

Congestive heart failure, adjunct in
(see also under Edema, congestive heart failure-induced, adjunctive therapy in; Edema, congestive heart failure-induced, treatment of)
Accupril Tablets (Quinapril Hydrochloride) Parke-Davis 1950
Altace Capsules (Ramipril) Hoechst Marion Roussel 1238
Bumex (Bumetanide) Roche Pharmaceuticals 2260
Diuril Sodium Intravenous (Chlorothiazide Sodium) Merck & Co., Inc. 1693
Isuprel Injection (Isoproterenol Hydrochloride) Sanofi Winthrop .. 2441
Midamor Tablets (Amiloride Hydrochloride) Merck & Co., Inc. 1746
Monopril Tablets (Fosinopril Sodium) Bristol-Myers Squibb 762
Prinivil Tablets (Lisinopril) Merck & Co., Inc. 1776
Vasotec Tablets (Enalapril Maleate) Merck & Co., Inc. 1816
Zestril Tablets (Lisinopril) Zeneca.... 2972

Conjunctival inflammation, bulbar, steroid-responsive
AK-CIDE (Prednisolone Acetate, Sulfacetamide Sodium) Akorn.... 203
AK-CIDE Ointment (Prednisolone Acetate, Sulfacetamide Sodium) Akorn 203
Blephamide Ointment (Sulfacetamide Sodium, Prednisolone Acetate) Allergan 234
Decadron Phosphate Sterile Ophthalmic Ointment (Dexamethasone Sodium Phosphate) Merck & Co., Inc. 1684
Decadron Phosphate Sterile Ophthalmic Solution (Dexamethasone Sodium Phosphate) Merck & Co., Inc. 1685
NeoDecadron Sterile Ophthalmic Ointment (Neomycin Sulfate, Dexamethasone Sodium Phosphate) Merck & Co., Inc. 1755
NeoDecadron Sterile Ophthalmic Solution (Neomycin Sulfate, Dexamethasone Sodium Phosphate) Merck & Co., Inc. 1756
Terra-Cortril Ophthalmic Suspension (Oxytetracycline Hydrochloride, Hydrocortisone Acetate) Pfizer Inc 2033

Conjunctival inflammation, palpebral, steroid-responsive
AK-CIDE (Prednisolone Acetate, Sulfacetamide Sodium) Akorn.... 203
AK-CIDE Ointment (Prednisolone Acetate, Sulfacetamide Sodium) Akorn 203
Blephamide Ointment (Sulfacetamide Sodium, Prednisolone Acetate) Allergan 234
Decadron Phosphate Sterile Ophthalmic Ointment (Dexamethasone Sodium Phosphate) Merck & Co., Inc. 1684
Decadron Phosphate Sterile Ophthalmic Solution (Dexamethasone Sodium Phosphate) Merck & Co., Inc. 1685
NeoDecadron Sterile Ophthalmic Ointment (Neomycin Sulfate, Dexamethasone Sodium Phosphate) Merck & Co., Inc. 1755
NeoDecadron Sterile Ophthalmic Solution (Neomycin Sulfate, Dexamethasone Sodium Phosphate) Merck & Co., Inc. 1756
Terra-Cortril Ophthalmic Suspension (Oxytetracycline Hydrochloride, Hydrocortisone Acetate) Pfizer Inc 2033

Conjunctivitis, allergic
AK-PRED (Prednisolone Sodium Phosphate) Akorn 204
Celestone Soluspan Suspension (Betamethasone Sodium Phosphate, Betamethasone Acetate) Schering 2484
Cortone Acetate Sterile Suspension (Cortisone Acetate) Merck & Co., Inc. 1663
Cortone Acetate Tablets (Cortisone Acetate) Merck & Co., Inc. 1664
Dalalone D.P. Injectable (Dexamethasone Acetate) Forest 1009
Decadron Elixir (Dexamethasone) Merck & Co., Inc. 1676
Decadron Phosphate Injection (Dexamethasone Sodium Phosphate) Merck & Co., Inc. 1680
Decadron Phosphate Sterile Ophthalmic Ointment (Dexamethasone Sodium Phosphate) Merck & Co., Inc. 1684
Decadron Phosphate Sterile Ophthalmic Solution (Dexamethasone Sodium Phosphate) Merck & Co., Inc. 1685
Decadron Tablets (Dexamethasone) Merck & Co., Inc. 1678
Decadron-LA Sterile Suspension (Dexamethasone Acetate) Merck & Co., Inc. 1687
Econopred & Econopred Plus Ophthalmic Suspensions (Prednisolone Acetate) Alcon Laboratories 216
HMS Liquifilm (Medrysone) Allergan 241
Hydeltrasol Injection, Sterile (Prednisolone Sodium Phosphate) Merck & Co., Inc. 1708
Hydrocortone Phosphate Injection, Sterile (Hydrocortisone Sodium Phosphate) Merck & Co., Inc. 1713
Hydrocortone Tablets (Hydrocortisone) Merck & Co., Inc. 1715
Livostin (Levocabastine Hydrochloride) CIBA Vision Ophthalmics 262
PBZ Tablets (Tripelennamine Hydrochloride) CibaGeneva 863
PBZ-SR Tablets (Tripelennamine Hydrochloride) CibaGeneva............ 862
Pediapred Oral Solution (Prednisolone Sodium Phosphate) Medeva 1618
Periactin (Cyproheptadine Hydrochloride) Merck & Co., Inc. 1767
Phenergan Suppositories (Promethazine Hydrochloride) Wyeth-Ayerst 2882
Phenergan Syrup (Promethazine Hydrochloride) Wyeth-Ayerst 2881
Phenergan Tablets (Promethazine Hydrochloride) Wyeth-Ayerst 2882
Prelone Syrup (Prednisolone) Muro 1834

Conjunctivitis, bacterial
Chibroxin Sterile Ophthalmic Solution (Norfloxacin) Merck & Co., Inc. 1657
Ciloxan Ophthalmic Solution (Ciprofloxacin Hydrochloride) Alcon Laboratories 468
Garamycin Ophthalmic (Gentamicin Sulfate) Schering 2501
Neosporin Ophthalmic Ointment Sterile (Polymyxin B Sulfate, Bacitracin Zinc, Neomycin Sulfate) Glaxo Wellcome 1130
Neosporin Ophthalmic Solution Sterile (Polymyxin B Sulfate, Neomycin Sulfate, Gramicidin) Glaxo Wellcome 1131
Ocuflox Ophthalmic Solution (Ofloxacin) Allergan 478
Polysporin Ophthalmic Ointment Sterile (Polymyxin B Sulfate, Bacitracin Zinc) Glaxo Wellcome .. 1140

(▣ Described in PDR For Nonprescription Drugs)   (◉ Described in PDR For Ophthalmology)

1511 Indications Index Corneal injury

Polytrim Ophthalmic Solution Sterile (Polymyxin B Sulfate, Trimethoprim Sulfate) Allergan 479

Conjunctivitis, fungal
Natacyn Antifungal Ophthalmic Suspension (Natamycin) Alcon Laboratories .... ⊚ 223

Conjunctivitis, granular (see under Trachoma)

Conjunctivitis, inclusion
Achromycin V Capsules (Tetracycline Hydrochloride) Lederle 1417
Declomycin Tablets (Demeclocycline Hydrochloride) Lederle 1421
Doryx Capsules (Doxycycline Hyclate) Parke-Davis 1970
DYNACIN Capsules (Minocycline Hydrochloride) Medicis 1627
Gantanol Tablets (Sulfamethoxazole) Roche Pharmaceuticals 2285
Gantrisin (Acetyl Sulfisoxazole) Roche Pharmaceuticals 2286
Minocin Intravenous (Minocycline Hydrochloride) Lederle 1428
Minocin Oral Suspension (Minocycline Hydrochloride) Lederle 1431
Minocin Pellet-Filled Capsules (Minocycline Hydrochloride) Lederle 1429
Monodox Capsules (Doxycycline Monohydrate) Oclassen 1858
Terramycin Intramuscular Solution (Oxytetracycline) Pfizer Inc 2034
Vibramycin (Doxycycline Calcium) Pfizer Inc 2038

Conjunctivitis, infective
AK-CIDE (Prednisolone Acetate, Sulfacetamide Sodium) Akorn .... ⊚ 203
AK-CIDE Ointment (Prednisolone Acetate, Sulfacetamide Sodium) Akorn .... ⊚ 203
AK-PRED (Prednisolone Sodium Phosphate) Akorn .... ⊚ 204
AK-Trol Ointment & Suspension (Dexamethasone, Neomycin Sulfate, Polymyxin B Sulfate) Akorn .... ⊚ 205
Blephamide Liquifilm Sterile Ophthalmic Suspension (Prednisolone Acetate, Sulfacetamide Sodium) Allergan 472
Blephamide Ointment (Sulfacetamide Sodium, Prednisolone Acetate) Allergan .... ⊚ 234
Decadron Phosphate Sterile Ophthalmic Ointment (Dexamethasone Sodium Phosphate) Merck & Co., Inc. 1684
Decadron Phosphate Sterile Ophthalmic Solution (Dexamethasone Sodium Phosphate) Merck & Co., Inc. 1685
Econopred & Econopred Plus Ophthalmic Suspensions (Prednisolone Acetate) Alcon Laboratories .... ⊚ 216
FML-S Liquifilm (Sulfacetamide Sodium, Fluorometholone) Allergan .... ⊚ 240
Maxitrol Ophthalmic Ointment and Suspension (Dexamethasone, Neomycin Sulfate, Polymyxin B Sulfate) Alcon Laboratories .... ⊚ 222
NeoDecadron Sterile Ophthalmic Ointment (Neomycin Sulfate, Dexamethasone Sodium Phosphate) Merck & Co., Inc. 1755
NeoDecadron Sterile Ophthalmic Solution (Neomycin Sulfate, Dexamethasone Sodium Phosphate) Merck & Co., Inc. 1756
Poly-Pred Liquifilm (Neomycin Sulfate, Polymyxin B Sulfate, Prednisolone Acetate) Allergan .. ⊚ 246
Pred-G Liquifilm Sterile Ophthalmic Suspension (Gentamicin Sulfate, Prednisolone Acetate) Allergan .... ⊚ 248
Pred-G S.O.P. Sterile Ophthalmic Ointment (Gentamicin Sulfate, Prednisolone Acetate) Allergan .. ⊚ 249
Terra-Cortril Ophthalmic Suspension (Oxytetracycline Hydrochloride, Hydrocortisone Acetate) Pfizer Inc 2033
TobraDex Ophthalmic Suspension and Ointment (Dexamethasone, Tobramycin) Alcon Laboratories .. 469

Conjunctivitis, neonatal
E-Mycin Tablets (Erythromycin) Knoll Laboratories 1388
Ery-Tab Tablets (Erythromycin) Abbott 426
Erythrocin Stearate Filmtab (Erythromycin Stearate) Abbott 429
Erythromycin Base Filmtab (Erythromycin) Abbott 430
Erythromycin Delayed-Release Capsules, USP (Erythromycin) Abbott 431
PCE Dispertab Tablets (Erythromycin) Abbott 453

Conjunctivitis, unspecified
Bleph-10 (Sulfacetamide Sodium) Allergan 472
Genoptic Sterile Ophthalmic Solution (Gentamicin Sulfate) Allergan .... ⊚ 241
Genoptic Sterile Ophthalmic Ointment (Gentamicin Sulfate) Allergan .... ⊚ 241
Gentak (Gentamicin Sulfate) Akorn .... ⊚ 209
Pred Mild (Prednisolone Acetate) Allergan .... ⊚ 250

Conjunctivitis, vernal
Alomide Ophthalmic Solution (Lodoxamide Tromethamine) Alcon Laboratories 465
Crolom (Cromolyn Sodium) Bausch & Lomb Pharmaceuticals .... ⊚ 254
HMS Liquifilm (Medrysone) Allergan .... ⊚ 241

Constipation, chronic
CITRUCEL Sugar Free Orange Flavor (Methylcellulose) SmithKline Beecham Consumer ▣ 770
DUPHALAC Solution (Lactulose) Solvay 2714
Konsyl Fiber Tablets (Calcium Polycarbophil) Konsyl .... ▣ 679
Konsyl Powder Sugar Free Unflavored (Psyllium Preparations) Konsyl .... ▣ 680
Metamucil (Psyllium Preparations) Procter & Gamble 2125
Perdiem Fiber (Psyllium Preparations) Ciba Self-Medication 889
Peri-Colace Capsules and Syrup (Casanthranol, Docusate Sodium) Roberts 2226
Senokot (Senna Concentrates) Purdue Frederick 2154
Senokot-S Tablets (Senna Concentrates, Docusate Sodium) Purdue Frederick 2154

Constipation, temporary
CITRUCEL Orange Flavor (Methylcellulose) SmithKline Beecham Consumer .... ▣ 770
Colace Capsules, Syrup, Liquid (Docusate Sodium) Roberts 2212
Colace Microenema (Docusate Sodium) Roberts 2213
Colace-T 50 mg Tablets (Docusate Sodium) Roberts 2213
Colace-T 100 mg Tablets (Docusate Sodium) Roberts 2213
Correctol Extra Gentle Stool Softener (Docusate Sodium) Schering-Plough HealthCare .... ▣ 762
Correctol Herbal Tea Laxative (Senna Concentrates) Schering-Plough HealthCare .... ▣ 761
Correctol Laxative Tablets & Caplets (Bisacodyl) Schering-Plough HealthCare .... ▣ 761
Dialose Tablets (Docusate Sodium) J&J•Merck Consumer 1358
Dialose Plus Tablets (Docusate Sodium, Phenolphthalein) J&J•Merck Consumer 1358
Doxidan Liqui-Gels (Docusate Calcium, Phenolphthalein) Upjohn .... ▣ 801
Dulcolax (Bisacodyl) Ciba Self-Medication 883
Ex-Lax Chocolated Laxative Tablets (Phenolphthalein) Sandoz Consumer .... ▣ 748
Extra Gentle Ex-Lax Laxative Pills (Docusate Sodium, Phenolphthalein) Sandoz Consumer .... ▣ 749
Maximum Relief Formula Ex-Lax Laxative Pills (Phenolphthalein) Sandoz Consumer .... ▣ 749
Regular Strength Ex-Lax Laxative Pills (Phenolphthalein) Sandoz Consumer .... ▣ 749
Ex-Lax Gentle Nature Laxative Pills (Senna Concentrates) Sandoz Consumer .... ▣ 749
FiberCon Caplets (Calcium Polycarbophil) Lederle Consumer .... ▣ 684
Fleet Babylax (Glycerin) Fleet 1000
Fleet Bisacodyl Enema (Bisacodyl) Fleet 1000
Fleet Enema (Sodium Phosphate, Dibasic, Sodium Phosphate, Monobasic) Fleet 1001
Fleet Glycerin Laxative Rectal Applicators (Glycerin) Fleet 1000
Fleet Mineral Oil Enema (Mineral Oil) Fleet 1001
Fleet Phospho-Soda (Sodium Phosphate, Dibasic, Sodium Phosphate, Monobasic) Fleet 1002
Fleet Sof-Lax (Docusate Sodium) Fleet 1003
Fleet Sof-Lax Overnight (Docusate Sodium, Casanthranol) Fleet 1003
Fletcher's Castoria (Senna Concentrates) Mentholatum .... ▣ 709
Fletcher's Cherry Flavor (Phenolphthalein) Mentholatum ▣ 710
Kondremul (Mineral Oil) Ciba Self-Medication .... ▣ 656
Maltsupex Liquid, Powder & Tablets (Malt Soup Extract) Wallace .... ▣ 803
Perdiem (Psyllium Preparations, Senna Concentrates) Ciba Self-Medication 889
Peri-Colace Capsules and Syrup (Casanthranol, Docusate Sodium) Roberts 2226
Phillips' Gelcaps (Docusate Sodium, Phenolphthalein) Bayer Consumer .... ▣ 627
Phillips' Milk of Magnesia Liquid (Magnesium Hydroxide) Bayer Consumer .... ▣ 627
Purge Concentrate (Castor Oil) Fleming .... ▣ 671
Senokot Children's Syrup (Senna) Purdue Frederick 2154
Senokot (Senna Concentrates) Purdue Frederick 2154
Senokot-S Tablets (Senna Concentrates, Docusate Sodium) Purdue Frederick 2154
Surfak Liqui-Gels (Docusate Calcium) Upjohn .... ▣ 803

Contact lenses, fitting of, adjunct in
Fluor-I-Strip (Fluorescein Sodium) Storz Ophthalmics .... ⊚ 319
Fluor-I-Strip A.T. (Fluorescein Sodium) Storz Ophthalmics .... ⊚ 320

Contraception (see under Pregnancy, prevention of)

Convulsions, reduction of the intensity of muscle contractions in
Metubine Iodide Vials (Metocurine Iodide) Dista 932

Convulsive disorders, adjunctive therapy in
Valium Tablets (Diazepam) Roche Products 2335

Convulsive episodes, control of
Nembutal Sodium Solution (Pentobarbital Sodium) Abbott 442

Corneal edema (see under Edema, corneal, temporary relief of)

Corneal erosions, recurrent
Lacrisert Sterile Ophthalmic Insert (Hydroxypropyl Cellulose) Merck & Co., Inc. 1730

Corneal inflammation, steroid-responsive
AK-PRED (Prednisolone Sodium Phosphate) Akorn .... ⊚ 204
AK-Trol Ointment & Suspension (Dexamethasone, Neomycin Sulfate, Polymyxin B Sulfate) Akorn .... ⊚ 205
Blephamide Liquifilm Sterile Ophthalmic Suspension (Prednisolone Acetate, Sulfacetamide Sodium) Allergan 472
Blephamide Ointment (Sulfacetamide Sodium, Prednisolone Acetate) Allergan .... ⊚ 234
Cortisporin Ophthalmic Ointment Sterile (Polymyxin B Sulfate, Bacitracin Zinc, Neomycin Sulfate, Hydrocortisone) Glaxo Wellcome 1074
Cortisporin Ophthalmic Suspension Sterile (Hydrocortisone, Polymyxin B Sulfate, Neomycin Sulfate) Glaxo Wellcome 1075
Decadron Phosphate Sterile Ophthalmic Ointment (Dexamethasone Sodium Phosphate) Merck & Co., Inc. 1684
Decadron Phosphate Sterile Ophthalmic Solution (Dexamethasone Sodium Phosphate) Merck & Co., Inc. 1685
Econopred & Econopred Plus Ophthalmic Suspensions (Prednisolone Acetate) Alcon Laboratories .... ⊚ 216
FML Forte Liquifilm (Fluorometholone) Allergan .... ⊚ 237
FML Liquifilm (Fluorometholone) Allergan .... ⊚ 238
FML S.O.P. (Fluorometholone) Allergan .... ⊚ 239
FML-S Liquifilm (Sulfacetamide Sodium, Fluorometholone) Allergan .... ⊚ 240
Maxitrol Ophthalmic Ointment and Suspension (Dexamethasone, Neomycin Sulfate, Polymyxin B Sulfate) Alcon Laboratories .... ⊚ 222
NeoDecadron Sterile Ophthalmic Ointment (Neomycin Sulfate, Dexamethasone Sodium Phosphate) Merck & Co., Inc. 1755
NeoDecadron Sterile Ophthalmic Solution (Neomycin Sulfate, Dexamethasone Sodium Phosphate) Merck & Co., Inc. 1756
Poly-Pred Liquifilm (Neomycin Sulfate, Polymyxin B Sulfate, Prednisolone Acetate) Allergan .. ⊚ 246
Pred Forte (Prednisolone Acetate) Allergan .... ⊚ 247
Pred-G Liquifilm Sterile Ophthalmic Suspension (Gentamicin Sulfate, Prednisolone Acetate) Allergan .... ⊚ 248
Pred-G S.O.P. Sterile Ophthalmic Ointment (Gentamicin Sulfate, Prednisolone Acetate) Allergan .. ⊚ 249
Terra-Cortril Ophthalmic Suspension (Oxytetracycline Hydrochloride, Hydrocortisone Acetate) Pfizer Inc 2033
TobraDex Ophthalmic Suspension and Ointment (Dexamethasone, Tobramycin) Alcon Laboratories .. 469

Corneal injury, chemical
AK-CIDE (Prednisolone Acetate, Sulfacetamide Sodium) Akorn .... ⊚ 203
AK-CIDE Ointment (Prednisolone Acetate, Sulfacetamide Sodium) Akorn .... ⊚ 203
AK-PRED (Prednisolone Sodium Phosphate) Akorn .... ⊚ 204
AK-Trol Ointment & Suspension (Dexamethasone, Neomycin Sulfate, Polymyxin B Sulfate) Akorn .... ⊚ 205
Blephamide Liquifilm Sterile Ophthalmic Suspension (Prednisolone Acetate, Sulfacetamide Sodium) Allergan 472
Blephamide Ointment (Sulfacetamide Sodium, Prednisolone Acetate) Allergan .... ⊚ 234
Cortisporin Ophthalmic Ointment Sterile (Polymyxin B Sulfate, Bacitracin Zinc, Neomycin Sul-

(▣ Described in PDR For Nonprescription Drugs) (⊚ Described in PDR For Ophthalmology)

Corneal injury | Indications Index | 1512

fate, Hydrocortisone) Glaxo Wellcome ... 1074
Cortisporin Ophthalmic Suspension Sterile (Hydrocortisone, Polymyxin B Sulfate, Neomycin Sulfate) Glaxo Wellcome ... 1075
Decadron Phosphate Sterile Ophthalmic Ointment (Dexamethasone Sodium Phosphate) Merck & Co., Inc. ... 1684
Decadron Phosphate Sterile Ophthalmic Solution (Dexamethasone Sodium Phosphate) Merck & Co., Inc. ... 1685
Econopred & Econopred Plus Ophthalmic Suspensions (Prednisolone Acetate) Alcon Laboratories ... ◉ 216
FML-S Liquifilm (Sulfacetamide Sodium, Fluorometholone) Allergan ... ◉ 240
Maxitrol Ophthalmic Ointment and Suspension (Dexamethasone, Neomycin Sulfate, Polymyxin B Sulfate) Alcon Laboratories ... ◉ 222
NeoDecadron Sterile Ophthalmic Ointment (Neomycin Sulfate, Dexamethasone Sodium Phosphate) Merck & Co., Inc. ... 1755
NeoDecadron Sterile Ophthalmic Solution (Neomycin Sulfate, Dexamethasone Sodium Phosphate) Merck & Co., Inc. ... 1756
Poly-Pred Liquifilm (Neomycin Sulfate, Polymyxin B Sulfate, Prednisolone Acetate) Allergan ... ◉ 246
Pred Mild (Prednisolone Acetate) Allergan ... ◉ 250
Pred-G Liquifilm Sterile Ophthalmic Suspension (Gentamicin Sulfate, Prednisolone Acetate) Allergan ... ◉ 248
Pred-G S.O.P. Sterile Ophthalmic Ointment (Gentamicin Sulfate, Prednisolone Acetate) Allergan ... ◉ 249
Terra-Cortril Ophthalmic Suspension (Oxytetracycline Hydrochloride, Hydrocortisone Acetate) Pfizer Inc ... 2033
TobraDex Ophthalmic Suspension and Ointment (Dexamethasone, Tobramycin) Alcon Laboratories ... 469

Corneal injury, foreign bodies
AK-CIDE (Prednisolone Acetate, Sulfacetamide Sodium) Akorn ... ◉ 203
AK-CIDE Ointment (Prednisolone Acetate, Sulfacetamide Sodium) Akorn ... ◉ 203
AK-PRED (Prednisolone Sodium Phosphate) Akorn ... ◉ 204
AK-Trol Ointment & Suspension (Dexamethasone, Neomycin Sulfate, Polymyxin B Sulfate) Akorn ... ◉ 205
Blephamide Liquifilm Sterile Ophthalmic Suspension (Prednisolone Acetate, Sulfacetamide Sodium) Allergan ... 472
Blephamide Ointment (Sulfacetamide Sodium, Prednisolone Acetate) Allergan ... ◉ 234
Cortisporin Ophthalmic Ointment Sterile (Polymyxin B Sulfate, Bacitracin Zinc, Neomycin Sulfate, Hydrocortisone) Glaxo Wellcome ... 1074
Cortisporin Ophthalmic Suspension Sterile (Hydrocortisone, Polymyxin B Sulfate, Neomycin Sulfate) Glaxo Wellcome ... 1075
Decadron Phosphate Sterile Ophthalmic Ointment (Dexamethasone Sodium Phosphate) Merck & Co., Inc. ... 1684
Decadron Phosphate Sterile Ophthalmic Solution (Dexamethasone Sodium Phosphate) Merck & Co., Inc. ... 1685
Econopred & Econopred Plus Ophthalmic Suspensions (Prednisolone Acetate) Alcon Laboratories ... ◉ 216
FML-S Liquifilm (Sulfacetamide Sodium, Fluorometholone) Allergan ... ◉ 240
FLURESS (Fluorescein Sodium, Benoxinate Hydrochloride) Akorn ... ◉ 208
Maxitrol Ophthalmic Ointment and Suspension (Dexamethasone, Neomycin Sulfate, Polymyxin B Sulfate) Alcon Laboratories ... ◉ 222
NeoDecadron Sterile Ophthalmic Ointment (Neomycin Sulfate, Dexamethasone Sodium Phosphate) Merck & Co., Inc. ... 1755
NeoDecadron Sterile Ophthalmic Solution (Neomycin Sulfate, Dexamethasone Sodium Phosphate) Merck & Co., Inc. ... 1756
Poly-Pred Liquifilm (Neomycin Sulfate, Polymyxin B Sulfate, Prednisolone Acetate) Allergan ... ◉ 246
Pred-G Liquifilm Sterile Ophthalmic Suspension (Gentamicin Sulfate, Prednisolone Acetate) Allergan ... ◉ 248
Pred-G S.O.P. Sterile Ophthalmic Ointment (Gentamicin Sulfate, Prednisolone Acetate) Allergan ... ◉ 249
Terra-Cortril Ophthalmic Suspension (Oxytetracycline Hydrochloride, Hydrocortisone Acetate) Pfizer Inc ... 2033
TobraDex Ophthalmic Suspension and Ointment (Dexamethasone, Tobramycin) Alcon Laboratories ... 469

Corneal injury, radiation
AK-CIDE (Prednisolone Acetate, Sulfacetamide Sodium) Akorn ... ◉ 203
AK-CIDE Ointment (Prednisolone Acetate, Sulfacetamide Sodium) Akorn ... ◉ 203
AK-PRED (Prednisolone Sodium Phosphate) Akorn ... ◉ 204
AK-Trol Ointment & Suspension (Dexamethasone, Neomycin Sulfate, Polymyxin B Sulfate) Akorn ... ◉ 205
Blephamide Liquifilm Sterile Ophthalmic Suspension (Prednisolone Acetate, Sulfacetamide Sodium) Allergan ... 472
Blephamide Ointment (Sulfacetamide Sodium, Prednisolone Acetate) Allergan ... ◉ 234
Cortisporin Ophthalmic Ointment Sterile (Polymyxin B Sulfate, Bacitracin Zinc, Neomycin Sulfate, Hydrocortisone) Glaxo Wellcome ... 1074
Cortisporin Ophthalmic Suspension Sterile (Hydrocortisone, Polymyxin B Sulfate, Neomycin Sulfate) Glaxo Wellcome ... 1075
Econopred & Econopred Plus Ophthalmic Suspensions (Prednisolone Acetate) Alcon Laboratories ... ◉ 216
FML-S Liquifilm (Sulfacetamide Sodium, Fluorometholone) Allergan ... ◉ 240
Maxitrol Ophthalmic Ointment and Suspension (Dexamethasone, Neomycin Sulfate, Polymyxin B Sulfate) Alcon Laboratories ... ◉ 222
NeoDecadron Sterile Ophthalmic Ointment (Neomycin Sulfate, Dexamethasone Sodium Phosphate) Merck & Co., Inc. ... 1755
NeoDecadron Sterile Ophthalmic Solution (Neomycin Sulfate, Dexamethasone Sodium Phosphate) Merck & Co., Inc. ... 1756
Poly-Pred Liquifilm (Neomycin Sulfate, Polymyxin B Sulfate, Prednisolone Acetate) Allergan ... ◉ 246
Pred-G Liquifilm Sterile Ophthalmic Suspension (Gentamicin Sulfate, Prednisolone Acetate) Allergan ... ◉ 248
Pred-G S.O.P. Sterile Ophthalmic Ointment (Gentamicin Sulfate, Prednisolone Acetate) Allergan ... ◉ 249
Terra-Cortril Ophthalmic Suspension (Oxytetracycline Hydrochloride, Hydrocortisone Acetate) Pfizer Inc ... 2033
TobraDex Ophthalmic Suspension and Ointment (Dexamethasone, Tobramycin) Alcon Laboratories ... 469

Corneal injury, thermal burns
AK-CIDE (Prednisolone Acetate, Sulfacetamide Sodium) Akorn ... ◉ 203
AK-CIDE Ointment (Prednisolone Acetate, Sulfacetamide Sodium) Akorn ... ◉ 203
AK-PRED (Prednisolone Sodium Phosphate) Akorn ... ◉ 204
AK-Trol Ointment & Suspension (Dexamethasone, Neomycin Sulfate, Polymyxin B Sulfate) Akorn ... ◉ 205
Blephamide Liquifilm Sterile Ophthalmic Suspension (Prednisolone Acetate, Sulfacetamide Sodium) Allergan ... 472
Blephamide Ointment (Sulfacetamide Sodium, Prednisolone Acetate) Allergan ... ◉ 234
Cortisporin Ophthalmic Ointment Sterile (Polymyxin B Sulfate, Bacitracin Zinc, Neomycin Sulfate, Hydrocortisone) Glaxo Wellcome ... 1074
Cortisporin Ophthalmic Suspension Sterile (Hydrocortisone, Polymyxin B Sulfate, Neomycin Sulfate) Glaxo Wellcome ... 1075
Decadron Phosphate Sterile Ophthalmic Ointment (Dexamethasone Sodium Phosphate) Merck & Co., Inc. ... 1684
Decadron Phosphate Sterile Ophthalmic Solution (Dexamethasone Sodium Phosphate) Merck & Co., Inc. ... 1685
Econopred & Econopred Plus Ophthalmic Suspensions (Prednisolone Acetate) Alcon Laboratories ... ◉ 216
FML-S Liquifilm (Sulfacetamide Sodium, Fluorometholone) Allergan ... ◉ 240
Maxitrol Ophthalmic Ointment and Suspension (Dexamethasone, Neomycin Sulfate, Polymyxin B Sulfate) Alcon Laboratories ... ◉ 222
NeoDecadron Sterile Ophthalmic Ointment (Neomycin Sulfate, Dexamethasone Sodium Phosphate) Merck & Co., Inc. ... 1755
NeoDecadron Sterile Ophthalmic Solution (Neomycin Sulfate, Dexamethasone Sodium Phosphate) Merck & Co., Inc. ... 1756
Poly-Pred Liquifilm (Neomycin Sulfate, Polymyxin B Sulfate, Prednisolone Acetate) Allergan ... ◉ 246
Pred Mild (Prednisolone Acetate) Allergan ... ◉ 250
Pred-G Liquifilm Sterile Ophthalmic Suspension (Gentamicin Sulfate, Prednisolone Acetate) Allergan ... ◉ 248
Pred-G S.O.P. Sterile Ophthalmic Ointment (Gentamicin Sulfate, Prednisolone Acetate) Allergan ... ◉ 249
Terra-Cortril Ophthalmic Suspension (Oxytetracycline Hydrochloride, Hydrocortisone Acetate) Pfizer Inc ... 2033
TobraDex Ophthalmic Suspension and Ointment (Dexamethasone, Tobramycin) Alcon Laboratories ... 469

Corneal marginal ulcers, allergic
Cortone Acetate Sterile Suspension (Cortisone Acetate) Merck & Co., Inc. ... 1663
Cortone Acetate Tablets (Cortisone Acetate) Merck & Co., Inc. ... 1664
Dalalone D.P. Injectable (Dexamethasone Acetate) Forest ... 1009
Decadron Elixir (Dexamethasone) Merck & Co., Inc. ... 1676
Decadron Phosphate Injection (Dexamethasone Sodium Phosphate) Merck & Co., Inc. ... 1680
Decadron Tablets (Dexamethasone) Merck & Co., Inc. ... 1678
Decadron-LA Sterile Suspension (Dexamethasone Acetate) Merck & Co., Inc. ... 1687
Hydeltrasol Injection, Sterile (Prednisolone Sodium Phosphate) Merck & Co., Inc. ... 1708
Hydrocortone Phosphate Injection, Sterile (Hydrocortisone Sodium Phosphate) Merck & Co., Inc. ... 1713
Hydrocortone Tablets (Hydrocortisone) Merck & Co., Inc. ... 1715
Pediapred Oral Solution (Prednisolone Sodium Phosphate) Medeva 1618
Prelone Syrup (Prednisolone) Muro 1834

Corneal sensitivity, decreased
Lacrisert Sterile Ophthalmic Insert (Hydroxypropyl Cellulose) Merck & Co., Inc. ... 1730

Corneal transplant, surgical aid in
AMO Vitrax Viscoelastic Solution (Sodium Hyaluronate) Allergan ... ◉ 229
Healon (Sodium Hyaluronate) Pharmacia & Upjohn ... ◉ 302
Healon GV (Sodium Hyaluronate) Pharmacia & Upjohn ... ◉ 303

Corneal ulcers
Bleph-10 (Sulfacetamide Sodium) Allergan ... 472
Celestone Soluspan Suspension (Betamethasone Sodium Phosphate, Betamethasone Acetate) Schering ... 2484
Ciloxan Ophthalmic Solution (Ciprofloxacin Hydrochloride) Alcon Laboratories ... 468
Garamycin Ophthalmic (Gentamicin Sulfate) Schering ... 2501
Genoptic Sterile Ophthalmic Solution (Gentamicin Sulfate) Allergan ... ◉ 241
Genoptic Sterile Ophthalmic Ointment (Gentamicin Sulfate) Allergan ... ◉ 241
Gentak (Gentamicin Sulfate) Akorn ... ◉ 209

Corns
(see under Hyperkeratosis skin disorders)

Coronary artery disease, reducing the risk of
Lopid Tablets (Gemfibrozil) Parke-Davis ... 1974
Zocor Tablets (Simvastatin) Merck & Co., Inc. ... 1821

Coronary atherosclerosis, to slow the progression of
(see also under Coronary artery disease, reducing the risk of)
Mevacor Tablets (Lovastatin) Merck & Co., Inc. ... 1742
Pravachol Tablets (Pravastatin Sodium) Bristol-Myers Squibb ... 770
Questran (Cholestyramine) Bristol-Myers Squibb ... 774

Coronary angioplasty or atherectomy, percutaneous transluminal, adjunct in
ReoPro Vials (Abciximab) Lilly ... 1526

Coronary events, primary prevention of
Pravachol Tablets (Pravastatin Sodium) Bristol-Myers Squibb ... 770

Corynebacterium diphtheriae
(see under C. diphtheriae infections)

Corynebacterium minutissimum
(see under C. minutissimum infections)

Coryza, acute
(see under Cold, common, symptomatic relief of)

Coughs and nasal congestion, symptomatic relief of
Alka-Seltzer Plus Cold & Cough Medicine (Aspirin, Chlorpheniramine Maleate, Dextromethorphan Hydrobromide, Phenylpropanolamine Bitartrate) Bayer Consumer ... ▣ 611
Benylin Multisymptom (Dextromethorphan Hydrobromide, Pseudoephedrine Hydrochloride, Guaifenesin) Warner Wellcome ... ▣ 816
Bromfed-DM Cough Syrup (Brompheniramine Maleate, Pseudoephedrine Hydrochloride, Dextromethorphan Hydrobromide) Muro ... 1832
Brontex (Codeine Phosphate, Guaifenesin) Procter & Gamble Pharmaceuticals ... 2130

(▣ Described in PDR For Nonprescription Drugs) (◉ Described in PDR For Ophthalmology)

Indications Index / Cough

Cerose DM (Chlorpheniramine Maleate, Dextromethorphan Hydrobromide, Phenylephrine Hydrochloride) Wyeth-Ayerst...... 853
Cheracol Plus Head Cold/Cough Formula (Phenylpropanolamine Hydrochloride, Dextromethorphan Hydrobromide, Chlorpheniramine Maleate) Roberts .. 741
Children's TYLENOL Cold Plus Cough Multi Symptom Chewable Tablets and Liquid (Acetaminophen, Chlorpheniramine Maleate, Dextromethorphan Hydrobromide, Pseudoephedrine Hydrochloride) McNeil Consumer 1560
Children's TYLENOL Flu Suspension Liquid (Acetaminophen, Chlorpheniramine Maleate, Dextromethorphan Hydrobromide, Pseudoephedrine Hydrochloride) McNeil Consumer 1560
Children's Vicks NyQuil Cold/Cough Relief (Chlorpheniramine Maleate, Dextromethorphan Hydrobromide, Pseudoephedrine Hydrochloride) Procter & Gamble 731
Codiclear DH Syrup (Guaifenesin, Hydrocodone Bitartrate) Central .. 808
Comtrex Multi-Symptom (Acetaminophen, Chlorpheniramine Maleate, Dextromethorphan Hydrobromide, Pseudoephedrine Hydrochloride) Bristol-Myers Products 638
Contac Severe Cold and Flu Formula Caplets (Acetaminophen, Chlorpheniramine Maleate, Dextromethorphan Hydrobromide, Phenylpropanolamine Hydrochloride) SmithKline Beecham Consumer 773
Deconsal II Tablets (Pseudoephedrine Hydrochloride, Guaifenesin) Medeva 1605
Dimetane-DC Cough Syrup (Brompheniramine Maleate, Phenylpropanolamine Hydrochloride, Codeine Phosphate) Robins 2232
Dimetane-DX Cough Syrup (Brompheniramine Maleate, Pseudoephedrine Hydrochloride, Dextromethorphan Hydrobromide) Robins.. 2233
Dimetapp Cold & Cough Liqui-Gels (Brompheniramine Maleate, Dextromethorphan Hydrobromide, Phenylpropanolamine Hydrochloride) Whitehall-Robins 839
Dimetapp DM Elixir (Brompheniramine Maleate, Dextromethorphan Hydrobromide) Whitehall-Robins 840
Dorcol Children's Cough Syrup (Pseudoephedrine Hydrochloride, Guaifenesin, Dextromethorphan Hydrobromide) Sandoz Consumer 748
Drixoral Cough + Congestion Liquid Caps (Dextromethorphan Hydrobromide, Pseudoephedrine Hydrochloride) Schering-Plough HealthCare 763
Duratuss HD Elixir (Hydrocodone Bitartrate, Pseudoephedrine Hydrochloride, Guaifenesin) UCB 2750
Guaifed (Guaifenesin, Pseudoephedrine Hydrochloride) Muro.... 1833
Histussin D Liquid (Hydrocodone Bitartrate, Pseudoephedrine Hydrochloride) Bock 670
Hycomine Compound Tablets (Hydrocodone Bitartrate, Chlorpheniramine Maleate, Acetaminophen, Phenylephrine Hydrochloride) DuPont 948
Hycomine (Hydrocodone Bitartrate, Phenylpropanolamine Hydrochloride) DuPont 947
Novahistine DMX (Dextromethorphan Hydrobromide, Guaifenesin, Pseudoephedrine Hydrochloride) SmithKline Beecham Consumer................ 782
Nucofed (Codeine Phosphate, Pseudoephedrine Hydrochloride, Guaifenesin) Roberts 2225
PediaCare (Pseudoephedrine Hydrochloride, Chlorpheniramine Maleate, Dextromethorphan Hydrobromide) McNeil Consumer............................... 1569
Pediatric Vicks 44d Cough & Head Congestion Relief (Dextromethorphan Hydrobromide, Pseudoephedrine Hydrochloride) Procter & Gamble.................... 736
Phenergan with Codeine (Codeine Phosphate, Promethazine Hydrochloride) Wyeth-Ayerst 2883
Phenergan with Dextromethorphan (Promethazine Hydrochloride, Dextromethorphan Hydrobromide) Wyeth-Ayerst 2885
Phenergan VC (Promethazine Hydrochloride, Phenylephrine Hydrochloride) Wyeth-Ayerst 2886
Phenergan VC with Codeine (Codeine Phosphate, Promethazine Hydrochloride, Phenylephrine Hydrochloride) Wyeth-Ayerst 2888
Robitussin Cold & Cough Liqui-Gels (Guaifenesin, Dextromethorphan Hydrobromide, Pseudoephedrine Hydrochloride) Whitehall-Robins 844
Robitussin Cold, Cough & Flu Liqui-Gels (Acetaminophen, Dextromethorphan Hydrobromide, Guaifenesin, Pseudoephedrine Hydrochloride) Whitehall-Robins 844
Robitussin Maximum Strength Cough & Cold (Dextromethorphan Hydrobromide, Pseudoephedrine Hydrochloride) Whitehall-Robins 847
Robitussin Pediatric Drops (Dextromethorphan Hydrobromide, Guaifenesin, Pseudoephedrine Hydrochloride) Whitehall-Robins 849
Robitussin-CF (Dextromethorphan Hydrobromide, Guaifenesin, Phenylpropanolamine Hydrochloride) Whitehall-Robins 846
Robitussin-DAC Syrup (Codeine Phosphate, Guaifenesin, Pseudoephedrine Hydrochloride) Robins 2249
Ryna (Chlorpheniramine Maleate, Codeine Phosphate, Pseudoephedrine Hydrochloride) Wallace 804
Rynatuss (Carbetapentane Tannate, Chlorpheniramine Tannate, Ephedrine Tannate, Phenylephrine Tannate) Wallace 2782
Sudafed Children's Cold & Cough Liquid Medication (Dextromethorphan Hydrobromide, Guaifenesin, Pseudoephedrine Hydrochloride) Warner Wellcome 825
Sudafed Cold and Cough Liquid Caps (Acetaminophen, Dextromethorphan Hydrobromide, Guaifenesin, Pseudoephedrine Hydrochloride) Warner Wellcome 826
Sunsource Cold Relief Tablets (Homeopathic Medications) Sunsource 792
Syn-Rx DM Tablets (Guaifenesin, Pseudoephedrine Hydrochloride, Dextromethorphan Hydrobromide) Medeva 1623
TheraFlu (Acetaminophen, Chlorpheniramine Maleate, Pseudoephedrine Hydrochloride) Sandoz Consumer 750
TheraFlu Maximum Strength, Non-Drowsy Formula Flu, Cold and Cough Caplets (Acetaminophen, Dextromethorphan Hydrobromide, Pseudoephedrine Hydrochloride) Sandoz Consumer............................ 752
Triaminic AM Cough and Decongestant Formula (Dextromethorphan Hydrobromide, Pseudoephedrine Hydrochloride) Sandoz Consumer 753
Triaminic Expectorant (Phenylpropanolamine Hydrochloride, Guaifenesin) Sandoz Consumer 753
Triaminic Night Time (Chlorpheniramine Maleate, Dextromethorphan Hydrobromide, Pseudoephedrine Hydrochloride) Sandoz Consumer.................... 754
Triaminic Triaminicol Cold & Cough (Phenylpropanolamine Hydrochloride, Chlorpheniramine Maleate, Dextromethorphan Hydrobromide) Sandoz Consumer.. 756
Triaminic DM Syrup (Phenylpropanolamine Hydrochloride, Dextromethorphan Hydrobromide) Sandoz Consumer.. 756
Tussend (Hydrocodone Bitartrate, Pseudoephedrine Hydrochloride, Chlorpheniramine Maleate) Monarch 1830
Tussend Expectorant (Hydrocodone Bitartrate, Pseudoephedrine Hydrochloride, Guaifenesin) Monarch 1831
TYLENOL Cold Medication, Multi-Symptom Formula Tablets and Caplets (Acetaminophen, Chlorpheniramine Maleate, Pseudoephedrine Hydrochloride, Dextromethorphan Hydrobromide) McNeil Consumer 1572
TYLENOL Cold Medication, Multi-Symptom Hot Liquid Packets (Acetaminophen, Chlorpheniramine Maleate, Pseudoephedrine Hydrochloride, Dextromethorphan Hydrobromide) McNeil Consumer 1572
TYLENOL Cold Medication, No Drowsiness Formula Caplets and Gelcaps (Acetaminophen, Pseudoephedrine Hydrochloride, Dextromethorphan Hydrobromide) McNeil Consumer 1572
TYLENOL Cold Severe Congestion Caplets (Acetaminophen, Dextromethorphan Hydrobromide, Guaifenesin, Pseudoephedrine Hydrochloride) McNeil Consumer 1573
TYLENOL Cough Medication with Decongestant, Multi Symptom (Dextromethorphan Hydrobromide, Acetaminophen, Pseudoephedrine Hydrochloride) McNeil Consumer 1574
TYLENOL Flu No Drowsiness Formula, Maximum Strength Gelcaps (Acetaminophen, Dextromethorphan Hydrobromide, Pseudoephedrine Hydrochloride) McNeil Consumer 1575
TYLENOL Flu NightTime, Maximum Strength Hot Medication Packets (Acetaminophen, Diphenhydramine Hydrochloride, Pseudoephedrine Hydrochloride) McNeil Consumer 1575
Vicks 44 LiquiCaps Non-Drowsy Cough & Cold Relief (Dextromethorphan Hydrobromide, Pseudoephedrine Hydrochloride) Procter & Gamble 729
Vicks 44D Cough & Head Congestion Relief (Dextromethorphan Hydrobromide, Pseudoephedrine Hydrochloride) Procter & Gamble 728
Vicks 44M Cough, Cold & Flu Relief (Acetaminophen, Dextromethorphan Hydrobromide, Chlorpheniramine Maleate, Pseudoephedrine Hydrochloride) Procter & Gamble 729
Vicks DayQuil LiquiCaps/Liquid Multi-Symptom Cold/Flu Relief (Acetaminophen, Dextromethorphan Hydrobromide, Pseudoephedrine Hydrochloride, Guaifenesin) Procter & Gamble 734
Vicks NyQuil LiquiCaps/Liquid Multi-Symptom Cold/Flu Relief, Original and Cherry Flavors (Acetaminophen, Pseudoephedrine Hydrochloride, Dextromethorphan Hydrobromide, Doxylamine Succinate) Procter & Gamble 736
Vicks VapoRub (Menthol, Camphor, Eucalyptus, Oil of) Procter & Gamble 739
Vicks VapoSteam (Camphor, Eucalyptus, Oil of, Menthol) Procter & Gamble 739

Cough, symptomatic relief of

Benadryl Allergy Liquid Medication (Diphenhydramine Hydrochloride) Warner Wellcome 813
Benylin Adult Formula Cough Suppressant (Dextromethorphan Hydrobromide) Warner Wellcome 817
Benylin Expectorant (Dextromethorphan Hydrobromide, Guaifenesin) Warner Wellcome .. 816
Benylin Pediatric Cough Suppressant (Dextromethorphan Hydrobromide) Warner Wellcome 817
Cheracol D Cough Formula (Dextromethorphan Hydrobromide, Guaifenesin) Roberts 740
Codiclear DH Syrup (Guaifenesin, Hydrocodone Bitartrate) Central .. 808
Coricidin Cough + Cold Tablets (Chlorpheniramine Maleate, Dextromethorphan Hydrobromide) Schering-Plough HealthCare 760
Cough-X Lozenges (Dextromethorphan Hydrobromide, Benzocaine) Ascher 606
Delsym Extended-Release Suspension (Dextromethorphan Polistirex) Fisons 670
Diabe-Tuss DM Syrup (Dextromethorphan Hydrobromide) Paddock .. 1948
Dilaudid Cough Syrup (Hydromorphone Hydrochloride) Knoll Laboratories 1383
Drixoral Cough Liquid Caps (Dextromethorphan Hydrobromide) Schering-Plough HealthCare 762
Drixoral Cough + Sore Throat Liquid Caps (Dextromethorphan Hydrobromide, Acetaminophen) Schering-Plough HealthCare 763
Halls Juniors Sugar Free Cough Suppressant Drops (Menthol) Warner-Lambert 806
Halls Mentho-Lyptus Cough Suppressant Drops (Menthol) Warner-Lambert 806
Halls Plus Maximum Strength Cough Suppressant Drops (Menthol) Warner-Lambert.......... 806
Halls Sugar Free Mentho-Lyptus Cough Suppressant Drops (Menthol) Warner-Lambert 806
Humibid (Guaifenesin, Dextromethorphan Hydrobromide) Medeva .. 1612
Hycodan Tablets and Syrup (Hydrocodone Bitartrate, Homatropine Methylbromide) DuPont 946
Hycotuss Expectorant Syrup (Hydrocodone Bitartrate, Guaifenesin) DuPont 950
Hyland's Cough Syrup with Honey (Ipecac) Standard Homeopathic...................................... 789
N'ICE Medicated Sugarless Sore Throat and Cough Lozenges (Menthol) SmithKline Beecham Consumer 781
Original Vicks Cough Drops, Menthol and Cherry Flavors (Menthol) Procter & Gamble 733
Pediatric Vicks 44e Cough & Chest Congestion Relief (Dextromethorphan Hydrobromide, Guaifenesin) Procter & Gamble 737
Pertussin Adult Extra Strength (Dextromethorphan Hydrobromide) Blairex 630
Pertussin Children's Strength (Dextromethorphan Hydrobromide) Blairex 630
Robitussin A-C Syrup (Codeine Phosphate, Guaifenesin) Robins ..2248
Robitussin Maximum Strength Cough Suppressant (Dextromethorphan Hydrobromide) Whitehall-Robins 847
Robitussin Pediatric Cough & Cold Formula (Dextromethorphan Hydrobromide, Pseudo-

(▣ Described in PDR For Nonprescription Drugs)   (● Described in PDR For Ophthalmology)

Cough

ephedrine Hydrochloride)
Whitehall-Robins 848
Robitussin Pediatric Cough
Suppressant (Dextromethor-
phan Hydrobromide)
Whitehall-Robins 848
Robitussin-DM (Dextromethor-
phan Hydrobromide,
Guaifenesin) Whitehall-Robins..... 846
Safe Tussin 30 Liquid (Dextro-
methorphan Hydrobromide,
Guaifenesin) Kramer 1413
Sucrets 4-Hour Cough
Suppressant (Dextromethor-
phan Hydrobromide)
SmithKline Beecham Consumer 785
Tessalon Perles (Benzonatate)
Forest 1018
TheraFlu Maximum Strength
Nighttime Flu, Cold & Cough
Medicine (Acetaminophen,
Dextromethorphan Hydrobro-
mide, Pseudoephedrine Hydro-
chloride, Chlorpheniramine
Maleate) Sandoz Consumer 751
Tussionex Pennkinetic
Extended-Release Suspension
(Hydrocodone Polistirex, Chlor-
pheniramine Polistirex) Medeva .. 1624
Tussi-Organidin DM NR Liquid and
DM-S NR Liquid (Guaifenesin,
Dextromethorphan
Hydrobromide) Wallace 2786
TYLENOL Cough Medication, Multi
Symptom (Dextromethorphan
Hydrobromide, Acetaminophen)
McNeil Consumer 1574
Vicks 44 Cough Relief (Dextro-
methorphan Hydrobromide)
Procter & Gamble 728
Vicks 44E Cough & Chest
Congestion Relief (Dextrometh-
orphan Hydrobromide,
Guaifenesin) Procter & Gamble ... 729
Vicks Chloraseptic Cough &
Throat Drops, Menthol, Cherry
and Honey Lemon Flavors
(Menthol) Procter & Gamble 732
Vicks Cough Drops, Menthol and
Cherry Flavors (Menthol)
Procter & Gamble 732
Vicodin Tuss Expectorant (Hydro-
codone Bitartrate, Guaifenesin)
Knoll Laboratories 1406

Cough, whooping
(see under Pertussis)

Cradle cap
(see under Dermatitis, seborrheic)

Cramps, abdominal, symptomatic relief of
Donnagel Liquid and Donnagel
Chewable Tablets (Attapulgite)
Wyeth-Ayerst 854
Gas-X Chewable Tablets
(Simethicone) Sandoz
Consumer 749
Levsin/Levsinex/Levbid (Hyoscya-
mine Sulfate) Schwarz 2549

Cramps, leg
(see under Leg muscle cramps)

Creeping eruptions
(see under Larva migrans, cutaneous)

Cretinism
(see under Hypothyroidism, replacement or supplemental therapy in)

Cryptitis, temporary relief of
Anusol-HC Suppositories (Hydrocortisone Acetate) Parke-Davis 1954

Cryptococcosis
Ancobon Capsules (Flucytosine)
Roche Pharmaceuticals 2254
Fungizone Intravenous (Amphoteri-
cin B) Apothecon 507

Cryptococcus meningitis
Ancobon Capsules (Flucytosine)
Roche Pharmaceuticals 2254
Diflucan Tablets, Injection, and
Oral Suspension (Fluconazole)
Pfizer Inc 2003

Cryptococcus strains pulmonary infections
Ancobon Capsules (Flucytosine)
Roche Pharmaceuticals 2254

Cryptococcus strains urinary tract infections
Ancobon Capsules (Flucytosine)
Roche Pharmaceuticals 2254

Cryptorchidism, prepubertal
Pregnyl for Injection (Chorionic
Gonadotropin) Organon 1878
Profasi (chorionic gonadotropin for
injection, USP) (Chorionic
Gonadotropin) Serono 2620

Cushing's syndrome
Cytadren Tablets
(Aminoglutethimide) CibaGeneva . 837

Cushing's syndrome, diagnosis of
(see under Adrenocortical hyperfunction, diagnostic testing of)

Cushing's syndrome, ACTH-dependent, differential diagnosis of
Acthrel for Injection (Corticorelin
Ovine Triflutate) Ferring 2990

Cuts, minor, infection from
(see under Infections, skin, bacterial, minor)

Cuts, minor, pain associated with
(see under Pain, topical relief of)

Cyclitis
AK-PRED (Prednisolone Sodium
Phosphate) Akorn 204
Decadron Phosphate Sterile
Ophthalmic Ointment (Dexa-
methasone Sodium Phosphate)
Merck & Co., Inc. 1684
Decadron Phosphate Sterile
Ophthalmic Solution (Dexameth-
asone Sodium Phosphate) Merck
& Co., Inc. 1685
Econopred & Econopred Plus
Ophthalmic Suspensions (Pred-
nisolone Acetate) Alcon
Laboratories 216

Cystic fibrosis
Chloromycetin Sodium Succinate
(Chloramphenicol Sodium
Succinate) Parke-Davis 1960

Cystic fibrosis, adjunctive therapy in
Pulmozyme Inhalation (Dornase
Alfa) Genentech 1054

Cystic tumors
Celestone Soluspan Suspension
(Betamethasone Sodium Phos-
phate, Betamethasone Acetate)
Schering 2484

Cystinuria
Cuprimine Capsules (Penicillamine)
Merck & Co., Inc. 1673
Depen Titratable Tablets
(Penicillamine) Wallace 2770

Cystitis
Azactam for Injection (Aztreonam)
Bristol-Myers Squibb 736
Ceclor Pulvules & Suspension
(Cefaclor) Lilly 1470
Cipro Tablets (Ciprofloxacin
Hydrochloride) Bayer
Pharmaceutical 584
Floxin I.V. (Ofloxacin) McNeil
Pharmaceutical 1580
Floxin Tablets (200 mg, 300 mg,
400 mg) (Ofloxacin) McNeil
Pharmaceutical 1577
Gantanol Tablets
(Sulfamethoxazole) Roche
Pharmaceuticals 2285
Gantrisin (Acetyl Sulfisoxazole)
Roche Pharmaceuticals 2286
Lorabid Suspension and Pulvules
(Loracarbef) Lilly 1513
Macrobid Capsules (Nitrofurantoin
Monohydrate) Procter & Gamble
Pharmaceuticals 2138
Maxaquin Tablets (Lomefloxacin
Hydrochloride) Searle 2593
Noroxin Tablets (Norfloxacin)
Merck & Co., Inc. 1758
Noroxin Tablets (Norfloxacin)
Roberts 2222
Penetrex Tablets (Enoxacin)
Rhone-Poulenc Rorer
Pharmaceuticals 2196
Urised Tablets (Atropine Sulfate,
Hyoscyamine, Methenamine,
Phenyl Salicylate) PolyMedica 2123
Uroqid-Acid No. 2 Tablets (Methe-
namine Mandelate, Sodium Acid
Phosphate) Beach 633
Vantin for Oral Suspension and
Vantin Tablets (Cefpodoxime
Proxetil) Pharmacia & Upjohn 2112

Cystitis, frequency and incontinence, symptomatic relief of
Urispas Tablets (Flavoxate
Hydrochloride) SmithKline
Beecham Pharmaceuticals 2710

Cystitis, hemorrhagic, prophylaxis
Mesnex Injection (Mesna)
Bristol-Myers Squibb
Oncology/Immunology 711

Cystitis, "Lacking substantial evidence of effectiveness" in
Urobiotic-250 Capsules (Oxytetra-
cycline Hydrochloride, Sulfamethizole, Phenazopyridine
Hydrochloride) Pfizer Inc 2038

Cytomegalovirus disease associated with renal transplantation, attenuation of
CytoGam (Cytomegalovirus Im-
mune Globulin) MedImmune 1630

Cytomegalovirus disease associated with transplant patients
Cytovene (Ganciclovir Sodium)
Roche Pharmaceuticals 2270

D

Dacryocystitis
Garamycin Ophthalmic (Gentami-
cin Sulfate) Schering 2501
Genoptic Sterile Ophthalmic
Solution (Gentamicin Sulfate)
Allergan 241
Genoptic Sterile Ophthalmic
Ointment (Gentamicin Sulfate)
Allergan 241
Gentak (Gentamicin Sulfate)
Akorn 209

Dandruff
(see also under Dermatitis, seborrheic)
Capitrol Shampoo (Chloroxine)
Westwood-Squibb 2791
DHS (Coal Tar) Persön & Covey 1989
Fototar Cream (Coal Tar) ICN 1300
Head & Shoulders Intensive
Treatment Dandruff and
Seborrheic Dermatitis Shampoo
(Selenium Sulfide) Procter &
Gamble 723
Nizoral 2% Shampoo
(Ketoconazole) Janssen 1344
Pentrax Shampoo (Coal Tar)
GenDerm 1042
Selsun Rx 2.5% Selenium Sulfide
Lotion, USP (Selenium Sulfide)
Ross 2345
Tegrin Dandruff Shampoo (Coal
Tar) Block...................................... 634

Dehydration, prevention of
Kao Lectrolyte (Electrolyte
Supplement) Pharmacia &
Upjohn 2099
Pedialyte Oral Electrolyte
Maintenance Solution (Electrolyte
Supplement) Ross 2340
Rehydralyte Oral Electrolyte
Rehydration Solution (Electrolyte
Supplement) Ross 2344

Dementia, Alzheimer's type
Cognex Capsules (Tacrine
Hydrochloride) Parke-Davis 1961

Dental caries, prophylaxis
Crest Sensitivity Protection
Toothpaste (Potassium Nitrate,
Sodium Fluoride) Procter &
Gamble 723
Luride Drops 50 ml (Sodium
Fluoride) Colgate Oral 891
Luride Lozi-Tabs Tablets (Sodium
Fluoride) Colgate Oral 892
Poly-Vi-Flor Drops (Vitamins with
Fluoride) Mead Johnson
Nutritionals 1600
Poly-Vi-Flor Tablets (Vitamins with
Fluoride) Mead Johnson
Nutritionals 1600
PreviDent 5000 Plus Cream (So-
dium Fluoride) Colgate Oral......... 893
Tri-Vi-Flor Drops (Vitamins with
Fluoride) Mead Johnson
Nutritionals 1601

Dental plaque, prevention of
Listerine Antiseptic (Eucalyptol,
Menthol, Methyl Salicylate)
Warner Wellcome 820
Baby Orajel Tooth & Gum
Cleanser (Simethicone) Del 668

Depression, atypical
(see under Depression, mental, nonendogenous)

Depression, bipolar
(see under Depression, manic-depressive)

Depression, major, without melancholia
Parnate Tablets (Tranylcypromine
Sulfate) SmithKline Beecham
Pharmaceuticals 2679

Depression, manic-depressive
Adapin Capsules (Doxepin
Hydrochloride) Lotus 1542
Depakote Tablets (Divalproex
Sodium) Abbott 418
Eskalith (Lithium Carbonate)
SmithKline Beecham
Pharmaceuticals 2658
Lithium Carbonate Capsules &
Tablets (Lithium Carbonate)
Roxane 2352
Lithonate/Lithotabs/Lithobid (Lith-
ium Carbonate) Solvay 2721
Ludiomil Tablets (Maprotiline
Hydrochloride) CibaGeneva......... 861
Sinequan (Doxepin Hydrochloride)
Pfizer Inc 2028
Thorazine (Chlorpromazine
Hydrochloride) SmithKline
Beecham Pharmaceuticals 2701

Depression, mental, nonendogenous
Nardil (Phenelzine Sulfate)
Parke-Davis................................... 1977

Depression, neurosis
Asendin Tablets (Amoxapine)
Lederle 1419
Ludiomil Tablets (Maprotiline
Hydrochloride) CibaGeneva 861

Depression, neurotic
(see under Depression, mental, nonendogenous)

Depression, relief of symptoms
Asendin Tablets (Amoxapine)
Lederle 1419
Desyrel and Desyrel Dividose
(Trazodone Hydrochloride)
Apothecon 504
Effexor (Venlafaxine
Hydrochloride) Wyeth-Ayerst 2825
Elavil (Amitriptyline Hydrochloride)
Zeneca 2945
Etrafon (Perphenazine, Amitripty-
line Hydrochloride) Schering 2495
Limbitrol (Chlordiazepoxide, Ami-
triptyline Hydrochloride) Roche
Products 2333
Ludiomil Tablets (Maprotiline
Hydrochloride) CibaGeneva 861
Norpramin Tablets (Desipramine
Hydrochloride) Hoechst Marion
Roussel 1273
Pamelor (Nortriptyline
Hydrochloride) Sandoz
Pharmaceuticals 2409
Paxil Tablets (Paroxetine
Hydrochloride) SmithKline
Beecham Pharmaceuticals 2681

Indications Index — Dermatoses

Prozac Pulvules & Liquid, Oral Solution (Fluoxetine Hydrochloride) Dista 935
Remeron Tablets (Mirtazapine) Organon 1878
Serzone Tablets (Nefazodone Hydrochloride) Bristol-Myers Squibb 776
Sinequan (Doxepin Hydrochloride) Pfizer Inc 2028
Surmontil Capsules (Trimipramine Maleate) Wyeth-Ayerst 2917
Tofranil Ampuls (Imipramine Hydrochloride) CibaGeneva 873
Tofranil Tablets (Imipramine Hydrochloride) CibaGeneva 875
Tofranil-PM Capsules (Imipramine Pamoate) CibaGeneva 876
Triavil Tablets (Perphenazine, Amitriptyline Hydrochloride) Merck & Co., Inc. 1800
Vivactil Tablets (Protriptyline Hydrochloride) Merck & Co., Inc. . 1820
Wellbutrin Tablets (Bupropion Hydrochloride) Glaxo Wellcome 1177
Zoloft Tablets (Sertraline Hydrochloride) Pfizer Inc 2051

Dermatitis, allergic contact, diagnosis of
T.R.U.E. Test (Allergens) Glaxo Wellcome 1162

Dermatitis, atopic
Celestone Soluspan Suspension (Betamethasone Sodium Phosphate, Betamethasone Acetate) Schering 2484
Cortaid Sensitive Skin Cream with Aloe (Hydrocortisone Acetate) Upjohn 800
Cortizone-5 Creme and Ointment (Hydrocortisone) Thompson Medical 795
Cortizone-10 Creme and Ointment (Hydrocortisone) Thompson Medical 795
Cortone Acetate Sterile Suspension (Cortisone Acetate) Merck & Co., Inc. 1663
Cortone Acetate Tablets (Cortisone Acetate) Merck & Co., Inc. 1664
Dalalone D.P. Injectable (Dexamethasone Acetate) Forest 1009
Decadron Elixir (Dexamethasone) Merck & Co., Inc. 1676
Decadron Phosphate Injection (Dexamethasone Sodium Phosphate) Merck & Co., Inc. 1680
Decadron Tablets (Dexamethasone) Merck & Co., Inc. 1678
Decadron-LA Sterile Suspension (Dexamethasone Acetate) Merck & Co., Inc. 1687
Hydeltrasol Injection, Sterile (Prednisolone Sodium Phosphate) Merck & Co., Inc. 1708
Hydrocortone Phosphate Injection, Sterile (Hydrocortisone Sodium Phosphate) Merck & Co., Inc. ... 1713
Hydrocortone Tablets (Hydrocortisone) Merck & Co., Inc. 1715
Mantadil Cream (Chlorcyclizine Hydrochloride) Glaxo Wellcome 1124
Pediapred Oral Solution (Prednisolone Sodium Phosphate) Medeva 1618
Prelone Syrup (Prednisolone) Muro 1834
Zonalon Cream (Doxepin Hydrochloride) GenDerm 1042

Dermatitis, contact
(see also under Dermatoses, corticosteroid-responsive)
Benadryl Itch Relief Stick Extra Strength (Diphenhydramine Hydrochloride, Zinc Acetate) Warner Wellcome 814
Benadryl Cream (Diphenhydramine Hydrochloride, Zinc Acetate) Warner Wellcome 814
Benadryl Gel (Diphenhydramine Hydrochloride, Zinc Acetate) Warner Wellcome 815
Benadryl Spray (Diphenhydramine Hydrochloride, Zinc Acetate) Warner Wellcome 815
Caladryl (Pramoxine Hydrochloride, Zinc Acetate) Warner Wellcome 817
Caldecort Anti-Itch Hydrocortisone Cream (Hydrocortisone Acetate) Ciba Self-Medication 651
Celestone Soluspan Suspension (Betamethasone Sodium Phosphate, Betamethasone Acetate) Schering 2484
Cortaid (Hydrocortisone Acetate) Upjohn 800
Cortizone-5 (Hydrocortisone) Thompson Medical 795
Cortizone-10 Creme and Ointment (Hydrocortisone) Thompson Medical 795
Cortone Acetate Sterile Suspension (Cortisone Acetate) Merck & Co., Inc. 1663
Cortone Acetate Tablets (Cortisone Acetate) Merck & Co., Inc. 1664
Dalalone D.P. Injectable (Dexamethasone Acetate) Forest 1009
Decadron Elixir (Dexamethasone) Merck & Co., Inc. 1676
Decadron Phosphate Injection (Dexamethasone Sodium Phosphate) Merck & Co., Inc. 1680
Decadron Tablets (Dexamethasone) Merck & Co., Inc. 1678
Decadron-LA Sterile Suspension (Dexamethasone Acetate) Merck & Co., Inc. 1687
Hydeltrasol Injection, Sterile (Prednisolone Sodium Phosphate) Merck & Co., Inc. 1708
Hydrocortone Phosphate Injection, Sterile (Hydrocortisone Sodium Phosphate) Merck & Co., Inc. ... 1713
Hydrocortone Tablets (Hydrocortisone) Merck & Co., Inc. 1715
Mantadil Cream (Chlorcyclizine Hydrochloride) Glaxo Wellcome 1124
Pediapred Oral Solution (Prednisolone Sodium Phosphate) Medeva 1618
Vistaril (Hydroxyzine Pamoate) Pfizer Inc 2042

Dermatitis, contact, infected
Garamycin 0.1% (Gentamicin Sulfate) Schering 2501

Dermatitis, corticosteroid-responsive, anal region
Analpram-HC Rectal Cream 1% and 2.5% (Hydrocortisone Acetate, Pramoxine Hydrochloride) Ferndale 993

Dermatitis, eczematoid
Zonalon Cream (Doxepin Hydrochloride) GenDerm 1042

Dermatitis, eczematoid, infected
Garamycin 0.1% (Gentamicin Sulfate) Schering 2501

Dermatitis, exfoliative
Celestone Soluspan Suspension (Betamethasone Sodium Phosphate, Betamethasone Acetate) Schering 2484
Cortone Acetate Sterile Suspension (Cortisone Acetate) Merck & Co., Inc. 1663
Cortone Acetate Tablets (Cortisone Acetate) Merck & Co., Inc. 1664
Dalalone D.P. Injectable (Dexamethasone Acetate) Forest 1009
Decadron Elixir (Dexamethasone) Merck & Co., Inc. 1676
Decadron Phosphate Injection (Dexamethasone Sodium Phosphate) Merck & Co., Inc. 1680
Decadron Tablets (Dexamethasone) Merck & Co., Inc. 1678
Decadron-LA Sterile Suspension (Dexamethasone Acetate) Merck & Co., Inc. 1687
Hydeltrasol Injection, Sterile (Prednisolone Sodium Phosphate) Merck & Co., Inc. 1708
Hydrocortone Phosphate Injection, Sterile (Hydrocortisone Sodium Phosphate) Merck & Co., Inc. ... 1713
Hydrocortone Tablets (Hydrocortisone) Merck & Co., Inc. 1715
Pediapred Oral Solution (Prednisolone Sodium Phosphate) Medeva 1618
Prelone Syrup (Prednisolone) Muro 1834

Dermatitis, herpetiformis
Dapsone Tablets USP (Dapsone) Jacobus 1331

Dermatitis, herpetiformis bullous
Celestone Soluspan Suspension (Betamethasone Sodium Phosphate, Betamethasone Acetate) Schering 2484
Cortone Acetate Sterile Suspension (Cortisone Acetate) Merck & Co., Inc. 1663
Cortone Acetate Tablets (Cortisone Acetate) Merck & Co., Inc. 1664
Dalalone D.P. Injectable (Dexamethasone Acetate) Forest 1009
Decadron Elixir (Dexamethasone) Merck & Co., Inc. 1676
Decadron Phosphate Injection (Dexamethasone Sodium Phosphate) Merck & Co., Inc. 1680
Decadron Tablets (Dexamethasone) Merck & Co., Inc. 1678
Decadron-LA Sterile Suspension (Dexamethasone Acetate) Merck & Co., Inc. 1687
Hydeltrasol Injection, Sterile (Prednisolone Sodium Phosphate) Merck & Co., Inc. 1708
Hydrocortone Phosphate Injection, Sterile (Hydrocortisone Sodium Phosphate) Merck & Co., Inc. ... 1713
Hydrocortone Tablets (Hydrocortisone) Merck & Co., Inc. 1715
Pediapred Oral Solution (Prednisolone Sodium Phosphate) Medeva 1618
Prelone Syrup (Prednisolone) Muro 1834

Dermatitis, lichenoid
Mantadil Cream (Chlorcyclizine Hydrochloride) Glaxo Wellcome 1124

Dermatitis, seborrheic
Aquanil HC Lotion (Hydrocortisone) Persön & Covey 1989
Capitrol Shampoo (Chloroxine) Westwood-Squibb 2791
Cortizone for Kids (Hydrocortisone) Thompson Medical 795
Cortizone-10 Creme and Ointment (Hydrocortisone) Thompson Medical 795
DHS Zinc Dandruff Shampoo (Pyrithione Zinc) Persön & Covey .. 1989
Fototar Cream (Coal Tar) ICN ... 1300
Head & Shoulders Intensive Treatment Dandruff and Seborrheic Dermatitis Shampoo (Selenium Sulfide) Procter & Gamble 723
Mantadil Cream (Chlorcyclizine Hydrochloride) Glaxo Wellcome 1124
Nizoral 2% Cream (Ketoconazole) Janssen 1344
Novacet Lotion (Sulfur, Sulfacetamide Sodium) GenDerm 1041
Pentrax Shampoo (Coal Tar) GenDerm 1042
Selsun Blue (Selenium Sulfide) Ross 746
Selsun Rx 2.5% Selenium Sulfide Lotion, USP (Selenium Sulfide) Ross 2345
Sulfacet-R Lotion (Sodium Sulfacetamide, Sulfur) Dermik 925
Sulfacet-R Tint Free Lotion (Sodium Sulfacetamide, Sulfur) Dermik 925
Tegrin Skin Cream & Tegrin Medicated Soap (Coal Tar) Block 634

Dermatitis, seborrheic, infected
Garamycin 0.1% (Gentamicin Sulfate) Schering 2501

Dermatitis, seborrheic, severe
Celestone Soluspan Suspension (Betamethasone Sodium Phosphate, Betamethasone Acetate) Schering 2484
Cortone Acetate Sterile Suspension (Cortisone Acetate) Merck & Co., Inc. 1663
Cortone Acetate Tablets (Cortisone Acetate) Merck & Co., Inc. 1664
Dalalone D.P. Injectable (Dexamethasone Acetate) Forest 1009
Decadron Elixir (Dexamethasone) Merck & Co., Inc. 1676
Decadron Phosphate Injection (Dexamethasone Sodium Phosphate) Merck & Co., Inc. 1680
Decadron Tablets (Dexamethasone) Merck & Co., Inc. 1678
Decadron-LA Sterile Suspension (Dexamethasone Acetate) Merck & Co., Inc. 1687
Hydeltrasol Injection, Sterile (Prednisolone Sodium Phosphate) Merck & Co., Inc. 1708
Hydrocortone Phosphate Injection, Sterile (Hydrocortisone Sodium Phosphate) Merck & Co., Inc. ... 1713
Hydrocortone Tablets (Hydrocortisone) Merck & Co., Inc. 1715
Pediapred Oral Solution (Prednisolone Sodium Phosphate) Medeva 1618
Prelone Syrup (Prednisolone) Muro 1834

Dermatomyositis, "possibly" effective in
Potaba Capsules, Envules, Powder, and Tablets (Aminobenzoate Potassium) Glenwood-Palisades .. 1234

Dermatomyositis, systemic
Cortone Acetate Sterile Suspension (Cortisone Acetate) Merck & Co., Inc. 1663
Cortone Acetate Tablets (Cortisone Acetate) Merck & Co., Inc. 1664
Hydeltrasol Injection, Sterile (Prednisolone Sodium Phosphate) Merck & Co., Inc. 1708
Hydrocortone Phosphate Injection, Sterile (Hydrocortisone Sodium Phosphate) Merck & Co., Inc. ... 1713
Hydrocortone Tablets (Hydrocortisone) Merck & Co., Inc. 1715
Pediapred Oral Solution (Prednisolone Sodium Phosphate) Medeva 1618
Prelone Syrup (Prednisolone) Muro 1834

Dermatoses, corticosteroid-responsive
(see also under Skin, inflammatory conditions)
Aclovate (Alclometasone Dipropionate) Glaxo Wellcome 1061
Cordran Lotion (Flurandrenolide) Oclassen 1854
Cordran Tape (Flurandrenolide) Oclassen 1855
Cormax Ointment (Clobetasol Propionate) Oclassen 1856
Cormax Scalp Application (Clobetasol Propionate) Oclassen 1857
Cortizone-10 (Hydrocortisone) Thompson Medical 795
Cutivate Cream (Fluticasone Propionate) Glaxo Wellcome 1078
Cutivate Ointment (Fluticasone Propionate) Glaxo Wellcome 1078
Decadron Phosphate Topical Cream (Dexamethasone Sodium Phosphate) Merck & Co., Inc. 1686
Decaspray Topical Aerosol (Dexamethasone) Merck & Co., Inc. 1689
Dermatop Emollient Cream 0.1% (Prednicarbate) Hoechst Marion Roussel 1264
DesOwen Cream, Ointment and Lotion (Desonide) Galderma 1032
Diprolene AF Cream 0.05% (Betamethasone Dipropionate) Schering 2489
Diprolene Gel 0.05% (Betamethasone Dipropionate) Schering 2490
Diprolene Ointment 0.05% (Betamethasone Dipropionate) Schering 2491
Elocon Cream 0.1% (Mometasone Furoate) Schering 2492
Elocon Lotion 0.1% (Mometasone Furoate) Schering 2493
Elocon Ointment 0.1% (Mometasone Furoate) Schering 2494
Epifoam (Hydrocortisone Acetate, Pramoxine Hydrochloride) Schwarz 2543
Florone/Florone E (Diflorasone Diacetate) Dermik 921

(▣ Described in PDR For Nonprescription Drugs)   (⊙ Described in PDR For Ophthalmology)

Dermatoses | Indications Index | 1516

Halog (Halcinonide) Westwood-Squibb 2795
Hytone (Hydrocortisone) Dermik 922
Hytone Ointment 2 ½ % (Hydrocortisone) Dermik 923
Lidex (Fluocinonide) Roche Pharmaceuticals 2299
Locoid Cream, Ointment and Topical Solution (Hydrocortisone Butyrate) Ferndale 994
Nupercainal Hydrocortisone 1% Cream (Hydrocortisone Acetate) Ciba Self-Medication .... ▣ 661
Pandel Cream, 0.1% (Hydrocortisone Buteprate) Savage 2475
Pramosone Cream, Lotion & Ointment (Hydrocortisone Acetate, Pramoxine Hydrochloride) Ferndale 995
Prelone Syrup (Prednisolone) Muro 1834
ProctoCream-HC 2.5% (Hydrocortisone) Schwarz 2552
ProctoFoam-HC (Hydrocortisone Acetate, Pramoxine Hydrochloride) Schwarz 2552
Psorcon Ointment 0.05% (Diflorasone Diacetate) Dermik 923
Synalar (Fluocinolone Acetonide) Roche Pharmaceuticals 2299
Temovate Cream (Clobetasol Propionate) Glaxo Wellcome 1152
Temovate E Emollient (Clobetasol Propionate) Glaxo Wellcome 1154
Temovate Gel (Clobetasol Propionate) Glaxo Wellcome 1153
Temovate Ointment (Clobetasol Propionate) Glaxo Wellcome 1152
Temovate Scalp Application (Clobetasol Propionate) Glaxo Wellcome 1153
Topicort Emollient Cream 0.25% (Desoximetasone) Hoechst Marion Roussel 1289
Topicort Gel 0.05% (Desoximetasone) Hoechst Marion Roussel 1290
Topicort LP Emollient Cream 0.05% (Desoximetasone) Hoechst Marion Roussel 1289
Topicort Ointment 0.25% (Desoximetasone) Hoechst Marion Roussel 1291
Tridesilon Cream 0.05% (Desonide) Bayer Pharmaceutical 609
Tridesilon Ointment 0.05% (Desonide) Bayer Pharmaceutical 610
Ultravate Cream 0.05% (Halobetasol Propionate) Westwood-Squibb 2797
Ultravate Ointment 0.05% (Halobetasol Propionate) Westwood-Squibb 2798
Westcort Cream 0.2% (Hydrocortisone Valerate) Westwood-Squibb 2799
Westcort Ointment 0.2% (Hydrocortisone Valerate) Westwood-Squibb 2800

Dermatoses, steroid-responsive, with secondary infection
Anusol-HC Cream 2.5% (Hydrocortisone) Parke-Davis 1953
Cortisporin Cream (Polymyxin B Sulfate, Neomycin Sulfate, Hydrocortisone Acetate) Glaxo Wellcome 1073
Cortisporin Ointment (Polymyxin B Sulfate, Bacitracin Zinc, Neomycin Sulfate, Hydrocortisone) Glaxo Wellcome 1074
NeoDecadron Topical Cream (Neomycin Sulfate, Dexamethasone Sodium Phosphate) Merck & Co., Inc. 1757

Dermographism
PBZ Tablets (Tripelennamine Hydrochloride) CibaGeneva 863
PBZ-SR Tablets (Tripelennamine Hydrochloride) CibaGeneva 862
Periactin (Cyproheptadine Hydrochloride) Merck & Co., Inc. 1767
Phenergan Suppositories (Promethazine Hydrochloride) Wyeth-Ayerst 2882
Phenergan Syrup (Promethazine Hydrochloride) Wyeth-Ayerst 2881
Phenergan Tablets (Promethazine Hydrochloride) Wyeth-Ayerst 2882

Diabetes insipidus
DDAVP Injection (Desmopressin Acetate) Rhone-Poulenc Rorer Pharmaceuticals 2178
DDAVP (Desmopressin Acetate) Rhone-Poulenc Rorer Pharmaceuticals 2180
DDAVP Tablets (Desmopressin Acetate) Rhone-Poulenc Rorer Pharmaceuticals 2182
Desmopressin Acetate Injection (Desmopressin Acetate) Ferring .. 996
Desmopressin Acetate Rhinal Tube (Desmopressin Acetate) Ferring .. 997

Diabetes mellitus, insulin-dependent
Humalog Injection (Insulin Lispro, Human) Lilly 1488
Humulin 50/50, 100 Units (Insulin, Human Isophane Suspension, Insulin, Human) Lilly 1491
Humulin 70/30, 100 Units (Insulin, Human Regular and Human NPH Mixture) Lilly 1492
Humulin L, 100 Units (Insulin, Human, Zinc Suspension) Lilly 1494
Humulin N, 100 Units (Insulin, Human NPH) Lilly 1495
Humulin R, 100 Units (Insulin, Human Regular) Lilly 1497
Humulin U, 100 Units (Insulin, Human, Zinc Suspension) Lilly 1498
Iletin I (Insulin, Zinc Suspension) Lilly 1501
Lente, 100 Units (Insulin, Zinc Suspension) Lilly 1501
NPH, 100 Units (Insulin, NPH) Lilly 1502
Regular, 100 Units (Insulin, Regular) Lilly 1503
Iletin II (Insulin, Zinc Suspension) Lilly 1504
Pork Lente, 100 Units (Insulin, Zinc Suspension) Lilly 1504
Pork NPH, 100 Units (Insulin, NPH) Lilly 1506
Pork Regular, 100 Units (Insulin, Regular) Lilly 1507
Pork Regular (Concentrated), 500 Units (Insulin, Regular) Lilly 1508
Novolin L Human Insulin 10 ml Vials (Insulin, Human, Zinc Suspension) Novo Nordisk 1846
Novolin N Human Insulin 10 ml Vials (Insulin, Human Isophane Suspension) Novo Nordisk 1846
Novolin N PenFill 1.5 ml Cartridges Durable Insulin Delivery System (Insulin, Human NPH) Novo Nordisk 1849
Novolin N Prefilled Syringe Disposable Insulin Delivery System (Insulin, Human NPH) Novo Nordisk 1850
Novolin 70/30 Human Insulin 10 ml Vials (Insulin, Human Regular and Human NPH Mixture) Novo Nordisk 1845
Novolin 70/30 PenFill 1.5 ml Cartridges Durable Insulin Delivery System (Insulin, Human Regular and Human NPH Mixture) Novo Nordisk 1848
Novolin 70/30 Prefilled Disposable Insulin Delivery System (Insulin, Human Regular and Human NPH Mixture) Novo Nordisk 1850
Novolin R Human Insulin 10 ml Vials (Insulin, Human Regular) Novo Nordisk 1846
Novolin R PenFill 1.5 ml Cartridges Durable Insulin Delivery System (Insulin, Human Regular) Novo Nordisk 1849
Novolin R Prefilled Syringe Disposable Insulin Delivery System (Insulin, Human Regular) Novo Nordisk 1850
Purified Pork Lente Insulin (Insulin, Zinc Suspension) Novo Nordisk 1852
Purified Pork NPH Isophane Insulin (Insulin, NPH) Novo Nordisk 1852
Purified Pork Regular Insulin (Insulin, Regular) Novo Nordisk 1852
Velosulin BR Human Insulin 10 ml Vials (Insulin, Human Regular) Novo Nordisk 1847

Diabetes mellitus, non-insulin-dependent
Amaryl Tablets (Glimepiride) Hoechst Marion Roussel 1241
DiaBeta Tablets (Glyburide) Hoechst Marion Roussel 1265
Diabinese Tablets (Chlorpropamide) Pfizer Inc 2002
Glucophage Tablets (Metformin Hydrochloride) Bristol-Myers Squibb 754
Glucotrol Tablets (Glipizide) Pfizer Inc 2011
Glucotrol XL Extended Release Tablets (Glipizide) Pfizer Inc 2012
Glynase PresTab Tablets (Glyburide) Pharmacia & Upjohn 2091
Micronase Tablets (Glyburide) Pharmacia & Upjohn 2099
Precose (Acarbose) Bayer Pharmaceutical 604

Diabetic nephropathy (see under Nephropathy, diabetic)

Diaper rash (see under Rash, diaper)

Diarrhea associated with vasoactive intestinal peptide tumors
Sandostatin Injection (Octreotide Acetate) Sandoz Pharmaceuticals 2421

Diarrhea, adjunctive therapy in
Imodium A-D Caplets and Liquid (Loperamide Hydrochloride) McNeil Consumer 1561
Kao Lectrolyte (Electrolyte Supplement) Pharmacia & Upjohn 2099
Lomotil (Diphenoxylate Hydrochloride, Atropine Sulfate) Searle 2591
Pedialyte Oral Electrolyte Maintenance Solution (Electrolyte Supplement) Ross 2340
Rehydralyte Oral Electrolyte Rehydration Solution (Electrolyte Supplement) Ross 2344

Diarrhea, bacterial (see under Diarrhea, infectious)

Diarrhea, E. coli-induced
Bactrim (Trimethoprim, Sulfamethoxazole) Roche Pharmaceuticals 2257
Cipro Tablets (Ciprofloxacin Hydrochloride) Bayer Pharmaceutical 584
Septra (Trimethoprim, Sulfamethoxazole) Glaxo Wellcome 1146

Diarrhea, infectious
Cipro Tablets (Ciprofloxacin Hydrochloride) Bayer Pharmaceutical 584
Furoxone (Furazolidone) Roberts 2221

Diarrhea, protozoal (see under Diarrhea, infectious)

Diarrhea, symptomatic relief of
Donnagel Liquid and Donnagel Chewable Tablets (Attapulgite) Wyeth-Ayerst .... ▣ 854
Imodium A-D Caplets and Liquid (Loperamide Hydrochloride) McNeil Consumer 1561
Imodium Capsules (Loperamide Hydrochloride) Janssen 1343
Kaopectate Concentrated Anti-Diarrheal, Peppermint Flavor (Attapulgite) Upjohn .... ▣ 802
Kaopectate Concentrated Anti-Diarrheal, Regular Flavor (Attapulgite) Upjohn .... ▣ 802
Kaopectate Children's Liquid (Attapulgite) Upjohn .... ▣ 802
Kaopectate Maximum Strength Caplets (Attapulgite) Upjohn .... ▣ 802
Maalox Anti-Diarrheal Caplets (Loperamide Hydrochloride) Ciba Self-Medication .... ▣ 658
Motofen Tablets (Atropine Sulfate, Difenoxin Hydrochloride) Carnrick 789
Pepto-Bismol Original Liquid, Original and Cherry Tablets and Easy-To-Swallow Caplets (Bismuth Subsalicylate) Procter & Gamble 2126
Pepto-Bismol Maximum Strength Liquid (Bismuth Subsalicylate) Procter & Gamble 2126
Pepto Diarrhea Control (Loperamide Hydrochloride) Procter & Gamble 2127
Rheaban Maximum Strength Fast Acting Caplets (Attapulgite, Activated) Pfizer Consumer .... ▣ 716

Diarrhea, traveler's
Bactrim (Trimethoprim, Sulfamethoxazole) Roche Pharmaceuticals 2257
Imodium A-D Caplets and Liquid (Loperamide Hydrochloride) McNeil Consumer 1561
Septra (Trimethoprim, Sulfamethoxazole) Glaxo Wellcome 1146

Digestive disorders, symptomatic relief of
Arco-Lase Plus Tablets (Amylase, Cellulase, Lipase, Protease, Hyoscyamine Sulfate, Phenobarbital) Arco 513
Arco-Lase Tablets (Amylase, Lipase, Cellulase, Protease) Arco 513
DDS-Acidophilus (Lactobacillus Acidophilus) UAS Laboratories .. ▣ 800
Kutrase Capsules (Hyoscyamine Sulfate, Phenyltoloxamine Citrate, Amylase, Cellulase, Lipase, Protease) Schwarz 2546
Ku-Zyme Capsules (Amylase, Lipase, Cellulase, Protease) Schwarz 2546

Digestive insufficiencies, symptomatic relief of
Arco-Lase Plus Tablets (Amylase, Cellulase, Lipase, Protease, Hyoscyamine Sulfate, Phenobarbital) Arco 513
Arco-Lase Tablets (Amylase, Lipase, Cellulase, Protease) Arco 513

Digoxin intoxication, life-threatening
Digibind (Digoxin Immune Fab (Ovine)) Glaxo Wellcome 1079

Diphtheria (see under C. diphtheriae infections)

Diphtheroid endocarditis
Vancocin HCl, Vials & ADD-Vantage (Vancomycin Hydrochloride) Lilly 1534

Diplococcus pneumoniae infections (see under S. pneumoniae infections)

Diuresis, induction of in edema due to lupus erythematosus
Cortone Acetate Sterile Suspension (Cortisone Acetate) Merck & Co., Inc. 1663
Cortone Acetate Tablets (Cortisone Acetate) Merck & Co., Inc. 1664
Dalalone D.P. Injectable (Dexamethasone Acetate) Forest 1009
Decadron Elixir (Dexamethasone) Merck & Co., Inc. 1676
Decadron Phosphate Injection (Dexamethasone Sodium Phosphate) Merck & Co., Inc. 1680
Decadron Tablets (Dexamethasone) Merck & Co., Inc. 1678
Decadron-LA Sterile Suspension (Dexamethasone Acetate) Merck & Co., Inc. 1687
Hydeltrasol Injection, Sterile (Prednisolone Sodium Phosphate) Merck & Co., Inc. 1708
Hydrocortone Phosphate Injection, Sterile (Hydrocortisone Sodium Phosphate) Merck & Co., Inc. 1713
Hydrocortone Tablets (Hydrocortisone) Merck & Co., Inc. 1715
Pediapred Oral Solution (Prednisolone Sodium Phosphate) Medeva 1618
Prelone Syrup (Prednisolone) Muro 1834

(▣ Described in PDR For Nonprescription Drugs) (◉ Described in PDR For Ophthalmology)

Diuresis, induction of in nephrotic syndrome
Cortone Acetate Sterile Suspension (Cortisone Acetate) Merck & Co., Inc. 1663
Cortone Acetate Tablets (Cortisone Acetate) Merck & Co., Inc. 1664
Dalalone D.P. Injectable (Dexamethasone Acetate) Forest 1009
Decadron Elixir (Dexamethasone) Merck & Co., Inc. 1676
Decadron Phosphate Injection (Dexamethasone Sodium Phosphate) Merck & Co., Inc. 1680
Decadron Tablets (Dexamethasone) Merck & Co., Inc. 1678
Decadron-LA Sterile Suspension (Dexamethasone Acetate) Merck & Co., Inc. 1687
Hydeltrasol Injection, Sterile (Prednisolone Sodium Phosphate) Merck & Co., Inc. 1708
Hydrocortone Phosphate Injection, Sterile (Hydrocortisone Sodium Phosphate) Merck & Co., Inc. 1713
Hydrocortone Tablets (Hydrocortisone) Merck & Co., Inc. 1715
Pediapred Oral Solution (Prednisolone Sodium Phosphate) Medeva 1618
Prelone Syrup (Prednisolone) Muro 1834

Donovania granulomatis infection
(see under Granuloma inguinale)

Drowsiness, symptomatic relief of
No Doz Maximum Strength Caplets (Caffeine) Bristol-Myers Products 644

Ductus arteriosus, patent, palliative maintenance
Indocin I.V. (Indomethacin Sodium Trihydrate) Merck & Co., Inc. 1727

Dukes' stage C colon cancer
(see under Carcinoma, colon, Dukes' stage C, adjunctive treatment in)

Duodenal ulcers, active, short-term treatment of
Axid Pulvules (Nizatidine) Lilly 1468
Carafate Suspension (Sucralfate) Hoechst Marion Roussel 1250
Carafate Tablets (Sucralfate) Hoechst Marion Roussel 1249
Pepcid Injection (Famotidine) Merck & Co., Inc. 1765
Pepcid (Famotidine) Merck & Co., Inc. 1763
Prevacid Delayed-Release Capsules (Lansoprazole) TAP 2746
Prilosec Delayed-Release Capsules (Omeprazole) Astra Merck 516
Tagamet (Cimetidine Hydrochloride) SmithKline Beecham Pharmaceuticals 2694
Zantac (Ranitidine Hydrochloride) Glaxo Wellcome 1182
Zantac Injection (Ranitidine Hydrochloride) Glaxo Wellcome 1180
Zantac Syrup (Ranitidine Hydrochloride) Glaxo Wellcome 1182

Duodenal ulcers, adjunctive therapy for
Donnatal (Phenobarbital, Belladonna Alkaloids) Robins 2234
Donnatal Extentabs (Phenobarbital, Belladonna Alkaloids) Robins 2234
Donnatal Tablets (Phenobarbital, Belladonna Alkaloids) Robins 2234

Duodenal ulcers, maintenance therapy for
Axid Pulvules (Nizatidine) Lilly 1468
Carafate Tablets (Sucralfate) Hoechst Marion Roussel 1249
Pepcid Injection (Famotidine) Merck & Co., Inc. 1765
Pepcid (Famotidine) Merck & Co., Inc. 1763
Tagamet (Cimetidine Hydrochloride) SmithKline Beecham Pharmaceuticals 2694
Zantac (Ranitidine Hydrochloride) Glaxo Wellcome 1182

Duodenal ulcers, to reduce the risk of recurrence
Prilosec Delayed-Release Capsules (Omeprazole) Astra Merck 516

Dysbetalipoproteinemia
Atromid-S Capsules (Clofibrate) Wyeth-Ayerst 2808

Dysentery, amoebic
(see under Amebiasis, acute intestinal)

Dysmenorrhea, primary
Anaprox/Naprosyn (Naproxen Sodium) Roche Pharmaceuticals .. 2277
Maximum Strength Ascriptin (Aspirin Buffered, Calcium Carbonate) Ciba Self-Medication 650
Extended-Release Bayer 8-Hour Aspirin (Aspirin) Bayer Consumer 616
Cataflam Tablets (Diclofenac Potassium) CibaGeneva 833
EC-Naprosyn Delayed-Release Tablets (Naproxen) Roche Pharmaceuticals 2277
IBU Tablets (Ibuprofen) Knoll Laboratories 1389
Motrin Ibuprofen Suspension, Oral Drops, Chewable Tablets, Caplets (Ibuprofen) McNeil Consumer 1563
Naprelan Tablets (Naproxen Sodium) Wyeth-Ayerst 2861
Anaprox/Naprosyn (Naproxen) Roche Pharmaceuticals 2277
Orudis Capsules (Ketoprofen) Wyeth-Ayerst 2874
Ponstel (Mefenamic Acid) Parke-Davis 1982

Dyspepsia
(see under Digestive disorders, symptomatic relief of)

Dysuria, symptomatic relief of
Urispas Tablets (Flavoxate Hydrochloride) SmithKline Beecham Pharmaceuticals 2710

E

E. cloacae gynecologic infections
Azactam for Injection (Aztreonam) Bristol-Myers Squibb 736
Timentin for Injection (Ticarcillin Disodium, Clavulanate Potassium) SmithKline Beecham Pharmaceuticals 2706

E. coli biliary tract infections
Ancef Injection (Cefazolin Sodium) SmithKline Beecham Pharmaceuticals 2632
Kefzol Vials, Faspak & ADD-Vantage (Cefazolin Sodium) Lilly 1511

E. coli bone and joint infections
Nebcin Vials, Hyporets & ADD-Vantage (Tobramycin Sulfate) Lilly 1518
Rocephin Injectable Vials, ADD-Vantage, Galaxy Container (Ceftriaxone Sodium) Roche Pharmaceuticals 2305

E. coli central nervous system infections
Claforan Sterile and Injection (Cefotaxime Sodium) Hoechst Marion Roussel 1259

E. coli genital infections
Ancef Injection (Cefazolin Sodium) SmithKline Beecham Pharmaceuticals 2632
Mefoxin (Cefoxitin Sodium) Merck & Co., Inc. 1734
Mefoxin Premixed Intravenous Solution (Cefoxitin Sodium) Merck & Co., Inc. 1737
Omnipen for Oral Suspension (Ampicillin) Wyeth-Ayerst 2873

E. coli gynecological infections
Azactam for Injection (Aztreonam) Bristol-Myers Squibb 736
Cefizox for Intramuscular or Intravenous Use (Ceftizoxime Sodium) Fujisawa 1025
Cefobid Intravenous/Intramuscular (Cefoperazone Sodium) Pfizer Inc 1996
Cefobid Pharmacy Bulk Package - Not for Direct Infusion (Cefoperazone Sodium) Pfizer Inc 1999
Cefotan (Cefotetan) Zeneca 2936
Ceptaz (Ceftazidime) Glaxo Wellcome 1070
Claforan Sterile and Injection (Cefotaxime Sodium) Hoechst Marion Roussel 1259
Fortaz (Ceftazidime) Glaxo Wellcome 1092
Mefoxin (Cefoxitin Sodium) Merck & Co., Inc. 1734
Mefoxin Premixed Intravenous Solution (Cefoxitin Sodium) Merck & Co., Inc. 1737
Mezlin (Mezlocillin Sodium) Bayer Pharmaceutical 594
Mezlin Pharmacy Bulk Package (Mezlocillin Sodium) Bayer Pharmaceutical 597
Primaxin I.M. (Cilastatin Sodium, Imipenem) Merck & Co., Inc. 1770
Primaxin I.V. (Cilastatin Sodium, Imipenem) Merck & Co., Inc. 1772
Tazicef for Injection (Ceftazidime) SmithKline Beecham Pharmaceuticals 2697
Tazidime Vials, Faspak & ADD-Vantage (Ceftazidime) Lilly .. 1531
Ticar for Injection (Ticarcillin Disodium) SmithKline Beecham Pharmaceuticals 2704
Timentin for Injection (Ticarcillin Disodium, Clavulanate Potassium) SmithKline Beecham Pharmaceuticals 2706
Unasyn (Ampicillin Sodium, Sulbactam Sodium) Pfizer Inc 2035
Zosyn (Piperacillin Sodium, Tazobactam Sodium) Lederle 1463

E. coli infections
Achromycin V Capsules (Tetracycline Hydrochloride) Lederle 1417
Amikacin Sulfate Injection, USP (Amikacin Sulfate) Astra 523
Amikacin Sulfate Injection, USP (Amikacin Sulfate) Elkins-Sinn 981
Amikin Injectable (Amikacin Sulfate) Apothecon 502
Amoxil (Amoxicillin Trihydrate) SmithKline Beecham Pharmaceuticals 2631
Ancef Injection (Cefazolin Sodium) SmithKline Beecham Pharmaceuticals 2632
Augmentin (Amoxicillin Trihydrate, Clavulanate Potassium) SmithKline Beecham Pharmaceuticals 2637
Augmentin Tablets (Amoxicillin Trihydrate, Clavulanate Potassium) SmithKline Beecham Pharmaceuticals 2640
Azactam for Injection (Aztreonam) Bristol-Myers Squibb 736
Bactrim DS Tablets (Trimethoprim, Sulfamethoxazole) Roche Pharmaceuticals 2257
Bactrim I.V. Infusion (Trimethoprim, Sulfamethoxazole) Roche Pharmaceuticals 2255
Bactrim (Trimethoprim, Sulfamethoxazole) Roche Pharmaceuticals 2257
Ceclor Pulvules & Suspension (Cefaclor) Lilly 1470
Cefizox for Intramuscular or Intravenous Use (Ceftizoxime Sodium) Fujisawa 1025
Cefobid Intravenous/Intramuscular (Cefoperazone Sodium) Pfizer Inc 1996
Cefobid Pharmacy Bulk Package - Not for Direct Infusion (Cefoperazone Sodium) Pfizer Inc 1999
Cefotan (Cefotetan) Zeneca 2936
Ceftin (Cefuroxime Axetil) Glaxo Wellcome 1067
Ceptaz (Ceftazidime) Glaxo Wellcome 1070
Cipro I.V. (Ciprofloxacin) Bayer Pharmaceutical 587
Cipro I.V. Pharmacy Bulk Package (Ciprofloxacin) Bayer Pharmaceutical 590
Cipro Tablets (Ciprofloxacin Hydrochloride) Bayer Pharmaceutical 584
Claforan Sterile and Injection (Cefotaxime Sodium) Hoechst Marion Roussel 1259
Declomycin Tablets (Demeclocycline Hydrochloride) Lederle 1421
Doryx Capsules (Doxycycline Hyclate) Parke-Davis 1970
Duricef Capsules, Tablets, and Oral Suspension (Cefadroxil) Bristol-Myers Squibb 750
DYNACIN Capsules (Minocycline Hydrochloride) Medicis 1627
Floxin I.V. (Ofloxacin) McNeil Pharmaceutical 1580
Floxin Tablets (200 mg, 300 mg, 400 mg) (Ofloxacin) McNeil Pharmaceutical 1577
Fortaz (Ceftazidime) Glaxo Wellcome 1092
Gantanol Tablets (Sulfamethoxazole) Roche Pharmaceuticals 2285
Gantrisin (Acetyl Sulfisoxazole) Roche Pharmaceuticals 2286
Garamycin Injectable (Gentamicin Sulfate) Schering 2502
Geocillin Tablets (Carbenicillin Indanyl Sodium) Pfizer Inc 2009
Keflex Pulvules & Oral Suspension (Cephalexin) Dista 930
Keftab Tablets (Cephalexin Hydrochloride) Dista 931
Kefurox Vials, Faspak & ADD-Vantage (Cefuroxime Sodium) Lilly 1509
Kefzol Vials, Faspak & ADD-Vantage (Cefazolin Sodium) Lilly 1511
Lorabid Suspension and Pulvules (Loracarbef) Lilly 1513
Macrobid Capsules (Nitrofurantoin Monohydrate) Procter & Gamble Pharmaceuticals 2138
Macrodantin Capsules (Nitrofurantoin) Procter & Gamble Pharmaceuticals 2140
Mandol Vials, Faspak & ADD-Vantage (Cefamandole Nafate) Lilly 1516
Maxaquin Tablets (Lomefloxacin Hydrochloride) Searle 2593
Maxipime for Injection (Cefepime Hydrochloride) Bristol-Myers Squibb 758
Mefoxin (Cefoxitin Sodium) Merck & Co., Inc. 1734
Mefoxin Premixed Intravenous Solution (Cefoxitin Sodium) Merck & Co., Inc. 1737
Merrem I.V. (Meropenem) Zeneca .. 2952
Mezlin (Mezlocillin Sodium) Bayer Pharmaceutical 594
Mezlin Pharmacy Bulk Package (Mezlocillin Sodium) Bayer Pharmaceutical 597
Minocin Intravenous (Minocycline Hydrochloride) Lederle 1428
Minocin Oral Suspension (Minocycline Hydrochloride) Lederle 1431
Minocin Pellet-Filled Capsules (Minocycline Hydrochloride) Lederle 1429
Monocid Injection (Cefonicid Sodium) SmithKline Beecham Pharmaceuticals 2674
Monodox Capsules (Doxycycline Monohydrate) Oclassen 1858
Nebcin Vials, Hyporets & ADD-Vantage (Tobramycin Sulfate) Lilly 1518
NegGram (Nalidixic Acid) Sanofi Winthrop 2453
Netromycin Injection 100 mg/ml (Netilmicin Sulfate) Schering 2516
Noroxin Tablets (Norfloxacin) Merck & Co., Inc. 1758
Noroxin Tablets (Norfloxacin) Roberts 2222
Omnipen Capsules (Ampicillin) Wyeth-Ayerst 2872
Omnipen for Oral Suspension (Ampicillin) Wyeth-Ayerst 2873
Penetrex Tablets (Enoxacin) Rhone-Poulenc Rorer Pharmaceuticals 2196
Pfizerpen for Injection (Penicillin G Potassium) Pfizer Inc 2022

Pipracil (Piperacillin Sodium) Lederle ... 1435
Primaxin I.M. (Cilastatin Sodium, Imipenem) Merck & Co., Inc. ... 1770
Primaxin I.V. (Cilastatin Sodium, Imipenem) Merck & Co., Inc. ... 1772
Proloprim Tablets (Trimethoprim) Glaxo Wellcome ... 1141
Rocephin Injectable Vials, ADD-Vantage, Galaxy Container (Ceftriaxone Sodium) Roche Pharmaceuticals ... 2305
Septra (Trimethoprim, Sulfamethoxazole) Glaxo Wellcome ... 1146
Septra I.V. Infusion (Trimethoprim, Sulfamethoxazole) Glaxo Wellcome ... 1142
Septra I.V. Infusion ADD-Vantage Vials (Trimethoprim, Sulfamethoxazole) Glaxo Wellcome ... 1144
Septra (Trimethoprim, Sulfamethoxazole) Glaxo Wellcome ... 1146
Seromycin Capsules (Cycloserine) Dura ... 975
Suprax (Cefixime) Lederle ... 1443
Tazicef for Injection (Ceftazidime) SmithKline Beecham Pharmaceuticals ... 2697
Tazidime Vials, Faspak & ADD-Vantage (Ceftazidime) Lilly ... 1531
Terramycin Intramuscular Solution (Oxytetracycline) Pfizer Inc ... 2034
Ticar for Injection (Ticarcillin Disodium) SmithKline Beecham Pharmaceuticals ... 2704
Timentin for Injection (Ticarcillin Disodium, Clavulanate Potassium) SmithKline Beecham Pharmaceuticals ... 2706
Trimpex Tablets (Trimethoprim) Roche Pharmaceuticals ... 2323
Unasyn (Ampicillin Sodium, Sulbactam Sodium) Pfizer Inc ... 2035
Vantin for Oral Suspension and Vantin Tablets (Cefpodoxime Proxetil) Pharmacia & Upjohn ... 2112
Vibramycin (Doxycycline Calcium) Pfizer Inc ... 2038
Vibramycin Hyclate Intravenous (Doxycycline Hyclate) Pfizer Inc ... 2040
Vibramycin (Doxycycline Monohydrate) Pfizer Inc ... 2038
Zinacef (Cefuroxime Sodium) Glaxo Wellcome ... 1184
Zosyn (Piperacillin Sodium, Tazobactam Sodium) Lederle ... 1463

E. coli infections, ocular

AK-CIDE (Prednisolone Acetate, Sulfacetamide Sodium) Akorn ... ◉ 203
AK-CIDE Ointment (Prednisolone Acetate, Sulfacetamide Sodium) Akorn ... ◉ 203
AK-Spore (Bacitracin Zinc, Neomycin Sulfate, Polymyxin B Sulfate) Akorn ... ◉ 205
AK-Trol Ointment & Suspension (Dexamethasone, Neomycin Sulfate, Polymyxin B Sulfate) Akorn ... ◉ 205
Blephamide Liquifilm Sterile Ophthalmic Suspension (Prednisolone Acetate, Sulfacetamide Sodium) Allergan ... 472
Blephamide Ointment (Sulfacetamide Sodium, Prednisolone Acetate) Allergan ... ◉ 234
Chloromycetin Ophthalmic Ointment, 1% (Chloramphenicol) Parke-Davis ... ◉ 298
Chloromycetin Ophthalmic Solution (Chloramphenicol) Parke-Davis ... ◉ 299
Chloroptic S.O.P. (Chloramphenicol) Allergan ... ◉ 236
Cortisporin Ophthalmic Ointment Sterile (Polymyxin B Sulfate, Bacitracin Zinc, Neomycin Sulfate, Hydrocortisone) Glaxo Wellcome ... 1074
Cortisporin Ophthalmic Suspension Sterile (Hydrocortisone, Polymyxin B Sulfate, Neomycin Sulfate) Glaxo Wellcome ... 1075
FML-S Liquifilm (Sulfacetamide Sodium, Fluorometholone) Allergan ... ◉ 240
Garamycin Ophthalmic (Gentamicin Sulfate) Schering ... 2501
Genoptic Sterile Ophthalmic Solution (Gentamicin Sulfate) Allergan ... ◉ 241
Genoptic Sterile Ophthalmic Ointment (Gentamicin Sulfate) Allergan ... ◉ 241
Gentak (Gentamicin Sulfate) Akorn ... ◉ 209
Maxitrol Ophthalmic Ointment and Suspension (Dexamethasone, Neomycin Sulfate, Polymyxin B Sulfate) Alcon Laboratories ... ◉ 222
NeoDecadron Sterile Ophthalmic Ointment (Neomycin Sulfate, Dexamethasone Sodium Phosphate) Merck & Co., Inc. ... 1755
NeoDecadron Sterile Ophthalmic Solution (Neomycin Sulfate, Dexamethasone Sodium Phosphate) Merck & Co., Inc. ... 1756
Poly-Pred Liquifilm (Neomycin Sulfate, Polymyxin B Sulfate, Prednisolone Acetate) Allergan ... ◉ 246
Pred-G Liquifilm Sterile Ophthalmic Suspension (Gentamicin Sulfate, Prednisolone Acetate) Allergan ... ◉ 248
Pred-G S.O.P. Sterile Ophthalmic Ointment (Gentamicin Sulfate, Prednisolone Acetate) Allergan ... ◉ 249
Terra-Cortril Ophthalmic Suspension (Oxytetracycline Hydrochloride, Hydrocortisone Acetate) Pfizer Inc ... 2033
TobraDex Ophthalmic Suspension and Ointment (Dexamethasone, Tobramycin) Alcon Laboratories ... 469

E. coli intra-abdominal infections

Azactam for Injection (Aztreonam) Bristol-Myers Squibb ... 736
Cefizox for Intramuscular or Intravenous Use (Ceftizoxime Sodium) Fujisawa ... 1025
Cefobid Intravenous/Intramuscular (Cefoperazone Sodium) Pfizer Inc ... 1996
Cefobid Pharmacy Bulk Package - Not for Direct Infusion (Cefoperazone Sodium) Pfizer Inc ... 1999
Cefotan (Cefotetan) Zeneca ... 2936
Ceptaz (Ceftazidime) Glaxo Wellcome ... 1070
Claforan Sterile and Injection (Cefotaxime Sodium) Hoechst Marion Roussel ... 1259
Fortaz (Ceftazidime) Glaxo Wellcome ... 1092
Mefoxin (Cefoxitin Sodium) Merck & Co., Inc. ... 1734
Mefoxin Premixed Intravenous Solution (Cefoxitin Sodium) Merck & Co., Inc. ... 1737
Merrem I.V. (Meropenem) Zeneca ... 2952
Mezlin (Mezlocillin Sodium) Bayer Pharmaceutical ... 594
Mezlin Pharmacy Bulk Package (Mezlocillin Sodium) Bayer Pharmaceutical ... 597
Nebcin Vials, Hyporets & ADD-Vantage (Tobramycin Sulfate) Lilly ... 1518
Netromycin Injection 100 mg/ml (Netilmicin Sulfate) Schering ... 2516
Omnipen for Oral Suspension (Ampicillin) Wyeth-Ayerst ... 2873
Pipracil (Piperacillin Sodium) Lederle ... 1435
Primaxin I.M. (Cilastatin Sodium, Imipenem) Merck & Co., Inc. ... 1770
Primaxin I.V. (Cilastatin Sodium, Imipenem) Merck & Co., Inc. ... 1772
Rocephin Injectable Vials, ADD-Vantage, Galaxy Container (Ceftriaxone Sodium) Roche Pharmaceuticals ... 2305
Tazicef for Injection (Ceftazidime) SmithKline Beecham Pharmaceuticals ... 2697
Tazidime Vials, Faspak & ADD-Vantage (Ceftazidime) Lilly ... 1531
Timentin for Injection (Ticarcillin Disodium, Clavulanate Potassium) SmithKline Beecham Pharmaceuticals ... 2706
Unasyn (Ampicillin Sodium, Sulbactam Sodium) Pfizer Inc ... 2035

E. coli lower respiratory tract infections

Azactam for Injection (Aztreonam) Bristol-Myers Squibb ... 736
Cefizox for Intramuscular or Intravenous Use (Ceftizoxime Sodium) Fujisawa ... 1025
Cefotan (Cefotetan) Zeneca ... 2936
Ceptaz (Ceftazidime) Glaxo Wellcome ... 1070
Cipro I.V. (Ciprofloxacin) Bayer Pharmaceutical ... 587
Cipro I.V. Pharmacy Bulk Package (Ciprofloxacin) Bayer Pharmaceutical ... 590
Cipro Tablets (Ciprofloxacin Hydrochloride) Bayer Pharmaceutical ... 584
Claforan Sterile and Injection (Cefotaxime Sodium) Hoechst Marion Roussel ... 1259
Fortaz (Ceftazidime) Glaxo Wellcome ... 1092
Kefurox Vials, Faspak & ADD-Vantage (Cefuroxime Sodium) Lilly ... 1509
Mefoxin (Cefoxitin Sodium) Merck & Co., Inc. ... 1734
Mefoxin Premixed Intravenous Solution (Cefoxitin Sodium) Merck & Co., Inc. ... 1737
Mezlin (Mezlocillin Sodium) Bayer Pharmaceutical ... 594
Mezlin Pharmacy Bulk Package (Mezlocillin Sodium) Bayer Pharmaceutical ... 597
Monocid Injection (Cefonicid Sodium) SmithKline Beecham Pharmaceuticals ... 2674
Nebcin Vials, Hyporets & ADD-Vantage (Tobramycin Sulfate) Lilly ... 1518
Netromycin Injection 100 mg/ml (Netilmicin Sulfate) Schering ... 2516
Pipracil (Piperacillin Sodium) Lederle ... 1435
Primaxin I.V. (Cilastatin Sodium, Imipenem) Merck & Co., Inc. ... 1772
Rocephin Injectable Vials, ADD-Vantage, Galaxy Container (Ceftriaxone Sodium) Roche Pharmaceuticals ... 2305
Tazicef for Injection (Ceftazidime) SmithKline Beecham Pharmaceuticals ... 2697
Tazidime Vials, Faspak & ADD-Vantage (Ceftazidime) Lilly ... 1531
Zinacef (Cefuroxime Sodium) Glaxo Wellcome ... 1184

E. coli meningitis

Rocephin Injectable Vials, ADD-Vantage, Galaxy Container (Ceftriaxone Sodium) Roche Pharmaceuticals ... 2305

E. coli peritonitis

Cefobid Intravenous/Intramuscular (Cefoperazone Sodium) Pfizer Inc ... 1996
Cefobid Pharmacy Bulk Package - Not for Direct Infusion (Cefoperazone Sodium) Pfizer Inc ... 1999
Ceptaz (Ceftazidime) Glaxo Wellcome ... 1070
Fortaz (Ceftazidime) Glaxo Wellcome ... 1092
Mandol Vials, Faspak & ADD-Vantage (Cefamandole Nafate) Lilly ... 1516
Mefoxin (Cefoxitin Sodium) Merck & Co., Inc. ... 1734
Mefoxin Premixed Intravenous Solution (Cefoxitin Sodium) Merck & Co., Inc. ... 1737
Merrem I.V. (Meropenem) Zeneca ... 2952
Mezlin (Mezlocillin Sodium) Bayer Pharmaceutical ... 594
Mezlin Pharmacy Bulk Package (Mezlocillin Sodium) Bayer Pharmaceutical ... 597
Nebcin Vials, Hyporets & ADD-Vantage (Tobramycin Sulfate) Lilly ... 1518
Netromycin Injection 100 mg/ml (Netilmicin Sulfate) Schering ... 2516
Tazidime Vials, Faspak & ADD-Vantage (Ceftazidime) Lilly ... 1531
Timentin for Injection (Ticarcillin Disodium, Clavulanate Potassium) SmithKline Beecham Pharmaceuticals ... 2706
Zosyn (Piperacillin Sodium, Tazobactam Sodium) Lederle ... 1463

E. coli prostatitis

Ancef Injection (Cefazolin Sodium) SmithKline Beecham Pharmaceuticals ... 2632
Floxin I.V. (Ofloxacin) McNeil Pharmaceutical ... 1580
Floxin Tablets (200 mg, 300 mg, 400 mg) (Ofloxacin) McNeil Pharmaceutical ... 1577
Geocillin Tablets (Carbenicillin Indanyl Sodium) Pfizer Inc ... 2009
Keflex Pulvules & Oral Suspension (Cephalexin) Dista ... 930
Keftab Tablets (Cephalexin Hydrochloride) Dista ... 931
Noroxin Tablets (Norfloxacin) Merck & Co., Inc. ... 1758
Noroxin Tablets (Norfloxacin) Roberts ... 2222

E. coli respiratory tract infections

Cefobid Intravenous/Intramuscular (Cefoperazone Sodium) Pfizer Inc ... 1996
Cefobid Pharmacy Bulk Package - Not for Direct Infusion (Cefoperazone Sodium) Pfizer Inc ... 1999
Ticar for Injection (Ticarcillin Disodium) SmithKline Beecham Pharmaceuticals ... 2704

E. coli septicemia

Ancef Injection (Cefazolin Sodium) SmithKline Beecham Pharmaceuticals ... 2632
Azactam for Injection (Aztreonam) Bristol-Myers Squibb ... 736
Cefizox for Intramuscular or Intravenous Use (Ceftizoxime Sodium) Fujisawa ... 1025
Cefobid Intravenous/Intramuscular (Cefoperazone Sodium) Pfizer Inc ... 1996
Cefobid Pharmacy Bulk Package - Not for Direct Infusion (Cefoperazone Sodium) Pfizer Inc ... 1999
Ceptaz (Ceftazidime) Glaxo Wellcome ... 1070
Cipro I.V. (Ciprofloxacin) Bayer Pharmaceutical ... 587
Claforan Sterile and Injection (Cefotaxime Sodium) Hoechst Marion Roussel ... 1259
Fortaz (Ceftazidime) Glaxo Wellcome ... 1092
Kefurox Vials, Faspak & ADD-Vantage (Cefuroxime Sodium) Lilly ... 1509
Kefzol Vials, Faspak & ADD-Vantage (Cefazolin Sodium) Lilly ... 1511
Mefoxin (Cefoxitin Sodium) Merck & Co., Inc. ... 1734
Mefoxin Premixed Intravenous Solution (Cefoxitin Sodium) Merck & Co., Inc. ... 1737
Mezlin (Mezlocillin Sodium) Bayer Pharmaceutical ... 594
Mezlin Pharmacy Bulk Package (Mezlocillin Sodium) Bayer Pharmaceutical ... 597
Monocid Injection (Cefonicid Sodium) SmithKline Beecham Pharmaceuticals ... 2674
Nebcin Vials, Hyporets & ADD-Vantage (Tobramycin Sulfate) Lilly ... 1518
Netromycin Injection 100 mg/ml (Netilmicin Sulfate) Schering ... 2516
Pfizerpen for Injection (Penicillin G Potassium) Pfizer Inc ... 2022
Primaxin I.V. (Cilastatin Sodium, Imipenem) Merck & Co., Inc. ... 1772
Rocephin Injectable Vials, ADD-Vantage, Galaxy Container (Ceftriaxone Sodium) Roche Pharmaceuticals ... 2305
Tazicef for Injection (Ceftazidime) SmithKline Beecham Pharmaceuticals ... 2697
Tazidime Vials, Faspak & ADD-Vantage (Ceftazidime) Lilly ... 1531
Ticar for Injection (Ticarcillin Disodium) SmithKline Beecham Pharmaceuticals ... 2704
Timentin for Injection (Ticarcillin Disodium, Clavulanate

(▣ Described in PDR For Nonprescription Drugs) (◉ Described in PDR For Ophthalmology)

Indications Index — Edema

Potassium) SmithKline Beecham Pharmaceuticals 2706
Zinacef (Cefuroxime Sodium) Glaxo Wellcome 1184

E. coli skin and skin structure infections
Amoxil (Amoxicillin Trihydrate) SmithKline Beecham Pharmaceuticals 2631
Augmentin (Amoxicillin Trihydrate, Clavulanate Potassium) SmithKline Beecham Pharmaceuticals 2637
Augmentin Tablets (Amoxicillin Trihydrate, Clavulanate Potassium) SmithKline Beecham Pharmaceuticals 2640
Azactam for Injection (Aztreonam) Bristol-Myers Squibb 736
Cefizox for Intramuscular or Intravenous Use (Ceftizoxime Sodium) Fujisawa 1025
Cefotan (Cefotetan) Zeneca 2936
Ceptaz (Ceftazidime) Glaxo Wellcome 1070
Cipro I.V. (Ciprofloxacin) Bayer Pharmaceutical 587
Cipro I.V. Pharmacy Bulk Package (Ciprofloxacin) Bayer Pharmaceutical 590
Cipro Tablets (Ciprofloxacin Hydrochloride) Bayer Pharmaceutical 584
Claforan Sterile and Injection (Cefotaxime Sodium) Hoechst Marion Roussel 1259
Fortaz (Ceftazidime) Glaxo Wellcome 1092
Kefurox Vials, Faspak & ADD-Vantage (Cefuroxime Sodium) Lilly 1509
Mandol Vials, Faspak & ADD-Vantage (Cefamandole Nafate) Lilly 1516
Mefoxin (Cefoxitin Sodium) Merck & Co., Inc. 1734
Mefoxin Premixed Intravenous Solution (Cefoxitin Sodium) Merck & Co., Inc. 1737
Mezlin (Mezlocillin Sodium) Bayer Pharmaceutical 594
Mezlin Pharmacy Bulk Package (Mezlocillin Sodium) Bayer Pharmaceutical 597
Nebcin Vials, Hyporets & ADD-Vantage (Tobramycin Sulfate) Lilly 1518
Netromycin Injection 100 mg/ml (Netilmicin Sulfate) Schering 2516
Pipracil (Piperacillin Sodium) Lederle 1435
Primaxin I.M. (Cilastatin Sodium, Imipenem) Merck & Co., Inc. 1770
Primaxin I.V. (Cilastatin Sodium, Imipenem) Merck & Co., Inc. 1772
Rocephin Injectable Vials, ADD-Vantage, Galaxy Container (Ceftriaxone Sodium) Roche Pharmaceuticals 2305
Tazicef for Injection (Ceftazidime) SmithKline Beecham Pharmaceuticals 2697
Tazidime Vials, Faspak & ADD-Vantage (Ceftazidime) Lilly .. 1531
Ticar for Injection (Ticarcillin Disodium) SmithKline Beecham Pharmaceuticals 2704
Timentin for Injection (Ticarcillin Disodium, Clavulanate Potassium) SmithKline Beecham Pharmaceuticals 2706
Unasyn (Ampicillin Sodium, Sulbactam Sodium) Pfizer Inc 2035
Zinacef (Cefuroxime Sodium) Glaxo Wellcome 1184

E. coli urinary tract infections
Ancef Injection (Cefazolin Sodium) SmithKline Beecham Pharmaceuticals 2632
Augmentin (Amoxicillin Trihydrate, Clavulanate Potassium) SmithKline Beecham Pharmaceuticals 2637
Augmentin Tablets (Amoxicillin Trihydrate, Clavulanate Potassium) SmithKline Beecham Pharmaceuticals 2640
Azactam for Injection (Aztreonam) Bristol-Myers Squibb 736

Bactrim DS Tablets (Trimethoprim, Sulfamethoxazole) Roche Pharmaceuticals 2257
Bactrim I.V. Infusion (Trimethoprim, Sulfamethoxazole) Roche Pharmaceuticals 2255
Bactrim (Trimethoprim, Sulfamethoxazole) Roche Pharmaceuticals 2257
Ceclor Pulvules & Suspension (Cefaclor) Lilly 1470
Cefizox for Intramuscular or Intravenous Use (Ceftizoxime Sodium) Fujisawa 1025
Cefobid Intravenous/Intramuscular (Cefoperazone Sodium) Pfizer Inc 1996
Cefobid Pharmacy Bulk Package - Not for Direct Infusion (Cefoperazone Sodium) Pfizer Inc 1999
Cefotan (Cefotetan) Zeneca 2936
Ceftin (Cefuroxime Axetil) Glaxo Wellcome 1067
Ceptaz (Ceftazidime) Glaxo Wellcome 1070
Cipro I.V. (Ciprofloxacin) Bayer Pharmaceutical 587
Cipro I.V. Pharmacy Bulk Package (Ciprofloxacin) Bayer Pharmaceutical 590
Cipro Tablets (Ciprofloxacin Hydrochloride) Bayer Pharmaceutical 584
Claforan Sterile and Injection (Cefotaxime Sodium) Hoechst Marion Roussel 1259
Duricef Capsules, Tablets, and Oral Suspension (Cefadroxil) Bristol-Myers Squibb 750
Floxin I.V. (Ofloxacin) McNeil Pharmaceutical 1580
Floxin Tablets (200 mg, 300 mg, 400 mg) (Ofloxacin) McNeil Pharmaceutical 1577
Fortaz (Ceftazidime) Glaxo Wellcome 1092
Gantanol Tablets (Sulfamethoxazole) Roche Pharmaceuticals 2285
Gantrisin (Acetyl Sulfisoxazole) Roche Pharmaceuticals 2286
Geocillin Tablets (Carbenicillin Indanyl Sodium) Pfizer Inc 2009
Keflex Pulvules & Oral Suspension (Cephalexin) Dista 930
Keftab Tablets (Cephalexin Hydrochloride) Dista 931
Kefurox Vials, Faspak & ADD-Vantage (Cefuroxime Sodium) Lilly 1509
Kefzol Vials, Faspak & ADD-Vantage (Cefazolin Sodium) Lilly 1511
Lorabid Suspension and Pulvules (Loracarbef) Lilly 1513
Macrobid Capsules (Nitrofurantoin Monohydrate) Procter & Gamble Pharmaceuticals 2138
Macrodantin Capsules (Nitrofurantoin) Procter & Gamble Pharmaceuticals 2140
Mandol Vials, Faspak & ADD-Vantage (Cefamandole Nafate) Lilly 1516
Maxaquin Tablets (Lomefloxacin Hydrochloride) Searle 2593
Maxipime for Injection (Cefepime Hydrochloride) Bristol-Myers Squibb 758
Mefoxin (Cefoxitin Sodium) Merck & Co., Inc. 1734
Mefoxin Premixed Intravenous Solution (Cefoxitin Sodium) Merck & Co., Inc. 1737
Mezlin (Mezlocillin Sodium) Bayer Pharmaceutical 594
Mezlin Pharmacy Bulk Package (Mezlocillin Sodium) Bayer Pharmaceutical 597
Monocid Injection (Cefonicid Sodium) SmithKline Beecham Pharmaceuticals 2674
Nebcin Vials, Hyporets & ADD-Vantage (Tobramycin Sulfate) Lilly 1518
NegGram (Nalidixic Acid) Sanofi Winthrop 2453
Netromycin Injection 100 mg/ml (Netilmicin Sulfate) Schering 2516
Noroxin Tablets (Norfloxacin) Merck & Co., Inc. 1758

Noroxin Tablets (Norfloxacin) Roberts 2222
Omnipen for Oral Suspension (Ampicillin) Wyeth-Ayerst 2873
Penetrex Tablets (Enoxacin) Rhone-Poulenc Rorer Pharmaceuticals 2196
Pipracil (Piperacillin Sodium) Lederle 1435
Primaxin I.V. (Cilastatin Sodium, Imipenem) Merck & Co., Inc. 1772
Proloprim Tablets (Trimethoprim) Glaxo Wellcome 1141
Rocephin Injectable Vials, ADD-Vantage, Galaxy Container (Ceftriaxone Sodium) Roche Pharmaceuticals 2305
Septra (Trimethoprim, Sulfamethoxazole) Glaxo Wellcome 1146
Septra I.V. Infusion (Trimethoprim, Sulfamethoxazole) Glaxo Wellcome 1142
Septra I.V. Infusion ADD-Vantage Vials (Trimethoprim, Sulfamethoxazole) Glaxo Wellcome 1144
Septra (Trimethoprim, Sulfamethoxazole) Glaxo Wellcome 1146
Seromycin Capsules (Cycloserine) Dura 975
Spectrobid Tablets (Bacampicillin Hydrochloride) Pfizer Inc 2030
Streptomycin Sulfate Injection (Streptomycin Sulfate) Pfizer Inc .. 2031
Suprax (Cefixime) Lederle 1443
Tazicef for Injection (Ceftazidime) SmithKline Beecham Pharmaceuticals 2697
Tazidime Vials, Faspak & ADD-Vantage (Ceftazidime) Lilly .. 1531
Ticar for Injection (Ticarcillin Disodium) SmithKline Beecham Pharmaceuticals 2704
Timentin for Injection (Ticarcillin Disodium, Clavulanate Potassium) SmithKline Beecham Pharmaceuticals 2706
Trimpex Tablets (Trimethoprim) Roche Pharmaceuticals 2323
Vantin for Oral Suspension and Vantin Tablets (Cefpodoxime Proxetil) Pharmacia & Upjohn .. 2112
Zinacef (Cefuroxime Sodium) Glaxo Wellcome 1184

E. coli-induced diarrhea
(see under Diarrhea, E. coli-induced)

Ear wax removal
(see under Cerumen, removal of)

Ear, infection
(see under Otitis externa; Otitis media, acute)

Ears, surgical procedures, irrigation of
AMO Endosol (Balanced Salt Solution) (Balanced Salt Solution) Allergan .... ⊚ 229

Echinococcus granulosus infections
Albenza Tablets (Albendazole) SmithKline Beecham Pharmaceuticals 2629

Ecthyma
Garamycin 0.1% (Gentamicin Sulfate) Schering 2501

Eczema, allergic
Mantadil Cream (Chlorcyclizine Hydrochloride) Glaxo Wellcome .. 1124

Eczema, nuchal
Mantadil Cream (Chlorcyclizine Hydrochloride) Glaxo Wellcome 1124

Eczema, nummular
Mantadil Cream (Chlorcyclizine Hydrochloride) Glaxo Wellcome 1124

Eczema, unspecified
(see under Skin, inflammatory conditions)

Eczemas, aid in evaluation of
T.R.U.E. Test (Allergens) Glaxo Wellcome 1162

Edema due to hyperaldosteronism, secondary
Dyrenium Capsules (Triamterene) SmithKline Beecham Pharmaceuticals 2655

Edema due to pathological causes in pregnancy
Aldactazide Tablets (Spironolactone, Hydrochlorothiazide) Searle 2556
Aldactone Tablets (Spironolactone) Searle 2558
Diucardin Tablets (Hydroflumethiazide) Wyeth-Ayerst 2824
Diuril Oral Suspension (Chlorothiazide) Merck & Co., Inc. 1694
Diuril Sodium Intravenous (Chlorothiazide Sodium) Merck & Co., Inc. 1693
Diuril Tablets (Chlorothiazide) Merck & Co., Inc. 1694
Dyazide Capsules (Triamterene, Hydrochlorothiazide) SmithKline Beecham Pharmaceuticals 2653
Dyrenium Capsules (Triamterene) SmithKline Beecham Pharmaceuticals 2655
HydroDIURIL Tablets (Hydrochlorothiazide) Merck & Co., Inc. 1716
Zaroxolyn Tablets (Metolazone) Medeva 1625

Edema, acute glomerulonephritis-induced
Diuril Oral Suspension (Chlorothiazide) Merck & Co., Inc. 1694
Diuril Sodium Intravenous (Chlorothiazide Sodium) Merck & Co., Inc. 1693
Diuril Tablets (Chlorothiazide) Merck & Co., Inc. 1694
Enduron Tablets (Methyclothiazide) Abbott 424
HydroDIURIL Tablets (Hydrochlorothiazide) Merck & Co., Inc. 1716
Oretic Tablets (Hydrochlorothiazide) Abbott 450
Thalitone (Chlorthalidone) Horus 1293

Edema, acute pulmonary
Edecrin Sodium Intravenous (Ethacrynate Sodium) Merck & Co., Inc. 1698

Edema, adjunctive therapy in
Diucardin Tablets (Hydroflumethiazide) Wyeth-Ayerst 2824
Enduron Tablets (Methyclothiazide) Abbott 424
Esidrix Tablets (Hydrochlorothiazide) CibaGeneva 839
Oretic Tablets (Hydrochlorothiazide) Abbott 450

Edema, cerebral
Decadron Phosphate Injection (Dexamethasone Sodium Phosphate) Merck & Co., Inc. .. 1680
Decadron Tablets (Dexamethasone) Merck & Co., Inc. 1678

Edema, chronic renal failure-induced
Bumex (Bumetanide) Roche Pharmaceuticals 2260
Demadex Tablets and Injection (Torsemide) Boehringer Mannheim 691
Diuril Oral (Chlorothiazide) Merck & Co., Inc. 1694
Enduron Tablets (Methyclothiazide) Abbott 424
HydroDIURIL Tablets (Hydrochlorothiazide) Merck & Co., Inc. 1716
Lasix Injection, Oral Solution and Tablets (Furosemide) Hoechst Marion Roussel 1267
Oretic Tablets (Hydrochlorothiazide) Abbott 450
Thalitone (Chlorthalidone) Horus 1293

(▨ Described in PDR For Nonprescription Drugs)   (⊚ Described in PDR For Ophthalmology)

Edema   Indications Index   1520

Edema, cirrhosis of the liver-induced, treatment of
- Aldactazide Tablets (Spironolactone, Hydrochlorothiazide) Searle ... 2556
- Aldactone Tablets (Spironolactone) Searle ... 2558
- Dyrenium Capsules (Triamterene) SmithKline Beecham Pharmaceuticals ... 2655
- Edecrin (Ethacrynate Sodium) Merck & Co., Inc. ... 1698
- Lasix Injection, Oral Solution and Tablets (Furosemide) Hoechst Marion Roussel ... 1267

Edema, congenital heart disease-induced, short-term management of
- Edecrin (Ethacrynate Sodium) Merck & Co., Inc. ... 1698

Edema, congestive heart failure-induced, adjunctive therapy in (see also under Congestive heart failure; Congestive heart failure, adjunct in)
- Aldactazide Tablets (Spironolactone, Hydrochlorothiazide) Searle ... 2556
- Aldactone Tablets (Spironolactone) Searle ... 2558
- Diamox (Acetazolamide Sodium) Storz Ophthalmics ... ⓞ 317
- Diucardin Tablets (Hydroflumethiazide) Wyeth-Ayerst ... 2824
- Diuril Oral Suspension (Chlorothiazide) Merck & Co., Inc. ... 1694
- Diuril Sodium Intravenous (Chlorothiazide Sodium) Merck & Co., Inc. ... 1693
- Diuril Tablets (Chlorothiazide) Merck & Co., Inc. ... 1694
- Enduron Tablets (Methyclothiazide) Abbott ... 424
- HydroDIURIL Tablets (Hydrochlorothiazide) Merck & Co., Inc. ... 1716
- Oretic Tablets (Hydrochlorothiazide) Abbott ... 450
- Thalitone (Chlorthalidone) Horus ... 1293

Edema, congestive heart failure-induced, treatment of (see also under Congestive heart failure; Congestive heart failure, adjunct in)
- Aldactazide Tablets (Spironolactone, Hydrochlorothiazide) Searle ... 2556
- Aldactone Tablets (Spironolactone) Searle ... 2558
- Bumex (Bumetanide) Roche Pharmaceuticals ... 2260
- Demadex Tablets and Injection (Torsemide) Boehringer Mannheim ... 691
- Dyrenium Capsules (Triamterene) SmithKline Beecham Pharmaceuticals ... 2655
- Edecrin (Ethacrynate Sodium) Merck & Co., Inc. ... 1698
- Lasix Injection, Oral Solution and Tablets (Furosemide) Hoechst Marion Roussel ... 1267
- Zaroxolyn Tablets (Metolazone) Medeva ... 1625

Edema, corneal, temporary relief of
- Muro 128 Ophthalmic Ointment (Sodium Chloride) Bausch & Lomb Pharmaceuticals ... ⓞ 256
- Muro 128 Solution 2% and 5% (Sodium Chloride) Bausch & Lomb Pharmaceuticals ... ⓞ 255
- Ophthalgan (Glycerin) Storz Ophthalmics ... ⓞ 323

Edema, corticosteroid therapy-induced, adjunctive therapy in
- Diucardin Tablets (Hydroflumethiazide) Wyeth-Ayerst ... 2824
- Diuril Oral Suspension (Chlorothiazide) Merck & Co., Inc. ... 1694
- Diuril Sodium Intravenous (Chlorothiazide Sodium) Merck & Co., Inc. ... 1693
- Diuril Tablets (Chlorothiazide) Merck & Co., Inc. ... 1694
- Enduron Tablets (Methyclothiazide) Abbott ... 424
- HydroDIURIL Tablets (Hydrochlorothiazide) Merck & Co., Inc. ... 1716
- Oretic Tablets (Hydrochlorothiazide) Abbott ... 450
- Thalitone (Chlorthalidone) Horus ... 1293

Edema, drug-induced
- Diamox (Acetazolamide Sodium) Storz Ophthalmics ... ⓞ 317

Edema, estrogen therapy-induced, adjunctive therapy in
- Diucardin Tablets (Hydroflumethiazide) Wyeth-Ayerst ... 2824
- Diuril Oral Suspension (Chlorothiazide) Merck & Co., Inc. ... 1694
- Diuril Sodium Intravenous (Chlorothiazide Sodium) Merck & Co., Inc. ... 1693
- Diuril Tablets (Chlorothiazide) Merck & Co., Inc. ... 1694
- Enduron Tablets (Methyclothiazide) Abbott ... 424
- HydroDIURIL Tablets (Hydrochlorothiazide) Merck & Co., Inc. ... 1716
- Oretic Tablets (Hydrochlorothiazide) Abbott ... 450
- Thalitone (Chlorthalidone) Horus ... 1293

Edema, hepatic cirrhosis-induced, adjunctive therapy in
- Bumex (Bumetanide) Roche Pharmaceuticals ... 2260
- Demadex Tablets and Injection (Torsemide) Boehringer Mannheim ... 691
- Diucardin Tablets (Hydroflumethiazide) Wyeth-Ayerst ... 2824
- Diuril Oral Suspension (Chlorothiazide) Merck & Co., Inc. ... 1694
- Diuril Sodium Intravenous (Chlorothiazide Sodium) Merck & Co., Inc. ... 1693
- Diuril Tablets (Chlorothiazide) Merck & Co., Inc. ... 1694
- Enduron Tablets (Methyclothiazide) Abbott ... 424
- HydroDIURIL Tablets (Hydrochlorothiazide) Merck & Co., Inc. ... 1716
- Oretic Tablets (Hydrochlorothiazide) Abbott ... 450
- Thalitone (Chlorthalidone) Horus ... 1293

Edema, idiopathic
- Dyrenium Capsules (Triamterene) SmithKline Beecham Pharmaceuticals ... 2655

Edema, idiopathic, ascites-induced
- Edecrin (Ethacrynate Sodium) Merck & Co., Inc. ... 1698

Edema, nephrotic syndrome-induced, treatment of
- Aldactazide Tablets (Spironolactone, Hydrochlorothiazide) Searle ... 2556
- Aldactone Tablets (Spironolactone) Searle ... 2558
- Bumex (Bumetanide) Roche Pharmaceuticals ... 2260
- Celestone Soluspan Suspension (Betamethasone Sodium Phosphate, Betamethasone Acetate) Schering ... 2484
- Demadex Tablets and Injection (Torsemide) Boehringer Mannheim ... 691
- Diuril Oral Suspension (Chlorothiazide) Merck & Co., Inc. ... 1694
- Diuril Sodium Intravenous (Chlorothiazide Sodium) Merck & Co., Inc. ... 1693
- Diuril Tablets (Chlorothiazide) Merck & Co., Inc. ... 1694
- Dyrenium Capsules (Triamterene) SmithKline Beecham Pharmaceuticals ... 2655
- Edecrin (Ethacrynate Sodium) Merck & Co., Inc. ... 1698
- Enduron Tablets (Methyclothiazide) Abbott ... 424
- HydroDIURIL Tablets (Hydrochlorothiazide) Merck & Co., Inc. ... 1716
- Lasix Injection, Oral Solution and Tablets (Furosemide) Hoechst Marion Roussel ... 1267
- Oretic Tablets (Hydrochlorothiazide) Abbott ... 450
- Thalitone (Chlorthalidone) Horus ... 1293
- Zaroxolyn Tablets (Metolazone) Medeva ... 1625

Edema, pulmonary, emergency treatment of
- Lasix Injection, Oral Solution and Tablets (Furosemide) Hoechst Marion Roussel ... 1267

Electrolytes, depletion of
- Kao Lectrolyte (Electrolyte Supplement) Pharmacia & Upjohn ... 2099
- Pedialyte Oral Electrolyte Maintenance Solution (Electrolyte Supplement) Ross ... 2340
- Rehydralyte Oral Electrolyte Rehydration Solution (Electrolyte Supplement) Ross ... 2344

Embolism, atrial fibrillation with (see under Atrial fibrillation with embolism)

Embolism, peripheral arterial
- Heparin Sodium Injection (Heparin Sodium) Wyeth-Ayerst ... 2832
- Heparin Sodium Vials (Heparin Sodium) Lilly ... 1486

Embolism, pulmonary
- Activase (Alteplase, Recombinant) Genentech ... 1045
- Coumadin (Warfarin Sodium) DuPont ... 941
- Heparin Sodium Vials (Heparin Sodium) Lilly ... 1486

Embolism, pulmonary, acute, lysis of
- Abbokinase (Urokinase) Abbott ... 403
- Activase (Alteplase, Recombinant) Genentech ... 1045
- Streptase for Infusion (Streptokinase) Astra ... 557

Embolism, pulmonary, postoperative
- Heparin Sodium Injection (Heparin Sodium) Wyeth-Ayerst ... 2832
- Lovenox Injection (Enoxaparin) Rhone-Poulenc Rorer Pharmaceuticals ... 2187

Embolism, pulmonary, prophylaxis of
- Coumadin (Warfarin Sodium) DuPont ... 941
- Heparin Sodium Vials (Heparin Sodium) Lilly ... 1486

Embolism, systemic, post-myocardial infarction, prophylaxis
- Coumadin (Warfarin Sodium) DuPont ... 941

Emphysema
- Atrovent Inhalation Aerosol (Ipratropium Bromide) Boehringer Ingelheim ... 674
- Brethine Ampuls (Terbutaline Sulfate) CibaGeneva ... 832
- Brethine Tablets (Terbutaline Sulfate) CibaGeneva ... 831
- Bricanyl Subcutaneous Injection (Terbutaline Sulfate) Hoechst Marion Roussel ... 1247
- Bricanyl Tablets (Terbutaline Sulfate) Hoechst Marion Roussel ... 1248
- Bronkometer Aerosol (Isoetharine) Sanofi Winthrop ... 2432
- Bronkosol Solution (Isoetharine) Sanofi Winthrop ... 2432
- Pima Syrup (Potassium Iodide) Fleming ... 1004
- Quadrinal Tablets (Ephedrine Hydrochloride, Phenobarbital, Potassium Iodide, Theophylline Calcium Salicylate) Knoll Laboratories ... 1398
- Respbid Tablets (Theophylline Anhydrous) Boehringer Ingelheim ... 687
- SSKI Solution (Potassium Iodide) Upsher-Smith ... 2767
- Slo-bid Gyrocaps (Theophylline Anhydrous) Rhone-Poulenc Rorer Pharmaceuticals ... 2201
- Uniphyl 400 mg and 600 mg Tablets (Theophylline Anhydrous) Purdue Frederick ... 2157

Emphysema, panacinar, due to congenital Alpha1-antitrypsin deficiency
- Prolastin Alpha$_1$-Proteinase Inhibitor (Human) (Alpha$_1$-Proteinase Inhibitor (Human)) Bayer Biological ... 629

Empyema
- Cleocin Phosphate Injection (Clindamycin Phosphate) Pharmacia & Upjohn ... 2068
- Flagyl 375 Capsules (Metronidazole) Searle ... 2587
- Flagyl I.V. (Metronidazole Hydrochloride) SCS ... 2373
- Pfizerpen for Injection (Penicillin G Potassium) Pfizer Inc ... 2022
- Ticar for Injection (Ticarcillin Disodium) SmithKline Beecham Pharmaceuticals ... 2704

Endocarditis, bacterial
- Ancef Injection (Cefazolin Sodium) SmithKline Beecham Pharmaceuticals ... 2632
- Flagyl 375 Capsules (Metronidazole) Searle ... 2587
- Flagyl I.V. (Metronidazole Hydrochloride) SCS ... 2373
- Garamycin Injectable (Gentamicin Sulfate) Schering ... 2502
- Kefzol Vials, Faspak & ADD-Vantage (Cefazolin Sodium) Lilly ... 1511
- Pfizerpen for Injection (Penicillin G Potassium) Pfizer Inc ... 2022
- Primaxin I.V. (Cilastatin Sodium, Imipenem) Merck & Co., Inc. ... 1772
- Vancocin HCl, Vials & ADD-Vantage (Vancomycin Hydrochloride) Lilly ... 1534

Endocarditis, bacterial, prophylaxis
- E.E.S. (Erythromycin Ethylsuccinate) Abbott ... 427
- E-Mycin Tablets (Erythromycin) Knoll Laboratories ... 1388
- ERYC (Erythromycin) Parke-Davis ... 1972
- EryPed (Erythromycin Ethylsuccinate) Abbott ... 425
- Ery-Tab Tablets (Erythromycin) Abbott ... 426
- Erythrocin Stearate Filmtab (Erythromycin Stearate) Abbott ... 429
- Erythromycin Base Filmtab (Erythromycin) Abbott ... 430
- Erythromycin Delayed-Release Capsules, USP (Erythromycin) Abbott ... 431
- Ilosone (Erythromycin Estolate) Dista ... 927
- PCE Dispertab Tablets (Erythromycin) Abbott ... 453
- Pfizerpen for Injection (Penicillin G Potassium) Pfizer Inc ... 2022
- Vancocin HCl, Vials & ADD-Vantage (Vancomycin Hydrochloride) Lilly ... 1534

Endocarditis, erysipeloid
- Pfizerpen for Injection (Penicillin G Potassium) Pfizer Inc ... 2022

Endocarditis, fungal
- Ancobon Capsules (Flucytosine) Roche Pharmaceuticals ... 2254

Endocarditis, gonorrheal
- Pfizerpen for Injection (Penicillin G Potassium) Pfizer Inc ... 2022

Endocrine adenomas, multiple (see also under Hypersecretory conditions, pathological)
- Pepcid Injection (Famotidine) Merck & Co., Inc. ... 1765
- Pepcid (Famotidine) Merck & Co., Inc. ... 1763
- Prilosec Delayed-Release Capsules (Omeprazole) Astra Merck ... 516

(⊞ Described in PDR For Nonprescription Drugs)   (ⓞ Described in PDR For Ophthalmology)

Indications Index — Enterobacter species

Tagamet (Cimetidine Hydrochloride) SmithKline Beecham Pharmaceuticals ... 2694

Endocrine disorders
Celestone Soluspan Suspension (Betamethasone Sodium Phosphate, Betamethasone Acetate) Schering ... 2484
Cortone Acetate Sterile Suspension (Cortisone Acetate) Merck & Co., Inc. ... 1663
Cortone Acetate Tablets (Cortisone Acetate) Merck & Co., Inc. ... 1664
Dalalone D.P. Injectable (Dexamethasone Acetate) Forest ... 1009
Decadron Elixir (Dexamethasone) Merck & Co., Inc. ... 1676
Decadron Phosphate Injection (Dexamethasone Sodium Phosphate) Merck & Co., Inc. ... 1680
Decadron Tablets (Dexamethasone) Merck & Co., Inc. ... 1678
Decadron-LA Sterile Suspension (Dexamethasone Acetate) Merck & Co., Inc. ... 1687
Hydeltrasol Injection, Sterile (Prednisolone Sodium Phosphate) Merck & Co., Inc. ... 1708
Hydrocortone Phosphate Injection, Sterile (Hydrocortisone Sodium Phosphate) Merck & Co., Inc. ... 1713
Hydrocortone Tablets (Hydrocortisone) Merck & Co., Inc. ... 1715
Pediapred Oral Solution (Prednisolone Sodium Phosphate) Medeva ... 1618
Prelone Syrup (Prednisolone) Muro ... 1834

Endometriosis
Aygestin Tablets (Norethindrone Acetate) ESI Lederle ... 990
Danocrine Capsules (Danazol) Sanofi Winthrop ... 2437
Lupron Depot 3.75 mg (Leuprolide Acetate) TAP ... 2739
Synarel Nasal Solution for Endometriosis (Nafarelin Acetate) Searle ... 2605
Zoladex (Goserelin Acetate) Zeneca 2976

Endometritis
(see also under Infections, gynecologic)
Azactam for Injection (Aztreonam) Bristol-Myers Squibb ... 736
Cefobid Intravenous/Intramuscular (Cefoperazone Sodium) Pfizer Inc ... 1996
Cefobid Pharmacy Bulk Package - Not for Direct Infusion (Cefoperazone Sodium) Pfizer Inc ... 1999
Ceptaz (Ceftazidime) Glaxo Wellcome ... 1070
Claforan Sterile and Injection (Cefotaxime Sodium) Hoechst Marion Roussel ... 1259
Cleocin Phosphate Injection (Clindamycin Phosphate) Pharmacia & Upjohn ... 2068
Flagyl 375 Capsules (Metronidazole) Searle ... 2587
Flagyl I.V. (Metronidazole Hydrochloride) SCS ... 2373
Fortaz (Ceftazidime) Glaxo Wellcome ... 1092
Mefoxin (Cefoxitin Sodium) Merck & Co., Inc. ... 1734
Mefoxin Premixed Intravenous Solution (Cefoxitin Sodium) Merck & Co., Inc. ... 1737
Mezlin (Mezlocillin Sodium) Bayer Pharmaceutical ... 594
Mezlin Pharmacy Bulk Package (Mezlocillin Sodium) Bayer Pharmaceutical ... 597
Pipracil (Piperacillin Sodium) Lederle ... 1435
Protostat Tablets (Metronidazole) Ortho Pharmaceutical ... 1939
Tazicef for Injection (Ceftazidime) SmithKline Beecham Pharmaceuticals ... 2697
Tazidime Vials, Faspak & ADD-Vantage (Ceftazidime) Lilly .. 1531
Ticar for Injection (Ticarcillin Disodium) SmithKline Beecham Pharmaceuticals ... 2704
Timentin for Injection (Ticarcillin Disodium, Clavulanate Potassium) SmithKline Beecham Pharmaceuticals ... 2706

Endometrial cancer
(see under Carcinoma, endometrium, palliative treatment of)

Endomyometritis
Flagyl 375 Capsules (Metronidazole) Searle ... 2587
Flagyl I.V. (Metronidazole Hydrochloride) SCS ... 2373
Primaxin I.M. (Cilastatin Sodium, Imipenem) Merck & Co., Inc. ... 1770
Protostat Tablets (Metronidazole) Ortho Pharmaceutical ... 1939

Entamoeba histolytica
(see under Amebiasis, acute intestinal)

Enteritis
Furoxone (Furazolidone) Roberts ... 2221
Septra (Trimethoprim, Sulfamethoxazole) Glaxo Wellcome ... 1146
Septra I.V. Infusion (Trimethoprim, Sulfamethoxazole) Glaxo Wellcome ... 1142
Septra I.V. Infusion ADD-Vantage Vials (Trimethoprim, Sulfamethoxazole) Glaxo Wellcome ... 1144
Septra (Trimethoprim, Sulfamethoxazole) Glaxo Wellcome ... 1146

Enteritis, regional, systemic therapy for
Celestone Soluspan Suspension (Betamethasone Sodium Phosphate, Betamethasone Acetate) Schering ... 2484
Cortone Acetate Sterile Suspension (Cortisone Acetate) Merck & Co., Inc. ... 1663
Cortone Acetate Tablets (Cortisone Acetate) Merck & Co., Inc. ... 1664
Dalalone D.P. Injectable (Dexamethasone Acetate) Forest ... 1009
Decadron Elixir (Dexamethasone) Merck & Co., Inc. ... 1676
Decadron Phosphate Injection (Dexamethasone Sodium Phosphate) Merck & Co., Inc. ... 1680
Decadron Tablets (Dexamethasone) Merck & Co., Inc. ... 1678
Decadron-LA Sterile Suspension (Dexamethasone Acetate) Merck & Co., Inc. ... 1687
Hydeltrasol Injection, Sterile (Prednisolone Sodium Phosphate) Merck & Co., Inc. ... 1708
Hydrocortone Phosphate Injection, Sterile (Hydrocortisone Sodium Phosphate) Merck & Co., Inc. ... 1713
Hydrocortone Tablets (Hydrocortisone) Merck & Co., Inc. ... 1715
Pediapred Oral Solution (Prednisolone Sodium Phosphate) Medeva ... 1618
Prelone Syrup (Prednisolone) Muro ... 1834

Enterobacter aerogenes infections
Achromycin V Capsules (Tetracycline Hydrochloride) Lederle ... 1417
Declomycin Tablets (Demeclocycline Hydrochloride) Lederle ... 1421
Doryx Capsules (Doxycycline Hyclate) Parke-Davis ... 1970
DYNACIN Capsules (Minocycline Hydrochloride) Medicis ... 1627
Floxin I.V. (Ofloxacin) McNeil Pharmaceutical ... 1580
Floxin Tablets (200 mg, 300 mg, 400 mg) (Ofloxacin) McNeil Pharmaceutical ... 1577
Minocin Intravenous (Minocycline Hydrochloride) Lederle ... 1428
Minocin Oral Suspension (Minocycline Hydrochloride) Lederle ... 1431
Minocin Pellet-Filled Capsules (Minocycline Hydrochloride) Lederle ... 1429
Monodox Capsules (Doxycycline Monohydrate) Oclassen ... 1858
Noroxin Tablets (Norfloxacin) Merck & Co., Inc. ... 1758
Noroxin Tablets (Norfloxacin) Roberts ... 2222
Pfizerpen for Injection (Penicillin G Potassium) Pfizer Inc ... 2022
Rocephin Injectable Vials, ADD-Vantage, Galaxy Container (Ceftriaxone Sodium) Roche Pharmaceuticals ... 2305
Terramycin Intramuscular Solution (Oxytetracycline) Pfizer Inc ... 2034
Vibramycin (Doxycycline Calcium) Pfizer Inc ... 2038
Vibramycin Hyclate Intravenous (Doxycycline Hyclate) Pfizer Inc.... 2040
Vibramycin (Doxycycline Monohydrate) Pfizer Inc ... 2038

Enterobacter aerogenes infections, ocular
Garamycin Ophthalmic (Gentamicin Sulfate) Schering ... 2501
Genoptic Sterile Ophthalmic Solution (Gentamicin Sulfate) Allergan ... ⊚ 241
Genoptic Sterile Ophthalmic Ointment (Gentamicin Sulfate) Allergan ... ⊚ 241
Gentak (Gentamicin Sulfate) Akorn ... ⊚ 209
Pred-G Liquifilm Sterile Ophthalmic Suspension (Gentamicin Sulfate, Prednisolone Acetate) Allergan ... ⊚ 248
Pred-G S.O.P. Sterile Ophthalmic Ointment (Gentamicin Sulfate, Prednisolone Acetate) Allergan.. ⊚ 249
TobraDex Ophthalmic Suspension and Ointment (Dexamethasone, Tobramycin) Alcon Laboratories .. 469

Enterobacter aerogenes lower respiratory tract infections
Rocephin Injectable Vials, ADD-Vantage, Galaxy Container (Ceftriaxone Sodium) Roche Pharmaceuticals ... 2305

Enterobacter aerogenes urinary tract infections
Floxin I.V. (Ofloxacin) McNeil Pharmaceutical ... 1580
Floxin Tablets (200 mg, 300 mg, 400 mg) (Ofloxacin) McNeil Pharmaceutical ... 1577
Noroxin Tablets (Norfloxacin) Merck & Co., Inc. ... 1758
Noroxin Tablets (Norfloxacin) Roberts ... 2222

Enterobacter cloacae bone and joint infections
Cipro I.V. (Ciprofloxacin) Bayer Pharmaceutical ... 587
Cipro I.V. Pharmacy Bulk Package (Ciprofloxacin) Bayer Pharmaceutical ... 590
Cipro Tablets (Ciprofloxacin Hydrochloride) Bayer Pharmaceutical ... 584

Enterobacter cloacae infections
Azactam for Injection (Aztreonam) Bristol-Myers Squibb ... 736
Cipro I.V. (Ciprofloxacin) Bayer Pharmaceutical ... 587
Cipro I.V. Pharmacy Bulk Package (Ciprofloxacin) Bayer Pharmaceutical ... 590
Cipro Tablets (Ciprofloxacin Hydrochloride) Bayer Pharmaceutical ... 584
Maxaquin Tablets (Lomefloxacin Hydrochloride) Searle ... 2593
Noroxin Tablets (Norfloxacin) Merck & Co., Inc. ... 1758
Noroxin Tablets (Norfloxacin) Roberts ... 2222
Penetrex Tablets (Enoxacin) Rhone-Poulenc Rorer Pharmaceuticals ... 2196
Primaxin I.M. (Cilastatin Sodium, Imipenem) Merck & Co., Inc. ... 1770
Rocephin Injectable Vials, ADD-Vantage, Galaxy Container (Ceftriaxone Sodium) Roche Pharmaceuticals ... 2305
Timentin for Injection (Ticarcillin Disodium, Clavulanate Potassium) SmithKline Beecham Pharmaceuticals ... 2706

Enterobacter cloacae infections, ocular
Ocuflox Ophthalmic Solution (Ofloxacin) Allergan ... 478

Enterobacter cloacae lower respiratory tract infections
Cipro I.V. (Ciprofloxacin) Bayer Pharmaceutical ... 587
Cipro I.V. Pharmacy Bulk Package (Ciprofloxacin) Bayer Pharmaceutical ... 590
Cipro Tablets (Ciprofloxacin Hydrochloride) Bayer Pharmaceutical ... 584

Enterobacter cloacae skin and skin structure infections
Cipro I.V. (Ciprofloxacin) Bayer Pharmaceutical ... 587
Cipro I.V. Pharmacy Bulk Package (Ciprofloxacin) Bayer Pharmaceutical ... 590
Cipro Tablets (Ciprofloxacin Hydrochloride) Bayer Pharmaceutical ... 584
Primaxin I.M. (Cilastatin Sodium, Imipenem) Merck & Co., Inc. ... 1770
Rocephin Injectable Vials, ADD-Vantage, Galaxy Container (Ceftriaxone Sodium) Roche Pharmaceuticals ... 2305

Enterobacter cloacae urinary tract infections
Azactam for Injection (Aztreonam) Bristol-Myers Squibb ... 736
Cipro I.V. (Ciprofloxacin) Bayer Pharmaceutical ... 587
Cipro I.V. Pharmacy Bulk Package (Ciprofloxacin) Bayer Pharmaceutical ... 590
Cipro Tablets (Ciprofloxacin Hydrochloride) Bayer Pharmaceutical ... 584
Maxaquin Tablets (Lomefloxacin Hydrochloride) Searle ... 2593
Noroxin Tablets (Norfloxacin) Merck & Co., Inc. ... 1758
Noroxin Tablets (Norfloxacin) Roberts ... 2222
Penetrex Tablets (Enoxacin) Rhone-Poulenc Rorer Pharmaceuticals ... 2196
Timentin for Injection (Ticarcillin Disodium, Clavulanate Potassium) SmithKline Beecham Pharmaceuticals ... 2706

Enterobacter species bone and joint infections
Ceptaz (Ceftazidime) Glaxo Wellcome ... 1070
Fortaz (Ceftazidime) Glaxo Wellcome ... 1092
Nebcin Vials, Hyporets & ADD-Vantage (Tobramycin Sulfate) Lilly ... 1518
Primaxin I.V. (Cilastatin Sodium, Imipenem) Merck & Co., Inc. ... 1772
Rocephin Injectable Vials, ADD-Vantage, Galaxy Container (Ceftriaxone Sodium) Roche Pharmaceuticals ... 2305
Tazicef for Injection (Ceftazidime) SmithKline Beecham Pharmaceuticals ... 2697
Tazidime Vials, Faspak & ADD-Vantage (Ceftazidime) Lilly .. 1531

Enterobacter species gynecologic infections
Azactam for Injection (Aztreonam) Bristol-Myers Squibb ... 736
Claforan Sterile and Injection (Cefotaxime Sodium) Hoechst Marion Roussel ... 1259
Mezlin (Mezlocillin Sodium) Bayer Pharmaceutical ... 594
Mezlin Pharmacy Bulk Package (Mezlocillin Sodium) Bayer Pharmaceutical ... 597
Primaxin I.V. (Cilastatin Sodium, Imipenem) Merck & Co., Inc. ... 1772
Timentin for Injection (Ticarcillin Disodium, Clavulanate Potassium) SmithKline Beecham Pharmaceuticals ... 2706

(⊠ Described in PDR For Nonprescription Drugs) (⊚ Described in PDR For Ophthalmology)

Enterobacter species infections

Enterobacter species infections
- Amikacin Sulfate Injection, USP (Amikacin Sulfate) Astra ... 523
- Amikacin Sulfate Injection, USP (Amikacin Sulfate) Elkins-Sinn ... 981
- Amikin Injectable (Amikacin Sulfate) Apothecon ... 502
- Ancef Injection (Cefazolin Sodium) SmithKline Beecham Pharmaceuticals ... 2632
- Augmentin (Amoxicillin Trihydrate, Clavulanate Potassium) SmithKline Beecham Pharmaceuticals ... 2637
- Augmentin Tablets (Amoxicillin Trihydrate, Clavulanate Potassium) SmithKline Beecham Pharmaceuticals ... 2640
- Azactam for Injection (Aztreonam) Bristol-Myers Squibb ... 736
- Bactrim DS Tablets (Trimethoprim, Sulfamethoxazole) Roche Pharmaceuticals ... 2257
- Bactrim I.V. Infusion (Trimethoprim, Sulfamethoxazole) Roche Pharmaceuticals ... 2255
- Bactrim (Trimethoprim, Sulfamethoxazole) Roche Pharmaceuticals ... 2257
- Cefizox for Intramuscular or Intravenous Use (Ceftizoxime Sodium) Fujisawa ... 1025
- Cefobid Intravenous/Intramuscular (Cefoperazone Sodium) Pfizer Inc ... 1996
- Cefobid Pharmacy Bulk Package - Not for Direct Infusion (Cefoperazone Sodium) Pfizer Inc ... 1999
- Ceptaz (Ceftazidime) Glaxo Wellcome ... 1070
- Claforan Sterile and Injection (Cefotaxime Sodium) Hoechst Marion Roussel ... 1259
- Fortaz (Ceftazidime) Glaxo Wellcome ... 1092
- Garamycin Injectable (Gentamicin Sulfate) Schering ... 2502
- Geocillin Tablets (Carbenicillin Indanyl Sodium) Pfizer Inc ... 2009
- Kefurox Vials, Faspak & ADD-Vantage (Cefuroxime Sodium) Lilly ... 1509
- Kefzol Vials, Faspak & ADD-Vantage (Cefazolin Sodium) Lilly ... 1511
- Macrodantin Capsules (Nitrofurantoin) Procter & Gamble Pharmaceuticals ... 2140
- Maxipime for Injection (Cefepime Hydrochloride) Bristol-Myers Squibb ... 758
- Mezlin (Mezlocillin Sodium) Bayer Pharmaceutical ... 594
- Mezlin Pharmacy Bulk Package (Mezlocillin Sodium) Bayer Pharmaceutical ... 597
- Nebcin Vials, Hyporets & ADD-Vantage (Tobramycin Sulfate) Lilly ... 1518
- NegGram (Nalidixic Acid) Sanofi Winthrop ... 2453
- Netromycin Injection 100 mg/ml (Netilmicin Sulfate) Schering ... 2516
- Pipracil (Piperacillin Sodium) Lederle ... 1435
- Primaxin I.V. (Cilastatin Sodium, Imipenem) Merck & Co., Inc. ... 1772
- Proloprim Tablets (Trimethoprim) Glaxo Wellcome ... 1141
- Rocephin Injectable Vials, ADD-Vantage, Galaxy Container (Ceftriaxone Sodium) Roche Pharmaceuticals ... 2305
- Septra (Trimethoprim, Sulfamethoxazole) Glaxo Wellcome ... 1146
- Septra I.V. Infusion (Trimethoprim, Sulfamethoxazole) Glaxo Wellcome ... 1142
- Septra I.V. Infusion ADD-Vantage Vials (Trimethoprim, Sulfamethoxazole) Glaxo Wellcome ... 1144
- Septra (Trimethoprim, Sulfamethoxazole) Glaxo Wellcome ... 1146
- Seromycin Capsules (Cycloserine) Dura ... 975
- Tazicef for Injection (Ceftazidime) SmithKline Beecham Pharmaceuticals ... 2697
- Tazidime Vials, Faspak & ADD-Vantage (Ceftazidime) Lilly ... 1531
- Timentin for Injection (Ticarcillin Disodium, Clavulanate Potassium) SmithKline Beecham Pharmaceuticals ... 2706
- Trimpex Tablets (Trimethoprim) Roche Pharmaceuticals ... 2323
- Unasyn (Ampicillin Sodium, Sulbactam Sodium) Pfizer Inc ... 2035
- Zinacef (Cefuroxime Sodium) Glaxo Wellcome ... 1184

Enterobacter species infections, ocular
- Pred-G S.O.P. Sterile Ophthalmic Ointment (Gentamicin Sulfate, Prednisolone Acetate) Allergan ... ◎ 249

Enterobacter species intra-abdominal infections
- Azactam for Injection (Aztreonam) Bristol-Myers Squibb ... 736
- Cefizox for Intramuscular or Intravenous Use (Ceftizoxime Sodium) Fujisawa ... 1025
- Mandol Vials, Faspak & ADD-Vantage (Cefamandole Nafate) Lilly ... 1516
- Nebcin Vials, Hyporets & ADD-Vantage (Tobramycin Sulfate) Lilly ... 1518
- Netromycin Injection 100 mg/ml (Netilmicin Sulfate) Schering ... 2516
- Primaxin I.V. (Cilastatin Sodium, Imipenem) Merck & Co., Inc. ... 1772
- Unasyn (Ampicillin Sodium, Sulbactam Sodium) Pfizer Inc ... 2035

Enterobacter species lower respiratory tract infections
- Azactam for Injection (Aztreonam) Bristol-Myers Squibb ... 736
- Cefizox for Intramuscular or Intravenous Use (Ceftizoxime Sodium) Fujisawa ... 1025
- Ceptaz (Ceftazidime) Glaxo Wellcome ... 1070
- Claforan Sterile and Injection (Cefotaxime Sodium) Hoechst Marion Roussel ... 1259
- Fortaz (Ceftazidime) Glaxo Wellcome ... 1092
- Maxipime for Injection (Cefepime Hydrochloride) Bristol-Myers Squibb ... 758
- Nebcin Vials, Hyporets & ADD-Vantage (Tobramycin Sulfate) Lilly ... 1518
- Primaxin I.V. (Cilastatin Sodium, Imipenem) Merck & Co., Inc. ... 1772
- Tazicef for Injection (Ceftazidime) SmithKline Beecham Pharmaceuticals ... 2697
- Tazidime Vials, Faspak & ADD-Vantage (Ceftazidime) Lilly ... 1531

Enterobacter species prostatitis
- Geocillin Tablets (Carbenicillin Indanyl Sodium) Pfizer Inc ... 2009

Enterobacter species respiratory tract infections
- Cefobid Intravenous/Intramuscular (Cefoperazone Sodium) Pfizer Inc ... 1996
- Cefobid Pharmacy Bulk Package - Not for Direct Infusion (Cefoperazone Sodium) Pfizer Inc ... 1999
- Ceptaz (Ceftazidime) Glaxo Wellcome ... 1070

Enterobacter species septicemia
- Azactam for Injection (Aztreonam) Bristol-Myers Squibb ... 736
- Mezlin (Mezlocillin Sodium) Bayer Pharmaceutical ... 594
- Mezlin Pharmacy Bulk Package (Mezlocillin Sodium) Bayer Pharmaceutical ... 597
- Netromycin Injection 100 mg/ml (Netilmicin Sulfate) Schering ... 2516
- Pipracil (Piperacillin Sodium) Lederle ... 1435
- Primaxin I.V. (Cilastatin Sodium, Imipenem) Merck & Co., Inc. ... 1772

Enterobacter species skin and skin structure infections
- Azactam for Injection (Aztreonam) Bristol-Myers Squibb ... 736
- Cefizox for Intramuscular or Intravenous Use (Ceftizoxime Sodium) Fujisawa ... 1025
- Ceptaz (Ceftazidime) Glaxo Wellcome ... 1070
- Claforan Sterile and Injection (Cefotaxime Sodium) Hoechst Marion Roussel ... 1259
- Fortaz (Ceftazidime) Glaxo Wellcome ... 1092
- Kefurox Vials, Faspak & ADD-Vantage (Cefuroxime Sodium) Lilly ... 1509
- Mandol Vials, Faspak & ADD-Vantage (Cefamandole Nafate) Lilly ... 1516
- Mezlin (Mezlocillin Sodium) Bayer Pharmaceutical ... 594
- Mezlin Pharmacy Bulk Package (Mezlocillin Sodium) Bayer Pharmaceutical ... 597
- Nebcin Vials, Hyporets & ADD-Vantage (Tobramycin Sulfate) Lilly ... 1518
- Netromycin Injection 100 mg/ml (Netilmicin Sulfate) Schering ... 2516
- Primaxin I.V. (Cilastatin Sodium, Imipenem) Merck & Co., Inc. ... 1772
- Tazicef for Injection (Ceftazidime) SmithKline Beecham Pharmaceuticals ... 2697
- Tazidime Vials, Faspak & ADD-Vantage (Ceftazidime) Lilly ... 1531
- Unasyn (Ampicillin Sodium, Sulbactam Sodium) Pfizer Inc ... 2035
- Zinacef (Cefuroxime Sodium) Glaxo Wellcome ... 1184

Enterobacter species urinary tract infections
- Ancef Injection (Cefazolin Sodium) SmithKline Beecham Pharmaceuticals ... 2632
- Augmentin (Amoxicillin Trihydrate, Clavulanate Potassium) SmithKline Beecham Pharmaceuticals ... 2637
- Augmentin Tablets (Amoxicillin Trihydrate, Clavulanate Potassium) SmithKline Beecham Pharmaceuticals ... 2640
- Azactam for Injection (Aztreonam) Bristol-Myers Squibb ... 736
- Bactrim DS Tablets (Trimethoprim, Sulfamethoxazole) Roche Pharmaceuticals ... 2257
- Bactrim I.V. Infusion (Trimethoprim, Sulfamethoxazole) Roche Pharmaceuticals ... 2255
- Bactrim (Trimethoprim, Sulfamethoxazole) Roche Pharmaceuticals ... 2257
- Ceptaz (Ceftazidime) Glaxo Wellcome ... 1070
- Claforan Sterile and Injection (Cefotaxime Sodium) Hoechst Marion Roussel ... 1259
- Fortaz (Ceftazidime) Glaxo Wellcome ... 1092
- Gantanol Tablets (Sulfamethoxazole) Roche Pharmaceuticals ... 2285
- Gantrisin (Acetyl Sulfisoxazole) Roche Pharmaceuticals ... 2286
- Geocillin Tablets (Carbenicillin Indanyl Sodium) Pfizer Inc ... 2009
- Kefzol Vials, Faspak & ADD-Vantage (Cefazolin Sodium) Lilly ... 1511
- Macrodantin Capsules (Nitrofurantoin) Procter & Gamble Pharmaceuticals ... 2140
- Mandol Vials, Faspak & ADD-Vantage (Cefamandole Nafate) Lilly ... 1516
- Mezlin (Mezlocillin Sodium) Bayer Pharmaceutical ... 594
- Mezlin Pharmacy Bulk Package (Mezlocillin Sodium) Bayer Pharmaceutical ... 597
- Nebcin Vials, Hyporets & ADD-Vantage (Tobramycin Sulfate) Lilly ... 1518
- NegGram (Nalidixic Acid) Sanofi Winthrop ... 2453
- Netromycin Injection 100 mg/ml (Netilmicin Sulfate) Schering ... 2516
- Primaxin I.V. (Cilastatin Sodium, Imipenem) Merck & Co., Inc. ... 1772
- Proloprim Tablets (Trimethoprim) Glaxo Wellcome ... 1141
- Septra (Trimethoprim, Sulfamethoxazole) Glaxo Wellcome ... 1146
- Septra I.V. Infusion (Trimethoprim, Sulfamethoxazole) Glaxo Wellcome ... 1142
- Septra I.V. Infusion ADD-Vantage Vials (Trimethoprim, Sulfamethoxazole) Glaxo Wellcome ... 1144
- Septra (Trimethoprim, Sulfamethoxazole) Glaxo Wellcome ... 1146
- Seromycin Capsules (Cycloserine) Dura ... 975
- Tazicef for Injection (Ceftazidime) SmithKline Beecham Pharmaceuticals ... 2697
- Tazidime Vials, Faspak & ADD-Vantage (Ceftazidime) Lilly ... 1531
- Trimpex Tablets (Trimethoprim) Roche Pharmaceuticals ... 2323

Enterobiasis
- Mintezol (Thiabendazole) Merck & Co., Inc. ... 1747
- Pin-X Pinworm Treatment (Pyrantel Pamoate) Effcon ... ⊞ 670
- Vermox Chewable Tablets (Mebendazole) Janssen ... 1357

Enterobius vermicularis infestation (see under Enterobiasis)

Enterococci infections (see under Streptococci group D infections)

Enterococci species genital infections
- Ancef Injection (Cefazolin Sodium) SmithKline Beecham Pharmaceuticals ... 2632

Enterococci species gynecologic infections
- Claforan Sterile and Injection (Cefotaxime Sodium) Hoechst Marion Roussel ... 1259

Enterococci species skin and skin structure infections
- Claforan Sterile and Injection (Cefotaxime Sodium) Hoechst Marion Roussel ... 1259

Enterococci species urinary tract infections
- Ancef Injection (Cefazolin Sodium) SmithKline Beecham Pharmaceuticals ... 2632
- Claforan Sterile and Injection (Cefotaxime Sodium) Hoechst Marion Roussel ... 1259
- Geocillin Tablets (Carbenicillin Indanyl Sodium) Pfizer Inc ... 2009
- Macrodantin Capsules (Nitrofurantoin) Procter & Gamble Pharmaceuticals ... 2140

Enterocolitis, acute, "possibly" effective in, adjunctive therapy
- Cystospaz (Hyoscyamine) PolyMedica ... 2123
- Donnatal (Phenobarbital, Belladonna Alkaloids) Robins ... 2234
- Donnatal Extentabs (Phenobarbital, Belladonna Alkaloids) Robins ... 2234
- Donnatal Tablets (Phenobarbital, Belladonna Alkaloids) Robins ... 2234
- Librax Capsules (Chlordiazepoxide Hydrochloride, Clidinium Bromide) Roche Products ... 2330

Enterocolitis, staphylococcal
- Vancocin HCl, Oral Solution & Pulvules (Vancomycin Hydrochloride) Lilly ... 1536
- Vancocin HCl, Vials & ADD-Vantage (Vancomycin Hydrochloride) Lilly ... 1534

Enuresis, childhood, temporary adjunctive therapy in
- Hyland's Bedwetting Tablets (Homeopathic Medications) Standard Homeopathic ... ⊞ 788
- Tofranil Tablets (Imipramine Hydrochloride) CibaGeneva ... 875

(⊞ Described in PDR For Nonprescription Drugs)   (◎ Described in PDR For Ophthalmology)

1523 **Indications Index** **Eyes**

Enuresis, nocturnal, primary
DDAVP (Desmopressin Acetate) Rhone-Poulenc Rorer Pharmaceuticals 2180
Desmopressin Acetate Rhinal Tube (Desmopressin Acetate) Ferring .. 997

Envenomation, pit viper
Antivenin (Crotalidae) Polyvalent (Antivenin (Crotalidae) Polyvalent) Wyeth-Ayerst 2803

Ependymoma, palliative therapy in
BiCNU (Carmustine (BCNU)) Bristol-Myers Squibb Oncology/Immunology 696

Epicondylitis
Celestone Soluspan Suspension (Betamethasone Sodium Phosphate, Betamethasone Acetate) Schering 2484
Cortone Acetate Sterile Suspension (Cortisone Acetate) Merck & Co., Inc. 1663
Cortone Acetate Tablets (Cortisone Acetate) Merck & Co., Inc. 1664
Dalalone D.P. Injectable (Dexamethasone Acetate) Forest 1009
Decadron Elixir (Dexamethasone) Merck & Co., Inc. 1676
Decadron Phosphate Injection (Dexamethasone Sodium Phosphate) Merck & Co., Inc. 1680
Decadron Tablets (Dexamethasone) Merck & Co., Inc. 1678
Decadron-LA Sterile Suspension (Dexamethasone Acetate) Merck & Co., Inc. 1687
Hydeltrasol Injection, Sterile (Prednisolone Sodium Phosphate) Merck & Co., Inc. 1708
Hydeltra-T.B.A. Sterile Suspension (Prednisolone Tebutate) Merck & Co., Inc. 1710
Hydrocortone Acetate Sterile Suspension (Hydrocortisone Acetate) Merck & Co., Inc. 1712
Hydrocortone Phosphate Injection, Sterile (Hydrocortisone Sodium Phosphate) Merck & Co., Inc. 1713
Hydrocortone Tablets (Hydrocortisone) Merck & Co., Inc. 1715
Pediapred Oral Solution (Prednisolone Sodium Phosphate) Medeva 1618
Prelone Syrup (Prednisolone) Muro 1834

Epidermophyton floccosum infections
Exelderm Cream 1.0% (Sulconazole Nitrate) Westwood-Squibb 2794
Exelderm Solution 1.0% (Sulconazole Nitrate) Westwood-Squibb 2795
Fulvicin P/G Tablets (Griseofulvin) Schering 2499
Fulvicin P/G 165 & 330 Tablets (Griseofulvin) Schering 2500
Grifulvin V (griseofulvin tablets) Microsize (griseofulvin oral suspension) Microsize (Griseofulvin) Ortho Dermatological 1944
Gris-PEG Tablets, 125 mg & 250 mg (Griseofulvin) Allergan 476
Lamisil Cream 1% (Terbinafine Hydrochloride) Sandoz Pharmaceuticals 2393
Loprox 1% Cream and Lotion (Ciclopirox Olamine) Hoechst Marion Roussel 1269
Lotrimin (Clotrimazole) Schering..... 2514
Lotrisone Cream (Clotrimazole, Betamethasone Dipropionate) Schering 2515
Monistat Dual-Pak (Miconazole Nitrate) Ortho Pharmaceutical 1906
Monistat-Derm (miconazole nitrate 2%) Cream (Miconazole Nitrate) Ortho Dermatological 1944
Naftin Cream 1% (Naftifine Hydrochloride) Allergan..... 477
Naftin Gel 1% (Naftifine Hydrochloride) Allergan..... 477
Nizoral 2% Cream (Ketoconazole) Janssen..... 1344
Oxistat Lotion (Oxiconazole Nitrate) Glaxo Wellcome 1139
Spectazole (econazole nitrate 1%) Cream (Econazole Nitrate) Ortho Dermatological..... 1947

Epididymitis
Ancef Injection (Cefazolin Sodium) SmithKline Beecham Pharmaceuticals 2632

Epilepsy, centrencephalic (see under Seizures, centrencephalic)

Epilepsy, generalized (see under Seizures, generalized, tonic-clonic)

Epilepsy, grand mal (see under Seizures, generalized, tonic-clonic)

Epilepsy, petit mal (see under Seizures, generalized, absence)

Epilepticus, status
Cerebyx Injection (Fosphenytoin Sodium) Parke-Davis 1956
Dizac (diazepam injectable emulsion) CIV (Diazepam) Ohmeda 1862
Nembutal Sodium Solution (Pentobarbital Sodium) Abbott 442
Valium Injectable (Diazepam) Roche Products..... 2336

Epinephrine sensitivity, ocular, treatment of
HMS Liquifilm (Medrysone) Allergan ..... ⊙ 241

Episcleritis
HMS Liquifilm (Medrysone) Allergan ..... ⊙ 241

Episiotomy, topical debriding in (see under Wounds, debridement of)

Erectile dysfunction, male
Caverject Injection (Alprostadil) Pharmacia & Upjohn..... 2064
Yocon Tablets (Yohimbine Hydrochloride) Glenwood-Palisades..... 1235
Yohimex Tablets (Yohimbine Hydrochloride) Kramer 1414

Erectile dysfuncton, male, diagnosis of
Caverject Injection (Alprostadil) Pharmacia & Upjohn..... 2064

Erysipelas
Bicillin C-R Injection (Penicillin G Procaine, Penicillin G Benzathine) Wyeth-Ayerst 2810
Bicillin C-R 900/300 Injection (Penicillin G Procaine, Penicillin G Benzathine) Wyeth-Ayerst 2812
Duricef Capsules, Tablets, and Oral Suspension (Cefadroxil) Bristol-Myers Squibb 750
Mezlin (Mezlocillin Sodium) Bayer Pharmaceutical 594
Mezlin Pharmacy Bulk Package (Mezlocillin Sodium) Bayer Pharmaceutical 597
Pen•Vee K (Penicillin V Potassium) Wyeth-Ayerst 2879

Erysipeloid
Pfizerpen for Injection (Penicillin G Potassium) Pfizer Inc 2022

Erysipelothrix insidiosa infections
Pfizerpen for Injection (Penicillin G Potassium) Pfizer Inc 2022

Erythema multiforme, severe (see under Stevens-Johnson syndrome)

Erythrasma
E.E.S. (Erythromycin Ethylsuccinate) Abbott..... 427
E-Mycin Tablets (Erythromycin) Knoll Laboratories 1388
ERYC (Erythromycin) Parke-Davis .. 1972
EryPed (Erythromycin Ethylsuccinate) Abbott..... 425
Ery-Tab Tablets (Erythromycin) Abbott 426
Erythrocin Stearate Filmtab (Erythromycin Stearate) Abbott 429
Erythromycin Base Filmtab (Erythromycin) Abbott 430
Erythromycin Delayed-Release Capsules, USP (Erythromycin) Abbott 431
Ilosone (Erythromycin Estolate) Dista..... 927
Ilotycin Gluceptate, IV, Vials (Erythromycin Gluceptate) Dista 929
PCE Dispertab Tablets (Erythromycin) Abbott 453

Erythroblastopenia
Celestone Soluspan Suspension (Betamethasone Sodium Phosphate, Betamethasone Acetate) Schering 2484
Cortone Acetate Sterile Suspension (Cortisone Acetate) Merck & Co., Inc. 1663
Cortone Acetate Tablets (Cortisone Acetate) Merck & Co., Inc. 1664
Dalalone D.P. Injectable (Dexamethasone Acetate) Forest 1009
Decadron Elixir (Dexamethasone) Merck & Co., Inc. 1676
Decadron Phosphate Injection (Dexamethasone Sodium Phosphate) Merck & Co., Inc. 1680
Decadron Tablets (Dexamethasone) Merck & Co., Inc. 1678
Decadron-LA Sterile Suspension (Dexamethasone Acetate) Merck & Co., Inc. 1687
Hydeltrasol Injection, Sterile (Prednisolone Sodium Phosphate) Merck & Co., Inc. 1708
Hydrocortone Phosphate Injection, Sterile (Hydrocortisone Sodium Phosphate) Merck & Co., Inc. 1713
Hydrocortone Tablets (Hydrocortisone) Merck & Co., Inc. 1715
Pediapred Oral Solution (Prednisolone Sodium Phosphate) Medeva 1618
Prelone Syrup (Prednisolone) Muro 1834

Erythroblastosis fetalis, prevention of
HypRho-D Full Dose Rho (D) Immune Globulin (Human) (Immune Globulin (Human)) Bayer Biological 623

Escherichia coli (see under E. coli infections)

Esophagitis, erosive (see also under Gastroesophageal reflux disease)
Axid Pulvules (Nizatidine) Lilly 1468
Prevacid Delayed-Release Capsules (Lansoprazole) TAP..... 2746
Prilosec Delayed-Release Capsules (Omeprazole) Astra Merck..... 516
Tagamet (Cimetidine Hydrochloride) SmithKline Beecham Pharmaceuticals..... 2694
Zantac (Ranitidine Hydrochloride) Glaxo Wellcome..... 1182

Esophageal varices, hemorrhage from
Ethamolin Injection (Ethanolamine Oleate) Schwarz 2544

Esotropia, accommodative
Humorsol Sterile Ophthalmic Solution (Demecarium Bromide) Merck & Co., Inc. 1707

Espundia (see under Leishmaniasis, American)

Estrogen, deficiency (see under Hypoestrogenism)

Eubacterium species infections
Flagyl 375 Capsules (Metronidazole) Searle..... 2587
Flagyl I.V. (Metronidazole Hydrochloride) SCS..... 2373
Primaxin I.V. (Cilastatin Sodium, Imipenem) Merck & Co., Inc. 1772

Eubacterium species intra-abdominal infections
Flagyl 375 Capsules (Metronidazole) Searle..... 2587
Flagyl I.V. (Metronidazole Hydrochloride) SCS..... 2373
Primaxin I.V. (Cilastatin Sodium, Imipenem) Merck & Co., Inc. 1772
Protostat Tablets (Metronidazole) Ortho Pharmaceutical 1939

Eubacterium species peritonitis
Flagyl 375 Capsules (Metronidazole) Searle..... 2587
Protostat Tablets (Metronidazole) Ortho Pharmaceutical 1939

Eustachian tube congestion, symptomatic relief of
Fedahist Gyrocaps (Pseudoephedrine Hydrochloride, Chlorpheniramine Maleate) Schwarz 2545
Novahistine Elixir (Chlorpheniramine Maleate, Phenylephrine Hydrochloride) SmithKline Beecham Consumer..... ▣ 782
Trinalin Repetabs Tablets (Azatadine Maleate, Pseudoephedrine Sulfate) Key 1373

Ewing's sarcoma, palliative treatment of
Cosmegen Injection (Dactinomycin) Merck & Co., Inc. 1666

Excoriations, infected
Garamycin 0.1% (Gentamicin Sulfate) Schering 2501

Extrapyramidal reactions, drug-induced
Akineton (Biperiden Hydrochloride) Knoll Laboratories 1380
Artane (Trihexyphenidyl Hydrochloride) Lederle 1418
Cogentin (Benztropine Mesylate) Merck & Co., Inc. 1661
Symmetrel Capsules (Amantadine Hydrochloride) DuPont 965
Symmetrel Syrup (Amantadine Hydrochloride) DuPont 963

Eye and its adnexa, external infections of
AK-Spore (Bacitracin Zinc, Neomycin Sulfate, Polymyxin B Sulfate) Akorn ..... ⊙ 205
Genoptic Sterile Ophthalmic Solution (Gentamicin Sulfate) Allergan..... ⊙ 241
Genoptic Sterile Ophthalmic Ointment (Gentamicin Sulfate) Allergan..... ⊙ 241
Neosporin Ophthalmic Ointment Sterile (Polymyxin B Sulfate, Bacitracin Zinc, Neomycin Sulfate) Glaxo Wellcome 1130
Neosporin Ophthalmic Solution Sterile (Polymyxin B Sulfate, Neomycin Sulfate, Gramicidin) Glaxo Wellcome..... 1131
Polysporin Ophthalmic Ointment Sterile (Polymyxin B Sulfate, Bacitracin Zinc) Glaxo Wellcome .. 1140
Tobrex Ophthalmic Ointment and Solution (Tobramycin) Alcon Laboratories ..... ⊙ 226

Eye, anterior segment inflammation (see under Inflammation, anterior segment)

Eyelids, cleansing of
Lid Wipes-SPF (Peg-200 Glyceryl Monotallowate) Akorn..... ⊙ 210

Eyes, anterior segment, staining of
Fluor-I-Strip (Fluorescein Sodium) Storz Ophthalmics ..... ⊙ 319
Fluor-I-Strip A.T. (Fluorescein Sodium) Storz Ophthalmics ..... ⊙ 320

Eyes, burning, reduction of
Eye-Stream Eye Irrigating Solution (Balanced Salt Solution) Alcon Laboratories..... 469
Similasan Eye Drops #2 (Homeopathic Medications) Similasan ⊙ 316
Tears Naturale II (Dextran 70, Hydroxypropyl Methylcellulose) Alcon Laboratories..... 469

Eyes — Indications Index

Eyes, cleansing of
- Collyrium for Fresh Eyes (Boric Acid, Sodium Borate) Storz Ophthalmics .... ⊚ 316
- Lavoptik Eye Wash (Isotonic Solution) Lavoptik .... 🅜 681

Eyes, diagnostic procedures, adjunct in
- FLUORACAINE (Fluorescein Sodium, Proparacaine Hydrochloride) Akorn .... ⊚ 208
- Fluor-I-Strip (Fluorescein Sodium) Storz Ophthalmics .... ⊚ 319
- Fluor-I-Strip A.T. (Fluorescein Sodium) Storz Ophthalmics .... ⊚ 320

Eyes, dry
(see under Keratoconjunctivitis sicca)

Eyes, emergency flushing of foreign bodies
- FLURESS (Fluorescein Sodium, Benoxinate Hydrochloride) Akorn .... ⊚ 208

Eyes, external infections of
- AKTOB (Tobramycin) Akorn .... ⊚ 207
- Genoptic Sterile Ophthalmic Solution (Gentamicin Sulfate) Allergan .... ⊚ 241
- Genoptic Sterile Ophthalmic Ointment (Gentamicin Sulfate) Allergan .... ⊚ 241

Eyes, goniscopic examinations, adjunct in
- FLURESS (Fluorescein Sodium, Benoxinate Hydrochloride) Akorn .... ⊚ 208

Eyes, inflammation
(see under Ocular inflammation)

Eyes, irrigation of
(see also under Eyes, cleansing of)
- Betadine 5% Sterile Ophthalmic Prep Solution (Povidone Iodine) Escalon Medical .... ⊚ 266
- Eye-Stream Eye Irrigating Solution (Balanced Salt Solution) Alcon Laboratories 469

Eyes, irritation, symptomatic relief of
- Clear Eyes CLR Soothing Drops (Hydroxypropyl Methylcellulose) Ross .... ⊚ 315
- Murine Tears Lubricant Eye Drops (Polyvinyl Alcohol, Povidone) Ross .... ⊚ 315
- Murine Tears Plus Lubricant Redness Reliever Eye Drops (Polyvinyl Alcohol, Povidone, Tetrahydrozoline Hydrochloride) Ross .... ⊚ 315
- Tears Naturale II (Dextran 70, Hydroxypropyl Methylcellulose) Alcon Laboratories 469
- Visine A.C. Seasonal Relief From Pollen and Dust (Tetrahydrozoline Hydrochloride, Zinc Sulfate) Pfizer Consumer .... ⊚ 301
- Visine Moisturizing Eye Drops (Tetrahydrozoline Hydrochloride, Polyethylene Glycol) Pfizer Consumer .... ⊚ 301
- Visine Original Eye Drops (Tetrahydrozoline Hydrochloride) Pfizer Consumer .... ⊚ 301
- Viva-Drops (Polysorbate 80) Vision Pharmaceuticals .... ⊚ 326

Eyes, itching, reduction of
- Allergy-Sinus Comtrex Multi-Symptom Allergy-Sinus Formula Tablets and Caplets (Acetaminophen, Chlorpheniramine Maleate, Pseudoephedrine Hydrochloride) Bristol-Myers Products .... 🅜 639
- Contac Night Allergy/Sinus Caplets (Acetaminophen, Pseudoephedrine Hydrochloride, Diphenhydramine Hydrochloride) SmithKline Beecham Consumer .... 🅜 771
- Ryna Liquid (Chlorpheniramine Maleate, Pseudoephedrine Hydrochloride) Wallace .... 🅜 804
- Similasan Eye Drops #2 (Homeopathic Medications) Similasan .... ⊚ 316
- Sinulin Tablets (Acetaminophen, Phenylpropanolamine Hydrochloride, Chlorpheniramine Maleate) Carnrick 792
- Triaminic Syrup (Phenylpropanolamine Hydrochloride, Chlorpheniramine Maleate) Sandoz Consumer .... 🅜 755
- TYLENOL Severe Allergy Medication Caplets (Acetaminophen, Chlorpheniramine Maleate, Pseudoephedrine Hydrochloride) McNeil Consumer 1571
- Vasocon-A (Antazoline Phosphate, Naphazoline Hydrochloride) CIBA Vision Ophthalmics .... ⊚ 263

Eyes, light occlusion therapy for
- Coverlet Eye Occlusor (Eye Occlusor) Beiersdorf .... ⊚ 257

Eyes, lubrication of
(see also under Keratoconjunctivitis sicca)
- HypoTears Lubricant Eye Drops (Polyvinyl Alcohol) CIBA Vision Ophthalmics .... ⊚ 262
- HypoTears Ointment (Petrolatum, White) CIBA Vision Ophthalmics .... ⊚ 262
- HypoTears PF Lubricant Eye Drops (Polyvinyl Alcohol) CIBA Vision Ophthalmics .... ⊚ 262
- Tears Renewed Ointment (Petrolatum, White) Akorn .... ⊚ 210

Eyes, red
(see under Ocular redness)

Eyes, surgery, adjunct to
- AMO Vitrax Viscoelastic Solution (Sodium Hyaluronate) Allergan .... ⊚ 229
- AMVISC Plus (Sodium Hyaluronate) Chiron Vision .... ⊚ 327
- Betadine 5% Sterile Ophthalmic Prep Solution (Povidone Iodine) Escalon Medical .... ⊚ 266
- Healon (Sodium Hyaluronate) Pharmacia & Upjohn .... ⊚ 302
- Miochol-E with Iocare Steri-Tags and Miochol-E System Pak (Acetylcholine Chloride) CIBA Vision Ophthalmics .... ⊚ 263
- OcuCoat (Hydroxypropyl Methylcellulose) Storz Ophthalmics .... ⊚ 321

Eyes, surgical procedures, irrigation of
(see also under Eyes, cleansing of)
- AMO Endosol (Balanced Salt Solution) (Balanced Salt Solution) Allergan .... ⊚ 229

Eyes, watery
(see under Lacrimation, symptomatic relief of)

F

Fatigue, symptomatic relief of
- No Doz Maximum Strength Caplets (Caffeine) Bristol-Myers Products .... 🅜 644

Febrile episodes, in immunosuppressed patients with granulocytopenia
- Mezlin (Mezlocillin Sodium) Bayer Pharmaceutical 594
- Mezlin Pharmacy Bulk Package (Mezlocillin Sodium) Bayer Pharmaceutical 597

Factor IX, deficiency of
- Konyne 80 Factor IX Complex (Factor IX Complex) Bayer Biological 627
- Mononine, Coagulation Factor IX (Human), Monoclonal Antibody Purified (Factor IX (Human)) Centeon 804

Fecal incontinence, adjunct
- Derifil Tablets (Chlorophyllin Copper Complex) Rystan 2371

Female castration
(see under Ovaries, castration of)

Fetal circulation, persistent
(see under Hypertension, pulmonary, persistent, of the newborn)

Fever associated with common cold
- Advil Cold and Sinus Caplets and Tablets (Ibuprofen, Pseudoephedrine Hydrochloride) Whitehall-Robins .... 🅜 837
- Regular Strength Ascriptin Tablets (Aspirin Buffered, Calcium Carbonate) Ciba Self-Medication .... 🅜 650
- BC Cold Powder Multi-Symptom Formula (Cold-Sinus-Allergy) (Aspirin, Phenylpropanolamine Hydrochloride, Chlorpheniramine Maleate) Block .... 🅜 631
- BC Cold Powder Non-Drowsy Formula (Cold-Sinus) (Aspirin, Phenylpropanolamine Hydrochloride) Block .... 🅜 631
- Children's TYLENOL Cold Multi-Symptom Chewable Tablets and Liquid (Acetaminophen, Chlorpheniramine Maleate, Pseudoephedrine Hydrochloride) McNeil Consumer 1559
- Contac Severe Cold and Flu Formula Caplets (Acetaminophen, Chlorpheniramine Maleate, Dextromethorphan Hydrobromide, Phenylpropanolamine Hydrochloride) SmithKline Beecham Consumer .... 🅜 773
- Sinulin Tablets (Acetaminophen, Phenylpropanolamine Hydrochloride, Chlorpheniramine Maleate) Carnrick 792
- TheraFlu Flu and Cold Medicine (Acetaminophen, Chlorpheniramine Maleate, Pseudoephedrine Hydrochloride) Sandoz Consumer .... 🅜 750
- TYLENOL Cold Medication, Multi-Symptom Formula Tablets and Caplets (Acetaminophen, Chlorpheniramine Maleate, Pseudoephedrine Hydrochloride, Dextromethorphan Hydrobromide) McNeil Consumer 1572
- TYLENOL Cold Medication, Multi-Symptom Hot Liquid Packets (Acetaminophen, Chlorpheniramine Maleate, Pseudoephedrine Hydrochloride, Dextromethorphan Hydrobromide) McNeil Consumer 1572
- TYLENOL Cold Medication, No Drowsiness Formula Caplets and Gelcaps (Acetaminophen, Pseudoephedrine Hydrochloride, Dextromethorphan Hydrobromide) McNeil Consumer 1572

Fever blisters
(see under Herpetic manifestations, oral, symptomatic relief of)

Fever, reduction of
- Actron Caplets and Tablets (Ketoprofen) Bayer Consumer .... 🅜 608
- Advil Ibuprofen Tablets, Caplets and Gel Caplets (Ibuprofen) Whitehall-Robins .... 🅜 836
- Aleve (Naproxen Sodium) Procter & Gamble 2124
- Maximum Strength Ascriptin (Aspirin Buffered, Calcium Carbonate) Ciba Self-Medication .... 🅜 650
- BC Powder (Aspirin, Salicylamide, Caffeine) Block .... 🅜 631
- Genuine Bayer Aspirin Tablets & Caplets (Aspirin) Bayer Consumer .... 🅜 618
- Extra Strength Bayer Aspirin Caplets & Tablets (Aspirin) Bayer Consumer .... 🅜 617
- Extra Strength Bayer Plus Aspirin Caplets (Aspirin, Calcium Carbonate) Bayer Consumer .... 🅜 617
- Aspirin Regimen Bayer Children's Chewable Aspirin (Aspirin) Bayer Consumer .... 🅜 616
- Bufferin Analgesic Tablets (Aspirin) Bristol-Myers Products .... 🅜 636
- Extra Strength Bufferin Analgesic Tablets (Aspirin) Bristol-Myers Products .... 🅜 637
- Children's Motrin Ibuprofen Oral Suspension (Ibuprofen) McNeil Consumer 1558
- Children's TYLENOL acetaminophen Chewable Tablets, Elixir, Suspension Liquid, and Suspension Drops (Acetaminophen) McNeil Consumer 1559
- Empirin Aspirin Tablets (Aspirin) Warner Wellcome .... 🅜 818
- Goody's Extra Strength Headache Powders (Aspirin, Acetaminophen, Caffeine) Block .... 🅜 632
- Goody's Extra Strength Pain Relief Tablets (Aspirin, Acetaminophen, Caffeine) Block .... 🅜 632
- Ibuprohm (Ibuprofen) Ohm .... 🅜 713
- Infants' TYLENOL acetaminophen Suspension Drops (Acetaminophen) McNeil Consumer 1559
- Junior Strength TYLENOL acetaminophen Coated Caplets and Chewable Tablets (Acetaminophen) McNeil Consumer 1562
- Mobigesic Tablets (Magnesium Salicylate, Phenyltoloxamine Citrate) Ascher .... 🅜 607
- Motrin IB Caplets, Tablets, and Gelcaps (Ibuprofen) Upjohn .... 🅜 802
- Motrin Ibuprofen Suspension, Oral Drops, Chewable Tablets, Caplets (Ibuprofen) McNeil Consumer 1563
- Nuprin Ibuprofen/Analgesic Tablets & Caplets (Ibuprofen) Bristol-Myers Products .... 🅜 645
- Orudis KT (Ketoprofen) Whitehall-Robins .... 🅜 842
- Panadol Tablets and Caplets (Acetaminophen) SmithKline Beecham Consumer .... 🅜 783
- Children's Panadol Chewable Tablets, Liquid, Infant's Drops (Acetaminophen) SmithKline Beecham Consumer .... 🅜 783
- Percogesic Analgesic Tablets (Acetaminophen, Phenyltoloxamine Citrate) Procter & Gamble .... 🅜 727
- St. Joseph Adult Chewable Aspirin (81 mg.) (Aspirin) Schering-Plough HealthCare .... 🅜 768
- Trilisate (Choline Magnesium Trisalicylate) Purdue Frederick 2155
- Tylenol (Acetaminophen) McNeil Consumer 1570
- Vanquish Analgesic Caplets (Acetaminophen, Aspirin, Caffeine, Aluminum Hydroxide Gel, Magnesium Hydroxide) Bayer Consumer .... 🅜 627

Fever, San Joaquin
(see under Coccidioidomycosis)

Fever, valley
(see under Coccidioidomycosis)

Fiber, deficiency of
- Unifiber (Cellulose) Niché 1845

Flatulence, relief of
- Arco-Lase Tablets (Amylase, Lipase, Cellulase, Protease) Arco 513
- Beano (Alpha Galactosidase Enzyme) AK Pharma .... 🅜 602
- CharcoCaps (Sulfur, Charcoal, Activated, Cinchona Officinalis, Lycopodium Clavatum) Requa .... 🅜 740
- Di-Gel Antacid/Anti-Gas (Calcium Carbonate, Magnesium Hydroxide, Simethicone) Schering-Plough HealthCare .... 🅜 762
- Gas-X (Simethicone) Sandoz Consumer .... 🅜 749
- Gelusil Antacid-Anti-gas Liquid (Aluminum Hydroxide, Magnesium Hydroxide, Simethicone) Warner Wellcome .... 🅜 819

(🅜 Described in PDR For Nonprescription Drugs)   (⊚ Described in PDR For Ophthalmology)

Indications Index — Gingivitis

Gelusil Antacid-Anti-gas Tablets (Aluminum Hydroxide, Magnesium Hydroxide, Simethicone) Warner Wellcome 819
Hyland's Colic Tablets (Homeopathic Medications) Standard Homeopathic 789
Kutrase Capsules (Hyoscyamine Sulfate, Phenyltoloxamine Citrate, Amylase, Cellulase, Lipase, Protease) Schwarz 2546
Ku-Zyme Capsules (Amylase, Lipase, Cellulase, Protease) Schwarz 2546
Maalox Antacid/Anti-Gas Tablets (Aluminum Hydroxide, Magnesium Hydroxide, Simethicone) Ciba Self-Medication 889
Maalox Anti-Gas Tablets, Regular Strength (Simethicone) Ciba Self-Medication 658
Maalox Anti-Gas Tablets, Extra Strength (Simethicone) Ciba Self-Medication 658
Extra Strength Maalox Antacid/Anti-Gas Liquid and Tablets (Aluminum Hydroxide, Magnesium Hydroxide, Simethicone) Ciba Self-Medication 888
Mylanta Gas Relief (Simethicone) J&J•Merck Consumer 1360
Fast-Acting Mylanta Liquid Antacid (Aluminum Hydroxide, Magnesium Hydroxide, Simethicone) J&J•Merck Consumer 1359
Mylicon Infants' Drops (Simethicone) J&J•Merck Consumer 1358
Phazyme Drops (Simethicone) Block 633
Phazyme-95 Tablets (Simethicone) Block 633
Phazyme-125 Chewable Tablets (Simethicone) Block 633
Phazyme-125 Softgels Maximum Strength (Simethicone) Block 633

Flatus, postoperative retention of
Phazyme-125 Chewable Tablets (Simethicone) Block 633

Fluoride and calcium, deficiency of
Florical Capsules and Tablets (Sodium Fluoride, Calcium Carbonate) Mericon Industries 1825
Monocal Tablets (Calcium Carbonate, Sodium Monofluorophosphate) Mericon Industries 1825

"Flu" symptoms
(see under Influenza syndrome, symptomatic relief of)

Folic acid antagonists, overdosage of
Leucovorin Calcium for Injection, Wellcovorin Brand (Leucovorin Calcium) Glaxo Wellcome Oncology/HIV 1203
Leucovorin Calcium for Injection (Leucovorin Calcium) Immunex ... 1313
Leucovorin Calcium Tablets, Wellcovorin Brand (Leucovorin Calcium) Glaxo Wellcome Oncology/HIV 1204
Leucovorin Calcium Tablets (Leucovorin Calcium) Immunex 1315

Folic acid deficiency, prevention of
Fero-Folic-500 Filmtab (Ferrous Sulfate, Folic Acid, Vitamin C) Abbott 433
Iberet-Folic-500 Filmtab (Vitamin B Complex With Vitamin C, Ferrous Sulfate) Abbott 433
Slow Fe with Folic Acid (Ferrous Sulfate, Folic Acid) Ciba Self-Medication 890

Folliculitis barbae
Fulvicin P/G Tablets (Griseofulvin) Schering 2499
Fulvicin P/G 165 & 330 Tablets (Griseofulvin) Schering 2500
Grifulvin V (griseofulvin tablets) Microsize (griseofulvin oral suspension) Microsize (Griseofulvin) Ortho Dermatological 1944

Gris-PEG Tablets, 125 mg & 250 mg (Griseofulvin) Allergan 476

Folliculitis, superficial
Garamycin 0.1% (Gentamicin Sulfate) Schering 2501

Francisella tularensis infections
Achromycin V Capsules (Tetracycline Hydrochloride) Lederle 1417
Declomycin Tablets (Demeclocycline Hydrochloride) Lederle 1421
Doryx Capsules (Doxycycline Hyclate) Parke-Davis 1970
DYNACIN Capsules (Minocycline Hydrochloride) Medicis 1627
Minocin Intravenous (Minocycline Hydrochloride) Lederle 1428
Minocin Oral Suspension (Minocycline Hydrochloride) Lederle 1431
Minocin Pellet-Filled Capsules (Minocycline Hydrochloride) Lederle 1429
Monodox Capsules (Doxycycline Monohydrate) Oclassen 1858
Streptomycin Sulfate Injection (Streptomycin Sulfate) Pfizer Inc 2031
Terramycin Intramuscular Solution (Oxytetracycline) Pfizer Inc 2034
Vibramycin (Doxycycline Calcium) Pfizer Inc 2038
Vibramycin Hyclate Intravenous (Doxycycline Hyclate) Pfizer Inc.... 2040
Vibramycin (Doxycycline Monohydrate) Pfizer Inc 2038

Fungal infection, skin
(see under Infections, mycotic, cutaneous)

Furunculosis
Garamycin 0.1% (Gentamicin Sulfate) Schering 2501

Furunculosis, symptomatic relief of
Panafil Ointment (Papain, Chlorophyllin Copper Complex, Urea) Rystan 2372
Panafil-White Ointment (Papain, Urea) Rystan 2372

Fusobacterium fusiformisans spirochete infections
Pfizerpen for Injection (Penicillin G Potassium) Pfizer Inc 2022

Fusobacterium nucleatum gynecologic infections
Claforan Sterile and Injection (Cefotaxime Sodium) Hoechst Marion Roussel 1259

Fusobacterium nucleatum infections
Claforan Sterile and Injection (Cefotaxime Sodium) Hoechst Marion Roussel 1259

Fusobacterium species gynecologic infections
Cefotan (Cefotetan) Zeneca 2936
Claforan Sterile and Injection (Cefotaxime Sodium) Hoechst Marion Roussel 1259

Fusobacterium species infections
Cefotan (Cefotetan) Zeneca 2936
Claforan Sterile and Injection (Cefotaxime Sodium) Hoechst Marion Roussel 1259
Flagyl 375 Capsules (Metronidazole) Searle 2587
Flagyl I.V. (Metronidazole Hydrochloride) SCS 2373
Primaxin I.M. (Cilastatin Sodium, Imipenem) Merck & Co., Inc. 1770
Primaxin I.V. (Cilastatin Sodium, Imipenem) Merck & Co., Inc. 1772
Protostat Tablets (Metronidazole) Ortho Pharmaceutical 1939

Fusobacterium species intra-abdominal infections
Primaxin I.M. (Cilastatin Sodium, Imipenem) Merck & Co., Inc. 1770
Primaxin I.V. (Cilastatin Sodium, Imipenem) Merck & Co., Inc. 1772

Fusobacterium species skin and skin structure infections
Flagyl 375 Capsules (Metronidazole) Searle 2587

Flagyl I.V. (Metronidazole Hydrochloride) SCS 2373
Primaxin I.V. (Cilastatin Sodium, Imipenem) Merck & Co., Inc. 1772

Fusospirochetosis
Achromycin V Capsules (Tetracycline Hydrochloride) Lederle 1417
Declomycin Tablets (Demeclocycline Hydrochloride) Lederle 1421
Doryx Capsules (Doxycycline Hyclate) Parke-Davis 1970
DYNACIN Capsules (Minocycline Hydrochloride) Medicis 1627
Minocin Intravenous (Minocycline Hydrochloride) Lederle 1428
Minocin Oral Suspension (Minocycline Hydrochloride) Lederle 1431
Minocin Pellet-Filled Capsules (Minocycline Hydrochloride) Lederle 1429
Monodox Capsules (Doxycycline Monohydrate) Oclassen 1858
Pen•Vee K (Penicillin V Potassium) Wyeth-Ayerst 2879
Pfizerpen for Injection (Penicillin G Potassium) Pfizer Inc 2022
Terramycin Intramuscular Solution (Oxytetracycline) Pfizer Inc 2034
Vibramycin (Doxycycline Calcium) Pfizer Inc 2038
Vibramycin Hyclate Intravenous (Doxycycline Hyclate) Pfizer Inc.... 2040
Vibramycin (Doxycycline Monohydrate) Pfizer Inc 2038

G

Gag reflex, suppression
Cetacaine Topical Anesthetic (Benzocaine, Tetracaine Hydrochloride, Butyl Aminobenzoate) Cetylite 812
Dyclone 0.5% and 1% Topical Solutions, USP (Dyclonine Hydrochloride) Astra 535

Gallstones
(see under Biliary calculi, chemical dissolution of)

Gardnerella vaginalis infections
MetroGel-Vaginal (Metronidazole) Curatek 917
Primaxin I.V. (Cilastatin Sodium, Imipenem) Merck & Co., Inc. 1772

Gardnerella vaginalis vaginitis
(see under H. vaginalis vaginitis)

Gastric acid secretory function, diagnosis of
Peptavlon (Pentagastrin) Wyeth-Ayerst 2997

Gastric emptying, delayed
Reglan (Metoclopramide Hydrochloride) Robins 2243

Gastric hyperacidity
(see under Hyperacidity, gastric)

Gastric stasis, diabetic
Reglan (Metoclopramide Hydrochloride) Robins 2243

Gastric ulcers, active, benign, short-term treatment of
Axid Pulvules (Nizatidine) Lilly 1468
Pepcid Injection (Famotidine) Merck & Co., Inc. 1765
Pepcid (Famotidine) Merck & Co., Inc. 1763
Tagamet (Cimetidine Hydrochloride) SmithKline Beecham Pharmaceuticals 2694
Zantac (Ranitidine Hydrochloride) Glaxo Wellcome 1182

Gastric ulcers, nonsteroidal anti-inflammatory drug-induced, prevention of
Cytotec (Misoprostol) Searle 2576

Gastroesophageal reflux disease
Axid Pulvules (Nizatidine) Lilly 1468
Pepcid Injection (Famotidine) Merck & Co., Inc. 1765
Pepcid (Famotidine) Merck & Co., Inc. 1763
Prilosec Delayed-Release Capsules (Omeprazole) Astra Merck 516

Tagamet (Cimetidine Hydrochloride) SmithKline Beecham Pharmaceuticals 2694
Zantac (Ranitidine Hydrochloride) Glaxo Wellcome 1182

Gastroesophageal reflux, symptomatic
Propulsid (Cisapride) Janssen 1346
Reglan (Metoclopramide Hydrochloride) Robins 2243

Gastrointestinal hypermotility, symptomatic relief of
Arco-Lase Plus Tablets (Amylase, Cellulase, Lipase, Protease, Hyoscyamine Sulfate, Phenobarbital) Arco 513
Bellergal-S Tablets (Phenobarbital, Ergotamine Tartrate, Belladonna Alkaloids) Sandoz Pharmaceuticals 2375
Levsin/Levsinex/Levbid (Hyoscyamine Sulfate) Schwarz 2549

Gastrointestinal tract, smooth muscle spasm
(see under Spasm, smooth muscle)

Gastroparesis, diabetic
(see also under Gastric stasis, diabetic; Gastric emptying, delayed)
Reglan (Metoclopramide Hydrochloride) Robins 2243

Gaucher disease, type 1, long-term enzyme replacement therapy for
Ceredase (Alglucerase) Genzyme 1055
Cerezyme (Imiglucerase) Genzyme 1056

Gelineau's syndrome
(see under Narcolepsy)

Genital warts
(see under Condylomata acuminata)

Genitourinary tract, smooth muscle spasm
(see under Spasm, smooth muscle)

GERD
(see under Gastroesophageal reflux disease)

German measles
(see under Rubella, prophylaxis)

Gestational trophoblastic disease, non-metastatic
Prostin E2 Suppository (Dinoprostone) Pharmacia & Upjohn 2109

Giardiasis
Furoxone Liquid (Furazolidone) Roberts 2221

Gibraltar fever
(see under Brucellosis)

Gilchrist's disease
(see under Blastomycosis)

Gingivitis, necrotizing ulcerative
(see under Fusospirochetosis)

Gingivitis, prevention of
Listerine Antiseptic (Eucalyptol, Menthol, Methyl Salicylate) Warner Wellcome 820
Cool Mint Listerine (Thymol, Eucalyptol, Methyl Salicylate, Menthol) Warner Wellcome 820
FreshBurst Listerine (Thymol, Eucalyptol, Methyl Salicylate, Menthol) Warner Wellcome 820
Peridex (Chlorhexidine Gluconate) Procter & Gamble 2127
Periogard Oral Rinse (Chlorhexidine Gluconate) Colgate Oral 892

Gingivitis, treatment of
Cool Mint Listerine (Thymol, Eucalyptol, Methyl Salicylate, Menthol) Warner Wellcome 820

(▣ Described in PDR For Nonprescription Drugs)   (◉ Described in PDR For Ophthalmology)

Gingivitis

Peridex (Chlorhexidine Gluconate) Procter & Gamble ... 2127
Periogard Oral Rinse (Chlorhexidine Gluconate) Colgate Oral ... 892

Glaucoma, acute attack

ISMOTIC 45% w/v Solution (Isosorbide) Alcon Laboratories ... 221
OSMOGLYN Oral Osmotic Agent (Glycerin) Alcon Laboratories ... 225

Glaucoma, angle-closure, acute

Daranide Tablets (Dichlorphenamide) Merck & Co., Inc. ... 1676
Diamox Intravenous (Acetazolamide Sodium) Storz Ophthalmics ... 317
Diamox Sequels (Sustained Release) (Acetazolamide) Storz Ophthalmics ... 318
Diamox Tablets (Acetazolamide) Storz Ophthalmics ... 317
GlaucTabs (Methazolamide) Akorn ... 209
Neptazane Tablets (Methazolamide) Storz Ophthalmics ... 320

Glaucoma, angle-closure, acute, preoperative

Diamox (Acetazolamide Sodium) Storz Ophthalmics ... 317

Glaucoma, angle-closure, chronic

Phospholine Iodide (Echothiophate Iodide) Storz Ophthalmics ... 323

Glaucoma, angle-closure, subacute

Phospholine Iodide (Echothiophate Iodide) Storz Ophthalmics ... 323

Glaucoma, aphakic

Phospholine Iodide (Echothiophate Iodide) Storz Ophthalmics ... 323

Glaucoma, chronic open-angle

AKPRO (Dipivefrin Hydrochloride) Akorn ... 206
Betagan (Levobunolol Hydrochloride) Allergan ... 230
Betoptic Ophthalmic Solution (Betaxolol Hydrochloride) Alcon Laboratories ... 465
Betoptic S Ophthalmic Suspension (Betaxolol Hydrochloride) Alcon Laboratories ... 467
Daranide Tablets (Dichlorphenamide) Merck & Co., Inc. ... 1676
Diamox Intravenous (Acetazolamide Sodium) Storz Ophthalmics ... 317
Diamox Sequels (Sustained Release) (Acetazolamide) Storz Ophthalmics ... 318
Diamox Tablets (Acetazolamide) Storz Ophthalmics ... 317
EPIFRIN (Epinephrine) Allergan ... 237
GlaucTabs (Methazolamide) Akorn ... 209
Neptazane Tablets (Methazolamide) Storz Ophthalmics ... 320
Ocupress Ophthalmic Solution, 1% Sterile (Carteolol Hydrochloride) Otsuka America ... 297
OptiPranolol (Metipranolol 0.3%) Sterile Ophthalmic Solution (Metipranolol Hydrochloride) Bausch & Lomb Pharmaceuticals ... 256
Phospholine Iodide (Echothiophate Iodide) Storz Ophthalmics ... 323
PROPINE with C CAP Compliance Cap (Dipivefrin Hydrochloride) Allergan ... 251
Timoptic in Ocudose (Timolol Maleate) Merck & Co., Inc. ... 1796
Timoptic Sterile Ophthalmic Solution (Timolol Maleate) Merck & Co., Inc. ... 1794
Timoptic-XE (Timolol Maleate) Merck & Co., Inc. ... 1798

Glaucoma, open-angle

Humorsol Sterile Ophthalmic Solution (Demecarium Bromide) Merck & Co., Inc. ... 1707

Trusopt Sterile Ophthalmic Solution (Dorzolamide Hydrochloride) Merck & Co., Inc. ... 1803
Xalatan (Latanoprost) Pharmacia & Upjohn ... 304

Glaucoma, secondary

Daranide Tablets (Dichlorphenamide) Merck & Co., Inc. ... 1676
Diamox Intravenous (Acetazolamide Sodium) Storz Ophthalmics ... 317
Diamox Sequels (Sustained Release) (Acetazolamide) Storz Ophthalmics ... 318
Diamox Tablets (Acetazolamide) Storz Ophthalmics ... 317
GlaucTabs (Methazolamide) Akorn ... 209
Neptazane Tablets (Methazolamide) Storz Ophthalmics ... 320
Phospholine Iodide (Echothiophate Iodide) Storz Ophthalmics ... 323

Glaucoma, unspecified

Isopto Carbachol Ophthalmic Solution (Carbachol) Alcon Laboratories ... 221

Glaucoma filtration, surgical aid in

AMO Vitrax Viscoelastic Solution (Sodium Hyaluronate) Allergan ... 229
Healon (Sodium Hyaluronate) Pharmacia & Upjohn ... 302
Healon GV (Sodium Hyaluronate) Pharmacia & Upjohn ... 303

Glioblastoma, palliative therapy in

BiCNU (Carmustine (BCNU)) Bristol-Myers Squibb Oncology/Immunology ... 696

Glioma, brainstem, palliative therapy in

BiCNU (Carmustine (BCNU)) Bristol-Myers Squibb Oncology/Immunology ... 696

Glomerulonephritis, acute, prophylaxis

Bicillin L-A Injection (Penicillin G Benzathine) Wyeth-Ayerst ... 2813

Goiter, euthyroid, treatment or prevention of

Cytomel Tablets (Liothyronine Sodium) SmithKline Beecham Pharmaceuticals ... 2647
Levothyroxine Sodium, USP for Injection (Levothyroxine Sodium) Astra ... 546
Synthroid (Levothyroxine Sodium) Knoll Pharmaceutical ... 1410

Goiter, suppression of pituitary TSH in

Cytomel Tablets (Liothyronine Sodium) SmithKline Beecham Pharmaceuticals ... 2647
Eltroxin Tablets (Levothyroxine Sodium) Roberts ... 2214
Levothroid Tablets (Levothyroxine Sodium) Forest ... 1015
Levothyroxine Sodium, USP for Injection (Levothyroxine Sodium) Astra ... 546
Synthroid (Levothyroxine Sodium) Knoll Pharmaceutical ... 1410

Gonococcal arthritis-dermatitis syndrome

Doryx Capsules (Doxycycline Hyclate) Parke-Davis ... 1970

Gonococcal infections, uncomplicated

Doryx Capsules (Doxycycline Hyclate) Parke-Davis ... 1970
Mefoxin Premixed Intravenous Solution (Cefoxitin Sodium) Merck & Co., Inc. ... 1737
Mezlin (Mezlocillin Sodium) Bayer Pharmaceutical ... 594
Mezlin Pharmacy Bulk Package (Mezlocillin Sodium) Bayer Pharmaceutical ... 597
Pipracil (Piperacillin Sodium) Lederle ... 1435
Rocephin Injectable Vials, ADD-Vantage, Galaxy Container

(Ceftriaxone Sodium) Roche Pharmaceuticals ... 2305
Vantin for Oral Suspension and Vantin Tablets (Cefpodoxime Proxetil) Pharmacia & Upjohn ... 2112
Vibramycin (Doxycycline Calcium) Pfizer Inc ... 2038
Zinacef (Cefuroxime Sodium) Glaxo Wellcome ... 1184

Gonorrhea

(see also under N. gonorrhoeae infections)
Amoxil (Amoxicillin Trihydrate) SmithKline Beecham Pharmaceuticals ... 2631
Cefizox for Intramuscular or Intravenous Use (Ceftizoxime Sodium) Fujisawa ... 1025
Claforan Sterile and Injection (Cefotaxime Sodium) Hoechst Marion Roussel ... 1259
E-Mycin Tablets (Erythromycin) Knoll Laboratories ... 1388
Kefurox Vials, Faspak & ADD-Vantage (Cefuroxime Sodium) Lilly ... 1509
Mefoxin (Cefoxitin Sodium) Merck & Co., Inc. ... 1734
Mefoxin Premixed Intravenous Solution (Cefoxitin Sodium) Merck & Co., Inc. ... 1737
Mezlin (Mezlocillin Sodium) Bayer Pharmaceutical ... 594
Mezlin Pharmacy Bulk Package (Mezlocillin Sodium) Bayer Pharmaceutical ... 597
Rocephin Injectable Vials, ADD-Vantage, Galaxy Container (Ceftriaxone Sodium) Roche Pharmaceuticals ... 2305
Spectrobid Tablets (Bacampicillin Hydrochloride) Pfizer Inc ... 2030
Zinacef (Cefuroxime Sodium) Glaxo Wellcome ... 1184

Gonorrhea, cervical/urethral

Cefizox for Intramuscular or Intravenous Use (Ceftizoxime Sodium) Fujisawa ... 1025
Ceftin for Oral Suspension (Cefuroxime Axetil) Glaxo Wellcome ... 1067
Cipro Tablets (Ciprofloxacin Hydrochloride) Bayer Pharmaceutical ... 584
Floxin I.V. (Ofloxacin) McNeil Pharmaceutical ... 1580
Floxin Tablets (200 mg, 300 mg, 400 mg) (Ofloxacin) McNeil Pharmaceutical ... 1577
Noroxin Tablets (Norfloxacin) Merck & Co., Inc. ... 1758
Noroxin Tablets (Norfloxacin) Roberts ... 2222
Penetrex Tablets (Enoxacin) Rhone-Poulenc Rorer Pharmaceuticals ... 2196
Rocephin Injectable Vials, ADD-Vantage, Galaxy Container (Ceftriaxone Sodium) Roche Pharmaceuticals ... 2305
Vantin for Oral Suspension and Vantin Tablets (Cefpodoxime Proxetil) Pharmacia & Upjohn ... 2112

Gonorrhea, pharyngeal

Rocephin Injectable Vials, ADD-Vantage, Galaxy Container (Ceftriaxone Sodium) Roche Pharmaceuticals ... 2305

Gonorrhea, rectal

Rocephin Injectable Vials, ADD-Vantage, Galaxy Container (Ceftriaxone Sodium) Roche Pharmaceuticals ... 2305

Gonorrhea, uncomplicated

Cefizox for Intramuscular or Intravenous Use (Ceftizoxime Sodium) Fujisawa ... 1025
Ceftin Tablets (Cefuroxime Axetil) Glaxo Wellcome ... 1067
Cipro Tablets (Ciprofloxacin Hydrochloride) Bayer Pharmaceutical ... 584
Mefoxin (Cefoxitin Sodium) Merck & Co., Inc. ... 1734
Monodox Capsules (Doxycycline Monohydrate) Oclassen ... 1858
Noroxin Tablets (Norfloxacin) Merck & Co., Inc. ... 1758

Noroxin Tablets (Norfloxacin) Roberts ... 2222
Penetrex Tablets (Enoxacin) Rhone-Poulenc Rorer Pharmaceuticals ... 2196
Rocephin Injectable Vials, ADD-Vantage, Galaxy Container (Ceftriaxone Sodium) Roche Pharmaceuticals ... 2305
Suprax Tablets (Cefixime) Lederle ... 1443

Gout, acute

Anaprox/Naprosyn (Naproxen Sodium) Roche Pharmaceuticals ... 2277
ColBENEMID Tablets (Probenecid, Colchicine) Merck & Co., Inc. ... 1662
Naprelan Tablets (Naproxen Sodium) Wyeth-Ayerst ... 2861
Anaprox/Naprosyn (Naproxen) Roche Pharmaceuticals ... 2277
Zyloprim Tablets (Allopurinol) Glaxo Wellcome ... 1194

Gout, management of signs and symptoms

Zyloprim Tablets (Allopurinol) Glaxo Wellcome ... 1194

Grand mal epilepsy

(see under Seizures, generalized, tonic-clonic)

Granuloma annulare, infiltrated inflammatory lesions of

Celestone Soluspan Suspension (Betamethasone Sodium Phosphate, Betamethasone Acetate) Schering ... 2484
Decadron Phosphate Injection (Dexamethasone Sodium Phosphate) Merck & Co., Inc. ... 1680
Decadron-LA Sterile Suspension (Dexamethasone Acetate) Merck & Co., Inc. ... 1687
Hydeltrasol Injection, Sterile (Prednisolone Sodium Phosphate) Merck & Co., Inc. ... 1708
Hydrocortone Acetate Sterile Suspension (Hydrocortisone Acetate) Merck & Co., Inc. ... 1712

Granuloma inguinale

Achromycin V Capsules (Tetracycline Hydrochloride) Lederle ... 1417
Declomycin Tablets (Demeclocycline Hydrochloride) Lederle ... 1421
Doryx Capsules (Doxycycline Hyclate) Parke-Davis ... 1970
DYNACIN Capsules (Minocycline Hydrochloride) Medicis ... 1627
Minocin Intravenous (Minocycline Hydrochloride) Lederle ... 1428
Minocin Oral Suspension (Minocycline Hydrochloride) Lederle ... 1431
Minocin Pellet-Filled Capsules (Minocycline Hydrochloride) Lederle ... 1429
Monodox Capsules (Doxycycline Monohydrate) Oclassen ... 1858
Streptomycin Sulfate Injection (Streptomycin Sulfate) Pfizer Inc ... 2031
Terramycin Intramuscular Solution (Oxytetracycline) Pfizer Inc ... 2034
Vibramycin (Doxycycline Calcium) Pfizer Inc ... 2038
Vibramycin Hyclate Intravenous (Doxycycline Hyclate) Pfizer Inc ... 2040
Vibramycin (Doxycycline Monohydrate) Pfizer Inc ... 2038

Granulomatous disease, chronic

Actimmune (Interferon Gamma-1B) Genentech ... 1043

Growth failure, chronic renal insufficiency-induced in children

Nutropin (Somatropin) Genentech ... 1049
Nutropin AQ Injection (Somatropin) Genentech ... 1051

Growth hormone secretion, evaluation of the secreting capability of

Geref (sermorelin acetate for injection) (Sermorelin Acetate) Serono ... 2995

Growth hormone secretion, inadequate

Genotropin Injection (Somatropin) Pharmacia & Upjohn ... 2090
Humatrope Vials (Somatropin) Lilly ... 1490

1527 **Indications Index** **H. influenzae**

Nutropin (Somatropin) Genentech .. 1049
Nutropin AQ Injection (Somatropin) Genentech 1051
Protropin (Somatrem) Genentech 1053

Gums, sore (see under Pain, dental)

H

H. aegypticus infections, ocular
TERAK Ointment (Oxytetracycline Hydrochloride, Polymyxin B Sulfate) Akorn .... ⊙ 210
Terramycin with Polymyxin B Sulfate Ophthalmic Ointment (Oxytetracycline Hydrochloride, Polymyxin B Sulfate) Pfizer Inc 2035
TobraDex Ophthalmic Suspension and Ointment (Dexamethasone, Tobramycin) Alcon Laboratories .. 469

H. ducreyi infections
Achromycin V Capsules (Tetracycline Hydrochloride) Lederle 1417
Declomycin Tablets (Demeclocycline Hydrochloride) Lederle 1421
Doryx Capsules (Doxycycline Hyclate) Parke-Davis 1970
DYNACIN Capsules (Minocycline Hydrochloride) Medicis 1627
Minocin Intravenous (Minocycline Hydrochloride) Lederle 1428
Minocin Oral Suspension (Minocycline Hydrochloride) Lederle 1431
Minocin Pellet-Filled Capsules (Minocycline Hydrochloride) Lederle 1429
Monodox Capsules (Doxycycline Monohydrate) Oclassen 1858
Streptomycin Sulfate Injection (Streptomycin Sulfate) Pfizer Inc 2031
Terramycin Intramuscular Solution (Oxytetracycline) Pfizer Inc 2034
Vibramycin (Doxycycline Calcium) Pfizer Inc 2038
Vibramycin Hyclate Intravenous (Doxycycline Hyclate) Pfizer Inc.... 2040
Vibramycin (Doxycycline Monohydrate) Pfizer Inc 2038

H. influenzae bacteremia
Ceptaz (Ceftazidime) Glaxo Wellcome 1070

H. influenzae bronchitis
Bactrim (Trimethoprim, Sulfamethoxazole) Roche Pharmaceuticals 2257
Biaxin (Clarithromycin) Abbott 406
Cedax (Ceftibuten Dihydrate) Schering 2480
Ceftin (Cefuroxime Axetil) Glaxo Wellcome 1067
Cefzil Tablets and Oral Suspension (Cefprozil) Bristol-Myers Squibb .. 747
Floxin I.V. (Ofloxacin) McNeil Pharmaceutical 1580
Lorabid Suspension and Pulvules (Loracarbef) Lilly 1513
Maxaquin Tablets (Lomefloxacin Hydrochloride) Searle 2593
Septra (Trimethoprim, Sulfamethoxazole) Glaxo Wellcome 1146
Spectrobid Tablets (Bacampicillin Hydrochloride) Pfizer Inc 2030
Suprax Tablets (Cefixime) Lederle .. 1443
Vantin for Oral Suspension and Vantin Tablets (Cefpodoxime Proxetil) Pharmacia & Upjohn 2112

H. influenzae infections
Achromycin V Capsules (Tetracycline Hydrochloride) Lederle 1417
Amoxil (Amoxicillin Trihydrate) SmithKline Beecham Pharmaceuticals 2631
Ancef Injection (Cefazolin Sodium) SmithKline Beecham Pharmaceuticals 2632
Augmentin (Amoxicillin Trihydrate, Clavulanate Potassium) SmithKline Beecham Pharmaceuticals 2637
Augmentin Tablets (Amoxicillin Trihydrate, Clavulanate Potassium) SmithKline Beecham Pharmaceuticals 2640
Azactam for Injection (Aztreonam) Bristol-Myers Squibb 736
Bactrim (Trimethoprim, Sulfamethoxazole) Roche Pharmaceuticals 2257
Biaxin (Clarithromycin) Abbott 406
Ceclor Pulvules & Suspension (Cefaclor) Lilly 1470
Cedax (Ceftibuten Dihydrate) Schering 2480
Cefizox for Intramuscular or Intravenous Use (Ceftizoxime Sodium) Fujisawa 1025
Cefotan (Cefotetan) Zeneca 2936
Ceftin (Cefuroxime Axetil) Glaxo Wellcome 1067
Cefzil Tablets and Oral Suspension (Cefprozil) Bristol-Myers Squibb .. 747
Ceptaz (Ceftazidime) Glaxo Wellcome 1070
Cipro I.V. (Ciprofloxacin) Bayer Pharmaceutical 587
Cipro Tablets (Ciprofloxacin Hydrochloride) Bayer Pharmaceutical 584
Claforan Sterile and Injection (Cefotaxime Sodium) Hoechst Marion Roussel 1259
Declomycin Tablets (Demeclocycline Hydrochloride) Lederle 1421
Doryx Capsules (Doxycycline Hyclate) Parke-Davis 1970
DYNACIN Capsules (Minocycline Hydrochloride) Medicis 1627
E.E.S. (Erythromycin Ethylsuccinate) Abbott 427
E-Mycin Tablets (Erythromycin) Knoll Laboratories 1388
ERYC (Erythromycin) Parke-Davis .. 1972
Ery-Tab Tablets (Erythromycin) Abbott 426
Erythrocin Stearate Filmtab (Erythromycin Stearate) Abbott 429
Erythromycin Base Filmtab (Erythromycin) Abbott 430
Erythromycin Delayed-Release Capsules, USP (Erythromycin) Abbott 431
Floxin I.V. (Ofloxacin) McNeil Pharmaceutical 1580
Floxin Tablets (200 mg, 300 mg, 400 mg) (Ofloxacin) McNeil Pharmaceutical 1577
Fortaz (Ceftazidime) Glaxo Wellcome 1092
Ilotycin Gluceptate, IV, Vials (Erythromycin Gluceptate) Dista 929
Keflex Pulvules & Oral Suspension (Cephalexin) Dista 930
Kefurox Vials, Faspak & ADD-Vantage (Cefuroxime Sodium) Lilly 1509
Kefzol Vials, Faspak & ADD-Vantage (Cefazolin Sodium) Lilly 1511
Lorabid Suspension and Pulvules (Loracarbef) Lilly 1513
Maxaquin Tablets (Lomefloxacin Hydrochloride) Searle 2593
Mefoxin (Cefoxitin Sodium) Merck & Co., Inc. 1734
Mefoxin Premixed Intravenous Solution (Cefoxitin Sodium) Merck & Co., Inc. .. 1737
Merrem I.V. (Meropenem) Zeneca .. 2952
Mezlin (Mezlocillin Sodium) Bayer Pharmaceutical 594
Mezlin Pharmacy Bulk Package (Mezlocillin Sodium) Bayer Pharmaceutical 597
Minocin Intravenous (Minocycline Hydrochloride) Lederle 1428
Minocin Oral Suspension (Minocycline Hydrochloride) Lederle 1431
Minocin Pellet-Filled Capsules (Minocycline Hydrochloride) Lederle 1429
Monocid Injection (Cefonicid Sodium) SmithKline Beecham Pharmaceuticals 2674
Monodox Capsules (Doxycycline Monohydrate) Oclassen 1858
Omnipen Capsules (Ampicillin) Wyeth-Ayerst 2872
Omnipen for Oral Suspension (Ampicillin) Wyeth-Ayerst 2873
PCE Dispertab Tablets (Erythromycin) Abbott 453
Pipracil (Piperacillin Sodium) Lederle 1435
Primaxin I.M. (Cilastatin Sodium, Imipenem) Merck & Co., Inc. 1770
Primaxin I.V. (Cilastatin Sodium, Imipenem) Merck & Co., Inc. 1772
Rocephin Injectable Vials, ADD-Vantage, Galaxy Container (Ceftriaxone Sodium) Roche Pharmaceuticals 2305
Septra (Trimethoprim, Sulfamethoxazole) Glaxo Wellcome 1146
Spectrobid Tablets (Bacampicillin Hydrochloride) Pfizer Inc 2030
Suprax (Cefixime) Lederle 1443
Tazicef for Injection (Ceftazidime) SmithKline Beecham Pharmaceuticals 2697
Tazidime Vials, Faspak & ADD-Vantage (Ceftazidime) Lilly .. 1531
TERAK Ointment (Oxytetracycline Hydrochloride, Polymyxin B Sulfate) Akorn .... ⊙ 210
Timentin for Injection (Ticarcillin Disodium, Clavulanate Potassium) SmithKline Beecham Pharmaceuticals 2706
Vantin for Oral Suspension and Vantin Tablets (Cefpodoxime Proxetil) Pharmacia & Upjohn 2112
Zinacef (Cefuroxime Sodium) Glaxo Wellcome 1184
Zithromax (Azithromycin) Pfizer Inc 2043
Zithromax Tablets (Azithromycin) Pfizer Inc 2046
Zosyn (Piperacillin Sodium, Tazobactam Sodium) Lederle 1463

H. influenzae infections, ocular
AK-CIDE (Prednisolone Acetate, Sulfacetamide Sodium) Akorn .... ⊙ 203
AK-CIDE Ointment (Prednisolone Acetate, Sulfacetamide Sodium) Akorn .... ⊙ 203
AK-Spore (Bacitracin Zinc, Neomycin Sulfate, Polymyxin B Sulfate) Akorn .... ⊙ 205
AK-Trol Ointment & Suspension (Dexamethasone, Neomycin Sulfate, Polymyxin B Sulfate) Akorn .... ⊙ 205
Blephamide Liquifilm Sterile Ophthalmic Suspension (Prednisolone Acetate, Sulfacetamide Sodium) Allergan 472
Blephamide Ointment (Sulfacetamide Sodium, Prednisolone Acetate) Allergan .... ⊙ 234
Chibroxin Sterile Ophthalmic Solution (Norfloxacin) Merck & Co., Inc. 1657
Chloromycetin Ophthalmic Ointment, 1% (Chloramphenicol) Parke-Davis ⊙ 298
Chloromycetin Ophthalmic Solution (Chloramphenicol) Parke-Davis .... ⊙ 299
Chloroptic S.O.P. (Chloramphenicol) Allergan .... ⊙ 236
Ciloxan Ophthalmic Solution (Ciprofloxacin Hydrochloride) Alcon Laboratories 468
Cortisporin Ophthalmic Ointment Sterile (Polymyxin B Sulfate, Bacitracin Zinc, Neomycin Sulfate, Hydrocortisone) Glaxo Wellcome 1074
Cortisporin Ophthalmic Suspension Sterile (Hydrocortisone, Polymyxin B Sulfate, Neomycin Sulfate) Glaxo Wellcome 1075
FML-S Liquifilm (Sulfacetamide Sodium, Fluorometholone) Allergan .... ⊙ 240
Garamycin Ophthalmic (Gentamicin Sulfate) Schering 2501
Genoptic Sterile Ophthalmic Solution (Gentamicin Sulfate) Allergan .... ⊙ 241
Genoptic Sterile Ophthalmic Ointment (Gentamicin Sulfate) Allergan .... ⊙ 241
Gentak (Gentamicin Sulfate) Akorn .... ⊙ 209
Maxitrol Ophthalmic Ointment and Suspension (Dexamethasone, Neomycin Sulfate, Polymyxin B Sulfate) Alcon Laboratories .... ⊙ 222
NeoDecadron Sterile Ophthalmic Ointment (Neomycin Sulfate, Dexamethasone Sodium Phosphate) Merck & Co., Inc. 1755
NeoDecadron Sterile Ophthalmic Solution (Neomycin Sulfate, Dexamethasone Sodium Phosphate) Merck & Co., Inc. 1756
Ocuflox Ophthalmic Solution (Ofloxacin) Allergan 478
Poly-Pred Liquifilm (Neomycin Sulfate, Polymyxin B Sulfate, Prednisolone Acetate) Allergan.. ⊙ 246
Polytrim Ophthalmic Solution Sterile (Polymyxin B Sulfate, Trimethoprim Sulfate) Allergan 479
Pred-G Liquifilm Sterile Ophthalmic Suspension (Gentamicin Sulfate, Prednisolone Acetate) Allergan .... ⊙ 248
Pred-G S.O.P. Sterile Ophthalmic Ointment (Gentamicin Sulfate, Prednisolone Acetate) Allergan.. ⊙ 249
TERAK Ointment (Oxytetracycline Hydrochloride, Polymyxin B Sulfate) Akorn .... ⊙ 210
Terramycin with Polymyxin B Sulfate Ophthalmic Ointment (Oxytetracycline Hydrochloride, Polymyxin B Sulfate) Pfizer Inc .. 2035
TobraDex Ophthalmic Suspension and Ointment (Dexamethasone, Tobramycin) Alcon Laboratories .. 469

H. influenzae infections, treatment adjunct
Streptomycin Sulfate Injection (Streptomycin Sulfate) Pfizer Inc 2031

H. influenzae lower respiratory tract infections
Amoxil (Amoxicillin Trihydrate) SmithKline Beecham Pharmaceuticals 2631
Augmentin (Amoxicillin Trihydrate, Clavulanate Potassium) SmithKline Beecham Pharmaceuticals 2637
Augmentin Tablets (Amoxicillin Trihydrate, Clavulanate Potassium) SmithKline Beecham Pharmaceuticals 2640
Azactam for Injection (Aztreonam) Bristol-Myers Squibb 736
Biaxin (Clarithromycin) Abbott 406
Ceclor Pulvules & Suspension (Cefaclor) Lilly 1470
Cefizox for Intramuscular or Intravenous Use (Ceftizoxime Sodium) Fujisawa 1025
Cefobid Intravenous/Intramuscular (Cefoperazone Sodium) Pfizer Inc 1996
Cefobid Pharmacy Bulk Package - Not for Direct Infusion (Cefoperazone Sodium) Pfizer Inc 1999
Cefotan (Cefotetan) Zeneca 2936
Cefzil Tablets and Oral Suspension (Cefprozil) Bristol-Myers Squibb .. 747
Ceptaz (Ceftazidime) Glaxo Wellcome 1070
Cipro I.V. (Ciprofloxacin) Bayer Pharmaceutical 587
Cipro I.V. Pharmacy Bulk Package (Ciprofloxacin) Bayer Pharmaceutical 590
Cipro Tablets (Ciprofloxacin Hydrochloride) Bayer Pharmaceutical 584
Claforan Sterile and Injection (Cefotaxime Sodium) Hoechst Marion Roussel 1259
Floxin I.V. (Ofloxacin) McNeil Pharmaceutical 1580
Floxin Tablets (200 mg, 300 mg, 400 mg) (Ofloxacin) McNeil Pharmaceutical 1577
Fortaz (Ceftazidime) Glaxo Wellcome 1092
Kefurox Vials, Faspak & ADD-Vantage (Cefuroxime Sodium) Lilly 1509
Lorabid Suspension and Pulvules (Loracarbef) Lilly 1513
Mandol Vials, Faspak & ADD-Vantage (Cefamandole Nafate) Lilly 1516
Mefoxin (Cefoxitin Sodium) Merck & Co., Inc. 1734
Mefoxin Premixed Intravenous Solution (Cefoxitin Sodium) Merck & Co., Inc. 1737
Mezlin (Mezlocillin Sodium) Bayer Pharmaceutical 594

(▣ Described in PDR For Nonprescription Drugs) (⊙ Described in PDR For Ophthalmology)

H. influenzae

Mezlin Pharmacy Bulk Package (Mezlocillin Sodium) Bayer Pharmaceutical 597
Monocid Injection (Cefonicid Sodium) SmithKline Beecham Pharmaceuticals 2674
Pipracil (Piperacillin Sodium) Lederle 1435
Primaxin I.M. (Cilastatin Sodium, Imipenem) Merck & Co., Inc. ... 1770
Primaxin I.V. (Cilastatin Sodium, Imipenem) Merck & Co., Inc. ... 1772
Rocephin Injectable Vials, ADD-Vantage, Galaxy Container (Ceftriaxone Sodium) Roche Pharmaceuticals 2305
Spectrobid Tablets (Bacampicillin Hydrochloride) Pfizer Inc 2030
Tazicef for Injection (Ceftazidime) SmithKline Beecham Pharmaceuticals 2697
Tazidime Vials, Faspak & ADD-Vantage (Ceftazidime) Lilly .. 1531
Timentin for Injection (Ticarcillin Disodium, Clavulanate Potassium) SmithKline Beecham Pharmaceuticals 2706
Vantin for Oral Suspension and Vantin Tablets (Cefpodoxime Proxetil) Pharmacia & Upjohn ... 2112
Zinacef (Cefuroxime Sodium) Glaxo Wellcome 1184
Zithromax (Azithromycin) Pfizer Inc 2043
Zithromax Tablets (Azithromycin) Pfizer Inc 2046
Zosyn (Piperacillin Sodium, Tazobactam Sodium) Lederle 1463

H. influenzae meningitis

Cefizox for Intramuscular or Intravenous Use (Ceftizoxime Sodium) Fujisawa 1025
Chloromycetin Sodium Succinate (Chloramphenicol Sodium Succinate) Parke-Davis 1960
Fortaz (Ceftazidime) Glaxo Wellcome 1092
Merrem I.V. (Meropenem) Zeneca .. 2952
Rocephin Injectable Vials, ADD-Vantage, Galaxy Container (Ceftriaxone Sodium) Roche Pharmaceuticals 2305
Tazicef for Injection (Ceftazidime) SmithKline Beecham Pharmaceuticals 2697
Tazidime Vials, Faspak & ADD-Vantage (Ceftazidime) Lilly .. 1531
Zinacef (Cefuroxime Sodium) Glaxo Wellcome 1184

H. influenzae otitis media

Augmentin (Amoxicillin Trihydrate, Clavulanate Potassium) SmithKline Beecham Pharmaceuticals 2637
Augmentin Tablets (Amoxicillin Trihydrate, Clavulanate Potassium) SmithKline Beecham Pharmaceuticals 2640
Bactrim (Trimethoprim, Sulfamethoxazole) Roche Pharmaceuticals 2257
Biaxin (Clarithromycin) Abbott 406
Ceclor Pulvules & Suspension (Cefaclor) Lilly 1470
Cedax (Ceftibuten Dihydrate) Schering 2480
Ceftin (Cefuroxime Axetil) Glaxo Wellcome 1067
Cefzil Tablets and Oral Suspension (Cefprozil) Bristol-Myers Squibb .. 747
Keflex Pulvules & Oral Suspension (Cephalexin) Dista 930
Lorabid Suspension and Pulvules (Loracarbef) Lilly 1513
Pediazole Suspension (Erythromycin Ethylsuccinate, Sulfisoxazole Acetyl) Ross 2340
Septra (Trimethoprim, Sulfamethoxazole) Glaxo Wellcome 1146
Suprax (Cefixime) Lederle 1443
Vantin for Oral Suspension and Vantin Tablets (Cefpodoxime Proxetil) Pharmacia & Upjohn 2112
Zithromax (Azithromycin) Pfizer Inc 2043

H. influenzae otitis media, adjunctive therapy in

Gantanol Tablets (Sulfamethoxazole) Roche Pharmaceuticals 2285
Gantrisin (Acetyl Sulfisoxazole) Roche Pharmaceuticals 2286

H. influenzae respiratory tract infections

Achromycin V Capsules (Tetracycline Hydrochloride) Lederle 1417
Ancef Injection (Cefazolin Sodium) SmithKline Beecham Pharmaceuticals 2632
Cefobid Intravenous/Intramuscular (Cefoperazone Sodium) Pfizer Inc 1996
Cefobid Pharmacy Bulk Package - Not for Direct Infusion (Cefoperazone Sodium) Pfizer Inc 1999
Declomycin Tablets (Demeclocycline Hydrochloride) Lederle 1421
Doryx Capsules (Doxycycline Hyclate) Parke-Davis 1970
DYNACIN Capsules (Minocycline Hydrochloride) Medicis 1627
Kefzol Vials, Faspak & ADD-Vantage (Cefazolin Sodium) Lilly 1511
Minocin Intravenous (Minocycline Hydrochloride) Lederle 1428
Minocin Oral Suspension (Minocycline Hydrochloride) Lederle 1431
Minocin Pellet-Filled Capsules (Minocycline Hydrochloride) Lederle 1429
Monodox Capsules (Doxycycline Monohydrate) Oclassen 1858
Omnipen for Oral Suspension (Ampicillin) Wyeth-Ayerst 2873
Streptomycin Sulfate Injection (Streptomycin Sulfate) Pfizer Inc 2031
Terramycin Intramuscular Solution (Oxytetracycline) Pfizer Inc 2034
Vibramycin (Doxycycline Calcium) Pfizer Inc 2038
Vibramycin Hyclate Intravenous (Doxycycline Hyclate) Pfizer Inc.... 2040
Vibramycin (Doxycycline Monohydrate) Pfizer Inc 2038

H. influenzae septicemia

Ceptaz (Ceftazidime) Glaxo Wellcome 1070
Fortaz (Ceftazidime) Glaxo Wellcome 1092
Kefurox Vials, Faspak & ADD-Vantage (Cefuroxime Sodium) Lilly 1509
Rocephin Injectable Vials, ADD-Vantage, Galaxy Container (Ceftriaxone Sodium) Roche Pharmaceuticals 2305
Tazicef for Injection (Ceftazidime) SmithKline Beecham Pharmaceuticals 2697
Tazidime Vials, Faspak & ADD-Vantage (Ceftazidime) Lilly .. 1531
Zinacef (Cefuroxime Sodium) Glaxo Wellcome 1184

H. influenzae sinusitis

Augmentin (Amoxicillin Trihydrate, Clavulanate Potassium) SmithKline Beecham Pharmaceuticals 2637
Augmentin Tablets (Amoxicillin Trihydrate, Clavulanate Potassium) SmithKline Beecham Pharmaceuticals 2640
Biaxin (Clarithromycin) Abbott 406
Ceftin (Cefuroxime Axetil) Glaxo Wellcome 1067
Lorabid Suspension and Pulvules (Loracarbef) Lilly 1513

H. influenzae upper respiratory tract infections

Cefobid Intravenous/Intramuscular (Cefoperazone Sodium) Pfizer Inc 1996
Cefobid Pharmacy Bulk Package - Not for Direct Infusion (Cefoperazone Sodium) Pfizer Inc 1999
E.E.S. (Erythromycin Ethylsuccinate) Abbott 427
E-Mycin Tablets (Erythromycin) Knoll Laboratories 1388
ERYC (Erythromycin) Parke-Davis .. 1972
EryPed (Erythromycin Ethylsuccinate) Abbott 425
Ery-Tab Tablets (Erythromycin) Abbott 426
Erythrocin Stearate Filmtab (Erythromycin Stearate) Abbott 429
Erythromycin Base Filmtab (Erythromycin) Abbott 430
Erythromycin Delayed-Release Capsules, USP (Erythromycin) Abbott 431
Ilosone (Erythromycin Estolate) Dista 927
Ilotycin Gluceptate, IV, Vials (Erythromycin Gluceptate) Dista 929
PCE Dispertab Tablets (Erythromycin) Abbott 453
Septra (Trimethoprim, Sulfamethoxazole) Glaxo Wellcome 1146
Spectrobid Tablets (Bacampicillin Hydrochloride) Pfizer Inc 2030

H. influenzae, central nervous system infections

Ceptaz (Ceftazidime) Glaxo Wellcome 1070
Claforan Sterile and Injection (Cefotaxime Sodium) Hoechst Marion Roussel 1259
Fortaz (Ceftazidime) Glaxo Wellcome 1092
Tazicef for Injection (Ceftazidime) SmithKline Beecham Pharmaceuticals 2697
Tazidime Vials, Faspak & ADD-Vantage (Ceftazidime) Lilly .. 1531

H. influenzae, skin and skin structure infections

Mandol Vials, Faspak & ADD-Vantage (Cefamandole Nafate) Lilly 1516

H. parainfluenzae bronchitis

Ceftin (Cefuroxime Axetil) Glaxo Wellcome 1067

H. parainfluenzae infections

Ceftin (Cefuroxime Axetil) Glaxo Wellcome 1067
Cipro I.V. Pharmacy Bulk Package (Ciprofloxacin) Bayer Pharmaceutical 590
Cipro Tablets (Ciprofloxacin Hydrochloride) Bayer Pharmaceutical 584
Claforan Sterile and Injection (Cefotaxime Sodium) Hoechst Marion Roussel 1259
Primaxin I.V. (Cilastatin Sodium, Imipenem) Merck & Co., Inc. 1772
Rocephin Injectable Vials, ADD-Vantage, Galaxy Container (Ceftriaxone Sodium) Roche Pharmaceuticals 2305

H. parainfluenzae lower respiratory tract infections

Cipro I.V. (Ciprofloxacin) Bayer Pharmaceutical 587
Cipro I.V. Pharmacy Bulk Package (Ciprofloxacin) Bayer Pharmaceutical 590
Cipro Tablets (Ciprofloxacin Hydrochloride) Bayer Pharmaceutical 584
Claforan Sterile and Injection (Cefotaxime Sodium) Hoechst Marion Roussel 1259
Primaxin I.V. (Cilastatin Sodium, Imipenem) Merck & Co., Inc. 1772
Rocephin Injectable Vials, ADD-Vantage, Galaxy Container (Ceftriaxone Sodium) Roche Pharmaceuticals 2305
Suprax for Oral Suspension (Cefixime) Lederle 1443

H. pylori infection and duodenal ulcer, adjunct in

Biaxin (Clarithromycin) Abbott 406
Helidac Therapy (Tetracycline Hydrochloride, Bismuth Subsalicylate, Metronidazole) Procter & Gamble Pharmaceuticals 2135
Prilosec Delayed-Release Capsules (Omeprazole) Astra Merck 516

H. vaginalis vaginitis

MetroGel-Vaginal (Metronidazole) Curatek 917

Sultrin (Sulfathiazole, Sulfacetamide, Sulfabenzamide) Ortho Pharmaceutical 1941

Haemophilus influenzae
(see under H. influenzae infections)

Hair, cleansing of

Bio-Complex 5000 Revitalizing Conditioner (Cleanser) Wellness International .... ▣ 830
Bio-Complex 5000 Revitalizing Shampoo (Cleanser) Wellness International .... ▣ 830
Concept Antimicrobial Skin Cleanser (Chloroxylenol) Care-Tech .... ▣ 646

Hairy cell leukemias
(see under Leukemia, hairy cell)

Halitosis, adjunctive therapy in

Breath + Plus (Vitamin A, Vitamin E) AML Laboratories .... ▣ 603
Cēpacol/Cēpacol Mint Antiseptic Mouthwash/Gargle (Cetylpyridinium Chloride) J.B. Williams .. ▣ 849
Listerine Antiseptic (Eucalyptol, Menthol, Methyl Salicylate) Warner Wellcome .... ▣ 820
FreshBurst Listerine (Thymol, Eucalyptol, Methyl Salicylate, Menthol) Warner Wellcome .... ▣ 820
Listermint (Sodium Lauryl Sulfate, Sodium Benzoate, Zinc Chloride) Warner Wellcome .... ▣ 820
Salix SST Lozenges Saliva Stimulant (Sorbitol, Malic Acid, Sodium Citrate, Citric Acid, Dicalcium Phosphate) Scandinavian Natural .... ▣ 757

Hansen's disease
(see under Leprosy)

Hashimoto's thyroiditis

Cytomel Tablets (Liothyronine Sodium) SmithKline Beecham Pharmaceuticals 2647
Levothyroxine Sodium, USP for Injection (Levothyroxine Sodium) Astra 546
Synthroid (Levothyroxine Sodium) Knoll Pharmaceutical 1410

Haverhill fever
(see under Streptobacillus moniliformis infections)

Hay fever
(see under Pollinosis)

Headache

Actron Caplets and Tablets (Ketoprofen) Bayer Consumer .. ▣ 608
Alka-Seltzer Cherry Effervescent Antacid and Pain Reliever (Aspirin, Sodium Bicarbonate, Citric Acid) Bayer Consumer ...... ▣ 609
Alka-Seltzer Extra Strength Effervescent Antacid and Pain Reliever (Aspirin, Sodium Bicarbonate, Citric Acid) Bayer Consumer .... ▣ 609
Alka-Seltzer Fast Relief Caplets (Acetaminophen, Calcium Carbonate) Bayer Consumer ...... ▣ 610
Alka-Seltzer Lemon Lime Effervescent Antacid and Pain Reliever (Aspirin, Sodium Citrate) Bayer Consumer .... ▣ 609
Alka-Seltzer Original Effervescent Antacid and Pain Reliever (Aspirin, Citric Acid, Sodium Bicarbonate) Bayer Consumer .. ▣ 609
Maximum Strength Ascriptin (Aspirin Buffered, Calcium Carbonate) Ciba Self-Medication .... ▣ 650
BC Powder (Aspirin, Salicylamide, Caffeine) Block .... ▣ 631
Genuine Bayer Aspirin Tablets & Caplets (Aspirin) Bayer Consumer .... ▣ 618
Extra Strength Bayer Aspirin Caplets & Tablets (Aspirin) Bayer Consumer .... ▣ 617
Extended-Release Bayer 8-Hour Aspirin (Aspirin) Bayer Consumer .... ▣ 616

1529 Indications Index Hemorrhoids

Extra Strength Bayer Plus Aspirin Caplets (Aspirin, Calcium Carbonate) Bayer Consumer ▣ 617
Aspirin Regimen Bayer Children's Chewable Aspirin (Aspirin) Bayer Consumer ▣ 616
Bufferin Analgesic Tablets (Aspirin) Bristol-Myers Products ▣ 636
Extra Strength Bufferin Analgesic Tablets (Aspirin) Bristol-Myers Products ▣ 637
Children's Motrin Ibuprofen Oral Suspension (Ibuprofen) McNeil Consumer 1558
Ecotrin (Aspirin) SmithKline Beecham 2625
Empirin Aspirin Tablets (Aspirin) Warner Wellcome ▣ 818
Aspirin Free Excedrin Analgesic Caplets and Geltabs (Acetaminophen, Caffeine) Bristol-Myers Products 734
Excedrin Extra-Strength Analgesic Tablets, Caplets, and Geltabs (Acetaminophen, Aspirin, Caffeine) Bristol-Myers Products 734
Excedrin P.M. Analgesic/Sleeping Aid Tablets, Caplets, Liquigels (Acetaminophen, Diphenhydramine Citrate) Bristol-Myers Products 735
Goody's Extra Strength Headache Powders (Aspirin, Acetaminophen, Caffeine) Block ▣ 632
Goody's Extra Strength Pain Relief Tablets (Aspirin, Acetaminophen, Caffeine) Block ▣ 632
Hyland's Headache Tablets (Homeopathic Medications, Ipecac, Belladonna Alkaloids) Standard Homeopathic ▣ 790
Ibuprohm (Ibuprofen) Ohm ▣ 713
Junior Strength TYLENOL acetaminophen Coated Caplets and Chewable Tablets (Acetaminophen) McNeil Consumer 1562
Maximum Strength Midol Teen Multi-Symptom Formula (Acetaminophen, Pamabrom) Bayer Consumer ▣ 621
Mobigesic Tablets (Magnesium Salicylate, Phenyltoloxamine Citrate) Ascher ▣ 607
Motrin IB Caplets, Tablets, and Gelcaps (Ibuprofen) Upjohn ▣ 802
Nuprin Ibuprofen/Analgesic Tablets & Caplets (Ibuprofen) Bristol-Myers Products ▣ 645
Orudis KT (Ketoprofen) Whitehall-Robins ▣ 842
Panodol Tablets and Caplets (Acetaminophen) SmithKline Beecham Consumer ▣ 783
Children's Panadol Chewable Tablets, Liquid, Infant's Drops (Acetaminophen) SmithKline Beecham Consumer ▣ 783
Percogesic Analgesic Tablets (Acetaminophen, Phenyltoloxamine Citrate) Procter & Gamble ▣ 727
St. Joseph Adult Chewable Aspirin (81 mg.) (Aspirin) Schering-Plough HealthCare ▣ 768
Tylenol (Acetaminophen) McNeil Consumer 1570
Vanquish Analgesic Caplets (Acetaminophen, Aspirin, Caffeine, Aluminum Hydroxide Gel, Magnesium Hydroxide) Bayer Consumer ▣ 627

Headache accompanied by insomnia
Extra Strength Bayer PM Aspirin Plus Sleep Aid (Aspirin, Diphenhydramine Hydrochloride) Bayer Consumer ▣ 617
Excedrin P.M. Analgesic/Sleeping Aid Tablets, Caplets, Liquigels (Acetaminophen, Diphenhydramine Citrate) Bristol-Myers Products 735
TYLENOL PM Pain Reliever/Sleep Aid, Extra Strength Gelcaps, Caplets, Geltabs (Acetaminophen, Diphenhydramine Hydrochloride) McNeil Consumer 1576
Unisom With Pain Relief-Nighttime Sleep Aid and Pain Reliever (Diphenhydramine Hydrochloride, Acetaminophen) Pfizer Consumer 1991

Headache associated with common cold (see also under Sinus headache)
Advil Cold and Sinus Caplets and Tablets (Ibuprofen, Pseudoephedrine Hydrochloride) Whitehall-Robins ▣ 837
Children's TYLENOL Cold Multi-Symptom Chewable Tablets and Liquid (Acetaminophen, Chlorpheniramine Maleate, Pseudoephedrine Hydrochloride) McNeil Consumer 1559

Headache with gastric hyperacidity
Alka-Seltzer Cherry Effervescent Antacid and Pain Reliever (Aspirin, Sodium Bicarbonate, Citric Acid) Bayer Consumer ▣ 609
Alka-Seltzer Extra Strength Effervescent Antacid and Pain Reliever (Aspirin, Sodium Bicarbonate, Citric Acid) Bayer Consumer ▣ 609
Alka-Seltzer Fast Relief Caplets (Acetaminophen, Calcium Carbonate) Bayer Consumer ▣ 610
Alka-Seltzer Lemon Lime Effervescent Antacid and Pain Reliever (Aspirin, Sodium Citrate) Bayer Consumer ▣ 609
Alka-Seltzer Original Effervescent Antacid and Pain Reliever (Aspirin, Citric Acid, Sodium Bicarbonate) Bayer Consumer ▣ 609
TYLENOL Headache Plus Pain Reliever with Antacid, Extra Strength Caplets (Acetaminophen, Calcium Carbonate) McNeil Consumer ▣ 705

Headache with upset stomach
Alka-Seltzer Cherry Effervescent Antacid and Pain Reliever (Aspirin, Sodium Bicarbonate, Citric Acid) Bayer Consumer ▣ 609
Alka-Seltzer Extra Strength Effervescent Antacid and Pain Reliever (Aspirin, Sodium Bicarbonate, Citric Acid) Bayer Consumer ▣ 609
Alka-Seltzer Lemon Lime Effervescent Antacid and Pain Reliever (Aspirin, Sodium Citrate) Bayer Consumer ▣ 609
Alka-Seltzer Original Effervescent Antacid and Pain Reliever (Aspirin, Citric Acid, Sodium Bicarbonate) Bayer Consumer ▣ 609

Headache, cluster (see under Cephalalgia, histaminic)

Headache, migraine
Cafergot (Ergotamine Tartrate, Caffeine) Sandoz Pharmaceuticals 2376
D.H.E. 45 Injection (Dihydroergotamine Mesylate) Sandoz Pharmaceuticals 2381
Imitrex Injection (Sumatriptan Succinate) Glaxo Wellcome 1095
Imitrex Tablets (Sumatriptan Succinate) Glaxo Wellcome 1099
Wigraine Tablets (Ergotamine Tartrate, Caffeine) Organon 1884

Headache, migraine, "possibly" effective in
Midrin Capsules (Isometheptene Mucate, Dichloralphenazone, Acetaminophen) Carnrick 788

Headache, migraine, prevention or reduction of intensity and frequency of
Cafergot (Ergotamine Tartrate, Caffeine) Sandoz Pharmaceuticals 2376
D.H.E. 45 Injection (Dihydroergotamine Mesylate) Sandoz Pharmaceuticals 2381
Ergomar Tablets (Ergotamine Tartrate) Lotus 1543
Sansert Tablets (Methysergide Maleate) Sandoz Pharmaceuticals 2424

Headache, migraine, prophylaxis of (see also under Headache, migraine, prevention or reduction of intensity and frequency of)
Blocadren Tablets (Timolol Maleate) Merck & Co., Inc. 1654
Depakote Tablets (Divalproex Sodium) Abbott 418
Inderal (Propranolol Hydrochloride) Wyeth-Ayerst 2834
Inderal LA Long Acting Capsules (Propranolol Hydrochloride) Wyeth-Ayerst 2836

Headache, sinus, symptomatic relief of (see under Sinus headache)

Headache, tension (see also under Pain, unspecified; Pain with anxiety and tension)
Axocet Capsules (Acetaminophen, Butalbital) Savage 2469
Esgic-plus Capsules (Butalbital, Acetaminophen, Caffeine) Forest 1012
Esgic-plus Tablets (Butalbital, Acetaminophen, Caffeine) Forest 1012
Fioricet Tablets (Butalbital, Acetaminophen, Caffeine) Sandoz Pharmaceuticals 2386
Fioricet with Codeine Capsules (Butalbital, Acetaminophen, Caffeine, Codeine Phosphate) Sandoz Pharmaceuticals 2387
Fiorinal Capsules (Butalbital, Aspirin, Caffeine) Sandoz Pharmaceuticals 2388
Fiorinal with Codeine Capsules (Codeine Phosphate, Butalbital, Caffeine, Aspirin) Sandoz Pharmaceuticals 2390
Fiorinal Tablets (Butalbital, Aspirin, Caffeine) Sandoz Pharmaceuticals 2388
Phrenilin (Butalbital, Acetaminophen) Carnrick 790
Sedapap Tablets 50 mg/650 mg (Acetaminophen, Butalbital) Merz 1826

Headache, vascular (see under Headache, migraine)

Heart block, mild or transient episodes of
Isuprel Injection (Isoproterenol Hydrochloride) Sanofi Winthrop 2441

Heart block, serious episodes of
Isuprel Injection (Isoproterenol Hydrochloride) Sanofi Winthrop 2441

Heart failure (see under Congestive heart failure)

Heart failure, congestive (see under Congestive heart failure)

Heart, allogeneic transplants, prophylaxis of organ rejection in
Neoral (Cyclosporine) Sandoz Pharmaceuticals 2405
Orthoclone OKT3 Sterile Solution (Muromonab-CD3) Ortho Biotech 1892
Sandimmune (Cyclosporine) Sandoz Pharmaceuticals 2416

Heartburn (see under Hyperacidity, gastric, symptomatic relief of)

Hemolytic disease, Rh, prevention of (see under Erythroblastosis fetalis, prevention of)

Hemophilia A
Bioclate, Antihemophilic Factor (Recombinant) (Antihemophilic Factor (Recombinant)) Centeon 797
DDAVP Injection (Desmopressin Acetate) Rhone-Poulenc Rorer Pharmaceuticals 2178
DDAVP Injection 15 mcg/mL (Desmopressin Acetate) Rhone-Poulenc Rorer Pharmaceuticals 2179
Desmopressin Acetate Injection (Desmopressin Acetate) Ferring 996
Helixate, Antihemophilic Factor (Recombinant) (Antihemophilic Factor (Recombinant)) Centeon 799
Humate-P, Antihemophilic Factor (Human), Dried Pasteurized (Antihemophilic Factor (Human)) Centeon 801
Koāte-HP Antihemophilic Factor (Human) (Antihemophilic Factor (Human)) Bayer Biological 624
KOGENATE Antihemophilic Factor (Recombinant) (Antihemophilic Factor (Recombinant)) Bayer Biological 626
Monoclate-P, Factor VIII:C Pasteurized, Monoclonal Antibody Purified Antihemophilic Factor (Human) (Antihemophilic Factor (Human)) Centeon 802
Stimate, (desmopressin acetate) Nasal Spray, 1.5 mg/mL (Desmopressin Acetate) Centeon 806

Hemophilia B
Konȳne 80 Factor IX Complex (Factor IX Complex) Bayer Biological 627
Mononine, Coagulation Factor IX (Human), Monoclonal Antibody Purified (Factor IX (Human)) Centeon 804

Hemophilia, congenital with antibodies to Factor VIII:C
KOGENATE Antihemophilic Factor (Recombinant) (Antihemophilic Factor (Recombinant)) Bayer Biological 626

Hemorrhage, coumarin anticoagulant-induced, reversal of
Konȳne 80 Factor IX Complex (Factor IX Complex) Bayer Biological 627

Hemorrhage, postpartum, control of
AquaMEPHYTON Injection (Phytonadione) Merck & Co., Inc. 1648
Methergine (Methylergonovine Maleate) Sandoz Pharmaceuticals 2401
Syntocinon Injection (Oxytocin) Sandoz Pharmaceuticals 2425

Hemorrhage, subarachnoid, resulting in neurological deficits
Nimotop Capsules (Nimodipine) Bayer Pharmaceutical 603

Hemorrhoidal pain (see under Pain, anorectal)

Hemorrhoids
Americaine Hemorrhoidal Ointment (Benzocaine) Ciba Self-Medication ▣ 649
Anusol (Pramoxine Hydrochloride, Zinc Oxide, Mineral Oil) Warner Wellcome ▣ 810
Anusol-HC Suppositories (Hydrocortisone Acetate) Parke-Davis 1954
Hemorid (Petrolatum, White, Mineral Oil, Pramoxine Hydrochloride, Phenylephrine Hydrochloride) Thompson Medical ▣ 797
Nupercainal Hemorrhoidal and Anesthetic Ointment (Dibucaine) Ciba Self-Medication ▣ 661
Nupercainal Suppositories (Cocoa Butter, Zinc Oxide) Ciba Self-Medication ▣ 661
Preparation H (Glycerin, Petrolatum, Phenylephrine Hydrochloride, Shark Liver Oil) Whitehall-Robins ▣ 842
Tronolane Anesthetic Cream for Hemorrhoids (Pramoxine Hydrochloride) Ross ▣ 746
Tronolane Hemorrhoidal Suppositories (Fat, Hard, Zinc Oxide) Ross ▣ 747
Tucks Clear Hemorrhoidal Gel (Witch Hazel, Glycerin) Warner Wellcome ▣ 829

(▣ Described in PDR For Nonprescription Drugs) (◉ Described in PDR For Ophthalmology)

Hemorrhoids

Tucks Pads (Witch Hazel) Warner Wellcome 830
Wyanoids Relief Factor Hemorrhoidal Suppositories (Liver, Desiccated, Shark Liver Oil) Wyeth-Ayerst 856

Hemostasis, an aid in
Amicar Syrup, Tablets, and Injection (Aminocaproic Acid) Immunex 1312
DDAVP Injection (Desmopressin Acetate) Rhone-Poulenc Rorer Pharmaceuticals 2178
Desmopressin Acetate Injection (Desmopressin Acetate) Ferring .. 996
Trasylol (Aprotinin) Bayer Pharmaceutical 607

Heparin overdose, treatment of
Protamine Sulfate Vials (Protamine Sulfate) Lilly 1526

Hepatitis, chronic, Non-A, Non-B/C
Intron A for Injection (Interferon alfa-2B, Recombinant) Schering .. 2506

Hepatitis B virus, postexposure prophylaxis
HyperHep Hepatitis B Immune Globulin (Human) (Hepatitis B Immune Globulin (Human)) Bayer Biological 619

Hepatitis A, prophylaxis
Vaqta (Hepatitis A Vaccine, Inactivated) Merck & Co., Inc......... 1805

Hepatitis B, chronic, treatment of
Intron A for Injection (Interferon alfa-2B, Recombinant) Schering ..2506

Hepatitis B virus infection, immunization against
Recombivax HB (Hepatitis B Vaccine) Merck & Co., Inc............. 1787

Herellea vaginicola
(see under Acinetobacter calcoaceticus infections, ocular)

Herpes, genital, initial and recurrent episodes
Famvir Tablets (Famciclovir) SmithKline Beecham Pharmaceuticals 2660
Zovirax Capsules (Acyclovir) Glaxo Wellcome 1187
Zovirax Sterile Powder (Acyclovir Sodium) Glaxo Wellcome 1191
Zovirax (Acyclovir) Glaxo Wellcome 1187

Herpes genitalis
Valtrex Caplets (Valacyclovir Hydrochloride) Glaxo Wellcome... 1167
Zovirax Capsules (Acyclovir) Glaxo Wellcome 1187
Zovirax Ointment 5% (Acyclovir) Glaxo Wellcome 1190
Zovirax Sterile Powder (Acyclovir Sodium) Glaxo Wellcome 1191
Zovirax (Acyclovir) Glaxo Wellcome 1187

Herpes simplex infections, ocular
Vira-A Ophthalmic Ointment, 3% (Vidarabine) Parke-Davis 299
Viroptic Ophthalmic Solution, 1% Sterile (Trifluridine) Glaxo Wellcome 1177

Herpes simplex keratitis
Viroptic Ophthalmic Solution, 1% Sterile (Trifluridine) Glaxo Wellcome 1177

Herpes simplex virus encephalitis
Zovirax Sterile Powder (Acyclovir Sodium) Glaxo Wellcome 1191

Herpes simplex virus infections
Zovirax Ointment 5% (Acyclovir) Glaxo Wellcome 1190
Zovirax Sterile Powder (Acyclovir Sodium) Glaxo Wellcome 1191

Herpes simplex virus mucocutaneous infection
Foscavir Injection (Foscarnet Sodium) Astra 541

Zovirax Ointment 5% (Acyclovir) Glaxo Wellcome 1190
Zovirax Sterile Powder (Acyclovir Sodium) Glaxo Wellcome 1191

Herpes zoster infections
Famvir Tablets (Famciclovir) SmithKline Beecham Pharmaceuticals 2660
Valtrex Caplets (Valacyclovir Hydrochloride) Glaxo Wellcome... 1167
Zovirax (Acyclovir) Glaxo Wellcome 1187

Herpes zoster ophthalmicus
Celestone Soluspan Suspension (Betamethasone Sodium Phosphate, Betamethasone Acetate) Schering 2484
Cortone Acetate Sterile Suspension (Cortisone Acetate) Merck & Co., Inc. 1663
Cortone Acetate Tablets (Cortisone Acetate) Merck & Co., Inc. 1664
Dalalone D.P. Injectable (Dexamethasone Acetate) Forest 1009
Decadron Elixir (Dexamethasone) Merck & Co., Inc. 1676
Decadron Phosphate Injection (Dexamethasone Sodium Phosphate) Merck & Co., Inc. 1680
Decadron Tablets (Dexamethasone) Merck & Co., Inc. 1678
Decadron-LA Sterile Suspension (Dexamethasone Acetate) Merck & Co., Inc. 1687
Hydeltrasol Injection, Sterile (Prednisolone Sodium Phosphate) Merck & Co., Inc. 1708
Hydrocortone Phosphate Injection, Sterile (Hydrocortisone Sodium Phosphate) Merck & Co., Inc. ... 1713
Hydrocortone Tablets (Hydrocortisone) Merck & Co., Inc. 1715
Pediapred Oral Solution (Prednisolone Sodium Phosphate) Medeva 1618
Prelone Syrup (Prednisolone) Muro 1834

Herpetic manifestations, oral, symptomatic relief of
Herpecin-L Cold Sore Lip Balm Stick (Allantoin) Chattem 812
Orajel CoverMed Tinted Cold Sore Medicine (Allantoin, Dyclonine Hydrochloride) Del 668
Orajel Mouth-Aid for Canker and Cold Sores (Benzocaine, Benzalkonium Chloride, Zinc Chloride) Del 668
Tanac Medicated Gel (Dyclonine Hydrochloride, Allantoin) Del...... 669
Tanac No Sting Liquid (Benzocaine, Benzalkonium Chloride) Del 669
Zilactin/Dermafilm (Benzyl Alcohol) Zila Pharmaceuticals 856

Hiccup
Thorazine (Chlorpromazine Hydrochloride) SmithKline Beecham Pharmaceuticals 2701

Histoplasmosis
Fungizone Intravenous (Amphotericin B) Apothecon 507
Nizoral Tablets (Ketoconazole) Janssen 1345
Sporanox Capsules (Itraconazole) Janssen 1352

HIV infection
(see under Infection, human immunodeficiency virus)

Hodgkin's disease
Adriamycin PFS (Doxorubicin Hydrochloride) Pharmacia & Upjohn 2056
Adriamycin RDF (Doxorubicin Hydrochloride) Pharmacia & Upjohn 2056
Blenoxane (Bleomycin Sulfate) Bristol-Myers Squibb Oncology/Immunology......... 697
Cytoxan (Cyclophosphamide) Bristol-Myers Squibb Oncology/Immunology......... 700
Doxorubicin Astra (Doxorubicin Hydrochloride) Astra 531
Leukeran Tablets (Chlorambucil) Glaxo Wellcome Oncology/HIV 1205

Oncovin Solution Vials & Hyporets (Vincristine Sulfate) Lilly 1521
Rubex for Injection (Doxorubicin Hydrochloride) Bristol-Myers Squibb Oncology/Immunology 721
Thioplex (Thiotepa For Injection) (Thiotepa) Immunex 1329
Velban Vials (Vinblastine Sulfate) Lilly 1537

Hodgkin's disease, adjunctive therapy in
Leukine (Sargramostim) Immunex .. 1317

Hodgkin's disease, secondary line therapy in
BiCNU (Carmustine (BCNU)) Bristol-Myers Squibb Oncology/Immunology 696
CeeNU Capsules (Lomustine (CCNU)) Bristol-Myers Squibb Oncology/Immunology 699
DTIC-Dome (Dacarbazine) Bayer Pharmaceutical 593
Matulane Capsules (Procarbazine Hydrochloride) Roche Pharmaceuticals 2300

Hodgkin's disease, stages III and IV, palliative treatment of
Matulane Capsules (Procarbazine Hydrochloride) Roche Pharmaceuticals 2300
Mustargen (Mechlorethamine Hydrochloride) Merck & Co., Inc. 1752

Hookworm infections
(see under Ancylostoma duodenale infections)

Hookworm, American
(see under Necator americanus infections)

Hormonal imbalance, male
Halotestin Tablets (Fluoxymesterone) Pharmacia & Upjohn 2095

Horton's headache
(see under Cephalalgia, histaminic)

Hydatid disease, cystic
Albenza Tablets (Albendazole) SmithKline Beecham Pharmaceuticals 2629

Hydatidiform mole
Methotrexate Sodium Tablets, Injection, for Injection and LPF Injection (Methotrexate Sodium) Immunex 1322

Hyperacidity, gastric, symptomatic relief of
Alka-Mints Chewable Antacid (Calcium Carbonate) Bayer Consumer 609
Alka-Seltzer Gold Effervescent Antacid (Citric Acid, Potassium Bicarbonate, Sodium Bicarbonate) Bayer Consumer .. 611
ALternaGEL Liquid (Aluminum Hydroxide) J&J•Merck Consumer 1358
Amphojel (Aluminum Hydroxide Gel) Wyeth-Ayerst 2802
Arm & Hammer Pure Baking Soda (Sodium Bicarbonate) Church & Dwight 648
Basaljel (Aluminum Carbonate) Wyeth-Ayerst 2810
Bicitra (Sodium Citrate, Citric Acid) Baker Norton 573
Di-Gel Antacid/Anti-Gas (Calcium Carbonate, Magnesium Hydroxide, Simethicone) Schering-Plough HealthCare 762
Gaviscon Antacid Tablets (Aluminum Hydroxide Gel, Magnesium Trisilicate) SmithKline Beecham Consumer 778
Gaviscon-2 Antacid Tablets (Aluminum Hydroxide Gel, Magnesium Trisilicate) SmithKline Beecham Consumer 779
Gaviscon Extra Strength Relief Formula Antacid Tablets (Aluminum Hydroxide, Magnesium

Carbonate) SmithKline Beecham Consumer......... 778
Gaviscon Extra Strength Relief Formula Liquid Antacid (Aluminum Hydroxide, Magnesium Carbonate) SmithKline Beecham Consumer......... 779
Gaviscon Liquid Antacid (Aluminum Hydroxide, Magnesium Carbonate) SmithKline Beecham Consumer......... 779
Gelusil Antacid-Anti-gas Liquid (Aluminum Hydroxide, Magnesium Hydroxide, Simethicone) Warner Wellcome......... 819
Gelusil Antacid-Anti-gas Tablets (Aluminum Hydroxide, Magnesium Hydroxide, Simethicone) Warner Wellcome......... 819
Maalox Antacid Caplets (Calcium Carbonate, Magnesium Carbonate) Ciba Self-Medication 657
Maalox Antacid/Anti-Gas Tablets (Aluminum Hydroxide, Magnesium Hydroxide, Simethicone) Ciba Self-Medication 889
Maalox Heartburn Relief Suspension (Aluminum Hydroxide, Magnesium Carbonate) Ciba Self-Medication 658
Maalox Antacid Liquid (Magnesium Hydroxide, Aluminum Hydroxide) Ciba Self-Medication 888
Extra Strength Maalox Antacid/Anti-Gas Liquid and Tablets (Aluminum Hydroxide, Magnesium Hydroxide, Simethicone) Ciba Self-Medication 888
Mag-Ox 400 (Magnesium Oxide) Blaine......... 666
Marblen (Calcium Carbonate, Magnesium Carbonate) Fleming 671
Mylanta Fast-Acting (Calcium Carbonate, Magnesium Hydroxide) J&J•Merck Consumer 1359
Mylanta Gelcaps Antacid (Calcium Carbonate, Magnesium Hydroxide) J&J•Merck Consumer......... 678
Fast-Acting Mylanta Liquid Antacid (Aluminum Hydroxide, Magnesium Hydroxide, Simethicone) J&J•Merck Consumer 1359
Mylanta Soothing Lozenges (Calcium Carbonate) J&J•Merck Consumer 1360
Maximum-Strength Fast-Acting Mylanta Liquid Antacid (Aluminum Hydroxide, Magnesium Hydroxide, Simethicone) J&J•Merck Consumer 1359
Nephrox Suspension (Aluminum Hydroxide Gel, Mineral Oil) Fleming 671
Pepcid AC Acid Controller (Famotidine) J&J•Merck Consumer 1360
Phillips' Milk of Magnesia Liquid (Magnesium Hydroxide) Bayer Consumer......... 627
Rolaids Antacid Tablets (Calcium Carbonate, Magnesium Hydroxide) Warner-Lambert 807
Rolaids Antacid Calcium Rich/Sodium Free Tablets (Calcium Carbonate) Warner-Lambert 807
Tagamet HB Tablets (Cimetidine) SmithKline Beecham Consumer 786
Tempo Soft Antacid (Calcium Carbonate, Aluminum Hydroxide, Magnesium Hydroxide, Simethicone) Thompson Medical 799
Titralac (Calcium Carbonate) 3M 686
Titralac Plus (Calcium Carbonate, Simethicone) 3M 687
Tums Antacid/Calcium Supplement Tablets (Calcium Carbonate) SmithKline Beecham Consumer 787
Tums Anti-gas/Antacid Formula Tablets, Assorted Fruit (Calcium Carbonate, Simethicone) SmithKline Beecham Consumer 788
Tums (Calcium Carbonate) SmithKline Beecham Consumer 787
Uro-Mag (Magnesium Oxide) Blaine 666

(▣ Described in PDR For Nonprescription Drugs)   (◉ Described in PDR For Ophthalmology)

1531 **Indications Index** **Hypertension**

Hyperaldosteronism, primary
Aldactone Tablets (Spironolactone) Searle ... 2558

Hyperbetalipoproteinemia (see under Hyperlipoproteinemia, types IIa and IIb, adjunct to diet)

Hypercalcemia associated with cancer
Aredia for Injection (Pamidronate Disodium) CibaGeneva ... 827
Celestone Soluspan Suspension (Betamethasone Sodium Phosphate, Betamethasone Acetate) Schering ... 2484
Cortone Acetate Sterile Suspension (Cortisone Acetate) Merck & Co., Inc. ... 1663
Cortone Acetate Tablets (Cortisone Acetate) Merck & Co., Inc. ... 1664
Dalalone D.P. Injectable (Dexamethasone Acetate) Forest ... 1009
Decadron Elixir (Dexamethasone) Merck & Co., Inc. ... 1676
Decadron Phosphate Injection (Dexamethasone Sodium Phosphate) Merck & Co., Inc. ... 1680
Decadron Tablets (Dexamethasone) Merck & Co., Inc. ... 1678
Decadron-LA Sterile Suspension (Dexamethasone Acetate) Merck & Co., Inc. ... 1687
Ganite (Gallium Nitrate) SoloPak ... 2711
Hydeltrasol Injection, Sterile (Prednisolone Sodium Phosphate) Merck & Co., Inc. ... 1708
Hydrocortone Phosphate Injection, Sterile (Hydrocortisone Sodium Phosphate) Merck & Co., Inc. ... 1713
Hydrocortone Tablets (Hydrocortisone) Merck & Co., Inc. ... 1715
Mithracin (Plicamycin) Bayer Pharmaceutical ... 599
Pediapred Oral Solution (Prednisolone Sodium Phosphate) Medeva 1618
Prelone Syrup (Prednisolone) Muro 1834

Hypercalcemia of malignancy, adjunct
Didronel I.V. Infusion (Etidronate Disodium (Biphosphonate)) MGI .. 1545

Hypercalcemic emergencies, adjunct in
Calcimar Injection, Synthetic (Calcitonin, Synthetic) Rhone-Poulenc Rorer Pharmaceuticals ... 2176
Miacalcin Injection (Calcitonin, Synthetic) Sandoz Pharmaceuticals ... 2402

Hypercalciuria associated with cancer
Mithracin (Plicamycin) Bayer Pharmaceutical ... 599

Hypercapnia, acute, with COPD (see under Respiratory insufficiency, acute, with chronic obstructive pulmonary disease)

Hypercholesterolemia, primary, adjunct to diet
Colestid (Colestipol Hydrochloride) Pharmacia & Upjohn ... 2073
Lescol Capsules (Fluvastatin Sodium) Sandoz Pharmaceuticals 2395
Mevacor Tablets (Lovastatin) Merck & Co., Inc. ... 1742
Pravachol Tablets (Pravastatin Sodium) Bristol-Myers Squibb ... 770
Questran (Cholestyramine) Bristol-Myers Squibb ... 774
Zocor Tablets (Simvastatin) Merck & Co., Inc. ... 1821

Hyperglycemia, control of, adjunct to diet (see also under Diabetes mellitus, insulin-dependent; Diabetes mellitus, non-insulin-dependent)
Amaryl Tablets (Glimepiride) Hoechst Marion Roussel ... 1241
DiaBeta Tablets (Glyburide) Hoechst Marion Roussel ... 1265
Diabinese Tablets (Chlorpropamide) Pfizer Inc ... 2002
Glucophage Tablets (Metformin Hydrochloride) Bristol-Myers Squibb ... 754
Glucotrol Tablets (Glipizide) Pfizer Inc ... 2011
Glucotrol XL Extended Release Tablets (Glipizide) Pfizer Inc ... 2012
Glynase PresTab Tablets (Glyburide) Pharmacia & Upjohn 2091
Micronase Tablets (Glyburide) Pharmacia & Upjohn ... 2099
Precose (Acarbose) Bayer Pharmaceutical ... 604

Hyperhidrosis associated with Parkinsonism
Levsin/Levsinex/Levbid (Hyoscyamine Sulfate) Schwarz ... 2549

Hyperhidrosis, topical relief of
Cruex Antifungal Powder (Calcium Undecylenate) Ciba Self-Medication ... ■ 652
Desenex Foot & Sneaker Deodorant Spray (Aluminum Chlorohydrate) Ciba Self-Medication ... ■ 653
Drysol Solution (Aluminum Chloride) Persōn & Covey ... 1989
Xerac AC Solution (Aluminum Chloride) Persōn & Covey ... 1990

Hyperkalemia
Kayexalate (Sodium Polystyrene Sulfonate) Sanofi Winthrop ... 2444
Sodium Polystyrene Sulfonate Suspension (Sodium Polystyrene Sulfonate) Roxane ... 2367

Hyperkeratosis skin disorders
Bichloracetic Acid Kahlenberg (Dichloroacetic Acid) Glenwood-Palisades ... 1233
Lac-Hydrin 12% Lotion (Ammonium Lactate) Westwood-Squibb .. 2796

Hyperlipidemia (see under Hyperlipoproteinemia, adjunct to diet)

Hyperlipoproteinemia, adjunct to diet (see also under Hypercholesterolemia, primary, adjunct to diet)
Atromid-S Capsules (Clofibrate) Wyeth-Ayerst ... 2808

Hyperlipoproteinemia, type III, adjunct to diet
Atromid-S Capsules (Clofibrate) Wyeth-Ayerst ... 2808

Hyperlipoproteinemia, types IIa and IIb, adjunct to diet
Lescol Capsules (Fluvastatin Sodium) Sandoz Pharmaceuticals 2395
Mevacor Tablets (Lovastatin) Merck & Co., Inc. ... 1742
Pravachol Tablets (Pravastatin Sodium) Bristol-Myers Squibb ... 770
Zocor Tablets (Simvastatin) Merck & Co., Inc. ... 1821

Hyperlipoproteinemia, types IV and V, adjunct to diet
Atromid-S Capsules (Clofibrate) Wyeth-Ayerst ... 2808
Lopid Tablets (Gemfibrozil) Parke-Davis ... 1974

Hyperphosphatemia
Basaljel (Aluminum Carbonate) Wyeth-Ayerst ... 2810
PhosLo Tablets (Calcium Acetate) Braintree ... 695

Hyperpigmentation, mottled, adjunct in
Renova (tretinoin emollient cream) 0.05% (Tretinoin) Ortho Dermatological ... 1945

Hyperpigmentation, skin, bleaching of
Eldopaque/Eldoquin/Solaquin/Viquin (Hydroquinone) ICN ... 1299
Melanex Topical Solution (Hydroquinone) Neutrogena ... 1842
Eldopaque/Eldoquin/Solaquin/Viquin (Hydroquinone) ICN ... 1299
Viquin Forte 4% Cream (Hydroquinone, Dioxybenzone, Oxybenzone, Padimate O (Octyl Dimethyl Paba)) ICN ... 1299

Hyperprolactinemia-associated dysfunctions
Parlodel (Bromocriptine Mesylate) Sandoz Pharmaceuticals ... 2411

Hypersecretory conditions, diagnosis of
Peptavlon (Pentagastrin) Wyeth-Ayerst ... 2997

Hypersecretory conditions, pathological
Pepcid Injection (Famotidine) Merck & Co., Inc. ... 1765
Pepcid (Famotidine) Merck & Co., Inc. ... 1763
Prevacid Delayed-Release Capsules (Lansoprazole) TAP ... 2746
Prilosec Delayed-Release Capsules (Omeprazole) Astra Merck ... 516
Tagamet (Cimetidine Hydrochloride) SmithKline Beecham Pharmaceuticals ... 2694
Zantac (Ranitidine Hydrochloride) Glaxo Wellcome ... 1182
Zantac Injection (Ranitidine Hydrochloride) Glaxo Wellcome ... 1180
Zantac Syrup (Ranitidine Hydrochloride) Glaxo Wellcome ... 1182

Hypersecretory conditions, pre-operative, symptomatic relief of
Levsin/Levsinex/Levbid (Hyoscyamine Sulfate) Schwarz ... 2549
Robinul Injectable (Glycopyrrolate) Robins ... 2247

Hypersensitivity, delayed, skin testing of
MSTA Mumps Skin Test Antigen (Mumps Skin Test Antigen) Connaught ... 2988

Hypersensitivity reactions, drug-induced
Celestone Soluspan Suspension (Betamethasone Sodium Phosphate, Betamethasone Acetate) Schering ... 2484
Cortone Acetate Sterile Suspension (Cortisone Acetate) Merck & Co., Inc. ... 1663
Cortone Acetate Tablets (Cortisone Acetate) Merck & Co., Inc. ... 1664
Dalalone D.P. Injectable (Dexamethasone Acetate) Forest ... 1009
Decadron Elixir (Dexamethasone) Merck & Co., Inc. ... 1676
Decadron Phosphate Injection (Dexamethasone Sodium Phosphate) Merck & Co., Inc. ... 1680
Decadron Tablets (Dexamethasone) Merck & Co., Inc. ... 1678
Decadron-LA Sterile Suspension (Dexamethasone Acetate) Merck & Co., Inc. ... 1687
EpiPen (Epinephrine) Center ... 808
Hydeltrasol Injection, Sterile (Prednisolone Sodium Phosphate) Merck & Co., Inc. ... 1708
Hydrocortone Phosphate Injection, Sterile (Hydrocortisone Sodium Phosphate) Merck & Co., Inc. ... 1713
Hydrocortone Tablets (Hydrocortisone) Merck & Co., Inc. ... 1715
Pediapred Oral Solution (Prednisolone Sodium Phosphate) Medeva 1618
Prelone Syrup (Prednisolone) Muro 1834

Hypertension
Accupril Tablets (Quinapril Hydrochloride) Parke-Davis ... 1950
Adalat CC (Nifedipine) Bayer Pharmaceutical ... 582
Aldactazide Tablets (Spironolactone, Hydrochlorothiazide) Searle 2556
Aldactone Tablets (Spironolactone) Searle ... 2558
Aldoclor Tablets (Methyldopa, Chlorothiazide) Merck & Co., Inc. 1638
Aldomet Ester HCl Injection (Methyldopate Hydrochloride) Merck & Co., Inc. ... 1642
Aldomet Oral (Methyldopa) Merck & Co., Inc. ... 1640
Aldoril Tablets (Methyldopa, Hydrochlorothiazide) Merck & Co., Inc. ... 1644
Altace Capsules (Ramipril) Hoechst Marion Roussel ... 1238
Apresazide Capsules (Hydralazine Hydrochloride, Hydrochlorothiazide) CibaGeneva 824
Apresoline Hydrochloride Tablets (Hydralazine Hydrochloride) CibaGeneva ... 826
Blocadren Tablets (Timolol Maleate) Merck & Co., Inc. ... 1654
Calan SR Caplets (Verapamil Hydrochloride) Searle ... 2571
Calan Tablets (Verapamil Hydrochloride) Searle ... 2568
Capoten Tablets (Captopril) Bristol-Myers Squibb ... 740
Capozide Tablets (Captopril, Hydrochlorothiazide) Bristol-Myers Squibb ... 744
Cardene Capsules (Nicardipine Hydrochloride) Roche Pharmaceuticals ... 2261
Cardene I.V. (Nicardipine Hydrochloride) Wyeth-Ayerst ... 2815
Cardene SR Capsules (Nicardipine Hydrochloride) Roche Pharmaceuticals ... 2264
Cardizem CD Capsules (Diltiazem Hydrochloride) Hoechst Marion Roussel ... 1251
Cardizem SR Capsules (Diltiazem Hydrochloride) Hoechst Marion Roussel ... 1255
Cardura Tablets (Doxazosin Mesylate) Pfizer Inc ... 1993
Cartrol Tablets (Carteolol Hydrochloride) Abbott ... 413
Catapres Tablets (Clonidine Hydrochloride) Boehringer Ingelheim ... 679
Catapres-TTS (Clonidine) Boehringer Ingelheim ... 680
Combipres Tablets (Clonidine Hydrochloride, Chlorthalidone) Boehringer Ingelheim ... 682
Covera-HS Tablets (Verapamil Hydrochloride) Searle ... 2573
Cozaar Tablets (Losartan Potassium) Merck & Co., Inc. ... 1668
Demadex Tablets and Injection (Torsemide) Boehringer Mannheim ... 691
Dilacor XR Extended-release Capsules (Diltiazem Hydrochloride) Rhone-Poulenc Rorer Pharmaceuticals ... 2183
Diucardin Tablets (Hydroflumethiazide) Wyeth-Ayerst ... 2824
Diupres Tablets (Reserpine, Chlorothiazide) Merck & Co., Inc. 1691
Diuril Oral (Chlorothiazide) Merck & Co., Inc. ... 1694
Dyazide Capsules (Triamterene, Hydrochlorothiazide) SmithKline Beecham Pharmaceuticals ... 2653
DynaCirc Capsules (Isradipine) Sandoz Pharmaceuticals ... 2381
DynaCirc CR Tablets (Isradipine) Sandoz Pharmaceuticals ... 2383
Enduron Tablets (Methyclothiazide) Abbott ... 424
Esidrix Tablets (Hydrochlorothiazide) CibaGeneva ... 839
Esimil Tablets (Guanethidine Monosulfate, Hydrochlorothiazide) CibaGeneva ... 840
Hydralazine Hydrochloride Injection USP (Hydralazine Hydrochloride) SoloPak ... 2712
HydroDIURIL Tablets (Hydrochlorothiazide) Merck & Co., Inc. ... 1716
Hydropres Tablets (Reserpine, Hydrochlorothiazide) Merck & Co., Inc. ... 1718
Hylorel Tablets (Guanadrel Sulfate) Medeva ... 1613
Hytrin Capsules (Terazosin Hydrochloride) Abbott ... 434

Hypertension — Indications Index

Hypertension
- Hyzaar Tablets (Losartan Potassium, Hydrochlorothiazide) Merck & Co., Inc. ... 1720
- Inderal (Propranolol Hydrochloride) Wyeth-Ayerst ... 2834
- Inderal LA Long Acting Capsules (Propranolol Hydrochloride) Wyeth-Ayerst ... 2836
- Inderide Tablets (Propranolol Hydrochloride, Hydrochlorothiazide) Wyeth-Ayerst ... 2838
- Inderide LA Long Acting Capsules (Propranolol Hydrochloride, Hydrochlorothiazide) Wyeth-Ayerst ... 2840
- Inversine Tablets (Mecamylamine Hydrochloride) Merck & Co., Inc. 1729
- Ismelin Tablets (Guanethidine Monosulfate) CibaGeneva ... 845
- Isoptin Oral Tablets (Verapamil Hydrochloride) Knoll Laboratories ... 1393
- Isoptin SR Tablets (Verapamil Hydrochloride) Knoll Laboratories ... 1395
- Kerlone Tablets (Betaxolol Hydrochloride) Searle ... 2588
- Lasix Injection, Oral Solution and Tablets (Furosemide) Hoechst Marion Roussel ... 1267
- Levatol Tablets (Penbutolol Sulfate) Schwarz ... 2547
- Lopressor (Metoprolol Tartrate) CibaGeneva ... 848
- Lopressor HCT Tablets (Metoprolol Tartrate, Hydrochlorothiazide) CibaGeneva ... 850
- Lotensin Tablets (Benazepril Hydrochloride) CibaGeneva ... 852
- Lotensin HCT Tablets (Benazepril Hydrochloride, Hydrochlorothiazide) CibaGeneva ... 855
- Lotrel Capsules (Amlodipine Besylate, Benazepril Hydrochloride) CibaGeneva ... 858
- Mavik Tablets (Trandolapril) Knoll Pharmaceutical ... 1407
- Minipress Capsules (Prazosin Hydrochloride) Pfizer Inc ... 2015
- Minizide Capsules (Prazosin Hydrochloride, Polythiazide) Pfizer Inc ... 2016
- Moduretic Tablets (Amiloride Hydrochloride, Hydrochlorothiazide) Merck & Co., Inc. ... 1748
- Monopril Tablets (Fosinopril Sodium) Bristol-Myers Squibb ... 762
- Mykrox Tablets (Metolazone) Medeva ... 1617
- Normodyne Injection (Labetalol Hydrochloride) Schering ... 2519
- Normodyne Tablets (Labetalol Hydrochloride) Schering ... 2522
- Norvasc Tablets (Amlodipine Besylate) Pfizer Inc ... 2020
- Oretic Tablets (Hydrochlorothiazide) Abbott ... 450
- Plendil Extended-Release Tablets (Felodipine) Astra Merck ... 514
- Prinivil Tablets (Lisinopril) Merck & Co., Inc. ... 1776
- Prinzide Tablets (Lisinopril, Hydrochlorothiazide) Merck & Co., Inc. ... 1780
- Procardia XL Extended Release Tablets (Nifedipine) Pfizer Inc ... 2026
- Sectral Capsules (Acebutolol Hydrochloride) Wyeth-Ayerst ... 2914
- Ser-Ap-Es Tablets (Hydralazine Hydrochloride, Hydrochlorothiazide, Reserpine) CibaGeneva ... 867
- Sular Tablets (Nisoldipine) Zeneca .. 2961
- Tenex Tablets (Guanfacine Hydrochloride) Robins ... 2249
- Tenoretic Tablets (Atenolol, Chlorthalidone) Zeneca ... 2963
- Tenormin Tablets and I.V. Injection (Atenolol) Zeneca ... 2965
- Thalitone (Chlorthalidone) Horus 1293
- Tiazac Capsules (Diltiazem Hydrochloride) Forest ... 1019
- Timolide Tablets (Timolol Maleate, Hydrochlorothiazide) Merck & Co., Inc. ... 1791
- Toprol-XL Tablets (Metoprolol Succinate) Astra ... 560
- Trandate (Labetalol Hydrochloride) Glaxo Wellcome ... 1158
- Univasc Tablets (Moexipril Hydrochloride) Schwarz ... 2553
- Vaseretic Tablets (Enalapril Maleate, Hydrochlorothiazide) Merck & Co., Inc. ... 1810
- Vasotec I.V. (Enalaprilat) Merck & Co., Inc. ... 1814
- Vasotec Tablets (Enalapril Maleate) Merck & Co., Inc. ... 1816
- Verelan Capsules (Verapamil Hydrochloride) Lederle ... 1455
- Visken Tablets (Pindolol) Sandoz Pharmaceuticals ... 2428
- Zaroxolyn Tablets (Metolazone) Medeva ... 1625
- Zebeta Tablets (Bisoprolol Fumarate) Lederle ... 1457
- Zestoretic Tablets (Lisinopril, Hydrochlorothiazide) Zeneca ... 2968
- Zestril Tablets (Lisinopril) Zeneca 2972
- Ziac (Bisoprolol Fumarate, Hydrochlorothiazide) Lederle ... 1459

Hypertension associated with anesthesia
- Brevibloc (esmolol HCl) Injection (Esmolol Hydrochloride) Ohmeda 1860

Hypertension associated with intratracheal intubation
- Brevibloc (esmolol HCl) Injection (Esmolol Hydrochloride) Ohmeda 1860

Hypertension associated with surgical procedures
- Brevibloc (esmolol HCl) Injection (Esmolol Hydrochloride) Ohmeda 1860
- Nitro-Bid IV (Nitroglycerin) Hoechst Marion Roussel ... 1270

Hypertension, adjunctive treatment
- Aldactone Tablets (Spironolactone) Searle ... 2558
- Dyazide Capsules (Triamterene, Hydrochlorothiazide) SmithKline Beecham Pharmaceuticals ... 2653
- Enduron Tablets (Methyclothiazide) Abbott ... 424
- Midamor Tablets (Amiloride Hydrochloride) Merck & Co., Inc. 1746
- Oretic Tablets (Hydrochlorothiazide) Abbott 450

Hypertension, essential
(see under Hypertension)

Hypertension, malignant
- Hyperstat I.V. Injection (Diazoxide) Schering ... 2504
- Inversine Tablets (Mecamylamine Hydrochloride) Merck & Co., Inc. 1729

Hypertension, non-malignant
- Hyperstat I.V. Injection (Diazoxide) Schering ... 2504

Hypertension, ocular
(see also under Glaucoma, aphakic; Glaucoma, chronic open-angle; Glaucoma, secondary)
- Betagan (Levobunolol Hydrochloride) Allergan ... ⊚ 230
- Betimol 0.25%, 0.5% (Timolol Hemihydrate) CIBA Vision Ophthalmics ... ⊚ 259
- Betoptic Ophthalmic Solution (Betaxolol Hydrochloride) Alcon Laboratories ... 465
- Betoptic S Ophthalmic Suspension (Betaxolol Hydrochloride) Alcon Laboratories ... 467
- Isopto Carbachol Ophthalmic Solution (Carbachol) Alcon Laboratories ... ⊚ 221
- Isopto Carpine Ophthalmic Solution (Pilocarpine Hydrochloride) Alcon Laboratories ... ⊚ 221
- Ocupress Ophthalmic Solution, 1% Sterile (Carteolol Hydrochloride) Otsuka America ⊚ 297
- Ocusert Pilo-20 and Pilo-40 Ocular Therapeutic Systems (Pilocarpine) Alza ... ⊚ 252
- OptiPranolol (Metipranolol 0.3%) Sterile Ophthalmic Solution (Metipranolol Hydrochloride) Bausch & Lomb Pharmaceuticals ... ⊚ 256
- Pilagan (Pilocarpine Nitrate) Allergan ... ⊚ 245
- Pilopine HS Ophthalmic Gel (Pilocarpine Hydrochloride) Alcon Laboratories ... ⊚ 224
- Timoptic in Ocudose (Timolol Maleate) Merck & Co., Inc. ... 1796
- Timoptic Sterile Ophthalmic Solution (Timolol Maleate) Merck & Co., Inc. ... 1794
- Timoptic-XE (Timolol Maleate) Merck & Co., Inc. ... 1798
- Trusopt Sterile Ophthalmic Solution (Dorzolamide Hydrochloride) Merck & Co., Inc. 1803
- Xalatan (Latanoprost) Pharmacia & Upjohn ... ⊚ 304

Hypertension, ocular, diagnostic agent for
- FLURESS (Fluorescein Sodium, Benoxinate Hydrochloride) Akorn ... ⊚ 208

Hypertension, ocular, post-surgical
- IOPIDINE Sterile Ophthalmic Solution (Apraclonidine Hydrochloride) Alcon Laboratories ... ⊚ 218
- MIOSTAT Intraocular Solution (Carbachol) Alcon Laboratories ⊚ 222

Hypertension, ocular, short-term reduction of
- Iopidine 0.5% (Apraclonidine Hydrochloride) Alcon Laboratories ... ⊚ 219
- ISMOTIC 45% w/v Solution (Isosorbide) Alcon Laboratories ⊚ 221
- OSMOGLYN Oral Osmotic Agent (Glycerin) Alcon Laboratories .... ⊚ 225

Hypertension, pulmonary
- Flolan for Injection (Epoprostenol Sodium) Glaxo Wellcome ... 1085

Hypertension, pulmonary, persistent, of the newborn
- Priscoline Hydrochloride Ampuls (Tolazoline Hydrochloride) CibaGeneva ... 864

Hypertension, renal
- Ismelin Tablets (Guanethidine Monosulfate) CibaGeneva ... 845

Hypertension, secondary to amyloidosis
- Ismelin Tablets (Guanethidine Monosulfate) CibaGeneva ... 845

Hypertension, secondary to pyelonephritis
- Ismelin Tablets (Guanethidine Monosulfate) CibaGeneva ... 845

Hypertension, secondary to renal artery stenosis
- Ismelin Tablets (Guanethidine Monosulfate) CibaGeneva ... 845

Hypertension, severe, acute
- Hyperstat I.V. Injection (Diazoxide) Schering ... 2504

Hypertensive episodes, control of, in pheochromocytoma
(see also under Pheochromocytoma, adjunctive therapy)
- Dibenzyline Capsules (Phenoxybenzamine Hydrochloride) SmithKline Beecham Pharmaceuticals ... 2650
- Regitine Vials (Phentolamine Mesylate) CibaGeneva ... 864

Hyperthermia, malignant, prophylaxis
- Dantrium Capsules (Dantrolene Sodium) Procter & Gamble Pharmaceuticals ... 2131
- Dantrium Intravenous (Dantrolene Sodium) Procter & Gamble Pharmaceuticals ... 2132

Hyperthermia, malignant, treatment adjunct
- Dantrium Intravenous (Dantrolene Sodium) Procter & Gamble Pharmaceuticals ... 2132

Hyperthyroidism
- Tapazole Tablets (Methimazole) Jones Medical Industries ... 1361

Hypertriglyceridemia, adjunct to diet
(see also under Dysbetalipoproteinemia)
- Atromid-S Capsules (Clofibrate) Wyeth-Ayerst ... 2808

Hyperuricemia associated with gout
- Benemid Tablets (Probenecid) Merck & Co., Inc. ... 1651

Hyperuricemia associated with gouty arthritis
- Benemid Tablets (Probenecid) Merck & Co., Inc. ... 1651

Hypnotic
(see under Sleep, induction of)

Hypocalcemia
- Calci-Chew Tablets (Calcium Carbonate) R&D ... 2168
- Calci-Mix Capsules (Calcium Carbonate) R&D ... 2168
- Calphosan Injection (Calcium Glycerophosphate, Calcium Lactate) Glenwood-Palisades ... 1234
- Caltrate 600 (Calcium Carbonate) Lederle Consumer .. ⊠ 681
- Caltrate PLUS (Calcium Carbonate, Vitamin D) Lederle Consumer ... ⊠ 681
- Citracal Tablets (Calcium Citrate) Mission ... 1828
- Nephro-Calci Tablets (Calcium Carbonate) R&D ... 2168
- One-A-Day Calcium Plus (Calcium Carbonate, Magnesium Carbonate, Vitamin D) Bayer Consumer ... ⊠ 625
- Rocaltrol Capsules (Calcitriol) Roche Pharmaceuticals ... 2303
- Tums 500 Calcium Supplement (Calcium Carbonate) SmithKline Beecham Consumer ⊠ 788

Hypocalcemia associated with chronic renal failure
- Calcijex Injection (Calcitriol) Abbott 412
- Rocaltrol Capsules (Calcitriol) Roche Pharmaceuticals ... 2303

Hypocalcemia with vitamin D, deficiency of
- Caltrate 600 + D (Calcium Carbonate, Vitamin D) Lederle Consumer ... ⊠ 681
- Dical-D Tablets & Wafers (Calcium Phosphate, Dibasic, Vitamin D) Abbott ... 424

Hypoestrogenism
- Climara Transdermal System (Estradiol) Berlex ... 640
- Ogen Tablets (Estropipate) Pharmacia & Upjohn ... 2103
- Ortho-Est (Estropipate) Ortho Pharmaceutical ... 1925
- Premarin Tablets (Estrogens, Conjugated) Wyeth-Ayerst ... 2896
- Vivelle Transdermal System (Estradiol) CibaGeneva ... 880

Hypogammaglobulinemia, prevention of bacterial infections
- Gammar-P I.V., Immune Globulin Intravenous (Human) (Globulin, Immune (Human)) Centeon ... 798

Hypoglycemia due to hyperinsulinism
- Glucagon for Injection Vials and Emergency Kit (Glucagon) Lilly 1485
- Proglycem (Diazoxide) Baker Norton ... 575

Hypoglycemia due to insulin shock therapy
- Glucagon for Injection Vials and Emergency Kit (Glucagon) Lilly .. 1485

Hypogonadism, female
- Estrace Cream and Tablets (Estradiol) Bristol-Myers Squibb .. 751
- Estraderm Transdermal System (Estradiol) CibaGeneva ... 842

(⊠ Described in PDR For Nonprescription Drugs)   (⊚ Described in PDR For Ophthalmology)

ESTRATAB Tablets (0.3, 0.625, 1.25, 2.5 mg) (Estrogens, Esterified) Solvay 2715
Menest Tablets (Estrogens, Esterified) SmithKline Beecham Pharmaceuticals 2671
Ogen Tablets (Estropipate) Pharmacia & Upjohn 2103
Ortho-Est (Estropipate) Ortho Pharmaceutical 1925

Hypogonadism, hypogonadotropic, in males
Androderm Testosterone Transdermal System (Testosterone) SmithKline Beecham Pharmaceuticals 2634
Android Capsules, 10 mg (Methyltestosterone) ICN 1297
Halotestin Tablets (Fluoxymesterone) Pharmacia & Upjohn 2095
Humegon for Injection (Menotropins) Organon 1873
Pergonal (menotropins for injection, USP) (Menotropins) Serono 2618
Pregnyl for Injection (Chorionic Gonadotropin) Organon 1878
Profasi (chorionic gonadotropin for injection, USP) (Chorionic Gonadotropin) Serono 2620
Testoderm Testosterone Transdermal System (Testosterone) Alza 486
Testred Capsules, 10 mg (Methyltestosterone) ICN 1308

Hypogonadism, hypogonadotropic, secondary, adjunctive therapy in
Humegon for Injection (Menotropins) Organon 1873
Pergonal (menotropins for injection, USP) (Menotropins) Serono 2618

Hypogonadism, male, primary
Androderm Testosterone Transdermal System (Testosterone) SmithKline Beecham Pharmaceuticals 2634
Android Capsules, 10 mg (Methyltestosterone) ICN 1297
Halotestin Tablets (Fluoxymesterone) Pharmacia & Upjohn 2095
Testoderm Testosterone Transdermal System (Testosterone) Alza 486

Hypokalemia with certain diarrheal states, prevention of
Micro-K (Potassium Chloride) Robins 2237
Micro-K LS Packets (Potassium Chloride) Robins 2238
Slow-K Extended-Release Tablets (Potassium Chloride) CibaGeneva 869

Hypokalemia with metabolic acidosis
Micro-K (Potassium Chloride) Robins 2237
Micro-K LS Packets (Potassium Chloride) Robins 2238
Slow-K Extended-Release Tablets (Potassium Chloride) CibaGeneva 869

Hypokalemia with metabolic alkalosis
K-Dur Microburst Release System (potassium chloride, USP) E.R. Tablets (Potassium Chloride) Key 1364
K-Lor Powder Packets (Potassium Chloride) Abbott 438
K-Norm Capsules (Potassium Chloride) Medeva 1615
K-Tab Filmtab (Potassium Chloride) Abbott 439
Micro-K (Potassium Chloride) Robins 2237
Slow-K Extended-Release Tablets (Potassium Chloride) CibaGeneva 869

Hypokalemia with significant cardiac arrhythmias
K-Dur Microburst Release System (potassium chloride, USP) E.R. Tablets (Potassium Chloride) Key 1364
K-Lor Powder Packets (Potassium Chloride) Abbott 438
K-Tab Filmtab (Potassium Chloride) Abbott 439
Slow-K Extended-Release Tablets (Potassium Chloride) CibaGeneva 869

Hypokalemia without metabolic alkalosis
K-Dur Microburst Release System (potassium chloride, USP) E.R. Tablets (Potassium Chloride) Key 1364
K-Lor Powder Packets (Potassium Chloride) Abbott 438
K-Norm Capsules (Potassium Chloride) Medeva 1615
K-Tab Filmtab (Potassium Chloride) Abbott 439
Micro-K (Potassium Chloride) Robins 2237
Micro-K LS Packets (Potassium Chloride) Robins 2238

Hypokalemia, digitalis intoxication-induced
K-Dur Microburst Release System (potassium chloride, USP) E.R. Tablets (Potassium Chloride) Key 1364
K-Lor Powder Packets (Potassium Chloride) Abbott 438
K-Norm Capsules (Potassium Chloride) Medeva 1615
K-Tab Filmtab (Potassium Chloride) Abbott 439
Micro-K (Potassium Chloride) Robins 2237
Micro-K LS Packets (Potassium Chloride) Robins 2238
Rum-K Syrup (Potassium Chloride) Fleming 1004
Slow-K Extended-Release Tablets (Potassium Chloride) CibaGeneva 869

Hypokalemia, digitalis-induced, prophylaxis of
Aldactone Tablets (Spironolactone) Searle 2558

Hypokalemia, drug-induced
K-Dur Microburst Release System (potassium chloride, USP) E.R. Tablets (Potassium Chloride) Key 1364
Micro-K (Potassium Chloride) Robins 2237
Micro-K LS Packets (Potassium Chloride) Robins 2238
Rum-K Syrup (Potassium Chloride) Fleming 1004
Slow-K Extended-Release Tablets (Potassium Chloride) CibaGeneva 869

Hypokalemia, drug-induced in congestive heart failure, prevention of
Micro-K (Potassium Chloride) Robins 2237
Micro-K LS Packets (Potassium Chloride) Robins 2238
Rum-K Syrup (Potassium Chloride) Fleming 1004
Slow-K Extended-Release Tablets (Potassium Chloride) CibaGeneva 869

Hypokalemia, hepatic cirrhosis with ascites-induced, prevention of
Micro-K (Potassium Chloride) Robins 2237
Micro-K LS Packets (Potassium Chloride) Robins 2238
Slow-K Extended-Release Tablets (Potassium Chloride) CibaGeneva 869

Hypokalemia, potassium-losing nephropathy-induced, prevention of
Slow-K Extended-Release Tablets (Potassium Chloride) CibaGeneva 869

Hypokalemia, unspecified
Aldactone Tablets (Spironolactone) Searle 2558
K-Dur Microburst Release System (potassium chloride, USP) E.R. Tablets (Potassium Chloride) Key 1364

Hypomagnesemia
Mag-Carb Capsules (Magnesium Carbonate) R&D 2168
Magonate Tablets and Liquid (Magnesium Gluconate) Fleming 1003
Mag-Ox 400 (Magnesium Oxide) Blaine 666
MagTab SR Caplets (Magnesium Lactate) Niché 1844
Uro-Mag (Magnesium Oxide) Blaine 666

Hypoparathyroidism, unspecified
DHT (Dihydrotachysterol) Tablets & Intensol (Dihydrotachysterol) Roxane 2351

Hypophosphatemia
K-Phos Neutral Tablets (Potassium Phosphate, Monobasic, Sodium Phosphate, Monobasic, Sodium Phosphate, Dibasic) Beach 633

Hypopigmentation, skin
Benoquin Cream 20% (Monobenzone) ICN 1298
8-MOP Capsules (Methoxsalen) ICN 1294
Oxsoralen Lotion 1% (Methoxsalen) ICN 1301
Trisoralen Tablets (Trioxsalen) ICN 1309

Hypoproteinemia
Albuminar-5, Albumin (Human) U.S.P. 5% (Albumin (Human)) Centeon 795
Albuminar-25, Albumin (Human) U.S.P. 25% (Albumin (Human)) Centeon 796
Plasma-Plex, Plasma Protein Fraction (Human) U.S.P. 5% Solution Heat-Treated (Plasma Protein Fraction (Human)) Centeon 806

Hypoprothrombinemia due to antibacterial therapy
AquaMEPHYTON Injection (Phytonadione) Merck & Co., Inc. 1648

Hypoprothrombinemia, drug-induced
AquaMEPHYTON Injection (Phytonadione) Merck & Co., Inc. 1648
Mephyton Tablets (Phytonadione) Merck & Co., Inc. 1739

Hypoprothrombinemia, salicylate-induced
AquaMEPHYTON Injection (Phytonadione) Merck & Co., Inc. 1648
Mephyton Tablets (Phytonadione) Merck & Co., Inc. 1739

Hypoprothrombinemia, secondary factors-induced
AquaMEPHYTON Injection (Phytonadione) Merck & Co., Inc. 1648
Mephyton Tablets (Phytonadione) Merck & Co., Inc. 1739

Hypotension
Neo-Synephrine Hydrochloride 1% Carpuject (Phenylephrine Hydrochloride) Sanofi Winthrop .. 2455
Neo-Synephrine Hydrochloride 1% Injection (Phenylephrine Hydrochloride) Sanofi Winthrop .. 2455

Hypotension associated with hemorrhage, adjunct to
Aramine Injection (Metaraminol Bitartrate) Merck & Co., Inc. 1649

Hypotension associated with spinal anesthesia
Aramine Injection (Metaraminol Bitartrate) Merck & Co., Inc. 1649
Levophed Bitartrate Injection (Norepinephrine Bitartrate) Sanofi Winthrop 2445

Hypotension due to drug reactions, adjunct to
Aramine Injection (Metaraminol Bitartrate) Merck & Co., Inc. 1649
Levophed Bitartrate Injection (Norepinephrine Bitartrate) Sanofi Winthrop 2445

Hypotension due to surgical complications, adjunct to
Aramine Injection (Metaraminol Bitartrate) Merck & Co., Inc. 1649

Hypotension, acute
Levophed Bitartrate Injection (Norepinephrine Bitartrate) Sanofi Winthrop 2445
Vasoxyl Injection (Methoxamine Hydrochloride) Glaxo Wellcome 1169

Hypotension, controlled, production of during surgical procedures
Nitro-Bid IV (Nitroglycerin) Hoechst Marion Roussel 1270

Hypotension, shock associated with brain damage due to trauma, adjunct to
Aramine Injection (Metaraminol Bitartrate) Merck & Co., Inc. 1649

Hypotension, shock associated with brain damage due to tumor, adjunct to
Aramine Injection (Metaraminol Bitartrate) Merck & Co., Inc. 1649

Hypothalamic-pituitary gonadotropic function, diagnostic evaluation of
Factrel (Gonadorelin Hydrochloride) Wyeth-Ayerst 2996

Hypothyroidism, ordinary
(see under Hypothyroidism, replacement or supplemental therapy in)

Hypothyroidism, primary
(see under Hypothyroidism, replacement or supplemental therapy in)

Hypothyroidism, replacement or supplemental therapy in
Cytomel Tablets (Liothyronine Sodium) SmithKline Beecham Pharmaceuticals 2647
Eltroxin Tablets (Levothyroxine Sodium) Roberts 2214
Levothroid Tablets (Levothyroxine Sodium) Forest 1015
Levothyroxine Sodium, USP for Injection (Levothyroxine Sodium) Astra 546
Levoxyl Tablets (Levothyroxine Sodium) Daniels 918
Synthroid (Levothyroxine Sodium) Knoll Pharmaceutical 1410

Hypothyroidism, secondary
(see under Hypothyroidism, replacement or supplemental therapy in)

Hypothyroidism, tertiary
(see under Hypothyroidism, replacement or supplemental therapy in)

Hypovolemia
Hespan Injection (Hetastarch) DuPont 945

Hypovolemic shock, treatment adjunct
Isuprel Injection (Isoproterenol Hydrochloride) Sanofi Winthrop .. 2441

Hysteria, acute
Vistaril Intramuscular Solution (Hydroxyzine Hydrochloride) Pfizer Inc 2042

Hysterosalpingography, diagnostic aid in
Ethiodol Injection (Ethiodized Oil) Savage 2472

I

Ichthyosis vulgaris
Lac-Hydrin 12% Lotion (Ammonium Lactate) Westwood-Squibb .. 2796

Idiopathic thrombocytopenic purpura
(see under Purpura, idiopathic thrombocytopenic)

Ileostomies, reducing the volume of discharge
Imodium Capsules (Loperamide Hydrochloride) Janssen ... 1343

Ileostomies, reduction in odor, adjunct to
Devrom Chewable Tablets (Bismuth Subgallate) Parthenon ... 714

Immunization, cholera
Cholera Vaccine (Cholera Vaccine) Wyeth-Ayerst ... 2818

Immunization, diphtheria and tetanus
Diphtheria & Tetanus Toxoids Adsorbed Purogenated (Diphtheria & Tetanus Toxoids Adsorbed, (For Pediatric Use)) Lederle ... 1422
Tetanus & Diphtheria Toxoids Adsorbed Purogenated (Tetanus & Diphtheria Toxoids Adsorbed) Lederle ... 1446

Immunization, diphtheria, tetanus and pertussis
Acel-Imune Diphtheria and Tetanus Toxoids and Acellular Pertussis Vaccine Adsorbed (Diphtheria & Tetanus Toxoids and Acellular Pertussis Vaccine) Lederle ... 1415
Diphtheria and Tetanus Toxoids and Pertussis Vaccine Adsorbed (Diphtheria & Tetanus Toxoids and Pertussis Vaccine Adsorbed) SmithKline Beecham Pharmaceuticals ... 2650
Tri-Immunol Adsorbed (Diphtheria & Tetanus Toxoids and Pertussis Vaccine Adsorbed) Lederle ... 1452
Tripedia (Diphtheria & Tetanus Toxoids w/Pertussis Vaccine Combined, Aluminum Potassium Sulfate Adsorbed) Connaught ... 908

Immunization, diphtheria, tetanus, pertussis, and haemophilus influenzae type B
ActHIB (Haemophilus B Conjugate Vaccine) Connaught ... 893
Tetramune (Diphtheria & Tetanus Toxoids and Pertussis with Hemophilus B Conjugate Vaccine) Lederle ... 1449

Immunization, Haemophilus influenzae type b
ActHIB (Haemophilus B Conjugate Vaccine) Connaught ... 893
HibTITER (Haemophilus B Conjugate Vaccine) Lederle ... 1423
OmniHIB (Haemophilus B Conjugate Vaccine) SmithKline Beecham Pharmaceuticals ... 2676
PedvaxHIB (Haemophilus B Conjugate Vaccine) Merck & Co., Inc. ... 1761

Immunization, hepatitis A virus
Havrix (Hepatitis A Vaccine, Inactivated) SmithKline Beecham Pharmaceuticals ... 2663

Immunization, hepatitis B virus
Engerix-B Unit-Dose Vials (Hepatitis B Vaccine) SmithKline Beecham Pharmaceuticals ... 2656

Immunization, hepatitis B virus, post-exposure
Hep-B-Gammagee (Hepatitis B Immune Globulin (Human)) Merck & Co., Inc. ... 1706

Immunization, influenza virus, types A and B
Fluvirin (Influenza Virus Vaccine) (Influenza Virus Vaccine) Medeva 1608
Influenza Virus Vaccine, Trivalent, Types A and B (chromatograph- and filter-purified subviron antigen) FluShield, 1996-1997 Formula (Influenza Virus Vaccine) Wyeth-Ayerst ... 2842

Immunization, Japanese encephalitis
JE-VAX (Japanese Encephalitis Vaccine Inactivated) Connaught ... 904

Immunization, poliovirus 1, 2, and 3
IPOL Poliovirus Vaccine Inactivated (Poliovirus Vaccine Inactivated, Trivalent Types 1,2,3) Connaught ... 903
Orimune (Poliovirus Vaccine, Live, Oral, Trivalent, Types 1,2,3 (Sabin)) Lederle ... 1433

Immunization, rabies
Imovax Rabies Vaccine (Rabies Vaccine) Connaught ... 899
Rabies Vaccine Adsorbed (Rabies Vaccine) SmithKline Beecham Pharmaceuticals ... 2686
Rabies Vaccine, Imovax Rabies I.D. (Rabies Vaccine) Connaught ... 901

Immunization, tetanus
Hyper-Tet Tetanus Immune Globulin (Human) (Tetanus Immune Globulin (Human)) Bayer Biological ... 621
Tetanus Toxoid Adsorbed Purogenated (Tetanus Toxoid, Adsorbed) Lederle ... 1447

Immunization, typhoid fever
Typhim Vi (Typhoid Vi Polysaccharide Vaccine) Connaught ... 914
Typhoid Vaccine (Typhoid Vaccine) Wyeth-Ayerst ... 2929
Vivotif Berna (Typhoid Vaccine Live Oral TY21a) Berna ... 660

Immunization, varicella
Varivax (Varicella Virus Vaccine Live) Merck & Co., Inc. ... 1807

Immunodeficiencies, primary
Gamimune N, 5% Immune Globulin Intravenous (Human), 5% (Globulin, Immune (Human)) Bayer Biological ... 612

Immunodeficiencies, primary, maintenance treatment of
Gammagard S/D, Immune Globulin, Intravenous (Human) (Globulin, Immune (Human)) Baxter Healthcare ... 577
Sandoglobulin I.V. (Globulin, Immune (Human)) Sandoz Pharmaceuticals ... 2419

Immunodeficiencies, severe, combined
Gamimune N, 5% Immune Globulin Intravenous (Human), 5% (Globulin, Immune (Human)) Bayer Biological ... 612
Gamimune N, 10% Immune Globulin Intravenous (Human), 10% (Globulin, Immune (Human)) Bayer Biological ... 615
Gammagard S/D, Immune Globulin, Intravenous (Human) (Globulin, Immune (Human)) Baxter Healthcare ... 577
Sandoglobulin I.V. (Globulin, Immune (Human)) Sandoz Pharmaceuticals ... 2419

Immunodeficiency disease, severe combined
(see under Adenosine deaminase, enzyme replacement therapy for)

Immunodeficiency, common variable
Gamimune N, 5% Immune Globulin Intravenous (Human), 5% (Globulin, Immune (Human)) Bayer Biological ... 612
Gamimune N, 10% Immune Globulin Intravenous (Human), 10% (Globulin, Immune (Human)) Bayer Biological ... 615
Sandoglobulin I.V. (Globulin, Immune (Human)) Sandoz Pharmaceuticals ... 2419

Immunodeficiency, primary humoral
Gamimune N, 10% Immune Globulin Intravenous (Human), 10% (Globulin, Immune (Human)) Bayer Biological ... 615

Immunodeficiency, x-linked with hyper IgM
Gamimune N, 5% Immune Globulin Intravenous (Human), 5% (Globulin, Immune (Human)) Bayer Biological ... 612
Gamimune N, 10% Immune Globulin Intravenous (Human), 10% (Globulin, Immune (Human)) Bayer Biological ... 615
Sandoglobulin I.V. (Globulin, Immune (Human)) Sandoz Pharmaceuticals ... 2419

Impetigo contagiosa
Bactroban Ointment (Mupirocin) SmithKline Beecham Pharmaceuticals ... 2642
Ceftin for Oral Suspension (Cefuroxime Axetil) Glaxo Wellcome ... 1067
Garamycin 0.1% (Gentamicin Sulfate) Schering ... 2501

Impotence, male
(see under Erectile dysfunction, male)

Indigestion
(see under Digestive disorders, symptomatic relief of)

Infection, acquired immunodeficiency syndrome-related complex
Biaxin (Clarithromycin) Abbott ... 406
Crixivan Capsules (Indinavir Sulfate) Merck & Co., Inc. ... 1670
Cytovene (Ganciclovir Sodium) Roche Pharmaceuticals ... 2270
DaunoXome (Daunorubicin Citrate) NeXstar ... 1842
Doxil (Doxorubicin Hydrochloride) Sequus ... 2613
Foscavir Injection (Foscarnet Sodium) Astra ... 541
Gamimune N, 5% Immune Globulin Intravenous (Human), 5% (Globulin, Immune (Human)) Bayer Biological ... 612
Gamimune N, 10% Immune Globulin Intravenous (Human), 10% (Globulin, Immune (Human)) Bayer Biological ... 615
Intron A for Injection (Interferon alfa-2B, Recombinant) Schering .. 2506
Marinol (Dronabinol) Capsules (Dronabinol) Roxane ... 2353
Mycobutin Capsules (Rifabutin) Pharmacia & Upjohn ... 2101
Neutrexin for Injection (Trimetrexate Glucuronate) U.S. Bioscience 2761
Retrovir Capsules (Zidovudine) Glaxo Wellcome Oncology/HIV ... 1216
Retrovir I.V. Infusion (Zidovudine) Glaxo Wellcome Oncology/HIV ... 1221
Retrovir Syrup (Zidovudine) Glaxo Wellcome Oncology/HIV ... 1216
Septra (Trimethoprim, Sulfamethoxazole) Glaxo Wellcome ... 1146
Sporanox Capsules (Itraconazole) Janssen ... 1352
Vistide Injection (Cidofovir) Gilead Sciences ... 1057
WinRho SD (Rh₀(D) Immune Globulin (Human)) NABI ... 1840

Infection, human immunodeficiency virus
Epivir (Lamivudine) Glaxo Wellcome Oncology/HIV ... 1200
Hivid Tablets (Zalcitabine) Roche Pharmaceuticals ... 2287
Invirase Capsules (Saquinavir Mesylate) Roche Pharmaceuticals ... 2291
Norvir (Ritonavir) Abbott ... 447
Retrovir Capsules (Zidovudine) Glaxo Wellcome Oncology/HIV ... 1216
Retrovir I.V. Infusion (Zidovudine) Glaxo Wellcome Oncology/HIV ... 1221
Retrovir Syrup (Zidovudine) Glaxo Wellcome Oncology/HIV ... 1216
Videx Tablets, Powder for Oral Solution, & Pediatric Powder for Oral Solution (Didanosine) Bristol-Myers Squibb Oncology/Immunology ... 2980
Viramune Tablets (Nevirapine) Roxane ... 2368
Zerit Capsules (Stavudine) Bristol-Myers Squibb Oncology/Immunology ... 731

Infections, human immunodeficiency virus, in combination with protease inhibitors
Hivid Tablets (Zalcitabine) Roche Pharmaceuticals ... 2287

Infection, human immunodeficiency virus, maternal-fetal transmission
Retrovir Capsules (Zidovudine) Glaxo Wellcome Oncology/HIV ... 1216
Retrovir I.V. Infusion (Zidovudine) Glaxo Wellcome Oncology/HIV ... 1221
Retrovir Syrup (Zidovudine) Glaxo Wellcome Oncology/HIV ... 1216

Infections, human immunodeficiency virus, advanced, in combination with zidovudine
Hivid Tablets (Zalcitabine) Roche Pharmaceuticals ... 2287

Infections, aerobic organisms
Cefizox for Intramuscular or Intravenous Use (Ceftizoxime Sodium) Fujisawa ... 1025
Ceptaz (Ceftazidime) Glaxo Wellcome ... 1070
Fortaz (Ceftazidime) Glaxo Wellcome ... 1092
Mefoxin (Cefoxitin Sodium) Merck & Co., Inc. ... 1734
Mefoxin Premixed Intravenous Solution (Cefoxitin Sodium) Merck & Co., Inc. ... 1737
Mezlin (Mezlocillin Sodium) Bayer Pharmaceutical ... 594
Mezlin Pharmacy Bulk Package (Mezlocillin Sodium) Bayer Pharmaceutical ... 597
Tazicef for Injection (Ceftazidime) SmithKline Beecham Pharmaceuticals ... 2697
Tazidime Vials, Faspak & ADD-Vantage (Ceftazidime) Lilly .. 1531

Infections, anaerobic cocci
Cefizox for Intramuscular or Intravenous Use (Ceftizoxime Sodium) Fujisawa ... 1025
Claforan Sterile and Injection (Cefotaxime Sodium) Hoechst Marion Roussel ... 1259
Pipracil (Piperacillin Sodium) Lederle ... 1435

Infections, anaerobic organisms
Cefobid Intravenous/Intramuscular (Cefoperazone Sodium) Pfizer Inc ... 1996
Cefobid Pharmacy Bulk Package - Not for Direct Infusion (Cefoperazone Sodium) Pfizer Inc ... 1999
Ceptaz (Ceftazidime) Glaxo Wellcome ... 1070
Cleocin Phosphate Injection (Clindamycin Phosphate) Pharmacia & Upjohn ... 2068
Flagyl 375 Capsules (Metronidazole) Searle ... 2587
Flagyl I.V. (Metronidazole Hydrochloride) SCS ... 2373
Fortaz (Ceftazidime) Glaxo Wellcome ... 1092
Garamycin Injectable (Gentamicin Sulfate) Schering ... 2502
Mefoxin (Cefoxitin Sodium) Merck & Co., Inc. ... 1734
Mefoxin Premixed Intravenous Solution (Cefoxitin Sodium) Merck & Co., Inc. ... 1737
Mezlin (Mezlocillin Sodium) Bayer Pharmaceutical ... 594
Mezlin Pharmacy Bulk Package (Mezlocillin Sodium) Bayer Pharmaceutical ... 597
Pipracil (Piperacillin Sodium) Lederle ... 1435
Primaxin I.V. (Cilastatin Sodium, Imipenem) Merck & Co., Inc. ... 1772
Tazicef for Injection (Ceftazidime) SmithKline Beecham Pharmaceuticals ... 2697
Tazidime Vials, Faspak & ADD-Vantage (Ceftazidime) Lilly .. 1531

1535 Indications Index Infections

Ticar for Injection (Ticarcillin Disodium) SmithKline Beecham Pharmaceuticals ... 2704

Infections, beta-lactamase producing organisms
Augmentin (Amoxicillin Trihydrate, Clavulanate Potassium) SmithKline Beecham Pharmaceuticals ... 2637
Augmentin Tablets (Amoxicillin Trihydrate, Clavulanate Potassium) SmithKline Beecham Pharmaceuticals ... 2640
Ceftin (Cefuroxime Axetil) Glaxo Wellcome ... 1067
Cefzil Tablets and Oral Suspension (Cefprozil) Bristol-Myers Squibb .. 747
Lorabid Suspension and Pulvules (Loracarbef) Lilly ... 1513
Merrem I.V. (Meropenem) Zeneca .. 2952
Unasyn (Ampicillin Sodium, Sulbactam Sodium) Pfizer Inc ... 2035
Vantin for Oral Suspension and Vantin Tablets (Cefpodoxime Proxetil) Pharmacia & Upjohn ... 2112
Zosyn (Piperacillin Sodium, Tazobactam Sodium) Lederle ... 1463

Infections, biliary tract
Ancef Injection (Cefazolin Sodium) SmithKline Beecham Pharmaceuticals ... 2632
Kefzol Vials, Faspak & ADD-Vantage (Cefazolin Sodium) Lilly ... 1511
Pipracil (Piperacillin Sodium) Lederle ... 1435

Infections, bone and joint
Amikacin Sulfate Injection, USP (Amikacin Sulfate) Astra ... 523
Amikacin Sulfate Injection, USP (Amikacin Sulfate) Elkins-Sinn ... 981
Amikin Injectable (Amikacin Sulfate) Apothecon ... 502
Ancef Injection (Cefazolin Sodium) SmithKline Beecham Pharmaceuticals ... 2632
Cefizox for Intramuscular or Intravenous Use (Ceftizoxime Sodium) Fujisawa ... 1025
Cefotan (Cefotetan) Zeneca ... 2936
Ceptaz (Ceftazidime) Glaxo Wellcome ... 1070
Cipro I.V. (Ciprofloxacin) Bayer Pharmaceutical ... 587
Cipro I.V. Pharmacy Bulk Package (Ciprofloxacin) Bayer Pharmaceutical ... 590
Cipro Tablets (Ciprofloxacin Hydrochloride) Bayer Pharmaceutical ... 584
Claforan Sterile and Injection (Cefotaxime Sodium) Hoechst Marion Roussel ... 1259
Cleocin Phosphate Injection (Clindamycin Phosphate) Pharmacia & Upjohn ... 2068
Flagyl 375 Capsules (Metronidazole) Searle ... 2587
Flagyl I.V. (Metronidazole Hydrochloride) SCS ... 2373
Fortaz (Ceftazidime) Glaxo Wellcome ... 1092
Garamycin Injectable (Gentamicin Sulfate) Schering ... 2502
Keflex Pulvules & Oral Suspension (Cephalexin) Dista ... 930
Keftab Tablets (Cephalexin Hydrochloride) Dista ... 931
Kefurox Vials, Faspak & ADD-Vantage (Cefuroxime Sodium) Lilly ... 1509
Kefzol Vials, Faspak & ADD-Vantage (Cefazolin Sodium) Lilly ... 1511
Mandol Vials, Faspak & ADD-Vantage (Cefamandole Nafate) Lilly ... 1516
Mefoxin (Cefoxitin Sodium) Merck & Co., Inc. ... 1734
Mefoxin Premixed Intravenous Solution (Cefoxitin Sodium) Merck & Co., Inc. ... 1737
Monocid Injection (Cefonicid Sodium) SmithKline Beecham Pharmaceuticals ... 2674
Nebcin Vials, Hyporets & ADD-Vantage (Tobramycin Sulfate) Lilly ... 1518
Pipracil (Piperacillin Sodium) Lederle ... 1435
Primaxin I.V. (Cilastatin Sodium, Imipenem) Merck & Co., Inc. ... 1772
Rocephin Injectable Vials, ADD-Vantage, Galaxy Container (Ceftriaxone Sodium) Roche Pharmaceuticals ... 2305
Tazicef for Injection (Ceftazidime) SmithKline Beecham Pharmaceuticals ... 2697
Tazidime Vials, Faspak & ADD-Vantage (Ceftazidime) Lilly .. 1531
Timentin for Injection (Ticarcillin Disodium, Clavulanate Potassium) SmithKline Beecham Pharmaceuticals ... 2706
Zinacef (Cefuroxime Sodium) Glaxo Wellcome ... 1184

Infections, burn wound (see also under Infections, skin, bacterial, minor)
Amikacin Sulfate Injection, USP (Amikacin Sulfate) Astra ... 523
Amikacin Sulfate Injection, USP (Amikacin Sulfate) Elkins-Sinn ... 981
Amikin Injectable (Amikacin Sulfate) Apothecon ... 502
Azactam for Injection (Aztreonam) Bristol-Myers Squibb ... 736
Garamycin Injectable (Gentamicin Sulfate) Schering ... 2502
SSD (Silver Sulfadiazine) Knoll Laboratories ... 1402

Infections, central nervous system
Amikacin Sulfate Injection, USP (Amikacin Sulfate) Astra ... 523
Amikacin Sulfate Injection, USP (Amikacin Sulfate) Elkins-Sinn ... 981
Amikin Injectable (Amikacin Sulfate) Apothecon ... 502
Ceptaz (Ceftazidime) Glaxo Wellcome ... 1070
Claforan Sterile and Injection (Cefotaxime Sodium) Hoechst Marion Roussel ... 1259
Flagyl 375 Capsules (Metronidazole) Searle ... 2587
Flagyl I.V. (Metronidazole Hydrochloride) SCS ... 2373
Fortaz (Ceftazidime) Glaxo Wellcome ... 1092
Garamycin Injectable (Gentamicin Sulfate) Schering ... 2502
Nebcin Vials, Hyporets & ADD-Vantage (Tobramycin Sulfate) Lilly ... 1518
Protostat Tablets (Metronidazole) Ortho Pharmaceutical ... 1939
Tazicef for Injection (Ceftazidime) SmithKline Beecham Pharmaceuticals ... 2697
Tazidime Vials, Faspak & ADD-Vantage (Ceftazidime) Lilly .. 1531

Infections, cutaneous dermatophyte, severe recalcitrant
Nizoral Tablets (Ketoconazole) Janssen ... 1345

Infections, fenestration cavities
Coly-Mycin S Otic w/Neomycin & Hydrocortisone (Colistin Sulfate, Neomycin Sulfate, Hydrocortisone Acetate) Parke-Davis ... 1965
Cortisporin Otic Suspension Sterile (Polymyxin B Sulfate, Neomycin Sulfate, Hydrocortisone) Glaxo Wellcome ... 1077
Pediotic Suspension Sterile (Polymyxin B Sulfate, Neomycin Sulfate, Hydrocortisone) Glaxo Wellcome ... 1140

Infections, fungal, severe systemic
Fungizone Intravenous (Amphotericin B) Apothecon ... 507

Infections, fungal, systemic
Diflucan Tablets, Injection, and Oral Suspension (Fluconazole) Pfizer Inc ... 2003

Infections, genitourinary tract
Ancef Injection (Cefazolin Sodium) SmithKline Beecham Pharmaceuticals ... 2632
Claforan Sterile and Injection (Cefotaxime Sodium) Hoechst Marion Roussel ... 1259
E-Mycin Tablets (Erythromycin) Knoll Laboratories ... 1388
Keflex Pulvules & Oral Suspension (Cephalexin) Dista ... 930
Keftab Tablets (Cephalexin Hydrochloride) Dista ... 931
Kefzol Vials, Faspak & ADD-Vantage (Cefazolin Sodium) Lilly ... 1511
Mefoxin (Cefoxitin Sodium) Merck & Co., Inc. ... 1734
Omnipen for Oral Suspension (Ampicillin) Wyeth-Ayerst ... 2873
Pfizerpen for Injection (Penicillin G Potassium) Pfizer Inc ... 2022
Spectrobid Tablets (Bacampicillin Hydrochloride) Pfizer Inc ... 2030
Ticar for Injection (Ticarcillin Disodium) SmithKline Beecham Pharmaceuticals ... 2704

Infections, genitourinary tract, "lacking substantial evidence of effectiveness" in
Urobiotic-250 Capsules (Oxytetracycline Hydrochloride, Sulfamethizole, Phenazopyridine Hydrochloride) Pfizer Inc ... 2038

Infections, gram-negative bacteria
Amikacin Sulfate Injection, USP (Amikacin Sulfate) Astra ... 523
Amikacin Sulfate Injection, USP (Amikacin Sulfate) Elkins-Sinn ... 981
Amikin Injectable (Amikacin Sulfate) Apothecon ... 502
Amoxil (Amoxicillin Trihydrate) SmithKline Beecham Pharmaceuticals ... 2631
Cefizox for Intramuscular or Intravenous Use (Ceftizoxime Sodium) Fujisawa ... 1025
Cefobid Intravenous/Intramuscular (Cefoperazone Sodium) Pfizer Inc ... 1996
Cefobid Pharmacy Bulk Package - Not for Direct Infusion (Cefoperazone Sodium) Pfizer Inc ... 1999
Chloromycetin Sodium Succinate (Chloramphenicol Sodium Succinate) Parke-Davis ... 1960
Doryx Capsules (Doxycycline Hyclate) Parke-Davis ... 1970
Garamycin Injectable (Gentamicin Sulfate) Schering ... 2502
Mefoxin (Cefoxitin Sodium) Merck & Co., Inc. ... 1734
Mefoxin Premixed Intravenous Solution (Cefoxitin Sodium) Merck & Co., Inc. ... 1737
Mezlin (Mezlocillin Sodium) Bayer Pharmaceutical ... 594
Mezlin Pharmacy Bulk Package (Mezlocillin Sodium) Bayer Pharmaceutical ... 597
Minocin Oral Suspension (Minocycline Hydrochloride) Lederle ... 1431
Monodox Capsules (Doxycycline Monohydrate) Oclassen ... 1858
Netromycin Injection 100 mg/ml (Netilmicin Sulfate) Schering ... 2516
Ocuflox Ophthalmic Solution (Ofloxacin) Allergan ... 478
Primaxin I.V. (Cilastatin Sodium, Imipenem) Merck & Co., Inc. ... 1772
Seromycin Capsules (Cycloserine) Dura ... 975
Ticar for Injection (Ticarcillin Disodium) SmithKline Beecham Pharmaceuticals ... 2704

Infections, gram-positive anaerobic cocci
Cefobid Intravenous/Intramuscular (Cefoperazone Sodium) Pfizer Inc ... 1996
Cefobid Pharmacy Bulk Package - Not for Direct Infusion (Cefoperazone Sodium) Pfizer Inc ... 1999
Cefotan (Cefotetan) Zeneca ... 2936
Mefoxin (Cefoxitin Sodium) Merck & Co., Inc. ... 1734
Mefoxin Premixed Intravenous Solution (Cefoxitin Sodium) Merck & Co., Inc. ... 1737

Infections, gram-positive bacteria
Amoxil (Amoxicillin Trihydrate) SmithKline Beecham Pharmaceuticals ... 2631
Doryx Capsules (Doxycycline Hyclate) Parke-Davis ... 1970
Mezlin (Mezlocillin Sodium) Bayer Pharmaceutical ... 594
Mezlin Pharmacy Bulk Package (Mezlocillin Sodium) Bayer Pharmaceutical ... 597
Minocin Oral Suspension (Minocycline Hydrochloride) Lederle ... 1431
Monodox Capsules (Doxycycline Monohydrate) Oclassen ... 1858
Ocuflox Ophthalmic Solution (Ofloxacin) Allergan ... 478
Omnipen Capsules (Ampicillin) Wyeth-Ayerst ... 2872
Omnipen for Oral Suspension (Ampicillin) Wyeth-Ayerst ... 2873
Primaxin I.V. (Cilastatin Sodium, Imipenem) Merck & Co., Inc. ... 1772
Seromycin Capsules (Cycloserine) Dura ... 975

Infections, gynecologic
Azactam for Injection (Aztreonam) Bristol-Myers Squibb ... 736
Cefobid Intravenous/Intramuscular (Cefoperazone Sodium) Pfizer Inc ... 1996
Cefobid Pharmacy Bulk Package - Not for Direct Infusion (Cefoperazone Sodium) Pfizer Inc ... 1999
Cefotan (Cefotetan) Zeneca ... 2936
Ceptaz (Ceftazidime) Glaxo Wellcome ... 1070
Claforan Sterile and Injection (Cefotaxime Sodium) Hoechst Marion Roussel ... 1259
Cleocin Phosphate Injection (Clindamycin Phosphate) Pharmacia & Upjohn ... 2068
E-Mycin Tablets (Erythromycin) Knoll Laboratories ... 1388
ERYC (Erythromycin) Parke-Davis .. 1972
Ery-Tab Tablets (Erythromycin) Abbott ... 426
Erythrocin Stearate Filmtab (Erythromycin Stearate) Abbott ... 429
Erythromycin Base Filmtab (Erythromycin) Abbott ... 430
Erythromycin Delayed-Release Capsules, USP (Erythromycin) Abbott ... 431
Flagyl 375 Capsules (Metronidazole) Searle ... 2587
Flagyl I.V. (Metronidazole Hydrochloride) SCS ... 2373
Fortaz (Ceftazidime) Glaxo Wellcome ... 1092
Mefoxin (Cefoxitin Sodium) Merck & Co., Inc. ... 1734
Mefoxin Premixed Intravenous Solution (Cefoxitin Sodium) Merck & Co., Inc. ... 1737
Mezlin (Mezlocillin Sodium) Bayer Pharmaceutical ... 594
Mezlin Pharmacy Bulk Package (Mezlocillin Sodium) Bayer Pharmaceutical ... 597
PCE Dispertab Tablets (Erythromycin) Abbott ... 453
Pipracil (Piperacillin Sodium) Lederle ... 1435
Primaxin I.M. (Cilastatin Sodium, Imipenem) Merck & Co., Inc. ... 1770
Primaxin I.V. (Cilastatin Sodium, Imipenem) Merck & Co., Inc. ... 1772
Tazicef for Injection (Ceftazidime) SmithKline Beecham Pharmaceuticals ... 2697
Tazidime Vials, Faspak & ADD-Vantage (Ceftazidime) Lilly .. 1531
Ticar for Injection (Ticarcillin Disodium) SmithKline Beecham Pharmaceuticals ... 2704
Timentin for Injection (Ticarcillin Disodium, Clavulanate Potassium) SmithKline Beecham Pharmaceuticals ... 2706
Unasyn (Ampicillin Sodium, Sulbactam Sodium) Pfizer Inc ... 2035
Vantin for Oral Suspension and Vantin Tablets (Cefpodoxime Proxetil) Pharmacia & Upjohn ... 2112
Zosyn (Piperacillin Sodium, Tazobactam Sodium) Lederle ... 1463

(▣ Described in PDR For Nonprescription Drugs) (◉ Described in PDR For Ophthalmology)

Infections — Indications Index

Infections, intra-abdominal
- Amikacin Sulfate Injection, USP (Amikacin Sulfate) Astra 523
- Amikacin Sulfate Injection, USP (Amikacin Sulfate) Elkins-Sinn 981
- Amikin Injectable (Amikacin Sulfate) Apothecon 502
- Azactam for Injection (Aztreonam) Bristol-Myers Squibb 736
- Cefizox for Intramuscular or Intravenous Use (Ceftizoxime Sodium) Fujisawa 1025
- Cefobid Intravenous/Intramuscular (Cefoperazone Sodium) Pfizer Inc 1996
- Cefobid Pharmacy Bulk Package - Not for Direct Infusion (Cefoperazone Sodium) Pfizer Inc 1999
- Cefotan (Cefotetan) Zeneca 2936
- Ceptaz (Ceftazidime) Glaxo Wellcome 1070
- Claforan Sterile and Injection (Cefotaxime Sodium) Hoechst Marion Roussel 1259
- Cleocin Phosphate Injection (Clindamycin Phosphate) Pharmacia & Upjohn 2068
- Flagyl 375 Capsules (Metronidazole) Searle 2587
- Flagyl I.V. (Metronidazole Hydrochloride) SCS 2373
- Fortaz (Ceftazidime) Glaxo Wellcome 1092
- Garamycin Injectable (Gentamicin Sulfate) Schering 2502
- Mefoxin (Cefoxitin Sodium) Merck & Co., Inc. 1734
- Mefoxin Premixed Intravenous Solution (Cefoxitin Sodium) Merck & Co., Inc. 1737
- Merrem I.V. (Meropenem) Zeneca 2952
- Mezlin (Mezlocillin Sodium) Bayer Pharmaceutical 594
- Mezlin Pharmacy Bulk Package (Mezlocillin Sodium) Bayer Pharmaceutical 597
- Nebcin Vials, Hyporets & ADD-Vantage (Tobramycin Sulfate) Lilly 1518
- Netromycin Injection 100 mg/ml (Netilmicin Sulfate) Schering 2516
- Omnipen for Oral Suspension (Ampicillin) Wyeth-Ayerst 2873
- Pipracil (Piperacillin Sodium) Lederle 1435
- Primaxin I.M. (Cilastatin Sodium, Imipenem) Merck & Co., Inc. 1770
- Primaxin I.V. (Cilastatin Sodium, Imipenem) Merck & Co., Inc. 1772
- Rocephin Injectable Vials, ADD-Vantage, Galaxy Container (Ceftriaxone Sodium) Roche Pharmaceuticals 2305
- Tazicef for Injection (Ceftazidime) SmithKline Beecham Pharmaceuticals 2697
- Tazidime Vials, Faspak & ADD-Vantage (Ceftazidime) Lilly .. 1531
- Ticar for Injection (Ticarcillin Disodium) SmithKline Beecham Pharmaceuticals 2704
- Timentin for Injection (Ticarcillin Disodium, Clavulanate Potassium) SmithKline Beecham Pharmaceuticals 2706
- Unasyn (Ampicillin Sodium, Sulbactam Sodium) Pfizer Inc 2035

Infections, lacrimal sac
(see under Dacryocystitis)

Infections, liver flukes
(see under Clonorchiasis)

Infections, lower respiratory tract
- Amoxil (Amoxicillin Trihydrate) SmithKline Beecham Pharmaceuticals 2631
- Augmentin (Amoxicillin Trihydrate, Clavulanate Potassium) SmithKline Beecham Pharmaceuticals 2637
- Augmentin Tablets (Amoxicillin Trihydrate, Clavulanate Potassium) SmithKline Beecham Pharmaceuticals 2640
- Azactam for Injection (Aztreonam) Bristol-Myers Squibb 736
- Biaxin (Clarithromycin) Abbott 406
- Ceclor Pulvules & Suspension (Cefaclor) Lilly 1470
- Cefizox for Intramuscular or Intravenous Use (Ceftizoxime Sodium) Fujisawa 1025
- Cefotan (Cefotetan) Zeneca 2936
- Cefzil Tablets and Oral Suspension (Cefprozil) Bristol-Myers Squibb .. 747
- Ceptaz (Ceftazidime) Glaxo Wellcome 1070
- Cipro I.V. (Ciprofloxacin) Bayer Pharmaceutical 587
- Cipro I.V. Pharmacy Bulk Package (Ciprofloxacin) Bayer Pharmaceutical 590
- Cipro Tablets (Ciprofloxacin Hydrochloride) Bayer Pharmaceutical 584
- Claforan Sterile and Injection (Cefotaxime Sodium) Hoechst Marion Roussel 1259
- Cleocin Phosphate Injection (Clindamycin Phosphate) Pharmacia & Upjohn 2068
- E.E.S. (Erythromycin Ethylsuccinate) Abbott 427
- E-Mycin Tablets (Erythromycin) Knoll Laboratories 1388
- ERYC (Erythromycin) Parke-Davis .. 1972
- EryPed (Erythromycin Ethylsuccinate) Abbott 425
- Ery-Tab Tablets (Erythromycin) Abbott 426
- Erythrocin Stearate Filmtab (Erythromycin Stearate) Abbott 429
- Erythromycin Base Filmtab (Erythromycin) Abbott 430
- Erythromycin Delayed-Release Capsules, USP (Erythromycin) Abbott 431
- Flagyl 375 Capsules (Metronidazole) Searle 2587
- Flagyl I.V. (Metronidazole Hydrochloride) SCS 2373
- Floxin I.V. (Ofloxacin) McNeil Pharmaceutical 1580
- Floxin Tablets (200 mg, 300 mg, 400 mg) (Ofloxacin) McNeil Pharmaceutical 1577
- Fortaz (Ceftazidime) Glaxo Wellcome 1092
- Ilosone (Erythromycin Estolate) Dista 927
- Ilotycin Gluceptate, IV, Vials (Erythromycin Gluceptate) Dista 929
- Kefurox Vials, Faspak & ADD-Vantage (Cefuroxime Sodium) Lilly 1509
- Lorabid Suspension and Pulvules (Loracarbef) Lilly 1513
- Mandol Vials, Faspak & ADD-Vantage (Cefamandole Nafate) Lilly 1516
- Maxaquin Tablets (Lomefloxacin Hydrochloride) Searle 2593
- Mefoxin (Cefoxitin Sodium) Merck & Co., Inc. 1734
- Mefoxin Premixed Intravenous Solution (Cefoxitin Sodium) Merck & Co., Inc. 1737
- Mezlin (Mezlocillin Sodium) Bayer Pharmaceutical 594
- Mezlin Pharmacy Bulk Package (Mezlocillin Sodium) Bayer Pharmaceutical 597
- Monocid Injection (Cefonicid Sodium) SmithKline Beecham Pharmaceuticals 2674
- Nebcin Vials, Hyporets & ADD-Vantage (Tobramycin Sulfate) Lilly 1518
- Netromycin Injection 100 mg/ml (Netilmicin Sulfate) Schering 2516
- PCE Dispertab Tablets (Erythromycin) Abbott 453
- Pfizerpen for Injection (Penicillin G Potassium) Pfizer Inc 2022
- Pipracil (Piperacillin Sodium) Lederle 1435
- Primaxin I.M. (Cilastatin Sodium, Imipenem) Merck & Co., Inc. 1770
- Primaxin I.V. (Cilastatin Sodium, Imipenem) Merck & Co., Inc. 1772
- Rocephin Injectable Vials, ADD-Vantage, Galaxy Container (Ceftriaxone Sodium) Roche Pharmaceuticals 2305
- Spectrobid Tablets (Bacampicillin Hydrochloride) Pfizer Inc 2030
- Tazicef for Injection (Ceftazidime) SmithKline Beecham Pharmaceuticals 2697
- Tazidime Vials, Faspak & ADD-Vantage (Ceftazidime) Lilly .. 1531
- Ticar for Injection (Ticarcillin Disodium) SmithKline Beecham Pharmaceuticals 2704
- Timentin for Injection (Ticarcillin Disodium, Clavulanate Potassium) SmithKline Beecham Pharmaceuticals 2706
- Vantin for Oral Suspension and Vantin Tablets (Cefpodoxime Proxetil) Pharmacia & Upjohn 2112
- Zinacef (Cefuroxime Sodium) Glaxo Wellcome 1184
- Zithromax (Azithromycin) Pfizer Inc 2043
- Zithromax Tablets (Azithromycin) Pfizer Inc 2046
- Zosyn (Piperacillin Sodium, Tazobactam Sodium) Lederle 1463

Infections, lower respiratory tract, RSV-induced
- Virazole (Ribavirin) ICN 1310

Infections, lower respiratory tract, RSV-induced, prevention of
- RespiGam (Immune Globulin Intravenous (Human)) MedImmune 1631

Infections, mastoidectomy
- Coly-Mycin S Otic w/Neomycin & Hydrocortisone (Colistin Sulfate, Neomycin Sulfate, Hydrocortisone Acetate) Parke-Davis 1965
- Cortisporin Otic Suspension Sterile (Polymyxin B Sulfate, Neomycin Sulfate, Hydrocortisone) Glaxo Wellcome 1077
- Pediotic Suspension Sterile (Polymyxin B Sulfate, Neomycin Sulfate, Hydrocortisone) Glaxo Wellcome 1140

Infections, mucomycotic
- Fungizone Intravenous (Amphotericin B) Apothecon 507

Infections, mycotic, cutaneous
- Mycostatin Cream & Topical Powder (Nystatin) Westwood-Squibb 2797
- Nystop (Nystatin Topical Powder, USP) (Nystatin) Paddock 1948

Infections, mycotic, mucocutaneous
- Mycostatin Cream & Topical Powder (Nystatin) Westwood-Squibb 2797
- Nystop (Nystatin Topical Powder, USP) (Nystatin) Paddock 1948

Infections, ocular, bacterial
- AK-Spore (Bacitracin Zinc, Neomycin Sulfate, Polymyxin B Sulfate) Akorn ..... ⊚ 205
- Bleph-10 (Sulfacetamide Sodium) Allergan 472
- Chloromycetin Ophthalmic Ointment, 1% (Chloramphenicol) Parke-Davis ..... ⊚ 298
- Chloromycetin Ophthalmic Solution (Chloramphenicol) Parke-Davis ..... ⊚ 299
- Chloroptic S.O.P. (Chloramphenicol) Allergan ..... ⊚ 236
- Chloroptic Sterile Ophthalmic Solution (Chloramphenicol) Allergan ..... ⊚ 236
- Cortisporin Ophthalmic Ointment Sterile (Polymyxin B Sulfate, Bacitracin Zinc, Neomycin Sulfate, Hydrocortisone) Glaxo Wellcome 1074
- Cortisporin Ophthalmic Suspension Sterile (Hydrocortisone, Polymyxin B Sulfate, Neomycin Sulfate) Glaxo Wellcome 1075
- Garamycin Ophthalmic (Gentamicin Sulfate) Schering 2501
- Gentak (Gentamicin Sulfate) Akorn ..... ⊚ 209
- Ilotycin Ophthalmic Ointment (Erythromycin) Dista 928
- NeoDecadron Sterile Ophthalmic Ointment (Neomycin Sulfate, Dexamethasone Sodium Phosphate) Merck & Co., Inc. 1755
- NeoDecadron Sterile Ophthalmic Solution (Neomycin Sulfate, Dexamethasone Sodium Phosphate) Merck & Co., Inc. 1756
- Neosporin Ophthalmic Ointment Sterile (Polymyxin B Sulfate, Bacitracin Zinc, Neomycin Sulfate) Glaxo Wellcome 1130
- Neosporin Ophthalmic Solution Sterile (Polymyxin B Sulfate, Neomycin Sulfate, Gramicidin) Glaxo Wellcome 1131
- Ocuflox Ophthalmic Solution (Ofloxacin) Allergan 478
- Polysporin Ophthalmic Ointment Sterile (Polymyxin B Sulfate, Bacitracin Zinc) Glaxo Wellcome .. 1140
- Polytrim Ophthalmic Solution Sterile (Polymyxin B Sulfate, Trimethoprim Sulfate) Allergan 479
- TERAK Ointment (Oxytetracycline Hydrochloride, Polymyxin B Sulfate) Akorn ..... ⊚ 210
- Terra-Cortril Ophthalmic Suspension (Oxytetracycline Hydrochloride, Hydrocortisone Acetate) Pfizer Inc 2033
- Terramycin with Polymyxin B Sulfate Ophthalmic Ointment (Oxytetracycline Hydrochloride, Polymyxin B Sulfate) Pfizer Inc .. 2035

Infections, perioperative, reduction of the incidence of
- Amikacin Sulfate Injection, USP (Amikacin Sulfate) Astra 523
- Amikacin Sulfate Injection, USP (Amikacin Sulfate) Elkins-Sinn 981
- Amikin Injectable (Amikacin Sulfate) Apothecon 502
- Ancef Injection (Cefazolin Sodium) SmithKline Beecham Pharmaceuticals 2632
- Cefotan (Cefotetan) Zeneca 2936
- Claforan Sterile and Injection (Cefotaxime Sodium) Hoechst Marion Roussel 1259
- Flagyl I.V. (Metronidazole Hydrochloride) SCS 2373
- Kefurox Vials, Faspak & ADD-Vantage (Cefuroxime Sodium) Lilly 1509
- Kefzol Vials, Faspak & ADD-Vantage (Cefazolin Sodium) Lilly 1511
- Mandol Vials, Faspak & ADD-Vantage (Cefamandole Nafate) Lilly 1516
- Mefoxin (Cefoxitin Sodium) Merck & Co., Inc. 1734
- Mefoxin Premixed Intravenous Solution (Cefoxitin Sodium) Merck & Co., Inc. 1737
- Mezlin (Mezlocillin Sodium) Bayer Pharmaceutical 594
- Mezlin Pharmacy Bulk Package (Mezlocillin Sodium) Bayer Pharmaceutical 597
- Pipracil (Piperacillin Sodium) Lederle 1435
- Rocephin Injectable Vials, ADD-Vantage, Galaxy Container (Ceftriaxone Sodium) Roche Pharmaceuticals 2305
- Zinacef (Cefuroxime Sodium) Glaxo Wellcome 1184

Infections, polymicrobic
- Ceptaz (Ceftazidime) Glaxo Wellcome 1070
- Fortaz (Ceftazidime) Glaxo Wellcome 1092
- Primaxin I.V. (Cilastatin Sodium, Imipenem) Merck & Co., Inc. 1772
- Tazicef for Injection (Ceftazidime) SmithKline Beecham Pharmaceuticals 2697
- Tazidime Vials, Faspak & ADD-Vantage (Ceftazidime) Lilly .. 1531

Infections, post-colorectal surgery, reduction of the incidence of
- Flagyl I.V. (Metronidazole Hydrochloride) SCS 2373
- Mezlin (Mezlocillin Sodium) Bayer Pharmaceutical 594
- Mezlin Pharmacy Bulk Package (Mezlocillin Sodium) Bayer Pharmaceutical 597

Infections, respiratory tract
- Amikacin Sulfate Injection, USP (Amikacin Sulfate) Astra 523
- Amikacin Sulfate Injection, USP (Amikacin Sulfate) Elkins-Sinn 981

(▣ Described in PDR For Nonprescription Drugs)   (⊚ Described in PDR For Ophthalmology)

1537 Indications Index Infections

Amikin Injectable (Amikacin Sulfate) Apothecon ... 502
Ancef Injection (Cefazolin Sodium) SmithKline Beecham Pharmaceuticals ... 2632
Cefobid Intravenous/Intramuscular (Cefoperazone Sodium) Pfizer Inc ... 1996
Cefobid Pharmacy Bulk Package - Not for Direct Infusion (Cefoperazone Sodium) Pfizer Inc ... 1999
DYNACIN Capsules (Minocycline Hydrochloride) Medicis ... 1627
ERYC (Erythromycin) Parke-Davis .. 1972
Erythrocin Stearate Filmtab (Erythromycin Stearate) Abbott ... 429
Erythromycin Base Filmtab (Erythromycin) Abbott ... 430
Erythromycin Delayed-Release Capsules, USP (Erythromycin) Abbott ... 431
Garamycin Injectable (Gentamicin Sulfate) Schering ... 2502
Keflex Pulvules & Oral Suspension (Cephalexin) Dista ... 930
Keftab Tablets (Cephalexin Hydrochloride) Dista ... 931
Kefzol Vials, Faspak & ADD-Vantage (Cefazolin Sodium) Lilly ... 1511
Minocin Oral Suspension (Minocycline Hydrochloride) Lederle ... 1431
Monodox Capsules (Doxycycline Monohydrate) Oclassen ... 1858
Omnipen for Oral Suspension (Ampicillin) Wyeth-Ayerst ... 2873
PCE Dispertab Tablets (Erythromycin) Abbott ... 453
Pen•Vee K (Penicillin V Potassium) Wyeth-Ayerst ... 2879
Pfizerpen for Injection (Penicillin G Potassium) Pfizer Inc ... 2022
Ticar for Injection (Ticarcillin Disodium) SmithKline Beecham Pharmaceuticals ... 2704
Vibramycin Hyclate Capsules (Doxycycline Hyclate) Pfizer Inc ... 2038

Infections, skin and skin structure

Amikacin Sulfate Injection, USP (Amikacin Sulfate) Astra ... 523
Amikacin Sulfate Injection, USP (Amikacin Sulfate) Elkins-Sinn ... 981
Amikin Injectable (Amikacin Sulfate) Apothecon ... 502
Amoxil (Amoxicillin Trihydrate) SmithKline Beecham Pharmaceuticals ... 2631
Ancef Injection (Cefazolin Sodium) SmithKline Beecham Pharmaceuticals ... 2632
Augmentin (Amoxicillin Trihydrate, Clavulanate Potassium) SmithKline Beecham Pharmaceuticals ... 2637
Augmentin Tablets (Amoxicillin Trihydrate, Clavulanate Potassium) SmithKline Beecham Pharmaceuticals ... 2640
Azactam for Injection (Aztreonam) Bristol-Myers Squibb ... 736
Biaxin (Clarithromycin) Abbott ... 406
Bicillin C-R Injection (Penicillin G Procaine, Penicillin G Benzathine) Wyeth-Ayerst ... 2810
Bicillin C-R 900/300 Injection (Penicillin G Procaine, Penicillin G Benzathine) Wyeth-Ayerst ... 2812
Ceclor Pulvules & Suspension (Cefaclor) Lilly ... 1470
Cefizox for Intramuscular or Intravenous Use (Ceftizoxime Sodium) Fujisawa ... 1025
Cefobid Intravenous/Intramuscular (Cefoperazone Sodium) Pfizer Inc ... 1996
Cefobid Pharmacy Bulk Package - Not for Direct Infusion (Cefoperazone Sodium) Pfizer Inc ... 1999
Cefotan (Cefotetan) Zeneca ... 2936
Ceftin (Cefuroxime Axetil) Glaxo Wellcome ... 1067
Cefzil Tablets and Oral Suspension (Cefprozil) Bristol-Myers Squibb .. 747
Ceptaz (Ceftazidime) Glaxo Wellcome ... 1070
Cipro I.V. (Ciprofloxacin) Bayer Pharmaceutical ... 587
Cipro I.V. Pharmacy Bulk Package (Ciprofloxacin) Bayer Pharmaceutical ... 590
Cipro Tablets (Ciprofloxacin Hydrochloride) Bayer Pharmaceutical ... 584
Claforan Sterile and Injection (Cefotaxime Sodium) Hoechst Marion Roussel ... 1259
Cleocin Phosphate Injection (Clindamycin Phosphate) Pharmacia & Upjohn ... 2068
Duricef Capsules, Tablets, and Oral Suspension (Cefadroxil) Bristol-Myers Squibb ... 750
Dynabac (Dirithromycin) Bock ... 668
DYNACIN Capsules (Minocycline Hydrochloride) Medicis ... 1627
E.E.S. (Erythromycin Ethylsuccinate) Abbott ... 427
E-Mycin Tablets (Erythromycin) Knoll Laboratories ... 1388
ERYC (Erythromycin) Parke-Davis .. 1972
EryPed (Erythromycin Ethylsuccinate) Abbott ... 425
Ery-Tab Tablets (Erythromycin) Abbott ... 426
Erythrocin Stearate Filmtab (Erythromycin Stearate) Abbott ... 429
Erythromycin Base Filmtab (Erythromycin) Abbott ... 430
Erythromycin Delayed-Release Capsules, USP (Erythromycin) Abbott ... 431
Flagyl 375 Capsules (Metronidazole) Searle ... 2587
Flagyl I.V. (Metronidazole Hydrochloride) SCS ... 2373
Floxin I.V. (Ofloxacin) McNeil Pharmaceutical ... 1580
Floxin Tablets (200 mg, 300 mg, 400 mg) (Ofloxacin) McNeil Pharmaceutical ... 1577
Fortaz (Ceftazidime) Glaxo Wellcome ... 1092
Garamycin Cream 0.1% (Gentamicin Sulfate) Schering ... 2501
Garamycin Injectable (Gentamicin Sulfate) Schering ... 2502
Garamycin Ointment 0.1% (Gentamicin Sulfate) Schering ... 2501
Ilosone (Erythromycin Estolate) Dista ... 927
Ilotycin Gluceptate, IV, Vials (Erythromycin Gluceptate) Dista ... 929
Keflex Pulvules & Oral Suspension (Cephalexin) Dista ... 930
Keftab Tablets (Cephalexin Hydrochloride) Dista ... 931
Kefurox Vials, Faspak & ADD-Vantage (Cefuroxime Sodium) Lilly ... 1509
Kefzol Vials, Faspak & ADD-Vantage (Cefazolin Sodium) Lilly ... 1511
Lorabid Suspension and Pulvules (Loracarbef) Lilly ... 1513
Mandol Vials, Faspak & ADD-Vantage (Cefamandole Nafate) Lilly ... 1516
Maxipime for Injection (Cefepime Hydrochloride) Bristol-Myers Squibb ... 758
Mefoxin (Cefoxitin Sodium) Merck & Co., Inc. ... 1734
Mefoxin Premixed Intravenous Solution (Cefoxitin Sodium) Merck & Co., Inc. ... 1737
Mezlin (Mezlocillin Sodium) Bayer Pharmaceutical ... 594
Mezlin Pharmacy Bulk Package (Mezlocillin Sodium) Bayer Pharmaceutical ... 597
Minocin Oral Suspension (Minocycline Hydrochloride) Lederle ... 1431
Monocid Injection (Cefonicid Sodium) SmithKline Beecham Pharmaceuticals ... 2674
Monodox Capsules (Doxycycline Monohydrate) Oclassen ... 1858
Nebcin Vials, Hyporets & ADD-Vantage (Tobramycin Sulfate) Lilly ... 1518
Netromycin Injection 100 mg/ml (Netilmicin Sulfate) Schering ... 2516
PCE Dispertab Tablets (Erythromycin) Abbott ... 453
Pen•Vee K (Penicillin V Potassium) Wyeth-Ayerst ... 2879
Pipracil (Piperacillin Sodium) Lederle ... 1435
Primaxin I.M. (Cilastatin Sodium, Imipenem) Merck & Co., Inc. ... 1770
Primaxin I.V. (Cilastatin Sodium, Imipenem) Merck & Co., Inc. ... 1772
Rocephin Injectable Vials, ADD-Vantage, Galaxy Container (Ceftriaxone Sodium) Roche Pharmaceuticals ... 2305
Spectrobid Tablets (Bacampicillin Hydrochloride) Pfizer Inc ... 2030
Tazicef for Injection (Ceftazidime) SmithKline Beecham Pharmaceuticals ... 2697
Tazidime Vials, Faspak & ADD-Vantage (Ceftazidime) Lilly .. 1531
Ticar for Injection (Ticarcillin Disodium) SmithKline Beecham Pharmaceuticals ... 2704
Timentin for Injection (Ticarcillin Disodium, Clavulanate Potassium) SmithKline Beecham Pharmaceuticals ... 2706
Unasyn (Ampicillin Sodium, Sulbactam Sodium) Pfizer Inc ... 2035
Vantin for Oral Suspension and Vantin Tablets (Cefpodoxime Proxetil) Pharmacia & Upjohn ... 2112
Zinacef (Cefuroxime Sodium) Glaxo Wellcome ... 1184
Zithromax (Azithromycin) Pfizer Inc ... 2043
Zithromax Tablets (Azithromycin) Pfizer Inc ... 2046
Zosyn (Piperacillin Sodium, Tazobactam Sodium) Lederle ... 1463

Infections, skin, bacterial, minor

Bactroban Ointment (Mupirocin) SmithKline Beecham Pharmaceuticals ... 2642
Betadine Brand First Aid Antibiotics & Moisturizer Ointment (Polymyxin B Sulfate, Bacitracin Zinc) Purdue Frederick ... 2144
Betadine First Aid Cream (Povidone Iodine) Purdue Frederick ... 2144
Betadine Ointment (Povidone Iodine) Purdue Frederick ... 2145
Betadine Solution (Povidone Iodine) Purdue Frederick ... 2145
Clorpactin WCS-90 (Sodium Oxychlorosene) Guardian ... 1236
Furacin Soluble Dressing (Nitrofurazone) Roberts ... 2220
Furacin Topical Cream (Nitrofurazone) Roberts ... 2220
Garamycin Injectable (Gentamicin Sulfate) Schering ... 2502
Medi-Quik (Benzalkonium Chloride, Lidocaine) Mentholatum ... ▣ 710
Mycitracin (Bacitracin Zinc, Neomycin Sulfate, Lidocaine, Polymyxin B Sulfate) Upjohn ... ▣ 803
Neosporin Ointment (Bacitracin Zinc, Neomycin Sulfate, Polymyxin B Sulfate) Warner Wellcome ... ▣ 821
Neosporin Plus Maximum Strength Cream (Polymyxin B Sulfate, Neomycin Sulfate, Lidocaine) Warner Wellcome ... ▣ 821
Neosporin Plus Maximum Strength Ointment (Polymyxin B Sulfate, Bacitracin Zinc, Neomycin Sulfate, Lidocaine) Warner Wellcome ... ▣ 822
Polysporin Ointment (Bacitracin Zinc, Polymyxin B Sulfate) Warner Wellcome ... ▣ 822
Polysporin Powder (Bacitracin Zinc, Polymyxin B Sulfate) Warner Wellcome ... ▣ 823

Infections, skin, secondary

Garamycin 0.1% (Gentamicin Sulfate) Schering ... 2501

Infections, soft tissues (see under Infections, skin and skin structure)

Infections, superficial, external auditory canal (see under Otitis externa)

Infections, tapeworm (see also under Taenia saginata infections; Diphyllobothrium latum infections; Hymenolepis nana infections)

Albenza Tablets (Albendazole) SmithKline Beecham Pharmaceuticals ... 2629

Infections, upper respiratory tract

Amoxil (Amoxicillin Trihydrate) SmithKline Beecham Pharmaceuticals ... 2631
Biaxin (Clarithromycin) Abbott ... 406
Bicillin C-R Injection (Penicillin G Procaine, Penicillin G Benzathine) Wyeth-Ayerst ... 2810
Bicillin C-R 900/300 Injection (Penicillin G Procaine, Penicillin G Benzathine) Wyeth-Ayerst ... 2812
Bicillin L-A Injection (Penicillin G Benzathine) Wyeth-Ayerst ... 2813
Ceclor Pulvules & Suspension (Cefaclor) Lilly ... 1470
Cedax (Ceftibuten Dihydrate) Schering ... 2480
Cefzil Tablets and Oral Suspension (Cefprozil) Bristol-Myers Squibb .. 747
Duricef Capsules, Tablets, and Oral Suspension (Cefadroxil) Bristol-Myers Squibb ... 750
DYNACIN Capsules (Minocycline Hydrochloride) Medicis ... 1627
E.E.S. (Erythromycin Ethylsuccinate) Abbott ... 427
E-Mycin Tablets (Erythromycin) Knoll Laboratories ... 1388
ERYC (Erythromycin) Parke-Davis .. 1972
EryPed (Erythromycin Ethylsuccinate) Abbott ... 425
Ery-Tab Tablets (Erythromycin) Abbott ... 426
Erythrocin Stearate Filmtab (Erythromycin Stearate) Abbott ... 429
Erythromycin Base Filmtab (Erythromycin) Abbott ... 430
Erythromycin Delayed-Release Capsules, USP (Erythromycin) Abbott ... 431
Ilosone (Erythromycin Estolate) Dista ... 927
Ilotycin Gluceptate, IV, Vials (Erythromycin Gluceptate) Dista ... 929
Lorabid Suspension and Pulvules (Loracarbef) Lilly ... 1513
Minocin Oral Suspension (Minocycline Hydrochloride) Lederle ... 1431
Monodox Capsules (Doxycycline Monohydrate) Oclassen ... 1858
PCE Dispertab Tablets (Erythromycin) Abbott ... 453
Pen•Vee K (Penicillin V Potassium) Wyeth-Ayerst ... 2879
Septra (Trimethoprim, Sulfamethoxazole) Glaxo Wellcome ... 1146
Spectrobid Tablets (Bacampicillin Hydrochloride) Pfizer Inc ... 2030
Suprax (Cefixime) Lederle ... 1443
Vantin for Oral Suspension and Vantin Tablets (Cefpodoxime Proxetil) Pharmacia & Upjohn ... 2112
Vibramycin Hyclate Capsules (Doxycycline Hyclate) Pfizer Inc ... 2038
Zithromax (Azithromycin) Pfizer Inc ... 2043
Zithromax Tablets (Azithromycin) Pfizer Inc ... 2046

Infections, urinary bladder, prophylaxis of

Neosporin G.U. Irrigant Sterile (Neomycin Sulfate, Polymyxin B Sulfate) Glaxo Wellcome ... 1130

Infections, urinary tract

Amikacin Sulfate Injection, USP (Amikacin Sulfate) Astra ... 523
Amikacin Sulfate Injection, USP (Amikacin Sulfate) Elkins-Sinn ... 981
Amikin Injectable (Amikacin Sulfate) Apothecon ... 502
Amoxil (Amoxicillin Trihydrate) SmithKline Beecham Pharmaceuticals ... 2631
Ancef Injection (Cefazolin Sodium) SmithKline Beecham Pharmaceuticals ... 2632
Augmentin (Amoxicillin Trihydrate, Clavulanate Potassium) SmithKline Beecham Pharmaceuticals ... 2637
Augmentin Tablets (Amoxicillin Trihydrate, Clavulanate Potassium) SmithKline Beecham Pharmaceuticals ... 2640

(▣ Described in PDR For Nonprescription Drugs) (◉ Described in PDR For Ophthalmology)

Infections

- Azactam for Injection (Aztreonam) Bristol-Myers Squibb ... 736
- Bactrim DS Tablets (Trimethoprim, Sulfamethoxazole) Roche Pharmaceuticals ... 2257
- Bactrim I.V. Infusion (Trimethoprim, Sulfamethoxazole) Roche Pharmaceuticals ... 2255
- Bactrim (Trimethoprim, Sulfamethoxazole) Roche Pharmaceuticals ... 2257
- Ceclor Pulvules & Suspension (Cefaclor) Lilly ... 1470
- Cefizox for Intramuscular or Intravenous Use (Ceftizoxime Sodium) Fujisawa ... 1025
- Cefobid Intravenous/Intramuscular (Cefoperazone Sodium) Pfizer Inc ... 1996
- Cefobid Pharmacy Bulk Package - Not for Direct Infusion (Cefoperazone Sodium) Pfizer Inc ... 1999
- Cefotan (Cefotetan) Zeneca ... 2936
- Ceftin (Cefuroxime Axetil) Glaxo Wellcome ... 1067
- Ceptaz (Ceftazidime) Glaxo Wellcome ... 1070
- Cipro I.V. (Ciprofloxacin) Bayer Pharmaceutical ... 587
- Cipro I.V. Pharmacy Bulk Package (Ciprofloxacin) Bayer Pharmaceutical ... 590
- Cipro Tablets (Ciprofloxacin Hydrochloride) Bayer Pharmaceutical ... 584
- Duricef Capsules, Tablets, and Oral Suspension (Cefadroxil) Bristol-Myers Squibb ... 750
- DYNACIN Capsules (Minocycline Hydrochloride) Medicis ... 1627
- Floxin I.V. (Ofloxacin) McNeil Pharmaceutical ... 1580
- Floxin Tablets (200 mg, 300 mg, 400 mg) (Ofloxacin) McNeil Pharmaceutical ... 1577
- Fortaz (Ceftazidime) Glaxo Wellcome ... 1092
- Gantanol Tablets (Sulfamethoxazole) Roche Pharmaceuticals ... 2285
- Gantrisin (Acetyl Sulfisoxazole) Roche Pharmaceuticals ... 2286
- Garamycin Injectable (Gentamicin Sulfate) Schering ... 2502
- Geocillin Tablets (Carbenicillin Indanyl Sodium) Pfizer Inc ... 2009
- Kefurox Vials, Faspak & ADD-Vantage (Cefuroxime Sodium) Lilly ... 1509
- Kefzol Vials, Faspak & ADD-Vantage (Cefazolin Sodium) Lilly ... 1511
- Lorabid Suspension and Pulvules (Loracarbef) Lilly ... 1513
- Macrobid Capsules (Nitrofurantoin Monohydrate) Procter & Gamble Pharmaceuticals ... 2138
- Macrodantin Capsules (Nitrofurantoin) Procter & Gamble Pharmaceuticals ... 2140
- Mandol Vials, Faspak & ADD-Vantage (Cefamandole Nafate) Lilly ... 1516
- Maxaquin Tablets (Lomefloxacin Hydrochloride) Searle ... 2593
- Maxipime for Injection (Cefepime Hydrochloride) Bristol-Myers Squibb ... 758
- Mefoxin (Cefoxitin Sodium) Merck & Co., Inc. ... 1734
- Mefoxin Premixed Intravenous Solution (Cefoxitin Sodium) Merck & Co., Inc. ... 1737
- Mezlin (Mezlocillin Sodium) Bayer Pharmaceutical ... 594
- Mezlin Pharmacy Bulk Package (Mezlocillin Sodium) Bayer Pharmaceutical ... 597
- Minocin Oral Suspension (Minocycline Hydrochloride) Lederle ... 1431
- Monocid Injection (Cefonicid Sodium) SmithKline Beecham Pharmaceuticals ... 2674
- Monodox Capsules (Doxycycline Monohydrate) Oclassen ... 1858
- Nebcin Vials, Hyporets & ADD-Vantage (Tobramycin Sulfate) Lilly ... 1518
- NegGram (Nalidixic Acid) Sanofi Winthrop ... 2453
- Netromycin Injection 100 mg/ml (Netilmicin Sulfate) Schering ... 2516
- Noroxin Tablets (Norfloxacin) Merck & Co., Inc. ... 1758
- Noroxin Tablets (Norfloxacin) Roberts ... 2222
- Penetrex Tablets (Enoxacin) Rhone-Poulenc Rorer Pharmaceuticals ... 2196
- Pipracil (Piperacillin Sodium) Lederle ... 1435
- Primaxin I.V. (Cilastatin Sodium, Imipenem) Merck & Co., Inc. ... 1772
- Proloprim Tablets (Trimethoprim) Glaxo Wellcome ... 1141
- Rocephin Injectable Vials, ADD-Vantage, Galaxy Container (Ceftriaxone Sodium) Roche Pharmaceuticals ... 2305
- Septra (Trimethoprim, Sulfamethoxazole) Glaxo Wellcome ... 1146
- Septra I.V. Infusion (Trimethoprim, Sulfamethoxazole) Glaxo Wellcome ... 1142
- Septra I.V. Infusion ADD-Vantage Vials (Trimethoprim, Sulfamethoxazole) Glaxo Wellcome ... 1144
- Septra (Trimethoprim, Sulfamethoxazole) Glaxo Wellcome ... 1146
- Seromycin Capsules (Cycloserine) Dura ... 975
- Spectrobid Tablets (Bacampicillin Hydrochloride) Pfizer Inc ... 2030
- Suprax (Cefixime) Lederle ... 1443
- Tazicef for Injection (Ceftazidime) SmithKline Beecham Pharmaceuticals ... 2697
- Tazidime Vials, Faspak & ADD-Vantage (Ceftazidime) Lilly ... 1531
- Ticar for Injection (Ticarcillin Disodium) SmithKline Beecham Pharmaceuticals ... 2704
- Timentin for Injection (Ticarcillin Disodium, Clavulanate Potassium) SmithKline Beecham Pharmaceuticals ... 2706
- Trimpex Tablets (Trimethoprim) Roche Pharmaceuticals ... 2323
- Urised Tablets (Atropine Sulfate, Hyoscyamine, Methenamine, Phenyl Salicylate) PolyMedica ... 2123
- Uroqid-Acid No. 2 Tablets (Methenamine Mandelate, Sodium Acid Phosphate) Beach ... 633
- Vantin for Oral Suspension and Vantin Tablets (Cefpodoxime Proxetil) Pharmacia & Upjohn ... 2112
- Zinacef (Cefuroxime Sodium) Glaxo Wellcome ... 1184

Infections, urinary tract, systemic candidal

- Diflucan Tablets, Injection, and Oral Suspension (Fluconazole) Pfizer Inc ... 2003

Infections, vaginal cuff, post-surgical

- Cleocin Phosphate Injection (Clindamycin Phosphate) Pharmacia & Upjohn ... 2068
- Flagyl 375 Capsules (Metronidazole) Searle ... 2587
- Flagyl I.V. (Metronidazole Hydrochloride) SCS ... 2373
- Protostat Tablets (Metronidazole) Ortho Pharmaceutical ... 1939

Infections, venereal
(see also under Bejel; Yaws; Pinta; Gonorrhea)

- Bicillin L-A Injection (Penicillin G Benzathine) Wyeth-Ayerst ... 2813

Infections, vulvovaginal mycotic, Candida species

- AVC (Sulfanilamide) Hoechst Marion Roussel ... 1245
- Mycelex-G 500 mg Vaginal Tablets (Clotrimazole) Bayer Pharmaceutical ... 602

Infectious diarrhea
(see under Diarrhea, infectious)

Inflammation, anorectal

- Analpram-HC Rectal Cream 1% and 2.5% (Hydrocortisone Acetate, Pramoxine Hydrochloride) Ferndale ... 993
- Anusol-HC Suppositories (Hydrocortisone Acetate) Parke-Davis ... 1954
- Cortizone-5 Creme and Ointment (Hydrocortisone) Thompson Medical ... ■ 795
- Cortizone-10 Creme and Ointment (Hydrocortisone) Thompson Medical ... ■ 795
- Hemorid (Petrolatum, White, Mineral Oil, Pramoxine Hydrochloride, Phenylephrine Hydrochloride) Thompson Medical ... ■ 797
- ProctoFoam-HC (Hydrocortisone Acetate, Pramoxine Hydrochloride) Schwarz ... 2552
- Tronolane Anesthetic Cream for Hemorrhoids (Pramoxine Hydrochloride) Ross ... ■ 746

Inflammation, anterior segment

- AK-CIDE (Prednisolone Acetate, Sulfacetamide Sodium) Akorn ... ⊚ 203
- AK-CIDE Ointment (Prednisolone Acetate, Sulfacetamide Sodium) Akorn ... ⊚ 203
- AK-PRED (Prednisolone Sodium Phosphate) Akorn ... ⊚ 204
- AK-Trol Ointment & Suspension (Dexamethasone, Neomycin Sulfate, Polymyxin B Sulfate) Akorn ... ⊚ 205
- Blephamide Liquifilm Sterile Ophthalmic Suspension (Prednisolone Acetate, Sulfacetamide Sodium) Allergan ... 472
- Blephamide Ointment (Sulfacetamide Sodium, Prednisolone Acetate) Allergan ... ⊚ 234
- Celestone Soluspan Suspension (Betamethasone Sodium Phosphate, Betamethasone Acetate) Schering ... 2484
- Cortisporin Ophthalmic Ointment Sterile (Polymyxin B Sulfate, Bacitracin Zinc, Neomycin Sulfate, Hydrocortisone) Glaxo Wellcome ... 1074
- Cortisporin Ophthalmic Suspension Sterile (Hydrocortisone, Polymyxin B Sulfate, Neomycin Sulfate) Glaxo Wellcome ... 1075
- Cortone Acetate Sterile Suspension (Cortisone Acetate) Merck & Co., Inc. ... 1663
- Cortone Acetate Tablets (Cortisone Acetate) Merck & Co., Inc. ... 1664
- Dalalone D.P. Injectable (Dexamethasone Acetate) Forest ... 1009
- Decadron Elixir (Dexamethasone) Merck & Co., Inc. ... 1676
- Decadron Phosphate Injection (Dexamethasone Sodium Phosphate) Merck & Co., Inc. ... 1680
- Decadron Phosphate Sterile Ophthalmic Ointment (Dexamethasone Sodium Phosphate) Merck & Co., Inc. ... 1684
- Decadron Phosphate Sterile Ophthalmic Solution (Dexamethasone Sodium Phosphate) Merck & Co., Inc. ... 1685
- Decadron Tablets (Dexamethasone) Merck & Co., Inc. ... 1678
- Decadron-LA Sterile Suspension (Dexamethasone Acetate) Merck & Co., Inc. ... 1687
- Econopred & Econopred Plus Ophthalmic Suspensions (Prednisolone Acetate) Alcon Laboratories ... ⊚ 216
- FML Forte Liquifilm (Fluorometholone) Allergan ... ⊚ 237
- FML Liquifilm (Fluorometholone) Allergan ... ⊚ 238
- FML S.O.P. (Fluorometholone) Allergan ... ⊚ 239
- FML-S Liquifilm (Sulfacetamide Sodium, Fluorometholone) Allergan ... ⊚ 240
- Hydeltrasol Injection, Sterile (Prednisolone Sodium Phosphate) Merck & Co., Inc. ... 1708
- Hydrocortone Phosphate Injection, Sterile (Hydrocortisone Sodium Phosphate) Merck & Co., Inc. ... 1713
- Hydrocortone Tablets (Hydrocortisone) Merck & Co., Inc. ... 1715
- Maxitrol Ophthalmic Ointment and Suspension (Dexamethasone, Neomycin Sulfate, Polymyxin B Sulfate) Alcon Laboratories ... ⊚ 222
- NeoDecadron Sterile Ophthalmic Ointment (Neomycin Sulfate, Dexamethasone Sodium Phosphate) Merck & Co., Inc. ... 1755
- NeoDecadron Sterile Ophthalmic Solution (Neomycin Sulfate, Dexamethasone Sodium Phosphate) Merck & Co., Inc. ... 1756
- Pediapred Oral Solution (Prednisolone Sodium Phosphate) Medeva ... 1618
- Poly-Pred Liquifilm (Neomycin Sulfate, Polymyxin B Sulfate, Prednisolone Acetate) Allergan ... ⊚ 246
- Pred Forte (Prednisolone Acetate) Allergan ... ⊚ 247
- Pred-G Liquifilm Sterile Ophthalmic Suspension (Gentamicin Sulfate, Prednisolone Acetate) Allergan ... ⊚ 248
- Pred-G S.O.P. Sterile Ophthalmic Ointment (Gentamicin Sulfate, Prednisolone Acetate) Allergan ... ⊚ 249
- Prelone Syrup (Prednisolone) Muro ... 1834
- Terra-Cortril Ophthalmic Suspension (Oxytetracycline Hydrochloride, Hydrocortisone Acetate) Pfizer Inc ... 2033
- TobraDex Ophthalmic Suspension and Ointment (Dexamethasone, Tobramycin) Alcon Laboratories ... 469

Influenza A virus, respiratory tract illness, chemoprophylaxis of

- Flumadine Tablets & Syrup (Rimantadine Hydrochloride) Forest ... 1013
- Symmetrel Capsules (Amantadine Hydrochloride) DuPont ... 965
- Symmetrel Syrup (Amantadine Hydrochloride) DuPont ... 963

Influenza A virus, respiratory tract illness, treatment of

- Flumadine Tablets & Syrup (Rimantadine Hydrochloride) Forest ... 1013
- Symmetrel Capsules (Amantadine Hydrochloride) DuPont ... 965
- Symmetrel Syrup (Amantadine Hydrochloride) DuPont ... 963

Influenza syndrome, symptomatic relief of

- Actifed Sinus Daytime/Nighttime Tablets and Caplets (Acetaminophen, Diphenhydramine Hydrochloride, Pseudoephedrine Hydrochloride) Warner Wellcome ... ■ 809
- Advil Cold and Sinus Caplets and Tablets (Ibuprofen, Pseudoephedrine Hydrochloride) Whitehall-Robins ... ■ 837
- Alka-Seltzer Plus Cold Medicine Liqui-Gels (Chlorpheniramine Maleate, Pseudoephedrine Hydrochloride, Acetaminophen) Bayer Consumer ... ■ 612
- Alka-Seltzer Plus Cold & Cough Medicine (Aspirin, Chlorpheniramine Maleate, Dextromethorphan Hydrobromide, Phenylpropanolamine Bitartrate) Bayer Consumer ... ■ 611
- Alka-Seltzer Plus Cold & Cough Medicine Liqui-Gels (Dextromethorphan Hydrobromide, Chlorpheniramine Maleate, Pseudoephedrine Hydrochloride, Acetaminophen) Bayer Consumer ... ■ 612
- Alka-Seltzer Plus Flu & Body Aches Effervescent Tablets (Acetaminophen, Chlorpheniramine Maleate, Dextromethorphan Hydrobromide, Phenylpropanolamine Hydrochloride) Bayer Consumer ... ■ 612
- Alka-Seltzer Plus Flu & Body Aches Liqui-Gels Non-Drowsy Formula (Acetaminophen, Dextromethorphan Hydrobromide, Pseudoephedrine Hydrochloride) Bayer Consumer ... ■ 613

(■ Described in PDR For Nonprescription Drugs) (⊚ Described in PDR For Ophthalmology)

1539 Indications Index Intubation

Alka-Seltzer Plus Night-Time Cold Medicine (Aspirin, Phenylpropanolamine Bitartrate, Doxylamine Succinate, Dextromethorphan Hydrobromide) Bayer Consumer ■ 611
Alka-Seltzer Plus Night-Time Cold Medicine Liqui-Gels (Dextromethorphan Hydrobromide, Doxylamine Succinate, Pseudoephedrine Hydrochloride, Acetaminophen) Bayer Consumer ■ 612
Atrohist Pediatric Capsules (Chlorpheniramine Maleate, Pseudoephedrine Hydrochloride) Medeva 1603
Benadryl Allergy (Diphenhydramine Hydrochloride) Warner Wellcome ■ 811
Benadryl Dye-Free Allergy Liquid Medication (Diphenhydramine Hydrochloride) Warner Wellcome ■ 814
Benylin Multisymptom (Dextromethorphan Hydrobromide, Pseudoephedrine Hydrochloride, Guaifenesin) Warner Wellcome ■ 816
Bromfed-DM Cough Syrup (Brompheniramine Maleate, Pseudoephedrine Hydrochloride, Dextromethorphan Hydrobromide) Muro 1832
Children's TYLENOL acetaminophen Chewable Tablets, Elixir, Suspension Liquid, and Suspension Drops (Acetaminophen) McNeil Consumer 1559
Children's Vicks NyQuil Cold/Cough Relief (Chlorpheniramine Maleate, Dextromethorphan Hydrobromide, Pseudoephedrine Hydrochloride) Procter & Gamble ■ 731
Comtrex Non-Drowsy (Acetaminophen, Dextromethorphan Hydrobromide, Pseudoephedrine Hydrochloride) Bristol-Myers Products ■ 640
Contac Day & Night (Acetaminophen, Pseudoephedrine Hydrochloride, Dextromethorphan Hydrobromide) SmithKline Beecham Consumer ■ 772
Contac Severe Cold and Flu Formula Caplets (Acetaminophen, Chlorpheniramine Maleate, Dextromethorphan Hydrobromide, Phenylpropanolamine Hydrochloride) SmithKline Beecham Consumer ■ 773
Contac Severe Cold & Flu Non-Drowsy (Acetaminophen, Dextromethorphan Hydrobromide, Pseudoephedrine Hydrochloride) SmithKline Beecham Consumer ■ 774
Dimetapp Cold & Allergy Chewable Tablets (Brompheniramine Maleate, Phenylpropanolamine Hydrochloride) Whitehall-Robins ■ 838
Dorcol Children's Cough Syrup (Pseudoephedrine Hydrochloride, Guaifenesin, Dextromethorphan Hydrobromide) Sandoz Consumer ■ 748
Drixoral Cold and Flu Extended-Release Tablets (Acetaminophen, Dexbrompheniramine Maleate, Pseudoephedrine Sulfate) Schering-Plough HealthCare ■ 764
Drixoral Cough + Sore Throat Liquid Caps (Dextromethorphan Hydrobromide, Acetaminophen) Schering-Plough HealthCare ■ 763
Duratuss HD Elixir (Hydrocodone Bitartrate, Pseudoephedrine Hydrochloride, Guaifenesin) UCB 2750
Empirin Aspirin Tablets (Aspirin) Warner Wellcome ■ 818
Entex PSE Tablets (Pseudoephedrine Hydrochloride, Guaifenesin) Dura 973
Excedrin Extra-Strength Analgesic Tablets, Caplets, and Geltabs (Acetaminophen, Aspirin, Caffeine) Bristol-Myers Products 734
Exgest LA Tablets (Phenylpropanolamine Hydrochloride, Guaifenesin) Carnrick 787
Extendryl (Chlorpheniramine Maleate, Methscopolamine Nitrate, Phenylephrine Hydrochloride) Fleming 1003
Fedahist Gyrocaps (Pseudoephedrine Hydrochloride, Chlorpheniramine Maleate) Schwarz 2545
Infants' TYLENOL acetaminophen Suspension Drops (Acetaminophen) McNeil Consumer 1559
Kronofed-A (Chlorpheniramine Maleate, Pseudoephedrine Hydrochloride) Ferndale 994
Novahistine DMX (Dextromethorphan Hydrobromide, Guaifenesin, Pseudoephedrine Hydrochloride) SmithKline Beecham Consumer ■ 782
Nucofed (Codeine Phosphate, Pseudoephedrine Hydrochloride, Guaifenesin) Roberts 2225
Ornade Spansule Capsules (Phenylpropanolamine Hydrochloride, Chlorpheniramine Maleate) SmithKline Beecham Pharmaceuticals 2678
Oscillococcinum (Homeopathic Medications) Boiron ■ 635
PediaCare NightRest Cough-Cold Liquid (Chlorpheniramine Maleate, Dextromethorphan Hydrobromide, Pseudoephedrine Hydrochloride) McNeil Consumer 1569
Pediatric Vicks 44m Cough & Cold Relief (Chlorpheniramine Maleate, Dextromethorphan Hydrobromide, Pseudoephedrine Hydrochloride) Procter & Gamble ■ 737
Phenergan with Codeine (Codeine Phosphate, Promethazine Hydrochloride) Wyeth-Ayerst 2883
Phenergan with Dextromethorphan (Promethazine Hydrochloride, Dextromethorphan Hydrobromide) Wyeth-Ayerst 2885
Phenergan VC (Promethazine Hydrochloride, Phenylephrine Hydrochloride) Wyeth-Ayerst 2886
Phenergan VC with Codeine (Codeine Phosphate, Promethazine Hydrochloride, Phenylephrine Hydrochloride) Wyeth-Ayerst 2888
Pyrroxate Caplets (Acetaminophen, Chlorpheniramine Maleate, Phenylpropanolamine Hydrochloride) Roberts ■ 742
Robitussin Cold, Cough & Flu Liqui-Gels (Acetaminophen, Dextromethorphan Hydrobromide, Guaifenesin, Pseudoephedrine Hydrochloride) Whitehall-Robins ■ 844
Robitussin Night-Time Cold Formula (Acetaminophen, Dextromethorphan Hydrobromide, Doxylamine Succinate, Phenylpropanolamine Hydrochloride) Whitehall-Robins ■ 847
Ryna (Chlorpheniramine Maleate, Pseudoephedrine Hydrochloride) Wallace ■ 804
Rynatan-S Pediatric Suspension (Phenylephrine Tannate, Chlorpheniramine Tannate, Pyrilamine Tannate) Wallace 2781
Sinarest Extra Strength Caplets (Acetaminophen, Chlorpheniramine Maleate, Pseudoephedrine Hydrochloride) Ciba Self-Medication ■ 663
Sudafed Cold and Cough Liquid Caps (Acetaminophen, Dextromethorphan Hydrobromide, Guaifenesin, Pseudoephedrine Hydrochloride) Warner Wellcome ■ 826
Sudafed Severe Cold Formula Caplets (Acetaminophen, Dextromethorphan Hydrobromide, Pseudoephedrine Hydrochloride) Warner Wellcome ■ 828
Sudafed Severe Cold Formula Tablets (Acetaminophen, Dextromethorphan Hydrobromide, Pseudoephedrine Hydrochloride) Warner Wellcome ■ 828
Sunsource Flu Relief Tablets (Homeopathic Medications) Sunsource ■ 792
Teldrin 12 Hour Antihistamine/Nasal Decongestant Allergy Relief Capsules (Chlorpheniramine Maleate, Phenylpropanolamine Hydrochloride) SmithKline Beecham Consumer ■ 786
TheraFlu Flu and Cold Medicine (Acetaminophen, Chlorpheniramine Maleate, Pseudoephedrine Hydrochloride) Sandoz Consumer ■ 750
Theraflu Maximum Strength Flu and Cold Medicine For Sore Throat (Acetaminophen, Chlorpheniramine Maleate, Pseudoephedrine Hydrochloride) Sandoz Consumer ■ 751
TheraFlu Maximum Strength Nighttime Flu, Cold & Cough Medicine (Acetaminophen, Dextromethorphan Hydrobromide, Pseudoephedrine Hydrochloride, Chlorpheniramine Maleate) Sandoz Consumer ■ 751
TheraFlu Maximum Strength Non-Drowsy Formula Flu, Cold & Cough Medicine (Acetaminophen, Dextromethorphan Hydrobromide, Pseudoephedrine Hydrochloride) Sandoz Consumer ■ 751
TheraFlu Maximum Strength, Non-Drowsy Formula Flu, Cold and Cough Caplets (Acetaminophen, Dextromethorphan Hydrobromide, Pseudoephedrine Hydrochloride) Sandoz Consumer ■ 752
Triaminic Sore Throat Formula (Acetaminophen, Dextromethorphan Hydrobromide, Pseudoephedrine Hydrochloride) Sandoz Consumer ■ 755
Triaminic Triaminicol Cold & Cough (Phenylpropanolamine Hydrochloride, Chlorpheniramine Maleate, Dextromethorphan Hydrobromide) Sandoz Consumer ■ 756
Trinalin Repetabs Tablets (Azatadine Maleate, Pseudoephedrine Sulfate) Key 1373
Tussionex Pennkinetic Extended-Release Suspension (Hydrocodone Polistirex, Chlorpheniramine Polistirex) Medeva 1624
TYLENOL Allergy Sinus NightTime, Maximum Strength Caplets (Acetaminophen, Pseudoephedrine Hydrochloride, Diphenhydramine Hydrochloride) McNeil Consumer 1571
TYLENOL Cold Medication, Multi-Symptom Formula Tablets and Caplets (Acetaminophen, Chlorpheniramine Maleate, Pseudoephedrine Hydrochloride, Dextromethorphan Hydrobromide) McNeil Consumer 1572
TYLENOL Cold Medication, Multi-Symptom Hot Liquid Packets (Acetaminophen, Chlorpheniramine Maleate, Pseudoephedrine Hydrochloride, Dextromethorphan Hydrobromide) McNeil Consumer 1572
TYLENOL Cold Medication, No Drowsiness Formula Caplets and Gelcaps (Acetaminophen, Pseudoephedrine Hydrochloride, Dextromethorphan Hydrobromide) McNeil Consumer 1572
TYLENOL Flu No Drowsiness Formula, Maximum Strength Gelcaps (Acetaminophen, Dextromethorphan Hydrobromide, Pseudoephedrine Hydrochloride) McNeil Consumer 1575
TYLENOL Flu NightTime, Maximum Strength Gelcaps (Acetaminophen, Pseudoephedrine Hydrochloride, Diphenhydramine Hydrochloride) McNeil Consumer 1575
TYLENOL Flu NightTime, Maximum Strength Hot Medication Packets (Acetaminophen, Diphenhydramine Hydrochloride, Pseudoephedrine Hydrochloride) McNeil Consumer 1575
Vicks 44 LiquiCaps Cough, Cold & Flu Relief (Dextromethorphan Hydrobromide, Pseudoephedrine Hydrochloride, Chlorpheniramine Maleate, Acetaminophen) Procter & Gamble ■ 728
Vicks 44M Cough, Cold & Flu Relief (Acetaminophen, Dextromethorphan Hydrobromide, Chlorpheniramine Maleate, Pseudoephedrine Hydrochloride) Procter & Gamble ■ 729
Vicks DayQuil Allergy Relief 12-Hour Extended Release Tablets (Phenylpropanolamine Hydrochloride, Brompheniramine Maleate) Procter & Gamble ■ 733
Vicks DayQuil Allergy Relief 4-Hour Tablets (Phenylpropanolamine Hydrochloride, Brompheniramine Maleate) Procter & Gamble ■ 733
Vicks DayQuil LiquiCaps/Liquid Multi-Symptom Cold/Flu Relief (Acetaminophen, Dextromethorphan Hydrobromide, Pseudoephedrine Hydrochloride, Guaifenesin) Procter & Gamble ■ 734
Vicks DayQuil SINUS Pressure & PAIN Relief with IBUPROFEN (Ibuprofen, Pseudoephedrine Hydrochloride) Procter & Gamble ■ 735
Vicks Nyquil Hot Therapy (Acetaminophen, Pseudoephedrine Hydrochloride, Dextromethorphan Hydrobromide, Doxylamine Succinate) Procter & Gamble ■ 735
Vicks NyQuil LiquiCaps/Liquid Multi-Symptom Cold/Flu Relief, Original and Cherry Flavors (Acetaminophen, Pseudoephedrine Hydrochloride, Dextromethorphan Hydrobromide, Doxylamine Succinate) Procter & Gamble ■ 736

Insect bites, pain due to
(see under Pain, topical relief of)

Insomnia
(see under Sleep, induction of)

Intermittent claudication
(see under Claudication, intermittent)

Intertrigo
(see under Skin, inflammatory conditions)

Intracranial pressure, elevation
(see under Hypertension, cerebral, in neurosurgery)

Intraocular pressure elevation
(see under Hypertension, ocular)

Intravascular device, maintenance of patency
Abbokinase (Urokinase) Abbott 403
Abbokinase Open-Cath (Urokinase) Abbott 405
Heparin Lock Flush Solution (Heparin Sodium) Wyeth-Ayerst 2831

Intubation, endotracheal
Anectine (Succinylcholine Chloride) Glaxo Wellcome 1062
Mivacron (Mivacurium Chloride) Glaxo Wellcome 1125
Nimbex Injection (Cisatracurium Besylate) Glaxo Wellcome 1131
Norcuron for Injection (Vecuronium Bromide) Organon 1875
Nuromax Injection (Doxacurium Chloride) Glaxo Wellcome 1136
Tracrium Injection (Atracurium Besylate) Glaxo Wellcome 1155

(■ Described in PDR For Nonprescription Drugs) (◉ Described in PDR For Ophthalmology)

Indications Index

Intubation
Zemuron Injection (Rocuronium Bromide) Organon ... 1885

Intubation, small bowel
Reglan (Metoclopramide Hydrochloride) Robins ... 2243

Iridectomy, post-, adjunct
Humorsol Sterile Ophthalmic Solution (Demecarium Bromide) Merck & Co., Inc. ... 1707

Iridocyclitis
Celestone Soluspan Suspension (Betamethasone Sodium Phosphate, Betamethasone Acetate) Schering ... 2484
Cortone Acetate Sterile Suspension (Cortisone Acetate) Merck & Co., Inc. ... 1663
Cortone Acetate Tablets (Cortisone Acetate) Merck & Co., Inc. ... 1664
Dalalone D.P. Injectable (Dexamethasone Acetate) Forest ... 1009
Decadron Elixir (Dexamethasone) Merck & Co., Inc. ... 1676
Decadron Phosphate Injection (Dexamethasone Sodium Phosphate) Merck & Co., Inc. ... 1680
Decadron Tablets (Dexamethasone) Merck & Co., Inc. ... 1678
Decadron-LA Sterile Suspension (Dexamethasone Acetate) Merck & Co., Inc. ... 1687
Hydeltrasol Injection, Sterile (Prednisolone Sodium Phosphate) Merck & Co., Inc. ... 1708
Hydrocortone Phosphate Injection, Sterile (Hydrocortisone Sodium Phosphate) Merck & Co., Inc. ... 1713
Hydrocortone Tablets (Hydrocortisone) Merck & Co., Inc. ... 1715
Pediapred Oral Solution (Prednisolone Sodium Phosphate) Medeva 1618
Prelone Syrup (Prednisolone) Muro 1834

Iritis
AK-PRED (Prednisolone Sodium Phosphate) Akorn ... ⊙ 204
Celestone Soluspan Suspension (Betamethasone Sodium Phosphate, Betamethasone Acetate) Schering ... 2484
Cortone Acetate Sterile Suspension (Cortisone Acetate) Merck & Co., Inc. ... 1663
Cortone Acetate Tablets (Cortisone Acetate) Merck & Co., Inc. ... 1664
Dalalone D.P. Injectable (Dexamethasone Acetate) Forest ... 1009
Decadron Elixir (Dexamethasone) Merck & Co., Inc. ... 1676
Decadron Phosphate Injection (Dexamethasone Sodium Phosphate) Merck & Co., Inc. ... 1680
Decadron Phosphate Sterile Ophthalmic Ointment (Dexamethasone Sodium Phosphate) Merck & Co., Inc. ... 1684
Decadron Phosphate Sterile Ophthalmic Solution (Dexamethasone Sodium Phosphate) Merck & Co., Inc. ... 1685
Decadron Tablets (Dexamethasone) Merck & Co., Inc. ... 1678
Decadron-LA Sterile Suspension (Dexamethasone Acetate) Merck & Co., Inc. ... 1687
Econopred & Econopred Plus Ophthalmic Suspensions (Prednisolone Acetate) Alcon Laboratories ... ⊙ 216
Hydeltrasol Injection, Sterile (Prednisolone Sodium Phosphate) Merck & Co., Inc. ... 1708
Hydrocortone Phosphate Injection, Sterile (Hydrocortisone Sodium Phosphate) Merck & Co., Inc. ... 1713
Hydrocortone Tablets (Hydrocortisone) Merck & Co., Inc. ... 1715
Pediapred Oral Solution (Prednisolone Sodium Phosphate) Medeva 1618
Prelone Syrup (Prednisolone) Muro 1834

Iron deficiency
Feosol Caplets (Iron) SmithKline Beecham ... 2626
Feosol Capsules (Ferrous Sulfate) SmithKline Beecham Consumer ▣ 777
Feosol Elixir (Ferrous Sulfate) SmithKline Beecham ... 2627
Feosol Tablets (Ferrous Sulfate) SmithKline Beecham ... 2627
Fero-Folic-500 Filmtab (Ferrous Sulfate, Folic Acid, Vitamin C) Abbott ... 433
Fero-Grad-500 Filmtab (Ferrous Sulfate, Vitamin C) Abbott ... 434
Fero-Gradumet Filmtab (Ferrous Sulfate) Abbott ... 434
Ferro-Sequels (Ferrous Fumarate) Lederle Consumer ... ▣ 684
Iberet Tablets (Vitamin B Complex With Vitamin C, Ferrous Sulfate) Abbott ... 437
Iberet-500 Liquid (Vitamin B Complex With Vitamin C, Ferrous Sulfate) Abbott ... 438
Iberet-Folic-500 Filmtab (Vitamin B Complex With Vitamin C, Ferrous Sulfate) Abbott ... 433
Iberet-Liquid (Vitamin B Complex With Vitamin C, Ferrous Sulfate) Abbott ... 438
INFeD (Iron Dextran Injection, USP) (Iron Dextran) Schein ... 2478
Irospan (Ferrous Sulfate, Vitamin C) Fielding ... 1000
Nephro-Fer Tablets (Ferrous Fumarate) R&D ... 2168
Nephro-Fer Rx Tablets (Ferrous Fumarate, Folic Acid) R&D ... 2168
Niferex-150 Forte Capsules (Polysaccharide-Iron Complex, Folic Acid, Cyanocobalamin) Central ... 811
Slow Fe Tablets (Ferrous Sulfate) Ciba Self-Medication ... 889

Iron intoxication, acute
Desferal Vials (Deferoxamine Mesylate) CibaGeneva ... 838

Iron overload, chronic
Desferal Vials (Deferoxamine Mesylate) CibaGeneva ... 838

Irritable bowel syndrome
(see under Bowel, irritable, syndrome)

Ischemic attacks, recurrent transient, in men
Regular Strength Ascriptin Tablets (Aspirin Buffered, Calcium Carbonate) Ciba Self-Medication ... ▣ 650
Genuine Bayer Aspirin Tablets & Caplets (Aspirin) Bayer Consumer ... ▣ 618
Bayer Enteric Aspirin (Aspirin, Enteric Coated) Bayer Consumer ... ▣ 613
Bufferin Analgesic Tablets (Aspirin) Bristol-Myers Products ... ▣ 636
Ecotrin (Aspirin) SmithKline Beecham ... 2625

Isoimmunization, prevention of in Rho(D) negative individuals
HypRho-D Full Dose Rho (D) Immune Globulin (Human) (Immune Globulin (Human)) Bayer Biological ... 623

Isoimmunization, prevention of in Rho(D) negative women
HypRho-D Mini-Dose Rho (D) Immune Globulin (Human) (Immune Globulin (Human)) Bayer Biological ... 622
MICRhoGAM Rh₀(D) Immune Globulin (Human) (Immune Globulin (Human)) Ortho Diagnostic ... 1902
RhoGAM Rh₀(D) Immune Globulin (Human) (Immune Globulin (Human)) Ortho Diagnostic ... 1902
WinRho SD (Rh₀(D) Immune Globulin (Human)) NABI ... 1839

Itching, skin
(see under Pruritus, topical relief of)

Itching, sunburn
(see under Pruritus, topical relief of)

J

Jock itch
(see under Tinea cruris infections)

Joint pain
(see under Pain, arthritic, minor)

K

K. pneumoniae bacteremia
Rocephin Injectable Vials, ADD-Vantage, Galaxy Container (Ceftriaxone Sodium) Roche Pharmaceuticals ... 2305

K. pneumoniae bone and joint infections
Rocephin Injectable Vials, ADD-Vantage, Galaxy Container (Ceftriaxone Sodium) Roche Pharmaceuticals ... 2305

K. pneumoniae central nervous system infections
Claforan Sterile and Injection (Cefotaxime Sodium) Hoechst Marion Roussel ... 1259

K. pneumoniae genitourinary tract infections
Keflex Pulvules & Oral Suspension (Cephalexin) Dista ... 930

K. pneumoniae gynecologic infections
Azactam for Injection (Aztreonam) Bristol-Myers Squibb ... 736
Primaxin I.M. (Cilastatin Sodium, Imipenem) Merck & Co., Inc. ... 1770
Timentin for Injection (Ticarcillin Disodium, Clavulanate Potassium) SmithKline Beecham Pharmaceuticals ... 2706

K. pneumoniae infections
Azactam for Injection (Aztreonam) Bristol-Myers Squibb ... 736
Cefobid Intravenous/Intramuscular (Cefoperazone Sodium) Pfizer Inc ... 1996
Cefobid Pharmacy Bulk Package - Not for Direct Infusion (Cefoperazone Sodium) Pfizer Inc ... 1999
Cefotan (Cefotetan) Zeneca ... 2936
Ceftin Tablets (Cefuroxime Axetil) Glaxo Wellcome ... 1067
Cipro I.V. (Ciprofloxacin) Bayer Pharmaceutical ... 587
Cipro I.V. Pharmacy Bulk Package (Ciprofloxacin) Bayer Pharmaceutical ... 590
Cipro Tablets (Ciprofloxacin Hydrochloride) Bayer Pharmaceutical ... 584
Claforan Sterile and Injection (Cefotaxime Sodium) Hoechst Marion Roussel ... 1259
Floxin I.V. (Ofloxacin) McNeil Pharmaceutical ... 1580
Floxin Tablets (200 mg, 300 mg, 400 mg) (Ofloxacin) McNeil Pharmaceutical ... 1577
Keflex Pulvules & Oral Suspension (Cephalexin) Dista ... 930
Maxaquin Tablets (Lomefloxacin Hydrochloride) Searle ... 2593
Maxipime for Injection (Cefepime Hydrochloride) Bristol-Myers Squibb ... 758
Merrem I.V. (Meropenem) Zeneca ... 2952
Mezlin (Mezlocillin Sodium) Bayer Pharmaceutical ... 594
Mezlin Pharmacy Bulk Package (Mezlocillin Sodium) Bayer Pharmaceutical ... 597
Monocid Injection (Cefonicid Sodium) SmithKline Beecham Pharmaceuticals ... 2674
Netromycin Injection 100 mg/ml (Netilmicin Sulfate) Schering ... 2516
Noroxin Tablets (Norfloxacin) Merck & Co., Inc. ... 1758
Noroxin Tablets (Norfloxacin) Roberts ... 2222
Penetrex Tablets (Enoxacin) Rhone-Poulenc Rorer Pharmaceuticals ... 2196
Primaxin I.M. (Cilastatin Sodium, Imipenem) Merck & Co., Inc. ... 1770
Prolorim Tablets (Trimethoprim) Glaxo Wellcome ... 1141
Rocephin Injectable Vials, ADD-Vantage, Galaxy Container (Ceftriaxone Sodium) Roche Pharmaceuticals ... 2305
Suprax for Oral Suspension (Cefixime) Lederle ... 1443
Timentin for Injection (Ticarcillin Disodium, Clavulanate Potassium) SmithKline Beecham Pharmaceuticals ... 2706
Trimpex Tablets (Trimethoprim) Roche Pharmaceuticals ... 2323
Unasyn (Ampicillin Sodium, Sulbactam Sodium) Pfizer Inc ... 2035
Vantin for Oral Suspension and Vantin Tablets (Cefpodoxime Proxetil) Pharmacia & Upjohn ... 2112

K. pneumoniae infections, ocular
Garamycin Ophthalmic (Gentamicin Sulfate) Schering ... 2501
Genoptic Sterile Ophthalmic Solution (Gentamicin Sulfate) Allergan ... ⊙ 241
Genoptic Sterile Ophthalmic Ointment (Gentamicin Sulfate) Allergan ... ⊙ 241
Gentak (Gentamicin Sulfate) Akorn ... ⊙ 209
Pred-G S.O.P. Sterile Ophthalmic Ointment (Gentamicin Sulfate, Prednisolone Acetate) Allergan ... ⊙ 249

K. pneumoniae intra-abdominal infections
Azactam for Injection (Aztreonam) Bristol-Myers Squibb ... 736
Cefotan (Cefotetan) Zeneca ... 2936
Merrem I.V. (Meropenem) Zeneca ... 2952
Netromycin Injection 100 mg/ml (Netilmicin Sulfate) Schering ... 2516
Primaxin I.M. (Cilastatin Sodium, Imipenem) Merck & Co., Inc. ... 1770
Rocephin Injectable Vials, ADD-Vantage, Galaxy Container (Ceftriaxone Sodium) Roche Pharmaceuticals ... 2305
Timentin for Injection (Ticarcillin Disodium, Clavulanate Potassium) SmithKline Beecham Pharmaceuticals ... 2706
Unasyn (Ampicillin Sodium, Sulbactam Sodium) Pfizer Inc ... 2035

K. pneumoniae lower respiratory tract infections
Azactam for Injection (Aztreonam) Bristol-Myers Squibb ... 736
Cefotan (Cefotetan) Zeneca ... 2936
Cipro I.V. (Ciprofloxacin) Bayer Pharmaceutical ... 587
Cipro I.V. Pharmacy Bulk Package (Ciprofloxacin) Bayer Pharmaceutical ... 590
Cipro Tablets (Ciprofloxacin Hydrochloride) Bayer Pharmaceutical ... 584
Maxipime for Injection (Cefepime Hydrochloride) Bristol-Myers Squibb ... 758
Mezlin (Mezlocillin Sodium) Bayer Pharmaceutical ... 594
Mezlin Pharmacy Bulk Package (Mezlocillin Sodium) Bayer Pharmaceutical ... 597
Monocid Injection (Cefonicid Sodium) SmithKline Beecham Pharmaceuticals ... 2674
Netromycin Injection 100 mg/ml (Netilmicin Sulfate) Schering ... 2516
Rocephin Injectable Vials, ADD-Vantage, Galaxy Container (Ceftriaxone Sodium) Roche Pharmaceuticals ... 2305

K. pneumoniae pneumonia, treatment, adjunct
Streptomycin Sulfate Injection (Streptomycin Sulfate) Pfizer Inc 2031

K. pneumoniae prostatitis
Keflex Pulvules & Oral Suspension (Cephalexin) Dista ... 930

K. pneumoniae respiratory tract infections
Cefobid Intravenous/Intramuscular (Cefoperazone Sodium) Pfizer Inc ... 1996

(▣ Described in PDR For Nonprescription Drugs)   (⊙ Described in PDR For Ophthalmology)

K. pneumoniae septicemia
Azactam for Injection (Aztreonam) Bristol-Myers Squibb ... 736
Cefobid Intravenous/Intramuscular (Cefoperazone Sodium) Pfizer Inc ... 1996
Cefobid Pharmacy Bulk Package - Not for Direct Infusion (Cefoperazone Sodium) Pfizer Inc ... 1999
Netromycin Injection 100 mg/ml (Netilmicin Sulfate) Schering ... 2516
Rocephin Injectable Vials, ADD-Vantage, Galaxy Container (Ceftriaxone Sodium) Roche Pharmaceuticals ... 2305

K. pneumoniae skin and skin structure infections
Azactam for Injection (Aztreonam) Bristol-Myers Squibb ... 736
Cefotan (Cefotetan) Zeneca ... 2936
Cipro I.V. (Ciprofloxacin) Bayer Pharmaceutical ... 587
Cipro I.V. Pharmacy Bulk Package (Ciprofloxacin) Bayer Pharmaceutical ... 590
Cipro Tablets (Ciprofloxacin Hydrochloride) Bayer Pharmaceutical ... 584
Netromycin Injection 100 mg/ml (Netilmicin Sulfate) Schering ... 2516
Primaxin I.M. (Cilastatin Sodium, Imipenem) Merck & Co., Inc. ... 1770
Rocephin Injectable Vials, ADD-Vantage, Galaxy Container (Ceftriaxone Sodium) Roche Pharmaceuticals ... 2305
Unasyn (Ampicillin Sodium, Sulbactam Sodium) Pfizer Inc ... 2035

K. pneumoniae urinary tract infections
Azactam for Injection (Aztreonam) Bristol-Myers Squibb ... 736
Cefotan (Cefotetan) Zeneca ... 2936
Ceftin Tablets (Cefuroxime Axetil) Glaxo Wellcome ... 1067
Cipro I.V. (Ciprofloxacin) Bayer Pharmaceutical ... 587
Cipro I.V. Pharmacy Bulk Package (Ciprofloxacin) Bayer Pharmaceutical ... 590
Cipro Tablets (Ciprofloxacin Hydrochloride) Bayer Pharmaceutical ... 584
Floxin I.V. (Ofloxacin) McNeil Pharmaceutical ... 1580
Floxin Tablets (200 mg, 300 mg, 400 mg) (Ofloxacin) McNeil Pharmaceutical ... 1577
Maxaquin Tablets (Lomefloxacin Hydrochloride) Searle ... 2593
Maxipime for Injection (Cefepime Hydrochloride) Bristol-Myers Squibb ... 758
Monocid Injection (Cefonicid Sodium) SmithKline Beecham Pharmaceuticals ... 2674
Netromycin Injection 100 mg/ml (Netilmicin Sulfate) Schering ... 2516
Noroxin Tablets (Norfloxacin) Merck & Co., Inc. ... 1758
Noroxin Tablets (Norfloxacin) Roberts ... 2222
Penetrex Tablets (Enoxacin) Rhone-Poulenc Rorer Pharmaceuticals ... 2196
Proloprim Tablets (Trimethoprim) Glaxo Wellcome ... 1141
Rocephin Injectable Vials, ADD-Vantage, Galaxy Container (Ceftriaxone Sodium) Roche Pharmaceuticals ... 2305
Streptomycin Sulfate Injection (Streptomycin Sulfate) Pfizer Inc ... 2031
Trimpex Tablets (Trimethoprim) Roche Pharmaceuticals ... 2323
Vantin for Oral Suspension and Vantin Tablets (Cefpodoxime Proxetil) Pharmacia & Upjohn ... 2112

Kaposi's sarcoma
Velban Vials (Vinblastine Sulfate) Lilly ... 1537

Kaposi's sarcoma, AIDS-related
DaunoXome (Daunorubicin Citrate) NeXstar ... 1842

Doxil (Doxorubicin Hydrochloride) Sequus ... 2613
Intron A for Injection (Interferon alfa-2B, Recombinant) Schering .. 2506
Roferon-A Injection (Interferon alfa-2A, Recombinant) Roche Pharmaceuticals ... 2308

Keloids
Celestone Soluspan Suspension (Betamethasone Sodium Phosphate, Betamethasone Acetate) Schering ... 2484
Decadron Phosphate Injection (Dexamethasone Sodium Phosphate) Merck & Co., Inc. ... 1680
Decadron-LA Sterile Suspension (Dexamethasone Acetate) Merck & Co., Inc. ... 1687
Hydeltrasol Injection, Sterile (Prednisolone Sodium Phosphate) Merck & Co., Inc. ... 1708
Hydrocortone Acetate Sterile Suspension (Hydrocortisone Acetate) Merck & Co., Inc. ... 1712

Keratitis
Celestone Soluspan Suspension (Betamethasone Sodium Phosphate, Betamethasone Acetate) Schering ... 2484
Cortone Acetate Sterile Suspension (Cortisone Acetate) Merck & Co., Inc. ... 1663
Cortone Acetate Tablets (Cortisone Acetate) Merck & Co., Inc. ... 1664
Decadron Elixir (Dexamethasone) Merck & Co., Inc. ... 1676
Decadron Phosphate Injection (Dexamethasone Sodium Phosphate) Merck & Co., Inc. ... 1680
Decadron Tablets (Dexamethasone) Merck & Co., Inc. ... 1678
Decadron-LA Sterile Suspension (Dexamethasone Acetate) Merck & Co., Inc. ... 1687
Garamycin Ophthalmic (Gentamicin Sulfate) Schering ... 2501
Genoptic Sterile Ophthalmic Solution (Gentamicin Sulfate) Allergan ... ⊚ 241
Genoptic Sterile Ophthalmic Ointment (Gentamicin Sulfate) Allergan ... ⊚ 241
Gentak (Gentamicin Sulfate) Akorn ... ⊚ 209
Hydeltrasol Injection, Sterile (Prednisolone Sodium Phosphate) Merck & Co., Inc. ... 1708
Hydrocortone Phosphate Injection, Sterile (Hydrocortisone Sodium Phosphate) Merck & Co., Inc. ... 1713
Hydrocortone Tablets (Hydrocortisone) Merck & Co., Inc. ... 1715
Neosporin Ophthalmic Ointment Sterile (Polymyxin B Sulfate, Bacitracin Zinc, Neomycin Sulfate) Glaxo Wellcome ... 1130
Neosporin Ophthalmic Solution Sterile (Polymyxin B Sulfate, Neomycin Sulfate, Gramicidin) Glaxo Wellcome ... 1131
Pediapred Oral Solution (Prednisolone Sodium Phosphate) Medeva 1618
Polysporin Ophthalmic Ointment Sterile (Polymyxin B Sulfate, Bacitracin Zinc) Glaxo Wellcome .. 1140
Prelone Syrup (Prednisolone) Muro 1834

Keratitis sicca
(see under Keratoconjunctivitis sicca)

Keratitis, bullous, diagnostic aid in
Ophthalgan (Glycerin) Storz Ophthalmics ... ⊚ 323

Keratitis, dendritic
Vira-A Ophthalmic Ointment, 3% (Vidarabine) Parke-Davis ... ⊚ 299
Viroptic Ophthalmic Solution, 1% Sterile (Trifluridine) Glaxo Wellcome ... 1177

Keratitis, exposure
Lacrisert Sterile Ophthalmic Insert (Hydroxypropyl Cellulose) Merck & Co., Inc. ... 1730

Keratitis, fungal
Natacyn Antifungal Ophthalmic Suspension (Natamycin) Alcon Laboratories ... ⊚ 223

Keratitis, Fusarium solani
Natacyn Antifungal Ophthalmic Suspension (Natamycin) Alcon Laboratories ... ⊚ 223

Keratitis, herpes zoster
AK-PRED (Prednisolone Sodium Phosphate) Akorn ... ⊚ 204
Decadron Phosphate Sterile Ophthalmic Ointment (Dexamethasone Sodium Phosphate) Merck & Co., Inc. ... 1684
Decadron Phosphate Sterile Ophthalmic Solution (Dexamethasone Sodium Phosphate) Merck & Co., Inc. ... 1685
Econopred & Econopred Plus Ophthalmic Suspensions (Prednisolone Acetate) Alcon Laboratories ... ⊚ 216

Keratitis, punctate, superficial
AK-PRED (Prednisolone Sodium Phosphate) Akorn ... ⊚ 204
Decadron Phosphate Sterile Ophthalmic Ointment (Dexamethasone Sodium Phosphate) Merck & Co., Inc. ... 1684
Decadron Phosphate Sterile Ophthalmic Solution (Dexamethasone Sodium Phosphate) Merck & Co., Inc. ... 1685
Econopred & Econopred Plus Ophthalmic Suspensions (Prednisolone Acetate) Alcon Laboratories ... ⊚ 216

Keratitis, recurrent epithelial
(see under Keratitis, dendritic)

Keratitis, vernal
Alomide Ophthalmic Solution (Lodoxamide Tromethamine) Alcon Laboratories ... 465
Crolom (Cromolyn Sodium) Bausch & Lomb Pharmaceuticals ... ⊚ 254

Keratoconjunctivitis sicca
Bion Tears (Lubricant) Alcon Laboratories ... ⊚ 214
Celluvisc Lubricant Eye Drops (Carboxymethylcellulose Sodium) Allergan ... ⊚ 236
Clear Eyes ACR Astringent/Lubricant Eye Redness Reliever Eye Drops (Zinc Sulfate, Naphazoline Hydrochloride) Ross ... ⊚ 314
Collagen Plugs (Intracanalicular) (Collagen, bovine) Lacrimedics .. ⊚ 275
Collyrium Fresh (Tetrahydrozoline Hydrochloride, Glycerin) Storz Ophthalmics ... ⊚ 316
Herrick Lacrimal Plugs (Silicone) Lacrimedics ... ⊚ 275
HypoTears Lubricant Eye Drops (Polyvinyl Alcohol) CIBA Vision Ophthalmics ... ⊚ 262
HypoTears Ointment (Petrolatum, White) CIBA Vision Ophthalmics ... ⊚ 262
HypoTears PF Lubricant Eye Drops (Polyvinyl Alcohol) CIBA Vision Ophthalmics ... ⊚ 262
Lacrisert Sterile Ophthalmic Insert (Hydroxypropyl Cellulose) Merck & Co., Inc. ... 1730
OcuCoat and OcuCoat PF Eye Drops (Dextran 70, Hydroxypropyl Methylcellulose) Storz Ophthalmics ... ⊚ 322
Refresh Plus Lubricant Eye Drops (Carboxymethylcellulose Sodium) Allergan ... ⊚ 252
Refresh PM Lubricant Eye Ointment (Petrolatum, White, Mineral Oil) Allergan ... ⊚ 252
Similasan Eye Drops #1 (Belladonna Alkaloids, Homeopathic Medications) Similasan ... ⊚ 316
Tears Naturale II (Dextran 70, Hydroxypropyl Methylcellulose) Alcon Laboratories ... 469
TheraTears ATF Formula (Carboxymethylcellulose Sodium) Advanced Vision Research ... ⊚ 201

Viva-Drops (Polysorbate 80) Vision Pharmaceuticals ... ⊚ 326

Keratoconjunctivitis, acute
Vira-A Ophthalmic Ointment, 3% (Vidarabine) Parke-Davis ... ⊚ 299

Keratoconjunctivitis, primary
Viroptic Ophthalmic Solution, 1% Sterile (Trifluridine) Glaxo Wellcome ... 1177

Keratoconjunctivitis, unspecified
Garamycin Ophthalmic (Gentamicin Sulfate) Schering ... 2501
Genoptic Sterile Ophthalmic Solution (Gentamicin Sulfate) Allergan ... ⊚ 241
Genoptic Sterile Ophthalmic Ointment (Gentamicin Sulfate) Allergan ... ⊚ 241
Gentak (Gentamicin Sulfate) Akorn ... ⊚ 209
Neosporin Ophthalmic Ointment Sterile (Polymyxin B Sulfate, Bacitracin Zinc, Neomycin Sulfate) Glaxo Wellcome ... 1130
Neosporin Ophthalmic Solution Sterile (Polymyxin B Sulfate, Neomycin Sulfate, Gramicidin) Glaxo Wellcome ... 1131
Polysporin Ophthalmic Ointment Sterile (Polymyxin B Sulfate, Bacitracin Zinc) Glaxo Wellcome .. 1140

Keratoconjunctivitis, vernal
Alomide Ophthalmic Solution (Lodoxamide Tromethamine) Alcon Laboratories ... 465
Crolom (Cromolyn Sodium) Bausch & Lomb Pharmaceuticals ... ⊚ 254

Keratosis palmaris
(see under Hyperkeratosis skin disorders)

Keratosis pilaris
(see under Hyperkeratosis skin disorders)

Keratosis plantaris
(see under Hyperkeratosis skin disorders)

Keratosis, actinic
Efudex (Fluorouracil) Roche Pharmaceuticals ... 2280
Fluoroplex Topical Solution & Cream 1% (Fluorouracil) Allergan ... 475

Keratosis, solar
Efudex (Fluorouracil) Roche Pharmaceuticals ... 2280

Klebsiella oxytoca infections
Azactam for Injection (Aztreonam) Bristol-Myers Squibb ... 736
Rocephin Injectable Vials, ADD-Vantage, Galaxy Container (Ceftriaxone Sodium) Roche Pharmaceuticals ... 2305

Klebsiella oxytoca skin and structure infections
Rocephin Injectable Vials, ADD-Vantage, Galaxy Container (Ceftriaxone Sodium) Roche Pharmaceuticals ... 2305

Klebsiella pneumoniae infections
(see under K. pneumoniae infections)

Klebsiella species bacteremia
Ceptaz (Ceftazidime) Glaxo Wellcome ... 1070

Klebsiella species biliary tract infections
Ancef Injection (Cefazolin Sodium) SmithKline Beecham Pharmaceuticals ... 2632
Kefzol Vials, Faspak & ADD-Vantage (Cefazolin Sodium) Lilly ... 1511

Klebsiella species bone and joint infections
Ceptaz (Ceftazidime) Glaxo Wellcome ... 1070

(⊠ Described in PDR For Nonprescription Drugs)   (⊚ Described in PDR For Ophthalmology)

Klebsiella species

Fortaz (Ceftazidime) Glaxo Wellcome ... 1092
Nebcin Vials, Hyporets & ADD-Vantage (Tobramycin Sulfate) Lilly ... 1518
Tazicef for Injection (Ceftazidime) SmithKline Beecham Pharmaceuticals ... 2697
Tazidime Vials, Faspak & ADD-Vantage (Ceftazidime) Lilly .. 1531

Klebsiella species genital tract infections

Ancef Injection (Cefazolin Sodium) SmithKline Beecham Pharmaceuticals ... 2632
Mefoxin (Cefoxitin Sodium) Merck & Co., Inc. ... 1734
Mefoxin Premixed Intravenous Solution (Cefoxitin Sodium) Merck & Co., Inc. ... 1737

Klebsiella species gynecologic infections

Claforan Sterile and Injection (Cefotaxime Sodium) Hoechst Marion Roussel ... 1259
Mezlin (Mezlocillin Sodium) Bayer Pharmaceutical ... 594
Mezlin Pharmacy Bulk Package (Mezlocillin Sodium) Bayer Pharmaceutical ... 597
Primaxin I.V. (Cilastatin Sodium, Imipenem) Merck & Co., Inc. ... 1772

Klebsiella species infections

Achromycin V Capsules (Tetracycline Hydrochloride) Lederle ... 1417
Amikacin Sulfate Injection, USP (Amikacin Sulfate) Astra ... 523
Amikacin Sulfate Injection, USP (Amikacin Sulfate) Elkins-Sinn ... 981
Amikin Injectable (Amikacin Sulfate) Apothecon ... 502
Ancef Injection (Cefazolin Sodium) SmithKline Beecham Pharmaceuticals ... 2632
Augmentin (Amoxicillin Trihydrate, Clavulanate Potassium) SmithKline Beecham Pharmaceuticals ... 2637
Augmentin Tablets (Amoxicillin Trihydrate, Clavulanate Potassium) SmithKline Beecham Pharmaceuticals ... 2640
Bactrim DS Tablets (Trimethoprim, Sulfamethoxazole) Roche Pharmaceuticals ... 2257
Bactrim I.V. Infusion (Trimethoprim, Sulfamethoxazole) Roche Pharmaceuticals ... 2255
Bactrim (Trimethoprim, Sulfamethoxazole) Roche Pharmaceuticals ... 2257
Ceclor Pulvules & Suspension (Cefaclor) Lilly ... 1470
Cefizox for Intramuscular or Intravenous Use (Ceftizoxime Sodium) Fujisawa ... 1025
Cefobid Intravenous/Intramuscular (Cefoperazone Sodium) Pfizer Inc ... 1996
Cefobid Pharmacy Bulk Package - Not for Direct Infusion (Cefoperazone Sodium) Pfizer Inc ... 1999
Cefotan (Cefotetan) Zeneca ... 2936
Ceptaz (Ceftazidime) Glaxo Wellcome ... 1070
Claforan Sterile and Injection (Cefotaxime Sodium) Hoechst Marion Roussel ... 1259
Declomycin Tablets (Demeclocycline Hydrochloride) Lederle ... 1421
Doryx Capsules (Doxycycline Hyclate) Parke-Davis ... 1970
Duricef Capsules, Tablets, and Oral Suspension (Cefadroxil) Bristol-Myers Squibb ... 750
DYNACIN Capsules (Minocycline Hydrochloride) Medicis ... 1627
Fortaz (Ceftazidime) Glaxo Wellcome ... 1092
Garamycin Injectable (Gentamicin Sulfate) Schering ... 2502
Kefurox Vials, Faspak & ADD-Vantage (Cefuroxime Sodium) Lilly ... 1509
Kefzol Vials, Faspak & ADD-Vantage (Cefazolin Sodium) Lilly ... 1511

Macrodantin Capsules (Nitrofurantoin) Procter & Gamble Pharmaceuticals ... 2140
Mefoxin (Cefoxitin Sodium) Merck & Co., Inc. ... 1734
Mefoxin Premixed Intravenous Solution (Cefoxitin Sodium) Merck & Co., Inc. ... 1737
Mezlin (Mezlocillin Sodium) Bayer Pharmaceutical ... 594
Mezlin Pharmacy Bulk Package (Mezlocillin Sodium) Bayer Pharmaceutical ... 597
Minocin Intravenous (Minocycline Hydrochloride) Lederle ... 1428
Minocin Oral Suspension (Minocycline Hydrochloride) Lederle ... 1431
Minocin Pellet-Filled Capsules (Minocycline Hydrochloride) Lederle ... 1429
Monodox Capsules (Doxycycline Monohydrate) Oclassen ... 1858
Nebcin Vials, Hyporets & ADD-Vantage (Tobramycin Sulfate) Lilly ... 1518
NegGram (Nalidixic Acid) Sanofi Winthrop ... 2453
Pipracil (Piperacillin Sodium) Lederle ... 1435
Primaxin I.V. (Cilastatin Sodium, Imipenem) Merck & Co., Inc. ... 1772
Septra (Trimethoprim, Sulfamethoxazole) Glaxo Wellcome ... 1146
Septra I.V. Infusion (Trimethoprim, Sulfamethoxazole) Glaxo Wellcome ... 1142
Septra I.V. Infusion ADD-Vantage Vials (Trimethoprim, Sulfamethoxazole) Glaxo Wellcome ... 1144
Septra (Trimethoprim, Sulfamethoxazole) Glaxo Wellcome ... 1146
Tazicef for Injection (Ceftazidime) SmithKline Beecham Pharmaceuticals ... 2697
Tazidime Vials, Faspak & ADD-Vantage (Ceftazidime) Lilly .. 1531
Terramycin Intramuscular Solution (Oxytetracycline) Pfizer Inc ... 2034
Timentin for Injection (Ticarcillin Disodium, Clavulanate Potassium) SmithKline Beecham Pharmaceuticals ... 2706
Unasyn (Ampicillin Sodium, Sulbactam Sodium) Pfizer Inc ... 2035
Vibramycin (Doxycycline Calcium) Pfizer Inc ... 2038
Vibramycin Hyclate Intravenous (Doxycycline Hyclate) Pfizer Inc ... 2040
Vibramycin (Doxycycline Monohydrate) Pfizer Inc ... 2038
Zinacef (Cefuroxime Sodium) Glaxo Wellcome ... 1184

Klebsiella species intra-abdominal infections

Azactam for Injection (Aztreonam) Bristol-Myers Squibb ... 736
Cefizox for Intramuscular or Intravenous Use (Ceftizoxime Sodium) Fujisawa ... 1025
Cefotan (Cefotetan) Zeneca ... 2936
Ceptaz (Ceftazidime) Glaxo Wellcome ... 1070
Claforan Sterile and Injection (Cefotaxime Sodium) Hoechst Marion Roussel ... 1259
Fortaz (Ceftazidime) Glaxo Wellcome ... 1092
Mefoxin (Cefoxitin Sodium) Merck & Co., Inc. ... 1734
Mefoxin Premixed Intravenous Solution (Cefoxitin Sodium) Merck & Co., Inc. ... 1737
Mezlin (Mezlocillin Sodium) Bayer Pharmaceutical ... 594
Mezlin Pharmacy Bulk Package (Mezlocillin Sodium) Bayer Pharmaceutical ... 597
Nebcin Vials, Hyporets & ADD-Vantage (Tobramycin Sulfate) Lilly ... 1518
Primaxin I.V. (Cilastatin Sodium, Imipenem) Merck & Co., Inc. ... 1772
Tazicef for Injection (Ceftazidime) SmithKline Beecham Pharmaceuticals ... 2697
Tazidime Vials, Faspak & ADD-Vantage (Ceftazidime) Lilly .. 1531

Unasyn (Ampicillin Sodium, Sulbactam Sodium) Pfizer Inc ... 2035

Klebsiella species lower respiratory tract infections

Cefizox for Intramuscular or Intravenous Use (Ceftizoxime Sodium) Fujisawa ... 1025
Cefotan (Cefotetan) Zeneca ... 2936
Ceptaz (Ceftazidime) Glaxo Wellcome ... 1070
Claforan Sterile and Injection (Cefotaxime Sodium) Hoechst Marion Roussel ... 1259
Fortaz (Ceftazidime) Glaxo Wellcome ... 1092
Mandol Vials, Faspak & ADD-Vantage (Cefamandole Nafate) Lilly ... 1516
Mefoxin (Cefoxitin Sodium) Merck & Co., Inc. ... 1734
Mefoxin Premixed Intravenous Solution (Cefoxitin Sodium) Merck & Co., Inc. ... 1737
Mezlin (Mezlocillin Sodium) Bayer Pharmaceutical ... 594
Mezlin Pharmacy Bulk Package (Mezlocillin Sodium) Bayer Pharmaceutical ... 597
Nebcin Vials, Hyporets & ADD-Vantage (Tobramycin Sulfate) Lilly ... 1518
Pipracil (Piperacillin Sodium) Lederle ... 1435
Primaxin I.V. (Cilastatin Sodium, Imipenem) Merck & Co., Inc. ... 1772
Tazicef for Injection (Ceftazidime) SmithKline Beecham Pharmaceuticals ... 2697
Tazidime Vials, Faspak & ADD-Vantage (Ceftazidime) Lilly .. 1531
Timentin for Injection (Ticarcillin Disodium, Clavulanate Potassium) SmithKline Beecham Pharmaceuticals ... 2706
Zinacef (Cefuroxime Sodium) Glaxo Wellcome ... 1184

Klebsiella species prostatitis

Ancef Injection (Cefazolin Sodium) SmithKline Beecham Pharmaceuticals ... 2632
Keftab Tablets (Cephalexin Hydrochloride) Dista ... 931

Klebsiella species respiratory tract infections

Achromycin V Capsules (Tetracycline Hydrochloride) Lederle ... 1417
Ancef Injection (Cefazolin Sodium) SmithKline Beecham Pharmaceuticals ... 2632
Ceptaz (Ceftazidime) Glaxo Wellcome ... 1070
Doryx Capsules (Doxycycline Hyclate) Parke-Davis ... 1970
DYNACIN Capsules (Minocycline Hydrochloride) Medicis ... 1627
Kefzol Vials, Faspak & ADD-Vantage (Cefazolin Sodium) Lilly ... 1511
Minocin Intravenous (Minocycline Hydrochloride) Lederle ... 1428
Minocin Oral Suspension (Minocycline Hydrochloride) Lederle ... 1431
Minocin Pellet-Filled Capsules (Minocycline Hydrochloride) Lederle ... 1429
Monodox Capsules (Doxycycline Monohydrate) Oclassen ... 1858
Terramycin Intramuscular Solution (Oxytetracycline) Pfizer Inc ... 2034
Vibramycin (Doxycycline Calcium) Pfizer Inc ... 2038
Vibramycin Hyclate Intravenous (Doxycycline Hyclate) Pfizer Inc ... 2040
Vibramycin (Doxycycline Monohydrate) Pfizer Inc ... 2038

Klebsiella species septicemia

Ancef Injection (Cefazolin Sodium) SmithKline Beecham Pharmaceuticals ... 2632
Cefizox for Intramuscular or Intravenous Use (Ceftizoxime Sodium) Fujisawa ... 1025
Ceptaz (Ceftazidime) Glaxo Wellcome ... 1070
Claforan Sterile and Injection (Cefotaxime Sodium) Hoechst Marion Roussel ... 1259

Fortaz (Ceftazidime) Glaxo Wellcome ... 1092
Kefurox Vials, Faspak & ADD-Vantage (Cefuroxime Sodium) Lilly ... 1509
Kefzol Vials, Faspak & ADD-Vantage (Cefazolin Sodium) Lilly ... 1511
Mefoxin (Cefoxitin Sodium) Merck & Co., Inc. ... 1734
Mefoxin Premixed Intravenous Solution (Cefoxitin Sodium) Merck & Co., Inc. ... 1737
Mezlin (Mezlocillin Sodium) Bayer Pharmaceutical ... 594
Mezlin Pharmacy Bulk Package (Mezlocillin Sodium) Bayer Pharmaceutical ... 597
Nebcin Vials, Hyporets & ADD-Vantage (Tobramycin Sulfate) Lilly ... 1518
Pipracil (Piperacillin Sodium) Lederle ... 1435
Primaxin I.V. (Cilastatin Sodium, Imipenem) Merck & Co., Inc. ... 1772
Tazicef for Injection (Ceftazidime) SmithKline Beecham Pharmaceuticals ... 2697
Tazidime Vials, Faspak & ADD-Vantage (Ceftazidime) Lilly .. 1531
Timentin for Injection (Ticarcillin Disodium, Clavulanate Potassium) SmithKline Beecham Pharmaceuticals ... 2706
Zinacef (Cefuroxime Sodium) Glaxo Wellcome ... 1184

Klebsiella species skin and skin structure infections

Augmentin (Amoxicillin Trihydrate, Clavulanate Potassium) SmithKline Beecham Pharmaceuticals ... 2637
Augmentin Tablets (Amoxicillin Trihydrate, Clavulanate Potassium) SmithKline Beecham Pharmaceuticals ... 2640
Cefizox for Intramuscular or Intravenous Use (Ceftizoxime Sodium) Fujisawa ... 1025
Ceptaz (Ceftazidime) Glaxo Wellcome ... 1070
Claforan Sterile and Injection (Cefotaxime Sodium) Hoechst Marion Roussel ... 1259
Fortaz (Ceftazidime) Glaxo Wellcome ... 1092
Kefurox Vials, Faspak & ADD-Vantage (Cefuroxime Sodium) Lilly ... 1509
Mefoxin (Cefoxitin Sodium) Merck & Co., Inc. ... 1734
Mefoxin Premixed Intravenous Solution (Cefoxitin Sodium) Merck & Co., Inc. ... 1737
Mezlin (Mezlocillin Sodium) Bayer Pharmaceutical ... 594
Mezlin Pharmacy Bulk Package (Mezlocillin Sodium) Bayer Pharmaceutical ... 597
Nebcin Vials, Hyporets & ADD-Vantage (Tobramycin Sulfate) Lilly ... 1518
Pipracil (Piperacillin Sodium) Lederle ... 1435
Primaxin I.V. (Cilastatin Sodium, Imipenem) Merck & Co., Inc. ... 1772
Tazicef for Injection (Ceftazidime) SmithKline Beecham Pharmaceuticals ... 2697
Tazidime Vials, Faspak & ADD-Vantage (Ceftazidime) Lilly .. 1531
Timentin for Injection (Ticarcillin Disodium, Clavulanate Potassium) SmithKline Beecham Pharmaceuticals ... 2706
Unasyn (Ampicillin Sodium, Sulbactam Sodium) Pfizer Inc ... 2035
Zinacef (Cefuroxime Sodium) Glaxo Wellcome ... 1184

Klebsiella species urinary tract infections

Achromycin V Capsules (Tetracycline Hydrochloride) Lederle ... 1417
Ancef Injection (Cefazolin Sodium) SmithKline Beecham Pharmaceuticals ... 2632
Augmentin (Amoxicillin Trihydrate, Clavulanate Potassium)

(▣ Described in PDR For Nonprescription Drugs) (⊙ Described in PDR For Ophthalmology)

Indications Index

SmithKline Beecham Pharmaceuticals 2637
Augmentin Tablets (Amoxicillin Trihydrate, Clavulanate Potassium) SmithKline Beecham Pharmaceuticals 2640
Bactrim DS Tablets (Trimethoprim, Sulfamethoxazole) Roche Pharmaceuticals 2257
Bactrim I.V. Infusion (Trimethoprim, Sulfamethoxazole) Roche Pharmaceuticals 2255
Bactrim (Trimethoprim, Sulfamethoxazole) Roche Pharmaceuticals 2257
Ceclor Pulvules & Suspension (Cefaclor) Lilly 1470
Cefizox for Intramuscular or Intravenous Use (Ceftizoxime Sodium) Fujisawa 1025
Cefotan (Cefotetan) Zeneca 2936
Ceptaz (Ceftazidime) Glaxo Wellcome 1070
Claforan Sterile and Injection (Cefotaxime Sodium) Hoechst Marion Roussel 1259
Declomycin Tablets (Demeclocycline Hydrochloride) Lederle 1421
Doryx Capsules (Doxycycline Hyclate) Parke-Davis 1970
Duricef Capsules, Tablets, and Oral Suspension (Cefadroxil) Bristol-Myers Squibb 750
DYNACIN Capsules (Minocycline Hydrochloride) Medicis 1627
Fortaz (Ceftazidime) Glaxo Wellcome 1092
Gantanol Tablets (Sulfamethoxazole) Roche Pharmaceuticals 2285
Gantrisin (Acetyl Sulfisoxazole) Roche Pharmaceuticals 2286
Keftab Tablets (Cephalexin Hydrochloride) Dista 931
Kefurox Vials, Faspak & ADD-Vantage (Cefuroxime Sodium) Lilly 1509
Kefzol Vials, Faspak & ADD-Vantage (Cefazolin Sodium) Lilly 1511
Macrodantin Capsules (Nitrofurantoin) Procter & Gamble Pharmaceuticals 2140
Mandol Vials, Faspak & ADD-Vantage (Cefamandole Nafate) Lilly 1516
Mefoxin (Cefoxitin Sodium) Merck & Co., Inc. 1734
Mefoxin Premixed Intravenous Solution (Cefoxitin Sodium) Merck & Co., Inc. 1737
Mezlin (Mezlocillin Sodium) Bayer Pharmaceutical 594
Mezlin Pharmacy Bulk Package (Mezlocillin Sodium) Bayer Pharmaceutical 597
Minocin Intravenous (Minocycline Hydrochloride) Lederle 1428
Minocin Oral Suspension (Minocycline Hydrochloride) Lederle 1431
Minocin Pellet-Filled Capsules (Minocycline Hydrochloride) Lederle 1429
Monodox Capsules (Doxycycline Monohydrate) Oclassen 1858
Nebcin Vials, Hyporets & ADD-Vantage (Tobramycin Sulfate) Lilly 1518
NegGram (Nalidixic Acid) Sanofi Winthrop 2453
Primaxin I.V. (Cilastatin Sodium, Imipenem) Merck & Co., Inc. 1772
Septra (Trimethoprim, Sulfamethoxazole) Glaxo Wellcome 1146
Septra I.V. Infusion (Trimethoprim, Sulfamethoxazole) Glaxo Wellcome 1142
Septra I.V. Infusion ADD-Vantage Vials (Trimethoprim, Sulfamethoxazole) Glaxo Wellcome 1144
Septra (Trimethoprim, Sulfamethoxazole) Glaxo Wellcome 1146
Tazicef for Injection (Ceftazidime) SmithKline Beecham Pharmaceuticals 2697
Tazidime Vials, Faspak & ADD-Vantage (Ceftazidime) Lilly .. 1531
Terramycin Intramuscular Solution (Oxytetracycline) Pfizer Inc 2034
Timentin for Injection (Ticarcillin Disodium, Clavulanate Potassium) SmithKline Beecham Pharmaceuticals 2706
Vibramycin (Doxycycline Calcium) Pfizer Inc 2038
Vibramycin Hyclate Intravenous (Doxycycline Hyclate) Pfizer Inc.... 2040
Vibramycin (Doxycycline Monohydrate) Pfizer Inc 2038
Zinacef (Cefuroxime Sodium) Glaxo Wellcome 1184

Klebsiella-Enterobacter species infections, ocular

AK-CIDE (Prednisolone Acetate, Sulfacetamide Sodium) Akorn.... ⊚ 203
AK-CIDE Ointment (Prednisolone Acetate, Sulfacetamide Sodium) Akorn .... ⊚ 203
AK-Spore (Bacitracin Zinc, Neomycin Sulfate, Polymyxin B Sulfate) Akorn .... ⊚ 205
AK-Trol Ointment & Suspension (Dexamethasone, Neomycin Sulfate, Polymyxin B Sulfate) Akorn .... ⊚ 205
Blephamide Liquifilm Sterile Ophthalmic Suspension (Prednisolone Acetate, Sulfacetamide Sodium) Allergan 472
Blephamide Ointment (Sulfacetamide Sodium, Prednisolone Acetate) Allergan .... ⊚ 234
Chloromycetin Ophthalmic Ointment, 1% (Chloramphenicol) Parke-Davis ⊚ 298
Chloromycetin Ophthalmic Solution (Chloramphenicol) Parke-Davis .... ⊚ 299
Chloroptic S.O.P. (Chloramphenicol) Allergan .... ⊚ 236
Cortisporin Ophthalmic Ointment Sterile (Polymyxin B Sulfate, Bacitracin Zinc, Neomycin Sulfate, Hydrocortisone) Glaxo Wellcome 1074
Cortisporin Ophthalmic Suspension Sterile (Hydrocortisone, Polymyxin B Sulfate, Neomycin Sulfate) Glaxo Wellcome 1075
FML-S Liquifilm (Sulfacetamide Sodium, Fluorometholone) Allergan .... ⊚ 240
Gantanol Tablets (Sulfamethoxazole) Roche Pharmaceuticals 2285
Gantrisin (Acetyl Sulfisoxazole) Roche Pharmaceuticals 2286
Maxitrol Ophthalmic Ointment and Suspension (Dexamethasone, Neomycin Sulfate, Polymyxin B Sulfate) Alcon Laboratories .... ⊚ 222
NeoDecadron Sterile Ophthalmic Ointment (Neomycin Sulfate, Dexamethasone Sodium Phosphate) Merck & Co., Inc. 1755
NeoDecadron Sterile Ophthalmic Solution (Neomycin Sulfate, Dexamethasone Sodium Phosphate) Merck & Co., Inc. 1756
Poly-Pred Liquifilm (Neomycin Sulfate, Polymyxin B Sulfate, Prednisolone Acetate) Allergan .... ⊚ 246
Pred-G Liquifilm Sterile Ophthalmic Suspension (Gentamicin Sulfate, Prednisolone Acetate) Allergan .... ⊚ 248
TobraDex Ophthalmic Suspension and Ointment (Dexamethasone, Tobramycin) Alcon Laboratories .. 469

Klebsiella-Enterobacter urinary tract infections

Gantanol Tablets (Sulfamethoxazole) Roche Pharmaceuticals 2285
Gantrisin (Acetyl Sulfisoxazole) Roche Pharmaceuticals 2286

Koch-Weeks bacillus infections, ocular

(see under H. aegypticus infections, ocular)

L

Labor and delivery, routine management of
Methergine (Methylergonovine Maleate) Sandoz Pharmaceuticals 2401

Labor, induction of
Syntocinon Injection (Oxytocin) Sandoz Pharmaceuticals 2425

Labor, preterm, management of
Yutopar Intravenous Injection (Ritodrine Hydrochloride) Astra .. 566

Labor, stimulation of
Syntocinon Injection (Oxytocin) Sandoz Pharmaceuticals 2425

Lacrimation, symptomatic relief of
Benadryl Allergy Liquid Medication (Diphenhydramine Hydrochloride) Warner Wellcome .... ⊞ 813
Benadryl Allergy (Diphenhydramine Hydrochloride) Warner Wellcome .... ⊞ 811
Benadryl Allergy Sinus Headache Caplets (Diphenhydramine Hydrochloride, Pseudoephedrine Hydrochloride, Acetaminophen) Warner Wellcome .... ⊞ 813
Chlor-Trimeton Allergy Tablets (Chlorpheniramine Maleate) Schering-Plough HealthCare .. ⊞ 758
Allergy-Sinus Comtrex Multi-Symptom Allergy-Sinus Formula Tablets and Caplets (Acetaminophen, Chlorpheniramine Maleate, Pseudoephedrine Hydrochloride) Bristol-Myers Products .... ⊞ 639
Contac Night Allergy/Sinus Caplets (Acetaminophen, Pseudoephedrine Hydrochloride, Diphenhydramine Hydrochloride) SmithKline Beecham Consumer............ ⊞ 771
Dimetapp Cold & Allergy Chewable Tablets (Brompheniramine Maleate, Phenylpropanolamine Hydrochloride) Whitehall-Robins .... ⊞ 838
Dimetapp Elixir (Brompheniramine Maleate, Phenylpropanolamine Hydrochloride) Whitehall-Robins .... ⊞ 840
Dimetapp Extentabs (Brompheniramine Maleate, Phenylpropanolamine Hydrochloride) Whitehall-Robins .... ⊞ 841
Dimetapp Tablets/Liqui-Gels (Brompheniramine Maleate, Phenylpropanolamine Hydrochloride) Whitehall-Robins .... ⊞ 841
Nolahist Tablets (Phenindamine Tartrate) Carnrick 790
Ryna Liquid (Chlorpheniramine Maleate, Pseudoephedrine Hydrochloride) Wallace .... ⊞ 804
Seldane Tablets (Terfenadine) Hoechst Marion Roussel 1284
Seldane-D Extended-Release Tablets (Pseudoephedrine Hydrochloride, Terfenadine) Hoechst Marion Roussel 1286
Similasan Eye Drops #2 (Homeopathic Medications) Similasan ⊚ 316
Tavist Syrup (Clemastine Fumarate) Sandoz Pharmaceuticals 2426
Tavist Tablets (Clemastine Fumarate) Sandoz Pharmaceuticals 2427
TYLENOL Severe Allergy Medication Caplets (Acetaminophen, Chlorpheniramine Maleate, Pseudoephedrine Hydrochloride) McNeil Consumer 1571

Lactose intolerance
Lactaid Drops (Lactase (beta-d-Galactosidase)) McNeil Consumer 1562
Lactaid (Lactase (beta-d-Galactosidase)) McNeil Consumer 1562

Lactobacillus acidophilus, deficiency of
DDS-Acidophilus (Lactobacillus Acidophilus) UAS Laboratories .. ⊞ 800
FLORAjen (Lactobacillus Acidophilus) American Lifeline .. ⊞ 602

Larva migrans, cutaneous
Mintezol (Thiabendazole) Merck & Co., Inc. 1747

Larva migrans, visceral
Mintezol (Thiabendazole) Merck & Co., Inc. 1747

Laryngeal edema, acute noninfectious, adjunctive therapy in
Celestone Soluspan Suspension (Betamethasone Sodium Phosphate, Betamethasone Acetate) Schering 2484
Cortone Acetate Sterile Suspension (Cortisone Acetate) Merck & Co., Inc. 1663
Decadron Phosphate Injection (Dexamethasone Sodium Phosphate) Merck & Co., Inc. .. 1680
Hydeltrasol Injection, Sterile (Prednisolone Sodium Phosphate) Merck & Co., Inc. 1708
Hydrocortone Phosphate Injection, Sterile (Hydrocortisone Sodium Phosphate) Merck & Co., Inc. 1713

LDL cholesterol, elevation
(see under Hyperlipoproteinemia, types IIa and IIb, adjunct to diet)

Lead encephalopathy
Calcium Disodium Versenate Injection (Calcium Disodium Edetate) 3M Pharmaceuticals........ 1548

Lead poisoning
Calcium Disodium Versenate Injection (Calcium Disodium Edetate) 3M Pharmaceuticals........ 1548
Chemet Capsules (Succimer) Bock 666

Leg muscle cramps
Hyland's Leg Cramps Tablets (Homeopathic Medications) Standard Homeopathic............ ⊞ 790

Legionella pneumophila infections
(see under Legionnaires' disease)

Legionnaires' disease
Dynabac (Dirithromycin) Bock 668
E.E.S. (Erythromycin Ethylsuccinate) Abbott 427
E-Mycin Tablets (Erythromycin) Knoll Laboratories 1388
ERYC (Erythromycin) Parke-Davis .. 1972
EryPed (Erythromycin Ethylsuccinate) Abbott 425
Ery-Tab Tablets (Erythromycin) Abbott 426
Erythrocin Stearate Filmtab (Erythromycin Stearate) Abbott 429
Erythromycin Base Filmtab (Erythromycin) Abbott 430
Erythromycin Delayed-Release Capsules, USP (Erythromycin) Abbott 431
Ilosone (Erythromycin Estolate) Dista 927
Ilotycin Gluceptate, IV, Vials (Erythromycin Gluceptate) Dista 929
PCE Dispertab Tablets (Erythromycin) Abbott 453

Leishmaniasis, American
Fungizone Intravenous (Amphotericin B) Apothecon 507

Lennox-Gastaut syndrome
Felbatol (Felbamate) Wallace 2774
Klonopin Tablets (Clonazepam) Roche Pharmaceuticals 2294

Lens, intraocular, implantation of, surgical aid in
AMO Vitrax Viscoelastic Solution (Sodium Hyaluronate) Allergan.. ⊚ 229
Healon (Sodium Hyaluronate) Pharmacia & Upjohn .... ⊚ 302
OcuCoat (Hydroxypropyl Methylcellulose) Storz Ophthalmics .... ⊚ 321

(⊞ Described in PDR For Nonprescription Drugs)   (⊚ Described in PDR For Ophthalmology)

Leprosy

Leprosy
- Dapsone Tablets USP (Dapsone) Jacobus ... 1331

Leprosy, lepromatous
- Lamprene Capsules (Clofazimine) CibaGeneva ... 846

Leprosy, lepromatous, complicated by erythema nodosum leprosum
- Lamprene Capsules (Clofazimine) CibaGeneva ... 846

Leprosy, lepromatous, dapsone-resistant
- Lamprene Capsules (Clofazimine) CibaGeneva ... 846

Letterer-Siwe disease
- Velban Vials (Vinblastine Sulfate) Lilly ... 1537

Leukapheresis, adjunct to
- Hespan Injection (Hetastarch) DuPont ... 945
- Pentaspan Injection (Pentastarch) DuPont ... 954

Leukemia, acute
- Oncovin Solution Vials & Hyporets (Vincristine Sulfate) Lilly ... 1521

Leukemia, acute erythroid
- Cerubidine for Injection (Daunorubicin Hydrochloride) Bedford ... 634

Leukemia, acute lymphoblastic
- Adriamycin PFS (Doxorubicin Hydrochloride) Pharmacia & Upjohn ... 2056
- Adriamycin RDF (Doxorubicin Hydrochloride) Pharmacia & Upjohn ... 2056
- Cytoxan (Cyclophosphamide) Bristol-Myers Squibb Oncology/Immunology ... 700
- Doxorubicin Astra (Doxorubicin Hydrochloride) Astra ... 531
- Oncaspar (Pegaspargase) Rhone-Poulenc Rorer Pharmaceuticals ... 2194
- Purinethol Tablets (Mercaptopurine) Glaxo Wellcome Oncology/HIV ... 1214
- Rubex for Injection (Doxorubicin Hydrochloride) Bristol-Myers Squibb Oncology/Immunology ... 721
- Vumon for Injection (Teniposide) Bristol-Myers Squibb Oncology/Immunology ... 729

Leukemia, acute lymphocytic
- Cerubidine for Injection (Daunorubicin Hydrochloride) Bedford ... 634
- Cytosar-U Sterile Powder (Cytarabine) Pharmacia & Upjohn ... 2077
- Elspar (Asparaginase) Merck & Co., Inc. ... 1700
- Purinethol Tablets (Mercaptopurine) Glaxo Wellcome Oncology/HIV ... 1214

Leukemia, acute monocytic
- Cerubidine for Injection (Daunorubicin Hydrochloride) Bedford ... 634
- Cytoxan (Cyclophosphamide) Bristol-Myers Squibb Oncology/Immunology ... 700

Leukemia, acute myeloblastic
- Adriamycin PFS (Doxorubicin Hydrochloride) Pharmacia & Upjohn ... 2056
- Adriamycin RDF (Doxorubicin Hydrochloride) Pharmacia & Upjohn ... 2056
- Doxorubicin Astra (Doxorubicin Hydrochloride) Astra ... 531
- Rubex for Injection (Doxorubicin Hydrochloride) Bristol-Myers Squibb Oncology/Immunology ... 721

Leukemia, acute myelogenous
- Cerubidine for Injection (Daunorubicin Hydrochloride) Bedford ... 634
- Cytoxan (Cyclophosphamide) Bristol-Myers Squibb Oncology/Immunology ... 700

- Idamycin Injection (Idarubicin Hydrochloride) Pharmacia & Upjohn ... 2096

Leukemia, acute nonlymphocytic
- Cerubidine for Injection (Daunorubicin Hydrochloride) Bedford ... 634
- Cytosar-U Sterile Powder (Cytarabine) Pharmacia & Upjohn ... 2077
- Novantrone for Injection (Mitoxantrone Hydrochloride) Immunex ... 1327
- Thioguanine Tablets, Tabloid Brand (Thioguanine) Glaxo Wellcome Oncology/HIV ... 1225

Leukemia, acute, palliative management of in childhood
- Cortone Acetate Sterile Suspension (Cortisone Acetate) Merck & Co., Inc. ... 1663
- Cortone Acetate Tablets (Cortisone Acetate) Merck & Co., Inc. ... 1664
- Dalalone D.P. Injectable (Dexamethasone Acetate) Forest ... 1009
- Decadron Elixir (Dexamethasone) Merck & Co., Inc. ... 1676
- Decadron Phosphate Injection (Dexamethasone Sodium Phosphate) Merck & Co., Inc. ... 1680
- Decadron Tablets (Dexamethasone) Merck & Co., Inc. ... 1678
- Decadron-LA Sterile Suspension (Dexamethasone Acetate) Merck & Co., Inc. ... 1687
- Hydeltrasol Injection, Sterile (Prednisolone Sodium Phosphate) Merck & Co., Inc. ... 1708
- Hydrocortone Phosphate Injection, Sterile (Hydrocortisone Sodium Phosphate) Merck & Co., Inc. ... 1713
- Hydrocortone Tablets (Hydrocortisone) Merck & Co., Inc. ... 1715
- Pediapred Oral Solution (Prednisolone Sodium Phosphate) Medeva 1618
- Prelone Syrup (Prednisolone) Muro 1834

Leukemia, acute, promyelocytic
- Vesanoid Capsules (Tretinoin) Roche Pharmaceuticals ... 2327

Leukemia, adjunctive therapy in
- Zyloprim Tablets (Allopurinol) Glaxo Wellcome ... 1194

Leukemia, chronic granulocytic
- Cytoxan (Cyclophosphamide) Bristol-Myers Squibb Oncology/Immunology ... 700

Leukemia, chronic lymphocytic
- Cytoxan (Cyclophosphamide) Bristol-Myers Squibb Oncology/Immunology ... 700
- Leukeran Tablets (Chlorambucil) Glaxo Wellcome Oncology/HIV ... 1205
- Methotrexate Sodium Tablets, Injection, for Injection and LPF Injection (Methotrexate Sodium) Immunex ... 1322
- Mustargen (Mechlorethamine Hydrochloride) Merck & Co., Inc. 1752

Leukemia, chronic lymphocytic, B-cell
- Fludara for Injection (Fludarabine Phosphate) Berlex ... 658

Leukemia, chronic lymphocytic, B-cell, prevention of bacterial infection in
- Gammagard S/D, Immune Globulin, Intravenous (Human) (Globulin, Immune (Human)) Baxter Healthcare ... 577

Leukemia, chronic myelocytic
- Cytosar-U Sterile Powder (Cytarabine) Pharmacia & Upjohn ... 2077
- Hydrea Capsules (Hydroxyurea) Bristol-Myers Squibb Oncology/Immunology ... 705
- Mustargen (Mechlorethamine Hydrochloride) Merck & Co., Inc. 1752

Leukemia, chronic myelogenous
- Myleran Tablets (Busulfan) Glaxo Wellcome Oncology/HIV ... 1209

- Roferon-A Injection (Interferon alfa-2A, Recombinant) Roche Pharmaceuticals ... 2308

Leukemia, hairy cell
- Intron A for Injection (Interferon alfa-2B, Recombinant) Schering .. 2506
- Leustatin (Cladribine) Ortho Biotech ... 1889
- Roferon-A Injection (Interferon alfa-2A, Recombinant) Roche Pharmaceuticals ... 2308

Leukemia, hairy cell, alpha-interferon-refractory
- Nipent for Injection (Pentostatin) SuperGen ... 2733

Leukemia, lymphoblastic, adjunctive therapy in
- Leukine (Sargramostim) Immunex .. 1317

Leukemia, meningeal, prophylaxis of
- Cytosar-U Sterile Powder (Cytarabine) Pharmacia & Upjohn ... 2077
- Methotrexate Sodium Tablets, Injection, for Injection and LPF Injection (Methotrexate Sodium) Immunex ... 1322

Leukemia, meningeal, treatment of
- Methotrexate Sodium Tablets, Injection, for Injection and LPF Injection (Methotrexate Sodium) Immunex ... 1322

Leukemias, palliative management of
- Celestone Soluspan Suspension (Betamethasone Sodium Phosphate, Betamethasone Acetate) Schering ... 2484
- Cortone Acetate Sterile Suspension (Cortisone Acetate) Merck & Co., Inc. ... 1663
- Cortone Acetate Tablets (Cortisone Acetate) Merck & Co., Inc. ... 1664
- Dalalone D.P. Injectable (Dexamethasone Acetate) Forest ... 1009
- Decadron Elixir (Dexamethasone) Merck & Co., Inc. ... 1676
- Decadron Phosphate Injection (Dexamethasone Sodium Phosphate) Merck & Co., Inc. ... 1680
- Decadron Tablets (Dexamethasone) Merck & Co., Inc. ... 1678
- Decadron-LA Sterile Suspension (Dexamethasone Acetate) Merck & Co., Inc. ... 1687
- Hydeltrasol Injection, Sterile (Prednisolone Sodium Phosphate) Merck & Co., Inc. ... 1708
- Hydrocortone Phosphate Injection, Sterile (Hydrocortisone Sodium Phosphate) Merck & Co., Inc. ... 1713
- Hydrocortone Tablets (Hydrocortisone) Merck & Co., Inc. ... 1715
- Pediapred Oral Solution (Prednisolone Sodium Phosphate) Medeva 1618
- Prelone Syrup (Prednisolone) Muro 1834

Lice, body
(see under Pediculosis, human)

Lice, head
(see under Pediculosis, human)

Lice, pubic
(see under Pediculosis, human)

Lichen planus
- Celestone Soluspan Suspension (Betamethasone Sodium Phosphate, Betamethasone Acetate) Schering ... 2484
- Decadron Phosphate Injection (Dexamethasone Sodium Phosphate) Merck & Co., Inc. ... 1680
- Decadron-LA Sterile Suspension (Dexamethasone Acetate) Merck & Co., Inc. ... 1687
- Hydeltrasol Injection, Sterile (Prednisolone Sodium Phosphate) Merck & Co., Inc. ... 1708
- Hydrocortone Acetate Sterile Suspension (Hydrocortisone Acetate) Merck & Co., Inc. ... 1712

Lichen simplex chronicus
- Celestone Soluspan Suspension (Betamethasone Sodium Phosphate, Betamethasone Acetate) Schering ... 2484
- Decadron Phosphate Injection (Dexamethasone Sodium Phosphate) Merck & Co., Inc. ... 1680
- Decadron-LA Sterile Suspension (Dexamethasone Acetate) Merck & Co., Inc. ... 1687
- Hydeltrasol Injection, Sterile (Prednisolone Sodium Phosphate) Merck & Co., Inc. ... 1708
- Hydrocortone Acetate Sterile Suspension (Hydrocortisone Acetate) Merck & Co., Inc. ... 1712
- Mantadil Cream (Chlorcyclizine Hydrochloride) Glaxo Wellcome .. 1124
- Zonalon Cream (Doxepin Hydrochloride) GenDerm ... 1042

Lips, dry
(see under Cheilitis, actinic)

Listeria monocytogenes infections
- Achromycin V Capsules (Tetracycline Hydrochloride) Lederle ... 1417
- Declomycin Tablets (Demeclocycline Hydrochloride) Lederle ... 1421
- Doryx Capsules (Doxycycline Hyclate) Parke-Davis ... 1970
- DYNACIN Capsules (Minocycline Hydrochloride) Medicis ... 1627
- E.E.S. (Erythromycin Ethylsuccinate) Abbott ... 427
- E-Mycin Tablets (Erythromycin) Knoll Laboratories ... 1388
- ERYC (Erythromycin) Parke-Davis .. 1972
- EryPed (Erythromycin Ethylsuccinate) Abbott ... 425
- Ery-Tab Tablets (Erythromycin) Abbott ... 426
- Erythrocin Stearate Filmtab (Erythromycin Stearate) Abbott ... 429
- Erythromycin Base Filmtab (Erythromycin) Abbott ... 430
- Erythromycin Delayed-Release Capsules, USP (Erythromycin) Abbott ... 431
- Ilosone (Erythromycin Estolate) Dista ... 927
- Ilotycin Gluceptate, IV, Vials (Erythromycin Gluceptate) Dista ... 929
- Minocin Intravenous (Minocycline Hydrochloride) Lederle ... 1428
- Minocin Oral Suspension (Minocycline Hydrochloride) Lederle ... 1431
- Minocin Pellet-Filled Capsules (Minocycline Hydrochloride) Lederle ... 1429
- Monodox Capsules (Doxycycline Monohydrate) Oclassen ... 1858
- Pfizerpen for Injection (Penicillin G Potassium) Pfizer Inc ... 2022
- Terramycin Intramuscular Solution (Oxytetracycline) Pfizer Inc ... 2034
- Vibramycin (Doxycycline Calcium) Pfizer Inc ... 2038
- Vibramycin Hyclate Intravenous (Doxycycline Hyclate) Pfizer Inc.... 2040
- Vibramycin (Doxycycline Monohydrate) Pfizer Inc ... 2038

Listeriosis
- DYNACIN Capsules (Minocycline Hydrochloride) Medicis ... 1627
- Minocin Oral Suspension (Minocycline Hydrochloride) Lederle ... 1431
- Minocin Pellet-Filled Capsules (Minocycline Hydrochloride) Lederle ... 1429
- Monodox Capsules (Doxycycline Monohydrate) Oclassen ... 1858

Liver abscess, amebic
(see under Amebic liver abscess)

Liver, allogeneic transplants, prophylaxis of organ rejection in
- Neoral (Cyclosporine) Sandoz Pharmaceuticals ... 2405
- Orthoclone OKT3 Sterile Solution (Muromonab-CD3) Ortho Biotech 1892
- Prograf (Tacrolimus) Fujisawa ... 1028
- Sandimmune (Cyclosporine) Sandoz Pharmaceuticals ... 2416

Lou Gehrig's disease
(see under Sclerosis, amyotrophic lateral)

(■ Described in PDR For Nonprescription Drugs)   (⊚ Described in PDR For Ophthalmology)

1545 Indications Index Malassezia furfur

Loeffler's syndrome
Celestone Soluspan Suspension (Betamethasone Sodium Phosphate, Betamethasone Acetate) Schering ... 2484
Cortone Acetate Sterile Suspension (Cortisone Acetate) Merck & Co., Inc. ... 1663
Cortone Acetate Tablets (Cortisone Acetate) Merck & Co., Inc. ... 1664
Dalalone D.P. Injectable (Dexamethasone Acetate) Forest ... 1009
Decadron Elixir (Dexamethasone) Merck & Co., Inc. ... 1676
Decadron Phosphate Injection (Dexamethasone Sodium Phosphate) Merck & Co., Inc. ... 1680
Decadron Tablets (Dexamethasone) Merck & Co., Inc. ... 1678
Decadron-LA Sterile Suspension (Dexamethasone Acetate) Merck & Co., Inc. ... 1687
Hydeltrasol Injection, Sterile (Prednisolone Sodium Phosphate) Merck & Co., Inc. ... 1708
Hydrocortone Phosphate Injection, Sterile (Hydrocortisone Sodium Phosphate) Merck & Co., Inc. ... 1713
Hydrocortone Tablets (Hydrocortisone) Merck & Co., Inc. ... 1715
Pediapred Oral Solution (Prednisolone Sodium Phosphate) Medeva 1618
Prelone Syrup (Prednisolone) Muro 1834

Lown-Ganong-Levine syndrome
Isoptin Injectable (Verapamil Hydrochloride) Knoll Laboratories ... 1391

Lubrication, sexual (see under Coitus, adjunct in)

Lung abscess (see under Abscess, lung)

Lupus erythematosus discoides
Celestone Soluspan Suspension (Betamethasone Sodium Phosphate, Betamethasone Acetate) Schering ... 2484
Decadron Phosphate Injection (Dexamethasone Sodium Phosphate) Merck & Co., Inc. ... 1680
Decadron-LA Sterile Suspension (Dexamethasone Acetate) Merck & Co., Inc. ... 1687
Hydeltrasol Injection, Sterile (Prednisolone Sodium Phosphate) Merck & Co., Inc. ... 1708
Hydrocortone Acetate Sterile Suspension (Hydrocortisone Acetate) Merck & Co., Inc. ... 1712
Plaquenil Sulfate Tablets (Hydroxychloroquine Sulfate) Sanofi Winthrop ... 2459

Lupus erythematosus, systemic
Extra Strength Bayer Arthritis Pain Regimen Formula (Aspirin, Enteric Coated) Bayer Consumer ... ▣ 615
Celestone Soluspan Suspension (Betamethasone Sodium Phosphate, Betamethasone Acetate) Schering ... 2484
Cortone Acetate Sterile Suspension (Cortisone Acetate) Merck & Co., Inc. ... 1663
Cortone Acetate Tablets (Cortisone Acetate) Merck & Co., Inc. ... 1664
Dalalone D.P. Injectable (Dexamethasone Acetate) Forest ... 1009
Decadron Elixir (Dexamethasone) Merck & Co., Inc. ... 1676
Decadron Phosphate Injection (Dexamethasone Sodium Phosphate) Merck & Co., Inc. ... 1680
Decadron Tablets (Dexamethasone) Merck & Co., Inc. ... 1678
Decadron-LA Sterile Suspension (Dexamethasone Acetate) Merck & Co., Inc. ... 1687
Ecotrin (Aspirin) SmithKline Beecham ... 2625
Hydeltrasol Injection, Sterile (Prednisolone Sodium Phosphate) Merck & Co., Inc. ... 1708
Hydrocortone Phosphate Injection, Sterile (Hydrocortisone Sodium Phosphate) Merck & Co., Inc. ... 1713
Hydrocortone Tablets (Hydrocortisone) Merck & Co., Inc. ... 1715
Pediapred Oral Solution (Prednisolone Sodium Phosphate) Medeva 1618
Plaquenil Sulfate Tablets (Hydroxychloroquine Sulfate) Sanofi Winthrop ... 2459
Prelone Syrup (Prednisolone) Muro 1834

Lyme disease (see under Borrelia burgdorferi infection)

Lymphogranuloma venereum
Achromycin V Capsules (Tetracycline Hydrochloride) Lederle ... 1417
Declomycin Tablets (Demeclocycline Hydrochloride) Lederle ... 1421
Doryx Capsules (Doxycycline Hyclate) Parke-Davis ... 1970
DYNACIN Capsules (Minocycline Hydrochloride) Medicis ... 1627
Minocin Intravenous (Minocycline Hydrochloride) Lederle ... 1428
Minocin Oral Suspension (Minocycline Hydrochloride) Lederle ... 1431
Minocin Pellet-Filled Capsules (Minocycline Hydrochloride) Lederle ... 1429
Monodox Capsules (Doxycycline Monohydrate) Oclassen ... 1858
Terramycin Intramuscular Solution (Oxytetracycline) Pfizer Inc ... 2034
Vibramycin (Doxycycline Calcium) Pfizer Inc ... 2038
Vibramycin Hyclate Intravenous (Doxycycline Hyclate) Pfizer Inc ... 2040
Vibramycin (Doxycycline Monohydrate) Pfizer Inc ... 2038

Lymphogranuloma-psittacosis group infections
Chloromycetin Sodium Succinate (Chloramphenicol Sodium Succinate) Parke-Davis ... 1960

Lymphography, diagnostic aid in
Ethiodol Injection (Ethiodized Oil) Savage ... 2472

Lymphoma, Burkitt's
Cytoxan (Cyclophosphamide) Bristol-Myers Squibb Oncology/Immunology ... 700

Lymphoma, cutaneous T-cell
8-MOP Capsules (Methoxsalen) ICN ... 1294

Lymphoma, hystiocytic
Cytoxan (Cyclophosphamide) Bristol-Myers Squibb Oncology/Immunology ... 700
Oncovin Solution Vials & Hyporets (Vincristine Sulfate) Lilly ... 1521
Velban Vials (Vinblastine Sulfate) Lilly ... 1537

Lymphoma, lymphocytic
Cytoxan (Cyclophosphamide) Bristol-Myers Squibb Oncology/Immunology ... 700
Oncovin Solution Vials & Hyporets (Vincristine Sulfate) Lilly ... 1521
Velban Vials (Vinblastine Sulfate) Lilly ... 1537

Lymphoma, mixed cell type
Cytoxan (Cyclophosphamide) Bristol-Myers Squibb Oncology/Immunology ... 700
Oncovin Solution Vials & Hyporets (Vincristine Sulfate) Lilly ... 1521

Lymphomas, giant follicular
Leukeran Tablets (Chlorambucil) Glaxo Wellcome Oncology/HIV ... 1205

Lymphomas, Hodgkin's (see under Hodgkin's disease)

Lymphomas, malignant
Adriamycin PFS (Doxorubicin Hydrochloride) Pharmacia & Upjohn ... 2056
Adriamycin RDF (Doxorubicin Hydrochloride) Pharmacia & Upjohn ... 2056
Cytoxan (Cyclophosphamide) Bristol-Myers Squibb Oncology/Immunology ... 700
Leukeran Tablets (Chlorambucil) Glaxo Wellcome Oncology/HIV ... 1205
Oncovin Solution Vials & Hyporets (Vincristine Sulfate) Lilly ... 1521
Rubex for Injection (Doxorubicin Hydrochloride) Bristol-Myers Squibb Oncology/Immunology ... 721

Lymphomas, non-Hodgkin's
BiCNU (Carmustine (BCNU)) Bristol-Myers Squibb Oncology/Immunology ... 696
Blenoxane (Bleomycin Sulfate) Bristol-Myers Squibb Oncology/Immunology ... 697
Doxorubicin Astra (Doxorubicin Hydrochloride) Astra ... 531
Leukeran Tablets (Chlorambucil) Glaxo Wellcome Oncology/HIV ... 1205
Methotrexate Sodium Tablets, Injection, for Injection and LPF Injection (Methotrexate Sodium) Immunex ... 1322
Mustargen (Mechlorethamine Hydrochloride) Merck & Co., Inc. 1752
Thioplex (Thiotepa For Injection) (Thiotepa) Immunex ... 1329

Lymphomas, non-Hodgkin's, adjunctive therapy in
Leukine (Sargramostim) Immunex .. 1317
Oncovin Solution Vials & Hyporets (Vincristine Sulfate) Lilly ... 1521

Lymphomas, palliative management of in adults
Celestone Soluspan Suspension (Betamethasone Sodium Phosphate, Betamethasone Acetate) Schering ... 2484
Cortone Acetate Sterile Suspension (Cortisone Acetate) Merck & Co., Inc. ... 1663
Cortone Acetate Tablets (Cortisone Acetate) Merck & Co., Inc. ... 1664
Dalalone D.P. Injectable (Dexamethasone Acetate) Forest ... 1009
Decadron Elixir (Dexamethasone) Merck & Co., Inc. ... 1676
Decadron Phosphate Injection (Dexamethasone Sodium Phosphate) Merck & Co., Inc. ... 1680
Decadron Tablets (Dexamethasone) Merck & Co., Inc. ... 1678
Decadron-LA Sterile Suspension (Dexamethasone Acetate) Merck & Co., Inc. ... 1687
Hydeltrasol Injection, Sterile (Prednisolone Sodium Phosphate) Merck & Co., Inc. ... 1708
Hydrocortone Phosphate Injection, Sterile (Hydrocortisone Sodium Phosphate) Merck & Co., Inc. ... 1713
Hydrocortone Tablets (Hydrocortisone) Merck & Co., Inc. ... 1715
Pediapred Oral Solution (Prednisolone Sodium Phosphate) Medeva 1618
Prelone Syrup (Prednisolone) Muro 1834

Lymphosarcoma (see under Lymphomas, non-Hodgkin's)

M

M. catarrhalis infections
Augmentin (Amoxicillin Trihydrate, Clavulanate Potassium) SmithKline Beecham Pharmaceuticals ... 2637
Augmentin Tablets (Amoxicillin Trihydrate, Clavulanate Potassium) SmithKline Beecham Pharmaceuticals ... 2640
Biaxin (Clarithromycin) Abbott ... 406
Cedax (Ceftibuten Dihydrate) Schering ... 2480
Ceftin (Cefuroxime Axetil) Glaxo Wellcome ... 1067
Cefzil Tablets and Oral Suspension (Cefprozil) Bristol-Myers Squibb .. 747
Dynabac (Dirithromycin) Bock ... 668
Keflex Pulvules & Oral Suspension (Cephalexin) Dista ... 930
Lorabid Suspension and Pulvules (Loracarbef) Lilly ... 1513
Maxaquin Tablets (Lomefloxacin Hydrochloride) Searle ... 2593
Suprax (Cefixime) Lederle ... 1443
Vantin for Oral Suspension and Vantin Tablets (Cefpodoxime Proxetil) Pharmacia & Upjohn ... 2112
Zithromax (Azithromycin) Pfizer Inc ... 2043
Zithromax Tablets (Azithromycin) Pfizer Inc ... 2046

M. catarrhalis lower respiratory tract infections
Augmentin (Amoxicillin Trihydrate, Clavulanate Potassium) SmithKline Beecham Pharmaceuticals ... 2637
Augmentin Tablets (Amoxicillin Trihydrate, Clavulanate Potassium) SmithKline Beecham Pharmaceuticals ... 2640
Biaxin (Clarithromycin) Abbott ... 406
Cefzil Tablets and Oral Suspension (Cefprozil) Bristol-Myers Squibb .. 747
Dynabac (Dirithromycin) Bock ... 668
Lorabid Suspension and Pulvules (Loracarbef) Lilly ... 1513
Maxaquin Tablets (Lomefloxacin Hydrochloride) Searle ... 2593
Vantin for Oral Suspension and Vantin Tablets (Cefpodoxime Proxetil) Pharmacia & Upjohn ... 2112
Zithromax (Azithromycin) Pfizer Inc ... 2043
Zithromax Tablets (Azithromycin) Pfizer Inc ... 2046

M. catarrhalis sinusitis
Augmentin (Amoxicillin Trihydrate, Clavulanate Potassium) SmithKline Beecham Pharmaceuticals ... 2637
Augmentin Tablets (Amoxicillin Trihydrate, Clavulanate Potassium) SmithKline Beecham Pharmaceuticals ... 2640
Biaxin (Clarithromycin) Abbott ... 406
Lorabid Suspension and Pulvules (Loracarbef) Lilly ... 1513

M. catarrhalis, otitis media
Augmentin (Amoxicillin Trihydrate, Clavulanate Potassium) SmithKline Beecham Pharmaceuticals ... 2637
Augmentin Tablets (Amoxicillin Trihydrate, Clavulanate Potassium) SmithKline Beecham Pharmaceuticals ... 2640
Biaxin (Clarithromycin) Abbott ... 406
Cedax (Ceftibuten Dihydrate) Schering ... 2480
Ceftin Tablets (Cefuroxime Axetil) Glaxo Wellcome ... 1067
Cefzil Tablets and Oral Suspension (Cefprozil) Bristol-Myers Squibb .. 747
Keflex Pulvules & Oral Suspension (Cephalexin) Dista ... 930
Lorabid Suspension and Pulvules (Loracarbef) Lilly ... 1513
Suprax (Cefixime) Lederle ... 1443
Vantin for Oral Suspension and Vantin Tablets (Cefpodoxime Proxetil) Pharmacia & Upjohn ... 2112
Zithromax (Azithromycin) Pfizer Inc ... 2043

Magnesium deficiency (see under Hypomagnesemia)

Malaria (see under P. vivax infections; P. malariae infections; P. ovale infections; P. falciparum infections)

Malaria, prophylaxis of
Fansidar Tablets (Sulfadoxine, Pyrimethamine) Roche Pharmaceuticals ... 2281
Lariam Tablets (Mefloquine Hydrochloride) Roche Pharmaceuticals ... 2295
Vibramycin Hyclate Capsules (Doxycycline Hyclate) Pfizer Inc ... 2038

Malassezia furfur (see under Pityrosporon orbiculare infections)

(▣ Described in PDR For Nonprescription Drugs) (◉ Described in PDR For Ophthalmology)

Malignant effusion, serosal cavities
Thioplex (Thiotepa For Injection) (Thiotepa) Immunex 1329

Manic episodes associated with bipolar disorder
Depakote Tablets (Divalproex Sodium) Abbott 418
Eskalith (Lithium Carbonate) SmithKline Beecham Pharmaceuticals 2658
Lithonate/Lithotabs/Lithobid (Lithium Carbonate) Solvay 2721

Mastocytosis, systemic
Gastrocrom Capsules (Cromolyn Sodium) Medeva 1611
Gastrocrom Oral Concentrate (Cromolyn Sodium) Medeva 1611
Prilosec Delayed-Release Capsules (Omeprazole) Astra Merck 516
Tagamet (Cimetidine Hydrochloride) SmithKline Beecham Pharmaceuticals 2694
Zantac (Ranitidine Hydrochloride) Glaxo Wellcome 1182

Measles, prophylaxis
Attenuvax (Measles Virus Vaccine Live) Merck & Co., Inc. 1650
M-M-R II (Measles, Mumps & Rubella Virus Vaccine Live) Merck & Co., Inc. 1730
M-R-VAX II (Measles & Rubella Virus Vaccine Live) Merck & Co., Inc. 1732

Meibomianitis, acute
Garamycin Ophthalmic (Gentamicin Sulfate) Schering 2501
Genoptic Sterile Ophthalmic Solution (Gentamicin Sulfate) Allergan ...... ⊚ 241
Genoptic Sterile Ophthalmic Ointment (Gentamicin Sulfate) Allergan ...... ⊚ 241
Gentak (Gentamicin Sulfate) Akorn ...... ⊚ 209

Melanin hyperpigmentation
(see under Hyperpigmentation, skin, bleaching of)

Melanoma, malignant
Hydrea Capsules (Hydroxyurea) Bristol-Myers Squibb Oncology/Immunology 705
Intron A for Injection (Interferon alfa-2B, Recombinant) Schering .. 2506

Melanoma, metastatic malignant
DTIC-Dome (Dacarbazine) Bayer Pharmaceutical 593

Melasma
(see under Hyperpigmentation, skin, bleaching of)

Meningitis
Amikacin Sulfate Injection, USP (Amikacin Sulfate) Astra 523
Amikacin Sulfate Injection, USP (Amikacin Sulfate) Elkins-Sinn 981
Amikin Injectable (Amikacin Sulfate) Apothecon 502
Cefizox for Intramuscular or Intravenous Use (Ceftizoxime Sodium) Fujisawa 1025
Ceptaz (Ceftazidime) Glaxo Wellcome 1070
Claforan Sterile and Injection (Cefotaxime Sodium) Hoechst Marion Roussel 1259
Flagyl 375 Capsules (Metronidazole) Searle 2587
Flagyl I.V. (Metronidazole Hydrochloride) SCS 2373
Fortaz (Ceftazidime) Glaxo Wellcome 1092
Garamycin Injectable (Gentamicin Sulfate) Schering 2502
Kefurox Vials, Faspak & ADD-Vantage (Cefuroxime Sodium) Lilly 1509
Merrem I.V. (Meropenem) Zeneca .. 2952
Nebcin Vials, Hyporets & ADD-Vantage (Tobramycin Sulfate) Lilly 1518
Omnipen for Oral Suspension (Ampicillin) Wyeth-Ayerst 2873
Pfizerpen for Injection (Penicillin G Potassium) Pfizer Inc 2022

Rocephin Injectable Vials, ADD-Vantage, Galaxy Container (Ceftriaxone Sodium) Roche Pharmaceuticals 2305
Tazicef for Injection (Ceftazidime) SmithKline Beecham Pharmaceuticals 2697
Tazidime Vials, Faspak & ADD-Vantage (Ceftazidime) Lilly .. 1531
Zinacef (Cefuroxime Sodium) Glaxo Wellcome 1184

Meningitis, gram-negative bacteria-induced
Chloromycetin Sodium Succinate (Chloramphenicol Sodium Succinate) Parke-Davis 1960

Meningitis, meningococcal, prophylaxis of
Gantanol Tablets (Sulfamethoxazole) Roche Pharmaceuticals 2285
Gantrisin (Acetyl Sulfisoxazole) Roche Pharmaceuticals 2286

Meningitis, meningococcal, treatment of
Gantrisin (Acetyl Sulfisoxazole) Roche Pharmaceuticals 2286
Pfizerpen for Injection (Penicillin G Potassium) Pfizer Inc 2022

Meningitis, tuberculous
Celestone Soluspan Suspension (Betamethasone Sodium Phosphate, Betamethasone Acetate) Schering 2484
Cortone Acetate Sterile Suspension (Cortisone Acetate) Merck & Co., Inc. 1663
Cortone Acetate Tablets (Cortisone Acetate) Merck & Co., Inc. 1664
Decadron Elixir (Dexamethasone) Merck & Co., Inc. 1676
Decadron Phosphate Injection (Dexamethasone Sodium Phosphate) Merck & Co., Inc. 1680
Decadron Tablets (Dexamethasone) Merck & Co., Inc. 1678
Hydeltrasol Injection, Sterile (Prednisolone Sodium Phosphate) Merck & Co., Inc. 1708
Hydrocortone Phosphate Injection, Sterile (Hydrocortisone Sodium Phosphate) Merck & Co., Inc. 1713
Hydrocortone Tablets (Hydrocortisone) Merck & Co., Inc. 1715
Pediapred Oral Solution (Prednisolone Sodium Phosphate) Medeva 1618
Prelone Syrup (Prednisolone) Muro 1834

Menopause, management of the manifestations of
PMB 200 and PMB 400 (Estrogens, Conjugated, Meprobamate) Wyeth-Ayerst 2890

Menopause, vasomotor symptoms of
Climara Transdermal System (Estradiol) Berlex 640
Estrace Cream and Tablets (Estradiol) Bristol-Myers Squibb .. 751
Estraderm Transdermal System (Estradiol) CibaGeneva 842
ESTRATAB Tablets (0.3, 0.625, 1.25, 2.5 mg) (Estrogens, Esterified) Solvay 2715
Estratest (Estrogens, Esterified, Methyltestosterone) Solvay 2718
Estring Vaginal Ring (Estradiol) Pharmacia & Upjohn 2086
Menest Tablets (Estrogens, Esterified) SmithKline Beecham Pharmaceuticals 2671
Ogen Tablets (Estropipate) Pharmacia & Upjohn 2103
Ortho-Est (Estropipate) Ortho Pharmaceutical 1925
PMB 200 and PMB 400 (Estrogens, Conjugated, Meprobamate) Wyeth-Ayerst 2890
Premarin Tablets (Estrogens, Conjugated) Wyeth-Ayerst 2896
Premphase (Estrogens, Conjugated, Medroxyprogesterone Acetate) Wyeth-Ayerst 2900

Prempro (Estrogens, Conjugated, Medroxyprogesterone Acetate) Wyeth-Ayerst 2905
Vivelle Transdermal System (Estradiol) CibaGeneva 880

Menstrual cramps
(see under Pain, menstrual)

Menstrual syndrome, pre-, management of
Lurline PMS Tablets (Acetaminophen, Pamabrom) Fielding 1000
Maximum Strength Multi-Symptom Formula Midol (Acetaminophen, Caffeine, Pyrilamine Maleate) Bayer Consumer ...... ⊞ 621
PMS Multi-Symptom Formula Midol (Acetaminophen, Pamabrom, Pyrilamine Maleate) Bayer Consumer ...... ⊞ 622

Mental capacity, idiopathic, decline in, symptomatic relief of
Hydergine (Ergoloid Mesylates) Sandoz Pharmaceuticals 2392

Methotrexate toxicity
(see under Folic acid antagonists, overdosage of)

Microsporum audouinii infections
Fulvicin P/G Tablets (Griseofulvin) Schering 2499
Fulvicin P/G 165 & 330 Tablets (Griseofulvin) Schering 2500
Grifulvin V (griseofulvin tablets) Microsize (griseofulvin oral suspension) Microsize (Griseofulvin) Ortho Dermatological 1944
Gris-PEG Tablets, 125 mg & 250 mg (Griseofulvin) Allergan 476
Spectazole (econazole nitrate 1%) Cream (Econazole Nitrate) Ortho Dermatological 1947

Microsporum canis infections
Exelderm Cream 1.0% (Sulconazole Nitrate) Westwood-Squibb 2794
Exelderm Solution 1.0% (Sulconazole Nitrate) Westwood-Squibb 2795
Fulvicin P/G Tablets (Griseofulvin) Schering 2499
Fulvicin P/G 165 & 330 Tablets (Griseofulvin) Schering 2500
Grifulvin V (griseofulvin tablets) Microsize (griseofulvin oral suspension) Microsize (Griseofulvin) Ortho Dermatological 1944
Gris-PEG Tablets, 125 mg & 250 mg (Griseofulvin) Allergan 476
Loprox 1% Cream and Lotion (Ciclopirox Olamine) Hoechst Marion Roussel 1269
Lotrimin (Clotrimazole) Schering 2514
Lotrisone Cream (Clotrimazole, Betamethasone Dipropionate) Schering 2515
Spectazole (econazole nitrate 1%) Cream (Econazole Nitrate) Ortho Dermatological 1947

Microsporum gypseum infections
Fulvicin P/G Tablets (Griseofulvin) Schering 2499
Fulvicin P/G 165 & 330 Tablets (Griseofulvin) Schering 2500
Grifulvin V (griseofulvin tablets) Microsize (griseofulvin oral suspension) Microsize (Griseofulvin) Ortho Dermatological 1944
Gris-PEG Tablets, 125 mg & 250 mg (Griseofulvin) Allergan 476
Spectazole (econazole nitrate 1%) Cream (Econazole Nitrate) Ortho Dermatological 1947

Migraine headache
(see under Headache, migraine)

Miliaria
Moisturel Cream (Dimethicone, Petrolatum) Westwood-Squibb .. 2796

Mima-Herellea species infections
(see under Acinetobacter species infections)

Miosis, intraoperative, inhibition of
Ocufen (Flurbiprofen Sodium) Allergan ...... ⊚ 242

Miosis, production of
Carbastat Intraocular Solution (Carbachol) CIBA Vision Ophthalmics ...... ⊚ 260
Humorsol Sterile Ophthalmic Solution (Demecarium Bromide) Merck & Co., Inc. 1707
Isopto Carpine Ophthalmic Solution (Pilocarpine Hydrochloride) Alcon Laboratories ...... ⊚ 221
Miochol-E with Iocare Steri-Tags and Miochol-E System Pak (Acetylcholine Chloride) CIBA Vision Ophthalmics ...... ⊚ 263
MIOSTAT Intraocular Solution (Carbachol) Alcon Laboratories ⊚ 222
Ocusert Pilo-20 and Pilo-40 Ocular Therapeutic Systems (Pilocarpine) Alza ...... ⊚ 252
Pilagan (Pilocarpine Nitrate) Allergan ...... ⊚ 245
Pilopine HS Ophthalmic Gel (Pilocarpine Hydrochloride) Alcon Laboratories ...... ⊚ 224
Rev-Eyes Ophthalmic Eyedrops 0.5% (Dapiprazole Hydrochloride) Storz Ophthalmics ...... ⊚ 324

Moraxella catarrhalis
(see under M. catarrhalis infections)

Moraxella lacunata infections, ocular
Chloromycetin Ophthalmic Ointment, 1% (Chloramphenicol) Parke-Davis ⊚ 298
Chloromycetin Ophthalmic Solution (Chloramphenicol) Parke-Davis ...... ⊚ 299
Chloroptic S.O.P. (Chloramphenicol) Allergan ...... ⊚ 236
TobraDex Ophthalmic Suspension and Ointment (Dexamethasone, Tobramycin) Alcon Laboratories .. 469

Morganella morganii infections
Bactrim DS Tablets (Trimethoprim, Sulfamethoxazole) Roche Pharmaceuticals 2257
Bactrim I.V. Infusion (Trimethoprim, Sulfamethoxazole) Roche Pharmaceuticals 2255
Bactrim (Trimethoprim, Sulfamethoxazole) Roche Pharmaceuticals 2257
Cefizox for Intramuscular or Intravenous Use (Ceftizoxime Sodium) Fujisawa 1025
Cefotan (Cefotetan) Zeneca 2936
Ceptaz (Ceftazidime) Glaxo Wellcome 1070
Cipro I.V. (Ciprofloxacin) Bayer Pharmaceutical 587
Cipro I.V. Pharmacy Bulk Package (Ciprofloxacin) Bayer Pharmaceutical 590
Cipro Tablets (Ciprofloxacin Hydrochloride) Bayer Pharmaceutical 584
Claforan Sterile and Injection (Cefotaxime Sodium) Hoechst Marion Roussel 1259
Fortaz (Ceftazidime) Glaxo Wellcome 1092
Geocillin Tablets (Carbenicillin Indanyl Sodium) Pfizer Inc 2009
Mefoxin (Cefoxitin Sodium) Merck & Co., Inc. 1734
Mefoxin Premixed Intravenous Solution (Cefoxitin Sodium) Merck & Co., Inc. 1737
Mezlin (Mezlocillin Sodium) Bayer Pharmaceutical 594
Mezlin Pharmacy Bulk Package (Mezlocillin Sodium) Bayer Pharmaceutical 597
Monocid Injection (Cefonicid Sodium) SmithKline Beecham Pharmaceuticals 2674

(⊞ Described in PDR For Nonprescription Drugs)

(⊚ Described in PDR For Ophthalmology)

Indications Index — Mycosis fungoides

Nebcin Vials, Hyporets & ADD-Vantage (Tobramycin Sulfate) Lilly 1518
Primaxin I.V. (Cilastatin Sodium, Imipenem) Merck & Co., Inc. .. 1772
Rocephin Injectable Vials, ADD-Vantage, Galaxy Container (Ceftriaxone Sodium) Roche Pharmaceuticals 2305
Septra (Trimethoprim, Sulfamethoxazole) Glaxo Wellcome 1146
Septra I.V. Infusion (Trimethoprim, Sulfamethoxazole) Glaxo Wellcome 1142
Septra I.V. Infusion ADD-Vantage Vials (Trimethoprim, Sulfamethoxazole) Glaxo Wellcome 1144
Septra (Trimethoprim, Sulfamethoxazole) Glaxo Wellcome 1146
Tazicef for Injection (Ceftazidime) SmithKline Beecham Pharmaceuticals 2697
Ticar for Injection (Ticarcillin Disodium) SmithKline Beecham Pharmaceuticals 2704

Morganella morganii infections, ocular
TobraDex Ophthalmic Suspension and Ointment (Dexamethasone, Tobramycin) Alcon Laboratories .. 469

Morganella morganii skin and skin structure infections
Cipro I.V. (Ciprofloxacin) Bayer Pharmaceutical 587
Cipro I.V. Pharmacy Bulk Package (Ciprofloxacin) Bayer Pharmaceutical 590
Cipro Tablets (Ciprofloxacin Hydrochloride) Bayer Pharmaceutical 584
Claforan Sterile and Injection (Cefotaxime Sodium) Hoechst Marion Roussel 1259
Mezlin (Mezlocillin Sodium) Bayer Pharmaceutical 594
Mezlin Pharmacy Bulk Package (Mezlocillin Sodium) Bayer Pharmaceutical 597
Primaxin I.V. (Cilastatin Sodium, Imipenem) Merck & Co., Inc. .. 1772
Rocephin Injectable Vials, ADD-Vantage, Galaxy Container (Ceftriaxone Sodium) Roche Pharmaceuticals 2305
Tazicef for Injection (Ceftazidime) SmithKline Beecham Pharmaceuticals 2697
Tazidime Vials, Faspak & ADD-Vantage (Ceftazidime) Lilly .. 1531

Morganella morganii urinary tract infections
Bactrim DS Tablets (Trimethoprim, Sulfamethoxazole) Roche Pharmaceuticals 2257
Bactrim I.V. Infusion (Trimethoprim, Sulfamethoxazole) Roche Pharmaceuticals 2255
Bactrim (Trimethoprim, Sulfamethoxazole) Roche Pharmaceuticals 2257
Cefizox for Intramuscular or Intravenous Use (Ceftizoxime Sodium) Fujisawa 1025
Cefotan (Cefotetan) Zeneca 2936
Ceptaz (Ceftazidime) Glaxo Wellcome 1070
Cipro I.V. (Ciprofloxacin) Bayer Pharmaceutical 587
Cipro I.V. Pharmacy Bulk Package (Ciprofloxacin) Bayer Pharmaceutical 590
Cipro Tablets (Ciprofloxacin Hydrochloride) Bayer Pharmaceutical 584
Claforan Sterile and Injection (Cefotaxime Sodium) Hoechst Marion Roussel 1259
Geocillin Tablets (Carbenicillin Indanyl Sodium) Pfizer Inc 2009
Mefoxin (Cefoxitin Sodium) Merck & Co., Inc. 1734
Mefoxin Premixed Intravenous Solution (Cefoxitin Sodium) Merck & Co., Inc. 1737

(▣ Described in PDR For Nonprescription Drugs)

Mezlin (Mezlocillin Sodium) Bayer Pharmaceutical 594
Mezlin Pharmacy Bulk Package (Mezlocillin Sodium) Bayer Pharmaceutical 597
Monocid Injection (Cefonicid Sodium) SmithKline Beecham Pharmaceuticals 2674
Primaxin I.V. (Cilastatin Sodium, Imipenem) Merck & Co., Inc. .. 1772
Rocephin Injectable Vials, ADD-Vantage, Galaxy Container (Ceftriaxone Sodium) Roche Pharmaceuticals 2305
Septra (Trimethoprim, Sulfamethoxazole) Glaxo Wellcome 1146
Septra I.V. Infusion (Trimethoprim, Sulfamethoxazole) Glaxo Wellcome 1142
Septra I.V. Infusion ADD-Vantage Vials (Trimethoprim, Sulfamethoxazole) Glaxo Wellcome 1144
Septra (Trimethoprim, Sulfamethoxazole) Glaxo Wellcome 1146
Tazicef for Injection (Ceftazidime) SmithKline Beecham Pharmaceuticals 2697
Tazidime Vials, Faspak & ADD-Vantage (Ceftazidime) Lilly .. 1531

Morphea, "possibly" effective in
Potaba Capsules, Envules, Powder, and Tablets (Aminobenzoate Potassium) Glenwood-Palisades .. 1234

Motion sickness
Antivert, Antivert/25 Tablets, & Antivert/50 Tablets (Meclizine Hydrochloride) Pfizer Inc 1992
Benadryl Injection (Diphenhydramine Hydrochloride) Parke-Davis 1955
Bonine Tablets (Meclizine Hydrochloride) Pfizer Consumer .. 1990
Dramamine Chewable Tablets (Dimenhydrinate) Upjohn .... ▣ 801
Children's Dramamine Liquid (Dimenhydrinate) Upjohn .... ▣ 801
Dramamine Tablets (Dimenhydrinate) Upjohn .... ▣ 801
Dramamine II Tablets (Meclizine Hydrochloride) Upjohn .... ▣ 801
Phenergan Injection (Promethazine Hydrochloride) Wyeth-Ayerst .. 2880
Phenergan Suppositories (Promethazine Hydrochloride) Wyeth-Ayerst 2882
Phenergan Syrup (Promethazine Hydrochloride) Wyeth-Ayerst .. 2881
Phenergan Tablets (Promethazine Hydrochloride) Wyeth-Ayerst .. 2882
Transderm Scōp Transdermal Therapeutic System (Scopolamine) Ciba Self-Medication 890

Mountain sickness, acute
Diamox Intravenous (Acetazolamide Sodium) Storz Ophthalmics ◎ 317
Diamox Sequels (Sustained Release) (Acetazolamide) Storz Ophthalmics .... ◎ 318
Diamox Tablets (Acetazolamide) Storz Ophthalmics .... ◎ 317

Mouth, dry
(see under Hyposalivation)

Mucormycosis
(see under Zygomycosis)

Multiple sclerosis, acute exacerbations of
(see under Sclerosis, multiple, acute exacerbations of)

Mumps and rubella immunization
(see under Rubella and mumps, prophylaxis)

Mumps, prophylaxis
M-M-R II (Measles, Mumps & Rubella Virus Vaccine Live) Merck & Co., Inc. 1730
Mumpsvax (Mumps Virus Vaccine, Live) Merck & Co., Inc. 1751

Muscle spasm
(see under Spasticity, muscle, symptomatic alleviation of)

Muscles, skeletal, relaxation, preoperative
Anectine (Succinylcholine Chloride) Glaxo Wellcome 1062
Metubine Iodide Vials (Metocurine Iodide) Dista 932
Mivacron (Mivacurium Chloride) Glaxo Wellcome 1125
Nimbex Injection (Cisatracurium Besylate) Glaxo Wellcome 1131
Norcuron for Injection (Vecuronium Bromide) Organon 1875
Nuromax Injection (Doxacurium Chloride) Glaxo Wellcome 1136
Tracrium Injection (Atracurium Besylate) Glaxo Wellcome 1155
Zemuron Injection (Rocuronium Bromide) Organon 1885

Musculo-skeletal discomfort, adjunct in
Flexeril Tablets (Cyclobenzaprine Hydrochloride) Merck & Co., Inc. .. 1701
Norflex (Orphenadrine Citrate) 3M Pharmaceuticals 1554
Norgesic (Orphenadrine Citrate, Aspirin) 3M Pharmaceuticals 1554
Parafon Forte DSC Caplets (Chlorzoxazone) McNeil Pharmaceutical 1590
Robaxin Injectable (Methocarbamol) Robins 2245
Robaxin Tablets (Methocarbamol) Robins 2246
Robaxisal Tablets (Methocarbamol, Aspirin) Robins 2246
Skelaxin Tablets (Metaxalone) Carnrick 793
Soma Compound w/Codeine Tablets (Carisoprodol, Aspirin, Codeine Phosphate) Wallace 2784
Soma Compound Tablets (Carisoprodol, Aspirin) Wallace 2783

Myalgia
(see under Pain, muscular, temporary relief of)

Myalgia, topical relief of
(see under Pain, topical relief of)

Myasthenia gravis, differential diagnosis of
Tensilon Injectable (Edrophonium Chloride) ICN 1307

Myasthenia gravis, treatment of
Mestinon Injectable (Pyridostigmine Bromide) ICN 1300
Mestinon (Pyridostigmine Bromide) ICN 1300
Prostigmin Injectable (Neostigmine Methylsulfate) ICN 1305
Prostigmin Tablets (Neostigmine Bromide) ICN 1306
Tensilon Injectable (Edrophonium Chloride) ICN 1307

Mycobacterium avium complex, (MAC) disease, disseminated
Biaxin (Clarithromycin) Abbott 406
Mycobutin Capsules (Rifabutin) Pharmacia & Upjohn 2101
Zithromax Tablets (Azithromycin) Pfizer Inc 2046

Mycobacterium avium complex (MAC) disease, disseminated, prophylaxis of
Biaxin (Clarithromycin) Abbott 406

Mycobacterium intracellulare infections
Biaxin (Clarithromycin) Abbott 406

Mycobacterium leprae infections
(see under Leprosy)

Mycobacterium marinum infections
DYNACIN Capsules (Minocycline Hydrochloride) Medicis 1627
Minocin Oral Suspension (Minocycline Hydrochloride) Lederle .. 1431
Minocin Pellet-Filled Capsules (Minocycline Hydrochloride) Lederle 1429

Mycobacterium tuberculosis infection
Capastat Sulfate Injection (Capreomycin Sulfate) Dura 968
Streptomycin Sulfate Injection (Streptomycin Sulfate) Pfizer Inc 2031
Trecator-SC Tablets (Ethionamide) Wyeth-Ayerst 2919

Mycoplasma pneumoniae infection
Achromycin V Capsules (Tetracycline Hydrochloride) Lederle 1417
Biaxin (Clarithromycin) Abbott 406
Declomycin Tablets (Demeclocycline Hydrochloride) Lederle 1421
Doryx Capsules (Doxycycline Hyclate) Parke-Davis 1970
Dynabac (Dirithromycin) Bock 668
DYNACIN Capsules (Minocycline Hydrochloride) Medicis 1627
E.E.S. (Erythromycin Ethylsuccinate) Abbott 427
E-Mycin Tablets (Erythromycin) Knoll Laboratories 1388
ERYC (Erythromycin) Parke-Davis .. 1972
EryPed (Erythromycin Ethylsuccinate) Abbott 425
Ery-Tab Tablets (Erythromycin) Abbott 426
Erythrocin Stearate Filmtab (Erythromycin Stearate) Abbott 429
Erythromycin Base Filmtab (Erythromycin) Abbott 430
Erythromycin Delayed-Release Capsules, USP (Erythromycin) Abbott 431
Ilosone (Erythromycin Estolate) Dista 927
Ilotycin Gluceptate, IV, Vials (Erythromycin Gluceptate) Dista 929
Minocin Intravenous (Minocycline Hydrochloride) Lederle 1428
Minocin Oral Suspension (Minocycline Hydrochloride) Lederle 1431
Minocin Pellet-Filled Capsules (Minocycline Hydrochloride) Lederle 1429
Monodox Capsules (Doxycycline Monohydrate) Oclassen 1858
PCE Dispertab Tablets (Erythromycin) Abbott 453
Terramycin Intramuscular Solution (Oxytetracycline) Pfizer Inc 2034
Vibramycin (Doxycycline Calcium) Pfizer Inc 2038
Vibramycin Hyclate Intravenous (Doxycycline Hyclate) Pfizer Inc.. 2040
Vibramycin (Doxycycline Monohydrate) Pfizer Inc 2038

Mycoplasma pneumoniae respiratory tract infections
Biaxin (Clarithromycin) Abbott 406
Dynabac (Dirithromycin) Bock 668
DYNACIN Capsules (Minocycline Hydrochloride) Medicis 1627
E.E.S. (Erythromycin Ethylsuccinate) Abbott 427
E-Mycin Tablets (Erythromycin) Knoll Laboratories 1388
ERYC (Erythromycin) Parke-Davis .. 1972
EryPed (Erythromycin Ethylsuccinate) Abbott 425
Ery-Tab Tablets (Erythromycin) Abbott 426
Erythrocin Stearate Filmtab (Erythromycin Stearate) Abbott 429
Erythromycin Base Filmtab (Erythromycin) Abbott 430
Erythromycin Delayed-Release Capsules, USP (Erythromycin) Abbott 431
Ilosone (Erythromycin Estolate) Dista 927
Ilotycin Gluceptate, IV, Vials (Erythromycin Gluceptate) Dista 929
Monodox Capsules (Doxycycline Monohydrate) Oclassen 1858
PCE Dispertab Tablets (Erythromycin) Abbott 453

Mycosis fungoides
Celestone Soluspan Suspension (Betamethasone Sodium Phosphate, Betamethasone Acetate) Schering 2484
Cortone Acetate Sterile Suspension (Cortisone Acetate) Merck & Co., Inc. 1663
Cortone Acetate Tablets (Cortisone Acetate) Merck & Co., Inc. .. 1664

(◎ Described in PDR For Ophthalmology)

Mycosis fungoides | Indications Index | 1548

Cytoxan (Cyclophosphamide) Bristol-Myers Squibb Oncology/Immunology 700
Dalalone D.P. Injectable (Dexamethasone Acetate) Forest 1009
Decadron Elixir (Dexamethasone) Merck & Co., Inc. 1676
Decadron Phosphate Injection (Dexamethasone Sodium Phosphate) Merck & Co., Inc. 1680
Decadron Tablets (Dexamethasone) Merck & Co., Inc. 1678
Decadron-LA Sterile Suspension (Dexamethasone Acetate) Merck & Co., Inc. 1687
Hydeltrasol Injection, Sterile (Prednisolone Sodium Phosphate) Merck & Co., Inc. 1708
Hydrocortone Phosphate Injection, Sterile (Hydrocortisone Sodium Phosphate) Merck & Co., Inc. 1713
Hydrocortone Tablets (Hydrocortisone) Merck & Co., Inc. 1715
Methotrexate Sodium Tablets, Injection, for Injection and LPF Injection (Methotrexate Sodium) Immunex 1322
Mustargen (Mechlorethamine Hydrochloride) Merck & Co., Inc. 1752
Pediapred Oral Solution (Prednisolone Sodium Phosphate) Medeva 1618
Prelone Syrup (Prednisolone) Muro 1834
Velban Vials (Vinblastine Sulfate) Lilly 1537

Mydriasis, production of
Neo-Synephrine Hydrochloride (Ophthalmic) (Phenylephrine Hydrochloride) Sanofi Winthrop .. 2456
Paremyd (Hydroxyamphetamine Hydrobromide, Tropicamide) Allergan .... ⊙ 244

Mydriasis, production of, in uveitis
Neo-Synephrine Hydrochloride (Ophthalmic) (Phenylephrine Hydrochloride) Sanofi Winthrop .. 2456

Mydriasis, reversal of
Isopto Carpine Ophthalmic Solution (Pilocarpine Hydrochloride) Alcon Laboratories .... ⊙ 221
Pilagan (Pilocarpine Nitrate) Allergan .... ⊙ 245

Myeloid recovery, acceleration of
Leukine (Sargramostim) Immunex .. 1317

Myeloma, multiple
Alkeran Tablets (Melphalan) Glaxo Wellcome Oncology/HIV 1198
Cytoxan (Cyclophosphamide) Bristol-Myers Squibb Oncology/Immunology 700

Myeloma, multiple, adjunct in
Alkeran for Injection (Melphalan Hydrochloride) Glaxo Wellcome Oncology/HIV 1196
Aredia for Injection (Pamidronate Disodium) CibaGeneva 827
BiCNU (Carmustine (BCNU)) Bristol-Myers Squibb Oncology/Immunology 696

Myocardial infarction, acute
Activase (Alteplase, Recombinant) Genentech 1045
Ecotrin (Aspirin) SmithKline Beecham 2625
Eminase (Anistreplase) Roberts 2215
Streptase for Infusion (Streptokinase) Astra 557

Myocardial infarction, post, left ventricular dysfunction
Capoten Tablets (Captopril) Bristol-Myers Squibb 740

Myocardial infarction, to reduce the risk of non-fatal
Pravachol Tablets (Pravastatin Sodium) Bristol-Myers Squibb 770
Zocor Tablets (Simvastatin) Merck & Co., Inc. 1821

Myocardial infarction, treatment adjunct
Altace Capsules (Ramipril) Hoechst Marion Roussel 1238
Prinivil Tablets (Lisinopril) Merck & Co., Inc. 1776
Zestril Tablets (Lisinopril) Zeneca 2972

Myocardial perfusion imaging, thallium, adjunct in
Adenoscan (Adenosine) Fujisawa 1022

Myocardial reinfarction, prophylaxis
Alka-Seltzer Cherry Effervescent Antacid and Pain Reliever (Aspirin, Sodium Bicarbonate, Citric Acid) Bayer Consumer .... ▣ 609
Alka-Seltzer Lemon Lime Effervescent Antacid and Pain Reliever (Aspirin, Sodium Citrate) Bayer Consumer .... ▣ 609
Alka-Seltzer Original Effervescent Antacid and Pain Reliever (Aspirin, Citric Acid, Sodium Bicarbonate) Bayer Consumer .. ▣ 609
Regular Strength Ascriptin Tablets (Aspirin Buffered, Calcium Carbonate) Ciba Self-Medication .... ▣ 650
Genuine Bayer Aspirin Tablets & Caplets (Aspirin) Bayer Consumer .... ▣ 618
Bayer Enteric Aspirin (Aspirin, Enteric Coated) Bayer Consumer .... ▣ 613
Blocadren Tablets (Timolol Maleate) Merck & Co., Inc. 1654
Bufferin Analgesic Tablets (Aspirin) Bristol-Myers Products .... ▣ 636
Coumadin (Warfarin Sodium) DuPont 941
Ecotrin (Aspirin) SmithKline Beecham 2625
Halfprin Tablets (Aspirin) Kramer 1413
Inderal (Propranolol Hydrochloride) Wyeth-Ayerst 2834
Lopressor Tablets (Metoprolol Tartrate) CibaGeneva 848
St. Joseph Adult Chewable Aspirin (81 mg.) (Aspirin) Schering-Plough HealthCare .... ▣ 768
Tenormin Tablets and I.V. Injection (Atenolol) Zeneca 2965

Myocardial revascularization procedures, to reduce the risk of
Pravachol Tablets (Pravastatin Sodium) Bristol-Myers Squibb 770
Zocor Tablets (Simvastatin) Merck & Co., Inc. 1821

Myxedema (see under Hypothyroidism, replacement or supplemental therapy in)

Myxedema coma/precoma (see also under Hypothyroidism, replacement or supplemental therapy in)
Triostat Injection (Liothyronine Sodium) SmithKline Beecham Pharmaceuticals 2708

N

N. gonorrhoeae endocervical infections
Cefizox for Intramuscular or Intravenous Use (Ceftizoxime Sodium) Fujisawa 1025
Ceftin (Cefuroxime Axetil) Glaxo Wellcome 1067
Cipro Tablets (Ciprofloxacin Hydrochloride) Bayer Pharmaceutical 584
Noroxin Tablets (Norfloxacin) Merck & Co., Inc. 1758
Noroxin Tablets (Norfloxacin) Roberts 2222
Rocephin Injectable Vials, ADD-Vantage, Galaxy Container (Ceftriaxone Sodium) Roche Pharmaceuticals 2305
Vantin for Oral Suspension and Vantin Tablets (Cefpodoxime Proxetil) Pharmacia & Upjohn 2112

N. gonorrhoeae epididymo-orchitis, acute
Doryx Capsules (Doxycycline Hyclate) Parke-Davis 1970
Monodox Capsules (Doxycycline Monohydrate) Oclassen 1858

N. gonorrhoeae gynecologic infections
Cefobid Intravenous/Intramuscular (Cefoperazone Sodium) Pfizer Inc 1996
Cefobid Pharmacy Bulk Package - Not for Direct Infusion (Cefoperazone Sodium) Pfizer Inc 1999
Cefotan (Cefotetan) Zeneca 2936
DYNACIN Capsules (Minocycline Hydrochloride) Medicis 1627
Erythrocin Stearate Filmtab (Erythromycin Stearate) Abbott 429
Erythromycin Base Filmtab (Erythromycin) Abbott 430
Erythromycin Delayed-Release Capsules, USP (Erythromycin) Abbott 431
Floxin I.V. (Ofloxacin) McNeil Pharmaceutical 1580
Floxin Tablets (200 mg, 300 mg, 400 mg) (Ofloxacin) McNeil Pharmaceutical 1577
Mefoxin (Cefoxitin Sodium) Merck & Co., Inc. 1734
Mefoxin Premixed Intravenous Solution (Cefoxitin Sodium) Merck & Co., Inc. 1737
Mezlin (Mezlocillin Sodium) Bayer Pharmaceutical 594
Mezlin Pharmacy Bulk Package (Mezlocillin Sodium) Bayer Pharmaceutical 597
Minocin Pellet-Filled Capsules (Minocycline Hydrochloride) Lederle 1429
Noroxin Tablets (Norfloxacin) Merck & Co., Inc. 1758
Noroxin Tablets (Norfloxacin) Roberts 2222
PCE Dispertab Tablets (Erythromycin) Abbott 453

N. gonorrhoeae infections
Achromycin V Capsules (Tetracycline Hydrochloride) Lederle 1417
Amoxil (Amoxicillin Trihydrate) SmithKline Beecham Pharmaceuticals 2631
Cefizox for Intramuscular or Intravenous Use (Ceftizoxime Sodium) Fujisawa 1025
Cefobid Intravenous/Intramuscular (Cefoperazone Sodium) Pfizer Inc 1996
Cefobid Pharmacy Bulk Package - Not for Direct Infusion (Cefoperazone Sodium) Pfizer Inc 1999
Cefotan (Cefotetan) Zeneca 2936
Ceftin (Cefuroxime Axetil) Glaxo Wellcome 1067
Ceptaz (Ceftazidime) Glaxo Wellcome 1070
Cipro Tablets (Ciprofloxacin Hydrochloride) Bayer Pharmaceutical 584
Claforan Sterile and Injection (Cefotaxime Sodium) Hoechst Marion Roussel 1259
Declomycin Tablets (Demeclocycline Hydrochloride) Lederle 1421
DYNACIN Capsules (Minocycline Hydrochloride) Medicis 1627
E-Mycin Tablets (Erythromycin) Knoll Laboratories 1388
ERYC (Erythromycin) Parke-Davis .. 1972
Ery-Tab Tablets (Erythromycin) Abbott 426
Erythrocin Stearate Filmtab (Erythromycin Stearate) Abbott 429
Erythromycin Base Filmtab (Erythromycin) Abbott 430
Erythromycin Delayed-Release Capsules, USP (Erythromycin) Abbott 431
Floxin I.V. (Ofloxacin) McNeil Pharmaceutical 1580
Floxin Tablets (200 mg, 300 mg, 400 mg) (Ofloxacin) McNeil Pharmaceutical 1577
Fortaz (Ceftazidime) Glaxo Wellcome 1092
Ilotycin Gluceptate, IV, Vials (Erythromycin Gluceptate) Dista 929
Kefurox Vials, Faspak & ADD-Vantage (Cefuroxime Sodium) Lilly 1509
Mefoxin (Cefoxitin Sodium) Merck & Co., Inc. 1734
Mefoxin Premixed Intravenous Solution (Cefoxitin Sodium) Merck & Co., Inc. 1737
Mezlin (Mezlocillin Sodium) Bayer Pharmaceutical 594
Mezlin Pharmacy Bulk Package (Mezlocillin Sodium) Bayer Pharmaceutical 597
Minocin Intravenous (Minocycline Hydrochloride) Lederle 1428
Minocin Oral Suspension (Minocycline Hydrochloride) Lederle 1431
Minocin Pellet-Filled Capsules (Minocycline Hydrochloride) Lederle 1429
Monodox Capsules (Doxycycline Monohydrate) Oclassen 1858
Noroxin Tablets (Norfloxacin) Merck & Co., Inc. 1758
Noroxin Tablets (Norfloxacin) Roberts 2222
Omnipen Capsules (Ampicillin) Wyeth-Ayerst 2872
Omnipen for Oral Suspension (Ampicillin) Wyeth-Ayerst 2873
PCE Dispertab Tablets (Erythromycin) Abbott 453
Penetrex Tablets (Enoxacin) Rhone-Poulenc Rorer Pharmaceuticals 2196
Pfizerpen for Injection (Penicillin G Potassium) Pfizer Inc 2022
Pipracil (Piperacillin Sodium) Lederle 1435
Rocephin Injectable Vials, ADD-Vantage, Galaxy Container (Ceftriaxone Sodium) Roche Pharmaceuticals 2305
Spectrobid Tablets (Bacampicillin Hydrochloride) Pfizer Inc 2030
Suprax Tablets (Cefixime) Lederle .. 1443
Tazicef for Injection (Ceftazidime) SmithKline Beecham Pharmaceuticals 2697
Tazidime Vials, Faspak & ADD-Vantage (Ceftazidime) Lilly .. 1531
Terramycin Intramuscular Solution (Oxytetracycline) Pfizer Inc 2034
Vantin for Oral Suspension and Vantin Tablets (Cefpodoxime Proxetil) Pharmacia & Upjohn 2112
Vibramycin (Doxycycline Calcium) Pfizer Inc 2038
Vibramycin Hyclate Intravenous (Doxycycline Hyclate) Pfizer Inc 2040
Vibramycin (Doxycycline Monohydrate) Pfizer Inc 2038
Zinacef (Cefuroxime Sodium) Glaxo Wellcome 1184

N. gonorrhoeae infections, ocular
Garamycin Ophthalmic (Gentamicin Sulfate) Schering 2501
Genoptic Sterile Ophthalmic Solution (Gentamicin Sulfate) Allergan .... ⊙ 241
Genoptic Sterile Ophthalmic Ointment (Gentamicin Sulfate) Allergan .... ⊙ 241
Gentak (Gentamicin Sulfate) Akorn .... ⊙ 209
Ilotycin Ophthalmic Ointment (Erythromycin) Dista 928
Pred-G Liquifilm Sterile Ophthalmic Suspension (Gentamicin Sulfate, Prednisolone Acetate) Allergan .... ⊙ 248
Pred-G S.O.P. Sterile Ophthalmic Ointment (Gentamicin Sulfate, Prednisolone Acetate) Allergan .. ⊙ 249

N. gonorrhoeae neonatal ophthalmia, prophylaxis of
Ilotycin Ophthalmic Ointment (Erythromycin) Dista 928

N. gonorrhoeae pelvic inflammatory disease
Cefizox for Intramuscular or Intravenous Use (Ceftizoxime Sodium) Fujisawa 1025
Cefobid Intravenous/Intramuscular (Cefoperazone Sodium) Pfizer Inc 1996
Cefobid Pharmacy Bulk Package - Not for Direct Infusion (Cefoperazone Sodium) Pfizer Inc 1999
ERYC (Erythromycin) Parke-Davis .. 1972
Ery-Tab Tablets (Erythromycin) Abbott 426
Mefoxin (Cefoxitin Sodium) Merck & Co., Inc. 1734

(▣ Described in PDR For Nonprescription Drugs) (⊙ Described in PDR For Ophthalmology)

N. gonorrhoeae pharyngeal infections

- Mefoxin Premixed Intravenous Solution (Cefoxitin Sodium) Merck & Co., Inc. 1737
- Mezlin (Mezlocillin Sodium) Bayer Pharmaceutical 594
- Mezlin Pharmacy Bulk Package (Mezlocillin Sodium) Bayer Pharmaceutical 597
- Rocephin Injectable Vials, ADD-Vantage, Galaxy Container (Ceftriaxone Sodium) Roche Pharmaceuticals 2305

N. gonorrhoeae pharnygeal infections
- Rocephin Injectable Vials, ADD-Vantage, Galaxy Container (Ceftriaxone Sodium) Roche Pharmaceuticals 2305

N. gonorrhoeae rectal infections
- Rocephin Injectable Vials, ADD-Vantage, Galaxy Container (Ceftriaxone Sodium) Roche Pharmaceuticals 2305
- Vantin for Oral Suspension and Vantin Tablets (Cefpodoxime Proxetil) Pharmacia & Upjohn 2112

N. gonorrhoeae urethral infections
- Ceftin (Cefuroxime Axetil) Glaxo Wellcome 1067
- Cipro Tablets (Ciprofloxacin Hydrochloride) Bayer Pharmaceutical 584
- DYNACIN Capsules (Minocycline Hydrochloride) Medicis 1627
- Floxin I.V. (Ofloxacin) McNeil Pharmaceutical 1580
- Minocin Oral Suspension (Minocycline Hydrochloride) Lederle 1431
- Noroxin Tablets (Norfloxacin) Merck & Co., Inc. 1758
- Noroxin Tablets (Norfloxacin) Roberts 2222
- Rocephin Injectable Vials, ADD-Vantage, Galaxy Container (Ceftriaxone Sodium) Roche Pharmaceuticals 2305
- Vantin for Oral Suspension and Vantin Tablets (Cefpodoxime Proxetil) Pharmacia & Upjohn 2112

N. gonorrhoeae urinary tract infections
- Claforan Sterile and Injection (Cefotaxime Sodium) Hoechst Marion Roussel 1259
- Kefurox Vials, Faspak & ADD-Vantage (Cefuroxime Sodium) Lilly 1509
- Mefoxin (Cefoxitin Sodium) Merck & Co., Inc. 1734
- Mefoxin Premixed Intravenous Solution (Cefoxitin Sodium) Merck & Co., Inc. 1737
- Spectrobid Tablets (Bacampicillin Hydrochloride) Pfizer Inc 2030

N. meningitidis central nervous system infections
- Claforan Sterile and Injection (Cefotaxime Sodium) Hoechst Marion Roussel 1259
- Tazicef for Injection (Ceftazidime) SmithKline Beecham Pharmaceuticals 2697

N. meningitidis infections
- Ceptaz (Ceftazidime) Glaxo Wellcome 1070
- Claforan Sterile and Injection (Cefotaxime Sodium) Hoechst Marion Roussel 1259
- Fortaz (Ceftazidime) Glaxo Wellcome 1092
- Merrem I.V. (Meropenem) Zeneca .. 2952
- Minocin Intravenous (Minocycline Hydrochloride) Lederle 1428
- Minocin Oral Suspension (Minocycline Hydrochloride) Lederle 1431
- Minocin Pellet-Filled Capsules (Minocycline Hydrochloride) Lederle 1429
- Omnipen for Oral Suspension (Ampicillin) Wyeth-Ayerst 2873
- Rocephin Injectable Vials, ADD-Vantage, Galaxy Container (Ceftriaxone Sodium) Roche Pharmaceuticals 2305
- Tazicef for Injection (Ceftazidime) SmithKline Beecham Pharmaceuticals 2697
- Tazidime Vials, Faspak & ADD-Vantage (Ceftazidime) Lilly .. 1531
- Vibramycin Hyclate Intravenous (Doxycycline Hyclate) Pfizer Inc.... 2040
- Zinacef (Cefuroxime Sodium) Glaxo Wellcome 1184

N. meningitidis meningitis
- Ceptaz (Ceftazidime) Glaxo Wellcome 1070
- Fortaz (Ceftazidime) Glaxo Wellcome 1092
- Kefurox Vials, Faspak & ADD-Vantage (Cefuroxime Sodium) Lilly 1509
- Merrem I.V. (Meropenem) Zeneca .. 2952
- Omnipen for Oral Suspension (Ampicillin) Wyeth-Ayerst 2873
- Rocephin Injectable Vials, ADD-Vantage, Galaxy Container (Ceftriaxone Sodium) Roche Pharmaceuticals 2305
- Tazicef for Injection (Ceftazidime) SmithKline Beecham Pharmaceuticals 2697
- Tazidime Vials, Faspak & ADD-Vantage (Ceftazidime) Lilly .. 1531
- Zinacef (Cefuroxime Sodium) Glaxo Wellcome 1184

N. meningitidis, asymptomatic carriers of
- Minocin Oral Suspension (Minocycline Hydrochloride) Lederle 1431
- Rifadin (Rifampin) Hoechst Marion Roussel 1276
- Rimactane Capsules (Rifampin) CibaGeneva 865

Narcolepsy
- Adderall Tablets (Amphetamine Aspartate, Amphetamine Sulfate, Dextroamphetamine Saccharate, Dextroamphetamine Sulfate) Richwood 2209
- Dexedrine (Dextroamphetamine Sulfate) SmithKline Beecham Pharmaceuticals 2648
- DextroStat-Dextroamphetamine Sulfate Tablets (Dextroamphetamine Sulfate) Richwood.......... 2211
- Ritalin (Methylphenidate Hydrochloride) CibaGeneva 866

Narcotic addiction, detoxification treatment of
- Methadone Hydrochloride Oral Concentrate (Methadone Hydrochloride) Roxane 2356
- Methadone Hydrochloride Oral Solution & Tablets (Methadone Hydrochloride) Roxane 2357
- Orlaam Oral Solution (Levomethadyl Acetate Hydrochloride) Roxane 2361

Narcotic addiction, maintenance therapy for
- Methadone Hydrochloride Oral Concentrate (Methadone Hydrochloride) Roxane 2356
- Methadone Hydrochloride Oral Solution & Tablets (Methadone Hydrochloride) Roxane 2357
- Orlaam Oral Solution (Levomethadyl Acetate Hydrochloride) Roxane 2361

Nasal congestion, symptomatic relief of
- Actifed Allergy Daytime/Nighttime Caplets (Diphenhydramine Hydrochloride, Pseudoephedrine Hydrochloride) Warner Wellcome 808
- Actifed Cold & Allergy Tablets (Pseudoephedrine Hydrochloride, Triprolidine Hydrochloride) Warner Wellcome 807
- Actifed Cold & Sinus Caplets and Tablets (Acetaminophen, Pseudoephedrine Hydrochloride, Triprolidine Hydrochloride) Warner Wellcome 808
- Afrin (Oxymetazoline Hydrochloride) Schering-Plough HealthCare 757
- Alka-Seltzer Plus Sinus Medicine (Phenylpropanolamine Bitartrate, Aspirin, Brompheniramine Maleate) Bayer Consumer 611
- Allerest Maximum Strength (Chlorpheniramine Maleate, Pseudoephedrine Hydrochloride) Ciba Self-Medication 649
- Allerest No Drowsiness (Acetaminophen, Pseudoephedrine Hydrochloride) Ciba Self-Medication 649
- Allerest Sinus Pain Formula (Acetaminophen, Chlorpheniramine Maleate, Pseudoephedrine Hydrochloride) Ciba Self-Medication 649
- Atrohist Pediatric Suspension (Chlorpheniramine Tannate, Phenylephrine Tannate, Pyrilamine Tannate) Medeva 1604
- Atrohist Pediatric Suspension Dye-Free (Chlorpheniramine Tannate, Phenylephrine Tannate, Pyrilamine Tannate) Medeva 1604
- Atrohist Plus Tablets (Chlorpheniramine Maleate, Phenylpropanolamine Hydrochloride, Phenylephrine Hydrochloride, Hyoscyamine Sulfate, Atropine Sulfate, Scopolamine Hydrobromide) Medeva .. 1605
- BC Cold Powder Multi-Symptom Formula (Cold-Sinus-Allergy) (Aspirin, Phenylpropanolamine Hydrochloride, Chlorpheniramine Maleate) Block 631
- BC Cold Powder Non-Drowsy Formula (Cold-Sinus) (Aspirin, Phenylpropanolamine Hydrochloride) Block.......... 631
- Benadryl Allergy/Cold Tablets (Acetaminophen, Diphenhydramine Hydrochloride, Pseudoephedrine Hydrochloride) Warner Wellcome 811
- Benadryl Allergy Decongestant Liquid Medication (Diphenhydramine Hydrochloride, Pseudoephedrine Hydrochloride) Warner Wellcome 812
- Benadryl Allergy Decongestant Tablets (Diphenhydramine Hydrochloride, Pseudoephedrine Hydrochloride) Warner Wellcome 812
- Benadryl Allergy Sinus Headache Caplets (Diphenhydramine Hydrochloride, Pseudoephedrine Hydrochloride, Acetaminophen) Warner Wellcome 813
- Bromfed (Brompheniramine Maleate, Pseudoephedrine Hydrochloride) Muro 1832
- Children's TYLENOL Flu Suspension Liquid (Acetaminophen, Chlorpheniramine Maleate, Dextromethorphan Hydrobromide, Pseudoephedrine Hydrochloride) McNeil Consumer 1560
- Children's Vicks DayQuil Allergy Relief (Chlorpheniramine Maleate, Pseudoephedrine Hydrochloride) Procter & Gamble 730
- Chlor-Trimeton Allergy Decongestant Tablets (Chlorpheniramine Maleate, Pseudoephedrine Sulfate) Schering-Plough HealthCare 759
- Allergy-Sinus Comtrex Multi-Symptom Allergy-Sinus Formula Tablets and Caplets (Acetaminophen, Chlorpheniramine Maleate, Pseudoephedrine Hydrochloride) Bristol-Myers Products 639
- Congess (Guaifenesin, Pseudoephedrine Hydrochloride) Fleming 1003
- Contac Continuous Action Nasal Decongestant/Antihistamine 12 Hour Capsules (Chlorpheniramine Maleate, Phenylpropanolamine Hydrochloride) SmithKline Beecham Consumer 773
- Contac Maximum Strength Continuous Action Decongestant/Antihistamine 12 Hour Caplets (Chlorpheniramine Maleate, Phenylpropanolamine Hydrochloride) SmithKline Beecham Consumer 772
- Coricidin 'D' Decongestant Tablets (Acetaminophen, Chlorpheniramine Maleate, Phenylpropanolamine Hydrochloride) Schering-Plough HealthCare 760
- Deconsal II Tablets (Pseudoephedrine Hydrochloride, Guaifenesin) Medeva 1605
- Dimetapp Cold & Fever Suspension (Acetaminophen, Brompheniramine Maleate, Pseudoephedrine Hydrochloride) Whitehall-Robins 839
- Dimetapp Decongestant Pediatric Drops (Pseudoephedrine Hydrochloride) Whitehall-Robins 840
- Dimetapp Elixir (Brompheniramine Maleate, Phenylpropanolamine Hydrochloride) Whitehall-Robins 840
- Dimetapp Extentabs (Brompheniramine Maleate, Phenylpropanolamine Hydrochloride) Whitehall-Robins 841
- Dimetapp Tablets (Brompheniramine Maleate, Phenylpropanolamine Hydrochloride) Whitehall-Robins 841
- Drixoral Cold and Allergy Sustained-Action Tablets (Dexbrompheniramine Maleate, Pseudoephedrine Sulfate) Schering-Plough HealthCare 763
- Drixoral Cold and Flu Extended-Release Tablets (Acetaminophen, Dexbrompheniramine Maleate, Pseudoephedrine Sulfate) Schering-Plough HealthCare 764
- Drixoral Non-Drowsy Formula Extended-Release Tablets (Pseudoephedrine Sulfate) Schering-Plough HealthCare 764
- Drixoral Allergy/Sinus Extended Release Tablets (Acetaminophen, Pseudoephedrine Sulfate, Dexbrompheniramine Maleate) Schering-Plough HealthCare 765
- Duration 12 Hour Nasal Spray (Oxymetazoline Hydrochloride) Schering-Plough HealthCare 766
- Duratuss Tablets (Pseudoephedrine Hydrochloride, Guaifenesin) UCB 2750
- Dura-Vent Tablets (Phenylpropanolamine Hydrochloride, Guaifenesin) Dura 971
- Efidac/24 (Pseudoephedrine Hydrochloride) Ciba Self-Medication 655
- Entex PSE Tablets (Pseudoephedrine Hydrochloride, Guaifenesin) Dura 973
- Exgest LA Tablets (Phenylpropanolamine Hydrochloride, Guaifenesin) Carnrick 787
- 4-Way Fast Acting Nasal Spray (regular & mentholated) (Naphazoline Hydrochloride, Phenylephrine Hydrochloride, Pyrilamine Maleate) Bristol-Myers Products 644
- Fedahist Gyrocaps (Pseudoephedrine Hydrochloride, Chlorpheniramine Maleate) Schwarz .. 2545
- Guaimax-D Tablets (Pseudoephedrine Hydrochloride, Guaifenesin) Central 809
- Infants' TYLENOL Cold Decongestant & Fever-Reducer Drops (Acetaminophen, Pseudoephedrine Hydrochloride) McNeil Consumer 1561
- Kronofed-A (Chlorpheniramine Maleate, Pseudoephedrine Hydrochloride) Ferndale 994
- Mentholatum Cherry Chest Rub for Kids (Camphor, Eucalyptus, Oil of, Menthol) Mentholatum 710
- Mentholatum Ointment (Camphor, Menthol) Mentholatum 711

(▣ Described in PDR For Nonprescription Drugs)   (◉ Described in PDR For Ophthalmology)

Nasal congestion / Indications Index

Nasal congestion (cont.)

- Neo-Synephrine Maximum Strength 12 Hour Nasal Spray (Oxymetazoline Hydrochloride) Bayer Consumer ... 624
- Neo-Synephrine 12 Hour (Oxymetazoline Hydrochloride) Bayer Consumer ... 624
- Neo-Synephrine (Phenylephrine Hydrochloride) Bayer Consumer ... 624
- Nolamine Timed-Release Tablets (Phenindamine Tartrate, Phenylpropanolamine Hydrochloride, Chlorpheniramine Maleate) Carnrick ... 790
- 12 Hour Nōstrilla (Oxymetazoline Hydrochloride) Ciba Self-Medication ... 660
- Novahistine Elixir (Chlorpheniramine Maleate, Phenylephrine Hydrochloride) SmithKline Beecham Consumer ... 782
- Ornade Spansule Capsules (Phenylpropanolamine Hydrochloride, Chlorpheniramine Maleate) SmithKline Beecham Pharmaceuticals ... 2678
- Otrivin (Xylometazoline Hydrochloride) Ciba Self-Medication ... 662
- PediaCare Infants' Decongestant Drops (Pseudoephedrine Hydrochloride) McNeil Consumer 1569
- Privine (Naphazoline Hydrochloride) Ciba Self-Medication ... 663
- Propagest Tablets (Phenylpropanolamine Hydrochloride) Carnrick ... 791
- Robitussin Pediatric Cough & Cold Formula (Dextromethorphan Hydrobromide, Pseudoephedrine Hydrochloride) Whitehall-Robins ... 848
- Robitussin Severe Congestion Liqui-Gels (Guaifenesin, Pseudoephedrine Hydrochloride) Whitehall-Robins ... 845
- Robitussin-PE (Guaifenesin, Pseudoephedrine Hydrochloride) Whitehall-Robins ... 846
- Ryna Liquid (Chlorpheniramine Maleate, Pseudoephedrine Hydrochloride) Wallace ... 804
- Rynatan (Chlorpheniramine Tannate, Pyrilamine Tannate, Phenylephrine Tannate) Wallace ... 2781
- Salinex Nasal Mist and Drops (Sodium Chloride) Muro ... 713
- Seldane-D Extended-Release Tablets (Pseudoephedrine Hydrochloride, Terfenadine) Hoechst Marion Roussel ... 1286
- Semprex-D Capsules (Acrivastine, Pseudoephedrine Hydrochloride) Medeva ... 1620
- Sine-Off No Drowsiness Formula Caplets (Acetaminophen, Pseudoephedrine Hydrochloride) SmithKline Beecham Consumer ... 784
- Sine-Off Sinus Medicine (Acetaminophen, Chlorpheniramine Maleate, Pseudoephedrine Hydrochloride) SmithKline Beecham Consumer ... 784
- Singlet Tablets (Acetaminophen, Chlorpheniramine Maleate, Pseudoephedrine Hydrochloride) SmithKline Beecham Consumer ... 785
- Sinulin Tablets (Acetaminophen, Phenylpropanolamine Hydrochloride, Chlorpheniramine Maleate) Carnrick ... 792
- Sinutab Sinus Allergy Medication, Maximum Strength Tablets and Caplets (Acetaminophen, Chlorpheniramine Maleate, Pseudoephedrine Hydrochloride) Warner Wellcome ... 823
- Sinutab Sinus Medication, Maximum Strength Without Drowsiness Formula, Tablets & Caplets (Acetaminophen, Pseudoephedrine Hydrochloride) Warner Wellcome ... 824
- Sudafed Children's Nasal Decongestant Liquid Medication (Pseudoephedrine Hydrochloride) Warner Wellcome ... 826
- Sudafed Nasal Decongestant Tablets, 30 mg (Pseudoephedrine Hydrochloride) Warner Wellcome ... 825
- Sudafed Nasal Decongestant Tablets, 60 mg (Pseudoephedrine Hydrochloride) Warner Wellcome ... 825
- Sudafed Non-Drying Sinus Liquid Caps (Pseudoephedrine Hydrochloride, Guaifenesin) Warner Wellcome ... 827
- Sudafed Pediatric Nasal Decongestant Liquid Oral Drops (Pseudoephedrine Hydrochloride) Warner Wellcome ... 827
- Sudafed Sinus Caplets (Acetaminophen, Pseudoephedrine Hydrochloride) Warner Wellcome ... 829
- Sudafed Sinus Tablets (Acetaminophen, Pseudoephedrine Hydrochloride) Warner Wellcome ... 829
- Sudafed 12 Hour Caplets (Pseudoephedrine Hydrochloride) Warner Wellcome ... 824
- Sunsource Sinus Relief Tablets (Homeopathic Medications) Sunsource ... 793
- Syn-Rx Tablets (Pseudoephedrine Hydrochloride, Guaifenesin) Medeva ... 1622
- Tavist-D 12 Hour Relief Tablets (Clemastine Fumarate, Phenylpropanolamine Hydrochloride) Sandoz Consumer ... 750
- Teldrin 12 Hour Antihistamine/Nasal Decongestant Allergy Relief Capsules (Chlorpheniramine Maleate, Phenylpropanolamine Hydrochloride) SmithKline Beecham Consumer ... 786
- Triaminic AM Decongestant Formula (Pseudoephedrine Hydrochloride) Sandoz Consumer ... 753
- Triaminic Infant Oral Decongestant Drops (Pseudoephedrine Hydrochloride) Sandoz Consumer ... 754
- Triaminicin Tablets (Acetaminophen, Chlorpheniramine Maleate, Phenylpropanolamine Hydrochloride) Sandoz Consumer ... 756
- Trinalin Repetabs Tablets (Azatadine Maleate, Pseudoephedrine Sulfate) Key ... 1373
- TYLENOL Allergy Sinus, Maximum Strength Caplets and Gelcaps (Acetaminophen, Chlorpheniramine Maleate, Pseudoephedrine Hydrochloride) McNeil Consumer 1571
- Vicks DayQuil Allergy Relief 12-Hour Extended Release Tablets (Phenylpropanolamine Hydrochloride, Brompheniramine Maleate) Procter & Gamble ... 733
- Vicks DayQuil Allergy Relief 4-Hour Tablets (Phenylpropanolamine Hydrochloride, Brompheniramine Maleate) Procter & Gamble ... 733
- Vicks DayQuil SINUS Pressure & CONGESTION Relief (Guaifenesin, Phenylpropanolamine Hydrochloride) Procter & Gamble ... 734
- Vicks DayQuil SINUS Pressure & PAIN Relief with IBUPROFEN (Ibuprofen, Pseudoephedrine Hydrochloride) Procter & Gamble ... 735
- Vicks Sinex 12-Hour Nasal Decongestant Spray and Ultra Fine Mist (Oxymetazoline Hydrochloride) Procter & Gamble ... 738
- Vicks Sinex Nasal Spray and Ultra Fine Mist (Phenylephrine Hydrochloride) Procter & Gamble ... 738

Nasal irritation, symptomatic relief of

- Afrin Saline Mist (Sodium Chloride) Schering-Plough HealthCare ... 758
- Atrohist Plus Tablets (Chlorpheniramine Maleate, Phenylpropanolamine Hydrochloride, Phenylephrine Hydrochloride, Hyoscyamine Sulfate, Atropine Sulfate, Scopolamine Hydrobromide) Medeva ... 1605
- Ryna-CX Liquid (Codeine Phosphate, Guaifenesin, Pseudoephedrine Hydrochloride) Wallace ... 804
- Salinex Nasal Mist and Drops (Sodium Chloride) Muro ... 713

Nausea
(see also under Motion sickness)

- Tigan (Trimethobenzamide Hydrochloride) Roberts ... 2231
- Torecan (Thiethylperazine Malate) Roxane ... 2367
- Vistaril Intramuscular Solution (Hydroxyzine Hydrochloride) Pfizer Inc ... 2042

Nausea, emetogenic, cancer chemotherapy-induced

- Kytril Injection (Granisetron Hydrochloride) SmithKline Beecham Pharmaceuticals ... 2667
- Kytril Tablets (Granisetron Hydrochloride) SmithKline Beecham Pharmaceuticals ... 2669
- Marinol (Dronabinol) Capsules (Dronabinol) Roxane ... 2353
- Reglan (Metoclopramide Hydrochloride) Robins ... 2243
- Zofran Injection (Ondansetron Hydrochloride) Glaxo Wellcome Oncology/HIV ... 1227
- Zofran Tablets (Ondansetron Hydrochloride) Glaxo Wellcome Oncology/HIV ... 1231

Nausea, emetogenic, radiation therapy-induced

- Zofran Tablets (Ondansetron Hydrochloride) Glaxo Wellcome Oncology/HIV ... 1231

Nausea, postoperative

- Emete-con Intramuscular/Intravenous (Benzquinamide Hydrochloride) Pfizer Inc ... 2007
- Phenergan Injection (Promethazine Hydrochloride) Wyeth-Ayerst ... 2880
- Phenergan Suppositories (Promethazine Hydrochloride) Wyeth-Ayerst ... 2882
- Phenergan Syrup (Promethazine Hydrochloride) Wyeth-Ayerst ... 2881
- Phenergan Tablets (Promethazine Hydrochloride) Wyeth-Ayerst ... 2882
- Reglan (Metoclopramide Hydrochloride) Robins ... 2243
- Zofran Injection (Ondansetron Hydrochloride) Glaxo Wellcome Oncology/HIV ... 1227
- Zofran Tablets (Ondansetron Hydrochloride) Glaxo Wellcome Oncology/HIV ... 1231

Nausea, severe, control of

- Compazine (Prochlorperazine) SmithKline Beecham Pharmaceuticals ... 2644
- Thorazine (Chlorpromazine Hydrochloride) SmithKline Beecham Pharmaceuticals ... 2701
- Trilafon (Perphenazine) Schering ... 2532

Necator americanus infections

- Mintezol (Thiabendazole) Merck & Co., Inc. ... 1747
- Vermox Chewable Tablets (Mebendazole) Janssen ... 1357

Necrobiosis lipoidica diabeticorum

- Celestone Soluspan Suspension (Betamethasone Sodium Phosphate, Betamethasone Acetate) Schering ... 2484
- Decadron Phosphate Injection (Dexamethasone Sodium Phosphate) Merck & Co., Inc. ... 1680
- Decadron-LA Sterile Suspension (Dexamethasone Acetate) Merck & Co., Inc. ... 1687
- Hydeltrasol Injection, Sterile (Prednisolone Sodium Phosphate) Merck & Co., Inc. ... 1708
- Hydrocortone Acetate Sterile Suspension (Hydrocortisone Acetate) Merck & Co., Inc. ... 1712

Necrosis, dermal

- Regitine Vials (Phentolamine Mesylate) CibaGeneva ... 864

Neisseria gonorrhoeae
(see under N. gonorrhoeae infections)

Neisseria meningitidis
(see under N. gonorrhoeae infections)

Neisseria species infections, ocular

- AK-Spore (Bacitracin Zinc, Neomycin Sulfate, Polymyxin B Sulfate) Akorn ... 205
- AK-Trol Ointment & Suspension (Dexamethasone, Neomycin Sulfate, Polymyxin B Sulfate) Akorn ... 205
- Chloromycetin Ophthalmic Ointment, 1% (Chloramphenicol) Parke-Davis ... 298
- Chloromycetin Ophthalmic Solution (Chloramphenicol) Parke-Davis ... 299
- Chloroptic S.O.P. (Chloramphenicol) Allergan ... 236
- Cortisporin Ophthalmic Ointment Sterile (Polymyxin B Sulfate, Bacitracin Zinc, Neomycin Sulfate, Hydrocortisone) Glaxo Wellcome ... 1074
- Cortisporin Ophthalmic Suspension Sterile (Hydrocortisone, Polymyxin B Sulfate, Neomycin Sulfate) Glaxo Wellcome ... 1075
- Maxitrol Ophthalmic Ointment and Suspension (Dexamethasone, Neomycin Sulfate, Polymyxin B Sulfate) Alcon Laboratories ... 222
- NeoDecadron Sterile Ophthalmic Ointment (Neomycin Sulfate, Dexamethasone Sodium Phosphate) Merck & Co., Inc. ... 1755
- NeoDecadron Sterile Ophthalmic Solution (Neomycin Sulfate, Dexamethasone Sodium Phosphate) Merck & Co., Inc. ... 1756
- Poly-Pred Liquifilm (Neomycin Sulfate, Polymyxin B Sulfate, Prednisolone Acetate) Allergan ... 246
- Pred-G Liquifilm Sterile Ophthalmic Suspension (Gentamicin Sulfate, Prednisolone Acetate) Allergan ... 248
- Terra-Cortril Ophthalmic Suspension (Oxytetracycline Hydrochloride, Hydrocortisone Acetate) Pfizer Inc ... 2033
- TobraDex Ophthalmic Suspension and Ointment (Dexamethasone, Tobramycin) Alcon Laboratories ... 469

Nephroblastoma
(see under Wilms' tumor)

Nephrolithiasis, calcium

- Urocit-K Tablets (Potassium Citrate) Mission ... 1828

Nephropathy, diabetic

- Capoten Tablets (Captopril) Bristol-Myers Squibb ... 740

Nephrotic syndrome, biopsy proven "minimal change", treatment of

- Cytoxan (Cyclophosphamide) Bristol-Myers Squibb Oncology/Immunology ... 700

Neuralgia
(see under Pain, neurogenic)

Neuralgia, glossopharyngeal

- Atretol Tablets (Carbamazepine) Athena ... 569
- Tegretol/Tegretol-XR (Carbamazepine) CibaGeneva ... 870

(▩ Described in PDR For Nonprescription Drugs) (◉ Described in PDR For Ophthalmology)

Neuralgia, trigeminal
Atretol Tablets (Carbamazepine) Athena 569
Sarapin (Sarracenia purpurea, Pitcher Plant Distillate) High Chemical 1237
Tegretol/Tegretol-XR (Carbamazepine) CibaGeneva 870

Neuritis, peripheral, acute
(see under Pain, neurogenic)

Neuroblastoma
Adriamycin PFS (Doxorubicin Hydrochloride) Pharmacia & Upjohn 2056
Adriamycin RDF (Doxorubicin Hydrochloride) Pharmacia & Upjohn 2056
Cytoxan (Cyclophosphamide) Bristol-Myers Squibb Oncology/Immunology 700
Doxorubicin Astra (Doxorubicin Hydrochloride) Astra 531
Oncovin Solution Vials & Hyporets (Vincristine Sulfate) Lilly 1521
Rubex for Injection (Doxorubicin Hydrochloride) Bristol-Myers Squibb Oncology/Immunology 721

Neurocysticercosis
Albenza Tablets (Albendazole) SmithKline Beecham Pharmaceuticals 2629

Neurodermatitis
(see under Lichen simplex chronicus)

Neurological deficits, post-SAH, improvement of
Nimotop Capsules (Nimodipine) Bayer Pharmaceutical 603

Neurological procedures, destructive, alternative therapy in
Lioresal Intrathecal (Baclofen) Medtronic Neurological 1634

Neuromuscular blockade, nondepolarizing, reversal of
Prostigmin Injectable (Neostigmine Methylsulfate) ICN 1305
Tensilon Injectable (Edrophonium Chloride) ICN 1307

Neutropenia, chemotherapy-induced
Neupogen for Injection (Filgrastim) Amgen 495

Neutropenia, febrile, to decrease the incidence of infection
Neupogen for Injection (Filgrastim) Amgen 495

Neutropenia, post-bone marrow transplant
Neupogen for Injection (Filgrastim) Amgen 495

Neutropenia-related clinical sequelae, post-bone marrow transplant
Neupogen for Injection (Filgrastim) Amgen 495

Niacin, deficiency of
Nicotinex Elixir (Niacin) Fleming 671
Slo-Niacin Tablets (Niacin) Upsher-Smith 2767

Nicolas-Favre disease
(see under Lymphogranuloma venereum)

Nocardia asteroides infections
(see under Nocardiosis)

Nocardiosis
Gantanol Tablets (Sulfamethoxazole) Roche Pharmaceuticals 2285
Gantrisin (Acetyl Sulfisoxazole) Roche Pharmaceuticals 2286

Nocturia, symptomatic relief of
Urispas Tablets (Flavoxate Hydrochloride) SmithKline Beecham Pharmaceuticals 2710

Nose, itchy
(see under Pruritus, rhinopharyngeal, symptomatic relief of)

Nose, runny
(see under Rhinorrhea)

Nose, surgical procedures, irrigation of
AMO Endosol (Balanced Salt Solution) (Balanced Salt Solution) Allergan .... ⊙ 229

Nutrients, deficiency of
AC Slim Cap (Nutritional Supplement) AC Laboratory 461
Advera Specialized Complete Nutrition (Nutritional Beverage) Ross 2337
Natural MD BASIC Rx (Vitamins, Multiple) AML Laboratories 602
AlitraQ Specialized Elemental Nutrition With Glutamine (L-Glutamine, Nutritional Supplement) Ross 2337
Aminoplex Capsules (Amino Acid Preparations) Tyson 2749
Aminotate Capsules (Amino Acid Preparations) Tyson 2749
Beelith Tablets (Magnesium Oxide, Vitamin B$_6$) Beach 632
Bio-Ginkgo (Ginkgo Biloba) Pharmanex 2984
BioLean (Nutritional Supplement) Wellness International 830
BioLean Accelerator (Nutritional Supplement) Wellness International 831
BioLean Free (Amino Acid Preparations, Nutritional Supplement) Wellness International 831
BioLean LipoTrim (Nutritional Supplement) Wellness International 832
BioLean Meal (Nutritional Beverage) Wellness International 832
Catemine Enteric Tablets (Tyrosine) (L-Tyrosine) Tyson 2750
Cholestin Capsules (Homeopathic Medications) Pharmanex 2985
Coenzyme Q10 200mg, 100mg & 60mg Chewable Wafers, and 200mg, 60mg & 25mg Tablets (Coenzyme Q-10) Vitaline 2768
Comtrex Multi-Symptom (Acetaminophen, Chlorpheniramine Maleate, Dextromethorphan Hydrobromide, Pseudoephedrine Hydrochloride) Bristol-Myers Products 638
CordyMax Cs-4 Capsules (Dietary Supplement) Pharmanex 2985
DIA-Reliever Tablets (Nutritional Supplement) AC Laboratory 461
Ensure Complete Balanced Nutrition (Nutritional Supplement) Ross 2338
Ensure High Protein Complete Balanced Nutrition (Nutritional Beverage) Ross 2337
Ensure Light Complete, Balanced Nutrition (Nutritional Supplement) Ross 2338
Ensure Plus High Calorie Complete Nutrition (Nutritional Supplement) Ross 2338
Ensure With Fiber Complete, Balanced Nutrition (Nutritional Supplement) Ross 2338
Food for Thought (Nutritional Beverage) Wellness International 833
Garlique (Garlic Extract) Sunsource 791
Ginkoba (Ginkgo Biloba) Pharmaton 721
Ginkgo Biloba Plus (Garlic Extract, Ginseng) Kyolic Ltd. 680
Ginsana (Ginseng) Pharmaton 721
Glucerna Specialized Nutrition with Fiber for Patients with Abnormal Glucose Tolerance (Nutritional Supplement) Ross 2338
Jevity Isotonic Liquid Nutrition with Fiber (Nutritional Supplement) Ross 2339
Jevity Plus 1.2 Cal/mL, High-Nitrogen Liquid Nutrition With Patented Fiber Blend (Nutritional Supplement) Ross 2339
Kyo-Chrome (Chromium Picolinate, Garlic Extract, Niacin) Kyolic Ltd. 680
Kyolic Aged Garlic Extract Caplets (Garlic Extract) Kyolic Ltd. 680
Lumitene (Beta Carotene) Tishcon 799
Marlyn Formula 50 Capsules (Amino Acid Preparations, Vitamin B$_6$) Marlyn 1558
Melatonex (Melatonin, Vitamin B$_6$) Sunsource 791
Melatonin Tablets (Melatonin) AC Laboratory 461
NephrAmine Injection (Amino Acid Preparations) R&D 2169
Nepro Specialized Liquid Nutrition (Nutritional Supplement) Ross 2339
One-A-Day Garlic Softgels (Garlic Extract) Bayer Consumer 626
One-A-Day Men's (Vitamins, Multiple) Bayer Consumer 626
Osmolite Isotonic Liquid Nutrition (Nutritional Supplement) Ross 2339
Osmolite HN High Nitrogen Isotonic Liquid Nutrition (Nutritional Supplement) Ross 2339
Osmolite HN Plus 1.2 Cal/mL, High-Nitrogen Liquid Nutrition (Nutritional Supplement) Ross 2340
PediaSure Complete Liquid Nutrition (Nutritional Supplement) Ross 2342
PediaSure With Fiber Complete Liquid Nutrition (Nutritional Supplement) Ross 2343
Perative Specialized Liquid Nutrition (Nutritional Beverage) Ross 2343
PhosChol (Phosphatidylcholine) American Lecithin 488
Phyto-Vite (Vitamins with Minerals) Wellness International 835
Polycose Glucose Polymers (Glucose Polymers) Ross 2343
Pro-Hepatone Capsules (Vitamins with Minerals, Amino Acid Preparations) Marlyn 1558
Promote High Protein Liquid Nutrition (Nutritional Supplement) Ross 2343
Promote With Fiber, High-Protein Liquid Nutrition (Nutritional Beverage) Ross 2343
Similac Toddler's Best Nutritional Beverage with Iron (Nutritional Beverage) Ross 746
StePHan Clarity (Nutritional Supplement) Wellness International 834
StePHan Elasticity (Nutritional Supplement) Wellness International 834
StePHan Elixir (Nutritional Supplement) Wellness International 834
StePHan Essential (Nutritional Supplement) Wellness International 834
StePHan Feminine (Nutritional Supplement) Wellness International 834
StePHan Flexibility (Nutritional Supplement) Wellness International 834
StePHan Lovpil (Nutritional Supplement) Wellness International 834
StePHan Masculine (Nutritional Supplement) Wellness International 835
StePHan Protector (Nutritional Supplement) Wellness International 835
StePHan Relief (Nutritional Supplement) Wellness International 836
StePHan Tranquility (Nutritional Supplement) Wellness International 836
SuperEPA (Docosahexaenoic Acid (DHA)) Advanced Nutritional 462
Suplena Specialized Liquid Nutrition (Nutritional Supplement) Ross 2346
Tēgreen 97 Capsules (Homeopathic Medications) Pharmanex 2985
Venolax (Vitamin B$_6$, Vitamin C) Lenes 686
Vital High Nitrogen Nutritionally Complete Partially Hydrolyzed Diet (Nutritional Supplement) Ross 2348
Winrgy (Nutritional Beverage) Wellness International 836

Nutrients, deficiency of, in respiratory insufficiency
Pulmocare Specialized Nutrition for Pulmonary Patients (Nutritional Supplement) Ross 2344

Nutrients, deficiency of, stress-induced
(see under Nutrients, deficiency of)

Nutrients, deficiency of, surgery-induced
(see under Nutrients, deficiency of)

Nutrition, infant
(see under Breast milk, replacement of or supplement to)

O

Obesity, exogenous
Adipex-P Tablets and Capsules (Phentermine Hydrochloride) Gate 1035
Bontril Slow-Release Capsules (Phendimetrazine Tartrate) Carnrick 786
Desoxyn Gradumet Tablets (Methamphetamine Hydrochloride) Abbott 422
Dexedrine (Dextroamphetamine Sulfate) SmithKline Beecham Pharmaceuticals 2648
Fastin Capsules (Phentermine Hydrochloride) SmithKline Beecham Pharmaceuticals 2662
Ionamin Capsules (Phentermine Resin) Medeva 1615
Pondimin Tablets (Fenfluramine Hydrochloride) Robins 2239
Prelu-2 Timed Release Capsules (Phendimetrazine Tartrate) Boehringer Ingelheim 687
Redux Capsules (Dexfenfluramine Hydrochloride) Wyeth-Ayerst 2911
Sanorex Tablets (Mazindol) Sandoz Pharmaceuticals 2423

Obsessive compulsive disorder
Anafranil Capsules (Clomipramine Hydrochloride) CibaGeneva 819
LUVOX Tablets (Fluvoxamine Maleate) Solvay 2723
Paxil Tablets (Paroxetine Hydrochloride) SmithKline Beecham Pharmaceuticals 2681
Prozac Pulvules & Liquid, Oral Solution (Fluoxetine Hydrochloride) Dista 935

Ocular congestion, symptomatic relief of
Albalon Solution with Liquifilm (Naphazoline Hydrochloride) Allergan .... ⊙ 229
Neo-Synephrine Hydrochloride (Ophthalmic) (Phenylephrine Hydrochloride) Sanofi Winthrop .. 2456

Ocular inflammation
AK-PRED (Prednisolone Sodium Phosphate) Akorn .... ⊙ 204
Econopred & Econopred Plus Ophthalmic Suspensions (Prednisolone Acetate) Alcon Laboratories .... ⊙ 216
Poly-Pred Liquifilm (Neomycin Sulfate, Polymyxin B Sulfate, Prednisolone Acetate) Allergan . ⊙ 246
Pred Mild (Prednisolone Acetate) Allergan .... ⊙ 250

Ocular inflammation with bacterial infection, steroid-responsive
AK-CIDE (Prednisolone Acetate, Sulfacetamide Sodium) Akorn .... ⊙ 203
AK-CIDE Ointment (Prednisolone Acetate, Sulfacetamide Sodium) Akorn .... ⊙ 203

(▣ Described in PDR For Nonprescription Drugs)   (⊙ Described in PDR For Ophthalmology)

Ocular inflammation Indications Index 1552

AK-Trol Ointment & Suspension (Dexamethasone, Neomycin Sulfate, Polymyxin B Sulfate) Akorn ◉ 205
Blephamide Liquifilm Sterile Ophthalmic Suspension (Prednisolone Acetate, Sulfacetamide Sodium) Allergan 472
Blephamide Ointment (Sulfacetamide Sodium, Prednisolone Acetate) Allergan ◉ 234
Cortisporin Ophthalmic Ointment Sterile (Polymyxin B Sulfate, Bacitracin Zinc, Neomycin Sulfate, Hydrocortisone) Glaxo Wellcome 1074
Cortisporin Ophthalmic Suspension Sterile (Hydrocortisone, Polymyxin B Sulfate, Neomycin Sulfate) Glaxo Wellcome 1075
FML-S Liquifilm (Sulfacetamide Sodium, Fluorometholone) Allergan ◉ 240
Maxitrol Ophthalmic Ointment and Suspension (Dexamethasone, Neomycin Sulfate, Polymyxin B Sulfate) Alcon Laboratories ◉ 222
NeoDecadron Sterile Ophthalmic Ointment (Neomycin Sulfate, Dexamethasone Sodium Phosphate) Merck & Co., Inc. 1755
NeoDecadron Sterile Ophthalmic Solution (Neomycin Sulfate, Dexamethasone Sodium Phosphate) Merck & Co., Inc. 1756
Poly-Pred Liquifilm (Neomycin Sulfate, Polymyxin B Sulfate, Prednisolone Acetate) Allergan ◉ 246
Pred-G Liquifilm Sterile Ophthalmic Suspension (Gentamicin Sulfate, Prednisolone Acetate) Allergan ◉ 248
Pred-G S.O.P. Sterile Ophthalmic Ointment (Gentamicin Sulfate, Prednisolone Acetate) Allergan ◉ 249
Terra-Cortril Ophthalmic Suspension (Oxytetracycline Hydrochloride, Hydrocortisone Acetate) Pfizer Inc 2033
TobraDex Ophthalmic Suspension and Ointment (Dexamethasone, Tobramycin) Alcon Laboratories 469

Ocular inflammation, postoperative
Vexol 1% Ophthalmic Suspension (Rimexolone) Alcon Laboratories ◉ 227
Voltaren Ophthalmic Sterile Ophthalmic Solution (Diclofenac Sodium) CIBA Vision Ophthalmics ◉ 264

Ocular inflammation, steroid-responsive
Decadron Phosphate Sterile Ophthalmic Ointment (Dexamethasone Sodium Phosphate) Merck & Co., Inc. 1684
Decadron Phosphate Sterile Ophthalmic Solution (Dexamethasone Sodium Phosphate) Merck & Co., Inc. 1685
Econopred & Econopred Plus Ophthalmic Suspensions (Prednisolone Acetate) Alcon Laboratories ◉ 216
Eflone Sterile Ophthalmic Suspension (Fluorometholone Acetate) CIBA Vision Ophthalmics ◉ 261
FML Liquifilm (Fluorometholone) Allergan ◉ 238
Flarex Ophthalmic Suspension (Fluorometholone Acetate) Alcon Laboratories ◉ 217
Pred Forte (Prednisolone Acetate) Allergan ◉ 247

Ocular redness
Clear Eyes ACR Astringent/Lubricant Eye Redness Reliever Eye Drops (Zinc Sulfate, Naphazoline Hydrochloride) Ross ◉ 314
Clear Eyes Lubricant Eye Redness Reliever (Glycerin, Naphazoline Hydrochloride) Ross ◉ 314
Collyrium Fresh (Tetrahydrozoline Hydrochloride, Glycerin) Storz Ophthalmics ◉ 316
Murine Tears Plus Lubricant Redness Reliever Eye Drops (Polyvinyl Alcohol, Povidone, Tetrahydrozoline Hydrochloride) Ross ◉ 315
Naphcon-A Ophthalmic Solution (Naphazoline Hydrochloride, Pheniramine Maleate) Alcon Laboratories 469
OcuHist (Naphazoline Hydrochloride, Pheniramine Maleate) Pfizer Consumer ◉ 300
Similasan Eye Drops #1 (Belladonna Alkaloids, Homeopathic Medications) Similasan ◉ 316
Similasan Eye Drops #2 (Homeopathic Medications) Similasan ◉ 316
Vasocon-A (Antazoline Phosphate, Naphazoline Hydrochloride) CIBA Vision Ophthalmics ◉ 263
Visine A.C. Seasonal Relief From Pollen and Dust (Tetrahydrozoline Hydrochloride, Zinc Sulfate) Pfizer Consumer ◉ 301
Visine Moisturizing Eye Drops (Tetrahydrozoline Hydrochloride, Polyethylene Glycol) Pfizer Consumer ◉ 301
Visine Original Eye Drops (Tetrahydrozoline Hydrochloride) Pfizer Consumer ◉ 301
Visine L.R. Eye Drops (Oxymetazoline Hydrochloride) Pfizer Consumer ◉ 301

Onychomycosis (see under Tinea unguium infections)

Oocytes, multiple, stimulation of the development of
Metrodin (urofollitropin for injection) (Urofollitropin) Serono 2616

Ophthalmia neonatorum, prophylaxis of
Ilotycin Ophthalmic Ointment (Erythromycin) Dista 928

Ophthalmia, Egyptian (see under Trachoma)

Ophthalmia, sympathetic
Celestone Soluspan Suspension (Betamethasone Sodium Phosphate, Betamethasone Acetate) Schering 2484
Cortone Acetate Sterile Suspension (Cortisone Acetate) Merck & Co., Inc. 1663
Cortone Acetate Tablets (Cortisone Acetate) Merck & Co., Inc. 1664
Dalalone D.P. Injectable (Dexamethasone Acetate) Forest 1009
Decadron Elixir (Dexamethasone) Merck & Co., Inc. 1676
Decadron Phosphate Injection (Dexamethasone Sodium Phosphate) Merck & Co., Inc. 1680
Decadron Tablets (Dexamethasone) Merck & Co., Inc. 1678
Decadron-LA Sterile Suspension (Dexamethasone Acetate) Merck & Co., Inc. 1687
Hydeltrasol Injection, Sterile (Prednisolone Sodium Phosphate) Merck & Co., Inc. 1708
Hydrocortone Phosphate Injection, Sterile (Hydrocortisone Sodium Phosphate) Merck & Co., Inc. 1713
Hydrocortone Tablets (Hydrocortisone) Merck & Co., Inc. 1715
Pediapred Oral Solution (Prednisolone Sodium Phosphate) Medeva 1618
Prelone Syrup (Prednisolone) Muro 1834

Opioids, acute overdosage, diagnosis of
Narcan Injection (Naloxone Hydrochloride) DuPont 950
Revex (nalmefene hydrochloride injection) (Nalmefene Hydrochloride) Ohmeda 1863

Opioids, blockade of the pharmacological effects
Narcan Injection (Naloxone Hydrochloride) DuPont 950
ReVia Tablets (Naltrexone Hydrochloride) DuPont 957
Revex (nalmefene hydrochloride injection) (Nalmefene Hydrochloride) Ohmeda 1863

Optic neuritis
Celestone Soluspan Suspension (Betamethasone Sodium Phosphate, Betamethasone Acetate) Schering 2484
Cortone Acetate Sterile Suspension (Cortisone Acetate) Merck & Co., Inc. 1663
Cortone Acetate Tablets (Cortisone Acetate) Merck & Co., Inc. 1664
Dalalone D.P. Injectable (Dexamethasone Acetate) Forest 1009
Decadron Elixir (Dexamethasone) Merck & Co., Inc. 1676
Decadron Phosphate Injection (Dexamethasone Sodium Phosphate) Merck & Co., Inc. 1680
Decadron Tablets (Dexamethasone) Merck & Co., Inc. 1678
Decadron-LA Sterile Suspension (Dexamethasone Acetate) Merck & Co., Inc. 1687
Hydeltrasol Injection, Sterile (Prednisolone Sodium Phosphate) Merck & Co., Inc. 1708
Hydrocortone Phosphate Injection, Sterile (Hydrocortisone Sodium Phosphate) Merck & Co., Inc. 1713
Hydrocortone Tablets (Hydrocortisone) Merck & Co., Inc. 1715
Pediapred Oral Solution (Prednisolone Sodium Phosphate) Medeva 1618
Prelone Syrup (Prednisolone) Muro 1834

Ornithosis (see under Chlamydia psittaci infection)

Ossification, heterotopic
Didronel Tablets (Etidronate Disodium (Diphosphonate)) Procter & Gamble Pharmaceuticals 2133

Osteitis deformans (see under Paget's disease of bone)

Osteitis fibrosa (see under Osteodystrophy)

Osteoarthritis
Anaprox/Naprosyn (Naproxen Sodium) Roche Pharmaceuticals 2277
Arthritis Pain Ascriptin (Aspirin Buffered, Calcium Carbonate) Ciba Self-Medication ▣ 650
Extra Strength Bayer Arthritis Pain Regimen Formula (Aspirin, Enteric Coated) Bayer Consumer ▣ 615
Cataflam Tablets (Diclofenac Potassium) CibaGeneva 833
Celestone Soluspan Suspension (Betamethasone Sodium Phosphate, Betamethasone Acetate) Schering 2484
Clinoril Tablets (Sulindac) Merck & Co., Inc. 1658
Daypro Caplets (Oxaprozin) Searle 2578
Disalcid (Salsalate) 3M Pharmaceuticals 1549
Dolobid Tablets (Diflunisal) Merck & Co., Inc. 1695
EC-Naprosyn Delayed-Release Tablets (Naproxen) Roche Pharmaceuticals 2277
Ecotrin (Aspirin) SmithKline Beecham 2625
Feldene Capsules (Piroxicam) Pfizer Inc 2008
IBU Tablets (Ibuprofen) Knoll Laboratories 1389
Indocin (Indomethacin) Merck & Co., Inc. 1723
Lodine Capsules and Tablets (Etodolac) Wyeth-Ayerst 2849
Mono-Gesic Tablets (Salsalate) Central 810
Motrin Ibuprofen Suspension, Oral Drops, Chewable Tablets, Caplets (Ibuprofen) McNeil Consumer 1563
Nalfon 200 Pulvules & Nalfon Tablets (Fenoprofen Calcium) Dista 933
Naprelan Tablets (Naproxen Sodium) Wyeth-Ayerst 2861
Anaprox/Naprosyn (Naproxen) Roche Pharmaceuticals 2277
Orudis Capsules (Ketoprofen) Wyeth-Ayerst 2874
Oruvail Capsules (Ketoprofen) Wyeth-Ayerst 2874
Relafen Tablets (Nabumetone) SmithKline Beecham Pharmaceuticals 2688
Salflex Tablets (Salsalate) Carnrick 791
Tolectin (200, 400 and 600 mg) (Tolmetin Sodium) McNeil Pharmaceutical 1591
Trilisate (Choline Magnesium Trisalicylate) Purdue Frederick 2155
Cataflam/Voltaren/Voltaren-XR (Diclofenac Sodium) CibaGeneva 833

Osteoarthritis, post-traumatic
Cortone Acetate Sterile Suspension (Cortisone Acetate) Merck & Co., Inc. 1663
Cortone Acetate Tablets (Cortisone Acetate) Merck & Co., Inc. 1664
Dalalone D.P. Injectable (Dexamethasone Acetate) Forest 1009
Decadron Elixir (Dexamethasone) Merck & Co., Inc. 1676
Decadron Phosphate Injection (Dexamethasone Sodium Phosphate) Merck & Co., Inc. 1680
Decadron Tablets (Dexamethasone) Merck & Co., Inc. 1678
Decadron-LA Sterile Suspension (Dexamethasone Acetate) Merck & Co., Inc. 1687
Hydeltrasol Injection, Sterile (Prednisolone Sodium Phosphate) Merck & Co., Inc. 1708
Hydeltra-T.B.A. Sterile Suspension (Prednisolone Tebutate) Merck & Co., Inc. 1710
Hydrocortone Acetate Sterile Suspension (Hydrocortisone Acetate) Merck & Co., Inc. 1712
Hydrocortone Phosphate Injection, Sterile (Hydrocortisone Sodium Phosphate) Merck & Co., Inc. 1713
Hydrocortone Tablets (Hydrocortisone) Merck & Co., Inc. 1715
Pediapred Oral Solution (Prednisolone Sodium Phosphate) Medeva 1618
Prelone Syrup (Prednisolone) Muro 1834

Osteoarthritis, synovitis of
Celestone Soluspan Suspension (Betamethasone Sodium Phosphate, Betamethasone Acetate) Schering 2484
Cortone Acetate Sterile Suspension (Cortisone Acetate) Merck & Co., Inc. 1663
Cortone Acetate Tablets (Cortisone Acetate) Merck & Co., Inc. 1664
Dalalone D.P. Injectable (Dexamethasone Acetate) Forest 1009
Decadron Elixir (Dexamethasone) Merck & Co., Inc. 1676
Decadron Phosphate Injection (Dexamethasone Sodium Phosphate) Merck & Co., Inc. 1680
Decadron Tablets (Dexamethasone) Merck & Co., Inc. 1678
Decadron-LA Sterile Suspension (Dexamethasone Acetate) Merck & Co., Inc. 1687
Hydeltrasol Injection, Sterile (Prednisolone Sodium Phosphate) Merck & Co., Inc. 1708
Hydeltra-T.B.A. Sterile Suspension (Prednisolone Tebutate) Merck & Co., Inc. 1710
Hydrocortone Acetate Sterile Suspension (Hydrocortisone Acetate) Merck & Co., Inc. 1712
Hydrocortone Phosphate Injection, Sterile (Hydrocortisone Sodium Phosphate) Merck & Co., Inc. 1713
Hydrocortone Tablets (Hydrocortisone) Merck & Co., Inc. 1715
Pediapred Oral Solution (Prednisolone Sodium Phosphate) Medeva 1618
Prelone Syrup (Prednisolone) Muro 1834

(▣ Described in PDR For Nonprescription Drugs) (◉ Described in PDR For Ophthalmology)

Indications Index — P. aeruginosa infections

Osteodystrophy
Rocaltrol Capsules (Calcitriol) Roche Pharmaceuticals 2303

Osteodystrophy, renal
Calcijex Injection (Calcitriol) Abbott 412

Osteolytic bone lesions, multiple myeloma-induced
Aredia for Injection (Pamidronate Disodium) CibaGeneva 827

Osteomalacia
(see under Osteodystrophy)

Osteomyelitis, acute hematogenous
Cleocin Phosphate Injection (Clindamycin Phosphate) Pharmacia & Upjohn 2068

Osteoporosis
Estrace Cream and Tablets (Estradiol) Bristol-Myers Squibb .. 751
Estraderm Transdermal System (Estradiol) CibaGeneva 842
Fosamax Tablets (Alendronate Sodium) Merck & Co., Inc. 1703
Miacalcin Nasal Spray (Calcitonin-Salmon) Sandoz Pharmaceuticals 2403
Ogen Tablets (Estropipate) Pharmacia & Upjohn 2103
Ortho-Est (Estropipate) Ortho Pharmaceutical 1925
Premarin Tablets (Estrogens, Conjugated) Wyeth-Ayerst 2896
Premphase (Estrogens, Conjugated, Medroxyprogesterone Acetate) Wyeth-Ayerst 2900
Prempro (Estrogens, Conjugated, Medroxyprogesterone Acetate) Wyeth-Ayerst 2905

Osteoporosis, postmenopausal, treatment adjunct
Calcimar Injection, Synthetic (Calcitonin, Synthetic) Rhone-Poulenc Rorer Pharmaceuticals 2176
Miacalcin Injection (Calcitonin, Synthetic) Sandoz Pharmaceuticals 2402

Osteosarcoma, nonmetastatic
Methotrexate Sodium Tablets, Injection, for Injection and LPF Injection (Methotrexate Sodium) Immunex 1322

Otitis externa
Coly-Mycin S Otic w/Neomycin & Hydrocortisone (Colistin Sulfate, Neomycin Sulfate, Hydrocortisone Acetate) Parke-Davis 1965
Pediotic Suspension Sterile (Polymyxin B Sulfate, Neomycin Sulfate, Hydrocortisone) Glaxo Wellcome 1140
VōSol (Acetic Acid, Hydrocortisone) Wallace 2786

Otitis externa with inflammation
Cortisporin Otic Solution Sterile (Polymyxin B Sulfate, Neomycin Sulfate, Hydrocortisone) Glaxo Wellcome 1076
Cortisporin Otic Suspension Sterile (Polymyxin B Sulfate, Neomycin Sulfate, Hydrocortisone) Glaxo Wellcome 1077
Decadron Phosphate Sterile Ophthalmic Solution (Dexamethasone Sodium Phosphate) Merck & Co., Inc. 1685
VōSol HC Otic Solution (Acetic Acid, Hydrocortisone) Wallace 2786

Otitis externa, symptomatic relief of
Americaine Otic Topical Anesthetic Ear Drops (Benzocaine) Medeva .. 1603
Otic Domeboro Solution (Acetic Acid) Bayer Pharmaceutical 604
Star-Otic Ear Solution (Acetic Acid, Boric Acid, Burow's Solution) Stellar ..... ▣ 790

Otitis media, acute
Amoxil (Amoxicillin Trihydrate) SmithKline Beecham Pharmaceuticals 2631
Augmentin (Amoxicillin Trihydrate, Clavulanate Potassium) SmithKline Beecham Pharmaceuticals 2637
Augmentin Tablets (Amoxicillin Trihydrate, Clavulanate Potassium) SmithKline Beecham Pharmaceuticals 2640
Bactrim (Trimethoprim, Sulfamethoxazole) Roche Pharmaceuticals 2257
Biaxin (Clarithromycin) Abbott 406
Bicillin C-R Injection (Penicillin G Procaine, Penicillin G Benzathine) Wyeth-Ayerst 2810
Bicillin C-R 900/300 Injection (Penicillin G Procaine, Penicillin G Benzathine) Wyeth-Ayerst 2812
Ceclor Pulvules & Suspension (Cefaclor) Lilly 1470
Cedax (Ceftibuten Dihydrate) Schering 2480
Ceftin (Cefuroxime Axetil) Glaxo Wellcome 1067
Cefzil Tablets and Oral Suspension (Cefprozil) Bristol-Myers Squibb .. 747
E.E.S. (Erythromycin Ethylsuccinate) Abbott 427
EryPed (Erythromycin Ethylsuccinate) Abbott 425
Ery-Tab Tablets (Erythromycin) Abbott 426
Erythrocin Stearate Filmtab (Erythromycin Stearate) Abbott 429
Erythromycin Base Filmtab (Erythromycin) Abbott 430
Keflex Pulvules & Oral Suspension (Cephalexin) Dista 930
Lorabid Suspension and Pulvules (Loracarbef) Lilly 1513
Pediazole Suspension (Erythromycin Ethylsuccinate, Sulfisoxazole Acetyl) Ross 2340
Septra (Trimethoprim, Sulfamethoxazole) Glaxo Wellcome 1146
Suprax (Cefixime) Lederle 1443
Vantin for Oral Suspension and Vantin Tablets (Cefpodoxime Proxetil) Pharmacia & Upjohn 2112
Zithromax (Azithromycin) Pfizer Inc 2043

Otitis media, acute, adjuvant therapy
Americaine Otic Topical Anesthetic Ear Drops (Benzocaine) Medeva .. 1603
Auralgan Otic Solution (Antipyrine, Benzocaine, Glycerin) Wyeth-Ayerst 2810
Congess (Guaifenesin, Pseudoephedrine Hydrochloride) Fleming 1003
Fedahist Gyrocaps (Pseudoephedrine Hydrochloride, Chlorpheniramine Maleate) Schwarz 2545
Gantanol Tablets (Sulfamethoxazole) Roche Pharmaceuticals 2285
Gantrisin (Acetyl Sulfisoxazole) Roche Pharmaceuticals 2286
Tympagesic Ear Drops (Antipyrine, Benzocaine, Phenylephrine Hydrochloride) Savage 2476

Otitis media, H. influenzae-induced
(see under H. influenzae otitis media)

Otitis media, S. pneumoniae-induced
(see under S. pneumoniae otitis media)

Otitis media, S. pyogenes-induced
(see under S. pyogenes otitis media)

Otitis media, Staphylococci-induced
(see under Staphylococci otitis media)

Ovarian failure, primary
Estrace Cream and Tablets (Estradiol) Bristol-Myers Squibb .. 751
Estraderm Transdermal System (Estradiol) CibaGeneva 842
ESTRATAB Tablets (0.3, 0.625, 1.25, 2.5 mg) (Estrogens, Esterified) Solvay 2715
Menest Tablets (Estrogens, Esterified) SmithKline Beecham Pharmaceuticals 2671
Ogen Tablets (Estropipate) Pharmacia & Upjohn 2103
Ortho-Est (Estropipate) Ortho Pharmaceutical 1925
Premarin Tablets (Estrogens, Conjugated) Wyeth-Ayerst 2896
Vivelle Transdermal System (Estradiol) CibaGeneva 880

Ovaries, castration of
Estrace Cream and Tablets (Estradiol) Bristol-Myers Squibb .. 751
Estraderm Transdermal System (Estradiol) CibaGeneva 842
ESTRATAB Tablets (0.3, 0.625, 1.25, 2.5 mg) (Estrogens, Esterified) Solvay 2715
Menest Tablets (Estrogens, Esterified) SmithKline Beecham Pharmaceuticals 2671
Ogen Tablets (Estropipate) Pharmacia & Upjohn 2103
Ortho-Est (Estropipate) Ortho Pharmaceutical 1925
Premarin Tablets (Estrogens, Conjugated) Wyeth-Ayerst 2896
Vivelle Transdermal System (Estradiol) CibaGeneva 880

Ovary, adenocarcinoma
(see under Carcinoma, ovary)

Ovulation, induction of
Clomid (Clomiphene Citrate) Hoechst Marion Roussel 1262
Humegon for Injection (Menotropins) Organon 1873
Metrodin (urofollitropin for injection) (Urofollitropin) Serono 2616
Pergonal (menotropins for injection, USP) (Menotropins) Serono 2618
Pregnyl for Injection (Chorionic Gonadotropin) Organon 1878
Profasi (chorionic gonadotropin for injection, USP) (Chorionic Gonadotropin) Serono 2620
Serophene (clomiphene citrate tablets, USP) (Clomiphene Citrate) Serono 2621

Oxyuriasis
(see under Enterobiasis)

P

P. aeruginosa bacteremia
Ceptaz (Ceftazidime) Glaxo Wellcome 1070

P. aeruginosa bone and joint infections
Ceptaz (Ceftazidime) Glaxo Wellcome 1070
Cipro I.V. (Ciprofloxacin) Bayer Pharmaceutical 587
Cipro I.V. Pharmacy Bulk Package (Ciprofloxacin) Bayer Pharmaceutical 590
Cipro Tablets (Ciprofloxacin Hydrochloride) Bayer Pharmaceutical 584
Claforan Sterile and Injection (Cefotaxime Sodium) Hoechst Marion Roussel 1259
Fortaz (Ceftazidime) Glaxo Wellcome 1092
Nebcin Vials, Hyporets & ADD-Vantage (Tobramycin Sulfate) Lilly 1518
Pipracil (Piperacillin Sodium) Lederle 1435
Primaxin I.V. (Cilastatin Sodium, Imipenem) Merck & Co., Inc. 1772
Tazicef for Injection (Ceftazidime) SmithKline Beecham Pharmaceuticals 2697
Tazidime Vials, Faspak & ADD-Vantage (Ceftazidime) Lilly .. 1531

P. aeruginosa infections
Amikacin Sulfate Injection, USP (Amikacin Sulfate) Astra 523
Amikacin Sulfate Injection, USP (Amikacin Sulfate) Elkins-Sinn 981
Amikin Injectable (Amikacin Sulfate) Apothecon 502
Azactam for Injection (Aztreonam) Bristol-Myers Squibb 736
Cefizox for Intramuscular or Intravenous Use (Ceftizoxime Sodium) Fujisawa 1025
Cefobid Intravenous/Intramuscular (Cefoperazone Sodium) Pfizer Inc 1996
Cefobid Pharmacy Bulk Package - Not for Direct Infusion (Cefoperazone Sodium) Pfizer Inc 1999
Ceptaz (Ceftazidime) Glaxo Wellcome 1070
Cipro I.V. (Ciprofloxacin) Bayer Pharmaceutical 587
Cipro I.V. Pharmacy Bulk Package (Ciprofloxacin) Bayer Pharmaceutical 590
Cipro Tablets (Ciprofloxacin Hydrochloride) Bayer Pharmaceutical 584
Claforan Sterile and Injection (Cefotaxime Sodium) Hoechst Marion Roussel 1259
Cortisporin Ophthalmic Ointment Sterile (Polymyxin B Sulfate, Bacitracin Zinc, Neomycin Sulfate, Hydrocortisone) Glaxo Wellcome 1074
Cortisporin Ophthalmic Suspension Sterile (Hydrocortisone, Polymyxin B Sulfate, Neomycin Sulfate) Glaxo Wellcome 1075
Floxin I.V. (Ofloxacin) McNeil Pharmaceutical 1580
Floxin Tablets (200 mg, 300 mg, 400 mg) (Ofloxacin) McNeil Pharmaceutical 1577
Fortaz (Ceftazidime) Glaxo Wellcome 1092
Garamycin Injectable (Gentamicin Sulfate) Schering 2502
Maxaquin Tablets (Lomefloxacin Hydrochloride) Searle 2593
Maxipime for Injection (Cefepime Hydrochloride) Bristol-Myers Squibb 758
Merrem I.V. (Meropenem) Zeneca .. 2952
Mezlin (Mezlocillin Sodium) Bayer Pharmaceutical 594
Mezlin Pharmacy Bulk Package (Mezlocillin Sodium) Bayer Pharmaceutical 597
Nebcin Vials, Hyporets & ADD-Vantage (Tobramycin Sulfate) Lilly 1518
Netromycin Injection 100 mg/ml (Netilmicin Sulfate) Schering 2516
Noroxin Tablets (Norfloxacin) Merck & Co., Inc. 1758
Noroxin Tablets (Norfloxacin) Roberts 2222
Penetrex Tablets (Enoxacin) Rhone-Poulenc Rorer Pharmaceuticals 2196
Pipracil (Piperacillin Sodium) Lederle 1435
Primaxin I.M. (Cilastatin Sodium, Imipenem) Merck & Co., Inc. 1770
Primaxin I.V. (Cilastatin Sodium, Imipenem) Merck & Co., Inc. 1772
Rocephin Injectable Vials, ADD-Vantage, Galaxy Container (Ceftriaxone Sodium) Roche Pharmaceuticals 2305
Tazicef for Injection (Ceftazidime) SmithKline Beecham Pharmaceuticals 2697
Tazidime Vials, Faspak & ADD-Vantage (Ceftazidime) Lilly .. 1531
TERAK Ointment (Oxytetracycline Hydrochloride, Polymyxin B Sulfate) Akorn ..... ◉ 210
Ticar for Injection (Ticarcillin Disodium) SmithKline Beecham Pharmaceuticals 2704
Timentin for Injection (Ticarcillin Disodium, Clavulanate Potassium) SmithKline Beecham Pharmaceuticals 2706

P. aeruginosa infections, ocular
AK-Spore (Bacitracin Zinc, Neomycin Sulfate, Polymyxin B Sulfate) Akorn ..... ◉ 205
AK-Trol Ointment & Suspension (Dexamethasone, Neomycin Sulfate, Polymyxin B Sulfate) Akorn ..... ◉ 205
Ciloxan Ophthalmic Solution (Ciprofloxacin Hydrochloride) Alcon Laboratories 468
Garamycin Ophthalmic (Gentamicin Sulfate) Schering 2501
Genoptic Sterile Ophthalmic Solution (Gentamicin Sulfate) Allergan ..... ◉ 241

(▣ Described in PDR For Nonprescription Drugs)   (◉ Described in PDR For Ophthalmology)

P. aeruginosa infections

Genoptic Sterile Ophthalmic Ointment (Gentamicin Sulfate) Allergan ... ⊚ 241
Gentak (Gentamicin Sulfate) Akorn ... ⊚ 209
Ocuflox Ophthalmic Solution (Ofloxacin) Allergan ... 478
Poly-Pred Liquifilm (Neomycin Sulfate, Polymyxin B Sulfate, Prednisolone Acetate) Allergan .. ⊚ 246
Polytrim Ophthalmic Solution Sterile (Polymyxin B Sulfate, Trimethoprim Sulfate) Allergan 479
Pred-G Liquifilm Sterile Ophthalmic Suspension (Gentamicin Sulfate, Prednisolone Acetate) Allergan ... ⊚ 248
Pred-G S.O.P. Sterile Ophthalmic Ointment (Gentamicin Sulfate, Prednisolone Acetate) Allergan .. ⊚ 249
TERAK Ointment (Oxytetracycline Hydrochloride, Polymyxin B Sulfate) Akorn ... ⊚ 210
Terramycin with Polymyxin B Sulfate Ophthalmic Ointment (Oxytetracycline Hydrochloride, Polymyxin B Sulfate) Pfizer Inc 2035
TobraDex Ophthalmic Suspension and Ointment (Dexamethasone, Tobramycin) Alcon Laboratories . 469

P. aeruginosa intra-abdominal infections

Azactam for Injection (Aztreonam) Bristol-Myers Squibb ... 736
Cefobid Intravenous/Intramuscular (Cefoperazone Sodium) Pfizer Inc ... 1996
Cefobid Pharmacy Bulk Package - Not for Direct Infusion (Cefoperazone Sodium) Pfizer Inc ... 1999
Merrem I.V. (Meropenem) Zeneca .. 2952
Netromycin Injection 100 mg/ml (Netilmicin Sulfate) Schering ... 2516
Pipracil (Piperacillin Sodium) Lederle ... 1435
Primaxin I.M. (Cilastatin Sodium, Imipenem) Merck & Co., Inc. ... 1770
Primaxin I.V. (Cilastatin Sodium, Imipenem) Merck & Co., Inc. ... 1772

P. aeruginosa lower respiratory tract infections

Azactam for Injection (Aztreonam) Bristol-Myers Squibb ... 736
Ceptaz (Ceftazidime) Glaxo Wellcome ... 1070
Cipro I.V. (Ciprofloxacin) Bayer Pharmaceutical ... 587
Cipro I.V. Pharmacy Bulk Package (Ciprofloxacin) Bayer Pharmaceutical ... 590
Cipro Tablets (Ciprofloxacin Hydrochloride) Bayer Pharmaceutical ... 584
Claforan Sterile and Injection (Cefotaxime Sodium) Hoechst Marion Roussel ... 1259
Fortaz (Ceftazidime) Glaxo Wellcome ... 1092
Maxipime for Injection (Cefepime Hydrochloride) Bristol-Myers Squibb ... 758
Mezlin (Mezlocillin Sodium) Bayer Pharmaceutical ... 594
Mezlin Pharmacy Bulk Package (Mezlocillin Sodium) Bayer Pharmaceutical ... 597
Nebcin Vials, Hyporets & ADD-Vantage (Tobramycin Sulfate) Lilly ... 1518
Netromycin Injection 100 mg/ml (Netilmicin Sulfate) Schering ... 2516
Pipracil (Piperacillin Sodium) Lederle ... 1435
Tazicef for Injection (Ceftazidime) SmithKline Beecham Pharmaceuticals ... 2697
Tazidime Vials, Faspak & ADD-Vantage (Ceftazidime) Lilly .. 1531

P. aeruginosa meningitis

Ceptaz (Ceftazidime) Glaxo Wellcome ... 1070
Fortaz (Ceftazidime) Glaxo Wellcome ... 1092
Tazicef for Injection (Ceftazidime) SmithKline Beecham Pharmaceuticals ... 2697
Tazidime Vials, Faspak & ADD-Vantage (Ceftazidime) Lilly .. 1531

P. aeruginosa respiratory tract infections

Cefobid Intravenous/Intramuscular (Cefoperazone Sodium) Pfizer Inc ... 1996
Cefobid Pharmacy Bulk Package - Not for Direct Infusion (Cefoperazone Sodium) Pfizer Inc ... 1999
Ticar for Injection (Ticarcillin Disodium) SmithKline Beecham Pharmaceuticals ... 2704

P. aeruginosa septicemia

Azactam for Injection (Aztreonam) Bristol-Myers Squibb ... 736
Cefobid Intravenous/Intramuscular (Cefoperazone Sodium) Pfizer Inc ... 1996
Cefobid Pharmacy Bulk Package - Not for Direct Infusion (Cefoperazone Sodium) Pfizer Inc ... 1999
Ceptaz (Ceftazidime) Glaxo Wellcome ... 1070
Fortaz (Ceftazidime) Glaxo Wellcome ... 1092
Nebcin Vials, Hyporets & ADD-Vantage (Tobramycin Sulfate) Lilly ... 1518
Netromycin Injection 100 mg/ml (Netilmicin Sulfate) Schering ... 2516
Pipracil (Piperacillin Sodium) Lederle ... 1435
Primaxin I.V. (Cilastatin Sodium, Imipenem) Merck & Co., Inc. ... 1772
Tazicef for Injection (Ceftazidime) SmithKline Beecham Pharmaceuticals ... 2697
Tazidime Vials, Faspak & ADD-Vantage (Ceftazidime) Lilly .. 1531
Ticar for Injection (Ticarcillin Disodium) SmithKline Beecham Pharmaceuticals ... 2704
Timentin for Injection (Ticarcillin Disodium, Clavulanate Potassium) SmithKline Beecham Pharmaceuticals ... 2706

P. aeruginosa skin and skin structure infections

Azactam for Injection (Aztreonam) Bristol-Myers Squibb ... 736
Cefobid Intravenous/Intramuscular (Cefoperazone Sodium) Pfizer Inc ... 1996
Cefobid Pharmacy Bulk Package - Not for Direct Infusion (Cefoperazone Sodium) Pfizer Inc ... 1999
Ceptaz (Ceftazidime) Glaxo Wellcome ... 1070
Cipro I.V. (Ciprofloxacin) Bayer Pharmaceutical ... 587
Cipro I.V. Pharmacy Bulk Package (Ciprofloxacin) Bayer Pharmaceutical ... 590
Cipro Tablets (Ciprofloxacin Hydrochloride) Bayer Pharmaceutical ... 584
Fortaz (Ceftazidime) Glaxo Wellcome ... 1092
Nebcin Vials, Hyporets & ADD-Vantage (Tobramycin Sulfate) Lilly ... 1518
Netromycin Injection 100 mg/ml (Netilmicin Sulfate) Schering ... 2516
Pipracil (Piperacillin Sodium) Lederle ... 1435
Primaxin I.M. (Cilastatin Sodium, Imipenem) Merck & Co., Inc. ... 1770
Primaxin I.V. (Cilastatin Sodium, Imipenem) Merck & Co., Inc. ... 1772
Rocephin Injectable Vials, ADD-Vantage, Galaxy Container (Ceftriaxone Sodium) Roche Pharmaceuticals ... 2305
Tazicef for Injection (Ceftazidime) SmithKline Beecham Pharmaceuticals ... 2697
Tazidime Vials, Faspak & ADD-Vantage (Ceftazidime) Lilly .. 1531
Ticar for Injection (Ticarcillin Disodium) SmithKline Beecham Pharmaceuticals ... 2704
Timentin for Injection (Ticarcillin Disodium, Clavulanate Potassium) SmithKline Beecham Pharmaceuticals ... 2706

P. aeruginosa urinary tract infections

Azactam for Injection (Aztreonam) Bristol-Myers Squibb ... 736
Cefizox for Intramuscular or Intravenous Use (Ceftizoxime Sodium) Fujisawa ... 1025
Cefobid Intravenous/Intramuscular (Cefoperazone Sodium) Pfizer Inc ... 1996
Cefobid Pharmacy Bulk Package - Not for Direct Infusion (Cefoperazone Sodium) Pfizer Inc ... 1999
Ceptaz (Ceftazidime) Glaxo Wellcome ... 1070
Cipro I.V. (Ciprofloxacin) Bayer Pharmaceutical ... 587
Cipro I.V. Pharmacy Bulk Package (Ciprofloxacin) Bayer Pharmaceutical ... 590
Cipro Tablets (Ciprofloxacin Hydrochloride) Bayer Pharmaceutical ... 584
Claforan Sterile and Injection (Cefotaxime Sodium) Hoechst Marion Roussel ... 1259
Floxin I.V. (Ofloxacin) McNeil Pharmaceutical ... 1580
Floxin Tablets (200 mg, 300 mg, 400 mg) (Ofloxacin) McNeil Pharmaceutical ... 1577
Fortaz (Ceftazidime) Glaxo Wellcome ... 1092
Maxaquin Tablets (Lomefloxacin Hydrochloride) Searle ... 2593
Nebcin Vials, Hyporets & ADD-Vantage (Tobramycin Sulfate) Lilly ... 1518
Netromycin Injection 100 mg/ml (Netilmicin Sulfate) Schering ... 2516
Noroxin Tablets (Norfloxacin) Merck & Co., Inc. ... 1758
Noroxin Tablets (Norfloxacin) Roberts ... 2222
Penetrex Tablets (Enoxacin) Rhone-Poulenc Rorer Pharmaceuticals ... 2196
Primaxin I.V. (Cilastatin Sodium, Imipenem) Merck & Co., Inc. ... 1772
Tazicef for Injection (Ceftazidime) SmithKline Beecham Pharmaceuticals ... 2697
Tazidime Vials, Faspak & ADD-Vantage (Ceftazidime) Lilly .. 1531
Ticar for Injection (Ticarcillin Disodium) SmithKline Beecham Pharmaceuticals ... 2704
Timentin for Injection (Ticarcillin Disodium, Clavulanate Potassium) SmithKline Beecham Pharmaceuticals ... 2706

P. falciparum infections

Aralen Hydrochloride Injection (Chloroquine Hydrochloride) Sanofi Winthrop ... 2430
Aralen Phosphate Tablets (Chloroquine Phosphate) Sanofi Winthrop ... 2431
Daraprim Tablets (Pyrimethamine) Glaxo Wellcome Oncology/HIV ... 1199
Fansidar Tablets (Sulfadoxine, Pyrimethamine) Roche Pharmaceuticals ... 2281
Lariam Tablets (Mefloquine Hydrochloride) Roche Pharmaceuticals ... 2295
Plaquenil Sulfate Tablets (Hydroxychloroquine Sulfate) Sanofi Winthrop ... 2459
Vibramycin Hyclate Capsules (Doxycycline Hyclate) Pfizer Inc... 2038

P. falciparum infections, adjunct in

Gantanol Tablets (Sulfamethoxazole) Roche Pharmaceuticals ... 2285
Gantrisin (Acetyl Sulfisoxazole) Roche Pharmaceuticals ... 2286

P. inconstans group B urinary tract infections

Claforan Sterile and Injection (Cefotaxime Sodium) Hoechst Marion Roussel ... 1259

P. malariae infections

Aralen Hydrochloride Injection (Chloroquine Hydrochloride) Sanofi Winthrop ... 2430
Aralen Phosphate Tablets (Chloroquine Phosphate) Sanofi Winthrop ... 2431
Daraprim Tablets (Pyrimethamine) Glaxo Wellcome Oncology/HIV ... 1199
Plaquenil Sulfate Tablets (Hydroxychloroquine Sulfate) Sanofi Winthrop ... 2459

P. mirabilis biliary tract infections

Ancef Injection (Cefazolin Sodium) SmithKline Beecham Pharmaceuticals ... 2632
Kefzol Vials, Faspak & ADD-Vantage (Cefazolin Sodium) Lilly ... 1511

P. mirabilis bone and joint infections

Cefizox for Intramuscular or Intravenous Use (Ceftizoxime Sodium) Fujisawa ... 1025
Claforan Sterile and Injection (Cefotaxime Sodium) Hoechst Marion Roussel ... 1259
Keflex Pulvules & Oral Suspension (Cephalexin) Dista ... 930
Keftab Tablets (Cephalexin Hydrochloride) Dista ... 931
Rocephin Injectable Vials, ADD-Vantage, Galaxy Container (Ceftriaxone Sodium) Roche Pharmaceuticals ... 2305

P. mirabilis genitourinary tract infections

Ancef Injection (Cefazolin Sodium) SmithKline Beecham Pharmaceuticals ... 2632
Azactam for Injection (Aztreonam) Bristol-Myers Squibb ... 736
Keflex Pulvules & Oral Suspension (Cephalexin) Dista ... 930
Keftab Tablets (Cephalexin Hydrochloride) Dista ... 931
Mefoxin (Cefoxitin Sodium) Merck & Co., Inc. ... 1734
Mefoxin Premixed Intravenous Solution (Cefoxitin Sodium) Merck & Co., Inc. ... 1737
Omnipen for Oral Suspension (Ampicillin) Wyeth-Ayerst ... 2873

P. mirabilis gynecologic infections

Cefotan (Cefotetan) Zeneca ... 2936
Claforan Sterile and Injection (Cefotaxime Sodium) Hoechst Marion Roussel ... 1259
Mezlin (Mezlocillin Sodium) Bayer Pharmaceutical ... 594
Mezlin Pharmacy Bulk Package (Mezlocillin Sodium) Bayer Pharmaceutical ... 597

P. mirabilis infections

Amoxil (Amoxicillin Trihydrate) SmithKline Beecham Pharmaceuticals ... 2631
Ancef Injection (Cefazolin Sodium) SmithKline Beecham Pharmaceuticals ... 2632
Azactam for Injection (Aztreonam) Bristol-Myers Squibb ... 736
Bactrim (Trimethoprim, Sulfamethoxazole) Roche Pharmaceuticals ... 2257
Ceclor Pulvules & Suspension (Cefaclor) Lilly ... 1470
Cefizox for Intramuscular or Intravenous Use (Ceftizoxime Sodium) Fujisawa ... 1025
Cefobid Intravenous/Intramuscular (Cefoperazone Sodium) Pfizer Inc ... 1996
Cefobid Pharmacy Bulk Package - Not for Direct Infusion (Cefoperazone Sodium) Pfizer Inc ... 1999
Cefotan (Cefotetan) Zeneca ... 2936
Ceptaz (Ceftazidime) Glaxo Wellcome ... 1070
Cipro I.V. (Ciprofloxacin) Bayer Pharmaceutical ... 587
Cipro I.V. Pharmacy Bulk Package (Ciprofloxacin) Bayer Pharmaceutical ... 590
Cipro Tablets (Ciprofloxacin Hydrochloride) Bayer Pharmaceutical ... 584
Claforan Sterile and Injection (Cefotaxime Sodium) Hoechst Marion Roussel ... 1259
Duricef Capsules, Tablets, and Oral Suspension (Cefadroxil) Bristol-Myers Squibb ... 750
Floxin I.V. (Ofloxacin) McNeil Pharmaceutical ... 1580
Floxin Tablets (200 mg, 300 mg, 400 mg) (Ofloxacin) McNeil Pharmaceutical ... 1577
Fortaz (Ceftazidime) Glaxo Wellcome ... 1092

Gantanol Tablets (Sulfamethoxazole) Roche Pharmaceuticals ... 2285
Gantrisin (Acetyl Sulfisoxazole) Roche Pharmaceuticals ... 2286
Geocillin Tablets (Carbenicillin Indanyl Sodium) Pfizer Inc ... 2009
Keflex Pulvules & Oral Suspension (Cephalexin) Dista ... 930
Keftab Tablets (Cephalexin Hydrochloride) Dista ... 931
Kefzol Vials, Faspak & ADD-Vantage (Cefazolin Sodium) Lilly ... 1511
Maxaquin Tablets (Lomefloxacin Hydrochloride) Searle ... 2593
Maxipime for Injection (Cefepime Hydrochloride) Bristol-Myers Squibb ... 758
Mefoxin (Cefoxitin Sodium) Merck & Co., Inc. ... 1734
Mefoxin Premixed Intravenous Solution (Cefoxitin Sodium) Merck & Co., Inc. ... 1737
Mezlin (Mezlocillin Sodium) Bayer Pharmaceutical ... 594
Mezlin Pharmacy Bulk Package (Mezlocillin Sodium) Bayer Pharmaceutical ... 597
Monocid Injection (Cefonicid Sodium) SmithKline Beecham Pharmaceuticals ... 2674
Netromycin Injection 100 mg/ml (Netilmicin Sulfate) Schering ... 2516
Noroxin Tablets (Norfloxacin) Merck & Co., Inc. ... 1758
Noroxin Tablets (Norfloxacin) Roberts ... 2222
Omnipen Capsules (Ampicillin) Wyeth-Ayerst ... 2872
Omnipen for Oral Suspension (Ampicillin) Wyeth-Ayerst ... 2873
Penetrex Tablets (Enoxacin) Rhone-Poulenc Rorer Pharmaceuticals ... 2196
Pfizerpen for Injection (Penicillin G Potassium) Pfizer Inc ... 2022
Pipracil (Piperacillin Sodium) Lederle ... 1435
Proloprim Tablets (Trimethoprim) Glaxo Wellcome ... 1141
Rocephin Injectable Vials, ADD-Vantage, Galaxy Container (Ceftriaxone Sodium) Roche Pharmaceuticals ... 2305
Septra (Trimethoprim, Sulfamethoxazole) Glaxo Wellcome ... 1146
Spectrobid Tablets (Bacampicillin Hydrochloride) Pfizer Inc ... 2030
Suprax (Cefixime) Lederle ... 1443
Tazicef for Injection (Ceftazidime) SmithKline Beecham Pharmaceuticals ... 2697
Tazidime Vials, Faspak & ADD-Vantage (Ceftazidime) Lilly .. 1531
Trimpex Tablets (Trimethoprim) Roche Pharmaceuticals ... 2323
Unasyn (Ampicillin Sodium, Sulbactam Sodium) Pfizer Inc ... 2035
Vantin for Oral Suspension and Vantin Tablets (Cefpodoxime Proxetil) Pharmacia & Upjohn ... 2112

P. mirabilis infections, ocular

Chibroxin Sterile Ophthalmic Solution (Norfloxacin) Merck & Co., Inc. ... 1657
Ocuflox Ophthalmic Solution (Ofloxacin) Allergan ... 478
TobraDex Ophthalmic Suspension and Ointment (Dexamethasone, Tobramycin) Alcon Laboratories .. 469

P. mirabilis intra-abdominal infections

Claforan Sterile and Injection (Cefotaxime Sodium) Hoechst Marion Roussel ... 1259
Mezlin (Mezlocillin Sodium) Bayer Pharmaceutical ... 594
Mezlin Pharmacy Bulk Package (Mezlocillin Sodium) Bayer Pharmaceutical ... 597
Netromycin Injection 100 mg/ml (Netilmicin Sulfate) Schering ... 2516
Omnipen for Oral Suspension (Ampicillin) Wyeth-Ayerst ... 2873

P. mirabilis lower respiratory tract infections

Azactam for Injection (Aztreonam) Bristol-Myers Squibb ... 736
Cefizox for Intramuscular or Intravenous Use (Ceftizoxime Sodium) Fujisawa ... 1025
Cefotan (Cefotetan) Zeneca ... 2936
Ceptaz (Ceftazidime) Glaxo Wellcome ... 1070
Cipro I.V. (Ciprofloxacin) Bayer Pharmaceutical ... 587
Cipro I.V. Pharmacy Bulk Package (Ciprofloxacin) Bayer Pharmaceutical ... 590
Cipro Tablets (Ciprofloxacin Hydrochloride) Bayer Pharmaceutical ... 584
Claforan Sterile and Injection (Cefotaxime Sodium) Hoechst Marion Roussel ... 1259
Fortaz (Ceftazidime) Glaxo Wellcome ... 1092
Mandol Vials, Faspak & ADD-Vantage (Cefamandole Nafate) Lilly ... 1516
Mezlin (Mezlocillin Sodium) Bayer Pharmaceutical ... 594
Mezlin Pharmacy Bulk Package (Mezlocillin Sodium) Bayer Pharmaceutical ... 597
Netromycin Injection 100 mg/ml (Netilmicin Sulfate) Schering ... 2516
Rocephin Injectable Vials, ADD-Vantage, Galaxy Container (Ceftriaxone Sodium) Roche Pharmaceuticals ... 2305
Tazicef for Injection (Ceftazidime) SmithKline Beecham Pharmaceuticals ... 2697
Tazidime Vials, Faspak & ADD-Vantage (Ceftazidime) Lilly .. 1531

P. mirabilis prostatitis

Ancef Injection (Cefazolin Sodium) SmithKline Beecham Pharmaceuticals ... 2632
Geocillin Tablets (Carbenicillin Indanyl Sodium) Pfizer Inc ... 2009
Keflex Pulvules & Oral Suspension (Cephalexin) Dista ... 930
Keftab Tablets (Cephalexin Hydrochloride) Dista ... 931

P. mirabilis respiratory tract infections

Cefobid Intravenous/Intramuscular (Cefoperazone Sodium) Pfizer Inc ... 1996
Cefobid Pharmacy Bulk Package - Not for Direct Infusion (Cefoperazone Sodium) Pfizer Inc ... 1999

P. mirabilis septicemia

Ancef Injection (Cefazolin Sodium) SmithKline Beecham Pharmaceuticals ... 2632
Azactam for Injection (Aztreonam) Bristol-Myers Squibb ... 736
Kefzol Vials, Faspak & ADD-Vantage (Cefazolin Sodium) Lilly ... 1511
Netromycin Injection 100 mg/ml (Netilmicin Sulfate) Schering ... 2516
Pipracil (Piperacillin Sodium) Lederle ... 1435

P. mirabilis skin and skin structure infections

Azactam for Injection (Aztreonam) Bristol-Myers Squibb ... 736
Cefizox for Intramuscular or Intravenous Use (Ceftizoxime Sodium) Fujisawa ... 1025
Ceptaz (Ceftazidime) Glaxo Wellcome ... 1070
Cipro I.V. (Ciprofloxacin) Bayer Pharmaceutical ... 587
Cipro I.V. Pharmacy Bulk Package (Ciprofloxacin) Bayer Pharmaceutical ... 590
Cipro Tablets (Ciprofloxacin Hydrochloride) Bayer Pharmaceutical ... 584
Claforan Sterile and Injection (Cefotaxime Sodium) Hoechst Marion Roussel ... 1259
Floxin I.V. (Ofloxacin) McNeil Pharmaceutical ... 1580
Floxin Tablets (200 mg, 300 mg, 400 mg) (Ofloxacin) McNeil Pharmaceutical ... 1577
Fortaz (Ceftazidime) Glaxo Wellcome ... 1092
Mandol Vials, Faspak & ADD-Vantage (Cefamandole Nafate) Lilly ... 1516
Mefoxin (Cefoxitin Sodium) Merck & Co., Inc. ... 1734
Mefoxin Premixed Intravenous Solution (Cefoxitin Sodium) Merck & Co., Inc. ... 1737
Mezlin (Mezlocillin Sodium) Bayer Pharmaceutical ... 594
Mezlin Pharmacy Bulk Package (Mezlocillin Sodium) Bayer Pharmaceutical ... 597
Netromycin Injection 100 mg/ml (Netilmicin Sulfate) Schering ... 2516
Pipracil (Piperacillin Sodium) Lederle ... 1435
Rocephin Injectable Vials, ADD-Vantage, Galaxy Container (Ceftriaxone Sodium) Roche Pharmaceuticals ... 2305
Tazicef for Injection (Ceftazidime) SmithKline Beecham Pharmaceuticals ... 2697
Tazidime Vials, Faspak & ADD-Vantage (Ceftazidime) Lilly .. 1531
Unasyn (Ampicillin Sodium, Sulbactam Sodium) Pfizer Inc ... 2035

P. mirabilis urinary tract infections

Ancef Injection (Cefazolin Sodium) SmithKline Beecham Pharmaceuticals ... 2632
Azactam for Injection (Aztreonam) Bristol-Myers Squibb ... 736
Bactrim (Trimethoprim, Sulfamethoxazole) Roche Pharmaceuticals ... 2257
Ceclor Pulvules & Suspension (Cefaclor) Lilly ... 1470
Cefizox for Intramuscular or Intravenous Use (Ceftizoxime Sodium) Fujisawa ... 1025
Cefotan (Cefotetan) Zeneca ... 2936
Ceptaz (Ceftazidime) Glaxo Wellcome ... 1070
Cipro I.V. (Ciprofloxacin) Bayer Pharmaceutical ... 587
Cipro I.V. Pharmacy Bulk Package (Ciprofloxacin) Bayer Pharmaceutical ... 590
Cipro Tablets (Ciprofloxacin Hydrochloride) Bayer Pharmaceutical ... 584
Claforan Sterile and Injection (Cefotaxime Sodium) Hoechst Marion Roussel ... 1259
Duricef Capsules, Tablets, and Oral Suspension (Cefadroxil) Bristol-Myers Squibb ... 750
Floxin I.V. (Ofloxacin) McNeil Pharmaceutical ... 1580
Floxin Tablets (200 mg, 300 mg, 400 mg) (Ofloxacin) McNeil Pharmaceutical ... 1577
Fortaz (Ceftazidime) Glaxo Wellcome ... 1092
Gantanol Tablets (Sulfamethoxazole) Roche Pharmaceuticals ... 2285
Gantrisin (Acetyl Sulfisoxazole) Roche Pharmaceuticals ... 2286
Geocillin Tablets (Carbenicillin Indanyl Sodium) Pfizer Inc ... 2009
Keflex Pulvules & Oral Suspension (Cephalexin) Dista ... 930
Keftab Tablets (Cephalexin Hydrochloride) Dista ... 931
Kefzol Vials, Faspak & ADD-Vantage (Cefazolin Sodium) Lilly ... 1511
Maxaquin Tablets (Lomefloxacin Hydrochloride) Searle ... 2593
Maxipime for Injection (Cefepime Hydrochloride) Bristol-Myers Squibb ... 758
Mefoxin (Cefoxitin Sodium) Merck & Co., Inc. ... 1734
Mefoxin Premixed Intravenous Solution (Cefoxitin Sodium) Merck & Co., Inc. ... 1737
Mezlin (Mezlocillin Sodium) Bayer Pharmaceutical ... 594
Mezlin Pharmacy Bulk Package (Mezlocillin Sodium) Bayer Pharmaceutical ... 597
Monocid Injection (Cefonicid Sodium) SmithKline Beecham Pharmaceuticals ... 2674
Netromycin Injection 100 mg/ml (Netilmicin Sulfate) Schering ... 2516
Noroxin Tablets (Norfloxacin) Merck & Co., Inc. ... 1758
Noroxin Tablets (Norfloxacin) Roberts ... 2222
Penetrex Tablets (Enoxacin) Rhone-Poulenc Rorer Pharmaceuticals ... 2196
Proloprim Tablets (Trimethoprim) Glaxo Wellcome ... 1141
Rocephin Injectable Vials, ADD-Vantage, Galaxy Container (Ceftriaxone Sodium) Roche Pharmaceuticals ... 2305
Septra (Trimethoprim, Sulfamethoxazole) Glaxo Wellcome ... 1146
Spectrobid Tablets (Bacampicillin Hydrochloride) Pfizer Inc ... 2030
Suprax (Cefixime) Lederle ... 1443
Tazicef for Injection (Ceftazidime) SmithKline Beecham Pharmaceuticals ... 2697
Tazidime Vials, Faspak & ADD-Vantage (Ceftazidime) Lilly .. 1531
Trimpex Tablets (Trimethoprim) Roche Pharmaceuticals ... 2323
Vantin for Oral Suspension and Vantin Tablets (Cefpodoxime Proxetil) Pharmacia & Upjohn ... 2112

P. ovale infections

Aralen Hydrochloride Injection (Chloroquine Hydrochloride) Sanofi Winthrop ... 2430
Aralen Phosphate Tablets (Chloroquine Phosphate) Sanofi Winthrop ... 2431
Daraprim Tablets (Pyrimethamine) Glaxo Wellcome Oncology/HIV ... 1199
Plaquenil Sulfate Tablets (Hydroxychloroquine Sulfate) Sanofi Winthrop ... 2459

P. vivax infections

Aralen Hydrochloride Injection (Chloroquine Hydrochloride) Sanofi Winthrop ... 2430
Aralen Phosphate Tablets (Chloroquine Phosphate) Sanofi Winthrop ... 2431
Daraprim Tablets (Pyrimethamine) Glaxo Wellcome Oncology/HIV ... 1199
Lariam Tablets (Mefloquine Hydrochloride) Roche Pharmaceuticals ... 2295
Plaquenil Sulfate Tablets (Hydroxychloroquine Sulfate) Sanofi Winthrop ... 2459

P. vulgaris infections

Bactrim (Trimethoprim, Sulfamethoxazole) Roche Pharmaceuticals ... 2257
Cefizox for Intramuscular or Intravenous Use (Ceftizoxime Sodium) Fujisawa ... 1025
Cefotan (Cefotetan) Zeneca ... 2936
Cipro I.V. (Ciprofloxacin) Bayer Pharmaceutical ... 587
Cipro I.V. Pharmacy Bulk Package (Ciprofloxacin) Bayer Pharmaceutical ... 590
Cipro Tablets (Ciprofloxacin Hydrochloride) Bayer Pharmaceutical ... 584
Claforan Sterile and Injection (Cefotaxime Sodium) Hoechst Marion Roussel ... 1259
Gantanol Tablets (Sulfamethoxazole) Roche Pharmaceuticals ... 2285
Gantrisin (Acetyl Sulfisoxazole) Roche Pharmaceuticals ... 2286
Geocillin Tablets (Carbenicillin Indanyl Sodium) Pfizer Inc ... 2009
Mefoxin (Cefoxitin Sodium) Merck & Co., Inc. ... 1734
Mefoxin Premixed Intravenous Solution (Cefoxitin Sodium) Merck & Co., Inc. ... 1737
Mezlin (Mezlocillin Sodium) Bayer Pharmaceutical ... 594
Monocid Injection (Cefonicid Sodium) SmithKline Beecham Pharmaceuticals ... 2674
Noroxin Tablets (Norfloxacin) Merck & Co., Inc. ... 1758

P. vulgaris infections — Indications Index — 1556

Noroxin Tablets (Norfloxacin) Roberts ... 2222
Primaxin I.V. (Cilastatin Sodium, Imipenem) Merck & Co., Inc. ... 1772
Rocephin Injectable Vials, ADD-Vantage, Galaxy Container (Ceftriaxone Sodium) Roche Pharmaceuticals ... 2305
Septra (Trimethoprim, Sulfamethoxazole) Glaxo Wellcome ... 1146

P. vulgaris infections, ocular
TobraDex Ophthalmic Suspension and Ointment (Dexamethasone, Tobramycin) Alcon Laboratories ... 469

P. vulgaris skin and skin structure infections
Cipro I.V. (Ciprofloxacin) Bayer Pharmaceutical ... 587
Cipro I.V. Pharmacy Bulk Package (Ciprofloxacin) Bayer Pharmaceutical ... 590
Cipro Tablets (Ciprofloxacin Hydrochloride) Bayer Pharmaceutical ... 584
Claforan Sterile and Injection (Cefotaxime Sodium) Hoechst Marion Roussel ... 1259
Mezlin (Mezlocillin Sodium) Bayer Pharmaceutical ... 594
Mezlin Pharmacy Bulk Package (Mezlocillin Sodium) Bayer Pharmaceutical ... 597
Primaxin I.V. (Cilastatin Sodium, Imipenem) Merck & Co., Inc. ... 1772

P. vulgaris urinary tract infections
Bactrim (Trimethoprim, Sulfamethoxazole) Roche Pharmaceuticals ... 2257
Cefizox for Intramuscular or Intravenous Use (Ceftizoxime Sodium) Fujisawa ... 1025
Cefotan (Cefotetan) Zeneca ... 2936
Claforan Sterile and Injection (Cefotaxime Sodium) Hoechst Marion Roussel ... 1259
Gantanol Tablets (Sulfamethoxazole) Roche Pharmaceuticals ... 2285
Gantrisin (Acetyl Sulfisoxazole) Roche Pharmaceuticals ... 2286
Geocillin Tablets (Carbenicillin Indanyl Sodium) Pfizer Inc ... 2009
Mefoxin (Cefoxitin Sodium) Merck & Co., Inc. ... 1734
Mefoxin Premixed Intravenous Solution (Cefoxitin Sodium) Merck & Co., Inc. ... 1737
Monocid Injection (Cefonicid Sodium) SmithKline Beecham Pharmaceuticals ... 2674
Noroxin Tablets (Norfloxacin) Merck & Co., Inc. ... 1758
Noroxin Tablets (Norfloxacin) Roberts ... 2222
Primaxin I.V. (Cilastatin Sodium, Imipenem) Merck & Co., Inc. ... 1772
Rocephin Injectable Vials, ADD-Vantage, Galaxy Container (Ceftriaxone Sodium) Roche Pharmaceuticals ... 2305
Septra (Trimethoprim, Sulfamethoxazole) Glaxo Wellcome ... 1146

Paget's disease of bone
Aredia for Injection (Pamidronate Disodium) CibaGeneva ... 827
Calcimar Injection, Synthetic (Calcitonin, Synthetic) Rhone-Poulenc Rorer Pharmaceuticals ... 2176
Didronel Tablets (Etidronate Disodium (Diphosphonate)) Procter & Gamble Pharmaceuticals ... 2133
Fosamax Tablets (Alendronate Sodium) Merck & Co., Inc. ... 1703
Miacalcin Injection (Calcitonin, Synthetic) Sandoz Pharmaceuticals ... 2402

Pain associated with arthritis, topical (see under Pain, topical relief of)

Pain associated with sports injuries (see under Pain, topical relief of)

Pain associated with upper respiratory infection
Advil Cold and Sinus Caplets and Tablets (Ibuprofen, Pseudoephedrine Hydrochloride) Whitehall-Robins ... ▣ 837
BC Cold Powder Multi-Symptom Formula (Cold-Sinus-Allergy) (Aspirin, Phenylpropanolamine Hydrochloride, Chlorpheniramine Maleate) Block ... ▣ 631
BC Cold Powder Non-Drowsy Formula (Cold-Sinus) (Aspirin, Phenylpropanolamine Hydrochloride) Block ... ▣ 631
Bufferin Analgesic Tablets (Aspirin) Bristol-Myers Products ... ▣ 636
Extra Strength Bufferin Analgesic Tablets (Aspirin) Bristol-Myers Products ... ▣ 637
Children's Motrin Ibuprofen Oral Suspension (Ibuprofen) McNeil Consumer ... 1558
Children's TYLENOL Cold Multi-Symptom Chewable Tablets and Liquid (Acetaminophen, Chlorpheniramine Maleate, Pseudoephedrine Hydrochloride) McNeil Consumer ... 1559
Contac Severe Cold and Flu Formula Caplets (Acetaminophen, Chlorpheniramine Maleate, Dextromethorphan Hydrobromide, Phenylpropanolamine Hydrochloride) SmithKline Beecham Consumer ... ▣ 773
Coricidin Cold + Flu Tablets (Acetaminophen, Chlorpheniramine Maleate) Schering-Plough HealthCare ... ▣ 760
Coricidin 'D' Decongestant Tablets (Acetaminophen, Chlorpheniramine Maleate, Phenylpropanolamine Hydrochloride) Schering-Plough HealthCare ... ▣ 760
Dimetapp Allergy Sinus Caplets (Acetaminophen, Brompheniramine Maleate, Phenylpropanolamine Hydrochloride) Whitehall-Robins ... ▣ 838
Drixoral Cold and Flu Extended-Release Tablets (Acetaminophen, Dexbrompheniramine Maleate, Pseudoephedrine Sulfate) Schering-Plough HealthCare ... ▣ 764
Infants' TYLENOL Cold Decongestant & Fever-Reducer Drops (Acetaminophen, Pseudoephedrine Hydrochloride) McNeil Consumer ... 1561
Mobigesic Tablets (Magnesium Salicylate, Phenyltoloxamine Citrate) Ascher ... ▣ 607
Pyrroxate Caplets (Acetaminophen, Chlorpheniramine Maleate, Phenylpropanolamine Hydrochloride) Roberts ... ▣ 742
Sine-Off No Drowsiness Formula Caplets (Acetaminophen, Pseudoephedrine Hydrochloride) SmithKline Beecham Consumer ... ▣ 784
Sinulin Tablets (Acetaminophen, Phenylpropanolamine Hydrochloride, Chlorpheniramine Maleate) Carnrick ... 792
Sinutab Sinus Allergy Medication, Maximum Strength Tablets and Caplets (Acetaminophen, Chlorpheniramine Maleate, Pseudoephedrine Hydrochloride) Warner Wellcome ... ▣ 823
Sinutab Sinus Medication, Maximum Strength Without Drowsiness Formula, Tablets & Caplets (Acetaminophen, Pseudoephedrine Hydrochloride) Warner Wellcome ... ▣ 824
TheraFlu Flu and Cold Medicine (Acetaminophen, Chlorpheniramine Maleate, Pseudoephedrine Hydrochloride) Sandoz Consumer ... ▣ 750
TYLENOL Cold Medication, Multi-Symptom Formula Tablets and Caplets (Acetaminophen, Chlorpheniramine Maleate, Pseudoephedrine Hydrochloride, Dextromethorphan Hydrobromide) McNeil Consumer ... 1572
TYLENOL Cold Medication, No Drowsiness Formula Caplets and Gelcaps (Acetaminophen, Pseudoephedrine Hydrochloride, Dextromethorphan Hydrobromide) McNeil Consumer ... 1572

Pain due to common cold (see under Pain associated with upper respiratory infection)

Pain with gastric hyperacidity
Alka-Seltzer Cherry Effervescent Antacid and Pain Reliever (Aspirin, Sodium Bicarbonate, Citric Acid) Bayer Consumer ... ▣ 609
Alka-Seltzer Extra Strength Effervescent Antacid and Pain Reliever (Aspirin, Sodium Bicarbonate, Citric Acid) Bayer Consumer ... ▣ 609
Alka-Seltzer Fast Relief Caplets (Acetaminophen, Calcium Carbonate) Bayer Consumer ... ▣ 610
Alka-Seltzer Lemon Lime Effervescent Antacid and Pain Reliever (Aspirin, Sodium Citrate) Bayer Consumer ... ▣ 609
Alka-Seltzer Original Effervescent Antacid and Pain Reliever (Aspirin, Citric Acid, Sodium Bicarbonate) Bayer Consumer ... ▣ 609
TYLENOL Headache Plus Pain Reliever with Antacid, Extra Strength Caplets (Acetaminophen, Calcium Carbonate) McNeil Consumer ... ▣ 705

Pain, anal (see under Pain, anorectal)

Pain, anogenital
Americaine Hemorrhoidal Ointment (Benzocaine) Ciba Self-Medication ... ▣ 649
Dyclone 0.5% and 1% Topical Solutions, USP (Dyclonine Hydrochloride) Astra ... 535
Preparation H (Glycerin, Petrolatum, Phenylephrine Hydrochloride, Shark Liver Oil) Whitehall-Robins ... ▣ 842

Pain, anorectal
Fleet Pain Relief Pads (Pramoxine Hydrochloride) Fleet ... 1001
Tronolane Anesthetic Cream for Hemorrhoids (Pramoxine Hydrochloride) Ross ... ▣ 746
Wyanoids Relief Factor Hemorrhoidal Suppositories (Liver, Desiccated, Shark Liver Oil) Wyeth-Ayerst ... ▣ 856

Pain, arthritic, minor
Actron Caplets and Tablets (Ketoprofen) Bayer Consumer ... ▣ 608
Advil Ibuprofen Tablets, Caplets and Gel Caplets (Ibuprofen) Whitehall-Robins ... ▣ 836
Aleve (Naproxen Sodium) Procter & Gamble ... 2124
ArthriCare Odor Free Rub (Capsaicin, Menthol, Methyl Nicotinate) Del ... ▣ 667
ArthriCare Triple Medicated Rub (Menthol, Methyl Nicotinate, Methyl Salicylate) Del ... ▣ 667
Regular Strength Ascriptin Tablets (Aspirin Buffered, Calcium Carbonate) Ciba Self-Medication ... ▣ 650
Arthritis Strength BC Powder (Aspirin, Salicylamide, Caffeine) Block ... ▣ 631
BC Powder (Aspirin, Salicylamide, Caffeine) Block ... ▣ 631
Genuine Bayer Aspirin Tablets & Caplets (Aspirin) Bayer Consumer ... ▣ 618
Extra Strength Bayer Arthritis Pain Regimen Formula (Aspirin, Enteric Coated) Bayer Consumer ... ▣ 615
Extra Strength Bayer Aspirin Caplets & Tablets (Aspirin) Bayer Consumer ... ▣ 617
Extended-Release Bayer 8-Hour Aspirin (Aspirin) Bayer Consumer ... ▣ 616
Extra Strength Bayer Plus Aspirin Caplets (Aspirin, Calcium Carbonate) Bayer Consumer ... ▣ 617
Bayer Enteric Aspirin (Aspirin, Enteric Coated) Bayer Consumer ... ▣ 613
Bufferin Analgesic Tablets (Aspirin) Bristol-Myers Products ... ▣ 636
Arthritis Strength Bufferin Analgesic Caplets (Aspirin) Bristol-Myers Products ... ▣ 637
Extra Strength Bufferin Analgesic Tablets (Aspirin) Bristol-Myers Products ... ▣ 637
Ecotrin (Aspirin) SmithKline Beecham ... 2625
Empirin Aspirin Tablets (Aspirin) Warner Wellcome ... ▣ 818
Aspirin Free Excedrin Analgesic Caplets and Geltabs (Acetaminophen, Caffeine) Bristol-Myers Products ... 734
Excedrin Extra-Strength Analgesic Tablets, Caplets, and Geltabs (Acetaminophen, Aspirin, Caffeine) Bristol-Myers Products ... 734
Goody's Extra Strength Headache Powders (Aspirin, Acetaminophen, Caffeine) Block ... ▣ 632
Goody's Extra Strength Pain Relief Tablets (Aspirin, Acetaminophen, Caffeine) Block ... ▣ 632
Ibuprohm (Ibuprofen) Ohm ... ▣ 713
Mobigesic Tablets (Magnesium Salicylate, Phenyltoloxamine Citrate) Ascher ... ▣ 607
Motrin IB Caplets, Tablets, and Gelcaps (Ibuprofen) Upjohn ... ▣ 802
Nuprin Ibuprofen/Analgesic Tablets & Caplets (Ibuprofen) Bristol-Myers Products ... ▣ 645
Orudis KT (Ketoprofen) Whitehall-Robins ... ▣ 842
Panodol Tablets and Caplets (Acetaminophen) SmithKline Beecham Consumer ... ▣ 783
Percogesic Analgesic Tablets (Acetaminophen, Phenyltoloxamine Citrate) Procter & Gamble ... ▣ 727
Sunsource Arthritis Relief Tablets (Homeopathic Medications) Sunsource ... ▣ 792
Traumeel Injection Solution (Homeopathic Medications) Heel/BHI ... 1237
Tylenol (Acetaminophen) McNeil Consumer ... 1570
Vanquish Analgesic Caplets (Acetaminophen, Aspirin, Caffeine, Aluminum Hydroxide Gel, Magnesium Hydroxide) Bayer Consumer ... ▣ 627

Pain, dental
Actron Caplets and Tablets (Ketoprofen) Bayer Consumer ... ▣ 608
Aleve (Naproxen Sodium) Procter & Gamble ... 2124
Arthritis Strength BC Powder (Aspirin, Salicylamide, Caffeine) Block ... ▣ 631
BC Powder (Aspirin, Salicylamide, Caffeine) Block ... ▣ 631
Genuine Bayer Aspirin Tablets & Caplets (Aspirin) Bayer Consumer ... ▣ 618
Extra Strength Bayer Aspirin Caplets & Tablets (Aspirin) Bayer Consumer ... ▣ 617
Extended-Release Bayer 8-Hour Aspirin (Aspirin) Bayer Consumer ... ▣ 616
Extra Strength Bayer Plus Aspirin Caplets (Aspirin, Calcium Carbonate) Bayer Consumer ... ▣ 617
Aspirin Regimen Bayer Children's Chewable Aspirin (Aspirin) Bayer Consumer ... ▣ 616
Bufferin Analgesic Tablets (Aspirin) Bristol-Myers Products ... ▣ 636
Extra Strength Bufferin Analgesic Tablets (Aspirin) Bristol-Myers Products ... ▣ 637
Children's Motrin Ibuprofen Oral Suspension (Ibuprofen) McNeil Consumer ... 1558
Children's TYLENOL acetaminophen Chewable

(▣ Described in PDR For Nonprescription Drugs) (⊙ Described in PDR For Ophthalmology)

Tablets, Elixir, Suspension Liquid, and Suspension Drops (Acetaminophen) McNeil Consumer 1559
Children's Vicks Chloraseptic Sore Throat Spray (Phenol) Procter & Gamble ▣ 730
Dyclone 0.5% and 1% Topical Solutions, USP (Dyclonine Hydrochloride) Astra 535
Empirin Aspirin Tablets (Aspirin) Warner Wellcome ▣ 818
Aspirin Free Excedrin Analgesic Caplets and Geltabs (Acetaminophen, Caffeine) Bristol-Myers Products 734
Excedrin Extra-Strength Analgesic Tablets, Caplets, and Geltabs (Acetaminophen, Aspirin, Caffeine) Bristol-Myers Products 734
Gly-Oxide Liquid (Carbamide Peroxide) SmithKline Beecham Consumer ▣ 779
Goody's Extra Strength Pain Relief Tablets (Aspirin, Acetaminophen, Caffeine) Block ▣ 632
Hyland's Teething Tablets (Calcium Phosphate, Homeopathic Medications) Standard Homeopathic ▣ 790
Ibuprohm (Ibuprofen) Ohm ▣ 713
Infants' TYLENOL acetaminophen Suspension Drops (Acetaminophen) McNeil Consumer 1559
Mobigesic Tablets (Magnesium Salicylate, Phenyltoloxamine Citrate) Ascher ▣ 607
Motrin IB Caplets, Tablets, and Gelcaps (Ibuprofen) Upjohn ▣ 802
Nuprin Ibuprofen/Analgesic Tablets & Caplets (Ibuprofen) Bristol-Myers Products ▣ 645
Baby Orajel Teething Pain Medicine (Benzocaine) Del ▣ 667
Orajel Maximum Strength Toothache Medication (Benzocaine) Del ▣ 668
Orajel Mouth-Aid for Canker and Cold Sores (Benzocaine, Benzalkonium Chloride, Zinc Chloride) Del ▣ 668
Orudis KT (Ketoprofen) Whitehall-Robins ▣ 842
Panodol Tablets and Caplets (Acetaminophen) SmithKline Beecham Consumer ▣ 783
Children's Panadol Chewable Tablets, Liquid, Infant's Drops (Acetaminophen) SmithKline Beecham Consumer ▣ 783
Percogesic Analgesic Tablets (Acetaminophen, Phenyltoloxamine Citrate) Procter & Gamble ▣ 727
Red Cross Toothache Medication (Eugenol) Mentholatum ▣ 711
Tylenol (Acetaminophen) McNeil Consumer 1570
Vanquish Analgesic Caplets (Acetaminophen, Aspirin, Caffeine, Aluminum Hydroxide Gel, Magnesium Hydroxide) Bayer Consumer ▣ 627

Pain, ear
Americaine Otic Topical Anesthetic Ear Drops (Benzocaine) Medeva 1603
Children's Panadol Chewable Tablets, Liquid, Infant's Drops (Acetaminophen) SmithKline Beecham Consumer ▣ 783
Tympagesic Ear Drops (Antipyrine, Benzocaine, Phenylephrine Hydrochloride) Savage 2476

Pain, general
Advil Ibuprofen Tablets, Caplets and Gel Caplets (Ibuprofen) Whitehall-Robins ▣ 836
Aleve (Naproxen Sodium) Procter & Gamble 2124
Alka-Seltzer Cherry Effervescent Antacid and Pain Reliever (Aspirin, Sodium Bicarbonate, Citric Acid) Bayer Consumer ▣ 609
Alka-Seltzer Extra Strength Effervescent Antacid and Pain Reliever (Aspirin, Sodium Bicarbonate, Citric Acid) Bayer Consumer ▣ 609
Alka-Seltzer Lemon Lime Effervescent Antacid and Pain Reliever (Aspirin, Sodium Citrate) Bayer Consumer ▣ 609
Alka-Seltzer Original Effervescent Antacid and Pain Reliever (Aspirin, Citric Acid, Sodium Bicarbonate) Bayer Consumer ▣ 609
Regular Strength Ascriptin Tablets (Aspirin Buffered, Calcium Carbonate) Ciba Self-Medication ▣ 650
Backache Caplets (Magnesium Salicylate) Bristol-Myers Products ▣ 635
Genuine Bayer Aspirin Tablets & Caplets (Aspirin) Bayer Consumer ▣ 618
Extra Strength Bayer Aspirin Caplets & Tablets (Aspirin) Bayer Consumer ▣ 617
Extended-Release Bayer 8-Hour Aspirin (Aspirin) Bayer Consumer ▣ 616
Extra Strength Bayer PM Aspirin Plus Sleep Aid (Aspirin, Diphenhydramine Hydrochloride) Bayer Consumer ▣ 617
Aspirin Regimen Bayer Adult Low Strength 81 mg Tablets (Aspirin, Enteric Coated) Bayer Consumer ▣ 613
Aspirin Regimen Bayer Children's Chewable Aspirin (Aspirin) Bayer Consumer ▣ 616
Aspirin Regimen Bayer Regular Strength 325 mg Caplets (Aspirin, Enteric Coated) Bayer Consumer ▣ 613
Children's Motrin Ibuprofen Oral Suspension (Ibuprofen) McNeil Consumer 1558
Children's TYLENOL acetaminophen Chewable Tablets, Elixir, Suspension Liquid, and Suspension Drops (Acetaminophen) McNeil Consumer 1559
Aspirin Free Excedrin Analgesic Caplets and Geltabs (Acetaminophen, Caffeine) Bristol-Myers Products 734
Ibuprohm (Ibuprofen) Ohm ▣ 713
Infants' TYLENOL acetaminophen Suspension Drops (Acetaminophen) McNeil Consumer 1559
Junior Strength TYLENOL acetaminophen Coated Caplets and Chewable Tablets (Acetaminophen) McNeil Consumer 1562
Levoprome (Methotrimeprazine) Immunex 1321
Children's Panadol Chewable Tablets, Liquid, Infant's Drops (Acetaminophen) SmithKline Beecham Consumer ▣ 783
St. Joseph Adult Chewable Aspirin (81 mg.) (Aspirin) Schering-Plough HealthCare ▣ 768
Traumeel Injection Solution (Homeopathic Medications) Heel/BHI 1237
Trilisate (Choline Magnesium Trisalicylate) Purdue Frederick 2155
Tylenol (Acetaminophen) McNeil Consumer 1570
TYLENOL PM Pain Reliever/Sleep Aid, Extra Strength Gelcaps, Caplets, Geltabs (Acetaminophen, Diphenhydramine Hydrochloride) McNeil Consumer 1576
Vanquish Analgesic Caplets (Acetaminophen, Aspirin, Caffeine, Aluminum Hydroxide Gel, Magnesium Hydroxide) Bayer Consumer ▣ 627

Pain, hemorrhoidal (see under Pain, anorectal)

Pain, intractable chronic (see also under Pain, severe)
Infumorph 200 and Infumorph 500 Sterile Solutions (Morphine Sulfate) Elkins-Sinn 985

Pain, menstrual
Actron Caplets and Tablets (Ketoprofen) Bayer Consumer ▣ 608
Advil Ibuprofen Tablets, Caplets and Gel Caplets (Ibuprofen) Whitehall-Robins ▣ 836
Aleve (Naproxen Sodium) Procter & Gamble 2124
BC Powder (Aspirin, Salicylamide, Caffeine) Block ▣ 631
Genuine Bayer Aspirin Tablets & Caplets (Aspirin) Bayer Consumer ▣ 618
Extra Strength Bayer Aspirin Caplets & Tablets (Aspirin) Bayer Consumer ▣ 617
Extra Strength Bayer Plus Aspirin Caplets (Aspirin, Calcium Carbonate) Bayer Consumer ▣ 617
Bufferin Analgesic Tablets (Aspirin) Bristol-Myers Products ▣ 636
Extra Strength Bufferin Analgesic Tablets (Aspirin) Bristol-Myers Products ▣ 637
Empirin Aspirin Tablets (Aspirin) Warner Wellcome ▣ 818
Aspirin Free Excedrin Analgesic Caplets and Geltabs (Acetaminophen, Caffeine) Bristol-Myers Products 734
Excedrin Extra-Strength Analgesic Tablets, Caplets, and Geltabs (Acetaminophen, Aspirin, Caffeine) Bristol-Myers Products 734
Goody's Extra Strength Pain Relief Tablets (Aspirin, Acetaminophen, Caffeine) Block ▣ 632
Ibuprohm (Ibuprofen) Ohm ▣ 713
Maximum Strength Multi-Symptom Formula Midol (Acetaminophen, Caffeine, Pyrilamine Maleate) Bayer Consumer ▣ 621
PMS Multi-Symptom Formula Midol (Acetaminophen, Pamabrom, Pyrilamine Maleate) Bayer Consumer ▣ 622
Motrin IB Caplets, Tablets, and Gelcaps (Ibuprofen) Upjohn ▣ 802
Nuprin Ibuprofen/Analgesic Tablets & Caplets (Ibuprofen) Bristol-Myers Products ▣ 645
Orudis KT (Ketoprofen) Whitehall-Robins ▣ 842
Panodol Tablets and Caplets (Acetaminophen) SmithKline Beecham Consumer ▣ 783
Percogesic Analgesic Tablets (Acetaminophen, Phenyltoloxamine Citrate) Procter & Gamble ▣ 727
St. Joseph Adult Chewable Aspirin (81 mg.) (Aspirin) Schering-Plough HealthCare ▣ 768
Tylenol (Acetaminophen) McNeil Consumer 1570
Vanquish Analgesic Caplets (Acetaminophen, Aspirin, Caffeine, Aluminum Hydroxide Gel, Magnesium Hydroxide) Bayer Consumer ▣ 627

Pain, mild
Actron Caplets and Tablets (Ketoprofen) Bayer Consumer ▣ 608
Advil Ibuprofen Tablets, Caplets and Gel Caplets (Ibuprofen) Whitehall-Robins ▣ 836
Aleve (Naproxen Sodium) Procter & Gamble 2124
Maximum Strength Ascriptin (Aspirin Buffered, Calcium Carbonate) Ciba Self-Medication ▣ 650
Aspirin Regimen Bayer 81 mg Tablets with Calcium (Aspirin, Calcium Carbonate) Bayer Consumer ▣ 615
Arthritis Strength Bufferin Analgesic Caplets (Aspirin) Bristol-Myers Products ▣ 637
Cama Arthritis Pain Reliever (Aspirin, Aluminum Hydroxide, Magnesium Oxide) Sandoz Consumer ▣ 748
Ecotrin (Aspirin) SmithKline Beecham 2625
Excedrin Extra-Strength Analgesic Tablets, Caplets, and Geltabs (Acetaminophen, Aspirin, Caffeine) Bristol-Myers Products 734
Goody's Extra Strength Headache Powders (Aspirin, Acetaminophen, Caffeine) Block ▣ 632
Goody's Extra Strength Pain Relief Tablets (Aspirin, Acetaminophen, Caffeine) Block ▣ 632
Junior Strength TYLENOL acetaminophen Coated Caplets and Chewable Tablets (Acetaminophen) McNeil Consumer 1562
Orudis KT (Ketoprofen) Whitehall-Robins ▣ 842
Panodol Tablets and Caplets (Acetaminophen) SmithKline Beecham Consumer ▣ 783
Tylenol (Acetaminophen) McNeil Consumer 1570

Pain, mild to moderate
Anaprox/Naprosyn (Naproxen Sodium) Roche Pharmaceuticals 2277
Darvon-N/Darvocet-N (Propoxyphene Napsylate, Acetaminophen) Lilly 1473
Darvon (Propoxyphene Hydrochloride, Aspirin, Caffeine) Lilly 1475
Darvon-N Suspension & Tablets (Propoxyphene Napsylate) Lilly 1473
Dolobid Tablets (Diflunisal) Merck & Co., Inc. 1695
Easprin (Aspirin) Parke-Davis 1971
IBU Tablets (Ibuprofen) Knoll Laboratories 1389
Motrin Ibuprofen Suspension, Oral Drops, Chewable Tablets, Caplets (Ibuprofen) McNeil Consumer 1563
Nalfon 200 Pulvules & Nalfon Tablets (Fenoprofen Calcium) Dista 933
Naprelan Tablets (Naproxen Sodium) Wyeth-Ayerst 2861
Anaprox/Naprosyn (Naproxen) Roche Pharmaceuticals 2277
Orudis Capsules (Ketoprofen) Wyeth-Ayerst 2874
Talacen Caplets (Pentazocine Hydrochloride) Sanofi Winthrop 2464
Trilisate (Choline Magnesium Trisalicylate) Purdue Frederick 2155
Tylenol with Codeine Elixir (Acetaminophen, Codeine Phosphate) McNeil Pharmaceutical 1592
Wygesic Tablets (Propoxyphene Hydrochloride, Acetaminophen) Wyeth-Ayerst 2930

Pain, mild to moderate, acute musculo-skeletal
Norgesic (Orphenadrine Citrate, Aspirin) 3M Pharmaceuticals 1554
Parafon Forte DSC Caplets (Chlorzoxazone) McNeil Pharmaceutical 1590
Soma Compound w/Codeine Tablets (Carisoprodol, Aspirin, Codeine Phosphate) Wallace 2784
Soma Compound Tablets (Carisoprodol, Aspirin) Wallace 2783
Soma Tablets (Carisoprodol) Wallace 2782

Pain, moderate
Ponstel (Mefenamic Acid) Parke-Davis 1982
Talwin Compound (Pentazocine Hydrochloride, Aspirin) Sanofi Winthrop 2466

Pain, moderate to moderately severe
DHCplus Capsules (Dihydrocodeine Bitartrate, Acetaminophen, Caffeine) Purdue Frederick 2148
Lorcet 10/650 Tablets (Hydrocodone Bitartrate, Acetaminophen) Forest 1016
Lortab (Hydrocodone Bitartrate, Acetaminophen) UCB 2751
OxyIR Capsules (Oxycodone Hydrochloride) Purdue Pharma 2167
Percocet Tablets (Oxycodone Hydrochloride, Acetaminophen) DuPont 955
Percodan Tablets (Oxycodone Hydrochloride, Oxycodone Terephthalate, Aspirin) DuPont 955
Percodan-Demi Tablets (Oxycodone Hydrochloride, Oxycodone Terephthalate, Aspirin) DuPont 956
Roxicodone Tablets, Oral Solution & Intensol (Oxycodone) (Oxycodone Hydrochloride) Roxane 2366
Toradol (Ketorolac Tromethamine) Roche Pharmaceuticals 2319
Tylenol with Codeine Phosphate Tablets (Acetaminophen, Co-

Pain — Indications Index

deine Phosphate) McNeil Pharmaceutical 1592
Tylox Capsules (Oxycodone Hydrochloride, Acetaminophen) McNeil Pharmaceutical 1593
Ultram Tablets (50 mg) (Tramadol Hydrochloride) McNeil Pharmaceutical 1594
Vicodin Tablets (Hydrocodone Bitartrate, Acetaminophen) Knoll Laboratories 1404
Vicodin ES Tablets (Hydrocodone Bitartrate, Acetaminophen) Knoll Laboratories 1405
Vicodin HP Tablets (Hydrocodone Bitartrate, Acetaminophen) Knoll Laboratories 1403
Zydone Capsules (Hydrocodone Bitartrate, Acetaminophen) DuPont 967

Pain, moderate to severe
Astramorph/PF Injection, USP (Preservative-Free) (Morphine Sulfate) Astra 526
Buprenex Injectable (Buprenorphine) Reckitt & Colman 2170
Dalgan Injection (Dezocine) Astra 529
Demerol (Meperidine Hydrochloride) Sanofi Winthrop .. 2438
Dilaudid Ampules (Hydromorphone Hydrochloride) Knoll Laboratories 1382
Dilaudid-HP Injection (Hydromorphone Hydrochloride) Knoll Laboratories 1384
Dilaudid-HP Lyophilized Powder 250 mg (Hydromorphone Hydrochloride) Knoll Laboratories 1384
Dilaudid (Hydromorphone Hydrochloride) Knoll Laboratories 1382
Dilaudid Oral Liquid (Hydromorphone Hydrochloride) Knoll Laboratories 1386
Dilaudid (Hydromorphone Hydrochloride) Knoll Laboratories 1382
Dilaudid Tablets - 8 mg (Hydromorphone Hydrochloride) Knoll Laboratories 1386
Duragesic Transdermal System (Fentanyl) Janssen 1336
Duramorph Injection (Morphine Sulfate) Elkins-Sinn 983
Hydrocet Capsules (Acetaminophen, Hydrocodone Bitartrate) Carnrick 787
Kadian Capsules (Morphine Sulfate) Zeneca 2948
Levo-Dromoran (Levorphanol Tartrate) Roche Pharmaceuticals 2297
Levoprome (Methotrimeprazine) Immunex 1321
MS Contin Tablets (Morphine Sulfate) Purdue Frederick 2149
MSIR (Morphine Sulfate) Purdue Frederick 2152
Nubain Injection (Nalbuphine Hydrochloride) DuPont 952
Numorphan Injection (Oxymorphone Hydrochloride) DuPont 953
Numorphan Suppositories (Oxymorphone Hydrochloride) DuPont 953
OxyContin Tablets (Oxycodone Hydrochloride) Purdue Pharma 2163
Stadol (Butorphanol Tartrate) Bristol-Myers Squibb 779
Talwin Injection (Pentazocine Lactate) Sanofi Winthrop 2465
Talwin Nx Tablets (Pentazocine Hydrochloride, Naloxone Hydrochloride) Sanofi Winthrop .. 2467

Pain, muscular, temporary relief of
Aleve (Naproxen Sodium) Procter & Gamble 2124
Alka-Seltzer Cherry Effervescent Antacid and Pain Reliever (Aspirin, Sodium Bicarbonate, Citric Acid) Bayer Consumer 609
Alka-Seltzer Extra Strength Effervescent Antacid and Pain Reliever (Aspirin, Sodium Bicarbonate, Citric Acid) Bayer Consumer 609
Alka-Seltzer Lemon Lime Effervescent Antacid and Pain

Reliever (Aspirin, Sodium Citrate) Bayer Consumer 609
Alka-Seltzer Original Effervescent Antacid and Pain Reliever (Aspirin, Citric Acid, Sodium Bicarbonate) Bayer Consumer .. 609
Aspercreme Creme, Lotion Analgesic Rub (Trolamine Salicylate) Thompson Medical 794
Extra Strength Bayer Aspirin Caplets & Tablets (Aspirin) Bayer Consumer 617
Extra Strength Bayer Plus Aspirin Caplets (Aspirin, Calcium Carbonate) Bayer Consumer 617
Bayer Enteric Aspirin (Aspirin, Enteric Coated) Bayer Consumer 613
Bufferin Analgesic Tablets (Aspirin) Bristol-Myers Products 636
Extra Strength Bufferin Analgesic Tablets (Aspirin) Bristol-Myers Products 637
Empirin Aspirin Tablets (Aspirin) Warner Wellcome 818
Aspirin Free Excedrin Analgesic Caplets and Geltabs (Acetaminophen, Caffeine) Bristol-Myers Products 734
Excedrin Extra-Strength Analgesic Tablets, Caplets, and Geltabs (Acetaminophen, Aspirin, Caffeine) Bristol-Myers Products 734
Fluori-Methane (Dichlorodifluoromethane, Trichloromonofluoromethane) Gebauer 1040
Ibuprohm (Ibuprofen) Ohm 713
Junior Strength TYLENOL acetaminophen Coated Caplets and Chewable Tablets (Acetaminophen) McNeil Consumer 1562
Maximum Strength Midol Teen Multi-Symptom Formula (Acetaminophen, Pamabrom) Bayer Consumer 621
Mobigesic Tablets (Magnesium Salicylate, Phenyltoloxamine Citrate) Ascher 607
Motrin IB Caplets, Tablets, and Gelcaps (Ibuprofen) Upjohn 802
Nuprin Ibuprofen/Analgesic Tablets & Caplets (Ibuprofen) Bristol-Myers Products 645
St. Joseph Adult Chewable Aspirin (81 mg.) (Aspirin) Schering-Plough HealthCare 768
Therapeutic Mineral Ice, Pain Relieving Gel (Menthol) Bristol-Myers Products 645
Traumeel Injection Solution (Homeopathic Medications) Heel/BHI 1237
Tylenol (Acetaminophen) McNeil Consumer 1570
Vanquish Analgesic Caplets (Acetaminophen, Aspirin, Caffeine, Aluminum Hydroxide Gel, Magnesium Hydroxide) Bayer Consumer 627

Pain, neurogenic
Maximum Strength Ascriptin (Aspirin Buffered, Calcium Carbonate) Ciba Self-Medication 650
Atretol Tablets (Carbamazepine) Athena 569
Arthritis Strength BC Powder (Aspirin, Salicylamide, Caffeine) Block 631
BC Powder (Aspirin, Salicylamide, Caffeine) Block 631
Sarapin (Sarracenia purpurea, Pitcher Plant Distillate) High Chemical 1237
Tegretol/Tegretol-XR (Carbamazepine) CibaGeneva 870
Vanquish Analgesic Caplets (Acetaminophen, Aspirin, Caffeine, Aluminum Hydroxide Gel, Magnesium Hydroxide) Bayer Consumer 627
Zostrix/Zostrix-HP (Capsaicin) GenDerm 1043

Pain, neurogenic, post-herpes zoster infections, topical relief of
Zostrix/Zostrix-HP (Capsaicin) GenDerm 1043

Pain, obstetrical
Demerol (Meperidine Hydrochloride) Sanofi Winthrop .. 2438
Nubain Injection (Nalbuphine Hydrochloride) DuPont 952
Sufenta Injection (Sufentanil Citrate) Janssen 1355

Pain, oral mucosal and gingival
Cēpacol Maximum Spray (Dyclonine Hydrochloride) J.B. Williams 849
Cetacaine Topical Anesthetic (Benzocaine, Tetracaine Hydrochloride, Butyl Aminobenzoate) Cetylite 812

Pain, pre- and postoperative, adjunct to
Phenergan Injection (Promethazine Hydrochloride) Wyeth-Ayerst 2880
Sublimaze Injection (Fentanyl Citrate) Akorn 463

Pain, pre- and postoperative, relief of
Alfenta Injection (Alfentanil Hydrochloride) Janssen 1334
Demerol (Meperidine Hydrochloride) Sanofi Winthrop .. 2438
Ethyl Chloride, U.S.P. (Chloroethane, Ethyl Chloride) Gebauer 1040
Levo-Dromoran (Levorphanol Tartrate) Roche Pharmaceuticals 2297
Mepergan Injection (Meperidine Hydrochloride, Promethazine Hydrochloride) Wyeth-Ayerst 2859
Nubain Injection (Nalbuphine Hydrochloride) DuPont 952
Sufenta Injection (Sufentanil Citrate) Janssen 1355
Talwin Injection (Pentazocine Lactate) Sanofi Winthrop 2465
Toradol (Ketorolac Tromethamine) Roche Pharmaceuticals 2319

Pain, prepartum
(see under Pain, obstetrical)

Pain, severe
Astramorph/PF Injection, USP (Preservative-Free) (Morphine Sulfate) Astra 526
Duramorph Injection (Morphine Sulfate) Elkins-Sinn 983
Kadian Capsules (Morphine Sulfate) Zeneca 2948
Methadone Hydrochloride Oral Solution & Tablets (Methadone Hydrochloride) Roxane 2357
Oramorph SR (Morphine Sulfate Sustained Release Tablets) (Morphine Sulfate) Roxane 2359
RMS Suppositories CII (Morphine Sulfate) Upsher-Smith 2766
Roxanol (Morphine Sulfate) Roxane 2365

Pain, short-term management of
Toradol (Ketorolac Tromethamine) Roche Pharmaceuticals 2319

Pain, suprapubic, symptomatic relief of
Urispas Tablets (Flavoxate Hydrochloride) SmithKline Beecham Pharmaceuticals 2710

Pain, teething
(see under Pain, dental)

Pain, topical relief of
Americaine (Benzocaine) Ciba Self-Medication 649
ArthriCare Odor Free Rub (Capsaicin, Menthol, Methyl Nicotinate) Del 667
ArthriCare Triple Medicated Rub (Menthol, Methyl Nicotinate, Methyl Salicylate) Del 667
Aspercreme Creme, Lotion Analgesic Rub (Trolamine Salicylate) Thompson Medical 794
Benadryl Cream (Diphenhydramine Hydrochloride, Zinc Acetate) Warner Wellcome 814
Benadryl Gel (Diphenhydramine Hydrochloride, Zinc Acetate) Warner Wellcome 815
Benadryl Spray (Diphenhydramine Hydrochloride, Zinc Acetate) Warner Wellcome 815

BenGay External Analgesic Products (Menthol, Methyl Salicylate) Pfizer Consumer 714
BiCozene Creme (Benzocaine, Resorcinol) Sandoz Consumer .. 747
Caladryl Cream For Kids (Calamine, Pramoxine Hydrochloride) Warner Wellcome 817
Capsagel (Capsaicin) Iyata 674
Capzasin-P (Capsaicin) Thompson Medical 794
Chloresium (Chlorophyllin Copper Complex) Rystan 2371
Dolorac Cream (Capsaicin) GenDerm 1041
EMLA Cream (Prilocaine, Lidocaine) Astra 536
Ethyl Chloride, U.S.P. (Chloroethane, Ethyl Chloride) Gebauer 1040
Eucalyptamint Arthritis Pain Reliever (External Analgesic) (Menthol) Ciba Self-Medication.. 656
Eucalyptamint Muscle Pain Relief Formula (Menthol) Ciba Self-Medication 656
Fluori-Methane (Dichlorodifluoromethane, Trichloromonofluoromethane) Gebauer 1040
Hyland's Arnicaid Tablets (Homeopathic Medications) Standard Homeopathic 788
Itch-X (Pramoxine Hydrochloride, Benzyl Alcohol) Ascher 607
Mantadil Cream (Chlorcyclizine Hydrochloride) Glaxo Wellcome 1124
Mentholatum Deep Heating Extra Strength Formula Rub (Menthol, Methyl Salicylate) Mentholatum 710
Mentholatum Menthacin (Capsaicin, Menthol) Mentholatum 711
Maximum Strength Midol Teen Multi-Symptom Formula (Acetaminophen, Pamabrom) Bayer Consumer 621
Mobisyl Analgesic Creme (Trolamine Salicylate) Ascher 607
Myoflex External Analgesic Creme (Trolamine Salicylate) Ciba Self-Medication 660
Nupercainal Hemorrhoidal and Anesthetic Ointment (Dibucaine) Ciba Self-Medication 661
Sportscreme External Analgesic Rub Cream & Lotion (Trolamine Salicylate) Thompson Medical 798
Sunsource Arthritis Relief Cream (Homeopathic Medications) Sunsource 793
Sunsource Sports Injury Relief Cream (Homeopathic Medications) Sunsource 794
Thera-Gesic (Methyl Salicylate, Menthol) Mission 1830
Therapeutic Mineral Ice, Pain Relieving Gel (Menthol) Bristol-Myers Products 645
Unguentine Plus (Lidocaine Hydrochloride, Phenol) Mentholatum 712
Vicks VapoRub (Menthol, Camphor, Eucalyptus, Oil of) Procter & Gamble 739
Xylocaine 2.5% Ointment (Lidocaine) Astra 608
Zilactin-B Medicated Gel with Benzocaine (Benzocaine) Zila Pharmaceuticals 856
Zostrix/Zostrix-HP (Capsaicin) GenDerm 1043

Pain, unspecified
Extra Strength Bayer Plus Aspirin Caplets (Aspirin, Calcium Carbonate) Bayer Consumer 617
Cataflam Tablets (Diclofenac Potassium) CibaGeneva 833
Ecotrin (Aspirin) SmithKline Beecham 2625
Lodine Capsules and Tablets (Etodolac) Wyeth-Ayerst 2849

Pain, urinary tract
Prodium (Phenazopyridine Hydrochloride) Breckenridge 695
Pyridium (Phenazopyridine Hydrochloride) Parke-Davis 1985

(■ Described in PDR For Nonprescription Drugs)   (● Described in PDR For Ophthalmology)

Palpebral conjunctiva inflammation
AK-PRED (Prednisolone Sodium Phosphate) Akorn ... ⊚ 204
AK-Trol Ointment & Suspension (Dexamethasone, Neomycin Sulfate, Polymyxin B Sulfate) Akorn ... ⊚ 205
Blephamide Liquifilm Sterile Ophthalmic Suspension (Prednisolone Acetate, Sulfacetamide Sodium) Allergan ... 472
Cortisporin Ophthalmic Ointment Sterile (Polymyxin B Sulfate, Bacitracin Zinc, Neomycin Sulfate, Hydrocortisone) Glaxo Wellcome ... 1074
Cortisporin Ophthalmic Suspension Sterile (Hydrocortisone, Polymyxin B Sulfate, Neomycin Sulfate) Glaxo Wellcome ... 1075
Econopred & Econopred Plus Ophthalmic Suspensions (Prednisolone Acetate) Alcon Laboratories ... ⊚ 216
FML Forte Liquifilm (Fluorometholone) Allergan ... ⊚ 237
FML Liquifilm (Fluorometholone) Allergan ... ⊚ 238
FML S.O.P. (Fluorometholone) Allergan ... ⊚ 239
FML-S Liquifilm (Sulfacetamide Sodium, Fluorometholone) Allergan ... ⊚ 240
Maxitrol Ophthalmic Ointment and Suspension (Dexamethasone, Neomycin Sulfate, Polymyxin B Sulfate) Alcon Laboratories ... ⊚ 222
Poly-Pred Liquifilm (Neomycin Sulfate, Polymyxin B Sulfate, Prednisolone Acetate) Allergan .. ⊚ 246
Pred Forte (Prednisolone Acetate) Allergan ... ⊚ 247
Pred-G Liquifilm Sterile Ophthalmic Suspension (Gentamicin Sulfate, Prednisolone Acetate) Allergan ... ⊚ 248
Pred-G S.O.P. Sterile Ophthalmic Ointment (Gentamicin Sulfate, Prednisolone Acetate) Allergan ... ⊚ 249
TobraDex Ophthalmic Suspension and Ointment (Dexamethasone, Tobramycin) Alcon Laboratories .. 469

Pancreas, disseminated adenocarcinoma
(see under Carcinoma, pancreas)

Pancreatic cells, cytopathologic examination, adjunct in
Secretin-Ferring (Secretin) Ferring .. 2991

Pancreatic cystic fibrosis
Cotazym Capsules (Pancrelipase) Organon ... 1866
Creon (Pancrelipase) Solvay ... 2714
Ku-Zyme HP Capsules (Pancrelipase) Schwarz ... 2547
Pancrease Capsules (Pancrelipase) McNeil Pharmaceutical ... 1589
Pancrease MT Capsules (Pancrelipase) McNeil Pharmaceutical ... 1589
Viokase (Pancrelipase) Robins ... 2251
Zymase Capsules (Pancrelipase) Organon ... 1889

Pancreatic exocrine disease, diagnosis of
Secretin-Ferring (Secretin) Ferring .. 2991

Pancreatic insufficiency
Cotazym Capsules (Pancrelipase) Organon ... 1866
Creon (Pancrelipase) Solvay ... 2714
Donnazyme Tablets (Pancreatin) Robins ... 2235
Ku-Zyme HP Capsules (Pancrelipase) Schwarz ... 2547
Pancrease Capsules (Pancrelipase) McNeil Pharmaceutical ... 1589
Pancrease MT Capsules (Pancrelipase) McNeil Pharmaceutical ... 1589
Ultrase Capsules (Pancrelipase) Scandipharm ... 2476
Ultrase MT Capsules (Pancrelipase) Scandipharm ... 2477
Viokase (Pancrelipase) Robins ... 2251
Zymase Capsules (Pancrelipase) Organon ... 1889

Panic disorder with or without agoraphobia
Paxil Tablets (Paroxetine Hydrochloride) SmithKline Beecham Pharmaceuticals ... 2681
Xanax Tablets (Alprazolam) Pharmacia & Upjohn ... 2115

Papillitis
(see under Optic neuritis)

Paracoccidioidomycosis
Nizoral Tablets (Ketoconazole) Janssen ... 1345

Paralysis agitans
(see under Parkinson's disease)

Paralysis, familial periodic, hypokalemic
K-Dur Microburst Release System (potassium chloride, USP) E.R. Tablets (Potassium Chloride) Key 1364
K-Lor Powder Packets (Potassium Chloride) Abbott ... 438
K-Tab Filmtab (Potassium Chloride) Abbott ... 439
Micro-K (Potassium Chloride) Robins ... 2237
Micro-K LS Packets (Potassium Chloride) Robins ... 2238
Slow-K Extended-Release Tablets (Potassium Chloride) CibaGeneva ... 869

Paralytic ileus
(see under Ileus, paralytic)

Paralytic ileus, post-surgery, prophylaxis
(see under Ileus, paralytic, post-surgery)

Parkinson's disease
Artane (Trihexyphenidyl Hydrochloride) Lederle ... 1418
Atamet Tablets (Carbidopa, Levodopa) Athena ... 567
Benadryl Injection (Diphenhydramine Hydrochloride) Parke-Davis 1955
Parlodel (Bromocriptine Mesylate) Sandoz Pharmaceuticals ... 2411
Sinemet Tablets (Carbidopa, Levodopa) DuPont ... 959
Sinemet CR Tablets (Carbidopa, Levodopa) DuPont ... 961
Symmetrel Capsules (Amantadine Hydrochloride) DuPont ... 965
Symmetrel Syrup (Amantadine Hydrochloride) DuPont ... 963

Parkinson's disease, adjunctive therapy in
Akineton (Biperiden Hydrochloride) Knoll Laboratories ... 1380
Cogentin (Benztropine Mesylate) Merck & Co., Inc. ... 1661
Eldepryl Capsules (Selegiline Hydrochloride) Somerset ... 2729
Levsin/Levsinex/Levbid (Hyoscyamine Sulfate) Schwarz ... 2549
Permax Tablets (Pergolide Mesylate) Athena ... 571

Parkinson's disease, idiopathic
Artane (Trihexyphenidyl Hydrochloride) Lederle ... 1418
Atamet Tablets (Carbidopa, Levodopa) Athena ... 567
Kemadrin Tablets (Procyclidine Hydrochloride) Glaxo Wellcome 1105
Larodopa Tablets (Levodopa) Roche Pharmaceuticals ... 2296
Parlodel (Bromocriptine Mesylate) Sandoz Pharmaceuticals ... 2411
Sinemet Tablets (Carbidopa, Levodopa) DuPont ... 959
Sinemet CR Tablets (Carbidopa, Levodopa) DuPont ... 961

Parkinsonism, arteriosclerotic
Artane (Trihexyphenidyl Hydrochloride) Lederle ... 1418
Kemadrin Tablets (Procyclidine Hydrochloride) Glaxo Wellcome 1105
Larodopa Tablets (Levodopa) Roche Pharmaceuticals ... 2296

Parkinsonism, postencephalitic
Artane (Trihexyphenidyl Hydrochloride) Lederle ... 1418
Atamet Tablets (Carbidopa, Levodopa) Athena ... 567
Kemadrin Tablets (Procyclidine Hydrochloride) Glaxo Wellcome 1105
Larodopa Tablets (Levodopa) Roche Pharmaceuticals ... 2296
Parlodel (Bromocriptine Mesylate) Sandoz Pharmaceuticals ... 2411
Sinemet Tablets (Carbidopa, Levodopa) DuPont ... 959
Sinemet CR Tablets (Carbidopa, Levodopa) DuPont ... 961
Symmetrel Capsules (Amantadine Hydrochloride) DuPont ... 965
Symmetrel Syrup (Amantadine Hydrochloride) DuPont ... 963

Parkinsonism, symptomatic, following carbon monoxide intoxication
Atamet Tablets (Carbidopa, Levodopa) Athena ... 567
Larodopa Tablets (Levodopa) Roche Pharmaceuticals ... 2296
Sinemet Tablets (Carbidopa, Levodopa) DuPont ... 959
Sinemet CR Tablets (Carbidopa, Levodopa) DuPont ... 961
Symmetrel Capsules (Amantadine Hydrochloride) DuPont ... 965
Symmetrel Syrup (Amantadine Hydrochloride) DuPont ... 963

Parkinsonism, symptomatic, following manganese intoxication
Atamet Tablets (Carbidopa, Levodopa) Athena ... 567
Larodopa Tablets (Levodopa) Roche Pharmaceuticals ... 2296
Sinemet Tablets (Carbidopa, Levodopa) DuPont ... 959
Sinemet CR Tablets (Carbidopa, Levodopa) DuPont ... 961

Pasteurella pestis
(see under Yersinia pestis infections)

Pasteurella tularensis
(see under Francisella tularensis infections)

PCP
(see under Pneumocystis carinii pneumonia)

Pediculosis capitis infestation
Kwell Shampoo (Lindane) Reedco 2173
Lindane Shampoo USP 1% (Lindane) Alpharma ... 483
Nix Creme Rinse (Permethrin) Warner Wellcome ... ■ 822

Pediculosis pubis infestation
Kwell Shampoo (Lindane) Reedco 2173
Lindane Shampoo USP 1% (Lindane) Alpharma ... 483

Pediculosis, human
A-200 Lice Killing Gel (Piperonyl Butoxide, Pyrethrum Extract) Hogil ... ■ 672
A-200 Lice Killing Shampoo (Piperonyl Butoxide, Pyrethrum Extract) Hogil ... ■ 672
InnoGel Plus (Pyrethrum Extract, Piperonyl Butoxide) Hogil ... ■ 673
Pronto Lice Killing Shampoo & Conditioner in One Kit (Pyrethrins, Piperonyl Butoxide) Del .. ■ 669
Rid Lice Killing Shampoo (Pyrethrum Extract, Piperonyl Butoxide) Pfizer Consumer ... ■ 717

Pediculosis, human, adjunct in
A-200 Lice Control Spray (Permethrin) Hogil ... ■ 672
Rid Lice Control Spray (Permethrin) Pfizer Consumer .. ■ 716

Pelvic cellulitis
(see also under Infections, gynecologic)
Azactam for Injection (Aztreonam) Bristol-Myers Squibb ... 736
Ceptaz (Ceftazidime) Glaxo Wellcome ... 1070
Claforan Sterile and Injection (Cefotaxime Sodium) Hoechst Marion Roussel ... 1259
Cleocin Phosphate Injection (Clindamycin Phosphate) Pharmacia & Upjohn ... 2068
Fortaz (Ceftazidime) Glaxo Wellcome ... 1092
Mefoxin (Cefoxitin Sodium) Merck & Co., Inc. ... 1734
Mefoxin Premixed Intravenous Solution (Cefoxitin Sodium) Merck & Co., Inc. ... 1737
Mezlin (Mezlocillin Sodium) Bayer Pharmaceutical ... 594
Mezlin Pharmacy Bulk Package (Mezlocillin Sodium) Bayer Pharmaceutical ... 597
Pipracil (Piperacillin Sodium) Lederle ... 1435
Tazicef for Injection (Ceftazidime) SmithKline Beecham Pharmaceuticals ... 2697
Tazidime Vials, Faspak & ADD-Vantage (Ceftazidime) Lilly .. 1531

Pelvic inflammatory disease
(see also under Infections, gynecologic)
Cefizox for Intramuscular or Intravenous Use (Ceftizoxime Sodium) Fujisawa ... 1025
Cefobid Intravenous/Intramuscular (Cefoperazone Sodium) Pfizer Inc ... 1996
Cefobid Pharmacy Bulk Package - Not for Direct Infusion (Cefoperazone Sodium) Pfizer Inc ... 1999
Claforan Sterile and Injection (Cefotaxime Sodium) Hoechst Marion Roussel ... 1259
E-Mycin Tablets (Erythromycin) Knoll Laboratories ... 1388
Ilotycin Glucpetate, IV, Vials (Erythromycin Gluceptate) Dista ... 929
Mefoxin (Cefoxitin Sodium) Merck & Co., Inc. ... 1734
Mefoxin Premixed Intravenous Solution (Cefoxitin Sodium) Merck & Co., Inc. ... 1737
Mezlin (Mezlocillin Sodium) Bayer Pharmaceutical ... 594
Mezlin Pharmacy Bulk Package (Mezlocillin Sodium) Bayer Pharmaceutical ... 597
Pipracil (Piperacillin Sodium) Lederle ... 1435
Rocephin Injectable Vials, ADD-Vantage, Galaxy Container (Ceftriaxone Sodium) Roche Pharmaceuticals ... 2305
Ticar for Injection (Ticarcillin Disodium) SmithKline Beecham Pharmaceuticals ... 2704

Pemphigus
Celestone Soluspan Suspension (Betamethasone Sodium Phosphate, Betamethasone Acetate) Schering ... 2484
Cortone Acetate Sterile Suspension (Cortisone Acetate) Merck & Co., Inc. ... 1663
Cortone Acetate Tablets (Cortisone Acetate) Merck & Co., Inc. ... 1664
Dalalone D.P. Injectable (Dexamethasone Acetate) Forest ... 1009
Decadron Elixir (Dexamethasone) Merck & Co., Inc. ... 1676
Decadron Phosphate Injection (Dexamethasone Sodium Phosphate) Merck & Co., Inc. ... 1680
Decadron Tablets (Dexamethasone) Merck & Co., Inc. ... 1678
Decadron-LA Sterile Suspension (Dexamethasone Acetate) Merck & Co., Inc. ... 1687
Hydeltrasol Injection, Sterile (Prednisolone Sodium Phosphate) Merck & Co., Inc. ... 1708
Hydrocortone Phosphate Injection, Sterile (Hydrocortisone Sodium Phosphate) Merck & Co., Inc. ... 1713
Hydrocortone Tablets (Hydrocortisone) Merck & Co., Inc. ... 1715
Pediapred Oral Solution (Prednisolone Sodium Phosphate) Medeva 1618
Prelone Syrup (Prednisolone) Muro 1834

Pemphigus, "possibly" effective in
Potaba Capsules, Envules, Powder, and Tablets (Aminobenzoate Potassium) Glenwood-Palisades ... 1234

(■ Described in PDR For Nonprescription Drugs)   (⊚ Described in PDR For Ophthalmology)

Penicillin group Indications Index 1560

Penicillin group of antibiotics, therapy adjunct
Benemid Tablets (Probenecid) Merck & Co., Inc. 1651

Penicillin therapy, an adjuvant to
PCE Dispertab Tablets (Erythromycin) Abbott 453

Peptic ulcer, adjunctive therapy in
Cystospaz (Hyoscyamine) PolyMedica 2123
Levsin Drops (Hyoscyamine Sulfate) Schwarz 2549
Pro-Banthine Tablets (Propantheline Bromide) Roberts 2226
Robinul Forte Tablets (Glycopyrrolate) Robins 2247
Robinul Injectable (Glycopyrrolate) Robins 2247
Robinul Tablets (Glycopyrrolate) Robins 2247

Peptic ulcer, "possibly" effective in, adjunctive therapy
Librax Capsules (Chlordiazepoxide Hydrochloride, Clidinium Bromide) Roche Products 2330

Peptococcus niger infections
Cefotan (Cefotetan) Zeneca 2936
Flagyl 375 Capsules (Metronidazole) Searle 2587

Peptococcus niger gynecologic infections
Cefotan (Cefotetan) Zeneca 2936
Flagyl 375 Capsules (Metronidazole) Searle 2587

Peptococcus niger skin and skin structure infections
Cefotan (Cefotetan) Zeneca 2936
Flagyl 375 Capsules (Metronidazole) Searle 2587

Peptococcus species bone and joint infections
Cefizox for Intramuscular or Intravenous Use (Ceftizoxime Sodium) Fujisawa 1025

Peptococcus species endomyometritis
Flagyl I.V. (Metronidazole Hydrochloride) SCS 2373
Protostat Tablets (Metronidazole) Ortho Pharmaceutical 1939

Peptococcus species gynecologic infections
Claforan Sterile and Injection (Cefotaxime Sodium) Hoechst Marion Roussel 1259
Flagyl I.V. (Metronidazole Hydrochloride) SCS 2373
Mefoxin (Cefoxitin Sodium) Merck & Co., Inc. 1734
Mefoxin Premixed Intravenous Solution (Cefoxitin Sodium) Merck & Co., Inc. 1737
Mezlin (Mezlocillin Sodium) Bayer Pharmaceutical 594
Mezlin Pharmacy Bulk Package (Mezlocillin Sodium) Bayer Pharmaceutical 597
Primaxin I.V. (Cilastatin Sodium, Imipenem) Merck & Co., Inc. 1772
Protostat Tablets (Metronidazole) Ortho Pharmaceutical 1939

Peptococcus species infections
Cefizox for Intramuscular or Intravenous Use (Ceftizoxime Sodium) Fujisawa 1025
Claforan Sterile and Injection (Cefotaxime Sodium) Hoechst Marion Roussel 1259
Flagyl I.V. (Metronidazole Hydrochloride) SCS 2373
Mefoxin (Cefoxitin Sodium) Merck & Co., Inc. 1734
Mefoxin Premixed Intravenous Solution (Cefoxitin Sodium) Merck & Co., Inc. 1737
Mezlin (Mezlocillin Sodium) Bayer Pharmaceutical 594
Mezlin Pharmacy Bulk Package (Mezlocillin Sodium) Bayer Pharmaceutical 597
Primaxin I.V. (Cilastatin Sodium, Imipenem) Merck & Co., Inc. 1772

Peptococcus species intra-abdominal infections
Cefizox for Intramuscular or Intravenous Use (Ceftizoxime Sodium) Fujisawa 1025
Claforan Sterile and Injection (Cefotaxime Sodium) Hoechst Marion Roussel 1259
Flagyl I.V. (Metronidazole Hydrochloride) SCS 2373
Mezlin (Mezlocillin Sodium) Bayer Pharmaceutical 594
Mezlin Pharmacy Bulk Package (Mezlocillin Sodium) Bayer Pharmaceutical 597
Primaxin I.M. (Cilastatin Sodium, Imipenem) Merck & Co., Inc. 1770
Primaxin I.V. (Cilastatin Sodium, Imipenem) Merck & Co., Inc. 1772
Protostat Tablets (Metronidazole) Ortho Pharmaceutical 1939

Peptococcus species peritonitis
Flagyl I.V. (Metronidazole Hydrochloride) SCS 2373
Mezlin (Mezlocillin Sodium) Bayer Pharmaceutical 594
Mezlin Pharmacy Bulk Package (Mezlocillin Sodium) Bayer Pharmaceutical 597
Protostat Tablets (Metronidazole) Ortho Pharmaceutical 1939

Peptococcus species skin and skin structure infections
Cefizox for Intramuscular or Intravenous Use (Ceftizoxime Sodium) Fujisawa 1025
Claforan Sterile and Injection (Cefotaxime Sodium) Hoechst Marion Roussel 1259
Flagyl I.V. (Metronidazole Hydrochloride) SCS 2373
Mefoxin (Cefoxitin Sodium) Merck & Co., Inc. 1734
Mefoxin Premixed Intravenous Solution (Cefoxitin Sodium) Merck & Co., Inc. 1737
Mezlin (Mezlocillin Sodium) Bayer Pharmaceutical 594
Mezlin Pharmacy Bulk Package (Mezlocillin Sodium) Bayer Pharmaceutical 597
Primaxin I.V. (Cilastatin Sodium, Imipenem) Merck & Co., Inc. 1772
Protostat Tablets (Metronidazole) Ortho Pharmaceutical 1939

Peptococcus species tubo-ovarian abscess
Flagyl I.V. (Metronidazole Hydrochloride) SCS 2373
Protostat Tablets (Metronidazole) Ortho Pharmaceutical 1939

Peptococcus species vaginal cuff infection, post-surgical
Flagyl I.V. (Metronidazole Hydrochloride) SCS 2373
Protostat Tablets (Metronidazole) Ortho Pharmaceutical 1939

Peptostreptococcus species bone and joint infections
Cefizox for Intramuscular or Intravenous Use (Ceftizoxime Sodium) Fujisawa 1025

Peptostreptococcus species endometritis
Flagyl 375 Capsules (Metronidazole) Searle 2587
Flagyl I.V. (Metronidazole Hydrochloride) SCS 2373
Mefoxin (Cefoxitin Sodium) Merck & Co., Inc. 1734
Mefoxin Premixed Intravenous Solution (Cefoxitin Sodium) Merck & Co., Inc. 1737
Mezlin (Mezlocillin Sodium) Bayer Pharmaceutical 594
Mezlin Pharmacy Bulk Package (Mezlocillin Sodium) Bayer Pharmaceutical 597
Protostat Tablets (Metronidazole) Ortho Pharmaceutical 1939

Peptostreptococcus species endomyometritis
Flagyl 375 Capsules (Metronidazole) Searle 2587
Flagyl I.V. (Metronidazole Hydrochloride) SCS 2373
Protostat Tablets (Metronidazole) Ortho Pharmaceutical 1939

Peptostreptococcus species gynecologic infections
Cefotan (Cefotetan) Zeneca 2936
Claforan Sterile and Injection (Cefotaxime Sodium) Hoechst Marion Roussel 1259
Flagyl 375 Capsules (Metronidazole) Searle 2587
Flagyl I.V. (Metronidazole Hydrochloride) SCS 2373
Mefoxin (Cefoxitin Sodium) Merck & Co., Inc. 1734
Mefoxin Premixed Intravenous Solution (Cefoxitin Sodium) Merck & Co., Inc. 1737
Mezlin (Mezlocillin Sodium) Bayer Pharmaceutical 594
Mezlin Pharmacy Bulk Package (Mezlocillin Sodium) Bayer Pharmaceutical 597
Primaxin I.M. (Cilastatin Sodium, Imipenem) Merck & Co., Inc. 1770
Primaxin I.V. (Cilastatin Sodium, Imipenem) Merck & Co., Inc. 1772
Protostat Tablets (Metronidazole) Ortho Pharmaceutical 1939

Peptostreptococcus species infections
Cefizox for Intramuscular or Intravenous Use (Ceftizoxime Sodium) Fujisawa 1025
Cefotan (Cefotetan) Zeneca 2936
Claforan Sterile and Injection (Cefotaxime Sodium) Hoechst Marion Roussel 1259
Flagyl 375 Capsules (Metronidazole) Searle 2587
Flagyl I.V. (Metronidazole Hydrochloride) SCS 2373
Mefoxin (Cefoxitin Sodium) Merck & Co., Inc. 1734
Mefoxin Premixed Intravenous Solution (Cefoxitin Sodium) Merck & Co., Inc. 1737
Merrem I.V. (Meropenem) Zeneca .. 2952
Mezlin (Mezlocillin Sodium) Bayer Pharmaceutical 594
Mezlin Pharmacy Bulk Package (Mezlocillin Sodium) Bayer Pharmaceutical 597
Primaxin I.M. (Cilastatin Sodium, Imipenem) Merck & Co., Inc. 1770
Primaxin I.V. (Cilastatin Sodium, Imipenem) Merck & Co., Inc. 1772
Rocephin Injectable Vials, ADD-Vantage, Galaxy Container (Ceftriaxone Sodium) Roche Pharmaceuticals 2305

Peptostreptococcus species intra-abdominal infections
Cefizox for Intramuscular or Intravenous Use (Ceftizoxime Sodium) Fujisawa 1025
Claforan Sterile and Injection (Cefotaxime Sodium) Hoechst Marion Roussel 1259
Flagyl 375 Capsules (Metronidazole) Searle 2587
Flagyl I.V. (Metronidazole Hydrochloride) SCS 2373
Merrem I.V. (Meropenem) Zeneca .. 2952
Mezlin (Mezlocillin Sodium) Bayer Pharmaceutical 594
Mezlin Pharmacy Bulk Package (Mezlocillin Sodium) Bayer Pharmaceutical 597
Primaxin I.M. (Cilastatin Sodium, Imipenem) Merck & Co., Inc. 1770
Primaxin I.V. (Cilastatin Sodium, Imipenem) Merck & Co., Inc. 1772
Protostat Tablets (Metronidazole) Ortho Pharmaceutical 1939
Rocephin Injectable Vials, ADD-Vantage, Galaxy Container (Ceftriaxone Sodium) Roche Pharmaceuticals 2305

Peptostreptococcus species peritonitis
Flagyl 375 Capsules (Metronidazole) Searle 2587
Flagyl I.V. (Metronidazole Hydrochloride) SCS 2373
Merrem I.V. (Meropenem) Zeneca .. 2952
Mezlin (Mezlocillin Sodium) Bayer Pharmaceutical 594
Mezlin Pharmacy Bulk Package (Mezlocillin Sodium) Bayer Pharmaceutical 597
Protostat Tablets (Metronidazole) Ortho Pharmaceutical 1939

Peptostreptococcus species skin and skin structure infections
Cefizox for Intramuscular or Intravenous Use (Ceftizoxime Sodium) Fujisawa 1025
Cefotan (Cefotetan) Zeneca 2936
Claforan Sterile and Injection (Cefotaxime Sodium) Hoechst Marion Roussel 1259
Flagyl 375 Capsules (Metronidazole) Searle 2587
Flagyl I.V. (Metronidazole Hydrochloride) SCS 2373
Mefoxin (Cefoxitin Sodium) Merck & Co., Inc. 1734
Mefoxin Premixed Intravenous Solution (Cefoxitin Sodium) Merck & Co., Inc. 1737
Primaxin I.V. (Cilastatin Sodium, Imipenem) Merck & Co., Inc. 1772
Protostat Tablets (Metronidazole) Ortho Pharmaceutical 1939
Rocephin Injectable Vials, ADD-Vantage, Galaxy Container (Ceftriaxone Sodium) Roche Pharmaceuticals 2305

Peptostreptococcus tubo-ovarian abscess
Flagyl 375 Capsules (Metronidazole) Searle 2587
Flagyl I.V. (Metronidazole Hydrochloride) SCS 2373
Protostat Tablets (Metronidazole) Ortho Pharmaceutical 1939

Peptostreptococcus species vaginal cuff infection, post-surgical
Flagyl 375 Capsules (Metronidazole) Searle 2587
Flagyl I.V. (Metronidazole Hydrochloride) SCS 2373
Protostat Tablets (Metronidazole) Ortho Pharmaceutical 1939

Peritonitis (see also under Infections, intra-abdominal)
Amikacin Sulfate Injection, USP (Amikacin Sulfate) Astra 523
Amikacin Sulfate Injection, USP (Amikacin Sulfate) Elkins-Sinn 981
Amikin Injectable (Amikacin Sulfate) Apothecon 502
Azactam for Injection (Aztreonam) Bristol-Myers Squibb 736
Cefobid Intravenous/Intramuscular (Cefoperazone Sodium) Pfizer Inc 1996
Cefobid Pharmacy Bulk Package - Not for Direct Infusion (Cefoperazone Sodium) Pfizer Inc 1999
Ceptaz (Ceftazidime) Glaxo Wellcome 1070
Claforan Sterile and Injection (Cefotaxime Sodium) Hoechst Marion Roussel 1259
Cleocin Phosphate Injection (Clindamycin Phosphate) Pharmacia & Upjohn 2068
Diflucan Tablets, Injection, and Oral Suspension (Fluconazole) Pfizer Inc 2003
Flagyl 375 Capsules (Metronidazole) Searle 2587
Flagyl I.V. (Metronidazole Hydrochloride) SCS 2373
Fortaz (Ceftazidime) Glaxo Wellcome 1092
Garamycin Injectable (Gentamicin Sulfate) Schering 2502
Mandol Vials, Faspak & ADD-Vantage (Cefamandole Nafate) Lilly 1516
Mefoxin (Cefoxitin Sodium) Merck & Co., Inc. 1734
Mefoxin Premixed Intravenous Solution (Cefoxitin Sodium) Merck & Co., Inc. 1737
Mezlin (Mezlocillin Sodium) Bayer Pharmaceutical 594

(▣ Described in PDR For Nonprescription Drugs) (◉ Described in PDR For Ophthalmology)

1561 Indications Index Pneumonia

Mezlin Pharmacy Bulk Package (Mezlocillin Sodium) Bayer Pharmaceutical 597
Nebcin Vials, Hyporets & ADD-Vantage (Tobramycin Sulfate) Lilly 1518
Netromycin Injection 100 mg/ml (Netilmicin Sulfate) Schering 2516
Tazicef for Injection (Ceftazidime) SmithKline Beecham Pharmaceuticals 2697
Tazidime Vials, Faspak & ADD-Vantage (Ceftazidime) Lilly .. 1531
Ticar for Injection (Ticarcillin Disodium) SmithKline Beecham Pharmaceuticals 2704
Timentin for Injection (Ticarcillin Disodium, Clavulanate Potassium) SmithKline Beecham Pharmaceuticals 2706

Peritonitis, candidal
Diflucan Tablets, Injection, and Oral Suspension (Fluconazole) Pfizer Inc 2003

Pertussis
E.E.S. (Erythromycin Ethylsuccinate) Abbott 427
E-Mycin Tablets (Erythromycin) Knoll Laboratories 1388
ERYC (Erythromycin) Parke-Davis .. 1972
EryPed (Erythromycin Ethylsuccinate) Abbott 425
Ery-Tab Tablets (Erythromycin) Abbott 426
Erythrocin Stearate Filmtab (Erythromycin Stearate) Abbott 429
Erythromycin Base Filmtab (Erythromycin) Abbott 430
Erythromycin Delayed-Release Capsules, USP (Erythromycin) Abbott 431
PCE Dispertab Tablets (Erythromycin) Abbott 453

Petit mal epilepsy (see under Seizures, generalized, absence)

Petriellidiosis (see under Pseudoallescheriosis)

Peyronie's disease, "possibly" effective in
Potaba Capsules, Envules, Powder, and Tablets (Aminobenzoate Potassium) Glenwood-Palisades .. 1234

Pharyngitis, symptomatic relief of
Aspirin Regimen Bayer Children's Chewable Aspirin (Aspirin) Bayer Consumer .... ▣ 616
Benadryl Allergy/Cold Tablets (Acetaminophen, Diphenhydramine Hydrochloride, Pseudoephedrine Hydrochloride) Warner Wellcome .... ▣ 811
Celestial Seasonings Soothers Herbal Throat Drops (Menthol, Pectin) Warner-Lambert .... ▣ 805
Cēpacol Maximum Strength Sore Throat Lozenges, Cherry Flavor (Benzocaine, Menthol) J.B. Williams .... ▣ 850
Cēpacol Maximum Strength Sore Throat Lozenges, Original Mint Flavor (Benzocaine, Menthol) J.B. Williams .... ▣ 850
Cēpacol Regular Strength Sore Throat Lozenges, Cherry Flavor (Menthol) J.B. Williams .... ▣ 850
Cēpacol Regular Strength Sore Throat Lozenges, Original Mint Flavor (Menthol) J.B. Williams .... ▣ 850
Cēpacol Maximum Spray (Dyclonine Hydrochloride) J.B. Williams .... ▣ 849
Cepastat (Phenol) SmithKline Beecham Consumer .... ▣ 770
Children's TYLENOL Cold Plus Cough Multi Symptom Chewable Tablets and Liquid (Acetaminophen, Chlorpheniramine Maleate, Dextromethorphan Hydrobromide, Pseudoephedrine Hydrochloride) McNeil Consumer 1560
Children's Vicks Chloraseptic Sore Throat Lozenges (Benzocaine) Procter & Gamble ▣ 730
Children's Vicks Chloraseptic Sore Throat Spray (Phenol) Procter & Gamble .... ▣ 730
Dura-Vent Tablets (Phenylpropanolamine Hydrochloride, Guaifenesin) Dura 971
Entex LA Tablets (Phenylpropanolamine Hydrochloride, Guaifenesin) Dura 972
Exgest LA Tablets (Phenylpropanolamine Hydrochloride, Guaifenesin) Carnrick 787
Humibid DM Tablets (Guaifenesin, Dextromethorphan Hydrobromide) Medeva 1612
N'ICE Medicated Sugarless Sore Throat and Cough Lozenges (Menthol) SmithKline Beecham Consumer .... ▣ 781
Original Vicks Cough Drops, Menthol and Cherry Flavors (Menthol) Procter & Gamble .... ▣ 733
Sucrets Maximum Strength (Dyclonine Hydrochloride) SmithKline Beecham Consumer ▣ 785
Sucrets Regular Strength Wild Cherry, Regular Strength Original Mint, Regular Strength Vapor Lemon Sore Throat Lozenges (Dyclonine Hydrochloride) SmithKline Beecham Consumer .... ▣ 785
TheraFlu Flu and Cold Medicine (Acetaminophen, Chlorpheniramine Maleate, Pseudoephedrine Hydrochloride) Sandoz Consumer .... ▣ 750
Theraflu Maximum Strength Flu and Cold Medicine For Sore Throat (Acetaminophen, Chlorpheniramine Maleate, Pseudoephedrine Hydrochloride) Sandoz Consumer .... ▣ 751
Triaminic Sore Throat Formula (Acetaminophen, Dextromethorphan Hydrobromide, Pseudoephedrine Hydrochloride) Sandoz Consumer .... ▣ 755
TYLENOL Cold Medication, Multi-Symptom Formula Tablets and Caplets (Acetaminophen, Chlorpheniramine Maleate, Pseudoephedrine Hydrochloride, Dextromethorphan Hydrobromide) McNeil Consumer 1572
TYLENOL Cold Medication, Multi-Symptom Hot Liquid Packets (Acetaminophen, Chlorpheniramine Maleate, Pseudoephedrine Hydrochloride, Dextromethorphan Hydrobromide) McNeil Consumer 1572
TYLENOL Cold Medication, No Drowsiness Formula Caplets and Gelcaps (Acetaminophen, Pseudoephedrine Hydrochloride, Dextromethorphan Hydrobromide) McNeil Consumer 1572
TYLENOL Cold Severe Congestion Caplets (Acetaminophen, Dextromethorphan Hydrobromide, Guaifenesin, Pseudoephedrine Hydrochloride) McNeil Consumer 1573
Tylenol Cough/Decongestant (Dextromethorphan Hydrobromide, Acetaminophen) McNeil Consumer 1574
TYLENOL Severe Allergy Medication Caplets (Acetaminophen, Chlorpheniramine Maleate, Pseudoephedrine Hydrochloride) McNeil Consumer 1571
Vicks Chloraseptic Cough & Throat Drops, Menthol, Cherry and Honey Lemon Flavors (Menthol) Procter & Gamble .... ▣ 732
Vicks Chloraseptic Sore Throat Lozenges, Menthol and Cherry Flavors (Benzocaine, Menthol) Procter & Gamble .... ▣ 732
Vicks Chloraspetic Sore Throat Spray, Gargle and Mouth Rinse, Menthol and Cherry Flavors (Phenol) Procter & Gamble .... ▣ 732

Pharyngitis, treatment of
Biaxin (Clarithromycin) Abbott 406
Ceclor Pulvules & Suspension (Cefaclor) Lilly 1470
Cedax (Ceftibuten Dihydrate) Schering 2480
Ceftin (Cefuroxime Axetil) Glaxo Wellcome 1067
Cefzil Tablets and Oral Suspension (Cefprozil) Bristol-Myers Squibb .. 747
Duricef Capsules, Tablets, and Oral Suspension (Cefadroxil) Bristol-Myers Squibb 750
Dynabac (Dirithromycin) Bock 668
E.E.S. (Erythromycin Ethylsuccinate) Abbott 427
E-Mycin Tablets (Erythromycin) Knoll Laboratories 1388
EryPed (Erythromycin Ethylsuccinate) Abbott 425
Ery-Tab Tablets (Erythromycin) Abbott 426
Erythrocin Stearate Filmtab (Erythromycin Stearate) Abbott 429
Erythromycin Base Filmtab (Erythromycin) Abbott 430
Ilosone (Erythromycin Estolate) Dista 927
Ilotycin Gluceptate, IV, Vials (Erythromycin Gluceptate) Dista 929
Lorabid Suspension and Pulvules (Loracarbef) Lilly 1513
PCE Dispertab Tablets (Erythromycin) Abbott 453
Suprax (Cefixime) Lederle 1443
Vantin for Oral Suspension and Vantin Tablets (Cefpodoxime Proxetil) Pharmacia & Upjohn 2112
Zithromax (Azithromycin) Pfizer Inc 2043
Zithromax Tablets (Azithromycin) Pfizer Inc 2046

Pheochromocytoma
Demser Capsules (Metyrosine) Merck & Co., Inc. 1690
Dibenzyline Capsules (Phenoxybenzamine Hydrochloride) SmithKline Beecham Pharmaceuticals 2650

Pheochromocytoma, adjunctive therapy
Demser Capsules (Metyrosine) Merck & Co., Inc. 1690
Inderal (Propranolol Hydrochloride) Wyeth-Ayerst 2834
Regitine Vials (Phentolamine Mesylate) CibaGeneva 864

Pheochromocytoma, diagnosis of
Regitine Vials (Phentolamine Mesylate) CibaGeneva 864

Phosphorus deficiency (see under Hypophosphatemia)

Photophobia
Voltaren Ophthalmic Sterile Ophthalmic Solution (Diclofenac Sodium) CIBA Vision Ophthalmics .... ◉ 264

Phycomycosis (see under Zygomycosis)

Piles (see under Hemorrhoids)

Pinta
Bicillin L-A Injection (Penicillin G Benzathine) Wyeth-Ayerst 2813

Pinworm infestation (see under Enterobiasis)

Pityrosporon orbiculare infections
Exelderm Cream 1.0% (Sulconazole Nitrate) Westwood-Squibb 2794
Exelderm Solution 1.0% (Sulconazole Nitrate) Westwood-Squibb 2795
Loprox 1% Cream and Lotion (Ciclopirox Olamine) Hoechst Marion Roussel 1269
Lotrimin (Clotrimazole) Schering 2514
Monistat Dual-Pak (Miconazole Nitrate) Ortho Pharmaceutical 1906
Monistat-Derm (miconazole nitrate 2%) Cream (Miconazole Nitrate) Ortho Dermatological 1944
Nizoral 2% Cream (Ketoconazole) Janssen 1344
Selsun Rx 2.5% Selenium Sulfide Lotion, USP (Selenium Sulfide) Ross 2345
Spectazole (econazole nitrate 1%) Cream (Econazole Nitrate) Ortho Dermatological 1947

Plague
DYNACIN Capsules (Minocycline Hydrochloride) Medicis 1627
Minocin Oral Suspension (Minocycline Hydrochloride) Lederle 1431
Minocin Pellet-Filled Capsules (Minocycline Hydrochloride) Lederle 1429
Monodox Capsules (Doxycycline Monohydrate) Oclassen 1858

Plasmodium infection (see under P. vivax infections; P. malariae infections; P. ovale infections; P. falciparum infections)

PMS (see under Menstrual syndrome, pre-, management of)

Pleural effusion, malignant
Blenoxane (Bleomycin Sulfate) Bristol-Myers Squibb Oncology/Immunology 697

Pleural effusions, recurrent, prevention of
Blenoxane (Bleomycin Sulfate) Bristol-Myers Squibb Oncology/Immunology 697

Pneumococcal disease, immunization against
Pneumovax 23 (Pneumococcal Vaccine, Polyvalent) Merck & Co., Inc. 1768
Pnu-Imune 23 (Pneumococcal Vaccine, Polyvalent) Lederle 1437

Pneumococci species infections (see under Pneumococcosis)

Pneumococcosis
Omnipen Capsules (Ampicillin) Wyeth-Ayerst 2872
Omnipen for Oral Suspension (Ampicillin) Wyeth-Ayerst 2873
Pen•Vee K (Penicillin V Potassium) Wyeth-Ayerst 2879
TERAK Ointment (Oxytetracycline Hydrochloride, Polymyxin B Sulfate) Akorn .... ◉ 210

Pneumocystis carinii pneumonia
Bactrim DS Tablets (Trimethoprim, Sulfamethoxazole) Roche Pharmaceuticals 2257
Bactrim I.V. Infusion (Trimethoprim, Sulfamethoxazole) Roche Pharmaceuticals 2255
Bactrim (Trimethoprim, Sulfamethoxazole) Roche Pharmaceuticals 2257
Mepron Suspension (Atovaquone) Glaxo Wellcome Oncology/HIV 1206
Neutrexin for Injection (Trimetrexate Glucuronate) U.S. Bioscience 2761
Septra (Trimethoprim, Sulfamethoxazole) Glaxo Wellcome 1146
Septra I.V. Infusion (Trimethoprim, Sulfamethoxazole) Glaxo Wellcome 1142
Septra I.V. Infusion ADD-Vantage Vials (Trimethoprim, Sulfamethoxazole) Glaxo Wellcome 1144
Septra (Trimethoprim, Sulfamethoxazole) Glaxo Wellcome 1146

Pneumonia (see also under Infections, lower respiratory tract)
Azactam for Injection (Aztreonam) Bristol-Myers Squibb 736
Biaxin (Clarithromycin) Abbott 406
Bicillin C-R Injection (Penicillin G Procaine, Penicillin G Benzathine) Wyeth-Ayerst 2810
Bicillin C-R 900/300 Injection (Penicillin G Procaine, Penicillin G Benzathine) Wyeth-Ayerst 2812
Ceclor Pulvules & Suspension (Cefaclor) Lilly 1470

Pneumonia — Indications Index

Pneumonia
- Ceptaz (Ceftazidime) Glaxo Wellcome 1070
- Claforan Sterile and Injection (Cefotaxime Sodium) Hoechst Marion Roussel 1259
- Cleocin Phosphate Injection (Clindamycin Phosphate) Pharmacia & Upjohn 2068
- Dynabac (Dirithromycin) Bock 668
- E.E.S. (Erythromycin Ethylsuccinate) Abbott 427
- EryPed (Erythromycin Ethylsuccinate) Abbott 425
- Ery-Tab Tablets (Erythromycin) Abbott 426
- Erythrocin Stearate Filmtab (Erythromycin Stearate) Abbott 429
- Erythromycin Base Filmtab (Erythromycin) Abbott 430
- Flagyl 375 Capsules (Metronidazole) Searle 2587
- Flagyl I.V. (Metronidazole Hydrochloride) SCS 2373
- Fortaz (Ceftazidime) Glaxo Wellcome 1092
- Ilosone (Erythromycin Estolate) Dista 927
- Ilotycin Gluceptate, IV, Vials (Erythromycin Gluceptate) Dista 929
- Kefurox Vials, Faspak & ADD-Vantage (Cefuroxime Sodium) Lilly 1509
- Lorabid Suspension and Pulvules (Loracarbef) Lilly 1513
- Mandol Vials, Faspak & ADD-Vantage (Cefamandole Nafate) Lilly 1516
- Maxipime for Injection (Cefepime Hydrochloride) Bristol-Myers Squibb 758
- Mefoxin (Cefoxitin Sodium) Merck & Co., Inc. 1734
- Mefoxin Premixed Intravenous Solution (Cefoxitin Sodium) Merck & Co., Inc. 1737
- Mezlin (Mezlocillin Sodium) Bayer Pharmaceutical 594
- Mezlin Pharmacy Bulk Package (Mezlocillin Sodium) Bayer Pharmaceutical 597
- Pfizerpen for Injection (Penicillin G Potassium) Pfizer Inc 2022
- Tao Capsules (Troleandomycin) Pfizer Inc 2033
- Tazicef for Injection (Ceftazidime) SmithKline Beecham Pharmaceuticals 2697
- Tazidime Vials, Faspak & ADD-Vantage (Ceftazidime) Lilly .. 1531
- Vantin for Oral Suspension and Vantin Tablets (Cefpodoxime Proxetil) Pharmacia & Upjohn 2112
- Vibramycin Hyclate Intravenous (Doxycycline Hyclate) Pfizer Inc 2040
- Zinacef (Cefuroxime Sodium) Glaxo Wellcome 1184
- Zithromax (Azithromycin) Pfizer Inc 2043
- Zithromax Tablets (Azithromycin) Pfizer Inc 2046

Pneumonia, candidal
- Diflucan Tablets, Injection, and Oral Suspension (Fluconazole) Pfizer Inc 2003

Pneumonia, nosocomial (see also under Infections, lower respiratory tract)
- Zosyn (Piperacillin Sodium, Tazobactam Sodium) Lederle 1463

Pneumonia, pneumocystis carinii (see under Pneumocystis carinii pneumonia)

Pneumonitis, anaerobic
- Ticar for Injection (Ticarcillin Disodium) SmithKline Beecham Pharmaceuticals 2704

Pneumonitis, aspiration
- Celestone Soluspan Suspension (Betamethasone Sodium Phosphate, Betamethasone Acetate) Schering 2484
- Cortone Acetate Sterile Suspension (Cortisone Acetate) Merck & Co., Inc. 1663
- Cortone Acetate Tablets (Cortisone Acetate) Merck & Co., Inc. 1664
- Dalalone D.P. Injectable (Dexamethasone Acetate) Forest 1009
- Decadron Elixir (Dexamethasone) Merck & Co., Inc. 1676
- Decadron Phosphate Injection (Dexamethasone Sodium Phosphate) Merck & Co., Inc. 1680
- Decadron Tablets (Dexamethasone) Merck & Co., Inc. 1678
- Decadron-LA Sterile Suspension (Dexamethasone Acetate) Merck & Co., Inc. 1687
- Hydeltrasol Injection, Sterile (Prednisolone Sodium Phosphate) Merck & Co., Inc. 1708
- Hydrocortone Phosphate Injection, Sterile (Hydrocortisone Sodium Phosphate) Merck & Co., Inc. 1713
- Hydrocortone Tablets (Hydrocortisone) Merck & Co., Inc. 1715
- Pediapred Oral Solution (Prednisolone Sodium Phosphate) Medeva 1618
- Prelone Syrup (Prednisolone) Muro 1834

Poison ivy (see under Dermatitis, contact)

Poison oak (see under Dermatitis, contact)

Poison sumac (see under Dermatitis, contact)

Poisoning, acute, unspecified, emergency treatment of
- CharcoAid 2000 (Charcoal, Activated) Requa 740

Poisoning, pesticides and chemicals of organophosphate class
- Protopam Chloride for Injection (Pralidoxime Chloride) Wyeth-Ayerst 2909

Poliomyelitis, prevention of (see under Immunization, poliovirus 1, 2, and 3)

Pollinosis (see also under Rhinitis, seasonal allergic)
- Actifed Allergy Daytime/Nighttime Caplets (Diphenhydramine Hydrochloride, Pseudoephedrine Hydrochloride) Warner Wellcome 808
- Actifed Cold & Allergy Tablets (Pseudoephedrine Hydrochloride, Triprolidine Hydrochloride) Warner Wellcome 807
- Actifed Sinus Daytime/Nighttime Tablets and Caplets (Acetaminophen, Diphenhydramine Hydrochloride, Pseudoephedrine Hydrochloride) Warner Wellcome 809
- Afrin (Oxymetazoline Hydrochloride) Schering-Plough HealthCare 757
- Alka-Seltzer Plus Sinus Medicine (Phenylpropanolamine Bitartrate, Aspirin, Brompheniramine Maleate) Bayer Consumer 611
- Benadryl Allergy Chewables (Diphenhydramine Hydrochloride) Warner Wellcome 811
- Benadryl Allergy Decongestant Tablets (Diphenhydramine Hydrochloride, Pseudoephedrine Hydrochloride) Warner Wellcome 812
- Benadryl Allergy Liquid Medication (Diphenhydramine Hydrochloride) Warner Wellcome 813
- Benadryl Allergy Sinus Headache Caplets (Diphenhydramine Hydrochloride, Pseudoephedrine Hydrochloride, Acetaminophen) Warner Wellcome 813
- Benadryl Dye-Free Allergy Liqui-gel Softgels (Diphenhydramine Hydrochloride) Warner Wellcome 813
- Benadryl Dye-Free Allergy Liquid Medication (Diphenhydramine Hydrochloride) Warner Wellcome 814
- Chlor-Trimeton Allergy Decongestant Tablets (Chlorpheniramine Maleate, Pseudoephedrine Sulfate) Schering-Plough HealthCare 759
- Chlor-Trimeton Allergy Tablets (Chlorpheniramine Maleate) Schering-Plough HealthCare 758
- Allergy-Sinus Comtrex Multi-Symptom Allergy-Sinus Formula Tablets and Caplets (Acetaminophen, Chlorpheniramine Maleate, Pseudoephedrine Hydrochloride) Bristol-Myers Products 639
- Contac Continuous Action Nasal Decongestant/Antihistamine 12 Hour Capsules (Chlorpheniramine Maleate, Phenylpropanolamine Hydrochloride) SmithKline Beecham Consumer 773
- Dimetapp Allergy Dye-Free Elixir (Brompheniramine Maleate) Whitehall-Robins 838
- Dimetapp Cold & Allergy Chewable Tablets (Brompheniramine Maleate, Phenylpropanolamine Hydrochloride) Whitehall-Robins 838
- Dimetapp Elixir (Brompheniramine Maleate, Phenylpropanolamine Hydrochloride) Whitehall-Robins 840
- Dimetapp Extentabs (Brompheniramine Maleate, Phenylpropanolamine Hydrochloride) Whitehall-Robins 841
- Dimetapp Tablets/Liqui-Gels (Brompheniramine Maleate, Phenylpropanolamine Hydrochloride) Whitehall-Robins 841
- Drixoral Cold and Allergy Sustained-Action Tablets (Dexbrompheniramine Maleate, Pseudoephedrine Sulfate) Schering-Plough HealthCare 763
- 4-Way Fast Acting Nasal Spray (regular & mentholated) (Naphazoline Hydrochloride, Phenylephrine Hydrochloride, Pyrilamine Maleate) Bristol-Myers Products 644
- 4-Way 12 Hour Nasal Spray (Oxymetazoline Hydrochloride) Bristol-Myers Products 644
- Kronofed-A (Chlorpheniramine Maleate, Pseudoephedrine Hydrochloride) Ferndale 994
- Neo-Synephrine Maximum Strength 12 Hour Nasal Spray (Oxymetazoline Hydrochloride) Bayer Consumer 624
- Neo-Synephrine Maximum Strength 12 Hour Nasal Spray Pump (Oxymetazoline Hydrochloride) Bayer Consumer 624
- Neo-Synephrine (Phenylephrine Hydrochloride) Bayer Consumer 624
- Nolahist Tablets (Phenindamine Tartrate) Carnrick 790
- Nolamine Timed-Release Tablets (Phenindamine Tartrate, Phenylpropanolamine Hydrochloride, Chlorpheniramine Maleate) Carnrick 790
- Novahistine Elixir (Chlorpheniramine Maleate, Phenylephrine Hydrochloride) SmithKline Beecham Consumer 782
- PediaCare Cough-Cold Chewable Tablets and Liquid (Pseudoephedrine Hydrochloride, Chlorpheniramine Maleate, Dextromethorphan Hydrobromide) McNeil Consumer 1569
- Propagest Tablets (Phenylpropanolamine Hydrochloride) Carnrick 791
- Sine-Off No Drowsiness Formula Caplets (Acetaminophen, Pseudoephedrine Hydrochloride) SmithKline Beecham Consumer 784
- Sinulin Tablets (Acetaminophen, Phenylpropanolamine Hydrochloride, Chlorpheniramine Maleate) Carnrick 792
- Sudafed Cold & Allergy Tablets (Chlorpheniramine Maleate, Pseudoephedrine Hydrochloride) Warner Wellcome 826
- Sunsource Allergy Relief Tablets (Homeopathic Medications) Sunsource 792
- Tavist-1 12 Hour Relief Tablets (Clemastine Fumarate) Sandoz Consumer 749
- Tavist-D 12 Hour Relief Tablets (Clemastine Fumarate, Phenylpropanolamine Hydrochloride) Sandoz Consumer 750
- Teldrin 12 Hour Antihistamine/Nasal Decongestant Allergy Relief Capsules (Chlorpheniramine Maleate, Phenylpropanolamine Hydrochloride) SmithKline Beecham Consumer 786
- TYLENOL Severe Allergy Medication Caplets (Acetaminophen, Chlorpheniramine Maleate, Pseudoephedrine Hydrochloride) McNeil Consumer 1571
- Vicks Sinex 12-Hour Nasal Decongestant Spray and Ultra Fine Mist (Oxymetazoline Hydrochloride) Procter & Gamble 738
- Vicks Sinex Nasal Spray and Ultra Fine Mist (Phenylephrine Hydrochloride) Procter & Gamble 738

Polycythemia vera
- Mustargen (Mechlorethamine Hydrochloride) Merck & Co., Inc. 1752

Polydipsia, temporary, management of
- DDAVP (Desmopressin Acetate) Rhone-Poulenc Rorer Pharmaceuticals 2180
- Desmopressin Acetate Rhinal Tube (Desmopressin Acetate) Ferring 997

Polymyositis (see under Dermatomyositis, systemic)

Polyps, nasal, prevention of recurrence
- Beconase (Beclomethasone Dipropionate) Glaxo Wellcome 1065
- Dexacort Phosphate in Turbinaire (Dexamethasone Sodium Phosphate) Medeva 1607
- Vancenase AQ Nasal Spray 0.042% (Beclomethasone Dipropionate) Schering 2535
- Vancenase AQ Double Strength Nasal Spray 0.084% (Beclomethasone Dipropionate) Schering 2536
- Vancenase PocketHaler Nasal Inhaler (Beclomethasone Dipropionate) Schering 2534

Polyuria, temporary, management of
- DDAVP (Desmopressin Acetate) Rhone-Poulenc Rorer Pharmaceuticals 2180
- Desmopressin Acetate Rhinal Tube (Desmopressin Acetate) Ferring 997

Porphyria, acute intermittent, adjunctive therapy in
- Thorazine (Chlorpromazine Hydrochloride) SmithKline Beecham Pharmaceuticals 2701

Porphyria, acute intermittent, amelioration of recurrent attacks of
- Panhematin (Hemin For Injection) Abbott 452

Porphyria variegata
- Panhematin (Hemin For Injection) Abbott 452

Portal-systemic encephalopathy (see under Hepatic encephalopathy)

(▣ Described in PDR For Nonprescription Drugs) (◉ Described in PDR For Ophthalmology)

Postnasal drip
(see under Cold, common, symptomatic relief of)

Pregnancy, diagnosis of
e.p.t. Pregnancy Test (HCG Monoclonal Antibody) Warner Wellcome .... ▣ 818

Pregnancy, prevention of
All-Flex Arcing Spring Diaphragm (See also Ortho Diaphragm Kits) (Diaphragm) Ortho Pharmaceutical 1921
Brevicon (Norethindrone, Ethinyl Estradiol) Searle 2563
Demulen (Ethynodiol Diacetate, Ethinyl Estradiol) Searle 2580
Depo-Provera Contraceptive Injection (Medroxyprogesterone Acetate) Pharmacia & Upjohn 2079
Desogen Tablets (Desogestrel, Ethinyl Estradiol) Organon 1867
Encare Vaginal Contraceptive Suppositories (Nonoxynol-9) Thompson Medical .... ▣ 797
Levlen/Tri-Levlen (Levonorgestrel, Ethinyl Estradiol) Berlex 646
Lo/Ovral Tablets (Norgestrel, Ethinyl Estradiol) Wyeth-Ayerst 2852
Lo/Ovral-28 Tablets (Norgestrel, Ethinyl Estradiol) Wyeth-Ayerst 2857
Micronor Tablets (Norethindrone) Ortho Pharmaceutical 1903
Modicon (Norethindrone, Ethinyl Estradiol) Ortho Pharmaceutical .. 1928
Nordette-21 Tablets (Levonorgestrel, Ethinyl Estradiol) Wyeth-Ayerst 2863
Nordette-28 Tablets (Levonorgestrel, Ethinyl Estradiol) Wyeth-Ayerst 2866
Norinyl (Ethinyl Estradiol, Norethindrone) Searle 2563
Norplant System (Levonorgestrel) Wyeth-Ayerst 2868
Nor-Q D Tablets (Norethindrone) Searle 2598
Ortho-Cept (Desogestrel, Ethinyl Estradiol) Ortho Pharmaceutical .. 1907
Ortho-Cyclen/Ortho-Tri-Cyclen (Norgestimate, Ethinyl Estradiol) Ortho Pharmaceutical 1914
Ortho Diaphragm Kits—All-Flex Arcing Spring; Ortho Coil Spring; Ortho-White Flat Spring (Diaphragm) Ortho Pharmaceutical 1921
Ortho Diaphragm Kit-Coil Spring (Diaphragm) Ortho Pharmaceutical 1921
Ortho-Novum (Norethindrone, Ethinyl Estradiol) Ortho Pharmaceutical 1928
Ortho-Cyclen/Ortho Tri-Cyclen (Norgestimate, Ethinyl Estradiol) Ortho Pharmaceutical 1914
Ortho-White Diaphragm Kit-Flat Spring (See also Ortho Diaphragm Kits) (Diaphragm) Ortho Pharmaceutical 1921
Ovcon (Norethindrone, Ethinyl Estradiol) Bristol-Myers Squibb 765
Ovral Tablets (Norgestrel, Ethinyl Estradiol) Wyeth-Ayerst 2877
Ovral-28 Tablets (Norgestrel, Ethinyl Estradiol) Wyeth-Ayerst 2878
Ovrette Tablets (Norgestrel) Wyeth-Ayerst 2878
ParaGard T 380A Intrauterine Copper Contraceptive (Intrauterine device) Ortho Pharmaceutical 1936
Levlen/Tri-Levlen (Levonorgestrel, Ethinyl Estradiol) Berlex 646
Tri-Norinyl (Norethindrone, Ethinyl Estradiol) Searle 2607
Triphasil-21 Tablets (Levonorgestrel, Ethinyl Estradiol) Wyeth-Ayerst 2919
Triphasil-28 Tablets (Levonorgestrel, Ethinyl Estradiol) Wyeth-Ayerst 2924

Pregnancy, termination of, from 12th through the 20th gestational week
Prostin E2 Suppository (Dinoprostone) Pharmacia & Upjohn 2109

Pregnancy, vitamin supplement for
(see under Vitamin deficiency, postpartum; Vitamin deficiency, prenatal)

Premenstrual syndrome
(see under Menstrual syndrome, pre-, management of)

Prickly heat
(see under Miliaria)

Prinzmetal's angina
(see under Angina, Prinzmetal's)

Proctitis
ROWASA Rectal Suspension Enema 4.0 grams/unit (60 mL) (Mesalamine) Solvay 2727

Proctitis, active ulcerative
ROWASA Rectal Suppositories, 500 mg (Mesalamine) Solvay 2727

Proctitis, temporary relief of
Anusol-HC Suppositories (Hydrocortisone Acetate) Parke-Davis 1954

Proctitis, ulcerative, adjunctive therapy in
CORTENEMA (Hydrocortisone) Solvay 2713
Cortifoam (Hydrocortisone Acetate) Schwarz 2540

Proctosigmoiditis
ROWASA Rectal Suspension Enema 4.0 grams/unit (60 mL) (Mesalamine) Solvay 2727

Proctosigmoiditis, ulcerative, adjunctive therapy in
CORTENEMA (Hydrocortisone) Solvay 2713

Propionibacterium species gynecologic infections
Primaxin I.V. (Cilastatin Sodium, Imipenem) Merck & Co., Inc. 1772

Propionibacterium species infections
Primaxin I.V. (Cilastatin Sodium, Imipenem) Merck & Co., Inc. 1772

Propionibacterium species intra-abdominal infections
Primaxin I.V. (Cilastatin Sodium, Imipenem) Merck & Co., Inc. 1772

Prostatic cancer
(see under Carcinoma, prostate)

Prostatic cancer, palliative treatment of
(see under Carcinoma, prostatic, palliative treatment of)

Prostatic hyperplasia, benign, symptomatic treatment
Cardura Tablets (Doxazosin Mesylate) Pfizer Inc 1993
Hytrin Capsules (Terazosin Hydrochloride) Abbott 434
Proscar Tablets (Finasteride) Merck & Co., Inc. 1784

Prostatitis
Ancef Injection (Cefazolin Sodium) SmithKline Beecham Pharmaceuticals 2632
Floxin I.V. (Ofloxacin) McNeil Pharmaceutical 1580
Floxin Tablets (200 mg, 300 mg, 400 mg) (Ofloxacin) McNeil Pharmaceutical 1577
Geocillin Tablets (Carbenicillin Indanyl Sodium) Pfizer Inc 2009
Keflex Pulvules & Oral Suspension (Cephalexin) Dista 930
Keftab Tablets (Cephalexin Hydrochloride) Dista 931
Noroxin Tablets (Norfloxacin) Merck & Co., Inc. 1758
Noroxin Tablets (Norfloxacin) Roberts 2222

Prostatitis, frequency and incontinence, symptomatic relief of
Urispas Tablets (Flavoxate Hydrochloride) SmithKline Beecham Pharmaceuticals 2710

Prostatitis, "lacking substantial evidence of effectiveness" in
Urobiotic-250 Capsules (Oxytetracycline Hydrochloride, Sulfamethizole, Phenazopyridine Hydrochloride) Pfizer Inc 2038

Proteinuria, remission of in nephrotic syndrome
Celestone Soluspan Suspension (Betamethasone Sodium Phosphate, Betamethasone Acetate) Schering 2484
Cortone Acetate Sterile Suspension (Cortisone Acetate) Merck & Co., Inc. 1663
Cortone Acetate Tablets (Cortisone Acetate) Merck & Co., Inc. 1664
Dalalone D.P. Injectable (Dexamethasone Acetate) Forest 1009
Decadron Elixir (Dexamethasone) Merck & Co., Inc. 1676
Decadron Phosphate Injection (Dexamethasone Sodium Phosphate) Merck & Co., Inc. 1680
Decadron Tablets (Dexamethasone) Merck & Co., Inc. 1678
Decadron-LA Sterile Suspension (Dexamethasone Acetate) Merck & Co., Inc. 1687
Hydeltrasol Injection, Sterile (Prednisolone Sodium Phosphate) Merck & Co., Inc. 1708
Hydrocortone Phosphate Injection, Sterile (Hydrocortisone Sodium Phosphate) Merck & Co., Inc. .. 1713
Hydrocortone Tablets (Hydrocortisone) Merck & Co., Inc. 1715
Pediapred Oral Solution (Prednisolone Sodium Phosphate) Medeva 1618
Prelone Syrup (Prednisolone) Muro 1834

Proteus mirabilis
(see under P. mirabilis infections)

Proteus species bone and joint infections
Nebcin Vials, Hyporets & ADD-Vantage (Tobramycin Sulfate) Lilly 1518

Proteus species gynecologic infections
Primaxin I.V. (Cilastatin Sodium, Imipenem) Merck & Co., Inc. 1772

Proteus species infections
Amikacin Sulfate Injection, USP (Amikacin Sulfate) Astra 523
Amikacin Sulfate Injection, USP (Amikacin Sulfate) Elkins-Sinn 981
Amikin Injectable (Amikacin Sulfate) Apothecon 502
Bactrim I.V. Infusion (Trimethoprim, Sulfamethoxazole) Roche Pharmaceuticals 2255
Cefobid Intravenous/Intramuscular (Cefoperazone Sodium) Pfizer Inc 1996
Cefobid Pharmacy Bulk Package - Not for Direct Infusion (Cefoperazone Sodium) Pfizer Inc 1999
Cefotan (Cefotetan) Zeneca 2936
Ceptaz (Ceftazidime) Glaxo Wellcome 1070
Fortaz (Ceftazidime) Glaxo Wellcome 1092
Garamycin Injectable (Gentamicin Sulfate) Schering 2502
Monocid Injection (Cefonicid Sodium) SmithKline Beecham Pharmaceuticals 2674
Nebcin Vials, Hyporets & ADD-Vantage (Tobramycin Sulfate) Lilly 1518
NegGram (Nalidixic Acid) Sanofi Winthrop 2453
Netromycin Injection 100 mg/ml (Netilmicin Sulfate) Schering 2516
Pipracil (Piperacillin Sodium) Lederle 1435

Primaxin I.V. (Cilastatin Sodium, Imipenem) Merck & Co., Inc. 1772
Septra I.V. Infusion (Trimethoprim, Sulfamethoxazole) Glaxo Wellcome 1142
Septra I.V. Infusion ADD-Vantage Vials (Trimethoprim, Sulfamethoxazole) Glaxo Wellcome 1144
Tazicef for Injection (Ceftazidime) SmithKline Beecham Pharmaceuticals 2697
Tazidime Vials, Faspak & ADD-Vantage (Ceftazidime) Lilly .. 1531
TERAK Ointment (Oxytetracycline Hydrochloride, Polymyxin B Sulfate) Akorn .... ◎ 210
Ticar for Injection (Ticarcillin Disodium) SmithKline Beecham Pharmaceuticals 2704

Proteus species infections, ocular
TERAK Ointment (Oxytetracycline Hydrochloride, Polymyxin B Sulfate) Akorn .... ◎ 210
Terramycin with Polymyxin B Sulfate Ophthalmic Ointment (Oxytetracycline Hydrochloride, Polymyxin B Sulfate) Pfizer Inc ... 2035

Proteus species infections, ocular, indole-negative
Pred-G Liquifilm Sterile Ophthalmic Suspension (Gentamicin Sulfate, Prednisolone Acetate) Allergan .... ◎ 248

Proteus species intra-abdominal infections
Netromycin Injection 100 mg/ml (Netilmicin Sulfate) Schering......... 2516
Primaxin I.V. (Cilastatin Sodium, Imipenem) Merck & Co., Inc. 1772

Proteus species lower respiratory tract infections
Netromycin Injection 100 mg/ml (Netilmicin Sulfate) Schering......... 2516
Ticar for Injection (Ticarcillin Disodium) SmithKline Beecham Pharmaceuticals 2704

Proteus species septicemia
Cefobid Intravenous/Intramuscular (Cefoperazone Sodium) Pfizer Inc 1996
Cefobid Pharmacy Bulk Package - Not for Direct Infusion (Cefoperazone Sodium) Pfizer Inc 1999
Ticar for Injection (Ticarcillin Disodium) SmithKline Beecham Pharmaceuticals 2704

Proteus species skin and skin structure infections
Ceptaz (Ceftazidime) Glaxo Wellcome 1070
Fortaz (Ceftazidime) Glaxo Wellcome 1092
Nebcin Vials, Hyporets & ADD-Vantage (Tobramycin Sulfate) Lilly 1518
Netromycin Injection 100 mg/ml (Netilmicin Sulfate) Schering......... 2516
Tazicef for Injection (Ceftazidime) SmithKline Beecham Pharmaceuticals 2697
Tazidime Vials, Faspak & ADD-Vantage (Ceftazidime) Lilly .. 1531
Ticar for Injection (Ticarcillin Disodium) SmithKline Beecham Pharmaceuticals 2704

Proteus species urinary tract infections
Bactrim I.V. Infusion (Trimethoprim, Sulfamethoxazole) Roche Pharmaceuticals 2255
Cefotan (Cefotetan) Zeneca 2936
Ceptaz (Ceftazidime) Glaxo Wellcome 1070
Fortaz (Ceftazidime) Glaxo Wellcome 1092
Mandol Vials, Faspak & ADD-Vantage (Cefamandole Nafate) Lilly 1516
Monocid Injection (Cefonicid Sodium) SmithKline Beecham Pharmaceuticals 2674
Nebcin Vials, Hyporets & ADD-Vantage (Tobramycin Sulfate) Lilly 1518

(▣ Described in PDR For Nonprescription Drugs)   (◎ Described in PDR For Ophthalmology)

Proteus species

- NegGram (Nalidixic Acid) Sanofi Winthrop ... 2453
- Netromycin Injection 100 mg/ml (Netilmicin Sulfate) Schering ... 2516
- Septra I.V. Infusion (Trimethoprim, Sulfamethoxazole) Glaxo Wellcome ... 1142
- Septra I.V. Infusion ADD-Vantage Vials (Trimethoprim, Sulfamethoxazole) Glaxo Wellcome ... 1144
- Streptomycin Sulfate Injection (Streptomycin Sulfate) Pfizer Inc ... 2031
- Tazicef for Injection (Ceftazidime) SmithKline Beecham Pharmaceuticals ... 2697
- Tazidime Vials, Faspak & ADD-Vantage (Ceftazidime) Lilly ... 1531

Proteus vulgaris
(see under P. vulgaris infections)

Proteus, indole-positive, infections
(see under Morganella morganii infections)

Prothrombin deficiency, anticoagulant-induced

- AquaMEPHYTON Injection (Phytonadione) Merck & Co., Inc. ... 1648
- Mephyton Tablets (Phytonadione) Merck & Co., Inc. ... 1739

Providencia rettgeri infections

- Amikacin Sulfate Injection, USP (Amikacin Sulfate) Astra ... 523
- Amikacin Sulfate Injection, USP (Amikacin Sulfate) Elkins-Sinn ... 981
- Amikin Injectable (Amikacin Sulfate) Apothecon ... 502
- Cefizox for Intramuscular or Intravenous Use (Ceftizoxime Sodium) Fujisawa ... 1025
- Cefotan (Cefotetan) Zeneca ... 2936
- Cipro I.V. (Ciprofloxacin) Bayer Pharmaceutical ... 587
- Cipro I.V. Pharmacy Bulk Package (Ciprofloxacin) Bayer Pharmaceutical ... 590
- Cipro Tablets (Ciprofloxacin Hydrochloride) Bayer Pharmaceutical ... 584
- Claforan Sterile and Injection (Cefotaxime Sodium) Hoechst Marion Roussel ... 1259
- Geocillin Tablets (Carbenicillin Indanyl Sodium) Pfizer Inc ... 2009
- Mefoxin (Cefoxitin Sodium) Merck & Co., Inc. ... 1734
- Mefoxin Premixed Intravenous Solution (Cefoxitin Sodium) Merck & Co., Inc. ... 1737
- Mezlin (Mezlocillin Sodium) Bayer Pharmaceutical ... 594
- Mezlin Pharmacy Bulk Package (Mezlocillin Sodium) Bayer Pharmaceutical ... 597
- Monocid Injection (Cefonicid Sodium) SmithKline Beecham Pharmaceuticals ... 2674
- Primaxin I.V. (Cilastatin Sodium, Imipenem) Merck & Co., Inc. ... 1772

Providencia rettgeri skin and skin structure infections

- Claforan Sterile and Injection (Cefotaxime Sodium) Hoechst Marion Roussel ... 1259
- Mezlin (Mezlocillin Sodium) Bayer Pharmaceutical ... 594
- Mezlin Pharmacy Bulk Package (Mezlocillin Sodium) Bayer Pharmaceutical ... 597
- Primaxin I.V. (Cilastatin Sodium, Imipenem) Merck & Co., Inc. ... 1772

Providencia rettgeri urinary tract infections

- Cefizox for Intramuscular or Intravenous Use (Ceftizoxime Sodium) Fujisawa ... 1025
- Cefotan (Cefotetan) Zeneca ... 2936
- Cipro I.V. (Ciprofloxacin) Bayer Pharmaceutical ... 587
- Cipro I.V. Pharmacy Bulk Package (Ciprofloxacin) Bayer Pharmaceutical ... 590
- Cipro Tablets (Ciprofloxacin Hydrochloride) Bayer Pharmaceutical ... 584

- Claforan Sterile and Injection (Cefotaxime Sodium) Hoechst Marion Roussel ... 1259
- Geocillin Tablets (Carbenicillin Indanyl Sodium) Pfizer Inc ... 2009
- Mefoxin (Cefoxitin Sodium) Merck & Co., Inc. ... 1734
- Mefoxin Premixed Intravenous Solution (Cefoxitin Sodium) Merck & Co., Inc. ... 1737
- Monocid Injection (Cefonicid Sodium) SmithKline Beecham Pharmaceuticals ... 2674
- Primaxin I.V. (Cilastatin Sodium, Imipenem) Merck & Co., Inc. ... 1772

Providencia species infections

- Amikacin Sulfate Injection, USP (Amikacin Sulfate) Astra ... 523
- Amikacin Sulfate Injection, USP (Amikacin Sulfate) Elkins-Sinn ... 981
- Amikin Injectable (Amikacin Sulfate) Apothecon ... 502
- Mefoxin (Cefoxitin Sodium) Merck & Co., Inc. ... 1734
- Mefoxin Premixed Intravenous Solution (Cefoxitin Sodium) Merck & Co., Inc. ... 1737
- Nebcin Vials, Hyporets & ADD-Vantage (Tobramycin Sulfate) Lilly ... 1518

Providencia species urinary tract infections

- Mefoxin (Cefoxitin Sodium) Merck & Co., Inc. ... 1734
- Nebcin Vials, Hyporets & ADD-Vantage (Tobramycin Sulfate) Lilly ... 1518

Providencia stuartii infections

- Amikacin Sulfate Injection, USP (Amikacin Sulfate) Astra ... 523
- Amikacin Sulfate Injection, USP (Amikacin Sulfate) Elkins-Sinn ... 981
- Amikin Injectable (Amikacin Sulfate) Apothecon ... 502
- Cipro I.V. (Ciprofloxacin) Bayer Pharmaceutical ... 587
- Cipro I.V. Pharmacy Bulk Package (Ciprofloxacin) Bayer Pharmaceutical ... 590
- Cipro Tablets (Ciprofloxacin Hydrochloride) Bayer Pharmaceutical ... 584

Providencia stuartii skin and skin structure infections

- Cipro I.V. (Ciprofloxacin) Bayer Pharmaceutical ... 587
- Cipro I.V. Pharmacy Bulk Package (Ciprofloxacin) Bayer Pharmaceutical ... 590
- Cipro Tablets (Ciprofloxacin Hydrochloride) Bayer Pharmaceutical ... 584

Pruritus ani
(see also under Pruritus, anogenital)

- Anusol-HC Suppositories (Hydrocortisone Acetate) Parke-Davis ... 1954
- PrameGel (Pramoxine Hydrochloride) GenDerm ... 1042
- Preparation H Hydrocortisone 1% Cream (Hydrocortisone) Whitehall-Robins ... 843

Pruritus associated with partial biliary obstruction

- Questran (Cholestyramine) Bristol-Myers Squibb ... 774

Pruritus, anogenital

- Americaine Hemorrhoidal Ointment (Benzocaine) Ciba Self-Medication ... 649
- Analpram-HC Rectal Cream 1% and 2.5% (Hydrocortisone Acetate, Pramoxine Hydrochloride) Ferndale ... 993
- Caldecort Anti-Itch Hydrocortisone Cream (Hydrocortisone Acetate) Ciba Self-Medication ... 651
- Cortaid (Hydrocortisone Acetate) Upjohn ... 800
- Cortizone-5 (Hydrocortisone) Thompson Medical ... 795
- Cortizone-10 (Hydrocortisone) Thompson Medical ... 795

- Mantadil Cream (Chlorcyclizine Hydrochloride) Glaxo Wellcome ... 1124
- Nupercainal Hydrocortisone 1% Cream (Hydrocortisone Acetate) Ciba Self-Medication ... 661
- Preparation H (Glycerin, Petrolatum, Phenylephrine Hydrochloride, Shark Liver Oil) Whitehall-Robins ... 842
- ProctoFoam-HC (Hydrocortisone Acetate, Pramoxine Hydrochloride) Schwarz ... 2552
- Tronolane Anesthetic Cream for Hemorrhoids (Pramoxine Hydrochloride) Ross ... 746
- Tronolane Hemorrhoidal Suppositories (Fat, Hard, Zinc Oxide) Ross ... 747
- Tucks Pads (Witch Hazel) Warner Wellcome ... 830
- Wyanoids Relief Factor Hemorrhoidal Suppositories (Liver, Desiccated, Shark Liver Oil) Wyeth-Ayerst ... 856

Pruritus, ocular

- Acular Sterile Ophthalmic Solution (Ketorolac Tromethamine) Allergan ... 470
- Naphcon-A Ophthalmic Solution (Naphazoline Hydrochloride, Pheniramine Maleate) Alcon Laboratories ... 469
- OcuHist (Naphazoline Hydrochloride, Pheniramine Maleate) Pfizer Consumer ... 300

Pruritus, rhinopharyngeal, symptomatic relief of

- Benadryl Allergy Decongestant Tablets (Diphenhydramine Hydrochloride, Pseudoephedrine Hydrochloride) Warner Wellcome ... 812
- Benadryl Allergy Liquid Medication (Diphenhydramine Hydrochloride) Warner Wellcome ... 813
- Benadryl Allergy (Diphenhydramine Hydrochloride) Warner Wellcome ... 811
- Benadryl Allergy Sinus Headache Caplets (Diphenhydramine Hydrochloride, Pseudoephedrine Hydrochloride, Acetaminophen) Warner Wellcome ... 813
- Nolahist Tablets (Phenindamine Tartrate) Carnrick ... 790
- Novahistine Elixir (Chlorpheniramine Maleate, Phenylephrine Hydrochloride) SmithKline Beecham Consumer ... 782
- Sinulin Tablets (Acetaminophen, Phenylpropanolamine Hydrochloride, Chlorpheniramine Maleate) Carnrick ... 792
- Tavist Syrup (Clemastine Fumarate) Sandoz Pharmaceuticals ... 2426
- Triaminic Syrup (Phenylpropanolamine Hydrochloride, Chlorpheniramine Maleate) Sandoz Consumer ... 755
- TYLENOL Severe Allergy Medication Caplets (Acetaminophen, Chlorpheniramine Maleate, Pseudoephedrine Hydrochloride) McNeil Consumer ... 1571

Pruritus, systemic relief of

- Atarax Tablets & Syrup (Hydroxyzine Hydrochloride) Pfizer Inc ... 1992
- Itch-X (Pramoxine Hydrochloride, Benzyl Alcohol) Ascher ... 607
- Seldane Tablets (Terfenadine) Hoechst Marion Roussel ... 1284
- Seldane-D Extended-Release Tablets (Pseudoephedrine Hydrochloride, Terfenadine) Hoechst Marion Roussel ... 1286
- Vistaril Capsules (Hydroxyzine Pamoate) Pfizer Inc ... 2042
- Vistaril Intramuscular Solution (Hydroxyzine Hydrochloride) Pfizer Inc ... 2042
- Vistaril Oral Suspension (Hydroxyzine Pamoate) Pfizer Inc ... 2042

Pruritus, topical relief of
(see also under Pruritus, systemic relief of)

- Aclovate (Alclometasone Dipropionate) Glaxo Wellcome ... 1061
- Americaine (Benzocaine) Ciba Self-Medication ... 649
- Anusol HC-1 Hydrocortisone Anti-Itch Ointment (Hydrocortisone Acetate) Warner Wellcome ... 810
- Anusol-HC Cream 2.5% (Hydrocortisone) Parke-Davis ... 1953
- Benadryl Itch Relief Stick Extra Strength (Diphenhydramine Hydrochloride, Zinc Acetate) Warner Wellcome ... 814
- Benadryl Cream (Diphenhydramine Hydrochloride, Zinc Acetate) Warner Wellcome ... 814
- Benadryl Gel (Diphenhydramine Hydrochloride, Zinc Acetate) Warner Wellcome ... 815
- Benadryl Spray (Diphenhydramine Hydrochloride, Zinc Acetate) Warner Wellcome ... 815
- BiCozene Creme (Benzocaine, Resorcinol) Sandoz Consumer ... 747
- Caladryl Cream For Kids (Calamine, Pramoxine Hydrochloride) Warner Wellcome ... 817
- Caldecort Anti-Itch Hydrocortisone Cream (Hydrocortisone Acetate) Ciba Self-Medication ... 651
- Cordran Lotion (Flurandrenolide) Oclassen ... 1854
- Cordran Tape (Flurandrenolide) Oclassen ... 1855
- Cortizone-5 Creme and Ointment (Hydrocortisone) Thompson Medical ... 795
- Cortizone-10 Creme and Ointment (Hydrocortisone) Thompson Medical ... 795
- Cutivate Cream (Fluticasone Propionate) Glaxo Wellcome ... 1078
- Cutivate Ointment (Fluticasone Propionate) Glaxo Wellcome ... 1078
- Decadron Phosphate Topical Cream (Dexamethasone Sodium Phosphate) Merck & Co., Inc. ... 1686
- Decaspray Topical Aerosol (Dexamethasone) Merck & Co., Inc. ... 1689
- Dermatop Emollient Cream 0.1% (Prednicarbate) Hoechst Marion Roussel ... 1264
- DesOwen Cream, Ointment and Lotion (Desonide) Galderma ... 1032
- Diprolene AF Cream 0.05% (Betamethasone Dipropionate) Schering ... 2489
- Diprolene Lotion 0.05% (Betamethasone Dipropionate) Schering ... 2491
- Diprolene Ointment 0.05% (Betamethasone Dipropionate) Schering ... 2491
- Elocon Cream 0.1% (Mometasone Furoate) Schering ... 2492
- Elocon Lotion 0.1% (Mometasone Furoate) Schering ... 2493
- Elocon Ointment 0.1% (Mometasone Furoate) Schering ... 2494
- Epifoam (Hydrocortisone Acetate, Pramoxine Hydrochloride) Schwarz ... 2543
- Eurax Cream & Lotion (Crotamiton) Westwood-Squibb ... 2794
- Florone/Florone E (Diflorasone Diacetate) Dermik ... 921
- Halog (Halcinonide) Westwood-Squibb ... 2795
- Hytone (Hydrocortisone) Dermik ... 922
- Hytone Ointment 2 ½% (Hydrocortisone) Dermik ... 923
- Lac-Hydrin 12% Lotion (Ammonium Lactate) Westwood-Squibb ... 2796
- Lidex (Fluocinonide) Roche Pharmaceuticals ... 2299
- Locoid Cream, Ointment and Topical Solution (Hydrocortisone Butyrate) Ferndale ... 994
- Mantadil Cream (Chlorcyclizine Hydrochloride) Glaxo Wellcome ... 1124
- Massengill Medicated Soft Cloth Towelettes (Hydrocortisone) SmithKline Beecham ... 2628
- PrameGel (Pramoxine Hydrochloride) GenDerm ... 1042
- Pramosone Cream, Lotion & Ointment (Hydrocortisone Acetate, Pramoxine Hydrochloride) Ferndale ... 995

1565 **Indications Index** **Purpura**

Preparation H Hydrocortisone 1% Cream (Hydrocortisone) Whitehall-Robins ▣ 843
Psorcon Ointment 0.05% (Diflorasone Diacetate) Dermik 923
Synalar (Fluocinolone Acetonide) Roche Pharmaceuticals 2299
Temovate Gel (Clobetasol Propionate) Glaxo Wellcome 1153
Temovate Scalp Application (Clobetasol Propionate) Glaxo Wellcome 1153
Topicort Emollient Cream 0.25% (Desoximetasone) Hoechst Marion Roussel 1289
Topicort Gel 0.05% (Desoximetasone) Hoechst Marion Roussel 1290
Topicort LP Emollient Cream 0.05% (Desoximetasone) Hoechst Marion Roussel 1289
Topicort Ointment 0.25% (Desoximetasone) Hoechst Marion Roussel 1291
Tridesilon Cream 0.05% (Desonide) Bayer Pharmaceutical 609
Tridesilon Ointment 0.05% (Desonide) Bayer Pharmaceutical 610
Ultravate Cream 0.05% (Halobetasol Propionate) Westwood-Squibb 2797
Ultravate Ointment 0.05% (Halobetasol Propionate) Westwood-Squibb 2798
Unguentine Plus (Lidocaine Hydrochloride, Phenol) Mentholatum ▣ 712
Westcort Cream 0.2% (Hydrocortisone Valerate) Westwood-Squibb 2799
Westcort Ointment 0.2% (Hydrocortisone Valerate) Westwood-Squibb 2800
Xylocaine 2.5% Ointment (Lidocaine) Astra ▣ 608
Zonalon Cream (Doxepin Hydrochloride) GenDerm 1042

Pruritus, vaginal
Betadine Medicated Douche (Povidone Iodine) Purdue Frederick 2144
Betadine Medicated Gel (Povidone Iodine) Purdue Frederick 2144
Betadine Medicated Vaginal Suppositories (Povidone Iodine) Purdue Frederick 2145
Cortaid (Hydrocortisone Acetate) Upjohn ▣ 800

Pseudomonas aeruginosa infections (see under P. aeruginosa infections)

Pseudomonas species bone and joint infections
Claforan Sterile and Injection (Cefotaxime Sodium) Hoechst Marion Roussel 1259

Pseudomonas species infections
Amikacin Sulfate Injection, USP (Amikacin Sulfate) Astra 523
Amikacin Sulfate Injection, USP (Amikacin Sulfate) Elkins-Sinn 981
Amikin Injectable (Amikacin Sulfate) Apothecon 502
Cefizox for Intramuscular or Intravenous Use (Ceftizoxime Sodium) Fujisawa 1025
Ceptaz (Ceftazidime) Glaxo Wellcome 1070
Claforan Sterile and Injection (Cefotaxime Sodium) Hoechst Marion Roussel 1259
Fortaz (Ceftazidime) Glaxo Wellcome 1092
Geocillin Tablets (Carbenicillin Indanyl Sodium) Pfizer Inc 2009
Mezlin (Mezlocillin Sodium) Bayer Pharmaceutical 594
Mezlin Pharmacy Bulk Package (Mezlocillin Sodium) Bayer Pharmaceutical 597
Pipracil (Piperacillin Sodium) Lederle 1435
Tazicef for Injection (Ceftazidime) SmithKline Beecham Pharmaceuticals 2697
Tazidime Vials, Faspak & ADD-Vantage (Ceftazidime) Lilly 1531

Pseudomonas species infections, ocular
AK-CIDE (Prednisolone Acetate, Sulfacetamide Sodium) Akorn ⊙ 203
AK-CIDE Ointment (Prednisolone Acetate, Sulfacetamide Sodium) Akorn ⊙ 203
Blephamide Liquifilm Sterile Ophthalmic Suspension (Prednisolone Acetate, Sulfacetamide Sodium) Allergan 472
Chibroxin Sterile Ophthalmic Solution (Norfloxacin) Merck & Co., Inc. 1657
Maxitrol Ophthalmic Ointment and Suspension (Dexamethasone, Neomycin Sulfate, Polymyxin B Sulfate) Alcon Laboratories ⊙ 222

Pseudomonas species lower respiratory tract infections
Claforan Sterile and Injection (Cefotaxime Sodium) Hoechst Marion Roussel 1259
Mezlin (Mezlocillin Sodium) Bayer Pharmaceutical 594
Mezlin Pharmacy Bulk Package (Mezlocillin Sodium) Bayer Pharmaceutical 597
Tazicef for Injection (Ceftazidime) SmithKline Beecham Pharmaceuticals 2697
Tazidime Vials, Faspak & ADD-Vantage (Ceftazidime) Lilly 1531

Pseudomonas species septicemia
Mezlin (Mezlocillin Sodium) Bayer Pharmaceutical 594
Mezlin Pharmacy Bulk Package (Mezlocillin Sodium) Bayer Pharmaceutical 597
Timentin for Injection (Ticarcillin Disodium, Clavulanate Potassium) SmithKline Beecham Pharmaceuticals 2706

Pseudomonas species skin and skin structure infections
Claforan Sterile and Injection (Cefotaxime Sodium) Hoechst Marion Roussel 1259
Mezlin (Mezlocillin Sodium) Bayer Pharmaceutical 594
Mezlin Pharmacy Bulk Package (Mezlocillin Sodium) Bayer Pharmaceutical 597

Pseudomonas species urinary tract infections
Cefizox for Intramuscular or Intravenous Use (Ceftizoxime Sodium) Fujisawa 1025
Claforan Sterile and Injection (Cefotaxime Sodium) Hoechst Marion Roussel 1259
Geocillin Tablets (Carbenicillin Indanyl Sodium) Pfizer Inc 2009
Mezlin (Mezlocillin Sodium) Bayer Pharmaceutical 594
Mezlin Pharmacy Bulk Package (Mezlocillin Sodium) Bayer Pharmaceutical 597
Timentin for Injection (Ticarcillin Disodium, Clavulanate Potassium) SmithKline Beecham Pharmaceuticals 2706

Psittacosis (see under Chlamydia psittaci infection)

Psoriasis
Cortizone-5 (Hydrocortisone) Thompson Medical ▣ 795
DHS (Coal Tar) Persōn & Covey 1989
Dovonex Cream 0.005% (Calcipotriene) Westwood-Squibb 2792
Dovonex Ointment 0.005% (Calcipotriene) Westwood-Squibb 2793
Drithocreme 0.1%, 0.25%, 0.5%, 1.0% (HP) (Anthralin) Dermik 920
Dritho-Scalp 0.25%, 0.5% (Anthralin) Dermik 921
Fototar Cream (Coal Tar) ICN 1300
MG 217 (Coal Tar) Triton Consumer ▣ 800
Oxsoralen-Ultra Capsules (Methoxsalen) ICN 1302
Pentrax Shampoo (Coal Tar) GenDerm 1042
Tegrin Dandruff Shampoo (Coal Tar) Block ▣ 634
Tegrin Skin Cream & Tegrin Medicated Soap (Coal Tar) Block ▣ 634

Psoriasis, erythrodermic
Tegison Capsules (Etretinate) Roche Pharmaceuticals 2314

Psoriasis, generalized pustular
Tegison Capsules (Etretinate) Roche Pharmaceuticals 2314

Psoriasis, pustular
Garamycin 0.1% (Gentamicin Sulfate) Schering 2501
Tegison Capsules (Etretinate) Roche Pharmaceuticals 2314

Psoriasis, severe
Celestone Soluspan Suspension (Betamethasone Sodium Phosphate, Betamethasone Acetate) Schering 2484
Cortone Acetate Sterile Suspension (Cortisone Acetate) Merck & Co., Inc. 1663
Cortone Acetate Tablets (Cortisone Acetate) Merck & Co., Inc. 1664
Dalalone D.P. Injectable (Dexamethasone Acetate) Forest 1009
Decadron Elixir (Dexamethasone) Merck & Co., Inc. 1676
Decadron Phosphate Injection (Dexamethasone Sodium Phosphate) Merck & Co., Inc. 1680
Decadron Tablets (Dexamethasone) Merck & Co., Inc. 1678
Decadron-LA Sterile Suspension (Dexamethasone Acetate) Merck & Co., Inc. 1687
Hydeltrasol Injection, Sterile (Prednisolone Sodium Phosphate) Merck & Co., Inc. 1708
Hydrocortone Phosphate Injection, Sterile (Hydrocortisone Sodium Phosphate) Merck & Co., Inc. 1713
Hydrocortone Tablets (Hydrocortisone) Merck & Co., Inc. 1715
Pediapred Oral Solution (Prednisolone Sodium Phosphate) Medeva 1618
Prelone Syrup (Prednisolone) Muro 1834

Psoriasis, severe recalcitrant
Methotrexate Sodium Tablets, Injection, for Injection and LPF Injection (Methotrexate Sodium) Immunex 1322
8-MOP Capsules (Methoxsalen) ICN 1294
Tegison Capsules (Etretinate) Roche Pharmaceuticals 2314

Psoriatic arthritis (see under Arthritis, psoriatic)

Psoriatic plaques
Celestone Soluspan Suspension (Betamethasone Sodium Phosphate, Betamethasone Acetate) Schering 2484
Decadron Phosphate Injection (Dexamethasone Sodium Phosphate) Merck & Co., Inc. 1680
Decadron-LA Sterile Suspension (Dexamethasone Acetate) Merck & Co., Inc. 1687
Dovonex Cream 0.005% (Calcipotriene) Westwood-Squibb 2792
Dovonex Ointment 0.005% (Calcipotriene) Westwood-Squibb 2793
Hydeltrasol Injection, Sterile (Prednisolone Sodium Phosphate) Merck & Co., Inc. 1708
Hydrocortone Acetate Sterile Suspension (Hydrocortisone Acetate) Merck & Co., Inc. 1712

Psychotic disorders with depressive symptoms
Etrafon (Perphenazine, Amitriptyline Hydrochloride) Schering 2495
Triavil Tablets (Perphenazine, Amitriptyline Hydrochloride) Merck & Co., Inc. 1800

Psychotic disorders, management of the manifestations in severely ill
Clozaril Tablets (Clozapine) Sandoz Pharmaceuticals 2377

Psychotic disorders, management of the manifestations of (see also under Psychotic disorders, management of the manifestations in severely ill)
Compazine (Prochlorperazine) SmithKline Beecham Pharmaceuticals 2644
Haldol Decanoate (Haloperidol Decanoate) McNeil Pharmaceutical 1587
Haldol Injection, Tablets and Concentrate (Haloperidol) McNeil Pharmaceutical 1585
Loxitane (Loxapine Hydrochloride) Lederle 1426
Mellaril (Thioridazine Hydrochloride) Sandoz Pharmaceuticals 2398
Moban Tablets and Concentrate (Molindone Hydrochloride) Gate 1036
Navane Capsules and Concentrate (Thiothixene) Pfizer Inc 2018
Navane Intramuscular (Thiothixene) Pfizer Inc 2019
Prolixin (Fluphenazine Decanoate) Apothecon 510
Risperdal Tablets (Risperidone) Janssen 1348
Serentil (Mesoridazine Besylate) Boehringer Ingelheim 689
Stelazine (Trifluoperazine Hydrochloride) SmithKline Beecham Pharmaceuticals 2692
Thorazine (Chlorpromazine Hydrochloride) SmithKline Beecham Pharmaceuticals 2701
Trilafon (Perphenazine) Schering 2532

Puberty, central precocious
Lupron Depot-PED 7.5 mg, 11.25 mg and 15 mg (Leuprolide Acetate) TAP 2744
Lupron Injection Pediatric (Leuprolide Acetate) TAP 2737
Supprelin Injection (Histrelin Acetate) Roberts 2230
Synarel Nasal Solution for Central Precocious Puberty (Nafarelin Acetate) Searle 2603

Puberty, delayed, in male
Android Capsules, 10 mg (Methyltestosterone) ICN 1297
Halotestin Tablets (Fluoxymesterone) Pharmacia & Upjohn 2095
Testred Capsules, 10 mg (Methyltestosterone) ICN 1308

Pulmonary disease, obstruction, exacerbation of
Zithromax (Azithromycin) Pfizer Inc 2043
Zithromax Tablets (Azithromycin) Pfizer Inc 2046

Pulmonary emphysema (see under Emphysema)

Pupil, dilatation of (see under Mydriasis, production of)

Purpura, idiopathic thrombocytopenic
Cortone Acetate Tablets (Cortisone Acetate) Merck & Co., Inc. 1664
Dalalone D.P. Injectable (Dexamethasone Acetate) Forest 1009
Decadron Elixir (Dexamethasone) Merck & Co., Inc. 1676
Decadron Phosphate Injection (Dexamethasone Sodium Phosphate) Merck & Co., Inc. 1680
Decadron Tablets (Dexamethasone) Merck & Co., Inc. 1678
Gamimune N, 5% Immune Globulin Intravenous (Human), 5% (Globulin, Immune (Human)) Bayer Biological 612
Gamimune N, 10% Immune Globulin Intravenous (Human),

(▣ Described in PDR For Nonprescription Drugs) (⊙ Described in PDR For Ophthalmology)

Purpura

10% (Globulin, Immune (Human)) Bayer Biological 615
Gammagard S/D, Immune Globulin, Intravenous (Human) (Globulin, Immune (Human)) Baxter Healthcare 577
Hydeltrasol Injection, Sterile (Prednisolone Sodium Phosphate) Merck & Co., Inc. 1708
Hydrocortone Phosphate Injection, Sterile (Hydrocortisone Sodium Phosphate) Merck & Co., Inc. 1713
Hydrocortone Tablets (Hydrocortisone) Merck & Co., Inc. 1715
Pediapred Oral Solution (Prednisolone Sodium Phosphate) Medeva 1618
Prelone Syrup (Prednisolone) Muro 1834
Sandoglobulin I.V. (Globulin, Immune (Human)) Sandoz Pharmaceuticals 2419
WinRho SD (Rho(D) Immune Globulin (Human)) NABI 1840

Pyelitis

Gantanol Tablets (Sulfamethoxazole) Roche Pharmaceuticals 2285
Gantrisin (Acetyl Sulfisoxazole) Roche Pharmaceuticals 2286
Uroqid-Acid No. 2 Tablets (Methenamine Mandelate, Sodium Acid Phosphate) Beach 633

Pyelitis, "lacking substantial evidence of effectiveness" in

Urobiotic-250 Capsules (Oxytetracycline Hydrochloride, Sulfamethizole, Phenazopyridine Hydrochloride) Pfizer Inc 2038

Pyelonephritis

Azactam for Injection (Aztreonam) Bristol-Myers Squibb 736
Ceclor Pulvules & Suspension (Cefaclor) Lilly 1470
Gantanol Tablets (Sulfamethoxazole) Roche Pharmaceuticals 2285
Gantrisin (Acetyl Sulfisoxazole) Roche Pharmaceuticals 2286
Lorabid Suspension and Pulvules (Loracarbef) Lilly 1513
Maxipime for Injection (Cefepime Hydrochloride) Bristol-Myers Squibb 758
Uroqid-Acid No. 2 Tablets (Methenamine Mandelate, Sodium Acid Phosphate) Beach 633

Pyelonephritis, "lacking substantial evidence of effectiveness" in

Urobiotic-250 Capsules (Oxytetracycline Hydrochloride, Sulfamethizole, Phenazopyridine Hydrochloride) Pfizer Inc 2038

Pyoderma gangrenosum

Garamycin 0.1% (Gentamicin Sulfate) Schering 2501

Q

Q fever

Achromycin V Capsules (Tetracycline Hydrochloride) Lederle 1417
Declomycin Tablets (Demeclocycline Hydrochloride) Lederle 1421
Doryx Capsules (Doxycycline Hyclate) Parke-Davis 1970
DYNACIN Capsules (Minocycline Hydrochloride) Medicis 1627
Minocin Intravenous (Minocycline Hydrochloride) Lederle 1428
Minocin Oral Suspension (Minocycline Hydrochloride) Lederle 1431
Minocin Pellet-Filled Capsules (Minocycline Hydrochloride) Lederle 1429
Monodox Capsules (Doxycycline Monohydrate) Oclassen 1858
Terramycin Intramuscular Solution (Oxytetracycline) Pfizer Inc 2034
Vibramycin (Doxycycline Calcium) Pfizer Inc 2038
Vibramycin Hyclate Intravenous (Doxycycline Hyclate) Pfizer Inc... 2040
Vibramycin (Doxycycline Monohydrate) Pfizer Inc 2038

R

Rabies, postexposure prophylaxis

Hyperab Rabies Immune Globulin (Human) (Rabies Immune Globulin (Human)) Bayer Biological 618
Imogam Rabies Immune Globulin (Human) (Rabies Immune Globulin (Human)) Connaught 897
Imovax Rabies Vaccine (Rabies Vaccine) Connaught 899
Rabies Vaccine Adsorbed (Rabies Vaccine) SmithKline Beecham Pharmaceuticals 2686

Radiography, gastrointestinal tract, adjunct in

Glucagon for Injection Vials and Emergency Kit (Glucagon) Lilly 1485
Reglan (Metoclopramide Hydrochloride) Robins 2243

Rash, diaper

A and D Medicated Diaper Rash Ointment (Petrolatum, White, Zinc Oxide) Schering-Plough HealthCare............ ⊞ 757
A and D Ointment (Petrolatum, Lanolin) Schering-Plough HealthCare............ ⊞ 757
Balmex Ointment (Zinc Oxide) Block............ ⊞ 631
Borofax Skin Protectant Ointment (Zinc Oxide, Petrolatum, White) Warner Wellcome............ ⊞ 817
Caldesene (Petrolatum, White, Zinc Oxide) Ciba Self-Medication............ ⊞ 652
Daily Care from DESITIN (Zinc Oxide) Pfizer Consumer............ ⊞ 715
Desitin Cornstarch Baby Powder (Zinc Oxide, Corn Starch) Pfizer Consumer............ ⊞ 715
Desitin Ointment (Cod Liver Oil, Zinc Oxide) Pfizer Consumer...... ⊞ 715
Impregon Concentrate (Tetrachlorosalicylanilide) Fleming 1003
Moisturel Cream (Dimethicone, Petrolatum) Westwood-Squibb... 2796

Rash, unspecified
(see under Skin, inflammatory conditions)

Rat-bite fever
(see under Streptobacillus moniliformis infections; Spirillum minus infections)

RDS
(see under Respiratory distress syndrome)

Regional enteritis
(see under Enteritis, protozoal)

Reiter's syndrome

Extra Strength Bayer Arthritis Pain Regimen Formula (Aspirin, Enteric Coated) Bayer Consumer............ ⊞ 615
Ecotrin (Aspirin) SmithKline Beecham 2625

Relapsing fever
(see under Borrelia recurrentis infection)

Renal calculi, calcium oxalate, recurrence, management of

Zyloprim Tablets (Allopurinol) Glaxo Wellcome............ 1194

Renal homotransplantation, adjunct for the prevention of rejection in

Azathioprine Tablets (Azathioprine) Roxane 2349
Imuran (Azathioprine) Glaxo Wellcome 1103

Renal plasma flow, estimation of

Aminohippurate Sodium Injection (Aminohippurate Sodium) Merck & Co., Inc. 1646

Renal toxicity, cumulative, cisplatin-induced

Ethyol (amifostine) for Injection (Amifostine) Alza 485

Renal transplantation, prevention of rejection in

CellCept Capsules (Mycophenolate Mofetil) Roche Pharmaceuticals .. 2265
Neoral (Cyclosporine) Sandoz Pharmaceuticals 2405
Orthoclone OKT3 Sterile Solution (Muromonab-CD3) Ortho Biotech 1892
Sandimmune (Cyclosporine) Sandoz Pharmaceuticals............ 2416

Renal tubular acidosis, management of

Urocit-K Tablets (Potassium Citrate) Mission............ 1828

Renal tubular secretory mechanism, measurement of the functional capacity of

Aminohippurate Sodium Injection (Aminohippurate Sodium) Merck & Co., Inc. 1646

Respiratory depression, curare overdosage-induced, treatment adjunct

Mestinon Injectable (Pyridostigmine Bromide) ICN 1300

Respiratory depression, post-anesthesia

Dopram Injectable (Doxapram Hydrochloride) Robins 2235
Tensilon Injectable (Edrophonium Chloride) ICN 1307

Respiratory distress syndrome

Exosurf Neonatal for Intratracheal Suspension (Colfosceril Palmitate) Glaxo Wellcome 1081
Survanta Beractant Intratracheal Suspension (Beractant) Ross 2346

Respiratory insufficiency, acute, with chronic obstructive pulmonary disease

Dopram Injectable (Doxapram Hydrochloride) Robins 2235

Respiratory symptoms, upper, relief of
(see under Influenza syndrome, symptomatic relief of)

Respiratory syncytial virus (RSV) infections
(see under Infections, lower respiratory tract, RSV-induced)

Retinal attachment, surgical aid in

Healon (Sodium Hyaluronate) Pharmacia & Upjohn .... ⊙ 302

Retinal detachment, adjunctive management of

AdatoSil 5000 (Silicone Oil) Escalon Medical .... ⊙ 265
ISPAN Perfluoropropane (Perfluoropropane) Escalon Medical .... ⊙ 267
ISPAN Sulfur Hexafluoride (Sulfur Hexafluoride) Escalon Medical .. ⊙ 266

Retinitis, cytomegalovirus

Cytovene (Ganciclovir Sodium) Roche Pharmaceuticals 2270
Foscavir Injection (Foscarnet Sodium) Astra 541
Vistide Injection (Cidofovir) Gilead Sciences 1057

Retinoblastoma

Cytoxan (Cyclophosphamide) Bristol-Myers Squibb Oncology/Immunology 700

Rhabdomyosarcoma

Cosmegen Injection (Dactinomycin) Merck & Co., Inc. 1666
Oncovin Solution Vials & Hyporets (Vincristine Sulfate) Lilly 1521

Rheumatic carditis, acute

Celestone Soluspan Suspension (Betamethasone Sodium Phosphate, Betamethasone Acetate) Schering 2484
Cortone Acetate Sterile Suspension (Cortisone Acetate) Merck & Co., Inc. 1663
Cortone Acetate Tablets (Cortisone Acetate) Merck & Co., Inc. 1664
Dalalone D.P. Injectable (Dexamethasone Acetate) Forest 1009
Decadron Elixir (Dexamethasone) Merck & Co., Inc. 1676
Decadron Phosphate Injection (Dexamethasone Sodium Phosphate) Merck & Co., Inc. .. 1680
Decadron Tablets (Dexamethasone) Merck & Co., Inc. 1678
Decadron-LA Sterile Suspension (Dexamethasone Acetate) Merck & Co., Inc. 1687
Hydeltrasol Injection, Sterile (Prednisolone Sodium Phosphate) Merck & Co., Inc. 1708
Hydrocortone Phosphate Injection, Sterile (Hydrocortisone Sodium Phosphate) Merck & Co., Inc. .. 1713
Hydrocortone Tablets (Hydrocortisone) Merck & Co., Inc. 1715
Pediapred Oral Solution (Prednisolone Sodium Phosphate) Medeva 1618
Prelone Syrup (Prednisolone) Muro 1834

Rheumatic disorders, unspecified

Regular Strength Ascriptin Tablets (Aspirin Buffered, Calcium Carbonate) Ciba Self-Medication .... ⊞ 650
Mono-Gesic Tablets (Salsalate) Central 810
Salflex Tablets (Salsalate) Carnrick 791

Rheumatic fever, prophylaxis of

Bicillin L-A Injection (Penicillin G Benzathine) Wyeth-Ayerst 2813
E-Mycin Tablets (Erythromycin) Knoll Laboratories 1388
ERYC (Erythromycin) Parke-Davis .. 1972
Erythromycin Base Filmtab (Erythromycin) Abbott 430
Erythromycin Delayed-Release Capsules, USP (Erythromycin) Abbott 431
Ilosone (Erythromycin Estolate) Dista 927
Ilotycin Gluceptate, IV, Vials (Erythromycin Gluceptate) Dista 929
PCE Dispertab Tablets (Erythromycin) Abbott 453
Pen•Vee K (Penicillin V Potassium) Wyeth-Ayerst 2879

Rheumatic heart disease, prophylaxis

E-Mycin Tablets (Erythromycin) Knoll Laboratories 1388

Rheumatoid arthritis

Anaprox/Naprosyn (Naproxen Sodium) Roche Pharmaceuticals.. 2277
Arthritis Pain Ascriptin (Aspirin Buffered, Calcium Carbonate) Ciba Self-Medication .... ⊞ 650
Azathioprine Tablets (Azathioprine) Roxane 2349
Extra Strength Bayer Arthritis Pain Regimen Formula (Aspirin, Enteric Coated) Bayer Consumer............ ⊞ 615
Bayer Enteric Aspirin (Aspirin, Enteric Coated) Bayer Consumer............ ⊞ 613
Cataflam Tablets (Diclofenac Potassium) CibaGeneva 833
Celestone Soluspan Suspension (Betamethasone Sodium Phosphate, Betamethasone Acetate) Schering 2484
Clinoril Tablets (Sulindac) Merck & Co., Inc. 1658
Cortone Acetate Sterile Suspension (Cortisone Acetate) Merck & Co., Inc. 1663
Cortone Acetate Tablets (Cortisone Acetate) Merck & Co., Inc. 1664
Cuprimine Capsules (Penicillamine) Merck & Co., Inc. 1673
Dalalone D.P. Injectable (Dexamethasone Acetate) Forest 1009
Daypro Caplets (Oxaprozin) Searle 2578
Decadron Elixir (Dexamethasone) Merck & Co., Inc. 1676
Decadron Phosphate Injection (Dexamethasone Sodium Phosphate) Merck & Co., Inc. .. 1680

(⊞ Described in PDR For Nonprescription Drugs)   (⊙ Described in PDR For Ophthalmology)

Indications Index — Rhinitis

Decadron Tablets (Dexamethasone) Merck & Co., Inc. 1678
Decadron-LA Sterile Suspension (Dexamethasone Acetate) Merck & Co., Inc. 1687
Depen Titratable Tablets (Penicillamine) Wallace 2770
Disalcid (Salsalate) 3M Pharmaceuticals 1549
Dolobid Tablets (Diflunisal) Merck & Co., Inc. 1695
Easprin (Aspirin) Parke-Davis 1971
EC-Naprosyn Delayed-Release Tablets (Naproxen) Roche Pharmaceuticals 2277
Ecotrin (Aspirin) SmithKline Beecham 2625
Feldene Capsules (Piroxicam) Pfizer Inc 2008
Hydeltrasol Injection, Sterile (Prednisolone Sodium Phosphate) Merck & Co., Inc. 1708
Hydeltra-T.B.A. Sterile Suspension (Prednisolone Tebutate) Merck & Co., Inc. 1710
Hydrocortone Acetate Sterile Suspension (Hydrocortisone Acetate) Merck & Co., Inc. 1712
Hydrocortone Phosphate Injection, Sterile (Hydrocortisone Sodium Phosphate) Merck & Co., Inc. 1713
Hydrocortone Tablets (Hydrocortisone) Merck & Co., Inc. 1715
IBU Tablets (Ibuprofen) Knoll Laboratories 1389
Imuran (Azathioprine) Glaxo Wellcome 1103
Indocin (Indomethacin) Merck & Co., Inc. 1723
Lodine Capsules and Tablets (Etodolac) Wyeth-Ayerst 2849
Methotrexate Sodium Tablets, Injection, for Injection and LPF Injection (Methotrexate Sodium) Immunex 1322
Mono-Gesic Tablets (Salsalate) Central 810
Motrin Ibuprofen Suspension, Oral Drops, Chewable Tablets, Caplets (Ibuprofen) McNeil Consumer 1563
Myochrysine Injection (Gold Sodium Thiomalate) Merck & Co., Inc. 1754
Nalfon 200 Pulvules & Nalfon Tablets (Fenoprofen Calcium) Dista 933
Naprelan Tablets (Naproxen Sodium) Wyeth-Ayerst 2861
Anaprox/Naprosyn (Naproxen) Roche Pharmaceuticals 2277
Orudis Capsules (Ketoprofen) Wyeth-Ayerst 2874
Oruvail Capsules (Ketoprofen) Wyeth-Ayerst 2874
Pediapred Oral Solution (Prednisolone Sodium Phosphate) Medeva 1618
Plaquenil Sulfate Tablets (Hydroxychloroquine Sulfate) Sanofi Winthrop 2459
Prelone Syrup (Prednisolone) Muro 1834
Relafen Tablets (Nabumetone) SmithKline Beecham Pharmaceuticals 2688
Ridaura Capsules (Auranofin) SmithKline Beecham Pharmaceuticals 2691
Salflex Tablets (Salsalate) Carnrick 791
Solganal Suspension (Aurothioglucose) Schering 2530
Tolectin (200, 400 and 600 mg) (Tolmetin Sodium) McNeil Pharmaceutical 1591
Trilisate (Choline Magnesium Trisalicylate) Purdue Frederick 2155
Cataflam/Voltaren/Voltaren-XR (Diclofenac Sodium) CibaGeneva 833

Rheumatoid arthritis, juvenile

Extra Strength Bayer Arthritis Pain Regimen Formula (Aspirin, Enteric Coated) Bayer Consumer ..... ▣ 615
Celestone Soluspan Suspension (Betamethasone Sodium Phosphate, Betamethasone Acetate) Schering 2484
Cortone Acetate Sterile Suspension (Cortisone Acetate) Merck & Co., Inc. 1663

Cortone Acetate Tablets (Cortisone Acetate) Merck & Co., Inc. 1664
Dalalone D.P. Injectable (Dexamethasone Acetate) Forest 1009
Decadron Elixir (Dexamethasone) Merck & Co., Inc. 1676
Decadron Phosphate Injection (Dexamethasone Sodium Phosphate) Merck & Co., Inc. 1680
Decadron Tablets (Dexamethasone) Merck & Co., Inc. 1678
Decadron-LA Sterile Suspension (Dexamethasone Acetate) Merck & Co., Inc. 1687
Ecotrin (Aspirin) SmithKline Beecham 2625
Hydeltrasol Injection, Sterile (Prednisolone Sodium Phosphate) Merck & Co., Inc. 1708
Hydrocortone Phosphate Injection, Sterile (Hydrocortisone Sodium Phosphate) Merck & Co., Inc. 1713
Hydrocortone Tablets (Hydrocortisone) Merck & Co., Inc. 1715
Myochrysine Injection (Gold Sodium Thiomalate) Merck & Co., Inc. 1754
Pediapred Oral Solution (Prednisolone Sodium Phosphate) Medeva 1618
Prelone Syrup (Prednisolone) Muro 1834
Tolectin (200, 400 and 600 mg) (Tolmetin Sodium) McNeil Pharmaceutical 1591
Trilisate (Choline Magnesium Trisalicylate) Purdue Frederick 2155

Rhinitis, acute, "drying agent" in

Levsin/Levsinex/Levbid (Hyoscyamine Sulfate) Schwarz 2549

Rhinitis, allergic

Actifed Cold & Allergy Tablets (Pseudoephedrine Hydrochloride, Triprolidine Hydrochloride) Warner Wellcome ..... ▣ 807
Atrohist Pediatric Suspension Dye-Free (Chlorpheniramine Tannate, Phenylephrine Tannate, Pyrilamine Tannate) Medeva 1604
Atrovent Nasal Spray 0.03% (Ipratropium Bromide) Boehringer Ingelheim 676
Bromfed (Brompheniramine Maleate, Pseudoephedrine Hydrochloride) Muro 1832
D.A. II Tablets (Chlorpheniramine Maleate, Methscopolamine Nitrate, Phenylephrine Hydrochloride) Dura 972
D.A. Chewable Tablets (Chlorpheniramine Maleate, Phenylephrine Hydrochloride, Methscopolamine Nitrate) Dura 970
Dimetapp Elixir (Brompheniramine Maleate, Phenylpropanolamine Hydrochloride) Whitehall-Robins ..... ▣ 840
Dimetapp Extentabs (Brompheniramine Maleate, Phenylpropanolamine Hydrochloride) Whitehall-Robins ..... ▣ 841
Dura-Tap/PD Capsules (Chlorpheniramine Maleate, Pseudoephedrine Hydrochloride) Dura 970
Dura-Vent/DA Tablets (Chlorpheniramine Maleate, Phenylephrine Hydrochloride, Methscopolamine Nitrate) Dura 972
Efidac 24 Chlorpheniramine (Chlorpheniramine Maleate) Ciba Self-Medication ..... ▣ 655
Extendryl (Chlorpheniramine Maleate, Methscopolamine Nitrate, Phenylephrine Hydrochloride) Fleming 1003
Nasalcrom Nasal Solution (Cromolyn Sodium) Rhone-Poulenc Rorer Pharmaceuticals 2192
Nolahist Tablets (Phenindamine Tartrate) Carnrick 790
Novahistine Elixir (Chlorpheniramine Maleate, Phenylephrine Hydrochloride) SmithKline Beecham Consumer ..... ▣ 782
Ocean Nasal Mist (Sodium Chloride) Fleming ..... ▣ 671
PBZ Tablets (Tripelennamine Hydrochloride) CibaGeneva 863

PBZ-SR Tablets (Tripelennamine Hydrochloride) CibaGeneva 862
Phenergan Suppositories (Promethazine Hydrochloride) Wyeth-Ayerst 2882
Phenergan Syrup (Promethazine Hydrochloride) Wyeth-Ayerst 2881
Phenergan Tablets (Promethazine Hydrochloride) Wyeth-Ayerst 2882
Ryna Liquid (Chlorpheniramine Maleate, Pseudoephedrine Hydrochloride) Wallace ..... ▣ 804
Rynatan (Chlorpheniramine Tannate, Pyrilamine Tannate, Phenylephrine Tannate) Wallace 2781
Semprex-D Capsules (Acrivastine, Pseudoephedrine Hydrochloride) Medeva 1620
Tavist Syrup (Clemastine Fumarate) Sandoz Pharmaceuticals 2426
Tavist Tablets (Clemastine Fumarate) Sandoz Pharmaceuticals 2427
Trinalin Repetabs Tablets (Azatadine Maleate, Pseudoephedrine Sulfate) Key 1373
Vancenase AQ Double Strength Nasal Spray 0.084% (Beclomethasone Dipropionate) Schering 2536

Rhinitis medicamentosa

Ayr (Sodium Chloride) Ascher ..... ▣ 606

Rhinitis, perennial allergic

Atrohist Pediatric Capsules (Chlorpheniramine Maleate, Pseudoephedrine Hydrochloride) Medeva 1603
Atrovent Nasal Spray 0.03% (Ipratropium Bromide) Boehringer Ingelheim 676
Beconase (Beclomethasone Dipropionate) Glaxo Wellcome 1065
Celestone Soluspan Suspension (Betamethasone Sodium Phosphate, Betamethasone Acetate) Schering 2484
Cortone Acetate Sterile Suspension (Cortisone Acetate) Merck & Co., Inc. 1663
Cortone Acetate Tablets (Cortisone Acetate) Merck & Co., Inc. 1664
Dalalone D.P. Injectable (Dexamethasone Acetate) Forest 1009
Decadron Elixir (Dexamethasone) Merck & Co., Inc. 1676
Decadron Phosphate Injection (Dexamethasone Sodium Phosphate) Merck & Co., Inc. 1680
Decadron Tablets (Dexamethasone) Merck & Co., Inc. 1678
Decadron-LA Sterile Suspension (Dexamethasone Acetate) Merck & Co., Inc. 1687
Dexacort Phosphate in Turbinaire (Dexamethasone Sodium Phosphate) Medeva 1607
Fedahist Gyrocaps (Pseudoephedrine Hydrochloride, Chlorpheniramine Maleate) Schwarz 2545
Flonase Nasal Spray (Fluticasone Propionate) Glaxo Wellcome 1088
Hydeltrasol Injection, Sterile (Prednisolone Sodium Phosphate) Merck & Co., Inc. 1708
Hydrocortone Phosphate Injection, Sterile (Hydrocortisone Sodium Phosphate) Merck & Co., Inc. 1713
Hydrocortone Tablets (Hydrocortisone) Merck & Co., Inc. 1715
Nasacort AQ Nasal Spray (Triamcinolone Acetonide) Rhone-Poulenc Rorer Pharmaceuticals 2191
Nasacort Nasal Inhaler (Triamcinolone Acetonide) Rhone-Poulenc Rorer Pharmaceuticals 2189
Nasalide Nasal Solution 0.025% (Flunisolide) Roche Pharmaceuticals 2301
Nasarel Nasal Solution (Flunisolide) Roche Pharmaceuticals 2302
Ornade Spansule Capsules (Phenylpropanolamine Hydrochloride, Chlorpheniramine Maleate) SmithKline Beecham Pharmaceuticals 2678
Pediapred Oral Solution (Prednisolone Sodium Phosphate) Medeva 1618

Periactin (Cyproheptadine Hydrochloride) Merck & Co., Inc. 1767
Prelone Syrup (Prednisolone) Muro 1834
Rhinocort Nasal Inhaler (Budesonide) Astra 552
Rondec Oral Drops (Carbinoxamine Maleate, Pseudoephedrine Hydrochloride) Dura 974
Rondec Syrup (Carbinoxamine Maleate, Pseudoephedrine Hydrochloride) Dura 974
Rondec Tablet (Carbinoxamine Maleate, Pseudoephedrine Hydrochloride) Dura 974
Rondec Chewable Tablets (Brompheniramine Maleate, Pseudoephedrine Hydrochloride) Dura 974
Rondec-TR Tablet (Carbinoxamine Maleate, Pseudoephedrine Hydrochloride) Dura 974
Trinalin Repetabs Tablets (Azatadine Maleate, Pseudoephedrine Sulfate) Key 1373
Vancenase AQ Nasal Spray 0.042% (Beclomethasone Dipropionate) Schering 2535
Vancenase PocketHaler Nasal Inhaler (Beclomethasone Dipropionate) Schering 2534
Zyrtec Tablets (Cetirizine Hydrochloride) Pfizer Inc 2053

Rhinitis, seasonal allergic

Atrohist Pediatric Capsules (Chlorpheniramine Maleate, Pseudoephedrine Hydrochloride) Medeva 1603
Beconase (Beclomethasone Dipropionate) Glaxo Wellcome 1065
Benadryl Allergy Decongestant Liquid Medication (Diphenhydramine Hydrochloride, Pseudoephedrine Hydrochloride) Warner Wellcome ..... ▣ 812
Benadryl Allergy Decongestant Tablets (Diphenhydramine Hydrochloride, Pseudoephedrine Hydrochloride) Warner Wellcome ..... ▣ 812
Benadryl Allergy Liquid Medication (Diphenhydramine Hydrochloride) Warner Wellcome ..... ▣ 813
Benadryl Allergy Sinus Headache Caplets (Diphenhydramine Hydrochloride, Pseudoephedrine Hydrochloride, Acetaminophen) Warner Wellcome ..... ▣ 813
Bromfed Syrup (Brompheniramine Maleate, Pseudoephedrine Hydrochloride) Muro ..... ▣ 712
Celestone Soluspan Suspension (Betamethasone Sodium Phosphate, Betamethasone Acetate) Schering 2484
Claritin Tablets (Loratadine) Schering 2485
Claritin-D Tablets (Loratadine, Pseudoephedrine Sulfate) Schering 2487
Cortone Acetate Sterile Suspension (Cortisone Acetate) Merck & Co., Inc. 1663
Cortone Acetate Tablets (Cortisone Acetate) Merck & Co., Inc. 1664
Dalalone D.P. Injectable (Dexamethasone Acetate) Forest 1009
Decadron Elixir (Dexamethasone) Merck & Co., Inc. 1676
Decadron Phosphate Injection (Dexamethasone Sodium Phosphate) Merck & Co., Inc. 1680
Decadron Tablets (Dexamethasone) Merck & Co., Inc. 1678
Decadron-LA Sterile Suspension (Dexamethasone Acetate) Merck & Co., Inc. 1687
Dexacort Phosphate in Turbinaire (Dexamethasone Sodium Phosphate) Medeva 1607
Fedahist Gyrocaps (Pseudoephedrine Hydrochloride, Chlorpheniramine Maleate) Schwarz 2545
Flonase Nasal Spray (Fluticasone Propionate) Glaxo Wellcome 1088
Hismanal Tablets (Astemizole) Janssen 1341

(▣ Described in PDR For Nonprescription Drugs) (◉ Described in PDR For Ophthalmology)

Indications Index

Rhinitis

Hydeltrasol Injection, Sterile (Prednisolone Sodium Phosphate) Merck & Co., Inc. ... 1708
Hydrocortone Phosphate Injection, Sterile (Hydrocortisone Sodium Phosphate) Merck & Co., Inc. ... 1713
Hydrocortone Tablets (Hydrocortisone) Merck & Co., Inc. ... 1715
Nasacort AQ Nasal Spray (Triamcinolone Acetonide) Rhone-Poulenc Rorer Pharmaceuticals ... 2191
Nasacort Nasal Inhaler (Triamcinolone Acetonide) Rhone-Poulenc Rorer Pharmaceuticals ... 2189
Nasalide Nasal Solution 0.025% (Flunisolide) Roche Pharmaceuticals ... 2301
Nasarel Nasal Solution (Flunisolide) Roche Pharmaceuticals ... 2302
Ornade Spansule Capsules (Phenylpropanolamine Hydrochloride, Chlorpheniramine Maleate) SmithKline Beecham Pharmaceuticals ... 2678
Pediapred Oral Solution (Prednisolone Sodium Phosphate) Medeva 1618
Periactin (Cyproheptadine Hydrochloride) Merck & Co., Inc. ... 1767
Prelone Syrup (Prednisolone) Muro 1834
Rhinocort Nasal Inhaler (Budesonide) Astra ... 552
Rondec Oral Drops (Carbinoxamine Maleate, Pseudoephedrine Hydrochloride) Dura ... 974
Rondec Syrup (Carbinoxamine Maleate, Pseudoephedrine Hydrochloride) Dura ... 974
Rondec Tablet (Carbinoxamine Maleate, Pseudoephedrine Hydrochloride) Dura ... 974
Rondec Chewable Tablets (Brompheniramine Maleate, Pseudoephedrine Hydrochloride) Dura ... 974
Rondec-TR Tablet (Carbinoxamine Maleate, Pseudoephedrine Hydrochloride) Dura ... 974
Seldane Tablets (Terfenadine) Hoechst Marion Roussel ... 1284
Seldane-D Extended-Release Tablets (Pseudoephedrine Hydrochloride, Terfenadine) Hoechst Marion Roussel ... 1286
Sinulin Tablets (Acetaminophen, Phenylpropanolamine Hydrochloride, Chlorpheniramine Maleate) Carnrick ... 792
Sinutab Sinus Allergy Medication, Maximum Strength Tablets and Caplets (Acetaminophen, Chlorpheniramine Maleate, Pseudoephedrine Hydrochloride) Warner Wellcome ... 823
Sinutab Sinus Medication, Maximum Strength Without Drowsiness Formula, Tablets & Caplets (Acetaminophen, Pseudoephedrine Hydrochloride) Warner Wellcome ... 824
Sunsource Allergy Relief Tablets (Homeopathic Medications) Sunsource ... 792
Vancenase AQ Nasal Spray 0.042% (Beclomethasone Dipropionate) Schering ... 2535
Vancenase PocketHaler Nasal Inhaler (Beclomethasone Dipropionate) Schering ... 2534
Zyrtec Tablets (Cetirizine Hydrochloride) Pfizer Inc ... 2053

Rhinitis sicca

Afrin Saline Mist (Sodium Chloride) Schering-Plough HealthCare ... 758
Ayr (Sodium Chloride) Ascher ... 606
Nasal Moist (Sodium Chloride) Blairex ... 630
Salinex Nasal Mist and Drops (Sodium Chloride) Muro ... 713

Rhinitis, vasomotor

Beconase AQ Nasal Spray (Beclomethasone Dipropionate) Glaxo Wellcome ... 1065
Bromfed (Brompheniramine Maleate, Pseudoephedrine Hydrochloride) Muro ... 1832
D.A. II Tablets (Chlorpheniramine Maleate, Methscopolamine Nitrate, Phenylephrine Hydrochloride) Dura ... 972
D.A. Chewable Tablets (Chlorpheniramine Maleate, Phenylephrine Hydrochloride, Methscopolamine Nitrate) Dura ... 970
Dura-Tap/PD Capsules (Chlorpheniramine Maleate, Pseudoephedrine Hydrochloride) Dura ... 970
Dura-Vent/DA Tablets (Chlorpheniramine Maleate, Phenylephrine Hydrochloride, Methscopolamine Nitrate) Dura ... 972
Fedahist Gyrocaps (Pseudoephedrine Hydrochloride, Chlorpheniramine Maleate) Schwarz ... 2545
Ornade Spansule Capsules (Phenylpropanolamine Hydrochloride, Chlorpheniramine Maleate) SmithKline Beecham Pharmaceuticals ... 2678
PBZ Tablets (Tripelennamine Hydrochloride) CibaGeneva ... 863
PBZ-SR Tablets (Tripelennamine Hydrochloride) CibaGeneva ... 862
Periactin (Cyproheptadine Hydrochloride) Merck & Co., Inc. 1767
Phenergan Suppositories (Promethazine Hydrochloride) Wyeth-Ayerst ... 2882
Phenergan Syrup (Promethazine Hydrochloride) Wyeth-Ayerst ... 2881
Phenergan Tablets (Promethazine Hydrochloride) Wyeth-Ayerst ... 2882
Rondec Oral Drops (Carbinoxamine Maleate, Pseudoephedrine Hydrochloride) Dura ... 974
Rondec Syrup (Carbinoxamine Maleate, Pseudoephedrine Hydrochloride) Dura ... 974
Rondec Tablet (Carbinoxamine Maleate, Pseudoephedrine Hydrochloride) Dura ... 974
Rondec Chewable Tablets (Brompheniramine Maleate, Pseudoephedrine Hydrochloride) Dura ... 974
Rondec-TR Tablet (Carbinoxamine Maleate, Pseudoephedrine Hydrochloride) Dura ... 974
Vancenase AQ Double Strength Nasal Spray 0.084% (Beclomethasone Dipropionate) Schering ... 2536

Rhinorrhea

Actifed Allergy Daytime/Nighttime Caplets (Diphenhydramine Hydrochloride, Pseudoephedrine Hydrochloride) Warner Wellcome ... 808
Atrovent Nasal Spray 0.03% (Ipratropium Bromide) Boehringer Ingelheim ... 676
Atrovent Nasal Spray 0.06% (Ipratropium Bromide) Boehringer Ingelheim ... 678
Benadryl Allergy Chewables (Diphenhydramine Hydrochloride) Warner Wellcome ... 811
Benadryl Allergy Decongestant Tablets (Diphenhydramine Hydrochloride, Pseudoephedrine Hydrochloride) Warner Wellcome ... 812
Benadryl Allergy Liquid Medication (Diphenhydramine Hydrochloride) Warner Wellcome ... 813
Benadryl Allergy (Diphenhydramine Hydrochloride) Warner Wellcome ... 811
Benadryl Allergy Sinus Headache Caplets (Diphenhydramine Hydrochloride, Pseudoephedrine Hydrochloride, Acetaminophen) Warner Wellcome ... 813
Benadryl Dye-Free Allergy Liqui-gel Softgels (Diphenhydramine Hydrochloride) Warner Wellcome ... 813
Benadryl Dye-Free Allergy Liquid Medication (Diphenhydramine Hydrochloride) Warner Wellcome ... 814
Cheracol Plus Head Cold/Cough Formula (Phenylpropanolamine Hydrochloride, Dextromethorphan Hydrobromide, Chlorpheniramine Maleate) Roberts ... 741
Chlor-Trimeton Allergy Decongestant Tablets (Chlorpheniramine Maleate, Pseudoephedrine Sulfate) Schering-Plough HealthCare ... 759
Chlor-Trimeton Allergy Tablets (Chlorpheniramine Maleate) Schering-Plough HealthCare ... 758
Allergy-Sinus Comtrex Multi-Symptom Allergy-Sinus Formula Tablets and Caplets (Acetaminophen, Chlorpheniramine Maleate, Pseudoephedrine Hydrochloride) Bristol-Myers Products ... 639
Contac Night Allergy/Sinus Caplets (Acetaminophen, Pseudoephedrine Hydrochloride, Diphenhydramine Hydrochloride) SmithKline Beecham Consumer ... 771
Dimetapp Allergy Dye-Free Elixir (Brompheniramine Maleate) Whitehall-Robins ... 838
Dimetapp Cold & Allergy Chewable Tablets (Brompheniramine Maleate, Phenylpropanolamine Hydrochloride) Whitehall-Robins ... 838
Dimetapp Cold & Fever Suspension (Acetaminophen, Brompheniramine Maleate, Pseudoephedrine Hydrochloride) Whitehall-Robins ... 839
Dimetapp Elixir (Brompheniramine Maleate, Phenylpropanolamine Hydrochloride) Whitehall-Robins ... 840
Dimetapp Extentabs (Brompheniramine Maleate, Phenylpropanolamine Hydrochloride) Whitehall-Robins ... 841
Dimetapp Tablets/Liqui-Gels (Brompheniramine Maleate, Phenylpropanolamine Hydrochloride) Whitehall-Robins ... 841
Efidac 24 Chlorpheniramine (Chlorpheniramine Maleate) Ciba Self-Medication ... 655
Hyland's C-Plus Cold Tablets (Homeopathic Medications) Standard Homeopathic ... 789
Nolahist Tablets (Phenindamine Tartrate) Carnrick ... 790
Novahistine Elixir (Chlorpheniramine Maleate, Phenylephrine Hydrochloride) SmithKline Beecham Consumer ... 782
Ornade Spansule Capsules (Phenylpropanolamine Hydrochloride, Chlorpheniramine Maleate) SmithKline Beecham Pharmaceuticals ... 2678
PediaCare Cough-Cold Chewable Tablets and Liquid (Pseudoephedrine Hydrochloride, Chlorpheniramine Maleate, Dextromethorphan Hydrobromide) McNeil Consumer ... 1569
Ryna (Chlorpheniramine Maleate, Pseudoephedrine Hydrochloride) Wallace ... 804
Seldane Tablets (Terfenadine) Hoechst Marion Roussel ... 1284
Seldane-D Extended-Release Tablets (Pseudoephedrine Hydrochloride, Terfenadine) Hoechst Marion Roussel ... 1286
Sinulin Tablets (Acetaminophen, Phenylpropanolamine Hydrochloride, Chlorpheniramine Maleate) Carnrick ... 792
Tavist Syrup (Clemastine Fumarate) Sandoz Pharmaceuticals ... 2426
Tavist Tablets (Clemastine Fumarate) Sandoz Pharmaceuticals ... 2427
Tavist-1 12 Hour Relief Tablets (Clemastine Fumarate) Sandoz Consumer ... 749
Triaminic Syrup (Phenylpropanolamine Hydrochloride, Chlorpheniramine Maleate) Sandoz Consumer ... 755
TYLENOL Allergy Sinus, Maximum Strength Caplets and Gelcaps (Acetaminophen, Chlorpheniramine Maleate, Pseudoephedrine Hydrochloride) McNeil Consumer 1571
TYLENOL Severe Allergy Medication Caplets (Acetaminophen, Chlorpheniramine Maleate, Pseudoephedrine Hydrochloride) McNeil Consumer 1571

Rickets

Rocaltrol Capsules (Calcitriol) Roche Pharmaceuticals ... 2303

Rickettsiae

Achromycin V Capsules (Tetracycline Hydrochloride) Lederle ... 1417
Chloromycetin Sodium Succinate (Chloramphenicol Sodium Succinate) Parke-Davis ... 1960
Declomycin Tablets (Demeclocycline Hydrochloride) Lederle ... 1421
Doryx Capsules (Doxycycline Hyclate) Parke-Davis ... 1970
DYNACIN Capsules (Minocycline Hydrochloride) Medicis ... 1627
Minocin Intravenous (Minocycline Hydrochloride) Lederle ... 1428
Minocin Oral Suspension (Minocycline Hydrochloride) Lederle ... 1431
Minocin Pellet-Filled Capsules (Minocycline Hydrochloride) Lederle ... 1429
Monodox Capsules (Doxycycline Monohydrate) Oclassen ... 1858
Terramycin Intramuscular Solution (Oxytetracycline) Pfizer Inc ... 2034
Vibramycin (Doxycycline Calcium) Pfizer Inc ... 2038
Vibramycin Hyclate Intravenous (Doxycycline Hyclate) Pfizer Inc ... 2040
Vibramycin (Doxycycline Monohydrate) Pfizer Inc ... 2038

Rickettsialpox

Achromycin V Capsules (Tetracycline Hydrochloride) Lederle ... 1417
Declomycin Tablets (Demeclocycline Hydrochloride) Lederle ... 1421
Doryx Capsules (Doxycycline Hyclate) Parke-Davis ... 1970
DYNACIN Capsules (Minocycline Hydrochloride) Medicis ... 1627
Minocin Intravenous (Minocycline Hydrochloride) Lederle ... 1428
Minocin Oral Suspension (Minocycline Hydrochloride) Lederle ... 1431
Minocin Pellet-Filled Capsules (Minocycline Hydrochloride) Lederle ... 1429
Monodox Capsules (Doxycycline Monohydrate) Oclassen ... 1858
Terramycin Intramuscular Solution (Oxytetracycline) Pfizer Inc ... 2034
Vibramycin (Doxycycline Calcium) Pfizer Inc ... 2038
Vibramycin Hyclate Intravenous (Doxycycline Hyclate) Pfizer Inc ... 2040
Vibramycin (Doxycycline Monohydrate) Pfizer Inc ... 2038

Ringworm infections of the body (see under Tinea corporis infections)

Ringworm infections of the feet (see under Tinea pedis infections)

Ringworm infections of the groin (see under Tinea cruris infections)

Ringworm infections of the nails (see under Tinea unguium infections)

Ringworm infections of the scalp (see under Tinea capitis infections)

Rocky Mountain spotted fever

Achromycin V Capsules (Tetracycline Hydrochloride) Lederle ... 1417
Declomycin Tablets (Demeclocycline Hydrochloride) Lederle ... 1421
Doryx Capsules (Doxycycline Hyclate) Parke-Davis ... 1970
DYNACIN Capsules (Minocycline Hydrochloride) Medicis ... 1627
Minocin Intravenous (Minocycline Hydrochloride) Lederle ... 1428
Minocin Oral Suspension (Minocycline Hydrochloride) Lederle ... 1431

Minocin Pellet-Filled Capsules (Minocycline Hydrochloride) Lederle ... 1429
Monodox Capsules (Doxycycline Monohydrate) Oclassen ... 1858
Terramycin Intramuscular Solution (Oxytetracycline) Pfizer Inc ... 2034
Vibramycin (Doxycycline Calcium) Pfizer Inc ... 2038
Vibramycin Hyclate Intravenous (Doxycycline Hyclate) Pfizer Inc ... 2040
Vibramycin (Doxycycline Monohydrate) Pfizer Inc ... 2038

Rosacea
MetroCream (Metronidazole) Galderma ... 1034
MetroGel (Metronidazole) Galderma ... 1034

Roundworm, common (see under Ascaris lumbricoides infections)

Rubella and mumps, prophylaxis
Biavax II (Rubella & Mumps Virus Vaccine Live) Merck & Co., Inc. ... 1653

Rubella, prophylaxis
M-M-R II (Measles, Mumps & Rubella Virus Vaccine Live) Merck & Co., Inc. ... 1730
M-R-VAX II (Measles & Rubella Virus Vaccine Live) Merck & Co., Inc. ... 1732
Meruvax II (Rubella Virus Vaccine Live) Merck & Co., Inc. ... 1740

S

S. agalactiae gynecologic infections
Cefobid Intravenous/Intramuscular (Cefoperazone Sodium) Pfizer Inc ... 1996
Cefobid Pharmacy Bulk Package - Not for Direct Infusion (Cefoperazone Sodium) Pfizer Inc ... 1999
Cefotan (Cefotetan) Zeneca ... 2936

S. agalactiae infections
Cefizox for Intramuscular or Intravenous Use (Ceftizoxime Sodium) Fujisawa ... 1025
Cefobid Intravenous/Intramuscular (Cefoperazone Sodium) Pfizer Inc ... 1996
Cefobid Pharmacy Bulk Package - Not for Direct Infusion (Cefoperazone Sodium) Pfizer Inc ... 1999
Cefotan (Cefotetan) Zeneca ... 2936
Monocid Injection (Cefonicid Sodium) SmithKline Beecham Pharmaceuticals ... 2674
Noroxin Tablets (Norfloxacin) Merck & Co., Inc. ... 1758
Noroxin Tablets (Norfloxacin) Roberts ... 2222
Zithromax (Azithromycin) Pfizer Inc ... 2043
Zithromax Tablets (Azithromycin) Pfizer Inc ... 2046

S. agalactiae pelvic inflammatory disease
Cefizox for Intramuscular or Intravenous Use (Ceftizoxime Sodium) Fujisawa ... 1025
Cefobid Intravenous/Intramuscular (Cefoperazone Sodium) Pfizer Inc ... 1996
Cefobid Pharmacy Bulk Package - Not for Direct Infusion (Cefoperazone Sodium) Pfizer Inc ... 1999

S. agalactiae septicemia
Cefobid Intravenous/Intramuscular (Cefoperazone Sodium) Pfizer Inc ... 1996
Cefobid Pharmacy Bulk Package - Not for Direct Infusion (Cefoperazone Sodium) Pfizer Inc ... 1999

S. agalactiae skin and skin structure infections
Monocid Injection (Cefonicid Sodium) SmithKline Beecham Pharmaceuticals ... 2674
Zithromax (Azithromycin) Pfizer Inc ... 2043
Zithromax Tablets (Azithromycin) Pfizer Inc ... 2046

S. agalactiae urinary tract infections
Noroxin Tablets (Norfloxacin) Merck & Co., Inc. ... 1758
Noroxin Tablets (Norfloxacin) Roberts ... 2222

S. aureus biliary tract infections
Ancef Injection (Cefazolin Sodium) SmithKline Beecham Pharmaceuticals ... 2632
Kefzol Vials, Faspak & ADD-Vantage (Cefazolin Sodium) Lilly ... 1511

S. aureus bone and joint infections
Ancef Injection (Cefazolin Sodium) SmithKline Beecham Pharmaceuticals ... 2632
Cefizox for Intramuscular or Intravenous Use (Ceftizoxime Sodium) Fujisawa ... 1025
Cefotan (Cefotetan) Zeneca ... 2936
Ceptaz (Ceftazidime) Glaxo Wellcome ... 1070
Claforan Sterile and Injection (Cefotaxime Sodium) Hoechst Marion Roussel ... 1259
Cleocin Phosphate Injection (Clindamycin Phosphate) Pharmacia & Upjohn ... 2068
Fortaz (Ceftazidime) Glaxo Wellcome ... 1092
Keftab Tablets (Cephalexin Hydrochloride) Dista ... 931
Kefurox Vials, Faspak & ADD-Vantage (Cefuroxime Sodium) Lilly ... 1509
Kefzol Vials, Faspak & ADD-Vantage (Cefazolin Sodium) Lilly ... 1511
Mandol Vials, Faspak & ADD-Vantage (Cefamandole Nafate) Lilly ... 1516
Mefoxin (Cefoxitin Sodium) Merck & Co., Inc. ... 1734
Mefoxin Premixed Intravenous Solution (Cefoxitin Sodium) Merck & Co., Inc. ... 1737
Monocid Injection (Cefonicid Sodium) SmithKline Beecham Pharmaceuticals ... 2674
Nebcin Vials, Hyporets & ADD-Vantage (Tobramycin Sulfate) Lilly ... 1518
Primaxin I.V. (Cilastatin Sodium, Imipenem) Merck & Co., Inc. ... 1772
Rocephin Injectable Vials, ADD-Vantage, Galaxy Container (Ceftriaxone Sodium) Roche Pharmaceuticals ... 2305
Tazicef for Injection (Ceftazidime) SmithKline Beecham Pharmaceuticals ... 2697
Tazidime Vials, Faspak & ADD-Vantage (Ceftazidime) Lilly .. 1531
Timentin for Injection (Ticarcillin Disodium, Clavulanate Potassium) SmithKline Beecham Pharmaceuticals ... 2706
Zinacef (Cefuroxime Sodium) Glaxo Wellcome ... 1184

S. aureus endocarditis
Ancef Injection (Cefazolin Sodium) SmithKline Beecham Pharmaceuticals ... 2632
Kefzol Vials, Faspak & ADD-Vantage (Cefazolin Sodium) Lilly ... 1511
Primaxin I.V. (Cilastatin Sodium, Imipenem) Merck & Co., Inc. ... 1772

S. aureus gynecologic infections
Cefotan (Cefotetan) Zeneca ... 2936
Primaxin I.V. (Cilastatin Sodium, Imipenem) Merck & Co., Inc. ... 1772
Timentin for Injection (Ticarcillin Disodium, Clavulanate Potassium) SmithKline Beecham Pharmaceuticals ... 2706

S. aureus infections
Achromycin V Capsules (Tetracycline Hydrochloride) Lederle ... 1417
Ancef Injection (Cefazolin Sodium) SmithKline Beecham Pharmaceuticals ... 2632
Augmentin (Amoxicillin Trihydrate, Clavulanate Potassium) SmithKline Beecham Pharmaceuticals ... 2637
Augmentin Tablets (Amoxicillin Trihydrate, Clavulanate Potassium) SmithKline Beecham Pharmaceuticals ... 2640
Bactroban Ointment (Mupirocin) SmithKline Beecham Pharmaceuticals ... 2642
Biaxin (Clarithromycin) Abbott ... 406
Ceclor Pulvules & Suspension (Cefaclor) Lilly ... 1470
Cefizox for Intramuscular or Intravenous Use (Ceftizoxime Sodium) Fujisawa ... 1025
Cefobid Intravenous/Intramuscular (Cefoperazone Sodium) Pfizer Inc ... 1996
Cefobid Pharmacy Bulk Package - Not for Direct Infusion (Cefoperazone Sodium) Pfizer Inc ... 1999
Cefotan (Cefotetan) Zeneca ... 2936
Ceftin (Cefuroxime Axetil) Glaxo Wellcome ... 1067
Cefzil Tablets and Oral Suspension (Cefprozil) Bristol-Myers Squibb .. 747
Ceptaz (Ceftazidime) Glaxo Wellcome ... 1070
Cipro I.V. (Ciprofloxacin) Bayer Pharmaceutical ... 587
Cipro Tablets (Ciprofloxacin Hydrochloride) Bayer Pharmaceutical ... 584
Claforan Sterile and Injection (Cefotaxime Sodium) Hoechst Marion Roussel ... 1259
Cleocin Phosphate Injection (Clindamycin Phosphate) Pharmacia & Upjohn ... 2068
Declomycin Tablets (Demeclocycline Hydrochloride) Lederle ... 1421
Dynabac (Dirithromycin) Bock ... 668
DYNACIN Capsules (Minocycline Hydrochloride) Medicis ... 1627
E.E.S. (Erythromycin Ethylsuccinate) Abbott ... 427
E-Mycin Tablets (Erythromycin) Knoll Laboratories ... 1388
ERYC (Erythromycin) Parke-Davis .. 1972
EryPed (Erythromycin Ethylsuccinate) Abbott ... 425
Ery-Tab Tablets (Erythromycin) Abbott ... 426
Erythrocin Stearate Filmtab (Erythromycin Stearate) Abbott ... 429
Erythromycin Base Filmtab (Erythromycin) Abbott ... 430
Erythromycin Delayed-Release Capsules, USP (Erythromycin) Abbott ... 431
Floxin I.V. (Ofloxacin) McNeil Pharmaceutical ... 1580
Floxin Tablets (200 mg, 300 mg, 400 mg) (Ofloxacin) McNeil Pharmaceutical ... 1577
Fortaz (Ceftazidime) Glaxo Wellcome ... 1092
Ilosone (Erythromycin Estolate) Dista ... 927
Ilotycin Glucepate, IV, Vials (Erythromycin Glucepate) Dista ... 929
Keftab Tablets (Cephalexin Hydrochloride) Dista ... 931
Kefurox Vials, Faspak & ADD-Vantage (Cefuroxime Sodium) Lilly ... 1509
Kefzol Vials, Faspak & ADD-Vantage (Cefazolin Sodium) Lilly ... 1511
Lorabid Suspension and Pulvules (Loracarbef) Lilly ... 1513
Macrodantin Capsules (Nitrofurantoin) Procter & Gamble Pharmaceuticals ... 2140
Mandol Vials, Faspak & ADD-Vantage (Cefamandole Nafate) Lilly ... 1516
Maxipime for Injection (Cefepime Hydrochloride) Bristol-Myers Squibb ... 758
Mefoxin (Cefoxitin Sodium) Merck & Co., Inc. ... 1734
Mefoxin Premixed Intravenous Solution (Cefoxitin Sodium) Merck & Co., Inc. ... 1737
Minocin Intravenous (Minocycline Hydrochloride) Lederle ... 1428
Minocin Oral Suspension (Minocycline Hydrochloride) Lederle ... 1431
Minocin Pellet-Filled Capsules (Minocycline Hydrochloride) Lederle ... 1429
Monocid Injection (Cefonicid Sodium) SmithKline Beecham Pharmaceuticals ... 2674
Monodox Capsules (Doxycycline Monohydrate) Oclassen ... 1858
Nebcin Vials, Hyporets & ADD-Vantage (Tobramycin Sulfate) Lilly ... 1518
Netromycin Injection 100 mg/ml (Netilmicin Sulfate) Schering ... 2516
Noroxin Tablets (Norfloxacin) Merck & Co., Inc. ... 1758
Noroxin Tablets (Norfloxacin) Roberts ... 2222
PCE Dispertab Tablets (Erythromycin) Abbott ... 453
Primaxin I.M. (Cilastatin Sodium, Imipenem) Merck & Co., Inc. ... 1770
Primaxin I.V. (Cilastatin Sodium, Imipenem) Merck & Co., Inc. ... 1772
Rocephin Injectable Vials, ADD-Vantage, Galaxy Container (Ceftriaxone Sodium) Roche Pharmaceuticals ... 2305
Tazicef for Injection (Ceftazidime) SmithKline Beecham Pharmaceuticals ... 2697
Tazidime Vials, Faspak & ADD-Vantage (Ceftazidime) Lilly .. 1531
Timentin for Injection (Ticarcillin Disodium, Clavulanate Potassium) SmithKline Beecham Pharmaceuticals ... 2706
Unasyn (Ampicillin Sodium, Sulbactam Sodium) Pfizer Inc ... 2035
Vantin for Oral Suspension and Vantin Tablets (Cefpodoxime Proxetil) Pharmacia & Upjohn ... 2112
Zinacef (Cefuroxime Sodium) Glaxo Wellcome ... 1184
Zithromax (Azithromycin) Pfizer Inc ... 2043
Zithromax Tablets (Azithromycin) Pfizer Inc ... 2046
Zosyn (Piperacillin Sodium, Tazobactam Sodium) Lederle ... 1463

S. aureus infection, eradication of nasal colonization of
Bactroban Nasal (Mupirocin Calcium) SmithKline Beecham Pharmaceuticals ... 2643

S. aureus infections, ocular
AK-CIDE (Prednisolone Acetate, Sulfacetamide Sodium) Akorn .... ◉ 203
AK-CIDE Ointment (Prednisolone Acetate, Sulfacetamide Sodium) Akorn ... ◉ 203
AK-Spore (Bacitracin Zinc, Neomycin Sulfate, Polymyxin B Sulfate) Akorn ... ◉ 205
AK-Trol Ointment & Suspension (Dexamethasone, Neomycin Sulfate, Polymyxin B Sulfate) Akorn ... ◉ 205
Blephamide Liquifilm Sterile Ophthalmic Suspension (Prednisolone Acetate, Sulfacetamide Sodium) Allergan ... 472
Blephamide Ointment (Sulfacetamide Sodium, Prednisolone Acetate) Allergan ... ◉ 234
Chibroxin Sterile Ophthalmic Solution (Norfloxacin) Merck & Co., Inc. ... 1657
Chloromycetin Ophthalmic Ointment, 1% (Chloramphenicol) Parke-Davis ... ◉ 298
Chloromycetin Ophthalmic Solution (Chloramphenicol) Parke-Davis ... ◉ 299
Chloroptic S.O.P. (Chloramphenicol) Allergan ... ◉ 236
Ciloxan Ophthalmic Solution (Ciprofloxacin Hydrochloride) Alcon Laboratories ... 468
Cortisporin Ophthalmic Ointment Sterile (Polymyxin B Sulfate, Bacitracin Zinc, Neomycin Sulfate, Hydrocortisone) Glaxo Wellcome ... 1074
Cortisporin Ophthalmic Suspension Sterile (Hydrocortisone, Polymyxin B Sulfate, Neomycin Sulfate) Glaxo Wellcome ... 1075
FML-S Liquifilm (Sulfacetamide Sodium, Fluorometholone) Allergan ... ◉ 240
Garamycin Ophthalmic (Gentamicin Sulfate) Schering ... 2501

(▩ Described in PDR For Nonprescription Drugs)   (◉ Described in PDR For Ophthalmology)

S. aureus infections

Genoptic Sterile Ophthalmic
Solution (Gentamicin Sulfate)
Allergan .... ⊚ 241
Genoptic Sterile Ophthalmic
Ointment (Gentamicin Sulfate)
Allergan .... ⊚ 241
Gentak (Gentamicin Sulfate)
Akorn .... ⊚ 209
Maxitrol Ophthalmic Ointment
and Suspension (Dexamethasone, Neomycin Sulfate, Polymyxin B Sulfate) Alcon
Laboratories .... ⊚ 222
NeoDecadron Sterile Ophthalmic
Ointment (Neomycin Sulfate,
Dexamethasone Sodium
Phosphate) Merck & Co., Inc. 1755
NeoDecadron Sterile Ophthalmic
Solution (Neomycin Sulfate, Dexamethasone Sodium Phosphate)
Merck & Co., Inc. 1756
Ocuflox Ophthalmic Solution
(Ofloxacin) Allergan 478
Poly-Pred Liquifilm (Neomycin
Sulfate, Polymyxin B Sulfate,
Prednisolone Acetate) Allergan ... ⊚ 246
Polytrim Ophthalmic Solution
Sterile (Polymyxin B Sulfate,
Trimethoprim Sulfate) Allergan 479
Pred-G Liquifilm Sterile
Ophthalmic Suspension (Gentamicin Sulfate, Prednisolone
Acetate) Allergan .... ⊚ 248
Pred-G S.O.P. Sterile Ophthalmic
Ointment (Gentamicin Sulfate,
Prednisolone Acetate) Allergan ... ⊚ 249
Terra-Cortril Ophthalmic
Suspension (Oxytetracycline
Hydrochloride, Hydrocortisone
Acetate) Pfizer Inc 2033
TobraDex Ophthalmic Suspension
and Ointment (Dexamethasone,
Tobramycin) Alcon Laboratories .. 469

S. aureus intra-abdominal infections

Ceptaz (Ceftazidime) Glaxo
Wellcome 1070
Fortaz (Ceftazidime) Glaxo
Wellcome 1092
Netromycin Injection 100 mg/ml
(Netilmicin Sulfate) Schering 2516
Primaxin I.V. (Cilastatin Sodium,
Imipenem) Merck & Co., Inc. 1772
Tazicef for Injection (Ceftazidime)
SmithKline Beecham
Pharmaceuticals 2697
Tazidime Vials, Faspak &
ADD-Vantage (Ceftazidime) Lilly .. 1531

S. aureus lower respiratory tract infections

Cefizox for Intramuscular or
Intravenous Use (Ceftizoxime
Sodium) Fujisawa 1025
Cefotan (Cefotetan) Zeneca 2936
Ceptaz (Ceftazidime) Glaxo
Wellcome 1070
Claforan Sterile and Injection
(Cefotaxime Sodium) Hoechst
Marion Roussel 1259
Cleocin Phosphate Injection (Clindamycin Phosphate) Pharmacia
& Upjohn 2068
Fortaz (Ceftazidime) Glaxo
Wellcome 1092
Mefoxin (Cefoxitin Sodium) Merck
& Co., Inc. 1734
Nebcin Vials, Hyporets &
ADD-Vantage (Tobramycin
Sulfate) Lilly 1518
Netromycin Injection 100 mg/ml
(Netilmicin Sulfate) Schering 2516
Primaxin I.V. (Cilastatin Sodium,
Imipenem) Merck & Co., Inc. 1772
Rocephin Injectable Vials,
ADD-Vantage, Galaxy Container
(Ceftriaxone Sodium) Roche
Pharmaceuticals 2305
Tazicef for Injection (Ceftazidime)
SmithKline Beecham
Pharmaceuticals 2697
Tazidime Vials, Faspak &
ADD-Vantage (Ceftazidime) Lilly .. 1531
Timentin for Injection (Ticarcillin
Disodium, Clavulanate
Potassium) SmithKline Beecham
Pharmaceuticals 2706
Zinacef (Cefuroxime Sodium)
Glaxo Wellcome 1184
Zosyn (Piperacillin Sodium, Tazobactam Sodium) Lederle 1463

S. aureus meningitis

Kefurox Vials, Faspak &
ADD-Vantage (Cefuroxime
Sodium) Lilly 1509
Zinacef (Cefuroxime Sodium)
Glaxo Wellcome 1184

S. aureus respiratory tract infections

Ancef Injection (Cefazolin Sodium)
SmithKline Beecham
Pharmaceuticals 2632
Cefobid Intravenous/Intramuscular
(Cefoperazone Sodium) Pfizer
Inc 1996
Cefobid Pharmacy Bulk Package -
Not for Direct Infusion (Cefoperazone Sodium) Pfizer Inc 1999
Kefzol Vials, Faspak &
ADD-Vantage (Cefazolin Sodium)
Lilly 1511

S. aureus skin and skin structure infections

Achromycin V Capsules (Tetracycline Hydrochloride) Lederle 1417
Ancef Injection (Cefazolin Sodium)
SmithKline Beecham
Pharmaceuticals 2632
Augmentin (Amoxicillin Trihydrate,
Clavulanate Potassium)
SmithKline Beecham
Pharmaceuticals 2637
Augmentin Tablets (Amoxicillin
Trihydrate, Clavulanate
Potassium) SmithKline Beecham
Pharmaceuticals 2640
Bactroban Ointment (Mupirocin)
SmithKline Beecham
Pharmaceuticals 2642
Biaxin (Clarithromycin) Abbott 406
Ceclor Pulvules & Suspension
(Cefaclor) Lilly 1470
Cefizox for Intramuscular or
Intravenous Use (Ceftizoxime
Sodium) Fujisawa 1025
Cefobid Intravenous/Intramuscular
(Cefoperazone Sodium) Pfizer
Inc 1996
Cefobid Pharmacy Bulk Package -
Not for Direct Infusion (Cefoperazone Sodium) Pfizer Inc 1999
Cefotan (Cefotetan) Zeneca 2936
Ceftin (Cefuroxime Axetil) Glaxo
Wellcome 1067
Cefzil Tablets and Oral Suspension
(Cefprozil) Bristol-Myers Squibb .. 747
Ceptaz (Ceftazidime) Glaxo
Wellcome 1070
Cipro I.V. (Ciprofloxacin) Bayer
Pharmaceutical 587
Cipro I.V. Pharmacy Bulk Package
(Ciprofloxacin) Bayer
Pharmaceutical 590
Cipro Tablets (Ciprofloxacin
Hydrochloride) Bayer
Pharmaceutical 584
Claforan Sterile and Injection
(Cefotaxime Sodium) Hoechst
Marion Roussel 1259
Cleocin Phosphate Injection (Clindamycin Phosphate) Pharmacia
& Upjohn 2068
Dynabac (Dirithromycin) Bock 668
DYNACIN Capsules (Minocycline
Hydrochloride) Medicis 1627
E.E.S. (Erythromycin
Ethylsuccinate) Abbott 427
E-Mycin Tablets (Erythromycin)
Knoll Laboratories 1388
ERYC (Erythromycin) Parke-Davis .. 1972
EryPed (Erythromycin
Ethylsuccinate) Abbott 425
Ery-Tab Tablets (Erythromycin)
Abbott 426
Erythrocin Stearate Filmtab (Erythromycin Stearate) Abbott 429
Erythromycin Base Filmtab
(Erythromycin) Abbott 430
Erythromycin Delayed-Release
Capsules, USP (Erythromycin)
Abbott 431
Floxin I.V. (Ofloxacin) McNeil
Pharmaceutical 1580
Floxin Tablets (200 mg, 300 mg,
400 mg) (Ofloxacin) McNeil
Pharmaceutical 1577
Fortaz (Ceftazidime) Glaxo
Wellcome 1092
Ilosone (Erythromycin Estolate)
Dista 927
Ilotycin Gluceptate, IV, Vials (Erythromycin Gluceptate) Dista 929
Keftab Tablets (Cephalexin
Hydrochloride) Dista 931
Kefurox Vials, Faspak &
ADD-Vantage (Cefuroxime
Sodium) Lilly 1509
Kefzol Vials, Faspak &
ADD-Vantage (Cefazolin Sodium)
Lilly 1511
Lorabid Suspension and Pulvules
(Loracarbef) Lilly 1513
Mandol Vials, Faspak &
ADD-Vantage (Cefamandole
Nafate) Lilly 1516
Maxipime for Injection (Cefepime
Hydrochloride) Bristol-Myers
Squibb 758
Mefoxin (Cefoxitin Sodium) Merck
& Co., Inc. 1734
Mefoxin Premixed Intravenous
Solution (Cefoxitin Sodium)
Merck & Co., Inc. 1737
Minocin Intravenous (Minocycline
Hydrochloride) Lederle 1428
Minocin Oral Suspension (Minocycline Hydrochloride) Lederle 1431
Minocin Pellet-Filled Capsules
(Minocycline Hydrochloride)
Lederle 1429
Monocid Injection (Cefonicid
Sodium) SmithKline Beecham
Pharmaceuticals 2674
Monodox Capsules (Doxycycline
Monohydrate) Oclassen 1858
Nebcin Vials, Hyporets &
ADD-Vantage (Tobramycin
Sulfate) Lilly 1518
Netromycin Injection 100 mg/ml
(Netilmicin Sulfate) Schering 2516
PCE Dispertab Tablets
(Erythromycin) Abbott 453
Primaxin I.M. (Cilastatin Sodium,
Imipenem) Merck & Co., Inc. 1770
Primaxin I.V. (Cilastatin Sodium,
Imipenem) Merck & Co., Inc. 1772
Rocephin Injectable Vials,
ADD-Vantage, Galaxy Container
(Ceftriaxone Sodium) Roche
Pharmaceuticals 2305
Tazicef for Injection (Ceftazidime)
SmithKline Beecham
Pharmaceuticals 2697
Tazidime Vials, Faspak &
ADD-Vantage (Ceftazidime) Lilly .. 1531
Timentin for Injection (Ticarcillin
Disodium, Clavulanate
Potassium) SmithKline Beecham
Pharmaceuticals 2706
Unasyn (Ampicillin Sodium, Sulbactam Sodium) Pfizer Inc 2035
Vantin for Oral Suspension and
Vantin Tablets (Cefpodoxime
Proxetil) Pharmacia & Upjohn 2112
Zinacef (Cefuroxime Sodium)
Glaxo Wellcome 1184
Zithromax (Azithromycin) Pfizer
Inc 2043
Zithromax Tablets (Azithromycin)
Pfizer Inc 2046
Zosyn (Piperacillin Sodium, Tazobactam Sodium) Lederle 1463

S. aureus septicemia

Ancef Injection (Cefazolin Sodium)
SmithKline Beecham
Pharmaceuticals 2632
Cefizox for Intramuscular or
Intravenous Use (Ceftizoxime
Sodium) Fujisawa 1025
Cefobid Intravenous/Intramuscular
(Cefoperazone Sodium) Pfizer
Inc 1996
Cefobid Pharmacy Bulk Package -
Not for Direct Infusion (Cefoperazone Sodium) Pfizer Inc 1999
Ceptaz (Ceftazidime) Glaxo
Wellcome 1070
Claforan Sterile and Injection
(Cefotaxime Sodium) Hoechst
Marion Roussel 1259
Cleocin Phosphate Injection (Clindamycin Phosphate) Pharmacia
& Upjohn 2068
Fortaz (Ceftazidime) Glaxo
Wellcome 1092
Kefurox Vials, Faspak &
ADD-Vantage (Cefuroxime
Sodium) Lilly 1509
Kefzol Vials, Faspak &
ADD-Vantage (Cefazolin Sodium)
Lilly 1511
Mefoxin (Cefoxitin Sodium) Merck
& Co., Inc. 1734
Mefoxin Premixed Intravenous
Solution (Cefoxitin Sodium)
Merck & Co., Inc. 1737
Primaxin I.V. (Cilastatin Sodium,
Imipenem) Merck & Co., Inc. 1772
Rocephin Injectable Vials,
ADD-Vantage, Galaxy Container
(Ceftriaxone Sodium) Roche
Pharmaceuticals 2305
Tazicef for Injection (Ceftazidime)
SmithKline Beecham
Pharmaceuticals 2697
Tazidime Vials, Faspak &
ADD-Vantage (Ceftazidime) Lilly .. 1531
Timentin for Injection (Ticarcillin
Disodium, Clavulanate
Potassium) SmithKline Beecham
Pharmaceuticals 2706
Zinacef (Cefuroxime Sodium)
Glaxo Wellcome 1184

S. aureus urinary tract infections

Cefizox for Intramuscular or
Intravenous Use (Ceftizoxime
Sodium) Fujisawa 1025
Claforan Sterile and Injection
(Cefotaxime Sodium) Hoechst
Marion Roussel 1259
Macrodantin Capsules
(Nitrofurantoin) Procter &
Gamble Pharmaceuticals 2140
Nebcin Vials, Hyporets &
ADD-Vantage (Tobramycin
Sulfate) Lilly 1518
Netromycin Injection 100 mg/ml
(Netilmicin Sulfate) Schering 2516
Noroxin Tablets (Norfloxacin)
Merck & Co., Inc. 1758
Noroxin Tablets (Norfloxacin)
Roberts 2222
Primaxin I.V. (Cilastatin Sodium,
Imipenem) Merck & Co., Inc. 1772
Timentin for Injection (Ticarcillin
Disodium, Clavulanate
Potassium) SmithKline Beecham
Pharmaceuticals 2706

S. aureus (non-penicillinase producing) infections

Cefotan (Cefotetan) Zeneca 2936
Claforan Sterile and Injection
(Cefotaxime Sodium) Hoechst
Marion Roussel 1259
Mefoxin (Cefoxitin Sodium) Merck
& Co., Inc. 1734
Mefoxin Premixed Intravenous
Solution (Cefoxitin Sodium)
Merck & Co., Inc. 1737
Primaxin I.V. (Cilastatin Sodium,
Imipenem) Merck & Co., Inc. 1772

S. aureus (penicillinase and non-penicillinase producing strains) skin and skin structure infections

Mandol Vials, Faspak &
ADD-Vantage (Cefamandole
Nafate) Lilly 1516
Mefoxin (Cefoxitin Sodium) Merck
& Co., Inc. 1734
Mefoxin Premixed Intravenous
Solution (Cefoxitin Sodium)
Merck & Co., Inc. 1737
Nebcin Vials, Hyporets &
ADD-Vantage (Tobramycin
Sulfate) Lilly 1518
Zinacef (Cefuroxime Sodium)
Glaxo Wellcome 1184

S. aureus (penicillinase-producing) infections

Cefotan (Cefotetan) Zeneca 2936
Cefzil Tablets and Oral Suspension
(Cefprozil) Bristol-Myers Squibb .. 747
Claforan Sterile and Injection
(Cefotaxime Sodium) Hoechst
Marion Roussel 1259
Kefzol Vials, Faspak &
ADD-Vantage (Cefazolin Sodium)
Lilly 1511
Lorabid Suspension and Pulvules
(Loracarbef) Lilly 1513
Mefoxin (Cefoxitin Sodium) Merck
& Co., Inc. 1734
Mefoxin Premixed Intravenous
Solution (Cefoxitin Sodium)
Merck & Co., Inc. 1737
Primaxin I.M. (Cilastatin Sodium,
Imipenem) Merck & Co., Inc. 1770

(▣ Described in PDR For Nonprescription Drugs)   (⊚ Described in PDR For Ophthalmology)

Indications Index — **S. pneumoniae infections**

S. bovis endocarditis
Vancocin HCl, Vials & ADD-Vantage (Vancomycin Hydrochloride) Lilly ... 1534

S. epidermis bone and joint infections
Primaxin I.V. (Cilastatin Sodium, Imipenem) Merck & Co., Inc. ... 1772

S. epidermis endocarditis, early-onset prosthetic valve
Vancocin HCl, Vials & ADD-Vantage (Vancomycin Hydrochloride) Lilly ... 1534

S. epidermis gynecologic infections
Cefobid Intravenous/Intramuscular (Cefoperazone Sodium) Pfizer Inc ... 1996
Cefobid Pharmacy Bulk Package - Not for Direct Infusion (Cefoperazone Sodium) Pfizer Inc ... 1999
Cefotan (Cefotetan) Zeneca ... 2936
Claforan Sterile and Injection (Cefotaxime Sodium) Hoechst Marion Roussel ... 1259
Primaxin I.V. (Cilastatin Sodium, Imipenem) Merck & Co., Inc. ... 1772
Timentin for Injection (Ticarcillin Disodium, Clavulanate Potassium) SmithKline Beecham Pharmaceuticals ... 2706

S. epidermis infections
Cefizox for Intramuscular or Intravenous Use (Ceftizoxime Sodium) Fujisawa ... 1025
Cefobid Intravenous/Intramuscular (Cefoperazone Sodium) Pfizer Inc ... 1996
Cefobid Pharmacy Bulk Package - Not for Direct Infusion (Cefoperazone Sodium) Pfizer Inc ... 1999
Cefotan (Cefotetan) Zeneca ... 2936
Cipro I.V. (Ciprofloxacin) Bayer Pharmaceutical ... 587
Cipro I.V. Pharmacy Bulk Package (Ciprofloxacin) Bayer Pharmaceutical ... 590
Cipro Tablets (Ciprofloxacin Hydrochloride) Bayer Pharmaceutical ... 584
Claforan Sterile and Injection (Cefotaxime Sodium) Hoechst Marion Roussel ... 1259
Mefoxin (Cefoxitin Sodium) Merck & Co., Inc. ... 1734
Mefoxin Premixed Intravenous Solution (Cefoxitin Sodium) Merck & Co., Inc. ... 1737
Monocid Injection (Cefonicid Sodium) SmithKline Beecham Pharmaceuticals ... 2674
Noroxin Tablets (Norfloxacin) Merck & Co., Inc. ... 1758
Noroxin Tablets (Norfloxacin) Roberts ... 2222
Penetrex Tablets (Enoxacin) Rhone-Poulenc Rorer Pharmaceuticals ... 2196
Primaxin I.V. (Cilastatin Sodium, Imipenem) Merck & Co., Inc. ... 1772
Rocephin Injectable Vials, ADD-Vantage, Galaxy Container (Ceftriaxone Sodium) Roche Pharmaceuticals ... 2305
Timentin for Injection (Ticarcillin Disodium, Clavulanate Potassium) SmithKline Beecham Pharmaceuticals ... 2706
Vancocin HCl, Vials & ADD-Vantage (Vancomycin Hydrochloride) Lilly 1534

S. epidermis infections, ocular
Chibroxin Sterile Ophthalmic Solution (Norfloxacin) Merck & Co., Inc. ... 1657
Ciloxan Ophthalmic Solution (Ciprofloxacin Hydrochloride) Alcon Laboratories ... 468
Garamycin Ophthalmic (Gentamicin Sulfate) Schering ... 2501
Genoptic Sterile Ophthalmic Solution (Gentamicin Sulfate) Allergan ... ⊚ 241
Genoptic Sterile Ophthalmic Ointment (Gentamicin Sulfate) Allergan ... ⊚ 241
Gentak (Gentamicin Sulfate) Akorn ... ⊚ 209
Ocuflox Ophthalmic Solution (Ofloxacin) Allergan ... 478
Polytrim Ophthalmic Solution Sterile (Polymyxin B Sulfate, Trimethoprim Sulfate) Allergan ... 479
TobraDex Ophthalmic Suspension and Ointment (Dexamethasone, Tobramycin) Alcon Laboratories .. 469

S. epidermis intra-abdominal infections
Cefizox for Intramuscular or Intravenous Use (Ceftizoxime Sodium) Fujisawa ... 1025
Primaxin I.V. (Cilastatin Sodium, Imipenem) Merck & Co., Inc. ... 1772

S. epidermis pelvic inflammatory disease
Cefobid Intravenous/Intramuscular (Cefoperazone Sodium) Pfizer Inc ... 1996
Cefobid Pharmacy Bulk Package - Not for Direct Infusion (Cefoperazone Sodium) Pfizer Inc ... 1999

S. epidermis meningitis
Rocephin Injectable Vials, ADD-Vantage, Galaxy Container (Ceftriaxone Sodium) Roche Pharmaceuticals ... 2305

S. epidermis skin and skin structure infections
Cefizox for Intramuscular or Intravenous Use (Ceftizoxime Sodium) Fujisawa ... 1025
Cefotan (Cefotetan) Zeneca ... 2936
Cipro I.V. (Ciprofloxacin) Bayer Pharmaceutical ... 587
Cipro I.V. Pharmacy Bulk Package (Ciprofloxacin) Bayer Pharmaceutical ... 590
Cipro Tablets (Ciprofloxacin Hydrochloride) Bayer Pharmaceutical ... 584
Claforan Sterile and Injection (Cefotaxime Sodium) Hoechst Marion Roussel ... 1259
Mefoxin (Cefoxitin Sodium) Merck & Co., Inc. ... 1734
Mefoxin Premixed Intravenous Solution (Cefoxitin Sodium) Merck & Co., Inc. ... 1737
Monocid Injection (Cefonicid Sodium) SmithKline Beecham Pharmaceuticals ... 2674
Primaxin I.V. (Cilastatin Sodium, Imipenem) Merck & Co., Inc. ... 1772
Rocephin Injectable Vials, ADD-Vantage, Galaxy Container (Ceftriaxone Sodium) Roche Pharmaceuticals ... 2305

S. epidermis urinary tract infections
Cipro I.V. (Ciprofloxacin) Bayer Pharmaceutical ... 587
Cipro I.V. Pharmacy Bulk Package (Ciprofloxacin) Bayer Pharmaceutical ... 590
Cipro Tablets (Ciprofloxacin Hydrochloride) Bayer Pharmaceutical ... 584
Claforan Sterile and Injection (Cefotaxime Sodium) Hoechst Marion Roussel ... 1259
Mandol Vials, Faspak & ADD-Vantage (Cefamandole Nafate) Lilly ... 1516
Noroxin Tablets (Norfloxacin) Merck & Co., Inc. ... 1758
Noroxin Tablets (Norfloxacin) Roberts ... 2222
Penetrex Tablets (Enoxacin) Rhone-Poulenc Rorer Pharmaceuticals ... 2196

S. faecalis gynecologic infections
Pipracil (Piperacillin Sodium) Lederle ... 1435

S. faecalis infections
Amoxil (Amoxicillin Trihydrate) SmithKline Beecham Pharmaceuticals ... 2631
Cipro I.V. (Ciprofloxacin) Bayer Pharmaceutical ... 587
Cipro Tablets (Ciprofloxacin Hydrochloride) Bayer Pharmaceutical ... 584
Geocillin Tablets (Carbenicillin Indanyl Sodium) Pfizer Inc ... 2009
Mezlin (Mezlocillin Sodium) Bayer Pharmaceutical ... 594
Mezlin Pharmacy Bulk Package (Mezlocillin Sodium) Bayer Pharmaceutical ... 597
Noroxin Tablets (Norfloxacin) Merck & Co., Inc. ... 1758
Noroxin Tablets (Norfloxacin) Roberts ... 2222
Pipracil (Piperacillin Sodium) Lederle ... 1435
Spectrobid Tablets (Bacampicillin Hydrochloride) Pfizer Inc ... 2030
Ticar for Injection (Ticarcillin Disodium) SmithKline Beecham Pharmaceuticals ... 2704

S. faecalis urinary tract infections
Cipro I.V. (Ciprofloxacin) Bayer Pharmaceutical ... 587
Cipro Tablets (Ciprofloxacin Hydrochloride) Bayer Pharmaceutical ... 584
Mezlin (Mezlocillin Sodium) Bayer Pharmaceutical ... 594
Mezlin Pharmacy Bulk Package (Mezlocillin Sodium) Bayer Pharmaceutical ... 597
Noroxin Tablets (Norfloxacin) Merck & Co., Inc. ... 1758
Noroxin Tablets (Norfloxacin) Roberts ... 2222
Spectrobid Tablets (Bacampicillin Hydrochloride) Pfizer Inc ... 2030
Ticar for Injection (Ticarcillin Disodium) SmithKline Beecham Pharmaceuticals ... 2704

S. faecalis, endocardial infections, treatment adjunct
Vancocin HCl, Vials & ADD-Vantage (Vancomycin Hydrochloride) Lilly 1534

S. pneumoniae bone and joint infections
Rocephin Injectable Vials, ADD-Vantage, Galaxy Container (Ceftriaxone Sodium) Roche Pharmaceuticals ... 2305

S. pneumoniae bronchitis
Bactrim (Trimethoprim, Sulfamethoxazole) Roche Pharmaceuticals ... 2257
Biaxin (Clarithromycin) Abbott ... 406
Cedax (Ceftibuten Dihydrate) Schering ... 2480
Ceftin (Cefuroxime Axetil) Glaxo Wellcome ... 1067
Dynabac (Dirithromycin) Bock ... 668
Floxin I.V. (Ofloxacin) McNeil Pharmaceutical ... 1580
Lorabid Suspension and Pulvules (Loracarbef) Lilly ... 1513
Septra (Trimethoprim, Sulfamethoxazole) Glaxo Wellcome ... 1146
Spectrobid Tablets (Bacampicillin Hydrochloride) Pfizer Inc ... 2030
Suprax (Cefixime) Lederle ... 1443
Vantin for Oral Suspension and Vantin Tablets (Cefpodoxime Proxetil) Pharmacia & Upjohn ... 2112

S. pneumoniae central nervous system infections
Claforan Sterile and Injection (Cefotaxime Sodium) Hoechst Marion Roussel ... 1259
Fortaz (Ceftazidime) Glaxo Wellcome ... 1092
Tazicef for Injection (Ceftazidime) SmithKline Beecham Pharmaceuticals ... 2697
Tazidime Vials, Faspak & ADD-Vantage (Ceftazidime) Lilly .. 1531

S. pneumoniae infections
Achromycin V Capsules (Tetracycline Hydrochloride) Lederle ... 1417
Amoxil (Amoxicillin Trihydrate) SmithKline Beecham Pharmaceuticals ... 2631
Ancef Injection (Cefazolin Sodium) SmithKline Beecham Pharmaceuticals ... 2632
Augmentin Chewable Tablets (Amoxicillin Trihydrate, Clavulanate Potassium) SmithKline Beecham Pharmaceuticals ... 2637
Augmentin Tablets (Amoxicillin Trihydrate, Clavulanate Potassium) SmithKline Beecham Pharmaceuticals ... 2640
Bactrim (Trimethoprim, Sulfamethoxazole) Roche Pharmaceuticals ... 2257
Biaxin (Clarithromycin) Abbott ... 406
Bicillin C-R Injection (Penicillin G Procaine, Penicillin G Benzathine) Wyeth-Ayerst ... 2810
Bicillin C-R 900/300 Injection (Penicillin G Procaine, Penicillin G Benzathine) Wyeth-Ayerst ... 2812
Ceclor Pulvules & Suspension (Cefaclor) Lilly ... 1470
Cedax (Ceftibuten Dihydrate) Schering ... 2480
Cefizox for Intramuscular or Intravenous Use (Ceftizoxime Sodium) Fujisawa ... 1025
Cefobid Intravenous/Intramuscular (Cefoperazone Sodium) Pfizer Inc ... 1996
Cefobid Pharmacy Bulk Package - Not for Direct Infusion (Cefoperazone Sodium) Pfizer Inc ... 1999
Cefotan (Cefotetan) Zeneca ... 2936
Ceftin (Cefuroxime Axetil) Glaxo Wellcome ... 1067
Cefzil Tablets and Oral Suspension (Cefprozil) Bristol-Myers Squibb .. 747
Ceptaz (Ceftazidime) Glaxo Wellcome ... 1070
Cipro I.V. (Ciprofloxacin) Bayer Pharmaceutical ... 587
Cipro I.V. Pharmacy Bulk Package (Ciprofloxacin) Bayer Pharmaceutical ... 590
Cipro Tablets (Ciprofloxacin Hydrochloride) Bayer Pharmaceutical ... 584
Claforan Sterile and Injection (Cefotaxime Sodium) Hoechst Marion Roussel ... 1259
Cleocin Phosphate Injection (Clindamycin Phosphate) Pharmacia & Upjohn ... 2068
Declomycin Tablets (Demeclocycline Hydrochloride) Lederle ... 1421
Doryx Capsules (Doxycycline Hyclate) Parke-Davis ... 1970
Dynabac (Dirithromycin) Bock ... 668
DYNACIN Capsules (Minocycline Hydrochloride) Medicis ... 1627
E.E.S. (Erythromycin Ethylsuccinate) Abbott ... 427
E-Mycin Tablets (Erythromycin) Knoll Laboratories ... 1388
ERYC (Erythromycin) Parke-Davis .. 1972
EryPed (Erythromycin Ethylsuccinate) Abbott ... 425
Ery-Tab Tablets (Erythromycin) Abbott ... 426
Erythrocin Stearate Filmtab (Erythromycin Stearate) Abbott ... 429
Erythromycin Base Filmtab (Erythromycin) Abbott ... 430
Erythromycin Delayed-Release Capsules, USP (Erythromycin) Abbott ... 431
Floxin I.V. (Ofloxacin) McNeil Pharmaceutical ... 1580
Floxin Tablets (200 mg, 300 mg, 400 mg) (Ofloxacin) McNeil Pharmaceutical ... 1577
Fortaz (Ceftazidime) Glaxo Wellcome ... 1092
Ilosone (Erythromycin Estolate) Dista ... 927
Ilotycin Gluceptate, IV, Vials (Erythromycin Gluceptate) Dista ... 929
Keflex Pulvules & Oral Suspension (Cephalexin) Dista ... 930
Keftab Tablets (Cephalexin Hydrochloride) Dista ... 931
Kefurox Vials, Faspak & ADD-Vantage (Cefuroxime Sodium) Lilly ... 1509
Kefzol Vials, Faspak & ADD-Vantage (Cefazolin Sodium) Lilly ... 1511
Lorabid Suspension and Pulvules (Loracarbef) Lilly ... 1513
Maxipime for Injection (Cefepime Hydrochloride) Bristol-Myers Squibb ... 758
Mefoxin (Cefoxitin Sodium) Merck & Co., Inc. ... 1734

(▩ Described in PDR For Nonprescription Drugs)   (⊚ Described in PDR For Ophthalmology)

S. pneumoniae infections — Indications Index — 1572

Mefoxin Premixed Intravenous Solution (Cefoxitin Sodium) Merck & Co., Inc. ... 1737
Merrem I.V. (Meropenem) Zeneca ... 2952
Mezlin (Mezlocillin Sodium) Bayer Pharmaceutical ... 594
Mezlin Pharmacy Bulk Package (Mezlocillin Sodium) Bayer Pharmaceutical ... 597
Minocin Intravenous (Minocycline Hydrochloride) Lederle ... 1428
Minocin Oral Suspension (Minocycline Hydrochloride) Lederle ... 1431
Minocin Pellet-Filled Capsules (Minocycline Hydrochloride) Lederle ... 1429
Monocid Injection (Cefonicid Sodium) SmithKline Beecham Pharmaceuticals ... 2674
Monodox Capsules (Doxycycline Monohydrate) Oclassen ... 1858
PCE Dispertab Tablets (Erythromycin) Abbott ... 453
Pfizerpen for Injection (Penicillin G Potassium) Pfizer Inc ... 2022
Pipracil (Piperacillin Sodium) Lederle ... 1435
Primaxin I.M. (Cilastatin Sodium, Imipenem) Merck & Co., Inc. ... 1770
Primaxin I.V. (Cilastatin Sodium, Imipenem) Merck & Co., Inc. ... 1772
Rocephin Injectable Vials, ADD-Vantage, Galaxy Container (Ceftriaxone Sodium) Roche Pharmaceuticals ... 2305
Spectrobid Tablets (Bacampicillin Hydrochloride) Pfizer Inc ... 2030
Suprax (Cefixime) Lederle ... 1443
Tao Capsules (Troleandomycin) Pfizer Inc ... 2033
Tazicef for Injection (Ceftazidime) SmithKline Beecham Pharmaceuticals ... 2697
Tazidime Vials, Faspak & ADD-Vantage (Ceftazidime) Lilly ... 1531
Terramycin Intramuscular Solution (Oxytetracycline) Pfizer Inc ... 2034
Vantin for Oral Suspension and Vantin Tablets (Cefpodoxime Proxetil) Pharmacia & Upjohn ... 2112
Vibramycin Hyclate Capsules (Doxycycline Hyclate) Pfizer Inc ... 2038
Vibramycin Hyclate Intravenous (Doxycycline Hyclate) Pfizer Inc ... 2040
Zinacef (Cefuroxime Sodium) Glaxo Wellcome ... 1184
Zithromax (Azithromycin) Pfizer Inc ... 2043
Zithromax Tablets (Azithromycin) Pfizer Inc ... 2046

S. pneumoniae infections, ocular

AK-CIDE (Prednisolone Acetate, Sulfacetamide Sodium) Akorn ... ◉ 203
AK-CIDE Ointment (Prednisolone Acetate, Sulfacetamide Sodium) Akorn ... ◉ 203
AK-Spore (Bacitracin Zinc, Neomycin Sulfate, Polymyxin B Sulfate) Akorn ... ◉ 205
Blephamide Liquifilm Sterile Ophthalmic Suspension (Prednisolone Acetate, Sulfacetamide Sodium) Allergan ... 472
Blephamide Ointment (Sulfacetamide Sodium, Prednisolone Acetate) Allergan ... ◉ 234
Chibroxin Sterile Ophthalmic Solution (Norfloxacin) Merck & Co., Inc. ... 1657
Chloromycetin Ophthalmic Ointment, 1% (Chloramphenicol) Parke-Davis ... ◉ 298
Chloromycetin Ophthalmic Solution (Chloramphenicol) Parke-Davis ... ◉ 299
Chloroptic S.O.P. (Chloramphenicol) Allergan ... ◉ 236
Ciloxan Ophthalmic Solution (Ciprofloxacin Hydrochloride) Alcon Laboratories ... 468
Cortisporin Ophthalmic Ointment Sterile (Polymyxin B Sulfate, Bacitracin Zinc, Neomycin Sulfate, Hydrocortisone) Glaxo Wellcome ... 1074
FML-S Liquifilm (Sulfacetamide Sodium, Fluorometholone) Allergan ... ◉ 240
Garamycin Ophthalmic (Gentamicin Sulfate) Schering ... 2501
Genoptic Sterile Ophthalmic Solution (Gentamicin Sulfate) Allergan ... ◉ 241
Genoptic Sterile Ophthalmic Ointment (Gentamicin Sulfate) Allergan ... ◉ 241
Gentak (Gentamicin Sulfate) Akorn ... ◉ 209
Ocuflox Ophthalmic Solution (Ofloxacin) Allergan ... 478
Polytrim Ophthalmic Solution Sterile (Polymyxin B Sulfate, Trimethoprim Sulfate) Allergan ... 479
Pred-G Liquifilm Sterile Ophthalmic Suspension (Gentamicin Sulfate, Prednisolone Acetate) Allergan ... ◉ 248
Pred-G S.O.P. Sterile Ophthalmic Ointment (Gentamicin Sulfate, Prednisolone Acetate) Allergan ... ◉ 249
Terra-Cortril Ophthalmic Suspension (Oxytetracycline Hydrochloride, Hydrocortisone Acetate) Pfizer Inc ... 2033
Terramycin with Polymyxin B Sulfate Ophthalmic Ointment (Oxytetracycline Hydrochloride, Polymyxin B Sulfate) Pfizer Inc ... 2035
TobraDex Ophthalmic Suspension and Ointment (Dexamethasone, Tobramycin) Alcon Laboratories ... 469

S. pneumoniae lower respiratory tract infections

Biaxin (Clarithromycin) Abbott ... 406
Ceclor Pulvules & Suspension (Cefaclor) Lilly ... 1470
Cefizox for Intramuscular or Intravenous Use (Ceftizoxime Sodium) Fujisawa ... 1025
Cefotan (Cefotetan) Zeneca ... 2936
Cefzil Tablets and Oral Suspension (Cefprozil) Bristol-Myers Squibb ... 747
Ceptaz (Ceftazidime) Glaxo Wellcome ... 1070
Cipro I.V. (Ciprofloxacin) Bayer Pharmaceutical ... 587
Cipro I.V. Pharmacy Bulk Package (Ciprofloxacin) Bayer Pharmaceutical ... 590
Cipro Tablets (Ciprofloxacin Hydrochloride) Bayer Pharmaceutical ... 584
Claforan Sterile and Injection (Cefotaxime Sodium) Hoechst Marion Roussel ... 1259
Cleocin Phosphate Injection (Clindamycin Phosphate) Pharmacia & Upjohn ... 2068
E.E.S. (Erythromycin Ethylsuccinate) Abbott ... 427
E-Mycin Tablets (Erythromycin) Knoll Laboratories ... 1388
ERYC (Erythromycin) Parke-Davis ... 1972
EryPed (Erythromycin Ethylsuccinate) Abbott ... 425
Ery-Tab Tablets (Erythromycin) Abbott ... 426
Erythrocin Stearate Filmtab (Erythromycin Stearate) Abbott ... 429
Erythromycin Base Filmtab (Erythromycin) Abbott ... 430
Erythromycin Delayed-Release Capsules, USP (Erythromycin) Abbott ... 431
Floxin I.V. (Ofloxacin) McNeil Pharmaceutical ... 1580
Floxin Tablets (200 mg, 300 mg, 400 mg) (Ofloxacin) McNeil Pharmaceutical ... 1577
Fortaz (Ceftazidime) Glaxo Wellcome ... 1092
Ilosone (Erythromycin Estolate) Dista ... 927
Ilotycin Gluceptate, IV, Vials (Erythromycin Gluceptate) Dista ... 929
Keftab Tablets (Cephalexin Hydrochloride) Dista ... 931
Kefurox Vials, Faspak & ADD-Vantage (Cefuroxime Sodium) Lilly ... 1509
Lorabid Suspension and Pulvules (Loracarbef) Lilly ... 1513
Mandol Vials, Faspak & ADD-Vantage (Cefamandole Nafate) Lilly ... 1516
Maxipime for Injection (Cefepime Hydrochloride) Bristol-Myers Squibb ... 758
Mefoxin (Cefoxitin Sodium) Merck & Co., Inc. ... 1734
Mefoxin Premixed Intravenous Solution (Cefoxitin Sodium) Merck & Co., Inc. ... 1737
Monocid Injection (Cefonicid Sodium) SmithKline Beecham Pharmaceuticals ... 2674
PCE Dispertab Tablets (Erythromycin) Abbott ... 453
Primaxin I.M. (Cilastatin Sodium, Imipenem) Merck & Co., Inc. ... 1770
Rocephin Injectable Vials, ADD-Vantage, Galaxy Container (Ceftriaxone Sodium) Roche Pharmaceuticals ... 2305
Spectrobid Tablets (Bacampicillin Hydrochloride) Pfizer Inc ... 2030
Tao Capsules (Troleandomycin) Pfizer Inc ... 2033
Tazicef for Injection (Ceftazidime) SmithKline Beecham Pharmaceuticals ... 2697
Tazidime Vials, Faspak & ADD-Vantage (Ceftazidime) Lilly ... 1531
Vantin for Oral Suspension and Vantin Tablets (Cefpodoxime Proxetil) Pharmacia & Upjohn ... 2112
Zinacef (Cefuroxime Sodium) Glaxo Wellcome ... 1184
Zithromax (Azithromycin) Pfizer Inc ... 2043
Zithromax Tablets (Azithromycin) Pfizer Inc ... 2046

S. pneumoniae meningitis

Cefizox for Intramuscular or Intravenous Use (Ceftizoxime Sodium) Fujisawa ... 1025
Ceptaz (Ceftazidime) Glaxo Wellcome ... 1070
Fortaz (Ceftazidime) Glaxo Wellcome ... 1092
Kefurox Vials, Faspak & ADD-Vantage (Cefuroxime Sodium) Lilly ... 1509
Merrem I.V. (Meropenem) Zeneca ... 2952
Rocephin Injectable Vials, ADD-Vantage, Galaxy Container (Ceftriaxone Sodium) Roche Pharmaceuticals ... 2305
Tazicef for Injection (Ceftazidime) SmithKline Beecham Pharmaceuticals ... 2697
Tazidime Vials, Faspak & ADD-Vantage (Ceftazidime) Lilly ... 1531
Zinacef (Cefuroxime Sodium) Glaxo Wellcome ... 1184

S. pneumoniae otitis media

Bactrim (Trimethoprim, Sulfamethoxazole) Roche Pharmaceuticals ... 2257
Biaxin (Clarithromycin) Abbott ... 406
Bicillin C-R Injection (Penicillin G Procaine, Penicillin G Benzathine) Wyeth-Ayerst ... 2810
Bicillin C-R 900/300 Injection (Penicillin G Procaine, Penicillin G Benzathine) Wyeth-Ayerst ... 2812
Ceclor Pulvules & Suspension (Cefaclor) Lilly ... 1470
Ceftin (Cefuroxime Axetil) Glaxo Wellcome ... 1067
Cefzil Tablets and Oral Suspension (Cefprozil) Bristol-Myers Squibb ... 747
E.E.S. (Erythromycin Ethylsuccinate) Abbott ... 427
EryPed (Erythromycin Ethylsuccinate) Abbott ... 425
Ery-Tab Tablets (Erythromycin) Abbott ... 426
Erythrocin Stearate Filmtab (Erythromycin Stearate) Abbott ... 429
Erythromycin Base Filmtab (Erythromycin) Abbott ... 430
Ilosone (Erythromycin Estolate) Dista ... 927
Ilotycin Gluceptate, IV, Vials (Erythromycin Gluceptate) Dista ... 929
Keflex Pulvules & Oral Suspension (Cephalexin) Dista ... 930
Lorabid Suspension and Pulvules (Loracarbef) Lilly ... 1513
Septra (Trimethoprim, Sulfamethoxazole) Glaxo Wellcome ... 1146
Suprax (Cefixime) Lederle ... 1443
Vantin for Oral Suspension and Vantin Tablets (Cefpodoxime Proxetil) Pharmacia & Upjohn ... 2112
Zithromax (Azithromycin) Pfizer Inc ... 2043

S. pneumoniae pharyngitis

Biaxin (Clarithromycin) Abbott ... 406
EryPed (Erythromycin Ethylsuccinate) Abbott ... 425
Ery-Tab Tablets (Erythromycin) Abbott ... 426
Erythrocin Stearate Filmtab (Erythromycin Stearate) Abbott ... 429
Erythromycin Base Filmtab (Erythromycin) Abbott ... 430
Erythromycin Delayed-Release Capsules, USP (Erythromycin) Abbott ... 431
Ilosone (Erythromycin Estolate) Dista ... 927
Ilotycin Gluceptate, IV, Vials (Erythromycin Gluceptate) Dista ... 929
PCE Dispertab Tablets (Erythromycin) Abbott ... 453

S. pneumoniae respiratory tract infections

Ancef Injection (Cefazolin Sodium) SmithKline Beecham Pharmaceuticals ... 2632
Cefobid Intravenous/Intramuscular (Cefoperazone Sodium) Pfizer Inc ... 1996
Cefobid Pharmacy Bulk Package - Not for Direct Infusion (Cefoperazone Sodium) Pfizer Inc ... 1999
Dynabac (Dirithromycin) Bock ... 668
Keflex Pulvules & Oral Suspension (Cephalexin) Dista ... 930
Kefzol Vials, Faspak & ADD-Vantage (Cefazolin Sodium) Lilly ... 1511

S. pneumoniae septicemia

Ancef Injection (Cefazolin Sodium) SmithKline Beecham Pharmaceuticals ... 2632
Cefizox for Intramuscular or Intravenous Use (Ceftizoxime Sodium) Fujisawa ... 1025
Cefobid Intravenous/Intramuscular (Cefoperazone Sodium) Pfizer Inc ... 1996
Cefobid Pharmacy Bulk Package - Not for Direct Infusion (Cefoperazone Sodium) Pfizer Inc ... 1999
Ceptaz (Ceftazidime) Glaxo Wellcome ... 1070
Claforan Sterile and Injection (Cefotaxime Sodium) Hoechst Marion Roussel ... 1259
Fortaz (Ceftazidime) Glaxo Wellcome ... 1092
Kefurox Vials, Faspak & ADD-Vantage (Cefuroxime Sodium) Lilly ... 1509
Kefzol Vials, Faspak & ADD-Vantage (Cefazolin Sodium) Lilly ... 1511
Mefoxin (Cefoxitin Sodium) Merck & Co., Inc. ... 1734
Mefoxin Premixed Intravenous Solution (Cefoxitin Sodium) Merck & Co., Inc. ... 1737
Monocid Injection (Cefonicid Sodium) SmithKline Beecham Pharmaceuticals ... 2674
Pipracil (Piperacillin Sodium) Lederle ... 1435
Rocephin Injectable Vials, ADD-Vantage, Galaxy Container (Ceftriaxone Sodium) Roche Pharmaceuticals ... 2305
Tazicef for Injection (Ceftazidime) SmithKline Beecham Pharmaceuticals ... 2697
Tazidime Vials, Faspak & ADD-Vantage (Ceftazidime) Lilly ... 1531
Zinacef (Cefuroxime Sodium) Glaxo Wellcome ... 1184

S. pneumoniae sinusitis

Biaxin (Clarithromycin) Abbott ... 406
Ceftin (Cefuroxime Axetil) Glaxo Wellcome ... 1067

S. pneumoniae upper respiratory tract infections

Biaxin (Clarithromycin) Abbott ... 406
DYNACIN Capsules (Minocycline Hydrochloride) Medicis ... 1627
E.E.S. (Erythromycin Ethylsuccinate) Abbott ... 427
E-Mycin Tablets (Erythromycin) Knoll Laboratories ... 1388
ERYC (Erythromycin) Parke-Davis ... 1972

(▣ Described in PDR For Nonprescription Drugs) (◉ Described in PDR For Ophthalmology)

1573 **Indications Index** **S. saprophyticus**

EryPed (Erythromycin Ethylsuccinate) Abbott 425
Ery-Tab Tablets (Erythromycin) Abbott 426
Erythrocin Stearate Filmtab (Erythromycin Stearate) Abbott 429
Erythromycin Base Filmtab (Erythromycin) Abbott 430
Erythromycin Delayed-Release Capsules, USP (Erythromycin) Abbott 431
Ilosone (Erythromycin Estolate) Dista 927
Ilotycin Gluceptate, IV, Vials (Erythromycin Gluceptate) Dista 929
Keftab Tablets (Cephalexin Hydrochloride) Dista 931
Minocin Oral Suspension (Minocycline Hydrochloride) Lederle 1431
Minocin Pellet-Filled Capsules (Minocycline Hydrochloride) Lederle 1429
Monodox Capsules (Doxycycline Monohydrate) Oclassen 1858
PCE Dispertab Tablets (Erythromycin) Abbott 453
Spectrobid Tablets (Bacampicillin Hydrochloride) Pfizer Inc 2030
Vibramycin Hyclate Capsules (Doxycycline Hyclate) Pfizer Inc 2038

S. pyogenes bone and joint infections

Claforan Sterile and Injection (Cefotaxime Sodium) Hoechst Marion Roussel 1259

S. pyogenes infections

Bactroban Ointment (Mupirocin) SmithKline Beecham Pharmaceuticals 2642
Biaxin (Clarithromycin) Abbott 406
Ceclor Pulvules & Suspension (Cefaclor) Lilly 1470
Cedax (Ceftibuten Dihydrate) Schering 2480
Cefizox for Intramuscular or Intravenous Use (Ceftizoxime Sodium) Fujisawa 1025
Cefobid Intravenous/Intramuscular (Cefoperazone Sodium) Pfizer Inc 1996
Cefobid Pharmacy Bulk Package - Not for Direct Infusion (Cefoperazone Sodium) Pfizer Inc 1999
Cefotan (Cefotetan) Zeneca 2936
Ceftin (Cefuroxime Axetil) Glaxo Wellcome 1067
Cefzil Tablets and Oral Suspension (Cefprozil) Bristol-Myers Squibb .. 747
Ceptaz (Ceftazidime) Glaxo Wellcome 1070
Cipro I.V. (Ciprofloxacin) Bayer Pharmaceutical 587
Cipro I.V. Pharmacy Bulk Package (Ciprofloxacin) Bayer Pharmaceutical 590
Cipro Tablets (Ciprofloxacin Hydrochloride) Bayer Pharmaceutical 584
Claforan Sterile and Injection (Cefotaxime Sodium) Hoechst Marion Roussel 1259
Cleocin Phosphate Injection (Clindamycin Phosphate) Pharmacia & Upjohn 2068
Dynabac (Dirithromycin) Bock 668
E.E.S. (Erythromycin Ethylsuccinate) Abbott 427
E-Mycin Tablets (Erythromycin) Knoll Laboratories 1388
ERYC (Erythromycin) Parke-Davis .. 1972
EryPed (Erythromycin Ethylsuccinate) Abbott 425
Ery-Tab Tablets (Erythromycin) Abbott 426
Erythrocin Stearate Filmtab (Erythromycin Stearate) Abbott 429
Erythromycin Base Filmtab (Erythromycin) Abbott 430
Erythromycin Delayed-Release Capsules, USP (Erythromycin) Abbott 431
Floxin I.V. (Ofloxacin) McNeil Pharmaceutical 1580
Floxin Tablets (200 mg, 300 mg, 400 mg) (Ofloxacin) McNeil Pharmaceutical 1577
Fortaz (Ceftazidime) Glaxo Wellcome 1092
Keflex Pulvules & Oral Suspension (Cephalexin) Dista 930
Kefurox Vials, Faspak & ADD-Vantage (Cefuroxime Sodium) Lilly 1509
Lorabid Suspension and Pulvules (Loracarbef) Lilly 1513
Maxipime for Injection (Cefepime Hydrochloride) Bristol-Myers Squibb 758
Monocid Injection (Cefonicid Sodium) SmithKline Beecham Pharmaceuticals 2674
PCE Dispertab Tablets (Erythromycin) Abbott 453
Primaxin I.M. (Cilastatin Sodium, Imipenem) Merck & Co., Inc. 1770
Rocephin Injectable Vials, ADD-Vantage, Galaxy Container (Ceftriaxone Sodium) Roche Pharmaceuticals 2305
Spectrobid Tablets (Bacampicillin Hydrochloride) Pfizer Inc 2030
Suprax (Cefixime) Lederle 1443
Tao Capsules (Troleandomycin) Pfizer Inc 2033
Tazicef for Injection (Ceftazidime) SmithKline Beecham Pharmaceuticals 2697
Tazidime Vials, Faspak & ADD-Vantage (Ceftazidime) Lilly .. 1531
Vantin for Oral Suspension and Vantin Tablets (Cefpodoxime Proxetil) Pharmacia & Upjohn 2112
Zinacef (Cefuroxime Sodium) Glaxo Wellcome 1184
Zithromax (Azithromycin) Pfizer Inc 2043
Zithromax Tablets (Azithromycin) Pfizer Inc 2046

S. pyogenes infections, ocular

Garamycin Ophthalmic (Gentamicin Sulfate) Schering 2501
Genoptic Sterile Ophthalmic Solution (Gentamicin Sulfate) Allergan .... ⊚ 241
Genoptic Sterile Ophthalmic Ointment (Gentamicin Sulfate) Allergan .... ⊚ 241
Gentak (Gentamicin Sulfate) Akorn .... ⊚ 209
Pred-G S.O.P. Sterile Ophthalmic Ointment (Gentamicin Sulfate, Prednisolone Acetate) Allergan .. ⊚ 249

S. pyogenes lower respiratory tract infections

Ceclor Pulvules & Suspension (Cefaclor) Lilly 1470
Claforan Sterile and Injection (Cefotaxime Sodium) Hoechst Marion Roussel 1259
E.E.S. (Erythromycin Ethylsuccinate) Abbott 427
E-Mycin Tablets (Erythromycin) Knoll Laboratories 1388
ERYC (Erythromycin) Parke-Davis .. 1972
EryPed (Erythromycin Ethylsuccinate) Abbott 425
Ery-Tab Tablets (Erythromycin) Abbott 426
Erythrocin Stearate Filmtab (Erythromycin Stearate) Abbott 429
Erythromycin Base Filmtab (Erythromycin) Abbott 430
Erythromycin Delayed-Release Capsules, USP (Erythromycin) Abbott 431
Ilosone (Erythromycin Estolate) Dista 927
Ilotycin Gluceptate, IV, Vials (Erythromycin Gluceptate) Dista 929
Kefurox Vials, Faspak & ADD-Vantage (Cefuroxime Sodium) Lilly 1509
PCE Dispertab Tablets (Erythromycin) Abbott 453
Spectrobid Tablets (Bacampicillin Hydrochloride) Pfizer Inc 2030
Zinacef (Cefuroxime Sodium) Glaxo Wellcome 1184

S. pyogenes otitis media

Ceclor Pulvules & Suspension (Cefaclor) Lilly 1470
Cedax (Ceftibuten Dihydrate) Schering 2480
Ceftin (Cefuroxime Axetil) Glaxo Wellcome 1067
Lorabid Suspension and Pulvules (Loracarbef) Lilly 1513
Suprax (Cefixime) Lederle 1443

S. pyogenes pharyngitis

Biaxin (Clarithromycin) Abbott 406
Ceclor Pulvules & Suspension (Cefaclor) Lilly 1470
Cedax (Ceftibuten Dihydrate) Schering 2480
Ceftin (Cefuroxime Axetil) Glaxo Wellcome 1067
Cefzil Tablets and Oral Suspension (Cefprozil) Bristol-Myers Squibb .. 747
Dynabac (Dirithromycin) Bock 668
Lorabid Suspension and Pulvules (Loracarbef) Lilly 1513
Suprax (Cefixime) Lederle 1443
Vantin for Oral Suspension and Vantin Tablets (Cefpodoxime Proxetil) Pharmacia & Upjohn 2112
Zithromax (Azithromycin) Pfizer Inc 2043
Zithromax Tablets (Azithromycin) Pfizer Inc 2046

S. pyogenes respiratory tract infections

Cefobid Intravenous/Intramuscular (Cefoperazone Sodium) Pfizer Inc 1996
Cefobid Pharmacy Bulk Package - Not for Direct Infusion (Cefoperazone Sodium) Pfizer Inc 1999
Keflex Pulvules & Oral Suspension (Cephalexin) Dista 930

S. pyogenes skin and skin structure infections

Biaxin (Clarithromycin) Abbott 406
Ceclor Pulvules & Suspension (Cefaclor) Lilly 1470
Cefizox for Intramuscular or Intravenous Use (Ceftizoxime Sodium) Fujisawa 1025
Cefobid Intravenous/Intramuscular (Cefoperazone Sodium) Pfizer Inc 1996
Cefobid Pharmacy Bulk Package - Not for Direct Infusion (Cefoperazone Sodium) Pfizer Inc 1999
Cefotan (Cefotetan) Zeneca 2936
Ceftin (Cefuroxime Axetil) Glaxo Wellcome 1067
Cefzil Tablets and Oral Suspension (Cefprozil) Bristol-Myers Squibb .. 747
Ceptaz (Ceftazidime) Glaxo Wellcome 1070
Cipro I.V. (Ciprofloxacin) Bayer Pharmaceutical 587
Cipro I.V. Pharmacy Bulk Package (Ciprofloxacin) Bayer Pharmaceutical 590
Cipro Tablets (Ciprofloxacin Hydrochloride) Bayer Pharmaceutical 584
Claforan Sterile and Injection (Cefotaxime Sodium) Hoechst Marion Roussel 1259
Cleocin Phosphate Injection (Clindamycin Phosphate) Pharmacia & Upjohn 2068
E.E.S. (Erythromycin Ethylsuccinate) Abbott 427
E-Mycin Tablets (Erythromycin) Knoll Laboratories 1388
ERYC (Erythromycin) Parke-Davis .. 1972
EryPed (Erythromycin Ethylsuccinate) Abbott 425
Ery-Tab Tablets (Erythromycin) Abbott 426
Erythrocin Stearate Filmtab (Erythromycin Stearate) Abbott 429
Erythromycin Base Filmtab (Erythromycin) Abbott 430
Erythromycin Delayed-Release Capsules, USP (Erythromycin) Abbott 431
Floxin I.V. (Ofloxacin) McNeil Pharmaceutical 1580
Floxin Tablets (200 mg, 300 mg, 400 mg) (Ofloxacin) McNeil Pharmaceutical 1577
Fortaz (Ceftazidime) Glaxo Wellcome 1092
Ilosone (Erythromycin Estolate) Dista 927
Ilotycin Gluceptate, IV, Vials (Erythromycin Gluceptate) Dista 929
Lorabid Suspension and Pulvules (Loracarbef) Lilly 1513
Mandol Vials, Faspak & ADD-Vantage (Cefamandole Nafate) Lilly 1516
Maxipime for Injection (Cefepime Hydrochloride) Bristol-Myers Squibb 758
Monocid Injection (Cefonicid Sodium) SmithKline Beecham Pharmaceuticals 2674
PCE Dispertab Tablets (Erythromycin) Abbott 453
Primaxin I.M. (Cilastatin Sodium, Imipenem) Merck & Co., Inc. 1770
Rocephin Injectable Vials, ADD-Vantage, Galaxy Container (Ceftriaxone Sodium) Roche Pharmaceuticals 2305
Tazicef for Injection (Ceftazidime) SmithKline Beecham Pharmaceuticals 2697
Tazidime Vials, Faspak & ADD-Vantage (Ceftazidime) Lilly .. 1531
Vantin for Oral Suspension and Vantin Tablets (Cefpodoxime Proxetil) Pharmacia & Upjohn 2112
Zinacef (Cefuroxime Sodium) Glaxo Wellcome 1184
Zithromax (Azithromycin) Pfizer Inc 2043
Zithromax Tablets (Azithromycin) Pfizer Inc 2046

S. pyogenes tonsillitis

Biaxin (Clarithromycin) Abbott 406
Ceclor Pulvules & Suspension (Cefaclor) Lilly 1470
Cedax (Ceftibuten Dihydrate) Schering 2480
Ceftin (Cefuroxime Axetil) Glaxo Wellcome 1067
Cefzil Tablets and Oral Suspension (Cefprozil) Bristol-Myers Squibb .. 747
Dynabac (Dirithromycin) Bock 668
Lorabid Suspension and Pulvules (Loracarbef) Lilly 1513
Suprax (Cefixime) Lederle 1443
Vantin for Oral Suspension and Vantin Tablets (Cefpodoxime Proxetil) Pharmacia & Upjohn 2112
Zithromax (Azithromycin) Pfizer Inc 2043
Zithromax Tablets (Azithromycin) Pfizer Inc 2046

S. pyogenes upper respiratory tract infections

Biaxin (Clarithromycin) Abbott 406
Ceclor Pulvules & Suspension (Cefaclor) Lilly 1470
E.E.S. (Erythromycin Ethylsuccinate) Abbott 427
E-Mycin Tablets (Erythromycin) Knoll Laboratories 1388
ERYC (Erythromycin) Parke-Davis .. 1972
EryPed (Erythromycin Ethylsuccinate) Abbott 425
Ery-Tab Tablets (Erythromycin) Abbott 426
Erythrocin Stearate Filmtab (Erythromycin Stearate) Abbott 429
Erythromycin Base Filmtab (Erythromycin) Abbott 430
Erythromycin Delayed-Release Capsules, USP (Erythromycin) Abbott 431
Ilosone (Erythromycin Estolate) Dista 927
Ilotycin Gluceptate, IV, Vials (Erythromycin Gluceptate) Dista 929
PCE Dispertab Tablets (Erythromycin) Abbott 453
Spectrobid Tablets (Bacampicillin Hydrochloride) Pfizer Inc 2030
Suprax (Cefixime) Lederle 1443
Tao Capsules (Troleandomycin) Pfizer Inc 2033
Zithromax (Azithromycin) Pfizer Inc 2043
Zithromax Tablets (Azithromycin) Pfizer Inc 2046

S. saprophyticus urinary tract infections

Cipro Tablets (Ciprofloxacin Hydrochloride) Bayer Pharmaceutical 584
Lorabid Suspension and Pulvules (Loracarbef) Lilly 1513
Macrobid Capsules (Nitrofurantoin Monohydrate) Procter & Gamble Pharmaceuticals 2138
Maxaquin Tablets (Lomefloxacin Hydrochloride) Searle 2593
Noroxin Tablets (Norfloxacin) Merck & Co., Inc. 1758

(▣ Described in PDR For Nonprescription Drugs)

(⊚ Described in PDR For Ophthalmology)

S. saprophyticus

S. saprophyticus
- Noroxin Tablets (Norfloxacin) Roberts ... 2222
- Penetrex Tablets (Enoxacin) Rhone-Poulenc Rorer Pharmaceuticals ... 2196
- Proloprim Tablets (Trimethoprim) Glaxo Wellcome ... 1141
- Trimpex Tablets (Trimethoprim) Roche Pharmaceuticals ... 2323
- Vantin for Oral Suspension and Vantin Tablets (Cefpodoxime Proxetil) Pharmacia & Upjohn ... 2112

S. typhi infections, acute
- Chloromycetin Sodium Succinate (Chloramphenicol Sodium Succinate) Parke-Davis ... 1960

S. viridans endocarditis
- Erythrocin Stearate Filmtab (Erythromycin Stearate) Abbott ... 429
- Erythromycin Base Filmtab (Erythromycin) Abbott ... 430
- Vancocin HCl, Vials & ADD-Vantage (Vancomycin Hydrochloride) Lilly 1534

S. warnerii infections, ocular
- Chibroxin Sterile Ophthalmic Solution (Norfloxacin) Merck & Co., Inc. ... 1657

SAH
(see under Hemorrhage, subarachnoid, resulting in neurological deficits)

Salmonella species infections
- Chloromycetin Sodium Succinate (Chloramphenicol Sodium Succinate) Parke-Davis ... 1960
- Omnipen Capsules (Ampicillin) Wyeth-Ayerst ... 2872
- Omnipen for Oral Suspension (Ampicillin) Wyeth-Ayerst ... 2873
- Pfizerpen for Injection (Penicillin G Potassium) Pfizer Inc ... 2022

Salmonella species infections, serious
- Pfizerpen for Injection (Penicillin G Potassium) Pfizer Inc ... 2022

Salmonella typhi infections
- Cipro Tablets (Ciprofloxacin Hydrochloride) Bayer Pharmaceutical ... 584

Salpingitis
- Ticar for Injection (Ticarcillin Disodium) SmithKline Beecham Pharmaceuticals ... 2704

Salt, substitute for
- Chlor-3 Condiment (Potassium Chloride) Fleming ... 1003

Sarcoidosis, symptomatic
- Celestone Soluspan Suspension (Betamethasone Sodium Phosphate, Betamethasone Acetate) Schering ... 2484
- Cortone Acetate Sterile Suspension (Cortisone Acetate) Merck & Co., Inc. ... 1663
- Cortone Acetate Tablets (Cortisone Acetate) Merck & Co., Inc. ... 1664
- Dalalone D.P. Injectable (Dexamethasone Acetate) Forest ... 1009
- Decadron Elixir (Dexamethasone) Merck & Co., Inc. ... 1676
- Decadron Phosphate Injection (Dexamethasone Sodium Phosphate) Merck & Co., Inc. ... 1680
- Decadron Tablets (Dexamethasone) Merck & Co., Inc. ... 1678
- Decadron-LA Sterile Suspension (Dexamethasone Acetate) Merck & Co., Inc. ... 1687
- Hydeltrasol Injection, Sterile (Prednisolone Sodium Phosphate) Merck & Co., Inc. ... 1708
- Hydrocortone Phosphate Injection, Sterile (Hydrocortisone Sodium Phosphate) Merck & Co., Inc. ... 1713
- Hydrocortone Tablets (Hydrocortisone) Merck & Co., Inc. ... 1715
- Pediapred Oral Solution (Prednisolone Sodium Phosphate) Medeva 1618
- Prelone Syrup (Prednisolone) Muro 1834

Sarcoma botryoides
- Cosmegen Injection (Dactinomycin) Merck & Co., Inc. ... 1666

Sarcoma, idiopathic multiple hemorrhagic
(see under Kaposi's sarcoma)

Sarcomas, soft tissue and bone
- Adriamycin PFS (Doxorubicin Hydrochloride) Pharmacia & Upjohn ... 2056
- Adriamycin RDF (Doxorubicin Hydrochloride) Pharmacia & Upjohn ... 2056
- Doxorubicin Astra (Doxorubicin Hydrochloride) Astra ... 531
- Rubex for Injection (Doxorubicin Hydrochloride) Bristol-Myers Squibb Oncology/Immunology ... 721

Sarcoptes scabiei infestations
- Elimite (permethrin) 5% Cream (Permethrin) Allergan ... 475
- Eurax Cream & Lotion (Crotamiton) Westwood-Squibb 2794
- Kwell Cream & Lotion (Lindane) Reedco ... 2172
- Lindane Lotion USP 1% (Lindane) Alpharma ... 481

Scabies
(see under Sarcoptes scabiei infestations)

Scarlatina
- Bicillin C-R Injection (Penicillin G Procaine, Penicillin G Benzathine) Wyeth-Ayerst ... 2810
- Bicillin C-R 900/300 Injection (Penicillin G Procaine, Penicillin G Benzathine) Wyeth-Ayerst ... 2812
- Pen•Vee K (Penicillin V Potassium) Wyeth-Ayerst ... 2879

Scarlet fever
(see under Scarlatina)

Schistosoma haematobium infections
- Biltricide Tablets (Praziquantel) Bayer Pharmaceutical ... 584

Schistosoma japonicum infections
- Biltricide Tablets (Praziquantel) Bayer Pharmaceutical ... 584

Schistosoma mansoni infections
- Biltricide Tablets (Praziquantel) Bayer Pharmaceutical ... 584

Schistosoma mekongi infections
- Biltricide Tablets (Praziquantel) Bayer Pharmaceutical ... 584

Schizophrenia
(see under Psychotic disorders, management of the manifestations of)

Schizophrenia with depression
(see under Psychotic disorders with depressive symptoms)

Sciatica, temporary relief of
- Arthritis Strength BC Powder (Aspirin, Salicylamide, Caffeine) Block ... 631
- BC Powder (Aspirin, Salicylamide, Caffeine) Block ... 631
- Sarapin (Sarracenia purpurea, Pitcher Plant Distillate) High Chemical ... 1237

Scleroderma, "possibly" effective in
- Potaba Capsules, Envules, Powder, and Tablets (Aminobenzoate Potassium) Glenwood-Palisades .. 1234

Scleroderma, linear, "possibly" effective in
- Potaba Capsules, Envules, Powder, and Tablets (Aminobenzoate Potassium) Glenwood-Palisades .. 1234

Sclerosis, amyotrophic lateral
- Rilutek Tablets (Riluzole) Rhone-Poulenc Rorer Pharmaceuticals ... 2198

Sclerosis, multiple, acute exacerbations of
- Pediapred Oral Solution (Prednisolone Sodium Phosphate) Medeva 1618

Sclerosis, multiple, alleviation of signs and symptoms
- Lioresal Tablets (Baclofen) CibaGeneva ... 847

Sclerosis, multiple, relapsing-remitting
- Avonex (Interferon Beta-1a) Biogen 662
- Betaseron for SC Injection (Interferon Beta-1b) Berlex ... 653

Seborrhea
(see also under Dandruff)
- MG 217 (Coal Tar) Triton Consumer ... 800
- Tegrin Dandruff Shampoo (Coal Tar) Block ... 634

Sedation
(see also under Sleep, induction of)
- Nembutal Sodium Capsules (Pentobarbital Sodium) Abbott ... 440
- Nembutal Sodium Solution (Pentobarbital Sodium) Abbott ... 442
- Nembutal Sodium Suppositories (Pentobarbital Sodium) Abbott ... 444
- Phenergan Injection (Promethazine Hydrochloride) Wyeth-Ayerst ... 2880
- Phenergan Suppositories (Promethazine Hydrochloride) Wyeth-Ayerst ... 2882
- Phenergan Syrup (Promethazine Hydrochloride) Wyeth-Ayerst ... 2881
- Phenergan Tablets (Promethazine Hydrochloride) Wyeth-Ayerst ... 2882

Sedation, benzodiazepine-induced, complete or partial reversal of
- Romazicon (Flumazenil) Roche Pharmaceuticals ... 2311

Sedation conscious, prediagnostic procedures
- Versed Injection (Midazolam Hydrochloride) Roche Pharmaceuticals ... 2324

Sedation, conscious, pre-endoscopic or therapeutic procedures
- Versed Injection (Midazolam Hydrochloride) Roche Pharmaceuticals ... 2324

Sedation, obstetric
- Levoprome (Methotrimeprazine) Immunex ... 1321
- Phenergan Injection (Promethazine Hydrochloride) Wyeth-Ayerst ... 2880
- Phenergan Suppositories (Promethazine Hydrochloride) Wyeth-Ayerst ... 2882
- Phenergan Syrup (Promethazine Hydrochloride) Wyeth-Ayerst ... 2881
- Phenergan Tablets (Promethazine Hydrochloride) Wyeth-Ayerst ... 2882

Sedation, postoperative
- Vistaril (Hydroxyzine Pamoate) Pfizer Inc ... 2042

Sedation, preoperative
- Atarax Tablets & Syrup (Hydroxyzine Hydrochloride) Pfizer Inc ... 1992
- Ativan Injection (Lorazepam) Wyeth-Ayerst ... 2805
- Inapsine Injection (Droperidol) Akorn ... 462
- Mepergan Injection (Meperidine Hydrochloride, Promethazine Hydrochloride) Wyeth-Ayerst ... 2859
- Versed Injection (Midazolam Hydrochloride) Roche Pharmaceuticals ... 2324
- Vistaril (Hydroxyzine Pamoate) Pfizer Inc ... 2042

Seizures, absence, adjunctive therapy in
- Depakene (Valproic Acid) Abbott ... 416
- Depakote Tablets (Divalproex Sodium) Abbott ... 418

Seizures, akinetic
- Klonopin Tablets (Clonazepam) Roche Pharmaceuticals ... 2294

Seizures, centrencephalic
(see also under Seizures, generalized, tonic-clonic; Seizures, generalized, absence)
- Diamox (Acetazolamide Sodium) Storz Ophthalmics ... 317

Seizures, convulsive, severe recurrent, adjunct in
- Dizac (diazepam injectable emulsion) CIV (Diazepam) Ohmeda ... 1862
- Valium Injectable (Diazepam) Roche Products ... 2336

Seizures, focal
- Atretol Tablets (Carbamazepine) Athena ... 569
- Felbatol (Felbamate) Wallace ... 2774
- Mesantoin Tablets (Mephenytoin) Sandoz Pharmaceuticals ... 2400
- Mysoline (Primidone) Wyeth-Ayerst 2860
- Phenobarbital Elixir and Tablets (Phenobarbital) Lilly ... 1523
- Tegretol/Tegretol-XR (Carbamazepine) CibaGeneva ... 870
- Tranxene T-TAB Tablets (Clorazepate Dipotassium) Abbott ... 459

Seizures, focal, adjunctive therapy in
- Felbatol (Felbamate) Wallace ... 2774
- Lamictal Tablets (Lamotrigine) Glaxo Wellcome ... 1105
- Neurontin Capsules (Gabapentin) Parke-Davis ... 1978
- Tranxene (Clorazepate Dipotassium) Abbott ... 459

Seizures, generalized, absence
- Celontin Kapseals (Methsuximide) Parke-Davis ... 1955
- Depakene (Valproic Acid) Abbott ... 416
- Depakote Tablets (Divalproex Sodium) Abbott ... 418
- Diamox (Acetazolamide Sodium) Storz Ophthalmics ... 317
- Klonopin Tablets (Clonazepam) Roche Pharmaceuticals ... 2294
- Mebaral Tablets (Mephobarbital) Sanofi Winthrop ... 2452
- Zarontin Capsules (Ethosuximide) Parke-Davis ... 1986
- Zarontin Syrup (Ethosuximide) Parke-Davis ... 1986

Seizures, generalized, tonic-clonic
- Atretol Tablets (Carbamazepine) Athena ... 569
- Diamox (Acetazolamide Sodium) Storz Ophthalmics ... 317
- Dilantin Infatabs (Phenytoin) Parke-Davis ... 1967
- Dilantin Kapseals (Phenytoin Sodium) Parke-Davis ... 1965
- Dilantin-125 Suspension (Phenytoin) Parke-Davis ... 1969
- Mebaral Tablets (Mephobarbital) Sanofi Winthrop ... 2452
- Mesantoin Tablets (Mephenytoin) Sandoz Pharmaceuticals ... 2400
- Mysoline (Primidone) Wyeth-Ayerst 2860
- Peganone Tablets (Ethotoin) Abbott ... 455
- Phenobarbital Elixir and Tablets (Phenobarbital) Lilly ... 1523
- Tegretol/Tegretol-XR (Carbamazepine) CibaGeneva ... 870

Seizures, Jacksonian
- Mesantoin Tablets (Mephenytoin) Sandoz Pharmaceuticals ... 2400

Seizures, multiple, adjunctive therapy in
- Depakene (Valproic Acid) Abbott ... 416
- Depakote Tablets (Divalproex Sodium) Abbott ... 418

Seizures, myoclonic
- Klonopin Tablets (Clonazepam) Roche Pharmaceuticals ... 2294

Seizures, neurosurgery-induced
- Cerebyx Injection (Fosphenytoin Sodium) Parke-Davis ... 1956
- Dilantin Infatabs (Phenytoin) Parke-Davis ... 1967

(⊡ Described in PDR For Nonprescription Drugs)

(⊚ Described in PDR For Ophthalmology)

1575 Indications Index Serratia species

Dilantin Kapseals (Phenytoin Sodium) Parke-Davis 1965

Seizures, neurosurgery-induced, prophylaxis of
Cerebyx Injection (Fosphenytoin Sodium) Parke-Davis 1956
Dilantin Infatabs (Phenytoin) Parke-Davis 1967
Dilantin Kapseals (Phenytoin Sodium) Parke-Davis 1965

Seizures, partial (see under Seizures, focal)

Seizures, psychomotor
Dilantin Infatabs (Phenytoin) Parke-Davis 1967
Dilantin Kapseals (Phenytoin Sodium) Parke-Davis 1965
Dilantin-125 Suspension (Phenytoin) Parke-Davis 1969
Mesantoin Tablets (Mephenytoin) Sandoz Pharmaceuticals 2400
Mysoline (Primidone) Wyeth-Ayerst 2860
Peganone Tablets (Ethotoin) Abbott 455
Phenurone Tablets (Phenacemide) Abbott 455
Tegretol-XR Tablets (Carbamazepine) CibaGeneva 870

Senile lentigines (see under Hyperpigmentation, skin, bleaching of)

Sepsis, bacterial, neonatal
Amikacin Sulfate Injection, USP (Amikacin Sulfate) Astra 523
Amikacin Sulfate Injection, USP (Amikacin Sulfate) Elkins-Sinn 981
Amikin Injectable (Amikacin Sulfate) Apothecon 502
Garamycin Injectable (Gentamicin Sulfate) Schering 2502

Sepsis, burn wound
SSD (Silver Sulfadiazine) Knoll Laboratories 1402
Silvadene Cream 1% (Silver Sulfadiazine) Hoechst Marion Roussel 1288

Septic shock (see under Bacterial shock, treatment adjunct)

Septicemia, anaerobic bacterial
Cefobid Intravenous/Intramuscular (Cefoperazone Sodium) Pfizer Inc 1996
Cefobid Pharmacy Bulk Package - Not for Direct Infusion (Cefoperazone Sodium) Pfizer Inc 1999

Septicemia, bacterial
Amikacin Sulfate Injection, USP (Amikacin Sulfate) Astra 523
Amikacin Sulfate Injection, USP (Amikacin Sulfate) Elkins-Sinn 981
Amikin Injectable (Amikacin Sulfate) Apothecon 502
Ancef Injection (Cefazolin Sodium) SmithKline Beecham Pharmaceuticals 2632
Azactam for Injection (Aztreonam) Bristol-Myers Squibb 736
Cefizox for Intramuscular or Intravenous Use (Ceftizoxime Sodium) Fujisawa 1025
Cefobid Intravenous/Intramuscular (Cefoperazone Sodium) Pfizer Inc 1996
Cefobid Pharmacy Bulk Package - Not for Direct Infusion (Cefoperazone Sodium) Pfizer Inc 1999
Ceptaz (Ceftazidime) Glaxo Wellcome 1070
Chloromycetin Sodium Succinate (Chloramphenicol Sodium Succinate) Parke-Davis 1960
Cipro I.V. (Ciprofloxacin) Bayer Pharmaceutical 587
Claforan Sterile and Injection (Cefotaxime Sodium) Hoechst Marion Roussel 1259
Cleocin Phosphate Injection (Clindamycin Phosphate) Pharmacia & Upjohn 2068
Flagyl 375 Capsules (Metronidazole) Searle 2587
Flagyl I.V. (Metronidazole Hydrochloride) SCS 2373
Fortaz (Ceftazidime) Glaxo Wellcome 1092
Garamycin Injectable (Gentamicin Sulfate) Schering 2502
Kefurox Vials, Faspak & ADD-Vantage (Cefuroxime Sodium) Lilly 1509
Kefzol Vials, Faspak & ADD-Vantage (Cefazolin Sodium) Lilly 1511
Mandol Vials, Faspak & ADD-Vantage (Cefamandole Nafate) Lilly 1516
Maxipime for Injection (Cefepime Hydrochloride) Bristol-Myers Squibb 758
Mefoxin (Cefoxitin Sodium) Merck & Co., Inc. 1734
Mefoxin Premixed Intravenous Solution (Cefoxitin Sodium) Merck & Co., Inc. 1737
Merrem I.V. (Meropenem) Zeneca .. 2952
Mezlin (Mezlocillin Sodium) Bayer Pharmaceutical 594
Mezlin Pharmacy Bulk Package (Mezlocillin Sodium) Bayer Pharmaceutical 597
Monocid Injection (Cefonicid Sodium) SmithKline Beecham Pharmaceuticals 2674
Nebcin Vials, Hyporets & ADD-Vantage (Tobramycin Sulfate) Lilly 1518
Netromycin Injection 100 mg/ml (Netilmicin Sulfate) Schering...... 2516
Pfizerpen for Injection (Penicillin G Potassium) Pfizer Inc 2022
Pipracil (Piperacillin Sodium) Lederle 1435
Primaxin I.V. (Cilastatin Sodium, Imipenem) Merck & Co., Inc. 1772
Protostat Tablets (Metronidazole) Ortho Pharmaceutical 1939
Rocephin Injectable Vials, ADD-Vantage, Galaxy Container (Ceftriaxone Sodium) Roche Pharmaceuticals 2305
Tazicef for Injection (Ceftazidime) SmithKline Beecham Pharmaceuticals 2697
Tazidime Vials, Faspak & ADD-Vantage (Ceftazidime) Lilly .. 1531
Ticar for Injection (Ticarcillin Disodium) SmithKline Beecham Pharmaceuticals 2704
Timentin for Injection (Ticarcillin Disodium, Clavulanate Potassium) SmithKline Beecham Pharmaceuticals 2706
Vancocin HCl, Vials & ADD-Vantage (Vancomycin Hydrochloride) Lilly 1534
Zinacef (Cefuroxime Sodium) Glaxo Wellcome 1184

Septicemia, candida
Ancobon Capsules (Flucytosine) Roche Pharmaceuticals 2254

Septicemia, cryptococcus
Ancobon Capsules (Flucytosine) Roche Pharmaceuticals 2254

Septicemia, fungal
Ancobon Capsules (Flucytosine) Roche Pharmaceuticals 2254

Septicemia, gram-negative bacillary, treatment adjunct
Streptomycin Sulfate Injection (Streptomycin Sulfate) Pfizer Inc 2031

Serratia marcescens bone and joint infections
Cipro I.V. (Ciprofloxacin) Bayer Pharmaceutical 587
Cipro I.V. Pharmacy Bulk Package (Ciprofloxacin) Bayer Pharmaceutical 590
Cipro Tablets (Ciprofloxacin Hydrochloride) Bayer Pharmaceutical 584

Serratia marcescens infections
Amikacin Sulfate Injection, USP (Amikacin Sulfate) Astra 523
Amikacin Sulfate Injection, USP (Amikacin Sulfate) Elkins-Sinn 981
Amikin Injectable (Amikacin Sulfate) Apothecon 502
Azactam for Injection (Aztreonam) Bristol-Myers Squibb 736
Cefizox for Intramuscular or Intravenous Use (Ceftizoxime Sodium) Fujisawa 1025
Cefotan (Cefotetan) Zeneca...... 2936
Cipro I.V. (Ciprofloxacin) Bayer Pharmaceutical 587
Cipro I.V. Pharmacy Bulk Package (Ciprofloxacin) Bayer Pharmaceutical 590
Cipro Tablets (Ciprofloxacin Hydrochloride) Bayer Pharmaceutical 584
Claforan Sterile and Injection (Cefotaxime Sodium) Hoechst Marion Roussel 1259
Noroxin Tablets (Norfloxacin) Merck & Co., Inc. 1758
Noroxin Tablets (Norfloxacin) Roberts 2222
Primaxin I.V. (Cilastatin Sodium, Imipenem) Merck & Co., Inc. 1772
Rocephin Injectable Vials, ADD-Vantage, Galaxy Container (Ceftriaxone Sodium) Roche Pharmaceuticals 2305
Timentin for Injection (Ticarcillin Disodium, Clavulanate Potassium) SmithKline Beecham Pharmaceuticals 2706

Serratia marcescens infections, ocular
Chibroxin Sterile Ophthalmic Solution (Norfloxacin) Merck & Co., Inc. 1657
Ciloxan Ophthalmic Solution (Ciprofloxacin Hydrochloride) Alcon Laboratories 468
Garamycin Ophthalmic (Gentamicin Sulfate) Schering 2501
Genoptic Sterile Ophthalmic Solution (Gentamicin Sulfate) Allergan ...... ◉ 241
Genoptic Sterile Ophthalmic Ointment (Gentamicin Sulfate) Allergan ...... ◉ 241
Gentak (Gentamicin Sulfate) Akorn ...... ◉ 209
Ocuflox Ophthalmic Solution (Ofloxacin) Allergan 478
Pred-G Liquifilm Sterile Ophthalmic Suspension (Gentamicin Sulfate, Prednisolone Acetate) Allergan ...... ◉ 248
Pred-G S.O.P. Sterile Ophthalmic Ointment (Gentamicin Sulfate, Prednisolone Acetate) Allergan.. ◉ 249

Serratia marcescens lower respiratory tract infections
Azactam for Injection (Aztreonam) Bristol-Myers Squibb 736
Cefotan (Cefotetan) Zeneca...... 2936
Claforan Sterile and Injection (Cefotaxime Sodium) Hoechst Marion Roussel 1259
Primaxin I.V. (Cilastatin Sodium, Imipenem) Merck & Co., Inc. 1772
Rocephin Injectable Vials, ADD-Vantage, Galaxy Container (Ceftriaxone Sodium) Roche Pharmaceuticals 2305

Serratia marcescens skin and skin structure infections
Azactam for Injection (Aztreonam) Bristol-Myers Squibb 736
Claforan Sterile and Injection (Cefotaxime Sodium) Hoechst Marion Roussel 1259
Rocephin Injectable Vials, ADD-Vantage, Galaxy Container (Ceftriaxone Sodium) Roche Pharmaceuticals 2305

Serratia marcescens urinary tract infections
Azactam for Injection (Aztreonam) Bristol-Myers Squibb 736
Cefizox for Intramuscular or Intravenous Use (Ceftizoxime Sodium) Fujisawa 1025
Cipro I.V. (Ciprofloxacin) Bayer Pharmaceutical 587
Cipro Tablets (Ciprofloxacin Hydrochloride) Bayer Pharmaceutical 584
Claforan Sterile and Injection (Cefotaxime Sodium) Hoechst Marion Roussel 1259
Noroxin Tablets (Norfloxacin) Merck & Co., Inc. 1758
Noroxin Tablets (Norfloxacin) Roberts 2222
Timentin for Injection (Ticarcillin Disodium, Clavulanate Potassium) SmithKline Beecham Pharmaceuticals 2706

Serratia species infections
Amikacin Sulfate Injection, USP (Amikacin Sulfate) Astra 523
Amikacin Sulfate Injection, USP (Amikacin Sulfate) Elkins-Sinn 981
Amikin Injectable (Amikacin Sulfate) Apothecon 502
Azactam for Injection (Aztreonam) Bristol-Myers Squibb 736
Cefizox for Intramuscular or Intravenous Use (Ceftizoxime Sodium) Fujisawa 1025
Ceptaz (Ceftazidime) Glaxo Wellcome 1070
Fortaz (Ceftazidime) Glaxo Wellcome 1092
Garamycin Injectable (Gentamicin Sulfate) Schering 2502
Mezlin (Mezlocillin Sodium) Bayer Pharmaceutical 594
Mezlin Pharmacy Bulk Package (Mezlocillin Sodium) Bayer Pharmaceutical 597
Nebcin Vials, Hyporets & ADD-Vantage (Tobramycin Sulfate) Lilly 1518
Netromycin Injection 100 mg/ml (Netilmicin Sulfate) Schering...... 2516
Pipracil (Piperacillin Sodium) Lederle 1435
Primaxin I.V. (Cilastatin Sodium, Imipenem) Merck & Co., Inc. 1772
Tazicef for Injection (Ceftazidime) SmithKline Beecham Pharmaceuticals 2697
Tazidime Vials, Faspak & ADD-Vantage (Ceftazidime) Lilly .. 1531

Serratia species lower respiratory tract infections
Cefizox for Intramuscular or Intravenous Use (Ceftizoxime Sodium) Fujisawa 1025
Ceptaz (Ceftazidime) Glaxo Wellcome 1070
Fortaz (Ceftazidime) Glaxo Wellcome 1092
Nebcin Vials, Hyporets & ADD-Vantage (Tobramycin Sulfate) Lilly 1518
Netromycin Injection 100 mg/ml (Netilmicin Sulfate) Schering...... 2516
Tazicef for Injection (Ceftazidime) SmithKline Beecham Pharmaceuticals 2697
Tazidime Vials, Faspak & ADD-Vantage (Ceftazidime) Lilly .. 1531

Serratia species septicemia
Azactam for Injection (Aztreonam) Bristol-Myers Squibb 736
Cefizox for Intramuscular or Intravenous Use (Ceftizoxime Sodium) Fujisawa 1025
Ceptaz (Ceftazidime) Glaxo Wellcome 1070
Claforan Sterile and Injection (Cefotaxime Sodium) Hoechst Marion Roussel 1259
Fortaz (Ceftazidime) Glaxo Wellcome 1092
Netromycin Injection 100 mg/ml (Netilmicin Sulfate) Schering...... 2516
Pipracil (Piperacillin Sodium) Lederle 1435
Primaxin I.V. (Cilastatin Sodium, Imipenem) Merck & Co., Inc. 1772
Tazicef for Injection (Ceftazidime) SmithKline Beecham Pharmaceuticals 2697
Tazidime Vials, Faspak & ADD-Vantage (Ceftazidime) Lilly .. 1531

Serratia species skin and skin structure infections
Cefizox for Intramuscular or Intravenous Use (Ceftizoxime Sodium) Fujisawa 1025
Ceptaz (Ceftazidime) Glaxo Wellcome 1070
Fortaz (Ceftazidime) Glaxo Wellcome 1092

(▣ Described in PDR For Nonprescription Drugs) (◉ Described in PDR For Ophthalmology)

Serratia species — Indications Index — 1576

Netromycin Injection 100 mg/ml (Netilmicin Sulfate) Schering ... 2516
Pipracil (Piperacillin Sodium) Lederle ... 1435
Primaxin I.V. (Cilastatin Sodium, Imipenem) Merck & Co., Inc. ... 1772
Tazicef for Injection (Ceftazidime) SmithKline Beecham Pharmaceuticals ... 2697
Tazidime Vials, Faspak & ADD-Vantage (Ceftazidime) Lilly ... 1531

Serratia species urinary tract infections
Cefizox for Intramuscular or Intravenous Use (Ceftizoxime Sodium) Fujisawa ... 1025
Cipro I.V. Pharmacy Bulk Package (Ciprofloxacin) Bayer Pharmaceutical ... 590
Mezlin (Mezlocillin Sodium) Bayer Pharmaceutical ... 594
Mezlin Pharmacy Bulk Package (Mezlocillin Sodium) Bayer Pharmaceutical ... 597
Nebcin Vials, Hyporets & ADD-Vantage (Tobramycin Sulfate) Lilly ... 1518
Netromycin Injection 100 mg/ml (Netilmicin Sulfate) Schering ... 2516

Serum sickness
Celestone Soluspan Suspension (Betamethasone Sodium Phosphate, Betamethasone Acetate) Schering ... 2484
Cortone Acetate Sterile Suspension (Cortisone Acetate) Merck & Co., Inc. ... 1663
Cortone Acetate Tablets (Cortisone Acetate) Merck & Co., Inc. ... 1664
Dalalone D.P. Injectable (Dexamethasone Acetate) Forest ... 1009
Decadron Elixir (Dexamethasone) Merck & Co., Inc. ... 1676
Decadron Phosphate Injection (Dexamethasone Sodium Phosphate) Merck & Co., Inc. ... 1680
Decadron Tablets (Dexamethasone) Merck & Co., Inc. ... 1678
Decadron-LA Sterile Suspension (Dexamethasone Acetate) Merck & Co., Inc. ... 1687
Hydeltrasol Injection, Sterile (Prednisolone Sodium Phosphate) Merck & Co., Inc. ... 1708
Hydrocortone Phosphate Injection, Sterile (Hydrocortisone Sodium Phosphate) Merck & Co., Inc. ... 1713
Hydrocortone Tablets (Hydrocortisone) Merck & Co., Inc. ... 1715
Pediapred Oral Solution (Prednisolone Sodium Phosphate) Medeva 1618
Prelone Syrup (Prednisolone) Muro 1834

Shigella flexneri enteritis
Bactrim DS Tablets (Trimethoprim, Sulfamethoxazole) Roche Pharmaceuticals ... 2257
Bactrim I.V. Infusion (Trimethoprim, Sulfamethoxazole) Roche Pharmaceuticals ... 2255
Bactrim (Trimethoprim, Sulfamethoxazole) Roche Pharmaceuticals ... 2257
Septra (Trimethoprim, Sulfamethoxazole) Glaxo Wellcome ... 1146
Septra I.V. Infusion (Trimethoprim, Sulfamethoxazole) Glaxo Wellcome ... 1142
Septra I.V. Infusion ADD-Vantage Vials (Trimethoprim, Sulfamethoxazole) Glaxo Wellcome ... 1144
Septra (Trimethoprim, Sulfamethoxazole) Glaxo Wellcome ... 1146

Shigella flexneri infectious diarrhea
Cipro Tablets (Ciprofloxacin Hydrochloride) Bayer Pharmaceutical ... 584

Shigella sonnei enteritis
Bactrim DS Tablets (Trimethoprim, Sulfamethoxazole) Roche Pharmaceuticals ... 2257
Bactrim I.V. Infusion (Trimethoprim, Sulfamethoxazole) Roche Pharmaceuticals ... 2255
Bactrim (Trimethoprim, Sulfamethoxazole) Roche Pharmaceuticals ... 2257
Septra (Trimethoprim, Sulfamethoxazole) Glaxo Wellcome ... 1146
Septra I.V. Infusion (Trimethoprim, Sulfamethoxazole) Glaxo Wellcome ... 1142
Septra I.V. Infusion ADD-Vantage Vials (Trimethoprim, Sulfamethoxazole) Glaxo Wellcome ... 1144
Septra (Trimethoprim, Sulfamethoxazole) Glaxo Wellcome ... 1146

Shigella sonnei infectious diarrhea
Cipro Tablets (Ciprofloxacin Hydrochloride) Bayer Pharmaceutical ... 584

Shigella species infections
Achromycin V Capsules (Tetracycline Hydrochloride) Lederle ... 1417
Declomycin Tablets (Demeclocycline Hydrochloride) Lederle ... 1421
Doryx Capsules (Doxycycline Hyclate) Parke-Davis ... 1970
DYNACIN Capsules (Minocycline Hydrochloride) Medicis ... 1627
Minocin Intravenous (Minocycline Hydrochloride) Lederle ... 1428
Minocin Oral Suspension (Minocycline Hydrochloride) Lederle ... 1431
Minocin Pellet-Filled Capsules (Minocycline Hydrochloride) Lederle ... 1429
Monodox Capsules (Doxycycline Monohydrate) Oclassen ... 1858
Omnipen Capsules (Ampicillin) Wyeth-Ayerst ... 2872
Omnipen for Oral Suspension (Ampicillin) Wyeth-Ayerst ... 2873
Pfizerpen for Injection (Penicillin G Potassium) Pfizer Inc ... 2022
Septra I.V. Infusion ADD-Vantage Vials (Trimethoprim, Sulfamethoxazole) Glaxo Wellcome ... 1144
Terramycin Intramuscular Solution (Oxytetracycline) Pfizer Inc ... 2034
Vibramycin (Doxycycline Calcium) Pfizer Inc ... 2038
Vibramycin Hyclate Intravenous (Doxycycline Hyclate) Pfizer Inc ... 2040
Vibramycin (Doxycycline Monohydrate) Pfizer Inc ... 2038

Shigellosis
Bactrim DS Tablets (Trimethoprim, Sulfamethoxazole) Roche Pharmaceuticals ... 2257
Bactrim I.V. Infusion (Trimethoprim, Sulfamethoxazole) Roche Pharmaceuticals ... 2255
Bactrim (Trimethoprim, Sulfamethoxazole) Roche Pharmaceuticals ... 2257
Septra (Trimethoprim, Sulfamethoxazole) Glaxo Wellcome ... 1146
Septra I.V. Infusion (Trimethoprim, Sulfamethoxazole) Glaxo Wellcome ... 1142
Septra I.V. Infusion ADD-Vantage Vials (Trimethoprim, Sulfamethoxazole) Glaxo Wellcome ... 1144
Septra (Trimethoprim, Sulfamethoxazole) Glaxo Wellcome ... 1146

Shingles (see under Herpes zoster infections)

Shock, emergency treatment of
Albuminar-5, Albumin (Human) U.S.P. 5% (Albumin (Human)) Centeon ... 795
Albuminar-25, Albumin (Human) U.S.P. 25% (Albumin (Human)) Centeon ... 796
Plasma-Plex, Plasma Protein Fraction (Human) U.S.P. 5% Solution Heat-Treated (Plasma Protein Fraction (Human)) Centeon ... 806

Shock, suspected adrenocortical insufficiency
Celestone Soluspan Suspension (Betamethasone Sodium Phosphate, Betamethasone Acetate) Schering ... 2484
Cortone Acetate Sterile Suspension (Cortisone Acetate) Merck & Co., Inc. ... 1663
Decadron Phosphate Injection (Dexamethasone Sodium Phosphate) Merck & Co., Inc. ... 1680
Hydrocortone Phosphate Injection, Sterile (Hydrocortisone Sodium Phosphate) Merck & Co., Inc. ... 1713

Shoulder, acute painful (see under Bursitis, subacromial, acute, symptomatic relief of)

Sialorrhea associated with Parkinsonism
Levsin/Levsinex/Levbid (Hyoscyamine Sulfate) Schwarz ... 2549

Sinus congestion, symptomatic relief of
Actifed Cold & Sinus Caplets and Tablets (Acetaminophen, Pseudoephedrine Hydrochloride, Triprolidine Hydrochloride) Warner Wellcome ... ▣ 808
Actifed Sinus Daytime/Nighttime Tablets and Caplets (Acetaminophen, Diphenhydramine Hydrochloride, Pseudoephedrine Hydrochloride) Warner Wellcome ... ▣ 809
Afrin (Oxymetazoline Hydrochloride) Schering-Plough HealthCare ... ▣ 757
Alka-Seltzer Plus Cold Medicine (Chlorpheniramine Maleate, Aspirin, Phenylpropanolamine Bitartrate) Bayer Consumer ... ▣ 611
Children's Vicks DayQuil Allergy Relief (Chlorpheniramine Maleate, Pseudoephedrine Hydrochloride) Procter & Gamble ... ▣ 730
Chlor-Trimeton Allergy Decongestant Tablets (Chlorpheniramine Maleate, Pseudoephedrine Sulfate) Schering-Plough HealthCare ... ▣ 759
Allergy-Sinus Comtrex Multi-Symptom Allergy-Sinus Formula Tablets and Caplets (Acetaminophen, Chlorpheniramine Maleate, Pseudoephedrine Hydrochloride) Bristol-Myers Products ... ▣ 639
Contac Day & Night (Acetaminophen) SmithKline Beecham Consumer ... ▣ 771
Coricidin 'D' Decongestant Tablets (Acetaminophen, Chlorpheniramine Maleate, Phenylpropanolamine Hydrochloride) Schering-Plough HealthCare ... ▣ 760
Dimetapp Elixir (Brompheniramine Maleate, Phenylpropanolamine Hydrochloride) Whitehall-Robins ... ▣ 840
Dimetapp Extentabs (Brompheniramine Maleate, Phenylpropanolamine Hydrochloride) Whitehall-Robins ... ▣ 841
Drixoral Allergy/Sinus Extended Release Tablets (Acetaminophen, Pseudoephedrine Sulfate, Dexbrompheniramine Maleate) Schering-Plough HealthCare ... ▣ 765
Novahistine DMX (Dextromethorphan Hydrobromide, Guaifenesin, Pseudoephedrine Hydrochloride) SmithKline Beecham Consumer ... ▣ 782
Sine-Aid Maximum Strength Sinus Headache Gelcaps, Caplets and Tablets (Acetaminophen, Pseudoephedrine Hydrochloride) McNeil Consumer ... 1570
Sine-Off No Drowsiness Formula Caplets (Acetaminophen, Pseudoephedrine Hydrochloride) SmithKline Beecham Consumer ... ▣ 784
Sine-Off Sinus Medicine (Acetaminophen, Chlorpheniramine Maleate, Pseudoephedrine Hydrochloride) SmithKline Beecham Consumer ... ▣ 784
Sinulin Tablets (Acetaminophen, Phenylpropanolamine Hydrochloride, Chlorpheniramine Maleate) Carnrick ... 792
Sinutab Non-Drying Liquid Caps (Pseudoephedrine Hydrochloride, Guaifenesin) Warner Wellcome ... ▣ 823
Sinutab Sinus Allergy Medication, Maximum Strength Tablets and Caplets (Acetaminophen, Chlorpheniramine Maleate, Pseudoephedrine Hydrochloride) Warner Wellcome ... ▣ 823
Sinutab Sinus Medication, Maximum Strength Without Drowsiness Formula, Tablets & Caplets (Acetaminophen, Pseudoephedrine Hydrochloride) Warner Wellcome ... ▣ 824
Theraflu Maximum Strength Sinus Non-Drowsy Formula Caplets (Acetaminophen, Pseudoephedrine Hydrochloride) Sandoz Consumer ... ▣ 752
Tylenol Allergy Sinus (Acetaminophen, Chlorpheniramine Maleate, Pseudoephedrine Hydrochloride) McNeil Consumer 1571
TYLENOL Sinus, Maximum Strength Geltabs, Gelcaps, Caplets and Tablets (Acetaminophen, Pseudoephedrine Hydrochloride) McNeil Consumer 1576
Vicks DayQuil SINUS Pressure & CONGESTION Relief (Guaifenesin, Phenylpropanolamine Hydrochloride) Procter & Gamble ... ▣ 734
Vicks Sinex 12-Hour Nasal Decongestant Spray and Ultra Fine Mist (Oxymetazoline Hydrochloride) Procter & Gamble ... ▣ 738
Vicks Sinex Nasal Spray and Ultra Fine Mist (Phenylephrine Hydrochloride) Procter & Gamble ... ▣ 738

Sinus headache
Actifed Sinus Daytime/Nighttime Tablets and Caplets (Acetaminophen, Diphenhydramine Hydrochloride, Pseudoephedrine Hydrochloride) Warner Wellcome ... ▣ 809
Alka-Seltzer Plus Cold Medicine (Chlorpheniramine Maleate, Aspirin, Phenylpropanolamine Bitartrate) Bayer Consumer ... ▣ 611
Alka-Seltzer Plus Sinus Medicine (Phenylpropanolamine Bitartrate, Aspirin, Brompheniramine Maleate) Bayer Consumer ▣ 611
Allergy-Sinus Comtrex Multi-Symptom Allergy-Sinus Formula Tablets and Caplets (Acetaminophen, Chlorpheniramine Maleate, Pseudoephedrine Hydrochloride) Bristol-Myers Products ... ▣ 639
Contac Day & Night (Acetaminophen) SmithKline Beecham Consumer ... ▣ 771
Coricidin 'D' Decongestant Tablets (Acetaminophen, Chlorpheniramine Maleate, Phenylpropanolamine Hydrochloride) Schering-Plough HealthCare ... ▣ 760
Drixoral Allergy/Sinus Extended Release Tablets (Acetaminophen, Pseudoephedrine Sulfate, Dexbrompheniramine Maleate) Schering-Plough HealthCare ... ▣ 765
Sinarest (Acetaminophen, Chlorpheniramine Maleate, Pseudoephedrine Hydrochloride) Ciba Self-Medication ... ▣ 663
Sine-Aid Maximum Strength Sinus Headache Gelcaps, Caplets and Tablets (Acetaminophen, Pseudoephedrine Hydrochloride) McNeil Consumer ... 1570

Sine-Off Sinus Medicine (Acetaminophen, Chlorpheniramine Maleate, Pseudoephedrine Hydrochloride) SmithKline Beecham Consumer 784
Singlet Tablets (Acetaminophen, Chlorpheniramine Maleate, Pseudoephedrine Hydrochloride) SmithKline Beecham Consumer 785
Sinutab Sinus Allergy Medication, Maximum Strength Tablets and Caplets (Acetaminophen, Chlorpheniramine Maleate, Pseudoephedrine Hydrochloride) Warner Wellcome 823
Sinutab Sinus Medication, Maximum Strength Without Drowsiness Formula, Tablets & Caplets (Acetaminophen, Pseudoephedrine Hydrochloride) Warner Wellcome 824
Sudafed Sinus Caplets (Acetaminophen, Pseudoephedrine Hydrochloride) Warner Wellcome 829
Sudafed Sinus Tablets (Acetaminophen, Pseudoephedrine Hydrochloride) Warner Wellcome 829
Sunsource Sinus Relief Tablets (Homeopathic Medications) Sunsource 793
Theraflu Maximum Strength Sinus Non-Drowsy Formula Caplets (Acetaminophen, Pseudoephedrine Hydrochloride) Sandoz Consumer 752
Tylenol Allergy Sinus (Acetaminophen, Chlorpheniramine Maleate, Pseudoephedrine Hydrochloride) McNeil Consumer 1571
TYLENOL Sinus, Maximum Strength Geltabs, Gelcaps, Caplets and Tablets (Acetaminophen, Pseudoephedrine Hydrochloride) McNeil Consumer 1576
Vicks DayQuil SINUS Pressure & PAIN Relief with IBUPROFEN (Ibuprofen, Pseudoephedrine Hydrochloride) Procter & Gamble 735

Sinusitis, adjunctive therapy
Advil Cold and Sinus Caplets and Tablets (Ibuprofen, Pseudoephedrine Hydrochloride) Whitehall-Robins 837
Afrin (Oxymetazoline Hydrochloride) Schering-Plough HealthCare 757
Alka-Seltzer Plus Sinus Medicine (Phenylpropanolamine Bitartrate, Aspirin, Brompheniramine Maleate) Bayer Consumer 611
Allerest Maximum Strength (Chlorpheniramine Maleate, Pseudoephedrine Hydrochloride) Ciba Self-Medication 649
Allerest No Drowsiness (Acetaminophen, Pseudoephedrine Hydrochloride) Ciba Self-Medication 649
Allerest Sinus Pain Formula (Acetaminophen, Chlorpheniramine Maleate, Pseudoephedrine Hydrochloride) Ciba Self-Medication 649
Allergy-Sinus Comtrex Multi-Symptom Allergy-Sinus Formula Tablets and Caplets (Acetaminophen, Chlorpheniramine Maleate, Pseudoephedrine Hydrochloride) Bristol-Myers Products 639
Congess (Guaifenesin, Pseudoephedrine Hydrochloride) Fleming 1003
Contac Continuous Action Nasal Decongestant/Antihistamine 12 Hour Capsules (Chlorpheniramine Maleate, Phenylpropanolamine Hydrochloride) SmithKline Beecham Consumer 773
D.A. II Tablets (Chlorpheniramine Maleate, Methscopolamine Nitrate, Phenylephrine Hydrochloride) Dura 972

D.A. Chewable Tablets (Chlorpheniramine Maleate, Phenylephrine Hydrochloride, Methscopolamine Nitrate) Dura 970
Dimetapp Allergy Sinus Caplets (Acetaminophen, Brompheniramine Maleate, Phenylpropanolamine Hydrochloride) Whitehall-Robins 838
Dimetapp Cold & Fever Suspension (Acetaminophen, Brompheniramine Maleate, Pseudoephedrine Hydrochloride) Whitehall-Robins 839
Drixoral Cold and Flu Extended-Release Tablets (Acetaminophen, Dexbrompheniramine Maleate, Pseudoephedrine Sulfate) Schering-Plough HealthCare 764
Dura-Tap/PD Capsules (Chlorpheniramine Maleate, Pseudoephedrine Hydrochloride) Dura 970
Dura-Vent/DA Tablets (Chlorpheniramine Maleate, Phenylephrine Hydrochloride, Methscopolamine Nitrate) Dura 972
Dura-Vent Tablets (Phenylpropanolamine Hydrochloride, Guaifenesin) Dura 971
Entex LA Tablets (Phenylpropanolamine Hydrochloride, Guaifenesin) Dura 972
Excedrin Extra-Strength Analgesic Tablets, Caplets, and Geltabs (Acetaminophen, Aspirin, Caffeine) Bristol-Myers Products 734
Exgest LA Tablets (Phenylpropanolamine Hydrochloride, Guaifenesin) Carnrick 787
4-Way Fast Acting Nasal Spray (regular & mentholated) (Naphazoline Hydrochloride, Phenylephrine Hydrochloride, Pyrilamine Maleate) Bristol-Myers Products 644
Fedahist Gyrocaps (Pseudoephedrine Hydrochloride, Chlorpheniramine Maleate) Schwarz 2545
Humibid DM Tablets (Guaifenesin, Dextromethorphan Hydrobromide) Medeva 1612
Kronofed-A (Chlorpheniramine Maleate, Pseudoephedrine Hydrochloride) Ferndale 994
Neo-Synephrine Maximum Strength 12 Hour Nasal Spray (Oxymetazoline Hydrochloride) Bayer Consumer 624
Neo-Synephrine Maximum Strength 12 Hour Nasal Spray Pump (Oxymetazoline Hydrochloride) Bayer Consumer 624
Neo-Synephrine (Phenylephrine Hydrochloride) Bayer Consumer 624
Nolamine Timed-Release Tablets (Phenindamine Tartrate, Phenylpropanolamine Hydrochloride, Chlorpheniramine Maleate) Carnrick 790
Propagest Tablets (Phenylpropanolamine Hydrochloride) Carnrick 791
Rynatan (Chlorpheniramine Tannate, Pyrilamine Tannate, Phenylephrine Tannate) Wallace 2781
Sinarest (Acetaminophen, Chlorpheniramine Maleate, Pseudoephedrine Hydrochloride) Ciba Self-Medication 663
Sine-Off No Drowsiness Formula Caplets (Acetaminophen, Pseudoephedrine Hydrochloride) SmithKline Beecham Consumer 784
Sine-Off Sinus Medicine (Acetaminophen, Chlorpheniramine Maleate, Pseudoephedrine Hydrochloride) SmithKline Beecham Consumer 784
Sinulin Tablets (Acetaminophen, Phenylpropanolamine Hydrochloride, Chlorpheniramine Maleate) Carnrick 792
Sinutab Sinus Allergy Medication, Maximum Strength Tablets and Caplets (Acetaminophen, Chlorpheniramine Maleate, Pseudo-

ephedrine Hydrochloride) Warner Wellcome 823
Sinutab Sinus Medication, Maximum Strength Without Drowsiness Formula, Tablets & Caplets (Acetaminophen, Pseudoephedrine Hydrochloride) Warner Wellcome 824
Sudafed Non-Drying Sinus Liquid Caps (Pseudoephedrine Hydrochloride, Guaifenesin) Warner Wellcome 827
Sudafed Sinus Caplets (Acetaminophen, Pseudoephedrine Hydrochloride) Warner Wellcome 829
Sudafed Sinus Tablets (Acetaminophen, Pseudoephedrine Hydrochloride) Warner Wellcome 829
Syn-Rx Tablets (Pseudoephedrine Hydrochloride, Guaifenesin) Medeva 1622
Teldrin 12 Hour Antihistamine/Nasal Decongestant Allergy Relief Capsules (Chlorpheniramine Maleate, Phenylpropanolamine Hydrochloride) SmithKline Beecham Consumer 786
Triaminicin Tablets (Acetaminophen, Chlorpheniramine Maleate, Phenylpropanolamine Hydrochloride) Sandoz Consumer 756
TYLENOL Allergy Sinus, Maximum Strength Caplets and Gelcaps (Acetaminophen, Chlorpheniramine Maleate, Pseudoephedrine Hydrochloride) McNeil Consumer 1571

Sinusitis, treatment of
Augmentin (Amoxicillin Trihydrate, Clavulanate Potassium) SmithKline Beecham Pharmaceuticals 2637
Augmentin Tablets (Amoxicillin Trihydrate, Clavulanate Potassium) SmithKline Beecham Pharmaceuticals 2640
Biaxin (Clarithromycin) Abbott 406
Ceftin (Cefuroxime Axetil) Glaxo Wellcome 1067
Dimetapp Cold & Allergy Chewable Tablets (Brompheniramine Maleate, Phenylpropanolamine Hydrochloride) Whitehall-Robins 838
Lorabid Suspension and Pulvules (Loracarbef) Lilly 1513

Skin grafting, treatment adjunct
Furacin Soluble Dressing (Nitrofurazone) Roberts 2220
Furacin Topical Cream (Nitrofurazone) Roberts 2220

Skin infections, bacterial, minor
(see under Infections, skin, bacterial, minor)

Skin lacerations, infected
(see under Infections, skin and skin structure)

Skin, bactericidal/virucidal cleansing of
Betadine Skin Cleanser (Povidone Iodine) Purdue Frederick 2145
Betadine Surgical Scrub (Povidone Iodine) Purdue Frederick 2145

Skin, bacteriostatic cleansing of
Barri-Care Antimicrobial Barrier Ointment (Chloroxylenol) Care-Tech 646
Betasept Surgical Scrub (Chlorhexidine Gluconate) Purdue Frederick 2145
Care Creme Antimicrobial Cream (Chloroxylenol) Care-Tech 646
Clinical Care Dermal Wound Cleanser (Benzethonium Chloride) Care-Tech 646
Hibiclens Antimicrobial Skin Cleanser (Chlorhexidine Gluconate) Zeneca 2947
Hibistat (Chlorhexidine Gluconate) Zeneca 2948
Lever 2000 Antibacterial Bar and Liquid (Triclosan) Lever 686

Orchid Fresh II Perineal/Ostomy Cleanser (Benzethonium Chloride) Care-Tech 647
pHisoHex (Hexachlorophene) Sanofi Winthrop 2458
Satin Antimicrobial Skin Cleanser for Diabetic/Cancer Patient Care (Chloroxylenol) Care-Tech 647
Techni-Care Surgical Scrub and Wound Cleanser (Chloroxylenol) Care-Tech 647

Skin, dry, moisturization of
Alpha Keri Moisture Rich Body Oil (Lanolin Oil) Bristol-Myers Products 635
Aquaphor Healing Ointment (Petrolatum, Mineral Oil) Beiersdorf .. 636
Aquaphor Healing Ointment, Original Formula (Mineral Oil, Petrolatum) Beiersdorf 636
Cetaphil Moisturizing Cream (Moisturizing formula) Galderma 1032
Cetaphil Moisturizing Lotion (Moisturizing formula) Galderma 1032
Curel Lotion and Cream (Moisturizing formula) Bausch & Lomb Personal 608
DML Facial Moisturizer with Sunscreen (Glycerin, Hyaluronic Acid, Octyl Methoxycinnamate, Oxybenzone) Persön & Covey ... 1989
Eucerin Original Moisturizing Creme (Unscented) (Mineral Oil, Petrolatum) Beiersdorf 636
Eucerin Facial Moisturizing Lotion SPF 25 (Phenylbenzimidazole-5-Sulfonic Acid, Titanium Dioxide, 2-Ethylhexyl-p-Methoxycinnamate, 2-Ethylhexyl Salicylate) Beiersdorf 636
Eucerin Original Moisturizing Lotion (Isopropyl Myristate, Mineral Oil) Beiersdorf 636
Eucerin Plus Dry Skin Care Moisturizing Lotion (Mineral Oil, Urea) Beiersdorf 636
Eucerin Plus Moisturizing Creme (Urea, Mineral Oil) Beiersdorf ... 636
Keri Lotion (Mineral Oil) Bristol-Myers Products 644
Lac-Hydrin 12% Lotion (Ammonium Lactate) Westwood-Squibb .. 2796
Lubriderm Bath and Shower Oil (Emollient, Mineral Oil) Warner Wellcome 821
Lubriderm Dry Skin Care Lotion (Emollient) Warner Wellcome 820
Lubriderm Moisture Recovery Alpha Hydroxy Cream and Lotion (Moisturizing formula) Warner Wellcome 821
Lubriderm Moisture Recovery GelCreme (Cetyl Alcohol, Glycerin, Mineral Oil) Warner Wellcome 821
Lubriderm Seriously Sensitive Lotion (Glycerin, Mineral Oil, Petrolatum) Warner Wellcome .. 821
Moisturel Cream (Dimethicone, Petrolatum) Westwood-Squibb .. 2796
Moisturel Lotion (Dimethicone) Westwood-Squibb 2797
Prophyllin CCC Topical Emollient Ointment (Petrolatum, White) Rystan 2372
StePHan Bio-Nutritional Daytime Hydrating Creme (Chamomile) Wellness International 833
StePHan Bio-Nutritional Eye-Firming Concentrate (Chamomile) Wellness International 833
StePHan Bio-Nutritional Nightime Moisture Creme (Moisturizing formula) Wellness International 833
StePHan Bio-Nutritional Ultra Hydrating Fluid (Moisturizing formula) Wellness International 833

Skin, emollient cleansing of
Bio-Complex 5000 Gentle Foaming Cleanser (Aloe Vera) Wellness International 830
Cetaphil Gentle Cleansing Bar (Cleanser) Galderma 1032
Cetaphil Skin Cleanser (Cetyl Alcohol) Galderma 1032
Dove Bar (Original, Unscented, and Sensitive Skin Formula) (Sodium Tallowate) Lever 686

Skin / Indications Index

Skin
Dove Moisturizing Body Wash (Sodium Cocoyl Isethionate) Lever 686
Liquid Dove Beauty Wash (Sodium Tallowate) Lever 686
Eucerin Dry Skin Therapy Cleansing Bar (Eucerite) Beiersdorf 636
StePHan Bio-Nutritional Refreshing Moisture Gel (Moisturizing formula) Wellness International 833

Skin, facial, tactile roughness of, adjunct in
Renova (tretinoin emollient cream) 0.05% (Tretinoin) Ortho Dermatological 1945

Skin, fine wrinkles, mitigation of
Renova (tretinoin emollient cream) 0.05% (Tretinoin) Ortho Dermatological 1945

Skin, hyperpigmentation
(see under Hyperpigmentation, skin, bleaching of)

Skin, increased tolerance to sunlight
Eucerin Facial Moisturizing Lotion SPF 25 (Phenylbenzimidazole-5-Sulfonic Acid, Titanium Dioxide, 2-Ethylhexyl-p-Methoxycinnamate, 2-Ethylhexyl Salicylate) Beiersdorf 636
Solbar PF Ultra Cream SPF 50 (PABA Free) (Oxybenzone) Persön & Covey 1989
Trisoralen Tablets (Trioxsalen) ICN 1309

Skin, inflammatory conditions
(see also under Rash, diaper; Dermatitis, contact; Dermatoses, corticosteroid-responsive)
Acid Mantle Creme (Petrolatum, White) Sandoz Consumer 747
Aquanil HC Lotion (Hydrocortisone) Persön & Covey 1989
Caldecort Anti-Itch Hydrocortisone Cream (Hydrocortisone Acetate) Ciba Self-Medication 651
Chloresium (Chlorophyllin Copper Complex) Rystan 2371
Cortizone-5 (Hydrocortisone) Thompson Medical 795
Cutivate Cream (Fluticasone Propionate) Glaxo Wellcome 1078
Cutivate Ointment (Fluticasone Propionate) Glaxo Wellcome 1078
Dermatop Emollient Cream 0.1% (Prednicarbate) Hoechst Marion Roussel 1264
Diprolene Gel 0.05% (Betamethasone Dipropionate) Schering 2490
Diprolene Lotion 0.05% (Betamethasone Dipropionate) Schering 2491
Mantadil Cream (Chlorcyclizine Hydrochloride) Glaxo Wellcome 1124
ProctoCream-HC 2.5% (Hydrocortisone) Schwarz 2552
Psorcon Cream 0.05% (Diflorasone Diacetate) Dermik 924
Sunsource Psoriasis/Eczema Relief Cream (Homeopathic Medications) Sunsource 793

Skin, irritation, minor, pain associated with
(see under Pain, topical relief of)

Skin, irritation, minor, temporary relief of
Caladryl Clear Lotion (Pramoxine Hydrochloride, Zinc Acetate) Warner Wellcome 817
Desitin Cornstarch Baby Powder (Zinc Oxide, Corn Starch) Pfizer Consumer 715
Domeboro Astringent (Aluminum Acetate, Calcium Acetate) Bayer Consumer 620
Formula Magic Antibacterial Powder (Benzethonium Chloride) Care-Tech 647
Moisturel Cream (Dimethicone, Petrolatum) Westwood-Squibb 2796
Moisturel Lotion (Dimethicone) Westwood-Squibb 2797
Nupercainal Pain Relief Cream (Dibucaine) Ciba Self-Medication 661

Sleep, induction of
(see also under Sedation)
Ambien Tablets (Zolpidem Tartrate) Searle 2559
Butisol Sodium Elixir & Tablets (Butabarbital Sodium) Wallace 2768
Dalmane Capsules (Flurazepam Hydrochloride) Roche Products 2329
Doral Tablets (Quazepam) Wallace 2773
Halcion Tablets (Triazolam) Pharmacia & Upjohn 2093
Hyland's Calms Forté Tablets (Homeopathic Medications) Standard Homeopathic 788
Mebaral Tablets (Mephobarbital) Sanofi Winthrop 2452
Nembutal Sodium Capsules (Pentobarbital Sodium) Abbott 440
Nembutal Sodium Solution (Pentobarbital Sodium) Abbott 442
Nembutal Sodium Suppositories (Pentobarbital Sodium) Abbott 444
Maximum Strength Nytol Caplets (Doxylamine Succinate) Block 632
Nytol QuickCaps Caplets (Diphenhydramine Hydrochloride) Block 632
Phenobarbital Elixir and Tablets (Phenobarbital) Lilly 1523
Placidyl Capsules (Ethchlorvynol) Abbott 456
ProSom Tablets (Estazolam) Abbott 457
Restoril Capsules (Temazepam) Sandoz Pharmaceuticals 2413
Seconal Sodium Pulvules (Secobarbital Sodium) Lilly 1529
Sleepinal Night-time Sleep Aid Capsules and Softgels (Diphenhydramine Hydrochloride) Thompson Medical 798
Sunsource Insomnia Relief Tablets (Homeopathic Medications) Sunsource 793
Maximum Strength Unisom Sleepgels (Diphenhydramine Hydrochloride) Pfizer Consumer 1990
Unisom Nighttime Sleep Aid (Doxylamine Succinate) Pfizer Consumer 1990
Versed Injection (Midazolam Hydrochloride) Roche Pharmaceuticals 2324

Smoking cessation, temporary aid to
Habitrol Nicotine Transdermal System (Nicotine) Ciba Self-Medication 884
Nicotrol NS Nicotine Nasal Spray (Nicotine) McNeil Consumer 1565
Nicotrol Nicotine Transdermal System (Nicotine) McNeil Consumer 1568
Prostep (nicotine transdermal system) (Nicotine) Lederle 1439

Sneezing
Benadryl Allergy Decongestant Tablets (Diphenhydramine Hydrochloride, Pseudoephedrine Hydrochloride) Warner Wellcome 812
Benadryl Allergy Liquid Medication (Diphenhydramine Hydrochloride) Warner Wellcome 813
Benadryl Allergy (Diphenhydramine Hydrochloride) Warner Wellcome 811
Benadryl Allergy Sinus Headache Caplets (Diphenhydramine Hydrochloride, Pseudoephedrine Hydrochloride, Acetaminophen) Warner Wellcome 813
Benadryl Dye-Free Allergy Liqui-gel Softgels (Diphenhydramine Hydrochloride) Warner Wellcome 813
Benadryl Dye-Free Allergy Liquid Medication (Diphenhydramine Hydrochloride) Warner Wellcome 814
Chlor-Trimeton Allergy Tablets (Chlorpheniramine Maleate) Schering-Plough HealthCare 758
Allergy-Sinus Comtrex Multi-Symptom Allergy-Sinus Formula Tablets and Caplets (Acetaminophen, Chlorpheniramine Maleate, Pseudoephedrine Hydrochloride) Bristol-Myers Products 639
Contac Night Allergy/Sinus Caplets (Acetaminophen, Pseudoephedrine Hydrochloride, Diphenhydramine Hydrochloride) SmithKline Beecham Consumer 771
Dimetapp Cold & Allergy Chewable Tablets (Brompheniramine Maleate, Phenylpropanolamine Hydrochloride) Whitehall-Robins 838
Dimetapp Elixir (Brompheniramine Maleate, Phenylpropanolamine Hydrochloride) Whitehall-Robins 840
Dimetapp Extentabs (Brompheniramine Maleate, Phenylpropanolamine Hydrochloride) Whitehall-Robins 841
Dimetapp Tablets/Liqui-Gels (Brompheniramine Maleate, Phenylpropanolamine Hydrochloride) Whitehall-Robins 841
Hyland's C-Plus Cold Tablets (Homeopathic Medications) Standard Homeopathic 789
Ryna (Chlorpheniramine Maleate, Pseudoephedrine Hydrochloride) Wallace 804
Seldane Tablets (Terfenadine) Hoechst Marion Roussel 1284
Seldane-D Extended-Release Tablets (Pseudoephedrine Hydrochloride, Terfenadine) Hoechst Marion Roussel 1286
Sinulin Tablets (Acetaminophen, Phenylpropanolamine Hydrochloride, Chlorpheniramine Maleate) Carnrick 792
Sinutab Sinus Allergy Medication, Maximum Strength Tablets and Caplets (Acetaminophen, Chlorpheniramine Maleate, Pseudoephedrine Hydrochloride) Warner Wellcome 823
Tavist Syrup (Clemastine Fumarate) Sandoz Pharmaceuticals 2426
Tavist Tablets (Clemastine Fumarate) Sandoz Pharmaceuticals 2427
TYLENOL Severe Allergy Medication Caplets (Acetaminophen, Chlorpheniramine Maleate, Pseudoephedrine Hydrochloride) McNeil Consumer 1571

Sour stomach
(see under Hyperacidity, gastric, symptomatic relief of)

Spasm, skeletal muscle
Dizac (diazepam injectable emulsion) CIV (Diazepam) Ohmeda 1862
Flexeril Tablets (Cyclobenzaprine Hydrochloride) Merck & Co., Inc. 1701
Valium Injectable (Diazepam) Roche Products 2336
Valium Tablets (Diazepam) Roche Products 2335

Spasm, smooth muscle
Papaverine Hydrochloride Vials and Ampoules (Papaverine Hydrochloride) Lilly 1523

Spasticity, cerebral palsy-induced
(see under Spasticity, upper motor neuron disorder-induced)

Spasticity, multiple sclerosis-induced
(see under Spasticity, upper motor neuron disorder-induced)

Spasticity, muscle, symptomatic alleviation of
Flexeril Tablets (Cyclobenzaprine Hydrochloride) Merck & Co., Inc. 1701

Spasticity
Lioresal Tablets (Baclofen) CibaGeneva 847

Spasticity, spinal cord injury-induced
(see under Spasticity, upper motor neuron disorder-induced)

Spasticity, stroke-induced
(see under Spasticity, upper motor neuron disorder-induced)

Spasticity, upper motor neuron disorder-induced
Dantrium Capsules (Dantrolene Sodium) Procter & Gamble Pharmaceuticals 2131
Dizac (diazepam injectable emulsion) CIV (Diazepam) Ohmeda 1862
Lioresal Intrathecal (Baclofen) Medtronic Neurological 1634
Lioresal Tablets (Baclofen) CibaGeneva 847
Valium Injectable (Diazepam) Roche Products 2336
Valium Tablets (Diazepam) Roche Products 2335

Spasticity of spinal cord, severe
Lioresal Intrathecal (Baclofen) Medtronic Neurological 1634

Spermatogenesis, stimulation of, adjunctive therapy in
Humegon for Injection (Menotropins) Organon 1873

Spirillum minus infections
Pfizerpen for Injection (Penicillin G Potassium) Pfizer Inc 2022

Spirochetes species infections
(see also under Borrelia recurrentis infection)
Minocin Intravenous (Minocycline Hydrochloride) Lederle 1428
Minocin Oral Suspension (Minocycline Hydrochloride) Lederle 1431
Minocin Pellet-Filled Capsules (Minocycline Hydrochloride) Lederle 1429
Terramycin Intramuscular Solution (Oxytetracycline) Pfizer Inc 2034
Vibramycin Hyclate Intravenous (Doxycycline Hyclate) Pfizer Inc. 2040

Sporothrix schenckii infections
(see under Sporotrichosis)

Sporotrichosis
Fungizone Intravenous (Amphotericin B) Apothecon 507

Sprains, topical relief of
(see under Pain, topical relief of)

Staphylococcal enterocolitis
(see under Enterocolitis, staphylococcal)

Staphylococci bone and joint infections
Keflex Pulvules & Oral Suspension (Cephalexin) Dista 930
Vancocin HCl, Vials & ADD-Vantage (Vancomycin Hydrochloride) Lilly 1534

Staphylococci endocarditis
Vancocin HCl, Vials & ADD-Vantage (Vancomycin Hydrochloride) Lilly 1534

Staphylococci lower respiratory tract infections
Vancocin HCl, Vials & ADD-Vantage (Vancomycin Hydrochloride) Lilly 1534

Staphylococci otitis media
Ceclor Pulvules & Suspension (Cefaclor) Lilly 1470
Keflex Pulvules & Oral Suspension (Cephalexin) Dista 930

Staphylococci septicemia
Vancocin HCl, Vials & ADD-Vantage (Vancomycin Hydrochloride) Lilly 1534

Staphylococci skin and skin structure infections
Duricef Capsules, Tablets, and Oral Suspension (Cefadroxil) Bristol-Myers Squibb 750

Described in PDR For Nonprescription Drugs   *Described in PDR For Ophthalmology*

Keflex Pulvules & Oral Suspension
(Cephalexin) Dista 930
Spectrobid Tablets (Bacampicillin
Hydrochloride) Pfizer Inc 2030
Vancocin HCl, Vials & ADD-Vantage
(Vancomycin Hydrochloride) Lilly 1534

Staphylococci, coagulase-negative, infections, ocular
Pred-G Liquifilm Sterile
Ophthalmic Suspension (Genta-
micin Sulfate, Prednisolone
Acetate) Allergan.................... ⊚ 248
TobraDex Ophthalmic Suspension
and Ointment (Dexamethasone,
Tobramycin) Alcon Laboratories .. 469

Staphylococci, coagulase-positive, infections, ocular
Pred-G Liquifilm Sterile
Ophthalmic Suspension (Genta-
micin Sulfate, Prednisolone
Acetate) Allergan.................... ⊚ 248
TobraDex Ophthalmic Suspension
and Ointment (Dexamethasone,
Tobramycin) Alcon Laboratories .. 469

Staphylococci, nonpenicillinase-producing, infections
Amoxil (Amoxicillin Trihydrate)
SmithKline Beecham
Pharmaceuticals 2631
Spectrobid Tablets (Bacampicillin
Hydrochloride) Pfizer Inc 2030

Staphylococci, nonpenicillinase-producing, respiratory tract infections
Omnipen for Oral Suspension
(Ampicillin) Wyeth-Ayerst........... 2873
Spectrobid Tablets (Bacampicillin
Hydrochloride) Pfizer Inc 2030

Staphylococci, penicillinase-producing, infections
Mefoxin (Cefoxitin Sodium) Merck
& Co., Inc. 1734
Mefoxin Premixed Intravenous
Solution (Cefoxitin Sodium)
Merck & Co., Inc. 1737
Mezlin (Mezlocillin Sodium) Bayer
Pharmaceutical 594
Mezlin Pharmacy Bulk Package
(Mezlocillin Sodium) Bayer
Pharmaceutical 597

Staphylococci, urinary tract infections
Gantanol Tablets
(Sulfamethoxazole) Roche
Pharmaceuticals 2285
Gantrisin (Acetyl Sulfisoxazole)
Roche Pharmaceuticals 2286
Proloprim Tablets (Trimethoprim)
Glaxo Wellcome 1141

Staphylococcus aureus
(see under S. aureus infections)

Staphylococcus epidermidis
(see under S. epidermis infections)

Staphylococcus species infections
Amikacin Sulfate Injection, USP
(Amikacin Sulfate) Astra 523
Amikacin Sulfate Injection, USP
(Amikacin Sulfate) Elkins-Sinn ... 981
Amikin Injectable (Amikacin
Sulfate) Apothecon.................. 502
Ceclor Pulvules & Suspension
(Cefaclor) Lilly 1470
Duricef Capsules, Tablets, and Oral
Suspension (Cefadroxil)
Bristol-Myers Squibb 750
Gantanol Tablets
(Sulfamethoxazole) Roche
Pharmaceuticals 2285
Gantrisin (Acetyl Sulfisoxazole)
Roche Pharmaceuticals 2286
Garamycin Injectable (Gentamicin
Sulfate) Schering 2502
Keflex Pulvules & Oral Suspension
(Cephalexin) Dista 930
Nebcin Vials, Hyporets &
ADD-Vantage (Tobramycin
Sulfate) Lilly 1518

Pfizerpen for Injection (Penicillin G
Potassium) Pfizer Inc 2022
TERAK Ointment (Oxytetracycline
Hydrochloride, Polymyxin B
Sulfate) Akorn .... ⊚ 210
Vancocin HCl, Vials & ADD-Vantage
(Vancomycin Hydrochloride) Lilly 1534

Staphylococcus species infections, ocular
TERAK Ointment (Oxytetracycline
Hydrochloride, Polymyxin B
Sulfate) Akorn .... ⊚ 210
Terramycin with Polymyxin B
Sulfate Ophthalmic Ointment
(Oxytetracycline Hydrochloride,
Polymyxin B Sulfate) Pfizer Inc 2035

Staphylococcus species, coagulase-negative, infections
Ceclor Pulvules & Suspension
(Cefaclor) Lilly 1470
Garamycin Injectable (Gentamicin
Sulfate) Schering 2502
Trimpex Tablets (Trimethoprim)
Roche Pharmaceuticals 2323

Staphylococcus species, coagulase-positive, infections
Garamycin Injectable (Gentamicin
Sulfate) Schering 2502

Status epilepticus
(see under Epilepticus, status)

Steatorrhea, adjunctive therapy in
Cotazym Capsules (Pancrelipase)
Organon 1866
Ku-Zyme HP Capsules
(Pancrelipase) Schwarz 2547
Ultrase MT Capsules
(Pancrelipase) Scandipharm 2477
Zymase Capsules (Pancrelipase)
Organon 1889

Stenosis, hypertrophic subaortic
Inderal (Propranolol
Hydrochloride) Wyeth-Ayerst 2834
Inderal LA Long Acting Capsules
(Propranolol Hydrochloride)
Wyeth-Ayerst 2836

Stevens-Johnson syndrome
Celestone Soluspan Suspension
(Betamethasone Sodium Phos-
phate, Betamethasone Acetate)
Schering............................... 2484
Cortone Acetate Sterile Suspension
(Cortisone Acetate) Merck & Co.,
Inc. 1663
Cortone Acetate Tablets (Cortisone
Acetate) Merck & Co., Inc. 1664
Dalalone D.P. Injectable (Dexa-
methasone Acetate) Forest 1009
Decadron Elixir (Dexamethasone)
Merck & Co., Inc. 1676
Decadron Phosphate Injection
(Dexamethasone Sodium
Phosphate) Merck & Co., Inc. 1680
Decadron Tablets
(Dexamethasone) Merck & Co.,
Inc. 1678
Decadron-LA Sterile Suspension
(Dexamethasone Acetate) Merck
& Co., Inc. 1687
Hydeltrasol Injection, Sterile (Pred-
nisolone Sodium Phosphate)
Merck & Co., Inc. 1708
Hydrocortone Phosphate Injection,
Sterile (Hydrocortisone Sodium
Phosphate) Merck & Co., Inc. 1713
Hydrocortone Tablets
(Hydrocortisone) Merck & Co.,
Inc. 1715
Pediapred Oral Solution (Predniso-
lone Sodium Phosphate) Medeva 1618
Prelone Syrup (Prednisolone) Muro 1834

Stiff-man syndrome, adjunctive therapy in
Dizac (diazepam injectable
emulsion) CIV (Diazepam)
Ohmeda 1862
Valium Injectable (Diazepam)
Roche Products 2336
Valium Tablets (Diazepam) Roche
Products 2335

Stomach, disseminated adenocarcinoma
(see under Carcinoma, stomach)

Stomach, sour
(see under Hyperacidity, gastric, symptomatic relief of)

Stomach, upset
(see under Digestive disorders, symptomatic relief of)

Stomatitis, recurrent aphthous, symptomatic relief of
Children's Vicks Chloraseptic
Sore Throat Lozenges
(Benzocaine) Procter & Gamble ▣ 730
Children's Vicks Chloraseptic
Sore Throat Spray (Phenol)
Procter & Gamble................... ▣ 730
Dyclone 0.5% and 1% Topical
Solutions, USP (Dyclonine
Hydrochloride) Astra 535
Gly-Oxide Liquid (Carbamide
Peroxide) SmithKline Beecham
Consumer .... ▣ 779
Orajel Perioseptic Oxygenating
Liquid (Carbamide Peroxide)
Del .... ▣ 669
Vicks Chloraseptic Sore Throat
Lozenges, Menthol and Cherry
Flavors (Benzocaine, Menthol)
Procter & Gamble................... ▣ 732
Vicks Chloraseptic Sore Throat
Spray, Gargle and Mouth Rinse,
Menthol and Cherry Flavors
(Phenol) Procter & Gamble ...... ▣ 732
Zilactin Medicated Gel (Benzyl
Alcohol) Zila Pharmaceuticals ... ▣ 856
Zilactin-B Medicated Gel with
Benzocaine (Benzocaine) Zila
Pharmaceuticals .... ▣ 856

Strabismus
BOTOX (Botulinum Toxin Type A)
Purified Neurotoxin Complex
(Botulinum Toxin Type A)
Allergan 473

Strabismus, accommodative convergent
(see under Esotropia, accommodative)

Strep throat
(see under Streptococci species upper respiratory tract infections)

Streptococcal pharyngitis
Duricef Capsules, Tablets, and Oral
Suspension (Cefadroxil)
Bristol-Myers Squibb 750
E.E.S. (Erythromycin
Ethylsuccinate) Abbott 427
Ilosone (Erythromycin Estolate)
Dista 927
Ilotycin Gluceptate, IV, Vials (Eryth-
romycin Gluceptate) Dista 929
Suprax (Cefixime) Lederle 1443
Vantin for Oral Suspension and
Vantin Tablets (Cefpodoxime
Proxetil) Pharmacia & Upjohn 2112

Streptococci biliary tract infections
Kefzol Vials, Faspak &
ADD-Vantage (Cefazolin Sodium)
Lilly 1511

Streptococci group A beta-hemolytic endocarditis
Ancef Injection (Cefazolin Sodium)
SmithKline Beecham
Pharmaceuticals 2632

Streptococci group A beta-hemolytic infections
(see also under Erysipelas)
Ancef Injection (Cefazolin Sodium)
SmithKline Beecham
Pharmaceuticals 2632
Ceclor Pulvules & Suspension
(Cefaclor) Lilly 1470
Doryx Capsules (Doxycycline
Hyclate) Parke-Davis................ 1970
Kefzol Vials, Faspak &
ADD-Vantage (Cefazolin Sodium)
Lilly 1511
Mandol Vials, Faspak &
ADD-Vantage (Cefamandole
Nafate) Lilly 1516
Mezlin (Mezlocillin Sodium) Bayer
Pharmaceutical 594

Mezlin Pharmacy Bulk Package
(Mezlocillin Sodium) Bayer
Pharmaceutical 597
Primaxin I.V. (Cilastatin Sodium,
Imipenem) Merck & Co., Inc. 1772

Streptococci group A beta-hemolytic otitis media
Ceclor Pulvules & Suspension
(Cefaclor) Lilly 1470

Streptococci group A beta-hemolytic skin and skin structure infections
Ceclor Pulvules & Suspension
(Cefaclor) Lilly 1470
Ceptaz (Ceftazidime) Glaxo
Wellcome 1070
Fortaz (Ceftazidime) Glaxo
Wellcome 1092
Ilotycin Gluceptate, IV, Vials (Eryth-
romycin Gluceptate) Dista 929
Kefzol Vials, Faspak &
ADD-Vantage (Cefazolin Sodium)
Lilly 1511
Mandol Vials, Faspak &
ADD-Vantage (Cefamandole
Nafate) Lilly 1516
Primaxin I.V. (Cilastatin Sodium,
Imipenem) Merck & Co., Inc. 1772
Tazicef for Injection (Ceftazidime)
SmithKline Beecham
Pharmaceuticals 2697
Tazidime Vials, Faspak &
ADD-Vantage (Ceftazidime) Lilly .. 1531

Streptococci group A beta-hemolytic species infections, ocular
Pred-G Liquifilm Sterile
Ophthalmic Suspension (Genta-
micin Sulfate, Prednisolone
Acetate) Allergan.................... ⊚ 248
Pred-G S.O.P. Sterile Ophthalmic
Ointment (Gentamicin Sulfate,
Prednisolone Acetate) Allergan.. ⊚ 249
TobraDex Ophthalmic Suspension
and Ointment (Dexamethasone,
Tobramycin) Alcon Laboratories .. 469

Streptococci group A beta-hemolytic upper respiratory tract infections
Ceclor Pulvules & Suspension
(Cefaclor) Lilly 1470
Duricef Capsules, Tablets, and Oral
Suspension (Cefadroxil)
Bristol-Myers Squibb 750
ERYC (Erythromycin) Parke-Davis .. 1972
Ilotycin Gluceptate, IV, Vials (Eryth-
romycin Gluceptate) Dista 929
Keftab Tablets (Cephalexin
Hydrochloride) Dista 931
PCE Dispertab Tablets
(Erythromycin) Abbott 453
Spectrobid Tablets (Bacampicillin
Hydrochloride) Pfizer Inc 2030
Tao Capsules (Troleandomycin)
Pfizer Inc 2033

Streptococci group B infections
Mefoxin (Cefoxitin Sodium) Merck
& Co., Inc. 1734
Mefoxin Premixed Intravenous
Solution (Cefoxitin Sodium)
Merck & Co., Inc. 1737
Primaxin I.V. (Cilastatin Sodium,
Imipenem) Merck & Co., Inc. 1772

Streptococci group D bone and joint infections
Primaxin I.V. (Cilastatin Sodium,
Imipenem) Merck & Co., Inc. 1772

Streptococci group D endocarditis, adjunct in
Garamycin Injectable (Gentamicin
Sulfate) Schering 2502

Streptococci group D genitourinary tract infections
Omnipen for Oral Suspension
(Ampicillin) Wyeth-Ayerst........... 2873
Primaxin I.V. (Cilastatin Sodium,
Imipenem) Merck & Co., Inc. 1772

Streptococci group D gynecologic infections
Primaxin I.M. (Cilastatin Sodium,
Imipenem) Merck & Co., Inc. 1770

(▣ Described in PDR For Nonprescription Drugs) (⊚ Described in PDR For Ophthalmology)

Streptococci group — Indications Index — 1580

Streptococci group D infections
Ancef Injection (Cefazolin Sodium) SmithKline Beecham Pharmaceuticals 2632
Claforan Sterile and Injection (Cefotaxime Sodium) Hoechst Marion Roussel 1259
Garamycin Injectable (Gentamicin Sulfate) Schering 2502
Mandol Vials, Faspak & ADD-Vantage (Cefamandole Nafate) Lilly 1516
Mezlin Pharmacy Bulk Package (Mezlocillin Sodium) Bayer Pharmaceutical 597
Omnipen Capsules (Ampicillin) Wyeth-Ayerst 2872
Omnipen for Oral Suspension (Ampicillin) Wyeth-Ayerst 2873
Pipracil (Piperacillin Sodium) Lederle 1435
Primaxin I.V. (Cilastatin Sodium, Imipenem) Merck & Co., Inc. 1772
Spectrobid Tablets (Bacampicillin Hydrochloride) Pfizer Inc 2030

Streptococci group D intra-abdominal infections
Omnipen for Oral Suspension (Ampicillin) Wyeth-Ayerst 2873
Pipracil (Piperacillin Sodium) Lederle 1435
Primaxin I.M. (Cilastatin Sodium, Imipenem) Merck & Co., Inc. 1770
Primaxin I.V. (Cilastatin Sodium, Imipenem) Merck & Co., Inc. 1772

Streptococci group D septicemia
Primaxin I.V. (Cilastatin Sodium, Imipenem) Merck & Co., Inc. 1772

Streptococci group D skin and skin structure infections
Primaxin I.M. (Cilastatin Sodium, Imipenem) Merck & Co., Inc. 1770
Primaxin I.V. (Cilastatin Sodium, Imipenem) Merck & Co., Inc. 1772

Streptococci group D urinary tract infections
Mandol Vials, Faspak & ADD-Vantage (Cefamandole Nafate) Lilly 1516

Streptococci infections, ocular
AK-Spore (Bacitracin Zinc, Neomycin Sulfate, Polymyxin B Sulfate) Akorn 205
Chloromycetin Ophthalmic Ointment, 1% (Chloramphenicol) Parke-Davis 298
Chloromycetin Ophthalmic Solution (Chloramphenicol) Parke-Davis 299
Cortisporin Ophthalmic Ointment Sterile (Polymyxin B Sulfate, Bacitracin Zinc, Neomycin Sulfate, Hydrocortisone) Glaxo Wellcome 1074
TERAK Ointment (Oxytetracycline Hydrochloride, Polymyxin B Sulfate) Akorn 210
Terra-Cortril Ophthalmic Suspension (Oxytetracycline Hydrochloride, Hydrocortisone Acetate) Pfizer Inc 2033
Terramycin with Polymyxin B Sulfate Ophthalmic Ointment (Oxytetracycline Hydrochloride, Polymyxin B Sulfate) Pfizer Inc 2035
TobraDex Ophthalmic Suspension and Ointment (Dexamethasone, Tobramycin) Alcon Laboratories .. 469

Streptococci skin and skin structure infections
Cefizox for Intramuscular or Intravenous Use (Ceftizoxime Sodium) Fujisawa 1025
Cefotan (Cefotetan) Zeneca 2936
Duricef Capsules, Tablets, and Oral Suspension (Cefadroxil) Bristol-Myers Squibb 750
Keflex Pulvules & Oral Suspension (Cephalexin) Dista 930
Kefzol Vials, Faspak & ADD-Vantage (Cefazolin Sodium) Lilly 1511
Mefoxin (Cefoxitin Sodium) Merck & Co., Inc. 1734
Mefoxin Premixed Intravenous Solution (Cefoxitin Sodium) Merck & Co., Inc. 1737

Streptococci species otitis media
Keflex Pulvules & Oral Suspension (Cephalexin) Dista 930

Streptococci species upper respiratory tract infections
Bicillin C-R Injection (Penicillin G Procaine, Penicillin G Benzathine) Wyeth-Ayerst 2810
Bicillin C-R 900/300 Injection (Penicillin G Procaine, Penicillin G Benzathine) Wyeth-Ayerst 2812
Bicillin L-A Injection (Penicillin G Benzathine) Wyeth-Ayerst 2813
Ceftin for Oral Suspension (Cefuroxime Axetil) Glaxo Wellcome 1067
Pen•Vee K (Penicillin V Potassium) Wyeth-Ayerst 2879
Suprax (Cefixime) Lederle 1443

Streptococci (viridans group) infections, ocular
AK-CIDE (Prednisolone Acetate, Sulfacetamide Sodium) Akorn 203
AK-CIDE Ointment (Prednisolone Acetate, Sulfacetamide Sodium) Akorn 203
Blephamide Liquifilm Sterile Ophthalmic Suspension (Prednisolone Acetate, Sulfacetamide Sodium) Allergan 472
Ciloxan Ophthalmic Solution (Ciprofloxacin Hydrochloride) Alcon Laboratories 468
FML-S Liquifilm (Sulfacetamide Sodium, Fluorometholone) Allergan 240
Polytrim Ophthalmic Solution Sterile (Polymyxin B Sulfate, Trimethoprim Sulfate) Allergan 479

Streptococci non-hemolytic species infections, ocular
Pred-G Liquifilm Sterile Ophthalmic Suspension (Gentamicin Sulfate, Prednisolone Acetate) Allergan 248
TobraDex Ophthalmic Suspension and Ointment (Dexamethasone, Tobramycin) Alcon Laboratories .. 469

Streptococci, alpha-hemolytic (viridans group), infections
Ilosone (Erythromycin Estolate) Dista 927

Streptococcus agalactiae infections
(see under S. agalactiae infections)

Streptococcus faecalis
(see under S. faecalis infections)

Streptococcus pneumoniae
(see under S. pneumoniae infections)

Streptococcus pyogenes
(see under S. pyogenes infections)

Streptococcus species bone and joint infections
Cefizox for Intramuscular or Intravenous Use (Ceftizoxime Sodium) Fujisawa 1025
Claforan Sterile and Injection (Cefotaxime Sodium) Hoechst Marion Roussel 1259

Streptococcus species gynecologic infections
Cefotan (Cefotetan) Zeneca 2936
Claforan Sterile and Injection (Cefotaxime Sodium) Hoechst Marion Roussel 1259

Streptococcus species infections
Achromycin V Capsules (Tetracycline Hydrochloride) Lederle 1417
Amoxil (Amoxicillin Trihydrate) SmithKline Beecham Pharmaceuticals 2631
Bactroban Ointment (Mupirocin) SmithKline Beecham Pharmaceuticals 2642
Cefizox for Intramuscular or Intravenous Use (Ceftizoxime Sodium) Fujisawa 1025
Cefotan (Cefotetan) Zeneca 2936
Claforan Sterile and Injection (Cefotaxime Sodium) Hoechst Marion Roussel 1259
Cleocin Phosphate Injection (Clindamycin Phosphate) Pharmacia & Upjohn 2068
Declomycin Tablets (Demeclocycline Hydrochloride) Lederle 1421
Duricef Capsules, Tablets, and Oral Suspension (Cefadroxil) Bristol-Myers Squibb 750
Garamycin Injectable (Gentamicin Sulfate) Schering 2502
Kefzol Vials, Faspak & ADD-Vantage (Cefazolin Sodium) Lilly 1511
Mezlin (Mezlocillin Sodium) Bayer Pharmaceutical 594
Mezlin Pharmacy Bulk Package (Mezlocillin Sodium) Bayer Pharmaceutical 597
Minocin Intravenous (Minocycline Hydrochloride) Lederle 1428
Netromycin Injection 100 mg/ml (Netilmicin Sulfate) Schering 2516
Pen•Vee K (Penicillin V Potassium) Wyeth-Ayerst 2879
Pfizerpen for Injection (Penicillin G Potassium) Pfizer Inc 2022
Spectrobid Tablets (Bacampicillin Hydrochloride) Pfizer Inc 2030
Suprax (Cefixime) Lederle 1443
TERAK Ointment (Oxytetracycline Hydrochloride, Polymyxin B Sulfate) Akorn 210
Terramycin Intramuscular Solution (Oxytetracycline) Pfizer Inc 2034
Vibramycin Hyclate Intravenous (Doxycycline Hyclate) Pfizer Inc 2040

Streptococcus species intra-abdominal infections
Cefizox for Intramuscular or Intravenous Use (Ceftizoxime Sodium) Fujisawa 1025
Cefotan (Cefotetan) Zeneca 2936
Claforan Sterile and Injection (Cefotaxime Sodium) Hoechst Marion Roussel 1259

Streptococcus species lower respiratory tract infections
Cefizox for Intramuscular or Intravenous Use (Ceftizoxime Sodium) Fujisawa 1025

Streptococcus species respiratory tract infections
Cleocin Phosphate Injection (Clindamycin Phosphate) Pharmacia & Upjohn 2068

Streptococcus species septicemia
Cefizox for Intramuscular or Intravenous Use (Ceftizoxime Sodium) Fujisawa 1025
Claforan Sterile and Injection (Cefotaxime Sodium) Hoechst Marion Roussel 1259
Cleocin Phosphate Injection (Clindamycin Phosphate) Pharmacia & Upjohn 2068

Streptococcus tonsillitis
(see under Streptococci species upper respiratory tract infections)

Streptococcus viridans group infections
Blephamide Ointment (Sulfacetamide Sodium, Prednisolone Acetate) Allergan 234
Merrem I.V. (Meropenem) Zeneca .. 2952
Primaxin I.M. (Cilastatin Sodium, Imipenem) Merck & Co., Inc. 1770
Rocephin Injectable Vials, ADD-Vantage, Galaxy Container (Ceftriaxone Sodium) Roche Pharmaceuticals 2305
Streptomycin Sulfate Injection (Streptomycin Sulfate) Pfizer Inc 2031

Stroke, thrombotic, to reduce the risk of
Genuine Bayer Aspirin Tablets & Caplets (Aspirin) Bayer Consumer 618
Coumadin (Warfarin Sodium) DuPont 941
Ticlid Tablets (Ticlopidine Hydrochloride) Roche Pharmaceuticals 2317

Strongyloidiasis
Mintezol (Thiabendazole) Merck & Co., Inc. 1747

Sty
(see under Hordeolum)

Subinvolution, routine management of
Methergine (Methylergonovine Maleate) Sandoz Pharmaceuticals 2401

Sunburn, acute, prophylaxis
Coppertone Skin Selects Sunscreen Lotion SPF 15 For Dry Skin (Ethylhexyl p-Methoxycinnamate, Oxybenzone) Schering-Plough HealthCare 759
Coppertone Skin Selects Sunscreen Lotion SPF 15 For Oily Skin (Ethylhexyl p-Methoxycinnamate, Oxybenzone) Schering-Plough HealthCare 760
Coppertone Skin Selects Sunscreen Lotion SPF 15 For Sensitive Skin (Ethylhexyl p-Methoxycinnamate, Titanium Dioxide) Schering-Plough HealthCare 760
Moisturel Cream (Dimethicone, Petrolatum) Westwood-Squibb .. 2796
Oil of Olay Daily UV Protectant SPF 15 Beauty Fluid-Original and Fragrance Free (Olay Co. Inc.) (Octyl Methoxycinnamate, Phenylbenzimidazole-5-Sulfonic Acid) Procter & Gamble 725
Shade Gel SPF 30 Sunblock (Ethylhexyl p-Methoxycinnamate, Oxybenzone, Homosalate) Schering-Plough HealthCare 767
Shade Lotion SPF 45 Sunblock (Ethylhexyl p-Methoxycinnamate, Oxybenzone, 2-Ethylhexyl Salicylate, Homosalate) Schering-Plough HealthCare 767
Shade UVAGUARD SPF 15 Suncreen Lotion (Octyl Methoxycinnamate, Avobenzone, Oxybenzone) Schering-Plough HealthCare 768
Solbar PF Ultra Liquid SPF 30 (Octyl Methoxycinnamate, Oxybenzone) Persōn & Covey 1989

Sunburn, pain associated with
(see under Pain, topical relief of)

Sweating disorders
(see under Miliaria)

Sycosis barbae
Garamycin 0.1% (Gentamicin Sulfate) Schering 2501

Sympathetic ophthalmia
(see under Ophthalmia, sympathetic)

Synechial formation
Humorsol Sterile Ophthalmic Solution (Demecarium Bromide) Merck & Co., Inc. 1707

Syphilis
(see under T. pallidum infections)

T

T. pallidum infections
Achromycin V Capsules (Tetracycline Hydrochloride) Lederle 1417
Bicillin L-A Injection (Penicillin G Benzathine) Wyeth-Ayerst 2813
Declomycin Tablets (Demeclocycline Hydrochloride) Lederle 1421
Doryx Capsules (Doxycycline Hyclate) Parke-Davis 1970
DYNACIN Capsules (Minocycline Hydrochloride) Medicis 1627

(■ Described in PDR For Nonprescription Drugs)   (⊙ Described in PDR For Ophthalmology)

Indications Index — **Thrush**

E.E.S. (Erythromycin
 Ethylsuccinate) Abbott 427
E-Mycin Tablets (Erythromycin)
 Knoll Laboratories 1388
ERYC (Erythromycin) Parke-Davis .. 1972
EryPed (Erythromycin
 Ethylsuccinate) Abbott 425
Ery-Tab Tablets (Erythromycin)
 Abbott 426
Erythrocin Stearate Filmtab (Eryth-
 romycin Stearate) Abbott 429
Erythromycin Base Filmtab
 (Erythromycin) Abbott 430
Erythromycin Delayed-Release
 Capsules, USP (Erythromycin)
 Abbott 431
Ilosone (Erythromycin Estolate)
 Dista 927
Minocin Intravenous (Minocycline
 Hydrochloride) Lederle 1428
Minocin Oral Suspension (Minocy-
 cline Hydrochloride) Lederle 1431
Minocin Pellet-Filled Capsules
 (Minocycline Hydrochloride)
 Lederle 1429
Monodox Capsules (Doxycycline
 Monohydrate) Oclassen 1858
PCE Dispertab Tablets
 (Erythromycin) Abbott 453
Pfizerpen for Injection (Penicillin G
 Potassium) Pfizer Inc 2022
Terramycin Intramuscular Solution
 (Oxytetracycline) Pfizer Inc 2034
Vibramycin (Doxycycline Calcium)
 Pfizer Inc 2038
Vibramycin Hyclate Intravenous
 (Doxycycline Hyclate) Pfizer Inc .. 2040
Vibramycin (Doxycycline
 Monohydrate) Pfizer Inc 2038

T. vaginalis infections
Betadine Medicated Douche (Povi-
 done Iodine) Purdue Frederick ... 2144
Betadine Medicated Gel (Povidone
 Iodine) Purdue Frederick 2144
Flagyl 375 Capsules
 (Metronidazole) Searle 2587
Protostat Tablets (Metronidazole)
 Ortho Pharmaceutical 1939

**Tachyarrhythmias,
catecholamine-induced, during
anesthesia**
Inderal (Propranolol
 Hydrochloride) Wyeth-Ayerst 2834

Tachyarrhythmias, digitalis-induced
Inderal (Propranolol
 Hydrochloride) Wyeth-Ayerst 2834

Tachycardia, atrial, paroxysmal
Lanoxicaps (Digoxin) Glaxo
 Wellcome 1110
Lanoxin Elixir Pediatric (Digoxin)
 Glaxo Wellcome 1113
Lanoxin Injection (Digoxin) Glaxo
 Wellcome 1116
Lanoxin Injection Pediatric
 (Digoxin) Glaxo Wellcome 1119
Lanoxin Tablets (Digoxin) Glaxo
 Wellcome 1121

**Tachycardia, noncompensatory
sinus**
Brevibloc (esmolol HCl) Injection
 (Esmolol Hydrochloride) Ohmeda 1860

**Tachycardia, paroxysmal
supraventricular**
Adenocard Injection (Adenosine)
 Fujisawa 1021
Cardizem Injectable (Diltiazem
 Hydrochloride) Hoechst Marion
 Roussel 1253
Inderal (Propranolol
 Hydrochloride) Wyeth-Ayerst 2834
Isoptin Injectable (Verapamil
 Hydrochloride) Knoll
 Laboratories 1391
Neo-Synephrine Hydrochloride 1%
 Carpuject (Phenylephrine
 Hydrochloride) Sanofi Winthrop .. 2455
Neo-Synephrine Hydrochloride 1%
 Injection (Phenylephrine
 Hydrochloride) Sanofi Winthrop .. 2455
Tambocor Tablets (Flecainide
 Acetate) 3M Pharmaceuticals 1555

**Tachycardia, paroxysmal
supraventricular associated with
Lown-Ganong-Levine syndrome
(see under Lown-Ganong-Levine
syndrome)**

**Tachycardia, paroxysmal
supraventricular associated with
Wolff-Parkinson-White syndrome
(see under Wolff-Parkinson-White
syndrome)**

**Tachycardia, repetitive paroxysmal
supraventricular, prophylaxis of**
Calan Tablets (Verapamil
 Hydrochloride) Searle 2568
Isoptin Oral Tablets (Verapamil
 Hydrochloride) Knoll
 Laboratories 1393

Tachycardia, supraventricular
Brevibloc (esmolol HCl) Injection
 (Esmolol Hydrochloride) Ohmeda 1860
Tambocor Tablets (Flecainide
 Acetate) 3M Pharmaceuticals 1555

Tachycardia, ventricular
Betapace Tablets (Sotalol
 Hydrochloride) Berlex 637
Inderal (Propranolol
 Hydrochloride) Wyeth-Ayerst 2834
Quinaglute Dura-Tabs Tablets
 (Quinidine Gluconate) Berlex 644
Tambocor Tablets (Flecainide
 Acetate) 3M Pharmaceuticals 1555
Tonocard Tablets (Tocainide
 Hydrochloride) Astra Merck 519

**Tachycardia, ventricular, recurrent
hemodynamically unstable**
Cordarone Intravenous (Amioda-
 rone Hydrochloride)
 Wyeth-Ayerst 2821
Cordarone Tablets (Amiodarone
 Hydrochloride) Wyeth-Ayerst 2818

Tachycardia, ventricular, sustained
Cardioquin Tablets (Quinidine
 Polygalacturonate) Purdue
 Frederick 2146
Ethmozine Tablets (Moricizine
 Hydrochloride) Roberts 2217
Mexitil Capsules (Mexiletine
 Hydrochloride) Boehringer
 Ingelheim 684
Norpace (Disopyramide
 Phosphate) Searle 2596
Procanbid Extended-Release
 Tablets (Procainamide
 Hydrochloride) Parke-Davis 1983
Quinidex Extentabs (Quinidine
 Sulfate) Robins 2240
Rythmol Tablets—150mg, 225mg,
 300mg (Propafenone
 Hydrochloride) Knoll
 Laboratories 1399
Tambocor Tablets (Flecainide
 Acetate) 3M Pharmaceuticals 1555

**Tachycardias due to thyrotoxicosis,
adjunct**
Inderal (Propranolol
 Hydrochloride) Wyeth-Ayerst 2834

**Tachycardias, paroxysmal atrial
(see under Tachycardia,
paroxysmal supraventricular)**

Tachycardias, sinus, persistent
Inderal (Propranolol
 Hydrochloride) Wyeth-Ayerst 2834

Tachycardias, supraventricular
Crystodigin Tablets (Digitoxin) Lilly 1472
Vasoxyl Injection (Methoxamine
 Hydrochloride) Glaxo Wellcome .. 1169

Taenia solium infections
Albenza Tablets (Albendazole)
 SmithKline Beecham
 Pharmaceuticals 2629

**Tapeworm infections
(see under Infections, tapeworm)**

**Tapeworm, dwarf
(see under Hymenolepis nana
infections)**

**Tapeworm, fish
(see under Diphyllobothrium
latum infections)**

Tendinitis
Anaprox/Naprosyn (Naproxen
 Sodium) Roche Pharmaceuticals .. 2277
Clinoril Tablets (Sulindac) Merck &
 Co., Inc. 1658
Indocin (Indomethacin) Merck &
 Co., Inc. 1723
Naprelan Tablets (Naproxen
 Sodium) Wyeth-Ayerst 2861
Anaprox/Naprosyn (Naproxen)
 Roche Pharmaceuticals 2277
Traumeel Injection Solution (Home-
 opathic Medications) Heel/BHI ... 1237

Tenosynovitis, acute nonspecific
Celestone Soluspan Suspension
 (Betamethasone Sodium Phos-
 phate, Betamethasone Acetate)
 Schering 2484
Cortone Acetate Sterile Suspension
 (Cortisone Acetate) Merck & Co.,
 Inc. 1663
Cortone Acetate Tablets (Cortisone
 Acetate) Merck & Co., Inc. 1664
Dalalone D.P. Injectable (Dexa-
 methasone Acetate) Forest 1009
Decadron Elixir (Dexamethasone)
 Merck & Co., Inc. 1676
Decadron Phosphate Injection
 (Dexamethasone Sodium
 Phosphate) Merck & Co., Inc. 1680
Decadron Phosphate with
 Xylocaine Injection, Sterile (Dexa-
 methasone Sodium Phosphate,
 Lidocaine Hydrochloride) Merck
 & Co., Inc. 1683
Decadron Tablets
 (Dexamethasone) Merck & Co.,
 Inc. 1678
Decadron-LA Sterile Suspension
 (Dexamethasone Acetate) Merck
 & Co., Inc. 1687
Hydeltrasol Injection, Sterile (Pred-
 nisolone Sodium Phosphate)
 Merck & Co., Inc. 1708
Hydeltra-T.B.A. Sterile Suspension
 (Prednisolone Tebutate) Merck &
 Co., Inc. 1710
Hydrocortone Acetate Sterile
 Suspension (Hydrocortisone
 Acetate) Merck & Co., Inc. 1712
Hydrocortone Phosphate Injection,
 Sterile (Hydrocortisone Sodium
 Phosphate) Merck & Co., Inc. 1713
Hydrocortone Tablets
 (Hydrocortisone) Merck & Co.,
 Inc. 1715
Pediapred Oral Solution (Predniso-
 lone Sodium Phosphate) Medeva 1618
Prelone Syrup (Prednisolone) Muro 1834

**Testis, advanced carcinoma of
(see under Carcinoma, testis,
advanced)**

**Testosterone, deficiency of
(see under Androgen, absence or
deficiency of)**

Tetanus
Hyper-Tet Tetanus Immune
 Globulin (Human) (Tetanus Im-
 mune Globulin (Human)) Bayer
 Biological 621
Pfizerpen for Injection (Penicillin G
 Potassium) Pfizer Inc 2022

Tetanus, treatment adjunct
Dizac (diazepam injectable
 emulsion) CIV (Diazepam)
 Ohmeda 1862
Thorazine (Chlorpromazine
 Hydrochloride) SmithKline
 Beecham Pharmaceuticals 2701
Valium Injectable (Diazepam)
 Roche Products 2336

Tetany, idiopathic
DHT (Dihydrotachysterol) Tablets
 & Intensol (Dihydrotachysterol)
 Roxane 2351

Tetany, postoperative
DHT (Dihydrotachysterol) Tablets
 & Intensol (Dihydrotachysterol)
 Roxane 2351

**Threadworm infestations
(see under Strongyloidiasis)**

**Throat, itchy
(see under Pruritus,
rhinopharyngeal, symptomatic
relief of)**

**Throat, sore
(see under Pharyngitis,
symptomatic relief of)**

**Throat, surgical procedures,
irrigation of**
AMO Endosol (Balanced Salt
 Solution) (Balanced Salt
 Solution) Allergan .... ⊚ 229

Thrombocytopenia, secondary
Celestone Soluspan Suspension
 (Betamethasone Sodium Phos-
 phate, Betamethasone Acetate)
 Schering 2484
Cortone Acetate Tablets (Cortisone
 Acetate) Merck & Co., Inc. 1664
Dalalone D.P. Injectable (Dexa-
 methasone Acetate) Forest 1009
Decadron Elixir (Dexamethasone)
 Merck & Co., Inc. 1676
Decadron Phosphate Injection
 (Dexamethasone Sodium
 Phosphate) Merck & Co., Inc. 1680
Decadron Tablets
 (Dexamethasone) Merck & Co.,
 Inc. 1678
Decadron-LA Sterile Suspension
 (Dexamethasone Acetate) Merck
 & Co., Inc. 1687
Hydeltrasol Injection, Sterile (Pred-
 nisolone Sodium Phosphate)
 Merck & Co., Inc. 1708
Hydrocortone Phosphate Injection,
 Sterile (Hydrocortisone Sodium
 Phosphate) Merck & Co., Inc. 1713
Hydrocortone Tablets
 (Hydrocortisone) Merck & Co.,
 Inc. 1715
Pediapred Oral Solution (Predniso-
 lone Sodium Phosphate) Medeva 1618
Prelone Syrup (Prednisolone) Muro 1834

Thromboembolic complications
Coumadin (Warfarin Sodium)
 DuPont 941

**Thromboembolism, postoperative,
adjunct in**
Persantine Tablets (Dipyridamole)
 Boehringer Ingelheim 686

**Thrombosis, coronary artery, acute,
lysis of**
Abbokinase (Urokinase) Abbott 403
Activase (Alteplase, Recombinant)
 Genentech 1045
Eminase (Anistreplase) Roberts 2215
Streptase for Infusion
 (Streptokinase) Astra 557

Thrombosis, venous
Coumadin (Warfarin Sodium)
 DuPont 941
Heparin Sodium Injection (Heparin
 Sodium) Wyeth-Ayerst 2832
Heparin Sodium Vials (Heparin
 Sodium) Lilly 1486
Streptase for Infusion
 (Streptokinase) Astra 557

Thrombosis, venous, prophylaxis of
Coumadin (Warfarin Sodium)
 DuPont 941
Fragmin Injection (Dalteparin
 Sodium) Pharmacia & Upjohn 2088
Heparin Sodium Vials (Heparin
 Sodium) Lilly 1486
Lovenox Injection (Enoxaparin)
 Rhone-Poulenc Rorer
 Pharmaceuticals 2187

**Thrush
(see under Candidiasis,
oropharyngeal)**

(▣ Described in PDR For Nonprescription Drugs)　　　　　　　　　　　　　　　　　　　　　　　　　　　　(⊚ Described in PDR For Ophthalmology)

Thyroid function — Indications Index — 1582

Thyroid function, aid in the diagnosis of
Cytomel Tablets (Liothyronine Sodium) SmithKline Beecham Pharmaceuticals ... 2647
Eltroxin Tablets (Levothyroxine Sodium) Roberts ... 2214
Levothroid Tablets (Levothyroxine Sodium) Forest ... 1015
Levothyroxine Sodium, USP for Injection (Levothyroxine Sodium) Astra ... 546
Synthroid (Levothyroxine Sodium) Knoll Pharmaceutical ... 1410
THYREL TRH (Protirelin) Ferring ... 2992

Thyroid uptake, blocking of in a radiation emergency
Thyro-Block Tablets (Potassium Iodide) Wallace ... 2785

Thyroiditis, chronic lymphocytic (see under Hashimoto's thyroiditis)

Thyroiditis, nonsuppurative
Celestone Soluspan Suspension (Betamethasone Sodium Phosphate, Betamethasone Acetate) Schering ... 2484
Cortone Acetate Sterile Suspension (Cortisone Acetate) Merck & Co., Inc. ... 1663
Cortone Acetate Tablets (Cortisone Acetate) Merck & Co., Inc. ... 1664
Dalalone D.P. Injectable (Dexamethasone Acetate) Forest ... 1009
Decadron Elixir (Dexamethasone) Merck & Co., Inc. ... 1676
Decadron Phosphate Injection (Dexamethasone Sodium Phosphate) Merck & Co., Inc. ... 1680
Decadron Tablets (Dexamethasone) Merck & Co., Inc. ... 1678
Decadron-LA Sterile Suspension (Dexamethasone Acetate) Merck & Co., Inc. ... 1687
Hydeltrasol Injection, Sterile (Prednisolone Sodium Phosphate) Merck & Co., Inc. ... 1708
Hydrocortone Phosphate Injection, Sterile (Hydrocortisone Sodium Phosphate) Merck & Co., Inc. ... 1713
Hydrocortone Tablets (Hydrocortisone) Merck & Co., Inc. ... 1715
Pediapred Oral Solution (Prednisolone Sodium Phosphate) Medeva 1618
Prelone Syrup (Prednisolone) Muro 1834

Tick fevers
Achromycin V Capsules (Tetracycline Hydrochloride) Lederle ... 1417
Declomycin Tablets (Demeclocycline Hydrochloride) Lederle ... 1421
Doryx Capsules (Doxycycline Hyclate) Parke-Davis ... 1970
DYNACIN Capsules (Minocycline Hydrochloride) Medicis ... 1627
Minocin Intravenous (Minocycline Hydrochloride) Lederle ... 1428
Minocin Oral Suspension (Minocycline Hydrochloride) Lederle ... 1431
Minocin Pellet-Filled Capsules (Minocycline Hydrochloride) Lederle ... 1429
Monodox Capsules (Doxycycline Monohydrate) Oclassen ... 1858
Terramycin Intramuscular Solution (Oxytetracycline) Pfizer Inc ... 2034
Vibramycin (Doxycycline Calcium) Pfizer Inc ... 2038
Vibramycin Hyclate Intravenous (Doxycycline Hyclate) Pfizer Inc ... 2040
Vibramycin (Doxycycline Monohydrate) Pfizer Inc ... 2038

Tinea barbae (see under Folliculitis barbae)

Tinea capitis infections
Fulvicin P/G Tablets (Griseofulvin) Schering ... 2499
Fulvicin P/G 165 & 330 Tablets (Griseofulvin) Schering ... 2500
Grifulvin V (griseofulvin tablets) Microsize (griseofulvin oral suspension) Microsize (Griseofulvin) Ortho Dermatological ... 1944
Gris-PEG Tablets, 125 mg & 250 mg (Griseofulvin) Allergan ... 476

Tinea corporis infections
Desenex Prescription (Clotrimazole) Ciba Self-Medication ... ▣ 653
Exelderm Cream 1.0% (Sulconazole Nitrate) Westwood-Squibb ... 2794
Exelderm Solution 1.0% (Sulconazole Nitrate) Westwood-Squibb ... 2795
Fulvicin P/G Tablets (Griseofulvin) Schering ... 2499
Fulvicin P/G 165 & 330 Tablets (Griseofulvin) Schering ... 2500
Grifulvin V (griseofulvin tablets) Microsize (griseofulvin oral suspension) Microsize (Griseofulvin) Ortho Dermatological ... 1944
Gris-PEG Tablets, 125 mg & 250 mg (Griseofulvin) Allergan ... 476
Lamisil Cream 1% (Terbinafine Hydrochloride) Sandoz Pharmaceuticals ... 2393
Loprox 1% Cream and Lotion (Ciclopirox Olamine) Hoechst Marion Roussel ... 1269
Lotrimin (Clotrimazole) Schering ... 2514
Lotrimin AF Antifungal Cream, Lotion and Solution (Clotrimazole) Schering-Plough HealthCare ... ▣ 766
Lotrimin AF Antifungal Spray Liquid, Spray Powder, Spray Deodorant Powder, Powder and Jock Itch Spray Powder (Miconazole Nitrate) Schering-Plough HealthCare ... ▣ 766
Lotrisone Cream (Clotrimazole, Betamethasone Dipropionate) Schering ... 2515
Monistat Dual-Pak (Miconazole Nitrate) Ortho Pharmaceutical ... 1906
Monistat-Derm (miconazole nitrate 2%) Cream (Miconazole Nitrate) Ortho Dermatological ... 1944
Mycelex OTC Cream Antifungal (Clotrimazole) Bayer Consumer ▣ 622
Naftin Cream 1% (Naftifine Hydrochloride) Allergan ... 477
Naftin Gel 1% (Naftifine Hydrochloride) Allergan ... 477
Nizoral 2% Cream (Ketoconazole) Janssen ... 1344
Oxistat (Oxiconazole Nitrate) Glaxo Wellcome ... 1139
Spectazole (econazole nitrate 1%) Cream (Econazole Nitrate) Ortho Dermatological ... 1947
Ting Antifungal Spray Powder (Miconazole Nitrate) Ciba Self-Medication ... ▣ 666

Tinea cruris infections
Cruex (Undecylenic Acid, Zinc Undecylenate) Ciba Self-Medication ... ▣ 652
Prescription Strength Desenex AF Cream (Clotrimazole) Ciba Self-Medication ... ▣ 653
Exelderm Cream 1.0% (Sulconazole Nitrate) Westwood-Squibb ... 2794
Exelderm Solution 1.0% (Sulconazole Nitrate) Westwood-Squibb ... 2795
Fulvicin P/G Tablets (Griseofulvin) Schering ... 2499
Fulvicin P/G 165 & 330 Tablets (Griseofulvin) Schering ... 2500
Grifulvin V (griseofulvin tablets) Microsize (griseofulvin oral suspension) Microsize (Griseofulvin) Ortho Dermatological ... 1944
Gris-PEG Tablets, 125 mg & 250 mg (Griseofulvin) Allergan ... 476
Lamisil Cream 1% (Terbinafine Hydrochloride) Sandoz Pharmaceuticals ... 2393
Loprox 1% Cream and Lotion (Ciclopirox Olamine) Hoechst Marion Roussel ... 1269
Lotrimin (Clotrimazole) Schering ... 2514
Lotrimin AF Antifungal Cream, Lotion and Solution (Clotrimazole) Schering-Plough HealthCare ... ▣ 766
Lotrimin AF Antifungal Spray Liquid, Spray Powder, Spray Deodorant Powder, Powder and Jock Itch Spray Powder (Miconazole Nitrate) Schering-Plough HealthCare ... ▣ 766
Lotrisone Cream (Clotrimazole, Betamethasone Dipropionate) Schering ... 2515
Monistat Dual-Pak (Miconazole Nitrate) Ortho Pharmaceutical ... 1906
Mycelex OTC Cream Antifungal (Clotrimazole) Bayer Consumer ▣ 622
Naftin Cream 1% (Naftifine Hydrochloride) Allergan ... 477
Naftin Gel 1% (Naftifine Hydrochloride) Allergan ... 477
Nizoral 2% Cream (Ketoconazole) Janssen ... 1344
Oxistat (Oxiconazole Nitrate) Glaxo Wellcome ... 1139
Spectazole (econazole nitrate 1%) Cream (Econazole Nitrate) Ortho Dermatological ... 1947
Ting (Tolnaftate) Ciba Self-Medication ... ▣ 666
Ting Antifungal Spray Powder (Miconazole Nitrate) Ciba Self-Medication ... ▣ 666

Tinea pedis infections
Desenex (Undecylenic Acid, Zinc Undecylenate) Ciba Self-Medication ... ▣ 652
Desenex Prescription (Clotrimazole) Ciba Self-Medication ... ▣ 653
Exelderm Cream 1.0% (Sulconazole Nitrate) Westwood-Squibb ... 2794
Fulvicin P/G Tablets (Griseofulvin) Schering ... 2499
Fulvicin P/G 165 & 330 Tablets (Griseofulvin) Schering ... 2500
Grifulvin V (griseofulvin tablets) Microsize (griseofulvin oral suspension) Microsize (Griseofulvin) Ortho Dermatological ... 1944
Gris-PEG Tablets, 125 mg & 250 mg (Griseofulvin) Allergan ... 476
Lamisil Cream 1% (Terbinafine Hydrochloride) Sandoz Pharmaceuticals ... 2393
Loprox 1% Cream and Lotion (Ciclopirox Olamine) Hoechst Marion Roussel ... 1269
Lotrimin (Clotrimazole) Schering ... 2514
Lotrimin AF Antifungal Cream, Lotion and Solution (Clotrimazole) Schering-Plough HealthCare ... ▣ 766
Lotrimin AF Antifungal Spray Liquid, Spray Powder, Spray Deodorant Powder, Powder and Jock Itch Spray Powder (Miconazole Nitrate) Schering-Plough HealthCare ... ▣ 766
Lotrisone Cream (Clotrimazole, Betamethasone Dipropionate) Schering ... 2515
Monistat Dual-Pak (Miconazole Nitrate) Ortho Pharmaceutical ... 1906
Mycelex OTC Cream Antifungal (Clotrimazole) Bayer Consumer ▣ 622
Naftin Cream 1% (Naftifine Hydrochloride) Allergan ... 477
Naftin Gel 1% (Naftifine Hydrochloride) Allergan ... 477
Oxistat (Oxiconazole Nitrate) Glaxo Wellcome ... 1139
Spectazole (econazole nitrate 1%) Cream (Econazole Nitrate) Ortho Dermatological ... 1947
Ting (Tolnaftate) Ciba Self-Medication ... ▣ 666
Ting Antifungal Spray Powder (Miconazole Nitrate) Ciba Self-Medication ... ▣ 666

Tinea unguium infections
Fulvicin P/G Tablets (Griseofulvin) Schering ... 2499
Fulvicin P/G 165 & 330 Tablets (Griseofulvin) Schering ... 2500
Grifulvin V (griseofulvin tablets) Microsize (griseofulvin oral suspension) Microsize (Griseofulvin) Ortho Dermatological ... 1944
Gris-PEG Tablets, 125 mg & 250 mg (Griseofulvin) Allergan ... 476
Lamisil Tablets (Terbinafine Hydrochloride) Sandoz Pharmaceuticals ... 2394
Sporanox Capsules (Itraconazole) Janssen ... 1352

Tinea versicolor infections (see under Pityrosporon orbiculare infections)

Toenails, ingrown, pain (see under Pain, unguis aduncus, temporary relief of)

Tonometry, Goldman (see under Hypertension, ocular, diagnostic agent for)

Tonsillitis
Biaxin (Clarithromycin) Abbott ... 406
Ceclor Pulvules & Suspension (Cefaclor) Lilly ... 1470
Cedax (Ceftibuten Dihydrate) Schering ... 2480
Ceftin (Cefuroxime Axetil) Glaxo Wellcome ... 1067
Cefzil Tablets and Oral Suspension (Cefprozil) Bristol-Myers Squibb .. 747
Duricef Capsules, Tablets, and Oral Suspension (Cefadroxil) Bristol-Myers Squibb ... 750
Dynabac (Dirithromycin) Bock ... 668
Lorabid Suspension and Pulvules (Loracarbef) Lilly ... 1513
PCE Dispertab Tablets (Erythromycin) Abbott ... 453
Suprax (Cefixime) Lederle ... 1443
Vantin for Oral Suspension and Vantin Tablets (Cefpodoxime Proxetil) Pharmacia & Upjohn ... 2112
Zithromax (Azithromycin) Pfizer Inc ... 2043
Zithromax Tablets (Azithromycin) Pfizer Inc ... 2046

Tooth, hypersensitivity of
Crest Sensitivity Protection Toothpaste (Potassium Nitrate, Sodium Fluoride) Procter & Gamble ... ▣ 723
Promise Sensitive Toothpaste (Potassium Nitrate, Sodium Monofluorophosphate) Block ... ▣ 633
Cool Gel Sensodyne (Potassium Nitrate, Sodium Fluoride) Block ▣ 634
Fresh Mint Sensodyne Toothpaste (Potassium Nitrate, Sodium Monofluorophosphate) Block ... ▣ 634
Original Formula Sensodyne-SC Toothpaste (Strontium Chloride Hexahydrate) Block ... ▣ 634
Sensodyne with Baking Soda (Potassium Nitrate, Sodium Fluoride) Block ... ▣ 634

Torulosis (see under Cryptococcosis)

Tourette, Gilles de la, syndrome
Haldol Injection, Tablets and Concentrate (Haloperidol) McNeil Pharmaceutical ... 1585
Orap Tablets (Pimozide) Gate ... 1037

Toxicity, anticholinergic agents, reversal of
Antilirium Injectable (Physostigmine Salicylate) Forest ... 1007

Toxoplasmosis, adjunctive therapy in
Daraprim Tablets (Pyrimethamine) Glaxo Wellcome Oncology/HIV ... 1199
Gantanol Tablets (Sulfamethoxazole) Roche Pharmaceuticals ... 2285
Gantrisin (Acetyl Sulfisoxazole) Roche Pharmaceuticals ... 2286

Tracheal lavage
Sodium Chloride Sterile Water for Inhalation, Arm-a-Vial (Sodium Chloride) Astra ... 557

Trachoma
Achromycin V Capsules (Tetracycline Hydrochloride) Lederle ... 1417
Declomycin Tablets (Demeclocycline Hydrochloride) Lederle ... 1421
Doryx Capsules (Doxycycline Hyclate) Parke-Davis ... 1970

(▣ Described in PDR For Nonprescription Drugs) (◉ Described in PDR For Ophthalmology)

DYNACIN Capsules (Minocycline Hydrochloride) Medicis ... 1627
Gantanol Tablets (Sulfamethoxazole) Roche Pharmaceuticals ... 2285
Gantrisin (Acetyl Sulfisoxazole) Roche Pharmaceuticals ... 2286
Minocin Intravenous (Minocycline Hydrochloride) Lederle ... 1428
Minocin Oral Suspension (Minocycline Hydrochloride) Lederle ... 1431
Minocin Pellet-Filled Capsules (Minocycline Hydrochloride) Lederle ... 1429
Monodox Capsules (Doxycycline Monohydrate) Oclassen ... 1858
Terramycin Intramuscular Solution (Oxytetracycline) Pfizer Inc ... 2034
Vibramycin (Doxycycline Calcium) Pfizer Inc ... 2038
Vibramycin Hyclate Intravenous (Doxycycline Hyclate) Pfizer Inc ... 2040
Vibramycin (Doxycycline Monohydrate) Pfizer Inc ... 2038

Trachoma, adjunct in
Bleph-10 (Sulfacetamide Sodium) Allergan ... 472

Tremor, essential
Inderal (Propranolol Hydrochloride) Wyeth-Ayerst ... 2834

Treponema pallidum
(see under T. pallidum infections)

Treponema pertenue infections
(see under Yaws)

Trichinosis
Mintezol (Thiabendazole) Merck & Co., Inc. ... 1747

Trichinosis with myocardial involvement
Celestone Soluspan Suspension (Betamethasone Sodium Phosphate, Betamethasone Acetate) Schering ... 2484
Cortone Acetate Sterile Suspension (Cortisone Acetate) Merck & Co., Inc. ... 1663
Cortone Acetate Tablets (Cortisone Acetate) Merck & Co., Inc. ... 1664
Dalalone D.P. Injectable (Dexamethasone Acetate) Forest ... 1009
Decadron Elixir (Dexamethasone) Merck & Co., Inc. ... 1676
Decadron Phosphate Injection (Dexamethasone Sodium Phosphate) Merck & Co., Inc. ... 1680
Decadron Tablets (Dexamethasone) Merck & Co., Inc. ... 1678
Decadron-LA Sterile Suspension (Dexamethasone Acetate) Merck & Co., Inc. ... 1687
Hydeltrasol Injection, Sterile (Prednisolone Sodium Phosphate) Merck & Co., Inc. ... 1708
Hydrocortone Phosphate Injection, Sterile (Hydrocortisone Sodium Phosphate) Merck & Co., Inc. ... 1713
Hydrocortone Tablets (Hydrocortisone) Merck & Co., Inc. ... 1715
Pediapred Oral Solution (Prednisolone Sodium Phosphate) Medeva ... 1618
Prelone Syrup (Prednisolone) Muro ... 1834

Trichinosis with neurologic involvement
Celestone Soluspan Suspension (Betamethasone Sodium Phosphate, Betamethasone Acetate) Schering ... 2484
Cortone Acetate Sterile Suspension (Cortisone Acetate) Merck & Co., Inc. ... 1663
Cortone Acetate Tablets (Cortisone Acetate) Merck & Co., Inc. ... 1664
Dalalone D.P. Injectable (Dexamethasone Acetate) Forest ... 1009
Decadron Elixir (Dexamethasone) Merck & Co., Inc. ... 1676
Decadron Phosphate Injection (Dexamethasone Sodium Phosphate) Merck & Co., Inc. ... 1680
Decadron Tablets (Dexamethasone) Merck & Co., Inc. ... 1678

Decadron-LA Sterile Suspension (Dexamethasone Acetate) Merck & Co., Inc. ... 1687
Hydeltrasol Injection, Sterile (Prednisolone Sodium Phosphate) Merck & Co., Inc. ... 1708
Hydrocortone Phosphate Injection, Sterile (Hydrocortisone Sodium Phosphate) Merck & Co., Inc. ... 1713
Hydrocortone Tablets (Hydrocortisone) Merck & Co., Inc. ... 1715
Pediapred Oral Solution (Prednisolone Sodium Phosphate) Medeva ... 1618
Prelone Syrup (Prednisolone) Muro ... 1834

Trichomoniasis, asymptomatic
Flagyl 375 Capsules (Metronidazole) Searle ... 2587
Protostat Tablets (Metronidazole) Ortho Pharmaceutical ... 1939

Trichomoniasis, symptomatic
Flagyl 375 Capsules (Metronidazole) Searle ... 2587
Protostat Tablets (Metronidazole) Ortho Pharmaceutical ... 1939

Trichophyton crateriform infections
Fulvicin P/G Tablets (Griseofulvin) Schering ... 2499
Fulvicin P/G 165 & 330 Tablets (Griseofulvin) Schering ... 2500
Grifulvin V (griseofulvin tablets) Microsize (griseofulvin oral suspension) Microsize (Griseofulvin) Ortho Dermatological ... 1944
Gris-PEG Tablets, 125 mg & 250 mg (Griseofulvin) Allergan ... 476

Trichophyton gallinae infections
Fulvicin P/G Tablets (Griseofulvin) Schering ... 2499
Fulvicin P/G 165 & 330 Tablets (Griseofulvin) Schering ... 2500
Grifulvin V (griseofulvin tablets) Microsize (griseofulvin oral suspension) Microsize (Griseofulvin) Ortho Dermatological ... 1944
Gris-PEG Tablets, 125 mg & 250 mg (Griseofulvin) Allergan ... 476

Trichophyton interdigitalis infections
Fulvicin P/G Tablets (Griseofulvin) Schering ... 2499
Fulvicin P/G 165 & 330 Tablets (Griseofulvin) Schering ... 2500
Grifulvin V (griseofulvin tablets) Microsize (griseofulvin oral suspension) Microsize (Griseofulvin) Ortho Dermatological ... 1944
Gris-PEG Tablets, 125 mg & 250 mg (Griseofulvin) Allergan ... 476

Trichophyton megnini infections
Fulvicin P/G Tablets (Griseofulvin) Schering ... 2499
Fulvicin P/G 165 & 330 Tablets (Griseofulvin) Schering ... 2500
Grifulvin V (griseofulvin tablets) Microsize (griseofulvin oral suspension) Microsize (Griseofulvin) Ortho Dermatological ... 1944
Gris-PEG Tablets, 125 mg & 250 mg (Griseofulvin) Allergan ... 476

Trichophyton mentagrophytes infections
Exelderm Cream 1.0% (Sulconazole Nitrate) Westwood-Squibb ... 2794
Exelderm Solution 1.0% (Sulconazole Nitrate) Westwood-Squibb ... 2795
Fulvicin P/G Tablets (Griseofulvin) Schering ... 2499
Fulvicin P/G 165 & 330 Tablets (Griseofulvin) Schering ... 2500
Grifulvin V (griseofulvin tablets) Microsize (griseofulvin oral suspension) Microsize (Griseofulvin) Ortho Dermatological ... 1944
Gris-PEG Tablets, 125 mg & 250 mg (Griseofulvin) Allergan ... 476
Lamisil Cream 1% (Terbinafine Hydrochloride) Sandoz Pharmaceuticals ... 2393

Loprox 1% Cream and Lotion (Ciclopirox Olamine) Hoechst Marion Roussel ... 1269
Lotrimin (Clotrimazole) Schering ... 2514
Lotrisone Cream (Clotrimazole, Betamethasone Dipropionate) Schering ... 2515
Monistat Dual-Pak (Miconazole Nitrate) Ortho Pharmaceutical ... 1906
Monistat-Derm (miconazole nitrate 2%) Cream (Miconazole Nitrate) Ortho Dermatological ... 1944
Naftin Cream 1% (Naftifine Hydrochloride) Allergan ... 477
Naftin Gel 1% (Naftifine Hydrochloride) Allergan ... 477
Nizoral 2% Cream (Ketoconazole) Janssen ... 1344
Oxistat (Oxiconazole Nitrate) Glaxo Wellcome ... 1139
Spectazole (econazole nitrate 1%) Cream (Econazole Nitrate) Ortho Dermatological ... 1947

Trichophyton rubrum infections
Exelderm Cream 1.0% (Sulconazole Nitrate) Westwood-Squibb ... 2794
Exelderm Solution 1.0% (Sulconazole Nitrate) Westwood-Squibb ... 2795
Fulvicin P/G Tablets (Griseofulvin) Schering ... 2499
Fulvicin P/G 165 & 330 Tablets (Griseofulvin) Schering ... 2500
Grifulvin V (griseofulvin tablets) Microsize (griseofulvin oral suspension) Microsize (Griseofulvin) Ortho Dermatological ... 1944
Gris-PEG Tablets, 125 mg & 250 mg (Griseofulvin) Allergan ... 476
Lamisil Cream 1% (Terbinafine Hydrochloride) Sandoz Pharmaceuticals ... 2393
Loprox 1% Cream and Lotion (Ciclopirox Olamine) Hoechst Marion Roussel ... 1269
Lotrimin (Clotrimazole) Schering ... 2514
Lotrisone Cream (Clotrimazole, Betamethasone Dipropionate) Schering ... 2515
Monistat Dual-Pak (Miconazole Nitrate) Ortho Pharmaceutical ... 1906
Monistat-Derm (miconazole nitrate 2%) Cream (Miconazole Nitrate) Ortho Dermatological ... 1944
Naftin Cream 1% (Naftifine Hydrochloride) Allergan ... 477
Naftin Gel 1% (Naftifine Hydrochloride) Allergan ... 477
Nizoral 2% Cream (Ketoconazole) Janssen ... 1344
Oxistat (Oxiconazole Nitrate) Glaxo Wellcome ... 1139
Spectazole (econazole nitrate 1%) Cream (Econazole Nitrate) Ortho Dermatological ... 1947

Trichophyton schoenleini infections
Fulvicin P/G Tablets (Griseofulvin) Schering ... 2499
Fulvicin P/G 165 & 330 Tablets (Griseofulvin) Schering ... 2500
Grifulvin V (griseofulvin tablets) Microsize (griseofulvin oral suspension) Microsize (Griseofulvin) Ortho Dermatological ... 1944
Gris-PEG Tablets, 125 mg & 250 mg (Griseofulvin) Allergan ... 476

Trichophyton sulfureum infections
Fulvicin P/G Tablets (Griseofulvin) Schering ... 2499
Fulvicin P/G 165 & 330 Tablets (Griseofulvin) Schering ... 2500
Grifulvin V (griseofulvin tablets) Microsize (griseofulvin oral suspension) Microsize (Griseofulvin) Ortho Dermatological ... 1944
Gris-PEG Tablets, 125 mg & 250 mg (Griseofulvin) Allergan ... 476

Trichophyton tonsurans infections
Fulvicin P/G Tablets (Griseofulvin) Schering ... 2499
Fulvicin P/G 165 & 330 Tablets (Griseofulvin) Schering ... 2500
Grifulvin V (griseofulvin tablets) Microsize (griseofulvin oral

suspension) Microsize (Griseofulvin) Ortho Dermatological ... 1944
Gris-PEG Tablets, 125 mg & 250 mg (Griseofulvin) Allergan ... 476
Naftin Gel 1% (Naftifine Hydrochloride) Allergan ... 477
Spectazole (econazole nitrate 1%) Cream (Econazole Nitrate) Ortho Dermatological ... 1947

Trichophyton verrucosum infections
Fulvicin P/G Tablets (Griseofulvin) Schering ... 2499
Fulvicin P/G 165 & 330 Tablets (Griseofulvin) Schering ... 2500
Grifulvin V (griseofulvin tablets) Microsize (griseofulvin oral suspension) Microsize (Griseofulvin) Ortho Dermatological ... 1944
Gris-PEG Tablets, 125 mg & 250 mg (Griseofulvin) Allergan ... 476

Trichuris trichiura infections
Vermox Chewable Tablets (Mebendazole) Janssen ... 1357

Trichuriasis, as secondary therapy
Mintezol (Thiabendazole) Merck & Co., Inc. ... 1747

Triglyceride levels, elevated
(see under Hypertriglyceridemia, adjunct to diet)

Trigonitis
Urised Tablets (Atropine Sulfate, Hyoscyamine, Methenamine, Phenyl Salicylate) PolyMedica ... 2123

Tuberculin-sensitivity, detection of
PPD Tine Test (Tuberculin, Purified Protein Derivative, Multiple Puncture Device) Lederle ... 2993
Tuberculin, Old, Tine Test (Tuberculin, Old) Lederle ... 2994

Tuberculosis, diagnostic aid in
Tubersol (Tuberculin Purified Protein Derivative (Mantoux)) (Tuberculin, Purified Protein Derivative For Mantoux Test) Connaught ... 2988

Tuberculosis meningitis, adjunctive therapy in
(see under Meningitis, tuberculous)

Tuberculosis, pulmonary
Capastat Sulfate Injection (Capreomycin Sulfate) Dura ... 968
Myambutol Tablets (Ethambutol Hydrochloride) Lederle ... 1432
Rifadin (Rifampin) Hoechst Marion Roussel ... 1276
Rifamate Capsules (Rifampin, Isoniazid) Hoechst Marion Roussel ... 1278
Rifater (Rifampin, Isoniazid, Pyrazinamide) Hoechst Marion Roussel ... 1280
Rimactane Capsules (Rifampin) CibaGeneva ... 865
Seromycin Capsules (Cycloserine) Dura ... 975
Streptomycin Sulfate Injection (Streptomycin Sulfate) Pfizer Inc ... 2031

Tuberculosis, pulmonary, disseminated
Celestone Soluspan Suspension (Betamethasone Sodium Phosphate, Betamethasone Acetate) Schering ... 2484
Cortone Acetate Sterile Suspension (Cortisone Acetate) Merck & Co., Inc. ... 1663
Cortone Acetate Tablets (Cortisone Acetate) Merck & Co., Inc. ... 1664
Decadron Elixir (Dexamethasone) Merck & Co., Inc. ... 1676
Decadron Phosphate Injection (Dexamethasone Sodium Phosphate) Merck & Co., Inc. ... 1680
Decadron Tablets (Dexamethasone) Merck & Co., Inc. ... 1678
Hydeltrasol Injection, Sterile (Prednisolone Sodium Phosphate) Merck & Co., Inc. ... 1708

Tuberculosis Indications Index 1584

Hydrocortone Phosphate Injection, Sterile (Hydrocortisone Sodium Phosphate) Merck & Co., Inc. 1713
Hydrocortone Tablets (Hydrocortisone) Merck & Co., Inc. 1715
Pediapred Oral Solution (Prednisolone Sodium Phosphate) Medeva 1618
Prelone Syrup (Prednisolone) Muro 1834

Tuberculosis, pulmonary, fulminating
Celestone Soluspan Suspension (Betamethasone Sodium Phosphate, Betamethasone Acetate) Schering 2484
Cortone Acetate Sterile Suspension (Cortisone Acetate) Merck & Co., Inc. 1663
Cortone Acetate Tablets (Cortisone Acetate) Merck & Co., Inc. 1664
Decadron Elixir (Dexamethasone) Merck & Co., Inc. 1676
Decadron Phosphate Injection (Dexamethasone Sodium Phosphate) Merck & Co., Inc. 1680
Decadron Tablets (Dexamethasone) Merck & Co., Inc. 1678
Hydeltrasol Injection, Sterile (Prednisolone Sodium Phosphate) Merck & Co., Inc. 1708
Hydrocortone Phosphate Injection, Sterile (Hydrocortisone Sodium Phosphate) Merck & Co., Inc. 1713
Hydrocortone Tablets (Hydrocortisone) Merck & Co., Inc. 1715
Pediapred Oral Solution (Prednisolone Sodium Phosphate) Medeva 1618
Prelone Syrup (Prednisolone) Muro 1834

Tuberculosis, pulmonary, prophylaxis of
TICE BCG, USP (BCG Vaccine) Organon 1881

Tuberculosis, treatment
Myambutol Tablets (Ethambutol Hydrochloride) Lederle 1432
Nydrazid Injection (Isoniazid) Apothecon 509
Pyrazinamide Tablets (Pyrazinamide) Lederle 1442
Rifadin (Rifampin) Hoechst Marion Roussel 1276
Rifamate Capsules (Rifampin, Isoniazid) Hoechst Marion Roussel 1278
Rimactane Capsules (Rifampin) CibaGeneva 865
Seromycin Capsules (Cycloserine) Dura 975
Streptomycin Sulfate Injection (Streptomycin Sulfate) Pfizer Inc 2031
Trecator-SC Tablets (Ethionamide) Wyeth-Ayerst 2919

Tuberculosis, treatment adjunct
PASER Granules (Aminosalicylic Acid) Jacobus 1333
Pyrazinamide Tablets (Pyrazinamide) Lederle 1442

Tularemia
DYNACIN Capsules (Minocycline Hydrochloride) Medicis 1627
Minocin Oral Suspension (Minocycline Hydrochloride) Lederle 1431
Minocin Pellet-Filled Capsules (Minocycline Hydrochloride) Lederle 1429
Monodox Capsules (Doxycycline Monohydrate) Oclassen 1858
Vibramycin Hyclate Capsules (Doxycycline Hyclate) Pfizer Inc.... 2038

Tumors, brain, metastatic
CeeNU Capsules (Lomustine (CCNU)) Bristol-Myers Squibb Oncology/Immunology 699

Tumors, brain, metastatic, palliative therapy in
BiCNU (Carmustine (BCNU)) Bristol-Myers Squibb Oncology/Immunology 696

Tumors, brain, palliative therapy in
BiCNU (Carmustine (BCNU)) Bristol-Myers Squibb Oncology/Immunology 696

Tumors, brain, primary
CeeNU Capsules (Lomustine (CCNU)) Bristol-Myers Squibb Oncology/Immunology 699

Tumors, carcinoid, symptomatic relief of
Sandostatin Injection (Octreotide Acetate) Sandoz Pharmaceuticals 2421

Typhus fever
Achromycin V Capsules (Tetracycline Hydrochloride) Lederle 1417
Declomycin Tablets (Demeclocycline Hydrochloride) Lederle 1421
Doryx Capsules (Doxycycline Hyclate) Parke-Davis 1970
DYNACIN Capsules (Minocycline Hydrochloride) Medicis 1627
Minocin Intravenous (Minocycline Hydrochloride) Lederle 1428
Minocin Oral Suspension (Minocycline Hydrochloride) Lederle 1431
Minocin Pellet-Filled Capsules (Minocycline Hydrochloride) Lederle 1429
Monodox Capsules (Doxycycline Monohydrate) Oclassen 1858
Terramycin Intramuscular Solution (Oxytetracycline) Pfizer Inc 2034
Vibramycin (Doxycycline Calcium) Pfizer Inc 2038
Vibramycin Hyclate Intravenous (Doxycycline Hyclate) Pfizer Inc.... 2040
Vibramycin (Doxycycline Monohydrate) Pfizer Inc 2038

Typhus group infection
Achromycin V Capsules (Tetracycline Hydrochloride) Lederle 1417
Declomycin Tablets (Demeclocycline Hydrochloride) Lederle 1421
Doryx Capsules (Doxycycline Hyclate) Parke-Davis 1970
DYNACIN Capsules (Minocycline Hydrochloride) Medicis 1627
Minocin Intravenous (Minocycline Hydrochloride) Lederle 1428
Minocin Oral Suspension (Minocycline Hydrochloride) Lederle 1431
Minocin Pellet-Filled Capsules (Minocycline Hydrochloride) Lederle 1429
Monodox Capsules (Doxycycline Monohydrate) Oclassen 1858
Terramycin Intramuscular Solution (Oxytetracycline) Pfizer Inc 2034
Vibramycin Hyclate Capsules (Doxycycline Hyclate) Pfizer Inc.... 2038
Vibramycin Hyclate Intravenous (Doxycycline Hyclate) Pfizer Inc.... 2040

U

Ulcerative colitis (see under Colitis, ulcerative, systemic therapy for)

Ulcers, decubitus, adjunctive therapy in
Chloresium (Chlorophyllin Copper Complex) Rystan 2371
Granulex (Trypsin, Balsam Peru, Castor Oil) Dow Hickam 940
Panafil Ointment (Papain, Chlorophyllin Copper Complex, Urea) Rystan 2372
Panafil-White Ointment (Papain, Urea) Rystan 2372

Ulcers, decubitus, reduction of possible occurrence of
Betadine Solution (Povidone Iodine) Purdue Frederick 2145

Ulcers, dermal
Primaxin I.M. (Cilastatin Sodium, Imipenem) Merck & Co., Inc. 1770

Ulcers, diabetic, adjunctive therapy in
Accuzyme Ointment (Papain, Urea) Healthpoint 1236
Panafil Ointment (Papain, Chlorophyllin Copper Complex, Urea) Rystan 2372
Panafil-White Ointment (Papain, Urea) Rystan 2372

Ulcers, varicose, adjunctive therapy in
Accuzyme Ointment (Papain, Urea) Healthpoint 1236
Panafil Ointment (Papain, Chlorophyllin Copper Complex, Urea) Rystan 2372
Panafil-White Ointment (Papain, Urea) Rystan 2372

Immunization, meningococcal
Menomune-A/C/Y/W-135 (Meningococcal Polysaccharide Vaccine) Connaught 906

Uncinariasis, as secondary therapy
Mintezol (Thiabendazole) Merck & Co., Inc. 1747

Ureaplasma urealyticum urethritis
E.E.S. (Erythromycin Ethylsuccinate) Abbott 427
EryPed (Erythromycin Ethylsuccinate) Abbott 425
Minocin Oral Suspension (Minocycline Hydrochloride) Lederle 1431

Ureaplasma urealyticum urethritis, nongonococcal
Doryx Capsules (Doxycycline Hyclate) Parke-Davis 1970
DYNACIN Capsules (Minocycline Hydrochloride) Medicis 1627
ERYC (Erythromycin) Parke-Davis .. 1972
Minocin Oral Suspension (Minocycline Hydrochloride) Lederle 1431
Minocin Pellet-Filled Capsules (Minocycline Hydrochloride) Lederle 1429
Monodox Capsules (Doxycycline Monohydrate) Oclassen 1858
PCE Dispertab Tablets (Erythromycin) Abbott 453
Vibramycin (Doxycycline Calcium) Pfizer Inc 2038

Urethritis
E.E.S. (Erythromycin Ethylsuccinate) Abbott 427
EryPed (Erythromycin Ethylsuccinate) Abbott 425
PCE Dispertab Tablets (Erythromycin) Abbott 453
Urised Tablets (Atropine Sulfate, Hyoscyamine, Methenamine, Phenyl Salicylate) PolyMedica 2123
Zithromax (Azithromycin) Pfizer Inc 2043
Zithromax Tablets (Azithromycin) Pfizer Inc 2046

Urethritis, atrophic
Premarin Tablets (Estrogens, Conjugated) Wyeth-Ayerst 2896

Urethritis, Chlamydia trachomatis, nongonococcal
Doryx Capsules (Doxycycline Hyclate) Parke-Davis 1970
Floxin I.V. (Ofloxacin) McNeil Pharmaceutical 1580
Monodox Capsules (Doxycycline Monohydrate) Oclassen 1858
Vibramycin (Doxycycline Calcium) Pfizer Inc 2038
Zithromax (Azithromycin) Pfizer Inc 2043
Zithromax Tablets (Azithromycin) Pfizer Inc 2046

Urethritis, frequency and incontinence, symptomatic relief of
Urispas Tablets (Flavoxate Hydrochloride) SmithKline Beecham Pharmaceuticals 2710

Urethritis, "lacking substantial evidence of effectiveness" in
Urobiotic-250 Capsules (Oxytetracycline Hydrochloride, Sulfamethizole, Phenazopyridine Hydrochloride) Pfizer Inc 2038

Urethritis, uncomplicated gonococcal
DYNACIN Capsules (Minocycline Hydrochloride) Medicis 1627
Minocin Oral Suspension (Minocycline Hydrochloride) Lederle 1431
Minocin Pellet-Filled Capsules (Minocycline Hydrochloride) Lederle 1429
Pipracil (Piperacillin Sodium) Lederle 1435

Urethrocystitis, frequency and incontinence, symptomatic relief of
Urispas Tablets (Flavoxate Hydrochloride) SmithKline Beecham Pharmaceuticals 2710

Urethrotrigonitis, frequency and incontinence, symptomatic relief of
Urispas Tablets (Flavoxate Hydrochloride) SmithKline Beecham Pharmaceuticals 2710

Uric acid lithiasis (see under Urolithiasis, management of)

Urinary bladder with retention, neurogenic atony of
Urecholine (Bethanechol Chloride) Merck & Co., Inc. 1804

Urinary bladder, reflex neurogenic, symptomatic relief of
Ditropan (Oxybutynin Chloride) Hoechst Marion Roussel 1267

Urinary frequency, symptomatic relief of
Prodium (Phenazopyridine Hydrochloride) Breckenridge 695
Pyridium (Phenazopyridine Hydrochloride) Parke-Davis 1985

Urinary incontinence, adjunct
Hyland's EnurAid Tablets (Homeopathic Medications) Standard Homeopathic .... ▣ 789

Urinary retention, acute postoperative
Prostigmin Injectable (Neostigmine Methylsulfate) ICN 1305
Urecholine (Bethanechol Chloride) Merck & Co., Inc. 1804

Urinary retention, postpartum nonobstructive
Urecholine (Bethanechol Chloride) Merck & Co., Inc. 1804

Urinary tract pain, relief of (see under Pain, urinary tract)

Urinary tract, burning, symptomatic relief of
Prodium (Phenazopyridine Hydrochloride) Breckenridge 695
Pyridium (Phenazopyridine Hydrochloride) Parke-Davis 1985

Urinary tract, hypermotility, control of symptoms
Levsin/Levsinex/Levbid (Hyoscyamine Sulfate) Schwarz 2549

Urinary tract, lower, hypermotility disorders
Cystospaz (Hyoscyamine) PolyMedica 2123
Urised Tablets (Atropine Sulfate, Hyoscyamine, Methenamine, Phenyl Salicylate) PolyMedica 2123

Urinary urgency, symptomatic relief of
Prodium (Phenazopyridine Hydrochloride) Breckenridge 695
Pyridium (Phenazopyridine Hydrochloride) Parke-Davis 1985
Urispas Tablets (Flavoxate Hydrochloride) SmithKline Beecham Pharmaceuticals 2710

Urinary voiding, irritable, symptomatic relief of
Ditropan (Oxybutynin Chloride) Hoechst Marion Roussel 1267

Urine, acidification of
K-Phos Original Formula 'Sodium Free' Tablets (Potassium Acid Phosphate) Beach 633

Urine, alkalinization of
Bicitra (Sodium Citrate, Citric Acid) Baker Norton ... 573
Polycitra Syrup (Potassium Citrate, Sodium Citrate, Citric Acid) Baker Norton ... 574
Polycitra-K Crystals (Potassium Citrate, Citric Acid) Baker Norton ... 574
Polycitra-K Oral Solution (Potassium Citrate, Citric Acid) Baker Norton ... 575
Polycitra-LC (Potassium Citrate, Citric Acid, Sodium Citrate) Baker Norton ... 574

Urticaria, chronic
(see also under Urticarial manifestations, relief of)
Atarax Tablets & Syrup (Hydroxyzine Hydrochloride) Pfizer Inc ... 1992
Claritin Tablets (Loratadine) Schering ... 2485
Hismanal Tablets (Astemizole) Janssen ... 1341
Vistaril (Hydroxyzine Pamoate) Pfizer Inc ... 2042
Zyrtec Tablets (Cetirizine Hydrochloride) Pfizer Inc ... 2053

Urolithiasis, management of
Urocit-K Tablets (Potassium Citrate) Mission ... 1828

Urticaria, cold
Periactin (Cyproheptadine Hydrochloride) Merck & Co., Inc. 1767

Urticarial manifestations, relief of
(see also under Urticaria, chronic)
Extendryl (Chlorpheniramine Maleate, Methscopolamine Nitrate, Phenylephrine Hydrochloride) Fleming ... 1003
PBZ Tablets (Tripelennamine Hydrochloride) CibaGeneva ... 863
PBZ-SR Tablets (Tripelennamine Hydrochloride) CibaGeneva ... 862
Periactin (Cyproheptadine Hydrochloride) Merck & Co., Inc. 1767
Phenergan Suppositories (Promethazine Hydrochloride) Wyeth-Ayerst ... 2882
Phenergan Syrup (Promethazine Hydrochloride) Wyeth-Ayerst ... 2881
Phenergan Tablets (Promethazine Hydrochloride) Wyeth-Ayerst ... 2882
Tavist Syrup (Clemastine Fumarate) Sandoz Pharmaceuticals ... 2426
Tavist Tablets (Clemastine Fumarate) Sandoz Pharmaceuticals ... 2427
Vistaril Intramuscular Solution (Hydroxyzine Hydrochloride) Pfizer Inc ... 2042

Urticarial transfusion reactions
Celestone Soluspan Suspension (Betamethasone Sodium Phosphate, Betamethasone Acetate) Schering ... 2484
Cortone Acetate Sterile Suspension (Cortisone Acetate) Merck & Co., Inc. ... 1663
Dalalone D.P. Injectable (Dexamethasone Acetate) Forest ... 1009
Decadron Phosphate Injection (Dexamethasone Sodium Phosphate) Merck & Co., Inc. ... 1680
Decadron-LA Sterile Suspension (Dexamethasone Acetate) Merck & Co., Inc. ... 1687
Hydeltrasol Injection, Sterile (Prednisolone Sodium Phosphate) Merck & Co., Inc. ... 1708
Hydrocortone Phosphate Injection, Sterile (Hydrocortisone Sodium Phosphate) Merck & Co., Inc. ... 1713

Uterine atony, postpartum
Methergine (Methylergonovine Maleate) Sandoz Pharmaceuticals ... 2401

Uterine bleeding, abnormal
Amen Tablets (Medroxyprogesterone Acetate) Carnrick ... 785
Aygestin Tablets (Norethindrone Acetate) ESI Lederle ... 990
Climara Transdermal System (Estradiol) Berlex ... 640

Cycrin Tablets (Medroxyprogesterone Acetate) ESI Lederle ... 991
Premarin Intravenous (Estrogens, Conjugated) Wyeth-Ayerst ... 2893
Provera Tablets (Medroxyprogesterone Acetate) Pharmacia & Upjohn ... 2110

Uterine cavity, hysteroscopic aid in
Hyskon Hysteroscopy Fluid (Dextran 70) Medisan ... 1633

Uterine contents, evacuation of
Prostin E2 Suppository (Dinoprostone) Pharmacia & Upjohn ... 2109

Uveitis, chronic anterior, steroid-responsive
AK-CIDE (Prednisolone Acetate, Sulfacetamide Sodium) Akorn ... ⊚ 203
AK-CIDE Ointment (Prednisolone Acetate, Sulfacetamide Sodium) Akorn ... ⊚ 203
AK-Trol Ointment & Suspension (Dexamethasone, Neomycin Sulfate, Polymyxin B Sulfate) Akorn ... ⊚ 205
Blephamide Liquifilm Sterile Ophthalmic Suspension (Prednisolone Acetate, Sulfacetamide Sodium) Allergan ... 472
Blephamide Ointment (Sulfacetamide Sodium, Prednisolone Acetate) Allergan ... ⊚ 234
Cortisporin Ophthalmic Ointment Sterile (Polymyxin B Sulfate, Bacitracin Zinc, Neomycin Sulfate, Hydrocortisone) Glaxo Wellcome ... 1074
Cortisporin Ophthalmic Suspension Sterile (Hydrocortisone, Polymyxin B Sulfate, Neomycin Sulfate) Glaxo Wellcome ... 1075
FML-S Liquifilm (Sulfacetamide Sodium, Fluorometholone) Allergan ... ⊚ 240
Maxitrol Ophthalmic Ointment and Suspension (Dexamethasone, Neomycin Sulfate, Polymyxin B Sulfate) Alcon Laboratories ... ⊚ 222
NeoDecadron Sterile Ophthalmic Ointment (Neomycin Sulfate, Dexamethasone Sodium Phosphate) Merck & Co., Inc. ... 1755
NeoDecadron Sterile Ophthalmic Solution (Neomycin Sulfate, Dexamethasone Sodium Phosphate) Merck & Co., Inc. ... 1756
Poly-Pred Liquifilm (Neomycin Sulfate, Polymyxin B Sulfate, Prednisolone Acetate) Allergan .. ⊚ 246
Pred-G Liquifilm Sterile Ophthalmic Suspension (Gentamicin Sulfate, Prednisolone Acetate) Allergan ... ⊚ 248
Pred-G S.O.P. Sterile Ophthalmic Ointment (Gentamicin Sulfate, Prednisolone Acetate) Allergan .. ⊚ 249
Terra-Cortril Ophthalmic Suspension (Oxytetracycline Hydrochloride, Hydrocortisone Acetate) Pfizer Inc ... 2033
TobraDex Ophthalmic Suspension and Ointment (Dexamethasone, Tobramycin) Alcon Laboratories .. 469
Vexol 1% Ophthalmic Suspension (Rimexolone) Alcon Laboratories ... ⊚ 227

Uveitis, diffuse posterior
Celestone Soluspan Suspension (Betamethasone Sodium Phosphate, Betamethasone Acetate) Schering ... 2484
Cortone Acetate Sterile Suspension (Cortisone Acetate) Merck & Co., Inc. ... 1663
Cortone Acetate Tablets (Cortisone Acetate) Merck & Co., Inc. ... 1664
Dalalone D.P. Injectable (Dexamethasone Acetate) Forest ... 1009
Decadron Elixir (Dexamethasone) Merck & Co., Inc. ... 1676
Decadron Phosphate Injection (Dexamethasone Sodium Phosphate) Merck & Co., Inc. ... 1680
Decadron Tablets (Dexamethasone) Merck & Co., Inc. ... 1678

Decadron-LA Sterile Suspension (Dexamethasone Acetate) Merck & Co., Inc. ... 1687
Hydeltrasol Injection, Sterile (Prednisolone Sodium Phosphate) Merck & Co., Inc. ... 1708
Hydrocortone Phosphate Injection, Sterile (Hydrocortisone Sodium Phosphate) Merck & Co., Inc. ... 1713
Hydrocortone Tablets (Hydrocortisone) Merck & Co., Inc. ... 1715
Pediapred Oral Solution (Prednisolone Sodium Phosphate) Medeva 1618
Prelone Syrup (Prednisolone) Muro 1834

V

Vagina, cleansing of
Hemorid For Women Cleanser (Cleanser) Thompson Medical.... ⊞ 797
Massengill Disposable Douche (Vinegar) SmithKline Beecham ... 2627
Massengill Feminine Cleansing Wash (Cleanser) SmithKline Beecham ... 2628
Massengill (Povidone Iodine) SmithKline Beecham ... 2627

Vaginal acidity, restoration of, adjunctive therapy for
Aci-Jel Therapeutic Vaginal Jelly (Acetic Acid, Oxyquinoline Sulfate) Ortho Pharmaceutical ... 1903

Vaginal and anogenital areas, external, cleansing of
Betadine Medicated Douche (Povidone Iodine) Purdue Frederick 2144
Betadine Solution (Povidone Iodine) Purdue Frederick ... 2145
Massengill Fragrance-Free Soft Cloth Towelette & Baby Powder Scent (Lactic Acid, Potassium Sorbate, Sodium Lactate) SmithKline Beecham ... 2628
Tucks Pads (Witch Hazel) Warner Wellcome ... ⊞ 830

Vaginal atrophy
Premphase (Estrogens, Conjugated, Medroxyprogesterone Acetate) Wyeth-Ayerst ... 2900
Prempro (Estrogens, Conjugated, Medroxyprogesterone Acetate) Wyeth-Ayerst ... 2905
Vivelle Transdermal System (Estradiol) CibaGeneva ... 880

Vaginal moisture, replenishing of
Replens Vaginal Moisturizer (Glycerin, Lubricant) Warner Wellcome ... ⊞ 823

Vaginosis, bacterial
Cleocin Vaginal Cream (Clindamycin Phosphate) Pharmacia & Upjohn ... 2070
MetroGel-Vaginal (Metronidazole) Curatek ... 917
Sultrin (Sulfathiazole, Sulfacetamide, Sulfabenzamide) Ortho Pharmaceutical ... 1941

Vaginitis
(see under Vaginosis, bacterial)

Vaginitis, atrophic
Climara Transdermal System (Estradiol) Berlex ... 640
Estrace Cream and Tablets (Estradiol) Bristol-Myers Squibb .. 751
Estraderm Transdermal System (Estradiol) CibaGeneva ... 842
ESTRATAB Tablets (0.3, 0.625, 1.25, 2.5 mg) (Estrogens, Esterified) Solvay ... 2715
Estring Vaginal Ring (Estradiol) Pharmacia & Upjohn ... 2086
Menest Tablets (Estrogens, Esterified) SmithKline Beecham Pharmaceuticals ... 2671
Ogen Tablets (Estropipate) Pharmacia & Upjohn ... 2103
Ogen Vaginal Cream (Estropipate) Pharmacia & Upjohn ... 2106
Ortho Dienestrol Cream (Dienestrol) Ortho Pharmaceutical ... 1922
Ortho-Est (Estropipate) Ortho Pharmaceutical ... 1925
Premarin Tablets (Estrogens, Conjugated) Wyeth-Ayerst ... 2896

Premarin Vaginal Cream (Estrogens, Conjugated) Wyeth-Ayerst .. 2898

Vaginitis, symptomatic relief of irritation and itching
Betadine Medicated Douche (Povidone Iodine) Purdue Frederick 2144
Betadine Medicated Gel (Povidone Iodine) Purdue Frederick.............. 2144
Betadine Pre-Mixed Medicated Disposable Douche (Povidone Iodine) Purdue Frederick........... 2144
Massengill Medicated Disposable Douche (Povidone Iodine) SmithKline Beecham ... 2628
Massengill Medicated Soft Cloth Towelettes (Hydrocortisone) SmithKline Beecham ... 2628

Varicella, acute, treatment of
Zovirax (Acyclovir) Glaxo Wellcome 1187

Varicose veins
(see under Veins, varicose, obliteration of)

Vascular failure
Neo-Synephrine Hydrochloride 1% Carpuject (Phenylephrine Hydrochloride) Sanofi Winthrop .. 2455
Neo-Synephrine Hydrochloride 1% Injection (Phenylephrine Hydrochloride) Sanofi Winthrop .. 2455

Vasopressin-sensitive diabetes insipidus
(see under Diabetes insipidus)

Veins, varicose, obliteration of
Scleromate Injection (Morrhuate Sodium) Glenwood-Palisades 1234
Sotradecol (Sodium Tetradecyl Sulfate Injection) (Sodium Tetradecyl Sulfate) Elkins-Sinn ... 987

Ventilation, mechanical, facilitation of
Anectine (Succinylcholine Chloride) Glaxo Wellcome ... 1062
Mivacron (Mivacurium Chloride) Glaxo Wellcome ... 1125
Nimbex Injection (Cisatracurium Besylate) Glaxo Wellcome ... 1131
Norcuron for Injection (Vecuronium Bromide) Organon ... 1875
Nuromax Injection (Doxacurium Chloride) Glaxo Wellcome ... 1136
Tracrium Injection (Atracurium Besylate) Glaxo Wellcome ... 1155
Zemuron Injection (Rocuronium Bromide) Organon ... 1885

Ventricular arrhythmias
(see under Arrhythmias, ventricular)

Ventricular dysfunction, left, asymptomatic
(see also under Myocardial infarction, post, left ventricular dysfunction)
Vasotec Tablets (Enalapril Maleate) Merck & Co., Inc. ... 1816

Ventricular extrasystoles, premature
Inderal (Propranolol Hydrochloride) Wyeth-Ayerst ... 2834

Ventricular fibrillation
Cordarone Intravenous (Amiodarone Hydrochloride) Wyeth-Ayerst ... 2821
Cordarone Tablets (Amiodarone Hydrochloride) Wyeth-Ayerst ... 2818

Ventricular tachycardia, sustained
(see under Tachycardia, ventricular, sustained)

Ventriculitis
(see also under Infections, central nervous system)
Claforan Sterile and Injection (Cefotaxime Sodium) Hoechst Marion Roussel ... 1259

Verrucae plantaris
(see under Warts, plantar, removal of)

(⊞ Described in PDR For Nonprescription Drugs)   (⊚ Described in PDR For Ophthalmology)

Verrucae vulgaris infection — Indications Index — 1586

Verrucae vulgaris infection
(see under Warts, common, removal of)

Vertigo, auditory
(see under Meniere's disease)

Vertigo, labyrinthine
(see under Meniere's disease)

Vertigo, "possibly" effective in
Antivert, Antivert/25 Tablets, & Antivert/50 Tablets (Meclizine Hydrochloride) Pfizer Inc ... 1992

Vibrio cholerae infections
Achromycin V Capsules (Tetracycline Hydrochloride) Lederle ... 1417
Declomycin Tablets (Demeclocycline Hydrochloride) Lederle ... 1421
Doryx Capsules (Doxycycline Hyclate) Parke-Davis ... 1970
DYNACIN Capsules (Minocycline Hydrochloride) Medicis ... 1627
Minocin Intravenous (Minocycline Hydrochloride) Lederle ... 1428
Minocin Oral Suspension (Minocycline Hydrochloride) Lederle ... 1431
Minocin Pellet-Filled Capsules (Minocycline Hydrochloride) Lederle ... 1429
Monodox Capsules (Doxycycline Monohydrate) Oclassen ... 1858
Terramycin Intramuscular Solution (Oxytetracycline) Pfizer Inc ... 2034
Vibramycin (Doxycycline Calcium) Pfizer Inc ... 2038
Vibramycin Hyclate Intravenous (Doxycycline Hyclate) Pfizer Inc ... 2040
Vibramycin (Doxycycline Monohydrate) Pfizer Inc ... 2038

Vibrio comma
(see under Vibrio cholerae infections)

Vibrio fetus infections
(see under Campylobacter fetus infections)

Vincent's gingivitis
(see under Fusospirochetosis)

Vincent's infection
(see under Fusospirochetosis)

Vincent's pharyngitis
(see under Fusospirochetosis)

Vitamin and mineral, multiple, deficiency of
Akorn AntiOxidants (Vitamins with Minerals) Akorn ... ◉ 206
Berocca Plus Tablets (Vitamins with Minerals) Roche Pharmaceuticals ... 2259
Bugs Bunny Complete Children's Chewable Vitamins + Minerals with Iron and Calcium (Sugar Free) (Vitamins with Minerals) Bayer Consumer ... ■ 620
Bugs Bunny With Extra C Children's Chewable Vitamins (Sugar Free) (Vitamins with Minerals) Bayer Consumer ... ■ 621
Bugs Bunny Plus Iron Children's Chewable Vitamins (Sugar Free) (Vitamins with Iron) Bayer Consumer ... ■ 619
Centrum (Vitamins with Minerals) Lederle Consumer ... ■ 682
Centrum, Jr. (Children's Chewable) + Extra C (Vitamins with Minerals) Lederle Consumer ... ■ 682
Centrum, Jr. (Children's Chewable) + Extra Calcium (Vitamins with Minerals) Lederle Consumer ... ■ 682
Centrum, Jr. (Children's Chewable) + Iron (Vitamins with Minerals) Lederle Consumer ... ■ 683
Centrum Silver (Vitamins with Minerals) Lederle Consumer ... ■ 683
Complete for Men (Vitamins with Minerals) AML Laboratories ... ■ 603
Complete for Women (Vitamins with Minerals) AML Laboratories ... ■ 603
Common Sense Complete (Vitamins with Minerals) AML Laboratories ... ■ 604
Common Sense Complete with Extra Calcium and Iron (Vitamins with Minerals) AML Laboratories ... ■ 604
Natural MD Complete Rx (Vitamins with Minerals) AML Laboratories ... ■ 605
DIA-Reliever Tablets (Nutritional Supplement) AC Laboratory ... 461
DiabeVite Tablets (Vitamins with Minerals) R&D ... 2168
Flintstones Children's Chewable Vitamins (Vitamins with Minerals) Bayer Consumer ... ■ 619
Flintstones Children's Chewable Vitamins Plus Extra C (Vitamins with Minerals) Bayer Consumer ■ 621
Flintstones Children's Chewable Vitamins Plus Iron (Vitamins with Iron) Bayer Consumer ... ■ 619
Flintstones Complete With Calcium, Iron & Minerals Children's Chewable Vitamins (Vitamins with Minerals) Bayer Consumer ... ■ 620
Flintstones Plus Calcium Children's Chewable Vitamins (Vitamins with Minerals) Bayer Consumer ... ■ 620
Gerimed Tablets (Vitamins with Minerals) Fielding ... 1000
Heplive Capsules (Vitamins with Minerals) AC Laboratory ... 461
MDR Fitness Tabs for Men and Women (Vitamins with Minerals) MDR Fitness ... 1544
May-Vita Elixir (Vitamins with Minerals) Merz ... 1826
Megadose (Vitamins with Minerals) Arco ... 513
Nestabs FA Tablets (Vitamins with Minerals) Fielding ... 1000
Ocuvite Vitamin and Mineral Supplement (Vitamins with Minerals) Storz Ophthalmics ... ◉ 322
Ocuvite Extra Vitamin and Mineral Supplement (Vitamins with Minerals) Storz Ophthalmics ... ◉ 322
One-A-Day Essential Vitamins with Beta Carotene (Vitamins with Minerals) Bayer Consumer ■ 625
One-A-Day Maximum (Vitamins with Minerals) Bayer Consumer ■ 626
One-A-Day Women's (Vitamins with Minerals) Bayer Consumer ■ 626
One-A-Day 55 Plus (Vitamins with Minerals) Bayer Consumer ■ 624
Phyto-Vite (Vitamins with Minerals) Wellness International ■ 835
Rejuvex (Vitamins with Minerals) Sunsource ... ■ 791
Stress Gum (Vitamins with Minerals) AML Laboratories ... ■ 606
Stresstabs (Vitamin B Complex With Vitamin C) Lederle Consumer ... ■ 685
Stresstabs + Iron (Vitamins with Iron) Lederle Consumer ... ■ 685
Sunkist Children's Chewable Multivitamins - Complete (Vitamins with Minerals) Ciba Self-Medication ... ■ 665
Sunkist Vitamin C (Vitamin C) Ciba Self-Medication ... ■ 666
Theragran-M Tablets (Vitamins with Minerals) Mead Johnson Nutritionals ... ■ 709
Vicon Forte Capsules (Vitamins with Minerals) UCB ... 2760

Vitamin A, deficiency of
Aquasol A Vitamin A Capsules, USP (Vitamin A) Astra ... 525
Aquasol A Parenteral (Vitamin A) Astra ... 526

Vitamin and mineral deficiency due to burns
Berocca Plus Tablets (Vitamins with Minerals) Roche Pharmaceuticals ... 2259

Vitamin B complex and C, deficiency of
Berocca Tablets (Vitamin B Complex With Vitamin C) Roche Pharmaceuticals ... 2259
Cefol Filmtab (Vitamin B Complex With Vitamin C, Vitamin E, Folic Acid) Abbott ... 415
Iberet-Liquid (Vitamin B Complex With Vitamin C, Ferrous Sulfate) Abbott ... 438
Nephrocaps (Vitamins, Multiple) Fleming ... 1004

Vitamin B complex, C and iron, deficiency of
Iberet Tablets (Vitamin B Complex With Vitamin C, Ferrous Sulfate) Abbott ... 437
Iberet-500 Liquid (Vitamin B Complex With Vitamin C, Ferrous Sulfate) Abbott ... 438
Iberet-Folic-500 Filmtab (Vitamin B Complex With Vitamin C, Ferrous Sulfate) Abbott ... 433

Vitamin B complex, deficiency of
Eldertonic (Vitamins with Minerals) Merz ... 1826
Mega-B (Vitamin B Complex) Arco ... 513

Vitamin C, deficiency of
Ester-C Mineral Ascorbates Powder (Calcium Ascorbate) Inter-Cal ... ■ 673
Halls Vitamin C Drops (Vitamin C) Warner-Lambert ... ■ 807

Vitamin deficiency, postpartum
Materna Tablets (Vitamins, Prenatal) Lederle ... 1427
Natalins Rx Tablets (Vitamins, Prenatal) Mead Johnson Nutritionals ... 1599
Niferex-PN Tablets (Vitamins with Iron) Central ... 811
Precare Prenatal Multi-Vitamin/Mineral (Vitamins with Minerals) UCB ... 2753
Advanced Formula ZENATE Tablets (Vitamins with Minerals) Solvay ... 2728

Vitamin deficiency, prenatal
Berocca Plus Tablets (Vitamins with Minerals) Roche Pharmaceuticals ... 2259
Materna Tablets (Vitamins, Prenatal) Lederle ... 1427
Natalins Rx Tablets (Vitamins, Prenatal) Mead Johnson Nutritionals ... 1599
Niferex-PN Tablets (Vitamins with Iron) Central ... 811
Precare Prenatal Multi-Vitamin/Mineral (Vitamins with Minerals) UCB ... 2753
Advanced Formula ZENATE Tablets (Vitamins with Minerals) Solvay ... 2728

Vitamin E, deficiency of
Nutr-E-Sol (Vitamin E) Advanced Nutritional ... 461
Unique E Vitamin E Capsules (Vitamin E) A.C. Grace ... 1236

Vitamin, multiple, deficiency of
Natural MD BASIC Rx (Vitamins, Multiple) AML Laboratories ... ■ 602
Cefol Filmtab (Vitamin B Complex With Vitamin C, Vitamin E, Folic Acid) Abbott ... 415
Fat Burning Factors (Vitamins, Multiple) AML Laboratories ... ■ 605
Healthy Heart (Vitamins, Multiple) Odyssey ... 1860
Hep-Forte Capsules (Vitamins with Minerals) Marlyn ... 1558
Nephro-Vite + Fe Tablets (Vitamins, Multiple, Ferrous Fumarate) R&D ... 2170
Nephro-Vite Rx Tablets (Vitamins with Minerals) R&D ... 2170
Pro-Hepatone Capsules (Vitamins with Minerals, Amino Acid Preparations) Marlyn ... 1558
Stresstabs + Zinc (Vitamins with Minerals) Lederle Consumer ... ■ 685
Sunkist Children's Chewable Multivitamins - Plus Extra C (Vitamins, Multiple) Ciba Self-Medication ... ■ 665
Sunkist Children's Chewable Multivitamins - Regular (Vitamins, Multiple) Ciba Self-Medication ... ■ 664
Theragran Tablets (Vitamin B Complex With Vitamin C, Vitamins with Minerals) Mead Johnson Nutritionals ... ■ 709

Vitamins and calcium deficiency
(see under Hypocalcemia with vitamin deficiency)

Vitamins and iron, deficiency of
Fero-Folic-500 Filmtab (Ferrous Sulfate, Folic Acid, Vitamin C) Abbott ... 433
Sunkist Children's Chewable Multivitamins - Plus Iron (Vitamins with Iron) Ciba Self-Medication ... ■ 665

Vitamins A, C and E and zinc deficiency
One-A-Day Antioxidant Plus (Vitamin A, Vitamin C, Vitamin E, Zinc Oxide) Bayer Consumer ... ■ 625

Vitamin C, E, beta carotene with selenium, deficiency of
ACES Antioxidant Soft Gels (Beta Carotene, Vitamin C, Vitamin E, Selenium) Carlson ... ■ 647

Vitamins, C, E, beta carotene with zinc, deficiency of
Protegra Antioxidant Vitamin & Mineral Supplement (Vitamin C, Vitamin E, Beta Carotene) Lederle Consumer ... ■ 685

Vitiligo
(see under Hypopigmentation, skin)

Vomiting
(see also under Motion sickness)
Tigan (Trimethobenzamide Hydrochloride) Roberts ... 2231
Torecan (Thiethylperazine Malate) Roxane ... 2367
Vistaril Intramuscular Solution (Hydroxyzine Hydrochloride) Pfizer Inc ... 2042

Vomiting, emetogenic, cancer chemotherapy-induced
Kytril Injection (Granisetron Hydrochloride) SmithKline Beecham Pharmaceuticals ... 2667
Kytril Tablets (Granisetron Hydrochloride) SmithKline Beecham Pharmaceuticals ... 2669
Marinol (Dronabinol) Capsules (Dronabinol) Roxane ... 2353
Reglan (Metoclopramide Hydrochloride) Robins ... 2243
Zofran Injection (Ondansetron Hydrochloride) Glaxo Wellcome Oncology/HIV ... 1227
Zofran Tablets (Ondansetron Hydrochloride) Glaxo Wellcome Oncology/HIV ... 1231

Vomiting, emetogenic, radiation therapy-induced
Zofran Tablets (Ondansetron Hydrochloride) Glaxo Wellcome Oncology/HIV ... 1231

Vomiting, postoperative
Emete-con Intramuscular/Intravenous (Benzquinamide Hydrochloride) Pfizer Inc ... 2007
Phenergan Injection (Promethazine Hydrochloride) Wyeth-Ayerst ... 2880
Phenergan Suppositories (Promethazine Hydrochloride) Wyeth-Ayerst ... 2882
Phenergan Syrup (Promethazine Hydrochloride) Wyeth-Ayerst ... 2881
Phenergan Tablets (Promethazine Hydrochloride) Wyeth-Ayerst ... 2882
Reglan (Metoclopramide Hydrochloride) Robins ... 2243
Vistaril Intramuscular Solution (Hydroxyzine Hydrochloride) Pfizer Inc ... 2042
Zofran Injection (Ondansetron Hydrochloride) Glaxo Wellcome Oncology/HIV ... 1227
Zofran Tablets (Ondansetron Hydrochloride) Glaxo Wellcome Oncology/HIV ... 1231

(■ Described in PDR For Nonprescription Drugs) (◉ Described in PDR For Ophthalmology)

Indications Index — Zygomycosis

Vomiting, postpartum, adjunctive therapy in
Vistaril Intramuscular Solution (Hydroxyzine Hydrochloride) Pfizer Inc 2042

Vomiting, severe, control of
Compazine (Prochlorperazine) SmithKline Beecham Pharmaceuticals 2644
Thorazine (Chlorpromazine Hydrochloride) SmithKline Beecham Pharmaceuticals 2701
Trilafon (Perphenazine) Schering 2532

Vulvae, kraurosis
Climara Transdermal System (Estradiol) Berlex 640
Estrace Cream and Tablets (Estradiol) Bristol-Myers Squibb .. 751
Estraderm Transdermal System (Estradiol) CibaGeneva 842
ESTRATAB Tablets (0.3, 0.625, 1.25, 2.5 mg) (Estrogens, Esterified) Solvay 2715
Estring Vaginal Ring (Estradiol) Pharmacia & Upjohn 2086
Menest Tablets (Estrogens, Esterified) SmithKline Beecham Pharmaceuticals 2671
Ogen Tablets (Estropipate) Pharmacia & Upjohn 2103
Ogen Vaginal Cream (Estropipate) Pharmacia & Upjohn 2106
Ortho Dienestrol Cream (Dienestrol) Ortho Pharmaceutical 1922
Ortho-Est (Estropipate) Ortho Pharmaceutical 1925
Premarin Vaginal Cream (Estrogens, Conjugated) Wyeth-Ayerst .. 2898

Vulvar atrophy
Premphase (Estrogens, Conjugated, Medroxyprogesterone Acetate) Wyeth-Ayerst 2900
Prempro (Estrogens, Conjugated, Medroxyprogesterone Acetate) Wyeth-Ayerst 2905
Vivelle Transdermal System (Estradiol) CibaGeneva 880

Vulvovaginal candidiasis
(see under Candidiasis, vaginal)

Vulvovaginitis
AVC (Sulfanilamide) Hoechst Marion Roussel 1245
Mycelex-G 500 mg Vaginal Tablets (Clotrimazole) Bayer Pharmaceutical 602

VIPomas diarrhea
(see under Diarrhea associated with vasoactive intestinal peptide tumors)

von Willebrand's disease, type 1
DDAVP Injection (Desmopressin Acetate) Rhone-Poulenc Rorer Pharmaceuticals 2178
DDAVP Injection 15 mcg/mL (Desmopressin Acetate) Rhone-Poulenc Rorer Pharmaceuticals 2179
Desmopressin Acetate Injection (Desmopressin Acetate) Ferring .. 996
Stimate, (desmopressin acetate) Nasal Spray, 1.5 mg/mL (Desmopressin Acetate) Centeon 806

W

Warts, common, removal of
DuoFilm Liquid Wart Remover (Salicylic Acid) Schering-Plough HealthCare 765
DuoFilm Patch Wart Remover (Salicylic Acid) Schering-Plough HealthCare 765
DuoPlant Gel Plantar Wart Remover (Salicylic Acid) Schering-Plough HealthCare 765
Occlusal-HP (Salicylic Acid) GenDerm 1041
Wart-Off Wart Remover (Salicylic Acid) Pfizer Consumer 720

Warts, genital
(see under Condylomata acuminata)

Warts, plantar, removal of
DuoFilm Liquid Wart Remover (Salicylic Acid) Schering-Plough HealthCare 765
DuoPlant Gel Plantar Wart Remover (Salicylic Acid) Schering-Plough HealthCare 765
Occlusal-HP (Salicylic Acid) GenDerm 1041
Wart-Off Wart Remover (Salicylic Acid) Pfizer Consumer 720

Water, body, depletion of
(see under Dehydration, prevention of)

Weight, body, management of
Dexatrim Plus Vitamins Caplets (Phenylpropanolamine Hydrochloride, Vitamins with Minerals) Thompson Medical 796
Oxandrin (Oxandrolone) Bio-Technology General 783

Wheezing, symptomatic relief of
(see also under Bronchial asthma)
Primatene Mist (Epinephrine) Whitehall-Robins 843

Whipworm infection
(see under Trichuris trichiura infections)

Whooping cough
(see under Pertussis)

Wilms' tumor
Adriamycin PFS (Doxorubicin Hydrochloride) Pharmacia & Upjohn 2056
Adriamycin RDF (Doxorubicin Hydrochloride) Pharmacia & Upjohn 2056
Cosmegen Injection (Dactinomycin) Merck & Co., Inc. 1666
Doxorubicin Astra (Doxorubicin Hydrochloride) Astra 531
Oncovin Solution Vials & Hyporets (Vincristine Sulfate) Lilly 1521
Rubex for Injection (Doxorubicin Hydrochloride) Bristol-Myers Squibb Oncology/Immunology 721

Wilson's disease
Cuprimine Capsules (Penicillamine) Merck & Co., Inc. 1673
Depen Titratable Tablets (Penicillamine) Wallace 2770
Syprine Capsules (Trientine Hydrochloride) Merck & Co., Inc. 1790

Wiskott-Aldrich syndrome
Gamimune N, 5% Immune Globulin Intravenous (Human), 5% (Globulin, Immune (Human)) Bayer Biological 612
Gamimune N, 10% Immune Globulin Intravenous (Human), 10% (Globulin, Immune (Human)) Bayer Biological 615
Gammagard S/D, Immune Globulin, Intravenous (Human) (Globulin, Immune (Human)) Baxter Healthcare 577

Wolff-Parkinson-White syndrome
Adenocard Injection (Adenosine) Fujisawa 1021
Isoptin Injectable (Verapamil Hydrochloride) Knoll Laboratories 1391

Wound care, adjunctive therapy in
Betasept Surgical Scrub (Chlorhexidine Gluconate) Purdue Frederick 2145
Desitin Ointment (Cod Liver Oil, Zinc Oxide) Pfizer Consumer 715
Granulex (Trypsin, Balsam Peru, Castor Oil) Dow Hickam 940
Matrix Microclysmic Gel (Propylene Glycol, Glycerin) Care-Tech 647
Orajel Perioseptic Oxygenating Liquid (Carbamide Peroxide) Del 669
Panafil Ointment (Papain, Chlorophyllin Copper Complex, Urea) Rystan 2372
Panafil-White Ointment (Papain, Urea) Rystan 2372
Tucks Pads (Witch Hazel) Warner Wellcome 830

Wounds, debridement of
Accuzyme Ointment (Papain, Urea) Healthpoint 1236
Collagenase Santyl Ointment (Collagenase) Knoll Laboratories .. 1381
Granulex (Trypsin, Balsam Peru, Castor Oil) Dow Hickam 940
Panafil Ointment (Papain, Chlorophyllin Copper Complex, Urea) Rystan 2372
Panafil-White Ointment (Papain, Urea) Rystan 2372

Wounds, deodorization of
Chloresium (Chlorophyllin Copper Complex) Rystan 2371

Wounds, removal of exudates, aids in
Panafil Ointment (Papain, Chlorophyllin Copper Complex, Urea) Rystan 2372
Panafil-White Ointment (Papain, Urea) Rystan 2372

Wrinkles, fine
(see under Skin, fine wrinkles, mitigation of)

X

Xerosis, symptomatic relief of pruritus associated with
Lac-Hydrin 12% Lotion (Ammonium Lactate) Westwood-Squibb .. 2796

Xerostomia, radiotherapy-induced
Salagen Tablets (Pilocarpine Hydrochloride) MGI 1546

Y

Yaws
Achromycin V Capsules (Tetracycline Hydrochloride) Lederle 1417
Bicillin L-A Injection (Penicillin G Benzathine) Wyeth-Ayerst 2813
Declomycin Tablets (Demeclocycline Hydrochloride) Lederle 1421
Doryx Capsules (Doxycycline Hyclate) Parke-Davis 1970
DYNACIN Capsules (Minocycline Hydrochloride) Medicis 1627
Minocin Intravenous (Minocycline Hydrochloride) Lederle 1428
Minocin Oral Suspension (Minocycline Hydrochloride) Lederle 1431
Minocin Pellet-Filled Capsules (Minocycline Hydrochloride) Lederle 1429
Monodox Capsules (Doxycycline Monohydrate) Oclassen 1858
Terramycin Intramuscular Solution (Oxytetracycline) Pfizer Inc 2034
Vibramycin (Doxycycline Calcium) Pfizer Inc 2038
Vibramycin Hyclate Intravenous (Doxycycline Hyclate) Pfizer Inc.... 2040
Vibramycin (Doxycycline Monohydrate) Pfizer Inc 2038

Yersinia pestis infections
Achromycin V Capsules (Tetracycline Hydrochloride) Lederle 1417
Declomycin Tablets (Demeclocycline Hydrochloride) Lederle 1421
Doryx Capsules (Doxycycline Hyclate) Parke-Davis 1970
DYNACIN Capsules (Minocycline Hydrochloride) Medicis 1627
Minocin Intravenous (Minocycline Hydrochloride) Lederle 1428
Minocin Oral Suspension (Minocycline Hydrochloride) Lederle 1431
Minocin Pellet-Filled Capsules (Minocycline Hydrochloride) Lederle 1429
Monodox Capsules (Doxycycline Monohydrate) Oclassen 1858
Streptomycin Sulfate Injection (Streptomycin Sulfate) Pfizer Inc 2031
Terramycin Intramuscular Solution (Oxytetracycline) Pfizer Inc 2034
Vibramycin (Doxycycline Calcium) Pfizer Inc 2038
Vibramycin Hyclate Intravenous (Doxycycline Hyclate) Pfizer Inc.... 2040
Vibramycin (Doxycycline Monohydrate) Pfizer Inc 2038

Z

Zollinger-Ellison syndrome
Pepcid Injection (Famotidine) Merck & Co., Inc. 1765
Pepcid (Famotidine) Merck & Co., Inc. 1763
Prevacid Delayed-Release Capsules (Lansoprazole) TAP 2746
Prilosec Delayed-Release Capsules (Omeprazole) Astra Merck 516
Tagamet (Cimetidine Hydrochloride) SmithKline Beecham Pharmaceuticals 2694
Zantac (Ranitidine Hydrochloride) Glaxo Wellcome 1182

Zollinger-Ellison tumor, diagnosis of
Peptavlon (Pentagastrin) Wyeth-Ayerst 2997
Secretin-Ferring (Secretin) Ferring .. 2991

Zygomycosis
Fungizone Intravenous (Amphotericin B) Apothecon 507

(▣ Described in PDR For Nonprescription Drugs)   (◉ Described in PDR For Ophthalmology)

SECTION 5

CONTRAINDICATIONS INDEX

This section lists in alphabetical order every medical condition cited as a contraindication in *PDR* and its companion volumes, with cross-references to all product entries in which the contraindication is found. Page numbers refer to the 1997 editions of *PDR* and *PDR For Ophthalmology* and the 1996 edition of *PDR For Nonprescription Drugs*, which is published later in the year. A key to the symbols denoting the companion volumes appears in the bottom margin.

These listings will enable you to quickly identify drugs that generally threaten to be inappropriate in the presence of a given complication. However, a drug's suitability is sometimes affected by the severity of the complicating condition, the age or gender of the patient, and the drug's route of administration. In ambiguous situations, a quick review of the underlying *PDR* text may therefore prove helpful.

Note, too, that the index does not list other drugs and dietary items whose use would present a contraindication. Contraindicated combinations can be found in the Interactions Index and the Food Interactions Cross-Reference. Hypersensitivity to the product's ingredients—an almost universal contraindication—also has not been indexed here. If the clinical picture includes the risk of allergic reaction, be sure to check individual product labeling for additional information.

A

Abortion, infected
ParaGard T 380A Intrauterine
  Copper Contraceptive 1936

Abortion, missed
Amen Tablets 785
Aygestin Tablets 990
Cycrin Tablets 991
Premphase 2900
Provera Tablets 2110

Abortion, threatened
Coumadin for Injection 941
Coumadin Tablets 941

Abscess, intestinal
Cortifoam 2540

Achalasia, esophageal
Fosamax Tablets 1703

Achalasia, unspecified
Cystospaz 2123
Donnatal 2234
Donnatal Extentabs 2234
Donnatal Tablets 2234
Kutrase Capsules 2546
Levsin/Levsinex/Levbid 2549
Norgesic 1554
Pro-Banthine Tablets 2226
Robinul Forte Tablets 2247
Robinul Injectable 2247
Robinul Tablets 2247
Urispas Tablets 2710

Acid base imbalance, uncorrected
(see also under Acidosis, hyperchloremic; Acidosis, metabolic, unspecified; Amino acid metabolism disorders; Ketoacidosis, diabetic)
NephrAmine Injection 2169

Acidosis, hyperchloremic
Daranide Tablets 1676

GlaucTabs .... ⊙ 209

Acidosis, metabolic, unspecified
(see also under Ketoacidosis, diabetic)
Glucophage Tablets 754

Acquired immune deficiency syndrome
(see also under Human immunodeficiency virus)
Attenuvax 1650
Biavax II 1653
M-M-R II 1730
M-R-VAX II 1732
Meruvax II 1740
Mumpsvax 1751
ParaGard T 380A Intrauterine
  Copper Contraceptive 1936
TICE BCG, USP 1881
Varivax 1807

Actinomycosis, genital
ParaGard T 380A Intrauterine
  Copper Contraceptive 1936

Adams-Stokes syndrome
Cerebyx Injection 1956

Addison's disease, untreated
Polycitra Syrup 574
Polycitra-K Crystals 574
Polycitra-K Oral Solution 575
Polycitra-LC 574
Rum-K Syrup 1004

Adenoma, hepatic
Brevicon 2563
Desogen Tablets 1867
Levlen/Tri-Levlen 646
Lo/Ovral Tablets 2852
Lo/Ovral-28 Tablets 2857
Modicon 1928
Nor-Q D Tablets 2598
Nordette-21 Tablets 2863
Nordette-28 Tablets 2866
Norinyl 2563

Ortho Tri-Cyclen 21 Tablets 1914
Ortho Tri-Cyclen 28 Tablets 1914
Ortho-Cept 21 Tablets 1907
Ortho-Cept 28 Tablets 1907
Ortho-Cyclen 21 Tablets 1914
Ortho-Cyclen 28 Tablets 1914
Ortho-Novum 1928
Ovcon 765
Ovral Tablets 2877
Ovral-28 Tablets 2878
Ovrette Tablets 2878
Levlen/Tri-Levlen 646
Tri-Norinyl 2607
Triphasil-21 Tablets 2919
Triphasil-28 Tablets 2924

Adrenal cortical insufficiency
(see under Addison's disease, untreated; Adrenal insufficiency, uncorrected; Adrenal insufficiency, unspecified)

Adrenal dysfunction, uncorrected
(see also under Adrenal insufficiency, uncorrected)
Clomid 1262
Humegon for Injection 1873
Metrodin (urofollitropin for
  injection) 2616
Pergonal (menotropins for
  injection, USP) 2618
Serophene (clomiphene citrate
  tablets, USP) 2621

Adrenal gland failure
(see under Adrenal insufficiency, unspecified)

Adrenal insufficiency, uncorrected
(see also under Addison's disease, untreated; Adrenal dysfunction, uncorrected)
Cytomel Tablets 2647
Eltroxin Tablets 2214

Levothroid Tablets 1015
Levothyroxine Sodium, USP for
  Injection 546
Levoxyl Tablets 918
Synthroid 1410
Triostat Injection 2708

Adrenal insufficiency, unspecified
Daranide Tablets 1676
GlaucTabs .... ⊙ 209
Urocit-K Tablets 1828

Adrenocortical insufficiency
(see under Adrenal insufficiency, uncorrected; Adrenal insufficiency, unspecified)

Adynamia episodica hereditaria
Polycitra-K Crystals 574
Polycitra-K Oral Solution 575

Agammaglobulinemia
Orimune 1433

Agitated states
(see under Agitation)

Agitation
Adderall Tablets 2209
Adipex-P Tablets and Capsules 1035
Bontril Slow-Release Capsules 786
Desoxyn Gradumet Tablets 422
Dexedrine 2648
DextroStat-Dextroamphetamine
  Sulfate Tablets 2211
Fastin Capsules 2662
Ionamin Capsules 1615
Ritalin 866
Sanorex Tablets 2423

Agranulocytosis
Solganal Suspension 2530

Agranulocytosis, history of
Clozaril Tablets 2377
Cuprimine Capsules 1673
Depen Titratable Tablets 2770

(⊞ Described in PDR For Nonprescription Drugs) (⊙ Described in PDR For Ophthalmology)

Contraindications Index

AIDS
(see under Acquired immune deficiency syndrome)

Albinism
- 8-MOP Capsules 1294
- Flagyl 375 Capsules 2587
- Oxsoralen-Ultra Capsules ... 1302

Alcoholism
- Methotrexate Sodium Tablets, Injection, for Injection and LPF Injection 1322
- Pondimin Tablets 2239
- RMS Suppositories CII 2766
- Roxanol 2365
- Seromycin Capsules 975

Alcoholism, unsupervised
- Coumadin for Injection 941
- Coumadin Tablets 941

Allograft
(see under Bone marrow transplantation; Organ allograft)

Amino acid metabolism disorders
(see also under Electrolyte imbalance, uncorrected)
- NephrAmine Injection 2169

Amniocentesis, genetic
- MICRhoGAM Rh₀(D) Immune Globulin (Human) 1902

Anastomosis, unspecified
(see also under Ileocolostomy)
- Cortifoam 2540
- RMS Suppositories CII 2766
- Roxanol 2365
- Urecholine 1804

Anemia, aplastic, history of
- Cuprimine Capsules 1673
- Depen Titratable Tablets 2770

Anemia, hemolytic, history of
- Skelaxin Tablets 793

Anemia, megaloblastic, unspecified
(see also under Anemia, pernicious)
- Bactrim DS Tablets 2257
- Bactrim I.V. Infusion 2255
- Bactrim 2257
- Daraprim Tablets 1199
- Fansidar Tablets 2281
- Leucovorin Calcium for Injection ... 1313
- Leucovorin Calcium for Injection, Wellcovorin Brand 1203
- Leucovorin Calcium for Injection ... 1315
- Leucovorin Calcium Tablets, Wellcovorin Brand 1204
- Proloprim Tablets 1141
- Septra 1146
- Septra I.V. Infusion 1142
- Septra I.V. Infusion ADD-Vantage Vials 1144
- Septra 1146
- Trimpex Tablets 2323

Anemia, non-iron deficiency, unspecified
- INFeD (Iron Dextran Injection, USP) 2478

Anemia, pernicious
- Chromagen FA Capsules 2471
- Chromagen Forte Capsules 2471
- Fero-Folic-500 Filmtab 433
- Iberet-Folic-500 Filmtab 433
- Leucovorin Calcium for Injection ... 1313
- Leucovorin Calcium for Injection, Wellcovorin Brand 1203
- Leucovorin Calcium for Injection ... 1315
- Leucovorin Calcium Tablets, Wellcovorin Brand 1204

Anemia, sickle cell
- Caverject Injection 2064

Anemia, unspecified
- Albuminar-5, Albumin (Human) U.S.P. 5% 795
- Albuminar-25, Albumin (Human) U.S.P. 25% 796
- Hydrea Capsules 705
- Methotrexate Sodium Tablets, Injection, for Injection and LPF Injection 1322
- Nitrostat Tablets 1981

- Plasma-Plex, Plasma Protein Fraction (Human), 5% Solution Heat-Treated 806

Anemia, unspecified, history of
- Skelaxin Tablets 793

Anesthesia, general
- Levophed Bitartrate Injection ... 2445
- Nardil 1977
- Parnate Tablets 2679
- Pondimin Tablets 2239
- Sus-Phrine Injection 1017

Anesthesia, local
(see also under Anesthesia, major regional lumbar block; Anesthesia, obstetrical, paracervical block; Denervation, skeletal muscle)
- Nardil 1977
- Parnate Tablets 2679
- Pondimin Tablets 2239
- Sus-Phrine Injection 1017

Anesthesia, major regional lumbar block
- Coumadin for Injection 941
- Coumadin Tablets 941

Anesthesia, obstetrical, paracervical block
- Marcaine 2446
- Sensorcaine 554
- Sensorcaine-MPF Injection ... 554
- Sensorcaine-MPF with Epinephrine Injection 554

Anesthesia, obstetrical, unspecified
- Fluothane 2830

Aneurysm
(see also under Cerebrovascular accident)
- Abbokinase 403
- Abbokinase Open-Cath 405
- Activase 1045
- Coumadin for Injection 941
- Coumadin Tablets 941
- Eminase 2215
- Neo-Synephrine Hydrochloride (Ophthalmic) 2456
- ReoPro Vials 1526

Angina pectoris
- Imitrex Injection 1095
- Imitrex Tablets 1099
- Isuprel Injection 2441

Angina, Prinzmetal's
- Imitrex Injection 1095
- Imitrex Tablets 1099

Angina, unspecified
- Regitine Vials 864

Angina, unspecified, history of
- Proleukin for Injection 812

Angina, unstable
- D.H.E. 45 Injection 2381

Angina, vasospastic, unspecified
- D.H.E. 45 Injection 2381

Angulation, penile
- Caverject Injection 2064

Anorexia nervosa
- Wellbutrin Tablets 1177

Anorexia nervosa, history of
- Wellbutrin Tablets 1177

Anovulation, non-hypothalamic
- Lutrepulse for Injection 998

Antepartum prophylaxis
- MICRhoGAM Rh₀(D) Immune Globulin (Human) 1902

Anuria
- Aldactazide Tablets 2556
- Aldactone Tablets 2558
- Aldoclor Tablets 1638
- Aldoril Tablets 1644
- Apresazide Capsules 824
- Bumex 2260
- Calcium Disodium Versenate Injection 1548
- Capozide Tablets 744
- Combipres Tablets 682
- Demadex Tablets and Injection .. 691
- Desferal Vials 838

- Diucardin Tablets 2824
- Diupres Tablets 1691
- Diuril Oral Suspension 1694
- Diuril Sodium Intravenous ... 1693
- Diuril Tablets 1694
- Dyazide Capsules 2653
- Dyrenium Capsules 2655
- Edecrin 1698
- Enduron Tablets 424
- Esidrix Tablets 839
- Esimil Tablets 840
- Hespan Injection 945
- HydroDIURIL Tablets 1716
- Hydropres Tablets 1718
- Hyzaar Tablets 1720
- Inderide LA Long Acting Capsules .. 2840
- Inderide Tablets 2838
- Ionamin Capsules 1615
- ISMOTIC 45% w/v Solution ... ⊞ 221
- Lasix Injection, Oral Solution and Tablets 1267
- Lopressor HCT Tablets 850
- Lotensin HCT Tablets 855
- Macrobid Capsules 2138
- Macrodantin Capsules 2140
- Midamor Tablets 1746
- Minizide Capsules 2016
- Moduretic Tablets 1748
- Mykrox Tablets 1617
- OSMOGLYN Oral Osmotic Agent ⊙ 225
- Pentaspan Injection 954
- Polycitra-K Crystals 574
- Polycitra-K Oral Solution 575
- Prinzide Tablets 1780
- Ser-Ap-Es Tablets 867
- Tenoretic Tablets 2963
- Thalitone 1293
- Timolide Tablets 1791
- Vaseretic Tablets 1810
- Zaroxolyn Tablets 1625
- Zestoretic Tablets 2968
- Ziac 1459

Anxiety
- Ritalin 866
- Seromycin Capsules 975

Aortic coarctation
(see under Stenosis, aortic)

Aortic stenosis
(see under Stenosis, aortic)

Aphakia
- 8-MOP Capsules 1294
- Oxsoralen-Ultra Capsules ... 1302

Apnea, sleep
(see under Sleep apnea)

Apoplexy, cerebral
(see under Cerebrovascular accident)

Appendicitis
- Dulcolax Suppositories 883
- Dulcolax Tablets .... ⊞ 654

Arrhythmia, cardiac, history of
- Proleukin for Injection 812

Arrhythmia, cardiac, unspecified
(see also under Arrhythmia, ventricular, unspecified; Bradycardia, sinus; Bradycardia, unspecified; Fibrillation, atrial; Fibrillation, ventricular; Flutter, atrial; Heart block, first degree; Heart block, greater than first degree; Heart block, sinoatrial; Heart block, unspecified; Lown-Ganong-Levine syndrome; PR Syndrome, short; Q-T interval prolongation; Sick sinus syndrome; Sinus node dysfunction, unspecified; Tachycardia, unspecified; Tachycardia, ventricular; Tachycardia, ventricular, history of; Torsade de pointes; Wolff-Parkinson-White syndrome)
- Cardioquin Tablets 2146
- Flexeril Tablets 1701
- Isuprel Hydrochloride Solution 2443
- Isuprel Injection 2441
- Isuprel Mistometer 2442

- Metaproterenol Sulfate Inhalation Solution, USP, Arm-a-Med ... 547
- Norisodrine with Calcium Iodide Syrup 446
- Quinidex Extentabs 2240
- RMS Suppositories CII 2766
- Roxanol 2365
- Rythmol Tablets–150mg, 225mg, 300mg 1399
- Yutopar Intravenous Injection ... 566

Arrhythmia, ventricular, unspecified
(see also under Fibrillation, ventricular; Tachycardia, ventricular; Tachycardia, ventricular, history of; Ventricular dysfunction, left)
- Isuprel Injection 2441
- Quinidex Extentabs 2240

Arterial disease, unspecified
(see also under Angina pectoris; Angina, Prinzmetal's; Angina, unspecified; Angina, unstable; Arteriosclerosis, cerebral; Arteriosclerosis, unspecified; Arteriovenous malformation; Arteritis, luetic; Coronary artery disease; Coronary artery disease, history of; Coronary artery vasospasm; Stenosis, aortic; Stenosis, subaortic)
- Scleromate Injection 1234

Arteriosclerosis, cerebral
- Ana-Kit Anaphylaxis Emergency Treatment Kit 611
- Sus-Phrine Injection 1017

Arteriosclerosis, unspecified
(see also under Coronary artery disease; Stenosis, aortic; Stenosis, subaortic)
- Adderall Tablets 2209
- Adipex-P Tablets and Capsules ... 1035
- Bontril Slow-Release Capsules .. 786
- Desoxyn Gradumet Tablets ... 422
- Dexedrine 2648
- DextroStat-Dextroamphetamine Sulfate Tablets 2211
- Fastin Capsules 2662
- Ionamin Capsules 1615
- Prelu-2 Timed Release Capsules .. 687

Arteriovenous malformation
- Abbokinase 403
- Abbokinase Open-Cath 405
- Activase 1045
- Eminase 2215
- ReoPro Vials 1526

Arteritis, luetic
- Ergomar Tablets 1543

Asthma, acute
(see also under Status asthmaticus)
- Astramorph/PF Injection, USP (Preservative-Free) 526
- Atrohist Pediatric Capsules ... 1603
- Azmacort Oral Inhaler 2175
- Beclovent Inhalation Aerosol and Refill 1063
- Bromfed 1832
- D.A. Chewable Tablets 970
- D.A. II Tablets 972
- Dopram Injectable 2235
- Dura-Tap/PD Capsules 970
- Dura-Vent/DA Tablets 972
- Duramorph Injection 983
- Fedahist Gyrocaps 2545
- Kadian Capsules 2948
- MS Contin Tablets 2149
- MSIR 2152
- Oramorph SR (Morphine Sulfate Sustained Release Tablets) ... 2359
- OxyContin Tablets 2163
- RMS Suppositories CII 2766
- Rondec Chewable Tablets 974
- Rondec 974
- Roxanol 2365
- Urecholine 1804
- Vanceril Inhaler 2538

Asthma, history of
- Betagan .... ⊙ 230
- Betimol 0.25%, 0.5% .... ⊙ 259
- Blocadren Tablets 1654

(⊞ Described in PDR For Nonprescription Drugs) (⊙ Described in PDR For Ophthalmology)

1591 **Contraindications Index** **Blood dyscrasias**

Ocupress Ophthalmic Solution, 1% Sterile ⊙ 297
OptiPranolol (Metipranolol 0.3%) Sterile Ophthalmic Solution ⊙ 256
Timolide Tablets 1791
Timoptic in Ocudose 1796
Timoptic Sterile Ophthalmic Solution ⊙ 286
Timoptic-XE 1798

Asthma, uncontrolled
Sotradecol (Sodium Tetradecyl Sulfate Injection) 987

Asthma, unspecified
Adenoscan 1022
Antilirium Injectable 1007
Atrohist Plus Tablets 1605
Betagan ⊙ 230
Betapace Tablets 637
Betimol 0.25%, 0.5% ⊙ 259
Blocadren Tablets 1654
Bromfed-DM Cough Syrup 1832
Brontex 2130
Cartrol Tablets 413
Dimetane-DC Cough Syrup 2232
Dimetane-DX Cough Syrup 2233
Inderal Injectable 2834
Inderal LA Long Acting Capsules 2836
Inderal Tablets 2834
Inderide LA Long Acting Capsules 2840
Inderide Tablets 2838
Kadian Capsules 2948
Levatol Tablets 2547
Mestinon Syrup 1300
MS Contin Tablets 2149
MSIR 2152
Normodyne Injection 2519
Normodyne Tablets 2522
Novahistine Elixir ▣ 782
Ocupress Ophthalmic Solution, 1% Sterile ⊙ 297
OptiPranolol (Metipranolol 0.3%) Sterile Ophthalmic Solution ⊙ 256
Oramorph SR (Morphine Sulfate Sustained Release Tablets) 2359
OxyContin Tablets 2163
PBZ Tablets 863
PBZ-SR Tablets 862
Phenergan Suppositories 2882
Phenergan Syrup 2881
Phenergan Tablets 2882
Phenergan VC 2886
Phenergan VC with Codeine 2888
Phenergan with Codeine 2883
Phenergan with Dextromethorphan 2885
Salagen Tablets 1546
Scleromate Injection 1234
Tavist Tablets 2427
Timolide Tablets 1791
Timoptic in Ocudose 1796
Timoptic Sterile Ophthalmic Solution ⊙ 286
Timoptic-XE 1798
Trandate 1158
Trinalin Repetabs Tablets 1373
Urecholine 1804
Visken Tablets 2428
Yutopar Intravenous Injection 566

Asthmatic attack
(see under Asthma, acute)

Atony, intestinal
Cystospaz 2123
Ditropan 1267
Donnatal 2234
Donnatal Extentabs 2234
Donnatal Tablets 2234
Kutrase Capsules 2546
Levsin/Levsinex/Levbid 2549
Pro-Banthine Tablets 2226
Robinul Forte Tablets 2247
Robinul Injectable 2247
Robinul Tablets 2247

Atresia, pulmonary
Indocin I.V. 1727

Atrial fibrillation
(see under Fibrillation, atrial)

Atrial flutter
(see under Flutter, atrial)

Atrioventricular block
(see under Heart block, first degree; Heart block, greater than first degree; Heart block, unspecified)

AV block
(see under Heart block, first degree; Heart block, greater than first degree; Heart block, unspecified)

Azotemia
(see also under Uremia)
Edecrin 1698
Polycitra Syrup 574
Polycitra-K Crystals 574
Polycitra-K Oral Solution 575
Polycitra-LC 574

B

Bacterial endocarditis
(see under Endocarditis, bacterial)

Bedridden
(see under Debilitation)

Beriberi
Crystodigin Tablets 1472

Biliary obstruction
(see under Obstruction, biliary tract)

Birthmarks
Podocon-25 1949

Bladder neck obstruction
(see under Obstruction, bladder neck)

Bleeding disorders, unspecified
(see also under Bleeding tendencies; Hemophilia; Hypoprothrombinemia; Thrombasthenia; Thrombocytopathy, unspecified; Thrombocytopenia, unspecified; Thrombocytopenic purpura, history of)
Easprin 1971
Hespan Injection 945
Indocin I.V. 1727
Mithracin 599
Mutamycin for Injection 712
Pentaspan Injection 954
Soma Compound Tablets 2783
Soma Compound w/Codeine Tablets 2784
Ticlid Tablets 2317

Bleeding tendencies
Abbokinase 403
Abbokinase Open-Cath 405
Activase 1045
Astramorph/PF Injection, USP (Preservative-Free) 526
Coumadin for Injection 941
Coumadin Tablets 941
Eminase 2215
Fiorinal Capsules 2388
Fiorinal with Codeine Capsules 2390
Mithracin 599
Mutamycin for Injection 712
ReoPro Vials 1526
Solganal Suspension 2530
Toradol 2319

Bleeding, abnormal, unspecified
(see also under Hematuria)
Indocin I.V. 1727
Pergonal (menotropins for injection, USP) 2618

Bleeding, antepartum
Yutopar Intravenous Injection 566

Bleeding, cerebrovascular
(see under Bleeding, intracranial; Cerebrovascular accident)

Bleeding, gastrointestinal
Easprin 1971
Indocin I.V. 1727
Propulsid 1346
Reglan 2243
ReoPro Vials 1526
Ticlid Tablets 2317
Toradol 2319
Urispas Tablets 2710

Bleeding, gastrointestinal, history of
Proleukin for Injection 812
Toradol 2319

Bleeding, genital, abnormal
(see also under Bleeding, genitourinary)
Amen Tablets 785
Aygestin Tablets 990
Brevicon 2563
Cervidil 1008
Climara Transdermal System 640
Clomid 1262
Cycrin Tablets 991
Danocrine Capsules 2437
Demulen 2580
Depo-Provera Contraceptive Injection 2079
Depo-Provera Sterile Aqueous Suspension 2083
Desogen Tablets 1867
Diethylstilbestrol Tablets 1477
Estrace Cream and Tablets 751
Estraderm Transdermal System 842
ESTRATAB Tablets (0.3, 0.625, 1.25, 2.5 mg) 2715
Estratest 2718
Estring Vaginal Ring 2086
Humegon for Injection 1873
Levlen/Tri-Levlen 646
Lo/Ovral Tablets 2852
Lo/Ovral-28 Tablets 2857
Lupron Depot 3.75 mg 2739
Menest Tablets 2671
Metrodin (urofollitropin for injection) 2616
Micronor Tablets 1903
Modicon 1928
Nor-Q D Tablets 2598
Nordette-21 Tablets 2863
Nordette-28 Tablets 2866
Norinyl 2563
Norplant System 2868
Ogen Tablets 2103
Ogen Vaginal Cream 2106
Ortho Dienestrol Cream 1922
Ortho Tri-Cyclen 21 Tablets 1914
Ortho Tri-Cyclen 28 Tablets 1914
Ortho-Cept 21 Tablets 1907
Ortho-Cept 28 Tablets 1907
Ortho-Cyclen 21 Tablets 1914
Ortho-Cyclen 28 Tablets 1914
Ortho-Est 1925
Ortho-Novum 1928
Ovcon 765
Ovral Tablets 2877
Ovral-28 Tablets 2878
Ovrette Tablets 2878
ParaGard T 380A Intrauterine Copper Contraceptive 1936
Pergonal (menotropins for injection, USP) 2618
PMB 200 and PMB 400 2890
Premarin Intravenous 2893
Premarin Tablets 2896
Premarin Vaginal Cream 2898
Premphase 2900
Prempro 2905
Prepidil Gel 2108
Provera Tablets 2110
Serophene (clomiphene citrate tablets, USP) 2621
Synarel Nasal Solution for Central Precocious Puberty 2603
Synarel Nasal Solution for Endometriosis 2605
Levlen/Tri-Levlen 646
Tri-Norinyl 2607
Triphasil-21 Tablets 2919
Triphasil-28 Tablets 2924
Vivelle Transdermal System 880

Bleeding, genitourinary
(see also under Bleeding, genital, abnormal)
ReoPro Vials 1526

Bleeding, history of
Oncaspar 2194

Bleeding, internal, unspecified
(see also under Hematuria)
Abbokinase 403
Abbokinase Open-Cath 405
Activase 1045
Eminase 2215
ReoPro Vials 1526
Streptase for Infusion 557

Bleeding, intracranial
Coumadin for Injection 941
Coumadin Tablets 941
Indocin I.V. 1727
Ticlid Tablets 2317
Toradol 2319
Trental Tablets 1291

Bleeding, rectal
Dulcolax Suppositories 883
Dulcolax Tablets ▣ 654
Indocin Suppositories 1723

Bleeding, retinal
Trental Tablets 1291

Bleeding, unspecified
(see also under Bleeding, internal, unspecified; Hematuria; Hemorrhagic shock; Hemostasis, incomplete)
Coumadin for Injection 941
Coumadin Tablets 941
Fragmin Injection 2088
Heparin Lock Flush Solution 2831
Heparin Sodium Injection 2832
Heparin Sodium Vials 1486
Humegon for Injection 1873
Lovenox Injection 2187
Nicotinex Elixir ▣ 671
Paraplatin for Injection 713
Ticlid Tablets 2317

Bleeding, uterine
(see under Bleeding, genital, abnormal)

Bleeding, vaginal, abnormal
(see under Bleeding, genital, abnormal)

Blood circulation, poor
Podocon-25 1949

Blood dyscrasias, history of
Anturane 823
Felbatol 2774
Torecan 2367

Blood dyscrasias, unspecified
(see also under Agranulocytosis; Agranulocytosis, history of; Anemia, aplastic, history of; Anemia, hemolytic, history of; Anemia, megaloblastic, unspecified; Anemia, non-iron deficiency, unspecified; Anemia, pernicious; Anemia, sickle cell; Anemia, unspecified; Anemia, unspecified, history of; Bleeding disorders, unspecified; Granulocytopenia; Granulocytopenia, history of; Hemophilia; Hypoprothrombinemia; Leukopenia; Neutropenia; Thrombocytopathy, unspecified; Thrombocytopenia, unspecified; Thrombocytopenic purpura, history of)
Anturane 823
Attenuvax 1650
Benemid Tablets 1651
Biavax II 1653
ColBENEMID Tablets 1662
Coumadin for Injection 941
Coumadin Tablets 941
Etrafon 2495
Fansidar Tablets 2281
M-M-R II 1730
M-R-VAX II 1732
Meruvax II 1740
Methotrexate Sodium Tablets, Injection, for Injection and LPF Injection 1322
Mumpsvax 1751
Navane Capsules and Concentrate 2018
Navane Intramuscular 2019
Peganone Tablets 455
Prolixin 510
Ridaura Capsules 2691
Scleromate Injection 1234
Solganal Suspension 2530
Sotradecol (Sodium Tetradecyl Sulfate Injection) 987

(▣ Described in PDR For Nonprescription Drugs)

(⊙ Described in PDR For Ophthalmology)

Blood dyscrasias — **Contraindications Index** — **1592**

Stelazine 2692
Ticlid Tablets 2317
Trilafon 2532
Varivax 1807

Blood volume, decreased (see under Hypovolemia)

Bone marrow aplasia (see under Bone marrow depression)

Bone marrow damage (see under Bone marrow depression)

Bone marrow depression
Adriamycin PFS 2056
Adriamycin RDF 2056
Cytoxan 700
Doxorubicin Astra 531
Etrafon 2495
Fluorouracil Injection 2282
Hexalen Capsules 2760
Hycamtin for Injection 2665
Hydrea Capsules 705
IFEX 706
Matulane Capsules 2300
Methotrexate Sodium Tablets, Injection, for Injection and LPF Injection 1322
Mithracin 599
Paraplatin for Injection 713
Platinol for Injection 717
Platinol-AQ Injection 719
Ridaura Capsules 2691
Rubex for Injection 721
Stelazine 2692
Sterile FUDR 2284
Thioplex (Thiotepa For Injection) 1329
Triavil Tablets 1800
Trilafon 2532

Bone marrow depression, history of
Atretol Tablets 569
Tegretol/Tegretol-XR 870
Tegretol-XR Tablets 870

Bone marrow function impairment (see under Bone marrow depression)

Bone marrow hypoplasia (see under Bone marrow depression)

Bone marrow transplantation
Adagen (pegademase bovine) Injection 988

Bowel disease, inflammatory (see under Inflammation, gastrointestinal tract)

Bowel ischemia, history of
Proleukin for Injection 812

Bowel obstruction (see under Bowel ischemia, history of; Obstruction, gastrointestinal tract)

Bowel perforation (see under Perforation, gastrointestinal tract)

Bowel perforation, history of (see under Perforation, gastrointestinal tract, history of)

Bradycardia, sinus
Adenoscan 1022
Betagan ⊙ 230
Betapace Tablets 637
Betimol 0.25%, 0.5% ⊙ 259
Betoptic Ophthalmic Solution 465
Betoptic S Ophthalmic Suspension 467
Blocadren Tablets 1654
Brevibloc (esmolol HCl) Injection 1860
Cerebyx Injection 1956
Cordarone Intravenous 2821
Cordarone Tablets 2818
Inderal Injectable 2834
Inderal LA Long Acting Capsules 2836
Inderal Tablets 2834
Inderide LA Long Acting Capsules 2840
Inderide Tablets 2838
Kerlone Tablets 2588
Levatol Tablets 2547
Lopressor 848
Lopressor HCT Tablets 850
Ocupress Ophthalmic Solution, 1% Sterile ⊙ 297
OptiPranolol (Metipranolol 0.3%) Sterile Ophthalmic Solution ⊙ 256
Tenoretic Tablets 2963
Tenormin Tablets and I.V. Injection 2965
Timolide Tablets 1791
Timoptic in Ocudose 1796
Timoptic Sterile Ophthalmic Solution ⊙ 286
Timoptic-XE 1798
Toprol-XL Tablets 560
Zebeta Tablets 1457
Ziac 1459

Bradycardia, unspecified
Cartrol Tablets 413
Cordarone Tablets 2818
Normodyne Injection 2519
Normodyne Tablets 2522
Rythmol Tablets–150mg, 225mg, 300mg 1399
Sectral Capsules 2914
Trandate 1158
Urecholine 1804
Visken Tablets 2428

Brain damage (see also under Hypothalamic damage; Motor neuron injury)
Ana-Kit Anaphylaxis Emergency Treatment Kit 611
Etrafon 2495
Prolixin 510
Trilafon 2532

Brain tumor (see under Tumor, pituitary, unspecified)

Breast cancer (see under Carcinoma, breast, history of; Carcinoma, breast, male; Carcinoma, breast, unspecified)

Breastfeeding
Atrohist Pediatric Capsules 1603
Atrohist Pediatric Suspension 1604
Atrohist Pediatric Suspension Dye-Free 1604
Atromid-S Capsules 2808
Bactrim DS Tablets 2257
Bactrim I.V. Infusion 2255
Bactrim 2257
Bellergal-S Tablets 2375
Benadryl Injection 1955
Bentyl 1246
Bromfed-DM Cough Syrup 1832
Cholestin Capsules 2985
Cuprimine Capsules 1673
Danocrine Capsules 2437
Depen Titratable Tablets 2770
D.H.E. 45 Injection 2381
Dimetane-DC Cough Syrup 2232
Dimetane-DX Cough Syrup 2233
Duratuss HD Elixir 2750
Entex PSE Tablets 973
Estratest 2718
Fansidar Tablets 2281
Fedahist Gyrocaps 2545
Furoxone 2221
Gantanol Tablets 2285
Gantrisin 2286
Guaifed 1833
Guaimax-D Tablets 809
Helidac Therapy 2135
Hycamtin for Injection 2665
Lescol Capsules 2395
Lupron Depot 3.75 mg 2739
Methotrexate Sodium Tablets, Injection, for Injection and LPF Injection 1322
Mevacor Tablets 1742
Novahistine DMX ◘ 782
Novahistine Elixir ◘ 782
Ornade Spansule Capsules 2678
Orthoclone OKT3 Sterile Solution 1892
PBZ Tablets 863
PBZ-SR Tablets 862
Pediazole Suspension 2340
Periactin 1767
Pravachol Tablets 770
Rynatan 2781
Rynatuss Pediatric Suspension 2782
Seldane-D Extended-Release Tablets 1286
Septra 1146
Septra I.V. Infusion 1142
Septra I.V. Infusion ADD-Vantage Vials 1144
Septra 1146
Sultrin 1941
Supprelin Injection 2230
Synarel Nasal Solution for Central Precocious Puberty 2603
Synarel Nasal Solution for Endometriosis 2605
Tapazole Tablets 1361
Tavist Syrup 2426
Tavist Tablets 2427
TICE BCG, USP 1881
Toradol 2319
Unisom Nighttime Sleep Aid 1990
Unisom With Pain Relief-Nighttime Sleep Aid and Pain Reliever 1991
Zocor Tablets 1821
Zoladex 2976

Breathing difficulty (see under Dyspnea)

Breathing problems, unspecified (see under Pulmonary disorders, unspecified; Respiratory illness, febrile; Respiratory illness, unspecified)

Bronchial asthma (see under Asthma, acute; Asthma, history of; Asthma, unspecified)

Bronchitis, chronic
Bonine Tablets 1990
Unisom Nighttime Sleep Aid 1990
Unisom With Pain Relief-Nighttime Sleep Aid and Pain Reliever 1991

Bronchography
Ethiodol Injection 2472

Bronchospastic disorders, unspecified (see also under Asthma, acute; Asthma, history of; Asthma, unspecified; Bronchitis, chronic; Emphysema)
Rythmol Tablets–150mg, 225mg, 300mg 1399

Bulimia
Wellbutrin Tablets 1177

Bulimia, history of
Wellbutrin Tablets 1177

Bundle branch block (see under Heart block, unspecified)

Burns
Anectine 1062
pHisoHex 2458

Bypass, cardiopulmonary
Plasma-Plex, Plasma Protein Fraction (Human), 5% Solution Heat-Treated 806

C

CAD (see under Coronary artery disease)

Cancer (see under Carcinoma, breast, history of; Carcinoma, breast, male; Carcinoma, breast, unspecified; Carcinoma, cervical; Carcinoma, endometrium; Carcinoma, female reproductive organs; Carcinoma, female reproductive organs, history of; Carcinoma, genital, unspecified; Carcinoma, hepatic; Carcinoma, hepatic, history of; Carcinoma, prostate; Carcinoma, skin, unspecified; Carcinoma, uterine; Lesions, malignant, unspecified; Malignancy, generalized; Metastasis, bone; Neoplasm, bone marrow system, malignant; Neoplasm, lymphatic system, malignant)

Cancer, prevention of
TheraCys BCG Live (Intravesical) 911

Carcinoma, breast, history of
Demulen 2580

Carcinoma, breast, male (see also under Carcinoma, breast, unspecified)
Androderm Testosterone Transdermal System 2634
Android Capsules, 10 mg 1297
Halotestin Tablets 2095
Oxandrin 783
Teslac Tablets 727
Testoderm Testosterone Transdermal System 486
Winstrol Tablets 2468

Carcinoma, breast, unspecified (see also under Carcinoma, breast, history of; Carcinoma, breast, male; Neoplasm, estrogen dependent)
Amen Tablets 785
Aygestin Tablets 990
Brevicon 2563
Climara Transdermal System 640
Cycrin Tablets 991
Demulen 2580
Depo-Provera Contraceptive Injection 2079
Depo-Provera Sterile Aqueous Suspension 2083
Desogen Tablets 1867
Diethylstilbestrol Tablets 1477
Estrace Cream and Tablets 751
Estraderm Transdermal System 842
ESTRATAB Tablets (0.3, 0.625, 1.25, 2.5 mg) 2715
Estratest 2718
Estring Vaginal Ring 2086
Levlen/Tri-Levlen 646
Lo/Ovral Tablets 2852
Lo/Ovral-28 Tablets 2857
Menest Tablets 2671
Micronor Tablets 1903
Modicon 1928
Nor-Q D Tablets 2598
Nordette-21 Tablets 2863
Nordette-28 Tablets 2866
Norinyl 2563
Norplant System 2868
Ogen Tablets 2103
Ogen Vaginal Cream 2106
Ortho Dienestrol Cream 1922
Ortho Tri-Cyclen 21 Tablets 1914
Ortho Tri-Cyclen 28 Tablets 1914
Ortho-Cept 21 Tablets 1907
Ortho-Cept 28 Tablets 1907
Ortho-Cyclen 21 Tablets 1914
Ortho-Cyclen 28 Tablets 1914
Ortho-Est 1925
Ortho-Novum 1928
Ovcon 765
Ovral Tablets 2877
Ovral-28 Tablets 2878
Ovrette Tablets 2878
Oxandrin 783
PMB 200 and PMB 400 2890
Premarin Intravenous 2893
Premarin Tablets 2896
Premarin Vaginal Cream 2898
Premphase 2900
Prempro 2905
Provera Tablets 2110
Levlen/Tri-Levlen 646
Tri-Norinyl 2607
Triphasil-21 Tablets 2919
Triphasil-28 Tablets 2924
Vivelle Transdermal System 880
Winstrol Tablets 2468

Carcinoma, cervical (see also under Carcinoma, female reproductive organs; Carcinoma, genital, unspecified)
ParaGard T 380A Intrauterine Copper Contraceptive 1936

Carcinoma, endometrium (see also under Carcinoma, female reproductive organs; Carcinoma, uterine)
Brevicon 2563
Desogen Tablets 1867

(◘ Described in PDR For Nonprescription Drugs) (⊙ Described in PDR For Ophthalmology)

1593 **Contraindications Index** **Cerebral vascular disease**

Levlen/Tri-Levlen ... 646
Lo/Ovral Tablets ... 2852
Lo/Ovral-28 Tablets ... 2857
Modicon ... 1928
Nor-Q D Tablets ... 2598
Nordette-21 Tablets ... 2863
Nordette-28 Tablets ... 2866
Norinyl ... 2563
Ortho Tri-Cyclen 21 Tablets ... 1914
Ortho Tri-Cyclen 28 Tablets ... 1914
Ortho-Cept 21 Tablets ... 1907
Ortho-Cept 28 Tablets ... 1907
Ortho-Cyclen 21 Tablets ... 1914
Ortho-Cyclen 28 Tablets ... 1914
Ortho-Novum ... 1928
Ovcon ... 765
Ovral Tablets ... 2877
Ovral-28 Tablets ... 2878
Ovrette Tablets ... 2878
Levlen/Tri-Levlen ... 646
Tri-Norinyl ... 2607
Triphasil-21 Tablets ... 2919
Triphasil-28 Tablets ... 2924

Carcinoma, female reproductive organs (see also under Carcinoma, cervical; Carcinoma, endometrium; Carcinoma, genital, unspecified; Carcinoma, uterine)
Demulen ... 2580

Carcinoma, female reproductive organs, history of
Demulen ... 2580

Carcinoma, genital, unspecified (see also under Carcinoma, cervical; Carcinoma, female reproductive organs; Carcinoma, prostate)
Amen Tablets ... 785
Cycrin Tablets ... 991
Provera Tablets ... 2110

Carcinoma, hepatic
Brevicon ... 2563
Demulen ... 2580
Desogen Tablets ... 1867
Levlen/Tri-Levlen ... 646
Lo/Ovral Tablets ... 2852
Lo/Ovral-28 Tablets ... 2857
Micronor Tablets ... 1903
Modicon ... 1928
Nor-Q D Tablets ... 2598
Nordette-21 Tablets ... 2863
Nordette-28 Tablets ... 2866
Norinyl ... 2563
Norplant System ... 2868
Ortho Tri-Cyclen 21 Tablets ... 1914
Ortho Tri-Cyclen 28 Tablets ... 1914
Ortho-Cept 21 Tablets ... 1907
Ortho-Cept 28 Tablets ... 1907
Ortho-Cyclen 21 Tablets ... 1914
Ortho-Cyclen 28 Tablets ... 1914
Ortho-Novum ... 1928
Ovcon ... 765
Ovral Tablets ... 2877
Ovral-28 Tablets ... 2878
Ovrette Tablets ... 2878
Levlen/Tri-Levlen ... 646
Tri-Norinyl ... 2607
Triphasil-21 Tablets ... 2919
Triphasil-28 Tablets ... 2924

Carcinoma, hepatic, history of
Demulen ... 2580

Carcinoma, ovarian (see under Carcinoma, female reproductive organs)

Carcinoma, prostate (see also under Carcinoma, genital, unspecified; Neoplasm, androgen dependent)
Androderm Testosterone Transdermal System ... 2634
Android Capsules, 10 mg ... 1297
Halotestin Tablets ... 2095
Oxandrin ... 783
Pregnyl for Injection ... 1878
Profasi (chorionic gonadotropin for injection, USP) ... 2620
Testoderm Testosterone Transdermal System ... 486
Winstrol Tablets ... 2468

Carcinoma, skin, unspecified (see also under Melanoma, history of)
Oxsoralen Lotion 1% ... 1301

Carcinoma, squamous cell, unspecified
8-MOP Capsules ... 1294
Flagyl 375 Capsules ... 2587
Oxsoralen-Ultra Capsules ... 1302

Carcinoma, uterine (see also under Carcinoma, endometrium; Carcinoma, female reproductive organs)
ParaGard T 380A Intrauterine Copper Contraceptive ... 1936

Cardiac arrhythmia (see under Arrhythmia, cardiac, unspecified)

Cardiac decompensation (see under Heart failure, unspecified)

Cardiac dilation
Ana-Kit Anaphylaxis Emergency Treatment Kit ... 611
Daranide Tablets ... 1676

Cardiac disease (see under Cardiovascular disorders, unspecified)

Cardiac dysfunction (see under Cardiovascular disorders, unspecified)

Cardiac failure (see under Heart failure, unspecified)

Cardiac insufficiency (see under Cardiovascular disorders, unspecified)

Cardiac rhythm disturbances, unspecified (see under Arrhythmia, cardiac, unspecified)

Cardiogenic shock
Ana-Kit Anaphylaxis Emergency Treatment Kit ... 611
Betagan ... ⊙ 230
Betapace Tablets ... 637
Betimol 0.25%, 0.5% ... ⊙ 259
Betoptic Ophthalmic Solution ... 465
Betoptic S Ophthalmic Suspension ... 467
Blocadren Tablets ... 1654
Brevibloc (esmolol HCl) Injection ... 1860
Calan SR Caplets ... 2571
Calan Tablets ... 2568
Cardizem Injectable ... 1253
Cardizem Lyo-Ject Syringe ... 1253
Cartrol Tablets ... 413
Cordarone Intravenous ... 2821
Covera-HS Tablets ... 2573
Ethmozine Tablets ... 2217
Inderal Injectable ... 2834
Inderal LA Long Acting Capsules ... 2836
Inderal Tablets ... 2834
Inderide LA Long Acting Capsules ... 2840
Inderide Tablets ... 2838
Isoptin Injectable ... 1391
Isoptin Oral Tablets ... 1393
Isoptin SR Tablets ... 1395
Kerlone Tablets ... 2588
Levatol Tablets ... 2547
Lopressor ... 848
Lopressor HCT Tablets ... 850
Mexitil Capsules ... 684
Normodyne Injection ... 2519
Normodyne Tablets ... 2522
Norpace ... 2596
Ocupress Ophthalmic Solution, 1% Sterile ... ⊙ 297
OptiPranolol (Metipranolol 0.3%) Sterile Ophthalmic Solution ... ⊙ 256
Rythmol Tablets–150mg, 225mg, 300mg ... 1399
Sectral Capsules ... 2914
Tambocor Tablets ... 1555
Tenoretic Tablets ... 2963
Tenormin Tablets and I.V. Injection ... 2965
Timolide Tablets ... 1791
Timoptic in Ocudose ... 1796
Timoptic Sterile Ophthalmic Solution ... ⊙ 286
Timoptic-XE ... 1798
Toprol-XL Tablets ... 560
Trandate ... 1158
Visken Tablets ... 2428
Zebeta Tablets ... 1457
Ziac ... 1459

Cardiomyopathy, restrictive
Nitro-Bid IV ... 1270

Cardiopulmonary resuscitation
Abbokinase ... 403
Abbokinase Open-Cath ... 405

Cardiospasm
Norflex ... 1554
Urised Tablets ... 2123

Cardiovascular collapse (see under Shock, unspecified)

Cardiovascular disorders, history of, postpartum period
Parlodel ... 2411

Cardiovascular disorders, unspecified (see also under Adams-Stokes syndrome; Angina pectoris; Angina, Prinzmetal's; Angina, unspecified; Angina, unstable; Angina, vasospastic, unspecified; Arrhythmia, cardiac, unspecified; Cardiogenic shock; Cardiomyopathy, restrictive; Cardiospasm; Carotid sinus syndrome; Congestive heart failure, uncontrolled; Congestive heart failure, unspecified; Cor pulmonale; Coronary artery disease; Coronary artery disease, history of; Coronary occlusion; ECG changes, history of; Endocarditis, bacterial; Heart disease, ischemic; Heart disease, mitral valvular, rheumatic; Heart failure, unspecified; Hypertension, unspecified; Hypovolemia; Myocardial infarction; Myocardial infarction, history of; Pericardial effusion; Pericardial tamponade)
Adderall Tablets ... 2209
Adipex-P Tablets and Capsules ... 1035
Antabuse Tablets ... 2802
Antilirium Injectable ... 1007
Bellergal-S Tablets ... 2375
Bontril Slow-Release Capsules ... 786
Cafergot ... 2376
Cortifoam ... 2540
Crystodigin Tablets ... 1472
Danocrine Capsules ... 2437
Desoxyn Gradumet Tablets ... 422
Dexedrine ... 2648
DextroStat-Dextroamphetamine Sulfate Tablets ... 2211
Dopram Injectable ... 2235
Doxorubicin Astra ... 531
Ergomar Tablets ... 1543
Extendryl ... 1003
Fastin Capsules ... 2662
Halotestin Tablets ... 2095
Hycomine Compound Tablets ... 948
Hycomine ... 947
Imitrex Injection ... 1095
Indocin I.V. ... 1727
Ionamin Capsules ... 1615
Kronofed-A ... 994
Levoprome ... 1321
Lithium Carbonate Capsules & Tablets ... 2352
Marax Tablets & DF Syrup ... 2015
Mellaril ... 2398
Midrin Capsules ... 788
Parnate Tablets ... 2679
Polycitra Syrup ... 574
Polycitra-K Crystals ... 574
Polycitra-K Oral Solution ... 575
Polycitra-LC ... 574
Prelu-2 Timed Release Capsules ... 687
Prostin E2 Suppository ... 2109
Regitine Vials ... 864
Sansert Tablets ... 2424
Sus-Phrine Injection ... 1017
Wigraine Tablets ... 1884
Yutopar Intravenous Injection ... 566

Cardiovascular status, unstable in acute hemorrhage
Bentyl ... 1246
Cystospaz ... 2123
Ditropan ... 1267
Donnatal ... 2234
Donnatal Extentabs ... 2234
Donnatal Tablets ... 2234
Kutrase Capsules ... 2546
Levsin/Levsinex/Levbid ... 2549
Pro-Banthine Tablets ... 2226
Robinul Forte Tablets ... 2247
Robinul Injectable ... 2247
Robinul Tablets ... 2247

Carotid sinus syndrome
Crystodigin Tablets ... 1472

Cavernosal fibrosis (see under Fibrosis, cavernosal)

Cellular immune deficiency (see under Immunodeficiency, unspecified)

Cellulitis
Sansert Tablets ... 2424
Sotradecol (Sodium Tetradecyl Sulfate Injection) ... 987

Central nervous system depression
Clozaril Tablets ... 2377
Compazine ... 2644
Etrafon ... 2495
Haldol Decanoate ... 1587
Haldol Injection, Tablets and Concentrate ... 1585
Loxitane ... 1426
Mellaril ... 2398
Moban Tablets and Concentrate ... 1036
Navane Capsules and Concentrate ... 2018
Navane Intramuscular ... 2019
Orap Tablets ... 1037
Phenergan Injection ... 2880
Prolixin ... 510
RMS Suppositories CII ... 2766
Roxanol ... 2365
Serentil ... 689
Stelazine ... 2692
Thorazine ... 2701
Torecan ... 2367
Triavil Tablets ... 1800
Trilafon ... 2532

Cephalopelvic disproportion
Cervidil ... 1008
Prepidil Gel ... 2108
Syntocinon Injection ... 2425

Cerebral apoplexy (see under Cerebrovascular accident)

Cerebral vascular accident (see under Cerebrovascular accident)

Cerebral vascular disease (see also under Arteriosclerosis, cerebral; Bleeding, intracranial; Cerebrovascular accident)
Brevicon ... 2563
Demulen ... 2580
Depo-Provera Contraceptive Injection ... 2079
Depo-Provera Sterile Aqueous Suspension ... 2083
Desogen Tablets ... 1867
Levlen/Tri-Levlen ... 646
Lo/Ovral Tablets ... 2852
Lo/Ovral-28 Tablets ... 2857
Modicon ... 1928
Nor-Q D Tablets ... 2598
Nordette-21 Tablets ... 2863
Nordette-28 Tablets ... 2866
Norinyl ... 2563
Ortho Tri-Cyclen 21 Tablets ... 1914
Ortho Tri-Cyclen 28 Tablets ... 1914
Ortho-Cept 21 Tablets ... 1907
Ortho-Cept 28 Tablets ... 1907
Ortho-Cyclen 21 Tablets ... 1914
Ortho-Cyclen 28 Tablets ... 1914
Ortho-Novum ... 1928
Ovcon ... 765
Ovral Tablets ... 2877
Ovral-28 Tablets ... 2878
Ovrette Tablets ... 2878

(▣ Described in PDR For Nonprescription Drugs)
(⊙ Described in PDR For Ophthalmology)

Contraindications Index

Cerebral vascular disease
- Parnate Tablets ... 2679
- Levlen/Tri-Levlen ... 646
- Tri-Norinyl ... 2607
- Triphasil-21 Tablets ... 2919
- Triphasil-28 Tablets ... 2924

Cerebral vascular disease, history of
(see also under Cerebrovascular accident, history of)
- Demulen ... 2580

Cerebrospinal diseases, unspecified
(see also under Meningitis; Syphilis)
- Novocain Hydrochloride for Spinal Anesthesia ... 2457

Cerebrospinal pressure, increased
- Roxanol ... 2365

Cerebrovascular accident
(see also under Bleeding, intracranial)
- Amen Tablets ... 785
- Aygestin Tablets ... 990
- Cycrin Tablets ... 991
- Dopram Injectable ... 2235
- Premphase ... 2900
- Prempro ... 2905
- Provera Tablets ... 2110
- ReoPro Vials ... 1526
- Streptase for Infusion ... 557

Cerebrovascular accident, history of
- Abbokinase ... 403
- Abbokinase Open-Cath ... 405
- Activase ... 1045
- Amen Tablets ... 785
- Aygestin Tablets ... 990
- Cycrin Tablets ... 991
- Eminase ... 2215
- Premphase ... 2900
- Prempro ... 2905
- Provera Tablets ... 2110
- ReoPro Vials ... 1526

Cerebrovascular defects
(see under Cerebral vascular disease)

Cerebrovascular disorders, unspecified
(see under Cerebral vascular disease; Neurological disorders, unspecified)

Cerebrovascular hemorrhage
(see under Bleeding, intracranial; Cerebrovascular accident)

Cervicitis, untreated
- ParaGard T 380A Intrauterine Copper Contraceptive ... 1936

Cesarean section, history of
- Cervidil ... 1008
- Prepidil Gel ... 2108

Charcot-Marie-Tooth syndrome
- Oncovin Solution Vials & Hyporets .. 1521

Chest pain, unspecified, history of
(see also under Angina, unspecified, history of)
- Proleukin for Injection ... 812

CHF
(see under Congestive heart failure, uncontrolled; Congestive heart failure, unspecified)

Chicken pox
(see under Varicella)

Cholangitis
- Actigall Capsules ... 818

Cholecystitis
- Actigall Capsules ... 818

Chorioamnionitis
- Yutopar Intravenous Injection ... 566

Chronic obstructive pulmonary disease
(see also under Asthma, history of; Asthma, uncontrolled; Asthma, unspecified; Bronchitis, chronic; Emphysema)
- Betagan ... ⊙ 230
- Betimol 0.25%, 0.5% ... ⊙ 259
- Blocadren Tablets ... 1654
- Dilaudid Ampules ... 1382
- Dilaudid Cough Syrup ... 1383
- Dilaudid ... 1382
- Novahistine Elixir ... ⊠ 782
- Ocupress Ophthalmic Solution, 1% Sterile ... ⊙ 297
- OptiPranolol (Metipranolol 0.3%) Sterile Ophthalmic Solution ... ⊙ 256
- Timolide Tablets ... 1791
- Timoptic in Ocudose ... 1796
- Timoptic Sterile Ophthalmic Solution ... ⊙ 286
- Timoptic-XE ... 1798

Circulatory collapse
(see under Shock, unspecified)

Cirrhosis, primary biliary
- Atromid-S Capsules ... 2808
- Lopid Tablets ... 1974

Cirrhosis, unspecified
- Aldoclor Tablets ... 1638
- Aldomet Ester HCl Injection ... 1642
- Aldomet Oral ... 1640
- Aldoril Tablets ... 1644
- Dantrium Capsules ... 2131
- GlaucTabs ... ⊙ 209
- Precose ... 604

Coagulation disorders
(see under Bleeding disorders, unspecified; Hemophilia)

Coagulation, intravascular, active
- Amicar Syrup, Tablets, and Injection ... 1312

Colitis, toxic
- Colyte and Colyte-flavored ... 2540
- GoLYTELY ... 694
- NuLYTELY ... 694
- Tri-Levlen 28 Tablets ... 646

Colitis, ulcerative
- Bentyl ... 1246
- Cystospaz ... 2123
- Ditropan ... 1267
- Diupres Tablets ... 1691
- Donnatal ... 2234
- Donnatal Extentabs ... 2234
- Donnatal Tablets ... 2234
- Hydropres Tablets ... 1718
- Kutrase Capsules ... 2546
- Levsin/Levsinex/Levbid ... 2549
- Precose ... 604
- Pro-Banthine Tablets ... 2226
- Robinul Forte Tablets ... 2247
- Robinul Injectable ... 2247
- Robinul Tablets ... 2247
- Ser-Ap-Es Tablets ... 867

Colitis, ulcerative, history of
- Cleocin T Topical ... 2072
- Cleocin Vaginal Cream ... 2070

Colitis, unspecified
(see also under Colitis, ulcerative; Enterocolitis, necrotizing; Enterocolitis, pseudomembranous)
- Ditropan ... 1267
- Solganal Suspension ... 2530

Colitis, unspecified, history of
- Cleocin T Topical ... 2072
- Cleocin Vaginal Cream ... 2070

Collagen diseases, unspecified
(see also under Lupus erythematosus)
- Sansert Tablets ... 2424

Colonic ulceration
(see under Colitis, ulcerative)

Coma, diabetic
- Amaryl Tablets ... 1241
- DiaBeta Tablets ... 1265
- Diabinese Tablets ... 2002
- Glucophage Tablets ... 754
- Glucotrol Tablets ... 2011
- Glucotrol XL Extended Release Tablets ... 2012
- Glynase PresTab Tablets ... 2091

Coma, hepatic
- Bumex ... 2260
- Mykrox Tablets ... 1617
- Zaroxolyn Tablets ... 1625

Coma, unspecified
- Clozaril Tablets ... 2377
- Compazine ... 2644
- Etrafon ... 2495
- Haldol Decanoate ... 1587
- Haldol Injection, Tablets and Concentrate ... 1585
- Levoprome ... 1321
- Loxitane ... 1426
- Mellaril ... 2398
- Moban Tablets and Concentrate ... 1036
- Navane Capsules and Concentrate .. 2018
- Navane Intramuscular ... 2019
- Orap Tablets ... 1037
- Phenergan Injection ... 2880
- Prolixin ... 510
- Serentil ... 689
- Stelazine ... 2692
- Thorazine ... 2701
- Torecan ... 2367
- Trilafon ... 2532

Coma, unspecified, history of
- Proleukin for Injection ... 812

Comatose states
(see under Coma, diabetic; Coma, hepatic; Coma, unspecified)

Conduction disorders, cardiac
(see under Arrhythmia, cardiac, unspecified)

Conduction disturbances
(see under Arrhythmia, cardiac, unspecified)

Congestive heart failure, uncontrolled
- Betapace Tablets ... 637
- Rythmol Tablets—150mg, 225mg, 300mg ... 1399
- Solganal Suspension ... 2530

Congestive heart failure, unspecified
- Cartrol Tablets ... 413
- Esimil Tablets ... 840
- Flexeril Tablets ... 1701
- Flolan for Injection ... 1085
- Hespan Injection ... 945
- Hylorel Tablets ... 1613
- Inderal Injectable ... 2834
- Inderal LA Long Acting Capsules ... 2836
- Inderal Tablets ... 2834
- Inderide LA Long Acting Capsules .. 2840
- Inderide Tablets ... 2838
- Ismelin Tablets ... 845
- Isoptin Injectable ... 1391
- Nardil ... 1977
- Pentaspan Injection ... 954

Convulsions, history of
(see under Convulsive disorders, history of; Seizure disorders, history of)

Convulsive disorders
(see also under Adams-Stokes syndrome; Seizure disorders, unspecified)
- Dopram Injectable ... 2235
- RMS Suppositories CII ... 2766
- Roxanol ... 2365

Convulsive disorders, history of
(see also under Seizure disorders, history of)
- Acel-Imune Diphtheria and Tetanus Toxoids and Acellular Pertussis Vaccine Adsorbed ... 1415
- NegGram ... 2453
- Tetramune ... 1449
- Tri-Immunol Adsorbed ... 1452

COPD
(see under Chronic obstructive pulmonary disease)

Cor pulmonale
- Dilaudid Ampules ... 1382
- Dilaudid Cough Syrup ... 1383
- Dilaudid ... 1382

Cord presentation
- Syntocinon Injection ... 2425

Cord prolapse
- Syntocinon Injection ... 2425

Corneal foreign body removal
- AK-CIDE ... ⊙ 203
- AK-Trol Ointment & Suspension ... ⊙ 205
- Blephamide Liquifilm Sterile Ophthalmic Suspension ... 472
- Isoptin SR Tablets ... 1395
- Poly-Pred Liquifilm ... ⊙ 246
- Pred-G S.O.P. Sterile Ophthalmic Ointment ... ⊙ 249
- Terra-Cortril Ophthalmic Suspension ... 2033
- TobraDex Ophthalmic Suspension and Ointment ... 469

Coronary artery disease
(see also under Coronary artery vasospasm; Stenosis, aortic; Stenosis, subaortic)
- Apresazide Capsules ... 824
- Apresoline Hydrochloride Tablets 826
- Atrohist Pediatric Capsules ... 1603
- Brevicon ... 2563
- Bromfed Capsules (Extended-Release) ... 1832
- Bromfed-DM Cough Syrup ... 1832
- Bromfed ... 1832
- Claritin-D Tablets ... 2487
- Cortifoam ... 2540
- D.A. Chewable Tablets ... 970
- D.A. II Tablets ... 972
- Deconsal II Tablets ... 1605
- Demulen ... 2580
- Desogen Tablets ... 1867
- D.H.E. 45 Injection ... 2381
- Dimetane-DC Cough Syrup ... 2232
- Dimetane-DX Cough Syrup ... 2233
- Dura-Tap/PD Capsules ... 970
- Dura-Vent ... 971
- Dura-Vent/DA Tablets ... 972
- Duratuss HD Elixir ... 2750
- Entex PSE Tablets ... 973
- Fedahist Gyrocaps ... 2545
- Guaifed ... 1833
- Guaimax-D Tablets ... 809
- Histussin D Liquid ... 670
- Hydralazine Hydrochloride Injection USP ... 2712
- Levlen/Tri-Levlen ... 646
- Lo/Ovral Tablets ... 2852
- Lo/Ovral-28 Tablets ... 2857
- Modicon ... 1928
- Nor-Q D Tablets ... 2598
- Nordette-21 Tablets ... 2863
- Nordette-28 Tablets ... 2866
- Norinyl ... 2563
- Novahistine DMX ... ⊠ 782
- Novahistine Elixir ... ⊠ 782
- Ortho Tri-Cyclen 21 Tablets ... 1914
- Ortho Tri-Cyclen 28 Tablets ... 1914
- Ortho-Cept 21 Tablets ... 1907
- Ortho-Cept 28 Tablets ... 1907
- Ortho-Cyclen 21 Tablets ... 1914
- Ortho-Cyclen 28 Tablets ... 1914
- Ortho-Novum ... 1928
- Ovcon ... 765
- Ovral Tablets ... 2877
- Ovral-28 Tablets ... 2878
- Ovrette Tablets ... 2878
- Regitine Vials ... 864
- Rondec Chewable Tablets ... 974
- Rondec ... 974
- Sansert Tablets ... 2424
- Seldane-D Extended-Release Tablets ... 1286
- Semprex-D Capsules ... 1620
- Ser-Ap-Es Tablets ... 867
- Syn-Rx DM Tablets ... 1623
- Syn-Rx Tablets ... 1622
- Levlen/Tri-Levlen ... 646
- Tri-Norinyl ... 2607
- Trinalin Repetabs Tablets ... 1373
- Triphasil-21 Tablets ... 2919
- Triphasil-28 Tablets ... 2924
- Urecholine ... 1804

Coronary artery disease, history of
- Demulen ... 2580

Coronary artery disease, history of, postpartum period
- Parlodel ... 2411

(⊠ Described in PDR For Nonprescription Drugs)   (⊙ Described in PDR For Ophthalmology)

1595 **Contraindications Index** **Eye surgery**

Coronary artery vasospasm (see also under Angina pectoris; Angina, Prinzmetal's; Angina, unspecified; Angina, unstable)
Imitrex Injection 1095

Coronary heart disease (see under Cardiovascular disorders, unspecified)

Coronary insufficiency (see under Cardiovascular disorders, unspecified)

Coronary occlusion (see also under Myocardial infarction)
Antabuse Tablets 2802

Cramps, heat (see under Heat cramps)

Crying, inconsolable, history of
Tri-Immunol Adsorbed 1452

Cysticercosis, ocular
Biltricide Tablets 584

Cysts, ovarian
Clomid 1262
Humegon for Injection 1873
Lutrepulse for Injection 998
Metrodin (urofollitropin for injection) 2616
Pergonal (menotropins for injection, USP) 2618
Serophene (clomiphene citrate tablets, USP) 2621

D

Dacryocystitis, chronic
Collagen Plugs (Intracanalicular) .. ⊙ 275
Herrick Lacrimal Plugs .... ⊙ 275

Debilitation
Lithium Carbonate Capsules & Tablets 2352
Myochrysine Injection 1754
Orimune 1433
Periactin 1767
Sansert Tablets 2424
Scleromate Injection 1234
Solganal Suspension 2530
Sotradecol (Sodium Tetradecyl Sulfate Injection) 987

Deep vein incompetence (see under Occlusion, deep vein)

Deep vein thrombophlebitis, history of (see under Thrombophlebitis, history of)

Dehydration
ISMOTIC 45% w/v Solution .... ⊙ 221
Lithium Carbonate Capsules & Tablets 2352
OSMOGLYN Oral Osmotic Agent .. ⊙ 225
Polycitra-K Crystals 574
Polycitra-K Oral Solution 575
Rum-K Syrup 1004
Urocit-K Tablets 1828
Uroqid-Acid No. 2 Tablets 633

Delirium tremens
RMS Suppositories CII 2766
Roxanol 2365

Delivery, traumatic, history of
Prepidil Gel 2108

Delivery, unspecified
Dilaudid-HP Injection 1384
Dilaudid-HP Lyophilized Powder 250mg 1384
Dilaudid Tablets and Liquid 1386
Macrobid Capsules 2138
Macrodantin Capsules 2140
Toradol 2319

Delivery, vaginal
Prepidil Gel 2108
Syntocinon Injection 2425

Dendritic keratitis (see under Herpes simplex keratitis)

Denervation, skeletal muscle
Anectine 1062

Depression, mental
Hydropres Tablets 1718
Ser-Ap-Es Tablets 867
Seromycin Capsules 975

Depression, mental, history of
Diupres Tablets 1691
Hydropres Tablets 1718
Ser-Ap-Es Tablets 867

Dermatitis (see also under Inflammation, local; Intertrigo; Rash)
Ridaura Capsules 2691
Solganal Suspension 2530
T.R.U.E. Test 1162

Diabetes mellitus
Urocit-K Tablets 1828

Diabetes mellitus, type I, sole therapy
Glynase PresTab Tablets 2091
Micronase Tablets 2099

Diabetes mellitus, uncontrolled
Scleromate Injection 1234
Solganal Suspension 2530
Sotradecol (Sodium Tetradecyl Sulfate Injection) 987
Yutopar Intravenous Injection 566

Diabetes, unspecified
Antilirium Injectable 1007
Cortifoam 2540
Hycomine Compound Tablets 948
Hycomine 947
Podocon-25 1949
Sotradecol (Sodium Tetradecyl Sulfate Injection) 987

Diabetic gastroparesis (see under Gastroparesis, diabetic)

Diabetic ketoacidosis (see under Ketoacidosis, diabetic)

Diabetic nephropathy (see under Nephropathy, diabetic)

Diarrhea, infectious
Lomotil 2591
Motofen Tablets 789

Diarrhea, severe
Edecrin 1698

Diet, low galactose
DUPHALAC Solution 2714

Diet, sodium restricted
Bicitra 573
Fleet Phospho-Soda 1002

Discharge, mucopurulent
Collagen Plugs (Intracanalicular) .. ⊙ 275
Herrick Lacrimal Plugs .... ⊙ 275

Discharge, otic
Americaine Otic Topical Anesthetic Ear Drops 1603
Tympagesic Ear Drops 2476

Disease, infectious, unspecified
Mustargen 1752

Disease, systemic, uncontrolled
Sotradecol (Sodium Tetradecyl Sulfate Injection) 987

Dissecting aorta
Coumadin for Injection 941
Coumadin Tablets 941

Diverticulitis
Cortifoam 2540

Drug abuse, history of
Adderall Tablets 2209
Adipex-P Tablets and Capsules 1035
Bontril Slow-Release Capsules 786
Desoxyn Gradumet Tablets 422
Dexedrine 2648
DextroStat-Dextroamphetamine Sulfate Tablets 2211
Fastin Capsules 2662
Ionamin Capsules 1615
Prelu-2 Timed Release Capsules 687
Sanorex Tablets 2423

Drug abuse, unspecified
ParaGard T 380A Intrauterine Copper Contraceptive 1936

Dysgammaglobulinemia
Attenuvax 1650
Biavax II 1653
M-M-R II 1730
M-R-VAX II 1732
Meruvax II 1740
Mumpsvax 1751
Varivax 1807

Dyspnea
Novahistine Elixir .... ■ 782
Phenobarbital Elixir and Tablets 1523
Seconal Sodium Pulvules 1529

E

Ear infection, fungal (see under Infection, otic, fungal)

Eardrum perforation (see under Tympanic membrane perforation)

ECG changes, history of
Proleukin for Injection 812

Eclampsia
Coumadin for Injection 941
Coumadin Tablets 941
Parlodel 2411
Yutopar Intravenous Injection 566

Eczema
Solganal Suspension 2530

Edema, pulmonary
ISMOTIC 45% w/v Solution .... ⊙ 221
OSMOGLYN Oral Osmotic Agent .. ⊙ 225

Effusion, pericardial (see under Pericardial effusion)

Electrocardiogram changes (see under ECG changes, history of)

Electroconvulsive therapy (see under Electroshock therapy)

Electrolyte depletion (see under Electrolyte imbalance, uncorrected)

Electrolyte disturbances (see under Electrolyte imbalance, uncorrected)

Electrolyte imbalance, uncorrected (see also under Hypercalcemia; Hyperkalemia; Hyperphosphatemia; Hypocalcemia; Hypokalemia; Hyponatremia)
Bumex 2260
Edecrin 1698
NephrAmine Injection 2169
Rythmol Tablets–150mg, 225mg, 300mg 1399

Electroshock therapy
Diupres Tablets 1691
Hydropres Tablets 1718

Emergency, obstetric
Prepidil Gel 2108
Syntocinon Injection 2425

Emphysema
Bonine Tablets 1990
Dilaudid Ampules 1382
Dilaudid Cough Syrup 1383
Dilaudid 1382
Novahistine Elixir .... ■ 782
Unisom Nighttime Sleep Aid 1990
Unisom With Pain Relief-Nighttime Sleep Aid and Pain Reliever 1991

Encephalopathy, history of
Acel-Imune Diphtheria and Tetanus Toxoids and Acellular Pertussis Vaccine Adsorbed 1415
Diphtheria and Tetanus Toxoids and Pertussis Vaccine Adsorbed .. 2650
Tetramune 1449
Tri-Immunol Adsorbed 1452

Endocarditis, bacterial
Coumadin for Injection 941
Coumadin Tablets 941

Endometrial cancer (see under Carcinoma, endometrium)

Endometritis, postpartum
ParaGard T 380A Intrauterine Copper Contraceptive 1936

Enteritis, history of
Cleocin T Topical 2072
Cleocin Vaginal Cream 2070

Enterocolitis, necrotizing
Indocin I.V. 1727
Ridaura Capsules 2691

Enterocolitis, pseudomembranous
Lomotil 2591

Epilepsy
Dopram Injectable 2235
Reglan 2243
Seromycin Capsules 975
Urecholine 1804

Epilepsy, uncontrolled (see also under Status epilepticus)
Clozaril Tablets 2377
Tri-Immunol Adsorbed 1452

Epiphora
Collagen Plugs (Intracanalicular) .. ⊙ 275
Herrick Lacrimal Plugs .... ⊙ 275

Epiphyses, closed
Genotropin Injection 2090
Humatrope Vials 1490
Nutropin 1049
Nutropin AQ Injection 1051
Protropin 1053

Epiphyses, fused (see under Epiphyses, closed)

Epithelial herpes simplex keratitis (see under Herpes simplex keratitis)

Esophageal abnormalities, unspecified (see also under Achalasia, esophageal; Esophageal compression; Esophagitis, reflux; Stricture, esophageal)
Fosamax Tablets 1703

Esophageal achalasia (see under Achalasia, esophageal)

Esophageal compression
K-Dur Microburst Release System (potassium chloride, USP) E.R. Tablets 1364
K-Norm Capsules 1615
Micro-K 2237
Micro-K LS Packets 2238
Slow-K Extended-Release Tablets 869

Esophageal stricture (see under Stricture, esophageal)

Esophagitis, reflux
Bentyl 1246
Donnatal 2234
Donnatal Extentabs 2234
Donnatal Tablets 2234

Exanthematous conditions (see under Rash)

Exercise, strenuous physical
Urocit-K Tablets 1828

Eye infection (see under Cysticercosis, ocular; Dacryocystitis, chronic; Infection, ophthalmic, fungal; Infection, ophthalmic, mycobacterial; Infection, ophthalmic, viral; Inflammation, eyelid; Iritis, acute)

Eye surgery (see under Surgery, ophthalmic)

(■ Described in PDR For Nonprescription Drugs)

(⊙ Described in PDR For Ophthalmology)

Contraindications Index

F

Fallot's tetralogy
(see under Tetralogy of Fallot)

Febrile illness
(see under Fever; Infection, febrile; Respiratory illness, febrile)

Fecal impaction
CITRUCEL Orange Flavor	770
CITRUCEL Sugar Free Orange Flavor	770
Konsyl Fiber Tablets	679
Konsyl Powder Sugar Free Unflavored	680
Metamucil	2125
Unifiber	1845

Fetal death, intrauterine
Yutopar Intravenous Injection	566

Fetal distress, non-imminent delivery
Cervidil	1008
Prepidil Gel	2108
Syntocinon Injection	2425

Fetal positions, unfavorable
Syntocinon Injection	2425

Fever
(see also under Infection, febrile; Respiratory illness, febrile)
Acel-Imune Diphtheria and Tetanus Toxoids and Acellular Pertussis Vaccine Adsorbed	1415
Biavax II	1653
Diphtheria & Tetanus Toxoids Adsorbed Purogenated	1422
Diphtheria and Tetanus Toxoids and Pertussis Vaccine Adsorbed	2650
Fluvirin (Influenza Virus Vaccine)	1608
Imovax Rabies Vaccine	899
Influenza Virus Vaccine, Trivalent, Types A & B (chromatograph- and filter-purified subvirion antigen) FluShield, 1996-1997 Formula	2842
IPOL Poliovirus Vaccine Inactivated	903
Pnu-Imune 23	1437
Rabies Vaccine, Imovax Rabies I.D.	901
Tetanus & Diphtheria Toxoids Adsorbed Purogenated	1446
Tetanus Toxoid Adsorbed Purogenated	1447
Tetramune	
TheraCys BCG Live (Intravesical)	911
TICE BCG, USP	1881
Tri-Immunol Adsorbed	1452
Tripedia	908

Fibrillation, atrial
Calan SR Caplets	2571
Calan Tablets	2568
Cardizem Injectable	1253
Cardizem Lyo-Ject Syringe	1253
Covera-HS Tablets	2573
Isoptin Injectable	1391
Isoptin Oral Tablets	1393
Isoptin SR Tablets	1395
Verelan Capsules	1455

Fibrillation, ventricular
Lanoxicaps	1110
Lanoxin Elixir Pediatric	1113
Lanoxin Injection	1116
Lanoxin Injection Pediatric	1119
Lanoxin Tablets	1121

Fibrosis, cavernosal
Caverject Injection	2064

Fibrosis, pulmonary
(see under Pulmonary fibrosis)

Fibrosis, unspecified
(see also under Fibrosis, cavernosal; Pulmonary fibrosis)
Sansert Tablets	2424

Fibrotic processes
(see under Fibrosis, cavernosal; Fibrosis, unspecified; Pulmonary fibrosis)

Fistula
Actigall Capsules	818
Cortifoam	2540

Flail chest
Dopram Injectable	2235

Fluid overload
Orthoclone OKT3 Sterile Solution	1892

Flutter, atrial
Calan SR Caplets	2571
Calan Tablets	2568
Cardizem Injectable	1253
Cardizem Lyo-Ject Syringe	1253
Covera-HS Tablets	2573
Isoptin Injectable	1391
Isoptin Oral Tablets	1393
Isoptin SR Tablets	1395
Verelan Capsules	1455

Fungal infections
(see under Actinomycosis, genital; Infection, fungal, unspecified; Infection, nasal, fungal; Infection, ophthalmic, fungal; Infection, otic, fungal; Infection, systemic, fungal; Lesions, skin, fungal)

G

Gallbladder disease, unspecified
(see also under Cholangitis; Cholecystitis; Obstruction, biliary tract)
Lopid Tablets	1974

Gangrene
Antilirium Injectable	1007

Gastric retention
Colyte and Colyte-flavored	2540
GoLYTELY	694
NuLYTELY	694
Tri-Levlen 28 Tablets	646

Gastroenteritis
Dulcolax Suppositories	883
Dulcolax Tablets	654

Gastrointestinal disorders
(see under Bleeding, gastrointestinal; Esophageal abnormalities, unspecified; Gastric retention; Gastroparesis, diabetic; Hernia, hiatal; Inflammation, gastrointestinal tract; Intestinal disorders, unspecified; Obstruction, gastrointestinal tract; Perforation, gastrointestinal tract; Spasms, gastrointestinal; Ulcer, gastrointestinal)

Gastrointestinal obstruction
(see under Obstruction, gastrointestinal tract)

Gastrointestinal perforation
(see under Perforation, gastrointestinal tract)

Gastroparesis, diabetic
K-Dur Microburst Release System (potassium chloride, USP) E.R. Tablets	1364
K-Tab Filmtab	439
K-Norm Capsules	1615
Micro-K	2237

General anesthesia
(see under Anesthesia, general)

Genital bleeding
(see under Bleeding, genital, abnormal)

Glaucoma, angle closure
Akineton	1380
Albalon Solution with Liquifilm	229
Ana-Kit Anaphylaxis Emergency Treatment Kit	611
Atamet Tablets	567
Ativan Injection	2805
Ativan Tablets	2807
Atrohist Pediatric Capsules	1603
Bromfed	1832
Claritin-D Tablets	2487
D.A. Chewable Tablets	970
D.A. II Tablets	972
Dizac (diazepam injectable emulsion) CIV	1862
Dura-Tap/PD Capsules	970
Dura-Vent/DA Tablets	972
EPIFRIN	237
Fedahist Gyrocaps	2545
GlaucTabs	209
Kemadrin Tablets	1105
Klonopin Tablets	2294
Larodopa Tablets	2296
Neo-Synephrine Hydrochloride (Ophthalmic)	2456
Novahistine Elixir	782
Paremyd	244
PBZ Tablets	863
PBZ-SR Tablets	862
Periactin	1767
Phospholine Iodide	323
Rondec Chewable Tablets	974
Rondec	974
Salagen Tablets	1546
Sinemet CR Tablets	961
Sinemet Tablets	959
Sus-Phrine Injection	1017
Tranxene	459
Trinalin Repetabs Tablets	1373
Valium Injectable	2336
Valium Tablets	2335
Versed Injection	2324
Xanax Tablets	2115

Glaucoma, angle closure, untreated
Ditropan	1267
Zonalon Cream	1042

Glaucoma, narrow angle
(see under Glaucoma, angle closure)

Glaucoma, open angle, untreated
Dizac (diazepam injectable emulsion) CIV	1862
Klonopin Tablets	2294
Valium Injectable	2336
Valium Tablets	2335
Versed Injection	2324
Xanax Tablets	2115

Glaucoma, pupillary block
Isopto Carpine Ophthalmic Solution	221

Glaucoma, unspecified
Adapin Capsules	1542
Adderall Tablets	2209
Adipex-P Tablets and Capsules	1035
Arco-Lase Plus Tablets	513
Atrohist Plus Tablets	1605
Bellergal-S Tablets	2375
Bentyl	1246
Bonine Tablets	1990
Bontril Slow-Release Capsules	786
Cystospaz	2123
Desoxyn Gradumet Tablets	422
Dexedrine	2648
DextroStat-Dextroamphetamine Sulfate Tablets	2211
Donnatal	2234
Donnatal Extentabs	2234
Donnatal Tablets	2234
Extendryl	1003
Fastin Capsules	2662
Inversine Tablets	1729
Ionamin Capsules	1615
ISPAN Perfluoropropane	267
ISPAN Sulfur Hexafluoride	266
Kutrase Capsules	2546
Levsin/Levsinex/Levbid	2549
Librax Capsules	2330
Midrin Capsules	788
Norflex	1554
Norgesic	1554
Ocusert Pilo-20 and Pilo-40 Ocular Therapeutic Systems	252
Pondimin Tablets	2239
Prelu-2 Timed Release Capsules	687
Pro-Banthine Tablets	2226
Ritalin	866
Robinul Forte Tablets	2247
Robinul Injectable	2247
Robinul Tablets	2247
Sanorex Tablets	2423
Sinequan	2028
Transderm Scōp Transdermal Therapeutic System	890
Unisom Nighttime Sleep Aid	1990
Unisom With Pain Relief-Nighttime Sleep Aid and Pain Reliever	1991
Urised Tablets	2123

Glomerulonephritis
Cortifoam	2540

Goiter
Quadrinal Tablets	1398

Gout, acute
Benemid Tablets	1651
ColBENEMID Tablets	1662
Pyrazinamide Tablets	1442
Rifater	1280

Granulocytopenia
Velban Vials	1537

Granulocytopenia, history of
Clozaril Tablets	2377

Guillain-Barre syndrome, history of
Influenza Virus Vaccine, Trivalent, Types A & B (chromatograph- and filter-purified subvirion antigen) FluShield, 1996-1997 Formula	2842

H

Head injury
(see also under Trauma, intracranial)
Dopram Injectable	2235
RMS Suppositories CII	2766
Roxanol	2365

Headache
(see under Headache, history of; Migraine, basilar; Migraine, hemiplegic)

Headache, history of
Parnate Tablets	2679

Hearing impairment
Platinol for Injection	717
Platinol-AQ Injection	719

Heart attack
(see under Myocardial infarction)

Heart block, first degree
Lopressor	848

Heart block, greater than first degree
Adenocard Injection	1021
Adenoscan	1022
Betagan	230
Betapace Tablets	637
Betimol 0.25%, 0.5%	259
Betoptic Ophthalmic Solution	465
Betoptic S Ophthalmic Suspension	467
Blocadren Tablets	1654
Brevibloc (esmolol HCl) Injection	1860
Calan SR Caplets	2571
Calan Tablets	2568
Cardizem CD Capsules	1251
Cardizem Injectable	1253
Cardizem Lyo-Ject Syringe	1253
Cardizem SR Capsules	1255
Cardizem Tablets	1257
Cartrol Tablets	413
Cerebyx Injection	1956
Cordarone Intravenous	2821
Cordarone Tablets	2818
Covera-HS Tablets	2573
Dilacor XR Extended-release Capsules	2183
Ethmozine Tablets	2217
Inderal Injectable	2834
Inderal LA Long Acting Capsules	2836
Inderal Tablets	2834
Inderide LA Long Acting Capsules	2840
Inderide Tablets	2838
Isoptin Injectable	1391
Isoptin Oral Tablets	1393
Isoptin SR Tablets	1395
Kerlone Tablets	2588
Levatol Tablets	2547
Lopressor	848
Lopressor HCT Tablets	850
Mexitil Capsules	684
Normodyne Injection	2519
Normodyne Tablets	2522
Norpace	2596
Ocupress Ophthalmic Solution, 1% Sterile	297
OptiPranolol (Metipranolol 0.3%) Sterile Ophthalmic Solution	256
Sectral Capsules	2914
Tambocor Tablets	1555
Tenoretic Tablets	2963
Tenormin Tablets and I.V. Injection	2965
Tiazac Capsules	1019
Timolide Tablets	1791
Timoptic in Ocudose	1796

Contraindications Index — **Hypertension**

Timoptic Sterile Ophthalmic
  Solution .... ⊙ 286
Timoptic-XE 1798
Tonocard Tablets 519
Toprol-XL Tablets 560
Trandate 1158
Verelan Capsules 1455
Visken Tablets 2428
Zebeta Tablets 1457
Ziac 1459

Heart block, sinoatrial
Cerebyx Injection 1956
Rythmol Tablets–150mg, 225mg,
  300mg 1399

Heart block, unspecified
Cardioquin Tablets 2146
Cerebyx Injection 1956
Decadron Phosphate with
  Xylocaine Injection, Sterile 1683
Ethmozine Tablets 2217
Flexeril Tablets 1701
Isuprel Injection 2441
Papaverine Hydrochloride Vials
  and Ampoules 1523
Primaxin I.M. 1770
Procanbid Extended-Release
  Tablets 1983
Quinaglute Dura-Tabs Tablets 644
Quinidex Extentabs 2240
Rythmol Tablets–150mg, 225mg,
  300mg 1399
Tambocor Tablets 1555

Heart damage
  (see under Cardiovascular
  disorders, unspecified)

Heart disease, ischemic
  (see also under Angina pectoris;
  Angina, unspecified; Ischemia,
  silent; Myocardial infarction)
Imitrex Injection 1095
Imitrex Tablets 1099

**Heart disease, mitral valvular,
rheumatic**
Apresazide Capsules 824
Apresoline Hydrochloride Tablets 826
Hydralazine Hydrochloride
  Injection USP 2712
Sansert Tablets 2424
Ser-Ap-Es Tablets 867

Heart disease, unspecified
  (see under Cardiovascular
  disorders, unspecified)

Heart disease, valvular
  (see also under Heart disease,
  mitral valvular, rheumatic)
Sansert Tablets 2424

Heart failure, unspecified
  (see also under Congestive heart
  failure, unspecified)
Albuminar-5, Albumin (Human)
  U.S.P. 5% 795
Albuminar-25, Albumin (Human)
  U.S.P. 25% 796
Betagan .... ⊙ 230
Betimol 0.25%, 0.5% .... ⊙ 259
Betoptic Ophthalmic Solution 465
Betoptic S Ophthalmic Suspension... 467
Blocadren Tablets 1654
Brevibloc (esmolol HCl) Injection ... 1860
Inversine Tablets 1729
ISMOTIC 45% w/v Solution .... ⊙ 221
Kerlone Tablets 2588
Lopressor 848
Lopressor HCT Tablets 850
Normodyne Injection 2519
Normodyne Tablets 2522
Ocupress Ophthalmic Solution,
  1% Sterile .... ⊙ 297
OptiPranolol (Metipranolol 0.3%)
  Sterile Ophthalmic Solution ..... ⊙ 256
Orthoclone OKT3 Sterile Solution ... 1892
OSMOGLYN Oral Osmotic Agent ... ⊙ 225
Plasma-Plex, Plasma Protein
  Fraction (Human),
  5% Solution Heat-Treated 806
RMS Suppositories CII 2766
Roxanol 2365
Sectral Capsules 2914
Tenoretic Tablets 2963
Tenormin Tablets and I.V. Injection 2965
Timolide Tablets 1791
Timoptic in Ocudose 1796

Timoptic Sterile Ophthalmic
  Solution .... ⊙ 286
Timoptic-XE 1798
Toprol-XL Tablets 560
Trandate 1158
Visken Tablets 2428
Zebeta Tablets 1457
Ziac 1459

Heat cramps
Polycitra-K Crystals 574
Polycitra-K Oral Solution 575
Rum-K Syrup 1004

Hematologic disorders
  (see under Bleeding disorders,
  unspecified; Blood dyscrasias,
  unspecified)

Hematopoietic disorders
  (see under Blood dyscrasias,
  unspecified; Bone marrow
  depression)

Hematuria
TICE BCG, USP 1881

Hemochromatosis
Chromagen Capsules 2470
Chromagen FA Capsules 2471
Chromagen Forte Capsules 2471
Natalins Rx Tablets 1599
Niferex 811
Niferex-150 Capsules 811
Trinsicon Capsules 2759

Hemophilia
Easprin 1971
Fiorinal Capsules 2388
Fiorinal with Codeine Capsules 2390

Hemorrhage
  (see under Bleeding disorders,
  unspecified; Bleeding tendencies;
  Bleeding, abnormal, unspecified;
  Bleeding, antepartum; Bleeding,
  gastrointestinal; Bleeding,
  gastrointestinal, history of;
  Bleeding, genital, abnormal;
  Bleeding, genitourinary; Bleeding,
  history of; Bleeding, internal,
  unspecified; Bleeding,
  intracranial; Bleeding, rectal;
  Bleeding, retinal; Bleeding,
  unspecified; Cardiovascular
  status, unstable in acute
  hemorrhage)

Hemorrhagic diathesis
  (see under Bleeding tendencies)

Hemorrhagic shock
Ana-Kit Anaphylaxis Emergency
  Treatment Kit 611

Hemosiderosis
Chromagen Capsules 2470
Chromagen FA Capsules 2471
Chromagen Forte Capsules 2471
Niferex 811
Niferex-150 Capsules 811
Trinsicon Capsules 2759

Hemostasis, incomplete
Toradol 2319

Hemostatic disorders
  (see under Bleeding disorders,
  unspecified)

Hepatic adenoma
  (see under Adenoma, hepatic)

Hepatic cancer
  (see under Carcinoma, hepatic)

Hepatic coma
  (see under Coma, hepatic)

Hepatic damage
  (see under Liver dysfunction)

Hepatic disease
  (see under Liver disease,
  unspecified)

Hepatic dysfunction
  (see under Liver dysfunction)

Hepatic failure
  (see under Liver failure)

Hepatic impairment
  (see under Liver dysfunction)

Hepatic injury
  (see under Liver dysfunction)

Hepatic insufficiency
  (see under Liver dysfunction)

Hepatic precoma
  (see under Precoma, hepatic)

Hepatitis
Aldoclor Tablets 1638
Aldomet Ester HCl Injection 1642
Aldomet Oral 1640
Aldoril Tablets 1644
Calcium Disodium Versenate
  Injection 1548
Dantrium Capsules 2131
Prodium 695
ReVia Tablets 957

Hepatitis, history of
Rifamate Capsules 1278
Solganal Suspension 2530

Hepatocellular failure
  (see under Liver failure)

Hernia, hiatal
Donnatal 2234
Donnatal Extentabs 2234
Donnatal Tablets 2234

Herpes genitalia
Prepidil Gel 2108

Herpes simplex keratitis
AK-CIDE .... ⊙ 203
AK-CIDE Ointment .... ⊙ 203
AK-PRED .... ⊙ 204
AK-Trol Ointment & Suspension ... ⊙ 205
Blephamide Liquifilm Sterile
  Ophthalmic Suspension 472
Blephamide Ointment .... ⊙ 234
Cortifoam 2540
Cortisporin Ophthalmic Ointment
  Sterile 1074
Cortisporin Ophthalmic Suspension
  Sterile 1075
Decadron Phosphate Sterile
  Ophthalmic Ointment 1684
Decadron Phosphate Sterile
  Ophthalmic Solution 1685
Dexacort Phosphate in Turbinaire... 1607
Econopred & Econopred Plus
  Ophthalmic Suspensions .... ⊙ 216
Eflone Sterile Ophthalmic
  Solution .... ⊙ 261
Flarex Ophthalmic Suspension .... ⊙ 217
FML Forte Liquifilm .... ⊙ 237
FML Liquifilm .... ⊙ 238
FML-S Liquifilm .... ⊙ 240
FML S.O.P. .... ⊙ 239
HMS Liquifilm .... ⊙ 241
Maxitrol Ophthalmic Ointment
  and Suspension .... ⊙ 222
NeoDecadron Sterile Ophthalmic
  Ointment 1755
NeoDecadron Sterile Ophthalmic
  Solution 1756
Poly-Pred Liquifilm .... ⊙ 246
Pred Forte .... ⊙ 247
Pred Mild .... ⊙ 250
Pred-G Liquifilm Sterile
  Ophthalmic Suspension .... ⊙ 248
Pred-G S.O.P. Sterile Ophthalmic
  Ointment .... ⊙ 249
Terra-Cortril Ophthalmic
  Suspension 2033
TobraDex Ophthalmic Suspension
  and Ointment 469
Vexol 1% Ophthalmic
  Suspension .... ⊙ 227

Herpes simplex, unspecified
Coly-Mycin S Otic w/Neomycin &
  Hydrocortisone 1965
Cortisporin Cream 1073
Cortisporin Ointment 1074
Cortisporin Otic Solution Sterile 1076
Cortisporin Otic Suspension Sterile 1077
Mantadil Cream 1124
Pediotic Suspension Sterile 1140
VoSoL HC Otic Solution 2786

Herpes zoster
Cosmegen Injection 1666

Hiatal hernia
  (see under Hernia, hiatal)

HIV
  (see under Human
  immunodeficiency virus)

Human immunodeficiency virus
  (see also under Acquired immune
  deficiency syndrome)
Attenuvax 1650
Biavax II 1653
M-R-VAX II 1732
Mumpsvax 1751
Orimune 1433
TICE BCG, USP 1881
Varivax 1807

Hyperammonemia
NephrAmine Injection 2169

Hypercalcemia
Calcijex Injection 412
Calphosan Injection 1234
DHT (Dihydrotachysterol) Tablets
  & Intensol 2351
Dovonex Cream 0.005% 2792
Dovonex Ointment 0.005% 2793
Ester-C Mineral Ascorbates
  Powder .... ▣ 673
Oxandrin 783
PhosLo Tablets 695
Rocaltrol Capsules 2303
Winstrol Tablets 2468

Hypercarbia
Levophed Bitartrate Injection 2445
OxyContin Tablets 2163

Hyperkalemia
Aldactazide Tablets 2556
Aldactone Tablets 2558
Dyazide Capsules 2653
Dyrenium Capsules 2655
K-Dur Microburst Release System
  (potassium chloride, USP) E.R.
  Tablets 1364
K-Lor Powder Packets 438
K-Phos Original Formula 'Sodium
  Free' Tablets 633
K-Tab Filmtab 439
K-Norm Capsules 1615
Micro-K 2237
Micro-K LS Packets 2238
Midamor Tablets 1746
Moduretic Tablets 1748
Polycitra-K Crystals 574
Polycitra-K Oral Solution 575
Rum-K Syrup 1004
Slow-K Extended-Release Tablets ... 869
Urocit-K Tablets 1828

Hyperphosphatemia
K-Phos Neutral Tablets 633
K-Phos Original Formula 'Sodium
  Free' Tablets 633
Uroqid-Acid No. 2 Tablets 633

Hypertension, compensatory
Hyperstat I.V. Injection 2504

**Hypertension, intracranial, history
of**
Norplant System 2868

Hypertension, malignant
Coumadin for Injection 941
Coumadin Tablets 941

Hypertension, pulmonary
Redux Capsules 2911
Yutopar Intravenous Injection 566

Hypertension, uncontrolled
Abbokinase 403
Abbokinase Open-Cath 405
Activase 1045
D.H.E. 45 Injection 2381
Eminase 2215
Epogen for Injection 489
Imitrex Tablets 1099
Parlodel 2411
Procrit for Injection 1896
ReoPro Vials 1526
Streptase for Infusion 557
Yutopar Intravenous Injection 566

Hypertension, unspecified
  (see also under Hypertensive
  disorders of pregnancy,
  unspecified)
Adderall Tablets 2209

(▣ Described in PDR For Nonprescription Drugs)   (⊙ Described in PDR For Ophthalmology)

Contraindications Index

Hypertension
- Adipex-P Tablets and Capsules ... 1035
- Atrohist Pediatric Capsules ... 1603
- Bellergal-S Tablets ... 2375
- Bontril Slow-Release Capsules ... 786
- Bromfed Capsules (Extended-Release) ... 1832
- Bromfed-DM Cough Syrup ... 1832
- Bromfed ... 1832
- Cafergot ... 2376
- Claritin-D Tablets ... 2487
- Cortifoam ... 2540
- D.A. Chewable Tablets ... 970
- D.A. II Tablets ... 972
- Deconsal II Tablets ... 1605
- Desoxyn Graduret Tablets ... 422
- Dexedrine ... 2648
- DextroStat-Dextroamphetamine Sulfate Tablets ... 2211
- Dimetane-DC Cough Syrup ... 2232
- Dimetane-DX Cough Syrup ... 2233
- Dopram Injectable ... 2235
- Dura-Tap/PD Capsules ... 970
- Dura-Vent Tablets ... 971
- Dura-Vent/DA Tablets ... 972
- Duratuss HD Elixir ... 2750
- Duratuss Tablets ... 2750
- Entex LA Tablets ... 972
- Entex PSE Tablets ... 973
- Ergomar Tablets ... 1543
- Exgest LA Tablets ... 787
- Extendryl ... 1003
- Fastin Capsules ... 2662
- Fedahist Gyrocaps ... 2545
- Guaifed ... 1833
- Guaimax-D Tablets ... 809
- Histussin D Liquid ... 670
- Hycomine Compound Tablets ... 948
- Hycomine ... 947
- Imitrex Injection ... 1095
- Inversine Tablets ... 1729
- Ionamin Capsules ... 1615
- Kronofed-A ... 994
- Marax Tablets & DF Syrup ... 2015
- Methergine ... 2401
- Midrin Capsules ... 788
- Neo-Synephrine Hydrochloride 1% Carpuject ... 2455
- Neo-Synephrine Hydrochloride 1% Injection ... 2455
- Novahistine DMX ... 782
- Novahistine Elixir ... 782
- Parnate Tablets ... 2679
- Phenergan VC ... 2886
- Phenergan VC with Codeine ... 2888
- Prelu-2 Timed Release Capsules ... 687
- Rondec Chewable Tablets ... 974
- Rondec ... 974
- Sansert Tablets ... 2424
- Seldane-D Extended-Release Tablets ... 1286
- Semprex-D Capsules ... 1620
- Solganal Suspension ... 2530
- Syn-Rx DM Tablets ... 1623
- Syn-Rx Tablets ... 1622
- Trinalin Repetabs Tablets ... 1373
- Vasoxyl Injection ... 1169
- Wigraine Tablets ... 1884

Hypertensive disorders of pregnancy, unspecified
- Parlodel ... 2411

Hyperthermia, malignant, history of
- Anectine ... 1062
- Suprane (desflurane, USP) ... 1865

Hyperthyroidism
(see also under Goiter; Thyrotoxicosis; Thyrotoxicosis, untreated)
- Adderall Tablets ... 2209
- Adipex-P Tablets and Capsules ... 1035
- Bontril Slow-Release Capsules ... 786
- Cortifoam ... 2540
- Desoxyn Graduret Tablets ... 422
- Dexedrine ... 2648
- DextroStat-Dextroamphetamine Sulfate Tablets ... 2211
- Extendryl ... 1003
- Fastin Capsules ... 2662
- Flexeril Tablets ... 1701
- Hycomine Compound Tablets ... 948
- Hycomine ... 947
- Ionamin Capsules ... 1615
- Marax Tablets & DF Syrup ... 2015
- Metrodin (urofollitropin for injection) ... 2616
- Prelu-2 Timed Release Capsules ... 687
- Trinalin Repetabs Tablets ... 1373
- Urecholine ... 1804
- Yutopar Intravenous Injection ... 566

Hypervitaminosis A
- Aquasol A Parenteral ... 526
- Aquasol A Vitamin A Capsules, USP ... 525

Hypervitaminosis D
(see also under Toxicity, vitamin D)
- DHT (Dihydrotachysterol) Tablets & Intensol ... 2351

Hypocalcemia
- Fosamax Tablets ... 1703

Hypogammaglobulinemia
(see also under Immunodeficiency, unspecified)
- Attenuvax ... 1650
- Biavax II ... 1653
- M-M-R II ... 1730
- M-R-VAX II ... 1732
- Meruvax II ... 1740
- Mumpsvax ... 1751
- Orimune ... 1433
- Varivax ... 1807

Hypoglycemia, functional
- Proglycem Suspension ... 575

Hypoglycemia, unspecified
- Humalog Injection ... 1488

Hypokalemia
- Daranide Tablets ... 1676
- Kayexalate ... 2444
- Sodium Polystyrene Sulfonate Suspension ... 2367

Hyponatremia
- Daranide Tablets ... 1676
- Lithium Carbonate Capsules & Tablets ... 2352

Hypoprothrombinemia
- Fiorinal Capsules ... 2388
- Fiorinal with Codeine Capsules ... 2390

Hypotension, history of
- Mivacron ... 1125

Hypotension, unspecified
- Calan SR Caplets ... 2571
- Calan Tablets ... 2568
- Cardizem CD Capsules ... 1251
- Cardizem Injectable ... 1253
- Cardizem Lyo-Ject Syringe ... 1253
- Cardizem SR Capsules ... 1255
- Cardizem Tablets ... 1257
- Covera-HS Tablets ... 2573
- Dilacor XR Extended-release Capsules ... 2183
- Isoptin Injectable ... 1391
- Isoptin Oral Tablets ... 1393
- Isoptin SR Tablets ... 1395
- Levoprome ... 1321
- Nicotinex Elixir ... 671
- Normodyne Injection ... 2519
- Normodyne Tablets ... 2522
- Rythmol Tablets–150mg, 225mg, 300mg ... 1399
- Tiazac Capsules ... 1019
- Trandate ... 1158
- Urecholine ... 1804
- Verelan Capsules ... 1455

Hypothalamic damage
- Etrafon ... 2495
- Trilafon ... 2532

Hypovolemia
(see also under Shock, unspecified)
- Levophed Bitartrate Injection ... 2445
- NephrAmine Injection ... 2169
- Yutopar Intravenous Injection ... 566

Hypoxia
- Levophed Bitartrate Injection ... 2445

I

IgA deficiencies, selective
(see under Immunoglobulin A deficiency)

Ileocolostomy
- Activase ... 1045
- CORTENEMA ... 2713
- Eminase ... 2215

Ileus, paralytic
- Cystospaz ... 2123
- Ditropan ... 1267
- Donnatal ... 2234
- Donnatal Extentabs ... 2234
- Donnatal Tablets ... 2234
- Kadian Capsules ... 2948
- Kutrase Capsules ... 2546
- Levsin/Levsinex/Levbid ... 2549
- MS Contin Tablets ... 2149
- MSIR ... 2152
- Oramorph SR (Morphine Sulfate Sustained Release Tablets) ... 2359
- OxyContin Tablets ... 2163
- Pro-Banthine Tablets ... 2226
- Robinul Forte Tablets ... 2247
- Robinul Injectable ... 2247
- Robinul Tablets ... 2247

Ileus, unspecified
(see also under Ileus, paralytic)
- Colyte and Colyte-flavored ... 2540
- GoLYTELY ... 694
- Tri-Levlen 28 Tablets ... 646
- Urispas Tablets ... 2710

Illness, unspecified
- Cholera Vaccine ... 2818

Immunodeficiency, family history of
- M-M-R II ... 1730
- Meruvax II ... 1740
- Mumpsvax ... 1751
- Orimune ... 1433

Immunodeficiency, history of
- Attenuvax ... 1650
- Biavax II ... 1653
- M-R-VAX II ... 1732
- Varivax ... 1807

Immunodeficiency, unspecified
(see also under Acquired immune deficiency syndrome; Dysgammaglobulinemia; Human immunodeficiency virus; Hypogammaglobulinemia; Immunodeficiency, family history of; Immunodeficiency, history of; Immunoglobulin A deficiency; Immunosuppression)
- Attenuvax ... 1650
- Biavax II ... 1653
- M-M-R II ... 1730
- M-R-VAX II ... 1732
- Meruvax II ... 1740
- Methotrexate Sodium Tablets, Injection, for Injection and LPF Injection ... 1322
- Mumpsvax ... 1751
- Orimune ... 1433
- Parlodel SnapTabs ... 2411
- TheraCys BCG Live (Intravesical) ... 911
- TICE BCG, USP ... 1881
- Varivax ... 1807
- Vivotif Berna ... 660

Immunodeficient state
(see under Immunodeficiency, unspecified)

Immunoglobulin A deficiency
- CytoGam ... 1630
- Gamimune N, 5% Immune Globulin Intravenous (Human), 5% ... 612
- Gamimune N, 10% Immune Globulin Intravenous (Human), 10% ... 615
- Gammar-P I.V., Immune Globulin Intravenous (Human) ... 798
- RespiGam ... 1631
- Sandoglobulin I.V. ... 2419

Immunosuppression
- Attenuvax ... 1650
- Biavax II ... 1653
- M-M-R II ... 1730
- M-R-VAX II ... 1732
- Meruvax II ... 1740
- Mumpsvax ... 1751
- Orimune ... 1433
- Pneumovax 23 ... 1768
- Solganal Suspension ... 2530
- TheraCys BCG Live (Intravesical) ... 911
- TICE BCG, USP ... 1881
- Varivax ... 1807
- Vivotif Berna ... 660

Impotence, treatment of
- Papaverine Hydrochloride Vials and Ampoules ... 1523

Impulse generation disorders
(see under Arrhythmia, cardiac, unspecified)

Increased intracranial pressure
(see under Intracranial pressure, increased)

Infants, newborn
- Atrohist Pediatric Suspension ... 1604
- Atrohist Pediatric Suspension Dye-Free ... 1604
- Bactrim DS Tablets ... 2257
- Bactrim I.V. Infusion ... 2255
- Bactrim ... 2257
- Benadryl Injection ... 1955
- Bentyl ... 1246
- Bromfed-DM Cough Syrup ... 1832
- Cardizem Injectable ... 1253
- Cardizem Lyo-Ject Syringe ... 1253
- Caverject Injection ... 2064
- Dimetane-DC Cough Syrup ... 2232
- Dimetane-DX Cough Syrup ... 2233
- Dopram Injectable ... 2235
- Fansidar Tablets ... 2281
- Fedahist Gyrocaps ... 2545
- Furoxone ... 2221
- Gantanol Tablets ... 2285
- Gantrisin ... 2286
- Lindane Shampoo USP 1% ... 483
- Macrobid Capsules ... 2138
- Macrodantin Capsules ... 2140
- Neo-Synephrine Hydrochloride (Ophthalmic) ... 2456
- Ornade Spansule Capsules ... 2678
- PBZ Tablets ... 863
- PBZ-SR Tablets ... 862
- Pediazole Suspension ... 2340
- Periactin ... 1767
- Robinul Injectable ... 2247
- Rynatan ... 2781
- Rynatuss Pediatric Suspension ... 2782
- Septra ... 1146
- Septra I.V. Infusion ... 1142
- Septra I.V. Infusion ADD-Vantage Vials ... 1144
- Septra ... 1146
- SSD ... 1402
- Tavist Syrup ... 2426
- Tigan Suppositories ... 2231

Infants, premature
- Benadryl Injection ... 1955
- Bromfed-DM Cough Syrup ... 1832
- Dimetane-DC Cough Syrup ... 2232
- Dimetane-DX Cough Syrup ... 2233
- Fedahist Gyrocaps ... 2545
- Kwell Cream & Lotion ... 2172
- Kwell Shampoo ... 2173
- Lindane Lotion USP 1% ... 481
- Ornade Spansule Capsules ... 2678
- PBZ Tablets ... 863
- PBZ-SR Tablets ... 862
- Periactin ... 1767
- SSD ... 1402
- Tavist Syrup ... 2426
- Tigan Suppositories ... 2231

Infection, bacterial, unspecified
(see also under Endocarditis, bacterial; Infection, skin, bacterial)
- Velban Vials ... 1537

Infection, febrile
- Attenuvax ... 1650
- Biavax II ... 1653
- M-M-R II ... 1730
- M-R-VAX II ... 1732
- Meruvax II ... 1740
- Mumpsvax ... 1751
- TheraCys BCG Live (Intravesical) ... 911
- Varivax ... 1807

Infection, fungal
(see under Actinomycosis, genital; Infection, fungal, unspecified; Infection, nasal, fungal; Infection, ophthalmic, fungal; Infection, otic, fungal; Infection, systemic, fungal; Lesions, skin, fungal)

Infection, fungal, unspecified
(see also under Actinomycosis, genital)
- Cortifoam ... 2540
- Eflone Sterile Ophthalmic Solution ... 261

(■ Described in PDR For Nonprescription Drugs)   (● Described in PDR For Ophthalmology)

Contraindications Index

Flarex Ophthalmic Suspension ...... ⊙ 217

Infection, mycobacterial
(see under Infection, ophthalmic, mycobacterial; Tuberculosis, unspecified)

Infection, nasal, fungal
Dexacort Phosphate in Turbinaire.... 1607

Infection, nasal, untreated
Nasarel Nasal Solution 2302

Infection, nasal, viral
Dexacort Phosphate in Turbinaire.... 1607

Infection, ophthalmic, cysticercosis
(see under Cysticercosis, ocular)

Infection, ophthalmic, fungal
AK-CIDE	⊙ 203
AK-CIDE Ointment	⊙ 203
AK-PRED	⊙ 204
AK-Trol Ointment & Suspension...	⊙ 205
Blephamide Liquifilm Sterile Ophthalmic Suspension	472
Blephamide Ointment	⊙ 234
Cortisporin Ophthalmic Ointment Sterile	1074
Cortisporin Ophthalmic Suspension Sterile	1075
Decadron Phosphate Sterile Ophthalmic Ointment	1684
Decadron Phosphate Sterile Ophthalmic Solution	1685
Econopred & Econopred Plus Ophthalmic Suspensions	⊙ 216
FML Forte Liquifilm	⊙ 237
FML Liquifilm	⊙ 238
FML-S Liquifilm	⊙ 240
FML S.O.P.	⊙ 239
HMS Liquifilm	⊙ 241
Maxitrol Ophthalmic Ointment and Suspension	⊙ 222
NeoDecadron Sterile Ophthalmic Ointment	1755
NeoDecadron Sterile Ophthalmic Solution	1756
Poly-Pred Liquifilm	⊙ 246
Pred Forte	⊙ 247
Pred Mild	⊙ 250
Pred-G Liquifilm Sterile Ophthalmic Suspension	⊙ 248
Pred-G S.O.P. Sterile Ophthalmic Ointment	⊙ 249
Terra-Cortril Ophthalmic Suspension	2033
TobraDex Ophthalmic Suspension and Ointment	469
Vexol 1% Ophthalmic Suspension	⊙ 227

Infection, ophthalmic, mycobacterial
(see also under Tuberculosis, unspecified)
AK-CIDE	⊙ 203
AK-CIDE Ointment	⊙ 203
AK-Trol Ointment & Suspension....	⊙ 205
Blephamide Liquifilm Sterile Ophthalmic Suspension	472
Blephamide Ointment	⊙ 234
Cortisporin Ophthalmic Ointment Sterile	1074
Cortisporin Ophthalmic Suspension Sterile	1075
Decadron Phosphate Sterile Ophthalmic Ointment	1684
Decadron Phosphate Sterile Ophthalmic Solution	1685
Econopred & Econopred Plus Ophthalmic Suspensions	⊙ 216
FML Forte Liquifilm	⊙ 237
FML Liquifilm	⊙ 238
FML S.O.P.	⊙ 239
HMS Liquifilm	⊙ 241
Maxitrol Ophthalmic Ointment and Suspension	⊙ 222
NeoDecadron Sterile Ophthalmic Ointment	1755
NeoDecadron Sterile Ophthalmic Solution	1756
Poly-Pred Liquifilm	⊙ 246
Pred Forte	⊙ 247
Pred Mild	⊙ 250
Pred-G Liquifilm Sterile Ophthalmic Suspension	⊙ 248
Pred-G S.O.P. Sterile Ophthalmic Ointment	⊙ 249
Terra-Cortril Ophthalmic Suspension	2033
TobraDex Ophthalmic Suspension and Ointment	469
Vexol 1% Ophthalmic Suspension	⊙ 227

Infection, ophthalmic, unspecified
(see under Cysticercosis, ocular; Dacryocystitis, chronic; Inflammation, eyelid; Iritis, acute)

Infection, ophthalmic, untreated
Flarex Ophthalmic Suspension	⊙ 217
Pred Forte	⊙ 247
Pred Mild	⊙ 250

Infection, ophthalmic, viral
(see also under Herpes simplex keratitis)
AK-CIDE	⊙ 203
AK-CIDE Ointment	⊙ 203
AK-PRED	⊙ 204
AK-Trol Ointment & Suspension...	⊙ 205
Blephamide Liquifilm Sterile Ophthalmic Suspension	472
Blephamide Ointment	⊙ 234
Cortisporin Ophthalmic Ointment Sterile	1074
Cortisporin Ophthalmic Suspension Sterile	1075
Decadron Phosphate Sterile Ophthalmic Ointment	1684
Decadron Phosphate Sterile Ophthalmic Solution	1685
Dexacort Phosphate in Turbinaire....	1607
Econopred & Econopred Plus Ophthalmic Suspensions	⊙ 216
Eflone Sterile Ophthalmic Solution	⊙ 261
Flarex Ophthalmic Suspension	⊙ 217
FML Forte Liquifilm	⊙ 237
FML Liquifilm	⊙ 238
FML S.O.P.	⊙ 239
HMS Liquifilm	⊙ 241
Maxitrol Ophthalmic Ointment and Suspension	⊙ 222
NeoDecadron Sterile Ophthalmic Ointment	1755
NeoDecadron Sterile Ophthalmic Solution	1756
Poly-Pred Liquifilm	⊙ 246
Pred Forte	⊙ 247
Pred Mild	⊙ 250
Pred-G Liquifilm Sterile Ophthalmic Suspension	⊙ 248
Pred-G S.O.P. Sterile Ophthalmic Ointment	⊙ 249
Terra-Cortril Ophthalmic Suspension	2033
TobraDex Ophthalmic Suspension and Ointment	469
Vexol 1% Ophthalmic Suspension	⊙ 227

Infection, otic
(see under Infection, otic, fungal; Otitis media)

Infection, otic, fungal
Decadron Phosphate Sterile Ophthalmic Solution 1685

Infection, penicillinase-producing organisms
Omnipen for Oral Suspension.......... 2873

Infection, respiratory
(see also under Bronchitis, chronic; Respiratory illness, febrile; Respiratory illness, unspecified; Tuberculosis, unspecified)
Typhoid Vaccine 2929

Infection, scalp
| Cormax Scalp Application | 1857 |
| Temovate Scalp Application | 1153 |

Infection, skin, bacterial
Mantadil Cream 1124

Infection, skin, fungal
(see under Lesions, skin, fungal)

Infection, skin, unspecified
Sotradecol (Sodium Tetradecyl Sulfate Injection)................................ 987

Infection, systemic, fungal
Celestone Soluspan Suspension	2484
CORTENEMA	2713
Cortifoam	2540

Infection, unspecified
Cortone Acetate Sterile Suspension	1663
Cortone Acetate Tablets	1664
Dalalone D.P. Injectable	1009
Decadron Elixir	1676
Decadron Phosphate Injection	1680
Decadron Phosphate with Xylocaine Injection, Sterile	1683
Decadron Tablets	1678
Decadron-LA Sterile Suspension	1687
Dexacort Phosphate in Respihaler	1606
Dexacort Phosphate in Turbinaire	1607
Florinef Acetate Tablets	506
Hydeltra-T.B.A. Sterile Suspension	1710
Hydeltrasol Injection, Sterile	1708
Hydrocortone Acetate Sterile Suspension	1712
Hydrocortone Phosphate Injection, Sterile	1713
Hydrocortone Tablets	1715
Pediapred Oral Solution	1618
Prelone Syrup	1834

Infection, unspecified
Astramorph/PF Injection, USP (Preservative-Free)	526
Cortifoam	2540
Diphtheria & Tetanus Toxoids Adsorbed Purogenated	1422
Diphtheria and Tetanus Toxoids and Pertussis Vaccine Adsorbed	2650
Fluorouracil Injection	2282
Sansert Tablets	2424
Scleromate Injection	1234
Sotradecol (Sodium Tetradecyl Sulfate Injection)	987
Sterile FUDR	2284
Tetanus & Diphtheria Toxoids Adsorbed Purogenated	1446
Tetanus Toxoid Adsorbed Purogenated	1447
Tetramune	1449
Tri-Immunol Adsorbed	1452
Tripedia	908
Typhoid Vaccine	2929

Infection, untreated
(see also under Infection, nasal, untreated; Infection, ophthalmic, untreated)
Eflone Sterile Ophthalmic Solution	⊙ 261
Flarex Ophthalmic Suspension	⊙ 217
Indocin I.V.	1727
Maxitrol Ophthalmic Ointment and Suspension	⊙ 222
Vexol 1% Ophthalmic Suspension	⊙ 227

Infection, urinary tract
(see also under Glomerulonephritis; Nephritis)
| TheraCys BCG Live (Intravesical) | 911 |
| TICE BCG, USP | 1881 |

Infection, vaginal
(see under Cervicitis, untreated; Vaginitis, untreated; Vaginosis, bacterial, untreated)

Infection, viral
(see under Herpes genitalia; Herpes simplex keratitis; Herpes simplex, unspecified; Herpes zoster; Human immunodeficiency virus; Infection, nasal, viral; Infection, ophthalmic, viral; Lesions, skin, viral; Varicella)

Infertility, non-anovulatory
Humegon for Injection	1873
Metrodin (urofollitropin for injection)	2616
Pergonal (menotropins for injection, USP)	2618

Infertility, non-hypogonadotropic
| Humegon for Injection | 1873 |
| Pergonal (menotropins for injection, USP) | 2618 |

Infertility, treatment of
Eltroxin Tablets	2214
Levothyroxine Sodium, USP for Injection	546
Synthroid	1410

Inflammation, eyelid
| Collagen Plugs (Intracanalicular) | ⊙ 275 |
| Herrick Lacrimal Plugs | ⊙ 275 |

Iritis

Inflammation, gastrointestinal tract
(see also under Abscess, intestinal; Colitis, toxic; Colitis, ulcerative; Colitis, ulcerative, history of; Colitis, unspecified; Colitis, unspecified, history of; Diverticulitis; Enteritis, history of; Enterocolitis, necrotizing; Enterocolitis, pseudomembranous; Esophagitis, reflux; Gastroenteritis; Ulcer, gastrointestinal)
Anturane	823
Ponstel	1982
Precose	604

Inflammation, local
Sarapin 1237

Inflammation, uveal
(see under Uveitis)

Inflammatory bowel disease
(see under Inflammation, gastrointestinal tract)

Intertriginous areas
(see under Intertrigo)

Intertrigo
Cordran Tape 1855

Intestinal atony
(see under Atony, intestinal)

Intestinal disorders, unspecified
(see also under Atony, intestinal; Bowel ischemia, history of; Inflammation, gastrointestinal tract; Megacolon, toxic; Megacolon, unspecified; Obstruction, gastrointestinal tract; Perforation, gastrointestinal tract)
Precose... 604

Intestinal obstruction
(see under Obstruction, gastrointestinal tract)

Intoxication, unspecified
Ultram Tablets (50 mg) 1594

Intracranial pressure, increased
Codiclear DH Syrup	808
Dilaudid Ampules	1382
Dilaudid Cough Syrup	1383
Dilaudid	1382
Hycomine Compound Tablets	948
Hycomine	947
Hycotuss Expectorant Syrup	950
Nitrostat Tablets	1981
RMS Suppositories CII	2766
Romazicon	2311
Roxanol	2365
Vicodin Tuss Expectorant	1406

Intracranial trauma
(see under Trauma, intracranial)

Intraspinal pressure, increased
RMS Suppositories CII 2766

Intravascular clotting process, active
(see under Coagulation, intravascular, active)

Intubation, history of
Proleukin for Injection 812

Iodism, history of
Norisodrine with Calcium Iodide Syrup 446

Iridocyclitis
(see also under Uveitis)
Humorsol Sterile Ophthalmic Solution 1707

Iritis, acute
(see also under Iridocyclitis; Uveitis)
Isopto Carbachol Ophthalmic Solution .... ⊙ 221

(▣ Described in PDR For Nonprescription Drugs)   (⊙ Described in PDR For Ophthalmology)

Contraindications Index

Iritis
- Isopto Carpine Ophthalmic Solution .... ⊙ 221
- Pilopine HS Ophthalmic Gel .... ⊙ 224
- Rev-Eyes Ophthalmic Eyedrops 0.5% .... ⊙ 324
- Salagen Tablets 1546

Ischemia, silent
- Imitrex Tablets 1099

Ischemia, unspecified
- Imitrex Injection 1095

Ischemic heart disease
(see under Heart disease, ischemic)

Ischemic myocardial disease
(see under Heart disease, ischemic)

J

Jaundice, cholestatic of pregnancy, history of
- Anturane Tablets 823
- Brevicon 2563
- Demulen 2580
- Desogen Tablets 1867
- Levlen/Tri-Levlen 646
- Lo/Ovral Tablets 2852
- Lo/Ovral-28 Tablets 2857
- Modicon 1928
- Nor-Q D Tablets 2598
- Nordette-21 Tablets 2863
- Nordette-28 Tablets 2866
- Norinyl 2563
- Ortho Tri-Cyclen 21 Tablets 1914
- Ortho Tri-Cyclen 28 Tablets 1914
- Ortho-Cept 21 Tablets 1907
- Ortho-Cept 28 Tablets 1907
- Ortho-Cyclen 21 Tablets 1914
- Ortho-Cyclen 28 Tablets 1914
- Ortho-Novum 1928
- Ovcon 765
- Ovral Tablets 2877
- Ovral-28 Tablets 2878
- Ovrette Tablets 2878
- Levlen/Tri-Levlen 646
- Tri-Norinyl 2607
- Triphasil-21 Tablets 2919
- Triphasil-28 Tablets 2924

Jaundice, history of
- Augmentin Chewable Tablets 2637
- Augmentin Powder for Oral Suspension 2637
- Augmentin Tablets 2640
- Brevicon 2563
- Cognex Capsules 1961
- Demulen 2580
- Desogen Tablets 1867
- Levlen/Tri-Levlen 646
- Lo/Ovral Tablets 2852
- Lo/Ovral-28 Tablets 2857
- Modicon 1928
- Nor-Q D Tablets 2598
- Nordette-21 Tablets 2863
- Nordette-28 Tablets 2866
- Norinyl 2563
- Ortho Tri-Cyclen 21 Tablets 1914
- Ortho Tri-Cyclen 28 Tablets 1914
- Ortho-Cept 21 Tablets 1907
- Ortho-Cept 28 Tablets 1907
- Ortho-Cyclen 21 Tablets 1914
- Ortho-Cyclen 28 Tablets 1914
- Ortho-Novum 1928
- Ovcon 765
- Ovral Tablets 2877
- Ovral-28 Tablets 2878
- Ovrette Tablets 2878
- Torecan 2367
- Levlen/Tri-Levlen 646
- Tri-Norinyl 2607
- Triphasil-21 Tablets 2919
- Triphasil-28 Tablets 2924

Jaundice, unspecified
- Lomotil 2591
- Motofen Tablets 789

K

Keratitis, dendritic
(see under Herpes simplex keratitis)

Ketoacidosis, diabetic
- Amaryl Tablets 1241
- DiaBeta Tablets 1265
- Diabinese Tablets 2002
- Glucophage Tablets 754
- Glucotrol Tablets 2011
- Glucotrol XL Extended Release Tablets 2012
- Glynase PresTab Tablets 2091
- Micronase Tablets 2099
- Precose 604

Kidney damage
(see under Renal dysfunction)

Kidney disease
(see under Renal disease, unspecified)

Kidney failure
(see under Renal failure)

Kidney stones, uric acid
- Benemid Tablets 1651
- ColBENEMID Tablets 1662

Kyphoscoliosis
- Dilaudid Ampules 1382
- Dilaudid Cough Syrup 1383
- Dilaudid 1382

L

Labor
- Dilaudid-HP Injection 1384
- Dilaudid-HP Lyophilized Powder 250mg 1384
- Dilaudid Tablets and Liquid 1386
- Macrobid Capsules 2138
- Macrodantin Capsules 2140
- Sus-Phrine Injection 1017
- Toradol 2319

Labor, difficult, history of
- Prepidil Gel 2108

Labored breathing
(see under Dyspnea)

Lactation
(see under Breastfeeding)

Left ventricular dysfunction
(see under Ventricular dysfunction, left)

Lesions, gastrointestinal, unspecified
(see also under Colitis, ulcerative; Colitis, ulcerative, history of; Ulcer, gastrointestinal)
- Fiorinal Capsules 2388
- Fiorinal with Codeine Capsules 2390
- Urecholine 1804
- Urispas Tablets 2710

Lesions, intracranial, unspecified
(see also under Prolactinoma, pituitary; Tumor, intracranial, unspecified; Tumor, pituitary, unspecified)
- Clomid 1262
- Dilaudid Ampules 1382
- Dilaudid Cough Syrup 1383
- Dilaudid 1382
- Genotropin Injection 2090
- Humatrope Vials 1490
- Humegon for Injection 1873
- Hycomine Compound Tablets 948
- Hycomine 947
- Hycotuss Expectorant Syrup 950
- Metrodin (urofollitropin for injection) 2616
- Pergonal (menotropins for injection, USP) 2618
- Serophene (clomiphene citrate tablets, USP) 2621
- Vicodin Tuss Expectorant 1406

Lesions, malignant, unspecified
(see also under Carcinoma, breast, history of; Carcinoma, breast, male; Carcinoma, breast, unspecified; Carcinoma, cervical; Carcinoma, endometrium; Carcinoma, female reproductive organs; Carcinoma, female reproductive organs, history of; Carcinoma, genital, unspecified; Carcinoma, hepatic; Carcinoma, prostate; Carcinoma, skin, unspecified; Carcinoma, squamous cell, unspecified; Melanoma, history of; Melanoma, unspecified; Neoplasm, bone marrow system, malignant; Neoplasm, lymphatic system, malignant)
- Bichloracetic Acid Kahlenberg 1233

Lesions, premalignant
- Bichloracetic Acid Kahlenberg 1233

Lesions, skin, fungal
- Cortisporin Cream 1073
- Cortisporin Ointment 1074

Lesions, skin, unspecified
(see also under Birthmarks; Burns; Melanoma, unspecified; Moles; Warts, atypical)
- Atamet Tablets 567
- Cordran Tape 1855
- Larodopa Tablets 2296
- Sinemet CR Tablets 961
- Sinemet Tablets 959

Lesions, skin, viral
(see also under Herpes genitalia; Herpes simplex, unspecified; Herpes zoster; Varicella)
- Cortisporin Cream 1073
- Cortisporin Ointment 1074

Leukemia, acute
- Myleran Tablets 1209

Leukemia, chronic lymphocytic
- Myleran Tablets 1209

Leukemia, chronic myelogenous, blastic crisis
- Myleran Tablets 1209

Leukemia, unspecified
- Attenuvax 1650
- Biavax II 1653
- Caverject Injection 2064
- M-M-R II 1730
- M-R-VAX II 1732
- Meruvax II 1740
- Mumpsvax 1751
- Orimune 1433
- ParaGard T 380A Intrauterine Copper Contraceptive 1936
- TICE BCG, USP 1881
- Varivax 1807

Leukoderma, infectious
- Trisoralen Tablets 1309

Leukopenia
- Hydrea Capsules 705
- Methotrexate Sodium Tablets, Injection, for Injection and LPF Injection 1322

Liver adenoma
(see under Adenoma, hepatic)

Liver cancer
(see under Carcinoma, hepatic)

Liver damage
(see under Liver dysfunction)

Liver disease, history of
(see also under Hepatitis, history of; Liver dysfunction, history of)
- Nardil 1977

Liver disease, unspecified
(see also under Cirrhosis, primary biliary; Cirrhosis, unspecified; Hepatitis; Liver dysfunction)
- Aldoclor Tablets 1638
- Aldomet Ester HCl Injection 1642
- Aldomet Oral 1640
- Aldoril Tablets 1644
- Amen Tablets 785
- Aygestin Tablets 990
- Cholestin Capsules 2985
- Clomid 1262
- Cycrin Tablets 991
- Dantrium Capsules 2131
- Depakene 416
- Depakote Tablets 418
- Depo-Provera Contraceptive Injection 2079
- Depo-Provera Sterile Aqueous Suspension 2083
- Dyrenium Capsules 2655
- GlaucTabs .... ⊙ 209
- Halotestin Tablets 2095
- Klonopin Tablets 2294
- Lescol Capsules 2395
- Levoprome 1321
- Methotrexate Sodium Tablets, Injection, for Injection and LPF Injection 1322
- Mevacor Tablets 1742
- Micronor Tablets 1903
- Midrin Capsules 788
- Norplant System 2868
- Nydrazid Injection 509
- Pravachol Tablets 770
- Premphase 2900
- Prempro 2905
- Prostin E2 Suppository 2109
- Provera Tablets 2110
- Rifamate Capsules 1278
- Rifater 1280
- Serophene (clomiphene citrate tablets, USP) 2621
- Uroqid-Acid No. 2 Tablets 633
- Zocor Tablets 1821

Liver disorders, history of
- Aldoclor Tablets 1638
- Aldomet Ester HCl Injection 1642
- Aldomet Oral 1640
- Aldoril Tablets 1644
- Augmentin Chewable Tablets 2637
- Augmentin Powder for Oral Suspension 2637
- Felbatol 2774

Liver disorders, unspecified
(see under Liver dysfunction)

Liver dysfunction
(see also under Jaundice, cholestatic of pregnancy, history of; Jaundice, history of; Jaundice, unspecified; Liver disease, unspecified; Liver failure; Obstruction, biliary tract; Serum transaminase elevation)
- Amen Tablets 785
- Atromid-S Capsules 2808
- Aygestin Tablets 990
- Bellergal-S Tablets 2375
- Cafergot 2376
- Cycrin Tablets 991
- Cylert Tablets 415
- Danocrine Capsules 2437
- Daranide Tablets 1676
- Depakene 416
- Depakote Tablets 418
- Depo-Provera Contraceptive Injection 2079
- Depo-Provera Sterile Aqueous Suspension 2083
- D.H.E. 45 Injection 2381
- Ergomar Tablets 1543
- Estratest 2718
- Etrafon 2495
- Fansidar Tablets 2281
- Fiorinal with Codeine Capsules 2390
- GlaucTabs .... ⊙ 209
- Helidac Therapy 2135
- Lopid Tablets 1974
- Nydrazid Injection 509
- Peganone Tablets 455
- Phenobarbital Elixir and Tablets 1523
- Premphase 2900
- Prempro 2905
- Prolixin 510
- Provera Tablets 2110
- Pyrazinamide Tablets 1442
- Rifater 1280
- Sansert Tablets 2424
- Seconal Sodium Pulvules 1529
- Seldane Tablets 1284
- Seldane-D Extended-Release Tablets 1286
- Skelaxin Tablets 793
- Solganal Suspension 2530
- Stelazine 2692
- Thioplex (Thiotepa For Injection) 1329
- Ticlid Tablets 2317
- Trecator-SC Tablets 2919
- Trilafon 2532
- Wigraine Tablets 1884
- Yodoxin Tablets 1235

(▣ Described in PDR For Nonprescription Drugs)   (⊙ Described in PDR For Ophthalmology)

1600

1601 **Contraindications Index** **Neoplasm**

Liver dysfunction, history of (see also under Liver disease, history of)
Augmentin Tablets 2640
Clomid 1262
Nydrazid Injection 509
Rifamate Capsules 1278
Serophene 2621

Liver failure (see also under Coma, hepatic; Liver dysfunction; Precoma, hepatic)
Aldactazide Tablets 2556
Fulvicin P/G 165 & 330 Tablets 2500
Fulvicin P/G Tablets 2499
Grifulvin V Microsize 1944
Gris-PEG Tablets 476
ReVia Tablets 957

Liver function tests, abnormal (see under Serum transaminase elevation)

Liver insufficiency (see under Liver dysfunction)

Liver tumor (see under Adenoma, hepatic; Carcinoma, hepatic; Tumor, liver, benign; Tumor, liver, benign, history of)

Local anesthesia (see under Anesthesia, local)

Lown-Ganong-Levine syndrome
Calan SR Caplets 2571
Calan Tablets 2568
Covera-HS Tablets 2573
Isoptin Injectable 1391
Isoptin Oral Tablets 1393
Isoptin SR Tablets 1395
Verelan Capsules 1455

Lung disease, unspecified (see under Pulmonary disorders, unspecified)

Lupus erythematosus
8-MOP Capsules 1294
Flagyl 375 Capsules 2587
Fototar Cream 1300
Myochrysine Injection 1754
Oxsoralen Lotion 1% 1301
Oxsoralen-Ultra Capsules 1302
Procanbid Extended-Release Tablets 1983
Solganal Suspension 2530
Trisoralen Tablets 1309

Lymphoma (see also under Neoplasm, lymphatic system, malignant)
Attenuvax 1650
Biavax II 1653
M-M-R II 1730
M-R-VAX II 1732
Meruvax II 1740
Mumpsvax 1751
Orimune 1433
TICE BCG, USP 1881
Varivax 1807

M

Malignancy (see under Carcinoma, breast, history of; Carcinoma, breast, male; Carcinoma, breast, unspecified; Carcinoma, endometrium; Carcinoma, hepatic; Carcinoma, hepatic, history of; Carcinoma, prostate; Carcinoma, skin, unspecified; Hypertension, malignant; Hyperthermia, malignant, history of; Lesions, malignant, unspecified; Leukemia, unspecified; Lymphoma; Malignancy, generalized; Melanoma, history of; Melanoma, unspecified; Metastasis, bone; Neoplasm, bone marrow system, malignant; Neoplasm, lymphatic system, malignant)

Malignancy, generalized
Orimune 1433

Malignant lesions, unspecified (see under Lesions, malignant, unspecified)

Malnutrition
Fluorouracil Injection 2282
Sterile FUDR 2284

Mechanical disorders of ventilation (see under Asthma, acute; Asthma, history of; Asthma, unspecified; Flail chest; Obstruction, respiratory tract; Paresis, respiratory; Pneumothorax; Pulmonary fibrosis)

Megacolon, toxic
Colyte and Colyte-flavored 2540
Cystospaz 2123
Ditropan 1267
Donnatal 2234
Donnatal Extentabs 2234
Donnatal Tablets 2234
GoLYTELY 694
Kutrase Capsules 2546
Levsin/Levsinex/Levbid 2549
NuLYTELY 694
Pro-Banthine Tablets 2226
Robinul Injectable 2247
Tri-Levlen 28 Tablets 646

Megacolon, unspecified
Akineton 1380
Ditropan 1267

Megaloblastic anemia (see under Anemia, megaloblastic, unspecified)

Melanoma, history of
8-MOP Capsules 1294
Atamet Tablets 567
Flagyl 375 Capsules 2587
Larodopa Tablets 2296
Oxsoralen Lotion 1% 1301
Oxsoralen-Ultra Capsules 1302
Sinemet CR Tablets 961

Melanoma, unspecified
8-MOP Capsules 1294
Flagyl 375 Capsules 2587
Oxsoralen Lotion 1% 1301
Oxsoralen-Ultra Capsules 1302
Sinemet Tablets 959

Meningitis
Novocain Hydrochloride for Spinal Anesthesia 2457

Mental depression (see under Depression, mental; Depression, mental, history of)

Metabolic acidosis (see under Acidosis, hyperchloremic; Acidosis, metabolic, unspecified; Ketoacidosis, diabetic)

Metastasis, bone
Calphosan Injection 1234

Migraine, basilar
Imitrex Injection 1095

Migraine, hemiplegic
Imitrex Injection 1095

Moles
Podocon-25 1949

Motor neuron injury
Anectine 1062

Multipara, grand
Prepidil Gel 2108

Multipara, unspecified
Cervidil 1008

Myasthenia gravis
Bentyl 1246
Cardioquin Tablets 2146
Cortifoam 2540
Cystospaz 2123
Ditropan 1267
Donnatal 2234
Donnatal Extentabs 2234
Donnatal Tablets 2234
Kutrase Capsules 2546
Levsin/Levsinex/Levbid 2549
Norflex 1554
Norgesic 1554
Pro-Banthine Tablets 2226
Quinaglute Dura-Tabs Tablets 644
Quinidex Extentabs 2240
Robinul Forte Tablets 2247
Robinul Injectable 2247
Robinul Tablets 2247

Mycobacterial infection (see under Infection, ophthalmic, mycobacterial; Tuberculosis, unspecified)

Myeloid blasts, leukemic (see also under Leukemia, chronic myelogenous, blastic crisis)
Leukine 1317

Myeloma, multiple
Caverject Injection 2064

Myeloproliferative disorders (see also under Leukemia, acute; Leukemia, chronic lymphocytic; Leukemia, chronic myelogenous, blastic crisis; Leukemia, unspecified; Myeloma, multiple)
Clozaril Tablets 2377

Myelosuppression (see under Bone marrow depression)

Myocardial damage (see under Cardiovascular disorders, unspecified)

Myocardial disease (see under Cardiovascular disorders, unspecified)

Myocardial infarction
Anafranil Capsules 819
Asendin Tablets 1419
Cardizem CD Capsules 1251
Cardizem SR Capsules 1255
Cardizem Tablets 1257
Demulen 2580
Dilacor XR Extended-release Capsules 2183
Elavil 2945
Etrafon 2495
Flexeril Tablets 1701
Inversine Tablets 1729
Levothroid Tablets 1015
Levoxyl Tablets 918
Limbitrol 2333
Ludiomil Tablets 861
Nitrostat Tablets 1981
Norpramin Tablets 1273
Pamelor 2409
Regitine Vials 864
Surmontil Capsules 2917
Tiazac Capsules 1019
Tofranil Ampuls 873
Tofranil Tablets 875
Tofranil-PM Capsules 876
Triavil Tablets 1800
Vivactil Tablets 1820

Myocardial infarction, history of
Demulen 2580
Imitrex Injection 1095
Imitrex Tablets 1099
Proleukin for Injection 812
Regitine Vials 864

Myopathy, skeletal muscle, history of
Anectine 1062

N

Narcotic dependence
ReVia Tablets 957

Narcotic withdrawal, acute
ReVia Tablets 957

Narrow angle glaucoma (see under Glaucoma, angle closure)

Narrow angles
AKPRO ⊙ 206
Ditropan 1267
Paremyd ⊙ 244
PROPINE with C CAP Compliance Cap ⊙ 251

Necrosis (see also under Enterocolitis, necrotizing; Gangrene)
Urocit-K Tablets 1828

Neonates (see under Infants, newborn)

Neonates, premature (see under Infants, premature)

Neoplasia, estrogen dependent (see under Neoplasm, estrogen dependent)

Neoplasia, hepatic (see under Adenoma, hepatic; Carcinoma, hepatic; Tumor, liver, benign)

Neoplasia, unspecified (see under Neoplasm, unspecified)

Neoplasm, androgen dependent (see also under Carcinoma, prostate; Tumor, hormone dependent)
Pregnyl for Injection 1878
Profasi (chorionic gonadotropin for injection, USP) 2620

Neoplasm, bone marrow system, malignant (see also under Myeloid blasts, leukemic; Myeloma, multiple)
Attenuvax 1650
Biavax II 1653
M-M-R II 1730
M-R-VAX II 1732
Meruvax II 1740
Mumpsvax 1751
Varivax 1807

Neoplasm, estrogen dependent (see also under Carcinoma, breast, male; Carcinoma, breast, unspecified; Tumor, hormone dependent)
Brevicon 2563
Climara Transdermal System 640
Demulen 2580
Desogen Tablets 1867
Diethylstilbestrol Tablets 1477
Estrace Cream and Tablets 751
Estraderm Transdermal System 842
ESTRATAB Tablets (0.3, 0.625, 1.25, 2.5 mg) 2715
Estratest 2718
Estring Vaginal Ring 2086
Levlen/Tri-Levlen 646
Lo/Ovral Tablets 2852
Lo/Ovral-28 Tablets 2857
Menest Tablets 2671
Modicon 1928
Nor-Q D Tablets 2598
Nordette-21 Tablets 2863
Nordette-28 Tablets 2866
Norinyl 2563
Ogen Tablets 2103
Ogen Vaginal Cream 2106
Ortho Dienestrol Cream 1922
Ortho Tri-Cyclen 21 Tablets 1914
Ortho Tri-Cyclen 28 Tablets 1914
Ortho-Cept 21 Tablets 1907
Ortho-Cept 28 Tablets 1907
Ortho-Cyclen 21 Tablets 1914
Ortho-Cyclen 28 Tablets 1914
Ortho-Est 1925
Ortho-Novum 1928
Ovcon 765
Ovral Tablets 2877
Ovral-28 Tablets 2878
Ovrette Tablets 2878
PMB 200 and PMB 400 2890
Premarin Intravenous 2893

(▣ Described in PDR For Nonprescription Drugs) (⊙ Described in PDR For Ophthalmology)

Neoplasm — Contraindications Index — 1602

Neoplasm
Premarin Tablets	2896
Premarin Vaginal Cream	2898
Premphase	2900
Prempro	2905
Levlen/Tri-Levlen	646
Tri-Norinyl	2607
Triphasil-21 Tablets	2919
Triphasil-28 Tablets	2924
Vivelle Transdermal System	880

Neoplasm, estrogen dependent, history of
(see also under Carcinoma, breast, history of)
Demulen	2580

Neoplasm, hepatic, history of
(see under Carcinoma, hepatic, history of; Tumor, liver, benign, history of)

Neoplasm, hepatic, unspecified
(see under Adenoma, hepatic; Carcinoma, hepatic; Carcinoma, hepatic, history of; Tumor, liver, benign; Tumor, liver, benign, history of)

Neoplasm, intracranial
(see under Tumor, intracranial, unspecified)

Neoplasm, lymphatic system, malignant
(see also under Lymphoma)
Attenuvax	1650
Biavax II	1653
M-M-R II	1730
M-R-VAX II	1732
Meruvax II	1740
Mumpsvax	1751
Varivax	1807

Neoplasm, ovarian
(see under Cysts, ovarian)

Neoplasm, unspecified
Nutropin	1049
Nutropin AQ Injection	1051
Protropin	1053
Scleromate Injection	1234
Sotradecol (Sodium Tetradecyl Sulfate Injection)	987

Neoplastic activity, unspecified
(see under Neoplasm, unspecified; Tumor activity, unspecified)

Nephritis
(see also under Glomerulonephritis)
Winstrol Tablets	2468

Nephropathy, diabetic
Midamor Tablets	1746
Moduretic Tablets	1748

Nephrosis
Oxandrin	783
Winstrol Tablets	2468

Neuritis, optic
Myambutol Tablets	1432

Neurologic toxicity
(see under Toxicity, neurologic)

Neurological disorders, unspecified
(see also under Central nervous system depression; Cerebral vascular disease; Cerebral vascular disease, history of; Cerebrovascular accident; Cerebrovascular accident, history of; Charcot-Marie-Tooth syndrome; Convulsive disorders; Convulsive disorders, history of; Depression, mental; Depression, mental, history of; Encephalopathy, history of; Epilepsy; Epilepsy, uncontrolled; Guillain-Barre syndrome, history of; Intracranial pressure, increased; Myasthenia gravis; Parkinsonism; Psychosis; Psychosis, toxic, history of; Psychosis, unsupervised; Seizure disorders, history of; Seizure disorders, unspecified; Seizure disorders, untreated; Senility; Senility, unsupervised; Tourette's syndrome; Toxicity, neurologic; Vagotonia)
Fluvirin (Influenza Virus Vaccine)	1608

Neurological signs, unspecified, history of
Acel-Imune Diphtheria and Tetanus Toxoids and Acellular Pertussis Vaccine Adsorbed	1415
Diphtheria & Tetanus Toxoids Adsorbed Purogenated	1422
Fluvirin (Influenza Virus Vaccine)	1608
Pnu-Imune 23	1437
Tetanus & Diphtheria Toxoids Adsorbed Purogenated	1446
Tetanus Toxoid Adsorbed Purogenated	1447
Tetramune	1449
Tri-Immunol Adsorbed	1452
Tripedia	908

Neurological symptoms, unspecified, history of
Acel-Imune Diphtheria and Tetanus Toxoids and Acellular Pertussis Vaccine Adsorbed	1415
Diphtheria & Tetanus Toxoids Adsorbed Purogenated	1422
Fluvirin (Influenza Virus Vaccine)	1608
Pnu-Imune 23	1437
Tetanus & Diphtheria Toxoids Adsorbed Purogenated	1446
Tetanus Toxoid Adsorbed Purogenated	1447
Tetramune	1449
Tri-Immunol Adsorbed	1452
Tripedia	908

Neutropenia
Taxol Injection	723
Ticlid Tablets	2317

Nursing mothers
(see under Breastfeeding)

O

Obesity, therapy of
Eltroxin Tablets	2214
Levothyroxine Sodium, USP for Injection	546
Synthroid	1410

Obstetric emergency
(see under Emergency, obstetric)

Obstetrics
(see under Delivery, unspecified; Labor)

Obstruction, biliary tract
(see also under Jaundice, cholestatic of pregnancy, history of; Jaundice, history of; Jaundice, unspecified)
Actigall Capsules	818
Questran	774

Obstruction, bladder neck
Cystospaz	2123
Donnatal	2234
Donnatal Extentabs	2234
Donnatal Tablets	2234
Levsin/Levsinex/Levbid	2549
Librax Capsules	2330
Norflex	1554
Norgesic	1554
PBZ Tablets	863
PBZ-SR Tablets	862
Periactin	1767
Pro-Banthine Tablets	2226
Robinul Forte Tablets	2247
Robinul Injectable	2247
Robinul Tablets	2247
Urecholine	1804
Urised Tablets	2123

Obstruction, gastrointestinal tract
(see also under Achalasia, esophageal; Achalasia, unspecified; Bowel ischemia, history of; Fecal impaction; Ileus, paralytic; Ileus, unspecified; Obstruction, pyloroduodenal; Stenosis, pyloric; Stenosis, pyloroduodenal; Stricture, esophageal)
Akineton	1380
Antilirium Injectable	1007
Azulfidine	2059
Bentyl	1246
CITRUCEL Orange Flavor	■□ 770
CITRUCEL Sugar Free Orange Flavor	■□ 770
Colyte and Colyte-flavored	2540
Cortifoam	2540
Cystospaz	2123
Ditropan	1267
Donnatal	2234
Donnatal Extentabs	2234
Donnatal Tablets	2234
Dulcolax Suppositories	883
GoLYTELY	694
K-Norm Capsules	1615
Konsyl Fiber Tablets	■□ 679
Konsyl Powder Sugar Free Unflavored	■□ 680
Kutrase Capsules	2546
Levsin/Levsinex/Levbid	2549
Mestinon Injectable	1300
Mestinon	1300
Metamucil	2125
Micro-K	2237
Norflex	1554
Norgesic	1554
NuLYTELY	694
PBZ Tablets	863
PBZ-SR Tablets	862
Precose	604
Pro-Banthine Tablets	2226
Propulsid	1346
Prostigmin Injectable	1305
Prostigmin Tablets	1306
Reglan	2243
Robinul Forte Tablets	2247
Robinul Injectable	2247
Robinul Tablets	2247
Slow-K Extended-Release Tablets	869
Tensilon Injectable	1307
Tri-Levlen 28 Tablets	646
Unifiber	1845
Urecholine	1804
Urised Tablets	2123
Urispas Tablets	2710

Obstruction, pulmonary
Daranide Tablets	1676

Obstruction, pyloroduodenal
Periactin	1767

Obstruction, respiratory tract
(see also under Obstruction, pulmonary)
Astramorph/PF Injection, USP (Preservative-Free)	526
Daranide Tablets	1676
Dopram Injectable	2235
Duramorph Injection	983
Phenobarbital Elixir and Tablets	1523
Seconal Sodium Pulvules	1529

Obstruction, urinary tract
(see also under Obstruction, bladder neck; Obstruction, urogenital tract; Prostatic hypertrophy; Urinary retention)
Azulfidine	2059
Bentyl	1246
Cystospaz	2123
Ditropan	1267
Donnatal	2234
Donnatal Extentabs	2234
Donnatal Tablets	2234
Kutrase Capsules	2546
Levsin/Levsinex/Levbid	2549
Mestinon Injectable	1300
Mestinon	1300
Pro-Banthine Tablets	2226
Prostigmin Injectable	1305
Prostigmin Tablets	1306
Robinul Forte Tablets	2247
Robinul Injectable	2247
Robinul Tablets	2247
Tensilon Injectable	1307
Urecholine	1804
Urispas Tablets	2710

Obstruction, urogenital tract
(see also under Obstruction, urinary tract)
Antilirium Injectable	1007

Obstructive uropathy
(see under Obstruction, urinary tract)

Obtundation
Etrafon	2495
Trilafon	2532

Occlusion, coronary
(see under Coronary occlusion)

Occlusion, deep vein
Scleromate Injection	1234
Sotradecol (Sodium Tetradecyl Sulfate Injection)	987

Ocular herpes simplex
(see under Herpes simplex keratitis)

Oliguria
Edecrin	1698
Hespan Injection	945
Macrobid Capsules	2138
Macrodantin Capsules	2140
Pentaspan Injection	954
Polycitra Syrup	574
Polycitra-K Crystals	574
Polycitra-K Oral Solution	575
Polycitra-LC	574

Ophthalmic changes
(see under Retinal changes; Visual field changes)

Opioid dependence
(see under Narcotic dependence)

Opioid withdrawal
(see under Narcotic withdrawal, acute)

Optic neuritis
(see under Neuritis, optic)

Organ allograft
Proleukin for Injection	812

Organic brain damage
(see under Brain damage)

Organic heart disease
(see under Cardiovascular disorders, unspecified; Heart disease, ischemic; Heart disease, mitral valvular, rheumatic)

Osteoporosis
Cortifoam	2540

Otic infection, fungal
(see under Infection, otic, fungal)

Otitis media
Cerumenex Drops	2148

Ovarian enlargement, unspecified
Clomid	1262
Humegon for Injection	1873
Metrodin (urofollitropin for injection)	2616
Pergonal (menotropins for injection, USP)	2618
Serophene (clomiphene citrate tablets, USP)	2621

Ovarian failure, primary
Humegon for Injection	1873
Metrodin (urofollitropin for injection)	2616
Pergonal (menotropins for injection, USP)	2618

Overt cardiac failure
(see under Heart failure, unspecified)

P

Pain, acute
Duragesic Transdermal System	1336

Pain, intermittent
Duragesic Transdermal System	1336

(■□ Described in PDR For Nonprescription Drugs)   (◉ Described in PDR For Ophthalmology)

1603 Contraindications Index Pregnancy

Pain, mild
Duragesic Transdermal System 1336

Pain, post operative
Duragesic Transdermal System 1336

Pancreatic diseases, unspecified
Pancrease MT Capsules 1589
Ultrase Capsules 2476
Ultrase MT Capsules 2477

Pancreatitis
Actigall Capsules 818
CREON 5 Capsules 2714
CREON 10 Capsules 2714
CREON 20 Capsules 2714
Elspar 1700
Oncaspar 2194
Pancrease MT Capsules 1589
Secretin-Ferring 2991
Ultrase Capsules 2476
Ultrase MT Capsules 2477

Pancreatitis, history of
Elspar 1700
Oncaspar 2194

Pap smear abnormality
ParaGard T 380A Intrauterine Copper Contraceptive 1936

Paracervical block anesthesia (see under Anesthesia, obstetrical, paracervical block)

Paralytic ileus (see under Ileus, paralytic)

Paresis, respiratory
Dopram Injectable 2235

Parkinson's disease (see under Parkinsonism)

Parkinsonism
Haldol Decanoate 1587
Haldol Injection, Tablets and Concentrate 1585
Urecholine 1804

Pelvic inflammatory disease
ParaGard T 380A Intrauterine Copper Contraceptive 1936
Prostin E2 Suppository 2109

Pelvic inflammatory disease, history of
ParaGard T 380A Intrauterine Copper Contraceptive 1936

Penile deformation (see under Angulation, penile; Fibrosis, cavernosal; Peyronie's disease)

Peptic ulcer (see under Ulcer, peptic)

Perforation, gastrointestinal tract (see also under Ulcer, gastrointestinal)
Colyte and Colyte-flavored 2540
Cortifoam 2540
GoLYTELY 694
NuLYTELY 694
Propulsid 1346
Reglan 2243
Toradol 2319
Tri-Levlen 28 Tablets 646

Perforation, gastrointestinal tract, history of
Proleukin for Injection 812

Perforation, intestinal (see under Perforation, gastrointestinal tract)

Pericardial effusion
Coumadin for Injection 941
Coumadin Tablets 941

Pericardial tamponade
Nitro-Bid IV 1270

Pericardial tamponade, history of
Proleukin for Injection 812

Pericarditis, constrictive
Nitro-Bid IV 1270

Pericarditis, unspecified
Coumadin for Injection 941
Coumadin Tablets 941

Peripheral arterial disease (see under Peripheral vascular disease)

Peripheral vascular disease (see also under Arteriosclerosis, unspecified; Arteritis, luetic; Raynaud's disease; Thromboangiitis obliterans; Thrombophlebitis)
Bellergal-S Tablets 2375
Cafergot 2376
D.H.E. 45 Injection 2381
Ergomar Tablets 1543
Ethyl Chloride, U.S.P. 1040
Fluori-Methane 1040
Phenergan VC 2886
Phenergan VC with Codeine 2888
Sansert Tablets 2424
Wigraine Tablets 1884

Peripheral vascular insufficiency (see under Peripheral vascular disease)

Peritonitis
Cortifoam 2540
Prostigmin Injectable 1305
Prostigmin Tablets 1306
Urecholine 1804

Pernicious anemia (see under Anemia, pernicious)

Peyronie's disease
Caverject Injection 2064

Pheochromocytoma
Esimil Tablets 840
Glucagon for Injection Vials and Emergency Kit 1485
Hylorel Tablets 1613
Ismelin Tablets 845
Nardil 1977
Parnate Tablets 2679
Reglan 2243
Yutopar Intravenous Injection 566

Phlebitis (see also under Thrombophlebitis)
Sansert Tablets 2424
Sotradecol (Sodium Tetradecyl Sulfate Injection) 987

Phosphate stones, infected
K-Phos Neutral Tablets 633
K-Phos Original Formula 'Sodium Free' Tablets 633

Photosensitivity diseases, unspecified (see also under Albinism; Lupus erythematosus; Porphyria cutanea tarda; Porphyria, acute; Porphyria, erythropoietic; Porphyria, unspecified; Xeroderma pigmentosum)
8-MOP Capsules 1294
Flagyl 375 Capsules 2587
Fototar Cream 1300
Oxsoralen Lotion 1% 1301
Oxsoralen-Ultra Capsules 1302
Trisoralen Tablets 1309

Photosensitivity, history of
pHisoHex 2458

Pituitary function, normal, male
Humegon for Injection 1873
Pergonal (menotropins for injection, USP) 2618

Placenta previa
Prepidil Gel 2108
Syntocinon Injection 2425

Platelet dysfunction, unspecified (see under Thrombocytopathy, unspecified)

Pneumothorax
Dopram Injectable 2235

Poliomyelitis outbreak
Diphtheria & Tetanus Toxoids Adsorbed Purogenated 1422
Diphtheria and Tetanus Toxoids and Pertussis Vaccine Adsorbed .. 2650
Tetanus & Diphtheria Toxoids Adsorbed Purogenated 1446
Tetanus Toxoid Adsorbed Purogenated 1447
Tetramune 1449
Tri-Immunol Adsorbed 1452
Tripedia 908

Poor nutritional state (see under Electrolyte imbalance, uncorrected; Malnutrition)

Porphyria cutanea tarda
8-MOP Capsules 1294
Flagyl 375 Capsules 2587
Oxsoralen-Ultra Capsules 1302

Porphyria, acute
Donnatal 2234
Donnatal Extentabs 2234
Donnatal Tablets 2234
Miltown Tablets 2780
PMB 200 and PMB 400 2890
Soma Compound Tablets 2783
Soma Compound w/Codeine Tablets 2784
Soma Tablets 2782

Porphyria, erythropoietic
8-MOP Capsules 1294
Flagyl 375 Capsules 2587
Oxsoralen-Ultra Capsules 1302

Porphyria, history of
Phenobarbital Elixir and Tablets 1523
Seconal Sodium Pulvules 1529

Porphyria, unspecified
Axocet Capsules 2469
Azulfidine 2059
Bellergal-S Tablets 2375
Butisol Sodium Elixir & Tablets 2768
Danocrine Capsules 2437
Esgic-plus 1012
Fioricet Tablets 2386
Fioricet with Codeine Capsules 2387
Fiorinal Capsules 2388
Fiorinal with Codeine Capsules 2390
Fulvicin P/G 165 & 330 Tablets 2500
Fulvicin P/G Tablets 2499
Grifulvin V (griseofulvin tablets) Microsize (griseofulvin oral suspension) Microsize 1944
Gris-PEG Tablets, 125 mg & 250 mg 476
Mebaral Tablets 2452
Mysoline 2860
Nembutal Sodium Capsules 440
Nembutal Sodium Solution 442
Nembutal Sodium Suppositories 444
Oxsoralen Lotion 1% 1301
Phrenilin 790
Placidyl Capsules 456
Trisoralen Tablets 1309

Porphyria, variegate
8-MOP Capsules 1294
Flagyl 375 Capsules 2587
Oxsoralen-Ultra Capsules 1302

PR Syndrome, short
Cardizem Injectable 1253
Cardizem Lyo-Ject Syringe 1253

Precocious puberty
Pregnyl for Injection 1878
Profasi (chorionic gonadotropin for injection, USP) 2620

Precoma, hepatic
Mykrox Tablets 1617
Zaroxolyn Tablets 1625

Preeclampsia
Coumadin for Injection 941
Coumadin Tablets 941
Parlodel 2411
Yutopar Intravenous Injection 566

Pregnancy
Accutane Capsules 2252
Android Capsules, 10 mg 1297
Aquasol A Parenteral 526
Atarax Tablets & Syrup 1992
Atrohist Plus Tablets 1605
Atromid-S Capsules 2808
Attenuvax 1650
Azathioprine Tablets 2349
Bactrim DS Tablets 2257
Bactrim I.V. Infusion 2255
Bactrim 2257
Bellergal-S Tablets 2375
Biavax II 1653
Brevicon 2563
Cafergot 2376
Casodex Tablets 2934
Cholestin Capsules 2985
Climara Transdermal System 640
Clomid 1262
ColBENEMID Tablets 1662
Cortifoam 2540
Coumadin for Injection 941
Coumadin Tablets 941
Cuprimine Capsules 1673
Cytotec 2576
Dalmane Capsules 2329
Danocrine Capsules 2437
Demulen 2580
Depen Titratable Tablets 2770
Depo-Provera Contraceptive Injection 2079
Depo-Provera Sterile Aqueous Suspension 2083
Desogen Tablets 1867
D.H.E. 45 Injection 2381
Diethylstilbestrol Tablets 1477
Doral Tablets 2773
Efudex 2280
Ergomar Tablets 1543
Estrace Cream and Tablets 751
Estraderm Transdermal System 842
ESTRATAB Tablets (0.3, 0.625, 1.25, 2.5 mg) 2715
Estratest 2718
Estring Vaginal Ring 2086
Fansidar Tablets 2281
Flagyl 375 Capsules 2587
Fluoroplex Topical Solution & Cream 1% 475
Fulvicin P/G 165 & 330 Tablets 2500
Fulvicin P/G Tablets 2499
Gantanol Tablets 2285
Gantrisin 2286
Grifulvin V (griseofulvin tablets) Microsize (griseofulvin oral suspension) Microsize 1944
Gris-PEG Tablets, 125 mg & 250 mg 476
Guaifed 1833
Halcion Tablets 2093
Halotestin Tablets 2095
Helidac Therapy 2135
Humegon for Injection 1873
Humorsol Sterile Ophthalmic Solution 1707
Hycamtin for Injection 2665
Imuran Injection 1103
Imuran Tablets 1103
Lescol Capsules 2395
Levlen/Tri-Levlen 646
Lo/Ovral Tablets 2852
Lo/Ovral-28 Tablets 2857
Lupron Depot 3.75 mg 2739
Lupron Depot 7.5 mg 2741
Lupron Depot--3 Month 22.5 mg 2743
Lupron Depot-PED 7.5 mg, 11.25 mg and 15 mg 2744
Lupron Injection 2736
Lupron Injection Pediatric 2737
M-M-R II 1730
M-R-VAX II 1732
Macrobid Capsules 2138
Macrodantin Capsules 2140
Marax Tablets & DF Syrup 2015
Megace Oral Suspension 708
Menest Tablets 2671
Menomune-A/C/Y/W-135 906
Meruvax II 1740
Methergine 2401
Methotrexate Sodium Tablets, Injection, for Injection and LPF Injection 1322
Metrodin (urofollitropin for injection) 2616
Mevacor Tablets 1742
Micronor Tablets 1903
Mithracin 599
Modicon 1928
Mumpsvax 1751
Nor-Q D Tablets 2598
Nordette-21 Tablets 2863
Nordette-28 Tablets 2866
Norinyl 2563
Norisodrine with Calcium Iodide Syrup 446
Norplant System 2868
Ogen Tablets 2103
Ogen Vaginal Cream 2106
Ortho Dienestrol Cream 1922
Ortho Tri-Cyclen 21 Tablets 1914
Ortho Tri-Cyclen 28 Tablets 1914
Ortho-Cept 21 Tablets 1907
Ortho-Cept 28 Tablets 1907

Pregnancy — Contraindications Index — 1604

Ortho-Cyclen 21 Tablets ... 1914
Ortho-Cyclen 28 Tablets ... 1914
Ortho-Est ... 1925
Ortho-Novum ... 1928
Orthoclone OKT3 Sterile Solution ... 1892
Ovcon ... 765
Ovral Tablets ... 2877
Ovral-28 Tablets ... 2878
Ovrette Tablets ... 2878
Oxandrin ... 783
ParaGard T 380A Intrauterine Copper Contraceptive ... 1936
Parlodel ... 2411
Pediazole Suspension ... 2340
Pergonal (menotropins for injection, USP) ... 2618
PMB 200 and PMB 400 ... 2890
Podocon-25 ... 1949
Pravachol Tablets ... 770
Premarin Intravenous ... 2893
Premarin Tablets ... 2896
Premarin Vaginal Cream ... 2898
Premphase ... 2900
Prempro ... 2905
Profasi (chorionic gonadotropin for injection, USP) ... 2620
Proscar Tablets ... 1784
ProSom Tablets ... 457
Protostat Tablets ... 1939
Quadrinal Tablets ... 1398
Restoril Capsules ... 2413
Sansert Tablets ... 2424
Septra ... 1146
Septra I.V. Infusion ... 1142
Septra I.V. Infusion ADD-Vantage Vials ... 1144
Septra ... 1146
Serophene (clomiphene citrate tablets, USP) ... 2621
Eldopaque/Eldoquin/Solaquin/Viquin ... 1299
Solganal Suspension ... 2530
SSD ... 1402
Sultrin ... 1941
Supprelin Injection ... 2230
Synarel Nasal Solution for Central Precocious Puberty ... 2603
Synarel Nasal Solution for Endometriosis ... 2605
Tegison Capsules ... 2314
Testoderm Testosterone Transdermal System ... 486
TICE BCG, USP ... 1881
Torecan ... 2367
Levlen/Tri-Levlen ... 646
Tri-Norinyl ... 2607
Triphasil-21 Tablets ... 2919
Triphasil-28 Tablets ... 2924
Unisom Nighttime Sleep Aid ... 1990
Unisom With Pain Relief-Nighttime Sleep Aid and Pain Reliever ... 1991
Urobiotic-250 Capsules ... 2038
Varivax ... 1807
Viquin Forte 4% Cream ... 1299
Virazole ... 1310
Vistaril Capsules ... 2042
Vistaril Intramuscular Solution ... 2042
Vistaril Oral Suspension ... 2042
Vivelle Transdermal System ... 880
Wigraine Tablets ... 1884
Winstrol Tablets ... 2468
Zocor Tablets ... 1821
Zoladex ... 2976
Zoladex 3-month ... 2978

Pregnancy, diagnostic test for
Amen Tablets ... 785
Aygestin Tablets ... 990
Cycrin Tablets ... 991
Depo-Provera Contraceptive Injection ... 2079
Depo-Provera Sterile Aqueous Suspension ... 2083
Megace Oral Suspension ... 708
Megace Tablets ... 710
Premphase ... 2900
Prempro ... 2905
Provera Tablets ... 2110

Presentation, non-vertex
Prepidil Gel ... 2108

Presentation, unfavorable
Syntocinon Injection ... 2425

Proctitis, history of
Indocin Suppositories ... 1723

Prolactinoma, pituitary (see also under Tumor, intracranial, unspecified)
Lutrepulse for Injection ... 998

Proliferative vitreoretinopathy
ISPAN Perfluoropropane ... ◉ 267
ISPAN Sulfur Hexafluoride ... ◉ 266

Prostate enlargement (see under Prostatic hypertrophy)

Prostatic hypertrophy
Arco-Lase Plus Tablets ... 513
Bonine Tablets ... 1990
Congess ... 1003
Donnatal ... 2234
Donnatal Extentabs ... 2234
Donnatal Tablets ... 2234
Entex PSE Tablets ... 973
Guaimax-D Tablets ... 809
Librax Capsules ... 2330
Norflex ... 1554
Norgesic ... 1554
PBZ Tablets ... 863
PBZ-SR Tablets ... 862
Periactin ... 1767
Pro-Banthine Tablets ... 2226
Robinul Forte Tablets ... 2247
Robinul Injectable ... 2247
Robinul Tablets ... 2247
Unisom Nighttime Sleep Aid ... 1990
Unisom With Pain Relief-Nighttime Sleep Aid and Pain Reliever ... 1991

Protoporphyria (see under Porphyria, erythropoietic)

Pruritus
Ergomar Tablets ... 1543

Pseudomembranous enterocolitis (see under Enterocolitis, pseudomembranous)

Psoriasis, acute
Dritho-Scalp 0.25%, 0.5% ... 921
Drithocreme 0.1%, 0.25%, 0.5%, 1.0% (HP) ... 920

Psoriatic eruptions, acute (see under Psoriasis, acute)

Psychic disturbances (see under Psychosis)

Psychosis
Antabuse Tablets ... 2802
Cortifoam ... 2540
Hydergine ... 2392
Pondimin Tablets ... 2239
Serax Capsules ... 2916
Serax Tablets ... 2916
Seromycin Capsules ... 975

Psychosis, toxic, history of
Proleukin for Injection ... 812

Psychosis, unsupervised
Coumadin for Injection ... 941
Coumadin Tablets ... 941

Pulmonary atresia (see under Atresia, pulmonary)

Pulmonary congestion (see also under Edema, pulmonary)
Cardizem CD Capsules ... 1251
Cardizem SR Capsules ... 1255
Cardizem Tablets ... 1257
Dilacor XR Extended-release Capsules ... 2183
Tiazac Capsules ... 1019

Pulmonary disorders, unspecified (see also under Asthma, acute; Asthma, unspecified; Atresia, pulmonary; Bronchitis, chronic; Chronic obstructive pulmonary disease; Cor pulmonale; Dyspnea; Edema, pulmonary; Emphysema; Hypertension, pulmonary; Obstruction, pulmonary; Pulmonary congestion; Pulmonary fibrosis; Pulmonary function test, abnormal; Respiratory tract conditions, lower; Tuberculosis, unspecified)
Adenoscan ... 1022
Novahistine Elixir ... ▣ 782
Prostin E2 Suppository ... 2109
Sansert Tablets ... 2424

Pulmonary edema (see under Edema, pulmonary)

Pulmonary emphysema (see under Emphysema)

Pulmonary fibrosis
Dopram Injectable ... 2235
Ridaura Capsules ... 2691

Pulmonary function test, abnormal
Proleukin for Injection ... 812

Pulmonary hypertension (see under Hypertension, pulmonary)

Pyloroduodenal obstruction (see under Obstruction, pyloroduodenal)

Pyloroduodenal stenosis (see under Stenosis, pyloroduodenal)

Q

Q-T interval prolongation
Betapace Tablets ... 637
Norpace ... 2596
Orap Tablets ... 1037

R

Radiation therapy
Leukine ... 1317
Orimune ... 1433
Pneumovax 23 ... 1768
Solganal Suspension ... 2530
TICE BCG, USP ... 1881

Radiotherapy (see under Radiation therapy)

Rash (see also under Dermatitis)
Cortifoam ... 2540

Raynaud's disease
Ergomar Tablets ... 1543

Rectal bleeding (see under Bleeding, rectal)

Renal decompensation (see under Renal failure)

Renal disease, unspecified (see also under Glomerulonephritis; Nephritis; Nephropathy, diabetic; Nephrosis; Renal dysfunction)
Calcium Disodium Versenate Injection ... 1548
Desferal Vials ... 838
Dyrenium Capsules ... 2655
Fleet Phospho-Soda ... 1002
GlaucTabs ... ◉ 209
Glucophage Tablets ... 754
Halotestin Tablets ... 2095
Hespan Injection ... 945
Levoprome ... 1321
Lithium Carbonate Capsules & Tablets ... 2352
Midrin Capsules ... 788
Novacet Lotion ... 1041
PASER Granules ... 1333
Pentaspan Injection ... 954
Ponstel ... 1982
Prostin E2 Suppository ... 2109
Robaxin Injectable ... 2245
Solganal Suspension ... 2530
Sulfacet-R Lotion ... 925
Sulfacet-R Tint Free Lotion ... 925
Sultrin ... 1941
Yocon Tablets ... 1235
Yohimex Tablets ... 1414

Renal dysfunction (see also under Anuria; Oliguria; Renal disease, unspecified; Renal failure; Uremia)
Aldactazide Tablets ... 2556
Aldactone Tablets ... 2558
Atromid-S Capsules ... 2808
Bellergal-S Tablets ... 2375
Bicitra ... 573
Cafergot ... 2376
Cuprimine Capsules ... 1673
Danocrine Capsules ... 2437
Depen Titratable Tablets ... 2770
D.H.E. 45 Injection ... 2381
Didronel I.V. Infusion ... 1545
Dyazide Capsules ... 2653
Dyrenium Capsules ... 2655
Ergomar Tablets ... 1543
Fansidar Tablets ... 2281
Ganite ... 2711
GlaucTabs ... ◉ 209
Glucophage Tablets ... 754
Helidac Therapy ... 2135
Indocin I.V. ... 1727
Inversine Tablets ... 1729
K-Phos Neutral Tablets ... 633
K-Phos Original Formula 'Sodium Free' Tablets ... 633
Lopid Tablets ... 1974
Macrobid Capsules ... 2138
Macrodantin Capsules ... 2140
Midamor Tablets ... 1746
Moduretic Tablets ... 1748
Nalfon 200 Pulvules & Nalfon Tablets ... 933
Platinol for Injection ... 717
Platinol-AQ Injection ... 719
Polycitra Syrup ... 574
Polycitra-K Crystals ... 574
Polycitra-K Oral Solution ... 575
Polycitra-LC ... 574
Prodium ... 695
Pyridium ... 1985
Robaxin Injectable ... 2245
Rum-K Syrup ... 1004
Sansert Tablets ... 2424
Seromycin Capsules ... 975
Skelaxin Tablets ... 793
Thioplex (Thiotepa For Injection) ... 1329
Toradol ... 2319
Uroqid-Acid No. 2 Tablets ... 633
Wigraine Tablets ... 1884

Renal dysfunction, history of
Cuprimine Capsules ... 1673
Proleukin for Injection ... 812

Renal excretory function impairment (see under Renal dysfunction)

Renal failure (see also under Renal dysfunction)
Daranide Tablets ... 1676
Oretic Tablets ... 450
Urocit-K Tablets ... 1828

Renal impairment (see under Renal dysfunction)

Renal insufficiency (see under Renal dysfunction)

Respiratory depression
Codiclear DH Syrup ... 808
Dilaudid Ampules ... 1382
Dilaudid Cough Syrup ... 1383
Dilaudid-HP Injection ... 1384
Dilaudid-HP Lyophilized Powder 250mg ... 1384
Dilaudid ... 1382
Dilaudid Oral Liquid ... 1386
Dilaudid ... 1382
Dilaudid Tablets - 8 mg ... 1386
Dilaudid Tablets 2 mg and 4 mg ... 1382
Hycomine Compound Tablets ... 948
Hycomine ... 947
Hycotuss Expectorant Syrup ... 950
Kadian Capsules ... 2948
MS Contin Tablets ... 2149
MSIR ... 2152
Oramorph SR (Morphine Sulfate Sustained Release Tablets) ... 2359
OxyContin Tablets ... 2163
RMS Suppositories CII ... 2766
Roxanol ... 2365
Vicodin Tuss Expectorant ... 1406

Respiratory depression, history of
Mivacron ... 1125

Respiratory disease, unspecified (see under Respiratory illness, febrile; Respiratory illness, unspecified)

Respiratory disorders (see under Bronchospastic disorders, unspecified; Infection,

(▣ Described in PDR For Nonprescription Drugs) (◉ Described in PDR For Ophthalmology)

1605 **Contraindications Index** **Surgery**

respiratory; Obstruction, respiratory tract; Pulmonary disorders, unspecified; Respiratory depression; Respiratory illness, unspecified; Respiratory tract conditions, lower)

Respiratory distress (see under Asthma, acute; Dyspnea; Respiratory depression)

Respiratory illness, febrile
Attenuvax 1650
Biavax II 1653
M-M-R II 1730
M-R-VAX II 1732
Meruvax II 1740
Mumpsvax 1751
Varivax 1807

Respiratory illness, unspecified (see also under Infection, respiratory; Pulmonary disorders, unspecified; Respiratory illness, febrile)
Adenoscan 1022
Bonine Tablets 1990
Dopram Injectable 2235
Phenobarbital Elixir and Tablets 1523
Scleromate Injection 1234
Seconal Sodium Pulvules 1529
Sotradecol (Sodium Tetradecyl Sulfate Injection) 987
Unisom Nighttime Sleep Aid 1990
Unisom With Pain Relief-Nighttime Sleep Aid and Pain Reliever 1991

Respiratory insufficiency, unspecified (see also under Obstruction, respiratory tract; Pulmonary disorders, unspecified; Respiratory illness, febrile; Respiratory illness, unspecified)
Roxanol 2365

Respiratory obstruction (see under Obstruction, respiratory tract)

Respiratory tract conditions, lower (see also under Pulmonary disorders, unspecified)
Bromfed-DM Cough Syrup 1832
Dimetane-DC Cough Syrup 2232
Dimetane-DX Cough Syrup 2233
PBZ Tablets 863
PBZ-SR Tablets 862
Phenergan Suppositories 2882
Phenergan Syrup 2881
Phenergan Tablets 2882
Phenergan VC 2886
Phenergan VC with Codeine 2888
Phenergan with Codeine 2883
Phenergan with Dextromethorphan 2885
Tavist Tablets 2427
Trinalin Repetabs Tablets 1373

Retinal changes
Aralen Hydrochloride Injection 2430
Aralen Phosphate Tablets 2431
Plaquenil Sulfate Tablets 2459

Retinal degeneration, peripheral
ISPAN Perfluoropropane .... ◉ 267
ISPAN Sulfur Hexafluoride .... ◉ 266

S

SA block (see under Heart block, sinoatrial)

Sarcoidosis
Calphosan Injection 1234

Scabies, Norwegian
Kwell Cream & Lotion 2172
Lindane Lotion USP 1% 481

Seizure disorders, history of (see also under Convulsive disorders, history of)
Acel-Imune Diphtheria and Tetanus Toxoids and Acellular Pertussis Vaccine Adsorbed 1415
Diphtheria and Tetanus Toxoids and Pertussis Vaccine Adsorbed .. 2650
Orthoclone OKT3 Sterile Solution 1892
Proleukin for Injection 812
Tetramune 1449
Tri-Immunol Adsorbed 1452

Seizure disorders, unspecified (see also under Convulsive disorders; Epilepsy; Epilepsy, uncontrolled; Status epilepticus)
Kwell Cream & Lotion 2172
Kwell Shampoo 2173
Lindane Lotion USP 1% 481
Lindane Shampoo USP 1% 483
Ludiomil Tablets 861
Reglan 2243
Wellbutrin Tablets 1177

Seizure disorders, untreated (see also under Epilepsy, uncontrolled)
Quibron 2227
Respbid Tablets 687
Slo-bid Gyrocaps 2201
Theo-Dur Extended-Release Tablets 1367
Theo-X Extended-Release Tablets 793
Uni-Dur Extended-Release Tablets .. 1374

Seizures, history of (see under Seizure disorders, history of)

Senility
Scleromate Injection 1234

Senility, unsupervised
Coumadin for Injection 941
Coumadin Tablets 941

Sepsis (see also under Toxemia)
Bellergal-S Tablets 2375
Cafergot 2376
D.H.E. 45 Injection 2381
Ergomar Tablets 1543
Novocain Hydrochloride for Spinal Anesthesia 2457
Scleromate Injection 1234
Sotradecol (Sodium Tetradecyl Sulfate Injection) 987
Wigraine Tablets 1884

Septicemia (see under Sepsis)

Serum transaminase elevation (see also under Liver dysfunction)
Lescol Capsules 2395
Mevacor Tablets 1742
Nardil 1977
Pravachol Tablets 770
Zocor Tablets 1821

Severe left ventricular dysfunction (see under Ventricular dysfunction, left)

Shingles (see under Herpes zoster)

Shock, cardiogenic (see under Cardiogenic shock)

Shock, hemorrhagic (see under Hemorrhagic shock)

Shock, history of
IPOL Poliovirus Vaccine Inactivated 903
Tri-Immunol Adsorbed 1452

Shock, traumatic (see under Traumatic shock)

Shock, unspecified (see also under Cardiogenic shock; Hemorrhagic shock; Traumatic shock)
Decadron Phosphate with Xylocaine Injection, Sterile 1683
D.H.E. 45 Injection 2381
Navane Capsules and Concentrate .. 2018
Navane Intramuscular 2019
Primaxin I.M. 1770
Sus-Phrine Injection 1017

Shortness of breath (see under Dyspnea)

Sick sinus node syndrome (see under Sick sinus syndrome)

Sick sinus syndrome
Adenocard Injection 1021
Adenoscan 1022
Calan SR Caplets 2571
Calan Tablets 2568
Cardizem CD Capsules 1251
Cardizem Injectable 1253
Cardizem Lyo-Ject Syringe 1253
Cardizem SR Capsules 1255
Cardizem Tablets 1257
Covera-HS Tablets 2573
Dilacor XR Extended-release Capsules 2183
Isoptin Injectable 1391
Isoptin Oral Tablets 1393
Isoptin SR Tablets 1395
Rythmol Tablets–150mg, 225mg, 300mg 1399
Tiazac Capsules 1019
Verelan Capsules 1455

Sickle cell anemia (see under Anemia, sickle cell)

Sino-atrial block (see under Heart block, first degree; Heart block, greater than first degree; Heart block, unspecified)

Sinus node disease (see under Bradycardia, sinus; Sick sinus syndrome; Sinus node dysfunction, unspecified)

Sinus node dysfunction, unspecified
Adenoscan 1022
Cordarone Tablets 2818

Sinus tracts, intestinal
Cortifoam 2540

Skin disorders, unspecified (see also under Dermatitis; Eczema; Infection, skin, bacterial; Infection, skin, unspecified; Intertrigo; Lesions, skin, fungal; Lesions, skin, unspecified; Lesions, skin, viral; Leukoderma, infectious; Melanoma, history of; Melanoma, unspecified; Psoriasis, acute; Rash; Skin, denuded; Xeroderma pigmentosum)
Scleromate Injection 1234
Sotradecol (Sodium Tetradecyl Sulfate Injection) 987

Skin lesions (see under Lesions, skin, fungal; Lesions, skin, unspecified; Lesions, skin, viral)

Skin, burned (see under Burns)

Skin, denuded
pHisoHex 2458

Sleep apnea
Doral Tablets 2773

Sodium depletion (see under Hyponatremia)

Spasms, gastrointestinal
Urecholine 1804

Spasms, infantile, history of
Tri-Immunol Adsorbed 1452

Spinal puncture
Coumadin for Injection 941
Coumadin Tablets 941

Status asthmaticus
AeroBid Inhaler System 1004
Aerobid-M Inhaler System 1004
Azmacort Oral Inhaler 2175
Beclovent Inhalation Aerosol and Refill 1063
Dilaudid Ampules 1382
Dilaudid Cough Syrup 1383
Dilaudid-HP Injection 1384
Dilaudid-HP Lyophilized Powder 250mg 1384
Dilaudid 1382
Dilaudid Oral Liquid 1386
Dilaudid 1382
Dilaudid Tablets - 8 mg 1386
Dilaudid Tablets 2 mg and 4 mg 1382
Vanceril Inhaler 2538

Status epilepticus
Romazicon 2311

Stenosis, aortic
Cardene Capsules 2261
Cardene I.V. 2815
Cardene SR Capsules 2264
Indocin I.V. 1727
Inversine Tablets 1729

Stenosis, pyloric (see also under Stenosis, pyloroduodenal)
Inversine Tablets 1729

Stenosis, pyloroduodenal
Cystospaz 2123
Donnatal 2234
Donnatal Extentabs 2234
Donnatal Tablets 2234
Kutrase Capsules 2546
Levsin/Levsinex/Levbid 2549
Norflex 1554
Norgesic 1554
Pro-Banthine Tablets 2226
Robinul Forte Tablets 2247
Robinul Injectable 2247
Robinul Tablets 2247
Urispas Tablets 2710

Stenosis, subaortic
Dobutrex Solution Vials 1480

Stokes-Adams syndrome (see under Adams-Stokes syndrome)

Stones, bile pigment
Actigall Capsules 818

Stones, calcified cholesterol
Actigall Capsules 818

Stones, radiopaque
Actigall Capsules 818

Stress test, abnormal
Proleukin for Injection 812

Stricture, esophageal
Fosamax Tablets 1703

Stroke (see under Cerebrovascular accident)

Stroke, history of (see under Cerebrovascular accident, history of)

Suicidal tendencies
Diupres Tablets 1691
Hydropres Tablets 1718
Ser-Ap-Es Tablets 867

Superficial herpes simplex keratitis (see under Herpes simplex keratitis)

Surgery, abdominal (see also under Surgery, gastrointestinal)
Dulcolax Suppositories 883
RMS Suppositories CII 2766
Roxanol 2365
Senna X-Prep Bowel Evacuant Liquid 1236

Surgery, biliary tract
RMS Suppositories CII 2766
Roxanol 2365

Surgery, bladder
Urecholine 1804

Surgery, central nervous system (see also under Surgery, intracranial; Surgery, intraspinal)
Coumadin for Injection 941
Coumadin Tablets 941

Surgery, elective
Nardil 1977
Parnate Tablets 2679

(Described in PDR For Nonprescription Drugs) (◉ Described in PDR For Ophthalmology)

Surgery **Contraindications Index** 1606

Surgery, gastrointestinal
Urecholine 1804

Surgery, intracranial
Abbokinase 403
Abbokinase Open-Cath 405
Activase 1045
Eminase 2215
Streptase for Infusion 557

Surgery, intraspinal
Abbokinase 403
Abbokinase Open-Cath 405
Activase 1045
Eminase 2215
Streptase for Infusion 557

Surgery, ophthalmic
Coumadin for Injection 941
Coumadin Tablets 941

Surgery, pediatric
Compazine 2644

Surgery, traumatic
Coumadin for Injection 941
Coumadin Tablets 941

Surgery, unspecified
ReoPro Vials 1526

Surgery, uterine, history of (see also under Cesarean section, history of)
Cervidil 1008
Prepidil Gel 2108

Surgery, vascular
D.H.E. 45 Injection 2381

Surgical abdomen (see under Surgery, abdominal)

Syncope
Cordarone Tablets 2818

Syphilis
Novocain Hydrochloride for Spinal Anesthesia 2457

Systemic lupus erythematosus (see under Lupus erythematosus)

T

Tachyarrhythmia (see under Arrhythmia, cardiac, unspecified; Tachycardia, unspecified)

Tachycardia, unspecified
Alupent 672
Isuprel Hydrochloride Solution 2443
Isuprel Injection 2441
Isuprel Mistometer 2442
Metaproterenol Sulfate Inhalation Solution, USP, Arm-a-Med 547
Yutopar Intravenous Injection 566

Tachycardia, ventricular
Cardizem Injectable 1253
Cardizem Lyo-Ject Syringe 1253
Crystodigin Tablets 1472
Isoptin Injectable 1391
Neo-Synephrine Hydrochloride 1% Carpuject 2455
Neo-Synephrine Hydrochloride 1% Injection 2455

Tachycardia, ventricular, history of
Proleukin for Injection 812

Tendinitis, history of
Noroxin Tablets 1758
Noroxin Tablets 2222
Penetrex Tablets 2196

Tendon rupture, history of
Noroxin Tablets 1758
Noroxin Tablets 2222
Penetrex Tablets 2196

Tension
Ritalin 866

Testicular failure, primary
Humegon for Injection 1873
Pergonal (menotropins for injection, USP) 2618

Tetralogy of Fallot
Indocin I.V. 1727

Thallium stress test, abnormal (see under Stress test, abnormal)

Thrombasthenia
Fiorinal Capsules 2388
Fiorinal with Codeine Capsules 2390

Thromboangiitis obliterans
Ergomar Tablets 1543

Thrombocytopathy, unspecified (see also under Thrombasthenia; Thrombocytopenia, unspecified; Thrombocytopenic purpura, history of)
Fiorinal Capsules 2388
Fiorinal with Codeine Capsules 2390
Mithracin 599

Thrombocytopenia, unspecified
Adagen (pegademase bovine) Injection 988
Fiorinal Capsules 2388
Fiorinal with Codeine Capsules 2390
Fragmin Injection 2088
Heparin Lock Flush Solution 2831
Heparin Sodium Injection 2832
Heparin Sodium Vials 1486
Hydrea Capsules 705
Indocin I.V. 1727
Lovenox Injection 2187
Methotrexate Sodium Tablets, Injection, for Injection and LPF Injection 1322
Mithracin 599
Mutamycin for Injection 712
ReoPro Vials 1526
Ticlid Tablets 2317

Thrombocytopenic purpura, history of
Cardioquin Tablets 2146
Quinaglute Dura-Tabs Tablets 644
Quinidex Extentabs 2240

Thromboembolic disorders (see also under Cerebrovascular accident)
Amen Tablets 785
Aygestin Tablets 990
Brevicon 2563
Climara Transdermal System 640
Cycrin Tablets 991
Demulen 2580
Depo-Provera Contraceptive Injection 2079
Depo-Provera Sterile Aqueous Suspension 2083
Desogen Tablets 1867
Diethylstilbestrol Tablets 1477
Emcyt Capsules 2085
Estrace Cream and Tablets 751
Estraderm Transdermal System 842
ESTRATAB Tablets (0.3, 0.625, 1.25, 2.5 mg) 2715
Estratest 2718
Levlen/Tri-Levlen 646
Lo/Ovral Tablets 2852
Lo/Ovral-28 Tablets 2857
Menest Tablets 2671
Modicon 1928
Nor-Q D Tablets 2598
Nordette-21 Tablets 2863
Nordette-28 Tablets 2866
Norinyl 2563
Norplant System 2868
Ogen Tablets 2103
Ogen Vaginal Cream 2106
Ortho Dienestrol Cream 1922
Ortho Tri-Cyclen 21 Tablets 1914
Ortho Tri-Cyclen 28 Tablets 1914
Ortho-Cept 21 Tablets 1907
Ortho-Cept 28 Tablets 1907
Ortho-Cyclen 21 Tablets 1914
Ortho-Cyclen 28 Tablets 1914
Ortho-Est 1925
Ortho-Novum 1928
Ovcon 765
Ovral Tablets 2877
Ovral-28 Tablets 2878
Ovrette Tablets 2878
PMB 200 and PMB 400 2890
Premarin Intravenous 2893
Premarin Tablets 2896
Premarin Vaginal Cream 2898
Premphase 2900
Prempro 2905
Provera Tablets 2110
Levlen/Tri-Levlen 646
Tri-Norinyl 2607
Triphasil-21 Tablets 2919
Triphasil-28 Tablets 2924
Vivelle Transdermal System 880

Thromboembolic disorders, history of (see also under Cerebrovascular accident, history of)
Amen Tablets 785
Aygestin Tablets 990
Brevicon 2563
Cycrin Tablets 991
Demulen 2580
Depo-Provera Contraceptive Injection 2079
Depo-Provera Sterile Aqueous Suspension 2083
Desogen Tablets 1867
Diethylstilbestrol Tablets 1477
Estratest 2718
Levlen/Tri-Levlen 646
Lo/Ovral Tablets 2852
Lo/Ovral-28 Tablets 2857
Menest Tablets 2671
Modicon 1928
Nor-Q D Tablets 2598
Nordette-21 Tablets 2863
Nordette-28 Tablets 2866
Norinyl 2563
Ortho Dienestrol Cream 1922
Ortho Tri-Cyclen 21 Tablets 1914
Ortho Tri-Cyclen 28 Tablets 1914
Ortho-Cept 21 Tablets 1907
Ortho-Cept 28 Tablets 1907
Ortho-Cyclen 21 Tablets 1914
Ortho-Cyclen 28 Tablets 1914
Ortho-Novum 1928
Ovcon 765
Ovral Tablets 2877
Ovral-28 Tablets 2878
Ovrette Tablets 2878
PMB 200 and PMB 400 2890
Premarin Intravenous 2893
Premarin Vaginal Cream 2898
Premphase 2900
Prempro 2905
Provera Tablets 2110
Levlen/Tri-Levlen 646
Tri-Norinyl 2607
Triphasil-21 Tablets 2919
Triphasil-28 Tablets 2924

Thrombophlebitis
Amen Tablets 785
Aygestin Tablets 990
Brevicon 2563
Climara Transdermal System 640
Cortifoam 2540
Cycrin Tablets 991
Demulen 2580
Depo-Provera Contraceptive Injection 2079
Depo-Provera Sterile Aqueous Suspension 2083
Desogen Tablets 1867
Diethylstilbestrol Tablets 1477
Emcyt Capsules 2085
Ergomar Tablets 1543
Estrace Cream and Tablets 751
Estraderm Transdermal System 842
ESTRATAB Tablets (0.3, 0.625, 1.25, 2.5 mg) 2715
Estratest 2718
Levlen/Tri-Levlen 646
Lo/Ovral Tablets 2852
Lo/Ovral-28 Tablets 2857
Menest Tablets 2671
Modicon 1928
Nor-Q D Tablets 2598
Nordette-21 Tablets 2863
Nordette-28 Tablets 2866
Norinyl 2563
Norplant System 2868
Ogen Tablets 2103
Ogen Vaginal Cream 2106
Ortho Dienestrol Cream 1922
Ortho Tri-Cyclen 21 Tablets 1914
Ortho Tri-Cyclen 28 Tablets 1914
Ortho-Cept 21 Tablets 1907
Ortho-Cept 28 Tablets 1907
Ortho-Cyclen 21 Tablets 1914
Ortho-Cyclen 28 Tablets 1914
Ortho-Est 1925
Ortho-Novum 1928
Ovcon 765
Ovral Tablets 2877
Ovral-28 Tablets 2878
Ovrette Tablets 2878
PMB 200 and PMB 400 2890
Premarin Intravenous 2893
Premarin Tablets 2896
Premarin Vaginal Cream 2898
Premphase 2900
Prempro 2905
Provera Tablets 2110
Sclеromate Injection 1234
Sotradecol (Sodium Tetradecyl Sulfate Injection) 987
Levlen/Tri-Levlen 646
Tri-Norinyl 2607
Triphasil-21 Tablets 2919
Triphasil-28 Tablets 2924
Vivelle Transdermal System 880

Thrombophlebitis, history of
Amen Tablets 785
Aygestin Tablets 990
Brevicon 2563
Cycrin Tablets 991
Demulen 2580
Desogen Tablets 1867
Diethylstilbestrol Tablets 1477
Estratest 2718
Levlen/Tri-Levlen 646
Lo/Ovral Tablets 2852
Lo/Ovral-28 Tablets 2857
Menest Tablets 2671
Modicon 1928
Nor-Q D Tablets 2598
Nordette-21 Tablets 2863
Nordette-28 Tablets 2866
Norinyl 2563
Ortho Dienestrol Cream 1922
Ortho Tri-Cyclen 21 Tablets 1914
Ortho Tri-Cyclen 28 Tablets 1914
Ortho-Cept 21 Tablets 1907
Ortho-Cept 28 Tablets 1907
Ortho-Cyclen 21 Tablets 1914
Ortho-Cyclen 28 Tablets 1914
Ortho-Novum 1928
Ovcon 765
Ovral Tablets 2877
Ovral-28 Tablets 2878
Ovrette Tablets 2878
PMB 200 and PMB 400 2890
Premarin Intravenous 2893
Premarin Vaginal Cream 2898
Premphase 2900
Prempro 2905
Provera Tablets 2110
Levlen/Tri-Levlen 646
Tri-Norinyl 2607
Triphasil-21 Tablets 2919
Triphasil-28 Tablets 2924

Thrombosis
Levophed Bitartrate Injection 2445

Thrombosis, history of
Diethylstilbestrol Tablets 1477
Estratest 2718
Menest Tablets 2671
Ortho Dienestrol Cream 1922
PMB 200 and PMB 400 2890
Premarin Intravenous 2893
Premarin Vaginal Cream 2898

Thymic abnormalities
Orimune 1433

Thyroid dysfunction, uncontrolled
Clomid 1262
Humegon for Injection 1873
Metrodin (urofollitropin for injection) 2616
Pergonal (menotropins for injection, USP) 2618
Serophene (clomiphene citrate tablets, USP) 2621

Thyroid enlargement (see under Goiter)

Thyrotoxicosis
Levoxyl Tablets 918
Scleromate Injection 1234

Thyrotoxicosis, untreated
Cytomel Tablets 2647
Eltroxin Tablets 2214
Levothroid Tablets 1015
Levothyroxine Sodium, USP for Injection 546
Sotradecol (Sodium Tetradecyl Sulfate Injection) 987
Synthroid 1410
Triostat Injection 2708

Tics, motor
Ritalin 866

Tics, non-Tourette's disorder
Orap Tablets 1037

(◘ Described in PDR For Nonprescription Drugs) (◉ Described in PDR For Ophthalmology)

1607 **Contraindications Index** Varicella

Tissue breakdown
(see under Necrosis)

Torsade de pointes
Procanbid Extended-Release Tablets ... 1983

Tourette's syndrome
Ritalin ... 866

Tourette's syndrome, history of
Ritalin ... 866

Toxemia
Methergine ... 2401

Toxemia, prolonged use
Syntocinon Injection ... 2425

Toxic megacolon
(see under Megacolon, toxic)

Toxic shock syndrome, history of
All-Flex Arcing Spring Diaphragm (See also Ortho Diaphragm Kits) .. 1921
Ortho Diaphragm Kit-Coil Spring ... 1921
Ortho Diaphragm Kits—All-Flex Arcing Spring; Ortho Coil Spring; Ortho-White Flat Spring ... 1921
Ortho-White Diaphragm Kit-Flat Spring (See also Ortho Diaphragm Kits) ... 1921

Toxicity, neurologic
Hexalen Capsules ... 2760

Toxicity, vitamin D
Calcijex Injection ... 412
Dovonex Cream 0.005% ... 2792
Dovonex Ointment 0.005% ... 2793
Rocaltrol Capsules ... 2303

Transaminases elevation, serum
(see under Serum transaminase elevation)

Transplant
(see under Bone marrow transplantation; Organ allograft)

Transverse lies
Syntocinon Injection ... 2425

Trauma, intracranial
(see also under Cerebrovascular accident; Head injury)
Activase ... 1045
Eminase ... 2215

Trauma, intraspinal
Activase ... 1045
Eminase ... 2215

Trauma, unspecified
Abbokinase ... 403
Abbokinase Open-Cath ... 405
Anectine ... 1062
ReoPro Vials ... 1526

Traumatic shock
Ana-Kit Anaphylaxis Emergency Treatment Kit ... 611

Tuberculin positive reactors
Tubersol (Tuberculin Purified Protein Derivative (Mantoux)) ... 2988

Tuberculosis, prevention of
TheraCys BCG Live (Intravesical) ... 911

Tuberculosis, untreated
Attenuvax ... 1650
Biavax II ... 1653
M-M-R II ... 1730
M-R-VAX II ... 1732
Meruvax II ... 1740
Mumpsvax ... 1751
Sotradecol (Sodium Tetradecyl Sulfate Injection) ... 987
Varivax ... 1807

Tuberculosis, unspecified
(see also under Infection, ophthalmic, mycobacterial)
AK-PRED ... ⊙ 204
Cortifoam ... 2540
Cortisporin Cream ... 1073
Cortisporin Ointment ... 1074
Dexacort Phosphate in Turbinaire ... 1607
Eflone Sterile Ophthalmic Solution ... ⊙ 261
Flarex Ophthalmic Suspension ... ⊙ 217
HMS Liquifilm ... ⊙ 241
Mantadil Cream ... 1124
Scleromate Injection ... 1234
TICE BCG, USP ... 1881

Tumor activity, unspecified
Genotropin Injection ... 2090
Humatrope Vials ... 1490

Tumor, adrenal
(see under Pheochromocytoma)

Tumor, breast, malignant
(see under Carcinoma, breast, history of; Carcinoma, breast, male; Carcinoma, breast, unspecified)

Tumor, hepatic
(see under Adenoma, hepatic; Carcinoma, hepatic; Tumor, liver, benign)

Tumor, hormone dependent
(see also under Neoplasm, androgen dependent; Neoplasm, estrogen dependent)
Lutrepulse for Injection ... 998

Tumor, intracranial, unspecified
(see also under Lesions, intracranial, unspecified; Prolactinoma, pituitary; Tumor, pituitary, unspecified)
Abbokinase ... 403
Abbokinase Open-Cath ... 405
Activase ... 1045
Eminase ... 2215
Pergonal (menotropins for injection, USP) ... 2618
ReoPro Vials ... 1526
RMS Suppositories CII ... 2766
Roxanol ... 2365
Streptase for Infusion ... 557

Tumor, liver, benign
Brevicon ... 2563
Demulen ... 2580
Nor-Q D Tablets ... 2598
Norinyl ... 2563
Norplant System ... 2868
Tri-Norinyl ... 2607

Tumor, liver, benign, history of
Demulen ... 2580

Tumor, liver, malignant
(see under Carcinoma, hepatic; Carcinoma, hepatic, history of)

Tumor, pituitary, unspecified
(see also under Prolactinoma, pituitary; Tumor, intracranial, unspecified)
Clomid ... 1262
Humegon for Injection ... 1873
Metrodin (urofollitropin for injection) ... 2616
Pergonal (menotropins for injection, USP) ... 2618
Serophene (clomiphene citrate tablets, USP) ... 2621

Tumor, unspecified
(see under Neoplasm, unspecified)

Tympanic membrane perforation
Americaine Otic Topical Anesthetic Ear Drops ... 1603
Auralgan Otic Solution ... 2810
Cerumenex Drops ... 2148
Cortisporin Cream ... 1073
Cortisporin Ointment ... 1074
Decadron Phosphate Sterile Ophthalmic Solution ... 1685
Otic Domeboro Solution ... 604
Tympagesic Ear Drops ... 2476
VoSol ... 2786

U

Ulcer, gastrointestinal
(see also under Lesions, gastrointestinal, unspecified; Perforation, gastrointestinal tract; Ulcer, peptic)
Anturane ... 823
Fiorinal with Codeine Capsules ... 2390
Ponstel ... 1982

Ulcer, peptic
Anturane ... 823
Atrohist Pediatric Capsules ... 1603
Bromfed ... 1832
Cortifoam ... 2540
D.A. Chewable Tablets ... 970
D.A. II Tablets ... 972
Diupres Tablets ... 1691
Dura-Tap/PD Capsules ... 970
Dura-Vent/DA Tablets ... 972
Fedahist Gyrocaps ... 2545
Fiorinal Capsules ... 2388
Fiorinal with Codeine Capsules ... 2390
Hydropres Tablets ... 1718
Norflex ... 1554
Novahistine Elixir ... ▣ 782
PBZ Tablets ... 863
PBZ-SR Tablets ... 862
Periactin ... 1767
Quibron ... 2227
Respbid Tablets ... 687
Robinul Injectable ... 2247
Rondec Chewable Tablets ... 974
Rondec ... 974
Ser-Ap-Es Tablets ... 867
Slo-bid Gyrocaps ... 2201
Theo-Dur Extended-Release Tablets ... 1367
Theo-X Extended-Release Tablets ... 793
Toradol ... 2319
Uni-Dur Extended-Release Tablets .. 1374
Urecholine ... 1804

Ulcer, peptic, history of
Toradol ... 2319

Ulcer, unspecified
(see under Ulceration, unspecified)

Ulceration, unspecified
Coumadin for Injection ... 941
Coumadin Tablets ... 941
Scleromate Injection ... 1234

Ulcerative colitis
(see under Colitis, ulcerative)

Unstable cardiovascular status in acute hemorrhage
(see under Cardiovascular status, unstable in acute hemorrhage)

Uremia
(see also under Azotemia)
Inversine Tablets ... 1729

Urinary obstruction
(see under Obstruction, urinary tract)

Urinary retention
(see also under Obstruction, urinary tract)
Adapin Capsules ... 1542
Atrohist Pediatric Capsules ... 1603
Bonine Tablets ... 1990
Bromfed ... 1832
Claritin-D Tablets ... 2487
D.A. Chewable Tablets ... 970
D.A. II Tablets ... 972
Dura-Tap/PD Capsules ... 970
Dura-Vent/DA Tablets ... 972
Fedahist Gyrocaps ... 2545
Novahistine Elixir ... ▣ 782
Rondec Chewable Tablets ... 974
Rondec ... 974
Sinequan ... 2028
Trinalin Repetabs Tablets ... 1373
Unisom Nighttime Sleep Aid ... 1990
Unisom With Pain Relief-Nighttime Sleep Aid and Pain Reliever ... 1991
Zonalon Cream ... 1042

Urinary tract disorders
(see under Infection, urinary tract; Obstruction, urinary tract; Renal disease, unspecified; Renal dysfunction)

Urogenital obstruction
(see under Obstruction, urogenital tract)

Uropathy, obstructive
(see under Obstruction, urinary tract; Obstruction, urogenital tract)

Urticaria
(see under Dermatitis)

Uterine abnormalities, unspecified
ParaGard T 380A Intrauterine Copper Contraceptive ... 1936

Uterine cavity distortion
ParaGard T 380A Intrauterine Copper Contraceptive ... 1936

Uterine inertia, prolonged use
Syntocinon Injection ... 2425

Uterine patterns, hypertonic
Prepidil Gel ... 2108
Syntocinon Injection ... 2425

Uveitis
Humorsol Sterile Ophthalmic Solution ... 1707
ISPAN Perfluoropropane ... ⊙ 267
ISPAN Sulfur Hexafluoride ... ⊙ 266
Phospholine Iodide ... ⊙ 323

V

Vaccinia
AK-CIDE ... ⊙ 203
AK-CIDE Ointment ... ⊙ 203
AK-PRED ... ⊙ 204
AK-Trol Ointment & Suspension ... ⊙ 205
Blephamide Liquifilm Sterile Ophthalmic Suspension ... 472
Blephamide Ointment ... ⊙ 234
Coly-Mycin S Otic w/Neomycin & Hydrocortisone ... 1965
Cortisporin Cream ... 1073
Cortisporin Ointment ... 1074
Cortisporin Ophthalmic Ointment Sterile ... 1074
Cortisporin Ophthalmic Suspension Sterile ... 1075
Cortisporin Otic Solution Sterile ... 1076
Cortisporin Otic Suspension Sterile 1077
Decadron Phosphate Sterile Ophthalmic Ointment ... 1684
Decadron Phosphate Sterile Ophthalmic Solution ... 1685
Econopred & Econopred Plus Ophthalmic Suspensions ... ⊙ 216
Eflone Sterile Ophthalmic Solution ... ⊙ 261
Flarex Ophthalmic Suspension ... ⊙ 217
FML Forte Liquifilm ... ⊙ 237
FML Liquifilm ... ⊙ 238
FML-S Liquifilm ... ⊙ 240
FML S.O.P. ... ⊙ 239
Mantadil Cream ... 1124
Maxitrol Ophthalmic Ointment and Suspension ... ⊙ 222
NeoDecadron Sterile Ophthalmic Ointment ... 1755
NeoDecadron Sterile Ophthalmic Solution ... 1756
Pediotic Suspension Sterile ... 1140
Poly-Pred Liquifilm ... ⊙ 246
Pred Forte ... ⊙ 247
Pred Mild ... ⊙ 250
Pred-G Liquifilm Sterile Ophthalmic Suspension ... ⊙ 248
Pred-G S.O.P. Sterile Ophthalmic Ointment ... ⊙ 249
Terra-Cortril Ophthalmic Suspension ... 2033
TobraDex Ophthalmic Suspension and Ointment ... 469
Vexol 1% Ophthalmic Suspension ... ⊙ 227
VoSoL HC Otic Solution ... 2786

Vaginal bleeding, abnormal
(see under Bleeding, genital, abnormal)

Vaginitis, untreated
ParaGard T 380A Intrauterine Copper Contraceptive ... 1936

Vaginosis, bacterial, untreated
ParaGard T 380A Intrauterine Copper Contraceptive ... 1936

Vagotonia
Antilirium Injectable ... 1007
Urecholine ... 1804

Valvular incompetence
Sotradecol (Sodium Tetradecyl Sulfate Injection) ... 987

Varicella
AK-CIDE ... ⊙ 203
AK-CIDE Ointment ... ⊙ 203

(▣ Described in PDR For Nonprescription Drugs) (⊙ Described in PDR For Ophthalmology)

Varicella — Contraindications Index — 1608

Varicella
- AK-PRED .... ⊚ 204
- AK-Trol Ointment & Suspension .... ⊚ 205
- Blephamide Liquifilm Sterile Ophthalmic Suspension 472
- Blephamide Ointment .... ⊚ 234
- Coly-Mycin S Otic w/Neomycin & Hydrocortisone 1965
- Cortisporin Cream 1073
- Cortisporin Ointment 1074
- Cortisporin Ophthalmic Ointment Sterile 1074
- Cortisporin Ophthalmic Suspension Sterile 1075
- Cortisporin Otic Solution Sterile 1076
- Cortisporin Otic Suspension Sterile . 1077
- Cosmegen Injection 1666
- Decadron Phosphate Sterile Ophthalmic Ointment 1684
- Decadron Phosphate Sterile Ophthalmic Solution 1685
- Econopred & Econopred Plus Ophthalmic Suspensions .... ⊚ 216
- Eflone Sterile Ophthalmic Solution .... ⊚ 261
- Flarex Ophthalmic Suspension ..... ⊚ 217
- FML Forte Liquifilm .... ⊚ 237
- FML Liquifilm .... ⊚ 238
- FML S.O.P. .... ⊚ 239
- Mantadil Cream 1124
- Maxitrol Ophthalmic Ointment and Suspension .... ⊚ 222
- NeoDecadron Sterile Ophthalmic Ointment 1755
- NeoDecadron Sterile Ophthalmic Solution 1756
- Pediotic Suspension Sterile 1140
- Poly-Pred Liquifilm .... ⊚ 246
- Pred Forte .... ⊚ 247
- Pred Mild .... ⊚ 250
- Pred-G Liquifilm Sterile Ophthalmic Suspension .... ⊚ 248
- Pred-G S.O.P. Sterile Ophthalmic Ointment .... ⊚ 249
- Terra-Cortril Ophthalmic Suspension 2033
- TobraDex Ophthalmic Suspension and Ointment 469
- Vexol 1% Ophthalmic Suspension .... ⊚ 227
- VoSoL HC Otic Solution 2786

Variscosity, tumor induced
- Scleromate Injection 1234
- Sotradecol (Sodium Tetradecyl Sulfate Injection) 987

Vasa previa
- Prepidil Gel 2108
- Syntocinon Injection 2425

Vasculitis, history of
- ReoPro Vials 1526

Vasomotor instability
- Urecholine 1804

Vasospasm, coronary artery
(see under Coronary artery vasospasm)

Ventilatory function depression
(see under Respiratory depression)

Ventricular arrythmia
(see under Arrhythmia, ventricular, unspecified)

Ventricular dysfunction, left
- Calan SR Caplets 2571
- Calan Tablets 2568
- Covera-HS Tablets 2573
- Flolan for Injection 1085
- Isoptin Oral Tablets 1393
- Isoptin SR Tablets 1395
- Verelan Capsules 1455

Ventricular fibrillation
(see under Fibrillation, ventricular)

Viral infections
(see under Herpes genitalia; Herpes simplex keratitis; Herpes simplex, unspecified; Herpes zoster; Human immunodeficiency virus; Infection, nasal, viral; Infection, ophthalmic, viral; Lesions, skin, viral; Varicella)

Visual field changes
- Aralen Hydrochloride Injection 2430
- Aralen Phosphate Tablets 2431
- Plaquenil Sulfate Tablets 2459

Vitamin D toxicity
(see under Toxicity, vitamin D)

Vitamin K, deficiency of
- Fiorinal Capsules 2388
- Fiorinal with Codeine Capsules 2390

Vitreoretinopathy, proliferative
(see under Proliferative vitreoretinopathy)

Von Willebrand's disease
- Fiorinal Capsules 2388
- Fiorinal with Codeine Capsules 2390

W

Warts, atypical
- Podocon-25 1949

Wilson's disease
- Natalins Rx Tablets 1599
- ParaGard T 380A Intrauterine Copper Contraceptive 1936

Wolff-Parkinson-White syndrome
- Calan SR Caplets 2571
- Calan Tablets 2568
- Cardizem Injectable 1253
- Cardizem Lyo-Ject Syringe 1253
- Covera-HS Tablets 2573
- Isoptin Injectable 1391
- Isoptin Oral Tablets 1393
- Isoptin SR Tablets 1395
- Verelan Capsules 1455

X

Xeroderma pigmentosum
- 8-MOP Capsules 1294
- Flagyl 375 Capsules 2587
- Oxsoralen Lotion 1% 1301
- Oxsoralen-Ultra Capsules 1302

(▣ Described in PDR For Nonprescription Drugs)   (⊚ Described in PDR For Ophthalmology)

VACCINE ADVERSE EVENT REPORTING SYSTEM

24 Hour Toll-free information line 1-800-822-7967
P.O. Box 1100, Rockville, MD 20849-1100
PATIENT IDENTITY KEPT CONFIDENTIAL

For CDC/FDA Use Only

VAERS Number _____

Date Received _____

Patient Name:

Last _____ First _____ M.I. ____

Address _____

_____

City _____ State ____ Zip _____

Telephone no. (___) _____

Vaccine administered by (Name): _____

Responsible Physician _____

Facility Name/Address _____

_____

City _____ State ____ Zip _____

Telephone no. (___) _____

Form completed by (Name): _____

Relation to Patient: ☐ Vaccine Provider ☐ Patient/Parent ☐ Manufacturer ☐ Other

Address *(if different from patient or provider)*

_____

City _____ State ____ Zip _____

Telephone no. (___) _____

1. State	2. County where administered	3. Date of birth mm/dd/yy	4. Patient age	5. Sex ☐ M ☐ F	6. Date form completed mm/dd/yy

7. Describe adverse event(s) (symptoms, signs, time course) and treatment, if any

8. Check all appropriate:
☐ Patient died (date ___/___/___)
☐ Life threatening illness
☐ Required emergency room/doctor visit
☐ Required hospitalization (_____ days)
☐ Resulted in prolongation of hospitalization
☐ Resulted in permanent disability
☐ None of the above

9. Patient recovered ☐ YES ☐ NO ☐ UNKNOWN

10. Date of vaccination ___/___/___ Time ____ AM/PM

11. Adverse event onset ___/___/___ Time ____ AM/PM

12. Relevant diagnostic tests/laboratory data

13. Enter all vaccines given on date listed in no. 10

	Vaccine (type)	Manufacturer	Lot number	Route/Site	No. Previous doses
a.					
b.					
c.					
d.					

14. Any other vaccinations within 4 weeks prior to the date listed in no. 10

	Vaccine (type)	Manufacturer	Lot number	Route/Site	No. Previous doses	Date given
a.						
b.						

15. Vaccinated at:
☐ Private doctor's office/hospital ☐ Military clinic/hospital
☐ Public health clinic/hospital ☐ Other/unknown

16. Vaccine purchased with:
☐ Private funds ☐ Military funds
☐ Public funds ☐ Other/unknown

17. Other medications

18. Illness at time of vaccination (specify)

19. Pre-existing physician-diagnosed allergies, birth defects, medical conditions (specify)

20. Have you reported this adverse event previously?
☐ No
☐ To doctor
☐ To health department
☐ To manufacturer

Only for children 5 and under

22. Birth weight ____ lb. ____ oz.

23. No. of brothers and sisters

21. Adverse event following prior vaccination (check all applicable, specify)

	Adverse Event	Onset Age	Type Vaccine	Dose no. in series
☐ In patient				
☐ In brother or sister				

Only for reports submitted by manufacturer/immunization project

24. Mfr. / imm. proj. report no.

25. Date received by mfr. / imm. proj.

26. 15 day report? ☐ Yes ☐ No

27. Report type ☐ Initial ☐ Follow-Up

Health care providers and manufacturers are required by law (42 USC 300aa-25) to report reactions to vaccines listed in the Table of Reportable Events Following Immunization. Reports for reactions to other vaccines are voluntary except when required as a condition of immunization grant awards.

Form VAERS -1

Vaccine Adverse Event Reporting System

Health care providers and manufacturers are required by law (42 USC 300aa-25) to report reactions to vaccines listed in the Vaccine Injury Table. Reports for reactions to other vaccines are voluntary except when required as a condition of immunization grant awards.

The form appears overleaf and may be photocopied for submission.

DIRECTIONS FOR COMPLETING FORM
(Additional pages may be attached if more space is needed.)

GENERAL

- Use a separate form for each patient. Complete the form to the best of your abilities. Items 3, 4, 7, 8, 10, 11, and 13 are considered essential and should be completed whenever possible. Parents/Guardians may need to consult the facility where the vaccine was administered for some of the information (such as manufacturer, lot number or laboratory data.)
- Refer to the Reportable Events Table (RET) for events mandated for reporting by law. Reporting for other serious events felt to be related but not on the RET is encouraged.
- Health care providers other than the vaccine administrator (VA) treating a patient for a suspected adverse event should notify the VA and provide the information about the adverse event to allow the VA to complete the form to meet the VA's legal responsibility.
- These data will be used to increase understanding of adverse events following vaccination and will become part of CDC Privacy Act System 09-20-0136, "Epidemiologic Studies and Surveillance of Disease Problems". Information identifying the person who received the vaccine or that person's legal representative will not be made available to the public, but may be available to the vaccinee or legal representative.
- Postage will be paid by addressee. Forms may be photocopied (must be front & back on same sheet).

SPECIFIC INSTRUCTIONS

Form Completed By: To be used by parents/guardians, vaccine manufacturers/distributors, vaccine administrators, and/or the person completing the form on behalf of the patient or the health professional who administered the vaccine.

Item 7: Describe the suspected adverse event. Such things as temperature, local and general signs and symptoms, time course, duration of symptoms diagnosis, treatment and recovery should be noted.

Item 9: Check "YES" if the patient's health condition is the same as it was prior to the vaccine, "NO" if the patient has not returned to the pre-vaccination state of health, or "UNKNOWN" if the patient's condition is not known.

Item 10: Give dates and times as specifically as you can remember. If you do not know the exact time, please
and 11: indicate "AM" or "PM" when possible if this information is known. If more than one adverse event, give the onset date and time for the most serious event.

Item 12: Include "negative" or "normal" results of any relevant tests performed as well as abnormal findings.

Item 13: List ONLY those vaccines given on the day listed in Item 10.

Item 14: List any other vaccines that the patient received within 4 weeks prior to the date listed in Item 10.

Item 16: This section refers to how the person who gave the vaccine purchased it, not to the patient's insurance.

Item 17: List any prescription or non-prescription medications the patient was taking when the vaccine(s) was given.

Item 18: List any short term illnesses the patient had on the date the vaccine(s) was given (i.e., cold, flu, ear infection).

Item 19: List any pre-existing physician-diagnosed allergies, birth defects, medical conditions (including developmental and/or neurologic disorders) for the patient.

Item 21: List any suspected adverse events the patient, or the patient's brothers or sisters, may have had to previous vaccinations. If more than one brother or sister, or if the patient has reacted to more than one prior vaccine, use additional pages to explain completely. For the onset age of a patient, provide the age in months if less than two years old.

Item 26: This space is for manufacturers' use only.

TABLE OF REPORTABLE EVENTS FOLLOWING VACCINATION

Vaccine/Toxoid	Event	Interval from Vaccination
DTP, DTaP, DTP-HiB, P, DT, Td, TT.	A. Anaphylaxis or anaphylactic shock B. Encephalopathy (or encephalitis) C. Any sequela (including death) of above events D. Events described in manufacturer's package insert as contraindications to additional doses of vaccine	7 days 7 days No limit See package insert
Measles & mumps in any combination; MMR, MR, M.	A. Anaphylaxis or anaphylactic shock B. Encephalopathy (or encephalitis) C. Residual seizure disorder D. Any sequela (including death) of above events E. Events described in manufacturer's package insert as contraindications to additional doses of vaccine	7 days 15 days 15 days No limit See package insert
Rubella in any combination; MMR, MR, R.	A. Chronic arthritis B. Anaphylaxis or anaphylactic shock C. Encephalopathy (or encephalitis) D. Residual seizure disorder E. Any sequela (including death) of above events F. Events described in manufacturer's package insert as contraindications to additional doses of vaccine	42 days 7 days 15 days 15 days No limit See package insert

Oral Polio (OPV)	A. Paralytic polio
	   —in a non-immunodeficient recipient
	   —in an immunodeficient recipient
	   —in a vaccine-associated community case
	B. Any sequela (including death) of above events
	C. Events described in manufacturer's package insert as contraindications to additional doses of vaccine
		
		30 days
		6 months
		No limit
		No limit
		See package insert

Inactivated Polio (IPV)	A. Anaphylaxis or anaphylactic shock D. Any sequela (including death) of the above events E. Events described in manufacturer's package insert as contraindications to additional doses of vaccine	7 days No limit See package insert

The Reportable Events Table (RET) reflects what is reportable by law (42 USC 300aa-25) to the Vaccine Adverse Event Reporting System (VAERS) including conditions found in the manufacturers package insert. In addition, individuals are encouraged to report **ANY** clinically significant or unexpected events (even if you are not certain the vaccine caused the event) for **ANY** vaccine, whether or not it is listed on the RET. Manufacturers are also required by regulation (21CFR 600.80) to report to the VAERS program all adverse events made known to them for any vaccine.

Effective March 1995. Revised 21 May 1996.